Anal abscess and fistula II
Anorectal fistula I
Anorexia II
Appendicitis I
Ascariasis I
Ascites I
Autoimmune hepatitis I
Bacterial overgrowth, small intestine II
Barrett's esophagus I
Bile duct, dilated II
Bleeding, gastrointestinal, algorithm III
Bleeding, rectal II
Bleeding, variceal III
Budd-Chiari syndrome I
Calcifications, liver on x-ray II
Calcifications, pancreas on x-ray II
Calcifications, spleen on x-ray II
Celiac disease I
Cholangiocarcinoma I
Cholangitis I
Cholecystitis I
Choledocholithiasis I
Cholelithiasis I
Chronic pancreatitis I
Cirrhosis I
Cirrhosis, primary biliary I
Colic, acute abdominal II
Colorectal cancer I
Colostridium difficile infection I
Constipation, adult patient II
Constipation, algorithm III
Crohn's disease I
Cryptosporidium infection I
Delayed passage of meconium II
Diarrhea, acute III
Diarrhea, acute watery and bloody II
Diarrhea, chronic III
Diarrhea, chronic, in patients with HIV infection, III
  algorithm
Diarrhea, infectious II
Diarrhea, non-infectious II
Diverticular disease (diverticulosis, I
  diverticulitis)
Drug-induced liver injury I
Dyspepsia III
Dyspepsia, nonulcerative I
Dysphagia, oropharyngeal II
Echinococcosis I
Epigastric pain II
Esophageal tumors I
Esophageal varices I
Esophagitis II
Familial adenomatous polyps and Gardner's I
  syndrome
Fetal alcohol syndrome I
Food poisoning, bacterial I
Functional gallbladder disorder I
Gastric cancer I
Gastric dilatation II
Gastric emptying, delayed II
Gastritis I
Gastroenteritis I
Gastroesophageal reflux disease I
Giardiasis I
Gilbert's disease I
Glossitis I
Glossodynia II
Helicobacter pylori infection I
Hematemesis II
Hemochromatosis I
Hemoperitoneum II
Hemoptysis I
Hepatic encephalopathy I
Hepatitis A I
Hepatitis, acute II
Hepatitis B I
Hepatitis B prophylaxis V
Hepatitis C I
Hepatitis D I
Hepatitis E I
Hepatitis, viral III
Hepatomegaly, algorithm III
Hepatomegaly, by shape of liver II
Hepatopulmonary syndrome I
Hepatorenal syndrome I
Hookworm I
Hypergastrinemia II
Hypersplenism, associated conditions II
Hypoglycemia II
Incontinence, fecal II
Irritable bowel syndrome I
Ischemia, colon III
Ischemic hepatitis I
Jaundice, classification II
Jaundice in the adult patient I
Jaundice, neonatal II
Jaundice, neonatal, algorithm III
Lactose intolerance I
Large bowel stricture II
Liver abscess I

Liver disease, pregnancy II
Liver lesions, benign II
Liver transplantation I
Lynch syndrome I
Malabsorption II
Malabsorption algorithm III
Mallory-Weiss tear I
Nonalcoholic fatty liver disease I
Nutrition assessment and intervention in cancer III
  patient
Odynophagia II
Pancreatic calcifications II
Pancreatic cancer (exocrine) I
Pancreatitis, drug-induced II
Peptic ulcer disease I
Perianal pain I
Peritonitis, secondary I
Peutz-Jeghers syndrome and other polyposis
  syndromes
Pinworms I
Pneumatosis intestinalis in neonate and older child II
Portal hypertension I
Portal vein thrombosis I
Primary sclerosing cholangitis I
Rectal mass, palpable II
Retropharyngeal abscess I
Shigellosis I
Short bowel syndrome I
Small bowel masses II
Small bowel obstruction I
Small intestinal bacterial overgrowth I
Small intestine ulceration II
Spontaneous bacterial peritonitis I
Tapeworm infestation I
Toxic megacolon I
Traveler's diarrhea I
Ulcerative colitis I
Vitamin deficiency (hypovitaminosis) I

GYNECOLOGY AND OBSTETRICS
Abruptio placentae I
Acute fatty liver of pregnancy I
Amniotic fluid alpha-fetoprotein elevation II
Bartholin gland abscess I
Bleeding, early pregnancy III
Bleeding neonate III
Bleeding, vaginal III
Bone mineral density, increased II
Breast cancer I
Breastfeeding difficulties III
Breast, nipple discharge evaluation III
Breast, radiologic evaluation III
Breast, routine screen or palpable mass evaluation III
Cervical cancer I
Cervical dysplasia I
Cervicitis I
Chlamydia genital infections I
Condyloma acuminatum I
Contraception I
Cystitis, acute III
Delayed passage of meconium II
Dysfunctional uterine bleeding I
Dysmenorrhea I
Dyspareunia I
Dysuria and/or urethral/vaginal discharge III
Eclampsia I
Ectopic pregnancy I
Endometrial cancer I
Endometriosis I
Endometritis I
Erosions, genitalia I
Fibrocystic breast disease I
Genital lesions or ulcers, algorithm III
Gonococcal urethritis I
Gonorrhea I
Groin masses II
Heart failure, pregnancy II
Hereditary breast and ovarian cancer syndrome I
Herpes simplex I
Hot flashes I
Hyperemesis gravidarum I
Hypoactive sexual desire disorder I
Hypogonadism III
Immunizations during pregnancy V
Incontinence (urinary) I
Infertility I
Mastitis I
Mastodynia I
Meigs' syndrome I
Menopause I
Menorrhagia I
Molar pregnancy I
Nipple lesions II
Nongonococcal urethritis I
Ovarian cancer I
Ovarian neoplasm, benign I
Paget's disease of the breast I
Pelvic abscess I
Pelvic inflammatory disease I
Pelvic mass, algorithm III

Pelvic organ I
Pelvic pain I
Pelvic pain I
Perirectal a I
Placenta previa I
Polycystic ovary syndrome I
Postpartum depression I
Postpartum hemorrhage I
Preeclampsia I
Premature rupture of membranes I
Premenstrual syndrome I
Preterm labor I
Primary ovarian insufficiency I
Pruritus, pregnant patient III
Pruritus vulvae I, II
Rh incompatibility I
Sexual assault I
Sexual dysfunction III
Sexual dysfunction in women I, II
Spontaneous miscarriage I
Syphilis I
Thrombocytopenia, in pregnancy II
Toxic shock syndrome I
Urinary tract infection I
Uterine fibroids I
Uterine malignancy I
Vaginal bleeding during pregnancy I
Vaginal discharge, algorithm III
Vaginal fistulas I
Vaginal malignancy I
Vaginal prolapse III
Vaginismus I
Vaginitis, estrogen-deficient I
Vaginitis, fungal I
Vaginitis, prepubescent I
Vaginitis, *Trichomonas* I
Vaginosis, bacterial I

HEMATOLOGY/ONCOLOGY
Acute lymphoblastic leukemia I
Acute myelogenous leukemia I
Anemia, algorithm III
Anemia, aplastic I, II
Anemia, aplastic due to drugs and chemicals II
Anemia, autoimmune hemolytic I
Anemia, hypochromic I
Anemia, inflammatory I
Anemia in newborn III
Anemia, iron deficiency I
Anemia, macrocytic III
Anemia, microcytic III
Anemia, pernicious I
Anemia with reticulocytosis III
Antiphospholipid antibody syndrome I
Astrocytoma I
Atypical lymphocytosis, heterophil negative, II
  infectious causes
Basal cell carcinoma I
Bladder cancer I
Bleeding, congenital disorder III
Bleeding neonate III
Bleeding time (modified Ivy method) IV
Bone marrow failure syndromes, inherited II
Bone tumor, primary malignant I
Brain metastases I
Brain neoplasm I
Brain neoplasm, benign I
Brain neoplasm, glioblastoma I
Breast cancer I
Cancer of unknown primary site I
Cervical cancer I
Chemotherapy-induced nausea and vomiting I
Cholangiocarcinoma I
Chronic lymphocytic leukemia I
Chronic myelogenous leukemia I
Chylothorax II
Cobalamin deficiency II
Colorectal cancer I
Conjunctival neoplasm II
Cryoglobulinemia I
Deep vein thrombosis I
Disseminated intravascular coagulation I
Endometrial cancer I
Erythrocytosis II
Erythrocytosis, acquired III
Esophageal tumors I
Eyelid neoplasm II
Fetal alcohol syndrome I
Fever and neutropenia, pediatric patient III
Fever, non-infectious causes II
Folate deficiency II
Gastric cancer I
Groin masses II
Head and neck squamous cell carcinoma I
Hemolysis, mechanical II
Hemolytic-uremic syndrome I
Hemophilia I
Hemoptysis I
Henoch-Schönlein purpura I
Heparin-induced thrombocytopenia I

Hepatocellular carcinoma | I
Hereditary breast and ovarian cancer syndrome | I
Hodgkin's lymphoma | I
Hypercalcemia, malignancy-induced | II
Hypercoagulable state | I
Hypercoagulable state, associated disorders | II
Hypersplenism | I
Hypersplenism, associated conditions | II
Immune thrombocytopenic purpura | I
Intraocular neoplasm | II
Iron overload | II
Kaposi's sarcoma | I
Lead poisoning | I
Liver lesions, benign | II
Lung cancer, occupational causes | II
Lung neoplasms, primary | I
Lymphadenopathy, generalized, algorithm | III
Lymphocytes | IV
Lymphocytosis, atypical | II
Lymphoma, non-Hodgkin | I
Macrothrombocytopenia, inherited | II
Meigs' syndrome | I
Melanoma | I
Meningioma | I
Menorrhagia | I
Mesothelioma, malignant | I
Monoclonal gammopathy of undetermined significance | I
Monocytosis | II
Mononucleosis, monospot negative | II
Multiple myeloma | I
Myelodysplastic syndrome | I
Neutropenia | II
Neutropenia with decreased marrow reserve | II
Neutrophilia | II
Nutrition assessment and intervention in cancer patient | III
Ovarian cancer | I
Ovarian neoplasm, benign | I
Paget's disease of the breast | I
Pancreatic cancer (exocrine) | I
Pancreatic islet cell tumors | III
Pancytopenia | II
Paraneoplastic neurologic syndromes | II
Pericardial effusion, malignant | III
Pheochromocytoma | I
Pigmenturia | II
Pituitary adenoma | I
Pituitary region tumors | II
Pleural effusion, malignant | III
Pleural effusions, malignancy-associated | II
Polycythemia | II
Polycythemia, algorithm | III
Polycythemia, relative versus absolute | II
Polycythemia vera | I
Postthrombotic syndrome | I
Prolactinoma | I
Prostate cancer | I
Pulmonary infiltrates, immunocompromised host | II
Purpura, nonpalpable | II
Purpura, non-purpuric disorders simulating purpura | II
Purpura, palpable | II
Renal cell adenocarcinoma | I
Reticulocyte count | IV
Retinoblastoma | I
Rh incompatibility | I
Salivary gland neoplasms | I
Sickle cell disease | I
Spine tumor | III
Splenomegaly, algorithm | III
Splenomegaly and hepatomegaly | II
Splenomegaly, children | II
Squamous cell carcinoma | I
Superior vena cava syndrome | I
Testicular cancer | I
Thalassemias | I
Thrombocytopenia, differential diagnosis | II
Thrombocytopenia, inherited disorders | II
Thrombocytopenia, in pregnancy | II
Thrombocytosis | I
Thrombosis or thrombotic diathesis | II
Thrombotic thrombocytopenic purpura | I
Thyroid carcinoma | I
Transfusion reaction, hemolytic | I
Tumor lysis syndrome | I
Tumor markers elevation | II
Upper extremity deep vein thrombosis | I
Uterine malignancy | I
Vaginal malignancy | I
Von Willebrand's disease | I
Waldenström's macroglobulinemia | I

INFECTIOUS DISEASES
Acquired immunodeficiency syndrome | I
Acute bronchitis | I
Amebiasis | I
Anaerobic infections | I
Anal abscess and fistula | II
Ascariasis | I

Aspergillosis | I
Aspiration, oral contents | III
Atypical lymphocytosis, heterophil negative, infectious causes | II
Babesiosis | I
Bacterial overgrowth, small intestine | II
Bacterial pneumonia | I
Balanitis | I
Bartholin gland abscess | I
Bedbug bite | I
Bite wounds | I
Botulism | I
Brain abscess | I
Breast abscess | I
Candidiasis, cutaneous | I
Candidiasis, invasive | I
Cat-scratch disease | I
Cavernous sinus thrombosis | I
Cellulitis | I
Cervicitis | I
Childhood and adolescent immunizations | V
Chlamydia genital infections | I
Cholangitis | I
Cholecystitis | I
Clostridium difficile infection | I
Condyloma acuminatum | I
Conjunctivitis | I
Cryptococcosis | I
Cryptosporidium infection | I
Cysticercosis | I
Cytomegalovirus infection | I
Diarrhea, infectious | II
Ear pain | III
Echinococcosis | I
Ehrlichiosis | I
Empyema | I
Encephalitis, acute viral | I
Endocarditis, infective | I
Endocarditis prophylaxis | V
Endometritis | I
Epididymitis | I
Epidural abscess | I
Epiglottitis | I
Epstein-Barr virus infection | I
Erysipelas | I
Esophagitis | II
Fever and infection in high-risk patient without obvious source | III
Fever and neutropenia, pediatric patient | III
Fever of undetermined origin | I
Fifth disease (parvovirus infection) | I
Folliculitis | I
Food poisoning, bacterial | I
Foot lesion, ulcerating | II
Genital lesions or ulcers | III
Giardiasis | I
Gonococcal urethritis | I
Granulomatous dermatitides | II
Groin masses | I
Hand-foot-mouth disease | I
Helicobacter pylori infection | I
Hepatitis A | I
Hepatitis, acute | II
Hepatitis B | I
Hepatitis C | I
Hepatitis D | I
Hepatitis E | I
Hepatitis, viral | III
Herpes simplex | I
Herpes zoster | I
Histoplasmosis | I
HIV cognitive dysfunction | I
HIV: Recommended immunization schedule for HIV-infected children | V
Hookworm | I
Human immunodeficiency virus | I
Impetigo | I
Immunization schedule, childhood, accelerated if necessary for travel | V
Immunization schedule, childhood and adolescence | V
Immunization schedule, contraindications and precautions | V
Immunization schedule, HIV-infected children | V
Immunizations for adults | V
Immunizations during pregnancy | V
Immunizations for immunocompromised infants and children | V
Immunizing agents and immunization schedules for health-care workers | V
Influenza | I
Ischemic hepatitis | I
Kaposi's sarcoma | I
Laryngitis | I
Laryngotracheobronchitis | I
Listeriosis | I
Liver abscess | I
Lung abscess | I
Lyme disease | I

Lymphangitis | I
Lymphocytosis, atypical | II
Malaria | I
Mastoiditis | I
Mediastinitis | I
Mediastinitis, acute | II
Meningitis, bacterial | I
Meningitis, viral | I
Meningitis, recurrent | II
Mesenteric adenitis | I
Methicillin resistant Staphylococcus aureus (MRSA) | I
Microsporidiosis | I
Molluscum contagiosum | I
Mononucleosis | I
Mononucleosis, monospot negative | II
Mucormycosis | I
Multidrug-resistant gram-negative rods (MRD-GNRs) | I
Mumps | I
Necrotizing fasciitis | I
Necrotizing pneumonias | II
Nongonococcal urethritis | I
Orchitis | I
Osteomyelitis | I
Otitis externa | I
Otitis media | I
Paronychia | I
Pediculosis | I
Pelvic abscess | I
Pelvic inflammatory disease | I
Perirectal abscess | I
Peritonitis, secondary | I
Pertussis | I
Pharyngitis/tonsillitis | I
Pinworms | I
Pneumonia, aspiration | I
Pneumonia, mycoplasma | I
Pneumonia, pnuemocystis jiroveci | I
Pneumonia, viral | I
Prostatitis | I
Pyelonephritis | I
Reiter's syndrome (reactive arthritis) | I
Renal abscess | I
Rocky Mountain spotted fever | I
Roseola | I
Salmonellosis | I
Scabies | I
Scarlet fever | I
Sepsis | I
Septic arthritis | I
Shigellosis | I
Sialadenitis | I
Sinusitis | I
Sore throat | II
Spinal epidural abscess | I
Spontaneous bacterial peritonitis | I
Stomatitis | I
Stye (hordeolum) | I
Syphilis | I
Tapeworm infestation | I
Thrombophlebitis, superficial | I
Tinea corporis | I
Tinea cruris | I
Tinea unguium | I
Tinea versicolor | I
Toxoplasmosis | I
Tuberculosis, miliary | I
Tuberculosis, pulmonary | I
Urinary tract infection | I
Urosepsis | II
Vaccinations for international travel | V
Vaccinations, recommendations for persons with medical conditions | V
Vaginitis, fungal | I
Vaginitis, Trichomonas | I
Vancomycin resistant Enterococcus (VRE) | I
Varicella | I
Zika virus | I

MISCELLANEOUS
Abdominal wall masses | II
Anaphylaxis | I
Anorexia | II
Cyanosis | II
Deep vein thrombosis | I
Dehydration correction, pediatric patient | III
Delayed passage of meconium | II
Drowning | I
Familial Mediterranean Fever | I
Fever, non-infectious causes | II
Food allergies | I
Groin lump | II
Iliac fossa pain, left sided | II
Iliac fossa pain, right sided | II
Lactic acidosis | I
Malignant hyperthermia | I
Mediastinitis | I
Mediastinal compartments, anatomy and pathology | II

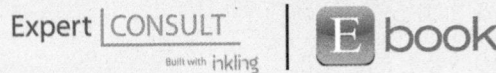

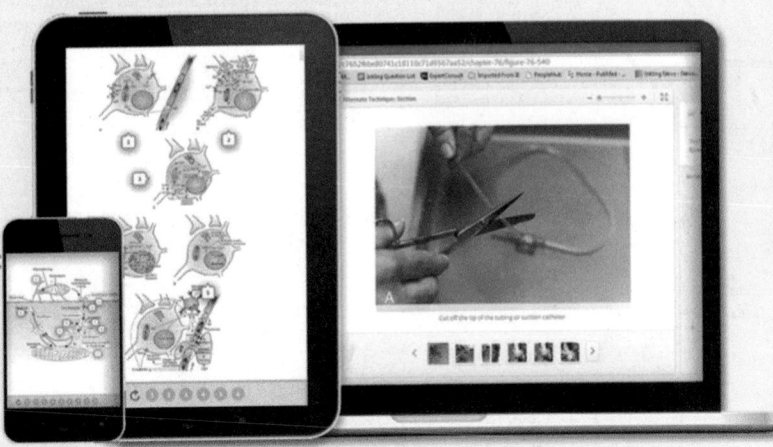

Any screen.
Any time.
Anywhere.

Activate the eBook version
of this title at no additional charge.

Expert Consult eBooks give you the power to browse and find content,
view enhanced images, share notes and highlights—both online and offline.

Unlock your eBook today.

1. Visit **expertconsult.inkling.com/redeem**
2. Scratch off your code
3. Type code into "Enter Code" box
4. Click "Redeem"
5. Log in or Sign up
6. Go to "My Library"

It's that easy!

Scan this QR code to redeem your
eBook through your mobile device:

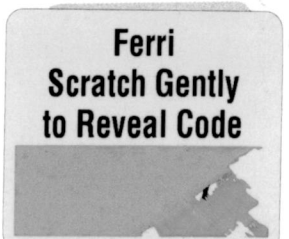

Ferri
**Scratch Gently
to Reveal Code**

For technical assistance:
email expertconsult.help@elsevier.com
call 1-800-401-9962 (inside the US)
call +1-314-447-8200 (outside the US)

ELSEVIER

2018

Ferri's CLINICAL ADVISOR

5 BOOKS IN 1

FRED F. FERRI, M.D., F.A.C.P.
Clinical Professor
The Warren Alpert Medical School
Brown University
Providence, Rhode Island

ELSEVIER

ELSEVIER

1600 John F. Kennedy Blvd.
Ste 1800
Philadelphia, PA 19103-2899

Senior Content Strategist: Sarah Barth
Content Development Specialist: Jennifer Horigan
Publishing Services Manager: Catherine Jackson
Project Manager: Kate Mannix
Design Direction: Paula Catalano
Illustrations Manager: Nichole Beard

Printed in the United States

Last digit is the print number: 9 8 7 6 5 4 3 2 1

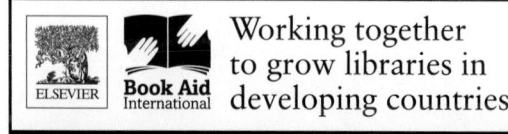

Working together to grow libraries in developing countries

www.elsevier.com • www.bookaid.org

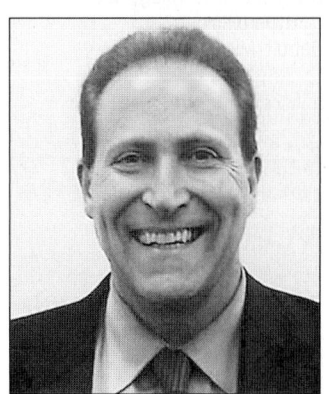

FRED F. FERRI, M.D., F.A.C.P.
Clinical Professor
The Warren Alpert Medical School
Brown University
Providence, Rhode Island

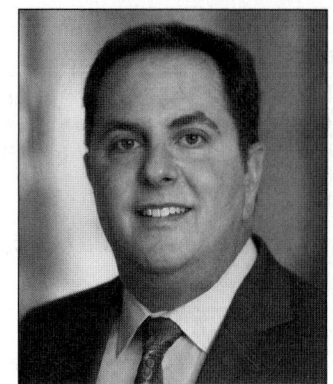

JOSEPH S. KASS, M.D., J.D., F.A.A.N.
Director, Alzheimer's Disease and
    Memory Disorders Center
Associate Professor
Department of Neurology
Menninger Department of
    Psychiatry & Behavioral Sciences
Center for Medical Ethics & Health
    Policy
Baylor College of Medicine;
Chief of Neurology
Director, Comprehensive Stroke
    Center
Ben Taub General Hospital
Houston, Texas

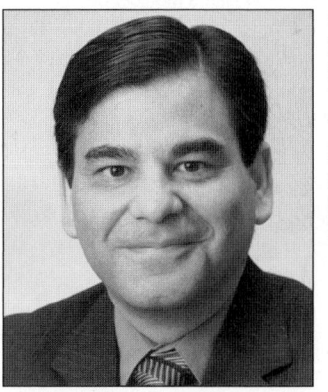

GLENN G. FORT, M.D., M.P.H., F.A.C.P., F.I.D.S.A.
Clinical Associate Professor of
    Medicine
The Warren Alpert Medical School
Brown University;
Chief, Infectious Diseases
Our Lady of Fatima Hospital
Providence, Rhode Island

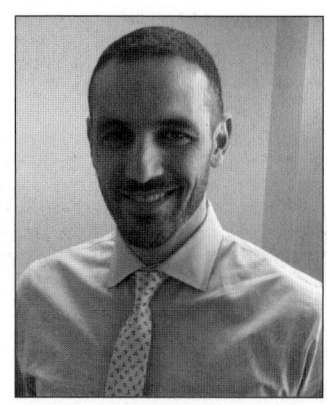

SAMAAN RAFEQ, M.D.
Assistant Professor of Medicine
Tufts Medical School;
Director, Interventional Pulmonary
    Services
Division of Pulmonary, Critical Care,
    and Sleep Medicine
Associate Program Director, Internal
    Medicine Residency Training
    Program
Department of Internal Medicine
St. Elizabeth's Medical Center
Boston, Massachusetts

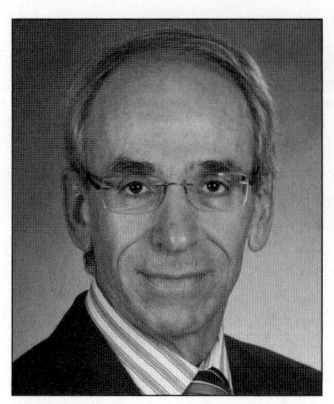

RICHARD J. GOLDBERG, M.D., M.S.
Psychiatrist-in-Chief
Rhode Island Hospital;
The Miriam Hospital;
Professor, Department of Psychiatry
    and Human Behavior
The Warren Alpert Medical School
Brown University
Providence, Rhode Island

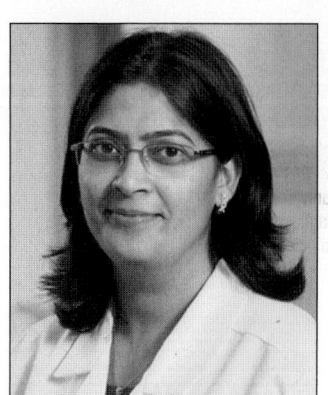

BHARTI RATHORE, M.D.
Program Director, Hematology/
    Oncology Fellowship
Roger Williams Medical Center
Providence, Rhode Island;
Assistant Professor of Medicine
Boston University School of
    Medicine
Boston, Massachusetts

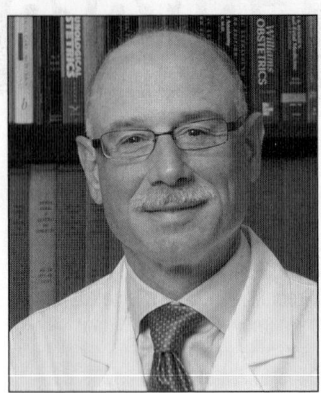

ANTHONY SCISCIONE, D.O.
Professor
Department of Obstetrics and
    Gynecology
Jefferson Medical College
Philadelphia, Pennsylvania;
Residency Program Director
Director, Maternal-Fetal Medicine
Department of Obstetrics and
    Gynecology
Christiana Care Health System
Newark, Delaware

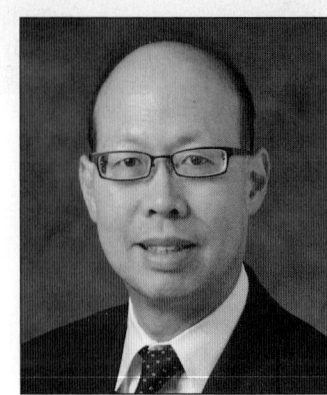

JERRY YEE, M.D.
Clinical Professor of Medicine
Department of Internal Medicine
Wayne State University School of
    Medicine;
Senior Staff Physician
Henry Ford Hospital
Division of Nephrology and
    Hypertension
Detroit, Michigan

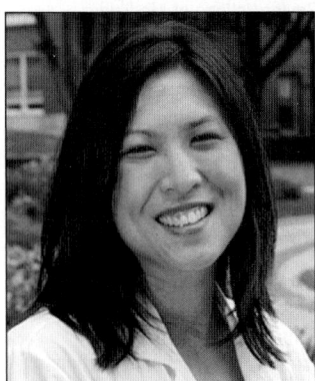

IRIS L. TONG, M.D.
Assistant Professor
Department of Medicine
The Warren Alpert Medical School
Brown University;
Director
Women's Primary Care
Women's Medicine Collaborative
Providence, Rhode Island

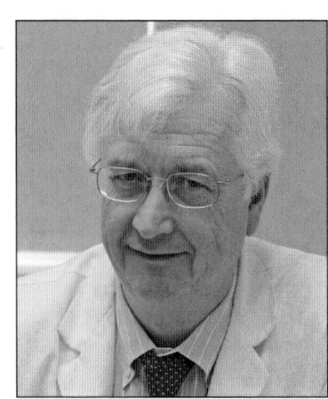

**BERNARD ZIMMERMANN,
M.D.**
Associate Professor Emeritus
Department of Medicine
Boston University
Boston, Massachusetts;
Rheumatologist
Department of Medicine
Division of Rheumatology
Roger Williams Medical Center
Providence, Rhode Island

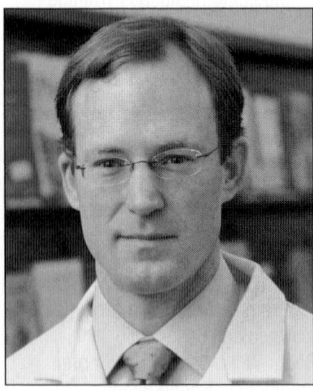

JOHN WYLIE, M.D., F.A.C.C.
Director, Cardiac Electrophysiology
Steward Health Care System;
Assistant Professor of Medicine
Tufts University School of Medicine
Boston, Massachusetts

NICHOLAS J. ABBOTT, M.D.
Fellow, Cardiovascular Disease
Division of Cardiology
University of California Irvine Medical Center
Irvine, California

SONYA S. ABDEL-RAZEQ, M.D.
Assistant Professor
Department of Obstetrics, Gynecology, and Reproductive Sciences
Yale University;
Yale–New Haven Hospital
New Haven, Connecticut

TONY ABDO, M.D.
Internal Medicine Resident
Roger Williams Medical Center
Boston University School of Medicine
Providence, Rhode Island

MAXWELL EYRAM AFARI, M.D.
Cardiovascular Medicine Fellow
Cardiovascular Medicine
St. Elizabeth's Medical Center
Brighton, Massachusetts

SANDEEP AGARWAL, M.D.
Assistant Professor of Medicine
Department of Medicine
Division of Nephrology
Departments of Medicine and Nephrology
Hahnemann University Hospital
Drexel University College of Medicine;
Senior Design Advisor
Biomedical Engineering
Drexel University School of Biomedical Engineering, Science and Health
    Systems
Philadelphia, Pennsylvania

BAHA AL-ABID, M.D.
Fellow
Department of Internal Medicine
Division of Nephrology and Hypertension
Henry Ford Hospital
Detroit, Michigan

TANYA ALI, M.D.
Clinical Assistant Professor of Medicine
Department of Medicine
The Warren Alpert Medical School
Brown University
Providence, Rhode Island

PHILIP J. ALIOTTA, M.D.
Clinical Instructor
Department of Urology
State University of New York at Buffalo School of Medicine and
    Biomedical Sciences
Buffalo, New York;
Medical Director
Center for Urologic Research of Western New York
Williamsville, New York

STEPHANIE MICHELLE ALLEN, M.SC.
Baylor College of Medicine
Houston, Texas

MONZR M. AL MALKI, M.D.
Instructor
Department of Hematology and Hematopoietic Cell Transplantation
City of Hope National Medical Center
Duarte, California

ROWENA ALMEIDA, M.D., F.R.C.P.C.
PGY 5, Gastroenterology
Division of Gastroenterology
University of Toronto
Toronto, Ontario, Canada

RASHA B. ALQADI, M.D.
Rheumatology Fellow
Department of Medicine
Boston University School of Medicine
Boston, Massachusetts;
Rheumatology Fellow
Department of Medicine
Division of Rheumatology
Roger Williams Medical Center
Providence, Rhode Island

RUBEN ALVERO, M.D.
Professor
Obstetrics and Gynecology
Director
Assisted Reproductive Technologies
Section Head
Reproductive Endocrinology and Infertility
Vice Chair for Education
University of Colorado Denver
Aurora, Colorado

MEL L. ANDERSON, M.D.
Assistant Professor of Medicine
University of Colorado School of Medicine
Denver Veterans Affairs Medical Center
Denver, Colorado

THOMAS J.T. ANDERSON, M.D.
Clinical Fellow
Harvard Medical School;
Diagnostic Radiology
Beth Israel Deaconess Medical Center
Boston, Massachusetts

LAURA M. ANDOLINA, M.S.
Clinical Instructor of Pediatrics
State University of New York at Buffalo School of Medicine and
    Biomedical Sciences
Buffalo, New York

Contributors

GEORGE F. ANDOSCIA, B.S.
Clinical Research Assistant
Rhode Island Hospital
Providence, Rhode Island

KATHRYN TAYLOR ANILOWSKI, M.S., P.T., C.L.T.-L.A.N.A.
Physical Therapist
Kinder Touch Lymphedema Center
Saratoga Springs, New York

ANNGENE ANTHONY, M.D., M.P.H., F.A.A.F.P.
Clinical Assistant Professor
Family Medicine
Rutgers New Jersey Medical School
Newark, New Jersey;
Active Staff
Family Medicine
Morristown Memorial Hospital
Morristown, New Jersey

ETSUKO AOKI, M.D., PH.D.
Assistant Professor
Departments of Leukemia and General Internal Medicine
University of Texas M.D. Anderson Cancer Center
Houston, Texas

NAIM AOUN, M.D.
Departments of Pulmonary, Critical Care, and Sleep Medicine
St. Joseph Hospital
Nashua, New Hampshire

GRAYSON W. ARMSTRONG, M.D., M.P.H.
The Warren Alpert Medical School
Brown University
Providence, Rhode Island;
Masters of Public Health Candidate
Health Policy and Management
Harvard School of Public Health
Boston, Massachusetts

ZUHAL ARZOMAND, M.D.
Department of Medicine
Boston University School of Medicine
Boston, Massachusetts;
Resident in Medicine
Roger Williams Medical Center
Providence, Rhode Island

DANIEL K. ASIEDU, M.D., PH.D.
Clinical Instructor of Medicine
The Warren Alpert Medical School
Brown University
Providence, Rhode Island;
Attending Physician
Department of Medicine
Coastal Medical, Inc.
Lincoln, Rhode Island

ARIF ASIF, M.D.
Professor of Medicine
Department of Medicine
Hackensack-Meridian Seton Hall School of Medicine;
Chairman
Department of Medicine
Hackensack-Meridian Health System
Neptune, New Jersey

SUDEEP K. AULAKH, M.D.
Assistant Professor of Medicine
Department of Medicine
Tufts University School of Medicine
Boston, Massachusetts;
Director, Ambulatory Education, Baystate Internal Medicine Residency
Co-Director, Baystate Primary Care Program
Department of Medicine
Baystate Health
Springfield, Massachusetts;
Medical Director, Physician Assistant Program
Bay Path University
Longmeadow, Massachusetts

RUPALI AVASARE, M.D.
Assistant Professor of Medicine
Department of Medicine
Division of Nephrology
Oregon Health and Science University
Portland, Oregon

TANIA B. BABAR, M.D.
Assistant Professor
Department of Electrophysiology
West Virginia University
Charleston, West Virginia

EMELIA ARGYROPOULOS BACHMAN, M.D., F.A.C.O.G.
Director of Fertility Preservation
Reproductive Associates of Delaware;
Department of Obstetrics and Gynecology
Christiana Hospital
Newark, Delaware

CRISOSTOMO R. BALIOG, JR., M.D.
Assistant Professor
Department of Internal Medicine
University of South Alabama College of Medicine
Mobile, Alabama

PRIYA BANSAL, M.D., M.P.H.
Physician
Department of Internal Medicine
Miriam Hospital
Rhode Island Hospital
Providence, Rhode Island

LUKE BARRÉ, M.D.
Instructor
Department of Medicine
Boston University School of Medicine;
Medical Resident
Department of Medicine
Roger Williams Medical Center
Providence, Rhode Island

TRACE BARRETT, M.D.
Departments of Internal Medicine and Cardiology
University of Vermont Medical Center
Burlington, Vermont

CRAIG L. BASMAN, M.D.
Department of Cardiology
Lenox Hill Hospital
New York, New York

DEANNA BENNER, A.P.R.N., C.R.N.P.
Women's Health Nurse Practitioner
Department of Obstetrics and Gynaecology
Christiana Care Health System
Newark, Delaware

ARNALDO A. BERGES, M.D.
Assistant Clinical Professor
Department of Psychiatry and Human Behavior
The Warren Alpert Medical School
Brown University;
Rhode Island Hospital
Providence, Rhode Island

VICKY H. BHAGAT, M.D., M.P.H.
Women's Gastroenterology Health Fellow
Women & Infants Hospital;
The Warren Alpert Medical School
Brown University
Providence, Rhode Island

HARIKRASHNA B. BHATT, M.D.
Assistant Professor of Medicine
Department of Medicine
Brown University
Providence, Rhode Island

DANISH BHATTI, M.D.
Assistant Professor
Department of Neurological Sciences
University of Nebraska Medical Center
Omaha, Nebraska

RACHAEL M. BIANCUZZO, D.O.
Department of Internal Medicine
Roger Williams Medical Center
Providence, Rhode Island

COURTNEY CLARK BILODEAU, M.D.
Assistant Professor
Department of Obstetric Medicine
The Warren Alpert Medical School
Brown University;
Attending Physician
Internal Medicine, Women's Medicine Collaborative
Miriam Hospital
Providence, Rhode Island

CRAIG BLAKENEY, M.D.
Resident Physician
The University of Tennessee College of Medicine
Memphis, Tennessee

CHRISTOPHER P. BLOMBERG, D.O.
Clinical Instructor
Department of Medicine
Tufts Medical Center;
Cardiology Fellow
Department of Cardiology
Steward St. Elizabeth's Medical Center
Boston, Massachusetts

TRAVIS D. BLOOD, M.D.
Department of Orthopaedic Surgery
Brown University
Providence, Rhode Island

STEVEN L. BOKSHAN, M.D.
Orthopedic Surgery Resident
Department of Orthopedics
The Warren Alpert Medical School
Brown University
Providence, Rhode Island

MARK ELIOT BOROWSKY, M.D., F.A.C.O.G., F.A.C.S.
Director, Division of Gynecologic Oncology
Department of Obstetrics and Gynecology
Helen F. Graham Cancer Center
Christiana Care Health System
Newark, Delaware;
Clinical Associate Professor
Sidney Kimmel Medical College
Thomas Jefferson University
Philadelphia, Pennsylvania

ALEXANDRA BOSKE, M.D.
Director of Inpatient Neurology
Stroke Program Director
Saint David's Round Rock Medical Center
Round Rock, Texas

TARA C. BOUTON, M.D., M.P.H.&T.M.
Division of Infectious Diseases
The Warren Alpert Medical School
Brown University
Providence, Rhode Island

LYNN A. BOWLBY, M.D., F.A.C.P.
Medical Director, Duke Outpatient Clinic
Duke University
Durham, North Carolina

MADALENE I. BOYLE, M.D.
Resident Physician
Emergency Medicine
Brown University
Providence, Rhode Island

MARK F. BRADY, M.D., M.P.H., M.M.S.
Attending Physician
Emergency Medicine
Baptist Memorial Hospital
Memphis, Tennessee

TINA BRAR, M.D.
Fellow
Department of Rheumatology
Brown University
Providence, Rhode Island

KEITH BRENNAN, M.D.
Geriatric Medicine
Stony Brook University
Stony Brook, New York;
Winthrop University Hospital
Mineola, New York

ELIZABETH BROWN, M.D.
Assistant Clinical Instructor of Family Medicine
Memorial Hospital of Rhode Island
Pawtucket, Rhode Island;
The Warren Alpert Medical School
Brown University
Providence, Rhode Island

GAVIN BROWN, M.D.
General Neurologist
Laureate Medical Group at Northside Hospital
Atlanta, Georgia

KIMBERLY M. BROWN, M.D., M.P.H.
Resident Physician
The University of Tennessee College of Medicine
Memphis, Tennessee

VICTORIA BROWN, M.D.
Chief Resident in Quality and Safety
The Warren Alpert Medical School
Brown University
Providence, Rhode Island

JENNIFER BUCKLEY, M.D.
Clinical Instructor of Family Medicine
Department of Family Medicine
The Warren Alpert Medical School
Brown University
Providence, Rhode Island;
Memorial Hospital of Rhode Island
Pawtucket, Rhode Island;
Kent Memorial Hospital
Warwick, Rhode Island

ALEXANDRA BUFFIE, M.D.
Baylor College of Medicine
Houston, Texas

JONATHAN BURNS, M.A., M.D.
Geriatrician
Division of Geriatrics
Department of Medicine
Cambridge Hospital
Cambridge, Massachusetts

D. BRANDON BURTIS, D.O.
Assistant Professor
Neurology
University of Florida
Gainesville, Florida

DOUGLAS BURTT, M.D.
Clinical Assistant Professor of Medicine
Division of Cardiology
The Warren Alpert Medical School
Brown University
Providence, Rhode Island

TAMARA BYSTRAK, PHARM.D. CANDIDATE
Yale New Haven Health
New Haven, Connecticut

CLAUDIA RODRIGUEZ CABRERA, M.D.
Department of Medicine
Universidad Tecnológica de Santiago;
Hospital Regional Universitario de José María Cabral y Báez
Santiago, Dominican Republic

KATE CAHILL, M.D.
Assistant Professor of Medicine (Clinical)
Division of General Internal Medicine
The Warren Alpert Medical School
Brown University
Providence, Rhode Island

SARA CAPOBIANCO, B.S.
College of Osteopathic Medicine
University of New England
Biddeford, Maine

ANDREW CARAGANIS, M.D.
Internal Medicine
Boston University School of Medicine;
Roger Williams Medical Center
Providence, Rhode Island

AAKRITI CARRUBBA, M.D.
Resident Physician
Obstetrics and Gynecology
University of Colorado Anschutz Medical Campus
Aurora, Colorado

JORGE J. CASTILLO, M.D.
Division of Hematologic Malignancies
Dana-Farber Cancer Institute;
Assistant Professor
Harvard Medical School
Boston, Massachusetts

ANDREEA M. CATANA, M.D.
Instructor in Medicine
Departments of Gastroenterology and Hepatology
Harvard Medical School;
Departments of Gastroenterology and Hepatology
Beth Israel Deaconess Medical Center
Boston, Massachusetts

FREDERIC CELESTIN, M.D.
Clinical Associate
Tufts Medical School
Tufts University;
Pulmonary and Critical Care Fellow
Department of Pulmonary and Critical Care
Steward St. Elizabeth's Medical Center
Boston, Massachusetts

CAROLINA S. CEREZO, M.D., F.A.A.P.
Department of Pediatrics
Rhode Island Hospital;
Assistant Professor of Pediatrics
The Warren Alpert Medical School
Brown University
Providence, Rhode Island

JOSHUA CHALKELY, M.S., D.O.
Department of Neurology
University of Kentucky Medical Center
Lexington, Kentucky

PAUL D. CHAMBERLAIN, B.S.
Department of Neurology
Baylor College of Medicine;
Ben Taub General Hospital
Houston, Texas

PHILIP A. CHAN, M.D., M.S.
Assistant Professor
Department of Medicine
Brown University;
Attending Physician
Infectious Diseases
The Miriam Hospital;
Consultant Medical Director
Center for HIV/AIDS, TB, STDs, and Viral Hepatitis
Rhode Island Department of Health
Providence, Rhode Island

ARLENE CHAPMAN, M.D.
Professor of Medicine
Department of Medicine
University of Chicago
Chicago, Illinois

LILY CHEN, M.D.
Resident Physician
Internal Medicine
University of California at Davis Medical Center
Sacramento, California

VICKY CHENG, M.D.
Assistant Professor
Department of Medicine
Division of Endocrinology
The Warren Alpert Medical School
Brown University;
Staff Endocrinologist
Department of Medicine
Division of Endocrinology
Rhode Island Hospital
Providence, Rhode Island

SARAH L. CHISHOLM, M.D.
Resident Physician
Department of Obstetrics and Gynecology
University of Colorado Hospital
Denver, Colorado

GEORGE CHOLANKERIL, M.D.
Transplant Hepatology
University of Tennessee Health Science Center
Memphis, Tennessee

ROSANN CHOLANKERIL
Boston University School of Medicine
Boston, Massachusetts;
Roger Williams Medical Center
Providence, Rhode Island

LINDSEY CILIA, M.D.
Resident, Internal Medicine
Brown University
Providence, Rhode Island

LISA COHEN, M.D.
Assistant Professor
Department of Medicine
Division of Nephrology
Oakland University School of Medicine
Rochester, Michigan;
William Beaumont Hospital
Royal Oak, Michigan

KAILA COMPTON, M.D., PH.D.
Attending Psychiatrist
Alta Bates Summit Medical Center
Herrick Hospital
Berkeley, California

EDDIE L. COPELIN II, M.D., M.H.A.
Medical Doctor
Department of Internal Medicine
Boston University School of Medicine;
Roger Williams Medical Center
Providence, Rhode Island

MEAGAN CRAMER, M.D.
Resident Physician
Departments of Obstetrics/Gynecology and Urogynecology
Christiana Care Health System
Newark, Delaware

PATRICIA CRISTOFARO, M.D.
Assistant Professor of Medicine
The Warren Alpert Medical School
Brown University;
Physician
Providence Veteran's Administration Medical Center
Providence, Rhode Island

JOANNE SZCZYGIEL CUNHA, M.D.
Assistant Professor of Medicine
Division of Rheumatology
The Warren Alpert Medical School
Brown University;
Department of Medicine
Division of Rheumatology
Rhode Island Hospital;
Departments of Medicine and Rheumatology
Providence Veterans Administration Medical Center
Providence, Rhode Island

KARLENE CUNNINGHAM, PH.D.
Clinical Assistant Professor
Department of Psychiatry and Behavioral Medicine
Brody School of Medicine at East Carolina University
Greenville, North Carolina

STEPHANIE A. CURRY, M.D.
Endocrinologist
Department of Medicine
Our Lady of Fatima Hospital;
Roger Williams Medical Center
Providence, Rhode Island

ALICIA J. CURTIN, PH.D.
Assistant Professor
Division of Geriatrics
The Warren Alpert Medical School
Brown University
Providence, Rhode Island

KAUSTUBH C. DABHADKAR, M.D., M.P.H.
Fellow in Cardiovascular Diseases
Division of Cardiology
Department of Medicine
Brown University;
Rhode Island Hospital;
Providence Veteran's Administration Medical Center
Providence, Rhode Island

Contributors

GANARY DABIRI, M.D., PH.D.
Dermatology Resident
Department of Dermatology
Boston University School of Medicine
Boston, Massachusetts;
Roger Williams Medical Center
Providence, Rhode Island

DEEPAN DALAL, M.D.
Assistant Professor of Medicine (Clinical)
The Warren Alpert Medical School
Brown University;
Division of Rheumatology
Rhode Island Hospital
Providence, Rhode Island

KRISTY L. DALRYMPLE, PH.D.
Assistant Professor (Research)
The Warren Alpert Medical School
Brown University;
Staff Psychologist
Rhode Island Hospital
Providence, Rhode Island

SHIVANG U. DANAK, M.D.
St. George's University
Detroit, Michigan

RITUPARNA DAS, M.D.
Assistant Professor
Department of Neurology
Baylor College of Medicine;
Baylor St. Luke's Medical Center
Houston, Texas

KATIA A. DASILVA, B.A.
Research Assistant
Department of Orthopedics
The Warren Alpert Medical School
Brown University;
Rhode Island Hospital
Providence, Rhode Island

MANUEL F. DASILVA, M.D.
Director, Medical Student Education
Assistant Professor of Orthopedics
Department of Orthopaedics
The Warren Alpert Medical School
Brown University;
Attending Physician
Orthopaedics
Rhode Island Hospital
Providence, Rhode Island

CATHERINE D'AVANZATO, PH.D.
Psychology Fellow
Rhode Island Hospital;
Department of Psychiatry and Human Behavior
The Warren Alpert Medical School
Brown University
Providence, Rhode Island

MELISSA L. DAWSON, D.O., M.S.
Fellow, Division of Female Pelvic Medicine and Reconstructive Surgery
Department of Obstetrics and Gynecology
Drexel University College of Medicine
Philadelphia, Pennsylvania;
Obstetrics and Gynecology
Christiana Health System
Newark, Delaware

STEVEN F. DEFRODA, M.D., M.ENG.
Resident in Orthopaedics
Department of Orthopaedics
The Warren Alpert Medical School
Brown University;
Rhode Island Hospital
Providence, Rhode Island

ALEXANDRA DEGENHARDT, M.D., M.M.SC.
Director
Multiple Sclerosis Center
Pen Bay Medical Center
Rockport, Maine

ANDRE LUIZ DE SOUZA, M.D.
Fellow
Hematology and Oncology
Roger Williams Medical Center
Providence, Rhode Island

JOSEPH A. DIAZ, M.D., M.P.H.
Associate Professor of Medicine
Department of Medicine
The Warren Alpert Medical School
Brown University
Providence, Rhode Island;
Department of Medicine
Memorial Hospital of Rhode Island
Pawtucket, Rhode Island

EMILY DIONNE, PHARM.D. CANDIDATE
Department of Pharmacy
University of Rhode Island
Kingston, Rhode Island

AMANDA C. DORAN, M.D., PH.D.
Cardiology Fellow
Department of Medicine
Division of Cardiology
Columbia University;
New York Presbyterian Hospital
New York, New York

ANDREW P. DUKER, M.D.
Movement Disorders Division Director
Associate Professor
Department of Neurology and Rehabilitation Medicine
University of Cincinnati College of Medicine
Cincinnati, Ohio

CHRISTINE EISENHOWER, PHARM.D.
Clinical Assistant Professor
Pharmacy Practice
University of Rhode Island College of Pharmacy
Kingston, Rhode Island

GREGORY ELIA, M.D.
Resident
Orthopaedic Surgery
The Warren Alpert Medical School
Brown University;
Rhode Island Hospital
Providence, Rhode Island

PAMELA ELLSWORTH, M.D.
Chief, Division of Pediatric Urology
Department of Urology
UMass Memorial Medical Center
University of Massachusetts Medical School
Worcester, Massachusetts

ALAN EPSTEIN, M.D.
Assistant Professor of Medicine
Boston University School of Medicine
Providence, Rhode Island

JUAN A. ESCARFULLER, M.D.
Assistant Clinical Professor
Department of Internal Medicine
Division of Cardiology
Albert Einstein College of Medicine;
Montefiore Hospital
New York, New York

MICHAEL A. ESKANDER, M.D.
Fellow, Cardiovascular Disease
Division of Cardiology
University of California Irvine Medical Center
Irvine, California

PATRICIO SEBASTIAN ESPINOSA, M.D., M.P.H.
Associate Professor
Departments of Neurology and Clinical Biomedical Science
Charles E. Schmidt College of Medicine
Florida Atlantic University;
Chief of Neurology
Director of Epilepsy
Boca Raton Regional Hospital;
Chairman and CEO
International Neurology Foundation
Boca Raton, Florida

RANIA ESTEITIE, M.D.
Clinical Instructor
Tufts School of Medicine
Tufts University;
Pulmonary Fellow, PGY5
Pulmonary Critical Care
Tufts Medical Center
Boston, Massachusetts

DANYELLE EVANS, M.D.
Baylor College of Medicine
Houston, Texas

MARK D. FABER, M.D.
Associate Professor of Medicine
Department of Internal Medicine
Wayne State University School of Medicine;
Senior Staff Physician
Division of Nephrology and Hypertension
Henry Ford Hospital
Detroit, Michigan

VALERIA FABRE, M.D.
Clinical Instructor
Department of Medicine
Brown University
Providence, Rhode Island;
Department of Medicine
Memorial Hospital of Rhode Island
Pawtucket, Rhode Island

MATTHEW J. FAGAN, M.D., F.A.C.O.G.
Director of Undergraduate Medical Education
Attending Physician
Obstetrics and Gynceology
Christianacare Health System
Newark, Delaware

FAHAD FAROOQ, M.D.
Clinical Associate
Tufts Medical School
Tufts University;
Pulmonary and Critical Care Fellow
Department of Pulmonary and Critical Care
Steward St. Elizabeth's Medical Center
Boston, Massachusetts

MUHAMMAD FAROOQ, M.D.
Nephrology Fellow
Department of Internal Medicine
Division of Nephrology and Hypertension
Henry Ford Hospital
Detroit, Michigan

TIMOTHY W. FARRELL, M.D., A.G.S.F.
Associate Professor of Medicine
Adjunct Associate Professor of Family Medicine
Department of Medicine
Division of Geriatrics
University of Utah School of Medicine;
Physician Investigator
Veteran's Affairs Salt Lake City Geriatric Research, Education, and Clinical Center (GRECC)
Veteran's Affairs Salt Lake City
Salt Lake City, Utah

MARIAM FAYEK, M.D.
Gastroenterology Attending Physician
Women & Infants Hospital
The Warren Alpert Medical School
Brown University
Providence, Rhode Island

JASON D. FERREIRA, M.D.
Instructor in Medicine
Department of Gastroenterology
Brown University;
Miriam Hospital;
Rhode Island Hospital;
Roger Williams Medical Center
Providence, Rhode Island

FRED F. FERRI, M.D., F.A.C.P.
Clinical Professor
The Warren Alpert Medical School
Brown University
Providence, Rhode Island

HEATHER FERRI, D.O.
Department of Medicine
The Warren Alpert Medical School
Brown University
Rhode Island Hospital
Providence, Rhode Island

Contributors

AMBER N. FONTENOT FERRISS, M.D.
Physician
Department of Obstetrics and Gynecology
Exempla Lutheran Medical Center
Wheat Ridge, Colorado;
Westside Women's Care
Arvada, Colorado

BARRY FINE, M.D., PH.D.
Fellow in Cardiovascular Medicine
Department of Cardiology
Columbia University;
Clinical Fellow
Department of Medicine
New York Presbyterian Hospital
New York, New York

GLEN FINNEY, M.D.
Neurologist
Geisinger Medical Center
Danville, Pennsylvania

STACI A. FISCHER, M.D.
Associate Professor of Medicine
The Warren Alpert Medical School
Brown University
Providence, Rhode Island

TAMARA G. FONG, M.D., PH.D.
Assistant Professor of Neurology
Harvard Medical School;
Staff Neurologist
Beth Israel Deaconess Medical Center;
Assistant Scientist
Aging Brain Center
Institute for Aging Research
Hebrew SeniorLife
Boston, Massachusetts

MICHELLE FORCIER, M.D., M.P.H.
Associate Professor of Pediatrics
Division of Adolescent Medicine
The Warren Alpert Medical School
Brown University
Providence, Rhode Island

FRANK G. FORT, M.D., F.A.C.S., R.PH.S.
Medical Director
Capital Region Vein Centre
Schenectady, New York

GLENN G. FORT, M.D., M.P.H.
Clinical Associate Professor of Medicine
The Warren Alpert Medical School
Brown University;
Chief, Infectious Diseases
Our Lady of Fatima Hospital
Providence, Rhode Island

JUSTIN F. FRASER, M.D.
Assistant Professor of Cerebrovascular, Endovascular, and Skull Base
    Surgery
Department of Neurosurgery
University of Kentucky
Lexington, Kentucky

MICHAEL FRIEDMAN, M.D.
Rhode Island Hospital;
The Miriam Hospital;
The Warren Alpert Medical School
Brown University
Providence, Rhode Island

DANIEL R. FRISCH, M.D.
Associate Professor of Medicine
Electrophysiology Section
Division of Cardiology
Thomas Jefferson University Hospital
Philadelphia, Pennsylvania

SAINATH GADDAM, M.D.
Fellow
Preventive Cardiology
Providence Veteran's Affairs Medical Center;
The Warren Alpert Medical School
Brown University
Providence, Rhode Island

ANTHONY GALLO, M.D.
Assistant Clinical Professor of Psychiatry
The Warren Alpert Medical School
Brown University
Providence, Rhode Island

MICHAL GANZ, M.D.
Gastroenterology Fellow
Department of Gastroenterology
Brown University;
Rhode Island Hospital
Providence, Rhode Island

MARINA GARAS, D.O.
Department of Anesthesia
Tufts Medical Center
Boston, Massachusetts

LEANNA R. GARBUS, O.M.S. III
University of New England College of Osteopathic Medicine
Biddeford, Maine

EDITH GARNEAU, M.D., M.SC.
Rheumatologist
Department of Medicine
Division of Rheumatology
Roger Williams Medical Center
Providence, Rhode Island

SARA W.F. GEFFERT, M.D., M.S., M(A.S.C.P.)
Infectious Diseases
The Warren Alpert Medical School
Brown University
Providence, Rhode Island

SAMANTHA L. GELFAND, M.D.
Physician
Department of Internal Medicine
Yale University School of Medicine
New Haven, Connecticut

PAUL F. GEORGE, M.D, M.H.P.E.
Associate Professor of Family Medicine
Associate Professor of Medical Science
Department of Family Medicine
Section on Medical Education
The Warren Alpert Medical School
Brown University
Providence, Rhode Island

JOYDEEP GHOSH, M.D., F.A.C.C., F.H.R.S.
Assistant Professor of Medicine
Department of Cardiology
Columbia University Medical Center
New York, New York

KATARZYNA GILEK-SEIBERT, M.D., RH.M.U.S.
Associate Program Director, Rheumatology Fellowship
Division of Rheumatology
Roger Williams Medical Center
Providence, Rhode Island

DIMITRI GITELMAKER, M.D.
Internal Medicine Resident
Roger Williams Medical Center
Boston University School of Medicine
Providence, Rhode Island

KIMBERLY A. GITTINGS, PHARM.D.
Xcenda Post-Doctoral Fellow
Health Outcomes and Market Access
Tampa, Florida

RICHARD J. GOLDBERG, M.D., M.S.
Psychiatrist-in-Chief
Rhode Island Hospital;
The Miriam Hospital;
Professor
Department of Psychiatry and Human Behavior
The Warren Alpert Medical School
Brown University
Providence, Rhode Island

ALLA GOLDBURT, M.D.
Clinical Assistant Professor
Department of Family Medicine
The Warren Alpert Medical School
Brown University
Providence Rhode Island

JESSE GOLDMAN, M.D., F.A.S.H.
Associate Professor of Medicine
Departments of Medicine and Nephrology
Drexel University;
Hahnemann University Hospital
Philadelphia, Pennsylvania

PAUL GORDON, M.D.
Clinical Assistant Professor of Medicine
Division of Cardiology
The Warren Alpert Medical School
Brown University
Providence, Rhode Island

NANCY R. GRAFF, M.D.
Professor of Pediatrics
University of California, San Diego
San Diego, California

FRAZER GRANT, M.D.
Resident
Department of Emergency Medicine
The University of Tennessee College of Medicine
Memphis, Tennessee

JOHN A. GRAY, M.D., PH.D.
Assistant Professor
Department of Neurology
Center for Neuroscience
University of California, Davis
Davis, California

NADIA GRILLER, M.D., F.R.C.P.
Department of Gastroenterology
University of Toronto
Toronto, Ontario, Canada

SIMON GRINGUT, M.D.
Cardiology Fellow
Department of Cardiology
St. Elizabeth's Medical Center
Brighton, Massachusetts

STEPHEN L. GRUPKE, M.D., M.S.
Assistant Professor
Department of Neurosurgery
University of Kentucky
Lexington, Kentucky

PATAN GULTAWATVICHAI, M.D.
Hematology/Oncology Fellow
Departments of Hematology and Oncology
University of Massachusetts Medical School
Worcester, Massachusetts

CANTING GUO, M.D.
Department of Internal Medicine
Rhode Island Hospital
Providence, Rhode Island

PRIYA SARIN GUPTA, M.D, M.P.H.
Adolescent Medicine Fellow
Department of Pediatrics
Division of General Pediatrics and Adolescent Medicine
Johns Hopkins Hospital
Baltimore, Maryland

NAWAZ K.A. HACK, M.D.
Assistant Professor of Neurology
Department of Neurology
F. Edward Hébert School of Medicine
Uniformed Services University of the Health Sciences
Bethesda, Maryland;
Movement Disorders Fellowship Trained
Department of Neurology
University of Florida
Gainesville, Florida

DENISA HAGAU, M.D.
Non-Invasive Cardiologist
Mercy Heart Center and Vascular Institute
Mason City Clinic
Mason City, Iowa

GREGORY M. HAIDEMENOS, M.D.
Boston University School of Medicine
Boston, Massachusetts;
Internal Medicine Department
Roger Williams Medical Center
Providence, Rhode Island

MOTI HAIM, M.D.
Associate Professor
Department of Cardiology
Faculty of Health Sciences
Ben-Gurion University;
Director of Cardiac Electrophysiology and Pacing
Department of Cardiology
Soroka Medical Center
Beer-Sheva, Israel

LEO HAN, M.D., M.P.H.
Instructor
Department of Obstetrics and Gynecology
Oregon Health and Science University
Portland, Oregon

SAJEEV HANDA, M.D., S.F.H.M.
Clinical Assistant Professor
Departments of Medicine and Neurology
The Warren Alpert Medical School
Brown University;
Director, Division of Hospital Medicine
Department of Medicine
Rhode Island Hospital
Providence, Rhode Island

NIKOLAS HARBORD, M.D.
Assistant Professor
Departments of Medicine and Nephrology
Icahn School of Medicine
New York, New York

ERICA HARDY, M.D., M.M.S.
Assistant Professor of Medicine (Clinical)
Department of Medicine
The Warren Alpert Medical School
Brown University;
Associate Director of Women's Infectious Disease Consultation Service
Department of Infectious Disease and Obstetric Medicine
Women & Infants Hospital
Providence, Rhode Island

ANDREW PAUL HARRIS, M.D.
Resident in Orthopaedic Surgery
Department of Orthopaedic Surgery
The Warren Alpert Medical School
Brown University;
Rhode Island Hospital
Providence, Rhode Island

TAYLOR HARRISON, M.D.
Assistant Professor of Neurology
Department of Neurology
Emory University
Atlanta, Georgia

NAOMI HAUSER, M.P.H., M.D.
Medical Resident
Department of Medicine
Boston University School of Medicine
Boston, Massachusetts;
Medical Resident
Internal Medicine
Roger Williams Medical Center
Providence, Rhode Island

DON HAYES, JR., M.D., M.S., M.ED.
Professor
Departments of Pediatrics, Internal Medicine, Surgery, and Epidemiology
The Ohio State University;
Section of Pulmonary Medicine
Nationwide Children's Hospital;
Division of Pulmonary, Allergy, Critical Care, and Sleep Medicine
The Ohio State University Wexner Medical Center
Columbus, Ohio

DWAYNE R. HEITMILLER, M.D.
Assistant Professor of Psychiatry and Human Behavior (Clinical)
Rhode Island Hospital;
The Miriam Hospital
Providence, Rhode Island

EMILY Z. HEJAZI, M.D., M.S.
Research Fellow
Department of Dermatology
University of Pennsylvania;
Hospital of the University of Pennsylvania
Philadelphia, Pennsylvania

MICHAEL HEUNG, M.D., M.S.
Clinical Associate Professor
Internal Medicine–Nephrology
University of Michigan;
Medical Director, Acute Dialysis Program
Department of Internal Medicine–Nephrology
University of Michigan Health System
Ann Arbor, Michigan

MARGARET R. HINES, M.D.
Resident
Department of Obstetrics/Gynecology
Christiana Care Health System
Newark, Delaware

BRIAN HOCHMAN, D.P.M.
Resident in Podiatry
Department of Podiatry
Boston University School of Medicine
Boston, Massachusetts;
Roger Williams Medical Center
Providence, Rhode Island

JONATHAN D. HODAX, M.D., M.S.
Resident
Department of Orthopaedic Surgery
Brown University
Providence, Rhode Island

R. SCOTT HOFFMAN, M.D.
Assistant Clinical Professor
Department of Ophthalmology and Visual Sciences
University of Louisville;
Ophthalmologist
Doctors Eye Institute
Louisville, Kentucky

DAWN HOGAN, M.D.
Clinical Assistant Professor of Family Medicine
The Warren Alpert Medical School
Brown University
Providence, Rhode Island

N. WILSON HOLLAND, M.D.
Associate Professor of Medicine
Division of Geriatrics and Gerontology
Emory University School of Medicine;
Acting Designated Learning Officer
Atlanta Veterans Administration Medical Center
Atlanta, Georgia

ANNE L. HUME, PHARM.D., F.C.C.P., B.C.P.S.
Professor of Pharmacy
Department of Pharmacy Practice
University of Rhode Island
Kingston, Rhode Island;
Adjunct Professor
Department of Family Medicine
Memorial Hospital of Rhode Island
Pawtucket, Rhode Island

DONNY V. HUYNH, M.D.
Hematology Oncology Fellow
Division of Hematology Oncology
Roger Williams Medical Center;
Boston University School of Medicine
Providence, Rhode Island

TERRI Q. HUYNH, M.D.
Minimally Invasive Gynecologic Surgery Fellow
Department of Obstetrics and Gynecology
Division of Minimally Invasive Gynecologic Surgery
Christiana Care Health Systems
Newark, Delaware

LOUIS INSALACO, M.D.
Otolaryngology Resident
Boston University School of Medicine
Boston, Massachusetts

AHMAD M. ISMAIL, M.D.
Pulmonary and Critical Care Fellow
East Carolina University
Greenville, North Carolina

VANITA B.D. JAIN, M.D.
Medical Director, Perinatal Special Care Unit and High Risk Clinic
Department of Obstetrics and Gynecology
Division of Maternal Fetal Medicine
Christiana Care Health Services
Newark, Delaware

ROBERT H. JANIGIAN, M.D.
Clinical Assistant Professor of Surgery
The Warren Alpert Medical School
Brown University
Providence, Rhode Island

NOELLE MARIE C. JAVIER, M.D.
Assistant Professor of Medicine
Geriatrics and Palliative Medicine
Icahn School of Medicine at Mount Sinai
New York, New York

COURTNY JOHNSON, D.P.M., M.S.H.S.
Podiatry Resident
Department of Podiatry
Boston University
Boston, Massachusetts;
Roger Williams Medical Center
Providence, Rhode Island

MICHAEL P. JOHNSON, M.D.
Associate Professor
Department of Medicine
The Warren Alpert Medical School;
Rhode Island Hospital
Providence, Rhode Island

STACEY M. JOLLEY, M.D.
Cleveland Clinic
Cleveland, Ohio

ANGAD JOLLY
Baylor College of Medicine
Houston, Texas

KIMBERLY JONES, M.D.
Associate Professor of Child Neurology
Department of Neurology
University of Kentucky
Lexington, Kentucky

SHYAM JOSHI, M.D.
Rhode Island Hospital;
Department of Internal Medicine
Brown University
Providence, Rhode Island

NAVEEN KACHROO, M.D. PH.D.
Urology Resident
Vattikuti Urology Institute
Henry Ford Hospital
Detroit, Michigan

LUCY KALANITHI, M.D., F.A.C.P.
Stanford Clinical Excellence Research Center
Stanford University School of Medicine
Stanford, California

SIDDHARTH KAPOOR, M.D.
Director, Headache Medicine
Program Director, Fellowship in Headache Medicine
Assistant Professor of Neurology
Department of Neurology
University of Kentucky College of Medicine
Lexington, Kentucky

JOSEPH S. KASS, M.D., J.D., F.A.A.N.
Director, Alzheimer's Disease and Memory Disorders Center
Associate Professor
Department of Neurology
Menninger Department of Psychiatry & Behavioral Sciences
Center for Medical Ethics & Health Policy
Baylor College of Medicine;
Chief of Neurology
Director, Comprehensive Stroke Center
Ben Taub General Hospital
Houston, Texas

EMILY R. KATZ, M.D.
Assistant Professor (Clinical)
Department of Psychiatry & Human Behavior
The Warren Alpert Medical School
Brown University;
Director, Child & Adolescent Psychiatry Consultation-Liaison Service
Hasbro Children's Hospital/Rhode Island Hospital
Providence, Rhode Island

HIRO KAWATA, M.D.
Fellow, Cardiovascular Disease
Division of Cardiology
University of California Irvine Medical Center
Irvine, California

ALI KAZIM, M.D.
Clinical Associate Professor
Department of Psychiatry
David Geffen School of Medicine at the University of California, Los
  Angeles
Los Angeles, California;
Associate Chief of Mental Health
Sepulveda Veterans Administration Ambulatory Health Care
Sepulveda, California

SACHIN KEDAR, M.B.B.S., M.D.
Associate Professor
Department of Neurological Sciences, Ophthalmology and Visual Sciences
University of Nebraska Medical School
Truhlsen Eye Institute
Omaha, Nebraska

ELLIE KELEPOURIS, M.D., F.A.H.A.
Professor and Interim Chair, Department of Medicine
Chief, Division of Nephrology and Hypertension
Drexel University College of Medicine
Philadelphia, Pennsylvania

PAUL S. KELLERMAN, M.D.
Professor of Medicine
Department of Internal Medicine
William Beaumont School of Medicine
Oakland University;
Section Head, Nephrology
Department of Internal Medicine
William Beaumont Health System
Royal Oak, Michigan

SUSAN KELLY, M.D.
Department of Obstetrics and Gynecology
Christiana Care Health System
Newark, Delaware

CHRISTOPHER R. KERN, D.O.
Physician
Department of Nephrology
Hahnemann University Hospital
Philadelphia, Pennsylvania

NAUSHABA ISHRATH KHALID, M.D.
Fellow
Division of Nephrology and Hypertension
Henry Ford Hospital
Detroit, Michigan

A. BASIT KHAN, B.A.
Baylor College of Medicine
Houston, Texas

BYUNG KIM, M.D.
Internal Medicine Chief Resident
Roger Williams Medical Center
Boston University School of Medicine
Boston, Massachusetts

BRANDI KIMBLE, D.P.M.
Doctor of Podiatric Medicine
Department of Podiatry
Roger Williams Medical Center
Providence, Rhode Island

ROBERT M. KIRCHNER, M.D.
Fellow, Cardiology
Division of Cardiology
The Warren Alpert Medical School
Brown University
Providence, Rhode Island

JORDAN KLEBANOFF, M.D.
Department of Obstetrics and Gynecology
Christiana Care Health System
Newark, Delaware

ROBERT KOHN, M.D.
Professor
Department of Psychiatry and Human Behavior
The Warren Alpert Medical School
Brown University
Providence, Rhode Island

ARAVIND RAO KOKKIRALA, M.D., F.A.C.C., R.P.V.I.
Cardiology Staff
Department of Cardiology
Brown University School of Medicine;
Rhode Island Hospital;
Providence Veteran's Affairs Medical Center
Providence, Rhode Island

DHAVAL KOLTE, M.D., PH.D.
Division of Cardiology
Brown University
Providence, Rhode Island

YUVAL KONSTANTINO, M.D.
Faculty of Health Sciences
Ben Gurion University of the Negev;
Department of Cardiology
Soroka University Medical Center
Beer Sheva, Israel

NELSON KOPYT, D.O.
Clinical Professor of Medicine
Department of Medicine
Morsani College of Medicine
Tampa, Florida;
Chief of Nephrology
Department of Medicine
Lehigh Valley Hospital
Allentown, Pennsylvania

KATHERINE KOSTROUN, B.S.
Baylor College of Medicine
Houston, Texas

GEORGE KOVALEVSKY, M.D.
Department of Obstetrics and Gynecology
Christiana Hospital;
Director of Academic Affairs
Reproductive Associates of Delaware
Newark, Delaware

PRASHANTH KRISHNAMOHAN, M.B.B.S., M.D.
Department of Neurocritical Care
Stanford University
Palo Alto, California

DAVID I. KURSS, M.D., F.A.C.O.G., N.C.M.P.
Department of Obstetrics and Gynecology
State University of New York at Buffalo School of Medicine
Buffalo, New York;
Private Practice
Women's Wellness Center of Western New York
Suburban Obstetrics and Gynecology—Invision Health
Williamsville, New York

PETER LACAMERA, M.D.
Chief, Pulmonary and Critical Care Medicine
St. Elizabeth's Medical Center;
Assistant Professor of Clinical Medicine
Tufts University School of Medicine
Boston, Massachusetts

ANN S. LACASCE, M.D., M.M.SC.
Associate Professor of Medicine
Harvard Medical School;
Department of Medical Oncology
Dana-Farber Cancer Institute
Boston, Massachusetts

ALISHA LAKHANI, M.D., M.P.H.
Department of Medicine
The Warren Alpert Medical School
Brown University;
Physician
Department of Medicine
Rhode Island Hospital
Providence, Rhode Island

ASHLEY LAKIN, D.O., M.A.
Assistant Professor of Family Medicine (Clinical)
Department of Family Medicine
The Warren Alpert Medical School
Brown University
Providence, Rhode Island

UYEN T. LAM, M.D.
Cardiology Fellow
Department of Cardiovascular Medicine
St. Elizabeth's Medical Center
Boston, Massachusetts

SYED R. LATIF, M.D.
Clinical Fellow, Cardiovascular Medicine
Department of Internal Medicine
University of California, Davis Medical Center
Sacramento, California

DAVID A. LEAVITT, M.D.
Associate Director of Endourology
Director of Laser Surgery
Vattikuti Urology Institute
Henry Ford Health System
Detroit, Michigan

KACHIU C. LEE, M.D., M.P.H.
Assistant Clinical Professor
Department of Dermatology
Brown University;
Rhode Island Hospital
Providence, Rhode Island

PAUL LEIS, D.O.
Professor of Biomedical Engineering
Johns Hopkins University
Baltimore, Maryland

BETH HILARY LEOPOLD, M.D.
Resident, PGY1
Department of Obstetrics and Gynecology
Christiana Care Health System
Newark, Delaware

ANDRE LEVCHENKO, PH.D.
John C. Malone Professor of Biomedical Engineering
Yale School of Engineering and Applied Science
New Haven, Connecticut;
Research Professor
Professor of Biomedical Engineering
Johns Hopkins Biomedical Engineering
Baltimore, Maryland

JIAN LI, M.D., PH.D.
Assistant Professor of Medicine
Department of Internal Medicine
Wayne State University School of Medicine;
Senior Staff Physician
Division of Nephrology and Hypertension
Henry Ford Hospital
Detroit, Michigan

DONITA DILLON LIGHTNER, M.D.
Assistant Professor of Pediatric Neurology
Department of Neurology
University of Kentucky
Lexington, Kentucky

PATRICIA W. LO, M.D.
Obstetrics/Gynecology Physician
Department of Obstetrics and Gynecology
Christiana Care Hospital
Newark, Delaware

RICHARD LONG, M.D.
Director of Maternal and Child Health
Associate Professor of Family Medicine
Department of Family Medicine
Boston University School of Medicine;
Department of Family Medicine
Boston Medical Center
Boston, Massachusetts

ELIZABETH A. LOWENHAUPT, M.D.
Associate Training Director
Child Psychiatry Fellowship & Triple Board Residency
Director, Medical Student Education in Child & Adolescent Psychiatry
Director of Psychiatric Services
Rhode Island Training School;
Clinical Assistant Professor
Department of Psychiatry and Human Behavior
Rhode Island Hospital;
Brown University
Providence, Rhode Island

RANDY L. LUCIANO, M.D., PH.D.
Assistant Professor of Medicine
Department of Medicine
Section of Nephrology
Yale University School of Medicine
New Haven, Connecticut

LAYOLA LUNGHAR, M.D.
Division of Pulmonary, Critical Care and Sleep Medicine
Norwood Hospital
Norwood, Massachusetts

MICHELLE C. MACIAG, M.D.
Physician
Departments of Internal Medicine and Pediatrics
Brown University;
Rhode Island Hospital;
Hasbro Children's Hospital
Providence, Rhode Island

SUSANNA R. MAGEE, M.D., M.P.H.
Assistant Professor
Department of Family Medicine
The Warren Alpert Medical School
Brown University
Providence, Rhode Island

DURKHANI MAHBOOB, M.D.
Rheumatology Fellow
Department of Medicine
Boston University School of Medicine
Boston, Massachusetts;
Rheumatology Fellow
Division of Rheumatology
Department of Medicine
Roger Williams Medical Center
Providence, Rhode Island

MARTA MAJCZAK, M.D.
Clinical Assistant Professor of Psychiatry and Human Behavior
Brown University
Providence, Rhode Island

SHEFALI MAJMUDAR, D.O.
Rheumatologist
Department of Internal Medicine
University of California San Francisco, Fresno;
Departments of Rheumatology and Internal Medicine
Community Regional Medical Center
Fresno, California

GRETCHEN MAKAI, M.D.
Director, Division of Minimally Invasive Gynecologic Surgery
Department of Obstetrics and Gynecology
Christiana Care Health System
Newark, Delaware

PIEUSHA MALHOTRA, M.D., M.P.H.
Rheumatology Fellow
Department of Medicine
Division of Rheumatology
Boston University
Boston, Massachusetts;
Roger Williams Medical Center
Providence, Rhode Island

EISHITA MANJREKAR, PH.D.
Postdoctoral Fellow
The Warren Alpert Medical School
Brown University;
Rhode Island Methods to Improve Diagnostic Assessment and Services
   (MIDAS) Project
Providence, Rhode Island

ABIGAIL K. MANSFIELD, PH.D.
Department of Psychiatry
Rhode Island Hospital
Providence, Rhode Island

MICHAEL C. MARIORENZI, M.S., M.D.
Resident Physician
Department of Orthopedic Surgery
The Warren Alpert Medical School
Brown University;
Rhode Island Hospital
Providence, Rhode Island

KELLY L. MATSON, B.S.N.U.T.R., PHARM.D.
Clinical Associate Professor
Department of Pharmacy Practice
University of Rhode Island
Kingston, Rhode Island;
Pediatric Clinical Specialist
UMass Memorial Children's Medical Center
Worcester, Massachusetts

MAITREYI MAZUMDAR, M.D., M.P.H., M.SC.
Assistant Professor of Neurology
Harvard Medical School;
Staff Physician
Department of Neurology
Boston's Children's Hospital;
Assistant Professor
Department of Environmental Health
Harvard School of Public Health
Boston, Massachusetts

NADINE MBUYI, M.D.
Rheumatology Fellow
Division of Rheumatology
Brown University
Rhode Island Hospital
Providence, Rhode Island

RUSSELL J. MCCULLOH, M.D.
Assistant Professor
Pediatric Infectious Diseases
University of Missouri-Kansas City
Kansas City, Missouri;
University of Kansas School of Medicine
Kansas City, Kansas

BARBARA MCGUIRK, M.D.
Reproductive Endocrinology and Infertility
Christiana Care Health System;
Director of Minimally Invasive Surgey
Reproductive Associates of Delaware
Newark, Delaware

ERIN E. MEDLIN, M.D.
Instructor
Department of Obstetrics, Gynecology, and Women's Health
University of Louisville School of Medicine
Louisville, Kentucky

JOSEPH MEHARG, M.D.
Assistant Professor of Medicine
Department of Medicine
Boston University School of Medicine
Boston, Massachusetts;
Director, Intensive Care Unit
Director, Division of Pulmonary & Critical Care Medicine
Department of Medicine
Roger Williams Medical Center
Providence, Rhode Island

AKANKSHA MEHTA, M.D., M.S.
Assistant Professor of Urology
Emory University School of Medicine
Atlanta, Georgia

JENNIFER B. MERRIMAN, M.D.
Department of Obstetrics & Gynecology
Division of Maternal Fetal Medicine
Christiana Care Health System;
Delaware Center for Maternal & Fetal Medicine of Christiana Care
Newark, Delware

GAETANE MICHAUD, M.D.
Associate Professor of Medicine and Cardiothoracic Surgery
Department of Medicine
New York University School of Medicine;
Section Chief, Interventional Pulmonology
Department of Medicine
Division of Pulmonary, Critical Care & Sleep Medicine
New York University Langone Medical Center
New York, New York

TARO MINAMI, M.D., F.A.C.P., F.C.C.P.
Assistant Professor of Medicine (Clinical)
Division of Pulmonary, Critical Care and Sleep Medicine
The Warren Alpert Medical School
Brown University
Providence, Rhode Island;
Director, Simulation and Ultrasound Training
Division of Pulmonary, Critical Care and Sleep Medicine
Memorial Hospital of Rhode Island
Pawtucket, Rhode Island

HASSAN M. MINHAS, M.D.
Child and Adolescent Psychiatry Chief Fellow
The Warren Alpert Medical School
Brown University
Providence, Rhode Island

FARHAN A. MIRZA, M.B.B.S.
Department of Neurosurgery
University of Kentucky
Lexington, Kentucky

NAUSHABA MOHIUDDIN, M.D.
Fellow
Department of Internal Medicine
Division of Nephrology and Hypertension
Henry Ford Hospital
Detroit, Michigan

THERESA A. MORGAN, PH.D.
Resident in Clinical Psychology
The Warren Alpert Medical School
Brown University;
Department of Psychiatry
Rhode Island Hospital
Providence, Rhode Island

ALEEM MUGHAL, M.D.
Clinical Fellow, Cardiac Electrophysiology
Department of Cardiac Electrophysiology
Steward St. Elizabeth's Medical Center;
Tufts University
Boston, Massachusetts

SHIVA KUMAR R. MUKKAMALLA, M.D., M.P.H.
Clinical Fellow
Department of Internal Medicine
Division of Hematology/Oncology
Roger Williams Medical Center
Providence, Rhode Island;
Boston University School of Medicine
Boston, Massachusetts

CATHERINE E. NAJEM, M.D.
Fellow
Division of Rheumatology
University of Pennsylvania Perelman School of Medicine;
Department of Biostatistics and Epidemiology
University of Pennsylvania
Philadelphia, Pennsylvania

BILAL H. NAQVI, M.D.
Hematologist/Oncologist
Marshfield Clinic Regional Cancer Center
Eau Claire, Wisconsin

HUSSAIN MOHAMMAD H. NASERI, M.D.
Fellow, Hematology/Oncology
Roger Williams Medical Center
Providence, Rhode Island;
Boston University
Boston, Massachusetts

UZMA NASIR, M.D.
Assistant Professor
Department of Clinical Anesthesia and Pain Management
State University of New York at Stony Brook University Hospital
Stony Brook, New York;
Veteran's Affairs Hospital
Northport, New York

SHAW NATAN, M.D.
Cardiac Electrophysiologist
St Elizabeth's Medical Center
Boston, Massachusetts;
Assistant Professor of Medicine
Tufts University
Boston, Massachusetts

ALI NAYER, M.D.
Nephrologist
Department of Medicine
Mercy Hospital;
Founder, Miami Renal Institute
Miami, Florida

LAMA NAZZAL, M.D., M.SC.
Clinical Instructor
New York University School of Medicine
New York, New York

ADRIENNE B. NEITHARDT, M.D.
Physician
Department of Obstetrics and Gynecology
Division of Reproductive Endocrinology and Infertility
Christiana Care Health System;
Associate Physician
Reproductive Endocrinology and Infertility
Reproductive Associates of Delaware
Newark, Delaware

MELISSA NOTHNAGLE, M.D., M.SC.
Associate Professor
Department of Family Medicine
The Warren Alpert Medical School
Brown University
Providence, Rhode Island;
Family Medicine Residency Director
Department of Family Medicine
Memorial Hospital of Rhode Island
Pawtucket, Rhode Island

JAMES E. NOVAK, M.D., PH.D.
Associate Clinical Professor
Department of Internal Medicine
Wayne State University;
Program Director, Nephrology Fellowship
Division of Nephrology and Hypertension
Henry Ford Hospital
Detroit, Michigan

ADAM M. NOYES, M.D.
Department of Cardiology
The Warren Alpert Medical School
Brown University;
Clinical Fellow
Department of Cardiology
Cardiovascular Institute of Rhode Island
Providence, Rhode Island

PATRICK NSEREKO, M.D.
Department of Medicine
Boston University School of Medicine
Boston, Massachusetts;
Medical Doctor/Resident Internal Medicine
Department of Medicine
Roger Williams Medical Center
Providence, Rhode Island

CHLOE MANDER NUNNELEY, M.D.
Baylor College of Medicine
Houston, Texas

GAIL M. O'BRIEN, M.D.
Martha's Vineyard Hospital
Oak Bluffs, Massachusetts

DANIEL W. OESTERLE, B.S.
Research Assistant
Department of Psychiatry
Rhode Island Hospital
Providence, Rhode Island

ALEXANDER B. OLAWAIYE, M.D.
Fellow
Vincent Department of Obstetrics
Division of Gynecologic Oncology
Gynecology and Reproductive Biology
Massachusetts General Hospital;
Harvard Medical School
Boston, Massachusetts

ADAM J. OLSZEWSKI, M.D.
Assistant Professor of Medicine
The Warren Alpert Medical School
Brown University
Rhode Island Hospital
Providence, Rhode Island

LINDSAY M. ORCHOWSKI, PH.D.
Staff Psychologist
Rhode Island Hospital;
Assistant Professor
Department of Psychiatry
The Warren Alpert Medical School
Brown University
Providence, Rhode Island

PAOLO G. PACE, M.A.SC., M.D.
Resident Physician
Department of Internal Medicine
Roger Williams Medical Center
Providence, Rhode Island

CRISTINA ANTONIO PACHECO, M.D
Clinical Assistant Professor
Department of Family Medicine
The Warren Alpert Medical School
Brown University
Providence, Rhode Island

CHRIS W. PAN, M.D., M.B.A., M.S.
Interventional Cardiology Fellow
Division of Cardiology
Department of Medicine
University of California, Irvine
Orange, California

LISA K. PAPPAS-TAFFER, M.D.
Assistant Professor of Dermatology
The University of Pennsylvania;
Perelman Center for Advanced Medicine;
The Hospital of the University of Pennsylvania;
Veterans Affairs Hospital;
Philadelphia, Pennsylvania

SARIKA PARIKH, D.P.M.
Podiatrist
Podiatric Surgery
Agnesian Health Care
Fond du Lac, Wisconsin

BHAVIN C. PATEL, M.D.
Department of Nephrology and Hypertension
Henry Ford Hospital
Detroit, Michigan

BIRJU B. PATEL, M.D.
Assistant Professor of Medicine
Department of Medicine
Division of Geriatrics and Gerontology
Emory University School of Medicine;
Atlanta Veterans Affairs Medical Center;
Director
Co-Consultant, Network Geriatrics and Extended Care
Bronze Geriatric Outpatient Clinic
Atlanta, Georgia

JANAKI PATEL, M.D.
Rheumatology Fellow–PGY4
Department of Rheumatology
Brown University;
Roger Williams Medical Center;
Rhode Island Hospital
Providence, Rhode Island

NIMA R. PATEL, M.D., M.S.
Associate Fellowship Director, Division of Minimally Invasive Gynecologic
    Surgery
Associate Program Director, Department of Obstetrics & Gynecology
Department of Obstetrics and Gynecology
Division of Minimally Invasive Gynecologic Surgery
Christiana Care Health System
Newark, Delaware

PRANAV M. PATEL, M.D., F.A.C.C., F.S.C.A.I.
Chief, Division of Cardiology
University of California, Irvine;
Director of Cardiac Cath Lab & Cardiac Care Unit
Departments of Cardiology and Medicine
University of California, Irvine Medical Center
Orange, California

SAAGAR N. PATEL, B.A., B.S.
Baylor College of Medicine
Houston, Texas

BRETT PATRICK, M.D.
University of Tennessee College of Medicine
Memphis, Tennessee

ALISON PATTERSON, M.D.
Resident in Obstetrics and Gynecology
Department of Obstetrics and Gynecology
University of Colorado
Aurora, Colorado

GRACE REBECCA PAUL, M.B.B.S., M.D.
Assistant Professor of Pediatrics
Division of Pulmonary and Sleep Medicine
Nationwide Children's Hospital
Columbus, Ohio

LYNN PESTA, M.D.
Attending Physician
Women's Medicine Collaborative
Miriam Hospital
Providence, Rhode Island

KATHARINE A. PHILLIPS, M.D.
Professor of Psychiatry and Human Behavior
The Warren Alpert Medical School
Brown University;
Director of Research for Adult Psychiatry
Director, Body Dysmorphic Disorder Program
Rhode Island Hospital
Providence, Rhode Island

TONI PICERNO, D.O.
Resident
Department of Obstetrics and Gynecology
Christiana Care Health System
Newark, Delaware

CHRISTOPHER PICKETT, M.D.
Director of Clinical Cardiology
Associate Professor of Medicine
Calhoun Cardiology Center
University of Connecticut Health Center
Farmington, Connecticut

WENDY A. PLANTE, PH.D.
Clinical Assistant Professor of Psychiatry and Human Behavior
The Warren Alpert Medical School
Brown University;
Rhode Island Hospital;
Hasbro Children's Research Center
Providence, Rhode Island

KEVIN V. PLUMLEY, M.D., M.P.H.
Roger Williams Medical Center
Boston University
Providence, Rhode Island

MICHAEL POHLEN, M.D.
Baylor College of Medicine
Houston, Texas

SHARON S. HARTMAN POLENSEK, M.D., PH.D.
Assistant Professor of Neurology
Center for Dizziness and Balance Disorders
Emory University
Atlanta, Georgia;
Chief
Audiology and Speech Pathology
Atlanta Veterans Affairs Medical Center
Decatur, Georgia

DONN POSNER, PH.D., C.B.S.M.
Clinical/Research Psychologist
Palo Alto Veterans Institute for Research
Veterans Affairs Palo Alto Health Care System
Palo Alto, California

AMANDA PRESSMAN, M.D.
Director of the Program in Pelvic Floor Disorders
Gastroenterologist
Department of Gastroenterology
Women's Medicine Collaborative;
Director of Motility
Department of Gastroenterology
Lifespan
Providence, Rhode Island

KITTICHAI PROMRAT, M.D.
Assistant Professor
Division of Gastroenterology
Department of Medicine
The Warren Alpert Medical School
Brown University;
Chief
Gastroenterology Section
Providence Veterans Affairs Medical Center
Providence, Rhode Island

SHAHNAZ PUNJANI, M.D.
Fellow, Preventive Cardiology
Providence Veterans Affairs Medical Center
The Warren Alpert Medical School
Brown University
Providence, Rhode Island

IMRANA QAWI, M.D.
Assistant Professor, Medicine
Pulmonary/Critical Care
Tufts Medical Center
Boston, Massachusetts;
Attending Physician
Critical Care
Lowell General Hospital
Lowell, Massachusetts

HEIDI RADLINSKI, M.D., M.P.H.
Clinical Instructor
Department of Family Medicine
University of Washington
Seattle, Washington;
Maternal Child Health Director
Department of Family Medicine
Peacehealth Southwest Medical Center
Vancouver, Washington;
Oregon Health & Science University
Portland, Oregon

WILLIAM M. RAFELSON, M.D., M.B.A.
Department of Internal Medicine
Rhode Island Hospital;
The Warren Alpert Medical School
Brown University
Providence, Rhode Island

SAMAAN RAFEQ, M.D.
Assistant Professor of Medicine
Tufts Medical School;
Director, Interventional Pulmonary Services
Division of Pulmonary, Critical Care, and Sleep Medicine
Associate Program Director, Internal Medicine Residency Training Program
Department of Internal Medicine
St. Elizabeth's Medical Center
Boston, Massachusetts

RESHMA RAMAKRISHNAN, M.D.
Endocrinology Fellow
Division of Endocrinology, Diabetes, Bone & Mineral Disorders
Henry Ford Health System
Detroit, Michigan

MEGHANA RAO, M.D.
Department of Cardiology
The Warren Alpert Medical School
Brown University;
Cardiology Fellow
Department of Cardiology
Rhode Island Hospital;
The Miriam Hospital;
Providence, Rhode Island

SOMWAIL RASLA, M.D.
Internal Medicine Department
Memorial Hospital of Rhode Island
Pawtucket, Rhode Island;
Department of Internal Medicine
Memorial Hospital of Rhode Island;
The Warren Alpert Medical School
Brown University
Providence, Rhode Island

BHARTI RATHORE, M.D.
Program Director, Hematology/Oncology Fellowship
Roger Williams Medical Center
Providence, Rhode Island;
Assistant Professor of Medicine
Boston University School of Medicine
Boston, Massachusetts

RITESH RATHORE, M.D.
Director, Division of Hematology/Oncology
Director, Cancer Protocol Office
Roger Williams Medical Center
Providence, Rhode Island;
Associate Professor of Medicine
Boston University School of Medicine
Boston, Massachusetts

NEHA P. RAUKAR, M.D., M.S.
Associate Professor
Department of Emergency Medicine
Brown University
Providence, Rhode Island

JOHN L. REAGAN, M.D.
Assistant Professor
Department of Medicine
The Warren Alpert Medical School
Brown University;
Attending Physician
Department of Medicine
Rhode Island Hospital
The Miriam Hospital
Providence, Rhode Island

BHARATHI V. REDDY, M.D.
Assistant Professor of Medicine
Department of Medicine
University of Chicago
Chicago, Illinois

CHAKRAVARTHY REDDY, M.D.
Associate Professor
Department of Pulmonary and Critical Care
University of Utah
Salt Lake City, Utah

SNIGDHA T. REDDY, M.D.
Senior Staff Physician
Division of Nephrology and Hypertension
Henry Ford Hospital
Detroit, Michigan

ANTHONY M. REGINATO, PH.D., M.D.
Director, Rheumatology Research and Musculoskeletal Ultrasound
Director, Rheumatology Fellowship Program
Associate Professor in Medicine
The Warren Alpert Medical School
Brown University;
Chief, Division of Rheumatology
Providence Veterans Affairs Medical Center
Providence, Rhode Island

RICHARD REGNANTE, M.D.
Division of Cardiovascular Medicine
The Warren Alpert Medical School
Brown University
Providence, Rhode Island

DANIEL BRIAN CARLIN REID, M.D., M.P.H.
Orthopedic Surgery Resident
Department of Orthopedics
Brown University;
Orthopedic Surgery Resident
Department of Orthopedics
Lifespan
Providence, Rhode Island

VICTOR I. REUS, M.D.
Professor
Department of Psychiatry
University of California, San Francisco;
Weill Institute of Neurosciences
University of California, San Francisco School of Medicine
San Francisco, California

MELISSA RICCI, D.P.M., M.B.S.
Podiatry Resident
Department of Surgery
Roger Williams Medical Center
Providence, Rhode Island

HARLAN G. RICH, M.D., F.A.C.P., A.G.A.F
Associate Professor of Medicine
Department of Medicine
The Warren Alpert Medical School
Brown University;
Director of Endoscopy
Department of Medicine
Division of Gastroenterology
Rhode Island Hospital;
Staff Physician
Division of Gastroenterology
University Medicine Foundation, Inc.
Providence, Rhode Island

ROCCO J. RICHARDS, M.D.
Department of Internal Medicine
Roger Williams Medical Center
Providence, Rhode Island;
Boston University School of Medicine
Boston, Massachusetts

GIULIA RIGHI, PH.D.
Staff Psychologist
Emma Pendleton Bradley Hospital;
Assistant Professor (Research)
The Warren Alpert Medical School
Brown University
Providence, Rhode Island

REBECCA RINKO, D.O.
Department of Obstetrics and Gynecology
Drexel University College of Medicine;
Hahnemann University Hospital
Philadelphia, Pennsylvania;
Christiana Care
Newark, Delaware

PETER RINTELS, M.D.
Kent Hospital
Warwick, Rhode Island;
Hematology & Oncology Associates of Rhode Island
Cranston, Rhode Island

ALVARO M. RIVERA, M.D.
Department of Internal Medicine
Roger Williams Medical Center
Providence, Rhode Island

NICOLE A. ROBERTS, M.D.
Resident
Obstetrics and Gynecology
Christiana Care Health System
Newark, Delaware

NICOLETTE J. RODRIGUEZ, M.D., M.P.H.
Resident Physician
Department of Internal Medicine
Yale University;
Yale-New Haven Hospital
New Haven, Connecticut

JAMISON ROGERS, M.D.
Program Director of Forensic Psychiatry Fellowship
Clinical Assistant Professor of Psychiatry and Human Behavior
The Warren Alpert Medical School
Brown University
Providence, Rhode Island

JULIE L. ROTH, M.D.
Assistant Professor
Department of Neurology
The Warren Alpert Medical School
Brown University;
Director of Women's Neurology
Department of Neurology
Rhode Island Hospital
Providence, Rhode Island

STEVEN ROUGAS, M.D., M.S.
Assistant Professor of Emergency Medicine
The Warren Alpert Medical School
Brown University
Providence, Rhode Island

AMITY RUBEOR, D.O., C.A.Q.S.M.
Assistant Professor
Department of Family Medicine
The Warren Alpert Medical School
Brown University;
Team Physician
Women's Ice Hockey
Providence College
Providence, Rhode Island;
Associate Fellowship Director
Brown University-Memorial Hospital of Rhode Island Primary Care Sports
    Medicine Fellowship
Pawtucket, Rhode Island

THOMAS M. RUENGER, M.D., PH.D.
Professor of Dermatology, Pathology and Laboratory Medicine
Boston University School of Medicine
Boston, Massachusetts

KELLY RUHSTALLER, M.D.
Maternal Fetal Medicine
Christiana Care
Newark, Delaware

HAYLEY RYAN, D.O.
Clinical Instructor in Family Medicine
Brown University
Providence, Rhode Island

IMMAD SADIQ, M.D.
Clinical Assistant Professor of Medicine
Division of Cardiology
The Warren Alpert Medical School
Brown University
Providence, Rhode Island

TANMAY SAHAI, M.D.
Roger Williams Medical Center
Providence, Rhode Island;
Boston University School of Medicine
Boston, Massachusetts

EMILY K. SAKS, M.D., M.S.C.E.
Adjunct Clinical Assistant Professor of Obstetrics and Gynecology
Department of Obstetrics and Gynecology
Drexel University College of Medicine
Philadelphia, Pennsylvania;
Department of Obstetrics/Gynecology—Urogynecology
Center for Urogynecology and Pelvic Surgery
Christiana Care Health System
Newark, Delaware

RADHIKA SAMPAT, D.O.
Instructor
Department of Neurology
Neuromuscular Division
Emory University School of Medicine;
Emory University Hospital;
Medical Director of the Grady Neurology Clinic
Grady Memorial Hospital;
Atlanta, Georgia

SONIA R. SAMTANI, M.D.
Fellow, Cardiovascular Disease
Division of Cardiology
University of California Irvine Medical Center
Irvine, California

HEMANT K. SATPATHY, M.D.
Fellow
Division of Maternal Fetal Medicine
Department of Obstetrics and Gynecology
Emory University
Atlanta, Georgia

RUBY K. SATPATHY, M.D.
Fellow, Cardiology
Department of Internal Medicine
Creighton University
Omaha, Nebraska

SYEDA M. SAYEED, M.D.
Clinical Instructor of Medicine
The Warren Alpert Medical School
Brown University
Providence Rhode Island

DAPHNE SCARAMANGAS-PLUMLEY, M.D.
Fellow, Rheumatology
Cedars-Sinai Medical Center
Los Angeles, California

HEIKO SCHMITT, M.D., PH.D.
Associate Professor
Department of Medicine
Division of Cardiology
John Dempsey Hospital
Farmington, Connecticut

CLAIRE SCHULTZ, M.D.
Resident Physician
Department of Obstetrics and Gynecology
University of Colorado;
University of Colorado Anschutz Medical Center
Denver, Colorado

ANTHONY SCISCIONE, D.O.
Professor
Department of Obstetrics and Gynecology
Jefferson Medical College
Philadelphia, Pennsylvania;
Residency Program Director
Director, Maternal-Fetal Medicine
Department of Obstetrics and Gynecology
Christiana Care Health System
Newark, Delaware

PETER J. SELL, D.O., F.A.A.P.
Associate Professor
Department of Pediatrics
University of Massachusetts Medical School;
Pediatric Hospitalist
Department of Pediatrics
Divisions of Critical Care and Child Protection
UMass Memorial Medical Center
Worcester, Massachusetts;
Adjunct Assistant Professor
Department of Family Medicine
The Warren Alpert Medical School
Brown University
Providence, Rhode Island

STEVEN M. SEPE, M.D., PH.D.
Chair of the Department of Medicine
Roger Williams Medical Center
Providence, Rhode Island;
Clinical Professor of Medicine
Assistant Dean of Clinical Affairs
Boston University School of Medicine
Boston, Massachusetts

CLAUDIA SERRANO, M.D.
Assistant Clinical Professor
Department of Internal Medicine
Division of Cardiology
New York University
New York, New York

REBECCA KURNIK SESHASAI, M.D., M.S.H.P.
Assistant Professor of Medicine
Department of Medicine
Division of Nephrology and Hypertension
Drexel University College of Medicine
Philadelphia, Pennsylvania

KALPIT N. SHAH, M.D.
Resident Physician
Department of Orthopaedic Surgery
Brown University;
Rhode Island Hospital
Providence, Rhode Island

SANJEEV R. SHAH, M.D.
Assistant Professor of Clinical Medicine
Renal Electrolyte and HTN Division
Perelman School of Medicine
Philadelphia, Pennsylvania

SHIVANI SHAH, M.D.
Resident
Department of Obstetrics and Gynecology
Christiana Care Health System
Newark, Delaware

JESSICA E. SHILL, M.D.
Senior Staff Physician, Endocrinologist
Division of Endocrinology, Diabetes, Bone & Mineral Disorders
Henry Ford Health System
Detroit, Michigan

ALEXANDRA SHINGINA, M.D.C.M.
Department of Gastroenterology
University of Toronto
Toronto, Ontario, Canada

PHILIP A. SHLOSSMAN, M.D.
Associate Director, Maternal & Fetal Medicine
Department of Obstetrics and Gynecology
Christiana Hospital
Newark, Delaware

ASHA SHRESTHA, M.D.
Fellow
Division of Rheumatology
Albert Einstein College of Medicine;
Montefiore Medical Center
Bronx, New York

MARK SIGMAN, M.D.
Kristhamurthi Family Professor and Chief of Urology
Department of Surgery (Urology)
The Warren Alpert Medical School
Brown University;
Chief of Urology
Department of Surgery (Urology)
Rhode Island Hospital;
The Miriam Hospital
Providence, Rhode Island

JARED A. SILVERSTEIN, M.D.
Pediatric Gastroenterology
Women & Infants Hospital
Providence, Rhode Island

JOANNE M. SILVIA, M.D.
Clinical Assistant Professor of Family Medicine
Department of Family Medicine
The Warren Alpert Medical School
Brown University
Providence, Rhode Island

JAMES F. SIMON, M.D.
Assistant Professor
Lerner College of Medicine;
Staff Nephrologist
Nephrology and Hypertension
Cleveland Clinic
Cleveland, Ohio

REDDY SINGASANI, M.D.
Fellow
Department of Internal Medicine
Division of Nephrology and Hypertension
Henry Ford Hospital
Detroit, Michigan

DIVYA SINGHAL, M.D.
Director, Resident Longitudinal Clinic
Vice Chair, Women's Issues in Neurology
American Academy of Neurology
Assistant Professor of Neurology
University of Oklahoma;
Epileptologist
Department of Neurology/Rehabilitation Services
Oklahoma City Veterans Affairs Medical Center
Oklahoma City, Oklahoma

JON SKALECKI, M.D.
Department of Internal Medicine
Roger Williams Medical Center
Providence, Rhode Island

IRINA A. SKYLAR-SCOTT, M.D.
Resident Physician
Department of Neurology
Harvard Medical School;
Resident Physician
Department of Neurology
Beth Israel Deaconess Medical Center
Boston, Massachusetts

JOHN SLADKY, M.D.
Staff Neurologist
Associate Program Director
Wilford Hall Medical Center
San Antonio, Texas

ARLENE J. SMALLS, M.D.
OB/GYN Generalist
Department of Obstetrics and Gynecology
Christiana Care Health System
Newark, Delaware

ERIN SMITH, M.D.
Physician
Obstetrics and Gynecology
Christiana Care Health System
Newark, Delaware

Contributors

JEANETTE G. SMITH, M.D.
Assistant Professor of Medicine
Department of Gastroenterology
The Warren Alpert Medical School
Brown University
Providence, Rhode Island

JONATHAN H. SMITH, M.D.
Assistant Professor
Department of Neurology
University of Kentucky
Lexington, Kentucky

THOMAS SMITH, M.D.
Assistant Clinical Professor, Cardiovascular Medicine
Department of Internal Medicine
University of California, Davis Medical Center
Sacramento, California

ANDREW D. SOBEL, M.D.
Chief Resident in Orthopaedic Surgery
Department of Orthopaedic Surgery
The Warren Alpert Medical School
Brown University;
Chief Resident in Orthopaedic Surgery
Department of Orthopaedic Surgery
Rhode Island Hospital
Providence, Rhode Island

U. SHIVRAJ SOHUR, M.D., PH.D.
Assistant Professor of Neurology
Harvard Medical School
Boston, Massachusetts

REBECCA SOINSKI, M.D.
Rhode Island Hospital;
The Miriam Hospital
Providence, Rhode Island

MARIA E. SOLER, M.D., M.P.H., M.B.A.
Director of Education Division
Medical Director of Triage
Department of Obstetrics and Gyncology
Christiana Care Health System
Newark, Delaware

SANDEEP SOMAN, M.D.
Clinical Associate Professor
Internal Medicine
Wayne State University School of Medicine;
Associate Division Head
Internal Medicine, Nephrology
Henry Ford Hospital
Detroit, Michigan

SCOTT M. SOUTHER, M.D.
Resident, Internal Medicine
Boston University
Boston, Massachusetts;
Roger Williams Medical Center
Providence, Rhode Island

PETER L. STEINBERG, M.D.
Assistant Professor
Department of Surgery (Urology)
Harvard Medical School;
Director of Endourology
Department of Surgery (Urology)
Beth Israel Deaconess Medical Center
Boston, Massachusetts

JOHANNES STEINER, M.D.
Assistant Professor of Medicine
Department of Cardiology
University of Vermont Medical Center
Burlington, Vermont;
Clinical Instructor
Department of Cardiology
Massachusetts General Hospital
Boston, Massachusetts

PHILIP STOCKWELL, M.D.
Department of Cardiology
Brown University School of Medicine;
Rhode Island Hospital
Providence, Rhode Island

LARA STONE, D.P.M.
Doctor of Podiatric Medicine
Department of Podiatry
Roger Williams Medical Center
Providence, Rhode Island

PADMAJA SUDHAKAR, M.B.B.S.
Assistant Professor
Department of Neurology
University of Kentucky
Lexington, Kentucky

ELIZABETH SUSHEREBA, M.S.N., C.N.M.
Faculty
Department of Obstetrics and Gynecology
Christiana Care Health Systems
Newark, Delaware

MARY BETH SUTTER, M.D.
Assistant Professor
Family and Community Medicine
University of New Mexico Health Sciences Center
Albuquerque, New Mexico

ARUN SWAMINATHAN, M.B.B.S.
Resident
Department of Neurology
University of Kentucky College of Medicine
University of Kentucky Hospital
Lexington, Kentucky

JOSEPH SWEENEY, M.D., F.A.C.P., F.R.C.PATH.
Professor
Laboratory Medicine and Pathology
Brown University;
Director, Coagulation and Transfusion Medicine
Department of Pathology
Lifespan;
Medical Director, Blood Bank
Roger Williams Hospital
Providence, Rhode Island

WAJIH A. SYED, M.D.
Department of Cardiology
St Elizabeth Medical Center
Boston, Massachusetts

MAHER TABBA, M.D., F.A.C.P., F.C.C.P.
Associate Professor of Medicine
Department of Pulmonary & Critical Care Medicine and Sleep Disorders
Tufts Medical Center
Boston, Massachusetts

DOMINICK TAMMARO, M.D.
The Warren Alpert Medical School
Brown University;
Rhode Island Hospital
Providence, Rhode Island

TAHIR TELLIOGLU, M.D.
Assistant Professor of Psychiatry and Human Behavior
The Warren Alpert Medical School
Brown University;
Director, Substance Abuse Division
Department of Psychiatry
Rhode Island Hospital
Providence, Rhode Island

JIGISHA P. THAKKAR, M.D.
Chief Resident
Department of Neurology
University of Kentucky;
Department of Neurology
University of Kentucky Medical Center, Chandler Hospital
Lexington, Kentucky

ANTHONY G. THOMAS, D.O., F.A.C.P.
Clinical Assistant Professor of Medicine
Department of Internal Medicine
The Warren Alpert Medical School
Brown University
Providence, Rhode Island;
Chief, Hematology/Oncology
Director, Cancer Center
Memorial Hospital of Rhode Island
Pawtucket, Rhode Island

ANDREW P. THOME, JR., M.D.
Resident, Orthopaedic Surgery
Brown University
Providence, Rhode Island

ERIN TIBBETTS, PHARM.D.
Eastern Maine Medical Center
Bangor, Maine

ALEXANDRA MEYER TIEN, M.D.
Clinical Assistant Professor of Family Medicine
The Warren Alpert Medical School
Brown University
Providence, Rhode Island

DAVID ROBBINS TIEN, M.D.
Clinical Associate Professor of Surgery (Ophthalmology)
The Warren Alpert Medical School
Brown University
Providence, Rhode Island

IRIS L. TONG, M.D.
Assistant Professor
Department of Medicine
The Warren Alpert Medical School
Brown University;
Director
Women's Primary Care
Women's Medicine Collaborative
Providence, Rhode Island

STEVEN P. TREON, M.D., PH.D.
Associate Professor, Medicine
Harvard Medical School;
Director
Bing Center for Waldenstrom's Macroglobulinemia
Adult Oncology
Dana-Farber Cancer Institute
Boston, Massachusetts

HIRSH D. TRIVEDI, M.D.
Department of Hepatology
Beth Israel Deaconess Medical Center
Harvard Medical School
Boston, Massachusetts

MARGARET TRYFOROS, M.D.
Assistant Professor of Family Medicine (Clinical)
Family Medicine
The Warren Alpert Medical School
Brown University
Providence, Rhode Island;
Clinical Team Leader
Family Medicine
Memorial Hospital of Rhode Island
Pawtucket, Rhode Island

HISASHI TSUKADA, M.D., PH.D.
Interventional Pulmonologist
Department of Thoracic Surgery
Brigham and Women's Hospital
Boston, Massachusetts

JOSEPH R. TUCCI, M.D.
Professor of Medicine
Department of Medicine
Boston University School of Medicine
Boston, Massachusetts;
Adjunct Professor of Medicine
Department of Medicine
The Warren Alpert Medical School
Brown University;
Director, Division of Endocrinology
Director, Bone & Mineral Unit
Department of Medicine
Roger Williams Medical Center
Providence, Rhode Island

MELISSA H. TUKEY, M.D., M.SC.
Assistant Professor of Medicine
Department of Pulmonary, Critical Care and Sleep
The Warren Alpert Medical School
Brown University;
Director of Interventional Pulmonology
Rhode Island Hospital;
The Miriam Hospital;
Providence, Rhode Island

JUNIOR UDUMAN, M.D.
Senior Staff Physician
Department of Internal Medicine
Division of Nephrology and Hypertension
Henry Ford Hospital
Detroit, Michigan

SEAN H. UITERWYK, M.D.
Clinical Assistant Professor of Community and Family Medicine
Geisel School of Medicine at Dartmouth
Hanover, New Hampshire;
White River Family Practice
White River Junction, Vermont

NICOLE J. ULLRICH, M.D., PH.D.
Associate Professor of Neurology
Harvard Medical School
Director of Neurologic Neuro-oncology
Boston Children's Hospital
Boston, Massachusetts

KAUSIK UMANATH, M.D., M.S.
Assistant Professor
Department of Internal Medicine
Division of Nephrology
Wayne State University;
Section Head, Clinical Trials Research
Departments of Nephrology and Hypertension
Henry Ford Hospital
Detroit, Michigan

BABAK VAKILI, M.D.
Clinical Associate Professor
Obstetrics and Gynecology
Drexel University College of Medicine
Philadelphia, Pennsylvania;
Medical Director, Center for Urogynecology and Pelvic Surgery
Obstetrics and Gynecology
Christiana Care Health System
Newark, Delaware

EMILY VAN KIRK, M.D.
Third Year Internal Medicine Resident
Department of Medicine
Roger Williams Medical Center
Providence, Rhode Island

DANNY H. VANVALKINBURGH, M.D.
Resident, Department of Emergency Medicine
The University of Tennessee College of Medicine
Memphis, Tennessee

JENNIFER E. VAUGHAN, M.D.
Fellow
Department of Neurology and Rehabilitation Medicine
University of Cincinnati College of Medicine;
University of Cincinnati Medical Center
Cincinnati, Ohio

POOJA VERMA, M.D.
Roger Williams Medical Center
Providence, Rhode Island

JORGE A. VILLAFUERTE, M.D.
Clinical Instructor in Orthopedic Surgery
Harvard Medical School;
Assistant Professor in Orthopedic Surgery
Boston University Medical School;
Acting Chief of Orthopedic Surgery
Veterans Affairs Boston HealthCare System
Boston, Massachusetts

MARC PAUL WAASE, M.D., PH.D
Cardiology Fellow
Department of Cardiology
Columbia University;
New York Presbyterian
New York, New York

JOEL P. WADDELL, D.O.
Fellow, Pediatric Infectious Diseases
Mercy Children's Hospital and Clinics
Kansas City, Missouri

BRENT T. WAGNER, M.D.
School of Medicine
University of Texas Health Science Center at San Antonio
San Antonio, Texas

ADAM J. WEINBERG, M.D.
Resident, Internal Medicine
Boston University Medical Center
Boston, Massachusetts

EMMA H. WEISS, B.B.A.
Baylor College of Medicine
Houston, Texas

MARY-BETH WELESKO, M.S., A.P.R.N.-B.C., W.C.C.
Teaching Associate
Department of Geriatrics and Palliative Medicine
The Warren Alpert Medical School
Brown University;
Rhode Island Hospital
Providence, Rhode Island

DENNIS M. WEPPNER, M.D.
Associate Professor of Clinical Gynecology/Obstetrics
State University of New York at Buffalo;
Clinical Chief
Department of Gynecology/Obstetrics
Millard Fillmore Hospital
Buffalo, New York

HILARY B. WHITLATCH, M.D.
Assistant Professor of Medicine
The Warren Alpert Medical School
Brown University;
Chief of Endocriniology Section
Providence Veterans Affairs Medical Center;
Staff Endocriniologist
Rhode Island Hospital
Providence, Rhode Island

ESTELLE H. WHITNEY, M.D.
Clinical Instructor
Department of Obstetrics and Gynecology
Christianacare Health Systems
Newark, Delaware

MATTHEW P. WICKLUND, M.D.
Professor
Department of Neurology
Penn State College of Medicine;
Vice-Chair for Education
Department of Neurology
Milton S. Hershey Medical Center
Hershey, Pennsylvania

JAMES F. WINCHESTER, M.D.
Professor of Medicine
Department of Medicine
Icahn School of Medicine at Mount Sinai
New York, New York

JEFFREY P. WINCZE, PH.D.
Department of Psychiatry
Rhode Island Hospital;
Clinical Assistant Professor
Department of Psychiatry and Human Behavior
The Warren Alpert Medical School
Brown University
Providence, Rhode Island

JOHN P. WINCZE, PH.D
Clinical Professor
Department of Psychiatry and Human Behavior
The Warren Alpert Medical School
Brown University;
Associate Director
The Men's Health Center
The Miriam Hospital
Providence, Rhode Island

MARLENE FISHMAN WOLPERT, M.P.H., C.I.C., F.A.P.I.C.
Director, Infection Prevention and Control
Our Lady of Fatima Hospital
Providence, Rhode Island

TZU-CHING (TEDDY) WU, M.D., M.P.H.
Assistant Professor of Neurology
University of Texas Medical School at Houston;
Director of Telemedicine
Mischer Neuroscience Institute
Houston, Texas

JOHN WYLIE, M.D., F.A.C.C.
Director, Cardiac Electrophysiology
Steward Health Care System;
Assistant Professor of Medicine
Tufts University School of Medicine
Boston, Massachusetts

NICOLE B. YANG, M.D.
Rheumatology Fellow
Brigham and Women's Hospital
Boston, Massachusetts

JERRY YEE, M.D.
Clinical Professor of Medicine
Department of Internal Medicine
Wayne State University School of Medicine;
Senior Staff Physician
Division of Nephrology and Hypertension
Henry Ford Hospital
Detroit, Michigan

LENAR TATIOS YESSAYAN, M.D., M.S.
Associate Professor of Medicine
Department of Internal Medicine
Division of Nephrology
University of Michigan
Ann Arbor, Michigan

AGUSTIN G. YIP, M.D., PH.D.
Clinical Assistant Professor
Butler Hospital;
Department of Psychiatry and Human Behavior
Brown University
Providence, Rhode Island

JOHN Q. YOUNG, M.D., M.P.P.
Associate Professor and Vice Chair
Department of Psychiatry
Hofstra North Shore-LIJ School of Medicine
Hempstead, New York

KATHERINE M. YU, M.D.
Cardiology Fellow
Department of Cardiology
University of California, Irvine
Orange, California;
Fellow, Cardiovascular Disease
Division of Cardiology
University of California Irvine Medical Center
Irvine, California

CANDICE YUVIENCO, M.D., RH.M.S.U.S.
Assistant Clinical Professor of Medicine
Department of Internal Medicine
Division of Rheumatology
University of California, San Francisco
San Francisco, California;
Rheumatologist
Department of Internal Medicine/Rheumatology
Community Regional Medical Center;
Veterans Affairs Medical Center
Fresno, California

ELIZABETH ZADZIELSKI, M.D., M.B.A., N.C.M.P.
Associate Clinical Lead, Women and Children's Service Line
Obstetrics and Gynecology
Christiana Care Health System
Newark, Delaware

FARIHA ZAHEER, M.D.
Assistant Professor of Neurology
Baylor College of Medicine;
Michael. E. DeBakey VA Medical Center
Houston, Texas

TALIA ZENLEA, M.D.
Assistant Professor
Department of Medicine
University of Toronto;
Division of Gastroenterology
Women's College Hospital
Toronto, Ontario, Canada

MARK ZIMMERMAN, M.D.
Director, Outpatient Psychiatry at Rhode Island Hospital, Rhode Island Methods to Improve Diagnostic Assessment and Services (MIDAS) project
The Warren Alpert Medical School
Brown University
Providence, Rhode Island

BERNARD ZIMMERMANN, M.D.
Associate Professor Emeritus
Department of Medicine
Boston University
Boston, Massachusetts;
Rheumatologist
Department of Medicine
Division of Rheumatology
Roger Williams Medical Center
Providence, Rhode Island

RYAN W. ZUZEK, M.D.
Fellow, Clinical Cardiology
Division of Cardiology
The Warren Alpert Medical School
Brown University
Providence, Rhode Island

To my sons, Dr. Vito F. Ferri and Dr. Christopher A. Ferri, and my daughter-in-law,
Dr. Heather A. Ferri, for their help and constant support, and to my wife, Christina, for her
patience during manuscript preparation. A special thanks to all the readers who have
personally commented on the merits of this book and through their suggestions have helped
make this product a bestseller in the medical field.

Fred F. Ferri, M.D., F.A.C.P.
Clinical Professor
The Warren Alpert Medical School
Brown University
Providence, Rhode Island

This book is intended to be a clear and concise reference for physicians and allied health professionals. Its user-friendly format was designed to provide a fast and efficient way to identify important clinical information and to offer practical guidance in patient management. The book is divided into five sections and an appendix, each with emphasis on clinical information.

The tremendous success of the previous editions and the enthusiastic comments from numerous colleagues have brought about several positive changes. Each section has been significantly expanded from prior editions, bringing the total number of medical topics covered in this book to more than 1200. 480 new illustrations, tables, and boxes have been added to this edition to enhance recollection of clinically important facts. The expedited claims submission and reimbursement ICD-10CM codes are included in all the topics.

Section I describes in detail 900 medical disorders. Thirty-five new topics have been added to the 2018 edition. Each medical topic in this section is arranged alphabetically, and the material in each topic is presented in outline format for ease of retrieval. Topics with an accompanying algorithm are identified with an algorithm symbol (ALG). Similarly, if topics also have a Patient Teaching Guide (PTG) available online, this has been noted. Throughout the text, key quick-access information is consistently highlighted, clinical photographs are used to further illustrate selected medical conditions, and relevant ICD-10CM codes are listed. Most references focus on current peer-reviewed journal articles rather than outdated textbooks and old review articles. Evidence-based medicine data have been added to relevant topics.

Topics in Section I use the following structured approach:

1. Basic Information (Definition, Synonyms, ICD-10CM Codes, Epidemiology & Demographics, Physical Findings & Clinical Presentation, Etiology)
2. Diagnosis (Differential Diagnosis, Workup, Laboratory Tests, Imaging Studies)
3. Treatment (Nonpharmacologic Therapy, Acute General Rx, Chronic Rx, Disposition, Referral)
4. Pearls & Considerations (Comments, Suggested Readings)
5. Evidence-Based Data and References

Section II includes the differential diagnosis, etiology, and classification of signs and symptoms. This section has been significantly expanded for the 2018 edition with the addition of 64 new topics. It is a practical section that allows the user investigating a physical complaint or abnormal laboratory value to follow a "workup" leading to a diagnosis. The physician can then easily look up the presumptive diagnosis in Section I for the information specific to that illness.

Section III includes clinical algorithms to guide and expedite the patient's workup and therapy. Thirty-three new algorithms have been added for the 2018 edition. Many physicians describe this section as particularly valuable in today's managed-care environment.

Section IV includes normal laboratory values and interpretation of results of commonly ordered laboratory tests. Several new illustrations and tables have been added to this section. By providing interpretation of abnormal results, this section facilitates the diagnosis of medical disorders and further adds to the comprehensive, "one-stop" nature of our text.

Section V focuses on preventive medicine. Information in this section includes recommendations for the periodic health examination, screening for major diseases and disorders, patient counseling, and immunization and chemoprophylaxis recommendations.

The **Appendix** has been divided into six major sections. Section I contains extensive information on complementary and alternative medicine (CAM). With the material in this appendix, we hope to lessen the current scarcity of exposure of allopathic and osteopathic physicians to the diversity of CAM therapies. Appendix II focuses on nutrition, with an emphasis on dietary supplements, vitamins, and minerals. Appendix III deals with diagnosis and treatment of acute poisoning. Appendix IV is a guide on impairment and disability evaluation. Appendix V, available online, contains an extensive section on primary care procedures. Appendix VI contains Patient Teaching Guides, including several not linked to Section I topics.

As clinicians, we all realize the importance of patient education and the need for clear communication with our patients. Toward that end, practical patient instruction sheets, organized alphabetically and covering the majority of the topics in this book, are available online and can be easily customized and printed from any computer. They represent a valuable addition to patient care and are useful for improving physician-patient communication, patient satisfaction, and quality of care.

I believe that we have produced a state-of-the-art information system with significant differences from existing texts. It contains five sections and patient education guides that could be sold separately based on their content, yet are available under a single cover, offering the reader a tremendous value. I hope that the *Clinical Advisor*'s user-friendly approach, numerous unique features, and yearly updates will make this book a valuable medical reference, not only to primary care physicians but also to physicians in other specialties, medical students, and allied health professionals.

Fred F. Ferri, M.D., F.A.C.P.

Note: Comments from readers are always appreciated and can be forwarded directly to Dr. Ferri at fred_ferri@brown.edu.

EVALUATION OF EVIDENCE

Ferri's Clinical Advisor evaluates all evidence based on a rating system published by the American Academy of Family Physicians. In order to indicate the strength of the supporting evidence, each summary statement is accorded one of three levels:

LEVEL A

- Systematic reviews of randomized controlled trials, including meta-analyses
- Good-quality randomized controlled trials

LEVEL B

- Good-quality nonrandomized clinical trials
- Systematic reviews not in Level A
- Lower-quality randomized controlled trials not in Level A
- Other types of study: case-control studies, clinical cohort studies, cross-sectional studies, retrospective studies, and uncontrolled studies

LEVEL C

- Evidence-based consensus statements and expert guidelines

SOURCES OF EVIDENCE

Evidence is summarized principally from three critically evaluated, very highly regarded sources:

- **Cochrane Systematic Reviews** are respected throughout the world as one of the most rigorous searches of medical journals for randomized controlled trials. They provide highly structured systematic reviews, with evidence included or excluded on the basis of explicit quality-related criteria, and they often use meta-analyses to increase the power of the findings of numerous studies.
- *Clinical Evidence* is produced by the BMJ Publishing Group. It provides synopses of the best currently available evidence on the treatment and prevention of many clinical conditions, based on searches and appraisals of the available literature.
- **The National Guideline Clearinghouse™** is a comprehensive database of evidence-based clinical practice guidelines and related documents produced by the Agency for Healthcare Research and Quality in partnership with the American Medical Association and the American Association of Health Plans.

In addition, where evidence exists that has not yet been critically reviewed in one of the three sites mentioned previously, the evidence is summarized briefly, categorized, and fully referenced. Guidelines are also sourced from government and professional bodies.

Ferri's Clinical Advisor 2018 — How to Use This Book

 Mouse icon – Indicates content with additional references, figures, or tables available at ExpertConsult.com

(PTG) PTG icon – indicates an accompanying Patient Teaching Guide available at ExpertConsult.com. There are also many additional PTGs online not linked to a topic in Section I.

(ALG) ALG icon – indicates a topic with an accompanying Algorithm

 EBM icon – indicates evidence-based medicine data added to relevant topics available at ExpertConsult.com

SECTION I   **Diseases and Disorders,** 1

SECTION II   **Differential Diagnosis,** 1385

SECTION III   **Clinical Algorithms,** 1547

SECTION IV   **Laboratory Tests and Interpretation of Results,** 1769

SECTION V   **Clinical Practice Guidelines,** 1845

APPENDIX I   **Complementary and Alternative Medicine,** 1913

APPENDIX II   **Nutrition,** 1927

APPENDIX III   **Acute Poisoning,** 1939

APPENDIX IV   **Impairment and Disability Issues,** 1947

APPENDIX V   **Primary Care Procedures, available online**

APPENDIX VI   **Patient Teaching Guides, available online**

SECTION I Diseases and Disorders

Abdominal Aortic Aneurysm, 3
Abdominal Compartment Syndrome, 7
Abruptio Placentae, 9
Acetaminophen Poisoning, 11
Achalasia, 12
Acne Vulgaris, 14
Acoustic Neuroma, 16
Acquired Immunodeficiency
    Syndrome, 17
Actinic Keratosis, 25
Acute Bronchitis, 27
Acute Colonic Pseudo-Obstruction
    (Ogilvie's Syndrome), 29
Acute Coronary Syndrome, 31
Acute Kidney Injury, 37
Acute Liver Failure, 42
Acute Respiratory Distress Syndrome, 45
Acute Stress Disorder, 49
Acute Urinary Retention (AUR), 51
Adrenal Insufficiency, 52
Adult-Onset Still's Disease, 54
Alcohol Abuse, 55
Alcoholic Hepatitis, 59
Aldosteronism (Hyperaldosteronism,
    Primary), 61
Allergic Rhinitis, 63
Alopecia, 64
Alpha-1-Antitrypsin Deficiency, 67
Alzheimer's Disease, 68
Amaurosis Fugax, 70
Amblyopia, 71
Amebiasis, 72
Amenorrhea, 73
Amyotrophic Lateral Sclerosis, 77
Anaerobic Infections, 78
Anaphylaxis, 79
Anemia, Aplastic, 80
Anemia, Autoimmune Hemolytic, 82
Anemia, Inflammatory, 85
Anemia, Iron Deficiency, 87
Anemia, Pernicious, 89
Angina Pectoris, 91
Angioedema, 97
Angular Cheilitis, 99
Ankylosing Spondylitis, 100
Anorectal Fistula, 102
Anorexia Nervosa, 103
Anoxic Brain Injury, 105
Antiphospholipid Antibody Syndrome, 107
Anxiety (Generalized Anxiety Disorder), 110
Aortic Coarctation, 111
Aortic Dissection, 113

Aortic Regurgitation, 116
Aortic Stenosis, 118
Appendicitis, 121
Arrhythmogenic Right Ventricular
    Dysplasia, 123
Asbestosis, 125
Ascariasis, 126
Ascites, 127
Aspergillosis, 130
Asthma, 132
Asthma-COPD Overlap Syndrome, 142
Astrocytoma, 144
Atelectasis, 146
Atopic Dermatitis, 147
Atrial Fibrillation, 149
Atrial Flutter, 153
Atrial Myxoma, 155
Atrial Septal Defect, 156
Atrioventricular Dissociation, 159
Attention Deficit Hyperactivity
    Disorder, 160
Autism Spectrum Disorder, 162
AV Malformations, Cerebral, 164
Avascular Necrosis, 166
Babesiosis, 169
Balanitis, 171
Barrett Esophagus, 172
Bartholin's Gland Cyst and Abscess, 175
Basal Cell Carcinoma, 177
Basic Calcium Phosphate Crystal
    Deposition Disease, 179
Bedbug Bite, 181
Bell Palsy, 183
Benign Paroxysmal Positional Vertigo, 185
Binge Eating Disorder (BED), 188
Bipolar Disorder, 190
Bite Wounds, 192
Bites and Stings, Arachnids, 194
Bites and Stings, Insect, 195
Bites, Snake, 197
Bladder Cancer, 200
Body Dysmorphic Disorder, 203
Bone Tumor, Primary Malignant, 204
Botulism, 206
Brain Abscess, 207
Brain Metastases, 209
Brain Neoplasm, Benign, 211
Brain Neoplasm, Glioblastoma, 213
Breast Abscess, 214
Breast Cancer, 215
Bronchiectasis, 219
Brugada Syndrome, 221

Budd-Chiari Syndrome, 223
Bulimia Nervosa, 225
Burns, 227
Calcium-Alkali Syndrome, 230
Cancer of Unknown Primary, 231
Candidiasis, Cutaneous, 234
Candidiasis, Invasive, 236
Carbon Monoxide Poisoning, 238
Cardiac Tamponade, 240
Cardiomyopathy, Chemical-Induced, 242
Cardiomyopathy, Dilated, 244
Cardiomyopathy, Hypertrophic, 246
Cardiomyopathy, Restrictive, 250
Cardiorenal Syndrome, 253
Carotid Sinus Syndrome, 255
Carotid Stenosis, 257
Carpal Tunnel Syndrome, 259
Cat-Scratch Disease, 260
Cavernous Sinus Thrombosis, 261
Celiac Disease, 263
Cellulitis, 265
Cervical Cancer, 267
Cervical Dysplasia, 269
Cervicitis, 272
Charcot Joint, 273
Charcot-Marie-Tooth Disease, 275
Chemotherapy-Induced Nausea and
    Vomiting, 276
Child Abuse, 277
Chlamydia Genital Infections, 280
Cholangiocarcinoma, 283
Cholangitis, 286
Cholecystitis, 287
Choledocholithiasis, 288
Cholelithiasis, 290
Chronic Fatigue Syndrome, 291
Chronic Inflammatory Demyelinating
    Polyneuropathy, 292
Chronic Kidney Disease, 294
Chronic Obstructive Pulmonary
    Disease, 299
Cirrhosis, 304
Claudication, 307
Clostridium difficile Infection, 310
Cocaine Overdose, 312
Colorectal Cancer, 314
Compartment Syndrome, 317
Complex Regional Pain Syndrome, 320
Concussion, 321
Conduct Disorder, 323
Condyloma Acuminatum, 324
Conjunctivitis, 326

Contact Dermatitis, 329
Contraception, 330
Contrast-Induced Acute Kidney Injury (CI-AKI), 333
Cor Pulmonale, 335
Corneal Abrasion, 338
Coronary Artery Disease, 339
Costochondritis, 343
Crohn's Disease, 344
Cryoglobulinemia, 346
Cryptococcosis, 347
Cryptosporidium Infection, 348
Cushing's Disease and Syndrome, 349
Cystic Fibrosis, 351
Cysticercosis, 353
Cytomegalovirus Infection, 355
De Quervain's Tenosynovitis, 356
Deep Vein Thrombosis, 357
Delayed Puberty, 361
Delirium, 364
Delirium Tremens, 367
Dementia with Lewy Bodies, 368
Dependent Personality Disorder, 370
Depression, Major, 371
Dermatitis Herpetiformis, 373
Diabetes Insipidus, 375
Diabetes Mellitus, 376
Diabetic Foot, 384
Diabetic Ketoacidosis, 386
Diabetic Polyneuropathy, 389
Diabetic Retinopathy, 392
Diffuse Idiopathic Skeletal Hyperostosis, 394
Discoid Lupus, 396
Disseminated Intravascular Coagulation, 398
Dissociative Disorders, 400
Diverticular Disease (Diverticulosis, Diverticulitis), 402
Drowning, 404
Drug Abuse, 405
Drug-Induced Liver Injury, 408
Drug-Induced Parenchymal Lung Disease (DILD), 411
Dysfunctional Uterine Bleeding, 413
Dysmenorrhea, 415
Dyspareunia, 416
Dyspepsia, Nonulcerative, 419
Dysphagia, 420
Dystonia, 422
Early Repolarization, 424
Echinococcosis, 427
Eclampsia, 429
Ectopic Pregnancy, 430
Ehrlichiosis and Anaplasmosis, 432
Ejaculation and Orgasm Disorders, 435
Elder Abuse, 437
Electrical and Lightning Injury, 439
Empyema, 441
Encephalitis, Acute Viral, 442
Encephalopathy, 444
Endocarditis, Infective, 446

Endometrial Cancer, 450
Endometriosis, 452
Endometritis, 454
Enteropathic Arthritis, 455
Enuresis, 457
Epididymitis, 459
Epidural Abscess, 460
Epidural Hematoma, 461
Epiglottitis, 463
Epstein-Barr Virus Infection, 464
Erectile Dysfunction, 466
Erysipelas, 468
Erythema Elevatum Diutinum, 469
Erythema Multiforme, 470
Erythema Nodosum, 471
Esophageal Tumors, 472
Esophageal Varices, 475
Essential Tremor, 476
Factitious Disorder (Including Munchausen Syndrome), 477
Failure to Thrive (Pediatric), 478
Falls in the Elderly, 480
Familial Adenomatous Polyposis and Gardner's Syndrome, 482
Familial Mediterranean Fever (FMF), 484
Fatty Liver of Pregnancy, Acute, 485
Fetal Alcohol Syndrome, 486
Fever of Undetermined Origin, 488
Fibrocystic Breast Disease, 490
Fibromyalgia, 491
Fifth Disease (Parvovirus B19 Infection), 493
Folliculitis, 495
Food Allergies, 496
Food Poisoning, Bacterial, 500
Frostbite, 502
Functional Gallbladder Disorder, 504
Galactorrhea, 505
Gastric Cancer, 506
Gastritis, 508
Gastroenteritis, 509
Gastroesophageal Reflux Disease (GERD), 511
Gestational Diabetes Mellitus (GDM), 513
Giant Cell Arteritis, 515
Giardiasis, 517
Gilbert's Syndrome, 518
Glaucoma, Open-Angle, 519
Glaucoma, Primary Angle-Closure, 521
Glomerulonephritis, Acute, 522
Glossitis, 525
Gonorrhea, 526
Goodpasture Disease, 528
Gout, 529
Granuloma Annulare, 531
Granulomatosis with Polyangiitis, 532
Graves' Disease, 535
Guillain-Barré Syndrome, 537
Gynecomastia, 539
Hand-Foot-Mouth Disease, 540
Head and Neck Squamous Cell Carcinoma, 541
Headache, Cluster, 543

Headache, Migraine, 545
Headache, Tension-Type, 548
Heart Block, Complete, 549
Heart Block, Second-Degree, 551
Heart Failure, 553
Heat Exhaustion and Heat Stroke, 561
Helicobacter pylori Infection, 563
Hemochromatosis, 565
Hemolytic-Uremic Syndrome, 567
Hemophilia, 569
Hemoptysis, 571
Henoch-Schönlein Purpura, 573
Heparin-Induced Thrombocytopenia, 575
Hepatic Encephalopathy, 577
Hepatitis A, 580
Hepatitis B, 582
Hepatitis C, 586
Hepatitis D, 590
Hepatitis E, 593
Hepatitis, Autoimmune, 595
Hepatocellular Carcinoma, 597
Hepatopulmonary Syndrome, 599
Hepatorenal Syndrome, 600
Hereditary Breast and Ovarian Cancer, 602
Herpes Simplex, 605
Herpes Zoster, 608
Hidradenitis Suppurativa, 610
High-Altitude Sickness, 612
Hip Fracture, 614
Hirsutism, 616
Histoplasmosis, 619
HIV-Associated Cognitive Dysfunction, 621
Hodgkin Lymphoma, 623
Hookworm, 627
Horner's Syndrome, 628
Hot Flashes, 629
Human Immunodeficiency Virus, 630
Huntington's Disease, 639
Hydrocele, 640
Hydrocephalus, Normal Pressure, 641
Hydronephrosis, 643
Hypercholesterolemia, 645
Hypercoagulable State, 648
Hyperemesis Gravidarum, 651
Hyperglycemic Hyperosmolar Syndrome, 652
Hyperlipoproteinemia, Primary, 654
Hyperparathyroidism, 655
Hypersensitivity Pneumonitis, 657
Hypersplenism, 659
Hypertension, 660
Hyperthyroidism, 666
Hypertrophic Osteoarthropathy, 668
Hyperuricemia, 670
Hypoactive Sexual Desire Disorder (HSDD), 672
Hypoaldosteronism, 674
Hypocomplementemic Urticarial Vasculitis, 675
Hypogonadism, Male, 677
Hyponatremia, 680
Hypoparathyroidism, 683

Hypopituitarism, 685
Hypothermia, 688
Hypothyroidism, 690
Idiopathic Pulmonary Fibrosis, 691
IgA Nephropathy, 693
Immune Thrombocytopenic Purpura, 695
Impetigo, 697
Inclusion Body Myositis, 698
Incontinence, Bowel, Elderly Patient, 699
Incontinence, Urinary, 700
Infertility, 702
Inflammatory Myopathies, 704
Influenza, 707
Insomnia, 710
Interstitial Cystitis, 713
Interstitial Lung Disease, 715
Interstitial Nephritis, 718
Intraventricular Conduction Delay
  (IVCD), 720
Irritable Bowel Syndrome, 722
Ischemic Hepatitis, 726
Ischemic Optic Neuropathy, 727
Jaundice in the Adult Patient, 729
Juvenile Idiopathic Arthritis, 732
Kaposi's Sarcoma, 735
Labyrinthitis, 736
Lactic Acidosis, 737
Lactose Intolerance, 738
Laryngitis, 739
Lead Poisoning, 740
Legg-Calvé-Perthes Disease, 742
Leukemia, Acute Lymphoblastic, 743
Leukemia, Acute Myelogenous, 746
Leukemia, Chronic Lymphocytic, 750
Leukemia, Chronic Myelogenous, 753
Leukoplakia, Oral Hairy, 755
Lichen Planus, 756
Lichen Sclerosus, 757
Lichen Simplex Chronicus, 758
Listeriosis, 759
Liver Abscess, 760
Liver Transplantation, 762
Long QT Syndrome, 764
Lung Abscess, 767
Lung Neoplasms, Primary, 769
Lyme Disease, 774
Lymphangitis, 776
Lymphedema, 777
Lymphoma, Non-Hodgkin's, 779
Lynch Syndrome, 782
Macular Degeneration, 783
Malabsorption, 785
Malaria, 787
Malignant Hyperthermia, 792
Mallory-Weiss Tear, 795
Mastitis, 796
Mastocytosis, 798
Mastodynia, 800
Mastoiditis, 801
Mediastinitis, 802
Meigs' Syndrome, 804
Melanoma, 805
Ménière's Disease, 808

Meningioma, 809
Meningitis, Bacterial, 811
Meningitis, Viral, 814
Menopause, 815
Menorrhagia, 817
Mesenteric Adenitis, 818
Mesenteric Ischemia, Acute, 819
Mesenteric Venous Thrombosis, 821
Mesothelioma, Malignant, 822
Metabolic Syndrome, 824
Methanol and Ethylene Glycol
  Poisoning, 826
Methicillin-Resistant *Staphylococcus
  aureus* (MRSA), 828
Microscopic Polyangiitis, 829
Microsporidiosis, 831
Mild Cognitive Impairment, 832
Mitral Regurgitation, 833
Mitral Stenosis, 836
Mitral Valve Prolapse, 839
Molar Pregnancy, 841
Molluscum Contagiosum, 843
Monoclonal Gammopathy of Undetermined
  Significance (MGUS), 844
Mononucleosis, 846
Motion Sickness, 847
Mucormycosis, 848
Multidrug-Resistant Gram-Negative Rods
  (MDR-GNRs), 849
Multifocal Atrial Tachycardia, 850
Multiple Myeloma, 851
Multiple Sclerosis, 855
Mumps, 858
Muscular Dystrophy, 860
Mushroom Poisoning, 862
Myasthenia Gravis, 863
Myelodysplastic Syndrome, 864
Myocardial Infarction, 867
Myocarditis, 875
Myoclonus, 878
Myofascial Pain Syndrome, 879
Myotonia, 881
Narcissistic Personality Disorder, 882
Narcolepsy, 883
Nasal Polyps, 885
Necrotizing Autoimmune Myopathy
  (NAM), 886
Necrotizing Fasciitis, 887
Nephrotic Syndrome, 889
Neurocognitive Disorders, 892
Neurofibromatosis, 894
Neuroleptic Malignant Syndrome, 896
Neuropathic Pain, 897
Neuropathy, Hereditary, 900
Nonalcoholic Fatty Liver Disease, 902
Nonallergic Rhinitis, 904
Obesity, 906
Obsessive-Compulsive Disorder (OCD), 910
Opioid Dependence, 911
Optic Neuritis, 914
Oral Cancer, 915
Orchitis, 917
Orthostatic Hypotension, 918

Osgood-Schlatter Disease, 920
Osteoarthritis, 921
Osteomyelitis, 923
Osteoporosis, 925
Otitis Externa, 928
Otitis Media, 930
Ovarian Cancer, 932
Ovarian Neoplasm, Benign, 934
Paget's Disease of Bone, 935
Paget's Disease of the Breast, 936
Pain Management in Chronic Pain, 937
Pancreatic Cancer (Exocrine), 941
Pancreatitis, Acute, 943
Pancreatitis, Chronic, 947
Panic Disorder, with or without
  Agoraphobia, 949
Panniculitis, 951
Paraneoplastic Syndromes, 953
Parkinson's Disease, 956
Paronychia, 958
Patent Ductus Arteriosus, 959
Pediculosis, 961
Pelvic Abscess, 962
Pelvic Inflammatory Disease, 963
Pelvic Organ Prolapse, 965
Pemphigus Vulgaris, 968
Peptic Ulcer Disease, 970
Pericarditis, 972
Peripheral Arterial Disease, 975
Perirectal Abscess, 978
Peritonitis, Secondary, 979
Peritonitis, Spontaneous Bacterial, 980
Peritonsillar Abscess, 981
Pertussis, 983
Peutz-Jeghers Syndrome and Other
  Polyposis Syndromes, 985
Peyronie's Disease, 987
Pharyngitis/Tonsillitis, 989
Pheochromocytoma, 991
Phobias, 993
Pilonidal Disease, 995
Pinworms, 996
Pituitary Adenoma, 997
Pityriasis Rosea, 1000
Placenta Previa, 1001
Plantar Fasciitis, 1003
Pleurisy, 1005
Pneumonia, Aspiration, 1006
Pneumonia, Bacterial, 1007
Pneumonia, Mycoplasma, 1011
Pneumonia, *Pneumocystis jiroveci
  (carinii)*, 1013
Pneumonia, Viral, 1015
Pneumothorax, Spontaneous, 1017
Poison Ivy Dermatitis, 1020
Polyarteritis Nodosa, 1021
Polycystic Kidney Disease, 1023
Polycystic Ovary Syndrome, 1025
Polycythemia Vera, 1029
Polymyalgia Rheumatica, 1031
Portal Hypertension, 1032
Portal Vein Thrombosis, 1034
Postconcussive Syndrome, 1035

Postherpetic Neuralgia, 1037
Postpartum Depression, 1039
Postpartum Hemorrhage, 1040
Postthrombotic Syndrome, 1042
Posttraumatic Stress Disorder, 1043
Precocious Puberty, 1045
Preeclampsia, 1049
Premature Rupture of Membranes, 1052
Premenstrual Syndrome, 1054
Pressure Injury, 1056
Preterm Labor, 1059
Primary Angiitis of the Central Nervous
    System, 1061
Primary Biliary Cholangitis, 1063
Primary Ovarian Insufficiency, 1066
Primary Sclerosing Cholangitis, 1067
Prolactinoma, 1069
Prostate Cancer, 1071
Prostatic Hyperplasia, Benign, 1075
Prostatitis, 1077
Pseudogout, 1078
Psoriasis, 1080
Psoriatic Arthritis, 1082
Psychosis, 1084
Pulmonary Edema, 1086
Pulmonary Embolism, 1088
Pulmonary Hypertension, 1092
Pulseless Electrical Activity, 1096
Pyelonephritis, 1097
Ramsay Hunt Syndrome, 1101
Raynaud's Phenomenon, 1102
Reiter's Syndrome (Reactive Arthritis), 1105
Renal Abscess, 1106
Renal Artery Stenosis, 1107
Renal Cell Carcinoma, 1111
Renal Tubular Acidosis, 1113
Renal Vein Thrombosis, 1115
Restless Legs Syndrome, 1116
Retropharyngeal Abscess, 1117
Rh Incompatibility, 1119
Rhabdomyolysis, 1122
Rheumatoid Arthritis, 1125
Rocky Mountain Spotted Fever, 1129
Rosacea, 1131
Roseola, 1133
Salivary Gland Neoplasms, 1134
Salmonellosis, 1135
Sarcoidosis, 1137
Sarcoma, 1139
Scabies, 1141
Scarlet Fever, 1143
Schizophrenia, 1144
Scleritis, 1146
Scleroderma (Systemic Sclerosis), 1147
Scoliosis, 1150
Seborrheic Dermatitis (SD), 1152
Seizures, Absence, 1153
Seizures, Febrile, 1154
Seizures, Generalized Tonic Clonic, 1156
Seizures, Partial, 1157
Sepsis, 1158
Septic Arthritis, 1161
Serotonin Syndrome, 1163

Sexual Assault, 1165
Sexual Dysfunction in Women, 1168
Shaken Baby Syndrome, 1171
Shigellosis, 1172
Short Bowel Syndrome, 1173
Short QT Syndrome, 1174
Sialadenitis, 1176
Sialolithiasis, 1177
Sick Sinus Syndrome, 1178
Sickle Cell Disease, 1179
Silicosis, 1183
Sinusitis, 1184
Sjögren's Syndrome, 1186
Sleep Apnea, 1189
Small Bowel Obstruction, 1192
Small Bowel Bacterial Overgrowth
    (SIBO), 1194
Somatic Symptom Disorder, 1195
Spasticity, 1196
Spinal Cord Compression, 1197
Spinal Epidural Abscess, 1200
Spinal Stenosis, Lumbar, 1202
Spontaneous Miscarriage, 1204
Squamous Cell Carcinoma, 1206
Statin-Induced Muscle Syndromes, 1208
Status Epilepticus, 1210
Stevens-Johnson Syndrome, 1213
Stomatitis/Mucositis, 1214
Stroke, Acute Ischemic, 1215
Stroke, Hemorrhagic, 1219
Stroke, Secondary Prevention, 1221
Stye (Hordeolum), 1223
Subarachnoid Hemorrhage, 1224
Subclavian Steal Syndrome, 1226
Subdural Hematoma, 1227
Superior Vena Cava Syndrome, 1228
Supraventricular Tachycardia, 1230
Syncope, 1233
Syndrome of Inappropriate
    Antidiuresis, 1235
Syphilis, 1238
Systemic Lupus Erythematosus, 1240
Takayasu's Arteritis, 1244
Takotsubo Cardiomyopathy, 1247
Tapeworm Infestation, 1249
Tardive Dyskinesia, 1251
Temporomandibular Joint Syndrome, 1252
Testicular Cancer, 1253
Testicular Torsion, 1255
Thalassemias, 1256
Thoracic Outlet Syndrome, 1258
Thrombocytosis, 1260
Thrombophlebitis, Superficial Venous, 1262
Thrombotic Thrombocytopenic
    Purpura, 1263
Thyroid Carcinoma, 1264
Thyroid Nodule, 1266
Thyroiditis, 1268
Tinea Capitis, 1269
Tinea Corporis, 1271
Tinea Cruris, 1272
Tinea Pedis, 1273
Tinea Unguium, 1274

Tinea Versicolor, 1276
Tinnitus, 1277
Torsade de Pointes, 1278
Tourette's Syndrome, 1281
Toxic Megacolon, 1283
Toxic Shock Syndrome, 1285
Toxoplasmosis, 1287
Transfusion Reaction, Hemolytic, 1291
Transient Global Amnesia, 1293
Transient Ischemic Attack, 1294
Transverse Myelitis, 1296
Traumatic Brain Injury, 1297
Traveler's Diarrhea, 1300
Trigeminal Neuralgia, 1302
Trochanteric Pain Syndrome (Trochanteric
    Bursitis), 1303
Tuberculosis, Miliary, 1304
Tuberculosis, Pulmonary, 1306
Tubular Necrosis, Acute, 1309
Tumor Lysis Syndrome, 1310
Ulcerative Colitis, 1313
Upper Extremity Deep Vein
    Thrombosis, 1316
Urethritis, Gonococcal, 1318
Urethritis, Nongonococcal, 1319
Urinary Tract Infection, 1320
Urolithiasis (Nephrolithiasis), 1323
Urticaria, 1326
Urticaria, Chronic, 1328
Uterine Fibroids, 1331
Uterine Malignancy, 1333
Uveitis, 1334
Vaginal Bleeding During Pregnancy, 1335
Vaginal Fistulas, 1336
Vaginal Malignancy, 1338
Vaginismus, 1339
Vaginitis, Estrogen-Deficient, 1340
Vaginitis, Fungal, 1341
Vaginitis, Prepubescent, 1342
Vaginitis, *Trichomonas*, 1343
Vaginosis, Bacterial, 1345
Vancomycin-Resistant *Enterococcus*
    (VRE), 1346
Varicella, 1347
Varicose Veins, 1348
Vasculitis, Systemic, 1350
Venous Insufficiency, Chronic, 1352
Venous Ulcers, 1354
Ventricular Fibrillation, 1356
Ventricular Septal Defect, 1358
Ventricular Tachycardia, 1361
Vertebral Compression Fractures, 1363
Vestibular Neuronitis, 1365
Vitamin D Deficiency, 1366
Vitamin Deficiency (Hypovitaminosis),
    1368
Vitiligo, 1370
Von Willebrand's Disease, 1371
Waldenström Macroglobulinemia, 1373
Warts, 1375
Wolff-Parkinson-White Syndrome, 1377
Zika Virus, 1379

Additional Topics Available at www.expertconsult.com

Achilles Tendon Rupture
Acromegaly
Actinomycosis
Amyloidosis
Anal Fissure
Anemia, Sideroblastic
Ankle Fracture
Ankle Sprain
Anthrax
Ataxia
Ataxia Telangiectasia
Baker's Cyst
Bartter Syndrome
Behçet's Disease
Biceps Tendonitis
Bisphosphonate-Related Osteonecrosis of
    the Jaw
Blastomycosis
Blepharitis
Borderline Personality Disorder
Breech Birth
Brucellosis
Bruxism
Bullous Pemphigoid
Burning Mouth Syndrome
Bursitis
Carcinoid Syndrome
Cataracts
Cerebral Palsy
Cerebral Vasculitis
Cervical Disc Syndromes
Cervical Insufficiency
Cervical Polyps
Chagas' Disease
Chancroid
Cholera
Chorea
Coccidioidomycosis
Cogan's Syndrome
Colorado Tick Fever
Congenital Adrenal Hyperplasia
Conversion Disorder
Corneal Ulceration
Craniopharyngioma
Creutzfeldt-Jakob Disease
Croup (Laryngotracheobronchitis)
Cryptorchidism
Cubital Tunnel Syndrome
Cutaneous Larva Migrans
Cyclic Vomiting Syndrome
Delusional Parasitosis
Dengue Fever
Digoxin Overdose
Diphtheria
Down Syndrome
Dumping Syndrome
Dupuytren's Contracture
Ehlers-Danlos Syndrome
Emergency Contraception
Encopresis

Eosinophilic Fasciitis
Eosinophilic Granulomatosis with Polyangiitis
Eosinophilic Pneumonias
Epicondylitis
Epiploic Appendagitis
Episcleritis
Epistaxis
Felty's Syndrome
Filariasis
Friedreich's Ataxia
Frozen Shoulder
Ganglia
Gastrinoma
Gender Dysphoria Disorder and Gender
    Nonconformity
Gingivitis
Gingivitis, Necrotizing Ulcerative (NUG)
Glenohumeral Dislocation
Granuloma Inguinale
Granulomatous Arthritis
Grief, Complicated or Prolonged
Hantavirus Pulmonary Syndrome
Health Care-Associated Infections
    (HAIs)
HELLP Syndrome
Hemorrhoids
Herpangina
Hiatal Hernia
Histocytosis X (Langerhans Cell
    Histocytosis)
Histrionic Personality Disorder
Hoarding Disorder
Hypereosinophilic Syndrome
Hypochondriasis (Illness Anxiety
    Disorder)
Hypospadias
ID Reaction
Idiopathic Intracranial Hypertension
Infantile Hypotonia
Influenza, Avian
Insulinoma
Intermittent Explosive Disorder
Kawasaki Disease
Keloid
Klinefelter's Syndrome
Korsakoff's Psychosis
Lambert-Eaton Myasthenic Syndrome
Laryngeal Carcinoma
Leishmaniasis
Leprosy
Leptospirosis
Leukemia, Hairy Cell
Lumbar Disk Syndrome
Lymphogranuloma Venereum
Marfan's Syndrome
Measles (Rubeola)
Meckel Diverticulum
Meningitis, Fungal
Meningomyelocele
Meralgia Paresthetica

Metatarsalgia
Mixed Connective Tissue Disease
Morton Neuroma
Multiple System Atrophy
Mycosis Fungoides
Myxedema Coma
Nephroblastoma
Nephrogenic Systemic Fibrosis
Neuroblastoma
Nocardiosis
Ocular Foreign Body
Oppositional Defiant Disorder (ODD)
Optic Atrophy
Osler-Rendu-Weber Syndrome
Osteochondritis Dissecans
Otosclerosis (Otospongiosis)
Over-the-Counter Medication Use in
    Pregnancy
Paranoid Personality Disorder
Paraphilic Disorders
Paroxysmal Cold Hemoglobinuria
Paroxysmal Nocturnal Hemoglobinuria
Patellofemoral Pain Syndrome
Patent Foramen Ovale
Pediatric Medication Errors
Pedophilic Disorder
Piriformis Syndrome
Poliomyelitis
Polypharmacy
Postpoliomyelitis Syndrome
Postural Orthostatic Tachycardia Syndrome
    (POTS)
Premenstrual Dysphoric Disorder
Preoperative Evaluation
Priapism
Primary Immunodeficiency Disease
Primary Myelofibrosis
Progressive Multifocal
    Leukoencephalopathy (PML)
Progressive Supranuclear Palsy
Pronator Syndrome
Pruritus Ani
Pruritus Vulvae
Psittacosis
Pure Red Cell Aplasia
Pyoderma Gangrenosum
Pyogenic Granuloma
Q Fever
Quadrilateral Space Syndrome
Rabies
Radiation Exposure
Rectal Prolapse
Respiratory Syncytial Virus
Retinal Detachment
Retinal Hemorrhage
Retinitis Pigmentosa
Retinoblastoma
Retroperitoneal Fibrosis
Reye's Syndrome
Rheumatic Fever

Rickets
Rotator Cuff Disease
Rubella
Schistosomiasis
Seasonal Affective Disorder
Severe Acute Respiratory Syndrome
Sheehan's Syndrome
Slipped Capital Femoral Epiphysis (SCFE)
Smallpox
Social Anxiety Disorder
Spina Bifida
Spinocerebellar Ataxia
Sporotrichosis
Strabismus
Sturge-Weber Syndrome
Stuttering

Suicide
Syringomyelia
Tabes Dorsalis
Tarsal Tunnel Syndrome
Tetanus
Tetralogy of Fallot
Thromboangitis Obliterans
Thyrotoxic Storm
Torticollis
Toxic Epidermal Necrolysis
Tracheitis
Trichinosis
Tricuspid Regurgitation
Tricuspid Stenosis
Tricyclic Antidepressant Overdose
Trigger Finger

Tropical Sprue
Tuberous Sclerosis
Tularemia
Turner Syndrome
Typhoid Fever
Varicocele
Von Hippel-Lindau Disease
Vulvar Cancer
Wernicke Syndrome
West Nile Virus Infection
Whiplash
Whipple's Disease
Wilson's Disease
Yellow Fever
Zenker's (Pharyngoesophageal)
   Diverticulum

SECTION II   Differential Diagnosis

Abdominal Distention, 1387
Abdominal Pain, Adolescence, 1387
Abdominal Pain, Childhood, 1387
Abdominal Pain, Chronic Lower, 1387
Abdominal Pain, Diffuse, 1387
Abdominal Pain, Epigastric, 1387
Abdominal Pain, Extraabdominal and
   Systemic Causes, 1387
Abdominal Pain, Infancy, 1388
Abdominal Pain, Left Lower Quadrant, 1388
Abdominal Pain, Left Upper Quadrant, 1388
Abdominal Pain, Nonsurgical Causes, 1388
Abdominal Pain, Periumbilical, 1388
Abdominal Pain, Poorly Localized, 1388
Abdominal Pain, Post-Cholecystectomy,
   1389
Abdominal Pain, Pregnancy, 1389
Abdominal Pain, Right Lower
   Quadrant, 1389
Abdominal Pain, Right Upper Quadrant, 1389
Abdominal Pain, Right Upper Quadrant,
   Differential Diagnosis in Pregnancy, 1389
Abdominal Pain, Suprapubic, 1389
Abdominal Wall Masses, 1389
Abortion, Recurrent, 1390
Aches and Pains, Diffuse, 1390
Acidosis, Hyperchloric Metabolic, 1390
Acidosis, Lactic, 1390
Acidosis, Metabolic, 1390
Acidosis, Respiratory, 1390
Acute Kidney Injury and Liver Disease,
   Causes, 1391
Acute Kidney Injury Due to Intrinsic Renal
   Diseases, 1391
Acute Kidney Injury, HIV Patient,
   Causes, 1391
Acute Kidney Injury in Specific Clinical
   Settings, 1391
Acute Kidney Injury, Pigment Induced, 1392
Acute Lung Injury, Disease and Disorders
   Associations, 1392

Acute Scrotum, 1392
Adnexal Mass, 1392
Adrenal Calcifications, 1393
Adrenal Cystic Lesions, 1393
Adrenal Masses, 1393
Adrenal Pseudomasses, 1393
Adrenocortical Hyperfunction, 1393
Adrenocortical Hypofunction, 1393
Adverse Food Reactions, Differential
   Diagnosis, 1394
Adynamic Ileus, 1394
Aerophagia (Belching, Eructation), 1394
Air-Space Opacification on X-Ray, 1394
Airway Obstruction, Pediatric Age, 1394
Akinetic/Rigid Syndrome, 1395
Alcohol-Related Seizures, 1395
Alkalosis, Metabolic, 1395
Alkalosis, Respiratory, 1395
Alopecia, 1395
Alopecia and Hypotrichosis, in Children
   and Adolescents, 1396
Alopecia, Drug-Induced, 1396
Alveolar Consolidation, 1396
Alveolar Hemorrhage, 1396
Amenorrhea, 1397
Amnesia, 1397
Amniotic Fluid α-Fetoprotein Elevation, 1397
Anal Abscess and Fistula, 1397
Anal Incontinence, 1397
Anaphylaxis, 1397
Anaphylaxis Mimics, 1398
Anaphylaxis, Pathophysiologic
   Classification, 1398
Anaphylactoid Syndrome of Pregnancy, 1398
Androgen Excess, Reproductive-Age
   Woman, 1398
Androgen Resistance, 1398
Anemia, Aplastic, 1398
Anemia, Aplastic, Due to Drugs and
   Chemicals, 1398
Anemia, Causes in Pregnancy, 1399

Anemia, Drug-Induced, 1399
Anemia, Hypochromic, 1399
Anemia, Low Reticulocyte Count, 1400
Anemia, Megaloblastic, 1400
Anemia, Microcytic, Hypochromic,
   Differential Diagnosis, 1401
Anergy, Cutaneous, 1401
Aneurysms, Thoracic Aorta, 1401
Anhidrosis, 1401
Anion Gap Acidosis, 1401
Anion Gap Increase, 1401
Anisocoria, 1401
Anorectal Disease, AIDS Patient, 1402
Anorexia, 1402
Anovulation, 1402
Appendicitis, Differential Diagnosis in
   Pregnancy, 1402
Appetite Loss in Infants and Children, 1402
Arterial Occlusion, 1403
Arthritis and Abdominal Pain, 1403
Arthritis and Diarrhea, 1403
Arthritis and Eye Lesions, 1403
Arthritis and Heart Murmur, 1403
Arthritis and Muscle Weakness, 1403
Arthritis and Rash, 1403
Arthritis and Subcutaneous Nodules, 1403
Arthritis and Weight Loss, 1403
Arthritis or Extremity Pain, in Children and
   Adolescents, 1403
Arthritis, Axial Skeleton, 1404
Arthritis, Chronic, Monoarticular or
   Oligoarticular, Infectious Causes, 1404
Arthritis, Fever, and Rash, 1404
Arthritis, Monoarticular and
   Oligoarticular, 1404
Arthritis, Pediatric Age, 1405
Arthritis, Polyarticular, 1405
Ascites, 1405
Aspiration Lung Injury, Children, 1405
Asthenia, 1406
Asthma, Childhood, 1406

Ataxia, 1406
Ataxia, Acute or Recurrent, 1406
Ataxia, Cerebellar, Adult Onset, 1406
Ataxia, Cerebellar, Children, 1407
Ataxia, Chronic or Progressive, 1407
Atelectasis, 1407
Atrial Enlargement, Left Atrium, 1407
Atrial Enlargement, Right Atrium, 1407
Atypical Lymphocytosis, Heterophil
    Negative, Infectious Causes, 1407
AV Nodal Block, 1407
Back Pain, 1407
Back Pain, Children and Adolescents, 1408
Back Pain, Low, Acute, 1408
Back Pain, Viscerogenic Origin, 1408
Bacterial Overgrowth, Small Intestine, 1408
Ballism, 1408
Bile Duct, Dilated, 1408
Biliary Obstruction, 1409
Biliary Tree, Reflux of Gas or Bowel, 1409
Bladder (Urinary) Wall Thickening, 1409
Bleeding, Lower GI, 1409
Bleeding, Lower GI, Pediatric, 1409
Bleeding, Rectal, 1410
Bleeding, Third Trimester, 1410
Bleeding, Upper GI, 1410
Bleeding, Upper GI, Pediatric, 1410
Bleeding, Vaginal, Non-Pregnant
    Female, 1410
Blindness, Geriatric Age, 1410
Blindness, Monocular, Transient, 1410
Blindness, Pediatric Age, 1410
Blisters, Subepidermal, 1411
Bone and/or Soft Tissue Hypertrophy, 1411
Bone Density, Decreased, Generalized, 1411
Bone Density, Decreased, Localized, 1412
Bone Lesions, Preferential Site of
    Origin, 1412
Bone Marrow Failure Syndromes,
    Inherited, 1412
Bone Marrow Fibrosis, 1412
Bone Mass, Low, 1413
Bone Mineral Density, Increased, 1413
Bone Pain, 1413
Bone Resorption, 1413
Bowel Wall Thickening, 1413
Bow Legs (Genu Varum), Classification, 1413
Bradycardia, Sinus, 1414
Brain Mass, 1414
Breast Inflammatory Lesion, 1414
Breast Mass, 1414
Breath Odor, 1414
Breathing, Noisy, 1414
Bronchial Obstruction, 1414
Bronchopleural Fistula, 1414
Brown Urine, 1414
Bruising, 1415
Bullous Diseases, 1415
Café-Au-Lait Spots, 1415
Calcification on Chest X-Ray, 1415
Calcifications, Abdominal, Nonvisceral on
    X-Ray, 1415
Calcifications, Adrenal Gland on X-Ray, 1415

Calcifications, Cardiac on X-Ray, 1415
Calcifications, Cutaneous, 1416
Calcifications, Genital Tract, Female on
    X-Ray, 1416
Calcifications, Liver on X-Ray, 1416
Calcifications, Pancreas on X-Ray, 1416
Calcifications, Spleen on X-Ray, 1416
Calcifications, Valvular on X-Ray, 1416
Calcium Stones, 1416
Cardiac Arrest, Nontraumatic, 1417
Cardiac Death, Sudden, 1417
Cardiac Enlargement, 1417
Cardiac Murmurs, 1417
Cardiac Tumors, 1417
Cardioembolism, 1417
Cardiogenic Shock, 1418
Cataracts, Pediatric Age, 1418
Cavitary Lesion on Chest X-Ray, 1418
Cerebral Infarction Secondary to Inherited
    Disorders, 1418
Cerebral Vasculitis, Causes, 1419
Cerebrovascular Disease, Ischemic, 1419
Cervical Instability, Pediatric, 1419
Chest Pain, Children, 1419
Chest Pain, Nonpleuritic, 1419
Chest Pain, Pleuritic, 1420
Chest Wall Tumors, Primary, 1420
Chiasmal Disease, 1420
Childhood Eosinophilia, 1420
Cholangitis, Acute, 1420
Cholestasis, 1421
Cholestasis, Neonatal and Infantile,
    Differential Diagnosis, 1421
Cholestatic Liver Enzyme Elevation,
    Extrahepatic Causes, 1421
Cholestatic Liver Enzyme Elevation,
    Intrahepatic Causes, 1421
Chorea, 1422
Choreoathetosis, 1422
Chylothorax, 1422
Cloudy Urine, 1422
Clubbing, 1422
Cobalamin Deficiency, 1422
Colic, Acute Abdominal, 1423
Colon Ischemia, 1423
Color Changes, Cutaneous, 1423
Coma, 1424
Coma, Normal Computed Tomography, 1424
Coma, Pediatric Population, 1424
Congestive Heart Failure and
    Cardiomyopathy, 1425
Congestive Heart Failure, Infant, 1425
Conjunctival Neoplasm, 1425
Consciousness Impairment, Acute, in
    Critically Ill Patient, 1425
Constipation, 1425
Constipation, Adult Patient, 1425
COPD Decompensation, 1426
Corneal Sensation, Decreased, 1426
Cough, 1426
Cough, Chronic, Adult Patient, 1426
Cutaneous Infections, Athletes, 1427
Cyanosis, 1427

Cyanosis, Neonatal, 1427
Daytime Sleepiness, 1427
Delayed Passage of Meconium, 1427
Delirium, 1427
Delirium and Agitation, Drug-Induced, 1428
Delirium, Agitated, 1428
Delirium, Dialysis Patient, 1428
Demyelinating Diseases, 1428
Diaphragm Elevation, Bilateral,
    Symmetrical, 1428
Diaphragm Elevation, Unilateral, 1428
Diarrhea, Acute Watery and Bloody, 1429
Diarrhea, Infectious, 1429
Diarrhea, Noninfectious, 1429
Diarrhea, Tube-Fed Patient, 1430
Diplopia, Binocular, 1430
Diplopia, Monocular, 1430
Diplopia, Vertical, 1430
Dysentery and Inflammatory
    Enterocolitis, 1430
Dizziness, 1430
Dry Eye, 1431
Dyslipoproteinemias, Secondary
    Causes, 1431
Dyspareunia, 1431
Dyspepsia and Pyrosis, Differential
    Diagnosis During Pregnancy, 1431
Dysphagia, 1431
Dysphagia, Esophageal, 1431
Dysphagia, Oropharyngeal, 1432
Dyspnea, 1432
Dysuria, 1432
Earache, 1432
Ectopic ACTH Secretion, 1432
Edema, Children, 1432
Edema, Generalized, 1432
Edema, Leg, Unilateral, 1433
Edema of Lower Extremities, 1433
Ejection Sound or Click, 1433
Elbow Pain, 1433
Elevated Hemidiaphragm, 1433
Emboli, Arterial, 1433
Emesis, Pediatric Age, 1433
Encephalomyelitis, Nonviral Causes, 1433
Encephalopathy, Hypertensive, 1434
Encephalopathy, Metabolic, 1434
Endometrial Thickening, 1434
Enthesopathy, 1434
Eosinophilia, Disease Associations, 1434
Eosinophilia, GI, 1435
Eosinophilic Lung Disease, 1435
Eosinophilia, Parasitic Causes, 1435
Epigastric Pain, 1435
Epilepsy, 1435
Epistaxis, 1435
Erectile Dysfunction, Organic, 1436
Erosions, Genitalia, 1436
Erythematous Annular Skin Lesions, 1436
Erythrocytosis, 1436
Erythroderma, 1436
Esophageal Perforation, 1436
Esophageal Strictures, 1436
Esophageal Tumors, Benign, 1436

Esophagitis, 1437
Esophagus, Systemic Diseases, 1437
Esotropia, 1437
Exanthems, 1437
Eyelid Neoplasm, 1437
Eyelid Retraction, 1437
Eye Pain, 1437
Facial Pain, 1437
Facial Paralysis, 1438
Failure to Thrive, 1438
Fatigue, 1438
Fatigue, Chronic, 1438
Fatty Liver, 1439
Fever And Cardiopulmonary Failure, 1439
Fever and Jaundice, 1439
Fever and Lymphadenopathy, 1439
Fever and Rash, 1439
Fever and Rash in ICU, 1439
Fever, After Travel to the Tropics, 1440
Fever, Drug-Induced, 1440
Fever, Hospital Associated, 1440
Fever in Returning Travelers and
    Immigrants, 1441
Fever, Noninfectious Causes, 1441
Fever, Postpartum, 1441
Fever, Periodic, 1441
Fever, Pediatric, Acute, 1441
Fever, Recurrent or Periodic, in
    Children, 1442
Fever with Maculopapular or Petechial
    Rash, 1442
Finger Lesions, Inflammatory, 1442
Flaccid Paralysis, Acute, Differential
    Diagnosis, 1442
Flatulence and Bloating, 1442
Flushing, 1443
Folate Deficiency, 1443
Foot and Ankle Pain, 1443
Foot and Ankle Pain, in Different Age
    Groups, 1443
Foot Dermatitis, 1444
Footdrop, 1444
Foot Lesion, Ulcerating, 1444
Foot Pain, 1444
Foot Pain by Age, 1444
Forearm and Hand Pain, 1444
Forearm Fractures, 1444
Gait Abnormality, 1445
Galactorrhea, 1445
Gallbladder Sonographic
    Non-visualization, 1445
Gallbladder Wall Thickening, 1445
Gastric Dilatation, 1445
Gastric Emptying, Delayed, 1445
Gastric Emptying, Rapid, 1445
Genital Discharge, Female, 1445
Genital Lesions, Infectious Causes, 1446
Genital Lesions, Noninfectious Causes, 1446
Genital Sores, 1446
Glomerulonephritis Associated with
    Malignancy, 1446
Glomerulonephritis, Rapidly
    Progressive, 1446

Glomerulopathies, Thrombotic,
    Microangiopathic, 1446
Glomerulosclerosis, Focal Segmental, 1446
Glossodynia, 1446
Glucocorticoid Deficiency, 1447
Goiter, 1447
Granulomatous Dermatitides, 1447
Granulomatous Disorders, 1447
Granulomatous Liver Disease, 1448
Green or Blue Urine, 1448
Groin Lump, 1448
Groin Masses, 1448
Groin Pain, 1448
Groin Pain, Active Patient, 1448
Gynecomastia, 1449
Hair Loss, 1449
Halitosis, 1449
Hand Pain and Swelling, 1449
Headache, 1449
Headache, Acute, 1450
Headache and Facial Pain, 1450
Headache, Chronic, 1450
Head and Neck, Soft Tissue Masses, 1450
Hearing Loss, Acute, 1450
Heartburn and Indigestion, 1451
Heart Failure with Preserved Left
    Ventricular Ejection Fraction, 1451
Heart Failure, Acute, 1451
Heart Failure, Chronic, 1451
Heart Failure, Congenital Heart Disease
    Causes, 1451
Heart Failure, Pathogenic Causes, 1451
Heart Failure, Pregnancy, 1452
Heat Stroke, 1452
Heel Pain, 1452
Heel Pain, Plantar, 1452
Hemarthrosis, 1452
Hematemesis, 1452
Hematuria, 1452
Hematuria, Differential Based on Age and
    Sex, 1453
Hematuria, in Children, 1453
Hemiparesis/Hemiplegia, 1453
Hemolysis and Hemoglobinuria, 1453
Hemolysis, Intravascular, 1453
Hemolysis, Mechanical, 1453
Hemoperitoneum, 1453
Hemoptysis, 1453
Hemorrhagic Cystitis, 1454
Hepatic Cysts, 1454
Hepatic Granulomas, 1454
Hepatitis, Acute, 1454
Hepatitis, Chronic, 1454
Hepatitis, in Children, 1454
Hepatomegaly, 1455
Hepatomegaly, by Shape of Liver, 1455
Hermaphroditism, 1455
Hiccups, 1456
Hilar and Mediastinal Lymph Node
    Enlargement, 1456
Hip Pain, Children, 1456
Hip Pain, Differential Diagnosis, 1456
Hip Pain, in Different Age Groups, 1456

Hip Pain Without Obvious Fracture, 1457
Hirsutism, 1457
HIV Infection, Anorectal Lesions, 1457
HIV Infection, Chest Radiographic
    Abnormalities, 1457
HIV Infection, Cognitive Impairment, 1457
HIV Infection, Cutaneous
    Manifestations, 1458
HIV Infection, Esophageal Disease, 1458
HIV Infection, Hepatic Disease, 1458
HIV Infection, Lower GI Tract Disease, 1458
HIV Infection, Musculoskeletal
    Disorders, 1458
HIV Infection, Ocular Manifestations, 1459
HIV Infection, Pulmonary Disease, 1459
Hoarseness, 1460
Hydrocephalus, 1460
Hypercalcemia, 1460
Hypercalcemia, Malignancy-Induced, 1460
Hypercapnia, Persistent, 1460
Hypercoagulable State, Associated
    Disorders, 1460
Hypergastrinemia, 1460
Hyperhidrosis, 1460
Hyperkalemia, 1461
Hyperkalemia, Drug-Induced, 1461
Hyperkalemia in Children, 1461
Hyperkinetic Movement Disorders, 1461
Hypermagnesemia, 1461
Hyperostosis, Cortical Bone, 1461
Hyperphosphatemia, 1462
Hyperphosphatemia in Children, 1462
Hyperpigmentation, 1462
Hyperprolactinemia, 1462
Hypersplenism, Associated Conditions, 1463
Hypertension, Adrenocortical Causes, 1463
Hypertension, Endocrine Causes, 1463
Hypertension, in Children, 1463
Hypertension, Resistant, 1463
Hypertensive Crisis Syndromes, 1464
Hypertrichosis, 1464
Hypertrophic Osteoarthropathy, 1464
Hyperventilation, Persistent, 1464
Hypocalcemia, 1464
Hypocalcemia in Pediatric Patients, 1465
Hypocapnia, 1465
Hypoglycemia, 1465
Hypoglycemia, in Infants and Children, 1465
Hypogonadism, 1466
Hypokalemia, 1466
Hypokalemia in Pediatric Patients, 1466
Hypomagnesemia, 1466
Hypomagnesemia in Pediatric Patients, 1467
Hyponatremia, 1467
Hypophosphatemia, 1467
Hypophosphatemia in Pediatric
    Patients, 1467
Hypopigmentation, 1467
Hypotension, Postural, 1467
Hypothyroidism, Congenital, 1468
Hypotonia, Infantile, Differential
    Diagnosis, 1468
Hypotonic Polyuria, 1468

Hypovolemia, 1469
Hypovolemic Shock, Pediatric
    Population, 1469
Hypoxemia and Hypercapnic Respiratory
    Failure, 1469
Iliac Fossa Pain, Left Sided, 1469
Iliac Fossa Pain, Right Sided, 1469
Immunodeficiency, Congenital
    (Primary), 1470
Impotence, 1470
Incontinence, Fecal, 1470
Infectious Diarrhea in Tropics, 1470
Infertility, Female, 1470
Infertility, Male, 1470
Insomnia, 1471
Intestinal Pseudoobstruction, 1471
Intraabdominal Mass Lesion, Neonatal, 1471
Intracerebral Hemorrhage,
    Nonhypertensive Causes, 1471
Intracranial Lesion, 1471
Intraocular Neoplasm, 1471
Iron Overload, 1471
Ischemia, Upper Extremity, Causes, 1472
Ischemic Bowel Disease, 1472
Ischemic Colitis, Nonocclusive, 1472
Ischemic Necrosis of Cartilage and
    Bone, 1472
Jaundice, 1472
Jaundice, Classification, 1473
Jaundice, Neonatal, 1473
Joint and Periarticular Pain, Acute, 1473
Joint Pain, Anterior Hip, Medial Thigh,
    Knee, 1473
Joint Pain, Hip, Lateral Thigh, 1474
Joint Pain, Polyarticular, 1474
Joint Pain, Posterior Hips, Thigh,
    Buttocks, 1474
Joint Swelling, 1474
Jugular Venous Distention, 1474
Keratitis, Noninfectious, 1474
Kidney Cystic Disease, 1474
Kidney Enlargement, Unilateral, 1474
Kidney Injury, Cancer Patients, 1475
Knee Pain, 1475
Knee Pain, in Different Age Groups, 1475
Large Bowel Stricture, 1475
Left Axis Deviation, 1476
Left Bundle Branch Block, 1476
Leg Cramps, Nocturnal, 1476
Leg Length Discrepancies, 1476
Leg Movement when Standing,
    Involuntary, 1476
Leg Pain with Exercise, 1476
Leg Swelling, 1476
Leg Ulcers, 1476
Leptomeningeal Lesions, 1477
Leukocoria, 1477
Lid Retraction, Causes, 1477
Light-Near Dissociation, 1477
Limb Ischemia, Acute, Nontraumatic, 1477
Limp, 1477
Limping, Pediatric Age, 1477
Livedo Reticularis, 1477

Liver Disease, Pregnancy, 1478
Liver Lesions, Benign, Often Confused with
    Malignancy, 1478
Low-Voltage ECG, 1478
Lung Cancer, Occupational Causes, 1478
Lung Disease and Gastrointestinal and
    Liver Involvement, 1478
Lung Disease and Renal Involvement, 1478
Lung Disease and Skin and Subcutaneous
    Lesions, 1478
Lung Disease with Bone, Joint, Nerve, and
    Muscle Involvement, 1479
Lung Tumors, Benign, 1480
Lung Volumes in Diffuse Lung Disease, 1480
Lymphadenopathy, 1480
Lymphangitis, 1480
Lymphedema, 1480
Lymphocytosis, Atypical, 1480
Macrothrombocytopenia, Inherited, 1481
Macular Crystals, 1481
Madarosis, 1481
Malabsorption, 1481
Malabsorption Syndrome in Tropics, 1481
Malnutrition, Causes in Early Life, 1481
Mediastinal Compartments, Anatomy and
    Pathology, 1481
Mediastinal Masses or Widening on Chest
    X-Ray, 1482
Mediastinal Masses, Sites of Origin, 1482
Mediastinitis, Acute, 1482
Melanonychia, 1483
Memory Loss Symptoms, Elderly
    Patients, 1483
Meningitis, Chronic, 1483
Meningitis, Recurrent, 1483
Mental Status Changes and Coma, 1483
Mental Status Changes and Coma,
    Structural Causes, 1484
Mental Status Changes and Coma,
    Metabolic and Systemic Causes, 1484
Mesenteric Arterial Embolism, Associated
    Factors, 1485
Mesenteric Ischemia, Nonocclusive, 1485
Mesenteric Venous Thrombosis, 1485
Metastatic Neoplasms, 1485
Methaemoglobinaemia, Drug Induced, 1485
Microcephaly, 1485
Micropenis, 1485
Miosis, 1485
Monoarthritis, Acute, 1486
Monocytosis, 1486
Mononeuropathy, 1486
Mononeuropathy, Isolated, 1486
Mononeuropathy Multiplex, 1486
Mononucleosis, Monospot Negative, 1486
Muscle Disease, 1486
Muscle Weakness, 1487
Muscle Weakness, Lower Motor Neuron
    Versus Upper Motor Neuron, 1487
Musculoskeletal Benign Tumors and
    Tumor-Like Lesions, 1487
Musculoskeletal Malignant Tumors and
    Tumor-Like Lesions, 1487

Mydriasis, 1487
Myelin Disorders, 1487
Myelopathy and Myelitis, 1487
Myocardial Ischemia, 1487
Myoclonus, 1488
Myopathic Syndromes, Drug-Induced, 1488
Myopathies Associated with Rest Pain, 1488
Myopathies, HIV Associated, 1488
Myopathies, Infectious, 1488
Myopathies, Inflammatory, 1488
Myopathies, Metabolic, 1488
Myopathies, Toxic, 1489
Myositis, Infectious Causes, 1489
Myositis, Inflammatory, 1489
Nail Clubbing, 1489
Nail, Horizontal White Lines
    (Beau's Lines), 1489
Nail Koilonychia, 1489
Nail Onycholysis, 1489
Nail Pitting, 1490
Nail Splinter Hemorrhage, 1490
Nail Striations, 1490
Nail Telangiectasia, 1490
Nail Whitening (Terry's Nails), 1490
Nail Yellowing, 1490
Nasal and Paranasal Sinus Tumors, 1490
Nasal Masses, Congenital, 1490
Nausea and Vomiting, 1490
Nausea and Vomiting, Causes During
    Pregnancy, 1490
Nausea and Vomiting, Chronic, 1490
Neck and Arm Pain, 1491
Neck Mass, 1491
Neck Pain, 1491
Neck Pain from Rheumatologic
    Disorders, 1491
Necrotizing Pneumonias, 1491
Nephritic Syndrome, Acute, 1491
Nephrocalcinosis, 1491
Nephropathy, Obstructive, 1491
Neurogenic Bladder, 1492
Neurologic Deficit, Focal, 1492
Neurologic Deficit, Multifocal, 1492
Neuromuscular Junction Dysfunction, 1492
Neuronopathies, Sensory
    (Ganglionopathies), 1492
Neuropathic Bladder, 1493
Neuropathies with Facial Nerve
    Involvement, 1493
Neuropathies, Autonomic, 1493
Neuropathies, Autonomic, Peripheral,
    Causes, 1493
Neuropathies, Painful, 1493
Neuropathies, Peripheral, Asymmetrical
    Proximal/Distal, 1493
Neuropathies, Toxic and Metabolic, 1494
Neutropenia, Drug-Induced, 1494
Neutropenia with Decreased Marrow
    Reserve, 1494
Neutropenia with Normal Marrow
    Reserve, 1494
Neutropenia, in Childhood, 1494
Neutrophilia, 1494

Nipple Lesions, 1495
Nodular Lesions, Skin, 1495
Nodules, Painful, 1495
Nystagmus, 1495
Nystagmus, Monocular, 1495
Odynophagia, 1495
Opacification of Hemidiaphragm on
   X-Ray, 1495
Ophthalmoplegia, 1495
Opsoclonus, 1495
Optic Atrophy, 1495
Optic Disc Elevation, 1496
Oral Mucosa, Erythematous Lesions, 1496
Oral Mucosa, Pigmented Lesions, 1496
Oral Mucosa, Punctate Erosive Lesions, 1496
Oral Mucosa, White Lesions, 1496
Oral Ulcers, Acute, 1496
Oral Vesicles and Ulcers, 1496
Orbital Inflammation, 1496
Orbital Lesions, Calcified, 1497
Orbital Lesions, Cystic, 1497
Orgasm Dysfunction, 1497
Orofacial Pain, 1497
Osteolytic Benign Bone Lesions,
   Multiple, 1497
Osteoporosis in Children, 1497
Osteoporosis, Secondary Causes, 1497
Osteosclerosis, Diffuse, 1497
Osteosclerotic Benign Bone Lesions,
   Multiple, 1497
Ovulatory Dysfunction, 1497
Pain, Midfoot, 1498
Pain, Plantar Aspect, Heel, 1498
Pain, Posterior Heel, 1498
Palindromic Rheumatism, 1498
Palmoplantar Hyperkeratosis, 1498
Palpitations, 1498
Pancreatic Calcifications, 1498
Pancreatic Cystic Lesions, 1499
Pancreatic Solid Lesions, 1499
Pancreatitis, Acute, in Children, 1499
Pancreatitis, Drug-Induced, 1499
Pancytopenia, 1500
Pancytopenia Syndrome, Inherited, 1500
Papilledema, 1500
Papulosquamous Diseases, 1500
Paraneoplastic Neurologic Syndromes, 1500
Paraneoplastic Syndromes, Endocrine, 1500
Paraneoplastic Syndromes,
   Nonendocrine, 1500
Paraparesis, Acute or Subacute, 1500
Paraparesis, Chronic Progressive, 1501
Paraplegia, 1501
Parasellar Masses, 1501
Paresthesias, 1501
Parkinsonism-Plus Syndromes, 1501
Parotid Swelling, 1502
Pelvic Avulsion Fractures, 1502
Pelvic Mass, 1502
Pelvic Pain, Causes in Women, 1502
Pelvic Pain, Chronic, 1502
Pelvic Pain, Genital Origin, 1503
Pelvic Pain, Non-Pregnant Female, 1503

Penile Rash, 1503
Perianal Pain, 1503
Pericardial Effusion, 1503
Periodic Paralysis, Hyperkalemic, 1503
Periodic Paralysis, Hypokalemic, 1503
Peritoneal Carcinomatosis, 1504
Peritoneal Effusion, 1504
Periumbilical Swelling, 1504
Pharyngeal Obstruction, Causes, 1504
Pheochromocytoma-Type spells, 1504
Photodermatoses, 1504
Photosensitivity, 1504
Pigmenturia, 1504
Pituitary Region Tumors, 1505
Pleural Effusions, 1505
Pleural Effusions, Malignancy-Associated,
   1505
Pleural Hyperplasia, 1505
Pleural Masses, 1505
Pneumatosis Intestinalis in Neonate and
   Older Child, 1505
Pneumonia, Chronic, 1505
Pneumonia Mimics, 1506
Pneumonia, Nonresponding, Causes, 1506
Pneumonia, Recurrent, 1506
Pneumoperitoneum, Neonatal, 1506
Pneumothorax, in Children, 1507
Poliosis, 1507
Polycythemia, 1507
Polycythemias, Differential Diagnosis, 1507
Polycythemia, Relative Versus Absolute, 1507
Polymyalgias, 1508
Polyneuropathy, 1508
Polyneuropathy, Demyelinating, 1508
Polyneuropathy, Distal Sensorimotor, 1508
Polyneuropathy, Drug-Induced, 1508
Polyneuropathy, Symmetric, 1509
Polyuria, 1509
Popliteal Swelling, 1509
Portal Hypertension, 1509
Postmenopausal Bleeding, 1509
Postural Hypotension, Nonneurologic
   Causes, 1509
Premature Graying, Scalp Hair, 1509
Premature Ventricular Contractions and
   Ventricular Tachycardia, 1509
Presacral Masses in Children, 1510
Prolonged QT Syndromes, 1510
Proptosis, 1510
Proptosis and Palatal Necrotic Ulcers, 1510
Protein-Losing Enteropathy,
   Pediatric Age, 1510
Proteinuria, 1510
Pruritus, 1510
Pruritus ANI, 1511
Pruritus Vulvae, 1511
Pseudocyanosis, Etiology, 1511
Pseudohermaphroditism, Female, 1511
Pseudohermaphroditism, Male, 1511
Pseudoinfarction, 1511
Psychosis, 1511
Psychosis, Medical Disorders-Induced, 1512
Psychosis, Medication-Induced, 1512

Ptosis, 1512
Puberty, Delayed, 1512
Puberty, Precocious, 1512
Pulmonary Crackles, 1512
Pulmonary Cysts on X-Ray, 1513
Pulmonary Edema, Noncardiogenic, 1513
Pulmonary Eosinophilia, 1513
Pulmonary Hemorrhage, Focal, 1513
Pulmonary Hemorrhage, Pediatric Age, 1514
Pulmonary Hemorrhagic Syndromes,
   Diffuse, 1514
Pulmonary Infiltrates,
   Immunocompromised Host, 1514
Pulmonary Lesions, 1514
Pulmonary Mass, Solitary, Causes, 1514
Pulmonary Mass, Solitary, Mimics, 1514
Pulmonary Nodule, Solitary, 1514
Pulmonary–Renal Syndromes,
   Causes, 1515
Pulseless Electrical Activity, 1515
Pupillary Dilatation, Poor Response to
   Darkness, 1515
Purpura, 1515
Purpura, Nonpalpable, 1515
Purpura, Nonpurpuric Disorders Simulating
   Purpura, 1515
Purpura, Palpable, 1516
QT Interval Prolongation, 1516
Radiation-Induced Neoplasms, 1516
Rectal Mass, Palpable, 1516
Rectal Pain, 1516
Red Blood Cell Aplasia, Acquired,
   Etiology, 1516
Red Blood Cell Fragmentation Hemolysis,
   Causes, 1516
Red Eye, 1516
Red Eye, Acute, 1517
Red Hot Joint, 1517
Red Urine, 1517
Renal Allograft Dysfunction, 1517
Renal Artery Occlusion, Causes, 1517
Renal Colic, 1517
Renal Cystic Disorders, 1517
Renal Disease, Skin Manifestations, 1517
Renal Failure, Acute, Pigment-Induced, 1518
Renal Failure, Chronic, 1518
Renal Failure, Intrinsic or Parenchymal
   Causes, 1518
Renal Failure, Postrenal Causes, 1518
Renal Failure, Prerenal Causes, 1518
Renal Infarction, 1519
Renal Parenchymal Disease, Chronic, 1519
Renal Vein Thrombosis, Causes, 1519
Respiratory Distress in the Newborn,
   Causes, 1519
Respiratory Failure, Hypoventilatory, 1519
Respiratory Muscle Weakness, 1520
Retinopathy, Hypertensive, 1520
Rhinitis, 1520
Rhinitis, Chronic, 1520
Rhinosinusitis, Differential Diagnosis, 1520
Rib Defects on X-Ray, 1520
Rib Notching on X-Ray, 1521

Right Axis Deviation, 1521
Salivary Gland Enlargement, 1521
Salivary Gland Secretion, Decreased, 1521
Scleroderma-Like Syndromes, 1521
Scrotal Calcifications, 1521
Scrotal Masses, Boys and Adolescents, 1521
Scrotal Pain, 1521
Scrotal Pain, Adolescent or Pediatric
    Patient, 1521
Scrotal Swelling, 1522
Seizure, 1522
Seizure, Pediatric, 1522
Seizure Mimics, 1522
Sexual Differentiation Abnormalities, 1522
Sexual Dysfunction, Female, 1523
Sexually Transmitted Diseases, Anorectal
    Region, 1523
Sexual Precocity, 1523
Shoulder Pain, 1523
Shoulder Pain by Location, 1523
Shoulder Pain, in Different Age Groups, 1523
Sinus Node Dysfunction, 1524
Sinus Ostial Obstruction, 1524
Sinus Tachycardia, 1524
Skin and Renal, 1524
Skin Induration, Chronic, 1524
Small Bowel Masses, 1525
Small Bowel Obstruction, 1525
Small Intestine Ulceration, 1525
Smell Disturbance, 1525
Sodium Retention, Renal Causes, 1525
Soft Tissue Mass Mimicking
    Malignancy, 1525
Soft Tissue Tumors, Pediatric Patients, 1525
Sore Throat, 1526
Spastic Paraplegias, 1526
Spinal Cord Compression, Epidural, 1526
Spinal Cord Dysfunction, 1526
Spinal Cord Dysfunction, Nontraumatic, 1526
Spinal Cord Ischemic Syndromes, 1526
Spinal Tumors, 1526
Splenic Cysts, Classification, 1527
Splenic Masses, Focal Solid, 1527
Splenic Nodules, 1527
Splenic Tumors, Classification, 1527
Splenomegaly, 1527
Splenomegaly and Hepatomegaly, 1527
Splenomegaly, Children, 1527
Spontaneous Pneumothorax, 1528
Statural Overgrowth, 1528
Steatohepatitis, 1528
Stomatitis, Bullous, 1528
Stridor in Neonates, 1528
Stridor, Pediatric Age, 1528

Stroke, 1529
Stroke, Pediatric Age, 1529
Stroke, Young Adult, Causes, 1529
ST-Segment Depression, Noncoronary
    Causes, 1529
ST-Segment Elevation, 1529
ST Segment Elevations, Nonischemic, 1530
Sudden Death, Pediatric Age, 1530
Sudden Death, Young Athlete, 1530
Swollen Limb, 1530
Tall Stature, 1530
Tardive Dyskinesia, 1530
Taste and Smell Loss, 1530
Telangiectasia, 1531
Tendinopathy, 1531
Testicular Cystic Lesions, 1531
Testicular Failure, 1531
Testicular Pain, 1531
Testicular Size Variations, 1531
Tetanus, 1532
Thrombocytopenia, 1532
Thrombocytopenia, In Pregnancy, 1532
Thrombocytopenia, Inherited Disorders, 1532
Thrombocytopenia in Newborns,
    Differential Diagnosis, 1532
Thrombocytosis, 1532
Thrombosis or Thrombotic Diathesis, 1532
Thymic Masses, 1533
Thymoma, Diseases Associations, 1533
Thyromegaly, 1533
Thyrotoxicosis, 1533
Tick-Related Infections, 1533
Tics, 1533
Torsades de Pointes, 1533
Toxic Megacolon, Causes, 1533
Tracheobronchial Narrowing On X-Ray, 1534
Tremor, 1534
Tremor, in Children, Causes, 1534
Trichomegaly, 1534
Tubulointerstitial Disease, Acute, 1534
Tubulointerstitial Kidney Disease, 1535
Tumor Markers Elevation, 1535
Uremic Encephalopathy, Differential
    Diagnosis, 1535
Ureteral Colic, 1535
Ureteral Stricture, 1535
Ureteric Obstruction, Congenital, 1536
Urethral Bleeding, 1536
Urethral Discharge and Dysuria, 1536
Urethral Obstruction, Children, 1536
Uric Acid Stones, 1536
Urinary Incontinence, Children, 1536
Urinary Retention, 1536
Urinary Retention, Acute, 1536

Urinary Tract Bleeding, Upper, 1536
Urinary Tract Obstruction, 1537
Urinary Tract Obstruction, Congenital
    Causes, 1537
Urine Casts, 1537
Urine Color Abnormalities, 1537
Urine, Red, 1538
Urolithiasis-Like Pain, 1538
Uropathy, Obstructive, 1538
Urosepsis, 1538
Uterine Bleeding, Abnormal, 1539
Uveitis, Pediatric Age, 1539
Vaginal Bleeding, Pregnancy, 1539
Vaginal Discharge, Prepubertal Girls, 1539
Valvular Heart Disease, 1539
Vascular Lesions of GI Tract, 1539
Vasculitis, Classification, 1540
Vasculitis (Diseases that Mimic
    Vasculitis), 1540
Vegetative State, Persistent, 1540
Ventilation–Perfusion Mismatch on Lung
    Scan, 1540
Ventricular Failure, 1540
Verrucous Lesions, 1540
Vertigo, 1541
Vertigo, Central, 1541
Vesiculobullous Diseases, 1541
Vision Loss, Acute, Painful, 1541
Vision Loss, Acute, Painless, 1541
Vision Loss After Diving, 1541
Vision Loss, Children, 1541
Vision Loss, Chronic, Progressive, 1542
Vision Loss, Monocular, Transient, 1542
Vitreous Hemorrhage, 1542
Vocal Cord Paralysis, 1542
Volume Depletion, 1542
Volume Excess, 1542
Vomiting, 1542
Vomiting, Neonatal, 1542
Vulvar Lesions, 1543
Weakness, Acute, Emergent, 1543
Weakness, Gradual Onset, 1543
Weakness, Nonneuromuscular
    Causes, 1543
Weight Gain, 1544
Weight Loss, 1544
Wheezing, 1544
Wheezing, Pediatric Age, 1544
Wrist and Hand Pain, in Different Age
    Groups, 1544
Wrist Pain, 1544
Xerophthalmia, 1545
Xerostomia, 1545
Yellow Urine, 1545

SECTION III **Clinical Algorithms**

Abdominal Abscess, 1550
Abdominal Pain, Acute, 1551
Abdominal Pain, Right Upper Quadrant, 1552

Acid-Base Homeostasis, 1553
Acidosis, Metabolic, 1555
Acidosis, Respiratory, Acute, 1556

Acidosis, Respiratory, Chronic, 1557
Adrenal Mass, 1558
Airway Obstruction, Malignant, 1559

Alcohol Poisoning, 1560
Allergic Reaction to Vaccines, 1561
Alkalosis, Metabolic, 1562
Alkalosis, Respiratory Treatment, 1563
Altered Mental Status and Coma, 1564
Alveolar Hemorrhage, 1565
Ambiguous Genitalia, 1567
Anemia, 1568
Anemia, Macrocytic, 1569
Anemia, Microcytic, 1570
Anisocoria, 1571
Anorectal Complaints, 1573
Anorexia, 1574
Anticholinergic Poisoning, 1575
Arthralgia Limited to One or Few
    Joints, 1576
Ataxia, Progressive, 1577
Azoospermia, 1578
Back Pain, 1579
Bleeding Disorders, 1580
Bleeding, Gastrointestinal, 1581
Bleeding, Vaginal, 1583
Bradycardia, 1585
Breast, Nipple Discharge Evaluation, 1586
Breast, Routine Screen or Palpable Mass
    Evaluation, 1588
Cardiac Arrest, 1590
Cardiomegaly on Chest X-Ray, 1591
Cardiomyopathy, 1592
Cerebral Ischemia, 1594
Chest Pain, 1595
Chest X-Ray Abnormality (Suspected), 1596
Connective Tissue Disorder,
    Suspected, 1597
Constipation, 1598
Cough, Chronic, 1600
Cyanosis, 1602
Cystitis, Acute, 1603
Defecation Disorder, Pediatric Age, 1604
Diarrhea, Acute, 1605
Diarrhea, Chronic, 1606
Diplopia, 1607
Diverticular Hemorrhage, 1609
Dyspnea, 1610
Dysuria and/or Urethral/Vaginal
    Discharge, 1614
Ear Pain, 1615
Eating Disorder, 1616
Edema, Generalized, 1617
Edema, Regional, 1618
Erythrocytosis, Acquired, 1619
Esophageal Foreign Body, 1620
Fatigue, 1622
Fecal Incontinence, 1623
Fever and Neutropenia, 1626
Fever Pediatric Patient, 1627
Food Reaction, 1628
Genital Lesions or Ulcers, 1629
Glomerulonephritis, 1630

Goiter, 1631
Granuloma, 1632
Hearing Loss, 1633
Hematuria, Asymptomatic, 1636
Hemoptysis, 1638
Hepatic Mass, 1639
Hepatitis, Viral, 1640
Hepatomegaly, 1641
HIV-Positive Patient with CNS Mass
    Lesions, 1643
HIV-positive patient with CNS Signs and
    Symptoms, 1644
Hypercalcemia, 1645
Hypercapnia, 1646
Hyperkalemia, 1647
Hypermagnesemia, 1648
Hypernatremia, 1649
Hyperpigmentation, 1650
Hyperphosphatemia, 1653
Hypocalcemia, 1654
Hypoglycemia, 1655
Hypogonadism, 1656
Hypokalemia, 1657
Hypomagnesemia, 1658
Hyponatremia, 1659
Hypophosphatemia, 1660
Hypotension, 1661
Hypotension, Postoperative, 1662
Hypovolemic Shock, 1663
Hypoxemia, Postoperative, 1664
Infections of Soft Tissue, Joints, and
    Bone, 1665
Infectious Diarrhea, 1666
Inflammatory Arthritis, 1667
Intraabdominal Infection, Suspected, 1668
Jaundice, 1669
Jaundice, Neonatal, 1670
Joint Effusion, 1671
Joint Pain and Swelling, 1672
Knee Pain, Anterior, 1673
Leg Ulcer, 1674
Liver Function Test Elevations, 1675
Low Back and/or Leg Pain, 1676
Lymphadenopathy, Generalized, 1677
Malabsorption, 1678
Malar Eruption, 1680
Mechanical Ventilation, Distressed
    Patient, 1681
Mental Status Change, Elderly Patient,
    1682
Murmur, Diastolic, 1683
Murmur, Systolic, 1684
Muscle Cramps and Aches, 1685
Muscle Weakness, 1686
Musculoskeletal Complaints, 1687
Nausea and Vomiting, 1688
Neck Mass, 1693
Neck Pain, 1694
Nystagmus, 1695

Occupational Asthma, 1700
Oliguria, 1702
Palpitations, Dizziness, and/or Syncope,
    1703
Pancreatic Mass, 1704
Patient with Ill-Defined Physical
    Complaints, 1705
Pelvic Mass, 1706
Pelvic Pain, Women, Diagnostic
    Evaluation, 1707
Pelvic Pain, Women, Management, 1709
Peripheral Neuropathy, 1710
Pituitary Tumor, 1711
Pleural Effusion, 1712
Pneumothorax, Traumatic, 1714
Poisoning, Acute, 1715
Proteinuria, 1720
Pruritus, Generalized, 1721
Pulmonary Hypertension, Chronic,
    Thromboembolic, 1722
Pulmonary Nodule, 1723
Purpura, Palpable, 1726
Renal Colic, 1727
Renal Mass, 1728
Renal Trauma, 1729
Scrotal Mass, 1730
Shock, 1731
Shoulder Pain, 1732
Skin and Soft Tissue Infections, 1735
Sleep Disorders, 1737
Sleep Disorders Associated with
    Pregnancy, 1740
Sleep-Related Movement Disorders, 1741
Sore Throat, 1742
Splenomegaly, 1743
Spondyloarthropathy, Diagnosis, 1744
Spondyloarthropathy, Treatment, 1745
Tachycardia, Diagnostic Approach, 1746
Tachycardia, Narrow Complex, 1747
Tachycardia, Wide Complex, 1748
Testicular Mass, 1749
Thyroid, Painful, 1750
Thyrotoxicosis, 1751
Trauma in Pregnancy, 1752
Traumatic Aortic Injury, 1753
Urinary Incontinence, Sphincteric, Male
    Patient, 1754
Urinary Tract Obstruction, 1755
Vaginal Discharge, Evaluation, 1756
Vaginitis, Pediatric, 1757
Ventricular Fibrillation or Pulseless
    Ventricular Tachycardia, 1758
Vertigo, 1759
Vomiting, 1761
Vomiting, Acute, Management, 1762
Weakness, 1763
Weakness, Neuromuscular, 1765
Weight Gain, 1766
Weight Loss, Unintentional, 1767

Additional Algorithms Available at ExpertConsult.com

Adrenal Incidentaloma (Fig. E11)
Anemia in Newborn (Fig. E25)
Anemia with Reticulocytosis (Fig. E28)
Aspiration, Gastric Contents (Fig. E36)
Aspiration, Oral Contents (Fig. E37)
Bleeding and Bruising Problems (Fig. E42)
Bleeding Disorder, Congenital (Fig. E43)
Bleeding, Early Pregnancy (Fig. E45)
Bleeding, Neonate (Fig. E47)
Bleeding, Variceal (Fig. E50)
Bradycardia, Pediatric Patient (Fig. E52)
Breast, Radiologic Evaluation (Fig. E54)
Breastfeeding Difficulties (Fig. E57)
Bullae on Lower Extremities (Fig. E58)
Cardiomyopathy, Ischemic (Fig. E64)
Convulsive Disorder, Suspected, Pediatric Patient (Fig. E70)
Corneal Disorders (Fig. E71)
Cutaneous Microvascular Occlusion Syndromes (Fig. E73, Tables E8 and E9)
Dehydration Correction, Pediatric Patient (Fig. E79, Tables E10 to E13)
Dementia, Management (Fig. E80, Table E14)
Developmental Delay (Fig. E81)
Diarrhea, Chronic, in Patients with HIV Infection (Fig. E84, Table E15)
Diarrhea, Watery (Fig. E85)
Dilated Pupil (Fig. E86)
Dyspepsia (Fig. E90)
Eosinophilic Dermatoses (Fig. E99)
Erythroderma (Fig. E101, Table E20)
Fever and Infection in High-Risk Hematology Patient without Obvious Source (Fig. E106)

Fever and Neutropenia, Pediatric Patient (Fig. E108)
Flushing (Fig. E110)
Foreign Body, in Wound (Fig. E112)
Fracture, Bone (Fig. E113)
Genitalia, Ambiguous (Fig. E115)
GI Bleeding, Pediatric Patient (Fig. E116)
Goiter Evaluation and Management (Fig. E119)
Hematochezia, Management (Fig. E122)
Hematuria, Pediatric Patient (Fig. E124)
HIV Detection, Patients at Risk (Fig. E130)
Intubation, Pediatric Patient Fig. E159, Table E31)
Ischemia, Colon Management (Fig. E160)
Knee Dislocation Treatment (Fig. E165)
Liver Mass, Solid (Fig. E169)
Lymphadenopathy, Axillary (Fig. E171)
Lymphadenopathy, Cervical (Fig. E172)
Lymphadenopathy, Epitrochlear (Fig. E173)
Lymphadenopathy, Inguinal (Fig. E175)
Myocardial Ischemia, Suspected (Fig. E186)
Myositis (Fig. E187)
Nail Dystrophy (Fig. E188)
Nutrition Assessment and Intervention in Cancer Patients (Fig. E193)
Nutritional Support (Fig. E194, Box E9)
Onycholysis (Fig. E203)
Pancreatic Islet Cell Tumors (Fig. E205)
Papulosquamous Disorders, Pediatric Patient (Fig. E207)
Pericardial Effusion, Malignant (Fig. E214)
Photosensitivity (Fig. E216)

Pleural Effusion, Malignant (Fig. E220)
Polycythemia (Fig. E224)
Pruritus, Pregnant Patient (Fig. E227)
Pseudohermaphroditism (Fig. E228)
Reactive Erythema, Pediatric Patient (Fig. E232)
Renal Disease, Ischemic, Management (Fig. E234)
Respiratory Distress (Fig. E239)
Rhinorrhea (Fig. E240)
Sexual Dysfunction Evaluation (Fig. E242)
Sexual Precocity, Female Breast Development (Fig. E243)
Sexual Precocity, Female Public Hair Development (Fig. E244, Table E54)
Sexual Precocity, Male (Fig. E245, Table E55)
Shin Splints (Fig. E246)
Short Stature (Fig. E248)
Skin Blisters (Fig. E252, Table E57)
Spine Tumor (Fig. E258)
Spondylosis, Cervical (Fig. E262)
Stroke (Fig. E263)
Subcutaneous Ossification, Evaluation (Fig. E264)
Tachycardia, Pediatric Patient (Fig. E268)
Thrombotic Microangiopathies, Differential Diagnosis (Fig. E272)
Unconscious Patient (Fig. E277)
Vaginal Prolapse/Pelvic Organ Prolapse (Fig. E281)

SECTION IV Laboratory Tests and Interpretation of Results

ACE Level, 1771
Acetone (serum or plasma), 1771
Acetylcholine Receptor (AChR) Antibody, 1771
Acid-Base Reference Values, 1771
Acid Phosphatase (serum), 1771
Acid Serum Test, 1771
Activated Clotting Time (ACT), 1771
Activated Partial Thromboplastin Time (APTT, aPTT), 1771
Adrenocorticotropic Hormone, 1771
Alanine Aminopeptidase, 1771
Alanine Aminotransferase (ALT, SGPT), 1771
Albumin (serum), 1773
Alcohol Dehydrogenase, 1773
Aldolase (serum), 1773
Aldosterone, 1773
Alkaline Phosphatase (ALP) (serum), 1774
Alpha-1-Antitrypsin (serum), 1774
Alpha-1-Fetoprotein (serum), 1774
ALT, 1774
Aluminum (serum), 1774

AMA, 1774
Amebiasis Serologic Test, 1774
Aminolevulinic Acid (δ-ALA) (24-hr urine collection), 1774
Ammonia (serum), 1774
Amylase (serum), 1774
Amylase, Urine, 1774
Amyloid A Protein (serum), 1774
ANA, 1774
ANCA, 1774
Androstenedione (serum), 1774
Angiotensin II, 1775
Angiotensin-Converting Enzyme (ACE level), 1775
ANH, 1775
Anion Gap, 1775
Anticardiolipin Antibody (ACA), 1775
Anticoagulant, 1775
Antidiuretic Hormone, 1775
Anti-DNA, 1776
ANTI-DS DNA, 1776
Antiglobulin Test, 1776

Antiglomerular Basement Antibody, 1776
Antihistone, 1776
Antimitochondrial Antibody (AMA, Mitochondrial antibody), 1776
Antineutrophil Cytoplasmic Antibody (ANCA), 1776
Antinuclear Antibody (ANA), 1776
Anti-RNP Antibody, 1777
ANTI-SCL-70, 1777
Anti-SM (anti-Smith) Antibody, 1777
Anti-Smooth Muscle Antibody, 1777
Antistreptolysin O Titer (Streptozyme, ASLO titer), 1777
Antithrombin III, 1777
Apolipoprotein A-1 (Apo A-1), 1777
Apolipoprotein B (Apo B), 1777
Arterial Blood Gases, 1777
Arthrocentesis Fluid, 1778
ASLO Titer, 1778
Aspartate Aminotransferase (AST, SGOT), 1778
Atrial Natriuretic Hormone (ANH), 1778

B-Type Natriuretic Peptide (BNP), 1779
Basophil Count, 1779
Bicarbonate, 1779
Bile, Urine, 1779
Bilirubin, Direct (conjugated bilirubin), 1779
Bilirubin, Indirect (unconjugated bilirubin), 1779
Bilirubin, Total, 1779
Bilirubin, Urine, 1779
Bladder Tumor Associated Antigen, 1779
Bleeding Time (modified Ivy method), 1779
Blood Volume, Total, 1781
BNP, 1781
Bordetella pertussis Serology, 1781
BRCA Analysis, 1781
Breath Hydrogen Test (hydrogen breath test), 1781
BUN, 1781
C282Y and H63D Mutation Analysis, 1781
C3, 1781
C4, 1781
Calcitonin (serum), 1781
Calcium (serum), 1782
Calcium, Urine, 1782
Cancer Antigen 15-3 (CA 15-3), 1782
Cancer Antigen 27-29 (CA 27-29), 1784
Cancer Antigen 72-4 (CA 72-4), 1784
Cancer Antigen 125 (CA 125), 1784
Captopril Stimulation Test, 1784
Carbamazepine (Tegretol), 1784
Carbohydrate Antigen 19-9, 1784
Carbon Dioxide, Partial Pressure, 1784
Carbon Monoxide, 1784
Carboxyhemoglobin, 1784
Carcinoembryonic Antigen (CEA), 1784
Carotene (serum), 1784
Catecholamines, Urine, 1784
CBC, 1784
CD40 Ligand, 1784
CD4+ T-Lymphocyte Count (CD4+ T-cells), 1784
CEA, 1784
Cerebrospinal Fluid (CSF), 1784
Ceruloplasmin (serum), 1785
Chlamydia Group Antibody Serologic Test, 1785
Chlamydia Trachomatis PCR, 1785
Chloride (serum), 1785
Chloride (sweat), 1785
Chloride, Urine, 1785
Cholecystokinin-Pancreozymin (CCK, CCK-PZ), 1785
Cholesterol, High-Density Lipoprotein, 1785
Cholesterol, Low-Density Lipoprotein, 1785
Cholesterol, Total, 1785
Chorionic Gonadotropins, Human (serum) (HCG), 1785
Chymotrypsin, 1788
Circulating Anticoagulant (lupus anticoagulant), 1788
CK, 1789
Clonidine Suppression Test, 1789

Clostridium difficile Toxin Assay (stool), 1789
CO, 1789
Coagulation Factors, 1789
Cobalamin, Serum, 1789
Cold Agglutinins Titer, 1789
Complement, 1790
Complement Deficiency, 1790
Complete Blood Count (CBC), 1790
Conjugated Bilirubin, 1792
Copper (serum), 1792
Copper, Urine, 1792
Corticotropin Releasing Hormone (CRH) Stimulation Test, 1792
Cortisol, Plasma, 1793
C-Peptide, 1793
Coombs Direct, 1793
Coombs Indirect, 1793
CPK, 1793
C-Reactive Protein, 1793
C-Reactive Protein, High Sensitivity (hs-CRP, cardio-CRP), 1793
Creatine Kinase (CK, CPK), 1793
Creatine Kinase Isoenzymes, 1794
Creatinine (serum), 1794
Creatinine Clearance, 1795
Creatinine, Urine, 1795
Cryoglobulins (serum), 1795
Cryptosporidium Antigen By EIA (stool), 1795
CSF, 1795
Cystatin C, 1795
Cystic Fibrosis PCR, 1795
Cytomegalovirus by PCR, 1795
d-Dimer, 1795
Dehydroepiandrosterone Sulfate, 1795
Dehydrotestosterone (serum, urine), 1795
Deoxycorticosterone (11-deoxycorticosterone, DOC) (serum), 1795
Dexamethasone Suppression Test, Overnight, 1795
Digoxin, 1795
Dilantin, 1796
Direct Antiglobulin (Coombs Direct), 1796
Disaccharide Absorption Tests, 1796
DOC, 1796
Donath-Landsteiner (D-L) Test For Paroxysmal Cold Hemoglobinuria, 1796
Dopamine, 1796
d-Xylose Absorption, 1796
d-Xylose Absorption Test, 1796
Electrophoresis, Hemoglobin, 1796
Electrophoresis, Protein, 1796
ENA Complex, 1796
Endomysial Antibodies, 1796
Eosinophil Count, 1796
Epinephrine, Plasma, 1797
Epstein-Barr Virus Serology, 1797
Erythrocyte Sedimentation Rate (ESR, sed rate, sedimentation rate), 1797
Erythropoietin (EP), 1797
Estradiol (serum), 1798

Estrogen, 1798
Ethanol (blood), 1798
Extractable Nuclear Antigen (ENA complex, anti-RNP antibody, anti-SM, anti-Smith), 1798
Factor V Leiden, 1799
Fasting Blood Sugar, 1799
FBS, 1799
FDP, 1799
Fecal Fat, Quantitative (72-hr collection), 1799
Fecal Globin Immunochemical Test, 1799
Ferritin (serum), 1799
α-1 Fetoprotein, 1799
Fibrin Degradation Product (FDP), 1800
Fibrinogen, 1800
Folate (folic acid), 1800
Follicle-Stimulating Hormone (FSH), 1800
Free T4, 1800
Free Thyroxine Index, 1800
FTA-ABS (serum), 1800
Furosemide Stimulation Test, 1801
Gamma-Glutamyl Transferase (GGT), 1801
Gastrin (serum), 1801
Gastrin Stimulation Test, 1801
Gliadin Antibodies, IgA and IgG, 1801
Glomerular Basement Membrane (GBM) Antibody, 1801
Glomerular Filtration Rate, 1801
Glucagon, 1801
Glucose, Fasting (FBS, fasting blood sugar), 1801
Glucose, Postprandial, 1801
Glucose Tolerance Test, 1801
Glucose-6-Phosphate Dehydrogenase (G6PD) screen (blood), 1802
γ-Glutamyl Transferase (GGT), 1802
Glycohemoglobin (glycated glycosylated hemoglobin), (HbA1c), 1802
Growth Hormone, 1802
Growth Hormone Releasing Hormone (GHRH), 1802
Growth Hormone Suppression Test (after glucose), 1802
Ham Test (acid serum test), 1802
Haptoglobin (serum), 1802
HBA_{1c}, 1802
HDL, 1802
Helicobacter pylori (serology, stool antigen), 1802
Hematocrit, 1802
Hemoglobin, 1803
Hemoglobin A_{1c}, 1803
Hemoglobin Electrophoresis, 1803
Hemoglobin, Glycated, 1803
Hemoglobin, Glycosylated, 1803
Hemoglobin H, 1803
Hemoglobin, Urine, 1804
Hemosiderin, Urine, 1804
Heparin-Induced Thrombocytopenia Antibodies, 1804
Hepatitis A Antibody, 1804

Detailed Contents

HAV-IgM Antibody, 1804
HAV Total Antibody, 1804
Hepatitis A Viral Infection, 1804
Hepatitis B Surface Antigen (HBsAg), 1804
Hepatitis B Viral Infection, 1804
Hepatitis C Viral Infection, 1805
Hepatitis C RNA, 1805
Hepatitis D Viral Infection, 1805
Delta Hepatitis Coinfection (acute HDV1 acute HBV) or Superinfection (acute HDV1 chronic HBV), 1805
HDV-Ag, 1806
HDV-Ab (IgM), 1806
HDV-Ab (total), 1806
HER-2/*NEU*, 1806
Herpes Simplex Virus (HSV), 1806
HFE Screen for Hereditary Hemochromatosis, 1806
Heterophil Antibody, 1806
High-Density Lipoprotein (HDL) Cholesterol, 1806
HLA Antigens, 1806
Homocysteine (plasma), 1806
Human Chorionic Gonadotropin (hCG), 1807
Human Herpes Virus 8 (HHV8), 1807
Human Immunodeficiency Virus Antibody, Type 1 (HIV-1), 1807
Human Immunodeficiency Virus Type 1 (HIV-1) Antigen (p24), Qualitative (p24 antigen), 1807
Human Immunodeficiency Virus Type 1 (HIV-1) Viral Load, 1809
Human Papilloma Virus (HPV), 1809
Huntington's Disease PCR, 1809
Hydrogen Breath Test, 1809
5-Hydroxyindole-Acetic Acid, Urine, 1809
Immune Complex Assay, 1809
Immunoglobulins, 1809
Indirect Antiglobulin (Coombs Indirect), 1809
Influenza A and B Tests, 1809
Insulin Autoantibodies, 1809
Insulin, Free, 1809
Insulin-Like Growth Factor-1 (IGF-1) (Serum), 1809
Insulin-Like Growth Factor-II, 1810
International Normalized Ratio (INR), 1810
Intrinsic Factor Antibodies, 1811
Iron (Serum), 1811
Iron-Binding Capacity, Total (TIBC), 1811
Iron Saturation (% Transferrin Saturation), 1811
Lactate (blood), 1812
Lactate Dehydrogenase (LDH), 1812
Lactate Dehydrogenase Isoenzymes, 1812
Lactose Tolerance Test (serum), 1812
Lap Score, 1812
Lead, 1812
LDH, 1812
LDL, 1812
Legionella pneumophila PCR, 1814
Legionella Titer, 1814
Leukocyte Alkaline Phosphatase (LAP), 1814
Leukocyte Count, 1814

Lipase, 1814
Lipoprotein(a), 1814
Lipoprotein Cholesterol, High-Density, 1814
Lipoprotein Cholesterol, Low-Density, 1814
Liver Kidney Microsome Type 1 Antibodies (LKM1), 1814
LKM1, 1814
Low-Density Lipoprotein (LDL) Cholesterol, 1814
Lupus Anticoagulant, 1814
Luteinizing Hormone, 1814
Lyme Disease Antibody Titer, 1814
Lymphocytes, 1815
Magnesium (Serum), 1816
Mean Corpuscular Volume (MCV), 1817
Metanephrines, Urine, 1817
Methylmalonic Acid (Serum), 1817
Mitochondrial Antibody (AMA), 1817
Monocyte Count, 1818
Mycoplasma Pneumoniae PCR, 1818
Myelin Basic Protein, Cerebrospinal Fluid, 1818
Myoglobin, Urine, 1818
Neisseria gonorrhoeae PCR, 1818
Neutrophil Count, 1818
Norepinephrine, 1818
5′-Nucleotidase, 1818
Osmolality (serum), 1818
Osmolality, Urine, 1819
Osmotic Fragility Test, 1819
Paracentesis Fluid, 1819
Parathyroid Hormone (PTH), 1820
Parietal Cell Antibodies, 1821
Partial Thromboplastin Time (PTT), Activated Partial Thromboplastin Time (APTT), 1821
Pepsinogen I, 1821
pH, Blood, 1821
pH, Urine, 1821
Phenobarbital, 1821
Phenytoin (Dilantin), 1821
Phosphatase, Acid, 1821
Phosphatase, Alkaline, 1821
Phosphate (serum), 1821
Plasminogen, 1821
Platelet Aggregation, 1821
Platelet Antibodies, 1822
Platelet Count, 1822
Platelet Function Analysis 100 Assay (PFA), 1822
Pleural Fluid, 1822
Potassium (serum), 1823
Potassium, Urine, 1824
Procainamide, 1824
Progesterone (serum), 1824
Prolactin, 1825
Prostate-Specific Antigen (PSA), 1825
Prostatic Acid Phosphatase, 1825
Protein (serum), 1825
Protein C Assay, 1825
Protein Electrophoresis (serum), 1825
Protein S Assay, 1826
Prothrombin Time (PT), 1826

Protoporphyrin (Free erythrocyte), 1826
PSA, 1826
PT, 1826
PTH, 1826
PTT, 1826
Rapid Plasma Reagin (RPR), 1827
RDW, 1827
Red Blood Cell (RBC) Count, 1827
Red Blood Cell Distribution Width (RDW), 1827
Red Blood Cell Folate, 1827
Red Blood Cell Mass (volume), 1827
Red Blood Cell Morphology, 1827
Renin (serum), 1827
Respiratory Syncytial Virus (RSV) Screen, 1827
Reticulocyte Count, 1827
Rheumatoid Factor, 1827
RNP, 1828
RPR, 1830
Rotavirus Serology, 1830
Sed Rate, 1830
Sedimentation Rate, 1830
Semen Analysis, 1830
SGOT, 1830
SGPT, 1830
Sickle Cell Test, 1830
Smooth Muscle Antibody, 1830
Sodium (serum), 1830
Streptozyme, 1831
Sucrose Hemolysis Test (sugar water test), 1831
Sudan III Stain (qualitative screening for fecal fat), 1831
Synovial Fluid Analysis, 1831
T_3 (triiodothyronine), 1832
T_3 Resin Uptake (T_3RU), 1832
T_4, Free (Free thyroxine), 1832
T_4, Serum T_4, 1832
Tegretol, 1833
Testosterone (total testosterone), 1833
Theophylline, 1833
Thoracentesis Fluid, 1833
Thrombin Time (TT), 1833
Thyroglobulin, 1833
Thyroid Microsomal Antibodies, 1833
Thyroid-Stimulating Hormone (TSH), 1833
Thyrotropin (TSH) Receptor Antibodies, 1835
Thyrotropin-Releasing Hormone (TRH) Stimulation Test, 1835
Thyroxine (T_4), 1835
TIBC, 1835
Tissue Transglutaminase Antibody, 1835
Transferrin, 1835
Triglycerides, 1835
Triiodothyronine, 1835
Troponins (serum), 1835
TSH, 1836
TT, 1836
Tuberculin Test (PPD), 1836
Unconjugated Bilirubin, 1836
Urea Nitrogen, Blood (BUN), 1836
Uric Acid (serum), 1836

Urinalysis, 1836
Urine Amylase, 1837
Urine Bile, 1837
Urine Calcium, 1837
Urine Camp, 1837
Urine Catecholamines, 1837
Urine Chloride, 1837
Urine Copper, 1837
Urine Cortisol, Free, 1837
Urine Creatinine (24 hr), 1838
Urine Crystals, 1838
Urine Eosinophils, 1838
Urine Glucose (qualitative), 1838
Urine Hemoglobin, Free, 1838

Urine Hemosiderin, 1838
Urine 5-Hydroxyindole-Acetic Acid (urine 5-HIAA), 1838
Urine Indican, 1838
Urine Ketones (semiquantitative), 1838
Urine Metanephrines, 1838
Urine Myoglobin, 1838
Urine Nitrite, 1838
Urine Occult Blood, 1838
Urine Osmolality, 1838
Urine pH, 1838
Urine Phosphate, 1839
Urine Potassium, 1839
Urine Protein (quantitative), 1839

Urine Sediment, 1839
Urine Sodium (quantitative), 1839
Urine Specific Gravity, 1841
Urine Vanillylmandelic Acid (VMA), 1841
Varicella-Zoster Virus (VZV) Serology, 1842
Vasoactive Intestinal Peptide (VIP), 1842
VDRL, 1842
Viscosity (serum), 1842
Vitamin B_{12} (cobalamin), 1842
Vitamin D, 1,25 Dihydroxy Calciferol, 1843
Vitamin K, 1843
Von Willebrand Factor, 1843

SECTION V Clinical Practice Guidelines

PART A • THE PERIODIC HEALTH EXAMINATION

Age-Specific Charts, 1849
TABLE 1 Birth to 10 years, 1849
TABLE 2 Ages 11 to 24 years, 1851
TABLE 3 Ages 25 to 64 years, 1853
TABLE 4 Ages 65 and older, 1855
TABLE 5 Pregnant women, 1857
TABLE 6 Cervical cancer screening guidelines, 1858

PART B • IMMUNIZATIONS AND CHEMOPROPHYLAXIS

Childhood and Adolescent Immunizations, 1859
TABLE 7 Recommended Immunization Schedule for Children and Adolescents Aged 18 Years or Younger—United States, 2017, 1859
TABLE 8 Catch-up Immunization Schedule for Persons Aged 4 Months Through 18 Years Who Start Late or Who Are More Than 1 Month Behind—United States, 2017, 1860
General Recommendations on Immunization, 1865
TABLE 9 Recommended and Minimum Ages and Intervals between Vaccine Doses, 1865
TABLE 10 Guidelines for Spacing of Live and Inactivated Antigens, 1866
TABLE 11 Guidelines for Administering Antibody-Containing Products and Vaccines, 1866
TABLE 12 Recommended Intervals between Administration of Antibody-Containing Products and Measles- or Varicella-Containing Vaccine, by Product and Indication for Vaccination, 1867
TABLE 13 Contraindications and Precautions to Commonly Used Vaccines, 1868

TABLE 14 Conditions Commonly Misperceived as Contraindications to Vaccination, 1870
Vaccine Administration, 1872
TABLE 15 Treatment of Anaphylaxis in Children and Adults with Drugs Administered Intramuscularly or Orally, 1872
TABLE 16 Vaccination of Persons with Primary and Secondary Immunodeficiencies, 1873
TABLE 17 Immunizations for Pediatric Oncology Patients, 1874
TABLE 18 Approaches to the Evaluation and Vaccination of Persons Vaccinated Outside the United States Who Have No (or Questionable) Vaccination Records, 1875
Immunizations for Adults, 1876
TABLE 19 Recommended Immunization Schedule for Adults Aged 19 Years or Older by Age Group, United States, 2017, 1877
TABLE 20A Recommended Immunization Schedule for Adults Aged 19 Years or Older by Medical Condition and Other Indications, United States, 2017, 1878
TABLE 20B Contraindications and Precautions for Vaccines Recommended for Adults Aged 19 Years or Older, 1882
TABLE 21 Immunization and Pregnancy, 1883
TABLE 22 Immunizing Agents and Immunization Schedules for Health Care Workers (HCWs), 1884
TABLE 23 Recommendations for Persons with Medical Conditions Requiring Special Vaccination Considerations, 1887
TABLE 24 Vaccinations for International Travel, 1888
Recommendations and Implementation Strategies for Hepatitis B Vaccination of Adults, 1889
BOX 1 Adults Recommended to Receive Hepatitis B Vaccination, 1889

BOX 2 Hepatitis B Vaccine Schedules for Adults (Aged ≥20 yr), 1889
TABLE 25 Recommended Doses of Currently Licensed Formulations of Adult Hepatitis B Vaccine by Group and Vaccine Type, 1890
TABLE 26 Recommended HIV/AIDS, Sexually Transmitted Disease (STD), and Viral Hepatitis Prevention Services by Risk Population, 1890
TABLE 27 Guidelines for Postexposure Prophylaxis of Persons with Nonoccupational Exposures to Blood or Body Fluids That Contain Blood by Exposure Type and Vaccination Status, 1891
TABLE 28 Typical Interpretation of Serologic Test Results for Hepatitis B Virus Infection, 1891
Hepatitis A Prophylaxis, 1892
TABLE 29 Recommended Dosages of Hepatitis A Immune Globulin, 1892
TABLE 30 Licensed Dosages of Hepatitis A Vaccines, 1892
Influenza Treatment and Prophylaxis, 1893
BOX 3 Summary of Seasonal Influenza Vaccination Recommendations, 1893
TABLE 31 Live, Attenuated Influenza Vaccine (LAIV) Compared with Inactivated Influenza Vaccine (TIV) for Seasonal Influenza, United States Formulations, 1894
Indications for Use of Antivirals, 1895
HIV Testing and Postexposure Prophylaxis, 1897
Recommendations for HIV Testing of Adults, Adolescents, and Pregnant Women, 1897
TABLE 32 HIV Exposure, Estimated Per-Act Risk, 1899
TABLE 33 Regimens for 28-Day Postexposure Prophylaxis for HIV Infection, 1900

TABLE 34 Antiretroviral Therapy Medications, Adult Dosage, and Side Effects, 1901

TABLE 35 Laboratory Tests Generally Recommended for Persons after Exposure to HIV, 1902

BOX 4 Situations for Which Expert Consultation for HIV Postexposure Prophylaxis Is Advised, 1902

BOX 5 Occupational Exposure Management Resources, 1903

BOX 6 Management of Occupational Blood Exposures, 1904

Endocarditis Prophylaxis, 1905

TABLE 36 Cardiac Conditions Associated with the Highest Risk of Adverse Outcome from Endocarditis for Which Prophylaxis with Dental Procedures Is Recommended, 1905

TABLE 37 Dental Procedures for Which Endocarditis Prophylaxis Is Recommended for Patients in Table 36, 1905

TABLE 38 Regimens for a Dental Procedure, 1905

TABLE 39 Summary of Major Changes in Updated Recommendations, 1906

Hepatitis C Testing, 1907

BOX 7 Recommendations for Prevention and Control of Hepatitis C Virus (HCV) Infection and HCV-Related Chronic Diseases, 1907

Hepatitis B Virus Postexposure Protection for Health Care Personnel, 1909

TABLE 40 Postexposure Management of Health Care Personnel After Occupational Percutaneous and Mucosal Exposure to Blood and Body Fluids, by Health Care Personnel HepB Vaccination and Response Status, 1909

APPENDIX I **Complementary and Alternative Medicine**

Ia Definitions of Complementary and Alternative Medicine Terms, 1913

Ib Relaxation Techniques, 1915

Ic Overview of Selected Natural Products, 1917

Id Natural Products and Drug Interactions, 1920

Ie Commonly Ingested Plants with Significant Toxic Potential, 1924

If Herbs Associated with Toxicity, 1925

Ig Websites Providing Data on Herbal Therapy Hazards, 1926

APPENDIX II **Nutrition**

IIa Dietary Supplements: What Every Primary Care Provider Should Know, 1927

IIb Vitamins and Their Functions, 1929

IIc Nutritional and Trace Elements and Their Clinical Implications, 1934

IId Summary of Vitamin and Mineral Deficiencies, 1937

APPENDIX III **Acute Poisoning**

IIIa Historical and Physical Findings in Poisoning, 1939

IIIb Recognizable Poison Symptoms, 1941

IIIc Antidotes and Their Indications for Use, 1942

APPENDIX IV **Impairment and Disability Issues, 1947**

APPENDIX V **Primary Care Procedures, available at ExpertConsult.com**

APPENDIX VI **Patient Teaching Guides, available at ExpertConsult.com**

Additional PTGs Available at ExpertConsult.com
Not Linked to Topics in Section I

Achilles Tendinitis
Acquired Polyneuropathy
Amphetamine Abuse
Anal Cancer
Aortic Valve Disease
Aspirin, Ibuprofen, and Other Pain
    Medication (Child)
Atypical Pneumonia
Back Pain
Bartholin Cyst
Blisters
Boils
Brain Trauma
Bundle Branch Block
Cardiac Pacemaker and Defibrillator
Cervical Radiculopathy
Cervical Spondylosis
Children's Vitamins
Chronic Renal Failure
Cleft Lip and Palate
Coarctation of the Aorta
Colic
Common Cold
Complications of Bariatric Surgery
Constipation
Coronary Artery Bypass Surgery
Cystitis
Dermatitis Herpetiformis
Diagnostic Heart Catheterization
Diaper Rash
Dietary Fiber
Dry Eye
Ear Ache
Elbow Dislocation
Ensuring Your Child's Safety
Eosinophilic Esophagitis
Epilepsy
Excessive Perspiration
Exercises and Cardiovascular Health
Femoral Hernia
Finger Sprain

Flu Vaccination
Food-Borne Intestinal Protozoan Infections
Forgetfulness
Gangrene
Gastroparesis and Gastric Motility Disorders
Gluten-Free Diet
Groin Strain
Halitosis
Hamstring Strain
Healthy Diet as a Teenager
Hearing Loss
Hernia
High Triglycerides
Hip Pain
Hydration (for athletes)
Hypoglycemia in Diabetes
Ingrown Toenail
Inguinal Hernia
Intussusception
Jellyfish and Other Marine Animals Stings
    and Bites
Kegel Exercises
Knee Sprain
Knee Swelling
Legionnaires' Disease
Lipoma
Liver Transplantation
Low Back Pain
Low Back Strain
Lumbosacral Radiculopathy
Microscopic Colitis
Mitral Valve Disease
Morning Sickness
Mouth and Tooth Care
Multivitamins
Neck Pain
Neck Strain
Night Terrors
Nutrition (for Athletes)
Osteorathritis of the Hip
Patellar Tendinitis

Percutaneous Coronary Intervention
Peripheral Neuropathy
Phymosis and Paraphymosis
Pneumoconiosis
Poor Circulation
Porphyria
Prediabetes
Premature Ventricular Contractions
Probiotics
Providing Your Child Good Nutrition
Puberty
Pulmonary Hypertension and
    Thromboembolic Disease
Pyloric Stenosis
Radial Neuropathy
Rectal Cancer
Rotavirus Infections
SARS
Sciatica
Shin Splints
Shoulder Dislocation
Sleep Disorder and Heart Disease
Slipped Disc
Smoke Inhalation
Smoking
Spinal Cord Trauma
Stress Test Used to Predict Heart Attack Risk
Sudden Infant Death Syndrome
Sun Poisoning
Surgical Site (Surgical Wound) Infections
Syndrome of Inappropriate Secretion of
    Diuretic Hormone
Tendinitis
Tinea Infections
Tuberculosis
Ulnar Neuropathy
Vaginal Dryness
Vertigo
Vomiting
Warfarin Therapy
Wrist Fracture

Diseases and Disorders

BASIC INFORMATION

DEFINITION

An abdominal aortic aneurysm (AAA) is a focal full-thickness dilation of the abdominal aortic artery to at least 1.5 times the diameter measured at the level of the renal arteries, or exceeding the normal diameter of the abdominal aorta by 50%. The normal diameter at the renal arteries is 2 cm (range 1.4-3.0 cm), and a diameter 3 cm or larger is generally considered aneurysmal.

ICD-10CM CODES
I71.4 Abdominal aortic aneurysm, without rupture
I71.3 Abdominal aortic aneurysm, ruptured

EPIDEMIOLOGY & DEMOGRAPHICS

- Approximately 15,000 deaths/year in the United States are attributed to AAA.
- AAA is predominantly a disease of older adults, affecting men more than women (4:1).
- The prevalence rate ranges from 4% to 9% in men in developed countries.
- Clinically important AAAs ≥4 cm are present in 1% of men between age 55 and 64; and the prevalence rate increases by 2% to 4% per decade thereafter.
- The peak incidence is among men approximately 70 years old.
- The frequency is much higher in smokers than in nonsmokers (8:1); and the risk decreases with smoking cessation.
- Risk factors for AAA are similar to those for other atherosclerotic cardiovascular diseases. They include age, Caucasian race, smoking, male gender, family history, hypertension, hyperlipidemia, peripheral vascular disease, and aneurysm of other large vessels.
- AAA is two to four times more common in first-degree male relatives of known AAA patients.
- A decreased risk of AAA is associated with female gender, non-Caucasian race, and diabetes.
- Rupture of the AAA occurs in 1% to 3% of men age 65 or older.
  1. Rupture is the 10th leading cause of death in men older than age 55.
  2. Mortality from rupture is 70% to 95%.
  3. Risk factors for rupture include cardiac or renal transplants, severe obstructive lung disease, uncontrolled blood pressure, female sex, and ongoing tobacco use.
- A recent decline in incidence and prevalence of AAA and related mortality has been attributed to reductions in tobacco use.

ETIOLOGY

- Exact etiology is unknown and is likely multifactorial.
  1) Degenerative:
     a. Alterations in vascular wall biology leading to a loss of vascular structural proteins and wall strength.
     b. The most common association is atherosclerosis. It is uncertain whether atherosclerosis causes or results from AAAs.
     c. Tobacco use: >90% of people who develop an AAA have smoked at some point in their lives.
  2) Inherited: Familial clusters are common. High familial prevalence rate is notable in male individuals. The nature of the genetic disorder is unclear but may be linked to alpha-1-antitrypsin deficiency or X-linked mutation. Connective tissue disorders, such as Marfan's syndrome and Ehlers-Danlos syndrome, have also been strongly associated with AAA.
  3) Inflammatory: AAA is a progressive inflammatory disease of the artery walls. Activated B lymphocytes promote AAA by producing immunoglobulins, cytokines, and matrix metalloproteinases (MMPs), resulting in the activation of macrophages, mast cells (MCs), and complement pathways that lead to the degradation of collagen and matrix proteins and to aortic wall remodeling.
  4) Infection, mycotic: syphilis, *Salmonella*.

NATURAL HISTORY

- AAAs tend to develop in the infrarenal aorta and to expand, on average, at a rate of 0.3 to 0.4 cm per year.
- The risk of aneurysmal rupture is largely influenced by aneurysm size, rate of expansion, and sex. Other factors associated with increased risk for rupture include continued smoking, uncontrolled hypertension, and increased wall stress.
- Higher tension in the abdominal aorta (together with histopathologic changes such as accumulation of foam cells, cholesterol crystals, and matrix metalloproteinases) renders the abdominal aortic wall more susceptible to dilation and subsequent rupture.
- The 5-year rupture rate of asymptomatic AAAs is 25% to 40% for aneurysms >5.0 cm in diameter, 1% to 7% for AAAs 4.0 to 5.0 cm, and nearly 0% for AAAs <4.0 cm. The likelihood that an aneurysm will rupture is increased in aneurysms with a diameter >5.5 cm; this size also demonstrates a faster rate of expansion (>0.5 cm over 6 months) and is more likely to be found in those who continue to smoke and in females.
- Mortality rate after rupture can be as high as 90% because most patients do not reach the hospital in time for surgical repair. Of those who reach the hospital, the mortality rate is still 50%, compared with the 1% to 4% mortality rate for elective repair of a nonruptured AAA. The U.S. Preventive Services Task Force (USPSTF) also concludes that the current evidence is insufficient to assess the balance of benefits and harms of screening for AAA in women aged 65 to 75 who ever smoked and recommends against routine screening in women who never smoked (most recent update in June 2014).

SCREENING AND MONITORING

- The USPSTF recommends one-time screening for AAA by ultrasonography in men ages 65 to 75 who have a history of smoking, and in those 60 years of age or older with a history of AAA in a parent or sibling. These populations have been shown to have a higher prevalence of AAA, and selectively screening this group has been shown to decrease AAA-specific mortality.
- The USPSTF has found little benefit in repeat screening in men with a negative ultrasound and has determined that men over the age of 75 are unlikely to benefit from screening. It was also concluded that the current evidence is insufficient to assess the balance of the harms and benefits of screening for AAA in women ages 65 to 75 who have ever smoked.
- Monitoring by ultrasound or CT scan should be performed every 6 to 12 months for patients with AAAs measuring 4.0 to 5.4 cm in diameter and by ultrasound every 2 years for those with AAAs measuring <4 cm.

PHYSICAL FINDINGS & CLINICAL PRESENTATION

- Most aneurysms are asymptomatic and incidentally discovered on imaging studies; however, symptomatic aneurysms are at an increased risk for rupture.
- Physical examination has a sensitivity of 76% for detecting AAAs >5 cm and only 29% for AAAs 3.0-3.9 cm. The accuracy of the physical examination is markedly diminished by obese body habitus.
- Symptomatic patients may present with abdominal, back, flank, or groin pain.
- A pulsatile epigastric mass that may or may not be tender may be present.
- Abdominal pain radiating to the back, flank, and groin.
- Abdominal bruits can be present in case of renal or visceral arterial stenosis.
- Common iliac arteries can be aneurysmal and palpable in the lower abdominal quadrants. In addition, prominent femoral and popliteal pulses warrant an abdominal ultrasound and lower extremity ultrasound.
- Early satiety, nausea, and vomiting may be caused by compression of adjacent bowel.
- Venous thrombosis or insufficiency may occur from iliocaval venous compression.
- Thromboembolization can cause lower extremity pain and discoloration.
- Ureteral obstruction and hydronephrosis can cause flank and groin pain and lead to obstructive renal failure.
- Rupture classically presents as a triad of abdominal or back pain, hypotension, and a pulsatile abdominal mass in 50% of patients.
- Acute blood loss may lead to myocardial infarction; arteriovenous fistulas may present as heart failure; aortoenteric fistulas may present as hematemesis or melena associated with abdominal and back pain.

DIAGNOSIS

DIFFERENTIAL DIAGNOSIS

Almost 75% of patients with AAA are asymptomatic, and the condition is discovered on routine examination or serendipitously when ordering studies for other symptoms. Diagnosis of AAA should be considered in the differential of the following symptoms: abdominal pain, back pain, and/or pulsatile abdominal mass.

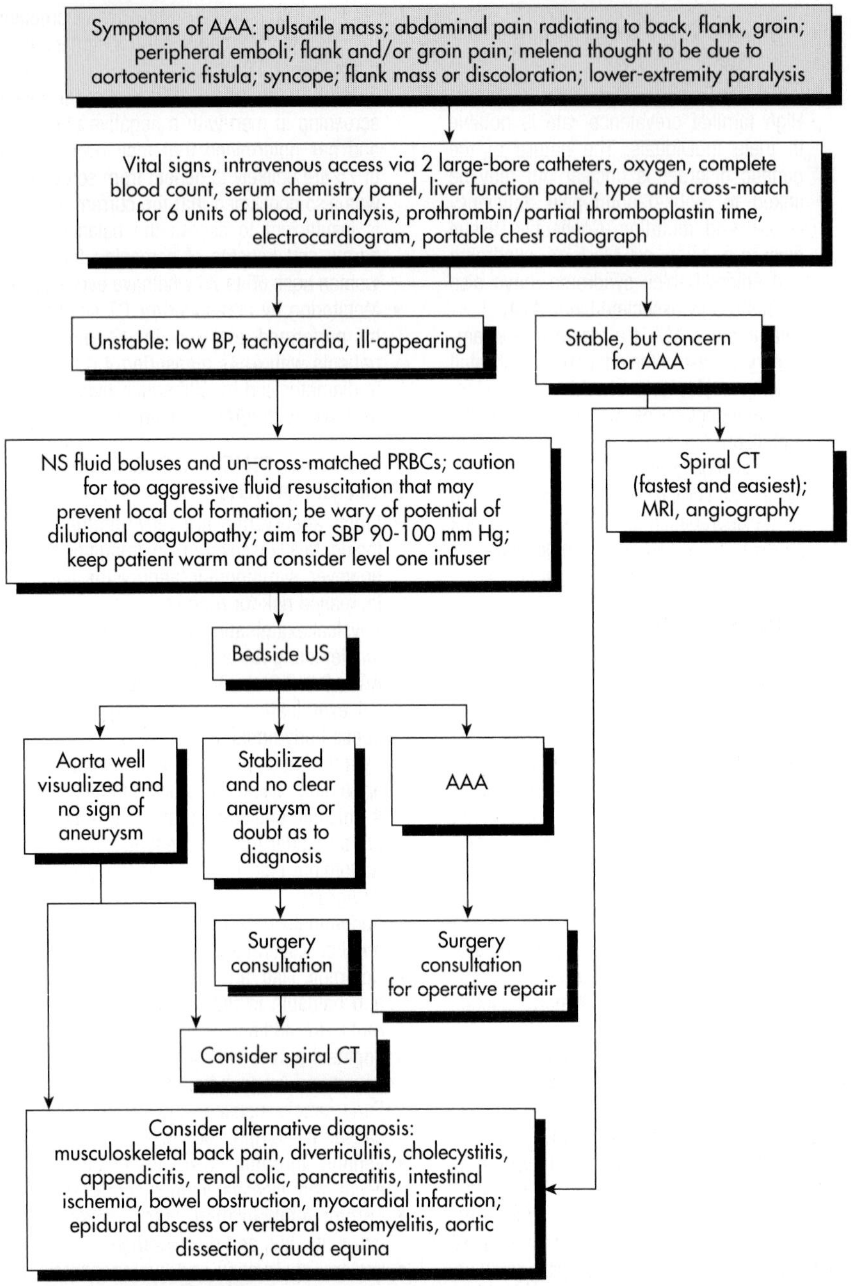

Symptoms of AAA: pulsatile mass; abdominal pain radiating to back, flank, groin; peripheral emboli; flank and/or groin pain; melena thought to be due to aortoenteric fistula; syncope; flank mass or discoloration; lower-extremity paralysis

Vital signs, intravenous access via 2 large-bore catheters, oxygen, complete blood count, serum chemistry panel, liver function panel, type and cross-match for 6 units of blood, urinalysis, prothrombin/partial thromboplastin time, electrocardiogram, portable chest radiograph

Unstable: low BP, tachycardia, ill-appearing

Stable, but concern for AAA

NS fluid boluses and un–cross-matched PRBCs; caution for too aggressive fluid resuscitation that may prevent local clot formation; be wary of potential of dilutional coagulopathy; aim for SBP 90-100 mm Hg; keep patient warm and consider level one infuser

Spiral CT (fastest and easiest); MRI, angiography

Bedside US

Aorta well visualized and no sign of aneurysm

Stabilized and no clear aneurysm or doubt as to diagnosis

AAA

Surgery consultation

Surgery consultation for operative repair

Consider spiral CT

Consider alternative diagnosis: musculoskeletal back pain, diverticulitis, cholecystitis, appendicitis, renal colic, pancreatitis, intestinal ischemia, bowel obstruction, myocardial infarction; epidural abscess or vertebral osteomyelitis, aortic dissection, cauda equina

FIG. 1 Algorithm for the diagnosis and treatment of abdominal aortic aneurysms (AAAs). *BP,* Blood pressure; *CT,* computed tomography; *MRI,* magnetic resonance imaging; *NS,* normal saline; *PRBCs,* packed red blood cells; *SBP,* systolic blood pressure; *US,* ultrasonography. (From Adams JG et al: *Emergency medicine, clinical essentials,* ed 2, Philadelphia, 2013, Elsevier.)

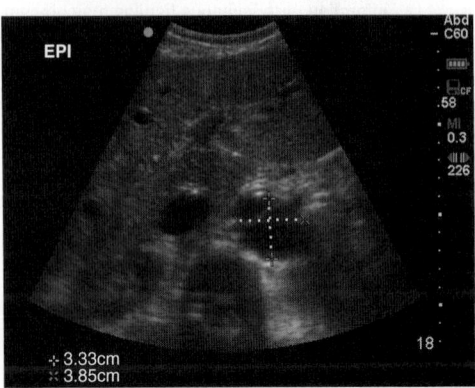

FIG. 2 Transverse image of an abdominal aortic aneurysm. Note the measurements of 3.35 × 3.85 cm. The inferior vena cava is seen to the patient's right of the aorta, and the vertebral body is seen below the two vessels. Note also that there appears to be an echogenic flap within the aorta, possibly representing an aortic dissection. (From Adams JG et al: *Emergency medicine, clinical essentials,* ed 2, Philadelphia, 2013, Elsevier.)

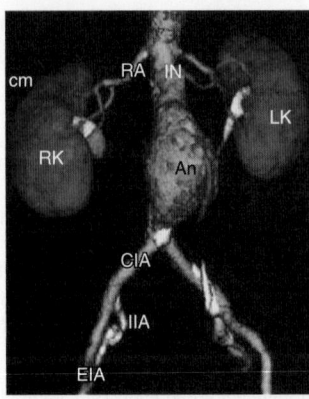

FIG. 3 Three-dimensional CT image illustrates the presence of an infrarenal abdominal aortic aneurysm. *An,* Aneurysm; *CIA,* common iliac artery; *EIA,* external iliac artery; *IIA,* internal iliac artery; *IN,* infrarenal neck; *LK,* left kidney; *RA,* renal artery; *RK,* right kidney. (From Townsend CM et al [eds]: *Sabiston textbook of surgery,* ed 17, Philadelphia, 2004, Saunders.)

LABORATORY TESTS

Not routinely indicated. For suspected infected or inflammatory aneurysms, WBC, ESR/CRP, and blood cultures can be considered. An elevated D-dimer may indicate a thrombus within the aneurysm. Fig. 1 describes an algorithm for the diagnosis and treatment of abdominal aortic aneurysms.

IMAGING STUDIES

- Abdominal ultrasound (Fig. 2) has nearly 100% sensitivity and specificity in identifying an aneurysm and estimating the size to within 0.3 to 0.4 cm. It is not accurate in estimating the extension to the renal arteries or the iliac arteries.
- Computed tomography (CT) (Fig. 3) scan is recommended for preoperative aneurysm imaging and estimates the size of the AAA to within 0.3 mm. There are no false-negative results, and the scan can localize the extent to renal vessels with more precision than ultrasound. It is the imaging modality of choice for symptomatic AAA. Intravenous contrast is not required to establish a diagnosis of ruptured AAA. CT can also detect the integrity of the wall (Fig. 4) and exclude rupture.
- Magnetic resonance angiography (MRA) may also be used and is at least as accurate as CT.
- Plain radiographs may show the outline of an aneurysm in calcified aortas. This is an insensitive test for diagnosing AAA.
- Diagnostic aortography has essentially been replaced by other noninvasive imaging modalities such as CT or MR angiography. Intraoperative angiography is still used for determining treatment options and post-procedure efficacy (Fig. 5).
- Endovascular aneurysm repair (EVAR) needs a close and lifelong imaging surveillance for a timely detection of possible complications, including endoleaks, graft migration, fractures, and enlargement of aneurysm sac size

with eventual rupture. Contrast-enhanced computed tomography (CTA) is considered the gold standard in EVAR follow-up, but it is accompanied with radiation burden and renal injury because of the use of contrast media. In the past 2 decades, several studies have shown the role of contrast-enhanced ultrasonography (CEUS) in post-EVAR surveillance, with very good diagnostic performance, absence of renal impairment, and no radiation, accompanied by low costs, in comparison with CTA. In numerous prospective studies and meta-analyses, the detection and characterization of endoleaks with CEUS is comparable to that of CTA imaging.

Rx TREATMENT

NONPHARMACOLOGIC THERAPY

- Despite lack of data substantiating reduction in expansion rate through treatment of cardiac risk factors, nonpharmacologic treatment continues to focus on risk factor modification (most importantly smoking cessation, diet, and exercise).

- Serial studies have shown that expansion rates are faster in current smokers than in former smokers. Patients with known AAA or a family history of aneurysms should be advised to stop smoking and be offered smoking cessation interventions.
- Definitive treatment depends on the size of the aneurysm (see "Chronic Rx").

ACUTE GENERAL Rx

- Acute symptomatic or ruptured AAA can be treated with open surgical or endovascular aneurysm repair (EVAR). The choice is determined by anatomic considerations, operative risks, and availability of regular patient follow-up for EVAR.
- Emergent open repair has been the traditional method of treatment. However, multiple trials including Impact of Managed Pharmaceutical care on Resource utilization and Outcomes in Veterans affairs medical centers (IMPROVE) study have shown lower mortality and shorter hospital stay with EVAR. More centers are increasingly using endovascular repair for patients who fit certain anatomic and physiologic criteria.
- The major limitations for EVAR include anatomical issues such as tortuosity or small caliber iliac arteries and inability to follow up of patients to exclude late failure of stents grafts and development of endoleaks.

CHRONIC Rx

- Blood pressure and fasting lipids should be monitored and controlled as recommended for patients with atherosclerotic disease. Statins are associated with decreased

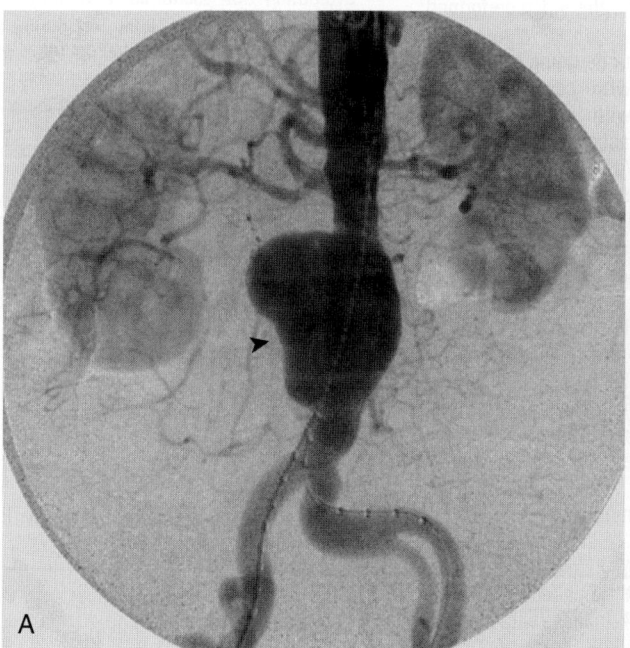

FIG. 4 Aneurysm of the abdominal aorta. A large aortic aneurysm is evident. The aorta exceeds 5 cm in diameter. A large amount of thrombus (T) partially surrounds the contrast-enhanced patent lumen (L). Note the atherosclerotic calcification (*arrowhead*) in the wall of the aneurysm.

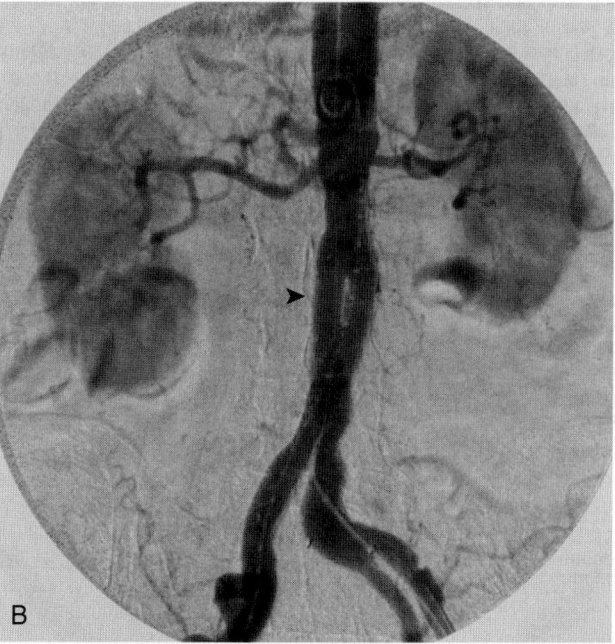

FIG. 5 A, Conventional catheter angiography with bilateral marked catheters in place demonstrates a large, lobulated, infrarenal aortic aneurysm (*arrowhead*) with a 4-cm proximal neck suitable for endovascular repair. **B,** An image after endovascular repair demonstrates complete exclusion of the aneurysm (*arrowhead*) with no endoleak and preservation of the renal and hypogastric arteries. (Soto JA, Lucey BC: *Emergency radiology: the requisites*, ed 2, Philadelphia, 2017, Elsevier.)

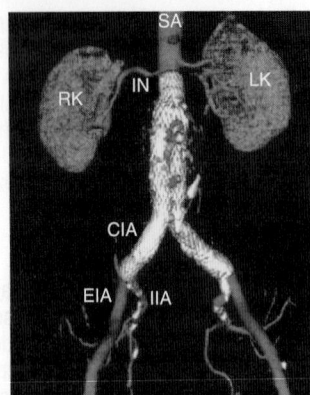

FIG. 6 Endovascular abdominal aortic aneurysm repair involves aneurysm exclusion with an endoluminal aortic stent-graft introduced remotely, usually through the femoral artery. An endovascular graft extends from the infrarenal aorta to both common iliac arteries, preserving the flow to the internal iliac arteries. *CIA,* Common iliac artery; *IIA,* internal iliac artery; *IN,* infrarenal aortic neck; *LK,* left kidney; *RK,* right kidney; *SA,* suprarenal aorta. (From Townsend CM et al [eds]: *Sabiston textbook of surgery,* ed 17, Philadelphia, 2004, Saunders.)

mortality after successful AAA repair, and are recommended for those with known AAA to reduce the progression of atherosclerosis.
- The most commonly used predictor of rupture is the maximum diameter of the AAA.
- Monitoring by ultrasound or CT scan should be performed every 6 to 12 months for patients with AAAs measuring 4.0 to 5.4 cm in diameter and by ultrasound every 2 years for those with AAAs measuring <4 cm.
- Long-term beta-blocker therapy has slowed the rate of aortic dilation and decreased the incidence of aortic complications in patients with Marfan's syndrome. Several studies have also suggested that beta-blocker therapy may reduce the rate of expansion and risk of rupture; however, conclusive evidence is lacking.
- A recent multicenter study of 5362 patients with AAA found no significant association between AAA progression and the use of statins, beta-blockers, angiotensin-converting enzyme inhibitors, or angiotensin II receptor blockers.
- Antibiotics such as doxycycline and roxithromycin have been shown to limit the expansion of small AAAs.
- Surgical repair to eliminate the risk for rupture should be performed for patients with infrarenal or juxtarenal AAA of approximately 5.5 cm or larger in diameter. All patients who are symptomatic should undergo repair, regardless of size.
- There is no clear advantage to early repair (open or endovascular) for small AAAs (less than 5.5 cm).
- Percutaneous, endovascular, stent-anchored grafts placed with the patient under local anesthesia have provided an alternative approach (Fig. 6) for patients with favorable

anatomy. In patients who have undergone endovascular repair, long-term surveillance is required to assess for an endoleak, stent migration, change in aneurysm size, and need for re-intervention.
- Fenestrated endovascular repair is an alternative to open repair in the management of juxtarenal aortic aneurysms (JRAs) and short-neck abdominal aortic aneurysms. Contemporary literature shows that it is a safe and efficacious treatment, particularly for those deemed surgically high risk. Growing experience and innovation of stent grafts are essential for the advancement of fenestrated grafting.
- Randomized trials have shown that endovascular repair of AAA is associated with a significantly lower operative mortality than open surgical repair but it has increased rates of graft-related complications and reintervention, and is more costly. There are no differences between endovascular repair and open surgical repair in total mortality or aneurysm-related mortality in the long term.
- Compared with open aneurysm repair, EVAR is associated with better health-related quality of life up to 12 months postoperatively.
- Most recent meta-analysis concludes that EVAR has lower rates of 30-day mortality, 30-day MI, and length of hospital stay in both elective and ruptured AAA repair.
- Based on current data, less than 1% of endovascular repairs require open conversion and approximately half of all early endoleaks resolve spontaneously within a period of 30 days.
- Open repair still represents a valuable solution for many patients with failed EVAR with relatively low mortality rates when performed electively.
- In high-risk patients undergoing AAA repair, specifically those with coronary artery disease or those with more than one clinical risk factor based on the American Heart Association (AHA) guidelines, preoperative administration of beta-blockers titrated to a goal heart rate of 60 have been shown to decrease incidence of death from cardiac causes or nonfatal myocardial infarctions.
- Patients with chronic obstructive pulmonary disease (COPD) are at higher risk for major clinical complications, particularly if the COPD is suboptimally managed or if it is present in conjunction with cardiac or renal disease. Smoking cessation for 2 months before surgery has also been shown to decrease pulmonary morbidity.
- Renal dysfunction is a strong predictor of mortality, showing up to as high as 41% mortality in those with impaired renal function compared with 6% in those without renal dysfunction.

REFERRAL
- Vascular surgical referral should be made in asymptomatic patients with AAAs that are approximately 4.5 cm.

- In patients with an expansion rate of 0.6-0.8 cm/year, it is reasonable to offer repair, although small studies have shown that using expansion as a criterion for surgical referral is of unclear benefit.
- It is important to optimize any comorbid conditions before surgical referral.

! PEARLS & CONSIDERATIONS
- Repairing asymptomatic AAAs smaller than 5.5 cm has not been shown to improve survival because the risk of rupture is lower than the risk of surgery.
- The results from multiple trials to date demonstrate no advantage to immediate repair for small AAA (4.0-5.5 cm), regardless of whether open or endovascular repair is used and, at least for open repair, regardless of patient age and AAA diameter. Thus, neither immediate open nor immediate endovascular repair of small AAAs is supported by the currently available evidence.
- Five-year survival remains poor after elective AAA repair despite advances in short-term outcomes and is associated with AAA diameter and patient age at the time of surgery. Research in this field should attempt to improve the life expectancy of patients with repaired AAA and to optimize patient selection.

COMMENTS
- Most AAAs are infrarenal.
- Surgical risk is increased in patients with coexisting coronary artery disease, pulmonary disease, or chronic renal failure. Evaluation for ischemia and aggressive perioperative hemodynamic monitoring help identify high-risk patients and decrease postoperative complications.
- It is estimated that AAAs at <5 cm expand at a rate of 0.3 to 0.4 cm/year.

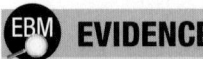 **EVIDENCE**

Available at www.expertconsult.com

SUGGESTED READINGS
Available at www.expertconsult.com

RELATED CONTENT
Abdominal Aortic Aneurysm (AAA) (Patient Information)

AUTHORS: **MICHAEL A. ESKANDER, M.D.,** and **PRANAV M. PATEL, M.D.**

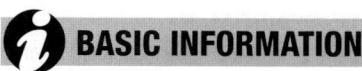

BASIC INFORMATION

DEFINITION

Abdominal compartment syndrome (ACS) is defined by the presence of organ dysfunction as a result of increased abdominal pressure or intraabdominal hypertension. The increased abdominal pressure reduces blood flow to internal organs, which can lead to multiple system failure and death if not promptly recognized and treated.

ICD-10CM CODES
M79.A3 Nontraumatic compartment
syndrome of abdomen

EPIDEMIOLOGY & DEMOGRAPHICS

INCIDENCE: Very few studies have examined the incidence of ACS outside of trauma patients, among whom it ranges from 1% to 14%, depending on the population and type of trauma studied. The incidence is the highest among critically ill patients.

RISK FACTORS: The biggest risk factor for developing ACS is critical illness stemming from a wide array of medical and surgical conditions (Table 1). In particular, any illness that requires a patient to undergo large volume intravenous fluid resuscitation can be associated with ACS; the third-spacing of fluid can lead to increased intraabdominal pressures secondary to tissue edema. Due to large volume fluid resuscitation, ACS is commonly seen in severe burns, trauma, post-surgical patients, and sepsis. Other conditions associated with ACS include intraabdominal and retroperitoneal pathologies such as significant bowel distention, liver transplantation, massive ascites, ruptured abdominal aortic aneurysm with resulting hemoperitoneum, pancreatitis, and abdominal surgery (Table 2).

PHYSICAL FINDINGS & CLINICAL PRESENTATION

- The most striking physical exam finding is often massive abdominal distention.
- Difficulty maintaining respiratory support and decreased urine output are also typical hallmarks.
- Other common findings include those associated with poor perfusion states and hypotension such as skin mottling, cool extremities, and obtundation. Patients will often have abdominal tenderness, signs of volume overload such as edema and elevated jugular venous pressures and may present with acute respiratory decompensation.

ETIOLOGY

- ACS can impact nearly every organ system. High intraabdominal pressures are associated with increased intracranial pressures, which can precipitate cerebral ischemia. Elevated abdominal pressures can cause cardiac compression by decreasing ventricular compliance and contractility as well as impairing inferior vena cava venous return, leading to increased central venous and pulmonary pressures. Due to elevation of the diaphragms, patients will often have reduced tidal volumes and lower chest wall compliance, which can lead to atelectasis, pneumonia, hypoxemia, and hypercarbia. Mechanically ventilated patients will also require increased airway pressures that can lead to barotrauma. In addition, renal vein compression and renal artery vasoconstriction lead to decreased urine output. Reduced mesenteric blood flow can lead to intestinal ischemia and lactic acidosis.

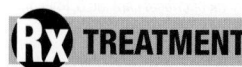

DIAGNOSIS

DIFFERENTIAL DIAGNOSIS

- Mesenteric ischemia
- Sepsis

- Shock
- Acute kidney injury
- Adult respiratory distress syndrome

WORKUP

- Measurement of intraabdominal pressure is required to make a definitive diagnosis. Bladder pressure is the most common surrogate used to estimate intraabdominal pressures and is measured using a bladder catheter. The most accurate measurements can be obtained with the patient in supine position at end expiration in the absence of abdominal contractions. The threshold abdominal pressure often set for research purposes to define ACS is >20 mm Hg, but patients may have ACS with pressures of >10 mm Hg and above. Oliguria tends to develop at a pressure of 15 mm Hg, and anuria occurs around 30 mm Hg. Intraabdominal pressures can also be estimated using intragastric, intracolonic, and inferior vena cava approaches (Table 3).

LABORATORY TEST(S)

- Laboratory testing is generally not helpful for the diagnosis of ACS. The presence of lactic acidosis suggests bowel ischemia, which portends a poorer prognosis.

IMAGING STUDIES

- Imaging alone has no diagnostic value in ACS, but chest imaging can be helpful to evaluate for diaphragmatic elevation and evidence of pulmonary complications (atelectasis, volume overload, pneumonia, etc.). Abdominal CT imaging will sometimes show renal displacement, inferior vena cava compression, abdominal wall thickening, or bowel injury related to ischemia but should not be relied upon to make the diagnosis of ACS.

TREATMENT

Supportive care and, when appropriate, surgical abdominal decompression are the mainstays of ACS treatment.

NONPHARMACOLOGIC THERAPY

- Supportive care, often with hemodynamic and ventilatory support, as well as techniques to improve abdominal wall compliance, are the foundations of ACS management.
- Severe burns to the abdomen leading to ACS will require surgical escharotomy to improve abdominal wall compliance.
- Patients with tense ascites leading to ACS will require large volume paracentesis to decrease intraabdominal pressures.
- Patients should be positioned supine if possible as any elevation of the head will increase abdominal pressures.
- Rectal and nasogastric decompression is required if ACS is due to massive bowel distention.
- Proper sedation and pain control can decrease intraabdominal pressures, and

TABLE 1 Causes of Intraabdominal Hypertension and Abdominal Compartment Syndrome

Increased Abdominal Contents	Decreased Abdominal Volume
Ascites	Reduction of large long-standing hernia
Hemoperitoneum	Direct closure of large, long-standing abdominal wall defect
Abdominal packs	
Peritonitis	
Retroperitoneal edema (pancreatitis)	Retroperitoneal edema (pancreatitis)
Large pelvic, retroperitoneal hematoma	Large pelvic, retroperitoneal hematoma
Intestinal obstruction	
Ileus	
Gastric distension (esophageal ventilation)	
Abdominal aortic aneurysm	
Severe constipation	
Large abdominal tumor (chronic)	
Morbid obesity (chronic)	
Pregnancy (chronic)	

From Vincent JL, et al. *Textbook of critical care*, ed 6, Philadelphia, 2011, Saunders.

TABLE 2 Independent Predictors of Postinjury Primary and Secondary Abdominal Compartment Syndrome

	ED Model	ICU Model
	Independent Predictors	**Independent Predictors**
Primary ACS	To OR <75 min	Temp ≤34°C
	Crystalloids ≥3 L	GAPco$_2$ ≥16
		Hb ≤8/dL
		BD ≥12 mEq/L
Secondary ACS	Crystalloids ≥3 L	GAPco$_2$ ≥16
	No urgent surgery	Crystalloids ≥7.5 L
	PRBC ≥3 units	UO ≤150 mL

From Vincent JL, et al. *Textbook of critical care,* ed 6, Philadelphia, 2011, Saunders.
ACS, Abdominal compartment syndrome; *BD,* arterial base deficit; *CI,* confidence interval; *ED,* emergency department; *GAPco$_2$,* carbon dioxide gap; *Hb,* hemoglobin concentration; *ICU,* intensive care unit; *OR,* operating room; *PRBC,* packed red blood cells; *Temp,* temperature; *UO,* urine output.

TABLE 3 Classification of Abdominal Compartment Syndrome

Basis of Classification	Subcategories
Time frame	Acute
	Chronic
Relation to peritoneal cavity	Primary
	Secondary
Etiology	Trauma
	Burn
	Postoperative
	Pancreatitis
	Bowel obstruction
	Ileus
	Abdominal aortic aneurysm
	Oncologic
	Gynecologic

From Vincent JL, et al. *Textbook of critical care,* ed 6, Philadelphia, 2011, Saunders.

some patients may require ventilatory support and chemical paralysis to maximize abdominal wall relaxation.

- Mechanical ventilation is often difficult due to the high pressures that need to be generated to overcome the increased intraabdominal pressures. Often a combination of low tidal volumes, permissive hypercapnia, chemical paralysis, and high PEEP are required to ensure adequate ventilatory support.
- Although there is little data to support its use, the administration of colloid may be superior to crystalloid if the patient requires further volume resuscitation. The administration of intravenous fluids will transiently increase renal blood flow, leading to increased urine output and improved organ perfusion and cardiac output. Pressors may also have a role to maintain perfusion pressures, but all of these measures are temporizing and supportive until definitive action through surgical decompression is performed.
- The threshold to perform surgical decompression for ACS has yet to be established; however, data suggest that early decompression prior to the development of ACS may lead to better outcomes. If appropriate, consensus dictates that surgical decompression should be performed on all patients with intraabdominal pressure >25 mm Hg; however, some surgeons are more aggressive and will consider decompression with pressures of 15-25 mm Hg in the right clinical setting. Surgical decompression by incising vertically through the linea alba can be performed at the bedside in emergent situations and most surgeons will then keep the abdomen open through the use of a temporary abdominal closure device that retains heat/fluid and prevents evisceration until the time is appropriate to attempt to close the abdomen again.

ACUTE GENERAL Rx

- There are no direct pharmacologic agents that treat ACS other than pressors, sedatives, pain medications, and paralytics required for supportive care as described above. Despite underlying volume overload, diuretics have no role in therapy. Definitive management is surgical decompression.

DISPOSITION

- Close inpatient monitoring, preferably in an intensive care setting, is indicated as mortality can be extremely high (>40%) with ACS.

REFERRAL

- Patients with ACS often require admission to an intensive care setting with surgical consultation in case decompression is required.

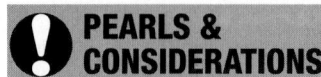

PEARLS & CONSIDERATIONS

COMMENTS

- ACS is seen in critically ill medical and surgical patients, and its diagnosis requires both the presence of intraabdominal hypertension and end organ dysfunction.
- ACS is truly a systemic illness that can lead to multisystem organ failure and is therefore associated with a high mortality.
- Definitive diagnosis of ACS requires measurement of intraabdominal pressure, which is most frequently estimated using bladder pressure as a surrogate.
- Supportive care, including hemodynamic support with colloids, pressors, and ventilatory support, is often required, but surgical decompression is the only definitive treatment.
- Surgical decompression is indicated for intraabdominal pressures >25 mm Hg; however, precise thresholds have not been established and earlier decompression may lead to better outcomes.

AUTHOR: **JASON D. FERREIRA, M.D.**

SUGGESTED READINGS
Available at www.expertconsult.com

BASIC INFORMATION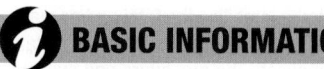

DEFINITION

Abruptio placentae is the separation of placenta from the uterine wall before delivery of the fetus. The condition occurs in approximately 1% of pregnancies. There are three classes of abruption based on maternal and fetal status, including an assessment of uterine contractions, quantity of bleeding, fetal heart rate monitoring, and abnormal coagulation studies (fibrinogen, prothrombin time, partial thromboplastin time).

- Grade I: mild vaginal bleeding, uterine irritability, stable vital signs, reassuring fetal heart rate, normal coagulation profile (fibrinogen 450 mg/dl). Approximately half of abruptions are grade I.
- Grade II: moderate vaginal bleeding, hypertonic uterine contractions, orthostatic blood pressure measurements, unfavorable fetal status, fibrinogen 150 to 250 mg. Approximately a quarter of abruptions are grade II.
- Grade III: severe bleeding (may be concealed), hypertonic uterine contractions, overt signs of hypovolemic shock, fetal death, thrombocytopenia, fibrinogen <150 mg/dl. Approximately a quarter of abruptions are grade III.

SYNONYM

Premature separation of placenta

ICD-10CM CODES

O45.8X9	Other premature separation of placenta, unspecified trimester
O45.8X1	Other premature separation of placenta, first trimester
O45.8X2	Other premature separation of placenta, second trimester
O45.8X3	Other premature separation of placenta, third trimester
O45.91	Premature separation of placenta, unspecified, first trimester
O45.92	Premature separation of placenta, unspecified, second trimester
O45.93	Premature separation of placenta, unspecified, third trimester

EPIDEMIOLOGY & DEMOGRAPHICS

INCIDENCE (IN U.S.): One in 86 to 206 births; 80% occur before the onset of labor
RISK FACTORS: Hypertension (greatest association), trauma, polyhydramnios, multifetal gestation, smoking, use of cocaine, chorioamnionitis, preterm premature rupture of membranes. Table 1 summarizes placental abruption risk factors.
RECURRENCE RATE: 5% to 17%, some studies showing a 5- to 10-fold increase in risk; with two prior episodes, 25%

PHYSICAL FINDINGS & CLINICAL PRESENTATION

- Triad of uterine bleeding (concealed or per vagina), hypertonic uterine contractions or signs of preterm labor, and evidence of fetal compromise exists.
- More than 80% of cases have external bleeding; 20% of cases have no bleeding but have indirect evidence of abruption, such as failed tocolysis for preterm labor.
- Tetanic uterine contractions are found in only 17%.

ETIOLOGY

- Primary etiology: unknown
- Hypertension: found in 40% to 50% of grade III abruptions
- Rapid decompression of uterine cavity, as can occur in polyhydramnios or multifetal gestation
- Blunt external trauma (motor vehicle accident, spousal abuse)

DIAGNOSIS

DIFFERENTIAL DIAGNOSIS

- Placenta previa
- Cervical or vaginal trauma
- Labor
- Cervical cancer
- Rupture of membranes
- The differential diagnosis of vaginal bleeding in pregnancy is described in Section III

TABLE 1 Placental Abruption Risk Factors

Increasing parity or maternal age
Cigarette smoking
Cocaine abuse
Trauma
Maternal hypertension
Preterm premature rupture of membranes
Rapid uterine decompression associated with multiple gestation and polyhydramnios
Inherited or acquired thrombophilia
Uterine malformations or fibroids
Placental abnormalities or ischemia
Prior abruption

From Gabbe, SG: *Obstetrics*, ed 6, Philadelphia, 2012, Saunders.

WORKUP

- Placental abruption is primarily a clinical diagnosis that is supported by laboratory, radiographic (Fig. 1), and pathologic studies.
- Initial assessment should evaluate for the source of bleeding, ruling out placenta previa that may contraindicate any type of vaginal examination (e.g., pelvic speculum examination).
- Continuous fetal heart monitoring is indicated for all viable gestations (60% incidence of fetal distress in labor); may show early signs of maternal hypovolemia (late decelerations or fetal tachycardia) before overt maternal vital sign changes.
- Actual amount of blood loss is often greater than initially perceived because of the possibility of concealed retroplacental bleeding and apparent "normal" vital signs. The relative hypervolemia of pregnancy initially protects the patient until late in the course of bleeding, when abrupt and sudden cardiovascular collapse can occur.

LABORATORY TESTS

- Baseline hemoglobin helps quantify blood loss and establish baseline values for serial comparisons during expectant management.
- Coagulation profile: platelets, fibrinogen, prothrombin, and partial thromboplastin time. Diffuse intravascular coagulation can develop with severe abruption. If fibrinogen is <150 mg/dl, estimated blood loss is approximately 2000 ml; if fibrinogen is <100 mg/dl, consider fresh frozen plasma to prevent further bleeding.
- Type and antibody screen is important to identify Rh-negative patients who need Rh immune globulin.

IMAGING STUDIES

Ultrasound should include fetal presentation and status, amniotic fluid volume, placental location,

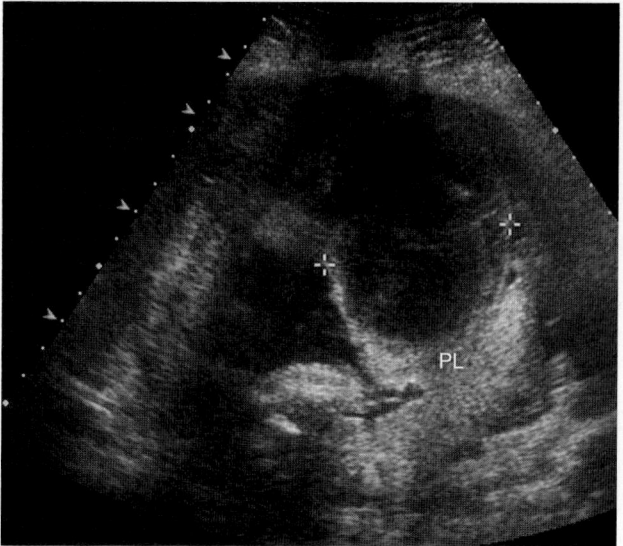

FIG. 1 Placental abruption. Transabdominal sonogram of the placenta *(PL)* with a hematoma *(calipers)* lifting the placenta away from the uterine wall. (From Rumack CM et al (eds): *Diagnostic ultrasound*, ed 4, Philadelphia, 2011, Mosby.)

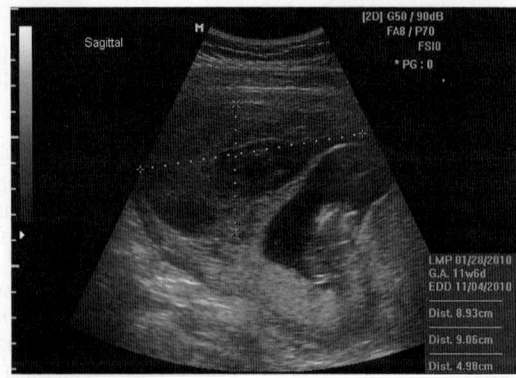

FIG. 2 Ultrasonic image of a subchorionic abruption. (Courtesy K. Francois; from Gabbe SG: *Obstetrics,* ed 6, Philadelphia, 2012, Saunders.)

as well as any evidence of hematoma (retroplacental, subchorionic, or preplacental) (Fig. 2).

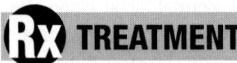

TREATMENT

ACUTE GENERAL Rx

- Stabilization of the mother is the first priority.
- Treatment depends on gestational age of the fetus, severity of the abruption, and maternal status.
- Initial assessment for signs of maternal hemodynamic compromise or hemorrhagic shock; large-bore intravenous access, with crystalloid fluid resuscitation using a replacement of 3 ml lactated Ringer's solution for every 1 ml estimated blood loss.
- Indwelling Foley catheter to monitor urine output and maternal volume status, with a goal of 30 ml/hr urine output.

- Assess fetal status and gestational age by sonogram and continuous fetal heart rate monitoring.
- Because of the unpredictable nature of abruptions, cross-matched blood should be made available during the initial resuscitation period.

CHRONIC Rx

- In the term fetus or when lung maturity has been documented, delivery is indicated.
- In the preterm fetus or a fetus with an immature lung profile, consider betamethasone 12.5 mg IM q24h for two doses and then delivery, depending on the severity of the abruption and the likelihood of fetal complications from preterm birth.
- Cesarean section should be reserved for cases of fetal distress or for standard obstetric indications. While cesarean delivery may

be needed to stabilize the fetal and/or maternal status, the mother's coagulation status may complicate the procedure and availability of blood products may be critical.
- In select cases, such as severe prematurity with a stable mother and mild contractions, magnesium sulfate can be used for tocolysis, 6 g IV loading dose then 3 g/hr maintenance, to allow for a course of steroids.

DISPOSITION

Because of the unpredictable nature of abruptions, expectant management should occur only under controlled circumstances and is rarely practiced.

REFERRAL

Abruptio placentae places mother and fetus in a high-risk situation and should be managed by a qualified obstetrician in a facility with capability for neonatal and maternal resuscitation, for supporting a preterm infant if delivery is indicated at an early gestational age, and for performing emergency cesarean sections.

RELATED CONTENT

Abruptio Placentae (Patient Information)
Premature Labor (Related Key Topic)
Vaginal Bleeding During Pregnancy (Related Key Topic)

AUTHOR: **ANTHONY SCISCIONE, D.O.**

BASIC INFORMATION

DEFINITION

Acetaminophen (APAP) poisoning is a disorder caused by excessive intake of APAP and is manifested by jaundice, nausea, vomiting, and potential death from hepatic necrosis if not treated appropriately.

SYNONYMS

Paracetamol poisoning

ICD-10CM CODES
T39.1 Poisoning by 4-aminophenol derivatives, accidental
X60 Intentional self-poisoning by 4-aminophenol derivatives

EPIDEMIOLOGY & DEMOGRAPHICS

- APAP is one of the most widely prescribed antipyretics and analgesics in the U.S. Potentially toxic ingestions, both intentional and unintentional, exceed 100,000 cases annually in the U.S.
- APAP toxicity is the number one cause of acute liver failure in the U.S.
- Death rate is approximately one in 1000 persons. Nearly 50% of exposures occur in children ≤6 yr.
- Hepatic necrosis is most likely to occur in people who are (1) chronically malnourished, (2) regularly abusing alcohol, and (3) using other potentially hepatotoxic medications.

PHYSICAL FINDINGS & CLINICAL PRESENTATION

- The physical examination may vary depending on the amount of time since ingestion.
- Phase I (0 to 24 hr): initial symptoms may be mild or absent and may consist of anorexia, diaphoresis, malaise, nausea, vomiting, lethargy, and a subclinical rise in transaminase levels.
- Phase II (24 to 72 hr): right upper quadrant pain, vomiting, somnolence, tachycardia, jaundice, hypotension, and continued increase in transaminases.
- Phase III (72 to 96 hr): hepatic necrosis with abdominal pain, jaundice, hepatic encephalopathy, coagulopathy, hypoglycemia, renal failure, fatality from multi-organ failure.
- Phase IV (4 days to 2 wk): complete resolution of symptoms and resolution of organ failure.
- Table E1 summarizes the four phases/stages of acetaminophen poisoning.

ETIOLOGY

- The amount of APAP necessary for hepatic toxicity varies with the patient's body size and hepatic function. It is recommended that APAP intake should not exceed 4 g for adults and 90 mg/kg in children within a 24-hr period.
- A standardized nomogram is used to determine potential hepatic toxicity by knowing the APAP plasma level and the number of hours after ingestion. See the APAP ingestion algorithm (Fig. E1).

DIAGNOSIS

DIFFERENTIAL DIAGNOSIS

- Liver disease from alcohol abuse or viral hepatitis
- Ingestion of other hepatotoxic substances
- Bacterial/viral gastroenteritis

WORKUP

Initial workup is aimed at confirming APAP overdose with plasma APAP level and assessment of hepatic damage. A careful history should elicit the time of APAP ingestion, amount, preparation (e.g., extended release) and possible co-ingestants (see "Laboratory Tests").

LABORATORY TESTS

- Initial laboratory evaluation should include an initial plasma APAP level with a second level drawn approximately 4 hr after the initial ingestion. Subsequent levels can be obtained every 2 to 4 hr until the levels stabilize or decline. These levels should be plotted on the Rumack-Matthew nomogram (see acetaminophen ingestion algorithm [Fig. E1] to calculate potential hepatic toxicity). The nomogram cannot be used with patients who present >24 hr after ingestion, took extended-release preparations, had chronic ingestions, or when the time of ingestion is unknown.
- Transaminases (AST, ALT), serum glucose, bilirubin level, lipase level, prothrombin time (INR), blood urea nitrogen, creatinine, EKG, and urinalysis should be initially obtained on all patients.
- Serum and urine toxicology screen for other potential toxic substances is also recommended on admission. Screening for infectious hepatitis should also be considered.
- Urine for β-hCG should be obtained from all women of childbearing age.

TREATMENT

NONPHARMACOLOGIC THERAPY

Consultation with a Poison Control Center is recommended for patients who have ingested a large amount of APAP and/or other toxic substances. A single toxic dose of APAP usually exceeds 7 g or 150 mg/kg adults.

ACUTE GENERAL Rx

- Hepatotoxicity is defined as any increase in alanine aminotransferase (ALT) or aspartate aminotransferase (AST) >1000 IU/L, and hepatic failure manifests as hepatotoxicity with hepatic encephalopathy. For those who cannot be risk stratified using the nomogram, the American College of Emergency Physicians recommends that N-acetylcysteine be administered without delay to those >12 yr and >8 hr after ingestion at presentation. This would include anyone with an ingestion of APAP over many days with an APAP level <20 μg/mL (with or without ALT elevation) or anyone with undetectable APAP levels with an elevated ALT and a history of excessive APAP intake.
- Administer activated charcoal 1g/kg PO if the patient is seen within 1 hr of ingestion or the clinician suspects polysubstance ingestion that delays gastric emptying.
- Determine blood levels 4 hr after ingestion; if in the toxic range based on the Rumack-Matthew nomogram, start N-acetylcysteine (NAC) either IV (Acetadote) or PO (Mucomyst). Acetylcysteine IV loading dose is 150 mg/kg ×1 diluted in 200 ml D5W over 15 to 60 min. Maintenance dose is 50 mg/kg diluted in 500 ml D5W over 4 hr, followed by 100 mg/kg diluted in 1000 ml D5W over 16 hr. The dose does not require adjustment for renal or hepatic impairment or for dialysis. Total administration time is 21 hours.
- Oral administration is 140 mg/kg PO as a loading dose, followed after 4 hr by 70 mg/kg PO q4h for a total of 18 doses. N-acetylcysteine therapy should be started within 24 hr of APAP overdose. Total administration time is 72 hours.
- Advantages of IV administration include more reliable absorption, fewer doses, and shorter duration of treatment. Disadvantages include cost and lower hepatic concentrations from first-pass flow as compared to oral acetylcysteine.
- Monitor APAP level; use Rumack-Matthew nomogram to trend hepatic toxicity. Repeat AST/ALT and APAP levels after 12 to 14 hr of IV acetylcysteine infusion and continue infusion longer than 16 hr if transaminases are elevated, if APAP concentration is still measurable, or if coagulopathy exists (INR >1.5-2.0). Patients with severe, irreversible liver failure may need to continue NAC until liver transplantation is available.
- Provide adequate IV hydration (e.g., $D_5\frac{1}{2}NS$ at 150 ml/hr).
- Patients on IV N-acetylcysteine with liver failure require frequent monitoring of vital signs, oxygen saturation by pulse oximetry, and frequent blood draws. Frequent reassessment for hypoglycemia and infection is also essential.
- If APAP level is nontoxic, N-acetylcysteine therapy may be discontinued.

DISPOSITION

All patients with confirmed APAP poisoning will require admission, usually to an intensive care unit. Most patients (90%) will recover fully without persisting hepatic abnormalities. Hepatic failure is particularly unusual in children <6 yr.

REFERRAL

Psychiatric referral is recommended after intentional ingestions.

RELATED CONTENT

Acetaminophen Overdose (Patient Information)

AUTHOR: **STEVEN ROUGAS, M.D., M.S.**

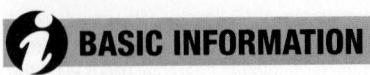

BASIC INFORMATION

DEFINITION

Achalasia is a motility disorder of the esophagus classically characterized by incomplete relaxation of the lower esophageal sphincter (LES) and aperistalsis of esophageal smooth muscle. The result is functional obstruction of the esophagus.

SYNONYMS

Achalasia and cardiospasm
Achalasia (of cardia)
Aperistalsis of esophagus
Megaesophagus
Esophageal achalasia
Esophageal cardiospasm

ICD-10CM CODES
K22.0 Achalasia of cardia

EPIDEMIOLOGY & DEMOGRAPHICS

- Annual incidence is approximately 0.5-1.0 in 100,000 persons.
- Prevalence is <10 per 100,000 persons.
- Although the onset of symptoms may occur at any age, incidence is typically bimodal, 20 to 40 yr, then after 60 yr, with greater incidence in the older group.
- Men and women are affected equally.

PHYSICAL FINDINGS & CLINICAL PRESENTATION

Symptoms:
- Dysphagia (most commonly with both solids and liquids)
- Difficulty belching
- Regurgitation
- Chest pain and/or heartburn
- Globus
- Frequent hiccups
- Vomiting of undigested food
- Symptoms of aspiration such as nocturnal cough; possible dyspnea and pneumonia
- Weight loss
Physical findings:
- Focal lung examination abnormalities and wheezing also possible

ETIOLOGY

- Etiology is poorly understood.
- Loss of myenteric nerve fibers in the LES and smooth muscle portion of the esophagus. This has been associated with lymphocytic and eosinophilic infiltrates and fibrosis in later stages of disease.
- Loss of intrinsic inhibitory neurons in the myenteric plexus as well as depletion of networks of interstitial cells of Cajal of the LES leads to incomplete relaxation of the LES secondary to loss of inhibitory neurotransmitters nitric oxide and vasoactive intestinal polypeptide.
- This disorder may be caused by autoimmune degeneration of the esophageal myenteric plexus in association with the HLA class II antigen DQw1. Antimyenteric plexus and other antineural autoantibodies have also been described.
- Abnormal immune reactions to neurotropic viruses such as varicella zoster, herpes simplex type 1, and measles viruses have been implicated, but the association has not been confirmed. A host T cell–mediated response may lead to neuronal injury; this has been suggested as the cause of types II and I achalasia (see Imaging Studies section).
- Achalasia is also seen in the rare autosomal recessive disorder, Allgrove syndrome (achalasia, alacrima, autonomic disturbance, and acetylcholine insensitivity), which has been linked to a gene mutation on chromosome 12q13. Neurons in this syndrome may be susceptible to oxidative injury.
- Recent studies suggest that type III achalasia (see Imaging Studies section) is associated with myenteric inflammation but not neuronal loss and that downregulation of nitric oxide synthase expression and increased cholinergic sensitivity are cytokine mediated.

DIAGNOSIS

DIFFERENTIAL DIAGNOSIS

- Primary achalasia:
  1. Idiopathic
- Secondary achalasia:
  1. Chagas disease
  2. Vagal injury or surgery, including fundoplication

  3. Achalasia-like esophageal dilation has been described after laparoscopic gastric banding
- Pseudoachalasia:
  1. Esophageal cancer
  2. Infiltrating gastric cancer
  3. Oat cell and bronchogenic lung cancer
  4. Lymphoma
  5. Amyloidosis
  6. Paraneoplastic syndrome
- Angina
- Bulimia
- Anorexia nervosa
- Gastric bezoar
- Gastritis
- Peptic ulcer disease
- Postvagotomy dysmotility
- Esophageal disease (Table 1):
  1. Gastroesophageal reflux disease
  2. Sarcoidosis
  3. Amyloidosis
  4. Esophageal stricture
  5. Esophageal webs and rings
  6. Scleroderma
  7. Barrett's esophagus
  8. Esophagitis
  9. Diffuse esophageal spasm

WORKUP

- Physical examination and laboratory analyses to rule out other causes and assess complications
- Imaging studies, manometry, and endoscopy (may be supportive or complementary)

LABORATORY TESTS

- Assessment of nutritional status
- Complete blood count, ECG, stress test if diagnosis is in doubt
- Serologic assays for *Trypanosoma cruzi* (Chagas disease) in appropriate individuals

IMAGING STUDIES

Barium swallow with fluoroscopy may demonstrate:
- Uncoordinated or absent esophageal contractions (loss of peristalsis)
- An acutely tapered contrast column ("bird's beak"; Fig. 1)
- Dilation of the distal (smooth muscle portion) esophagus

TABLE 1	Esophageal Motor Disorders		
	Achalasia	**Scleroderma**	**Diffuse Esophageal Spasm**
Symptoms	Dysphagia	Gastroesophageal reflux disease	Substernal chest pain (angina-like)
	Regurgitation of nonacidic material	Dysphagia	Dysphagia with pain
Radiographic appearance	Dilated, fluid-filled esophagus	Aperistaltic esophagus	Simultaneous noncoordinated contractions
	Distal *bird-beak* stricture	Free reflux	
		Peptic stricture	
Manometric findings			
Lower esophageal sphincter	High resting pressure	Low resting pressure	Normal pressure
	Incomplete or abnormal relaxation with swallow		
Body	Low-amplitude, simultaneous contractions after swallowing	Low-amplitude peristaltic contractions or no peristalsis	Some peristalsis
			Diffuse and simultaneous nonperistaltic contractions, occasionally high amplitude

From Andreoli TE et al: *Andreoli and Carpenter's Cecil essentials of medicine*, ed 8, Philadelphia, 2010, Saunders.

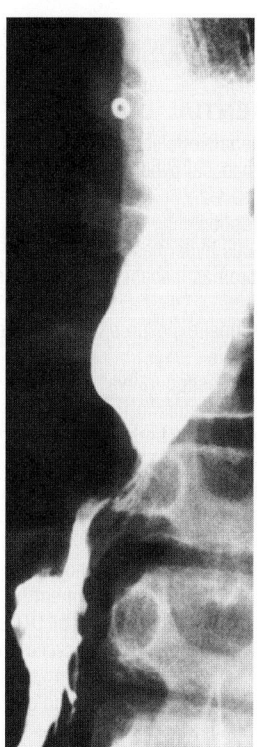

FIG. 1 Classic appearance of achalasia of the esophagus. The dilated esophagus ends in a narrow segment. (From Hoekelman R [ed]: *Primary pediatric care*, ed 3, St Louis, 1997, Mosby.)

- Esophageal air-fluid level with evidence of poor esophageal emptying
- Late-stage changes include tortuosity, angulation, dilated megaesophagus, retained food, and secretions

Manometry is generally considered to be the "gold standard" test to confirm the diagnosis. In classic achalasia, conventional manometric abnormalities are as follows:

- Low-amplitude disorganized contractions/aperistalsis, incomplete or absent LES relaxation (with residual pressure >10 mm Hg) after swallow, and high resting LES pressure
- A subset of patients with "vigorous achalasia" may have high-amplitude, long-duration, simultaneous esophageal contractions. This term is now felt to be imprecise because of a newer classification of the disease.
- High-resolution manometry (HRM), or high-resolution esophageal pressure topography (HREPT), has defined subsets of patients with achalasia who may have different responses to medical or surgical therapies. Unlike classic achalasia (type I), type II achalasia shows panesophageal pressurization to greater than 30 mm Hg with ≥20% of test swallows, and type III achalasia shows spastic lumen-obliterating contractions of the distal esophagus with ≥20% of swallows. This technique uses the integrated relaxation pressure (IRP) to define better the adequacy of esophagogastric junction relaxation.
- HREPT has also defined an achalasia variant described as esophagogastric junction outflow obstruction.
- Direct visualization by endoscopy, including careful visualization of the esophagogastric junction and cardia, should be performed to exclude other causes of dysphagia, including "functional esophagogastric junction obstruction," strictures, secondary causes of achalasia (including infiltrating cancers), and pseudoachalasia.

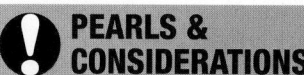

Rx TREATMENT

NONPHARMACOLOGIC THERAPY

- The goals of therapy are to decrease LES pressure to relieve the functional obstruction, relieve symptoms, and prevent progression to a dilated esophagus, sometimes referred to as a megaesophagus. Treatment does not improve esophageal peristalsis. Achalasia is treatable but incurable.
- Pneumatic dilation to disrupt the LES muscle fibers may benefit 65% to 90% of patients. Multiple sessions may be required, and most protocols use a graded dilation approach, starting with a 30-mm balloon, and repeating if required with a 35-mm or 40-mm balloon. Some studies suggest this may be more effective in women or older patients. Esophageal rupture or perforation is a rare complication (2% to 4%) that may be managed conservatively in some stable patients with a small perforation.
- Surgical: laparoscopic, or now less commonly open, (Heller's) esophagomyotomy is effective (90%). Approximately 35% of patients undergoing surgery will develop reflux disease. As a result, some surgeons will perform a "loose" or partial antireflux repair (fundoplication) as part of the surgical procedure. Some studies suggest this may be more effective in men and younger patients. An observational study has suggested that those who have had prior endoscopic treatment before myotomy may not do as well as those who have a primary myotomy.
- Studies suggest that type II patients respond better than type I patients, and type III patients have poorer treatment responses to these therapies.
- A large European study suggested that in experienced hands, patients may expect similar medium-term outcomes from myotomy and balloon dilation. A meta-analysis suggests better long-term durability of myotomy. Balloon dilation may be the more cost-effective treatment. A small percentage (20 to 30%) of patients undergoing either therapy may require re-treatment within 5 to 7 years.
- Assessment of esophagogastric junction distensibility by an endoscopic functional luminal imaging probe may help to better evaluate the efficacy of treatment.
- Endoscopic submucosal myotomy (POEM [per-oral endoscopic myotomy]) has been reported in several large series, with a high success rate comparable to laparoscopic Heller myotomy, few adverse events (which can include pneumomediastinum, pneumothorax, pneumoperitoneum, pleural effusion, and bleeding), and exceedingly rare mortality. Because no antireflux procedure is performed, there is a modest risk (up to 53%) of developing pathologic reflux. For now, it should only be performed at high-volume centers.

- Esophagectomy has been performed in patients with end-stage achalasia with a dilated, often sigmoid-shaped or megaesophagus, who have failed myotomy or pneumatic dilation.

GENERAL Rx

- Medications may be useful for short-term symptom relief and in patients with refractory chest pain. They should only be considered in patients unable to receive, or who are scheduled for, more definitive procedures. LES pressure may be lowered by up to 50% through sublingual use of long-acting nitrates (e.g., isosorbide dinitrate 5 to 20 mg) or calcium channel blockers (e.g., nifedipine 10 to 30 mg). Side effects are common and duration of relief tends to be short. Sildenafil was shown to be effective in a few small, short-term studies, but it is generally not recommended.
- Botulinum toxin injection will benefit up to 85% of patients by inhibiting acetylcholine release from cholinergic nerve endings, blocking the unopposed cholinergic stimulation of the LES, but having no impact on the myogenic tone; up to half of these patients will require repeat injections by 6 months. A few studies have suggested that repeated injections can lead to fibrosis, which may complicate subsequent attempts at surgical therapy.
- Many patients will require proton pump inhibitor therapy for gastroesophageal reflux after effective disruption of the LES.

! PEARLS & CONSIDERATIONS

COMMENTS

- Medication has a limited role in treatment.
- Botulinum toxin is transiently effective in improving symptoms. Pneumatic dilation, surgical myotomy, and POEM provide more durable long-term responses and are the treatment of choice for most patients. Botulinum toxin should be considered primarily in patients too elderly or ill to be considered for these other therapies.
- Patients with achalasia may be at long-term risk of squamous cell carcinoma of the esophagus and non–reflux-associated esophagitis. Treated patients may be at long-term risk for reflux esophagitis, Barrett's esophagus, and adenocarcinoma. Endoscopic surveillance is not routinely recommended in these patients.

EBM EVIDENCE

Available at www.expertconsult.com

SUGGESTED READINGS

Available at www.expertconsult.com

RELATED CONTENT

Achalasia (Patient Information)
Dysphagia (Related Key Topic)

AUTHOR: **HARLAN G. RICH, M.D.**

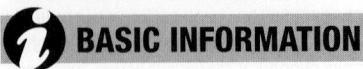

BASIC INFORMATION

DEFINITION

Acne vulgaris is a chronic disorder of the pilosebaceous apparatus caused by abnormal desquamation of follicular epithelium leading to obstruction of the pilosebaceous canal, resulting in inflammation and subsequent formation of papules, pustules, nodules, comedones, and scarring. Based on their appearance, the acne lesions can be divided into inflammatory (presence of papules, pustules, and nodules) or noninflammatory (open and closed comedones) For inflammatory acne, lesions can be classified as papulopustular, nodular, or both. The American Academy of Dermatology classification scheme for acne denotes the following three levels:

1. Mild acne: characterized by the presence of comedones (noninflammatory lesions), few papules and pustules (generally <10), but no nodules.
2. Moderate acne: presence of several to many papules and pustules (10 to 40) along with comedones (10 to 40). The presence of >40 papules and pustules along with larger, deeper nodular inflamed lesions (up to five) denotes moderately severe acne (Fig. 1).
3. Severe acne (Fig. 2): presence of numerous or extensive papules and pustules as well as many nodular lesions.

SYNONYMS

Acne

ICD-10CM CODES
L70.0 Acne vulgaris
L70.1 Acne conglobata
L70.2 Acne varioliformis
L70.3 Acne tropica
L70.4 Infantile acne
L70.5 Acne excoriee des jeunes filles
L70.8 Other acne
L70.9 Acne, unspecified
L73.0 Acne keloid

EPIDEMIOLOGY & DEMOGRAPHICS

- Acne is the most common skin disease in the U.S.
- It is most common in teenagers, with 85% of all teenagers being affected to some degree.
- Highest incidence between ages of 15 and 18 yr in both genders.
- Involution of the disease usually occurs before age 25 yr, but 12% of women and 3% of men will continue to have clinical acne until the mid-40s.

PHYSICAL FINDINGS & CLINICAL PRESENTATION

- Open comedones (blackheads), closed comedones (whiteheads)
- Greasiness (oily skin)
- Presence of scars from prior acne cysts
- Various stages of development and severity may be present concomitantly
- Common distribution of acne: face, back, and upper chest
- Inflammatory papules, pustules, and ectatic pores

ETIOLOGY

- Acne vulgaris is exclusively a follicular disease, with the principal abnormality being comedone formation.
- Overactivity of the sebaceous glands and blockage in the ducts. The obstruction leads to the formation of comedones, which can become inflamed because of overgrowth of *Propionibacterium acnes.*
- Exacerbated by environmental factors (hot, humid, tropical climate), medications (e.g., iodine in cough mixtures, hair greases), industrial exposure to halogenated hydrocarbons.
- Mechanical or frictional forces can aggravate existing acne (e.g., excessive washing by some patients to help rid them of their blackheads or oiliness).

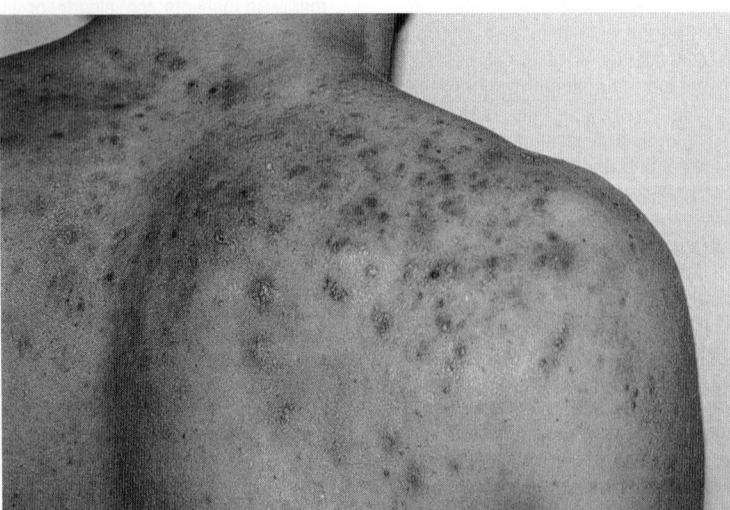

FIG. 1 Acne on back and shoulders. This acne is typically inflammatory and usually needs oral antibiotics or possibly isotretinoin, but the patient may apply topical medication as well. Heat and sweat may aggravate the condition. (From White GM, Cox NH [eds]: *Diseases of the skin,* ed 2, St Louis, 2006, Mosby.)

DIAGNOSIS

DIFFERENTIAL DIAGNOSIS

- Gram-negative folliculitis
- Staphylococcal pyoderma
- Acne rosacea
- Drug eruption
- Sebaceous hyperplasia
- Angiofibromas, basal cell carcinomas, osteoma cutis
- Occupational exposures to oils or grease
- Steroid acne
- Hidradenitis suppurativa
- Perioral dermatitis
- Pseudofolliculitis barbae
- Miliaria
- Seborrheic dermatitis

WORKUP

History and physical examination:
- Inquire about previous treatment
- Careful drug history (including all OTC products)
- Family history, history of cyclic menstrual flares
- History of use of cosmetics and cleansers
- Oral contraceptive use
- Use of medications that may worsen acne such as corticosteroids, anabolic steroids, lithium, neuroleptics, cyclosporine
- Consider the possibility of hyperandrogenic state in all women (hirsutism, irregular menses, androgenic alopecia) or children (seborrhea, acanthosis nigricans, onset of acne between ages 1 and 7 years and no obvious external factors)

LABORATORY TESTS

- Laboratory evaluation is generally not helpful. Patients who are candidates for therapy with isotretinoin should have baseline liver enzymes, cholesterol, and triglycerides checked because this medication may result in elevation of lipids and liver enzymes.
- A negative serum pregnancy test or two negative urine pregnancy tests should also be obtained in females 1 wk before initiation of isotretinoin; it is also imperative to maintain effective contraception during and 1 mo after therapy with isotretinoin ends because of its teratogenic effects. Pregnancy status should be rechecked at monthly visits.
- If hyperandrogenism is suspected in female patients, levels of dehydroepiandrosterone sulfate (DHEAS), testosterone (total and free), and androstenedione should be measured. For women with regular menstrual cycles, serum androgen measurements generally are not necessary.

TREATMENT

NONPHARMACOLOGIC THERAPY

- Blue light (ClearLight therapy system) can be used for treatment of moderate inflammatory acne vulgaris. Light in the violet/blue range can cause bacterial death by a photoreaction in which porphyrins react with oxygen to generate

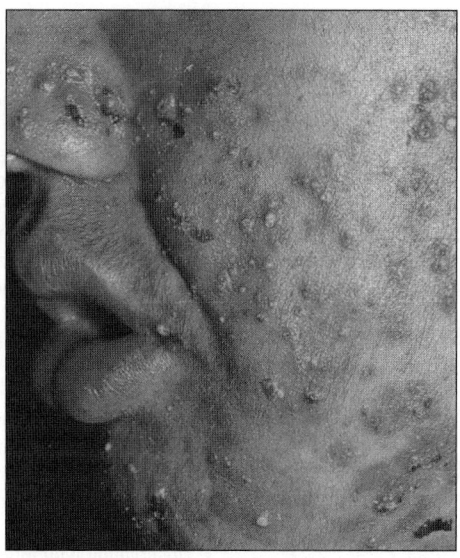

FIG. 2 Severe acne. Acne this severe on presentation should prompt the consideration of early use of isotretinoin. The dose should be low initially to prevent a severe flare. An oral tetracycline or erythromycin may be helpful to calm the acne before isotretinoin. (From White GM, Cox NH [eds]: *Diseases of the skin,* ed 2, St Louis, 2006, Mosby.)

reactive oxygen species, which damage the cell membranes of *P. acnes.* Treatment usually consists of 15-min exposures twice weekly for 4 wk. Phototherapy may be effective for short-term treatment of acne, but long-term efficacy and how it compares with conventional acne therapy is unclear.

- Diet: In obese patients, dietary counseling is recommended. A high-glycemic diet may worsen acne, although the strength of its influence is controversial.

ACUTE GENERAL Rx

Treatment generally varies with the type of lesions (comedones, papules, pustules, cystic lesions) and the severity of acne. Use of topical treatments for 6 to 8 weeks is required to judge their efficacy.

- Comedones (noninflammatory acne) can be treated with retinoids or retinoid analogs. Topical retinoids are comedolytic and work by normalizing follicular keratinization. Commonly available agents are Adapalene (Differin, 0.1% gel or cream, applied once or twice daily), tazarotene (Tazorac 0.1% cream or gel applied daily), tretinoin (Retin-A 0.1% cream or 0.025 gel applied once daily), tretinoin microsphere (Retin-A Micro, 0.1% gel, applied at bedtime). Tretinoin is inactivated by ultraviolet light and oxidized by benzoyl peroxide; therefore it should only be applied at night and not used concomitantly with benzoyl peroxide.
- Tretinoin is pregnancy category C and tazarotene is pregnancy category X. Salicylic acid preparations (e.g., Neutrogena 2% wash) have keratolytic and antiinflammatory properties and are also useful in the treatment of comedones. Large, open comedones (blackheads) should be expressed.
- Patients should be reevaluated after 4 to 6 wk. Benzoyl peroxide gel (2.5% or 5%) may be added if the comedones become inflamed

or form pustules. The most common adverse effects are dryness, erythema, and peeling. Topical antibiotics (erythromycin, clindamycin lotions or pads) can also be used in patients with significant inflammation. They reduce *P. acnes* in the pilosebaceous follicle and have some antiinflammatory effects. The combination of 5% benzoyl peroxide and 3% erythromycin (Benzamycin) or 1% clindamycin with 5% benzoyl peroxide (BenzaClin) is highly effective in patients who have a mixture of comedonal and inflammatory acne lesions.

- Fixed-dose combinations of clindamycin phosphate 1.2% and tretinoin 0.025% are available (Veltin gel, Ziana) and are more effective than either product used alone; however, they are much more expensive than the individual generic components.
- Pustular acne can be treated with tretinoin and benzoyl peroxide gel applied on alternate evenings; drying agents (sulfacetamide-sulfa lotions [Novacet, Sulfacet]) are also effective when used in combination with benzoyl peroxide; oral antibiotics (doxycycline 100 mg qd or erythromycin 1 g qd given in 2 to 3 divided doses) are effective in patients with moderate to severe pustular acne. Patients not responding well to these antibiotics can be switched to minocycline 50 to 100 mg bid; however, this medication is more expensive.
- Patients with nodular cystic acne and those with moderate to severe inflammatory acne unresponsive to topical drugs can be treated with systemic agents: antibiotics (erythromycin, tetracycline, doxycycline, minocycline), isotretinoin (available on a restricted basis), or oral contraceptives. Periodic intralesional triamcinolone (Kenalog) injections by a dermatologist are also effective. The possibility of endocrinopathy should be considered in patients responding poorly to therapy.

- Isotretinoin is the most effective drug available for treatment of severe nodulocystic acne. It is indicated for acne resistant to antibiotic therapy and severe acne. It inhibits *P. acne's* colonization by reducing sebum production and has antiinflammatory and keratolytic effects. It is available only on a restricted basis. Dosage is 0.5 to 1 mg/kg/day in 2 divided doses (maximum of 2 mg/kg/day); duration of therapy is generally 20 wk for a cumulative dose ≥120 mg/kg for severe cystic acne. Before using this medication patients should undergo baseline laboratory evaluation (see "Laboratory Tests"). This drug is absolutely contraindicated during pregnancy because of its teratogenicity. It should be used with caution in patients with history of depression. Physicians, distributors, pharmacies, and patients must register in the iPLEDGE program (http://www.ipledgeprogram.com) before using isotretinoin.
- Azelaic acid is a bacteriostatic dicarboxylic acid used to normalize keratinization and reduce inflammation. It can be used in pregnant women.
- Oral contraceptives reduce androgen levels and therefore sebum production. They represent a useful adjunctive therapy for all types of acne in women and adolescent girls. Commonly used agents are norgestimate/ethinyl estradiol (Ortho Tri-Cyclen) and drospirenone/ethinyl estradiol (Yasmin).

REFERRAL

Referral for intralesional injection and dermabrasion should be considered in patients with severe acne unresponsive to conventional therapy.

ⓘ PEARLS & CONSIDERATIONS

- Gram-negative folliculitis should be suspected if inflammatory acne worsens after several months of oral antibiotic therapy.
- Acne may worsen during the first 3 to 4 wk of retinoid therapy before improving.

COMMENTS

Indications for systemic therapy of acne are:
- Painful deep papules or nodules
- Extensive lesions
- Active acne with severe scarring or hyperpigmentation
- Patient's morale

Patients should be educated that in most cases acne can be controlled but not cured and that at least 4 to 6 wk of initial therapy should be required before significant improvement is noted.

SUGGESTED READINGS

Available at www.expertconsult.com

RELATED CONTENT

Acne (Patient Information)

AUTHOR: **FRED F. FERRI, M.D.**

A

Diseases and Disorders

BASIC INFORMATION

DEFINITION

Acoustic neuroma is a benign proliferation of the Schwann cells that cover the vestibular branch of the eighth cranial nerve (CN VIII). Symptoms are commonly a result of compression of the acoustic branch of CN VIII, the facial nerve (CN VII), and the trigeminal nerve (CN V). The glossopharyngeal nerve (CN IX) and vagus nerve (CN X) are less commonly involved. In extreme cases, compression of the brain stem may lead to obstruction of cerebrospinal fluid (CSF) outflow and elevated intracranial pressure (ICP).

SYNONYMS

Vestibular schwannoma

ICD-10CM CODES
D33.3 Benign neoplasm of cranial nerves

EPIDEMIOLOGY & DEMOGRAPHICS

Overall incidence is approximately 1.2 in 100,000 person-years, with a higher incidence in patients with neurofibromatosis type 2 (NF2). The prevalence is 2 in 10,000 people. The tumor most commonly presents in the fifth and sixth decades.

PHYSICAL FINDINGS & CLINICAL PRESENTATION

- Most frequently unilateral hearing loss and/or tinnitus. Also balance problems, vertigo, facial pain (trigeminal neuralgia) and weakness, difficulty swallowing, fullness or pain of the involved ear. Headache may occur.
- With elevated ICP, patients may also have vomiting, fever, and visual changes.
- Hearing loss is the most common presenting complaint and is usually high frequency.

ETIOLOGY

The etiology is incompletely understood, but long-term exposure to acoustic trauma has been implicated. Bilateral acoustic neuromas may be inherited in an autosomal-dominant manner as part of NF2. This disease is associated with a defect on chromosome 22q1. Childhood exposure to low-dose radiation for benign head and neck conditions may increase risk for acoustic neuromas. There is inconclusive evidence to link chronic exposure to radio-frequency radiation from cellular telephone use and the risk for developing brain tumors.

DIAGNOSIS

DIFFERENTIAL DIAGNOSIS

- Benign positional vertigo
- Ménière's disease
- Trigeminal neuralgia
- Cerebellar disease
- Normal-pressure hydrocephalus
- Presbycusis
- Glomus tumors
- Vertebrobasilar insufficiency
- Ototoxicity from medications
- Other tumors:
  1. Meningioma, glioma
  2. Facial nerve schwannoma
  3. Cavernous hemangioma
  4. Metastatic tumors

WORKUP

- A detailed neurologic examination with special attention to the cranial nerves is crucial.
- Otoscopic evaluation may help rule out other causes of hearing loss.

LABORATORY TESTS

- Audiometry is useful, often showing asymmetric, sensorineural, high-frequency hearing loss.
- CSF protein may be elevated.

IMAGING STUDIES

- MRI with gadolinium (Fig. 1) is the preferred test. It can detect tumors as small as 2 mm in diameter.
- High-resolution CT scan with and without contrast can detect tumors 1 cm in diameter or larger.
- Treatment decisions should be based on the size of the tumor, rate of growth (older patients tend to have slower-growing tumors), degree of neurologic deficit, desire to preserve hearing, life expectancy, age of the patient, and surgical risk. A combination of treatments can also be used.

TREATMENT

NONPHARMACOLOGIC THERAPY

- Surgery is the definitive treatment. Choice of approach (middle cranial fossa, translabyrinthine, or retromastoid suboccipital) may vary depending on the size of the tumor, amount of residual hearing desired, and degree of

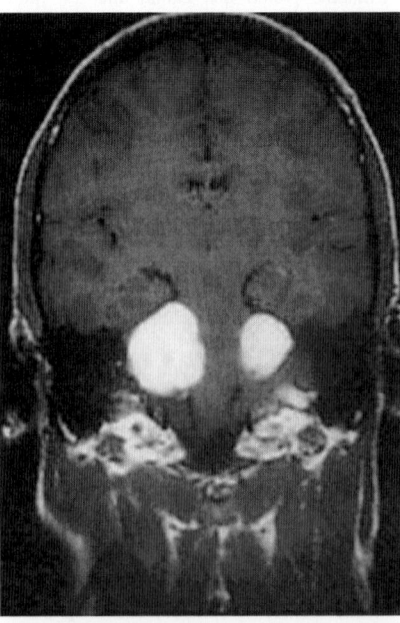

FIG. 1 MR with enhancement shows bilateral acoustic neuromas. Coronal view. (From Kanski JJ, Bowling B: *Clinical ophthalmology, a systematic approach*, ed 7, Philadelphia, 2011, Saunders.)

surgical risk that can be tolerated. Partial resection is sometimes undertaken to minimize the risk of injury to nearby structures. Intraoperative facial nerve monitoring is recommended.
- Radiation therapy (stereotactic radiotherapy, stereotactic radiosurgery, or proton beam radiotherapy) is useful for tumors <3 cm in diameter or for those in whom surgery is not an option. Radiotherapy after partial resection has also been used to minimize complications.
- Age alone is not a contraindication to surgery.

GENERAL Rx

- Bevacizumab, an antivascular endothelial growth factor (VEGF) monoclonal antibody, has been shown to improve hearing and reduce the volume of growing acoustic neuromas in some neurofibromatosis type 2 patients.
- Observation with MRI every 6 to 12 mo may be appropriate for frail patients with small tumors, but risk of unrecoverable hearing loss may increase if surgery is delayed. Also, progressive hearing loss may occur despite absence of growth on subsequent imaging.

DISPOSITION

Hearing can be preserved at near-preoperative levels in more than two thirds of patients with small- to medium-sized tumors. Occurrence of secondary radiation-related tumors following radiosurgery is rare. There are no standard posttreatment follow-up recommendations. Therefore, an individualized approach to follow-up imaging and audiometry is recommended.

REFERRAL

Prompt referral to an otolaryngologist or neurosurgeon who is facile with all three surgical approaches is recommended.

PEARLS & CONSIDERATIONS

COMMENTS

- Presents most commonly as unilateral, sensorineural hearing loss.
- Treatment outcomes are generally good, with cure rates approaching 90% at 5 years.
- Of those who are managed with observation only, approximately half have continued enlargement and approximately one fifth eventually have a surgical intervention.

PATIENT/FAMILY EDUCATION

Acoustic Neuroma Association: https://www.anausa.org/

SUGGESTED READINGS
Available at www.expertconsult.com

RELATED CONTENT

Acoustic Neuroma (Patient Information)
Tinnitus (Related Key Topic)

AUTHOR: **COURTNEY CLARK BILODEAU, M.D.**

ℹ️ BASIC INFORMATION

DEFINITION

Acquired immunodeficiency syndrome (AIDS) is a disorder caused by infection with the human immunodeficiency virus (HIV) and marked by progressive deterioration of the cellular immune system, leading to secondary (opportunistic) infections and/or malignancies.

SYNONYMS

AIDS

ICD-10CM CODES
B20 Human immunodeficiency virus [HIV] disease

EPIDEMIOLOGY & DEMOGRAPHICS

INCIDENCE (IN U.S.):
- The estimated number of persons diagnosed with AIDS in the U.S. exceeds 20,000/year.
- Almost 50% of new AIDS cases are in black/African Americans, 20% in Hispanics, and 25% in white Americans.
- Approximately 57% of all new AIDS diagnoses in 2014 were among gay, bisexual, or other men who have sex with men (MSM).

PREVALENCE (IN U.S.):
- The cumulative number of AIDS diagnoses in the U.S. exceeds 1.2 million.

PREDOMINANT SEX: Men constitute approximately 75% of incident AIDS diagnoses in the U.S.; more than 55% of AIDS diagnoses occur in MSM.

PREDOMINANT AGE: The predominant age group diagnosed with AIDS is 40-49 years of age, closely followed by 30-39 years of age.

PEAK INCIDENCE: Ages 45-49

GENETICS:
- Familial disposition: Although there is no proven genetic predisposition, individuals with deletions in the *CCR5* gene are immune from HIV infection with macrophage tropic virus (the predominant virus in sexual transmission) and may progress to AIDS more slowly.
- Congenital infection:
  1. HIV is transmittable from an infected mother to the fetus in utero in as many as 30% of pregnancies.
  2. No specific congenital malformations associated with infection; low birth weight and spontaneous abortion are possible.

PHYSICAL FINDINGS & CLINICAL PRESENTATION

- Nonspecific findings: fever, weight loss, anorexia.
- Specific syndromes:
  1. Seen in association with opportunistic infections and malignancies, so-called indicator diseases; these include:
     a. Opportunistic infections:
        - Disseminated strongyloidiasis
        - Disseminated toxoplasmosis, cryptococcosis, histoplasmosis, cytomegalovirus (CMV), herpes simplex, or mycobacterial disease
        - *Candida* esophagitis or bronchopulmonary disease
        - Chronic *Cryptosporidia* spp. diarrhea
        - *Pneumocystis jiroveci* pneumonia (PJP)
        - Extensive pulmonary and extrapulmonary tuberculosis
        - Recurrent bacterial pneumonia
        - Progressive multifocal leukoencephalopathy (PML)
     b. AIDS-related neoplasms:
        - Kaposi's sarcoma
        - Primary brain lymphoma
        - Invasive cervical carcinoma
        - High-grade B cell non-Hodgkin's lymphoma, Burkitt's lymphoma, undifferentiated non-Hodgkin's lymphoma, or immunoblastic lymphoma
  2. Most common:
     - Respiratory infections (*Pneumocystis jiroveci* [formerly known as *Pneumocystis carinii*] pneumonia, TB, bacterial pneumonia, fungal infection)
     - CNS infections (toxoplasmosis, TB)
     - GI (cryptosporidiosis, isosporiasis, CMV); Sections II and III describe organisms associated with diarrhea in patients with AIDS
     - Eye infections (CMV, toxoplasmosis)
     - Kaposi's sarcoma (cutaneous or visceral) or lymphoma (nodal or extranodal)
- Possibly asymptomatic.
- Diagnosis of AIDS if the CD4 cell count is <200 or <14% of total lymphocyte in the presence of proven HIV infection, even in the absence of other infections.
- The various manifestations of HIV infection are described in Section II.

ETIOLOGY

- Caused by infection with HIV-1 or HIV-2 (less common).
- HIV is transmitted by sexual contact, needle-sharing (during IV drug use), transfusion of contaminated blood or blood products, and from infected mother to fetus or neonate as described previously.

🔬 DIAGNOSIS

DIFFERENTIAL DIAGNOSIS

- Other wasting illnesses mimicking the non-specific features of AIDS:
  1. TB
  2. Neoplasms
  3. Disseminated fungal infection
  4. Malabsorption syndromes
  5. Depression
- Other disorders associated with dementia or demyelination producing encephalopathy, myelopathy, or neuropathy.

WORKUP

Prompt evaluation of respiratory, CNS, and GI complaints

LABORATORY TESTS

- HIV antibody testing. See "Human Immunodeficiency Virus" topic for the 2014 revised surveillance case definition for HIV infection.
- T-lymphocyte subset analysis: performed to determine the degree of immunodeficiency (i.e., CD4 cell count).
- Viral load assay: to plan long-term antiviral therapy and to follow progression and success of treatment (i.e., HIV RNA PCR).
- CSF examination: for meningitis (if indicated).
- Serologic tests for syphilis, hepatitis B, hepatitis C, and toxoplasmosis.
- Genotypic resistance testing: used to assess for primary resistance in naïve patients and secondary resistance in patients failing a regimen.
- Eye exam: to evaluate for CMV retinitis in patients with CD4 counts <50 cells/mm^3.
- Cryptococcal antigen: part of the evaluation in AIDS patients with CD4 counts <100 cells/mm^3 who have fever, diffuse pneumonia, or evidence of meningitis.
- Evaluation for infection with mycobacterium (TB or MAI) including PPD, sputum cultures, chest radiograph, and blood cultures for acid-fast bacteria, depending on clinical presentation.

IMAGING STUDIES

- MRI or CT of head for encephalopathy or focal CNS complications (e.g., toxoplasmosis, lymphoma).

Chest radiography or CT to aid in the diagnosis of *Pneumocystis jiroveci* (*P. carinii*) pneumonia, TB, or bacterial pneumonia.

℞ TREATMENT

The most important aspect in management of AIDS due to HIV infection is the timely initiation of antiretroviral therapy (see section on HIV treatment).

NONPHARMACOLOGIC THERAPY

- Maintain adequate caloric intake.
- Encourage good oral hygiene and regular dental care.
- Avoid high-risk behaviors that increase the risk of repeated exposure to HIV and other potential pathogens—use condoms, avoid sharing needles, etc.
- Update vaccines—particularly the pneumococcal and hepatitis A/B vaccine along with annual influenza vaccines.
- Avoid administration of any live attenuated vaccines that may be a risk to these immunocompromised patients (e.g., MMR, varicella). (See Section V for immunization schedules for HIV-infected children.)
- When feasible, avoid activities that might increase risk of exposure to opportunistic infections (e.g., cleaning out a cat litter box [toxoplasmosis], getting scratched by a cat [*Bartonella* infections], exposure to pet reptiles [salmonellosis], traveling to developing countries [cryptosporidiosis, tuberculosis], eating undercooked foods and drinking from unsafe water supplies, etc.).

ACUTE GENERAL Rx

Acute management of opportunistic infections is summarized in Table 1 and reviewed elsewhere in this text under specific AIDS-related disorders. For management of AIDS-related malignancies, please refer to the specific malignancy elsewhere in this text.

CHRONIC Rx

For all HIV-infected patients, particularly those meeting the case definition of AIDS:

- Preventive therapy for *Pneumocystis jiroveci* pneumonia and *Mycobacterium avium* (see specific chapters elsewhere in this text). With the advent of modern antiretroviral therapy, many patients have experienced substantial restoration of cellular immune function. It has become clear that preventive therapy for *Pneumocystis jiroveci* and *Mycobacterium avium* complex as well as suppressive therapy for CMV and cryptococcal infection can often be safely withdrawn if the CD4 cell count rises above 200 for at least six months.
- Based on the Department of Health and Human Services (DHHS) Guidelines, active antiretroviral therapy (ART) should be started regardless of CD4 cell count. Individuals with CD4 cell counts <350 and especially CD4 cell counts <200 should be strongly encouraged to start ART in a timely fashion.
- ART usually includes three-drug combinations of:
  1. Nucleoside reverse transcriptase inhibitors (NRTI): tenofovir disoproxil fumarate (TDF), tenofovir alafenamide fumarate (TAF), zidovudine (AZT), didanosine (DDI), lamivudine (3TC), emtricitabine (FTC), stavudine (D4T), and abacavir (ABC).
  2. Protease inhibitors (PI): saquinavir, amprenavir, indinavir, nelfinavir, agenerase, lopinavir/ritonavir, atazanavir, and darunavir.
  3. Nonnucleoside reverse transcriptase inhibitors (NNRTI): nevirapine, delavirdine, efavirenz (EFV), etravirine, and rilpivirine.
  4. Integrase inhibitors: raltegravir, elvitegravir, and dolutegravir.
  5. Others: maraviroc and enfuvirtide.

The protease inhibitors ritonavir or cobicistat should be used in combination with other protease inhibitors to obtain more sustained drug levels. Usual initial dosing regimens include two NRTIs and an NNRTI or PI or integrase inhibitor. Currently, integrase inhibitors are recommended as first-line drugs because of tolerability. Examples of initial regimens recommended by the guidelines:

1. Dolutegravir/abacavir/lamivudine (in patients who are HLA-B*5701 NEGATIVE)
2. Dolutegravir plus tenofovir/emtricitabine (tenofovir-based drugs can include either TDF or TAF)
3. Elvitegravir/cobicistat/tenofovir/emtricitabine
4. Raltegravir plus tenofovir/emtricitabine
5. Darunavir/ritonavir plus tenofovir/emtricitabine
   Previous first-line drugs, including efavirenz/tenofovir/emtricitabine and rilpivirine/tenofovir/emtricitabine, are now considered alternative regimens.

All these drugs have unique and class-specific side effects and require careful and expert follow-up to achieve optimal antiviral effects, ensure compliance, and maintain efficacy. Antiviral response should be monitored by baseline HIV viral load and CD4 count and repeat measurement at 2 weeks and 4 weeks into treatment and then periodically (every 3-6 months) to ensure viral suppression.

- An approach to evaluating chronic diarrhea in patients with HIV infection is described in Fig. E1, the approach to the acutely ill HIV-infected patient is outlined in Fig. E2, and the evaluation of HIV-positive patients with respiratory complaints is described in Figs. E3 and E4. The approach to a patient with a suspected CNS lesion is described in Figs. E5 and E6. Fig. E7 presents an approach to cardiac dysfunction.
- Genotypic resistance testing is strongly encouraged for all patients initiating treatment and for any patient failing antiretroviral therapy. Poor adherence to therapy, however, often underlies virologic failure.

DISPOSITION

The outlook for AIDS has changed radically since the advent of ART therapy from an essentially fatal disease to a chronic medical illness compatible with long-term survival and remarkably good quality of life. Patients should be aggressively treated for severe illnesses as outcomes following ICU admissions remain good. This is accomplished through expert and continuous follow-up, use of ART, and careful detail to compliance to medications and lifestyle modification.

Table 1 Treatment of AIDS-Associated Opportunistic Infections

Opportunistic Infection	Preferred Therapy	Alternative Therapy	Other Comments
PJP	Patients who develop PJP despite TMP-SMX prophylaxis can usually be treated with standard doses of TMP-SMX. Duration of PJP treatment: 21 days *For Moderate to Severe PJP:* TMP-SMX: (TMP 15-20 mg and SMX 75-100 mg/kg/day) IV given q6h or q8h, may switch to PO after clinical improvement. *For Mild to Moderate PJP:* TMP-SMX: (TMP 15-20 mg and SMX 75-100 mg/kg/day), given PO in 3 divided doses, *or* TMP-SMX: (160 mg/800 mg or DS) 2 tablets PO tid. *Secondary Prophylaxis, after completion of PJP treatment:* TMP-SMX DS: 1 tablet PO daily *or* TMP-SMX (80 mg/400 mg or SS): 1 tablet PO daily	*For Moderate to Severe PJP:* Pentamidine 4 mg/kg IV daily infused over ≥60 minutes; can reduce dose to 3 mg/kg IV daily because of toxicities, *or* Primaquine 30 mg (base) PO daily + (clindamycin 600 mg q6h IV or 900 mg IV q8h) or (clindamycin 300 mg PO q6h or 450 mg PO q8h). *For Mild to Moderate PJP:* Dapsone 100 mg PO daily + TMP 5 mg/kg PO tid, *or* Primaquine 30 mg (base) PO daily + (clindamycin 300 mg PO q6h or 450 mg PO q8h), *or* Atovaquone 750 mg PO bid with food. *Secondary Prophylaxis, after completion of PJP treatment:* TMP-SMX DS: 1 tablet PO tiw, *or* Dapsone 100 mg PO daily, *or* Dapsone 50 mg PO daily + (pyrimethamine 50 mg + leucovorin 25 mg) PO weekly, *or* (Dapsone 200 mg + pyrimethamine 75 mg + leucovorin 25 mg) PO weekly, *or* Aerosolized pentamidine 300 mg monthly via Respirgard II nebulizer, *or* Atovaquone 1500 mg PO daily, *or* (Atovaquone 1500 mg + pyrimethamine 25 mg + leucovorin 10 mg) PO daily.	*Indications for Adjunctive Corticosteroids:* Pa_{O_2} <70 mm Hg at room air, *or* Alveolar-arterial O_2 gradient >35 mm Hg *Prednisone Doses (beginning as early as possible and within 72 hours of PJP therapy):* Days 1-5: 40 mg PO bid Days 6-10: 40 mg PO daily Days 11-21: 20 mg PO daily IV methylprednisolone can be administered as 75% of prednisone dose. Benefit of corticosteroid if started after 72 hours of treatment is unknown, but some clinicians will use it for moderate-to-severe PJP. Whenever possible, patients should be tested for G6PD before use of dapsone or primaquine. Alternative therapy should be used in patients found to have G6PD deficiency. Patients who are receiving pyrimethamine/sulfadiazine for treatment or suppression of toxoplasmosis do not require additional PJP prophylaxis. If TMP-SMX is discontinued because of a mild adverse reaction, reinstitution should be considered after the reaction resolves. The dose can be increased gradually (desensitization) or be reduced, or the frequency can be modified. TMP-SMX should be permanently discontinued in patients with possible or definite Stevens-Johnson syndrome or toxic epidermal necrosis.

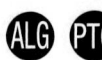
Table 1   Treatment of AIDS-Associated Opportunistic Infections—cont'd

Opportunistic Infection	Preferred Therapy	Alternative Therapy	Other Comments
Toxoplasma gondii encephalitis	*Treatment of Acute Infection:* Pyrimethamine 200 mg PO 1 time, followed by weight-based therapy: If <60 kg, pyrimethamine 50 mg PO once daily + sulfadiazine 1000 mg PO q6h + leucovorin 10-25 mg PO once daily. If ≥60 kg, pyrimethamine 75 mg PO once daily + sulfadiazine 1500 mg PO q6h + leucovorin 10-25 mg PO once daily. Leucovorin dose can be increased to 50 mg daily or bid. *Duration for Acute Therapy:* At least 6 weeks; longer duration if clinical or radiologic disease is extensive or response is incomplete at 6 weeks *Chronic Maintenance Therapy:* Pyrimethamine 25-50 mg PO daily + sulfadiazine 2000-4000 mg PO daily (in 2-4 divided doses) + leucovorin 10-25 mg PO daily (AI)	*Treatment of Acute Infection:* Pyrimethamine (leucovorin)* + clindamycin 600 mg IV or PO q6h *or* TMP-SMX (TMP 5 mg/kg and SMX 25 mg/kg) IV or PO bid, *or* Atovaquone 1500 mg PO bid with food + pyrimethamine (leucovorin), *or* Atovaquone 1500 mg PO bid with food + sulfadiazine 1000-1500 mg PO q6h (weight-based dosing, as in preferred therapy) *or* Atovaquone 1500 mg PO bid with food, *or* Pyrimethamine (leucovorin)* + azithromycin 900-1200 mg PO daily. *Chronic Maintenance Therapy:* Clindamycin 600 mg PO q8h + (pyrimethamine 25-50 mg + leucovorin 10-25 mg) PO daily or TMP-SMX DS 1 tablet bid, *or* Atovaquone 750-1500 mg PO bid + (pyrimethamine 25 mg + leucovorin 10 mg) PO daily, *or* Atovaquone 750-1500 mg PO bid + sulfadiazine 2000-4000 mg PO daily (in 2-4 divided doses), *or* Atovaquone 750-1500 mg PO bid with food *Pyrimethamine and leucovorin doses are the same as for preferred therapy.	Adjunctive corticosteroids (e.g., dexamethasone) should only be administered when clinically indicated to treat mass effect associated with focal lesions or associated edema; discontinue as soon as clinically feasible. Anticonvulsants should be administered to patients with a history of seizures and continued through acute treatment but should not be used as seizure prophylaxis. If clindamycin is used in place of sulfadiazine, additional therapy must be added to prevent PCP.
Mycobacterium tuberculosis disease (TB)	After collecting specimen for culture and molecular diagnostic tests, empiric TB treatment should be started in individuals with clinical and radiographic presentation suggestive of TB. *Initial Phase (2 months, given daily, 5-7 times/week by DOT):* INH + [RIF or RFB] + PZA + EMB *Continuation Phase:* INH + (RIF or RFB) daily (5-7 times/week) or tiw *Total Duration of Therapy (for drug-susceptible TB):* Pulmonary TB: 6 months Pulmonary TB and culture-positive after 2 months of TB treatment: 9 months Extrapulmonary TB with CNS infection: 9-12 months; Extrapulmonary TB with bone or joint involvement: 6 to 9 months; Extrapulmonary TB in other sites: 6 months Total duration of therapy should be based on number of doses received, not on calendar time.	*Treatment for Drug-Resistant TB* *Resistant to INH:* (RIF or RFB) + EMB + PZA + (moxifloxacin or levofloxacin) for 2 months; followed by (RIF or RFB) + EMB + (moxifloxacin or levofloxacin) for 7 months. *Resistant to Rifamycins ± Other Drugs:* Regimen and duration of treatment should be individualized based on resistance pattern, clinical and microbiologic responses, and in close consultation with experienced specialists.	Adjunctive corticosteroid improves survival for TB meningitis and pericarditis. See text for drug, dose, and duration recommendations. RIF *is not recommended* for patients receiving HIV PI because of its induction of PI metabolism. RFB is a less potent CYP3A4 inducer than RIF and is preferred in patients receiving PIs. Once-weekly rifapentine can result in development of rifamycin resistance in HIV-infected patients and *is not recommended.* Therapeutic drug monitoring should be considered in patients receiving rifamycin and interacting ART. Paradoxical IRIS that is not severe can be treated with NSAIDs without a change in TB or HIV therapy. For severe IRIS reaction, consider prednisone and taper over 4 weeks based on clinical symptoms. For example: *If receiving RIF:* prednisone 1.5 mg/kg/day for 2 weeks, then 0.75 mg/kg/day for 2 weeks *If receiving RFB:* Prednisone 1.0 mg/kg/day for 2 weeks, then 0.5 mg/kg/day for 2 weeks A more gradual tapering schedule over a few months may be necessary for some patients.
Disseminated MAC disease	*At Least 2 Drugs as Initial Therapy with:* Clarithromycin 500 mg PO bid + ethambutol 15 mg/kg PO daily, *or* azithromycin 500-600 mg + ethambutol 15 mg/kg PO daily if drug interaction or intolerance precludes the use of clarithromycin *Duration:* At least 12 months of therapy, can discontinue if no signs and symptoms of MAC disease and sustained (>6 months) CD4 count >100 cells/μl in response to ART	Addition of a third or fourth drug should be considered for patients with advanced immunosuppression (CD4 counts <50 cells/μl), high mycobacterial loads (>2 log CFU/ml of blood), or in the absence of effective ART. *Third or Fourth Drug Options May Include:* RFB 300 mg PO daily (dosage adjustment may be necessary based on drug interactions), Amikacin 10-15 mg/kg IV daily, *or* Streptomycin 1 g IV or IM daily, *or* Moxifloxacin 400 mg PO daily or levofloxacin 500 mg PO daily	Testing of susceptibility to clarithromycin and azithromycin is recommended. NSAIDs can be used for patients who experience moderate to severe symptoms attributed to IRIS. If IRIS symptoms persist, short-term (4-8 weeks) systemic corticosteroids (equivalent to 20-40 mg prednisone) can be used.

Table 1   Treatment of AIDS-Associated Opportunistic Infections—cont'd

Opportunistic Infection	Preferred Therapy	Alternative Therapy	Other Comments
Bacterial respiratory diseases *(with focus on pneumonia)*	Empiric antibiotic therapy should be initiated promptly for patients presenting with clinical and radiographic evidence consistent with bacterial pneumonia. The recommendations listed are suggested empiric therapy. The regimen should be modified as needed once microbiologic results are available. *Empiric Outpatient Therapy:* A PO β-lactam + a PO macrolide (azithromycin or clarithromycin) *Preferred β-lactams:* High-dose amoxicillin or amoxicillin/clavulanate *Alternative β-lactams:* Cefpodoxime or cefuroxime, *or* *For penicillin-allergic patients:* Levofloxacin 750 mg PO once daily, or moxifloxacin 400 mg PO once daily *Duration:* 7-10 days (a minimum of 5 days). Patients should be afebrile for 48-72 hours and clinically stable before stopping antibiotics. *Empiric Therapy for Non-ICU Hospitalized Patients:* An IV β-lactam + a macrolide (azithromycin or clarithromycin) *Preferred β-lactams:* ceftriaxone, cefotaxime, or ampicillin-sulbactam *For penicillin-allergic patients:* Levofloxacin, 750 mg IV once daily, *or* moxifloxacin, 400 mg IV once daily *Empiric Therapy for ICU Patients:* An IV β-lactam + IV azithromycin , *or* An IV β-lactam + (levofloxacin 750 mg IV once daily or moxifloxacin 400 mg IV once daily) *Preferred β-lactams:* ceftriaxone, cefotaxime, or ampicillin-sulbactam *Empiric Therapy for Patients at Risk of* Pseudomonas *Pneumonia:* An IV antipneumococcal, antipseudomonal β-lactam + ciprofloxacin 400 mg IV q8-12h or levofloxacin 750 mg IV once daily *Preferred β-lactams:* piperacillin-tazobactam, cefepime, imipenem, or meropenem *Empiric Therapy for Patients at Risk for Methicillin-Resistant* Staphylococcus aureus *Pneumonia:* Add vancomycin IV or linezolid (IV or PO) to the baseline regimen. Addition of clindamycin to vancomycin (but not to linezolid) can be considered for severe necrotizing pneumonia to minimize bacterial toxin production.	*Empiric Outpatient Therapy:* A PO β-lactam + PO doxycycline *Preferred β-lactams:* High-dose amoxicillin or amoxicillin/clavulanate *Alternative β-lactams:* Cefpodoxime or cefuroxime *Empiric Therapy for Non-ICU Hospitalized Patients:* An IV β-lactam + doxycycline *Empiric Therapy for ICU Patients:* *For penicillin-allergic patients:* Aztreonam IV + (levofloxacin 750 mg IV once daily or moxifloxacin 400 mg IV once daily) *Empiric Therapy for Patients at Risk of* Pseudomonas *Pneumonia:* An IV antipneumococcal, antipseudomonal β-lactam + an aminoglycoside + azithromycin, *or* above β-lactam + an aminoglycoside + (levofloxacin 750 mg IV once daily or moxifloxacin 400 mg IV once daily), *or* *For penicillin-allergic patients:* Replace the β-lactam with aztreonam	Fluoroquinolones should be used with caution in patients in whom TB is suspected but is not being treated. Empiric therapy with a macrolide alone is not routinely recommended because of increasing pneumococcal resistance. Patients receiving a macrolide for MAC prophylaxis should not receive macrolide monotherapy for empiric treatment of bacterial pneumonia. For patients begun on IV antibiotic therapy, switching to PO should be considered when they are clinically improved and able to tolerate oral medications. Chemoprophylaxis can be considered for patients with frequent recurrences of serious bacterial pneumonia. Clinicians should be cautious about using antibiotics to prevent recurrences because of the potential for developing drug resistance and drug toxicities.
Bacterial enteric infections *Empiric therapy pending definitive diagnosis*	Diagnostic fecal specimens should be obtained before initiation of empiric antibiotic therapy. Empiric antibiotic therapy is indicated for patients with advanced HIV (CD4 count <200 cells/μl or concomitant AIDS-defining illnesses), with clinically severe diarrhea (>6 stools/day), and/or accompanying fever or chills. *Empiric Therapy:* Ciprofloxacin 500-750 mg PO (or 400 mg IV) q12h. Therapy should be adjusted based on the results of diagnostic workup. For patients with chronic diarrhea (>14 days) without severe clinical signs, empiric antibiotics therapy is not necessary; can withhold treatment until a diagnosis is made.	*Empiric Therapy:* Ceftriaxone 1 g IV q24h, *or* Cefotaxime 1 g IV q8h	Hospitalization with IV antibiotics should be considered in patients with marked nausea, vomiting, diarrhea, electrolyte abnormalities, acidosis, and blood pressure instability. Oral or IV rehydration if indicated. Antimotility agents should be avoided if there is concern about inflammatory diarrhea, including *Clostridium difficile*–associated diarrhea. If no clinical response after 5-7 days, consider follow-up stool culture with antibiotic susceptibility testing or alternative diagnostic tests (e.g., toxin assays, molecular testing), alternative diagnosis, or antibiotic resistance.

Table 1 Treatment of AIDS-Associated Opportunistic Infections—cont'd

Opportunistic Infection	Preferred Therapy	Alternative Therapy	Other Comments
Salmonellosis	All HIV-infected patients with salmonellosis should be treated because of high risk of bacteremia. Ciprofloxacin 500-750 mg PO (or 400 mg IV) q12h, if susceptible *Duration of Therapy:* *For gastroenteritis without bacteremia:* If CD4 count ≥200 cells/μl: 7-14 days If CD4 count <200 cells/μl: 2-6 weeks *For gastroenteritis with bacteremia:* If CD4 count ≥200/μl: 14 days; longer duration if bacteremia persists or if the infection is complicated (e.g., if metastatic foci of infection are present) If CD4 count <200 cells/μl: 2-6 weeks *Secondary Prophylaxis Should Be Considered for:* Patients with recurrent *Salmonella* gastroenteritis ± bacteremia, *or* Patients with CD4 <200 cells/μl with severe diarrhea	Levofloxacin 750 mg (PO or IV) q24h, *or* Moxifloxacin 400 mg (PO or IV) q24h, *or* TMP, 160 mg-SMX 800 mg (PO or IV) q12h, *or* Ceftriaxone 1 g IV q24h, *or* Cefotaxime 1 g IV q8h	Oral or IV rehydration if indicated. Antimotility agents should be avoided. The role of long-term secondary prophylaxis in patients with recurrent *Salmonella* bacteremia is not well established. Must weigh benefit against risks of long-term antibiotic exposure. Effective ART may reduce the frequency, severity, and recurrence of *Salmonella* infections.
Mucocutaneous candidiasis	*For Oropharyngeal Candidiasis; Initial Episodes (for 7-14 days):* *Oral therapy* Fluconazole 100 mg PO daily, *or* *Topical therapy* Clotrimazole troches, 10 mg PO 5 times daily, or Miconazole mucoadhesive buccal 50-mg tablet—apply to mucosal surface over the canine fossa once daily (do not swallow, chew, or crush). *For Esophageal Candidiasis (for 14-21 days):* Fluconazole 100 mg (up to 400 mg) PO or IV daily, *or* Itraconazole oral solution 200 mg PO daily. *For Uncomplicated Vulvovaginal Candidiasis:* Oral fluconazole 150 mg for 1 dose, *or* Topical azoles (clotrimazole, butoconazole, miconazole, tioconazole, or terconazole) for 3-7 days *For Severe or Recurrent Vulvovaginal Candidiasis:* Fluconazole 100-200 mg PO daily for ≥7 days, *or* Topical antifungal ≥7 days	*For Oropharyngeal Candidiasis; Initial Episodes (for 7-14 days):* *Oral therapy* Itraconazole oral solution 200 mg PO daily, *or* Posaconazole oral solution 400 mg PO bid for 1 day, then 400 mg daily *Topical therapy* Nystatin suspension 4-6 ml qid or 1-2 flavored pastilles 4-5 times daily. *For Esophageal Candidiasis (for 14-21 days):* Voriconazole 200 mg PO or IV bid, *or* Posaconazole 400 mg PO bid, *or* Anidulafungin 100 mg IV 1 time, then 50 mg IV daily, *or* Caspofungin 50 mg IV daily, *or* Micafungin 150 mg IV daily, *or* Amphotericin B deoxycholate 0.6 mg/kg IV daily, *or* Lipid formulation of amphotericin B 3-4 mg/kg IV daily. *For Uncomplicated Vulvovaginal Candidiasis:* Itraconazole oral solution 200 mg PO daily for 3-7 days	Chronic or prolonged use of azoles may promote development of resistance. Higher relapse rate for esophageal candidiasis is seen with echinocandins than with fluconazole use. Suppressive therapy is usually not recommended unless patients have frequent or severe recurrences. *If Decision Is to Use Suppressive Therapy:* *Oropharyngeal Candidiasis:* Fluconazole 100 mg PO daily or tiw Itraconazole oral solution 200 mg PO daily *Esophageal Candidiasis:* Fluconazole 100-200 mg PO daily Posaconazole 400 mg PO bid *Vulvovaginal Candidiasis:* Fluconazole 150 mg PO once weekly
Cryptococcosis	*Cryptococcal Meningitis* *Induction Therapy (for at least 2 weeks, followed by consolidation therapy):* Liposomal amphotericin B 3-4 mg/kg IV daily + flucytosine 25 mg/kg PO qid (Note: Flucytosine dose should be adjusted in patients with renal dysfunction). *Consolidation Therapy (for at least 8 weeks followed by maintenance therapy):* Fluconazole 400 mg PO (or IV) daily. *Maintenance therapy:* Fluconazole 200 mg PO daily for at least 12 months. *For Non-CNS, Extrapulmonary Cryptococcosis and Diffuse Pulmonary Disease:* Treatment same as for cryptococcal meningitis. *Non-CNS Cryptococcosis with Mild to Moderate Symptoms and Focal Pulmonary Infiltrates:* Fluconazole, 400 mg PO daily for 12 months.	*Cryptococcal Meningitis* *Induction Therapy (for at least 2 weeks, followed by consolidation therapy):* Amphotericin B deoxycholate 0.7 mg/kg IV daily + flucytosine 25 mg/kg PO qid, *or* Amphotericin B lipid complex 5 mg/kg IV daily + flucytosine 25 mg/kg PO qid, *or* Liposomal amphotericin B 3-4 mg/kg IV daily + fluconazole 800 mg PO or IV daily, *or* Amphotericin B deoxycholate 0.7 mg/kg IV daily + fluconazole 800 mg PO or IV daily, *or* Fluconazole 400-800 mg PO or IV daily + flucytosine 25 mg/kg PO qid, *or* Fluconazole 1200 mg PO or IV daily *Consolidation Therapy (for at least 8 weeks followed by maintenance therapy):* Itraconazole 200 mg PO bid for 8 weeks—less effective than fluconazole *Maintenance therapy:* No alternative therapy recommendation	Addition of flucytosine to amphotericin B has been associated with more rapid sterilization of CSF and decreased risk for subsequent relapse. Patients receiving flucytosine should have either blood levels monitored (peak level 2 hours after dose should be 30-80 μg/ml) or close monitoring of blood counts for development of cytopenia. Dosage should be adjusted in patients with renal insufficiency. Opening pressure should always be measured when an LP is performed. Repeated LPs or CSF shunting are essential to effectively manage increased intracranial pressure. Corticosteroids and mannitol are ineffective in reducing intracranial pressure and are *not* recommended. Some specialists recommend a brief course of corticosteroid for management of severe IRIS symptoms.

Continued

Table 1   Treatment of AIDS-Associated Opportunistic Infections—cont'd

Opportunistic Infection	Preferred Therapy	Alternative Therapy	Other Comments
Histoplasmosis	*Moderately Severe to Severe Disseminated Disease Induction Therapy (for at least 2 weeks or until clinically improved):* Liposomal amphotericin B 3 mg/kg IV daily. *Maintenance Therapy:* Itraconazole 200 mg PO tid for 3 days, then 200 mg PO bid. *Less Severe Disseminated Disease Induction and Maintenance Therapy:* Itraconazole 200 mg PO tid for 3 days, then 200 mg PO bid. *Duration of Therapy:* At least 12 months. *Meningitis Induction Therapy (4-6 weeks):* Liposomal amphotericin B 5 mg/kg/day. *Maintenance Therapy:* Itraconazole 200 mg PO bid to tid for ≥1 year and until resolution of abnormal CSF findings. *Long-Term Suppression Therapy:* For patients with severe disseminated or CNS infection after completion of at least 12 months of therapy; and those who relapse despite appropriate therapy Itraconazole 200 mg PO daily.	*Moderately Severe to Severe Disseminated Disease Induction Therapy (for at least 2 weeks or until clinically improved):* Amphotericin B lipid complex 3 mg/kg IV daily, *or* Amphotericin B cholesteryl sulfate complete 3 mg/kg IV daily *Alternatives to Itraconazole for Maintenance Therapy or Treatment of Less Severe Disease:* Voriconazole 400 mg PO bid for 1 day, then 200 mg bid, *or* Posaconazole 400 mg PO bid Fluconazole 800 mg PO daily *Meningitis:* No alternative therapy recommendation *Long-Term Suppression Therapy:* Fluconazole 400 mg PO daily	Itraconazole, posaconazole, and voriconazole may have significant interactions with certain ARV agents. These interactions are complex and can be bidirectional. Therapeutic drug monitoring and dosage adjustment may be necessary to ensure triazole antifungal and ARV efficacy and to reduce concentration-related toxicities. Random serum concentration of itraconazole + hydroxyitraconazole should be >1 μg/ml. Clinical experience with voriconazole or posaconazole in the treatment of histoplasmosis is limited. Acute pulmonary histoplasmosis in HIV-infected patients with CD4 counts >300 cells/μl should be managed as nonimmunocompromised host.
Coccidioidomycosis	*Clinically Mild Infections (e.g., focal pneumonia):* Fluconazole 400 mg PO daily *or* Itraconazole 200 mg PO bid. *Severe, Nonmeningeal Infection (diffuse pulmonary infection or severely ill patients with extrathoracic, disseminated disease):* Amphotericin B deoxycholate 0.7-1.0 mg/kg IV daily Lipid formulation amphotericin B 4-6 mg/kg IV daily Duration of therapy: continue until clinical improvement, then switch to an azole. *Meningeal Infections:* Fluconazole 400-800 mg IV or PO daily. *Chronic Suppressive Therapy:* Fluconazole 400 mg PO daily, *or* Itraconazole 200 mg PO bid	*Mild Infections (focal pneumonia) for patients who failed to respond to fluconazole or itraconazole:* Posaconazole 200 mg PO bid, *or* Voriconazole 200 mg PO bid. *Severe, Nonmeningeal Infection (diffuse pulmonary infection or severely ill patients with extrathoracic, disseminated disease):* Some specialists will add a triazole (fluconazole or itraconazole, with itraconazole preferred for bone disease) 400 mg per day to amphotericin B therapy and continue triazole once amphotericin B is stopped. *Meningeal Infections:* Itraconazole 200 mg PO tid for 3 days, then 200 mg PO bid, *or* Posaconazole 200 mg PO bid, *or* Voriconazole 200-400 mg PO bid, *or* Intrathecal amphotericin B deoxycholate, when triazole antifungals are ineffective. *Chronic suppressive therapy:* Posaconazole 200 mg PO bid, *or* Voriconazole 200 mg PO bid	Some patients with meningitis may develop hydrocephalus and require CSF shunting. Therapy should be continued indefinitely in patients with diffuse pulmonary or disseminated diseases because relapse can occur in 25%-33% of HIV-negative patients. It can also occur in HIV-infected patients with CD4 counts >250 cells/μl. Therapy should be lifelong in patients with meningeal infections because relapse occurs in 80% of HIV-infected patients after discontinuation of triazole therapy. Itraconazole, posaconazole, and voriconazole may have significant interactions with certain ARV agents. These interactions are complex and can be bidirectional. Therapeutic drug monitoring and dosage adjustment may be necessary to ensure triazole antifungal and antiretroviral efficacy and to reduce concentration-related toxicities. Intrathecal amphotericin B should be given only in consultation with a specialist and should be administered by an individual with experience with the technique.
Aspergillosis, invasive	*Preferred Therapy:* Voriconazole 6 mg/kg IV q12h for 1 day, then 4 mg/kg IV q12h, followed by voriconazole 200 mg PO q12h after clinical improvement *Duration of Therapy:* Until CD4 cell count >200 cells/μl and the infection appears to be resolved	*Alternative Therapy:* Lipid formulation of amphotericin B 5 mg/kg IV daily, *or* Amphotericin B deoxycholate 1 mg/kg IV daily, *or* Caspofungin 70 mg IV 1 time, then 50 mg IV daily, *or* Micafungin 100-150 mg IV daily, *or* Anidulafungin 200 mg IV 1 time, then 100 mg IV daily, *or* Posaconazole 200 mg PO qid, then, after condition improved, 400 mg PO bid.	Potential for significant pharmacokinetic interactions between certain ARV agents and voriconazole; they should be used cautiously in these situations. Consider therapeutic drug monitoring and dosage adjustment if necessary.

Table 1 Treatment of AIDS-Associated Opportunistic Infections—cont'd

Opportunistic Infection	Preferred Therapy	Alternative Therapy	Other Comments
CMV disease	*CMV Retinitis Induction Therapy for Immediate Sight-Threatening Lesions (adjacent to the optic nerve or fovea)* *Consult ophthalmologist; ganciclovir implant no longer available:* Ganciclovir 5 mg/kg IV q12h for 14-21 days followed by Valganciclovir 900 mg PO bid *For Small Peripheral Lesions:* Valganciclovir 900 mg PO bid for 14-21 days One dose of intravitreal ganciclovir can be administered immediately after diagnosis until steady-state plasma ganciclovir concentration is achieved with oral valganciclovir *Chronic Maintenance (secondary prophylaxis):* Valganciclovir 900 mg PO daily (for small peripheral lesion). *CMV Esophagitis or Colitis:* Ganciclovir 5 mg/kg IV q12h; may switch to valganciclovir 900 mg PO q12h once patient can tolerate oral therapy Duration: 21-42 days or until symptoms have resolved. Maintenance therapy is usually not necessary but should be considered after relapses. *Well-Documented, Histologically Confirmed CMV Pneumonia:* Experience for treating CMV pneumonitis in HIV patients is limited. Use of IV ganciclovir or IV foscarnet is reasonable (doses same as for CMV retinitis). The optimal duration of therapy and the role of oral valganciclovir have not been established. *CMV Neurologic Disease* Note: Treatment should be initiated promptly. Ganciclovir 5 mg/kg IV q12h + (foscarnet 90 mg/kg IV q12h or 60 mg/kg IV q8h) to stabilize disease and maximize response; continue until symptomatic improvement and resolution of neurologic symptoms. The optimal duration of therapy and the role of oral valganciclovir have not been established.	*CMV Retinitis Induction Therapy:* Ganciclovir 5 mg/kg IV q12h for 14-21 days, *or* Foscarnet 90 mg/kg IV q12h or 60 mg q8h for 14-21 days, *or* Cidofovir 5 mg/kg/week IV for 2 weeks; saline hydration before and after therapy and probenecid, 2 g PO 3 hours before dose, followed by 1 g PO 2 hours and 8 hours after the dose (total of 4 g). (Note: This regimen should be avoided in patients with sulfa allergy because of cross-hypersensitivity with probenecid.) *Chronic Maintenance (secondary prophylaxis):* Ganciclovir 5 mg/kg IV 5-7 times weekly, *or* Foscarnet 90-120 mg/kg IV once daily, *or* Cidofovir 5 mg/kg IV every other week with saline hydration and probenecid as above. *CMV Esophagitis or Colitis:* Foscarnet 90 mg/kg IV q12h or 60 mg/kg q8h for patients with treatment-limiting toxicities to ganciclovir or with ganciclovir resistance, *or* Valganciclovir 900 mg PO q12h in milder disease and if able to tolerate PO therapy, *or* For mild cases, if ART can be initiated without delay, consider withholding CMV therapy. Duration: 21-42 days or until symptoms have resolved	The choice of therapy for CMV retinitis should be individualized, based on location and severity of the lesions, level of immunosuppression, and other factors (e.g., concomitant medications and ability to adhere to treatment). The choice of chronic maintenance therapy (route of administration and drug choices) should be made in consultation with an ophthalmologist. Considerations should include the anatomic location of the retinal lesion, vision in the contralateral eye, the patients' immunologic and virologic status, and response to ART. Patients with CMV retinitis who discontinue maintenance therapy should undergo regular eye examinations for early detection of relapse IRU—optimally every 3 months and then annually after immune reconstitution. IRU may develop in the setting of immune reconstitution. *Treatment of IRU:* Periocular corticosteroid or short courses of systemic steroid. Initial therapy in patients with CMV retinitis, esophagitis, colitis, and pneumonitis should include initiation or optimization of ART.
HSV disease	*Orolabial Lesions (for 5-10 days):* Valacyclovir 1 g PO bid *or* Famciclovir 500 mg PO bid *or* Acyclovir 400 mg PO tid. *Initial or Recurrent Genital HSV (for 5-14 days):* Valacyclovir 1 g PO bid, *or* Famciclovir 500 mg PO bid, *or* Acyclovir 400 mg PO tid *Severe Mucocutaneous HSV:* Initial therapy acyclovir 5 mg/kg IV q8h After lesions begin to regress, change to PO therapy as previously. Continue until lesions are completely healed. *Chronic Suppressive Therapy for Patients with Severe Recurrences of Genital Herpes or for Patients Who Want to Minimize Frequency of Recurrences:* Valacyclovir 500 mg PO bid Famciclovir 500 mg PO bid Acyclovir 400 mg PO bid Continue indefinitely regardless of CD4 cell count.	*For Acyclovir-Resistant HSV* *Preferred Therapy:* Foscarnet 80-120 mg/kg/day IV in 2-3 divided doses until clinical response. *Alternative Therapy* IV cidofovir (dosage as in CMV retinitis), *or* Topical trifluridine, *or* Topical cidofovir, *or* Topical imiquimod *Duration of Therapy:* 21-28 days or longer	Patients with HSV infections can be treated with episodic therapy when symptomatic lesions occur, or with daily suppressive therapy to prevent recurrences. Topical formulations of trifluridine and cidofovir are not commercially available. Extemporaneous compounding of topical products can be prepared using trifluridine ophthalmic solution and the IV formulation of cidofovir.

Continued

Table 1 Treatment of AIDS-Associated Opportunistic Infections—cont'd

Opportunistic Infection	Preferred Therapy	Alternative Therapy	Other Comments
VZV disease	*Primary Varicella Infection (Chickenpox): Uncomplicated Cases (for 5-7 days):* Valacyclovir 1 g PO tid *or* Famciclovir 500 mg PO tid. *Severe or Complicated Cases:* Acyclovir 10-15 mg/kg IV q8h for 7-10 days. May switch to oral valacyclovir, famciclovir, or acyclovir after defervescence if no evidence of visceral involvement. *Herpes Zoster (Shingles) Acute Localized Dermatomal:* For 7-10 days; consider longer duration if lesions are slow to resolve. Valacyclovir 1 g PO tid *or* Famciclovir 500 mg tid. *Extensive Cutaneous Lesion or Visceral Involvement:* Acyclovir 10-15 mg/kg IV q8h until clinical improvement is evident. May switch to PO therapy (valacyclovir, famciclovir, or acyclovir) after clinical improvement (i.e., when no new vesicle formation or improvement of signs and symptoms of visceral VZV), to complete a 10- to 14-day course. *Progressive Outer Retinal Necrosis:* Ganciclovir 5 mg/kg + foscarnet 90 mg/kg IV q12h + ganciclovir 2 mg/0.05 ml ± foscarnet 1.2 mg/0.05 ml intravitreal injection twice weekly *or* Initiate or optimize ART. *Acute Retinal Necrosis:* Acyclovir 10 mg/kg IV q8h for 10-14 days, followed by valacyclovir 1 g PO tid for 6 weeks.	*Primary Varicella Infection (Chickenpox): Uncomplicated Cases (for 5-7 days):* Acyclovir 800 mg PO 5 times/day *Herpes Zoster (Shingles) Acute Localized Dermatomal:* For 7-10 days; consider longer duration if lesions are slow to resolve. Acyclovir 800 mg PO 5 times/day	In managing VZV retinitis: Consultation with an ophthalmologist experienced in management of VZV retinitis is strongly recommended. Duration of therapy for VZV retinitis is not well defined and should be determined based on clinical, virologic, immunologic, and ophthalmologic responses. Optimization of ART is recommended for serious and difficult-to-treat VZV infections (e.g., retinitis, encephalitis).
Progressive multifocal leukoencephalopathy (JC virus infections)	There is no specific antiviral therapy for JC virus infection. The main treatment approach is to reverse the immunosuppression caused by HIV. Initiate ART immediately in ART-naïve patients. Optimize ART in patients who develop PML in phase of HIV viremia on ART.	None.	Corticosteroids may be used for PML-IRIS characterized by contrast enhancement, edema, or mass effect and with clinical deterioration.

ART, antiretroviral therapy; ARV, antiretroviral; bid, twice a day; CD4, CD4 T lymphocyte cell; CFU, colony-forming unit; CMV, cytomegalovirus; CNS, central nervous system; CSF, cerebrospinal fluid; CYP3A4, cytochrome P-450 3A4; DOT, directly observed therapy; DS, double strength; EMB, ethambutol; G6PD, glucose-6-phosphate dehydrogenase; GI, gastrointestinal; HSV, herpes simplex virus; ICU, intensive care unit; IM, intramuscular; INH, isoniazid; IRIS, immune reconstitution inflammatory syndrome; IV, intravenous; LP, lumbar puncture; MAC, *Mycobacterium avium* complex; mm Hg, millimeters of mercury; NSAID, nonsteroidal anti-inflammatory drugs; PCP, *Pneumocystis* pneumonia; PI, protease inhibitor; PML, progressive multifocal leukoencephalopathy; PO, oral; PZA, pyrazinamide; qid, four times a day; RFB, rifabutin; RIF, rifampin; SS, single strength; tid, three times daily; tiw, three times weekly; TMP-SMX, trimethoprim-sulfamethoxazole; VZV, varicella zoster virus.
Quality of Evidence for the Recommendation:
I: One or more randomized trials with clinical outcomes and/or validated laboratory endpoints
II: One or more well-designed, nonrandomized trials or observational cohort studies with long-term clinical outcomes
III: Expert opinion
Parrillo JE, Dellinger RP: *Critical care medicine: principles of diagnosis and management in the adult*, ed 2, Philadelphia, 2014, Elsevier.

REFERRAL

All patients with AIDS: to a physician knowledgeable and experienced in the management of the disease and its complications

SUGGESTED READINGS
Available at www.expertconsult.com

RELATED CONTENT

Acquired Immunodeficiency Syndrome (AIDS) (Patient Information)

Candidiasis, Cutaneous (Related Key Topic)
Candidiasis, Invasive (Related Key Topic)
Cryptosporidium Infection (Related Key Topic)
Cytomegalovirus Infection (Related Key Topic)
Herpes Simplex (Related Key Topic)
Histoplasmosis (Related Key Topic)
HIV Cognitive Dysfunction (Related Key Topic)
Human Immunodeficiency Virus (Related Key Topic)
Kaposi Sarcoma (Related Key Topic)
Pneumonia, *pneumocystis jiroveci (carinii)* (Related Key Topic)
Progressive Multifocal Leukoencephalopathy (Related Key Topic)

Toxoplasmosis (Related Key Topic)
Tuberculosis (Related Key Topic)

AUTHOR: **PHILIP A. CHAN, M.D., M.S.**

BASIC INFORMATION

DEFINITION

Actinic keratoses (AKs) are common skin lesions usually presenting as multiple erythematous or yellow-brown, dry, scaly lesions in the middle aged or elderly.

SYNONYMS

Solar keratosis
Senile keratosis
AK

ICD-10CM CODES
L57.0 Actinic keratosis

EPIDEMIOLOGY & DEMOGRAPHICS

INCIDENCE: In regions of the northern hemisphere, 11%-25% of adults have a minimum of one AK. In regions closer to the equator, 40%-60% of adults have a minimum of one AK.
PEAK INCIDENCE: The risk of squamous cell carcinoma in patients with AK is 6%-10%. Risk factors associated with increased risk of invasive squamous cell carcinoma arising from actinic keratosis include lesion location (lip, ear, extremities), lesion characteristics (ulceration, induration, hyperkeratotic, proliferative, inflamed, bleeding, large surface area and depth), pigmentation (any rapid changes in presentation, presence of multiple lesions, evidence of greater ultraviolet [UV]-induced skin damage), presence of concomitant illness (lymphoma, leukemia), and use of concomitant medications (immunosuppressive agents, medications that increase sun sensitivity)[1]
PREVALENCE:
- In the United States, 58.08 million per year.
- Highest prevalence in those with fair complexions with high sun exposure.
- Approximately 60% of predisposed individuals older than 40 years will have one AK.
- Caucasians' risk increases with age: at age 20-29 prevalence is <10%; at age 80-89, prevalence is approximately 75%.

PREDOMINANT SEX AND AGE: Males > females, age 65-74. Occurs most in those with fair complexions who burn rather than tan following sun exposure.
GENETICS: There is increased frequency of non-melanoma skin cancers connected to squamous cell cancers with the genetic conditions xeroderma pigmentosum, oculocutaneous albinism, epidermodysplasia verruciformis, dystrophic epidermolysis bullosa, Ferguson-Smith syndrome, and Muir-Torre syndrome.
RISK FACTORS:
- Immunosuppression, exposure to UV light, ionizing radiation, arsenic, human papillomavirus, cigarette smoke, chronic ulcers, thermal burns, chronic discoid lupus erythematosus, and nonhealing wounds.
- Lichen planus, lichen sclerosis, linear and classic porokeratosis, and disseminated superficial actinic porokeratosis.
- Age, gender, skin color, and mutations in p53 tumor suppressor gene.

PHYSICAL FINDINGS & CLINICAL PRESENTATION

- Typical lesions occur on sun-damaged skin, usually on the face and neck and the dorsal aspects of hands (Fig. 1) and forearms.
- Advanced lesions are characterized by a hard, spiky scale (Fig. 2) and usually measure 1 cm in diameter or less. Early lesions manifest with redness and minimal scale. With progression, scales become thicker and yellow and may resemble a small squamous cell carcinoma. On examinations, lesions are rough and gritty (Fig. 3).
- The surrounding skin frequently shows additional features of sun damage, including atrophy (Fig. 4), pigment changes, and telangiectasia.
- Classifications
  1. Hypertrophic AK with a cutaneous horn: Biopsy is necessary to distinguish the cutaneous horn from squamous cell carcinoma, seborrheic keratosis, verruca, and trichilemmoma and basal cell carcinoma. Hypertrophic AK has appearance of thick, scaling skin elevations.
  2. Lichenoid AK: Most commonly found on the torso and upper extremities. Must be distinguished from BCC due to pink and pearly characteristics.
  3. Proliferative AK: Often reappear after treatment and are characterized by a diameter >1 cm. Often occurs in same differential as Bowen's disease or SCC.
  4. Spreading pigmented AK: Must be biopsied to distinguish from lentigo maligna–type melanoma in situ as well as solar lentigo.
  5. Actinic cheilitis: Characterized by red and sometimes abrasive lesions around the border of the lips and skin.

ETIOLOGY

- Sun exposure, ionizing radiation.
- Arsenic, polycyclic hydrocarbon exposure.

DIAGNOSIS

DIFFERENTIAL DIAGNOSIS

- Heavily pigmented variants may be clinically mistaken for lentigo maligna.
- Basal cell or squamous cell carcinoma.
- Seborrheic keratosis.
- Eczema.
- Bowen disease (intraepithelial carcinoma).
- Wart.
- Lichenoid keratosis.
- Cutaneous lupus.

WORKUP

- History, physical, and lesion biopsy. Include risk assessment and family or personal history of skin cancers or previous skin lesions.

LABORATORY TESTS

- Skin biopsy in recurrent lesions or when diagnosis is unclear to rule out squamous cell or basal cell carcinoma.
- Microscopy reveals atypical keratinocytes in the lower epidermis basal layers. They are enlarged and often lack normal polarity. The thickness of the epidermis can be compromised with a distribution of atrophic to hyperplastic. Abnormal keratinocytes can cause parakeratosis of the overlying stratum corneum. Visible signs of an alternating orthohyperkeratosis can overlie the spared epithelium, causing the signature "flag sign." Additionally, there is a distinct margin between normal epidermis and the region of AK at lateral edges. Histologic subtypes are hypertrophic, acantholytic, lichenoid, and bowenoid, which are characterized by a thick stratum corneum, lack of intracellular

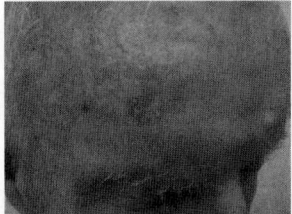

FIG. 4 Actinic keratosis (shown here on a patient's forehead) is often best appreciated by its rough, tactile quality, similar to that of sandpaper. (From Ferri F et al: *Ferri's fast facts in dermatology,* Philadelphia, 2010, Saunders.)

1. Rigel DS, Stein Goold LF: The importance of early diagnosis and treatment of actinic keratosis. *J Am Acad Dermatol* 68:S20-27, 2013.

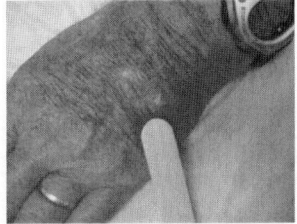

FIG. 1 Several scaly, adherent, yellow-brown lesions on the sun-exposed dorsum of the hand. (From Ferri F et al: *Ferri's fast facts in dermatology,* Philadelphia, 2010, Saunders.)

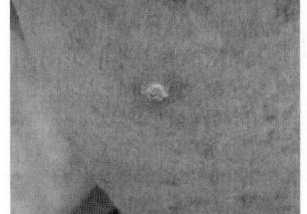

FIG. 2 Scaly, raised lesion on sun-exposed back. Pain was elicited when scraping this lesion. (From Ferri F et al: *Ferri's fast facts in dermatology,* Philadelphia, 2010, Saunders.)

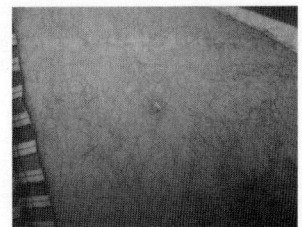

FIG. 3 Raised, rough, gritty actinic keratosis on the anterior thigh of an outdoorsman. (From Ferri F et al: *Ferri's fast facts in dermatology,* Philadelphia, 2010, Saunders.)

cohesion, presence of lymphocytic infiltrate in papillary dermis, and either lack of association of adnexal epithelium or full epithelial thickness with pleomorphic keratinocytes, respectively.

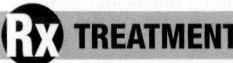 **TREATMENT**

NONPHARMACOLOGIC THERAPY

- Cryotherapy with liquid nitrogen: treatment of choice for most isolated, superficial AKs
- Carbon dioxide laser.
- Dermabrasion.
- Chemical peel.
- Curettage.
- Excision.
- Photodynamic therapy with 5-aminolevulinic acid and blue light (16 minutes) or methyl aminolevulinate and red light (7-10 minutes).

ACUTE GENERAL Rx

- Topical 5-fluorouracil (5-FU) bid for 4-6 weeks. Table 1 summarizes guidelines for duration of 5-FU therapy according to site.
- Topical diclofenac sodium 3% gel bid for 60-90 days.
- Topical imiquimod 5% cream bid for 3-4 months.
- Oral retinoids.
- Topical ingenol mebutate 0.05% gel applied for 2 days with exception of face—or 0.015% for 3 days. Combination medication therapy or nonpharmacologic therapy with pharmacologic therapy is common (especially in refractory AK).

- A 10% nanoemulsion gel formulation of the porphyrin-based photosensitizers aminolevulinic acid (Ameluz) is available for use in combination with a narrow-band red light photodynamic therapy (PDT) lamp (BF-RhodoLED) for mild to moderate severity AK on face and scalp.
- Table 2 describes preparations for treatment of actinic keratosis.

REFERRAL

- To a dermatologist for biopsy of suspicious lesions, then follow up minimum annually or semiannually.

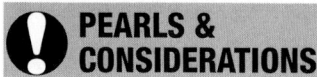 **PEARLS & CONSIDERATIONS**

COMMENTS

- AKs are of particular importance because they are a sensitive indicator of exposure to UV light and strongly predict the likelihood of developing cutaneous squamous cell carcinoma.
- The cumulative probability of development of invasive squamous cell carcinoma in patients with 10 or more AKs has been estimated at 14% in a 5-year period.
- It is estimated that up to 10% of AKs tend to progress to invasive carcinoma. Factors associated with increased risk of invasive squamous cell carcinoma include presence of multiple lesions, large surface area and depth, hyperkeratotic proliferative lesions, location on lip, ear, and extremities and concomitant illness (leukemia, lymphoma),

and use of immunosuppressive agents and agents that increase sun sensitivity.

PREVENTION

- Avoidance of sun exposure or tanning booths.
- Use of sunscreens.
- Routine self-skin examinations.
- Pharmaceutical prevention:
  1. Mild to moderate reduction of AK formation has been documented with the use of topical tretinoin, isotretinoin, and arotinoid methylsulfonyl.
  2. Nicotinamide as preventive rx has been documented to have a possible 30% relative reduction in AK.
  3. Decreased AK development has been documented with the use of high-SPF sunscreens.
  4. Decreased AK development has been seen in patients with xeroderma pigmentosum who used DNA repair enzymes.
  5. Decreased AK formation has been documented in high-risk patients (specifically those with xeroderma pigmentosum, nevoid basal cell carcinoma syndrome, and organ transplantation recipients) with the use of oral retinoids.

SUGGESTED READINGS

Available at www.expertconsult.com

AUTHORS: **FRED F. FERRI, M.D.,** and **HEATHER FERRI, D.O.**

TABLE 1   Guidelines for Duration of 5-Fluorouracil Therapy According to Site

Site	Early Signs of Inflammation (days)	Duration of Treatment (weeks)
Face, lips	3-5	2-4
Scalp	4-7	3-5
Neck	4-7	2-4
Arms, hands, legs	10-14	4-8
Back	10-14	4-6
Chest	10-14	4-6

From Habif TP: *Clinical dermatology*, ed 6, Philadelphia, 2016, Elsevier.

TABLE 2   Preparations for Treatment of Actinic Keratosis

Product	Active Ingredient	Packaging
Carac	0.5% fluorouracil	30-g cream
Efudex	2% fluorouracil	10-ml liquid
	5% fluorouracil	10-ml liquid
	5% fluorouracil	25-g cream
Fluoroplex	1% fluorouracil	30-ml solution, 30-g cream
	1% fluorouracil	
Aldara	5% imiquimod	Cream—box of 12 or 24 packets
Zyclara	2.5%, 3.75% imiquimod	Cream—box of 28 packets, 7.5- and 15-g pump bottle

From Habif TP: *Clinical dermatology*, ed 6, Philadelphia, 2016, Elsevier.

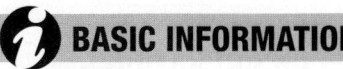 BASIC INFORMATION

DEFINITION
Acute bronchitis is a self-limited inflammation of trachea and bronchi.

SYNONYMS
Chest cold

ICD-10CM CODES
J20.9 Acute bronchitis, unspecified

EPIDEMIOLOGY & DEMOGRAPHICS
- Highest incidence in smokers, older adults, and young children and during winter months.
- In the U.S. there are nearly 30 million ambulatory visits annually for cough, leading to more than 12 million diagnoses of "bronchitis."
- Acute lower respiratory tract infection is the most common condition treated in primary care.

PHYSICAL FINDINGS & CLINICAL PRESENTATION
- In most cases, acute bronchitis begins with signs and symptoms typical of the common cold syndrome (nasal congestion, sore throat), followed shortly by the onset of cough
- Cough, usually worse in the morning, often productive; mainly caused by transient bronchial hyperresponsiveness
- Low-grade fever
- Substernal discomfort worsened by coughing
- Postnasal drip, pharyngeal injection
- Rhonchi that may clear after cough, occasional wheezing
- Various host factors (age, immune status, smoking, underlying medical conditions) can influence illness severity and clinical presentation
- In mild cases, the illness lasts only 7 to 10 days, whereas in others, cough may persist for up to 3 weeks or longer

ETIOLOGY
- Viral infections are the leading cause of bronchitis (rhinovirus, influenza virus, adenovirus, respiratory syncytial virus)
- Atypical organisms (Mycoplasma, Chlamydia pneumoniae)
- Bacterial infections (Bordetella pertussis, Haemophilus influenzae, Moraxella, Streptococcus pneumoniae)
- Table 1 summarizes viral and bacterial causes of acute bronchitis

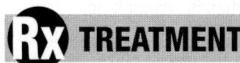 DIAGNOSIS

DIFFERENTIAL DIAGNOSIS
- Pneumonia
- Asthma
- Sinusitis
- Bronchiolitis
- Aspiration
- Cystic fibrosis
- Pharyngitis
- Cough secondary to medications
- Neoplasm (elderly patients)
- Influenza
- Allergic aspergillosis
- Gastroesophageal reflux disease
- Congestive heart failure (in elderly patients)
- Bronchogenic neoplasm

WORKUP
Seldom necessary (e.g., to rule out pneumonia, neoplasm)

LABORATORY TESTS
Laboratory tests are generally not necessary.

IMAGING STUDIES
Chest x-ray is usually reserved for patients with suspected pneumonia, influenza, or underlying chronic obstructive pulmonary disease (COPD) and no improvement with therapy.

TREATMENT

NONPHARMACOLOGIC THERAPY
- Avoidance of tobacco and other pulmonary irritants
- Increased fluid intake
- Use of vaporizer to increase room humidity

TABLE 1 Viral and Bacterial Causes of Acute Bronchitis

Pathogen	Seasonality	Comments
Influenza viruses	Winter	Local epidemics last 6-8 wk during which clinical illness of cough and fever has high predictive value; laboratory diagnosis readily available; early neuraminidase inhibitor therapy effective
Rhinoviruses	Fall and spring	Most frequent cause of common cold syndrome; immunity is serotype specific
Coronaviruses	Winter to spring	Cause common cold syndrome; newer strains are difficult to culture and require RT-PCR for diagnosis
Adenoviruses	Year round, winter epidemics	High attack rates in closed populations such as persons living in military barracks or college dormitories; serotype-specific immunity
Respiratory syncytial virus (RSV)	Late fall to early spring	Attack rates approach 75% in neonates, 3%-5% in adults; associated with wheezing in all age groups; rapid antigen test accurate in children but requires culture or RT-PCR to diagnose in adults
Human metapneumovirus (hMPV)	Winter to early spring	Associated with wheezing in adults and in infants; difficult to isolate in tissue culture and often requires RT-PCR
Parainfluenza viruses	Fall to winter	Similar to RSV and hMPV, parainfluenza viruses primarily pediatric pathogens but can cause severe acute disease in some adults
Measles virus	Year round	Can cause respiratory disease in malnourished children; illness causes transient immune suppression
Mycoplasma pneumoniae	Year round, fall outbreaks	Long incubation period (10-21 days) results in staggered epidemic pattern in families; nonproductive persistent cough typical; diagnosed by IgM serology; treated with macrolide, quinolone, or tetracycline antibiotics
Chlamydia pneumoniae	Year round	Associated with sinusitis; diagnosis by RT-PCR not readily available
Bordetella pertussis	Year round	Severe illness in nonimmunized children; illness milder in partially immune adults; can be associated with prolonged cough; adults often reservoir for epidemics; early therapy with antibiotics can reduce spread

From Bennett JE, Dolin R, Blaser MJ: *Mandell, Douglas, and Bennett's principles and practice of infectious diseases*, ed 8, Philadelphia, 2015, Saunders.
RT-PCR, Reverse-transcriptase polymerase chain reaction.

ACUTE GENERAL Rx

- Therapy is generally symptomatic and directed at relief of cough and wheezing.
- Inhaled bronchodilators (e.g., albuterol, metaproterenol) PRN for 1 to 2 wk in patients with wheezing or troublesome cough. Inhaled albuterol has been proven effective in reducing the duration of cough in adults with uncomplicated acute bronchitis.
- Cough suppression with dextromethorphan and guaifenesin is commonly recommended; addition of codeine for cough suppression if cough is severe and is significantly interrupting patient's sleep pattern.
- Use of antibiotics (TMP-SMX, amoxicillin, doxycycline, cefuroxime) for acute bronchitis is generally not indicated; should be considered only in patients with concomitant COPD and purulent sputum or in patients with suspected pertussis. In the few cases of acute bronchitis caused by *B. pertussis* or atypical bacteria such as *C. pneumoniae* or *Mycoplasma pneumoniae,* early use of macrolide antibiotics is reasonable.
- Antibiotics are overused in patients with acute bronchitis (70% to 90% of office visits for acute bronchitis result in treatment with antibiotics); this practice pattern is contributing to increases in resistant organisms.
- Trials have shown that there are no significant differences in patients receiving antibiotics compared with those receiving placebo in overall clinical improvements or limitations in work or other activities. There was a significant increase in adverse effects in the antibiotic group, particularly gastrointestinal symptoms.[1]

CHRONIC Rx

Avoidance of tobacco and other pulmonary irritants

DISPOSITION

- Complete recovery within 7 to 10 days in most patients.
- Patients should be informed to expect to have a cough for 10 to 14 days after the visit.

REFERRAL

For pulmonary function testing only in patients with recurrent bronchitis and suspected underlying pulmonary disease.

---

[1]Smith SM, Smucny J, Fahey T: Antibiotics for acute bronchitis, *JAMA* 312:2678, 2014.

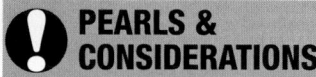

PEARLS & CONSIDERATIONS

COMMENTS

- Intervention studies reveal that patient and physician education are effective in reducing the use of antibiotic therapy. No offer or delayed offer of antibiotics for acute uncomplicated lower respiratory tract infection is acceptable, is associated with little difference in symptom resolution, and is likely to reduce antibiotic use and beliefs in the effectiveness of antibiotics.
- It is helpful to refer to acute bronchitis as a "chest cold." Patients should be informed that antibiotics are probably not going to be beneficial and may result in significant side effects.

SUGGESTED READINGS

Available at www.expertconsult.com

RELATED CONTENT

Acute Bronchitis (Patient Information)

AUTHOR: **FRED F. FERRI, M.D.**

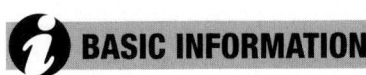

BASIC INFORMATION

DEFINITION

Ogilvie's syndrome is characterized by acute massive dilation of the cecum and right colon, with occasional extension to the rectum, in the absence of any mechanical obstruction. Oftentimes, acute colonic pseudo-obstruction occurs after surgery, and it can also be seen in patients with significant underlying medical illnesses. Cecal diameter on abdominal radiographs greater than nine centimeters is considered to be the threshold where spontaneous perforation becomes more likely. Medications such as opiates and anticholinergics also contribute to the development of this condition.

SYNONYMS

Ogilvie's syndrome
ACPO
Acute megacolon

ICD-10CM CODES
K56.6   Other and unspecified intestinal obstruction

EPIDEMIOLOGY & DEMOGRAPHICS

INCIDENCE: Unknown
PEAK INCIDENCE: Unknown
PREVALENCE: Unknown
PREDOMINANT SEX AND AGE: Although recent data is lacking, data from a retrospective study in 1986 suggested a male predominance with average age of onset in the 6th decade. In general, prevalence is thought to increase with age, although affected females tend to be younger because of the association of acute colonic pseudo-obstruction with obstetric complications.
GENETICS: None
RISK FACTORS: Elderly patients seem to be at greatest risk. Other risk factors include significant underlying medical illness, sepsis, electrolyte abnormalities, recent cardiac events, certain medications (opiates, anticholinergics, phenothiazines, benzodiazepines, calcium channel blockers, chemotherapeutic agents, and antiparkinsonian agents), and postoperative patients (Box 1).

PHYSICAL FINDINGS & CLINICAL PRESENTATION:

- Acute abdominal distention and crampy abdominal pain are the most common symptoms associated with Ogilvie's syndrome. The distention can be so severe that it may lead to labored breathing. Nausea, vomiting, obstipation, constipation, and, paradoxically, diarrhea, can also be seen but are not consistently present. It has been estimated that 40% to 50% of patients continue to pass flatus.
- Physical exam is significant for massive abdominal distention that is tympanic to percussion and varying degrees of abdominal pain or discomfort are also present. Hypoactive or hyperactive bowel sounds are often described. Peritoneal signs are often absent early on but their presence is concerning for imminent perforation.

ETIOLOGY:

- Colonic motor and secretory functions are mediated by the autonomic nervous system with the ascending colon receiving parasympathetic innervation from the medulla oblongata via the vagus nerve, which increases gut motility, and sympathetic innervation from the spinal cord, which decreases motility. It is thought that parasympathetic dysfunction is the main driving force that leads to Ogilvie's syndrome but the exact mechanism is unknown.

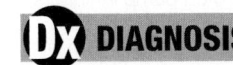

DIAGNOSIS

DIFFERENTIAL DIAGNOSIS

- Mechanical obstruction
- Volvulus
- Intussusception
- Ileus
- Toxic megacolon

WORKUP

- History should be focused on the perceived progression of distention and timing of most

---

BOX 1   Clinical Factors Predisposing to Ogilvie's Syndrome or Acute Colonic Pseudo-Obstruction

Cardiovascular
- Heart failure, stroke
- Gut ischemia
Critical illness
- Severe sepsis
- Acute pancreatitis
- Shock or hypoxemia
Postoperative state or trauma
- Intestinal manipulation
- Peritonitis
- Immobility and dehydration
- Vertebral, pelvic or hip fracture/surgery
- Retroperitoneal hematoma
Metabolic factors
- Hypokalemia and hyperglycemia
- Hypothyroidism, diabetes mellitus
- Liver or renal failure
- Amyloidosis
Drugs
- α-Adrenergic agonists, dopamine
- Clonidine and dexmedetomidine
- Opioids
- Anticholinergics, calcium channel antagonists
- Antipsychotics
- Antidepressants
- High-dose phosphodiesterase inhibitors
Gastrointestinal infections
- Cytomegalovirus, herpes zoster
- Tuberculosis
Neurologic
- Transection of the spinal cord
- Low spinal cord disease
- Parkinson's disease
Obstetric
- Caesarean section
- Normal delivery

From Vincent JL, Abraham E, Moore FA, Kochanek PM, Fink MP: *Textbook of critical care*, ed 6, Philadelphia, 2011, Saunders.

---

recent flatus or bowel movement as well as determining any predisposing factors such as recent surgery, severe illness, and recent medication changes. Physical examination should focus on assessing the degree of abdominal distention and percussion to evaluate for tympanic sounds, which is a hallmark of Ogilvie's syndrome. Serial abdominal exams should be performed to ensure no peritoneal signs such a rebound, guarding, or rigidity that would suggest impending or frank perforation.
- Laboratory evaluation should center on metabolic abnormalities as well as lactic acidosis and leukocytosis that can both be used as a barometer of the degree of the patient's underlying illness as well as a marker for impending perforation.
- Imaging of the abdomen with plain radiograph is important for tracking degree of distention.

LABORATORY TESTS

- Metabolic abnormalities such as hypocalcemia, hypomagnesemia, and hypokalemia are commonly present and should be corrected accordingly.
- Leukocytosis as well as lactic acidosis for markers of underlying disease and impending perforation.

IMAGING STUDIES

- Plain and upright abdominal radiographs (Fig. 1) are important to establish degree of colonic distention, which often involves the cecum but can also extend to the splenic flexure or rectum. Haustral markings are usually normal.
- CT scan or enema-enhanced radiograph is imperative to confirm the diagnosis and rule out underlying mechanical obstruction.

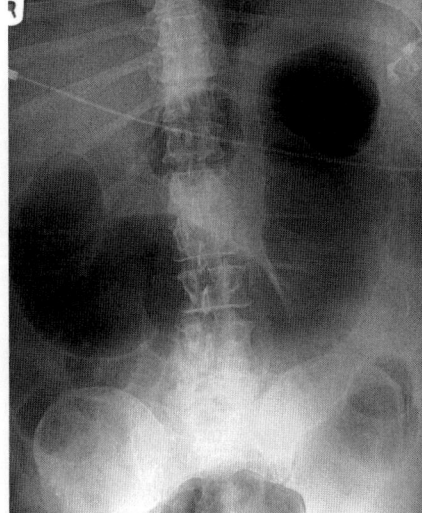

FIG. 1 Plain abdominal radiograph of patient with Ogilvie's syndrome 11 days after surgery for ruptured aneurysm of abdominal aorta. Dilation (probably due to ischemia) is present in both right and left colon. Syndrome resolved with vasodilators and intravenous neostigmine. (From Vincent JL, Abraham E, Moore FA, Kochanek PM, Fink MP: *Textbook of critical care*, ed 6, Philadelphia, 2011, Saunders.)

Rx TREATMENT

The goals of treatment are to decompress the colon in order to relieve the patient's abdominal discomfort and also mitigate the risk of developing intestinal ischemia or frank perforation.

NONPHARMACOLOGIC THERAPY

- Supportive care with plain radiographs every 12-24 hr, serial abdominal exams, elimination of potential precipitants (medications, treatment of underlying medical illness), correction of electrolyte abnormalities, restricting PO intake, gastric decompression with NG tube to intermittent suction, rectal decompression with rectal tube attached to gravity, IV fluids, encouraging ambulation if possible, and alternating the patient in bed between right and left lateral decubitus as well as prone positioning with hips elevated are all appropriate nonpharmacologic approaches that can be made initially in the absence of colonic distention >12 cm or significant abdominal pain.
- Colonoscopic decompression with or without placement of a decompression tube is often the next step in management although use of this technique remains controversial as some studies indicate that the majority of patients spontaneously resolve within 48 hr. The risk of complication with colonoscopy in this setting is 3%, with a quoted death rate of 1%. Other studies suggest a success rate of 69% to 90% with colonoscopic decompression.
- Colonoscopic decompression is indicated when supportive measures fail, there is clinical deterioration, or colonic diameter is between 11-13 cm. Placement of a decompression tube at the time of colonoscopy is thought to reduce the need for repeat colonoscopic decompression, which is required in about 40% of cases, but no trials have been done to compare rates of repeat decompression with and without decompression tube placement.
- Alternative minimally invasive options which are usually reserved for failed colonoscopic decompression include percutaneous tube cecostomy performed under radiologic guidance and percutaneous endoscopic colostomy, which are both techniques that grant percutaneous access to the colon for both decompression and irrigation to promote transit.
- Surgical management is reserved for those who have failed minimally invasive approaches or for patients with peritonitis or perforation. Surgical cecostomy tube or right hemicolectomy can be performed in the absence of perforation whereas ileostomy, colectomy, and Hartmann procedure can be performed in patients who have perforated or who have significant ischemia.

BOX 2   Strategies to Prevent Ogilvie's Syndrome in the Critically Ill

- Early resuscitation of the circulation
- Minimizing prolonged infusion of high doses of α-adrenergic drugs
- Minimizing the use of dopamine
- Minimizing the prolonged use of opioids
- Use of thoracic epidural anesthesia
- Minimally invasive or laparoscopic surgery
- Selective decontamination of the digestive tract
- Avoiding antibiotics that disrupt growth of anaerobic fecal bacteria
- Early oral or enteral feeding
- Avoidance of proton pump inhibitors
- Early mobilization and ambulation
- Promoting timely defecation with
  - Oral polyethylene glycol from day 3
  - Intravenous neostigmine from day 5

From Vincent JL, Abraham E, Moore FA, Kochanek PM, Fink MP: *Textbook of critical care*, ed 6, Philadelphia, 2011, Saunders.

ACUTE GENERAL Rx

- Neostigmine is an IV anticholinesterase inhibitor that induces rapid colonic decompression in 80% to 100% of appropriate candidates with a median response rate of 4 minutes at a starting dose of 2 mg, but requires close cardiovascular monitoring at the time of its administration and has several contraindications. Dose adjustments are required in chronic kidney disease and caution should be used in patients who have bradyarrhythmias, recent myocardial infarction, beta-blocker use, and asthma. Atropine should be made available at bedside and administration of glycopyrrolate, an anticholinergic agent, should be considered to decrease the risk of bradycardia and bronchoconstriction.
- Methylnaltrexone, a peripherally acting opiate receptor antagonist, can also be considered in cases thought to be precipitated by opiates but little data supports its use at this time.

CHRONIC Rx

- None

COMPLEMENTARY AND ALTERNATIVE MEDICINE

- None

DISPOSITION

- Close inpatient monitoring is indicated until there is return of spontaneous bowel function and resolution of abdominal distention.

REFERRAL

- Ogilvie's syndrome is best managed in a team approach involving both surgeons and gastroenterologists. Administration of neostigmine in proper candidates or decompressive colonoscopy should be pursued in patients with absence of peritoneal signs. If there is evidence of perforation, surgical management is indicated.

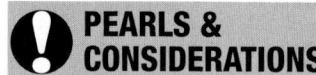

! PEARLS & CONSIDERATIONS

COMMENTS

- Maximal supportive care should be initiated for up to 48 hr barring any significant abdominal pain or massive distention >12 cm on imaging.
- Administration of neostigmine is suggested in appropriate candidates.
- Colonic decompression should be attempted with or without decompression tube placement in patients who fail neostigmine or those who have contraindications to its use.
- Minimally invasive fluoroscopic, endoscopic, or surgical approaches are rarely needed. Surgery is reserved for patients who show signs of perforation.
- Oral laxatives should be discontinued with diagnosis but should be restarted once decompression is achieved.

PREVENTION

Box 2 describes some prevention strategies for Ogilvie's Syndrome in the critically ill.

SUGGESTED READINGS

Available at www.expertconsult.com

AUTHOR: **JASON D. FERREIRA, M.D.**

BASIC INFORMATION

Acute coronary syndrome (ACS) represents a spectrum of clinical disorders that includes unstable angina (UA), non–ST-elevation myocardial infarction (NSTEMI), and ST-elevation myocardial infarction (STEMI). Although the severity of disease will vary between the three subsets of ACS, they share a common clinical presentation and pathophysiology. This syndrome is typically caused by atherosclerotic coronary artery disease (CAD). In this spectrum, UA and NSTEMI are represented electrocardiographically by the absence of ST-segment elevation in the appropriate clinical setting (i.e., chest discomfort). NSTEMI is represented by the addition of positive cardiac biomarkers. STEMI is characterized by ST-segment elevation or presumed new left bundle branch block on electrocardiogram (ECG). ACS should be thought of as a continuous spectrum as UA will often progress to a myocardial infarction if left untreated (Table 1). Because of this continuum, the 2014 American College of Cardiology/American Heart Association (ACC/AHA) guidelines have grouped UA and NSTEMI into a single category called non–ST-elevation ACS (NSTE-ACS).

SYNONYMS

Unstable angina
NSTEMI
STEMI
Acute myocardial infarction

ICD-10CM CODES

I20.0	Unstable angina
I21.0-I21.3	ST elevation (STEMI)
I21.4	non-ST elevation (NSTEMI) myocardial infarction
I24.9	Acute ischemic heart disease, unspecified

EPIDEMIOLOGY & DEMOGRAPHICS

INCIDENCE: In the U.S., there are more than 780,000 cases of ACS yearly. Approximately 70% of myocardial infarctions are listed as NSTEMI, with the remainder being listed as STEMI. Coronary heart disease accounted for approximately 1 out of every 7 deaths in the U.S. in 2015. Patients with NSTE-ACS have more cardiac and noncardiac comorbidities than patients with STEMI. The underlying etiology, atherosclerotic CAD, is the number one cause of mortality.

PREDOMINANT SEX AND AGE: In evaluating chest pain, male gender and older age are important clinical factors that can identify ACS as a potential cause. In a 2005-2011 study sponsored by National Heart, Lung, and Blood Institute, the average age-adjusted first MI or fatal coronary heart disease rates per 1000 population in patients age 35 to 84 years of age were 3.7 for white men, 5.9 for black men, 2.1 for white women, and 4.0 for black women. As noted in this study, heart disease affects African Americans disproportionately, with more than 39,000 deaths from heart disease

in 2013. Heart disease is the number one killer of women. It takes more lives than all forms of cancer combined.

RISK FACTORS: Hypertension, diabetes mellitus, dyslipidemia, tobacco use, family history of premature CAD (CAD in a male first-degree relative younger than 55 years or a female younger than 65 years). Refer to the topic "Angina Pectoris" for an extensive list of risk factors. Presence of these risk factors causes damage to the vascular endothelium and progression of atherosclerotic coronary artery plaques.

PHYSICAL FINDINGS & CLINICAL PRESENTATION

- Symptoms often, but not always, include chest discomfort described as a pressure that may radiate to the shoulders, neck, jaw, or back. Typical angina is substernal in location, brought on by emotional or physical stress, and relieved with rest and/or nitroglycerin.
- Women, diabetics, and the elderly often have an atypical presentation for ACS.
- Unstable angina has three typical presentations:
  - Rest angina: angina occurring at rest and prolonged usually for longer than 20 minutes.
  - New-onset angina: new-onset angina of at least Canadian Cardiovascular Society (CCS) class III symptoms (Table 2).
  - Increasing angina: previously diagnosed angina that has become distinctly more frequent, longer in duration, or lower in threshold (i.e., increased by ≥1 CCS class to at least CCS class III severity).
- "Anginal equivalents" may include dyspnea, nausea, vomiting, and fatigue.
- ECG for NSTE-ACS may reveal ST-segment depression and/or T-wave inversion. ECG for definition of STEMI will reveal at least 1-mm ST-segment elevation in two contiguous leads or new left bundle branch block in the appropriate clinical presentation.
- Physical exam findings alone are insufficient for the diagnosis of ACS. It is, however, important to assess the patient's hemodynamic stability and volume status. The patient may be diaphoretic and tachycardic. Signs of heart failure may be present, which include elevated jugular venous pressure (JVP), presence of an S3 gallop, and peripheral edema. The degree

of heart failure with MI can be represented by the Killip classification, with the greater the Killip classification, the greater the mortality noted:
- Killip Class 1 is no heart failure.
- Killip Class 2 includes individuals with rales, elevated JVP, and S3 on exam.
- Killip Class 3 includes individuals with frank pulmonary edema.
- Killip Class 4 describes individuals in cardiogenic shock or hypotension with evidence of vasoconstriction noted.

ETIOLOGY

Atherosclerotic CAD is the underlying etiology. The hallmark of ACS is the vulnerable atherosclerotic plaque, which typically has a thin fibrous cap and a large lipid core. This vulnerable plaque ultimately ruptures, which leads to platelet activation and aggregation, leading to thrombus formation. STEMI typically results from complete thrombotic occlusion of a coronary artery, whereas NSTE-ACS often has partial occlusion. Angiographically, it is often the intermediate coronary artery lesions (30% to 50% diameter vessel stenosis) that lead to subtotal or total vessel occlusion in two thirds of STEMI cases.

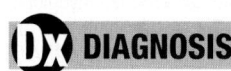 **DIAGNOSIS**

DIFFERENTIAL DIAGNOSIS

Chest pain mimicking ACS may be the result of various underlying disorders, some of which are also accompanied by ECG changes and/or cardiac biomarker release. Examples include acute pulmonary embolism, acute aortic dissection, pericarditis, myocarditis, costochondritis, pneumonia, tension pneumothorax, perforating ulcer, or Boerhaave syndrome. Refer to topics "Angina Pectoris," "Coronary Artery Disease," and "Myocardial Infarction" for extensive differential diagnoses of chest pain.

WORKUP

Focused history and physical exam, 12-lead ECG, cardiac biomarkers, and chest radiograph (CXR). Initial biomarkers may not be positive early in the disease process. Often serial biomarkers are drawn every 6 to 8 hours for a total of three sets for the purposes of ruling out myocardial infarction (MI), or until peak to determine the severity of an established MI. Echocardiogram may reveal

---

TABLE 1 Acute Coronary Syndromes

Spectrum of Acute Coronary Syndrome			
	Unstable Angina	**NSTEMI**	**STEMI**
Chest discomfort	1	1	1
Cardiac biomarkers	2	1	1
ECG changes	TWI and/or ST depression	TWI and/or ST depression	ST elevation or presumed new left bundle branch block
Pathophysiology	Partial/transient thrombotic occlusion	Partial/transient thrombotic occlusion	Complete thrombotic occlusion

NSTEMI, Non–ST-segment elevation myocardial infarction; *STEMI,* ST-segment myocardial infarction; *TWI,* T-wave inversion; *ECG,* electrocardiogram.

TABLE 2 Grading of Angina Pectoris According to CCS Classification

Class	Description of Stage
I	"Ordinary physical activity does not cause ... angina," such as walking or climbing stairs. Angina occurs with strenuous, rapid, or prolonged exertion at work or recreation.
II	"Slight limitation of ordinary activity." Angina occurs on walking or climbing stairs rapidly; walking uphill; walking or stair climbing after meals; in cold, in wind, or under emotional stress; or only during the few hours after awakening. Angina occurs on walking 0.2 blocks on the level and climbing 0.1 flight of ordinary stairs at a normal pace and under normal conditions.
III	"Marked limitations of ordinary physical activity." Angina occurs on walking 1 to 2 blocks on the level and climbing 1 flight of stairs under normal conditions and at a normal pace.
IV	"Inability to carry on any physical activity without discomfort—anginal symptoms may be present at rest."

Adapted with permission from Campeau L. Grading of angina pectoris (letter), Circulation 54:522–523, 1976. © 1976, American Heart Association, Inc.

From: Braunwald E et al.: ACC/AHA guidelines for the management of patients with unstable angina and non–ST-segment elevation myocardial infarction. A report of the American College of Cardiology/American Heart Association Task Force on Practice Guidelines (Committee on the Management of Patients With Unstable Angina), *J Am Coll Cardiol* 36:970-1062, 2000.

new regional wall motion abnormalities. Fig. 1 summarizes the evaluation of patients for acute coronary syndrome.

LABORATORY TESTS

- Cardiac biomarkers, which include creatine kinase (CK), its MB isoenzyme, myoglobin, and troponin I or T, will be positive in the setting of NSTEMI or STEMI. See Fig. 2, *A* for timing of release of each biomarker. Troponin I is the most sensitive biomarker for cardiac myocyte damage and also predicts 42-day mortality in ACS. Troponin I is considered the gold standard biomarker for diagnosis of myocardial infarction (Fig. 2, *B*).
- Testing for B-type natriuretic peptide (BNP) has a class IIb recommendation in the 2014 NSTE-ACS guidelines for use as a prognostic tool in patients presenting with an MI. BNP >80 portends a high risk of death at initial presentation of a STEMI.
- A complete fasting lipid panel and Hgb A1c should be obtained during the hospital admission.

RISK MODELS AND RISK SCORES

Risk models and scores such as TIMI (see "Risk Assessment" in "Myocardial Infarction" topic), PURSUIT, and GRACE based on clinical, ECG, and laboratory data at presentation help to discriminate patients at high risk versus low risk for short- and intermediate-term adverse outcomes (Fig. 2, *C*).

IMAGING STUDIES

- A CXR to assist in evaluating for volume status and for other possible causes of chest discomfort.
- In patients for whom ECG and cardiac biomarkers are nondiagnostic but the suspicion for ACS is high given the history, an echocardiogram may be helpful to assess left ventricular (LV) function and regional wall motion abnormalities.
- Coronary CT angiography can be performed in patients with possible ACS, a normal 12-lead EKG result, negative troponin results, and no history of coronary artery disease (Class IIa)

- Cardiac stress testing (treadmill ECG, imaging stress studies using echocardiography or nuclear modalities) may further help to diagnose and risk stratify these patients. (See Coronary Artery Disease topic in Section I.)
- Coronary angiogram/cardiac catheterization will reveal coronary artery luminal irregularities/stenotic lesions. In patients with ACS who undergo coronary angiography, approximately 25% will have one vessel disease, 25% will have two vessel disease, 25% will have three vessel disease, 10% will have left main disease, and 15% will have coronary stenosis of <50% or normal coronaries.

℞ TREATMENT

The overall goal for patients with NSTE-ACS is to relieve myocardial ischemia and to prevent recurrent cardiovascular events. Antithrombotic therapy is needed to reduce thrombus burden, prevent further thrombosis, and improve coronary artery flow. Revascularization is needed to prevent further events and improve flow within the coronary artery lumen. For patients with STEMI, the goal is immediate reperfusion therapy, whether it is chemical (i.e., thrombolysis) or mechanical (i.e., percutaneous coronary intervention [PCI]), and time from onset of ischemia to revascularization is an important prognostic factor. STEMI patients presenting to a hospital with PCI capability should be treated with primary PCI within 90 minutes of first medical contact (Figs. 3 and 4). At non–PCI-capable hospitals where the first medical contact to balloon time is more than 120 minutes, thrombolytic therapy should be given if no contraindications are present; thrombolytics should not be administered 24 hours after initial diagnosis of STEMI. Absolute contraindications to thrombolytic therapy include the following: history of hemorrhagic cerebrovascular accident (CVA), history of CVA, dementia or central nervous system damage within the past year, head trauma or brain surgery within the past 6 months, or intracranial neoplasm. Other contraindications include

suspected aortic dissection, internal bleeding within the past 6 weeks, active bleeding or known bleeding disorder, and traumatic CPR within the past 3 weeks.

NONPHARMACOLOGIC THERAPY

- STEMI is a medical emergency and requires immediate reperfusion therapy; the best outcomes are seen in cardiac catheterization with primary PCI. Guidelines call for a goal door-to-balloon time of ≤90 minutes.
- Patients with NSTE-ACS should be risk stratified in conjunction with the cardiology consult service. Risk scores such as the TIMI and GRACE scores can be used to decide between an early invasive strategy and an ischemia-guided strategy. Overall, an early invasive strategy is associated with better outcomes in patients with higher risk (i.e., TIMI score >3 or GRACE >140) and involves cardiac catheterization followed by revascularization with PCI or coronary artery bypass grafting (CABG) within 4 to 24 hours of presentation. An ischemia-guided strategy involves aggressive medical management and revascularization only if ischemia recurs or is documented on noninvasive testing. This should only be reserved for selected patients with low-risk scores (TIMI score 0-2). The early invasive strategy can be further stratified by timing:
  1. Immediate (within 2 hours): Patients with refractory or recurrent angina despite optimal initial treatment, signs or symptoms of heart failure, new or worsening mitral regurgitation, hemodynamic instability, sustained ventricular tachycardia or ventricular fibrillation
  2. Early (within 24 hours): No characteristics from the immediate category but new ST-segment depression, a GRACE risk score >140 or temporal change in troponin
  3. Delayed invasive: None of the immediate or early characteristics but renal insufficiency, left ventricular ejection fraction of <40%, early post-infarct angina, history of PCI within the past 6 months, prior coronary artery bypass graft, GRACE risk score of 109-140, or TIMI score of 2 or more.
- Bed rest and continuous ECG monitoring is recommended for all ACS patients. Supplemental oxygen should be administered to patients with arterial oxygen saturation of less than 90%, respiratory distress, or other high-risk features of hypoxemia. Finger pulse oximetry should be utilized to assess arterial oxygen saturation.

ACUTE GENERAL ℞

- All patients with ACS should receive full-dose non–enteric-coated chewable aspirin of 162 to 325 mg to establish a high blood level for its antiplatelet effects. Thereafter, daily dose of 81 to 325 mg are prescribed and continued indefinitely, with the lower dose of 81 mg showing lower bleeding risk with comparable efficacy.
- Antithrombotic therapy is critical in treating the underlying pathophysiology of ACS. This consists of administering antiplatelet and anticoagulant agents.

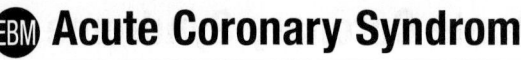

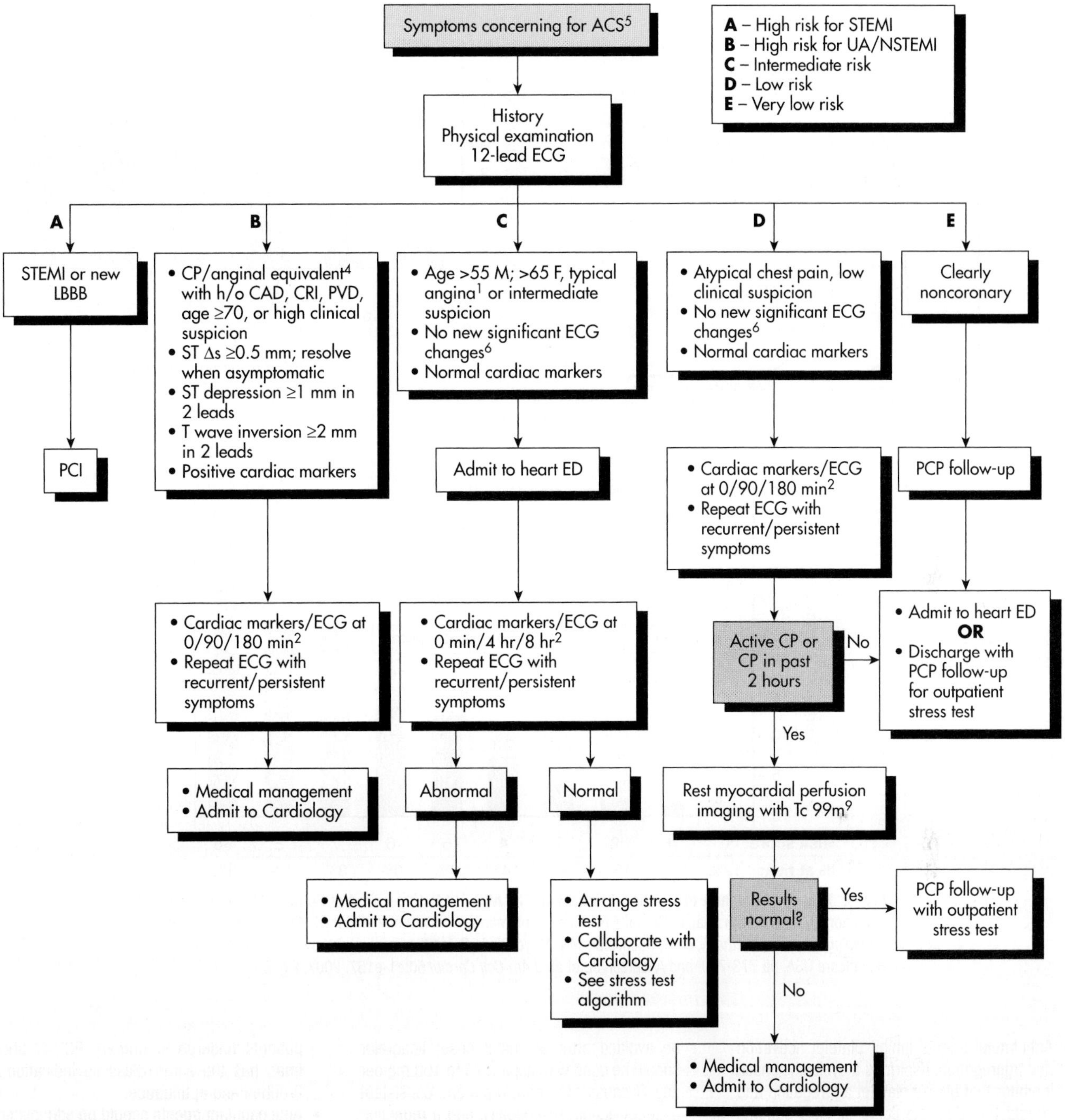

A

Diseases and Disorders

I

Symptoms concerning for ACS[5]

| A – High risk for STEMI |
| B – High risk for UA/NSTEMI |
| C – Intermediate risk |
| D – Low risk |
| E – Very low risk |

History
Physical examination
12-lead ECG

A

STEMI or new LBBB

↓

PCI

B

- CP/anginal equivalent[4] with h/o CAD, CRI, PVD, age ≥70, or high clinical suspicion
- ST Δs ≥0.5 mm; resolve when asymptomatic
- ST depression ≥1 mm in 2 leads
- T wave inversion ≥2 mm in 2 leads
- Positive cardiac markers

↓

- Cardiac markers/ECG at 0/90/180 min[2]
- Repeat ECG with recurrent/persistent symptoms

↓

- Medical management
- Admit to Cardiology

C

- Age >55 M; >65 F, typical angina[1] or intermediate suspicion
- No new significant ECG changes[6]
- Normal cardiac markers

↓

Admit to heart ED

↓

- Cardiac markers/ECG at 0 min/4 hr/8 hr[2]
- Repeat ECG with recurrent/persistent symptoms

↓

Abnormal →
- Medical management
- Admit to Cardiology

Normal →
- Arrange stress test
- Collaborate with Cardiology
- See stress test algorithm

D

- Atypical chest pain, low clinical suspicion
- No new significant ECG changes[6]
- Normal cardiac markers

↓

- Cardiac markers/ECG at 0/90/180 min[2]
- Repeat ECG with recurrent/persistent symptoms

↓

Active CP or CP in past 2 hours — No →
- Admit to heart ED **OR**
- Discharge with PCP follow-up for outpatient stress test

Yes ↓

Rest myocardial perfusion imaging with Tc 99m[9]

↓

Results normal? — Yes → PCP follow-up with outpatient stress test

No ↓

- Medical management
- Admit to Cardiology

E

Clearly noncoronary

↓

PCP follow-up

↓

- Admit to heart ED **OR**
- Discharge with PCP follow-up for outpatient stress test

DEFINITIONS:

[1]Typical angina:
1) Substernal chest pain or discomfort that is 2) provoked by exertion or emotional stress and 3) relieved by rest and/or nitroglycerin

[2]Cardiac marker timing: based on symptom onset; in cases of uncertainty assume symptom onset at ED arrival

[3]ECG normal: no significant ST depression/T wave inversions, BBB, LVH with repolarization, conduction defect, digoxin effect

[4]Anginal equivalent:
- Any symptoms that the physician feels may represent ACS
- Exertional dyspnea—most common anginal equivalent symptom

[5]ACS:
- STE-ACS—1 mm ST elevation in 2 leads
- NSTE-ACS
  - NSTEMI—positive cardiac biomarkers
  - Unstable angina—ischemia with negative biomarkers

[6]New significant ECG changes:
- ST Δs ≥0.5 mm; resolve when asymptomatic
- ST depression ≥1 mm in 2 leads
- T wave inversion ≥2 mm in 2 leads

[7]Regadenoson is preferred agent for chemical nuclear stress test. Technetium Tc-99m tetrofosmin is the preferred tracer.

FIG. 1 Evaluation of patients for acute coronary syndrome (ACS). *CAD,* Coronary artery disease; *CP,* chest pain; *CRI,* chronic renal insufficiency; *ECG,* electrocardiogram; *ED,* emergency department; *h/o,* history of; *LBBB,* left bundle branch block; *NSTE,* non–ST-segment elevation; *NSTEMI,* non–ST-segment elevation myocardial infarction; *PCP,* primary care physician; *PVD,* peripheral vascular disease; *STE,* ST-segment elevation; *STEMI,* ST-segment elevation myocardial infarction; *UA,* unstable angina. (From Adams JG et al: *Emergency medicine, clinical essentials,* ed 2, Philadelphia, 2013, Elsevier.)

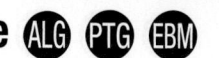
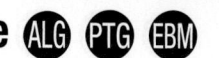

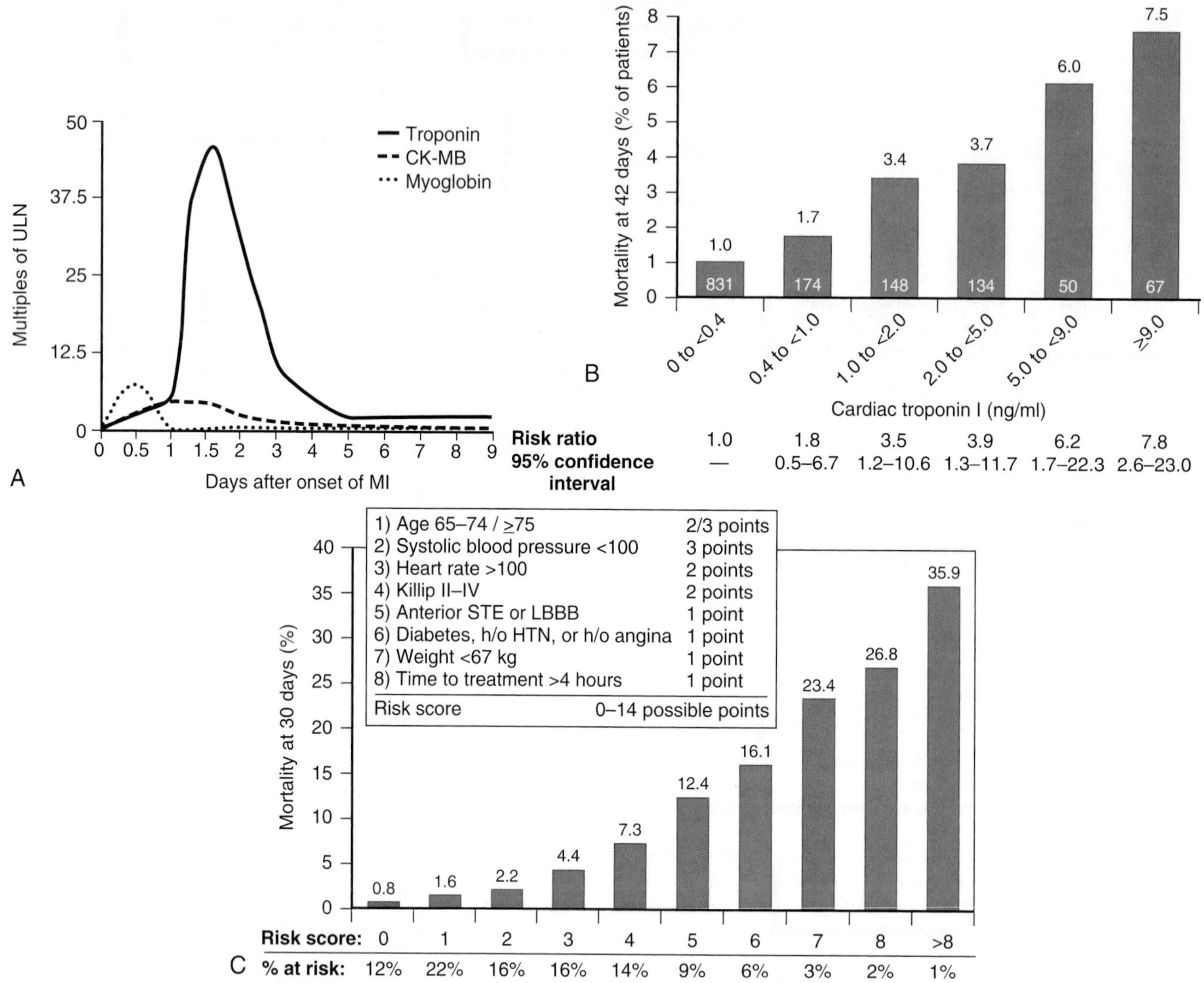

FIG. 2 Timing of release of cardiac biomarkers in ACS. *ULN,* Upper limit of normal; *MI,* myocardial infarction. (Modified from Shapiro BP, Jaffe AS: Cardiac biomarkers. In: Murphy JG, Lloyd MA [eds]: *Mayo Clinic cardiology: concise textbook,* ed 3, Rochester, MN: Mayo Clinic Scientific Press and New York, 2007, Informa Healthcare USA, pp 773-780; and Anderson JL et al: *J Am Coll Cardiol* 50:e1-e157, 2007, Fig. 5.)

- Antiplatelet agents inhibit platelet activation and aggregation. Aspirin is a cyclooxygenase inhibitor that blocks platelet aggregation and should be administered to all ACS patients without contraindications.
- Clopidogrel is a thienopyridine agent that inhibits platelet activation and aggregation. It should be administered in all ACS patients, with the timing dependent on the clinical scenario and management strategy. It requires a loading dose of 300 to 600 mg followed by 75 mg daily. It should be discontinued at least 5 days before CABG. If a patient is unable to take aspirin in the setting of hypersensitivity or major gastrointestinal intolerance, a loading dose of clopidogrel followed by daily maintenance should be started. Other antiplatelet agents that can be substituted instead of clopidogrel include prasugrel, ticlopidine, and ticagrelor. However, maintenance doses of aspirin above 100 mg reduce the effectiveness of ticagrelor and should

be avoided after an initial dose; ticagrelor should be used with aspirin 75 to 100 mg per day. Because of a more rapid and consistent onset of action, reversibility, and a reduction in death from vascular causes, MI, or stroke, ticagrelor is preferred over clopidogrel in patients with NSTE-ACS. Prasugrel is not recommended in ACS patients with stroke or transient ischemic attack (TIA), or those patients managed with fibrinolysis because of an increased risk of bleeding complications. As a rule, all ACS patients should have two antiplatelet agents initiated and should be continued up to 12 months regardless of ischemia-guided vs invasive strategy.
- GP IIB/III a inhibitors may be considered as an intravenous antiplatelet therapy in addition to aspirin for medium- or high-risk patients with NSTE-ACS in whom an invasive strategy is planned (Class IIb). Eptifibatide and tirofiban are preferred agents over abciximab for NSTE-ACS patients; however, for STEMI

patients undergoing primary PCI, IV abciximab has the same Class IIa indication as tirofiban and eptifibatide.
- Anticoagulant agents should be administered to all ACS patients. Options include either unfractionated heparin (UFH), or low-molecular-weight heparin (enoxaparin), or factor Xa inhibitors such as fondaparinux, or direct thrombin inhibitors such as bivalirudin.
- In the most recent guidelines, enoxaparin and UFH have both received Class I recommendations for use among ACS patients managed conservatively or invasively.
- For STEMI, fondaparinux can be used for anticoagulation. It has been shown to decrease bleeding complications as compared with either UFH or LMWH. However, it has a long half-life (15 hours), and thrombosis on catheters has been noted when using only fondaparinux in the cath lab; therefore, it is not recommended as a sole anticoagulation during primary PCI.

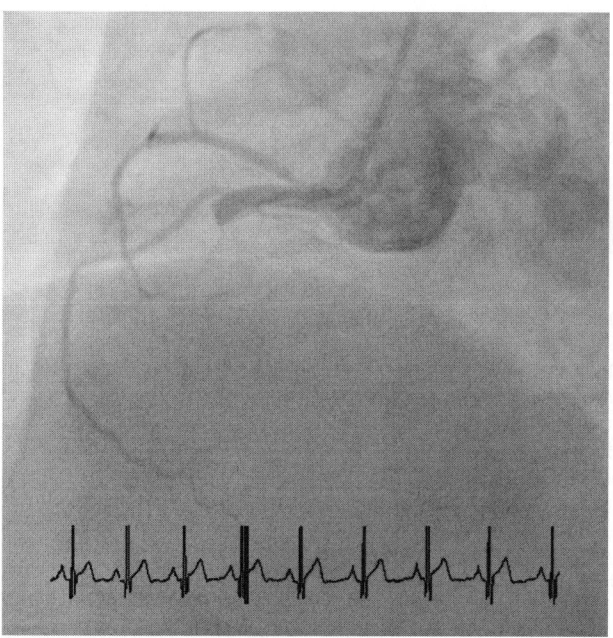

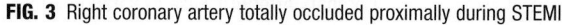

FIG. 3 Right coronary artery totally occluded proximally during STEMI.

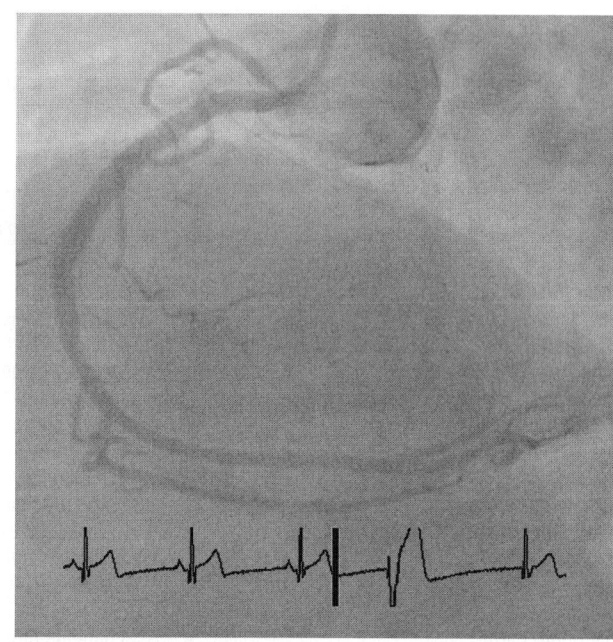

FIG. 4 Right coronary artery after successful percutaneous coronary artery stenting during STEMI.

- Bivalirudin is a reversible direct thrombin inhibitor and may be considered as an alternative to UFH and GP IIb/IIIa inhibitors in patients with STEMI (HORIZONS AMI trial) who are undergoing primary PCI (PPCI). When bivalirudin was compared to UFH plus a glycoprotein IIb/IIIa inhibitor in patients with STEMI and PCI, less bleeding and a short- and long-term reduction in cardiac events and overall mortality was observed. With bivalirudin, there is no risk of heparin-induced thrombocytopenia, less bleeding is observed, and the anticoagulant effect can be monitored during intervention by the activated clotting time. Similar results were reported in the use of bivalirudin alone in patients with UA/NSTEMI in the ACUITY trial when compared to enoxaparin/UFH with GP IIb/IIIa arms.
- Beta-blocker therapy reduces ischemia by decreasing myocardial oxygen demand and oral therapy should be initiated within 24 hours of onset of ACS unless signs or symptoms of heart failure and shock are present or arrhythmias preclude its use. Oral administration, titrated to a heart rate of 50-60 beats/min, is preferred. Intravenous beta-blockers can be administered to STEMI patients who are hypertensive or have ongoing ischemia; they should be avoided if the patients have any of the following:
  1. Signs of heart failure,
  2. Evidence of a low output state,
  3. Increased risk for cardiogenic shock, or
  4. Other relative contraindications to beta-blockade (PR interval >0.24 second, second- or third-degree heart block, active asthma, or reactive airway disease).
- Nitroglycerin is a vasodilator that should be administered to relieve chest discomfort in all ACS patients. It can be administered

sublingually at first, up to 3 doses, followed by intravenous administration if symptoms persist. In the setting of an inferior STEMI, it is necessary to rule out a right ventricular (RV) infarct with a right-sided ECG before the administration of nitroglycerin. This is because RV infarcts are preload dependent and nitroglycerin decreases preload through venodilation, which leads to hypotension in this setting. This can be corrected by discontinuing nitroglycerin and starting bolus intravenous fluids. Nitroglycerin provides no mortality benefit in ACS patients.
- Oxygen should be administered to patients with shortness of breath, signs of acute heart failure, cardiogenic shock, or an arterial oxyhemoglobin saturation of less than 90%. The 2014 ACC/AHA guidelines report no demonstrated benefit for routine use of supplemental oxygen in normoxic patients with NSTE-ACS; rather, emerging data suggest that routine use of oxygen can lead to adverse effects such as increased coronary vascular resistance, reduced coronary blood flow, and increased mortality rate.
- The 2014 ACC/AHA Guidelines for unstable NSTE-ACS have downgraded the recommendation for morphine use for uncontrolled ischemic chest discomfort from a Class IIa to a Class IIb recommendation due to reports linked to increased adverse events.
- Calcium channel blockers (nondihydropyridine) may be used in patients with persisting or recurrent symptoms, despite treatment with beta-blockers and nitroglycerin. They work by causing coronary vasodilation and decreasing myocardial oxygen demand. They are useful when beta-blockers are contraindicated and in patients with Prinzmetal variant angina. Calcium channel blockers should not be used in cases of severe LV

dysfunction, pulmonary edema, increased risk for cardiogenic shock or advanced heart blocks.
- Patients routinely taking nonsteroidal anti-inflammatory drugs (NSAIDs) (except for aspirin), both nonselective as well as COX-2 selective agents, before ACS should discontinue those agents at the time of presentation because of the increased risks of mortality, reinfarction, hypertension, heart failure, and myocardial rupture associated with their use.
- Angiotensin-converting enzyme (ACE) inhibitors may be added and should be used within 24 hours of onset of ACS in all patients with depressed LV function (ejection fraction [EF] <40%) or pulmonary vascular congestion. Angiotensin receptor blockers (ARBs) should be used in patients who are ACE inhibitor intolerant.
- Refer to topic "Cocaine Overdose" for treatment of cocaine-related ACS.

CHRONIC Rx

- Post-ACS medical therapy involves aspirin, statin, beta-blocker, and a second anti-platelet agent such as clopidogrel, ticagrelor, or prasugrel.
- In patients already on an oral anticoagulant for another diagnosis such as atrial fibrillation, the duration of triple therapy should be minimized. The WOEST trial showed that using clopidogrel along with an oral anticoagulant but without aspirin resulted in a significant reduction in bleeding complications with those patients on a triple therapy of oral anticoagulant, aspirin, and clopidogrel. It is a class IIB recommendation in those patients with atrial fibrillation and a CHADS-VASC score of 2 or greater after coronary revascularization to consider using clopidogrel concurrently with oral anticoagulant but without aspirin.

- Lipid lowering with statins has been evaluated in trials such as the MIRACL study, in which high-dose atorvastatin 80 mg reduced death, MI, and cardiac events at 16 weeks when administered early, within 24-96 hours after an ACS. The A-Z trial and PROVE IT-TIMI 22 trials demonstrated benefit of early high-intensity statin therapy with LDL targets <70 mg/dl in ACS.
- ACE inhibitors may be added to treat hypertension and should be used in all patients with depressed LV function (EF <40%) or pulmonary vascular congestion. ARBs should be used in patients who are ACE inhibitor intolerant.
- An aldosterone blocker should be used in post-MI patients without significant renal dysfunction or hyperkalemia who have an ejection fraction of less than 40% and are already on therapeutic doses of an ACE inhibitor and a beta-blocker.
- Cardiac rehabilitation and a monitored exercise program should be recommended at the time of discharge.
- Aggressive risk factor management, including smoking cessation, weight loss, diet and exercise, diabetes control, and so on, for secondary prevention of future events is crucial.

REFERRAL

- All ACS patients should be cared for in conjunction with the cardiology consult service.
- When appropriate, referral to a cardiac surgeon may be necessary for CABG.

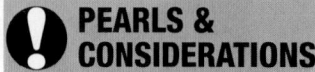

PEARLS & CONSIDERATIONS

COMMENTS

- ACS is common and a leading cause of mortality in the United States.
- The diagnosis hinges on the basics—history and physical, ECG, biomarkers, and CXR.
- Remember the potentially fatal non-ACS causes of chest discomfort, which include acute pulmonary embolism and acute ascending aortic dissection.
- STEMI patients presenting to a hospital with PCI capability should be treated with primary PCI within 90 minutes of first medical contact.
- STEMI patients presenting to a hospital without PCI capability and who cannot be transferred to a PCI center and undergo PCI within 90 minutes of first medical contact should be treated with fibrinolytic therapy within 30 minutes of hospital presentation unless fibrinolytic therapy is contraindicated.
- Refer to topics "Angina Pectoris" and "Myocardial Infarction" for additional discussion of this subject matter.

PREVENTION

- Primary prevention of ACS is based on recognizing the major risk factors for CAD and treating them as appropriate.
- Patients with depressed LV function (ejection fraction <35%) at least 40 days after an acute MI benefit from an implantable cardioverter defibrillator (ICD) for the prevention of sudden cardiac death.

SUGGESTED READINGS
Available at www.expertconsult.com

RELATED CONTENT
Acute Coronary Syndrome (Patient Information)
Angina (Related Key Topic)
Coronary Artery Disease (Related Key Topic)
Myocardial Infarction (Related Key Topic)

AUTHORS: **SONIA R. SAMTANI, M.D.,** and **PRANAV M. PATEL, M.D.**

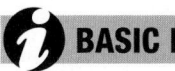

BASIC INFORMATION

DEFINITION

Acute kidney injury (AKI) is defined as a rapid (<48 hr) impairment in kidney function that results in retention of products in the blood that are normally excreted by the kidneys, and it is frequently manifested by concurrent extracellular fluid volume and acid-base and mineral metabolism dysregulation. Criteria and staging of AKI are described in Table 1.

SYNONYMS

AKI
Acute renal failure (ARF)
Acute renal insufficiency syndrome
Acute kidney failure

ICD-10-CM CODES
N17.9 Acute kidney failure, unspecified
N17.0 Acute kidney failure with tubular necrosis
N17.1 Acute kidney failure with acute cortical necrosis
N17.2 Acute kidney failure with medullary necrosis
N17.8 Other acute kidney failure
N99.0 Postprocedural (acute) (chronic) kidney failure
O90.4 Postpartum acute kidney failure

EPIDEMIOLOGY & DEMOGRAPHICS

- Incidence of AKI is 3 cases per 1000 persons in the general population. AKI that requires dialysis develops in 5 per 100,000 persons annually. Among hospitalized patients, approximately 20% develop AKI, and nearly 60% of intensive care unit patients incur AKI. AKI occurs in 20% of patients with moderate sepsis and in >50% of patients with septic shock and positive blood cultures. Greater than 40% of hospital-associated AKI is iatrogenic.
- Most common cause of AKI in hospitalized patients is intrinsic kidney failure caused by acute tubular necrosis (ATN) and prerenal disease.
- Risk factors for AKI include older age, preexisting chronic kidney disease, diabetes mellitus, and preexisting proteinuria.

PHYSICAL FINDINGS & CLINICAL PRESENTATION

- Early or mild AKI may be asymptomatic. Frequent presenting symptoms include weakness, anorexia, generalized malaise, and nausea.
- Oliguria is defined as <400 to 500 ml of urine per 24 hr. However, patients may develop nonoliguric kidney failure or anuria.
- Physical examination should focus on volume status. Findings vary with duration and rapidity of onset of renal failure and the underlying etiology for AKI.
- Peripheral edema resulting from volume overload, heart failure, liver failure, or nephrotic syndrome. Pulmonary rales may also be present.
- Arrhythmias due to electrolyte imbalances and acidosis
- Neurologic findings include altered mental status, delirium, lethargy, myoclonus, seizures, and flapping tremor (asterixis)
- Uremic odor, pruritus
- Flank pain, fasciculations, muscle cramps
- Pericardial effusion or pericardial rub (or both) from pericarditis
- The classic triad of fever, rash, and eosinophilia suggests allergic interstitial nephritis and should prompt a careful review of medications. However, the triad occurs uncommonly.

ETIOLOGY

- **Prerenal:** inadequate renal perfusion caused by hypovolemia, congestive heart failure (impaired cardiac output), cirrhosis (fluid third-spacing), sepsis (vasodilation), abdominal compartment syndrome. Sixty percent of community-acquired cases of AKI are from prerenal conditions.
- **Postrenal:** bladder outlet obstruction (prostatic enlargement, ureteral or urethral fibrosis), ureteral obstruction (stones, bladder masses, retroperitoneal fibrosis), or bilateral renal vein occlusion. With two functioning kidneys, bilateral obstruction is usually required to cause significant AKI. Postrenal causes of AKI account for 5% to 15% of community-acquired AKI.
- **Intrinsic renal:** ATN, glomerulonephritis, allergic interstitial nephritis (AIN). Common causes of ATN include ischemia (e.g., hypotension or shock, postcardiac bypass or aorta surgery), rhabdomyolysis, sepsis, drug toxicity (e.g., aminoglycosides), and iodinated radiocontrast nephropathy. Contrast-induced nephropathy is the third-most common cause of new-onset AKI in hospitalized patients. AIN can develop after exposure to a variety of medications, most commonly nonsteroidal antiinflammatory drugs, antibiotics, and proton pump inhibitors.
- Causes of AKI are described in Table 2.
- Nearly one third of cases of acute kidney injury may be prevented or mitigated by appropriate physician actions.

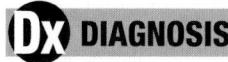 DIAGNOSIS

DIFFERENTIAL DIAGNOSIS

Refer to "Etiology." Diagnostic tests to distinguish prerenal and renal AKI are described in Table 3. A diagnostic approach to patients with suspected AKI is described in Fig. 1.

LABORATORY TESTS

- Elevated serum creatinine: rate of rise is approximately 1 mg/dl/day in complete kidney failure. Standard estimating equations for glomerular filtration rate (GFR) assume a steady-state creatinine level and are not recommended for use in evolving AKI.
- Elevated blood urea nitrogen (BUN): BUN/plasma creatinine ratio is commonly >20:1 in prerenal azotemia, postrenal azotemia, and acute glomerulonephritis. The ratio is <20:1 in acute interstitial nephritis and ATN (Table 4).
- Potassium and phosphate elevated; bicarbonate level, sodium, and calcium decreased; metabolic acidosis is frequent.
- Complete blood count may reveal anemia from decreased erythropoietin production. Hemoconcentration, hemolysis, or leukocytosis may imply the presence of infection.
- Urinalysis is an important first step in the diagnostic evaluation. Prerenal and postrenal AKI are typically characterized by a normal urinalysis. Conversely, abnormal findings should prompt further work-up for specific intrinsic renal causes of AKI that may require urgent intervention. Hematuria and proteinuria imply glomerulonephritis, heavy (>3+) proteinuria is associated with nephrotic syndrome, and pyuria may signify AIN. Microscopic examination of urine sediment may facilitate diagnosis: granular casts in ATN, dysmorphic red blood cells or red blood cell casts in acute glomerulonephritis, and white blood cell casts in acute interstitial nephritis.
- In oliguric patients, obtain urinary sodium and urinary creatinine to calculate fractional excretion of sodium [$FE_{Na} = 100\% \times (U_{Na} \times P_{Cr})/(P_{Na} \times U_{Cr})$]. FE_{Na} <1 is seen in prerenal AKI and >1 in intrinsic AKI when urine output <400 ml/day. FE_{Na} may be falsely elevated in patients taking diuretics or falsely low in several intrinsic renal conditions, including acute glomerulonephritis, contrast-induced nephropathy, and rhabdomyolysis.

TABLE 1 Kidney Disease: Improving Global Outcomes (KDIGO) Criteria for Diagnosis of Acute Kidney Injury

AKI Definition and Staging		
Stage	**Serum Creatinine Criteria**	**Urine Output Criteria**
1	$\Delta S_{Cr} \geq 0.3$ mg/dl (30 μmol/L) or S_{Cr} $\geq 1.5, <2.0 \times$ baseline*	UO <0.5 ml/kg/h × 6-12 h
2	S_{Cr} >2.0, <3.0 × baseline	UO <0.5 ml/kg/h >= 12 h
3	S_{Cr} >3.0 × baseline or	
	$S_{Cr} \geq 4.0$ mg/dl with an acute rise ≥ 0.5 mg/dl (50 μmol/L) or on renal replacement therapy	UO <0.3 ml/kg/h × 24 h or anuria × 12 h

SCr, serum creatinine; *UO*, urinary output.
*To meet criteria, rise of >=0.3mg/dl must be within 48 hours; or increase to ≥1.5 times baseline SCr is known or presumed to have occurred within previous 7 days.
Adapted from KDIGO Clinical Practice Guideline for Acute Kidney Injury, 2012.

TABLE 2 Etiologies of Acute Kidney Injury

Prerenal Causes (Decreased Renal Blood Flow)	Intrinsic Renal Causes	Postrenal Causes
Hypovolemia	**Vascular: Large and Small Vessels**	**Ureteral Obstruction**
Renal losses (diuretics, osmotic agents, polyuria)	Trauma	Calculus
Gastrointestinal losses (vomiting, diarrhea)	Renal vein obstruction (thrombosis, ventilation with high-level PEEP, abdominal compartment syndrome)	Tumor (intrinsic or extrinsic)
Cutaneous losses (burns, exfoliative syndromes)	Microangiopathy (thrombotic thrombocytopenic purpura, hemolytic-uremic syndrome, disseminated intravascular coagulation, preeclampsia)	Fibrosis
Hemorrhage		Ligation during pelvic surgery
Pancreatitis	Malignant hypertension	**Bladder Neck Obstruction**
Decreased Cardiac Output	Scleroderma renal crisis	Benign prostatic hypertrophy
Congestive heart failure	Transplant rejection	Prostate cancer
Pulmonary embolism	Atheroembolic disease	Neurogenic bladder
Acute myocardial infarction	**Glomerular**	Tricyclic antidepressants
Severe valvular heart disease	Antiglomerular basement membrane disease (Goodpasture syndrome)	Ganglionic blockers
Abdominal compartment syndrome	Antineutrophil cytoplasmic antibody-associated glomerulonephritis (Wegener granulomatosis)	Bladder tumor
Renal artery obstruction (stenosis, embolism, thrombosis, dissection)	Immune complex glomerulonephritis, systemic lupus erythematosus, postinfectious cryoglobulinemia, primary membranoproliferative glomerulonephritis	Calculus
Systemic Vasodilation		Hemorrhage/clot
Sepsis	**Tubular**	**Urethral Obstruction**
Anaphylaxis	Ischemic	Strictures
Anesthetics	Cytotoxic	Tumor
Drug overdose	Heme pigment (rhabdomyolysis, intravascular hemolysis)	Phimosis
Afferent Arteriolar Vasoconstriction	Crystals (tumor lysis syndrome, seizures, ethylene glycol poisoning, vitamin C megadose, acyclovir, indinavir, methotrexate)	Renal calcinosis
Hypercalcemia		Obstructed urinary catheter, ureteral stent, or ileal conduit
Drugs (NSAIDs, amphotericin B, calcineurin inhibitors, norepinephrine, radiocontrast agents, aminoglycosides)	Drugs (aminoglycosides, lithium, amphotericin B, pentamidine, cisplatin, ifosfamide, radiocontrast agents), synthetic cannabinoid use	Pelvic trauma, retroperitoneal hematoma
Hepatorenal syndrome	**Interstitial**	
Efferent arteriolar vasodilation (angiotensin converting enzyme inhibitors, aldosterone receptor blockers)	Drugs (penicillins, cephalosporins, NSAIDs, proton pump inhibitors, allopurinol, rifampin, indinavir, mesalamine, sulfonamides)	
	Infection (pyelonephritis, viral infection)	
	Systemic Disease	
	Sjögren syndrome, sarcoidosis, systemic lupus erythematosus, lymphoma, leukemia, tubulonephritis, uveitis	

NSAIDs, Nonsteroidal antiinflammatory drugs; *PEEP,* positive end-expiratory pressure.
Modified from Cameron JL, Cameron AM: *Current surgical therapy,* ed 10, Philadelphia, 2011, Saunders.

TABLE 3 Diagnostic Tests to Distinguish Between Prerenal and Renal Acute Kidney Injury

Index	Prerenal Causes	Renal Causes
FENa	<1%	>2%
Urine sodium	<10 mmol/L	>40 mmol/L
Urine/plasma osmolality	>1.5	1 to 1.5
Renal failure index	<1	>2
BUN/creatinine ratio	>20	<10

BUN, Blood urea nitrogen; *FENa,* fractional excretion of sodium. Calculation of FENa: (Urine sodium × Plasma creatinine)/(Plasma sodium × Serum creatinine) × 100. Renal failure index: (Urine sodium × Urine creatinine)/Plasma creatinine.
From Cameron JL, Cameron AM: *Current surgical therapy,* ed 10, Philadelphia, 2011, Saunders.

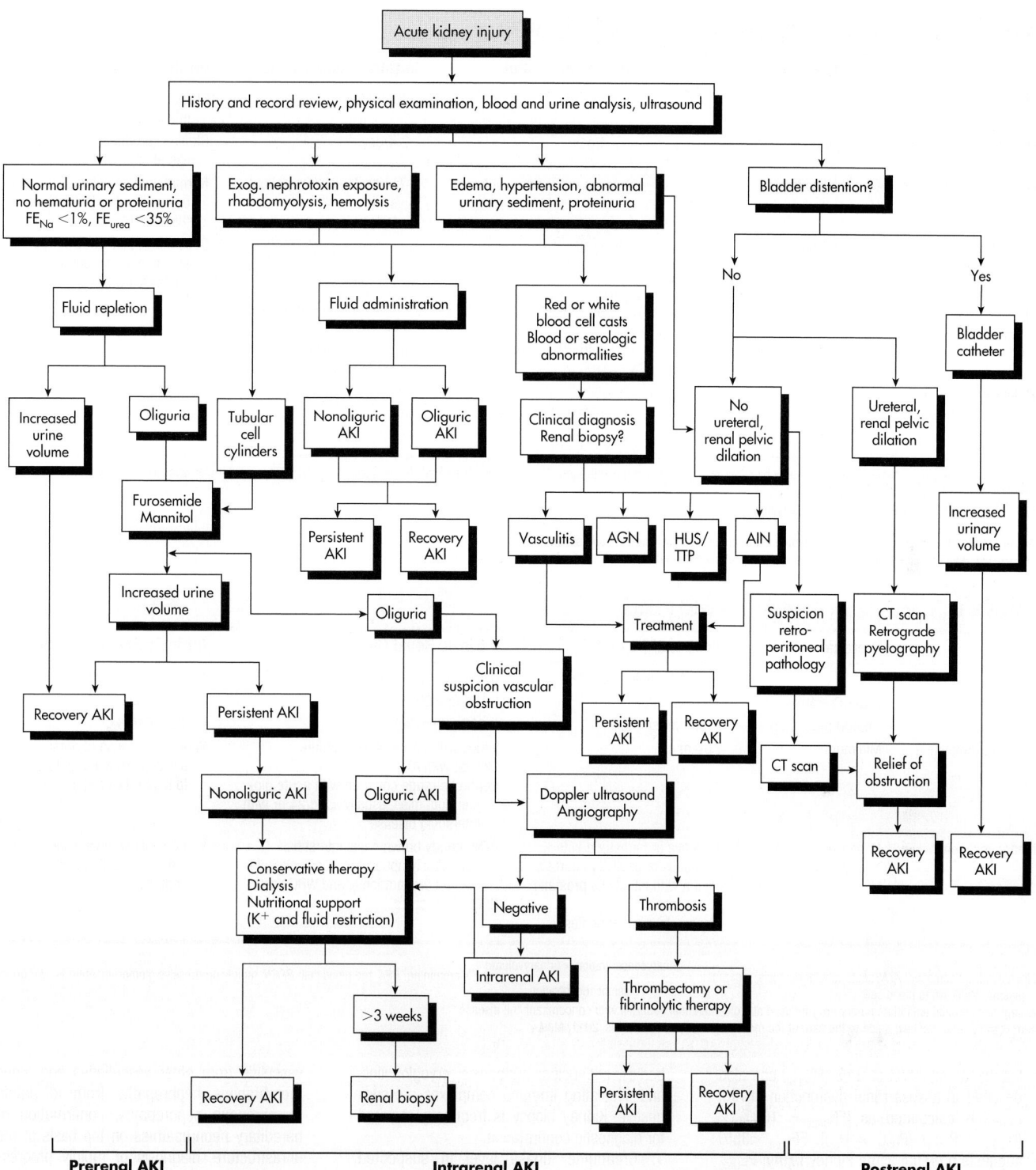

FIG. 1 Diagnostic approach to patients with suspected AKI. *AGN,* Acute glomerulonephritis; *AIN,* acute interstitial nephritis; *CT,* computed tomography; *Exog.,* exogenous; *HUS/TTP,* hemolytic-uremic syndrome/thrombotic thrombocytopenic purpura. (From Floege J et al: *Comprehensive clinical nephrology,* ed 4, Philadelphia, 2010, Saunders.)

TABLE 4 Serum and Radiographic Abnormalities in Renal Failure

	Prerenal	Postrenal (Acute)	Intrinsic Renal (Acute)	Intrinsic Renal (Chronic)
BUN	↑ 10:1 > Cr	↑ 20-40/day	↑ 20-40/day	Stable; ↑ varies with protein intake
Serum creatinine	N/moderate ↑	↑ 2-4/day	↑ 2-4/day	Stable ↑ (production equals excretion)
Serum potassium	N/moderate ↑	↑ varies with urinary volume	↑↑ (particularly when patient is oliguric) ↑↑↑ with rhabdomyolysis	Normal until end stage, unless tubular dysfunction (type 4 RTA)
Serum phosphate	N/moderate ↑	Moderate ↑	↑	Becomes significantly elevated when serum creatinine surpasses 3 mg/dl
		↑↑ with rhabdomyolysis	Poor correlation with duration of renal disease	
Serum calcium	N	N/↓ with $PO_4{}^{-3}$ retention	↓ (poor correlation with duration of renal failure)	Usually ↓
Renal size				
By ultrasonography	N/↑	↑ and dilated calyces	N/↑	↓ and with ↑ echogenicity
FE_{Na}*	<1	<1 → >1	>1[†]	1

↑, Increase; ↓, decrease; ↑↑, large increase; ↑↑↑, very high increase; *BUN*, blood urea nitrogen; *Cr*, creatinine; *N*, normal; *Na*, sodium; *P*, plasma; *RTA*, renal tubular acidosis; *U*, urine.

*FE_{Na} $\left[\dfrac{U/P_{Na}^{+}}{U/P_{Cr}} \times 100 \right]$ (useful only in oliguric patient).

[†]May be ≤1 in radiocontrast-induced myoglobinuric acute tubular necrosis and in early sepsis.

From Ferri FF (ed): Practical guide to the care of the medical patient, ed 8, St Louis, 2011, Mosby.

TABLE 5 Urinary Abnormalities in Renal Failure

	Prerenal	Postrenal (Acute)	Intrinsic Renal (Acute)	Intrinsic Renal (Chronic)
Urinary volume	↓	Absent-to-wide fluctuation	Oliguric or nonoliguric	1000 ml + until end stage
Urinary creatinine	↑ (U/P Cr 640)	↓ (U/P Cr 620)	↓ (U/P Cr <20)	↓ (U/P Cr <20)
Osmolarity	↑ (6400 mOsm/kg)	(<350 mOsm/kg)	(<350 mOsm/kg)	(<350 mOsm/kg)
Degree of proteinuria	Minimum	Absent	Varies with cause of renal failure: Modest with ATN. Nephrotic range common with acute glomerulopathies, usually <2 g/24 hr with interstitial disease*	Varies with cause of renal disease (from 1-2 g/day to nephrotic range)
Urinary sediment	Negative, or occasional hyaline cast	Negative or hematuria with stones or papillary necrosis Pyuria with infectious prostatic disease Nephrosis: oval fat bodies	ATN: muddy brown casts Interstitial nephritis: lymphocytes, eosinophils (in stained preparations), and WBC casts RPGN: RBC casts	Broad casts with variable renal "residual" acute findings

↑, Increased; ↓, decreased; *ATN*, acute tubular necrosis; clearance = $\dfrac{\text{urinary concentration} \times \text{urinary volume}}{\text{plasma concentration}}$; *Cr*, creatinine; *RBC*, red blood cell; *RPGN*, rapidly progressive glomerulonephritis; *U/P*, urine/plasma; *WBC*, white blood cell.

*Except nonsteroidal antiinflammatory drug-induced allergic interstitial nephritis with concomitant "nil disease."

From Ferri FF (ed): Practical guide to the care of the medical patient, ed 8, St Louis, 2011, Mosby.

- Fractional excretion of urea (FE_{Urea}) can also be used to assess renal dysfunction in AKI. FE_{Urea} is calculated as [FE_{Urea} = 100% × (U_{Urea} × P_{Cr}) / (P_{Urea} × U_{Cr})]. FE_{Urea} <35% suggests prerenal acute kidney injury; FE_{Urea} >50% indicates intrinsic AKI. FE_{Urea} is more useful than FE_{Na} during diuretic therapy.
- Urinary osmolarity is 250 to 300 mOsm/kg in ATN, <400 mOsm/kg in postrenal azotemia, and >500 mOsm/kg in prerenal azotemia and acute glomerulonephritis (Table 5)
- Blood cultures for suspected sepsis
- In cases of suspected glomerulonephritis (e.g., abnormal urinalysis, suggestive systemic clinical picture), additional serologic testing may be warranted: Abnormal liver function tests, decreased complement (C3, C4) levels, elevated anti–glomerular basement membrane antibody titers, antineutrophil cytoplasmic anti-

bodies, antinuclear antibodies, cryoglobulins, and circulating immune complexes are suggestive. Kidney biopsy is frequently required for diagnostic confirmation.

1. Creatinine kinase level in suspected rhabdomyolysis: A positive blood reaction on a urine dipstick with few or no red blood cells by urine microscopy is a clue to myoglobinuria from rhabdomyolysis, but it is not invariable.
2. Serum free light chains, serum and urine protein electrophoresis, and urine immuno-fixation electrophoresis for suspected multiple myeloma or other plasma cell dyscrasias.

- Kidney biopsy may be indicated in patients with intrinsic kidney failure when considering specific therapy. The major reasons for renal biopsy are for the differential diagnosis of nephrotic syndrome, distinguishing lupus

vasculitis from other vasculitides and lupus membranous nephropathy from idiopathic membranous nephropathy, confirmation of hereditary nephropathies on the basis of the ultrastructure, diagnosis of rapidly progressive glomerulonephritis, distinguishing allergic interstitial nephritis from ATN, and separation of primary glomerulonephritides. In addition to establishing a diagnosis, biopsy may illuminate renal prognosis and guide direction of management. Severe interstitial fibrosis is associated with poor renal outcomes.

- Biomarkers of kidney injury have been explored for earlier diagnosis of AKI or to separate intrinsic from prerenal causes. Early candidates included cystatin C, neutrophil gelatinase–associated lipocalin (NGAL), kidney-injury molecule 1 (KIM-1), and liver fatty acid binding protein (LFABP). To date, all these biomarkers are available in the United States for research purposes only. In 2014, tissue inhibitor of metalloproteinases and insulin-like growth-factor binding protein 7 (TIMP2*IGFBP7) became the first biomarker for AKI risk prediction approved in the U.S. However, the clinical role of this test remains undefined.

IMAGING STUDIES

- ECG for arrhythmia detection, especially in hyperkalemia: peaked T waves in precordial leads, widening QRS interval, and/or brady-cardia with AV nodal blockade
- Chest radiograph to detect signs of congestive heart failure and pulmonary renal syndromes often characterized by pulmonary alveolar hemorrhage (Goodpasture syndrome, small vessel vasculitis)
- Kidney ultrasonography to determine kidney sizes (distinguishes acute from chronic kidney disease), presence of obstruction, and renal vascular status (Doppler study)
- Computed tomography (CT) with radiocontrast administration is typically avoided in AKI. However, unenhanced CT scans may identify obstructing ureteral stones.

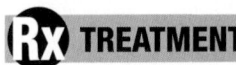 **TREATMENT**

Management of AKI depends on the underlying etiology. Some conditions (e.g., glomerulonephritis) require specific therapy, but the general focus of treatment for established AKI is supportive care and limiting additional injury.

NONPHARMACOLOGIC THERAPY

- Stop nephrotoxic medications
- Appropriate fluid balance, including balancing needs of resuscitation versus avoiding excessive fluid accumulation
- Dietary modification: (1) energy prescription of 120–150 KJ/kg/day, (2) potassium restriction (60 mEq/day), (3) sodium restriction (90 mEq/day), (4) phosphorus (800 mg/day), and (5) protein supplementation of 0.6 to 1.4 g/kg per day depending on requirement for dialysis
- Daily weight
- Modification of drug dosages or schedules of renally excreted medications. Dosing should take into account the trajectory of renal function (during evolving and recovering AKI), and it may require additional adjustment in patients who require dialysis.

ACUTE GENERAL Rx

- Correct electrolyte abnormalities and metabolic acidosis.
- Administer loop diuretics for volume overload.

- Administer vasopressors or vasodilators, when applicable, in congestive heart failure. Specific treatment is variable and dependent on etiology of AKI:
- Prerenal: IV volume expansion with isotonic solutions in hypovolemic patients or those with shock.
- Intrinsic kidney failure: discontinue all potential nephrotoxins and treat condition(s) causing kidney failure. In severe AIN cases, consider a trial of corticosteroids. For acute noninfectious glomerulonephritis, high-dose pulse corticosteroids are first-line therapy, typically in conjunction with other immunomodulatory therapy and plasma exchange, depending on the clinical scenario.
- Postrenal: Eliminate cause of obstruction. Immediate bladder catheter insertion for suspected bladder outlet obstruction and nephrostomy or ureteral stents for upper tract obstruction.
- Hyperkalemia-related ECG changes: IV calcium for cardiac membrane stabilization to prevent arrhythmias; IV insulin and glucose to shift potassium into cells; and IV bicarbonate therapy when metabolic acidosis is present to shift potassium into cells. These three treatments are temporary and definitive therapy requires bodily potassium removal via the gastrointestinal (potassium-binding agents) or urinary (diuretics) tracts or dialytic therapy.

ADJUNCTIVE Rx

- Monitoring of renal function parameters and electrolytes
- Renally excreted drugs are adjusted according to creatinine clearance or GFR to prevent further kidney damage or other medication-related toxicities.
- Prevent further renal insult with appropriate volume expansion, particularly before contrast administration, and avoid nephrotoxic agents. Volume expansion with isotonic solutions is more effective than hydration with hypotonic solutions. Isotonic saline or bicarbonate-containing solutions are effective, with or without concomitant *N*-acetylcysteine prophylaxis, which has shown conflicting results regarding its ability to reduce the risk of iodinated radiocontrast-induced nephropathy. See "Chronic Kidney Disease" entry for indications for initiation of dialysis.

DISPOSITION

- General indications for initiation of dialysis in AKI:
  1. Uremic symptoms (encephalopathy, pericarditis)

  2. Extracellular fluid volume overload refractory to medical management
  3. Severe acid-base imbalance refractory to medical management
  4. Significant electrolyte derangement in (e.g., hyperkalemia, hyponatremia) refractory to medical management
- Intermittent hemodialysis (IHD) and continuous renal replacement therapy (CRRT) have similar outcomes for patients with AKI. However, CRRT is associated with greater hemodynamic stability and fluid removal compared to conventional IHD. CRRT is the preferred modality in critically ill patients with hemodynamic instability.
- Renal function recovery (ability to discontinue dialysis) varies from 50% to 75% in AKI survivors.
- Overall mortality rate in AKI is nearly 25% and approaches 50% to 60% in patients who require acute dialysis.
- The combination of AKI and sepsis is associated with a 70% mortality rate.

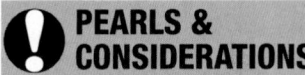 **PEARLS & CONSIDERATIONS**

- Patients with AKI are susceptible to infections and sepsis.
- In patients with community-acquired AKI, it is important to obtain a thorough medication history, including nonprescription medications or supplements.
- AKI survivors are at risk for development of CKD, and follow-up with monitoring of kidney function is essential even after apparent renal recovery.

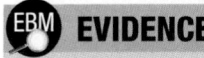 **EVIDENCE**

Available at www.expertconsult.com

SUGGESTED READINGS
Available at www.expertconsult.com

RELATED CONTENT

Acute Renal Failure (Patient Information)
Chronic Kidney Disease (Related Key Topic)

AUTHOR: **MICHAEL HEUNG, M.D., M.S.**

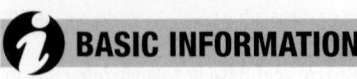

BASIC INFORMATION

DEFINITION

Acute liver failure (ALF) is defined as rapid development (<26 wk) of severe hepatic injury, coagulation abnormalities (international normalized ratio [INR] >1.5), and encephalopathy in a patient without preexisting liver disease, in the absence of acute alcoholic hepatitis. However, ALF can also be diagnosed in patients with preexisting Wilson disease, vertically acquired hepatitis B, and autoimmune hepatitis, provided that diagnosis of these conditions was made within the preceding 26 weeks.

SYNONYMS

Fulminant hepatic failure
Fulminant hepatitis
Fulminant hepatic necrosis
Acute hepatic necrosis
Acute and subacute necrosis of liver

ICD-10CM CODES
K72	Hepatic failure, not elsewhere classified
K72.0	Acute and subacute hepatic failure
K72.00	Acute and subacute hepatic failure without coma
K72.01	Acute and subacute hepatic failure with coma

EPIDEMIOLOGY & DEMOGRAPHICS

INCIDENCE (IN U.S.): Affects approximately 2000 people/year
PREDOMINANT SEX AND AGE: Seen more in women (90% of cases), average age 38 years
RISK FACTORS:
- Intentional or inadvertent drug overdose
- Intravenous drug use
- Previous alcohol use
- Occupational exposure to blood or body fluids
- Hepatotoxic medications
- Travel to endemic hepatitis areas
- Critical illness

PHYSICAL FINDINGS & CLINICAL PRESENTATION

- By definition, symptoms of ALF must include some degree of encephalopathy but otherwise are nonspecific, such as fatigue, lethargy, anorexia, and nausea/vomiting. Pruritus, jaundice, and abdominal pain may be present.
- Physical examination findings include some degree of encephalopathy (see Table 1) and may include jaundice, asterixis, hepatomegaly, decreased hepatic mass on percussion, and ascites. Multisystem organ failure can ensue. In rare cases, cerebral edema and increased intracranial pressure can occur, with abnormal pupillary exam findings, hypertension, bradycardia, respiratory depression (Cushing's triad), seizures, and loss of brain stem reflexes.

- Vesicular skin lesions are suggestive of herpes simplex virus (HSV).
- Family history of unexplained liver disease/cirrhosis should prompt ocular exam to look for Kayser-Fleischer rings (copper rings around the iris seen in Wilson disease).

ETIOLOGY

- Common causes in the Western world include:
  1. Acetaminophen toxicity (46%)
  2. Indeterminate (14%)
  3. Idiosyncratic drug reaction (12%)
  4. Viral hepatitis (A, B) (10%)
  Rarer causes include alcoholic hepatitis, autoimmune hepatitis, Wilson disease, ischemic hepatopathy, Budd-Chiari syndrome, acute fatty liver of pregnancy, venoocclusive disease, toxin ingestion (e.g., mushroom poisoning [Amanita phalloides]), sepsis, infiltrative malignancy (breast cancer, lymphoma, myeloma, melanoma, small cell lung cancer), and other viruses (adenovirus, hepatitis E, HSV).

DIAGNOSIS

DIFFERENTIAL DIAGNOSIS

- Severe acute hepatitis, also known as acute liver injury (including alcoholic hepatitis): jaundice and coagulopathy without encephalopathy
- Acute or chronic liver failure (in patients with liver disease duration >26 weeks)
- Cirrhosis (includes decompensated cirrhosis)
- Hepatocellular carcinoma

WORKUP (BOX 1)

- Fig. 1 describes an algorithm for evaluation of acute liver failure.
- Clinical history is critical and should include medication use (prescriptions, over-the-counter medications, herbal supplements), alcohol use, recreational drug use, prior symptoms of jaundice, onset of symptoms, history of suicide attempts, recent travel to endemic areas of viral hepatitis, and family history of liver failure/disease.
- Laboratory evaluation: complete blood count, liver function tests (LFTs) including prothrombin time and INR, chemistry panel

TABLE 1 Grades of Encephalopathy

Grade	Description
I	Changes in behavior with minimal change in level of consciousness
II	Gross disorientation, drowsiness, possibly asterixis, inappropriate behavior
III	Marked confusion, incoherent speech, sleeping most of the time but arousable to vocal stimuli
IV	Comatose, unresponsiveness to pain, decorticate or decerebrate posturing

(sodium, potassium, chloride, bicarbonate, BUN, creatinine, glucose, magnesium, phosphate, calcium), arterial blood gas, arterial lactate, blood type and screen, acetaminophen level, ethanol level, toxicology screen, viral hepatitis serologies (hepatitis A IgM, hepatitis B surface antigen, anti–hepatitis B core IgM, anti–hepatitis C antibody, hepatitis C viral load, anti–hepatitis E Ab, HSV-1 IgM, varicella zoster virus), ceruloplasmin level, pregnancy test, arterial ammonia level, autoimmune markers (ANA, ASMA, total IgG levels), HIV-1, HIV-2, amylase, lipase.

- Imaging: abdominal ultrasound with Doppler (hard to diagnose cirrhosis because liver may appear nodular in ALF due to massive necrosis), CT/MRI of the head.
- Prompt liver biopsy (via transjugular approach to decrease risk of bleeding) should be performed in cases in which:

BOX 1 Investigations in Fulminant Hepatic Failure

Baseline essential investigations
Biochemistry
  ○ Bilirubin, transaminases
  ○ Alkaline phosphatase
  ○ Albumin
  ○ Urea and electrolytes
  ○ Creatinine
  ○ Calcium, phosphate
  ○ Ammonia
  ○ Acid-base, lactate
  ○ Glucose
Hematology
  ○ Full blood count, platelets
  ○ PT, PTT
  ○ Factors V or VII
  ○ Blood group cross-match
Septic screen
Omitting lumbar puncture
  ○ Radiology
  ○ Chest radiograph
  ○ Abdominal ultrasound
  ○ Head CT scan or MRI
Neurophysiology
  ○ Electroencephalogram
Diagnostic investigations
Serum
  ○ Acetaminophen levels
  ○ Cu, ceruloplasmin (>3 yr)
  ○ Autoantibodies
  ○ Immunoglobulins
  ○ Amino acids
  ○ Lactate
  ○ Pyruvate
  ○ Hepatitis A, B, C, E
  ○ EBV, CMV, HSV
  ○ Other viruses
Urine
  ○ Toxic metabolites
  ○ Amino acids, succinylacetone
  ○ Organic acids
  ○ Reducing sugars

CMV, Cytomegalovirus; *EBV,* Epstein-Barr virus; *HSV,* herpes simplex virus; *PT,* prothrombin time; *PTT,* partial thromboplastin time.
From Fuhrman BP, Zimmerman JJ: *Fuhrman and Zimmerman's pediatric critical care,* ed 4, Philadelphia, 2011, Mosby.

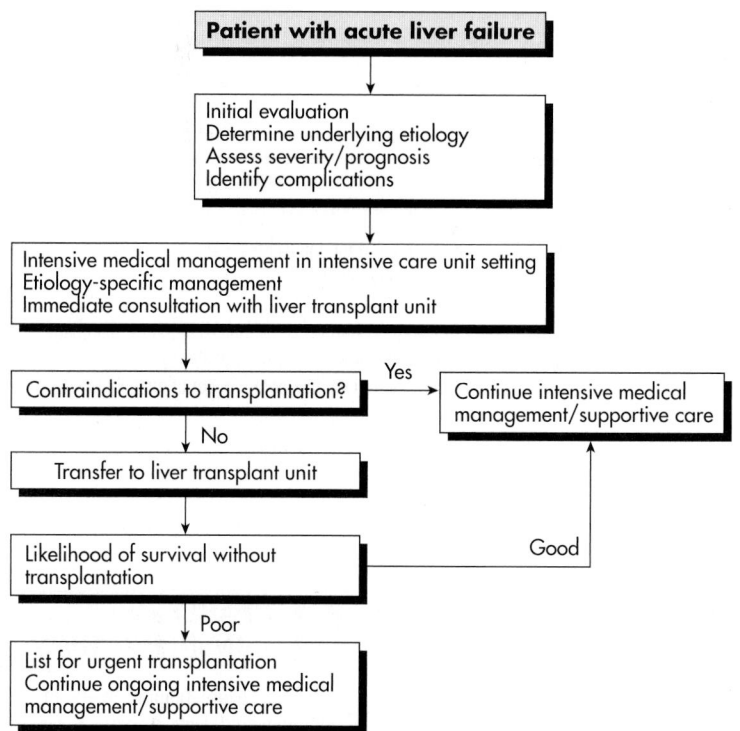

FIG. 1 Management of acute liver failure. (From Tally NJ: *Gastroenterology and hepatology*, Philadelphia, 2008, Churchill Livingston.)

Flowchart content:

Patient with acute liver failure
↓
Initial evaluation
Determine underlying etiology
Assess severity/prognosis
Identify complications
↓
Intensive medical management in intensive care unit setting
Etiology-specific management
Immediate consultation with liver transplant unit
↓
Contraindications to transplantation? — Yes → Continue intensive medical management/supportive care
↓ No
Transfer to liver transplant unit
↓
Likelihood of survival without transplantation — Good → Continue intensive medical management/supportive care
↓ Poor
List for urgent transplantation
Continue ongoing intensive medical management/supportive care

Diseases and Disorders

1. The etiology is thought to be secondary to autoimmune hepatitis, malignancy, or HSV

LABORATORY TESTS

- Patients with ALF typically have a prolonged prothrombin time (INR >1.5), elevated transaminases, elevated bilirubin, and may have a low platelet count (<150,000).
- Other possible lab findings can include an elevated BUN/creatinine (studies show 30% to 50% also have acute kidney injury), hypoglycemia (impairment of gluconeogenesis), hypophosphatemia, hypomagnesemia, hypokalemia, metabolic acidosis or respiratory alkalosis, elevated LDH, and elevated ammonia.

IMAGING STUDIES

- Abdominal ultrasound with Doppler should be ordered to evaluate for Budd-Chiari syndrome, portal hypertension, hepatic congestion, and hepatic steatosis.
- CT or MRI scan of the head should be considered to ensure no other causes for altered mental status.

COMPLICATIONS

Complications or progression of liver failure may result in cerebral edema due to increased intracranial pressure (in up to 40% of patients), high-output cardiac failure, hypoglycemia, lactic acidosis, acute respiratory distress syndrome, upper gastrointestinal hemorrhage (in 1.5% of patients), infectious disease from impaired leukocyte function (in nearly 80% patients), acute kidney injury, and pancreatitis (particularly in acetaminophen-induced ALF). Hypotension can occur due to decreased oral intake as well as extravasation of fluid into extravascular space.

Rx TREATMENT (BOXES 2 AND 3)

NONPHARMACOLOGIC THERAPY

- Initial treatment should focus on the patient's mental status.
  - Grade I/II encephalopathy may be managed on a medical ward (neuro vital signs q4h).
  - Grade III and IV encephalopathy should be managed in ICU (elevate head of the bed to 30 degrees).
  - Decrease stimulation (quiet room, no audible monitor alarms).
  - Avoid sedatives and opioids.
- A liver specialist should be notified urgently, and arrangements should be made for imminent transfer to a transplant center.
- Nutritional support should be initiated early. A daily intake goal of 60 g of protein is recommended to prevent catabolism of protein stores.
- Fluid support should be initiated if patient is not tolerating oral intake, or signs of hypoperfusion are present. Crystalloid solutions (normal saline in hypotensive patients, ½ normal saline + 75 mEq/L NaCO₃ in acidotic patients, normal saline + dextrose in hypoglycemic patients) can be used.

MONITORING

- Neuro exam q4h
- Patients with suspected acetaminophen toxicity should have LFTs monitored every 12 hr. Otherwise, LFTs can be monitored daily.
- Chemistry panels and PT/INR should be monitored every 8-12 hr. Correction of coagulopathy should be avoided because it can interfere with assessment of liver function. In

BOX 2 Management of Fulminant Hepatic Failure

No sedation except for procedures
Minimal handling
Enteric precautions until infection ruled out
Monitor:
  ○ Heart and respiratory rate
  ○ Arterial BP, CVP
  ○ Core/toe temperature
  ○ Neurologic observations
  ○ Gastric pH (>5.0)
  ○ Blood glucose (>4 mmol/L)
  ○ Acid-base
  ○ Electrolytes
  ○ PT, PTT
Fluid balance
  ○ 75% maintenance
  ○ Dextrose 10%-50% (provide 6-10 mg/kg/min)
  ○ Sodium (0.5-1 mmol/L)
  ○ Potassium (2-4 mmol/L)
Maintain circulating volume with colloid/FFP
Coagulation support only if required
Drugs
  ○ Vitamin K
  ○ H₂ antagonist
  ○ Antacids
  ○ Lactulose
  ○ N-acetylcysteine for acetaminophen toxicity
  ○ Broad-spectrum antibiotics
  ○ Antifungals
Nutrition
  ○ Enteral feeding (1-2 g protein/kg/day)
  ○ PN if ventilated

BP, Blood pressure; *CVP,* central venous pressure; *FFP,* fresh frozen plasma; *PN,* parenteral nutrition; *PT,* prothrombin time; *PTT,* partial thromboplastin time. From Fuhrman BP, Zimmerman JJ: *Fuhrman and Zimmerman's pediatric critical care,* ed 4, Philadelphia, 2011, Mosby.

the setting of life-threatening bleeding, fresh frozen plasma (FFP) and recombinant factor VIIa can be considered.

- Glucose finger sticks should be checked every 4 hr initially to evaluate for hypoglycemia. If hypoglycemia is detected, dextrose should be added to crystalloid solution.
- Because of the increased risk of infection, daily urine, sputum, and blood cultures should be checked in the absence of signs or symptoms of infection.

PHARMACOLOGIC TREATMENT

- If acetaminophen is the known or suspected cause, an IV acetylcysteine protocol must be initiated. *N*-acetylcysteine is not harmful and dramatically alters the course in acetaminophen toxicity, so there should be a low threshold to start, particularly in young patients or those with no known cause of ALF.
  ○ The 20-hr protocol is:
    1. Initial loading dose of 150 mg/kg IV given over 60 min followed by
    2. 12.5 mg/kg IV/hr over 4 hr followed by
    3. 6.25 mg/kg IV/hr for 16 hr

BOX 3 Hepatic Replacement Therapeutic Options Available to Patients with Fulminant Hepatic Failure

Liver Transplantation
Cadaveric transplantation
Whole liver
Reduced-size liver
Split liver
Auxiliary partial liver
Orthotopic position
Heterotopic position
Auxiliary whole liver
Heterotopic position
Living-related transplantation
Left lateral segment
Left lobe
Extended left lobe
Right lobe

Artificial Liver Assist Devices
Non–cell-based systems
Charcoal hemoperfusion
High-volume plasmapheresis
Continuous high-frequency hemodiafiltration
Molecular adsorbent recirculating system (MARS)
Cell-based systems (bioartificial liver assist devices)
Primary porcine hepatocytes
Human hepatoblastoma cells
Extracorporeal liver assist device (ELAD)

Hepatocyte Transplantation

From Vincent JL, Abraham E, Moore FA, et al: *Textbook of critical care,* ed 6, Philadelphia, 2011, Saunders.

- A repeat acetaminophen level and ALT should be checked at hour 18 of treatment. If either the acetaminophen level or the ALT is elevated, the 16-hour portion of treatment (6.25 mg/kg) should be extended and another ALT, INR, or acetaminophen level should be checked every 12 hr. The acetylcysteine can be stopped once the acetaminophen level is undetectable, INR <2, or ALT is shown to be either normal or decreasing. Additional information on acetaminophen overdose is available in the topic "Acetaminophen Poisoning."
- *N*-acetylcysteine therapy outside of acetaminophen poisoning has been investigated and may be beneficial; however, its routine use is not currently recommended by practice guidelines.(9)
- Patients should be placed on stress ulcer prophylaxis given the risk of gastrointestinal bleeding.
- Antibiotics should be started immediately if infection is suspected. Sources usually include respiratory, urinary, and blood; there is no evidence for empiric antibiotic treatment. Antifungals should be initiated if no initial improvement with antibiotics occurs.
- Norepinephrine is the initial vasopressor of choice; vasopressin can be added as a second pressor. Persistent hypotension despite fluid resuscitation and pressor support should prompt concern for adrenal insufficiency.
- Lactulose is not routinely recommended for encephalopathy treatment; neomycin should be avoided due to concerns of nephrotoxicity.

PROGNOSIS

- Overall mortality from ALF is 30% to 40% and improved significantly over the last 20 years.
- Transplant-free survival in ALF in the setting of acetaminophen, hepatitis A, shock liver, and pregnancy-related disease is >50%; for all other causes of ALF, transplant-free survival is <25%.
- Multiple models have been developed to predict spontaneous recovery in ALF patients (King's College criteria, Clichy criteria, MELD score, APACHE II score).
- The King's College criteria form the basis of the model most commonly used for prognostication (Table 2).
- Transplantation.
  - Contraindications to listing include: medical history of psychiatric illness severe enough to affect patients' survival or likelihood of compliance with medications, active sepsis, severe medical comorbidities, increasing dependence on ventilator/inotropic support, acute substance abuse, previous episodes of self-harm (>5 episodes), refractory mental illness.
  - Mortality on waiting list is 25%; 1-year and 5-year survival is 66% and 70%.

TABLE 2 King's College Hospital Criteria for Liver Transplantation in Acute Liver Failure

Acetaminophen-Induced Acute Liver Failure	Non–Acetaminophen-Induced Acute Liver Failure
Arterial pH <7.3 (irrespective of grade of encephalopathy) *OR* Grade III or IV encephalopathy *and* Prothrombin time >100 sec *and* Serum creatinine >3.4 mg/dL	Prothrombin time >100 seconds (irrespective of grade of encephalopathy *OR* Any of three of the following variables (irrespective of grade of encephalopathy): 1. Age <10 yr or >40 yr 2. Etiology: non–A hepatitis, non–B hepatitis, halothane hepatitis, idiosyncratic drug reactions 3. Duration of jaundice before onset of encephalopathy >7 days 4. Prothrombin time >50 sec 5. Serum bilirubin >18 mg/dL

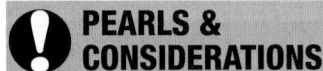

PEARLS & CONSIDERATIONS

- ALF is severe hepatic injury (as evidenced by elevated liver enzymes) with INR >1.5 and hepatic encephalopathy from a disease process that started <26 wk before presentation in a patient with no prior history of liver disease.
- Close to half of ALF is caused by drug ingestion, usually acetaminophen.
- Given the potential rapidity of deterioration, referral must be made as soon as possible to a liver transplant center.
- There should be a low threshold to start *N*-acetylcysteine.
- Do not correct coagulopathy unless life-threatening bleeding occurs or it is recommended by the liver transplant hepatologist.

SUGGESTED READINGS
Available at www.expertconsult.com

RELATED CONTENT
Acetaminophen Poisoning (Related Key Topic)
Ascites (Related Key Topic)
Encephalopathy (Related Key Topic)
Hepatopulmonary Syndrome (Related Key Topic)
Hepatorenal Syndrome (Related Key Topic)

AUTHOR: **TALIA ZENLEA, M.D.,** and **ALEXANDRA SHINGINA, M.D.C.M.**

BASIC INFORMATION

DEFINITION

Acute respiratory distress syndrome (ARDS) is a form of noncardiogenic pulmonary edema that results from acute damage to the alveoli. It is characterized by acute diffuse infiltrative lung lesions with resulting interstitial and alveolar edema, severe hypoxemia, and respiratory failure. The cardinal feature of ARDS, refractory hypoxemia, is caused by formation of protein-rich alveolar edema after damage to the integrity of the lung's alveolar-capillary barrier.

The definition of ARDS based on the American–European Consensus Conference (AECC) from 1994 included the following components:

1. The syndrome must present acutely
2. A ratio of Pao_2 to Fio_2 ≤200 regardless of the level of positive end expiratory pressure (PEEP)
3. The detection of bilateral pulmonary infiltrates on frontal chest radiograph
4. Absence of congestive heart failure (pulmonary artery wedge pressure [PAWP] ≤18 mm Hg or no clinical evidence of elevated left atrial pressure on the basis of chest radiograph or other clinical data)

The Berlin definition of ARDS adopted in 2011 addresses some of the limitations of the AECC definition and establishes the following criteria for ARDS:

- Timing: Within 1 week of a known clinical insult or new or worsening respiratory symptoms
- Chest imaging (chest x-ray or CT scan): Bilateral opacities, not fully explained by effusions, lobar/lung collapse, or nodules
- Origin of edema: Respiratory failure not fully explained by cardiac failure or fluid overload. Need objective assessment (e.g., echocardiography) to exclude hydrostatic edema if no risk factor present
- Oxygenation (if altitude is higher than 1000 m, the correction factor should be calculated as follows: $[Pao_2/Fio_2 \times \{$barometric pressure/760$\}]$)
- Mild: 200 mm Hg <Pao_2/Fio_2 ≤300 mm Hg with PEEP or CPAP ≥5 cm H_2O (this may be delivered noninvasively in the mild ARDS group)

- Moderate: 100 mm Hg <Pao_2/Fio_2 ≤200 mm Hg with PEEP or CPAP ≥5 cm H_2O
- Severe; Pao_2/Fio_2 ≤100 mm Hg with PEEP or CPAP ≥5 cm H_2O

SYNONYMS

ARDS
Adult respiratory distress syndrome

ICD-10CM CODES
J80 Acute respiratory distress syndrome

EPIDEMIOLOGY & DEMOGRAPHICS

- More than 150,000 ARDS cases per year in the U.S. 7.1% of all patients admitted to an ICU and 16.1% of all patients on mechanical ventilation develop ARDS.
- Incidence is 1.5 to 8.3 cases per 100,000 per year.
- Approximately 50% of patients who develop ARDS do so within 24 hours of the inciting event. Mortality rate is 40% to 50%.

PHYSICAL FINDINGS & CLINICAL PRESENTATION

- Signs and symptoms
  1. Dyspnea
  2. Chest discomfort
  3. Cough
  4. Anxiety
- Physical examination
  1. Tachypnea
  2. Tachycardia
  3. Hypertension
  4. Paradoxical breathing and use of accessory muscles
  5. Coarse crepitations or crackles of both lungs
  6. Fever may be present if infection is the underlying etiology

ETIOLOGY

- Sepsis (>40% of cases)
- Aspiration: near-drowning, aspiration of gastric contents (>30% of cases)
- Trauma (>20% of cases)
- Multiple transfusions, blood products
- Drugs (e.g., overdose of morphine, methadone, heroin; reaction to nitrofurantoin)
- Noxious inhalation (e.g., chlorine gas, high O_2 concentration)
- Post-resuscitation

- Cardiopulmonary bypass
- Pneumonia
- Burns
- Pancreatitis
- A history of chronic alcohol abuse significantly increases the risk of developing ARDS in critically ill patients.
- Table 1 describes risk factors associated with development of ARDS.

DIAGNOSIS

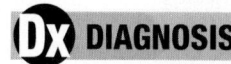

DIFFERENTIAL DIAGNOSIS

- Cardiogenic pulmonary edema
- Viral pneumonitis
- Lymphangitic carcinomatosis
- Transfusion-related lung injury
- Acute idiopathic interstitial lung disease (e.g., Hamman-Rich syndrome, acute eosinophilic pneumonitis)

WORKUP

The search for an underlying cause should focus on treatable causes (e.g., infections such as sepsis or pneumonia)

- Arterial blood gases (ABGs)
- Hemodynamic monitoring
- Bronchoalveolar lavage (selected patients)

LABORATORY TESTS

- ABGs:
  1. Initially: varying degrees of hypoxemia, generally resistant to supplemental oxygen
  2. Respiratory alkalosis, decreased Pco_2
  3. Widened alveolar-arterial gradient
  4. Hypercapnia as the disease progresses
- Bronchoalveolar lavage:
  1. The most prominent finding is an increased number of polymorphonucleocytes.
  2. The presence of eosinophilia has therapeutic implications because these patients respond to corticosteroids.
- Blood and urine cultures
- Blood work:
  1. Increased or reduced white blood cell count with left shift if concomitant infectious process
  2. Normal or mildly elevated B-type natriuretic peptide level
  3. Increased lactate level if concomitant sepsis or septic shock

IMAGING STUDIES

Chest radiograph (Fig. 1).
- The initial chest radiograph might be normal in the initial hours after the precipitating event.
- Bilateral interstitial infiltrates are usually seen within 24 hr; they often are more prominent in the bases and periphery.
- "White out" of both lung fields can be seen in advanced stages.
- CT scan of chest: diffuse consolidation with air bronchograms, bullae, pleural effusions. Pneumomediastinum and pneumothoraces may also be present and could result from ventilatory-associated barotrauma.

TABLE 1 Risk Factors Associated with Development of Acute Lung Injury and Acute Respiratory Distress Syndrome

Direct Lung Injury	Indirect Lung Injury
Pneumonia	Sepsis
Aspiration of gastric contents	Multiple trauma
Pulmonary contusion	Cardiopulmonary bypass
Fat, amniotic fluid, or air emboli	Drug overdose
Near-drowning	Acute pancreatitis
Inhalational injury	Transfusion of blood products
Reperfusion pulmonary edema	

From Vincent JL et al: *Textbook of critical care*, ed 6, Philadelphia, 2011, Saunders.

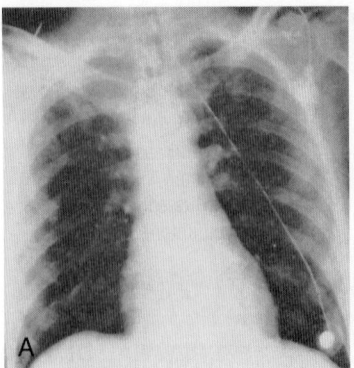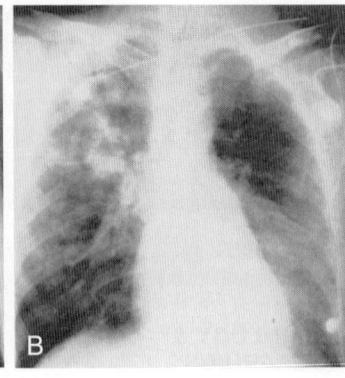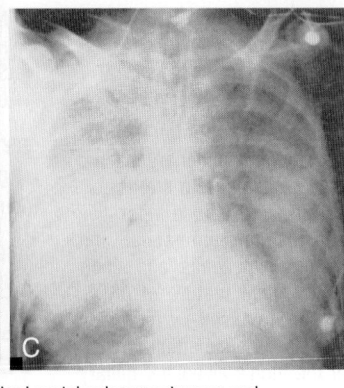

FIG. 1 Acute respiratory distress syndrome. X-ray of a young man who had sustained severe trauma and blood loss in a road traffic accident; the lungs cover a period of 5 days from a relatively normal x-ray **(A)**, to bilateral infiltrates **(B)**, to bilateral "white out" **(C)**, accompanied by severe hypoxemia. A Swan-Ganz catheter for measurement of pulmonary artery "wedge" pressure (as a reflection of left atrial pressure) can be seen *in situ* on the x-ray in **C**. The patient died shortly after the last film. (From Souhami RL, Moxham J: *Textbook of medicine*, ed 4, London, 2002, Churchill Livingstone.)

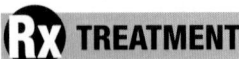 **TREATMENT**

NONPHARMACOLOGIC THERAPY

Treatment of ARDS is supportive.

Hemodynamic monitoring:

- Can be used for the initial evaluation of ARDS (in ruling out cardiogenic pulmonary edema) and its subsequent management. However, a pulmonary catheter is not indicated in the routine management of ARDS and trials have shown that clinical management involving the early use of pulmonary artery catheters in patients with ARDS did not significantly affect mortality and morbidity rates and may result in more complications as compared with a central venous catheter.
- Although no dynamic profile is diagnostic of ARDS, the presence of pulmonary edema, a high cardiac output, and a low pulmonary capillary wedge pressure (PCWP) is characteristic of ARDS.
- It is important to remember that partially treated intravascular volume overload and flash pulmonary edema can have the hemodynamic features of ARDS; filling pressures can also be elevated by increased intrathoracic pressures or with fluid administration; cardiac function can be depressed by acidosis, hypoxemia, or other factors associated with sepsis.

Ventilatory support:

Noninvasive positive-pressure ventilation (NIPPV) (i.e., BiPAP) should only be used in selected cases in patients with hypoxic respiratory failure. A recent randomized control study showed that high-flow oxygen by nasal cannula reduced ventilator-free days and mortality compared with NIPPV in patients with hypoxemic respiratory failure without hypercapnia. Either modality should not delay intubation and mechanical ventilation initiation in patients with rapidly progressing clinical deterioration.

Mechanical ventilation is generally necessary to maintain adequate gas exchange (Table 2). General recommendations for ventilator settings in ARDS are described in Table 3. A low tidal volume and low plateau pressure ventilator strategy are recommended to avoid ventilator-induced injury. Assist-control is generally preferred initially with the following ventilator settings:

- Fio_2 1.0 (until a lower value can be used to achieve adequate oxygenation). When possible, minimize oxygen toxicity by maintaining Fio_2 at <60%.
- Tidal volume: Set initial tidal volume at 6 ml/kg of predicted body weight (PBW 5 50.0 1 0.91 [height: 152.4 cm] for men, PBW 5 45.5 1 0.91 [height: 152.4 cm] for women). The concept of using PBW is based on the fact that lung size depends most strongly on height and sex; PBW normalizes the tidal volume to lung size. Aim to maintain plateau pressure (Pplat) at <30 mm Hg.
- PEEP 5 cm H_2O or greater (to increase lung volume and keep alveoli open). PEEP should be applied in small increments of 3 to 5 cm H_2O (see Table 2) to achieve acceptable arterial saturation (>0.9) with nontoxic Fio_2 values (<0.6) and acceptable airway plateau pressures (<30 to 35 cm H_2O). It is important to remember that an increase in PEEP may lower cardiac output and, despite improvement in Pao_2, may actually have a negative effect on tissue oxygenation (the major determinants of tissue oxygenation are hemoglobin, percent saturation, and cardiac output). The optimal level of PEEP remains unestablished. Although higher levels of PEEP may help prevent life-threatening hypoxemia and be associated with lower hospital mortality in patients meeting criteria for ARDS, such benefit is unlikely in patients with less severe lung injury (paO2/FiO2 >200) and a strategy of treating such patients with high PEEP levels may be harmful.
- Inspiratory flow: 60 L/min.
- Ventilatory rate: high ventilatory rates of up to 35 breaths/min are often necessary in patients with ARDS to achieve the desired minute ventilation because of their increased physiologic dead space and smaller lung volumes. Patients must be monitored for excessive intrathoracic gas trapping (auto-PEEP or intrinsic PEEP) that can depress cardiac output.
- Permissive hypercapnia: To maintain a low plateau pressure, a low tidal volume is frequently required, leading to a reduced minute ventilation and hypoventilation with consequently a respiratory acidosis (elevated PCO_2 and reduced pH). Most patients (excluding patients with cerebral edema, acute coronary syndrome, seizures, cardiac arrhythmias, and so on) can tolerate a low pH without major consequences. Bicarbonate replacement is suggested when the pH falls to below 7.20.
- Sedation: GABA receptor agonists (including propofol and benzodiazepines such as midazolam) have traditionally been the most commonly administered sedative drugs for ICU patients. Recent trials indicate that the alpha-2 agonist dexmedetomidine (Precedex) may have distinct advantages. At comparable sedation levels, dexmedetomidine-treated patients spent less time on ventilator, experienced less delirium, and developed less tachycardia and hypertension. The most notable adverse effect of dexmedetomidine was bradycardia. Preliminary trials involving early administration of the neuromuscular blocking agent cisatracurium in patients with severe ARDS have shown improvement in the adjusted 90-day survival and increase in the time off the ventilator without increase in muscle weakness. However, patients who receive continuous infusions of sedatives generally need to be on mechanical ventilation longer than those who receive intermittent dosing. Paralysis of patients with neuromuscular blockade (NMB) to facilitate controlled ventilation is associated with protracted mechanical ventilation and postparalysis weakness. It should ideally be conducted for a brief period, and limited to patients with severe ARDS. Daily interruption of sedation (daily awakening) in mechanically ventilated

TABLE 2 Management of Patients with ARDS

Calculate Predicted Body Weight (PBW)	• Males: PBW (kg) = 50 + 2.3[(height in inches) − 60] or 50 + 0.91[(height in cm) − 152.4]. • Females: PBW (kg) = 45.5 + 2.3[(height in inches) − 60] or 45.5 + 0.91[(height in cm) − 152.4].
Ventilator Mode	• Volume assist/control until weaning.
Tidal Volume (V_T)	• Initial V_T: 6 ml/kg predicted body weight. • Measure inspiratory plateau pressure (Pplat, 0.5 sec inspiratory pause) every 4 hours AND after each change in PEEP or V_T. • If Pplat >30 cm H_2O, decrease V_T to 5 or to ml/kg. • If Pplat <25 cm H_2O and V_T <6 ml/kg PBW, increase V_T by 1 ml/kg PBW.
Respiratory Rate (RR)	• With initial change in V_T, adjust RR to maintain minute ventilation. • Make subsequent adjustments to RR to maintain pH of 7.30-7.45, but do not exceed RR = 35/min, and do not increase set rate if Pa_{CO_2} <25 mm Hg.
I:E Ratio	• Acceptable range = 1:1 to 1:3 (no inverse ratio).
F_{IO_2}, Positive End-Expiratory Pressure (PEEP), and Arterial Oxygenation	• Maintain Pa_{O_2} = 55-80 mm Hg or Sp_{O_2} = 88%-95% using the following PEEP/F_{IO_2} combinations:

F_{IO_2}	0.3-0.4	0.4	0.5	0.6	0.7	0.8	0.9	1
PEEP	5-8	8-14	8-16	10-20	10-20	14-22	16-22	18-25

Acidosis Management	1. If pH <7.30, increase RR until pH ≥7.30 or RR = 35/min. 2. If pH remains <7.30 with RR = 35, consider bicarbonate infusion. 3. If pH <7.15, V_T may be increased (Pplat may exceed 30 cm H_2O).
Alkalosis Management	• If pH >7.45 and patient not triggering ventilator, decrease set RR but not below 6/min.
Fluid Management	• Once patients are out of shock, adopt a conservative fluid management strategy. • Use diuretics or fluids to target a central venous pressure (CVP) of <4 or a pulmonary artery occlusion pressure (PAOP) of <8.
Liberation from Mechanical Ventilation	• Daily interruption of sedation. • Daily screen for spontaneous breathing trial (SBT). • SBT when all of the following criteria are present: (a) F_{IO_2} <0.40 and PEEP <8 cm H_2O. (b) Not receiving neuromuscular blocking agents. (c) Patient awake and following commands. (d) Systolic arterial pressure >90 mm Hg without vasopressor support. (e) Tracheal secretions are minimal, and the patient has a good cough and gag reflex.
Spontaneous Breathing Trial	• Place patient on 5 mm Hg pressure support with 5 mm Hg PEEP or T-piece. • Monitor HR, RR, oxygen saturation for 30-90 minutes. • Extubate if there are no signs of distress (tachycardia, tachypnea, agitation, hypoxia, diaphoresis).

From Vincent JL, Abraham E, Moore FA, et al: *Textbook of critical care*, ed 6, Philadelphia, 2011, Elsevier Saunders.

TABLE 3 Recommendations for Ventilator Settings in ARDS

Conventional Mechanical Ventilation

Mode		Volume- or pressure-controlled "Airway pressure release ventilation" preferred when preservation of spontaneous ventilation is desired
Tidal volume	6-10 ml/kg	Permissive hypercapnia (increase <5 mm Hg/h) $PaCO_2$ 65-85 mm Hg well tolerated unless increased ICP Arterial pH >7.15
End-inspiratory plateau pressure	<30 cm H_2O	Above this limit, increased risks of barotrauma and air leaks
Positive end-expiratory pressure	10-15 cm H_2O	Lower PEEP levels, if heterogeneous lung injury Higher PEEP levels, if diffuse lung injury Consider early prone positioning (6-12 h)
Respiratory rate	20-60 beats/min	Adjusted to age; higher than normal may limit hypercapnia
Inspiratory/expiratory ratio	1:2 to 1:1	Check for inadvertent PEEP
FiO_2	<60%-80%	Depends on how the diseased lung may be recruited PaO_2 40-60 mm Hg, SpO_2 85%-95%

High-Frequency Oscillatory Ventilation

Amplitude pressure	30-50 cm H_2O	To achieve visible chest vibrations
Mean airway pressure	15-30 cm H_2O	To achieve adequate chest recruitment (7 to 9 ribs)
Respiratory rate	3-10 Hz	Decrease to increase tidal volume (usually not measured)
Inspiratory/expiratory ratio	1:3 to 1:1	1:1 more appropriate in diffuse lung injury
FiO_2	<60%-80%	Depends on whether the lung may be recruited

ICP, Intracranial pressure.
From Fuhrman BP et al: *Pediatric critical care*, ed 4, Philadelphia, 2011, Saunders.

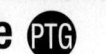
patients is safe and is associated with a shorter length of mechanical ventilation.

- The management of sedation and delirium can have important effects on the outcomes of patients in ICUs. The best outcomes are achieved with the use of a protocol in which the depth of sedation and the presence of pain and delirium are routinely monitored, pain is treated promptly and effectively, sedation is kept to the necessary minimum for the comfort and safety of the patient, and early mobilization is achieved whenever possible (Reade, Finfer, 2014).

ACUTE GENERAL Rx

Identify and treat precipitating conditions:

- Blood and urine cultures and trial of antibiotics in presumed sepsis (routine administration of antibiotics in all cases of ARDS is not recommended).
- Prompt repair of bone fractures in patients with major trauma.
- Crystalloid resuscitation in pancreatitis.
- Fluid management: In most patients with ARDS, fluid restriction is associated with better outcomes than a liberal fluid policy. Optimal fluid and hemodynamic management of patients with ARDS should be patient specific; in general, administration of crystalloids is recommended if a downward trend in PCWP is associated with diminished cardiac index, resulting in prerenal azotemia, oliguria, and relative tachycardia.
- Positioning the patient: changes in position can improve oxygenation by improving the distribution of perfusion to ventilated lung regions; repositioning (lateral decubitus positioning) should be attempted in patients with hypoxemia that is not responsive to other medical interventions. Placing patients with moderate and severe hypoxemia in a prone position may improve their oxygenation. A metaanalysis that included the recent trials by Guerin et al have shown that in patients with severe ARDS, early application of prolonged (over 16 hours/day) prone-positioning sessions significantly decreases 28-day and 90-day mortality.
- Corticosteroids: routine use of corticosteroids in ARDS is not recommended; corticosteroids may be beneficial in patients with many eosinophils in the bronchoalveolar lavage fluid or in patients with severe pneumonia. Systemic infections should be ruled out or adequately treated before administration of corticosteroids. Use of methylpred-

nisolone has not been shown to increase the rate of infectious complications but is associated with a higher rate of neuromuscular weakness. In addition, starting methylprednisolone therapy more than 2 wk after the onset of ARDS may increase the risk of death.

- Nutritional support: nutritional support, preferably administered by the enteral route, is necessary to maintain adequate colloid oncotic pressure and intravascular volume. The use of antioxidants and dietary oil supplements is still equivocal and cannot be recommended at this time.
- Tracheostomy: tracheostomy is warranted in patients requiring >2 wk of mechanical ventilation; discussion regarding tracheostomy should begin with patient (if alert and oriented) and/or family members/legal guardian after 5 to 7 days of ventilatory support. Early tracheostomy (within 4 days of admission to critical care) does not limit mortality and results in many unneeded procedures (Young et al, 2013).
- Some form of deep vein thrombosis prophylaxis is indicated in all patients with ARDS.
- Stress ulcer prophylaxis with sucralfate suspension (by nasogastric tube), or proton pump inhibitors (PO or IV) or H_2 blockers (PO or IV).
- The use of surfactant remains controversial. Patients who receive surfactant have a greater improvement in gas exchange in the initial 24-hour period than patients who receive standard therapy alone; however, the use of exogenous surfactant does not improve survival.

DISPOSITION

- Patients who survive ARDS are at risk of diminished functional capacity, mental illness, and decreased quality of life. Prognosis for ARDS varies with the underlying cause. Prognosis is worse in patients with chronic liver disease, nonpulmonary organ dysfunction, sepsis, and advanced age.
- Elevated values of dead space fraction ([$Paco_2$ $Peco_2$]/$Paco_2$; normal is <0.3) is associated with an increased risk of death.
- In ARDS, the percentage of potentially recruitable lung is variable and associated with the response to PEEP.
- Overall mortality rate varies between 32% and 45%. Most deaths are attributable to sepsis or multiorgan dysfunction rather than primary respiratory causes.

- Recent trials have shown that as compared with the current standard of care, a ventilator strategy using esophageal measures to estimate the transpulmonary pressure significantly improves oxygenation and compliance. Further trials will determine if this approach should be widely adapted.
- Strategies for treatment of life-threatening refractory hypoxemia (prone positioning, inhaled nitric acid, extracorporeal membrane oxygenation (ECMO), high-frequency oscillatory ventilation, recruitment maneuvers) may improve oxygenation, but their impact on mortality remains unproven. Use of ECMO in combination with lung-protective ventilation was found to be beneficial as a treatment strategy early in the course of ARDS related to H1N1 infection. Extracorporeal gas exchange may allow the use of low tidal volumes and lower levels of inspired oxygen and use of higher PEEP if desired. ECMO is costly and labor-intensive. The role and proper use of ECMO for patients with ARDS have not been clearly defined. General indications for venovenous ECMO in severe cases of ARDS are:
  1. Severe hypoxemia (e.g., ratio of PaO_2 to FiO_2 <80 despite the application of high levels of PEEP [typically 15 to 20 cm H_2O]) for at least 6 hr in patients with potentially reversible respiratory failure
  2. Uncompensated hypercapnia with acidemia (pH <7.15) despite the best accepted standard of care for management with a ventilator
  3. Excessively high end-inspiratory plateau pressure (>35 to 45 cm H_2O, according to the patient's body size) despite the best accepted standard of care for management with a ventilator

REFERRAL

Surgical referral for tracheostomy (see "Acute General Rx").

SUGGESTED READINGS

Available at www.expertconsult.com

RELATED CONTENT

Acute Respiratory Distress Syndrome (ARDS) (Patient Information)

AUTHOR: **NAIM AOUN, M.D.**

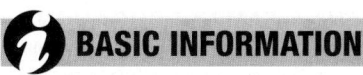

BASIC INFORMATION

DEFINITION

Acute stress disorder (ASD) includes severe acute stress reactions (ASRs) that occur between 3 days to 1 month after exposure to a traumatic event.

SYNONYMS

ASD
ASR

ICD-10CM CODES
F43.0   Acute stress reaction
F43.11 Post-traumatic stress disorder, acute

EPIDEMIOLOGY & DEMOGRAPHICS

PREVALENCE: Prevalence of ASD varies according to the nature of the traumatic event. Prevalence is estimated at less than 20% in cases that do not involve a personal assault and at 20% to 50% in cases of interpersonal trauma (e.g., sexual assault, witnessing a mass shooting).

PREDOMINANT AGE: ASD can be diagnosed at all ages. Children can manifest symptoms differently (e.g., frightening dreams that do not directly reflect the trauma). Young children may not report fear at the time of the trauma or when reexperiencing the trauma.

PREDOMINANT SEX: Females more than males

GENETICS: Differential function of the serotonin transporter may mediate differential responses to trauma. The 5-HTTLPR may constitute a genetic candidate region. Higher rates of ASD among women may be attributable to higher rates of violence against women and sex-linked neurobiological differences in the stress response.

RISK FACTORS:

- Greater perceived severity of the trauma (i.e., catastrophic interpretations of the event, exaggerated appraisals of future harm, hopelessness), high levels of negative affect, avoidant coping style, history of prior trauma, lack of social support, premorbid mental disorder (e.g., preexisting anxiety or depressive disorders)

PHYSICAL FINDINGS & CLINICAL PRESENTATION

DSM-5 criteria are met when the following criteria are satisfied:

A. Exposure to actual or threatened serious injury, death, or sexual violation in one or more of the following ways:
- Directly experiencing a traumatic event
- Witnessing a traumatic event as it occurred
- Learning that a traumatic event occurred to a family member or close friend
- Repeated or extreme exposure to traumatic details of an event

B. Presence of nine or more of the following symptoms from any of the following five categories: (1) intrusion, (2) negative mood, (3) dissociation, (4) avoidance, and (5) arousal

- Recurrent, distressing, involuntary memories of the trauma (intrusion)
- Recurrent distressing dreams relating to the trauma (intrusion)
- Flashbacks to the event, in which the individual feels/acts as if the event is recurring (intrusion)
- Intense or prolonged psychological distress or physiological reaction in response to cues that are reminiscent of the trauma (intrusion)
- Continual inability to experience positive emotions (negative mood)
- Altered sense of reality (dissociation)
- Inability to remember components of the trauma (dissociation)
- Avoidance of memories, thoughts, or feelings associated with the event (avoidance)
- Avoidance of external reminders of the event (avoidance)
- Sleep disturbance (arousal)
- Irritability and anger outbursts (arousal)
- Hypervigilance (arousal)
- Difficulties concentrating (arousal)
- Exaggerated startle response (arousal)

C. Symptoms typically begin immediately after the trauma and must persist for at least 3 days, and up to 1 month, following exposure to trauma. If symptoms persist for longer than 1 month, a diagnosis of posttraumatic stress disorder (PTSD) may be considered.

D. Exposure to trauma must result in clinically significant impairment in functioning.

E. Symptoms must not be attributable to a medical condition or substance use, and cannot be better explained by brief psychotic disorder.

ETIOLOGY

Factors predicting the development of ASD have not been established; however, multiple theoretical models have been proposed. Dissociative models propose that individuals minimize the emotional consequences of trauma by restricting awareness of the event to reduce fear. Cognitive perspectives propose that intentional cognitive processes (e.g., avoidance, distraction, dysfunctional appraisals, attribution of responsibility) result in pathological reactions to trauma. Biological theories focus on the immediate effects of trauma on neuronal function, including cortisol, catecholamines, glucocorticoids, serotonin, and endogenous opioids as mediating factors of the trauma response.

DIAGNOSIS

DIFFERENTIAL DIAGNOSIS

- Adjustment disorder
- Panic disorder
- Dissociative disorders
- PTSD
- Obsessive-compulsive disorder
- Psychotic disorders
- Traumatic brain injury

WORKUP

- Diagnosis is made based on individual interviews, including a history of past trauma, age at the time of the trauma, and duration of the trauma. Structured clinical interviews may be used and may be supplemented with standardized self-report measures. It should be noted that dissociative symptoms may prevent individuals from remembering components of the trauma, as well as remembering feelings of fear, helplessness, or horror. Collateral data from other sources (e.g., family, close friends, medical providers, therapists) may be useful.

LABORATORY TESTS

- None indicated

IMAGING STUDIES

- None indicated

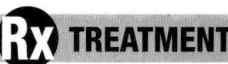 TREATMENT

- Early treatment should focus on establishing a therapeutic alliance and acknowledging fears about reexposure.
- Resilience-focused psychosocial interventions may focus on better tolerating the distress of trauma-related memories, reducing reexperiencing and reactivity to reminders of the trauma, reducing trauma-related avoidance and sleep disturbances and nightmares, increasing social support, decreasing behaviors that interfere with daily life, limiting generalization of the danger experienced, and altering maladaptive attributions and appraisals.
- Early behavioral and educational interventions also show small to moderate effects for reducing symptoms of psychological trauma.
- In cases of interpersonal trauma, safety planning is necessary for individuals who remain in unsafe situations or relationships.
- Pharmacological treatment is typically reserved for individuals who have already received psychotherapy. There are few controlled pharmacological treatment trials for ASD.
- There are currently no medications approved by the FDA for treatment of ASD. Clinicians may consider FDA-approved medications for PTSD, such as paroxetine and sertraline.

NONPHARMACOLOGIC THERAPY

- Cognitive behavioral therapy
- Prolonged exposure
- Cognitive processing therapy
- Relaxation and mindfulness

ACUTE GENERAL Rx

- Acute medication may be necessary when the individual is dangerous, agitated, or psychotic. In emergencies, short-acting benzodiazepines or neuroleptics with minimal side effects may be effective.
- Antiadrenergic agents may be useful for treatment of arousal.
- Brief, time-limited treatment using benzodiazepines may be useful for treating arousal, insomnia, and anxiety. It should be noted that prolonged use of benzodiazepines has been associated with higher rates of PTSD.
- Prazosin is recommended for treatment of nightmares.
- SSRIs and other antidepressants may be useful for reexperiencing symptoms, avoidance, and hyperarousal.

COMPLEMENTARY & ALTERNATIVE MEDICINE

- Patients may find activities that increase relaxation (i.e., yoga, mindfulness, meditation) useful.
- Eye movement desensitization and reprocessing (EMDR) has shown promise in alleviating symptoms in patients diagnosed with ASD; however, more research is needed to distinguish between the effects of EMDR treatment and the natural recovery from traumatic stress.

DISPOSITION

Treatment should be delivered in the least restrictive environment that can ensure patient safety. Most patients with ASD can be managed in an outpatient setting. Partial or inpatient hospitalization may be necessary for crisis management and may be considered for patients who have comorbid psychiatric/medical diagnoses; who are experiencing suicidal or homicidal ideation, plans, or intention; or who are severely ill.

REFERRAL

Patients are treated by a mental health clinician.

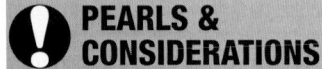

PEARLS & CONSIDERATIONS

COMMENTS

- Although many individuals with ASD go on to develop PTSD, many with ASD do not go on to develop PTSD. Available data at this time suggest that ASD criteria are not adequate for identifying individuals at risk for developing PTSD.
- There is evidence to suggest that the identification of subtypes of ASD, as well as a focus on high levels of arousal symptoms, could lead to better predictability of subsequent diagnoses of PTSD.
- Standardized assessment tools, such as the Structured Clinical Interview for DSM-5 Dissociative Disorders (SCID-D), Acute Stress Disorder Interview (ASDI), Stanford Acute Stress Reaction Questionnaire (SASRQ), and Acute Stress Disorder Scale (ASDS), may be helpful in the diagnosis of ASD or treatment monitoring.

PREVENTION

- Critical incident stress debriefing (CISD) after a trauma is typically administered in one 2- to 3-hour group session within 72 hours of the trauma, with the goals of allowing survivors to "vent." There is some evidence that CISD does not prevent PTSD and may contribute to poor recovery. Psychological first aid (PFA) is designed to improve outcomes after trauma by fostering safety, calmness, social connectedness, and optimism. Although PFA has received some empirical support, questions remain regarding the optimal format of administration.

PATIENT & FAMILY EDUCATION

- National Center for PTSD, Public Section, Information on Trauma and PTSD for Veterans, the General Public and Families: Acute Stress Disorder. (http://www.ptsd.va.gov/profession al/treatment/early/acute-stress-disorder.asp)

SUGGESTED READINGS

Available at www.expertconsult.com

RELATED CONTENT

Posttraumatic Stress Disorder (Related Key Topic)

AUTHORS: **LINDSAY M. ORCHOWSKI, PH.D.,** and **GEORGE F. ANDOSCIA, B.S.**

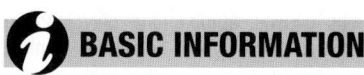

BASIC INFORMATION

DEFINITION

The acute cessation of urinary flow; inability to void.

SYNONYMS

AUR

ICD-10CM CODES
R33.8 Other retention of urine
R33.9 Retention of urine, unspecified

EPIDEMIOLOGY & DEMOGRAPHICS

INCIDENCE: It is the most common urologic emergency. May occur in any age group in either sex.

PEAK INCIDENCE: Males older than 60 years. Over a 5-year period, AUR will occur in 10% of men older than 70 years and in one third of men older than 80 years.

PREVALENCE: 40/100,000 in males and 3/100,000 in females. Prevalence has increased with longer average life spans.

PREDOMINANT SEX AND AGE: Men older than 60 years.

GENETICS: None known.

RISK FACTORS: Underlying causes of obstruction are the most common risk factors, including benign prostatic hyperplasia (BPH) and bladder, pelvic, and urethral masses. Acute trauma, surgery, medications (e.g., over-the-counter [OTC] antihistamines and α-agonists), neurologic disease, and infection can be contributing or precipitating factors, particularly when superimposed on obstructive risk factors.

PHYSICAL FINDINGS & CLINICAL PRESENTATION

- Patients will present with the acute inability to pass urine.
- Pain in the lower abdomen and suprapubic region is typical, but pain is not typically present with chronic urinary retention due to its more gradual onset.
- The bladder may be palpable on abdominal exam. Tenderness with deep palpation may be elicited.
- Patients with cognitive deficits may present with restlessness, discomfort, worsened confusion, or delirium and may not be able to provide a history of urinary retention.

ETIOLOGY

- Most commonly results from obstruction of various causes, including BPH and bladder and pelvic masses.
- Nonobstructive causes include medications, surgery, trauma, neurologic disease, and infection. Frequently multifactorial in older patients, with an underlying obstructive risk factor and an acute precipitant.
- In women, obstructive factors include benign tumors (especially fibroids); malignant tumors of pelvic, urethral, or vaginal origin; postpartum vulvar edema; and labial fusion.
- Infection such as prostatitis, urethritis, genital herpes, and herpes zoster may also produce AUR.
- Very common in the postoperative period when patients are less mobile, constipated, etc.

DIAGNOSIS

DIFFERENTIAL DIAGNOSIS

- AUR is typically self-evident to the cognitively intact patient and physician. Occasionally, a pelvic mass or fluid collection can be confused for a full bladder, but this is rare.

WORKUP

- History should focus on urologic symptoms, including dysuria, hematuria, history of retention, urologic surgery, and urologic cancer.
- History should include a complete list of prescribed and over-the-counter medications and recent changes in medications.
- Review of symptoms should include presence of fever, back pain, neurologic symptoms, and rash.
- Rectal exam for masses, fecal impaction, perineal sensation, and sphincter tone.
- Pelvic exam for female patients.
- Neurologic exam to rule out an underlying neurologic cause.

LABORATORY TESTS

- Serum creatinine level: In acute retention, level may not be elevated above baseline.
- Urinalysis and culture (obtained via bladder catheterization).
- Electrolytes, BUN.
- Prostate-specific antigen testing is not helpful in AUR and may be falsely elevated after catheter placement. This test should be checked acutely.

IMAGING STUDIES

- Bladder ultrasound or a bedside post-void residual urine scan ("bladder scanner") can be diagnostic.
- Abdominal ultrasound or computed tomography may be helpful if there is suspicion of a pelvic mass.
- Magnetic resonance imaging (MRI) is used when symptoms suggest spinal cord problems.
- Renal ultrasound may be obtained if there is associated renal impairment and hydronephrosis is suspected.
- Evaluation of bladder function may be considered after initial management, particularly in females with no evidence of anatomic obstruction.

TREATMENT

ACUTE GENERAL Rx

- Prompt bladder decompression and drainage is initial management of AUR, usually with an indwelling bladder catheter.
- Consultation with a urologist is advised when there has been recent genitourinary surgery.

CHRONIC Rx

- A voiding trial is reasonable in 5 to 7 days in most patients.
- α-blockers are effective for treatment of BPH symptoms in men and may increase the success of trials of early catheter removal and should be initiated, unless contraindicated.
- 5-α reductase inhibitors are not indicated for acute management when AUR is caused by BPH, due to slow decrease of prostatic volume.
- Where feasible, medications that increase the risk of AUR should be stopped.
- If a patient remains unable to void after 5 to 7 days of catheterization, urologic consultation is imperative. Plans to further evaluate the etiology of AUR are critical.

Patients unable to void after a voiding trial can either initiate clean intermittent catheterization every 4 to 6 hours or have the urinary bladder catheter replaced.

DISPOSITION

- To home if close follow-up can be ensured.
- Hospital admission may be needed, particularly in patients with sepsis associated with urinary tract infection, acute kidney injury due to retention, or electrolyte abnormalities, or when urinary retention is due to malignancy or spinal cord compression.

REFERRAL

- Request immediate urologic assistance when attempts at initial bladder catheterization are unsuccessful or when the patient has recently undergone urologic surgery, especially radical prostatectomy, transurethral radical prostatectomy, and other bladder/prostate surgeries.
- Urologic referral is appropriate for almost all cases, but it can be completed either after a successful voiding trial or after the catheter has been in a few days. This allows the urologist to perform the voiding trial and/or to assess baseline voiding function. Recurrent episodes of retention in men warrant urologic referral to consider transurethral resection of the prostate.
- Gynecologic referral is mandatory if a pelvic mass is found to be the cause of AUR in a woman.

PEARLS & CONSIDERATIONS

PREVENTION

Patients with BPH should be cautious regarding the use of medications that can precipitate acute retention, including antihistamines, sympathomimetics, sedatives, and others. Inhaled anticholinergic agents may increase the risk of AUR, and they should be used cautiously in patients with risk factors, especially BPH.

SUGGESTED READINGS

Available at www.expertconsult.com

RELATED CONTENT

Benign Prostatic Hypertrophy (Related Key Topic)

AUTHOR: **MARGARET TRYFOROS, M.D.**

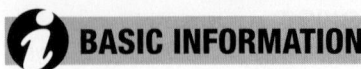

DEFINITION

Adrenal insufficiency is characterized by inadequate secretion of corticosteroids resulting from partial or complete destruction of the adrenal glands (primary adrenal failure). Inadequate secretion of cortisol from the adrenals due to critical illness and pituitary insufficiency is known as secondary cortisol deficiency.

SYNONYMS

Primary adrenocortical insufficiency
Addison disease

ICD-10CM CODES
E27.1 Primary adrenocortical insufficiency
E27.2 Addisonian crisis
E27.40 Unspecified adrenocortical
        insufficiency
E27.49 Other adrenocortical insufficiency
E27.3 Drug-induced adrenocortical
        insufficiency
E23.3 Hypopituitarism

EPIDEMIOLOGY & DEMOGRAPHICS

PREVALENCE: 10 to 15 per 100,000 persons
PREDOMINANT SEX: Female/male ratio of 2:1

PHYSICAL FINDINGS & CLINICAL PRESENTATION

- Adrenal insufficiency may present insidiously with nonspecific symptoms. A high index of suspicion is required for diagnosis. About half of patients may present acutely with adrenal crises. Table 1 summarizes the clinical features of primary adrenal insufficiency.
- Hyperpigmentation of skin (Figs. E1 and E2) and mucous membranes is a cardinal sign of adrenal insufficiency: more prominent in palmar creases, buccal mucosa, pressure points (elbows, knees, knuckles), perianal mucosa, and around areolas of nipples
- Hypotension, postural dizziness
- Generalized weakness, chronic fatigue, malaise, anorexia
- Amenorrhea and loss of axillary hair in females

ETIOLOGY

- Autoimmune destruction of the adrenal glands (80% of cases)
- Tuberculosis (TB) (7%-20% of cases)
- Carcinomatous destruction of the adrenal glands, lymphoma
- Adrenal hemorrhage (anticoagulants, trauma, coagulopathies, pregnancy, sepsis)
- Adrenal infarction (antiphospholipid syndrome, arteritis, thrombosis)
- AIDS (adrenal insufficiency develops in 30% of patients with AIDS, often cytomegalovirus [CMV] adrenalitis)
- Genetic causes: autoimmune polyglandular syndromes (APS) types 1 and 2, X-linked adrenoleukodystrophy, congenital adrenal hyperplasia
- Other: sarcoidosis, amyloidosis, hemochromatosis, Wegener's granulomatosis, postoperative, fungal infections (candidiasis, histoplasmosis)

DX DIAGNOSIS

DIFFERENTIAL DIAGNOSIS

Sepsis, hypovolemic shock, acute abdomen, apathetic hyperthyroidism in the elderly, myopathies, gastrointestinal malignancy, major depression, anorexia nervosa, hemochromatosis, salt-losing nephritis, chronic infection

WORKUP

- An early morning (8 am) serum cortisol <3 mcg/dl (82.8 mmol/L) is consistent with cortisol deficiency.
- If the clinical picture is highly suggestive of adrenocortical insufficiency, the diagnosis can be confirmed with the rapid adrenocorticotropic hormone (ACTH) test:
  1. Give 250 mcg ACTH (Sinachten, tetracosatrin) by IV push and measure cortisol levels at 0, 30, and 60 min.
  2. An increase in serum cortisol level to peak concentration >500 nmol/L (18 mcg/dl) indicates a normal response. Cortisol level <18 mcg/dl at 30 or 60 min is suggestive of adrenal insufficiency.
  3. Measure plasma ACTH. A high ACTH level (>200 pg/mL [44 pmol/L]) confirms primary adrenal insufficiency.
- Critical illness-related corticosteroid insufficiency (e.g., in sepsis) is best established with the 1-mcg ACTH stimulation test in which cortisol levels are measured at baseline and 30 min after administration of ACTH. A level <25 mcg/dl (690 nmol/L) or an increment over baseline of <9 mcg (250 nmol/L) represents an inadequate adrenal response.
- Secondary adrenocortical insufficiency (caused by pituitary dysfunction) can be distinguished from primary adrenal insufficiency by the following:
  1. Normal or low plasma ACTH level after rapid ACTH
  2. Absence of hyperpigmentation
  3. No significant impairment of aldosterone secretion (because aldosterone secretion is under control of the renin-angiotensin system)
  4. Additional evidence of hypopituitarism (e.g., hypogonadism, hypothyroidism)

LABORATORY TESTS

- Hyponatremia, hyperkalemia
- Decreased glucose
- Increased BUN/creatinine ratio (prerenal azotemia)
- Mild normocytic, normochromic anemia, neutropenia, lymphocytosis, eosinophilia (significant dehydration may mask hyponatremia and anemia), hypercalcemia, metabolic acidosis

---

TABLE 1   Clinical Features of Primary Adrenal Insufficiency

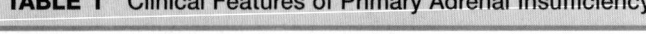

Feature	Frequency (%)
Symptoms	
Weakness, tiredness, fatigue	100
Anorexia	100
Gastrointestinal symptoms	92
Nausea	86
Vomiting	75
Constipation	33
Abdominal pain	31
Diarrhea	16
Salt craving	16
Postural dizziness	12
Muscle or joint pains	13
Signs	
Weight loss	100
Hyperpigmentation	94
Hypotension (<110 mm Hg systolic)	88-94
Vitiligo	10-20
Auricular calcification	5
Laboratory Findings	
Electrolyte disturbances	92
Hyponatremia	88
Hyperkalemia	64
Hypercalcemia	6
Azotemia	55
Anemia	40
Eosinophilia	17

From Melmed S, Polonsky KS, Larsen PR, Kronenberg HM: *Williams textbook of endocrinology,* ed 12, Philadelphia, 2011, Saunders.

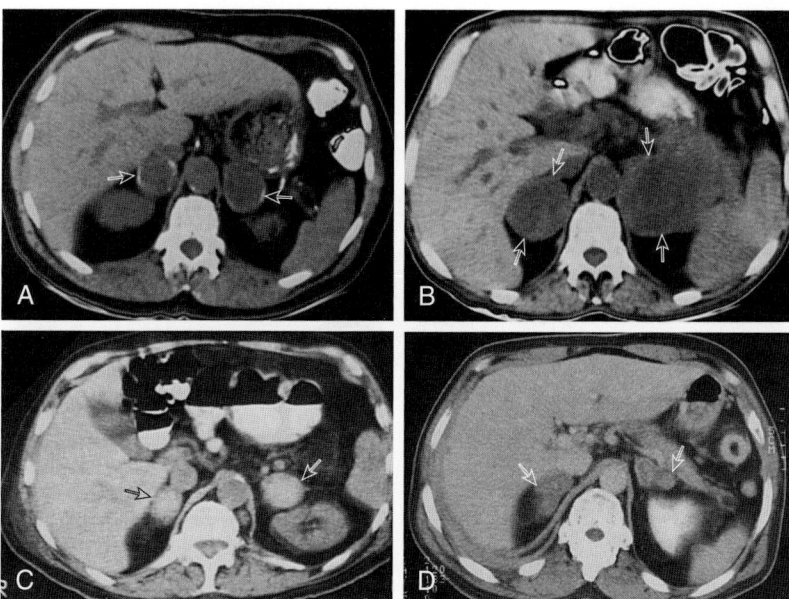

FIG. 3 Computed tomographic (CT) scans of patients with primary adrenal insufficiency. The affected adrenal glands are indicated by arrows. **A,** CT scan of a 59-year-old man with histoplasmosis. Notice the subcapsular calcium in both glands. **B,** CT scan of a 59-year-old man with metastatic melanoma. **C,** CT scan of an 80-year-old man with bilateral adrenal hemorrhage resulting from anticoagulation for pulmonary emboli. **D,** Bilateral adrenal tuberculomas in a 79-year-old man with tuberculosis affecting the urogenital tract. (**A** and **B** courtesy of Dr. William D. Salmon, Jr.; **C,** courtesy of Dr. Craig R. Sussman.) (From Melmed S, Polonsky KS, Larsen PR, Kronenberg HM: *Williams textbook of endocrinology,* ed 12, Philadelphia, 2011, Saunders.)

- A morning cortisol level >500 mmol/L (18 mcg/dl) generally excludes the diagnosis whereas a level <165 mmol/L (6 mcg/dl) is suggestive of Addison disease and a level <3 mcg/dl requires further evaluation (see "Workup")
- Useful tests in evaluating the cause of adrenal insufficiency are: PPD (rule out TB), adrenal cortex antibodies and 21-hydroxylase antibodies (rule out autoimmune Addison disease), plasma very-long-chain fatty acids (rule out adrenoleukodystrophy)

IMAGING STUDIES

- Imaging is not necessary for diagnosis but may help identify potential causes.
- Abdominal CT scan (Fig. 3): small adrenal glands generally indicate either idiopathic atrophy or longstanding TB, whereas enlarged glands are suggestive of early TB or potentially treatable diseases.
- Chest radiograph may reveal a small heart (Fig. E4).
- Abdominal radiograph: adrenal calcifications may be noted if the adrenocortical insufficiency is secondary to TB or fungal infection.

Rx TREATMENT

NONPHARMACOLOGIC THERAPY

- Perform periodic monitoring of serum electrolytes, vital signs, and body weight; liberal sodium intake is suggested.
- Periodic measurement of bone density may be helpful in identifying patients at risk for the development of osteoporosis.
- Patients should carry a MedicAlert bracelet and an emergency pack containing hydrocortisone 100-mg ampule, syringe, and needle.
- Patients and partners should be educated on how to give IM injection in case of vomiting or coma.

ACUTE GENERAL Rx

- Addisonian crisis is an acute complication of adrenal insufficiency characterized by circulatory collapse, dehydration, nausea, vomiting, hypoglycemia, and hyperkalemia.
  1. Draw plasma cortisol level; do not delay therapy while waiting for confirming laboratory results.
  2. Administer hydrocortisone 100 mg IV immediately, followed by 100 to 200 mg of hydrocortisone every 24 hours divided into 3 or 4 doses; if patient shows good clinical response, gradually taper dosage and change to oral maintenance dose (usually prednisone 7.5 mg/day).
  3. Provide adequate volume replacement with D_5NS solution until hypotension, dehydration, and hypoglycemia are completely corrected. Large volumes (2 to 3 L) under continuous cardiac monitoring may be necessary in the first 2 to 3 hr to correct the volume deficit and hypoglycemia and to avoid further hyponatremia.
- Identify and correct any precipitating factor (e.g., sepsis, hemorrhage).

CHRONIC Rx

- Give hydrocortisone 15 to 20 mg PO every morning and 5 to 10 mg in late afternoon or prednisone 5 mg in morning and 2.5 mg hs.
- Give oral fludrocortisone 0.05 mg/day to 0.20 mg/day: this mineralocorticoid is necessary if the patient has primary adrenocortical insufficiency. The dose is adjusted based on the serum sodium level and the presence of postural hypotension or marked orthostasis.
- Instruct patients to increase glucocorticoid replacement in times of stress and to receive parenteral glucocorticoids if diarrhea or vomiting occurs. Typical supplementation varies from 25 mg PO qd of hydrocortisone for minor medical and surgical stress to 50 to 100 mg IV hydrocortisone q8h for sepsis-induced hypotension or shock.
- The administration of dehydroepiandrosterone (DHEA) is controversial. It is not indicated in men but may be considered in women with primary adrenal failure. A dose of 50 mg PO qd may improve well-being and sexuality in women with adrenal insufficiency.
- Patients with concomitant hypothyroidism should be treated with glucocorticoids first before correcting hypothyroidism because correction of thyroid hormone deficiency will accelerate cortisol clearance and can precipitate adrenal crisis.

SUGGESTED READINGS

Available at www.expertconsult.com

RELATED CONTENT

Addison Disease (Patient Information)

AUTHOR: **FRED F. FERRI, M.D.**

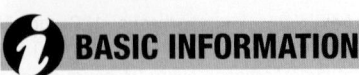

BASIC INFORMATION

DEFINITION

Adult-onset Still's disease (AOSD) is a rare systemic autoinflammatory disorder of unknown etiology. It is characterized mainly by daily high spiking fevers >102° F, arthritis or arthralgias, and an evanescent salmon-colored skin rash with an elevated serum ferritin. The temperature returns to normal between fever spikes and is usually the initial manifestation. Musculoskeletal symptoms are universal and eventually progress to destructive arthropathy, which is most commonly located in the knees, wrists, and ankles. As this is a systemic condition, there is a large variety of symptom presentations in affected individuals.

SYNONYMS

Adult Still's disease
Wissler's syndrome
Wissler-Fanconi syndrome
AOSD

ICD-10CM CODES
M06.1 Adult-onset Still disease

EPIDEMIOLOGY & DEMOGRAPHICS

INCIDENCE: 22/10,000,000 in men, 34/10,000,000 in women
PEAK INCIDENCE: Age 16 to 35
PREVALENCE: 1.5 cases per 100,000 to 1,000,000 population.
PREDOMINANT SEX AND AGE: Roughly equal sex distribution, bimodal age range 15 to 25 and 36 to 46
GENETICS: Relative risk ranging from 2.1 to 2.9 associated with HLA B17, B18, B35, and DR2. Cytokine production is thought to be implicated in the pathogenesis: IL6, IL2, interferon gamma, and tumor necrosis factor alpha (TNF-α)
RISK FACTORS: Stress is the only known risk factor.
PHYSICAL FINDINGS & CLINICAL PRESENTATION:
- Triad (occurring in 75%-95% of patients): High spiking fevers, characteristic rash, and arthritis/arthralgias.
- Fever is >102° F, transient, quotidian in pattern, usually in the late afternoon/early evening.
- Rash is typically evanescent, salmon pink, and maculopapular. It is usually located on the trunk and proximal extremities, but it can involve the palms and soles (and occasionally the face). The rash often accompanies fever and resolves when the patient is afebrile.
- Arthritis is symmetric and destructive, involving the wrists, knees, and ankles. Fusion of the wrist joints is characteristic of AOSD.
- Nonspecific symptoms: pharyngitis, myalgias, lymphadenopathy, splenomegaly, and serositis, including pleuritis and pericarditis.

ETIOLOGY
- None identified

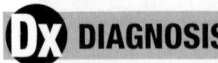

DIAGNOSIS

DIFFERENTIAL DIAGNOSIS
- Infection, malignancy, or autoimmune disorders
  1. Infection: Hepatitis, rubella, CMV, EBV, mumps, coxsackie virus, adenovirus
  2. Neoplasms: Leukemia, lymphoma, angioblastic T cell lymphoma, solid cancers, myeloproliferative disorders
  3. Autoinflammatory: Schnitzler syndrome, Sweet syndrome, sarcoid, hemophagocytic lymphohistiocytosis
  4. Rheumatologic: Rheumatoid arthritis, reactive arthritis, systemic lupus erythematosus, dermatomyositis/polymyositis, periarteritis nodosa (PAN)
  5. Periodic fever syndromes: Familial Mediterranean fever (FMF), TNF receptor–associated periodic syndrome (TRAPS)

DIAGNOSTIC CRITERIA

This is a diagnosis of exclusion made only in the absence of other clinical conditions that present in a similar fashion.

Multiple potential diagnostic criteria have been proposed in the evaluation of patients suspected of having adult-onset Still's disease. The Yamaguchi criteria are the most widely used and have 93.5% sensitivity.

Yamaguchi criteria

MAJOR CRITERIA:
- Arthralgia >2 weeks
- Fever >102.2° F; >1 week
- Nonpruritic salmon rash
- WBC >10,000 with 80% granulocytes

MINOR CRITERIA:
- Sore throat
- Lymphadenopathy
- Hepatomegaly/splenomegaly
- LFT abnormalities
- Negative ANA and RF

Exclusion criteria: infections, malignancies, and rheumatic diseases
Diagnosis: 5 criteria with at least 2 major criteria

LABORATORY TESTS
- CBC generally demonstrates leukocytosis with a predominance of polymorphonuclear leukocytes.
- ANA and RF results are usually within normal levels in AOSD, whereas ESR/CRP are often markedly elevated in virtually all patients.
- ALT/AST and LDH are elevated in at least 75% of patients.
- Ferritin can be markedly elevated beyond the level expected for a typical inflammatory process (as much as 70% of patients).
- Normocytic anemia with hemoglobin <10 g/dl and reactive thrombocytosis.

IMAGING STUDIES
- Radiographs are not helpful at early onset of symptoms; helpful if chronic.

- Early changes could show soft tissue swelling, joint effusions, and/or periarticular osteopenia.
- Classic finding is nonerosive narrowing of carpometacarpal (CMC) and intercarpal joint space of wrist. This can eventually lead to ankylosis.
- X-ray findings are seen in only 40% of patients, however.
- Radionuclide bone scan and MRI with gadolinium may be helpful for early diagnosis.

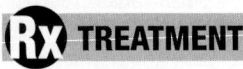

TREATMENT

ACUTE GENERAL Rx
- Aspirin and NSAIDs at full doses are used initially to control arthritic symptoms.
- Systemic glucocorticoids are often required to control systemic inflammation in more severe disease.

CHRONIC Rx
- In patients with persistent symptoms, steroid-sparing immunomodulatory agents are often required.
- Oral or injectable methotrexate is often added to control chronic disease, specifically the arthritis symptoms.
- TNF-inhibitors including etanercept and infliximab can be effective at controlling symptoms.
- Anti-IL6 (tocilizumab) and anti-IL1 (anakinra) may also be effective in controlling disease activity.

DISPOSITION
- Three distinct patterns of clinical course:
  1. Self-limited/monocyclic pattern: systemic symptoms of fever, rash, serositis, hepatosplenomegaly predominate for a few weeks to months; remission in 1 year
  2. Intermittent/polycyclic pattern: recurrent fevers with or without articular symptoms lasting from a few weeks up to 2 years; may have complete remission between flares that could be years apart
  3. Chronic articular pattern: severe articular presentation leading to joint destruction; more disability, worst prognosis

REFERRAL
- Rheumatology for diagnosis and treatment
- Dermatology for evaluation and possible biopsy of rash

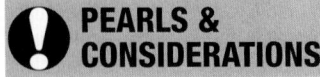

PEARLS & CONSIDERATIONS

COMMENTS
- AOSD is a diagnosis of exclusion.
- Evanescent rash often dissipates when the patient is afebrile; it is therefore important to do a skin exam while the patient is febrile.
- Suspect AOSD when ferritin levels >3000 ng/ml in clinical context when bacterial and viral infections are excluded.

AUTHOR: **JANAKI PATEL, M.D.**

BASIC INFORMATION

DEFINITION

Moderate drinking has been defined as two standard drinks (e.g., 12 oz of beer) per day and one drink per day for women and persons older than 65 yr. Although not generally included under the alcoholism topic, hazardous or at-risk drinking should also be considered. For men, *at-risk drinking* is defined as more than 14 drinks/wk or more than 4 drinks/occasion. For women, at-risk drinking is defined as approximately half that given for men.

The American Psychiatric Association defines diagnostic criteria for *alcohol withdrawal* as follows:

A. Cessation of (or reduction in) alcohol use that has been heavy and prolonged.

B. Two (or more) of the following, developing within several hours to a few days after criterion A:
1. Autonomic hyperactivity (e.g., sweating or pulse rate >100 beats/min)
2. Increased hand tremor
3. Insomnia
4. Nausea and vomiting
5. Transient visual, tactile, or auditory hallucinations or illusions
6. Psychomotor agitation
7. Anxiety
8. Grand mal seizures

C. The symptoms in criterion B cause clinically significant distress or impairment in social, occupational, or other important areas of functioning.

The symptoms are not attributable to a general medical condition and are not better accounted for by another mental disorder.

SYNONYMS

Alcohol abuse
Substance abuse

ICD-10CM CODES
F10	Mental and behavioral disorders due to use of alcohol
F10.1	Mental and behavioral disorders due to use of alcohol: harmful use
F10.2	Mental and behavioral disorders due to use of alcohol: dependence syndrome
F10.3	Mental and behavioral disorders due to use of alcohol: withdrawal state
F10.4	Mental and behavioral disorders due to use of alcohol: withdrawal state with delirium
F10.5	Mental and behavioral disorders due to use of alcohol: psychotic disorder
F10.6	Mental and behavioral disorders due to use of alcohol: amnesic syndrome

EPIDEMIOLOGY & DEMOGRAPHICS

INCIDENCE (IN U.S.):
- The clinical history suggests alcohol problems in 15% to 20% of patients in primary care and hospitalized patients. In the U.S., alcohol abuse generates nearly $223 billion in annual economic costs. An estimated 9% of adults in the U.S. have alcohol dependence.
- 20% achieve abstinence without help; 70% achieve sobriety for 1 yr.

PREVALENCE (IN U.S.): 7% of population ≥18 yr

PREDOMINANT SEX
- Lifetime risk for males 8% to 10%
- Lifetime risk for females 3% to 5%

PEAK INCIDENCE: 20 to 40 yr. The most common age range for initial treatment of alcohol dependence is 35 to 45 yr. However, the peak period for meeting alcohol dependence criteria is ≥10 years earlier.

GENETICS: More common with a family history of alcoholism and in patients of Irish, Scandinavian, and Native American descent

PHYSICAL FINDINGS & CLINICAL PRESENTATION

- Recurring minor trauma
- Gastrointestinal bleeding from gastritis and/or varices
- Pancreatitis (acute and chronic)
- Liver disease
- Odor of alcohol on breath
- Tremulousness
- Tachycardia
- Peripheral neuropathy
- Recent memory loss

ETIOLOGY

- Social and genetic factors important
- Risk factors:
  1. Broken homes
  2. Unemployment
  3. Divorce
  4. Recurrent depression
  5. Addiction to another substance, including tobacco
  6. Working long hours (≥55 hours/week)

DIAGNOSIS

WORKUP

- The USPSTF recommends that clinicians screen adults 18 years and older for alcohol misuse and provide persons engaged in risky or hazardous drinking with brief behavioral counseling interventions to reduce alcohol misuse. Several screening tests (CAGE, TWEAK, CRAFFT, AUDIT-C) are available. The four-item CAGE (feeling need to **C**ut down, **A**nnoyed by criticism, **G**uilty about drinking, and need for an **E**ye-opener in the morning) is the most popular screening test in primary care (Fig. E1). A positive response should lead to further questioning. The sensitivity of the CAGE ranges from 43% to 94% and its specificity ranges from 70% to 97%. The five-item TWEAK scale (**T**olerance, **W**orry, **E**ye-openers, **A**mnesia, [**K**] cut down) and the TACE questionnaire (**T**olerance, **A**nnoyance, **C**ut down, **E**ye-opener) are designed to screen pregnant women for alcohol misuse. They detect lower levels of alcohol consumption that may pose risks during pregnancy. The CRAFFT questionnaire (riding in **C**ar with someone who was drinking, using alcohol to **R**elax, using alcohol while **A**lone, **F**orgetfulness, criticism from **F**riends and **F**amily, **T**rouble) is useful as a screening tool for adolescents. Its sensitivity is 92% and specificity 64% for alcohol abuse. Single-question screening about alcohol consumption in a day ("When was the last time you had more than X drinks in a day?" [where X is 5 for men and 4 for women]) with the threshold set at "in the past 3 months" is 85% sensitive and 70% specific in men and 82% and 70% in women for unhealthy alcohol use. The 3-question AUDIT-C is a shorter form of the 10-item AUDIT, and the questions center on the quantity and frequency of alcohol use. It asks how often someone has had a drink containing alcohol, how many standard drinks containing alcohol one consumes on a typical day when one is drinking, and how often one has six or more drinks on one occasion. Scoring ranges from 0 to 4 on each question with a total score range of 0 to 12. A total score of 3 or higher for women and 4 or higher for men indicates alcohol use disorder and need for further assessment. Its sensitivity ranges from 85% in Hispanic women to 95% in white men.
- Laboratory evaluation (see below).

LABORATORY TESTS

- Lab tests alone do not accurately detect alcohol problems but can help identify medical complications related to alcohol use, such as pancreatitis or cirrhosis.
- Gamma-glutamyltransferase (GGTP), generally elevated
- Liver transaminases (alanine aminotransferase [ALT], aspartate aminotransferase [AST]), often elevated, may be normal or low in advanced liver disease.
- Low albumin level, hypophosphatemia, hypomagnesemia from malnutrition
- Complete blood count (CBC) reveals elevated mean corpuscular volume from toxic effect of alcohol on erythrocyte development in nutritional deficiencies.
- Stool for occult blood may be positive as a result of gastritis or variceal bleeding
- RBC folate, vitamin B_{12} level, vitamin B_6, vitamin B_1 level

IMAGING STUDIES

Indicated only with a history of trauma. CT or ultrasound of abdomen may reveal fatty liver or cirrhosis in advanced stages.

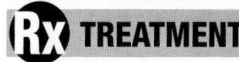 TREATMENT

NONPHARMACOLOGIC THERAPY

- Twelve-step facilitation, cognitive behavioral therapy, and motivational enhancement therapy improve the chances of recovery in patients with alcohol abuse and dependence.
- Depression, if present, should be treated at same time alcohol is withdrawn.

ACUTE GENERAL Rx

Alcohol withdrawal syndrome (AWS) occurs when a person stops ingesting alcohol after prolonged consumption. It can result in four possible clinical patterns depending on the severity of the patient's alcohol abuse and the time from the patient's previous alcohol ingestion. Fig. 2 illustrates typical symptoms depending on time course of alcohol withdrawal. Blood ethanol level decreases by ~20 mg/dl/hr (Fig. E3) in a normal person. Although discussed separately, these withdrawal states blend together in real life. Table 1 summarizes medications for the treatment of alcohol dependence.

1. **Tremulous state** (early alcohol withdrawal, "impending DTs," "shakes," "jitters").

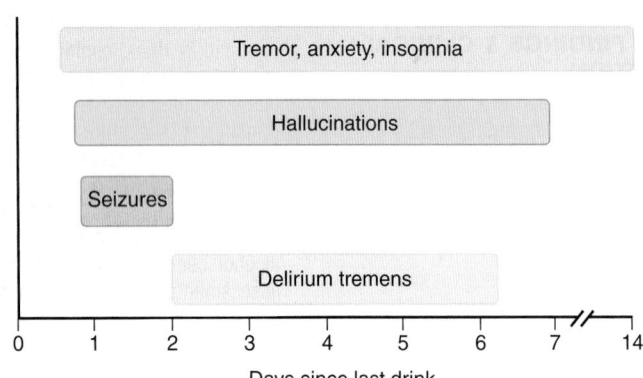

FIG. 2 Time course of alcohol withdrawal. (From Goldman L, Schafer AI: *Goldman's Cecil medicine,* ed 24, Philadelphia, 2012, Saunders.)

a. Time interval: usually occurs 6 to 8 hr after the last drink or 12 to 48 hr after reduction of alcohol intake; becomes most pronounced at 24 to 36 hr.
b. Manifestation: tremors, mild agitation, insomnia, tachycardia; symptoms are relieved by alcohol.
c. Detoxification can be in the outpatient (ambulatory) or inpatient setting. Candidates for outpatient detoxification should have a reasonable support system (e.g., reliable contact person) who can monitor progress and lack of any significant comorbid conditions (e.g., suicide risk, seizure disorder, coexisting benzodiazepine dependence, prior unsuccessful outpatient detoxification, pregnancy, cirrhosis) or risk factors for severe withdrawal (age >40 yr, drinking >100 g of ethanol daily [e.g., 1 pint of liquor or eight 12-oz cans of beer, random blood alcohol concentration >200 mg/dl]).
d. Inpatient treatment:
   (1) Admit to medical floor (private room); monitor vital signs q4h; institute seizure precautions; maintain adequate sedation.
   (2) Administer lorazepam as follows:
      (a) Day 1: 2 mg PO q4h while awake and not lethargic.
      (b) Day 2: 1 mg PO q4h while awake and not lethargic.
      (c) Day 3: 0.5 mg PO q4h while awake and not lethargic.
      (d) NOTE: Hold sedation for lethargy or abnormal vital or neurologic signs. The preceding doses are only guidelines; it is best to titrate the dose case by case.
   (3) In patients with mild to moderate withdrawal and without history of seizures, individualized benzodiazepine administration (rather than a fixed-dose regimen) results in lower benzodiazepine administration and avoids unnecessary sedation. The Clinical Institute Withdrawal Assessment Scale for Alcohol, Revised (CIWA-Ar) scale (Box 1) can be used to measure the severity of alcohol withdrawal. It consists of 10 items: nausea; tremor; autonomic hyperactivity; anxiety; agitation; tactile, visual, and auditory

TABLE 1	Medications for the Treatment of Alcohol Dependence*				
Medication	**Dose and Route**	**Frequency**	**Effects**		**Major Common Adverse Effects**
Alcohol Withdrawal					
			Benzodiazepines†		
Chlordiazepoxide*	25-100 mg, PO/IV/IM†	Every 4-6 hr	Decreased severity of withdrawal; stabilization of vital signs; prevention of seizures and delirium tremens		Confusion, oversedation, respiratory depression
Diazepam‡	5-10 mg, PO/IV/IM†	Every 6-8 hr			
Oxazepam‡	15-30 mg, PO†	Every 6-8 hr			
Lorazepam‡	1-4 mg, PO/IV/IM†	Every 4-8 hr			
			β-Blockers		
Atenolol	25-50 mg, PO	Once a day	Improvement in vital signs		Bradycardia, hypotension
Propranolol	10-40 mg, PO	Every 6-8 hr	Reduction in craving		
			α-Agonists		
Clonidine	0.1-0.2 mg, PO	Every 6 hr	Decreased withdrawal symptoms		Hypotension, fatigue
			Antiepileptics		
Carbamazepine	200 mg, PO	Every 6-8 hr	Decreased severity of withdrawal; prevention of seizures		Dizziness, fatigue, red blood cell abnormalities
			Prevention of Relapse		
Disulfiram‡	125-500 mg, PO	Daily	Decreased alcohol use among those who relapse		Disulfiram-alcohol reaction, rash, drowsiness, peripheral neuropathy
Naltrexone‡	50 mg, PO	Daily	Increased abstinence, decreased drinking days		Nausea, abdominal pain, myalgias-arthralgias
	380 mg, IM	Every 4 wk			
Acamprosate‡	666 mg, PO	Three times a day	Increased abstinence		Diarrhea

*Most commonly used medications listed.
†Currently approved by U.S. Food and Drug Administration for the indication noted.
‡Dose and routes given for standard fixed-dose regimens, which include dose tapers over time.
From Goldman L, Schafer AI: *Goldman's Cecil medicine,* ed 24, Philadelphia, 2012, Saunders.

disturbances; headache; and disorientation. Each item is assigned a score from 0 to 7. For example, in the "agitation" category 0 indicates normal activity, and 7 indicates that the patient constantly thrashes about. For the category of "tremor," 0 indicates that tremor is not present and 7 that tremor is severe, even with arms not extended. The maximum total score is 67. Patients with mild AWS symptoms (CIWA-Ar score <8 can be monitored on an outpatient basis. Benzodiazepines are beneficial for most patients with a CIWA-AR score ≥8 and are strongly recommended in patients with substantial withdrawal symptoms (CIWA-Ar score >12). Patients with CIWA-Ar score of ≥15 should be admitted to detox unit. In-patient treatment is also recommended for patients with history of withdrawal seizures and for those with suicidal ideation and significant comorbidities.

(4) Beta-adrenergic blockers: beta-blockers are useful for controlling blood pressure and tachyarrhythmias. However, they do not prevent progression to more serious symptoms of withdrawal and, if used, should not be administered alone but in conjunction with benzodiazepines. Beta-blockers should be avoided in patients with contraindications to their use (e.g., bronchospasm, bradycardia, or severe congestive heart failure). Centrally acting alpha-adrenergic agonists such as clonidine ameliorate symptoms in patients with mild to moderate withdrawal but do not reduce delirium or seizures.

(5) Vitamin replacement: thiamine 100 mg IV or IM for at least 5 days plus oral multivitamins. The IV administration of glucose can precipitate Wernicke's encephalopathy in alcoholics with thiamine deficiency; therefore thiamine administration should precede IV dextrose.

(6) Hydration PO or IV (high-caloric solution): if IV, glucose with Na^+, K^+, Mg^{2+}, and phosphate replacement prn.

(7) Laboratory studies.
   (a) CBC, platelet count, INR.
   (b) Electrolytes, glucose, blood urea nitrogen, creatinine.
   (c) GGTP, ALT, AST.
   (d) Phosphorus and magnesium.
   (e) Serum vitamin B_{12} and folic acid (if megaloblastic features in blood smear).

(8) Diagnostic imaging: generally not necessary; if subdural hematoma is suspected (evidence of trauma, persistent lethargy), a CT scan should be ordered.

(9) Social rehabilitation: group therapy such as Alcoholics Anonymous; identification and treatment of social and family problems should be initiated during the patient's hospital stay.

2. **Alcoholic hallucinosis:**
   a. Manifestations: hallucinations usually are auditory, but hallucinations occasionally are visual, tactile, or olfactory; usually there is no clouding of sensorium as in delirium (clinical presentation may be mistaken for an acute schizophrenic episode). Disordered perceptions become most pronounced after 24 to 36 hr of abstinence.
   b. Treatment: same as for DTs (see "Withdrawal seizures").

3. **Withdrawal seizures ("rum fits"):**
   a. Time interval: usually occurs 7 to 30 hr after cessation of drinking, with a peak incidence between 13 and 24 hr.
   b. Manifestations: generalized convulsions with loss of consciousness; focal signs are usually absent; consider further investigation with CT scan of head and electroencephalography if clearly indicated (e.g., presence of focal neurologic deficits, prolonged postictal confusion state). In addition, in a febrile patient who is having a seizure or altered mental state, a lumbar puncture is necessary.
   c. Treatment:
      (1) Diazepam 2.5 mg/min IV until seizure is controlled (check for respiratory depression or hypotension) may be beneficial for prolonged seizure

---

BOX 1 Alcohol Withdrawal Assessment Scoring Guidelines (Revised Clinical Institute Withdrawal Assessment for Alcohol Scale)

Nausea and Vomiting (0-7)
0, none; 1, mild nausea with no vomiting; 4, intermittent nausea; 7, constant nausea, frequent dry heaves and vomiting

Tremor (0-7)
0, no tremor; 1, not visible, but can be felt fingertip to fingertip; 4, moderate, with patient's arms extended; 7, severe, even with arms not extended

Paroxysmal Sweats (0-7)
0, no sweats; 1, barely perceptible sweating, palms moist; 4, beads of sweat obvious on forehead; 7, drenching sweats

Anxiety (0-7)
0, no anxiety, patient at ease; 1, mildly anxious; 4, moderately anxious or guarded, so anxiety is inferred; 7, equivalent to acute panic states seen in severe delirium or acute schizophrenic reactions

Agitation (0-7)
0, normal activity; 1, somewhat more than normal activity; 4, moderately fidgety and restless; 7, pacing back and forth during, or constantly thrashing about

Tactile Disturbances (0-7)
Ask, "Have you experienced any itching, pins and needles sensation, burning or numbness, or a feeling of bugs crawling on or under your skin?"
   0, none; 1, very mild itching, pins and needles, burning, or numbness; 2, mild itching, pins and needles, burning, or numbness; 3, moderate itching, pins and needles, burning, or numbness; 4, moderately severe tactile hallucinations; 5, severe hallucinations; 6, extremely severe hallucinations; 7, continuous hallucinations

Auditory Disturbances (0-7)
Ask, "Are you more aware of sounds around you? Are they harsh? Do they startle you? Do you hear anything that disturbs you or that you know isn't there?"
   0, not present; 1, very mild harshness or ability to startle; 2, mild harshness or ability to startle; 3, moderate harshness or ability to startle; 4, moderate hallucinations; 5, severe hallucinations; 6, extremely severe hallucinations; 7, continuous hallucinations

Visual Disturbances (0-7)
Ask, "Does the light appear to be too bright? Is its color different than normal? Does it hurt your eyes? Are you seeing anything that disturbs you?"
   0, not present; 1, very mild sensitivity to light; 2, mild sensitivity; 3, moderate sensitivity; 4, moderate hallucinations; 5, severe hallucinations; 6, extremely severe hallucinations; 7, continuous hallucinations

Headache (0-7)
0, not present; 1, very mild; 2, mild; 3, moderate; 4, moderately severe; 5, severe; 6, very severe; 7, extremely severe

Orientation and Clouding of Sensorium (0-4)
Ask, "What day is this? Where are you? Who am I?"
   0, oriented; 1, cannot do serial additions or is uncertain about date; 2, disoriented to date by no more than 2 calendar days; 3, disoriented to date by more than 2 calendar days; 4, disoriented to place and/or person

Total Score
0 to 9: absent or minimal withdrawal
10 to 19: mild to moderate withdrawal
More than 20: severe withdrawal

From Sullivan JT, Sykora K, Schneiderman J, et al: Assessment of alcohol withdrawal: the revised clinical institute withdrawal assessment for alcohol scale (CIWA-Ar). *Br J Addict* 84:1353-1357, 1989.

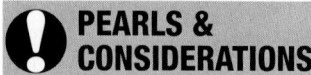
activity; IV lorazepam 1 to 2 mg q2h can be used in place of diazepam. Withdrawal seizures generally are self-limited and treatment is not required; the use of phenytoin or other anticonvulsants for short-term treatment of alcohol withdrawal seizures is not recommended.

(2) Thiamine 100 mg IV, followed by IV dextrose, should also be administered.

(3) Electrolyte imbalances (increased Mg^{2+}, decreased K^+, increased or decreased Na^+, decreased PO_4^{3-}) that may exacerbate seizures should be corrected.

4. **DTs:**

a. Time interval: variable; usually occurs within 1 wk after reduction or cessation of heavy alcohol intake and persists for 1 to 3 days. Peak incidence is 72 hr and 96 hr after the cessation of alcohol consumption.

b. Manifestations: profound confusion, tremors, vivid visual and tactile hallucinations, autonomic hyperactivity; this is the most serious clinical presentation of alcohol withdrawal (mortality rate is approximately 15% in untreated patients).

c. Treatment

(1) Admission to a detoxification unit where patient can be observed closely.

(2) Vital signs q30min (neurologic signs, if necessary).

(3) Use of lateral decubitus or prone position if restraints are necessary

(4) NPO: nasogastric tube for abdominal distention may be necessary but should not be routinely used.

(5) Laboratory studies: same as for early alcohol withdrawal.

(6) Vigorous hydration (4 to 6 L/day): IV with glucose (Na^+, K^+, PO_4^{3-} and Mg^{2+} replacement [if patient has hypophosphatemia or hypomagnesemia]).

(7) Vitamins: thiamine 100 mg IV qd. The initial dose of thiamine should precede the administration of IV dextrose; multivitamins (may be added to the hydrating solution).

(8) Sedation: control of agitation should be achieved with rapid-acting sedative-hypnotic agents in adequate doses to maintain light somnolence for the duration of delirium.

(a) Initially: lorazepam 2 to 5 mg IM/IV repeated prn.

(b) Maintenance (individualized dosage): chlordiazepoxide, 50 to 100 mg PO q4-6h, lorazepam 2 mg PO q4h, or diazepam 5 to 10 mg PO tid; withhold doses or decrease subsequent doses if signs of oversedation are apparent.

(c) Midazolam is also effective for managing DTs. Its rapid onset (sedation within 2 to 4 min of IV injection) and short duration of action (approximately 30 min)

make it an ideal agent for titration in continuous infusion.

(9) Treatment of seizures (as previously described).

(10) Diagnosis and treatment of concomitant medical, surgical, or psychiatric conditions.

CHRONIC Rx

- See "Referral."
- Pharmacotherapies for alcoholism include:

1. Acamprosate is a synthetic compound with a chemical structure similar to the neurotransmitter gamma-aminobutyric acid and the amino acid neuromodulator taurine. Its mechanism of action is not completely understood. It is indicated for the maintenance of abstinence from alcohol in patients with alcohol dependence who are abstinent at treatment initiation. It should be used only as part of a comprehensive psychosocial treatment program. It does not cause a disulfiram-like reaction as a result of ethanol ingestion. Dose is two 333-mg tablets tid. Treatment should be initiated as soon as possible after the period of alcohol withdrawal, when the patient has achieved abstinence, and should be maintained if the patient relapses.

2. The long-acting opiate antagonist naltrexone inhibits the rewarding effects of alcohol. The starting dose is 25 mg/day, increased to 50 mg PO qd after 1 wk. An extended-release, once-monthly injection of naltrexone is also available and can be used along with psychosocial support to maintain alcohol abstinence. In patients with opioid dependence, naltrexone can precipitate acute withdrawal syndrome and should not be used at least 7 days from last opioid use. There are no established guidelines on the appropriate length of naltrexone treatment for alcohol dependence. One study recommends at least 3 mo of treatment.

3. In a recent study, gabapentin showed a significant dose-response effect, and estimates of effect sizes were larger than those seen for naltrexone and acamprosate.[1]

4. Disulfiram (Antabuse). Dosage is 500 mg max qd for 1 to 2 wk, then 125 to 500 mg qd. It interferes with the metabolism of alcohol by inhibiting aldehyde dehydrogenase, causing an accumulation of acetaldehyde. It produces unpleasant symptoms (nausea, flushing, elevated blood pressure, headache, weakness) when alcohol is ingested. It is an older drug that is now rarely used.

DISPOSITION

See "Referral."

---

[1]Mason BJ et al: Gabapentin treatment for alcohol dependence: a randomized clinical trial, *JAMA Intern Med* 174:70-77, 2014.

REFERRAL

- To Alcoholics Anonymous or Adult Children of Alcoholics
- Family members to Al-Anon or Al-A-Teen
- Many cities have Salvation Army Adult Rehabilitation centers; all patients accepted, regardless of ability to pay

❗ PEARLS & CONSIDERATIONS

COMMENTS

- Relative indications for inpatient alcohol detoxification are as follows: history of DTs or withdrawal seizures, severe withdrawal symptoms, concomitant psychiatric or medical illness, pregnancy, multiple previous detoxifications, recent high levels of alcohol consumption, and lack of reliable support network.

- Detoxification is not a stand-alone treatment but should serve as a bridge to a formal treatment program for alcohol dependence.

- The cure rate for alcoholism is highly disappointing, regardless of the modality. Only those who want to be helped will be helped. An effective strategy for the primary care physician is a prominently displayed sign in the office that states, "If you think you consume too many alcoholic beverages, please discuss it with me." Those who do open up the discussion can be given the facts in a nonjudgmental way and often can be helped. All too often problem drinkers lie on the questionnaire until they face a life-threatening health issue—and even then denial often reigns supreme.

- In a recent clinical trial, patients receiving medical management with naltrexone (100 mg/day), combined behavioral intervention (CBI), or both fared better on drinking outcomes, whereas acamprosate showed no evidence of efficacy, with or without CBI. No combination produced better efficacy than naltrexone or CBI alone in the presence of medical management.

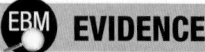 **EVIDENCE**

Available at www.expertconsult.com

SUGGESTED READINGS

Available at www.expertconsult.com

RELATED CONTENT

Alcohol Abuse (Patient Information)
Abuse, Drug (Related Key Topic)
Alcoholic Hepatitis (Related Key Topic)
Wernicke Syndrome (Related Key Topic)

AUTHOR: **FRED F. FERRI, M.D.**

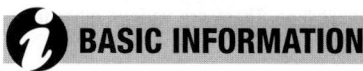

BASIC INFORMATION

DEFINITION

Alcoholic hepatitis (AH) is a severe, progressive, inflammatory, and cholestatic liver disease occurring in patients with long-term ethanol abuse.

SYNONYM

AH

ICD-10CM CODES
K70.10 Alcoholic hepatitis without ascites
K70.9 Alcoholic liver disease, unspecified

EPIDEMIOLOGY & DEMOGRAPHICS

- Approximately 2 million people in the U.S. (about 1% of the population) are affected by alcoholic liver disease.
- In 2007, alcoholic hepatitis accounted for 0.71% of all admissions in the U.S.
- Typical presentation age: 40 to 50 yr. Majority occurs before age 60.
- Patients with alcoholic hepatitis typically drink more than 80 g of alcohol daily for at least 5 years.

PREVALENCE: Approximately 25% to 30%

PREDOMINANT SEX AND AGE: The majority of patients are males. Males are two times as likely as women to abuse alcohol. However, women develop alcoholic hepatitis after a shorter time and smaller amount of alcoholic exposure than men.

GENETICS: No genetic predilection for any one race. In the U.S., however, there is increased incidence in minority groups.

RISK FACTORS: Drinking multiple alcohol types, drinking alcohol between meal times, poor nutrition, female gender, obesity, Hispanic ethnicity, long-term ingestion of >10 to 20 g/day of alcohol in women and >20 to 40 g/day in men

PHYSICAL FINDINGS & CLINICAL PRESENTATION

Common presenting symptoms include:
- Rapid onset of jaundice
- Nausea/vomiting
- Malaise
- Low-grade fever
- Anorexia
- Abdominal distention/pain
- Weight loss or malnourishment
- Complications of liver impairment (GI bleed; confusion, lethargy, ascites)
  Findings on physical examination include:
- Fever
- Tachycardia
- Hypotension
- Hepatomegaly, with tender liver on palpation
- Jaundice and ascites
- Splenomegaly
- Asterixis (a flapping tremor)
- Peripheral edema
- Abdominal distention with shifting dullness (ascites)
- Hepatic bruit

- With coexistent cirrhosis look for:
  1. Gynecomastia
  2. Proximal muscles wasting
  3. Spider angiomata
  4. Altered hair distribution

DIAGNOSIS

DIFFERENTIAL DIAGNOSIS

- Hepatitis B
- Hepatitis C
- Nonalcoholic steatohepatitis (NASH)
- Chronic pancreatitis
- Drug-induced liver injury
- Hemochromatosis
- Cholangitis

WORK-UP

- A thorough and detailed history is needed.
- Relevant questions may include:
  1. When patients started drinking
  2. Number of times patient drinks per day
  3. How many years of regular/daily drinking
  4. Types of alcohol
  5. Home or bar drinking?
  6. Rehabilitation for drinking?
  7. Social problems (e.g., arrest for public intoxication or driving under the influence, marital discord due to alcoholism)

LABORATORY TESTS

- Elevated transaminase (AST >45 U/L but <300 U/L; AST:ALT ratio >2.0) but some patients may not have elevations in ALT, AST in early phases
- S-bilirubin >2 mg/dl
- Increased prothrombin time (PT)
- Elevated gamma glutamyltransferase (GGT)
- Carbohydrate-deficient transferrin (CDT) is a reliable marker for chronic alcoholism
- Elevated C-reactive protein
- Electrolyte disorder (hypokalemia, hypomagnesemia, low zinc, hypophosphatemia)
- Hypoalbuminemia
- Hyperferritinemia
- CBC (may reveal leukocytosis with bandemia or anemia or thrombocytopenia); MCV may be elevated
- Screening tests to rule out other conditions include checking:
  1. Hepatitis B surface antigen (HBsAg)
  2. Anti–hepatic C
  3. Ferritin-transferrin saturation
  4. Alpha-fetoprotein
  5. Alkaline phosphatase
- The severity of AH can be calculated with the Maddrey Discriminant Function (MDF) score, which is calculated as follows:
  MDF = 4.6 × prothrombin time – control prothrombin time + total bilirubin (mg/dl)

IMAGING STUDIES

Ultrasonography is the preferred imaging study. The earliest histologic change in alcoholic liver disease is macrovesicular steatosis.

LIVER BIOPSY

- Liver biopsy is rarely needed.

- Useful to:
  1. Confirm the diagnosis.
  2. Evaluate the effect of coexisting disease.
  3. Rule out cirrhosis.
  4. Exclude other diagnosis (especially other causes of liver diseases).
- Typical finding include:
  1. Macrovascular steatosis
  2. Hepatocyte injury (ballooning degeneration and focal hepatocyte necrosis)
  3. Mallory's bodies (characteristic of alcoholic hepatitis)
  4. Perivenular fibrosis
  5. Portal and lobular inflammation

TREATMENT

An algorithm for the management of patients with alcoholic hepatitis is described in Fig. 1. Treatment can be divided into three main components:
1 Lifestyle modifications
2 Nutritional support
3 Pharmacologic therapy

LIFESTYLE MODIFICATIONS

- Abstinence from alcohol (this improves both short- and long-term survival). Fig. 2 describes the effect of subsequent alcohol intake on 5-year survival in patients with alcoholic hepatitis
- Smoking cessation (to decrease oxidative stress)
- Treatment of substance abuse

NUTRITIONAL SUPPORT

- Good nutrition is an essential part of treatment because many patients with alcoholic hepatitis are usually in a catabolic state.
- Nutritional support includes:
  1. Liberal vitamin supplementation (especially thiamine, folic acid, vitamin K)
  2. Mineral supplementation (**but not iron**)
  3. Calorie counting is essential. A high calorie intake (1.2 to 1.4 times the normal resting intake) may be required.
  4. Protein intake of 1.2 to 1.5 g/kg of ideal body weight per day will provide adequate support. **Exception: in patients with severe encephalopathy, protein restriction may be required.**

PHARMACOLOGIC THERAPY

Severe alcoholic hepatitis may require treatment. Severity can be assessed by calculating the Model for End-Stage Liver Disease (MELD) score or MDF or the Glasgow score.
- An MDF score >32 indicates significant or severe alcoholic hepatitis (30-day mortality of 50%).
- MELD score can easily be calculated (visit http://www.unos.org/resources/meldpeldcalculator.asp?index=98). This score predicts short-term survival in patients with cirrhosis. A score ≥20 predicts increased short-term mortality.
- Glasgow score: contains four variables (BUN, PT, WBC count, and bilirubin). A score ≥9 indicates increased mortality.

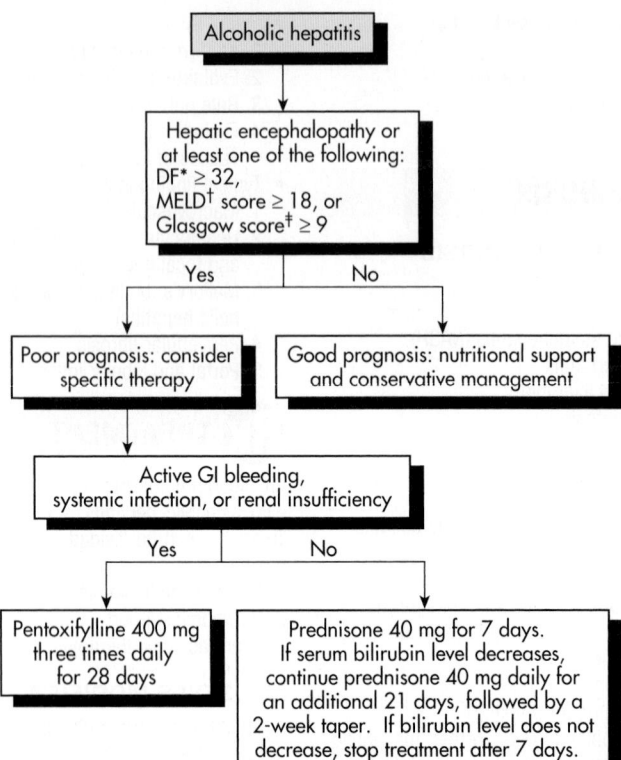

FIG. 1 Algorithm for the management of patients with alcoholic hepatitis. *The DF is calculated as follows: 4.6 (prothrombin time of patient − prothrombin time of control) + serum bilirubin level (in mg/dl). †The Model for End-Stage Liver Disease score is based on the serum bilirubin level, INR, and serum creatinine level. ‡The Glasgow alcoholic hepatitis score is based on the patient's age, white blood cell count, blood urea nitrogen level, ratio of prothrombin time to a control value, and serum bilirubin level. *DF*, Discriminant function. Online calculators for these various models are available at http://www.lillemodel.com. (Feldman M et al: *Sleisenger and Fortran's gastrointestinal and liver disease*, ed 10, Philadelphia, 2016, Elsevier.)

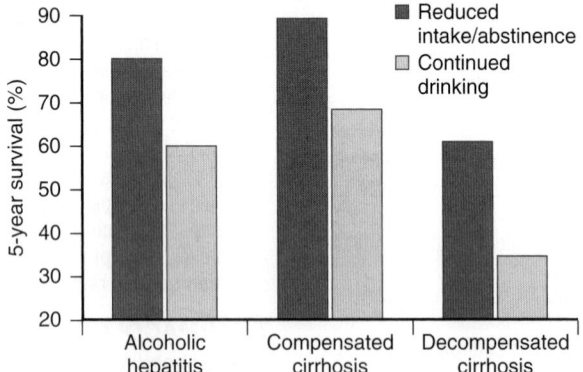

FIG. 2 Effect of subsequent alcohol intake on 5-year survival in patients with alcoholic hepatitis and cirrhosis. (From Day CP, Liver disorder part 1 of 2, *Medicine* 35(1), 2007, p 22–25.)

Indications for initiating therapy include:
- MDF >32
- MELD >20
- Glasgow score >8
- Hepatic encephalopathy

Patients with severe alcoholic hepatitis may be treated with glucocorticosteroids (predniso-lone 40 mg/day for 28 days with a 2-wk taper). Glucocorticosteroids reduce hepatic injury, suppress inflammation, and promote liver regeneration. An alternative first-line agent (especially for patients with contraindications to corticosteroids) in patients with severe alcoholic hepatitis is pentoxifylline. There are various other treatments, but these are mainly experimental.

LIVER TRANSPLANTATION
- Usually reserved for patients with end-stage liver disease. Patients whose hepatitis is not responding to medical therapy have a 6-month survival rate of approximately 30%. Since most hepatitis deaths occur within 2 months, early liver transplantation is attractive but controversial.
- Patients with alcoholic hepatitis must be sober for at least 6 mo before they can be eligible for consideration for liver transplantation.

REFERRAL
Severe acute alcoholic hepatitis may require ICU care and referral to different subspecialists:
- GI/hepatology (for patients with evidence of GI hemorrhage)
- Nutritional services
- Nephrology (for acute renal failure, hepatorenal syndrome)
- Neurology (for change in mental status, seizures)
- Infectious disease (for fever/leukocytosis)

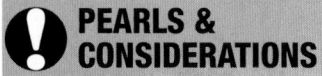

PEARLS & CONSIDERATIONS

COMMENTS
- Referral to substance abuse treatment programs may be helpful.
  1. Stress to patients that there are limited long-term drug treatments for alcoholic hepatitis.
  2. Maintaining good general nutrition is important.
  3. Advise patient about the risk of taking certain medications, especially acetaminophen.
- Periodic follow-up to monitor patient's response to check BMP and LFTs.
- Encourage alcohol abstinence. Abstinence improves long-term survival.
- If patient develops liver cirrhosis, check serum alpha-fetoprotein every 6 mo and liver ultrasound annually to rule out hepatocellular carcinoma.
- Vaccinate patient against hepatitis A and B viruses, pneumococci, influenza A virus, and routine adult vaccinations, if appropriate.

SUGGESTED READINGS
Available at www.expertconsult.com

RELATED CONTENT
Alcoholic Hepatitis (Patient Information)

AUTHORS: **DANIEL K. ASIEDU, M.D., PH.D.,** and **FRED F. FERRI, M.D.**

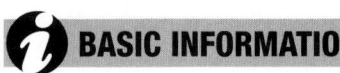
Diseases
and Disorders

BASIC INFORMATION

DEFINITION

Primary hyperaldosteronism is a clinical syndrome characterized by hypokalemia, hypertension, low plasma renin activity (PRA), and excessive aldosterone secretion.

SYNONYMS

Hyperaldosteronism
Primary aldosteronism
Conn's syndrome

ICD-10CM CODES
E26.0 Primary hyperaldosteronism
E26.1 Secondary hyperaldosteronism
E26.8 Other hyperaldosteronism
E26.9 Hyperaldosteronism, unspecified

EPIDEMIOLOGY & DEMOGRAPHICS

INCIDENCE: 1% to 2% of patients with hypertension
PREVALENCE: More common in females

PHYSICAL FINDINGS & CLINICAL PRESENTATION

- Generally asymptomatic
- If significant hypokalemia is present, possible muscle cramping, weakness, paresthesias
- Hypertension
- Polyuria, polydipsia

ETIOLOGY

- Aldosterone-producing adenoma (40%-60%)
- Idiopathic hyperaldosteronism (>30%)
- Glucocorticoid-suppressible hyperaldosteronism (<1%)
- Aldosterone-producing carcinoma (<1%)

DIAGNOSIS

DIFFERENTIAL DIAGNOSIS

- Diuretic use
- Hypokalemia from vomiting, diarrhea
- Renovascular hypertension
- Other endocrine neoplasm (pheochromocytoma, deoxycorticosterone-producing tumor, renin-secreting tumor)

WORKUP

Fig. 1 provides guidance on when to consider testing for primary aldosteronism. Fig. 2 describes a diagnostic approach to patients with suspected primary aldosteronism. CT, MRI, and adrenal vein sampling (AVS) are used to distinguish unilateral from bilateral increased aldosterone secretion. This distinction will dictate treatment options since unilateral primary aldosteronism is treated surgically rather than medically.

LABORATORY TESTS

Routine laboratory tests can be suggestive but are not diagnostic of primary aldosteronism. Common abnormalities are:

When to consider testing for primary aldosteronism:
- Hypertension and hypokalemia
- Resistant hypertension
- Adrenal incidentaloma and hypertension
- Onset of hypertension at a young age (<20 y)
- Severe hypertension (≥160 mm Hg systolic or ≥100 mm Hg diastolic)
- Whenever considering secondary hypertension

↓

Morning blood sample in seated ambulant patient
- Plasma aldosterone concentration (PAC)
- Plasma renin activity (PRA) or PRC

↓

↑ PAC (≥15 ng/dL)
↓ PRA (<1.0 ng/mL per hour) or
↓ PRC (<lower limit of detection for the assay)
and
PAC/PRA ratio ≥20 ng/dL per ng/mL per hour

↓

Investigate for primary aldosteronism

FIG. 1 Algorithm provides guidance on when to consider testing for primary aldosteronism and use of the ratio of plasma aldosterone concentration (PAC) to plasma renin activity (PRA) as a case-detection tool. *PRC*, Plasma renin concentration. (Melmed S, Polonsky KS, Larsen PR, Kronenberg HM: *Williams textbook of endocrinology,* ed 12, Philadelphia, 2011, Saunders.)

- Spontaneous hypokalemia or moderately severe hypokalemia while receiving conventional doses of diuretics
- Possible alkalosis and hypernatremia

IMAGING STUDIES

- Adrenal CT scans (Fig. E3) or MRI may be used to localize neoplasm.
- Adrenal scanning with iodocholesterol (NP-59) or 6-beta-iodomethyl-19-norcholesterol after dexamethasone suppression. The uptake of tracer is increased in those with aldosteronoma and absent in those with IHA and adrenal carcinoma.

TREATMENT

NONPHARMACOLOGIC THERAPY

- Regular monitoring and control of blood pressure
- Low-sodium diet, tobacco avoidance, maintenance of ideal body weight, and regular exercise

ACUTE GENERAL Rx

- Control of blood pressure and hypokalemia with eplerenone, spironolactone, or amiloride
- Surgery (unilateral adrenalectomy) for APA

CHRONIC Rx

Chronic medical therapy with spironolactone, eplerenone, or amiloride to control blood pressure and hypokalemia is necessary in all patients with bilateral IHA. Eplerenone causes less gynecomastia in men and menstrual irregularities in women because of greater mineralocorticoid receptor selectivity, but tends to be more expensive than spironolactone or amiloride and has less effective antihypertensive effect.

DISPOSITION

- Unilateral adrenalectomy normalizes hypertension and hypokalemia in 70% of patients with APA after 1 yr. After 5 yr, 50% of patients remain normotensive.
- Experimental animal studies have suggested that long-term exposure to increased aldosterone levels in untreated aldosteronism may result in renal structural damage. However, clinical trials have shown that primary aldosteronism is characterized by partially reversible renal dysfunction in which elevated albuminuria is a marker of a dynamic rather than structural renal defect.

REFERRAL

Surgical referral for unilateral adrenalectomy after confirmation of unilateral APA or carcinoma

PEARLS & CONSIDERATIONS

- Frequent monitoring of blood pressure and electrolytes postoperatively is necessary because normotension after unilateral adrenalectomy may take up to 4 mo.
- Recent investigations regarding serum aldosterone and the incidence of hypertension in nonhypertensive persons indicate that increased aldosterone levels within the physiologic range predispose to the development of hypertension.

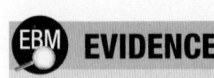

RELATED CONTENT

Aldosteronism (Patient Information)

AUTHOR: **FRED F. FERRI, M.D.**

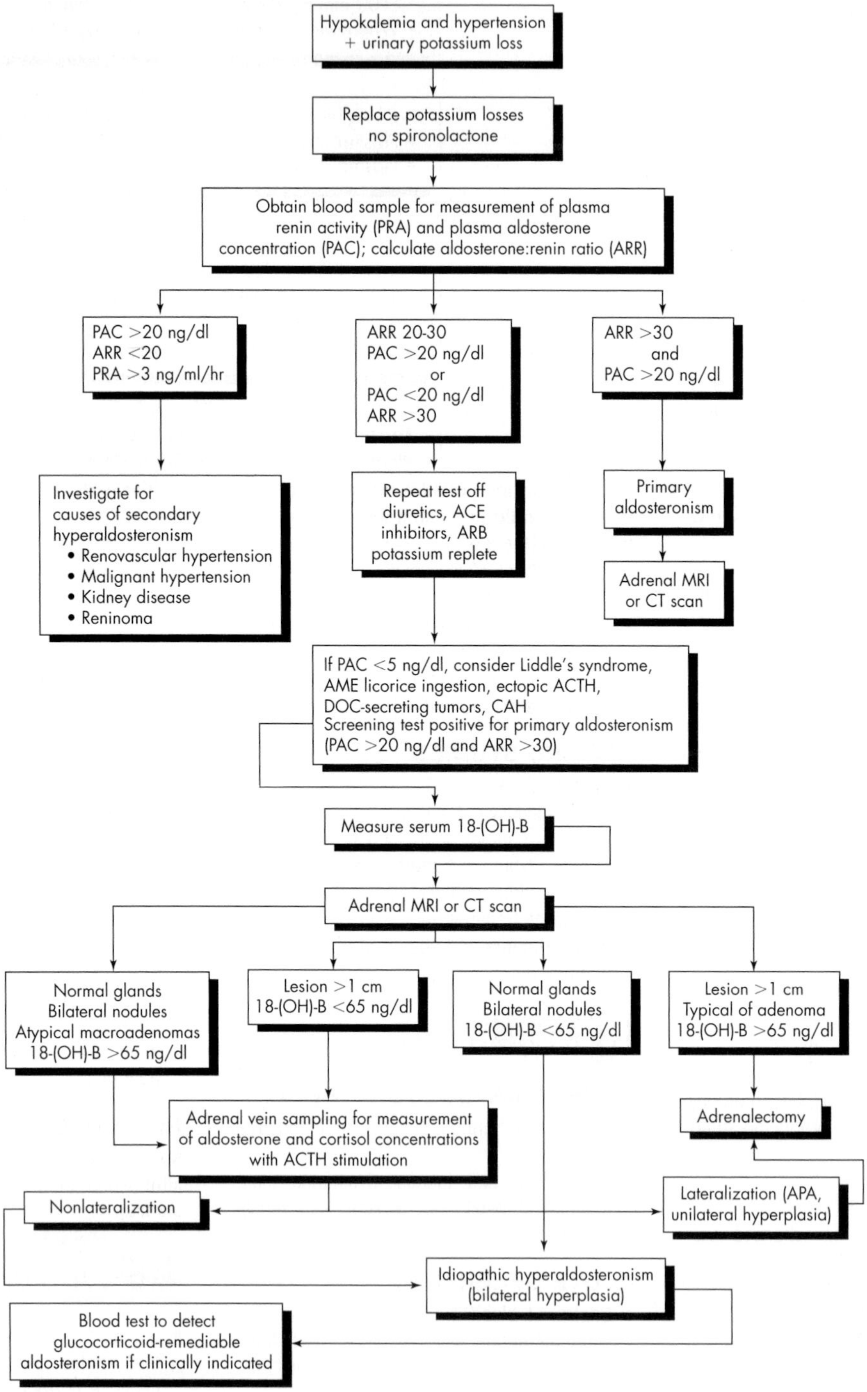

Hypokalemia and hypertension + urinary potassium loss

↓

Replace potassium losses no spironolactone

↓

Obtain blood sample for measurement of plasma renin activity (PRA) and plasma aldosterone concentration (PAC); calculate aldosterone:renin ratio (ARR)

PAC >20 ng/dl / ARR <20 / PRA >3 ng/ml/hr
→ Investigate for causes of secondary hyperaldosteronism
- Renovascular hypertension
- Malignant hypertension
- Kidney disease
- Reninoma

ARR 20-30 / PAC >20 ng/dl / or / PAC <20 ng/dl / ARR >30
→ Repeat test off diuretics, ACE inhibitors, ARB potassium replete
→ If PAC <5 ng/dl, consider Liddle's syndrome, AME licorice ingestion, ectopic ACTH, DOC-secreting tumors, CAH Screening test positive for primary aldosteronism (PAC >20 ng/dl and ARR >30)

ARR >30 / and / PAC >20 ng/dl
→ Primary aldosteronism → Adrenal MRI or CT scan

↓

Measure serum 18-(OH)-B

↓

Adrenal MRI or CT scan

Normal glands / Bilateral nodules / Atypical macroadenomas / 18-(OH)-B >65 ng/dl

Lesion >1 cm / 18-(OH)-B <65 ng/dl

Normal glands / Bilateral nodules / 18-(OH)-B <65 ng/dl

Lesion >1 cm / Typical of adenoma / 18-(OH)-B >65 ng/dl
→ Adrenalectomy

Adrenal vein sampling for measurement of aldosterone and cortisol concentrations with ACTH stimulation

Nonlateralization

Lateralization (APA, unilateral hyperplasia)

Idiopathic hyperaldosteronism (bilateral hyperplasia)

Blood test to detect glucocorticoid-remediable aldosteronism if clinically indicated

FIG. 2 Diagnostic approach to patients with suspected primary aldosteronism. Cortisol concentration ratio in an adrenal vein four times greater than that in the other adrenal vein and/or an aldosterone/cortisol concentration ratio from the vein of the unaffected adrenal that is less than the ratio in the vena cava. Urinary loss of potassium can be documented by measuring potassium excretion in a 24-hour collection of urine; excretion of more than 30 mEq per day in the presence of hypokalemia indicates potassium wasting. An alternative and simpler approach is to obtain a random sample of urine to calculate fractional excretion of potassium. A fractional excretion greater than 10% when hypokalemia is present indicates potassium wasting. *AME,* Syndrome of apparent mineralocorticoid excess; *APA,* aldosterone-producing adenoma; *CAH,* congenital adrenal hyperplasia; *CT,* computed tomography; *DOC,* deoxycorticosterone; *ectopic ACTH,* production of corticotrophin by a tumor outside the pituitary gland; *serum 18-(OH)-B,* serum concentration of 18-hydroxycorticosterone. (From Runge MS, Greganti MA: *Netter's internal medicine,* Philadelphia, 2008, Saunders.)

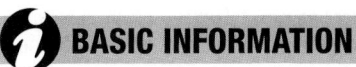

BASIC INFORMATION

DEFINITION

Allergic rhinitis is an IgE-mediated hypersensitivity response to nasally inhaled allergens that involves mucosal inflammation driven by type 2 helper T (Th2) cells that causes sneezing, rhinorrhea, nasal pruritus, and congestion. It may be seasonal or perennial.

SYNONYMS

Hay fever
IgE-mediated rhinitis
Seasonal allergic rhinitis
SAR

ICD-10CM CODES
J30.1 Allergic rhinitis due to pollen
J30.2 Other seasonal allergic rhinitis
J30.3 Other allergic rhinitis
J30.4 Allergic rhinitis, unspecified

EPIDEMIOLOGY & DEMOGRAPHICS

- Allergic rhinitis affects approximately 10% to 20% of the U.S. population and 40% of children.
- Mean age of onset is 8 to 12 yr.
- The prevalence of allergic rhinitis in patients presenting to their primary care provider with nasal symptoms is estimated to be 30% to 60%.

PHYSICAL FINDINGS & CLINICAL PRESENTATION

- Pale or violaceous mucosa of the turbinates caused by venous engorgement (this can distinguish it from erythema present in viral rhinitis)
- Nasal polyps
- Lymphoid hyperplasia in the posterior oropharynx with cobblestone appearance
- Erythema of the throat, conjunctival and scleral injection
- Clear nasal discharge
- Clinical presentation: usually consists of sneezing, nasal congestion, cough, postnasal drip, loss of or alteration of smell, and sensation of plugged ears

ETIOLOGY

- Pollens in the springtime, ragweed in fall, grasses in the summer
- Dust, mites, animal allergens
- Smoke or any irritants
- Perfumes, detergents, soaps
- Emotion, changes in atmospheric pressure or temperature

DIAGNOSIS

DIFFERENTIAL DIAGNOSIS

- Infections (sinusitis; viral, bacterial, or fungal rhinitis)
- Rhinitis medicamentosa (cocaine, sympathomimetic nasal drops)
- Vasomotor rhinitis (e.g., secondary to air pollutants)
- Septal obstruction (e.g., deviated septum), nasal polyps, nasal neoplasms
- Systemic diseases (e.g., Wegener's granulomatosis, hypothyroidism [rare])

WORKUP

- The initial strategy should be to determine whether patients should undergo diagnostic testing or receive empirical treatment.
- Workup is often unnecessary if the diagnosis is apparent. A detailed medical history is useful in identifying the culprit allergen.
- Selected patients with allergic rhinitis that is not controlled with standard therapy may benefit from allergy testing to target allergen avoidance measures or guide immunotherapy. Allergy testing can be performed using skin testing or radioallergosorbent (RAST) testing. Immunoglobulin E (IgE) testing using newest-generation assays is also an excellent tool for diagnosing the cause of symptoms related to rhinitis. Allergy testing with skin or blood testing is most useful as confirmatory tests when the patient's history is compatible with an IgE-mediated reaction and should generally be reserved for ambiguous or complicated cases.
- Examination of nasal smears for the presence of neutrophils to rule out infectious causes and the presence of eosinophils (suggestive of allergy) may be useful in selected patients.
- Peripheral blood eosinophil counts are not useful in allergy diagnosis.

TREATMENT

NONPHARMACOLOGIC THERAPY

- Maintain allergen-free environment by covering mattresses and pillows with allergen-proof casings, eliminating carpeting, eliminating animal products, and removing dust-collecting fixtures.
- Use of air purifiers and dust filters is helpful.
- Maintain humidity in the environment below 50% to prevent dust mites and mold.
- Use air conditioners, especially in the bedroom.
- Remove pets from homes of patients with suspected sensitivity to animal allergens.
- Use of acupuncture to treat seasonal allergic rhinitis is controversial. A recent trial showed that acupuncture led to statistically significant improvement in disease-specific quality of life and antihistamine use measures after 8 weeks of treatment compared with sham acupuncture and with rescue medication alone.

ACUTE GENERAL Rx

- Determine if the patient is troubled by swollen turbinates (best treated with decongestants) or blockages secondary to mucus (effectively treated by antihistamines).
- Topical nasal steroids are very effective and are preferred by many as first-line treatment for allergic rhinitis in adults. Patients should be instructed on proper use and informed that improvement might not occur for at least 1 wk after initiation of therapy. Commonly available inhalers follow.
- Beclomethasone dipropionate: one to two sprays in each nostril bid
- Fluticasone: initially two sprays in each nostril qd or one spray in each nostril bid, decreasing to one spray in each nostril qd based on response
- Flunisolide: initially two sprays in each nostril bid
- Budesonide: two sprays in each nostril bid or four sprays in each nostril qam
- Most first-generation antihistamines can cause considerable sedation and anticholinergic symptoms. The second-generation antihistamines (loratadine, fexofenadine, cetirizine, levocetirizine, desloratadine) are preferred because they do not have any significant anticholinergic or sedative effects.
- Montelukast, a leukotriene receptor antagonist commonly used for asthma, is also effective for allergic rhinitis. Usual adult dose is 10 mg qd.
- Azelastine is an antihistamine nasal spray effective for seasonal allergic rhinitis. Olopatadine is an intranasal H_1-antihistamine alternative to azelastine in mild to moderate seasonal allergic rhinitis.

CHRONIC Rx

- Cromolyn sodium: one spray to each nostril three to four times daily can be used for prophylaxis (mast cell stabilizer).
- Immunotherapy is generally reserved for patients responding poorly to the above treatments. Traditionally, immunotherapy consisted of subcutaneous injections of gradually increased doses of allergens. Recently, the FDA has approved 3 allergen extracts for sublingual administration as immunotherapy.

DISPOSITION

Most patients experience significant relief with avoidance of allergens and proper use of medications.

REFERRAL

Allergy testing in patients with severe symptoms who are unresponsive to therapy or when the diagnosis is uncertain

SUGGESTED READINGS
Available at www.expertconsult.com

RELATED CONTENT
Allergic Rhinitis (Patient Information)

AUTHOR: **FRED F. FERRI, M.D.**

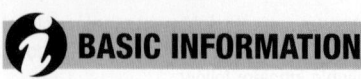

DEFINITION

Alopecia is the term used to describe involuntary hair loss, typically on the scalp but can occur anywhere over the body. *Nonscarring alopecia* is hair loss without clinically apparent scarring, inflammation, or skin atrophy. *Scarring alopecia* is characterized by permanent hair loss accompanied by tissue destruction in the form of scarring, inflammation, and/or skin atrophy.

SYNONYMS

Hair loss
Balding

ICD-10CM CODES
L63	Alopecia aerata
L63.0	Alopecia (capitis) totalis
L64	Androgenic alopecia
L64.0	Drug-induced androgenic alopecia
L64.8	Other androgenic alopecia
L64.9	Androgenic alopecia, unspecified
L65	Other nonscarring hair loss
L66	Cicatricial alopecia
L65.9	Nonscarring hair loss, unspecified
L63.8	Other alopecia areata
L65.0	Telogen effluvium

EPIDEMIOLOGY & DEMOGRAPHICS

INCIDENCE: Depends on etiology, for example:
- Alopecia areata affects 1% of the U.S. population by age 50 yr. There is a higher incidence at a younger age and both sexes are affected equally.
- Androgenetic alopecia affects males > females with 50% of Caucasian men affected by age 50 yr. Less common in Asians and African-American men, and often has later onset. By age 70, 40% of females are affected, with incidence increasing after menopause.

GENETICS: Depends on etiology, for example:
- Androgenetic alopecia is polygenic with variable penetrance and can be inherited from one or both parents.
- Certain scarring alopecias are more predominant in people with coarser hair.

ETIOLOGY

NONSCARRING:
- Failure of follicle production
- Hair shaft abnormality
- Pattern hair loss, i.e., androgenetic alopecia
- Hair breakage, i.e., trichotillomania, traction alopecia, cosmetic overprocessing
- Problem with cycling (excess shedding), i.e., telogen effluvium, anagen effluvium, loose chemotherapy anagen syndrome, alopecia areata, syphilis

SCARRING:
- Infectious: tinea capitis with inflammation (kerion), bacterial folliculitis as in dissecting folliculitis and folliculitis decalvans
- Neoplasm: alopecia mucinosa in cutaneous T-cell lymphoma or alopecia neoplastica due to metastatic carcinoma (breast cancer)

- Autoimmune: chronic cutaneous lupus erythematosus
- Congenital

CLINICAL FEATURES

HISTORY: A careful history must be taken and should include time course for hair loss, the pattern of hair loss, any recent change in life situation/stresses, any associated medical conditions, new medications, any family history of hair loss, diet, hair care practices, and other skin/nail symptoms.

PHYSICAL EXAMINATION:
- General: patient's emotional response to hair loss
- Hair/skin:
  1. Hair thinning/loss
  2. May have fine downy hairs also referred to as vellus hairs
  3. Skin may show changes consistent with inflammation, infection, and/or atrophy
  4. Women may show virilization (e.g., hirsutism)
  5. Exclamation-point hairs can be seen in alopecia areata
  6. Broken hairs of different length may be seen in traumatic alopecia
  7. Hairs that crack or crumble with palpation most often signify shaft damage due to overprocessing

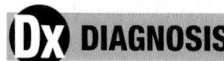 **DIAGNOSIS**

WORKUP

- Pull test—no shower for 24 hr, 60 hairs are gently pulled from the scalp, removal of 6 or more hairs is considered positive result and indicates telogen effluvium (active shedding). Look for telogen bulbs on recovered hairs to differentiate from breaking (blunt ends).
- Punch biopsy—Mandatory when suspecting scarring alopecia. Send two punches: one for vertical and one for horizontal sectioning for histopathologic analysis, preferably by a dermatopathologist.
- Trichogram—quantifies hair loss. Pull 25-50 hairs and measure proportion of anagen to catagen and telogen hairs under light microscopy. 10% to 20% telogen hairs is normal, >35% is highly suspicious for telogen effluvium.
- Fig. E1 describes the evaluation and treatment of alopecia in females.

LABORATORY TESTS

Initiate laboratory studies if not clear based on clinical presentation:
- CBC—rule out Fe deficiency
- Total Fe/ferritin—rule out subclinical Fe deficiency
- TSH—rule out underlying thyroid disease
- ANA—screen for autoimmune disease
- RPR—rule out cutaneous syphilis if history suggestive of increased risk

DIFFERENTIAL DIAGNOSIS

NONSCARRING:
- *Telogen effluvium:* This type of alopecia is usually diffuse thinning that follows significant life stress (death of loved one, high fever, severe infection, crash dieting) or change in hormones (postpartum, change in or cessation of oral contraceptives). Patient often presents with a bag of hair that has fallen out. This is caused by a large number of anagen (growing) hairs entering telogen (dying phase) simultaneously. Telogen effluvium is more common in women.
- *Androgenetic alopecia:* Gradual thinning of hair and a trend toward finer hair, which in men has a typical pattern of receding anterior bitemporal hairline resulting in an M-shaped pattern and hair loss at the vertex and in women has a typical pattern of thinning along vertex with or without frontotemporal thinning. This type of thinning is due to a combination of genetic predisposition and androgenic conversion of hair follicles into vellus-like follicles.
- *Alopecia areata:* Patches of acute hair loss (Fig. 2), typically 2 to 5 cm in diameter, with normal-appearing skin, black dots (cadaver hairs, point noir) from hair that breaks before reaching the skin's surface, and occasional "exclamation point hairs," which are evidence of hairs breaking off as they are pushed from the follicle. Fingernails may show fine pitting. On biopsy, lymphocytes surround the hair bulb and resemble a "swarm of bees," evidence of the autoimmune etiology. Patients often have positive family history.
  AA Universalis (AAU)—generalized loss of body hair
  AA Totalis (AAT)—complete loss of scalp hair
- *Tinea:* This type of hair loss is evident in round patches, possibly with scarring, erythema, and lymphadenopathy. This is the most common type of hair loss in children. Diagnosis can be made by scraping the erythematous edge and placing the scraping with KOH under a microscope to check for hyphae. Wood's lamp only fluoresces if tinea is caused by *Microsporum* spp.; however, the most common (in the U.S.) *Trichophyton* spp. does not fluoresce. If a kerion (severe alopecia associated with bogginess) is present, it may cause scarring.
- *Traumatic alopecia:* This type of hair loss is in a pattern consistent with breaking off of hairs due to traction (hair pulling) or chemical or heating agents (hair straightening or permanent). Etiology usually becomes apparent with careful history taking and visualizing the pattern of hair loss. In trichotillomania (Fig. 3) the alopecia area has an irregular shape, scalp excoriations may present, and hairs are broken at different lengths.

SCARRING:
- *Lichen planus:* The hair loss associated with LP is typically associated with scaling and atrophy of pruritic, painful skin underlying the hair loss. This hair loss is more common in middle-aged women. While there are numerous variations in clinical presentation, the general clinical picture is one of a chronic inflammatory condition of the skin, nails, mucous membranes, and/or hair. The typical skin lesions are flat topped, violaceous lesions with white lines (Wickham's striae), while the typical oral lesions are milky white.

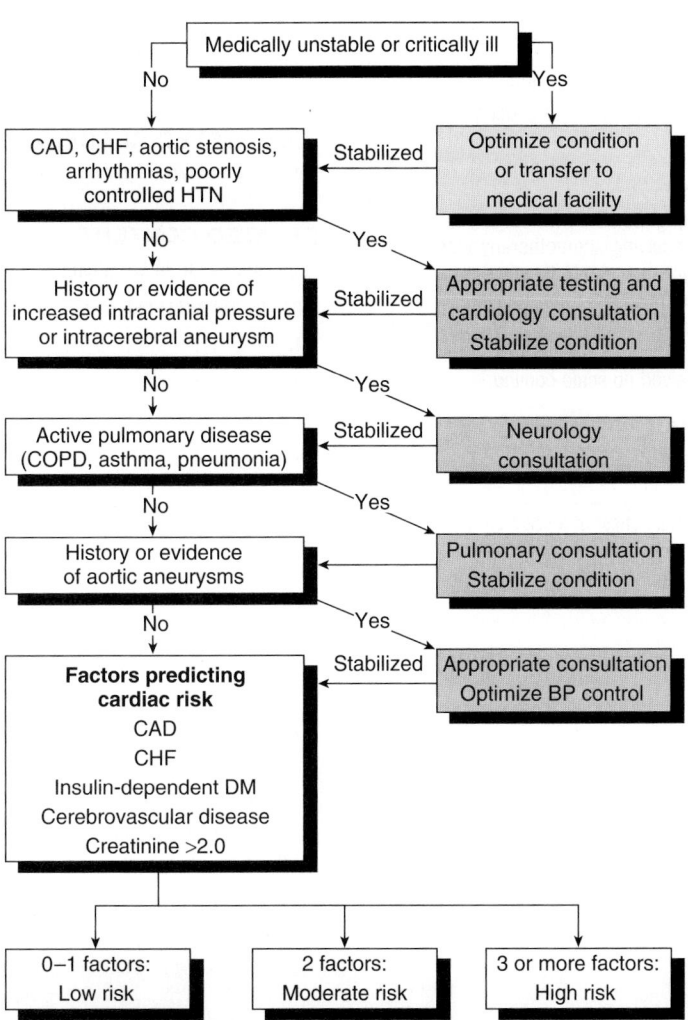

FIG. 2 Alopecia areata: patchy hair loss. The alopecic area is devoid of hairs, and the scalp does not present inflammatory changes. (From Goldman L, Schafer AI: *Goldman's Cecil medicine,* ed 24, Philadelphia, 2012, Saunders.)

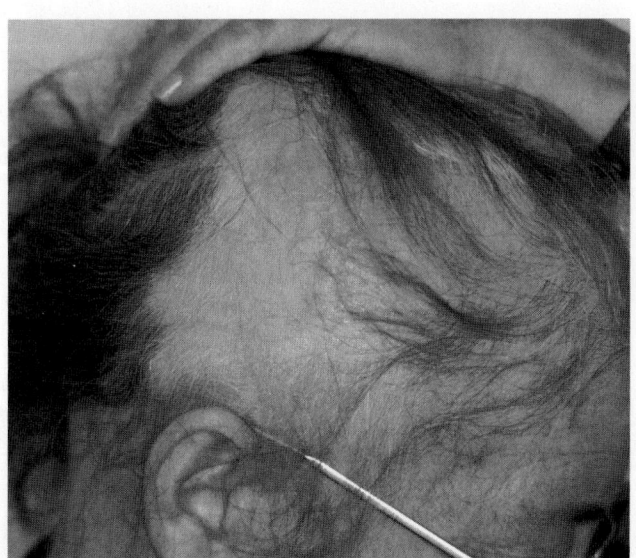

FIG. 3 Trichotillomania: patchy hair loss. The alopecic area has an irregular shape and present hairs are broken at different lengths. Also note scalp excoriations. (From Goldman L, Schafer AI: *Goldman's Cecil medicine,* ed 24, Philadelphia, 2012, Saunders.)

- *Chronic cutaneous (discoid) lupus erythematosus:* This type of hair loss frequently is evident in well-demarcated, erythematous plaques in chronically sun-exposed areas of skin. Lesions exhibit hypopigmentations or hyperpigmentations, atrophy, erythema, and scaling. It may be present concurrently with SLE or be the first presenting symptom of SLE, but in most cases it is a purely cutaneous condition.
- *Tinea with kerion:* A kerion represents an exuberant delayed-type hypersensitivity reaction to the tinea capitis, resulting in one (or many) inflamed boggy plaque(s) on the scalp depending on the severity of the infection.

Rx TREATMENT

- *Telogen effluvium:* Stop offending stress/ medication and in 3 to 4 months anagen recurs. Hair density should be normalized by 12 months. Multiple medications have been shown to be an inciting factor and one should consider stopping them (these include, but are not limited to, enalapril, colchicine, levodopa, metoprolol, propranolol, oral contraceptives, and lithium). Full regrowth is expected in most cases.
- *Androgenetic alopecia:* For men, the most likely first-line treatment is oral finasteride (type II 5α-reductase inhibitor) which leads to lower levels of dihydrotestosterone. This leads to hair regrowth in about 6 months, but with cessation, hair returns to pattern of loss within 6 to 9 months. Topical minoxidil has shown similar results to finasteride and can be useful in partially restoring lost hair in both men and women. Dutasteride (off-label) has been shown to be superior to finasteride in a randomized trial but requires higher doses than that used for BPH. Discontinuation of minoxidil will result in loss of regrown hair often over several months. Other options include surgical intervention with hair transplantation or hair flaps, camouflaging agents, the use of a hairpiece, or low-level light therapy. In women with elevated androgens, antiandrogens such as spironolactone, flutamide, and cimetidine may be considered.
- *Alopecia areata (AA):* Spontaneous remission occurs in patchy AA, but less commonly in AAT or AAU. Glucocorticoids (GCs) are the mainstay of treatment but have little effect on the long-term outcome of hair loss—topical GC for small patches, intralesional injection of high-potency GC, and even systemic steroids can all be temporarily effective but at the cost of glucocorticoid exposure. Induction of allergic contact dermatitis using short-contact anthralin therapy or squaric acid sensitization can be effective but tends to have significant local discomfort, thereby limiting its use. Photochemotherapy has shown some beneficial outcomes, although there is a high relapse rate after discontinuation.

- *Tinea capitis:* To effectively treat tinea capitis, oral antifungal agents must be used. Griseofulvin is considered the drug of choice in the U.S., and the recommended time course is 6 weeks to several months. Other oral agents to consider include terbinafine, itraconazole, fluconazole, and ketoconazole. If there is a kerion (area of boggy, purulent inflammation underlying the area of hair loss), the patient is at increased risk for scarring alopecia due to bacterial superinfection, and a short course of oral steroids and oral antibiotic must be considered.
- *Traumatic alopecia:* First priority is stopping inciting activity/agent, ideally leading to gradual resolution of hair loss and hair regrowth.
- *Lichen planus:* Associated hair loss is often permanent; however, for symptomatic control of itching and pain, topical or oral glucocorticoids may be considered.
- *Chronic cutaneous discoid erythematosus:* The best prevention is sun protection, with SPF lotion. Treatment options center around the cautious use of topical or intralesional glucocorticoids. Hydroxychloroquine and retinoids are also used with caution.
- *Chemotherapy-induced alopecia:* Scalp cooling devices may be effective in reducing chemotherapy-induced alopecia. In a recent trial among women with stage I to II breast cancer receiving chemotherapy with taxane, anthracycline, or both, those who underwent scalp cooling were significantly more likely to have less than 50% hair loss after the fourth chemotherapy cycle compared with those who received no scalp cooling.[1]

REFERRAL

Dermatology

---

[1]Nangia J, et al.: Effect of a scalp cooling device on alopecia in women undergoing chemotherapy for breast cancer. The SCALP randomized clinical trial, *JAMA* 317(6):596-605, 2017.

PATIENT/FAMILY EDUCATION

Alopecia areata: www.naaf.org

SUGGESTED READING

Available at www.expertconsult.com

RELATED CONTENT

Alopecia (Patient Information)

AUTHOR: **JON SKALECKI, M.D.**

BASIC INFORMATION

DEFINITION

Alpha-1-antitrypsin deficiency is a genetic deficiency of the protease inhibitor alpha-1-antitrypsin that results in a predisposition to pulmonary emphysema and hepatic cirrhosis.

SYNONYMS

AATD

ICD-10CM CODES
E88.01 Alpha-1-antitrypsin deficiency

EPIDEMIOLOGY & DEMOGRAPHICS

- Underrecognized by clinicians, but accounts for approximately 2% to 5% of chronic obstructive pulmonary disease (COPD) cases in Americans
- Prevalence is about 1 per 2000 to 5000 people in the United States
- Inherited as an autosomal co-dominant disorder
- Most frequent mutation is in the *SERPINA 1* gene (previously known as *PI* gene)
- Most common alleles are:
  1. normal "M" allele (95% frequency in the U.S.)
  2. deficient variant "Z" allele (1% to 2%)
  3. deficient variant "S" allele (2% to 3%)
- Severe deficiency is most commonly due to homozygotes ZZ
- Risk of lung disease is uncertain with MZ genotype, but increased with SZ genotype (especially in smokers)
- One in 10 individuals of European descent carries one of two mutations that may result in partial alpha-1-antitrypsin deficiency

PHYSICAL FINDINGS & CLINICAL PRESENTATION

- Physical findings and clinical presentation are varied and depend on phenotype (see "Etiology")
- Most often affects the lungs but can also involve liver and skin
- Classically associated with early-onset, severe, lower-lobe predominant panacinar emphysema; bronchiectasis may also be seen
- Symptoms are similar to "typical" COPD presentation (dyspnea, cough, sputum production)
- Liver involvement includes neonatal cholestasis, cirrhosis in children and adults, and primary carcinoma of the liver
- Panniculitis is the major dermatologic manifestation (Rare: 1 in 1000 AATD individuals)

ETIOLOGY

- Degree of alpha-1-antitrypsin deficiency depends on phenotype.
- "MM" represents the normal genotype and is associated with alpha-1-antitrypsin levels in the normal range.
- Mutation most commonly associated with emphysema is Z, with homozygote (ZZ) resulting in approximately 85% deficit in plasma alpha-1-antitrypsin concentrations.
- Development of emphysema is believed to result from an imbalance between the proteolytic enzyme elastase, produced by neutrophils, and alpha-1-antitrypsin, which normally protects lung elastin by inhibiting elastase.
- Deficiency of alpha-1-antitrypsin increases risk of early-onset emphysema, but not all alpha-1-antitrypsin deficient individuals will develop lung disease.
- Smoking increases risk and accelerates onset of COPD.
- Liver disease is caused by pathologic accumulation of alpha-1-antitrypsin in hepatocytes.
- Similar to lung disease, skin involvement is thought to be attributable to unopposed proteolysis in skin.

DIAGNOSIS

DIFFERENTIAL DIAGNOSIS

See "Chronic Obstructive Pulmonary Disease." See "Cirrhosis."

WORKUP

- Suspicion for alpha-1-antitrypsin deficiency usually results from emphysema developing at an early age (45 yr or younger) or emphysema without risk factors (e.g., smoking, dust exposure) and with basilar predominance of disease.

LABORATORY TESTS

- Serum level of alpha-1-antitrypsin can confirm or reject suspicion of deficiency.
- Investigate possibility of abnormal alleles with genotyping.
- Pulmonary function testing is generally consistent with "typical" COPD.

IMAGING STUDIES

- Chest x-ray shows characteristic emphysematous changes at lung bases.
- High-resolution chest CT usually confirms the basal-predominant emphysema (64%) and may also show significant bronchiectasis.

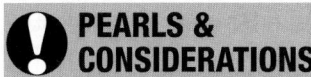

TREATMENT

NONPHARMACOLOGIC THERAPY

- Avoidance of smoking is paramount.
- Avoidance of other environmental and occupational exposures that may increase risk of COPD. Routine vaccinations are also recommended.

ACUTE GENERAL Rx

Acute exacerbations of COPD from alpha-1-antitrypsin deficiency are treated in a similar fashion to "typical" COPD exacerbations.

CHRONIC Rx

- The goal of treatment in alpha-1-antitrypsin deficiency is to increase serum alpha-1-antitrypsin levels above a minimum, "protective" threshold of 50 mg/dL.
- Although several therapeutic options are under investigation, IV administration of pooled human alpha-1-antitrypsin is currently the only approved method to raise serum alpha-1-antitrypsin levels. AAT augmentation therapy has been approved by the FDA for patients with AAT deficiency who have COPD. Augmentation therapy is expensive ($93,000 to $120,000/year) and requires lifelong treatment. However, given the cost and a lack of evidence of clinical benefit, a 2010 Cochrane Collaboration review noted that augmentation therapy with alpha-1-antitrypsin cannot be recommended.
- Organ transplantation for patients with end-stage lung or liver disease is also an option.

DISPOSITION

- Prognosis of patients with alpha-1-antitrypsin deficiency will depend on phenotype and level of deficiency.
- Among patients with severe alpha-1-antitrypsin deficiency, the most common underlying causes of death are respiratory failure (45% to 72%) and cirrhosis (10% to 13%).

REFERRAL

- Referral to specialists with experience in AAT deficiency is preferred
- Pulmonary and hepatology referrals for advanced lung and liver disease, or if replacement therapy is contemplated (e.g., moderate-severe lung disease)
- Lung and liver transplantation in suitable cases

PEARLS & CONSIDERATIONS

- The liver damage arising from the mutation is not from a deficiency in alpha-1-antitrypsin but from a pathologic accumulation of alpha-1-antitrypsin in hepatocytes.
- Strong association between PI*ZZ phenotypes and liver disease has prompted recommendations for AATD testing in individuals with unexplained liver disease.
- Consider alpha-1-antitrypsin deficiency in patients presenting with lower-lobe predominant emphysema; in most smokers without alpha-1-antitrypsin deficiency, emphysema predominates in the upper lobes.
- Alpha-1-antitrypsin deficiency is believed to be under-recognized.
- The American Thoracic Society and the European Respiratory Society recommend testing for AAT deficiency in all symptomatic patients with COPD, emphysema, or asthma with irreversible obstruction, whereas the Global Initiative for Chronic Obstructive Lung Disease only suggests testing for those with early-onset COPD (age <45 yr) with lower lobe emphysema.

SUGGESTED READINGS

Available at www.expertconsult.com

RELATED CONTENT

Alpha-1-Antitrypsin Deficiency (Patient Information)
Chronic Obstructive Pulmonary Disease (Related Key Topic)
Cirrhosis (Related Key Topic)

AUTHOR:**TARO MINAMI, M.D.**

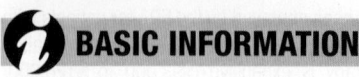

BASIC INFORMATION

DEFINITION

Dementia is a syndrome characterized by progressive loss of previously acquired cognitive skills including memory, language, insight, and judgment. Alzheimer's disease (AD) is believed to account for the majority (50%-75%) of all cases of dementia.

ICD-10CM CODES
G30.0 Alzheimer's disease with early onset
G30.1 Alzheimer's disease with late onset
G30.8 Other Alzheimer's disease
G30.9 Alzheimer's disease, unspecified

EPIDEMIOLOGY & DEMOGRAPHICS

INCIDENCE: Risk doubles every 5 years after the age of 65; above the age of 85, the annual incidence is about 8%.

PREVALENCE: Currently an estimated 5.4 million Americans have AD; 6% between the ages of 65 and 74, 44% between 75 and 84, and 46% at 85 years and older.

PREDOMINANT SEX: Female greater than male

PHYSICAL FINDINGS & CLINICAL PRESENTATION

- Spouse or other family member, usually not the patient, notes insidious memory impairment.
- Patients have difficulties learning and retaining new information and handling complex tasks (e.g., balancing the checkbook) and have impairments in reasoning, judgment, spatial ability, and orientation (e.g., difficulty driving, getting lost away from home).
- Behavioral changes, such as mood changes and apathy, may accompany memory impairment. In later stages, patients may develop agitation and psychosis.
- Atypical presentations include early and severe behavioral changes, focal findings on examination, parkinsonism, hallucinations, falls, or onset of symptoms younger than the age of 65.

DIAGNOSIS

There is no definitive imaging or laboratory test for the diagnosis of AD. Diagnosis is commonly made based on clinical history, a thorough physical and neurologic examination, and use of reliable and valid diagnostic criteria (i.e., DSM or NINDCS-ADRDA) such as the following:

- Loss of memory and one or more additional cognitive abilities (aphasia, apraxia, agnosia, or other disturbance in executive functioning)
- Impairment in social or occupational functioning that represents a decline from a previous level of functioning and results in significant disability

- Deficits that do not occur exclusively during the course of delirium
- Insidious onset and gradual progression of symptoms
- Cognitive loss documented by neuropsychologic tests
- No physical signs, neuroimaging, or laboratory evidence of other diseases that can cause dementia (i.e., metabolic abnormalities, medication or toxin effects, infection, stroke, Parkinson's disease, subdural hematoma, or tumors)

The National Institute on Aging (NIA) and the Alzheimer's Association (AA) recommended new diagnostic criteria and guidelines for AD in 2011. The NIA-AA criteria differ from prior DSM or NINDCS-ADRDA criteria in the following way: (1) they recommend AD be considered a disease well before the onset of symptoms by incorporating the biomarkers in diagnosis; and (2) they define three distinct stages of AD: (1) *preclinical* AD, in which there is measurable biologic evidence of AD pathology but no symptoms; (2) *mild cognitive impairment* (MCI) due to AD, in which there is mild memory loss but no functional impairment at home or work; and (3) *dementia due to AD.*

DIFFERENTIAL DIAGNOSIS

- Cancer (brain tumor, meningeal neoplasia)
- Infection (HIV-associated dementia, neurosyphilis, progressive multifocal leukoencephalopathy [PML])
- Toxic/metabolic (EtOH, hypothyroidism, vitamin B_{12} deficiency, mercury exposure, drug effects)
- Organ failure (dialysis dementia, Wilson's disease)
- Vascular disorder (multiple strokes, severe small vessel changes, chronic vasculitis, or chronic subdural hematoma)
- Depression (pseudodementia)

WORKUP

HISTORY & GENERAL PHYSICAL EXAMINATION:
- Medication lists should always be reviewed for drugs or home remedies that may cause mental status changes, especially anticholinergic medications, benzodiazepines, barbiturates, and neuroleptics.
- Patients should be screened for depression, because it can sometimes mimic dementia but also often occurs as a coexisting condition and should be treated.
- On examination, look for signs of metabolic disturbance, presence of psychiatric features, or focal neurologic deficits.

MENTAL STATUS TESTING: Brief mental status testing can be done easily and quickly in the office. Commonly used cognitive tests to detect dementia include the Mini-Mental State Examination (MMSE), the Mini-Cog test, and the Addenbrooke's Cognitive Examination-Revised (ACE-R) test. For detecting mild cognitive impairment and dementia, the Montreal Cognitive Assessment (MoCA, http://www.moca test.org/) is a highly sensitive 30-point test that takes approximately 10 minutes to administer.

Cognitive domains tested include visual-spatial, attention, verbal recall, language, abstraction, and orientation. A score of 25 points or less (26 points if the patient has less than 12 years of education) indicates cognitive impairment. The test is available in over 35 languages and dialects, and multiple forms in English allow for repeated assessments over time.

Mental status testing should include tests that assess the following cognitive functions:

- Orientation: ask the patient to give the day, date, month, year, and place and to name the current president.
- Attention: ask the patient to recite the months of the year forward and in reverse.
- Verbal recall: ask the patient to remember three items; test for recall after a 1- and 5-min delay.
- Language: ask the patient to write and then read a sentence; have the patient name both common and less common objects.
- Visual-spatial: ask the patient to draw a clock and to set the hands of the clock at 11:10.

Patients with AD typically have trouble with verbal recall plus visuospatial or language deficits. Attention is usually preserved until the late stages of AD, so consider alternate diagnoses in patients who perform poorly on tests of attention.

LABORATORY TESTS

- CBC
- Serum electrolytes
- Glucose
- BUN/creatinine
- Liver and thyroid function tests
- Serum vitamin B_{12}
- Syphilis serology (RPR), if supported by clinical history
- HIV screening as appropriate
- Lumbar puncture if history or signs of cancer, infectious process, or unusual clinical presentation (e.g., rapid progression of symptoms)
- EEG if there is history of seizures, episodic confusion, rapid clinical decline, or suspicion of Creutzfeldt-Jakob disease
- Measurement of apolipoprotein E genotyping, CSF tau and amyloid, and functional imaging including positron emission tomography (PET), single proton emission computed tomography (SPECT), or amyloid PET imaging using florbetapir (Amyvid) are not yet routinely indicated.
- Brain biopsy is usually reserved for diagnoses such as prion disease and cerebral vasculitis. Generally performed postmortem.

IMAGING STUDIES

- CT scan or MRI to rule out hydrocephalus, cerebrovascular disease, and mass lesions, including subdural hematoma
- Florbetapir-PET imaging of the brain correlates with the presence and density of beta-amyloid with high sensitivity and specificity of plaque detection, but is not covered by most payers. It is not part of routine clinical practice but can be considered on a case-by-case basis.

A

Rx TREATMENT

NONPHARMACOLOGIC THERAPY

- Patient safety, including risks associated with impaired driving, wandering behavior, leaving stoves unattended, and accidents, must be addressed with the patient and family early and appropriate measures implemented.
- Wandering, hoarding or hiding objects, repetitive questioning, withdrawal, and social inappropriateness often respond to behavioral therapies.

ACUTE GENERAL Rx

None

CHRONIC Rx

1. Symptomatic treatment of memory disturbance (Table 1):
   a. Cholinesterase inhibitors (ChEls): donepezil (Aricept), galantamine (Razadyne), and rivastigmine (Exelon)
      FDA approved for the treatment of mild to moderate AD with the exception of donepezil, which is approved for mild, moderate, and severe dementia. Common side effects including nausea, diarrhea, and anorexia may be bothersome enough to require a slower escalation of dosage or switching to another agent.
   b. NMDA receptor antagonist: memantine (Namenda)

FDA approved for the treatment of moderate to severe AD. Common side effects include constipation, dizziness, or headache. Memantine is contraindicated in patients with renal insufficiency or history of seizures.

2. Symptomatic treatment of neuropsychiatric and behavioral disturbances (Table 2).
3. Depression, agitation, delusions, or hallucinations may respond to medications.

DISPOSITION & REFERRAL

- Patients with complex or atypical presentations or challenging management issues should be referred to a neurologist or another specialist with expertise in dementia.
- Approximately 1 in 8 hospitalized patients with AD who develop delirium will have at least one adverse outcome (e.g., institutionalization, cognitive decline, death) associated with delirium.
- Family education and support may help reduce need for skilled nursing facility and reduce caregiver stress, depression, and burnout.

⊘ PEARLS & CONSIDERATIONS

The physician should make a thorough search for the treatable causes of dementia. Current American Academy of Neurology practice parameters recommend:
- Treat cognitive symptoms of AD with ChEls.

- Treat agitation, psychosis, and depression.
- Encourage caregivers to participate in educational programs and support groups.

COMMENTS

- Ginkgo biloba is marketed widely as effective in delaying cognitive impairment; however, trials have shown that it is not effective in reducing the incidence of Alzheimer dementia or dementia overall.
- Higher midlife fitness levels seem to be associated with lower hazards of developing all-cause dementia later in life independent of cerebrovascular disease. Exercise also may slow the rate of functional deterioration in mild AD.
- Lower plasma beta-amyloid 42/40 is associated with greater cognitive decline among elderly persons without dementia over 9 years, and this association is stronger among those with low measures of cognitive reserve.
- The *APOE* genotype provides information on the risk for AD, but the genotyping of patients raises ethical and emotional concerns. Because the benefits of genetic testing are often modest, and the tests themselves are often imprecise in identifying risk, the test is generally discouraged. Recent trials, however, reveal that the disclosure of *APOE* genotyping results to adult children of patients with AD did not result in significant short-term psychological risks. Test-related distress was reduced among those who learned that they were *APOE*4 negative. Persons with high levels of emotional distress before undergoing genetic testing are more likely to have emotional difficulties after disclosure.

For additional information for patients, families, and clinicians, contact the following organizations:
- Alzheimer's Association (www.alz.org; 800-272-3900)
- Alzheimer's Disease Education and Referral Center (http://www.nia.nih.gov/Alzheimers; 800-438-4380)

TABLE 1   Symptomatic Treatment of Memory Disturbance

	Initial Dose	Target Dose
Donepezil	5 mg qd for 4-6 weeks	10 mg qd
Rivastigmine	1.5 mg bid with food, increase by 1.5 mg bid weekly	3-6 mg bid
Galantamine	4 mg bid with food, increase by 4 mg bid every 4 weeks	8-12 mg bid
Memantine	5 mg qd, increase by 5 mg weekly	10 mg bid

TABLE 2   Treatment of Behavioral and Neuropsychiatric Symptoms

	Initial Dose	Maximum Dose
Atypical Antipsychotics		
Olanzapine	2.5 mg qd to bid, may increase by 2.5 mg as needed	7.5 mg bid
Quetiapine	25 mg bid, may increase by 25 mg every 2 days	250 mg tid
Antidepressants		
Sertraline	25-50 mg qd, may increase by 25 mg every week	200 mg qd
Citalopram	10 mg qd, may increase after 1 week	20 mg qd

SUGGESTED READINGS

Available at www.expertconsult.com

RELATED CONTENT

Alzheimer's Disease (Patient Information)
Dementia with Lewy Bodies (Related Key Topic)
Mild Cognitive Impairment (Related Key Topic)

AUTHORS: **TAMARA G. FONG, M.D., PH.D.,** and **IRINA A. SKYLAR-SCOTT, M.D.**

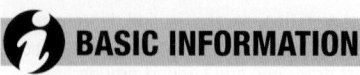
DEFINITION

Amaurosis fugax is a temporary loss of monocular vision caused by transient retinal ischemia.

ICD-10CM CODES
G45.3 Amaurosis fugax

EPIDEMIOLOGY & DEMOGRAPHICS

INCIDENCE (IN U.S.): An uncommon but important presentation of carotid artery disease
PEAK INCIDENCE: Approximately 55 yr

PHYSICAL FINDINGS & CLINICAL PRESENTATION

- Onset is sudden, typically lasting seconds to minutes, and often accompanied by scotomas such as a shade or curtain being pulled over the front of the eye (usually downward).
- Vision loss can be complete, hemianopic, or quadrantic.
- Acute stage: cholesterol emboli may be seen in retinal artery (*Hollenhorst plaque*); carotid bruits or other evidence of generalized atherosclerosis.
- If embolus is cardiac in origin, atrial fibrillation is often present.

ETIOLOGY

- Usually embolic from the internal carotid artery or the heart
- Giant cell arteritis causing inflammation of retinal arteries
- Hyperviscosity syndromes, such as sickle cell disease, which causes ischemia in the vascular territory of the ophthalmic artery
- Hypercoagulability states
- Transient vasospasm often associated with exercise

DX DIAGNOSIS

DIFFERENTIAL DIAGNOSIS

- Retinal migraine: in contrast to amaurosis, the onset of visual loss develops more slowly, usually over 15 to 20 min.
- Transient visual obscurations occur in the setting of papilledema; intermittent rises in intracranial pressure briefly compromise optic disc perfusion and cause transient visual loss lasting 1 to 2 seconds. The episodes may be binocular. If the visual loss persists at the time of evaluation (i.e., vision has not yet recovered), then the differential diagnosis should be broadened to include:
  1. Anterior ischemic optic neuropathy: arteritic (classically GCA) or nonarteritic
  2. Central retinal vein occlusion

WORKUP

- Workup should focus on embolic sources, but GCA should always be considered.

- Careful examination of retina; embolus may be visible and confirm the diagnosis (Fig. 1).
- Auscultation of arteries for carotid bruits.
- Examination of all pulses and for temporal artery tenderness.
- Inquire about symptoms of GCA (scalp tenderness, headache, fever, jaw claudication).
- Examine for signs of hemispheric stroke resulting from intracranial aneurysm (contralateral limb and facial weakness or sensory loss, aphasia, etc.).

LABORATORY TESTS

- Complete blood count with erythrocyte sedimentation rate and C-reactive protein.
- Serum chemistries, including lipid profile.
- Cardiac enzymes and ECG.
- Hypercoagulable workup is discretionary based on younger age and history.

IMAGING STUDIES

- Carotid Doppler imaging followed by MR or CT angiography as indicated.
- Transthoracic echocardiography is indicated to screen for sources of emboli in patients with evidence of heart disease and in patients without an evident source for transient neurologic deficit. Transesophageal echocardiography is more sensitive for detecting cardiac sources of emboli (ventricular mural thrombus, atrial appendage, patent foramen ovale, aortic arch).
- MRI of the brain with diffusion-weighted imaging to look for infarcts, especially those presenting with focal neurologic disturbances.

Rx TREATMENT

NONPHARMACOLOGIC THERAPY

- Diet (decrease saturated fatty acids and high-cholesterol foods)
- Exercise
- Cessation of tobacco use

ACUTE GENERAL Rx

- Investigate as an emergency.
- Aspirin if etiology is presumed embolic.

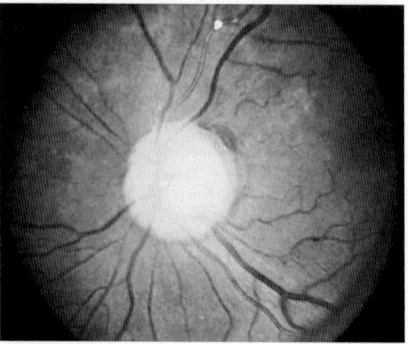

FIG. 1 A cholesterol crystal embolus lodged at an arterial bifurcation. (From Stein JH [ed]: *Internal medicine,* ed 5, St Louis, 1998, Mosby.)

- If GCA is suspected, start prednisone and refer for temporal artery biopsy within 48 hr (see "Giant Cell Arteritis" in Section I).

CHRONIC Rx

- Reduce risks by carotid endarterectomy or carotid stenting if stenosis >70%. Stenting may be performed in high-risk surgical candidates.
- Control hypertension and manage vascular risk factors.
- Antiplatelet therapy.
- Consider starting statin medication.

DISPOSITION

Among patients with >50% carotid stenosis who do not undergo carotid endarterectomy, those who present with transient monocular blindness have an approximate 10% risk of stroke in 3 years compared with an approximate 20% risk in patients who present with a hemispheric transient ischemic attack (TIA).

REFERRAL

- Recommend referral to a neurologist for evaluation and workup.
- If significant carotid stenosis, consider either carotid endarterectomy or carotid stenting for the following:
  1. High-grade (≥70%) stenosis
  2. Multiple TIAs despite medical therapy in the setting of high-grade or ulcerative disease

! PEARLS & CONSIDERATIONS

- Cholesterol emboli in retinal arteries on funduscopy confirm the diagnosis.
- Recognize that transient visual loss has multiple other causes.

RELATED CONTENT

Amaurosis Fugax (Patient Information)
Carotid Stenosis (Related Key Topic)
Giant Cell Arteritis (Related Key Topic)
Transient Ischemic Attack (Related Key Topic)

AUTHORS: **JOSEPH S. KASS, M.D., J.D.,** and **TZU-CHING (TEDDY) WU, M.D., M.P.H.**

ⓘ BASIC INFORMATION

DEFINITION

Amblyopia refers to decreased vision in one or both eyes as a result of insufficient stimulation of the developing visual system. The most common etiologies of amblyopia are ocular misalignment (strabismus) and unequal refractive error (anisometropia). Less commonly, amblyopia results from bilateral high refractive error (ametropic) or blockage of the ocular media (deprivation).

SYNONYMS

Deprivation amblyopia (formerly amblyopia ex anopsia)
Occlusion amblyopia
Strabismic amblyopia
Refractive amblyopia
Lazy eye

ICD-10CM CODES
H53.009	Unspecified amblyopia, unspecified eye
H53.001	Unspecified amblyopia, right eye
H53.002	Unspecified amblyopia, left eye
H53.009	Unspecified amblyopia, unspecified eye
H53.019	Deprivation amblyopia, unspecified eye
H53.011	Deprivation amblyopia, right eye
H53.012	Deprivation amblyopia, left eye
H53.013	Deprivation amblyopia, bilateral
H53.029	Refractive amblyopia, unspecified eye
H53.021	Refractive amblyopia, right eye
H53.022	Refractive amblyopia, left eye
H53.023	Refractive amblyopia, bilateral
H53.039	Strabismic amblyopia, unspecified eye
H53.031	Strabismic amblyopia, right eye
H53.032	Strabismic amblyopia, left eye
H53.033	Strabismic amblyopia, bilateral

EPIDEMIOLOGY & DEMOGRAPHICS

INCIDENCE (IN U.S.): 1% to 5% of the general population. Amblyopia is the leading cause of vision loss in children. It is also the cause of permanent vision loss in approximately 2.9% of adults.
PREVALENCE (IN U.S.): High incidence in premature infants with drug-dependent mothers and in neurologically impaired children. Children with a family history of strabismus, amblyopia, or high refractive errors are at increased risk.
PREDOMINANT SEX: None
PREDOMINANT AGE: Childhood
PEAK INCIDENCE: Childhood

PHYSICAL FINDINGS & CLINICAL PRESENTATION

Decreased vision using best refraction in the presence of normal retinal and optic nerve appearance (Fig. 1).

ETIOLOGY

- Refractive errors
- Strabismus
- Visual deprivation from congenital cataract, corneal opacities, ptosis or nystagmus
- Occlusion from patching (rare)
- Malnutrition or vitamin deficiency

ⓧ DIAGNOSIS

DIFFERENTIAL DIAGNOSIS

- Central nervous system (CNS) disease (i.e., cortical visual impairment)
- Optic nerve disorders
- Corneal or other eye diseases
- Retinal disorders
- Malingering or secondary gain (i.e., desire for glasses in children—more commonly girls)

WORKUP

- Complete eye examination to find the cause of decreased vision. Referral to an ophthalmologist is recommended for any child with a visual acuity in either eye of ≤20/40 at or a two-line difference in acuity between the eyes.
- Ocular motility evaluation.

LABORATORY TESTS

Usually none

IMAGING STUDIES

Usually not necessary unless central nervous system (CNS) lesion suspected

ⓡ TREATMENT

- Treatment depends on the age of the patient and etiology of the amblyopia.

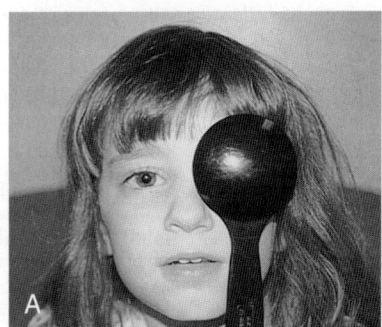
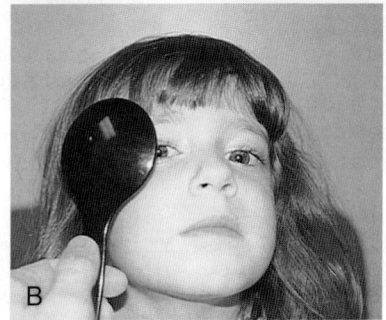

FIG. 1 A, This child happily fixes with her right eye and does not object if the left eye is covered. **B,** When the right eye is covered she moves her head away and tries to remove the cover, demonstrating a fixation preference for the right eye and amblyopia of the left eye. (From Hoekelman R [ed]: *Primary pediatric care,* ed 3, St Louis, 1997, Mosby.)

- Glasses to align eyes in certain types of strabismus and/or to correct significant refractive errors.
- Patching or atropine eye drops are both effective depending on the type of amblyopia. Penalization of the better-seeing eye with atropine 1% drops or patching are used for varying lengths of time, usually months, depending on patient age, response, and compliance. In general, younger patients (<age 5 yr) respond faster and more fully than older children. Older children (>10 yr) who have never been treated can sometimes still respond to amblyopia therapy.
- Surgery for deprivation amblyopia (i.e., congenital cataract, severe congenital ptosis).

CHRONIC Rx

- Maintenance treatment with glasses, patching, or atropine may be necessary until age 9 or 10 yr.
- Monitoring until visual maturity, which occurs around age 9 or 10 yr, is important to avoid relapses.

REFERRAL

To ophthalmologist if vision is compromised

❗ PEARLS & CONSIDERATIONS

COMMENTS

- The earlier the diagnosis, the better the outcome. Amblyopia is more responsive to treatment in children younger than 5 years of age. Although the average treatment response is weaker in children over age 5 years, some older children show response to treatment.
- The success of therapy is highly dependent on treatment compliance.
- Amblyopia recurs in 25% of children after patching is discontinued.

SUGGESTED READINGS

Available at www.expertconsult.com

AUTHORS: **DAVID ROBBINS TIEN, M.D.,** and **ALEXANDRA MEYER TIEN, M.D.**

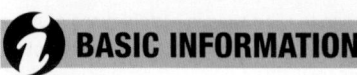

BASIC INFORMATION

DEFINITION

Amebiasis is an infection caused by the protozoal parasite *Entamoeba histolytica*. Although primarily an infection of the colon, amebiasis may cause extraintestinal disease, particularly liver abscess.

SYNONYMS

Amebic dysentery (when severe intestinal infection)

ICD-10CM CODES
A06.9 Amebiasis, unspecified
A06.1 Chronic intestinal amebiasis
A06.7 Cutaneous amebiasis

EPIDEMIOLOGY & DEMOGRAPHICS

INCIDENCE (IN U.S.): 1.2 cases per 100,000 U.S. population. Highest in institutionalized patients, and travelers to/immigrants from developing nations.
PREVALENCE (IN U.S.): 4% (80% of infections asymptomatic)
PREDOMINANT SEX:
- Equal sex distribution in general
- Striking male predominance of liver abscess
PREDOMINANT AGE: 2nd through 6th decades
PEAK INCIDENCE: Peaks at age 2 to 3 yr and >40 yr

PHYSICAL FINDINGS & CLINICAL PRESENTATION

- Often nonspecific
- Approximately 20% of cases symptomatic
  1. Diarrhea, which may be bloody
  2. Abdominal and back pain
- Abdominal tenderness in 83% of severe cases
- Fever in 38% of severe cases
- Hepatomegaly, right upper quadrant tenderness, and fever in almost all patients with liver abscess (may be absent in fulminant cases)

ETIOLOGY

- Caused by the protozoal parasite *E. histolytica*. *E. dispar* and *E. moshkovskii* are 10 times more common but nonpathogenic and difficult to distinguish from *E. histolytica*.
- Transmission by the fecal-oral route
- Infection usually localized to the large bowel, particularly the cecum where a localized mass lesion (ameboma) may form
- Extraintestinal infection in which the organism invades the bowel mucosa and gains access to the portal circulation

DIAGNOSIS

DIFFERENTIAL DIAGNOSIS

- Severe intestinal infection possibly confused with ulcerative colitis or other infectious enterocolitis syndromes, such as those caused by *Shigella, Salmonella, Campylobacter,* or invasive *Escherichia coli*
- In elderly patients: ischemic bowel possibly producing a similar picture

WORKUP

- Stool antigen testing is more sensitive than ova and parasite examination for the diagnosis of amebiasis
- Three stool specimens over a period of 7 to 10 days to search for cysts or trophozoites has a sensitivity of 85% to 95%, but microscopy cannot differentiate between the species
- Concentration and staining the specimen with Lugol's iodine or methylene blue to increase the diagnostic yield
- Fecal leukocytes not always present

LABORATORY TESTS

- Fecal ELISA antigen detection is specific for *E. histolytica* (87% percent sensitive) and also useful for diagnosis of liver abscess.
- PCR-based assays on stool: 90%-95% sensitive; 95%-100% specific.
- Mucosal biopsy is occasionally necessary to look for cysts or trophozoites.
- Serum antibody assays specific for *E. histolytica* are available and are particularly sensitive and specific for extraintestinal infection or severe intestinal disease but may not distinguish recent from remote infection.
- Aspiration of abscess fluid is used to distinguish amebic from bacterial abscesses.

IMAGING STUDIES

Abdominal imaging studies (sonography or CT scan) to diagnose liver abscess

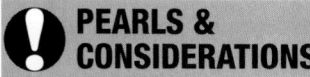

TREATMENT

ACUTE GENERAL Rx

- *Entamoeba histolytica* causes amoebic dysentery and requires treatment. Other species of *Entamoeba* may colonize the gastrointestinal tract but are not pathogenic and do not mandate treatment.

- Table 1 summarizes drug treatment options for amebiasis in adults and children.
- Liver abscess is generally responsive to medical management but surgical intervention indicated for extension of liver abscess into pericardium or for toxic megacolon.

DISPOSITION

Host immunity incomplete and reinfection rate high for patients remaining at risk

REFERRAL

- For consultation with infectious diseases specialist for extraintestinal infection or persistent or relapsing intestinal infection
- For surgical consultation:
  1. For toxic megacolon
  2. For impending rupture of or extension of liver abscess into adjacent structures

PEARLS & CONSIDERATIONS

COMMENTS

- Infection with other intestinal parasites, particularly *Giardia lamblia,* may coexist with amebiasis.
- There is a high prevalence of *E. dispar* in homosexual males, which is nonpathogenic but may be difficult to distinguish from the pathogen *E. histolytica*.

SUGGESTED READINGS

Available at www.expertconsult.com

RELATED CONTENT

Amebiasis (Patient Information)

AUTHOR: **GLENN G. FORT, M.D., M.P.H.**

TABLE 1 Drug Treatment for Amebiasis

Medication	Adult Dosage (Oral)	Pediatric Dosage (Oral)*
Invasive Disease		
Metronidazole	Colitis or liver abscess: 750 mg tid for 7-10 days	Colitis or liver abscess: 35-50 mg/kg/day in 3 divided doses for 7-10 days
or		
Tinidazole	Colitis: 2 g once daily for 3 days Liver abscess: 2 g once daily for 3-5 days	Colitis: 50 mg/kg/day once daily for 3 days Liver abscess: 50 mg/kg/day once daily for 3-5 days
Followed by:		
Paromomycin (preferred)	500 mg tid for 7 days	25-35 mg/kg/day in 3 divided doses for 7 days
or		
Diloxanide furoate† or	500 mg tid for 10 days	20 mg/kg/day in 3 divided doses for 7 days
Iodoquinol	650 mg tid for 20 days	30-40 mg/kg/day in 3 divided doses for 20 days
Asymptomatic Intestinal Colonization		
Paromomycin (preferred) or Diloxanide furoate† or Iodoquinol	As for invasive disease	As for invasive disease

*All pediatric dosages are up to a maximum of the adult dose.
†Not available in the United States.
From Kliegman RM et al: *Nelson textbook of pediatrics*, ed 19, Philadelphia, 2011, Saunders.

BASIC INFORMATION

DESCRIPTION

Amenorrhea means absence of menstruation. It is classified as either primary or secondary depending on whether the patient has had previous menstrual cycles.

- Primary amenorrhea is defined as the absence of menses by age 16 in the presence of secondary sexual characteristics. However, in the absence of these secondary sexual features by the age of 14 years, one should begin the workup for primary amenorrhea.
- Secondary amenorrhea is the absence of menses for more than six months in a patient who has had previous normal progesterone withdrawal cycles. The duration of amenorrhea required for the diagnosis of secondary amenorrhea varies somewhat depending on the source.

ICD-10CM CODES
N91.0 Primary amenorrhea
N91.1 Secondary amenorrhea
N91.2 Amenorrhea, unspecified

EPIDEMIOLOGY & DEMOGRAPHICS

- Incidence of primary amenorrhea and secondary amenorrhea in the U.S. is <1% and 5% to 7%, respectively.
- There is no racial or ethnic predilection.

ETIOLOGY

- Physiologic amenorrhea
  1. Pregnancy
  2. Lactation
  3. Menopause
- Pathologic amenorrhea
  A. Primary amenorrhea
    1. Hypergonadotropic hypogonadism
       a. Turner's syndrome
       b. Pure gonadal dysgenesis
       c. Autoimmune oophoritis
       d. 17,20-desmolase deficiency or 17-hydroxylase deficiency
       e. Galactosemia
       f. Müllerian agenesis
       g. Eugonadism
    2. Androgen insensitivity (Table 1)
       a. Müllerian agenesis
       b. Transverse vaginal septum
       c. Imperforate hymen
       d. Androgen insensitivity syndrome (AIS) (1%)
       e. 5-alpha reductase deficiency
       f. Polycystic ovarian syndrome (PCOS)
       g. Adult-onset congenital adrenal hyperplasia (CAH)
       h. Cushing's syndrome
       i. Hypothyroidism
    3. Hypogonadotropic hypogonadism
       a. Constitutional delay
       b. Hypothalamic disorders
       c. Pituitary diseases
       d. Other CNS diseases

- Secondary amenorrhea
  1. Ovarian diseases
     a. PCOS
     b. Iatrogenic (oophorectomy, S/P radiation, chemotherapy)
     c. Primary ovarian insufficiency (previously referred to as premature ovarian failure [POF]) and premature menopause; these terms should no longer be used)
     d. Ovarian tumors
  2. Hypothalamic dysfunction
     a. Functional (eating disorders, exercise, stress)
     b. Congenital GnRH deficiency
     c. Infiltrative diseases (sarcoidosis, histiocytosis, lymphoma)
  3. Pituitary diseases
     a. Hyperprolactinemia (drug induced, hypothyroidism, prolactinoma)
     b. Craniopharyngiomas
     c. Empty sella syndrome
     d. Sheehan's syndrome
     e. S/P radiation
     f. Infiltrative diseases
  4. Asherman's syndrome
  5. Others
  Hypothyroidism, Cushing's syndrome, adult-onset congenital adrenal hyperplasia, drug induced (e.g., Lupron Depot, Depo-Provera, levonorgestrel IUD, Danazol), chronic illnesses

PHYSICAL FINDINGS & CLINICAL PRESENTATION

- Turner's syndrome
  1. Usually presents with primary amenorrhea unless mosaic
  2. Short stature
  3. Epicanthic folds
  4. Low-set ears
  5. High-arched palate
  6. Micrognathia
  7. Sensorineural hearing loss
  8. Otitis media
  9. Webbing of the neck
  10. Pigmented nevi
  11. Square/shield chest
  12. Widely spaced nipples
  13. Absent breast development
  14. Bicuspid aortic valve
  15. Coarctation of aorta
  16. Cubit valgus
  17. Short fourth metacarpal
  18. Hyperconvex nails
  19. Leg edema
  20. Renal abnormalities
  21. Autoimmune disorders including thyroiditis
  22. Diabetes mellitus
- Pure gonadal dysgenesis
  1. Unlike Turner's syndrome has no dysmorphic features
- Müllerian agenesis
  1. Sporadic inheritance
  2. Primary amenorrhea
  3. Normal breast development
  4. Normal pubic and axillary hair
  5. Normal female external genitalia
  6. Absent uterus and upper part of vagina
  7. Ovaries present

  8. Renal and vertebral anomalies in some patients; renal agenesis should be evaluated
- Transverse vaginal septum and imperforate hymen
  1. Primary amenorrhea
  2. Progressive cyclic lower abdominal pain
  3. Imperforate hymen or transverse vaginal septum on pelvic examination
  4. Perirectal fullness from hematocolpos
  5. Imaging with MRI identifies level of obstruction
- Androgen insensitivity syndrome
  1. Primary amenorrhea
  2. X-linked recessive inheritance in some patients
  3. Normal breast development
  4. Absent pubic and axillary hair
  5. Testis may be present in the groin or inguinal canal
  6. Uterus and vagina absent
  7. No associated renal or vertebral anomalies
- Adult-onset congenital adrenal hyperplasia
  1. Commonly seen in Ashkenazi Jewish, Inuit Native American, French Canadian, Mexican population
  2. Mimics the presentation of PCOS
  3. Features of hyperandrogenism (virilization, hirsutism, acne)
  4. Hypertension
- 5-alpha reductase deficiency
  1. Primary amenorrhea
  2. Undergo striking virilization at puberty
- PCOS
  1. Usually presents with secondary amenorrhea and oligomenorrhea
  2. Features of hyperandrogenism
  3. Obesity (60% to 80% of PCOS patients)
  4. Infertility
  5. Insulin resistance, predisposition to type II diabetes mellitus
  6. Association with the metabolic syndrome
- Strict diagnosis may also require performance of pelvic ultrasonography
  1. Cushing's syndrome (rare disorder, prevalence 1/1,000,000)
  2. Secondary amenorrhea
  3. Features of hyperandrogenism
  4. Abnormal fat distribution (dorsocervical fat pad [buffalo hump], spider legs, significant central obesity)
  5. Abdominal striae due to weakening of skin integument
  6. Easy bruising
  7. Hypertension
  8. Proximal muscle weakness
- Hypothyroidism
  1. Secondary amenorrhea
  2. Lethargy
  3. Constipation
  4. Decreased appetite
  5. Weight gain
  6. Cold intolerance
  7. Hair loss
  8. Dry skin
  9. Hypotension
  10. Bradycardia
- Primary ovarian insufficiency (previously premature ovarian failure)

TABLE 1 Congenital Anatomic Causes of Primary Amenorrhea with Normal Breast Development*

Diagnosis	Müllerian Agenesis	Androgen Insensitivity (AI)	Transverse Vaginal Septum	Imperforate Hymen
Patients with primary amenorrhea[†]	15%	1%	3%	1%
Patients with primary amenorrhea and apparent obstruction or absence of vagina[†]	75%	5%	15%	5%
Chromosomes[‡]	46,XX	46,XY	46,XX	46,XX
Gonads	Ovaries	Testes	Ovaries	Ovaries
Serum testosterone[‡]	Normal female level	Normal male level (high)	Normal female level	Normal female level
Vagina	Absent or shallow	Absent or shallow	Obstructed by septum which may be thick or thin, high or low	Obstructed by thin membrane, which may look blue from hematocolpos
Axillary/pubic hair	+	Absent unless AI is incomplete	+	+
Cyclic pain	±	−	+	+
Uterus	Absent or rudimentary	−	+	+
Mass	−	−	+ Can present with acute urinary retention as hematocolpos mass obstructs urethra	+ Can present with acute urinary retention
Introitus bulges with Valsalva maneuver	−	−	−	+
Associated anomalies	Urinary tract and skeletal	Inguinal hernias; gonadal malignancy in adulthood	Major urinary tract abnormalities in 15%	Possibly some increase in urinary tract abnormalities
Treatment	Vaginal dilation or surgical neovagina	Gonadectomy after age 16-18 yr Vaginal dilation or surgical neovagina	Surgical approach depends on extent and location of septum; may be extensive; should be done as soon as possible	Excision of hymen as soon as possible; diagnostic needle aspiration contraindicated because of risk of infection
Fertility	Advanced reproductive technology required; in vitro fertilization surrogate with uterus to gestate pregnancy	Not fertile	Variable, low septa have a better prognosis than do high septa	Usually fertile

+, Present; −, absent; ±, may be present or absent.
*Cervix not visible on pelvic examination. Short vagina; may be absent or obstructed.
[†]Data from Reindollar RH, Byrd JR, McDonough PG: Delayed sexual development: a study of 252 patients, *Am J Obstet Gynecol* 140:371, 1981.
[‡]Sometimes useful in differentiating Müllerian agenesis from androgen insensitivity.
From Kliegman RM et al: *Practical strategies in pediatric diagnosis and therapy,* ed 2, Philadelphia, 2004, Elsevier.

1. Secondary amenorrhea prior to the age of 40 yr and elevated gonadotropins (FSH and LH)
2. History of oophorectomy or pelvic radiation or chemotherapy
3. Vasomotor symptoms
4. Dry, thin vaginal mucosa without rugosity
5. Associated autoimmune or karyotypic abnormalities possible

- Hyperprolactinemia
  1. Usually presents with secondary amenorrhea
  2. History of use of drugs such as antipsychotics, oral contraceptive (OC) pills, antidepressants, antihypertensives, H_2 blockers, opioids, etc.
  3. Pituitary adenomas may be associated with headache, vomiting, vision changes
  4. Galactorrhea
- Sheehan's syndrome
  1. History of secondary amenorrhea following postpartum hemorrhage
  2. Failure of lactation
  3. Other features of hypopituitarism

- Asherman's syndrome
  1. History of D&C
  2. Secondary amenorrhea
  3. Recurrent miscarriage/infertility
- Functional hypothalamic disorders
  1. Usually presents with secondary amenorrhea
  2. History of eating disorders, severe exercise or stress
  3. Use of street drugs
- Kallmann's syndrome
  1. Usually presents with anosmia, congenital defect of development of both the GnRH neurons and olfactory placode

Ⓓⓧ DIAGNOSIS

- First step in the workup of amenorrhea is to rule out pregnancy by serum/urine pregnancy test.
- Diagnostic workup depends on history and physical.
- Physical examination, determining the presence or absence of advanced breast Tanner stage and presence or absence of uterus can help

guide evaluation (e.g., presence of breasts but absence of uterus can only be Müllerian agenesis or androgen insensitivity syndrome).

- Primary amenorrhea (Fig. E1 and Box E1):
  1. Pelvic ultrasonography or MRI to detect any anatomic abnormalities of uterus, cervix, ovaries, or vagina. At times examination under anesthesia is needed to assess the pelvic organs.
  2. Karyotyping (46,XX in Müllerian agenesis; 46,XY in AIS; 45,XO in Turner's syndrome) is done when uterus is absent or Turner's syndrome is suspected.
  3. Serum FSH, TSH/FT4, prolactin, estradiol: FSH 40 mIU/ml along with estradiol <20 pg/ml is indicative of primary ovarian insufficiency.

  Prolactin >200 ng/ml is suggestive of prolactinoma. Lower levels may also be associated with prolactinoma. Threshold levels may vary by laboratory, and providers are advised to become familiar with their institution's normal range.

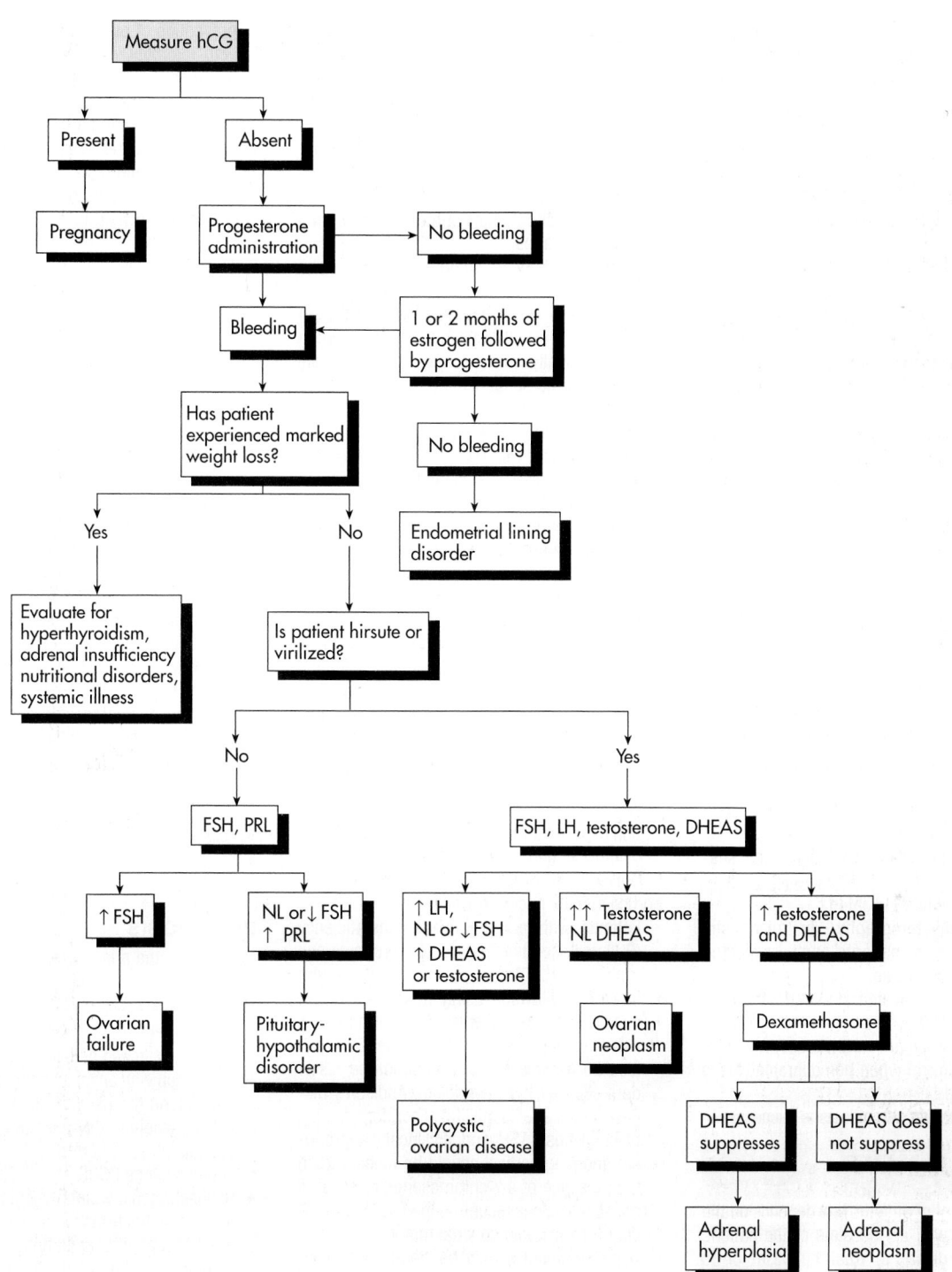

FIG. 2 Evaluation of secondary amenorrhea. *DHEAS,* Dehydroepiandrosterone-sulfate; *FSH,* follicle-stimulating hormone; *hCG,* human chorionic gonadotropin; *LH,* luteinizing hormone; *NL,* normal; *PRL,* prolactin; ↑, increased; ↑↑, markedly increased; ↓, decreased. (From Andreoli TE [ed]: *Cecil essentials of medicine,* ed 7, Philadelphia, 2008, Saunders.)

4. Check serum testosterone (male range in AIS; female range in Müllerian agenesis) when uterus is absent or in presence of features of hyperandrogenism.
5. 17-alpha hydroxyprogesterone level in presence of features of hyperandrogenism to rule out CAH. In addition to high level of 17 alpha hydroxyprogesterone due to compromised 21-hydroxylase activity, these patients have elevated level of serum progesterone and deoxycorticosterone, hypernatremia, and hypokalemia.
6. MRI of head in presence of:
• Primary hypogonadotrophic hypogonadism.
1. Hyperprolactinemia.
2. Visual field defects.
3. Headaches.
4. Signs of hypothalamic-pituitary dysfunction.

• Secondary amenorrhea (Fig. 2):
1. Serum FSH, TSH/FT4, prolactin, estradiol: Low serum FSH with low estradiol indicates hypogonadotropic hypogonadism. High serum FSH with low estradiol suggests hypergonadotropic hypogonadism.
Progesterone withdrawal bleeding.
10 mg medroxyprogesterone is given for 10 days.

Withdrawal bleeding suggests euestrogenic anovulation in presence of normal end organ (outflow tract) and ovarian function.
- Estrogen-progesterone withdrawal bleeding:
  In the absence of progesterone withdrawal bleeding, the patients are exposed to 25 to 35 days of estrogen (0.625 to 2.5 mg Premarin daily) followed by 10 days of medroxyprogesterone.
  Withdrawal bleeding indicates hypogonadism.
  Absence of bleeding suggests defects with end organ (e.g., Asherman's syndrome).
- Serum LH, testosterone and DHEA-S:
  When features of hyperandrogenism are seen these tests are ordered.
  Serum testosterone >200 ng/ml suggests androgen-producing adrenal or ovarian tumors (high index of suspicion with moderate elevation; threshold value not required in cases of ovarian or adrenal tumors). This level may be mildly elevated in patients with PCOS.
  DHEA-S >700 mcg/dl suggests adrenal origin over ovarian (high index of suspicion with moderate elevation; threshold value not required in cases of ovarian or adrenal tumors).
  LH/FSH ratio >2 may be present in patients with PCOS, although this is not part of diagnostic criteria according to the Rotterdam consensus conference.
- Pelvic ultrasound when PCOS or ovarian tumor suspected.
- Abdominal CT when adrenal tumor suspected.
- MRI of head when indicated.
- HSG, sonohysterography, or diagnostic hysteroscopy in patients with suspected Asherman's syndrome.
- Karyotyping is indicated when primary ovarian insufficiency occurs before the age of 40.
- Other tests which are rarely needed:
  Serum transferrin when hemochromatosis is suspected.
  Serum ACE when sarcoidosis is suspected.

Rx TREATMENT

- The treatment of amenorrhea depends on the etiology, as well as the aims of the patient, such as a desire to treat hirsutism or to become pregnant.
- In the absence of pregnancy, withdrawal bleeding may be induced in the majority of patients with amenorrhea using 5 to 10 mg of medroxyprogesterone for 10 days.
- Estrogen replacement along with calcium and vitamin D should be instituted in essentially every patient with hypogonadism to avoid osteoporosis. Women with a uterus require continuous or intermittent progesterone administration to protect against endometrial hyperplasia or cancer. Frequently, it is easiest to prescribe combination OC pills. For most patients, continuation until ~50 years, the usual age of menopause, seems reasonable. Young women in whom

secondary sex characteristics have failed to develop fully should be exposed initially to very low dose estrogen (0.3 mg of conjugated equine estrogen or equivalent) given unopposed daily for 6 mo with incremental dose increases at 6-mo intervals until the required maintenance dose is achieved. Cyclic progesterone therapy, 12 to 14 days per month, should be instituted once vaginal bleeding ensues.
- Most patients with anatomic abnormalities will require surgical correction. Creation of a new vagina for patients with Müllerian agenesis is usually delayed until the woman is emotionally mature and ready to participate in the serial dilation or postoperative care required to maintain vaginal patency. However, if adequate correction is impossible, pregnancy will often require a surrogate to carry a gestation. One should not forget to look for the associated urogenital anomalies, such as renal agenesis, in these patients and, when present, treat them appropriately.
- In patients with androgen insensitivity syndrome, the incidence of gonadal malignancy is 22%. However, it rarely occurs before the age of 20. Gonadectomy is performed by laparoscopy following breast development and the attainment of adult stature. In the absence of a uterus these individuals only need estrogen replacement without progesterone.
- Women with adult-onset CAH may be treated with low-dose corticosteroids in addition to sex steroids to partially block ACTH stimulation of adrenal function and thereby decrease overproduction of adrenal androgens.
  Universal treatment of adult-onset CAH with corticosteroids is controversial.
- Patients with primary ovarian insufficiency (POI) will need estrogen and progesterone replacement. These patients will require in vitro fertilization using donor oocytes to conceive. These patients have an increased risk of osteoporosis and heart disease. It can also be associated with autoimmune disorders such as hypothyroidism, Addison's disease, and diabetes mellitus. Therefore, fasting blood glucose, TSH, and, if clinically appropriate, morning cortisol should be measured. In the presence of a Y chromosome, removal of gonadal tissue is recommended at the time of diagnosis to avoid gonadal tumors.
- Hypothyroidism should be treated with thyroid replacement.
- Hyperprolactinemia is treated by avoiding the culprit drugs or by giving dopamine agonists, such as bromocriptine or cabergoline. Pituitary adenomas rarely require surgery but surgery may be performed if secondary deficits such as visual changes are observed, when they are resistant to medical therapy, or the lesion is rapidly growing.
- Treatment of hypothalamic amenorrhea depends on the etiology. Patients with eating disorders or who exercise excessively will require behavioral modification and nutritional counseling. Elite athletes may choose not to alter their exercise regimens and will therefore require estrogen treatment and

prevention of osteoporosis. When associated with infertility, ovulation induction with clomiphene citrate, exogenous gonadotropins, or pulsatile GnRH therapy should be offered.
- The primary treatment of PCOS is weight loss through diet and exercise. Other treatment options include:
  1. Use of OC pills or cyclic progestational agents to help maintain a normal endometrium.
  2. Insulin-sensitizing agents such as metformin to reduce insulin resistance and improve ovulatory function. Recent studies suggest that insulin-sensitizing agents may not be as effective in improving ovulatory effort.
  3. Oral contraceptives and/or spironolactone to treat hyperandrogenism.
  4. Clomiphene citrate or an aromatase inhibitor such as letrozole to induce ovulation.
- In patients with Asherman's syndrome, hysteroscopic lysis of intrauterine adhesions is followed by administration of long-term exogenous estrogen to stimulate regrowth of endometrial tissue.
- Geneticist consult is given in patients with hereditary causes of amenorrhea.
- Psychiatrist consult is needed in patients with major depression, anorexia nervosa, bulimia nervosa, or other major psychiatric disorders.

COMPLICATIONS

- Osteoporosis
- Endometrial hyperplasia and uterine cancer
- Infertility

PROGNOSIS

Depends on the primary cause of amenorrhea

PATIENT EDUCATION

- Patients with amenorrhea should be reassured that this is, in and of itself, not a concern.
- All women with an intact endometrium should understand the risks of unopposed estrogen action, whether the estrogen is exogenous such as through hormone therapy, or endogenous such as PCOS.
- Hypoestrogenic women should be counseled about the importance of estrogen replacement to protect against bone loss.
- Potential for future childbearing should be discussed.

SUGGESTED READINGS
Available at www.expertconsult.com

RELATED CONTENT

Hypothalamic Amenorrhea (Patient Information)
Infertility (Related Key Topic)
Pituitary Adenoma (Related Key Topic)
Polycystic Ovary Syndrome (Related Key Topic)
Prolactinoma (Related Key Topic)
Sheehan's Syndrome (Related Key Topic)
Turner Syndrome (Related Key Topic)

AUTHOR: **HEMANT K. SATPATHY, M.D.**

ℹ BASIC INFORMATION

DEFINITION

Amyotrophic lateral sclerosis (ALS) is a progressive, degenerative neuromuscular condition of undetermined etiology affecting corticospinal tracts and anterior horn cells, resulting in dysfunction of both upper motor neurons (UMN) and lower motor neurons (LMN), respectively.

SYNONYMS

Lou Gehrig's disease
ALS

ICD-10CM CODES
G12.21 Amyotrophic lateral sclerosis

EPIDEMIOLOGY & DEMOGRAPHICS

INCIDENCE:
- 3.9 cases per 100,000 persons.
- Onset is usually between the ages of 50 and 70 yr.
- Male/female ratio is 2:1.

PREVALENCE: Five in 100,000 persons

PHYSICAL FINDINGS & CLINICAL PRESENTATION

- LMN signs (weakness, hypotonia, wasting, fasciculations, hyporeflexia or areflexia).
- UMN signs (loss of fine motor dexterity, spasticity, extensor plantar responses, hyperreflexia, clonus).
- Preservation of extraocular movements, sensation, bowel and bladder function.
- Dysarthria, dysphagia, pseudobulbar affect, frontal lobe dysfunction.
- Respiratory insufficiency typically occurs late in the disease.
- ALS comprises approximately 90% of adult-onset motor neuron diseases. Other presentations of motor neuron disease include progressive muscular atrophy, primary lateral sclerosis, progressive bulbar palsy, progressive pseudobulbar palsy, and ALS-parkinsonism-dementia complex.

ETIOLOGY

- 90% to 95% of all cases are sporadic.
- 5% to 10% cases are familial; known genetic mutations include copper-zinc superoxide dismutase enzyme mutations (10%–20% of familial cases), TAR DNA-binding protein mutations (3%–10% of familial cases), FUS (5% of familial cases), ANG (which encodes angiogenin, ribonuclease, RNase A family, 5; 1% of familial cases), and C9ORF72.
- C9ORF72 hexanucleotide repeat expansion recently identified genetic cause, although the frequency is geographically variable; in the U.S., reported in up to 23% of familial ALS and 4% of sporadic ALS.
- TDP-43 and FUS mutations also associated with ALS and frontotemporal dementia.
- Increased risk factors in whites, nonHispanics, age >60 years. Family history of ALS, previous exposure to heavy metals, pesticides, BMAA.[1]

℞ DIAGNOSIS

DIFFERENTIAL DIAGNOSIS

- Multifocal motor neuropathy with conduction block
- Cervical spondylotic myelopathy with polyradiculopathy
- Spinal stenosis with compression of lumbosacral nerve roots
- Chronic inflammatory demyelinating polyneuropathy with central nervous system lesions
- Syringomyelia
- Syringobulbia
- Foramen magnum tumor
- Meningeal carcinomatosis
- Spinal muscular atrophy
- Polyglucosan body disease
- Bulbospinal muscular atrophy (Kennedy disease)
- Monomelic amyotrophy
- Lyme disease
- ALS-like syndromes have been reported in the setting of lead intoxication, HIV, hyperparathyroidism, hyperthyroidism, lymphoma, and vitamin B_{12} deficiency.

WORKUP

- Diagnosis is based on clinical findings, EMG results, and exclusion of alternative causes.
- Electromyography and nerve conduction studies (El Escorial criteria; see Table E1)
- Assessment of respiratory function (forced vital capacity [FVC], negative inspiratory force)

LABORATORY TESTS

- Vitamin B_{12}, thyroid function, parathyroid hormone, HIV may be considered.
- Serum protein and immunofixation electrophoresis.
- DNA studies for SMA or bulbospinal atrophy, hexosaminidase levels in pure LMN syndrome.
- 24-hour urine for heavy metals if indicated.

IMAGING STUDIES

- Craniospinal neuroimaging contingent on clinical scenario. MRI of the brain and spinal cord are useful to help exclude stroke and cervical cord compression.
- Modified barium swallow to evaluate aspiration risk

℞ TREATMENT

NONPHARMACOLOGIC THERAPY

- Noninvasive positive-pressure ventilation may improve quality of life and may increase tracheostomy-free survival in patients with respiratory difficulty (defined by orthopnea or FVC 50% of predicted).
- Percutaneous endoscopic gastrostomy (PEG) tube placement improves nutritional intake, promotes weight stabilization, and eases medication administration. Some studies suggest PEG placement may prolong life 1 to 4 mo, particularly when placed before FVC falls to ≤50% of predicted value.
- Nutrition, speech therapy, physical and occupational therapy services.
- Suction device for sialorrhea.
- Cough assist device for ineffective coughing and maintaining a clear airway.
- Communication may be eased with computerized assistive devices.
- Early discussion of living will, resuscitation orders, desire for PEG and tracheostomy, potential long-term care options.
- Encourage contact with local support groups.

ACUTE GENERAL Rx

Riluzole, a glutamate antagonist, is the only FDA-approved medication known to extend tracheostomy-free survival in patients with ALS. Dosage is 50 mg q12h, at least 1 hr before or 2 hr after meals. It is shown to prolong survival by 2 to 3 months. Manufacturer recommends checking alanine aminotransferase (ALT) once a month for 3 months initially, followed by once every 3 months until the first year of therapy is completed. ALT should be checked periodically thereafter.

CHRONIC Rx

- Sialorrhea may respond to either glycopyrrolate or amitriptyline (consider either propranolol or metoprolol if secretions are thick). Botulinum toxin may be effective in medically refractory cases.
- Spasticity may be treated pharmacologically with baclofen, tizanidine, clonazepam.
- Pseudobulbar affect may improve with amitriptyline, sertraline, or dextromethorphan/quinine.

DISPOSITION

- Mean duration of symptoms is 3 to 5 yr.
- Approximately 20% of patients survive >5 yr.

REFERRAL

- Referral to a neurologist experienced in neuromuscular disease is recommended to confirm the diagnosis. One prospective, population-based study suggested improved survival in subjects treated in a multidisciplinary clinic.
- Gastrointestinal referral for PEG placement is recommended while FVC remains >50% to minimize morbidity attributable to risks inherent to the procedure.

❗ PEARLS & CONSIDERATIONS

- Patient-physician communication is an integral and essential part in both the initial diagnosis and subsequent treatment of ALS.
- A multidisciplinary approach to supportive care may lead to an improved level of daily functioning and foster an increased sense of independence.

SUGGESTED READINGS

Available at www.expertconsult.com

RELATED CONTENT

Amyotrophic Lateral Sclerosis (Patient Information)

AUTHOR: **TAYLOR HARRISON, M.D.**

[1]Mehta P, et al.: Prevalence of ALS in USA, 2012–2013, *MMWR* 65(8), 2016.

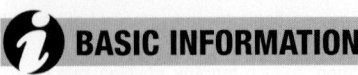

BASIC INFORMATION

DEFINITION

An anaerobic infection is caused by one of a group of bacteria that requires a reduced oxygen tension for growth.

ICD-10CM CODES
A41.4 Sepsis, anaerobic
A48 Cellulitis, anaerobic

PHYSICAL FINDINGS & CLINICAL PRESENTATION

- May occur at any site, but most are anatomically related to mucosal surfaces
- Should be suspected when there is foul-smelling tissue, soft tissue gas, necrotic tissue, or abscesses
- Head and neck
  1. Odontogenic infections from dental or soft tissue possibly progressing to periapical abscesses, at times extending to bone
  2. Both anaerobic and aerobic pathogens in chronic sinusitis, chronic mastoiditis, peritonsillar abscess, and chronic otitis media
  3. Complications: deep neck space infections, brain abscesses, mediastinitis
  4. Specific examples of anaerobic infections in head and neck:
     a. Ludwig's angina: bilateral infection of sublingual and submandibular spaces that causes swelling of the base of the tongue with potential airway compromise. Usually mixed aerobic and anaerobic flora
     b. Lemierre's syndrome: jugular vein suppurative thrombophlebitis caused by anaerobic bacteria: *Fusobacterium necrophorum*
- Pleuropulmonary
  1. May involve anaerobes present in the oropharynx
  2. Aspiration more common in persons with altered mental status or seizures
  3. Anaerobic bacteria more likely in those with gingivitis or periodontitis
  4. Manifestations: necrotizing pneumonia, empyema, lung abscess
- Intraabdominal
  1. Disruption of intestinal integrity leading to infection involving anaerobic bacteria
  2. Bacteria from colonic neoplasm, perforated appendicitis, diverticulitis, or bowel surgery, causing bacteremia, peritonitis, at times intraabdominal abscesses
  3. Resulting infections usually mixed, containing both anaerobes and aerobes
- Female genital tract
  1. Anaerobes in bacterial vaginosis, salpingitis, endometritis, pelvic abscesses, septic abortion; infections tend to be mixed
  2. Possible pelvic thrombophlebitis when resolving pelvic infection is accompanied by new or persistent fever
- Other anaerobic infections
  1. Skin and soft tissue infection at any site

  2. More commonly associated infections: synergistic gangrene, bite wound infections, infected decubitus ulcers
  3. Clinical significance of anaerobes in diabetic foot infections unclear
  4. Anaerobic bacteremia uncommon with source usually intraabdominal, followed by female genital tract, pleuropulmonary, and head and neck infections
  5. Osteomyelitis especially when associated with decubitus ulcers or vascular insufficiency
  6. Facial bone osteomyelitis from adjacent infections of the teeth or sinuses

ETIOLOGY

- Most commonly endogenous, arising from bacteria that normally line mucosal surfaces
- Disruption of mucosal barriers resulting from various conditions (trauma, ischemia, surgery, perforation), with infection occurring when organisms gain access to normally sterile sites, causing tissue destruction and abscess formation
- Synergy between different anaerobes or between anaerobes and aerobes important
- Examples of anaerobic bacteria include gram-negative bacteria such as *Bacteroides* species, *Fusobacterium* and *Prevotella* species; and gram-positive bacteria such as *Peptostreptococcus*, *Clostridium* species, and *Actinomyces* species

DIAGNOSIS

DIFFERENTIAL DIAGNOSIS

- Primary differential possibility is an aerobic bacterial infection without the presence of anaerobic bacteria.
- Ischemic necrosis without accompanying anaerobic infection (or "dry" gangrene [non-infected necrosis] vs. "wet" gangrene [infected tissue with anaerobic infection]).

WORKUP

- Specimens submitted for anaerobic culture should be processed within 30 min and may take up to 5 to 7 days to grow
- Large volume of material more likely to have significant growth; swabs less efficient for transporting infected material
- Blood cultures—preferably before antibiotic administration

LABORATORY TESTS

- Elevated WBC count, with extremely high WBC counts sometimes seen with pseudomembranous colitis
- Positive stool *C. difficile* by polymerase chain reaction (PCR) or nucleic acid amplification test (NAAT)
- Increased lactate levels in ischemia or perforation
- Possible positive blood or wound cultures, but failure to grow anaerobes in culture may be common, attributed to inadequate culturing techniques or fastidious organisms

IMAGING STUDIES

- Plain film of an affected area to show gas in tissues, free air resulting from a perforated viscus, or an air/fluid level inside an abscess
- Ultrasound, CT scan, or MRI to reveal abscesses or tissue destruction

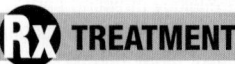 TREATMENT

NONPHARMACOLOGIC THERAPY

- Removal of necrotic tissue
- Drainage of abscesses (accomplished by CT scan–guided percutaneous drainage)

ACUTE GENERAL Rx

Oral antibiotics with anaerobic activity: clindamycin, metronidazole, and chloramphenicol
- Broader spectrum of activity with amoxicillin/clavulanate
- Penicillin VK in odontogenic infections
- Oral metronidazole for *C. difficile*–associated diarrhea, with oral vancomycin used for severe, recurrent, or recalcitrant infections

Parenteral antibiotics for more serious illness
- IV clindamycin, metronidazole, and chloramphenicol
- Cephalosporins (anaerobic or mixed infections): cefoxitin and cefotetan
- Extended-spectrum penicillins (e.g., piperacillin) and combination beta-lactamase plus beta-lactamase inhibitor drugs (e.g., clavulanic acid, sulbactam, tazobactam)
  1. Significant anaerobic activity, plus various degrees of broad-spectrum coverage
  2. Include ampicillin/sulbactam, ticarcillin/clavulanate, and piperacillin/tazobactam
- Imipenem or other carbapenems, such as meropenem, doripenem, or ertapenem, which are broad-spectrum agents with extensive anaerobic activity
- Actinomycosis treated with penicillin for 6 to 12 mo
- SMX/TMP and fluoroquinolones are generally ineffective, but some newer quinolones (e.g., moxifloxacin) have inhibitory activity against anaerobes

DISPOSITION

It is essential that all necrotic debris be removed when treating an anaerobic infection or it will recur; follow-up is critically important to ensure resolution of the process.

REFERRAL

Refer to a surgeon if drainage is required; infectious disease consultation may be useful in complicated patients or if treatment regimen is failing or slow to respond.

AUTHOR: **GLENN G. FORT, M.D., M.P.H.**

SUGGESTED READINGS
Available at www.expertconsult.com

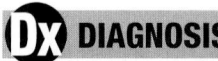 BASIC INFORMATION

DEFINITION

Anaphylaxis is a severe allergic reaction that is rapid in onset and life-threatening. It is characterized by respiratory, cardiovascular, gastrointestinal, and cutaneous manifestations, as well as vasodilatory hemodynamic changes in response to a particular allergen. Anaphylactoid reaction is an entity closely related to anaphylaxis and is caused by release of mast cells and basophil mediators triggered by non–IgE-mediated events.

SYNONYMS

Anaphylactoid reaction.

ICD-10CM CODES
T78.2	Anaphylactic shock, unspecified, initial encounter
T78.00XA	Anaphylactic reaction due to unspecified food, initial encounter
T80.52XA	Anaphylactic reaction due to vaccination, initial encounter
T50.904A	Poisoning by unspecified drugs, medicaments, and biologic substances, undetermined, initial encounter
T63.94XA	Toxic effect of contact with unspecified venomous animal, undetermined, initial encounter

EPIDEMIOLOGY & DEMOGRAPHICS

INCIDENCE: The incidence of anaphylaxis in the U.S. is 50 to 2000 episodes per 100,000 persons. Lifetime prevalence is 0.05% to 2%, with a mortality rate of 1%. Anaphylaxis rates are 0.0004% for food, 0.7% to 10% for penicillin, 0.22% to 1% for contrast media, and 0.5% to 5% after insect stings. Annual mortality is 500 to 1000 persons per year in the U.S.

PHYSICAL FINDINGS & CLINICAL PRESENTATION

- Urticaria, pruritus, skin flushing, angioedema (Table E1)
- Dyspnea, cough, wheezing, shortness of breath
- Nausea, vomiting, diarrhea, difficulty swallowing
- Hypotension, tachycardia, weakness, dizziness, malaise, vascular collapse (Table E2)

ETIOLOGY

Anaphylaxis results from a sudden systematic release of histamine and other inflammatory mediators from basophils and mast cells. This causes swelling of the mucus membranes and the urticarial rash on the skin. Virtually any substance may induce anaphylaxis.

- Foods and food additives: peanuts, tree nuts, eggs, shellfish, fish, cow's milk, fruits, soy
- Medications: antibiotics (especially penicillins), insulin, allergen extracts, opiates, vaccines, NSAIDs, contrast media, streptokinase
- Environmental exposures: bee or wasp sting, snake venom, fire ant venom
- Blood products: plasma, immunoglobulin, cryoprecipitate, whole blood
- Latex

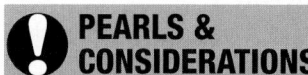 DIAGNOSIS

DIFFERENTIAL DIAGNOSIS

- Endocrine disorders (carcinoid, pheochromocytoma)
- Globus hystericus, anxiety disorder
- Systemic mastocytosis
- Pulmonary embolism, serum sickness, vasovagal reactions
- Severe asthma (the key clinical difference is the abrupt onset of symptoms in anaphylaxis versus a history of progressive worsening of symptoms)
- Septic shock or other form of vasodilatory shock
- Airway foreign body

WORKUP

Workup is aimed at ruling out other conditions that may mimic anaphylaxis.

LABORATORY TESTS

- Laboratory evaluation is generally not helpful because anaphylaxis is typically a clinical diagnosis.
- ABG analysis may be useful to help differentiate between pulmonary embolism, status asthmaticus, and foreign body aspiration.
- Elevated serum and urine histamine levels and serum tryptase levels can be useful for diagnosis of anaphylaxis, but these tests are not commonly available in the emergency setting.

IMAGING STUDIES

Generally not helpful.

- Chest radiography for evaluation of foreign body aspiration or pulmonary pathology is indicated in patients with acute respiratory compromise.
- Consider ECG in all patients with sudden loss of consciousness or reports of chest pain or dyspnea and in any elderly patient. ECG in anaphylaxis usually reveals sinus tachycardia.

TREATMENT

NONPHARMACOLOGIC THERAPY

- Establish and protect airway. Provide supplemental O₂ if indicated.
- IV access should be rapidly established, and IV fluids (i.e., normal saline) should be administered.
- Cardiac monitoring is recommended.

ACUTE GENERAL Rx

- Epinephrine should be rapidly administered as an IM injection at a dose of 0.3 mg of aqueous epinephrine for adults and children >30 kg. Epinephrine 0.15 mg should be given for children <30 kg (1:1000 concentration).

Intramuscular administration is preferred because it provides more reliable and quicker rise to effective plasma levels. The dose may be repeated after approximately 5 to 15 min if symptoms persist.

- Adjunct therapies include H_1 and H_2 receptor antagonists such as diphenhydramine 25 to 50 mg IV or IM (or PO in mild cases) and famotidine 20 to 40 mg IV (or PO in mild cases). Although useful to improve cutaneous erythema and pruritus, H_1 antagonists are not as effective as epinephrine, since onset of action is 1 to 2 hours and they are not effective in reversing upper airway obstruction or improving hypotension.
- Corticosteroids are not useful in the acute episode because of their slow onset of action; however, they should be administered in most cases to prevent prolonged or recurrent anaphylaxis. Commonly used agents are prednisone, methylprednisolone 40 to 250 mg IV in adults (1 to 2 mg/kg in children), or dexamethasone.
- Aerosolized β-agonists (e.g., albuterol, 2.5 mg, repeat prn 20 min) are useful to control bronchospasm.
- Vasopressor therapy with epinephrine (1:10,000), or dopamine is indicated in patients with refractory hypotension/cardiovascular collapse after crystalloid resuscitation.
- Table E3 summarizes drugs and other agents used in anaphylaxis therapy.

PEARLS & CONSIDERATIONS

COMMENTS

- Patient education regarding the nature of the illness and preventive measures is recommended. A documented history of previous anaphylactic episodes or known triggers is the most reliable method of identifying individuals at risk.
- Prescription for a prefilled epinephrine syringe (EpiPen or EpiPen Jr.) should be given, and the patient should be instructed on the use of this emergency kit, and to carry it on his/her person at all times. School-aged children should keep an additional EpiPen at school with the appropriate staff.
- Patients should also be advised to carry or wear a MedicAlert ID describing substances that have caused anaphylaxis.
- Avoidance of radiologic contrast is also recommended in those who have had a prior reaction. However, pretreatment regimens with methylprednisolone, diphenhydramine, or n-acetylcysteine exist for those who have had contrast reactions in the past.
- Venom immunotherapy immediately after a sting is effective and recommended for up to 5 yr after the anaphylactic incident.

SUGGESTED READINGS

Available at www.expertconsult.com

AUTHOR: **STEVEN ROUGAS, M.D., M.S.**

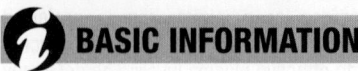

DEFINITION

Aplastic anemia (AA) refers to a bone marrow failure syndrome characterized by immune-mediated bone marrow destruction and peripheral blood pancytopenia. Severe aplastic anemia (SAA) is defined by the presence of two criteria from either neutrophil counts $<50 \times 10^9$/L, platelet counts $<20 \times 10^9$/L, or corrected reticulocyte count $<1\%$.

SYNONYMS

Aplastic anemia AA
Refractory anemia
Hypoplastic anemia

ICD-10CM CODES
D61.9	Aplastic anemia, unspecified
D60.9	Acquired pure red cell aplasia, unspecified
D60.8	Other acquired pure red cell aplasias
D61.09	Other constitutional aplastic anemia
D61.1	Drug-induced aplastic anemia
D61.2	Aplastic anemia due to other external agents
D61.3	Idiopathic aplastic anemia
D61.89	Other specified aplastic anemias and other bone marrow failure syndromes

EPIDEMIOLOGY & DEMOGRAPHICS

INCIDENCE: The annual incidence of aplastic anemia is 2 cases per million in the Western population and 2 to 3 times higher in Asia.

PREDOMINANT SEX AND AGE: The incidence has two peaks, with most patients presenting between ages 15 and 30 years or after 60 years.

PHYSICAL FINDINGS & CLINICAL PRESENTATION

- Fatigue, pallor, exertional shortness of breath, or palpitations are seen secondary to anemia.
- Mucosal bleeding, easy bruising, petechiae or heavy menstrual bleeding is seen secondary to thrombocytopenia.
- Infection is uncommon at clinical presentation, but severe neutropenia may lead to fever and sore throat.
- Various physical manifestations like short stature, skeletal or nail changes may be seen in congenital forms of aplastic anemia.

ETIOLOGY

- In most patients with idiopathic aplastic anemia, bone marrow failure results from immunologically mediated, active destruction of hematopoietic cells by lymphocytes.
- Mutations in *TERT*, the gene for the RNA component of telomerase, cause short telomerases in congenital aplastic anemia and in some cases of apparently acquired hematopoietic failure. In patients with severe aplastic anemia receiving immunosuppressive therapy (IST), telomere length is unrelated to response but is associated with risk of relapse, clonal evolution, and overall survival.
- Common etiologic factors in acquired aplastic anemia include:
  1. Toxins (e.g., benzene, insecticides)
  2. Drugs (e.g., felbamate , cimetidine, NSAIDs, antiepileptics, gold salts, chloramphenicol, sulfonamides, trimethadione, quinacrine, phenylbutazone). Table 1 describes a classification of drugs and chemicals associated with aplastic anemia.
  3. Ionizing radiation
  4. Infections (e.g., hepatitis C, HIV, Epstein-Barr virus, parvovirus B19)
- Inherited aplastic anemia
  1. Fanconi's anemia
  2. Reticular dysgenesis
  3. Dyskeratosis congenita
  4. Nonhematologic syndromes (Down syndrome, etc.)
  5. Shwachman-Diamond syndrome
- Pregnancy
- Idiopathic

DIFFERENTIAL DIAGNOSIS

- Bone marrow infiltration from lymphoma, carcinoma, myelofibrosis
- Severe infection
- Hypoplastic myelodysplastic syndrome
- Hypersplenism
- Hairy cell leukemia

WORKUP

- Diagnostic workup (Fig. E1) consists primarily of bone marrow aspiration and biopsy, and laboratory evaluation (CBC and examination of peripheral blood smear).
- Bone marrow examination generally shows paucity or absence of hematopoietic precursor cells (Figs. E2, *B* and *C*, and E3); patients with pure red cell aplasia demonstrate only absence of red blood cell (RBC) precursors in the marrow.

LABORATORY TESTS

- CBC reveals pancytopenia (Fig. E2, *A*). Macrocytosis and toxic granulation of

---

TABLE 1 Classification of Drugs and Chemicals Associated With Aplastic Anemia

I. Agents That Regularly Produce Bone Marrow Depression as a Major Toxic Effect When Used in Commonly Used Doses or Normal Exposures

Cytotoxic drugs used in cancer chemotherapy
Alkylating agents (busulfan, melphalan, cyclophosphamide)
Antimetabolites (antifolic compounds, nucleotide analogs) antimitotics (vincristine, vinblastine, colchicine)
Some antibiotics (daunorubicin, doxorubicin [Adriamycin])
Benzene (and less often benzene-containing chemicals: kerosene, carbon tetrachloride, Stoddard solvent, chlorophenols)

II. Agents Probably Associated With Aplastic Anemia but With a Relatively Low Probability Relative to Their Use

Chloramphenicol
Insecticides
Antiprotozoals (quinacrine and chloroquine)
Nonsteroidal antiinflammatory drugs (including phenylbutazone, indomethacin, ibuprofen, sulindac, diclofenac, naproxen, piroxicam, fenoprofen, fenbufen, aspirin)
Anticonvulsants (hydantoins, carbamazepine, phenacemide, ethosuximide)
Gold, arsenic, and other heavy metals such as bismuth and mercury
Sulfonamides as a class
Antithyroid medications (methimazole, methylthiouracil, propylthiouracil)
Antidiabetes drugs (tolbutamide, carbutamide, chlorpropamide)
Carbonic anhydrase inhibitors (acetazolamide, methazolamide, mesalazine)
D-Penicillamine
2-Chlorodeoxyadenosine

III. Agents More Rarely Associated With Aplastic Anemia

Antibiotics (streptomycin, tetracycline, methicillin, ampicillin, mebendazole and albendazole, sulfonamides, flucytosine, mefloquine, dapsone)
Antihistamines (cimetidine, ranitidine, chlorpheniramine)
Sedatives and tranquilizers (chlorpromazine, prochlorperazine, piperacetazine, chlordiazepoxide, meprobamate, methyprylon, remoxipride)
Antiarrhythmics (tocainide, amiodarone)
Allopurinol (can potentiate marrow suppression by cytotoxic drugs)
Ticlopidine
Methyldopa
Quinidine
Lithium
Guanidine
Canthaxanthin
Thiocyanate
Carbimazole
Cyanamide
Deferoxamine
Amphetamines

From Hoffman R: *Hematology, basic principles and practice,* 6th ed, Philadelphia, Saunders, 2013.

neutrophils may also be present. Isolated cytopenias may occur in the early stages.
- Reticulocytopenia can be seen.
- Additional laboratory evaluation should include Ham test and/or peripheral blood flow cytometry to exclude paroxysmal nocturnal hemoglobinuria (PNH) and testing for hepatitis C.

IMAGING STUDIES

MRI with spin-echo sequence is helpful in the study of bone marrow disease, and the high fat content of an aplastic marrow can be easily seen on MRI.

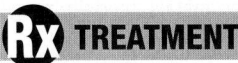 TREATMENT

NONPHARMACOLOGIC THERAPY

Discontinue any potential offending drugs or agents.

ACUTE GENERAL Rx

- Aggressive treatment of neutropenic fevers with empiric broad-spectrum antibiotics.
- Administer platelet and packed RBC transfusions as needed; however, it is important to avoid frequent transfusions in patients who are candidates for stem cell transplantation (SCT).
- Fig. 4 describes a treatment algorithm for aplastic anemia.

CHRONIC Rx

- Initial treatment can include observation and supportive care alone. Progression to transfusion dependence or to criteria meeting definition of SAA necessitates definitive treatment.
- The major treatment options for SAA are IST and allogeneic SCT. Treatment decisions are based on age, availability of histocompatible stem cell donor, and presence of comorbidities. Patients >40 years old are usually not considered for up-front stem cell transplant but are treated with immunosuppressive therapy only.
- Allogeneic SCT from a human leukocyte antigen (HLA)-matched sibling donor is potentially curative. Patients who do not have a matched sibling can be treated with a matched unrelated donor (MUD) SCT. Alternatively, there is increasing efficacy data with the use of haploidentical donor SCT when related donors are unavailable.
- Studies have shown an association between leukocyte telomere length and outcomes in MUD-SCT. Longer donor leukocyte telomere length was associated with increased 5-year survival.
- Patients who fail to respond to initial IST are candidates for alternative donor SCT or other immunosuppressive therapy such as Alemtuzumab (anti-CD52 monoclonal antibody).
- Other immunosuppressive agents such as cyclosporine, cyclophosphamide, or corticosteroids also have a role in the treatment of SAA.

- Androgens such as danazol are effective second-line agents.
- The oral thrombopoietin mimetic eltrombopag can improve platelet recovery in refractory SAA.

DISPOSITION

- The most recent retrospective analyses have revealed 5-year survival rates of 80% to 85% with allogeneic SCT, especially for younger patients <40 years old.
- Approximately 50% of patients treated with IST alone achieve long-term remissions and do not have disease relapse.
- Graft rejection and graft-versus-host disease are the major complications of allogeneic SCT.
- Approximately 10%–15% patients develop clonal evolution, which manifests as myelodysplastic syndrome or acute myeloid leukemia.

REFERRAL

Hematology referral is indicated in all patients with aplastic anemia.

SUGGESTED READINGS

Available at www.expertconsult.com

RELATED CONTENT

Aplastic Anemia (Patient Information)

AUTHOR: **RITESH RATHORE, M.D.**

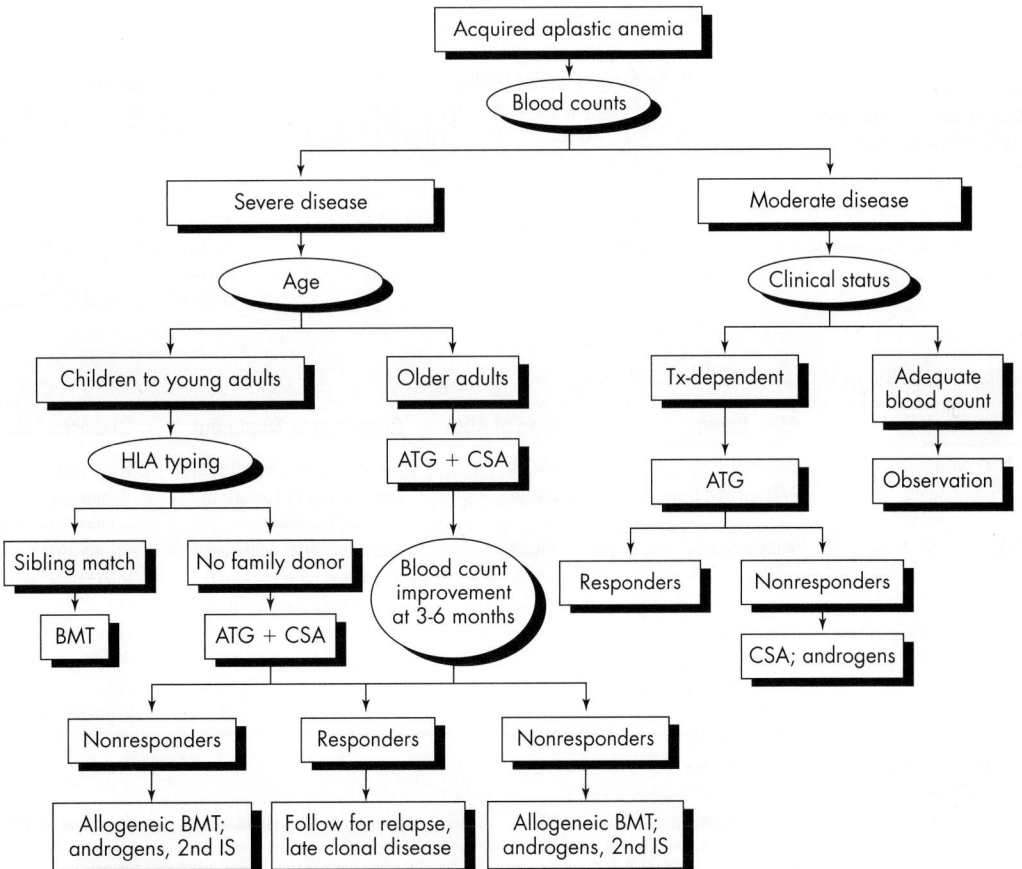

FIG. 4 Treatment algorithm in aplastic anemia. Algorithm-based selection of treatment for patients with aplastic anemia. *ATG,* Antithymocyte globulin; *BMT,* bone marrow transplantation; *CSA,* cyclosporine A; *HLA,* human leukocyte antigen; *IS,* immunosuppression; *Tx,* treatment. (From Hoffmann R et al: *Hematology, basic principles and practice,* ed 6, Philadelphia, 2013, Elsevier.)

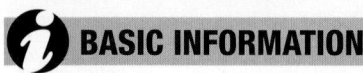

BASIC INFORMATION

DEFINITION

Autoimmune hemolytic anemia (AIHA) is anemia secondary to premature clearance of red blood cells (RBCs) caused by binding of autoantibodies and/or complement to RBCs. The classification of the hemolytic anemias is described in Table 1.

SYNONYMS

Autoimmune hemolytic anemia
Drug-induced hemolytic anemia
Cold agglutinin disease
Warm autoimmune hemolytic anemia

ICD-10CM CODES
D59.0 Drug-induced autoimmune hemolytic anemia
D59.1 Other autoimmune hemolytic anemias

TABLE 1 Classification of the Hemolytic Anemias

Acquired

Environmental factors
  Antibody: immunohemolytic anemias
  Mechanical trauma: TTP, HUS, heart valve
  Toxins, infectious agents: malaria, etc.
Membrane defects
  Paroxysmal nocturnal hemoglobinuria
  Spur cell anemia
Hereditary spherocytosis, etc.

Congenital

Defects of cell interior
  Hemoglobinopathies: sickle cell, thalassemia
  Enzymopathies: G6PD deficiency, etc.

G6PD, Glucose-6-phosphate dehydrogenase; HUS, hemolytic-uremic syndrome; TTP, thrombotic thrombocytopenic purpura.
From Goldman L, Schafer AI: Goldman's Cecil medicine, ed 24, Philadelphia, 2012, Saunders.

EPIDEMIOLOGY & DEMOGRAPHICS

The annual incidence is 3 cases per 100,000 persons, with 10% mortality; most common in women <50 years.

PHYSICAL FINDINGS & CLINICAL PRESENTATION

- Most common presentation is dyspnea and fatigue.
- Pallor, jaundice may be present.
- Tachycardia with a flow murmur may be present if anemia is pronounced.
- Patients with intravascular hemolysis may present with dark urine and back pain.
- The presence of hepatomegaly and/or lymphadenopathy suggests an underlying lymphoproliferative disorder or malignancy; splenomegaly may indicate hypersplenism as a cause of hemolysis.

ETIOLOGY

- Warm antibody mediated: IgG only (often idiopathic or associated with leukemia, lymphoma, thymoma, myeloma, viral infections, and collagen-vascular disease)
- Cold antibody mediated: IgM and complement in majority of cases (often idiopathic; at times associated with infections, lymphoma, or cold agglutinin disease)
- Il-33 may have a role in promoting increasing RBC autoantibodies in AIHA.
- Drug induced (Table 2): three major mechanisms:
  1. Antibody directed against Rh complex (e.g., methyldopa)
  2. Antibody directed against RBC-drug complex (hapten induced; e.g., penicillin)
  3. Antibody directed against complex formed by drug and plasma proteins; the drug-plasma protein-antibody complex causes destruction of RBCs (innocent bystander; e.g., quinidine)

DIAGNOSIS

DIFFERENTIAL DIAGNOSIS

- Hemolytic anemia caused by membrane defects (acquired: paroxysmal nocturnal hemoglobinuria, spur cell anemia, Wilson disease; inherited: spherocytosis, elliptosis), hemoglobinopathies, and enzyme deficiencies (G6PD, pyruvate kinase)
- Non–immune mediated (microangiopathic hemolytic anemias, hypersplenism, cardiac valve prosthesis, giant cavernous hemangiomas, march hemoglobinuria, physical agents, infections, heavy metals, certain drugs [nitrofurantoin, sulfonamides, ribavirin])

WORKUP

Evaluation consists primarily of laboratory evaluation to confirm hemolysis and exclude other causes of the anemia. Although most cases of AIHA are idiopathic, potential causes should always be sought.

LABORATORY TESTS

- The basic features of hemolytic anemia are reticulocytosis (if no concurrent bone marrow suppression), low haptoglobin levels, elevated indirect bilirubin, and elevated LDH.
- Initial laboratory tests: complete blood count (anemia), reticulocyte count (elevated; Fig. E1 describes the evaluation of anemia with increased reticulocytes), liver function studies (elevated indirect bilirubin, LDH), evaluation of peripheral smear (Fig. E2).
- A direct antiglobulin test (DAT, Coombs test) is initially performed with a polyspecific antibody to detect IgG or complement C3d bound to RBCs. If the DAT is positive, the diagnosis of autoimmune hemolytic anemia (AIHA) is confirmed. A positive direct Coombs test indicates presence of antibodies or complement on the surface of RBCs (Fig. 3); positive indirect Coombs test implies presence of anti-RBC antibodies freely circulating in the patient's serum (Fig. 4).

TABLE 2 Drug-Induced Autoimmune Hemolytic Anemia

Drug	Risk Factors	AIHA Onset	Type of AIHA	Response to Treatment	Diseases Treated
Methyldopa	Not known	Delayed	WAIHA	Resolution after withdrawal	Hypertension
INF-α	Pretherapeutic positive DAT	Delayed (8-11 mo)	WAIHA	Resolution spontaneous or after steroids	Hepatitis C Hematologic malignancies
Efazulimab	Not known	Many months	WAIHA	Resolution after withdrawal	Arthritis (rare)
Etanercept	Not known	Delayed	CAIHA	Resolution after rituximab	Rheumatoid arthritis (rare)
Fludarabine Cladribine Pentostatin	CLL Pretherapeutic positive DAT result	Early (median, 3-4 cycle) or delayed	WAIHA Mixed AIHA	Half of AIHA resolve after steroids	CLL Lymphomas* AML*
Bendamustine	CLL	No or only very low risk of AIHA			CLL Lymphomas
Chlorambucil	CLL	Delayed onset	WAIHA		CLL
Eculizumab	Patients with incomplete response	After treatment	CAIHA		PNH
Lenalidomide		During treatment	WAIHA	Resolution after withdrawal	One case treated for lymphoma

AML, Acute myeloid leukemia; CAIHA, cold autoimmune hemolytic anemia; CLL, chronic lymphocytic leukemia; INF, interferon; PNH, paroxysmal nocturnal hemoglobinuria; WAIHA, warm autoimmune hemolytic anemia.
*No or very low risk.
From Hoffman R: Hematology, basic principles and practice, 6th ed, Philadelphia, 2013, Saunders.

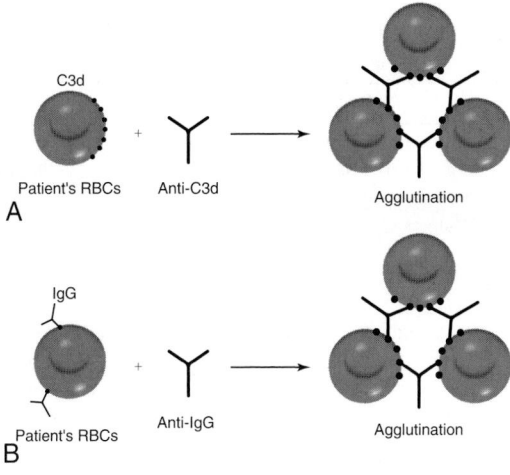

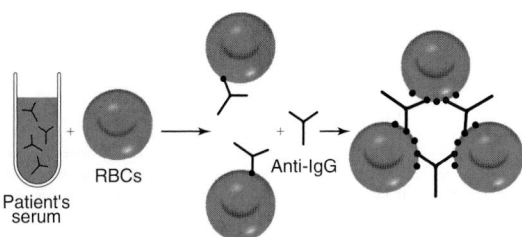

FIG. 3 Direct antiglobulin test for detection of **(A)** erythrocyte bound C3d or **(B)** IgG. Hemagglutination occurs when anti-C3d or anti-IgG can create a lattice structure by bridging sensitized red blood cells *(RBCs)*. (From Hoffman R et al: *Hematology, basic principles and practice,* ed 6, Philadelphia, 2013, Saunders.)

FIG. 4 Indirect antiglobulin test for detection of antierythrocyte antibodies in serum. The patient's serum is mixed with a panel of normal red blood cells *(RBCs),* some (or all) of which express the antigen(s) recognized by the serum antibodies. After the antibody-coated erythrocytes are washed, an anti-IgG reagent is added and hemagglutination occurs. (From Hoffman R et al: *Hematology, basic principles and practice,* ed 6, Philadelphia, 2013, Elsevier.)

- If the DAT is positive with IgG alone or with IgG + C3d, the AIHA is most likely due to warm antibody (WAIHA), whereas if the DAT is positive with C3d only it is most likely caused by a cold antibody (CAIHA).
- Hepatitis serology, antinuclear antibody.
- Urinary tests may reveal hemosiderinuria or hemoglobinuria.

IMAGING STUDIES
- Chest x-ray
- CT scan of chest, abdomen, and pelvis should be considered if underlying lymphoprolifera-tive disorder is suspected

Rx TREATMENT

NONPHARMACOLOGIC THERAPY
- Discontinuation of any potentially offensive drugs
- Plasmapheresis exchange transfusion for severe life-threatening cases only

- Avoid cold exposure in patients with cold antibody

ACUTE GENERAL Rx
- Prednisone 1 to 2 mg/kg/day in divided doses initially in warm antibody AIHA. Corticosteroids are generally ineffective in cold antibody AIHA. In cold agglutinin disease treatment, modalities consist of cold avoid-ance, therapy of underlying lymphoprolif-erative disorder, and use of rituximab and plasmapheresis in severe cases.
- Splenectomy in patients responding inad-equately to corticosteroids when RBC sequestration studies indicate splenic sequestration.
- Immunosuppressive drugs and/or immuno-globulins only after both corticosteroids and splenectomy (unless surgery is contraindi-cated) have failed to produce an adequate remission.

- Danazol, typically used in conjunction with corticosteroids (may be useful in warm anti-body AIHA).
- Immunosuppressive drugs (azathioprine, cyclophosphamide) may be useful in warm antibody AIHA but are indicated only after both corticosteroids and splenectomy (unless surgery is contraindicated) have failed to produce an adequate remission.
- Table 3 summarizes treatment options for primary and secondary warm autoimmune hemolytic anemia and cold autoimmune hemolytic anemia. Second-line treatment options after steroids are described in Table 4.

DISPOSITION
Prognosis is generally good unless anemia is associated with underlying disorder with a poor prognosis (e.g., leukemia, myeloma).

REFERRAL
- Hematology referral in all cases of AIHA
- Surgical referral for splenectomy in refractory cases

! PEARLS & CONSIDERATIONS

COMMENTS
- The direct antiglobulin test demonstrates the presence of antibodies or complement on the surface of RBCs and is the hallmark of autoimmune hemolysis.
- Warm AIHA is often associated with autoim-mune diseases, whereas cold AIHA often follows viral infections (e.g., mononucleosis) and *Mycoplasma pneumoniae* infections.
- HIV can induce both warm and cold AIHA.
- Hemolytic anemia is a common autoim-mune complication of hematopoietic stem cell transplantation occurring in up to 6% of patients as a late complication (median 202 days); it presents as either warm or cold AIHA.

SUGGESTED READINGS
Available at www.expertconsult.com

AUTHORS: **ANDRE LUIZ DE SOUZA, M.D.,** and **BHARTI RATHORE, M.D.**

TABLE 3 Treatment Options for Primary and Secondary Warm Autoimmune Hemolytic Anemia and Cold Autoimmune Hemolytic Anemia

Disease or Condition	First Line	Second Line	Beyond Second Line	Last Resort
Primary AIHA	Steroids	Splenectomy Rituximab	Azathioprine, MMF, cyclosporine, cyclophosphamide	High-dose cyclophospha-mide, alemtuzumab
B- and T-cell NHL	Steroids	Chemotherapy +/− rituximab (splenectomy in SMZL)		
Hodgkin's lymphoma	Steroids	Chemotherapy		
Solid tumors	Steroids Surgery			
Ovarian dermoid cyst	Ovariectomy			
SLE	Steroids	Azathioprine	MMF	Rituximab Autologous SCT
Ulcerative colitis	Steroids	Azathioprine		Total colectomy
CVID	Steroids + IgG replacement			
ALPD	Steroids	MMF	Sirolimus	
Wiskott Aldrich syndrome	Steroids	Allogeneic SCT		
Allogeneic SCT	Steroids	Rituximab*	Splenectomy T-cells infusion	
Organ transplantation	Reduction of immune suppression, steroids			
Drug induced	Withdrawal	Steroids		
Primary CAD	Protection from cold exposure	Rituximab Chlorambucil	Fludarabine + rituximab	Eculizumab,† bortezomib†
PCH	Supportive treatment (postinfectious)	Rituximab* (chronic)		

AIHA, Autoimmune hemolytic anemia; *ALPD*, autoimmune lymphoproliferative disorders; *CAD*, cold agglutinin disease; *CVID*, common variable immune deficiency; *IgG*, immunoglobulin G; *MMF*, mycophenolate mofetil; *NHL*, non-Hodgkin lymphoma; *PCH*, paroxysmal cold hemoglobinuria; *SCT*, stem cell transplantation; *SLE*, systemic lupus erythematosus; *SMZL*, splenic marginal zone lymphoma.
*Early second-line treatment because of known poor response to steroids.
†Off-label use in single cases.
From Hoffman R: *Hematology, basic principles and practice*, 6th ed, Philadelphia, 2013, Saunders.

TABLE 4 Second-Line Treatment Options After Steroids

Treatment	Dosing and Application	Side Effects	Precautions
Splenectomy (acute)	Preferentially laparoscopic	Infections, thrombosis	Postoperative thromboprophylaxis
Splenectomy (long term)	—	Infections Venous thrombosis	Vaccination, patient information
Rituximab	375 mg/m² on days 1, 8, 15, and 22 IV	Infusional reactions Infections	Premedication with antihistamines (and steroids)
Danazol	200-400/day PO	Hepatotoxicity	None
Cyclophosphamide	PO or IV Dose adjusted to neutrophil count	Neutropenia Mutagenesis	Neutrophil count monitoring, bladder protection after high doses
Azathioprine	2.0-3.mg/kg/day PO Dose adjusted to neutrophil count	Neutropenia	Neutrophil count monitoring; avoid interaction with other drugs (e.g., allopurinol)
Mycophenolate mofetil	1-2 × 1 g/d PO	Gastrointestinal	
Cyclosporine	PO Dose adjusted to blood levels of CyA Target level, 200-400 ng/mL	Nephrotoxicity Gum hyperplasia	Monitoring of CyA levels and creatinine
Alemtuzumab	SC (variable doses)	Neutropenia	Anti-infectious prophylaxis

CyA, Cyclosporine A; *IV*, intravenous; *PO*, oral; *SC*, subcutaneous.
From Hoffman R: *Hematology, basic principles and practice*, 6th ed, Philadelphia, 2013, Saunders.

BASIC INFORMATION

DEFINITION

Inflammatory anemia or anemia of chronic disease (ACD) is a disorder of iron homeostasis promoted by hepcidin-25 in response to an inflammatory condition.

Iron is carried in the bloodstream shelled by a hollow protein called transferrin (<0.2% of total iron body content) or at the core of hemoglobin in RBCs (60% of total iron body content).

Iron is stored (15%-30% of total iron body content), especially inside the liver, spleen, and skeletal muscle cytoplasm as ferritin (although released to the bloodstream), and in lysosomes as hemosiderin. The rest of the iron body content is trapped in myoglobin in skeletal muscle and cytochromes in mitochondrias. In clinical practice, ferritin is a surrogate for iron stores and TIBC a surrogate for transferrin and carrying capacity of iron.

Cells involved in the defense from the inflammatory insult release cytokines such as IL-6, which stimulates hepatic release of hepcidin-25. Hepcidin is a circulating protein that blocks ferroportin, an iron channel responsible for the exit of iron from enterocytes (and thus gastrointestinal absorption) and macrophages (which accumulate iron from engulfed senescent blood cells). IL-1 and TNF-alpha stimulate INF-gamma release by marrow stromal cells, which in turn suppress the erythroid response to erythropoietin (EPO). In chronic kidney disease, ACD is a consequence of decreased production of EPO and decreased renal clearance of hepcidin. The low availability of serum iron causes iron deficiency in the bone marrow compartment and decreased reticulocyte levels.

SYNONYMS

Inflammatory anemia
Anemia of chronic disease
ACD

ICD-10CM CODES
D63.8 Anemia in chronic diseases classified elsewhere
D63.0 Anemia in neoplastic disease
D64.8 Anemia, unspecified

EPIDEMIOLOGY & DEMOGRAPHICS

PREVALENCE:
- Second-most prevalent anemia after iron deficiency anemia
  1. Around 11% of men and 10% of women ages 65 to 85 years
  2. >20% of adults older than 85 years

CLINICAL PRESENTATION
- Besides fatigue, shortness of breath, and generalized weakness from the anemia itself, it is important to consider other complaints if the underlying diagnosis is unknown, such as weight loss (malignancy, chronic infections, connective tissue diseases), anorexia, nausea, paresthesias, pleuritic chest pain, weight gain (CKD), diarrhea, bloody stools, abdominal pain, oral ulcers (IBD), and fevers (HIV, chronic infections).
- Physical findings may include pallor, lymphadenopathy, stigmatas of connective tissue diseases (malar rash, sclerodactyly), palpable or visible masses, and localized findings for infection or malignancy.

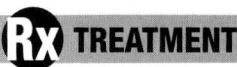

DIAGNOSIS

Isolated ACD:
CBC with differential: normocytic (MCV 80-100 fL), normochromic (<36 g/dL), moderate (Hb rarely <8 g/dL) anemia
Hypoproliferative anemia (low reticulocyte index; reticulocyte count corrected to hematocrit <2%).
Iron studies:
- Low iron concentration as in IDA (iron deficiency anemia)
- Normal/high ferritin (>35 mg/dL) in ACD as it is an acute phase reactant (Fig. 1).
- Low/normal TIBC (as opposed to IDA) and low transferrin saturation (as in IDA)
- Normal soluble transferrin receptor (sTfR, high in IDA)
Combined ACD/IDA
If normal to high ferritin, sTfR/log ferritin <1 defines isolated ACD, and >2 defines combined IDA/ACD

ETIOLOGY

Malignancy
CKD (patients with CKD stage IV [GFR<30 mL/min] should be screened for ACD)
CHF (ACD is the main cause of anemia in CHF patients)
Chronic infections
Anemia of critical illness (develops within days)
Connective tissue diseases

DIFFERENTIAL DIAGNOSIS

- Liver injury (increases ferritin)
  - Iron deficiency anemia
    - Other causes of normocytic anemia or microcytic anemia (Table 1)
      Red blood cell loss or destruction
        Acute blood loss
        Hypersplenism
        Hemolysis
    - Decreased red blood cell production
      Primary causes
        Bone marrow hypoplasia or aplasia
        Myeloproliferative disease
        Pure red blood cell aplasia
      Secondary causes
        Chronic renal failure
        Liver disease
        Endocrine deficiency states
        Sideroblastic anemia

WORKUP

- CBC, reticulocyte count, peripheral smear (Fig. E2, A), iron level, ferritin, TIBC. Table 2 summarizes characteristic findings in inflammatory anemia.

TREATMENT

Treat the underlying disorder/disease.

ACUTE GENERAL Rx

Blood transfusion is usually reserved for severe anemia (with Hb level <7 g/dl or <8 g/dl in patients with cardiac disease) especially if complicated with ongoing bleeding.

CHRONIC Rx

- Erythropoiesis-stimulating agents (ESA) (epoetin alfa and darbepoetin alfa) are FDA approved for use in patients with anemia resulting from:
  1. Chronic kidney disease
  2. Chemotherapy
  3. Zidovudine therapy.

Although a 1998 study called Normal Hematocrit Cardiac Trial (NHCT) showed a nonsignificant increase in the combined endpoint death and nonfatal MI in patients with goal hematocrit of 33% versus 27%, subsequent studies (CHOIR, CREATE, and TREAT) suggest that higher doses and higher hematocrit targets are associated with increased cardiovascular events.

ESA dose should be individualized for each patient, and the lowest sufficient dose to reduce blood transfusions should be used. A hemoglobin target of approximately 10 g% is widely acceptable. Iron deficiency should be ruled out before ESA is started. After starting ESA therapy, ASH/ASCO guidelines recommend periodic monitoring of iron status. When there is no or suboptimal response to oral therapy, parenteral iron therapy should be considered before concluding that a patient is nonresponsive to iron therapy.

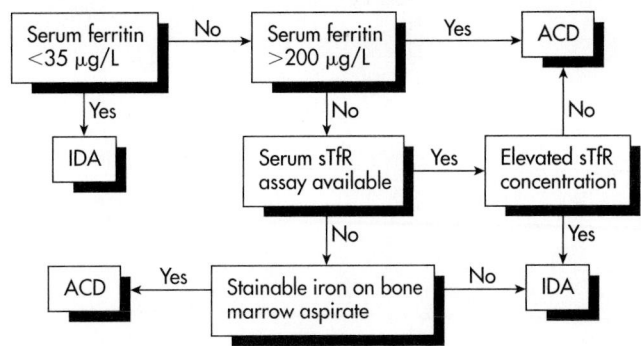

FIG. 1 Differential diagnosis of anemia with low serum iron. *ACD,* Anemia of chronic disease; *IDA,* iron deficiency anemia; *sTfR,* soluble transferrin receptor. (Modified from Young NS et al. [eds]: *Clinical hematology,* St Louis, 2006, Mosby.)

TABLE 1   Laboratory Features in Microcytic Hypochromic Anemias

	Serum Iron	Serum TIBC	% Saturation	MARROW % Sideroblasts	MARROW Iron Stores	Serum Ferritin	ZPP	Hb A$_2$	Hb F
Iron deficiency	↓	↑	↓	↓	↓	↓	↑	N-↓	N
β-Thalassemia trait	N (↑)	N	N	N	N-↑	N-↑	N	↑	N-↑
ACD	↓	N-↓	↓	↓	N-↑	N-↑	↑	N	N
Sideroblastic anemia	↑	↓	↑	↑	↑	↑	↑ (↓)	N	N-↑

ACD, Anemia of chronic disease; *N,* normal; *TIBC,* total iron-binding capacity; *ZPP,* zinc protoporphyrins; ↓, decreased; ↑, increased.
McPherson RA, Pincus MR: *Henry's clinical diagnosis and management by laboratory methods,* ed 23, Philadelphia, 2017, Elsevier.

TABLE 2   Laboratory Characteristics of ACD, IDA, and IDA With Inflammation

	Anemia of Chronic Disease (ACD)	Iron Deficiency Anemia (IDA)	IDA with Inflammation
Mean corpuscular volume (MCV)	72-100 fL	<85 fL	<100 fL
Mean corpuscular hemoglobin concentration (MCHC)	<36 g/dl	<32 g/dl	<32 g/dl
Serum iron	Decreased	Decreased	Decreased
Serum total iron-binding capacity (TIBC)	Typical below mid-normal range	Elevated	Less than upper limit of normal range
Transferrin saturation*	2%-20%	<15% (usually <10%)	<15%
Serum ferritin	>35 µg/L	<35 µg/L	>35 µg/L, <200µg/L
Serum soluble transferrin receptor concentration (sTfR)	Normal (may be increased if serum ferritin >200 µg/L)	Increased	Increased
TfR index (sTfR/log ferritin)	<1	>2	>2
Hepcidin	High	Low	Normal
Stainable iron in bone marrow	Present	Absent	Absent

*Serum iron/TIBC * 100.
From Young NS et al (eds): *Clinical hematology,* St Louis, 2006, Mosby.

Promising research on the hepcidin–ferroportin axis with novel therapeutics that inhibit the BMP6-HJV-SMAD and the IL-6-STAT3 pathways may lead to better management of ACD. New available therapies in clinical trials include a once-a-month erythropoietin-stimulating agent (peginesatide) and a hypoxia-inducible factor agent that increases erythropoiesis and decreases hepcidin (roxadustat).

SUGGESTED READINGS
Available at www.expertconsult.com

AUTHORS: **ANDRE LUIZ DE SOUZA, M.D.,** and **BHARTI RATHORE, M.D.**

BASIC INFORMATION

DEFINITION

Anemia is defined as a hemoglobin level 2 standard deviations below normal for age and sex. Iron deficiency anemia is anemia resulting from inadequate iron supplementation or excessive blood loss.

ICD-10CM CODES
D50.9	Iron deficiency anemia, unspecified
O99.019	Anemia complicating pregnancy, unspecified trimester
D50.0	Iron deficiency anemia secondary to blood loss (chronic)
D50.8	Other iron deficiency anemias

EPIDEMIOLOGY & DEMOGRAPHICS

- Dietary iron deficiency occurs often in infants as a result of unsupplemented milk diets. It is also commonly seen in women during their reproductive years, as a result of heavy menstrual periods, and during pregnancy (increased demand).
- Iron deficiency is the most common nutritional deficiency worldwide.
- The prevalence of iron deficiency is greatest among toddlers ages 1 to 2 yr (7%) from inadequate intake and female individuals ages 12 to 49 yr (9% to 16%) from menstrual losses.
- The prevalence of iron deficiency is 2% in adult men, 9% to 12% in non-Hispanic white women, and 20% in black and Mexican American women.
- GI cancer is diagnosed in 10% of elderly patients with iron deficiency anemia.

PHYSICAL FINDINGS & CLINICAL PRESENTATION

- Most patients have normal examination results.
- Skin pallor and conjunctival pallor may be present.
- Signs and symptoms specific for iron deficiency are koilonychias, pica, pagophagia, blue sclera, glossitis, and angular stomatitis (Fig. 1).

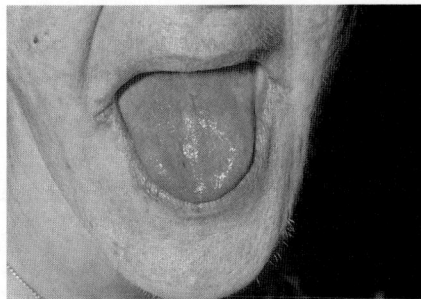

FIG. 1 Iron deficiency. (From White GM, Cox NH [eds]: *Diseases of the skin, a color atlas and text,* ed 2, St. Louis, 2006, Mosby.)

- Patients with severe anemia can have palpitations, headache, weakness, dizziness, and easy fatigability.

ETIOLOGY

- Blood loss from GI or menstrual bleeding (genitourinary blood loss less often the cause)
- Dietary iron deficiency (rare in adults)
- Poor iron absorption in patients with gastric or small-bowel surgery
- Repeated phlebotomy
- Increased requirements (e.g., during pregnancy)
- Other: traumatic hemolysis (abnormally functioning cardiac valves), idiopathic pulmonary hemosiderosis (iron sequestration in pulmonary macrophages), paroxysmal nocturnal hemoglobinuria (intravascular hemolysis)
- The most common cause worldwide is hookworm infection

DIAGNOSIS

DIFFERENTIAL DIAGNOSIS

- Anemia of chronic disease
- Sideroblastic anemia
- Thalassemia trait
- Lead poisoning

WORKUP

Diagnostic workup consists primarily of laboratory evaluation. Table 1 describes laboratory studies differentiating the most common microcytic anemias. Most patients with iron deficiency anemia are asymptomatic in the early stages. With progressive anemia, the major symptoms are fatigue, dizziness, exertional dyspnea, pagophagia (ice eating), and pica. Patient history may also suggest GI blood loss (melena, hematochezia, hemoptysis).

LABORATORY TESTS

- Laboratory results vary with the stage of deficiency.

- Absent iron marrow stores and decreased serum ferritin are the initial abnormalities.
- Decreased serum iron and increased total iron-binding capacity (TIBC) are the next abnormalities.
- Hypochromic microcytic anemia is present with significant iron deficiency.
- Peripheral smear in patients with iron deficiency generally reveals microcytic hypochromic red blood cells (Fig. 2) with a wide area of central pallor, anisocytosis, and poikilocytosis when severe.
- Laboratory abnormalities consistent with iron deficiency are low serum ferritin level, increased RBC distribution width with values generally >15, low mean corpuscular volume, low mean corpuscular hemoglobin, increased TIBC, and low serum iron.
- In patients diagnosed with iron deficiency anemia, a GI workup including an upper endoscopy and colonoscopy is recommended to look for source of iron loss.

TREATMENT

The goal of therapy is to supply sufficient iron to correct the low hemoglobin and replenish iron stores.

NONPHARMACOLOGIC THERAPY

Patients should be instructed to consume foods that contain large amounts of iron, such as liver, red meat, and legumes.

ACUTE GENERAL Rx

- Treatment consists of ferrous sulfate 325 mg PO daily for at least 6 mo. Doses higher than 325 mg/day are poorly tolerated. Calcium supplements can decrease iron absorption; therefore, these two medications should be staggered.
- Parenteral iron therapy is reserved for patients with poor tolerance, noncompliance with oral preparations, or malabsorption.
- Transfusion of packed RBCs is indicated in patients with severe symptomatic anemia.

TABLE 1 Laboratory Studies Differentiating the Most Common Microcytic Anemias

Study	Iron Deficiency Anemia	α or β Thalassemia	Anemia of Chronic Disease
Hemoglobin	Decreased	Decreased	Decreased
MCV	Decreased	Decreased	Normal-decreased
RDW	Increased	Normal	Normal-increased
RBC	Decreased	Normal-increased	Normal-decreased
Serum ferritin	Decreased	Normal	Increased
Total Fe binding capacity	Increased	Normal	Decreased
Transferrin saturation	Decreased	Normal	Decreased
FEP	Increased	Normal	Increased
Transferrin receptor	Increased	Normal	Increased
Reticulocyte hemoglobin concentration	Decreased	Normal	Normal-decreased

Fe, Ferritin; *FEP,* free erythrocyte protoporphyrin; *MCV,* mean corpuscular volume; *RBC,* red blood cell; *RDW,* red cell distribution width.
From Kliegman RM et al: *Nelson textbook of pediatrics,* ed 19, Philadelphia, 2011, Saunders.

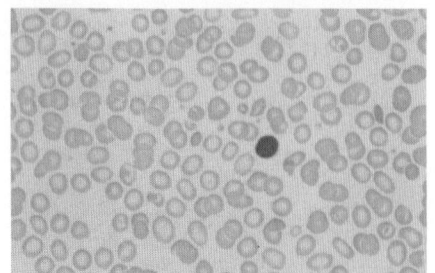

FIG. 2 Iron deficiency anemia. Many of these red blood cells are microcytic (smaller than the nucleus of the normal lymphocyte near the center of the field) and hypochromic (with central areas of pallor that exceed half the diameter of the cells). (From Goldman L, Schafer AI: *Goldman's Cecil medicine,* ed 24, Philadelphia, 2012, Saunders.)

CHRONIC Rx

Patients should be instructed to continue their iron supplements for at least 6 mo or longer to correct depleted body iron stores.

DISPOSITION

- Most patients respond rapidly to iron supplementation with improvement in CBC and general well-being (Table 2). GI side effects from oral iron therapy are common and may require decreased dosage to once every other day or to change to parenteral iron.
- A differential diagnosis of microcytic anemia that fails to respond to oral iron is described in Table 3.

REFERRAL

GI referral for evaluation of GI malignancy is recommended in all patients with iron deficiency and suspected GI blood loss.

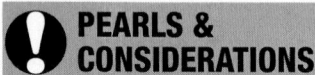

COMMENTS

- Iron deficiency may impair aerobic performance and worsen symptoms in patients with heart failure. Treatment with IV iron

TABLE 2 Responses to Iron Therapy in Iron Deficiency Anemia

Time after Iron Administration	Response
12-24 hr	Replacement of intracellular iron enzymes; subjective improvement; decreased irritability; increased appetite
36-48 hr	Initial bone marrow response; erythroid hyperplasia
48-72 hr	Reticulocytosis, peaking at 5–7 days
4-30 days	Increase in hemoglobin level
1-3 mo	Repletion of stores

From Kliegman RM et al: *Nelson textbook of pediatrics,* ed 19, Philadelphia, 2011, Saunders.

TABLE 3 Differential Diagnosis of Microcytic Anemia That Fails to Respond to Oral Iron

Poor compliance (true intolerance of iron is uncommon)

Incorrect dose or medication

Malabsorption of administered iron

Ongoing blood loss including gastrointestinal, menstrual, and pulmonary

Concurrent infection or inflammatory disorder inhibiting the response to iron

Concurrent vitamin B_{12} or folate deficiency

Diagnosis other than iron deficiency
- Thalassemias
- Hemoglobin C and E disorders
- Anemia of chronic disease
- Lead poisoning
- Sickle thalassemias, hemoglobin SC disease
- Rare microcytic anemias

From Kliegman RM et al: *Nelson textbook of pediatrics,* ed 19, Philadelphia, 2011, Saunders.

in patients with chronic heart failure and iron deficiency has been shown to improve symptoms, quality of life, and functional capacity.
- If the diagnosis of iron deficiency anemia is made, locating the suspected site of iron loss is mandatory.

SUGGESTED READINGS

Available at www.expertconsult.com

RELATED CONTENT

Algorithm for diagnosis of anemias (Algorithm in Section III)

Iron Deficiency Anemia (Patient Information)
Anemia (Patient Information)

AUTHORS: **BILAL H. NAQVI, M.D.,** and **BHARTI RATHORE, M.D.**

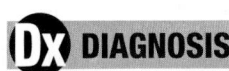 BASIC INFORMATION

DEFINITION

Pernicious anemia (PA) is an autoimmune disease resulting from antibodies against intrinsic factor and gastric parietal cells.

SYNONYMS

Megaloblastic anemia resulting from vitamin B_{12} deficiency

Addison-Biermer anemia

ICD-10CM CODES

D51.0 Vitamin B12 deficiency anemia due to intrinsic factor deficiency
D51.8 Other vitamin B12 deficiency anemias
D51.9 Vitamin B12 deficiency anemia, unspecified
D51.1 Vitamin B12 deficiency anemia due to selective vitamin B12 malabsorption with proteinuria

EPIDEMIOLOGY & DEMOGRAPHICS

- Increased incidence in females and older adults (40-70 years)
- More frequent in patients of northern European ancestry
- The overall prevalence of undiagnosed PA after age 60 years is 1.9%
- Prevalence is highest in women (2.7%), particularly in black women (4.3%)
- Associated with other autoimmune diseases (e.g., type 1 diabetes mellitus, Graves disease, Addison disease), along with possible *Helicobacter pylori* association

PHYSICAL FINDINGS & CLINICAL PRESENTATION

- Mucosal pallor and/or glossitis
- Peripheral sensory neuropathy with paresthesias initially and absent reflexes in advanced disease
- Delirium or dementia
- Worsening weakness and possible subacute combined degeneration of spinal cord
- Loss of proprioception and an unsteady gait
- Gastrointestinal symptoms including anorexia, pyrosis, nausea, and vomiting
- Possible splenomegaly and mild hepatomegaly

ETIOLOGY

- Parietal cell antibodies are present in >70% of patients, while intrinsic factor antibodies are noted in >50% of patients
- Atrophic gastric mucosa with achlorhydria
- Inborn errors of cobalamin-cofactor synthesis are rare. Fig. E1 illustrates the components and mechanism of cobalamin absorption. An etio-pathophysiologic classification of cobalamin deficiency is described in Section II.

Dx DIAGNOSIS

DIFFERENTIAL DIAGNOSIS

- Nutritional vitamin B_{12} deficiency
- Malabsorption (e.g., celiac disease)
- Chronic alcoholism (multifactorial)
- Chronic gastritis related to *H. pylori* infection
- Folic acid deficiency
- Myelodysplasia

- Thyroid abnormalities
- Atrophic gastritis

WORKUP

- The clinical presentation of PA varies with the stage. Initially, patients may be asymptomatic. In advanced stages patients may have impaired memory, depression, gait disturbances, paresthesias, and generalized weakness.
- Investigation consists primarily of laboratory evaluation. Table 1 describes a step-wise approach to the diagnosis of cobalamin and folate deficiency.
- Endoscopy and biopsy for atrophic gastritis may be performed in selected cases.
- Diagnosis is crucial because failure to treat may result in irreversible neurologic deficits.

LABORATORY TESTS

- Complete blood count generally reveals macrocytic anemia, thrombocytopenia, and mild leukopenia with hypersegmented neutrophils (Fig. E2).
- Mean corpuscular volume (MCV) is significantly elevated in advanced stages.
- Reticulocyte count is low to normal.
- False low serum cobalamin levels can occur in patients who are pregnant or taking oral contraceptives, have multiple myeloma, have transcobalamin I (TCI) deficiency, have severe folic acid deficiency, or are taking large doses of ascorbic acid. False high normal levels in patients with cobalamin deficiency can occur in several conditions including hepatomas, severe liver disease, or monoblastic leukemias (Table 2).
- The absence of anemia or macrocytosis does not exclude the diagnosis of cobalamin deficiency. Anemia is absent in 20% of patients with cobalamin deficiency, and macrocytosis is absent in >30% of patients at the time of diagnosis. Macrocytosis can be masked by concurrent iron deficiency, anemia of chronic disease, or thalassemia trait.
- Laboratory tests used for detecting cobalamin deficiency in patients with normal vitamin B_{12} levels include serum and urinary methylmalonic acid (MMA) level (elevated), total homocysteine level (elevated), and intrinsic factor antibody (positive). Cobalamin is a cofactor for the enzymes L-methylmalonyl coenzyme A mutase and methionine synthase. Inadequate levels of cobalamin will thus result in increased MMA and homocysteine levels. Plasma MMA levels can also be used to differentiate cobalamin deficiency from folate deficiency because patients with folate deficiency have normal or mild elevations of MMA levels.
- An increased concentration of plasma MMA does not predict clinical manifestations of vitamin B_{12} deficiency and should not be used as the only marker for diagnosis of B_{12} deficiency.
- Additional laboratory abnormalities can include elevated lactate dehydrogenase, direct hyperbilirubinemia, and decreased haptoglobin.

TABLE 1 Stepwise Approach to the Diagnosis of Cobalamin and Folate Deficiency

Megaloblastic Anemia or Neurologic-Psychiatric Manifestations Consistent With Cobalamin Deficiency *Plus* Test Results on Serum Cobalamin and Serum Folate

Cobalamin* (pg/mL)	Folate† (ng/mL)	Provisional Diagnosis	Proceed With Metabolites?‡
>300	>4	Cobalamin or folate deficiency is unlikely	No
<200	>4	Consistent with cobalamin deficiency	No
200-300	>4	Rule out cobalamin deficiency	Yes
>300	<2	Consistent with folate deficiency	No
<200	<2	Consistent with (1) combined cobalamin plus folate deficiency or (2) isolated folate deficiency	Yes
>300	2-4	Consistent with (1) folate deficiency or (2) an anemia unrelated to vitamin deficiency	Yes

Test Results on Metabolites: Serum Methylmalonic Acid and Total Homocysteine

Methylmalonic Acid (Normal, 70-270 nM)	Total Homocysteine (Normal, 5-14 μM)	Diagnosis
Increased	Increased	Cobalamin deficiency confirmed; folate deficiency still possible (i.e., combined cobalamin plus folate deficiency possible)
Normal	Increased	Folate deficiency is likely
Normal	Normal	Cobalamin and folate deficiency is excluded

*Serum cobalamin levels: abnormally low, less than 200 pg/mL; clinically relevant low-normal range, 200 to 300 pg/mL.
†Serum folate levels: abnormally low, less than 2 ng/mL; clinically relevant low-normal range, 2 to 4 ng/mL.
‡Any frozen-over sample from serum folate/cobalamin determination can be subjected to metabolite tests.
From Hoffman R: *Hematology, basic principles and practice*, ed 6, Philadelphia, 2013, Saunders.

TABLE 2 Serum Cobalamin: False-Positive and False-Negative Test Results

Falsely Low Serum Cobalamin in the Absence of True Cobalamin Deficiency

Folate deficiency (one-third of patients)
Multiple myeloma
TCI deficiency
Megadose vitamin C therapy
Pregnancy
Oral contraceptives

Falsely Raised Cobalamin Levels in the Presence of a True Deficiency*

Cobalamin binders (TCI and II) increased (e.g., myeloproliferative states, hepatomas, and fibrolamellar hepatic tumors)
TCII-producing macrophages are activated (e.g., autoimmune diseases, monoblastic leukemias and lymphomas)
Release of cobalamin from hepatocytes (e.g., active liver disease)
High serum anti-IF antibody titer

IF, Intrinsic factor; *TC,* transcobalamin.
*Although a low serum cobalamin level is not synonymous with cobalamin deficiency, 5% of patients with true cobalamin deficiency have low-normal cobalamin levels, a potentially serious problem because the patient's underlying cobalamin deficiency will progress if uncorrected.
From Hoffman R: *Hematology, basic principles and practice,* ed 6, Philadelphia, 2013, Saunders, 2013.

- Bone marrow aspirate is not necessary to diagnose cobalamin deficiency. It may show giant C-shaped neutrophil bands and megaloblastic normoblasts (Fig. E3).
- Schilling test: No longer available in most laboratories. It was historically used to identify the locus of cobalamin malabsorption and the cause of cobalamin deficiency.

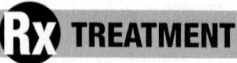 **TREATMENT**

NONPHARMACOLOGIC THERAPY

Avoid folic acid supplementation without proper vitamin B_{12} supplementation. Folic acid supplementation alone may result in hematologic remission in patients with vitamin B_{12} deficiency but will not treat or prevent neurologic manifestations.

ACUTE GENERAL Rx

Traditional therapy of cobalamin deficiency consists of intramuscular (IM) or deep subcutaneous (SC) injections of vitamin B_{12} 1000 mcg/day for 1 week, followed by 1000 mcg/month, indefinitely. Monitor response and increase dosing if serum B_{12} levels decline. Consider returning to IM vitamin B_{12} supplementation if decline recurs.

CHRONIC Rx

- Parenteral vitamin B_{12} 1000 mcg/month or intranasal cyanocobalamin 500 mcg/week for the remainder of life.
- In patients who have no nervous system involvement, intranasal cyanocobalamin may be used in place of parenteral cyanocobalamin after hematologic parameters have returned to normal range. The initial dose of intranasal cyanocobalamin (Nascobal) is 1 spray (500 mcg) in one nostril once per week. Nasal cyanocobalamin is expensive with costs generally exceeding $140/month.
- Oral cobalamin (1000-2000 mcg/day) has been reported as also being effective in mild cases of pernicious anemia because approximately 1% of an oral dose is absorbed by passive diffusion, a pathway that does not require intrinsic factor. Cost for 1 month of therapy is approximately $5.

DISPOSITION

Anemia generally resolves with appropriate cobalamin replacement therapy. Neurologic deficits, on the other hand, may be corrected only if treated early on.

REFERRAL

Gastroenterology referral for endoscopy on diagnosis of PA followed by periodic surveillance endoscopies to rule out gastric adenocarcinoma or carcinoid tumors.

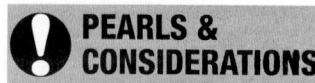 **PEARLS & CONSIDERATIONS**

COMMENTS

- Early manifestations of negative cobalamin balance are increased serum methylmalonic acid and total homocysteine levels. This occurs when the total cobalamin in serum is still in the low-normal range.
- Vitamin B_{12} deficiency that is allowed to progress for longer than 3 months may produce permanent degenerative lesions of the spinal cord (e.g., subacute combined degeneration of spinal cord).
- Vitamin B_{12} deficiency may suppress signs of polycythemia vera; treatment of B_{12} deficiency may unmask this disorder.
- Blunted or impeded therapeutic response to vitamin B_{12} may be due to concurrent iron or folic acid deficiency, uremia, infections, or use of drugs with bone marrow suppressant properties.
- Drugs that interfere with B_{12} absorption include metformin, colchicine, neomycin, and aminosalicylic acid.
- Patients must understand that cobalamin replacement therapy is lifelong.
- Self-injection of vitamin B_{12} may be taught in selected patients. Cost of monthly injections is less than $10.

SUGGESTED READINGS

Available at www.expertconsult.com

RELATED CONTENT

Pernicious Anemia (Patient Information)

AUTHORS: **SHIVA KUMAR R. MUKKAMALLA, M.D., M.P.H.,** and **BHARTI RATHORE, M.D.**

BASIC INFORMATION

DEFINITION

Angina pectoris is a term used to describe a clinical syndrome, typically characterized by chest, jaw, shoulder, back or arm discomfort that is caused by myocardial ischemia. This is most commonly related to atheromatous plaque in one or more than one large epicardial coronary artery; however, myocardial ischemia may occur in the absence of obstructive coronary artery disease (CAD), such as uncontrolled hypertension, valvular heart disease, hypertrophic cardiomyopathy, coronary spasm, or endothelial dysfunction. Any situation that causes an imbalance in myocardial oxygen supply and demand can cause an angina syndrome. Angina can be classified as follows:

1. Chronic stable ischemic heart disease (SIHD):
   ○ Predictable. Usually follows a precipitating event (e.g., climbing stairs, sexual intercourse, a heavy meal, emotional stress, cold weather).
   ○ Generally has the same severity as previous attacks; relieved by rest or by the customary dose of sublingual nitroglycerin.
   ○ Caused by a fixed coronary artery obstruction secondary to atherosclerosis. The presence of one or more obstructions in major coronary arteries is likely; the severity of stenosis is usually >70%.
2. Unstable (rest, recent onset, crescendo, acute coronary syndrome; will be reviewed under Acute Coronary Syndrome):
   ○ Rest angina: Angina occurring at rest and usually prolonged >20 min, occurring within 1 week of presentation
   ○ Recent onset. Angina of at least CCS Class III severity occurring less than 2 months after the onset of the symptoms.
   ○ Crescendo angina: Previously diagnosed angina that is distinctly more frequent, longer in duration, or lower in threshold (i.e., increased by >1 CCS class within 2 months of initial presentation to at least CCS Class III severity)
3. Prinzmetal's variant:
   ○ Occurs at rest.
   ○ Cyclical in nature.
   ○ Manifests electrocardiographically as episodic ST-segment elevations.
   ○ Caused by coronary artery spasms with or without superimposed CAD.
   ○ Patients also more likely to develop ventricular arrhythmias.
4. Microvascular angina (syndrome X):
   ○ Refers to patients with angina symptoms, positive exercise test, normal coronary angiograms and no coronary spasm. Defective endothelium-dependent dilation in the coronary microcirculation contributes to the altered regulation of myocardial perfusion and the ischemic manifestations in these patients.
   ○ Patients with chest pain and normal or nonobstructive coronary angiograms are predominantly women, and many have

a prognosis that is not as benign as commonly thought (2% risk of death or myocardial infarction [MI] at 30 days of follow-up).
5. Refractory angina:
   ○ Refers to patients whom, despite optimal medical therapy with at least maximal doses, or as tolerated of 2 antianginal medications, in addition to aspirin, aggressive risk factor modification, such as smoking cessation, adequate control of hypertension, diabetes, and hyperlipidemia, still have both angina and objective evidence of ischemia.
6. Other:
   ○ Angina due to aortic stenosis and idiopathic hypertrophic subaortic stenosis, cocaine-induced coronary vasoconstriction.

FUNCTIONAL CLASSIFICATION

Stable angina should be classified using a grading system. The most commonly adopted is that of the Canadian Cardiovascular Society:

- Class I: Ordinary physical activity, such as walking or climbing stairs, does not cause angina. Angina occurs with strenuous, rapid, or prolonged exertion at work or recreation.
- Class II: Slight limitation of ordinary activity. Angina occurs on walking or climbing stairs rapidly; walking uphill; walking or stair climbing after meals, in cold, in wind, or under emotional stress; or only during the few hours after awakening. Angina occurs on walking more than two level blocks and climbing more than one flight of ordinary stairs at a normal pace and in normal conditions.
- Class III: Marked limitations of ordinary physical activity. Angina occurs on walking one to two level blocks and climbing one flight of stairs in normal conditions and at a normal pace.
- Class IV: Inability to carry on any physical activity without discomfort; anginal symptoms may be present at rest.

ICD-10CM CODES

I20.8	Other forms of angina pectoris
I20.9	Angina pectoris, unspecified
I20.1	Angina pectoris with documented spasm
I25.110	Atherosclerotic heart disease of native coronary artery with unstable angina pectoris
I25.111	Atherosclerotic heart disease of native coronary artery with angina pectoris with documented spasm
I25.118	Atherosclerotic heart disease of native coronary artery with other forms of angina pectoris
I25.119	Atherosclerotic heart disease of native coronary artery with unspecified angina pectoris
I25.700	Atherosclerosis of coronary artery bypass graft(s), unspecified, with unstable angina pectoris
I25.790	Atherosclerosis of other coronary artery bypass graft(s) with unstable angina pectoris
I25.791	Atherosclerosis of other coronary artery bypass graft(s) with angina pectoris with documented spasm
I25.798	Atherosclerosis of other coronary artery bypass graft(s) with other forms of angina pectoris
I25.799	Atherosclerosis of other coronary artery bypass graft(s) with unspecified angina pectoris

EPIDEMIOLOGY & DEMOGRAPHICS

- It is estimated that 1 in 3 adults in the United States (about 81 million) has some form of cardiovascular disease. Based on the NHANES survey 2007-2010, an estimated 15.4 million have coronary heart disease of which 7.8 million have angina.
- Angina is most common in middle-aged and elderly men. Among persons 60 to 79 years of age, approximately 25% of men and 16% of women have coronary heart disease, and these figures rise to 37% and 23% among men and women >80 years of age, respectively
- The incidence of coronary heart disease and angina in women after menopause is similar to that of men.
- Although the survival rate has steadily improved over time, SIHD remains the number one cause of death in men and women (27% of deaths).
- The initial manifestation of ischemic heart disease is angina pectoris in 50%, and about 50% of patients presenting to the hospital with acute coronary syndrome have preceding angina.
- Two older population-based studies from Olmstead County, MN, and Framingham, MA, showed annual rate of myocardial infarction in patients with symptomatic angina of 3 to 3.5%/year.
- Within 12 months of initial diagnosis, 10% to 20% of patients with diagnosis of stable angina progress to MI or unstable angina.

PHYSICAL FINDINGS & CLINICAL PRESENTATION

- The assessment of chest pain should include quality, location, severity, and duration of pain; radiation; associated symptoms; provocative factors; and alleviating factors. Anginal pain can be described as "squeezing," "griplike," "suffocating," and "heavy," but it is rarely sharp or stabbing and typically does not vary with position or respiration. The classic Levine's sign is placing a clenched fist over the precordium to describe the pain. Many patients do not, however, describe angina as frank pain but as tightness, pressure, or discomfort. Other patients, in particular women and older adults, can present with atypical symptoms such as nausea, vomiting, midepigastric discomfort, sharp (atypical) chest pain, dizziness, or syncope.
- Ischemic pain of more than 20 minutes' duration should raise concern for possible MI.

- Women are more likely than men to report atypical chest pain or discomfort (65% reported on Women's Ischemic Syndrome Evaluation [WISE] study).
- Elderly and diabetics may report symptoms other than chest pain, such as dyspnea, fatigue, or diaphoresis.

ETIOLOGY

RISK FACTORS:
- Advanced age.
- Male sex.
- Genetic predisposition, family history of premature coronary artery disease (CAD) in first-degree relatives (men younger than 55 years of age, and women younger than 65 years of age).
- Smoking (risk of first MI is increased by near threefold)
- Hypertension (risk is double if systolic blood pressure is >180 mm Hg).
- Hyperlipidemia (prevalence remained unchanged from 2002-2008).
- Impaired glucose tolerance or diabetes mellitus (prevalence decreased from 2002-2008).
- History of stroke or peripheral arterial disease.
- Chronic kidney disease (CKD).
- Metabolic syndrome.
- Physical inactivity.
- Obesity (body mass index >30% over ideal). A higher body mass index during childhood is also associated with an increased risk of coronary heart disease (CHD) in adulthood.
- Entities that cause increased oxygen demand include hyperthermia (particularly if accompanied by volume contraction), hyperthyroidism, and cocaine or methamphetamine abuse..
- Cocaine is used by >5 million Americans regularly and is responsible for >64,000 emergency department (ED) evaluations yearly to rule out myocardial ischemia. Cocaine causes sympathomimetic toxicity and not only increases myocardial oxygen demand but also induces coronary vasospasm and can cause infarction in young patients. Long-term cocaine use can cause premature development of SIHD.
- Increased myocardial oxygen demand and decreased subendocardial perfusion are caused by severe uncontrolled hypertension that increases LV wall tension. Hypertrophic cardiomyopathy and aortic stenosis can induce even more severe LV hypertrophy and resultant wall tension.
- Other causes of increased myocardial oxygen demand are ventricular or supraventricular tachycardias, but when paroxysmal, these are difficult to diagnose.
- Entities that limit myocardial oxygen supply such as anemia where the cardiac output rises when the hemoglobin drops to <9 g/dl and ST-T-wave changes (depression or inversion) can occur at levels <7 g/dl.
- Hypoxemia resulting from pulmonary disease (e.g., pneumonia, asthma, chronic obstructive pulmonary disease, pulmonary

hypertension, interstitial fibrosis, or obstructive sleep apnea) can also precipitate angina.
- Polycythemia, leukemia, thrombocytosis, and hypergammaglobulinemia.
- Oral contraceptive and HRT use.
- Coronary artery calcium is associated with an increased risk of MI.
- Long-term use of nonsteroidal antiinflammatory drugs (NSAIDs).
- Exposure to air pollution from traffic (dilute diesel exhaust) promotes myocardial ischemia and is associated with adverse cardiovascular events.
- Low serum folate levels required for conversion of homocysteine to methionine are associated with an increased risk of fatal CHD. Hyperhomocysteinemia has a toxic effect on vascular endothelium and interferes with proliferation of arterial wall smooth muscle cells. Elevated plasma homocysteine level is a strong and independent risk factor for CHD events, especially in patients with type 2 diabetes mellitus.
- Elevated levels of highly sensitive C-reactive protein (hs-CRP, cardio CRP), suggesting that diseases associated with systemic inflammation can lead to accelerated atherosclerosis.
- Depression.
- Vasculitis.
- Elevated levels of lipoprotein-associated phospholipase A_2.
- Elevated fibrinogen levels.
- Low level of red blood cell glutathione peroxidase-1 activity.
- Radiation therapy.

(Dx) DIAGNOSIS

DIFFERENTIAL DIAGNOSIS

Nonischemic Cardiovascular: Aortic dissection, pericarditis
Pulmonary: Pulmonary embolism, pneumothorax, pneumonia, pleuritis
Gastrointestinal: Esophageal, esophagitis, spasm, reflux, biliary colic, cholecystitis, choledocholithiasis, cholangitis, peptic ulcer, pancreatitis
Chest Wall: Costochondritis, fibrositis, rib fracture, sternoclavicular arthritis, herpes zoster (before the rash)
Psychiatric: Anxiety disorders, hyperventilation, panic disorder, primary anxiety, affective disorders (i.e., depression), somatoform disorders, thought disorders (i.e., fixed delusions)

WORKUP

- In patients with chest pain, the probability of CAD should be estimated on the basis of patient age, sex, cardiovascular risk factors, and pain characteristics.
- The most important diagnostic factor is the history. Chest pain or left arm pain or discomfort occurring with exertion and relieved by rest in a patient with cardiovascular risk factors is consistent with a high likelihood of CAD.
- In assessing the likelihood of underlying SIHD it is helpful to classify the chest pain

as typical angina, atypical angina, and/or noncardiac chest pain.
- Typical angina, (definite) will have the following three features: (1) substernal chest discomfort with a characteristic quality and duration, (2) provoked by exertion or emotional stress, and (3) relieved by rest and/or sublingual nitroglycerin (NTG).
- Atypical angina, (probable) will have two of the above listed three features.
- Noncardiac chest pain will have one of the above listed features.
- Physical examination may be completely normal in many patients; however, certain findings may be helpful in the assessment of the patient with suspected SIHD. Some findings may identify consequences of ischemia or possible causes of the anginal syndrome other than CAD. The presence of hypertension, arcus senilis, xanthelasma, carotid or peripheral bruits, and a prominent S4 are all physical signs that could raise concern for the presence of CAD. A murmur of mitral regurgitation may be a marker of an ischemic cardiomyopathy or transient ischemia. A murmur suggestive of hypertrophic cardiomyopathy or aortic stenosis may suggest a cause of angina other than CAD.

LABORATORY TESTS

- Initial laboratory tests in patients with chronic SIHD should include a hemoglobin, fasting glucose, and fasting lipid panel.
- Cardiovascular screening: Measurement of total cholesterol, low-density lipoprotein cholesterol (LDL-C), high-density lipoprotein cholesterol (HDL-C), and fasting serum triglycerides. Also, measurement of Non–HDL-C, the ratio of total cholesterol to HDL-C, and apolipoprotein fractions (e.g., apolipoprotein B100, apolipoprotein A1).
- Electrocardiogram should be obtained during pain and when the patient is free of any discomfort. A normal resting electrocardiogram is not unusual in patients with SIHD; in patients who present with chest pain, 1% to 6% who have an acute MI will have a normal or nondiagnostic electrocardiogram.
- Chest x-ray PA and lateral, to rule out heart failure, valvular disease, pericardial disease, aortic aneurysm/dissection.
- Cardio-CRP (hs-CRP): Its elevation is a relatively moderate predictor of CHD, and it adds prognostic information to that conveyed by the Framingham risk score.

EXERCISE TESTING AND IMAGING STUDIES

- The value of further testing is greatest in patients who have an intermediate risk of CAD (10%-90% pretest likelihood).
- Exercise testing is used for the purpose of diagnosis as well as prognosis. If the patient is physically capable to perform at least moderate physical exercise, exercise stress testing (Fig. 1) is useful because of the important prognostic information obtained from exercise performance and the hemodynamic response. Patients who have an

STRESS TEST ALGORITHM

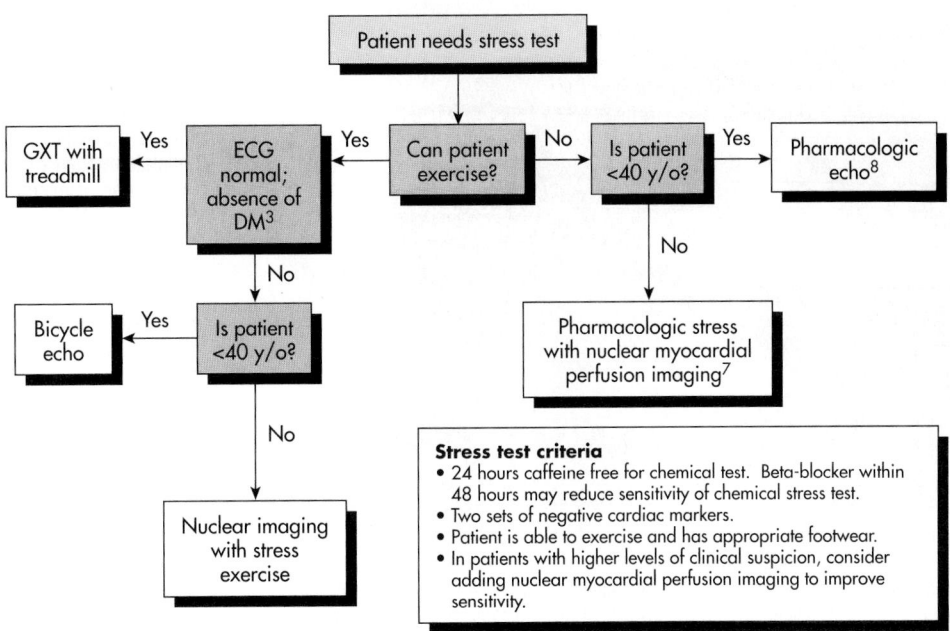

FIG. 1 **Stress test algorithm.** *ACS,* Acute coronary syndrome; *BBB,* bundle branch block; *DM,* diabetes mellitus; *ECG,* electrocardiogram; *echo,* echocardiography; *ED,* emergency department; *GTX,* graded exercise test; *LVH,* left ventricular hypertrophy; *NSTE,* non–ST-segment elevation; *NSTEMI,* NSTE myocardial infarction; *STE,* ST-segment elevation; *y/o,* years old. (From Adams JG et al: *Emergency medicine: clinical essentials,* ed 2, Philadelphia, 2013, Saunders.)

intermediate risk of CAD, as patients in a low-risk or high-risk category are more likely to have a false-positive or false-negative result, respectively. Risk assessment is also indicated in patients with SIHD who are being considered for revascularization of known coronary stenosis of unclear physiological significance.

- Stress echocardiography or stress testing with myocardial perfusion imaging may be employed when baseline electrocardiographic abnormalities are present that render the

electrocardiographic response to exercise uninterpretable, such as >1 mm ST segment depression, LBBB, preexcitation, paced ventricular rhythm, digoxin treatment with ST segment changes. Stress echocardiography has the advantage of higher specificity and a lower cost. Stress radionuclide perfusion imaging has a higher sensitivity, particularly for single-vessel coronary disease, and has a higher technical success rate. When the patient is unable to exercise adequately, pharmacologic testing (i.e., dobutamine,

adenosine, regadenoson) may be used with these imaging modalities

- A very good predictor of risk for a patient with stable angina is the Duke treadmill score, which incorporates the patient's functional status (METS or time in minutes during the Bruce protocol), ST-segment depression in millimeters, and an angina index (yes or no). Patients with favorable Duke scores (>5) have a 5-year survival rate of >97%; this is independent of other factors such as coronary anatomy and LV function.

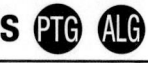
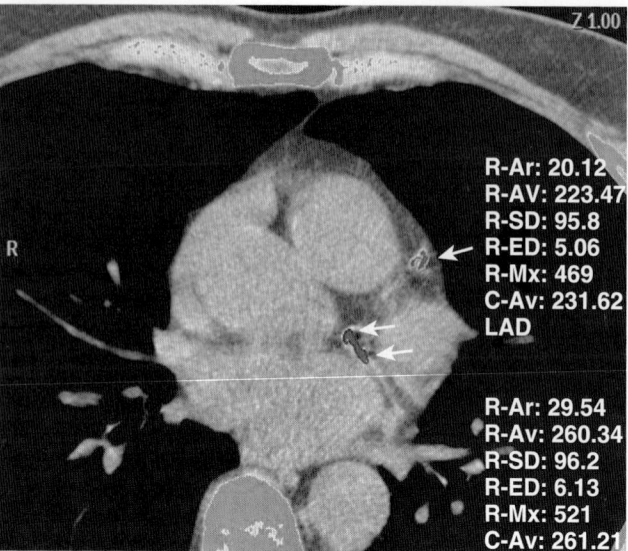

R-Ar: 20.12
R-AV: 223.47
R-SD: 95.8
R-ED: 5.06
R-Mx: 469
C-Av: 231.62
LAD

R-Ar: 29.54
R-Av: 260.34
R-SD: 96.2
R-ED: 6.13
R-Mx: 521
C-Av: 261.21

FIG. 2 Example of coronary artery calcium scoring in which calcified foci are identified within the left anterior descending (*orange; single arrow*) and left circumflex (*pink outlined in blue; double arrow*) coronary arteries. The region's area (R-Ar) and its average density in Hounsfield units (R-Av) are displayed and used in the area-density calcium scoring calculation. (From Bonow RO et al: *Heart disease,* ed 9, Philadelphia, 2012, Saunders.)

- Echocardiography is indicated in patients with murmurs suggestive of aortic stenosis, hypertrophic cardiomyopathy, mitral regurgitation, mitral valve prolapse, previous MI, pathological Q waves, complex ventricular arrhythmias, heart failure, hypertension, diabetes, and abnormal EKG.
- Cardiac computed tomography (CCTA; Fig. 2) is useful for the detection of subclinical CAD in asymptomatic patients with an intermediate Framingham 10-year risk estimate of 10% to 20%. Detects and quantifies coronary calcium and evaluates the lumen and wall of the coronary artery. CCTA can be useful as a first-line test for risk assessment in patients with SIHD who are unable to exercise to an adequate workload regardless of interpretability of ECG. Also can be used when a functional test has an indeterminate result and to assess bypass graft patency or patency of previous stents >3 mm diameter. CCTA CT cost and radiation exposure are limiting factors to recommending widespread routine use of this marker.
- Coronary artery calcium (CAC) score is a strong predictor of incidence of CAD and provides predictive information in patients with low to intermediate pretest probability of CAD beyond that provided by standard risk factors. A score below 100 indicates low risk, and a score above 400 high risk.
- Cardiac magnetic resonance imaging (CMRA), in addition to its use for diagnosis of arrhythmogenic right ventricular dysplasia, can also be used to assess myocardial perfusion and viability as well as function in patients unable to exercise. Additional studies are needed to determine the cost effectiveness of these studies in patients with ischemic cardiomyopathy.
- Invasive coronary angiography remains the gold standard for the identification of clinically significant CAD. Angiography is performed to define the location and extent of coronary disease; indicated in selected patients who are candidates for coronary revascularization (either coronary artery bypass graft [CABG] surgery or angioplasty).

Rx TREATMENT

FIVE FUNDAMENTAL OVERLAPPING STRATEGIES ARE RECOMMENDED

- Patient education: To support active participation of patients in the decision-making process of their treatment.
- Management of comorbid conditions that contribute or worsen SIHD.
- Aggressive modification of preventable risk factors such as smoking cessation, weight reduction in obese patients, regular aerobic exercise program (at least 30 to 60 min/day), correction of folate deficiency, reduced intake of saturated fats (to <7% of total calories), trans fatty acids (to <1% of total calories), cholesterol (to <200 mg/day), low-sodium diet (<2 g/day), and teaching importance of medication adherence. Whole grains as the main form of carbohydrates, an abundance of fruits and vegetables, and adequate omega-3 fatty acids are optimal for prevention of SIHD.
- Evidence-based pharmacologic management to improve quality of life and survival.
- Use appropriate revascularization procedures to improve survival and long-term outcomes in selected patients.

PHARMACOLOGIC THERAPY

Treatment can be classified based on medications that prevent MI and death.

- Aspirin reduces cardiovascular mortality and morbidity rates by 20% to 25% among patients with CAD. Its dose is 75 to 162 mg/day in the absence of contraindications. It inhibits the enzyme cyclooxygenase and synthesis of thromboxane A2 and reduces the risk of adverse cardiovascular events by 33% in patients with unstable angina. Patients intolerant to aspirin can be treated with other antiplatelet agents (see below).
- Clopidogrel irreversibly blocks the P2Y12 adenosine diphosphate receptor on the platelet surface, thereby interrupting platelet activation and aggregation. Clopidogrel can be combined with ASA in high-risk patients with SIHD or can be given alone in patients that are aspirin intolerant. Its dose is 75 mg/day.
- Ticagrelor, the newest CTPT inhibitor (P2Y12 antagonist), in the Pegasus-TIMI-54 reduced the risk of death, cardiovascular MI, or stroke in patients after 1 year of MI. However, it is associated with a slight increased risk of bleeding when compared to placebo.
- Dipyridamole is not recommended as an antiplatelet therapy for the treatment of patients with SIHD.
- Beta-adrenergic blockers, which prevent MI and death, are first-line therapy in the management of angina pectoris. They achieve their major antianginal effect by decreasing myocardial oxygen demand in reducing heart rate and systolic blood pressure product, AV nodal conduction, and myocardial contractility, in this manner contributing to a reduction in angina onset, with improvement in the ischemic threshold during exercise and during the usual daily activities. Absent contraindications, they should be regarded as initial therapy for stable angina for all patients. Their dose should generally be adjusted to reduce the resting heart rate to 55 to 60 beats/min. Despite the difference among the available beta blockers, they all seem to be equally efficacious in SIHD.
- Nitrates cause venodilation and relaxation of vascular smooth muscle; the decreased venous return from venodilation decreases diastolic ventricular wall tension (preload) and thereby reduces mechanical activity (and myocardial oxygen consumption) during systole. Relaxation of vascular smooth muscle increases coronary blood flow and reduces systemic pressure. Dilatation of the arterial wall will not be affected by plaque, but independent of an intact endothelium, leads to reduced resistance across the obstructed lumen. Nitroglycerin contributes to coronary blood flow redistribution by augmenting collateral flow and lowering ventricular diastolic pressure from areas of normal perfusion to ischemic zones. Nitroglycerin also has demonstrated antithrombotic and antiplatelet effects. Sublingual nitroglycerin or nitroglycerin spray should be prescribed to all patients with SIHD for immediate angina relief. Tolerance to nitrates can be minimized by avoiding sustained blood levels with a daily nitrate-free period (e.g., omission of bedtime dose of oral isosorbide dinitrate or 12 hr on/12 hr off transdermal nitroglycerin therapy). Nitrates are relatively

contraindicated in patients with hypertrophic obstructive cardiomyopathy, and should also be avoided in patients with severe aortic stenosis. Nitrates should not be used within 24 hr of sildenafil (Viagra) or vardenafil (Levitra) or within 48 hr of tadalafil (Cialis) because of the potential for hypotension.

- Calcium channel blockers are antiischemic medications that have no proven mortality benefit in SIHD. They improve myocardial oxygen supply by decreasing coronary vascular resistance and augmenting epicardial conduit vessel and systemic arterial blood flow. Myocardial demand is decreased by a reduction in myocardial contractility, systemic vascular resistance, and arterial pressure. They are first-line treatment when beta-blockers are contraindicated. They play a major role in preventing and terminating myocardial ischemia induced by coronary artery spasm. They are particularly effective in treating microvascular angina. All classes of calcium channel blockers reduce anginal episodes, increase exercise duration, and reduce use of sublingual nitroglycerin in patients with effort-induced angina. Short-acting calcium channel blockers should be avoided. Calcium channel blockers (particularly nondihydropyridine) should generally also be avoided in patients with CHF secondary to systolic dysfunction due to its negative inotropic effect.

- Ranolazine, which has been tested in four different studies with a total of 1737 patients (MARISA, CARISA, RANO80, and ERICA), inhibits the late inward sodium current, indirectly reducing the sodium-dependent calcium current during ischemic conditions and leading to improvement in ventricular diastolic tension and oxygen consumption. It seems to increase the efficiency of energy production in the heart, maintaining cardiac function. Its antianginal and antiischemic effects do not depend on reductions in heart rate or blood pressure. It is indicated for treatment of chronic angina that is inadequately controlled with other antianginals. It represents a new class of drugs known as metabolic modulators and can be useful when prescribed as substitute for beta-blockers or in combination with them for relief of symptoms when initial treatment with beta-blockers is not successful or is contraindicated. Side effects include prolongation of QT interval. Low doses of diltiazem and verapamil should be used with ranolazine. The extended-release preparation reduces the frequency of angina, improves exercise performance, and delays the development of exercise-induced angina and ST-segment depression.

- Angiotensin-converting enzyme (ACE) inhibition through changes in the physiologic balance between angiotensin II and bradykinin could contribute to the reductions in LV and vascular hypertrophy, atherosclerosis progression, plaque rupture, and thrombosis; the favorable changes in cardiac hemodynamics;

and the improved myocardial oxygen supply/demand. It has been shown to be effective in reducing cardiovascular death, MI, and stroke in patients who are at risk for or who had vascular disease. They are indicated in patients with hypertension, diabetes, LVEF <40%, and CKD. Angiotensin receptor blockers (ARBs) can be given to patients with SIHD who are intolerant to ACEI and qualify for them.

- Use of lipid-lowering drugs is recommended in patients with CAD and in patients with hyperlipidemia refractory to diet and exercise. Among patients who have recently had an acute coronary syndrome, an intensive lipid-lowering statin regimen to reduce LDL cholesterol to <70 mg/dl is a reasonable treatment objective. Statins also decrease the level of the inflammatory marker hs-CRP independently of the magnitude of change in lipid parameters.

- Influenza vaccine is recommended for patients with SIHD on annual basis to prevent all-cause mortality, morbidity, and hospitalization caused by the exacerbation of underlying medical conditions produced by influenza.

NEW MODALITIES FOR THE TREATMENT OF CHRONIC STABLE ANGINA PECTORIS

- Although a significant amount of progress has been made in the management of CAD with percutaneous coronary intervention (PCI) and CABG, many patients with the condition require additional therapeutic modalities for relief of symptoms and improvement in quality of life. This group of patients includes those with diffuse CAD who are not suitable for revascularization, patients with previous multiple PCIs or CABG limiting the chances for further revascularization, the lack of vascular conduits for CABG, severe left ventricular systolic dysfunction in patients with previous CABG or PCI, and comorbidities that would render the patients at high risk for revascularization.

- The following pharmacologic agents have been used for the management of stable angina in combination with the standard protocol of nitrates, beta-blockers, calcium channel blockers, and ranolazine: high-dose statin therapy, trimetazidine, perhexiline, nicorandil, allopurinol, ivabradine, fasudil, and testosterone.

- Other, nonpharmacologic modalities that are highly experimental include stem cell therapy, therapeutic angiogenesis, and mechanical therapies like external counterpulsation, spinal cord stimulation, transmyocardial laser revascularization, and coronary sinus reducing device.

- Allopurinol, a xanthine oxidase inhibitor, was shown to reduce myocardial oxygen demand per unit of cardiac output in patients with heart failure in a small crossover study of 65 patients given 600 mg of allopurinol daily for 6 weeks. Allopurinol increased the median time to ST depression from 232 seconds at

baseline to 393 seconds. Further and larger studies are necessary to recommend allopurinol as an adjunctive therapy for stable angina.

- Testosterone improves endothelial dysfunction and may be an effective antiangina agent. However, given the potential side effects, additional trials are necessary to recommend testosterone as an adjunctive drug for chronic angina.

The value of enhanced external counterpulsation, or EECP, was assessed with the MUST-EECP trial, which randomly assigned 139 outpatients with angina, documented CAD, and a positive stress test to 35 hours of active EECP. The results indicated the following regarding EECP: (1) was well tolerated; (2) exercise duration increased in both groups; (3) active EECP patients had a significant increase in time to 1-mm ST-segment depression, while there was no change in the inactive group; (4) more patients undergoing active EECP had a decrease in angina episodes, and fewer had an increase in angina symptoms compared with the active group. These data corroborate similar data from multicenter registries. The American Heart Association, American College of Cardiology, Society for Cardiovascular Angiography and Interventions, American Thoracic Society, and Society of Thoracic Surgeons focused update states that EECP may be considered for relief of refractory angina.

The following treatments have NOT been shown to be beneficial in reducing cardiovascular risk or improving clinical outcomes: estrogen therapy, vitamin C, vitamin E, and beta-carotene supplementation; treatment of elevated homocysteine with folate or vitamins B_6 and B_{12}; chelation therapy; garlic; coenzyme Q10; selenium; and chromium.

REFERRAL

Revascularization:

- Revascularization methods should be formulated taking into consideration improved survival or improved symptoms. Revascularization includes either percutaneous coronary intervention (balloon angioplasty and stenting) or CABG. However, note that although the role of PCI is unquestionable in the presence of an acute myocardial infarction, its role is not so clear in stable CAD. The utilization of PCI for stable CAD was reduced by 51.7% from 2007 to 2011, and hospitals with higher volumes of PCI had the largest reduction of these procedures.

- **To improve survival:**

  1. Perform CABG for patients with significant (>50% diameter stenosis) left main coronary artery stenosis, more than 70% diameter stenosis in proximal left anterior descending artery (LAD), or more than 70% diameter stenosis in three major epicardial vessels, >70% diameter stenosis in two major coronary arteries with severe or extensive myocardial ischemia, and in patients with mild to moderate LV systolic dysfunction (EF 35% to 50%) and significant multivessel CAD. Left internal mammary artery (LIMA) graft improves survival when used to bypass a proximal

LAD artery stenosis. CABG is recommended in preference to PCI to improve survival in patients with multivessel CAD and diabetes, particularly if a LIMA graft to LAD is used.
2. PCI is reasonable as an alternative to CABG in selected stable patients with unprotected left main CAD, low risk of PCI procedural complications, and a high likelihood of good long-term outcome *and* clinical characteristics that predict a significantly increased risk of adverse surgical outcomes (e.g., STS-predicted risk of operative mortality >5).
- **To improve symptoms:**
  1. CABG or PCI to improve symptoms is beneficial in patients with one or more significant (>70% diameter) coronary artery stenosis amenable to revascularization and unacceptable angina despite maximal medical treatment, or in whom increasing medical therapy cannot be implemented because of medication contraindications, adverse effects, or patient preferences.
  2. Hybrid coronary revascularization: LIMA-to-LAD artery grafting and of >1 non-LAD coronary artery can be used in patients who have an unfavorable aorta, have poor target vessels for CABG, have unsuitable graft conduits, or have unfavorable LAD for PCI.
- Compared with percutaneous coronary intervention (PCI), CABG is more effective in relieving angina and leads to fewer repeated revascularizations but has a higher risk for procedural stroke. Survival to 10 years is similar for both procedures.

Angioplasty and coronary stents (Fig. E3):

- PCI has an established place in treating angina but is not superior to intensive medical therapy to prevent MI and death in symptomatic or asymptomatic patients. Patients selected for PCI should also be candidates for CABG. Approximately 80% of patients show immediate benefit after PCI. The development of coronary stents has increased the number of patients who can be treated in the cardiac laboratory. Cardiac stents (Fig. E4) are currently used in nearly 95% of all patients with PCI lesions. The rate of restenosis is reduced by placing a stent electively in primary atheromatous lesions. The major limitations of stenting are subacute thrombosis, restenosis within the stent, bleeding complications when antiplatelets are used after stenting, and higher cost. The combination of aspirin and P2Y12 antagonists is effective in preventing coronary stent thrombosis and the duration of therapy depends on whether bare metal stents (BMS) or drug-eluting stents (DES) are used. Duration of dual antiplatelet therapy can be as short as 4 weeks for BMS, but 12 months of therapy is generally required for DES. This difference in duration is due to the lack of endothelium proliferation in DES initially. New drug-eluting stents with thin struts releasing Limus-family analogs from durable polymers have lowered the risk of stent thrombosis compared with early-generation stents releasing sirolimus or paclitaxel. Current evidence supports the use of drug-eluting stents in most clinical settings without safety concerns (unless there are contraindications to use of dual antiplatelet therapy). Recent data has shown that extending clopidogrel therapy beyond 6 months after stent placement does not reduce death or ischemic events, and it increases the risk of bleeding complications.

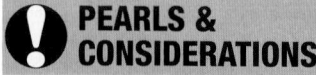

PEARLS & CONSIDERATIONS

COMMENTS

- Although nitrate responsiveness is usually an integral part of a diagnostic strategy for SIHD, recent reports question its value and conclude that in a general population admitted for chest pain, relief of pain after nitroglycerin treatment does not predict active CAD and should not be used to guide diagnosis in the acute care setting.
- CABG is associated with higher long-term survival rates and lower rates of repeat revascularization than PCI and stenting; however, patients often prefer stenting because it is less invasive, involves a shorter hospital stay, and has a lower in-hospital mortality rate.

SUGGESTED READINGS
Available at www.expertconsult.com

RELATED CONTENT
Angina (Patient Information)
Unstable Angina (Patient Information)
Acute Coronary Syndrome (Related Key Topic)
Coronary Artery Disease (Related Key Topic)
Myocardial Infarction (Related Key Topic)

AUTHORS: **JUAN A. ESCARFULLER, M.D.,** and **CLAUDIA SERRANO, M.D.**

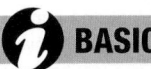 BASIC INFORMATION

DEFINITION

- The mucocutaneous swelling caused by the release of vasoactive mediators is called urticaria and angioedema.
- Urticaria causes edema of the superficial dermis.
- Angioedema involves the deep layers of the dermis and the subcutaneous tissue.

SYNONYMS

Angioneurotic edema
HAE (hereditary angioedema)

ICD-10CM CODES
T78.3 Angioedema
D84.1 Angioedema, hereditary

EPIDEMIOLOGY & DEMOGRAPHICS

INCIDENCE: 100 to 3000/100,000 persons (for urticaria and angioedema)
LIFETIME PREVALENCE: Approximately 20% of the population experiences urticaria and/ or angioedema at some time during life. The prevalence of hereditary angioedema is 1 case per 50,000 persons.
DEMOGRAPHICS:
Race: Slightly more common among African Americans.
Sex: More occurrences in women than men.
Angioedema commonly occurs after adolescence in the third decade of life.
Angioedema can occur together with urticaria (40%) or alone (20%); the remaining 40% have urticaria alone.

PHYSICAL FINDINGS & CLINICAL PRESENTATION

- Angioedema may be acute or chronic.
  1. Acute angioedema is defined as symptoms lasting 6 wk.
  2. Chronic angioedema is defined as symptoms lasting >6 wk.
- Urticaria is commonly known as "hives" and is:
  1. Pruritic
  2. Palpable and well demarcated
  3. Erythematous
  4. Millimeters to centimeters in size
  5. Multiple in number
  6. Fades within 12 to 24 hr
  7. Reappears at other sites
- Angioedema is characterized by the following:
  1. Nonpruritic
  2. Burning
  3. Not well demarcated
  4. Involves eyelids (Fig. 1), lips, tongue, and extremities
  5. Can involve the upper airway, causing respiratory distress
  6. Can involve the gastrointestinal tract, leading to cyclic abdominal pain, nausea, vomiting, and diarrhea
  7. Resolves slowly

ETIOLOGY

- Angioedema, with or without urticaria, is classified as acquired (allergic or idiopathic) or hereditary.
- Angioedema is primarily caused by mast cell activation and degranulation with release of vasoactive mediators (e.g., histamine, serotonin, bradykinins), resulting in postcapillary venule inflammation, vascular leakage, and edema in the deep layers of the dermis and subcutaneous tissue.
- Pathologically, angioedema has both immunologic- and nonimmunologic-mediated mechanisms.
  1. Immunoglobulin E–mediated angioedema may result from antigen exposure (e.g., foods [milk, eggs, peanuts, shellfish, tomatoes, chocolate, sulfites] or drugs [penicillin, aspirin, nonsteroidal antiinflammatory drugs, phenytoin, sulfonamides, recombinant tissue plasminogen activator]).
  2. Complement-mediated angioedema involving immune complex mechanisms can also lead to mast cell activation that manifests as serum sickness.
  3. Hereditary angioedema is an autosomal-dominant disease caused by a deficiency of or mutation in C1 esterase inhibitor (C1-INH). C1-INH is a protease inhibitor normally present in high concentrations in the plasma. C1-INH serves many functions, one of which is to inhibit plasma kallikrein, a protease that cleaves kininogen and releases bradykinin. Deficient C1-INH activity results in excess concentration of kininogen and the subsequent release of kinin mediators.
  4. Acquired angioedema is usually associated with other diseases, most commonly B-cell lymphoproliferative disorders, but may also result from the formation of autoantibodies directed against C1 inhibitor protein.
  5. Other causes of angioedema include infection (e.g., herpes simplex, hepatitis B, Coxsackie A and B, *Streptococcus, Candida, Ascaris,* and *Strongyloides*), insect bites and stings, stress, physical factors (e.g., cold, exercise, pressure, and vibration), connective tissue diseases (e.g., systemic lupus erythematosus, Henoch-Schönlein purpura), and idiopathic causes. Angiotensin-converting enzyme (ACE) inhibitors can increase kinin activity and lead to angioedema.

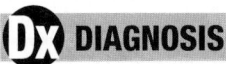 DIAGNOSIS

A detailed history and physical examination usually establish the diagnosis of angioedema. Extensive laboratory testing is of limited value.

DIFFERENTIAL DIAGNOSIS

- Cellulitis
- Arthropod bite
- Hypothyroidism
- Contact dermatitis
- Atopic dermatitis
- Mastocytosis
- Granulomatous cheilitis
- Bullous pemphigoid
- Urticaria pigmentosa
- Anaphylaxis
- Erythema multiforme
- Epiglottitis
- Peritonsillar abscess

WORKUP

- An extensive workup searching for the cause of angioedema is often unrevealing (90%).
- Workup, including diagnostic blood tests and allergy testing, is performed according to results of the history and physical examination. Fig. E2 illustrates a diagnostic algorithm for recurrent angioedema.

LABORATORY TESTS

- Complete blood count, erythrocyte sedimentation rate, and urinalysis are sometimes helpful as part of the initial evaluation.
- Stools for ova and parasites.
- Serology testing.
- C4 levels are usually reduced in acquired and hereditary angioedema (occurring without urticaria). If C4 levels are low, C1-INH levels and activity should be obtained. There are isolated reports of hereditary angioedema with normal C4 levels but reduced C1-INH levels.
- Skin and radioallergosorbent testing may be done if food allergies are suspected.
- Skin biopsy is usually done in patients with chronic angioedema refractory to corticosteroid treatment.

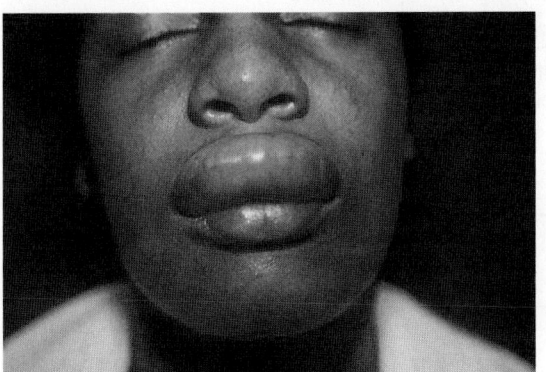

FIG. 1 Angioedema of the upper lip, with severe swelling of deeper tissues. (From Goldstein BG, Goldstein AO: *Practical dermatology,* ed 2, St Louis, 1997, Mosby.)

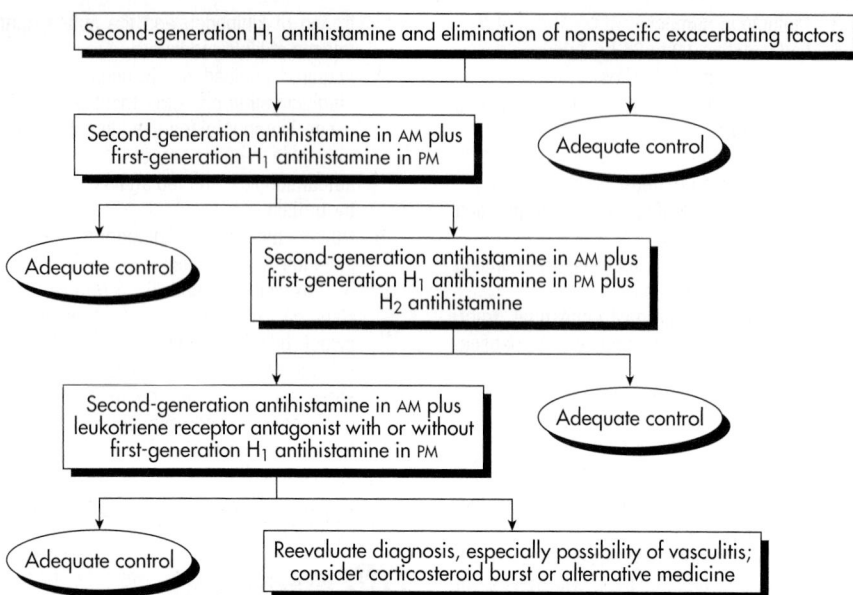

FIG. 3 Therapeutic algorithm for chronic urticaria/angioedema. (From Leung D, Sampson H, Geha R, Szefler S: Pediatric allergy: principles and practice, Chapter 55, 2010, Saunders, p 575-584.)

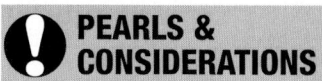 **TREATMENT**

NONPHARMACOLOGIC THERAPY
- Eliminate the offending agent
- Avoid triggering factors (e.g., cold, stress)
- Cold compresses to affected areas

ACUTE GENERAL Rx
- Acute life-threatening angioedema involving the larynx is treated with:
  1. Epinephrine 0.3 mg in a solution of 1:1000 given SC
  2. Diphenhydramine 25 to 50 mg IV or IM
  3. Cimetidine 300 mg IV or ranitidine 50 mg IV
  4. Methylprednisolone 125 mg IV
- Mainstay therapy in nonhereditary angioedema is H_1 antihistamines
  1. Diphenhydramine 25 to 50 mg q6h
  2. Chlorpheniramine 4 mg q6h
  3. Hydroxyzine 10 to 25 mg q6h
  4. Cetirizine 5 to 10 mg qd
  5. Loratadine 10 mg qd
  6. Fexofenadine 60 mg qd
- H_2 antihistamines can be added to H_1 antihistamines
  1. Ranitidine 150 mg bid
  2. Cimetidine 400 mg bid
  3. Famotidine 20 mg bid
- Tricyclic antidepressants
  1. Doxepin 25 to 50 mg qd

- Corticosteroids are rarely required for symptomatic relief of acute angioedema.
- Antihistamines are probably ineffective in acute hereditary angioedema.
- Purified plasma-derived C1-INH replacement therapy is effective and safe in treating acute attacks of hereditary angioedema caused by C1 inhibitor deficiency. Cost is a limiting factor. Acute attacks can be managed with plasma-derived or recombinant preparations of C1 inhibitor, with ecallantide, a specific plasma kallikrein inhibitor, or with the use of the B2 bradykinin-receptor antagonist icatibant.

CHRONIC Rx
- Chronic angioedema is treated as described under "Acute General Rx." Fig. 3 describes a therapeutic algorithm for chronic angioedema
- Corticosteroids are used more often in chronic nonhereditary angioedema.
- Prednisone 1 mg/kg/day for 5 days and then tapered over a period of weeks.
- Androgens (danazol, stanozolol, oxandrolone, methyltestosterone) and antifibrinolytic agents can be used for the treatment of chronic hereditary angioedema, which does not respond to antihistamines or corticosteroids but these agents are associated with many adverse effects. Long-term prophylaxis with plasma-derived C1 inhibitors (Cinryze,

Berinert) are safe and effective and may be used in patients who have frequent or severe attacks. Cost is a limiting factor. Icatibant is a new bradykinin-receptor antagonist effective in hereditary angioedema.
- Fig. E4 illustrates a hereditary angioedema treatment algorithm.
- Table E1 summarizes approved drugs used to treat hereditary angioedema attacks.

DISPOSITION
- Antihistamines achieve symptomatic relief in more than 80% of patients with nonhereditary acute angioedema.
- In chronic nonhereditary angioedema, corticosteroids are given in addition to antihistamines.
- A small percentage of people will have recurrence of symptoms after steroid treatment.
- Chronic angioedema can last for months and even years.

REFERRAL
Consultation with dermatologist and allergist is recommended in patients with chronic angioedema, hereditary angioedema, and recurring angioedema.

❗ PEARLS & CONSIDERATIONS

ACE inhibitors can cause angioedema up to many months after initiation. There are multiple case reports and case series of angiotensin receptor blocker (ARB)–induced angioedema, although the risk is substantially less than that of ACE inhibitors. (Incidence rates per 1000 person-years are 4.38 cases for ACE inhibitors, 1.66 cases for ARBs.) The incidence rate is also very high for the direct renin inhibitor aliskiren (4.67).

COMMENTS
- Identifying a cause for angioedema in patients is often difficult and met with frustration.
- Chronic angioedema, unlike acute angioedema, is rarely caused by an allergic reaction.

SUGGESTED READINGS
Available at www.expertconsult.com

RELATED CONTENT
Angioedema (Patient Information)

AUTHOR: **MEL L. ANDERSON, M.D.**

BASIC INFORMATION

DEFINITION

Angular cheilitis refers to inflammation of one, or both, of the corners of the mouth. Most commonly, it represents an infectious etiology, as an opportunistic fungal or bacterial pathogen, and leads to a spectrum of varying severities.

SYNONYM(S)

Angular cheilosis
Rhagades
Commissural cheilitis
Perleche
Angular stomatitis

ICD 10-CM CODE(S)
K13.0   Diseases of lips
B37.83 Candidal cheilitis

EPIDEMIOLOGY & DEMOGRAPHICS

INCIDENCE: Unknown
PEAK INCIDENCE: Advanced age
PREVALENCE: Suspected of causing 0.5% to 5% of lip infections in adults
PREDOMINANT SEX AND AGE: This form of lip inflammation has a predilection for the elderly, seen with denture use as an example.
GENETICS: No identified correlation
RISK FACTORS: These include dry mouth, nutritional deficiencies (B vitamins, iron), immunosuppression, or chronic irritation as with lip licking, drooling, oral hardware, or dentures.

PHYSICAL FINDINGS & CLINICAL PRESENTATION

- The majority of cases of this lip condition involve both sides of the mouth, which initially involves erythema and swelling (Fig. 1). Over time, the erythema and subsequent linear fissures, or rhagades, may become cracked or ulcerated. Skin thickening is common during the progression of inflammation. It is important to note that this progression may involve strictly the mucosa of the lips or may propagate to the facial dermis, crossing the vermillion border.

ETIOLOGY

- Microorganisms commonly represent underlying infectious causes. These include *Candida* species, *Staphylococcal aureus,* beta-hemolytic *Streptococcus* species, or polymicrobial findings. Another common cause of this condition includes direct irritation of saliva on the corners of the mouth with overclosure of the lower jaw, as evident in edentulous individuals and those who wear dentures. Nearly any condition that leads to chronic irritation or moisture settling in the corners of the mouth, including lip licking, drooling, or habits of oral fixation, may lead to this state. Nutritional deficiencies, specifically of iron, B vitamins, and zinc, are also associated with angular cheilitis. Varying levels of immunosuppression, as seen in diabetes mellitus, HIV, and so on, predispose to subacute infection as well. Patients on medications leading to xerostomia or hypersalivation can develop bilateral involvement.

DIAGNOSIS

DIFFERENTIAL DIAGNOSIS

- Oral candidiasis or oral-associated angular cheilitis; *S. aureus* infection or impetigo; contact dermatitis; angular herpes simplex

WORK-UP

- Primarily clinical in nature, taking into consideration full details of the patient's medical history and medications

LABORATORY TEST(S)

- If applicable, bacterial and fungal cultures may be beneficial to detect probable infectious component with routine lab testing, including CBC, HIV, BMP, iron, folate, and vitamin B_{12}, to be performed as well.

IMAGING STUDIES

- None needed

TREATMENT

The hallmark of treatment used in this condition revolves around proper identification and understanding of the etiology of the inflammation. With the highest prevalence of this condition seen in those with dentures, proper oral fit and dental hygiene are of the utmost importance.

Certainly, good oral hygiene also includes smoking and tobacco use cessation. Topical antifungal use is at the cornerstone of treatment (details follow). Proper identification may include the presence of *S. aureus, Streptococcus* species, and other pathogens, which will need focused treatment. Treatment-refractory cheilitis may require additional workup to identify possible systemic etiology.

NONPHARMACOLOGIC THERAPY

- Dental hygiene, specifically, with a focus on proper cleaning of dentures, plays a pivotal role in prevention. Alcohol or bleach-based solutions are commonly available OTC. If significant lag is noted in the corners of the mouth, surgery and collagen injections have been successful. Petrolatum jelly has been used for preventive measures as well.

ACUTE GENERAL Rx

- With the underlying pathology involving inflammation, topical corticosteroid creams are commonly used. If *S. aureus* has been implicated, topical mupirocin or fusidic acid has a role. Clotrimazole or ketoconazole can be used for combating *Candida albicans*, implicated in >50% of cases.

CHRONIC Rx

- Pending laboratory workup and identification of a nutritional deficiency, iron, B vitamins, or folate supplementation will likely lead to reduction. Proper alignment of dentures, involving possible surgical repair and fitment, may be needed.

DISPOSITION

- Outpatient workup and assessment

REFERRAL

- Dermatology assessment may be needed in refractory cases of angular cheilitis.

PEARLS & CONSIDERATIONS

COMMENTS

Identification of etiology is of utmost importance for further workup.

PREVENTION

See previously.

SUGGESTED READINGS

Available on www.expertconsult.com

AUTHOR: **GREGORY M. HAIDEMENOS, M.D.**

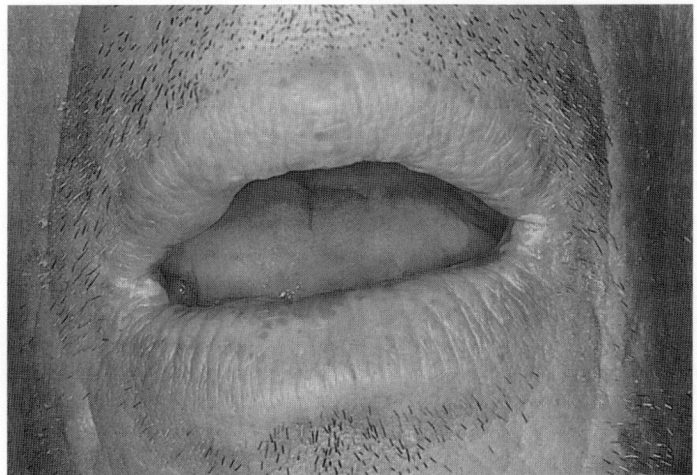

FIG. 1 Angular cheilitis. (From Swartz MH: *Textbook of physical diagnosis, history and examination,* ed 7, Philadelphia, 2014, Saunders.)

BASIC INFORMATION

DEFINITION

Ankylosing spondylitis is a type of inflammatory arthritis involving the sacroiliac joints and axial skeleton characterized by ankylosis and enthesitis (inflammation at tendon insertions). It is one of a family of overlapping syndromes called seronegative spondyloarthropathies (SpA) that includes reactive arthritis (formerly Reiter syndrome), psoriatic spondylitis, and enteropathic arthritis.

SYNONYMS

Marie-Strümpell disease

ICD-10CM CODES

M45.9   Ankylosing spondylitis of unspecified sites in spine
M08.1   Juvenile ankylosing spondylitis
M45.0   Ankylosing spondylitis of multiple sites in spine
M45.1   Ankylosing spondylitis of occipito-atlanto-axial region
M45.2   Ankylosing spondylitis of cervical region
M45.3   Ankylosing spondylitis of cervicothoracic region
M45.4   Ankylosing spondylitis of thoracic region
M45.5   Ankylosing spondylitis of thoracolumbar region
M45.6   Ankylosing spondylitis lumbar region
M45.7   Ankylosing spondylitis of lumbosacral region
M45.8   Ankylosing spondylitis sacral and sacrococcygeal region

EPIDEMIOLOGY & DEMOGRAPHICS

PREVALENCE: Between 0.1% and 1% of the population. Varies with prevalence of HLA-B27.
PREDOMINANT AGE AT ONSET: 15 to 35 years
PREDOMINANT SEX: Male/female ratio 2 to 3:1

PHYSICAL FINDINGS & CLINICAL PRESENTATION

- Prolonged morning back stiffness of insidious onset lasting more than 3 months
- Bilateral sacroiliac tenderness (sacroiliitis)
- Back pain often improves with exercise and is worse with rest
- Limited lumbar spine motion (Fig. 1)
- Tenderness at tendon insertion sites, especially the Achilles tendons and plantar fascia
- Loss of chest expansion reflecting rib cage involvement
- Peripheral joint arthritis, usually involving the large joints of the lower extremities, may be present
- In advanced cases the typical posture consists of compensatory hyperextension of neck, fixed flexion of hips, and compensatory flexion of knees (Fig. 2)
- There is an increased incidence of iritis and uveitis (30%-40% lifetime prevalence)
- Other extraskeletal manifestations include effects on the cardiovascular system (aortic insufficiency and cardiovascular disease) and lungs (pulmonary fibrosis). There is also an increased risk for osteoporosis.

ETIOLOGY

Genetic factors, particularly *HLA-B27*, play an important role in susceptibility to the spondyloarthropathies. Infectious triggers have been implicated in some cases. Tumor necrosis factor is important in the inflammatory response.

DIAGNOSIS

DIFFERENTIAL DIAGNOSIS

- Diffuse idiopathic skeletal hyperostosis (Forestier disease)
- Noninflammatory back pain (A clinical algorithm for the evaluation of back pain is described in Section III.)

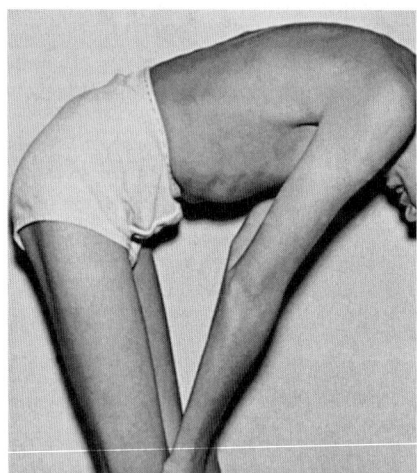

FIG. 1 Loss of lumbodorsal spine mobility in a boy with ankylosing spondylitis. The lower spine remains straight when the patient bends forward. (From Behrman RE: *Nelson textbook of pediatrics,* ed 17, Philadelphia, 2005, Saunders.)

- Table 1 compares ankylosing spondylitis and related disorders.

LABORATORY TESTS

- Elevated sedimentation rate, C-reactive protein
- Mild hyperchromic anemia
- Demonstration of inflammatory sacroiliitis by radiography or MRI is diagnostic for most patients, although some patients may meet criteria for "preradiographic spondyloarthropathy" based on compelling clinical evaluation.
- HLA/B27 antigen is not useful in the evaluation of noninflammatory back pain because it is present in up to 8% to 10% of the normal population.

IMAGING STUDIES

- Classic features are those of bilateral sacroiliitis on radiographs of the pelvis
- Vertebral bodies lose anterior concave shape and become square
- With progression, calcification of the annulus fibrosus and paravertebral ligaments develops, giving rise to the so-called *bamboo spine* and a "trolley track" appearance (Fig. 3).
- MRI (Fig. 4) may be useful in detecting early inflammatory lesions and is especially helpful when the history is suggestive but radiographs are equivocal.

TREATMENT

NONPHARMACOLOGIC THERAPY

- Exercises primarily to maintain flexibility and aerobic activity are important
- Postural training
  1. Patients must be instructed on spinal extension exercises to avoid fusion in a flexed position
  2. Sleeping should be in the supine position on a firm mattress; pillows should not be placed under the head or knees.

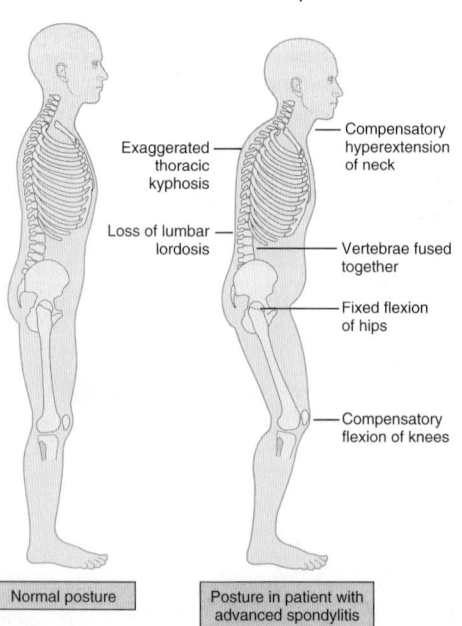

Normal posture

Posture in patient with advanced spondylitis

Exaggerated thoracic kyphosis

Loss of lumbar lordosis

Compensatory hyperextension of neck

Vertebrae fused together

Fixed flexion of hips

Compensatory flexion of knees

FIG. 2 Ankylosing spondylitis. Typical posture in advanced cases compared with normal posture. (From Ballinger A: *Kumar & Clark's essentials of clinical medicine,* ed 6, Edinburgh, 2012, Saunders.)

TABLE 1 Comparison of Ankylosing Spondylitis and Related Disorders

Feature	Ankylosing Spondylitis	Psoriatic Arthritis	Reactive Arthritis	Enteropathic Arthropathy
Gender (M:F)	2-3:1	1:1	8:1 (GU) [1:1 (GI)]	1:1
Age at onset	<40	35-55	20-40	Young adult
Sacroiliitis or spondylitis	100%	~20%	~40%	<20%
Symmetry of sacroiliitis	Symmetric	Asymmetric	Asymmetric	Symmetric
Peripheral arthritis	~25%	95%	90%	15%-20%
Distribution	Axial and lower limbs	Any joint	Lower limbs	Variable
HLA-B27	85%-95%	25%	30%-80%	7%
Uveitis	25%-40%	25%	25%	10%-36%

From Hochberg MC et al: *Rheumatology,* ed 5, St Louis, 2011, Mosby.

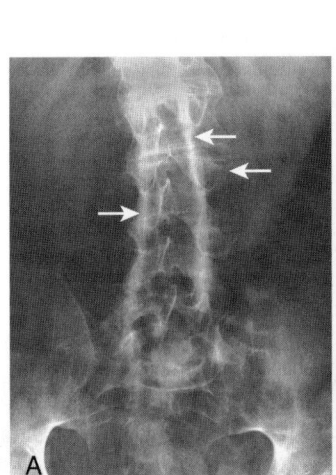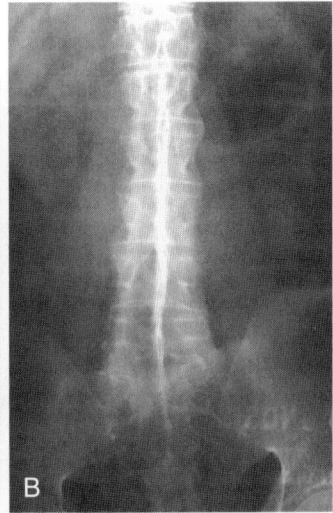

FIG. 3 Ankylosing spondylitis. A, Fusion of the facet joints and ossification of the adjacent soft tissue have produced a "trolley track" appearance *(arrows)*. The sacroiliac joints are fused, and syndesmophytes are present. **B,** In another patient, there is a prominent fusion of the interspinous ligaments producing a "saber sheath" appearance. (From Harris ED: *Kelley's textbook of rheumatology,* ed 7, Philadelphia, 2005, Saunders.)

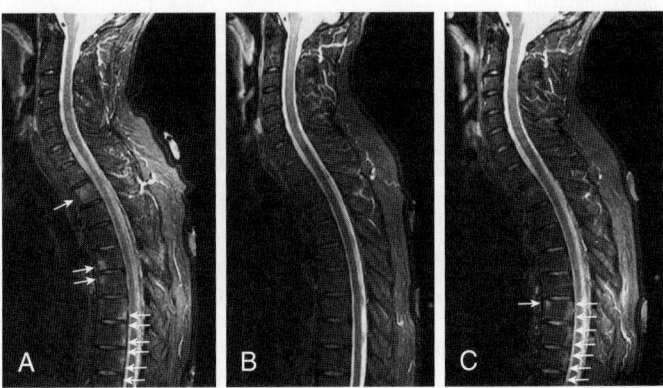

FIG. 4 Spine inflammation in ankylosing spondylitis (magnetic resonance imaging [MRI]). A 43-year-old man with HLA-B27–positive ankylosing spondylitis with deteriorating symptoms, including inflammatory back pain, had an MRI scan before starting biologic therapy. Baseline sagittal short tau inversion recovery (STIR) MRI **(A)** shows diffuse increased signal (edema) in the T2 vertebral body and multiple foci of corner inflammation anteriorly at T5 and T6, and posteriorly at T7, T8, T9, and T10 *(arrows)*. Other images confirmed extensive active inflammation in the spine. The patient responded very well, and after 6 months of therapy, a repeat STIR MRI **(B)** showed complete resolution of bone marrow inflammation. Subsequently, the patient experienced recurrence of symptoms, and a third MRI **(C)** was performed (2 months after anti-TNF therapy was stopped). This MRI shows no edema at T5-T6, a conspicuous new lesion anteriorly at T7, and recurrent inflammation posteriorly in the lower thoracic spine *(arrows)*. (From Firestein GS, et al: *Kelley's textbook of rheumatology,* ed 9, Philadelphia, 2013, Saunders.)

PHARMACOLOGIC THERAPY

- NSAIDs: Patients with ankylosing spondylitis should be prescribed full-dose continuous NSAID therapy. There is anecdotal evidence suggesting that indomethacin may be more effective than other NSAIDs, but other NSAIDs are efficacious and may be better tolerated. One study suggested that continuous NSAID therapy may retard the radiographic progression of ankylosing spondylitis, but conflicting data have been published.
- Sulfasalazine may be efficacious in some patients, especially for peripheral arthritis
- Tumor necrosis factor (TNF) antagonists such as etanercept, infliximab, and adalimumab have been shown to be very effective for relieving symptoms of spinal inflammatory arthritis in numerous controlled studies. Anti-TNF therapy should be recommended for patients whose symptoms are not completely controlled with NSAIDs, and it sometimes results in dramatic improvement in symptoms, range of motion of the spine, and quality of life for these patients. There is evidence suggesting that anti-TNF therapy slows the radiographic progression of the disease.
- Recent phase 3 trials with secukinumab, an anti-interleukin-17A monoclonal antibody, showed significant reductions in the signs and symptoms of ankylosing spondylitis.

DISPOSITION

Most patients have a normal life span but many suffer significant disability from loss of spinal mobility.

REFERRAL

All patients with seronegative spondyloarthropathy should be referred to a rheumatologist for consideration of anti-TNF therapy.

! PEARLS & CONSIDERATIONS

A family history of seronegative spondyloarthropathy increases the specificity of testing for HLA-B27. Surgical osteotomy may benefit selected patients with severe spinal deformity. Recent data suggest that men with AS have increased risk of vascular mortality.

SUGGESTED READINGS
Available at www.expertconsult.com

RELATED CONTENT
Fig. E260 Spondyloarthropathy, diagnosis (Algorithm)
Fig. 261 Spondyloarthropathy, treatment (Algorithm)
Ankylosing Spondylitis (Patient Information)

AUTHOR: **BERNARD ZIMMERMANN, M.D.**

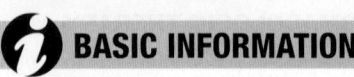

BASIC INFORMATION

DEFINITION

An anorectal fistula is an inflammatory tract with a secondary (external) opening in the perianal skin and a primary (internal) opening in the anal canal at the dentate line. Anorectal fistulae usually originate as a complication of a perianal abscess. Anorectal fistulae can be classified as follows (based on their relationship to the anal sphincter complex):

1. Intersphincteric: fistula track passes within the intersphincteric plane to the perianal skin (most common)
2. Transsphincteric: fistula track passes from the internal opening, through the internal and external sphincter, and into the ischiorectal fossa to the perianal skin (frequent)
3. Suprasphincteric: after passing through the internal sphincter, fistula tract passes above the puborectalis and then tracts downward, lateral to the external sphincter, into the ischiorectal space to the perianal skin (uncommon); if abscess cavity extends cephalad, a supralevator abscess possibly palpable on rectal examination
4. Extrasphincteric: fistula tract passes from the rectum, above the levators, through the levator muscles to the ischiorectal space and perianal skin (rare)
5. Submucosal: originate at the level of the dentate line in an infected crypt not involving the sphincter muscles

With a horseshoe fistula, the tract passes from one ischiorectal fossa to the other behind the rectum.

SYNONYM

Fistula-in-ano

ICD-10CM CODES
K60.3 Anal fistula
K60.5 Anorectal fistula

EPIDEMIOLOGY & DEMOGRAPHICS

- Common in all ages (average age is 39 years)
- Occurs twice as often in men as compared to women (12.1/100,000 vs. 5.5/100,000)
- Associated with inflammatory bowel disease and constipation
- Pediatric age group: more common in infants; boys more than girls

PHYSICAL FINDINGS & CLINICAL PRESENTATION

- Acute stage: perianal swelling, pain with defecation, and fever
- Chronic stage: history of rectal drainage or bleeding; previous abscess with drainage
- Tender external fistulous opening, within 2 to 3 cm of the anal verge, with purulent or serosanguineous drainage on compression; the greater the distance from the anal margin, the greater the probability of a complicated upward extension

- Goodsall's rule:
  1. Location of the internal opening related to the location of the external opening.
  2. With external opening anterior to an imaginary line drawn horizontally across the midpoint of the anus: fistulous tract runs radially into the anal canal.
  3. With opening posterior to the transanal line: tract is usually curvilinear, entering the anal canal in the posterior midline.
  4. Exception to this rule: an external anterior opening that is >3 cm from the anus. In this case the tract may curve posteriorly and end in the posterior midline.
- If perianal abscess recurs, presence of a fistula is suggested.

ETIOLOGY

- Most common: nonspecific cryptoglandular infection (skin or intestinal flora)
- Fistulas more common when intestinal microorganisms are cultured from the anorectal abscess
- Tuberculosis
- Lymphogranuloma venereum
- Actinomycosis
- Inflammatory bowel disease (IBD): Crohn's disease, ulcerative colitis
- Trauma: surgery (episiotomy, prostatectomy), foreign bodies, anal intercourse
- Malignancy: carcinoma, leukemia, lymphoma
- Treatment of malignancy: surgery, radiation

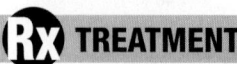

DIAGNOSIS

DIFFERENTIAL DIAGNOSIS

- Hidradenitis suppurativa
- Pilonidal sinus
- Bartholin's gland abscess or sinus
- Infected perianal sebaceous cysts

WORKUP

- Digital rectal examination:
  1. Assess sphincter tone and voluntary squeeze pressure
  2. Determine the presence of an extraluminal mass
  3. Identify an indurated fistula tract
  4. Palpate an internal opening or pit
- Gentle probing of external orifice to avoid creating a false tract; 50% do not have clinically detectable opening
- Anoscopy
- Proctosigmoidoscopy to exclude inflammatory or neoplastic disease
- All studies done under adequate anesthesia

LABORATORY TESTS

- Complete blood count
- Rectal biopsy if diagnosis of IBD or malignancy suspected; biopsy of external orifice is useless

IMAGING STUDIES

- Colonoscopy or barium enema if:
  1. Diagnosis of IBD or malignancy is suspected
  2. History of recurrent or multiple fistulas
  3. Patient <<25 yr

- Small bowel series: occasionally obtained for reasons similar to previously
- Fistulography: unreliable but may be helpful in complicated fistulas
- Endoanal ultrasound, MRI, or CT scan can be considered preoperatively

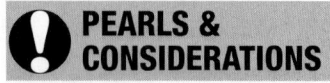

TREATMENT

NONPHARMACOLOGIC THERAPY

Sitz baths

PHARMACOLOGIC THERAPY (RARELY RECOMMENDED)

- Immunomodulators (Infliximab)

ACUTE GENERAL Rx

- Treatment of choice: surgery
- Broad-spectrum antibiotic given if:
  1. Cellulitis present
  2. Patient is immunocompromised
  3. Valvular heart disease present
  4. Prosthetic devices present
- Stool softener/laxative

CHRONIC Rx

- Surgery
- Surgical goals are as follows:
  1. Cure the fistula
  2. Prevent recurrence
  3. Preserve sphincter function
  4. Minimize healing time
- Methods for the management of anal fistulas: fistulotomy, fistulectomy, setons (maintains fistula patent for drainage while spontaneous healing occurs), fibrin glue (clot formation within the fistulous tract), fistula plugs (promote closure of fistula), LIFT procedure, rectal advancement flaps, and colostomy

DISPOSITION

Outpatient surgery

REFERRAL

Refer to a surgeon with expertise in this area.

PEARLS & CONSIDERATIONS

COMMENTS

- HIV-positive and diabetic patients with perirectal abscesses/fistulas are true surgical emergencies.
- Risk of septicemia, Fournier's gangrene, and other septic complications make immediate drainage imperative.

SUGGESTED READINGS

Available at www.expertconsult.com

RELATED CONTENT

Anal Fissure (Related Key Topic)
Hemorrhoids (Related Key Topic)

AUTHORS: **JORDAN KLEBANOFF, M.D.**, and **BABAK VAKILI, M.D.**

BASIC INFORMATION

DEFINITION

Anorexia nervosa is a psychiatric disorder characterized by abnormal eating behavior, severe self-induced weight loss, and a specific psychopathology (see "Workup").

ICD-10CM CODES
F50.00 Anorexia nervosa, unspecified
F50.01 Restricting type
F50.02 Binge-eating/purging type

EPIDEMIOLOGY & DEMOGRAPHICS

INCIDENCE/PREVALENCE (IN U.S.):
- Anorexia nervosa occurs in 0.2% to 1.3% of the general population, with an annual incidence of 5 to 10 cases per 100,000 persons.
- Participation in activities that promote thinness (athletics, modeling) is associated with a higher incidence of anorexia nervosa.

PREDOMINANT SEX: Female/male ratio is 9:1. Approximately 0.5% to 1% of women between the ages of 15 and 30 yr have anorexia nervosa.

PREDOMINANT AGE: Adolescence to young adulthood is the predominant age. Mean age of onset is 17 yr. Approximately 0.5% to 1% of college-aged women have anorexia nervosa.

PHYSICAL FINDINGS & CLINICAL PRESENTATION

Eating disorders can affect every organ system. Primary care physicians must be skilled at recognizing this disorder because patients with mild cases usually present with nonspecific symptoms such as asthenia, cold intolerance, lack of energy, or dizziness. Children and adolescents are at particular risk due to their active phase of growth and development. The physical examination may be normal in the early stages or in mild cases. Patients with moderate to severe anorexia have the following physical characteristics:
- Patient is emaciated and bundled in clothing.
- Skin is dry and has excessive growth of lanugo. Skin may also be yellow-tinged from carotenodermia.
- Brittle nails, thinning scalp hair are present.
- Bradycardia, hypotension, hypothermia, and bradypnea are common.
- Female fat distribution pattern is no longer evident.
- Axillary and pubic hair is preserved.
- Peripheral edema may be present.

ETIOLOGY

- Etiology is unknown, but probably multifactorial (sociocultural, psychological, familial, and genetic factors).
- A history of sexual abuse has been reported in as many as 50% of patients with anorexia nervosa.
- Psychological factors: anorexics often have an incompletely developed personal identity. They struggle to maintain a sense of control over their environment, they usually have a low self-esteem, and they lack the sense that they are valued and loved for themselves.

DIAGNOSIS

DIFFERENTIAL DIAGNOSIS

- Other eating disorders (bulimia nervosa, binge eating disorder [Table 1])
- Substance abuse
- Depression with loss of appetite
- Obsessive compulsive disorder
- Schizophrenia
- Conversion disorder
- Occult carcinoma, lymphoma
- Endocrine disorders: Addison disease, diabetes mellitus, hypothyroidism or hyperthyroidism, panhypopituitarism
- Gastrointestinal disorders: celiac disease, Crohn's disease, intestinal parasitosis
- Infectious disorders: AIDS, tuberculosis
- A clinical algorithm for the evaluation of anorexia is described in Section III

WORKUP

- A diagnosis can be made by using the following *DSM-5* diagnostic criteria for anorexia nervosa.
  - A. Restriction of energy intake relative to requirements, leading to a significantly low body weight in the context of age, sex, developmental trajectory, and physical health. Significantly low weight is defined as a weight that is less than minimally normal or, for children or adolescents, less than that minimally expected.
  - B. Intense fear of gaining weight or becoming fat, or persistent behavior that interferes with weight gain, even though at a significantly low weight.
  - C. Disturbance in the way in which one's body or shape is experienced, undue influence of body weight or shape on self-evaluation, or persistent lack of recognition of the seriousness of the current low body weight.

Specify type:

Restricting type: During the last 3 mo, the individual has not engaged in recurrent episodes of binge eating or purging behavior (i.e., self-

---

TABLE 1 Diagnostic Features of Eating Disorders

Anorexia nervosa	Body weight willfully maintained below normal level
	Abnormal perception of body morphology
	Intense fear of weight gain
	Amenorrhea
Bulimia nervosa	Large uncontrolled eating binges at least twice weekly
	Inappropriate compensatory behavior (e.g., vomiting, purging)
Binge eating disorder	Large uncontrolled eating binges at least twice weekly
	No regular inappropriate compensatory disorders
	Marked distress about binges

From Besser CM, Thorner MO: *Comprehensive clinical endocrinology*, ed 3, St Louis, 2002, Mosby.

---

induced vomiting or the misuse of laxatives, diuretics, or enemas). This subtype describes presentations in which weight loss is accomplished primarily through dieting, fasting, and/or excessive exercise.

Binge-eating/purging type: During the last 3 mo, the individual has engaged in recurrent episodes of binge eating or purging behavior (i.e., self-induced vomiting or the misuse of laxatives, diuretics, or enemas).

Severity level: see "Acute General Rx" section

The SCOFF questionnaire is a screening tool for eating disorders used in England. It consists of the following five questions:
1. Do you make yourself **s**ick because you feel full?
2. Have you lost **c**ontrol over how much you eat?
3. Have you lost more than **o**ne stone (approximately 6 kg) recently?
4. Do you believe yourself to be **f**at when others say you are thin?
5. Does **f**ood dominate your life?

A positive response to two or more questions has a reported sensitivity of 100% for anorexia and bulimia and an overall specificity of 87.5%.

In college-aged women a positive response to any of the following screening questions also warrants further evaluation:
1. How many diets have you been on in the past year?
2. Do you think you should be dieting?
3. Are you dissatisfied with your body size?
4. Does your weight affect the way you think about yourself?

Baseline ECG should be performed on all patients with anorexia nervosa. Routine monitoring of patients with prolonged QT interval is necessary; sudden death in these patients is often caused by ventricular arrhythmias related to QT interval prolongation.

A dual-energy x-ray absorptiometry (DEXA) scan to screen for osteopenia should be considered after 6 mo of amenorrhea in patients suspected of anorexia nervosa.

LABORATORY TESTS

- In mild cases, laboratory findings may be completely normal.
- Endocrine abnormalities:
  1. Decreased follicle-stimulating hormone, luteinizing hormone, T_4, T_3, estrogens, urinary 17-OH steroids, estrone, and estradiol
  2. Normal free T_4, thyroid-stimulating hormone
  3. Increased cortisol, growth hormone, rT_3, T_3RU
  4. Absence of cyclic surge of luteinizing hormone
- Leukopenia, thrombocytopenia, anemia, reduced erythrocyte sedimentation rate, reduced complement levels, and reduced CD4 and CD8 cells may be present.
- Metabolic alkalosis, hypocalcemia, hypokalemia, hypomagnesemia, hypercholesterolemia, and hypophosphatemia may be present.
- Increased plasma b-carotene levels are useful to distinguish these patients from others on starvation diets.

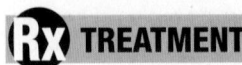 **TREATMENT**

NONPHARMACOLOGIC THERAPY

- A multidisciplinary approach with psychological, medical, and nutritional support is necessary.
- A goal weight should be set and the patient should be initially monitored at least once a week in the office setting. The target weight is 100% of ideal BW for teenagers and 90% to 100% for older patients.
- Weight gain should be gradual (1 to 3 lb/wk) to prevent gastric dilation. Begin with 800 to 1200 kcal in frequent small meals (to avoid bloating sensation), then increase calories to 1500 to 3000 depending on height and age.
- Add, as necessary, vitamin and mineral supplements.
- In severe cases, total parenteral nutrition must be used (starting at 800 to 1200 kcal/day).
- Electrolyte levels should be strictly monitored.
- Mealtime should be a time for social interaction, not confrontation.
- Postprandially, sedentary activities are recommended. The patient's access to a bathroom should be monitored to prevent purging.

ACUTE GENERAL Rx

- Criteria to decide on the appropriate initial course of treatment for patients with anorexia nervosa are usually based on the presence of complications, percentage of ideal BW, and severity of body image distortion. According to *DSM-5*,[1] the minimum level of severity is based, for adults, on current body mass index (BMI; see below) or, for children and adolescents, on BMI percentile. The level of severity may be increased to reflect clinical symptoms, the degree of functional disability, and need for supervision.
  - Mild: BMI ≥17 kg/m²
  - Moderate: BMI 16-16.99 kg/m²
  - Severe: BMI 15-15.99 kg/m²
  - Extreme: BMI <15 kg/m²
- Outpatient treatment is adequate for most patients.

[1]American Psychiatric Association: Desk Reference to the Diagnostic Criteria from DSM-5, Arlington, VA, 2013, American Psychiatric Association.

- Indications for hospitalization are described under "Referral" section and summarized in Table 2.
- Medically stable patients who are within 85% of ideal BW can be followed up by the primary care physician at 3- or 4-wk intervals, which can be lengthened as the patient improves.
- Pharmacologic treatment generally has no role in anorexia nervosa unless major depression or another psychiatric disorder is present. SSRIs can be used to alleviate the depressed mood and moderate obsessive-compulsive behavior in some individuals.

CHRONIC Rx

- Psychotherapy continued for years and focused specifically on self-image, family and peer interactions, and relapse prevention is an integral part of a successful recovery.
- Family therapy is also recommended, especially in younger patients.

TABLE 2 Indications for Inpatient Medical Hospitalization of Patients with Anorexia Nervosa

Physical and Laboratory

Heart rate <45 beats/min

Other cardiac rhythm disturbances

Blood pressure <80/50 mm Hg

Postural hypotension resulting in a >10 mm Hg drop or a >20 beats/min increase

Hypokalemia

Hypophosphatemia

Hypoglycemia

Dehydration

Body temperature <97° F

<80% healthy body weight

Hepatic, cardiac, or renal compromise

Psychiatric

Suicidal intent and plan

Very poor motivation to recover (in family and patient)

Preoccupation with ego-syntonic thoughts

Coexisting psychiatric disorders

Miscellaneous

Requires supervision after meals and while using the restroom

Failed day treatment

From Kliegman RM et al: *Nelson textbook of pediatrics*, ed 19, Philadelphia, 2011, Saunders.

DISPOSITION

- The long-term prognosis is generally poor and marked by recurrent exacerbations. The percentage of patients with anorexia nervosa who fully recover is modest. Most patients continue to have a distorted body image, disordered eating habits, and psychic difficulties.
- Most patients with anorexia nervosa will recover menses within 6 mo of reaching 90% of their ideal BW. It is important to note that patients with anorexia nervosa can become pregnant despite amenorrhea.
- Mortality rates vary from 5% to 20% and are six times that of peers without anorexia. Frequent causes of death are electrolyte abnormalities, starvation, or suicide.
- Factors that predict improved outcome in patients with eating disorders include early age at diagnosis, brief interval before initiation of treatment, good parent-child relationships, and having other healthy relationships with friends or therapists.
- A prolonged QT interval is a marker for risk of sudden death.

REFERRAL

Hospitalization should be considered in the following situations:
1. Severe dehydration or electrolyte imbalance
2. ECG abnormalities (prolonged QT interval, arrhythmias)
3. Significant physiologic instability (hypotension, orthostatic changes)
4. Intractable vomiting, purging, or bingeing
5. Suicidal thoughts
6. Weight loss exceeding 30% of ideal BW and unresponsiveness to outpatient treatment
7. Rapidly progressing weight loss (>2 lb in a week)
8. Failure to progress in nutritional rehabilitation in outpatient treatment

SUGGESTED READINGS
Available at www.expertconsult.com

RELATED CONTENT

Fig. 33 Evaluation of anorexia (Algorithm)
Anorexia Nervosa (Patient Information)
Binge-Eating Disorder (Related Key Topic)
Bulimia Nervosa (Related Key Topic)

AUTHOR: **FRED F. FERRI, M.D.**

BASIC INFORMATION

DEFINITION

Anoxic brain injury occurs when a decrease in either blood flow or oxygen causes cerebral ischemia. The inadequate delivery of nutrients and oxygen to cerebral tissue commonly reflects defects in either cardiac circulation or respiratory function, or defects in both.

SYNONYMS

Hypoxic-ischemic injury
Anoxic encephalopathy
Cerebral hypoxia
Hypoxia of brain
Perinatal or intrapartum asphyxia (pediatric)

ICD-10CM CODES
G93.1 Anoxic brain damage, not elsewhere classified

EPIDEMIOLOGY & DEMOGRAPHICS

INCIDENCE:
- Variable based on diagnostic criteria
- 424,000 out-of-hospital cardiac arrests per year in the U.S.

PREVALENCE:
- Sequelae of anoxic brain injury may include vegetative state, which varies in prevalence from 40 to 168 per 1 million population, depending on definition used.
- Recovery is rare after 3 months of vegetative state, with life expectancy of 2 to 5 years.

RISK FACTORS: Same as risk factors for cardiorespiratory arrest: age, race, HTN, hyperlipidemia, tobacco use, drug or alcohol abuse, and physical inactivity.

PHYSICAL FINDINGS & CLINICAL PRESENTATION

- Variable depending on degree of insult
- Patient typically initially in coma and then may either recover awareness and wakefulness with variable degrees of cognitive or physical impairment, may progress to a vegetative state or a minimally conscious state, or may die due to cardiopulmonary arrest or loss of whole brain function (brain death).
- Coma: eyes-closed state of both unconsciousness and unawareness with loss of sleep-wake cycles
- Minimally conscious state: altered state of awareness with normal sleep-wake cycles and intermittent interactivity with the environment; patient may intermittently follow simple commands and maintain visual tracking
- Vegetative state (also known as unresponsive wakefulness): altered state of awareness with normal sleep-wake cycles but with complete loss of both cognitive awareness and ability to interact with environment; persistent vegetative state is the term used for vegetative state after anoxic injury of between 1 and 3 months' duration, and permanent vegetative state is the term used for a vegetative state persisting beyond 3 months. A vegetative

state due to traumatic brain injury is permanent only after 12 months.
- Brain death: irreversible loss of both cortical and brainstem function manifesting as loss of awareness, cranial reflexes, and motor responses; brain death meets the legal criteria for death in U.S. jurisdictions. EEG is isoelectric; there is no intracerebral blood flow.

ETIOLOGY

- Ischemia (decreased cerebral perfusion): myocardial infarction, hemorrhage, shock, high intracranial pressure
- Hypoxia (decreased oxygenation): drowning, strangulation, aspiration, carbon monoxide poisoning
- Fig. 1 shows categories of mechanisms proposed to be involved in the evolution of secondary damage after severe traumatic brain injury in infants and children.

DIAGNOSIS

DIFFERENTIAL DIAGNOSIS

- Other causes of encephalopathy, including toxic, metabolic, infectious, or neoplastic causes; nonconvulsive status epilepticus; hypothermia
- Histotoxic hypoxia, the inability to utilize oxygen despite adequate delivery to cerebral tissue; i.e., cyanide poisoning

WORKUP

- Neurologic examination (coma examination) to ascertain level of encephalopathy
- Systemic evaluation for causes of cardiorespiratory failure
- Laboratory studies (listed in the following) to evaluate alternate causes of encephalopathy

- Imaging studies: MRI of brain or CT of head (if MRI cannot be obtained)

LABORATORY TESTS

Urine drug screen, serum metabolic profile, ammonia, complete blood count, coagulation panel, finger stick glucose, arterial blood gas, blood alcohol panel, serum neuron-specific enolase (if available)

IMAGING STUDIES

- Imaging is usually not revealing within first 24 hr of an anoxic event.
- Head CT without contrast (Fig. 2): repeat 24 hr after anoxic event to evaluate for stroke, trauma, hemorrhage, or cerebral edema.
- MRI of brain (Fig. 3): obtain if head CT scan unrevealing; may show cortical necrosis and infarcts of the basal ganglia

OTHER STUDIES

- EEG: to assess for non-convulsive status epilepticus
- Somatosensory evoked potentials (SSEP; aka, N20 response): obtain 24 to 72 hr after anoxic event

TREATMENT

NONPHARMACOLOGIC THERAPY

- Hypothermia: evidence suggests that inducing hypothermia 32° to 34° C for 24 hr following anoxic brain injury reduces metabolic need and may improve prognosis for recovery. However, recent meta-analysis suggests that the true risk-benefit of therapeutic hypothermia is unclear and a topic of debate.
- Complications from hypothermia include bradycardia, hemodynamic instability,

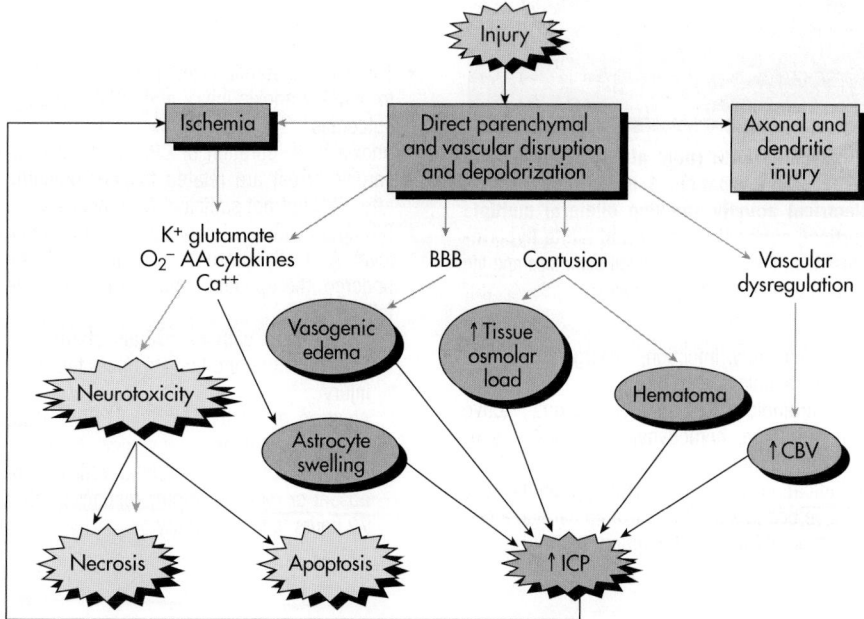

FIG. 1 Categories of mechanisms proposed to be involved in the evolution of secondary damage after severe traumatic brain injury in infants and children. Three major categories for these secondary mechanisms are (1) ischemia, excitotoxicity, energy failure, and cell death cascades; (2) cerebral swelling; and (3) axonal injury. (From Fuhrman BP: *Pediatric critical care*, ed 4, St. Louis, 2011, Mosby.)

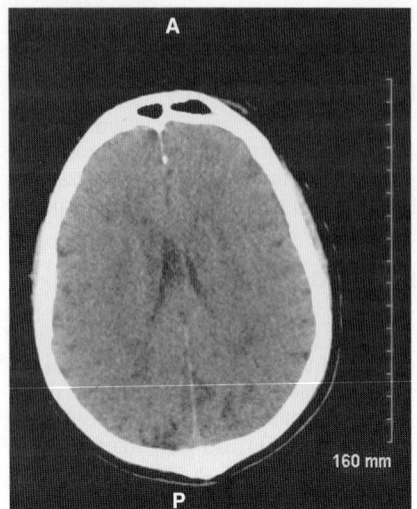

FIG. 2 CT without contrast of a patient 1 day after pulseless electrical activity showing diffuse sulci effacement and loss of gray-white matter differentiation indicating cerebral edema. Diffuse white and gray matter hypodensities are also present. The patient remained comatose and life support was eventually withdrawn.

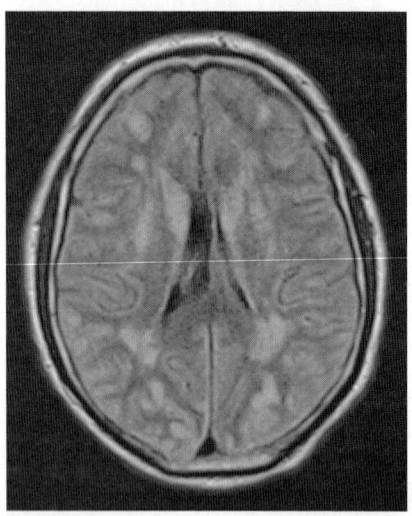

FIG. 3 MRI FLAIR (fluid attenuated inversion recovery) of a patient 1 day after pulseless electrical activity showing bilateral multiple cortical, subcortical, gray and white hyperintensities. The patient remained comatose and life support was eventually withdrawn.

coagulopathy, infection, hyperglycemia, and hypokalemia.
- Contraindications for hypothermia: active hemorrhage, hemodynamic instability, sepsis, or trauma
- Indication for hypothermia: patients who have been resuscitated from a cardiac arrest with VF/VT as the presenting rhythm

TABLE 1 Predictors of Good Prognosis

Time from Onset of Anoxic Event	Clinical Exam
Initial exam	Pupils react to light (reflex present), motor response flexor or extensor, and eye movements spontaneous roving conjugate or orienting
24 hr	Motor response withdrawal or better, and eye opening improved at least 2 grades
72 hr	Motor response withdrawal or better and normal spontaneous eye movements present
1 wk	Follows commands
2 wk	Normal oculocephalic response

Composed from data presented in Levy DE et al: Predicting outcome from hypoxic-ischemic coma, *JAMA* 253(10):1420-1426, 1985.

- Hyperbaric oxygen is used in carbon monoxide poisoning.

ACUTE GENERAL Rx
- Supportive care: ABCs, secure airway, cardiopulmonary support in the critical care unit
- Control seizures with antiepileptic medications (may need midazolam or propofol drip if severe uncontrolled seizures).
- Treat myoclonus with clonazepam 8 to 12 mg daily in divided doses; levetiracetam and divalproate may be used for myoclonic status epilepticus.

CHRONIC Rx
- Maintain adequate nutrition, infection precautions; provide DVT and gastric ulceration prophylaxis.
- Physical, occupational, and speech therapy as indicated per prognosis and patient ability
- May consider withdrawal of critical care and implementation of palliative care per prognosis, family consultation, and respect for autonomy and dignity of the patient

PROGNOSIS
- Out-of-hospital cardiopulmonary resuscitation (CPR) for cardiac arrest has a success rate of <10%.
- There is no standardized battery of testing to quantify anoxic injury and reliably predict outcomes.
- Anoxia time, duration of CPR, and cause of cardiac arrest are related to poor outcome after CPR but not sufficient for prognosis.
- Strong predictors of poor outcome (evidence level A or B) (assuming patient did not undergo therapeutic hypothermia) are the following:
  - ○ Presentation with myoclonus status epilepticus within the first 24 hours following injury
  - ○ Absence of bilateral cortical SSEPs (N20 response) anytime
  - ○ Absent papillary or corneal reflexes, or absent or extensor motor responses after 72 hours following injury
  - ○ Serum NSE levels >33 μg/L 24 to 72 hours following injury
- Neuroimaging and EEG are sensitive but not specific predictors of outcome.
- Burst-suppression pattern or flat-line EEG carries bad prognosis, while reactive EEG to noxious stimuli predicts favorable outcome. Refer to Table 1 for predictors of good prognosis.

DISPOSITION: Varies per extent of insult from long-term care facility to acute rehabilitation to return to home

REFERRAL: Referral to a neurologist is appropriate for definitive prognostication.

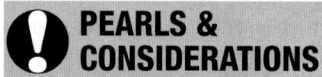 **PEARLS & CONSIDERATIONS**

COMMENTS
When assessing prognosis, use caution if patient is being treated with anesthetic agents or depressants including anticonvulsants. Thus serial neurologic exams are substantial and integral to best-practice care. When examining patients and determining prognosis, account for medications and illicit drugs that may depress consciousness and awareness as well as metabolic derangements that may affect the metabolism of pharmacologic agents or illicit drugs.

PREVENTION
CPR, risk factor modification, induced hypothermia

PATIENT/FAMILY EDUCATION
Consult with family members regularly and provide accurate assessment of prognosis.

SUGGESTED READINGS
Available at www.expertconsult.com

AUTHORS: **ANGAD JOLLY,** and **JOSEPH S. KASS, M.D., J.D.**

BASIC INFORMATION

DEFINITION

Antiphospholipid antibody syndrome (APS), the most common acquired thrombophilia, is characterized by clinical features of arterial or venous thrombosis and/or pregnancy morbidity *and* the presence of at least one type of antiphospholipid autoantibody (aPL). aPLs are antibodies directed against serum proteins bound to anionic phospholipids. Autoantibodies inhibit the fibrinolytic system and bind to antigenic anticoagulants, which activate endothelial cells, monocytes, and trophoblasts, resulting in complement-mediated thrombosis.

Three types of aPL have been characterized:
- Anticardiolipin antibodies—the most common
- Lupus anticoagulants
- Anti-β2-glycoprotein-1 antibodies

APS can be primary, or secondary to a rheumatic disease, the most common being systemic lupus erythematosus (SLE). APS can affect all organ systems and includes venous and arterial thrombosis, recurrent fetal losses, and thrombocytopenia.

ICD-10CM CODES
D68.61 Antiphospholipid syndrome

EPIDEMIOLOGY & DEMOGRAPHICS

PREVALENCE:
- Up to 5% of healthy individuals have positive aPLs
- Approximately 10% of patients with a deep venous thrombosis have aPLs
- Nearly 20% of women under 50 who have a cerebrovascular accident (CVA) test positive for aPLs
- 10% to 15% of women with recurrent miscarriages have aPLs
- Rule of 40s with systemic lupus erythematosus: 40% of patients with SLE have aPLs but only 40% of patients with antibodies will have thrombosis

---

TABLE 1 Other Features Suggesting the Presence of Antiphospholipid Antibodies

Clinical

Livedo reticularis

Thrombocytopenia (usually 50,000-100,000 platelets/mm^3)

Autoimmune hemolytic anemia

Cardiac valve disease (vegetations or thickening)

Multiple sclerosis–like syndrome, chorea, or other myelopathy

Laboratory

IgA anticardiolipin antibody

IgA anti–β2-glycoprotein I

From Firestein GS, et al: Kelly's *textbook of rheumatology*, ed 9, Philadelphia, 2013, Saunders.

- aPL without APS can be seen in patients with certain medications, infections, malignancies, and autoimmune conditions

PREDOMINANT AGE: Young to middle-aged adults

RISK FACTORS:
- Underlying SLE and collagen-vascular diseases; other autoimmune disorders, including rheumatoid arthritis, Sjögren's syndrome, Behçet's syndrome, primary immune thrombocytopenia (also known as idiopathic thrombocytopenic purpura); AIDS; hypertension (HTN).
- Most individuals are otherwise healthy and have no underlying medical condition.

PROGNOSIS:
- 91% survival at 10 years
- 73% success rate in pregnancy; prematurity and intrauterine growth restriction are common complications.

GENETICS: Some APS-positive families exist, and human leukocyte antigen (HLA) studies have suggested associations with HLA DR7, DR4, and Dqw7+Drw53.

PHYSICAL FINDINGS & CLINICAL PRESENTATION

No pathognomonic findings on examination; Table 1 summarizes other features suggesting the presence of antiphospholipid antibodies, abnormal findings consistent with ischemia or infarction.
- Thrombosis (Fig. 1):
  1. Patients with APS are at risk for both venous and arterial thromboses. Venous thromboses are more common, occurring as the initial manifestation of APS in approximately 30% of APS patients. Of

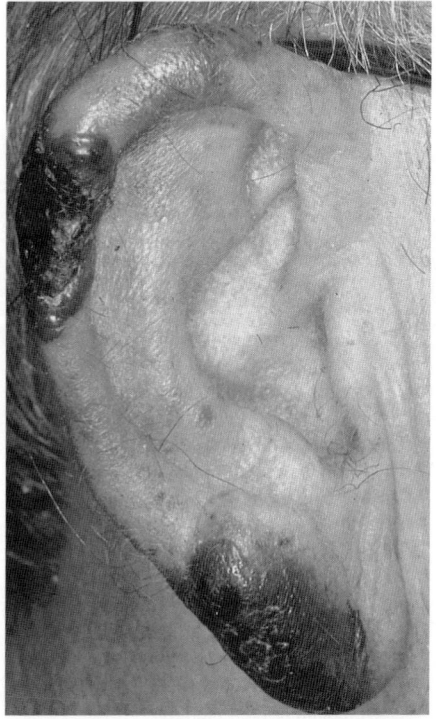

FIG. 1 Cutaneous thrombosis in antiphospholipid antibody syndrome. (From James WD et al: *Andrews' diseases of the skin*, ed 12, Philadelphia, 2016, Saunders.)

all patients with deep venous thrombosis, approximately 10% have aPL. The most common site for deep vein thrombosis is the calf, but thromboses may also occur in the renal, hepatic, axillary, subclavian, vena cava, and retinal veins. The most common site of arterial thrombosis is the cerebral vessels, followed by the coronary, renal, mesenteric, and bypass arteries. Recurrent thrombosis is common with APS.
- Commonly involved organ systems include:
  1. Central nervous system: stroke, transient ischemic attack, migraine, multi-infarct dementia, epilepsy, movement disorders, transverse myelopathy, depression, Guillain-Barré syndrome, and migraine.
  2. Pulmonary: pulmonary embolism and infarction; pulmonary hypertension; acute respiratory distress syndrome; intra-alveolar pulmonary hemorrhage (a postpartum syndrome characterized by fever, pleuritic chest pain, dyspnea, and patchy infiltrates with pleural effusion on chest radiograph).
  3. Cardiology: Libman-Sacks endocarditis, intracardiac thrombosis, coronary artery disease, myocardial infarction, valvulopathy, left ventricular diastolic dysfunction.
  4. Gastrointestinal: abdominal pain, gastrointestinal bleed secondary to ischemia, splenic or pancreatic infarction, hepatic vein thrombosis, Budd-Chiari syndrome (second-most common cause of Budd-Chiari syndrome).
  5. Renal: proteinuria, acute renal failure, hypertension, renal infarct, renal artery or vein thrombosis, post-partum hemolytic uremic syndrome.
  6. Hematology: thrombocytopenia, hemolytic anemia, thrombotic microangiopathic hemolytic anemias (HUS, TTP).
  7. Endocrine: Addison's disease secondary to adrenal hemorrhage and, less frequently, thrombosis.
  8. Cutaneous: livedo reticularis, cutaneous necrosis, skin ulcerations, phlegmasia cerulea dolens, gangrene of digits (Fig. 2).
  9. Obstetrics: recurrent spontaneous abortion, premature delivery or fetal growth retardation.
- **Catastrophic APS** (CAPS) (Table 2): CAPS is a rapidly progressive multi-organ thrombotic disease. Approximately 1% of APS is CAPS; approximately 45% of CAPS do not present as APS initially. A 50% mortality rate is seen in patients with CAPS. To make the diagnosis of catastrophic APS, four criteria must be satisfied:
  1. Evidence of involvement of three or more organs, systems, and/or tissues. The most common symptoms are abdominal pain, dyspnea, neurologic symptoms, chest pain, and skin rash.
  2. Development of manifestations simultaneously or in ≤1 week.
  3. Confirmation by histopathology of small-vessel occlusion in at least one organ or tissue.
  4. Laboratory confirmation of the presence of aPL.

ETIOLOGY

- aPLs react with negatively charged phospholipids.
- Possible mechanisms of thrombosis include effects of aPL on platelet membranes, endothelial cells, and clotting components such as prothrombin, protein C, or protein S. The mammalian target of rapamycin complex (mTORC) has been shown to be involved in the vascular lesions associated with the antiphospholipid syndrome, and mTOR inhibitors have shown to be beneficial in renal allograft recipients with APS nephropathy.
- Studies have recently shown that prephospholipids are not immunogenic and that a binding protein (β2-glycoprotein I) may be the key immunogen in the APS.
- APS patients exhibit dysfunctional HDL molecules that paradoxically inhibit both nitric oxide and anti-inflammatory pathways.

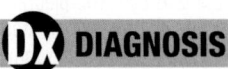 **DIAGNOSIS**

DIFFERENTIAL DIAGNOSIS

Other hypercoagulable states (inherited or acquired):
- Inherited: ATIII, protein C and protein, S deficiencies, factor V Leiden, prothrombin gene mutation.
- Acquired: heparin-induced thrombocytopenia, myeloproliferative syndromes, malignancy
- Nephrotic syndrome

WORKUP

Diagnostic criteria of APS include at least one clinical criterion and at least one laboratory criterion. A single clot may not be sufficient, especially with other thrombotic risk factors.
- Clinical:
  1. Venous, arterial, or small vessel thrombosis *or*
  2. Morbidity with pregnancy, defined as:
     1. Fetal death at ≥10 weeks' gestation *or*
     2. ≥1 premature births before 34 weeks' gestation secondary to eclampsia, preeclampsia, or severe placental insufficiency *or*
     3. ≥3 unexplained spontaneous abortions before 10 weeks' gestation.
- Laboratory (see Table 3):
- Screening tests
  1. Partial thromboplastin time (PTT): Elevated, indicating either the presence of a clotting factor deficiency, or the presence of an inhibitor such as a lupus anticoagulant.
  2. Mixing study: Elevated. Normal plasma is incubated with the patient's plasma. In cases of clotting factor deficiencies the PTT will correct. If an inhibitor is present as in the case with APS, the PTT will not correct.
  3. Dilute Russell viper venom time: Elevated. Laboratory clotting requires the addition of phospholipids and calcium to plasma samples. Antiphospholipid antibodies bind the phospholipids in the test tube, thereby preventing clot formation. The addition of Russell viper venom to plasma results in

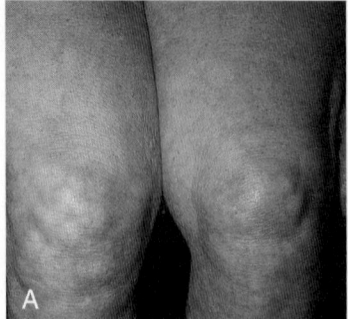 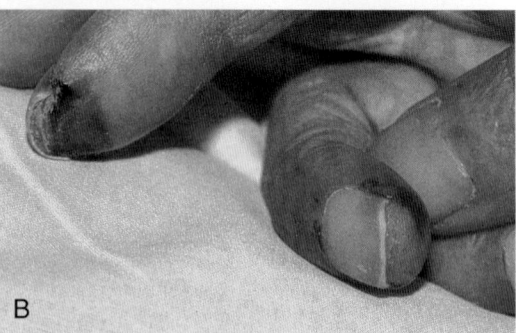

FIG. 2 Antiphospholipid syndrome. The clinical presentations of this disorder are protean and include those shown here. **A,** Broad bands of livedo around the knees in a patient with anticardiolipin antibodies. Physiologic livedo has a finer patterning and less obvious lesions. **B,** Digital infarcts, a nonspecific feature of several vascular occlusion disorders. (From White GM, Cox NH [eds]: *Diseases of the skin, a color atlas and text,* ed 2, St Louis, 2006, Mosby.)

TABLE 2 Differential Diagnosis of Catastrophic Antiphospholipid Syndrome (CAPS)

Laboratory Abnormalities	CAPS	TTP	DIC
Microangiopathic hemolytic anemia	−	+	+
Thrombocytopenia	+	+	+
Fibrinogen/FDP	Normal/Normal	Normal/Increased	Decreased/Increased
Anticardiolipin antibody	+	−	−
Lupus anticoagulant	+	−	−

TABLE 3 Assays Used to Confirm Diagnosis of Antiphospholipid Syndrome

Assay	Methodology
"Criteria" aPL Assays	
aCL	ELISA
Anti-β2-GPI	ELISA
LAC	Clotting/functional assays
"Noncriteria" aPL Assays	
Assays to detect antibodies to other phospholipids (i.e., phosphatidylserine, phosphatidylinositol, phosphatidic acid, phosphatidylglycerol, phosphatidylethanolamine, phosphatidylcholine)	ELISA
Annexin A5 resistance assay	Clotting/mechanistic assay
Assays to detect antibodies to prothrombin or prothrombin/phosphatidylserine	ELISA
Assays to detect antibodies to clotting proteins (i.e., protein C, protein S)	ELISA

aCL, Anticardiolipin; *aPL,* antiphospholipid antibody; *ELISA,* enzyme-linked immunosorbent assay; *LAC,* lupus anticoagulant.
From Hochberg MC et al: *Rheumatology,* ed 5, St Louis, 2011, Mosby.

immediate activation of Factor X (common pathway). It, therefore, will not be prolonged in intrinsic or extrinsic factor deficiencies but will be prolonged in the presence of an antiphospholipid antibody.
  4. The Lupus Anticoagulant screen is the addition of Russell viper venom to plasma. In the Lupus Anticoagulant confirmatory testing, massive doses of phospholipids are added to saturate the antiphospholipid antibody, thereby correcting the prolonged PTT.
- Initial testing for presence of aPL:
  1. Anticardiolipin (aCL) ELISA antibodies in medium or high titers *or*
  2. Lupus anticoagulant activity found *or*
  3. Anti-beta2-glycoprotein (anti-β2GPI) ELISA antibodies no more than 5 years from the clinical event.

- Confirmatory aPL testing: repeat testing after 12 weeks is required to confirm the persistence of a positive aCL, anti-β2GPI, or LA test because transient elevations of aCL can occur.

LABORATORY TESTS

Diagnostic evaluation of aCL and LA antibodies is indicated in:
- Patient with underlying SLE or collagen-vascular disease with thrombosis.
- Patient with recurrent, familial, or juvenile deep vein thrombosis (DVT) or thrombosis in an unusual location (mesenteric or cerebral).
- One or more unexplained thrombotic events. Do not test those at low risk, e.g., the elderly with clot and other risk factors.
- One or more specific pregnancy events.
- Unexplained thrombocytopenia.

A

- Patients with an elevated PTT.

Abnormal tests include:

- False-positive test for syphilis (RPR/VDRL)
- Lupus anticoagulant activity
- Presence of anticardiolipin antibodies (ELISA for anticardiolipin is the most sensitive and specific test [>80%]).
- Presence of anti-b$_2$-glycoprotein I antibody

Rx TREATMENT

ACUTE Rx

Treatment includes use of heparin, low-molecular-weight heparin (LMWH), warfarin, antiplatelet agents, acetylsalicylic acid (aspirin), clopidogrel, hydroxychloroquine. The efficacy of direct oral anticoagulants (DOACs), while promising, remains unproven.

- For a patient with positive aPL and venous or arterial thrombosis, treat as any other thrombosis.

  Anticoagulation with heparin or LMWH, then followed by indefinite warfarin treatment, with a target international normalized ratio (INR) of 2.0 to 3.0. There is conflicting evidence on the benefit of a higher INR target (>3.0) or the addition of other agents in patients with arterial clots, especially if they have recurrent events while taking warfarin. Any escalation of therapy should be weighed by the increased hemorrhage risk.
- Length of treatment needed is unknown, but likely indefinite barring no contraindication to anticoagulation, as the lifelong recurrence rate is 11% to 29%.
- Unfractionated heparin (UFH) is preferred if quick reversibility is needed.

PRIMARY PREVENTION

- Aspirin is of no benefit for prevention in patients with a prior clot.
- Aspirin may help patients without a history of clot.
- Patients with a previous history of venous thromboembolism and antiphospholipid antibodies are typically placed on an indefinite course of anticoagulation.
- Adding low-dose warfarin to aspirin for primary prevention seems to confer no benefit.
- Vascular risk factors, such as hypertension and hyperlipidemia, should be controlled.
- Hydroxychloroquine may be useful in those patients with SLE and aPL.
- Avoid oral contraceptive pills; modifiable risk factors for thrombosis such as smoking and immobility should also be addressed.
- For pregnant women with a positive test for aPL antibodies without a history of DVT or pregnancy loss, consider low-dose subcutaneous UFH or LMWH, aspirin 81 mg, or surveillance.

SECONDARY PREVENTION

- For pregnant women with previously diagnosed APS:
  1. Warfarin should be discontinued before pregnancy secondary to its teratogenic effects.
  2. Aspirin 81 mg and subcutaneous UFH or LMWH to therapeutic partial thromboplastin time (PTT) or factor Xa levels, respectively. This is superior to aspirin monotherapy. The evidence for UFH in APS and live birth is more robust than LMWH.
  3. Pregnant patients taking LMWH should be transitioned to unfractionated heparin before delivery due to reversibility.
  4. Intravenous immunoglobulin (IVIG), plasmapheresis, hydroxychloroquine, statins, clopidogrel, dipyridamole, and rituximab have been used when other treatments have failed.
  5. Some evidence shows a benefit for prednisolone in the first trimester; however, steroid-related adverse events are a concern.
  6. Hypertension, if present, should be controlled.
  7. For refractory obstetric APS, new studies suggest hydroxychloroquine to be promising therapy; however, randomized studies are lacking.
- For pregnant women with a positive test for aPL antibodies and a history of fewer than three spontaneous abortions:
  1. Low-dose aspirin at conception, followed by UFH, prophylactically or an intermediate dose at 7 weeks, continuing until 6 weeks' postpartum.
  2. A mid-interval PTT should be checked and should be normal or similar to baseline before therapy.
  3. LMWH can be used in place of unfractionated heparin and should be titrated to factor Xa levels in the recommended prophylactic range. The combination of aspirin (75 mg daily) plus LMWH has been associated with a higher live birth rate when compared with IVIG.

FOR CATASTROPHIC ANTIPHOSPHOLIPID ANTIBODY SYNDROME (CAPS)

- Represents fewer than 1% of all patients with APS; however, the mortality rate approaches 50%.
- Highest survival rates are achieved with the combination of anticoagulation, corticosteroids, and IVIG or plasma exchange.
- Case reports have shown both rituximab and the monoclonal antibody, eculizumab, which inhibits terminal complement activation, to be a successful therapy for patients with life-threatening thrombosis refractory to anticoagulation.

CHRONIC Rx

- Anticoagulation with warfarin therapy.
- Immunosuppressive agents such as corticosteroids and cyclophosphamide have not been shown to be effective.
- Limited data suggest that hydroxychloroquine may be effective in patients with APS and SLE.

DISPOSITION

- APS patients have a 20% to 70% risk for recurrent thrombosis.
- Initial arterial thrombosis tends to be followed by arterial events, and initial venous thrombosis tends to be followed by venous events.
- Catastrophic APS is associated with a high mortality rate, approaching 50%.
- Incidence of developing catastrophic APS is approximately 0.8% among APS patients.

REFERRAL

To hematology, rheumatology, and/or obstetric medicine when diagnosis is made.

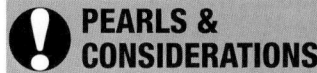 PEARLS & CONSIDERATIONS

COMMENTS

Cerebral features of SLE may be more related to thrombosis than inflammation and may respond better to anticoagulants than immunosuppression.

False-positive LAC tests have been reported in patients taking rivaroxaban and enoxaparin. For this reason thrombophilia testing should be delayed until two to four weeks after completion of anticoagulation.

PREVENTION

Prophylaxis for asymptomatic patients with positive aPL tests without previous thrombosis:

- No routine prophylaxis is recommended.
- Questionable whether low-dose aspirin is effective.
- Antithrombotic prophylaxis for major surgery, prolonged immobilization, and pregnancy.
- Avoid oral contraceptive pills in women with positive aPL test.

SUGGESTED READINGS
Available at www.expertconsult.com

RELATED CONTENT

Antiphospholipid Antibody Syndrome (Patient Information)
Deep Vein Thrombosis (Related Key Topic)
Hypercoagulable States (Related Key Topic)
Pulmonary Embolism (Related Key Topic)

AUTHORS: **WILLIAM M. RAFELSON, M.D., M.B.A.,** and **JOHN L. REAGAN, M.D.**

BASIC INFORMATION

DEFINITION

Generalized anxiety disorder (GAD) is most likely to present in combination with other psychiatric and medical conditions. Individuals with GAD commonly present with excessive and disproportionately high levels of anxiety, fear, or worry for most days over at least a 6-mo period in a number of areas. The worrying must be greater than would be expected given the situation, and it must cause significant interference in functioning. The subjective anxiety must be accompanied by at least three somatic symptoms in adults, and one in children (e.g., restlessness, irritability, sleep disturbance, muscle tension, difficulty concentrating, or fatigue). GAD cannot be diagnosed if it occurs only in the context of an active mood disorder, such as depression, or if the anxiety is better explained by another active anxiety disorder, such as PTSD or panic disorder.

SYNONYMS

Anxiety neurosis (former name for a subset of anxiety disorders)
Chronic anxiety
GAD

ICD-10CM CODES
F41.1 Generalized anxiety disorder

EPIDEMIOLOGY & DEMOGRAPHICS

INCIDENCE (IN U.S.): 6% to 9% per year in adult primary care clinics; 1-yr incident rate per 100 person-yr of 1.12
PEAK INCIDENCE: Peak incidence tends to occur later relative to other anxiety disorders, such as phobias; cumulative incidence of 4.3% by age 34 in a German community sample
PREVALENCE (IN U.S.):
- In general population: lifetime morbid risk of 9%; 12-month prevalence of 2.9%
- In primary care setting: 3% (the most common anxiety disorder in this setting)
PREDOMINANT SEX: Women are more frequently affected (2:1 ratio) but may present for treatment less often (3:2 female/male).
PREDOMINANT AGE:
- 30% report onset before age 11
- 50% have onset before age 18
- Median age of onset: 30 years
GENETICS: Concordance rates in dizygotic twins and monozygotic twins are not different (0% to 5%)

PHYSICAL FINDINGS & CLINICAL PRESENTATION

- Report of being "anxious" all of their lives.
- Excessive worry, usually regarding family, finances, work, or health.
- Sleep disturbance, particularly early insomnia.
- Muscle tension (typically in the muscles of neck and shoulders) or headache.
- Difficulty concentrating.
- Daytime fatigue.
- GI symptoms compatible with IBS (one third of patients).
- Physical symptoms are the usual reason for seeking medical attention.
- Comorbid psychiatric illness (e.g., dysthymia or major depression) and substance abuse (e.g., alcohol abuse) are frequent.

ETIOLOGY

- Hypotheses include models based on neurotransmitters (catecholamines, indolamines) and developmental psychology (e.g., behavioral inhibition, neuroticism, and harm avoidance).
- Prevalence increased with a family history, increase in stress, history of physical or emotional trauma, and medical illness.

DIAGNOSIS

DIFFERENTIAL DIAGNOSIS

- Wide range of psychiatric and medical conditions:
  1. Cardiovascular and pulmonary disease, such as cardiac arrhythmias or COPD
  2. Hyperthyroidism, hypoglycemia
  3. Substance abuse (e.g., cocaine, amphetamines, and PCP) or withdrawal (e.g., alcohol or benzodiazepines)
  4. Other anxiety disorders (e.g., social anxiety disorder), mood disorder

WORKUP

- Screening tests may enhance detection. A screening tool often used in primary care is the GAD-2. It asks, "During the past month, have you been bothered a lot by: (1) Nerves or feeling anxious or on edge? (2) Worrying about a lot of different things?" The response to each question is given a score of 0 (not at all), 1 (several days), 2 (more than half of the days), 3 (nearly every day). A score of ≥3 has a sensitivity of 86% and a specificity of 83% for detecting GAD. A simple 7-item in-office case finding instrument, the GAD-7, includes additional questions to assess symptom severity and can be used to monitor symptoms.
- Physical examination: additional laboratory and radiologic workup depend on presenting symptoms.
- Iatrogenic cause should be suspected if anxiety follows recent changes in medication.

TREATMENT

NONPHARMACOLOGIC THERAPY

- Cognitive-behavioral therapy
- Acceptance and commitment therapy
- Relaxation training
- Biofeedback
- Psychodynamic psychotherapy

PHARMACOLOGIC THERAPY

- SSRIs/SNRIs
- Azapirones (e.g., buspirone)
- Benzodiazepines (less favored)

ACUTE GENERAL Rx

- Acute treatment is rarely indicated because GAD is a chronic condition.
- If patients are in acute distress, the possibility of another cause, including another anxiety disorder such as panic disorder, should be considered.
- Caution in prescribing benzodiazepines because of the propensity for misuse and dependence. If used, the patient should be educated about the options and the risks.

CHRONIC Rx

- SSRIs and SNRIs (e.g., venlafaxine and duloxetine) are effective typical first-line treatment. Particularly useful if comorbid depression present.
- Buspirone can be effective with minimal potential for tolerance or abuse. May be less effective in patients with previous benzodiazepine exposure and may require a high-dose titration.
- Benzodiazepines can be effective under close supervision; however, they have fallen out of favor as a first-line treatment given their potential for functional impairment, abuse, and dependence.
- Sedating antidepressants, such as mirtazapine, may also be useful for initial insomnia secondary to anxious ruminations.

DISPOSITION

- GAD is chronic with periodic exacerbations.
- Treatment is given to reduce level of symptoms and improve functioning. Suicide risk is higher than in the general population.

REFERRAL

- For refractory symptoms.
- For comorbid psychiatric conditions.

SUGGESTED READINGS
Available at www.expertconsult.com

RELATED CONTENT
Anxiety (Patient Information)
Panic Disorder (Related Key Topic)
Social Anxiety Disorder (Related Key Topic)

AUTHOR: **KRISTY L. DALRYMPLE, PH.D.**

BASIC INFORMATION

DEFINITION

- Coarctation of the aorta is a narrowing of the aorta that occurs near the ligamentum arteriosum just distal to the origin of the left subclavian artery. It causes an outflow obstruction proximal to the site of the stenosis, which leads to left ventricular pressure overload, hypertrophy, and potentially heart failure. The stenosis can be discrete or long, and may have collateral vessels. It is commonly associated with other cardiac abnormalities such as a bicuspid aortic valve, patent ductus arteriosus, or ventricular septal defect.

SYNONYMS

Postductal coarctation of the aorta
Preductal coarctation of the aorta
Congenital hypoplasia of aortic arch
Coarctation of the aorta

ICD 10-CM CODES
Q25.1 Aortic coarctation

EPIDEMIOLOGY & DEMOGRAPHICS

INCIDENCE:
- Coarctation of the aorta occurs in 6%-8% of patients with congenital heart disease.

PREDOMINANT SEX AND AGE:
- Aortic coarctation affects predominantly males, with a male to female ratio of 1.7:1.

GENETICS:
- There have been case reports of coarctation occurring in families, which suggests heredity may play a role. Its association with a number of other conditions, such as Williams-Beuren and Sturge-Weber syndrome, also suggests a genetic predisposition. Most notably, up to 30% of patients with Turner syndrome also have coarctation of the aorta, and 5%-15% of girls with coarctation have Turner syndrome.

RISK FACTORS:
- Although most cases of aortic coarctation are congenital, it can be acquired through inflammatory conditions such as Takayasu arteritis.

PHYSICAL FINDINGS & CLINICAL PRESENTATION

- Clinical presentation
  - The clinical manifestations of coarctation of the aorta depend on the age of discovery, severity of the aortic narrowing, and adequacy of collateral circulation.
  - Neonates with severe coarctation may present with heart failure and/or shock when the ductus arteriosus closes. Neonates without severe aortic coarctation or with a persistent patent ductus arteriosus may be asymptomatic.
  - Beyond infancy, most patients are asymptomatic. Symptoms arise from severe hypertension, which may lead to headache, heart failure symptoms, or aortic dissection. Claudication of the lower extremities may also occur with physical exertion.

- Physical exam findings
  - "Brachial-femoral" delay characterized by diminished or delayed femoral pulses compared to the brachial pulses.
  - Upper extremity systolic hypertension.
  - Low or unobtainable blood pressure in the lower extremities.
  - Systolic ejection murmur at the left upper sternal border and left subscapular region.
  - A continuous murmur heard best posteriorly over the thoracic spine may be heard if there are large collaterals.
  - Systolic murmurs may be heard if there are coexisting cardiac defects (i.e., systolic ejection murmur with bicuspid aortic valve).

ETIOLOGY

- In aortic coarctation, the arterial wall of the aorta has several pathologic abnormalities. There is cystic medial necrosis, increased stiffness and less distensibility, and increased collagen and less smooth muscle mass in the prestenotic segment. The exact mechanism for these changes is unknown.
- The two main theories for potential mechanisms are reduced antegrade intrauterine flow leading to underdevelopment of the fetal aortic arch and abnormal extension of tissue from the ductus arteriosus into the wall of the fetal thoracic aorta. As stated previously, there may be genetic predispositions as well.

DIAGNOSIS

DIFFERENTIAL DIAGNOSIS

- Hypoplastic left heart syndrome
- Interrupted aortic arch
- Pseudocoarctation
- Left ventricular outflow tract obstruction, including subaortic and supravalvular aortic stenosis
- Critical aortic valve stenosis
- Obstructive peripheral arterial disease
- Aortic dissection

WORK-UP

- For patients with suspected aortic coarctation, the brachial and femoral pulses should be simultaneously palpated for intensity and timing to assess for the "brachial-femoral delay" of significant aortic coarctation.
- Bilateral arm and leg blood pressures should be measured to search for a differential pressure.
- An electrocardiogram may show left ventricular hypertrophy, ST-T wave abnormalities, and RV conduction delay.
- Transthoracic echocardiogram, including suprasternal notch acoustic windows, should be performed.
- Every patient with coarctation should have at least one cardiovascular MRI or CT scan for a complete evaluation of the thoracic aorta and intracranial vessels.

LABORATORY TESTS

- No specific laboratory tests are needed for coarctation of the aorta.

IMAGING STUDIES

- Box 1 summarizes important findings in the imaging evaluation of coarctation of the aorta. Anomalies associated with aortic coarctation are described in Box 2.
- Chest x-ray (Fig. E1)
  - Posterior rib notching of ribs 3-9 is due to bony erosion by large collateral arteries.
  - The "3" sign is formed by an enlarged aortic knob and subclavian artery forming the upper portion of the 3, the indentation of the aortic wall at the site of the coarctation forming the waist, and the lower portion is formed by the post-stenotic dilatation of the proximal descending aorta.
- Echocardiography
  - Aortic narrowing is visualized in the suprasternal notch view.
  - Color flow imaging and pulsed Doppler localizes the area of coarctation.
  - Continuous wave Doppler estimates the severity of coarctation.
  - Associated cardiac defects, chamber sizes and left ventricular function can be evaluated.
  - Generally, echocardiography is less useful for postoperative patients or for adult patients who may have less favorable acoustic windows compared with children.
- Magnetic resonance imaging/computed tomography
  - Per 2008 ACC/AHA adult congenital heart disease guidelines, every adult patient with coarctation should have at least one cardiovascular MRI (Figs. E2 and E3) or CT (Fig. E4) or a complete evaluation of the thoracic aorta.
  - The modalities have very high diagnostic accuracy (>95%) in detecting coarctation of the aorta and its associated abnormalities.
  - Both provide a large field of view and allow simultaneous visualization of the ascending aorta, aortic arch, descending aorta, aortic valve, and collaterals.
  - CT and MRI are indicated for serial follow up imaging after surgical repair to assess for aortic dilatation or aneurysm formation.
  - MRI is preferred to CT to decrease the lifetime exposure to radiation.
- Cardiac catheterization
  - Cardiac catheterization (Fig. E5) may be used to assess the peak gradient across the coarctation, but is usually performed in conjunction with a therapeutic intervention.

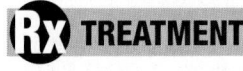 TREATMENT

NONPHARMACOLOGIC THERAPY

- Aortic coarctation can be repaired surgically or percutaneously by balloon angioplasty and/or stent placement. The choice of intervention is made on an individual basis based on aortic morphology and should be determined by a multidisciplinary team including cardiologists, interventionalists, and cardiac surgeons who are experienced in treating patients with congenital heart disease.

BOX 1 Imaging Evaluation of Coarctation of the Aorta

Patency of the Ductus Arteriosus
Closed
Patent
Flow from aorta to pulmonary artery (typically postductal coarctation)
Flow from pulmonary artery to aorta (preductal coarctation or pulmonary hypertension)

Collateral Pathways
Scarce (typical of patients under 2 years of age)
Abundant
Bridging the coarctated segment
Internal mammary to intercostal to distal aorta
Circumscapular pathways to distal aorta

Other Arch Anomalies and Stenoses
Arch interruption
Double aortic arch with stenosis in either or both arches
Coarctation proximal to left subclavian artery
Takayasu aortitis, rubella, Williams syndrome, neurofibromatosis, mucopolysaccharidosis, and other causes of stenoses not in the aortic isthmus

Subclavian Artery Anomalies
Atresia or stenosis of the left subclavian artery
Aberrant retroesophageal right subclavian artery
Proximal to the coarctation
Distal to the coarctation
Origin of both subclavian arteries distal to the coarctation

Associated Lesions
Cardiac, such as ventricular septal defect or bicuspid aortic valve
Aneurysms
In aorta adjacent to coarctation
In the ductus
In the intercostal arteries
In the circle of Willis

(Boxt LM, Abbara S: *Cardiac imaging: the requisites*, ed 4, Philadelphia, 2016, Elsevier.)

BOX 2 Anomalies Associated with Aortic Coarctation

Common
Bicuspid aortic valve with stenosis and regurgitation
Patent ductus arteriosus
Ventricular septal defects
Turner syndrome

Rare
Transposition of the great arteries
Double-outlet right ventricle
Shone's syndrome (parachute mitral valve, supramitral ring, aortic valve stenosis, and aortic coarctation)

(Boxt LM, Abbara S: *Cardiac imaging: the requisites*, ed 4, Philadelphia, 2016, Elsevier.)

- Repair should be performed in infancy or early childhood to prevent the common complications of unrepaired coarctation, including systemic hypertension, accelerated coronary artery disease, stroke, heart failure, and aortic dissection.
- The indications for intervention according to the 2008 ACC/AHA guidelines for the management of adults with congenital heart disease are:
  ○ Peak-to-peak coarctation gradient ≥20 mm Hg (Level of evidence C)
  ○ Peak-to-peak coarctation gradient <20 mm Hg in the presence of anatomic imaging evidence of significant coarctation with radiologic evidence of significant collateral flow (Level of evidence C)
- Surgery
  ○ Surgery compared with balloon angioplasty has been shown to be equally effective in reducing the peak systolic pressure gradient early after intervention.
  ○ Surgery is indicated in the presence of a long re-coarctation segment, aortic aneurysm or pseudoaneurysm, or aortic arch hypoplasia.
- Balloon angioplasty and/or stent placement
  ○ Balloon angioplasty is the preferred intervention for patients with recurrent, discrete stenosis.

  ○ Aortic stents placed in children will likely require a planned reintervention to dilate the stent as the child grows.
  ○ Potential complications of percutaneous intervention include immediate residual pressure gradients, re-coarctation, aneurysm formation, and femoral artery complications.

ACUTE GENERAL Rx

- Infants with critical coarctation are at risk for heart failure and death once the ductus arteriosus closes. Treatments include:
  ○ Intravenous infusion of prostaglandin E1 to keep the ductus arteriosus patent.
  ○ Dopamine and/or dobutamine to increase contractility for those with heart failure.
  ○ Surgical repair once the patient is stabilized.

CHRONIC Rx

- Systemic hypertension should be treated with ACE inhibitors, angiotensin-receptor blockers, or beta-blockers.
- All patients with aortic coarctation should have long-term follow up with a congenital heart disease specialist.
- After repair, a CT or MRI of the repair site should be obtained at one year postoperatively and then every 5 years or less depending on anatomy to detect long-term complications.

REFERRAL

- All patients with coarctation of the aorta, with or without repair, should be referred to a congenital heart specialist.
- Intervention should involve a multidisciplinary team of cardiologists, interventionalists, and surgeons at an adult congenital heart disease center.

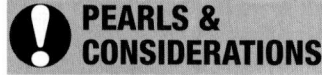 **PEARLS & CONSIDERATIONS**

COMMENTS

- Aortic coarctation is most commonly found distal to the origin of the left subclavian artery.
- The pathognomonic physical exam finding of aortic coarctation is the brachio-femoral delay.
- Systemic hypertension is the most common long-term complication of untreated aortic coarctation, but it is also associated with accelerated coronary artery disease, stroke, aortic dissection and heart failure.
- An adult congenital heart disease specialist should monitor all patients with aortic coarctation.

AUTHORS: **KATHERINE M. YU, M.D.**, and **PRANAV M. PATEL, M.D.**

ℹ BASIC INFORMATION

DEFINITION

Aortic dissection is part of a spectrum of aortic pathologies (acute aortic syndromes) that includes intramural hematomas and penetrating atherosclerotic ulcers. Aortic dissection occurs when blood passes through an intimal tear, separating the intima from the medial layers and creating a false lumen. Intramural hematoma (IMH) occurs when the vasa vasorum ruptures within the medial wall. IMH does not involve an intimal tearing unless a dissection develops. Seventeen percent of IMH will transform into aortic dissection. Penetrating atherosclerotic ulcers, which occur in the setting of extensive aortic atherosclerosis and hypertension, destroy the aortic intima and dissect into the aortic media. Rupture of atherosclerotic plaques with subsequent blood entry into the median wall forms a pseudoaneurysm. Fig. 1 illustrates acute aortic syndromes.

SYNONYMS

Dissecting aortic aneurysm
Acute aortic syndrome
AAS

ICD-10CM CODES
I71.00 Dissection of unspecified site of aorta
I71.01 Dissection of thoracic aorta
I71.02 Dissection of abdominal aorta
I71.03 Dissection of thoracoabdominal aorta

EPIDEMIOLOGY & DEMOGRAPHICS

INCIDENCE: 2.6-3.5 per 100,000 person-years
PREDOMINANT SEX AND AGE: Males (65%) females (35%), ages 60 to 80 yr; mean, 63 yr
RISK FACTORS:
- Hypertension (found in up to 77% of patients with aortic dissection)
- Atherosclerosis (found in up to 31% of patients with aortic dissection)

- Age (60 to 80 years)
- Family history of aortic aneurysms/dissection
- History of cardiac surgery, aortic valve replacement, intraaortic catheterization
- Disorders of collagen (Marfan's syndrome, Ehlers-Danlos syndrome)
- Vascular inflammation (giant cell arteritis, Takayasu arteritis, rheumatoid arthritis, syphilitic aortitis)
- Aortic coarctation, bicuspid aortic valve
- Turner's syndrome
- Cocaine abuse (usually within 12 hours of last use of cocaine)
- Trauma

CLASSIFICATION

Aortic dissection is generally classified according to anatomic location (Fig. 2):
- Stanford (more commonly used classification system): type A ascending aorta (proximal), type B descending aorta (distal) (Fig. 3)
- DeBakey: type I ascending and descending aorta, type II ascending aorta, type III descending aorta
- Aortic dissection can also be classified by acuity of presentation (acute or chronic), based on the time of onset.

PHYSICAL FINDINGS & CLINICAL PRESENTATION

- Sudden onset of severe sharp, tearing, or ripping chest pain. However, painless dissection occurs in approximately 6.4% of cases.
- Anterior chest pain (85% type A, 67% type B).
- Back pain, abdominal pain (43% type A, 70% type B).
- Syncope (19% type A, 3% type B), generally secondary to cardiac tamponade or stroke.
- Congestive heart failure (CHF).
- May present with hypertension (28% for type A, 66% in type B dissection), although 25% present with hypotension (systolic blood pressure <100 mm Hg), which can indicate bleeding, cardiac tamponade, or severe aortic regurgitation.

- Pulse and blood pressure differentials (>20 mm Hg between arms) in 19% to 31% of cases caused by partial compression of subclavian arteries.
- Aortic regurgitation in 18% to 50% of cases of proximal dissection, often with diastolic decrescendo murmur.
- Myocardial ischemia caused by coronary artery occlusion, most commonly involving the right coronary artery.
- Stroke in 5% to 10% of patients (secondary to dissection into or decreased blood flow to the carotids).
- Mesenteric ischemia occurs in 3% to 5% of cases, with external compression, flap prolapse, or involvement of arterial ostia.
- Horner syndrome (ptosis, miosis, anhidrosis).
- Vocal cord paralysis or hoarse voice (caused by compression of the left recurrent laryngeal nerve).

ETIOLOGY

Genetics, in addition to other risk factors listed previously, contribute to the development of aortic dissection.

Dx DIAGNOSIS

DIFFERENTIAL DIAGNOSIS

- Known as the great imitator: Pulmonary embolism, acute coronary syndrome, aortic stenosis/insufficiency, nondissecting aneurysm, pericarditis, cholecystitis, peptic ulcer disease, pancreatitis, musculoskeletal pain
- Consider aortic dissection in patients with unexplained stroke, chest pain, syncope, acute-onset CHF, abdominal pain, back pain, and malperfusion of extremities or internal organs.

LABORATORY TESTS

- ECG: helpful to rule out MI, although dissection can lead to coronary ischemia
- D-dimer has a 100% negative predictive value in dissection, but lacks specificity in the setting of acute aortic dissection.

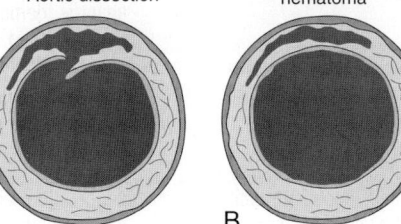
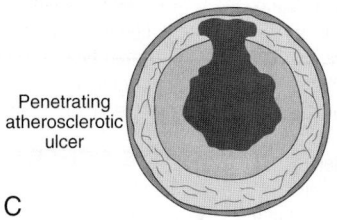

FIG. 1 Acute aortic syndromes A, Classic aortic dissection. **B,** Aortic intramural hematoma. **C,** Penetrating atherosclerotic aortic ulcer. (From Bonow RO, et al: *Heart disease*, ed 9, Philadelphia, 2012, Saunders.)

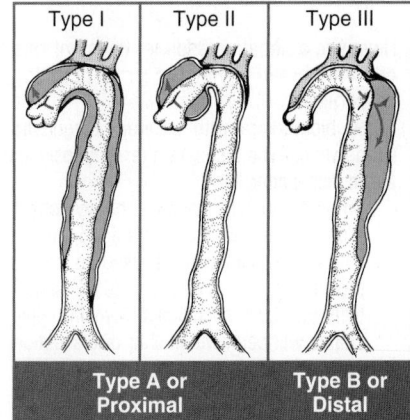

FIG. 2 Classification systems for aortic dissection. (From Isselbacher EM et al: Disease of the aorta. In Braunwald E [ed]: *Heart disease: a textbook of cardiovascular medicine*, ed 5, Philadelphia, 1997, Saunders.)

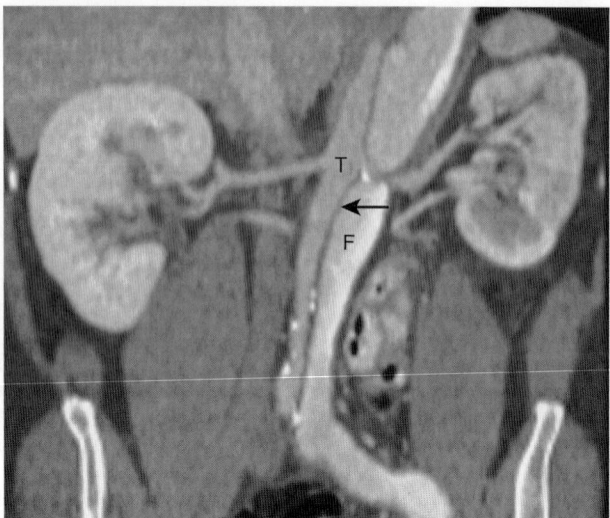

FIG. 3 Computed tomographic angiogram of the aorta shows type B aortic dissection. The intimal flap *(arrow)* separates the true lumen *(T)* from the false lumen *(F)* and compromises blood flow to the right kidney, causing renal atrophy and cortical thinning. (Image courtesy of Bart Domatch, M.D., Radiology Department, University of Texas Southwestern Medical Center, Dallas, TX; from Andreoli TE et al: *Andreoli and Carpenter's Cecil essentials of medicine,* ed 8, Philadelphia, 2010, Saunders.)

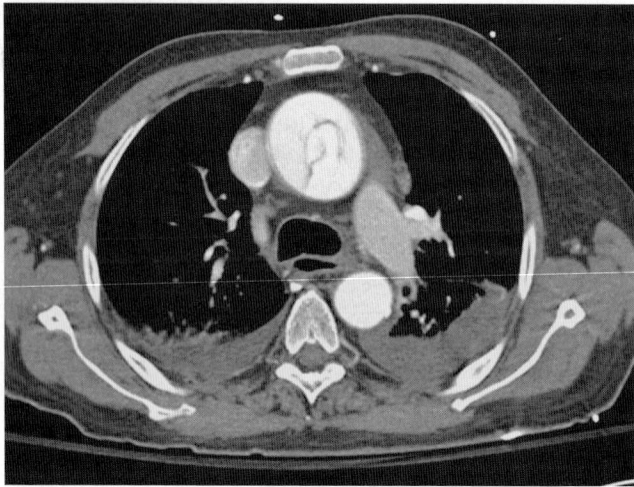

FIG. 4 Thin-slice CT image of a classic ascending dissection with aneurysmal dilation. (From Cameron JL, Cameron AM: *Current surgical therapy,* ed 10, Philadelphia, 2011, Saunders.)

However, a negative D-dimer does not rule out intramural hematoma or penetrating aortic ulcer.
- Three biomarkers with different diagnostic windows can be used in the diagnosis of aortic dissection:
  - Smooth muscle myosin heavy chain protein (released from damaged medial smooth muscle) can be used to detect proximal aortic dissections (91% sensitivity and 93% specificity). Myosin heavy chains will peak within 3 hr of dissection and clear within 24 hr of aortic injury.
  - CK-BB isoenzyme also peaks within 6 hr of dissection.
  - Calponin, a smooth muscle troponin counterpart, increases in aortic dissection with a wider diagnostic window when compared to smooth muscle myosin heavy chain and CK-BB.
  - C-reactive protein, fibrinogen, and soluble elastin fragments are under investigation.

IMAGING STUDIES
- Multidetector CT is considered the gold standard, but its use may be limited in patients with renal failure as it involves the use of IV contrast. Fig. 4 shows a thin-slice CT image of a classic ascending dissection with aneurysmal dilation.
- TEE, multidetector CT, and MRI are all highly sensitive (98%-100%) and specific (95%-98%). Test of choice depends on clinical circumstances and hospital availability.
- Transesophageal echocardiography (TEE) is study of choice in unstable patients with type A dissection but is operator dependent.
- MRI has high sensitivity and specificity but limited availability; not suitable for unstable patients; contraindicated with pacemakers, metal devices.

- With medium or high pretest probability, a second diagnostic test should be done if the first is negative.
- Coronary computed tomographic angiography (CTA) may be an alternative and useful diagnostic study when evaluating for pulmonary embolism, acute coronary syndrome, and aortic dissection.
- Aortography rarely done, as less sensitive than TEE, CT, or MRI.
- Chest radiograph may show widened mediastinum (52% in type A dissections and 39% in type B dissections) and displacement of aortic intimal calcium. It is normal in 29% to 36% of patients with aortic dissection.
- Although the diagnostic sensitivity of transthoracic echocardiography is suboptimal (31% to 55%), it is useful in assessing potential high-risk features or complications, such as pericardial effusion, and making other potential diagnoses. A negative transthoracic echocardiography, however, does not exclude aortic dissection.

Ⓡ TREATMENT

- Urgent surgical consultation should be obtained for all thoracic aortic dissection regardless of anatomic location.
- Proximal dissections (acute type A) require emergent surgery to prevent rupture or pericardial effusion.
- Distal dissections (Stanford type B) are usually treated medically unless distal organ involvement or impending rupture occurs.
  1. Surgical intervention for distal dissections is reserved for patients who have a complicated course, including occlusion of a major aortic branch, propagation of the dissection, enlarging aneurysm, and evidence of aortic rupture.
  2. Thoracic endovascular aortic repair (TEVAR) is a less invasive option for complicated type B aortic dissections and is associated with lower short- and midterm mortality than medical therapy. Retrospective analysis demonstrated lower in-hospital mortality and morbidity in complicated type B dissections undergoing endovascular repair rather than open surgery.
  3. Independent predictors of complication and mortality in distal dissections include periaortic hematoma and descending aortic diameter >5.5 cm, partial false lumen thrombosis, primary tear >10 mm, one entry tear, and false lumen >22 mm.
  4. There is ongoing debate about a possible beneficial role of TEVAR for uncomplicated type B dissections.

Fig. 5 describes an algorithm for the diagnosis and treatment of aortic dissection.

ACUTE GENERAL Rx
- Admit to ICU for monitoring.
- Target SBP 100 to 120 mm Hg or as low as tolerated; heart rate <60 beats/min to reduce aortic wall stress.

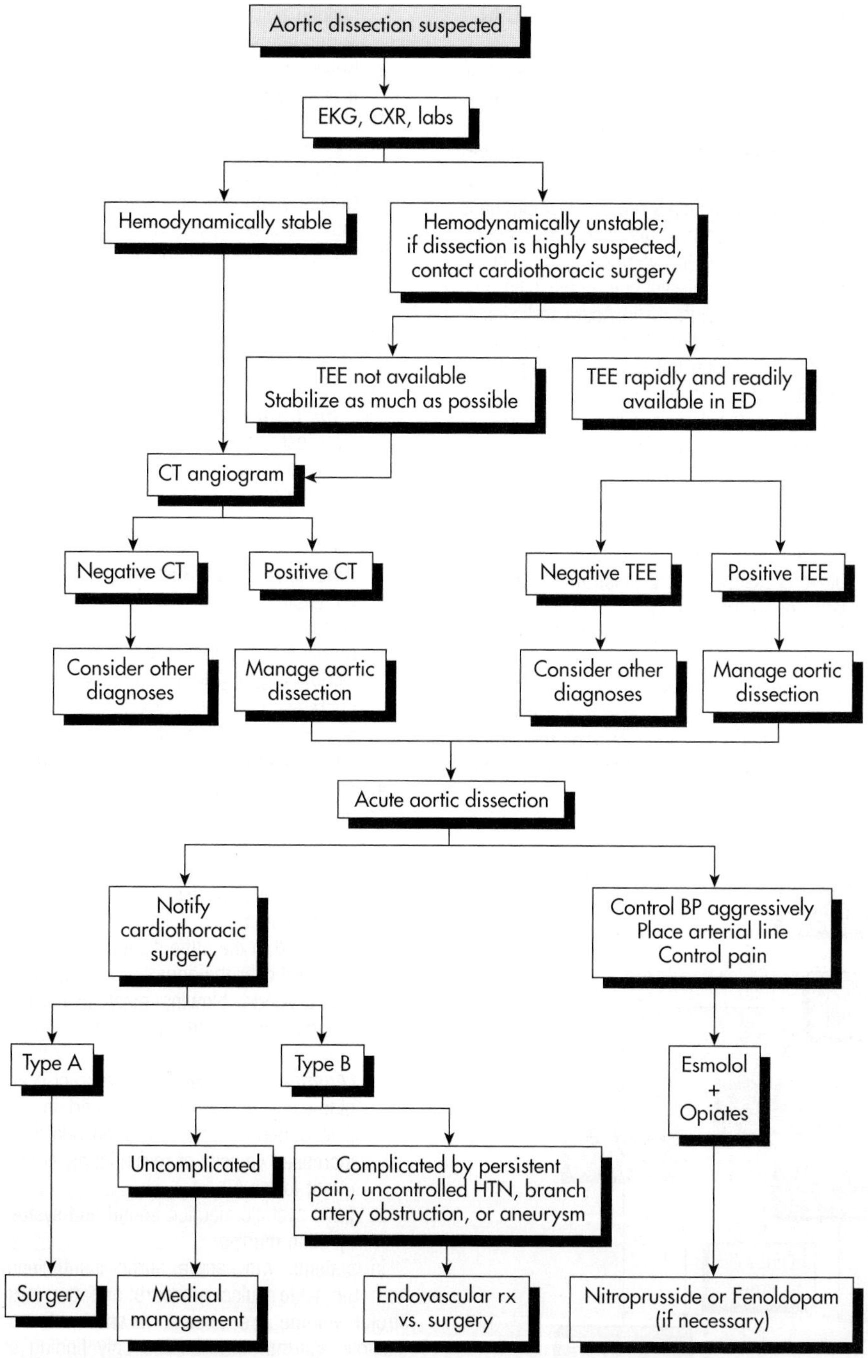

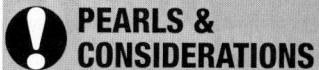

```
Aortic dissection suspected
            │
            ▼
    EKG, CXR, labs
       │         │
       ▼         ▼
Hemodynamically    Hemodynamically unstable;
   stable          if dissection is highly suspected,
                   contact cardiothoracic surgery
       │              │            │
       │              ▼            ▼
       │       TEE not available    TEE rapidly and readily
       │       Stabilize as much    available in ED
       │       as possible
       │         │                     │
       ▼         ▼                     │
    CT angiogram                       │
     │      │                    │           │
     ▼      ▼                    ▼           ▼
Negative  Positive          Negative    Positive
   CT       CT                TEE          TEE
   │         │                 │            │
   ▼         ▼                 ▼            ▼
Consider   Manage aortic   Consider    Manage aortic
 other     dissection       other       dissection
diagnoses                  diagnoses
            │                              │
            ▼                              ▼
           Acute aortic dissection
              │                    │
              ▼                    ▼
         Notify             Control BP aggressively
      cardiothoracic        Place arterial line
         surgery            Control pain
        │       │                   │
        ▼       ▼                   ▼
     Type A   Type B            Esmolol
        │       │                  +
        │       │               Opiates
        │    ┌──┴────┐
        │    ▼       ▼
        │ Uncomplicated  Complicated by persistent
        │               pain, uncontrolled HTN, branch
        │               artery obstruction, or aneurysm
        │    │                  │
     ┌──┴─┐  ▼                  ▼
     ▼    ▼                          ▼
  Surgery Medical        Endovascular rx    Nitroprusside or Fenoldopam
          management     vs. surgery        (if necessary)
```

FIG. 5 Algorithm for the diagnosis and treatment of aortic dissection. *BP*, Blood pressure; *CT*, computed tomography; *CXR*, chest radiograph; *ECG*, electrocardiography; *ED*, emergency department; *HTN*, hypertension; *labs*, laboratory tests; *TEE*, transesophageal echocardiography. (Adams JG et al: *Emergency medicine, clinical essentials*, ed 2, Philadelphia, 2013, Elsevier.)

- IV beta-blockers are cornerstones of treatment, but multiple medications may be needed.
  1. Propranolol 1 mg every 3 to 5 min, metoprolol 5 mg IV every 5 min, or labetalol 20 mg IV, then 20 to 80 mg every 10 min, followed by nitroprusside 0.3 to 10 mcg/kg/min.
  2. Vasodilators should not be used without beta-blockade because they can induce reflex sympathetic stimulation and increase aortic shear stress.
  3. IV calcium channel blockers with negative inotropy (i.e., verapamil, diltiazem) may be used if beta-blockers are contraindicated.

- Pain control, often with morphine.

CHRONIC Rx

- Chronic aortic dissection (>2 wk) managed with aggressive blood pressure control: target <120/80 mm Hg in most patients.
- Target low-density lipoprotein <70 mg/dl.
- Tobacco cessation.
- Minimize strenuous physical activity such as heavy lifting.
- Serial imaging of the aorta, with multidetector CT or MRI should be performed at presentation, at 1 wk, and at 6 wks given the higher risk of instability early on, followed by yearly clinical and imaging follow-up.
- As stated above, endovascular repair should be considered in complicated chronic type B dissections, i.e., when the aortic diameter exceeds 5.5 cm, when there is uncontrolled pain or blood pressure, or when there is rapid growth of the dissecting aneurysm (>4 mm per year).

DISPOSITION

- 90% mortality rate within 2 weeks for an untreated type A dissection.
- Proximal dissection is a surgical emergency. Time is critical; mortality rate is 1% to 3% per hour, approaching 70% after 48 hours.
- Overall, in-hospital mortality rate is 22% with proximal dissections (27% treated surgically and 56% treated medically) and 10% to 17% with distal dissections.

REFERRAL

For ICU management and surgical intervention

❶ PEARLS & CONSIDERATIONS

- Blood pressure control is essential; beta-blocker is first-line medication.
- Proximal dissection is a surgical emergency.
- Cardiac tamponade is not uncommon in patients with acute type A aortic dissection. Syncope, altered mental status, and a widened mediastinum on chest radiograph on presentation suggest tamponade, which warrants urgent operative therapy.
- Surgery for acute type A aortic dissection in patients ≥70 years old can be performed with acceptable outcomes.
- Because of the high mortality rate, AAS should be considered and diagnosed promptly in patients presenting with acute chest or back pain and high blood pressure. Computerized tomography, magnetic resonance imaging, and transesophageal echocardiography are reliable tools for diagnosing AAS. Available data suggest that open surgical repair is optimal for treating type A (ascending aorta) AAS, whereas thoracic endovascular aortic repair may be optimal for treating type B (descending aorta) AAS. However, evidence is limited by the paucity of randomized trials.

SUGGESTED READINGS

Available at www.expertconsult.com

RELATED CONTENT

Aortic Dissection (Patient Information)

AUTHORS: **MEGHANA RAO, M.D.,** and **PHILIP STOCKWELL, M.D.**

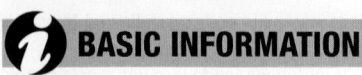

DEFINITION

Aortic regurgitation (AR) is retrograde blood flow into the left ventricle from the aorta as a result of an incompetent aortic valve.

SYNONYMS

Aortic insufficiency
AI
AR

ICD-10CM CODES

I35.1   Nonrheumatic aortic (valve) insufficiency
I35.2   Nonrheumatic aortic (valve) stenosis with insufficiency
Q23.1   Congenital insufficiency of aortic valve

EPIDEMIOLOGY & DEMOGRAPHICS

- Prevalence ranges from 4.9% to 10% and increases with age.
- The most common cause of isolated severe AR is aortic root dilation.
- Infectious endocarditis is the most frequent cause of acute AR.

PHYSICAL FINDINGS & CLINICAL PRESENTATION

The pathophysiology of AR is described in Fig. 1. The clinical presentation varies depending on whether aortic insufficiency is acute or chronic. Chronic aortic insufficiency is well tolerated (except when secondary to infective endocarditis), and the patients remain asymptomatic for years. Common manifestations after significant deterioration of left ventricular function are dyspnea on exertion, syncope, chest pain, and congestive heart failure (CHF). Acute aortic insufficiency manifests primarily with hypotension caused by a sudden fall in cardiac output and resultant cardiogenic shock. In addition, a rapid rise in left ventricular diastolic pressure results in a further decrease in coronary blood flow.

Physical findings in chronic aortic insufficiency include the following:

- Widened pulse pressure (markedly increased systolic blood pressure, decreased diastolic blood pressure). Fig. 2 illustrates characteristics of AR murmur.
- Findings associated with the widened pulse pressure:
  1. Bounding pulses, "water hammer" or collapsing pulse (*Corrigan's pulse*), can be palpated at the wrist or on the femoral artery and is caused by rapid rise and sudden collapse of the arterial pressure during late systole.
  2. Head "bobbing" with each systole (*de Musset's sign*).
  3. "Pistol shot femorals" (*Traube's sign*) is a term used to describe a loud sound over the femoral artery
  4. Capillary pulsations (*Quincke's sign*) may occur at the base of the nail beds.
- A to-and-fro Duroziez double intermittent femoral murmur may be heard over femoral arteries with slight compression with the edge of the stethoscope.
- Popliteal systolic pressure is increased more than 20 mm Hg over brachial systolic pressure (*Hill's sign*), with a 40 to 60 mm difference representing moderate AR and >60 mm difference severe AR.
- Other findings associated with AR, which are more of historical than practical interest, include:
  1. *Mueller's sign*—Systolic pulsations of the uvula.
  2. *Becker's sign*—Visible pulsations of the retinal arteries and pupils.
  3. *Mayne's sign*—More than a 15 mm Hg decrease in diastolic blood pressure with arm elevation from the value obtained with the arm in the standard position.
  4. *Rosenbach's sign*—Systolic pulsations of the liver.
  5. *Gerhard's sign*—Systolic pulsations of the spleen.
- Cardiac auscultation reveals:
  1. Displacement of cardiac impulse downward and to the patient's left
  2. S_3 heard over the apex
  3. Decrescendo, blowing diastolic murmur heard along left sternal border
  4. Low-pitched apical diastolic rumble (*Austin-Flint murmur*)—the precise etiology of the murmur is uncertain, but it is generally believed to be related to increased velocity of mitral inflow consequent to the AR.
  5. Early systolic ejection sound and systolic ejection murmur.

In patients with acute aortic insufficiency both the wide pulse pressure and the large stroke volume are absent. A short, blowing diastolic murmur may be the only finding on physical examination.

ETIOLOGY

- Leaflet abnormalities:
  1. Infective endocarditis
  2. Rheumatic fibrosis (most common cause in developing countries)
  3. Trauma with valvular rupture
  4. Congenital bicuspid aortic valve (most common cause in the United States)
  5. Myxomatous degeneration
  6. Fenfluramine, dexfenfluramine, pergolide, cabergoline
  7. Ankylosing spondylitis
- Aortic root or ascending aorta abnormalities:
  1. Annuloaortic ectasia
  2. Ehlers-Danlos syndrome
  3. Marfan's syndrome

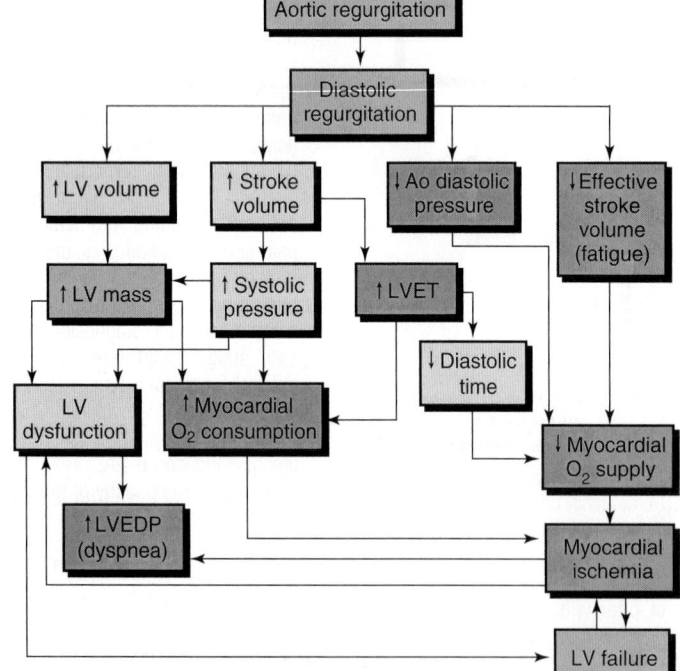

FIG. 1 Pathophysiology of aortic regurgitation. Aortic regurgitation results in an increased left ventricular *(LV)* volume, increased stroke volume, increased aortic *(Ao)* systolic pressure, and decreased effective stroke volume. Increased LV volume results in an increased LV mass, which may lead to LV dysfunction and failure. Increased LV stroke volume increases systolic pressure and prolongation of LV ejection time *(LVET)*. Increased LV systolic pressure results in a decrease in diastolic time. Decreased diastolic time (myocardial perfusion time), diastolic aortic pressure, and effective stroke volume reduce myocardial O_1 supply. Increased myocardial O_2 consumption and decreased myocardial O_2 supply produce myocardial ischemia, which further deteriorates LV function. *LVEDP*, LV end-diastolic pressure. (From Boudoulas H, Gravanis MB: Valvular heart disease. In Gravanis MB, ed: *Cardiovascular disorders: pathogenesis and pathophysiology*, St Louis, 1993, Mosby.)

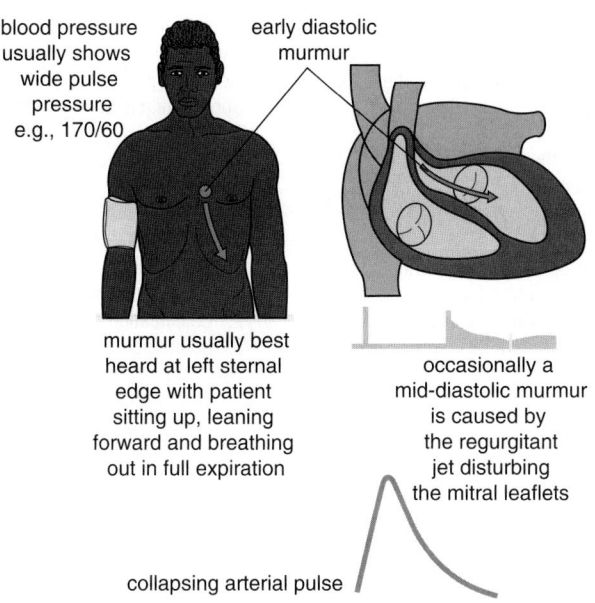

blood pressure usually shows wide pulse pressure e.g., 170/60

early diastolic murmur

murmur usually best heard at left sternal edge with patient sitting up, leaning forward and breathing out in full expiration

occasionally a mid-diastolic murmur is caused by the regurgitant jet disturbing the mitral leaflets

collapsing arterial pulse

FIG. 2 Aortic regurgitation as an example of an early diastolic murmur. (From Epstein O: *Pocket Guide to Clinical Examination,* ed 4, 2009.)

4. Trauma: ankylosing spondylitis
5. Syphilitic aortitis
6. Systemic hypertension
7. Aortic dissection

- Postprocedural aortic regurgitation, usually due to a paravalvular leak, occurs in 10% to 20% of patients undergoing transcatheter aortic valve replacement. Patients with more than mild aortic regurgitation after transcatheter aortic valve replacement have worse outcomes than those without aortic regurgitation.

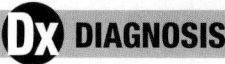 **DIAGNOSIS**

DIFFERENTIAL DIAGNOSIS

- Patent ductus arteriosus, pulmonary regurgitation, and other valvular abnormalities.
- The differential diagnosis of cardiac murmurs is described in Sections II and III.

WORKUP

- Echocardiogram, chest radiograph, electrocardiogram (ECG), and cardiac catheterization (selected patients).
- Medical history and physical examination focused on the following clinical manifestations:
  1. Dyspnea on exertion.
  2. Syncope.
  3. Chest pain.
  4. CHF.

IMAGING STUDIES

- Chest radiography:
  1. Left ventricular hypertrophy (LVH) (chronic AR).
  2. Aortic dilation.
  3. Normal cardiac silhouette with pulmonary edema: possible in patients with acute AR.
- ECG: LVH.
- Echocardiography (Fig. E3) is the main imaging modality to diagnose AR and assess left ventricular size and function. Quantification

of the severity of regurgitation can be made either qualitatively by Doppler vena contracta width (severe if >0.6 cm) or quantitatively by effective regurgitant orifice area (severe if >0.30 cm^2) and/or regurgitant volume (severe if >60 mL per/beat).
- Cardiac magnetic resonance is indicated (class 1) in patients with moderate or severe AR and suboptimal echocardiographic images for the assessment of AR severity as well as LV systolic function and volumes.
- Cardiac catheterization is indicated in selected patients to assess the degree of left ventricular dysfunction, to assess the degree of AR when echocardiographic parameters are inconclusive, and to determine if there is coexistent coronary artery disease.

Rx TREATMENT

NONPHARMACOLOGIC THERAPY

- Avoidance of competitive sports and heavy weight lifting if the AR is severe and associated with aortic root dilatation.
- Salt restriction.
- In 2007, the American Heart Association (AHA) guidelines for prevention of infectious endocarditis were revised; and routine antibiotic prophylaxis to undergo dental or other invasive procedures is no longer recommended, unless the patient has a prior history of endocarditis.

MEDICAL
ACUTE GENERAL RX:

- Afterload reduction: angiotensin-converting enzyme (ACE) inhibitors and vasodilators (i.e., nitroprusside) in acute AR; diuretics for pulmonary edema.
- Avoid beta-blockers that can prolong diastole.
- Emergent surgical referral for cardiogenic shock.

CHRONIC RX:

- Long-term vasodilator therapy with ACE inhibitors or nifedipine in patients who have concomitant hypertension. In one 1994 study (Scognamiglio et al) nifedipine delayed the need for aortic valve surgery compared to digoxin, but in a second randomized trial (Evangelista et al) comparing placebo to nifedipine and enalapril, there was no reduction in need for aortic valve surgery when followed up to 7 years. Therefore there is no current definitive indication of medical therapy with afterload reduction for aortic regurgitation other than hypertension control.
- Beta-blockers in combination with ACE inhibitors are reasonable in patients with symptomatic severe AR or LV dysfunction when surgery cannot be performed because of concomitant comorbidities. In a retrospective cohort study of 756 patients with chronic AR, beta-blocker therapy was associated with decreased mortality. Patients treated with beta-blockers were more likely to be taking ACE inhibitors and dihydropyridine calcium channel blockers as well (53% vs. 40%). In the same study, patients treated with beta-blockers and undergoing AVR were also noted to have a mortality benefit.
- Diuretics and sodium restriction for CHF.
- Comparable efficacy of losartan and atenolol was shown in curbing aortic root dilatation growth in children and young adults (6 mo-25 yr) with Marfan's syndrome, with similar outcomes of aortic regurgitation severity, surgery, aortic dissection, and death at 3 years.

SURGICAL RESERVED FOR: REFERRAL

Reserved for:
- Patients with acute severe AR (i.e., infective endocarditis) and cardiogenic shock.
- Symptomatic patients with severe AR regardless of LV systolic function (class I).
- Patients with hemodynamically stable severe AR undergoing CABG or surgery on the aorta or other heart valves.
- Evidence of systolic dysfunction with left ventricular ejection fraction of less than 50%.
- Asymptomatic patients with severe AR and left ventricular ejection fraction >50%, but with left ventricular dilation:
  1. Echocardiographic end-systolic dimension >50 mm (Class IIa level of evidence) *or*
  2. Echocardiographic end-diastolic dimension >65 mm with low surgical risk (Class IIb).

SUGGESTED READINGS
Available at www.expertconsult.com

RELATED CONTENT
Aortic Insufficiency (Patient Information)

AUTHOR: **DENISA HAGAU, M.D.**

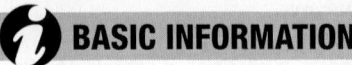

BASIC INFORMATION

DEFINITION

Aortic stenosis (AS) is obstruction to left ventricular systolic outflow across the aortic valve. Symptoms typically appear when the valve orifice decreases to <1 cm^2 (normal orifice is 3 to 4 cm^2). Criteria for severe AS include a valve area <1.0 cm^2, a mean gradient > 40 mm Hg, or a peak gradient > 4 m/s.

SYNONYMS

Aortic valvular stenosis
AS

ICD-10CM CODES
I35.0   Nonrheumatic aortic (valve) stenosis
I35.2   Nonrheumatic aortic (valve) stenosis with insufficiency
Q23.0   Congenital stenosis of aortic valve

EPIDEMIOLOGY & DEMOGRAPHICS

- Aortic stenosis is the most common valve lesion in adults in Western countries, affecting 3% of persons older than 65 years.
- Calcific stenosis (most common cause in patients >70 yr) occurs in 75% of patients.

PHYSICAL FINDINGS & CLINICAL PRESENTATION

- Harsh midsystolic, crescendo-decrescendo murmur (Fig. 1) best heard at base of heart and radiating into neck vessels; often associated with a thrill or ejection click; may also be heard well at the apex.
- Signs of severe AS include absent or diminished intensity of the second heart sound and/or late rising carotid upstroke with delayed amplitude (pulsus parvus et tardus), presence of S4, and a reverse splitting of the second heart sound.
- Classic symptoms include angina, syncope, and heart failure.
- Acquired von Willebrand disease is seen in approximately 20% of severe AS, which can lead to GI bleeding from angiodysplasia (Heyde's syndrome) that resolves after aortic valve replacement.

ETIOLOGY

- Idiopathic calcification of the aortic valve (most common cause, presents at ages 60 to 80)
- Progressive stenosis of congenital bicuspid valve (found in 1% to 2% of the population, presents at ages 40 to 60)
- Rheumatic heart disease
- Less common causes include congenital (major cause of AS in patients <30 yr), radiation, and obstructive vegetations (endocarditis)
- Genetic variation in the LPA locus, mediated by Lp(2) levels, is associated with aortic valve calcification across multiple ethnic groups and with incidental clinical aortic stenosis.

DIAGNOSIS

DIFFERENTIAL DIAGNOSIS

- Hypertrophic cardiomyopathy
- Mitral regurgitation

- Ventricular septal defect
- Aortic sclerosis. Aortic stenosis is distinguished from aortic sclerosis by the degree of valve impairment. In aortic sclerosis, the valve leaflets are abnormally thickened but obstruction to outflow is absent or minimal.
- Subvalvular membrane or supravalvular AS
- Stages of valvular AS
  - Stage A = at risk of AS
  - Stage B = progressive AS (formerly known as mild and moderate AS)
  - Stage C = asymptomatic severe AS
  - Stage D = symptomatic severe AS

WORKUP

- ECG: may demonstrate left ventricular hypertrophy and/or left atrial abnormality.
- Chest radiograph: may demonstrate cardiomegaly. Poststenotic dilation of the ascending aorta may also be evident.

- Echocardiography (see "Imaging Studies")
- Cardiac catheterization in selected patients (see "Imaging Studies")
- Dobutamine challenge (for low-gradient, low-flow AS)
- Fig. 2 describes an algorithm for evaluation of AS.

IMAGING STUDIES

- Chest x-ray:
  1. Poststenotic dilation of the ascending aorta
  2. Calcification of aortic cusps
  3. Rounding of left ventricle (LV) apex
- ECG:
  1. Left ventricular hypertrophy (found in 80% of patients)
  2. Left atrial enlargement
  3. Atrial fibrillation (in late disease)
- Doppler echocardiography: thickening of the left ventricular wall; allows calculation of both

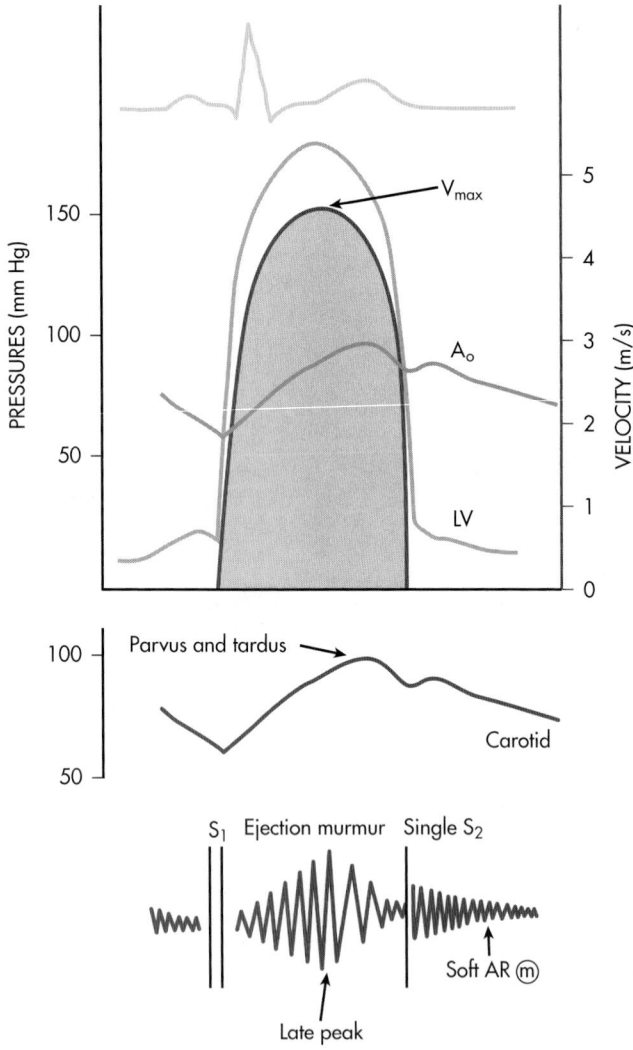

FIG. 1 Relationship between left ventricle (LV) and aortic (Ao) pressures and the Doppler aortic stenosis velocity curve (*in red*). The pressure difference between the LV and aorta in systole is four times the velocity squared (the Bernoulli equation). Thus, a maximum velocity (Vmax) of 4.3 m/sec corresponds to a maximum LV to Ao pressure difference of 74 mm Hg and a mean systolic gradient of 44 mm Hg. On physical examination, the slow rate of rise and delayed peak in the carotid pulse (or parvus and tardus) matches the contour of the aortic pressure waveform. The murmur corresponds to the Doppler velocity curve with a harsh crescendo-decrescendo late-peaking systolic murmur, best heard at the aortic region (upper right sternal border). Often, a soft, high-pitched diastolic decrescendo murmur of aortic regurgitation also is appreciated. (From Bonow et al [eds]: *Braunwald's heart disease*, ed 9, Philadelphia, 2012, Saunders.)

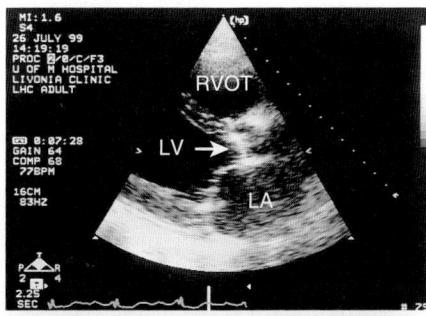

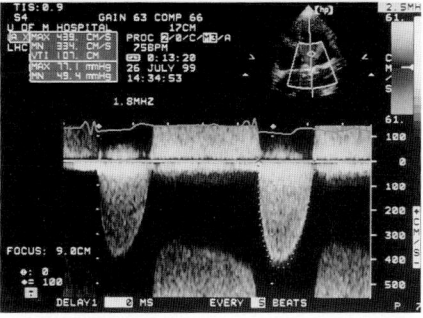

FIG. 3 Echocardiogram recorded in a patient with severe aortic stenosis. The *top panel* is a parasternal long-axis view recorded in systole. Left ventricular function is diminished. The aortic valve is markedly thickened and partially calcified. Its motion is markedly reduced, and in systole it appears that the valve occludes the orifice *(arrow).* The *lower panel* is a continuous-wave Doppler recorded from the apex of the left ventricle along a line aimed through the stenotic aortic valve. Note the aortic stenosis signal below the zero crossing line. The peak velocity is 430 cm/sec, which corresponds to a maximum gradient of 77 mm Hg and a mean gradient of 49.4 mm Hg. *LA,* Left atrium; *LV,* left ventricle; *RVOT,* right ventricular outflow tract. (From Zipes DP et al, eds: *Braunwauld's heart disease,* ed 7, Philadelphia, 2005, Saunders.)

aortic valve area and estimation of pressure gradients to determine severity of AS. (Fig. 3).
- Cardiac catheterization: indicated in symptomatic patients awaiting aortic valve replacement (AVR) in order to detect coexisting coronary artery stenosis that may need bypass at the same time as aortic valve replacement; also indicated in symptomatic patients when noninvasive tests are inconclusive or when there is a discrepancy between noninvasive tests and clinical findings regarding severity of AS because it confirms the diagnosis and the estimates of the severity of the valvular stenosis by directly measuring the gradient across the valve, allowing calculation of the valve area.
- A CT with contrast for imaging the aorta may be needed for annular sizing, aortic measurements, etc., if a transcatheter aortic valve replacement (TAVR) is planned.

Rx TREATMENT

NONPHARMACOLOGIC THERAPY
- Strenuous activity should be avoided in patients with moderate to severe AS
- Sodium restriction if CHF is present

GENERAL Rx
MEDICAL:
- Once symptomatic, AS is a surgical disease.
- Gentle diuresis for volume overload as preload dependent; control hypertension (HTN) but avoid vasodilators (nitrates), maintain sinus rhythm
- In 2007, the AHA guidelines for prevention of infectious endocarditis were revised and routine antibiotic prophylaxis to undergo dental or other invasive procedures is no longer recommended, unless the patient has prior endocarditis.

SURGICAL:
- Surgical valve replacement is the treatment of choice in symptomatic patients because there is a 50% mortality rate at 2 years with medical therapy alone. Valve replacement is a Class I indication for patients with (a) symptomatic severe AS, (b) asymptomatic severe AS with LV ejection fraction (EF) <50%, and (c) severe AS undergoing CABG or surgery on the aorta or other heart valves. Valve replacement is a class 2a indication for patients with (a) asymptomatic severe AS and abnormal blood pressure response (decrease in systolic blood pressure) or decreased exercise tolerance during exercise; (b) asymptomatic patients with very severe AS (peak velocity > 5 m/s or mean pressure gradient >60 mm Hg) with low surgical risk; (c) low flow-low gradient (with low ejection fraction <50%) with a positive low-dose dobutamine stress echo; (d) symptomatic patients with low-flow/low gradient severe AS with a **normal LVEF** ≥50%, a valve area ≤1.0 cm^2, and a stroke volume index <35 mL/m^2; and (e) patients with moderate AS who are undergoing cardiac surgery for other indications. Patients with asymptomatic severe AS with rapid disease progression and low surgical risk are a class 2b indication for valve replacement surgery.
- Percutaneous aortic balloon valvuloplasty serves best as palliative therapy in severely symptomatic patients who are not surgical candidates and as a bridge to surgery in hemodynamically unstable adult patients. It is not an option in patients who are good candidates for surgical valve replacement because restenosis occurs in most adult patients at 6 mo.
- For patients in whom transcatheter aortic valve replacement (TAVR) or high-risk surgical AVR is being considered, a heart valve team approach is a class I recommendation.
- TAVR is recommended (class I) in patients who have a prohibitive surgical risk and are predicted to survive >12 months after TAVR.
- Percutaneous heart valve replacement is a catheter-based technology that allows for implantation of a prosthetic valve without open heart surgery. TAVR has been shown to reduce mortality by 20% in patients with severe AS and coexisting conditions that exclude them as candidates for surgical replacement of the aortic valve. In a large randomized trial involving **high-risk patients** with severe AS who were candidates for surgery, TAVR was found to be noninferior to surgical valve replacement for short-term efficacy with similar all-cause mortality at

2 years. The surgical group had double the incidence of new-onset atrial fibrillation and major bleeding, but the TAVR group had a higher rate of paravalvular regurgitation, major stroke, and vascular complications. In **intermediate-risk patients**, TAVR was similar to surgical aortic valve replacement with respect to death or disabling stroke rates, as demonstrated by a large randomized multicenter trial involving 2032 patients followed for 2 years. The notable differences were that TAVR resulted in larger aortic valve areas and had a lower rate of acute kidney injury, severe bleeding, and new-onset atrial fibrillation, whereas surgery resulted in fewer major vascular complications and less paravalvular aortic regurgitation.

Possible predictors of stroke following TAVR were evaluated by a large systematic review and meta-analysis involving 64 studies including 72,318 patients that looked at rates of stroke at 30 days following TAVR. They concluded that female gender, chronic kidney disease, new atrial fibrillation following TAVR, and lower site experience were associated with increased risk of stroke post TAVR.

There also appears to be a risk of early thrombosis after transcatheter aortic valve implantation as demonstrated by a large multicenter study involving 460 patients. There was a 7% incidence of valve thrombosis after Sapien XT or Sapien 3 TAVR, suggesting that warfarin therapy reconsideration may be warranted.

DISPOSITION
- The presence of even mild symptoms is an indicator of poor survival for patients with AS. The average duration of symptoms before death is angina, 5 years; syncope, 3 years; CHF, 2 years.
- Approximately 75% of patients with symptomatic AS will die within 3 yr of symptom onset unless the aortic valve is replaced.

REFERRAL
- Surgical referral for valve replacement in all symptomatic AS patients. There are studies that are examining the presence of moderate or severe valvular calcification, together with a rapid increase in aortic jet velocity and elevated BNP, to identify patients with a very poor prognosis who should be considered for early valve replacement rather than have surgery delayed until symptoms develop. Additionally, patients with severe AS who are asymptomatic should be considered for exercise stress test to see if they are truly without symptoms (low exercise tolerance) or if the BP drops with exercise, both which would be indications for surgical referral. Surgical mortality rate for valve replacement is 3% to 5%; however, it varies with patient's age (>8% in patients >75 yr).
- In asymptomatic patients, Doppler echocardiography is recommended every 6 to 12 months for severe aortic stenosis, every 1 to 2 years for moderate disease, and every 3 to 5 years for mild disease.

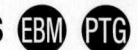

- Referral to cardiology should be considered in patient with low-flow, low-gradient (low ejection fraction) symptomatic aortic stenosis for further work-up (dobutamine stress echo).
- Balloon valvuloplasty is useful in infants and children or poor surgical candidates who do not have calcified valve apparatus; it can be done as an intermediate procedure to stabilize high-risk patients before surgery.
- Patients who are considered high risk for cardiac surgery or have contraindications (porcelain aorta) should be referred to a center with a transcatheter program for TAVR evaluation.

SUGGESTED READINGS

Available at www.expertconsult.com

RELATED CONTENT

Aortic Stenosis (Patient Information)

AUTHOR: **DENISA HAGAU, M.D.**

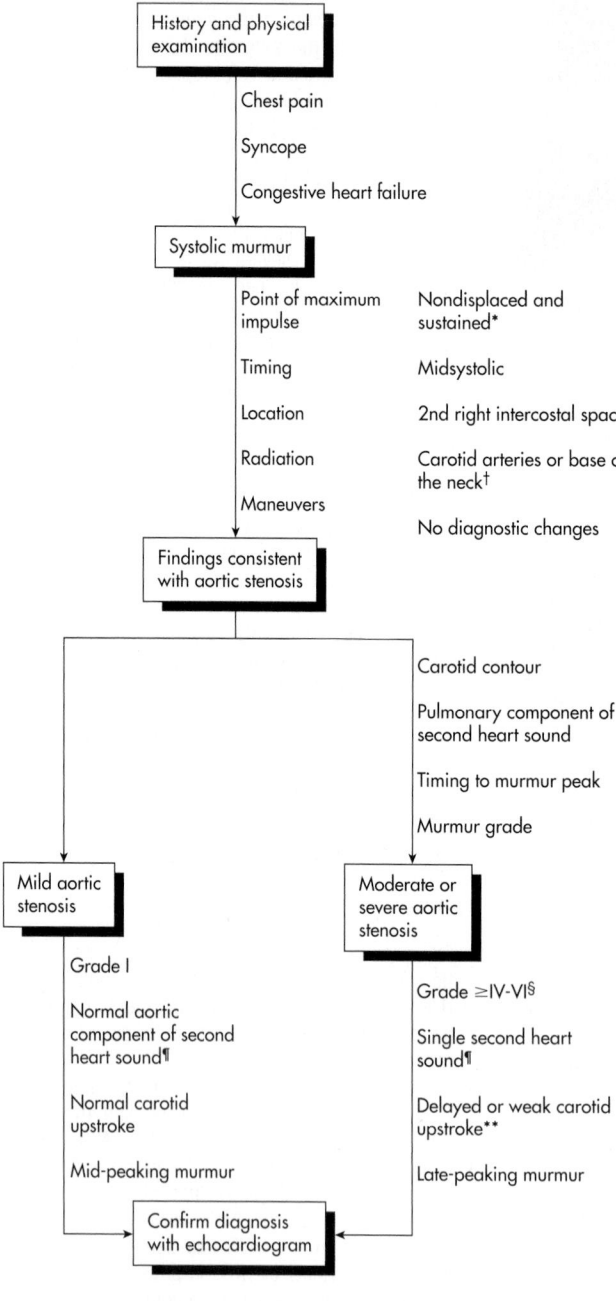

FIG. 2 Aortic stenosis, diagnostic approach. Initial diagnostic evaluation of patients with suspected aortic stenosis. (From Crawford MH et al, eds: *Cardiology*, ed 2, St Louis, 2004, Mosby.)

ℹ BASIC INFORMATION

DEFINITION

Appendicitis is the acute inflammation of the vermiform appendix.

ICD-10CM CODES
K35.2	Acute appendicitis with generalized peritonitis
K35.3	Acute appendicitis with localized peritonitis
K35.80	Unspecified acute appendicitis
K35.89	Other acute appendicitis
K36	Other appendicitis
K37	Unspecified appendicitis

EPIDEMIOLOGY & DEMOGRAPHICS

- Appendicitis occurs in 10% of the population, most commonly between the ages of 10 and 30 yr. Median age is 22 yr. Lifetime risk is 7% to 14%.
- Approximately 300,000 appendectomies are performed in the U.S. each year.
- It is the most common abdominal surgical emergency.
- Incidence of appendicitis has declined over the past 30 yr.
- Male/female ratio is 3:2 until mid-20s; it equalizes after age 30 yr.

PHYSICAL FINDINGS & CLINICAL PRESENTATION

- In children with abdominal pain, fever is the single most useful sign associated with appendicitis. Vomiting, rectal tenderness, and rebound tenderness along with fever are more indicative of appendicitis in children than in adults.
- Abdominal pain: initially the pain may be epigastric or periumbilical in nearly 50% of patients; it subsequently localizes to the right lower quadrant within 12 to 18 hr. Pain can be found in back or right flank if appendix is retrocecal or in other abdominal locations if there is malrotation of the appendix.
- Pain with right thigh extension *(psoas sign)*, low-grade fever: temperature may be >38° C if there is appendiceal perforation.
- Pain with internal rotation of the flexed right thigh *(obturator sign)* is present.
- Right lower quadrant (RLQ) pain on palpation of the left lower quadrant (LLQ) *(Rovsing's sign)*: physical examination may reveal right-sided tenderness in patients with pelvic appendix.
- Point of maximum tenderness is in the RLQ *(McBurney's point)*.
- Nausea, vomiting, tachycardia, cutaneous hyperesthesias at the level of T12 can be present.

ETIOLOGY

Obstruction of the appendiceal lumen with subsequent vascular congestion, inflammation, and edema; common causes of obstruction are:
- Fecaliths: 30% to 35% of cases (most common in adults)
- Foreign body: 4% (fruit seeds, pinworms, tapeworms, roundworms, calculi)
- Inflammation: 50% to 60% of cases (submucosal lymphoid hyperplasia [most common etiology in children, teens])
- Neoplasms: 1% (carcinoids, metastatic disease, carcinoma)

Dx DIAGNOSIS

DIFFERENTIAL DIAGNOSIS

- Intestinal: regional cecal enteritis, incarcerated hernia, cecal diverticulitis, intestinal obstruction, perforated ulcer, perforated cecum, Meckel's diverticulitis
- Reproductive: ectopic pregnancy, ovarian cyst, torsion of ovarian cyst, salpingitis, tubo-ovarian abscess, mittelschmerz, endometriosis, seminal vesiculitis
- Renal: renal and ureteral calculi, neoplasms, pyelonephritis
- Vascular: leaking aortic aneurysm
- Psoas abscess
- Trauma
- Cholecystitis
- Mesenteric adenitis

WORKUP

Patients with RLQ pain, nausea, vomiting, anorexia, and RLQ rebound tenderness should undergo prompt clinical and laboratory evaluation. Imaging studies are generally not necessary in typical appendicitis and generally reserved for patients with an equivocal likelihood of appendicitis. They are useful when the diagnosis is uncertain. Laparoscopy may be useful as both a diagnostic and a therapeutic modality.

LABORATORY TESTS

- Complete blood count with differential reveals leukocytosis with a left shift in 90% of patients with appendicitis. Total white blood cell (WBC) count is generally lower than 20,000/mm^3. Higher counts may be indicative of perforation. Less than 4% have a normal WBC and differential. A WBC count <10,000/mm^3 decreases the likelihood of appendicitis. Low hemoglobin and hematocrit levels in an older patient should raise suspicion for GI tract carcinoma.
- Microscopic hematuria and pyuria may occur in <20% of patients.
- HCG to rule out pregnancy in females of reproductive age.

IMAGING STUDIES

- Multidetector computed tomography (Fig. 1) is a useful test for routine evaluation of suspected appendicitis in adults. CT of the abdomen/pelvis without contrast has a sensitivity of >90% and an accuracy >94% for acute appendicitis. A distended appendix, periappendiceal inflammation, and a thickened appendiceal wall are indicative of appendicitis. Table 1 describes CT findings of appendicitis. In children and young adults, exposure to CT radiation is of particular concern. Trials with low-dose CT

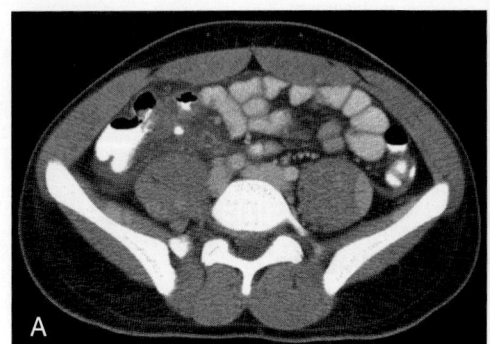
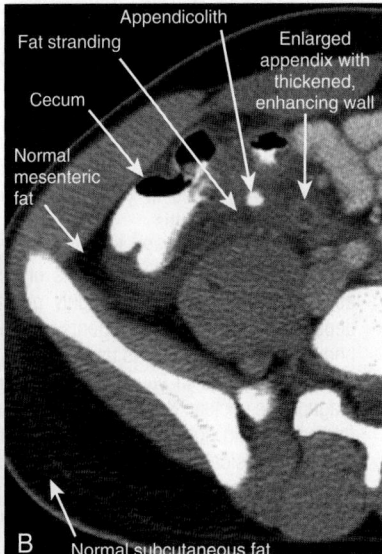

FIG. 1 Appendicitis, CT with IV and oral contrast. This CT demonstrates classic findings of appendicitis in an 18-year-old male with right lower quadrant pain, as seen with CT with IV and oral contrast. Studies suggest that CT without contrast has similar sensitivity and specificity. An enlarged appendix is seen near the cecum as a right lower quadrant tubular structure in short-axis cross section, giving it a circular appearance. The surrounding fat shows stranding, a smoky appearance indicating inflammation (compare with normal mesenteric and subcutaneous fat, which is nearly black). The appendiceal wall shows enhancement, a brightening after administration of IV contrast. This slice also shows an appendicolith, an occasional finding of appendicitis. It does not appear to be within the appendix in this slice, because the appendix bends in and out of the plane of this slice. An appendicolith usually appears as a calcified (white) rounded structure, visible without any contrast. **A,** Axial CT image. **B,** Close-up. (From Broder JS: *Diagnostic imaging for the emergency physician,* Philadelphia, 2011, Saunders.)

TABLE 1 CT Findings of Appendicitis: SCALPEL Mnemonic

Term	Description
Stranding	Fat stranding suggests regional inflammation, possibly because of appendicitis.
Cecum	The appendix originates from the cecum, which should be identified first to help localize the appendix. The cecum may show wall thickening, suggesting appendicitis.
Air	Air outside of the lumen of the appendix is pathologic and suggests perforation. Air within the appendiceal wall is also abnormal.
Large	The normal appendix is <6 mm; an enlarged appendix >6 mm suggests appendicitis. Wall thickening >1 mm also suggests appendicitis.
Phlegmon	Inflammatory changes surrounding the appendix suggest a perforated appendix. A heterogeneous collection called a phlegmon may be seen. If the appendix has ruptured, a pericecal phlegmon may be the only remaining evidence, because the appendix itself may not be seen.
Enhancement	The wall of an abnormal appendix enhances with IV contrast and appears brighter than the normal bowel or the normal psoas muscle.
Lith	An appendicolith is a calcified stone sometimes found in the lumen of an inflamed appendix.

From Broder JS: *Diagnostic imaging for the emergency physician,* Philadelphia, 2011, Saunders.

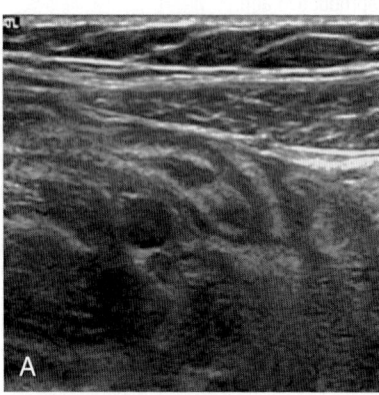 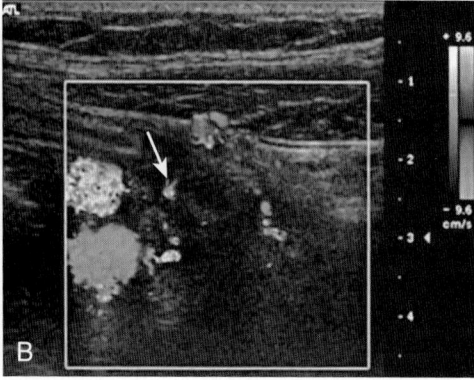

FIG. 2 Appendicitis. A, Transabdominal ultrasound using a linear transducer demonstrates a thick, tubular, noncompressible structure. **B,** Same imaging method with addition of color Doppler ultrasound shows increased vascularity within the luminal wall consistent with inflammation *(arrow).* (From Fielding JR et al: *Gynecologic imaging,* Philadelphia, 2011, Saunders.)

(116 mGy cm) have shown that low-dose CT is not inferior to standard-dose CT (521 mGy cm) with respect to negative (unnecessary) appendectomy rates in young adults with suspected appendicitis.

- Ultrasonography (Fig. 2) has a sensitivity of 75% to 90% for the diagnosis of acute appendicitis, although it is highly operator dependent and difficult in patients with large body habitus. Ultrasound is useful, especially in pregnancy and in younger women when diagnosis is unclear. Normal ultrasonographic findings should not deter surgery if the history and physical examination are indicative of appendicitis.
- MRI of the abdomen and pelvis can also be used to accurately diagnose acute appendicitis in pregnant patients (100% sensitivity, 93.6% specificity) without exposure to ionizing radiation.

TREATMENT

NONPHARMACOLOGIC THERAPY

- Nothing by mouth
- Do not administer analgesics until the diagnosis is made

ACUTE GENERAL Rx

- Urgent appendectomy (laparoscopic or open), correction of fluid and electrolyte imbalance with vigorous IV hydration and electrolyte replacement
- IV antibiotic prophylaxis to cover gram-negative bacilli and anaerobes (ampicillin/sulbactam 3 g IV q6h or piperacillin/tazobactam 4.5 g IV q8h in adults)

(!) PEARLS & CONSIDERATIONS

COMMENTS

- Perforation is common (20% in adult patients). Indicators of perforation are pain lasting >24 hr, leukocytosis >20,000/mm³, temperature >102° F, palpable abdominal mass, and peritoneal findings.
- In general, prognosis is excellent. Mortality rate is <1% in young adults without complications; however, it exceeds 10% in elderly patients with ruptured appendix.
- In approximately 20% of patients who undergo exploratory laparotomy because of suspected appendicitis, the appendix is normal.

- An increasing amount of evidence supports the use of antibiotics instead of surgery for treating patients with uncomplicated appendicitis. A recent trial assessing the feasibility of nonoperative management for uncomplicated acute appendicitis in children using either IV piperacillin-tazobactam or ciprofloxacin metronidazole therapy for at least 24 hours followed by oral antibiotics for 10 days revealed that 90% of children managed nonoperatively had no progression within 30 days.[1] Another trial among patients with CT-proven, uncomplicated appendicitis revealed that antibiotic treatment did not meet the prescribed criterion for noninferiority compared with appendectomy. Most patients randomized to antibiotic treatment for uncomplicated appendicitis did not require appendectomy during the 1-yr follow-up period, and those who required appendectomy did not experience significant complications.[2] It remains to be determined whether the benefits of potentially avoiding an operation with antibiotics-first approach are outweighed by the burden to the patient related to future appendicitis episodes, more days of antibiotic therapy, lingering symptoms, and uncertainty that may affect quality of life.[3]

(EBM) EVIDENCE

Available at www.expertconsult.com

SUGGESTED READINGS
Available at www.expertconsult.com

RELATED CONTENT
Appendicitis (Patient Information)

AUTHOR: **FRED F. FERRI, M.D.**

[1]Minneci PC et al: Feasibility of a nonoperative management strategy for uncomplicated acute appendicitis in children. *J Am Coll Surg* 219:272-279, 2014.
[2]Salminen P et al: Antibiotic therapy vs appendectomy for treatment of uncomplicated acute appendicitis, the APPAC Randomized trial. *JAMA* 313(23):2340-2348, 2015.
[3]Flum DR: Acute appendicitis—appendectomy or the "antibiotics first" strategy. *N Engl J Med* 372:1937-43, 2015.

ℹ️ BASIC INFORMATION

DEFINITION

Arrhythmogenic right ventricular dysplasia (ARVD) is a cardiomyopathy characterized by replacement of the normal myocardium with fibrofatty tissue, mainly of the right ventricle but also occasionally with involvement of the left ventricle. It is defined clinically by palpitations and syncope and potentially life-threatening ventricular arrhythmias.

SYNONYMS

Arrhythmogenic right ventricular cardiomyopathy
ARVC

ICD-10CM CODES
I42.8 Arrhythmogenic ventricular dysplasia

EPIDEMIOLOGY & DEMOGRAPHICS

PREVALENCE: 1:2000-5000 persons. It is one of the leading causes of arrhythmic cardiac arrest in young people and athletes
PREDOMINANT SEX AND AGE: Mean age, 31 yr (range, 12-50 yr), predominantly male
RISK FACTORS: Family history of ARVD (present in nearly 50% of affected patients)
GENETICS:
- Autosomal dominant (most common) with variable penetrance and polymorphic phenotypic expression.
- Autosomal recessive (rarely, e.g., Naxos disease).
- Several different gene mutations in desmosomal proteins.
- Gene mutations can be identified in 50% of affected individuals.

PHYSICAL FINDINGS & CLINICAL PRESENTATION

- ARVD can present with palpitations, syncope, and chest discomfort and less commonly sudden cardiac arrest and signs of right ventricular failure such as dyspnea, edema, and fatigue. Patients may be clinically asymptomatic for many years.
- Cardiac arrest after physical exertion may be the initial presentation.
- Physical examination will be normal in most patients. Widely split S2 is an important diagnostic clue.

ETIOLOGY

ARVD is characterized by progressive replacement of mainly the right ventricular myocardium with fibrofatty tissue after apoptotic myocardial cell death caused by mutations of desmosomal protein.

🆅🆇 DIAGNOSIS

- A major criteria equals 2 points; a minor criteria equals 1 point. The diagnosis of ARVD is considered definite if the patient has 4 points and probable with 3 points. See Table 1 for diagnostic criteria.

DIFFERENTIAL DIAGNOSIS

- Cardiomyopathy with involvement of the right ventricle
- Uhl's anomaly: rare anomaly that presents mainly in childhood with signs and symptoms of right heart failure and characterized by a paper-thin right ventricle resulting from death of the myocytes throughout the right ventricle
- Idiopathic RV tachycardia
- Sarcoidosis
- Right ventricular infarction

WORKUP

- Initial workup includes history with focus on sudden death in the family, resting ECG, 24-Holter ECG, signal-averaged ECG, and imaging studies with echocardiography and MRI.
- ECG will have diagnostic findings in 50% to 90% of patients with ARVD, including T-wave inversions in anterior precordial leads V_1-V_6, epsilon waves, and a QRS duration longer than 110 ms in V1 or >40 ms longer in V1 than v6. (Fig. 1)
- Ventricular tachycardia (VT) with left bundle branch block pattern and frequent PVCs (>500 in 24 h) might be detected by 24-hr Holter monitoring.
- An abnormal signal-averaged ECG is a minor diagnostic criteria.
- Echocardiography will show right ventricular dilation with regional wall motion abnormalities, aneurysms, and depressed RV function that varies with the severity of the disease.
- MRI is a noninvasive method to detect structural abnormalities (fibrofatty changes) and regional dysfunction. Cardiac MRI (CMR) is the most sensitive method to detect ARVD, but it has high false-positive rates. Cardiac CT angiogram (Fig. E2) will reveal thinning and aneurysmal dilation of the RV anterior wall and outflow tract.

If the routine tests are not conclusive, endomyocardial biopsy and electrophysiologic testing can be considered. However, biopsies and radionuclide ventriculography are rarely performed in the U.S.

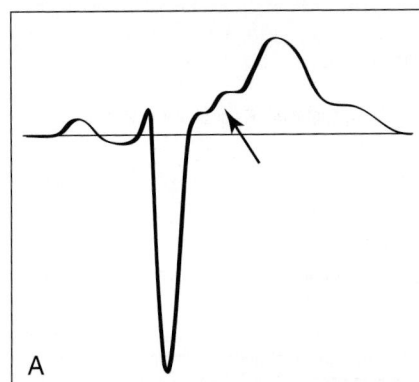

FIG. 1 Epsilon waves are small deflections just beyond the QRS complex. Best visualized in leads V_1-V_3. Any potential in leads V_1-V_3 that exceeds the QRS in leads V6 by more than 25 millisecond should be considered epsilon wave. (From Anderson EL: Arrhythmogenic right ventricular dysplasia, *Am Fam Physician* 73(8):1391-1398, 2006.)

℞ TREATMENT

No curative treatment is available. The treatment goal is focused on preventing sudden cardiac death, symptomatic treatment of right heart failure, and pharmacologic and invasive treatment of arrhythmias. Family members with a negative phenotype (either healthy gene carriers or those with an unknown genotype) do not need any specific treatment other than sports restriction; however, lifelong clinical assessment with the use of noninvasive tests at least every 2 years is warranted.[1]

NONPHARMACOLOGIC THERAPY

- Avoidance of activity that may trigger ventricular tachycardia and may lead to disease progression.
- ICD implantation needs to be considered in patients who have the definite diagnosis of ARVD. Patients with unexplained syncope, advanced disease, documented ventricular arrhythmias, or a family history of sudden cardiac death or who have been resuscitated from cardiac arrest are at high risk. A subcutaneous ICD might be an alternative option instead of transvenous implantation.
- Radiofrequency catheter ablation is used in cases of refractory VT or frequent tachycardia after defibrillator placement.
- Cardiac transplantation.

PHARMACOLOGIC TREATMENT

- Antiarrhythmic therapy with sotalol (first-line treatment) or amiodarone, often in combination with beta-blockers, is used for tachycardia suppression.

REFERRAL

- Early cardiology and electrophysiology referral
- Consider referring for genetic counseling

❗ PEARLS & CONSIDERATIONS

PREVENTION

All first-degree relatives should be tested if ARVD is confirmed. Sports activity increases the risk of sudden cardiac death among adolescents and young adults with ARVC. The estimated overall mortality ranges from 0.08% to 3.6% per year.[1]

SUGGESTED READINGS

Available at www.expertconsult.com

AUTHOR: **HEIKO SCHMITT, M.D., PH.D.**

[1]Corrado D, et al.: Arrhythmogenic right ventricular cardiomyopathy, *N Engl J Med* 376:61–72, 2017.

TABLE 1 Global or Regional Dysfunction and Structural Alterations

Major

2D echo criteria

Regional RV akinesia, dyskinesia, or aneurysm and one of the following measured at end diastole

PLAX RVOT ≥32 mm or

PSAX RVOT ≥36

Fractional area change ≤33%

MRI criteria

Regional RV akinesia or dyskinesia or dyssynchronous RV contraction and one of the following

Ratio of RV end-diastolic volume to BSA >100, <110 mL/m^2 (male) or >100

mL/m2

RV ejection fraction >40% ≤45%

RV angiography criteria

Regional RV akinesia, dyskinesia, or aneurysm

Minor

2D echo criteria

Regional RV akinesia or dyskinesia or dyssynchronous RV contraction and one of the following measured at end diastole

PLAX RVOT ≥29 <32 mm or

PSAX RVOT ≥32 <36

Fractional area change >33% ≤40%

MRI criteria

Regional RV akinesia or dyskinesia or dyssynchronous RV contraction and one of the following

Ratio of RV end-diastolic volume to BSA ≥110 mL/m^2 (male) or _≥100 mL/m^2

RV ejection fraction ≤40%

Tissue characterization of wall

Major

Residual myocytes <60% by morphometric analysis (or <50% if estimated) with fibrous replacement of the RV free wall myocardium in >1 sample, with or without fatty replacement of tissue on endomyocardial biopsy

Minor

Residual myocytes 60%-75% by morphometric analysis (or 50%-65% if estimated), with fibrous replacement of the RV free wall myocardium in >1 sample with or without fatty replacement of tissue on endomyocardial biopsy

Repolarization abnormalities

Major

Inverted T waves in right precordial leads (V1, V2, and V3) or beyond in individuals >14 y of age (in the absence of complete RBBB QRS ≥120 ms)

Minor

Inverted T waves in V1 and V2 in individuals >14 y of age (in the absence of complete RBBB) or in V4, V5, and V6

Inverted T waves in leads V1, V2, V3, and V4 in individuals >14 y of age in the presence of a complete RBBB

Depolarization or conduction abnormalities

Major

Epsilon wave (reproducible low-amplitude signals between end of QRS complex to onset of T wave) in the right precordial leads (V1-V3)

Minor

Late potentials by SAECG in ≥1 of 3 parameters in the absence of a QRSd of ≥110 ms on standard ECG

Filtered QRS ≥114 ms

Duration of terminal QRS <40 mV ≥38 ms

Root-mean-square voltage of terminal 40 ms ≤20 μV

Terminal activation duration ≥55 ms measured from the nadir of the end of the QRS, including R', in V1, V2, or V3 in absence of complete RBBB

Arrhythmias

Major

Nonsustained or sustained VT of LBBB morph with superior axis

Minor

Nonsustained or sustained VT of RVOT configuration, LBBB morph with inferior axis or of unknown axis

>500 PVCs per 24 h (Holter)

Family history

Major

ARVD/C in first-degree relative who meets Task Force criteria

ARVD/C confirmed pathologically at autopsy or surgery in first-degree relative

Identification of pathogenic mutation categorized as associated or probably associated with ARVD/C in the patient under evaluation

Minor

History of ARVD/C in first-degree relative in whom it is not possible to determine whether the family member meets Task Force criteria

Premature sudden death (<35 y of age) caused by suspected ARVD/C in a first-degree relative

ARVD/C confirmed pathologically or by current Task Force criteria in second-degree relative.

A major criteria equals 2 points, a minor criteria 1 point. The diagnosis of arrhythmogenic right ventricular dysplasia (ARVD) is considered definite if the patient has 4 points and probable with 3 points. *BSA*, body surface area; *MRI*, magnetic resonance imaging; *RBBB*, right bundle branch block; *RV*, right ventricle; *RVOT*, right ventricular outflow tract; *2D*, two dimensional; *VT*, ventricular tachycardia. From Marcus IM: Diagnosis of arrhythmogenic right ventricular cardiomyopathy/dysplasia proposed modification of the Task Force criteria. *Circulation* 121: 1533-1541, 2010.

BASIC INFORMATION

DEFINITION

Asbestosis is a slowly progressive diffuse interstitial fibrosis resulting from dose-related inhalation exposure to fibers of asbestos in miners, millers, workers of asbestos textiles, and insulators. Clinically, the lung involvement is characterized by bilateral diffuse interstitial fibrosis, more pronounced in the lower lobes, and pleural thickening, leading to shortness of breath and dry cough.

Asbestos exposure can lead to the spectrum of pulmonary pathology, including pulmonary fibrosis; asbestos-related pleural plaque (ARPD), both focal and diffuse; and malignancies (small cell carcinoma, non–small cell carcinoma, or mesothelioma).

ICD-10CM CODES
J61 Pneumoconiosis due to asbestos and other mineral fibers

EPIDEMIOLOGY & DEMOGRAPHICS

- Five to 10 new cases per 100,000 persons per year in the U.S.
- Prolonged interval (20 to 30 yr) between exposures to inhaled fibers and clinical manifestations of disease
- Most common in workers involved in the primary extraction of asbestos from rock deposits and in those involved in the fabrication and installation of products containing asbestos (e.g., naval shipyards in World War II; installation of floor tiles, ceiling tiles, acoustic ceiling coverings, wall insulation, and pipe coverings in public buildings)

PHYSICAL FINDINGS & CLINICAL PRESENTATION

- Insidious onset of shortness of breath with exertion is usually the first sign of asbestosis.
- Dyspnea becomes more severe as the disease advances; with time, progressively less exertion is tolerated.
- Cough is frequent and usually paroxysmal, dry, and nonproductive.
- Scant mucoid sputum may accompany the cough in the later stages of the disease.
- Fine end-respiratory crackles (rales, crepitations) are heard more predominantly in the lung bases.
- Digital clubbing, edema, jugular venous distention are present.

ETIOLOGY/PATHOGENESIS

Inhalation of asbestos fibers. Recent work has shown that pathogenesis of pulmonary interstitial inflammation and fibrosis is related to immune mechanisms. Asbestosis is known to be associated with positive serum antinuclear antibody (ANA) and rheumatoid factor (RF). Recently, an important role of interleukin-1beta (IL-1beta) in the pathogenesis of asbestosis and its systemic autoimmune manifestations has been reported.

DIAGNOSIS

DIFFERENTIAL DIAGNOSIS

- Silicosis
- Siderosis, other pneumonoconioses
- Lung cancer
- Atelectasis

WORKUP

Documentation of exposure history, diagnostic imaging, pulmonary function testing

LABORATORY TESTS

- Generally not helpful
- Possible mild elevation of erythrocyte sedimentation rate (ESR), positive antinuclear antibody (ANA), and rheumatoid factor (RF) (these tests are nonspecific and do not correlate with disease severity or activity)
- Pulmonary function testing: with decreased vital capacity (VC), decreased total lung capacity (TLC), decreased carbon monoxide gas transfer (DLco)
- FEV1 might be reduced in concomitant smokers
- Arterial blood gases: hypoxemia, hypercarbia in advanced stages

IMAGING STUDIES

Chest radiograph (Fig. E1):

Small, irregular shadows in lower lung zones.

The imaging findings vary from benign pleural disease (including discrete plaques, pleural calcification, diffuse pleural thickening with blunting of costophrenic angles, and thickening of the interlobar fissure) to asbestosis (diffuse interstitial pulmonary fibrosis).
- Thickened pleura, calcified plaques (present under diaphragm and lateral chest wall).
- CT scan of chest (Fig. E2) confirms diagnosis. Typical findings on high-resolution CT of the chest include increased interstitial markings found mainly at the bases. As the disease progresses, honeycombing is noted.

TREATMENT

NONPHARMACOLOGIC THERAPY

- Smoking cessation, proper nutrition, exercise program to maximize available lung function
- Home oxygen therapy PRN
- Removal of patient from further asbestos fiber exposure

GENERAL Rx

- Prompt identification and treatment of respiratory infections
- Supplemental oxygen on a PRN basis
- Annual influenza vaccination, pneumococcal vaccination

Some new data are coming out targeting IL-1 beta therapy on the progression of lung fibrosis that suggest a new perspective for the treatment of systemic autoimmune features of asbestosis and, possibly, of lung involvement.[1]

DISPOSITION

- There is no specific treatment for asbestosis.
- Death is usually from respiratory failure from cor pulmonale.
- Diffuse pleural thickening and asbestosis are associated with increased risks of malignant peritoneal mesothelioma beyond the risk calculated to be associated with the degree of asbestos exposure.[2]
- None of the benign pleural diseases or ARPD was associated with an increased risk of malignant pleural mesothelioma.
- Asbestos increases lung cancer mortality among nonsmokers.
- Asbestos exposure without asbestosis and smoking increases the risk of lung cancer. The joint effect of asbestos and smoking is additive and depends in part on the presence of asbestosis. Asbestos workers who stop smoking experience a dramatic decline in lung cancer risk, which approaches that of nonsmokers after 30 years.
- Low-dose chest CT scanning offers an excellent opportunity to detect early-stage lung cancers in asbestos-exposed workers.
- Computed tomography is more sensitive than radiography, computed tomography without contrast generally suffices for evaluation, and PET scan (fluorodeoxyglucose-positron emission tomography) may have utility in patients with mesothelioma.
- Survival in patients after development of mesothelioma is 4 to 6 yr.

SUGGESTED READINGS
Available at www.expertconsult.com

RELATED CONTENT
Asbestosis (Patient Information)

AUTHOR: **IMRANA QAWI, M.D.**

[1]Systemic autoimmune disease in asbestosis rapidly responding to anti-interleukin-1beta antibody canakinumab: a case report. *BMC Musculoskelet Disord* 14(16):146, 2015.
[2]The additional risk of malignant mesothelioma in former workers and residents of Wittenoom with benign pleural disease or asbestosis. *Occup Environ Med* 62:665-669, 2005.

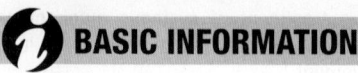

DEFINITION

Ascariasis is a parasitic infection caused by the nematode *Ascaris lumbricoides*. The majority of those infected are asymptomatic; however, clinical disease may arise from pulmonary hypersensitivity, intestinal obstruction, and secondary complications.

SYNONYMS

Round worms
Worms

ICD-10CM CODES
B77.9   Ascariasis, unspecified
B77.81 Ascariasis pneumonia
B77.0   Ascariasis with intestinal complications
B77.89 Ascariasis with other complications

EPIDEMIOLOGY & DEMOGRAPHICS

INCIDENCE (IN U.S.):
- Unknown. Worldwide, A. *lumbricoides* is the most common helminthic infection of humans, infecting as many as 1 billion or more persons. 71% of persons at risk for infection live in Asia and the Western Pacific.
- Three times the infection rates found in blacks as in whites

PEAK INCIDENCE: Unknown
PREVALENCE (IN U.S.): Estimated at 4 million, the majority of which live in the rural southeastern part of the country; ascariasis is associated with poor sanitation
PREDOMINANT SEX: Both sexes probably equally affected, with a possible slight female preponderance
PREDOMINANT AGE: Most common in children from ages 2 to 10 years old and decreases after age 15; infections tend to cluster in families
NEONATAL INFECTION: Probable transmission, though not specifically studied

PHYSICAL FINDINGS & CLINICAL PRESENTATION

- Most people infected with *Ascaris* are asymptomatic.
- Occurs approximately 9 to 12 days after ingestion of eggs (corresponding to the larval migration through the lungs)
- Nonproductive cough
- Substernal chest discomfort
- Fever
- In patients with large worm burdens, especially children, intestinal obstruction associated with perforation, volvulus, and intussusception
- Migration of worms into the biliary tree giving clinical appearance of biliary colic and pancreatitis as well as acute appendicitis with movement into that appendage
- Rarely, infection with *A. lumbricoides* producing interstitial nephritis and acute renal failure
- In endemic areas in Asia and Africa, malabsorption of dietary proteins and vitamins as a consequence of chronic worm intestinal

carriage; 1 billion people worldwide are infected with this nematode

ETIOLOGY

- Transmission is usually hand to mouth, but eggs may be ingested via transported vegetables grown in contaminated soil.
- Eggs are hatched in the small intestine, with larvae penetrating intestinal mucosa and migrating via the circulation to the lungs.
- Larval forms proceed through the alveoli, ascend the bronchial tree, and return to the intestines after swallowing, where they mature into adult worms.
- Estimated time until the female adult worm begins producing eggs is 2 to 3 mo.
- Eggs are passed out of the intestines with feces and can survive for years in warm, moist, shaded soil.
- Within human host, adult worm life span is 1 to 2 yr.

DIAGNOSIS

DIFFERENTIAL DIAGNOSIS

- Radiologic manifestations and eosinophilia to be distinguished from drug hypersensitivity and Löffler's syndrome.
- Table E1 compares features of major intestinal nematodes.

LABORATORY TESTS

- Examination of the stool for *Ascaris* ova (Fig. E1)
- Expectoration or fecal passage of adult worm
- Adult male worms: 10 to 30 cm long; adult female worms: larger than male, up to 40 cm
- Eosinophilia: most prominent early in the infection and subsides as the adult worm infestation established in the intestines; usually in 5% to 12% range but can be up to 50%
- Serology: patients develop IgG antibodies, but they cross react with antigens from other helminths and are not protective; thus serology is used more for epidemiologic purposes than for individual diagnosis

IMAGING STUDIES

- Chest x-ray to reveal bilateral oval or round infiltrates of varying size (Löffler's syndrome); NOTE: infiltrates are transient and eventually resolve.
- Plain films of the abdomen and contrast studies to reveal worm masses in loops of bowel.
- Ultrasonography and endoscopic retrograde cholangiopancreatography (ERCP) to identify worms in the pancreaticobiliary tract.
- CT scan with oral contrast can also assist in the detection of GI foreign bodies such as parasites.

TREATMENT

NONPHARMACOLOGIC THERAPY

Aggressive IV hydration, especially in children with fever, severe vomiting, and resultant dehydration

ACUTE GENERAL Rx

- All infected patients, including asymptomatic ones, should be treated

1. Albendazole: 400 mg PO × 3 days is the first-line agent. Single-dose albendazole is used in mass treatment campaigns.
2. Mebendazole 100 mg PO bid y × 3 days: not commercially available in the U.S.
- Cure rate with these agents is 95% to 100%, but they are contraindicated in pregnancy.
- Side effects: GI discomfort, headache, and rarely leukopenia
- Alternative agent or for use in pregnancy: pyrantel pamoate (Antiminth)
  1. Given at a dose of 11 mg/kg PO (maximum dose of 1 g/day)
  2. Considered safe for use in pregnant women
- Other alternative agents:
  1. Ivermectin: 150 to 200 mcg/kg orally once
  2. Nitazoxanide: cure rates in heavy worm burden are only 50% to 80%
  3. Piperazine citrate: no longer first-line agent due to toxicity but still used in cases of intestinal or biliary obstruction, as drug paralyzes the worm, helping its expulsion. Dose: 50 to 75 mg/kg once daily up to maximum of 3.5 g for 2 days.
  4. Levamisole: 2.5 mg/kg once orally is recommended by the WHO as alternative therapy, but not available in the U.S.
- Complete obstruction should be managed surgically.

DISPOSITION

Overall prognosis is good. Patients should be reevaluated in 2 to 3 months. Reinfection is common.

REFERRAL

- To gastroenterologist in cases of visualized pancreaticobiliary tract or appendiceal obstruction
- To surgeon in cases of complete obstruction or suspected secondary complication (e.g., perforation or volvulus)

PEARLS & CONSIDERATIONS

COMMENTS

- Hepatic abscess, containing both viable and dead worms, complicating *Ascaris*-induced biliary duct disease has been documented.
- Given the known transmission of the parasite, routine hand washing with soap and proper disposal of human waste would significantly decrease the prevalence of this disease.
- Other protective measures to avoid ingestion of worm eggs:
  1. Peel or cook food.
  2. Boil drinking water.
  3. Do not place small children directly on soil.

SUGGESTED READINGS

Available at www.expertconsult.com

RELATED CONTENT

Ascariasis (Patient Information)

AUTHOR: **GLENN G. FORT, M.D., M.P.H.**

BASIC INFORMATION

DEFINITION

Ascites is the accumulation of excess fluid (>25 mL) in the peritoneal cavity, most commonly caused by liver cirrhosis.

SYNONYMS

Fluid in peritoneal cavity
Hydroperitoneum
Hydroperitonia
Hydrops abdominis

ICD-10CM CODES

R18   Ascites
C78.6   Malignant ascites
K70.11   Alcoholic hepatitis with ascites
K70.31   Alcoholic cirrhosis of liver with ascites
K71.51   Toxic liver disease with chronic active hepatitis with ascites
R18.8   Other ascites

EPIDEMIOLOGY & DEMOGRAPHICS

Ascites is the most common complication of cirrhosis. Ascites occurs in 60% of individuals with cirrhosis within ten years of diagnosis. Cirrhosis is the cause of 75% of cases of ascites. Other causes include malignancy, heart failure, tuberculosis, pancreatitis, nephrotic syndrome, and Budd-Chiari syndrome.

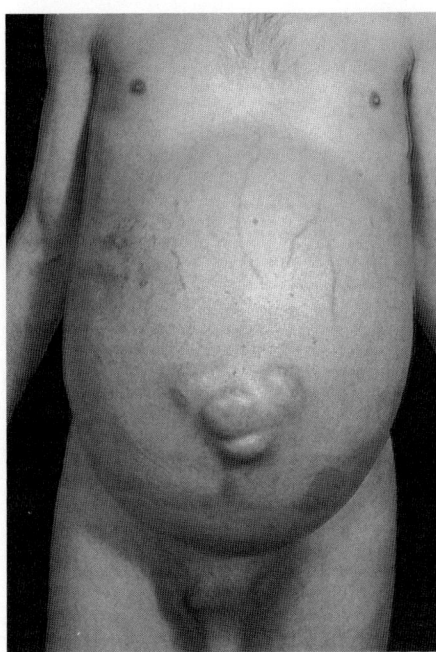

FIG. 1 Ascites in a patient with alcoholic cirrhosis showing distended abdomen; dilated superficial collateral veins; hemorrhagic scratch marks due to pruritus and coagulopathy; umbilical varices; and plaster in left iliac fossa indicating diagnostic paracentesis.
(From Forbes A et al [eds]: *Atlas of clinical gastroenterology*, ed 3, Oxford, 2005, Mosby.)

CLINICAL PRESENTATION

• Important information to elicit within history:
  1. History of viral hepatitis
  2. Alcoholism
  3. Increasing abdominal girth
  4. Increasing lower extremity edema
  5. Intravenous drug use
  6. Sexual history (i.e., men who have sex with men)
  7. History of transfusions
• Important physical exam findings:
  1. Bulging flanks
  2. Flank dullness to percussion
  3. Fluid wave on abdominal exam
  4. Lower extremity edema
  5. Shifting dullness on abdominal exam
  6. Physical signs associated with liver cirrhosis: spider angiomas, jaundice, loss of body hair, Dupuytren's contracture, muscle wasting, bruising, palmar erythema, gynecomastia, testicular atrophy, hemorrhoids, and caput medusae (Fig. 1)

ETIOLOGY

Pathophysiology of ascites (Fig. E2): increased hepatic resistance to portal flow leads to portal hypertension. The splanchnic vessels respond by increased secretion of nitric oxide, causing splanchnic artery vasodilation. Early in the disease increased plasma volume and increased cardiac output compensate for this vasodilation. However, as disease progresses the effective arterial blood volume decreases, causing sodium and fluid retention through activation of the renin-angiotensin system. The change in capillary pressure causes increased permeability and retention of fluid in the abdomen.

DIAGNOSIS

DIFFERENTIAL DIAGNOSIS

• Chronic parenchymal liver disease, leading to portal hypertension
• Peritoneal carcinomatosis
• Congestive heart failure
• Peritoneal tuberculosis
• Nephrotic syndrome
• Pancreatitis

LABORATORY TESTS

• Initial evaluation should always include:
  1. Diagnostic paracentesis (Fig. 3). Laboratory tests on this fluid should include a CBC with differential, albumin, total protein, culture, and Gram stain. A serum-ascites albumin gradient (SAAG) should be calculated in all patients.
     a. If the SAAG is greater than 1.1, the cause of ascites can be attributed to portal hypertension.
     b. If SAAG is less than 1.1, a non-portal hypertension etiology of ascites must be sought (see Table 1). Optional tests on paracentesis fluid include amylase, LDH, acid-fast bacilli, and glucose levels.
  2. AST, ALT, total and direct bilirubin, albumin, alkaline phosphatase, GGTP
  3. CBC, coagulation studies
  4. Electrolytes, BUN, creatinine

IMAGING STUDIES

• Abdominal ultrasound (Fig. 4) is the most sensitive measure for detecting ascitic fluid; a CT or MRI scan is a viable alternative.
• Endoscopy of the upper GI tract to evaluate for esophageal varices if ascites is secondary to portal hypertension.

TREATMENT

NONPHARMACOLOGIC THERAPY

• Sodium-restricted diet (<2 g/day).
• Fluid restriction to 1 L/day in patients with hyponatremia (sodium <130 mEq/L).

ACUTE GENERAL Rx

• Patients with moderate-volume ascites causing only moderate discomfort may be treated on an outpatient basis with the following diuretic regimen: spironolactone 50 to 200 mg daily or amiloride 5 to 10 mg daily. Add furosemide 20 to 40 mg/day in the first several days of treatment, monitoring renal function carefully for signs of prerenal azotemia (in patients without edema, goal weight loss is 300 to 500 g/day; in patients with edema it is 800 to 1000 g/day). Furosemide alone is not recommended.
• Patients with large-volume ascites causing marked discomfort or decrease in activities of daily living may also be treated as outpatients if there are no complications. There are two options for treatment in these patients:
  (1) large-volume paracentesis or
  (2) diuretic therapy until loss of fluid is noted (maximum spironolactone 400 mg daily and furosemide 160 mg daily).
No difference in long-term mortality rate was found; however, paracentesis is faster, more effective, and associated with fewer adverse effects.
• Table 2 summarizes primary medical therapy and adjunctive medications used to increase the efficacy of primary therapy in the treatment of ascites.

CHRONIC Rx

5% to 10% of patients with large-volume ascites will be refractory to high-dose diuretic treatment. Treatment strategies include repeated large-volume paracentesis with infusion of albumin every 2 to 4 weeks or placement of a transjugular intrahepatic portosystemic shunt (TIPS). Tolvaptan is reported to be effective in treating refractory ascites although no effect on prognosis has been reported. A treatment approach to patients with malignant ascites is described in Fig. E5.

DISPOSITION

Monitor closely for worsening liver function and development of spontaneous bacterial peritonitis (SBP).

REFERRAL

Referral to gastroenterology with ascites

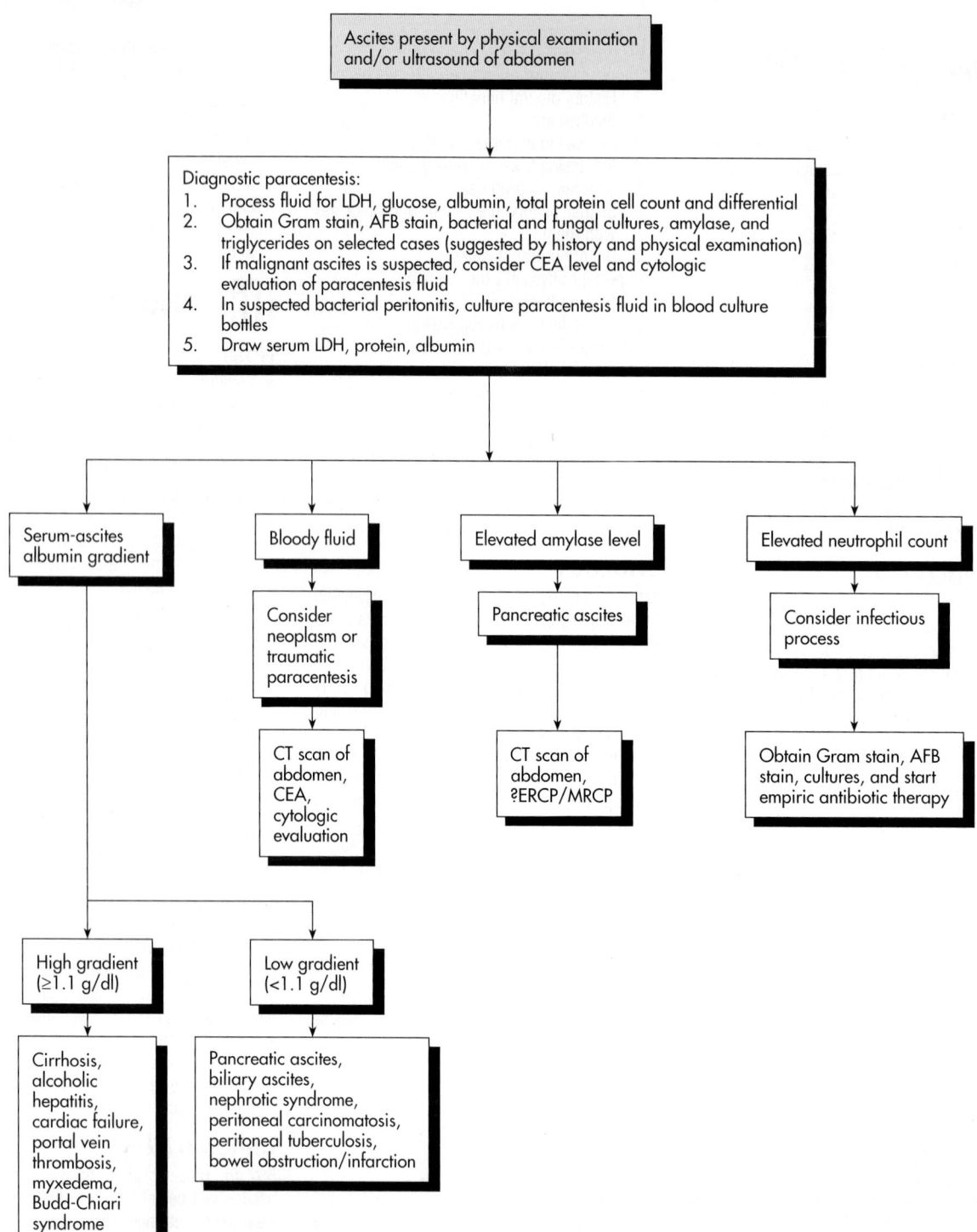

FIG. 3 Evaluation of ascites. *AFB,* Acid-fast bacillus; *CEA,* carcinoembryonic antigen; *CT,* computed tomography; *ERCP,* endoscopic retrograde cholangiopancreatography; *LDH,* lactate dehydrogenase; *MRCP,* magnetic resonance cholangiopancreatography.

TABLE 1 Using the Serum-Ascites Albumin Gradient and the Ascites Total Protein Level to Diagnose the Cause of Ascites

Condition	Serum-Ascites Albumin Gradient*	Ascites Total Protein Level†
Cirrhosis	High	Low
Malignant ascites	Low	High
Cardiac ascites	High	High

*High is greater than 1.1 g/dL; low is less than 1.1 g/dL.
†High is greater than 2.5 g/dL; low is less than 2.5 g/dL.
From Goldman L, Schafer AI: *Goldman's Cecil medicine,* ed 24, Philadelphia, 2012, Saunders.

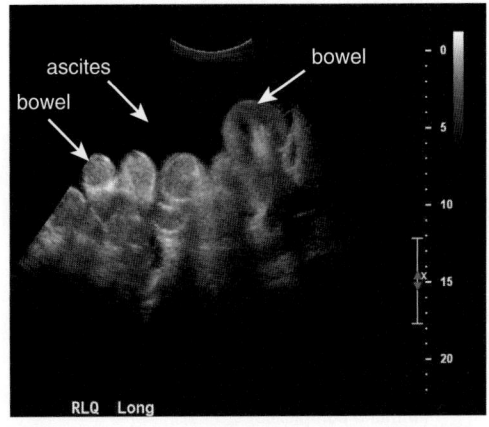

FIG. 4 Ascites, ultrasound. Ultrasound is useful for detection of ascites. Simple fluids such as ascites are excellent sound transmission media, reflecting almost no sound waves. As a consequence, they appear quite hypoechoic *(black)* on ultrasound. This view of the right lower quadrant shows loops of bowel surrounded by fluid. During the ultrasound, the bowel loops would be seen to undergo peristalsis and drift back and forth in the ascitic fluid with patient movement. Ultrasound cannot distinguish the composition of the fluid; ascites, liquid blood, liquid bile, urine, and infectious fluids have a similar appearance, with a few exceptions. Blood may coagulate and form septations within the fluid collection. Infectious fluids also frequently form loculated fluid collections that may be recognized on ultrasound, although the exact composition cannot be determined. (From Broder JS: *Diagnostic imaging for the emergency physician,* Philadelphia, 2011, Saunders.)

TABLE 2 Primary Medical Therapy and Adjunctive Medications Used to Increase the Efficacy of Primary Therapy in the Treatment of Ascites

Class	Medication	Dosing	Relevant Action	Notes
Diuretics	Spironolactone	400 mg + daily*	Aldosterone receptor antagonist	Primary therapy
	Furosemide	160 mg + daily*	Inhibits Na-K-2Cl symporter	Primary therapy
	Mannitol	20%*	Osmotic diuresis	Give dose just prior to furosemide and spironolactone
Vasoconstrictors	Octreotide	300 mcg bid*	Splanchnic vasoconstriction, inhibits RAAS	Also used in combination with midodrine to treat hepatorenal syndrome; given for first 5 days following variceal bleeding to decrease recurrence
	Midodrine	7.5 mg tid*	Inhibits RAAS	Also used in combination with octreotide and albumin to treat hepatorenal syndrome
α2-Agonist	Clonidine	0.075 mg bid*	Inhibits sympathetic outflow, inhibits RAAS	Increases sensitivity to spironolactone
Colloid	Albumin	25 g*	Increased oncotic pressure	Also utilized with large-volume paracentesis and in the treatment of hepatorenal syndrome
Aquaretics	None are FDA approved	N/A	Vasopressin receptor antagonist	May also treat hyponatremia

*The above doses have been derived from various studies and may not be suitable for all patients. Titration is always recommended.
From Cameron JL, Cameron AM: *Current surgical therapy,* ed 10, Philadelphia, 2011, Saunders.

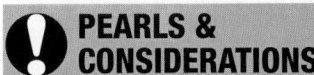 **PEARLS & CONSIDERATIONS**

COMMENTS

- Prevalence of SBP in patients with ascites ranges between 10% and 30%.
  - Presence of at least 250 neutrophils per cubic millimeter of ascitic fluid is diagnostic.
  - Gram negative bacteria such as *E. coli* are the most common isolates.
  - Third-generation cephalosporins are the treatment of choice.

- By 1 year, 70% of patients have recurrence of SBP and may be prophylaxed with trimethoprim/sulfamethoxazole DS 1 tab PO bid 5 days/wk or ciprofloxacin 750 mg PO once/wk.

PREVENTION

Prevention of liver cirrhosis through avoidance of long-term use of alcohol, immunization against hepatitis A and B, and treatment of hepatitis C.

SUGGESTED READINGS

Available at www.expertconsult.com

RELATED CONTENT

Ascites (Patient Information)
Cirrhosis (Related Key Topic)

AUTHORS: **JOANNE M. SILVIA, M.D.,** and **PAUL F. GEORGE, M.D, M.H.P.E.**

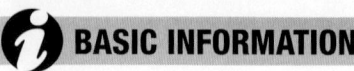

DEFINITION

Aspergillosis refers to several forms of a broad range of illnesses caused by infection with *Aspergillus* species.

ICD-10CM CODES
B44.0	Invasive pulmonary aspergillosis
B44.1	Other pulmonary aspergillosis
B44.2	Tonsillar aspergillosis
B44.7	Disseminated aspergillosis
B44.81	Allergic bronchopulmonary aspergillosis
B44.89	Other forms of aspergillosis
B44.9	Aspergillosis, unspecified

EPIDEMIOLOGY & DEMOGRAPHICS

INCIDENCE & PREVALENCE:

- *Aspergillus* species are ubiquitous in the environment internationally and occur as a mold found in soil.
- Cause a variety of illness from hypersensitivity pneumonitis to disseminated overwhelming infection in immunosuppressed patients.
- Frequently cultured from hospital wards from unfiltered outside air circulating through open windows as well as water sources.
- Reach the patient by airborne conidia (spores) that are small enough (2.5 to 3 μm) to reach the alveoli on inhalation.
- Can invade the nose, paranasal sinuses, external ear, or traumatized skin.

RISK FACTORS:

- The clinical syndrome depends on the underlying lung architecture, the host's immune response, and the degree of inoculum.
- Incidence of invasive aspergillosis is increasing with advances in the treatment of life-threatening diseases, such as aggressive chemotherapy or bone marrow and organ transplantation. It also can rarely occur in normal hosts, especially associated with influenza A. Liver and lung transplant recipients are at highest risk for pulmonary disease. Genetic deficiency of the soluble-pattern-recognition receptor known as long pentraxin 3 (PTX3) affects the antifungal capacity of neutrophils and may contribute to the risk of invasive aspergillosis in patients treated with hematopoietic stem-cell transplantation (HSCT).
- Patients with AIDS and a CD4 count <50/mm³ have an increased susceptibility to invasive aspergillosis, but it is otherwise uncommon in patients with HIV.
- Pandemic influenza A (H1N1) infection may predispose immunocompromised patients to invasive aspergillosis.

ETIOLOGY

- *A. fumigatus* is the usual cause.
- *A. flavus* is the second most important species, particularly in invasive disease of immunosuppressed patients and in lesions beginning in the nose and paranasal sinuses. *A. niger* can also cause invasive human infection.

ALLERGIC ASPERGILLOSIS:

- Is a hypersensitivity pneumonitis.
- Presents as cough, dyspnea, fever, chills, and malaise typically 4 to 8 hr after exposure.
- Repeated attacks can lead to granulomatous disease and pulmonary fibrosis.

ALLERGIC BRONCHOPULMONARY ASPERGILLOSIS (ABPA):

- Symptoms occur most commonly in atopic individuals during the third and fourth decades of life.
- Hypersensitivity reaction to *Aspergillus* fungal antigens present in the bronchial tree.
- Results from an initial type I (immediate hypersensitivity) and type III reactions (immune complexes).
- Underdiagnosed pulmonary disorder in patients with asthma and cystic fibrosis (reported prevalence in asthmatic patients varies from 6% to 28% and in cystic fibrosis 6% to 25%).

ASPERGILLOMAS ("FUNGUS BALLS"):

- In the absence of invasion or significant immune response, *Aspergillus* can colonize a preexisting cavity, causing pulmonary aspergilloma.
- Forms masses of tangled hyphal elements, fibrin, and mucus.
- Patients typically have a history of chronic lung disease, tuberculosis, sarcoidosis, or emphysema.
- Manifests commonly as hemoptysis.
- Many are asymptomatic.

INVASIVE ASPERGILLOSIS:

- Patients with prolonged and profound granulocytopenia or impaired phagocytic function are predisposed to rapidly progressive *Aspergillus* pneumonia.
- Typically a necrotizing bronchopneumonia, ranging from small areas of infiltrate to intensive bilateral hemorrhagic infarction.
- Most common presentation: unremitting fever and a new pulmonary infiltrate despite broad-spectrum antibiotic therapy in an immunosuppressed patient.
- Dyspnea and nonproductive cough are common; sudden pleuritic pain and tachycardia, sometimes with a pleural rub, may mimic pulmonary embolism; hemoptysis is uncommon.
- Chest radiograph (CXR) may reveal patchy bronchopneumonic, nodular densities, consolidation, or cavitation. High-resolution CT scan is more sensitive and specific than CXR in neutropenic patients.
- Immunocompromised patients: invasive pulmonary *Aspergillus* (IPA) generally is acute and evolves over days to weeks; less commonly, patients with normal or only mild abnormalities of the immune system may develop a more chronic, slowly progressive form of IPA.

EXTRAPULMONARY DISSEMINATION:

- Cerebral infarction from hematogenous dissemination may occur in immunosuppressed individuals.
- Abscess formation from direct extension or invasive disease in the sinuses.
- Esophageal or gastrointestinal ulcerations may occur in the immunosuppressed host.
- Fatal perforation of the viscus or bowel infarction may occur.
- Necrotizing skin ulcers involving the extremities (Fig. 1).
- Osteomyelitis.
- Endocarditis in patients who have recently undergone open heart surgery.
- Infection of an implantable cardioverter-defibrillator has been reported.

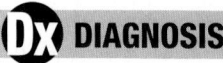 **DIAGNOSIS**

DIFFERENTIAL DIAGNOSIS

- Tuberculosis
- Cystic fibrosis
- Carcinoma of the lung
- Eosinophilic pneumonia
- Bronchiectasis
- Sarcoidosis
- Lung abscess

WORKUP

Physical examination and laboratory data

LABORATORY TESTS

ABPA:

- Peripheral blood eosinophilia and an elevated total serum immunoglobulin E (IgE) level.
- Skin test with *Aspergillus* antigenic extract is usually positive but nonspecific.
- *Aspergillus* serum precipitating antibody is present in 70% to 100% of cases.
- Sputum cultures may be positive for *Aspergillus* spp. but are nonspecific.

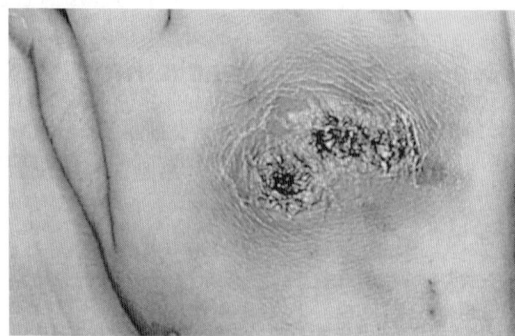

FIG. 1 Cutaneous aspergillosis in a patient with acute leukemia and marked neutropenia. The lesion developed at the site where a steel needle had been left for several days of intravenous infusion. (From Mandell GL [ed]: *Mandell, Douglas, and Bennett's principles and practice of infectious diseases,* ed 6, New York, 2005, Churchill Livingstone.)

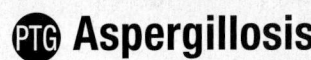

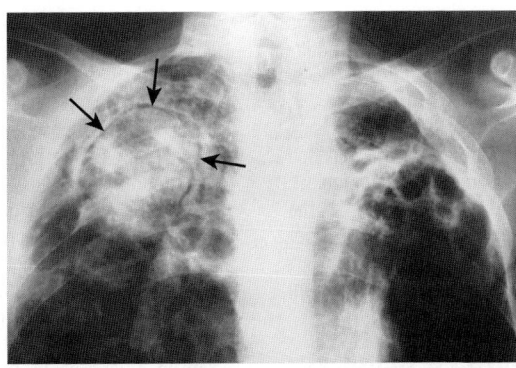

FIG. 2 Fungus ball or mycetoma caused by *Aspergillus*. Coned-down posteroanterior view of the chest of a patient with biapical fibrocavitary tuberculosis accompanied by volume loss. There is a mass in a large right upper-lobe cavity with air dissecting into the cavity producing "air crescents" *(arrows)*. (From McLoud TC: *Thoracic radiology: the requisites,* St Louis, 1998, Mosby.)

ASPERGILLOMAS:
- Sputum culture
- Serum precipitating antibody

Invasive aspergillosis: definitive diagnosis requires the demonstration of tissue invasion (i.e., septate, acute angle branching hyphae) or a positive culture from the tissue obtained by an invasive procedure such as transbronchial biopsy.
- Sputum and nasal cultures: in high-risk patients a positive culture is strongly suggestive of invasive aspergillosis.
- Serology: the *Platelia Aspergillus* ELISA assay detects a circulating fungal antigen, galactomannan. Galactomannan is a polysaccharide contained in the cell wall of *Aspergillus.* Its presence in serum or other body fluids is indicative of invasive infection, and it is recommended as an accurate marker for diagnosis in certain patient subpopulations (hematologic malignancy and hematopoietic stem cell transplantation). The β-D glucan assay can also be used to detect early infection, but is not specific for *Aspergillus* species.
- Blood cultures: usually negative.
- Lung biopsy is necessary for definitive diagnosis.
- Biopsy and culture of extrapulmonary lesions.
- Real-time polymerase chain reaction tests are investigational.

IMAGING STUDIES
ABPA:
- CXRs show a variety of abnormalities, from small, patchy, fleeting infiltrates (commonly in the upper lobes) to lobar consolidation or cavitation.
- A majority of patients eventually develop central bronchiectasis.

ASPERGILLOMAS: CXR or CT scans usually show the characteristic intracavity mass par-

tially surrounded by a crescent of air ("halo sign") (Fig. 2).

INVASIVE ASPERGILLOSIS: CXR and CT scanning may also reveal cavity formation and the halo sign. Air bronchograms typically disappear as they are filled with hemorrhagic fluid.

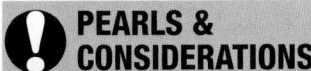 **TREATMENT**

ACUTE GENERAL Rx
ABPA:
- Prednisone (0.5 to 1 mg/kg PO) until the CXR has cleared, followed by alternate-day therapy at 0.5 mg/kg PO (3 to 6 mo).
- If a patient is corticosteroid dependent, prophylaxis for the prevention of *Pneumocystis jiroveci* infection and maintenance of bone mineralization should be considered.
- Bronchodilators and physiotherapy.
- Serial CXR and serum IgE is useful in guiding treatment.
- Itraconazole 200 mg PO bid for 4 to 6 mo, then taper over 4 to 6 mo may be considered as a steroid-sparing agent or if steroids are ineffective.

ASPERGILLOMAS:
- Controversial and problematic; the optimal treatment strategy is unknown.
- Up to 10% of aspergillomas may resolve clinically without overt pharmacologic or surgical intervention.
- Observation for asymptomatic patients.
- Surgical resection/arterial embolization for those patients with severe hemoptysis or life-threatening hemorrhage.
- For those patients at risk for marked hemoptysis with inadequate pulmonary reserve, consider itraconazole 200 to 400 mg/day PO.

INVASIVE ASPERGILLOSIS (IA):
- Voriconazole 6 mg/kg IV/PO bid on day 1 followed by 4 mg/kg IV/PO bid. Voriconazole

serum concentrations need to be monitored to achieve a target range of 1.0 to 5.5 mg/L (trough on day 4).
- Isavuconazole 200 mg (which equals 372 mg of prodrug isavuconazonium sulfate) IV/PO tid for six doses and then 200 mg PO/IV daily. Alternative Treatment:
- Amphotericin B lipid complex (ABLC) 5 mg/kg IV daily.
- Liposomal amphotericin B (L-AMB) 3 to 5 mg/kg IV daily.
- Posaconazole 200 delayed-release tabs 300 mg PO for two doses, then 300 mg PO daily or posaconazole 300 mg IV over 90 minutes bid for one day, then 300 mg IV daily.
- Because azoles and echinocandins target different cellular sites, combination therapy may have additive activity against *Aspergillus* species. Although still under investigation, some bone marrow transplant units use caspofungin and voriconazole as the preferred initial treatment, especially in patients receiving high-dose corticosteroids. Recent trials (Marr et al., 2015) have shown that compared with voriconazole monotherapy, combination therapy with anidulafungin, and echinocandin antifungal drug that blocks the synthesis of (13)β-D glucan led to higher survival in subgroups of patients with IA.

REFERRAL
To an infectious diseases specialist

! PEARLS & CONSIDERATIONS

- Unlike fluconazole, the potential for drug-drug interactions with voriconazole is high. Azoles may interact with drugs used for chemotherapy by increasing toxicity and/or by reducing efficacy.
- Agitation of hospital buildings by renovations or repairs may increase the incidence of *Aspergillus* infections in immunosuppressed individuals.
- Echinocandins should never be used as primary treatment of aspergillosis.

SUGGESTED READINGS
Available at www.expertconsult.com

RELATED CONTENT
Aspergillosis (Patient Information)

AUTHOR: **SAJEEV HANDA, M.D.**

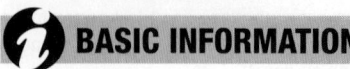
BASIC INFORMATION

DEFINITION

The National Asthma Education and Prevention Program (NAEPP) guidelines define asthma as "a chronic inflammatory disease of the airways in which many cells and cellular elements play a role: in particular mast cells, neutrophils, eosinophils, T lymphocytes, macrophages, and epithelial cells. In susceptible individuals, this inflammation causes recurrent episodes of coughing (particularly at night or early in the morning), wheezing, breathlessness, and chest tightness. The episodes are usually associated with widespread but variable airflow obstruction that is reversible either spontaneously or as a result of treatment."
Status asthmaticus, or acute severe asthma, is a refractory state that does not respond to standard therapy such as inhaled beta-agonists or subcutaneous epinephrine. It may persist for several hours.

SYNONYMS

Bronchospasm
Reactive airway disease
Asthmatic bronchitis

ICD-10CM CODES
J45.20	Mild intermittent asthma, uncomplicated
J45.21	Mild intermittent asthma with (acute) exacerbation
J45.22	Mild intermittent asthma with status asthmaticus
J45.30	Mild persistent asthma, uncomplicated
J45.31	Mild persistent asthma with (acute) exacerbation
J45.32	Mild persistent asthma with status asthmaticus
J45.40	Moderate persistent asthma, uncomplicated
J45.41	Moderate persistent asthma with (acute) exacerbation
J45.42	Moderate persistent asthma with status asthmaticus
J45.50	Severe persistent asthma, uncomplicated
J45.51	Severe persistent asthma with (acute) exacerbation
J45.52	Severe persistent asthma with status asthmaticus
J45.901	Unspecified asthma with (acute) exacerbation
J45.902	Unspecified asthma with status asthmaticus
J45.909	Unspecified asthma, uncomplicated
J45.991	Cough variant asthma
J45.998	Other asthma

EPIDEMIOLOGY & DEMOGRAPHICS

- Asthma affects more than 12% of the population in the United States, and its prevalence is steadily rising.
- It accounts for around 440,000 hospitalizations and 1.8 million emergency department visits yearly in the United States.
- It is more common in children, but the gap is closing because of a rapid increase in adult-onset asthma (9.5% of children vs 8.2% of adults).
- 50% to 80% of children with asthma develop symptoms before 5 yr of age. Early childhood risk factors for asthma are described in Table 1.
- The overall asthma mortality rate in the United States has slightly improved to 11 per 1 million persons.
- Seniors have a high level of mortality from their asthma.

PHYSICAL FINDINGS & CLINICAL PRESENTATION

Physical examination varies with the stage and severity of asthma and may reveal normal lung examination results in many patients. However, some degree of wheezing and prolonged expiratory phases of respiration are seen with persistent or acute disease. Physical examination during status asthmaticus may reveal:
- Tachycardia and tachypnea
- Use of accessory respiratory muscles
- Pulsus paradoxus (inspiratory decline in systolic blood pressure >10 mm Hg)
- Absence of wheezing (silent chest) or decreased wheezing can indicate worsening obstruction
- Mental status changes: generally secondary to hypoxia and hypercapnia and constitute an indication for urgent intubation
- Paradoxic abdominal and diaphragmatic movement on inspiration (detected by palpation over the upper part of the abdomen in a semirecumbent position) indicates diaphragmatic fatigue, another sign of impending respiratory crisis
- The following abnormalities in vital signs are indicative of severe asthma:
  1. Pulsus paradoxus >18 mm Hg
  2. Respiratory rate >30 breaths/min
  3. Tachycardia with heart rate >120 beats/min

ETIOLOGY

- The pathophysiology of asthma involves a complex interaction among various environmental and genetic factors.

TABLE 1 Early Childhood Risk Factors for Persistent Asthma

Parental asthma
Allergy:
 Atopic dermatitis (eczema)
 Allergic rhinitis
 Food allergy
 Inhalant allergen sensitization
 Food allergen sensitization
Severe lower respiratory tract infection:
 Pneumonia
 Bronchiolitis requiring hospitalization
Wheezing apart from colds
Male gender
Low birthweight
Environmental tobacco smoke exposure
Possible use of acetaminophen (paracetamol)
Exposure to chlorinated swimming pools
Reduced lung function at birth

From Kliegman RM et al: *Nelson textbook of pediatrics,* ed 19, Philadelphia, 2011, Saunders.

- Allergic (extrinsic) asthma is triggered by various aeroallergens or nonspecific (e.g., dust, cigarette smoke, fumes, cold air, exercise) exposures in patients who are prone to develop Ig E antibodies in response to various exposures.
- A recent study of a prebirth cohort observed that maternal intake of foods commonly considered allergenic (peanut and milk) was associated with a decrease in allergy and asthma in the offspring. No dietary changes during pregnancy are therefore recommended for prevention of allergies or asthma.
- A recent trial revealed that supplementation with n-3 long-chain polyunsaturated fatty acids (LCPUFAs, fish oil-derived fatty acids) in the third trimester of pregnancy reduced the absolute risk of persistent wheeze or asthma and infections of the lower respiratory tract in offspring by approximately 7 percentage points, or one third.[1]
- Nonallergic (intrinsic) asthma commonly manifests as adult-onset asthma in response to respiratory tract infection or psychological stress.
- Occupation exposure to certain organic or nonorganic agents can trigger asthma.
- Evidence suggests that dampness and mold contribute to the risk of developing asthma and that remediation of these in homes reduces asthma symptoms and medication use in adults.
- Exercise-induced asthma is seen most frequently in adolescents and manifests with bronchospasm after beginning of exercise and improves with discontinuation of exercise.
- Drug-induced asthma is associated with use of NSAIDs, β-blockers, sulfites, and certain foods and beverages.
- There is a strong association of the *ADAM 33* gene with asthma and bronchial hyper-responsiveness. Experimental, genetic, and clinical studies support an important role for Th2 immune pathways in the pathogenesis of severe asthma. Th2 cells are stimulated by dendritic cells to produce IL-5, IL-13, and IL-4, the latter driving IgE synthesis. This group is characterized by eosinophilia, and IL-5 is felt to be the most specific cytokine in eosinophil regulatory pathways.

DIAGNOSIS

DIFFERENTIAL DIAGNOSIS

- Postinfectious bronchitis
- Rhinitis with postnasal drip
- COPD
- GERD
- Pneumonia and other upper respiratory infections
- Foreign body aspiration (most frequent in younger patients)
- Anxiety disorder
- Diffuse interstitial lung disease
- Hypersensitivity pneumonitis
- CHF
- Pulmonary embolism (in adult and elderly patients)

---

[1]Bisgaard H, et al.: Fish oil-derived fatty acids in pregnancy and wheeze and asthma in offspring, *N Engl J Med* 375:2530-2539, 2016.

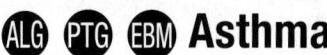

WORKUP

- Diagnosis of asthma requires documentation of airway obstruction and some degree of reversibility of the obstruction, if and when patient can participate.
- For symptomatic adults and children age >5 yr who can perform spirometry, pre- and postbronchodilator spirometry is the recommended test of choice.
- Airflow reversibility is defined as increase in forced expiratory volume in 1 sec (FEV_1 by at least 12% increase and 200 mL) after inhaling a short bronchodilator.
- The degree of reversibility measured by spirometry correlates with airway inflammation, and patients with a high degree of reversibility have a greater risk of irreversible airflow obstruction in subsequent years.
- For children age<5 yr, spirometry is generally not feasible. Young children with asthma symptoms should be treated as having suspected asthma after alternative diagnoses are ruled out.
- Negative spirometry results do not rule out asthma. Patients with high clinical suspicion should undergo bronchial challenge test using methacholine or other specific agents.
- The clinician should evaluate for environmental causes (e.g., house dust mites, indoor pets) and exposure to other allergens such as tobacco smoke. The degree of reversibility measured by spirometry correlates with airway inflammation, and patients with a high degree of

reversibility have a greater risk of irreversible airflow obstruction in subsequent years.
- In the absence of spirometry testing, variability of peak flow measurements by a handheld device can be used to diagnose asthma.
- After the diagnosis of asthma is confirmed, the clinician should evaluate for environmental triggers (e.g., house dust mites, indoor pets) and exposure to other allergens such as tobacco smoke.
- Fig. E1 describes an algorithm for diagnosing asthma.
  After diagnosis, the severity of asthma should be classified during the initial assessment before initiating therapy. Patients are divided into four groups based on the severity of their asthma symptoms and number of exacerbations (see Table 2).
- Once therapy is initiated, the emphasis for clinical management should gear toward achievement of asthma control. The level of asthma control should be used to guide decisions either to maintain or adjust therapy.
- Schedule visits at 2- to 6-wk intervals for patients who are just starting therapy or who require a step up in therapy to achieve or regain asthma control. Schedule visits at 6- to 12-mo intervals, after asthma control is achieved, to monitor whether asthma control is maintained. The interval will depend on factors such as the duration of asthma control or the level of treatment required. Consider scheduling visits at 3-mo intervals if step-down therapy is anticipated.

LABORATORY TESTS

Laboratory tests are usually not necessary and the results can be normal if obtained during a stable period.

- Arterial blood gases (ABGs) can be used during acute bronchospasm in staging the severity of an asthmatic attack:
  1. Mild: decreased PaO_2 and $PaCO_2$, increased pH
  2. Moderate: decreased PaO_2, normal $PaCO_2$, normal pH
  3. Severe: marked decreased PaO_2, increased $PaCO_2$, and decreased pH
- Complete blood count: leukocytosis with left shift may indicate the existence of bacterial infection. Elevated eosinophils point toward allergic component of asthma.
- Spirometry is recommended at the initial assessment and at least every 1 to 2 yr after treatment is initiated and when the symptoms and peak expiratory flow have stabilized. Spirometry as a monitoring measure may be performed more frequently, if indicated, based on severity of symptoms and the disease's lack of response to treatment.
- Peak expiratory flow rate (PEFR) can be used to assess severity of an acute exacerbation episode. Value should be compared with individual's personal best number (see asthma action plan).
- Serum IgE levels help guide treatment for patients with severe persistent asthma, and they also help monitor response to treatment in the same group.

TABLE 2 Classifying Asthma Severity and Initiating Treatment in Youths ≥12 Yr and Adults (Assessing severity and initiating treatment for patients who are not currently taking long-term control medications)

| | | | **CLASSIFICATION OF ASTHMA SEVERITY (≥12 yr)** | | |
| | | | | **PERSISTENT** | |
Components of Severity		**Intermittent**	**Mild**	**Moderate**	**Severe**
Impairment Normal FEV_1/ FVC: yr85% yr80% yr75% yr70%	Symptoms	≤2 days/wk	>2 days/wk but not daily	Daily	Throughout the day
	Nighttime awakenings	≤2x/mo	3-4x/mo	>1x/wk but not nightly	Often 7x/wk
	Short-acting beta₂-agonist use for symptom control (not prevention of EIB)	≤2 days/wk	>2 days/wk but not daily, and not more than 1x on any day	Daily	Several times per day
	Interference with normal activity	None	Minor limitation	Some limitation	Extremely limited
	Lung function	Normal FEV_1 between exacerbations			
		FEV_1>80% predicted	FEV_1>80% predicted	FEV_1>60% but <80% predicted	FEV_1<60% predicted
		FEV_1/FVC normal	FEV_1/FVC normal	FEV_1/FVC reduced 5%	FEV_1/FVC reduced>5%
Risk	Exacerbations requiring oral systemic corticosteroids	0-1 per yr	≥2 per yr		
		Consider severity and interval since last exacerbation. Frequency and severity may fluctuate over time for patients in any severity category. Relative annual risk of exacerbations may be related to FEV_1.			
Recommended Step for Initiating Therapy		Step 1	Step 2	Step 3	Step 4 or 5 and consider short course of oral systemic corticosteroids
		In 2-6 wk, evaluate level of asthma control that is achieved and adjust therapy accordingly.			

The stepwise approach is meant to assist, not replace, the clinical decision-making required to meet individual patient needs.
Level of severity is determined by assessment of both impairment and risk. Assess impairment domain by patient's/caregiver's recall of previous 2-4 wk and spirometry. Assign severity to the most severe category in which any feature occurs.
At present, there are inadequate data to correspond frequencies of exacerbations with different levels of asthma severity. In general, more frequent and intense exacerbations (e.g., requiring urgent, unscheduled care, hospitalization, or ICU admission) indicate greater underlying disease severity. For treatment purposes, patients who had ≥2 exacerbations requiring oral systemic corticosteroids in the past year may be considered the same as patients who have persistent asthma, even in the absence of impairment levels consistent with persistent asthma.
To access the complete *Expert Panel Report 3: Guidelines for the Diagnosis and Management of Asthma,* go to www.nhlbi.nih.gov/guidelines/asthma/asthgdln.pdf.
EIB, Exercise-induced bronchospasm; FEV_1, forced expiratory volume in 1 second; *FVC,* forced vital capacity; *ICU,* intensive care unit.
From National Asthma Education and Prevention Program: *Expert panel report 3: Guidelines for diagnosis and management of asthma,* National Institutes of Health, National Heart, Lung, and Blood Institute, August 2007, NIH publication 08-4051.

- Specific allergy testing may be helpful in a subgroup of patients.

IMAGING STUDIES

- Chest x-ray: usually normal, may show evidence of thoracic hyperinflation (e.g., flattening of the diaphragm, increased volume over the retrosternal air space).
- ECG: tachycardia, nonspecific ST-T wave changes are common during an asthma attack; may also show cor pulmonale, right bundle branch block, right axial deviation, counterclockwise rotation.

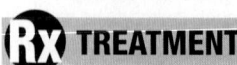 **TREATMENT**

NONPHARMACOLOGIC THERAPY

- Avoidance of triggering factors (e.g., salicylates, sulfites), environmental or occupational triggers

- Encouragement of regular exercise (e.g., swimming)
- Patient education regarding warning signs of an attack and proper use of medications (e.g., correct use of inhalers)

GENERAL Rx

The 2007 NAEPP guidelines (see Tables 2 to 10) provide treatment options by age groups: 0 to 4 yr, 5 to 11 yr, and >12 yr. A step-up approach is described based on the severity of symptoms.

An approach to home management of acute asthma is described in Fig. E2. Short-acting beta-selective adrenergic agonists (SABAs) administered by inhalation is the most effective therapy for quick relief of asthmatic symptoms. They are recommended for use only as needed for relief of symptoms or before anticipated exposure to known triggers such as exercise. They should not be use as a single agent except for intermittent asthma symptoms. When symptoms become more frequent or more severe, step-up treatment with maintenance inhalers is recommended (see Table 4). Inhaled steroid is the mainstay of treatment for maintenance therapy. Other treatment options include long-acting beta-agonist (LABA), combination of inhaled steroids and LABA, leukotriene receptor antagonist (LTRA), cromolyn, zileuton, and theophylline. Oral corticosteroids are reserved as a last resort for maintenance therapy for recalcitrant cases. Long-acting muscarinic antagonists (LAMAs) are only approved for treatment of COPD, but various studies have showed some degree of benefit when adding LAMA to ICS + LABA. There are several corticosteroid/LABA combination inhalers available (fluticasone/salmeterol [Advair], budesonide/formoterol [Symbicort], mometasone/formoterol [Dulera], and ICS/LABA fluticasone furoate 200 mcg and vilanterol 25

TABLE 3 Assessing Asthma Control and Adjusting Therapy in Youths ≥12 Yr and Adults

	Components of Control	CLASSIFICATION OF ASTHMA CONTROL (≥12 yr)		
		Well Controlled	**Not Well Controlled**	**Very Poorly Controlled**
Impairment	Symptoms	≤2 days/wk	>2 days/wk	Throughout the day
	Nighttime awakenings	≤2×/mo	1-3x/wk	≥4/wk
	Interference with normal activity	None	Some limitation	Extremely limited
	Short-acting beta$_2$-agonist use for symptom control (not prevention of EIB)	≤2 days/wk	>2 days/wk	Several times per day
	FEV$_1$ or peak flow	>80% predicted/personal best	60%-80% predicted/personal best	<60% predicted/personal best
	Validated questionnaires			
	ATAQ	0	1-2	3-4
	ACQ	≤0.75*	≥1.5	N/A
	ACT™	≥20	16-19	≤15
Risk	Exacerbations requiring oral systemic corticosteroids	0-1 per yr	≥2 per yr	
		Consider severity and interval since last exacerbation		
	Progressive loss of lung function	Evaluation requires long-term follow-up care		
	Treatment-related adverse effects	Medication side effects can vary in intensity from none to very troublesome and worrisome. The level of intensity does not correlate to specific levels of control but should be considered in the overall assessment of risk.		
Recommended Action for Treatment		Maintain current step. Regular follow-up every 1-6 mo to maintain control. Consider step down if well controlled for at least 3 mo.	Step up 1 step and reevaluate in 2-6 wk. For side effects, consider alternative treatment options.	Consider short course of oral systemic corticosteroids. Step up 1-2 steps. Reevaluate in 2 wk. For side effects, consider alternative treatment options.

The stepwise approach is meant to assist, not replace, the clinical decision-making required to meet individual patient needs.

The level of control is based on the most severe impairment or risk category. Assess impairment domain by patient's recall of previous 2-4 wk and by spirometry or peak flow measures.

Symptom assessment for longer periods should reflect a global assessment, such as inquiring whether the patient's asthma is better or worse since the last visit.

At present, there are inadequate data to correspond frequencies of exacerbations with different levels of asthma control. In general, more frequent and intense exacerbations (e.g., requiring urgent, unscheduled care, hospitalization, or ICU admission) indicate poorer disease control. For treatment purposes, patients who had ≥2 exacerbations requiring oral systemic corticosteroids in the past year may be considered the same as patients who have not-well-controlled asthma, even in the absence of impairment levels consistent with not-well-controlled asthma.

Validated questionnaires for the impairment domain (the questionnaires do not assess lung function or the risk domain)

    —ATAQ = Asthma Therapy Assessment Questionnaire

    —ACQ = Asthma Control Questionnaire (user package may be obtained at www.qoltech.co.uk or juniper@qoltech.co.uk)

    —ACT = Asthma Control Test™

    —Minimal Important Difference: 1.0 for the ATAQ; 0.5 for the ACQ; not determined for the ACT

Before step up in therapy:

    —Review adherence to medication, inhaler technique, environmental control, and comorbid conditions

    —If an alternative treatment option was used in a step, discontinue and use the preferred treatment for that step

EIB, Exercise-induced bronchospasm; *FEV$_1$*, forced expiratory volume in 1 second; *ICU*, intensive care unit.

The Asthma Control Test is a trademark of QualityMetric Incorporated.

*ACQ values of 0.76-1.4 are indeterminate regarding well-controlled asthma.

From National Asthma Education and Prevention Program: *Expert panel report 3: Guidelines for diagnosis and management of asthma*, National Institutes of Health, National Heart, Lung, and Blood Institute, August 2007, NIH publication 08-4051.

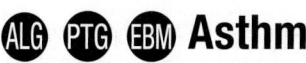
A

Diseases and Disorders

mcg inhalation powder [Breo Ellipta]) on the market. None of these combinations is indicated for the initial treatment of asthma or for acute therapy of asthma symptoms. There is no evidence that one product is more effective than the others.

IMMUNOLOGIC TARGETS

Omalizumab, an anti-IgE monoclonal antibody, is indicated for the treatment of moderate and severe persistent asthma with elevated IgE level, which is refractory to other treatment noted earlier. It is administered subcutaneously every 2 or 4 wk. This medicine is expensive ($10,000 to $30,000/yr). Patients should be closely monitored in the first month because omalizumab can result in allergic reactions (anaphylaxis) in 1 to 2 patients/1000. The NIH guidelines recommend considering omalizumab only after consultation with an asthma specialist. Recent trials (Wenzel et al) have also shown that in patients with persistent, moderate to severe asthma and elevated eosinophil levels who used inhaled glucocorticoids

and LABAs, therapy with the human monoclonal antibody dupilumab, as compared with placebo, was associated with fewer asthma exacerbations when LABAs and inhaled glucocorticoids were withdrawn, with improved lung function and reduced levels of Th2-associated inflammatory markers. Another recent trial evaluated the role of a novel DNA enzyme, which inactivates GATA3 messenger RNA and thus prevents transcription of various cytokines involved in the Th2 pathway. The study showed significant attenuation of both late and early asthmatic responses after allergen provocation in patients with allergic asthma who were treated with once-daily inhalation of this drug for 28 days.[1]

Since 2015, Mepolizumab (Nucala), an anti-interleukin-5 treatment, has been approved by the FDA as an add-on for patients aged ≥12 yr with severe eosinophilic asthma that is uncontrolled on Step 4 treatment. Mepolizumab is a monoclonal antibody to IL-5 that has been shown to reduce exacerbations in patients with severe asthma who

---
[1]N Engl J Med 2015;372:1987-1995.

have blood eosinophil counts of 150/μL or greater. Mepolizumab is administered subcutaneously into the upper arm, thigh, or abdomen, 100 mg every 4 weeks. Hypersensitivity reactions have been reported with mepolizumab. In addition, herpes zoster infections have led to the recommendation of the administration of the varicella zoster vaccine to adults ages 50 or older 4 weeks prior to initiation of mepolizumab (unless they are at risk for disseminated zoster).

Reslizumab, another anti-IL-5 monoclonal antibody, has a similar indication for eosinophilic asthma and uses a higher eosinophil cutoff (400) based on a greater predictive value for sputum eosinophilia.

Anti-IL-13: IL-13 promotes IgE production by B cells, generation of eosinophil chemoattractants, and contractility of airway smooth muscle cells and is therefore of interest as a potential target for asthma therapy. Preliminary clinical studies, however, have not documented a benefit to anti-IL-13 monoclonal antibodies such as lebrikizumab and tralokinumab.

TABLE 4 Stepwise Approach for Managing Asthma in Youths ≥12 Yr and Adults

Intermittent Asthma	Persistent Asthma: Daily Medication Consult with asthma specialist if step 4 care or higher is required. Consider consultation at step 3.

Step 1
Preferred:
SABA prn

Step 2
Preferred:
Low-dose ICS

Alternative:
Cromolyn, LTRA, nedocromil, or theophylline

Step 3
Preferred:
Low-dose ICS + LABA
OR
Medium-dose ICS

Alternative:
Low-dose ICS + either LTRA, theophylline, or zileuton

Step 4
Preferred:
Medium-dose ICS + LABA

Alternative:
Medium-dose ICS + either LTRA, theophylline, or zileuton

Step 5
Preferred:
High-dose ICS + LABA

AND

Consider omalizumab for patients who have allergies

Step 6
Preferred:
High-dose ICS + LABA + oral corticosteroid

AND

Consider omalizumab for patients who have allergies

Step up if needed
(first, check adherence, environmental control, and comorbid conditions)

Assess control

Step down if possible
(and asthma is well controlled at least 3 months)

Each step: Patient education, environmental control, and management of comorbidities
Steps 2-4: Consider subcutaneous allergen immunotherapy for patients who have allergic asthma

Quick-Relief Medication for All Patients
• SABA as needed for symptoms. Intensity of treatment depends on severity of symptoms: up to 3 treatments at 20-minute intervals as needed. Short course of oral systemic corticosteroids may be needed.
• Use of SABA >2 days a week for symptom relief (not prevention of EIB) generally indicates inadequate control and the need to step up treatment.

The stepwise approach is meant to assist, not replace, the clinical decision-making required to meet individual patient needs.
If alternative treatment is used and response is inadequate, discontinue it and use the preferred treatment before stepping up.
Zileuton is a less desirable alternative due to limited studies as adjunctive therapy and the need to monitor liver function. Theophylline requires monitoring of serum concentration levels. In step 6, before oral systemic corticosteroids are introduced, a trial of high-dose ICS + LABA + either LTRA, theophylline, or zileuton may be considered, although this approach has not been studied in clinical trials.
Steps 1, 2, and 3 preferred therapies are based on Evidence A; step 3 alternative therapy is based on Evidence A for LTRA, Evidence B for theophylline, and Evidence D for zileuton. Step 5 preferred therapy is based on Evidence B. Step 6 preferred therapy is based on (EPR-2 1997) and Evidence B for omalizumab.
Immunotherapy for steps 2-4 is based on Evidence B for house-dust mites, animal danders, and pollens; evidence is weak or lacking for molds and cockroaches. Evidence is strongest for immunotherapy with single allergens. The role of allergy in asthma is greater in children than in adults.
Clinicians who administer immunotherapy or omalizumab should be prepared and equipped to identify and treat anaphylaxis that may occur.
This information is directly abstracted from the 2007 NAEPP *Expert Panel Report 3: Guidelines for the Diagnosis and Management of Asthma* and is not intended to promote or endorse any of the listed products.
To access the complete *Expert Panel Report 3: Guidelines for the Diagnosis and Management of Asthma*, go to www.nhlbi.nih.gov/guidelines/asthma/asthgdln.pdf.
EIB, Exercise-induced bronchospasm; *ICS,* inhaled corticosteroid; *LABA,* inhaled long-acting beta₂-agonist; *LTRA,* leukotriene receptor antagonist; *SABA,* inhaled short-acting beta₂-agonist.
From National Asthma Education and Prevention Program: *Expert panel report 3: Guidelines for diagnosis and management of asthma*, National Institutes of Health, National Heart, Lung, and Blood Institute, August 2007, NIH publication 08-4051.

TABLE 5 Classifying Asthma Severity and Initiating Treatment in Children 5-11 Yr (Assessing severity and initiating treatment in children who are not currently taking long-term control medications)

		CLASSIFICATION OF ASTHMA SEVERITY (5-11 yr of age)			
		Intermittent	PERSISTENT		
Components of Severity			Mild	Moderate	Severe
Impairment	Symptoms	≤2 days/wk	>2 days/wk but not daily	Daily	Throughout the day
	Nighttime awakenings	≤23/mo	3-4×/mo	>1×/wk but not nightly	Often 7×/wk
	Short-acting beta$_2$-agonist use for symptom control (not prevention of EIB)	≤2 days/wk	>2 days/wk but not daily	Daily	Several times per day
	Interference with normal activity	None	Minor limitation	Some limitation	Extremely limited
	Lung function	Normal FEV$_1$ between exacerbations			
		FEV$_1$>80% predicted	FEV$_1$ = >80% predicted	FEV$_1$ 60%-80% predicted	FEV$_1$ <60% predicted
		FEV$_1$/FVC>85%	FEV$_1$/FVC>80%	FEV$_1$/FVC 75%-80%	FEV$_1$/FVC <75%
Risk	Exacerbations requiring oral systemic corticosteroids	0-1 per yr	≥2 per yr		
		Consider severity and interval since last exacerbation. Frequency and severity may fluctuate over time for patients in any severity category.			
		Relative annual risk of exacerbations may be related to FEV$_1$.			
Recommended Step for Initiating Therapy		Step 1	Step 2	Step 3, medium-dose ICS option	Step 3, medium-dose ICS option, or Step 4
					and consider short course of oral systemic corticosteroids
		In 2-6 wk, evaluate level of asthma control that is achieved and adjust therapy accordingly.			

The stepwise approach is meant to assist, not replace, the clinical decision-making required to meet individual patient needs.
Level of severity is determined by both impairment and risk. Assess impairment domain by patient's/caregiver's recall of previous 2-4 wk and spirometry. Assign severity to the most severe category in which any feature occurs.
At present, there are inadequate data to correspond frequencies of exacerbations with different levels of asthma severity. In general, more frequent and intense exacerbations (e.g., requiring urgent, unscheduled care, hospitalization, or ICU admission) indicate greater underlying disease severity. For treatment purposes, patients who had ≥2 exacerbations requiring oral systemic corticosteroids in the past year may be considered the same as patients who have persistent asthma, even in the absence of impairment levels consistent with persistent asthma.
EIB, Exercise-induced bronchospasm; *FEV$_1$,* forced expiratory volume in 1 second; *FVC,* forced vital capacity; *ICU,* intensive care unit.
From National Asthma Education and Prevention Program: *Expert panel report 3: Guidelines for diagnosis and management of asthma,* National Institutes of Health, National Heart, Lung, and Blood Institute, August 2007, NIH publication 08-4051.

TABLE 6 Assessing Asthma Control and Adjusting Therapy in Children 5-11 Yr

		CLASSIFICATION OF ASTHMA CONTROL (5-11 yr of age)		
Components of Control		Well Controlled	Not Well Controlled	Very Poorly Controlled
Impairment	Symptoms	≤2 days/wk but not more than once on each day	>2 days/wk or multiple times on ≤2 days/wk	Throughout the day
	Nighttime awakenings	≤1×/mo	≥2×/mo	≥2×/wk
	Interference with normal activity	None	Some limitation	Extremely limited
	Short-acting beta$_2$-agonist use for symptom control (not prevention of EIB)	≤2 days/wk	>2 days/wk	Several times per day
	Lung function			
	FEV$_1$ or peak flow	>80% predicted/personal best	60%-80% predicted/personal best	<60% predicted/personal best
	FEV$_1$/FVC	>80% predicted	75%-80%	<75% predicted
Risk	Exacerbations requiring oral systemic corticosteroids	0-1 per yr	≥2 per yr	
		Consider severity and interval since last exacerbation		
	Reduction in lung growth	Evaluation requires long-term follow-up care		
	Treatment-related adverse effects	Medication side effects can vary in intensity from none to very troublesome and worrisome. The level of intensity does not correlate to specific levels of control but should be considered in the overall assessment of risk.		
Recommended Action for Treatment		Maintain current step. Regular follow-up every 1-6 mo. Consider step down if well controlled for at least 3 mo.	Step up 1 step and reevaluate in 2-6 wk. For side effects, consider alternative treatment options.	Consider short course of oral systemic corticosteroids. Step up 1-2 steps. Reevaluate in 2 wk. For side effects, consider alternative treatment options.

The stepwise approach is meant to assist, not replace, the clinical decision-making required to meet individual patient needs.
The level of control is based on the most severe impairment or risk category. Assess impairment domain by patient's/caregiver's recall of previous 2-4 wk and by spirometry or peak flow measures. Symptom assessment for longer periods should reflect a global assessment such as inquiring whether the patient's asthma is better or worse since the last visit.
At present, there are inadequate data to correspond frequencies of exacerbations with different levels of asthma control. In general, more frequent and intense exacerbations (e.g., requiring urgent, unscheduled care, hospitalization, or ICU admission) indicate poorer disease control. For treatment purposes, patients who had ≥2 exacerbations requiring oral systemic corticosteroids in the past year may be considered the same as patients who have persistent asthma, even in the absence of impairment levels consistent with persistent asthma.
Before step up in therapy:
  −Review adherence to medications, inhaler technique, environmental control, and comorbid conditions.
  −If an alternative treatment option was used in a step, discontinue it and use preferred treatment for that step.
EIB, Exercise-induced bronchospasm; *FEV$_1$,* forced expiratory volume in 1 second; *ICU,* intensive care unit.
From National Asthma Education and Prevention Program: *Expert panel report 3: Guidelines for diagnosis and management of asthma,* National Institutes of Health, National Heart, Lung, and Blood Institute, August 2007, NIH publication 08-4051.

TABLE 7 Stepwise Approach for Managing Asthma in Children 5-11 Yr

Intermittent Asthma	**Persistent Asthma: Daily Medication** Consult with asthma specialist if step 4 care or higher is required. Consider consultation at step 3.

Step 1
Preferred:
SABA prn

Step 2
Preferred:
Low-dose ICS
Alternative:
Cromolyn, LTRA, nedocromil, or theophylline

Step 3
Preferred:
Low-dose ICS
+ either LABA, LTRA, or theophylline
OR
Medium-dose ICS

Step 4
Preferred:
Medium-dose ICS + LABA
Alternative:
Medium-dose ICS + either LTRA or theophylline

Step 5
Preferred:
High-dose ICS + LABA
Alternative:
High-dose ICS + either LTRA or theophylline

Step 6
Preferred:
High-dose ICS + LABA + oral corticosteroid
Alternative:
High-dose ICS + either LTRA or theophylline + oral systemic corticosteroid

Step up if needed
(first, check adherence, inhaler technique, environmental control, and comorbid conditions)

Assess control

Step down if possible
(and asthma is well controlled at least 3 months)

Each step: Patient education, environmental control, and management of comorbidities
Steps 2-4: Consider subcutaneous allergen immunotherapy for patients who have allergic asthma

Quick-Relief Medication for All Patients
- SABA as needed for symptoms. Intensity of treatment depends on severity of symptoms: up to 3 treatments at 20-minute intervals as needed. Short course of oral systemic corticosteroids may be needed.
- Caution: Increasing use of SABA or use >2 days a week for symptom relief (not prevention of EIB) generally indicates inadequate control and the need to step up treatment.

The stepwise approach is meant to assist, not replace, the clinical decision-making required to meet individual patient needs.
If alternative treatment is used and response is inadequate, discontinue it and use the preferred treatment before stepping up.
Theophylline is a less desirable alternative due to the need to monitor serum concentration levels.
Step 1 and step 2 medications are based on Evidence A. Step 3 ICS 1 adjunctive therapy and ICS are based on Evidence B for efficacy of each treatment and extrapolation from comparator trials in older children and adults—comparator trials are not available for this age group; steps 4-6 are based on expert opinion and extrapolation from studies in older children and adults. Immunotherapy for steps 2-4 is based on Evidence B for house-dust mites, animal danders, and pollens; evidence is weak or lacking for molds and cockroaches. Evidence is strongest for immunotherapy with single allergens. The role of allergy in asthma is greater in children than in adults. Clinicians who administer immunotherapy should be prepared and equipped to identify and treat anaphylaxis that may occur.
This information is directly abstracted from the 2007 NAEPP *Expert Panel Report 3: Guidelines for the Diagnosis and Management of Asthma* and is not intended to promote or endorse any of the listed products.
ICS, Inhaled corticosteroid; *LABA,* inhaled long-acting beta$_2$-agonist; *LTRA,* leukotriene receptor antagonist; *SABA,* inhaled short-acting beta$_2$-agonist.
From National Asthma Education and Prevention Program: *Expert panel report 3: Guidelines for diagnosis and management of asthma,* National Institutes of Health, National Heart, Lung, and Blood Institute, August 2007, NIH publication 08-4051.

BRONCHIAL THERMOPLASTY

Selected patients with severe persistent asthma who have failed medical treatment may benefit from bronchial thermoplasty. This requires the insertion of a catheter via bronchoscopy and use of radiofrequency heat to reduce bronchial smooth muscle. Long-term follow-up data showed persistent reduction in asthma exacerbation and fewer ED visits over a period of 5 years. FDA labeling is for "severe persistent asthma inadequately controlled on ICS + LABA."

OTHER MEDICATIONS

Tiotropium (Spiriva) has been used for decades as first-line treatment for COPD. This LAMA is now approved for a second indication for the treatment of asthma and is included in the most recent (2015) Global Initiative for Asthma (GINA) guidelines as a possible add-on at step 4.

Azithromycin: The AZISAST Trial randomized 109 patients on high-dose ICS/LABA (step 4 or 5 per GINA guidelines) to maintenance therapy with azithromycin or placebo. Overall, there was

BOX 1 Possible Indications for Referral to an Asthma Specialist

- Severe, acute asthma that has caused loss of consciousness, hypoxia, respiratory failure, convulsions, or near death
- Poorly controlled asthma as indicated by admission to a hospital, frequent need for emergency care, need for oral corticosteroids, absence from school or work, disruption of sleep, interference with quality of life
- Severe, persistent asthma requiring step 4 care (consider for patients who require step 3 care)
- Patient <3 yr who requires step 3 or 4 care (consider for patient <3 yr who requires step 2 care)
- Requirement for continuous oral corticosteroids or high-dose inhaled corticosteroids or more than two short courses of oral corticosteroids within 1 yr
- Need for additional diagnostic testing such as allergy skin testing, rhinoscopy, provocative challenge, complete pulmonary function testing, bronchoscopy
- Consideration for immunotherapy
- Need for additional education regarding asthma, complications of asthma and treatment of asthma, problems with adherence to management recommendations, or allergen avoidance
- Uncertainty of diagnosis
- Complications of asthma, including sinusitis, nasal polyposis, aspergillosis, severe rhinitis, vocal cord dysfunction, gastroesophageal reflux

Modified from National Asthma Education and Prevention Program, National Heart, Lung, and Blood Institute: *Expert Panel Report 2: guidelines for the diagnosis and management of asthma,* Bethesda, MD, 1997, National Institutes of Health, NIH publication No 97-4051.

TABLE 8 Classifying Asthma Severity and Initiating Treatment in Children 0-4 Yr (Assessing severity and initiating treatment in children who are not currently taking long-term control medications)

Components of Severity		Intermittent	PERSISTENT		
			Mild	Moderate	Severe
Impairment	Symptoms	≤2 days/wk	>2 days/wk but not daily	Daily	Throughout the day
	Nighttime awakenings	0	1-2×/mo	3-4×/mo	>1×/wk
	Short-acting beta$_2$-agonist use for symptom control (not prevention of EIB)	≤2 days/wk	>2 days/wk but not daily	Daily	Several times per day
	Interference with normal activity	None	Minor limitation	Some limitation	Extremely limited
Risk	Exacerbations requiring oral systemic corticosteroids	0-1 per yr	≥2 exacerbations in 6 mo requiring oral systemic corticosteroids, or ≥4 wheezing episodes/1 yr lasting >1 day AND risk factors for persistent asthma		
			Consider severity and interval since last exacerbation. Frequency and severity may fluctuate over time. Exacerbations of any severity may occur in patients in any severity category.		
Recommended Step for Initiating Therapy		Step 1	Step 2	Step 3 and consider short course of oral systemic corticosteroids	
			In 2-6 wk, depending on severity, evaluate level of asthma control that is achieved. If no clear benefit is observed in 4-6 wk, consider adjusting therapy or alternative diagnoses.		

The stepwise approach is meant to assist, not replace, the clinical decision-making required to meet individual patient needs.

Level of severity is determined by assessment of both impairment and risk. Assess impairment domain by patient's/caregiver's recall of previous 2-4 wk. Symptom assessment for longer periods should reflect a global assessment such as inquiring whether the patient's asthma is better or worse since the last visit. Assign severity to the most severe category in which any feature occurs.

At present, there are inadequate data to correspond frequencies of exacerbations with different levels of asthma severity. For treatment purposes, patients who had ≥2 exacerbations requiring oral systemic corticosteroids in the past six months, or ≥4 wheezing episodes in the past year, and who have risk factors for persistent asthma may be considered the same as patients who have persistent asthma, even in the absence of impairment levels consistent with persistent asthma.

To access the complete Expert Panel Report 3: Guidelines for the Diagnosis and Management of Asthma, go to www.nhlbi.nih.gov/guidelines/asthma/asthgdln.pdf.

EIB, Exercise-induced bronchospasm.

From National Asthma Education and Prevention Program: *Expert panel report 3: Guidelines for diagnosis and management of asthma*, National Institutes of Health, National Heart, Lung, and Blood Institute, August 2007, NIH publication 08-4051.

TABLE 9 Assessing Asthma Control and Adjusting Therapy in Children 0-4 Yr of Age

Components of Control		Classification Of Asthma Control (0-4 yr of age)		
		Well Controlled	Not Well Controlled	Very Poorly Controlled
Impairment	Symptoms	≤2 days/wk	>2 days/wk	Throughout the day
	Nighttime awakenings	≤13/mo	>1×/mo	>1×/wk
	Interference with normal activity	None	Some limitation	Extremely limited
	Short-acting beta$_2$-agonist use for symptom control (not prevention of EIB)	≤2 days/wk	>2 days/wk	Several times per day
Risk	Exacerbations requiring oral systemic corticosteroids	0-1 per yr	2-3 per yr	>3 per yr
	Treatment-related adverse effects	Medication side effects can vary in intensity from none to very troublesome and worrisome. The level of intensity does not correlate to specific levels of control but should be considered in the overall assessment of risk.		
Recommended Action for Treatment		Maintain current step. Regular follow-up every 1-6 mo. Consider step down if well controlled for at least 3 mo.	Step up 1 step. Reevaluate in 2-6 wk. If no clear benefit in 4-6 wk, consider alternative diagnoses or adjusting therapy. For side effects, consider alternative treatment options.	Consider short course of oral systemic corticosteroids. Step up 1-2 steps. Reevaluate in 2 wk. If no clear benefit in 4-6 wk, consider alternative diagnoses or adjusting therapy. For side effects, consider alternative treatment options.

The stepwise approach is meant to assist, not replace, the clinical decision-making required to meet individual patient needs.

The level of control is based on the most severe impairment or risk category. Assess impairment domain by caregiver's recall of previous 2-4 wk. Symptom assessment for longer periods should reflect a global assessment such as inquiring whether the patient's asthma is better or worse since the last visit.

At present, there are inadequate data to correspond frequencies of exacerbations with different levels of asthma control. In general, more frequent and intense exacerbations (e.g., requiring urgent, unscheduled care, hospitalization, or ICU admission) indicate poorer disease control. For treatment purposes, patients who had ≥2 exacerbations requiring oral systemic corticosteroids in the past year may be considered the same as patients who have not-well-controlled asthma, even in the absence of impairment levels consistent with not-well-controlled asthma.

Before step up in therapy:

   –Review adherence to medications, inhaler technique, and environmental control.

   –If an alternative treatment option was used in a step, discontinue it and use preferred treatment for that step.

EIB, Exercise-induced bronchospasm; *ICU*, intensive care unit.

From National Asthma Education and Prevention Program: *Expert panel report 3: Guidelines for diagnosis and management of asthma*, National Institutes of Health, National Heart, Lung, and Blood Institute, August 2007, NIH publication 08-4051.

TABLE 10 Stepwise Approach for Managing Asthma in Children 0-4 Yr

Intermittent Asthma	Persistent Asthma: Daily Medication
	Consult with asthma specialist if step 3 care or higher is required. Consider consultation at step 2.

Step 6
Preferred:
High-dose ICS
+ either LABA or
montelukast

Oral systemic
corticosteroid

Step 5
Preferred:
High-dose ICS
+ either LABA or
montelukast

Step 4
Preferred:
Medium-dose ICS
+ either LABA or
montelukast

Step 3
Preferred:
Medium-dose ICS

Step 2
Preferred:
Low-dose ICS

Alternative:
Cromolyn or
montelukast

Step 1
Preferred:
SABA prn

Step up if needed

(first, check
adherence, inhaler
technique, and
environmental
control)

**Assess
control**

Step down
if possible

(and asthma is
well controlled
at least 3 months)

Patient Education and Environmental Control at Each Step

Quick-Relief Medication for All Patients
- SABA as needed for symptoms. Intensity of treatment depends on severity of symptoms.
- With viral respiratory infection: SABA q 4-6 hours up to 24 hours (longer with physician consult). Consider short course of oral systemic corticosteroids if exacerbation is severe or patient has history of previous severe exacerbations.
- Caution: Frequent use of SABA may indicate the need to step up treatment. See text for recommendations on initiating daily long-term-control therapy.

The stepwise approach is meant to assist, not replace, the clinical decision-making required to meet individual patient needs. If alternative treatment is used and response is inadequate, discontinue it and use the preferred treatment before stepping up.

If clear benefit is not observed within 4-6 wk and patient/family medication technique and adherence are satisfactory, consider adjusting therapy or alternative diagnosis.

Studies on children 0-4 yr are limited. Step 2 preferred therapy is based on Evidence A. All other recommendations are based on expert opinion and extrapolation from studies in other children.

This information is directly abstracted from the 2007 NAEPP *Expert Panel Report 3: Guidelines for the Diagnosis and Management of Asthma* and is not intended to promote or endorse any of the listed products.

ICS, Inhaled corticosteroid; *LABA,* inhaled long-acting beta$_2$-agonist; *SABA,* inhaled short-acting beta$_2$-agonist.

From National Asthma Education and Prevention Program: *Expert panel report 3: Guidelines for diagnosis and management of asthma,* National Institutes of Health, National Heart, Lung, and Blood Institute, August 2007, NIH publication 08-4051.

no benefit seen with azithromycin therapy with regard to any of the outcomes tested. However, subgroup analysis showed that patients with noneosinophilic asthma had fewer exacerbations. More data are needed, but this result suggests azithromycin may be an effective option for the neutrophilic/Th-1 phenotype (COPD is also neutrophilic).

TREATMENT OF SEVERE ASTHMA (ETS/ETA GUIDELINES)

- The American Thoracic Society (ATS) classification of "severe asthma" refers to patients who require high-dose inhaled or near-continuous oral glucocorticoid treatment to maintain asthma control.
- In patients who do not achieve adequate control with the combination of a high-dose inhaled glucocorticoid and LABA, an additional controller medication such as an antileukotriene agent is recommended (tiotropium or theophylline).
- For patients with atopic severe asthma who have a serum IgE level of 30 to 700 IU/ml and documented sensitivity to a perennial allergen, recommend adding omalizumab.
- For patients with severe asthma, frequent exacerbations, and an eosinophilic phenotype despite guideline-based therapy,

consider add-on therapy with one of the anti-interleukin (IL)-5 antibodies, mepolizumab or reslizumab.
- Bronchial thermoplasty is approved for use in selected adults with severe asthma that is not well controlled with inhaled glucocorticoids and LABAs.
- Potential alternative and experimental therapies include immunomodulatory therapy and macrolide antibiotics.
- In the future, treatments tailored to asthma phenotypes may improve asthma outcomes.

Treatment of status asthmaticus is as follows:
- Oxygen generally started at 2 to 4 L/min by nasal cannula or Venti-Mask at 40% Fio$_2$; further adjustments are made according to oxygen saturations.
- Bronchodilators: Initiate treatment with high-dose SABA plus ipratropium bromide administered by means of a nebulizer every 20 min. Use of a metered-dose inhaler with valved holding chamber may be acceptable for patients with mild-to-moderate exacerbations.
- Albuterol nebulizer solution (0.63 mg/3 mL, 1.25 mg/3 mL, 2.5 mg/3 mL, or 5.0 mg/mL): 2.5 to 5 mg every 20 min over the first hr, then 2.5-10 mg every 1-4 hr as needed or 10-15 mg/hr continuously. Other useful

medications are levalbuterol nebulizer solution (0.31 mg/3 mL, 0.63 mg/3 mL, 1.25 mg/3 mL) and ipratropium nebulizer solution (0.25/mL [0.025%]).
- Corticosteroids:
1. Early administration is advised, particularly in patients using steroids at home.
2. Patients may be started on systemic corticosteroids: methylprednisolone, prednisone, or prednisolone may be used. Dose range is from 40-80 mg/day in one or two divided doses, generally given until peak expiratory flow reaches 70% of predicted value.
3. Generally for corticosteroid courses <1 week there is no need to taper the dose.
- IV hydration: judicious use is necessary to avoid congestive heart failure in elderly patients. Aggressive IV hydration is not recommended.
- IV antibiotics are indicated when there is suspicion of bacterial infection (e.g., infiltrate on chest radiograph, fever, or leukocytosis).
- Intubation and mechanical ventilation are indicated when previous measures fail to produce significant improvement (Fig. 3).
- Discharge home from the emergency department is appropriate if the FEV$_1$ or PEF after treatment is 70% or greater of the personal

best or predicted value and if there is sustained improvement in lung function and symptoms for at least 1 hr.

REFERRAL

Box 1 describes indications for referral to an asthma specialist.

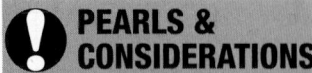 **PEARLS & CONSIDERATIONS**

COMMENTS

- The differentiation of asthma from COPD can be challenging. A history of atopy and intermittent, reactive symptoms points toward a diagnosis of asthma, whereas smoking and advanced age are more indicative of COPD. Spirometry is useful in distinguishing asthma from COPD.
- In all asthma patients it is important to treat or prevent comorbid conditions (e.g., rhinosinusitis, vocal cord dysfunction, gastroesophageal reflux disease). However, despite the presumed association between asthma and GERD, trials of PPIs in patients with poorly controlled asthma did not reveal any beneficial effects.
- Inhaled low-dose corticosteroids are the single most effective therapy for adult patients with asthma who require more than an occasional use of SABAs to control their asthma.
- Stepping down inhaled corticosteroids after asthma is well controlled now has level A evidence.
- Leukotriene modifiers/receptor agonists represent a reasonable alternative in adults unable or unwilling to use corticosteroids;

however, these agents are less effective than monotherapy with inhaled corticosteroids.

- Use of LABAs alone without use of a long-term asthma medication, such as an inhaled corticosteroid, is contraindicated. LABAs should also not be used in patients whose asthma is adequately controlled on low- or medium-dose inhaled corticosteroids. Continued use of LABAs may cause down-regulation of the beta-2 receptor with loss of the bronchoprotective effect from rescue therapy with a SABA.
- Patients who remain symptomatic despite inhaled corticosteroids benefit from the addition of LABAs. Trials in patients with poorly controlled asthma despite the use of inhaled glucocorticoids and LABAs have shown that the addition of tiotropium, a long-acting anticholinergic bronchodilator approved for treatment of COPD, increased the time to the first severe exacerbation and provided modest sustained bronchodilation.
- Therapy with systemic corticosteroids accelerates the resolution of acute asthma and reduces the risk of relapse. There is no evidence that doses >50-100 mg prednisone equivalent are beneficial.
- In patients with allergies and elevated serum immunoglobulin (Ig) E levels, use of anti-IgE therapy is beneficial.
- Bronchial thermoplasty should be considered in selective patients with severe persistent asthma with recurrent exacerbations or ED visits. Biologic modifiers of the Th2 immune pathways (neutralizing monoclonal antibodies, receptor antagonists, soluble receptors)

are potential options for the development of new treatments of severe asthma.

- The response to treatment for asthma is characterized by wide individual variability. A functional glucocorticoid-induced transcript 1 gene (GLCCI1) variant is associated with substantial decrements in the response to inhaled glucocorticoids in patients with asthma. Another potential cause of the variability in response to treatment is heterogeneity in the role of interleukin-13 expression in the clinical asthma phenotype. Patients with asthma who have a certain biochemical signature are more likely to respond to an anti–interleukin-13 monoclonal antibody than those without such a signature. Identification of genetic variants can eventually lead to personalized asthma treatment.

 EVIDENCE

Available at www.expertconsult.com

SUGGESTED READINGS
Available at www.expertconsult.com

RELATED CONTENT
Asthma (Patient Information)

AUTHORS: **RANIA ESTEITIE, M.D.,** and **SAMAAN RAFEQ, M.D.**

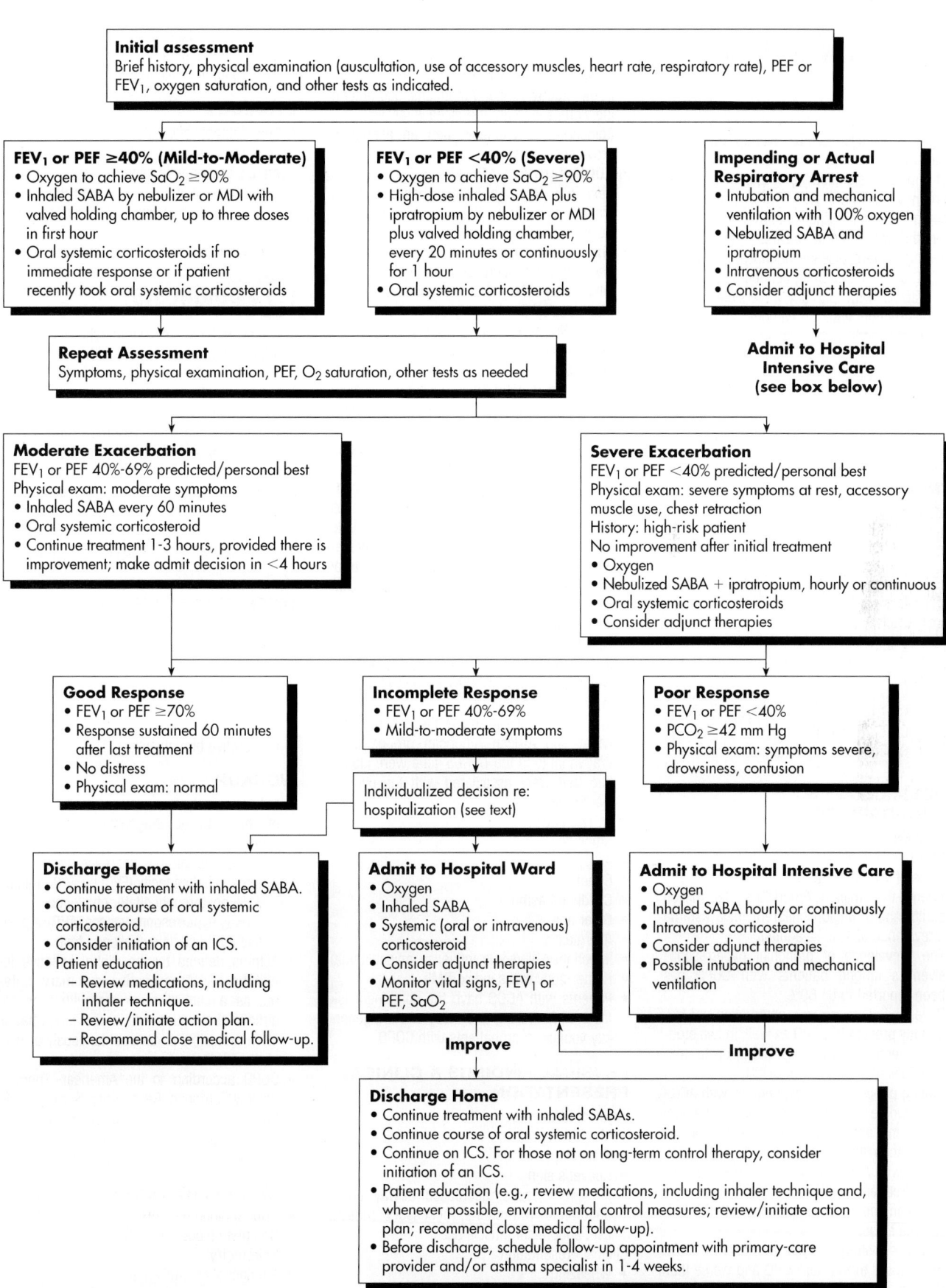

Initial assessment
Brief history, physical examination (auscultation, use of accessory muscles, heart rate, respiratory rate), PEF or FEV_1, oxygen saturation, and other tests as indicated.

FEV_1 or PEF ≥40% (Mild-to-Moderate)
- Oxygen to achieve SaO_2 ≥90%
- Inhaled SABA by nebulizer or MDI with valved holding chamber, up to three doses in first hour
- Oral systemic corticosteroids if no immediate response or if patient recently took oral systemic corticosteroids

FEV_1 or PEF <40% (Severe)
- Oxygen to achieve SaO_2 ≥90%
- High-dose inhaled SABA plus ipratropium by nebulizer or MDI plus valved holding chamber, every 20 minutes or continuously for 1 hour
- Oral systemic corticosteroids

Impending or Actual Respiratory Arrest
- Intubation and mechanical ventilation with 100% oxygen
- Nebulized SABA and ipratropium
- Intravenous corticosteroids
- Consider adjunct therapies

Admit to Hospital Intensive Care (see box below)

Repeat Assessment
Symptoms, physical examination, PEF, O_2 saturation, other tests as needed

Moderate Exacerbation
FEV_1 or PEF 40%-69% predicted/personal best
Physical exam: moderate symptoms
- Inhaled SABA every 60 minutes
- Oral systemic corticosteroid
- Continue treatment 1-3 hours, provided there is improvement; make admit decision in <4 hours

Severe Exacerbation
FEV_1 or PEF <40% predicted/personal best
Physical exam: severe symptoms at rest, accessory muscle use, chest retraction
History: high-risk patient
No improvement after initial treatment
- Oxygen
- Nebulized SABA + ipratropium, hourly or continuous
- Oral systemic corticosteroids
- Consider adjunct therapies

Good Response
- FEV_1 or PEF ≥70%
- Response sustained 60 minutes after last treatment
- No distress
- Physical exam: normal

Incomplete Response
- FEV_1 or PEF 40%-69%
- Mild-to-moderate symptoms

Individualized decision re: hospitalization (see text)

Poor Response
- FEV_1 or PEF <40%
- PCO_2 ≥42 mm Hg
- Physical exam: symptoms severe, drowsiness, confusion

Discharge Home
- Continue treatment with inhaled SABA.
- Continue course of oral systemic corticosteroid.
- Consider initiation of an ICS.
- Patient education
  - Review medications, including inhaler technique.
  - Review/initiate action plan.
  - Recommend close medical follow-up.

Admit to Hospital Ward
- Oxygen
- Inhaled SABA
- Systemic (oral or intravenous) corticosteroid
- Consider adjunct therapies
- Monitor vital signs, FEV_1 or PEF, SaO_2

Admit to Hospital Intensive Care
- Oxygen
- Inhaled SABA hourly or continuously
- Intravenous corticosteroid
- Consider adjunct therapies
- Possible intubation and mechanical ventilation

Improve   **Improve**

Discharge Home
- Continue treatment with inhaled SABAs.
- Continue course of oral systemic corticosteroid.
- Continue on ICS. For those not on long-term control therapy, consider initiation of an ICS.
- Patient education (e.g., review medications, including inhaler technique and, whenever possible, environmental control measures; review/initiate action plan; recommend close medical follow-up).
- Before discharge, schedule follow-up appointment with primary-care provider and/or asthma specialist in 1-4 weeks.

FIG. 3 Management of asthma exacerbations: emergency department and hospital-based care. *FEV₁*, Forced expiratory volume in 1 second; *ICS*, inhaled corticosteroid; *MDI*, metered-dose inhaler; *PCO₂*, partial pressure carbon dioxide; *PEF*, peak expiratory flow; *SABA*, short-acting beta₂-agonist; *SaO₂*, oxygen saturation. (From National Asthma Education and Prevention Program: *Guidelines for the diagnosis and management of asthma*, 2007, National Institutes of Health, National Heart, Lung, and Blood Institute.)

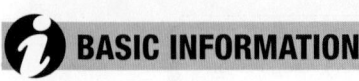

BASIC INFORMATION

DEFINITION

- The asthma and chronic obstructive pulmonary disease (COPD) overlap syndrome (ACOS) is a recently recognized clinical entity of important significance. It identifies a subgroup of smokers with COPD that shares some pathogenic and inflammatory characteristics with asthma and that tends to have a more severe disease phenotype than just COPD alone. It has been defined as either:
  - Asthma with partially reversible airflow obstruction with or without emphysema or reduced carbon monoxide diffusing capacity (DLco) to <80% predicted.
  - Chronic obstructive pulmonary disease (COPD) with emphysema accompanied by reversible or partially reversible airflow obstruction, with or without environmental allergies or reduced DLco.

SYNONYMS

Bronchospasm
Reactive airway disease
Asthmatic bronchitis
Hyperreactive airways
Chronic obstructive pulmonary disease

ICD10-CM CODES	
J45	Asthma
J42	Unspecified chronic bronchitis
J43	Emphysema
J44	COPD
J44.9	COPD, unspecified
M35.1	Other overlap syndromes

EPIDEMIOLOGY & DEMOGRAPHICS

PREVALENCE:

- COPD afflicts 14.2 million adults (a prevalence of 1 in 5) in the U.S.
- Twenty-five million Americans (18 million adults and 7 million children) have asthma (prevalence of 1 in 12 adults).
- The prevalence of bronchial hyperresponsiveness among patients with COPD has been reported to be 60%.
- Reversibility of airway obstruction is frequently present in COPD as well; in two studies, reversibility was observed in up to 44% and 50% of patients with COPD.
- Among published studies, persons with ACOS have worse lung function, more respiratory symptoms, and a lower health-related quality of life than those with either disease alone. Those with ACOS are reported to experience more frequent health care utilization and more severe impairment than persons with COPD or asthma alone.
- In a recent study, 15-year mortality for ACOS was similar to that for COPD and worse than that for asthma and healthy controls. ACOS had a significant impact on physical performance, functional ability, and health-related quality of life.

- The prevalence of ACOS is between 15% and 25% in an adult population of obstructive airway diseases. ACOS is also more prevalent in the elderly, African Americans, and among individuals with greater disease severity.
- Epidemiologic studies report an estimated prevalence of 20%.

PREDOMINANT SEX AND AGE:

- Sex: In a large, population-based sample, women were more likely than men to report ACOS.
- Age: The prevalence of overlap syndrome has been shown to increase with age (>60-70), which may reflect that with time asthmatics may develop fixed airway obstruction.
- Race: No published predilection for race/ethnicity noted.

GENETICS:

- No known genetic basis described. Genetic linkage studies and genome-wide association (GWA) studies have been of limited value in characterizing a link between asthma and COPD.
- Postma et al evaluated the paucity of GWA studies, assessing overlap syndrome and the focus on clearly defined outcomes that do not include overlap and that hamper the current insight that genetic studies provide. However, Hardin et al (2014) showed that the two most significant associations among non-Hispanic white overlap subjects include variants from the *CSMD1* gene, which has been associated with emphysema, and within the *SOX5* gene, which has previously been associated with COPD and may play a role in lung development.
- In a meta-analysis across the non-Hispanic white and African American groups, several variants in the *GPR65* gene were identified that were associated with the overlap syndrome.

RISK FACTORS:

- Smoking
- Atopy
- Genetics
- Childhood asthma
- Older age
- Allergies
- Infections (rhinovirus, influenza, mycoplasma)
- Higher body mass index (BMI)
- Patients with ACOS have the combined risk factors of smoking and atopy and are generally younger than patients with COPD.

PHYSICAL FINDINGS & CLINICAL PRESENTATION

Physical Examination
- May be normal
- Wheezing, rhonchi
- Hoover's sign
- In severe cases, decreased airway entry, abdominal retractions, accessory muscle use, abdominal muscle use

Clinical Presentation
- Wheezing
- Shortness of breath
- Chest tightness
- History of repeated respiratory infections
- Chronic cough (typically productive)

- Episodic symptoms instigated by certain triggers (odors, temperatures, allergens)
- Decreased exercise tolerance

ETIOLOGY

- The pathophysiology of asthma involves a complex interaction among various environmental and genetic factors.
- Cigarette smoking interacts with the inflammation and remodeling that occur in asthma and COPD.
- No genetic basis identified thus far.

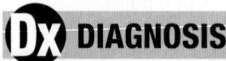

DIAGNOSIS

ACOS should be considered when "a similar number of features listed for asthma and COPD are present." This definition for ACOS is not yet very specific because it is recognized that a more detailed classification of patients with overlapping features of asthma and COPD is needed. Studies performed so far have generally based the diagnosis of ACOS on the pattern of symptoms, the presence of incompletely reversible airflow obstruction in ex- or current smokers or patients with asthma, the degree of bronchodilator reversibility, and bronchial hyperresponsiveness.

DIFFERENTIAL DIAGNOSIS

- Chronic obstructive pulmonary disease (COPD)
- Asthma
- Central airway obstruction
- Bronchiectasis
- Heart failure
- Obliterative bronchiolitis

WORKUP

- Patients must have demonstrated either one of these to be diagnosed with "overlap syndrome."
  - Reversible airflow: increase in FEV1 or forced vital capacity (FVC) by ≥200 ml and 12% postbronchodilator challenge
  - Airway hyperresponsiveness (AHR): a positive methacholine challenge test
- Asthma defined by the Global Initiative for Asthma (GINA) executive summary criteria, as a clinical syndrome with "variable airflow obstruction within the lung that is often reversible either spontaneously or with treatment."
- COPD according to the American Thoracic Society/European Respiratory Society (ATS/ERS) joint task force: "a preventable and treatable disease state characterized by airflow limitation that is not fully reversible."

LABORATORY TESTS

- Arterial blood gas (ABG)
- Complete blood count (CBC)
- Spirometry
- Methacholine challenge
- Peak expiratory flow rate (PEFR)
- Serum immunoglobulin E
- Sputum
- Allergy testing

IMAGING STUDIES

- Chest x-ray
- Chest CT scan
- ECG

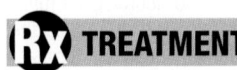

TREATMENT

There is little information about the response of ACOS patients to most of the current pharmacologic therapies because they have been systematically excluded from both COPD and asthma pharmacologic trials. The main interest in differentiating ACOS from COPD lies in the different response to inhaled corticosteroids (ICS). Some studies demonstrate that patients with COPD and eosinophilic inflammation treated with ICS present a significant improvement clinically and objectively by spirometry.

NONPHARMACOLOGIC THERAPY

- Avoidance of environmental or occupational trigger factors
- Patient education regarding warning signs of an attack and proper use of medications (e.g., correct use of inhalers)
- Pulmonary rehabilitation

ACUTE GENERAL Rx

- At present, there are no randomized clinical trial data to help guide therapeutic interventions in overlap syndrome.
- Treatment typically is directed toward management of symptoms.
- For dynamic obstruction and/or hyperinflation, bronchodilators may provide the greatest benefit.
- Whether long-acting muscarinic antagonists (LAMAs) alone or in combination with long-acting beta-agonists (LABAs) are appropriate in overlap syndrome remains to be elucidated.

- For patients in whom bronchospasm is demonstrated, bronchodilators and ICSs are reasonable options.
- Clinical trials have shown efficacy for fluticasone furoate/vilanterole combination (the first once-daily ICS/LABA) versus twice-daily fluticasone propionate/salmeterol; it can provide substantial improvement in lung functions in a population of ACOS, indicating that this combination should be considered for the regular treatment of ACOS.
- A more recent study showed some efficacy with the use of omalizumab as an effective and safe therapy for patients with ACOS. However, this study included only 3 patients; therefore, larger randomized trials are needed.

CHRONIC Rx

- Earlier screening of the overlap syndrome is important in current or former smokers in their fifth decade of life who have partially reversible airway obstruction and progressive exercise intolerance and who have variable or no response to guideline-recommended asthma treatments. Smoking cessation, oxygen supplementation, pulmonary rehabilitation, and vaccines are all reasonable interventions.
- As the prevalence of overlap syndrome increases with age, targeting nonrespiratory age-related changes that may influence respiratory disease is paramount. This includes targeting nasal obstruction symptoms (due to nonallergic or allergic rhinitis, mucosal dryness, or vasomotor symptoms) with nasal irrigation, nasal steroids, and/or nasal anticholinergics.
- Treating comorbidities such as heart failure or chronic aspiration is important, especially gastroesophageal reflux disease (GERD) or vocal cord dysfunction (VCD), which can be subclinical.

COMPLEMENTARY AND ALTERNATIVE MEDICINE

None

REFERRAL

- Referral for expert advice and further diagnostic evaluation is necessary in the following contexts:
  - Persistent symptoms and/or exacerbations
  - Diagnostic uncertainty
  - Patients with asthma/COPD with atypical/additional symptoms such as hemoptysis, weight loss, night sweats, fevers, signs of bronchiectasis
  - Comorbidities that may interfere with assessment and management
  - No response to treatment.

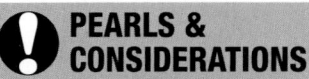

PEARLS & CONSIDERATIONS

PREVENTION

- Smoking cessation
- Avoidance of triggers

SUGGESTED READINGS

See www.expertconsult.com

RELATED TOPICS

Asthma (Related Key Topic)
Chronic Obstructive Pulmonary Disease (Related Key Topic)

AUTHORS: **RANIA ESTEITIE, M.D.,** and **SAMAAN RAFEQ, M.D.**

A

Diseases and Disorders

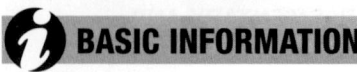
DEFINITION

Astrocytoma is a type of neuroepithelial tumor that arises from astrocytes, which are glial precursor cells. According to the current World Health Organization (WHO) classification astrocytoma is classified as below based on the histopathology:

- Grade I: Pilocytic astrocytoma
- Grade II: Diffuse astrocytoma
- Grade III: Anaplastic astrocytoma
- Grade IV: Glioblastoma
- Grades III and IV are considered high-grade astrocytomas (HGAs) or malignant.

The distinction of different grades of astrocytoma provides important clinical prognostic information.

SYNONYMS

Astroglial neoplasms

ICD-10CM CODES
C71.9 Malignant neoplasm of brain, unspecified

EPIDEMIOLOGY & DEMOGRAPHICS

According to SEER registry, the incidence of primary CNS tumor is 6.4 cases per 100,000 persons per year with age-adjusted death rate of 4.4 per 100,000. According to the Central Brain Tumor Registry of the United States (CBTRUS) astrocytomas constitute about 10% of the central nervous system neoplasms.

ETIOLOGY

- No agent has been definitely implicated in the causation of CNS tumors, and risk factors can be identified only in minority of patients. Farmers and petrochemical workers have been shown to have a higher incidence of primary brain tumors. Exposure to ionizing radiation is a known risk factor for a small percentage of astrocytomas.
- Different hereditary syndromes are associated with increased risk and high frequency of astrocytoma
  A) Neurofibromatosis type 1 is associated with increased frequency of astrocytoma.
  B) Li-Fraumeni syndrome (germ line mutation in one of p53 allele) is associated with increased frequency of malignant gliomas.

GENE AND CHROMOSOMAL ALTERATIONS IN ASTROCYTOMA:

- Alteration in p53, a tumor suppressor encoded by the TP53 gene on chromosome 17p plays a key role in the development of at least one third of all grades of astrocytoma. In addition, in high-grade astrocytomas, p53 function may be deregulated by alteration of other genes, including amplification of MDM2 or MDM4 and 9p deletions that result in loss of the p14 product of the CDKN2A gene.
- Recently mutations of isocitrate dehydrogenase 1 gene (IDH1) have been shown to occur in a large fraction of grade II and grade III astrocytomas as well as in other gliomas. Antibodies specific to mutant form of IDH1 protein can now be used reliably for glioma diagnosis on routine tissue sections.

PHYSICAL FINDINGS & CLINICAL PRESENTATION

The presenting symptoms of astrocytoma depend, in part, on the location of the lesion and its rate of growth. Astrocytomas classically present with any one or more of the following features:

- Headache (less frequent)
- New-onset partial or generalized seizures (>50%)
- Nausea and vomiting
- Focal neurologic deficit (cranial nerve palsy, hemiplegia, ataxia)
- Change in mental status
- Papilledema (rare)

A provisional diagnosis of astrocytoma is made on clinical grounds and radiographic imaging studies. Tissue pathology is needed to establish the diagnosis and to grade the astrocytoma.

DIFFERENTIAL DIAGNOSIS

The differential diagnosis is vast and includes any cause of headache, seizures, change in mental status, and focal neurologic deficits.

WORKUP

- The imaging modality of choice for most CNS tumors is contrast enhanced MRI which can demonstrate anatomy and pathological process in detail. CT scan is reserved for patients who are unable or unwilling to get MRI. Biopsy with histological confirmation is required to establish a diagnosis of astrocytoma.
- Stereotactic biopsy under CT or MRI guidance has been reserved for tumors that are deeply seated, multicentric tumors or diffuse nonfocal tumors where surgical resection is not practical. Major objectives of surgical resection are to maximally remove the tumor bulk, reduce tumor-associated mass effect and elevated intracranial pressure and provide tissue for pathological analysis. The surgical resection is carried out in a manner that minimizes the risk to neurological functioning. Surgery can also rapidly reduce the tumor bulk with potential benefits in terms of mass effect, edema, and hydrocephalus.

LABORATORY TESTS

There are no diagnostic or supportive blood tests for astrocytoma.

IMAGING STUDIES

- MRI (Fig. 1) is the diagnostic imaging study of choice. MRI with contrast and magnetic resonance angiography are used to locate the margins of the tumor, distinguish vascular masses from tumors, detect LGAs not seen by CT scan, and provide clear views of the posterior fossa.

ACUTE GENERAL Rx

- Corticosteroids (usually dexamethasone) need to be started immediately preoperatively in all primary CNS tumors unless CNS lymphoma is being suspected. Corticosteroids reduce cerebral edema and thus minimize secondary brain injury from cerebral retraction. Corticosteroids needs to be continued in the immediate postoperative period and tapered as quickly as possible. If there is increased intracranial pressure and impending herniation, patient should be started on IV mannitol, and mechanical ventilation with hyperventilation should be considered if there is depressed consciousness.
- The use of preoperative prophylactic anticonvulsants is less commonly indicated. The practice pattern in US seems to indicate its widespread use.

STAGE-SPECIFIC Rx

- Grade I astrocytoma are usually indolent and circumscribed tumors. Complete surgical

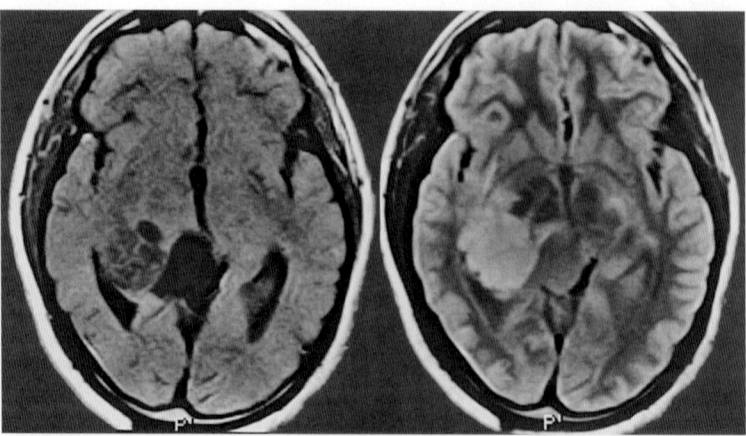

FIG. 1 MR image of a low-grade astrocytoma, demonstrating a hypointense right temporal lesion without contrast enhancement on T1 and hyperintense signal on T2. (From Goetz CG, Pappert EJ: *Textbook of clinical neurology,* Philadelphia, 1999, Saunders.)

resection, whenever feasible is curative and it is the mainstay therapy for these tumors. If complete surgical resection is not feasible due to location of tumor such as when the tumor is in optic pathway, hypothalamus, and in deep midline structures, asymptomatic patients can be observed in these cases until maximally safe resection is feasible upon progression. Unfortunately, despite aggressive near-total resection, delayed recurrence and eventual malignant transformation are common.

- In grade II astrocytoma, the extent of postoperative residual disease is an important variable for time to first relapse. The role of postoperative radiotherapy, in particular, timing is controversial. Observation with imaging is a reasonable option in patients who are young (<40) and had a gross tumor resection. In patients who have undergone subtotal resection and who are >40 years of age postoperative radiotherapy is recommended. Radiotherapy in this setting has been shown to improve progression-free survival (PFS) without improvement in overall survival.
- In Grade III anaplastic astrocytoma, surgical resection has shown to prolong survival but almost all of these tumors are characterized by postoperative residual disease. So, postoperative radiotherapy is used adjunctively. The role of adjunct chemotherapy is controversial. Most phase 3 clinical trials have demonstrated no benefit compared with radiation alone.
- In Grade IV glioblastoma, surgical resection has been shown to improve median survival. Multiple randomized trials have demonstrated survival benefit with radiotherapy following surgery. Use of chemotherapy as an adjunct to radiation therapy has been shown to improve the median survival in patients with glioblastoma in a randomized phase 3 clinical trial. Hence, radiation therapy concurrent with temozolomide (an alkylating agent) following surgical resection is the standard of care in Grade IV glioblastoma. Unfortunately, even with chemotherapy and radiation therapy, the 2-year survival in these patients is only 16%.

TREATMENT OF RECURRENT DISEASE

- For Grade 1 astrocytoma, re-resection should be considered. For patients who have tumors that are not amenable to resection, chemotherapy or radiotherapy can improve recurrence-free survival, although role of chemotherapy in adults remain controversial.
- For Grade 2 astrocytoma, radiation therapy can be considered in the relapsed setting if not given in the adjuvant setting. Data on use of chemotherapy in low-grade gliomas in adults is sparse. Although the results are encouraging, number of patients treated in these studies is small and there were a lot of methodological flaws in the studies. For recurrent Grade III anaplastic astrocytoma treated with radiation therapy in the past (Fig. 2), there is a role for chemotherapy. Nitrosoureas-based regimen and temozolomide (alkylating agent) have shown efficacy in this setting.
- Various targeted therapies are currently being studied in patients with recurrent glioblastoma. Irinotecan with bevacizumab or bevacizumab alone have been studied in a phase 2 trial, and a response rate of 38% and 28% respectively was reported in that study. Median survival was 8.7 months and 9.2 months respectively.

PROGNOSIS

- Grade 1 astrocytoma have a good prognosis and they are usually cured with surgical resection
- Grade 2 astrocytoma has a median survival of about 7.5 years with treatment.
- Grade 3 anaplastic astrocytoma has a median survival of approximately 5 years. The patients with 1p and 19q co deletion have superior survival compared to patients without deletion.
- Median survival of glioblastoma is approximately 14 months.

REFERRAL

A multidisciplinary consultation is indicated in patients diagnosed with astrocytoma. A neurosurgeon, radiation oncologist, and neurooncologist are needed to assist in establishing the diagnosis and to provide immediate and follow-up treatment.

SUGGESTED READINGS

Available at www.expertconsult.com

RELATED CONTENT

Astrocytoma (Patient Information)
Brain Cancer (Patient Information)
Brain Neoplasm, Benign (Related Key Topic)
Brain Neoplasm, Glioblastoma (Related Key Topic)

AUTHOR: **BHARTI RATHORE, M.D.**

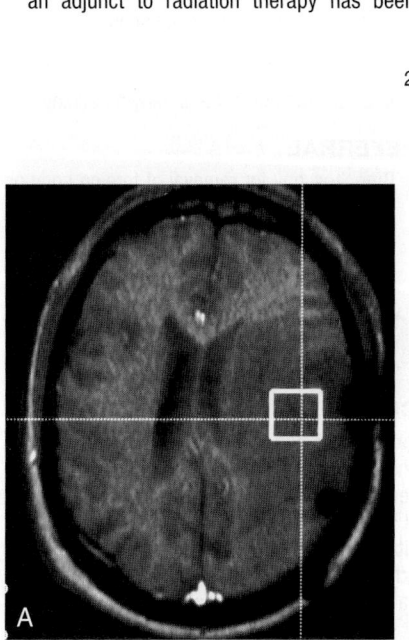
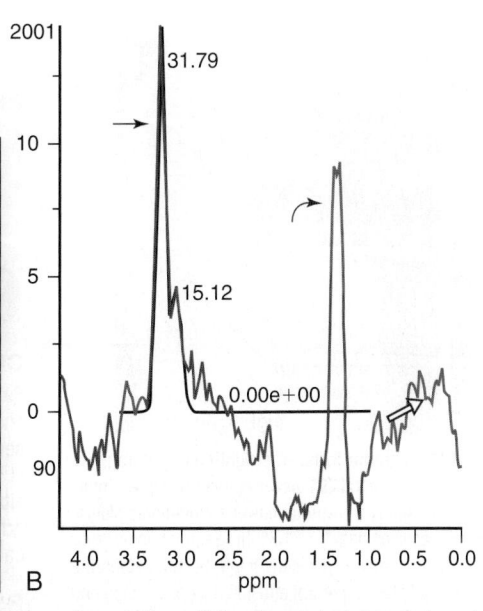

FIG. 2 Recurrent high-grade astrocytoma. Study performed after radiation therapy (not shown) showed increased edema and mass effect; differential diagnosis included recurrent tumor and radiation necrosis. **A,** Axial MRI scan shows volume of tissue *(box)* selected for spectroscopy. **B,** Proton spectroscopy reveals increase in choline peak *(arrow)*, decrease in N-acetyl aspartate peak *(curved arrow)*, and appearance of a lactate peak *(open arrow)*. This appearance is consistent with recurrent tumor, which was verified with repeat surgery and biopsy. (From Vincent JL et al: *Textbook of critical care*, ed 6, Philadelphia, 2011, Saunders.)

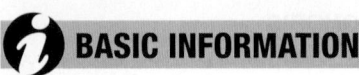

DEFINITION

Atelectasis is the collapse of lung with some degree of volume loss.

ICD-10CM CODES
J98.11 Atelectasis

EPIDEMIOLOGY & DEMOGRAPHICS

- Postoperative patients and patients with lung or chest wall injury are at increased risk of atelectasis.
- Asbestos exposure increases risk for an entity called "rounded atelectasis."
- Occurs frequently in patients receiving mechanical ventilation.
- Dependent regions of the lung are more prone to atelectasis: they are partially compressed, they are not as well ventilated, and there is no spontaneous drainage of secretions with gravity.

PHYSICAL FINDINGS & CLINICAL PRESENTATION

- Decreased or absent breath sounds
- Abnormal chest percussion
- Cough, dyspnea, decreased vocal fremitus and vocal resonance
- Diminished chest expansion, tachypnea, tachycardia

ETIOLOGY

- Trauma caused by shear force generated by repetitive expansion and collapse during positive-pressure ventilation (e.g., mechanical ventilation)
- Airway obstruction (e.g., endobronchial tumor, foreign bodies, mucus plug)
- Extrinsic bronchial compression (e.g., neoplasms, aneurysms of ascending aorta, enlarged left atrium)
- Pleural disease (e.g., pleural effusion, mesothelioma, rounded atelectasis, pneumothorax)
- Alveolar injury (e.g., toxic fumes, aspiration of gastric contents, infections, ARDS)
- Chest wall abnormalities (e.g. trauma, scoliosis, rib fracture, obesity)
- Impaired respiratory mechanics or decreased cough response (e.g., pain, postanesthetic effect, abdominal distention, neuromuscular disease)

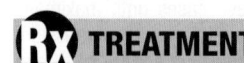 **DIAGNOSIS**

DIFFERENTIAL DIAGNOSIS

- Neoplasm
- Pneumonia
- Pleural effusion
- Abnormalities of brachiocephalic vein and the left pulmonary ligament

WORKUP

- Chest x-ray (Fig. 1)
- Thoracic ultrasonography
- CT scan and fiberoptic bronchoscopy (selected patients)

IMAGING STUDIES

- Chest radiograph suggests the diagnosis but fails to confirm the diagnosis in many cases.
- Ultrasonography helps differentiate atelectasis from effusion or consolidation.
- CT scan is useful in patients with suspected endobronchial neoplasm or extrinsic bronchial compression.
- Prone images help differentiate true consolidation from dependent atelectasis.
- Fiberoptic bronchoscopy (selected patients) is useful for removal of foreign body or evaluation of endobronchial and peribronchial lesions.

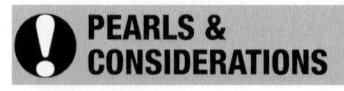 **TREATMENT**

NONPHARMACOLOGIC THERAPY

- Deep breathing, mobilization of the patient
- Incentive spirometry
- Handheld PEEP devices (e.g., PEEP valve, Acapella)
- Tracheal suctioning in select patients (e.g., mechanical ventilation and tracheostomy)
- Humidification
- Chest physiotherapy with percussion and postural drainage

ACUTE GENERAL Rx

- Positive-pressure breathing (continuous positive airway pressure by face mask, positive end-expiratory pressure for patients on mechanical ventilation)
- Use of mucolytic agents (e.g., acetylcysteine [Mucomyst])
- Recombinant human DNase (dornase alpha) in patients with cystic fibrosis
- Bronchodilator therapy in selected patients
- Pain control in postoperative and trauma cases
- Pleural drainages in cases of large effusions, hemothorax, or empyema

CHRONIC Rx

- Chest physiotherapy
- Humidification of inspired air
- Frequent nasotracheal suctioning

DISPOSITION

Prognosis varies with the underlying etiology

REFERRAL

- Bronchoscopy for removal of foreign body or plugs unresponsive to conservative treatment
- Surgical referral for removal of obstructing neoplasm

PEARLS & CONSIDERATIONS

COMMENTS

Patients should be educated that frequent changes of position are helpful in clearing secretions. Sitting the patient upright in a chair is recommended to increase both volume and vital capacity relative to the supine position. Adequate pain control is paramount after surgical intervention or rib fractures.

RELATED CONTENT

Atelectasis (Patient Information)

AUTHORS: **FREDERIC CELESTIN, M.D.,** and **SAMAAN RAFEQ, M.D.**

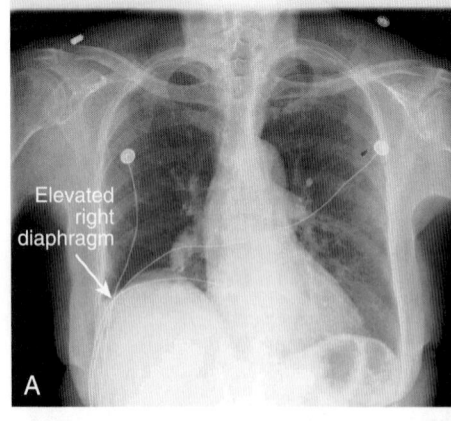
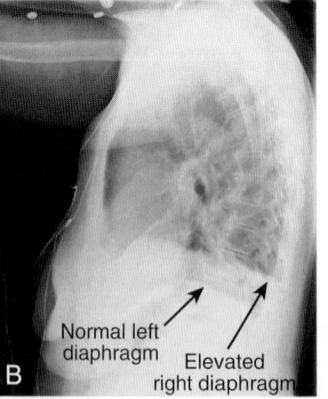

FIG. 1 Atelectasis with elevated diaphragm: an example of volume loss. The right hemidiaphragm in this patient appears elevated on both the posterior-anterior **(A)** and the lateral **(B)** views. Is this the correct interpretation of the x-ray, and if so, what is the cause? Consider the alternative interpretations. A subpulmonic pleural effusion would appear similar, as it would have the same density as liver, heart, and diaphragm and would layer over the diaphragm with the patient upright. This appears less likely in that a meniscus might be seen along the lateral chest wall with a pleural effusion but is not present here. In addition, a pleural effusion occupies space and might be expected to push the heart to the left, whereas in this case the heart may be slightly deviated to the right. Atelectasis of the lower right lung would result in volume loss, pulling the heart and hemidiaphragm into the space normally occupied by lung. This is consistent with the observed features. An infiltrate in this location could explain the x-ray findings but appears less likely for similar reasons to those cited for effusion. Some simple maneuvers could narrow the differential diagnosis. Chest ultrasound, decubitus x-ray views, or CT could identify an effusion. (From Broder JS: *Diagnostic imaging for the emergency physician,* Philadelphia, 2011, Saunders.)

BASIC INFORMATION

DEFINITION

Atopic dermatitis is a genetically determined eczematous eruption that is pruritic, symmetric, and associated with personal family history of allergic manifestations (atopy). Box 1 summarizes criteria for atopic dermatitis. Modified criteria for children with atopic dermatitis are described in Box 2.

SYNONYMS

Eczema
Atopic neurodermatitis
Atopic eczema

ICD-10CM CODES
L20.9 Atopic dermatitis, unspecified
L20.89 Other atopic dermatitis

EPIDEMIOLOGY & DEMOGRAPHICS

- Incidence is between 5 and 25 cases/1000 persons.
- Highest incidence is among children (10% to 20%). It accounts for 4% of acute care pediatric visits. It affects 1% to 3% of the adult population.
- Onset of disease before age 5 yr in 85% of patients.
- More than 50% of children with generalized atopic dermatitis develop asthma and allergic rhinitis by age 13 yr.
- Concordance in monozygotic twins is 77%.

PHYSICAL FINDINGS & CLINICAL PRESENTATION

- Atopic dermatitis presentation can be subdivided into three phases:
  1. Acute: vesicular, crusting, weeping eruption
  2. Subacute: dry, scaly, erythematous papules and plaques
  3. Chronic: lichenification from repeated scratching
- The lesions are typically on the neck, face, upper trunk, and bends of elbows and knees (symmetric on flexural surfaces of extremities) (Figs. 1 and E2). Atopic dermatitis lesions are usually discrete but vaguely delineated, scaly, and erythematous.
- There is dryness, thickening of the involved areas, discoloration, blistering, and oozing.
- Papular lesions are frequently found in the antecubital and popliteal fossae.
- In children, red scaling plaques are often confined to the cheeks and the perioral and perinasal areas.
- ***Hertoghe sign:*** loss of the outer eyebrow from chronic rubbing (Fig. 1, *B*).
- Constant scratching may result in areas of hypopigmentation or hyperpigmentation (more common in blacks).
- In adults, redness and scaling in the dorsal aspect of the hands or about the fingers are the most common expression of atopic dermatitis; oozing and crusting may be present.
- Secondary skin infections may be present (*Staphylococcus aureus,* dermatophytosis, herpes simplex).

ETIOLOGY

Unknown; elevated T-lymphocyte activation, defective cell immunity, and B-cell IgE overproduction may play a significant role.

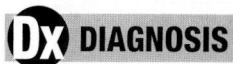 DIAGNOSIS

DIFFERENTIAL DIAGNOSIS

- Scabies
- Psoriasis
- Dermatitis herpetiform
- Contact dermatitis
- Photosensitivity
- Seborrheic dermatitis
- Candidiasis, tinea
- Lichen simplex chronicus
- Other: xerosis, impetigo, Wiskott-Aldrich syndrome, PKU, ichthyosis, HIV dermatitis, nonnummular eczema, histiocytosis X, malignancies (T-cell lymphoma/*Mycosis fungoides*, Letterer-Siwe disease), graft-versus-host disease, metabolic and nutritional deficiencies (zinc, niacin, pyridoxine deficiencies)

BOX 1 Criteria for Atopic Dermatitis

Major criteria
Must have three of the following:
- Pruritus
- Typical morphology and distribution
  - Flexural lichenification in adults
  - Facial and extensor involvement in infancy
- Chronic or chronically relapsing dermatitis
- Personal or family history of atopic disease (e.g., asthma, allergic rhinitis, atopic dermatitis)

Minor criteria
Must also have three of the following:
1. Xerosis
2. Ichthyosis or hyperlinear palms or keratosis pilaris
3. IgE reactivity (immediate skin test reactivity, RAST test positive)
4. Elevated serum IgE
5. Early age of onset
6. Tendency for cutaneous infections (especially *Staphylococcus aureus* and HSV)
7. Tendency to nonspecific hand/foot dermatitis
8. Nipple eczema
9. Cheilitis
10. Recurrent conjunctivitis
11. Dennie-Morgan infraorbital fold
12. Keratoconus
13. Anterior subcapsular cataracts
14. Orbital darkening
15. Facial pallor or facial erythema
16. Pityriasis alba
17. Itch when sweating
18. Intolerance to wool and lipid solvents
19. Perifollicular accentuation
20. Food hypersensitivity
21. Course influenced by environmental or emotional factors
22. White dermatographism or delayed blanch to cholinergic agents

HSV, Herpes simplex virus; *RAST,* radioallergosorbent assay.
From James WD et al: *Andrews' diseases of the skin,* ed 12, Philadelphia, 2016, Saunders.

BOX 2 Modified Criteria for Children with Atopic Dermatitis

Essential features
1. Pruritus
2. Eczema
   - Typical morphology and age-specific pattern
   - Chronic or relapsing history

Important features
1. Early age at onset
2. Atopy
3. Personal or family history
4. IgE reactivity
5. Xerosis

Associated features
1. Atypical vascular responses (e.g., facial pallor, white dermatographism)
2. Keratosis pilaris, ichthyosis, or hyperlinear palms
3. Orbital or periorbital changes
4. Other regional findings (e.g., perioral changes, periauricular lesions)
5. Perifollicular accentuation, lichenification, or prurigo lesions

From James WD et al: *Andrews' diseases of the skin,* ed 12, Philadelphia, 2016, Saunders.

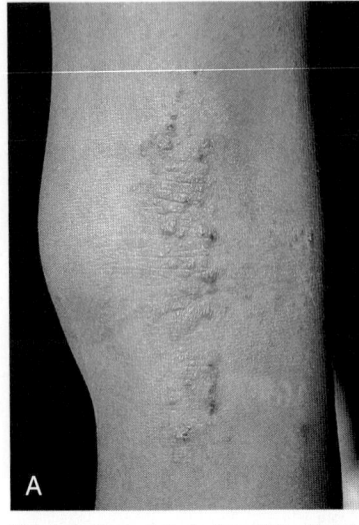
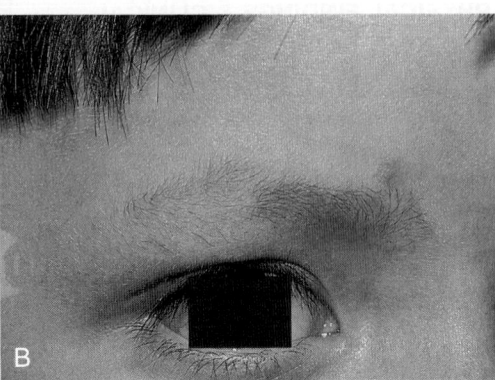

FIG. 1 A, Flexural atopic dermatitis with lichenification. Many of the skin changes are secondary to scratching. Linear lichenification, as shown here, and excoriations are typical. **B,** Hertoghe sign: loss of the outer eyebrow may occur in the atopic patient as a result of chronic rubbing. (From White GM, Cox NH [eds]: *Diseases of the skin, a color atlas and text,* ed 2, St Louis, 2006, Mosby.)

WORKUP

Diagnosis is based on the presence of three of the following major features and three minor features.

MAJOR FEATURES:
- Pruritus
- Personal or family history of atopy: asthma, allergic rhinitis, atopic dermatitis
- Facial and extensor involvement in infants and children
- Flexural lichenification in adults

MINOR FEATURES:
- Elevated IgE
- Eczema-perifollicular accentuation
- Recurrent conjunctivitis
- Ichthyosis
- Nipple dermatitis
- Wool intolerance
- Cutaneous *S. aureus* infections or herpes simplex infections
- Food intolerance
- Hand dermatitis (nonallergic irritant)
- Facial pallor, facial erythema
- Cheilitis
- White dermographism
- Early age of onset (after 2 mo of age)

LABORATORY TESTS

- Lab tests are generally not helpful.
- Elevated IgE levels are found in 80% to 90% of atopic dermatitis.

- Consider skin biopsy only in cases unresponsive to treatment.

℞ TREATMENT
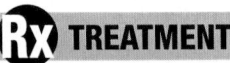

NONPHARMACOLOGIC THERAPY

- Clip nails to decrease abrasion of skin
  Avoidance of triggering factors:
- Sudden temperature changes, sweating, low humidity in the winter
- Contact with irritating substance (e.g., wool, cosmetics, some soaps and detergents, tobacco)
- Foods that provoke exacerbations (e.g., eggs, peanuts, fish, soy, wheat, milk)
- Stressful situations
- Allergens and dust
- Excessive hand washing

GENERAL Rx

- Emollients can be used to prevent dryness. Severely affected skin can be optimally hydrated by occlusion in addition to application of emollients.
- Low-potency topical corticosteroids (e.g., 1% to 2.5% hydrocortisone) may be helpful and are generally considered first-line therapy. Use intermediate-potency steroids (e.g., triamcinolone, fluocinolone) for more severe cases and limit potent corticosteroids (e.g.,

betamethasone, desoximetasone, clobetasol) to severe cases.
- Oral antihistamines (e.g., hydroxyzine, diphenhydramine) are effective in controlling pruritus and inducing sedation, restful sleep, and prevention of scratching during sleep. Doxepin and other tricyclic antidepressants also have antihistamine effect, induce sleep, and reduce pruritus.
- The topical immunomodulators pimecrolimus and tacrolimus are especially useful for treatment of the face and intertriginous sites, where steroid-induced atrophy may occur. However, due to concerns about carcinogenic potential, the FDA recommends limiting their use for short periods in patients who are intolerant or unresponsive to other treatments. Pimecrolimus cream 1% is applied bid and has antiinflammatory effects secondary to blockage of activated T-cell cytokine production. Tacrolimus ointment (0.03% or 0.1%) applied bid is a macrolide that suppresses humoral and cell-mediated immune responses.
- Oral prednisone, IM triamcinolone, Goeckerman regimen, PUVA are generally reserved for severe cases.
- Cyclosporine, azathioprine, mycophenolate, and interferon gamma are sometimes tried for recalcitrant disease in adults by physicians who specialize in severe inflammatory skin conditions.
- Clinical phase 3 trials have shown that the human monoclonal antibody dupilumab is effective in adults with moderate to severe atopic dermatitis. Trials of longer duration are needed to assess the long-term effectiveness and safety of dupilumab.[1]

DISPOSITION

- Resolution occurs in approximately 70% of patients by adulthood.
- Most patients have a course characterized by remissions and intermittent flares.

SUGGESTED READINGS
Available at www.expertconsult.com

RELATED CONTENT
Dermatitis (Patient Information)
Eczema (Patient Information)

AUTHOR: **FRED F. FERRI, M.D.**

[1]Bieber GL, et al.: Two phase 3 trials of dupilumab versus placebo in atopic dermatitis, *N Engl J Med* 375:2335–2348, 2016.

BASIC INFORMATION

DEFINITION

Atrial fibrillation (AF) is a supraventricular tachyarrhythmia characterized by disorganized and rapid atrial activation and uncoordinated atrial contraction. AF occurs when structural and/or electrophysiologic abnormalities alter atrial tissue to promote abnormal impulse formation and/or propagation. The ventricular rate is dependent on the conduction properties of the atrioventricular (AV) node, which can be influenced by vagal/sympathetic tone, medications, or disease of the AV node.

Multiple classification schemes have been used in the past to characterize AF. The current classification scheme (divided into three major types) used by the ACC/AHA guideline committee is as follows:

- Paroxysmal AF—more than one episode of AF that terminate spontaneously or with intervention within 7 days
- Persistent AF—episodes of AF that last longer than 7 days
- Long-standing persistent AF—AF that has persisted for longer than 1 yr, either because cardioversion has failed or because cardioversion has not been attempted
- Permanent AF: When patient and physician decide to stop pursuing restoring sinus rhythm
- In addition to the previous AF categories, which are mainly defined by episode timing and termination, the ACC/AHA/ESC guidelines describe additional AF categories in terms of other characteristics of the patient:
  ○ Lone atrial fibrillation (LAF)—generally refers to AF in younger patients without clinical or echocardiographic evidence of cardiopulmonary disease, diabetes, or hypertension
  ○ Nonvalvular AF—absence of rheumatic mitral valve disease, a mechanical or bioprosthetic heart valve, or mitral valve repair
  ○ Secondary AF—occurs in the setting of a primary condition that may be the cause of the AF, such as acute myocardial infarction, cardiac surgery, pericarditis, myocarditis, hyperthyroidism, pulmonary embolism, pneumonia, or other acute disease. It is considered separately because AF is less likely to recur once the precipitating condition has resolved.

SYNONYMS

AF
PAF
AFib

ICD-10CM CODES
I48.0	Paroxysmal atrial fibrillation
I48.1	Persistent atrial fibrillation
I48.2	Chronic atrial fibrillation
I48.91	Unspecified atrial fibrillation

EPIDEMIOLOGY & DEMOGRAPHICS

- The prevalence of AF increases with age, from 2% in adults <65 yr to 9% of those >65 yr.
- AF affects 2.7 million people in the United States. AF is uncommon in infants and children and, when present, almost always occurs in association with structural heart disease.
- The incidence of AF is significantly higher in men than in women in all age groups (1.1% versus 0.8%). AF appears to be more common in whites than in blacks, who may have lower awareness of the disease.
- Stroke due to thromboembolism is the most common and dreaded complication of AF. The rate of ischemic stroke in patients with non-rheumatic AF averages 5% a year, which is somewhere between two and seven times the rate of stroke in patients without AF. The risk of stroke is not due solely to AF; it increases substantially in the presence of other cardiovascular diseases. The attributable risk of stroke from AF is estimated to be 1.5% for those aged 50 to 59 yr, and it approaches 36% for those aged 80 to 89 yr.

PHYSICAL FINDINGS & CLINICAL PRESENTATION

Clinical presentation is variable:
- Palpitations, dizziness, or lightheadedness
- Fatigue, weakness, or impaired exercise tolerance
- Angina
- Dyspnea
- Some patients are asymptomatic
- Cardiac auscultation revealing irregularly irregular rhythm
- Thromboembolic phenomenon such as stroke

ETIOLOGY

- The most frequent change in AF is the loss of atrial muscle mass and atrial fibrosis.
- Fibrillation is presumed to be caused by multiple wandering wavelets, usually originating from the pulmonary veins. Both reentrant and focal mechanisms have been proposed.
- Vascular causes: hypertensive heart disease
- Valvular heart disease
- Pulmonary causes: pulmonary embolism, chronic obstructive pulmonary disease, obstructive sleep apnea, carbon monoxide poisoning
- Structural cardiac disease: hypertrophic cardiomyopathy, congestive heart failure, coronary artery disease, myocardial infarction, congenital heart disease (especially those that lead to atrial enlargement such as atrial septal defect)
- Pericarditis and myocarditis
- Arrhythmias: atrial tachycardias and atrial flutters have been associated with atrial fibrillation, as has Wolff-Parkinson-White syndrome
- Endocrine: thyrotoxicosis, hyperthyroidism or subclinical hyperthyroidism, pheochromocytoma, obesity
- Surgery: both cardiac and noncardiac
- Electrolytes: hypokalemia, hypomagnesemia
- Systemic stress: fever, anemia, hypoxia, sepsis, infections (e.g., pneumonia)
- Medications/toxins: digitalis, adenosine, theophylline, amphetamines, cocaine, antihistamines, alcohol abuse and/or withdrawal, caffeine, steroidal antiinflammatory drugs (SAIDs), nonsteroidal antiinflammatory drugs (NSAIDs)
- Frequency of vigorous exercise is associated with an increased risk of developing AF in young men and joggers
- Porphyrias have been associated with autonomic dysfunction and increased risk of AF
- Patients with metabolic syndrome, excessive vitamin D intake, or excessive niacin intake have a higher risk of AF

DIAGNOSIS

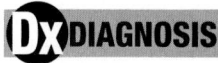

DIFFERENTIAL DIAGNOSIS

- Multifocal atrial tachycardia
- Atrial flutter
- Frequent atrial premature beats
- Atrial tachycardia
- AV nodal reentry tachycardia (AVNRT)
- Wolff-Parkinson-White syndrome

WORKUP

The evaluation of atrial fibrillation involves diagnosis, determination of the etiology, and classification of the arrhythmia. A minimal evaluation includes a history and physical examination, ECG, transthoracic echocardiogram, and case-specific laboratory work to rule out secondary AF.

LABORATORY TESTS

- Thyroid-stimulating hormone, free T_4
- Serum electrolytes
- Toxicity screen
- CBC count (looking for anemia, infection)
- Renal and hepatic function tests
- D-dimer/CT scan of chest PE protocol (if the patient has risk factors to merit a pulmonary embolism workup)

IMAGING STUDIES

- ECG (Fig. 1)
- Absence of P waves
- Fibrillatory or f waves at the isoelectric baseline with varying amplitude, morphology, and intervals
- Irregular ventricular rate
- Echocardiography to rule out structural heart disease (evaluate ventricular size, thickness, and function, atrial size, pericardial disease, and valve function)
- Chest radiography (if pulmonary disease or CHF is suspected)
- Transesophageal echocardiography (TEE): helpful to evaluate for left atrial thrombus (particularly in the LA appendage) to guide cardioversion or ablation (if thrombus is seen, cardioversion should be delayed)
- CT and MRI: in patients with a positive D-dimer result, chest CT angiogram may be necessary to rule out pulmonary embolus. Three-dimensional imaging technologies (CT scan or MRI) are often helpful to evaluate atrial anatomy if AF ablation is planned
- Six-minute walk test or exercise test: six-minute walk or exercise testing can help assess the adequacy of rate control. Exercise testing can also exclude ischemia prior to treatment of

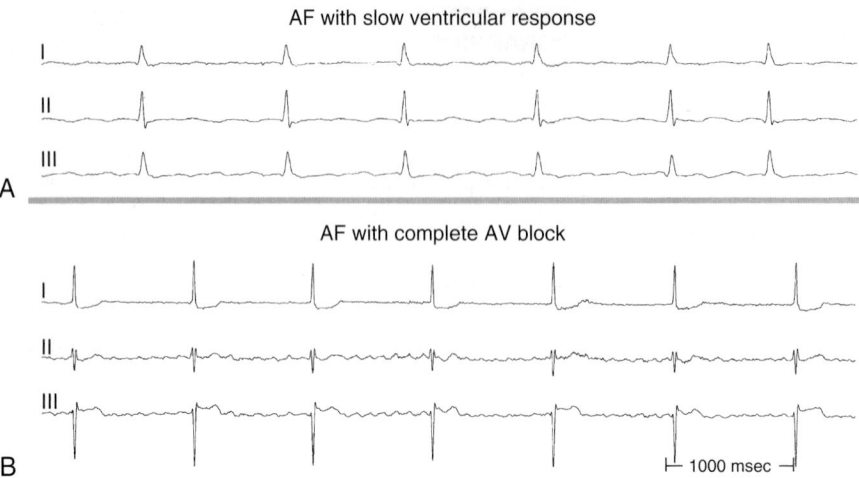

FIG. 1 Atrial fibrillation (AF) with slow ventricular rate. A, The ventricular rhythm is irregular, indicating that it is the result of conducted atrial beats. **B,** The ventricular rhythm is regular, consistent with the presence of complete atrioventricular *(AV)* block and a regular junctional escape rhythm. (From Issa Z et al: *Clinical arrhythmology and electrophysiology,* ed 2, Philadelphia.)

patients with class Ic antiarrhythmic drugs and can be used to reproduce exercise-induced AF
- Sleep study (if sleep apnea is suspected)
- Holter monitor or event recorder if the diagnosis of AF is in question and to assess AF burden
- Electrophysiologic study: when initiation of AF is secondary to a supraventricular tachycardia, such as AVNRT or Wolff-Parkinson-White syndrome

℞ TREATMENT

ACUTE TREATMENT

ACUTE GENERAL RX: New-onset AF:
- If the patient is hemodynamically unstable (hypotension, congestive heart failure, or angina), perform synchronized cardioversion after immediate conscious sedation with a rapid short-acting sedative (e.g., midazolam). The likelihood of cardioversion-related clinical thromboembolism is low in patients with AF lasting <48 hr. Patients with AF lasting >2 days have a 5% to 7% risk for clinical thromboembolism if cardioversion is not preceded by several weeks of anticoagulation therapy. However, if transesophageal echocardiography reveals no atrial thrombus, cardioversion may be performed safely after therapeutic anticoagulation has been achieved. Alternatively, patients can be safely anticoagulated for approximately 1 month and then undergo cardioversion without transesophageal echocardiogram. Anticoagulant therapy should be continued for at least 1 month after cardioversion to minimize the incidence of adverse thromboembolic events. It can be stopped after 1 month as long as AF has not recurred if the patient is deemed low risk of stroke using the CHA2DS2VASc scoring system (see the following).
- If the patient is hemodynamically stable, a rate-control strategy is typically pursued initially.
- Treatment options for rate control include the following:
  1. Diltiazem 0.25 mg/kg (maximum of 25 mg) given intravenously (IV) over 2 min

followed by a second dose of 0.35 mg/kg (maximum of 25 mg) 15 min later if the rate is not slowed to <100 beats/min. May then follow with IV infusion 10 mg/hr (range, 5-15 mg/h) to achieve a resting heart rate of <100 beats/min. Onset of action after IV administration is usually within 3 min, with peak effect most often occurring within 10 min. After the ventricular rate is slowed, the patient can be changed to oral diltiazem 60 to 90 mg q4 to 6h. High doses of calcium channel blockers can exacerbate heart failure and thus should be used with caution in patients presenting with symptoms of heart failure or depressed ejection fraction.
  2. Verapamil 2.5 to 5 mg IV initially, then 5 to 10 mg IV 10 min later if the rate is still not slowed to <100 beats/min. After the ventricular rate is slowed, the patient can be changed to oral verapamil 80 to 120 mg q6 to 8h. Main concern is hypotension and heart failure with this medication. Because of its poor safety profile, it is infrequently used.
  3. Esmolol, metoprolol, and atenolol are beta-blockers available in IV preparations that can be used in AF. High doses of β-blockers can have negative inotropic effects in heart failure and should be used with caution.
  4. Digoxin is not a potent AV nodal blocking agent and has a potential for toxicity and therefore cannot be relied on for acute control of the ventricular response, but it may be used in conjunction with beta-blockers and calcium channel blockers. However, it can be a useful adjunct to a beta-blocker in the hypotensive or heart failure patient, which is not infrequent. When used, give 0.5 mg IV loading dose (slow) and then 0.25 mg IV 6 hr later. A third dose may be needed after 6 to 8 hr; the daily dose varies from 0.125 to 0.25 mg (decrease dosage in patients with renal insufficiency and elderly patients) depending on the heart rate and signs or symptoms of digoxin toxicity.

Toxicity is manifested by GI and visual complaints, atrial tachyarrhythmias, heart block, and ventricular tachycardia.
  5. Amiodarone has a class IIa recommendation from the ACC/AHA/ESC for use as a rate-controlling agent for patients who are intolerant of or unresponsive to other agents, such as patients with heart failure who may otherwise not tolerate diltiazem or metoprolol. Caution should be exercised in those who are not receiving anticoagulation because amiodarone can promote cardioversion, thereby posing a thromboembolic risk.
- All AV nodal blocking agents should be avoided in patients with Wolff-Parkinson-White syndrome and AF because, by blocking the AV node, AF impulses may be transmitted exclusively down the accessory pathway, which can result in ventricular fibrillation. If this happens, the patient will require immediate defibrillation. Procainamide, flecainide, or amiodarone can be used instead if Wolff-Parkinson-White syndrome is suspected.
- In the acute setting, pharmacologic cardioversion (e.g., ibutilide, dofetilide) is less commonly used than electrical cardioversion. A major disadvantage with pharmacologic cardioversion is the risk of development of ventricular tachycardia and other serious arrhythmias, especially due to acute prolongation of the QT interval.

CHRONIC THERAPY

- Avoidance of alcohol in patients with suspected excessive alcohol use.
- Treatment of underlying source or cause, if any found.
- Per the AFFIRM and RACE trials, either rate control or rhythm control strategies show no difference in composite cardiovascular end points of death, CHF, bleeding, drug side effects, or thromboembolism. Both approaches have similar outcomes as long as appropriate anticoagulation is maintained based on the individual's stroke risk.

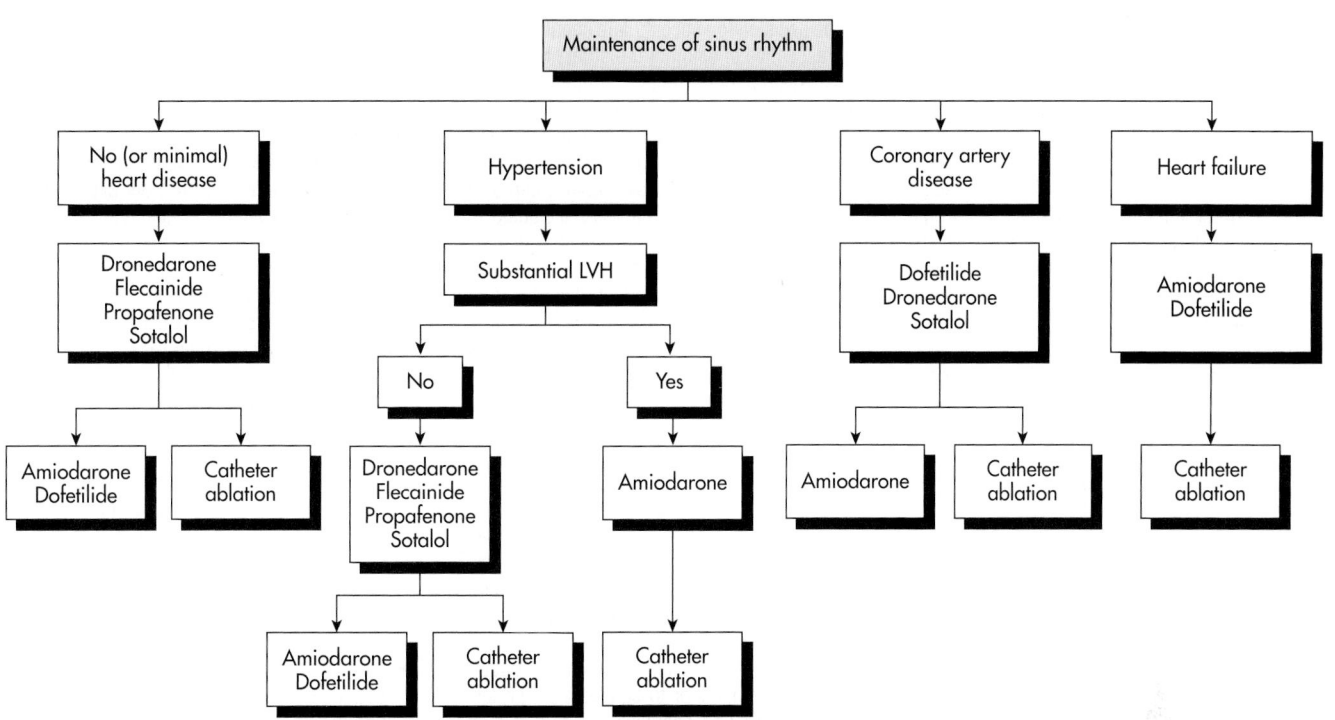

FIG. 2 Therapy to maintain sinus rhythm in patients with recurrent paroxysmal or persistent atrial fibrillation. Drugs are listed alphabetically and not in order of suggested use. The seriousness of heart disease progresses from left to right, and selection of therapy in patients with multiple conditions depends on the most serious condition present. *LVH,* Left ventricular hypertrophy. (From 2011 ACCF/AHA/HRS Focused Update on the Management of Patients With Atrial Fibrillation [Updating the 2006 Guideline]: A Report of the American College of Cardiology Foundation/American Heart Association Task Force on Practice Guidelines, *J Am Coll Cardiol* 57[2]:223-242, 2011.)

- For patients without symptomatic AF, a rate-control strategy with calcium channel blockers, beta-blockers, or digoxin is a reasonable option. The RACE 2 trial indicates that a lenient rate control strategy, with a target resting heart rate of <110 beats/min, is noninferior for a composite primary end point that included CV death, heart failure hospitalization, stroke, and other major events over a median 3-yr follow-up compared with a strict control strategy, with a target resting heart rate of <80 beats/min and an exercise heart rate of <110 beats/min. Most recent ACC/AHA guidelines, however, recommend targeting a HR <80 beats/min over a target of <110 beats/min.

- In patients with symptomatic AF, younger patients, or those with difficult to control heart rate, an attempt should be made to maintain sinus rhythm with antiarrhythmic agents. Options of antiarrhythmic agents include amiodarone, dronedarone, (paroxysmal atrial fibrillation only without heart failure), dofetilide, flecainide, propafenone (contraindicated with structural heart disease), procainamide, or sotalol. The decision of which strategy to follow should be best made in consultation with cardiology. Use of dronedarone should be avoided in patients with persistent or permanent atrial fibrillation because of worsened cardiovascular outcomes, especially in those with concomitant symptomatic heart failure (see Fig. 2 for a proposed algorithm to guide maintenance of sinus rhythm).

NONPHARMACOLOGIC THERAPY

- Catheter ablation of AF has become a common procedure for symptomatic drug-refractory or drug-intolerant patients. Sinus rhythm can be maintained long term in the majority of patients with PAF by circumferential pulmonary vein ablation performed in experienced centers. Established centers have reported success rates of 70% to 85% in patients with paroxysmal AF, but up to 50% of patients may require more than one ablation to achieve success. Complication rates are 4.5% in the largest international survey of hospitals performing this procedure. Success with persistent AF is much lower, with long-term success rates of 40% to 50% in many studies, and such patients often require more than one procedure. The most common techniques used to isolate the pulmonary veins are radiofrequency ablation and cryoballoon ablation, which have shown similar results for patients with PAF.

- Pulmonary vein isolation is being increasingly used to treat AF in patients with heart failure. Trials have shown that pulmonary vein isolation is superior to AV node ablation with biventricular pacing in patients with heart failure who have drug-refractory AF.

- AV nodal ablation with permanent pacemaker implantation may become necessary in some patients in whom rate and rhythm are difficult to control despite drugs and cardioversion, although it is generally used as a therapy of last resort.

- The Cox-Maze III surgical procedure, with its modifications creating electrical barriers to the macroreentrant circuits that are believed to underlie AF, is being performed with good results in some medical centers (preservation of sinus rhythm in 70% to 95% of patients without the use of long-term antiarrhythmic medication). Success rates are higher in paroxysmal than in persistent or permanent atrial fibrillation. Some centers perform surgical pulmonary vein isolation similar to this procedure using a mini-thoracotomy or video thoracoscopic "Mini-Maze" approach. Another surgical method is a pericardioscopic approach that allows extensive posterior wall ablation and, when combined with catheter ablation in a "hybrid" approach, has shown promising results for patients with persistent AF.

- It is important to understand that ablation therapy will not eliminate the need to take anticoagulant drugs. Even after ablation, patients with AF face increased risk of thromboembolic events and most electrophysiologists suggest lifelong anticoagulation for patients with elevated stroke risk score. Due the increasing success rate of ablation, catheter-based therapy is now considered an acceptable first-line alternative to cardioversion and pharmacologic management to *paroxysmal* atrial fibrillation in the most recent ACC/AHA Guidelines in 2014. It remains second-line therapy for patients in persistent and permanent atrial fibrillation.

STROKE PREVENTION

- The decision whether to pursue long-term anticoagulation must be made in light of the patient's risk for a cardioembolic event versus risk for a bleeding event. In nonvalvular AF, CHA2DS2-VASc has superseded the CHADS2 scoring system (C = congestive heart failure; H = hypertension; A = age [>75 years is 2 points]; D = diabetes; S = stroke, transient ischemic attack, or thromboembolic disease [2 points]; V = vascular disease, A = age 65-74 years; and

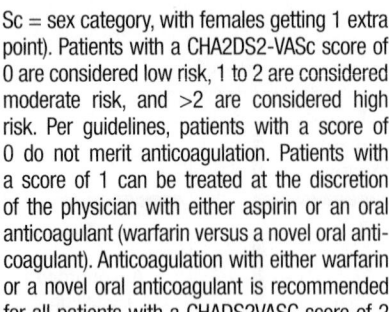

Sc = sex category, with females getting 1 extra point). Patients with a CHA2DS2-VASc score of 0 are considered low risk, 1 to 2 are considered moderate risk, and >2 are considered high risk. Per guidelines, patients with a score of 0 do not merit anticoagulation. Patients with a score of 1 can be treated at the discretion of the physician with either aspirin or an oral anticoagulant (warfarin versus a novel oral anticoagulant). Anticoagulation with either warfarin or a novel oral anticoagulant is recommended for all patients with a CHADS2VASC score of 2 or above.

- Increasing amounts of evidence now show that aspirin likely does not protect a person from stroke in AF and has recently been dropped from most of the ACC/AHA and European Atrial Fibrillation guidelines. Target INR for patients with a CHADS-VASc score of >1 is 2 to 3 and should be diligently monitored to avoid risk of stroke versus bleeding. Patients with hypertrophic cardiomyopathy or thyrotoxicosis with AF also have a high risk of stroke and should be anticoagulated irrespective of their CHADS-VASc score.

- Alternatives to warfarin now include several factor Xa inhibitors and a direct thrombin inhibitor.
  1. Dabigatran is an FDA-approved direct thrombin inhibitor indicated to reduce the risk of stroke and systemic embolism in patients with nonvalvular atrial fibrillation. In the RE-LY trial of 18,113 patients with mean CHADS2 score of 2.1, dabigatran 110 mg bid was noninferior to warfarin, and 150 mg bid was superior to warfarin in prevention of thromboembolic events. Bleeding risk was similar to that of warfarin for both doses. Idarucizumab has been approved as a dabigatran reversal agent. Onset is immediate, and it provides full reversal for at least 24 hours in most patients.
  2. Factor Xa inhibitors (apixaban, rivaroxaban, edoxaban) are also effective in reducing stroke and systemic embolism in patients with atrial fibrillation. The ARISTOTLE trial in patients at high risk for stroke (mean CHADS2 score 2.1) using apixaban, the ROCKET AF trial using rivaroxaban in patients with CHADS2 score 3.5, and the ENGAGE-AF trial using edoxaban in patients with a CHADS2 score of at least 2, showed that these anticoagulants reduce the risk of stroke, systemic embolism, and serious bleeding compared with warfarin. Rivaroxaban showed noninferior efficacy to warfarin in prevention of thromboembolism. Apixaban showed superior stroke reduction, reduced bleeding events, and an overall mortality benefit when compared with warfarin. Edoxaban showed noninferiority to warfarin with respect to stroke and systemic embolism prevention, with lower rates of bleeding and death from cardiovascular causes, but benefit was limited to patients with moderately impaired renal function. Rivaroxaban and edoxaban are dosed once a day, and apixaban is dosed twice a day. A factor Xa reversal agent, andexanet alfa, is available for reversing the anticoagulant effect of these agents.

- The decision to anticoagulate should be made irrespective of whether the atrial fibrillation is paroxysmal, persistent or permanent.
- For patients in whom anticoagulation with warfarin or other anticoagulants is contraindicated due to high bleeding risk, left atrial appendage exclusion is an alternative. Several methods can be used, including the Lariat procedure and the Atriclip, but these are still considered unproven for stroke prevention in AF. The Watchman device is a left atrial appendage occlusion device and is the only device approved by the FDA for stroke prevention specifically for patients with AF that require anticoagulation but have an appropriate reason to seek an alternative.
- Perioperative bridging anticoagulation in patients with AF: current guidelines advise perioperative continuation of warfarin in low-risk patients (CHADS2 score 0 to 2) and bridging anticoagulation in those at highest risk of thromboembolism (CHADS2 score 5 to 6). The recent BRIDGE Study found that for patients who require procedure-related warfarin interruption, forgoing bridging anticoagulation was noninferior to perioperative bridging with LMWH and decrease the risk of major bleeding. Based on this study, a no-bridging strategy is responsible for lower-risk AF and minor procedures but in patients having major surgery the answer remains debatable.

PROGNOSIS

- AF is associated with a 1.5- to 1.9-fold higher risk of death, which is in part due to the strong association between AF and thromboembolic events.
- AF is also independently associated with an increased risk of incident MI, especially in women and blacks.
- Development of AF predicts heart failure and is associated with a worse New York Heart Association Heart Failure classification. AF may also worsen heart failure in individuals who are dependent on the atrial component of the cardiac output.
- AF in the setting of acute myocardial infarction was associated with a 40% increase in mortality compared to patients in sinus rhythm.

DISPOSITION

Factors associated with maintenance of sinus rhythm after cardioversion include:
- Left atrium diameter <60 mm
- Absence of mitral valve disease
- Short duration of AF

REFERRAL

Refer to a cardiologist those patients in whom antiarrhythmic therapy or catheter-based/surgical intervention is being considered.

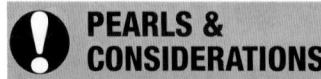

PEARLS & CONSIDERATIONS

COMMENTS

The number of patients anticoagulated in the United States is approximately half the amount

that should be anticoagulated for AF, resulting in a large burden of stroke. The exact burden of AF needed to trigger the need for anticoagulation is not known, though recent pacemaker trials have suggested that as little as 6 min confers significant stroke risk. Reversal agents for the new class of anticoagulation are now available: idarucizumab for reversal of dabigatran; andexanet alfa for reversal of apixaban and rivaroxaban.

The American Academy of Family Physicians and the American College of Physicians provide the following recommendations for the management of newly detected AF:

- Rate control with chronic anticoagulation is the recommended strategy for the majority of asymptomatic patients with chronic AF. Rhythm control has not been shown to be superior to rate control (with chronic anticoagulation) in reducing morbidity and mortality, and may be inferior in some patient subgroups to rate control. Rhythm control is appropriate when based on other special considerations, such as patient symptoms, exercise tolerance, and patient preference.
- Patients with AF should receive chronic anticoagulation, unless they are at low risk for stroke as stated earlier or have specific contraindications.
- For patients with AF, the following drugs are recommended for their demonstrated efficacy in rate control during exercise and while at rest: atenolol, metoprolol, diltiazem, and verapamil (drugs listed alphabetically by class). Digoxin is effective only for rate control at rest and, therefore, should be used only as a second-line agent for rate control in AF.
- For patients who elect to undergo acute cardioversion to achieve sinus rhythm in AF, both direct-current cardioversion and pharmacologic conversion are appropriate options in an otherwise healthy patient.
- Both transesophageal echocardiography with short-term prior anticoagulation followed by early acute cardioversion (in absence of intracardiac thrombus) with post-cardioversion anticoagulation vs. delayed cardioversion with preanticoagulation and postanticoagulation are appropriate management strategies for patients who elect to undergo cardioversion.
- Among patients with paroxysmal AF without previous antiarrhythmic drug treatment, ablation compared with antiarrhythmic drugs resulted in a lower rate of recurrent atrial tachyarrhythmias at 2 years. However, recurrence was frequent in both groups.

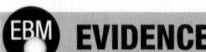 **EVIDENCE**

Available at www.expertconsult.com

SUGGESTED READINGS

Available at www.expertconsult.com

RELATED CONTENT

Atrial Fibrillation (Patient Information)

AUTHOR: **TANIA B. BABAR, M.D.**

BASIC INFORMATION

DEFINITION

Typical atrial flutter is the term commonly applied to the atrial macroreentrant circuit that circulates around the tricuspid annulus in the right atrium. The critical isthmus of the circuit is the tissue between the inferior vena cava and the tricuspid annulus, and a more precise name for this arrhythmia is *cavotricuspid isthmus-dependent atrial flutter*, or CTI flutter. Because of its anatomic and physiologic stability, the result is regular atrial depolarizations, typically at a rate of 250 to 350 beats/min. Regular, macroreentrant atrial arrhythmias at this rate that do not use the CTI are referred to as *atypical atrial flutter*. Because of the circuit's stability, conduction through the atrioventricular node (AVN) is often predictable at a common mathematical denominator. For example, when the flutter rate is 300 beats/min, 2:1 conduction results in a ventricular rate of 150 beats/min. By extension, 3:1 conduction results in a ventricular rate of 100 beats/min, 4:1 in a rate of 75 beats/min, and 5:1 in a rate of 60 beats/min. If the regular atrial impulses conduct at a variable rate through the AVN, the result may be an irregular QRS pattern.

ICD-10CM CODES
I48.3   Typical atrial flutter
I48.4   Atypical atrial flutter
I48.92 Unspecified atrial flutter

EPIDEMIOLOGY & DEMOGRAPHICS

- Atrial flutter is the second most common atrial tachyarrhythmia after atrial fibrillation, with an estimated 200,000 new cases annually in the United States.
- Atrial flutter is common in patients with congestive heart failure, COPD, or during the first week after open-heart surgery.
- Atrial flutter occurs more frequently with advancing age (5/10,0000 age <50 vs 587/100,000 age >80 yr) and 2.5 times more frequently in men than in women.
- Patients taking antiarrhythmics for chronic suppression of atrial fibrillation may convert to atrial flutter.
- Atrial flutter is typically seen in patients with underlying structural heart disease and is uncommon in children or young adults.
- More than 50% of patient with atrial flutter will develop atrial fibrillation in 3 years, and more than 80% will develop atrial fibrillation within 5 years.

CLASSIFICATION

Historically, the Wells classification designated atrial flutter as type I and type II. However, it is now recognized that tachycardias satisfying either of the definitions for type I or type II can be caused by reentrant circuits or to rapid focal atrial tachycardia, and this classification is infrequently used. Designating atrial flutter based on whether or not it is CTI dependent is more useful because of the management (i.e., ablation) options. Type I CTI-dependent atrial flutter, also known as common atrial flutter or typical atrial flutter, has an atrial rate of 240 to 350 beats/min. The reentrant loop circles the right atrium, passing through the CTI, a body of fibrous tissue in the lower atrium between the inferior vena cava and the tricuspid valve. CTI flutter can revolve around the tricuspid annulus in either direction (counterclockwise or clockwise) when viewing the tricuspid annulus *en face*.

- Counterclockwise atrial flutter is the more common type (~75%). The flutter waves are "sawtooth" and negative on the surface ECG leads II, III, and aVF; positive in V1; and negative in V6.
- Clockwise atrial flutter is less common (~25%): The reentry loop cycles in the opposite direction; thus, the flutter waves are upright in leads II, III, and aVF; negative in V1; and positive in V6.

Atypical atrial flutter is defined by absence of CTI dependence and may occur in patients with prior cardiac surgery, congenital heart disease, or prior radiofrequency ablation (especially left atrial ablation for atrial fibrillation) or may be idiopathic. One ECG feature is the lack of discordance between the inferior leads (leads II, III, and aVF) and V1.

PHYSICAL FINDINGS & CLINICAL PRESENTATION

- Palpitations
- Dizziness, lightheadedness, syncope, or near syncope
- Angina
- Congestive heart failure
- Embolic phenomena from intracardiac thrombus

ETIOLOGY

- Age-related degenerative changes
- Rheumatic heart disease
- Congenital heart disease
- Left ventricular dysfunction or congestive heart failure
- Acute myocardial infarction (rarely)
- Thyrotoxicosis
- Pulmonary embolism
- Mitral valve disease
- Cardiac surgery
- Chronic obstructive pulmonary disease
- Obesity
- Pericarditis
- Pulmonary hypertension
- Antiarrhythmic therapy use in patients with atrial fibrillation

DIAGNOSIS

DIFFERENTIAL DIAGNOSIS

- Atrial fibrillation
  Atrial tachycardia:
- Supraventricular tachycardia:
  - Atrioventricular node reentry
  - Orthodromic reciprocating tachycardia (using a concealed bypass tract)
  - Junctional ectopic tachycardia
  - Wolff-Parkinson-White syndrome
- Sinus tachycardia

WORKUP

- ECG
- Laboratory evaluation
- Assessment of CHA_2DS_2-VaSc score

LABORATORY TESTS

- Thyroid function studies
- Serum electrolytes, including renal and hepatic tests (anticipating antiarrhythmic therapy use)

IMAGING STUDIES

- ECG (Fig. 1):
  1. Absence of P waves.
  2. Regular, "sawtooth," or "F" (flutter)" wave pattern without an isoelectric baseline in leads II, III, and AVF (seen most commonly with counterclockwise typical CTI-flutter)
  3. There is rarely 1:1 atrioventricular (AV) conduction in atrial flutter (unless preexcitation is present). Rather, AV conduction is usually in a 2:1, 3:1, or 4:1 fashion, with corresponding usual ventricular rates of 150, 100, or 75 beats/min, respectively (assuming an atrial rate of 300 beats/min).
- Echocardiography (for new diagnoses) to evaluate for structural heart disease (ventricular size, thickness, and function; atrial size, and valve function).
- Transesophageal echocardiography: consider in patients with associated structural or functional heart disease to ascertain the presence of intracardiac thrombi, in the absence of an appropriate duration of anticoagulation.
- Holter monitoring or event recorder to assess for paroxysmal atrial flutter or rate control or to identify the arrhythmia if symptoms are nonspecific or to identify triggering events.
- Electrophysiologic studies: required for a precise diagnosis, for mapping pathway, and for ablation.

TREATMENT

NONPHARMACOLOGIC THERAPY

- Vagal maneuvers (e.g., the Valsalva maneuver or carotid sinus massage) may transiently slow the ventricular rate (by increasing AV block) and may make flutter waves more evident. Adenosine may be similarly helpful for diagnostic purposes, allowing the unmasking of the atrial rhythm in the absence of ventricular activity. Maneuvers that affect AV conduction would be unlikely to terminate atrial flutter.
- Direct current cardioversion is the treatment of choice for acute management of atrial flutter associated with hemodynamic instability or debilitating symptoms such as angina, congestive heart failure, or hypotension. Electrical cardioversion may be successful with energies as low as 25 joules, but because 100 joules is virtually always successful, this may

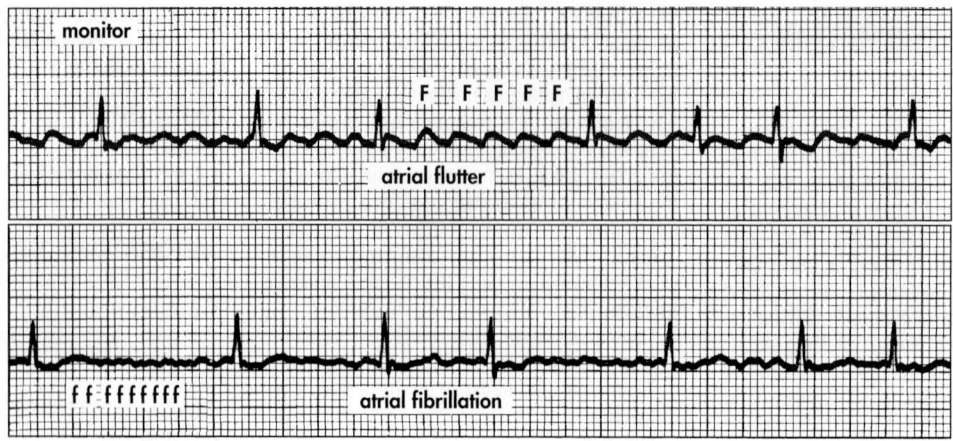

FIG. 1 Atrial flutter and fibrillation. Notice the sawtooth waves with atrial flutter (F) and the irregular fibrillatory waves with atrial fibrillation (f). (From Goldberger AL [ed]: *Clinical electrocardiography*, ed 5, St Louis, 1994, Mosby.)

Table 1 CHA$_2$DS$_2$-VASc Risk Score for Prediction of Stroke Risk in Atrial Fibrillation

Risk Factor	Points
CHF/LV dysfunction	1
Hypertension	1
Age ≥75 years	2
Diabetes mellitus	1
Stroke/TIA/embolism	2
Vascular disease	1
Age 64-74 years	1
Sex category (female)	1
Maximum score	9

CHF, congestive heart failure; *LV,* left ventricular; *TIA,* transient ischemic attack.

be a reasonable initial shock strength. If the electrical shock results in atrial fibrillation, a second shock at a higher energy level is used to restore normal sinus rhythm. Sedation of a conscious patient is highly recommended before cardioversion is performed. The use of external defibrillators with biphasic waveforms decreases the amount of energy required for cardioversion and improves cardioversion success rate. Patients should be therapeutically anticoagulated for at least a month or longer depending on their stroke risk (CHA$_2$DS$_2$-VASc score; Table 1).

- Overdrive pacing in the atrium may also terminate atrial flutter. This method is especially useful in patients who have recently undergone cardiac surgery and still have temporary atrial pacing wires and in patients who have an implanted pacemaker or defibrillator with an atrial lead.
- Radiofrequency ablation to interrupt the atrial flutter is highly effective for patients with chronic or recurring atrial flutter and is generally considered first-line therapy in those with recurrent episodes of atrial flutter and may be offered for a first-ever episode of atrial flutter. It has been shown to improve health-related quality of life. Despite successful ablation of atrial flutter, however, the risk of future atrial fibrillation remains.

ACUTE Rx

- Treatment choices are based on clinical circumstances. If the patient is unstable, proceed directly to electrical cardioversion.
- In the hemodynamically stable patient, proceed with rate control or rhythm control strategy.
- AV blocking agents such as calcium channel blockers, beta-blockers, and digitalis (second-line treatment) may all be used for rate control. Atrial flutter may spontaneously convert to normal sinus rhythm with this strategy.
- In general, atrial flutter is more difficult to rate-control than atrial fibrillation.
- The rate of recurrence of atrial flutter with cardioversion alone is difficult to determine because most published data combine atrial flutter with atrial fibrillation. However, the recurrence rate is substantial, perhaps 50% at 1 yr.
- Intravenous ibutilide is a first-line medication for pharmacologic cardioversion of atrial flutter in patients with normal systolic function and QT intervals. The success rate is approximately 60%, and it is more effective than procainamide, sotalol, or amiodarone.

CHRONIC Rx

- Few data exist to decide on the choice of rate control versus rhythm control in patients with atrial flutter. However, rate control may be difficult in atrial flutter, and ablation success exceeds 90%. Although ablation results in more durable freedom from atrial flutter recurrence, there are several pharmacologic options to help maintain sinus rhythm after cardioversion of atrial flutter, such as dofetilide, amiodarone, flecainide, propafenone, or sotalol. The choice of antiarrhythmic therapy is, in part, dictated by the presence or absence of underlying structural heart disease.
- Elective outpatient cardioversion or ablation can be performed either immediately preceded by TEE to evaluate the left atrium and the left atrial appendage for thrombus or after a period of at least 3 weeks of documented therapeutic anticoagulation before cardioversion. At least 4 weeks of anticoagulation should be performed after cardioversion, if not longer, depending on the overall thromboembolic risk of the patient as determined by the CHADS$_2$-VASC$_2$ score.

DISPOSITION

More than 85% of patients convert to regular sinus rhythm after cardioversion. Ablation success rates exceed 90%.

REFERRAL

Refer patients who are considered for rhythm control of atrial flutter to cardiologists, especially patients who are candidates for radiofrequency ablation.

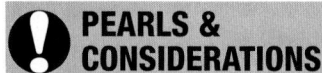 **PEARLS & CONSIDERATIONS**

COMMENTS

- The surface ECG is the best tool for recognizing atrial flutter and distinguishing atrial flutter from atrial fibrillation.
- Ablation for typical atrial flutter is highly effective, straightforward, and relatively safe. It should be considered for patients with recurrent episodes and even for a first-ever episode.
- Patients with atrial flutter carry a significant risk for subsequent development of atrial fibrillation.
- Anticoagulation should be considered for all patients whose CHA$_2$DS$_2$-VaSc score is ≥2. Anticoagulation is generally not recommended in patients with a CHA$_2$DS$_2$-VaSc score of zero. For patients with a CHA$_2$DS$_2$-VaSc score of 1, low-dose aspirin or oral anticoagulants (warfarin, dabigatran, rivaroxaban, apixaban, or edoxaban) are appropriate options.

SUGGESTED READINGS

Available at www.expertconsult.com

RELATED CONTENT

Atrial Flutter (Patient Information)
Atrial Fibrillation (Related Key Topic)

AUTHOR: **DANIEL R. FRISCH, M.D.**

BASIC INFORMATION

DEFINITION

Atrial myxoma is a benign neoplasm of mesenchymal origin and is the most common primary tumor of the heart.

SYNONYMS

Cardiac myxoma

ICD-10CM CODES
D15.1 Benign neoplasm of heart

EPIDEMIOLOGY & DEMOGRAPHICS

- Primary cardiac tumors are extremely rare, with an autopsy frequency of 0.001% to 0.03%. The most frequent cardiac tumors are metastases, occurring 30 times more frequently than primary tumors.
- Myxomas are the most common primary cardiac tumors, accounting for 30% to 50% of all benign neoplasms of the heart.
- 65% of cardiac myxomas occur in females. 4.5% to 10% of cardiac myxomas are familial (Carney syndrome).
- Average age of incidence of sporadic cases is 30 to 50 yr but can occur at any age.
- Average age of incidence of familial cases is 25 yr.
- Most arise in the left atrium (75%), but myxomas can also be found in the right atrium (18%), right ventricle (4%), and left ventricle (3%). They are usually pedunculated and attached to the intra-atrial septum.

PHYSICAL FINDINGS & CLINICAL PRESENTATION

Patients with atrial myxomas, when symptomatic, characteristically present in one of three ways:

1. Atrioventricular valve obstruction (e.g., mitral or tricuspid valve): may present with dyspnea, orthopnea, paroxysmal nocturnal dyspnea, wheezing, edema, dizziness, syncope, chest pain, atrial fibrillation, and sudden death (rare). A marked change in the severity of any symptom caused by a change in position of the patient, especially if recumbency relieves dyspnea, is suggestive of myxoma
2. Systemic embolization: leading to cerebrovascular accidents, pulmonary embolism, paradoxical embolism and acute coronary syndrome.
3. Constitutional symptoms: fever, weight loss, arthralgias and Raynaud's phenomenon.
4. Other rare manifestations include peripheral neuropathy, typical angina caused by coronary steal phenomenon (especially large vascularized atrial myxomas), and paraneoplastic syndromes.

On exam there may be widely split loud S1, secondary pulmonary hypertension, murmurs of regurgitation (holosystolic) or stenosis (rumbles), an early diastolic sound 80-120 milliseconds after A2 called "tumor plop" which may resemble an opening snap.

ETIOLOGY:

- Most cases (90%) of atrial myxomas are sporadic with no known cause
- Carney complex, transmitted in an autosomal dominant pattern, accounts for the majority of familial myxomas and as much as 7% of cardiac myxomas. Carney syndrome manifests as cardiac and extracardiac myxomas, pigmented skin discoloration, endocrine hyperactivity, and other tumors, such as schwannomas. There are at least three different genetic loci with two identified genes for this complex.

DIAGNOSIS

DIFFERENTIAL DIAGNOSIS

- Primary valvular diseases: mitral stenosis, mitral regurgitation, tricuspid stenosis, tricuspid regurgitation
- Pulmonary hypertension
- Endocarditis
- Vasculitis
- Atrial thrombus
- Pulmonary embolism
- Cerebrovascular accidents
- Collagen-vascular disease
- Carcinoid heart disease
- Benign tumors of the heart (papillary fibroelastoma, rhabdomyoma, fibroma, teratoma, and lipoma)
- Malignant tumors of the heart (angiosarcoma, rhabdosarcoma, fibrosarcoma, and leiomyosarcoma)
- Metastatic tumors to the heart (melanoma, lung, breast, renal, esophageal, and sarcomas)

WORKUP

A high index of suspicion is needed because the clinical manifestations are nonspecific and similar to many common cardiovascular and pulmonary diseases.

LABORATORY TESTS

Although not very specific, the following laboratory findings may be abnormal in patients with atrial myxomas:

- Complete blood count: anemia, polycythemia, thrombocytopenia may occur
- Erythrocyte sedimentation rate, C-reactive protein, and serum immunoglobulins are commonly elevated
- Electrocardiogram: left or right atrial enlargement, atrial fibrillation, premature ventricular depolarizations, or ventricular tachycardia

IMAGING STUDIES

- Transthoracic echocardiography: With 95% diagnostic sensitivity, it is the initial test of choice in suspected cases of atrial myxoma.
- Chest radiograph: about one third of patients have normal findings. Evidence of altered cardiac contour, pulmonary edema, and chamber enlargement may be present
- Transesophageal echocardiography: is the recommended measure for initial assessment and may better define cardiac masses not clearly visualized by transthoracic echocardiography.

- CT: often used for diagnosis; defines tumor extension and evaluates adjacent cardiac structures.
- MRI (Fig. E1): delineates size, shape, and tissue characteristics, helping distinguish thrombus from tumor.
- Cardiac catheterization: will show neovascularization in 50% of the cases and may be required to rule out concomitant coronary artery disease in anticipation of surgical excision.

TREATMENT

ACUTE GENERAL THERAPY

- Surgical excision is the treatment of choice
- Surgery should be done promptly because systemic embolization and/or sudden death can occur while waiting for the procedure

CHRONIC Rx

Postoperative arrhythmias and conduction abnormalities were present in 26% of patients and can be treated accordingly.

DISPOSITION

- Surgical results have reported a 95% survival rate after a follow-up of 3 yr.
- Careful follow-up is necessary because up to 5% of sporadic cases and 20% of familial cases of atrial myxoma may recur within the first 6 yr after surgery.
- Sudden death in untreated patients may occur in up to 15%, resulting from coronary or systemic embolization or obstruction of the mitral or tricuspid valve.

REFERRAL

- Consultation with a cardiologist is recommended.
- Once the presence of cardiac tumor is confirmed, consultation with a cardiovascular surgeon is needed for prompt surgical excision.

PEARLS & CONSIDERATIONS

- Approximately two thirds of patients present with cardiovascular symptoms, specifically dyspnea, often suggestive of valvular obstruction.
- Nearly one third of patients have evidence of systemic embolization.

COMMENTS

Annual echocardiograms should be performed to monitor for recurrence of atrial myxomas after surgical excision.

SUGGESTED READINGS
Available at www.expertconsult.com

RELATED CONTENT
Atrial Myxoma (Patient Information)

AUTHOR: **BARRY FINE, M.D., PH.D.**

BASIC INFORMATION

DEFINITION

An atrial septal defect (ASD) is a true deficiency in the interatrial septum that allows blood flow between the atria. It should be distinguished from patent foramen ovale (PFO), which is a defect caused by a failure of the septum primum to fuse to the superior limb of the septum secundum at the edge of the fossa ovalis in postnatal life, leaving a flaplike communication between the two atria. PFO occurs in approximately 20%-25% of the normal adult population. Fig. 1 illustrates the physiology of ASD. There are several forms of ASD (Fig. 2):

- Primum: This type of ASD occurs when there is failure of normal fusion of anterior and posterior endocardial cushions with the septum primum, with resultant deficiency in the inferior portion of the septum primum. The defect frequently coexists with abnormalities of the atrioventricular valves, commonly resulting in a cleft anterior mitral leaflet.
- Secundum: The most common form of ASD; it represents a true deficiency in the septum primum or a septum secundum, or both. This defect most often occurs in the region of the fossa ovalis.
- Sinus venosus defect: This defect is located at the junction of the right atrium and either the superior vena cava or inferior vena cava. In a sinus venosus defect, the wall separating the pulmonary veins and the right atrium is deficient, causing a left-to-right shunt. Most commonly this defect involves the right upper pulmonary vein, which is still anatomically connected to the left atrium but is deficient anteriorly and thus drains anomalously into the right atrium. Less commonly, the right lower pulmonary vein is involved.
- Coronary sinus septal defect (unroofed coronary sinus): This defect results when the wall separating the coronary sinus from the left atrium is deficient, causing a left-to-right shunt. This defect is often associated with a persistent left superior vena cava.

SYNONYMS

ASD
Interatrial septal defect

ICD-10CM CODES
Q21.1   Atrial septal defect
I23.1   Atrial septal defect as current complication following acute myocardial infarction

EPIDEMIOLOGY & DEMOGRAPHICS

- Secundum, 75%; primum, 15%-20%; sinus venosus, 5%-10%; coronary sinus, <1%
- Incidence is greater in females and in patients with Down syndrome
- Accounts for 8% to 10% of congenital heart abnormalities
- Prevalence is 1.6 per 1000 live births
- Holt-Oram syndrome is an autosomal dominant disorder that involves skeletal anomalies, such as absent radial bones in both arms, as well as ASD (generally secundum) and cardiac conduction disease, such as atrioventricular (AV) blocks.
- Association with other genetic syndromes (e.g., Noonan syndrome, Treacher Collins syndrome, and the thrombocytopenia-absent radii syndrome) has been described for secundum defects. Down syndrome (trisomy 21) is strongly associated with AV canal defects, but these patients also have an increased frequency of secundum defects.
- ASDs may occur as an isolated defect or as part of other congenital cardiac syndromes such as Ebstein's anomaly, Lutembacher syndrome, or fetal alcohol syndrome.

CLINICAL PRESENTATION

- Small ASDs or PFOs may close spontaneously during infancy. The majority of ASDs are small and do not cause any symptoms during infancy. These patients are usually diagnosed by the presence of a cardiac murmur during routine physical examination. Infants with large ASDs may presents with heart failure, recurrent respiratory infections, and failure to thrive.
- Exertional fatigue and dyspnea are usually the main presenting symptoms.
- On rare occasions, young adults may presents with ischemic stroke caused by paradoxical embolism through the ASD or PFO.
- Platypnea-orthodeoxia (characterized by dyspnea and deoxygenation when changing from a recumbent position to sitting or standing).
- Patients with ASDs caused by congenital syndromes may present with clinical features related to the underlying syndrome.

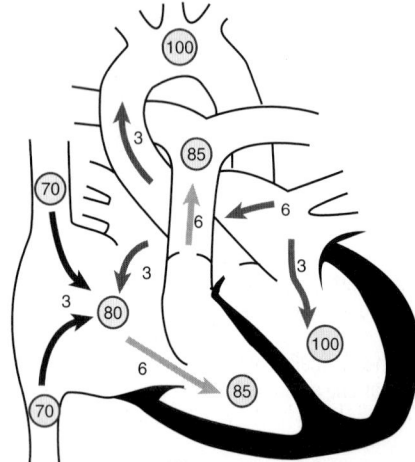

FIG. 1 Physiology of atrial septal defect (ASD). Circled numbers represent oxygen saturation values. The numbers next to the arrows represent volumes of blood flow (in L/min/m²). This illustration shows a hypothetical patient with a pulmonary-to-systemic blood flow ratio (Qp/Qs) of 2:1. Desaturated blood enters the right atrium from the venae cavae at a volume of 3 L/min/m² and mixes with an additional 3 L of fully saturated blood shunting left to right across the ASD; the result is an increase in oxygen saturation in the right atrium. Six liters of blood flow through the tricuspid valve and cause a mid-diastolic flow rumble. Oxygen saturation may be slightly higher in the RV because of incomplete mixing at the atrial level. The full 6 L flows across the RV outflow tract and causes a systolic ejection flow murmur. Six liters return to the left atrium, with 3 L shunting left to right across the defect and 3 L crossing the mitral valve to be ejected by the left ventricle into the ascending aorta (normal cardiac output). (From Kliegman RM et al: *Nelson textbook of pediatrics*, ed 19, Philadelphia, 2011, Saunders.)

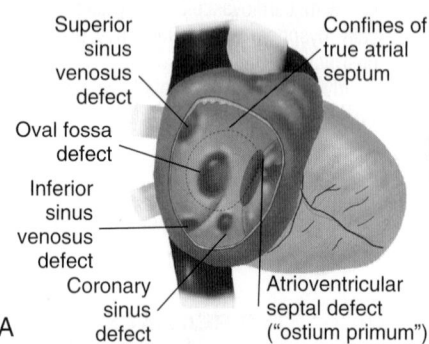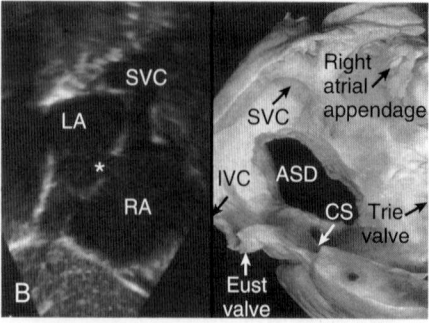

FIG. 2 A, Schematic diagram outlining the different types of interatrial shunting that can be encountered. Note that only the central defect is suitable for device closure. **B,** Subcostal right anterior oblique view of a secundum atrial septal defect *(ASD) (asterisk)* that is suitable for device closure. The right panel is a specimen as seen in a similar view, outlining the landmarks of defect. *CS,* Coronary sinus; *IVC,* inferior vena cava; *LA,* left atrium; *RA,* right atrium; *SVC,* superior vena cava. (From Zipes DP et al [eds]: *Braunwald's heart disease,* ed 7, Philadelphia, 2005, Saunders.)

Clinical Features:
- Cyanosis and clubbing (when abnormal right ventricular [RV] compliance has led to right-to-left shunting)
- Increased jugular venous pressure (with RV failure). Jugular venous pressure may also be a direct reflection of left atrial pressure if there is a significant ASD.
- Prominent RV impulse
- Visible and palpable pulmonary artery pulsations
- Wide fixed splitting of S_2
- An accentuated pulmonic component of S_2 if there is pulmonary hypertension
- Pansystolic murmur best heard at apex secondary to mitral regurgitation (ostium primum defect)
- Ejection systolic flow murmur (pulmonary valve flow murmur) (Fig. E3)
- Diastolic rumble (atrioventricular valve flow murmur)

DX DIAGNOSIS

DIFFERENTIAL DIAGNOSIS
- Primary pulmonary hypertension
- Pulmonary stenosis
- Rheumatic heart disease
- Mitral valve prolapse
- Cor pulmonale
- Anomalous pulmonary venous connection

WORKUP
- ECG:
  1. Ostium primum defect: extreme left axis deviation, incomplete or total right bundle branch block, prolongation of PR interval
  2. Sinus venosus defect: right axis deviation, abnormal P axis (suggesting an absent or deficient sinus node)
  3. Ostium secundum defect: right axis deviation, incomplete or total right bundle branch block, right atrial enlargement

IMAGING STUDIES
- Chest x-ray: cardiomegaly, right heart enlargement, increased pulmonary vascular pattern
- Echocardiography (Fig. 4): Transthoracic echocardiography has a high degree of sensitivity for diagnosing secundum and primum ASDs. Echocardiography with saline bubble contrast and Doppler flow studies may demonstrate the size of the defect, the direction of shunting, the presence of anomalous pulmonary return (in sinus venosus ASD), right heart volume overload, and elevated pulmonary artery pressures. It should be noted that sinus venosus defects are frequently missed.
- Transesophageal echocardiography: It is much more sensitive than transthoracic echocardiography in identifying sinus venosus defects and can be helpful for all forms of ASD when the transthoracic echo is nondiagnostic. It is also useful to determine defect size, proximity to other cardiac structures, and sizes of rims when determining suitability for device closure and is therefore used in the catheterization laboratory to assist with these issues.
- Cardiac catheterization: Invasive cardiac catheterization generally is not necessary for the diagnosis of ASDs since noninvasive modalities can generally identify and quantify the defect. Left heart catheterization is generally only useful when the coronary arteries need to be assessed before surgery. When performed, right heart catheterization will reveal a "step-up" in arterial oxygen saturation in the right atrium compared with the superior vena cava. This may not be the case in patients with partial anomalous pulmonary venous return associated with the sinus venosus type of ASD. Right heart catheterization can also aid in assessing shunt severity and the severity of pulmonary hypertension, and it can help to assess pulmonary vascular resistance (PVR) as well as pulmonary artery vasoreactivity in response to vasodilators.

- Cardiac MRI and CT: may be useful if echocardiography is not diagnostic; MRI is the gold standard for assessing RV size and function, and it can determine whether the right-sided chambers are, in fact, enlarged. MRI is also useful to assess anomalous pulmonary venous return and persistent left superior vena cava. Cardiac CT can offer similar information.

Rx TREATMENT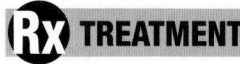

NONPHARMACOLOGIC THERAPY
- Symptomatic patients should avoid strenuous activity.
- Asymptomatic patients with small defects with shunts with a pulmonary to systemic flow ratio (Qp/Qs) of <1.5:1 without pulmonary artery hypertension (PAH) and normal RV size require no medical therapy and may be observed. Routine assessment of these patients includes assessment of symptoms, arrhythmias, and embolic events and serial echocardiography.
- A repeat echocardiogram should be obtained every 2 to 3 yr to assess RV size and function and pulmonary pressure; with increasing age, the degree of left-to-right shunting may increase due to progressive noncompliance of the left ventricle with age-related acquired heart disease.

GENERAL Rx
- Children and infants: Closure of ASD before age 10 yr is indicated if Qp/Qs is >2:1 (although many experts advocate closure for Qp/Qs >1.5:1), if ASD size is significantly >5 mm, or if there is evidence of RV dilation.
  1. Small ASDs with a diameter of <5 mm and no evidence of RV volume overload do not impact the natural history of the individual and thus may not require closure unless associated with paradoxic embolism.
  2. Closure of an ASD either percutaneously or surgically is indicated for right atrial and RV enlargement with or without symptoms.
  3. A sinus venosus, coronary sinus, or primum ASD should be repaired surgically rather than by percutaneous closure.
  4. Surgical closure of secundum ASD is appropriate when concomitant surgical repair/replacement of associated defects is needed or when the anatomy of the defect precludes the use of a percutaneous device.
- Adults: Closure of an ASD, either percutaneously or surgically, may be considered in the presence of net left-to-right shunting with Qp/Qs >1.5:1, right-sided chamber enlargement, symptoms, pulmonary hypertension with pulmonary artery pressure less than two-thirds systemic levels, PVR less than two-thirds systemic vascular resistance, or when pulmonary hypertension is responsive to either acute or chronic pulmonary

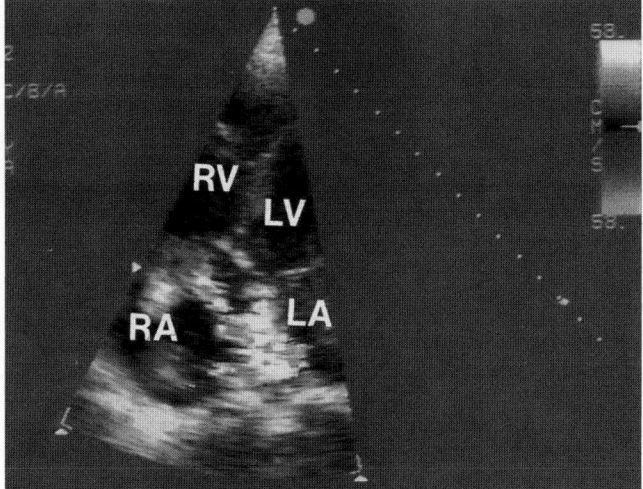

FIG. 4 Color flow Doppler apical four-chamber view showing blood flow from the left atrium (LA) to the right atrium (RA) through a moderately sized atrial septal defect. *LV,* Left ventricle; *RV,* right ventricle. (From Forbes CD, Jackson WF: *Color atlas and text of clinical medicine,* ed 3, London, 2003, Mosby.)

vasodilator therapy. These patients must be treated in conjunction with providers who have expertise in the management of adult congenital heart disease and pulmonary hypertension.

- Patients with severe irreversible PAH and no evidence of a left-to-right shunt should not undergo ASD closure.
- Closure of an ASD, either percutaneously or surgically, is reasonable in the presence of:
  1. Paradoxic embolism (Class 2a indication)
  2. Documented orthodeoxia-platypnea (Class 2a indication)
- Percutaneous catheter device closure is possible in many patients with secundum ASDs (if stretched diameter is <41 mm with adequate rims), with >95% success rate in appropriate candidates. The procedure is guided by fluoroscopy and transesophageal echocardiography. A combination of low-dose aspirin and clopidogrel is usually prescribed for 3-6 months after the procedure to prevent thrombus formation. Early complications include device thrombus formation, atrial arrhythmias, erosion, and device dislodgement. Potential mid- and long-term complications include late device erosion into the aortic root or pericardium, atrial dysrhythmias, and infective endocarditis. In one study the long-term outcomes of device closure using the Amplatzer septal occluder were excellent as evidenced by no deaths and minimal complication in 151 patients followed for 6.5 years after ASD closure. In October 2013 the Food and Drug Administration (FDA) began alerting health care providers and patients that in very rare instances, tissue surrounding the Amplatzer ASO can erode and result in life-threatening emergencies that require immediate surgery, especially when the rim adjacent to the aortic root is <5 mm. Based on published estimates, these events occur in approximately 1 to 3 of every 1,000 patients implanted with the Amplatzer device. Close clinical follow up and an echocardiogram is recommended predischarge, at 1 wk, at 6 mo, and at 12 mo after implant.
- Percutaneous closure is contraindicated in those with sinus venosus, primum, or unroofed coronary sinus defects. In addition, it is not suitable for secundum defects with unsuitable anatomy (too large; too close to coronary sinus, AV valves, or pulmonary veins; or inadequate rims), presence of sepsis, bleeding disorder, or intracardiac thrombi.
- In adult patients undergoing surgical closure, the surgical mortality should be <1%.

Surgical closure is generally accomplished with a pericardial or Dacron patch, and it can usually be performed through a minimally invasive approach with or without robotic system assistance. Surgical closure of ASD improves function status, exercise capacity, and patient survival; however, it does not prevent atrial fibrillation or stroke, especially if patients are operated on after age 40. Concomitant maze procedure may be considered for intermittent or chronic atrial fibrillation in adults with ASDs who are undergoing surgical repair.

DISPOSITION

- Mortality rate is elevated in patients with large ASDs if left untreated, with complications such as RV failure, arrhythmias, paradoxic embolism, and PAH leading to right-to-left shunting (Eisenmenger syndrome).
- Patients with small shunts (<1.5:1) have a normal life expectancy.
- A reduction in size or spontaneous closure is more likely in younger patients with small defects (<10 mm in diameter).
- Basic assessment for adult congenital heart disease patients should include systemic arterial oximetry, an ECG, chest radiograph, transthoracic echocardiography, and blood tests for full blood count and coagulation screen.
- Intracardiac shunts are considered moderate risk for preoperative evaluation for noncardiac procedure. High-risk features include severe systolic dysfunction (ejection fraction <35%), severe pulmonary hypertension whether primary or secondary, cyanotic heart disease, or severe left-side outlet obstruction.
- Annual clinical follow-up is recommended for patients postoperatively if their ASD was repaired as an adult to monitor for PAH, atrial arrhythmias, RV or left ventricular dysfunction, and coexisting valvular lesions.
- Preoperative atrial fibrillation is a risk factor for immediate postoperative and long-term atrial fibrillation. Patients with a repaired ASD still have an increased risk for development of atrial fibrillation that directly correlates with the age at which the defect is corrected (later correction poses greater risk).
  1. After closure, anticipated benefits include improved functional status and exercise capacity, improved survival after closure as a child, improved quality of life, prevention of right heart failure, and prevention of PAH.
  2. Potential mid- to long-term complications after ASD closure in adulthood include tachyarrhythmias (atrial fibrillation or atrial flutter), bradyarrhythmias (sinus node dysfunction or heart block), stroke (greater risk in older patients), residual ASDs (because of patch dehiscence or incomplete closure by device), right heart failure or PAH (risk is correlated with the size of the original defect and inversely related to age at time of closure), mitral valve regurgitation or subaortic stenosis (in patients with primum ASDs), device migration/erosion, and pulmonary venous congestion (uncommon).
  3. Pregnancy is usually well tolerated in women with ASDs. Follow-up during pregnancy is recommended because of small risk for paradoxic embolus, stroke, arrhythmia, and heart failure. If known, ASDs should be closed before pregnancy is indicated. The sole contraindication to pregnancy in women with an ASD is severe PAH.
  4. Scuba diving is generally contraindicated in patients with unrepaired ASDs because of the risk of paradoxical emboli. In addition, high-altitude climbing should be avoided because it can cause oxygen desaturation from right-to-left shunting in these patients.
- In regard to infective endocarditis prophylaxis for dental procedures:
  1. Prophylaxis is not indicated for an unrepaired ASD.
  2. Prophylaxis is indicated for a repaired ASD or any congenital heart disease with prosthetic material as part of the repair during the first 6 mo after the repair.
  3. Prophylaxis is indicated for a repaired ASD or any congenital heart defect in the presence of residual defects at the site or adjacent to the site of a prosthetic patch or prosthetic device (both of which inhibit endothelialization).

The estrogen-containing oral contraceptive pill is not recommended in acute congenital heart disease patients at risk of thromboembolism, such as those with cyanosis related to an intracardiac shunt, atrial fibrillation, severe PAH, or Fontan repair.

SUGGESTED READINGS

Available at www.expertconsult.com

RELATED CONTENT

Atrial Septal Defect (ASD) (Patient Information)

AUTHOR: **CRAIG L. BASMAN, M.D.**

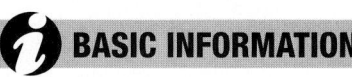

BASIC INFORMATION

DEFINITION

Atrioventricular (AV) dissociation is defined as a lack of association between the atria and the ventricles or independent function of the atria and ventricles. This simple definition will serve as a reminder that AV dissociation should be considered an umbrella rather than a diagnosis. AV dissociation may occur in the setting of bradycardic rhythms (complete heart block, as well as tachycardic rhythms [ventricular tachycardia, atrial rhythm with associated accelerated junctional rhythm (Fig. 1) or AV nodal reentrant tachycardia]).

SYNONYMS

Third-degree AV block
CHB
Complete AV block

ICD-10CM CODES
I44.2 Atrioventricular block, complete

EPIDEMIOLOGY & DEMOGRAPHICS

- The prevalence is the sum of the diagnoses that are characterized by AV dissociation

PHYSICAL FINDINGS & CLINICAL PRESENTATION

Physical examination findings may be normal unless the arrhythmia is causing hemodynamic compromise. If the right atrium contracts against a closed tricuspid valve during ventricular systole, Cannon A waves may be seen in the jugular vein. Patients may present with the following clinical manifestations:

- Dizziness, palpitations
- Syncope or presyncope (caused by reduced cardiac output)
- Fatigue, impaired exercise tolerance
- Mental status changes
- Congestive heart failure
- Angina pectoris
- Some patients may be asymptomatic

ETIOLOGY

- Slow rate of firing from sinus node
- Inappropriately fast pacemaker from the ventricle

- Iatrogenic: anesthesia, inotrope infusion, ventricular pacing, radiofrequency ablation of slow pathway, digoxin toxicity
- Sinus node disease, ischemia, hyperkalemia, overactive vagal drive
- Complete heart block: progressive fibrosis of the His-Purkinje system, medications, Lyme disease

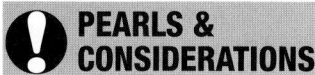

DIAGNOSIS

DIFFERENTIAL DIAGNOSIS

- The differential diagnosis should be targeted toward the diagnoses that include AV dissociation.
- Note: The atrium does not need to be faster than the ventricular rate in AV dissociation, as is the case in the definition of complete heart block.
  - Isorhythmic AV dissociation: Atrial and ventricular rates are the same but dissociated.
  - Interference dissociation: Similar atrial and ventricular rates but conduction occurs sometimes.

WORKUP

- Workup such as routine laboratory studies, cardiac biomarkers, and cardiac imaging should be dictated by the clinical circumstances.
  - Laboratory studies: particular attention to electrolyte abnormalities (potassium) and digoxin level
  - Lyme antibody titer in the case of complete heart block, particularly in the Northeastern U.S.

TREATMENT

ACUTE GENERAL Rx

- Initial treatment should focus on the hemodynamic stability and symptoms of the patient.
- Bradycardic rhythms
  - If necessary (i.e., symptoms or hemodynamic compromise), a temporary pacemaker is the most reliable therapy.
  - Hold AV-nodal blocking agents.
  - Chronotropic medications: Atropine, dopamine, dobutamine, or isoproterenol may be used as second-line agents while preparing for a temporary pacemaker.

- Tachycardic rhythms (ventricular tachycardia)
  - In the setting of hemodynamic compromise, cardioversion is the first-line therapy.
  - IV antiarrhythmic drugs: amiodarone or lidocaine to suppress the arrhythmia.
  - Treatment of the underlying cause of ventricular tachycardia: coronary angiogram if ischemia vs electrophysiology (EP) study +/− ablation.

REFERRAL

All patients with AV dissociation should be referred to a cardiologist for diagnostic evaluation of the rhythm.

PEARLS & CONSIDERATIONS

COMMENTS

- Recall that AV dissociation is merely an umbrella that includes multiple diagnoses, including both bradycardic and tachycardic arrhythmias.
- Specific considerations in regards to etiology, treatment, and disposition should be directed toward the rhythm that has caused AV dissociation.

SUGGESTED READINGS

Available at www.expertconsult.com

AUTHORS: **ALEEM MUGHAL, M.D.,** and **JOHN WYLIE, M.D.**

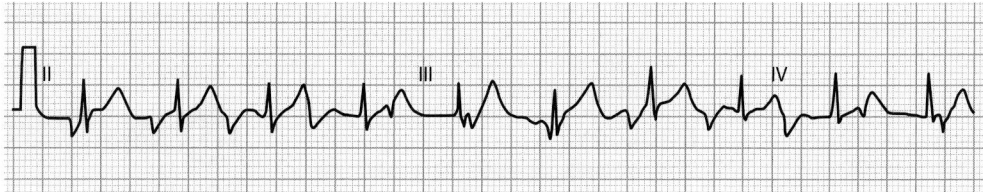

FIG. 1 Rhythm strip shows a low atrial rhythm at 100 beats/min with a nearly isorhythmic accelerated junctional rhythm at 95 beats/min in a patient with suspected endocarditis.

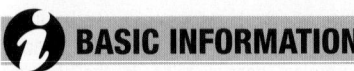 BASIC INFORMATION

DEFINITION

Attention deficit hyperactivity disorder (ADHD) is a chronic disorder of attention and/or hyperactivity-impulsivity. Symptoms must be present before 12 yr of age, last at least 6 mo, and cause functional impairment in multiple settings. The diagnostic keys for ADHD are described in Table 1.

SYNONYMS

Hyperactivity
Hyperkinetic disorder
Attention deficit disorder (ADD)
ADHD

ICD-10CM CODES
F90.0 Attention-deficit hyperactivity disorder, predominantly inattentive type
F90.1 Attention-deficit hyperactivity disorder, predominantly hyperactive type
F90.2 Attention-deficit hyperactivity disorder, combined type
F90.8 Attention-deficit hyperactivity disorder, other type
F90.9 Attention-deficit hyperactivity disorder, unspecified type
DSM-5 CODES
314.00, 314.01

EPIDEMIOLOGY & DEMOGRAPHICS

PEAK INCIDENCE: Diagnosis is usually first made in school-aged children (6 to 9 yr).
PREVALENCE: Five percent to 10% of school-aged children (most prevalent neurodevelopmental disorder among children) and 2% to 5% of adults. Children from families with low socioeconomic status and children with public insurance are diagnosed with ADHD at higher rates than their peers.
PREDOMINANT SEX: Among children, male predominance with ratio of 2:1 to 4:1. Among adults, ratio is closer to 1:1 (sex difference may reflect referral bias).
PREDOMINANT AGE: Some symptoms must occur before age 12 yr. Symptoms (especially motoric hyperactivity) tend to diminish with age. Up to 70% continue to meet criteria in adolescence, and an estimated 40% to 65% have some symptoms in adulthood.
GENETICS: Strong polygenetic component. First-degree relatives of ADHD patients have 5 times greater risk of ADHD relative to controls. Studies suggest potential involvement of several genes, including those associated with serotonin and glutamate transporters as well as dopamine metabolism.
RISK FACTORS: Possible risk factors include in utero tobacco/drug exposure or hypoxia, low birth weight, prematurity, pregnancy, lead exposure (though most children with elevated lead levels do not develop ADHD), head trauma in young children, family dysfunction, low socioeconomic status. Evidence supports possible association between dietary factors (e.g., refined sugar, food additives) and ADHD in a small percentage of patients. A causal link between environmental toxins and ADHD has not been clearly established.

PHYSICAL FINDINGS & CLINICAL PRESENTATION

- Three types:
  1. Predominantly inattentive: difficulty organizing, planning, remembering, concentrating, starting/completing tasks; symptoms may not be present during preferred activities.
  2. Predominantly hyperactive-impulsive: edgy/restless, talkative, disruptive/intrusive, disinhibited, impatient.
  3. Combined.
- Usually diagnosed in elementary school when achievement is compromised and behavioral problems are not tolerated. Children with academic underproductivity, problems with peer and family relations, or discipline issues are often referred for evaluation. Of the more than 4 million children in the U.S. who have ADHD, most have comorbid conditions (see the following) and nearly half use special education and mental health services.
- Up to 50% may have associated disorders such as psychiatric diagnoses (oppositional defiant disorder, conduct disorder, depression, anxiety, eating disorders), learning disabilities, or substance abuse.
- In adults, motoric hyperactivity is less common, but restlessness, edginess, and difficulty relaxing are often seen. Disorganization and difficulty completing tasks are other common complaints.

ETIOLOGY

Strongest evidence exists for genetic inheritance. Other theories include abnormal metabolism of brain catecholamines, structural brain abnormalities, reduced activation in the basal ganglia and anterior frontal lobe, as well as environmental factors (see earlier).

Table 1 Diagnostic Keys for Attention Deficit Hyperactivity Disorder

1. Inattention
   a. Careless mistakes in schoolwork, work, or other activities
   b. Seems not to listen when spoken to directly
   c. Poor follow-through on schoolwork or chores
   d. Difficulty organizing
   e. Easily distracted by extraneous stimuli and is forgetful
2. Hyperactivity
   a. Trouble sitting still
   b. May act as if "driven by a motor"
   c. May talk excessively
3. Impulsivity
   a. Trouble holding back in class
   b. Trouble taking turns
   c. Interrupts

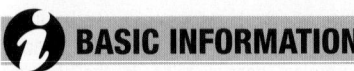 DIAGNOSIS

DIFFERENTIAL DIAGNOSIS

- Medical: visual/hearing impairment, seizure disorder, head injury, sleep disorder, medication interactions, mental retardation intellectual disability, specific learning disorder, autism spectrum disorder/development delay, thyroid abnormalities, lead toxicity, movement disorders.
- Psychiatric: depression, bipolar disorder, disruptive mood, dysregulation disorder, anxiety, obsessive-compulsive disorder, oppositional defiant disorder, intermittent explosive disorder, conduct disorder, posttraumatic stress disorder, reactive attachment disorder, and substance abuse.
- Psychosocial: mismatch of learning environment with ability, family dysfunction, abuse/neglect.

WORKUP

- Clinical interview should include assessment of symptoms and impact on work/school and relationships; developmental history; personal and family psychiatric history, including substance abuse; social history, including family dysfunction; medical history.
- Physical examination should be performed to investigate medical causes for symptoms, coexisting conditions, and contraindications to treatment. Special focus should be paid to evaluation of dysmorphic features; neurologic examination, including assessment for neurocutaneous findings; and assessment of hearing and vision.
- Information from collateral sources (parents, partners, teachers) is crucial to diagnosis. Many patients will not display symptoms during an office visit and may underreport or overreport symptoms.
- Self-rating scales and standardized symptom-specific questionnaires from collateral sources can help diagnose and assess response to treatment. The use of ADHD-specific rating scales over broadband behavioral scale is associated with improved sensitivity and specificity.
- Laboratory or imaging studies should be undertaken only if indicated by history or physical examination.
- The FDA has approved a quantitative EEG test to aid in the diagnosis of ADHD in children, but sufficient evidence to support its routine use is lacking.
- Ancillary testing (e.g., IQ/achievement testing, language evaluation, and mental health assessment) may be indicated based on clinical findings and may require referral.

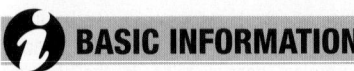 TREATMENT

NONPHARMACOLOGIC THERAPY

- The majority of studies comparing the efficacy of pharmacologic vs nonpharmacologic interventions demonstrate the superiority of pharmacologic treatments.

- Studies on combined treatments have not shown significant improvements in core ADHD symptoms when behavioral treatments are added to stimulant medications. However, improvements in related areas of concern such as parent-child relations, aggressiveness, teacher-rated social skills, and reaching achievement have been seen in combined treatment groups.
- Prevailing opinion favors a multimodal approach in which nonpharmacologic behavioral therapies including parent-child behavioral therapy and social skills training can be used to target comorbid conditions or behaviors that have not responded to medication.
- Behavioral therapy alone is often considered when children are under 6 yr, symptoms and impairment are mild, if parents are opposed to or patients cannot tolerate medications, or if there is uncertainty or disagreement about the diagnosis (e.g., between parents and teachers).
- Educational interventions are recommended, particularly in the setting of learning disabilities. Children with ADHD are entitled to reasonable educational accommodations under a 504 Plan or the Individuals with Disabilities Education Act.
- Behavioral interventions (e.g., goal setting and rewards systems) show short-term efficacy and are endorsed by most national organizations (e.g., American Academy of Pediatrics, American Medical Association). Time management and organizational skills appear useful. Social skills training may also be useful.
- Psychotherapy such as cognitive therapy, play therapy, or insight-oriented therapy are unlikely to be useful in addressing the core symptoms of ADHD. However, it may be beneficial in treating comorbid psychiatric conditions.
- Elimination diets are not routinely recommended.
- Many support and advocacy groups provide education and other resources (e.g., Children and Adolescents with ADHD, National ADD Association, American Academy of Child and Adolescent Psychiatry).

ACUTE GENERAL Rx

- Most studies on treatment of ADHD are performed in children; limited data available on adults.
- Mainstay of treatment is stimulant medications. Second-line therapies include antidepressants and alpha-agonists.
- Stimulants:
  1. Release or block uptake of dopamine and norepinephrine.
  2. Include short- and long-acting methylphenidate, dextroamphetamine, and dextroamphetamine/amphetamine combinations (mixed amphetamine salts). A methylphenidate patch (Daytrana) is available, as is a pro-drug form of dextroamphetamine, lisdexamfetamine (Vyvanse), which is designed to limit the abuse potential. A long-acting oral suspension of methylphenidate (Quillivant XR), a long-acting chewable tablet of methylphenidate (QuilliChew ER), and a long-acting liquid amphetamine preparation (Dyanavel XR) are now available.
  3. All stimulants equally effective; however, not all patients improve with stimulants. Patients who do not respond well to one stimulant may respond to another.
  4. Do not cause euphoria or lead to addiction when taken as directed.
  5. Improve cognition, inattention, impulsiveness/hyperactivity, and driving skills. Limited impact on academic performance, learning, and emotional problems.
  6. Side effects are usually mild, reversible, and dose dependent, including anorexia, weight loss, sleep disturbances, increased heart rate and blood pressure, irritability, moodiness, headache, onset or worsening of motor tics, reduction of growth velocity (but not adult height). Do not worsen seizures in patients on adequate anticonvulsant therapy. Rebound of symptoms can occur with withdrawal of medication.
  7. Stimulants have generally been associated with cardiovascular events and death. Patients should be carefully evaluated for cardiovascular disease before beginning therapy and be periodically monitored, including blood pressure checks, while they are treated. However, despite concerns regarding cardiovascular risk, these medications are generally safe. Recent studies have shown that among young and middle-aged adults, current or new use of ADHD medications, compared with nonuse or remote use, is not associated with an increased risk of serious cardiovascular events. Routine, pre-treatment screening with ECGs is not currently recommended by the American Academy of Pediatrics or the American Academy of Child and Adolescent Psychiatry.
- Atomoxetine (Strattera):
  1. Selective norepinephrine reuptake inhibitor.
  2. Generally felt to be less effective than stimulants, but a useful alternative in patients who have not tolerated or responded to stimulants or in the setting of patient or family substance abuse.
  3. Efficacy and safety of use beyond 2 years of treatment have not been studied. There have been reports of behavioral abnormalities and increased suicidality in children and adolescents.
  4. Side effects: gastrointestinal upset, sleep disturbance, decreased appetite, dizziness, sexual side effects in men. Cardiovascular side effects have also been reported.
  5. There have been rare reports of severe liver injury in adults and children.
- Antidepressants (bupropion, imipramine, desipramine, nortriptyline):
  1. May be useful in patients with coexisting psychiatric disorders.
  2. Studies comparing efficacy versus stimulants are inconclusive.
  3. Side effects: arrhythmias, anticholinergic effects, lowering of seizure threshold.
- Alpha-2-adrenergic agonists (clonidine, guanfacine)
  1. Appear to be less effective than stimulants, but may be particularly useful as an adjunctive treatment to stimulants, particularly in patients with a partial stimulant response or who experience side effects such as sleep disturbance or concurrent symptoms of overarousal, irritability, or aggression.
  2. Extended-release formulations of guanfacine (Intuniv) and clonidine (Kapvay) have been approved by the FDA for treatment of ADHD in children ages 6 to 17 yr. A transdermal clonidine patch is also available.
  3. Potential side effects include sedation, fatigue, headache, bradycardia, hypotension, and depression.
- Use of medications, particularly stimulants (which are monitored under the Controlled Substance Act), requires frequent monitoring.

DISPOSITION

- Although symptoms may change over time, for many patients ADHD represents a chronic condition that requires lifelong management.
- Patients are at higher risk for academic underachievement, lower socioeconomic status, work and relationship difficulties, high-risk behavior, and psychiatric comorbidities.

REFERRAL

- Diagnosis complicated by difficult-to-treat comorbid psychiatric conditions, developmental disorders, or mental retardation
- Lack of adequate response to stimulants/atomoxetine/alpha-adrenergic agents.

⚠ PEARLS & CONSIDERATIONS

- The World Health Organization's Adult Self-Report Scale (ASRS) v1.1 has good sensitivity and adaptability to the primary care setting.
- Among adults with persistent ADHD symptoms treated with medication, trials have shown that the use of cognitive behavioral therapy compared with relaxation with educational support resulted in improved ADHD symptoms, which were maintained at 12 mo.
- ADHD has been associated with criminal behavior in some studies. Data analysis has shown that among patients with ADHD, rates of criminality are lower during periods when they receive ADHD medication.
- Recommendations for the diagnosis and management of ADHD have been published by the Centers for Disease Control and Prevention (www.cdc.gov/ncbddd/adhd/treatment/treatment.html).

SUGGESTED READINGS
Available at www.expertconsult.com

RELATED CONTENT
Attention Deficit Hyperactivity Disorder (ADHD) (Patient Information)

AUTHOR: **EMILY R. KATZ, M.D.**

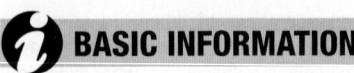

BASIC INFORMATION

DEFINITION

Autism spectrum disorder (ASD) encompasses a continuum of developmental disabilities characterized by marked social impairment. Table 1 describes the diagnostic keys. There is usually impairment in several additional domains integral to social functioning, including communication, language, and social interactions. Repetitive/stereotyped behaviors and interests as well as sensory issues (i.e., hypersensitivity, hyposensitivity) also are prominent. Comorbid intellectual disability, neurological and medical problems, and an increased risk of psychiatric disorders are frequently present in ASD. Both core and associated features can vary dramatically among individuals. In addition, timing of onset can differ, as about one quarter of children with ASD are noted to lose skills after developing normally for as long as 2 years, whereas others present with delays across most developmental domains within the first year of life. The diagnosis of ASD can accurately be made by 3 years of age. However, gender and cognitive, linguistic, and adaptive functioning impact ASD presentation and can affect age of diagnosis. DSM-5 criteria no longer differentiate separate disorders. Instead, an overarching diagnosis of ASD is given; severity levels (1, 2, or 3) have been introduced to identify the magnitude of social and behavioral impairment and the support required to ensure the safety and well-being of the individual. Specifiers have been added to capture associated features (e.g., intellectual disability, language impairment, medical or genetic conditions, and catatonia).

SYNONYMS

ASD
Autism
Autistic disorder
Early infantile autism
Childhood autism
Kanner's autism
Asperger's disorder
Pervasive developmental disorder
PDD NOS

Table 1 Diagnostic Keys for Autism Spectrum Disorder

1. Impairment in social interaction and communication
   a. Deficits in social-emotional reciprocity
   b. Deficits in nonverbal communicative behaviors
   c. Deficits in developing and maintaining age-appropriate relationships
2. Restricted/Repetitive behaviors
   a. Stereotyped or repetitive actions
   b. Insistence on sameness and/or ritualistic behaviors
   c. Highly restricted/fixated interests
   d. Hypo- or hyperreactivity to sensory stimuli

ICD-10CM CODES
F84.0   Autism spectrum disorder
DSM-5 CODE
299.00 Autism spectrum disorder

EPIDEMIOLOGY & DEMOGRAPHICS

INCIDENCE (IN U.S.): Autism spectrum disorder afflicts approximately 1% of children in the United States.
PREVALENCE: 1:68 (1:42 for boys, 1:189 for girls). It is unclear whether the increase in prevalence reflects an expansion of the diagnosis to include subthreshold cases, increased awareness of the disorder, improvement in diagnostic accuracy, changes in public policy related to special education eligibility, or a true increase in the frequency of autism spectrum disorder.
PREDOMINANT SEX: Male/female ratio of 4:1
PREDOMINANT AGE: Lifelong
PEAK INCIDENCE: Before age 3 yr
GENETICS:

- Autism spectrum disorder is highly inheritable with a heritability index of 82% to 90%.
- The concordance rate for ASD varies across studies and ranges from 36% to 95% for monozygotic twins; the concordance rate is estimated between 20% and 40% for dizygotic twins and between 10% and 20% for nontwin siblings.
- Copy number variants (CVNs) account for 10% to 20% of autism spectrum disorder cases. Single-gene disorders account for approximately 5% of the cases. Chromosomal abnormalities account for approximately 5% of the cases.
- In the remaining cases, the risk appears to be polygenic. Research has identified approximately 1000 gene mutations as being possibly contributory, but only about 20 of them have been associated with ASD with "high confidence."

PHYSICAL FINDINGS & CLINICAL PRESENTATION:

- Common triad of marked impairment in social interactions (poor social-emotional reciprocity), impaired and atypical verbal and nonverbal communication, and repetitive and unusual behavior or play.
- Marked impairment in the understanding and use of both verbal and nonverbal communication, including unchanging facial expression and lack of gestures during interactions.
- Stereotypic behavior (i.e., hand flapping, body rocking), or language (i.e., echolalia, palilalia).
- Perceptual hypersensitivity (i.e., auditory, tactile, olfactory, gustatory) and avoidance of novel stimuli; or perceptual hyposensitivity (e.g., abnormally high threshold for pain).
- Brain abnormalities have been identified at anatomical and functional levels. Abnormalities are detected as early as the first year of life and are accompanied by atypical brain maturation trajectories. However, no biomarkers have been identified.

ETIOLOGY:

- Majority of cases are not associated with a comorbid medical condition.
- High prevalence of comorbid seizure disorder (25%) and/or intellectual disability (up to 75%).
- Sometimes present in the context of neurologic conditions (e.g., encephalitis, cytomegalovirus, toxoplasmosis, tuberous sclerosis, phenylketonuria [PKU], fragile X syndrome, tuberous sclerosis complex, neurofibromatosis).
- Numerous studies have shown **no** association between immunizations (specifically MMR vaccine) or thimerosal-containing vaccines (i.e., DPT) and autism spectrum disorder.
- Prenatal and perinatal risk factors identified include hypoxia-related obstetric complications, gestational diabetes, maternal bleeding during pregnancy, and low gestational age. However, it is not clear whether these are causal factors.
- Maternal use of valproate has been associated with increased risk of ASD in offspring, even when accounting for seizure status.

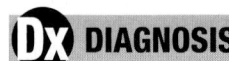 DIAGNOSIS

DIFFERENTIAL DIAGNOSIS

- Disorders that present with symptoms similar to ASD (i.e., Phelan-McDermid syndrome, Aicardi syndrome, Rett syndrome, Prader-Willi syndrome, Tourette syndrome, selective mutism, social phobia, expressive language disorder, mixed receptive-expressive language disorder, stereotypic movement disorder, intellectual disability).
- Social (pragmatic) communication disorder, introduced in DSM-5 and characterized by significant difficulties with verbal and nonverbal communication.
- Childhood-onset schizophrenia: follows period of normal development.
  Attachment disorders (reactive attachment disorder, disinhibited social engagement disorder); individuals with these disorders can present with language delays, cognitive delays, social difficulties, and stereotypies. Differences are notable before 5 years of age.

WORKUP

- Rule out underlying medical condition, including genetic syndromes.
- Validated autism spectrum disorder–specific screening tools are available for children age ≥18 mo. All children should be screened specifically for autism spectrum disorder at 18 and 24 mo. General developmental screening tools are currently used in children 9 to 18 mo.
- Gold standard assessment includes detailed developmental and family history, assessment of developmental/intellectual functioning, assessment of ASD symptomatology, and assessment of adaptive behaviors.
- Additional workup may include assessment of language functioning, neuropsychological functioning, and psychiatric presentation.

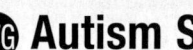

LABORATORY TESTS

- PKU screen (usually done at birth in the United States)
- Lead exposure screening
- Audiology testing for young children with autism spectrum disorder; school-based hearing screening may be sufficient in older children with autism spectrum disorders and without significant language or learning deficits
- Karyotype, microarray analysis, and DNA testing for fragile X syndrome in both boys and girls, as well as for different de novo copy number variants or de novo mutations in specific genes associated with the disorder.

IMAGING STUDIES

- EEG to diagnose coexisting seizure disorder if seizure is suspected or if language regression is present (i.e., Landau-Kleffner syndrome)
- Brain MRI if tuberous sclerosis or Aicardi syndrome (callosal agenesis) is suspected

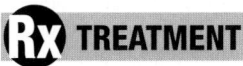 **TREATMENT**

NONPHARMACOLOGIC THERAPY

- Consistent behavioral training program in both the home and school environments
- A number of treatment programs have been developed; many are based on applied behavioral analysis (ABA) (e.g., Discrete Trial Training); others combine ABA procedures with social-emotional development (e.g., Pivotal Response Training, Floortime, Early Start Denver Model).
- Special educational program focused on language and communication skills, social and life skills development (e.g., TEACCH)
- Highly structured home environment
- Education for families and teachers; the Autism Speaks™ website may be helpful in this regard: http://www.autismspeaks.org/about_us.php

ACUTE GENERAL Rx

- Obsessive or ritualistic behaviors: selective serotonin reuptake inhibitors (SSRIs), atypical antipsychotics, valproic acid.

- Aggression, irritability, self-injury: atypical antipsychotic agents (e.g., risperidone), α-agonists, anticonvulsant mood stabilizers, SSRIs, beta-blockers, opiate antagonist (self-injury only).
- Hyperactivity, impulsivity, inattention: stimulants, alpha-agonists, atypical antipsychotics.
- Anxiety: SSRIs, buspirone, mirtazapine.
- Bipolar, mood lability: valproic acid, carbamazepine, lithium, aripiprazole.
- Depression: SSRIs, mirtazapine.

CHRONIC Rx

- Extended use of medications for acute management of comorbid psychiatric disorder.
- Pharmacotherapy is palliative, not curative of autism spectrum disorder.

DISPOSITION

- Most children will require some degree of assistance as adults.
- DSM-5 identifies 3 severity levels based on social communication and restricted, repetitive behaviors: Level 1 (requiring support), Level 2 (requiring substantial support), and Level 3 (requiring very substantial support).
- With early diagnosis and proper treatment/support, the prognosis for children without language and intellectual impairment is fair to very good despite lifelong symptoms.
- Poorer outcomes include a lack of joint attention by age 4 yr, a lack of functional speech by age 5 yr, intellectual disability, seizures, comorbid medical or psychiatric syndromes, and a pervasive lack of social relatedness.
- Best outcomes are associated with early identification and treatment, the development of oral communication skills, and the cognitive and behavioral capacity for inclusion in regular education settings with typically developing peers.

REFERRAL

Assistance may be needed in diagnosis (child psychiatrist, clinical psychologist, geneticist, pediatric neurologist, developmental pediatrician), management (speech language pathologist, occupational therapist, clinical psychologist), parental teaching (psychiatric social worker), or intervention with the school system (educational advocate, attorney).

PEARLS & CONSIDERATIONS

- There is no scientific evidence of a relation between childhood vaccination and the development of autism spectrum disorder.
- Evidence suggests that a disproportionate number of children with autism spectrum disorder suffer from a variety of medical problems including sleep difficulties, gastrointestinal problems, food allergies, and oral health problems.
- Psychiatric comorbidities are very prominent across the life span, with estimated prevalence ranging from 30% to 70%.
- The Center for Autism & Developmental Disabilities at Bradley Hospital, an affiliate of the Brown Medical School, is one of the largest and most comprehensive treatment programs in the U.S. for children with autism spectrum disorder and comorbid psychiatric illness (www.bradleyhospital.org).
- The new U.S. Preventive Services Task Force (USPSTF) recommendation on screening for autism spectrum disorder (ASD) in young children concludes that the current evidence is insufficient to assess the balance of benefits and harms of screening for ASD in young children for whom no concerns of ASD have been raised by their parents or a clinician.

SUGGESTED READINGS
Available at www.expertconsult.com

RELATED CONTENT
Autism (Patient Information)

AUTHOR: **GIULIA RIGHI, PH.D.**

DEFINITION

Cerebral arteriovenous malformations (AVMs) are congenital vascular lesions that are characterized by blood flow from high-pressure arterial vessels directly into thin-walled veins without passing through an intervening capillary/venule system (Fig. 1).

SYNONYMS

AVM
Brain AVM

ICD-10CM CODES
Q28.2 Arteriovenous malformations of cerebral vessels

EPIDEMIOLOGY & DEMOGRAPHICS

INCIDENCE:
- Detection rates in large prospective studies range from 1.1 to 1.4 per 100,000 person-years.
- Incidence of hemorrhage, the most common and often most clinically dangerous presentation, is estimated to be 2% to 4% per year.

PREVALENCE: Estimated about 1.3 per 100,000.

PREDOMINANT SEX AND AGE:
- There is a slight male preponderance; studies of varying populations show 1.04:1 to 1.2:1 M:F ratio.
- Peak age at time of hemorrhage occurrence is about 20 years, but it can occur in younger and older patients.

GENETICS:
- Cerebral AVMs are sporadic in most cases.
- AVMs are present in about 20% of cases of Osler-Weber-Rendu syndrome (also known as hereditary hemorrhagic telangiectasia [HHT]), an autosomal dominant disorder that results in abnormal blood vessel formation in the skin, lungs, liver, brain, and other organs.

RISK FACTORS:
- Male sex and presence of HHT are risk factors for AVM.
- The risk of hemorrhage is increased with prior hemorrhage, presence of a single draining vein, and diffuse nidus morphology.

PHYSICAL FINDINGS & CLINICAL PRESENTATION

- The most common presentation is hemorrhage; symptoms vary based on location and magnitude of hemorrhage.
- Patients may present with seizures or neurologic deficits related to mass effect of the AVM nidus.
- Headache and pulsatile tinnitus may be present.
- In infants, AVM may present as cyanotic heart failure, macrocephaly, or hydrocephalus.
- A bruit may be auscultated through the scalp or orbit.
- AVMs may also present with associated intracranial aneurysms that occur on distant, unrelated vessels, on a proximal artery that feeds the aneurism (flow-related aneurysm), or within the AVM nidus itself (intranidal aneurysm). Patients may present with a subarachnoid hemorrhage related to the aneurysm rather than to the AVM.

ETIOLOGY

In most cases, AVMs are congenital abnormalities caused by failure of formation of a capillary bed between embryonic arterial and venous vascular plexuses during the first trimester of gestation; however, de novo sporadic AVMs have been reported.

ⓓⓧ DIAGNOSIS

DIFFERENTIAL DIAGNOSIS

The differential diagnosis of cerebral AVMs includes other vascular lesions such as cavernous malformations, dural arteriovenous fistulas, and intracranial aneurysms. Table E1 compares vascular malformations, and Table E2 describes major differences between hemangiomas and vascular malformations.

LABORATORY TESTS

- CBC and BMP with renal function panel prior to contrast dye administration with CT angiography/cerebral angiogram.
- PT/INR/PTT should be drawn and corrected in the case of bleeding diathesis.

IMAGING STUDIES

- In the acute setting, a CT scan of the head to check for hemorrhage and a CT angiogram of the head for characterization of the lesion may be helpful (although calcification may be present and potentially pose as small acute blood).
- MRI of the brain delineates the nidus and its relationship to surrounding soft tissue structures better than a CT scan; however, in the setting of an acute hemorrhage these details will be obscured.
- Four-vessel cerebral angiogram (arteriogram) is the best study to evaluate AVM. Angiography in multiple projections helps identify the number and location of feeding and draining vessels for treatment planning (Fig. 2). High-resolution images of the nidus may also reveal other irregularities such as

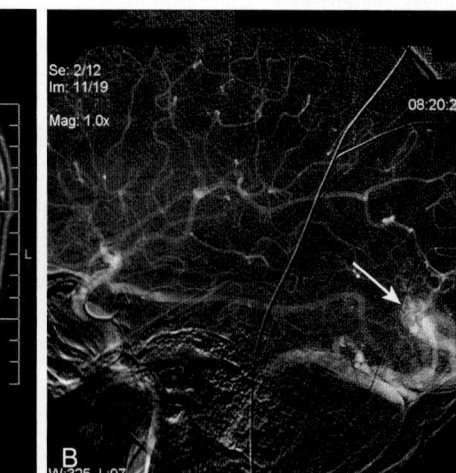
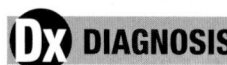
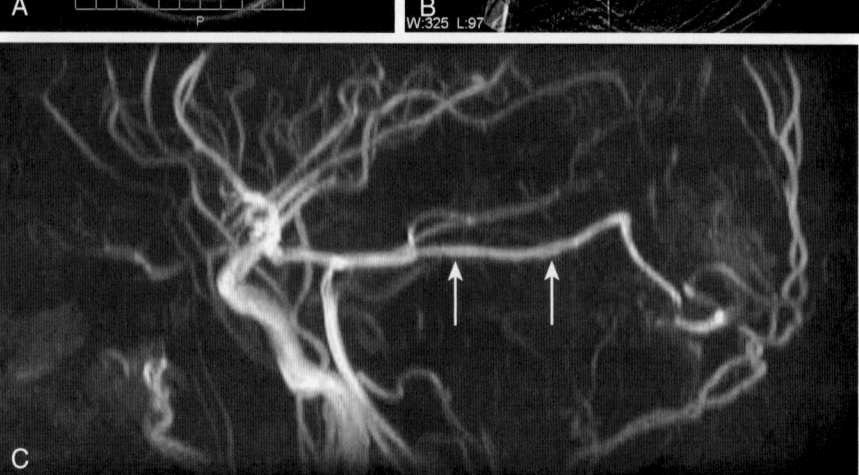

FIG. 1 A 14-year-old child with a left occipital arteriovenous malformation (AVM). A, MRI shows multiple flow voids in the left occipital lobe *(arrow).* **B,** Lateral view from catheter angiogram confirms the presence of an AVM *(arrow)* and early draining veins *(curved arrow).* **C,** Lateral maximum intensity projection image from an MR angiogram shows an enlarged posterior cerebral artery branch *(arrows),* which feeds the tangle of abnormal vessels. (From Fuhrman BP et al: *Pediatric critical care,* ed 4, Philadelphia, 2011, Saunders.)

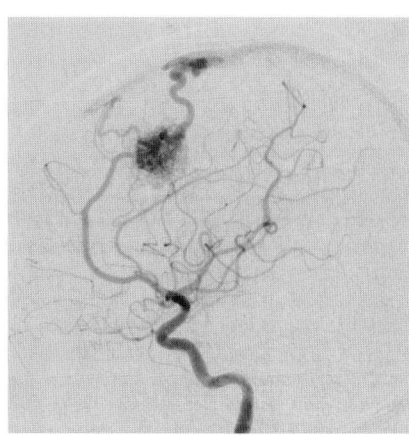

FIG. 2 Arteriovenous malformation of the frontal lobe. The anterior cerebral artery provides primary arterial supply with venous drainage superficially into the superior sagittal sinus.

aneurysms that often arise given the abnormal histology of the vessel walls and the high-pressure blood flow traversing them.

Rx TREATMENT

Pharmacologic management of seizures with antiepilepsy drugs and of headaches with oral analgesics can provide symptomatic relief.

NONPHARMACOLOGIC THERAPY

- Nonemergent outpatient setting: cerebral angiogram provides characterization of the lesion. Based on angiographic characteristics, the Spetzler-Martin AVM grading system may be used to help guide treatment. In general, grade 5 AVMs are considered unresectable; they are not treated because the risks of treatment likely outweigh the risk of hemorrhage. Current tools for the treatment of AVMs include surgical resection, radiosurgery, and endovascular embolization (with liquid glues or embolic agents).
- Surgical resection: in low-grade lesions by an experienced neurosurgeon yields a high cure rate (~95% in published studies). Resection should include removal of all of the nidus of the AVM; failure to remove the complete nidus may increase the risk of recurrence. An increasing Spetzler-Martin grading scale increases risk of neurologic complications. Intraoperative imaging techniques such as indocyanine-green in-field angiography and conventional digital subtraction angiography are used to verify complete resection.
- Radiosurgery: alternative definitive treatment for AVMs. Traditionally employed to treat AVMs in eloquent areas (e.g., brainstem); stereotactic radiosurgery is increasingly used for higher Spetzler-Martin grade AVM. Reported rates of confirmed radiographic obliteration after AVM radiosurgery range from 47% to 90%.
- Endovascular embolization involves transarterial superselective blockage of the AVM. It has become an important adjunctive tool. Currently recommended and approved for use before resection, preoperative embolization can reduce arterial flow and pressure within the AVM, assisting in speed and safety of surgical resection. In addition, embolization may often be used to treat intranidal or flow-related aneurysms in coordination with either resection or radiosurgery. Embolization alone in obliterating an AVM is not routinely recommended.
- Treatment decisions should take into consideration the morbidity associated with the treatment modality versus the risk of future hemorrhage or neurologic deterioration. Disability stemming from intractable seizures or severe headaches may make invasive definitive treatment a more attractive option.
- Acute cerebral hemorrhage: in the case of an acute hemorrhage, airway and breathing must be maintained, with intubation if necessary. Acute neurosurgical intervention for clot evacuation may be warranted. Microsurgical resection of the AVM may or may not be feasible in the acute setting and is controversial.

DISPOSITION

Whether the patient is receiving elective treatment of a known lesion or presenting with an acute hemorrhage, the patient should receive care in a progressive or intensive care unit with experience dealing with cerebrovascular disease. Once the patient is stabilized, appropriate rehabilitation should be arranged.

REFERRAL

- Cerebral AVMs should be managed by a qualified neurosurgeon.
- Referral to radiation medicine for adjuvant radiosurgery should be made when indicated.
- Referral to an interventional radiologist for endovascular treatment may be warranted.
- Treatment in a primary stroke center or other specialized center that offers all treatment modalities is recommended.

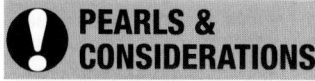

! PEARLS & CONSIDERATIONS

COMMENTS

No two AVMs are exactly the same; individualization of treatment decisions is the mainstay. Additionally, many AVMs could be effectively treated through one of several modalities or a combination thereof. Factors such as patient age, overall health status, radiographic characteristics, route of surgical access, and potential morbidities of each treatment modality are vital variables in consideration for treatment. The advisability of intervention for unruptured AVMs remains controversial. In a recent randomized trial comparing medical management with specific interventions to obliterate AVMs (neurosurgery, embolization, radiotherapy, or a combination) the rates of neurological disability were higher in the intervention group than with conservative treatment.[1]

PATIENT/FAMILY EDUCATION

If a patient with a known AVM suffers from acute-onset neurologic deficits or stroke-like symptoms, emergency medical attention is warranted for potential hemorrhage. Presence of AVMs, cerebral or otherwise, in family members should be disclosed to the patient's primary care physician because the presence of a genetic condition predisposing to cerebral AVMs should be considered.

SUGGESTED READINGS
Available at www.expertconsult.com

AUTHORS: **STEPHEN L. GRUPKE, M.D., M.S.,** and **JUSTIN F. FRASER, M.D.**

[1]Mohr JP et al: Medical management with or without interventional therapy for unruptured brain arteriovenous malformations (ARUBA): a multicentre non-blinded, randomized trial, *Lancet* 383:614-621, 2014.

A

Diseases and Disorders

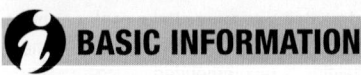

BASIC INFORMATION

DEFINITION

Avascular necrosis (AVN) is ischemic death of bone due to insufficient blood supply. It is not a specific disease entity but a final common pathway to several disorders that impair blood supply to the femoral head and other locations.

SYNONYMS

AVN
Osteonecrosis
Aseptic necrosis

ICD-10CM CODES
M87   Idiopathic aseptic necrosis of bone
M87.1   Osteonecrosis due to drugs
M87.2   Osteonecrosis due to previous trauma
M87.3   Other secondary osteonecrosis
M87.9   Osteonecrosis, unspecified

EPIDEMIOLOGY & DEMOGRAPHICS

- 15,000 new cases per year in the United States. It is most commonly associated with the hip and accounts for 10% of total hip replacements in the United States.
- Usually occurs in middle age and is more frequent in males than females
- Associated conditions:
  1. Corticosteroid treatment: 35%
  2. Alcohol abuse: 22%
  3. Idiopathic and other: 43%
  4. Hemoglobinopathies, pancreatitis, chronic renal failure, SLE, chemotherapy, decompression sickness
- Common sites involved
  1. Femoral head
  2. Femoral condyle
  3. Humeral head
  4. Navicular and lunate wrist bones
  5. Talus

PHYSICAL FINDINGS & CLINICAL PRESENTATION

- May be asymptomatic in early stages
- Pain in the involved area exacerbated by movement or weight bearing in later stages
- Decreased range of motion as the disease progresses
- Functional limitation

ETIOLOGY

Final common pathway of conditions that lead to impairment of the blood supply to the involved bone. Trauma disrupting the blood supply is the most common cause of AVN. Arterial factors are considered the most common cause of AVN. Table 1 describes proposed mechanism of disease of common conditions associated with osteonecrosis.

STAGING

Table 2 describes the Modified Steinberg Staging System for osteonecrosis.
Stages:
- Stage 0
  1. Asymptomatic
  2. Normal imaging
  3. Histologic findings only (i.e., silent osteonecrosis)

TABLE 2 Modified Steinberg Staging System for Osteonecrosis

Stage	Radiographic Appearance	Reversible
I	Normal radiographs, but abnormal bone scan or magnetic resonance image	Yes
II	Lucent and sclerotic changes	Yes
III	Subchondral fracture without flattening	No
IV	Subchondral fracture with flattening or segmental depression of femoral head	No
V	Joint space narrowing or acetabular changes	No
VI	Advanced degenerative changes	No

From Firestein GS, Budd RC, Gabriel SE, et al: *Kelly's textbook of rheumatology*, ed 9, Philadelphia, 2013, Saunders.

- Stage 1
  1. Asymptomatic or symptomatic
  2. Normal radiographs and CT scan
  3. Abnormal bone scan or MRI
- Stage 2
  1. Abnormal radiographs or CT scan, including linear sclerosis, focal bead mineralization, cysts; however, the overall architecture of the involved bone is normal
- Stage 3
  1. Early evidence of mechanical bone failure (subchondral fracture), but the overall shape of the bone is still intact
- Stage 4
  1. Flattening or collapse of the bone
- Stage 5
  1. Joint space narrowing
- Stage 6
  1. Extensive joint destruction

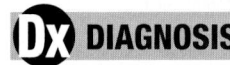 DIAGNOSIS

DIFFERENTIAL DIAGNOSIS

- None in late stages
- Early: any condition causing focal musculoskeletal pain, including arthritis, bursitis, tendinitis, myopathy, neoplastic bone and joint diseases, traumatic injuries, pathologic fractures

WORKUP

Fig. 1 describes a diagnostic algorithm for osteonecrosis.

IMAGING STUDIES (FIG. 2)

1. MRI: the most sensitive technology to diagnose early aseptic necrosis. The first sign is a margin of low signal. An inner border of high signal associated with a low-signal line is specific for aseptic necrosis ("double line sign"). Sensitivity is 75% to 100%.
2. Radiography: insensitive early in the course. The earliest changes include diffuse osteopenia, areas of radiolucency with sclerotic border, and linear sclerosis. Later, a subchondral lucency (crescent sign) indicates subchondral fracture. More advanced cases reveal flattening, collapsed bone, and abnormal bone contour. In late disease, osteoarthritic changes are seen.

TABLE 1 Proposed Mechanism of Disease of Common Conditions Associated with Osteonecrosis

Associated Condition	Mechanism of Osteonecrosis							
	Apoptosis	Osteoblast/ Osteoclast Homeostasis	Lipid Abnormalities	Coagulation Abnormalities	Oxidative Stress	Parathyroid/ Calcium Imbalance	Vascular Plugging	Vasoactive Substances
Corticosteroids	X	X	X	X	X			X
Bisphosphonates	X	X	X					
Alcohol abuse	X	X	X	X	X			
Trauma	X	X						X
Renal transplantation	X	X		X		X		
Dialysis						X		
Sickle cell disease							X	

From Firestein GS, Budd RC, Gabriel SE, et al: *Kelly's textbook of rheumatology*, ed 9, Philadelphia, 2013, Saunders.

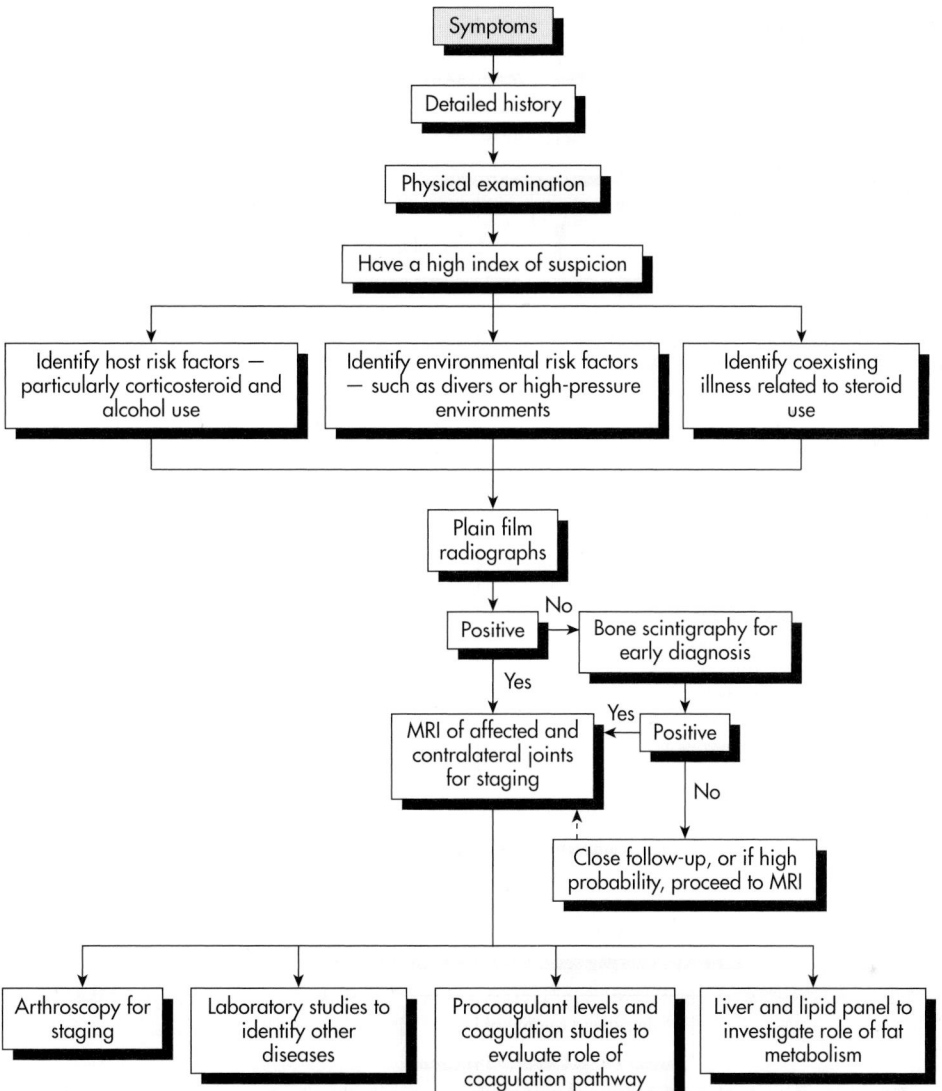

FIG. 1 Diagnostic algorithm for osteonecrosis. *MRI,* Magnetic resonance image. (From Firestein GS, Budd RC, Gabriel SE, et al: *Kelly's textbook of rheumatology,* ed 9, Philadelphia, 2013, Saunders.)

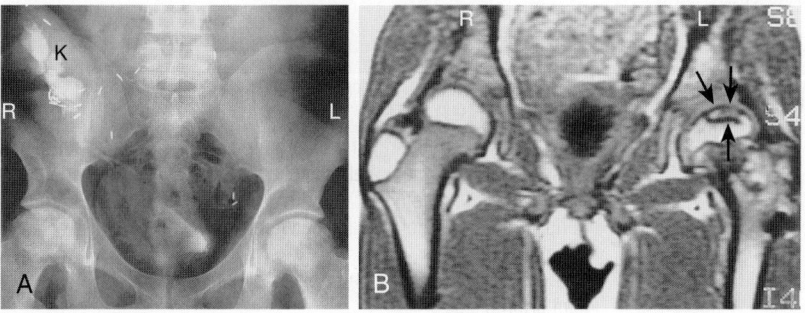

FIG. 2 Aseptic necrosis of the hips. A, Aseptic necrosis can occur from a number of causes, including trauma and steroid use. In this patient, an anteroposterior view of the pelvis shows a transplanted kidney *(K)* in the right iliac fossa. Use of steroids has caused this patient to have bilateral aseptic necrosis. The femoral heads are somewhat flattened, irregular, and increased in density. **B,** Aseptic necrosis in a different patient is demonstrated on an MRI scan as an area of decreased signal *(arrows)* in the left femoral head. This is the most sensitive method for detection of early aseptic necrosis. (From Mettler FA [ed]: *Primary care radiology,* Philadelphia, 2000, Saunders.)

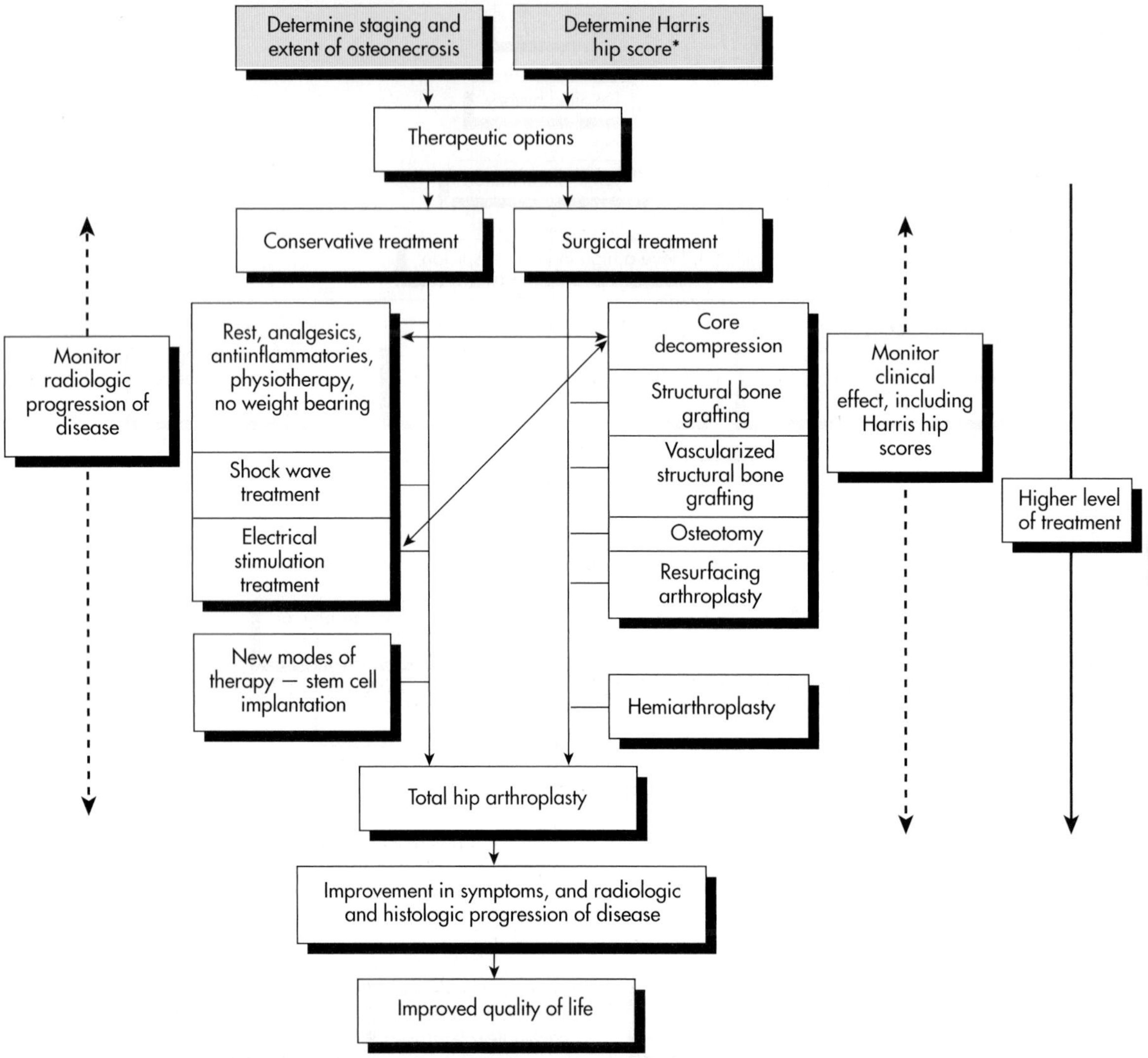

FIG. 3 Treatment algorithm for osteonecrosis. *www.ncbi.nlm.nih.gov/pubmed/22588745. (From Firestein GS, Budd RC, Gabriel SE, et al: *Kelly's textbook of rheumatology*, ed 9, Philadelphia, 2013, Saunders.)

3. Bone scan:
   - Early: "cold" area.
   - Later: increased radionuclide uptake as a result of remodeling.
   - Sensitivity in early disease is only 70% and specificity is poor.
4. CT scan: may reveal central necrosis and area of collapse before those are visible on radiographs.

Rx TREATMENT

PREVENTION
- Manage etiologic conditions
- Minimize corticosteroid use

NONPHARMACOLOGIC THERAPY
- Core decompression: effectiveness 35% to 95% in early phases
- Bone grafting
- Osteotomies
- Joint replacement

ACUTE GENERAL Rx
- Decrease weight bearing of affected area.
- Pulsing electromagnetic fields applied externally (still experimental).
- Peripheral vasodilators (e.g., dihydroergotamine) (unproven).
- Late-stage AVN is most often treated by total joint arthroplasty.
- A treatment algorithm for osteonecrosis is described in Fig. 3.

PROGNOSIS
- When diagnosed at an early stage treatment is appropriate in all cases because 85% to 90% can be expected to progress to a more advanced stage.
- Contralateral joint involvement is common (30% to 70%).

SUGGESTED READINGS
Available at www.expertconsult.com

RELATED CONTENT
Avascular Necrosis (Patient Information)

AUTHOR: **FRED F. FERRI, M.D.**

ℹ BASIC INFORMATION

DEFINITION
Babesiosis is a tick-transmitted protozoan disease of animals, caused by intraerythrocytic parasites of the genus *Babesia*. Humans are incidentally infected, resulting in a nonspecific febrile illness. The disease can be severe in immunocompromised hosts.

ICD-10CM CODES
B60.0 Babesiosis

EPIDEMIOLOGY & DEMOGRAPHICS
INCIDENCE (IN U.S.): Unknown
PREVALENCE (IN U.S.):
- In areas of high endemicity, seropositivity ranging from 9% (Rhode Island) to 21% (Connecticut)
- Highest number of reported cases in New York

PREDOMINANT SEX: Males (most likely through increased exposure to vectors during recreational or occupational activities)
PREDOMINANT AGE: Severity apparently increasing with age greater than 60 yr
PEAK INCIDENCE: Spring and summer months, May through September
GENETICS: None known
CONGENITAL INFECTION: Definite evidence of vertical transmission
NEONATAL INFECTION: Many cases of perinatal transmission
BLOOD TRANSFUSION: Many instances. Blood donation screening for antibodies to and DNA from *B. microti* has been shown to significantly decrease the risk of transfusion-transmitted babesiosis

PHYSICAL FINDINGS & CLINICAL PRESENTATION
- Incubation period 1 to 4 wk, or 6 to 9 wk in transfusion-associated disease

- Gradual onset of irregular fever, chills, diaphoresis, headache, myalgia, arthralgia, fatigue, and dark urine
- On physical examination: petechiae, frank or mild hepatosplenomegaly, and jaundice. Most patients have a normal physical exam.
- Infection with *B. divergens* (Europe) producing a more severe illness with a rapid onset of symptoms and increasing parasitemia progressing to massive intravascular hemolysis and renal failure

ETIOLOGY
- Vector: Deer tick, *Ixodes scapularis* (also known as *I. dammini*)
  1. Feeds on rodents during the spring and summer while in its larval and nymphal stages and on deer as an adult
  2. Requires a blood meal to mature to each stage, hence human infection
  3. During the warmer months in endemic areas, humans are readily infected while engaging in outdoor activities

---

TABLE 1 Causal Agents and Clinical Manifestations of Babesiosis

Babesia Species	Geographic Distribution	Tick Vectors	Animal Reservoirs	Epidemiology	Clinical Manifestations
B. divergens	United Kingdom, Western Europe, Eastern Europe, Sweden, Russia; not reported in United States	Ixodes ricinus	Cattle, reindeer	Incubation, 1-4 wk Occurs during summer months in cattle-raising regions Targets splenectomized or immunocompromised patients primarily	Fulminant course with high case-fatality rate Fever, rigors, headache, myalgia, jaundice, hemoglobinuria, hemolytic anemia, acute renal failure, multiorgan failure
B. microti	Parallels the U.S. Northeast endemic regions for *Borrelia burgdorferi*, especially the islands off New York, Massachusetts, Connecticut, and Rhode Island and focal areas in Connecticut, New Jersey, Wisconsin, and Minnesota	Deer ticks: *Ixodes dammini* and *Ixodes scapularis*	White-footed mouse (*Peromyscus leucopus*)	Incubation, 1-4 wk after tick bites or 4-9 wk after blood transfusions Transmission primarily by nymphal ticks Targets older, not necessarily immunocompromised patients, particularly severe in those immunocompromised by HIV infection, advanced age, coinfections with *B. burgdorferi* Seasonality parallels tick nymph activity; 80% of cases occur from May to August	Often asymptomatic in young, healthy patients Self-limited influenza-like febrile illness with onset of anorexia, malaise, and lethargy followed in 1 wk by high fever, diaphoresis, myalgias; mild splenomegaly, and rarely hepatomegaly Later hemolysis, hemolytic anemia, thrombocytopenia, jaundice, acute renal failure, especially in the splenectomized, older adults, or the immunocompromised Complications include ARDS and DIC Case-fatality rate, 5%
MO-1 (a relative or subspecies of B. divergens)	Rural Missouri and Kentucky	Ixodes dentatus (rabbit tick)	Rabbits, birds	Incubation, 1-4 wk after tick bites Spring to autumn seasonality Targets the splenectomized, like *B. divergens*	Same as above—often asymptomatic, except in the splenectomized, who will develop high parasitemias and multiorgan failure
WA-1 (a relative or subspecies of B. gibsoni)	Rural Washington State	Ixodid ticks, including *Ixodes dentatus*	Unknown—wild canids and ungulates suspected	Incubation, 1-4 wk Targets the splenectomized, older adults, immunocompromised, premature infants May be transmitted by blood transfusion	Same as above—often asymptomatic, except in the splenectomized, who will develop high parasitemias and multiorgan failure
CA-1, CA-2, etc. subspecies (relatives or subspecies of mule deer and bighorn sheep *Babesia* species)	U.S. Pacific coast, primarily rural and semirural areas of California	Ixodid ticks	Unknown—mule deer and bighorn sheep suspected	Incubation, 1-4 wk Targets the splenectomized, elderly, immunocompromised, and premature infants	Same as above—often asymptomatic, except in the splenectomized, who will develop high parasitemias and multiorgan failure

ARDS, Acute respiratory distress syndrome; *DIC*, disseminated intravascular coagulation.
From Bennett JE, Dolin R, Blaser MJ: Mandell, Douglas, and Bennett's principles and practice of infectious diseases, ed 8, Philadelphia, 2015, Saunders.

- *B. microti* and *B. divergens* account for most human infections. Table 1 compares causal agents and clinical manifestations of babesiosis.
- In the U.S., cases caused by *B. microti* are acquired on offshore islands of the northeastern coast, including Nantucket Island, Cape Cod, and Martha's Vineyard in Massachusetts; Block Island in Rhode Island; and Long Island, Fire Island, and Shelter Island in New York; as well as the nearby mainland including Connecticut, Rhode Island, and New Jersey.
- Sporadic cases reported from California, Georgia, Maryland, Minnesota, Virginia, Wisconsin, and most recently the WA-1 strain from Washington State and the MO-1 strain from Missouri.
- *B. divergens* is implicated in human disease in Europe, where the disease remains rare and predominantly associated with asplenia.
- Majority of cases are asymptomatic.
- May be transmissible by transfusion, through platelets and erythrocytes.
- Mixed infections (*B. microti* and *Borrelia burgdorferi,* the causative agent of Lyme disease) are estimated to occur in 10% (Rhode Island and Connecticut) to 60% (New York) of cases.

DIAGNOSIS

DIFFERENTIAL DIAGNOSIS
- Amebiasis
- Ehrlichiosis
- Hepatic abscess
- Leptospirosis
- Malaria
- Salmonellosis, including typhoid fever
- Acute viral hepatitis
- Hemorrhagic fevers
- Subacute bacterial endocarditis

WORKUP
Should be suspected in any febrile patient living or traveling in an endemic area, irrespective of exposure history to ticks or tick bites, especially if asplenic

LABORATORY TESTS
- The preferred method for diagnosing babesiosis is PCR using whole blood specimens.
- Babesial DNA by polymerase chain reaction (PCR) has comparable sensitivity and specificity to microscopic analysis of thin blood smears. PCR is more sensitive than smears at the onset of infection when parasite load may be minimal.
- Diagnosis achieved serologically by indirect immunofluorescence assay (IFA) is specific for *B. microti.*
  1. Assay is hampered by the inability to distinguish between exposed patients and those who are actively infected.
  2. IGG titer of ≥1:64 is indicative of seropositivity, whereas one ≥1:1024 is considered diagnostic of acute infection. IGM titer of 1:64 is considered indicative of acute infection.

3. Immunoglobulin M indirect immunofluorescent-antibody test may be highly sensitive and specific for diagnosis. IGM titer of 1:64 is considered indicative of acute infection.
- CBC to reveal mild to moderate thrombocytopenia and anemia. The WBC count may be normal, elevated, or low. Abnormally elevated serum chemistries, including creatinine, liver function profile, lactate dehydrogenase, and indirect and total bilirubin levels; haptoglobin is low.
- Urinalysis to reveal proteinuria and hemoglobinuria
- Examination of Giemsa- or Wright-stained thin blood films for intraerythrocytic parasites
  1. In its classic, though infrequently seen, form a "tetrad" or "Maltese cross" composed of four daughter cells attached by cytoplasmic strands is observed (Fig. 1).
  2. More commonly, smaller forms composed of a single chromatin dot are eccentrically located within bluish cytoplasm.
  3. Parasitized erythrocytes may be multiply infected but not enlarged.
  4. Extra-erythrocytic forms may be seen.

Rx TREATMENT

NONPHARMACOLOGIC THERAPY
Supportive care with adequate hydration

ACUTE GENERAL Rx
- In patients with intact spleens: predominantly asymptomatic or if symptomatic, generally self-limited
- Therapy reserved for the severely ill patient, especially if asplenic, elderly, or immunosuppressed. Therapy may be offered to any symptomatic patient.
- Combination of atovaquone 750 mg q12h and azithromycin 500 mg on day 1 and 250 mg per day thereafter for 7 to 10 days appears to be as effective as a regimen of clindamycin and quinine with fewer adverse reactions. This is the preferred regimen for mild disease.
- Combination of quinine sulfate 650 mg PO tid plus clindamycin 600 mg PO tid (600 mg parenterally qid) taken for 7 to 10 days: effective but may not eliminate parasites
- Severely ill patients are hospitalized and treated with clindamycin and quinine
- Exchange transfusions in addition to antimicrobial therapy: successful treatment for severe infections in asplenic patients associated with high levels of *B. microti* or *B. divergens* parasitemia. Exchange transfusion is recommended for patients with >10% parasitemia, but may be considered for any severely ill patient.
- Relapsed and immunocompromised patients require a longer duration of therapy.

DISPOSITION
Prognosis is usually good and fatal outcomes are rare.

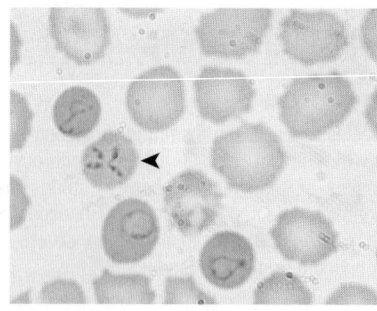

FIG. 1 Babesia spp. Single and multiple intraerythrocytic parasites can be seen. The *arrow* marks a typical Maltese cross. (From Cohen J, Powderly WG: *Infectious diseases,* ed 2, St Louis, 2004, Mosby.)

REFERRAL
- For prompt consultation with an infectious disease specialist if the diagnosis is acutely suspected, especially in the asplenic, elderly, or immunocompromised patient
- For hospitalization for the severely ill patient who may require exchange transfusions in addition to antibiotic therapy

! PEARLS & CONSIDERATIONS

COMMENTS
- Prevention of babesiosis in asplenic or immunocompromised hosts is best achieved by avoidance of areas where the vector is endemic, especially May through September.
- If residence or travel in endemic areas is unavoidable, advise patients to perform daily cutaneous self-examination, wear light-colored clothing (to facilitate removal of ticks), tuck pants into socks, and apply tick repellent (diethyltoluamide and dimethyl phthalate) to skin or clothing.
- Advise a daily inspection for ticks in family pets (e.g., cats and dogs).
- Infection with *B. divergens*, especially in the asplenic patient, is often fatal.
- Concurrent cases of babesiosis and Lyme disease have been documented—check for combined infection in severely ill patients.
- A combination of clindamycin and quinine has been successfully used to treat babesiosis during the third trimester of pregnancy without incurring apparent adverse effect on the fetus.
- In 2011 the CDC added babesiosis to the list of nationally notifiable diseases.

SUGGESTED READINGS
Available at www.expertconsult.com

RELATED CONTENT
Babesiosis (Patient Information)

AUTHOR: **PATRICIA CRISTOFARO, M.D.**

BASIC INFORMATION

DEFINITION

Balanitis is an inflammation of the superficial tissues of the penile head (glans penis). If the foreskin (prepuce) is involved, it is called *balanoposthitis*.

ICD-10CM CODES
B37.42 Candidal balanitis
N48.1 Balanitis

EPIDEMIOLOGY & DEMOGRAPHICS

INCIDENCE (IN U.S.): More common in uncircumcised males and in diabetic patients
PREVALENCE (IN U.S.): One study reports that 11% of adult men seen in a urology clinic and 3% of male children (mostly uncircumcised) have balanitis.
PREDOMINANT SEX: Almost exclusive to males but can affect clitoris
PEAK INCIDENCE: All ages, especially in sexually active men. It occurs in ¼ of male sex partners of women infected with *Candida*.

PHYSICAL FINDINGS & CLINICAL PRESENTATION

- Itching and tenderness
- Pain, dysuria, and local edema and erythema
- Rarely, ulceration and lymph node enlargement
- Severe ulcerations leading to superimposed bacterial infections
- Inability to void: unusual, but a more distressing and serious complication

ETIOLOGY

- Causes include infectious agents, skin disorders, or miscellaneous.
- Infectious diseases: *Candida species* (40%), *Neisseria gonorrhoeae,* HPV, herpes simplex, *Gardnerella vaginalis, Treponema pallidum* (syphilis), HIV, *Trichomonas, Staphylococcus aureus,* anaerobic bacteria

- Skin disorders: circinate balanitis of **Reiter's syndrome,** lichen sclerosis
- Miscellaneous: poor hygiene, causing erosion of tissue with erythema and promoting growth of *Candida albicans* (Fig. 1), trauma (zippers, urinary catheters), allergic reactions to condoms or medications

DIAGNOSIS

DIFFERENTIAL DIAGNOSIS

- Leukoplakia
- Nummular eczema
- Balanitis xerotica obliterans
- Psoriasis
- Carcinoma of the penis
- Plasma cell balanitis (noninfectious)
- Erythroplasia of Queyrat
- Nodular scabies
- Circinate balanitis (Reiter's syndrome)

WORKUP

- Sexually active males: assessment for evidence of other sexually transmitted diseases
- Biopsy if lesions do not heal

LABORATORY TESTS

- VDRL, HIV, NAATs for chlamydia and gonorrhea
- FBS, HBA$_{1C}$ to rule out diabetes
- Wet mount for *Trichomonas*
- KOH prep for yeast

TREATMENT

NONPHARMACOLOGIC THERAPY

- Maintenance of meticulous hygiene
- Retraction and bathing of prepuce several times a day
- Warm sitz baths to ease edema and erythema
- Consideration of circumcision, especially when symptoms are severe or recurrent
- With Foley catheters, strict catheter care strongly advised

ACUTE GENERAL Rx

- Metronidazole 2 g PO as a single dose or fluconazole 150 mg PO × 1 or itraconazole 200 mg PO bid × 1 day
- Clotrimazole 1% cream applied topically twice daily to affected areas
- Bacitracin or Neosporin ointment applied topically 4 times daily
- With more severe bacterial superinfection: cephalexin 500 mg PO qid
- Topical corticosteroids added 4 times daily if dermatitis severe
- Patients with suspected urinary tract infections: trimethoprim-sulfa DS twice daily or ciprofloxacin 500 mg PO bid after obtaining appropriate cultures

DISPOSITION

Balanitis is often self-limited and usually responds to conservative therapy; if it does not improve, consider circinate balanitis of Reiter's syndrome, nodular scabies, and primary skin lesions including skin carcinoma.

PEARLS & CONSIDERATIONS

Don't forget about nodular scabies involving the prepubic area—examine the region carefully for burrows and tracks of *Sarcoptes scabiei*.

REFERRAL

- For surgical evaluation for circumcision if symptoms are recurrent, especially if phimosis or meatitis occurs (note: Severe phimosis with an inability to void may require prompt slit drainage.)
- For biopsy to rule out other diagnoses such as premalignant or malignant lesions if lesions are not healing

SUGGESTED READINGS
Available at www.expertconsult.com

RELATED CONTENT
Balanitis (Patient Information)

AUTHOR: **GLENN G. FORT, M.D., M.P.H.**

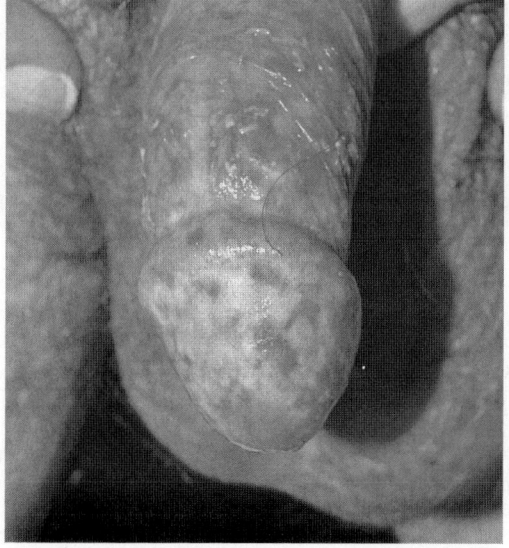

FIG. 1 Candidal balanitis. (From Swartz MH: Male genitalia and hernias. In Swartz MH [ed]: *Textbook of physical diagnosis: history and examination,* Philadelphia, 2014, Elsevier.)

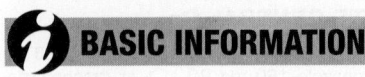

BASIC INFORMATION

DEFINITION

Barrett esophagus occurs when the squamocolumnar junction is displaced proximal to the gastroesophageal junction and the squamous lining of the lower esophagus is replaced by metaplastic columnar epithelium, which predisposes to the development of esophageal adenocarcinoma. While cardia-type epithelium has been shown to predispose to esophageal cancer, the presence of intestinalized epithelium is still considered essential for the diagnosis. Recent data show that the absolute annual risk for esophageal carcinoma in Barrett esophagus is 0.12%, which is much lower than the assumed risk of 0.5% that is the basis for current surveillance guidelines.

SYNONYMS

Barrett's esophagus
Esophagus, Barrett
Esophagus, columnar-lined
Ulcer, Barrett's

ICD-10CM CODES
K22.70	Barrett esophagus without dysplasia
K22.710	Barrett's esophagus with low grade dysplasia
K22.711	Barrett's esophagus with high grade dysplasia
K22.719	Barrett's esophagus with dysplasia, unspecified

EPIDEMIOLOGY & DEMOGRAPHICS

- Male/female ratio of 4:1.
- Mean age of onset is 40 yr, with a mean age range of diagnosis of 55 to 60 yr.
- Occurs more frequently in white and Hispanic individuals than in African American individuals, with a ratio of 10 to 20:1.
- Mean prevalence of 5% to 15% in patients undergoing endoscopy (EGD) for symptoms of gastroesophageal reflux disease (GERD).
- Independent risk factors include chronic reflux (>5 years), hiatal hernia, age >50 years, male gender, white ethnicity, smoking history, and intraabdominal obesity. A family history with at least one first-degree relative with Barrett esophagus or adenocarcinoma of the esophagus may also be a risk factor.
- It is estimated that 5.6% of adults in the United States have Barrett esophagus. Prevalence rate in asymptomatic cohorts ranges from 5% to 25%.

PHYSICAL FINDINGS & CLINICAL PRESENTATION

SYMPTOMS:
- Chronic heartburn
- Dysphagia with solid food
- May be an incidental finding on EGD in patients without reflux symptoms
- Less frequent: chest pain, hematemesis, melena
- Patients may be asymptomatic.

PHYSICAL FINDINGS:
- Nonspecific; can be completely normal
- Epigastric tenderness on palpation

ETIOLOGY

- Metaplasia is thought to result from reepithelialization of esophageal tissue injured as a result of chronic GERD.
- Patients with Barrett esophagus tend to have more severe esophageal motility disturbances (decreased lower esophageal sphincter pressure, ineffective peristalsis) and greater esophageal acid exposure on 24-hour pH monitoring. Table 1 lists some physiologic abnormalities that have been reported in Barrett patients and suggests how these abnormalities may contribute to GERD severity.
- Intraesophageal bile reflux may also play a role in the pathogenesis.
- Familial clustering of GERD and Barrett esophagus suggests a genetic predisposition, but no gene has yet been identified. Early data suggest that patients who develop Barrett are genetically predisposed to a severe inflammatory response to GERD. Candidate susceptibility loci include *CRTC1*, *BARX1*, and *FOXP1*.
- Progression from metaplasia to carcinoma is associated with changes in gene structure and expression, including the caudal-related homeobox family of transcription factors (CDX1 and CDX2) and the tumor suppressors p16 (CDKN2A) and TP53.

DIAGNOSIS

DIFFERENTIAL DIAGNOSIS

- GERD, uncomplicated
- Erosive esophagitis
- Gastritis
- Peptic ulcer disease
- Angina
- Malignancy
- Stricture or Schatzki's ring

WORKUP

- The American Gastroenterological Association Medical Position Panel gave a weak recommendation for screening patients with multiple risk factors, including age over 50, male sex, white race, chronic GERD, hiatal hernia, elevated body mass index, and intraabdominal distribution of body fat. An international consensus group suggested screening men over 60 with GERD symptoms for more than 10 years. An American College of Gastroenterology (ACG) Clinical Guideline suggested screening men with >5 years and/or frequent symptoms of GERD and two or more risk factors including age >50, Caucasian race, presence of central obesity, current or past history of smoking, and a confirmed family history of Barrett or esophageal adenocarcinoma. General population screening is not currently recommended. Although screening has become standard of practice in some communities, the effectiveness of screening using current techniques is controversial because it may not improve mortality rates from adenocarcinoma.
- EGD with biopsy is necessary for diagnosis. Ideally, this should be done via high-resolution white-light endoscopy with at least four biopsies for every 2-cm segment. If esophagitis is present, patients should be treated to heal esophagitis with repeat endoscopy and biopsies 8-12 weeks later to determine if underlying Barrett esophagus is present.
- Unsedated transnasal endoscopy and an esophageal cytology device called a *Cytosponge* may be acceptable alternatives to conventional endoscopy. Wireless esophageal capsule endoscopy may detect Barrett esophagus but with too low a sensitivity and specificity to be recommended. Imaging studies are not useful.
- Diagnosis requires the presence of metaplastic columnar epithelium at least 1 cm proximal to the gastroesophageal junction (Figs. 1 and 2). Longer-segment (≥3 cm) Barrett esophagus is more readily diagnosed (Fig. 3). Some endoscopists describe the extent of Barrett esophagus using the Prague criteria, describing the circumferential and maximal length via a C and M score. At least two expert gastrointestinal pathologists should concur if any grade of dysplasia is diagnosed.
- Intestinal metaplasia of the gastric cardia is not Barrett esophagus and does not have the same risk for malignancy.

TABLE 1 Proposed Physiologic Abnormalities Contributing to Gastroesophageal Reflux Disease in Patients With Barrett Esophagus

Abnormality	Potential Consequences
Extreme hypotension of the lower esophageal sphincter	Gastroesophageal reflux
Ineffective esophageal motility	Defective clearance of refluxed material
Gastric acid hypersecretion	Reflux of highly acidic gastric juice
Duodenogastric reflux	Esophageal injury caused by reflux of bile acids and pancreatic enzymes
Decreased salivary secretion of EGF	Delayed healing of reflux-damaged esophageal mucosa
Decreased esophageal pain sensitivity to refluxed caustic material	Failure to initiate therapy

EGF, Epidermal growth factor.
From Feldman M, et al: *Sleisenger and Fordtran's gastrointestinal and liver disease*, ed 10, Philadelphia, 2016, Saunders.

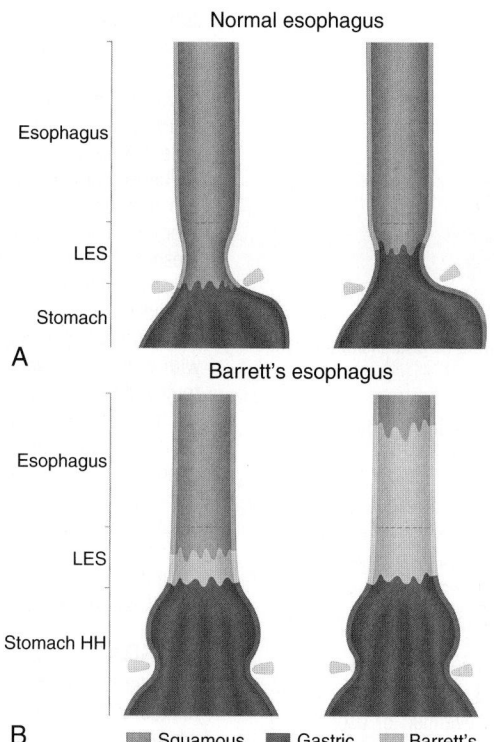

Normal esophagus

Esophagus

LES

Stomach

A

Barrett's esophagus

Esophagus

LES

Stomach HH

B

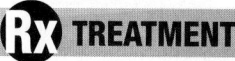
☐ Squamous ☐ Gastric ☐ Barrett's

FIG. 1 Anatomic landmarks of the normal LES region (A) and of Barrett esophagus (B). Note that gastric mucosa is very common and normal in the LES region and that in Barrett esophagus, the squamocolumnar junction is not only proximally displaced within the tubular esophagus, but that the intervening mucosa is composed of intestinalized Barrett's metaplastic epithelium. *HH,* Hiatal hernia. (From Silverburg SG: *Principles of practice of surgical pathology and cytopathology,* ed 4, New York, 2006, Churchill Livingstone.)

- Biomarkers and advanced imaging techniques such as chromoendoscopy, narrow band imaging, confocal laser endomicroscopy, and optical coherence tomography are being evaluated to assist with diagnosis and to better understand progression of disease, prediction of response to therapy, or prognosis.
- Screening for *Helicobacter pylori* infection in patients with GERD and Barrett esophagus is not recommended.

Rx TREATMENT

The goal is to control GERD symptoms and maintain healed mucosa.

NONPHARMACOLOGIC THERAPY

Nonpharmacologic therapy includes lifestyle modifications; elevating head of bed; and avoiding chocolate, tobacco, caffeine, mints, and certain drugs (see "Gastroesophageal Reflux Disease").

ACUTE GENERAL Rx

- Proton pump inhibitors are the most effective treatment for GERD. Therapy should be titrated to control symptoms and/or to promote healing of endoscopic signs of disease.
- If patient is asymptomatic and incidentally found to have Barrett esophagus, once-daily proton pump inhibitors should be prescribed, as they may reduce the risk of neoplastic progression.

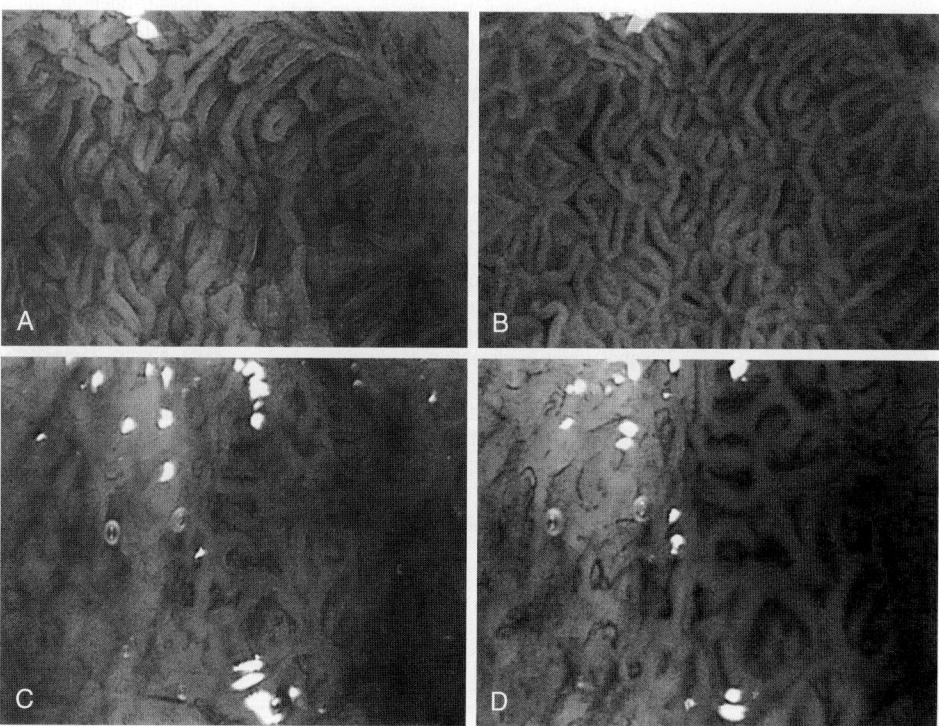

FIG. 2 Images of nondysplastic Barrett esophagus using a high-resolution endoscope without *(A)* and with *(B)* narrow band imaging. In the lower panels *(C, D)* an area of early intramucosal cancer in the background of high-grade dysplasia associated with Barrett esophagus is shown. Note the irregular and distorted pit and vascular pattern in the area of high-grade dysplasia or intramucosal cancer compared with the nondysplastic Barrett esophagus *(A, B),* which has a regular pit and vascular pattern. (From Feldman M, et al: *Sleisenger and Fordtran's gastrointestinal and liver disease,* ed 10, Philadelphia, 2016, Saunders.)

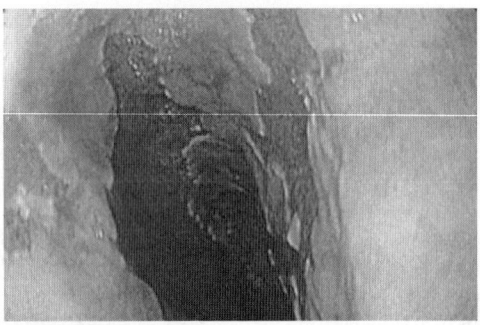

FIG. 3 Long-segment Barrett esophagus. (From Cameron JL, Cameron AM: *Current surgical therapy,* ed 10, Philadelphia, 2011, Saunders.)

CHRONIC Rx

- Chronic acid suppression is recommended to control symptoms, maintain healing, and reduce neoplastic progression.
- Antireflux surgery may be considered for management of GERD and associated sequelae, but it has not been proven to be superior to medical therapy. Patients continue to require endoscopic surveillance of their esophagus.
- When GERD is controlled by either medical or surgical therapy, ablation of metaplastic epithelium usually leads to replacement by normal squamous epithelium. Because only a minority of patients with Barrett esophagus progress to high-grade dysplasia or carcinoma, endoscopic eradication therapy is not recommended for the general population of patients with nondysplastic Barrett esophagus.
- Endoscopic eradication therapy is becoming the treatment of choice for low-grade dysplasia and is the treatment of choice for high-grade dysplasia. Radiofrequency ablation or photodynamic therapy, combined with endoscopic mucosal resection (EMR) or endoscopic submucosal dissection (ESD) of visible mucosal irregularities, should be performed in conjunction with aggressive surveillance and eradication of all remaining Barrett epithelium. Endoscopic therapy is preferred over surgical treatment in properly staged individuals. These therapies may even be considered for patients with focal intramucosal carcinoma, if properly staged (T1SM1 or lower). Cryotherapy is being evaluated for the complete eradication of both dysplasia and intestinal metaplasia and reduced risk for disease progression. All these options run the risk for residual or buried metaplasia.

- Surgical resection is definitive therapy and may be offered for multifocal high-grade dysplasia or carcinoma that has extended into the submucosa (T1 SM2 or 3), or for patients with poorly differentiated carcinomas or with evidence of lymphovascular invasion. Mortality appears to be lower with experienced surgeons operating in high-volume centers.
- Patients with cardiovascular risk factors may be considered for low-dose aspirin therapy for chemoprevention of esophageal adenocarcinoma.

DISPOSITION

- The relative risk of developing esophageal adenocarcinoma for a patient with Barrett esophagus, as compared with the general population, is 11.3, a substantial drop from the relative risk of 30 or 40 estimated in earlier reports. The risk is greater in men and in patients with longer ($\geq$8 cm) columnar-lined segments.
- The risk of progression from untreated Barrett with high-grade dysplasia to esophageal adenocarcinoma ranges from 6% to 19% per year.
- Frequency of monitoring is controversial. No prospective studies have proven that endoscopic surveillance is cost effective or increases life expectancy. Although some studies have suggested that close adherence to surveillance protocols is associated with higher rates of detection of dysplasia and cancer, a recent case-control study showed no reduction in mortality.
- Patients with Barrett esophagus currently undergo surveillance EGD and systematic four-quadrant biopsy at intervals determined by the presence and grade of dysplasia. Some

authors suggest that only high-risk individuals undergo surveillance. All mucosal abnormalities should undergo biopsy. Patients without dysplasia should have follow-up every 3 to 5 yr. Patients with low-grade dysplasia should have aggressive antisecretory (proton pump inhibitor) therapy and have endoscopic ablation therapy or extensive mucosal sampling every 12 months until dysplasia is no longer present. They then revert to a 3- to 5-year interval. Patients with high-grade dysplasia should have expert confirmation and extensive mucosal sampling. High-grade dysplasia with visible mucosal irregularities should be removed by EMR or ESD, followed by mucosal ablation. Consider intensive surveillance every 3 mo. Indefinite dysplasia requires aggressive medical therapy and close follow-up and resampling. Endoscopic treatment is preferred over intensive surveillance in patients with high-grade dysplasia.
- Patients should be treated aggressively for GERD before surveillance.

REFERRAL

- Consider EGD with biopsy in male or selected female patients with multiple risk factors who have not had previous EGD.
- Refer patients with GERD for evaluation if "red flag" symptoms are present (dysphagia, odynophagia, weight loss, vomiting, early satiety, GI bleeding, iron deficiency).
- Refer patients with biopsy-proved Barrett esophagus for surveillance.
- For those with low-grade or high-grade dysplasia, refer for ablative therapy with EMR or ESD if appropriate, followed by intensive surveillance. Esophageal resection may be considered.

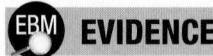

Available at www.expertconsult.com

SUGGESTED READINGS
Available at www.expertconsult.com

RELATED CONTENT

Barrett Esophagus (Patient Information)
Esophageal Tumors (Related Key Topic)
Gastroesophageal Reflux Disease (Related Key Topic)

AUTHOR: **HARLAN G. RICH, M.D.**

BASIC INFORMATION

DEFINITION

- The Bartholin's glands are located in the labia minora at 4 o'clock and 8 o'clock. They are nonpalpable and approximately 0.5 cm in diameter. The glands are used for lubrication and moisturizing the vaginal vestibular mucosa.

ETIOLOGY

- Cyst obstruction of the duct is normally due to inflammation or trauma. The cyst will fill with fluid and become distended due to continued glandular secretion following the obstruction. Cyst size can range from 1 to 3 cm. The patient with a cyst will present with a painless labial mass, no redness, no cellulitis.
- Patients with an abscess often present complaining of a tender, painful, fluid-filled mass in the labia. Sometimes they will report drainage but deny fever or illness. The cause of a Bartholin's abscess is rarely a sexually transmitted infection. Other pathogens responsible include *E. coli*, staphylococcus, and streptococcus.
- The Bartholin's abscess pain is significant. Following drainage and treatment the patient will experience immediate relief, although they may still may require oral analgesia for a few days following the procedure.

EPIDEMIOLOGY AND DEMOGRAPHICS

- In women of reproductive age, 2% may experience swelling of the Bartholin's gland.
- Primary gland infection or infected cyst would be the cause in a patient presenting with a Bartholin's abscess.
- 5% of vulvar carcinoma are of the Bartholin's gland. Missed diagnosis of malignancy may result in poorer outcome for those patients due to the extensive vascular and lymphatic vessels present in the vulva. Any patient presenting after age 40 or with a history of vulvar cancer should be evaluated by a gynecologist, and biopsy is recommended.

PHYSICAL FINDINGS AND CLINICAL PRESENTATION

- Patients may have a painless, unilateral labial mass without signs of surrounding cellulitis.
- Patients with abscess may present after having a painless cyst, but then new onset of symptoms will occur, including but not limited to:
  - Painful, acute swelling of unilateral labia, tender, fluctuant labial mass, erythema, edema, dyspareunia, pain while sitting or walking, or sudden discharge from abscess resulting in relief of pain. Fever is rare, but may be present in individuals who are immunocompromised.
- The provider will be able to visualize unilateral swelling of labia and palpate a fluctuant mass; tenderness with palpation, erythema, edema, and cellulitis surrounding the abscess may be present. Purulent discharge may be noted if the abscess is rupturing. Patients may present complaining of drainage of an abscess that has already ruptured; if completely drained, there may be no observation of a mass.

DIAGNOSIS

DIFFERENTIAL DIAGNOSIS

- Bartholin's gland malignancy/vulvar malignancy
- Folliculitis
- Garter duct cyst
- Genital warts
- Hernia
- Hidradenoma
- Lipoma
- Sebaceous cysts
- Skene duct cyst
- Syphilis/chancroid
- Vaginitis
- Vestibular mucous cysts
- Trauma/hematoma
- Vulvar lesion/HSV

WORKUP

- STI testing if indicated
- Biopsy in women over age 40, or with history of vulvar carcinoma
- Discuss the following treatment options with patient. Explain the risks, benefits, and possible complications. For medical legal purposes know the process for performing outpatient procedures in the facility.

TREATMENT

- Treatment depends on symptoms. Asymptomatic women <40 do not require treatment.
  1. **No treatment**: Patient is asymptomatic or cyst is not interfering with activities of daily living. Most tend to rupture spontaneously.
  2. **Sitz baths**: Recommended 3 times daily to promote spontaneous rupture of the cyst. Can use a warm, shallow bath or warm compress in place of sitz bath.
  3. **Simple needle aspiration**: Making a small incision with a needle insertion into the cyst to facilitate drainage. This technique has a high rate for reoccurrence.
  4. **Incision and drainage (I&D)**: Incision and drainage can be accomplished via a variety of techniques to promote facilitation of drainage and relief of pain from fluid collection. Local anesthesia is essential when draining abscess to promote patient tolerance and comfort with procedure. It is important to apply anesthesia to the tissue mucosa instead of the abscess. Anesthesia directed at the fluid collection will not provide proper pain relief for procedure. Performed in office or outpatient setting. Procedure: Following local anesthetic injection, a small 2- to 5-mm incision is made with #11 surgical blade into abscess. The contents are then manually expressed to promote drainage. Next, the area is flushed with sterile saline. The incisional site can then be packed with packing or left alone. If packing is placed, it should be removed 2 days after procedure. This technique provides immediate relief of discomfort but comes with high risk of reoccurrence.
  5. **Fistulization**: Creation of a new outflow tract by placing a drainage catheter, such as a Word catheter, into the incision following I&D. See procedure for I&D. Instead of gauze packing, a catheter is inserted into the abscess to promote continual drainage and to facilitate outflow tract development. Procedure: After incision is cleansed with sterile saline, the catheter is inserted. The bulb is inflated with 3 to 5 cc of saline. The catheter is then tucked in vagina for 4 to 6 weeks to create epithelium tract. In one study, a Word catheter as treatment was successful in 26 of 30 cases (87%) of Bartholin's cyst or abscess (Fig. 1).
  6. **Marsupialization**: For recurrent cysts that have failed fistulization. This surgical procedure is usually performed in outpatient surgical site when abscess is not present. Complications: infection and hematoma. Heals in approximately 2 weeks following surgery.
  7. **Surgical excision**: Reserved for recurrent cysts or suspicion of malignancy. This surgical procedure is rarely needed for treatment of uncomplicated abscesses.
  8. **Other treatment options**: CO_2 laser, silver nitrate application, and alcohol sclerotherapy.
- The goal is to develop tract to facilitate drainage of gland.
- Antibiotics are not necessary for uncomplicated abscesses.
- Common antibiotics when needed are: azithromycin, ceftriaxone, ciprofloxacin, and doxycycline. Women require antibiotics when reoccurrence, pregnancy, immunosuppression, MRSA, and concurrent gonorrhea or chlamydia infection occur.

SUGGESTED READINGS

Available at www.expertconsult.com

RELATED CONTENT

Vaginal Fistulas (Related Key Topic)

AUTHORS: **DEANNA BENNER, A.P.R.N., C.R.N.P,** and **ELIZABETH SUSHEREBA, M.S.N., C.N.M.**

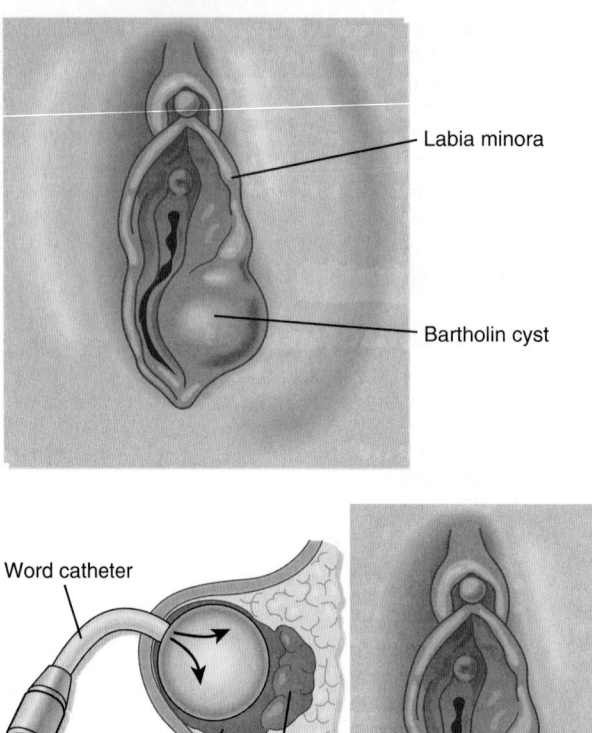

Labia minora

Bartholin cyst

Word catheter

Cyst cavity

Bartholin gland

A

Inflated balloon in cyst cavity

B

FIG. 1 A, Scalpel incision of a Bartholin duct cyst. **B,** Placement of a Word catheter in the cyst. (From Adams JG et al: *Emergency medicine: clinical essentials*, ed 2, Philadelphia, 2013, Saunders.)

BASIC INFORMATION

DEFINITION

Basal cell carcinoma (BCC) is a malignant tumor of the skin arising from basal cells of the lower epidermis and adnexal structures. It may be classified as one of six types: nodular, superficial, pigmented, cystic, sclerosing or morpheaform, and nevoid. The most common type is nodular (21%); the least common is morpheaform (1%). A mixed pattern is present in approximately 40% of cases. BCC advances by direct expansion and destroys normal tissue.

SYNONYMS

BCC

ICD-10CM CODES

C44.01	Basal cell carcinoma of skin of lip
C44.111	Basal cell carcinoma of skin of unspecified eyelid, including canthus
C44.112	Basal cell carcinoma of skin of right eyelid, including canthus
C44.119	Basal cell carcinoma of skin of left eyelid, including canthus
C44.211	Basal cell carcinoma of skin of unspecified ear and external auricular canal
C44.212	Basal cell carcinoma of skin of right ear and external auricular canal
C44.219	Basal cell carcinoma of skin of left ear and external auricular canal
C44.310	Basal cell carcinoma of skin of unspecified parts of face
C44.311	Basal cell carcinoma of skin of nose
C44.319	Basal cell carcinoma of skin of other parts of face
C44.41	Basal cell carcinoma of skin of scalp and neck
C44.510	Basal cell carcinoma of anal skin
C44.511	Basal cell carcinoma of skin of breast
C44.519	Basal cell carcinoma of skin of other part of trunk
C44.611	Basal cell carcinoma of skin of unspecified upper limb, including shoulder
C44.612	Basal cell carcinoma of skin of right upper limb, including shoulder
C44.619	Basal cell carcinoma of skin of left upper limb, including shoulder
C44.711	Basal cell carcinoma of skin of unspecified lower limb, including hip
C44.712	Basal cell carcinoma of skin of right lower limb, including hip
C44.719	Basal cell carcinoma of skin of left lower limb, including hip
C44.81	Basal cell carcinoma of overlapping sites of skin
C44.91	Basal cell carcinoma of skin, unspecified

EPIDEMIOLOGY & DEMOGRAPHICS

- Most common cutaneous neoplasm
- 85% of cases appear on the head and neck region
- Most common site: nose (30%)
- Increased incidence with age >40 yr
- Increased incidence in men
- Risk factors: fair skin, increased sun exposure, use of tanning salons with ultraviolet A or B radiation, history of irradiation (e.g., Hodgkin's disease), personal or family history of skin cancer, impaired immune system

PHYSICAL FINDINGS & CLINICAL PRESENTATION

Variable with the histologic type:
- Nodular: dome-shaped, painless lesion that may become multilobular and frequently ulcerates (rodent ulcer); prominent telangiectatic vessels are noted on the surface. Border is translucent, elevated, pearly white (Fig. 1). Some nodular BCCs may contain pigmentation, giving an appearance similar to a melanoma.
- Superficial: circumscribed, scaling, black appearance with a thin, raised, pearly-white border (Fig. 2); a crust and erosions may be present. Occurs most frequently on the trunk and extremities.
- Morpheaform: flat or slightly raised yellowish or white appearance (similar to localized scleroderma); appearance similar to scars; surface has a waxy consistency.

DIAGNOSIS

DIFFERENTIAL DIAGNOSIS

- Keratoacanthoma
- Melanoma (pigmented BCC)
- Xeroderma pigmentosa
- Basal cell nevus syndrome
- Molluscum contagiosum
- Sebaceous hyperplasia
- Psoriasis

WORKUP

Biopsy to confirm diagnosis

TREATMENT

Variable with tumor size, location, and cell type:
- Excision surgery: preferred method for large tumors with well-defined borders on the legs, cheeks, forehead, and trunk.
- Mohs' micrographic surgery: preferred for lesions in high-risk areas (e.g., nose, eyelid), very large primary tumors, recurrent BCCs, and tumors with poorly defined clinical margins.
- Electrodesiccation and curettage: useful for small (>6 mm) nodular BCCs.
- Cryosurgery with liquid nitrogen: useful in BCCs of the superficial and nodular types with clearly definable margins; no clear advantages over the other forms of therapy; generally reserved for uncomplicated tumors.
- Radiation therapy: generally used for BCCs in areas requiring preservation of normal surrounding tissues for cosmetic reasons (e.g., around lips); also useful in patients who cannot tolerate surgical procedures or for large lesions and surgical failures.
- Imiquimod 5% cream can be used for treatment of small, superficial BCCs of

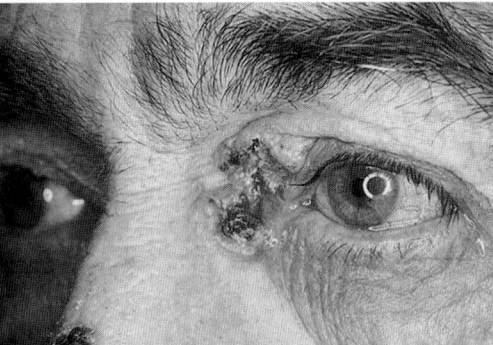

FIG. 1 Basal cell carcinoma. Note rolled translucent border and central ulceration in typical facial location. (From Noble J et al: *Textbook of primary care medicine,* ed 3, St Louis, 2001, Mosby.)

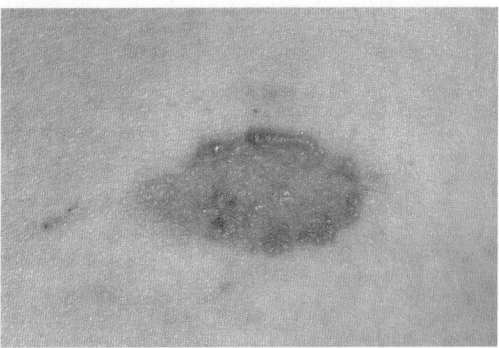

FIG. 2 Superficial variant of basal cell carcinoma. Multiple lesions are common with this variant, often on the trunk. Closer examination shows the typical raised pearly edge. (From White GM, Cox NH [eds]: *Diseases of the skin: a color atlas and text,*)

the trunk and extremities. Efficacy rate is approximately 80%. Its main advantage is lack of scarring, which must be weighed against higher cure rates with surgical intervention.

- Vismodegib and sonidegib are orally active hedgehog pathway inhibitors FDA approved for metastatic BCC, recurrent basal cell carcinoma post-surgery, and locally advanced BCC in patients who are not candidates for surgery or radiation.
- Table 1 summarizes advantages and disadvantages of BCC treatment options.

DISPOSITION

- More than 90% of patients are cured; however, periodic evaluation for at least 5 yr is necessary because of increased risk of recurrence of another BCC (<40% risk within 5 yr of treatment).
- A lesion is considered low risk if it is >1.5 cm in diameter, is nodular or cystic, is not in a difficult-to-treat area (H zone of face), and has not been previously treated.
- Nodular and superficial BCCs are the least aggressive.
- Morpheaform lesions have the highest incidence of positive tumor margins (<30%) and the greatest recurrence rate.

PREVENTION

Oral nicotinamide, a form of vitamin B_3 available without prescription (500 mg bid), has been reported to prevent development of new nonmelanoma skin cancer in high-risk patients.

SUGGESTED READINGS
Available at www.expertconsult.com

RELATED CONTENT

Basal Cell Skin Cancer (Patient Information)
Actinic Keratosis (Related Key Topic)
Melanoma (Related Key Topic)
Squamous Cell Carcinoma (Related Key Topic)

AUTHOR: **FRED F. FERRI, M.D.**

TABLE 1 Advantages and Disadvantages of Basal Cell Carcinoma Treatment Options

Modality	Advantages	Disadvantages
Mohs micrographic surgery	Complete margin analysis Well tolerated by elderly Gold standard treatment	Cost Longer procedure (stages)
Conventional surgical excision	Well tolerated by elderly	Cost Lack of complete margin analysis
Electrodesiccation and curettage	Shorter procedure Does not require return visit Patients can avoid surgery	Lack of histologic confirmation of malignancy removal Not appropriate for lesions with extension into deep dermis
Cryosurgery	Patients can avoid surgery	Higher recurrence rates than surgery Lack of histologic confirmation of malignancy removal Recurrent carcinoma could be extensive (can be obscured by fibrous scar tissue) Hypertropic scarring Postinflammatory pigment changes
Imiquimod	Patient self-administration Excellent cosmetic results	Local skin reactions Lack of histologic confirmation of malignancy removal Cost
Photodynamic therapy	Excellent cosmetic outcome	Higher recurrence rates than with surgery Lack of histologic confirmation of malignancy removal
5-FU	Patient self-administration	Higher recurrence rates than with surgery
Radiation therapy	Good option in patients who are not surgical candidates	Cost Higher recurrence rates than with surgery Scars tend to worsen with time Can require 15-30 visits Side effects are considerable
Vismodegib	Approved for metastatic BCC and locally advanced BCC that has recurred following surgery; option in patients who are not surgical or radiation therapy candidates	Cost
Observation	Patients can avoid surgery Cost	No standard as to length of time for which it is appropriate to monitor patients clinically More dangerous neoplasms may be missed (such as Merkel cell carcinoma or amelanotic melanoma)

BCC, Basal cell carcinoma; *5-FU*, 5-fluorouracil.
Wiznia LE, Federman DG: Treatment of basal cell carcinoma in the elderly; what nondermatologists need to know, *Am J Med* 129:655-660, 2016.

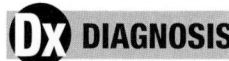

BASIC INFORMATION

DEFINITION

Basic calcium phosphate crystal deposition disease, commonly known as calcific periarthritis, refers to periarticular and intraarticular deposits of calcific material. Basic calcium phosphate (BCP) comprises crystals of partially carbonate-substituted hydroxyapatite (form of calcium phosphate), octacalcium phosphate, and tricalcium phosphate. BCP crystal deposits are often asymptomatic and found incidentally on plain radiograph. Acute attacks can be manifest as hot, swollen, tender joint symptoms appearing clinically similar to gout, pseudogout, and septic arthritis. BCP crystals are frequently found in the synovial fluid of patients with osteoarthritis, and are involved in the soft-tissue calcinosis seen in scleroderma and dermatomyositis.

SYNONYMS

Calcific periarthritis/calcific tendonitis
Hydroxyapatite deposition
Apatite-associated destructive arthritis
Idiopathic destructive arthritis of the shoulder
BCP crystal-associated destructive arthropathies
BCPCDD
Milwaukee shoulder syndrome

ICD10CM CODES
M11.0 Hydroxyapatite deposition disease
M11.8 Other specified crystal arthropathies

EPIDEMIOLOGY & DEMOGRAPHICS

PREVALENCE: Often asymptomatic and incidentally found. Prevalence not established.
PREDOMINANT SEX: Females > males
PREDOMINANT AGE: Middle age, 70+
GENETICS: Caucasian predominant
RISK FACTORS: Most cases spontaneous onset. May arise from trauma or overuse.

PHYSICAL FINDINGS & CLINICAL PRESENTATION

- Periarticular calcific deposits are often asymptomatic
- Acute attacks have sudden onset of severe pain, swelling, warmth, local tenderness, and associated loss of function. Reduced active ROM in all affected joints, sometimes associated with joint instability. Most present with spontaneous onset but may be preceded by mild trauma or overuse
- Commonly affects shoulder (dominant side usually although 60% bilateral). Hip, knee, elbow, wrist, ankle joints also common sites.
- Hydroxyapatite pseudopodagra – describes acute calcific arthritis at the first metatarsophalangeal joint usually in young women
- *Milwaukee shoulder syndrome* – describes destructive arthropathy of the shoulder from calcium deposits leading to disruption and loss of function in shoulder, usually in females older than 60 years (Fig. 1 and Table 1)

ETIOLOGY

- Idiopathic
- No known relationship to HLA specificity or other genetic markers even with known occurrence of familial cases

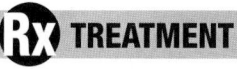

DIAGNOSIS

DIFFERENTIAL DIAGNOSIS OF ACUTE CALCIFIC PERIARTHRITIS

- Gouty arthritis
- Pseudogout
- Septic arthritis

DIFFERENTIAL DIAGNOSIS OF CHRONIC CALCIFIC PERIARTHRITIS

- Osteoarthritis (unusual sites of osteoarthritis such as shoulder, elbow, ankle joint should lead to further investigation)
- Seronegative polyarthritis
- CPPD
- Trauma, impingement
- Inflammatory arthritis

WORKUP

LABORATORY TESTS:
- Phosphate, calcium levels, and renal function for any metabolic causes
- Analysis of synovial or bursal fluid: low cell count, viscous, sometimes blood tinged in destructive arthropathies. BCP crystals are small, less than 0.1 μm long, needle shaped, nonbirefringent.
- Calcium stains: Alizarin Red S (highly sensitive – lacks specificity to qualify for routine use) or oxytetracycline stain with UV light
- Labeled diphosphonate binding

IMAGING STUDIES

- Plain radiograph—AP and lateral sufficient but internal or external rotation may be needed for retrohumeral deposits
  - Inert periarticular calcium deposits appear dense, homogenous, without trabeculations with well-defined borders
  - Acute calcific periarthritis attacks appear fluffy with poorly defined margins as crystals shed into surrounding tissues, with soft tissue swelling
- Ultrasonography
- Scanning and transmission electron microscope—due to small size (20-100 nm)
- MRI of affected joint (Fig. 2)

TREATMENT

Asymptomatic deposits—no treatment needed

NONPHARMACOLOGIC THERAPY

- Immobilization, heat application, range of motion exercises

ACUTE GENERAL Rx

- Analgesics, nonsteroidal antiinflammatory drugs, or colchicine
- Nonselective COX inhibitors (BCP crystals induce both COX-1 and COX-2)
- Needle aspiration of the deposits with or without irrigation
- Intraarticular steroids
- Pain relief with suprascapular nerve blocks, or transcutaneous nerve stimulation

CHRONIC Rx

- Physical therapy
- Pulsed ultrasonography—increased rate of resorption and reduced pain

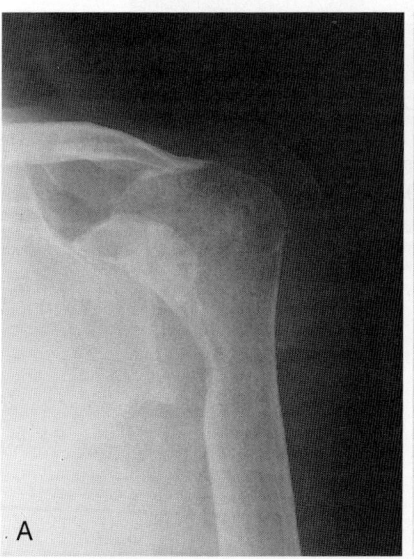
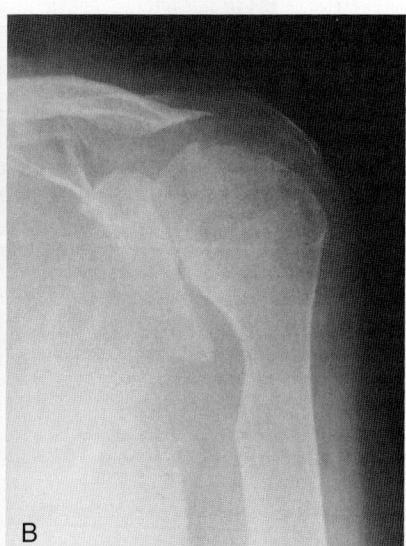

FIG. 1 Anteroposterior radiographs of a shoulder joint affected by basic calcium phosphate crystal–associated destructive arthritis (Milwaukee shoulder syndrome). The extensive destruction of periarticular tissues, including the rotator cuff, has led to instability of the shoulder. **A,** The upward subluxation of the humerus can be overcome by **B,** traction on the shoulder. Note the extensive atrophic destruction and loss of bone of both the acromion and the glenohumeral joint. (Hochberg MC, et al.: *Rheumatology*, ed 5, St Louis, 2011, Mosby)

TABLE 1 Clinical Syndromes That Can Be Associated With the Deposition of Basic Calcium Phosphate Crystals in and Around Joints

Subcutaneous deposits (e.g., calcification of hands in scleroderma)	Asymptomatic chance finding
	Acute and chronic inflammation
	Skin ulceration
	Secondary infection
	Pressing necrosis of surrounding tissues
	Mechanical interference with function
Periarticular deposits (e.g., calcification of supraspinatus tendon)	Asymptomatic chance finding
	Acute calcific periarthritis
	Chronic periarticular pain and/or dysfunction
Intraarticular deposits (e.g., synovial and cartilage deposits in damaged joints)	Asymptomatic chance finding
	Acute synovitis
	Severe osteoarthritis
	Destructive arthropathies of older people

BCP, basic calcium phosphate.
Hochberg MC, et al.: *Rheumatology*, ed 5, St Louis, 2011, Elsevier.

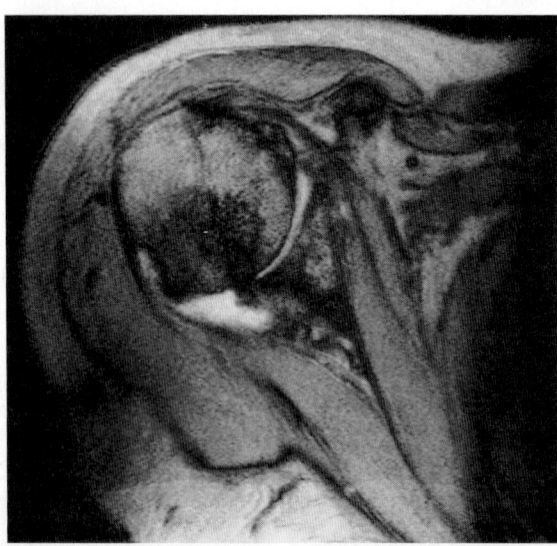

FIG. 2 Axial T2-weighted magnetic resonance imaging scan of a shoulder joint affected by basic calcium phosphate crystal–associated destructive arthritis (Milwaukee shoulder). There is advanced glenohumeral joint degeneration with loss of articular cartilage, truncation of the anterior and posterior labrum, narrowing of the joint space, osteophyte formation, muscle atrophy, and joint effusion. (Hochberg MC, et al.: *Rheumatology*, ed 5, St Louis, 2011, Mosby)

- Surgical therapy (arthroplasty or debridement) may be warranted for restoration of function and pain relief
- Disodium ethylenediamine tetraacetic acid (EDTA)—administered at painful site with mesotherapy

REFERRAL
- Rheumatology
- Orthopedic surgery if considering joint replacement

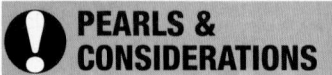 **PEARLS & CONSIDERATIONS**

COMMENTS
Basic calcium phosphate deposition should be considered in the differential diagnosis of acute polyarthritis, especially in the setting of chronic severe OA. Specific crystal identification is difficult with methods that are currently clinically available.

PREVENTION
None known

SUGGESTED READINGS
Available at www.expertconsult.com

RELATED CONTENT
Osteoarthritis (Related Key Topic)

AUTHOR: **ZUHAL ARZOMAND, M.D.**

BASIC INFORMATION

DEFINITION

A bedbug's bite is a wound caused by the penetration of the bedbug mouthpiece into the skin as the insect feeds on blood from vessels or extravasated blood from the damaged surrounding tissue. The saliva of the bedbug contains pharmacologically active substances responsible for a spectrum of undesirable skin reactions depending on the individual. The bugs typically feed during times when an individual is at rest and may feed without being detected. Typically feedings take 5 to 10 minutes.

SYNONYMS

Insect bite
Bedbug *Cimex lectularius* bite

ICD-10CM CODES
T00.9 Multiple superficial (insect bite) injuries, unspecified

EPIDEMIOLOGY & DEMOGRAPHICS

- Traditionally, bedbugs were considered more common in poorer areas, but they are now increasingly found in areas of frequent travel.
- Bedbug infestations may spread among multifamily and institutional facilities with shared walls and are consequently difficult to eradicate.
- Reports of bedbug infestations have increased dramatically in the U.S., as well as worldwide, likely because of the decreased use of pesticides and increased international travel.
- Bedbugs are attracted to carbon dioxide gas and warm bodies.
- Bedbugs do not have a preference for specific age groups, ethnicity, or sex.
- Persons at higher risk include those who have recently stayed overnight in a hotel, dorm room, hospital, or new home.
- Studies have shown increased sensitivity of cutaneous reaction in previous bite victims.

PHYSICAL FINDINGS AND CLINICAL PRESENTATION

- Bites typically occur at night on exposed areas of skin, most often the face, neck, arms, and legs.
- The bites are painless and so do not awaken the individual.
- Onset of signs and symptoms of bites can be immediately on awakening or up to 10 days after the bite.
- Firm, purpuric or erythematous macules, urticaria, papules (Fig. 1), or bullae may be present. Bites are often inflammatory and pruritic, although bedbug-naive individuals may be asymptomatic to their first bites.
- Bite may have a central hemorrhagic punctum.
- Victim may observe a linear series often consisting of three bites ("breakfast, lunch, and dinner").
- Bites are typically pruritic.

- The size, degree of itching, and propensity toward vesiculation all increase with repeated bedbug bites.
- Fig. 2 illustrates symptoms and behaviors resulting from bed bug bites.

ETIOLOGY

- The *Cimex lectularius* species, also known as the common bedbug (Fig. 3), have flat, oval bodies and retroverted mouth parts used for taking blood meals. It feeds on mammals and birds. *Cimex hemipterus* is a tropical species that bites mostly humans, and hybrid species of the two insects exist. Both generally feed nocturnally on the blood of sleeping humans. They hide in beds, the floor, or furniture crevices during the day and emerge at night. They go through a larva stage (Fig. 4) and have a life span from 4 months up to 1 year. The adult bedbug is wingless and about 5 to 7 mm in length. It has a modified mouthpart for piercing and sucking that usually leaves a bite mark of papular urticarial presentation to exposed areas of skin. Bedbugs have weak appendages for latching on to their hosts and are not usually transported from person to person.

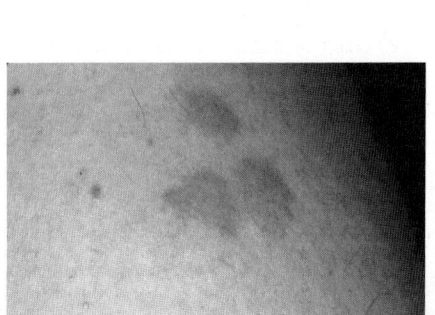

FIG. 1 Pruritic papules after bedbug bites. (From Kliegman RM et al: Nelson textbook of pediatrics, ed 19, Philadelphia, 2011, Saunders.)

- The saliva of the bedbug contains nitrophorin that enables vasodilation, an anticoagulant that interferes with production of coagulation factor Xa, a salivary apyrase that inhibits platelet aggregation, and an anesthetic. Consequently, the host often does not feel the bite until the effects have worn off.

DIAGNOSIS

DIFFERENTIAL DIAGNOSIS

Scabies, flea and mite bites, vesicular disorders, delusional parasitosis, dermatitis herpetiformis, pemphigus herpetiformis, ecthyma, drug eruptions

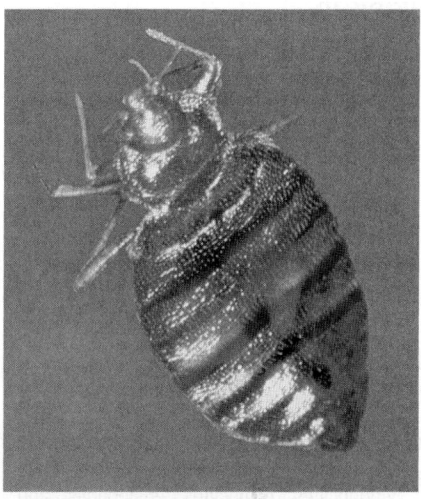

FIG. 3 Bedbug. (From James WD et al: *Andrews' diseases of the skin*, ed 12, Philadelphia, 2016, Saunders.)

Symptoms and behaviors resulting from bed bug attacks

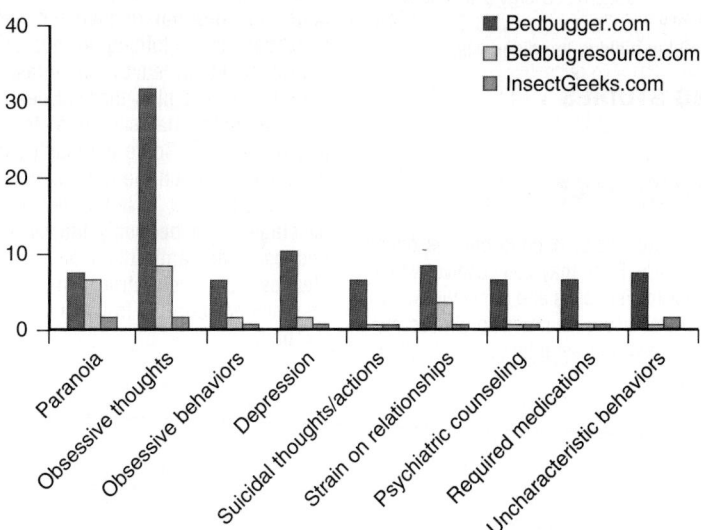

- Bedbugger.com
- Bedbugresource.com
- InsectGeeks.com

FIG. 2 Distribution of symptoms in 135 Internet reports describing effects of bed bug bites. (From Goddard J, de Shazo R: Psychological effects of bed bug attacks *(Cimex lectularius L.), Am J Med* 125:101-103, 2012.)

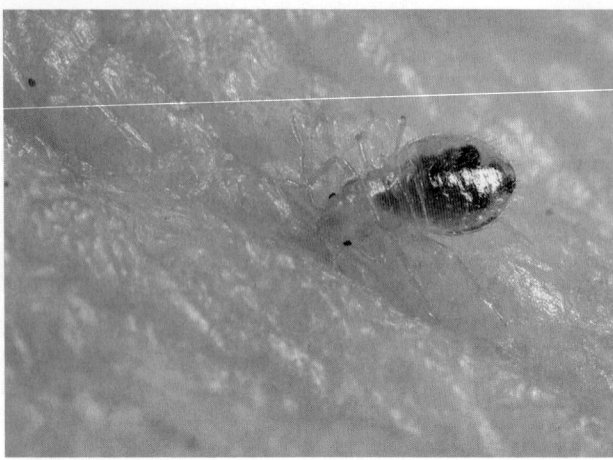

FIG. 4 Bedbug—second-stage larva. (Habif TP: *Clinical dermatology: a color guide to diagnosis and therapy*, ed 6, Philadelphia, 2016, Elsevier.)

WORKUP

- Workup begins with history and physical for clinical symptoms and environmental findings suggestive of insect bites.
- Victims should carefully scrutinize the bedroom for signs of bedbug infestation. One may encounter fecal smears or flecks of blood on bed linens, inside furniture cracks and crevices, and behind peeling wallpaper. Bedbugs may travel as far as 20 feet for a meal. Densely infested rooms may also have a distinctive, pungent, soda syrup–like odor.

LABORATORY TESTS

- No specific tests recommended except for identification of the insect.
- The histology of bedbug bites is similar to other insect bites. Perivascular infiltrate of lymphocytes, histiocytes, eosinophils, and mast cells is seen within the upper dermis. One may also observe collagen bundles with interstitial eosinophils, dermal edema, and extravasated erythrocytes.
- Hypersensitivity to bedbug salivary proteins may be tested via intradermal allergy skin testing.
- Skin biopsy results are nonspecific and are not helpful in making the diagnosis.

IMAGING STUDIES

None

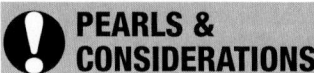

- Specific treatment of bedbug bites is often not necessary. Bites may self-resolve within a week for milder cases and a few weeks for more severe cases. Treatment regimens are based on resolving symptoms of the bites, mainly pruritus.

- To prevent infection, avoid scratching the area.
- Topical glucocorticoids or systemic antihistamines are appropriate in patients with severe pruritus from the bedbug bite.
  1. Triamcinolone cream 0.1%; apply thin film to affected areas bid
  2. Chlorpheniramine 4 mg PO at bedtime (adults), 2 mg PO at bedtime (children)
- Insecticides may be effective in eradicating the bedbug, but growing resistance has been seen and multi-insecticide therapy is recommended.
  1. Use permethrin spray for clothing and bedsheets or bed nets
  2. Diethyltoluamide (DEET): Be wary of toxic levels in children when used at high concentrations.
  3. Deltamethrin and chlorfenapyr are two common insecticides used.
  4. Please consult a pest control professional for safe eradication.

NONPHARMACOLOGIC THERAPY

Vacuuming is effective in removing bedbugs but does not remove the eggs. Wash bedsheets and clothing in hot water with detergent with at least 20 minutes in a dryer. Bedbugs have a high thermal death point of 45° C and also may survive at temperatures as low as 7° C. Some companies perform a treatment in which the room is heated above 50° C, which is a lethal temperature for all stages of a bedbug's life cycle. Coating bedposts with antifriction or adhesive substances such as petrolatum or duct tape may hinder bedbugs from gaining access to the bed.

ACUTE GENERAL Rx

Immunologic response is dependent on immunocompetence and individual sensitivity to the salivary components of the bedbug bite. Often, patients with papular urticaria have IgG antibodies to specific bedbug proteins. IgE antibodies may also mediate bullae formation. Anaphylaxis and death from bites is rare but documented in literature.

DISPOSITION

Patient may resume normal activity and lifestyle. Travelers should inspect their clothing and suitcases before returning home.

BEDBUGS AS POTENTIAL VECTORS

The bedbug has been studied extensively as a potential vector for human pathogens such as HIV, hepatitis B, hepatitis C, and Chagas' disease. To date, there is no evidence of transmission from an infected bedbug to a human.

❗ PEARLS & CONSIDERATIONS

COMMENTS

- Bedbugs are an increasing source of anguish and frustration for humans, and clinicians should evaluate for signs of stress and depression.
- A combination of chemical and physical intervention is often necessary for complete eradication. All hiding areas must be carefully inspected and cleaned. Treatment may include pesticides, laundering, heat, freezing, vacuuming, and hiring a professional service to eradicate bedbugs.

SUGGESTED READINGS

Available at www.expertconsult.com

RELATED CONTENT

Bedbugs (Patient Information)
Bites and Stings, Insect (Related Key Topic)

AUTHOR: **SCOTT M. SOUTHER, M.D.**

BASIC INFORMATION

DEFINITION
Acute peripheral facial nerve (cranial nerve VII) palsy

SYNONYMS
Idiopathic facial paralysis
Facial nerve palsy

ICD-10CM CODES
G51.0 Bell palsy

EPIDEMIOLOGY & DEMOGRAPHICS
INCIDENCE: 20-30 cases per 100,000.
PEAK INCIDENCE: Patients less than 70 years old and pregnant females, especially during the third trimester and first postpartum week.
PREDOMINANT SEX AND AGE: Sexes are equally affected. The median age is age 40.
RISK FACTORS: Diabetes and pregnancy.

PHYSICAL FINDINGS & CLINICAL PRESENTATION
- Patients present with acute or subacute (hours to days) onset of unilateral facial paralysis with maximal weakness at 3 wk. Clinical findings are dependent on the location of facial nerve injury and involvement of associated branches (Fig. 1). One third of patients demonstrate incomplete paralysis, and the remaining two thirds have complete paralysis. Recovery usually occurs within the first 6 mo.
- Patients may also present with variable involvement of taste over the anterior two thirds of the tongue and/or altered secretion of the lacrimal and salivary glands

ETIOLOGY
Most cases of Bell palsy are thought to be secondary to either a viral inflammatory or immune injury. Herpes simplex virus is thought to be the most common viral pathogen followed by herpes zoster. Other infectious causes include Epstein-Barr virus, cytomegalovirus, adenovirus, rubella, and mumps.

DIAGNOSIS

DIFFERENTIAL DIAGNOSIS
- Cortical stroke: forehead and periorbital muscles are spared in stroke patients because of bilateral innervation of the upper face.
- Brainstem stroke: ipsilateral weakness in the upper and lower muscles of facial expression due to a stroke affecting the nucleus or fascicle of the seventh nerve.
- Lyme disease: facial nerve palsy is the most common cranial neuropathy associated with Lyme disease. In Lyme meningitis, facial nerve palsy may be unilateral or bilateral.
- HIV.
- Ramsay Hunt syndrome: facial nerve paralysis associated with ipsilateral zoster oticus.
- Parotid gland tumors.
- Trauma/temporal bone fracture.
- Meningeal processes
  1. Infectious: Lyme disease, HIV, syphilis, leprosy, tuberculosis meningitis, fungal meningitis.
  2. Inflammatory: Sarcoidosis, Sjögren syndrome, and Guillain-Barré syndrome and its variants.
  3. Leptomeningeal carcinomatosis or lymphomatosis: breast cancer, lung cancer, and lymphoma are most common.

- Möbius syndrome
- Melkersson-Rosenthal syndrome

WORKUP
- Bell palsy is a clinical diagnosis.
- Additional workup may be necessary in patients with an uncertain diagnosis, complete seventh nerve injury, evidence of neurologic dysfunction in addition to seventh nerve injury, and lack of recovery.

LABORATORY TESTS
Laboratory tests are not typically recommended. However, if the diagnosis of Bell palsy is in question (e.g., bilateral facial nerve palsy, concern for a secondary etiology), then it is reasonable to pursue the following tests:
- Lyme antibody followed by Western blot for positive cases for confirmation. Consider lumbar puncture for CSF analysis for Lyme serologies.
- ACE level
- Glycosylated hemoglobin (HgA1C)
- HIV
- RPR and VDRL in CSF
- ESR

ELECTRODIAGNOSTIC TESTING
Electrodiagnostic testing may be performed 2 wk after the onset of symptoms to assess the integrity of a motor unit and the degree of nerve damage. Facial motor response remains normal for the first 3 days following an injury and then rapidly decreases depending on the severity of the lesion. A facial motor study may be performed at 10 days and compared to the contralateral side. A motor response that is 10% the amplitude of the unaffected side on electrodiagnostic testing corresponds with 90% motor axon degeneration. One study found that patient recovery was poor when this critical value was reached.

IMAGING STUDIES
Imaging studies are not usually indicated.
- Brain MRI is indicated in certain cases, such as an upper motor neuron pattern (able to wrinkle forehead) where the temporalis branch of the facial nerve is spared.
- Brain MRI with gadolinium is indicated either when other cranial nerve palsies are present or when a meningeal process is suspected.
- CT temporal bone is indicated in cases of either trauma or complete facial paralysis in which the surgeon is considering decompression.

TREATMENT

NONPHARMACOLOGIC THERAPY
- Reassurance that most patients will have a full recovery and that the patient did not sustain a stroke.
- Eye patch to prevent corneal drying/abrasion and subsequent ulceration. Patients may protect their eyes with Lacri-Lube at night and artificial tears during the day.

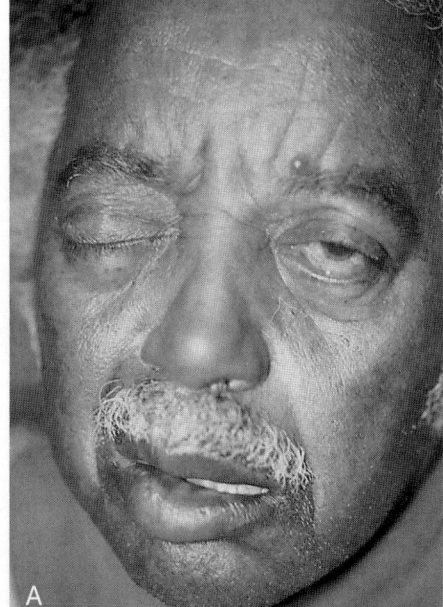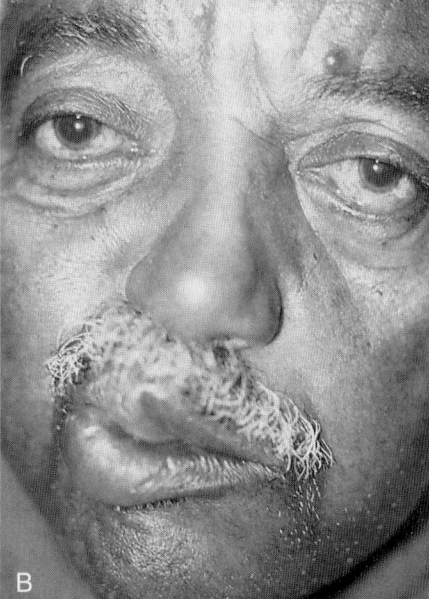

FIG. 1 A patient with a lesion of the facial nerve. A, The patient has difficulty in closing his left eye, and the left corner of his mouth droops. **B,** The latter defect is especially evident when the patient attempts to purse his lips. (From Haines DE: *Fundamental neuroscience for basic and clinical applications,* ed 3, Philadelphia, 2006, Churchill Livingstone.)

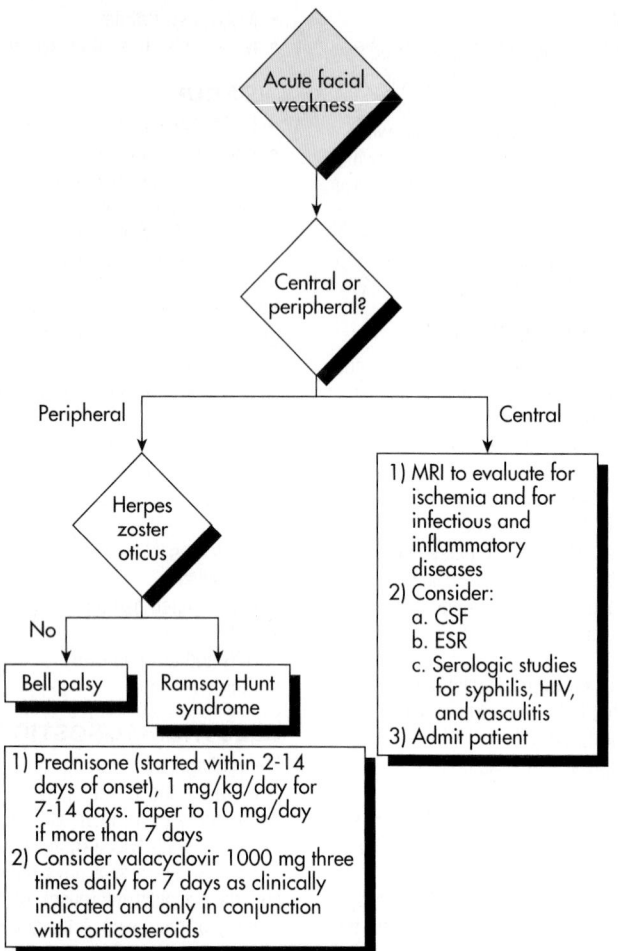

FIG. 2 Algorithm outlining the treatment of patients with Bell palsy. *CSF*, Cerebrospinal fluid; *ESR*, erythrocyte sedimentation rate; *HIV*, human immunodeficiency virus; *MRI*, magnetic resonance imaging. (Modified from Adams JG et al: *Emergency medicine, clinical essentials*, ed 2, St Louis, 2013, Elsevier.)

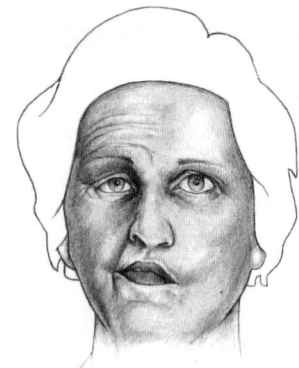

FIG. 3 Bell palsy. The patient with Bell palsy (facial nerve palsy) will demonstrate an unwrinkled forehead, widely opened eyes (with weakness of eyelid color), flattening of the nasolabial fold, and a droop of the corner of the mouth. (From Remmel KS et al: *Handbook of symptom-oriented neurology*, ed 3, St Louis, 2002, Mosby.)

CHRONIC Rx

Botulinum toxin may be used in cases of hemifacial spasm.

DISPOSITION

- 71% of patients with Bell palsy have a complete recovery.
- 85% show recovery after 3 wk. Prognosis is favorable if recovery is seen during this timeframe.
- 13% have slight sequelae, and 16% have residual weakness, synkinesis, or contracture.
- Recurrence rate is 7%, and the average time to recurrence is 10 yr.

REFERRAL

- Neurologist if clinical diagnosis is in question.
- Ophthalmologist if concern for corneal abrasion or ulceration.

❗ PEARLS & CONSIDERATIONS

COMMENTS

- Assess wrinkling of forehead (Fig. 3). If present on affected side, ensure that the facial weakness is not central.
- Assess for other cranial nerve deficits or long-tract signs because brainstem fascicular lesions of the seventh nerve can show peripheral facial pattern of weakness.

SUGGESTED READINGS

Available at www.expertconsult.com

RELATED CONTENT

Bell Palsy (Facial Palsy) (Patient Information)

AUTHORS: **ALEXANDRA BUFFIE, M.D.,**
JOSEPH KASS, M.D., J.D., and
JOHN SLADKY, M.D.

- Acupuncture with needle manipulation and strong stimulation has been shown to improve recovery after Bell palsy when compared to acupuncture without needle manipulation.[1]

ACUTE GENERAL Rx

- Corticosteroids started within 72 hr will expedite speed and rate of recovery in most patients. Antiviral therapy alone has no benefit.
  1. Two high-quality randomized trials assessed efficacy of early (<72 hr) treatment with glucocorticoids alone, antiviral therapy alone, and combination therapy in the treatment of Bell palsy. Glucocorticoids alone were effective, while antiviral therapy showed no benefit when given either alone or with concomitant glucocorticoid therapy.
  2. The largest study compared groups receiving the following treatments: (a) 60 mg prednisolone daily, (b) 1000 mg valacyclovir three times daily for 1 wk, (c) combination therapy, and (d) placebo. All interventions were administered within 72 hr of presentation.

[1]Xu SB et al: Effectiveness of strengthened stimulation during acupuncture for the treatment of Bell palsy: a randomized controlled trial, *CMAJ* 185:473-479, 2013.

3. Time to recovery, determined at a 1-year follow-up appointment, was shortest in the group treated with prednisolone monotherapy. The efficacy of valacyclovir monotherapy did not differ from placebo, and no added benefit was seen with combination therapy.
- Treatment guidelines recommend prednisone 60 to 80 mg daily for 1 wk.
  1. Despite the lack of strong clinical evidence, some authors still recommend treatment with valacyclovir (1000 mg 3 times daily for 1 wk) in severe cases (i.e., level IV or greater on the House-Brackmann grading system).
- Surgical decompression is not currently recommended.
  1. The 2001 American Academy of Neurology Practice Parameter concluded there was insufficient evidence to make any recommendation regarding surgical decompression for Bell palsy.
  2. This conclusion was further substantiated by a 2011 Cochrane systematic review, which looked at two additional studies, again citing insufficient evidence regarding surgical decompression for Bell palsy.
- Fig. 2 describes an algorithm for the treatment of patients with Bell palsy.

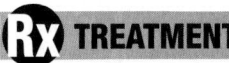 BASIC INFORMATION

DEFINITION

Benign paroxysmal positional vertigo (BPPV) is a labyrinthine disorder and is the most common cause of vertigo. It is characterized by paroxysms of brief spinning sensation accompanied by nystagmus that usually lasts less than a minute. These paroxysms are generally induced by changes in head position with respect to gravity.

SYNONYMS

BPPV

ICD-10 CM CODES
H81.1 Benign paroxysmal vertigo

EPIDEMIOLOGY & DEMOGRAPHICS

Higher prevalence seen in elderly and women.
INCIDENCE: Incidence increases with advancing age. Unrecognized BPPV can be found in about 10% of certain geriatric populations, and there is a cumulative incidence of nearly 10% by age 80 yr.
PREVALENCE: Lifetime prevalence is 2.4%. Reported prevalence is 10.7 and 64 cases per 100,000 population. BPPV is by far the most common type of vertigo.
PREDOMINANT SEX AND AGE: Female (2:1 to 3:1 ratio); peak onset: 50-60 years.
GENETICS: Unknown
RISK FACTORS: Head trauma, inner ear surgery, viral labyrinthitis, Meniere's disease, migraine. The majority are idiopathic.

PHYSICAL FINDINGS & CLINICAL PRESENTATION

- Brief paroxysms of vertigo and nystagmus with certain head positions are seen in 70%.
- Episodes are typically triggered by head position changes such as while getting in or out of bed, rolling over in bed, forward head tilt, or bending forward.
- Episodes are brief, usually lasting 30 to 40 seconds but can recur for several days or months.
- Usually no hearing abnormalities are present.
- Direction of nystagmus depends on the canal affected with reversal of direction being seen while sitting up, and fatigability with repeated testing.
- Rarely persistent vertigo and disequilibrium may be seen.

POSTERIOR SEMICIRCULAR CANAL (PCC)

While posterior, horizontal or superior semicircular canal can be affected as isolated or in different combinations, PCC involvement is commonest (60%-90%) and will be discussed in the following sections. Nystagmus is up-beating and torsional and can be elicited by the Dix Hallpike maneuver.
DIX-HALLPIKE MANEUVER: With head turned to one side at an angle of 45 degrees, patient is moved from sitting to supine position with head hanging below the end of the table at an angle of 20 deg. The posterior semicircular canal comes into the sagittal plane and the free floating otolith debris moves down and away from the ampulla. An up-beating and torsional nystagmus will be seen with the top poles of the eye beating towards the lower ear.

HORIZONTAL SEMICIRCULAR CANAL

Involvement may be underestimated as it may remit spontaneously. It produces either geotropic nystagmus beating towards the ground or apogeotropic nystagmus beating towards the ceiling when the head is turned to either side in the supine position. The nystagmus beats stronger towards the affected ear.
HEAD ROLL TEST FOR THE RIGHT HORIZONTAL SEMICIRCULAR CANAL (INDUCING GEOTROPIC NYSTAGMUS): Patient is moved from sitting to supine position, then head is rolled 90 degrees to the left. The otolithic debris moves away from the cupula of horizontal semicircular canal, a left beating geotropic nystagmus (towards the ground) is seen. Next the head is turned 90 degrees to the right—a right-beating stronger geotropic nystagmus is seen as otolithic debris moves towards the cupula of the right horizontal semicircular canal.
SUPINE HEAD ROLL TEST FOR THE RIGHT HORIZONTAL SEMICIRCULAR CANAL (INDUCING APOGEOTROPIC NYSTAGMUS): Patient is moved from sitting to supine position, then head is rolled 90 degrees to the left. This induces deflection of the cupula of the right horizontal semicircular canal due to otolithic debris near or attached to the cupula. A strong, right-beating apogeotropic nystagmus (towards the ceiling) is induced. Next, the head is turned 90 degrees in the opposite direction. Now the right horizontal semicircular canal cupula is deflected in the opposite direction and a weak, left-beating apogeotropic nystagmus results.

ANTERIOR SEMICIRCULAR CANAL

Involvement is rare as it is located uppermost in the labyrinth and so otolithic debris is unlikely to become trapped. A downbeat and torsional nystagmus where the top poles of the eye beat towards the lower ear is seen. Evaluating for central lesions is a must in these cases.

ETIOLOGY

The fundamental pathologic process is believed to be the movement of otolithic debris in the endolymph of the inner ear. The debris may be present in the cupula (cupulolithiasis) or free floating within the semicircular canal near the cupula (canalithiasis). Static head position changes with respect to gravity, causing the debris to move within the semicircular canal and creating a false sense of rotation.

DX DIAGNOSIS

Elicitation of a typical nystagmus with Dix-Hall pike is the standard for diagnosing posterior canal BPPV. However, 25% of symptomatic patients may not exhibit nystagmus. Appropriate referral to a neurologist or neuro-otologist should be considered in these cases.

Fig. 1 shows a diagnostic algorithm for vertigo and dizziness.

DIFFERENTIAL DIAGNOSIS

- Vestibular neuritis
- Vestibular migraine
- Meniere's disease
- Stroke
- Box 1 lists causes of vertigo with and without hearing loss.
- Table 1 describes the differential diagnosis of true vertigo

WORK-UP

None; BPPV is a clinical diagnosis

IMAGING STUDIES

- To be obtained only when stroke remains high in the differential diagnosis.

Rx TREATMENT

- BPPV usually resolves without treatment in 2-4 weeks. Recurrences are common in the first year, and long-term recurrence rates range from 30% to 50%.
- Nausea and vomiting may be treated symptomatically with medications.
- Canalith repositioning maneuvers (Epley's and Semont's maneuvers for the posterior canal) are effective. They are designed to "flush" otolithic debris out of the semicircular canals into the vestibule where they are resorbed. Epley's maneuver for BPPV of the posterior canal is recommended as standard of care by the American Academy of Neurology and American Academy of Otolaryngology-Head and Neck Surgery. When patients do not respond, it may be related to the technique, or they may be

BOX 1 Causes of Vertigo With and Without Hearing Loss

Hearing Loss
Conductive
  Otitis media with effusion
  Chronic suppurative otitis media or
    cholesteatoma should be considered

Sensorineural
  Perilymphatic fistula
  Tumor
  Ménière's disease
  Migraine headache
  Genetic syndromes
  Temporal bone fracture
  Vestibular concussion

No Hearing Loss
Acute Vertigo
  Perilymphatic fistula
  Benign positional vertigo
  Seizure
  Labyrinthitis

Recurrent or Chronic Vertigo
  Acoustic neuroma
  Multiple sclerosis

From Marx JA et al: *Rosen's emergency medicine: concepts and clinical practice*, ed 7, Philadelphia, 2010, Elsevier.

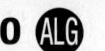

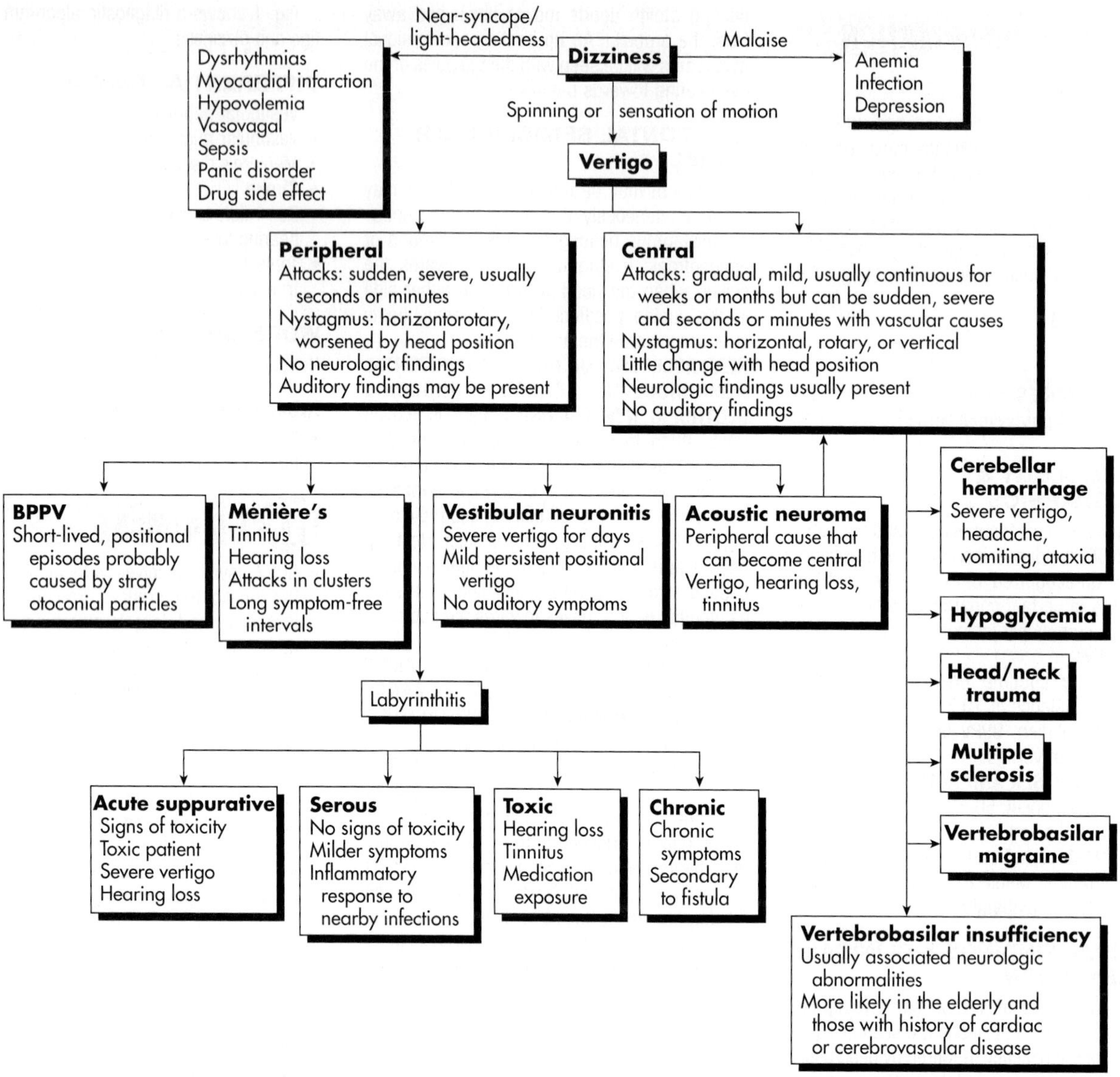

Near-syncope/
light-headedness   **Dizziness**   Malaise

Dysrhythmias
Myocardial infarction
Hypovolemia
Vasovagal
Sepsis
Panic disorder
Drug side effect

Anemia
Infection
Depression

Spinning or | sensation of motion

Vertigo

Peripheral
Attacks: sudden, severe, usually
  seconds or minutes
Nystagmus: horizontorotary,
  worsened by head position
No neurologic findings
Auditory findings may be present

Central
Attacks: gradual, mild, usually continuous for
  weeks or months but can be sudden, severe
  and seconds or minutes with vascular causes
Nystagmus: horizontal, rotary, or vertical
Little change with head position
Neurologic findings usually present
No auditory findings

BPPV
Short-lived, positional
  episodes probably
  caused by stray
  otoconial particles

Ménière's
Tinnitus
Hearing loss
Attacks in clusters
Long symptom-free
  intervals

Vestibular neuronitis
Severe vertigo for days
Mild persistent positional
  vertigo
No auditory symptoms

Acoustic neuroma
Peripheral cause that
  can become central
Vertigo, hearing loss,
  tinnitus

**Cerebellar
hemorrhage**
Severe vertigo,
  headache,
  vomiting, ataxia

Hypoglycemia

**Head/neck
trauma**

Labyrinthitis

**Multiple
sclerosis**

Acute suppurative
Signs of toxicity
Toxic patient
Severe vertigo
Hearing loss

Serous
No signs of toxicity
Milder symptoms
Inflammatory
  response to
  nearby infections

Toxic
Hearing loss
Tinnitus
Medication
  exposure

Chronic
Chronic
  symptoms
Secondary
  to fistula

**Vertebrobasilar
migraine**

Vertebrobasilar insufficiency
Usually associated neurologic
  abnormalities
More likely in the elderly and
  those with history of cardiac
  or cerebrovascular disease

FIG. 1 Diagnostic algorithm for dizziness and vertigo. *BPPV,* benign paroxysmal positional vertigo. (From Marx JA et al: *Rosen's emergency medicine: concepts and clinical practice,* ed 7, Philadelphia, 2010, Elsevier.)

refractory. There is no clear consensus on how many times the maneuver should be performed at a single visit. Many prefer to do it two or three times if nystagmus is still present with the second maneuver. Other maneuvers such as Barbecue, Vannucchi, and Gufoni are used to reposition debris in the horizontal semicircular canal and will not be discussed here.

EPLEY'S MANEUVER:
• Head is turned 90 degrees towards unaffected side. The head and trunk are then turned an additional 90 degrees in the same direction, so that the patient lies on the unaffected side with head pointing towards the floor. The otolithic debris moves in the same direction, producing a brief nystagmus. The patient is then moved to a sitting position, which allows the debris to fall out of the canal into the utricle through the common crus.
• Each position should be maintained for 30 seconds or until the nystagmus or

vertigo resolves. Sometimes nystagmus in the opposite direction is seen. It is prudent for patients to sit still in the upright position for about 15 minutes and then to walk cautiously.

NONPHARMACOLOGIC THERAPY
Transection of the ampullary nerve (singular nerve) and plugging of the involved canal are rarely performed for intractable and treatment-resistant cases.

ACUTE GENERAL Rx
Canalith repositioning

CHRONIC Rx
If multiple treatments are needed, patients should be instructed to perform the maneuvers at home.

REFERRAL
To a neuro-otologist, otolaryngologist, neurologist

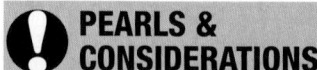

BPPV is a benign and self-limiting condition but can be disabling.
  Diagnosis is clinical and canalith repositioning maneuvers are effective.

PATIENT/FAMILY EDUCATION
• Reassurance
• Fall precautions

RELATED CONTENT
Meniere's Disease (Related Key Topic)
Vestibular Neuritis (Related Key Topic)

SUGGESTED READINGS
Available at www.expertconsult.com

AUTHORS: **PADMAJA SUDHAKAR, M.B.B.S.,** and **SACHIN KEDAR, M.B.B.S., M.D.**

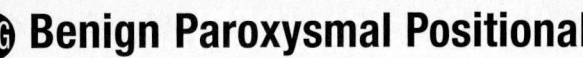

B

I

TABLE 1 Differential Diagnosis of Patients with True Vertigo

Cause	History	Associated Symptoms	Physical
Peripheral			
1. Benign paroxysmal positional vertigo	Short-lived, positional, fatigable episodes	Nausea, vomiting	Single position can precipitate vertigo. Horizontorotary nystagmus often can be induced at bedside.
2. Labyrinthitis			
A. Serous	Mild to severe positional symptoms. Usually coexisting or antecedent infection of ear, nose, throat, or meninges	Mild to severe hearing loss can occur	Usually nontoxic patient with minimal fever elevation
A. Acute suppurative	Coexisting acute exudative infection of the inner ear. Severe symptoms	Usually severe hearing loss, nausea, vomiting	Febrile patient showing signs of toxicity. Acute otitis media
I. Toxic	Gradually progressive symptoms: Patients on medication causing toxicity	Hearing loss that may become rapid and severe, nausea and vomiting	Hearing loss. Ataxia common feature in chronic phase
3. Ménière's disease	Recurrent episodes of severe rotational vertigo usually lasting hours. Onset usually abrupt. Attacks may occur in clusters. Long symptom-free remissions	Nausea, vomiting, tinnitus, hearing loss	Positional nystagmus not present
4. Vestibular neuronitis	Sudden onset of severe vertigo, increasing in intensity for hours, then gradually subsiding over several days. Mild positional vertigo often lasts weeks to months. Sometimes history of infection or toxic exposure that precedes initial attack. Highest incidence is found in third and fifth decades	Nausea, vomiting. Auditory symptoms do not occur	Spontaneous nystagmus toward the involved ear may be present.
5. Acoustic neuroma	Gradual onset and increase in symptoms. Neurologic signs in later stages. Most occur in women between 30 and 60	Hearing loss, tinnitus. True ataxia and neurologic signs as tumor enlarges	Unilateral decreased hearing. True truncal ataxia and other neurologic signs when tumor enlarges. May have diminution or absence of corneal reflex. Eighth cranial nerve deficit may be present.
Central			
1. Vascular disorders			
A. Vertebrobasilar insufficiency	Should be considered in any patient of advanced age with isolated new-onset vertigo without an obvious cause. More likely with history of atherosclerosis. Initial episode usually seconds to minutes	Often headache. Usually neurologic symptoms including dysarthria, ataxia, weakness, numbness, double vision. Tinnitus and deafness uncommon	Neurologic deficits usually present, but initially neurologic examination can be normal.
A. Cerebellar hemorrhage	Sudden onset of severe symptoms	Headache, vomiting, ataxia	Signs of toxicity. Dysmetria, true ataxia. Ipsilateral sixth cranial nerve palsy may be present.
I. Occlusion of posterior inferior cerebellar artery (Wallenberg's syndrome)	Vertigo associated with significant neurologic complaints	Nausea, vomiting, loss of pain and temperature sensation, ataxia, hoarseness	Loss of pain and temperature sensation on the side of the face ipsilateral to the lesion and on the opposite side of the body, paralysis of the palate, pharynx, and larynx. Horner's syndrome (ipsilateral ptosis, miosis, and decreased facial sweating)
I. Subclavian steal syndrome	Classic picture is syncopal attacks during exercise, but most cases present with more subtle symptoms.	Arm fatigue, cramps, mild light-headedness may be only other symptoms than vertigo	Diminished or absent radial pulses in affected side or systolic blood pressure differentials between the two areas occur in most patients.
2. Head trauma	Symptoms begin with or shortly after head trauma. Positional symptoms most common type after trauma. Self-limited symptoms that can persist weeks to months	Usually mild nausea	Occasionally, basilar skull fracture
3. Neck trauma	Usual onset 7–10 days after whiplash injury. Symptoms may last weeks to months. Episodes seconds to minutes when turning head	Neck pain	Neck tenderness, pain on movement, and positional nystagmus and vertigo when head is turned to side of the whiplash
4. Vertebrobasilar migraine	Vertigo almost always followed by headache. Patient has usually had similar episodes in past. Most patients have a family history of migraine. Syndrome usually begins in adolescence	Dysarthria, ataxia, visual disturbances, or paresthesias usually precede headache	No residual neurologic or otologic signs are present after attack.
5. Multiple sclerosis	Vertigo presenting symptoms in 7%–10% and appears in the course of the disease in a third. Onset may be severe and suggest labyrinth disease. Disease onset usually between ages 20 and 40. Often history of other attacks with varying neurologic signs or symptoms	Nausea and vomiting, which may be severe	May have horizontal, rotary, or vertical nystagmus. Nystagmus may persist after the vertiginous symptoms have subsided. Bilateral internuclear ophthalmoplegia and ataxic eye movements suggest multiple sclerosis.
6. Temporal lobe epilepsy	Can be initial or prominent symptom in some patients with the disorder	Memory impairment, hallucinations, trancelike states, seizures	May have aphasia or convulsions
7. Hypoglycemia	Should be considered in diabetics and any other patient with unexplained symptoms	Sweating, anxiety	Tachycardia, mental status change may be present.

From Marx JA et al: *Rosen's emergency medicine: concepts and clinical practice*, ed 7, Philadelphia, 2010, Elsevier.

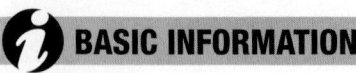

BASIC INFORMATION

DEFINITION

Binge eating disorder (BED) is characterized by recurrent binge eating episodes, during which an abnormally large amount of food is consumed in a short period of time, accompanied by a sense of loss of control. At least 3 of the following features need to be present in a binge eating episode:

1. Consuming food faster than normal
2. Consuming food until uncomfortably full
3. Consuming large amounts of food when not hungry
4. Consuming food alone due to embarrassment
5. Feeling disgusted, depressed, or guilty after eating a large amount of food

In order to meet criteria for BED, individuals must engage in binge eating episodes at least once per week for 3 months, feel significant distress with regard to their binge eating behaviors, and not utilize compensatory behaviors (e.g., induced vomiting, laxative misuse, over-exercising) seen in other eating disorders like bulimia nervosa.

SYNONYMS

Compulsive overeating
BED

ICD 10-CM CODES
F50.81 Binge eating disorder

EPIDEMIOLOGY & DEMOGRAPHICS

INCIDENCE: To our knowledge, no incidence studies on BED yet exist.
PREVALENCE (IN US): Approximately 2% lifetime prevalence in adult community samples was found (women 3.5 %; men 2.0 %). Lower lifetime prevalence rates among 13 to 18 year old adolescents (girls 2.3 %; boys 0.8 %) were found. The 12-month prevalence among adult women and men is 1.6 and 0.8%, respectively
PREDOMINANT AGE (IN US): Higher prevalence rates in females (1.75:1) were found among adults.
GENETICS:
- BED appears to aggregate in families and have a significant genetic component
- Family studies report odds ratios between 1.9 and 2.2 for the risk of BED in a relative of a proband with BED compared with relatives of controls
- Twin studies of BED have reported heritability estimates ranging from 41% to 57% for varying definitions of this disorder
RISK FACTORS:
- Mental health concerns and psychopathology (mood disorders, anxiety disorders, personality disorders, conduct problems, negative affectivity, substance abuse)
- Temperament and coping style (e.g., high avoidance motivation, low distress tolerance, low extraversion and self-directedness)
- Severe childhood obesity

- Experience of bullying/weight-related stigmas
- Lifestyle disruptions and deprivation
- Family weight and eating concerns (family dieting, family history of bulimia nervosa, family overeating)
- Quality of parenting (family discord, maternal/paternal problem parenting, parental separation/absence/death)
- Sexual and physical abuse

PHYSICAL FINDINGS & CLINICAL PRESENTATION

- Although not necessary for a diagnosis, individuals presenting with BED are often overweight or obese
- BED is highly comorbid with other forms of psychopathology, especially mood and anxiety disorders. Individuals seeking treatment with acute symptoms of other disorders might not initially report binging episodes, which underscores the importance of thorough initial assessment
- Males with BED are more likely to underreport symptoms
- Disordered eating symptoms can improve or worsen over time, and diagnostic labels might transition from BED to other eating disorders over time
- There is potential for higher suicide risk among individuals with BED, possibly because of comorbid psychopathology, and suicidal ideation/intent should be monitored
- General difficulty to cope with negative emotions and avoidance of aversive experiences/feelings might be apparent
- Significant shame and self-conscious emotions regarding bingeing behaviors might be present

ETIOLOGY

- Research suggests that individual factors (e.g., genetic, biologic, temperamental), environmental factors (e.g., family environment, external sources of stress), and their interactions each contribute.

DIAGNOSIS

DIFFERENTIAL DIAGNOSIS

- Important to establish the presence of objective binge eating episodes versus subjective binge eating episodes and non-binge forms of overeating.
- Important to establish that binge eating episodes are not associated with the recurrent use of inappropriate compensatory behaviors (e.g., purging, overexercising).
- Important to establish that binge eating episodes do not occur exclusively during the course of anorexia nervosa, bulimia nervosa, or avoidant/restrictive food intake disorder.

WORK-UP

- Careful medical and psychosocial history
- Physical examination reveals no specific diagnostic signs of BED
- Mental status examination

LABORATORY TESTS

- No laboratory tests are diagnostic. However, given that BED is frequently associated with overweight and obesity, tests examining associated medical problems (e.g., Type II diabetes, high triglycerides) might benefit an individual's overall treatment plan

IMAGING STUDIES

- Neuroimaging studies suggest there are corticostriatal circuitry alterations in BED similar to those observed in substance abuse, including altered function of prefrontal, insular, and orbitofrontal cortices and the striatum. Imaging is not recommended as part of routine evaluation.

TREATMENT

NONPHARMACOLOGIC THERAPY

- The primary goal of therapeutic approaches to BED is reduction and/or elimination of binge eating episodes and the associated symptoms of distress.
- Variations of cognitive behavior therapy (CBT) and interpersonal psychotherapy (IPT) remain the most established treatments for BED.
- Growing literature on other psychotherapeutic approaches to BED has also yielded empirical support for dialectical behavior therapy (DBT), and mindfulness-based therapies.
- Combining different interventions at the same time does not add significant advantages. Planning sequential treatments, with more specific interventions for non-responders, seems to be a more promising strategy.
- Behavioral weight loss (BWL) and self-help interventions evidenced some efficacy in patients with lower psychopathological features. Although BWL approaches have yielded weight loss in the short-term, long-term weight loss maintenance has not been typically achieved. Moreover, BWL approaches have not fared as well as CBT and IPT approaches in ameliorating disordered eating patterns.
- Morbidly obese patients with BED might be well-served by weight loss (bariatric) surgery, which has been found to be associated with sustained, substantial weight loss, as well as reduction in binge eating episodes. More research is needed in this area.
- Although further research is needed, preliminary findings regarding electronically delivered psychotherapeutic interventions (e.g., Internet-based CBT) for BED have yielded some empirical support. The utility of internet-based treatment compared to face-to-face treatment, has not yet been studied extensively with regard to BED.
- One of the limitations of existing literature on the psychotherapeutic approaches to BED is the predominant inclusion of female participants in RCTs.

ACUTE GENERAL Rx

- The pharmacotherapy literature on treating BED in the short-term has focused on achieving the following objectives: reducing the frequency of binge eating episodes, reducing weight, and improving associated psychopathology (e.g., depression/anxiety symptoms).
- Preliminary support for specific medications within the classes of antidepressants, anticonvulsants, and antiobesity agents has been found for treating symptoms associated with BED
- Antidepressants are thought to influence treatment outcomes by addressing the mood and anxiety symptoms that often co-occur with BED. Anticonvulsants have been examined in the treatment of BED because of their success in treating other impulse control disorders. Antiobesity agents have been used to address the overweight and obesity that usually accompanies BED.
- Lisdexamfetamine dimesylate (Vyvanse) is the only medication that has been approved by the Food and Drug Administration (FDA) for the treatment of BED. Two studies found that participants taking the medication experienced a decrease in the number of binge-eating days per week and had fewer obsessive-compulsive binge eating behaviors compared to those on placebo. Longer-term maintenance studies examining the treatment of BED have not yet been published.
- Exploratory work using substance use treatment agents to address BED symptoms is currently underway
- The existing literature on pharmacotherapy approaches to BED has several limitations, including short duration of RCTs, and lack of adequately sized RCTs

CHRONIC Rx

- The long-term treatment of BED using pharmacotherapy has not as yet been systematically investigated

COMPLEMENTARY & ALTERNATIVE MEDICINE

- One study found that hour-long, weekly yoga sessions were associated with reductions in binge eating, BMI, and hip and waist measurements, and an increase in physical activity. More follow-up research is needed in this area.

DISPOSITION

- Data on the long-term outcome of BED, including mortality, are scarce.
- Most outcome data on BED are derived from RCTs. In studies on the outcome of binge eating disorder with a follow-up duration over 3 years, remission rates in the samples treated with psychotherapy ranged from 19% to 65% across the studies.
- Prospective longitudinal studies with adolescents have found that girls with BED had a twofold risk of becoming overweight or obese, or developing high depressive symptoms compared with non-disordered girls. Among boys, weekly binges predicted drug use as well.
- Various factors may affect treatment response to BED. For instance, higher frequency of binges, increased comorbid psychopathology, and decreased social/family support have been found to be associated with worse treatment outcomes

REFERRAL

- Referral to mental health specialists: For diagnosis and symptom management (using psychotherapy, pharmacotherapy)
- Referral to nutrition, exercise specialist and/or bariatric surgeon: If patient with BED is morbidly obese, and has associated medical problems

⚠ PEARLS & CONSIDERATIONS

COMMENTS

- Individuals with BED who are overweight or obese and are interested in weight loss, should also be encouraged to engage in treatment for disordered eating. Although the psychological treatments for BED do not produce substantial weight loss, the elimination of binge eating protects against future weight gain.
- If possible, including family in treatment can be helpful for building social and environmental supports, especially for adolescent and young adult clients

PREVENTION

- There are no known ways to prevent BED (or other eating disorders). However, research suggests that involving education on weight stigma, healthy eating, and body confidence in interventions amongst school children might ameliorate future body dissatisfaction and disordered eating.

PATIENT/FAMILY EDUCATION

National Education Disorders Association (NEDA, https://www.nationaleatingdisorders.org/) provides patient, family, and professional information on eating disorders including BED.

Binge Eating Disorder Association (BEDA, http://bedaonline.com/) provides patient, and professional information on BED.

Additional, local and/or online support groups for BED are common and should be investigated.

SUGGESTED READINGS

Available at www.expertconsult.com.

RELATED TOPICS

Anorexia Nervosa (Related Key Topic)
Bulimia Nervosa (Related Key Topic)

AUTHORS: **EISHITA MANJREKAR, PH.D.,** and **MARK ZIMMERMAN, M.D.**

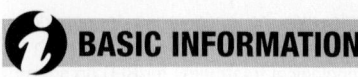

DEFINITION

Bipolar disorder is an episodic, recurrent, and frequently progressive condition in which the afflicted individual experiences at least one episode of mania, characterized by at least 1 wk of continuous symptoms of elevated, expansive, or irritable mood, in association with three or more of the following symptoms (four if irritability is the presenting mood):

- Decreased need for sleep
- Grandiosity or inflated self-esteem
- Pressured speech
- Flight of ideas or subjective sense of racing thoughts
- Distractibility
- Increased level of goal-directed activity
- Problematic behavior with a high potential for painful consequences

Most individuals with bipolar disorder also experience one or more episodes of major depression over their lifetimes or have symptoms of a depressive episode commingled with those of mania (mixed episode). Hypomanic episodes may also occur.

SYNONYMS

Manic-depression
Cycloid psychosis

ICD-10CM CODES
F42.0	Bipolar affective disorder, current episode hypomanic
F31.1	Bipolar affective disorder, current episode manic without psychotic symptoms
F31.2	Bipolar affective disorder, current episode manic with psychotic symptoms
F31.3	Bipolar affective disorder, current episode mild or moderate depression
F31.4	Bipolar affective disorder, current episode severe depression without psychotic symptoms
F31.5	Bipolar affective disorder, current episode severe depression with psychotic symptoms
F31.6	Bipolar affective disorder, current episode mixed
F31.8	Bipolar II disorder

EPIDEMIOLOGY & DEMOGRAPHICS

INCIDENCE: 0.016% to 0.021%
PREVALENCE (IN U.S.): 0.4% to 1.6% (lifetime); bipolar spectrum disorders: 2.8%; approximately 25% attempt suicide, 164 per 100,000 person-years, a rate 10× that of the general population.
PREDOMINANT SEX: Equal distribution among male and female
PREDOMINANT AGE: Lifelong condition with age of onset 14 to 30 yr
PEAK INCIDENCE: Onset in 20s
GENETICS:

- Concordance rates for monozygotic twins: 0.7 to 0.8; for dizygotic twins: 0.2
- Risk of affective disorder in offspring with one affected parent with bipolar disorder: 27% to 29%; with two affected parents: 50% to 74%
- Heritability estimate of 0.85
- No specific causal mutations have been identified, but cross-disorder studies indicate an overlap with genes associated with a risk for autism or schizophrenia. Genome-wide association analyses and exome sequencing have suggested a role for *CACNA1C, ANK3, TRANK1, ODZ4, ZNF 804A,* and *KDM5B,* among others, and have implicated ion channelopathies, immune and neuronal signaling, and histone methylation in pathogenesis of bipolar disorder. It remains unclear whether the high heritability is the result of the additive effect of many common risk variants or a few higher-risk rare variants.

PHYSICAL FINDINGS & CLINICAL PRESENTATION

- Mania associated with:
  1. Psychomotor activation that is usually goal directed but not necessarily productive
  2. Increase in goal-directed activity and excessive involvement in activities leading to unexpected adverse outcomes
  3. Elevated, euphoric, and frequently labile mood
  4. Decreased need for sleep
  5. Flight of ideas with rapid, loud, pressured speech
- Psychosis may occur, with delusions, hallucinations, and formal thought disorder.
- Depressive episodes resembling major depressive disorder (see "Depression, Major"); however, atypical features (hypersomnia, prominent anxiety, weight gain) may be present.
- Mixed states, characterized by activation, irritability, and dysphoria, also possible.

KEY DIAGNOSTIC CRITERIA DISTINGUISHING BIPOLAR I DISORDER FROM BIPOLAR II DISORDER[1]:

Manic episode (Bipolar I Disorder)

- Distinct period during which there is an abnormally and persistently elevated, expansive, or irritable mood and abnormally and persistently increased goal-directed activity or energy lasting at least 1 wk (or less if hospitalization is required)
- Must be accompanied by at least three of the following symptoms (four if mood is only irritable): inflated self-esteem or grandiosity, decreased need for sleep, pressured speech, racing thoughts, distractibility, increased involvement in goal-directed activity or psychomotor agitation, excessive involvement in pleasurable activities with a high potential for painful consequences
- Symptoms do not meet criteria for a mixed episode
- Disturbance must be sufficiently severe to cause marked impairment in social or occupational functioning or to require hospitalization, or it is characterized by the presence of psychotic features
- Symptoms not due to direct physiologic effect of medication, general medication condition, or substance abuse

[1]Criteria are from the American Psychiatric Association: *Diagnostic and statistic manual of mental disorders, fifth edition,* Washington, DC, 2013, American Psychiatric Association.

Hypomanic episode (Bipolar II Disorder)

- Distinct period during which there is an abnormally and persistently elevated, expansive, or irritable mood and abnormally and persistently elevated activity or energy lasting at least 4 consecutive days
- Must be accompanied by at least three of the following symptoms (four if mood is only irritable): inflated self-esteem or grandiosity, decreased need for sleep, pressured speech, racing thoughts, distractibility, increased involvement in goal-directed activity or psychomotor agitation, excessive involvement in pleasurable activities with a high potential for painful consequences
- Hypomanic episodes must be clearly different from the person's usual nondepressed mood, and there must be a clear change in functioning that is not characteristic of the person's usual functioning
- Changes in mood and functioning must be observable by others. In contrast to a manic episode, a hypomanic episode is not severe enough to cause marked impairment in social or occupational functioning or to require hospitalization, and there are no psychotic features
- Symptoms not due to direct physiologic effect of medication, general medication condition, or substance abuse

ETIOLOGY

Hypotheses:
1. Abnormalities of GABAA and G protein–coupled receptor and membrane function, calcium dysregulation
2. Alteration of cAMP, MAP kinase, protein kinase C, arachidonic acid cascade, and glycogen synthase kinase-3 signal transduction pathways; mitochondrial dysfunction
3. Alteration in cell survival pathways, glial and neuronal death and loss of neuroplasticity; proposed biomarkers include BDNF and measures of inflammation, oxidative stress, and endothelial function.

DX DIAGNOSIS

DIFFERENTIAL DIAGNOSIS

- Secondary manias caused by medical disorders (e.g., hyperthyroidism, AIDS, early dementia, stroke, Cushing syndrome) or pharmacologic treatment (e.g., steroids, stimulants).
- First onset of mania after age 50 yr suggestive of secondary mania.
- Less severe, and possibly distinct, conditions of bipolar type II and cyclothymia.
- Comorbid substance abuse or dependency occurs in 60% to 75% of patients and may confound diagnosis and treatment.
- Presentation can be confused with schizophrenia or paranoid psychosis.

WORKUP

- History
- Physical examination
- Mental status examination
- Mood Disorder Questionnaire (MDQ); Composite International Diagnostic Interview (CIDI) (3.0)

B

LABORATORY TESTS

Because of high rate of secondary manias, initial evaluation to confirm health of all major organ systems (routine chemistries, complete blood count, urinalysis, sedimentation rate)

IMAGING STUDIES

- Consider brain imaging if late onset or if neurologic examination is abnormal.
- Neuroimaging may show evidence of ventricular enlargement or increased white matter hyperintensities; decrements in prefrontal and temporal lobe cortical thickness also reported. Corresponding changes in neurocognition, including changes in executive function and processing speed, may occur.

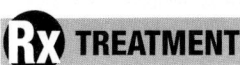 TREATMENT

NONPHARMACOLOGIC THERAPY

- Cognitive-behavioral and family-focused psychoeducational psychotherapy to help patients cope with consequences of the disease, improve adherence with medications, and identify possible environmental triggers
- Bright light therapy in the northern latitudes in individuals exhibiting a seasonal pattern of winter depression
- Lifestyle "regularization"; interpersonal and social rhythm therapy; integrated care management for chronic conditions
- Many smartphone mobile apps for bipolar disorder are available to provide information, help monitor symptoms, and deliver interventions.

ACUTE GENERAL Rx

- First-line agents for acute mania and mixed states: lithium 1500 to 1800 mg/day (0.8 to 1.2 mEq/L), valproate 1000 to 1500 mg/day (50 to 125 ng/ml), carbamazepine 600 to 800 mg/day (4 to 12 micrograms/ml), oxcarbazepine 900 to 2400 mg/day, olanzapine 10 to 20 mg/day, risperidone 2 to 4 mg/day, quetiapine 350 to 800 mg/day, ziprasidone 80 to 120 mg/day, asenapine 10 to 20 mg/day, or aripiprazole 10 to 30 mg/day. Treatment-resistant cases may respond to varying combinations of these agents or to the addition of clozapine.
- Useful adjuncts to acute treatment of mania: benzodiazepines: lorazepam 1 to 2 mg q4h, clonazepam 1 to 2 mg q4h.
- Traditional antidepressants can induce manic episodes and exacerbate mania in mixed episodes.

- First-line options for bipolar depression include lithium, lurasidone, quetiapine, lamotrigine, and olanzapine/fluoxetine combination. Bupropion may have a lower risk for triggering mania, and MAOIs or ECT may be efficacious in treatment-resistant cases.

CHRONIC Rx

- Goal of long-term treatment: prevention of relapse or episode recurrence
- Best agents for prophylaxis of mania: lithium, quetiapine, aripiprazole, and olanzapine (valproate, carbamazepine/oxcarbazepine possibly beneficial)
- Best agents for prophylaxis of depression: lamotrigine and lithium
- Risk/benefit of atypical antipsychotics versus traditional mood stabilizers in maintenance unclear
- Long-term use of antidepressants: frequently destabilizes patient and leads to more frequent relapses; depression outweighs mania as the most debilitating dimension over the life span; bipolar disorder accounts for 7% of all disease-related disability-adjusted life years.

DISPOSITION

- Course is variable.
- More than 90% of patients having a single manic episode are likely to experience others.
- Uncontrolled manic or depressive episodes can lead to additional episodes.
- Lithium shown to specifically decrease suicidal risk.
- Socioeconomic consequences of both mania and depression can be severe and disabling.

REFERRAL

- If use of antidepressant contemplated
- If patient is severely manic, rapid cycling, or suicidal or is in a bipolar, mixed episode

! PEARLS & CONSIDERATIONS

COMMENTS

- All patients presenting with depression should be asked about past personal and family history of mania and hypomania; 70% of bipolar patients have previously been misdiagnosed. Onset before age 25 and poor prior response to antidepressants are additional clues.
- Prompt recognition of the earliest signs of mania in a given individual (e.g., decreased need for sleep, increased rate of speech)

allows earlier intervention and a better likelihood of preventing a full episode.

- Bipolar disorder in children frequently manifests as episodic behavioral disinhibition, affective lability, and temper dysregulation, but current consensus indicates that the condition is overdiagnosed in this age group. Disruptive mood dysregulation disorder (DMDD) describes children who exhibit persistent irritability and severe temper outbursts on a frequent basis (at least three times/week for a year or more).
- Rapid cycling (greater than three episodes/year) is associated with a poorer prognosis, including a longer course, more treatment resistance, more substance use comorbidity, and increased suicidal risk.
- Patients treated with atypical antipsychotic agents should be carefully monitored for development of metabolic syndrome. Independent of medication effect, there is a higher prevalence of metabolic syndrome and abdominal obesity in those with bipolar disorder.
- Despite some variation in prevalence, the severity, impact, and patterns of comorbidity of bipolar disorder are similar in different countries in world health surveys.
- Bipolar disorder often co-occurs with anxiety disorders and attention deficit hyperactivity disorder (ADHD), making attribution of specific symptoms difficult.
- Patients receiving anticonvulsants or antidepressants should be monitored for a possible increase in suicidal thoughts or behavior.
- There is preliminary evidence that nutraceutical agents like omega-3 fatty acids and N-acetyl cysteine (NAC) may have efficacy in the treatment of bipolar disorder.
- Multiple studies show a correlation between bipolar disorder and heightened creativity.

PATIENT/FAMILY EDUCATION

Information available at www.NMHA.org/ and www.dbsalliance.org/.

SUGGESTED READINGS

Available at www.expertconsult.com

RELATED CONTENT

Bipolar Disorder (Patient Information)
Depression, Major (Related Key Topic)

AUTHOR: **VICTOR I. REUS, M.D.**

Diseases and Disorders

I

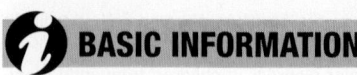

BASIC INFORMATION

DEFINITION

A bite wound can be animal or human, accidental, or intentional.

ICD-10CM CODES	
T14.1	Open wound of unspecified body region
T01.9	Multiple open wounds, unspecified
S31.000A	Unspecified open wound of lower back and pelvis without penetration into retroperitoneum, initial encounter
S41.159A	Open bite of unspecified upper arm, initial encounter

EPIDEMIOLOGY & DEMOGRAPHICS

- Bite wounds account for 1% of emergency department visits, and about 2% of patients need hospitalization.
- More than 1 million bites occur in human beings annually in the U.S.
- Dog bites account for 85% to 90% of all bites and result in 10 to 20 fatalities yearly in the U.S.; most dog bite victims are children. Cat bites account for 10% to 20%. The animal typically is owned by the victim.
- Infection rates are highest for cat bites (30%-50%), followed by human bites (15%-30%) and dog bites (5%).
- The extremities are involved in 75% of bites.

PHYSICAL FINDINGS & CLINICAL PRESENTATION

- The appearance of the bite wound is variable (e.g., puncture wound, tear, avulsion).
- Cellulitis, lymphangitis, and focal adenopathy may be present in infected bite wounds.
- Patient may have fever and chills.

ETIOLOGY

- Increased risk of infection: human and cat bites, closed-fist injuries, wounds involving joints, puncture wounds, face and lip bites, bites with skull penetration, bites in immunocompromised hosts
- Most frequent infecting organisms:
  1. *Pasteurella* spp.: responsible for majority of infections within 24 hr of dog (*P. canis*) and cat (*P. multocida, P. septica*) bites
  2. *Capnocytophaga canimorsus* (formerly DF-2 bacillus): a gram-negative organism responsible for late infection, usually after dog bites
  3. Gram-negative organisms (*Pseudomonas, Haemophilus*): often found in human bites
  4. *Streptococcus* spp., *Staphylococcus aureus*
  5. *Eikenella corrodens* in human bites

DIAGNOSIS

DIFFERENTIAL DIAGNOSIS

- Bite from a rabid animal (often the attack is unprovoked)
- Factitious injury

WORKUP

- Determination of the time elapsed since the patient was bitten, status of rabies immunization of the animal, and underlying medical conditions that might predispose the patient to infection (e.g., DM, immunodeficiency)
- Documentation of bite site, notification of appropriate authorities (e.g., police department, animal officer)

LABORATORY TESTS

- Generally not necessary
- Hct if there has been significant blood loss
- Wound cultures (aerobic and anaerobic) if there is evidence of sepsis or victim is immunocompromised; cultures should be obtained before irrigation of the wound but after superficial cleaning

IMAGING STUDIES

Radiographs are indicated when bony penetration is suspected or if there is suspicion of fracture or significant trauma; they are also useful for detecting foreign bodies (when suspected).

TREATMENT

NONPHARMACOLOGIC THERAPY

- Local care with debridement, vigorous cleansing, and saline irrigation of the wound; debridement of devitalized tissue
- High-pressure irrigation to clean bite wound and ensure removal of contaminants (e.g., use saline solution with a 30- to 35-mL syringe equipped with a 20-gauge needle or catheter with tip of syringe placed 2 to 3 cm above the wound)
- Avoid blunt probing of wounds (increased risk of infection)
- If the animal is suspected to be rabid: infiltrate wound edges with 1% procaine hydrochloride, swab wound surface vigorously with cotton swabs and 1% benzalcuronium solution or other soap, and rinse wound with normal saline

ACUTE GENERAL Rx

- Avoid suturing of hand wounds and any wounds that appear infected
- Clenched fist injuries that develop after a punch to another's mouth usually require hospitalization, IV antibiotics, and evaluation by a hand specialist.
- Puncture wounds should be left open
- Give antirabies therapy and tetanus immune globulin (250-500 units IM in limb contralateral to toxoid) and toxoid (adult or child older than 5 yr: 0.5 ml DT given IM, child <5 yr 0.5 mL DPT IM) as needed
- Use empiric antibiotic therapy in high-risk wounds (e.g., cat bite, hand bites, face bites, genital area bites, bites with joint or bone penetration, human bites, immunocompromised host): amoxicillin-clavulanate 875 to 1000 mg bid for 7 days or cefuroxime 500 mg bid for 7 days
- In hospitalized patients, IV antibiotics of choice are cefoxitin 1 to 2 g q6h,

ampicillin-sulbactam 1.5 to 3 g q6h, ticarcillin-clavulanate 3 g q6h, cefoxitin 2 g IV q8h, or ceftriaxone 1 to 2 g q24h
- Penicillin allergy: animal bite (doxycycline or moxifloxacin or trimethoprim/sulfamethoxazole with either clindamycin or metronidazole); human bite (moxifloxacin plus clindamycin, trimethoprim/sulfamethoxazole plus metronidazole)
- Prophylactic therapy for persons bitten by others with HIV and hepatitis B (see Section V)
- Table 1 summarizes the treatment of mammalian bites

DISPOSITION

- Prognosis is favorable with proper treatment.
- Important prognostic factors are type and depth of wound, which compartments are entered, and pathogenicity of inoculated bacteria.
- Punctures that are difficult to irrigate adequately, carnivore bites over vital structures (arteries, nerves, joints), and tissue crushing that cannot be debrided have a worse prognosis.
- In general, human bites have a higher complication and infection rate than do animal bites.
- Nearly 50% of the anaerobic gram-negative bacilli isolated from human bite wounds may be penicillin resistant and beta-lactamase positive.

PREVENTION

- Box 1 provides advice for avoiding the bites and attacks of common pets.

REFERRAL

- Hospitalization and IV antibiotic therapy for infected human bites; bites with injury to joints, nerves, or tendons; or any animal bites unresponsive to oral therapy.
- Human bites with tendon involvement should go to operating room for washout.
- In the outpatient setting, bite wounds should be reevaluated within 48 hr to assess for signs of infection.

SUGGESTED READINGS

Available at www.expertconsult.com

RELATED CONTENT

Animal and Human Bites (Patient Information)

AUTHOR: **FRED F. FERRI, M.D.**

TABLE 1 Treatment of Mammalian Bites

Type	Wound Care	Antibiotic PR	Tetanus PR	Rabies PR	HIV PR	Hepatitis PR
Human	High-pressure irrigation of the wound with normal saline or dilute (<1%) povidone-iodine solution; débride devitalized tissue or ragged edges	Amoxicillin-clavulanate, second-generation cephalosporin with anaerobic activity, penicillin plus dicloxacillin, clindamycin plus ciprofloxacin or trimethoprim-sulfamethoxazole	Tetanus immunoglobulin (250 units IM) and tetanus toxoid (0.5 mg IM) if never had a tetanus vaccine or have not had 3 doses of tetanus toxoid; tetanus toxoid (0.5 mg IM) if >5 yr since previous tetanus booster	None	ART therapy started within the first 48-72 hr and continued for 28 days or bite source tested HIV negative; refer to the hospital for the specific drugs used in ART therapy	HBIG (0.06 ml/kg IM); HBV given at separate site from HBIG
Cat	High-pressure irrigation of the wound with normal saline or dilute (<1%) povidone-iodine solution; débride devitalized tissue or ragged edges	Amoxicillin-clavulanate, second-generation cephalosporin with anaerobic activity, penicillin plus a first-generation cephalosporin, clindamycin plus a fluoroquinolone or trimethoprim-sulfamethoxazole	Tetanus immune globulin (250 units IM) and tetanus toxoid (0.5 mg IM) if never had a tetanus vaccine or have not had 3 doses of tetanus toxoid; tetanus toxoid (0.5 mg IM) if >5 yr since previous tetanus booster	HRIG (20 IU/kg) injected IM and/or around the bite site; rabies vaccine (1 mL IM) given in the deltoid in adults and in the thigh in children, on days 0, 3, 7, 14, and 28	None	None
Dog	High-pressure irrigation of the wound with normal saline or dilute (<1%) povidone-iodine solution; débride devitalized tissue or ragged edges	Amoxicillin-clavulanate, second-generation cephalosporin with anaerobic activity, penicillin plus a first-generation cephalosporin, clindamycin plus a fluoroquinolone or trimethoprim-sulfamethoxazole	Tetanus immune globulin (250 units IM) and tetanus toxoid (0.5 mg IM) if never had a tetanus vaccine or have not had 3 doses of tetanus toxoid; tetanus toxoid (0.5 mg IM) if >5 yr since previous tetanus booster	HRIG (20 IU/kg) injected IM and/or around the bite site; rabies vaccine (1 mL IM) given in the deltoid in adults and in the thigh in children, on days 0, 3, 7, 14, and 28	None	None

ART, Antiretroviral therapy; *HBIG,* hepatitis B immune globulin; *HBV,* hepatitis B vaccine; *HIV,* human immunodeficiency virus; *HRIG,* human rabies immune globulin; *IM,* intramuscularly; *PR,* prophylaxis.
From Adams JG et al: *Emergency medicine: clinical essentials*, ed 2, Philadelphia, 2013, Elsevier.

BOX 1 Advice for Avoiding the Bites and Attacks of Common Pets*

Dogs
- Do not leave a young child alone with a dog.
- Never approach or try to pet an unfamiliar dog, especially if it is tied up or confined.
- Always ask the dog's owners if you can pet the dog.
- Do not lean over a dog or pet it directly on the head.
- Do not kiss a dog.
- Avoid quick or sudden movements that may startle a dog.
- Never pet or step over a sleeping dog.
- Never try to take a bone or toy away from a dog (other than your own dog).
- Know the appearance of an angry dog: barking, growling, snarling with teeth showing, ears laid flat, legs stiff, tail up, and hair on the back standing up.
- Never step between two fighting dogs; if you need to separate them, use a bucket of water or a hose.
- Do not approach a female dog that is nursing her pups.
- Teach injury prevention advice to children from an early age.

Cats
- Be aware that some cats do not like prolonged petting.
- Know warning signs of an impending bite: twitching of the tail, restlessness, and "intention" bites (i.e., the cat moves to bite but does not bite).

Ferrets
- Do not sell or adopt a ferret that is known to bite.
- Do not push your fingers through the wires of a ferret cage.
- Reach for a ferret from the side with the palm upward rather than from above.
- Do not handle food and then handle young ferrets without washing your hands first.
- Do not poke a ferret or pull on its tail or ears.
- Never leave a ferret alone with a child or infant.
- If a ferret bites and locks on very tightly, pour cold and fast-running water over its face.

From Auerbach P: *Wilderness medicine, expert consult,* premium edition—Enhanced online features and print, Philadelphia, 2012, Elsevier.

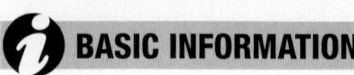

DEFINITION

There are two major classes of arthropods: insects and Arachnida. This chapter focuses on the class Arachnida. Arachnid bites consist of bites caused by:
- Spiders
- Scorpions
- Ticks

ICD-10CM CODES	
T63.301	Toxic effect of unspecified spider venom, accidental (unintentional), initial encounter
T63.2	Toxic effect of venom of scorpion, accidental (unintentional), initial encounter
E906	Bite of nonvenomous arthropod; insect bite NOS

EPIDEMIOLOGY & DEMOGRAPHICS

- Spiders—ubiquitous; only three types potentially significantly harmful:
  1. Sydney funnel web spider—Australia
  2. Black widow (Fig. E1)—worldwide (excluding Alaska)
  3. Brown recluse (Fig. E2)—most common (South Central U.S.)
- Scorpions—various warm climates: Africa, Central South America, Middle East, India; Texas, New Mexico, California, and Nevada in the U.S.
- Ticks—woodlands

PHYSICAL FINDINGS & CLINICAL PRESENTATION

Spiders:
- Sydney funnel web—atracotoxin toxin
  1. Piloerection, muscle spasms leading to tachycardia, hypertension, increased intracranial pressure, coma
- Black widow—females toxic
  1. Initial reaction: local swelling, redness (two fang marks) leading to local piloerection, edema, urticaria, diaphoresis, lymphangitis
  2. Pain in limb leading to rest of body (chest pain, abdominal pain), compartment syndrome
- Brown recluse
  1. Minor sting or burn.
  2. Wound may become pruritic and red with a blanched center with vesicle (Fig. E3). Can necrose, especially in fatty areas (Fig. E4). Leaves eschar, which sloughs and leaves ulcer; can take months to heal.
  3. Systemic symptoms: headache, fever, chills, gastrointestinal upset, hemolysis, renal tubular necrosis, disseminated intravascular coagulation possible.

Scorpions:
- Sting leading to sympathetic and parasympathetic stimulation: hypertension, bradycardia, vasoconstriction, pulmonary edema, reduced coronary blood flow, priapism, inhibition of insulin.
- Also possible: tachycardia, arrhythmia, vasodilation, bronchial relaxation, excessive salivation, vomiting, sweating, bronchoconstriction, pancreatitis.
- Clinically significant scorpion envenomation by *Centruroides sculpturatus* produces a severe neuromotor syndrome and respiratory insufficiency that often requires ICU admission.

Ticks: U.S., Europe, Asia
- Very small (<1 mm). Must be attached >36 hr to transmit disease.
- Lyme disease—most common (see "Lyme Disease")
  1. Early: erythema migrans in 60% to 80% of cases
  2. 7 to 10 days: mild to moderate constitutional symptoms; disseminated—secondary skin lesions, fever, adenopathy, constitutional symptoms, facial palsy, peripheral neuropathy, lymphocytic meningitis, meningoencephalitis, cardiac manifestations (heart block)
  3. Late: chronic arthritis, dermatitis, neuropathy, keratitis
- Babesiosis (see "Babesiosis")
- Ehrlichiosis/anaplasmosis (see "Ehrlichiosis and Anaplasmosis")

DIAGNOSIS

DIFFERENTIAL DIAGNOSIS

- Cellulitis
- Urticaria
  Other tick-borne illnesses:
- Babesiosis
- Tick-borne relapsing fever/*Borrelia miyamotoi*
- Tularemia
- Rocky Mountain spotted fever
- Ehrlichiosis/anaplasmosis
- Colorado tick fever
- Tick paralysis
- Community-acquired cutaneous methicillin-resistant *Staphylococcus aureus*

WORKUP

Physical examination: thorough skin examination may reveal fang marks, attached ticks, black eschar.

TREATMENT

ACUTE GENERAL Rx

Spiders:
- Sydney funnel web
  1. Pressure, immediate immobilization, supportive care, antivenin.
- Black widow
  1. Treatment based on severity of symptoms; bite is rarely fatal.
  2. All should receive oxygen, IV, cardiac monitor, tetanus prophylaxis.
  3. Symptomatic/supportive therapy.
  4. 10% calcium gluconate for muscle cramps (controversial).
  5. Antivenin only for more severe reactions; it carries a risk of anaphylaxis.
    1. Dose: one vial in 100 ml 0.9% saline over 20 to 30 min.
    2. Skin test before use.
    3. Give antihistamines with use.
- Brown recluse
  1. Pain management, tetanus, supportive treatment.
  2. No consensus regarding best treatment; some evidence for hyperbaric oxygen.

Scorpions:
- Fluids, supportive care, species-specific antivenin (equine based, risk of serum sickness) is controversial.
- IV administration of scorpion-specific F(ab')2 antivenin has been reported effective in resolving the clinical syndrome within 4 hours and reducing the need for concomitant sedation with midazolam and reducing the levels of circulating unbound venom.

Ticks:
- Prophylactic: tick >36 hr: single dose of doxycycline 200 mg
- Early localized disease
  1. Treatment of choice in children: amoxicillin for 14 days.
  2. Doxycycline preferred in patients with possible concurrent ehrlichiosis.
  3. Early disseminated: treatment depends on manifestation.
  4. Late disease: may require longer-term or IV therapy; controversial for neurologic disease (see "Lyme Disease").

DISPOSITION

- For patients with systemic reactions, send home with emergency epinephrine kit.
- If severe or anaphylactic reaction, admit and observe for 48 hr for cardiac, renal, or neurologic problems.

REFERRAL

For patients with systemic reactions, refer to allergist for immunotherapy; 95% to 98% effective in preventing anaphylaxis.

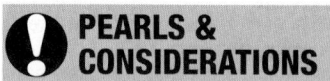

PEARLS & CONSIDERATIONS

Actual spider bites rare, need witnessed bite, patient should bring spider if possible for confirmation. Bites usually occur in settings of unusually close contact with spider. Bedbugs becoming more prevalent, repeated exposure increases severity of reaction.

SUGGESTED READINGS

Available at www.expertconsult.com

RELATED CONTENT

Bites and Stings (Patient Information)
Bites and Stings, Insect (Related Key Topic)

AUTHOR: **GAIL M. O'BRIEN, M.D.**

BASIC INFORMATION

DEFINITION

Most stinging insects belong to the Hymenoptera order and include honey bees, hornets, bumblebees, sweat bees, wasps (including yellow jackets), harvester ants, fire ants, and the Africanized honey bee ("killer bee"). Wasps cause 70% of all reactions to stings. Spiders, which are arachnids, not insects, are another cause of bites (Fig. 1) (see "Bites and Stings, Arachnids"). The venom of the Hymenoptera order contains vasoactive and proinflammatory mediators that can cause local reactions. A small number of those stung can develop a systemic hypersensitivity reaction. The usual local effect of a sting is intense pain, immediate erythema, edema, and pruritus from the injecting venom. Allergic reactions can be either local or generalized. Generalized reactions can lead to anaphylactic shock. The majority of reactions occur within the first 6 hr after the sting or bite, but a delayed reaction may occur up to 24 hr after the sting. Delayed reactions are rare and include serum sickness (fever, malaise, urticaria, and arthralgias).

SYNONYMS

Venom allergy

ICD-10CM CODES
T63.444 Toxic effect of venom of bees, undetermined, initial encounter
T63.464 Toxic effect of venom of wasps, undetermined, initial encounter
T63.424 Toxic effect of venom of ants, undetermined, initial encounter

EPIDEMIOLOGY & DEMOGRAPHICS

PREVALENCE (OF BEE STINGS AND INSECT BITES):
- Unknown prevalence, very underreported.
- Account for 2.3% of ED visits. 5% to 7.5% of the population is hypersensitive, with large local or systemic reactions to the venom of one or more stinging insects.
- Insect bites are the most common cause of anaphylaxis reactions.

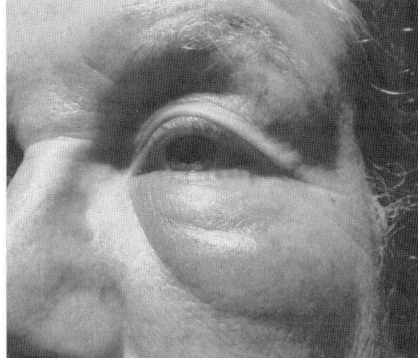

FIG. 1 Spider bite to lower eyelid. (From Swartz MH: *Textbook of physical diagnosis*, ed 7, Philadelphia, 2014, Elsevier.)

- Most anaphylactic reactions occur during summer months in those most likely to be exposed, including children, males, outdoor workers. There are no tests to predict reaction accurately; the reaction to a prior sting is still the best predictor. Anaphylaxis can occur after a number of uneventful stings.
- Approximately half of fatal reactions occur without prior allergic response.
- Bites by fire ants are less likely to cause systemic disease.
- Spider bites are rare; only a few of the thousands of spider species cause a reaction in humans. Observation and collection of the spider inflicting the bite is necessary (see Bites and Stings, Arachnids).

INCIDENCE (IN U.S.): Forty to 100 people die each year from insect sting anaphylaxis; anaphylaxis occurs most often within 10 to 30 min of a sting. Delayed reactions are rare, occurring only in <0.3% of stings.

PHYSICAL FINDINGS & CLINICAL PRESENTATION

Stings:
Local reactions:
- Cutaneous: the skin is the most common site of a local allergic reaction. Manifestations include flushing, urticaria, pruritus, and angioedema. Local reactions may last several days.

Systemic reactions:
- Local swelling greater than 10 cm is associated with increased risk of a systemic reaction with repeat exposure.
- Respiratory: This is the leading cause of anaphylactic death. Anaphylaxis as defined by consensus of the NIH 2006 as a severe life-threatening hypersensitivity reaction. Symptoms of upper and lower airway obstruction including hoarseness, choking, throat tightness or tingling that may progress to stridor, laryngeal edema, laryngospasm, and bronchoconstriction.
- Cardiovascular: Cardiac manifestations are the second leading cause of death from anaphylaxis; the most common reaction is hypotension that can progress to profound hypovolemic shock. Tachycardia and arrhythmia may occur. Myocardial infarction is rare.
- General symptoms: abdominal pain, nausea, vomiting, lightheadedness, and diarrhea.

Fire ant bites:
- Initial wheal and flare response.
- Subsequent development of circularly arrayed blisters within 24 hr (Fig. 2).
- Blisters may develop the appearance of pustules, but they are not infected.

ETIOLOGY

Stings:
- Most systemic reactions to insect stings are classic immunoglobulin E (IgE)–mediated reactions. Anaphylaxis can be the presenting sign of indolent mastocytosis.
- Reactions occur in previously sensitized patients who have produced high titers of IgE antibody to insect venom antigens.

- Sensitization to wasp venom can occur after a single sting but is more common after a few stings.
- Sensitization to bee venom occurs mainly in people who have been stung frequently by bees.
- Fig. E3 illustrates representative venomous hymenoptera

Bites:
- Fire ant venom contains proteins toxic to the skin.

DIAGNOSIS

DIFFERENTIAL DIAGNOSIS
- Stings: cellulitis, bites, rash
- Bites: stings, cellulitis

WORKUP

The history is essential for accurate diagnosis including timing of sting or bite and type of insect (bee, wasp, spider, or ant) if known.

LABORATORY TESTS (FOR HYPERSENSITIVITY REACTION)
- Skin test: either skin prick test or intradermal method with fire ant or hymenoptera venom.
- Venom skin tests and occasionally radioallergosorbent tests (RAST) to provide additional information, only for those with history of a systemic reaction.
- Venom-specific IgE tests
- Basophil activation tests and mast cell mediator testing are being developed to identify those with allergy and predict those who will have more severe reactions.

TREATMENT

ACUTE GENERAL Rx

Sting:
- Local Poison Control Center can be contacted.
- Removal of the stinger most easily performed with a flat tool such as a credit card within 30 seconds of the sting, followed by cleansing and application of ice.
- Venom may all be released within 20 seconds of bite or sting.
- Avoid squeezing, which may push venom out of the venom sac and into the tissue.
- Supportive care with oral antihistamines, nonsteroidal antiinflammatory medications/pain medications, topical corticosteroids, and cold compresses for limited reactions.
- Large local reactions (>10 cm) may benefit from oral steroids.
- Patients with previous reactions or multiple stings to the mouth or neck should be evaluated in an emergency department.
- Unusual reactions to multiple stings include acute kidney injury or cerebrovascular accident.
- Systemic reactions: Treat with intramuscular epinephrine (no contraindication for use). Increased risk of death if epinephrine delayed. The patient should be supine with 0.30 mg IM in anterior/lateral thigh. Patient should be observed for 4 to 8 hours.

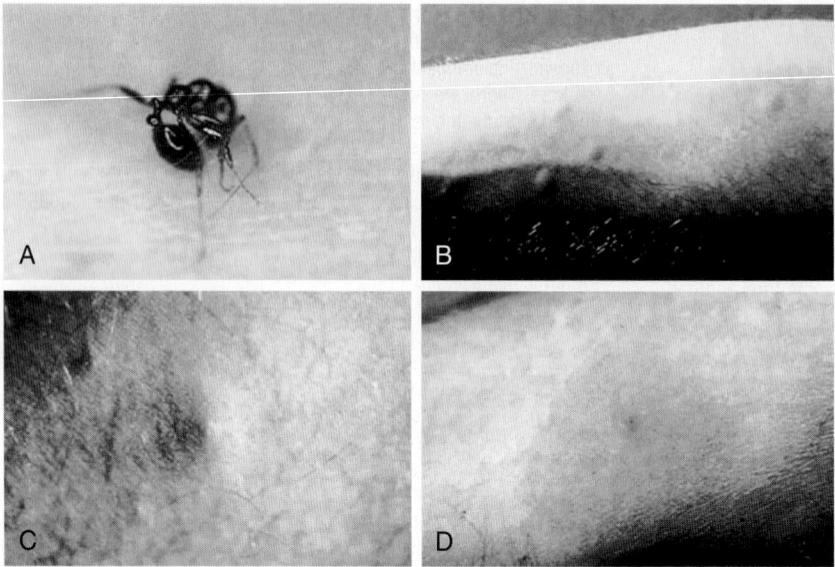

FIG. 2 A, Stinging fire ant (*Solenopsis invicta*). **B,** Wheal-and-flare reactions 5 minutes after multiple fire ant stings. **C,** Sterile pustule 24 hours after fire ant sting. **D,** Cutaneous late-phase allergic reaction 24 hours after fire ant sting. Excoriated sterile pustule in center of lesion. (From Kemp SF et al: Expanding habitat of the imported fire ant (*Solenopsis invicta*): a public health concern, *J Allergy Clin Immunol* 105(4):683-691, 2000.)

- H1- and H2-blockers, oxygen, IV glucocorticoids, beta-agonists, pressors, and IV fluids may also be beneficial for anaphylaxis. No data that glucocorticoids improve clinical outcomes.
- Patients should be given 2 units of self-injectable epinephrine pens for home use and referral to allergy indicated after a systemic reaction.

Bite:
- Supportive care—wash with soap and water
- Application of ice or cooling. Calamine lotion may be helpful.
- Surveillance for secondary infection

DISPOSITION

Sting:
- Prognosis for a limited reaction is excellent.
- Subsequent anaphylaxis may occur in up to 65% of patients stung again with history of prior systemic reaction. Large local reaction does not predict a systemic reaction.
- There is no evidence that the next sting will necessarily cause a more severe reaction. Variable outcome is due to the patient's age, comorbidities, time elapsed since prior exposure, dose of venom injected, and site of sting.
- Watch for secondary cellulitis.
- Patients who have a history of a severe systemic reaction:
  1. Should be educated to avoid stinging insects
  2. Carry 2 syringes preloaded with epinephrine for self-administration
  3. Undergo testing for serum levels of venom-specific IgE
  4. Refer to allergist for venom immunotherapy (VIT), which reduces chance of serious allergic reaction from 60% to <5%. VIT is typically needed for 3 to 5 yr.
  5. Carry medical identification for stinging insect hypersensitivity
  6. Baseline tryptase level for any patient with an anaphylactic reaction to a sting to evaluate the possibility of an underlying mast cell disorder. Patients with levels >20 ng/mL need further evaluation. VIT may benefit those with mastocytosis and wasp venom allergy.

Bite:
- Prognosis for fire ant bite is excellent.
- Large lesions from brown recluse spider bites may take months to heal.
- Watch for secondary cellulitis.

REFERRAL

- Consider a referral to an allergist for venom immunotherapy (VIT).
- Risk of subsequent anaphylaxis with immunotherapy falls to <3%.
- VIT for 3 to 5 yr induces long-term protection in most patients.

ⓘ PEARLS & CONSIDERATIONS

Hypersensitivity to stings is common. Reactions range from local nonallergic reaction to venom to life-threatening systemic reaction with anaphylaxis. This could indicate underlying mast cell disorder; tryptase level is indicated. Venom-specific immunotherapy is highly effective in decreasing subsequent anaphylaxis. Although venom immunotherapy is currently indicated only for systemic reactions, investigation is under way to assess efficacy for prevention of large local reactions, which can result in significant morbidity.

SUGGESTED READINGS
Available at www.expertconsult.com

RELATED CONTENT
Bites and Stings (Patient Information)
Bites and Stings, Arachnids (Related Key Topic)

AUTHOR: **LYNN A. BOWLBY, M.D.**

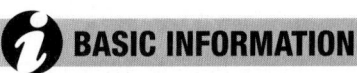

BASIC INFORMATION

DEFINITION
Injury resulting from a snake biting a human.

ICD-10CM CODES
T63.0   Toxic effect of snake venom
T63.001A Toxic effect of unspecified snake
            venom, accidental (unintentional),
            initial encounter

EPIDEMIOLOGY & DEMOGRAPHICS
- The CDC reports between 7000 and 9000 venomous snakebites annually in the United States, with <1% resulting in death. The highest incidence is reported in southern states, peaking during the warmer months of April through November. Worldwide, farm workers have the highest incidence of snakebites. In the U.S., most snakebites occur as a consequence of voluntary interaction with snakes. Snakebites frequently result from intentional provocation of wild snakes or in the setting of handling captive snakes. Men comprise the majority of snakebite victims, with white men ages 25 to 34 representing the group at highest risk of envenomation. Alcohol use and drug intoxication are implicated in many snakebites. Risk of death is highest in children, the elderly, and in those with delayed presentation to care.
- In the U.S., at least one species of poisonous snake (Fig. E1) has been identified in every state, with the exception of Alaska, Hawaii, and Maine. Table 1 summarizes medically important snake families.
- The Crotalinae subfamily (Viperidae family), commonly referred to as crotalids or pit vipers, includes rattlesnakes, copperheads, and cottonmouths (water moccasins). Crotalids are responsible for the vast majority of snake envenomations in the U.S. They are characterized by a prominent, diamond-shaped head, a heat-sensing pit between the eye and nostril, long retractable fangs, and, in the case of rattlesnakes, the telltale rattler. Crotalid bites are typically very painful.
- The Elapidae family includes mambas, cobras, and coral snakes. Coral snakes are the only member of the Elapidae family found in the U.S. Coral snakes are much less common than crotalids. Coral snakes are innately less aggressive and represent only 1% to 2% of venomous snakebites in the U.S. Elapids have smaller heads and shorter fangs, and they are identified by vibrant bands of yellow, red, and black. The popular saying "Red on yellow, kill a fellow; red on black, venom lack" is used to distinguish between venomous and nonvenomous snakes. Caution should be used when applying this axiom internationally, as some coral snakes within South America display red-on-black coloring and are in fact venomous. Elapid bites cause less local tissue destruction and are typically less painful, however, because elapids must "chew" in order to inject venom, victims may report difficulty dislodging the snake after the bite.
- Exotic, nonnative pets also account for 1% to 2% of snake envenomations.

PHYSICAL FINDINGS & CLINICAL PRESENTATION
The effects of envenomation vary by the type of snake but may include local tissue injury, coagulopathy, neurotoxicity, and cardiovascular instability as well as renal failure. Crotalids typically cause severe local effects as well as hematologic symptoms including primary consumptive coagulopathies. Neurologic complications are less common in crotalid bites. The exception is the Mojave rattlesnake bite, in which case local tissue destruction following envenomation is minimal, but severe neurologic symptoms can occur up to 12 hours after the bite. Elapid bites similarly cause less localized tissue damage but have more severe and often delayed neurotoxic manifestations.

CROTALINAE (PIT VIPERS): Local signs and symptoms
- Intense pain within 5 minutes
- Localized edema within 30 minutes
- Erythema, ecchymosis, and serous/hemorrhagic bullae can develop over hours (Fig. E2)
- Compartment syndrome may develop around the site of the bite from significant amounts of soft tissue swelling and subcutaneous tissue fluid accumulation.
- If edema or erythema does not occur within 8 hours of a confirmed crotalid snakebite, it is assumed envenomation did not occur ("dry bite"). Roughly 25% of crotalid bites are "dry bites."

Systemic manifestations
- Nonspecific: nausea, vomiting, diarrhea, lightheadedness, weakness, diaphoresis, chills
- Coagulopathy: epistaxis, bleeding from gums, internal hemorrhage
- Neurotoxicity: perioral paresthesias, metallic taste, tingling of fingers or toes (especially with rattlesnake bites), localized/generalized fasciculations, mental status change
- Nephrotoxicity: secondary to rhabdomyolysis
- Increased vascular permeability: severe hypotension, tachycardia, respiratory distress

ELAPIDAE (CORAL SNAKES): Local signs and symptoms
- Absent or minimal local effects, such as mild pain, swelling, or paresthesias at site of bite.

Systemic Manifestations
- May be delayed for up to 12 hours.

TABLE 1 Medically Important Snake Families

Family	Venomous?	Location	Examples	Toxin Effects/Other Comments
Colubridae	Some species	Most parts of the world	Garter snakes (*Thamnophis* spp.), king snakes and milk snakes (*Lampropeltis* spp.)	Largest family of snakes; most are considered harmless to humans; a few species are dangerously toxic (e.g., African boomslang [*Dispholidus typus*])
Boidae	None	Most parts of the world	*Boa* sp., *Python* sp.	Constrictors; unsupervised children should not be allowed access to large constrictors
Viperidae				
Subfamily Crotalinae (pit vipers)	All	Americas, Asia	Rattlesnakes (*Crotalus* spp.), cottonmouths and copperheads (*Agkistrodon* spp.), Lancehead pit vipers (*Bothrops* spp.)	Heat-sensing "pit" between each eye and nostril
Subfamily Viperinae (true vipers)	All	Europe, Africa, Middle East, Asia	Puff adder (*Bitis arietans*), Gaboon viper (*Bitis gabonica*)	No heat-sensing pits
Elapidae	All	Americas, Africa, Middle East, Asia	Cobras (*Naja* spp.), mambas (*Dendroaspis* spp.), kraits (*Bungarus* spp.), coral snakes (*Micrurus* spp.), and the venomous snakes of Australia	Highly variable venom effects—some largely neurotoxic, others causing severe local tissue damage
Hydrophiidae	All	Warm waters of the Pacific Ocean, Indian Ocean, and Oceania (none in the Atlantic Ocean)	Sea snakes including the pelagic sea snake (*Pelamis platurus*)	Neurotoxins and myotoxins; rarely bite humans unless provoked

From Kliegman RM et al: *Nelson textbook of pediatrics*, ed 19, Philadelphia, 2011, Saunders.

B

Diseases and Disorders

I

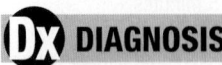

- Nonspecific: Nausea, vomiting, abdominal pain, dizziness
- Neurotoxic: Cranial neuropathies typically appear first including ptosis, ophthalmoplegia, dysphagia, drooling, and mydriasis with absent or prolonged pupillary light reflex. Descending paralysis and respiratory failure (due to diaphragmatic weakness) can be delayed many hours.

Dx DIAGNOSIS

DIFFERENTIAL DIAGNOSIS

- Bite: nonvenomous snakebite, "dry bite," scorpion bite, insect bite, cellulitis, laceration, puncture wound, necrotizing fasciitis
- Descending paralysis: myasthenia gravis, botulism, shellfish poisoning
- Rhabdomyolysis: crush injury, prolonged immobilization, marked exercise, hyperthermia, metabolic myopathies, drugs or toxins, infections, electrolyte disorders
- Coagulopathy: sepsis, multiple trauma, obstetrical complications, malignancy

WORKUP

1. Stabilize and resuscitate unstable patients.
2. Initial evaluation of the bite (as detailed in the following)
   a. Complete physical and neurologic examination
   b. Obtain past medical history, including any history of allergic reaction to horse serum in those previously treated for snakebite.
3. Labs and imaging (see the following)
4. Determine need for antivenom (see the following and Table 2)
5. Call Poison Control Hotline: 1-800-222-1222
6. Call local zoo when treating patients with envenomations from exotic pets or nonnative snakes
7. Serially reassess, including serial neurologic exams, all cases of suspected envenomation for 8 hours or longer if clinical status deteriorates

LABORATORY TESTS

- CBC with peripheral smear, electrolytes, BUN, creatinine, PT, INR, PTT, fibrinogen, d-dimer, creatine kinase, liver function tests (LFTs), sedimentation rate (ESR), arterial blood gas (ABG), type and crossmatch, urinalysis, and electrocardiogram (ECG).
- Repeat labs every 4 to 6 hours to monitor progression.

IMAGING

- Consider chest x-ray in cases of severe envenomation or in patients over 40 years old with underlying cardiopulmonary disease to rule out pulmonary edema
- Plain films of bite site for retained fangs (poor sensitivity)
- Computed tomography (CT) of head if concern for intracranial hemorrhage or if any cognitive/neurologic deficit is appreciated on exam
- CT abdomen or focused assessment with sonography in trauma (FAST) if concern for intraabdominal bleeding exists or if patient complains of abdominal pain or distention

Rx TREATMENT

ACUTE GENERAL Rx
IN THE FIELD:

- Transport immediately to nearest medical facility. No treatments in the field should delay transport to a facility able to administer antivenom if clinically indicated.
- Remove any constricting items including rings, watches, jewelry, or tight clothing.
- The affected part should be kept at the level of the heart. Keep the joint in a functional position to minimize disability should the limb or joint become severely swollen or immobile.
- Do _not_ apply a tourniquet, incise wound, apply mechanical or oral suction, attempt electrotherapy, or apply ice.
- In general, do _not_ apply a pressure dressing. Since most bites are from crotalids, a pressure dressing can exacerbate local tissue destruction and necrosis. However, if the bite is _known_ to be from a coral snake, applying a pressure dressing can prevent the spread of neurotoxin.
- Avoid alcohol, stimulants (caffeine), or agents that can suppress mental status.
- Do _not_ pick up a dead snake, as the strike reflexes remain intact and can still envenomate.
- When possible, a picture can be taken from a safe distance for later classification of the snake.

IN THE HOSPITAL:

- Assess airway, breathing, and circulation and intervene as needed. Patients with neurotoxic envenomation from elapids or Mojave rattlesnakes can develop respiratory failure (from diaphragmatic paralysis) and may require intubation. Be cautious and repeat the examination as neurotoxic symptoms may be delayed for many hours.

- Place on monitor, obtain vital signs, place 2 large-bore IVs and give crystalloid.
- Unstable patients should be given antivenom immediately. Administration should not be delayed for wound care of bite.
- If patient is stable, obtain a history, including the time of bite and description of snake.
- Inspect bite site for fang marks and local tissue injury. Clean bite site and remove any retained fangs. Bite may appear like two distinct puncture wounds or small scratches.
- Mark leading edge of erythema and edema, and obtain circumferential measurements every 15 minutes to assess for progression.
- Obtain initial labs and repeat every 4 to 6 hours.
- Determine need for antivenom and begin preparation. It can take up to 1 hour to reconstitute antivenom, so this process should be started as early as possible.
- Contact Poison Control at 1-800-222-1222, which will connect you to your local poison control center. They will provide guidance for treatment and use of antivenom, and also track snakebite incidence.
- Immunize against tetanus if no booster within the past 5 years. If never immunized, give immunoglobulin as well as toxoid.
- Prophylactic antibiotics are not recommended. Antibiotics should be given only if purulence or other signs of infection progress. When indicated, broad-spectrum antibiotics should be used to cover gram-negative bacteria (i.e., ampicillin-sulbactam or quinolone derivatives).
- Aggressive pain control with opioids. Avoid NSAIDs, as they increase risk of bleeding and platelet dysfunction and are nephrotoxic.

ANTIVENOM TREATMENT
CROTALID (RATTLESNAKE, COPPERHEAD, COTTONMOUTH) ENVENOMATIONS:

- CroFab (Crotalinae polyvalent ovine immune Fab), made from sheep serum, is the antivenom commercially available in the US for crotalid envenomations.
- Indications for antivenom administration include swelling, pain, and/or ecchymosis extending beyond area immediately adjacent to bite, any progression of local symptoms (≥2 cm of erythema spread), any systemic symptoms, any development of coagulation lab abnormalities, or abnormal bleeding.
- Patients with crotalid envenomation who have minimal or nonprogressive symptoms should _not_ be given CroFab and instead should be monitored for 8 to 12 hours.
- Dosing:
  - For moderate symptoms, reconstitute 4 to 6 vials of antivenom. Each vial should be mixed in 25 ml of normal saline. The 4 to 6 reconstituted vials should then be mixed in 250 ml normal saline and infused over 60 minutes. Infuse slowly over the first 10 minutes to monitor for allergic reaction.
  - For patients with shock or serious active bleeding, give an initial dose of 8 to 12 vials.
  - If no improvement after first round (defined as progression of local symptoms, persistent systemic symptoms, derangement of

---

TABLE 2 Indications for Snake Antivenom Administration

Evidence of Systemic Toxicity:	
Hemodynamic or respiratory instability	Hypotension, respiratory distress
Hemotoxicity	Clinically significant bleeding or abnormal coagulation studies
Neurotoxicity	Any evidence of toxicity: usually beginning with cranial nerve abnormalities and progressing to descending paralysis including the diaphragm
Evidence of local toxicity	_Progressive_ soft tissue swelling

From Kliegman RM et al: *Nelson textbook of pediatrics*, ed 19, Philadelphia, 2011, Saunders.

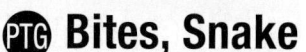

laboratory values, or continued bleeding), repeat the initial dose of antivenom.

- Between 4 and 18 vials of antivenom may be necessary to accomplish initial control of symptoms.
- After initial control of symptom progression, give scheduled dose of 2 vials every 6 hours for 3 doses to prevent recurrent toxicity.
- The manufacturer of CroFab maintains a 24/7 hotline: 877-377-3784
- A new Crotalinae antivenom, Anavip, was approved by the FDA in May 2015, with anticipated availability in October 2018. Anavip is approved for use against crotalid envenomations. Anavip is an equine antivenom that has venom specific F(ab')$_2$ fragments of immunoglobulin G (IgG), as opposed to two separate Fab fragments, increasing the half-life in the blood and leading to greater binding and therefore greater elimination of the venom. Because of the longer half-life, dosing with Anavip also eliminates the need for repeat outpatient antivenom dosing, as is required with CroFab. There is a low risk of adverse reactions and serum sickness because, similar to CroFab, these antivenoms lack the Fc component of the IgG.

ELAPID (CORAL SNAKE) ENVENOMATIONS:

- In the U.S., production of coral snake antivenom was discontinued in 2006, and only one lot of antivenom still exists. After its expiration, which was recently extended to April 30, 2017, the only option to obtain antivenom will be to seek compassionate release of expired stock in conjunction with your local Poison Control Center. If coral snake antivenom is not available, providers may consider contacting their local zoo to determine whether a provisional antivenom is available. Small-animal studies support the use of Mexican Coral Snake, Australian Tiger Snake, or anticoral antivenom for neutralization of North American coral snake venom. Many zoos caring for wild snake species stock these specific antivenoms. It is important to note that the effectiveness of these particular antivenoms in human snakebites by the North American coral snake has not been studied. If considering administering alternate antivenom, the provider should contact Poison Control to help orchestrate acquisition.
- A potent, safe, sheep-based antivenom for elapid bites exists and is being used internationally but is not yet approved in the U.S. The University of Arizona is currently sponsoring a clinical trial evaluating the use of a new F(ab')2 antivenom in management of coral snakebites in the U.S. The results of this study have not yet been published.
- In the U.S., only symptomatic patients with confirmed coral snake bites should receive antivenom. The initial dose is 3 to 5 vials given by slow intravenous push, although a higher dose may be necessary in children or in envenomations from large coral snakes.
- In the U.S., asymptomatic patients should not receive antivenom. They should be observed, and antivenom should be administered only if symptoms develop.

- There is a high risk of allergic reaction with horse serum-based elapid antivenom so epinephrine, diphenhydramine, IV corticosteroids, and albuterol should be readily available prior to giving antivenom.

NONNATIVE OR EXOTIC SNAKE ENVENOMATIONS:

- Contact the Poison Control Center or your local zoo, as zoos with exotic snakes are required to maintain a supply of snake-specific antivenom on their premises.

DISPOSITION

- All patients who are given antivenom must be admitted and monitored in an ICU for further observation and supportive care. Patients should be observed for 18 to 24 hours after initial control of symptom progression, and they are safe for discharge when symptom progression has resolved and laboratory values have normalized.
- Victims of crotalid envenomations with minimal to no toxicity and normal serial lab values should be observed for 8 to 12 hours. Patients are safe for discharge when symptom progression has resolved and labs have normalized. Children, the elderly, those with significant comorbidities, and patients who sustain bites to the legs, face, or neck may require observation for 24 hours.
- Suspected Mojave rattlesnake bites should be observed 12 to 24 hours as their venom predominantly causes neurotoxicity and symptoms may be delayed (similar to elapids).
- Asymptomatic patients with coral snakebites should be observed for 12 to 24 hours because neurotoxicity may be delayed.

FOLLOW-UP:

- All patients who receive antivenom should have repeat labs at 2 to 3 days and 5 to 7 days after discharge to evaluate for delayed hematologic complications or serum sickness.
- Return for worsening, nondependent swelling, abnormal bleeding, or signs of serum sickness, which include fatigue, rash, or arthralgias.
- Have patients adhere to bleeding precautions (no contact sports, dental extractions, elective surgery, etc.) for 2 weeks.

REFERRAL

Refer to a medical facility with an ICU for administration of antivenom. The approach to snakebites should be multidisciplinary and should include medical toxicology or other physician snakebite specialists, as well as hematology or nephrology if needed. All snakebites should be reported to Poison Control and the local health department for surveillance.

⊕ PEARLS & CONSIDERATIONS

OTHER CONSIDERATIONS

- Dosage of antivenom is based on typical envenomation rather than age or weight, so the dose is the same for children and adults.
- Antivenom is not contraindicated in pregnancy. There have been no adverse reactions to

mother or to fetus reported secondary to antivenom treatment. The potential coagulopathy associated with envenomation may place the fetus at higher risk for placental abruption, so prompt treatment with antivenom is prudent. Pregnant victims of snakebites have a significantly lower rate of miscarriage when compared with those who did not receive antivenom.

- Antivenom is most effective when given within 4 hours of the bite and least effective if delayed beyond 12 hours. Systemic symptoms (coagulopathy, CNS effects, etc.) respond better to treatment than do local symptoms (erythema/edema, bullae, etc.).
- Although local wound effects can be severe, wound management should not take precedence over antivenom administration. Some studies suggest that even in the case of compartment syndrome, antivenom may be more effective than fasciotomy, although both may be necessary.

COMPLICATIONS

- Hypersensitivity reactions and serum sickness can occur following any antivenom administration. These reactions are much more common with equine-derived antivenom than with ovine-derived antivenom. CroFab derived from sheep serum should be used preferentially over equine serum if available, given the decreased risk for adverse reaction. Elapid antivenom is derived from horse serum, so the risk for allergic reaction and anaphylaxis remains high.
- Anaphylaxis can occur within 30 minutes and should be treated by immediately stopping the infusion and managing the symptoms. Give epinephrine, diphenhydramine, and hydrocortisone as needed. If the anaphylaxis is well controlled and the envenomation is severe, the infusion can then be resumed.
- Delayed or recurrent hematologic complications are common and can manifest up to 2 weeks post treatment. Most bleeding is self-limited but can rarely be severe, necessitating close follow-up and occasionally repeat doses of antivenom.
- Serum sickness occurs 7 to 14 days after antivenom administration and is characterized by fever, rash, arthralgias, and lymphadenopathy. It can be treated with prednisone 60 mg PO daily, tapered over 7 to 10 days.

SUGGESTED READINGS
Available at www.expertconsult.com

RELATED CONTENT
Snakebites (Patient Information)

AUTHORS: **MADALENE I. BOYLE, M.D.,** and **NEHA P. RAUKAR, M.D., M.S.**

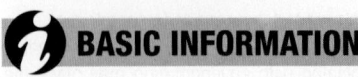

BASIC INFORMATION

DEFINITION

Bladder cancer is a heterogeneous spectrum of neoplasms ranging from non–life-threatening, low-grade, superficial papillary lesions to high-grade invasive tumors, which often have metastasized at the time of presentation. It is a field change disease in which the entire urothelium from the renal pelvis to the urethra may be susceptible to malignant transformation. The three types of bladder cancer are transitional cell carcinoma (TCCa), squamous cell carcinoma, and adenocarcinoma.

ICD-10CM CODES
C67.9	Malignant neoplasm of bladder, unspecified
C79.11	Secondary malignant neoplasm of bladder
D09.0	Carcinoma in situ of bladder
D30.3	Benign neoplasm of bladder
D41.4	Neoplasm of uncertain behavior of bladder
D49.4	Neoplasm of unspecified behavior of bladder

EPIDEMIOLOGY & DEMOGRAPHICS

Each year over 70,000 new cases are diagnosed and more than 14,000 deaths are attributed to bladder cancer. Overall, bladder cancer is the sixth most prevalent malignancy in the U.S. and the seventh leading cause of solid-cancer–related death.

Until 1990, the incidence of bladder cancer in the U.S. was rising. Since 1990, the incidence of bladder cancer is decreasing at a rate of 0.8% per year (1.2% among men and 0.4% among women).

PREDOMINANT SEX: In males, it is the fourth most common cancer, accounting for 10% of all cancers. In females, it is the tenth most common cancer, accounting for 4% of all cancers.

RISK: The lifetime risk of developing bladder cancer is 2.8% in white males, 0.9% in black males, 1% in white females, and 0.6% in black females.

Smoking:
- Users of "black" tobacco in place of "blond" tobacco have a twofold to threefold increase in developing bladder cancer.
- Smoking risk is based on consumption:
  1. A twofold to threefold increase for subjects smoking at least 10 cigarettes per day
  2. The risk increases again when the daily consumption rises above 40 to 60 cigarettes per day
- Smokers of low-tar and nicotine cigarettes have a lower risk when compared with higher tar and nicotine cigarettes.
- Those who smoke unfiltered cigarettes have a 50% increased risk of bladder cancer compared with those who smoke filtered cigarettes.
- Pipe smokers have a lower risk of bladder cancer compared with cigarette smokers.

- Cigars, snuff, and chewing tobacco, although implicated in nonurologic cancers, are not believed to influence bladder cancer risk.
  Diet:
- Diets rich in beef, pork, and animal fat increase risk of bladder cancer.
- There is no indication that consumption of non-beer alcoholic drinks contributes to bladder cancer development.
- Beer consumption has been linked to bladder cancer development as a result of the presence of nitrosamines in the beer. Nitrosamines have also been implicated in the development of rectal cancer.
- Drinking coffee is not believed to contribute to bladder cancer risk. There is additional evidence that coffee consumption is protective for colorectal cancers, possibly by diminishing fecal transit time.
  Medications: Long-term (>1 yr) use of pioglitazone and rosiglitazone

PEAK INCIDENCE: Incidence increases with age: higher after age 60 yr, uncommon younger than 40 yr.

GENETICS: It is thought to be multifactorial in etiology, involving both genetic and environmental interactions. Overall, approximately 20% to 25% of the male population in the U.S. with bladder cancer is estimated to have the disease as a result of occupational exposure.

DISTRIBUTION: In North America, transitional cell carcinomas comprise 93%, squamous cell carcinomas comprise 6%, and adenocarcinomas account for 1% of bladder cancers.

PATHOGENESIS: Two pathways exist for bladder cancer (TCCa):
1. Papillary superficial disease occasionally leading to invasive cancer (75%)
2. Carcinoma in situ (CIS) and solid invasive cancer with high risk of disease progression (25%)

Two distinct forms of "superficial cancer" exist:
1. T_a: Papillary low-grade tumor with a high rate of recurrence; disease progression occurs in 5%.
2. T_1: Higher-grade papillary tumor that infiltrates the lamina propria; often associated with flat CIS that may involve the urothelium diffusely. Disease progression occurs in 30% to 50%.

Subdivided into:
- T_{1a}: Penetration of tumor up to the muscularis mucosa; disease progression in 5.3%
- T_{1b}: Penetration of tumor through the muscularis mucosa; disease progression 53%

Flat CIS:
- Entirely different and separate pathway of cancer development whose mechanism is manifested by dysplasia, which leads to the occurrence of poorly differentiated malignant cells that replace or undermine the normal urothelium and extend along the plane of the bladder wall. It penetrates the basement membrane and lamina propria in 20% to 30% of cases and is associated with the development of solid tumor growth. A defect in chromosome 17p53 occurs in 50% of the cases.

At presentation, 72% of cancers are localized to the bladder, 20% of the cancers extend to the regional lymph nodes, and 3% present with distant metastases. Eighty percent of superficial TCCa recur, with up to 30% progressing to a higher stage or grade. Younger patients most commonly develop low-grade papillary noninvasive TCCa and are less likely to have recurrences when compared with older patients with similar lesions. Involvement of the upper tracts with tumor occurs in 25% to 50% of the cases.

STAGING (BASED ON THE TNM SYSTEM):
T_0	No tumor in specimen
T_{is}	CIS
T_a	Papillary TCCa noninvasive
T_1	Papillary TCCa into lamina propria
T_2	TCCa invasive of superficial muscle
T_{3a}	Invasive of deep muscle
T_{3b}	Invasive of perivesical fat
T_{4a}	Invasive of adjacent pelvic organ
T_{4b}	Invasive of pelvic wall with fixation

Invasive of nodal status
N_0	No nodal involvement
N_{1-3}	Pelvic nodes
N_4	Nodes above bifurcation
N_x	Unknown

Invasive of metastatic status
M_0	No distant metastases
M_1	Distant metastases
M_x	Unknown

MOLECULAR EPIDEMIOLOGY: TCCa is usually a field change disease with tumors arising at different times and sites in the urothelium, suggesting a polyclonal etiology of bladder cancer. Bladder cancers have been associated with abnormalities on chromosomes 1, 4, 11, 5, 7, 3, 9, 21, 18, 13, 8; with alterations in suppressor genes *P53*, retinoblastoma gene, and *P16*; and with alterations in oncogenes H-ras and epidermal growth factor receptor.

PHYSICAL FINDINGS & CLINICAL PRESENTATION

- Gross, painless hematuria
- Microhematuria
- Frequency, urgency, occasional dysuria
- With locally invasive to distant metastatic disease, the presentation can include:
  1. Abdominal pain
  2. Flank pain
  3. Lymphedema
  4. Renal failure
  5. Anorexia
  6. Bone pain

ETIOLOGY

Bladder cancer is a potentially preventable disease associated with specific etiologic factors:
- Cigarette smoking is associated with 25% to 65% of cases. The risk of developing a TCCa is two to four times higher in smokers than in nonsmokers, and that risk persists for many years, being equal to nonsmokers only after 12 to 15 yr of smoking abstinence. Smoking tobacco is associated with tumors that are characterized by higher histologic grade, increased tumor stage, increase in

the numbers of tumor present, and increased tumor size.

- Occupational exposures: dye workers, textile workers, tire and rubber workers, petroleum workers.
- Chemical exposure: O-toluidine, 2-naphthylamine, benzidine, 4-amino-biphenyl, and nitrosamines.
- Exposure to herpes papilloma virus type 16.

Squamous carcinomas are associated with:
- Schistosomiasis
- Urinary calculi
- Indwelling catheters
- Bladder diverticula

Miscellaneous causes:
- Phenacetin abuse
- Cyclophosphamide
- Pelvic irradiation
- Tuberculosis

Adenocarcinomas are associated with:
- Exstrophy
- Endometriosis
- Neurogenic bladder
- Urachal abnormalities
- As a secondary site for distant metastases from other organs (e.g., colon cancer)

Dx DIAGNOSIS

- History and physical examination.
- Urinalysis.
- Cystoscopy with bladder barbotage and biopsy. Fluorescence cystoscopy offers improvement in the detection of flat neoplastic lesions such as carcinoma in situ.
- Transurethral resection of bladder tumor(s).
- There is insufficient evidence to determine whether a decrease in mortality rate from bladder cancer occurs with hematuria testing, urinary cytology, or a variety of other tests on exfoliated urinary cells or other substances.
- In addition to urinary cytology and bladder barbotage, BTA, NMP22, and fibrin degradation products have been approved by the FDA as bladder cancer tumor markers. No marker has general, widespread acceptance because the results are affected by the presence of stents, recent urologic manipulation, stones, infection, bowel interposition, and prostatitis, creating false-positive results.
- Urinary biomarkers: six urinary biomarkers have been approved by the FDA for diagnosis on surveillance of bladder cancer
  - Quantitative nuclear matrix protein 22 (Alere NMP22)
  - Qualitative NMP22 (BladderChek)
  - Qualitative bladder tumor antigen (BTA stat)
  - Quantitative BTA (BTA TRAK)
  - Fluorescence in situ hybridization (FISH)
  - Fluorescent immunohistochemistry (ImmunoCyt)
- Generally urinary biomarkers miss a substantial proportion of patients with bladder cancer and are subject to false-positive results in

others. Accuracy is poor for low-stage and low-grade tumors.[1]

DIFFERENTIAL DIAGNOSIS

- Urinary tract infection
- Frequency-urgency syndrome
- Interstitial cystitis
- Stone disease
- Endometriosis
- Neurogenic bladder

LABORATORY TESTS

- Urine cytology.
- Urine telomerase: telomerase activity in voided urine or bladder washings determined by the telomeric repeat amplification protocol (TRAP) assay. This test has been reported to accurately detect the presence of bladder tumors in men. It represents a potentially useful noninvasive diagnostic innovation for bladder cancer detection in high-risk groups such as habitual smokers or in symptomatic patients.

RADIOLOGIC TESTS

- Renal ultrasound, retrograde pyelography, CT scan, and MRI.
- One or a combination of studies can be used. In the absence of skeletal symptoms, bone scan is not recommended.

Rx TREATMENT

NONPHARMACOLOGIC THERAPY

- Initially, transurethral resection of bladder tumor (TURBT) (Fig. 1)
- Loop biopsy of the prostatic urethra if high-grade TCCa is suspected
- If superficial disease, follow-up protocol with repeat TURBT and/or the use of intravesical agents is recommended
- For advanced bladder cancer, radical cystectomy with urethrectomy (unless orthotopic diversion is planned), and either ileal loop conduit or orthotopic diversion

BLADDER PRESERVATION APPROACHES: After cystectomy for muscle-invasive disease, 50% or more of the patients will develop metastases. Most patients develop metastases at distant sites; a third relapse locally. Bladder preservation management is offered in individuals who refuse surgery or who might not be suitable radical cystectomy patients. Bladder-sparing protocols include extensive TURBT or partial cystectomy with external-beam or interstitial radiotherapy and systemic chemotherapy. Radiotherapy as a single treatment modality is not effective. The best predictor of successful bladder preservation is a complete response after the combination of initial TURBT and two cycles of CMV (cisplatin, methotrexate, vinblastine) chemotherapy used with stages T_2 to T_{3a}.

---

[1]Chou R, et al.: Urinary biomarkers for diagnosis of bladder cancer: a systematic review and meta-analysis, *Ann Intern Med* 163:922-931, 2015.

INDICATIONS FOR PARTIAL CYSTECTOMY:
- Tumor within a bladder diverticulum
- Solitary, primary, and muscle-invasive or high-grade lesion of a region of the bladder that allows complete excision with adequate surgical margins
- Inability to adequately resect tumor by TURBT alone because of size or location
- Tumor overlying a ureteral orifice requiring ureteral reimplantation
- Biopsy of a radiation-induced ulceration
- Palliation of severe local symptoms
- Patient refusal of urinary diversion
- Poor-risk patient who is not a diversion candidate

CONTRAINDICATIONS:
- Multiple tumors
- CIS
- Cellular atypia on biopsy
- Prostatic invasion
- Invasion of the trigone
- Inability to achieve adequate surgical margins
- Prior radiotherapy
- Inability to maintain adequate bladder volume after resection
- Evidence of extravesical tumor extension
- Poor surgical risk

ACUTE GENERAL Rx
INDICATIONS FOR INTRAVESICAL CHEMOTHERAPY:
- High-grade tumor
- Tumor size >5 cm
- Multiple tumors
- Presence of CIS
- Positive urinary cytologic findings after a resection
- Incomplete tumor resection

Intravesical agents: thiotepa, Adriamycin, mitomycin C, AD-32, BCG, interferon, bropirimine, Epodyl, interleukin-2, and keyhole-limpet hemocyanin. Photodynamic therapy with hematoporphyrin derivatives has also been used.

INDICATIONS FOR CYSTECTOMY:
- Large tumors not amenable to complete TURBT
- High-grade tumor
- Multiple tumors with frequent recurrences
- Diffuse CIS not responsive to intravesical chemotherapy
- Prostatic urethra involvement
- Irritative bladder symptoms with upper tract deterioration
- Muscle-invasive disease
- Disease outside the bladder

SYSTEMIC CHEMOTHERAPY: Used as neoadjuvant and adjuvant therapy for systemic disease. The most effective agents are cisplatin, methotrexate, vinblastine, Adriamycin (MVAC). Other agents include mitoxantrone, vincristine, etoposide (VP16), 5-fluorouracil, ifosfamide, Taxol, gemcitabine, Piritrexim, mitomycin C, and gallium nitrate. Chemotherapy in combination can provide palliation and modest survival benefit.

RADIOTHERAPY: Conflicting reports suggest that superficial bladder cancer is more sensitive to radiotherapy. Squamous changes within the tumor and secretion of human chorionic gonadotropin by the lesion are associated with poor response to radiotherapy. Only 20% to 30% of patients with invasive bladder cancer can be cured by external-beam radiation therapy alone. It is used in combination with surgery or with systemic agents to treat bladder cancer primarily in patients who are not surgical candidates or who refuse surgery. Trials with synchronous chemotherapy with fluorouracil and mitomycin C combined with radiotherapy have shown significant improved locoregional control of bladder cancer, as compared with radiotherapy alone in patients with muscle-invasive bladder cancer.

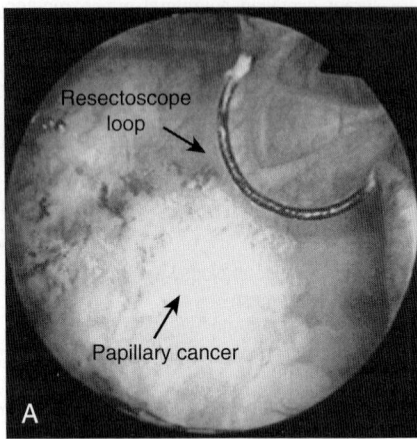
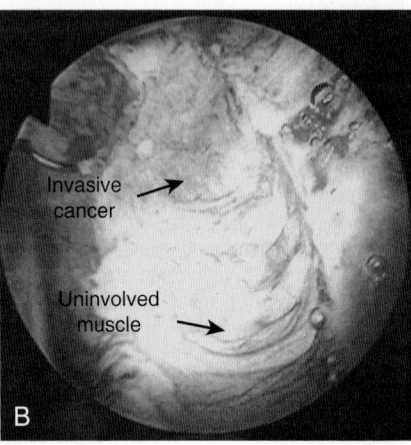

FIG 1 A, Papillary bladder cancer in right lower aspect of photo with resection loop poised to begin transurethral resection. **B,** Demonstration of grossly uninvolved muscularis propria *(bottom)* and cancer grossly invading the bladder wall *(top)*. (From Abeloff MD: *Clinical oncology,* ed 3, Philadelphia, 2004, Churchill Livingstone.)

BOX 1   American Urological Association Guideline Recommendations

For all index patients
- Standard: Physicians should discuss with the patient the treatment options and the benefits and harms, including side effects, of intravesical treatment.

For a patient who presents with an abnormal growth on the urothelium but who has not yet been diagnosed with bladder cancer
- Standard: If the patient does not have an established histologic diagnosis, a biopsy should be obtained for pathologic analysis.
- Standard: Under most circumstances, complete eradication of all visible tumors should be performed.
- Standard: If bladder cancer is confirmed, periodic surveillance cystoscopy should be performed.
- Option: An initial single dose of intravesical chemotherapy may be administered immediately postoperatively.

For a patient with small volume, low-grade Ta bladder cancer
- Recommendation: An initial single dose of intravesical chemotherapy may be administered immediately postoperatively.

For a patient with multifocal and/or large volume, histologically confirmed, low-grade Ta or a patient with recurrent low-grade Ta bladder cancer
- Recommendation: An induction course of intravesical therapy with bacillus Calmette-Guérin or mitomycin C is recommended for the treatment of these patients with the goal of preventing or delaying recurrence.
- Option: Maintenance bacillus Calmette-Guérin or mitomycin C may be considered.

For a patient with initial histologically confirmed high-grade Ta, T1, and/or carcinoma in situ bladder cancer
- Standard: For patients with lamina propria invasion (T1) but without muscularis propria in the specimen, repeat resection should be performed prior to additional intravesical therapy.
- Recommendation: An induction course of bacillus Calmette-Guérin followed by maintenance therapy is recommended for treatment of these patients.
- Option: Cystectomy should be considered for initial therapy in select patients.

For a patient with high-grade Ta, T1, and/or carcinoma in situ bladder cancer that has recurred after prior intravesical therapy
- Standard: For patients with lamina propria invasion (T1) but without muscularis propria in the specimen, repeat resection should be performed prior to additional intravesical therapy.
- Recommendation: Cystectomy should be considered as a therapeutic alternative for these patients.
- Option: Further intravesical therapy may be considered for these patients.

From the American Urological Association, Guideline Division, http://www.auanet.org.

CHRONIC Rx

FOLLOW-UP RECOMMENDATIONS FOR SUPERFICIAL BLADDER CANCER:
- Cystoscopy, bladder barbotage, and bimanual examination every 3 mo for 2 yr, then every 6 mo for 2 yr, and annually thereafter.
- Upper tract studies are based on the risk of upper tract tumor development, generally every 2 to 5 yr.

FOLLOW-UP RECOMMENDATIONS FOR ADVANCED DISEASE: Bladder preservation:
- Cystoscopy, barbotage, bimanual examination, biopsy (when indicated), every 3 mo for 2 yr, then every 6 mo for 2 yr, yearly thereafter
- CT scan of abdomen and pelvis every 6 mo for 2 yr in addition to chest x-ray examination, liver function testing, and serum creatinine

Cystectomy with ileal loop/orthotopic bladder:
- Neobladder endoscopy and IVP yearly
- CT scan of abdomen and pelvis every 6 mo for 2 yr in addition to chest x-ray examination, liver function tests, and serum creatinine
- Loopogram every 6 mo for 2 yr, then annually

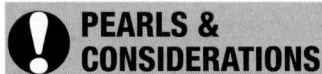

PEARLS & CONSIDERATIONS

COMMENTS
- The most useful prognostic parameters for bladder tumor recurrence and subsequent cancer progression are tumor grade, depth of tumor penetration, multifocal tumors, frequency of recurrence, tumor size, CIS, lymphatic invasion, papillary or solid tumor configuration.
- Box 1 describes the American Urological Association Guideline Recommendations for bladder cancer.

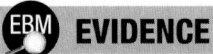 **EVIDENCE**

Available at www.expertconsult.com

SUGGESTED READINGS
Available at www.expertconsult.com

RELATED CONTENT
Bladder Cancer (Patient Information)

AUTHOR: **BHARTI RATHORE, M.D.**

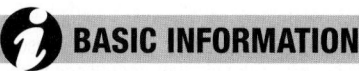 BASIC INFORMATION

DEFINITION

Body dysmorphic disorder (BDD) is classified as an obsessive-compulsive and related disorder. It is characterized by preoccupation with one or more perceived defects or flaws in physical appearance that are not observable or appear only slight to others, as well as repetitive behaviors (e.g., excessive grooming, mirror checking) in response to the appearance concerns. The preoccupations cause clinically significant distress or impairment in social, occupational, or other important areas of functioning. The appearance preoccupations are not better explained by concerns with body fat or weight in a person whose symptoms meet diagnostic criteria for an eating disorder.

SYNONYMS

Dysmorphophobia
BDD

ICD-10CM CODES
F45.22 Body dysmorphic disorder

EPIDEMIOLOGY & DEMOGRAPHICS

- Affects 1.7% to 2.4% of the general population (in nationwide epidemiologic studies)
- Weighted prevalence among general cosmetic surgery patients is 13.2%
- Weighted prevalence in rhinoplasty surgery settings is 20.1%
- Weighted prevalence among dermatology outpatients is 11.3%
- Slightly higher prevalence among females (but not in cosmetic surgery or dermatology settings)
- Onset most commonly in adolescence

PHYSICAL FINDINGS & CLINICAL PRESENTATION

- Excessive preoccupation (obsession) with one or more perceived defects in appearance that are not observable or appear slight to others. Patients believe they look abnormal, ugly, or deformed, whereas in reality they look normal. Any part of the body may be a focus of concern; skin, hair, and nose concerns are most common. Muscle dysmorphia is a form of BDD that occurs primarily in men and focuses on excessive concern that one's body build is too small or is insufficiently muscular. Most patients are preoccupied with multiple body areas.
- The body areas with which the patient is concerned appear physically normal; if a physical defect is present, it is slight, and the patient's reaction to it is excessive.
- Most patients have poor insight (i.e., are mostly convinced) or absent insight (i.e., delusional beliefs; are completely convinced) regarding the accuracy of their beliefs about the appearance of the perceived defects.
- Over the course of the disorder, all patients engage in repetitive behaviors such as frequent mirror checking, excessive grooming, skin picking to try to fix perceived skin flaws, reassurance seeking, and repeatedly measuring or feeling the perceived defect.

The intent of these behaviors is to check, try to improve, or gain reassurance about the appearance of the perceived flaws. Nearly all patients attempt to camouflage or hide the perceived defects—e.g., with makeup, a hat, hair, or body position.

- Nearly all experience impairment in psychosocial functioning and quality of life; impairment is usually substantial.
- Suicidal ideation, suicide attempts, and completed suicide appear common.
- Commonly co-occurring mental disorders are major depressive disorder, substance use disorders (including abuse of anabolic androgenic steroids in muscle dysmorphia), social anxiety disorder, obsessive-compulsive disorder (OCD), and personality disorder.

ETIOLOGY

Likely multifactorial, with both genetic and environmental risk factors (e.g., teasing). Neuropsychological and fMRI studies indicate abnormalities in visual processing consisting of excessive focus on details rather than on larger global and configural elements of visual stimuli.

Dx DIAGNOSIS

Psychiatric interview
Ask:
1. Are you very worried about your appearance in any way? *OR:* Are you unhappy with how you look?
2. Does this concern with your appearance preoccupy you? If you add up all the time you spend each day thinking about your appearance, how much time would you estimate it takes (at least an hour a day)?
3. How much distress does this concern cause you?
4. What effect does this concern have on your life?
5. Is there anything you feel an urge to do over and over again in response to your appearance concerns? (Give examples, such as mirror checking, comparing with others, skin picking to remove perceived skin flaws)
   - Determine that the perceived appearance defects are actually nonexistent or only slight

DIFFERENTIAL DIAGNOSIS

- Often undiagnosed because of patient's reluctance to divulge symptoms due to shame and fear of being misunderstood (e.g., considered vain)
- OCD
- Eating disorder
- Social anxiety disorder
- Major depressive disorder

WORKUP

Clinical evaluation focused on BDD symptoms and associated impairment in functioning.

Rx TREATMENT

NONPHARMACOLOGIC THERAPY

- CBT, with a focus on cognitive restructuring, exposure, and response prevention; CBT

must be specifically tailored to BDD's unique symptoms.
- Do not try to talk patients out of their concern; it is ineffective.
- Avoid cosmetic procedures; a majority of patients with BDD receive them, but such treatments do not appear effective for BDD. Dissatisfied patients may sue or even become violent toward the treating clinician.

CHRONIC Rx

- SRIs are medication of choice; relatively high doses often needed.
- Other agents (e.g., neuroleptics, tricyclic antidepressants other than clomipramine) do not appear as beneficial.
- CBT tailored specifically to BDD is recommended, with an SRI if BDD symptoms are more severe, the patient is suicidal because of BDD symptoms, or comorbidity is present that may benefit from an SRI.
- Support groups if available.
- More intensive BDD-focused treatment (e.g., intensive outpatient, residential treatment) if outpatient care is insufficient.

DISPOSITION

- Untreated BDD tends to be chronic and can lead to social isolation; school dropout; loss of employment; major depression; unnecessary surgery, dermatologic treatment, or other cosmetic treatment; and even suicide.
- With correct diagnosis and treatment, a majority improve.

! PEARLS & CONSIDERATIONS

- In clinical settings, more than 60% have co-occurring major depressive disorder.
- Reassurance that the patient looks normal is rarely helpful.
- Patients often have an unrealistic expectation of improvement with plastic surgery, dermatologic treatment, and other cosmetic procedures; these treatments do not appear to be effective.
- All patients should be screened and monitored for suicidality.

PATIENT/FAMILY EDUCATION

- Family support and encouragement of appropriate treatment is important.
- Phillips KA: *Understanding Body Dysmorphic Disorder: An Essential Guide.* Oxford University Press, 2009.
- www.RhodeIslandHospital.org/bdd

SUGGESTED READINGS
Available at www.expertconsult.com

RELATED CONTENT
Body Dysmorphic Disorder (Patient Information)
Obsessive Compulsive Disorder (Related Key Topic)

AUTHOR: **KATHARINE A. PHILLIPS, M.D.**

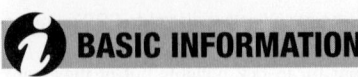

BASIC INFORMATION

DEFINITION
Primary malignant bone tumors are invasive and anaplastic and have the ability to metastasize. Most arise from the marrow (myeloma), but tumors may develop from bone, cartilage, fat, and fibrous tissues. Leukemia and lymphoma are excluded from this discussion.

FIBROSARCOMA AND LIPOSARCOMA: Extremely rare. They are similar to tumors arising in soft tissue.

OSTEOSARCOMA: A rare primary malignant tumor of bone characterized by malignant tumor cells that produce osteoid or bone. Several variants have been described: parosteal sarcoma, periosteal sarcoma, multicentric, and telangiectatic forms.

CHONDROSARCOMA: A malignant cartilage tumor that may develop primarily or secondarily from transformation of a benign osteocartilaginous exostosis or enchondroma.

EWING'S SARCOMA: A malignant tumor of unknown histogenesis.

MULTIPLE MYELOMA: A neoplastic proliferation of plasma cells.

SYNONYMS
Multiple myeloma:
1. Plasma cell myeloma
2. Plasmacytoma

ICD-10CM CODES
C41.9　Malignant neoplasm of bone and articular cartilage, unspecified
C40.00　Malignant neoplasm of scapula and long bones of unspecified upper limb
C40.01　Malignant neoplasm of scapula and long bones of right upper limb
C40.02　Malignant neoplasm of scapula and long bones of left upper limb
C40.10　Malignant neoplasm of short bones of unspecified upper limb
C40.11　Malignant neoplasm of short bones of right upper limb
C40.12　Malignant neoplasm of short bones of left upper limb
C40.20　Malignant neoplasm of long bones of unspecified lower limb
C40.21　Malignant neoplasm of long bones of right lower limb
C40.22　Malignant neoplasm of long bones of left lower limb
C40.30　Malignant neoplasm of short bones of unspecified lower limb
C40.31　Malignant neoplasm of short bones of right lower limb
C40.32　Malignant neoplasm of short bones of left lower limb
C40.80　Malignant neoplasm of overlapping sites of bone and articular cartilage of unspecified limb
C40.81　Malignant neoplasm of overlapping sites of bone and articular cartilage of right limb
C40.82　Malignant neoplasm of overlapping sites of bone and articular cartilage of left limb
C40.90　Malignant neoplasm of unspecified bones and articular cartilage of unspecified limb
C40.91　Malignant neoplasm of unspecified bones and articular cartilage of right limb
C40.92　Malignant neoplasm of unspecified bones and articular cartilage of left limb
C41.0　Malignant neoplasm of bones of skull and face
C41.4　Malignant neoplasm of pelvic bones, sacrum and coccyx
C41.9　Malignant neoplasm of bone and articular cartilage, unspecified

EPIDEMIOLOGY & DEMOGRAPHICS
Table 1 summarizes incidence, in decreasing order, of lesions that may present as a primary bone tumor.

MULTIPLE MYELOMA:
- The most common tumor in bone
- Age at onset: usually >40 yr
- Male/female ratio of 2:1

OSTEOGENIC SARCOMA:
- Average age at onset: 10 to 20 yr
- Males afflicted more often than females
- Parosteal sarcoma in older patients

CHONDROSARCOMA:
- Age at onset: 40 to 60 yr
- Male/female ratio of 2:1

EWING'S SARCOMA: Age at onset: 10 to 15 yr

PHYSICAL FINDINGS & CLINICAL PRESENTATION

MULTIPLE MYELOMA:
- May present as a systemic process or, less commonly, as a "solitary" lesion

- Early manifestations: anorexia, weight loss, and bone pain; majority of cases present initially with back pain that often leads to the detection of a destructive skeletal lesion
- Other organ systems eventually become involved, resulting in more bone pain, anemia, renal insufficiency, and/or bacterial infections, usually as a result of the dysproteinemia typical of this disorder
- Possible secondary amyloidosis, leading to cardiac failure or nephrotic syndrome

OSTEOSARCOMA:
- Most originating in the metaphysis
- 50% to 60% around the knee
- Possible pain and swelling, but otherwise healthy patient
- Osteosarcoma in conjunction with Paget's disease, manifested primarily as a sudden increase in bone pain

CHONDROSARCOMA:
- Tumor most commonly involving the pelvis, upper femur, and shoulder girdle
- Painful swelling

EWING'S SARCOMA:
- Painful soft tissue mass often present
- Possibly increased local heat
- Midshaft of a long bone usually affected (in contrast to other tumors)
- Weight loss, fever, and lethargy

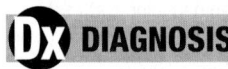 DIAGNOSIS

DIFFERENTIAL DIAGNOSIS
- Osteomyelitis
- Metastatic bone disease

LABORATORY TESTS
- Slightly elevated alkaline phosphatase in osteosarcoma

TABLE 1 Incidence, in Decreasing Order, of Lesions That May Present as a Primary Bone Tumor

Lesion	Incidence of All Tumors (%)[†,‡]
Osteosarcoma	17
Chondrosarcoma	11
Enchondroma*	6
Fibrous dysplasia*	6
Giant cell tumor	6
Nonossifying fibroma/fibrous cortical defect*	5
Ewing sarcoma	5
Malignant fibrous histiocytoma/fibrosarcoma	5
Osteochondroma*	4
Aneurysmal bone cyst	4
Metastasis	4
Osteomyelitis	4
Solitary bone cyst	3
Osteoid osteoma	3
Langerhans cell histiocytosis (eosinophilic granuloma)	3
Chondroblastoma	2
Others	12

*Lesions are often asymptomatic and therefore much more frequent than the table suggests.
[†]Benign tumors and tumor-like lesions in general are underreported in these frequency distributions.
[‡]Data are based on 6873 tumors on file in the Netherlands Committee on Bone Tumors.
Pope TL, Bloem HL et al: *Musculoskeletal imaging*, ed 2, Philadelphia, 2015, Elsevier.

TABLE 2 Systemic Approach in Diagnosing Osseous Tumors or Tumor-Like Lesions

1. Categorize the radiograph (normal, variant, tumor-like lesion, tumor).
2. Determine the prevalence of lesions in relation to the age of the patient.
3. Determine the prevalence of lesions in the affected bone.
4. Is the lesion solitary, or are there multiple lesions?
5. Determine the prevalence of osseous lesions in the affected part of the bone.
6. Analyze the radiograph in detail.
7. Analyze additional information (MR, CT, clinical and laboratory data, and so on).
8. Perform a biopsy, if needed, based on the comprehensive imaging findings.

From Pope TL, Bloem HL et al: *Musculoskeletal imaging*, ed 2, Philadelphia, 2015, Elsevier.

- In Ewing's sarcoma: reflective of systemic reaction; includes anemia, an increase in white blood cell count, and an elevated sedimentation rate
- In multiple myeloma:
  1. Bence Jones protein in the urine
  2. Anemia and elevated sedimentation rate
  3. Characteristic dysproteinemia on serum protein electrophoresis
  4. Diagnostic feature: peak in the electrophoretic pattern suggestive of a monoclonal gammopathy
  5. Rouleaux formation in the peripheral blood smear
  6. Often presence of hypercalcemia, but alkaline phosphatase levels usually normal

IMAGING STUDIES

- Table 2 summarizes a systemic approach in diagnosing osseous tumors or tumor-like lesions.
- Classic osteogenic sarcoma penetrates the cortex early in many cases.
  1. A blastic (dense), lytic (lucent), or mixed response may be seen in the affected bone (Fig. 1).

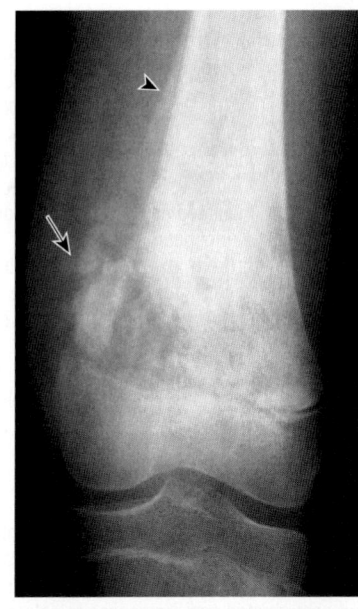

FIG. 1 Conventional central osteosarcoma. AP radiograph of the distal femur showing a classic osteosarcoma with mixed lytic and sclerotic areas, tumor bone formation in the extraosseous mass *(arrow)*, and a proximal Codman's triangle *(arrowhead)*. (From Adam A et al: *Grainger & Allison's diagnostic radiology*, ed 5, Philadelphia, 2008, Churchill Livingstone.)

  2. An aggressive perpendicular sunburst pattern may be present as a result of periosteal reaction, and peripheral Codman's triangles are often noted.
  3. Margins of the tumor are poorly defined.
- Speckled calcifications in a destructive radiolucent lesion are usually suggestive of chondrosarcoma.
- Ewing's sarcoma is characterized radiographically by mottled, irregular destructive changes with periosteal new bone formation. The latter may be multilayered, producing the typical "onion skin" appearance.
- Typical roentgenographic finding in multiple myeloma is the "punched out" lesion with sharply demarcated edges.

1. Multiple lesions are usual.
2. Diffuse osteoporosis may be the only finding in many cases.
3. Pathologic fractures are common.

Rx TREATMENT

The evaluation and treatment of malignant bone tumors are complicated. Diagnostic studies and treatment should be supervised by an orthopedic cancer specialist and oncologist.

DISPOSITION

- In the past 20 yr, dramatic improvements have been made in the treatment protocols for osteosarcoma with the use of adjuvant multidrug regimens and limb-sparing surgery.
- Prognosis of multiple myeloma remains poor despite new therapies.
- Prognosis for Ewing's sarcoma has improved with a combination of chemotherapy, local resection, and radiation therapy.
- Chondrosarcomas are not sensitive to chemotherapy or radiation, and prognosis depends on the grade of the tumor and the ability to obtain an adequate resection.

! PEARLS & CONSIDERATIONS

Early diagnosis is important because most tumors have not metastasized at the time of initial presentation.

SUGGESTED READINGS

Available at www.expertconsult.com

RELATED CONTENT

Multiple Myeloma (Related Key Topic)
Sarcoma (Related Key Topic)

AUTHOR: **BHARTI RATHORE, M.D.**

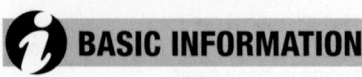

BASIC INFORMATION

DEFINITION

Botulism is an illness caused by a neurotoxin produced primarily by *Clostridium botulinum*. Five types of disease can occur: foodborne botulism, wound botulism, infant intestinal botulism, adult enteric botulism (similar to infant botulism), and inhalational botulism. Of note, inhalational botulism is exceedingly rare, but could occur as a result of bioterrorism.

SYNONYMS

Clostridium botulinum food poisoning
Botulinum toxin food poisoning
Wound botulism
Infantile botulism

ICD-10CM CODES
A05.1   Botulism food poisoning
A48.51   Infant botulism
A48.52   Wound botulism

EPIDEMIOLOGY & DEMOGRAPHICS

INCIDENCE (IN U.S.): An average of 110 cases of botulism are reported in the U.S. annually. One quarter of cases are due to food-borne botulism; nearly 70% of reported cases are infant botulism.

PHYSICAL FINDINGS & CLINICAL PRESENTATION

- Symptoms usually begin 12 to 36 hr following ingestion. Patients present with symmetric descending flaccid paralysis and prominent bulbar signs (diplopia, dysarthria, dysphonia, and dysphagia [the four "Ds"])
- Severity of illness is related to the quantity of toxin ingested.
- Significant findings:
  1. Acute, bilateral cranial nerve palsies, with ocular and bulbar manifestations being most frequent (diplopia, ophthalmoplegia, ptosis, dysphagia, dysarthria, fixed and dilated pupils, and dry mouth)
  2. Usually bilateral nerve involvement that may progress to a descending flaccid paralysis
  3. No sensory deficits, aside from possible blurred vision
  4. GI symptoms (dry mouth, nausea, vomiting, diarrhea, or cramps)
  5. Generally an absence of fever
  6. Normal heart rate to mild bradycardia with patient remaining normotensive
  7. Normal mental status
- Wound botulism
  1. Occurs primarily in injecting drug users (subcutaneous "black tar" heroin injection— "skin popping") or with traumatic injury.
  2. Presentation is similar to that of food-borne disease, except for a longer incubation period (4-14 days) and absence of GI symptoms.
  3. Fever is uncommon and if present may be due to wound infection, which is not always apparent.

ETIOLOGY

- Cause is one of several types of neurotoxins (usually A, B, E, or F) produced by *C. botulinum,* an anaerobic, gram-positive bacillus. Spore production guarantees survival of the organism in extreme conditions, and they are found in the environment worldwide. Botulinum toxin blocks acetylcholine-mediated neurotransmission and is the most powerful neurotoxin known.
- Disease results from absorption of toxin into the circulation from a mucosal surface or wound. Botulinum toxin does not penetrate intact skin.
- In foodborne variety, disease is caused by ingestion of preformed toxin. Although rapidly inactivated by heat, the toxin can survive the proteolytic environment of the stomach.
- In wound botulism, toxin is elaborated by organisms that contaminate a wound.
- In infant botulism (and probably adult botulism of unknown etiology), toxin is produced by organisms in the GI tract. Antibiotic use and achlorhydria can predispose to colonization by *C. botulinum* and elaboration of toxin.
- Inhalational botulism has been demonstrated experimentally in primates. Rare case reports of inhalational botulism from snorting contaminated cocaine have been reported, and there is concern for the potential use of manufactured aerosolized toxin as a bioterrorism agent.

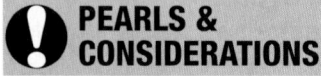

DIAGNOSIS

DIFFERENTIAL DIAGNOSIS

- Myasthenia gravis, Lambert-Eaton myasthenic syndrome
- Guillain-Barré syndrome or other acute inflammatory demyelinating polyneuropathy
- Tick paralysis
- CVA
- Other: polio, heavy metal intoxication, and shellfish poisoning

LABORATORY TESTS

- Treatment should start *before* laboratory confirmation in suspected cases, as laboratory testing may take several days.
- Anaerobic cultures of serum, of food, and/or stool.
- Food, serum, and stool are sent for toxin assay.
- Public health laboratories may perform mouse bioassay testing, which confirms toxin type in 75% of cases.

TREATMENT

NONPHARMACOLOGIC THERAPY

- Supportive care with intubation if respiratory failure occurs; may need to continue for prolonged period, as pharmacologic therapy halts disease progression only in the short term
- Debridement of the wound in wound botulism

ACUTE GENERAL Rx

- **For non-infants:** Give equine heptavalent botulinum antitoxin (HBAT), which contains antibodies for seven known botulism types (A through G), as early as possible. Once a clinical diagnosis is made, antitoxin should be administered before laboratory confirmation.
  1. The antitoxin (BAT, Cangene Corporation) is available from the Centers for Disease Control and Prevention (1-404-639-2206 Monday-Friday or 1-404-639-2888 evenings/weekends); it is derived from horse serum, so there is a significant incidence of serum sickness.
  2. Skin testing (conjunctival instillation and observation for 15 min), and possible desensitization, is recommended before treatment. Reported hypersensitivity rates range from 9% to 20%.
- Give wound botulism patients penicillin 2 million U IV q4h after antitoxin has been given. Use metronidazole 500 million U IV q8h as alternative for penicillin-allergic patients. Avoid aminoglycosides and tetracyclines, as they are ineffective and can worsen neuromuscular blockade.
- **For infants:** Give human botulinum immunoglobulin (BabyBIG) IV, single dose. Call 1-510-231-7600. Do not use equine antitoxin. Babies with infantile intestinal botulism may benefit from a cathartic to mechanically clear the number of *C. botulinum* vegetative forms and spores residing in the gastrointestinal tract. Avoid antibiotics in infant botulism because antimicrobials may lyse *C. botulinum* in the gut and increase toxin load.

DISPOSITION

- Highest mortality in the first cases in an outbreak, with subsequent cases receiving rapid treatment
- Complete recovery for most individuals (may take up to 1 year)

PEARLS & CONSIDERATIONS

COMMENTS

- Routine cooking inactivates the toxin, but spores are resistant to environmental factors. At room temperature, spores can germinate and produce toxin. Pressure cooking can kill spores.
- Most outbreaks are associated with home-canned foods, including fruits, vegetables, and fish.
- Patients must be closely monitored for progression to respiratory paralysis.
- Notify public health authorities immediately to alert other health care services of possible additional cases and to initiate investigation into cause and scope of outbreak.
- Immunity to botulism does not occur after toxin exposure/infection, and repeated botulism can occur.

SUGGESTED READINGS

Available at www.expertconsult.com

RELATED CONTENT

Botulism (Patient Information)

AUTHOR: **RUSSELL J. MCCULLOH, M.D.**

BASIC INFORMATION

DEFINITION

A brain abscess is a focal intracerebral infection that can arise as a complication from a bacterial, mycobacterial, fungal, or parasitic infection, surgery, or trauma.

ICD-10CM CODES
G06.0 Intracranial abscess and granuloma

EPIDEMIOLOGY & DEMOGRAPHICS

INCIDENCE: Uncommon (reported incidence 0.4 to 0.9 cases per 100,000 population; occurs about 2% as commonly as brain tumors)
PEAK INCIDENCE: Preadolescence and middle age (and depends on predisposing condition); increased rates in the immunocompromised host
PREDOMINANT AGE: Occurs at any age
PREDOMINANT SEX:
- Men affected more than women (ratio 2:1 to 3:1)

PHYSICAL FINDINGS & CLINICAL PRESENTATION

- Classic triad: fever, headache, and focal neurologic deficit (present in less than 50% of cases).
- Clinical presentation is often due to the manifestations of the space-occupying lesion rather than to signs of systemic infection.
- Fever is present in only 32% to 79% of patients.
- Headache is usually localized to the side of the abscess; onset can be gradual or severe; present in an average of 70% to 75% of cases.
- Focal neurologic findings (e.g., seizures, hemiparesis, aphasia, ataxia) depend on the location of the abscess and are seen in 23% to 66% of cases.
- Papilledema is present in 9% to 51% of cases.
- Presence of adjacent infections (dental abscess, otitis media, sinusitis, or postneurosurgical infection) may be a clue to the underlying diagnosis and should be sought in any suspected case.
- Time course from symptom onset to presentation ranges from hours in fulminant cases to more than 1 month; 75% present in the first 2 weeks.
- The nonspecific presentation of a brain abscess warrants that clinicians maintain a high index of suspicion. Table 1 describes common initial features of brain abscess.

ETIOLOGY

- Brain abscesses are classified based on the likely portal of entry and can arise from:
  Contiguous infection (e.g., dental abscess, otitis media, sinusitis, or post neurosurgical infection)
  Hematogenous spread from a remote site (e.g., endocarditis, bacteremia)
- Likely source of abscess and common organisms involved:
  A. Contiguous focus or primary infection (55% of all brain abscesses):

TABLE 1 Brain Abscess: Initial Features in 123 Cases

Headache	55%
Disturbed consciousness	48%
Fever	58%
Nuchal rigidity	29%
Nausea, vomiting	32%
Seizures	19%
Visual disturbance	15%
Dysarthria	20%
Hemiparesis	48%
Sepsis	17%

From Goldman L, Schafer AI: *Goldman's Cecil medicine*, ed 24, Philadelphia, 2012, Saunders.

1. Paranasal sinus: occur in frontal lobe; streptococci (especially microaerophilic and anaerobic streptococci), *Bacteroides*, *Haemophilus*, and *Fusobacterium* spp.
2. Otitis media/mastoiditis: occur in temporal lobe and cerebellum; aerobic and anaerobic streptococci, *Enterobacteriaceae*, *Bacteroides*, and *Pseudomonas* spp.
3. Dental sepsis: occur in frontal lobe; mixed *Fusobacterium*, *Bacteroides*, and *Streptococcus* spp. (especially *S. viridans* and anaerobic streptococci)
4. Penetrating head injury: site of abscess depends on site of wound; *Staphylococcus aureus*, aerobic streptococci, *Clostridium* spp., *Enterobacteriaceae*
5. Postoperative: *Staphylococcus epidermidis* and *S. aureus*, *Enterobacteriaceae*, and *Pseudomonas aeruginosa*

B. Hematogenous spread from a distant site of infection (25% of all brain abscesses): abscesses most commonly multiple, especially in middle cerebral artery distribution; infecting organism(s) depend on source.

1. Congenital heart disease: streptococci, *Haemophilus* spp.
2. Endocarditis: *S. aureus*, viridans streptococci
3. Urinary tract: Enterobacteriaceae, Pseudomonadaceae
4. Intraabdominal: streptococci, *Enterobacteriaceae*, anaerobes
5. Lung: streptococci, *Actinomyces* spp., *Fusobacterium* spp.
6. Immunocompromised host: *Toxoplasma* spp., *Enterobacteriaceae*, *Nocardia* spp., listeriosis, other fungi, tuberculosis
   a. Fungi are responsible for up to 90% of cerebral abscesses in solid organ transplant recipients.

C. Cryptogenic (unknown source): 20% of all brain abscesses

DIAGNOSIS

DIFFERENTIAL DIAGNOSIS

- Other parameningeal infections: subdural empyema, epidural abscess, thrombophlebitis

of the major dural venous sinuses and cortical veins
- Embolic strokes in patients with bacterial endocarditis
- Mycotic aneurysms with leakage
- Acute hemorrhagic leukoencephalitis
- Parasitic infections: toxoplasmosis, echinococcosis, cysticercosis
- Metastatic or primary brain tumors
- Cerebral infarction
- CNS vasculitis
- Chronic subdural hematoma

WORKUP

Physical examination, laboratory tests, and imaging studies

LABORATORY TESTS

- White blood cell counts are elevated in 60% of patients.
- Erythrocyte sedimentation rate is usually elevated but may be normal.
- Lumbar puncture is contraindicated because of the potential for increased intracranial pressure and the risk for herniation due to the space-occupying abscess. Lumbar puncture may be helpful only in those with suspicion for meningitis or abscess rupture into the ventricular system; however, the risk of herniation must be considered.
- The yield of gram stain and culture of material aspirated at time of surgical drainage is very high.
- Cultures of contiguous sites of infection should be considered (e.g., paranasal sinus, otitis, skin site abscess from a neurosurgical procedure). These sites of infection may need surgical drainage in order to control the infection.
- Blood cultures and cerebrospinal fluid cultures may identify the causative organism in up to 25% of patients.

IMAGING STUDIES

- CT scan with contrast enhancement or MRI with gadolinium can be used to detect brain abscess. CT is rapid and available in most medical settings. An MRI with gadolinium is able to provide more detailed images in order to differentiate between abscess and tumor or other mass.
- CT scan (Fig. 1) with intravenous contrast enhancement is still an excellent test (sensitivity 95%-99%).
- Serial CT or MRI scanning is recommended to follow the response to therapy.

TREATMENT

ACUTE GENERAL Rx

- Effective treatment involves a combination of empiric antibiotic therapy and timely excision or aspiration of the abscess.
- If evidence of edema or mass effect, treatment of elevated intracranial pressure is paramount.
  - Hyperventilation of mechanically ventilated patient.

- Dexamethasone initially in a dosage of 10 mg IV followed by 4 mg IV q6h until symptoms of cerebral edema subside. Steroids should be discontinued as soon as possible.
- Mannitol 0.25 to 1 g/kg IV over 20 to 30 min q6 to 8h; maximum of 6 g/kg in 24 hr.
- Medical therapy is never a substitute for surgical intervention to relieve increased intracranial pressure. Neurologic deterioration usually mandates surgical intervention.
- Steroids should be limited to patients with severe cerebral edema or midline shift.

MEDICAL Rx

If abscess <2.5 cm and patient is neurologically stable and conscious, may start antibiotics and observe. Empiric antibiotic therapy guided by:

- Abscess location
- Suspicion of primary source
- Presence of single or multiple abscesses
- Patient's underlying medical conditions (e.g., HIV, immunocompromised)
  Selection of empiric antibiotic therapy:
- Primary infection or contiguous source:
  1. Otitis media/mastoiditis, sinusitis: third-generation cephalosporin (cefotaxime 2 g q4h IV or ceftriaxone 2 g q12h IV) plus metronidazole 15 mg/kg IV as a loading dose, then 7.5 mg/kg q8h IV, not to exceed 4 g per day
  2. Dental infection: penicillin G (20 million to 24 million units per day IV in six divided doses) plus metronidazole (dose as above)
  3. Head trauma: third- or fourth-generation cephalosporin (cefotaxime 2 g IV q4h or ceftriaxone 2 g IV q12h or cefepime 2 g IV q8h) plus vancomycin (30 mg/kg IV in two divided doses adjusted for renal function)
  4. Postoperative neurosurgery: vancomycin (dose as above) plus ceftazidime (2 g IV q8h) or cefepime (2 g IV q8h), or meropenem (1 g IV q8h). Replace vancomycin with nafcillin (2g IV q4h) if susceptibility testing reveals methicillin-sensitive *Staphylococcus aureus.*
- Hematogenous spread (congenital heart disease, endocarditis, urinary tract, lung, intraabdominal): vancomycin (empiric therapy, dose as above) or nafcillin (if susceptibility testing reveals methicillin-sensitive *S. aureus,* dose as above) plus metronidazole plus third-generation cephalosporin (cefotaxime 2 g IV q4h or ceftriaxone 2 g IV q12h). Antibiotic therapy can be adjusted based on the etiology of the underlying infection, if known.
- HIV infected or immunocompromised patient: metronidazole plus a third-generation cephalosporin, antifungal, or antiparasitic agent
  Duration of antibiotic therapy is guided by the clinical course and by whether the abscess was surgically aspirated or excised; it is usually prolonged. Most recommend parenteral treatment for at least 4 to 8 weeks, with serial neuroimaging to ensure adequate resolution. (Imaging weekly could be considered for first 2 weeks of therapy, then every 2 weeks until resolution.) Surgical therapy may be required for clinical failure (i.e., increasing size of abscess on imaging despite antibiotic therapy).

SURGICAL Rx

- Three indications for surgical intervention:
  1. Collect specimens for culture and sensitivity
  2. Reduce mass effect
  3. Clinical failure with antibiotic therapy alone
- Stereotactic biopsy or aspirate of the abscess if surgically feasible
- Essential to selection of targeted antimicrobial coverage

- Timing and choice of surgery depends on:
  - Primary infection source
  - Number and location of the abscesses
  - Whether the procedure is diagnostic or therapeutic
  - Neurologic status of the patient

DISPOSITION

- Prompt diagnostic consideration, early institution of appropriate antimicrobial therapy, and advanced neuroradiologic imaging have reduced the mortality rate from brain abscesses from 40% to 80% in the preantibiotic era to 10% to 20% at present.
- Morbidity is usually manifest as persistent neurologic sequelae (seizures, intellectual or behavioral impairment, motor deficits).

REFERRAL

Consultation with a neurosurgeon is mandatory.

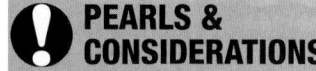

❗ PEARLS & CONSIDERATIONS

COMMENTS

- It is important to maintain a high index of suspicion because a brain abscess often presents with nonspecific symptoms.
- Rapid imaging and early institution of appropriate antimicrobial therapy improve patient morbidity and mortality.
- Neurosurgical consultation is mandatory.

PREVENTION

Because brain abscesses arise from either contiguous infections or hematogenously from a remote site, early and appropriate treatment of predisposing infections is paramount to prevent brain abscess.

SUGGESTED READINGS
Available at www.expertconsult.com

RELATED CONTENT
Brain Abscess (Patient Information)

AUTHOR: **ERICA HARDY, M.D., M.M.S.**

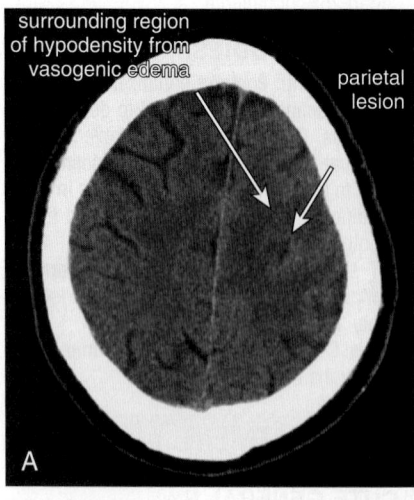
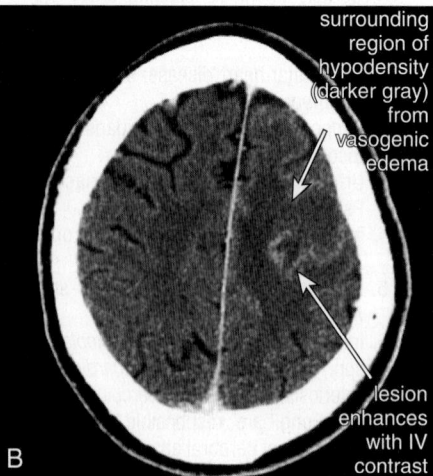

FIG. 1 Brain abscess. This 48-year-old male presented with status epilepticus. Computed tomography (CT) of the brain showed a parietal mass, which at brain biopsy was found to be an abscess. Cultures grew mixed gram-positive and gram-negative organisms and anaerobes. The patient was subsequently found to be human immunodeficiency virus positive. **A,** Noncontrast head CT, brain windows. **B,** CT with intravenous (IV) contrast moments later, brain windows. Abscesses and other infectious, inflammatory, or neoplastic lesions typically have surrounding hypodense regions representing vasogenic edema. When IV contrast is administered **(B),** the lesion may enhance peripherally, often referred to as ring enhancement. (From Broder JS: *Diagnostic imaging for the emergency physician,* Philadelphia, 2011, Saunders.)

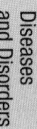
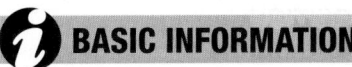

BASIC INFORMATION

DEFINITION

Brain metastases result from a spread of cancers originating in other organs to the brain and are devastating complications of cancer. Brain metastases are the most common intracranial tumors in adults and account for more than one half of brain tumors.

SYNONYMS

ICD-10CM CODES	
C80.0	Disseminated malignant neoplasm, unspecified
C80.9	Malignant neoplasm, unspecified
C79.89	Secondary malignant neoplasm of other specified sites

EPIDEMIOLOGY & DEMOGRAPHICS

INCIDENCE:

- Accurate data on the incidence of metastatic brain disease are not available. Population studies based on review of epidemiological data show an overall incidence of 8.3 to 14.3 per 100,000 population per year. However, these studies underestimate the true incidence of brain metastases because they rely on historical data from times when diagnostic imaging was poor. Autopsy-based studies are thought to show higher incidence of brain metastases because they identify asymptomatic brain metastases. However, autopsy-based data are now more than 20 years old. Ultimately, the incidence of metastatic brain malignancy is rising, likely due to improved detection and better control of extracerebral disease.
- In the U.S., an estimated 98,000 to 170,000 new cases occur each year, representing 24% to 45% of all cancer patients. The incidence is higher in autopsy series, where 20% of patients with systemic disease have brain metastases.

PREDOMINANT SEX AND AGE:

- In patients with systemic malignancies, brain metastases occur in 10% to 30% of adults and 6% to 10% of children. Of these, about 60% of patients are between the ages of 50 and 70 years.
- There is no definite gender predilection. Some data indicate that metastatic brain malignancy has a higher incidence in men because men have a higher incidence of primary lung cancer.

RISK FACTORS

- In adults, the cumulative incidence (CI) of metastases to the brain depends on the type of primary cancer as follows: lung cancer (16%-20% CI), renal cell carcinoma (7%-10% CI), melanoma (7% CI), breast cancer (5% CI), and colorectal cancers (1%-2% CI). Lymphoma is also known to metastasize to the brain. These metastatic lesions may or may not be present at the patient's initial presentation. The majority of patients with

metastases to the brain have greater than one metastasis. The cancers with the highest association of intracranial hemorrhage include renal cell carcinoma, melanoma, and the less common malignancies of thyroid carcinoma and choriocarcinoma.
- In children, metastatic disease is uncommon. The most common primary pediatric solid tumors associated with metastatic spread include sarcomas, neuroblastoma, and germ cell tumors. Leukemias are well known to seed the CNS. Metastatic disease is usually never seen when a child first presents with malignancy, with the occasional exception of leukemia. For solid tumors, metastatic disease is seen at the time of disease recurrence. Neuroblastoma CNS lesions have an association of tumoral hemorrhage.

PHYSICAL FINDINGS & CLINICAL PRESENTATION

- Clinical presentations vary depending on where the lesion is located. Brain metastases should be suspected in any cancer patient who develops acute neurologic signs or symptoms. Neurologic symptoms, however, are common in patients with systemic cancer. In an analysis of more than 800 patients with neurologic symptoms, brain metastases were found in only 16%.
- Symptoms:
  1. Headache occurs in 40% to 50% of patients with brain metastases. Frequency is higher with metastases located in the posterior fossa, which may result in obstructive hydrocephalus. The headache can be accompanied by nausea, vomiting, focal neurologic signs, and postural variation.
  2. Focal neurologic signs/symptoms are the presenting symptom in 20% to 40% of patients. Hemiparesis is the most frequent complaint. However, the specific neurologic dysfunction depends on the location of the brain metastases.
  3. Cognitive dysfunction, including memory problems or mood or personality changes, is the presenting problem in 30% to 45% of patients.
  4. Seizures are the presenting symptom for 10% to 20% of patients with metastatic brain tumors and indicate supratentorial metastases.
  5. Acute stroke secondary to hemorrhage into a metastasis, hypercoagulability, or local vascular invasion accounts for 5% to 10% of patients.

ETIOLOGY

The most common mechanism of metastasis to the brain is by hematogenous spread. The most common location is at the junction of the gray and white matter and metastases are more frequently seen in the cerebral hemispheres (almost 80%). The blood vessels decrease in diameter in these regions, which is thought to act like a trap for clumps of tumor cells. Different tumor types have a tendency to metastasize to different regions of the brain. For example, metastases of small cell lung carcinoma are equally distributed in all regions, whereas pelvic (prostate and uterine) and gastrointestinal tumors more commonly metastasize to the posterior fossa.

DIAGNOSIS

DIFFERENTIAL DIAGNOSIS

- Primary brain tumor
- Infection: bacterial abscess or fungal disease
- Progressive multifocal leukoencephalopathy
- Demyelinating disease: multiple sclerosis, postinfectious encephalomyelitis
- Cerebral infarction or bleeding
- Effects of treatment, such as radiation necrosis

LABORATORY TESTS

- Routine laboratory studies are not typically helpful.
- Lumbar puncture is generally contraindicated due to increased intracranial pressure and risk of herniation.
- Brain biopsy is necessary in some cases for a definitive diagnosis, particularly in the case of unknown primary tumor. Illustrating this is a study of cancer patients with solitary brain lesions that were presumed to be metastatic disease; in about 10% of study participants, the lesions were proved to be a different pathology.

IMAGING STUDIES

- MRI (Fig. 1) with and without contrast is the imaging study of choice. Important features on MRI that suggest brain metastases include: presence of multiple lesions, localization at the junction of the gray and white matter, circumscribed margins, or large amounts of vasogenic edema. CT of the head with contrast (Fig. E2) can be used when MRI is contraindicated.

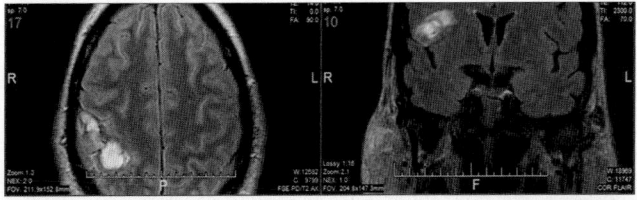

FIG. 1 Brain magnetic resonance imaging (axial and coronal fluid-attenuated inversion recovery sequences) showing hemorrhagic metastatic deposition in the inferior right frontoparietal lobe (lobulated high signal focus) in a 40-year-old woman with metastatic choriocarcinoma to the brain. (From Fielding JR et al: *Gynecologic imaging*, Philadelphia, 2011, Saunders.)

- MR spectroscopy and PET are useful to delineate tumor from other space-occupying lesions or from radiation necrosis.
- Newer experimental imaging studies, such as receptor-targeted and ligand-based molecular imaging, are on the horizon.
- In about 80% of patients, brain metastases develop after the diagnosis of systemic cancer. In the remaining patients, brain metastases are diagnosed simultaneously or before the primary tumor is found. In patients without a known primary tumor, the lung should be the primary focus of evaluation by chest radiograph and then CT scan. Other frequent sites include melanoma, colon cancer, and breast cancer. PET scan may be useful in these patients to help identify the primary tumor or to identify other sites of metastatic disease—these latter sites might also be more amenable to biopsy.

Rx TREATMENT

- Management of patients with brain metastases is influenced by the overall prognosis and may include treatments targeted at the metastases, management and prevention of complications (seizures, edema), and treatment of systemic malignancy, where appropriate.
- In patients considered to have a favorable prognosis (i.e., one to three metastases, good Karnofsky performance score, and controlled or absent systemic disease), treatment focuses on surgical resection and stereotactic radiation to eradicate or control the brain metastases. Whole-brain radiation (WBRT) is widely used but has significant side effects. A study through the European Organisation for Research and Treatment of Cancer (EORTC), along with prior randomized studies, has shown the addition of WBRT did not improve overall survival but seemed to reduce the rates of disease relapse. A meta-analysis of five randomized controlled trials found that WBRT decreased the relative risk of intracranial disease progression at 1 year by 53% but did not improve survival. Additionally, the individuals who did not receive WBRT after stereotactic radiosurgery or surgery had better quality of life scores. Unfortunately, few patients with metastatic disease are able to meet inclusion criteria for such studies.
- In patients with poor prognosis, treatment focuses on symptom control and WBRT.

ACUTE GENERAL Rx

- Steroids are used to reduce peritumoral edema and intracranial pressure.
- Antiepileptics are started for patients who present with seizures. Prophylactic treatment for seizure is not indicated in patients without prior history of seizure.
- Anticoagulants are sometimes used to prevent venous thromboembolic disease.

CHRONIC Rx

- Radiation therapy has become the mainstay of treatment for brain metastases, including whole brain radiation therapy and stereotactic radiosurgery (SRS).
- For highly chemosensitive tumors, chemotherapy has been integrated into the primary management of patients with disseminated disease.
- For other tumors (e.g., small cell and non-small cell lung cancers, breast cancer, melanoma) systemic chemotherapy or molecularly targeted agents may be of palliative value when surgery, whole brain radiation therapy, and SRS have failed or are inappropriate. In most cases, two to three agents in combination and in conjunction with whole brain radiation therapy are used. A phase II trial has shown combination treatment of lapatinib, an epidermal growth factor receptor inhibitor (EGFR-inhibitor), and capecitabine, an antimetabolite prodrug that is converted to 5-fluorouracil, as active for first-line treatment of *HER2*-positive breast brain metastases. Another phase II trial showed sagopilone (low-molecular-weight epothilone B analogue) as showing modest activity in patients with metastatic breast cancer. Additionally, dabrafenib, a tyrosine kinase inhibitor of BRAF, had some activity and acceptable safety profile for metastatic melanoma with BRAF^{V600E} mutations. Ipilimumab, a monoclonal antibody against cytotoxic T-lymphocyte antigen 4, was used for patients with metastatic melanoma and showed an improved median overall survival of 7 months in clinically asymptomatic lesions and 3.7 months in patients with neurologic symptoms. There are also other reports of its efficacy.

DISPOSITION

- The median survival of patients who receive supportive care and are treated with corticosteroids only is approximately 1 to 2 months.
- Key prognostic factors are performance status, extent of systemic disease, and age. Most favorable outcome is found in patients with Karnofsky performance score ≥70, age younger than 70 years, no systemic disease or local control of primary tumor without extracranial metastases, and female gender. In this group, median survival is estimated at 7.1 months.

REFERRAL

Treatment involves a multispecialty team. Consultations from oncology, neurosurgery, neurology, radiation oncology, psychiatry, and physical therapy are all warranted.

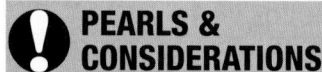

PEARLS & CONSIDERATIONS

COMMENTS

- Brain metastases are the most common intracranial tumors in adults, accounting for more than half of all brain tumors.
- Lung cancer, melanoma, renal cell carcinoma, and breast cancer are the most common primary tumors that metastasize to the brain.
- MRI is the most reliable imaging modality.
- Patient treatment depends upon the overall prognosis.

PATIENT/FAMILY EDUCATION

American Brain Tumor Association (http://www.abta.org)

National Brain Tumor Society (http://www.braintumor.org)

SUGGESTED READINGS

Available at www.expertconsult.com

RELATED CONTENT

Brain Cancer (Patient Information)

AUTHORS: **A. BASIT KHAN, B.A., JOSEPH S. KASS, M.D., J.D.,** and **NICOLE J. ULLRICH, M.D., PH.D.**

BASIC INFORMATION

DEFINITION

Brain neoplasms are a diverse group of primary (nonmetastatic) tumors arising from one of many different cell types within the central nervous system (CNS). Specific tumor subtypes and prognosis depend on the tumor cell of origin and pattern of growth. The diffuse low-grade gliomas (LGGs) include World Health Organization Grade II astrocytomas, oligodendrogliomas, and oligoastrocytomas.

SYNONYMS

Low-grade glioma (LGG)
Glioneuronal tumor
Meningioma
Primary brain tumor

ICD-10CM CODES
D33.2 Benign neoplasm of brain, unspecified

EPIDEMIOLOGY & DEMOGRAPHICS

INCIDENCE: U.S. incidence rate of a new brain tumor is approximately 6.4/100,000 persons per yr for all primary brain tumors (Table 1). One third of these are considered malignant and the remainder benign or borderline malignant. The incidence rate in children aged 0 to 19 years is lower (5.6 per 100,000 children). Primary brain neoplasms account for ~2% of all cancers, with a disproportionate share of cancer morbidity and mortality. It is the most common cause of cancer death in children up to 15 yr.
PEAK INCIDENCE: Depends on histology, though highest peak at ~age 50 yr
PREDOMINANT SEX AND AGE: Slight male predominance of malignant brain tumors (8.0 vs. 5.5/100,000 person/yr). Men account for slightly less than half of cases of both benign and malignant brain tumors, as meningiomas have a higher incidence in women.

GENETICS: Most primary CNS neoplasms are sporadic; 5% is associated with hereditary syndromes that predispose to neoplasia. The most common of these include:
- Li-Fraumeni syndrome: *p53* mutation on chromosome 17q13, gliomas
- Von Hippel-Lindau: VHL, chromosome 3p25, hemangioblastoma
- Tuberous sclerosis: TSC1/TSC2 (chromosome 9q34/16p13), subependymal giant cell astrocytoma
- Neurofibromatosis type 1: NF1, chromosome 17q11, neurofibroma, optic nerve glioma, low-grade glioma
- Neurofibromatosis type 2: NF2, chromosome 22q12, schwannoma, meningioma, ependymoma
- Retinoblastoma: pRB, chromosome 13q, retinoblastoma
- Gorlin's syndrome: PTCH, chromosome 9q31, desmoplastic medulloblastoma
- Hereditary nonpolyposis colorectal cancer (HNPCC): mismatch repair deficiency, high-grade gliomas

RISK FACTORS: Exposure to ionizing radiation has been implicated in meningiomas, gliomas, and nerve sheath tumors. No convincing evidence has shown a link with trauma, occupation, cellular phone use, diet, or electromagnetic fields.

PHYSICAL FINDINGS & CLINICAL PRESENTATION

- In general, the location, size, and rate of growth will determine the symptoms and signs of a brain tumor.
- Headache is common and is the worst symptom in nearly half of all patients. The headaches are usually dull, constant pain that is often worse at night. Symptoms of increased intracranial pressure may also be present, including nausea and vomiting, and may worsen with changes in body position that increase thoracic pressure (coughing, sneezing, Valsalva maneuver). Papilledema is suggestive of obstructive hydrocephalus.
- Seizures occur in 33% of patients and are among the most common symptoms, particularly with brain metastases and low-grade gliomas. The type of seizure and clinical presentation depend on the location of the brain tumor. Tumor-related seizures are typically repetitive and have similar presentation patterns. It is thought that patients with seizures typically have smaller tumors at the time of diagnosis compared with those with other symptoms, because the onset of seizures prompts an imaging study, leading to an earlier diagnosis.
- Focal neurologic signs and symptoms, including muscle weakness, sensory changes, or visual disturbances are also quite frequent. In addition, cognitive dysfunction, accompanied by changes in memory or personality change, may be recounted, often in retrospect.

ETIOLOGY

Most cases are idiopathic, though specific chromosomal abnormalities have been implicated in some tumor types.

DIAGNOSIS

- Diagnosis is typically based on clinical presentation and imaging characteristics. Specifically, neuroimaging is critical for preoperative planning and tumor etiology.
- Tumors are best seen on MRI; calcifications are sometimes present.
- Benign and low-grade tumors, typically in the glioma family, are heterogeneous and are generally seen as an infiltrating hemispheric lesion.

LABORATORY

- Ultimately, only histologic examination can provide the exact diagnosis. Additional features such as proliferative index, immunohistochemical stains, and electron microscopy can also be used to aid in diagnosis.
- The current classification schema for gliomas is based on pathologic and microscopic criteria. Tumor histology/histologic diagnosis (World Health Organization [WHO] grading system), includes number of mitoses, capillary endothelial proliferation, and necrosis. However, even tumors with benign histology can cause significant morbidity due to their location and effect on surrounding structures.
- Genetic analysis of tumors is rapidly becoming important for genetic classification, stratification of treatments, and predicting outcome. Different subtypes of gliomas have distinct gene-expression profiles, which can be distinguished from one another and from normal tissue; these differences typically involve pathways of cell proliferation, energy metabolism, and signal transduction. In adults, global expression profiling identified differences in 360 genes between low-grade and high-grade tumors.

TABLE 1 Frequency of Primary CNS Tumors

CHILDREN (0-14 YEARS)		ADULTS (≥15 YEARS)	
Type	**Percentage**	**Type**	**Percentage**
Glioblastoma	20	Glioblastoma	50
Astrocytoma	21	Astrocytoma	10
Ependymoma	7	Ependymoma	2
Oligodendroglioma	1	Oligodendroglioma	3
Medulloblastoma	24	Medulloblastoma	2
Neuroblastoma	3	Neurilemmoma	2
Neurilemmoma	1	Pituitary adenoma	4
Craniopharyngioma	5	Craniopharyngioma	1
Meningioma	5	Meningioma	17
Teratoma	2	Pinealoma	1
Pinealoma	2	Hemangioma	2
Hemangioma	3	Sarcoma	1
Sarcoma	1	Others	5
Others	5	TOTAL	100
TOTAL	100		

From Goetz CG, Pappert EJ: *Textbook of clinical neurology,* Philadelphia, 1999, Saunders.

DIFFERENTIAL DIAGNOSIS

- Stroke/cerebral hemorrhage
- Abscess/parasitic cyst
- Demyelinating disease: multiple sclerosis, postinfectious encephalomyelitis
- Metastatic tumors
- Primary CNS lymphoma

WORKUP

- Neuroimaging studies and pathologic sampling are the most important diagnostic modalities in evaluation of brain tumors and may be critical for preoperative planning.

IMAGING STUDIES

- MRI with gadolinium enhancement is highly sensitive and permits visualization of the tumor with relation to the surrounding tissue. Specifically, enhancing tumor can be distinguished from surrounding edema. Low-grade tumors often present as an infiltrating lesion without mass effect. MRI is superior to CT scanning for evaluating the meninges, subarachnoid space, and posterior fossa, and for defining relation to major intracranial vessels, although CT scanning is useful if calcification or hemorrhage is suspected (Fig. E1). Fig. E2 shows the appearance of astrocytoma in imaging studies.
- Magnetic resonance spectroscopy is increasingly being used as a diagnostic tool to help differentiate intracranial tumors from other intracranial processes using different chemical markers. For example, N-acetylaspartate is often decreased in brain tumors, whereas choline, a component of cell membranes, is often increased in brain tumors because of high cellular turnover.
- PET scan is helpful to distinguish neoplastic lesions (with high rate of metabolism) from other lesions such as demyelination or radiation necrosis (with a much lower metabolic rate). Such lesions take up greater amounts of glucose than surrounding tissues or tumors with slower metabolic rates. May be useful to help map functional areas of the brain before surgery or radiation.
- Functional MRI is now used as an adjunct in perioperative planning for patients whose lesion is in vital regions, such as those responsible for speech, language, and motor control.

Rx TREATMENT

NONPHARMACOLOGIC THERAPY

- Maximal surgical removal or debulking is the initial treatment of choice and provides tissue for diagnosis and molecular characterization. Maximal safe resection is often favored with a trend toward improved survival with this approach.
- Biopsy alone is performed if the tumor is located in eloquent regions of brain or is inaccessible; this is essential for histopathologic diagnosis. Biopsy can be performed under CT or MRI guidance using stereotactic localization.
- If the tumor is benign (e.g., meningioma, acoustic neuroma), often no further therapy is required.

ACUTE GENERAL Rx

Antiseizure medications have been used perioperatively and to control seizures resulting from focal lesions. Prophylactic use of anticonvulsants is not typically recommended without clear history of seizures.

CHRONIC Rx

- Chemotherapy (combination or single agent) may be used before, during, or after surgery and radiation therapy. In children, chemotherapy is often used to delay radiation therapy. A recent trial in patients with grade 2 glioma who were younger than 40 years of age and had undergone subtotal tumor resection or who were 40 years of age or older, progression-free survival and overall survival were longer among those who received combination chemotherapy in addition to radiation therapy than among those who received radiation therapy alone.[1]
- Radiation is useful for certain types of tumors and is often used if there is residual tumor after surgery; conventional radiation uses external beams over a period of weeks, whereas stereotactic radiosurgery delivers a single, high dose of radiation to a well-defined area (usually <1 cm). Long-term effects of radiation therapy include radiation necrosis (particularly of white matter), blood vessel hyalinization, and secondary tumors (usually meningiomas, sarcomas, and malignant astrocytomas). Radiosensitizers may help increase the therapeutic effect of radiation therapy.
- Experimental therapies are continually in development and target molecular characterization of tumors and small molecule blockers of signal transduction cascades involved in tumor growth. Some of these therapies involve antisense molecules, biologic agents, immunotherapies, or angiogenesis inhibitors. Intratumoral drug infusions and convection-enhanced delivery of novel agents are currently under study.

DISPOSITION

In general, younger age, high performance status, and lower pathologic grade have more favorable prognosis. For all histologic subtypes of brain tumors, pediatric and young adult patients have a better survival rate.

REFERRAL

- All cases warrant evaluation by an oncologist and neurosurgeon.
- Patients should be evaluated for physical and occupational therapy.
- Children should undergo neuropsychologic evaluations and screening for learning disabilities.

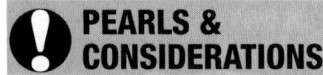 **PEARLS & CONSIDERATIONS**

COMMENTS

In general, younger age, high performance status, and lower pathologic grade have more favorable prognosis. For all histologic subtypes of brain tumors, pediatric and young adult patients have a better survival.

PATIENT/FAMILY EDUCATION

American Brain Tumor Association (http://www.abta.org)

National Brain Tumor Society (http://www.braintumor.org)

Pediatric Low Grade Astrocytoma (PLGA) (http://fightplga.org)

SUGGESTED READINGS
Available at www.expertconsult.com

RELATED CONTENT

Brain Cancer (Patient Information)
Astrocytoma (Related Key Topic)
Meningioma (Related Key Topic)

AUTHORS: **EMMA H. WEISS, B.B.A, NICOLE J. ULLRICH, M.D., PH.D.,** and **JOSEPH S. KASS, M.D., J.D.**

[1]Buckner JC, et al.: Radiation plus procarbazine, CCNU, and vincristine in low-grade glioma, *N Engl J Med* 374:1344–1355, 2016.

DEFINITION

Glioblastoma (GBM) is the most aggressive diffuse glioma of astrocytic lineage and corresponds to grade IV based on the World Health Organization's (WHO) Classification. GBM is the most common brain and central nervous system (CNS) malignancy, accounting for 45.2% of malignant primary brain and CNS tumors, 54% of all gliomas, and 16% of all primary brain and CNS tumors.

GBM represents a molecularly heterogeneous disease with numerous subclassifications. GBMs comprise primary and secondary subtypes that evolve through different genetic pathways, affect patients at different ages, and have differences in outcomes. Primary (de novo) GBMs account for 80% of GBMs and occur in older patients (mean age 62 years). Secondary GBMs develop from lower-grade astrocytoma or oligodendrogliomas and occur in younger patients (mean age 45 years).

ICD-10CM CODES
C71.9 Malignant neoplasm of brain, unspecified

EPIDEMIOLOGY & DEMOGRAPHICS

INCIDENCE: Based on the 2014 CBTRUS report, the average annual age-adjusted incidence rate (IR) of GBM is 3.19/100,000 population.

PREDOMINANT SEX AND AGE: GBM is primarily diagnosed at older ages, with the median age of diagnosis at 64 years. It is uncommon in children, accounting for ~3% of all brain and CNS tumors reported among infants to 19-year-olds. A higher incidence of GBM has been reported in men compared to women; the incidence rate is 1.6 times higher in males [3.97 versus 2.53]. Whites have the highest incidence rates for GBM compared to any other race in the US.

RISK FACTORS: Many genetic and environmental factors have been studied in GBM, but no risk factor that accounts for a large proportion of GBM has been identified. Like many cancers, the causes are sporadic. Factors associated with GBM risk are prior therapeutic radiation, decreased susceptibility to allergy, immune factors and immune genes, and some single nucleotide polymorphisms (SNPs) detected by genome-wide association studies (GWAS). There is no substantial evidence of GBM association with lifestyle characteristics such as cigarette smoking, alcohol consumption, drugs, or dietary exposure to N-nitroso compounds (cured or smoked meat or fish). Inconsistent and nondefinitive results have been published regarding the risk of glioma with use of mobile phones.

PHYSICAL FINDINGS & CLINICAL PRESENTATION

Patients present with a variety of symptoms, including headache, seizures, symptoms of increased intracranial pressure, and cognitive disturbances.

Dx DIAGNOSIS

IMAGING STUDIES

Initial work up includes imaging studies. MRI with and without contrast is the study of choice, and demonstrates a contrast-enhancing tumor. Functional MRI is now used as an adjunct modality in perioperative planning for patients whose lesion is in vital regions (eloquent regions), such as those responsible for speech, language, and motor control. Pathologically, GBM is a high-grade astrocytoma characterized by hypercellularity, mitotic activity, nuclear atypia, pseudopalisading necrosis, and microvascular proliferation. Various molecular markers have been identified that help distinguish it from other astrocytomas and between primary and secondary subtypes of GBM.

Rx TREATMENT

- GBM is an aggressive neoplasm which has a median survival of 3 months if untreated.
- Combined modality therapy with surgery, RT, and chemotherapy has significantly improved survival of GBM patients. Treatment is complex and initially consists of maximal-safe surgical resection followed by RT with concurrent temozolomide (TMZ) chemotherapy followed by six cycles of maintenance TMZ with tumor-treating fields.
- Surgical intervention has decompressive and cytoreductive effects, and there is increasing evidence of a significant survival advantage with complete resection.
- Various emerging treatment modalities under investigation seem promising, including immunotherapy. Regression of glioblastoma after chimeric antigen receptor T-cell therapy has been reported (see Brown CE, et al., in Suggested Readings).
- Symptomatic treatment includes corticosteroids to reduce cerebral edema, antiepileptic drugs for seizures, and painkillers for headache.

REFERRAL

Treatment involves a multidisciplinary team approach including oncology, neurosurgery, neurology, and radiation oncology.

PROGNOSIS

Survival: GBM has a poor prognosis with a low relative survival estimate; only a few patients reach long-term survival status of 2.5 years, and less than 5% of patients survive 5 years post-diagnosis. The relative survival for the first year after diagnosis is 35%, and it falls in the second year post-diagnosis to 13.7%, and continues to fall thereafter. Median survival of GBM post-diagnosis is 15 months following standard therapy. Several variables affect the prognosis of patients with GBM, including age, preoperative performance status, tumor location, preoperative imaging characteristics of the tumor, and the extent of resection.

Prognostic molecular markers in GBM: All GBMs are WHO grade IV but exhibit significant genetic heterogeneity, and tumor subtypes with genetic alterations exist within this larger homogeneous histologic category that carry prognostic significance. These markers include methylation status of the gene promoter for O^6-methylguanine-DNA methyltransferase (MGMT), isocitrate dehydrogenase enzyme 1/2 (IDH1/2) mutation, epidermal growth factor receptor (EGFR) overexpression and amplification, tumor protein (TP53) mutation, ATRX mutation and genetic losses of chromosomes.

- Primary GBMs show EGFR overexpression, phosphatase and tensin homolog gene (PTEN) mutations, and loss of heterozygosity (LOH) 10q, p16 deletions; less frequently shown are mouse double-minute 2 (MDM2) amplification, high frequency of telomerase reverse transcriptase (hTERT) promoter mutations, and absence of IDH1 mutation. The hallmark of secondary GBMs is TP53, alpha thalassemia/mental retardation syndrome X-linked (ATRX) and IDH1 mutations; additionally, they show LOH 10q.
- The MGMT promoter is methylated in approximately 50% of newly diagnosed GBMs. MGMT methylation is more common in secondary than primary GBM (75% versus 36%, respectively) and has prognostic and predictive significance of better overall survival in patients with GBM, irrespective of treatment choices.
- IDH1/2 mutations are far more common in grades II and III astrocytomas and oligodendrogliomas compared to GBMs, and more than 90% of the mutations involve IDH1. IDH1/2 mutations are a selective molecular marker of secondary GBMs, help distinguish them from primary GBMs, and are a marker of more favorable prognosis in high-grade gliomas.
- In GBMs, EGFR signaling promotes cell division, tumor invasiveness, and resistance to radiation therapy (RT) and chemotherapy. About 40% of all GBMs have EGFR amplification, and it is more common in primary as compared to secondary GBMs.
- Mutation of the *TP53* gene has been found in 60% to 70% of secondary GBMs and 25% to 30% of primary GBMs, and it occurs more frequently in younger patients. Studies of *TP53* mutations as a prognostic marker have not been definitive.
- *ATRX* is frequently mutated in grade II-III astrocytomas (71%), oligoastrocytomas (68%), and secondary GBMs (57%), but is infrequent in primary (4%) and pediatric GBMs (20%) as well as pure oligodendroglial tumors (14%). In a prospective cohort of patients with astrocytic tumors, those harboring *ATRX* loss had a significantly better prognosis than the ones that expressed *ATRX* and had IDH mutation.
- *TERT* mutation is one of the most frequent genetic alterations in primary adult GBMs and is significantly higher in these tumors as compared to secondary adult or any pediatric GBMs. GBMs with *TERT* mutation have a shorter survival than those without *TERT* mutations. However, when adjusted for GBM subtype (primary and secondary), they do not have a significant impact on survival.

SUGGESTED READINGS

Available at www.expertconsult.com

AUTHOR: **JIGISHA P. THAKKAR, M.D.**

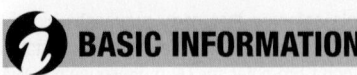

BASIC INFORMATION

DEFINITION

Breast abscess is an acute inflammatory process resulting in the formation of a collection of purulent material in breast tissue. Typically there is painful erythematous mass formation in the breast, occasionally draining through the overlying skin or nipple duct.

SYNONYMS

Subareolar abscess
Lactational or puerperal abscess

ICD-10CM CODES

O91.111 Abscess of breast associated with pregnancy, first trimester
O91.112 Abscess of breast associated with pregnancy, second trimester
O91.113 Abscess of breast associated with pregnancy, third trimester
O91.119 Abscess of breast associated with pregnancy, unspecified trimester
O91.12 Abscess of breast associated with the puerperium
O91.13 Abscess of breast associated with lactation

EPIDEMIOLOGY & DEMOGRAPHICS

INCIDENCE: 10% to 30% of all breast abscesses are lactational; acute mastitis occurs in 10% of nursing mothers, with one in 15 of these women developing abscess. A recent Cochrane review, however, found that as many as 30% of nursing mothers may have evidence of mastitis. Smoking and diabetes may be risk factors for nonpuerperal mastitis with abscess. More recently, nipple piercing may also be associated with infection.

PHYSICAL FINDINGS & CLINICAL PRESENTATION

Painful erythematous induration involving breast and leading to fluctuant abscess

ETIOLOGY

- Lactational abscess: milk stasis and bacterial infection leading to mastitis and then abscess, with *Staphylococcus aureus* the most common causative agent
- Subareolar abscess:
  1. Central ducts involved, with obstructive nipple duct changes leading to bacterial infection
  2. Cultured organisms mixed, including anaerobes, staphylococci, streptococci, and others

DIAGNOSIS

DIFFERENTIAL DIAGNOSIS

- Inflammatory carcinoma
- Advanced carcinoma with erythema, edema, and/or ulceration
- Tuberculous abscess (rare in the United States)
- Hidradenitis of breast skin
- Sebaceous cyst with infection

WORKUP

- Clinical examination. Fig. 1 illustrates the various areas where breast abscesses can develop.
- If abscess suspected, referral to surgeon for incision, drainage, and biopsy.

LABORATORY TESTS

- Perform culture and sensitivity test of abscess contents.
- If mammogram or ultrasound is required but prevented by discomfort, perform after treatment and subsequent resolution of abscess.

TREATMENT

NONPHARMACOLOGIC THERAPY

- Established abscess: incision and drainage
- Biopsy of abscess cavity wall to exclude carcinoma

ACUTE GENERAL Rx

- Antibiotics: generally staphylococci in lactational abscess. Recommended initial antibiotic therapy is nafcillin or oxacillin 2 g q4h IV or cefazolin 1 g q8h IV for 10 to 14 days. Alternative includes vancomycin 1 g IV q12h.
- If acute mastitis is identified and treated early without the development of an abscess, resolution without drainage is possible.
- Subareolar abscess: broad-spectrum antibiotic treatment (e.g., cephalexin 500 mg PO qid or cefazolin 1 g q8h IV for 10 to 14 days for more severe infection) and drainage (Fig. 1) are needed to control acute phase. If abscess is odoriferous, consider anaerobes as most likely etiology and add metronidazole 500 mg PO/IV tid.

CHRONIC Rx

Further surgical treatment for recurrences or fistula

DISPOSITION

- Lactational abscess: possible to continue breastfeeding without risk of infection to the infant
- Subareolar abscess:
  1. High risk for recurrence or complication of fistula formation
  2. Patient informed and referred to General Surgery for evaluation and treatment

REFERRAL

- If abscess drainage required.
- If subareolar abscess involved, refer to surgery.

SUGGESTED READINGS

Available at www.expertconsult.com

RELATED CONTENT

Breast Abscess (Patient Information)
Breast Cancer (Related Key Topic)
Mastodynia (Related Key Topic)

AUTHOR: **RUBEN ALVERO, M.D.**

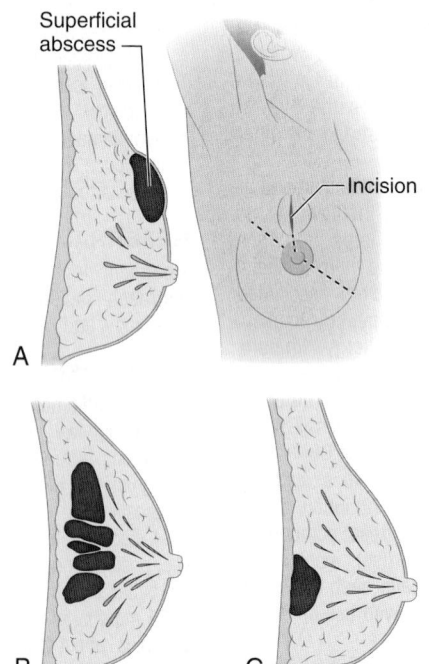

FIG. 1 A, A superficial breast abscess may be drained with a linear incision that radiates from the nipple. **B** and **C**, Diagrams of intramammary abscess (**B**) and retromammary abscess (**C**). Both require drainage under general anesthesia. The abscess itself may not be fully appreciated if it is deep seated, and the mistaken diagnosis of cellulitis may be made. (Redrawn from Wolcott MW: *Ferguson's surgery of the ambulatory patient*, 5th ed. Philadelphia, JB Lippincott, 1974. Reprinted with permission.)

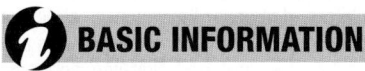

BASIC INFORMATION

DEFINITION

Breast cancer refers to both in situ and invasive carcinoma of the breast. Breast cancer can be of either ductal or lobular types.

SYNONYMS

Carcinoma of the breast

ICD-10CM CODES
C50.911 Malignant neoplasm of unspecified site of right female breast
C50.912 Malignant neoplasm of unspecified site of left female breast
C50.919 Malignant neoplasm of unspecified site of unspecified female breast
C50.921 Malignant neoplasm of unspecified site of right male breast
C50.922 Malignant neoplasm of unspecified site of left male breast
C50.929 Malignant neoplasm of unspecified site of unspecified male breast

EPIDEMIOLOGY & DEMOGRAPHICS

- In the U.S., there will be an estimated 249,260 new patients in 2016 and an estimated 40,890 deaths.
- The most common form of breast cancer is hormone-receptor positive; its incidence has increased particularly among young women. It is nearly exclusively the disease of women, with only 1% of breast cancers occurring in males.
- Table 1 enumerates risk factors for breast cancer.
- Genetically defined group of women with *BRCA-1* or *BRCA-2* genes identified to carry lifetime risk as high as 85%.

PHYSICAL FINDINGS & CLINICAL PRESENTATION

- Increasing number of small breast cancers are found by mammograms in which case patients are usually completely free of symptoms or physical findings.
- Palpable lump or mass which can be self-detected or physician-detected.
- Skin and/or nipple retraction and skin edema, erythema, ulcer, satellite nodule.
- Nodal enlargement in axilla and supraclavicular areas.
- Nipple discharge may be serous or bloody
- Generalized symptoms and signs, including fatigue, weight loss, jaundice, and anorexia, may be present in metastatic cases.

ETIOLOGY

- The precise mechanism of carcinogenesis is not understood. Endogenous and exogenous estrogen exposure is a key to the development of receptor-positive breast cancer.
- Breast cancer is no longer perceived as a single disease. Molecular classification based on gene expression profiling has shown breast cancer to be of the following types:
  1. Luminal A type: endocrine responsive with favorable prognosis
  2. Luminal B type: endocrine responsive with less favorable prognosis
  3. Normal type: resemble normal epithelium and prognosis similar to luminal B type
  4. HER-2 amplified type: HER-2 gene amplification
  5. Basal type: hormone receptor and *HER-2* negative cancers with poor prognosis
- Approximately 10% of all women with breast cancer have a germline mutation of *BRCA-1, BRCA-2, P53,* or other mutations.
- Possibly interaction of ovarian estrogen, non-ovarian estrogen, estrogens of exogenous origin with breast tissue of varied carcinogenic susceptibility to develop cancer
- Other known or suspected variables: childbearing, breastfeeding practice, diet, physical activity, body mass, alcohol intake

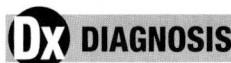

DIAGNOSIS

DIFFERENTIAL DIAGNOSIS

The following nonmalignant breast lesions can simulate breast cancer on both physical and mammogram examinations:
- Fibrocystic changes
- Fibroadenoma
- Hamartoma

TABLE 1 Risk Factors for Breast Cancer

Risk Factor	Relative Risk
Any benign breast disease	1.5
Postmenopausal hormone replacement	1.5
Menarche at <12 yr	1.1-1.9
Moderate alcohol intake (2-3 drinks/day)	1.1-1.9
Menopause at >55 yr	1.1-1.9
Increased bone density	1.1-1.9
Sedentary lifestyle and lack of exercise	1.1-1.9
Proliferative breast disease without atypia	2
Age at first birth >30 yr or nulliparous	2-4
First-degree relative with breast cancer	2-4
Postmenopausal obesity	2-4
Upper socioeconomic class	2-4
Personal history of endometrial or ovarian cancer	2-4
Significant radiation to chest	2-4
Increased breast density on mammogram	2-4
Older age	>4
Personal history of breast cancer (in situ or invasive)	>4
Proliferative breast disease with atypia	>4
Two first-degree relatives with breast cancer	5
Atypical hyperplasia and first-degree relative with breast cancer	10

From Goldman L, Schafer AI: *Goldman's Cecil medicine*, ed 24, Philadelphia, 2012, Saunders.

WORKUP

- Initial work-up:
  1. Mass assessment by medical professional.
  2. Diagnostic mammogram followed by breast ultrasound for suspicious lesions.
  3. MRI may detect suspicious lesions better than mammography alone in women with dense breasts or inherited predisposition to breast cancer.
- Diagnosis:
  1. Positive aspiration cytology on a clinically and mammographically suspicious mass is highly accurate, but it requires open biopsy confirmation.
  2. Stereotactic, ultrasound-guided core-needle biopsy procedures are accurate and have low complication rates.
  3. Excisional surgical biopsy establishes diagnosis.
- Breast radiologic evaluation and an algorithm for breast cancer screening and evaluation are described in Section III. The differential diagnosis of breast lumps is described in Section II.

STAGING

Table 2 describes the pathologic staging of breast cancer.

IMAGING STUDIES

Mammograms (Figs. 1 and E2): 30% to 50% of breast cancers are detected by screening mammograms as a spiculated mass, a mass with or without microcalcifications, or a cluster of microcalcifications. MRI is a modality that is particularly useful in patients with breast implants and when there is a strong family history of breast cancer. MRI is also better for assessing the response to neoadjuvant chemotherapy and is useful in identifying the primary tumor in patients who present with axillary adenopathy.

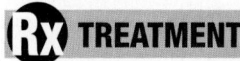

TREATMENT

NONPHARMACOLOGIC THERAPY

- These approaches include various types of surgical resection and reconstruction as well as adjuvant radiotherapy.
- For early breast cancer, the primary therapy is typically surgical. The choice is between modified mastectomy and breast-conserving treatment, which consists of lumpectomy, axillary staging with sentinel node biopsy, or axillary dissection.
- Table 3 compares ductal versus lobular carcinoma in situ. Adjuvant treatment guidelines for patients with early-stage invasive breast cancer are described in Table 4.
- Among patients with limited sentinel lymph nodes (SLN) who are treated with breast conservation and systemic therapy, the use of sentinel lymph node dissection (SLND) alone compared with axillary lymph node dissection (ALND) did not result in inferior survival.

TABLE 2 Pathological Staging of Breast Cancer*

Primary Tumor (pT)

pT0: No evidence of primary tumor

pTis (DCIS): Ductal carcinoma in situ

pT1: Tumor ≤20 mm in greatest dimension

pT1mi: Tumor ≤1 mm in greatest dimension (microinvasion)

pT1a: Tumor >1 mm but ≤5 mm in greatest dimension

pT1b: Tumor >5 mm but ≤10 mm in greatest dimension

pT1c: Tumor >10 mm but ≤20 mm in greatest dimension

pT2: Tumor >20 mm but ≤50 mm in greatest dimension

pT3: Tumor >50 mm in greatest dimension

pT4: Tumor of any size with direct extension to the chest wall and/or to the skin

pT4a: Extension to chest wall, not including only pectoralis muscle adherence/invasion

pT4b: Ulceration and/or ipsilateral satellite nodules and/or edema of the skin

pT4c: Both T4a and T4b

pT4d: Inflammatory carcinoma (a clinical-pathologic entity characterized by diffuse erythema and edema [peau d'orange] involving one-third or more of the skin of the breast; the skin changes are due to lymphedema caused by tumor emboli within dermal lymphatics)

Regional Lymph Nodes (pN)

pNX: Regional lymph nodes cannot be assessed (e.g., previously removed, or not removed)

pN0: No regional lymph node metastasis identified histologically

Note: Isolated tumor cell (ITC) clusters are defined as small clusters of cells not greater than 0.2 mm or single tumor cells, or a cluster of fewer than 200 cells in a single histologic section. ITCs may be detected by routine histology or by immunohistochemical (IHC) methods. Nodes containing only ITCs are excluded from the total positive node count for purposes of N classification but should be included in the total number of nodes evaluated.

pN0 (i-): No regional lymph node metastases histologically, negative IHC

pN0 (i+): Malignant cells in regional lymph node(s) no greater than 0.2 mm and no more than 200 cells (detected by H&E or IHC including ITC)

pN1mi: Micrometastases (greater than 0.2 mm and/or more than 200 cells, but none greater than 2.0 mm)

pN1a: Metastases in 1 to 3 axillary lymph nodes

pN2a: Metastases in 4 to 9 axillary lymph nodes

pN3a: Metastases in 10 or more axillary lymph nodes

Distant Metastasis (M)

pMX: Metastatic sites cannot be assessed

pM0: No metastases

pM1: Distant detectable metastasis

Stage Groupings in Breast Cancer

Stage	T	N	M
0	Tis	N0	M0
IA	T1	N0	M0
IB	T0-T1	N1mi	M0
IIA	T0-T1	N1	M0
	T2	N0	M0
IIB	T2	N1	M0
	T3	N0	M0
IIIA	T0-T2	N2	M0
	T3	N1-N2	M0
IIIB	T4	N0-N2	M0
IIIC	Any T	N3	M0
IV	Any T	Any N	M1

*AJCC 7th Edition

- DCIS: Local breast-conserving therapy (lumpectomy plus radiation therapy) or mastectomy followed by endocrine therapy in estrogen receptor-positive cases
- Invasive breast cancer: Mastectomy and sentinel lymph node evaluation *or* lumpectomy and sentinel lymph node evaluation plus whole breast radiation therapy
- Invasive breast cancer may require adjuvant endocrine therapy and chemotherapy. Endocrine therapy is recommended alone or after chemotherapy in patients with hormone-receptor positive tumors. Adjuvant hormone therapy with anti-estrogen drugs reduces disease recurrence and mortality in women with breast cancer. Aromatase inhibitors decrease the agonist effect of estrogen by inhibiting estrogen synthesis and have become preferred first-line hormonal treatment agents over the selective estrogen receptor modulator tamoxifen.
- Standard adjuvant chemotherapy regimens include first-generation regimens such as CMF (cyclophosphamide, methotrexate, and fluorouracil) and second-generation regimens such as AC (cyclophosphamide plus doxorubicin). Third-generation regimens such as ACT (standard doxorubicin and cyclophosphamide plus taxane) are also in routine use. Fig. E3 illustrates considerations for adjuvant chemotherapy in breast cancer.
- Neoadjuvant combination chemotherapy results in pathologic complete responses in significant number of cases, causes downstaging, provides an assessment of chemosensitivity, and provides no deleterious effect on survival.
- The benefit of adjuvant chemotherapy or hormone therapy can be assessed by commercially available multi-gene assays that have demonstrated utility in determining prognostic and predictive benefit with both hormonal therapy and chemotherapy in breast cancer.
- Metastatic breast cancer is approached based on the extent of bone-only or visceral disease sites as well as the rate of symptomatic progression. Typically, bone-only metastatic disease is approached with upfront, sequential hormonal therapy. The addition of the mTOR inhibitor everolimus or the CDK4/CDK6 inhibitor palbociclib to endocrine therapy has been associated with improvement in overall survival. Patients with progressive bone disease or those with visceral disease are treated with typically single-agent chemotherapy and occasionally with combination chemotherapy regimens. The chemotherapy agents are the same as those used in early stages of disease. Sequential chemotherapy with different classes of chemotherapy agents are usually used to provide palliation with improvement in survival and symptoms.
- Recent trials in patients with HER2-positive metastatic breast cancer have shown that the addition of pertuzumab to trastuzumab and docetaxel, as compared with the addition of placebo, significantly improved the median overall survival to 56.6 months and extended the results of previous analyses showing the efficacy of the drug combination.

CHRONIC Rx

Follow-up after treatment of early breast cancer stages includes:

- Regular clinical evaluations as delineated by medical oncologist or surgeon
- Annual mammograms and breast MRI as indicated
- Laboratory tests as indicated
- Tumor markers and CT scans for surveillance are not recommended
- Patient instruction in monthly breast self-examination

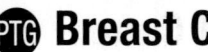

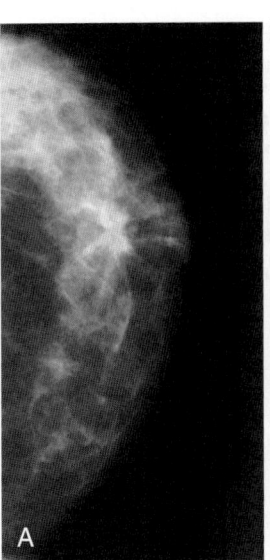 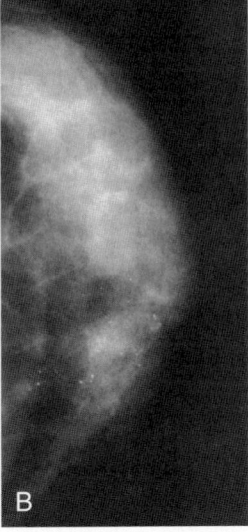 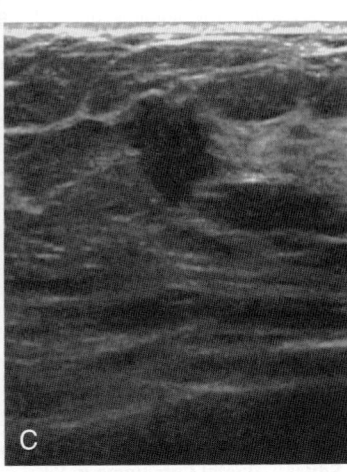

FIG. 1 Mammogram and ultrasound findings of breast disease. A, A stellate mass in the breast. The combination of a density with spiculated borders and distortion of surrounding breast architecture suggests a malignancy. **B,** Clustered microcalcification. Fine, pleomorphic, and linear calcifications that cluster together suggest the diagnosis of ductal carcinoma in situ (DCIS). **C,** An ultrasound image of breast cancer. The mass is solid, containing internal echoes, and displaying an irregular border. Most malignant lesions are taller than they are wide. (From Townsend CM et al [eds]: *Sabiston textbook of surgery*, ed 17, Philadelphia, 2004, Saunders.)

- Prognosis after curative therapy: depends on size of tumor, extent of nodal metastasis, and pathologic grade of tumor
- Systemic adjuvant therapy: improves prognosis significantly. Women who take tamoxifen for 10 yr lower their recurrence risk by 25% and their dying of breast cancer risk by 27% compared with those who took it for just 5 yr. Adjuvant therapy with an aromatase inhibitor improves survival outcomes, compared with tamoxifen, in postmenopausal women with hormone receptor–positive breast cancer. Recent trials have shown that in premenopausal women with hormone receptor–positive early breast cancer, adjuvant treatment with the aromatase inhibitor exemestane plus ovarian suppression, compared with tamoxifen plus ovarian suppression, significantly reduced recurrence.
- Isolated tumor cells or micrometastases in regional lymph nodes are associated with a reduced 5-yr rate of disease-free survival among women with favorable early-stage breast cancer who do not receive adjuvant therapy. Survival is improved in patients with isolated tumor cells or micrometastases who received adjuvant therapy.
- Retrospective analyses suggest that occult lymph-node metastases are an important prognostic factor for disease recurrence or survival among patients with breast cancer; however, recent trials indicate that the magnitude of the difference in outcome at 5 yr is small (1.2 percentage points). These data do not favor a clinical benefit of additional evaluation (including immunohistochemical analysis) of initially negative sentinel nodes in patients with breast cancer.
- The addition of zoledronic acid to adjuvant endocrine therapy improves disease-free survival in premenopausal patients with estrogen-responsive early breast cancer.

REFERRAL

Referral to a multidisciplinary team consisting of a breast surgeon, reconstructive surgeon, medical oncologist, and radiation oncologist is necessary as soon as breast cancer is suspected.

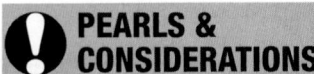 **PEARLS & CONSIDERATIONS**

BREAST CANCER IN PREGNANCY AND LACTATION

- Frequency in women 40 yr or younger reported to be 15%
- May carry worse prognosis because disease discovery delayed by engorged and nodular breast changes and/or because disease progression more rapid in pregnancy
- Survival rates similar to those for nonpregnant early-stage breast cancer patients in same age group
- Expedient workup recommended, including mammography and sonography
- Choice of mastectomy or lumpectomy with axillary dissection for treatment
- Adjuvant chemotherapy delayed until third trimester or after delivery
- Irradiation to breast after lumpectomy delayed until after delivery

DUCTAL CARCINOMA IN SITU (DCIS, INTRADUCTAL CARCINOMA) (SEE TABLE 3)

- Discovered by mammogram as cluster of microcalcifications and/or density
- Presents less often as a palpable mass or nipple discharge
- Before mammogram screening, DCIS accounted for 1% of all breast cancers
- Now 15% to 20% or even higher proportion have DCIS

- Treated with lumpectomy with cure rates 98% to 99%
- Higher-risk cases require breast radiation and adjuvant hormone therapy
- Mastectomy possibly required with multifocal and/or high-grade DCIS

INFLAMMATORY CARCINOMA

- Rare, rapidly progressive and often lethal form of breast cancer
- Presents as erythematous and edematous breast resembling mastitis
- Biopsy required, including that of the skin
- Treatment with upfront combination chemotherapy followed by surgery and radiotherapy
- Prognosis once dismal; now 5-yr disease-free survival approaches 50% (Fig. E4)

COMMENTS

- The U.S. Preventive Services Task Force (USPSTF) now recommends against automatic "routine" screening of younger women (age range 40 to 49). The task force recommends biennial screening mammography for all middle-aged women (age range 50 to 74). It also states that current evidence is insufficient to assess the benefits and harms of screening mammography in older women (aged 75 and older). The task force also discourages women from performing breast self-examination. Several other U.S. organizations, such as the American Congress of Obstetricians and Gynecologists, however, still recommend annual screening beginning at age 40 yr.
- The 2015 American Cancer Society guidelines for breast cancer screening are summarized in the following:
  1. Women with an average risk of breast cancer should undergo regular screening mammography starting at age 45 years. (Strong recommendation)
     a. Women aged 45 to 54 years should be screened annually. (Qualified recommendation)
     b. Women 55 years and older should transition to biennial screening or have the opportunity to continue screening annually. (Qualified recommendation)
     c. Women should have the opportunity to begin annual screening between the ages of 40 and 44 years. (Qualified recommendation)
  2. Women should continue screening mammography as long as their overall health is good and they have a life expectancy of 10 years or longer. (Qualified recommendation)
  3. The ACS does not recommend clinical breast examination for breast cancer screening among average-risk women at any age. (Qualified recommendation)
- Physicians should be familiar with the risks and benefits of various competing recommendations in order to better counsel patients.
- Breast radiologic evaluation, evaluation of nipple discharge, and evaluation of palpable mass are described in Section III.

- Exposure of the heart to ionizing radiation during breast cancer radiotherapy increases risk of ischemic heart disease. The increased rate of ischemic heart disease begins within a few years of exposure and continues for at least 20 yr. The increase is proportional to the mean radiation dose to the heart.

RISK REDUCTION STRATEGIES

- Prophylactic bilateral mastectomy reduces the risk for invasive breast cancer by > 90%.
- Selective estrogen receptor modulators (SERM) reduce the incidence of hormone receptor-positive invasive breast cancer by 50%.
- Ovarian failure is a common toxic effect of chemotherapy. Administration of the gonadotropin-releasing hormone (GnRH) agonist Goserelin appears to protect against ovarian failure, reducing the risk of early menopause and improving prospects for fertility.

(EBM) **EVIDENCE**

Available at www.expertconsult.com

SUGGESTED READINGS

Available at www.expertconsult.com

RELATED CONTENT

Breast Cancer (Patient Information)
Breast Cancer: For Men (Patient Information)
Breast Abscess (Related Key Topic)
Fibrocystic Breast Disease (Related Key Topic)

AUTHOR: **BHARTI RATHORE, M.D.**

TABLE 3 Carcinoma in Situ: Lobular Versus Ductal

Feature	Lobular Carcinoma in Situ	Ductal Carcinoma in Situ
Age	Younger	Older
Palpable mass	No	Uncommon
Mammographic appearance	Not detected on mammography	Microcalcifications, mass
Immunophenotype	E-cadherin negative	E-cadherin positive
Usual manifestation	Incidental finding on breast biopsy	Microcalcifications on mammography or breast mass
Bilateral involvement	Common	Uncertain
Risk and site of subsequent breast cancer	25% risk for invasive breast cancer in either breast over remaining lifespan	At site of initial lesion; 0.5% risk/yr of invasive breast cancer in opposite breast
Prevention	Consider tamoxifen or raloxifene	Consider tamoxifen or raloxifene if estrogen-receptor positive
Treatment	Yearly mammography and breast examination	Lumpectomy ± radiation; mastectomy for large or multifocal lesions

From Goldman L, Schafer AI: *Goldman's Cecil medicine,* ed 24, Philadelphia, 2012, Saunders.

TABLE 4 Adjuvant Treatment Guidelines for Patients with Early-Stage Invasive Breast Cancer

Patient Group	Treatment
Hormone Receptor-Positive and HER-2 Positive Breast Cancer	
<0.5 cm	Consider adjuvant endocrine therapy
0.6-1 cm	Adjuvant endocrine therapy Consider adjuvant chemotherapy and trastuzumab
>1 cm or node positive	Adjuvant endocrine therapy Adjuvant chemotherapy and trastuzumab
Hormone Receptor-Positive and HER-2 Negative Breast Cancer	
<0.5 cm	No adjuvant therapy
>0.5 cm	Adjuvant hormonal therapy Consider adjuvant chemotherapy based on 21-gene recurrence score
Node-positive	Adjuvant hormonal therapy + adjuvant chemotherapy
Hormone Receptor-Negative and HER-2 Positive Breast Cancer	
<0.5 cm	Consider adjuvant chemotherapy and trastuzumab
0.6-1 cm	Consider adjuvant chemotherapy and trastuzumab
>1 cm or node-positive	Adjuvant chemotherapy and trastuzumab
Hormone Receptor-Negative and HER-2 Negative Breast Cancer	
≤0.5 cm	No adjuvant therapy
0.6-1.0 cm	Consider adjuvant chemotherapy
>1 cm or node positive	Adjuvant chemotherapy

HER2, human epidermal growth factor receptor 2
Modified from National Comprehensive Cancer Network Guidelines. Available at www.nccn.org.

BASIC INFORMATION

DEFINITION

Bronchiectasis is an irreversible pathologic dilatation of the bronchi or bronchioles resulting from a variety of causes through an interplay of host factors (either anatomic or immune defense abnormality), respiratory pathogens, and environmental factors. Radiographically, it is often divided into cylindrical, varicose, and cystic varieties, although these variants have no significant etiologic or prognostic relevance.

ICD-10CM CODES
J47.0 Bronchiectasis with acute lower respiratory infection
J47.1 Bronchiectasis with (acute) exacerbation
J47.9 Bronchiectasis, uncomplicated
Q33.4 Congenital bronchiectasis

EPIDEMIOLOGY & DEMOGRAPHICS

- The exact prevalence of bronchiectasis is unknown.
- Cystic fibrosis is responsible for nearly 50% of all cases of bronchiectasis.
- Acquired primary bronchiectasis is uncommon because of rapid diagnosis of pulmonary infections and frequent use of antibiotics.
- Effective childhood immunizations have led to a significant decrease in the incidence of bronchiectasis resulting from pertussis.
- Declining incidence of pulmonary tuberculosis has also resulted in a decline in bronchiectasis without apparent causes.
- In developed countries, an increasing proportion of patients with an identifiable cause of bronchiectasis is being seen.
- Data on morbidity and mortality from bronchiectasis are limited because patients with the highest morbidity typically are not adequately represented in randomized controlled studies.

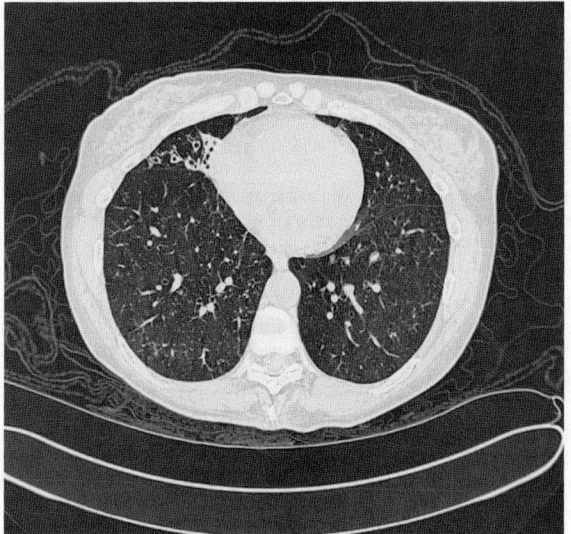

FIG. 1 High-resolution computed tomographic image of nodular bronchiectasis due to nontuberculous mycobacterium infection. (From Goldman L, Schafer AI: *Goldman's Cecil medicine,* ed 24, Philadelphia, 2012, Saunders.)

PHYSICAL FINDINGS & CLINICAL PRESENTATION

- Moist crackles at lung bases
- Chronic cough, typically with expectoration of large amount of purulent sputum
- Fever, night sweats, generalized malaise, weight loss
- Hemoptysis
- Halitosis, skin pallor
- Clubbing (infrequent)

ETIOLOGY

- Cystic fibrosis
- Lung infections (pneumonia, lung abscess, TB, nontubercular mycobacterial infections, fungal infections, viral infections)
- Impaired host defense (panhypogamma-globulinemia, primary ciliary dyskinesia/Kartagener's syndrome, AIDS, chemotherapy)
- Localized airway obstruction (congenital structural defects, foreign bodies, neoplasms)
- Inflammation (inflammatory pneumonitis, granulomatous lung disease, allergic aspergillosis)
- Rheumatoid arthritis, ulcerative colitis, and so on
- Congenital disorders such as tracheobronchomegaly (Mounier Kuhn syndrome), cartilage deficiency (Williams-Campbell syndrome)

DIAGNOSIS

DIFFERENTIAL DIAGNOSIS

- TB
- Asthma
- Chronic bronchitis or chronic rhinosinusitis
- Interstitial fibrosis
- Chronic lung abscess
- Foreign body aspiration
- Cystic fibrosis
- Lung carcinoma
- GERD

LABORATORY TESTS

- Sputum for Gram stain, culture and sensitivity, and acid-fast bacteria

- Complete blood count with differential (leukocytosis with left shift, anemia)
- Serum protein electrophoresis to evaluate for hypogammaglobulinemia
- Antibody test for aspergillosis
- Sweat test in patients with suspected cystic fibrosis
- Pulmonary function tests: mild to moderate airflow obstruction

IMAGING STUDIES

- Chest radiograph: hyperinflation, crowded lung markings, small cystic spaces at the base of the lungs.
- High-resolution CT scan of the chest (Fig. 1) has become the best tool to detect cystic lesions and exclude underlying obstruction from neoplasm with a sensitivity and specificity exceeding 90%. The CT study should be a noncontrast study with the use of 1- to 1.5-mm window every 1 cm with acquisition time of 1 sec. Typical findings on CT include enlarged internal bronchial diameter, bronchi appearing larger than accompanying artery, lack of tapering of an airway toward periphery, ballooned cysts at the end of bronchus, and varicose constrictions along airways.
- Bronchoscopy may be helpful to evaluate hemoptysis, rule out obstructive lesions, remove mucus plugs, and also obtain microbiologic data on respiratory pathogens.
- Table 1 summarizes diagnostic studies for the classification and management of patients with bronchiectasis.

TREATMENT

NONPHARMACOLOGIC THERAPY

- Postural drainage (reclining prone on a bed with the head down on the side) and chest percussion with use of inflatable vests/high-frequency chest wall oscillation or mechanical vibrators applied to the chest may enhance removal of respiratory secretions.
- Adequate hydration.
- Supplemental oxygen for hypoxemia.
- Inhaled hypertonic saline in conjunction with chest physiotherapy improves airway clearance.

ACUTE GENERAL Rx

- Antibiotic therapy is based on the results of sputum, Gram stain, and culture and sensitivity; in patients with inadequate or inconclusive results, empiric therapy with amoxicillin/clavulanate 500 to 875 mg q12h, TMP-SMX q12h, doxycycline 100 mg bid, or cefuroxime 250 mg bid for 10 to 14 days is recommended.
- Bronchodilators are useful in patients with demonstrable airflow obstruction.

CHRONIC Rx

- Avoidance of tobacco.
- Maintenance of proper nutrition and hydration.
- Prompt identification and treatment of infections.
- Pneumococcal vaccination and annual influenza vaccination.
- In patients with cystic fibrosis, using rhDNase and aerosolized antipseudomonal antibiotics should be considered.

- Specific immunoglobulin replacement in patients with selective immunoglobulin deficiency.

DISPOSITION
Prognosis is variable with severity of the disease and underlying etiology of bronchiectasis.

REFERRAL
- Surgical referral for partial lung resection in patients with localized, severe disease

unresponsive to medical therapy or in patients with massive hemoptysis. Surgical resection of localized bronchiectasis is safe and improves quality of life.
- Lung transplantation for bronchiectasis accounts for about 2% to 3% of all lung transplant candidates (*The Registry of the International Society for Heart and Lung Transplantation*).

SUGGESTED READINGS
Available at www.expertconsult.com

RELATED CONTENT
Bronchiectasis (Patient Information)

AUTHOR: **LAYOLA LUNGHAR, M.D.**

TABLE 1 Diagnostic Studies for the Classification and Management of Patients with Bronchiectasis

Test	Comments
Routine, Universal Studies	
Computed tomography lung scan (CTLS)	If bronchiectasis (BXSIS) is suspected, CTLS is the definitive test. Thin-section, high-resolution images may help detect subtle airway dilation before bronchial walls are grossly thickened. Contrast is generally not helpful and may, in fact, compromise the overall resolution of the study. CTLS may also identify esophageal abnormalities.
Pulmonary function tests (PFTs)	For patients with significant bronchiectasis, comprehensive PFTs, including spirometry, bronchodilator responsiveness, lung volumes, and diffusion capacity, are important studies that aid in management and prognosis. PFTs may also provide useful hints regarding predisposing conditions.
Complete blood count	Anemia may reflect effects of chronic infection or blood loss (consider inflammatory bowel disorders). Leukocytosis may mark severity of infection. Eosinophilia may suggest ABPA/M.
ESR, C-reactive protein	Nonspecific markers of inflammation; very high levels may suggest underlying connective tissue disease or vasculitis.
Routine sputum culture	Antibiotic therapy in bronchiectasis should generally be directed against specific pathogens and guided by in vitro susceptibility. The presence of mucoid strains of *Pseudomonas aeruginosa* and *Staphylococcus aureus* may raise suspicions for CF. *Stenotrophomonas maltophilia*, *Alcaligenes xylosoxidans*, and *Burkholderia cepacia* are gram-negative bacilli that may prove problematic pathogens in patients with long-standing bronchiectasis. Isolation of *B. cepacia* and *Helicobacter pylori* requires special laboratory techniques.
Mycobacterial sputum culture	Environmental mycobacteria such as *Mycobacterium avium* complex, *M. chelonae*, and *M. abscessus* appear to be increasingly common in contemporary bronchiectasis. May be commensal but often are pathogenic.
Fungal sputum culture	In patients with an asthmatic component, the presence of *Aspergillus* species (or other molds including Pseudallescheria or penicillium) may be suggestive of etiology.
CT scan of sinuses	Many patients with bronchiectasis also suffer chronic rhinosinusitis. The presence of extensive sinus involvement suggests possible CF, immunoglobulin deficiencies, or ciliary disorders. Also, optimal management often entails aggressive sinus care.
Specific, Directed Studies	
Sweat chloride, CF genotyping, and nasal potential differences	For bronchiectasis patients with bilateral disease, recurrent sinusitis, and no other identified risk factor, mild variants of CF appear to be relatively common. Sweat chloride is regarded as the primary screening test for CF, but a considerable portion of adults with CF have borderline or normal results. Nasal potential difference may be useful for identifying CF in equivocal cases.
Alpha$_1$-antitrypsin (AAT) levels and phenotype	AAT anomalies appear to be a substantial risk factor for bronchiectasis, especially with white females. Abnormal proteinase inhibitor (Pi) phenotypes, even heterozygous patterns such as MS, appear to confer risk even with normal levels of AAT. Repletion of AAT may enhance resistance to lower respiratory tract infections.
Immunoglobulin (Ig) levels	Deficiencies of IgG or IgA may promote bronchiectasis; IgG subclass deficiencies may also be a factor. Elevated levels of IgE may suggest ABPA/M or Job's syndrome. Hyper-IgM may be associated, as well, with chronic infections.
Ciliary morphology or function	For individuals with suggestive stories, a nasal ciliated epithelium biopsy with transmission electron microscopy may identify primary ciliary dyskinesia. Other studies including ex- vivo ciliary activity, the saccharine test, or spermatozoa analysis may aid in this diagnosis.
Nasal nitric oxide (NNO) levels	Patients with documented PCD have significantly lower levels of NNO than normal or patients with CF. Although not universally available, such testing may prove highly useful in identifying PCD. Paradoxically, exhaled NO levels have been elevated in bronchiectasis of diverse etiologies except CF.
Barium swallow (BaS)	The BaS may detect disturbed deglutition, esophageal diverticula, obstructing lesions (tumors or strictures), hypomotility, achalasia, hiatal hernias, or lower esophageal sphincter (LES) incompetence with reflux. The absence of reflux on a BaS, however, does not exclude this problem (see pH probe).
pH probe	For patients suspected of gastroesophageal reflux, an 18- to 24-hour study with a transnasal pH probe may identify, quantitate, and characterize reflux. Medications that inhibit acid production must be stopped before such tests.
Esophageal manometry	For patients being considered for surgical repair of the LES, manometry should be performed to determine that the esophagus generates sufficient pressure to propel food and liquids through the tightened sphincter.
Tailored hypopharyngography (TH)	TH is useful in detecting abnormalities of the initial phase of swallowing, deglutition. Persons particularly prone to problems include those with prior strokes, Parkinson's disease, bulbar disorders including postpolio syndrome, and those with prior laryngeal or pharyngeal surgery. Note that some patients have gross aspiration without clinical manifestations (choking, coughing); this may occur in individuals with none of the above risk factors.
Less Common, Exotic Studies	
Collagen vascular disease (CVD) serologies	Various CVDs may contribute to the risk for bronchiectasis, including RA, ankylosing spondylitis, and systemic lupus erythematosus. Thus, for patients with compatible histories or physical findings, assays for rheumatoid factor, HLA-B27, and ANA may provide insight into predisposing conditions. CVD serologies may also suggest the diagnosis of Sjögren's syndrome, particularly SSA/Ro and/or SSB/La.
Schirmer's test	For patients with histories suggestive of "sicca syndrome" (dry eyes, dry mouth, oral ulcers), a positive Schirmer's test may indicate the presence of either primary or secondary (associated with a CVD) Sjögren's syndrome.

ABPA/M, Allergic bronchopulmonary aspergillosis/other mycoses; *ANA*, antinuclear antibody; *CF*, cystic fibrosis; *ESR*, erythrocyte sedimentation rate; *HLA*, human leukocyte antigen; *PCD*, primary ciliary dyskinesia; *RA*, rheumatoid arthritis.
From Mason, RJ: *Murray & Nadel's textbook of respiratory medicine*, 5th ed, Philadelphia, 2010, Saunders.

BASIC INFORMATION

DEFINITION

Brugada syndrome (BRS) is an inherited disorder involving cardiac sodium channels characterized by typical electrocardiographic abnormalities. Patients with a Brugada pattern on ECG and symptoms such as palpitations, syncope, or sudden death are deemed to have BRS. BRS predisposes one to sudden cardiac death (SCD) secondary to polymorphic ventricular tachycardia (PVT)/ventricular fibrillation (VF) in the absence of structural heart disease.

SYNONYMS

Sudden unexpected nocturnal death syndrome (SUNDS)

ICD-10CM CODES
I49.9 Cardiac arrhythmia, unspecified
I47.2 Ventricular tachycardia

EPIDEMIOLOGY & DEMOGRAPHICS

INCIDENCE: The incidence ranges from 1 to 5:10,000 people in Europe and 12:10,000 in Southeast Asia.
PREVALENCE: It comprises 4% of SCD and 20% of SCD in structurally normal hearts. Although found in every population, the prevalence is much higher in Asian and Southeast Asian countries; in fact in some Southeast Asian countries, such as Laos and Thailand, it may be the most common form of natural death in younger males.
PREDOMINANT SEX AND AGE: BRS is more common in males (58% to 80% of patients). Mean age at presentation is 40 to 45.
GENETICS: The disease is autosomal dominant with variable expression (Table 1).
- *SCN5A*, the gene that encodes for the alpha subunit of the cardiac sodium channel, accounts for about 20% to 30% of cases of BRS.
- *SCN10a*, the gene that encodes the Nav1.8 subunit of the sodium channel, has been found in 17% of BRS patients, making it the second most common known mutation.
- Known genetic abnormalities are only found in half of patients; thus the impact of genetic testing is limited. When available, it may be useful in identifying silent carriers.
- In all genotypes, the basic abnormality is either a decrease in the inward sodium or calcium current or an increase in the outward potassium current.

RISK FACTORS:
- First-degree relatives with sudden death or known BRS

PHYSICAL FINDINGS & CLINICAL PRESENTATION
- Physical exam is usually benign.
- Classic ECG finding is a pattern of right bundle branch block (RBBB) with persistent ST elevation of cove-like morphology and T-wave inversion in the anterior leads (V_1-V_2)
- Often an incidental finding diagnosed from a typical ECG pattern

- Palpitations
- Nocturnal agonal respirations
- Syncope
- Sudden cardiac arrest (SCA)/SCD secondary to rapid PVT that frequently degenerates into VF more often at night
- Two ECG patterns were described. Type 1 is the most common and characteristic (Fig. 1).
- Type 1 ECG pattern is defined as an elevated ST segment ≥2 mm that descends in a coved pattern to an inverted T wave. This finding can be transient and may be provoked (sodium channel blockers, vagal maneuvers, increased alpha-adrenergic tone, beta-blockers, tricyclic or tetracyclic antidepressants, fever, hypokalemia, hyperkalemia, hypercalcemia, and alcohol and cocaine toxicity).
- Type 2 ECG pattern is not diagnostic of BRS but may be suggestive and warrant further testing. This pattern is a "saddle back" ST-T wave morphology with an upright or biphasic T wave. Type 2 (formerly known as types 2 and 3) can change to a type 1 pattern with the triggers noted above. Table 2 describes drugs used to unmask Brugada ECG pattern.

ETIOLOGY
- Autosomal dominant inheritance with variable penetration.

DIAGNOSIS

Diagnosis is made by the presence of a type 1 ECG and symptoms.
- ST segment elevation with type 1 morphology ≥2 mm in one or more right-sided leads (V_1-V_2), occurring either spontaneously or after provocative drug testing
- Type 2 ECG that converts into type 1 following sodium channel blocker (procainamide/flecainide/ajmaline) challenge (Fig. 1)

DIFFERENTIAL DIAGNOSIS

A number of diseases can lead to a BRS-like abnormality on the surface ECG, including the following:
- Atypical RBBB
- Early repolarization
- Acute pericarditis
- Acute myocardial infarction or ischemia

TABLE 1 Molecular Basis of the Brugada Syndrome

Disease	Gene	Protein	Ionic Current	Function	Inheritance
BrS type 1	*SCN5A*	Na$_v$1.5	Subunit alpha I$_{Na}$	Loss	Autosomal dominant
BrS type 2	*GPD1L*	G3PD1L	Interaction subunit alpha I$_{Na}$	Loss	Autosomal dominant
BrS type 3	*CACNA1C*	Ca$_v$1.2	Subunit alpha I$_{CaL}$	Loss	Autosomal dominant
BrS type 4	*CACNB2B*	Ca$_v$β$_2$	Subunit beta I$_{CaL}$	Loss	Autosomal dominant
BrS type 5	*SCN1B*	Na$_v$β$_1$/I$_{b1}$	Subunit beta I$_{Na}$	Loss	Autosomal dominant
BrS type 6	*KCNE3*	MiRP2	Subunit beta I$_{Ks}$/I$_{to}$	Gain	Autosomal dominant
BrS type 7	*SCN3B*	Na$_v$β$_3$	Subunit beta I$_{Na}$	Loss	Autosomal dominant

Issa ZF, et al.: *Clinical arrhythmology and electrophysiology: a companion to Braunwald's heart disease*, ed 2, Philadelphia, 2012, Saunders.

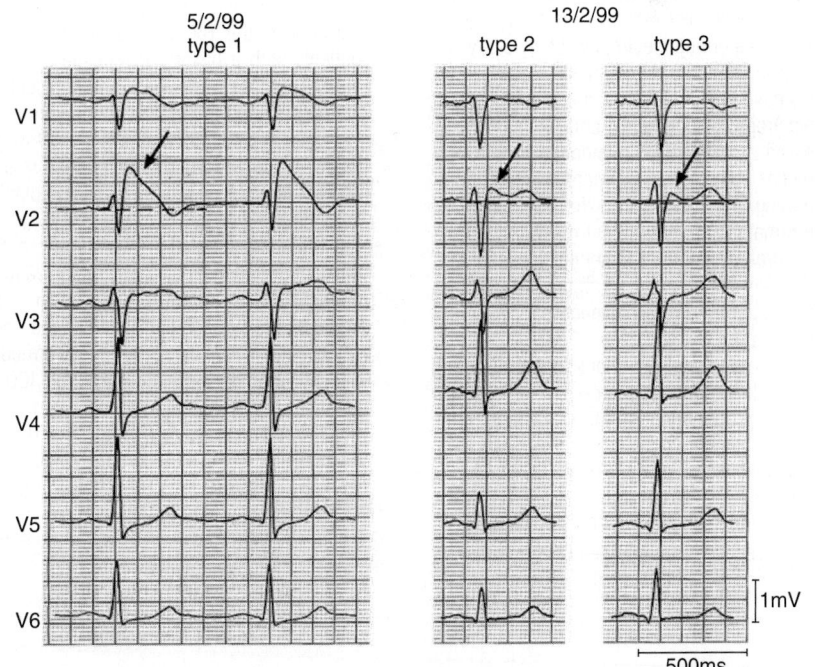

FIG. 1 ECG changes in Brugada syndrome. ST elevation occurs in the anterior precordial leads, leads V1 and V2. Type 1 (coved) ECGs with 1 mV of ST elevation have the most prognostic significance. (From Strickberger SA et al: AHA/ACCF scientific statement on the evaluation of syncope, *J Am Coll Cardiol* 47:473-484, 2006.)

TABLE 2 Drugs Used to Unmask Brugada ECG Pattern

Drug	Dose
Ajmaline	1-mg/kg IV infusion over 5 min
Flecainide	2-mg/kg IV infusion over 10 min, maximum 150 mg; or 400 mg PO
Procainamide	10-mg/kg IV infusion over 10 min
Pilsicainide	1-mg/kg IV infusion over 10 min

From Issa Z et al: *Clinical arrhythmology and electrophysiology*, ed 2, Philadelphia, 2012, Saunders.

- Pulmonary embolism
- Various central and autonomic system abnormalities
- Duchenne's muscular dystrophy
- Electrolyte abnormalities such as hyperkalemia and hypercalcemia
- Arrhythmogenic right ventricular cardiomyopathy
- Pectus excavatum

WORKUP

- Clinical history with special emphasis on syncope, palpitations, nocturnal agonal respirations, and family history.
- Echocardiography to rule out structural heart disease. While no structural heart disease is usually apparent, there are some recent reports indicating mild abnormalities in the right ventricle (RV) and left ventricle (LV).
- MRI, especially to rule out ARVC (arrhythmogenic right ventricular cardiomyopathy).
- Electrophysiology study. No consensus exists on the value of arrhythmia induction in predicting future clinical events in individual patients. However, findings such as HV (His ventricular) conduction interval >60 ms and VERP (ventricular effective refractory period) <200 ms during electrophysiology study can help in supporting a diagnosis. Repeated trials have failed to show a predictive power of electrophysiology study, and although it still exists as a IIb recommendation in the most recent consensus statement, the data supporting this practice are extremely limited, so it remains a matter of controversy.
- Laboratory tests are unhelpful. Genetic testing may be helpful for prognosis and family evaluation, but it is not necessary for diagnostic purposes.
- First-degree relatives should obtain ECG and be evaluated for symptoms.
- Risk stratification in the asymptomatic patient
- The following are considered indicators of high risk:
  1. Spontaneous type 1 ECG at baseline
  2. Presence of fragmented QRS on ECG

  3. RVERP (right ventricular effective refractory period) <200 ms on EPS
  4. Male sex
  5. Spontaneous atrial fibrillation

  Note that family history of sudden death is not considered a high-risk feature in BRS.

Rx TREATMENT

NONPHARMACOLOGIC THERAPY

- The only effective strategy that prevents sudden cardiac death in BRS is implantable cardioverter-defibrillator (ICD). Currently there are no class I recommendations for primary prevention because clinical events are extremely rare, even in high-risk patients. Fig. E2 depicts the algorithm for clinical decision making regarding recommendation of an ICD.
- Definitive candidates for ICD (class I) are patients who survived SCD or have had sustained VT (secondary prevention).
- ICD can be useful (class IIa) for patients who have type 1 ECG pattern in the absence of class IC drug test associated with history of syncope.
- ICD may be considered (class IIb) if there is inducible VF on electrophysiologic (EP) study, but the literature on EP study in patients with BRS does not support this practice.
- Patients with spontaneous type 1 ECG without syncope or inducible VF on EP study or asymptomatic patients with drug-induced type 1 ECG pattern are considered a lower risk group for SCD, and ICD is not indicated in these patients.

ACUTE GENERAL RX:

- Isoproterenol (class IIa) may be used for electrical storm.
- Quinidine, which blocks both Ito and IKr currents in the RV epicardium, is used in patients with a history of multiple appropriate ICD shocks, as well as for electrical storms and treatment of supraventricular tachycardia (SVT) in these patients. It is also useful in cases where the patient refuses an ICD implant or when an ICD implant is contraindicated.
- Radiofrequency ablation: There are a few published case reports of radiofrequency ablation of premature ventricular contractions (PVCs) leading to reduced clinical events. These have been performed in patients already implanted with an ICD. In addition, epicardial substrate ablation in the right ventricular outflow tract (RVOT) has been shown to prevent VF inducibility.

REFERRAL

Consultation with cardiology is strongly recommended if BRS is suspected.

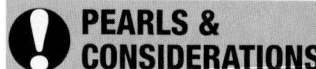 **PEARLS & CONSIDERATIONS**

COMMENTS

- The clinical manifestations, such as syncope and SCD, are rare in the pediatric group, but fever can acutely predispose to cardiac arrest. Mean age of presentation is 40 to 45 years.
- Cardiac events may occur during sleep, at rest, or after a large meal.
  BRS patients should be advised to avoid all drugs that may induce a type 1 ECG pattern and/or be known to trigger ventricular arrhythmias and avoid unnecessary use of drugs (a drug that is not yet identified as potentially dangerous for these patients does not make its use safe). For up-to-date information on this matter, a full list can be found at www.brugadadrugs.org.
- Fever may induce the appearance of a type 1 BRS ECG pattern and may trigger episodes of PVT/VF in BRS patients. In the case of fever, close ECG monitoring is appropriate in combination with lowering of the body temperature.
- The classic ECG changes in BRS can be transient with patients having normal ECGs in between highly abnormal ones.
- The appearance of syncope, seizures, or nocturnal agonal respiration must lead to prompt medical evaluation.
- Family screening for BRS in first-degree relatives is strongly recommended.
- Although participation in sports is not strictly prohibited, competitive training can lead to development of strong vagal tone and subsequent higher risk of clinical events. Hence, participation in sports at a competitive or professional level is not advised.
- Once diagnosed initially by an ECG pattern, all patients must be followed up on a regular basis by an electrophysiologist.

PREVENTION

Identification of patients with BRS, risk stratification, and appropriate screening of family members are paramount to the prevention of SCD. Patients with known BRS should have fevers aggressively treated with antipyretics and avoid drugs associated with drugs that induce a type 1 pattern.

PATIENT/FAMILY EDUCATION

Immediate family members should be notified and be screened for BRS.

SUGGESTED READINGS

Available at www.expertconsult.com

AUTHOR: **JOHN WYLIE, M.D**

BASIC INFORMATION

DEFINITION

Budd-Chiari syndrome (BCS) is an uncommon disorder defined by the obstruction of hepatic venous outflow anywhere from the small hepatic veins to the junction of the inferior vena cava (IVC) and the right atrium. Primary BCS is defined by endoluminal obstruction as seen in thromboses or webs. Secondary BCS occurs when the obstruction is caused by compression or invasion by a lesion originating outside the veins (tumor, abscess, cyst, etc.). It can also be a postoperative complication of orthotopic liver transplantation.

SYNONYMS

BCS
Hepatic vein thrombosis
Obliterative endophlebitis of the hepatic veins
IVC thrombosis (obliterative hepatocavopathy)
Chiari-Budd syndrome
Budd's syndrome
Chiari's disease
Rokitansky's disease

ICD-10CM CODE
I82.0 Budd-Chiari syndrome

EPIDEMIOLOGY & DEMOGRAPHICS

INCIDENCE: 1/2.5 million persons per yr
PREDOMINANT SEX: In Western countries, women are more commonly affected (approximately 2/3 of cases).

In Asia, men are slightly more affected.
PREDOMINANT AGE: In Western countries, presentation is usually in the third and fourth decades of life, with the median age being 35 yr.

In Asia, presentation is usually at a median age of 45 yr.

PHYSICAL FINDINGS & CLINICAL PRESENTATION

Clinical presentation and characteristics vary with geography. In Africa and South Asia, intravascular webs are more often associated with IVC thrombosis with a stronger association with subsequent hepatocellular carcinoma. In the United States, BCS is more commonly associated with primary myeloproliferative disorders and underlying hypercoagulable states. Underlying factors that contribute to BCS can be identified in ~85% of cases; multiple causative factors are identified in 50% of cases.
- Clinical manifestations can be caused by complete or partial occlusion of any or all of the three major hepatic veins or the inferior vena cava.
- Presentation is variable according to the degree, location, acuity of obstruction, and presence of collateral circulation:
  1. Fulminant/acute (20%): severe right upper quadrant abdominal pain, fever, nausea, vomiting, mild jaundice, hepatomegaly, transudative and intractable ascites, marked elevation in serum aminotransferases (ALT >5 times the upper limit of normal), elevation of alkaline phosphatase to 300 to 400 IU/L, increase

in the serum-ascitic fluid albumin gradient with total protein greater than 2.5 g/dl, decrease in coagulation factors, variceal bleeding, encephalopathy within 8 wk of onset of jaundice. Biopsy, if performed, would reveal hepatic necrosis. Early recognition and treatment are essential for survival; a slow decrease in ALT is associated with poor survival.
  2. Subacute/chronic (60%): vague abdominal discomfort, gradual progression to caudate lobe hypertrophy with atrophy of the rest of the liver, portal hypertension with or without cirrhosis and its sequelae, transudative ascites, lower-extremity edema, esophageal varices, splenomegaly, coagulopathy, hepatorenal syndrome in up to half of patients, hepatopulmonary syndrome in up to 28% of patients, and rarely, encephalopathy; biopsy, if performed, could reveal minimal hepatic necrosis.
  3. Asymptomatic (5% to 20%): usually discovered incidentally by abnormal liver function tests or imaging attained for other reasons

ETIOLOGY

84% have one prothrombotic risk factor, and 46% have multiple.
- Primary myeloproliferative diseases: 39% polycythemia vera, responsible for 10% to 40% of cases
  1. Essential thrombocythemia and idiopathic myelofibrosis are less common causes
  2. JAK2 mutations are implicated in cases of idiopathic BCS (identified in 30%-60% of cases)
  3. Rare but recently reported: idiopathic hypereosinophilia syndrome
- Hypercoagulable states (inherited and acquired) often coexist with other causes, 30% to 65%
  1. Anticardiolipin antibodies (15%-25%)
  2. Hyperhomocysteinemia (22%)
  3. Paroxysmal nocturnal hemoglobinuria (19%)
  4. Factor V Leiden (12%)
  5. Factor II gene mutation (5%)
- Protein C, protein S, and antithrombin III deficiency are difficult to interpret because the presence of liver disease may confound results. However, recent studies show that they account for 4.0%, 3.0%, and 3.0% of BCS, respectively.
- Heterozygosity for G20210A prothrombin gene mutation, methylene-tetrahydrofolate reductase (MTHFR) mutation, Tet methylcytosine dioxygenase 2 mutation, and calreticulin mutation may be seen in BCS.
- Pregnancy (6%) and oral contraceptive pills (33%; cases reported after <2 wk of use)
- Malignancy (up to 10% of cases, causing external compression or invasions of vascular structures)
  1. Most commonly due to hepatocellular carcinoma but also can be due to neoplasms of the kidney, adrenal gland, pancreas, stomach, and sarcomas of the right atrium, inferior vena cava, and hepatic veins
- Rare but reported: sickle cell anemia, infections with liver abscess, hydatid cyst

(echinococcosis), schistosomiasis, sarcoidosis, Behçet's disease, membranous webs of IVC or hepatic veins (more common in Africa and South Asia, can be congenital or acquired secondary to underlying myeloproliferative disorder), abdominal trauma, liver torsion, granulomatous venulitis, ulcerative colitis, celiac disease, systemic lupus erythematous, minimal change nephrotic syndrome, neurofibromatosis, alpha-1 antitrypsin deficiency, idiopathic (10%-20%)

DIAGNOSIS

DIFFERENTIAL DIAGNOSIS

- Hepatitis from ischemia, viral infection, toxin, alcohol
- Cholecystitis
- Hepatic venoocclusive disease (sinusoidal obstruction syndrome)
- Congestive hepatopathy, also known as cardiac cirrhosis, from tricuspid regurgitation, right atrial myxoma, constrictive pericarditis
- Cirrhosis from any etiology

LABORATORY TESTS

- Assessment of liver injury and function: serum aminotransferases, alkaline phosphatase, prothrombin time (PT), albumin, bilirubin
- Exclusion of another form of liver disease: viral hepatitis panel, autoantibodies (antinuclear antibody, anti–smooth muscle antibody, anti-mitochondrial antibody), serum iron, transferrin saturation, ferritin, ceruloplasmin, and α-1 antitrypsin
- Ascites protein content >3.0 g/dl and serum ascites albumin gradient ≥1.1 g/dl are suggestive of transudative ascites from BCS, cardiac, or pericardial disease
- Evaluation for underlying myeloproliferative disorder and hypercoagulable state: CBC, bone marrow biopsy, tests for hypercoagulable states (Factor V Leiden, prothrombin gene G20210A mutation, protein C, protein S, and antithrombin deficiencies, antiphospholipid antibodies, and paroxysmal nocturnal hemoglobinuria). Protein C, protein S, and antithrombin deficiencies may be difficult to interpret in the setting of liver dysfunction, but levels <20% of normal are suggestive of a true deficiency; thrombophilia screening for the JAK2 V617F mutation, hyperhomocysteinemia, and MTHFR C677T mutation may be useful if no other cause for myeloproliferative disorders/hypercoagulable states are identified.

IMAGING STUDIES

- Diagnosis of BCS is made by radiographic imaging.
- Ultrasound and color and pulsed Doppler are the first-line tests. Diagnostic sensitivity and specificity are 85% to 90%, respectively. Findings include large hepatic vein with an absent flow signal, or with reversed or turbulent flow; large intrahepatic or subcapsular collateral vessels; enlarged, stenotic, thickened, or tortuous hepatic veins; spiderweb pattern near hepatic vein ostia and associated absent flow in that region; caudate lobe

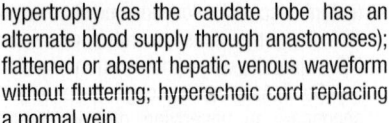

hypertrophy (as the caudate lobe has an alternate blood supply through anastomoses); flattened or absent hepatic venous waveform without fluttering; hyperechoic cord replacing a normal vein.

- MRI with gadolinium contrast is the second-line test. It is superior to contrast-enhanced CT (Fig. E1), with a sensitivity and specificity of approximately 90%. Findings include obstructed hepatic veins or IVC, large intrahepatic or subcapsular collaterals, and caudate lobe hypertrophy. MRI is beneficial to visualize the entire length of the IVC and distinguish between acute, subacute, and chronic BCS. Three-dimensional contrast-enhanced magnetic resonance angiography (MRA, see Fig. E2) rivals hepatic venography in sensitivity.
- Contrast-enhanced CT may reveal similar findings as Doppler ultrasound, as well as delayed or absent filling of the hepatic veins, parenchymal opacification of the liver, narrowing and/or compression of the inferior vena cava, and caudate lobe hypertrophy. Contrast enhancement localizes more centrally than peripherally and has a patchy and flea-bitten appearance. However, ultrasonography is more accurate than CT for detecting lesions in the hepatic veins and IVC.
- CT image reconstruction of vasculature is becoming available.
- Venography: not essential for diagnosis; it should be performed when other noninvasive imaging tests are nondiagnostic in the setting of strong clinical suspicion for BCS. Measurement of pressure gradients can help predict success of percutaneous or surgical shunt intervention and plan surgical intervention. Confirms the pathognomonic web pattern caused by collateral venous flow.
- Liver biopsy: not necessary to diagnose BCS but may be helpful in patients with cirrhosis in whom the diagnosis remains uncertain and is critical for differentiating from hepatic veno-occlusive disease or congestive hepatopathy. Findings include hepatic congestion, hepatocyte necrosis and fibrosis in centrilobular areas, and compensatory nodular regenerative hyperplasia with progression to fibrosis and cirrhosis. In advanced BCS, infarction caused by concomitant thrombosis of the intrahepatic, extrahepatic, and portal veins may be seen. There are conflicting studies regarding the association of histologic findings and prognosis.

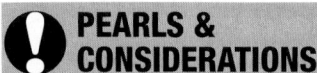 TREATMENT

NONPHARMACOLOGIC THERAPY
- Goal of therapy is decompression of hepatic congestion.
- In general, therapeutic procedures should be introduced by order of increasing invasiveness based on response/failure to therapy rather than disease severity.
- Hypercoagulable states should be investigated in all patients.

ACUTE GENERAL RX:
- Anticoagulation, first with low-molecular-weight heparin (LMWH), followed by warfarin, even in the absence of an underlying hypercoagulable disorder

- In situ thrombolysis: can be successful when performed in patients with recently thrombosed veins (clot less than 3 to 4 wk old) that are well defined on venography and do not involve the inferior vena cava or in patients with a large clot in the hepatic veins or intrahepatic vena cava. Mature clots are nonresponsive to thrombolysis, and bleeding risk is high if portal hypertension has developed.
- Balloon angioplasty: complicated by 31% to 50% restenosis rate; effective when membranous webs are the etiology.
- Stenting: may improve long-term patency rates to 90%, but if placed above the intrahepatic IVC, may complicate future liver transplantation.
- Transjugular intrahepatic portosystemic shunt (TIPS) has been increasingly used in recent years; usually performed in patients with no improvement on anticoagulation therapy or when a dilatable lesion cannot be found. TIPS has replaced surgical shunting as the most common invasive therapeutic procedure; recently, polytetrafluoroethylene (ePTFE)-coated stents have improved TIPS-patency rates, especially in patients with underlying hypercoagulable defects.
- Surgical portal systemic shunts: indicated when angioplasty and stenting have failed and when complications from portal hypertension are also present. This option does not have a survival benefit and is no longer common practice.
- Liver transplant may be indicated in patients with cirrhosis or fulminant hepatic failure and in patients who fail to respond to TIPS; 10-year survival is reported to range between 69% and 84%.
- Supportive measures

CHRONIC Rx
- Lifelong anticoagulation: Warfarin therapy with a target international normalized ratio (INR) of 2 to 3 lessens, but does not completely prevent, recurrence. Anticoagulation should be continued permanently unless the patient has an adverse event to anticoagulation, the obstruction is because of an anatomic cause that has been corrected, or anticoagulation is contraindicated.
- In patients with an underlying myeloproliferative disorder, first-line treatment is with hydroxyurea and aspirin.
- Treat liver dysfunction and complications related to portal hypertension, such as ascites and variceal bleeding (diuretics, low-sodium diet, and paracentesis if needed).
- Invasive interventions should be reserved for symptomatic patients who do not improve with medical therapy.
- Manage shunt thrombosis, which is a common complication.
- Liver transplantation is another treatment option; up to 27% recurrence of BCS after transplant has been recognized.
- Monitor for development of hepatocellular carcinoma and transformation of myeloproliferative disease in patients with longstanding, well-controlled BCS.

DISPOSITION
Prognosis is variable and depends on multiple factors, including time to recognition and treatment, etiology, acuity, the type of intervention, and the condition of the patient at the time of treatment. Overall mortality rates are decreasing with the use of anticoagulation and early diagnosis of asymptomatic cases. Given numerous therapeutic options, the survival rate is 87%, 82%, and 74% at 1, 2, and 5 yr from diagnosis. A prognostic index called the *Rotterdam BCS Index* has been described: $1.27 \times$ Encephalopathy $+ 1.04 \times$ Ascites $+ 0.72 \times$ PT $+ 0.004 \times$ Bilirubin. Encephalopathy and ascites are scored as 1 for present or 0 as absent, and PT is scored as greater (1) or less than (0) an INR of 2.3. An index of >1.1 correlates to low risk (5-yr survival rate, 89%), 1.1 to 1.5 with intermediate risk (5-yr survival rate, 74%), and <1.5 with high risk (5-yr survival rate, 42%).

REFERRAL
Fulminant presentations should immediately be referred to a center capable of liver transplantation. All cases benefit from referral to a hepatologist, a hematologist, an interventional radiologist, and a surgeon specializing in hepatobiliary disease.

❗ PEARLS & CONSIDERATIONS

COMMENTS
- Look for one or more underlying causes, especially hypercoagulable or hematologic disorders, and malignancies or space-occupying lesions that may compress or invade the hepatic outflow tract.
- Myeloproliferative disorders are most common.
- Diagnosis relies on imaging, beginning with Doppler ultrasound.
- Treatment with anticoagulation comes first, followed by invasive interventions as needed. Prophylaxis of portal hypertension can reduce the risk of major bleeding associated with anticoagulation therapy.
- Referral for liver transplantation may be necessary.
- Prognosis depends on the presence of ascites, encephalopathy, prothrombin time, and serum bilirubin levels.

PREVENTION
In the setting of known risk factors, such as a hypercoagulable state or myeloproliferative disorder, any additional risks, such as smoking or oral contraceptive therapy, should be avoided.

SUGGESTED READINGS
Available at www.expertconsult.com

RELATED CONTENT
Budd-Chiari Syndrome (Patient Information)
Hypercoagulable States (Related Key Topic)

AUTHORS: **JEANETTE G. SMITH, M.D.**, and
NICOLETTE J. RODRIGUEZ, M.D., M.P.H.

BASIC INFORMATION

DEFINITION

Bulimia nervosa is a prolonged illness characterized by a specific psychopathology. According to the *Diagnostic and Statistical Manual of Mental Disorders*, 5th edition, bulimia nervosa can be diagnosed by: (A) recurrent episodes of binge eating. An episode of binge eating is characterized by both of the following:

1. Eating, in a discrete period of time, an amount of food that is definitely larger than what most individuals would eat in a similar period of time under similar circumstances.
2. A sense of lack of control over eating during the episode.

(B) Recurrent inappropriate compensators/behaviors in order to prevent weight gain, such as self-induced vomiting; misuse of laxatives, diuretics, or other medications; fasting; or excessive exercise. (C) The binge eating and inappropriate compensatory behaviors both occur, on average, at least once a week for 3 mo. (D) Self-evaluation is unduly influenced by body shape and weight. (E) The disturbance does not occur exclusively during episodes of anorexia nervosa.

ICD-10CM CODES
F50.2 Bulimia nervosa

EPIDEMIOLOGY & DEMOGRAPHICS

INCIDENCE/PREVALENCE: Affects 1% to 3% of female adolescents and young adults
PREDOMINANT SEX: Female/male ratio of 10:1
PREDOMINANT AGE: Adolescence to young adulthood; mean age of onset: 17 yr

PHYSICAL FINDINGS & CLINICAL PRESENTATION

- Parotid and salivary gland swelling
- Scars on the back of the hand and knuckles (Russell sign) from rubbing against the upper incisors when inducing vomiting
- Eroded enamel, particularly on the lingual surface of the upper teeth; pyorrhea and other gum disorders possible
- Petechial hemorrhages of the cornea, soft palate, or face possibly noted after vomiting
- Loss of gag reflex, well-developed abdominal musculature
- Often no emaciation; normal physical examination possible

ETIOLOGY

- Etiology is unknown but likely multifactorial (sociocultural, psychological, familial factors).
- Bulimia is much more common in Western societies, where there is a strong cultural pressure to be slender.
- According to the American Psychiatric Association, patients with eating disorders display a broad range of symptoms that occur along a continuum between those of anorexia nervosa and bulimia.

DIAGNOSIS

DIFFERENTIAL DIAGNOSIS

- Schizophrenia
- Gastrointestinal disorders
- Neurologic disorders (seizures, Kleine-Levin syndrome, Klüver-Bucy syndrome)
- Brain neoplasms
- Psychogenic vomiting

WORKUP

- The following questions are useful to screen patients for bulimia:
  1. "Are you satisfied with your eating habits?"
  2. "Do you ever eat in secret?"
- Answering "no" to the first question and/or "yes" to the second question has 100% sensitivity and 90% specificity for bulimia. The SCOFF questionnaire can also be used as a screening tool for eating disorders (see "Anorexia Nervosa").
- According to the DSM-5, the level of severity is based on the frequency of inappropriate compensatory behaviors and may be increased to reflect other symptoms and degree of functional disability, as noted below:
  - Mild: An average of 1 to 3 episodes of inappropriate compensatory behaviors per week.
  - Moderate: An average of 4 to 7 episodes of inappropriate compensatory behaviors per week
  - Severe: An average of 8 to 13 episodes of inappropriate compensatory behaviors per week
  - Extreme: An average of ≥14 inappropriate compensatory behaviors per week
- Table 1 describes eating and weight control habits commonly found in children and adolescents with an eating disorder.

LABORATORY TESTS

- Electrolyte abnormalities from vomiting (hypokalemia and metabolic alkalosis) or diarrhea from laxative abuse (hypokalemia and hyperchloremic metabolic acidosis)
- Hyponatremia, hypocalcemia, hypomagnesemia (caused by laxative abuse)
- Elevated cortisol, decreased luteinizing hormone, decreased follicle-stimulating hormone

TREATMENT

NONPHARMACOLOGIC THERAPY

- Cognitive behavioral therapy, particularly interpersonal therapy to control abnormal behaviors
- Use of food diaries, nutritional counseling, and planning meals at least 1 day in advance are useful measures to counter abnormal eating behaviors
- Correction of electrolyte abnormalities

ACUTE GENERAL Rx

- Selective serotonin reuptake inhibitors are generally considered to be the safest medication option in these patients. They are useful in severely depressed patients and in those who do not benefit from cognitive behavioral therapy.
- Prompt recognition and treatment of complications:
  1. Ipecac cardiotoxicity from laxative abuse
  2. Electrolyte abnormalities (see "Laboratory Tests")
  3. Esophagitis and Mallory-Weiss tears; esophageal rupture from repeated vomiting
  4. Aspiration pneumonia and pneumomediastinum
  5. Menstrual irregularities (including amenorrhea)
  6. Gastrointestinal abnormalities: acute gastric dilation, pancreatitis, abdominal pain, constipation

CHRONIC Rx

- Psychotherapy continued for years and focused specifically on self-image and family and peer interactions is an integral part of successful recovery.
- Family therapy is also recommended, especially in younger patients.

DISPOSITION

Course is variable and marked by frequent recurrence of exacerbations.

REFERRAL

- In addition to the primary care physician, the multidisciplinary team should include a dietician, a psychiatrist, and a family therapist.
- Hospitalization should be considered for patients with severe electrolyte abnormalities or those with suicidal thoughts.

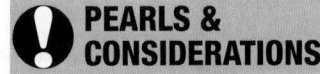

PEARLS & CONSIDERATIONS

COMMENTS

- Bulimia has a close association with depression, bipolar disorder, obsessive-compulsive disorder, alcoholism, and substance abuse.
- Bulimia should be considered in all patients (especially adolescents) with unexplained hypokalemia and metabolic alkalosis.

SUGGESTED READINGS
Available at www.expertconsult.com

RELATED CONTENT
Bulimia (Patient Information)
Anorexia Nervosa (Related Key Topic)
Binge-Eating Disorder (Related Key Topic)

AUTHOR: **FRED F. FERRI, M.D.**

TABLE 1 Eating and Weight Control Habits Commonly Found in Children and Adolescents with an Eating Disorder

	Prominent Features		Clinical Comments Regarding Eating Disorder Habits	
Habit	Anorexia Nervosa	Bulimia Nervosa	Anorexia Nervosa	Bulimia Nervosa
Overall intake	Inadequate energy (calories), although volume of food and beverages may be high due to very low caloric density of intake due to "diet" and nonfat choices	Variable, but calories normal to high; intake in binges often "forbidden" food or drink that differs from intake at meals	Consistent inadequate caloric intake leading to wasting of the body	Inconsistent balance of intake, exercise and vomiting, but severe caloric restriction is short-lived
Food	Counts and limits calories, especially from fat; emphasis on "healthy food choices" with reduced caloric density Monotonous, limited "good" food choices, often leading to vegetarian or vegan diet Strong feelings of guilt after eating more than planned leads to exercise and renewed dieting	Aware of calories and fat, but less regimented in avoidance than in AN Frequent dieting interspersed with overeating, often triggered by depression, isolation, or anger	Obsessive-compulsive attention to nutritional data on food labels and may have "logical" reasons for food choices in highly regimented pattern, such as sports participation or family history of lipid disorder	Choices less structured, with more frequent diets
Beverages	Water or other low- or no-calorie drinks; nonfat milk	Variable, diet soda common; may drink alcohol to excess	Fluids often restricted to avoid weight gain	Fluids ingested to aid vomiting or replace losses
Meals	Consistent schedule and structure to meal plan Reduced or eliminated caloric content, often starting with breakfast, then lunch, then dinner Volume can increase with fresh fruits, vegetables, and salads as primary food sources	Meals less regimented and planned than in AN; more likely impulsive and unregulated, often eliminated following a binge-purge episode	Rigid adherence to "rules" governing eating leads to sense of control, confidence, and mastery	Elimination of a meal following a binge-purge only reinforces the drive for binge later in the day
Snacks	Reduced or eliminated from meal plan	Often avoided in meal plans, but then impulsively eaten	Snack foods removed early because "unhealthy"	Snack "comfort foods" can trigger a binge
Dieting	Initial habit that becomes progressively restrictive, although often appearing superficially "healthy" Beliefs and "rules" about the patient's idiosyncratic nutritional requirements and response to foods are strongly held	Initial dieting gives way to chaotic eating, often interpreted by the patient as evidence of being "weak" or "lazy"	Distinguishing between healthy meal planning with reduced calories and dieting in ED may be difficult	Dieting tends to be impulsive and short-lived, with "diets" often resulting in unintended weight gain
Binge eating	None in restrictive subtype, but an essential feature in binge-purge subtype	Essential feature, often secretive Shame and guilt prominent afterward	Often "subjective" (more than planned but not large)	Relieves emotional distress, may be planned
Exercise	Characteristically obsessive-compulsive, ritualistic, and progressive May excel in dance, long-distance running	Less predictable May be athletic, or may avoid exercise entirely	May be difficult to distinguish active thin vs. ED	Males often use exercise as means of "purging"
Vomiting	Characteristic of binge-purge subtype May chew then spit out, rather than swallow, food as a variant	Most common habit intended to reduce effects of overeating Can occur after meal as well as a binge	Physiologic and emotional instability prominent	Strongly "addictive" and self-punishing, but does not eliminate calories ingested—many still absorbed
Laxatives	If used, generally to relieve constipation in restrictive subtype, but as a cathartic in binge-purge subtype	Second most common habit used to reduce or avoid weight gain, often used in increasing doses for cathartic effect	Physiologic and emotional instability prominent	Strongly "addictive," self-punishing, but ineffective means to reduce weight (calories are absorbed in the small intestine, but laxatives work in the colon)
Diet pills	Very rare, if used; more common in binge-purge subtype	Used to either reduce appetite or increase metabolism	Use of diet pills implies inability to control eating	Control over eating may be sought by any means

AN, Anorexia nervosa; *BN,* bulimia nervosa; *ED,* eating disorder.
From Kliegman RM et al: *Nelson textbook of pediatrics,* ed 19, Philadelphia, 2011, Saunders.

BASIC INFORMATION

DEFINITION

- Cutaneous burns can be classified by type of injury (e.g., thermal vs. chemical), burn depth (e.g., 1st, 2nd, 3rd degree), extent of burn (total burn surface area [TBSA]), and burn severity (e.g., minor vs. major). Types of burn injury include thermal (flames, scalds, hot contactants), chemical, electrical, and radiation burns. This chapter will focus on thermal and electrical burns.
- Burns can affect skin and respiratory, ocular, oral, and genital mucosa.

SYNONYMS

Thermal injury
Chemical injury
Electrical injury
Radiation injury

ICD-10CM CODES
T29.0 Burns of multiple regions, unspecified degree
T30.0 Burn of unspecified body region, unspecified degree
T30.1 Burn of first degree, body region unspecified
T30.2 Burn of second degree, body region unspecified
T30.3 Burn of third degree, body region unspecified
T31.0 Burns involving less than 10% of body surface
T31.1 Burns involving 10-19% of body surface
T31.2 Burns involving 20-29% of body surface
T31.3 Burns involving 30-39% of body surface
T31.4 Burns involving 40-49% of body surface
T31.5 Burns involving 50-59% of body surface

EPIDEMIOLOGY & DEMOGRAPHICS

PREVALENCE (IN U.S.):
- More than 1.2 million individuals experience burns in the U.S., and burn injuries account for approximately 500,000 emergency department visits, with 9% (45,000) requiring hospitalization and 0.8% (4000) resulting in death annually.
- Of thermal injury, scald burn from liquid is most common—followed by flame, flash burn, and then contact burn.

PREDOMINANT AGE & SEX:
- Children ages 2-4 years have the greatest frequency of burns (most commonly scald burns), with male adolescent and young adults ages 17 to 25 with second greatest frequency (most commonly from flammable liquids).

PHYSICAL FINDINGS & CLINICAL PRESENTATION

- It is important to note that burns occur unevenly—often with various depths (Table 1).
- 1st-degree (superficial) burns—penetrate epidermis only (minimal barrier loss)
  1. Very painful, intact, erythematous skin with minimal to no edema and no blistering.
- 2nd-degree (partial-thickness) burns—epidermis and part of dermis is affected.
  1. Moist, very painful skin with edema and blistering/blebs
  2. Superficial partial-thickness burns—cherry red with two-point discrimination intact, incredibly painful
  3. Deep partial-thickness burns—mottled white and cherry red; only the sensation of pressure is intact in these areas
- 3rd-degree (full-thickness) burns—entire epidermis and dermis are affected, with destruction of hair follicles and sweat glands.
  1. The skin is dry, charred, pale, painless, and leathery. Charred vessels may be visible beneath, little or no pain, and hair pulls out easily.

DIAGNOSIS

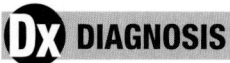

CLASSIFICATION

- Burns are classified by (1) depth of injury, (2) extent of injury, and (3) severity, according to the American Burn Association.
- Depth of injury (see Table 1)
  1. Indicates how the wound will heal and whether grafting will be needed
- Extent of TBSA
  1. The TBSA is best classified by using age-specific burn charts and the "rule of nines" (Fig. E1).
  2. For scattered burns, utilizing patient's palm including fingers to equate 1% body surface area can be helpful.
  3. TBSA indicates how aggressively the patient will need to be resuscitated.
- Severity—determined by burn depth, TBSA, age, location, type of injury, and presence/absence of coexisting conditions. Severity classification helps triage patients to outpatient, inpatient, or burn unit care (see Table 2).
  1. Minor burns—outpatient management.
  2. Moderate burns—admission to hospital with experience managing burns or burn center referral.
  3. Major burns—referral to burn center.

LABORATORY STUDIES (MODERATE OR MAJOR BURNS)

- CBC, electrolytes, BUN, creatinine, glucose, liver function tests, venous blood gas, blood coagulation, and type and screen in anticipation of blood transfusion
- *If smoke inhalation expected:* serial ABG carboxyhemoglobin and continuous ECG
- *If electrical burn or if concern for rhabdomyolysis:* urinalysis, urine myoglobin, and CPK levels
- *If severe lactic acidosis:* consider checking cyanide level

IMAGING STUDIES

- If smoke inhalation suspected: chest radiograph and bronchoscopy
- If high-voltage electrical burn: cardiac monitoring first 24 hours

---

TABLE 1 Categorization of Burn by Depth

Burn Type	Histologic Depth	Clinical Presentation	Treatment	Healing Time/Prognosis
1st degree	Epidermis	Erythematous but intact skin, no blisters, pain may range in severity	Topical salves, cold compresses, NSAIDs for pain control	2-5 days with no scarring
Superficial 2nd degree (partial thickness)	Papillary dermis	Erythematous with superficial blisters, intense pain	Topical antimicrobials with gauze dressing or biosynthetic dressing (if widespread), pain control	5-21 days with no grafting
Deep 2nd degree (partial thickness)	Reticular dermis	Erythematous with superficial/deep blisters, range of pain depending on nerve involvement	Same	21-35 days with no infection; if infected, converts to full-thickness burn
3rd degree (full thickness)	Through dermis to subcutaneous tissue. Can involve fascia, muscle and bone.	White or black, possible eschar, may or may not be painful depending on nerve damage	Usually requires grafting, may require resuscitation depending on TBSA affected, pain control	Large areas require grafting, but small areas may heal from the edges after weeks

From Kliegman RM et al: *Nelson textbook of pediatrics*, ed 19, Philadelphia, 2011, Saunders; and Kessides MC, Skelsey MK: Management of acute partial-thickness burns, *Cutis* 86:249-257, 2010.

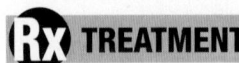

TREATMENT

DIFFERENTIAL DIAGNOSIS

Cultural practices leading to burn-like lesions in distinctive patterns (e.g., cupping, coining, moxibustion), cellulitis, Stevens-Johnson syndrome/toxic epidermolytic necrolysis

ACUTE GENERAL Rx

MINOR BURNS (1ST DEGREE BURNS AND 2ND/3RD DEGREE BURNS OF LIMITED TBSA):

- Outpatient management—"6 Cs"
  1. Clothing: Remove hot or burned clothing
  2. Cooling: Cool (approximately 54° F) for 10 to 30 minutes (under faucet or compress) to reduce edema/pain by conducting heat away from skin. Not recommended with extensive burns due to theoretical risk of hypothermia and shock. No ice packs.
  3. Cleaning: Wash gently with mild alcohol-free soap, then normal saline daily. Remove all old ointment and any loose skin. Blot dry. No evidence supports vigorous cleansing with antiseptic solutions. Embedded materials should be removed by copious irrigation using a large-gauge syringe.
  4. Chemoprophylaxis: Tetanus immunization (all deep 2nd and 3rd degree burns). Routine skin cultures are NOT recommended except when wound infection suspected, and prophylactic systemic antibiotics are NOT recommended. All 2nd and 3rd degree burns are treated with a topical antimicrobial agent. This may include silver sulfadiazine, bacitracin, bismuth-impregnated Vaseline gauze, or silver-impregnated synthetic dressings.
  5. Covering: All 2nd and 3rd degree burns should be covered with sterile dressing. If financial resources are limited, instead of gauze, can purchase cotton gloves, T-shirts, or similar at discount stores, wash, and reuse.
  6. Comfort: Analgesics (Tylenol and NSAIDs—alone or in combination with opioids) around the clock are recommended. Additional "rescue" analgesics before dressing changes and physical activity recommended.

MODERATE AND MAJOR BURNS (2ND/3RD DEGREE BURNS OF EXTENSIVE TBSA):

- Patients with moderate/major burns should be admitted to the hospital or referred to a burn center. Indications for hospitalization for burns are described in Table 2.
- Resuscitation (in addition to previous)
  1. Assessment of ABCs: Establish airway and assess breathing (inspect for inhalation injury and intubate for suspected airway edema, often seen 12 to 24 hours later); O_2; establish circulation (place two large-bore peripheral IV lines, ECG).
  2. IV fluid resuscitation—Parkland formula (Ringer's lactate at 2 to 4 ml/kg per % TBSA per 24 hours with half the calculated fluid given in the first 8 hours is an effective modality in severe burns)
  3. Baseline neurologic and vascular assessment
  4. Foley catheter and NG tube (20% of patients develop an ileus)—urine output 30 ml/hr
  5. Optimize nutritional support: Mayes equations to calculate energy requirements after burn (Box 1)
- Frequent reassessment in the first 24 to 72 hours, as wound depth can change significantly
- The four phases of burn care, with physiologic changes and objectives, are described in Table E3. Box 2 describes the modified Brooke resuscitation formula.

BURN WOUND CARE BY BURN DEPTH Rx

GENERAL:

- Vigilant wound care with dressings to prevent evaporation and minimize threat of wound colonization and infection of nonintact skin
- Daily activity necessary to maintain function of burned extremity, decrease pain and swelling, and promote healing
- 1st-degree burns (skin intact):
  1. Dressing: None required (except to protect from injury); topical antibacterial agents NOT recommended
  2. Other: Emollients, cool compresses (avoid ice), if pruritic, trial of antihistamines
  3. Prognosis: Heals within 1 week without scarring. May heal with pigmentary changes (limit by sunscreen and sun avoidance of area for 1 year).
- 2nd degree (superficial partial-thickness) burns without adherent exudate or eschar:
  1. Blisters: Sharp debridement of ruptured blisters; leave intact blisters. Quicker healing and reduced infections when intact blisters are not disturbed. Consider unroofing blisters that show no sign of resorption over several weeks or contain cloudy fluid.
  2. Dressing: Topical antimicrobial ointment (bacitracin) or A&D ointment with nonadherent dressing twice a day. Alternate: biosynthetic dressing (alginates, hydrofibers, or foam dressings)—many with silver as antimicrobial (absorb exudates, maintain moist environment, require fewer dressing changes, which reduces pain/anxiety)
  3. Prognosis: Heals with minimal scarring in 10 to 14 days. May heal with pigmentary changes (reduced with sunscreen and sun avoidance of area × 1 year)
- 2nd degree (deep partial-thickness) burns with adherent exudates; localized 3rd degree burns; cellulitic wounds:
  1. Dressing: Silver sulfadiazine 1%: broader spectrum, better penetration of necrotic tissue than bacitracin, but inhibits epithelialization. Must stop use once exudates and eschar have separated from wound. Alternative: enzymatic debrider (e.g., Santyl or Accuzyme)—chemically debrides devitalized tissue without harming healthy tissue.
  2. Referral: Burn specialist for consultation regarding need for excision and grafting.
  3. Prognosis: Deep 2nd degree burns heal with significant scarring, often take 3 to 4 weeks to heal. If infected, convert to 3rd degree burns. 3rd degree

TABLE 2	Classification of Burns by Severity and Indications for Hospitalization or Burn Center Referral		
Criteria	**Minor Burn**	**Moderate Burn**	**Major Burn**
Total body surface area (%)	• All 1st degree burns <10% adults <5% children or elderly • <2% for 3rd degree	• 2nd degree burns 10%-20% adults 5%-10% in children or elderly • 2%-5% 3rd degree	• All 1st degree burns >20% adults >10% children and elderly • >5% 3rd degree
Type of burn injury		• Low-voltage burn • Suspected inhalation injury	• High-voltage burn • Chemical burn • Known
Location		Circumferential burn	• Clinically significant burn to face, eyes, ears, genitalia, over joints
Coexisting conditions		• Concomitant medical problem predisposing to infection (e.g., diabetes, sickle cell anemia)	• Significant associated injuries (e.g., fracture, other major trauma)
	Outpatient management	Inpatient management—consider referral to burn center*	Referral to burn center

*Per the American Burn Association (ABA), any partial-thickness burn >10% total body surface area or any factors listed in moderate or major burn category warrant referral to burn center. Additional factors per the ABA include burned children in a hospital without qualified personnel or equipment for the care of children and burn injury in a patient who will require special social, emotional, or rehabilitative intervention (including suspected child abuse).

Modified from Singer AJ, Dagum AB: Current management of acute cutaneous wounds, *N Engl J Med* 359 (10):1037-1046, 2008; www.ameriburn.org.

BOX 1   Mayes Equations to Calculate Energy Requirement After a Burn

Mayes equation for a 5- to 10-year-old burn patient with injury < 50% TBSA:

$$818 + 37.4 \text{ (weight in kilograms)} + 9.3 \times \text{TBSA burn}$$

Mayes equation for a 5.5-year-old patient with a 45% TBSA scald burn weighing 20 kg:

$$818 + 37.4 \text{ (20kg)} + 9.3 \times 45 \text{ TBSA scald}$$

$$818 + 748 + 481.5 = 2047.5 \text{ calories/day}$$

From Fuhrman BP et al: *Pediatric critical care*, ed 4, Philadelphia, 2011, Saunders.

BOX 2   Modified Brooke Resuscitation Formula

0-24 Hours
Adults and Children >10 kg
Lactated Ringer's: 2 to 4 mL/kg/% burn/24 hr (first half in first 8 hr)
Colloid: none*

Children <10 kg
Lactated Ringer's: 2 to 3 mL/kg/% burn/24 hr (first half in first 8 hr)
Lactated Ringer's with 5% dextrose: 4 mL/kg/hr
Colloid: none

24-48 Hours
All Patients
Crystalloid: to maintain urine output. If silver nitrate is used, sodium leaching will mandate continued isotonic crystalloid. If other topical is used, free water requirement is significant. Serum sodium should be monitored closely. Nutritional support should begin, ideally by the enteral route.
Colloid: (5% albumin in lactated Ringer's):
  0% to 30% burn: none
  30% to 50% burn: 0.3 mL/kg/% burn/24 hr
  50% to 70% burn: 0.4 mL/kg/% burn/24 hr
  >70% burn: 0.5 mL/kg/% burn/24 hr. *Note:* The Modified Brooke formula is a common consensus formula that is only useful in individual patients if adjusted to physiologic endpoints. Like all resuscitative formulas, it is a helpful starting point, but optimal-quality resuscitation requires the bedside presence of a physician capable of regularly evaluating resuscitation endpoints.

From Vincent JL et al: *Textbook of critical care*, ed 6, Philadelphia, 2011, Saunders.

burns typically require skin graft, but small areas may heal from edges after weeks.

DISPOSITION/FOLLOW-UP CARE

- Outpatient: Evaluate next day to assess level of injury, level of pain, and ability to manage dressing changes on own. If insufficient, daily evaluation until complete wound epithelialization recommended. Epithelialization = tiny islands of epithelialization throughout wound. If no epithelialization after 2 weeks, or subsequent evaluation reveals 3rd degree burn, referral to burn surgeon recommended. Box E3 describes common complications in burn patients.

- Following re-epithelialization, visits every 4 to 6 weeks to monitor for hypertrophic scar formation (early referral to burn/scar specialist if occurs).
- Mortality rates higher in patients >60 yr of age, with burns >40% TBSA, or with inhalation injury. Long-term risk of developing squamous cell carcinoma of the skin within burn injury. Long-term skin monitoring necessary.

REFERRAL

Consultation of burn specialist or burn center referral per Table 2.

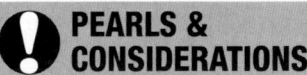 **PEARLS & CONSIDERATIONS**

COMMENTS

- In circumferential skin burns, look for compartment syndrome of limbs (e.g., tightening, progressive deterioration of peripheral motor and sensory exam findings, severe pain, and loss of arterial Doppler signals). Escharotomy may be necessary.
- If child abuse is suspected, social services at the hospital or child protective services must be contacted.
- Fig. E2 describes an algorithm for the treatment of chemical burns.

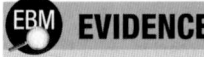 **EVIDENCE**

Available at www.expertconsult.com

SUGGESTED READINGS
Available at www.expertconsult.com

RELATED CONTENT

Burns (Patient Information)
Electrical and Lightning Injury (Related Key Topic)

AUTHOR: **LISA K. PAPPAS-TAFFER, M.D.**

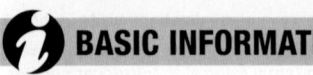

BASIC INFORMATION

DEFINITION

Calcium-alkali syndrome is the triad of hypercalcemia, metabolic alkalosis, and renal insufficiency due to consumption of large amounts of calcium and absorbable alkali. For conventional diagnostic purposes, only hypercalcemia with an appropriate history of ingestions must be present.

SYNONYMS

Milk-alkali syndrome

PRESENTATIONS

Calcium-alkali syndrome presents in one of three patterns:
1) Acute: This stage occurs after approximately 1 week of excessive calcium and alkali intake. Symptoms are due to hypercalcemia and include nausea, vomiting, weakness, and mental status depression or confusion. Metabolic alkalosis is present with a normal or elevated serum phosphorus level. An elevated serum creatinine reflects acute kidney injury. Cessation of exogenous calcium and alkali leads to resolution of signs and symptoms.
2) Subacute or intermediate *(Cope syndrome):* Patients typically are encountered after milk and alkali have been ingested intermittently for years. Affected patients demonstrate symptoms of acute and chronic hypercalcemia and respond to medication withdrawal with gradual improvement. Kidney function often is mildly and chronically impaired.
3) Chronic form *(Burnett's disease):* Patients present with symptoms of chronic hypercalcemia after a prolonged high calcium and alkali intake; polyuria, polydipsia, myalgias, or pruritus are present. Physical evidence of metastatic calcification is detectable: nephrocalcinosis and band keratopathy. Laboratory findings are similar to those found in the acute syndrome, but muscle aches and pruritus improve slowly as the plasma calcium concentration gradually improves. Minimal or no improvement in kidney function occurs due to irreversible chronic kidney disease.

ICD-10CM CODES
E83.52 Disorders of calcium metabolism

EPIDEMIOLOGY & DEMOGRAPHICS

In the early twentieth century, the calcium-alkali syndrome was associated with the Sippy antacid regimen for peptic ulcer disease that entailed ingestion of large amounts of calcium salts, particularly from milk, and absorbable bicarbonate compounds. Kidney injury and alkalosis were followed by hypercalcemia after its measurement became routine. Following the developments of type 2 histamine receptor blockers and proton pump inhibitors, the syndrome virtually disappeared. Since the 1980s, a resurgence of hypercalcemia associated with the use of calcium-containing products for osteoporosis prevention has occurred. In chronic kidney disease patients, the use of calcium carbonate instead of aluminum hydroxide as a phosphate binder has produced the "calcium-alkali" syndrome. The updated term, calcium-alkali syndrome, supplants the milk-alkali syndrome because milk is no longer the source of calcium. The calcium-alkali syndrome was the third-leading cause of hypercalcemia (12%) in hospitalized patients from 1990 to 1993, after hypercalcemia of malignancy and primary hyperparathyroidism.

PHYSICAL FINDINGS & CLINICAL PRESENTATION

- Asymptomatic hypercalcemia:
  1. Less than half of all cases are incidental findings of hypercalcemia on random laboratory testing.
- Symptomatic hypercalcemia:
  1. Symptoms: nausea, vomiting, anorexia, fatigue, vague abdominal pain, nephrolithiasis- and pancreatitis-related pain, constipation, myalgia, confusion, and psychosis. In chronic cases, polyuria and polydipsia may be reported.
  2. Physical examination and other testing: mental status changes include anxiety, depression, and cognitive dysfunction; also shortened QT segment interval.

ETIOLOGY

Overconsumption of supplemental calcium of 3 to 20 g daily in association with volume depletion, renal impairment, or thiazide diuretic use is the most common etiology. The resulting hypercalcemia reduces glomerular filtration of calcium and induces salt-wasting reducing extracellular fluid volume that further lowers glomerular filtration and increases bicarbonate reabsorption with metabolic alkalosis. Vomiting or diuretic-induced volume depletion worsen hypercalcemia and alkalosis. Elderly individuals experience greater bone loss and are prone to developing hypercalcemia in the presence of excess calcium supplements. Betel nut chewing, a practice in Asia and the South Pacific, is associated with calcium-alkali syndrome. The nuts are bitter and coated with a compound that is converted to bicarbonate, fostering metabolic alkalosis.

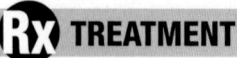

DIAGNOSIS

DIFFERENTIAL DIAGNOSIS

Hypercalcemia from other causes includes primary hyperparathyroidism, certain malignancies, and granulomatous disorders including tuberculosis, sarcoidosis, and silicosis.

LABORATORY TESTS

- Elevated serum ionized calcium (wide variation reported)
- Elevated BUN and serum creatinine from acute kidney injury or chronic kidney disease
- Elevated serum bicarbonate and arterial pH from metabolic alkalosis
- Parathyroid hormone, which usually is suppressed with calcium-alkali syndrome, may be elevated, particularly if evaluated after treatment initiation
- Serum phosphorus level is variable (historically high with milk ingestion but low with calcium carbonate ingestion due to gut phosphate binding)
- Hypomagnesemia occasionally

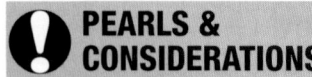

TREATMENT

NONPHARMACOLOGIC THERAPY

Hemodialysis is indicated rarely for severe renal dysfunction or markedly symptomatic hypercalcemia.

ACUTE GENERAL Rx

- Discontinuation of all calcium and bicarbonate supplementation
- Volume repletion with IV saline and furosemide administration
- Patient education to limit future calcium supplementation from over-the-counter calcium supplements (TUMS) and antacids containing calcium carbonate (Calcarb, CitraCal, Caltrate)

PROGNOSIS

Hypercalcemia and symptoms resolve with withdrawal of excess calcium supplementation and treatment of hypercalcemia. Acute cases typically resolve in 1 to 2 days while chronic cases take longer. Patients initially presenting with kidney failure may incur residual kidney damage.

DISPOSITION

Treatment is determined by degree of hypercalcemia and symptoms. Hospitalization is required for symptomatic patients or for patients whose total serum calcium is >11.5 mg/dl and who may require IV volume repletion and other intensive treatments for hypercalcemia.

REFERRAL

Endocrinology
Nephrology

PEARLS & CONSIDERATIONS

COMMENTS

Detailed history of dietary supplements and over-the-counter medications (see Table E1) can provide the most important clues. Many patients do not list dietary supplements as a medication.

SUGGESTED READINGS

Available at www.expertconsult.com

AUTHORS: **JESSE GOLDMAN, M.D., REBECCA KURNIK SESHASAI, M.D., M.S.H.P.,** and **ELLIE KELEPOURIS, M.D.**

BASIC INFORMATION

DEFINITION

Carcinoma of unknown primary (CUP) refers to a diverse group of malignancies for which the anatomic site of origin cannot be determined despite extensive investigations.

SYNONYMS

Cancer NOS
Cancer unspecified site
Malignancy unspecified site
CUP

ICD-10CM CODES
C80.1 Malignant (primary) neoplasm, unspecified

EPIDEMIOLOGY & DEMOGRAPHICS

- CUP accounts for about 5% of all cancers, and the annual incidence in the United States is 7-12 cases per 100,000 persons.
- It is the seventh most frequent common cause of cancer and the fourth most common cause of cancer death. It predominantly occurs in adults and is more common in males.
- In the United States, an estimated 34,170 new cases are expected in 2016.
- Most cases of CUP are carcinomas, which are divided into adenocarcinomas (90%), squamous cell carcinomas (5%), and undifferentiated carcinomas (5%). Box 1 describes primaries most commonly metastatic to the lung, and Box 2 indicates tumors with the highest predilection for pulmonary metastasis. Table 1 summarizes the most common sites of metastasis and the percentage with isolated disease.
- There is a variable rate of mutations detected in CUP (18%-30%). The tumor suppressor gene p-53 has overexpression rates (40%-50%) or mutation rates (25%-40%) that are comparable to that seen in other solid tumors. The evaluation of VEGF-A (vascular endothelial growth factor-A, angiogenesis factor) and matrix metalloproteinases (enzymes that degrade stroma) showed that these are universally expressed and active angiogenesis is present in CUP.

PHYSICAL FINDINGS & CLINICAL PRESENTATION

- Physical findings can be variable and include generalized and organ-specific findings.

- General findings can include cachexia, pallor, edema, icterus, edema, skin rash, muscle wasting among others.
- Organ-specific findings are related to the dysfunction of the underlying organ(s) involved with CUP.
- The clinical course is often highlighted by a short presentation history, with symptoms and signs associated with metastatic sites, early dissemination, aggressive clinical course, and occasionally an unpredictable metastatic pattern.
- Multiple organs are involved at diagnosis in up to half of patients.
- The clinicopathologic subsets comprising CUP are shown in Table 2.

DIAGNOSIS

WORKUP

- Comprehensive medical history
- Complete physical examination with particular attention to skin, lymph node sites, organ enlargement, and testes; also rectal examination and pelvic examination (in women) (Table 3).
- Histopathology review of biopsy specimens

LABORATORY TESTS

- Complete blood count
- Comprehensive chemistry panel
- Urine analysis
- Stool for occult blood
- Tumor markers (in selected cases): prostate-specific antigen (PSA), β-human chorionic gonadotrophin, α-fetoprotein.
- Adequate tissue biopsy with immunohistochemical (IHC) staining is done to guide broad diagnostic category assignments—carcinoma, melanoma, sarcoma, or lymphoma.
- Subtyping with IHC panels helps further classifying into adenocarcinoma, squamous carcinoma, germ cell tumor, neuroendocrine, thyroid, hepatocellular, or renal origin.
- Step-wise approach for IHC derived diagnosis of likely site of origin are depicted in Table 4.
- In up to 25% cases, a single site of origin can be narrowed down by IHC staining (e.g., TTF-1 positive and CK-1 positive lung cancer profile)
- Molecular diagnosis is carried out by commercially available multi-gene assays that utilize micro-array or polymerase chain

reaction assays and can assist in finalizing diagnosis in up to 70% cases.

IMAGING STUDIES

- CT scans of the chest, abdomen, and pelvis; also CT of the neck in case of neck lymphadenopathy
- For selected cases
  - PET scan
  - Mammography and/or breast MRI
  - Testicular ultrasonography

TREATMENT

- CUP patients often require early supportive care for their advanced cancer; also there is elevated psychosocial distress with the uncertainties of diagnosis and treatment options. Anxiety and depression are more common in CUP patients compared to patients with known primaries.
- Treatment is based according to the most likely site of origin for the cancer with systemic chemotherapy typically being the mainstay of therapy.
- Favorable and unfavorable CUP subsets are shown in Table 5.
- **Favorable CUP**
  - Women with peritoneal adenocarcinoma when treated as advanced ovarian cancer with surgical cytoreduction and adjuvant systemic chemotherapy can have median survivals in the 36-month range
  - Patients with a midline tumor characteristically treated as germ cell tumors have median survivals of 12 months.
  - Patients with poorly differentiated neuroendocrine cancers are treated with combination platinum-containing chemotherapy and median survivals are in the 15-month range
  - Women with axillary nodal adenocarcinoma are approached as breast cancers with treatment plans incorporating axillary and breast surgery followed by adjuvant chemotherapy, hormone therapy and radiotherapy; survival rates are comparable to similarly staged breast cancers.
  - Patients with metastatic squamous neck nodal cancer are treated as head–neck cancers with chemoradiotherapy and/or neck dissection
  - Patients with a colon adenocarcinoma profile are treated with systemic regimens as in metastatic colorectal cancers with median survivals in the 24-month range.
  - Men with blastic bone metastases and elevated prostate specific antigen are treated with initial androgen deprivation therapy and later on with systemic chemotherapy.
- **Unfavorable CUP**
  - Account for 75% to 80% of all CUP patients
  - The most common presentation is advanced visceral disease, often with liver metastases; median survivals with systemic platinum and taxane-containing chemotherapy are typically in the range of 6 to 7 months.

BOX 1 Primaries Most Commonly Metastatic to the Lung*

- Breast
- Colon
- Kidney
- Uterus
- Prostate
- Oropharyngeal carcinoma

*Most common because of greater prevalence.
Sellke FW, del Nido PJ, Swanson SJ: *Sabiston & Spencer surgery of the chest*, 9th ed, Philadelphia, 2016, Elsevier.

BOX 2 Tumors with the Highest Predilection for Pulmonary Metastasis

- Choriocarcinoma
- Osteosarcoma
- Testicular tumors
- Melanoma
- Ewing sarcoma
- Kaposi sarcoma

Sellke FW, del Nido PJ, Swanson SJ: *Sabiston & Spencer surgery of the chest*, 9th ed, Philadelphia, 2016, Elsevier.

TABLE 1   Most Common Site of Metastasis and Percentage with Isolated Disease

Histology	Most Common Site of Metastasis (%)	Second Most Common Site of Metastasis	Those with Isolated Pulmonary Metastases (% of All Patients)
Breast carcinoma	Lung (59-65)		22
Colorectal	Liver	Lung	2-4
Germ cell tumors	Lung		
Head and neck squamous cell carcinoma	Lung (75)		
Melanoma	Lung*† (18-36)		5
Osteosarcoma	Lung (85)		
Renal cell carcinoma	Lung		4
Soft tissue sarcoma	Lung (80-90)		20
All histologies	Liver	Lung	15-20

*Secondary to skin, subcutaneous, lymph nodes.
†In clinical series; however, 70% to 87% in autopsy series.
Sellke FW, del Nido PJ, Swanson SJ: *Sabiston & Spencer surgery of the chest*, 9th ed, Philadelphia, 2016, Elsevier.

TABLE 2   Clinicopathologic Subsets of Patients with CUP

	Median Age (Years)	Sex of Patients (M/F)	Histopathology
Lymph nodes			
Mediastinal retroperitoneal	<50	70%/30%	UDF or PDF
Axillary	52	0%/100%	Adenocarcinoma (WDF, MDF, or PDF)
Cervical	57-60	80%/20%	SCC
Inguinal	58	50%/50%	UDF, SCC, mixed SCC and adenocarcinoma
Peritoneal cavity			
Primary peritoneal in women	55-65	0%/100%	Adenocarcinoma (serous papillary)
Ascites of other unknown origin	–	–	Adenocarcinoma (MDF or PDF; mucin; with or without signet ring cells)
Neuroendocrine tumors	63	60%/40%	PDF with neuroendocrine features; low-grade neuroendocrine cancers; small-cell anaplastic cancers
Liver (mainly) or other organs, or both	62	61%39%	Adenocarcinoma (MDF or PDF)
Lungs			
Pulmonary metastases	–	–	Adenocarcinoma (WDF, MDF, or PDF)
Pleural effusions	–	–	Adenocarcinoma (MDF or PDF)
Bones (one or more)	–	–	Adenocarcinoma (WDF, MDF, or PDF)
Brain (one or more)	51-55	M>F	Adenocarcinoma (WDF, UDF, or PDF); SCC

F, women; *M,* men; *MDF,* moderately differentiated; *PDF,* poorly differentiated; *SCC,* squamous cell carcinoma; *UDF,* undifferentiated; *WDF,* well differentiated.
From Pavlidis N, Pentheroudakis G: Cancer of unknown primary site, *Lancet* 379(9824):1428-35, 2012.

TABLE 3   Recommended Evaluation Following Initial Light Microscopic Diagnosis

Diagnosis	Clinical Evaluation*	Special Pathologic Studies
Adenocarcinoma (or poorly differentiated adenocarcinoma)	PET CT of chest, abdomen Men: serum PSA Women: mammogram Additional directed radiologic or endoscopic studies to evaluate abnormal symptoms, signs, laboratory values	Men: PSA stain Women: estrogen and progesterone receptor stains (if clinical features suggest metastatic breast cancer)
Poorly differentiated carcinoma	PET CT of chest, abdomen Serum hCG, AFP Additional directed radiologic or endoscopic studies to evaluate abnormal symptoms, signs, laboratory values	Immunoperoxidase staining Electron microscopy (if immunoperoxidase stains indeterminate)
Squamous carcinoma, cervical nodes	PET Direct laryngoscopy with visualization; biopsy of nasopharynx, pharynx, hypopharynx, larynx Fiberoptic bronchoscopy (if laryngoscopy is negative)	—
Squamous carcinoma, inguinal nodes	PET Complete examination of perineal area (including pelvic examination) Anoscopy Cystoscopy	—

AFP, α-fetoprotein; *CT,* computed tomography; *hCG,* human chorionic gonadotropin; *PET,* positron emission tomography; *PSA,* prostate-specific antigen.
*In addition to a history, physical examination, complete blood cell counts, chemistry profile, and chest radiograph.
Goldman L, Schafer AI: *Goldman's Cecil medicine,* ed 24, Philadelphia, 2012, Saunders.

TABLE 4 Immunohistochemical Approaches for Diagnosis of CUP

	Diagnosis
Step One	
AE1 or AE3 pan-cytokeratin	Carcinoma
Common leukocyte antigen	Lymphoma
S100; HMB-45	Melanoma
S100; vimentin	Sarcoma
Step Two	
CK7 or CK20; PSA	Adenocarcinoma
PLAP; OCT4; AFP; human chorionic gonadotropin	Germ cell tumors
Hepatocyte paraffin1; canalicular pCEA, CD10, or CD13	Hepatocellular carcinoma
RCC; CD10	Renal cell carcinoma
TTF1; thyroglobulin	Thyroid carcinoma
Chromogranin; synaptophysin, PGP9.5; CD56	Neuroendocrine carcinoma
CK5 or CK6; p63	Squamous cell carcinoma
Step Three	
PSA; PAP	Prostate
TTF1	Lung
GCDFP-15; mammaglobin; ER	Breast
CDX2; CK20	Colon
CDX2 (intestinal epithelium); CK20; CK7	Pancreas or biliary
ER; CA-125; mesothelin; WT1	Ovary

Step one detects broad type of cancer. Step two detects subtype. Step three detects origin of adenocarcinoma. Positive results with any of these stains indicates a tumor is present, but without absolute certainty.

AFP, α-fetoprotein; *ER,* estrogen receptor; *OCT4,* octamer-binding transcription factor 4; *PAP,* prostatic acid phosphatase; *pCEA,* polyclonal carcinoembryonic antigen; *PLAP,* placental alkaline phosphatase; *PSA,* prostate-specific antigen; *RCC,* renal cell carcinoma antigen.

From Pavlidis N, Pentheroudakis G: Cancer of unknown primary site, *Lancet* 379(9824):1428-35, 2012.

TABLE 5 Prognostic Classification of CUP Patients

Favorable Subset

Women with papillary adenocarcinoma of the peritoneal cavity
Women with adenocarcinoma involving the axillary lymph nodes
Poorly differentiated carcinoma with midline distribution
Poorly differentiated neuroendocrine carcinoma
Squamous cell carcinoma involving cervical lymph nodes
Adenocarcinoma with a colon-cancer profile (CK20+, CK7−, CDX2+)
Men with blastic bone metastases and elevated prostate-specific antigen (adenocarcinoma)
Isolated inguinal adenopathy (squamous carcinoma)
Patients with one small, potentially resectable tumor

Unfavorable Subset

Adenocarcinoma metastatic to the liver or other organs
Nonpapillary malignant ascites (adenocarcinoma)
Multiple cerebral metastases (adenocarcinoma or squamous carcinoma)
Several lung or pleural metastases (adenocarcinoma)
Multiple metastatic lytic bone disease (adenocarcinoma)
Squamous cell carcinoma of the abdominopelvic cavity

From Pavlidis N, Pentheroudakis G: Cancer of unknown primary site, *Lancet* 379(9824):1428-35, 2012.

DISPOSITION

- Pathologic workup is critical, with detailed IHC staining. Molecular diagnosis utilizing commercially available multi-gene tissue of origin assays is a valuable tool for narrowing the likely site of cancer origin.
- Favorable subset CUP patients have a better outcome; multimodality therapy including chemotherapy results in improved survival
- Unfavorable CUP has poor outcomes with the use of systemic chemotherapy, with median survivals of 6 to 7 months

REFERRAL

To medical oncologist, surgeon and radiation oncologist.

SUGGESTED READINGS

Available at www.expertconsult.com

AUTHOR: **RITESH RATHORE, M.D.**

C

Diseases and Disorders

I

BASIC INFORMATION

DEFINITION

Infection caused by the species of the genus *Candida*, mainly *Candida albicans*. *Candida* species are ubiquitous. They are the most common fungal pathogens affecting mankind. Cutaneous candidiasis comprises superficial *Candida* infections of the skin and mucosal membranes.

Cutaneous candidiasis can be classified into two subgroups: cutaneous candidiasis syndromes and chronic mucocutaneous syndromes. Cutaneous candidiasis syndromes include:

- Generalized cutaneous candidiasis
- Intertrigo
- *Candida* folliculitis
- Paronychia/onychomycosis
- Perianal candidiasis
- Erosio interdigitalis blastomycetica
- Balanitis

Chronic mucocutaneous syndromes include:
- Oropharyngeal candidiasis
- Esophageal candidiasis
- Vulvovaginal candidiasis
- GI candidiasis (gastric/intestines/perianal)
- *Candida* cystitis

SYNONYMS

Yeast infection
Candidosis
Moniliasis
Oidiomycosis

ICD-10CM CODES
B37.2   Candidiasis of skin and nail
B37.8   Candidiasis, unspecified
B37.89   Other sites of candidiasis

EPIDEMIOLOGY & DEMOGRAPHICS

- *Candida* species: it is the most common fungal infection in immunocompromised people.
- Most females (75%) experience an episode of vulvovaginal candidiasis in their lifetime.

INCIDENCE: Estimated to be 50 cases per 100,000 persons

PREVALENCE: Colonizes more than 50% of U.S. population

PREDOMINANT SEX AND AGE:
- Female > male
- No predominant age, but neonates and the elderly (adults >65 yr) are susceptible to *Candida* colonization and to getting mucocutaneous candidiasis.

RISK FACTORS: Risk factors that allow *Candida* infection include:
- Age >65 yr
- Females in the third trimester
- Defects in the mucocutaneous barrier (e.g., wounds, burns, ulcerations)
- Decreased/defective granulocytes/monocytes
- Diseases of white blood cells (e.g., chronic granulomatous disease)
- Complement deficiency

- Certain diseases associated with cell-mediated immunity (e.g., HIV, DM)
- Use of certain medications (e.g., broad-spectrum antibiotics, high doses of corticosteroids)
- Increased skin pH due to panty liners and occlusive attire
- **Chronic mucocutaneous candidiasis** (CMC) is characterized by susceptibility to *Candida* infection of skin, nails (Fig. 1), and mucous membranes. Patients with recessive CMC and autoimmunity have mutations in the autoimmune regulator *AIRE*. Mutations in the CC domain of *STAT1* underlie autosomal-dominant CMC and lead to defective Th1 and Th17 responses, which may explain the increased susceptibility to fungal infections (van de Veerdonk et al).

Anatomical sites predisposed to *Candida* infection include:
- Axilla
- Beneath the breast, abdominal fold, intertriginous areas
- Periungual creases
- Inguinal creases
- Back and buttocks of bedridden persons

PHYSICAL FINDINGS & CLINICAL PRESENTATION

There are several clinical presentations of cutaneous candidiasis. A few are presented here.

A. Cutaneous candidiasis
- Presents as erythematous, sometimes shiny with flakes and fluid lesions at the edge of the redness (satellite pustules). It is itchy and the skin becomes inflamed. Pustules may be present in candidiasis of the scrotal and perineal skin.

B. Gastrointestinal tract candidiasis
1. Oropharyngeal candidiasis
   - Usually seen in diabetics, after exposure to inhaled steroids or broad-spectrum antibiotics and in immunosuppressed individuals (e.g., patients with a history of HIV infection).
   Symptoms include:
     - White thick patches on the oral mucosa (Fig. 2)
     - Dysphagia, mouth soreness, and pain
     - Tongue burning

2. Physical examination shows:
   - Erythema of the buccal mucosa
   - White patches on buccal cavity surfaces
   - Transverse fissuring
3. Esophageal candidiasis:
   - History of oropharyngeal candidiasis
   Symptoms include:
     - Dysphagia
     - Odynophagia
     - Epigastric pain
     - Retrosternal pain
   Physical examination shows:
     - Affects mainly the distal one third of the esophagus Endoscopy shows areas of the erythema and edema; scattered white patches or ulcers
4. Perianal candidiasis
   - Skin maceration
   - Itching
   - Frequently extends to the perineum

C. Paronychia/onychomycosis
- Fungal infection of the nail and surrounding tissues
- Associated with diabetes mellitus and immersion of hands or feet in water
- History: pain and redness around and beneath the nail and nail bed
- Physical exam: inflammation around the toe nail. There may also be nail thickening and discoloration (dystrophic nails). Nail loss may also occur.

D. Respiratory tract candidiasis
1. Usually seen in hospitalized patients
2. About 25% of outpatients have their respiratory tract colonized by *Candida* species

E. Genitourinary tract candidiasis
1. Vulvovaginal candidiasis
   - It causes itching, curdy white discharge, and occasionally dysuria and dyspareunia.
   - On examination the mucosa may be inflamed.
   - Painful erythema or itchy penile inflammation may occur in male sexual partners of affected females.
2. *Candida* balanitis
   - Usually acquired through sexual contact with a partner who has vulvovaginal candidiasis.
   - Symptoms include penile pruritus and white patches on penis.
   - Physical exam: dry, erythematous, and scaly patches on penis.

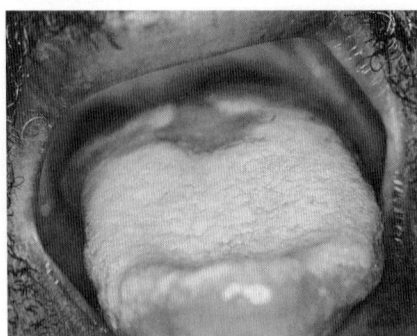

FIG. 1 Oral candidiasis. (From Swartz, MH: *Textbook of physical diagnosis,* ed 7, Philadelphia, 2014, Elsevier.)

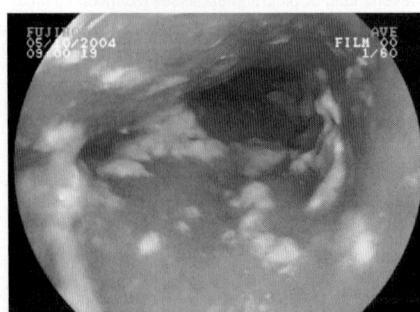

FIG. 2 Endoscopic appearance of esophageal candidiasis. (Courtesy Dr. B. Rembacken, Leeds, U.K.)

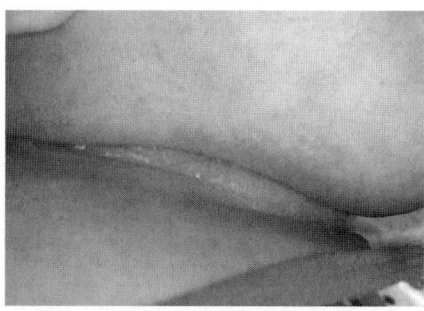

FIG. 3 Intertriginous candidosis of the neck. (From Kliegman RM et al: *Nelson textbook of pediatrics,* ed 19, Philadelphia, 2011, Saunders.)

F. Others
- Erosio interdigitalis blastomycetica: Denudating/macerating area commonly seen in third web space
- *Candida* folliculitis: Pustulous nodules in hairy areas
- Intertrigo: This occurs in folds of the skin and creases (Fig. 3). It is characterized by erosions, exudation, oozing, and maceration.

ETIOLOGY
The most common cause of cutaneous candidiasis is *Candida albicans.*

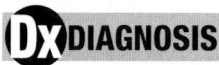**DIAGNOSIS**

DIFFERENTIAL DIAGNOSIS
Intertrigo
Seborrheic dermatitis
Psoriasis

WORK-UP
Mucocutaneous and cutaneous candidiasis
1. Obtain scrapings from the skin, oral, and vaginal mucosa or nails.
2. The presence of hyphae/pseudohyphae or budding yeast cells on wet smear, as well as confirmation by culture, is the recommended procedure to diagnose cutaneous candidiasis.
3. KOH smears are helpful.
Respiratory candidiasis
1. Sputum gram stain: shows yeast cells
2. Sputum cultures
3. Lung biopsy: establishes the diagnosis (Fig. 3)
Gastrointestinal candidiasis
1. Upper endoscopy with or without biopsy (Fig. 3)

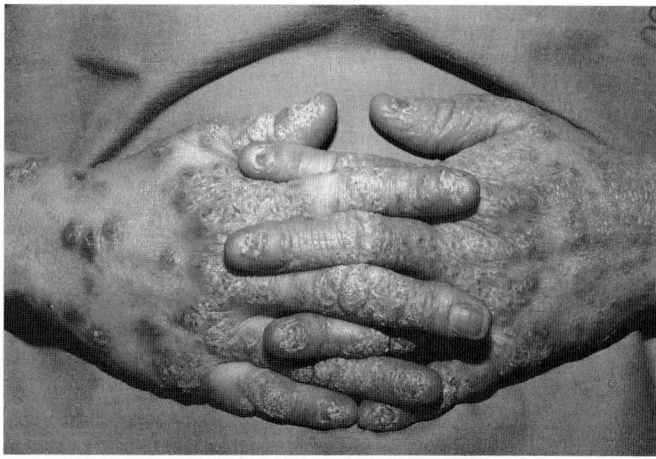

FIG. 4 Hand and nail involvement in chronic mucocutaneous candidiasis. (From James WD, et al: *Andrews' diseases of skin*, ed 12, Philadelphia, 2016, Saunders.)

Rx TREATMENT

PHARMACOLOGIC THERAPY
A. Cutaneous candidiasis
   1. Decrease/prevent moisture in area
   2. Apply antifungal agents (nystatin powder or cream with an azole or ciclopirox [e.g., clotrimazole, econazole, miconazole])
B. Gastrointestinal candidiasis
   1. Oropharyngeal candidiasis
      1. Treat with either
         1. Oral topical antifungal agent (e.g., nystatin swish and swallow) OR
         2. Systemic oral azoles (e.g., fluconazole)
      2. In HIV-positive patients, use high doses of fluconazole (100-200 mg PO qd for 7-14 days), itraconazole, or posaconazole.
C. *Candida* esophagitis
   1. Treat with systemic fluconazole for 2 to 3 wk.
   2. Treat with IV fluconazole if patient is unable to take oral medication.
D. Genitourinary tract candidiasis
   1. Vulvovaginal candidiasis: Treatment options for acute cases include:
      1. A single dose of oral fluconazole (fluconazole 150 mg PO × 1 dose) OR
      2. Topical antifungal agent
   2. For chronic or recurrent cases, treat with fluconazole 150 mg qod × 3 doses and then 150 mg/wk for 6 mo.

E. Chronic mucocutaneous candidiasis
   1. Treatment with azoles is effective (e.g., fluconazole 100-400 mg daily).
   2. When patient improves, follow with maintenance treatment with same azole for life.

FOLLOW-UP CARE
Mucocutaneous candidiasis
- Patient should be instructed to call or follow up if symptoms persist, recur, or worsen.
- For recurrent infections:
   1. Check HIV antibodies.
   2. Check FBS, HbA_{1c}.
   3. Rule out hematologic malignancy or solid organ malignancy.
   4. Refer to infectious disease specialist if no etiology is found.

PREVENTION
- Maintaining dry environment (e.g., by wearing cotton underwear)
- Decreased use of antibiotic
- No douching

SUGGESTED READINGS
Available at www.expertconsult.com

RELATED CONTENT
Candidiasis (Patient Information)

AUTHOR: **DANIEL K. ASIEDU, M.D., PH.D.**

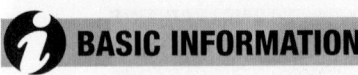

DEFINITION

Severe and invasive diseases are caused by *Candida* infection. The most common pathogen is *C. albicans*. Invasive candidiasis embodies a variety of diseases including candidemia, disseminated candidiasis, meningitis, and endophthalmitis. Invasive candidiasis is a significant cause of morbidity and mortality for certain groups of patients.

SYNONYMS

Systemic candidiasis

ICD-10CM CODES
B37.89 Other sites of candidiasis
B37.1 Pulmonary candidiasis
B37.2 Candidiasis of skin and nail
B37.5 Candidal meningitis
B37.6 Candidal endocarditis
B37.7 Candidal sepsis
B37.9 Candidiasis unspecified

EPIDEMIOLOGY & DEMOGRAPHICS

INCIDENCE: Invasive candidiasis is the most common fungal disease among hospitalized patients in the developed world. It affects over 250,000 people worldwide each year and causes more than 50,000 deaths.

In the U.S., *Candida* species cause 8% to 10% of nosocomial bloodstream infections (fourth most common bloodstream infection). Incidence rates of candidemia are between 2 and 14 cases/100,000 persons.

PREVALENCE: No data available

PREDOMINANT SEX AND AGE: Equal between males and females; all ages are susceptible.

RISK FACTORS: Prolonged hospitalization and ICU stay, use of broad-spectrum antibiotics, prolonged indwelling of catheters (especially central venous catheters), acute and chronic renal failure, surgery requiring general anesthesia, cancer (e.g., solid neoplasms), transplantation (bone marrow or solid organ), recent chemotherapy/radiation therapy, use of immunosuppressive drugs, parenteral alimentation, use of internal prosthetic devices, organ transplant, hemodialysis, mechanical, surgical procedures

PHYSICAL FINDINGS & CLINICAL PRESENTATION

1. History
   - Fever unresponsive to broad-spectrum antibiotics
   - History of prolonged indwelling IV catheter
   - A personal history of any of the risk factors listed earlier
2. Physical findings (general)
   - Fever
   - Hypotension
   - Generalized malaise
   - Tachycardia
   - Change in mental status
3. Specific diseases
   - Candidemia
     1. *Candida* species are isolated from at least one blood culture.
   2. Most common form of invasive candidiasis
   3. Physical exam may include fever, macronodular skin lesions, septic shock, *Candida* endophthalmitis.
   - Disseminated candidiasis
     1. Seen in patients with neutropenia
     2. Associated with multiple deep-organ infections or failure
     3. Blood culture negative
     4. Fever not responding to broad-spectrum antibiotics
     5. Physical exam: discrete erythematous or palpable rash, sepsis/septic shock
   - Endophthalmitis
     1. Iatrogenic/accidental fungal infection of the eye (exogenous) or hematogenous seeding of the eye (endogenous)
     2. Starts as choroidal lesion, progresses to vitreitis and endophthalmitis and eventually blindness
     3. Physical exam shows fever. Funduscopic examination shows large and off-white cotton ball–like lesions with indistinct borders.
   - *Candida* infection of the CNS
     1. Exogenous and endogenous forms
     2. Commonly found in long-term ICU patients
     3. May present as meningitis, mycotic aneurysms, change in mental status
     4. Physical examination reveals fever, neck rigidity, confusion, and coma.
   - Candidal musculoskeletal infections
     1. Previously uncommon; now relatively common probably due to increased frequency of candidemia and disseminated candidiasis
     2. Knee and vertebral column (especially lumbosacral vertebral disks and vertebral bodies) are involved.
     3. Physical exam is usually unremarkable but may show tenderness over involved area, fever, erythema, bone deformity, weight loss, and sometimes a draining fistulous tract.
   - Candidal infections of the heart
     1. May present as infective endocarditis, myocarditis, or pericarditis.
     2. Physical examination reveals fever, hypotension, tachycardia, new or changing murmur.
   - Hepatosplenic candidiasis (chronic systemic candidiasis)
     1. Seen in patients with hematologic malignancy and neutropenia; usually develops during recovery from a neutropenic state (normally after undergoing myeloablative chemotherapy)
     2. On examination, patients have low-grade fever, right upper quadrant pain, palpable/tender liver, splenomegaly, and rarely jaundice.
   - *Candida* peritonitis
     1. Associated with GI surgery, peritoneal dialysis
     2. Clinical manifestations include fever, chills, abdominal pain; nausea, vomiting, constipation.
     3. Physical examination reveals abdominal distention, abdominal pain, absent bowel sounds.
   - Other forms of invasive candidiasis
     1. *Candida* splenic abscess
     2. *Candida* cholecystitis
     3. Renal candidiasis

ETIOLOGY

- Several species of *Candida* exist in nature
- Medically significant include:
  1. *C. albicans:* together with *C. glabrata*, they account for 70% to 80% of *Candida* in invasive candidiasis.
  2. *C. glabrata:* together with *C. albicans*, they account for 70% to 80% of *Candida* in invasive candidiasis.
  3. *C. parapsilosis:* associated with indwelling vascular catheters and prosthetic devices
  4. *C. tropicalis:* especially in leukemic patients
  5. *C. krusei:* resistant to fluconazole and ketoconazole

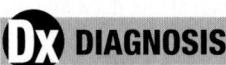

DIFFERENTIAL DIAGNOSIS

- Sepsis (bacterial)
- Septic shock
- Cryptococcosis
- Aspergillosis

WORKUP

LABORATORY TESTS:

- Laboratory studies are nonspecific. It is often necessary to perform several diagnostic tests to achieve maximum accuracy.
- High index of suspicion is needed.
- Candidemia/disseminated candidiasis: Candidemia represents the tip of the iceberg (Fig. 1) with respect to the more invasive forms of candidiasis. Central lines often contribute to the propagation of candidemia. From the blood, infection can spread to almost any organ.
  1. Blood cultures are the mainstay of diagnosis. They are helpful but have low positive yield.
  2. Diagnosis can also be made from normally sterile sites.
  3. Serum (1,3) beta-D-glucan detection assay: high specificity and high positive predictive value but it is relatively difficult to perform.
- Two commercial PCR tests are available (Septifast, Multiplex T2 candida panel) and have shown promising results.
- Hepatosplenic candidiasis (focal)
  1. Elevated serum alkaline phosphatase

IMAGING STUDIES:

- Imaging studies are generally not required or useful.
- Ultrasound is useful for diagnosing hepatosplenic abscess. "Bull's eye or target lesions" are observed in the liver and spleen.
- CT scanning may be used to diagnose hepatosplenic candidiasis, as well as intraabdominal/renal abscesses.
- ECHO is useful to rule in or rule out *Candida* endocarditis.

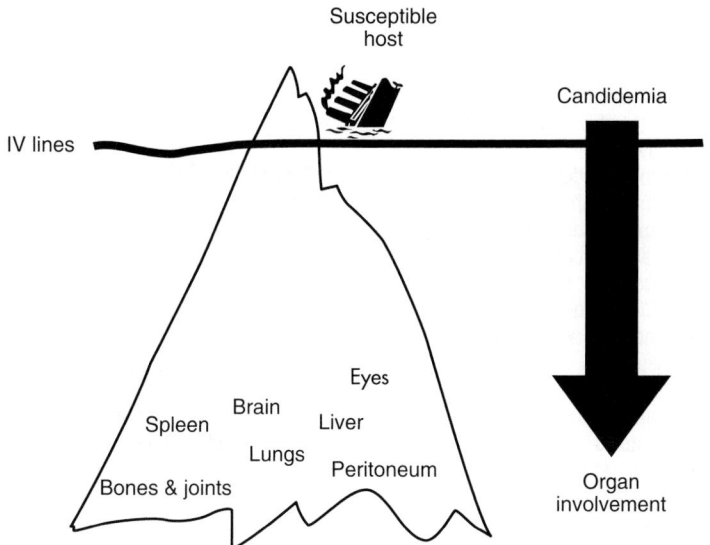

FIG. 1 Spectrum of disease of invasive candidiasis. Candidemia represents the tip of the iceberg with respect to the more invasive forms of candidiasis. Central lines often contribute to the propagation of candidemia. From the blood, infection can spread to almost any organ. (From Ostrosky-Zeichner L et al: Deeply invasive candidiasis, *Infect Dis Clin North Am* 16:821-835, 2002.)

Rx TREATMENT

- To successfully treat invasive *Candida* infection, it is important to start antifungal medication as early as possible. A small delay (approximately 12-24 hr) in starting treatment may result in a significantly excessive mortality rate.
  1. Do not dismiss *Candida* spp. as a contaminant when it is isolated in blood cultures or other sterile sites.
  2. Before treatment, also consider removal of an intravenous catheter.
- Antifungals available include:
  1. Azoles (e.g., fluconazole, posaconazole, itraconazole, voriconazole). They inhibit the synthesis of ergosterol, a fungal cell component.
  2. Echinocandins (e.g., caspofungin, micafungin, anidulafungin). These are glucan synthesis inhibitors. Glucan is an important component of fungal cell walls. Most studies have provided reasonable support for echinocandins as treatment of choice for the majority of patients with invasive candidiasis.
  3. Polyenes (e.g., amphotericin B, lipid formulation of amphotericin, nystatin). Broad spectrum. Their mechanism of action is to increase cytoplasmic permeability.
  4. Antimetabolites (e.g., flucytosine). Flucytosine is deaminated to 5-fluorouracil in fungal cell. 5-Fluorouracil inhibits RNA and protein synthesis.

TREATMENT PLANS
CANDIDEMIA:
- Treatment depends on whether the patient is neutropenic or not.
  1. Nonneutropenic adult patients: drug of choice is fluconazole; 800 mg as loading dose then 400 mg/day for at least 2 wk after clinical improvement or negative blood culture. Amphotericin B is equally efficacious.

  2. Neutropenic adult patients: an echinocandin is the drug of choice (e.g., caspofungin 70 mg IV loading dose then 50 mg/day IV or micafungin 100 mg/day IV or anidulafungin 200 mg IV loading dose then 100 mg IV all for at least 2 wk after clear blood culture and after clinical improvement.
DISSEMINATED CANDIDIASIS: Fluconazole is the drug of choice.
DISSEMINATED CANDIDIASIS WITH END-ORGAN INFECTION:
- Treatment is the same as for candidemia of nonneutropenic patients. In most cases, therapy is prolonged for at least 4 to 6 wk.
- The echinocandins are the first-line therapy.
OSTEOMYELITIS OR SEPTIC ARTHRITIS:
- Fluconazole 400 mg IV or PO *or*
- Lipid-based amphotericin B 3-5 mg/kg qd
ENDOCARDITIS:
- Caspofungin 50-150 mg/day or
- Micafungin 100-150 mg/day or
- Anidulafungin 100-200 mg/day
MYOCARDITIS:
- Lipid-based amphotericin B 3-5 mg/kg daily *or*
- Fluconazole 400-800 mg daily IV or PO
ESOPHAGITIS:
- Fluconazole 200-400 mg/day or
- Caspofungin 50 mg IV daily
PERICARDITIS:
- Lipid-based amphotericin B 3-5 mg/kg daily *or*
- Fluconazole 400-800 mg PO qd IV or PO
SURGICAL CARE: Include:
- Drainage
- Removal of any foreign bodies
- Surgical debridement
- Organ-specific care (e.g., valve replacement for endocarditis, splenectomy for splenic abscess, or vitrectomy for fungal endophthalmitis)

DISPOSITION
- Several factors affect prognosis: infection site, degree of immune suppression, and how quickly diagnosis and therapy is initiated

- Overall mortality rate: 30% to 40%

REFERRAL
- Always involve an infectious disease specialist.
- Referral to specialist will depend on the organ involved. For example:
  1. Endocarditis will require a cardiothoracic surgeon.
  2. Endophthalmitis will require an ophthalmologist.

FOLLOW-UP CARE
- Prolonged periods, mainly in the hospital, of antifungal treatment may be necessary.
- Closely monitor patients on amphotericin B because of the high incidence of side effects. Check basic metabolic panel, magnesium, and CBC at least twice a week.

❗ PEARLS & CONSIDERATIONS

PREVENTION
Basic preventive measures are similar to those used for nosocomial infections. This includes:
- Maximizing hand hygiene recommendations:
  1. Hand washing
  2. Using alcohol/chlorhexidine solution
- Adhering strictly to recommendations for placement and care of central lines and catheters.
- Judicious use of antimicrobials

PROPHYLAXIS
Antifungal prophylaxis should be limited to patients in whom it has proved beneficial: patients with gastrointestinal anastomotic leakage, patients undergoing transplantation of the pancreas or small bowel, selected patients undergoing liver transplantation who are at high risk for candidiasis and extremely low-birth-weight neonates in settings with a high incidence of neonatal candidiasis (Kullberg BJ, Arendrup MC: *NJEM* 373:1445-1456, 2015.)

PATIENT/FAMILY EDUCATION
- Inform them about the risk factors for invasive candidiasis.
- Inform them of the seriousness of the disease and the associated high morbidity/mortality rates, thus requiring aggressive treatment.
- Side effects and toxicities associated with treatment

SUGGESTED READINGS
Available at www.expertconsult.com

RELATED CONTENT
Candidiasis (Patient Information)
Candidiasis, Cutaneous (Related Key Topic)

AUTHOR: **DANIEL K. ASIEDU, M.D., PH.D.**

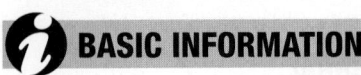

BASIC INFORMATION

DEFINITION

Carbon monoxide (CO) is a colorless, odorless, tasteless, nonirritating gas. When inhaled it produces toxicity by causing cellular hypoxia and damage.

ICD-10CM CODES
T68   Toxic effect of carbon monoxide
T58.01 Toxic effect of carbon monoxide from motor vehicle exhaust, accidental (unintentional), initial encounter

EPIDEMIOLOGY & DEMOGRAPHICS

- A leading cause of accidental and intentional poisoning in the U.S.
- Can occur because of acute toxicity or chronic exposure.
- CO poisoning is seen more frequently during the fall and winter months in cold climates. Frequently seen after storm-related power outages, mostly due to the use of portable gasoline-powered electrical generators.
- Most fatal cases of CO poisoning occur in the home.

PHYSICAL FINDINGS & CLINICAL PRESENTATION

- Depends on the severity and duration of exposure. The brain and heart are most sensitive to CO poisoning.
- Presentation is often nonspecific and may be mistaken for a flulike illness.
- Severity of poisoning does not correlate with carboxyhemoglobin (COHb) levels.
- Mild to moderate poisoning may present with headache, malaise, dizziness, nausea, dyspnea, difficulty concentrating, confusion, and blurred vision. Patients may have tachypnea and tachycardia.
- Severe poisoning may present with hypotension, arrhythmias, myocardial ischemia, pulmonary edema, lethargy, ataxia, loss of consciousness, seizure, coma, or rarely, cherry-red skin.
- Delayed neurologic sequelae may develop days to weeks after apparent recovery from acute poisoning. Patients may present with neurologic or psychiatric symptoms (cognitive deficits, memory loss, personality changes, movement disorders, Parkinson's, psychosis, neurologic deficits).

ETIOLOGY

- CO results from the incomplete combustion of carbon-containing compounds. CO poisoning occurs from inhaling smoke from fires, motor vehicle/motor boat exhaust, or the burning of fuel (oil, wood, coal, gasoline, natural gas) in poorly functioning or improperly ventilated devices (heating systems, stoves/grills, portable generators, etc.). Methylene chloride (paint stripper) fumes are converted to CO by the liver.

- CO toxicity results from tissue hypoxia and direct CO-mediated damage at the cellular level. This may explain why COHb levels alone are not predictive of clinical toxicity. The mechanisms of CO toxicity are not completely understood.
- CO impairs oxygen delivery. CO reversibly binds hemoglobin with an affinity 250 times greater than oxygen, displacing oxygen from hemoglobin and decreasing the oxygen-carrying capacity of blood. By binding to hemoglobin, CO changes the structure of the hemoglobin molecule and decreases oxygen release to tissue.
- CO may also interfere with peripheral oxygen utilization by binding to other heme-containing proteins including cytochromes and myoglobin. Cellular respiration may be depressed by inhibition of mitochondrial function. Neurologic toxicity is not explained by hypoxia alone and is related to the complex intracellular actions of CO. CO precipitates an inflammatory cascade that results in oxidative damage and brain lipid peroxidation.

DIAGNOSIS

DIFFERENTIAL DIAGNOSIS

- Viral syndromes
- Cyanide, hydrogen sulfide
- Methemoglobinemia
- Amphetamines and derivatives
- Cocaine, phencyclidine (PCP)
- Cyclic antidepressants
- Phenothiazines
- Theophylline

WORKUP

History (duration and source of CO exposure, loss of consciousness), physical examination (detailed neurologic examination), laboratory and imaging tests

LABORATORY TESTS

- COHb level (measured by CO-oximetry on arterial or venous blood). COHb level >3% in nonsmokers confirms exposure. Heavy smokers may have baseline levels of up to 10%. Levels may be low if the patient has already received supplemental oxygen or if delays occur between exposure and testing.
- NOTE: Pulse oximetry and arterial blood gas (ABG) may be falsely normal because neither measures oxygen saturation of hemoglobin directly. Pulse oximetry is inaccurate because of the similar absorption characteristics of oxyhemoglobin and COHb. An ABG is inaccurate because it measures oxygen dissolved in plasma (which is not affected by CO) and then calculates oxygen saturation of hemoglobin.
- Electrolytes, glucose, BUN, creatinine, cardiac biomarkers, ABG (lactic acidosis and rhabdomyolysis may develop), CBC

(polycythemia from hypoxia in chronic CO poisoning).
- ECG (ischemia, arrhythmia).
- Pregnancy test (fetus at high risk).
- Consider toxicology screen.

IMAGING STUDIES

- Chest x-ray (noncardiogenic edema)
- Brain CT, MRI if neurologic abnormalities are present

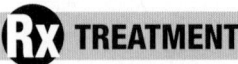 TREATMENT

ACUTE GENERAL Rx

- Remove from site of CO exposure.
- Ensure adequate airway.
- Continuous ECG monitor.
- Fetal monitoring if pregnant.
- 100% oxygen by nonrebreather mask or endotracheal tube (decreases half-life of COHb from 4 to 6 hr to 60 to 90 min) until COHb level is <10% and patient is asymptomatic. Table 1 describes the half-life of COHb.
- Hyperbaric oxygen (2.5 to 3 atm).
  1. Questionable beneficial effect over normobaric oxygen. Disparate findings in various studies: some suggest hyperbaric oxygen treatment reduces the incidence of neurologic sequelae, and others have found it worsens neurologic outcomes compared to normobaric oxygen treatment.
  2. Decreases half-life of COHb to 20 to 30 min; increases amount of oxygen dissolved in plasma. It also reduces CO binding to other heme-containing proteins.
  3. Consider for:
     1. Severe intoxication (COHb >25%, history of loss of consciousness, neurologic symptoms or signs, cardiovascular compromise, severe metabolic acidosis)
     2. Pregnant women with COHb >20% or signs of fetal distress. CO elimination is slower in fetus than mother, fetal Hgb has greater affinity for CO than adult Hgb
     3. Should be instituted quickly if deemed necessary
- Consider concomitant poisoning with other toxic/irritant gases that may be present in smoke (e.g., cyanide) or thermal injury to airway. Toxic effects of CO and cyanide are synergistic.

TABLE 1 Half-Life of COHb	
Oxygen Concentration	**Half-Life**
21% (room air)	4-5 hr
100% (mask or endotracheal)	60-90 min
100% (hyperbaric molecular oxygen)	20-30 min

From Fuhrman BP et al: *Pediatric critical care*, ed 4, Philadelphia, 2011, Saunders.

- Identify source of exposure and determine if poisoning was accidental (Fig. 1).

DISPOSITION

- Patients with mild accidental poisoning can be treated in an ambulatory setting. Those with moderate/severe poisoning or coexisting illness require hospitalization.
- Survivors of severe poisoning are at 14% to 40% risk for neurologic sequelae.

1. Deficits are usually apparent within 3 wk of poisoning but may present months later.
2. Risk of developing sequelae is greater if patient lost consciousness during acute poisoning and with older age.
3. Brain MRI and functional CT may reveal changes; damage is seen most often in the globus pallidus and deep white matter.

4. Recovery may occur over months to years.
- Severe CO poisoning is associated with increased long-term morbidity and mortality.
- High risk of fetal demise

REFERRAL

- American Association of Poison Control Centers: 1-800-222-1222
- Hyperbaric unit; accredited facilities are listed on the Undersea & Hyperbaric Medical Society website (www.uhms.org)
- Psychiatric evaluation if intentional poisoning

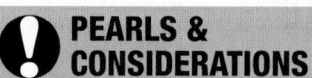

PEARLS & CONSIDERATIONS

- Severity of poisoning and prognosis do not correlate with COHb levels because hypoxia represents only a component of CO's toxic effect. New therapies to address CO toxicity are being proposed.
- Neuropsychometric testing is an objective measure of cognitive function but is not universally used.
- Imaging techniques and biomarkers to define severity of CO poisoning, early prediction of CNS damage and prognosis are being studied, but are not ready for application.
- Pulse CO-oximetry measurement of CO saturation has limited clinical use.
- Treatment with hydroxocobalamin (for cyanide toxicity) may make subsequent COHb testing unreliable.
- Contact local fire department to assess environment and identify source of CO.

SUGGESTED READINGS
Available at www.expertconsult.com

RELATED CONTENT
Carbon Monoxide Poisoning (Patient Information)

AUTHOR: **SUDEEP K. AULAKH, M.D.**

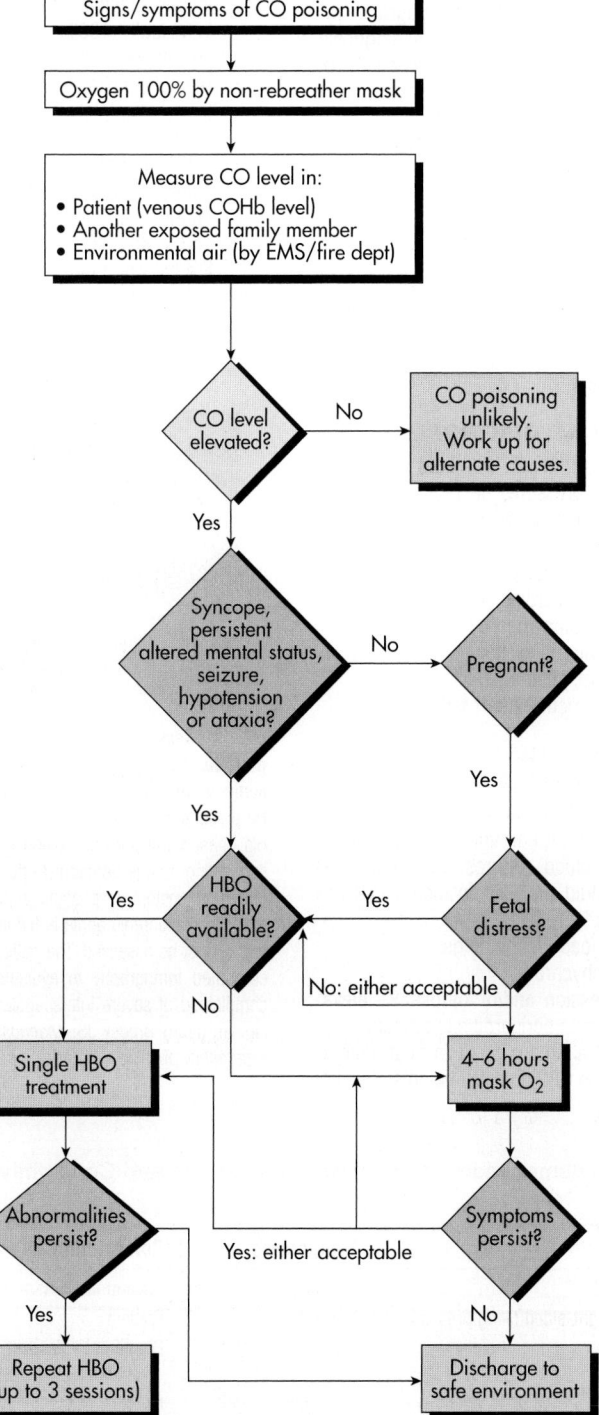

FIG. 1 Suggested management algorithm for carbon monoxide poisoning. (From Lavonas EJ: Carbon monoxide poisoning. In Shannon MW, Borron SW, Burns M (eds): *Haddad and Winchester's clinical management of poisoning and drug overdose*, Philadelphia, 2007, Elsevier.)

Diseases and Disorders

C

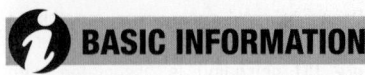

DEFINITION

Cardiac tamponade is a life-threatening condition where an accumulation of fluid within the pericardial sac causes equal elevation of atrial, end diastolic pressures in the ventricles, and pericardial pressures, as well as an exaggerated inspiratory decrease in arterial systolic pressure (pulsus paradoxus) along with arterial hypotension.

ICD-10CM CODES
I31.4 Cardiac tamponade

PHYSICAL FINDINGS & CLINICAL PRESENTATION

- Tachypnea/dyspnea
- Chest pain may be present
- Beck's triad
  1. Absolute or relative hypotension
  2. Elevated jugular venous pressure (with prominent *x* descent and blunted *y* descent)
  3. Muffled heart sounds
- Tachycardia (except in uremia or hypothyroid patients)
- Pulsus paradoxus (decrease in systolic arterial pressure of 10 mm Hg or more during normal inspiration while in normal sinus rhythm)
- Pericardial friction rub may or may not be present
- Reduced or absent apical cardiac impulse

ETIOLOGY

I. Acute (rapidly accumulating pericardial effusion leading to cardiac tamponade): does not need a large amount of effusion to cause tamponade; rather, it is the rapidity of fluid accumulation that leads to clinical tamponade. Clinical presentation typically resembles that of cardiogenic shock requiring urgent reduction of pericardial pressure. Causes for acute cardiac tamponade include:
  1. Penetrating trauma
  2. Aortic dissection (more commonly in Type A)
  3. Postinfarction myocardial rupture and/or hemorrhagic pericarditis
  4. Iatrogenic (central line and pacemaker insertions, cardiac ablation, post–coronary bypass surgery or post–percutaneous coronary intervention)
II. Subacute or chronic: occurs over days to weeks, and the effusion is usually large; causes include the following:
  1. Malignancy (e.g., lung, breast, lymphoma)
  2. Viral pericarditis (e.g., Coxsackie, human immunodeficiency virus, enterovirus, HSV 6, parvovirus, etc.)
  3. Bacterial, fungal, or tuberculous pericarditis
  4. Uremia
  5. Hypothyroidism/myxedema (rare)
  6. Collagen vascular disease (e.g., lupus, rheumatoid arthritis, scleroderma)
  7. Radiation
  8. Post–myocardial infarction or post–cardiac ablation inflammation
  9. Idiopathic
III. Regional cardiac tamponade occurs when the localized or loculated hematoma compresses only selected cardiac chambers.

DX DIAGNOSIS

Cardiac tamponade is a clinical diagnosis made at the bedside from history and physical examination. The echocardiogram will help confirm or reject the clinical diagnosis. Tamponade can be confirmed invasively by the measurement of elevated intrapericardial pressures with an intrapericardial catheter and right-sided heart catheterization. Typical findings are diastolic equalization of pressures, usually ranging from 10 to 30 mm Hg (diastolic pulmonary artery pressure = right ventricular diastolic pressure = right atrial pressure = intrapericardial pressure), and lowering of the intrapericardial pressure with fluid drainage. Thereafter, the underlying etiology must be determined with specific laboratory work (see "Laboratory Tests").

DIFFERENTIAL DIAGNOSIS

Other conditions that can also lead to elevated jugular venous pressure, decreased systemic pressure, and pulsus paradoxus include:
- Chronic obstructive pulmonary disease and asthma exacerbations
- Constrictive pericarditis (Table 1)
- Restrictive cardiomyopathy
- Right ventricular infarction
- Pulmonary embolism
- Chronic biventricular heart failure

LABORATORY TESTS

- Electrolytes, blood urea nitrogen, creatinine, erythrocyte sedimentation rate, thyroid function tests, antinuclear antibody, rheumatoid factor, PPD, blood cultures, viral titers, and pericardial fluid analysis including cytology and cultures
- Possible 12-lead ECG findings:
  1. Sinus tachycardia
  2. PR depression and/or diffuse ST elevations if acute pericarditis is present
  3. Electrical alternans (beat to beat alternations in the QRS complex heights) (Fig. E1)
  4. Low voltage if massive effusion is present. (QRS complex <0.5 mV in the limb leads and <1.0 mV in precordial leads)

IMAGING STUDIES

- Chest radiograph (enlarged cardiac silhouette with clear lung fields) (Fig. 2)
- Chest CT (may overestimate size of the effusion) (Fig. 3)
- Echocardiogram findings (Fig. 4):
  1. Pericardial effusion
  2. Diastolic collapse of the right atrium in late diastole (during atrial relaxation) is virtually 100% sensitive but has low specificity.
  3. Diastolic collapse of the right ventricle (early diastole) is pathognomonic and very specific.
  4. >25% mitral and >50% tricuspid valve inflow variation with respiration
  5. Plethoric inferior vena cava (IVC dilation and <50% decrease in the diameter of the IVC during inspiration)
  6. Left atrial collapse (high specificity)
- Cardiac catheterization as discussed earlier will see equalization of intracardiac diastolic

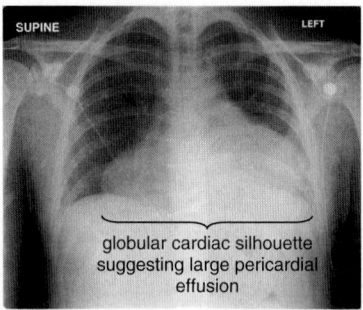
globular cardiac silhouette suggesting large pericardial effusion

FIG. 2 Massive pericardial effusion and tamponade. This 23-year-old male has a history of aortic valve replacement for infective endocarditis. He presented with increased chest pain and dyspnea. His chest x-ray shows a globular cardiac silhouette, suggesting a large pericardial effusion. The lung fields and right costophrenic angle appear clear, although the left costophrenic angle is hidden behind the heart and cannot be assessed. The patient underwent chest computed tomography to evaluate his aorta, as he complained of severe interscapular pain as well (see Fig. 3). (From Broder JS: *Diagnostic imaging for the emergency physician*, Philadelphia, 2011, Saunders.)

TABLE 1 Hemodynamics in Cardiac Tamponade and Constrictive Pericarditis

	Tamponade	Constriction
Paradoxical pulse	Usually present	Present in ~1/3
Equal left- and right-sided filling pressures	Present	Present
Systemic venous wave morphology	Absent *y* descent	Prominent *y* descent (M or W shape)
Inspiratory change in systemic venous pressure	Decrease (normal)	Increase or no change (Kussmaul sign)
"Square root" sign in ventricular pressure	Absent	Present

From Fuhrman BP et al: *Pediatric critical care*, ed 4, Philadelphia, 2011, Saunders.

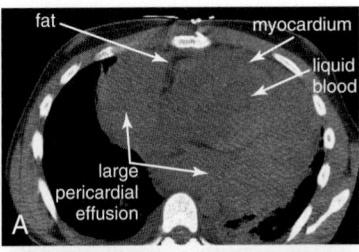

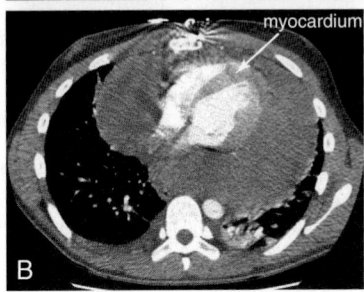

FIG. 3 Massive pericardial effusion. Same patient as Fig. 2. The patient underwent chest computed tomography (CT) without **(A)** and then with **(B)** intravenous contrast to evaluate his aorta, which was normal. However, the CT confirmed a massive pericardial effusion surrounding a normal-appearing heart. Without contrast, note that fluid blood within the chambers of the heart has a slightly lower density than the pericardial effusion, which has a density more similar to that of myocardium. When contrast is administered, the ventricular chambers fill completely, and the myocardium enhances and becomes somewhat brighter than the surrounding pericardial effusion. The heart itself is outlined by a thin stripe of fat, which appears nearly black on soft tissue windows. The patient developed hypotension, suggesting cardiac tamponade, and pericardial window was performed for drainage of the effusion. In the operating room, the effusion was found to be coagulated blood. (From Broder JS: *Diagnostic imaging for the emergency physician,* Philadelphia, 2011, Saunders.)

pressures and increase of right-sided pressures and reduction of left-sided pressures, which subsequently causes pulsus paradoxus (the pathognomonic finding on physical examination)

Rx TREATMENT

NONPHARMACOLOGIC THERAPY
- Cardiac tamponade should be treated emergently with removal of the pericardial fluid.
- Avoid drugs that reduce preload (e.g., nitrates, diuretics).
- Large pericardial effusions without hemodynamic compromise (tamponade) can be managed conservatively with careful monitoring, IV fluids, treatment of the underlying cause, clinical follow-up, and frequent serial surveillance echocardiography.

ACUTE GENERAL Rx
- Aggressive intravascular volume expansion (saline or blood).
- Emergency pericardial fluid removal by pericardiocentesis or surgical pericardiotomy by way of the subxiphoid pericardial window.

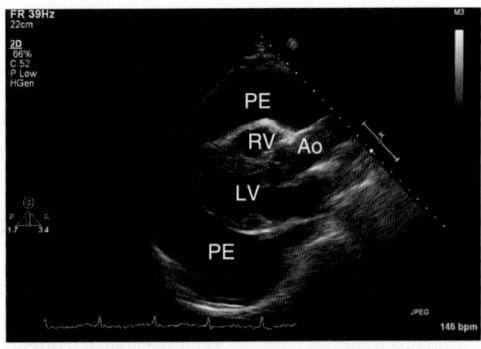

FIG. 4 Two-dimensional echocardiogram of a large, circumferential pericardial effusion (PE). *Ao,* Aorta; *LV,* left ventricle; *RV,* right ventricle. (From Kabbani SS, LeWinter M: Cardiac constriction and restriction. In Crawford MH, DiMarco JP [eds]: *Cardiology,* St Louis, 2001, Mosby.)

- Pericardiocentesis should be performed under fluoroscopic or echocardiographic guidance when available.
- Pericardiocentesis is an absolute contraindication if the etiology of the pericardial effusion is aortic dissection, wherein emergent surgical management is indicated.
- Inotropic or vasopressor support if above measures cannot be performed immediately.

CHRONIC Rx
- Depends on etiology. Patients with inflammatory causes of pericarditis leading to effusion should be treated with an extended course of colchicine.
- Pericardiocentesis with draining catheter: the catheter can be left inside the pericardium to allow continued drainage for 24 to 48 hr. If residual fluid still persists with hemodynamic compromise, surgical drainage should be considered. In the absence of hemodynamic compromise or significant residual fluid, discontinuation of the draining catheter can be done with periodic postprocedure echocardiographic monitoring for re-accumulation (e.g., 24 hr, 7 days, 30 days, 3 mo, 6 mo, 12 mo) depending on the etiology and the rate of reaccumulation.
- Other surgical drainage procedures include:
  1. Subxiphoid pericardiotomy drainage
  2. Pericardial window; draining the pericardial fluid into the left hemithorax
  3. Limited pericardiectomy
  4. Complete pericardiectomy, especially in patients with effusive-constrictive pericarditis, bacterial pericarditis, or tuberculous pericarditis. (see "Pearls & Considerations").

DISPOSITION
The prognosis of cardiac tamponade depends on the underlying cause.

REFERRAL
- Emergent cardiology consultation along with thorough echocardiographic exam should be made if cardiac tamponade is suspected.
- Cardiothoracic surgery or interventional cardiology consultation should also be considered if pericardial drainage is indicated.

⚠ PEARLS & CONSIDERATIONS
- Cardiac tamponade should always be considered during pulseless electrical activity arrest and may require emergent pericardiocentesis at the bedside.
- Evaluation for pulsus paradoxus should always be performed during normal respiration because deep inspiration may render a false-positive finding.
- Strong consideration should be given to performing early pericardiocentesis in patients who have pericardial effusion associated with bacterial pneumonia or empyema because the incidence of bacterial pericarditis is especially high in this clinical situation and the subsequent development of cardiac tamponade and severe chronic constrictive pericarditis are ominous complications.
- Pericardiocentesis is an absolute contraindication if the etiology of the pericardial effusion is due to aortic dissection extending into the pericardial sac.
- As little as 100 ml of fluid can lead to acute cardiac tamponade if the rate of accumulation is rapid, whereas with gradual accumulation, the pericardial sac can hold up to 5 L of fluid before tamponade occurs.

SUGGESTED READINGS
Available at www.expertconsult.com

RELATED CONTENT
Cardiac Tamponade (Patient Information)
Pericarditis (Related Key Topic)

AUTHORS: **ADAM M. NOYES, M.D.,** and **ARAVIND RAO KOKKIRALA, M.D.**

DEFINITION

Cardiomyopathy, chemical-induced (CMc), is the changes of cardiac structure and function caused by chemical compounds. Many chemicals, including environmental, prescription drugs, or illicit drugs, are associated with cardiomyopathy. These include (but are not limited to) alcohol, cocaine, amphetamine, synthetic cannabinoids, doxorubicin, 5-fluorouracil (5-FU), zidovudine, and trastuzumab.

SYNONYMS

Alcoholic cardiomyopathy (ACM)
Cocaine-induced cardiomyopathy (CM)
Anabolic steroid–induced CM
Anthracycline-induced CM
CMc

ICD-10CM CODES
I42.7 Cardiomyopathy due to drug and external agent

EPIDEMIOLOGY & DEMOGRAPHICS

- ACM occurs in about 10% of alcoholics. The prevalence ranges from 23% to 40% of non-ischemic cardiomyopathy.
- The risk of doxorubicin-induced heart failure increases with cumulative dose of anthracycline: 3% to 5% with 400 mg/m^2, 7% to 26% at 550 mg/m^{22}, and 18% to 48% at 700 mg/m^2.
- Addition of chemotherapeutic agent trastuzumab to traditional chemotherapy in breast cancer was associated with marginal increase in symptomatic heart failure events. However, long-term follow-up of the pivotal adjuvant trials has demonstrated the cardiac safety of trastuzumab with no substantial increase in cardiovascular events over 8 to 10 years.
- Other chemotherapeutic agents known to cause cardiomyopathy include epirubicin, docetaxel, mitomycin, cyclophosphamide, bortezomib, sunitinib, 5-fluorouracil [5-FU], and emerging reports of carfilzomib.

PREDOMINANT SEX AND AGE: Among ACM cases, men represent more than 80% and have higher mortality compared with women. In all races, blacks have higher death rates compared to whites. Anthracycline- and trastuzumab-induced cardiomyopathy is predominantly more common in those ages >50 years.

GENETICS:

- In patients with ACM, deletion (DD) genotype of ACE is more common than insertion (II) and deletion insertion (DI) genotypes. The underlying mechanism involves direct toxicity of ethanol to the myocardium through uncoupling of ATP.
- Anthracycline-induced cardiomyopathy is linked to an increase in cardiac oxidative stress via the pathways of mitochondria, nitric oxide synthesis, and nicotinamide adenine dinucleotide phosphate reduction.
- One study suggests that polymorphisms in the carbonyl reductase genes could be related to anthracycline-induced CM.

RISK FACTORS:

- Consumption of more than 80 g/day of alcohol for more than 5 years increases risk of ACM.
- The occurrence of chronic anthracycline-induced CM is correlated to cumulative dose, age, preexisting heart disease, concomitant chemotherapy, and history of mediastinal radiation therapy. Children are more susceptible to anthracycline-induced CM.
- Continuous infusions of chemotherapy pose a higher risk for cardiotoxicity, compared to bolus regimens.

PHYSICAL FINDINGS & CLINICAL PRESENTATION

The majority of clinical characteristics of CMc are similar to the dilated cardiomyopathy of other etiologies. Symptoms may develop either insidiously or acute in onset.

- The acute anthracycline-induced cardiotoxicity can start at anytime after the first dose and presents with arrhythmias, most commonly supraventricular tachycardia, ventricular dysfunction, and pericardial diseases. Typically the first manifestation of anthracycline-induced cardiotoxicity is subtle diastolic dysfunction noted on tissue Doppler. The subacute and chronic symptoms occur from 3 months after the last dose to 10 years later. Patients usually present with congestive heart failure (CHF). More recently, mortality has improved as a result of medical treatment with ACE inhibitors and beta-blockers. In fact, some recent trials including the Overcome Trial have demonstrated a possible benefit in preemptively treating patients with beta-blockers and ACE-inhibitors undergoing anthracycline therapy before the development of any CM.
- Cardiac symptoms after 5-FU treatment include angina (most common), myocardial infarction, arrhythmia, acute pulmonary edema, cardiac arrest, and pericarditis. The mortality of 5-FU–induced cardiotoxicity is 2% to 13%.
- The presentation of CHF may occur over 15 years of heavy drinking. In the presentation of arrhythmia, atrial fibrillation is most common with chronic ETOH abuse and can also be seen acutely with intoxication (holiday heart syndrome).
- Patients with cocaine CM may present with adrenergic symptoms (palpitations, pallor, diaphoresis, and anxiety), hypertension, angina, atrial and ventricular arrhythmia, and heart failure.
- Anabolic steroids can cause left ventricular hypertrophy and dilation, and can lead to heart failure, arrhythmia, myocardial infarction, hypertension, and sudden death.

ETIOLOGY

The underlying mechanism of chemotherapy is not well established. Several pathways have been proposed, including an increase in oxidative stress, free radical production, apoptosis, disturbance of DNA, RNA and protein synthesis, and vasospasm. Nutritional deficiency, such as thiamine deficiency, also plays a role in ACM.

Dx DIAGNOSIS

DIFFERENTIAL DIAGNOSIS

- Infectious cardiomyopathy: viral, HIV related, Lyme disease, Chagas disease
- Ischemic cardiomyopathy
- Dilated cardiomyopathy, related to valvular disease, hypertension, and causes other than chemicals
- Cirrhotic cardiomyopathy
- Tachycardia-induced cardiomyopathy

WORKUP

- The diagnosis is based on the history of chemical exposure and the clinical presentation of heart failure, arrhythmia, and angina pectoris.
- Electrocardiogram (ECG) and serum electrolytes, renal function, and hepatic function.
- Serum troponin and brain natriuretic peptide (BNP) levels.
- Transthoracic echocardiogram for the evaluation of heart structure and function.
- Rule out the diagnosis of coronary artery disease by coronary angiography.
- Cardiac magnetic resonance (CMR) imaging can be used to evaluate for myocardial scar and fibrosis.

LABORATORY TESTS

- There are no specific diagnostic tests to help differentiate CMc from other forms of CM, but the following laboratory tests are generally helpful.
- Serum electrolytes, renal function, hepatic function, thyroid-stimulating hormone, iron profile, and inflammatory factors
- Recent studies have suggested that early elevation of troponin I levels, BNP, and myeloperoxidase following chemotherapy may be an early predictor of future development of cardiomyopathy.

IMAGING STUDIES

- ECG
  1. ST deviation and atrial and ventricular arrhythmia in 5-FU toxicity
     1. Sinus tachycardia
     2. Nonspecific ST-T change
     3. Decreased QRS voltage
     4. Prolonged QT interval
- Echocardiogram
  1. Asymptomatic alcoholics may present with mild left ventricular (LV) hypertrophy, diastolic dysfunction, LV dilation, and decrease in left ventricular ejection fraction (LVEF).
  2. Baseline LVEF should be performed before initiation of doxorubicin-based chemotherapy with either serial echocardiograms or MUGA (multigated acquisition) scan.
     1. If baseline LVEF is >55%, then subsequent evaluation should be at the end of treatment if anthracycline dose is <200 mg/m^2 or serially at 200, 300, 350, and 400 mg/m^2 dose completion. Doxorubicin therapy should be discontinued if there is a >15% absolute drop or >10% drop below normal or symptomatic congestive heart failure develops.
     2. Peak systolic global longitudinal strain imaging (GLS) is an emerging echocardiographic measurement. A 10% to 15% early decrease in GLS by speckle tracking echocardiography during treatment seems to be the most useful parameter for the early detection of

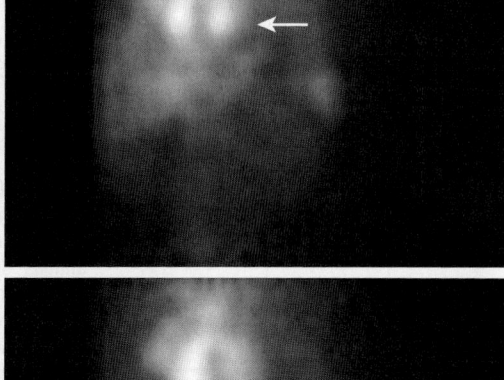

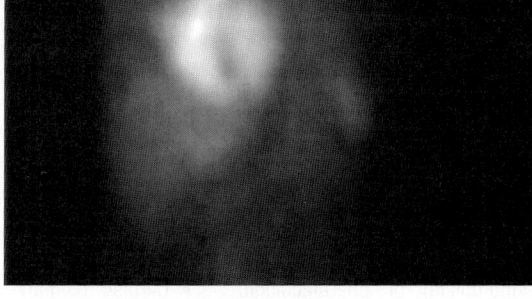

End-Diastole   End-Systole

FIG. 1 Technetium-99m-pertechnetate multigated acquisition scans in a 47-year-old woman with breast cancer treated with doxorubicin. The top scan was taken before initiation of doxorubicin and cyclophosphamide therapy in September 2009. The left ventricular ejection fraction (left ventricular end-diastolic counts minus left ventricular end-systolic counts/left ventricular end-diastolic counts 100) was calculated at 60%. The bottom scan was taken in March 2010 after treatment with a total doxorubicin dose of 451 mg/m². Left ventricular ejection fraction was calculated at 28%. Left ventricle (*white arrows*) during end-diastole and end-systole. (From Figueredo VM: Chemical cardiomyopathies: the negative effects of medications and nonprescribed drugs on the heart, *Am J Med* 124:480-488, 2011.)

cardiotoxicity. However, large population studies confirming the validity of GLS are still awaited.
- Radionuclide imaging (Fig. 1).
  1. If baseline LVEF ≤55%, the cardiac risks vs. oncological benefits should be discussed with the patient, cardiologist, and oncologist before initiating therapy. Cardio-protective agents such as ACE inhibitors and beta-blockers should be initiated and serial LVEF measurements done after each dose.
  2. Even after chemotherapy is completed, annual LVEF measurements with echocardiograms or MUGA scans should be done for 5 years to detect late anthracycline cardiotoxicity.

Rx TREATMENT

Prevention:
- The noninvasive assessment of LV function before, during, and after anthracycline-containing chemotherapy by means of echocardiograms and MUGA scan.
- To reduce the risk of anthracycline-induced cardiotoxicity, the lifetime cumulative dosage should be limited to <350 mg/m² in adults.
- Other approaches include the use of infusion other than bolus, liposomal encapsulated doxorubicin, less cardiotoxic analogs of doxorubicin such as epirubicin, and co-administration of protective agents such as dexrazoxane.
- Termination of 5-FU treatment if cardiac symptoms manifest and re-administration is not recommended

ACUTE GENERAL Rx
- Treat decompensated CHF with diuresis and inotropes if low cardiac output.
- For angina in acute cocaine intoxication, benzodiazepines, nitrites, and calcium channel blockers are the first line of therapy. Once myocardial infarction is indicated by ECG and serum troponin, patients should be evaluated by cardiac catheterization.

CHRONIC Rx
- Nitrates, beta-blockers, and calcium channel blockers for angina caused by 5-FU.
- Dexrazoxane is an ethylenediaminetetraacetic acid–like chelator that acts by binding to iron, which prevents anthracycline cardiotoxicity. Cardio-oncology experts suggest a 10:1 ratio of dexrazoxane to anthracycline, administered 15 to 30 minutes before doxorubicin administration. However, the routine use of the drug is currently not approved in adults except in cases of cumulative dose of doxorubicin of 300 mg/m² or greater.
- Those developing anthracycline cardiomyopathy should never be re-challenged with the drug as the cardiac damage is usually irreversible due to cell death (Type I cardiotoxicity). The cardiotoxicity from trastuzumab, however, is reversible (Type II cardiotoxicity).
- Beta-blocker: Carvedilol and nebivolol have been shown to have protective effects on left ventricular systolic function during anthracycline therapy.
- ACE inhibitor and angiotensin receptor blockers (ARBs) Enalapril, ramipril, and telmisartan

can protect myocardial contractility during doxorubicin or epirubicin treatment.
- Thiamine, folic acid, and multivitamins are adjunctive treatments for alcoholic cardiomyopathy. Abstinence can usually reverse the cardiomyopathy.

DISPOSITION
Prognosis depends on the dosage of chemicals and the severity of LV dysfunction.

REFERRAL
Close follow-up with cardiologist.

! PEARLS & CONSIDERATIONS

The presentation of chemotherapy-induced cardiac toxicity ranges from asymptomatic decline in LVEF to heart failure. The incidence is dose-dependent in the case of anthracyclines and may manifest itself up to 10 years after initial exposure. Therefore, a regular clinical follow-up of such patients is advised and echocardiographic surveillance is possibly indicated to detect late cardiotoxicity.

SUGGESTED READINGS
Available at www.expertconsult.com

AUTHORS: **KAUSTUBH C. DABHADKAR, M.D., M.P.H., SOMWAIL RASLA, M.D.,** and **ARAVIND RAO KOKKIRALA, M.D.**

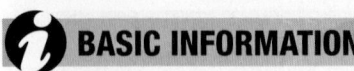

DEFINITION

Dilated cardiomyopathy describes a group of diseases involving the myocardium and characterized by myocardial dysfunction that is not wholly the result of hypertension, coronary atherosclerosis, valvular dysfunction, congenital, or other structural heart disease. As a result, the heart is enlarged and the ventricles are dilated with impaired systolic function.

SYNONYMS

Congestive cardiomyopathy
Idiopathic cardiomyopathy

ICD-10CM CODES

B33.24	Viral cardiomyopathy
I11.0	Hypertensive heart disease with heart failure
I42.0	Dilated cardiomyopathy (includes congestive cardiomyopathy)
I42.9	Cardiomyopathy, unspecified (includes cardiomyopathy [primary] [secondary] NOS)
I43	Cardiomyopathy in diseases classified elsewhere
I50.20 to I50.9	(Unspecified, Acute, Chronic, or Acute on Chronic) + (systolic, diastolic, or combined) (congestive) heart failure
O90.3	Peripartum cardiomyopathy

EPIDEMIOLOGY & DEMOGRAPHICS

- The estimated prevalence of dilated cardiomyopathy in the general adult population is approximately 1:2500. The incidence is approximately 4 to 8 per 100,000 persons per yr.
- The incidence of dilated cardiomyopathy is greatest in middle age and among men.
- African Americans have a three-fold increased risk for developing DCM, irrespective of comorbidities or socioeconomic factors, compared with whites.
- It is the most common cardiomyopathy and accounts for 25% of cases of congestive heart failure.

PHYSICAL FINDINGS & CLINICAL PRESENTATION

The patient will present with common symptoms of congestive heart failure, which may be of insidious or sudden onset. The patient may also be asymptomatic and the diagnosis made by the unexpected finding of cardiomegaly on a chest x-ray. The history should focus also on information that could help determine the etiology. Classical signs of heart failure may be absent. When present, findings are indistinguishable from other heart failure syndromes, including:

- Increased jugular venous pressure
- Narrow pulse pressure
- Pulmonary rales, hepatomegaly, peripheral edema
- S3, S4
- Mitral regurgitation, tricuspid regurgitation (less common)

ETIOLOGY

In approximate order of occurrence:

- Idiopathic (often a viral infection that cannot be confirmed)
- Infections (viral [human herpesvirus 6, influenza, echovirus, cytomegalovirus, Coxsackie B, adenovirus, parvovirus, HIV], rickettsial, mycobacterial, toxoplasmosis, trichinosis, Chagas' disease)
- Alcoholism (15% to 40% of all cases in Western countries)
- Uncontrolled tachyarrhythmia ("tachycardia-mediated")
- Sleep apnea–obstructive or nonobstructive
- Cirrhotic–not necessarily alcohol-induced
- End-stage renal disease–related
- Nutritional deficiencies–selenium, L-carnitine, thiamine
- Peripartum (greatest risk from last trimester of pregnancy to 6 months postpartum)
- Chemotherapeutic (anthracycline, doxorubicin, daunorubicin) or pharmacologic agents (antiretrovirals, phenothiazines) (see "Cardiomyopathy, Chemical-Induced")
- Substance abuse (cocaine, heroin, organic solvents "glue-sniffer's heart")
- Postmyocarditis
- Toxins (cobalt, lead, phosphorus, carbon monoxide, mercury) Collagen-vascular disease (systemic lupus, rheumatoid arthritis, polyarteritis, dermatomyositis, sarcoidosis)
- Heredofamilial neuromuscular disease (e.g., muscular dystrophy)
- Excess hormones (acromegaly, osteogenesis imperfecta, myxedema, thyrotoxicosis, diabetes)
- Hematologic (e.g., sickle cell anemia, hemochromatosis, hypereosinophilia)
- Stress-induced (i.e., takotsubo or broken heart syndrome)
- LV noncompaction
- TTN truncating mutations (mutations in TTN, the gene encoding the sarcomere protein titin) are a common cause of dilated cardiomyopathy, occurring in approximately 25% of familial cases of idiopathic dilated cardiomyopathy and in 18% of sporadic cases.

DX DIAGNOSIS

Dilated cardiomyopathy is a diagnosis of exclusion, made after ruling out other potential causes of myocardial dysfunction.

DIFFERENTIAL DIAGNOSIS

- Coronary atherosclerosis, that is, left ventricular dysfunction secondary to ischemia and/or myocardial infarction
- Valvular dysfunction (especially aortic and mitral regurgitation)
- Other cardiomyopathies (restrictive, hypertrophic)
- Pulmonary disease (embolism, obstructive, restrictive)
- Pericardial abnormalities (constrictive pericarditis, tamponade)
- Hypothyroidism/myxedema
- Athlete's heart

WORKUP

- Medical history: emphasis on symptoms of dyspnea, orthopnea, paroxysmal nocturnal dyspnea, weight gain, palpitations, or signs of systemic and pulmonary embolism, substance abuse history, possible toxin exposures (especially occupational)
- Physical exam (see "Physical Findings & Clinical Presentation")
- Testing (see "Laboratory Tests" and "Imaging Studies" for more detail): laboratory, chest x-ray, ECG, echocardiogram, cardiac catheterization; myocardial biopsy is not routinely recommended, unless acute myocarditis requiring immunosuppressive therapy is considered (e.g., giant cell myocarditis)

LABORATORY TESTS

- Chemistries/metabolites (deficiencies), renal function tests (renal dysfunction)
- Cardiac biomarkers (elevation of cardiac troponin or BNP)
  1. Persistently increased cardiac troponin T levels are a marker of poor outcome in cardiomyopathy patients
- Endocrine (particularly thyroid)
- Iron studies (hemochromatosis, deficiency)
- Rheumatologic and inflammatory (ANA, ESR, CRP)
- Others as indicated (HIV, Lyme, neurohormonal)

IMAGING STUDIES

Chest x-ray:

- Cardiac silhouette enlargement (particularly left ventricle)
- Pulmonary vascular redistribution and congestion (Kerley B lines, cephalization of vasculature), pleural effusion (may appear as unilateral, most often on the right side)

ECG:

- ECG findings are typically nonspecific, and sinus tachycardia is usually a reflection of underlying heart failure. Large voltage in precordial leads and low voltage in limb leads may be seen in advanced disease.
- Intraventricular conduction defects and left bundle branch block
- Arrhythmias (atrial fibrillation, premature ventricular or atrial contractions, ventricular tachycardia)

Echocardiogram (Fig. E1B):

- Low ejection fraction with global hypokinesis
- Four-chamber enlargement (LV enlargement usually predominates)
- Mitral or tricuspid regurgitation (tethering due to incomplete leaflet closure caused by ventricular dilation)

Cardiac catheterization:

- On initial presentation to exclude obstructive epicardial coronary artery disease

Cardiac magnetic resonance imaging (CMRI):

- Particularly if infiltrative or inflammatory etiology suspected

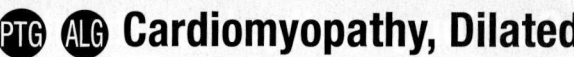

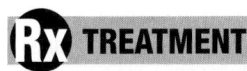 **TREATMENT**

NONPHARMACOLOGIC THERAPY

- Treatment of underlying disease (systemic lupus, alcoholism)
- Dietary sodium restriction (<2 g/day).
- Exercise training has been shown to be associated with reduced risk for hospitalization and death in patients with history of heart failure in limited trials; enrollment in a formal cardiac rehabilitation program may be beneficial in improving patient's functional status

ACUTE GENERAL Rx

- Identify and treat the etiology of the acute exacerbation, when able. A helpful mnemonic is FAILURE: **f**ailure to take medications, **a**nemia/**a**rrhythmia, **i**schemia/**i**nfection/**i**nfarction, **l**ifestyle (dietary indiscretion), **u**pregulation of cardiac output (hyperthyroidism or pregnancy), **r**enal failure, **e**mbolus (pulmonary).
- Diuretics are indicated for all patients with current symptoms or history of heart failure and reduced left ventricular ejection fraction (LVEF) with evidence of volume overload (see "Physical Findings and Clinical Presentation") to improve symptoms. It is important to note that diuretics have not been shown to improve mortality rates.
- Patients with associated coronary atherosclerosis (angina, ECG changes, reversible defects on myocardial perfusion imaging) may benefit from percutaneous or surgical revascularization.

CHRONIC Rx

- Diuretics and digoxin as noted in "Acute General Rx."
- ACE inhibitors (and angiotensin receptor blockers) have been shown to have favorable effects on ventricular remodeling in patients with cardiomyopathy and a demonstrable mortality benefit in these patients. They also reduce afterload and improve cardiac output. Therefore, they are recommended in all patients with reduced LV systolic function (EF ≤40%), regardless of symptoms unless specific contraindications exist.
- Beta-blockers work by inhibiting the adverse effects of the sympathetic nervous system in patients with ventricular systolic dysfunction (EF ≤40%). *Only* carvedilol, long-acting metoprolol succinate, and bisoprolol have shown a mortality benefit in patients with LV systolic dysfunction. Unless specifically contraindicated, they should be started after the acute exacerbation has resolved and titrated to the maximum tolerated dose.
- Aldosterone antagonists (spironolactone and eplerenone) have shown mortality benefit along with a decreased rate of hospitalization for heart failure in patients with symptomatic heart failure and reduced LV systolic function (EF ≤35%). They should be used following label guidelines and with close monitoring of renal function and potassium.
- Additional medical therapies (hydralazine/nitrates, digitalis) can be considered in certain patient subpopulations with persistent symptoms on otherwise optimal medical management.
- Digoxin has no mortality benefit but has been shown to improve patients' quality of life in appropriately selected patients.
- The angiotensin receptor-neprilysin inhibitor sacubitril/valsartan (LCZ696 or Entresto™) in place of an ACE inhibitor or angiotensin receptor blocker and on top of optimal medical therapy in patients with class II-IV heart failure and an EF of 40% or less was found to significantly reduce multiple heart failure end points, including death, hospitalizations, and CV death in comparison to enalapril. This medication was approved in the U.S. in 2015.
- Ivabradine was FDA approved in 2015 for patients with stable, symptomatic chronic heart failure with left ventricular ejection fraction ≤35% who are in sinus rhythm with resting heart rates ≥70 beats/min and either are on maximally tolerated doses of beta-blockers or have a contraindication to beta-blocker use. It acts by blocking the hyperpolarization-activated cyclic nucleotide-gated (HCN) channel responsible for the cardiac pacemaker I_f current, which regulates heart rate.

DISPOSITION

- Annual mortality rate is 20% in patients with moderate heart failure, and it exceeds 50% in patients with severe heart failure. Once symptomatic, hospitalizations are frequent and readmission rates are high (>50% at 3 mo). A multispecialty treatment approach (e.g., primary care, cardiology, nutrition, cardiac rehabilitation) is recommended.
- Factors associated with an adverse outcome in dilated cardiomyopathy are described in Table 1.

REFERRAL

- Implantation of a cardiac defibrillator for primary prevention of sudden cardiac death can be considered for patients with LVEF <35% on optimal medical therapy regardless of symptom status.

- Patients with LVEF <35%, left bundle branch block on ECG (QRS ≥0.13 sec), and persistent heart failure symptoms may benefit from cardiac resynchronization therapy via a biventricular pacemaker.
- Consider heart transplantation for relatively young patients (there is no precise age threshold) free of other significant comorbid conditions who are unresponsive to medical therapy. Dilated cardiomyopathy is the reason for 45% of all heart transplantations in the U.S.

! PEARLS & CONSIDERATIONS

COMMENTS

- Patients should be encouraged to restrict or eliminate alcohol and reduce sodium intake (<2 g daily).
- Patients may benefit from daily weight checks as a means of early detection of volume overload and decompensated heart failure.
- Vulnerability to cardiomyopathy among chronic alcohol abusers is partially genetic and related to the presence of the ACE DD genotype.
- Idiopathic dilated cardiomyopathy is often familial, and apparently healthy relatives may have latent, early, or undiagnosed disease. Echocardiographic evaluation of family members is recommended.
- Incorporation of sequencing approaches that detect TTN truncations into genetic testing for dilated cardiomyopathy may substantially increase test sensitivity and allow earlier diagnosis of dilated cardiomyopathy.

SUGGESTED READINGS

Available at www.expertconsult.com

RELATED CONTENT

Dilated Cardiomyopathy (Patient Information)

AUTHOR: **CHRISTOPHER P. BLOMBERG, D.O.**

TABLE 1 Factors Associated with an Adverse Outcome in Dilated Cardiomyopathy

Clinical	Noninvasive	Invasive
NYHA Class III/IV	Low LV ejection fraction	High LV filling pressures
Increasing age	Marked LV dilation	
Low exercise peak oxygen consumption	Low LV mass	
Marked intraventricular conduction delay	≥Moderate mitral regurgitation	
Complex ventricular arrhythmias	Abnormal diastolic function	
Abnormal signal-averaged ECG	Abnormal contractile reserve	
Evidence of excessive sympathetic stimulation	Right ventricular dilation or dysfunction	
Protodiastolic gallop (S₃)		
Elevated serum BNP		
Elevated uric acid		
Decreased serum sodium		

BNP, Brain natriuretic peptide; *ECG*, electrocardiogram; *LV*, left ventricular; *NYHA*, New York Heart Association.
From Hare JM: The dilated, restrictive, and infiltrative cardiomyopathies. In Bonow RO et al (eds): *Braunwald's heart disease—a textbook of cardiovascular medicine*, ed 9, St Louis, 2011, Saunders.

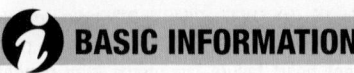

DEFINITION

Hypertrophic cardiomyopathy (HCM) is most commonly an autosomal dominant myocardial disorder characterized by disorganized myocyte architecture and marked thickening (hypertrophy) of the left ventricular wall (≥15 mm), without dilation, not explained by another cardiac or systemic disorder. The interventricular septum is the most common site of enlargement, though hypertrophy may involve other focal regions or may be concentric. HCM may result in hemodynamically significant obstruction within the left ventricular outflow tract (LVOT) and/or impairment of the diastolic function of the left ventricle. However, about one third of patients have no obstruction at rest or with provocation.

SYNONYMS

HCM
Hypertrophic cardiomyopathy
Idiopathic hypertrophic subaortic stenosis (IHSS)
Hypertrophic obstructive cardiomyopathy (HOCM)
Hypertrophic nonobstructive cardiomyopathy
Asymmetric septal hypertrophy (ASH)
Familial hypertrophic cardiomyopathy

ICD-10CM CODES
I42.1 Obstructive hypertrophic cardiomyopathy (Includes hypertrophic subaortic stenosis)
I42.2 Other hypertrophic cardiomyopathy (Includes nonobstructive hypertrophic cardiomyopathy)
I42.8 Other cardiomyopathies
I42.9 Cardiomyopathy, unspecified (includes cardiomyopathy [primary] [secondary] NOS)

EPIDEMIOLOGY & DEMOGRAPHICS

- Prevalence in the general population in the U.S., China, and Japan is estimated to be between 1/500 to 1/200 (the most common genetically transmitted cardiovascular disease).
- HCM is the most common cause of sudden cardiac death in young athletes (more commonly among blacks).
- There is equal prevalence in men and women (probably underdiagnosed in women).
- It occurs across ethnicities, perhaps underdiagnosed among blacks.
- Mortality rate is approximately 1%/yr, as high as to 2%/yr in children.
- The most common form of the disease is familial (60% to 70% of cases), and it follows an autosomal dominant inheritance pattern with variable expression.
- Spontaneous mutations can also occur, accounting for approximately 20% of cases. It is otherwise indistinguishable from the familial form.
- A variant form seen in the elderly (5%-10% of cases) has a better prognosis, and it is not typically associated with sudden cardiac death.

- The familial form is usually diagnosed in young patients. It is most often caused by a mutation in one of the contractile protein genes of the cardiac sarcomere. See "Etiology" or more details.
- Nonsarcomeric genetic mutations that cause storage disease (e.g., Fabry disease) have a very similar clinical presentation.
- Apical HCM is a variant more common among Asians: as many as 41% of Chinese HCM and 15% of Japanese HCM patients. Clinically there is no LVOT obstruction.

PHYSICAL FINDINGS & CLINICAL PRESENTATION

Patients may have subtle symptoms of progressive congestive heart failure (CHF). At time of diagnosis, most patients are asymptomatic, referred and diagnosed based on family history. HCM may be suspected on the basis of abnormalities found on physical examination. Classic findings include:

- Harsh, systolic, crescendo–decrescendo murmur at the left sternal border or apex. The murmur increases with maneuvers that decrease venous return or LV size (Valsalva, standing), and decreases with those that increase venous return or afterload (squatting, hand grip, post-Valsalva release).
- Paradoxical splitting of S2 (if left ventricular obstruction is present).
- S4 may be present.
- Double or triple LV apical impulse ("triple ripple": atrial contraction, early rapid ejection, and late slow ejection).
- Pulsus bisferiens (double pulsation on palpation of the carotid pulse).

Increased obstruction can occur with:
- Drugs: digitalis, β-adrenergic stimulators (isoproterenol, dopamine, epinephrine), nitroglycerin, vasodilators, diuretics, alcohol, inhalation of amyl nitrate
- Hypovolemia
- Tachycardia
- Valsalva maneuver
- Standing position

Decreased obstruction is seen with:
- Drugs: β-adrenergic blockers, calcium channel blockers, disopyramide, α-adrenergic stimulators
- Volume expansion
- Bradycardia
- Hand-grip exercise
- Squatting position
- Release phase of the Valsalva maneuver

Clinical manifestations are as follows:
- Syncope or presyncope (usually seen with exercise)
- Angina
- Palpitations
- Sudden cardiac death
- Heart failure (typically with advanced stages): dyspnea on exertion, orthopnea, edema, increased jugular venous pressure, paroxysmal nocturnal dyspnea

ETIOLOGY

- Genetic: Autosomal dominant trait with variable penetrance caused by mutations in

multiple genes encoding proteins of the cardiac sarcomere and calcium regulation. To date, >1400 mutations have been identified among at least 13 genes, with variable phenotypes, expressivity, and penetrance. The most vigorous evidence indicates that 8 genes are known to definitively cause HCM: beta myosin heavy chain, myosin binding protein C, troponin T, troponin I, tropomyosin alpha-1 chain, actin, regulatory light chain, and essential light chain. HCM may be caused by a single mutation in one of two alleles; however, 5% of patients have at least two mutations. Sarcomeric protein gene mutations account for up to 60% of cases of HCM.
- Metabolic: Most are autosomal recessive, but some are X-linked. Most commonly, they are due to Anderson-Fabry disease (a lysosomal storage disease). Other metabolic etiologies include the glycogen storage diseases Pompe and Danon, AMP-kinase (PRKAG2), and carnitine disorders.
- Mitochondrial: These comprise autosomal dominant, autosomal recessive, X-linked, and maternally inherited traits. Most frequently, they are due to mutations in the respiratory chain protein complexes. The age of onset and severity of involvement are variable.
- Neuromuscular: These are most commonly associated with Friedreich's ataxia, but they are also associated with FHLI.
- Malformation syndromes: These etiologies include Noonan, LEOPARD, Costello, and cardiofasciocutaneous.
- Amyloidosis: These include familial ATTR, wild-type TTR (senile), and amyloid light-chain (AL) amyloidosis.
- Drug-induced: Tacrolimus, hydroxychloroquine, and steroids.
- Sporadic occurrence.

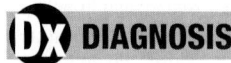 **DIAGNOSIS**

DIFFERENTIAL DIAGNOSIS

- Hypertensive heart disease
- Aortic stenosis
- Subaortic stenosis
- Athlete's heart
- Volume depletion

WORKUP

- Medical history: Unexplained "Clinical Manifestations" and/or family history of sudden death.
- Physical exam: See "Physical Findings & Clinical Presentation."
- Genetic counseling with or without testing.
- ECG is abnormal in 75% to 95% of patients, although there are no pathognomonic findings. Typical findings include:
  1. LV hypertrophy (abnormally tall R waves in the precordial leads) in up to 80% of patients
  2. Abnormal Q waves in lateral and inferior leads (Fig. 1)
  3. T wave inversions (associated with the apical hypertrophy predominant variant)

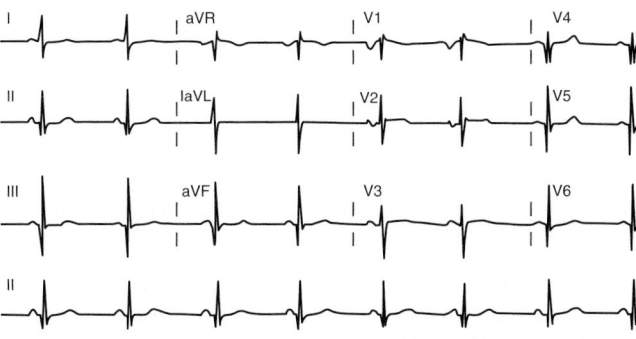

FIG. 1 Surface ECG in a patient with hypertrophic cardiomyopathy. Note the deep narrow Q waves in the inferolateral leads. (From Issa Z et al: *Clinical arrhythmology and electrophysiology,* ed 2, Philadelphia, 2012, Saunders.)

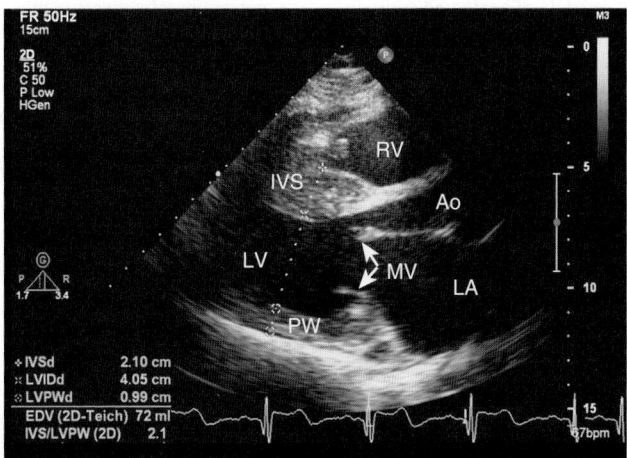

FIG. 2 Echocardiographic appearance of hypertrophic cardiomyopathy. Parasternal long-axis view from a patient with hypertrophic cardiomyopathy demonstrating asymmetrical septal hypertrophy. The interventricular septum (marked by *arrow*) measures 2.1 cm; the posterior wall measures 0.99 cm. *Ao,* Aorta; *IVS,* interventricular septum; *LA,* left atrium; *LV,* left ventricle; *MV,* mitral valve; *PW,* posterior wall; *RV,* right ventricle. (From Issa Z et al: *Clinical arrhythmology and electrophysiology,* ed 2, Philadelphia, 2012, Saunders.)

- Echocardiography (Fig. 2) is usually diagnostic as the majority of patients have significant LV hypertrophy (See "Imaging Studies" for details) and should be repeated every 12 to 24 months or as clinically needed.
- 24-hour Holter monitor to screen for potentially lethal ventricular arrhythmias (principal cause of syncope or sudden death in obstructive cardiomyopathy) should be performed at the initial diagnosis and in patients that subsequently develop palpitations, lightheadedness, or syncope. The presence of these arrhythmias identifies patients who are candidates for ICD therapy.
- In the absence of significant LVOT obstruction, exercise testing is indicated at diagnosis and annually thereafter to evaluate for symptoms and response to exercise. A drop in systolic blood pressure by at least 20 mm Hg or failure to augment by at least 20 mm Hg with exercise are markers of poor prognosis and are indicators for referral for myotomy/myomectomy. Cardiopulmonary exercise testing can provide objective evidence for worsening diseases, but need only be performed every 2 to 3 years.
- Biomarkers of myocardial fibrosis in HCM include BNP and high-sensitivity cardiac

troponin T and I. Other labs include CBC, BMP, LFTs, TSH, SPEP, UPEP, Kappa/Lambda.
- Screening for sarcomere protein gene mutations in family members of patients with HCM can identify a broad subgroup of patients with increased propensity toward long-term impairment of left ventricular function and adverse outcome, irrespective of the myofilament (thick, intermediate, or thin) involvement.
- In individuals with pathogenic mutations who do not express the HCM phenotype, it is recommended to perform serial electrocardiogram (ECG), transthoracic echocardiogram (TTE), and clinical assessment at periodic intervals (12 to 18 months in children and adolescents and about every 5 years in adults), based on the patient's age and change in clinical status.
- Endomyocardial biopsy may be helpful to rule out diseases other than HCM if a diagnosis remains inconclusive after extensive testing.

IMAGING STUDIES

- Chest x-ray may be normal or show cardiomegaly.

- Two-dimensional echocardiography is used to establish the diagnosis and assess the severity of obstruction when present. LV wall thickness will usually be ≥15 mm (although some may be genetically positive but phenotype negative), and most patients (up to 95%) will have asymmetric (ratio of septum thickness to left ventricular wall thickness >1.3:1) LV wall hypertrophy. Symmetric LV hypertrophy is less common. The septum is most often affected, followed by the left ventricular mid-cavity and apex. In addition, 25% to 30% of patients will manifest systolic anterior motion (SAM) of the anterior leaflet of the mitral valve, causing obstruction of the LVOT and mitral regurgitation. Two-dimensional strain imaging echocardiography is useful for differentiation of HCM and cardiac amyloidosis from other causes of ventricular wall thickening. Up to 80% of HCM patients will also have diastolic dysfunction as evidenced by pulsed mitral valve inflow pattern and tissue Doppler.
- Cardiac MRI or cardiac CT may be of diagnostic value when echocardiographic studies are technically inadequate. MRI is also useful in identifying unusual segmental hypertrophy undetectable by standard echocardiography and can detect myocardial replacement fibrosis (an independent predictor of adverse cardiac outcomes and ventricular arrhythmias) using late gadolinium enhancement. CMR evaluation may be considered every 5 years or every 2 to 3 years in patients with progressive disease.

Rx TREATMENT

NONPHARMACOLOGIC THERAPY

- Avoid volume depletion: HCM patients experience decrease in stroke volume and consequent increase in left ventricular outflow gradient with exercise. This may lead to hypotension, dizziness, and syncope.
- Exercise restriction: The risk of sudden cardiac death is increased by exercise in HCM patients. Participation in competitive sports and intense physical activity should be avoided. As a part of a healthy lifestyle, low-intensity aerobic exercise is reasonable.
- Avoidance of alcohol: Alcohol use (even in small amounts) may result in increased obstruction of the left ventricular outflow tract. Other stimulants such as cocaine and other sympathomimetic recreational drugs should also be avoided.

GENERAL Rx

- Therapy for HCM is directed at blocking the effect of catecholamines and avoiding vasodilator or diuretic agents that can exacerbate the dynamic left ventricular outflow tract obstruction.
- Beta-blockers' beneficial effects on symptoms (principally dyspnea and chest pain) and exercise tolerance appear to be largely a result of a decrease in the heart rate with consequent prolongation of diastole and increased passive

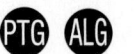
ventricular filling. By reducing the inotropic response, beta-blockers may also reduce myocardial oxygen demand and decrease the outflow gradient during exercise, when sympathetic tone is increased.

- Nondihydropyridine calcium channel blockers (e.g., verapamil, diltiazem) can also decrease left ventricular outflow obstruction through a mechanism similar to beta-blockers. However, they are mainly second-line agents used in patients who cannot tolerate beta-blockers as they also theoretically have vasodilatory properties that may worsen severe outflow tract gradients.
- Disopyramide is an antiarrhythmic that is also a negative inotrope, resulting in further decrease in outflow gradient. It is sometimes used in combination with beta-blockers.
- Prophylactic antibiotics before dental, GI, and genitourinary procedures are no longer recommended according to the 2007 American Heart Association (AHA) guidelines.
- Avoid use of digitalis, intravenous inotropes, dihydropyridine calcium channel blockers (e.g., nifedipine, amlodipine), nitrates, and vasodilators.
- Diuretics, angiotensin-converting enzyme inhibitors, and angiotensin receptor blockers should be used with caution.
- Intravenous phenylephrine (or another pure vasoconstricting agent) is recommended for the treatment of acute hypotension in patients with obstructive HCM who do not respond to fluid administration.
- Implantable cardiac defibrillators (ICDs) are a safe and effective therapy in HCM patients prone to ventricular arrhythmias. In their practice guidelines, the major cardiology societies (AHA/ACC/HRS) give a strong recommendation (Class I) for ICD implantation in all patients with HCM who have had an episode of sustained ventricular tachycardia or fibrillation. In addition, they endorse the prophylactic placement of an ICD (Class IIa recommendation) for patients with one or more of the major risk factors for sudden cardiac death (outlined in "Disposition").

- Dual-chamber pacing may provide symptomatic relief of symptoms attributable to LVOT obstruction and refractory to medical therapy.
- HCM patients are at an increased risk of atrial fibrillation (AF) as well as systemic thromboembolization. AF occurs in over 20% of the HCM population. AF is an important source of symptoms, morbidity, and mortality and correlates to a worse prognosis. AF therapy should aim for thromboembolic risk mitigation with a vitamin K antagonist (unless contraindicated) and symptom alleviation via rate or rhythm control. Direct thrombin and factor Xa inhibitor use has not yet reached societal guidelines for this population given the lack of data.
- Fig. 3 describes management strategies for subgroups of patients within the broad HCM clinical spectrum.

DISPOSITION

HCM is not a static disease. Some adults may experience subtle regression in wall thickness, whereas others (~5%-10%) paradoxically evolve

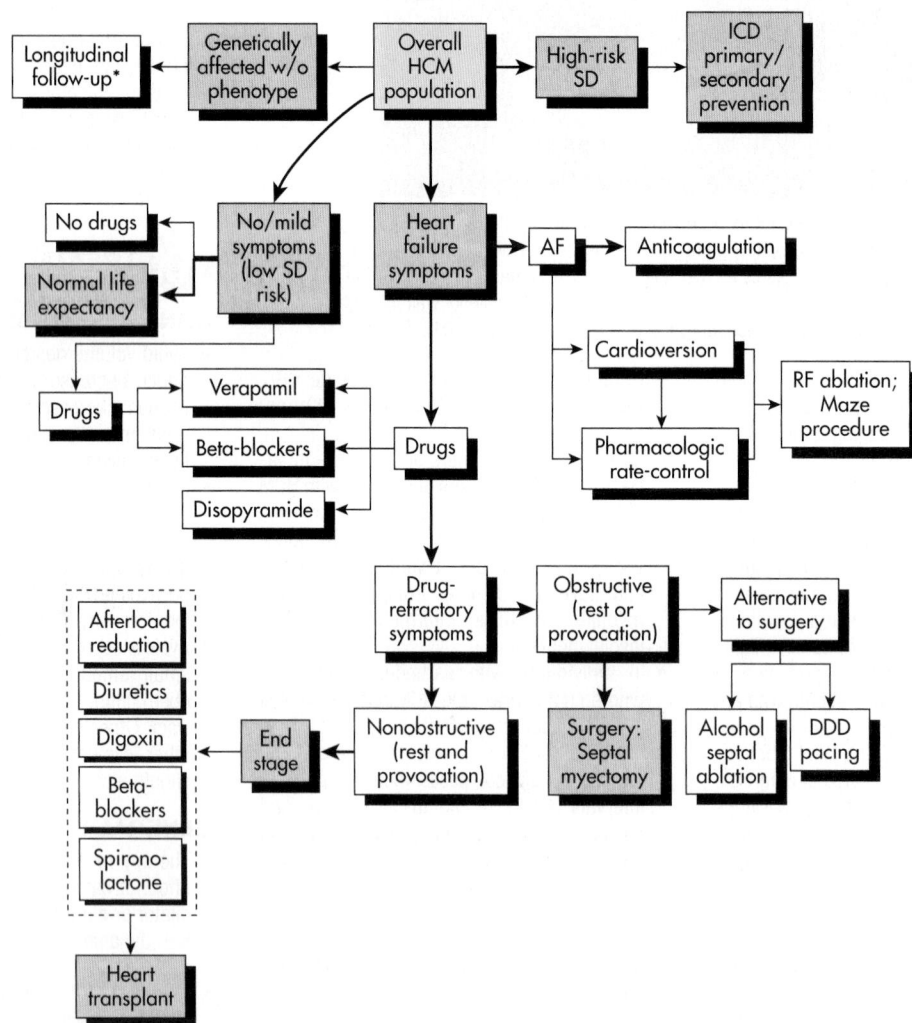

FIG. 3 Management strategies for subgroups of patients within the broad HCM clinical spectrum. *Generally no specific treatment or intervention indicated. *AF*, Atrial fibrillation; *DDD*, dual-chamber defibrillator; *ICD*, implanted cardioverter-defibrillator; *RF*, radiofrequency; *SD*, sudden death. (From Bonow RO et al: *Braunwald's heart disease—a textbook of cardiovascular medicine*, ed 9, St Louis, 2011, Saunders.)

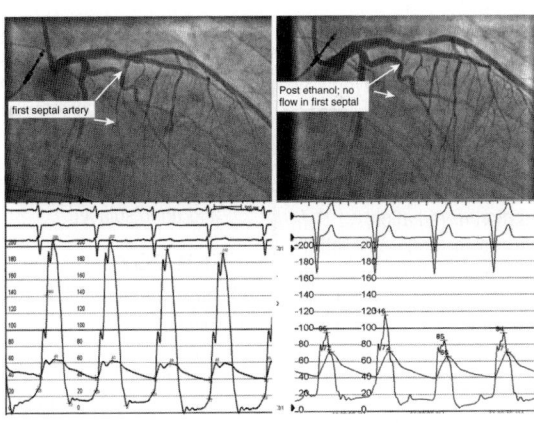

FIG. 4 Septal ablation for obstructive hypertrophic cardiomyopathy. *Left,* Large pressure gradient between the left ventricle and aorta. A large proximal septal perforating artery is identified. *Right,* Following selective injection of ethanol, there is no flow within the septal artery and the gradient is dramatically reduced. (From Bonow RO et al: *Braunwald's heart disease—a textbook of cardiovascular medicine,* ed 9, St Louis, 2011, Saunders.)

into an end-stage cardiomyopathy resembling dilated cardiomyopathy, characterized by cavity enlargement, left ventricular wall thinning, and systolic dysfunction. Patients with HCM are at increased risk for sudden death, especially if the onset of symptoms began during childhood. Severe left ventricular outflow obstruction at rest is also a strong, independent predictor of severe symptoms of heart failure and death. ICD implantation for primary prevention should be considered if patients (particularly the young) have any of the following high risk features:

- Personal history of sudden cardiac death or out of hospital cardiac arrest (major risk factor)
- Spontaneous sustained ventricular tachycardia or ventricular fibrillation (major risk factor)
- Family history of premature death in a first-degree relative possibly caused by HCM
- Unexplained syncope
- Nonsustained ventricular tachycardia during Holter monitoring
- Substantial septal hypertrophy (>30 mm)
- Abnormal blood pressure response during exercise
- Increased delayed gadolinium enhancement on cardiac magnetic resonance imaging is suggested in some recent studies as a marker of increased SCD risk

REFERRAL

- Surgical treatment (septal myectomy involving resection of the basal septum) is now the gold standard for relieving outflow tract obstruction in patients with large outflow gradient (≥50 mm Hg) and moderate to severe symptoms unresponsive to medical therapy. The risk for sudden death from arrhythmias is not altered by surgery. When this operation is performed by experienced surgeons in tertiary referral centers, the operative mortality rate is <1%, and many patients are able to achieve near-normal exercise capacity after surgery. Mitral valvuloplasty or plication in combination with myectomy may be necessary in <5% of patients. Risks of surgery include AV nodal block, ventricular septal defect, and aortic regurgitation (AR).
- Alcohol septal ablation is a nonsurgical alternative to reduce the size of the interventricular septum. This can be done in patients with HCM refractory to pharmacologic treatment, particularly in those who are not candidates for myectomy due to high surgical risk or patient preference. This technique involves the injection of ethanol in a septal perforator branch of the left anterior descending coronary artery (Fig. 4), producing a controlled myocardial infarction of the interventricular septum, and thereby reducing septal mass and consequently the left ventricular outflow tract gradient. This method may lead to improvement in both subjective and objective measures of exercise capacity, but results are not as effective as surgery because they are associated with a high incidence of heart block, requiring permanent pacing in approximately one fourth of patients, and/or recurrence of obstruction and symptoms. This should be done only at centers with experienced operators.
- Refractory end-stage HF symptoms can be treated with LVAD, BiVAD, or heart transplant.

⚠ PEARLS & CONSIDERATIONS

COMMENTS

- Clinical screening of first-degree relatives with two-dimensional echocardiography and ECG is indicated. Starting at the age of 12, periodic screening at 12- to 18-month intervals is recommended for children of patients with HCM and in competitive athletes. Periodic screening of first-degree adult family members not in competitive athletics is recommended at 5-yr intervals because hypertrophy may not be detected until the sixth decade of life. Genetic testing is not indicated in relatives of index patients who do not have a definite pathogenic mutation.
- Genetic counseling and screening is recommended in first-degree relatives of patients with HCM. Genetic screening of first-degree relatives can refine or eliminate the need for periodic clinical screening. At least 13 genes are known to cause HCM, among them: cardiac myosin binding protein-C, beta-myosin heavy chain, troponin T, troponin I, alpha tropomyosin, actin regulatory light chain, and essential light chain. Clinical predictors of positive genotype, such as the presence of ventricular arrhythmias, age at diagnosis, degree of left ventricular wall hypertrophy, and family history of HCM, may aid in patient selection for genetic testing and increase the yield of cardiac sarcomere gene screening. Currently a mutation can be identified in 40% to 60% of all cases, sporadic or familial.
- All HCM patients who wish to become pregnant should be given prenatal counseling about the risk of transmission (about 50%) to their offspring and should be followed at a tertiary care center that specializes in high-risk pregnancies. Most patients with HCM tolerate pregnancy well due to the higher circulating blood volume.
- The mortality rate in HCM is approximately 1% to 2% per yr.
- About one third of HCM patients will not have a resting or labile outflow gradient (i.e., nonobstructive form of HCM), but it is important to note that lethal ventricular arrhythmias can occur in the absence of obstruction or symptoms.
- Myocardial fibrosis is a hallmark of hypertrophic cardiomyopathy. Biomarkers of collagen metabolism such as serum C-terminal propeptide of type I procollagen (PICP) are significantly higher in mutation carriers without left ventricular hypertrophy and in subjects with overt hypertrophic cardiomyopathy than in controls, indicating that a probiotic state precedes the development of hypertrophy of fibrosis identifiable with cardiac MRI.

EBM **EVIDENCE**

Available at www.expertconsult.com

SUGGESTED READINGS

Available at www.expertconsult.com

RELATED CONTENT

Hypertrophic Cardiomyopathy (Patient Information)

AUTHORS: **CHRISTOPHER P. BLOMBERG, D.O.,** and **MARC PAUL WAASE, M.D., PH.D.**

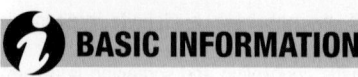
DEFINITION

Restrictive cardiomyopathy refers to either an idiopathic or a systemic myocardial disorder (in the absence of ischemic, hypertensive, valvular, or congenital heart disease) characterized by restrictive filling (Fig. 1), normal or reduced left ventricular (LV) and right ventricular (RV) volumes, and normal or near normal systolic LV and RV function. Pathophysiologically, the heart muscle is abnormally stiff, resulting in decreased compliance, abnormal relaxation in diastole, and increased filling pressures. Except for primary nonhypertrophic cardiomyopathy and a few infiltrative diseases, restrictive cardiomyopathies are secondary.

SYNONYMS

Idiopathic restrictive cardiomyopathy
Infiltrative cardiomyopathy

ICD-10CM CODES

D86.XX	Sarcoidosis-related codes
E83.11X	Hemochromatosis-related codes
E85.X	Amyloidosis-related codes
I42.5	Other restrictive cardiomyopathy
I42.8	Other cardiomyopathies
I43.1	Cardiomyopathy in metabolic diseases
I42.9	Cardiomyopathy, unspecified

EPIDEMIOLOGY & DEMOGRAPHICS

- A relatively uncommon cardiomyopathy, accounting for 5% of all primary myocardial diseases.
- Most frequently caused by amyloidosis or myocardial fibrosis (following open heart surgery, transplantation or radiation).
- Patients classified as having "idiopathic" restrictive cardiomyopathy may have mutations in the gene for cardiac troponin I, and restrictive cardiomyopathy may represent an overlap with hypertrophic cardiomyopathy in many familial cases.

PHYSICAL FINDINGS & CLINICAL PRESENTATION

Restrictive cardiomyopathy presents with symptoms of progressive left-sided and right-sided heart failure:

- Fatigue, weakness (caused by low output as patients are unable to augment cardiac output by increasing heart rate without compromising ventricular filling).
- Progressively worsening exercise intolerance and dyspnea.
- Anginal chest pain can be seen (particularly in patients with amyloidosis) from myocardial compression of small coronaries.
- Palpitations (atrial fibrillation is common), dizziness or syncope (from orthostasis, heart block, or malignant arrhythmia).
- Edema, ascites, hepatomegaly, distended neck veins (from elevated heart pressures).
- Kussmaul sign may be present (rise, or failure to fall, of the jugular veins on inspiration).
- On auscultation: murmurs of mitral or tricuspid regurgitation may be heard; an S3 may be present.
- Apical impulse may be palpable (can help distinguish it from constrictive pericarditis) and nondisplaced.

ETIOLOGY

Disease may be classified according to pathophysiologic processes:
Infiltrative:
1. Amyloidosis (most common overall): The main types include AA, AL, Aß (ß amyloid), and ATTR (transthyretin-mutated or wild type [commonly known as senile systemic]).
2. Sarcoidosis (usually results in a dilated cardiomyopathy with regional wall motion abnormalities)

Noninfiltrative:
1. Idiopathic (familial subtypes may have genetic overlap with hypertrophic cardiomyopathy)
2. Scleroderma
3. Diabetic cardiomyopathy
4. Pseudoxanthoma elasticum

Storage diseases:
1. Hemochromatosis (unusual as it is commonly associated with a dilated cardiomyopathy)
2. Glycogen or other storage diseases (Gaucher, Hurler, Fabry—all rare)

Endomyocardial:
1. Endomyocardial fibrosis
2. Hypereosinophilic syndrome (Loeffler's)

Carcinoid heart disease
Radiation
Metastatic cancers
Drug related (anthracyclines, serotonin, ergotamine, busulfan, methysergide)

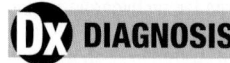
DIFFERENTIAL DIAGNOSIS

- Constrictive pericarditis (see Table E1)
- Valvular dysfunction (especially aortic stenosis)
- Hypertrophic cardiomyopathy
- Hypertensive heart disease

WORKUP

- Blood count (to identify eosinophilia), iron studies, serum renal function studies, chest x-ray, ECG, echocardiogram.
- Cardiac catheterization, magnetic resonance imaging, and computed tomography (selected cases).
- Aspiration biopsy of subcutaneous fat to detect amyloidosis.
- Endomyocardial biopsy if diagnostic confirmation needed.
- Brain natriuretic peptide (BNP) serum levels: there is data suggesting that BNP levels are markedly elevated in restrictive cardiomyopathy but near normal in patients with constrictive pericarditis, despite nearly identical clinical and hemodynamic features, most likely

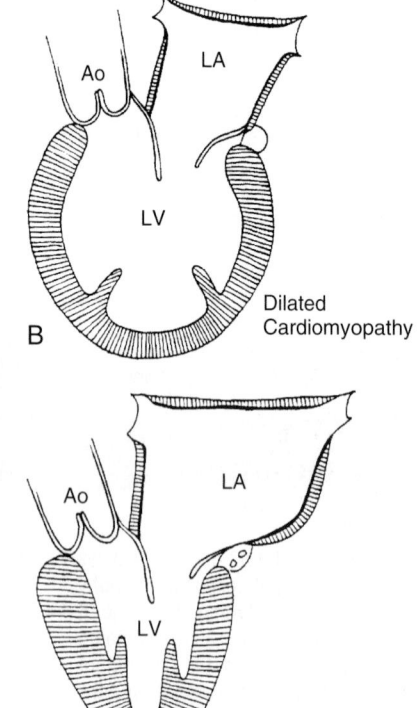

FIG. 1 Cardiomyopathies. **A,** Normal. **B,** Dilated. **C,** Hypertrophic. **D,** Restrictive. *Ao,* Aorta; *LA,* left atrium; *LV,* left ventricle. (Modified from Roberts WC, Ferrans VJ: Pathologic anatomy of the cardiomyopathies. *Hum Pathol* 6:289–342, 1975.)

resulting from the lack of myocardial stretching in constriction that is required for BNP release.
- Genetic testing.

IMAGING STUDIES

- Chest x-ray:
  1. Ranges from normal cardiomediastinal silhouette to moderate cardiomegaly (primarily because of biatrial enlargement).
  2. Evidence of heart failure may be present.
  3. Presence of pericardial calcification favors alternative diagnosis of constrictive pericarditis.
- ECG:
  1. Nonspecific ST-T wave abnormalities are the most common finding. Voltage may be low in infiltrative etiologies such as amyloidosis.
  2. Frequent atrial and ventricular ectopy are often present. Atrial fibrillation may be present.
  3. High-degree atrioventricular block, intraventricular conduction delay may be seen in advanced cases.
- Echocardiogram (Fig. 2):
  1. Biatrial enlargement almost always present.
  2. Wall thickness depends on etiology; often thickened in infiltrative disease such as amyloidosis.
  3. Myocardial appearance may be altered (speckled pattern suggestive of infiltration).
  4. Ventricular chamber sizes and systolic function are often normal or reduced.
  5. Echo Doppler shows evidence of diastolic dysfunction. Tissue Doppler demonstrates low mitral annular velocities.
- Cardiac catheterization:
  1. Characteristic hemodynamic findings are a dip and plateau, or square-root sign, in the left ventricular tracing where a deep and rapid decline in ventricular pressure at the onset of diastole is immediately followed by rapid rise and plateau in early diastolic phase.
  2. To distinguish restrictive cardiomyopathy from constrictive processes (Fig. 3):
     - Constrictive: Usually involves both ventricles and leads to equalization of diastolic pressures between all four cardiac chambers to within 5 mm Hg. There is discordance in RV and LV pressures generated during inspiration, which is due to increased ventricular interdependence and decreased left atrial filling (caused by a decreased gradient in inspiration between the pulmonary veins, which are outside the constrictive process and the left atrium).
     - Restrictive cardiomyopathy: Impairs the left ventricle more than the right, often with left-sided end-diastolic pressures of 5 mm Hg greater than the right. The presence of increased pulmonary arterial systolic pressures is also suggestive of restrictive disease. Simultaneous RV and LV pressure tracings demonstrate concordant patterns during the respiratory cycle.
- Cardiac computed tomographic scan may be helpful to identify a thickened and calcified pericardium, consistent with constrictive pericarditis.
- Cardiac magnetic resonance imaging (CMRI) may also be useful to distinguish restrictive cardiomyopathy from constrictive pericarditis (thickness of the pericardium greater than 4 mm in the latter). CMRI is particularly helpful in the diagnosis of the amyloid or sarcoid variants and may have value in other variants as well. Late gadolinium enhancement can be seen with infiltrative diseases.

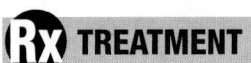 TREATMENT

NONPHARMACOLOGIC THERAPY

Congestive symptoms may respond to dietary sodium restriction (<2 g/day).

ACUTE GENERAL Rx

Treatment of volume overload and heart failure symptoms with diuretic therapy.

CHRONIC Rx

- Treatment involves management of the underlying disease if it exists:
  1. Hemochromatosis may respond to repeated phlebotomy and iron chelators to decrease iron deposition in the heart.
  2. Sarcoidosis may respond to corticosteroid therapy.
  3. Primary amyloidosis may respond to chemotherapy (high-dose melphalan with autologous stem cell therapy or bortezomib-based regimens). ATTR may be treated with liver transplant or other promising novel therapeutic agents that are currently being tested in clinical trials.
  4. Eosinophilic cardiomyopathy may respond to corticosteroid and cytotoxic drugs.
  5. There is no effective therapy for other causes of restrictive cardiomyopathy.
- Overall, the goal of treatment is to reduce symptoms by decreasing filling pressures while preserving cardiac output. Since there is currently no drug available to specifically act on myocardial relaxation, therapy centers on low-dose diuretics to lower the preload.
- Beta-blockers or calcium channel blockers have not been demonstrated to improve symptoms or alter the course of disease.
- ACE inhibitors (or angiotensin receptor blockers [ARBs]) and vasodilators should be avoided in patients with amyloidosis as they are poorly tolerated. Even small doses can trigger profound hypotension (probably due to associated autonomic neuropathy).
- Atrial fibrillation is common and patients with it or with a history of embolization should be anticoagulated. Tachycardia (of any cause) is poorly tolerated and a common cause of decompensation. Rate control is of paramount importance. Cardioversion in case of rapid atrial fibrillation should be considered. Of note, digoxin should be used with caution as it is potentially arrhythmogenic (particularly in patients with amyloidosis).
- Fibrosis of the cardiac conduction system may result in complete heart block presenting as dizziness or syncope (especially in amyloidosis) and pacemaker implantation may be required. The course of restrictive cardiomyopathy is variable and depends on the underlying etiology. Death usually results from heart failure or arrhythmias, and interventions aimed at addressing these are recommended.
  1. For the amyloid variant, an implantable cardiac defibrillator offers little prophylactic benefit beyond the ability to pace because the cause of sudden cardiac death is usually electromechanical disassociation.

DISPOSITION

Prognosis varies with the etiology of the cardiomyopathy but is poor overall as disease is rarely detected before advanced stages.

REFERRAL

Cardiac transplantation can be considered in patients with refractory symptoms and idiopathic or familial restrictive cardiomyopathies.

SUGGESTED READINGS

Available at www.expertconsult.com

RELATED CONTENT

Restrictive Cardiomyopathy (Patient Information)

AUTHORS: **CHRISTOPHER P. BLOMBERG, D.O.,** and **BARRY FINE, M.D., PH.D.**

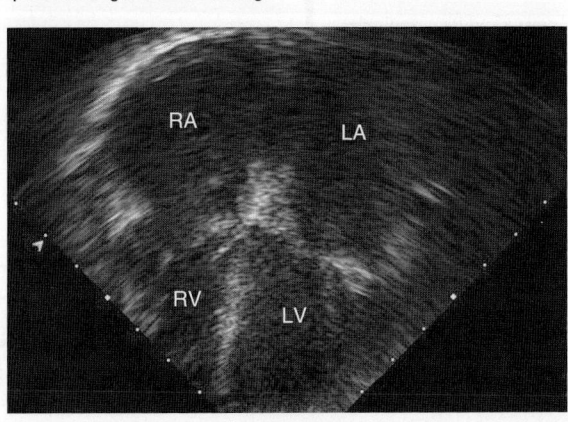

FIG. 2 Echocardiogram of a patient with restrictive cardiomyopathy. The optical four-chamber view shows the markedly enlarged right and left atria, compared to the normal-sized left and right ventricular chambers. *LA,* Left atrium; *LV,* left ventricle; *RA,* right atrium; *RV,* right ventricle. (From Kliegman RM et al: *Nelson textbook of pediatrics,* ed 19, Philadelphia, 2011, Saunders.)

DIFFERENTIATION OF RESTRICTIVE CARDIOMYOPATHY FROM CONSTRICTIVE PERICARDITIS

Heart failure by history and examination

Echocardiography

Left ventricular ejection fraction ≥50%

Left ventricular ejection fraction <40%

Rule out aortic stenosis, hypertension, hypertrophic cardiomyopathy

Nondilated left ventricle

Dilated left ventricle

Work-up for dilated cardiomyopathy

Doppler echocardiography
- Increased early diastolic filling velocity (E)
- Decreased atrial filling velocity (A)
- E/A ratio ≥1.5
- Decreased deceleration time
- Decreased isovolumetric relaxation time
- Absence of respiratory variation in mitral inflow pattern
- Marked decrease in ratio of systolic pulmonary venous flow to diastolic pulmonary venous flow
- Augmented atrial reversal velocity

Probable restrictive cardiomyopathy

Inconclusive

CT scan or MRI
- Increased pericardial thickness suggestive of constriction
- Gadolinium enhancement present in infiltrative cardiomyopathy

Inconclusive

Cardiac catheterization
- Right atrial pressures elevated with prominent *x* and *y* descents that show no respiratory variation
- Classic square-root sign (i.e., a prominent, early decrease in ventricular diastolic pressure followed by a rapid rise to a plateau)
- Right ventricular systolic pressures ≥50 mm Hg
- Right ventricular diastolic pressures less than one third of right ventricular systolic pressures
- Left ventricular EDP is typically greater than right ventricular EDP by 5 mm Hg or more
- Separation of left ventricular EDP from right ventricular EDP with volume challenge if equalization is present
- Absence of discordance in right ventricular and left ventricular systolic pressures during respiration

Probable restrictive cardiomyopathy

Inconclusive

Endomyocardial biopsy
- Diagnostic of specific restrictive cardiomyopathy

Inconclusive

Constrictive pericarditis or primary restrictive cardiomyopathy

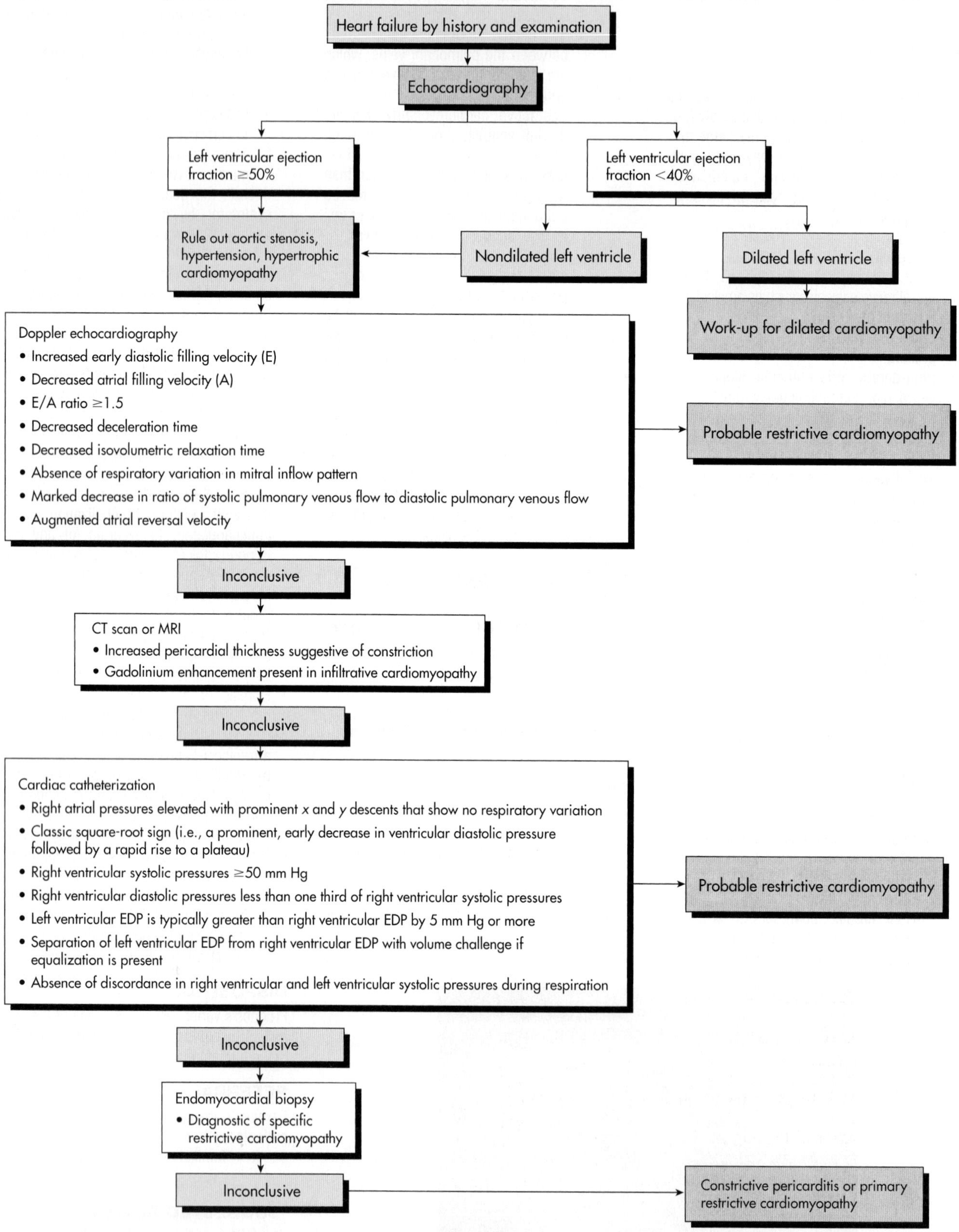

FIG. 3 Differentiation of restrictive cardiomyopathy from constrictive pericarditis. *CT,* Computed tomography; *MRI,* magnetic resonance imaging; *EDP,* end-diastolic pressure. (From Pereira NL, Dec GW: Restrictive and infiltrative cardiomyopathies. In Crawford MH et al: *Cardiology,* Philadelphia, 2010, Elsevier.)

BASIC INFORMATION

DEFINITION

Cardiorenal syndrome (CRS) is a pathophysiologic disorder whereby acute or chronic dysfunction of the heart or kidneys can induce acute or chronic dysfunction of the other organ. Another definition proposed by the National Heart, Lung, and Blood Institute (NHLBI) is one in which therapy to relieve congestive symptoms of heart failure is limited by progressive renal insufficiency. There are five types of CRS:

Type 1: Acute cardiorenal syndrome: acute cardiac dysfunction leading to acute kidney injury

Type 2: Chronic cardiorenal syndrome: chronic heart failure leading to renal dysfunction

Type 3: Acute renocardiac syndrome: acute kidney injury leading to or resulting in acute cardiac dysfunction

Type 4: Chronic renocardiac syndrome: chronic kidney disease (CKD) leading to cardiac dysfunction

Type 5: Secondary cardiorenal syndrome: systemic conditions that cause both cardiac and renal dysfunction

This section will focus on CRS types 1 and 2.

SYNONYM

CRS

ICD-10CM CODES

I13	Hypertensive heart and renal disease
I13.0	Hypertensive heart and renal disease with (congestive) heart failure
I13.2	Hypertensive heart and renal disease with both (congestive) heart failure and renal failure
I17.8	Other renal failure

EPIDEMIOLOGY & DEMOGRAPHICS

- CKD is present in 20% to 67% of patients with congestive heart failure (CHF).
  1. Females, the elderly, whites, and patients with diabetes or systolic blood pressure >160 mm Hg have an increased incidence.
  2. In general, mortality is increased in patients with heart failure and reduced glomerular filtration rate (GFR).
  3. Patients with CKD have an increased risk of atherosclerotic heart disease and heart failure.
  4. Cardiovascular disease is responsible for about 50% of deaths in patients with CKD.
- 20% to 30% of patients who are treated for acute or chronic CHF will develop acute kidney injury (AKI).
  1. In patients with acute CHF, the severity of AKI is increased with decreased left ventricular systolic function and baseline CKD.
  2. Only 9% of patients hospitalized with acute heart failure in the ADHERE trial had normal renal function with GFR >90 ml/min/1.73 m^2 on admission.
- Patients with acute heart failure experienced the highest occurrence rate of CRS, but the impact on mortality was greatest in patients who developed CRS in the setting of cardiac surgery.

PHYSICAL FINDINGS & CLINICAL PRESENTATION

- Acute/subacute decompensated heart failure (ADHF)
  1. Clinical symptoms:
     1. Dyspnea with exertion or at rest
     2. Orthopnea
     3. Paroxysmal nocturnal dyspnea
     4. Right upper quadrant pain
  2. Vital signs:
     1. Sinus tachycardia
     2. Hypertension or hypotension
     3. Elevated respiratory rate
     4. Narrow pulse pressure
     5. Pulsus alternans: poor prognostic indicator
  2. Physical exam findings:
     1. Elevated jugular venous pressures
     2. Peripheral edema
     3. Third heart sound (S3)
     4. Respiratory crackles
     5. Abdominal ascites
     6. Hepatomegaly and splenomegaly
- Chronic heart failure
  1. Clinical symptoms:
     1. Dyspnea
     2. Fatigue
     3. Anorexia: poor prognostic indicator
  2. Vital signs:
     1. Similar to ADHF, but sinus tachycardia may not be present, and hypotension may be present with a low cardiac output state.
     2. Physical exam findings:
        1. Similar to ADHF, but rales may be absent, reflecting the rapidity of the collection of fluid. In chronic heart failure, the pulmonary vasculature may store large fluid volumes in alveoli rather than the total volume of fluid.
- These findings of heart failure will be associated with laboratory findings of kidney disease (discussed later); in extreme cases, physical exam findings of severe kidney disease such as asterixis, uremic frost, uremic smell, and uremic pericarditis may be present.

ETIOLOGY

The etiology of CRS can be divided into four mechanisms (Figs. E1 and 2):
- Increased renal venous pressure
  1. Occurs secondary to elevated central venous pressure or elevated intraabdominal pressure.
  2. Frequency of worsening kidney function is lowest in patients with CVP <8 mm Hg.
  3. GFR increase may occur following diuretic therapy, which is most likely mediated by a reduction in renal venous pressure and/or a reduction in right ventricular dilation.
- Reduced renal perfusion
  1. Common cause of CRS type 1 (acute CHF results in AKI).
  2. Loop diuretic therapy can reduce ventricular preload and reduce cardiac output by as much as 20%.

- Right ventricular dilation and dysfunction
  1. Increases central venous pressure that increases renal venous pressure and reduces GFR.
  2. Right ventricular dilation and dysfunction reduce left ventricular filling and renal blood flow.
- Neurohormonal
  1. Activation of the renin-angiotensin-aldosterone system, sympathetic nervous system, antidiuretic hormone, and endothelin-1 increase salt and water retention, and systemic vasoconstriction decreases renal perfusion.
  2. Activation of the above systems overrides vasodilatory effects of natriuretic peptides, nitric oxide, prostaglandins, and bradykinin.

DIAGNOSIS

DIFFERENTIAL DIAGNOSIS

- Before establishing the diagnosis of CRS, rule out other causes of kidney failure:
  1. Prerenal causes
     1. Volume depletion (overdiuresis, gastrointestinal losses, or vomiting)
     2. Fluid overload states besides CHF (cirrhosis, nephrotic syndrome)
  2. Intrinsic renal disease
     1. Acute tubular necrosis
     2. Glomerular disease
- Nephrotic and nephritic syndromes
  1. Postrenal causes
     1. Obstruction

WORKUP

- Medical history is consistent with CHF symptoms and includes dyspnea, orthopnea, paroxysmal nocturnal dyspnea, edema, increasing abdominal girth, or weight gain. Laboratory results will show signs of kidney injury.
- Diagnostic workup includes chest radiograph, echocardiogram, kidney ultrasound, and laboratory tests.

LABORATORY TESTS

- Serum creatinine
  1. Patients with CRS had a mortality odds ratio of 1.48 for even mild increases in serum creatinine levels (0.3-0.5 mg/dl), with higher odds ratio for mortality with increases in serum creatinine >0.5 mg/dl.
     - For serum creatinine level increases of >0.5 mg/dl, the odds ratio for mortality increases to 3.22.
- Glomerular filtration rate (GFR)
  1. Evaluation of GFR using estimated GFR (eGFR) or calculated GFR as appropriate
- Blood urea nitrogen
  1. Admission levels >43 mg/dl are associated with a higher in-hospital mortality rate.
- Cystatin C
  1. GFR calculations are moderately less accurate than cystatin C assays.
- Beta natriuretic peptide (BNP)
  1. Initial admission values >480 pg/ml are associated with a 51% chance of death,

INTERACTIONS BETWEEN THE HEART AND THE KIDNEY IN CARDIORENAL SYNDROME

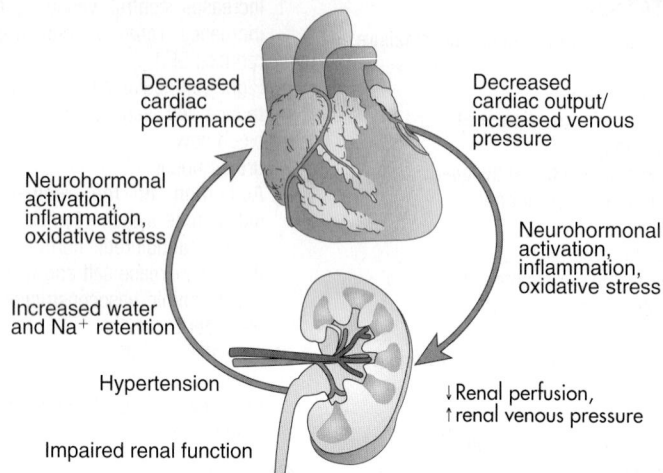

FIG. 2 Interactions between the heart and the kidney in cardiorenal syndrome. (From Pereira NL, Dec GW: Special problems in chronic heart failure. In Crawford MH et al [eds]: *Cardiology,* Philadelphia, 2010, Elsevier.)

hospital readmission, or an emergency department visit within 6 months compared to patients whose levels were <230 pg/ml.

- It may be difficult to distinguish between CKD and impaired kidney function due to cardiorenal syndrome, especially if prior renal function is unknown. Some patients have both underlying CKD and CRS. Findings that support underlying CKD include significant proteinuria (>1000 mg/day), urine sediment with hematuria and/or pyuria, cellular casts, and/or small echogenic kidneys on ultrasound

IMAGING STUDIES

- Chest radiograph
  1. May demonstrate signs of fluid overload, including pulmonary edema, effusions, or fluid in the fissures
- Echocardiogram
  1. Determines if there is underlying systolic or diastolic dysfunction and/or significant valvular disease present
- Kidney ultrasound
  1. Distinguishes between acute and chronic kidney disease and determines whether obstruction may be worsening kidney function

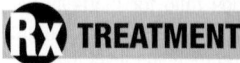 **TREATMENT**

NONPHARMACOLOGIC THERAPY

- Sodium and fluid restriction
- Hemodialysis/ultrafiltration
  - Used when there is insufficient response to pharmacologic treatment or when pharmacologic agents are limited by hemodynamics or worsening laboratory values

- Left ventricular assist device/cardiac resynchronization therapy (CRT)
  - Improves cardiac output and reverses cardiac dyssynchrony. CRT improves ejection fraction by 7% and CHF symptoms in patients with NYHA class II–IV heart failure with ejection fractions ≤35% and left bundle branch block morphology and QRS duration >150 msec.

ACUTE GENERAL Rx

There is no medical treatment that directly improves GFR in the setting of CRS, but improving cardiac function improves kidney function by alleviating any of the mechanisms of CRS listed previously.

- Diuretics
  1. Extracellular fluid volume reduction returns hemodynamics to a more optimal position on the Frank-Starling curve.
  2. Reducing volume overload improves renal perfusion pressure by decreasing central venous pressure, renal venous pressure, and right ventricular dilation, which improves right ventricular function and left ventricular performance.
  3. Twice-daily intravenous furosemide that is 2.5 times the daily oral furosemide equivalent dose is a reasonable starting point.
  4. High-dose intravenous bolus loop diuretic therapy improves cardiopulmonary congestion more effectively than low-dose loop diuretics. Continuous loop diuretic infusions are not more effective than frequently administered bolus loop diuretic regimens.
  5. Diuretic resistance is common, and a combination of diuretics with different sites of action may optimize treatment (e.g., furosemide and metolazone).

- Inhibitors of the renin-angiotensin-aldosterone system
  1. Angiotensin-converting enzyme (ACE) inhibitors, angiotensin II receptor blockers, aldosterone receptor antagonists, and direct renin inhibitors
     1. Use limited by worsening kidney function, especially when serum creatinine is greater than 2.5 mg/dl.
     2. Permits lesser diuretic dosages.
     3. Efficacy of anti-renin-angiotensin-aldosterone system therapy in the management of decompensated heart failure (HF) is established, but its role in CRS is unproven.
- Vasodilators
  1. Includes nitroglycerin and nitroprusside
     1. Increase renal perfusion pressure by improving Frank-Starling relationships and cardiac output
- Inotropic agents
  1. Include dobutamine, dopamine, and milrinone.
  2. Improve cardiac output and renal perfusion by vasodilation. Used to treat cardiogenic shock and low cardiac output states with normal blood pressure.
  3. Dobutamine and milrinone may lower systemic blood pressures, limiting therapeutic efficacy.
- Mechanical fluid removal such as extracorporeal ultrafiltration (UF) may be required to achieve control of fluid retention, particularly in patients resistant to diuretic therapy. UF removes plasma salt and water isotonically by convection through a highly permeable filter in an extracorporeal circuit and typically requires central venous catheterization. Newer technologies permit vascular access via peripheral veins. With slow continuous UF, the intravascular fluid volume remains stable as fluid shifts from the extravascular to intravascular space without inducing hypotension. UF may be indicated in highly refractory HF with diuretic resistance.

DISPOSITION

Based on improvements in heart failure and kidney function.

REFERRAL

Consultations by a cardiologist and nephrologist are recommended

SUGGESTED READINGS
Available at www.expertconsult.com

RELATED CONTENT
Acute Kidney Injury (Related Key Topic)
Heart Failure (Related Key Topic)

AUTHORS: **SANDEEP SOMAN, M.D.,** and **NAUSHABA MOHIUDDIN, M.D.**

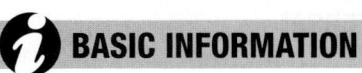 BASIC INFORMATION

DEFINITION

Light-headedness, dizziness, presyncope, or syncope in a patient with carotid sinus hypersensitivity is defined as carotid sinus syndrome (CSS). Carotid sinus hypersensitivity is the exaggerated response to carotid stimulation resulting in bradycardia, hypotension, or both. CSS is often considered a variant of neurocardiogenic syncope. The 2013 European Guidelines (ESC) defines CSS as syncope with reproduction of symptoms during carotid sinus massage of 10-second duration. There are two components of CSS: cardioinhibitory and vasodepressor.

SYNONYMS

Carotid sinus syncope
CSS
Carotid sinus hypersensitivity

ICD-10CM CODES
G90.01 Carotid sinus syncope
R55   Syncope and collapse

EPIDEMIOLOGY & DEMOGRAPHICS

- Carotid sinus hypersensitivity accounts for 1% of syncopal episodes (Fig. 1).
- Carotid sinus hypersensitivity is frequently associated with atherosclerosis and diabetes mellitus.
- Incidence increases with age, with an average age of onset at 61 to 74 yr. Fig. 2 illustrates age distribution of the patients with carotid sinus syndrome.
- Men are affected more often than women (2:1).
- CSS is rarely found in patients younger than 50 yr.

MECHANISM

- The carotid sinus is located in the internal carotid artery.
- There is a reflex loop between the mechanoreceptors of the carotid sinus and the vagal nucleus in the midbrain.
- There is an exaggerated cardioinhibitory and vasodepressor reaction caused by decreased sympathetic and increased parasympathetic outflow to the heart and vasculature, respectively.

PHYSICAL FINDINGS & CLINICAL PRESENTATION

- Often associated with sudden neck movements, especially rotation, neck palpation, shaving, or tight-fitting collars, but can occur in the absence of clear provocation.
- Mild form has symptoms such as fatigue, lightheadedness, nausea, warmth, pallor, or diaphoresis.
- More severe form of the condition has sudden abrupt loss of consciousness without prodrome.

Properly performed carotid sinus massage (CSM) at the bedside is diagnostic. The European Society of Cardiology recommends carotid sinus massage as part of the exam in patients with syncope of unknown etiology and age over 40. This maneuver can elicit three types of responses in patients with carotid sinus hypersensitivity (see "Diagnosis").

1. CSM should be performed with the patient in the supine and upright positions while monitoring the patient's blood pressure by cuff and heart rate by ECG.
2. CSM should be performed on both the right and left sides but on only one carotid artery at a time.
3. Vigorous pressure is applied over the carotid artery, directed posterior to compress the artery against the spinous process of the vertebrae, at the level of the cricoid cartilage for 10 to 30 seconds. Repeat on the opposite side if no effect is produced.
4. Contraindications to CSM include the presence of carotid artery bruits, documented carotid artery stenosis >70%, history of stroke or transient ischemic attack <3 mo, history of myocardial infarction <6 mo, history of serious ventricular arrhythmia, or prior carotid endarterectomy.
5. Complications of CSM are rare (0.1%-1%) and may include transient visual disturbance, transient paresis, tachyarrhythmias, or bradyarrhythmias.
6. False-positive results with carotid sinus massage may be relatively common in the elderly population. Thus alternative explanations for syncope should be investigated prior to attribution of symptoms to carotid sinus hypersensitivity.

ETIOLOGY

- Idiopathic
- Head and neck tumors (e.g., thyroid)
- Significant lymphadenopathy
- Carotid body tumors
- Prior neck surgery

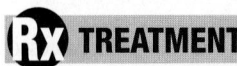 DIAGNOSIS

- The diagnosis of CSS is made in a patient with a history of syncope when carotid sinus hypersensitivity is demonstrated by CSM and no other cause of syncope is identified.
- CSM can elicit three types of responses diagnostic of carotid sinus hypersensitivity:
  1. Cardioinhibitory type: CSM producing (1) asystole for at least 3 sec in the absence of symptoms or (2) reproduction of symptoms occurring with a decline in heart rate of 30% to 40% or asystole of up to 2 sec in duration. Symptoms should not recur when CSM is repeated after atropine infusion.
  2. Vasodepressor type: CSM producing (1) a decrease in systolic blood pressure of 50 mm Hg in the absence of symptoms or 30 mm Hg in the presence of neurologic symptoms; (2) no evidence of asystole; or (3) neurologic symptoms that persist after infusion of atropine.
  3. Mixed type: CSM producing both types of responses.

DIFFERENTIAL DIAGNOSIS

All causes of syncope

WORKUP

- CSS is a diagnosis of exclusion.
- Exclude other causes of syncope or presyncope: detailed history, physical examination including orthostatic vital signs, ECG. Other tests should be considered depending on the clinical setting.

TREATMENT

NONPHARMACOLOGIC THERAPY

Reassurance and education are important. Avoid applying neck pressure from tight collars, shaving, or rapid head turning.

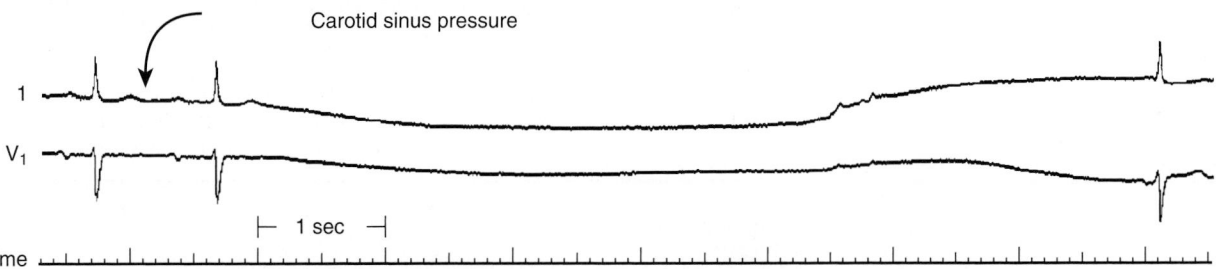

FIG. 1 Carotid sinus hypersensitivity. Two surface ECG leads are shown during carotid sinus pressure, as indicated. The PR interval is prolonged and followed by a 7.5-second sinus pause ended by a P wave and probable junctional escape complex. The patient was nearly syncopal during this period. (From Issa ZF et al: *Clinical arrhythmology and electrophysiology: a companion to Braunwald's heart disease*, ed 2, Philadelphia, 2012, Saunders.)

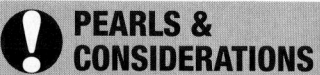

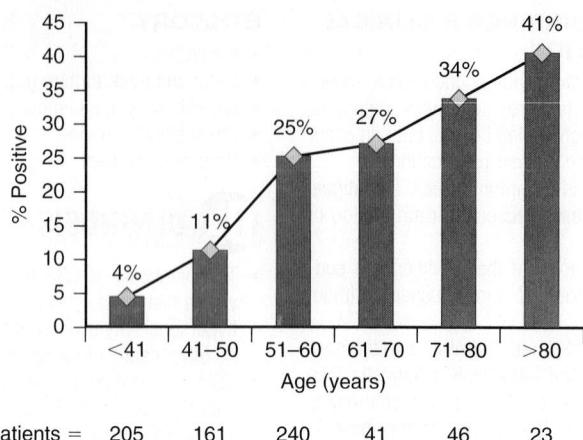

FIG. 2 Age distribution of patients with carotid sinus syndrome. (From Puggioni E et al: Results and complications of the carotid sinus massage performed according to the "method of symptoms," *Am J Cardiol* 89:599–601, 2002.)

| Patients = | 205 | 161 | 240 | 41 | 46 | 23 |

ACUTE GENERAL Rx

Treatment will vary according to the type of carotid hypersensitivity response and symptoms present (see "Chronic Rx").

CHRONIC Rx

Therapy is divided into three classes: medical, surgical (carotid denervation), and cardiac pacing.
- Surgical therapy has been largely abandoned except in cases of compressing tumors or masses responsible for CSS.
- For infrequent and mildly symptomatic carotid sinus hypersensitivity of either the cardioinhibitory or vasodepressor type, treatment is generally not necessary.
- Cardiac pacing is indicated in patients with recurrent syncope in whom CSM induces ventricular asystole of more than 3 seconds, especially if accompanied by reproduction of symptoms.

Permanent pacing is not indicated for carotid sinus hypersensitivity with no, or only vague, symptoms.
For symptomatic patients with a vasodepressor response to CSM:
- No medical treatment is proven to be effective

- Drugs, such as vasodilators, that would worsen the response should be discontinued or reduced if feasible
- Permissive hypertension
- Increased fluids (≥2 L) and salt intake (>6 g/day)
- Sympathomimetics: midodrine, titrate from 2.5 to 10 mg tid based on BP and therapeutic response (major side effect in urinary retention in elderly males)
- Serotonin-specific reuptake inhibitors
- Fludrocortisone
- Elastic knee-high or thigh-high stockings
- Carotid sinus denervation

For symptomatic patients with CSS with a mixed response to CSM:
- Combination of dual-chamber permanent pacemaker and agents used to treat vasodepressor response

DISPOSITION

- Up to 50% of the patients have recurrent symptoms.
- No increased mortality rate in patients with idiopathic CSS compared with the general population.

REFERRAL

Cardiology referral is indicated if pacemaker placement is being considered.

❗ PEARLS & CONSIDERATIONS

The most common type of CSS is cardioinhibitory, followed by mixed and vasodepressor responses.

Driving restrictions in the 2009 ESC syncope update and 2006 AHA/ACCF consensus document on syncope are stratified according to whether patients have mild or severe syncope.

Mild carotid sinus syndrome is defined as infrequent mild symptoms (without syncope), with clear precipitating causes (usually standing), warning signs, and infrequent occurrence. For patients with mild sinus hypersensitivity, no driving restrictions are recommended for private or commercial driving.

Severe carotid sinus syndrome is marked by syncope without warning occurring in any position, without precipitating causes and frequent occurrences. For patients with severe hypersensitivity, all driving is prohibited. If symptoms are controlled, driving is permitted 1 to 6 months after, based on the modality of treatment.

COMMENTS

Prognosis depends on the underlying cause.

SUGGESTED READINGS

Available at www.expertconsult.com

RELATED CONTENT

Syncope (Patient Information)
Orthostatic Hypotension (Related Key Topic)
Syncope (Related Key Topic)

AUTHORS: **CHRISTOPHER PICKETT, M.D.,** and **BARRY FINE, M.D., PH.D.**

BASIC INFORMATION

DEFINITION

Carotid stenosis is narrowing of the carotid arterial lumen, typically as a result of atherosclerosis.

SYNONYMS

Atherosclerotic disease of the carotid artery

ICD-10CM CODES
I65.29 Occlusion and stenosis of unspecified carotid artery
I65.21 Occlusion and stenosis of right carotid artery
I65.22 Occlusion and stenosis of left carotid artery
I65.23 Occlusion and stenosis of bilateral carotid arteries

EPIDEMIOLOGY & DEMOGRAPHICS

INCIDENCE: 2.2 to 8/1000 persons per year
PREVALENCE: 1.1 to 77/100,000 persons; it is estimated that 5/1000 persons aged 50 to 60 yr and 100/1000 persons >80 yr have carotid stenosis >50%. (*Note:* The incidence of carotid stenosis is unknown as screening is not routine. However, the incidence of transient ischemic attack [TIA], a common presenting symptom of carotid stenosis, is well known.)
PREDOMINANT SEX AND AGE: Male/female ratio of 2:1; more common in whites than African Americans and Asians
PEAK INCIDENCE: Peak incidence is between 50 and 60 years.
GENETICS: Multifactorial; twin studies (monozygotic versus dizygotic) suggest a familial influence.

RISK FACTORS: Hypertension, dyslipidemia, diabetes mellitus, and smoking are the four major risk factors.

PHYSICAL FINDINGS & CLINICAL PRESENTATION

Patients with carotid stenosis are often asymptomatic, but many have the presence of a carotid bruit or TIA.
- Carotid bruit: The presence of a carotid bruit is a better indicator of generalized atherosclerosis and thus is a better predictor of ischemic heart disease than future stroke.
- TIA: Carotid stenosis is classically heralded by ipsilateral transient monocular blindness (amaurosis fugax), contralateral numbness or weakness, contralateral homonymous hemianopsia, aphasia, or syncope (if bilateral disease is present).

ETIOLOGY

- Atherosclerosis (most common by far)
- Aneurysm
- Arteritis
- Carotid dissection
- Fibromuscular dysplasia
- Postradiation necrosis
- Vasospasm

DIAGNOSIS

DIFFERENTIAL DIAGNOSIS

Aneurysm, arteritis, and carotid dissection.

WORKUP

Systematic history, examination, and diagnostic studies to assess for carotid stenosis and other risk factors of TIA.

LABORATORY TESTS

CBC, basic metabolic panel, fasting lipid profile, PT/international normalized ratio, APTT, CRP.

IMAGING STUDIES

- Four imaging modalities are available for the evaluation of carotid stenosis (Table 1).
- Patients who have neurologic sequelae suggestive of carotid stenosis should be screened via carotid duplex. If carotid stenosis is suspected on carotid duplex, but inconclusive, magnetic resonance angiography, computed tomography angiography, or conventional angiography should be obtained to confirm the degree of stenosis (Fig. 1).
- Screening of asymptomatic patients without any risk factors for atherosclerosis is not routinely recommended.
- When required, carotid duplex is considered the imaging modality of choice for screening.
- Screening with carotid duplex may be considered in asymptomatic patients with carotid bruit, in those with multiple risk factors for atherosclerosis, or those with known atherosclerotic disease at other sites such as coronary artery disease, peripheral arterial disease, or abdominal aortic aneurysms.
- Patients identified to have >50% stenosis on carotid duplex may be re-imaged annually to assess progression.

TREATMENT

ACUTE GENERAL Rx

- General medical therapy should be aimed at risk factor reduction. As stated earlier, the major risk factors for carotid stenosis are hypertension, diabetes mellitus, dyslipidemia, and smoking (see "Stroke, Secondary Prevention").
- Antiplatelet therapy: Three antiplatelet options are available for patients with carotid stenosis: ASA, ASA plus dipyridamole, or clopidogrel.

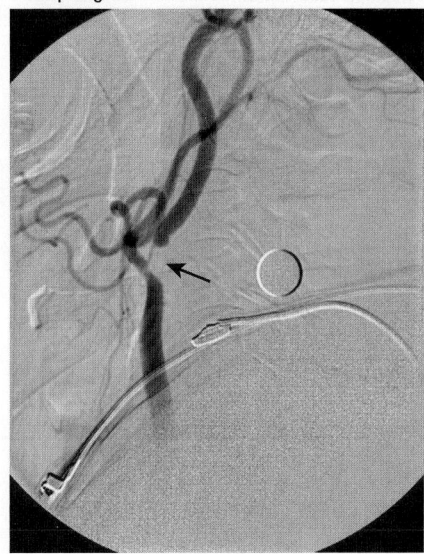

FIG. 1 Conventional angiography demonstrating severe stenosis of the internal carotid artery at the bifurcation.

TABLE 1 Imaging Modalities for Carotid Stenosis

Imaging Modality	Benefit	Drawback
Cerebral angiography	• Gold standard • Assesses plaque morphology • Assesses presence of collaterals	• Invasive • High cost • 4% incidence rate of complications • 1% incidence rate of serious complications or death
Carotid duplex	• Sensitive in detecting high-grade stenosis (>70%) • Less invasive • Lower cost	• Can be limited by body habitus • Technician dependent • Overestimates degree of stenosis
Magnetic resonance angiography (MRA)	• Sensitive in detecting high-grade stenosis (>70%) • Less operator dependent	• Overestimates degree of stenosis • Cannot be performed in patients who are critically ill, unable to tolerate supine positioning, have pacemaker or other ferromagnetic hardware, or are claustrophobic* • Expensive • Takes much longer to obtain compared with other modalities
Computed tomography angiography (CTA)	• Sensitive for high-grade stenosis	• Contraindicated in patients with serum creatinine concentration >1.5 mg/dl

*One study revealed that ~17% of patients are unable to tolerate MRA secondary to claustrophobia or are unable to lie still for procedure.

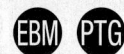

NONPHARMACOLOGIC THERAPY

Carotid endarterectomy (CEA) and carotid angioplasty and stenting (CAS) are the nonpharmacologic options available. The decision on which revascularization procedure to favor is dependent upon the presence or absence of symptoms, degree of stenosis, and medical comorbidities.

In a trial involving asymptomatic patients with severe carotid stenosis who were not at high risk for surgical complications, stenting was noninferior to endarterectomy with regard to the rate of the primary composite end point at 1 year. In analyses that included up to 5 years of follow-up, there were no significant differences between the study groups in the rates of nonprocedure-related stroke, all stroke, and survival.[1]

ASYMPTOMATIC CAROTID STENOSIS

The benefit of surgical revascularization of the carotids (CEA or CAS) in asymptomatic patients is not well established. In the United States, more than 90% of carotid artery interventions are performed in asymptomatic patients, even though evidence suggests that up to 90% of them will undergo an ultimately unnecessary and potentially harmful procedure. By contrast, the percentage of interventions that are performed for asymptomatic stenoses is approximately 60% in Germany and Italy, 15% in Canada and Australia, and 0% in Denmark.[2]

According to the most recent guidelines, revascularization procedures may be considered in asymptomatic patients with >70% stenosis if the anticipated perioperative risk is low, but this should be done only after considering their medical comorbidities, life expectancy, and after discussing the risks and benefits in detail with the patients. It is important to note that trials of CEA for asymptomatic carotid stenosis were performed prior to the era of aggressive medical management of vascular risk factors.

SYMPTOMATIC CAROTID STENOSIS

In patients who have suffered a non-disabling ischemic stroke or TIA in the preceding 6 months, surgical revascularization by CEA is recommended if the degree of stenosis is >70% by noninvasive imaging or >50% by catheter angiogram and if the anticipated rate of perioperative stroke or mortality is <6%.

All patients undergoing CEA should be started on aspirin (ASA; 81 or 325 mg daily) before surgery and this should be continued indefinitely.

CAS can be an alternative to CEA in select patients considered to be at high surgical risk or with unfavorable neck anatomy for surgery.

CEA is preferred over CAS in older patients.

For patients undergoing CAS, dual antiplatelet therapy is recommended for a minimum of 30 days.

When feasible, early revascularization within 14 days should be undertaken unless there are definite contraindications.

Surgical revascularization is not recommended in <50% stenosis, total occlusion, or in patients with major disabling strokes.

In patients who are considered high surgical risk for either CEA or CAS, the role of medical therapy alone compared with surgical revascularization is not well established.

DISPOSITION

Disposition and prognosis depend on several variables (Table 2): the degree of stenosis, the presence of symptoms, medication compliance, and the type of intervention (if any).

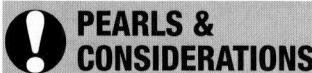

PEARLS & CONSIDERATIONS

There are ongoing studies concerning the best treatment of patients with carotid artery stenosis. Based on the results of these studies, guidelines may change rapidly.

SPECIAL CONSIDERATION

Some studies have shown that in patients with bilateral hemodynamically significant stenosis (>70%), blood pressure reduction resulted in worsened outcomes for stroke. These patients would likely be candidates for CEA.

Carotid artery occlusion (100% blockage), for which there is no routine treatment, was reexamined in the national Carotid Occlusion Surgery Study (http://www.cosstrial.org). Recently published results from the COSS trial demonstrate that superficial temporal artery to middle cerebral artery anastomosis does not provide an overall benefit for ipsilateral 2-year stroke recurrence when compared to medical therapy alone.

PREVENTION

Prevention of carotid stenosis should include pursuit of a healthy lifestyle and management of risk factors for atherosclerosis.

PATIENT/FAMILY EDUCATION

Patients should be counseled to pursue a healthy lifestyle including exercise and smoking cessation. In addition, patients should take an active role in controlling blood pressure and blood glucose. Further educational materials can be found online at: http://www.strokecenter.org/education.

SUGGESTED READINGS
Available at www.expertconsult.com

RELATED CONTENT
Carotid Stenosis (Patient Information)
Transient Ischemic Attack (Related Key Topic)

AUTHORS: **SAAGAR N. PATEL, B.A., B.S., JOSEPH S. KASS, M.D., J.D.,** and **PRASHANTH KRISHNAMOHAN, M.B.B.S., M.D.**

[1]Rosenfield K, Matsumura JS, Chaturvedi S, et al., for the ACT I Investigators: Randomized trial of stent versus surgery for asymptomatic carotid stenosis, *N Engl J Med* 374:1011–1020, 2016.
[2]Spence DJ, Naylor AR: Endarterectomy, stenting, or neither for asymptomatic carotid artery stenosis, *N Engl J Med* 374:1087–1088, 2016.

TABLE 2 Carotid Stenosis Management

Degree of Carotid Stenosis	<50%	50%-69%	70%-99%
Asymptomatic	• Medical management	• Medical management • Inconclusive evidence base to favor surgical treatment. May be considered in select patients with >60% stenosis.*	• Medical management • CEA in highly selected patients*
Symptomatic	• Medical management	• CEA • CAS can be an alternative	• CEA • CAS can be an alternative

CAS, Carotid artery stenting; *CEA,* carotid endarterectomy.
*CEA can be considered in asymptomatic patients with >70% stenosis if the anticipated rate of perioperative complications (stroke, myocardial infarction, and death) is low, their life expectancy is greater than 5 years, and the risks and benefits (including medical comorbidities) have been discussed thoroughly with the patients and their families.

BASIC INFORMATION

DEFINITION

Carpal tunnel syndrome (CTS) is a compression neuropathy of the median nerve as it passes under the transverse carpal ligament at the wrist (Figs. E1 and E2). It is the most common entrapment neuropathy.

SYNONYMS

CTS

ICD-10CM CODES
G56.0   Carpal tunnel syndrome, unspecified upper limb
G56.01   Carpal tunnel syndrome, right upper limb
G56.02   Carpal tunnel syndrome, left upper limb

EPIDEMIOLOGY & DEMOGRAPHICS

INCIDENCE: 3.8% of the general population (the most common entrapment neuropathy)
PREVALENT AGE: 30 to 60 years
PREVALENT SEX: Females are affected two to five times as often as males.

PHYSICAL FINDINGS & CLINICAL PRESENTATION

- Pain, paresthesia in 1st, 2nd, 3rd, and lateral ½ of 4th fingers, worse at night.
- *Tinel's sign* at wrist (Fig. 3): tapping lightly over the median nerve on the volar surface of the wrist produces a tingling sensation radiating from the wrist to the hand.
- *Phalen's sign* (Fig. 4): reproduction of symptoms after 1 min of gentle, unforced wrist flexion.

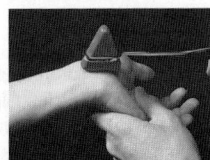

FIG. 3 Tinel's sign. The wrist is held in extension while gentle percussion is performed over and just proximal to the transverse carpal ligament. (From Hochberg MC et al: *Rheumatology,* ed 5, St Louis, 2011, Mosby.)

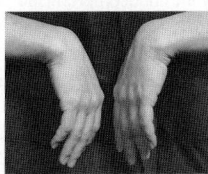

FIG. 4 Phalen's (wrist flexion) test. With the wrists held in unforced flexion for 30 to 60 seconds, a positive test reproduces or worsens the patient's symptoms. (From Hochberg MC et al: *Rheumatology,* ed 5, St Louis, 2011, Mosby.)

- Carpal compression test: direct pressure over the patient's carpal tunnel for 30 sec elicits symptoms.
- Thenar atrophy in longstanding cases with weakness of thumb abduction and opposition.
- Findings may be bilateral in up to 65% of patients.

ETIOLOGY

- Idiopathic in most cases—caused by increased intracarpal tunnel pressure
- Commonly associated with diabetes, obesity, female gender, advancing age, pregnancy, hypothyroidism, rheumatologic disorders, autoimmune disorders, and trauma
- Specific occupations with repetitive strain or job-related mechanical overuse

DIAGNOSIS

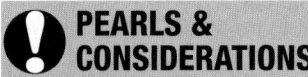

DIFFERENTIAL DIAGNOSIS

- Cervical radiculopathy
- Chronic tendinitis
- Pronator teres syndrome
- Anterior interosseous syndrome
- Complex regional pain syndrome
- Brachial plexopathy, thoracic outlet syndrome
- Polyneuropathy
- Other entrapment neuropathies
- Traumatic wrist injuries
- Vascular disorders (Raynaud syndrome)
- Cervical myelopathy

IMAGING STUDIES

Carpal tunnel syndrome is a clinical diagnosis but imaging may assist workup in uncertain situations. Ultrasound has been effective in supporting the diagnosis and may help identify the structural cause of nerve compression. X-ray or MRI may be helpful in ruling out other conditions.

ELECTRODIAGNOSTIC STUDIES

Nerve conduction velocity tests (NCS) demonstrate impaired sensory conduction across the carpal tunnel and may help guide treatment based on the severity of median nerve compression. Electromyography may show active denervation muscle potentials. Specificity of NCS and electromyography for CTS is >95%, and sensitivity is >85%.

TREATMENT

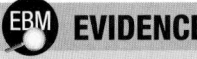

ACUTE GENERAL Rx

- Activity modification and ergonomic changes (desk, keyboard).
- Nocturnal wrist splint has been shown to be effective.
- No evidence for effectiveness of NSAIDs.
- Corticosteroid injection of carpal canal on ulnar side of palmaris longus tendon proximal to wrist crease (Figs. E5 and E6): can be done with palpation guidance or under ultrasound guidance. In different clinical studies,

injections have increased patient satisfaction and improved clinical symptoms, albeit temporarily.
- Low-dose oral corticosteroids are optional but usually not effective.
- Short-term benefit from ultrasound therapy (physical therapy modality).
- Carpal tunnel release if no response from nonoperative treatment.

DISPOSITION

Clinical course may have remissions and exacerbations. Some may progress from intermittent to persistent sensory complaints (numbness, tingling, paresthesia) and then to motor symptoms. In pregnancy, symptoms usually resolve spontaneously weeks after delivery.

REFERRAL

Surgical referral is needed if conservative treatment fails. Surgery (sectioning of transverse carpal ligament) is performed by open, endoscopic, or minimal incision techniques with good long-term results. Carpal tunnel release is one of the most common surgeries performed, with approximately 400,000 conducted per year.

PEARLS & CONSIDERATIONS

- The sensory changes of carpal tunnel syndrome spare the thenar eminence. This distinctive pattern occurs because the palmar sensory cutaneous branch of the median nerve arises proximal to the wrist, passing superficial to the tunnel.
- Role of repetitive hand or wrist use and workplace factors in the development of carpal tunnel syndrome remains controversial.

EVIDENCE

Available at www.expertconsult.com

SUGGESTED READINGS

Available at www.expertconsult.com

RELATED CONTENT

Carpal Tunnel Syndrome (Patient Information)

AUTHORS: **MANUEL F. DASILVA, M.D.,** and **KATIA A. DASILVA, B.A.**

BASIC INFORMATION

DEFINITION

Cat-scratch disease (CSD) is an infectious disease consisting of gradually enlarging regional lymphadenopathy occurring after contact with a feline. Atypical presentations are characterized by a variety of neurologic manifestations as well as granulomatous involvement of the eye, liver, spleen, and bone. The disease is usually self-limiting, and recovery is complete; however, patients with atypical presentations, especially if immunocompromised, may suffer significant morbidity and mortality.

SYNONYMS

Cat-scratch fever
Benign inoculation lymphoreticulosis
Nonbacterial regional lymphadenitis

ICD-10CM CODES
A28.1 Cat-scratch disease

EPIDEMIOLOGY & DEMOGRAPHICS

PREVALENCE: Unknown
INCIDENCE (IN U.S.):
- 9 to 10 cases per 100,000 persons per year (22,000 cases per year)
- Majority of reported cases occur in persons <21 yr

PEAK INCIDENCE: August through January

PHYSICAL FINDINGS & CLINICAL PRESENTATION

- Classic, most common finding: regional lymphadenopathy occurring within 2 wk of a scratch or contact with felines; usually a new kitten in the household
- Tender, swollen lymph nodes most commonly found in the head and neck (Fig. E1), followed by the axilla and the epitrochlear, inguinal, and femoral areas
- Erythematous overlying skin, showing signs of suppuration from involved lymph nodes
- On careful examination, evidence of cutaneous inoculation in the form of a nonpruritic, slightly tender pustule or papule
- Fever in most patients
- Malaise and headache in fewer than a third of patients
- Atypical presentations in fewer than 15% of cases
  1. Usually in association with lymphadenopathy and a low-grade or frank fever (>101 °F, >38.3 °C)
  2. Include granulomatous involvement of the conjunctiva (Parinaud's oculoglandular syndrome) and focal masses in the liver, spleen, and mesenteric nodes
- CNS involvement: neuroretinitis, encephalopathy, encephalitis, transverse myelitis, seizure activity, and coma
- Osteomyelitis in adults and children
- Can be a cause of culture-negative endocarditis
- In HIV-infected and other immunocompromised patients, *Bartonella henselae* is the cause of bacillary angiomatous and peliosis hepatis

ETIOLOGY

- Major cause: *Bartonella henselae,* possibly *Afipia felis* and *Bartonella clarridgeiae*
- Mode of transmission: predominantly by direct inoculation through the scratch, bite, or lick of a cat, especially a kitten
- Also can be transmitted by flea bite (with the flea obtaining the bacteria from a bacteremic cat); rarely after exposure to a dog, probably secondary to flea bites
- Approximately 2 wk after introduction of the bacteria into the host, regional lymphatic tissues displaying granulomatous infiltration associated with gradual hypertrophy
- Possible dissemination to distant sites (e.g., liver, spleen, and bone), usually characterized by focal masses or discrete parenchymal lesions

DIAGNOSIS

DIFFERENTIAL DIAGNOSIS

Granulomas of this syndrome must be differentiated from those associated with:
- Tularemia
- Tuberculosis or other mycobacterial infections
- Brucellosis
- Sarcoidosis
- Sporotrichosis or other fungal diseases
- Toxoplasmosis
- Lymphogranuloma venereum
- Benign and malignant tumors such as lymphoma

WORKUP

Diagnosis should be considered in patients who present with a predominant complaint of gradually enlarging regional (focal) lymphadenopathy, often with fever and a recent history of having contact with a cat. A primary ulcer at the site of the cat scratch may or may not be present at the time lymphadenopathy becomes manifest.

LABORATORY TESTS

- Serologies: An IFA or EIA *Bartonella* serology (titer ≥1:64) is diagnostic. A PCR assay on tissue or blood is also available.
- Lymph node biopsy: granulomatous inflammation consistent with CSD.
- Warthin-Starry silver stain on biopsy can identify the bacteria.
- Histopathologically, Warthin-Starry silver stain has been used to identify the bacillus.
- Culture: *B. henselae* is a fastidious, slow-growing, gram-negative rod that requires specific culture techniques for tissue or blood.
- Routine laboratory findings:
  1. Mild leukocytosis or leukopenia
  2. Infrequent eosinophilia
  3. Elevated ESR or CRP
- Abnormalities of bilirubin excretion and elevated hepatic transaminases are usually secondary to hepatic obstruction by granuloma, mass, or lymph node.
- In patients with neurologic manifestations, lumbar puncture usually reveals normal CSF, although there may be a mild pleocytosis and modest elevation in protein.
- CSD skin test is no longer used for clinical purposes.

TREATMENT

NONPHARMACOLOGIC THERAPY

- Warm compresses to the affected nodes
- In cases of encephalitis or coma: supportive care

ACUTE GENERAL Rx

- This disease is typically self-limited and generally resolves within 2 to 6 months. Most studies show no additional benefit from antibiotic therapy.
- It would be prudent to treat severely ill patients, especially if immunocompromised, with antibiotic therapy, because these patients tend to suffer dissemination of infection and increased morbidity.
- *Bartonella* is usually sensitive to a 5-day course of azithromycin (500 mg on day 1 followed by 250 mg for 4 days for weight >45.5 kg; 10 mg/kg on day 1 followed by 5 mg/kg for 4 days for weight <45.5 kg) or alternatively tetracycline, sulfa, and the quinolones can be used for 7 to 10 days.
- Hepatosplenic disease, neuroretinitis, and endocarditis require longer courses of therapy.
- Antipyretics and NSAIDs may also be used for lymphadenitis.

DISPOSITION

Overall prognosis is good.

REFERRAL

- For diagnostic aspiration or excision in presence of regional lymphadenopathy, bone lesions, and mesenteric lymph nodes and organs
- Infectious diseases specialist for organ involvement including endocarditis
- To ophthalmologist for ocular granulomas

PEARLS & CONSIDERATIONS

COMMENTS

- A presentation of this syndrome, especially in patients with HIV infection or impaired cellular immunity, may be fever of unknown origin.
- Hepatic and splenic granulomas, coronary valve infections may offer few physical clues to diagnosis, emphasizing the need for a complete history.
- CSD should be considered in the differential diagnosis of school-aged children presenting with status epilepticus.
- Chronically immunocompromised patients considering the acquisition of a young feline should be made aware of the possible risk of infection.
- No signs of illness may be apparent in bacteremic kittens.

SUGGESTED READINGS
Available at www.expertconsult.com

RELATED CONTENT

Cat-Scratch Disease (Patient Information)

AUTHOR: **GLENN G. FORT, M.D., M.P.H.**

BASIC INFORMATION

DEFINITION

Cavernous sinus thrombosis (CST) is a late complication of either facial or paranasal sinus infection, resulting in thrombosis of the cavernous sinus and inflammation of its surrounding anatomic structures, including cranial nerves III, IV, V (ophthalmic and maxillary branch), and VI, and the internal carotid artery.

SYNONYMS

Cavernous sinus thrombosis (CST)
Intracranial venous sinus thrombosis or thrombophlebitis
Dural sinus thrombosis

ICD-10CM CODES
G08   Intracranial and intraspinal phlebitis and thrombophlebitis

EPIDEMIOLOGY & DEMOGRAPHICS

- CST is rare in the post-antibiotic era.
- Before antibiotics the mortality rate was 80% to 100%.
- With antibiotics and early diagnosis, mortality rates have fallen to ~20%.
- Reported morbidity rates have also declined from between 50% and 70% to about 20% to 30% with advances in imaging modalities and aggressive medical care.

PHYSICAL FINDINGS & CLINICAL PRESENTATION

- Can be either an acute and fulminant disease or an indolent and subacute presentation.
- Septic cases of CST commonly present with high-grade fever (picket fence pattern) and signs of sepsis.
- Headache, although not specific, is the most common presenting symptom and may precede fever and periorbital edema by several days. Elderly patients, however, may only demonstrate alteration in mental status without antecedent headache. The triad of unilateral or bilateral progressive chemosis, periorbital edema, and proptosis with headache is a classical presentation in patients with CST. These signs and symptoms are related to the anatomic structures affected within the cavernous sinus, notably cranial nerves III to VI, as well as impaired venous drainage from the orbit and eye.

Other common signs and symptoms include:
- Ptosis.
- Cranial nerve palsies (III, IV, V, VI).
  1. Ophthalmoplegia caused by involvement of cranial nerves III, IV, and VI is present in most cases. Sixth nerve palsy can occur early in some cases of septic CST, especially when originating from the sphenoid sinus owing to its anatomic proximity.
  2. Hypoesthesia or hyperesthesia of the ophthalmic and maxillary branch of the fifth nerve is common. Periorbital sensory loss and impaired corneal reflex may be noted.

- Papilledema, retinal hemorrhages, and decreased visual acuity progressing to blindness may occur from venous congestion within the retina.
- Pupil may be dilated and sluggishly reactive.
- Headache with nuchal rigidity and changes in mental status may occur if the infection spreads intracranially to the meninges and brain parenchyma.
- Infection can spread to the contralateral cavernous sinus through the intercavernous sinuses within 24 to 48 hours of initial presentation.
- Patients may also develop signs and symptoms of pituitary insufficiency.

ETIOLOGY

- CST most commonly results from contiguous spread of an infection from either the sinuses (sphenoid, ethmoid, or frontal) or the medial third of the face (areas around the eyes and nose that drain to the ophthalmic vein). Nasal furuncles are the most common facial infection to produce this complication. Less-common primary sites of infection include dental abscess, tonsils, soft palate, middle ear, or orbit (orbital cellulitis).
- CST also can result from hematogenous spread of infection to the cavernous sinus by the superior and inferior ophthalmic veins or through the lateral and sigmoid sinuses. Depending on the pressure gradients, infection can spread in a retrograde direction because the dural sinuses are valveless.
- *Staphylococcus aureus* is the most commonly identified pathogen, found in 60% to 70% of the cases.
- *Streptococcus* is the second leading cause.
- Gram-negative rods and anaerobes may also lead to CST.
- Rarely, *Aspergillus fumigatus* and mucormycosis cause CST.
- Risk factors for dural sinus thrombosis include venous hypercoagulable disorders, infections (see previous), trauma, malignancies, systemic inflammatory disorders, pregnancy, and dehydration.

DIAGNOSIS

- The diagnosis of CST is made by clinical suspicion and confirmed by appropriate imaging studies.
- Proptosis, ptosis, chemosis, and cranial nerve palsy beginning in one eye and progressing to the other eye establish the diagnosis.

DIFFERENTIAL DIAGNOSIS

- Orbital or periorbital cellulitis.
- Internal carotid artery aneurysm or fistula.
- Cerebrovascular disease.
- Migraine headache.
- Allergic blepharitis.
- Thyroid ophthalmopathy.
- Orbital neoplasm.
- Meningitis.
- Epidural and subdural infections.
- Epidural and subdural hematoma.
- Subarachnoid hemorrhage.

- Acute angle-closure glaucoma.
- Trauma.

WORKUP

CST is a clinical diagnosis, with laboratory tests and imaging studies confirming the clinical impression.

LABORATORY TESTS

- Complete blood count, erythrocyte sedimentation rate, blood cultures, and sinus cultures help establish and identify an infectious primary source. Metabolic panel to look for electrolyte imbalances in cases of suspected pituitary involvement (DI/SIADH).
- Lumbar puncture (LP) helps to distinguish CST from more localized processes (e.g., sinusitis, orbital cellulitis). LP reveals inflammatory cells in 75% of cases. In half of these cases, the cerebrospinal fluid profile is typical for a parameningeal focus (high white blood cells with polymorphonuclear and/or mononuclear cells, normal glucose, normal protein, culture negative), and in one third may be similar to that of bacterial meningitis.

IMAGING STUDIES

- MRI with gadolinium, including magnetic resonance angiography and magnetic resonance venogram (Fig. 1), is more sensitive than CT scan and is the imaging study of choice to diagnose CST. Findings may include deformity of the internal carotid artery within the cavernous sinus and an obvious signal hyperintensity within thrombosed vascular sinuses.
- Noncontrast CT scan of the head and orbits may demonstrate increased density in the region of the cavernous sinus but has relatively low sensitivity. Contrast-enhanced CT scan may reveal underlying sinusitis, thickening of the superior ophthalmic vein, and irregular filling defects within the cavernous sinus; however, findings may be normal early in the disease course.

TREATMENT

NONPHARMACOLOGIC THERAPY

Recognizing the primary source of infection (i.e., facial cellulitis, middle ear, and sinus infections) and treating the primary source expeditiously is the best way to prevent CST.

ACUTE GENERAL Rx

- Appropriate therapy should take into account the primary source of infection as well as possible associated complications such as brain abscess, meningitis, or subdural empyema.
- Broad-spectrum intravenous antibiotics are used as empiric therapy until a definite pathogen is found. Treatment should include vancomycin to cover hospital or community-acquired methicillin-resistant *Staphylococcus aureus* or resistant *Streptococcus pneumoniae* plus a third- or fourth-generation cephalosporin:
  1. Vancomycin (1 g q12h with normal renal function) plus either ceftriaxone (2 g q12h) or cefepime (2 g q8 to 12h).

2. Metronidazole 500 mg IV q6h should be added if anaerobic bacterial infection is suspected (dental or sinus infection).

- Most experts recommend anticoagulation with heparin after the diagnosis is confirmed, unless surgical intervention is planned or there is evidence of an expanding hematoma. Spontaneous intracranial hemorrhage should first be ruled out before initiating heparin therapy. Early heparinization has been suggested in patients with unilateral CST to prevent clot propagation. Coumadin therapy should be avoided in the acute phase of the illness, but should ultimately be instituted to achieve an INR of 2 to 3 and continued until the infection, symptoms, and signs of CST have either resolved or significantly improved. Retrospective case reports and case series have demonstrated a favorable outcome in terms of decreased mortality and morbidity in the anticoagulated patients.

- Steroid therapy is also controversial but may prove helpful in reducing cranial nerve dysfunction or when progression to pituitary insufficiency occurs. Corticosteroids should only be instituted after appropriate antibiotic coverage. Dexamethasone 10 mg q6h is the treatment of choice.

- Emergent surgical drainage with sphenoidotomy is indicated if the primary site of infection is believed to be the sphenoid sinus.

CHRONIC Rx

- Patients with CST are usually treated with prolonged courses (3 to 4 weeks) of IV antibiotics. If there is evidence of complications such as intracranial suppuration, 6 to 8 weeks of total therapy may be warranted.
- All patients should be monitored for signs of complicated infection, continued sepsis, or septic emboli while antibiotic therapy is being administered. Relapse of septic CST can occur after an initial improvement weeks after stopping antibiotic treatment.

DISPOSITION

- CST can be a life-threatening, rapidly progressive infectious disease with high morbidity and mortality rates (30%) despite antibiotic use. Morbidity and mortality rates are increased in cases of sphenoid sinus infection.
- Complications of untreated CST include extension of thrombus to other dural sinuses, carotid thrombosis with concomitant strokes, subdural empyema, brain abscess, or meningitis. Septic embolization may also occur to the lungs, resulting in acute

respiratory distress syndrome, pulmonary abscess, empyema, and pneumothorax.

- Thirty percent of treated patients develop long-term sequelae, including cranial nerve palsies, blindness, pituitary insufficiency, and hemiparesis.

REFERRAL

If suspected, CST should be considered a medical emergency. Depending on source of infection, appropriate consultation should be made (i.e., ear-nose-throat, ophthalmology, and infectious disease).

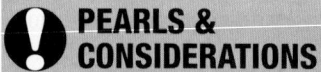

❗ PEARLS & CONSIDERATIONS

COMMENTS

CST is a medical emergency and should be suspected with progressing chemosis, proptosis, and cranial neuropathy in a patient with headaches with or without fever.

The anatomy of the cavernous sinus explains the clinical findings: The cavernous sinus lies just above and lateral to the sphenoid sinus and drains the middle portion of the face by the superior and inferior ophthalmic veins; cranial nerves III, IV, V, and VI pass alongside or through the cavernous sinus.

SUGGESTED READINGS

Available at www.expertconsult.com

RELATED CONTENT

Cavernous Sinus Thrombosis (Patient Information)

AUTHORS: **DANYELLE EVANS, M.D.,**
JOSEPH S. KASS, M.D., J.D., and
PRASHANTH KRISHNAMOHAN, M.B.B.S., M.D.

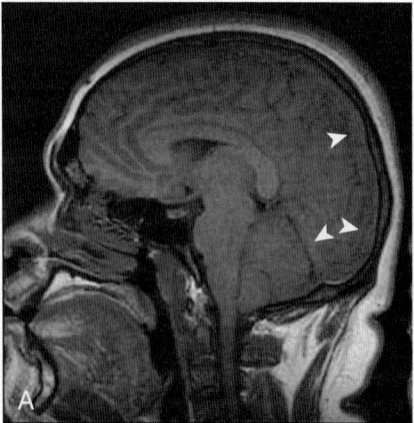
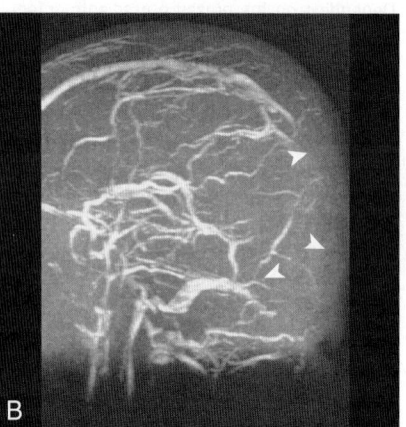
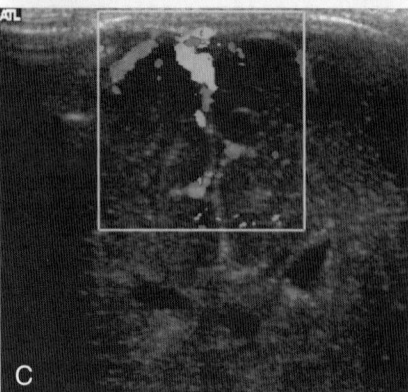

FIG. 1 Superior sagittal sinus (SSS) thrombosis on magnetic resonance venogram (MRV). Sagittal T1 magnetic resonance imaging **(A)** shows intermediate signal intensity in sagittal and straight sinuses *(arrowheads)*. No flow is seen on MRV **(B)** in these vessels *(arrowheads)*, which is consistent with thrombosis. Color Doppler evacuation **(C)** of the SSS in another 6-mo-old patient with suspected thrombosis demonstrated a patent SSS with normal draining cortical veins. (From Fuhrman BP et al: *Pediatric critical care*, ed 4, Philadelphia, 2011, Saunders.)

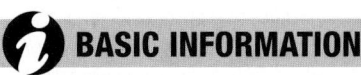

BASIC INFORMATION

DEFINITION

Celiac disease is a chronic autoimmune disease characterized by malabsorption and diarrhea precipitated by ingestion of food products containing gluten. Gluten is a protein complex found in wheat, rye, and barley.

SYNONYMS

Gluten-sensitive enteropathy
Celiac sprue
Nontropical sprue

ICD-10CM CODES
K90.0 Celiac disease

EPIDEMIOLOGY & DEMOGRAPHICS

- The prevalence of celiac disease is 0.5% to 1% in the general population in North America and Western Europe and 5% in high-risk groups such as first-degree relatives of persons with the disease. The prevalence of celiac disease in the U.S. has increased fourfold over the past three decades, but the trend is flattening. The decline in undiagnosed celiac disease may reflect greater public and professional attention to gluten-related issues. Worldwide celiac disease affects 0.6% to 1% of the population.

Celiac disease is significantly more common in persons with type 1 DM and is associated with greater risk of retinopathy and nephropathy in this population.
- Incidence is highest during infancy and the first 36 mo of life (after introduction of foods containing gluten), in the third decade (frequently associated with pregnancy and severe anemia during pregnancy), and in the seventh decade.
- There is a slight female predominance.
- The average age of diagnosis is in the fifth decade of life.
- The risk for celiac disease is 5% to 10% in newborn children of parents with the disease and nearly 20% in siblings.
- It is estimated that only 10% to 15% of persons with celiac disease in the U.S. have been diagnosed.

PHYSICAL FINDINGS & CLINICAL PRESENTATION

- Physical examination may be entirely within normal limits.
- Weight loss, dyspepsia, short stature, and failure to thrive may be noted in children and infants (Fig. 1).
- Weight loss, fatigue, and diarrhea are common in adults.
- Abdominal pain, nausea, and vomiting are unusual.
- Pallor as a result of iron-deficiency anemia is common.

- Atypical forms of the disease are being increasingly recognized and include osteoporosis, short stature, anemia, infertility, and neurologic problems. Manifestations of calcium deficiency, such as tetany and seizures, are rare and can be exacerbated by coexistent magnesium deficiency.
- Angular cheilitis, aphthous ulcers, atopic dermatitis, and dermatitis herpetiformis are frequently associated with celiac disease.
- Table 1 summarizes the clinical spectrum of celiac disease.

ETIOLOGY

- Celiac sprue is considered an autoimmune-type disease, with tissue transglutaminase (tTG) suggested as a major autoantigen. It results from an inappropriate T-cell–mediated immune response against ingested gluten in genetically predisposed individuals who carry either *HLA-DQ2* or *HLA-DQ8* genes. There is sensitivity to gliadin, a protein fraction of gluten found in wheat, rye, and barley. In patients with celiac disease, immune responses to gliadin fractions promote an inflammatory reaction, mainly in the upper small intestine, manifested by infiltration of the lamina propria and the epithelium with chronic inflammatory cells and villous atrophy.
- Seroconversion to celiac autoimmunity may occur at any time.
- Timing of introduction of gluten into the infant diet is associated with the appearance of celiac disease in children at risk. Children initially exposed to gluten in the first 3 mo of life have a fivefold increased risk. Current recommendations are to delay introduction of gluten into the diet of a genetically susceptible infant until 4 to 6 mo of age while the mother continues to breastfeed.

TABLE 1 Clinical Spectrum of Celiac Disease

Symptomatic

Frank malabsorption symptoms: chronic diarrhea, failure to thrive, weight loss

Extraintestinal manifestations: anemia, fatigue, hypertransaminasemia, neurologic disorders, short stature, dental enamel defects, arthralgia, aphthous stomatitis

Silent

No apparent symptoms in spite of histologic evidence of villous atrophy

In most cases identified by serologic screening in at-risk groups (see Laboratory Tests)

Latent

Subjects who have a normal histology, but at some other time, before or after, have shown a gluten-dependent enteropathy

Potential

Subjects with positive celiac disease serology but without evidence of altered jejunal histology

It might or might not be symptomatic

From Kliegman RM et al: *Nelson textbook of pediatrics*, ed 19, Philadelphia, 2011, Saunders.

FIG. 1 Gluten-sensitive enteropathy. Growth curve demonstrates initial normal growth from 0 to 9 mo, followed by onset of poor appetite with intermittent vomiting and diarrhea after initiation of gluten-containing diet *(single arrow)*. After biopsy-confirmed diagnosis and treatment with gluten-free diet *(double arrow)*, growth improves. (From Kliegman RM et al: *Nelson textbook of pediatrics*, ed 19, Philadelphia, 2011, Saunders.)

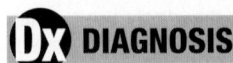

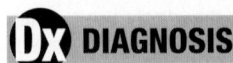 DIAGNOSIS

Diagnostic criteria for celiac disease require at least four out of five or three out of four if the *HLA* genotype is not performed:
1. Typical symptoms of celiac disease
2. Positivity of serum celiac disease Ig A class autoantibodies at high titer
3. *HLA-DQ2* or *HLA-DQ8* genotypes
4. Celiac enteropathy at the small intestinal biopsy
5. Response to gluten-free diet

DIFFERENTIAL DIAGNOSIS
- Inflammatory bowel disease
- Laxative abuse
- Intestinal parasitic infestations
- Lactose intolerance
- Other: irritable bowel syndrome, tropical sprue, chronic pancreatitis, Zollinger-Ellison syndrome, cystic fibrosis (children), lymphoma, eosinophilic gastroenteritis, short bowel syndrome, Whipple's disease
- Intestinal lymphoma, tuberculosis, radiation enteritis, HIV enteropathy

LABORATORY TESTS
- IgA anti-tTG antibody by enzyme-linked immunosorbent assay (tissue transglutaminase [tTG] test) is the best screening serologic test for celiac disease. IgA antiendomysial antibodies (EMA) test is also a good screening test for celiac disease but is best used as a confirmatory test in cases of borderline positive results. In patients with IgA deficiency, the IgG DPG test (deamidated gliadin peptides) can be used for diagnosis. Screening of close relatives is initially done with PCR testing for *HLA DQ2* or *HLA DQ8*. Those that are positive should then have serum tTG IgA screening. All diagnostic serologic testing for celiac disease should be performed before a gluten-free diet is initiated.
- CBC, ferritin level: Iron-deficiency anemia (microcytic anemia, low ferritin level) may be present.
- Celiac disease can lead to malabsorption: Screen for vitamin B_{12} level, folate level, vitamin D level, serum calcium, albumin, magnesium; vitamin B_{12} deficiency, vitamin D deficiency, hypomagnesemia, and hypocalcemia are not uncommon in celiac disease.
- Biopsy of the small bowel, considered the gold standard, has been questioned as a reliable and conclusive test in all cases. It may be reasonable in children with significant elevations of tTG levels (>100 U) to first try a gluten-free diet and consider biopsy in those who do not improve with diet. Repeat small-bowel biopsies are no longer required to show healing when there is a clear response to a gluten-free diet.
- The HLA-DQ2 allele is identified in >90% of patients with celiac disease, and HLA-DQ8 is identified in most of the remaining patients. These genes occur in only 30% to 40% of the general population. Their greatest diagnostic value is in their negative predictive value, making them useful when negative in ruling out the disease.

IMAGING STUDIES
- Consider bone density in newly diagnosed adult patients.
- Capsule endoscopy can be used to evaluate mucosa of the small intestine, especially if future innovations will allow mucosal biopsy.

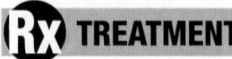 TREATMENT

NONPHARMACOLOGIC THERAPY
Patients should be instructed on a gluten-free diet (avoidance of wheat, rye, and barley). Safe grains (gluten-free) include rice, corn, oats, buckwheat, millet, amaranth, quinoa, sorghum, and teff (an Ethiopian cereal grain). The lowest amount of daily gluten that causes damage to the celiac intestinal mucosa is 10-15 mg/day. One slice of bread contains 1.6 g of gluten.

GENERAL Rx
- Correct nutritional deficiencies with iron, folic acid, calcium, vitamin D, and vitamin B_{12} as needed.
- Prednisone 20 to 60 mg qd gradually tapered is useful in refractory cases.
- Lifelong gluten-free diet is necessary. A referral to a nutritionist experienced in celiac disease and gluten-free diet is recommended at initial diagnosis.

DISPOSITION
- Prognosis is good with adherence to a gluten-free diet. Rapid improvement is usually seen within a few days of treatment. Healing of the intestinal damage typically occurs within 6 to 24 mo after initiation of the diet. Lack of response to gluten-free diet occurs in 5% of patients and is due to unintentional ingestion of gluten or presence of coexisting GI disorders such as IBD, lactose or other carbohydrate intolerance, and pancreatic insufficiency.
- Serial antigliadin or antiendomysial antibody tests can be used to monitor the patient's adherence to a gluten-free diet.
- Repeat small-bowel biopsy after treatment generally reveals significant improvement. It is also useful to evaluate for increased risk of small-bowel T-cell lymphoma in these patients, especially untreated patients. Some experts recommend a repeat biopsy only in selected patients who have an unsatisfactory response to a strict gluten-free diet; however, recent data (Lebwohl et al) show that the risk for lymphoproliferative malignancy (LPM) is affected by the results of follow-up intestinal biopsy performed to document mucosal healing. Increased risk for LPM in CD is associated with the follow-up biopsy results, with a higher risk among patients with persistent villous atrophy. Follow-up biopsy may effectively stratify patients with CD by risk for subsequent LPM.

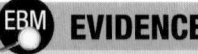 PEARLS & CONSIDERATIONS

COMMENTS
- The presence of dermatitis herpetiformis is pathognomonic for celiac disease.

- In close relatives, repeated serum tTG IgA testing may be useful in those with positive *HLA-DQ2* or *HLA-DQ8* tests because celiac disease may not manifest until later in life, and initial negative results do not preclude the possibility of future onset of celiac disease.
- Celiac disease should be considered in patients with unexplained metabolic bone disease, osteoporosis, transaminasemia, or hypocalcemia, because gastrointestinal symptoms are absent or mild. Clinicians should also consider testing children and young adults for celiac disease if unexplained weight loss, abdominal pain or distention, or chronic diarrhea is present.
- Screening for celiac disease is recommended in first-degree relatives. It should also be considered in patients with type 1 diabetes mellitus and in those with certain autoimmune disorders such as primary biliary cirrhosis, primary sclerosing cholangitis, autoimmune hepatitis, IBD, thyroid disease (hypothyroidism occurs in up to 15% of patients with celiac disease), SLE, RA, and Sjögren's syndrome due to increased risk of celiac disease in these populations. Screening persons with Down syndrome or Turner syndrome has also been recommended.
- The prevalence of celiac disease in patients with dyspepsia is twice that of the general population. Screening for celiac disease should be considered in all patients with persistent dyspepsia.
- Patients with celiac disease have an overall risk of cancer that is almost twice that of the general population. The risk of adenocarcinoma of the small intestine is increased manifold compared with the risk in the general population. Celiac disease is also associated with an increased risk for non-Hodgkin's lymphoma, especially of T-cell type and primarily localized in the gut. Lymphoma is 4 to 40 times more common, and death from lymphoma is 11 to 70 times more common in patients with celiac disease.
- Patients with celiac disease who have followed a gluten-free diet for prolonged periods may not experience relapse of symptoms for several months after gluten is reintroduced.

Trials involving randomized feeding intervention in infants at high risk for celiac disease have shown that as compared with placebo, the introduction of small quantities of gluten at 16 to 24 weeks of age did not reduce the risk of celiac disease by 3 years of age.

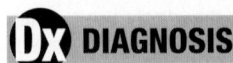 EVIDENCE

Available at www.expertconsult.com

SUGGESTED READINGS
Available at www.expertconsult.com

RELATED CONTENT
Celiac Disease (Patient Information)
Dermatitis Herpetiformis (Related Key Topic)
Malabsorption (Related Key Topic)

AUTHOR: **FRED F. FERRI, M.D.**

BASIC INFORMATION

DEFINITION

Cellulitis is an infection of the deep dermis and subcutaneous tissues characterized by erythema, warmth, and tenderness of the involved area.

SYNONYMS

Erysipelas (cellulitis generally caused by group A β-hemolytic streptococci [GABHS])
SSSIs (skin and skin structure infections)
ABSSSIs (acute bacterial skin and skin structure infections)

ICD-10CM CODES
H05.011	Cellulitis of right orbit
H05.012	Cellulitis of left orbit
H05.013	Cellulitis of bilateral orbits
H05.019	Cellulitis of unspecified orbit
H60.10	Cellulitis of external ear, unspecified ear
H60.11	Cellulitis of right external ear
H60.12	Cellulitis of left external ear
H60.13	Cellulitis of external ear, bilateral
K12.2	Cellulitis and abscess of mouth
L03.011	Cellulitis of right finger
L03.012	Cellulitis of left finger
L03.019	Cellulitis of unspecified finger
L03.031	Cellulitis of right toe
L03.032	Cellulitis of left toe
L03.039	Cellulitis of unspecified toe
L03.111	Cellulitis of right axilla
L03.112	Cellulitis of left axilla
L03.113	Cellulitis of right upper limb
L03.114	Cellulitis of left upper limb
L03.115	Cellulitis of right lower limb
L03.116	Cellulitis of left lower limb
L03.119	Cellulitis of unspecified part of limb
L03.211	Cellulitis of face
L03.221	Cellulitis of neck
L03.311	Cellulitis of abdominal wall
L03.312	Cellulitis of back [any part except buttock]
L03.313	Cellulitis of chest wall
L03.314	Cellulitis of groin
L03.315	Cellulitis of perineum
L03.316	Cellulitis of umbilicus
L03.317	Cellulitis of buttock
L03.319	Cellulitis of trunk, unspecified
L03.811	Cellulitis of head [any part, except face]
L03.818	Cellulitis of other sites
L03.90	Cellulitis, unspecified

EPIDEMIOLOGY & DEMOGRAPHICS

- Occurs most frequently in diabetics, immunocompromised hosts, and patients with venous and lymphatic compromise.
- Frequently found near skin breaks (trauma, surgical wounds [surgical site infections develop in 2% to 5% of all surgical procedures], ulcerations, tinea infections). Edema, animal or human bites, subadjacent osteomyelitis, and bacteremia are potential sources of cellulitis.
- Skin and soft-tissue infections account for >14 million outpatient visits per year and $3.7 billion in ambulatory care costs. They also are responsible for more than 650,000 admissions in the U.S./yr.

PHYSICAL FINDINGS & CLINICAL PRESENTATION

Variable with the causative organism:

- Erysipelas (Fig. E1): superficial-spreading, warm, erythematous lesion distinguished by indurated, elevated margin; lymphatic involvement, vesicle formation common.
- Staphylococcal cellulitis: area involved is erythematous, hot, and swollen; differentiated from erysipelas by nonelevated, poorly demarcated margin; local tenderness and regional adenopathy are common; up to 85% of cases occur on the legs and feet.
- *Haemophilus influenzae* cellulitis: area involved is a blue-red/purple-red color; occurs mainly in children; generally involves the face in children and the neck or upper chest in adults.
- *Vibrio vulnificus:* larger hemorrhagic bullae, cellulitis, lymphadenitis, myositis; often found in critically ill patients in septic shock.
- Table 1 describes anatomic variants of or predispositions to cellulitis. Typically, nonpurulent cellulitis is caused by β-hemolytic streptococci, whereas cellulitis with purulent drainage is caused by MRSA.

ETIOLOGY

- Group A β-hemolytic streptococci (may follow a streptococcal infection of the upper respiratory tract). β-hemolytic streptococci are implicated in most cases of nontraumatic cellulitis.
- Staphylococcal cellulitis: Diabetics, athletes, men who have sex with men, people living in public housing, and incarcerated men are at greater risk for methicillin-resistant *Staphylococcus aureus* (MRSA) infection. A community-acquired MRSA strain, USA 300, is replacing nosocomial strains of MRSA in hospitals.
- IV drug use: MRSA, *Pseudomonas aeruginosa.*
- *V. vulnificus:* higher incidence in patients with liver disease (75%) and in immunocompromised hosts. *V. vulnificus* infection is the leading cause of death related to seafood consumption in the U.S.
- *Erysipelothrix rhusiopathiae:* common in people handling poultry, fish, or meat.
- *Aeromonas hydrophila:* generally occurs in contaminated open wounds in fresh water.
- Fungi *(Cryptococcus neoformans):* in immunocompromised granulopenic patients.
- Gram-negative rods *(Serratia, Enterobacter, Proteus, Pseudomonas):* may be present in immunocompromised or granulopenic patients.
- Hot tub exposure: *P. aeruginosa*; fish tank exposure: *Mycobacterium marinum.*
- Bites: human *(Eikenella corrodens),* dog *(Pasteurella multocida, C. canimorsus),* cat *(P. multocida),* rat *(Streptobacillus moniliformis).*

DIAGNOSIS

DIFFERENTIAL DIAGNOSIS

- Necrotizing fasciitis (reddish-purple discoloration of skin, rapid increase in size, woody induration and pale appearance rather than erythema, violaceous bullae, pain out of proportion to appearance, sepsis)
- Deep vein thrombosis
- Peripheral vascular insufficiency
- Paget disease of the breast
- Thrombophlebitis
- Acute gout
- Psoriasis
- *Candida* intertrigo
- Pseudogout
- Osteomyelitis
- Insect bite
- Fixed drug eruption
- Lymphedema
- Contact dermatitis
- Olecranon bursa infection
- Herpetic whitlow, early herpes zoster (before blisters)
- Erythema migrans (Lyme disease)
- Rare: *Vaccinia* vaccination, Kawasaki disease, pyoderma gangrenosum, Sweet syndrome, carcinoma erysipeloides, anaerobic myonecrosis, erythromelalgia, eosinophilic cellulitis (Well's syndrome), familial Mediterranean fever

LABORATORY TESTS

- Gram stain, culture (aerobic and anaerobic):
  1. Aspirated material from:
     a. Advancing edge of cellulitis
     b. Any vesicles
  2. Swab of any drainage material
  3. Punch biopsy (in selected patients)
- Blood cultures in hospitalized patients, patients with cellulitis superimposed on lymphedema, patients with buccal or periorbital cellulitis, and patients suspected of having a salt- or fresh-water source of infection. Bacteremia uncommon in cellulitis (positive blood cultures in 4% of patients).
- Anti-streptolysin O (ASLO) titer (in suspected streptococcal disease)

The cause of cellulitis remains unidentified in most patients. Patients with recurrent lower-extremity cellulitis should be inspected for tinea pedis. If found it should be treated.

IMAGING STUDIES

CT or MRI in patients with suspected necrotizing fasciitis (deep-seated infection of the subcutaneous tissue that results in the progressive destruction of fascia and fat).

TREATMENT

NONPHARMACOLOGIC THERAPY

Immobilization and elevation of the involved limb. Cool sterile saline dressings to remove purulence from any open lesion. Support stockings in patients with peripheral edema.

ACUTE GENERAL Rx

Treatment should initially cover *Streptococcus* and methicillin-sensitive *S. aureus* and should be expanded for MRSA in patients with risk factors (e.g., IV drug users, residents of long-term care facilities, athletes, children, men who have sex with men, prisoners).

Erysipelas:
- PO: dicloxacillin 500 mg PO q6h

TABLE 1 Anatomic Variants of or Predispositions to Cellulitis

Anatomic Variant or Predisposition	Location	Likely Bacterial Cause
Periorbital cellulitis	Periorbital	*Staphylococcus aureus, Streptococcus pneumoniae,* group A streptococci
Buccal cellulitis	Cheek	*Haemophilus influenzae* type b
Cellulitis complicating body piercing	Ear, nose, umbilicus	*S. aureus,* group A streptococci
After mastectomy (with axillary node dissection)	Ipsilateral upper extremity	Non–group A β-hemolytic streptococci
After lumpectomy (with limited axillary node dissection, breast irradiation)	Ipsilateral breast	Non–group A β-hemolytic streptococci
After saphenous vein harvest for coronary artery bypass	Ipsilateral leg	Group A or non–group A β-hemolytic streptococci
After radical pelvic surgery, radiation therapy	Vulva, inguinal areas, legs	Group B and group G streptococci
After liposuction	Thigh, abdominal wall	Group A streptococci, peptostreptococci
Postoperative (very early) wound infection	Abdomen, chest, hip	Group A streptococci
Injection drug use ("skin popping")	Extremities, neck	*S. aureus,* streptococci (groups A, C, F, G)*
Perianal cellulitis	Perineum	Group A streptococcus

*Other bacteria to consider based on isolation from skin or abscesses in this setting include *Enterococcus faecalis,* viridans group streptococci, coagulase-negative staphylococci, anaerobes (including *Bacteroides* and *Clostridium* spp.), and Enterobacteriaceae.

From Bennett JE, Dolin R, Blaser MJ: *Mandell, Douglas, and Bennett's principles and practice of infectious diseases,* ed 8, Philadelphia, 2015, Saunders.

- IV: cefazolin 1 g q6 to 8h or nafcillin 1.0 or 1.5 g IV q4 to 6h
  NOTE: Use vancomycin 1 g IV q12h in patients allergic to penicillin.
  Staphylococcal cellulitis:
- PO: dicloxacillin 250 to 500 mg qid
- IV: nafcillin 1 to 2 g q4 to 6h
- Cephalosporins (cephalothin, cephalexin, cephradine) also provide adequate antistaphylococcal coverage, except for MRSA.
- Trimethoprim-sulfamethoxazole (160 mg/800 mg 1 PO bid) may be appropriate in mild MRSA infections. Use vancomycin 1.0 to 2.0 g IV qd or linezolid 0.6 g IV q12h in patients allergic to penicillin or cephalosporins and in patients with moderate/severe MRSA. Daptomycin (Cubicin), a cyclic lipopeptide, can be used as an alternative to vancomycin for complicated skin and skin structure infections. Usual dose is 4 mg/kg IV given over 30 min every 24 hr. Telavancin is a new glycopeptide derivative of vancomycin effective for gram-positive skin and skin structure infections, including those caused by MRSA. Tedizolid is an oxazolidinone effective in ABSSSI as an alternative to linezolid. Ceftaroline fosamil (Teflaro) is a newer IV cephalosporin also effective against MRSA. Dalbavancin and tedizolid are two new drugs recently FDA-approved for skin and skin

structure infections, including those caused by MRSA. Trials involving once-weekly IV dalbavancin have shown noninferiority to daily IV vancomycin in adults with acute bacterial skin and skin-structure infection (SSSI).[1]
H. influenzae cellulitis:
- PO: cefixime or cefuroxime
- IV: cefuroxime or ceftriaxone
  Vibrio vulnificus:
- Doxycycline 100 mg IV bid + ceftazidime 2 g IV q8h or IV ciprofloxacin 400 mg bid. Mild cases treated with oral antibiotics (doxycycline 100 mg bid + ciprofloxacin 750 mg bid).
- IV support and admission into intensive care unit (mortality rate >50% in septic shock).
  E. rhusiopathiae:
- Penicillin
  A. hydrophila:
- Aminoglycosides
- Chloramphenicol
- Complicated skin and skin structure infections in hospitalized patients can be treated with daptomycin (Cubicin) 4 mg/kg IV q24h

[1]Boucher HW, Wilcox M, Talbot GH et al: Once-weekly dalbavancin versus daily conventional therapy for skin infections. N Engl J Med 370: 2169-79, 2014

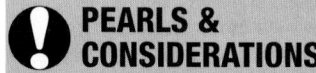

PEARLS & CONSIDERATIONS

- 16.6% of acute cellulitis cases are unresponsive to initial treatment mainly due to inappropriate antibiotic selection and dosing (weight-based dosing is preferred).
- Prophylactic antibiotics (e.g., dicloxacillin 500 mg bid or erythromycin 250 mg bid) are controversial but can be considered with patients with >4 episodes of cellulitis despite optimized control of risk factors. Recurrent cellulitis with no identifiable cause occurs in 22% of cases despite antibiotic prophylaxis.

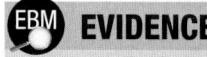 **EVIDENCE**

Available at www.expertconsult.com

SUGGESTED READINGS
Available at www.expertconsult.com

RELATED CONTENT

Cellulitis (Patient Information)
Erysipelas (Related Key Topic)
Necrotizing Fasciitis (Related Key Topic)

AUTHOR: **FRED F. FERRI, M.D.**

BASIC INFORMATION

DEFINITION

Cervical cancer is the penetration of the basement membrane and infiltration of the stroma of the uterine cervix by malignant cells.

ICD-10CM CODES

C53.8   Malignant neoplasm of overlapping sites of cervix uteri
C53.9   Malignant neoplasm of cervix uteri, unspecified
D06.7   Carcinoma in situ of other parts of cervix
D06.9   Carcinoma in situ of cervix, unspecified

EPIDEMIOLOGY & DEMOGRAPHICS

INCIDENCE: Approximately 12,000 new cases annually, with 4000 to 5000 associated deaths. Mean age at diagnosis is 48 years. U.S. has age-adjusted mortality rate of 2.6 per 100,000 persons.
PREDOMINANCE: Higher incidence rates occur in developing countries. Among the U.S. population, Hispanics have a higher incidence than African Americans, who likewise have a higher incidence than whites. Worldwide, cervical cancer is the third most common cancer in women.
RISK FACTORS: Smoking, early age at first intercourse, multiple sexual partners, immunocompromised state, nonbarrier methods of birth control, infection with high-risk human papillomavirus (HPV; types 16 and 18), and multiparity.

PHYSICAL FINDINGS & CLINICAL PRESENTATION

- Unusual vaginal bleeding, particularly postcoital (Fig. 1)
- Vaginal discharge and/or odor
- Advanced cases may present with lower-extremity edema or renal failure
- In early stages, there may be little or no obvious cervical lesion; more advanced cases may have large, bulky, friable lesions encompassing majority of vagina

ETIOLOGY

- Infection with high-risk HPV types is a necessary, although not sufficient, cause of almost all cases of cervical cancer. Persistent HPV infection leads to precancerous changes of cervix (cervical intraepithelial neoplasia [CIN]). CIN can progress to invasive cervical cancer.
- Both squamous cell and adenocarcinoma of cervix are associated with HPV infection.
- More than 40 HPV types can infect the cervix. Most cases are believed to be linked to presence of HPV 16, 18, 45, and 56 by interaction of E6 oncoprotein on *p53* gene product.
- There may be an association with past infection with *Chlamydia trachomatis*.

DIAGNOSIS

DIFFERENTIAL DIAGNOSIS

- Cervical polyp or prolapsed uterine fibroid
- Preinvasive cervical lesions
- Neoplasia metastatic from a separate primary neoplasia

WORKUP

- Thorough history and physical examination.
- Pelvic examination with careful rectovaginal examination.
- Compared with Pap testing, HPV testing has greater sensitivity for detection of CIN. Addition of HPV test for high-risk types to Pap test to screen women in mid-30s for cervical cancer reduces incidence of grade 2 or 3 CIN or cancer detected by subsequent screening examinations.
- Colposcopy with directed biopsy and endocervical curettage.
- FIGO staging described in Table 1.

LABORATORY TESTS

- Complete blood count, chemistry profile
- SCC antigen in research setting
- Carcinoembryonic antigen

IMAGING STUDIES

- Chest x-ray
- Depending on stage, may need CT scan, MRI (Fig. 2), PET/CT
- Intravenous pyelogram

TREATMENT

NONPHARMACOLOGIC THERAPY

- FIGO stage IA: cone biopsy or simple hysterectomy
- FIGO stage IB or IIA: type III radical hysterectomy and pelvic lymphadenectomy or pelvic radiation therapy
- Advanced or bulky disease: multimodality therapy (radiation, chemotherapy, and/or surgery); platinum use before radiation therapy

ACUTE GENERAL Rx

Table 1 summarizes treatment according to tumor stage. Chemotherapy is cisplatin-based. In advanced cases, cervical cancer may present with massive and acute vaginal bleeding requiring volume and blood replacement, vaginal packing or other hemostatic modalities, and/or high-dose local radiotherapy.

CHRONIC Rx

- Physical examination with Pap smear every 3 mo for 2 yr, every 6 mo for 3 to 5 yr, annually thereafter
- Chest x-ray annually (optional)
- Other imaging done only as clinically indicated
- Localized pelvic recurrence may be treated and cured with pelvic exenteration

DISPOSITION

Five-year survival varies by stage:
- Stage I: 90% to 95%

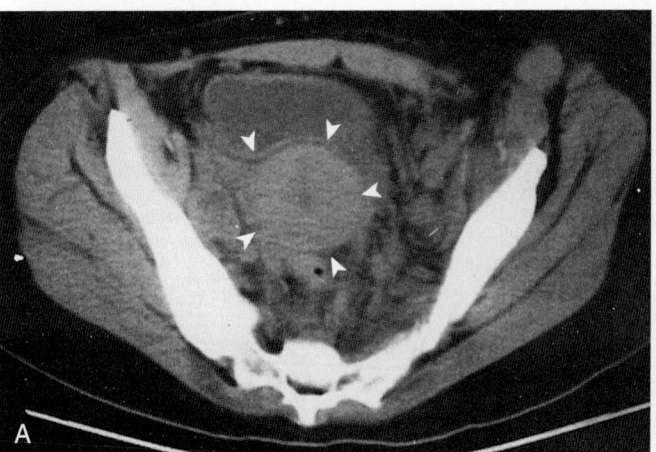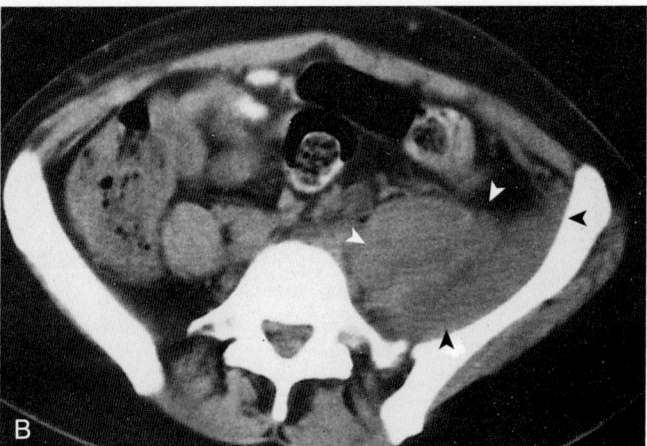

FIG. 1 Stage IIIb cervical carcinoma. A 27-year-old woman presented with increased vaginal bleeding, left leg swelling, and abdominal pain. Examination revealed a large, fixed pelvic mass. CT scan evaluation **(A)** confirms the mass *(arrowheads)* and **(B)** shows extension into the left psoas and iliacus muscles *(arrowheads)*. She also had hydronephrosis. Pathologic examination showed an adenosquamous carcinoma. (Skarin AT: *Atlas of diagnostic oncology,* ed 4, Philadelphia, 2010, Mosby.)

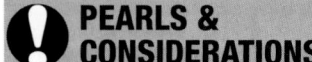
Table 1 FIGO Staging of Cervical Cancer

Stage	Invasion	Prognosis: 5-yr Survival	Treatment
1$_{A1}$	Depth of invasion ≤3 mm and width ≤7 mm (includes early stromal invasion of ≤1 mm)	84% to 90% if tumor <3 cm; 85% will have negative pelvic nodes, and 95% of these patients will be "cured"	Local excision; if margins of cone clear (i.e., no residual tumor or CIN), then conization is adequate, with no need for pelvic lymphadenectomy
1$_{A2}$	Depth of invasion between 3 and 5 mm (i.e., 3.1-5 mm) and width up to 7 mm		Simple hysterectomy and pelvic lymphadenectomy
1$_{B1}$	Tumor confined to cervix and diameter <4 cm	66% if tumor >3 cm	Radical hysterectomy or radiotherapy
1$_{B2}$	Tumor confined to cervix and diameter >4 cm		Radical hysterectomy or radiotherapy
II$_A$	Upper third of the vagina		Radical hysterectomy or radiotherapy
II$_B$	Upper two thirds of the vagina plus parametrial disease	62%	Radiotherapy ± chemotherapy
III$_A$	Lower third of the vagina		Radiotherapy ± chemotherapy
III$_B$	Pelvic sidewall and/or hydronephrosis	40%	Radiotherapy ± chemotherapy
IV$_A$	Bladder, rectum		Radiotherapy ± chemotherapy
IV$_B$	Beyond pelvis	15%	Radiotherapy ± chemotherapy

From Drife J, Magowan B: *Clinical obstetrics and gynecology*, Philadelphia, 2004, Saunders.

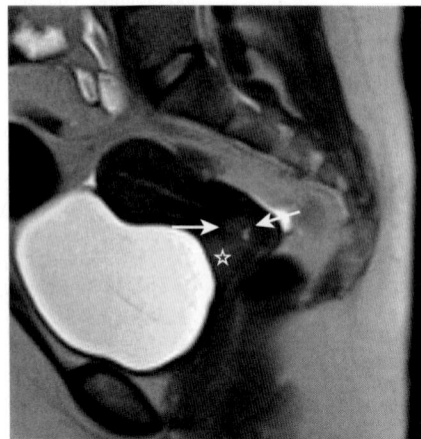

FIG. 2 Cervical carcinoma. T2-weighted sagittal image through the cervix shows an intermediate signal mass *(arrows)* disrupting the normally intense low signal ring of the cervical stroma with areas of high signal. The mass infiltrates the upper vagina *(star)*. (From Fielding JR et al: *Gynecologic imaging*, Philadelphia, 2011, Saunders.)

- Stage II: 40% to 80%
- Stage III: <60%
- Stage IV: <15%

Early detection by Pap smear is imperative for long-term improvements in survival.

REFERRAL
Gynecologic oncologist for all invasive disease

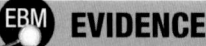

PEARLS & CONSIDERATIONS

- HPV vaccination is indicated in males and females age 9 to 26 yr for the prevention of cervical cancer caused by HPV types 6, 11, 16, and 18. HPV vaccination is over 90% effective in preventing infection and cervical cancer.
- Available evidence supports discontinuation of cervical cancer screening among women aged 65 yr or older who have had adequate screening and are not otherwise at high risk.
- Updated recommendations from the American College of Physicians on screening for cervical cancer in average-risk women are as follows.[1]
- Women should be screened with cervical cytology every 3 years beginning at age 21.
- After age 30, women can be screened with cytology and HPV testing every 5 years.
- Before age 21, women should not be scanned at all.
- Before age 30, women should not be screened with HPV testing.
- At age 65, screening can stop in women with three consecutive negative cytology results or two consecutive negative cytology results combined with a negative HPV test within the last 10 years (with the most recent test within 5 years).
- Women without a cervix should not be screened.

EBM EVIDENCE

Available at www.expertconsult.com

SUGGESTED READINGS
Available at www.expertconsult.com

RELATED CONTENT
Cervical Cancer (Patient Information)
Cervical Dysplasia (Related Key Topic)

AUTHOR: **ANTHONY SCISCIONE, D.O.**

[1]Sawaya GF, et al.: Cervical cancer screening in average-risk women: best practice advice from the Cervical Guidelines Committee of the American College of Physicians, *Ann Intern Med* 162(12):851-859, 2015.

BASIC INFORMATION

DEFINITION

Cervical dysplasia refers to atypical development of immature squamous epithelium that does not penetrate the basement epithelial membrane. Characteristics include increased cellularity, nuclear abnormalities, and increased nuclear/cytoplasmic ratio. A progressive loss of squamous differentiation exists beginning adjacent to the basement membrane and progressing to the most advanced stage (severe dysplasia), which encompasses the complete squamous epithelial layer thickness. The revised 2001 Bethesda System terminology was used in a National Institutes of Health consensus conference, sponsored by the American Society for Colposcopy and Cervical Pathology (ASCCP) and its partner professional organizations in 2006. The conference updated therapeutic options for women based on studies such as the **A**SC-US (atypical squamous cells of undetermined significance)/**L**SIL (low-grade squamous intraepithelial lesions) **T**riage **S**tudy (ALTS) that appeared after revision of the Bethesda classification. Fig. 1 provides a comparison of grading systems for cervical squamous dysplasia.

In 2012, the American Cancer Society (ACS), ASCCP, and American Society for Clinical Pathology (ASCP) published a new set of recommendations for lifetime assessment and early diagnosis of cervical dysplasia and cancer. The recommendations attempted to reduce the number of lifetime assessments, thereby reducing the possible morbidity associated with excess testing and also optimizing the co-evaluation with Pap smear and HPV testing. In brief, women younger than 21 yr of age should not have any screening. Women 21-29 yr of age should have testing every 3 yr with only cytology. With negative cytology or HPV-negative ASC-US, patients can repeat every 3 yr. For HPV-positive ASC-US or cytology with LG-SIL, follow-up is as per the 2006 guidelines (essentially a colposcopic examination as the initial step with follow-up steps depending on the findings). Women between the ages of 30 and 65 yr should have co-testing every 5 yr with both Pap cytology and HPV testing. Alternatively, it is also acceptable to perform cytology alone, but then the testing interval should be every 3 yr. With negative cytology or HPV-negative ASC-US, patients can repeat with co-testing every 5 yr. For HPV-positive ASC-US or cytology with LG-SIL, follow-up is as per the 2006 guidelines, as previously documented. For patients with positive HPV but negative cytology, the patient can repeat testing 12 months later with co-testing; patients can also specifically test for HPV 16 or HPV 16/18 genotypes and, if positive, should be referred for colposcopy. Patients with positive HPV but negative 16 and/or 18 should be retested in 12 months with co-testing.

Women older than the age of 65 yr and those with a history of hysterectomy (including removal of cervix) should no longer be tested unless they had previous diagnosis of cervical intraepithelial neoplasia (CIN) 2 or more severe; these women should be tested for at least 20 yr. Women who have been vaccinated for HPV should still use age-specific recommendations for screening.

BETHESDA 2001 UPDATED CLASSIFICATION:

The Bethesda 2001 System was the result of a year-long iterative process held to update the original 1991 system and to broaden participation in the consensus process, clarify reporting of abnormalities, and incorporate data that had been collected since the initial system was created.

The reporting system includes the following areas:

Specimen adequacy: The system defines the specimen as either satisfactory for evaluation or unsatisfactory and then specifies the reason for inadequacy if necessary.

General categorization (optional): This serves to triage the specimen into normal finding (negative for intraepithelial lesion or malignancy) or identifies it as an "epithelial abnormality." The descriptions are meant to be mutually exclusive.

Interpretation/result: Makes a distinction between "interpretation" and "diagnosis" of the specimen so that the interpretation may be incorporated into the overall clinical context for the particular patient being evaluated.

Negative for intraepithelial lesion or malignancy: In this screening test, no intraepithelial lesion or malignancy is identified. Non-neoplastic findings such as organisms or reactive cellular findings may be specified but are still considered to be a negative result.

Epithelial cell abnormalities:
  Squamous cell:
    Atypical squamous cell (ASC) of undetermined significance (ASC-US) emphasizing the unusual but still possible association with underlying CIN II/III and extremely rare possibility of squamous cell carcinoma
    ASC cannot exclude high-grade squamous intraepithelial lesion (HSIL) (ASC-H), suggesting a risk for CIN II/III that is intermediate between ASC-US and HSIL
    Low-grade squamous intraepithelial lesion (LSIL) suggests a transient viral infection with a greater likelihood for regression, more likely to encompass human papillomavirus (HPV) infection and CIN I histologically
    HSIL suggestive of a more persistent viral infection and with a greater risk for progressive disease, more likely to encompass CIN II/III and carcinoma in situ (CIS) histologically
  Squamous cell carcinoma
  Glandular cell
    Atypical glandular cells (should specify endocervical, endometrial, or not otherwise specified)
    Atypical glandular cell, favor neoplasia (should specify endocervical or not otherwise specified)
    Endocervical adenocarcinoma in situ (AIS)
    Adenocarcinoma
Other: Endometrial cells in a woman ≥>40 yr of age. Because menopausal status is sometimes uncertain, age was chosen to discriminate

Histological features	Traditional system	WHO system	British Society for Cervical Cytology	Bethesda system
Atypical squamous cells not meeting the criteria for dysplasia	Mild atypia	Mild atypia	Borderline nuclear abnormality	Atypical squamous cells (ASC)
Koilocytes plus mild atypia	HPV infection	HPV infection	HPV plus borderline change	Low-grade squamous intraepithelial lesion (SIL)
Dysplasia limited to lower third of epithelium	Mild dysplasia	CIN 1	Mild dyskaryosis (low-grade dyskaryosis)	Low-grade SIL
Dysplasia limited to lower two-thirds of epithelium	Moderate dysplasia	CIN 2	Moderate dyskaryosis (high-grade dyskaryosis)	High-grade SIL
Dysplasia extending into upper third of epithelium	Severe dysplasia	CIN 3	Severe dyskaryosis (high-grade dyskaryosis)	High-grade SIL
Dysplasia of full thickness of epithelium	Carcinoma in situ	CIN 3	Severe dyskaryosis (high-grade dyskaryosis)	High-grade SIL

FIG. 1 Comparison of grading systems (From Young B et al: Female reproductive system. In *Wheater's basic pathology*, Philadelphia, 2011, Elsevier, pp 216-315.)

women who might, with the findings of endometrial cells on cytology, warrant further evaluation with endometrial sampling

KEY POINTS:

1. The cytologic distinctions of low grade (LSIL) and high grade (HSIL) do not necessarily equate to the histologic classifications CIN I and CIN II/III.
2. The 2006 conference notes that one cytologic abnormality can have different histologic risk in different women and highlights "special populations" such as adolescent and young women, and those women who are pregnant. In young women, spontaneous HPV clearance rates are exceptionally high. The new testing recommendations essentially remove the possibility of testing women younger than 21 yr of age.
3. DNA testing for high-risk HPV types is incorporated into the evaluation and treatment algorithms for women with cytologic cervical abnormalities.

Histologically, a two-tiered system is developed in this guideline that distinguishes between the lower-risk CIN I and higher-risk CIN II/III diagnoses.

ICD-10CM CODES

N87.9	Dysplasia of cervix uteri, unspecified
R87.610	Atypical squamous cells of undetermined significance on cytologic smear of cervix (ASC-US)
R87.611	Atypical squamous cells cannot exclude high grade squamous intraepithelial lesion on cytologic smear of cervix (ASC-H)
R87.612	Low grade squamous intraepithelial lesion on cytologic smear of cervix (LGSIL)
R87.613	High grade squamous intraepithelial lesion on cytologic smear of cervix (HGSIL)
R87.614	Cytologic evidence of malignancy on smear of cervix
R87.615	Unsatisfactory cytologic smear of cervix
R87.618	Other abnormal cytological findings on specimens from cervix uteri
R87.619	Unspecified abnormal cytological findings in specimens from cervix uteri
Z12.4	Encounter for screening for malignant neoplasm of cervix

EPIDEMIOLOGY & DEMOGRAPHICS

PREDOMINANT AGE:

- Dysplasia: peak age, 26 yr (3600 cases/100,000 persons)
- CIS: peak age, 32 yr (1100 cases/100,000 persons)
- Invasive cancer: peak age <>60 yr (800 cases/100,000 persons)

PEAK INCIDENCE:

- Age 35 yr
- Abnormal Pap smear rate revealing dysplasia approximates 2% to 5% depending on

population risk factors and false-negative rate variance

- False-negative rate approaching 40%
- Average age-adjusted incidence of severe dysplasia is 35 cases/100,000 persons
- Approximately half of the cases of new cervical cancer had never been screened, and another 10% had not been screened in more than 5 yr. Many of these women come from underserved or underresourced communities. The single biggest impact in reducing the morbidity and mortality from cervical cancer would come from appropriately addressing these health disparities.

PHYSICAL FINDINGS & CLINICAL PRESENTATION

- Cervical lesions associated with dysplasia often are not visible to the naked eye; therefore, physical findings are best viewed by colposcopy of a 3% acetic acid–prepared cervix.
- Patients evaluated by colposcopy are identified by abnormal cervical cytology screening from Pap smear screening.
- Colposcopic findings:
  1. Leukoplakia (white lesion seen by the unaided eye that may represent condyloma, dysplasia, or cancer)
  2. Acetowhite epithelium with or without associated punctation, mosaicism, abnormal vessels
  3. Abnormal transformation zone (abnormal iodine uptake, "cuffed" gland openings)

ETIOLOGY

- Strongly associated and initiated by oncogenic HPV infection (high-risk HPV types are 16, 18, 31, 33, 35, 45, 51, 52, 56, and 58; low-risk HPV types are 6, 11, 42, 43, and 44)
- Risk factors:
  1. HPV
  2. Any heterosexual coitus
  3. Coitus during puberty (transformation-zone metaplasia peak)
  4. Diethylstilbestrol exposure
  5. Multiple sexual partners
  6. Lack of prior Pap smear screening
  7. History of STD
  8. Other genital tract neoplasia
  9. HIV
  10. Tuberculosis
  11. Substance abuse
  12. "High-risk" male partner (HPV)
  13. Low socioeconomic status
  14. Early first pregnancy
  15. Tobacco use

🅳🆇 DIAGNOSIS

DIFFERENTIAL DIAGNOSIS

- Metaplasia
- Hyperkeratosis
- Condyloma
- Microinvasive carcinoma
- Glandular epithelial abnormalities
- Vulvar intraepithelial neoplasm
- Vaginal intraepithelial neoplasm
- Metastatic tumor involvement of the cervix

WORKUP

- Periodic history and physical examination (including cytologic screening) depending on age, risk factors, and history of preinvasive cervical lesions
- Consider screening for sexually transmitted disease (gonorrhea, *Chlamydia,* herpes, HIV, HPV)
- Abnormal cytology (HSIL/LSIL, initial ASC/ASC-US/ASC-H in high-risk patients, recurrent in low-risk/postmenopausal patients) and grossly evident suspicious lesions; refer for colposcopy and possible directed biopsy/endocervical curettage (ECC; examination should include cervix, vagina, vulva, and anus)
- For glandular cell abnormalities (AGCs): refer for colposcopy and possible directed biopsy/ECC, and consider endometrial sampling
- In pregnancy: abnormal cytology followed by colposcopy in the first trimester and at 28 to 32 wk; only high-grade lesions suspicious for carcinoma biopsied; ECC is contraindicated

LABORATORY TESTS

- Gonorrhea, chlamydia to rule out STD
- Pap cytology screening (requires appropriate sampling, preparation, cytologist interpretation, and reporting)
- Colposcopy and directed biopsy, ECC for indications (see "Workup")
- HPV DNA typing if identified abnormal cytology
- As compared with Pap testing, HPV testing has greater sensitivity for the detection of intraepithelial neoplasia

IMAGING STUDIES

- Cervicography
- Computer-enhanced Pap cytology screening (e.g., PAPNET)

MANAGEMENT

Refer to the literature for a more comprehensive approach. The following treatment paradigms in Table 1 give a general outline for care.

DISPOSITION

- Because of the large number of women in high-risk groups, the prevalence of HPV, and the high false-negative Pap smear rate, routine Pap smear screening should be strongly encouraged for all women, especially those with a history of cervical dysplasia. The addition of an HPV test to the Pap test reduces the incidence of CIN II or III, or cancer detected by subsequent screening.
- Success rates for treatment approach 80% to 90%.
- Detection of persistence of recurrence requires careful follow-up.
- Cervical treatment possibly results in infertility (cervical stenosis or incompetence), which requires careful consideration and discretion for use of LEEP and cone biopsy.
- Appropriate counseling and informed consent are needed when considering any form of management of cervical dysplasia.

C

TABLE 1 Summary of Recommendations

Population	Recommended Screening Method	Management of Screen Results	Comments
<21 yr	No screening		
21-29 yr	Cytology alone every 3 yr	HPV-positive ASC-US or cytology of LSIL or more severe: Refer to ASCCP Guidelines Cytology Negative or HPV-Negative ASC-USRe-screen with cytology in 3 yr	
30-65 yr	HPV and cytology "co-testing" every 5 yr (preferred)	HPV-positive ASC-US or cytology of LSIL or more severe: Refer to ASCCP guidelines	Screening by HPV testing alone is not recommended for most clinical settings.
		HPV positive, cytology negative:Option 1: Y 12-month follow-up with co-testing	
		Option 2: Y test for HPV16 or HPV16/18 genotypes. If HPV16 or HPV16/18 positive, refer to colposcopy. If HPV16 or HPV16/18 negative, 12-mo follow-up with co-testing	
		Co-test negative or HPV-negative ASC-US: Rescreen with co-testing in 5 yr	
	Cytology alone every 3 yr (acceptable)	HPV-positive ASC-US or cytology of LSIL or more severe: Refer to ASCCP guidelines	
		Cytology negative or HPV-negative ASC-US: Rescreen with cytology in 3 yr	
>65 yr	No screening following adequate negative prior screening		Women with a history of CIN2 or a more severe diagnosis should continue routine screening for at least 20 yr
After hysterectomy	No screening		Applies to women without a cervix and without a history of CIN2 or a more severe diagnosis in the past 20 yr or cervical cancer ever.
HPV vaccinated	Follow age-specific recommendations (same as unvaccinated women)		

ASCCP, American Society for Colposcopy and Cervical Pathology; *ASC-US,* atypical squamous cells of undetermined significance; *CIN,* cervical intraepithelial neoplasia; *HPV,* human papillomavirus; *LSIL,* low-grade squamous intraepithelial lesions.
Modified from Saslow D et al: American Cancer Society, American Society for Colposcopy and Cervical Pathology, and American Society for Clinical Pathology screening guidelines for the prevention and early detection of cervical cancer, *J Low Gen Tract Dis* 16(3):175-204, 2012.

REFERRAL

- Patients with abnormal Pap cytology should be referred to a provider, likely a trained obstetrician/gynecologist, who can appropriately treat the patient in an age-specific manner and also perform a colposcopy if indicated as part of the new recommendations. Given the morbidity associated with both underevaluating and treating as well as reacting excessively to cytologic findings, a provider who is intimately familiar with ASCCP guidelines should be sought.
- If treatment is required, patient should be referred to a gynecologist or gynecologic oncologist skilled in the diagnosis and treatment of preinvasive cervical disease.

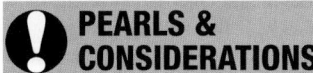

PEARLS & CONSIDERATIONS

COMMENTS

- Testing for human papillomavirus by Hybrid capture 2 DNA test will identify 91% of the small proportion of women with post-treatment residual or recurrent disease, but 30% of all women who are tested will test positive and need colposcopy.
- HPV vaccination is recommended for males and females from ages 9 to 26.

SUGGESTED READINGS

Available at www.expertconsult.com

RELATED CONTENT

Cervical Dysplasia (Patient Information)
Pap Smear Abnormalities (Patient Information)
Cervical Cancer (Related Key Topic)
Cervical Polyps (Related Key Topic)

AUTHOR: **ANTHONY SCISCIONE, D.O.**

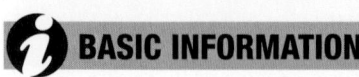

BASIC INFORMATION

DEFINITION

Cervicitis is an inflammation of the cervix. It may result from direct infection of the cervix, secondary to a uterine or vaginal infection, or due to an exposure to a local irritation.

SYNONYMS

Endocervicitis
Ectocervicitis
Mucopurulent cervicitis

ICD-10CM CODES
N72	Inflammatory disease of cervix uteri
A54.03	Gonococcal cervicitis, unspecified
A74.89	Other chlamydial diseases
A60.03	Herpesviral cervicitis
O86.11	Cervicitis following delivery

EPIDEMIOLOGY & DEMOGRAPHICS

Cervicitis accounts for 20% to 25% of patients who present with complaints of abnormal vaginal discharge. It is most common in women aged 15 to 24 but it can occur in any sexually active woman. Women who have had sex without condoms or sex with multiple partners are at increased risk of developing cervicitis as well as other sexually transmitted diseases (STDs).

PHYSICAL FINDINGS & CLINICAL PRESENTATION

Cervicitis is usually asymptomatic or associated with mild symptoms. Copious purulent or mucopurulent vaginal discharge (Fig. E1), pelvic pain, and dyspareunia may be present if cervicitis is severe. The cervix can be erythematous and tender on palpation during bimanual examination. The cervix may also bleed easily when obtaining cultures or a Pap smear. Patients may have postcoital or intermenstrual bleeding. The CDC emphasizes that the two diagnostic signs are either mucopurulent discharge or sustained cervical bleeding with gentle trauma.

INFECTIOUS ETIOLOGY

- *Chlamydia trachomatis*
- *Neisseria gonorrhoeae*
- *Trichomonas*
- Herpes simplex
- *T. vaginalis*
- Human papillomavirus

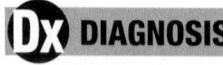 DIAGNOSIS

DIFFERENTIAL DIAGNOSIS

- Carcinoma of the cervix
- Cervical erosion (from tampons or other intravaginal devices)
- Cervical metaplasia
- Cervical ectropion
- Cervical and vaginal irritation due to chemicals or hormonal imbalance

WORKUP

The patient usually presents with complaints of vaginal discharge or postcoital bleeding. Otherwise, the patient may be asymptomatic and diagnosed during routine gynecologic examination. On speculum examination, there is gross visualization of yellow, mucopurulent material extruding from the cervix or abnormal bleeding when touched with a cotton swab. Abnormal discharge extruding from or coating the vagina may also be seen.

LABORATORY TESTS

A finding of leucorrhea (>10 WBC per high-power field on microscopic examination of vaginal fluid) has been associated with chlamydial and gonococcal infection of the cervix. Positive Gram stain is found. Nucleic acid amplification tests (NAAT) should be used for diagnosing *C. trachomatis* and *N. gonorrhoeae* in women with cervicitis; this testing can be performed on vaginal, cervical, or urinary samples. Use a wet mount to look for evidence of bacterial vaginitis (BV) and trichomonads, but because the sensitivity of microscopy to detect *T. vaginalis* is relatively low (~50%), symptomatic women with cervicitis and negative microscopy for BV and trichomonads should receive further testing with NAAT or culture if there is concern for resistant infection. HIV testing is recommended in all patients with supposed cervicitis. Although HSV-2 infection has been associated with cervicitis, the utility of specific testing (i.e., culture or serologic testing) for HSV-2 in this setting is not recommended unless there are clinical findings suggestive of herpes infection.

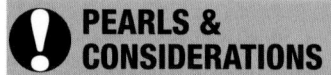 TREATMENT

NONPHARMACOLOGIC THERAPY

- The patient's history of hygiene habits, which may increase her risk for cervicitis, should be obtained including history of douching, tampon usage, and other potential chemical exposures to vaginal irritants.
- Uncomplicated cervicitis is typically treated as an outpatient.
- Safe sex should be recommended including monogamous relationships and the consistent use of condoms (male and female).
- Sexual partners should be offered treatment in all cases of STD infection proven by culture.

ACUTE GENERAL Rx

Because *Chlamydia* and *N. gonorrhoeae* cause 50% of cases of infectious cervicitis, if either of these infections is suspected, then treatment should be initiated without waiting for the test results. Administer ceftriaxone 250 mg IM single dose followed by azithromycin 1 g single dose or doxycycline 100 mg PO bid for 7 days. If the patient is pregnant, treat with azithromycin 1 g single dose instead of using doxycycline, which is contraindicated in pregnant or nursing mothers. If *Trichomonas* is the etiologic agent, treat with metronidazole or tinidazole 2 g single dose. For herpes infection, treat with acyclovir 200 mg PO five times daily for 7 days.

DISPOSITION

Bacterial cervicitis responds well to antibiotics. Possible complications to watch for include subsequent pelvic inflammatory disease (PID) and infertility (found in 5%-10% of patients with increasing rates with repeat episodes of PID). Repeat cervical cultures should be performed after treatment. Sexual relations can be resumed after negative cultures.

REFERRAL

If subsequent PID develops, consider hospital admission for IV antibiotics.

PEARLS & CONSIDERATIONS

COMMENTS

- Management of sex partners of women tested for cervicitis should be appropriate for the identified or suspected STD.
- Repeat testing 3 to 6 months after treatment is recommended for all women diagnosed with chlamydia or gonorrhea, and all sex partners in the preceding 60 days should be evaluated and treated for the STDs for which the index patient received treatment.
- Limited data indicate that infection with *M. genitalium* or BV and frequent douching might cause cervicitis.
- *M. genitalium* might be considered for cases of clinically significant cervicitis that persist after azithromycin or doxycycline therapy in which reexposure to an infected partner or medical nonadherence is unlikely. If *M. genitalium* infection is confirmed, treatment is with moxifloxacin.

SUGGESTED READING
Available at www.expertconsult.com

RELATED CONTENT
Cervicitis (Patient Information)
Chlamydia Genital Infections (Related Key Topic)
Gonorrhea (Related Key Topic)
Nongonococcal Urethritis (Related Key Topic)

AUTHOR: **ARLENE J. SMALLS, M.D.**

BASIC INFORMATION

DEFINITION

In 1708, William Musgrave was the first person who coined the term *Charcot* to describe arthralgia associated with neuropathic joints caused by venereal disease. In 1868, Jean-Martin Charcot described Charcot with neuropathic disease caused by syphilis. Charcot arthropathy is a progressive condition that within the past few years has become better represented in the literature. Some of the hallmark features of this condition include pathologic fractures, dislocations, and gross foot and ankle deformities that can lead to ulceration, infection, and possible amputation. Charcot arthropathy is commonly associated with diabetes and diabetic peripheral neuropathy. Early recognition and diagnosis are imperative to avoid severe and irreversible foot deformities that may lead to ulceration and amputation.

SYNONYMS

Neuropathic arthropathy
Charcot osteoarthropathy
Charcot neuropathic osteoarthropathy
Charcot arthropathy
Charcot foot
Charcot's joint

ICD-10CM CODES
M14.671 Charcot's joint, right ankle and foot
M14.672 Charcot's joint, left ankle and foot

EPIDEMIOLOGY & DEMOGRAPHICS
PREVALENCE:
- The estimated prevalence of Charcot arthropathy is 8% to 16% in the general population.
- Charcot arthropathy is seen in ~29% of diabetics with sensory neuropathy and loss of protective sensation.
- Bilateral presentation is seen in 10% to 35% of patients.
- The midfoot is involved 70% of the time, followed by the forefoot and rear foot, each accounting for 15%.
- Patients with type 1 diabetes mellitus have a higher predisposition to Charcot arthropathy than patients with type 2 diabetes mellitus.
- Observed in the fifth decade in diabetes mellitus Type 1; observed in the sixth decade in diabetes mellitus Type 2.
- Unknown sex predilection and ethnic distribution.

PHYSICAL FINDINGS & CLINICAL PRESENTATION
- Acute phase: Erythema, edema, and calor. There is at least a 2° C temperature difference between the involved limb and the contralateral foot. May present with mild pain or discomfort. Bounding pedal pulses. Typically no radiologic osseous abnormalities are seen during the early acute phase.
- The tarsometatarsal joints are most commonly involved, followed by the forefoot and rear foot; a deformity in the foot may lead to an unstable foot architecture.

- As Charcot arthropathy progresses in the untreated state, joint dislocation/subluxation occurs.
- During the coalescence phase, there is a reduction in warmth, edema, and calor. Coalescence of osseous fragments, ankylosis of joints, and new bone formation also take place during this phase.
- In the remodeling phase, a fixed deformity classically known as the "rocker bottom" foot occurs.
- Ulcerations may appear at any time during the acute and chronic stages of Charcot arthropathy.

ETIOLOGY

The most common cause of Charcot arthropathy is peripheral neuropathy associated with diabetes mellitus (Fig. 1). Less common conditions associated with Charcot arthropathy include syphilis, alcoholism, spina bifida, poliomyelitis, Charcot-Marie-Tooth disease, leprosy, familial amyloid neuropathy, CNS/PNS tumors, pernicious anemia, cerebral vascular accident, lead poisoning, rheumatoid arthritis, multiple sclerosis, and trauma. Currently, three theories contribute to the etiology involved in this disease:

1. Neurotraumatic theory: Unperceived trauma or injury to an insensate foot. Osseous destruction is the result of unperceived sensory neuropathy with continued ambulation and repetitive stress. This repetitive microtrauma can lead to extensive bone destruction resulting in joint subluxation, dislocation, and pedal deformity.
2. Neurovascular theory: Autonomic neuropathy, particularly sympathetic denervation, leads to arteriovenous shunting. This increase of blood flow into the bone causes demineralization of the bone and stimulates osteoclastic activity that causes bone destruction, leading to osteopenia.
3. Inflammatory theory: During the acute inflammation phase that is seen in Charcot arthropathy, the inflammatory cytokines, tumor necrosis factor-alpha, IL-1, and IL-6 are present. The role of these inflammatory cytokines is bone resorption by promoting osteoclastic proliferation and differentiation. Receptor activator of nuclear factor-kappa B ligand (RANKL) is responsible for activating osteoclasts in Charcot arthropathy. Osteopro-

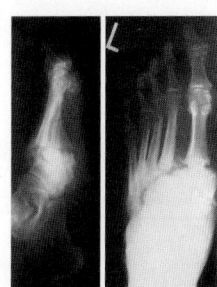

FIG. 1 Diabetes mellitus and neuropathic arthritis. Note lateral displacement of metatarsals *(left)* and fragmentation and osseous debris *(right)*. (From Goldman L, Ausiello D [eds]: *Cecil textbook of medicine,* ed 22, Philadelphia, 2004, Saunders.)

tegrin is the antagonist of RANKL, and thus when this pathway is disrupted, osteoclastic activity predominates. The production of calcitonin gene-related peptide, which also antagonizes RANKL expression, is reduced in peripheral and autonomic neuropathy. Nitric oxide, which suppresses osteoclastic activity, has also been found to be dramatically decreased in Charcot arthropathy. Furthermore, advanced glycation end products are associated with increased RANKL activation. Hyperglycemia is the triggering factor for production of advanced glycation end products.

DIAGNOSIS

DIFFERENTIAL DIAGNOSIS
- Abscess
- Osteomyelitis
- Cellulitis
- Gout
- Deep vein thrombosis
- Infectious arthritis/septic joint
- Osteoarthritis
- Complex regional pain syndrome
- Peripheral vascular disease
- Trauma

WORKUP

A thorough history and physical examination is the key to recognition of Charcot arthropathy. Early diagnosis requires an astute physician to be aware of the signs associated with acute Charcot, including but not limited to edema, erythema, and calor, which play a role in the inflammatory cascade. Testing for peripheral neuropathy should be performed utilizing methods such as electromyography, nerve conduction velocity tests, nerve biopsy if warranted, biothesiometer, and Semmes-Weinstein monofilament testing.

LABORATORY TESTS

Laboratory testing can be utilized to rule in or rule out diagnoses that may present with manifestations similar to those of Charcot arthropathy.
- The following labs may be ordered if warranted: complete blood count with differential, basic metabolic panel, vitamin B_{12}, folate, RPR, ESR, CRP, uric acid, rheumatoid panel, joint aspiration, and bone biopsy.

IMAGING STUDIES

Plain x-rays
- Plain x-rays may or may not show evidence of early osteomyelitis. Osseous findings will depend on the stage (inflammatory, development, coalescence, remodeling) of presentation of Charcot arthropathy.
- MRI can detect subtle changes in the early stages of active Charcot arthropathy.
- Three-phase bone scan: Results are less accurate in the setting of diminished blood flow; thus, labeled white blood cell scanning can improve specificity (Armstrong et al, p. 2125).
- Positron emission tomography is currently being researched for an additional imaging modality to detect Charcot arthropathy.

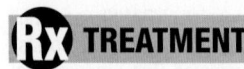 **TREATMENT**

ACUTE GENERAL Rx

The most instrumental aspect of medical treatment of Charcot arthropathy is offloading. Offloading is accomplished with the use of total contact cast for approximately 12 to 18 weeks pending clinical and radiographic assessment.

Once the acute phase has transpired, custom-molded Plastazote insoles in accommodative diabetic shoe gear, Charcot restraint orthotic walker, and customized braces, just to name a few, can be utilized.

SURGERY: There is equivocal evidence to support whether surgical intervention is recommended during the acute phase of Charcot arthropathy. The general consensus for podiatric surgical intervention is for when there is acute fracture dislocation or infection, or when there is continued recurrence of ulceration. Arthrodesis is recommended for unstable pedal construct, and Achilles tendon lengthening to reduce forefoot pressure improves the overall pedal alignment.

PHARMACOLOGIC THERAPY

Studies are currently being conducted to determine the efficacy of bisphosphonates whose mechanism of action is to decrease osteoclastic resorption and symptoms in active Charcot arthropathy.

DISPOSITION

Early recognition of Charcot arthropathy is essential in preventing the devastating complications associated with this disease.

REFERRAL

Podiatrist with expertise in Charcot arthropathy
Endocrinology for diabetic blood glucose control

RELATED CONTENT

Charcot Joint (Patient Information)

SUGGESTED READINGS

Available at www.expertconsult.com

AUTHOR: **BRANDI KIMBLE, D.P.M.**

BASIC INFORMATION

DEFINITION

Charcot-Marie-Tooth disease (CMT) is a heterogeneous group of noninflammatory inherited peripheral neuropathies characterized by chronic motor and sensory polyneuropathy. It is the most common inherited neuromuscular disorder (see also "Neuropathy, Hereditary").

SYNONYMS

Peroneal muscular atrophy
Hereditary motor and sensory neuropathy (HMSN)
CMT

EPIDEMIOLOGY & DEMOGRAPHICS

PREVALENCE: 1:2500; CMT type 1 and type 2 are the major divisions with an estimated prevalence of 40 per 100,000
PREDOMINANT AGE: Onset usually 10 to 20 yr; may present in infants
GENETICS: Transmission may be autosomal dominant, autosomal recessive, or X-linked, with some sporadic cases reported. Duplication of *peripheral myelin protein 22* (PMP22) is the most common cause of CMT. CMT is classified into types 1 through 7 and is genetically heterogeneous with at least 43 CMT genes known.

PHYSICAL FINDINGS & CLINICAL PRESENTATION

- Wide variation in clinical presentation, but affected individuals in a family tend to have similar symptoms.
- Symmetric, slowly progressive distal motor neuropathy resulting in weakness and atrophy in legs, often progresses to involve hands.
- High-arched feet (pes cavus), claw toe deformities (Fig. 1), and hammer toes.
- Atrophy of the lower legs producing a stork-like appearance (muscle wasting does not involve the upper legs) (Fig. 2).
- Nerve enlargement.
- Mild to moderate distal sensory loss; uncommonly can have painful paresthesias.
- Decreased proprioception and weakness of ankle dorsiflexors often interfere with balance and gait (steppage gait).
- Depressed or absent deep tendon reflexes in many cases.

- Hearing loss and hip dysplasia are under-recognized manifestations.
- Ambulation usually maintained throughout life.
- CMT has been reported to be associated with renal diseases, mostly focal segmental glomerulosclerosis (FSGS).

ETIOLOGY

Genetic abnormalities cause defects in either peripheral nerve myelination, or result in axonal degeneration. Mutations in one of several myelin genes result in defects in myelin structure, maintenance, and formation. Duplication of the PMP22 gene causes CMT1A, the most common type of hereditary motor sensory neuropathy (~40% overall). INF_2 mutations appear to cause many cases of FSGS-associated CMT.

DIAGNOSIS

DIFFERENTIAL DIAGNOSIS

- Other inherited neuropathies.
- Acquired peripheral neuropathies such as toxic, metabolic, infectious, endocrine, inflammatory, immune-mediated, and nutritional polyneuropathies.

WORKUP

- Clinical diagnosis is based on family history, characteristic presentation, and findings on detailed physical and neurologic examination.
- Electrophysiologic studies are often diagnostic and may help define various subtypes of CMT.
- Occasionally, sural nerve biopsy is helpful in establishing diagnosis.

TREATMENT

ACUTE GENERAL Rx

- Symptomatic and supportive, managed by multidisciplinary team including physical and occupational therapy.
- Special shoes with good ankle support, ankle/foot orthoses.
- Some require crutches/cane for gait stability; <5% need wheelchair.
- Daily heel cord stretching exercises and hand grip exercises.
- Musculoskeletal pain may respond to acetaminophen or NSAIDs; neuropathic pain may respond to tricyclic antidepressants or drugs such as carbamazepine or gabapentin.

CHRONIC Rx

Occasionally, orthopedic surgery is required to correct severe pes cavus deformity or hip dysplasia. Avoiding obesity is essential as this makes walking difficult; avoiding potentially neurotoxic medications is also important, particularly *Vinca* alkaloids.

DISPOSITION

- Disability is usually compatible with a long life.
- 10% to 20% of patients are asymptomatic.

REFERRAL

- Orthopedic consultation for bracing and surgical treatment of deformity.
- Genetic counseling and family planning.

PEARLS & CONSIDERATIONS

COMMENTS

Patient information on CMT disease is available from the Muscular Dystrophy Association, 3300 East Sunrise Drive, Tucson, AZ 85718; (520) 529-2000.

SUGGESTED READINGS

Available at www.expertconsult.com

RELATED CONTENT

Charcot-Marie-Tooth Disease (Patient Information)

AUTHOR: **CANDICE YUVIENCO, M.D., RH.M.S.U.S.**

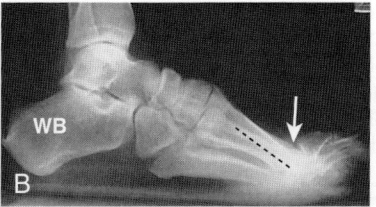

FIG. 1 A, Non–weight-bearing view of cavus and claw toe deformities in a patient with Charcot-Marie-Tooth disease. **B,** On weight-bearing view, plantar flexion of first ray is less noticeable, but clawed hallux remains, indicating fixed extension contracture at first metatarsophalangeal joint. (From Canale ST, Beaty JH: *Campbell's operative orthopedics*, ed 11, Philadelphia, 2007, Mosby.)

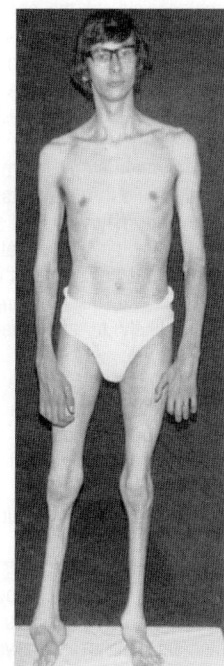

FIG. 2 Patient with Charcot-Marie-Tooth disease showing marked wasting of calf muscles and intrinsic foot muscles. (From Dubowitz V: *Muscle disorders in childhood*, London, 1995, Saunders.)

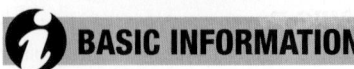

DEFINITION

Chemotherapy-induced nausea and vomiting (CINV) refers to adverse emetic effects associated with the use of drugs used to treat cancer. There are five recognized subtypes:

- Acute-phase CINV: nausea and vomiting start within minutes to hours after receiving chemotherapy.
- Delayed-phase CINV: nausea and vomiting begin or return 24 hours or more after receiving chemotherapy.
- Breakthrough CINV: Occurring despite appropriate prophylactic treatment
- Anticipatory CINV: symptoms begin before receiving therapy as a conditioned response in patients who have developed significant nausea and vomiting during previous chemotherapy.
- Refractory CINV: Recurring in subsequent cycles of therapy, excluding anticipatory CINV

SYNONYMS

Drug-induced nausea and vomiting
Chemotherapy-induced emesis
CINV

ICD-10CM CODES
R11.2 Nausea with vomiting, unspecified
R11.0 Nausea
R11.10 Vomiting, unspecified
Z51.11 Encounter for antineoplastic chemotherapy

EPIDEMIOLOGY & DEMOGRAPHICS

- The patient's risk for development of nausea and vomiting is most strongly dependent on the emetogenicity of the chemotherapy agent(s) being used.
- Emetogenicity is classified into four categories: highly emetic (>90%), moderately emetic (>30%–90%), low emetic (10%–30%), and minimally emetic (0%–10%).
- With certain chemotherapy regimens, CINV will occur in the majority of patients. However, patients' tolerance may vary, and symptoms may occur in as low as 10% of patients.
- Symptoms may be dose dependent (the higher the dose, the greater the risk for symptoms).
- CINV is more likely to affect female and younger patients.
- Patients expecting CINV before receiving therapy (anticipatory emesis) are at greater risk of experiencing symptoms.
- Patients with a history of alcohol consumption are at lower risk.
- Patients with a history of motion sickness are at greater risk.

INCIDENCE: The highest incidence is before or during the first cycle of chemotherapy.
GENETICS: Some rapid metabolizers of certain 5-HT3 receptor antagonists and polymorphisms in the 5-HT3 receptor confer greater risk for CINV.
RISK FACTORS:
- Previous history of CINV.
- History of motion sickness or vestibular dysfunction.
- Higher levels of anxiety.
- History of alcohol use decreases risk.

PHYSICAL FINDINGS & CLINICAL PRESENTATION

- Symptoms may include anxiety and lightheadedness.
- The most common physical findings are elevated pulse and abnormal blood pressure (elevated if the person is highly anxious, reduced if the patient is dehydrated).
- Symptoms such as diarrhea, fever, headache, and abdominal pain may suggest an alternative diagnosis; physical examination findings such as increased blood pressure, abdominal tenderness, or focal neurologic deficits may suggest symptoms caused by cancer progression or other acute illness such as infection.

PATHOPHYSIOLOGY

CINV is probably the result of chemotherapy drugs acting in two places: directly in the gastrointestinal tract and in the vomiting center of the brain. In both areas, nausea and vomiting are mediated by the actions of certain neurotransmitters, with serotonin, dopamine, and neurokinin-1 being the most important.

DIAGNOSIS

DIFFERENTIAL DIAGNOSIS

- The two main considerations are progression of cancer and infection
- Intestinal/gastric: obstruction or partial obstruction of the digestive tract from tumor
- Neurologic: metastases to the brain causing vomiting; metastatic infiltration of nerves affecting the digestive tract
- Infectious: acute bacterial, viral, or parasitic infections of the digestive tract causing symptoms (can be associated with diarrhea or pain)
- Renal: dehydration leading to acute kidney injury and failure, causing worsening of nausea and vomiting

WORKUP

No workup is indicated if patient's symptoms and onset of nausea and vomiting fit the usual presentation for CINV. If other symptoms or unexpected physical examination findings are present, then other causes need to be ruled out. A combination of blood work and imaging may be helpful.

LABORATORY TESTS

- If the onset of symptoms is not typical for CINV, then blood tests such as a CBC, liver function tests, and kidney function tests may be indicated.
- Stool studies looking for infections from bacteria or parasites may be ordered if diarrhea is also present.

IMAGING STUDIES

- Abdominal radiographs may be ordered to look for obstruction of the digestive tract but will not provide any information about tumor progression.
- Abdominal CT scan may provide more detailed information about local cancer progression/invasion in the proximity of the digestive tract and whether obstruction of the digestive tract is present.
- Brain CT scan or magnetic resonance imaging (MRI) may provide information about possible metastases to the brain.

TREATMENT

- Choice and duration of antiemetic use are dependent on the chemotherapy regimen used.
- For chemotherapy agents with high emetogenic potential, the use of multidrug antiemetic regimens has proven to be highly effective in symptom prevention.
- The most common treatment combination includes a serotonin-receptor antagonist (ondansetron, granisetron, dolasetron, or palonosetron), a corticosteroid (methylprednisolone or dexamethasone), and a neurokinin-1 receptor antagonist (aprepitant, rolapitant, or fosaprepitant).
- Many other adjunct drugs are available, such as olanzapine, prochlorperazine, metoclopramide, haloperidol, and marinol, but they are less effective and have greater potential for adverse effects.
- Benzodiazepines (usually lorazepam) may help in patients with significant anxiety levels that lead to anticipatory CINV.
- Patients with uncontrolled symptoms may require hospitalization for supportive care including intravenous medications and fluids.

NONPHARMACOLOGIC THERAPY

For those patients with a significant anxiety component to their CINV, cognitive behavioral therapy may help.

DISPOSITION

Although CINV is one of the most feared complications of cancer therapy, its treatment has been revolutionized in the last 20 years, with most patients achieving adequate symptom control.

PEARLS & CONSIDERATIONS

COMMENTS

- Aggressive symptom control in the acute phase of CINV is the key initial therapeutic approach. Prevention of the acute phase has led to much improved control of the delayed phase and has greatly decreased the incidence of anticipatory CINV.
- Prevention of symptoms is much easier to achieve than controlling or treating active symptoms.

SUGGESTED READINGS

Available at www.expertconsult.com

AUTHORS: **BYUNG KIM, M.D.,** and **BHARTI RATHORE, M.D.**

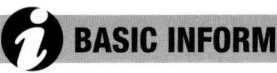 **BASIC INFORMATION**

DEFINITION

Definition from the Federal Child Abuse Prevention and Treatment Act (CAPTA): any recent act or failure to act on the part of a parent or caretaker that results in death, serious physical or emotional harm, sexual abuse or exploitation of a child; or an act or failure to act that presents an imminent risk of serious harm to a child. More specific definitions may be found in individual state criminal statutes.

- Neglect: failure to provide for the basic needs of a child
  1. Physical neglect: failure to provide necessary food, shelter, and supervision
  2. Medical neglect: failure to provide necessary medical or mental health care
  3. Educational neglect: failure to meet educational needs
  4. Emotional neglect: failure to attend to emotional needs, exposure to domestic violence
- Physical abuse: physical injury inflicted by a parent or caregiver intentionally or in the course of excessive discipline
- Sexual abuse: sexual act inflicted by parent or caretaker; includes exploitation and pornography
- Emotional/psychological abuse: pattern of behavior of caretaker toward a child that impairs emotional development. This includes verbal abuse, cruelty, and threats. Difficult to prove. Almost always present when other forms of abuse occur.
- Abandonment: child left and parents' whereabouts unknown.
- Substance abuse: includes: prenatal exposure to mother's use of illicit drugs; manufacture of drugs, e.g., methamphetamine in the presence of a child; selling or giving drugs to a child; use of mood-altering substance by caregivers that impairs their ability to provide care for their child.

SYNONYMS

Child maltreatment syndrome
Physical abuse
Sexual abuse
Battered child syndrome
Shaken baby syndrome
Shaken impact syndrome
Abusive head trauma

ICD-10 CM CODES
T74	Adult and child abuse, neglect or other maltreatment, confirmed
T74.02	Child neglect or abandonment, confirmed
T74.12	Child physical abuse, confirmed
T74.32	Child psychological abuse, confirmed
T74.22	Child sexual abuse, confirmed
Z62.810	Personal history of physical and sexual abuse in childhood
Z62.811	Personal history of psychological abuse in childhood
Z62.819	Personal history of unspecified abuse in childhood
T76.32XA	Child psychological abuse, suspected, initial encounter
T76.22XA	Child sexual abuse, suspected, initial encounter
T76.12XA	Child physical abuse, suspected, initial encounter

EPIDEMIOLOGY & DEMOGRAPHICS

INCIDENCE (IN U.S.): Any reports of incidence are underestimates because many cases are not recognized or reported. The following data are based on Child Protective Services (CPS) state aggregate as reported in *Child Maltreatment 2014*. In 2014 roughly 702,000 unique children were determined to be victims of abuse or neglect. This is a rate of 9.4 unduplicated victims per 1000 children.

- Types of abuse by percentage (note the total is greater than 100% since children are often victims of more than one type of abuse).
  1. Neglect: 75%
  2. Physical abuse: 17%
  3. Sexual abuse: 8.3%
  4. Psychological abuse: 6%
  5. Medical neglect: 2.2%
  6. Other: 6.8% (e.g., abandonment, threats of harm, congenital drug addiction)
- For 2014, an estimated 1580 child deaths were caused by abuse or neglect.
  1. Overall annual death rate resulting from abuse or neglect is estimated to be 2.13 deaths/100,000 children.
  2. 72% of these deaths were due to neglect alone or in combination with other forms of abuse; 41% were due to physical abuse, alone or in combination.
  3. 70.7% of these children were younger than 3 yr of age with 44% less than 1 yr old.
  4. Most fatalities were directly caused by one or both parents (79.3%).
  5. 58% were male. Boys die at a higher rate than girls, regardless of age.
  6. Many child abuse fatalities are underreported because of misdiagnosis or variations in state definitions and coding.
- 91.6% of abused children were victimized by one or both of their parents.
- One fifth of adult women report history of molestation or sexual assault as a child or adolescent.

PREDOMINANT SEX: There is a slight predominance of girls as victims. However, rates vary by age. Boys 5 and under have a higher rate of abuse, whereas girls 6 to 17 have higher rates of abuse. At all ages, boys have a higher child fatality rate than girls (2.48/100,000 for boys and 1.82/100,000 for girls).

PREDOMINANT AGE: Youngest children (0 to 3 yr old) have the highest rates of victimization with 27% being younger than the age of 3.

GENETICS: No known genetic factors.

ETIOLOGY

- Parent
  1. Substance abuse
  2. Mental illness
  3. Intellectual impairment
  4. Parental history of being abused as a child
  5. Young age of parent
  6. Poor knowledge of child development leading to unrealistic expectations
- Child
  1. Low birth weight or prematurity
  2. Chronic physical disability or illness
  3. Prior CPS report
  4. Unplanned, unwanted child
- Family
  1. Social isolation
  2. Poor parent-child bonding
  3. Stress: unemployment, chronic illness, eviction, arrest, poverty, military deployment
  4. Domestic violence
  5. Nonbiologically related adult male living in household
- Community/society
  1. Limited transportation
  2. Limited day care
  3. Unsafe neighborhoods
  4. Poverty

DX DIAGNOSIS

Careful documentation of any statements regarding origin of injuries or history of abuse is crucial. Careful history of behavior before and after the event and activities leading up to the event are also critical, especially in infants and toddlers. Chart and photographic documentation of injuries is also essential. The following are keys to the final diagnosis:

- Patterned bruising (e.g., loop-shaped, square, oval) is indicative of being struck with an object (Fig. E1).
- Bruising to nonbony areas: torso, ears, face, neck and upper arms, especially in children younger than the age of 4 yr.
- Injury observed is incompatible with the history provided.
- History of injury provided is incompatible with the developmental capabilities of the child.
- Delay in seeking care for a significant injury (e.g., callus formation on a fracture, eschar formation on a burn).
- Any injury (bruise, mouth injury, fracture, internal hemorrhage) is rare in healthy preambulatory infants and warrants further investigation.
- Multiple significant injuries of different ages.
- Infant with clinically significant head trauma attributed to a trivial cause (e.g., a short fall). Often associated with retinal hemorrhages and skeletal fractures, which are indicative of shaken baby syndrome or abusive head trauma.
- No history or explanation in a child with significant injury.
- Changing histories as investigation continues.
- Certain fractures in infants without a history of significant trauma (e.g., motor vehicle accident) are characteristic of abuse: metaphyseal, rib, sternum, scapula, vertebral body.
- Inflicted contact burns are indicated by an impression of the burning object: lighter, iron, cigarette (Fig. E2).

- Inflicted immersion burns are indicated by "stocking" burns of the feet or "glove" burns of the hands. Stocking burns are often associated with buttocks/perineal burns from immersion of a minor in a flexed position.
- Most sexual abuse victims will have a normal or nonspecific genital examination. A normal genital examination does not mean the child was not abused. History is the most important part of the diagnosis. Forensic interview by a trained professional is recommended, as is an examination by a health care provider experienced in sexual abuse evaluations.
- The identification of a sexually transmitted disease in a prepubertal child who is beyond the neonatal period is highly suspicious and, in some instances, diagnostic of sexual abuse. Reporting and further careful investigation are mandatory. Consult current CDC guidelines and a child sexual abuse expert for further guidance.

DIFFERENTIAL DIAGNOSIS

In all categories, accidental injury is the most common entity to be distinguished from abuse. Accidental injuries are most common over bony prominences: forehead, elbows, knees, shins; soft, fleshy areas are more common for inflicted injury: buttocks, thighs, upper arms. Neck and ears are also more common locations for inflicted injury. Table 1 describes patterns of injury.

BRUISING:
- Bleeding disorder (idiopathic thrombocytopenic purpura, hemophilia, leukemia, hemorrhagic disease of the newborn, von Willebrand's disease)
- Connective tissue disorder (Ehlers-Danlos syndrome, vasculitis)
- Pigments (Mongolian spots)
- Dermatitis (phytophotodermatitis, nickel allergy)
- Folk treatment (coining, cupping)

BURNS:
- Chemical burn
- Impetigo
- Folk treatment (moxibustion)
- Dermatitis (phytophotodermatitis)

INTRACRANIAL HEMORRHAGE:
- Bleeding disorder
- Perinatal trauma (should resolve by 4 wk)
- Arteriovenous malformation rupture
- Glutaric aciduria

TABLE 1 Patterns of Injury

Accidental	Nonaccidental
Unilateral	Bilateral/symmetrical
Isolated injury	Multiple injuries
Amorphous shape	Well-defined shape
Prominent bone areas	Soft tissue areas
Posterior aspect of body	Anterior aspect of body
One age of injury	Multiple ages of injury

From Fuhrman BP et al: *Pediatric critical care*, ed 4, Philadelphia, 2011, Saunders.

FRACTURES:
- Osteogenesis imperfecta
- Rickets
- Congenital syphilis
- Very low birth weight (osteopenia of prematurity)

SEXUAL ABUSE:
- Normal variants
- Lichen sclerosis et atrophicus
- Congenital abnormalities
- Urethral prolapse
- Hemangioma
- Nonsexually acquired infection (group A *Streptococcus, Shigella*)

WORKUP (FIG. E3)

History and physical examination:
- Careful history from all caretakers and child.
- Scene investigation may be necessary.
- Complete physical examination.
- Sexual abuse: forensic interview and magnified examinations by trained professionals are the standard for evaluation and evidence collection. This is especially important to avoid further psychological or physical trauma to the child.

Laboratory tests to assess for bleeding disorder in the case of children with suspicious bruising. These tests may not be necessary if the abuse was witnessed or if the child has clear patterned bruising or other indicators of physical abuse:
- CBC with differential and platelets.
- Prothrombin time, activated partial thromboplastin time.
- Von Willebrand factor antigen and activity
- Factor VIII and IX levels
- Alanine aminotransferase, amylase, urinalysis should be considered in infants or other children with abdominal bruising to look for evidence of internal injury to the liver, pancreas, or kidneys.

Laboratory tests to assess for bleeding disorder in the case of children with suspicious ICH. These tests may not be necessary if the abuse was witnessed or if the child has clear patterned bruising or other indicators of physical abuse:
- CBC with differential and platelets.
- Prothrombin time, activated partial thromboplastin time.
- Factor VIII and IX levels
- DIC Panel
- Consultation with a child abuse expert physician should be strongly considered in children with suspicion of abusive head trauma.

Laboratory tests for sexual abuse:
- If within 72 hr of acute sexual assault/abuse, swabs are obtained from the oropharynx, areas of skin exposure (use an alternate light source to ID), genitalia, and rectum to send to the crime lab for DNA and other testing. Also collect samples of foreign hair, blood, saliva, or other tissue if present. A wet mount from cervical/vaginal specimen should be done to look for motile sperm.
- Per current CDC recommendations, adolescent victims of acute assault should have appropriate specimens collected from sites of penetration or attempted penetration for *Neisseria gonorrhoeae* and *Chlamydia.*

Nucleic acid amplification tests (NAATs) may be used and are preferred. In females, wet mount and culture or POC testing of vaginal swab for *T. vaginalis* should also be done. If there is itching, vaginal discharge or malodor present, wet mount for bacterial vaginosis and *Candida* should also be done. Serum should be obtained for HIV, hepatitis B, and syphilis testing acutely. If negative, HIV and syphilis testing should be repeated 6, 12, and 24 wk after the assault.

- Child victims (i.e., prepubertal) should have specimens collected if considered high risk for a sexually transmitted infection (STI) per current CDC recommendations. Cervical specimens are not collected and vaginal specimens must be collected with care by an experienced provider to avoid further trauma to the child. Gonorrhea and *Chlamydia* culture is the gold standard for diagnosis and legal purposes. However, many providers now analyze specimens using urine or vaginal NAAT followed by culture confirmation or 2nd NAAT if any positive results are obtained. However, extragenital sites should have cultures obtained when assessing for gonorrhea and *Chlamydia.* Any culture testing positive for *N. gonorrhoeae* should be confirmed by at least two laboratory tests that are based on different principles. Specimens should be collected for gonorrhea and *Chlamydia,* wet mount, and blood for serologic testing (HIV, hepatitis B, syphilis) in the following cases:
  1. Child has a past or current symptom of an STI, such as vaginal discharge, genital ulcer, or vaginal pain or currently diagnosed STI
  2. Alleged assailant is known to have an STI or be at high risk for an STI
  3. A sibling or adult in the same household has a known STI
  4. Evidence of ejaculation or of oral, genital, and/or anal penetration is present on the examination
  5. Child was assaulted by a stranger
  6. Child lives in an area with a high rate of STI
  7. Child or parent requests testing

IMAGING STUDIES

Physical abuse:
- Radiographic skeletal survey for all children with suspicious injuries up to 2 yr. Additionally, any twin of an abused infant or toddler younger than 2 yr or a child younger than 2 yr of an abused sibling. For children 2 to 5 yr, done only for severe abuse. Consider repeat skeletal survey in 2 wk if severe physical injury is present. Adjunct imaging (MRI, ultrasound, bone scan) may be useful to further define suspicious lesions seen on plain films. Skeletal survey should conform to American College of Radiology Standards.
- Noncontrast head CT scan or MRI for all children <1 yr; for children over 1 yr, clinical judgment should be used.

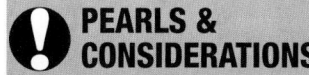
- Head MRI for children with significant abusive head trauma. This is used as an adjunct a few days after initial head CT.
- Abdominal CT scan if indicated by clinical examination or laboratory evaluation.
- Box 1 describes the specificity of radiologic findings for child abuse.

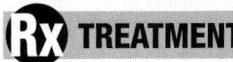 **TREATMENT**

ACUTE GENERAL Rx

- Stabilize and treat acute medical injuries.
- Report to Child Protective Services. HIPAA allows reports for suspected child abuse without parental authorization.
- Early report to law enforcement for suspected physical abuse or sexual abuse to allow scene investigation.
- Disposition, once medically stable, is dependent on CPS. The child cannot be returned home if the environment is not safe.
- Physician should remain available to discuss with investigators. This is often critical to determining the outcome of the case and placement of the child.
- Because follow-up of adolescent sexual assault victims can be difficult, many experts

---

BOX 1 Specificity of Radiologic Findings for Child Abuse

High Specificity
Classic metaphyseal lesions
Rib fractures, especially posterior
Scapular fractures
Spinous process fractures
Sternal fractures

Moderate Specificity
Multiple fractures, especially bilateral
Fractures of different ages
Epiphyseal separations
Vertebral body fractures and subluxations
Digital fractures
Complex skull fractures

Common but Low Specificity
Subperiosteal new bone formation
Clavicular fractures
Long bone shaft fractures
Linear skull fractures

From Manaster BJ: *Musculoskeletal imaging—the requisites,* ed 3, Philadelphia, Mosby, 2006.

---

recommend offering empiric treatment for STIs: gonorrhea, *Chlamydia, Trichomonas,* and bacterial vaginosis. Pregnancy prophylaxis should also be offered. Hepatitis B immunization should be offered if not previously given. HIV prophylaxis is offered in certain situations depending on local epidemiology and type of assault. Consult local infectious disease experts for current recommendations. Repeat examination should be done in 2 wk for all victims of sexual assault, especially if they declined empiric treatment. If empiric treatment was not done, STI testing should be repeated at the 2-week follow-up visit.

- Empiric treatment of child victims of sexual abuse is generally not recommended. This is especially important if NAATs are used for screening for STIs because confirmation is necessary for any positive results. Careful follow-up within 2 wk and treatment based on culture results are indicated. HIV prophylaxis is offered in certain circumstances according to local epidemiology and risk. Consult with a local infectious disease expert for further recommendations.

CHRONIC Rx

- Often depends on CPS and court-ordered interventions
- Treatment of parental mental illness
- Treatment of parental substance abuse, including requirements for random drug testing
- Instruction for parents in behavior management skills, including appropriate limit setting and discipline
- Anger management classes for parents
- Trauma-focused cognitive-behavioral therapy is an evidence-based practice for victims of sexual abuse and exposure to domestic violence; useful to include nonoffending parent/caregiver
- Ongoing individual and family therapy
  1. Parent-child interactive therapy is an evidence-based practice that is used with young children with behavioral problems and parent-child relationship problems
  2. Child-parent psychotherapy is an evidence-based practice that is for young children (<5 yr) who have experienced a trauma and their caregivers

- May need long-term placement in foster care before it is safe to return home. In extreme cases of abuse, parental rights may be terminated without offering services.

OUTCOMES

- Victims of chronic abuse and neglect:
  1. Have higher rates of mental illness (depression, suicide, posttraumatic stress disorder, eating disorders)
  2. Have more cognitive difficulties, often impaired academic performance
  3. Are more likely to become aggressive
  4. Are more likely as adults to have adverse physical health outcomes (cardiovascular disease, cancer, STDs)
- Victims of abusive head trauma:
  1. One third die, one third have severe disability, one third appear normal in the short term.

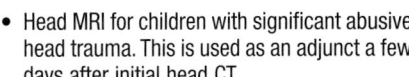 **PEARLS & CONSIDERATIONS**

PREVENTION

- Home visitation by a specially trained nurse to high-risk families during pregnancy and infancy has shown positive outcomes (Nurse-Family Partnership).
- Anticipatory guidance at health visits to teach normal developmental expectations and appropriate discipline.
- Screening to identify at-risk or abused children.
- Targeted education in the newborn nursery for shaken baby prevention has been shown to be effective.
- Substance abuse prevention and treatment.
- Identification and intervention for domestic violence before children are born.

SUGGESTED READINGS

Available at www.expertconsult.com

RELATED CONTENT

Protecting Children from Abuse (Patient Information)

AUTHOR: **NANCY R. GRAFF, M.D.**

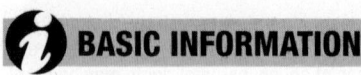

BASIC INFORMATION

DEFINITION

Genital infection with *Chlamydia trachomatis* (CT) is the most prevalent sexually transmitted disease in the U.S. Chlamydia infection can result in cervicitis, acute urethral syndrome, endometritis, pelvic inflammatory disease, ectopic pregnancy, infertility, and chronic pelvic pain in women (see "Pelvic Inflammatory Disease"). In men, CT infection may cause mucopurulent discharge, urethritis, epididymitis, and prostatitis. Newborns born via an infected birth canal are at risk for conjunctivitis and pneumonia. A majority of the men and women affected with CT are asymptomatic. Thus, screening tests play a very important role in detection of this infection to initiate treatment, impede disease sequelae, and prevent further transmissions.

ICD-10CM CODES
A56.2	Chlamydial infection of genitourinary tract, unspecified
A56	Other sexually transmitted chlamydial diseases
A56.0	Chlamydial infection of lower genitourinary tract
A56.00	Chlamydial infection of lower genitourinary tract, unspecified
A56.01	Chlamydial cystitis and urethritis
A56.02	Chlamydia vulvovaginitis
A56.09	Other chlamydial infection of lower genitourinary tract
A56.1	Chlamydial infection of pelviperitoneum and other genitourinary organs
A56.19	Other chlamydial genitourinary infection
A56.2	Chlamydial infection of genitourinary tract, unspecified
A56.3	Chlamydial infection of anus and rectum
A56.4	Chlamydial infection of pharynx
A56.8	Sexually transmitted chlamydial infection of other sites

EPIDEMIOLOGY & DEMOGRAPHICS

- *C. trachomatis* is the most common sexually transmitted disease in the U.S., with more than 1.4 million cases reported annually to the Centers for Disease Control and Prevention. However, it is thought that this number is an underestimate since many cases of CT infection are asymptomatic and potentially can remain undiagnosed.
- Age is a strong predictor for risk of CT infection. Individuals less than 25 years old are the largest age group affected by *C. trachomatis*. Chlamydia infections are 10 times more prevalent than gonococcal infections in young women between the ages of 18 and 26 years.
- Chlamydia conjunctivitis occurs in 18% to 44% of infants, and chlamydial pneumonia occurs in 3% to 16% of infants who are delivered by mothers with untreated CT infection at the time of delivery.
- Pelvic inflammatory disease develops in 10% to 15% of women with untreated CT infections.
- Untreated CT increases a person's risk of acquiring HIV.
- In men, 15% to 55% of nongonococcal urethritis cases are caused by *C. trachomatis*.
- Table 1 summarizes clinical characteristics of common *C. trachomatis* infections.

PHYSICAL FINDINGS & CLINICAL PRESENTATION

Clinical manifestations in symptomatic women affected with *C. trachomatis* are vaginal discharge or irregular vaginal bleeding. Purulent discharge or cervicitis may be visualized on speculum exam. Easily induced endocervical bleeding can be noted on exam and is caused by inflammation of endocervical columnar epithelium. Untreated infection can ascend the reproductive tract, causing pelvic inflammatory disease. Clinical signs of pelvic inflammatory disease are cervical, uterine, or adnexal tenderness on exam. Complications of pelvic disease are ectopic pregnancy, infertility, and chronic pelvic pain.

Most men are asymptomatic, but when they do experience symptoms, it is usually dysuria or a mucopurulent penile discharge. A complication that can arise from CT infection in men is epididymitis, which manifests as unilateral testicular pain, hydrocele, or swelling of the epididymis. An untreated CT infection can also cause prostatitis in men. Prostatitis may present as urinary dysfunction, pain with ejaculation, and pelvic pain.

Chlamydial conjunctivitis can be experienced by both men and women and is the result of conjunctiva exposed to infected genital secretions. CT infection can also cause proctitis or infection of the rectum in men and women. This usually presents with rectal pain, discharge, or bleeding. CT infection of the throat is usually asymptomatic in both men and women and not a usual cause of pharyngitis. Less frequent manifestations of CT infection may include perihepatitis (Fitz-Hugh–Curtis syndrome) or reactive arthritis (Reiter's syndrome).

ETIOLOGY

- *C. trachomatis* consists of 15 serotypes
- Obligate, intracellular bacteria

Dx DIAGNOSIS

DIFFERENTIAL DIAGNOSIS

Differential diagnosis depends on presenting symptoms. Some of the common differentials are listed in the following:
Candidiasis
Conjunctivitis
Ectopic pregnancy
Endometriosis
Gonorrhea
Mycoplasma infection
Pelvic inflammatory disease
Trichomonas
Urethritis
Urinary tract infection

WORKUP

- Individuals with signs and symptoms mentioned previously should be screened for CT infection. Since the majority of CT infections are asymptomatic, routine screening should be offered to individuals at risk for CT infection. Annual screening of all sexually active women less than 25 years and women at any age at risk for sexually transmitted diseases is recommended. Risk factors include a new sexual partner, more than one sexual partner, individuals not in a mutually monogamous relationship, a previous or concurrent sexually transmitted disease, or working in the sex industry for profit. Screening interval is determined by any new risk for exposure since the last negative screening. The CDC recommends CT screening for all pregnant women under the age of 25 and for any pregnant woman over the age of 25 who is at increased risk for acquiring CT. These same pregnant women should be screened again during the third trimester.

LABORATORY TESTS

- Nucleic acid amplification tests (NAATs) are the gold standard for diagnosis because of their high sensitivity and specificity for the detection of CT infection. The FDA has approved these tests for male and female urine collection and for provider-collected endocervical, vaginal, and male urethral specimens.
- Rectal and pharyngeal collection site specimens may be taken from individuals who engage in receptive anal and oral intercourse, but these collection sites are not FDA approved.
- For best results, urine collection should be completed with a first-void urine sample.
- Self-collected vaginal swab samples for women have the same sensitivity and specificity as provider-collected samples.
- The same specimen can be used to test for chlamydia and gonorrhea.
- Sexual partners of a person testing positive for CT infection should be treated if they had sexual contact with that individual within 60 days prior to onset of symptoms or CT diagnosis.
- Microscopy should not be used for chlamydia diagnosis; however, greater than 10 white blood cells per high-power field with a mucopurulent discharge can be a presumptive diagnosis.

Rx TREATMENT

ACUTE GENERAL Rx

Nongonococcal urethritis, urethritis, cervicitis, conjunctivitis (except for lymphogranuloma venereum):
- Azithromycin 1 g PO ×single dose therapy *or*
- Doxycycline 100 mg PO bid for 7 days

TABLE 1 Clinical Characteristics of Common *Chlamydia trachomatis* Infections

	Infection	Symptoms and Signs	Presumptive Diagnosis	Definitive Diagnosis	Treatment
Men	Nongonococcal urethritis	Urethral discharge, dysuria	Urethral leukocytosis; no gonococci seen	Urine or urethral NAAT	Azithromycin, 1 g PO (single dose) *or* Doxycycline, 100 mg PO bid, for 7 days
	Epididymitis	Unilateral epididymal tenderness, swelling; pain; fever, presence of NGU	Urine or urethral NAAT	Urethral leukocytosis; pyuria on urinalysis	STI likely: Ceftriaxone 250 mg IM plus doxycycline, 100 mg PO bid, for 10 days *History of insertive anal intercourse:* Ceftriaxone, 250 mg IM, plus levofloxacin, 500 mg bid for 10 days
	Proctitis (non-LGV)	Rectal pain, discharge and bleeding; history of receptive anal intercourse	≥1 PMN/OIF on rectal Gram stain; no gonococci seen	Urine or urethral NAAT; rectal culture or NAAT	Doxycycline, 100 mg PO bid, for 7 days
	LGV	Painful, tender inguinal lymphadenopathy, fever	"Groove sign"	Urine, urethral, lymph node or rectal NAAT; rectal or lymph node culture; LGV-specific testing if available	Doxycycline, 100 mg PO bid, for 21 days
	LGV proctitis	Rectal pain, discharge, and bleeding in MSM; absence of inguinal lymphadenopathy	≥1 PMN/OIF on rectal Gram stain; no gonococci seen	Urine, urethral, or rectal NAAT; rectal culture; LGV-specific testing if available	Doxycycline, 100 mg PO bid, for 21 days
	Conjunctivitis	Ocular pain, redness, discharge; simultaneous genital infection	Gram stain of conjunctival swab negative for bacterial pathogens; PMNs on smear	Rectal culture or NAAT; NAAT of conjunctivae	Azithromycin, 1 g PO (single dose) *or* Doxycycline, 100 mg PO bid, for 7 days
Women	Cervicitis	Mucopurulent cervical discharge; ectopy, easily induced bleeding	≥20 PMN/OIF on cervical Gram stain	Urine or cervical NAAT	Azithromycin, 1 g PO (single dose) *or* Doxycycline, 100 mg PO bid, for 7 days
	Urethritis	Dysuria, frequency; no hematuria	Pyuria on UA; negative urine Gram stain and culture	Urine, cervical, or urethral NAAT	Azithromycin, 1 g PO (single dose) *or* Doxycycline, 100 mg PO bid for 7 days
	Pelvic inflammatory disease	Lower abdominal pain, adnexal pain, cervical motion tenderness	Evidence of mucopurulent cervicitis	Urine or cervical NAAT	Outpatient: Ceftriaxone 250 mg IM as a single dose, plus doxycycline 100 mg PO bid for 14 days, with or without metronidazole, 500 mg PO bid for 14 days
Adults	Conjunctivitis	Ocular pain, redness, discharge; simultaneous genital infection	Gram stain of conjunctival swab negative for bacterial pathogens; PMNs on smear	DFA or NAAT on conjunctival swab	Azithromycin, 1 g PO (single dose) *or* Doxycycline, 100 mg PO bid for 7 days
Newborns	Conjunctivitis	Ocular pain, redness, discharge; simultaneous genital infection	Gram stain of conjunctival swab negative for bacterial pathogens; PMNs on smear	DFA or NAAT on conjunctival swab; vagina, rectum, pharynx also often positive	Erythromycin base 50 mg/kg/day, orally divided into four doses daily for 14 days; evaluate and treat parents as well
	Pneumonia	Staccato cough, tachypnea, hyperinflation	Diffuse interstitial infiltrate, eosinophilia	Nasopharyngeal NAATs or culture; MIF serology (IgM)	Erythromycin base 50 mg/kg/day, orally divided into four doses daily for 14 days; evaluate and treat parents as well

DFA, Direct fluorescent antibody; *IgM,* immunoglobulin M; *LGV,* lymphogranuloma venereum; *MIF,* microimmunofluorescence; *MSM,* men who have sex with men; *NAAT,* nucleic acid amplification test; *NGU,* nongonococcal urethritis; *OIF,* oil immersion field; *PMN,* polymorphonuclear neutrophil; *STI,* sexually transmitted infection; *UA,* urinalysis.
From Bennett JE, Dolin R, Blaser MJ. *Mandell, Douglas, and Bennett's principles and practice of infectious diseases,* ed 8, Philadelphia, 2015, Saunders.

Diseases and Disorders

- Alternatives
  1. Erythromycin base 500 mg PO qid for 7 days *or*
  2. Erythromycin ethylsuccinate 800 mg PO qid for 7 days *or*
  3. Levofloxacin 500 mg PO qd for 7 days *or*
  4. Ofloxacin 300 mg PO bid for 7 days

  Infection in pregnancy:
- Azithromycin 1 gm PO single-dose therapy

  Alternatives:
- Amoxicillin 500 mg PO tid for 7 days *or*
- Erythromycin 500 mg PO qid for 7 days *or*
- Erythromycin base 250 mg PO qid for 7 days *or*
- Erythromycin ethylsuccinate 800 mg PO qid for 7 days
- Erythromycin ethylsuccinate 400 mg PO qid for 14 days

  NOTE: Azithromycin (Pregnancy Risk Category B) is generally considered safe and effective for treatment of CT infection during pregnancy and with lactation. Erythromycin base (Pregnancy Risk Category B) is an acceptable alternate agent for treatment of CT infection in pregnancy. Doxycycline and ofloxacin are contraindicated in pregnancy. Erythromycin estolate is contraindicated in pregnancy because of drug-related hepatotoxicity.

FOLLOW-UP:

- Observed single-dose therapy should be offered to individuals for whom compliance is a concern.
- To minimize disease transmission to partners, affected persons should be advised to refrain from sexual intercourse for 7 days after single-dose therapy, until completion of 7-day therapy, or until resolution of symptoms.
- To prevent reinfection, affected individuals should refrain from sexual intercourse until all of their partners have been treated.
- Test of cure to detect treatment failure is not needed.
- Re-collection by NAAT method in less than 3 weeks from treatment can yield a false-positive result due to the sensitivity of this testing method.
- Both men and women treated for chlamydia should be retested at approximately 3 months after treatment to screen for reinfection. If patients do not return to clinical settings within 3 months, rescreen the patient at the next presentation for clinical care.
- Pregnant women with CT infection should have a test of cure 3 to 4 weeks after treatment and should then be retested within 3 months.

  Refer partners for evaluation and treatment.

RECURRENT AND PERSISTENT URETHRITIS: Retreat noncompliant patients with the above regimens. If patient was initially compliant, recommended regimens: metronidazole 2 g PO in single dose plus erythromycin base 500 mg PO qid for 7 days or erythromycin ethylsuccinate 800 mg PO qid for 7 days.

REFERRAL

Refer to infectious disease specialist if persistent infection or gynecologist if salpingitis is suspected.

SUGGESTED READINGS

Available at www.expertconsult.com

RELATED CONTENT

Cervicitis (Related Key Topic)
Gonococcal Urethritis (Related Key Topic)
Gonorrhea (Related Key Topic)
Nongonococcal Urethritis (Related Key Topic)
Pelvic Inflammatory Disease (Related Key Topic)

AUTHOR: **RUBEN ALVERO, M.D.,** and **DEANNA L. BENNER, A.P.R.N., C.R.N.P.**

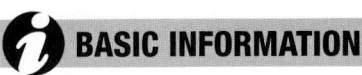

BASIC INFORMATION

DEFINITION

Cholangiocarcinoma is a cancer that originates from the epithelial lining of bile ducts. Most commonly an adenocarcinoma, this tumor is classified based on its location within the biliary tree as intrahepatic, perihilar, or extrahepatic.

SYNONYMS

Bile duct carcinoma

ICD-10CM CODES
C22.1 Intrahepatic bile duct carcinoma
C24.0 Malignant neoplasm of extrahepatic bile duct

EPIDEMIOLOGY & DEMOGRAPHICS

INCIDENCE:

- The incidence rate of cholangiocarcinoma is 1-2 per 100,000
- Incidence rate of intrahepatic cholangiocarcinoma appears to be increasing
- Higher incidence in Hispanic and Asian populations

PREDOMINANT SEX AND AGE:

- Slightly more common in men
- Most often diagnosed between 50 and 70 years of age
- Patients with primary sclerosing cholangitis (PSC) can present as early as 30 years old

RISK FACTORS:

- PSC causes inflammation of the bile ducts leading to fibrosis and stricturing of the biliary tree. PSC is the most common risk factor for development of cholangiocarcinoma, with a lifetime risk of up to 15%
- Other risk factors include infection with hepatitis B and C, liver cirrhosis, chronic hepatolithiasis, choledochal cysts, and parasitic infections of the liver.

PHYSICAL FINDINGS & CLINICAL PRESENTATION

- With early-stage cholangiocarcinoma, the patient may be completely asymptomatic, and diagnosis is made incidentally on imaging or during the workup for elevation of liver enzymes.
- Later-stage cholangiocarcinoma may present as biliary obstruction.
- The clinical presentation is also dependent on the location of the tumor. Cholangiocarcinoma involving the intrahepatic ducts tends to cause nonspecific symptoms of dull, aching right upper quadrant pain and weight loss. A tumor of the extrahepatic ducts most often causes symptoms of biliary obstruction including jaundice, pale stools, and dark urine.
- Findings on physical examination may include jaundice, pain on palpation of the right upper quadrant, hepatomegaly, and fever.

DIAGNOSIS

DIFFERENTIAL DIAGNOSIS

The differential diagnosis includes other conditions that may cause right upper quadrant pain, fever, and symptoms of biliary obstruction or those that present with a mass on imaging.

- Primary sclerosing cholangitis
- Cholecystitis
- Acute cholangitis
- Liver metastases

WORKUP

Fig. 1 describes an algorithm for the diagnosis of intrahepatic cholangiocarcinoma. The approach to the diagnosis of perihilar cholangiocarcinoma is summarized in Fig. 2.

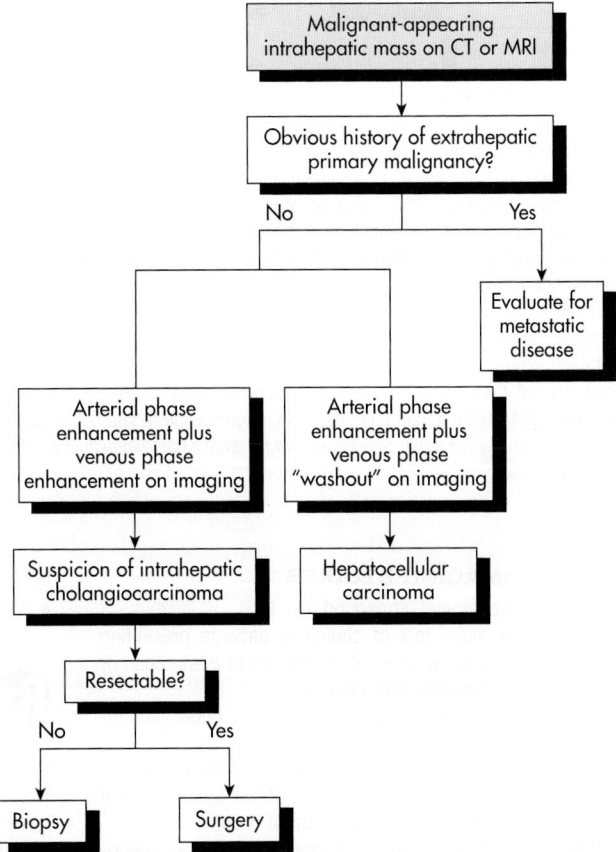

FIG. 1 Algorithm for the diagnosis of intrahepatic cholangiocarcinoma. In cases of an intrahepatic mass lesion and in the absence of known extrahepatic primary malignancy, dynamic imaging with either CT or MRI of the liver should be performed. Contrast enhancement throughout the arterial phase with "washout" in the portal venous phase indicates a hepatocellular carcinoma. Contrast enhancement throughout the arterial and portal venous phases should raise the suspicion of an intrahepatic cholangiocarcinoma; in such cases, the resectability of the tumor should be determined. If the lesion is deemed resectable, the patient should be referred for surgical resection without biopsy. If an intrahepatic cholangiocarcinoma is deemed unresectable, a biopsy should be performed to confirm the diagnosis and guide appropriate treatment. (From Feldman M et al [eds]: *Sleisenger and Fordtran's gastrointestinal and liver disease*, ed 10, Philadelphia, 2016, Saunders.)

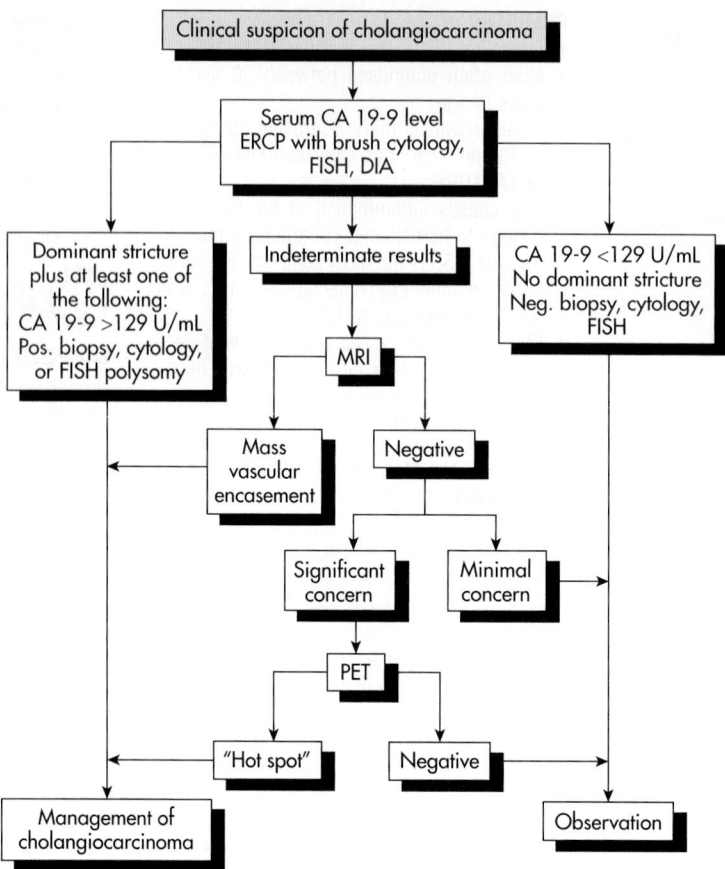

FIG. 2 Algorithm for the diagnosis of perihilar cholangiocarcinoma. In cases of clinically suspected perihilar cholangiocarcinoma, a serum CA 19-9 level, ERCP, and conventional as well as molecular cytologic analysis of endoscopically obtained biliary brushings of malignant-appearing areas should be performed. If the results of these tests are normal or negative, close follow-up of the patient is recommended. Management of cholangiocarcinoma should be prompted by identification of a dominant stricture, a serum CA 19-9 level above 129 U/mL, or a biopsy or cytology result that is positive for carcinoma or polysomy. In indeterminate cases, gadolinium-enhanced MRI of the liver is recommended. If a mass lesion or vascular encasement is identified, management of cholangiocarcinoma should be initiated. If the MRI study is negative but clinical concern about cholangiocarcinoma persists, PET can be performed. If "hot spots" are identified on PET (positive result), treatment for cholangiocarcinoma should be initiated. If the result of the PET scan is negative, close follow-up of the patient is recommended. If MRI is negative and cholangiocarcinoma is considered unlikely, the patient can be followed expectantly. *DIA,* digital image analysis; *FISH,* fluorescence in situ hybridization; *neg.,* negative; *pos.,* positive. (From Feldman M et al [eds]: *Sleisenger and Fordtran's gastrointestinal and liver disease,* ed 10, Philadelphia, 2016, Saunders.)

LABORATORY TESTS

- Liver enzymes
- INR
- Bilirubin
  Blood work may reveal an "obstructive pattern" with predominant elevation of alkaline phosphatase and bilirubin.
  Tumor markers
- CEA
- CA19-9
  It is important to note that these tumor markers may be elevated even in the setting of benign inflammation of the biliary tree, for example, during an episode of acute cholangitis. These markers are neither sensitive nor specific for cholangiocarcinoma, but if they are elevated at the time of diagnosis, they may be helpful in tracking response to therapy or in monitoring for disease recurrence.

IMAGING STUDIES

Abdominal ultrasound (Fig. E3)

- Initial test of choice in patients presenting with nonspecific symptoms of obstruction or elevated liver enzymes.
  CT scan/magnetic resonance cholangiopancreatography (MRCP)
- Improved visualization of the biliary tree to allow for identification of the tumor, level of obstruction, and extent of disease.
  Endoscopic retrograde cholangiopancreatography (ERCP) (Fig. E4)
- Can be used to obtain brushings of the biliary tree for cytology, but diagnostic yield is poor, and there is a risk of cholangitis in patients with significant obstruction of bile drainage.
  Endoscopic ultrasound (EUS)
- Allows fine-needle aspiration of distal biliary duct tumors and involved lymph nodes.

STAGING

- Tables E1 to E3 describe staging systems for cholangiocarcinoma.

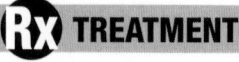 **TREATMENT**

ACUTE GENERAL Rx

- The only curative treatment option for cholangiocarcinoma is surgical extirpation. Eligibility for surgical resection with curative intent is based both on the location of the tumor and the stage of disease. Box 1 summarizes criteria for unresectability of perihilar cholangiocarcinoma.
- Surgical approaches include partial liver resection, pancreaticoduodenectomy, pancreaticojejunostomy, or even liver transplantation in carefully selected patients.

BOX 1   Criteria for Unresectability of Perihilar Cholangiocarcinoma

1. Atrophy of one liver lobe with encasement of the contralateral portal vein branch
2. Atrophy of one liver lobe with contralateral secondary biliary radical involvement
3. Bilateral portal vein branch encasement
4. Bilateral hepatic artery encasement
5. Distant lymph node metastases
6. Hilar cholangiocarcinoma, Bismuth-Corlette type IV
7. Intrahepatic or distant metastases
8. Primary sclerosing cholangitis
9. Significant comorbid conditions

From Feldman M et al [eds]: *Sleisenger and Fordtran's gastrointestinal and liver disease*, ed 10, Philadelphia, 2016, Saunders.

- Adjuvant chemotherapy has been shown to reduce mortality in patients with both positive margins post-resection and/or involved lymph nodes.
- The use of adjuvant radiation remains an area of controversy, but there is evidence of improved survival in nonoperable patients with localized disease.

DISPOSITION

- Surveillance imaging for recurrence is recommended every 6 months for a total of 2 years.
- Recurrence can occur locally or as metastatic disease, most commonly to liver, lung, or peritoneum.
- Five-year survival rates vary between 15% and 60% based on the stage of disease.

Unfortunately, even those patients with node-negative disease who undergo resection with curative intent have a high rate of disease recurrence.

REFERRAL

Referral should be made to a hepatobiliary surgeon for consideration of surgical resection and to a medical oncologist for possible adjuvant chemotherapy.

SUGGESTED READINGS

Available at www.expertconsult.com

RELATED CONTENT

Primary Sclerosing Cholangitis (Related Key Topic)

AUTHORS: **TALIA ZENLEA, M.D.,** and **NADIA GRILLER, M.D.**

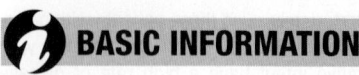

BASIC INFORMATION

DEFINITION

Cholangitis refers to an inflammation and/or infection of the hepatic and common bile ducts associated with obstruction of the common bile duct.

SYNONYMS

Biliary sepsis
Ascending cholangitis
Suppurative cholangitis

ICD-10CM CODES
K83.0 Cholangitis

EPIDEMIOLOGY & DEMOGRAPHICS

INCIDENCE (IN U.S.): Complicates approximately 1% of cases of cholelithiasis
PEAK INCIDENCE: Seventh decade
PREVALENCE (IN U.S.): 2 cases/1000 hospital admissions
PREDOMINANT SEX:
- Females, for cholangitis secondary to gallstones
- Males, for cholangitis secondary to malignant obstruction and HIV infection

PREDOMINANT AGE: Seventh decade and older; unusual <50 yr of age

PHYSICAL FINDINGS & CLINICAL PRESENTATION

- Usually acute onset of fever, abdominal pain (RUQ), and jaundice (Charcot's triad)
- All signs and symptoms in only 50% to 85% of patients
- Often, dark coloration of the urine resulting from bilirubinuria
- Complications:
  1. Bacteremia (50%) and septic shock
  2. Hepatic abscess and pancreatitis

ETIOLOGY

Obstruction of the common bile duct causing rapid proliferation of bacteria in the biliary tree
- Most common cause of common bile duct obstruction: stones, usually migrated from the gallbladder
- Other causes: prior biliary tract surgery with secondary stenosis, tumor (usually arising from the pancreas or biliary tree), and parasitic infections from *Ascaris lumbricoides* or *Fasciola hepatica*
- Iatrogenic after contamination of an obstructed biliary tree by endoscopic retrograde cholangiopancreatoscopy (ERCP) or percutaneous transhepatic cholangiography (PTC)
- Primary sclerosing cholangitis (PSC)
- HIV-associated sclerosing cholangitis: associated with infection by CMV, *Cryptosporidium,* Microsporida, and *Mycobacterium avium* complex

DIAGNOSIS

DIFFERENTIAL DIAGNOSIS

- Biliary colic
- Acute cholecystitis
- Liver abscess
- Peptic ulcer disease (PUD)
- Pancreatitis
- Intestinal obstruction
- Right kidney stone
- Hepatitis
- Pyelonephritis

WORKUP

- Blood cultures
- CBC
- Liver function tests

LABORATORY TESTS

- Usually, elevated WBC count with a predominance of polymorphonuclear forms
- Elevated alkaline phosphatase and bilirubin in chronic obstruction
- Elevated transaminases in acute obstruction
- Positive blood cultures in 50% of cases, typically with enteric gram-negative aerobes (e.g., *Escherichia coli, Klebsiella pneumoniae*), enterococci, or anaerobes

IMAGING STUDIES

- Ultrasound:
  1. Allows visualization of the gallbladder and bile ducts to differentiate extrahepatic obstruction from intrahepatic cholestasis
  2. Insensitive but specific for visualization of common duct stones
- CT scan:
  1. Less accurate for gallstones
  2. More sensitive than ultrasound for visualization of the distal part of the common bile duct
  3. Also allows better definition of neoplasm
- ERCP:
  1. Confirms obstruction and its level
  2. Allows collection of specimens for culture and cytology
  3. Indicated for diagnosis if ultrasound and CT scan are inconclusive
  4. May be indicated in therapy (see "Treatment")

TREATMENT

NONPHARMACOLOGIC THERAPY

Biliary decompression
- May be urgent in severely ill patients or those unresponsive to medical therapy within 12 to 24 hr
- May also be performed semielectively in patients who respond
- Options:
  1. ERCP with or without sphincterotomy or placement of a draining stent.

  2. Percutaneous transhepatic biliary drainage for the acutely ill patient who is a poor surgical candidate.
  3. Recently, endoscopic ultrasound–guided biliary drainage has been proven as an alternative to percutaneous transhepatic biliary drainage in specialized centers when ERCP fails or is not available.
  4. Surgical exploration of the common bile duct.

ACUTE GENERAL Rx

- Nothing by mouth
- Intravenous hydration
- Broad-spectrum antibiotics directed at gram-negative enteric organisms, anaerobes, and enterococcus such as carbapenems (meropenem: 1 g q8h or imipenem: 500 mg IV q6h if life threatening), piperacillin/tazobactam: 3.375 or 4.5 g IV q6h, or ampicillin-sulbactam, or ticarcillin-clavulanate; if infection is nosocomial, post-ERCP, or the patient is in shock, broaden antibiotic coverage.

CHRONIC Rx

Repeated decompression may be necessary, particularly when obstruction is related to neoplasm.

DISPOSITION

Excellent prognosis if obstruction is amenable to definitive surgical therapy; otherwise relapses are common.

REFERRAL

- To biliary endoscopist if obstruction is from stones or a stent needs to be placed
- To interventional radiologist if external drainage is necessary
- To a general surgeon in all other cases
- To an infectious disease specialist if blood cultures are positive or the patient is in shock or otherwise severely ill

PEARLS & CONSIDERATIONS

- Cholangitis is a life-threatening form of intra-abdominal sepsis, though it may appear to be rather innocuous at its onset.
- Antibiotics alone will not resolve cholangitis in the presence of biliary obstruction because high intrabiliary pressures prevent antibiotic delivery. Decompression and drainage of the biliary tract to alleviate the obstruction with antimicrobial therapy is the therapy of choice.

SUGGESTED READINGS

Available at www.expertconsult.com

AUTHOR: **GLENN G. FORT, M.D., M.P.H.**

BASIC INFORMATION

DEFINITION

Cholecystitis is acute or chronic inflammation of the gallbladder generally caused by gallstones (>95% of cases).

SYNONYMS

Gallbladder attack

ICD-10CM CODES
K81.9   Acute cholecystitis
K80.00 Calculus of gallbladder with acute cholecystitis without obstruction
K81.9   Cholecystitis, unspecified

EPIDEMIOLOGY & DEMOGRAPHICS

- Acute cholecystitis occurs most commonly in women during the fifth and sixth decades. Approximately 120,000 cholecystectomies are performed for acute cholecystitis annually in the U.S.
- The incidence of gallstones is 0.6% in the general population and much higher in certain ethnic groups (>75% of Native Americans by age 60 yr). Most patients with gallstones are asymptomatic. Of such patients, biliary colic develops in 1% to 4% annually.

PHYSICAL FINDINGS & CLINICAL PRESENTATION

- Pain and tenderness in the right hypochondrium or epigastrium; pain possibly radiating to the infrascapular region
- Palpation of the right upper quadrant (RUQ) eliciting marked tenderness and stoppage of inspired breath (**Murphy's sign**)
- Guarding
- Fever (33%)
- Jaundice (25% to 50% of patients)
- Palpable gallbladder (20% of cases)
- Nausea and vomiting (>70% of patients)
- Fever and chills (>25% of patients)
- Medical history often revealing ingestion of large, fatty meals before onset of pain in the epigastrium and RUQ

ETIOLOGY

- Gallstones (>95% of cases)
- Ischemic damage to the gallbladder, critically ill patient (acalculous cholecystitis)
- Infectious agents, especially in patients with AIDS (cytomegalovirus, *Cryptosporidium*)
- Strictures of the bile duct
- Neoplasms, primary or metastatic
- Risk factors for cholelithiasis include age, obesity, female sex, rapid weight loss, ethnicity/race (Native American), use of contraceptives, pregnancy, diabetes mellitus, hemolysis, total parenteral nutrition, biliary parasites

DIAGNOSIS

DIFFERENTIAL DIAGNOSIS

- Hepatic: hepatitis, abscess, hepatic congestion, neoplasm, trauma
- Biliary: neoplasm, stricture, sphincter of Oddi dysfunction
- Gastric: pelvic ulcer disease, neoplasm, alcoholic gastritis, hiatal hernia, non-ulcer dyspepsia
- Pancreatic: pancreatitis, neoplasm, stone in the pancreatic duct or ampulla
- Renal: calculi, infection, inflammation, neoplasm, ruptured kidney
- Pulmonary: pneumonia, pulmonary infarction, right-sided pleurisy
- Intestinal: retrocecal appendicitis, intestinal obstruction, high fecal impaction, irritable bowel syndrome (IBS), inflammatory bowel disease (IBD)
- Cardiac: myocardial ischemia (particularly involving the inferior wall), pericarditis
- Cutaneous: herpes zoster
- Trauma
- Fitz-Hugh–Curtis syndrome (perihepatitis), ruptured ectopic pregnancy
- Subphrenic abscess
- Dissecting aneurysm
- Nerve root irritation caused by osteoarthritis of the spine

WORKUP

Workup consists of detailed history and physical examination coupled with laboratory evaluation and imaging studies. No single clinical finding or laboratory test is sufficient to establish or exclude cholecystitis without further testing.

LABORATORY TESTS

- Leukocytosis (12,000 to 20,000) is present in >70% of patients.
- Elevated alkaline phosphatase, ALT, AST, bilirubin; bilirubin elevation >4 mg/dl is unusual and suggests presence of choledocholithiasis.
- Elevated amylase may be present (consider pancreatitis if serum amylase elevation exceeds 500 U).

IMAGING STUDIES

- Ultrasound of the gallbladder (Fig. E1) is the preferred initial test; it will demonstrate the presence of stones and also dilated gallbladder with thickened wall and surrounding edema in patients with acute cholecystitis.
- Nuclear imaging (HIDA scan) (Fig. E2) is useful for diagnosis of cholecystitis when sonogram is inconclusive: sensitivity and specificity exceed 90% for acute cholecystitis. This test is only reliable when bilirubin is <5 mg/dl. A positive test result (absence of gallbladder filling within 60 min after the administration of tracer) will demonstrate obstruction of the cystic or common hepatic duct; the test will not demonstrate the presence of stones.
- CT scan of abdomen is useful in cases of suspected abscess, neoplasm, or pancreatitis.
- Plain radiograph of the abdomen generally is not useful because <25% of stones are radiopaque.

TREATMENT

NONPHARMACOLOGIC THERAPY

Provide IV hydration; withhold oral feedings.

ACUTE GENERAL Rx

- Laparoscopic (percutaneous) cholecystectomy (PC) is considered the treatment of choice for most patients. The rate of conversion to open cholecystectomy is higher when laparoscopic cholecystectomy (CCY) is performed for acute cholecystitis rather than for uncomplicated cholelithiasis; conservative management with IV fluids and antibiotics (ampicillin-sulbactam 3 g IV q6h or piperacillin-tazobactam 4.5 g IV q8h) may be justified in some high-risk patients to convert an emergency procedure into an elective one with a lower mortality rate.
- Endoscopic retrograde cholangiopancreatography with sphincterectomy and stone extraction can be performed in conjunction with laparoscopic cholecystectomy for patients with choledochal lithiasis; approximately 7% to 15% of patients with cholelithiasis also have stones in the common bile duct.

DISPOSITION

- Prognosis is good; elective laparoscopic cholecystectomy can be performed as outpatient procedure.
- Hospital stay (when necessary) varies from overnight with laparoscopic cholecystectomy to 4 to 7 days with open cholecystectomy.
- Complication rate is approximately 1% (hemorrhage and bile leak) for laparoscopic cholecystectomy and <0.5% (infection) with open cholecystectomy.

REFERRAL

Surgical referral in all patients with acute cholecystitis

PEARLS & CONSIDERATIONS

COMMENTS

- Patients should be instructed that stones may recur in bile ducts.
- Gallbladder aspiration, in which all fluid visualized by ultrasound is aspirated, represents a nonsurgical treatment when patients who are at high operative risk develop acute cholecystitis. Salvage cholecystectomy is reserved for nonresponders.

SUGGESTED READINGS

Available at www.expertconsult.com

RELATED CONTENT

Gallbladder Attack (Cholecystitis) (Patient Information)
Cholelithiasis (Related Key Topic)
Cholangitis (Related Key Topic)

AUTHOR: **FRED F. FERRI, M.D.**

DEFINITION

Choledocholithiasis is a derivation from the Greek words of *choli* (bile), *docheion* (container), and *lithos* (stone) and refers to the presence of gallstones within the common bile duct (CBD).

SYNONYMS

Common bile duct stone(s)

ICD-10CM CODES
K80.50 Calculus of bile duct

EPIDEMIOLOGY & DEMOGRAPHICS

- While the exact incidence and prevalence are unknown, an estimated 10% to 20% of patients are found to have choledocholithiasis at the time of cholecystectomy.
- Passage of gallstones into the CBD occurs in approximately 10% to 15% of those with cholelithiasis, and the incidence is known to increase with age.
- Risk factors for gallstone formation include nonmodifiable factors such age, female sex, family history, ethnic background, and genetic predilection, while modifiable factors are centripetal obesity and metabolic syndrome, rapid weight loss, ileal Crohn's disease, cirrhosis, total parenteral nutrition, and medications such as estrogen replacement therapy.

PHYSICAL FINDINGS & CLINICAL PRESENTATION

- Uncomplicated choledocholithiasis presents with biliary colic; it is classically described as intense and constant pain in the right upper quadrant or epigastric region, associated with nausea and vomiting.
- Occasionally patients may remain asymptomatic, but resolution of pain more often reflects passage of stone into the bowel.
- Physical examination demonstrates right upper quadrant or epigastric tenderness and occasionally jaundice.
- Courvoisier's sign for a palpable gallbladder is more typically associated with malignant obstruction of the CBD, but it has been reported with choledocholithiasis.
- Other clinical findings of fever (Charcot's triad), hypotension, and altered mental status (Reynolds' pentad) are found only when choledocholithiasis is complicated by acute cholangitis.
- Choledocholithiasis can also be complicated by acute pancreatitis.

ETIOLOGY

- The majority of cases are due to passage of cholesterol stones from the gallbladder into the common bile duct.
- De novo formation of choledocholithiasis (primary choledocholithiasis) is uncommon but is seen amongst those with increased propensity for pigment stone formation due to chronic recurrent pyogenic cholangitis from trematodes, congenital biliary duct anomalies, dilated or strictured ducts or *MDR3* gene defects causing impairments in biliary phospholipid secretions, or biliary stasis such as from cystic fibrosis.

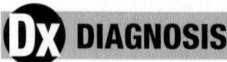 DIAGNOSIS

DIFFERENTIAL DIAGNOSIS

- Acute cholecystitis
- Sphincter of Oddi dysfunction
- Functional gallbladder disorder

WORKUP

- The constellation of symptomatic cholelithiasis with elevated liver enzymes should prompt a transabdominal ultrasound (US) of the right upper quadrant to evaluate for a stone in the CBD, which is the most reliable predictor of choledocholithiasis.
- Clinical predictors may be utilized to risk-stratify patients and to inform the next step in management. For instance, strong predictors for high-risk choledocholithiasis are a CBD stone or dilated CBD seen on transabdominal US, clinical or biochemical evidence of cholangitis, and elevated bilirubin (>1.8 mg/dl).
- See Fig. 1 for the ASGE guideline for a proposed risk-stratification model.

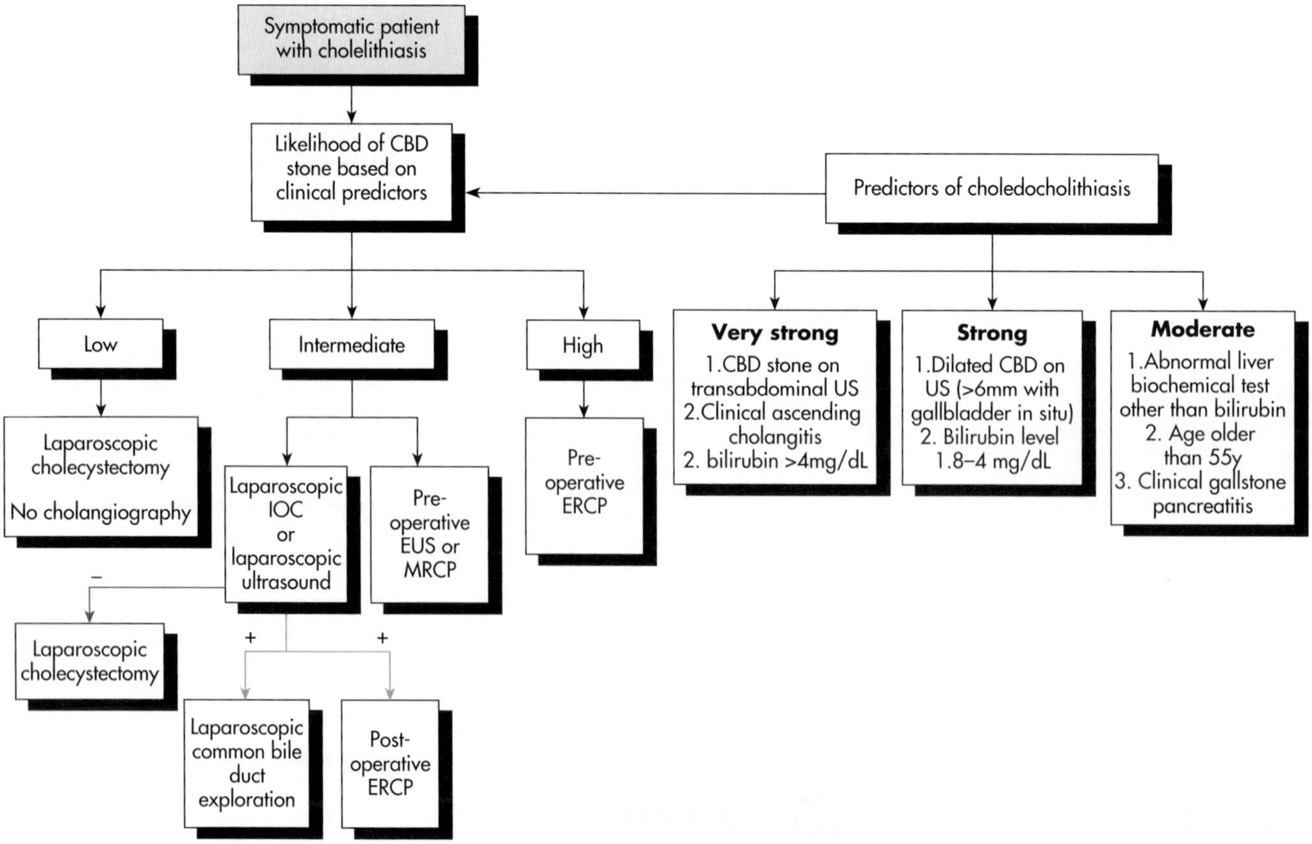

FIG. 1 Algorithm for the management of patients with symptomatic cholelithiasis. (Adapted from Tse et al and ASGE 2010.)

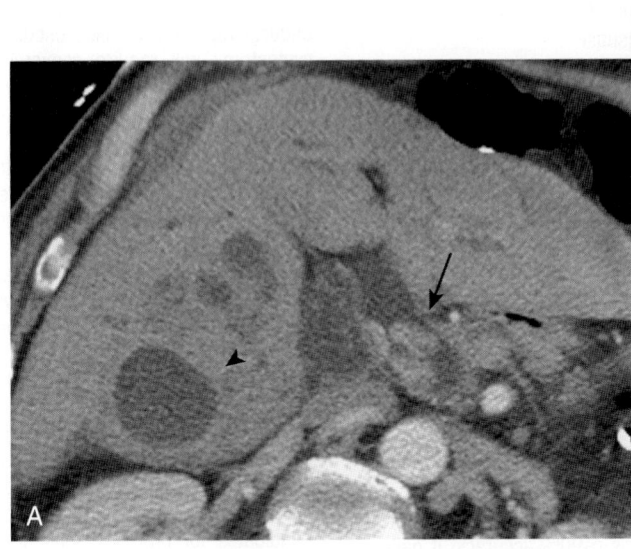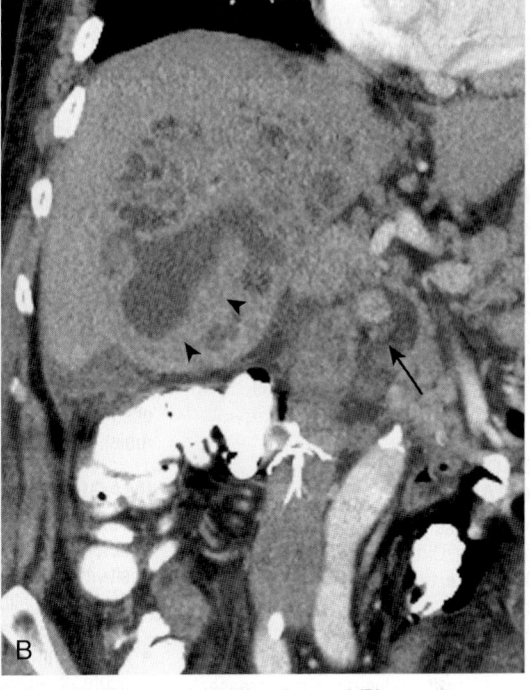

FIG. 2 A 70-year-old man with choledocholithiasis and a hepatic abscess. Axial **(A)** and coronal **(B)** portal venous phase computed tomography images demonstrate large bile duct stones *(arrows)* with a focal intrahepatic fluid collection *(arrowheads)* consistent with the patient's known pyogenic abscess. (From Soto JA, Lucey BC: *Emergency radiology: the requisites*, ed 2, Philadelphia, 2017, Elsevier.)

LABORATORY TESTS

- Elevations in serum alanine aminotransferase (ALT) and aspartate aminotransferase (AST) reflect early biliary obstruction; followed by a disproportionate increase in serum bilirubin, alkaline phosphatase (ALP), and gamma-glutamyl transpeptidase (GGT), which are independent predictors of a CBD stone.
- An isolated and transient increase in alanine transaminase or amylase reflects passage of the gallstone.
- In addition, patients with choledocholithiasis complicated by acute pancreatitis and cholangitis have elevated serum amylase or lipase (>3 times upper limit of normal), and leukocytosis, respectively.

IMAGING STUDIES

- Ultrasound of the gallbladder has a relatively poor sensitivity (22%-55%) for stone detection but is relied upon for CBD dilation, which is associated with choledocholithiasis.
- The finding of CBD dilation >8 mm (sensitivity 77%-87%, negative predictive value 95%-96%) with an intact gallbladder is indicative of biliary obstruction. Multiple small gallbladder stones (<5 mm) portend a fourfold higher risk of passage of stones into the CBD.

- Other imaging modalities such as helical CT (Fig. 2), magnetic resonance cholangiopancreatography, and CT cholangiography have improved performance characteristics for CBD stone detection; however, their use as first-line diagnostic tools is contingent on diagnostic uncertainty, patient factors, and availability.
- Magnetic resonance cholangiopancreatography should be considered in intermediate-risk patients or in those with prior cholecystectomy.
- High-risk patients should proceed directly to endoscopic retrograde cholangiopancreatography (ERCP) for diagnosis and treatment.

Rx TREATMENT

ACUTE GENERAL Rx

- The mainstay is removal of CBD stones via ERCP and papillotomy either before or at the time of laparoscopic or open cholecystectomy.
- Failure of ERCP to clear the biliary duct warrants biliary stenting for drainage as a temporary measure in the event of acute cholangitis.

CHRONIC Rx

- Patients with recurrent choledocholithiasis from cholesterol gallstones after cholecystectomy might be considered for chronic treatment with ursodeoxycholic acid to facilitate reduction of cholesterol saturation of bile.

REFERRAL

- Gastroenterology
- General surgery

SUGGESTED READINGS

Available at www.expertconsult.com

RELATED CONTENT

Cholangiocarcinoma (Related Key Topic)
Cholelithiasis (Related Key Topic)
Cholecystitis (Related Key Topic)

AUTHORS: **ROWENA ALMEIDA, M.D.,** and **TALIA ZENLEA, M.D.**

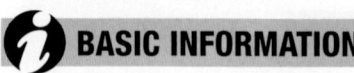

BASIC INFORMATION

DEFINITION

Cholelithiasis is the presence of stones in the gallbladder

SYNONYMS

Gallstones

ICD-10CM CODES
K80.80 Other cholelithiasis without obstruction
K80.81 Other cholelithiasis with obstruction
K91.86 Retained cholelithiasis following cholecystectomy

EPIDEMIOLOGY & DEMOGRAPHICS

- Gallstone disease can be found in 12% of the U.S. population. Of these, 2% to 3% (500,000 to 600,000) are treated with cholecystectomies each year.
- Annual medical expenditures for gallbladder surgeries in the U.S. exceed $5 billion.
- Incidence of gallbladder disease increases with age. Highest incidence is in the fifth and sixth decades. Predisposing factors for gallstones are female sex, pregnancy, age >40 yr, family history of gallstones, obesity, ileal disease, oral contraceptives, diabetes mellitus, rapid weight loss, estrogen replacement therapy. Risk factors for the development of cholelithiasis are described in Table E1.
- Patients with gallstones have a 20% chance of developing biliary colic or its complications at the end of a 20-yr period. Significant predictors of gallstone-related events are large stone (>10 mm), presence of multiple stones, and female sex.

PHYSICAL FINDINGS & CLINICAL PRESENTATION

- Physical examination is entirely normal unless patient is having biliary colic; 80% of gallstones are asymptomatic.
- Typical symptoms of obstruction of the cystic duct include intermittent, severe, cramping pain affecting the right upper quadrant.
- Pain occurs mostly at night and may radiate to the back or right shoulder. It can last from a few minutes to several hours.

ETIOLOGY

- 75% of gallstones contain cholesterol and are usually associated with obesity, female sex, and diabetes mellitus; mixed stones are most common (80%); pure cholesterol stones account for only 10% of stones.
- 25% of gallstones are pigment stones (bilirubin, calcium, and variable organic material) associated with hemolysis and cirrhosis. These tend to be black-pigmented stones that are refractory to medical therapy.
- 50% of mixed-type stones are radiopaque.

DIAGNOSIS

DIFFERENTIAL DIAGNOSIS

- Peptic ulcer disease
- Gastroesophageal reflux disease
- Irritable bowel disease
- Pancreatitis
- Neoplasms
- Nonnuclear dyspepsia
- Inferior wall myocardial infarction
- Hepatic abscess

LABORATORY TESTS

Generally normal unless patient has biliary obstruction (elevated alkaline phosphatase, bilirubin).

IMAGING STUDIES

- Ultrasound of the gallbladder (Fig. E1) will detect small stones and biliary sludge (sensitivity, 95%; specificity, 90%); the presence of dilated gallbladder with thickened wall is suggestive of acute cholecystitis.
- Nuclear imaging (HIDA scan) can confirm acute cholecystitis (>90% accuracy) if gallbladder does not visualize within 4 hr of injection and the radioisotope is excreted in the common bile duct.
- Common bile duct stones can be detected noninvasively by magnetic resonance cholangiopancreatography or invasively by endoscopic retrograde cholangiopancreatography (ERCP) and intraoperative cholangiography.

TREATMENT

NONPHARMACOLOGIC THERAPY

Lifestyle changes (avoidance of diets high in polyunsaturated fats, weight loss in obese patients; however, avoid rapid weight loss)

ACUTE GENERAL Rx

- The management of gallstones is affected by the clinical presentation.
- Asymptomatic patients do not require therapeutic intervention. Proposed criteria for prophylactic cholecystectomy are described in Table 2.

TABLE 2 Proposed Criteria for Prophylactic Cholecystectomy

Life expectancy >20 years

Calculi >2 cm in diameter

Calculi >3 mm and patent cystic duct

Radiopaque calculi

Gallbladder polyps >15 mm

Nonfunctioning or calcified gallbladder ("porcelain" gallbladder)

Women <60 years

Patients in areas with high prevalence of gallbladder cancer

From Cameron JL, Cameron AM: *Current surgical therapy*, ed 10, Philadelphia, 2011, Saunders.

- Surgical intervention is generally the ideal approach for symptomatic patients. Laparoscopic cholecystectomy is preferred over open cholecystectomy because of the shorter recovery period and lower mortality rate. Between 5% and 26% of patients undergoing elective laparoscopic cholecystectomy will require conversion to an open procedure. Most common reason is the inability to clearly identify the biliary anatomy.
- Laparoscopic cholecystectomy after endoscopic sphincterectomy is recommended for patients with common bile duct stones and residual gallbladder stones. Where possible, single-stage laparoscopic treatments with removal of duct stones and cholecystectomy during the same procedure are preferable. Percutaneous cholecystectomy is an alternative for patients who are critically ill with gallbladder empyema and sepsis.
- Patients who are not appropriate candidates for surgery because of coexisting illness or patients who refuse surgery can be treated with oral bile salts: ursodiol or chenodiol. Candidates for oral bile salts are patients with cholesterol stones (radiolucent, noncalcified stones), with a diameter of ≤15 mm and having three or fewer stones. Candidates for medical therapy must have a functioning gallbladder and must have absence of calcifications on CT scans.
- Extracorporeal shock wave lithotripsy (ESWL) is another form of medical therapy. It can be used in patients with stone diameter of ≤3 cm and having three or fewer stones.

DISPOSITION

- Complicated gallstone events develop in 8% of patients with incidentally discovered gallstones after 17 years (Shabanzadeh DM, et al: *Gastroenterology* 150:156, 2016).
- After ESWL, stones recur in approximately 20% of patients after 4 yr.
- Patients with at least one gallstone <5 mm in diameter have a greater than fourfold increased risk of presenting with acute biliary pancreatitis. A policy of watchful waiting in such cases is generally warranted.
- A potential serious complication of gallstones is acute cholangitis. ERCP and endoscopic sphincterectomy followed by interval laparoscopic cholecystectomy are effective in acute cholangitis.

SUGGESTED READINGS

Available at www.expertconsult.com

RELATED CONTENT

Gallstones (Patient Information)
Cholecystitis (Related Key Topic)
Choledocholithiasis (Related Key Topic)

AUTHOR: **FRED F. FERRI, M.D.**

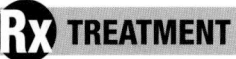

BASIC INFORMATION

DEFINITION

Chronic fatigue syndrome (CFS), also known as myalgic encephalomyelitis/chronic fatigue syndrome (ME/CFS) is characterized by at least three of the following symptoms, present concurrently for at least 6 mo:
- Impaired memory or concentration (cognitive impairment)
- Sore throat
- Tender cervical or axillary lymph nodes
- Muscle pain
- Multijoint pain
- New headaches
- Unrefreshing sleep
- Postexertion malaise for longer than 24 hr
- Orthostatic intolerance

There are currently several sets of clinical criteria to define ME/CFS, yet there is no consensus regarding which set of criteria best identifies patients with this condition.

SYNONYMS

Yuppie flu
CFS
Chronic Epstein-Barr syndrome
Myalgic encephalomyelitis/chronic fatigue syndrome (ME/CFS)
Systemic exertion intolerance disease (SEID)

ICD-10CM CODES	
R53.82	Chronic fatigue, unspecified
F45.8	Other somatoform disorders

EPIDEMIOLOGY & DEMOGRAPHICS

PREVALENCE IN U.S.: Prevalence rates of CFS in the U.S. range from 0.3% to 2.5%. It is estimated that 800,000 to 2.5 million Americans have CFS.
PREDOMINANT AGE: Young adulthood and middle age
PREDOMINANT SEX: Females affected more often than males
ECONOMICS: The estimated annual cost of lost productivity is estimated to be between $17 billion and $24 billion annually.

PHYSICAL FINDINGS & CLINICAL PRESENTATION

- There are no physical findings specific for CFS.
- The physical examination may be useful to identify fibromyalgia and other rheumatologic conditions that may coexist with CFS.

ETIOLOGY

- The etiology of CFS is unknown.
- Some theorize that a viral illness may trigger certain immune responses that lead to the various symptoms. Most patients often report the onset of their symptoms with a flulike illness.

- The presence of numerous psychiatric comorbidities in CFS have led some experts to question the existence of any organic etiology.

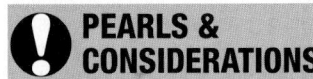

DIAGNOSIS

DIFFERENTIAL DIAGNOSIS

- Psychosocial depression, dysthymia, anxiety-related disorders, and other psychiatric diseases
- Sleep apnea
- Infectious diseases (subacute bacterial endocarditis, Lyme disease, fungal diseases, mononucleosis, HIV, chronic hepatitis B or C, tuberculosis (TB), chronic parasitic infections)
- Autoimmune diseases: systemic lupus erythematosus, myasthenia gravis, multiple sclerosis, thyroiditis, rheumatoid arthritis
- Endocrine abnormalities: hypothyroidism, hypopituitarism, adrenal insufficiency, Cushing's syndrome, diabetes mellitus, hyperparathyroidism, pregnancy, reactive hypoglycemia
- Occult malignant disease
- Substance abuse
- Systemic disorders: chronic renal failure, chronic obstructive pulmonary disease, cardiovascular disease, anemia, electrolyte abnormalities, liver disease
- Other: inadequate rest, sleep apnea, narcolepsy, fibromyalgia, sarcoidosis, medications, toxic agent exposure, Wegener's granulomatosis, vitamin deficiency

LABORATORY TESTS

- No specific laboratory tests exist for diagnosing CFS. Initial laboratory tests are useful to exclude other conditions that may mimic or may be associated with CFS.
  1. Screening laboratory tests: CBC, ESR, ALT, total protein, albumin, globulin, alkaline phosphatase, calcium, phosphorus, glucose, BUN, creatinine, electrolytes, TSH, and urinalysis are useful.
  2. Serologic tests for Epstein-Barr virus, *Candida albicans,* human herpesvirus 6, and other studies for immune cellular abnormalities are not useful; these tests are expensive and generally not recommended.
- Other tests may be indicated depending on the history and physical examination (e.g., ANA, RF in patients presenting with joint complaints or abnormalities on physical examination, Lyme titer in areas where Lyme disease is endemic).

IMAGING STUDIES

Generally not recommended unless history and physical examination indicate specific abnormalities (e.g., chest radiography in any patient suspected of TB or sarcoidosis)

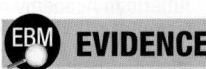

TREATMENT

NONPHARMACOLOGIC THERAPY

- Patients should be reassured that the illness is not fatal and that most patients improve over time.
- An initially supervised exercise program to preserve and increase strength is beneficial for most patients and can improve symptoms.
- Cognitive behavioral therapy trials have shown positive effects on fatigue levels, work, depression/anxiety, and social adjustment.

GENERAL Rx

Therapy is generally palliative. The following medications may be helpful; however, evidence is conflicting:
- Antidepressants: The choice of antidepressant varies with the desired side effects. Patients with difficulty sleeping or fibromyalgia-like symptoms may benefit from low-dose trazodone 50 mg hs. When sedation is not desirable, low-dose SSRIs (fluoxetine 20 mg qd) often help alleviate fatigue and associated symptoms.
- NSAIDs can be used to relieve muscle and joint pain and headaches.

"Alternative" medications (herbs, multivitamins, nutritional supplements) are very popular with many CFS patients but are generally not very helpful.

PEARLS & CONSIDERATIONS

COMMENTS

- In CFS the symptoms are serious enough to reduce daily activities by >50% in the absence of any other medically identifiable disorders.
- The suicide rate is nearly sevenfold higher in people with CFS.
- Moderate to complete recovery at 1 yr occurs in 22% to 60% of patients with CFS.

EVIDENCE

Available at www.expertconsult.com

SUGGESTED READINGS

Available at www.expertconsult.com

RELATED CONTENT

Evaluation of Fatigue (Algorithm, Section III)
Chronic Fatigue Syndrome (Patient Information)

AUTHOR: **FRED F. FERRI, M.D.**

BASIC INFORMATION

DEFINITION

Chronic inflammatory demyelinating polyneuropathy (CIDP) is a chronic autoimmune neuropathy manifesting with symmetric proximal and distal weakness with associated sensory loss along with reduced or absent reflexes. By definition, the symptoms reach nadir no earlier than 8 weeks after onset.

SYNONYMS

Chronic inflammatory demyelinating polyradiculoneuropathy
CIDP

ICD-10CM CODES
G61.81 Chronic inflammatory demyelinating polyneuritis

EPIDEMIOLOGY & DEMOGRAPHICS

PREVALENCE: 0.5/100,000 children; 1 to 2/100,000 adults
PREDOMINANT SEX AND AGE: Slightly higher in males
RISK FACTORS: It is associated with certain systemic medical conditions (see under "Differential Diagnosis"), but the association is unclear.

PHYSICAL FINDINGS & CLINICAL PRESENTATION

- Symmetrical weakness in both proximal and distal muscles that peaks after at least 8 weeks; onset may appear acute in a minority of patients, and the disease course may be either relapsing or progressive.
- Impaired sensation with distal paresthesias, poor balance, and/or impaired proprioception.
- Reduced or absent deep tendon reflexes.
- Facial, oropharyngeal, and ocular involvement in a small minority of patients.
- Autonomic dysfunction occurs very infrequently compared with Guillain-Barré syndrome.

ETIOLOGY

Immune-mediated disorder emerging from interplay of both cell-mediated and humoral immune responses directed against incompletely characterized peripheral nerve antigens. May also be associated with antecedent illness, although no infectious etiologies have been consistently linked with disease occurrence.

DIAGNOSIS

There is no universal consensus regarding diagnostic criteria for CIDP. The three most widely used criteria are the American Academy of Neurology (AAN), Saperstein, and Inflammatory Neuropathy Cause and Treatment (INCAT) criteria. See Table 1 for a complete review of differences. Of note are the following:

- The AAN and INCAT criteria are the least stringent regarding clinical criteria and require assessment of motor and sensory function in one limb. The Saperstein criteria are more stringent, requiring both symmetrical proximal and distal weakness. Therefore, a patient with distal acquired demyelinating symmetric neuropathy (DADS) could fulfill AAN and INCAT criteria for CIDP.
- All require cerebrospinal fluid analysis to assess for albuminocytologic dissociation.
- All require some features of demyelination evident on nerve conduction studies, including prolonged distal latencies and F-waves, slowed conduction velocities, and at least one nerve demonstrating partial conduction block, a feature of acquired demyelination.
- INCAT criteria do not require a nerve biopsy.

DIFFERENTIAL DIAGNOSIS

- Other demyelinating neuropathies such as the following:
  1. Distal acquired demyelinating symmetric neuropathy (DADS)
  2. Multifocal motor neuropathy (MMN)
  3. Multifocal acquired demyelinating sensory and motor neuropathy (MADSAM; Lewis-Sumner syndrome)
- Inherited neuropathies: Charcot-Marie-Tooth subtypes
- Metabolic neuropathies: diabetes, uremia
- Paraneoplastic and neoplastic neuropathies: lymphoma and carcinoma
- Neuropathy associated with monoclonal gammopathy:
  1. Polyneuropathy, organomegaly, endocrinopathy, monoclonal gammopathy, and skin changes (POEMS) syndrome
  2. Multiple myeloma
  3. Monoclonal gammopathy of undetermined significance (MGUS)
  4. Waldenström's macroglobulinemia
- Neuropathy associated with infectious diseases: HIV and leprosy
- Neuropathy associated with systemic inflammatory or immune-mediated diseases:
  1. Sarcoidosis
  2. Amyloidosis
  3. Vasculitis: PAN, Behçet's, Sjögren's, cryoglobulinemia, lupus, Castleman's disease, granulomatosis with polyangiitis (formerly Wegener's granulomatosis), and eosinophilic granulomatosis with polyangiitis (formerly Churg-Strauss)
- Toxic neuropathies: ETOH, acrylamide, drugs (platinum-based agents, amiodarone, tacrolimus, perhexiline)

WORKUP

Nerve conduction studies and EMG to assess for demyelinating polyneuropathy with features of acquired demyelination (temporal dispersion) and conduction block (Fig. 1)

LABORATORY TESTS

- CSF analysis to assess for albuminocytologic dissociation (i.e., elevated protein with normal cell count), along with appropriate laboratory studies to exclude associated conditions.

TABLE 1 Diagnostic Criteria

Feature	American Academy of Neurology (AAN) Criteria	Saperstein Criteria	Inflammatory Neuropathy Cause and Treatment Criteria
Clinical involvement	Motor dysfunction, sensory dysfunction of >1 limb or both	Major: Symmetric proximal and distal weakness; minor: exclusively symmetrical distal weakness or sensory loss	Progressive or relapsing motor and sensory dysfunction of >1 limb
Time course	≥2 mo	≥2 mo	≥2 mo
Reflexes	Reduced or absent	Reduced or absent	Reduced or absent
Electro-diagnostics	Any 3 of the following 4 criteria: partial conduction block of ≥1 motor nerve, reduced velocity of ≥2 motor nerves, prolonged distal latency of ≥2 motor nerves, or prolonged F-waves of ≥2 motor nerves	2 of the 4 AAN electrodiagnostic criteria	Partial conduction block of ≥2 motor nerves and abnormal conduction velocity or distal latency or F-wave latency in 1 other nerve; or, in the absence of partial conduction block, abnormal conduction velocity, distal latency, or F-wave latency in 3 motor nerves; or electrodiagnostic abnormalities indicating demyelination in 2 nerves and histologic evidence of demyelination
CSF analysis	WBC count <10, negative CSF VDRL, and elevated protein (supportive)	Protein >45, WBC <10 (supportive)	CSF recommended but not mandatory
Biopsy findings	Evidence of demyelination and remyelination	Predominant features of demyelination; inflammation (not required)	Not mandatory (except in cases with electrodiagnostic abnormalities in only 2 motor nerves)

- Nerve biopsy specimens (rarely done now) also reveal signs of demyelination with variable degrees of inflammation and secondary axonal loss.

IMAGING STUDIES

MRI with/without gadolinium may show enlargement and enhancement of the proximal nerve root segments (Figs. 2 and 3).

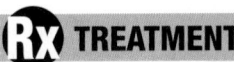 TREATMENT

Therapies are directed at blocking the underlying immune processes to arrest demyelination and inflammation and to prevent secondary axonal degeneration. The first-line agents for immunomodulatory therapy are intravenous immunoglobulin (IVIg), plasmapheresis and corticosteroids. There is no difference in efficacy between these three treatment modalities. Azathioprine, mycophenolate mofetil, cyclophosphamide, rituximab, and cyclosporine may be used as secondary agents.

NONPHARMACOLOGIC THERAPY

Orthotics or braces may be useful for significant distal weakness.

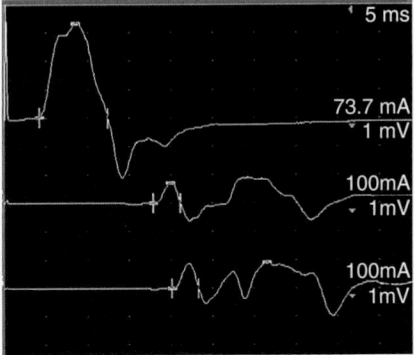

FIG. 1 Conduction block.

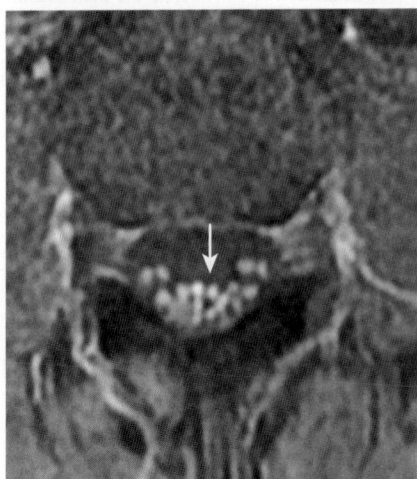

FIG. 2 Contrast-enhanced MRI shows enhancement of nerve roots.

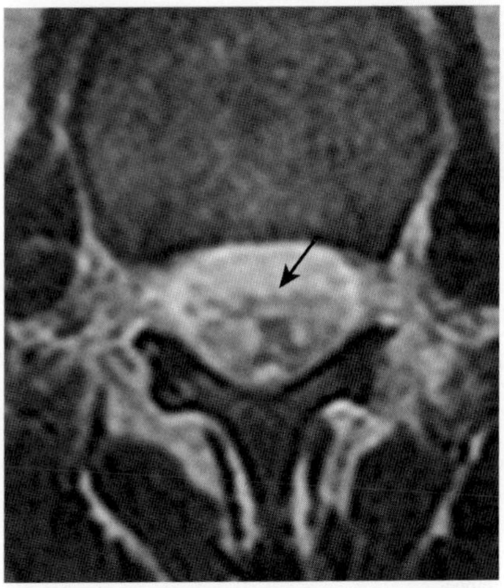

ACUTE GENERAL Rx

- Prednisone 60 mg per day or 100 mg every other day
- IVIg 2 g/kg divided over 2 to 5 days
- Plasmapheresis (5 to 6 exchanges)

CHRONIC Rx

- Oral prednisone: 1 mg/kg daily starting dose, typically changed to every other day after 1 month or when strength plateaus. Reduce by 10 mg per month until dose reaches 20 mg every other day; then reduce by 5 mg per month. Supplement calcium and vitamin D. Patients should receive a tuberculin skin test prior to administration as well as surveillance exams for cataracts, glaucoma, diabetes, and gastroesophageal reflux.
- Dexamethasone: PREDICT study compared dexamethasone 40 mg daily for 4 days per month with prednisone 60 mg daily for 2 months and then tapered over 27 weeks. No difference in efficacy was found between the two groups. However, pulse steroids were associated with less weight gain, fewer cushingoid features, and more sleep and psychological disturbances.
- Pulse Solu-Medrol: no standard regimen. However, 1000 mg for 3 days can be used, followed by 1000 mg per week with the goal of reduced frequency to every 2 to 12 weeks.
- IVIg: 0.4 to 1 g/kg administered every 2 to 3 weeks, with adjustment based on therapeutic response. Baseline IgA level, renal function, and coagulation studies should be assessed.
- Mycophenolate mofetil: Initial dose of 500 mg every other day; increase to 2 g orally divided twice daily in 2 to 4 weeks. Complete blood counts and liver panel should be assessed monthly for the first 3 months, then every 3 months thereafter. May cause GI upset.
- Azathioprine: Initial dose of 25 to 50 mg every other day; increase to 100 mg twice daily in 4 weeks. Complete blood counts and liver panel should be assessed for first 3 months, then every 3 months thereafter. Idiosyncratic reaction of fever and GI upset may occur.

FIG. 3 T2-weighted axial MRI shows enlarged nerve roots.

- Cyclophosphamide: used for severe cases. 1000 mg/m^2 monthly for 6 months (moderate dose) or 50 mg/kg daily for 4 days (high dose).
- Other treatments used (case reports/anecdotal evidence): etanercept, rituximab, tacrolimus, interferon beta-1a.

PROGNOSIS

- Although available data on the long-term prognosis of patients are limited, the majority of patients improve and reach stability. Relapses may occur in 50% of patients. A small minority of patients remain severely disabled, and up to 11% die from the disease.
- Patients with CIDP associated with IgM monoclonal gammopathy often respond poorly to treatment.
- Younger age, female gender, and relapsing-remitting course may portend a more favorable prognosis. Four-limb weakness at onset and prominent axonal loss on EMG may signify poor prognosis.

REFERRAL

- Neurologist, physical therapy/occupational therapy, orthotics

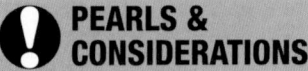 PEARLS & CONSIDERATIONS

- Patients are compliant with azathioprine treatment if MCV >100.
- Always place PPD prior to initiation of steroid treatment.
- Consider trimethoprim-sulfamethoxazole 3 times weekly in patients taking steroids and other immunosuppressant agents for *Pneumocystis* pneumonia prophylaxis (especially in patients with coexisting lung disease).
- Look for acquired features of demyelination on nerve conduction studies (conduction block and temporal dispersion).
- Examine CSF for albuminocytologic dissociation (high CSF protein with normal cell count).
- CIDP can present like Guillain-Barré syndrome. Sensory symptoms and proximal weakness are more common in CIDP, and symptoms continue to evolve over more than 8 weeks.

PATIENT/FAMILY EDUCATION

CIDP is a chronic illness usually characterized by a relapsing-remitting course that typically responds well to treatment. Early referral to a neurologist is important, and education on steroid side effects and mitigating factors is paramount.

SUGGESTED READINGS

Available at www.expertconsult.com

AUTHORS: **CHLOE MANDER NUNNELEY, M.D.**, **JOSEPH S. KASS, M.D., J.D**, and **JOHN SLADKY, M.D.**

C

Diseases and Disorders

I

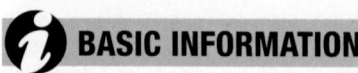

BASIC INFORMATION

DEFINITION

Chronic kidney disease (CKD) is diagnosed when there is evidence for more than 3 months of **kidney damage** (urine albumin >30 mg/g creatinine, hematuria, or parenchymal abnormalities) and/or **decreased kidney function** (glomerular filtration rate, GFR <60 ml/min/1.73 m^2). CKD is characterized by accumulation of metabolic waste products in blood, electrolyte abnormalities, mineral and bone disorders, and anemia. The manifestations of CKD are summarized in Table 1.

SYNONYMS

CKD
Chronic renal failure
CRF
Chronic renal insufficiency
CRI

ICD-10CM CODES
N18.1 Chronic kidney disease, stage 1
N18.2 Chronic kidney disease, stage 2
N18.3 Chronic kidney disease, stage 3
N18.4 Chronic kidney disease, stage 4
N18.5 Chronic kidney disease, stage 5
N18.6 End-stage renal disease
N18.9 Chronic kidney disease, unspecified

EPIDEMIOLOGY & DEMOGRAPHICS

- Prevalence of CKD in the U.S. is approximately 13%. More than 26 million Americans have CKD stages 1 through 5.
- Incidence of end-stage renal disease (ESRD) is 7% to 9% per year in the U.S., primarily due to diabetes mellitus and hypertension, the leading risk factors for CKD. Annually, 3 in 10,000 persons develop ESRD, and more than 100,000 patients begin dialysis each year.
- In the U.S., nearly 400,000 people per year receive dialysis treatments for ESRD with an annual average cost per patient of approximately $70,000.
- Kidney transplantation is the best option for kidney replacement therapy, but many patients are not eligible for transplantation.

PHYSICAL FINDINGS & CLINICAL PRESENTATION

- Skin pallor, ecchymosis.
- Sleep disorder.
- Hypertension.
- Edema, leg cramps, restless legs, peripheral neuropathy.
- Emotional lability, depression, decreased cognitive function.
- Clinical presentation varies with the degree of kidney disease and its underlying etiology. Common symptoms are generalized fatigue, nausea, anorexia, pruritus (Fig. E1), sleep disturbances, smell and taste disturbances, hiccups, and seizures.
- Manifestations of uremic encephalopathy are described in Table 2.

ETIOLOGY

- Diabetes (43.2%), hypertension (23%), chronic glomerulonephritis (12.3%)
- Failed kidney transplant
- Polycystic kidney disease (2.9%)
- Interstitial nephritis (e.g., drug hypersensitivity, analgesic nephropathy)
- Obstructive nephropathies (e.g., nephrolithiasis, prostatic disease)
- Vascular diseases (renal artery stenosis, hypertensive nephrosclerosis)
- Autoimmune diseases

Dx DIAGNOSIS

- Although GFR is considered the best overall index of kidney function, it is not the only measure of kidney health that should be considered. When applying estimated glomerular filtration rate (eGFR) equations, one

---

TABLE 1 Pathophysiology of Chronic Kidney Disease

Manifestation	Mechanisms
Accumulation of nitrogenous waste products	Decrease in glomerular filtration rate
Acidosis	Decreased ammonia synthesis Impaired bicarbonate reabsorption Decreased net acid excretion
Sodium retention	Excessive renin production Oliguria
Sodium wasting	Solute diuresis Tubular damage
Urinary concentrating defect	Solute diuresis Tubular damage
Hyperkalemia	Decrease in glomerular filtration rate Metabolic acidosis Excessive potassium intake Hyporeninemic hypoaldosteronism
Renal osteodystrophy	Impaired renal production of 1,25-dihydroxycholecalciferol Hyperphosphatemia Hypocalcemia Secondary hyperparathyroidism
Growth retardation	Inadequate caloric intake Renal osteodystrophy Metabolic acidosis Anemia Growth hormone resistance
Anemia	Decreased erythropoietin production Iron deficiency Folate deficiency Vitamin B$_{12}$ deficiency Decreased erythrocyte survival
Bleeding tendency	Defective platelet function
Infection	Defective granulocyte function Impaired cellular immune functions Indwelling dialysis catheters
Neurologic symptoms (fatigue, poor concentration, headache, drowsiness, memory loss, seizures, peripheral neuropathy)	Uremic factor(s) Aluminum toxicity Hypertension
Gastrointestinal symptoms (feeding intolerance, abdominal pain)	Gastroesophageal reflux Decreased gastrointestinal motility
Hypertension	Volume overload Excessive renin production
Hyperlipidemia	Decreased plasma lipoprotein lipase activity
Pericarditis, cardiomyopathy	Uremic factor(s) Hypertension Fluid overload
Glucose intolerance	Tissue insulin resistance

From Kliegman RM et al: *Nelson textbook of pediatrics*, ed 19, Philadelphia, 2011, Saunders.

TABLE 2 Criteria for Definition of Chronic Kidney Disease

Kidney damage for ≥3 months, as defined by structural or functional abnormalities of the kidney, with or without decreased GFR, that can lead to decreased GFR, manifest by either:
- Pathologic abnormalities
- Markers of kidney damage, including abnormalities in the composition of blood or urine, or abnormalities in imaging tests
- GFR <60 ml/min/1.73 m^2 for ≥3 months, with or without kidney damage

GFR, Glomerular filtration rate.
From Floege J et al: *Comprehensive clinical nephrology*, ed 5, Philadelphia, 2015, Saunders.

must appreciate that CKD is defined over a 3-month interval. Therefore, the serum creatinine must be repeated and trended to establish a diagnosis of CKD in individuals who must also be in a steady state of creatinine generation or production.

WORKUP

- Laboratory evaluation and imaging studies can identify reversible causes of acute GFR decline (e.g., volume depletion, urinary tract obstruction, heart failure)
- Ultrasound evaluation of the kidneys often reveals small kidneys (<9 cm sagittal length) with increased echogenicity

- Kidney biopsy is generally not considered when kidneys are small or CKD is advanced.

LABORATORY TESTS

- Elevated blood urea nitrogen (BUN), creatinine, and low GFR, are the best overall indicators of kidney function. GFR is estimated by multivariable (creatinine, age, sex, race) prediction equations normalized to body surface area. GFR calculators are available online (http://www.kidney.org/kls/professionals/gfr_calculator.cfm).
- Urinalysis may reveal proteinuria, hematuria, or formed elements such as casts.

- Serum chemistries: elevated BUN and creatinine, hyperkalemia, hyperuricemia, hypocalcemia, hyperphosphatemia, hyperglycemia, decreased bicarbonate.
- Urinary protein excretion. A urine total protein-to-creatinine ratio >1000 mg/g generally indicates glomerular disease.
- Special studies: serum and urine immunoelectrophoresis (multiple myeloma), antinuclear antibody (i.e., systemic lupus erythematosus).
- Cystatin C measurement or direct glomerular filtration clearance methods may confirm CKD in situations when serum creatinine–based GFR equations are less accurate (e.g., HIV, malnutrition) or more precise measurement is desired (e.g., kidney transplant organ donation).

IMAGING STUDIES

- Ultrasound of kidneys for size measurements and to rule out obstruction.
- Plain radiographs of the aorta and extremities ordered for other reasons may reveal vascular and extraskeletal calcification (Fig. E2).

CLASSIFICATION

The 2012 Kidney Disease: International Global Outcomes classifies CKD with a CGA format: **C**ause (etiology), **G**FR (G1 to G5), and **A**lbuminuria (A1 to A3) by urine albumin-to-creatinine ratio (Table 3). This format is now recommended when documenting and discussing CKD. Table 4 depicts how CKD prognosis worsens with either increasing levels of proteinuria or declining GFR.

Diseases and Disorders

I

TABLE 3 Classification of Chronic Kidney Disease Based on GFR

CKD Stage	Definition
1	Normal or increased GFR; some evidence of kidney damage reflected by microalbuminuria, proteinuria, and hematuria as well as radiologic or histologic changes
2	Mild decrease in GFR (89 to 60 ml/min per 1.73 m^2) with some evidence of kidney damage reflected by albuminuria, proteinuria, and hematuria as well as radiologic or histologic changes
3	GFR 59 to 30 ml/min per 1.73 m^2
3A	GFR 59 to 45 ml/min per 1.73 m^2
3B	GFR 44 to 30 ml/min per 1.73 m^2
4	GFR 29 to 15 ml/min per 1.73 m^2
5	GFR <15 ml/min per 1.73 m^2; when renal replacement therapy in the form of dialysis or transplantation must be considered to sustain life

Classification and prognosis of chronic kidney disease from 2012 KDIGO guidelines.
CKD, Chronic kidney disease; *GFR,* glomerular filtration rate; *KDIGO,* Kidney Disease: Improving Global Outcomes.
From Floege J et al: *Comprehensive clinical nephrology,* ed 5, Philadelphia, 2010, Saunders.

TABLE 4 KDOQI US Commentary on the 2012 KDIGO Clinical Practice Guideline for the Evaluation and Management of CKD

Prognosis of CKD by GFR and albuminuria categories: KDIGO 2012			Persistent albuminuria categories description and range		
			A1	**A2**	**A3**
			Normal to mildly increased	Moderately increased	Severely increased
			<30 mg/g <3 mg/mmol	30–300 mg/g 3–30 mg/mmol	>300 mg/g >30 mg/mmol
GFR categories (ml/min/ 1.73 m^2) description and range	**G1**	Normal or high	90			
	G2	Mildly decreased	60–89			
	G3a	Mildly to moderately decreased	45–59			
	G3b	Moderately to severely decreased	30–44			
	G4	Severely decreased	15–29			
	G5	Kidney failure	<15			

Green, low risk (if no other markers of kidney disease, no CKD); *Yellow,* moderately increased risk; *Orange,* high risk; *Red,* very high risk.
American Journal of Kidney Diseases. Inker LA, Astor BC, Fox, CH, et al. 63(5):713-735, 2014.

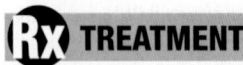
Rx TREATMENT

Management varies according to stage (Table 5).

NONPHARMACOLOGIC THERAPY

- Provide adequate nutrition and calories (147–168 kJ/kg/day energy intake, mainly from carbohydrate and polyunsaturated fats). Table 6 describes nutritional recommendations in CKD. Referral to a dietitian for nutritional therapy for patients with GFR <50 ml/min/1.73 m^2 is recommended and is a Medicare-covered service.

- Dietary restriction of sodium (~100 mmol/day), potassium (≤60 mmol/day), and phosphorus (<800 mg/day).
- Blood pressure: Target blood pressure of ≤140/90 mm Hg if CKD (diabetic and nondiabetic) and urine albumin excretion ≤30 mg/24 hr. If CKD (diabetic and nondiabetic) and albumin excretion >30 mg/24 hr are present, consider a target blood pressure ≤130/80 mm Hg.
- Adjust medication doses for reduced GFR.
- Restrict fluid intake if significant edema or hyponatremia (serum Na <130 mEq/L) is present.

- Resistance exercise training can preserve lean body mass, improve nutritional status, and muscle function in patients with moderate CKD.
- Avoid radiocontrast agents. Prophylactic volume expansion with sodium chloride or sodium bicarbonate before dye exposure is equally effective.
- Smoking cessation.
- Prompt referral to a nephrologist is helpful. Late evaluation of patients with CKD is associated with greater burden and severity of comorbid disease and complications

---

TABLE 5 Management Plan for Patients with Chronic Kidney Disease, According to Stage

KDOQI Classification	GFR (ml/min)	Typical Serum Creatinine in 65-kg Subject	Consequences	Actions to Consider
3	30-59	2 mg/dl (170 μmol/L)	Hypertension, secondary hyperparathyroidism	6 monthly eGFR initially 12 monthly eGFR if stable Annual Hb, K$^+$, Ca, P Treat hypertension Immunize against hepatitis B
4	15-29	4 mg/dl (350 μmol/L)	*Plus* anemia, hyperphosphatemia	3 monthly eGFR initially 6 monthly eGFR if stable 6 monthly Hb, K$^+$, Ca, P, and PTH Start phosphate-restricted diet and phosphate binders Correct vitamin D deficiency Start vitamin D analogue Plan renal replacement therapy, including vascular access
5	<15	8 mg/dl (700 μmol/L)	*Plus* sodium and water retention, anorexia, vomiting, reduced higher mental function	Plan elective start of dialysis or pre-emptive renal transplant
5	<5	17 mg/dl (1500 μmol/L)	*Plus* pulmonary edema, coma, fits, metabolic acidosis, hyperkalemia, death	Start dialysis or provide palliative care

The table gives a rough guide to the level of serum creatinine corresponding to each stage of CKD in a typical 65-kg subject and shows the approximate timing of the anticipated clinical problems and interventions required as CKD progresses. At each stage, the action plan for the previous CKD stage should be followed if it has not already been initiated. *eGFR,* Estimated glomerular filtration rate; *PTH,* parathyroid hormone.

From Floege J et al: *Comprehensive clinical nephrology,* ed 4, Philadelphia, 2010, Saunders.

TABLE 6 Nutritional Recommendations in Renal Disease

Daily Intake	Predialysis CKD	Hemodialysis	Peritoneal Dialysis
Protein (g/kg ideal BW) (see KDOQI for estimation of adjusted edema-free body weight)	0.6-1.0 Level depends on the view of the nephrologist 1.0 for nephrotic syndrome	1.1-1.2	1.0-1.3
		This is a broad recommendation as protein intake would be individualized for the patient's nutritional status, serum phosphate levels, and dialysis adequacy	
Energy (kcal/kg BW)	35 (<60 yr) 30-35 (>60 yr)	35 (<60 yr) 30-35 (>60 yr)	35 including dialysate calories (<60 yr) 30-35 including dialysate calories (<60 yr)
Sodium (mmol)	<100 (more if salt wasting)	<100	<100
Potassium	Reduce if hyperkalemic	Reduce if hyperkalemic	Reduce if hyperkalemic; potassium restriction is generally not required
	If hyperkalemic, advice will take the form of decreasing certain foods (e.g., some fruits and vegetables) and giving information about cooking methods		
Phosphorus	Reduce; level dependent on protein intake		
	Advice will take the form of reducing certain foods (e.g., dairy, offal, some shellfish) and giving information about the timing of binders with high-phosphorus meals and snacks		
Calcium	In CKD stages 3-5, total intake of elemental calcium (including dietary calcium) should not exceed 2000 mg/day	Total intake of elemental calcium (including dietary calcium) should not exceed 2000 mg/day	Total intake of elemental calcium (including dietary calcium) should not exceed 2000 mg/day

Recommendations are for typical patients but should always be individualized on the basis of clinical, biochemical, and anthropometric indices.

BW, Body weight; *CKD,* chronic kidney disease; *CRF,* chronic renal failure; *KDOQI,* Kidney Disease Outcomes Quality Initiative.

From Floege J et al: *Comprehensive clinical nephrology,* ed 5, Philadelphia, 2015, Saunders.

TABLE 7 Suggested Criteria for Referral of Patients with Chronic Kidney Disease to a Nephrologist

New Diagnosis	Stage 3	Stage 4
eGFR <30 ml/min/per 1.73 m²	eGFR falling by >4 ml/min per year	eGFR <20 ml/min per 1.73 m²
Hemoglobin <11 g/dl	eGFR <50 ml/min in patient younger than 50 years	eGFR falling by >4 ml/min per year
K⁺ >6 mmol/L	Hemoglobin <11 g/dl	Hemoglobin <11 g/dl
Ca <2.1 mmol/L	K⁺ >6 mmol/L	K⁺ >6 mmol/L
Pi >1.5 mmol/L	Ca <2.1 mmol/L	Ca <2.1 mmol/L
PTH >3× upper limit normal	Pi >1.5 mmol/L	Pi >1.5 mmol/L
Hematuria		PTH >3× upper limit normal
Urine ACR >30 mg/mmol		
Suspected renovascular disease		

ACR, Albumin to creatinine ratio; *eGFR*, estimated glomerular filtration rate; *PTH*, parathyroid hormone.
From Floege J et al: *Comprehensive clinical nephrology*, ed 5, Philadelphia, 2015, Saunders.

TABLE 8 When to Initiate Dialysis

Indications for early start on dialysis
- Intractable fluid overload
- Intractable hyperkalemia
- Malnutrition due to uremia
- Uremic neurologic dysfunction
- Uremic serositis
- Functional deterioration otherwise unexplained

Uremic cognitive dysfunction can affect learning

Therefore, home-based self-dialysis may need to start earlier than center-assisted dialysis.

Start of dialysis may be delayed if patient is

asymptomatic, awaiting imminent kidney transplant, awaiting imminent placement of permanent HD or PD access, or, after appropriate education, has chosen conservative therapy.

If start of dialysis is delayed,

patient should be reevaluated regularly to see if dialysis has become necessary.

Patients who choose PD

should not be required to have HD access placed, but venous sites for possible future HD access in arms should be preserved since HD may be required in the future.

Incremental start on PD may be considered if there is significant residual renal function.

Nephrologists should consider conservative (non dialysis) treatment of kidney failure an integral part of their clinical practice.

HD, Hemodialysis; *PD*, peritoneal dialysis.
Modified from NKF KDOQI Clinical Practice Guideline for initiation of dialysis. http://www.kidney.org/professional/Kdoqi/guideline_upHD_PD_VA/pd_rec1.htm. From Floege J et al: *Comprehensive clinical nephrology*, ed 5, Philadelphia, 2015, Saunders.

and lesser survival. Suggested criteria for nephrology referral are described in Table 7.
- Referral for kidney transplantation in selected patients.

GENERAL Rx

Angiotensin–converting-enzyme inhibitors (ACEIs) and angiotensin II receptor blockers (ARBs) reduce proteinuria and slow progression of CKD, especially in hypertensive diabetic patients. The combination of ACEI and ARB is not recommended due to increased risks of hyperkalemia, hypotension, and acute kidney injury. Increases of serum creatinine of up to 30% greater than baseline within 3 months of initiating ACEI or ARB therapy may be acceptable.
- Addition of chlorthalidone to CKD patients with difficult-to-treat hypertension may reduce blood pressure and proteinuria. Consistent with loop diuretic therapy, successful blood pressure–lowering is associated with weight loss and the complication of hypokalemia.
- Initiation of dialysis:
  1. Urgent indications: uremic pericarditis, neuropathy, neuromuscular abnormalities, CHF, hyperkalemia, seizures
  2. Other indications: GFR 10–15 mL/min; progressive anorexia, weight loss, disordered sleep, pruritus, uncontrolled fluid gain with hypertension and signs of heart failure.
  3. General indications for initiation of dialysis are summarized in Table 8. Suggested steps for resolving conflict in the shared decision-making process regarding dialysis initiation are described (Fig. 3). Early initiation of dialysis when the GFR is 10–15 mL/min per 1.73 m² does not enhance survival compared with a symptom-driven strategy for initiation of dialysis at eGFR <8–10 ml/min per 1.73 m².
- Erythropoiesis-stimulating agents (e.g., epoetins alfa and beta, darbepoetin alfa) are administered to reduce transfusions in anemic CKD patients. A target hemoglobin of 9–11 g/dl is reasonable to avoid premature and excessive ESA use. Higher hemoglobin values have been associated with adverse cardiovascular events. Iron sufficiency should be present, defined as transferrin saturation >20% and ferritin >100 ng/ml, before ESA therapy is initiated.
- Diuretics for edema or cardiopulmonary congestion.
- ACEIs or ARBs retard progression of CKD and lower blood pressure, but may reduce GFR and renal potassium excretion.

- Treat metabolic acidosis with oral sodium bicarbonate to attain a goal serum HCO₃ level of 22 to 26 mEq/L.
- Statin or a combination of statin and ezetimibe is recommended in adults aged ≥50 years with eGFRs <60 mL/min/1.73 m². Lipid management focuses on absolute risk for coronary events, and there are no target cholesterol levels.
- Therapy of mineral and bone disease in CKD is geared toward normalizing serum phosphorus concentration. Calcitriol and vitamin D analogs should be reserved for patients with CKD stages 4-5 and severe and progressive hyperparathyroidism.
- Dietary phosphate restriction is recommended for nearly all CKD patients. For additional management of hyperphosphatemia, phosphorus binders are recommended. Calcium-based phosphate binders, although inexpensive, should be restricted if total serum calcium is >10.2 mg/dl. Sevelamer carbonate and lanthanum carbonate are effective as phosphate binders but are more expensive. Two iron-based phosphate-binding agents have recently been approved by the FDA.
- General considerations in the continuing assessment of the CKD patient are described in Table 9.
- A sequential approach to the uremic patient with pruritus is described in Fig. E4.

DISPOSITION

- Prognosis is influenced by CKD stage and burden of comorbid illness. Late referral of patients to a nephrologist is associated with greater morbidity and mortality. Despite recommendations for early referral, nearly two thirds of CKD patients are referred late.
- Genetic susceptibility for CKD is prominent in African Americans. Apolipoprotein E2 allele status predicts CKD progression, independent of diabetes, race, lipid, and nonlipid factors.
- Kidney transplantation in selected patients improves survival. Whereas the 2-year kidney graft survival rate for living related donor transplantations is >80%, the 2-year graft survival rate for cadaveric donor transplantation is nearly 70%.
- Principles underlying withdrawal from dialysis treatment are described in Table 10.

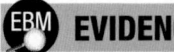 **EVIDENCE**

Available at www.expertconsult.com

SUGGESTED READINGS

Available at www.expertconsult.com

AUTHORS: **SNIGDHA T. REDDY, M.D., BHAVIN C. PATEL, M.D.,** and **JERRY YEE, M.D.**

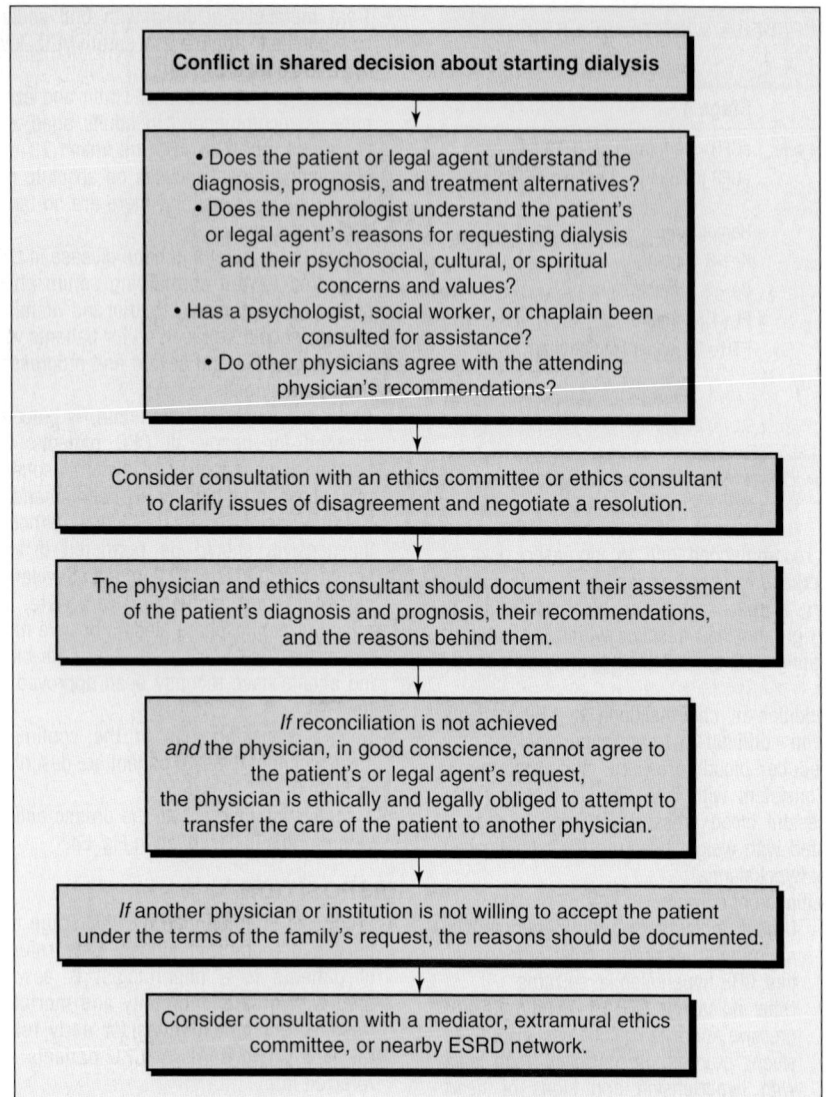

FIG. 3 Suggested steps for resolving conflict in the shared decision about starting dialysis. (From Floege J et al: *Comprehensive clinical nephrology*, ed 5, Philadelphia, 2015, Saunders.)

TABLE 9 Continuing Assessment of the Chronic Kidney Disease Patient

Kidney Function

Has kidney function declined?

Has kidney function declined at the predicted rate?

If not, are there exacerbating factors?

Should dialysis be started?

Are there life-threatening complications?
Pericarditis
Fluid overload
Resistant hypertension
Hyperkalemia
Uncompensated metabolic acidosis

Should access be created or transplantation planned?

Supportive Treatment

Can salt, potassium, and fluid balance be improved by diet or diuretics?

Is the phosphate controlled?

Is the dose of vitamin D compound appropriate?

Should erythropoietin (EPO) be prescribed?

Are nutritional supplements needed?

Does the patient need counseling?

Questions to be posed in evaluation of the patient.
From Floege J et al: *Comprehensive clinical nephrology*, ed 5, Philadelphia, 2010, Saunders.

TABLE 10 Principles Underlying Withdrawal of Dialysis

The ultimate responsibility for the decision rests with the physician, not the relative.

The patient's interests and dignity should be protected at all times.

The process should not be rushed. If there is any doubt about the correctness of the decision, treatment should continue.

There should be an open discussion among the multidisciplinary team to avoid any damaging disagreements.

The psychological needs of the health care team should not be overlooked.

Palliative care must be given in the most appropriate environment, e.g., a hospice or, ideally, the patient's own home.

From Floege J et al: *Comprehensive clinical nephrology*, ed 5, Philadelphia, 2010, Saunders.

BASIC INFORMATION

DEFINITION

Chronic obstructive pulmonary disease (COPD) is an inflammatory respiratory disease usually caused by exposure to tobacco smoke. It is characterized by the presence of airflow limitation that is not fully reversible. The pathophysiology of COPD is related to enhanced inflammatory response to noxious particles and gases, chronic airway irritation, mucus production, and pulmonary scarring and changes in pulmonary vasculature.

Acute exacerbations and comorbidities contribute to the overall severity and prognosis of the disease in individual patients.

Traditionally, COPD was described as encompassing *emphysema*, characterized by loss of lung elasticity and destruction of lung parenchyma with enlargement of air spaces, and *chronic bronchitis*, characterized by obstruction of small airways and productive cough >3 months for more than 2 successive years. These terms are no longer included in the formal definition of COPD, although they are still used clinically. Although emphysema and chronic bronchitis are commonly associated with COPD, neither is required to make the diagnosis.

An overlap syndrome known as ACOS (asthma-COPD overlap syndrome), characterized by persistent airflow limitation with several features associated with asthma and several features associated with COPD, has been gaining recognition and may have treatment and mortality implications (Global Initiative for Chronic Obstructive Lung Disease (GOLD) and Global Initiative for Asthma (GINA) consensus statement).

SYNONYMS

COPD
Emphysema
Chronic bronchitis

ICD-10CM CODES
J44.9 Chronic obstructive pulmonary
disease, unspecified
J43.9 Emphysema, unspecified

EPIDEMIOLOGY & DEMOGRAPHICS

- COPD affects 14% of U.S. adults aged 40 to 79 years.
- Between 10% and 20% of COPD in the U.S. is due to occupational or other exposure to chemical vapors, irritants, and fumes; 80% to 90% is due to cigarette smoking.
- COPD is the third leading cause of death in the U.S.
- Highest incidence is in males >40 yr.
- 16 million office visits, 500,000 hospitalizations, 120,000 deaths annually, and >$18 billion in direct health care costs annually can be attributed to COPD.
- Patients with COPD living in isolated rural areas of the U.S. are at greater risk for COPD exacerbation-related mortality than those living in urban areas, independent of hospital rurality and volume.

PHYSICAL FINDINGS & CLINICAL PRESENTATION

- Patients with COPD have historically been classically subdivided in two major groups based on their phenotype
  1. *Blue bloaters* are patients with chronic bronchitis; the name is derived from the bluish tinge of the skin (as a result of chronic hypoxemia and hypercapnia) and from the frequent presence of peripheral edema (from cor pulmonale); chronic cough with production of large amounts of sputum is characteristic.
  2. *Pink puffers* are patients with emphysema; they have a cachectic appearance but pink skin color (adequate oxygen saturation); shortness of breath is manifested by pursed-lip breathing and use of accessory muscles of respiration.
- COPD may present with combinations of the following signs and symptoms:
  1. Cyanosis, chronic cough (usually productive but may be intermittent and may be unproductive), tachypnea, tachycardia.
  2. Dyspnea (persistent, progressive), pursed-lip breathing with use of accessory muscles for respiration, decreased breath sounds, wheezing.
  3. Chronic sputum production.
  4. Chest wall abnormalities (hyperinflation, "barrel chest," protruding abdomen).
  5. Flattening of diaphragm.
- Systemic manifestations and comorbidities of COPD are described in Table 1.
- Acute exacerbation of COPD is mainly a clinical diagnosis and generally manifests with worsening dyspnea, increase in sputum purulence, and increase in sputum volume. Respiratory symptom status, however, is not a reliable indicator of the presence of airflow obstruction. Individuals with normal spirometric values may report respiratory symptoms, whereas individuals who have severe to very severe airflow obstruction by spirometry may report no symptoms.

TABLE 1 Systemic Manifestations and Comorbidities of COPD

Cardiovascular	Infarction
	Arrhythmia
	Congestive heart failure
	Aortic aneurysm
Hypercoagulability	Stroke
	Pulmonary embolism
	Deep vein thrombosis
	Atrophy
Systemic	Weight loss
	Osteoporosis
	Skin wrinkling
	Anemia
	Fluid retention
Lung cancer	Depression

From Mason RJ: *Murray & Nadel's textbook of respiratory medicine*, 5th ed, Philadelphia, 2010, Saunders.

Individuals with sedentary lifestyles may underestimate their symptoms and careful history taking is important to elicit symptoms suggestive of COPD.

ETIOLOGY

- Tobacco exposure
- Occupational exposure to pulmonary toxins (e.g., dust, noxious gases, vapors, fumes, cadmium, coal, silica). The industries with the highest exposure risk are plastics, leather, rubber, and textiles.
- Atmospheric pollution.
- Alpha-1-antitrypsin deficiency (rare; <1% of COPD patients).

DIAGNOSIS

DIFFERENTIAL DIAGNOSIS

- Heart failure (HF)
- Asthma
- Tuberculosis, other respiratory infections
- Bronchiectasis
- Anemia
- Cystic fibrosis
- Neoplasm
- Pulmonary embolism
- Obliterative bronchiolitis
- Diffuse panbronchiolitis
- Sleep apnea, obstructive
- Hypothyroidism <50% predicted
- Neuromuscular disease

DIAGNOSTIC WORKUP

Chest x-ray is seldom diagnostic but useful to visualize significant hyperinflation and to exclude alternative diagnosis (e.g., CHF, TB).

Pulmonary function testing (spirometry).

Oxygen saturation and arterial blood gases (useful in selected patients with FEV_1 <50% predicted, with acute exacerbation or hypoxia by pulse oximetry).

Alpha-1-antitrypsin deficiency screening may be useful in whites with suspected COPD and no clear risk factors.

LABORATORY TESTS

- CBC: generally not helpful, may reveal leukocytosis with left shift during acute exacerbation and secondary polycythemia in COPD with significant, chronic hypoxia. Recent trials have shown that eosinophilia in COPD patients predicts response to corticosteroids. Eosinophilia may also be found in an acute exacerbation in an asthma-COPD overlap syndrome.
- Sputum may be purulent with bacterial respiratory tract infections. Sputum staining and cultures are usually reserved for cases refractory to antibiotic therapy.
- Arterial blood gases: normocapnia, mild to moderate hypoxemia may be present. ABGs and pulse oximetry are usually used to determine if a patient is a candidate for long-term oxygen therapy or if hypercapnia is present (ABGs).
- Spirometry pulmonary function testing (PFT) with measurement of forced vital

capacity (FVC) and forced expiratory volume in 1 s (FEV_1). Spirometry should be obtained to diagnose airflow obstruction in clinically stable patients with respiratory symptoms. It should not be used to screen for airflow obstruction in individuals without respiratory symptoms. Spirometry reveals that the primary physiologic abnormality in COPD is an accelerated decline in FEV_1 from the normal rate in adults >30 yr of approximately 30 mL/yr to nearly 60 mL/yr. PFT results in COPD reveal abnormal diffusing capacity, increased total lung capacity and/or residual volume, and fixed reduction in FEV_1 in patients with emphysema; normal diffusing capacity and reduced FEV_1 are found in patients with chronic bronchitis. Stage and severity of COPD according to postbronchodilator spirometry are described in Table 2. It is important to note that FEV_1 does not correlate well with individual patients' severity of dyspnea, exercise limitations, or health status. Evaluation of patients should also focus on symptom control and risk for adverse events in addition to FEV_1.

- Patients with COPD can generally be distinguished from asthmatics by their incomplete response to short-acting beta agonist (change in FEV_1 <200 ml and 12%) and absence of an abnormal bronchoconstrictor response to methacholine or other stimuli. Nearly 40% of patients with COPD will, however, respond to bronchodilators. Similarly, patients without a smoking history but with chronic asthmatic bronchitis may have airflow obstruction that is not completely reversible.

ASSESSMENT

- The global initiative for chronic obstructive lung disease (GOLD) assigns patients with COPD into four groups (A, B, C, D) based on (1) the degree of airflow restriction (Table 2), (2) a patient symptom score using one of two symptom questionnaires (CAT or mMRC), or (3) the number of COPD exacerbations in one year.[1]

IMAGING STUDIES

Chest x-ray:
- Hyperinflation with flattened diaphragm, tenting of the diaphragm at the rib, and increased retrosternal chest space (Fig. 1)
- Decreased vascular markings and bullae in patients with emphysema
- Thickened bronchial markings and enlarged right side of the heart in patients with chronic bronchitis
- Computed tomography: Emphysematous lung, tracheobronchomalacia

Rx TREATMENT

NONPHARMACOLOGIC THERAPY

- Avoidance of tobacco and elimination of air pollutants.

[1]Lee H, Kim J, Tagmazyan K: Treatment of stable chronic obstructive pulmonary disease: the GOLD guidelines, *Am Fam Physician* 88(10):655-663, 2013.

- Supplemental oxygen, usually through a face mask/nasal cannula, to ensure oxygen saturation >90% as measured by pulse oximetry. Continuous oxygen therapy should be prescribed for patients with COPD who have arterial partial pressure of oxygen 55 mm Hg or less, or oxygen saturation 88% or less as measured by pulse oximetry. Pulmonary secretion clearance: careful nasotracheal suction is indicated only in patients with excessive secretions and an inability to expectorate. Mechanical percussion of the chest as applied by a physical or respiratory therapist is ineffective with acute exacerbations of COPD.
- Pulmonary rehabilitation should be considered in COPD patients who remain

TABLE 2 Stage and Severity of COPD According to Postbronchodilator Spirometry

GOLD Stage and Severity	Definition
I: Mild	FEV_1/FVC <0.70, FEV_1 ≥80% of predicted
II: Moderate	FEV_1/FVC <0.70, 50%≤FEV_1 <80% of predicted
III: Severe	FEV_1/FVC <0.70, 30%≤FEV_1 <50% of predicted
IV: Very severe	FEV_1/FVC <0.70, FEV_1 <30% of predicted or FEV_1 <50% of predicted plus chronic respiratory failure

Data from the Global Initiative for Chronic Obstructive Lung Disease. Goldman L, Schafer AI: *Goldman's Cecil medicine,* ed 24, Philadelphia, 2012, Saunders.

symptomatic despite optimal medical management. Medicare will cover up to 36 sessions of pulmonary rehabilitation in COPD patients.
- Weight loss in obese patients.
- Identification of depression in patients newly diagnosed with COPD is important, as it may be associated with decreased adherence to maintenance therapy of COPD (Albrecht JS, et al: *Ann Am Thorac Soc* 13(9):1497-1594, 2016).
- Preliminary trials involving lung volume reduction using bronchoscopic treatment with nitinol coils have shown improved exercise capacity in patients with severe emphysema (Deslee G, et al: *JAMA* 315(2):175-184, 2016).
- Endobronchial valve (EBV) placement via bronchoscopy to reduce lung volume with one-way valves that are allowed to leave but not enter a lung segment has been used in Europe but is not yet approved in the U.S. (Klooster K, et al: *NEJM* 373:2325, 2015).

GENERAL Rx

- Pharmacologic treatment should be administered in a stepwise approach according to the severity of disease and patient's tolerance for specific drugs. Fig. E2 describes general management approaches for COPD. When using the COLD assessment criteria, pulmonary rehabilitation is recommended for patients in groups B, C, and D. Those in group A should receive a short-acting anticholinergic or short-acting β_2-agonist for mild intermittent symptoms. For patients in group B, long-acting anticholinergics or long-acting β_2-agonists should be added. Patients in group C or D are at high risk of exacerbations and should

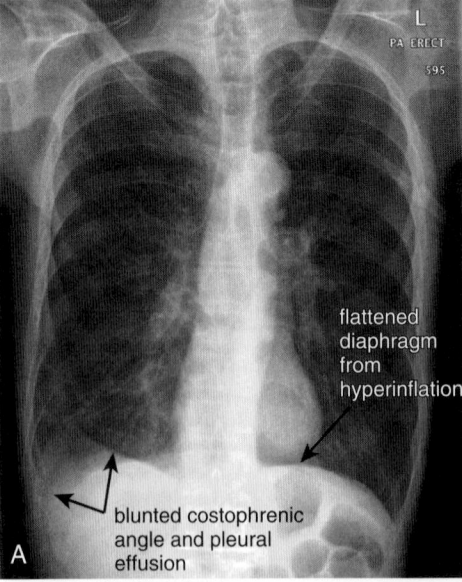
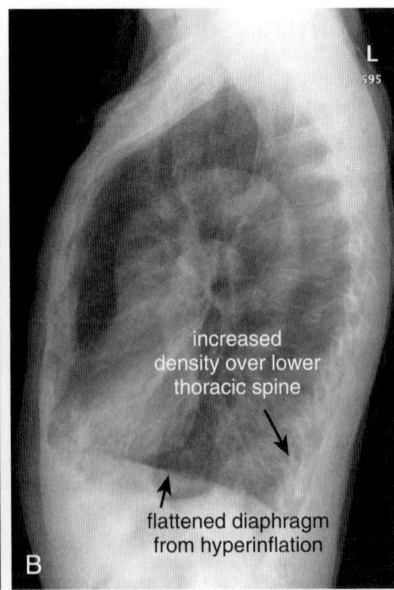

FIG. 1 Chronic obstructive pulmonary disease (COPD). A, Posterior-anterior (PA) upright chest x-ray. **B,** Lateral upright chest x-ray. This 63-year-old man with a history of COPD presented with 2 weeks of worsening cough with yellow sputum and dyspnea. His oxygen saturation was 87% in the emergency room. He has evidence of hyperinflation with flat diaphragms (particularly evident on the lateral x-ray, **(B)**. The patient also has a blunted right costophrenic angle with an apparent effusion and increased densities in both the right and the left lung base **(A)**. The lateral x-ray also shows increased density overlying the inferior thoracic spine, an abnormal spine sign. (From Broder JS: *Diagnostic imaging for the emergency physician,* Philadelphia, 2011, Saunders.)

C

receive a long-acting anticholinergic or a combination of an inhaled corticosteroid and a long-acting β_2-agonist.

1. Bronchodilators improve symptoms, quality of life, and exercise tolerance and decrease incidence of exacerbations. Inhaled bronchodilators *may be used* for stable COPD patients with respiratory symptoms and FEV_1 between 60% and 80% of predicted. They are *recommended* for stable COPD patients with respiratory symptoms and FEV_1 <60% of predicted. Recent guidelines from ACP, ACCP, ATS, and ERS recommend that clinicians prescribe monotherapy using either long-acting inhaled anticholinergics or long-acting inhaled β-agonists for symptomatic patients with COPD and FEV_1 <60% of predicted. Clinicians should base the choice of specific monotherapy on patient preference, cost, and adverse effect profile.

2. Short-acting β_2-agonists (e.g., albuterol metered-dose inhaler 1 to 2 puffs q4 to 6h prn) or short-acting anticholinergic agents (e.g., ipratropium inhaler 2 puffs qid) are acceptable in patients with mild, variable symptoms. Anticholinergics are also effective and are available in combination with albuterol (e.g., Combivent). Long-acting inhaled agents are preferred in patients with mild to moderate or continuous symptoms. Tiotropium is an excellent long-acting bronchodilator. It is very effective for long-term, once-a-day use. It has been shown to be superior to salmeterol, an inhaled long-acting β-agonist (LABA) in patients with moderate to severe COPD and may possibly slow the rate of decline in FEV1. Some recent trials, however, have shown higher hospitalization rates and mortality with tiotropium compared to LABAs. Indacaterol, umeclinidium, olodaterol, and vilanterol are other available LABAs for long-term maintenance treatment of bronchospasm associated with COPD. Indacaterol provides the convenience of once-daily dosing. Aclidinium, unlike tiotropium, is another long-acting anticholinergic that is predominantly renally excreted, can be used safely in renal impairment. Olodaterol is also for once-a-day use. As with other LABAs, these medications should not be used with other sympathomimetic drugs, medications that can prolong the QT interval, or beta-blockers. LABA and long-acting anticholinergics in different combinations are now available in the market. A combination of Umeclidinium and vilanterol in once-a-day dosing was found to achieve greater increases in trough FEV_1 and mean peak FEV_1 over the 6 hours after dosing compared with monotherapy or placebo.

3. Addition of inhaled steroids (fluticasone, budesonide, triamcinolone) is used to reduce exacerbations in patients with moderate to severe COPD. Inhaled steroids are reserved for patients with either ≥2 exacerbations annually or FEV_1 <50% of predicted. The role of inhaled corticosteroids (ICS) in COPD is controversial. Although some trials have demonstrated mild improvement in patients' symptoms and decreased frequency of exacerbations, most pulmonologists believe that these drugs are ineffective in most patients with COPD but should be considered for patients with moderate to severe airflow limitation who have persistent symptoms despite optimal bronchodilator therapy. ICS therapy does not affect 1-yr all-cause mortality among patients with COPD and is associated with a higher risk of pneumonia.

4. Roflumilast is a selective oral PDE4 inhibitor useful to reduce the risk of COPD exacerbations in patients with severe COPD associated with chronic bronchitis and a history of exacerbations. It is not a bronchodilator and is not indicated for the relief of acute bronchospasm.

5. Recent guidelines from ACP (American College of Physicians), ACCP (American College of Chest Physicians), ATS (American Thoracic Society), and ERS (European Respiratory Society) suggest that clinicians may administer combination inhaled therapies for symptomatic patients with stable COPD and FEV_1 <60% predicted. They also recommend that clinicians should prescribe pulmonary rehabilitation for symptomatic patients with an FEV_1 <50% predicted and continuous oxygen therapy in patients with COPD who have resting hypoxemia (Pa_{O_2} <55 mm Hg or Sp_{O_2} <88%).

6. Chronic antibiotic therapy: Chronic antibiotic therapy, specifically macrolide, should be considered in patients with frequent acute exacerbations of COPD despite optimal therapy with bronchodilators and antiinflammatory agents.

7. Systemic glucocorticoid therapy: Chronic systemic glucocorticoid therapy is generally not recommended even in severe COPD due to associated increase in mortality and morbidity.

• Acute exacerbation of COPD (increase in sputum volume and purulence, worsening dyspnea) can be treated with:

1. Aerosolized β_2-agonists (e.g., metaproterenol nebulizer solution 5% 0.3 ml or albuterol nebulized 5% solution 2.5 to 5 mg).

2. Anticholinergic agents, which have equivalent efficacy to inhaled beta-adrenergic agonists. Inhalant solution of ipratropium bromide 0.5 mg can be administered every 4 to 8 hr.

3. Short courses of systemic corticosteroids have been shown to improve spirometric and clinical outcomes. Treatment failure occurs less often in patients who receive low-dose steroids than in those receiving high-dose parenteral steroids. Oral prednisone 40 mg/day for 5 to 14 days is generally effective. Courses of treatment that are extended for >14 days confer no added benefit and increase the risk of adverse events. Recent trials[2] have shown that in patients with acute COPD exacerbations, systemic glucocorticoid treatment for 5 days is not inferior to treatment for 14 days.

4. Use of noninvasive positive pressure ventilation (NIPPV) decreases the risk of endotracheal intubation and decreases intensive care unit admission rates. Contraindications to its use are uncooperative patient, decreased level of consciousness, hemodynamic instability, inadequate mask fit, and severe respiratory acidosis. Increased airway pressure can be delivered by using inspiratory positive airway pressure, continuous positive airway pressure, or bilevel positive airway pressure, which combines the other modalities. When using NIPPV, the nasal mask is usually tolerated the best; however, patients must be instructed to keep their mouths closed while breathing with the nasal apparatus. Oxygen can be delivered at 10 to 15 L/min and started in spontaneous ventilation mode with an initial expiratory positive airway pressure setting of 3 to 5 cm H_2O and an inspiratory positive airway pressure setting of up to 10 cm H_2O. Adjustments in these settings should be made in 2-cm H_2O increments. It is important to monitor patients with frequent vital signs measurements, arterial blood gases, or pulse oximetry. Intubation and mechanical ventilation may be necessary if previous measures fail to provide improvement.

5. IV aminophylline administration is controversial and generally not recommended. When used in patients with refractory symptoms, serum levels should be closely monitored (keep level 8 to 12 mcg/ml) to minimize risks of tachyarrhythmias.

• Approximately 50% of COPD exacerbations are caused by bacterial infection. Antibiotics are indicated in suspected bacterial respiratory infection (e.g., increased purulence and volume of phlegm).

1. *Haemophilus influenzae* and *Streptococcus pneumoniae* are frequent causes of acute bronchitis.

2. Oral antibiotics of choice are azithromycin, levofloxacin, amoxicillin-clavulanate, trimethoprim-sulfamethoxazole, doxycycline, and cefuroxime.

3. The two best predictors of potential benefit from antibiotics are purulent sputum and C-reactive protein (CRP) level >40 mg/L.[3]

[2]Leuppi JD et al: Short-term vs conventional glucocorticoid therapy in acute exacerbations of chronic obstructive pulmonary disease: the REDUCE randomized clinical trial, *JAMA* 309:2223-2231, 2013.
[3]Miravilles M et al: Is it possible to identify exacerbations of mild to moderate COPD that do not require antibiotic treatment? *Chest* 144:1571, 2013.

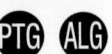

Table 3 Guideline Recommendations for Hospital Management of COPD Exacerbations

	Global Initiative for Chronic Obstructive Lung Disease*	American Thoracic Society/ European Respiratory Society[†]	National Institute for Clinical Excellence[‡]
Date of statement	2010	2004	2010
Diagnostic testing	Chest radiograph, oximetry, ABGs, and ECG. Other testing as warranted by clinical indication.	Chest radiograph, oxygen saturation, ABGs, ECG, sputum Gram stain and culture.	Chest radiograph, ABG, ECG, complete blood count, sputum smear and culture, blood cultures if febrile.
Bronchodilator therapy	Inhaled short-acting β_2-agonist is recommended. Consider ipratropium if inadequate clinical response. Consider theophylline or aminophylline as second-line intravenous therapy.	Inhaled short-acting β_2-agonist and/or ipratropium with spacer or nebulizer, as needed.	Administer inhaled drugs by nebulizer or handheld inhaler. Specific agents and dosing regimens not specified. Consider theophylline if inadequate response to inhaled bronchodilators.
Antibiotics	Recommended if (1) increases in dyspnea, sputum volume, and sputum purulence all are present; (2) increase in sputum purulence along with increase in either dyspnea or sputum volume; or (3) need for assisted ventilation. See original document for complex treatment algorithm.	Base choice on local bacterial resistance patterns. Consider amoxicillin/clavulanate or respiratory fluoroquinolones. If *Pseudomonas* species and/or other Enterobacteriaceae are suspected, consider combination therapy.	Administer only if history of purulent sputum. Initiate with an aminopenicillin, a macrolide, or a tetracycline, taking into account local bacterial resistance patterns. Adjust therapy according to sputum and blood cultures.
Systemic corticosteroids	Daily prednisolone 30-40 mg (or its equivalent) orally for 7-10 days.	Daily prednisone 30-40 mg orally for 10-14 days. Equivalent dose intravenously if unable to tolerate oral intake. Consider inhaled corticosteroids.	Daily prednisolone 30 mg (or its equivalent) orally for 7-14 days.
Supplemental oxygen	Maintain oxygen saturation >90%. Monitor ABGs for hypercapnia and acidosis.	Maintain oxygen saturation >90%. Monitor ABGs for hypercapnia and acidosis.	Maintain oxygen saturation within the individualized target range. Monitor ABGs.
Assisted ventilation	Indications for NPPV include severe dyspnea, acidosis (pH ≤7.35) and/or hypercapnia (PCO_2 >45 mm Hg), and respiratory rate >25 breaths/min. Contraindications to NPPV include respiratory arrest, hemodynamic instability, impaired mental status, copious bronchial secretions, and extreme obesity. Intubate if contraindication to NPPV or failure of NPPV (worsening ABGs or clinical status). Consider likelihood of recovery and patient's wishes and expectations before intubation.	Consider with pH <7.35 and PCO_2 >45-60 mm Hg and respiratory rate >24 breaths/min. Institute NPPV in a controlled environment, unless there are contraindications (e.g., respiratory arrest, hemodynamic instability, impaired mental status, copious bronchial secretions, and extreme obesity). Intubate if contraindication to NPPV or failure of NPPV (worsening ABGs or clinical status).	NPPV treatment of choice for persistent hypercapnic respiratory failure. Consider functional status, body mass index, home oxygen, comorbidities, prior ICU admissions, age, and FEV_1 when assessing suitability for intubation and ventilation.

ABGs, Arterial blood gases; *ECG,* electrocardiogram; *ICU,* intensive care unit; *NPPV,* noninvasive positive pressure ventilation.
*Data from http://www.goldcopd.com.
[†]Data from MacNee W. Standards for the diagnosis and treatment of patients with COPD: a summary of the ATS/ERS position paper. *Eur Respir J* 23:932-946, 2004.
[‡]Data from http://www.nice.org.uk.
From Goldman L, Schafer AI: *Goldman's Cecil medicine,* ed 24, Philadelphia, 2012, Saunders.

- Guaifenesin may improve cough symptoms and mucus clearance; however, mucolytic medications are generally ineffective. Their benefits may be greatest in patients with more advanced disease.
- Guideline recommendations for hospital management of COPD exacerbations are described in Table 3. Indications for invasive mechanical ventilation are described in Box 1.
- Lung volume reduction surgery has been proposed as a palliative treatment for severe emphysema. Overall it increases the chance of improved exercise capacity but does not confer a survival advantage over medical therapy. It is most beneficial in patients with both predominantly upper-lobe emphysema and low baseline exercise capacity.
- Single-lung transplantation should be considered a surgical option in patients with end-stage emphysema who have an FEV_1 <25% of predicted normal value after administration

of bronchodilator and additional complications such as severe hypoxemia, hypercapnia, and pulmonary hypertension.
- Trials involving endobronchial valves that allow air to escape from a pulmonary lobe but not to enter it have been done to improve lung function by reducing lobar volume in patients with advanced heterogeneous emphysema. Results have shown modest improvements in lung function, symptoms, and exercise tolerance, but more frequent exacerbations of COPD, Other complications included pneumonia and hemoptysis postimplantation.

DISPOSITION

- After the initial episode of respiratory failure, 5-yr survival is approximately 25%.
- Development of cor pulmonale or hypercapnia and persistent tachycardia are poor prognostic indicators.

- The need for oxygen at rest may be the strongest predictor of mortality in chronic respiratory failure from COPD.

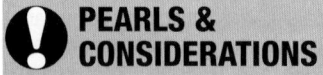 **PEARLS & CONSIDERATIONS**

COMMENTS

- All patients with COPD should receive pneumococcal vaccine and yearly influenza vaccine.
- Early antibiotic administration is associated with improved outcomes among patients hospitalized for acute exacerbations of COPD regardless of the risk of treatment failure.
- In assessing the severity of COPD, the FEV_1 is limited by the fact that it does not take into account the systemic manifestations of COPD. The BODE index (body mass index, degree of obstruction, dyspnea, and exercise capacity)

BOX 1 Indications for Invasive Mechanical Ventilation

Severe dyspnea, with use of accessory muscles and paradoxical abdominal motion
Respiratory frequency >35 breaths/min
Life-threatening hypoxemia (Pao_2 <40 mm Hg or Pao_2/Fio_2 <200 mm Hg)
Severe acidosis (pH <7.25) and hypercapnia ($Paco_2$ >60 mm Hg)
Respiratory arrest
Somnolence, impaired mental status
Cardiovascular complications (hypotension, shock, heart failure)
Other complications: metabolic abnormalities, sepsis, pneumonia, pulmonary embolism, barotrauma, massive pleural effusion
Noninvasive positive-pressure ventilation failure (or exclusion criteria)

Fio$_2$, Inspired oxygen fraction; *Pao$_2$*, partial pressure of carbon dioxide in arterial blood; *Pao$_2$*, partial pressure of oxygen in arterial blood.
From Vincent JL et al: *Textbook of critical care*, ed 6, Philadelphia, 2011, Saunders.

has been proposed as a multidimensional scale to better assess the morbidity and mortality associated with COPD. It is better than the FEV$_1$ alone at predicting the risk of death from any cause and from respiratory causes among patients with COPD. In the BODE index, obstruction is measured by FEV$_1$ and dyspnea is measured by the modified Medical Research Council (MMRC) dyspnea questionnaire in a 6-minute walk test. A score of 0 on the MMRC indicates that the individual is not troubled with breathlessness except with strenuous exercise, 1 indicates shortness of breath when hurrying or walking up a slight hill, and 2 means the individual walks slower than people of the same age due to breathlessness or has to stop for breath when walking at own pace on level ground. A score of 3 means severe dyspnea because the person has to stop for breath after walking approximately 100 meters or after a few minutes on level ground, and a score of 4 indicates very severe dyspnea and is given when the individual is too breathless to leave the house or is breathless when dressing or undressing.

- Pulmonary artery enlargement as determined by a ratio of the diameter of the pulmonary artery to the diameter of the aorta [PA:A ratio] of >1 detected by CT is associated with severe exacerbations of COPD.

- The average person with COPD has one or two acute exacerbations each year. Prophylactic use of macrolide antibiotics (azithromycin 250 mg/day) has been shown to decrease the frequency of exacerbations and improve quality of life among selected patients with COPD; however, it leads to hearing decrements in a small percentage of patients and increased prevalence of macrolide-resistant bacteria colonizing the airway and is therefore not recommended.

C

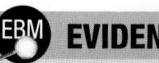 **EVIDENCE**

Available at www.expertconsult.com

SUGGESTED READINGS

Available at www.expertconsult.com

RELATED CONTENT

Chronic Obstructive Pulmonary Disease (Patient Information)
Asthma-COPD Overlap Syndrome (Related Key Topic)
Emphysema (Patient Information)

AUTHOR: **LAYOLA LUNGHAR, M.D.**

Diseases and Disorders

I

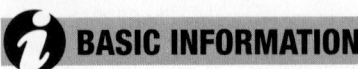
DEFINITION

Cirrhosis is defined histologically as the presence of irreversible fibrosis in the liver. It can be classified as micronodular, macronodular, or mixed; however, each form may be seen in the same patient at different stages of the disease. Cirrhosis manifests clinically with portal hypertension, hepatic encephalopathy, and variceal bleeding.

ICD-10CM CODES
K70.30 Alcoholic cirrhosis of liver without ascites
K70.31 Alcoholic cirrhosis of liver with ascites
K71.7 Toxic liver disease with fibrosis and cirrhosis of liver
K74.3 Primary biliary cirrhosis
K74.4 Secondary biliary cirrhosis
K74.5 Biliary cirrhosis, unspecified
K74.60 Unspecified cirrhosis of liver
K74.69 Other cirrhosis of liver
P78.81 Congenital cirrhosis (of liver)

EPIDEMIOLOGY & DEMOGRAPHICS

- Cirrhosis is the eighth-leading cause of death in the U.S. and the thirteenth-leading cause of death globally.
- Alcohol abuse, viral hepatitis, and nonalcoholic steatohepatitis are the major causes of cirrhosis in the U.S.
- Economic burden of cirrhosis in the U.S. exceeds $2 billion in direct costs and over $10 billion in indirect costs.

PHYSICAL FINDINGS & CLINICAL PRESENTATION

SKIN: Jaundice, palmar erythema (alcohol abuse), spider angiomata, ecchymosis (thrombocytopenia or coagulation factor deficiency), dilated superficial periumbilical vein (caput medusae), increased pigmentation (hemochromatosis), xanthomas (primary biliary cirrhosis), and needle tracks (viral hepatitis). Cutaneous lesions often accompany cirrhosis and can be found in >40% of people with chronic alcoholism.
EYES: Kayser-Fleischer rings (corneal copper deposition seen in Wilson's disease; best diagnosed with slit lamp examination), scleral icterus
BREATH: Fetor hepaticus (musty odor of breath and urine found in cirrhosis with hepatic failure)
CHEST: Possible gynecomastia in men
ABDOMEN: Tender hepatomegaly (congestive hepatomegaly), small, nodular liver (cirrhosis), palpable, nontender gallbladder (neoplastic extrahepatic biliary obstruction), palpable spleen (portal hypertension), venous hum auscultated over periumbilical veins (portal hypertension), ascites (portal hypertension, hypoalbuminemia)
RECTAL EXAMINATION: Hemorrhoids (portal hypertension), guaiac-positive stools (alcoholic gastritis, bleeding esophageal varices, peptic ulcer disease, bleeding hemorrhoids)
GENITALIA: Testicular atrophy in males (chronic liver disease, hemochromatosis)

EXTREMITIES: Pedal edema (hypoalbuminemia, failure of right side of the heart), arthropathy (hemochromatosis)
NEUROLOGIC: Flapping tremor, asterixis (hepatic encephalopathy), choreoathetosis, dysarthria (Wilson's disease)

ETIOLOGY

- Chronic hepatitis B virus (HBV) and hepatitis C virus (HCV) infection
- Alcoholism
- Nonalcoholic steatohepatitis
- Secondary biliary cirrhosis, obstruction of the common bile duct (stone, stricture, pancreatitis, neoplasm, sclerosing cholangitis)
- Drugs (e.g., acetaminophen, isoniazid, methotrexate, methyldopa)
- Hepatic congestion (e.g., CHF, constrictive pericarditis, tricuspid insufficiency, thrombosis of the hepatic vein, obstruction of the vena cava)
- Primary biliary cirrhosis
- Hemochromatosis
- Wilson's disease
- Alpha-1-antitrypsin deficiency
- Infiltrative diseases (amyloidosis, glycogen storage diseases, hemochromatosis)
- Nutritional: jejunoileal bypass
- Others: parasitic infections (schistosomiasis), idiopathic portal hypertension, congenital hepatic fibrosis, systemic mastocytosis, autoimmune hepatitis, inflammatory bowel disease (IBD)

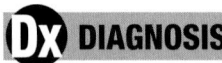 **DIAGNOSIS**

WORKUP

In addition to an assessment of liver function, the evaluation of patients with cirrhosis should also include an assessment of renal and circulatory function. Diagnostic workup is aimed primarily at identifying the most likely cause of cirrhosis. The history is extremely important:
- Alcohol abuse: alcoholic liver disease
- History of hepatitis B or hepatitis C
- Obesity, type 2 diabetes mellitus, hyperlipidemia (nonalcoholic steatohepatitis)
- History of IBD (primary sclerosing cholangitis)
- History of pruritus, hyperlipoproteinemia, and xanthomas in a middle-aged or elderly woman (primary biliary cirrhosis)
- Impotence, diabetes mellitus, hyperpigmentation, arthritis (hemochromatosis)
- Neurologic disturbances (Wilson's disease, hepatolenticular degeneration)
- Family history of "liver disease" (hemochromatosis [positive family history in 25% of patients], alpha-1-antitrypsin deficiency)
- History of recurrent episodes of right upper quadrant pain (biliary tract disease)
- History of blood transfusions, IV drug abuse (hepatitis C)
- History of hepatotoxic drug exposure
- Coexistence of other diseases with immune or autoimmune features (immune thrombocytopenic purpura, myasthenia gravis, thyroiditis, autoimmune hepatitis)

LABORATORY TESTS

- Decreased hemoglobin and hematocrit, elevated mean corpuscular volume, increased blood urea nitrogen (BUN) and creatinine (the BUN may also be "normal" or low if the patient has severely diminished liver function), decreased sodium (dilutional hyponatremia), and decreased potassium (as a result of secondary aldosteronism or urinary losses). Evaluation of renal function should also include measurement of urinary sodium and urinary protein from 24-hr urine collection.
- Decreased glucose in a patient with liver disease, indicating severe liver damage.
- Other laboratory abnormalities:
  1. Alcoholic hepatitis and cirrhosis: possible mild elevation of alanine aminotransferase (ALT) and aspartate aminotransferase (AST), usually <500 IU; AST >ALT (ratio >2:3).
  2. Extrahepatic obstruction: possible moderate elevations of ALT and AST to levels <500 IU.
  3. Viral, toxic, or ischemic hepatitis: extreme elevations (>500 IU) of ALT and AST.
  4. Transaminases may be normal despite significant liver disease in patients with jejunoileal bypass operations or hemochromatosis or after methotrexate administration.
  5. Alkaline phosphatase elevation can occur with extrahepatic obstruction, primary biliary cholangitis, and primary sclerosing cholangitis.
  6. Serum lactate dehydrogenase is significantly elevated in metastatic disease of the liver; lesser elevations are seen with hepatitis, cirrhosis, extrahepatic obstruction, and congestive hepatomegaly.
  7. Serum gamma-glutamyl transpeptidase is elevated in alcoholic liver disease and may also be elevated with cholestatic disease (primary biliary cholangitis, primary sclerosing cholangitis).
  8. Serum bilirubin may be elevated; urinary bilirubin can be present in hepatitis, hepatocellular jaundice, and biliary obstruction.
  9. Serum albumin: significant liver disease results in hypoalbuminemia. Malnutrition occurs in 20% to 60% of patients with cirrhosis.
  10. Prothrombin time/INR: elevation in patients with liver disease indicates severe liver damage and poor prognosis.
  11. Presence of hepatitis B surface antigen implies acute or chronic hepatitis B.
  12. Presence of antimitochondrial antibody suggests primary biliary cholangitis, chronic hepatitis.
  13. Elevated serum copper, decreased serum ceruloplasmin, and elevated 24-hr urine may be diagnostic of Wilson's disease.
  14. Protein immunoelectrophoresis may reveal decreased α-1 globulins (alpha-1-antitrypsin deficiency), increased IgA (alcoholic cirrhosis), increased IgM (primary biliary cirrhosis), increased IgG (chronic hepatitis, cryptogenic cirrhosis).

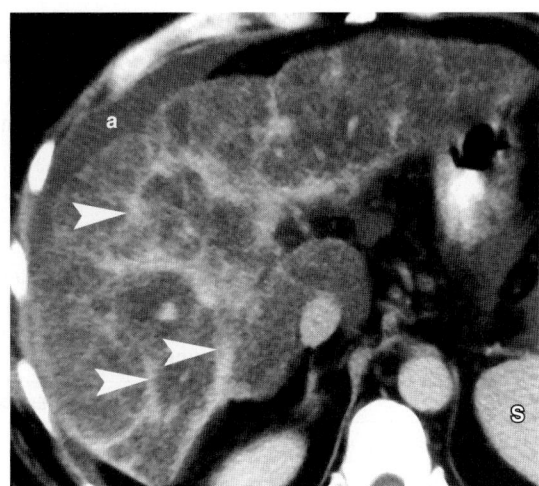

FIG. 1 Advanced cirrhosis with fatty infiltration. Delayed portal venous–phase computed tomography reveals that the liver is misshapen and nodular in contour. Parenchymal density that is significantly lower than that of the spleen *(S)* is indicative of fatty infiltration and continuing liver injury. Prominent scars and bands of fibrosis *(arrowheads)* are seen throughout the liver. Ascites *(a)* is present. (From Webb WR et al: *Fundamentals of body CT*, ed 4, Philadelphia, 2015, Saunders.)

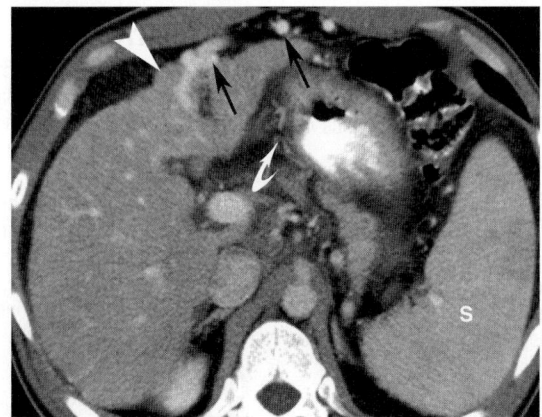

FIG. 2 Cirrhosis with portal hypertension. Postcontrast computed tomography reveals a liver that is nodular in contour *(arrowhead)* with patent enlarged paraumbilical veins *(blue arrows)* and splenomegaly *(S)*, findings indicative of portal hypertension. Mildly enlarged portosystemic collateral vessels *(curved arrow)* are also evident in the gastrohepatic ligament. (From Webb WR et al: *Fundamentals of body CT*, ed 4, Philadelphia, 2015, Saunders.)

15. An elevated serum ferritin and increased transferrin saturation are suggestive of hemochromatosis.
16. An elevated blood ammonia suggests hepatocellular dysfunction; serial values, however, are generally not useful in monitoring patients with hepatic encephalopathy because there is poor correlation between blood ammonia level and degree of hepatic encephalopathy.
17. Serum cholesterol is elevated in cholestatic disorders.
18. Antinuclear antibodies (ANA) may be found in autoimmune hepatitis.
19. Alpha fetoprotein: levels >1000 pg/ml are highly suggestive of primary liver cell carcinoma.
20. Hepatitis C viral testing identifies patients with chronic hepatitis C infection.
21. Elevated level of serum globulin (especially gamma-globulins) and positive ANA test may occur with autoimmune hepatitis.
22. End-stage liver disease is characterized by decreased levels of most procoagulant factors with the notable exceptions of factor VIII and von Willebrand factor, which are elevated.

IMAGING STUDIES

- Ultrasonography is the procedure of choice for detecting gallstones and dilation of common bile ducts. The use of sonography on a periodic basis to screen for hepatocellular carcinoma in patients with cirrhosis has been questioned and should be avoided until additional data are available.
- CT scan (Figs. 1 and 2) is useful for detecting mass lesions in liver and pancreas, assessing hepatic fat content, identifying idiopathic hemochromatosis, diagnosing Budd-Chiari syndrome early, assessing dilation of intrahepatic bile ducts, and detecting varices and splenomegaly.
- MRI can be used to identify hemangiomas.

- Transient elastography (Fibroscan) is useful to quantify liver fibrosis.
- Technetium-99m sulfur colloid scanning is rarely used but can be useful for diagnosing cirrhosis (there is a shift of colloid uptake to the spleen and bone marrow), identifying hepatic adenomas (cold defect is noted), and diagnosing Budd-Chiari syndrome (there is increased uptake by the caudate lobe).
- Endoscopic retrograde cholangiopancreatography can be used for diagnosing periampullary carcinoma and common duct stones; it is also useful in diagnosing primary sclerosing cholangitis.
- Percutaneous transhepatic cholangiography is useful when evaluating patients with cholestatic jaundice and dilated intrahepatic ducts by ultrasonography; presence of intrahepatic strictures and focal dilation is suggestive of primary sclerosing cholangitis.
- Percutaneous liver biopsy is useful in evaluating hepatic filling defects; diagnosing hepatocellular disease or hepatomegaly; evaluating persistently abnormal liver function tests; and diagnosing hemachromatosis, primary biliary cirrhosis, Wilson's disease, glycogen storage diseases, chronic hepatitis, autoimmune hepatitis, infiltrative diseases, alcoholic liver disease, drug-induced liver disease, and primary or secondary carcinoma.

Rx TREATMENT

NONPHARMACOLOGIC THERAPY

- Avoid any hepatotoxins (e.g., ethanol, acetaminophen), improve nutritional status.
- Transjugular intrahepatic portosystemic shunt (TIPS) in patients with recurrent variceal hemorrhage despite optical medical therapy (Fig. 3). Early use of TIPS is associated with significant reductions in treatment failure and in mortality in patients with cirrhosis who are hospitalized for acute variceal bleeding and are at high risk for treatment failure.
- Correction of malnutrition: daily protein intake of 1.0 to 1.5 g per kg of body weight.

GENERAL Rx

- Beta-blockers with or without nitrates in patients with cirrhosis and variceal hemorrhage. Use with caution in patients with severe alcoholic hepatitis, decompensated cirrhosis with refractory ascites, and spontaneous bacterial peritonitis.
- Pruritus due to liver disease may be treated with cholestyramine 4 g/day initially. Dose can be increased to 24 g/day as needed.
- Pain management: Avoid opiates (may precipitate or aggravate hepatic encephalopathy) and NSAIDs (increased risk of gastrointestinal bleeding and renal failure). Low-dose tramadol and lidocaine patches are generally well tolerated.
- Sedatives: Benzodiazepines (lorazepam or oxazepam) may be used for alcohol withdrawal but should be avoided in patients with hepatic encephalopathy.

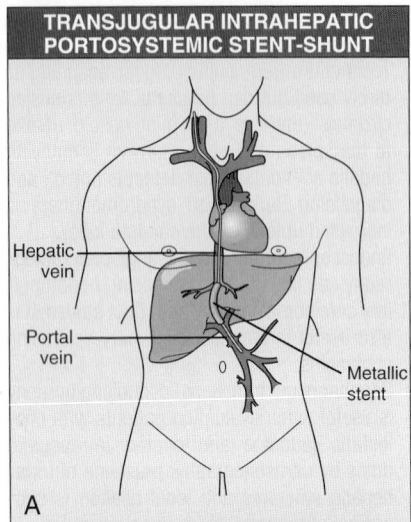

TRANSJUGULAR INTRAHEPATIC PORTOSYSTEMIC STENT-SHUNT

Hepatic vein
Portal vein
Metallic stent

A

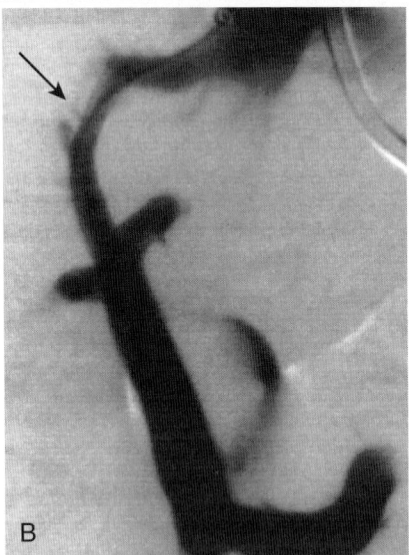

B

FIG. 3 Transjugular intrahepatic portosystemic stent shunt. A, An intrahepatic track has been created between the right hepatic vein and the right portal vein. **B,** The track is dilated *(arrow)* and stented, creating a shunt as demonstrated on shuntogram. (Courtesy Dr. W. K. Tso, Queen Mary Hospital, Hong Kong.)

- Statins: Can be safely started and continued in patients with hyperlipidemia and/or nonalcoholic fatty liver disease.
- Proton pump inhibitors: Not routinely indicated; their use in patients with cirrhosis is associated with excess risk for spontaneous bacterial peritonitis and hepatic encephalopathy; avoid indiscriminate use of PPIs in patients with cirrhosis.
- Liver transplantation may be indicated in otherwise healthy patients (ages <65 yr) with sclerosing cholangitis, chronic hepatitis cirrhosis, or primary biliary cholangitis, with prognostic information suggesting <20% chance of survival without transplantation. Contraindications

Table 1 Child-Pugh Staging Criteria

CHILD-PUGH SCORE			
Criteria	1 Point	2 Points	3 Points
Total serum bilirubin (mg/dl)	<2	2-3	>3
Serum albumin (g/dl)	>3.5	2.8-3.5	<2.8
INR	<1.70	1.71-2.20	>2.20
Ascites	No ascites	Ascites controlled	Ascites not controlled
Encephalopathy	No encephalopathy	Encephalopathy controlled	Encephalopathy not controlled

INTERPRETATION OF CHILD-PUGH SCORES			
	Points	Life Expectancy	Perioperative Mortality
Child Class A	5-6	15-20 yr	10%
Child Class B	7-9	Candidate for liver transplant	30%
Child Class C	10-15	1-3 yr	82%

to liver transplantation are AIDS, most metastatic malignancies, active substance abuse, uncontrolled sepsis, and uncontrolled cardiac or pulmonary disease.
- Treatment of complications of portal hypertension (ascites, esophagogastric varices, hepatic encephalopathy, and hepatorenal syndrome; refer to these individual topics in Section I).

TREATMENT BASED ON SPECIFIC CAUSE OF CIRRHOSIS

- Remove excess body iron with phlebotomy and deferoxamine in patients with hemochromatosis.
- Remove copper deposits with D-penicillamine in patients with Wilson's disease.
- Long-term ursodiol therapy will slow the progression of primary biliary cirrhosis. It is, however, ineffective in primary sclerosing cholangitis.
- Glucocorticoids (prednisone 20 to 30 mg/day initially or combination therapy or prednisone and azathioprine) are useful in autoimmune hepatitis.
- Antivirals in chronic hepatitis C.

DISPOSITION

- Prognosis varies with the etiology of the patient's cirrhosis and whether there is ongoing hepatic injury. Regression of cirrhosis has been demonstrated after antiviral therapy in some patients with chronic hepatitis C. Regression is associated with decreased disease-related morbidity and improved survival. Mortality rate exceeds 80% in patients with hepatorenal syndrome.
- If advanced cirrhosis is present and transplantation is not feasible, survival is 1 to 2 yr.
- Cirrhosis is associated with an increased risk for hepatocellular carcinoma. However, the risk is low (1% 5-year cumulative risk in alcoholic cirrhosis).

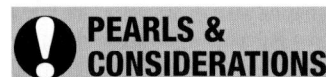

PEARLS & CONSIDERATIONS

COMMENTS

- Thrombocytopenia and advanced Child-Pugh cases (Table 1) are associated with the presence of varices. These factors are useful to identify cirrhotic patients who benefit most from referral for endoscopic screening for varices.
- A combination of endoscopic and drug therapy reduces overall and variceal rebleeding in cirrhosis more than either therapy alone.
- PPI use, but not H_2RA use, is associated with risk for serious infections in patients with decompensated cirrhosis.

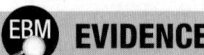 **EVIDENCE**

Available at www.expertconsult.com

SUGGESTED READINGS

Available at www.expertconsult.com

RELATED CONTENT

Cirrhosis (Patient Information)
Ascites (Related Key Topic)
Esophageal Varices (Related Key Topic)
Hepatic Encephalopathy (Related Key Topic)
Hepatopulmonary Syndrome (Related Key Topic)
Hepatorenal Syndrome (Related Key Topic)
Peritonitis, Spontaneous Bacterial (Related Key Topic)
Primary Biliary Cholangitis (Related Key Topic)

AUTHOR: **FRED F. FERRI, M.D.**

BASIC INFORMATION

DEFINITION

Claudication refers to reproducible pain in a muscle group that is brought on by exertion and is relieved with rest. The pain experienced results from inadequate blood flow to the target muscle group, which is not able to meet increased metabolic demand. Claudication is therefore a supply and demand mismatch and is due to peripheral arterial disease (PAD). Intermittent vascular claudication is more common in the lower extremities but can also affect the upper extremities.

SYNONYMS

• Intermittent claudication

ICD-10CM CODES
I70.211 Atherosclerosis of native arteries of extremities with intermittent claudication, right leg
I70.212 Atherosclerosis of native arteries of extremities with intermittent claudication, left leg
I70.213 Atherosclerosis of native arteries of extremities with intermittent claudication, bilateral legs
I70.219 Atherosclerosis of native arteries of extremities with intermittent claudication, unspecified extremity
I70.311 Atherosclerosis of unspecified type of bypass graft(s) of the extremities with intermittent claudication, right leg
I70.312 Atherosclerosis of unspecified type of bypass graft(s) of the extremities with intermittent claudication, left leg
I70.313 Atherosclerosis of unspecified type of bypass graft(s) of the extremities with intermittent claudication, bilateral legs
I70.319 Atherosclerosis of unspecified type of bypass graft(s) of the extremities with intermittent claudication, unspecified extremity
I70.719 Atherosclerosis of other type of bypass graft(s) of the extremities with intermittent claudication, unspecified extremity

EPIDEMIOLOGY & DEMOGRAPHICS

• Symptomatic claudication in Western countries affects 5% of patients between the ages of 55 and 74.
• Lower-extremity PAD, which includes both symptomatic claudication and asymptomatic disease, is present in 13% of patients over the age of 50. This finding demonstrates that a large portion of patients is at risk of developing claudication.
• Risk factors associated with development of PAD are similar to coronary atherosclerosis (CAD) and include increasing age, cigarette smoking, hypertension, diabetes mellitus, and dyslipidemia. In addition, patients with chronic kidney disease, metabolic syndrome,

and elevated levels of C-reactive protein, lipoprotein(a), and homocysteine are at increased risk. Nontraditional risk factors include race/ethnicity, with African American patients being at higher risk. Hispanics also have similar to slightly higher rates of PAD compared to non-Hispanic whites.
• There is a strong correlation among PAD, CAD, carotid artery stenosis, and generalized cerebrovascular disease.
• The American College of Cardiology/American Heart Association (ACC/AHA) guidelines suggested the following distribution of clinical presentation of PAD in patients 50 yr of age or older:
  1. Asymptomatic: 20% to 50%
  2. Atypical leg pain: 40% to 50%
  3. Classic claudication: 10% to 35%
  4. Critical limb ischemia with threatened limb: 1% to 2%

PHYSICAL FINDINGS & CLINICAL PRESENTATION

• The severity of symptoms varies with degree of PAD, collateral blood supply, and exertional demands.
• Classic symptoms include exertional calf pain, which limits the patient's activity and self-resolves with rest within 10 minutes. Claudication can also typically present in the buttock and hip, thigh, calf, or foot, with one or more of the following signs or symptoms, depending on the level and degree of peripheral stenosis:
  1. Diminished or absent pedal pulses
  2. Bruit over the distal aorta, iliac, or femoral arteries
  3. Pallor of the distal extremities on elevation with cooling to the touch
  4. Rubor with prolonged capillary refill on dependency
  5. Trophic changes, including hair/nail loss and muscle atrophy
  6. Non-healing ulcers, necrotic tissue, and gangrene
  7. Weakness, numbness, or heaviness in the lower extremities
• True vascular claudication must be distinguished from "pseudoclaudication," which can be caused by severe venous obstruction or insufficiency, chronic compartment

syndrome, spinal stenosis, osteoarthritis, and inflammatory muscle diseases. The characteristic features of pseudoclaudication that distinguish it from claudication are summarized in Table 1. Table 2 illustrates the differential diagnosis of intermittent claudication.
• Location of pain usually corresponds to analogous anatomy:
  1. Buttock and hip: aortic or iliac disease
  2. Thigh: aorta, iliac, or common femoral artery
  3. Upper two thirds of calf: superficial femoral artery
  4. Lower one third of calf: popliteal artery
  5. Foot: tibial or peroneal artery
• Asymptomatic PAD is typically diagnosed by screening studies (exercise ankle brachial index, lower-extremity ultrasound) or incidentally on physical exam. Patients who are at significant risk for PAD often have multiple comorbidities that can alter their presentation. In the PARTNERS program report, 47% of those with a new diagnosis of PAD had no history of leg symptoms, 47% had atypical symptoms, and only 6% had classic symptoms.
• Symptoms of intermittent claudication classically start distally within a muscle group (below the stenosis) and then ascend with continued activity.
• Rest pain that occurs with leg elevation and is paradoxically relieved by walking may suggest severe PAD.
• Critical limb ischemia may present as tissue ulceration and gangrene, which require prompt intervention.

ETIOLOGY

The primary cause of claudication is peripheral atherosclerosis, resulting in a stenosis that impedes blood flow beyond the level necessary to meet the metabolic demand of limb muscles first with activity and then ultimately at rest.

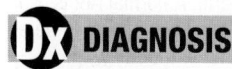 DIAGNOSIS

DIFFERENTIAL DIAGNOSIS

• Spinal stenosis (neurogenic or pseudoclaudication)
• Musculoskeletal disorders: arthritis or myositis

TABLE 1 Characteristic Features of Pseudoclaudication that Distinguish it from Claudication

	Claudication	Pseudoclaudication
Characteristics	Limb cramping, tightness, fatigue	Similar to claudication with numbness
Location of discomfort	Lower extremity involving buttock, hip, thigh, calf, foot	Similar to claudication
Induced by exercise	Yes	Variable
Reproducible with distance walked	Consistent	Variable
Occurs with standing	No	Yes
Actions which provide relief	Stand	Sit
Time to relief	<5 min	≥30 min

TABLE 2 Differential Diagnosis of Intermittent Claudication

	Intermittent Claudication	Venous Claudication	Neurogenic Claudication
Quality of pain	Cramping	Aching, heaviness, tightness	"Pins and needles" sensation going down the leg, weakness
Onset	Gradual, consistent	Gradual; can, however, be immediate	Can be immediate
Relieved by	Stopping walking	Activity, elevation of leg	Sitting down, stooping, flexion at the waist
Location	Muscle groups (e.g., buttocks, thigh, calf)	Whole leg	Poorly localized, but can affect whole leg
Legs affected	Usually one	Usually one	Often both

From Swartz, MH: *Textbook of physical diagnosis*, ed 7, Philadelphia, 2014, Saunders.

- Degenerative osteoarthritic joint disease, predominantly of the lumbar spine and hips
- Compartment or popliteal artery entrapment syndrome
- Peripheral neuropathy
- Atheromatous embolization and deep venous thrombosis
- Vasculitis: thromboangiitis obliterans, Takayasu, or giant cell arteritis

WORKUP

History and physical findings suggest the diagnosis of claudication and noninvasive studies help confirm the diagnosis.

- Measurement of resting ankle–brachial index (ABI) should be considered in patients at risk for PAD and may be repeated at least once every 5 yr. At-risk patients include:
    1. Patients with exertional leg symptoms.
    2. Non-healing lower-extremity wounds.
    3. Asymptomatic patients 50 yr or older with a history of smoking or diabetes.
    4. Patients younger than the age of 50 yr with diabetes and an additional cardiovascular risk factor (smoking, dyslipidemia, hypertension, or homocysteinemia).

    All patients age 65 yr or older.
- An ABI is the ratio of highest ankle systolic pressure to the highest brachial systolic pressure of either arm. A normal ABI is 1.00 to 1.40. A low ABI has been shown to be an independent predictor of mortality.
- The severity of PAD is based on the resting ABI. The absolute value of the ABI correlates with the severity of the disease but does not define its exact level.
    1. Borderline disease: ABI at rest 0.91 to 0.99
    2. Mild disease: ABI at rest 0.71 to 0.90
    3. Moderate disease: ABI at rest 0.41 to 0.70
    4. Severe disease: ABI at rest <0.40 or >1.4
- Segmental systolic pressures are measured at the level of the thigh, calf, ankle, metatarsal, and toes. Normally, successive segments have <20 mm Hg difference in pressures. If the gradient is >20 mm Hg, a significant stenosis is suspected in the interval vascular segment.
- ABI >1.3 may represent significant PAD caused by heavy calcification. In such cases, measuring a toe–brachial index can increase the sensitivity of testing, as highly calcified arteries are incompressible and may have an elevated ABI. A toe–brachial index <0.7 is considered abnormal.

- Progression of PAD is considered to have occurred if a decrease in ABI of 0.15 occurs while the patient is in treatment.
- If a patient has a history concerning for PAD but a normal ABI, and if the clinician is concerned about a potential false-negative finding, performing an exercise stress ABI can potentially demonstrate lower-extremity PAD.
- If after exercise an ABI reading decreases by more than 20% or an ankle pressure decreases by 30 mm Hg, the patient should be considered to have significant PAD.

IMAGING STUDIES

- Duplex ultrasound can be used to assess occlusion location, length, and patency of the distal arterial system or prior grafts; it is a good choice for initial imaging.
- Ultrasound is an excellent noninvasive modality for surveillance monitoring after revascularization.
- In patients with prior infrainguinal bypass grafts, the long-term patency should be evaluated at regular intervals using a duplex ultrasound. The 2011 ACC guidelines recommend routine surveillance using a duplex ultrasound at approximately 3, 6, and 12 months after graft placement and then yearly.
- Magnetic resonance angiography (MRA) and CT angiography (CTA) are effective for imaging of the aorta and peripheral lower-extremity arteries above the knee. MRA has almost replaced catheter-based angiography, with 90% sensitivity and 97% specificity in identification of hemodynamically significant stenosis in the lower extremities.
- MRA and CTA are useful to define the anatomy and assist in planning percutaneous and surgical revascularization; however, the utility of each is decreased by necessity of gadolinium contrast and non-iodinated contrast agents, respectively.
- CTA of occlusive aortoiliac disease with fractional flow reserve (FFR) has been correlated with invasive angiographic evaluation with FFR and demonstrated, although in a small sample of people the correlation is excellent. One may then surmise that the patients could benefit from noninvasive CTA to plan and evaluate any potential areas of disease amenable to revascularization.
- Angiography (Fig. E1) remains the gold standard for diagnosing PAD, particularly below the knee.

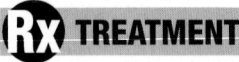 **TREATMENT**

NONPHARMACOLOGIC THERAPY

- Smoking cessation is of paramount importance. Smokers and former smokers should be asked about tobacco use status on each visit. Assistance and counseling for smoking cessation should be addressed thoroughly.
- Aggressive risk factor modification for hypertension, dyslipidemia, and diabetes mellitus, including diet, weight loss, and lifestyle counseling, is recommended.
- Supervised exercise training should be performed as a first-line therapy for a minimum of 30 to 45 minutes, in sessions performed at least 3 times per week for a minimum of 12 weeks.
- Supervised exercise training has been shown to increase maximal walking distance, pain-free walking distance, and the 6-minute walking distance.
- Home-based walking exercise program combined with group-mediated cognitive behavioral intervention can significantly improve endurance and physical activity for patients unable or unwilling to participate in supervised exercise training.
- Lifestyle therapy in conjunction with exercise can be as or more effective than pharmacologic therapy and in some cases more effective than stent revascularization, as shown by the CLEVER Study.
- Intermittent pneumatic compression may hold promise as an adjunctive therapy.

ACUTE GENERAL Rx

Revascularization by an endovascular or surgical approach is usually reserved for patients with symptoms refractory to medical therapy or those with impending critical limb ischemia.

CHRONIC Rx

- Aspirin 81 to 325 mg daily is standard therapy.
- Thienopyridine medications such as clopidogrel may be considered as an alternative to aspirin, especially for those intolerant of aspirin.
- Current data do not support combination treatment with aspirin and clopidogrel (CHARISMA trial).
- Hydroxymethyl glutaryl (HMG) coenzyme-A reductase inhibitor (statin) medications are indicated for all patients with PAD.

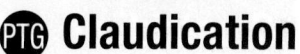

C

Diseases and Disorders

I

1. LDL cholesterol level of less than 100 mg/dl is recommended.
2. A goal LDL cholesterol level of less than 70 mg/dl is recommended for patients with PAD and high risk for coronary atherosclerotic disease.
3. Although new lipid guidelines have been published, the guidelines did not specifically address patients with PAD; therefore, the numerical targets can be considered. In those unable to reach the targets, a reduction in LDL >50% should be approached at a minimum.

- Antihypertensive therapy with beta-adrenergic blocking drugs and/or ACE inhibitors should be administered to all hypertensive patients with PAD to reduce the risk of MI, stroke, congestive heart failure, and cardiovascular death.
  1. In non-diabetics, the target blood pressure is <140 mm Hg systolic over 90 mm Hg diastolic.
  2. In diabetics or patients with chronic renal disease, the target blood pressure is <130 mm Hg systolic over 80 mm Hg diastolic.
  3. Recent hypertension guidelines have raised the targets for some diseases; however, they do not address the higher risk posed by multiple comorbidities.
- Cilostazol 100 mg bid may be used in conjunction with aspirin or clopidogrel. It has been shown to increase walking distance by 50% to 67% in symptomatic patients.
- Among patients with intermittent claudication, a single randomized controlled trial has shown a 24-week treatment with ramipril resulted in significant increases in pain-free and maximum treadmill walking times compared with placebo. Furthermore, the use of ACE inhibitors may be considered in patients with PAD to reduce the risk of cardiovascular events.
- Pentoxifylline 400 mg three times per day may be considered as second-line alternative therapy to cilostazol to improve walking. However, the clinical effectiveness of pentoxifylline as therapy for claudication is not well established.
- In patients with type II diabetes, a secondary analysis of the BARI 2D trial showed that an insulin-sensitizing approach (metformin, glitazones) reduces the risk of developing PAD when compared to insulin-providing therapy (glipizide, insulin). These patients also have lower rates of revascularization and amputation.
- Patients who are tobacco smokers should be offered either varenicline or bupropion along with nicotine replacement therapy in the absence of any contraindications.
- Revascularization through either a percutaneous or surgical approach is indicated in patients with refractory rest pain or claudication that is lifestyle limiting. It is also indicated in those with non-healing ulcers or

gangrene and in select patients with functional disability. Before such revascularization, each patient should have:
1. Been provided information regarding supervised claudication exercise therapy and pharmacotherapy
2. Received comprehensive risk factor modification and antiplatelet therapy
3. Significant disability with either the inability to perform normal work or a serious impairment of other activities important to the patient
4. Lower-extremity PAD lesion anatomy amenable to revascularization, defined by a low risk and a high probability of initial and long-term success

Common procedures include:
1. Aorto-iliofemoral reconstruction or bypass or infrainguinal bypass (e.g., femoropopliteal, femorotibial).
2. Percutaneous balloon angioplasty, often with stenting, is primarily used on discrete stenotic lesions in the iliac or femoropopliteal arteries.
3. Endovascular intervention is recommended as the preferred revascularization technique for iliac and femoropopliteal arterial lesions.
4. Stenting is effective primary therapy for common and external iliac artery stenosis and occlusions. However, it is not recommended in the femoral, popliteal, or tibial arteries due to a low success rate except to salvage suboptimal balloon dilatation.

COMPLEMENTARY & ALTERNATIVE MEDICINE

- A meta-analysis found that over 12 to 24 weeks, *Ginkgo biloba* increased pain-free walking distance by 34 m compared with placebo, although the benefit is not well established according to ACC/AHA guidelines.
- Naftidrofuryl, a serotonin receptor inhibitor, available in Europe and other parts of the world, has shown some efficacy in improving claudication symptoms.
- Estrogen replacement therapy, propionyl-L-carnitine, L-arginine, oral vasodilators, prostaglandins, and chelation therapy are ineffective in the treatment of intermittent claudication.

DISPOSITION

- It is unusual for intermittent claudication to progress to ischemic leg or limb loss, especially with aggressive use of conservative treatments, risk factor modification, exercise, and smoking cessation.
- The 5-yr risk for development of ischemic ulceration in patients treated for diabetes and with ABI <0.5 was 30% compared with only 5% in patients without either characteristic.

REFERRAL

Consultation with physicians specializing in vascular medicine is recommended for the patient with threatened limb loss, rest pain, non-healing ulcers, functional disability from pain, and gangrene.

⚠ PEARLS & CONSIDERATIONS

- Approximately 70% of patients with peripheral vascular disease will have concomitant coronary artery disease.
- Beta-blockers may worsen claudication symptoms in some patients, although their underuse is associated with excess cardiovascular death. Patients with intermittent claudication are less likely to receive beta-blocker therapy after a myocardial infarction. Those who do not receive post-MI beta-blockers have at least a threefold higher mortality.
- Patients with peripheral vascular disease may benefit from secondary cardiovascular prevention with clopidogrel versus aspirin more so than other high-risk patients (CAPRIE trial).
- Often, PAD can be asymptomatic or with atypical symptoms, and a thorough history, physical exam and clinical suspicion based on medical comorbidities may help guide therapy before lifestyle-limiting claudication or limb ischemia develops.

COMMENTS

- Claudication is a marker for generalized atherosclerosis. Patients have a higher risk of death from cardiovascular events than from limb loss. Patients with PAD experience diminished overall quality of life similar to patients with diagnosed coronary artery or cerebrovascular disease.
- The ABI is more closely associated with exercise tolerance and severity of disease in persons with PAD than intermittent claudication or other leg symptoms.

SUGGESTED READINGS
Available at www.expertconsult.com

RELATED CONTENT
Poor Circulation (Claudication) (Patient Information)
Peripheral Arterial Disease (PAD) (Related Key Topic)

AUTHORS: **NICHOLAS J. ABBOTT, M.D.,** and **PRANAV M. PATEL, M.D.**

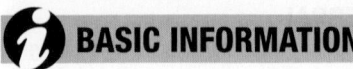

BASIC INFORMATION

DEFINITION

Clostridium difficile infection (CDI) is the occurrence of diarrhea and bowel inflammation associated with antibiotic use caused by *C. difficile*, an anaerobic gram-positive, spore-forming, toxin-producing bacillus transmitted through the fecal–oral route. CDI can manifest clinically in several forms ranging from fulminant diarrhea and leukocytosis associated with pseudomembranous colitis, mild to severe acute diarrhea, short-term colonization seen typically in health care facilities, and recurrent CDI within 60 days after initial treatment occurring in 20% to 30% of cases.

SYNONYMS

Antibiotic-induced colitis
Pseudomembranous colitis
CDI

ICD-10CM CODES
A04.7 Enterocolitis due to *Clostridium difficile*

EPIDEMIOLOGY & DEMOGRAPHICS

- Cephalosporins are the most frequent offending agent in CDI because of their high rates of use.
- The antibiotic with the highest incidence is clindamycin (10% incidence of CDI with its use).
- Since 1996, the incidence of CDI has more than doubled. Severity of CDI has also increased due to the emergence of an epidemic virulent strain (NAP1/BI/027). CDI is the most common infectious cause of healthcare-associated diarrhea in adults. In 2011, *C. difficile* was responsible for nearly half a million infections and was associated with approximately 29,000 deaths.
- Nosocomial CDI quadruples the cost of hospitalizations and increases annual expenditures by $1.5 billion in the U.S.
- Asymptomatic carriage of *C. difficile* is identified in more than 20% of patients hospitalized without diarrhea.

PHYSICAL FINDINGS & CLINICAL PRESENTATION

- Abdominal tenderness (generalized or lower abdominal)
- Fever
- In patients with prolonged diarrhea, poor skin turgor, dry mucous membranes, and other signs of dehydration may be present

ETIOLOGY

C. difficile colonizes the large intestines and releases 2 protein exotoxins (TcdA and TcdB) that cause colitis. Infection is transmitted by spores that are resistant to antibiotics, heat, and acid. The NAP1 strain is predominant among patients with *C. difficile* infection, whereas asymptomatic patients are more likely to be colonized with other strains. Risk factors for *C. difficile* (the major identifiable agent of antibiotic-induced diarrhea and colitis):

- Administration of antibiotics: can occur with any antibiotic, but occurs most frequently with clindamycin, ampicillin, cephalosporins, and fluoroquinolone
- Prolonged hospitalization
- Advanced age
- Abdominal surgery
- Underlying disease (malignancy, renal failure, debilitated status)
- Hospitalized, tube-fed patients are at risk for *C. difficile*–associated diarrhea. Clinicians should consider testing for *C. difficile* in tube-fed patients with diarrhea unrelated to the feeding solution.
- PPI and H_2 blocker therapy increases risk of CDI and recurrent CDI. Risk is 1.7-fold higher with PPIs.

DIAGNOSIS

The clinical signs of CDI generally include diarrhea, fever, and abdominal cramps after use of antibiotics. Although a history of recent antibiotic use is common, it is not a requirement for diagnosis.

DIFFERENTIAL DIAGNOSIS

- Gastrointestinal bacterial infections (e.g., *Salmonella, Shigella, Campylobacter, Yersinia*)
- Enteric parasites (e.g., *Cryptosporidium, Entamoeba histolytica*)
- Inflammatory bowel disease
- Celiac sprue
- Irritable bowel syndrome
- Ischemic colitis
- Antibiotic intolerance

WORKUP

- All patients with diarrhea accompanied by current or recent antibiotic use should be tested for *C. difficile* (see later discussion). *C. difficile* stool tests are positive in 3% of outpatients and up to 29% of inpatients without signs of infection. Testing and treatment for CDI is not recommended in asymptomatic individuals.
- Sigmoidoscopy (without cleansing enema) may be necessary when the clinical and laboratory diagnosis is inconclusive and the diarrhea persists.
- In antibiotic-induced pseudomembranous colitis, the sigmoidoscopy often reveals raised white-yellow exudative plaques adherent to the colonic mucosa pseudomembranes. These are seen more commonly in severe CDI (Fig. 1).

LABORATORY TESTS

- Stool test for *C. difficile* toxin: enzyme-linked immunosorbent assay for *C. difficile* toxins A and B. The latter is used most widely in the clinical setting. It has a sensitivity of 85% and a specificity of 100%.
- *C. difficile* toxin can be detected by cytotoxin tissue-culture assay (cytotoxin assay, gold standard for identifying *C. difficile* toxin in stool

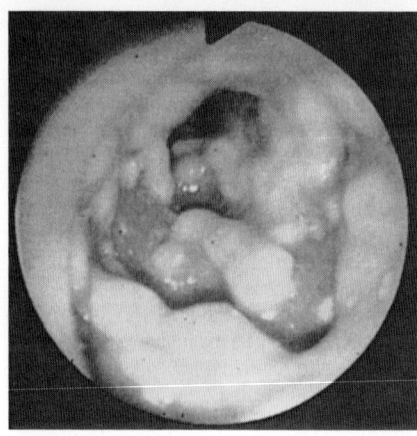

FIG. 1 Pseudomembranous plaques seen with colonoscopy in a patient with *Clostridium difficile*–associated pseudomembranous colitis. (From Gorbach SL: *Infectious diseases,* ed 2, Philadelphia, 1998, Saunders.)

specimen). This test is difficult to perform and results are not available for 24 to 48 hr.
- Fecal leukocytes (assessed by microscopy or lactoferrin assay) are generally present in stool samples.
- Complete blood count usually reveals leukocytosis. A sudden increase in white blood cells to >30,000/mm^3 may be indicative of fulminant colitis.
- Laboratory indicators of **severe CDI** are leukocyte count >15,000/mm^3, serum creatinine ≥1.5 times baseline level, serum albumin <2.5 g/dL.

IMAGING STUDIES

Abdominal film (flat plate and upright) is useful in patients with abdominal pain or evidence of obstruction on physical examination.

TREATMENT

NONPHARMACOLOGIC THERAPY

- Discontinue offending antibiotic.
- Fluid hydration and correction of electrolyte abnormalities
- Probiotics to restore natural defense mechanisms may be useful as adjuvant therapy; however, evidence is limited. Probiotic trials have failed to show benefit in preventing *C. difficile*–associated diarrhea
- Fecal microbiota transplantation (FMT) is an excellent treatment modality for recurrent CDI. It replaces the altered gut flora to allow colonization resistance. Trials have shown that it is more effective than vancomycin and may become standard treatment for recurrent CDI. Recent trials have shown that donor stool administered via colonoscopy are safe and more efficacious than autologous FMT in preventing further CDI episodes.

ACUTE GENERAL Rx

- Metronidazole 500 mg PO qid for 10 to 14 days is indicated in patients with mild to moderate disease. A significant rise in clinical failure has been seen with metronidazole over the past decade, especially in patients with the BI/NAP/027 strain.

- Vancomycin 125 mg PO qid for 10 to 14 days in cases resistant to metronidazole. However, vancomycin may be considered as first-line therapy in hospitalized patients who are seriously ill.
- When parenteral therapy is necessary (e.g., patient with paralytic ileus), IV metronidazole 500 mg qid can be used. It can also be supplemented with vancomycin 500 mg by nasogastric tube with intermittent clamping or retention enema.
- Fidaxomicin, has shown non-inferiority to vancomycin and a lower rate of CDI recurrence (25% with vancomycin vs. 15% with fidaxomicin); however, its higher cost and the fact that a lower risk of recurrence was not seen among patients infected with the BI/NAP1/027 strain (found in 38% of isolates) has limited its use.
- IV tigecycline (a broad-spectrum antibiotic used for skin or soft-tissue infection) can be used as adjunctive or alternative therapy for severe refractory *C. difficile* toxin infection.
- The addition of monoclonal antibodies against *C. difficile* toxins to antibiotic agents has been shown to reduce the recurrence of *C. difficile* infection.
- Fecal microbiota transplantation (FMT): When standard treatment has failed, intestinal microbiota transplantation (IMT) is an effective alternative therapy (eradication rate is 94%). It involves infusing intestinal microorganisms (in a suspension of healthy donor stool) into the intestine of a sick patient via enema, gastroscope/colonoscope, or nasojejunal tube to restore the microbiota. Trials comparing fresh versus frozen fecal microbiota transplantation have shown equal efficacy.
- Trials using the human monoclonal antibody bezlotoxumab for prevention of recurrent CDI have shown efficacy and favorable safety profile. Cost is a limiting factor.

SURGICAL MANAGEMENT OF CDI

- Indications: CDI unresponsive to medical therapy, fulminant colitis
- Clinical features: colonic distention, severe abdominal pain/tenderness, systemic inflammatory response syndrome. Diarrhea may be absent because of ileus.
- Surgical approaches:
  1. Traditional (subtotal or total colectomy), high mortality (50%)
  2. Colon-sparing (loop ileostomy with intraoperative colonic lavage using warmed polyethylene glycol solution via the

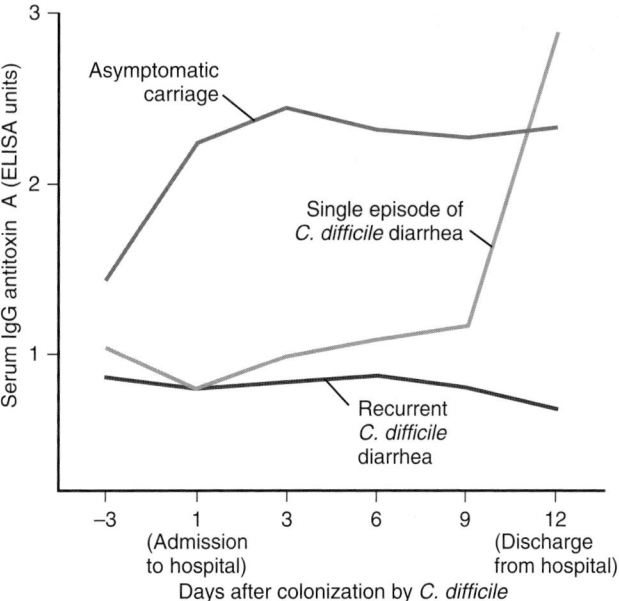

FIG. 2 Serum immunoglobulin G (IgG) antitoxin A antibody response and clinical outcome of infection with *Clostridium difficile*. Patients with nosocomial *C. difficile* diarrhea were studied prospectively, and serum IgG antitoxin A antibody concentrations were measured by enzyme-linked immunosorbent assay (ELISA) at regular intervals. A correlation was observed between the IgG response to toxin A and the clinical outcome of infection. Asymptomatic carriers mounted an early memory immune response to toxin A. By contrast, no significant increase was found in serum IgG antitoxin A of patients who experienced recurrent *C. difficile* diarrhea. In those who had a single episode of diarrhea, IgG antitoxin A levels generally were increased on day 12 of their first episode. Thus, a serum antibody response to toxin A during *C. difficile* infection is associated with protection against symptoms and against recurrent diarrhea. (From Feldman M et al (eds): *Sleisenger and Fordtran's gastrointestinal and liver disease*, ed 10, Philadelphia, 2016, Saunders.)

ileostomy and instillations of postoperative vancomycin flushes via the ileostomy); lower mortality compared to traditional approach

CHRONIC Rx

- Judicious future use of antibiotics to prevent recurrences (e.g., avoid prolonged antibiotic therapy)
- Probiotics have been shown mildly effective in reducing the risk for CDI among patients prescribed antibiotics.
- Alcohol-based hand gels are inadequate for eradication of spores. They are inferior to soap and water for eradication of spores.

DISPOSITION

- Most patients recover completely with appropriate therapy. Fever resolves within 48 hr and diarrhea within 4 to 5 days. Overall mortality rate is 1% to 2.5% but exceeds 10% in untreated patients. CDI recurrence after an initial episode is 20% to 25% regardless of initial treatment with metronidazole or vancomycin. Each recurrence increases risk of repeat episodes (65% chance of recurrence

after 3 CDI episodes). Recurrent CDI usually represents relapse rather than reinfection, no matter how long between episodes (Fig. 2). Recurrent episodes are best treated with a prolonged course of oral vancomycin tapered off over several weeks to months.
- Hospital-acquired CDI is independently associated with an increased risk of in-hospital death. All hospitalized patients with CDI should be placed in contact isolation at least until resolution of diarrhea.

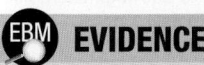 **EVIDENCE**

Available at www.expertconsult.com

SUGGESTED READINGS
Available at www.expertconsult.com

RELATED CONTENT
Clostridium difficile Infection (Patient Information)
Pseudomembranous Colitis (Patient Information)

AUTHOR: **FRED F. FERRI, M.D.**

BASIC INFORMATION

DEFINITION

Cocaine is an alkaloid derived from the coca plant *Erythroxylum coca,* native to South America, which contains approximately 0.5% to 1% cocaine. The drug produces physiologic and behavioral effects when administered orally, intranasally, intravenously, or by inhalation after smoking. Cocaine has potent pharmacologic effects on dopamine, norepinephrine, and serotonin neurons in the central nervous system (CNS) involving alteration and blockade of cellular membrane transport and prevention of reuptake. Cocaine's second action involves the blockage of voltage-gated sodium ion membrane channels, which is responsible for its anesthetic effect. Table 1 describes the pharmacokinetics of cocaine according to route of administration.

SYNONYMS

Cocaine hydrochloride: topical solution (FDA approved as a topical anesthetic)

Crack: this is produced when the hydrochloride molecule is removed by ether extraction, which frees the basic cocaine molecule or "free base." Heating does not destroy the free base; rather, it melts at 98° F and vaporizes at higher temperatures allowing it to be smoked.

Freebase: aqueous solution of cocaine hydrochloride converted to a more volatile base state by the addition of alkali, thereby extracting the cocaine base in a residue or precipitate.

Street names include Bernice, Blow, C, Carrie, Cecil, Charlie, Coke, Dust, Dynamite, Flake, Gin, Girl, Gold dust, Green gold, Jet, Powder, Star dust, Paradise, Pimp's drug, Snow, Stardust, White girl, Yay, Yayo

Liquid lady: alcohol + cocaine

Speedball: heroin + cocaine

Street measures: hit (2 to 200 mg), snort, line, dose, spoon (approximately 1 g)

ICD-10CM CODES
T40.5   Poisoning, cocaine
F14.20 Cocaine dependence, uncomplicated

EPIDEMIOLOGY & DEMOGRAPHICS

- The National Survey on Drug Use and Health (NSDUH) reported in 2012 that there were 1.6 million individuals ages 12 yr or older who had dependence on or had abused cocaine in the preceding year compared with 1.4 million in 2011.

PHYSICAL FINDINGS & CLINICAL PRESENTATION

PHASE I:
- CNS: euphoria, agitation, headache, vertigo, twitching, bruxism, unintentional tremor
- Nausea, vomiting, fever, hypertension, tachycardia

PHASE II:
- CNS: lethargy, hyperreactive deep tendon reflexes, seizures (status epilepticus)
- Sympathetic overdrive: tachycardia, hypertension, hyperthermia
- Incontinence

PHASE III:
- CNS: flaccid paralysis, coma, fixed dilated pupils, loss of reflexes
- Pulmonary edema
- Cardiopulmonary arrest

Psychological dependence manifests with habituation, paranoia, and hallucinations (cocaine "bugs").

CNS: Cerebral ischemia and infarction, cerebral arterial spasm, cerebral vasculitis, cerebral vascular thrombosis, subarachnoid hemorrhage, intraparenchymal hemorrhage, seizures, cerebral atrophy, movement disorders, and hyperthermia

Cardiac: Acute myocardial ischemia and infarction (Fig. E1 and Table 2), arrhythmias (Table 3), and sudden death, dilated cardiomyopathy and myocarditis, infective endocarditis, aortic rupture, acceleration of coronary atherosclerosis

Pulmonary: Inhalation injuries (secondary to smoking crack cocaine): cartilage and nasal septal perforation, oropharyngeal ulcers; immunologically mediated diseases: hypersensitivity pneumonitis, bronchiolitis obliterans; pulmonary vascular lesions and hemorrhage, pulmonary infarction, pulmonary edema secondary to left ventricular failure, pneumomediastinum, and pneumothorax

Gastrointestinal: Gastroduodenal ulceration and perforation; intestinal infarction or perforation, colitis

Renal: Acute renal failure secondary to rhabdomyolysis and myoglobinuria; renal infarction; focal segmental glomerulosclerosis

Obstetric: Placental abruption, low infant weight, prematurity, microcephaly

Psychiatric: Anxiety, depression, paranoia, delirium, psychosis, suicide

Adulterants such as levamisole (an immuno-modulator) and clenbuterol (a beta-adrenergic agonist) have been found mixed with cocaine. Levamisole can cause agranulocytosis, leukoencephalopathy, and cutaneous vasculitis leading to necrosis of the skin. Clenbuterol may cause tachycardia, hyperglycemia, and hypokalemia.

ETIOLOGY

Cocaine may be absorbed through different routes with varying degrees of speed:
- Nasal insufflation/snorting: 2.5 min
- Smoking: <30 sec
- Oral: 2 to 5 min
- Mucosal: <20 min
- Intravenous injection: <30 sec

TABLE 2   Characteristics of Patients with Cocaine-Induced Myocardial Infarction

Dose of Cocaine
Five or six lines (150 mg), up to 2 g
Serum concentration, 0.01-1.02 mg/liter

Frequency of Use
Reported in chronic, recreational, and first-time users

Route of Administration
Occurs with all routes of administration
75% of reported MIs occurred after intranasal use

Age
Mean, 34 yr (range, 17-71 yr)
20% younger than 25 yr

Sex
80%-90% male

Timing
Often within minutes of cocaine use
Reported as late as 5-15 hr after use

From Bonow RO et al: *Heart disease,* ed 9, Philadelphia, 2012, Saunders.

TABLE 3   Cardiac Dysrhythmias and Conduction Disturbances Reported with Cocaine Use

Sinus tachycardia
Sinus bradycardia
Supraventricular tachycardia
Bundle branch block
Complete heart block
Accelerated idioventricular rhythm
Ventricular tachycardia
Ventricular fibrillation
Asystole
Torsades de pointes
Brugada pattern (right bundle branch block with ST-segment elevation in leads V_1, V_2, and V_3)

From Bonow RO et al: *Heart disease,* ed 9, Philadelphia, 2012, Saunders.

TABLE 1   Pharmacokinetics of Cocaine According to Route of Administration

Route of Administration	Onset of Action	Peak Effect	Duration of Action
Inhalation (smoking)	3-5 sec	1-3 min	5-15 min
Intravenous	10-60 sec	3-5 min	20-60 min
Intranasal or other mucosal	1-5 min	15-20 min	60-90 min

From Bonow RO et al: *Heart disease,* ed 9, Philadelphia, 2012, Saunders.

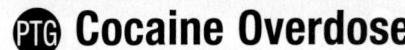

DIAGNOSIS

DIFFERENTIAL DIAGNOSIS

- Methamphetamine ("speed") abuse
- Methylenedioxyamphetamine ("ecstasy") abuse
- Cathinone ("khat") abuse
- Lysergic acid diethylamide (LSD) abuse

WORKUP

Physical examination and laboratory evaluation

LABORATORY TESTS

- Toxicology screen (urine): cocaine is metabolized within 2 hr by the liver to major metabolites, benzoylecgonine and ecgonine methyl ester, which are excreted in the urine. Metabolites can be identified in urine within 5 min of IV use and up to 48 hr after oral ingestion.
- Blood: CBC, electrolytes, glucose, BUN, creatinine, calcium
- Arterial blood gas analysis
- ECG
- Serum creatine kinase and troponin concentration

TREATMENT

There is no specific antidote, and at present, no drug therapy is uniquely effective in treating cocaine abuse and dependence. Modifying cocaine's pharmacokinetic properties by sequestering or hydrolyzing it in serum and limiting its access to its sites of action may prove helpful by using a bacterial cocaine esterase, currently investigational. Adulterants (such as levamisole and clenbuterol, discussed earlier), contaminants, and other drugs may be admixed with street cocaine and should be kept in mind with patients presenting with unusual manifestations. Amantadine may provide effective treatment for cocaine-dependent patients with severe cocaine withdrawal symptoms, as well as the other dopamine agonist bromocriptine (1.5 mg PO tid), which may alleviate some of the symptoms of craving associated with acute cocaine withdrawal.

ACUTE GENERAL Rx

Acute cocaine toxicity requires following advanced poisoning treatment and life support. A suspected "body packer" should have an abdominal radiograph to detect the continued presence of cocaine-containing condoms in the intestinal tract. If present, gentle catharsis with charcoal and mineral oil should be performed with ICU admission and monitoring.

SPECIFIC TREATMENT

INHALATION: Wash nasal passages
AGITATION:
- Check STAT glucose

- Diazepam 15 to 20 mg PO or 2 to 10 mg IM or IV for severe agitation

HYPERTHERMIA:
- Check rectal temperature, creatine kinase, electrolytes
- Monitor with continuous rectal probe; bring temperature down to 101° F within 30 to 45 min

RHABDOMYOLYSIS:
- Vigorous hydration with urine output at least 2 ml/kg
- Mannitol or bicarbonate for rhabdomyolysis resistant to hydration

SEIZURE MANAGEMENT (STATUS EPILEPTICUS):
- Diazepam 5 to 10 mg IV over 2 to 3 min; may be repeated every 10 to 15 min.
- Lorazepam 2 to 3 mg IV over 2 to 3 min; may be repeated.
- Phenytoin loading dose 15 to 18 mg/kg IV at a rate not to exceed 25 to 50 mg/min under cardiac monitoring.
- Phenobarbital loading dose 10 to 15 mg/kg IV at a rate of 25 mg/min; an additional 5 mg/kg may be given in 30 to 45 min if seizures are not controlled.
- For refractory seizures, consider:
  1. Pancuronium 0.1 mg/kg IV
  2. Halothane general anesthesia
  3. Both require EEG monitoring to determine brain seizure activity.

HYPERTENSION: Cocaine-induced hypertension usually responds to benzodiazepines. If this fails:
- Consider arterial line for continuous blood pressure monitoring.
- Avoid the use of calcium channel blockers because they may potentiate the incidence of seizures and death, especially in body packers.
- The use of beta-blockers may exacerbate cocaine-induced vasoconstriction and may cause paradoxical hypertension, worsening patient outcomes.
- Phentolamine (unopposed adrenergic effects) or nitroglycerin may be required.
- If diastolic pressure >120 mm Hg: hydralazine hydrochloride 25 mg IM or IV; may repeat q1h.
- If hypertension is uncontrolled or hypertensive encephalopathy is present: sodium nitroprusside initially at 0.5 mg/kg/min not to exceed 10 mg/kg/min.

CHEST PAIN:
- Chest radiograph, ECG, cardiac enzymes
- Benzodiazepines for agitation
- Acetylsalicylic acid and nitroglycerin for ischemic pain (Aspirin is contraindicated if dissection is suspected.)
- Percutaneous transluminal coronary angioplasty possibly better than thrombolysis for cocaine-associated myocardial infarction
- Phentolamine will reverse cocaine-induced vasoconstriction and may be administered 5 to 10 mg every 5 to 10 minutes.

- The use of beta-adrenergic blockers is not generally recommended for reasons highlighted earlier.
- If beta-blockers are to be used, this should be preceded by administration of phentolamine to prevent unopposed alpha-adrenergic stimulation. Many authors recommend not using beta-blockers until the cocaine has been systemically eliminated.

VENTRICULAR ARRHYTHMIAS (CONSIDERATIONS):
- The Advanced Cardiac Life Support (ACLS) protocol should be followed.
- Antiarrhythmic agents should be used with caution during the early period after cocaine exposure as a result of their proarrhythmic and proconvulsant effects.
- Termination of ventricular arrhythmias may be resistant to lidocaine and even cardioversion.
- In a cardiac arrest situation secondary to cocaine toxicity, vasopressin offers a theoretical advantage over epinephrine as it increases coronary blood flow and myocardial oxygen availability. In the 2015 ACLS update, however, vasopressin was removed from the treatment algorithm, so it may not be readily available.

DISPOSITION

Although many patients who use cocaine may not require treatment because of the short half-life of the drug, others may require specific treatment for possible cocaine-related complications.

REFERRAL

Consider psychotherapy or behavioral therapy once stable. There is some evidence that topiramate 300 mg orally daily added to cognitive behavioral therapy may be beneficial in patients with severe withdrawal symptoms.

PEARLS & CONSIDERATIONS

- Cocaine-induced vasoconstriction may be exacerbated by the use of selective and non-selective beta-adrenergic blocking agents.
- The use of lidocaine in treating ventricular arrhythmias may precipitate seizures and further arrhythmias.

SUGGESTED READINGS

Available at www.expertconsult.com

RELATED CONTENT

Cocaine Abuse and Dependence (Patient Information)
Drug Abuse (Patient Information)
Drug Abuse (Related Key Topic)

AUTHOR: **SAJEEV HANDA, M.D.**

Diseases and Disorders

C

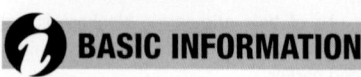

BASIC INFORMATION

DEFINITION

Colorectal cancer (CRC) is a neoplasm arising from the luminal surface of the large bowel; locations include descending colon (40% to 42%), rectosigmoid and rectum (30% to 33%), cecum and ascending colon (25% to 30%), and transverse colon (10% to 13%).

ICD-10CM CODES
C18	Malignant neoplasm of colon
C18.2	Malignant neoplasm of colon, ascending colon
C18.4	Malignant neoplasm of colon, transverse colon
C18.6	Malignant neoplasm of colon, descending colon
C18.7	Malignant neoplasm of colon, sigmoid colon
C19	Malignant neoplasm of rectosigmoid junction

EPIDEMIOLOGY & DEMOGRAPHICS

- Worldwide, CRC accounts for about 1.4 million new cases and almost 700,000 deaths annually. The highest incidence is in North America, Australasia, Europe, and South Korea.
- CRC is the third most common cancer and the third leading cause of cancer deaths in the U.S. (134,490 new cases and 49,190 deaths annually estimated for 2016).
- Peak incidence is in the seventh decade of life. The lifetime risk for development of CRC is 1 in 17, with 90% of cases occurring after age 50 yr.
- CRC accounts for 14% of all cases of cancer (excluding skin malignancies) and 8% of all yearly cancer deaths.
- Risk factors:
  1. Hereditary polyposis syndromes
  2. Familial polyposis (high risk)
  3. Gardner's syndrome (high risk)
  4. Turcot's syndrome (high risk)
  5. Peutz-Jeghers syndrome (low to moderate risk)
  6. Inflammatory bowel disease (IBD), both ulcerative colitis and Crohn's disease
  7. Family history of "cancer family syndrome"
  8. Heredofamilial breast cancer and colon carcinoma
  9. Pelvic irradiation history
  10. First-degree relatives with colorectal carcinoma
  11. Age >50 years
  12. Dietary factors (diet high in fat or red meat, alcohol use, low vegetable intake)
  13. Hereditary nonpolyposis colon cancer (HNPCC): autosomal dominant disorder characterized by early age of onset (mean age, 44 yr) and right-sided or proximal colon cancers, synchronous and metachronous colon cancers, mucinous and poorly differentiated colon cancers; accounts for 1% to 5% of all cases of CRC
  14. Previous endometrial or ovarian cancer, particularly when diagnosed at an early age

PHYSICAL FINDINGS & CLINICAL PRESENTATION

- Physical examination may be completely unremarkable.
- Digital rectal examination can detect approximately 50% of rectal cancers.
- Palpable abdominal masses may indicate metastasis or complications of colorectal carcinoma (abscess, intussusception, volvulus).
- Abdominal distention and tenderness are suggestive of colonic obstruction.
- Hepatomegaly is indicative of hepatic metastasis.

ETIOLOGY

CRC can arise through either of two mutational pathways: microsatellite instability or chromosomal instability. Germline genetic mutations are the basis of inherited colon cancer syndromes; an accumulation of somatic mutations in a cell is the basis of sporadic colon cancer.

DIAGNOSIS

DIFFERENTIAL DIAGNOSIS

- Diverticular disease
- Strictures or adhesions
- Inflammatory bowel disease (IBD)
- Infectious or inflammatory lesions
- Arteriovenous malformations
- Metastatic carcinoma
- Extrinsic masses (cysts, abscesses)

WORKUP

The clinical presentation of colorectal malignancies may consist of nonspecific symptoms (weight loss, anorexia, malaise) or of specific symptoms related to mass effect or bleeding. It is useful to divide colon cancer symptoms into those usually associated with the right- or left-sided cancers because the clinical presentation can vary with the location.

- Right side of colon:
  1. Anemia (from chronic blood loss).
  2. Abdominal pain may be present, or the patient may be completely asymptomatic.
  3. Rectal bleeding is often missed because blood is mixed with feces.
  4. Obstruction and constipation are unusual because of large lumen and more liquid stools.
- Left side of colon:
  1. Change in bowel habits (constipation, diarrhea, tenesmus, pencil-thin stools).
  2. Rectal bleeding (bright red blood coating the surface of the stool).
  3. Intestinal obstruction is frequent because of small lumen.

CLASSIFICATION AND STAGING

AJCC classification for CRC:
- **A.** Confined to the mucosa-submucosa (stage I)
- **B.** Invasion of muscularis propria (stage II)
- **C.** Local node involvement (stage III)
- **D.** Distant metastasis (stage IV)

TNM Classification:

Stage	TNM Classification
I	T1-2, N0, M0
IIA	T3, N0, M0
IIB	T4a, N0, M0
IIC	T4b, N0, M0
IIIA	T1-2, N1, M0T1, N2a, M0
IIIB	T3-4, N1, M0T2-3, N2a, M0T1-2, N2b, M0
IIIC	T4a, N2a, M0T3-4a, N2b, M0T4b, N1-2, M0
IVA	T(any), N(any), M1a
IVB	T(any), N(any), M1b

LABORATORY TESTS

- Positive fecal occult blood test (FOBT): Many primary care physicians use single digital FOBT as their primary screening test for CRC. Single FOBT has low specificity for detecting human hemoglobin, is a poor screening method for CRC (sensitivity, 4.9%), and is inappropriate as the only test because negative results do not decrease the odds of advanced neoplasia. The American College of Gastroenterology recommends fecal immunochemical test (FIT) as a replacement for guaiac-based FOBT for CRC detection. FIT measures intact human globin protein (as opposed to heme) in the stool. It detects more advanced adenomas than FOBT. Fecal DNA testing is a newer screening method that detects colonic cells shed into the fecal stream that possess specific genetic or epigenetic changes. The technique has a reported sensitivity of 97% and a specificity of 90% for CRC stages I-III. In trials involving asymptomatic persons at average risk for colorectal cancer, multitarget stool DNA testing detects significantly more cancers than FIT but has more false-positive results. High cost and rate of false positives are the main obstacles inhibiting broader adoption of fecal DNA testing. Microcytic anemia on CBC may be indicative of chronic blood loss.
- Molecular markers including abnormal DNA from cancerous cells can be detected in stool. FIT combined with stool DNA test (FIT-DNA) has been approved by the FDA for colorectal screening. One study showed that one-time FIT-DNA had a higher sensitivity for detection of colorectal cancer than one-time FIT alone (92.3% vs. 73.8%), but specificity was lower (86.6% vs. 94.9%).[1]
- Circulating methylated SEPT9 DNA: does not reliably detect precancerous neoplasia. Studies showing mortality benefit are lacking.
- Increased plasma carcinoembryonic antigen (CEA) level: CEA is not useful for screening because it can be increased in nonmalignant conditions (smoking, IBD, alcoholic liver disease). A normal CEA result does not exclude the diagnosis of CRC.

[1]Inadomi JM: Screening for colorectal neoplasia, *N Engl J Med* 376:149–156, 2017.

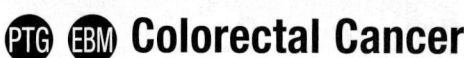

IMAGING STUDIES

- Colonoscopy with biopsy (primary assessment tool): The American College of Physicians (ACP) recommends that patients should be offered a colonoscopy beginning at age 50, and it should be repeated every 10 years in average-risk patients. Screening is recommended in African Americans beginning at age 45 yr. Persons with only one first-degree relative with CRC or advanced adenomas diagnosed at 60 yr or older may be screened as at average risk. The U.S. Preventive Services Task Force guidelines state that screening should not be routinely recommended in persons older than 75 yr, and it should not be recommended at all in persons older than 85 yr. If persons between the ages of 75 and 85 yr have never undergone screening, the decision about screening should be individualized according to health status. The ACP recommends that clinicians stop screening for colorectal cancer in adults over age 75 yr or in adults with a life expectancy of <10 yr. Table 1 describes CRC screening and surveillance recommendations.
- Computed tomography colonoscopy (CTC) virtual colonoscopy (VC) uses helical (spiral) CT scanning to generate a two- or three-dimensional virtual colorectal image (Fig. 1). CTC does not require sedation, but, like optical colonoscopy, it requires some bowel preparation (either bowel cathartics or ingestion of iodinated contrast medium with meals during the 48 hr before CT) and air insufflation. It also involves substantial exposure to radiation. In addition, patients with lesions detected by VC will require traditional colonoscopy. Compared with colonoscopy, CTC sensitivity for detection

of polyps >10 mm ranges from 70% to 96%, and specificity ranges from 72% to 96%. CTC has replaced double-contrast barium enema as the radiographic screening alternative when patients decline colonoscopy.
- Capsule endoscopy allows visualization of the colonic mucosa but is not recommended as a screening procedure because its sensitivity for detecting colonic lesions is low compared with colonoscopy.
- CT scanning of the abdomen (Fig. 2), pelvis, and chest assists in preoperative staging.
- PET scanning can display functional information and is accurate in the detection of CRC and its distant metastases. Colonography composed of a combined modality of PET and CT is a newer diagnostic modality that can provide whole-body tumor staging in a single session.

Rx TREATMENT

GENERAL Rx

- Surgical resection is the definitive and curative upfront treatment for stages I-III colon cancers. Selected patients (high-risk stage II, all stage III) are often recommended for adjuvant chemotherapy.
- The standard chemotherapy regimen for adjuvant therapy of resected CRC is the combination of oxaliplatin with a fluoropyrimidine (5-fluorouracil or capecitabine). Older patients and patients who are not considered candidates for aggressive therapy are recommended treatment with single-agent fluoropyrimidine therapy.
- The combination of neoadjuvant chemotherapy and radiation therapy is used to downsize and downstage rectal cancers before definitive resection and has been proven to

improve overall survival and local disease control in stage II-III cancers.
- The use of adjuvant chemotherapy in stage II disease (no nodal involvement) is estimated to provide an improvement in overall survival by 3% to 4% with current 5-yr survival rates in the 80% range. Given the modest benefit, current guidelines recommend consideration of adjuvant chemotherapy only in high-risk stage II patients. The magnitude of survival benefit is higher in stage III patients and combination chemotherapy regimen as above is associated with 5-year overall survival in the 70% range with wide variation in the subgroups.
- The outlook for patients with metastatic and relapsed CRC has improved dramatically in the past few years. Median overall survival is now expected in the 30+ month range with modern chemotherapeutic regimen usage. Patients with limited and resectable metastases in sites such as the liver have even better survivals with 5-year survival ranges in the 50% range.
- Current chemotherapy agents that are used in the metastatic setting include 5-fluorouracil (5-FU), capecitabine, irinotecan, oxaliplatin, and mitomycin. Two-drug chemotherapy regimens using a combination of antimetabolite (5-FU or capecitabine) in combination with either oxaliplatin or irinotecan form the backbone of systemic therapy approaches.
- Molecularly targeted therapy against the epidermal growth factor receptor (EGFR) and the angiogenesis pathway are used in combination with the chemotherapy backbone in metastatic CRC. Antiangiogenesis agents include monoclonal antibodies bevacizumab, aflibercept, and ramucirumab. Cetuximab and panitumumab are EGFR receptor blockers which are active in metastatic CRC patients whose tumors do not harbor mutated RAS oncogenes.
- The liver is generally the initial and most common site of CRC metastases. Resection of metastases limited to the liver followed by systemic chemotherapy is curative in more than 30% of selected patients. Metasectomy of limited pulmonary metastases can also be considered in selected cases.
- Unresectable multiple liver metastases are often approached by locoregional therapeutic approaches such as transarterial chemoembolization (TACE), selective internal radiation therapy (SIRT) using yttrium-90 brachytherapy, or hepatic arterial infusional chemotherapy.
- The oral multitargeted kinase inhibitor regorafenib and the oral antimetabolite drug TAS-102 provide modest survival benefit in patients who have failed standard chemotherapy approaches.
- In patients with pathologically confirmed microsatellite instability in their cancers, the role of checkpoint inhibitors (pembrolizumab, nivolumab) is being investigated and seems to be a potential effective option after failure of all standard therapies.

TABLE 1 Colorectal Cancer (CRC) Screening and Surveillance Recommendations*

Indication	Recommendations
Average risk	Beginning at age 50 yr:Colonoscopy every 10 yrComputed tomographic colonography every 5 yrFlexible sigmoidoscopy every 5 yrDouble-contrast barium enema every 5 yrStool blood testing annually or stool DNA testing acceptable but not preferred
One or two first-degree relatives with CRC at any age or adenoma at age <60 yr	Colonoscopy every 5 yr beginning at age 40 yr, or 10 yr younger than earliest diagnosis, whichever comes first
Hereditary nonpolyposis CRC	Genetic counseling and screening†Colonoscopy every 1 to 2 yr beginning at age 25 yr and then yearly after age 40 yr‡
Familial adenomatous polyposis and variants	Genetic counseling and testing†Flexible sigmoidoscopy yearly beginning at puberty‡
Personal history of CRC	Colonoscopy within 1 yr of curative resection; repeat at 3 yr and then every 5 yr if normal
Personal history of colorectal adenoma	Colonoscopy every 3 to 5 yr after removal of all index polyps
Inflammatory bowel disease	Colonoscopy every 1 to 2 yr beginning after 8 yr of pancolitis or after 15 yr if only left-sided disease

*Recommendations proposed by the American Cancer Society and U.S. Multi-Society Task Force on Colorectal Cancer; recommendations for average-risk patients also endorsed by the American College of Radiology.
†Whenever possible, affected relatives should be tested first because of potential false-negative results.
‡Screening recommendation for individuals with positive or indeterminate tests as well as for those who refuse genetic testing.
From Andreoli TE et al: *Andreoli and Carpenter's Cecil essentials of medicine*, ed 8, Philadelphia, 2010, Saunders.

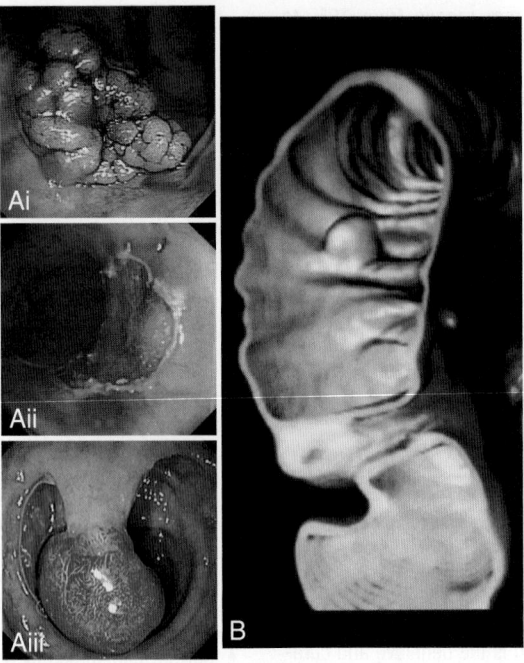

FIG. 1 Colon polyps seen at (Ai–iii) colonoscopy and (B) computed tomography (CT) colonography. Aii is after endoscopic resection of the polyps in Ai. (From Ballinger A: *Kumar & Clark's essentials of medicine*, ed 5, Edinburgh, 2012, Saunders.)

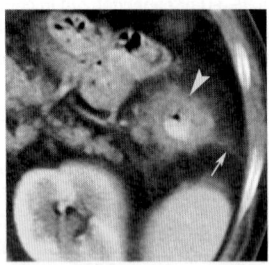

FIG. 2 Colon carcinoma: wall thickening. A carcinoma of the descending colon near the splenic flexure causes thickening of the colon wall (*arrowhead*) and narrowing of the lumen. Stranding densities (*arrow*) extending into the pericolonic fat suggest tumor extension through the bowel wall. (From Webb WR, Brant WE, Major NM: *Fundamentals of body CT*, ed 4, Philadelphia, 2015, Saunders.)

CHRONIC Rx

Follow-up is indicated with:
- Physician visits with a focus on clinical and disease-related history, directed physical examination, coordination of follow-up, and counseling every 3 to 4 mo for the first 3 yr and then every 6 months for 2 yr.
- Colonoscopy at end of first year, then after 3 yr and subsequently every 5 yr.
- Baseline CEA level, if elevated, can be used after surgery as a measure of completeness of tumor resection. It is used to monitor tumor recurrence and is obtained every 3 to 6 mo for up to 5 yr.

DISPOSITION

The 5-yr survival rate varies with the stage of the carcinoma:
- TNM stage:

Stage	5-yr Survival Rate (%)
I	>90
IIA-C	60-85
IIIA-C	25-65
IV	5-10

- Overall 5-yr disease-free survival rate has increased from 50% to 63% during the past two decades.
- High-frequency microsatellite instability in CRC is independently predictive of a relatively favorable outcome and reduces the likelihood of metastases.
- In patients with high-risk stage II and with stage III CRC, there is improved 5-yr survival among patients treated with adjuvant chemotherapy.
- Expression patterns of microRNA are systemically altered in colon adenocarcinomas. High miR-21 expression is associated with poor survival and poor therapeutic outcome.
- The optimal timing from surgery to initiation of adjuvant chemotherapy is 4 to 8 wk. A longer time to initiation of adjuvant chemotherapy is associated with worse survival rates.
- Regular aspirin use after the diagnosis of CRC has been reported to be associated with lower risk for CRC-specific and overall mortality, especially among individuals with tumors that overexpress cyclooxygenase-2. Regular aspirin use is associated with lower BRAF-wild type colorectal cancer but not with BRAF-mutated cancer risk. All aspirin doses starting with 75 mg daily had similar effects on CRC incidence and mortality.

REFERRAL

- Multidisciplinary referral to colorectal surgery or surgical oncology, medical oncology, radiation oncology

! PEARLS & CONSIDERATIONS

COMMENTS

- Metastases of tumor cells to regional lymph nodes is the single most important prognostic factor in patients with colon cancer.
- Decreased fat intake to 30% of total energy intake, increased fiber through fruit and vegetable consumption may reduce CRC risk.
- Chemoprophylaxis with aspirin (81 mg/day) reduces the incidence of colorectal adenomas in persons at risk.
- The National Cancer Institute has published consensus guidelines for universal screening for HNPCC in patients with newly diagnosed CRC. Tumors in mutation carriers of HNPCC typically exhibit microsatellite instability, a characteristic phenotype caused by expansion or contraction of short nucleotide repeat sequences. These guidelines (Bethesda Guidelines) are useful for selective patients for microsatellite instability testing. Screening patients with newly diagnosed CRC for HNPCC is cost effective, especially if the benefits to their immediate relatives are considered.
- The use of either annual or biennial FOBT significantly reduces the incidence of CRC.
- The detection of mutations in the *APC* gene from stool samples is a promising new modality for early detection of colorectal neoplasms.

SUGGESTED READINGS
Available at www.expertconsult.com

RELATED CONTENT

Colon Cancer (Patient Information)
Familial Adenomatous Polyposis and Gardner's Syndrome (Related Key Topic)
Lynch Syndrome (Related Key Topic)
Peutz-Jeghers Syndrome and Other Polyposis Syndromes (Related Key Topic)

AUTHOR: **RITESH RATHORE, M.D.**

BASIC INFORMATION

DEFINITION

Compartment syndrome is a condition that occurs when elevated pressure within a confined space compromises circulation and results in ischemia and end organ damage (i.e., tissue necrosis). Acute compartment syndrome is a surgical emergency necessitating prompt diagnosis and intervention.

ICD-10CM CODES: Code x Y (Y = encounter type: (A) initial, D (subsequent), S (sequelae)
T79.A0xA	Compartment syndrome, unspecified, initial encounter
T79.A0xD	Compartment syndrome, unspecified, subsequent encounter
T79.A0xS	Compartment syndrome, unspecified, sequelae
T79.A19xY	Traumatic compartment syndrome of unspecified upper extremity
T79.A11x Y	Traumatic compartment syndrome of the right upper extremity
T79.A12x Y	Traumatic compartment syndrome of the left upper extremity
T79.A29x Y	Traumatic compartment syndrome of unspecified lower extremity
T79.A21x Y	Traumatic compartment syndrome of right lower extremity
T79.A22x Y	Traumatic compartment syndrome of left lower extremity
T79.A9x Y	Traumatic compartment syndrome of other sites
M79.A19x Y	Nontraumatic compartment syndrome of unspecified upper extremity
M79.A11x Y	Nontraumatic compartment syndrome of the right upper extremity
M79.A12x Y	Nontraumatic compartment syndrome of the left upper extremity
M79.A29x Y	Nontraumatic compartment syndrome of unspecified lower extremity
M79.A21x Y	Nontraumatic compartment syndrome of right lower extremity
M79.A22x Y	Nontraumatic compartment syndrome of left lower extremity
M79.A9x Y	Nontraumatic compartment syndrome of other sites

EPIDEMIOLOGY & DEMOGRAPHICS

- Most commonly associated with acute trauma, comprising 70% of cases. Up to 30% of cases are not associated with a fracture.
- Typically occurs in persons <35 years of age with approximately 10× higher incidence in males.
- Can affect any compartment; most commonly in the distal lower extremity and forearm but may affect the thigh, foot, hand, buttock, or abdomen.

- Associated with up to 1/3 of tibial shaft fractures.
- Injuries commonly associated with compartment syndrome: fractures of the tibial shaft/plateau, distal radius, and femoral shaft as well as both bone forearm and pediatric supracondylar fractures.
- Other etiologies include significant soft-tissue injury, gunshot wound, crush injury, prolonged downtime, burns, IV fluid extravasation, reperfusion injury, bleeding disorders, and external forces such as circumferential cast or splint immobilization.

PATHOPHYSIOLOGY

Compartment syndrome occurs when the pressure within a compartment limits blood flow and results in tissue ischemia and necrosis. The perfusion pressure is defined as the difference between the diastolic and intracompartmental pressures. Under normal physiologic conditions, tissue perfusion decreases as intracompartmental pressure increases. Eventually, the pressure within the compartment exceeds capillary pressure and results in capillary bed collapse, venous congestion, and tissue hypoperfusion. Local tissue hypoperfusion results in hypoxia and cell death. Tissue perfusion has been shown to significantly decrease with intracompartmental pressures between 10 and 20 mm Hg. Decreased tissue perfusion can result in reversible neuropraxia within 1 hour. Cell death, myonecrosis, and other irreversible changes can occur within 4-6 hours.

A variety of clinical conditions have been associated with the development of compartment syndrome:

- Conditions that increase the volume within a compartment, such as bleeding from fracture, vascular injury, or diathesis. Other causes of significant soft-tissue swelling include reperfusion injury (e.g., following embolectomy or arterial bypass grafting), crush injury, high-energy soft-tissue injury (e.g., gunshot or ballistic injury), thermal or electrical burn injuries, extravasation of intravenous fluids, injection of recreational drugs, massive fluid resuscitation, and snake bites.
- Conditions that decrease the volume of a compartment via external forces, such as tight external dressings (e.g., fracture casts/splints), prolonged downtime, or external pressure seen in sedated or comatose patients who lie on an extremity for a prolonged period (e.g., drug overdose, ICU patients, and prolonged surgical procedures).

PHYSICAL FINDINGS & CLINICAL PRESENTATION

Signs and symptoms are usually apparent but can be unreliable in certain circumstances and may lead to delayed or missed diagnosis. Acute compartment syndrome can develop within hours; therefore, serial examinations are critical for patients with high risk. Patients with tense, painful compartments are considered to have acute compartment syndrome. In the majority of cases, compartment syndrome is a clinical diagnosis based on history and examination. The diagnosis may be confirmed with the use of intracompartmental pressure-measuring devices in the setting of comatose or unresponsive patients and in clinically equivocal cases.

Clinical signs and symptoms of compartment syndrome include:

- Pain out of proportion to a given injury or worsening pain despite adequate or increasing analgesia requirement (earliest sign).
- Pain with passive stretch of the muscles within the compartment. Patients typically endorse constant, deep pain that is severe and located to the compartment with passive stretch of the musculature (Fig. 1). Many trauma patients will complain of pain with any movement of the affected extremity, and it may be useful for providers to attempt to distract patients while testing for pain with passive stretch.
- Tense and swollen compartment (Figs. 2 and 3).
- Tingling or pins and needles or reduced sense of touch or sensation within the distribution of the nerve(s) traversing the compartment. Muscle weakness is a late finding suggestive of permanent muscle damage.
- Capillary refill can be sluggish or normal.
- Palpable peripheral pulses may be present even in late stages of the disease process due to collateral blood flow and reconstitution distal to the compartment of concern.
- Pediatric patients may demonstrate agitation, anxiety, and increasing analgesia requirement (the 3 As).

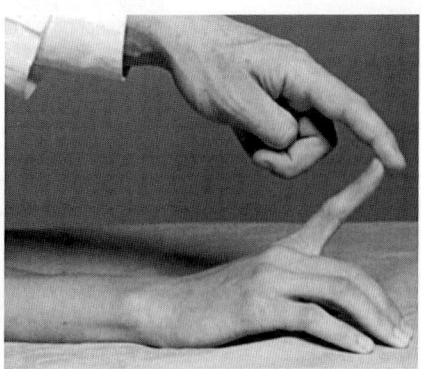

FIG. 1 Passive extension of the digit causes pain referred to the compartment. (From Browner BD et al [eds]: *Skeletal trauma: basic science, management, and reconstruction,* ed 4, Philadelphia, 2009, Saunders.)

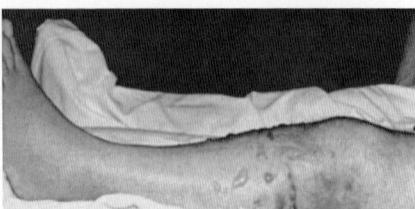

FIG. 2 Acute compartment syndrome of the leg. (From Browner BD et al [eds]: *Skeletal trauma,* ed 4, Philadelphia, 2009, Saunders.)

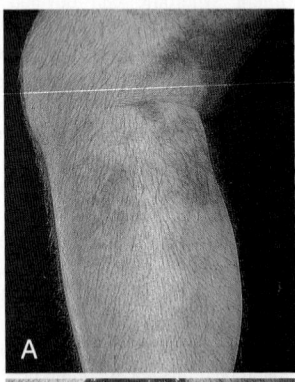

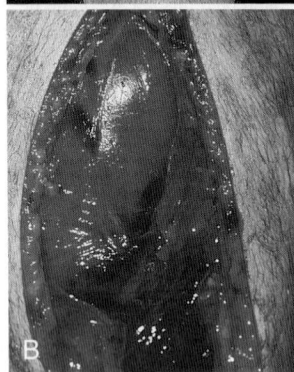

FIG. 3 A, Severe calf swelling due to anterior and posterior compartment syndromes after ischemia-reperfusion. **B,** Appearance after emergency fasciotomy. Note edematous muscle and hematoma. (Courtesy Michael J. Allen, FRCS, Leicester, UK. From Floege J et al: *Comprehensive clinical nephrology,* ed 4, Philadelphia, 2010, Saunders.)

- Comatose, nonresponsive, or unreliable patients may require intracompartmental pressure measurements.
- Compartment syndrome can develop in the setting of an open fracture.

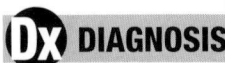 **DIAGNOSIS**

The diagnosis of compartment syndrome is based on clinical signs and symptoms with intracompartmental pressure measurements being reserved for comatose, unreliable, or nonresponsive patients.

DIFFERENTIAL DIAGNOSIS

- Physiologic soft-tissue edema or swelling
- Muscle strains or contusion
- Cellulitis
- Gangrene
- Peripheral vascular injury
- Necrotizing fasciitis
- Stress fractures
- Deep vein thrombosis and thrombophlebitis
- Tendinitis
- Tarsal tunnel or posterior ankle syndrome
- Popliteal artery impingement
- Claudication
- Tumor
- Venous insufficiency

LABORATORY TESTS

Diagnosis is based on clinical findings and intracompartmental pressures as needed. Laboratory values are not useful in the diagnosis of compartment syndrome but are important for other diagnoses or associated conditions. The exception to this is an INR or a coagulation panel in patients on anticoagulation (e.g., fall while on Coumadin).

- INR/PT and PTT to assess coagulation profile and bleeding diathesis
- CBC with differential for evaluation of infection
- Creatine phosphokinase (CK) levels, which can rise as muscle injury develops (e.g., crush injury)
- Metabolic panel for the assessment of electrolytes and renal function
- Urinalysis for rhabdomyolysis
- Urine and serum myoglobin levels

IMAGING STUDIES

- Radiography of the affected extremity should be obtained to evaluate for fracture or foreign body.
- Direct intracompartmental pressure measurement can be obtained as needed using handheld manometer, wick or slit catheter technique, or a simple needle manometer system. Compartment syndrome is diagnosed or confirmed when the difference between diastolic blood pressure and compartment pressure (Δ pressure) is ≤30 mm Hg.
- Ultrasonography or Doppler ultrasonography can be used to rule out deep vein thrombosis and evaluate blood flow to the extremity. Arteriography can be used to evaluate for arterial injury as well as blood flow within a compartment.
- Near-infrared spectroscopy and technetium-99m methoxyisobutylisonitrile scintigraphy can also be used.

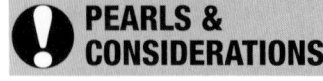 **TREATMENT**

The goal of treatment is to reduce the intracompartmental pressure and prevent tissue ischemia and necrosis (Fig. 4).

ACUTE GENERAL Rx

- Analgesics for pain control.
- Advanced trauma life support (hypotension can worsen tissue perfusion and ischemia).
- Remove circumferential dressings, cast, and all external pressure generators.
- The affected extremity should be elevated above the level of the heart to aid in resolution of swelling.
- Emergent fasciotomies and thorough debridement of nonviable tissue is the standard of care. This should be performed within 4-6 hours of symptom onset.
- Measurement of compartment pressure is not necessary to perform fasciotomy if clinical suspicion is high.
- Concomitant fractured bones should be stabilized with plating, external fixation, or intramedullary nailing.

CHRONIC Rx

- Patients should return to the operating room every 48 hours to assess for tissue viability and repeat debridement as needed.
- A negative pressure wound therapy system may be placed over fasciotomy wounds with delayed wound closure and skin grafting performed as needed.
- Opsite sheet and boot lace techniques may also be used for fasciotomy site closure.
- Local wound care should be emphasized to decrease the risk of infection.

DISPOSITION

With early diagnosis and prompt intervention, the prognosis and functional outcomes are excellent. The following are sequelae of delayed or undiagnosed compartment syndrome:

- Myonecrosis
- Permanent nerve damage and paralysis
- Muscle contracture (e.g., Volkmann's contracture in the forearm)
- Gangrene
- Infection and possible sepsis
- Amputation
- Rhabdomyolysis and possible renal failure
- Cardiac arrhythmias and possible death from reperfusion injury and electrolyte abnormalities

REFERRAL

Patients with suspected compartment syndrome should be promptly referred to an orthopedic and general surgeon.

! PEARLS & CONSIDERATIONS

- Compartment syndrome is a surgical emergency necessitating prompt diagnosis and intervention. It is commonly associated with fractures, most notably tibial shaft, both bones of the forearm, and supracondylar fractures of the distal humerus.
- Compartment syndrome is a clinical diagnosis, and intracompartmental pressures are not required to make the diagnosis.

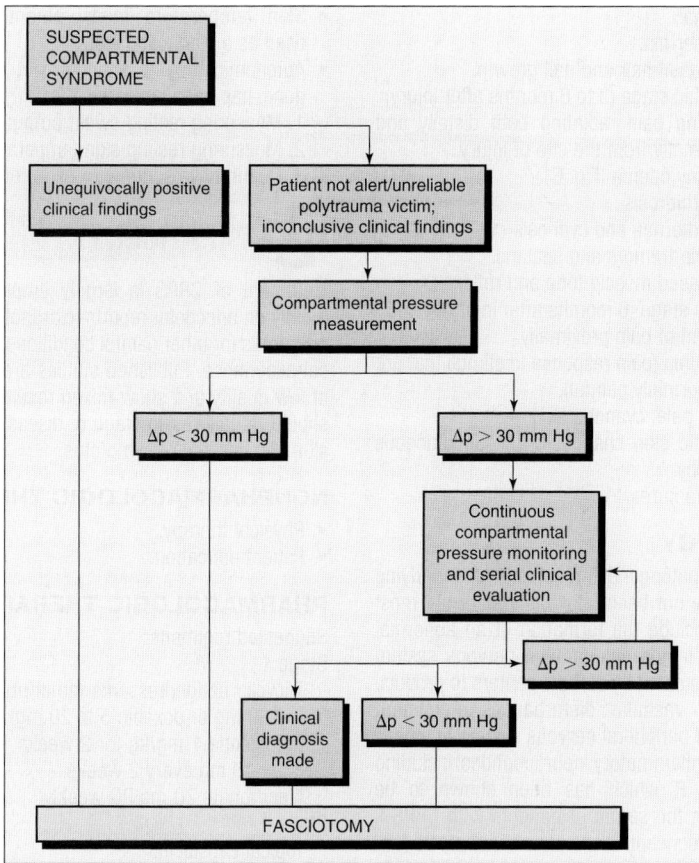

FIG. 4 Algorithm for management for a patient with suspected compartment syndrome. Δp is defined as the difference between the diastolic pressure and the measured compartment pressure in mm Hg as documented by McQueen and Court-Brown. (From Browner BD et al [eds]: *Skeletal trauma*, ed 4, Philadelphia, 2009, Saunders.)

- Pain with passive stretch, pain out of proportion to the injury, or increasing analgesia requirement should raise concern for compartment syndrome.
- The presence of palpable peripheral pulses does not rule out compartment syndrome.
- Compartment syndrome is a surgical emergency, and prompt surgical intervention is required.
- Universal precautions and aseptic measures are necessary for patients undergoing fasciotomy due to the elevated risk of local and systemic infection following the procedure (nonviable tissue is a nidus for infection).
- Patients with fracture treated with a cast should be informed about the risks of swelling and the signs and symptoms of compartment syndrome with instructions to go to the nearest emergency department if these symptoms develop.

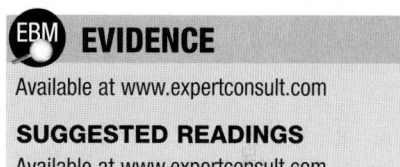

EBM EVIDENCE

Available at www.expertconsult.com

SUGGESTED READINGS

Available at www.expertconsult.com

RELATED CONTENT

Compartment Syndrome (Patient Information)

AUTHOR: **MICHAEL C. MARIORENZI, M.S., M.D.**

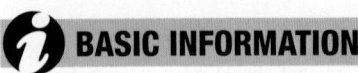
DEFINITION

Complex regional pain syndrome (CRPS) is a pain disorder characterized by constant and intense limb pain associated with vasomotor and neurosensory abnormalities, skin changes, and demineralization of bone. CRPS has been divided into type I, in which there is usually an initiating noxious event but no distinct nerve lesion, and type II, in which a definable (usually traumatic) nerve lesion exists. CRPS type I generally correlates with the syndrome formerly known as reflex sympathetic dystrophy (RSD), and CRPS type II equates with what was previously termed causalgia. The term *shoulder-hand syndrome* has been used to describe CRPS in the setting of myocardial infarction or ischemia.

SYNONYMS

Reflex sympathetic dystrophy
Shoulder hand syndrome
CRPS

ICD-10CM CODES	
M89.0	Algoneurodystrophy
G90.59	Complex regional pain syndrome I of other specified site
G90.511	Complex regional pain syndrome I of right upper limb
G90.512	Complex regional pain syndrome I of left upper limb
G90.513	Complex regional pain syndrome I of upper limb, bilateral
G90.519	Complex regional pain syndrome I of unspecified upper limb
G90.521	Complex regional pain syndrome I of right lower limb
G90.522	Complex regional pain syndrome I of left lower limb
G90.523	Complex regional pain syndrome I of lower limb, bilateral
G90.529	Complex regional pain syndrome I of unspecified lower limb
G90.59	Complex regional pain syndrome I of other specified site

EPIDEMIOLOGY & DEMOGRAPHICS

The incidence and prevalence of CRPS are not known. It occurs in adults and children. Common situations in which CRPS is seen include extremity trauma, burns, stroke, and orthopedic and podiatric procedures. Immobilization of the limb often precedes the development of symptoms. CRPS in the setting of myocardial infarction seems to be decreasing, presumably due to early mobilization and more effective pain control.

PHYSICAL FINDINGS & CLINICAL PRESENTATION

CRPS is divided into three stages:
1. Acute stage (occurring within hours to days after the injury).
   ○ Burning or aching pain occurring over the injured extremity.
   ○ Hyperalgesia (exaggerated response to nociceptive stimuli).
   ○ Edema.
   ○ Dysthermia.
   ○ Increased hair and nail growth.
2. Dystrophic stage (3 to 6 months after injury).
   ○ Burning pain radiating both distally and proximally from the site of injury.
   ○ Brawny edema (Fig. E1).
   ○ Hyperhidrosis.
   ○ Hypothermia and cyanosis.
   ○ Muscle tremors and spasms.
   ○ Increased muscle tone and reflexes.
3. Atrophic stage (6 months after injury).
   ○ Spread of pain proximally.
   ○ Allodynia (pain response to stimuli that are not normally painful).
   ○ Cold, pale, cyanotic skin.
   ○ Trophic skin changes with subcutaneous atrophy.
   ○ Contractures.

ETIOLOGY

The exact pathogenetic mechanisms underlying CRPS have not been fully elucidated, but most theories include the formation of an abnormal reflex arc in the sympathetic nervous system that is modulated by cortical centers to produce peripheral vascular disturbances. Persistent pain in the peripheral nervous system is modulated by inflammatory neuropeptides including substance P, which has been shown to be elevated in the serum of patients with CRPS-I. Increased concentrations of tumor necrosis factor and IL-6 have been demonstrated in the skin of patients with CRPS-I, and immune abnormalities such as reduced numbers of CD8-positive T lymphocytes have also been seen.

DIAGNOSIS

Criteria proposed for the diagnosis of CRPS type I include:
- An initiating noxious event, spontaneous pain or alloying/hyperalgesia disproportionate to the inciting event.
- Evidence of edema, skin blood flow, or sweating abnormality in the region of the pain.
- Absence of other conditions that could explain the symptoms.
  Tests such as nuclear medicine bone scanning, nerve conduction testing, and plain radiographs are often indicated to confirm the diagnosis and rule out other possibilities.

DIFFERENTIAL DIAGNOSIS

The differential diagnosis includes nerve entrapment syndromes such as cervical radiculopathy, myofascial pain syndromes, and fibromyalgia.

WORKUP

- Bone scintigraphy (Fig. E2) shows decreased perfusion of the affected areas if done soon after the onset of symptoms. If done after 6 weeks of symptoms, bone scan may show increased uptake in the region of the peripheral joints of the involved extremity.
- Electrophysiologic testing is useful to identify nerve injury in patients with type II CRPS.
- Plain radiographs show diffuse patchy osteopenia (Fig. E3).
- Skin temperature measurements can be used as a diagnostic test.
- Autonomic testing, although not commonly done, has been proposed.
  1. Measuring resting sweat output.
  2. Measuring resting skin temperature.
  3. Quantitative sudomotor axon reflex test.

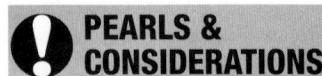 TREATMENT

Treatment of CRPS is largely empiric, based mostly on anecdotal reports, extrapolation from drug trials for other painful conditions, and clinical experience. Published studies are generally of low quality and show mixed results. Therapy should be tailored to stage of disease progression and severity of symptoms.

NONPHARMACOLOGIC THERAPY

- Physical therapy.
- Patient education.

PHARMACOLOGIC THERAPY

Suggested regimens:
Stage 1
    Tricyclic antidepressants (amitriptyline 25 to 150 mg or doxepin 5 to 20 mg).
    Prednisone 1 mg/kg for 2 weeks, then taper by 10 mg every 2 weeks.
    Alendronate 70 mg PO weekly.
Stage II
    Topical capsaicin.
    Gabapentin 300 mg tid.
    Regional nerve blocks.
Stage III
    Sympathetic ganglion blocks.
    Refer to multidisciplinary pain center.
    NOTE: High-dose vitamin C may decrease the incidence of CRPS following wrist fracture and foot and ankle surgery or trauma.

DISPOSITION

Spontaneous remission can occur after several weeks to months.

REFERRAL

Cases in which the diagnosis is not clear or there is suboptimal response to therapy should promptly be referred to a multidisciplinary pain clinic.

PEARLS & CONSIDERATIONS

COMMENTS

- CRPS is a common clinical entity without clear definition, pathophysiologic features, or treatment.
- Early mobilization in high-risk situations is important for prevention of CRPS.
- Prompt diagnosis and aggressive physical and pharmacologic therapy may prevent progression to chronic, intractable pain.

SUGGESTED READINGS

Available at www.expertconsult.com

AUTHOR: **BERNARD ZIMMERMANN, M.D.**

BASIC INFORMATION

DEFINITION

- Concussion is a mild traumatic brain injury that manifests with self-limited symptoms at the less severe end of the brain injury spectrum.
- The fourth International Conference on Concussion (2012) defines concussion as "a complex pathophysiological process affecting the brain, induced by traumatic biomechanical forces," characterized by the following features: (1) caused by a direct blow to the head or blow to the body that transmits an "impulsive" force to the head; (2) results in rapid onset of short-lived neurotic impairment that resolves spontaneously; (3) variable clinical symptoms that may not include loss of consciousness; (4) symptoms that largely reflect a functional disturbance rather than structural injury (thus, no abnormalities are seen on standard structural neuroimaging studies); and (5) symptom resolution that typically follows a sequential course but may be prolonged in a small percentage of cases.

SYNONYMS

Sports-related mild traumatic brain injury (mTBI)

ICD-10CM CODES
S06.0	Concussion
S06.0X0A	Concussion without loss of consciousness, initial encounter
S06.0X0D	Concussion without loss of consciousness, subsequent encounter
S06.0X0S	Concussion without loss of consciousness, sequela
S06.0X1A	Concussion with loss of consciousness of 30 minutes or less, initial encounter
S06.0X9A	Concussion with loss of consciousness of unspecified duration, initial encounter

EPIDEMIOLOGY & DEMOGRAPHICS

INCIDENCE: 3.8 million sports- and recreation-related concussions occur each year in the U.S. It is estimated that as many as 50% of concussions go unreported.

PREVALENCE: Each year, U.S. emergency departments treat an estimated 135,000 sports- and recreation-related TBIs, including concussions, among children ages 5 to 18.

PREDOMINANT SEX AND AGE:
- Children and teens are more likely to get a concussion and take longer to recover than adults.
- Limited studies have shown that in sports that are played by both men and women, women are at more risk of sustaining a concussion.

RISK FACTORS:
- Individuals engaged in high-impact sports and recreation are more likely to sustain a concussion.
- Individuals in organized sports are six times more likely to sustain a concussion than those involved in leisure physical activity.

- Individuals who have sustained a concussion previously are at a higher risk of sustaining another concussion.
- Athletes with a body mass index (BMI) >27 kg/m^2 and those who train <3 hr/wk are also at greater risk.
- Individuals who sustain a sports-related concussion and continue playing immediately after the injury require nearly twice as much time to recover as those who are removed immediately.

PHYSICAL FINDINGS & CLINICAL PRESENTATION

See Table 1.

ETIOLOGY

- Concussion occurs when rotational or angular acceleration forces are applied to the brain, resulting in shear strain of the underlying neural elements, including altered autonomic function and impaired control of cerebral blood flow.
- This may be associated with a blow to the skull; however, direct impact to the head is not required.

Table 1 Symptoms and Signs of Concussion

Mental Status Changes

Amnesia

Confusion

Disorientation

Easily distracted

Excessive drowsiness

Feeling dinged, stunned, or foggy

Impaired level of consciousness

Inappropriate play behaviors

Poor concentration and attention

Seeing stars or flashing lights

Slow to answer questions or to follow directions

Physical or Somatic

Ataxia or loss of balance

Blurry vision

Decreased performance or playing ability

Dizziness

Double vision

Fatigue

Headache

Lightheadedness

Nausea, vomiting

Poor coordination

Ringing in the ears

Seizures

Slurred, incoherent speech

Vacant stare/glassy-eyed

Vertigo

Behavior or Psychosomatic

Emotional lability

Irritability

Low frustration tolerance

Personality changes

Nervousness, anxiety

Sadness, depressed mood

From Patel DR et al: Sports Concussions in adolescents, *Pediatr Clin N Am* 57:652, 2010.

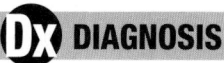

DIAGNOSIS

DIFFERENTIAL DIAGNOSIS

- Migraine
- Cervical strain
- Posttraumatic vestibular injury

WORKUP

- Sideline assessment:
  1. No athlete with a suspected concussion should return to play that day.
  2. Neurologic assessment using a standardized tool, such as s SCAT-3 (Sports Concussion Assessment Tool), which includes the BESS (Balance Error Scoring System), Maddocks Questions, and SAC (Standardized Assessment of Concussion) (Fig. 1).
  3. Monitor for deterioration; no athlete should be left alone.
- Office assessment:
  1. History focused on current symptoms. Consider using Postconcussion Symptom Checklist.
  2. Neurological exam
     a. Gait/balance testing. Consider the Balance Error Scoring System (BESS).
     b. Cerebellar coordination: finger-to-nose testing (tested on SCAT-3 card).
     c. Convergence of Accommodative Sufficiency.
- Neurocognitive testing:
  1. Computer-based programs, such as ImPACT, ANAM, CogSport
  2. Neuropsychiatric testing administered by a neuropsychologist
- When used in combination, symptom assessment, balance assessment, and neurocognitive testing provide a sensitivity of >90% for the identification of concussion.
- Consider the Buffalo Concussion Treadmill Test, which identifies physiologic dysfunction in concussion, rules out other diagnoses, and can quantify a safe level of activity in concussion recovery.

IMAGING STUDIES

- CT imaging is indicated in any athlete with a rapidly changing or focal neurologic exam or with a suspected intracranial bleed.
- Consider following PECARN guidelines.

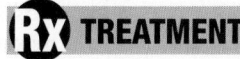

TREATMENT

ACUTE GENERAL Rx

- Removal from game
- Physical rest
  1. No return to play until asymptomatic for 24 hours.
  2. Follow the return-to-play guidelines (Table 2).
  3. There is no evidence to support prolonged rest in concussed athletes longer than several weeks (see "Post-Concussion Syndrome"). Prolonged inactivity after concussion has been linked to negative health effect. Light aerobic activity that avoids risk for reinjury decreases concussion symptoms, suggesting that low-level physical activity post-concussion might be beneficial.

NAME: _____

AGE: ____ SEX: ____ EXAMINER: _____

Nature of Injury: _____

Date of Exam: _____ Time: _____ No. _____

1) ORIENTATION:

Month: _____ 0   1
Date: _____ 0   1
Day of Week: _____ 0   1
Year: _____ 0   1
Time (within 1 hour): _____ 0   1

Orientation Total Score _____ /5

2) IMMEDIATE MEMORY: (all 3 trials are completed regardless of score on trials 1 & 2; score equals sum across all 3 trials)

LIST	TRIAL 1	TRIAL 2	TRIAL 3
Elbow	0 1	0 1	0 1
Apple	0 1	0 1	0 1
Carpet	0 1	0 1	0 1
Saddle	0 1	0 1	0 1
Bubble	0 1	0 1	0 1
Total			

Immediate Memory Score _____ /15

3) CONCENTRATION:

Digits Backward: (if correct, go to next string length. If incorrect, read trial 2. Stop after incorrect on both trials.)

4–9–3	6–2–9	0	1
3–8–1–4	3–2–7–9	0	1
6–2–9–7–1	1–5–2–8–6	0	1
7–1–8–4–6–2	5–3–9–1–4–8	0	1

Months in Reverse Order: (entire reverse sequence correct for 1 point)
DEC–NOV–OCT–SEP–AUG–JUL
JUN–MAY–APR–MAR–FEB–JAN   0   1

Concentration Total Score _____ /5

EXERTIONAL MANEUVERS (when appropriate):

5 jumping jacks   5 push-ups
5 sit-ups   5 knee-bends

4) DELAYED RECALL

Elbow	0	1
Apple	0	1
Carpet	0	1
Saddle	0	1
Bubble	0	1

Delayed Recall Score _____ /5

SUMMARY OF TOTAL SCORES:

Orientation   _____ /5
Immediate Memory   _____ /15
Concentration   _____ /5
Delayed Recall   _____ /5

OVERALL TOTAL SCORE _____ /30

FIG. 1 Standardized assessment of concussion (SAC). (Redrawn from McCrea M et al: Standard assessment of concussion in football players, *Neurology* 48:586–588, 1997.)

Table 2 Graduated Return to Play Protocol

Rehabilitation Stage	Functional Exercise at Each Stage of Rehabilitation	Objective of Each Stage
1. No activity	Complete physical and cognitive rest	Recovery
2. Light aerobic exercise	Walking, swimming, or stationary cycling, keeping intensity <70% maximum predicted heart rate. No resistance training	Increase heart rate
3. Sport-specific exercise	Skating drills in ice hockey, running drills in soccer. No head impact activities	Add movement
4. Noncontact training drills	Progression to more complex training drills, e.g., passing drills in football and ice hockey. May start progressive resistance training	Exercise, coordination, and cognitive load
5. Full contact practice	After medical clearance, participate in normal training activities	Restore confidence and assess functional skills by coaching staff
6. Return to play	Normal game play	

From Putukian M: The acute symptoms of sports-related concussion: diagnosis and on-field management, *Clin Sports Med* 30(58), 2011.

- Cognitive rest to limit symptoms
  1. Limit screen time to less than 2 hours per day.
  2. Academic accommodations at school. Consider return to school for half-days when tolerating 2 hours of work at home.
  3. Encourage good sleep hygiene.

CHRONIC Rx

See "Postconcussive Syndrome"

DISPOSITION

- Table 2 summarizes the American Academy of Neurology, American Medical Society for Sports Medicine, and International Conference on Concussion recommendations on returning to play after a concussion.
- If concussion symptoms occur with activity at one level, the athlete should stop the activity, rest until symptoms resolve, and then restart his or her progression at the level that did not elicit symptoms.
- There are no evidence-based guidelines for disqualifying or retiring an athlete from sport after a concussion. Each case should be individually considered.

REFERRAL

Sports-medicine physician, neuropsychology or concussion center

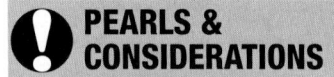

PEARLS & CONSIDERATIONS

PREVENTION

- Preparticipation evaluations for all athletes
- Preparticipation neurocognitive and balance testing to establish a baseline
- There is currently no evidence to support the use of concussion prevention headbands or mouth guards.

PATIENT/FAMILY EDUCATION

Centers for Disease Control and Prevention: www.cdc.gov/TraumaticBrainInjury/causes.html.

SUGGESTED READINGS

Available at www.expertconsult.com

RELATED CONTENT

Concussion (Patient Information)
Traumatic Brain Injury (Related Key Topic)
Post-Concussion Syndrome (Related Key Topic)

AUTHORS: **PETER J. SELL, D.O.,** and **AMITY RUBEOR, D.O.**

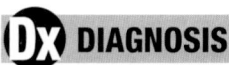 BASIC INFORMATION

DEFINITION

Conduct disorder (CD) is a repetitive and persistent pattern of behaviors in which either the basic rights of others are violated and/or major age-appropriate societal rules are violated. Classified under the DSM-5 category "disruptive, impulse control, and conduct disorders."

ICD-10CM CODES
F43.24 Adjustment disorder with disturbance of conduct
F43.25 Adjustment disorder with mixed disturbance of emotions and conduct
F91.0 Conduct disorder confined to family context
F91.1 Conduct disorder, childhood-onset type
F91.2 Conduct disorder, adolescent-onset type
F91.8 Other conduct disorders
F91.9 Conduct disorder, unspecified
I45.89 Other specified conduction disorders
I45.9 Conduction disorder, unspecified

EPIDEMIOLOGY & DEMOGRAPHICS

INCIDENCE: 1% (12 mo span, National Comorbidity Survey-Replication [NCS-R])
PREVALENCE: Approximately 2% to 10%; NCS-R: 9%. Disruptive behavior disorders are considered the most common reason for referral of children to mental health providers.
PREDOMINANT SEX: More common in males (4:1 preadolescence and 2:1 postadolescence). It is unclear if CD females are underrepresented because diagnostic criteria were validated on male samples. Nonconfrontational aggression and promiscuity are examples of possible gender-specific criteria that, at this time, have unknown predictive validity.
PREDOMINANT AGE: Most common onset in early adolescence. Median age of onset is 11 yr.
GENETICS: Risk increased if parent or sibling with disorder.
RISK FACTORS: There are various temperamental (including lower-than-average intelligence, especially verbal), family-level (including parental rejection or neglect, early institutional living, frequent caregiver changes, large family size, parental criminality or substance use), and community-level (including peer rejection, association with delinquent peer group, exposure to violence) risk factors.

PHYSICAL FINDINGS & CLINICAL PRESENTATION

- The DSM-5 lists 15 possible behavioral manifestations of CD, grouped into four categories: aggression to people and animals, destruction of property, deceitfulness or theft, and serious violations of rules. Three of the 15 behaviors are required to have occurred in the previous 12 mo, and one behavior must have occurred in the previous 6 mo.
- Specifiers describe the age of onset and the severity of the disorder.
- New to the DSM-5 is an additional specifier addressing issues relating to intent and reaction to the behaviors, including the following

options: "With limited prosocial emotions," "lack of remorse or guilt," "callous-lack of empathy," "unconcerned about performance," and "shallow or deficient affect."
- CD represents a heterogeneous group with respect to presentation, etiology, severity, and course.
- Symptom severity often progresses over time with age (i.e., lying and truancy to sexual assault and robbery).
- Aggressive youth are more likely to interpret as negative or hostile the intent of neutral others and are more likely to believe that conflict can be adequately resolved via aggression.
- Poor frustration tolerance, irritability, temper outbursts, and recklessness are often associated with CD.
- Slow resting heart rate associated with reduced autonomic response to fear is the most replicated of all biologic markers for conduct problems.

ETIOLOGY

Estimated population variance in antisocial behavior accounted for by:
1. Genes: 50%
2. Environmental factors shared among family members: 20%
3. Environmental factors unshared among family members: 20% to 30%

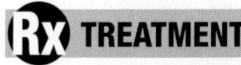 DIAGNOSIS

DIFFERENTIAL DIAGNOSIS

- Oppositional defiant disorder
- ADHD
- Mood disorder
- Adjustment disorder
- Substance use disorder, intoxication, or withdrawal
- Posttraumatic stress disorder
- Antisocial personality disorder (for those >18 yr)
- Adaptive behavior or subcultural delinquency
- Underlying neurological disorder (rare)

WORKUP

Diagnosis is made based on history, including individual and family interviews as well as collateral data from additional sources (e.g., parents, teachers, other medical providers, therapists).

LABORATORY TESTS

Consider urine toxicology for possible substance use comorbidity.

IMAGING STUDIES

None indicated; however, both structural and functional differences have been noted in certain areas of the brain in individuals with CD.

TREATMENT

Initial treatment of CD should include psychosocial and environmental interventions aimed at decreasing the frequency and severity of delinquent behaviors. If the interventions listed here are not effective or if serious concerns exist regarding safety or impairment in functioning, pharmacologic interventions targeting specific symptoms

(e.g., aggression) or comorbid disorders (e.g., ADHD, anxiety disorders, or mood disorders) may help. There are currently no medications approved by the FDA for the treatment of CD.

NONPHARMACOLOGIC THERAPY

- Parent management training.
- Cognitive problem-solving skills training (including elements of social skills, conflict resolution, anger management, impulse control, and vocational training).
- Multisystemic therapy (MST).
- Social skills training.
- Individual psychotherapy.
- Family psychotherapy.
- Higher levels of care such as a hospital or acute residential setting may be required for stabilization if acute safety concerns develop in the context of CD, such as severe aggression.
- Legal involvement or out-of-home-placements may be necessary to monitor safety of both the patient and the community.

PHARMACOLOGIC THERAPY

Medication may be considered as an adjunct to behavioral treatment or in cases in which comorbidity is a factor. There is some evidence for symptom improvement with trials of several classes of psychotropic medications—including stimulants, mood stabilizers, atypical antipsychotics, antidepressants, and alpha-2 agonists—all of which seem to target aggressive symptoms in particular; medication, however, should never be used alone or as first-line treatment for CD.

DISPOSITION

- Approximately half of those with early onset of CD persist with antisocial behaviors into adulthood. There is no reliable way to predict which 50% will persist.
- Approximately half of those with early onset of CD do not develop antisocial personality disorder in adulthood. This subgroup is at higher risk for depression, anxiety, and social isolation as adults.
- Approximately 85% of those with adolescent onset of CD do not demonstrate lifetime persistent violence, convictions, and incarcerations. However, adult prognosis may often include substance use and crimes that go largely undetected.

PEARLS & CONSIDERATIONS

COMMENTS

- Treatment noncompliance is common (expect 30% treatment noncompliance rate).
- Consider community-based resources (including unique strengths of patient and family) and recruit multiple multidisciplinary team members to create the most effective possible treatment plan.

SUGGESTED READINGS
Available at www.expertconsult.com

AUTHORS: **HASSAN M. MINHAS, M.D.,** and **ELIZABETH A. LOWENHAUPT, M.D.**

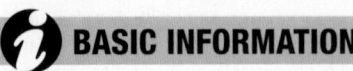

DEFINITION

Condyloma acuminatum is a sexually transmitted viral disease of the penis, vulva, vagina, cervix, perineum, and perianal area caused by the human papillomavirus (HPV). More than 100 subtypes of the HPV virus have been identified, yet 90% of genital warts are caused by HPV types 6 or 11.

SYNONYMS

Genital warts
Venereal warts
Anogenital warts

ICD-10CM CODES
A63.0 Anogenital (venereal) warts

EPIDEMIOLOGY & DEMOGRAPHICS

- Seen mostly in young adults, with peak age of onset of 16 to 25 yr
- A sexually transmitted disease spread by skin-to-skin contact
- Highly contagious, with 25% to 65% of sexual partners developing it
- Virus shed from both macroscopic and microscopic lesions
- Average incubation time is 2 months (range, 1 to 8 months)
- Predisposing conditions: diabetes, pregnancy, local trauma, and immunosuppression (e.g., transplant recipients, those with HIV infection)

PHYSICAL FINDINGS & CLINICAL PRESENTATION

- Usually found in genital area but can be present elsewhere on the body (larynx, oropharynx, trachea, and extremities)
- Lesions usually in similar positions on both sides of perineum
- Initial lesions are pedunculated, soft papules about 2 to 3 mm in diameter, 10 to 20 mm long; may occur as single papule or in clusters
- Size of lesions varies from pinhead to large cauliflower-like masses (Fig. 1)
- Usually asymptomatic, but if infected can cause pain, odor, or bleeding
- Vulvar condyloma more common than vaginal and cervical
- Four morphologic types: condylomatous, keratotic, papular, and flat warts
- Intra-anal warts are observed predominantly in persons who have had receptive anal intercourse.

ETIOLOGY

- HPV DNA types 6 and 11 usually found in exophytic warts and have no malignant potential. 90% of genital warts are caused by HPV 6 and 11.
- HPV types 16 and 18 usually found in flat warts and are associated with increased risk of malignancy
- Recurrence associated with persisting viral infection of adjacent normal skin in 25% to 50% of cases

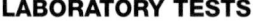 **DIAGNOSIS**

DIFFERENTIAL DIAGNOSIS

- Abnormal anatomic variants or skin tags around labia minora and introitus.
- Dysplastic warts.
- Table 1 summarizes sexually transmitted diseases of the anorectum.

WORKUP

- Colposcopic examination of lower genital tract from cervix to perianal skin with 3% to 5% acetic acid
- Biopsy of vulvar lesions that lack the classic appearance of warts and that become ulcerated or do not respond to treatment
- Biopsy of flat, white, or ulcerated cervical lesions

LABORATORY TESTS

- HPV tests are available to detect oncogenic types of HPV infection and are used in the context of cervical cancer screening and management or follow-up of abnormal cervical cytology or histology.
- Cervical cultures for *Neisseria gonorrhoeae* and Chlamydia
- Serologic test for syphilis
- HIV testing offered
- Wet mount or DNA testing for trichomoniasis, *Candida albicans*, and *Gardnerella vaginalis* (if patient has abnormal vaginal discharge)

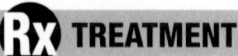 **TREATMENT**

NONPHARMACOLOGIC THERAPY

1. Cryotherapy with liquid nitrogen.
2. Surgical removal.

ACUTE GENERAL Rx

Factors that influence selection of treatment include wart size, wart number, anatomic site of wart, wart morphology, patient preference, cost of treatment, convenience, adverse effects, and provider experience.

Keratolytic agents:
- Podophyllin (Podofilox 0.5% solution or gel)
  1. Acts by poisoning mitotic spindle and causing intense vasospasm
  2. Applied by patient directly to lesion weekly and washed off in 6 hours
  3. Used in minimal vulvar or anal disease
  4. Applied cautiously to nonkeratinized epithelial surfaces
  5. Contraindicated in pregnancy
  6. Discontinued if lesions do not disappear in 6 weeks; switch to other treatment
- Sinecatechins 15% ointment (green tea flavonoid extracts)
  1. Applied by patient three time daily (0.5 cm strand of ointment to each wart)
  2. Should not be continued longer than 16 weeks
- Trichloroacetic acid (30% to 80% solution)
  1. Acts by destruction of the warty lesions through precipitation of surface proteins
  2. Applied weekly to lesion by a trained clinician
  3. Indicated for vulvar, anal, and vaginal lesions; can be used for cervical lesions
  4. Less painful and irritating to normal tissue than podophyllin
- 5-Fluorouracil
  1. Causes necrosis and sloughing of growing tissue
  2. Can be used intravaginally or for vulvar, anal, or urethral lesions
  3. Better tolerated; 3 g (two thirds of vaginal applicator) applied weekly for 12 weeks
  4. Possible vaginal ulceration and erythema
  5. Patient's vagina examined after four to six applications
  6. 80% cure rate

Physical agents:
- Cryotherapy with liquid nitrogen or cryoprobe
  1. Can be used weekly for 3 to 6 weeks
  2. 62% to 79% cure rate
  3. Not suitable for large warts
- Laser therapy
  1. Done by physician with necessary expertise and equipment
  2. Painful; requires anesthesia

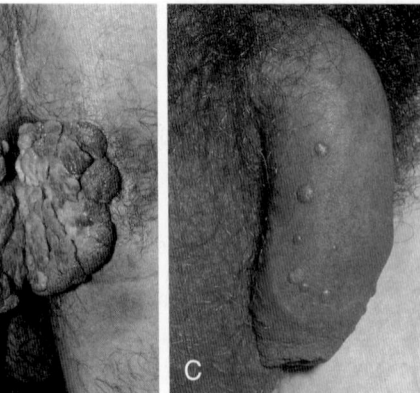

FIG. 1 Condyloma acuminatum. A, Scattered, flesh-colored or hyperpigmented, smooth or verrucous papules or erythematous macules along the shaft of the penis, scrotum, and perianal area are characteristic. The term *bowenoid papulosis* is used when the histologic picture of a lesion resembles Bowen's disease. **B,** Perianal condyloma acuminatum. The viral particles causing perianal condyloma may have originated from warts elsewhere on the body and been transmitted via the patient's own hands, or they may have been contracted during anal sex. **C,** Condyloma acuminatum. Multiple lesions on the shaft of the penis. (From White GM, Cox NH [eds]: *Diseases of the skin: a color atlas and text,* ed 2, St Louis, 2006, Mosby.)

TABLE 1 Sexually Transmitted Diseases of the Anorectum

Disease or Condition (With Specific Pathogen When Known)	Findings	Treatment
Ulcerative Conditions		
LGV	Unilateral inguinal adenopathy Fever, malaise Mucoid or bloody discharge	Doxycycline 100 mg PO bid × 21 days *For pregnant patients or those allergic to tetracyclines:* Erythromycin 500 mg PO qid × 21 days
HSV infection	Rectal pain, tenesmus, constipation Bloody mucoid discharge Vesicles and ulcerations Fever, malaise, myalgias, paresthesias	*First episode:* Acyclovir 400 mg PO tid 7-10 days *or* Acyclovir 200 mg PO 5×/day × 7-10 days *or* Famciclovir 250 mg PO bid × 7-10 days *or* Valacyclovir 1 g PO daily for 7-10 days
Early (primary) syphilis (*Treponema pallidum*)	Chancre Tenesmus, pain, mucoid drainage Inguinal lymphadenopathy	Benzathine penicillin G 2.4 million units IM once
Chancroid (*Haemophilus ducreyi*)	Inflammatory lesion progresses to ulcer Inguinal adenitis—bubo	Azithromycin 1 g PO once *or* Ceftriaxone 250 mg IM once *or* Ciprofloxacin 500 mg PO bid × 3 days *or* Erythromycin 500 mg PO tid × 7 days
Idiopathic (usually HIV positive)	Eccentric, deep, poor healing, multiple lesions	Symptomatic relief or surgical referral
Nonulcerative Conditions		
Condylomata acuminata (HPV)	Keratinized vegetative growths in anus or skin Asymptomatic, or pruritus ani, or bleeding	Podofilox 0.5% topically, or cryotherapy
Gonorrhea (*Neisseria gonorrhoeae*)	Pruritus ani Tenesmus Purulent yellow discharge	Ceftriaxone 250 mg IM once *or* cefixime 400 mg PO once
Chlamydial infection (*Chlamydia trachomatis*)	Mucoid or bloody discharge Tenesmus	Azithromycin 1 g PO once *or* Doxycycline 100 mg PO twice per day × 7 days
Syphilis (secondary)	Maculopapular rash Condyloma latum	Benzathine penicillin G 2.4 million units IM once

HIV, human immunodeficiency virus; *HPV,* human papillomavirus; *HSV,* herpes simplex virus; *IM,* intramuscularly; *LGV,* lymphogranuloma venereum; *PO,* orally.
From Marx J et al (eds): *Rosen's emergency medicine: concepts and clinical practice,* ed 7, Philadelphia, 2010, Saunders.

- Electrocautery or excision
  1. For recurrent, very large lesions
  2. Local anesthesia needed
- Immunotherapy:
- Interferon
  1. Injected intralesionally at a dose of 3 million U/m² three times weekly for 8 weeks
  2. Side effects: fever, chills, malaise, headache
- Imiquimod 5% cream:
  1. Applied by patient at night, 3 times per week; wash off after 6-10 hours
  2. Usage for 16 weeks maximum
  3. Increases wart clearance after 3 months

- 40% to 77% cure rate
- Interferon, topical: increases wart clearance at 4 weeks

DISPOSITION
- Follow-up exam every 6 to 12 months as needed.

PREVENTION
- Male and female condoms should be used consistently and correctly to lower the risks of acquiring and transmitting HPV. However, because HPV can infect areas not covered by a condom, condoms will not fully protect against HPV.
- New guidelines for the routine vaccination of young adolescents (females and males) ages 9 to 14 are 2 doses of the HPV vaccine given at a 6- to 12-month interval, which offers the same protection as the 3-dose vaccination.
- Young women from ages 15 to 26 should receive 3 doses of the HPV vaccine (the 9vHPV, 4vHPV, and 2vHPV are approved for females).
- Young males from ages 15 to 21 should receive 3 doses of the HPV vaccine. The age limit for male HPV vaccination may be extended up to age 26 (only the 4vHPV and 9vHPV vaccines are approved for males). For men who have sex with men (including young men who identify as gay and bisexual), for young transgender adults, and for young adults who are immunocompromised (secondary to HIV, chronic steroid usage, or prior history of transplant), HPV vaccination is recommended up to age 26. Three-dose HPV vaccination series are administered as IM injections over a 6-month period, with the second and third doses given 1 to 2 and 6 months after the first dose, respectively. The same vaccine type should be used for the entire 3-dosage series.
- 4vHPV (Gardasil) vaccinates against types 6, 11, 16, and 18, which account for 66% of all cervical cancers.
- 2vHPV (Cervarix) vaccinates against types 16 and 18 (licensed for females only).
- 9vHPV (Gardasil 9) vaccine is available for preventing infection against HPV types 6, 11, 16, 18, 31, 33, 45, 52, and 58. It offers protection against five additional types of HPV accounting for 15% of cervical cancers not covered by Gardasil or Cervarix.
- HPV vaccines are not recommended for use in pregnant women.

SUGGESTED READINGS
Available at www.expertconsult.com

RELATED CONTENT
Genital Warts (Patient Information)
Warts (Related Key Topic)

AUTHOR: **ARLENE J. SMALLS, M.D.**

C

I

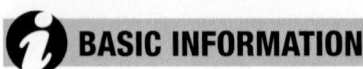

DEFINITION

The term *conjunctivitis* refers to an inflammation of the conjunctiva resulting from a variety of causes, including allergies and bacterial, viral, and chlamydial infections.

SYNONYMS

"Red eye"
Pink eye
Acute conjunctivitis
Subacute conjunctivitis
Chronic conjunctivitis
Purulent conjunctivitis
Pseudomembranous conjunctivitis
Papillary conjunctivitis
Follicular conjunctivitis
Newborn conjunctivitis

ICD-10CM CODES
H10.9 Unspecified conjunctivitis
B30 Viral conjunctivitis
H10.0 Mucopurulent conjunctivitis
H10.1 Acute atopic conjunctivitis
H10.4 Chronic conjunctivitis

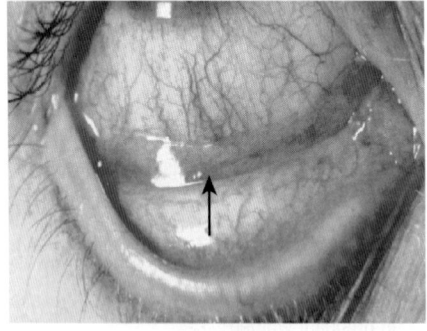

FIG. 1 Allergic conjunctivitis. *Arrow* indicates area of chemosis in the conjunctivitis. (From Adkinson NF Jr et al [eds]: *Middleton's allergy principles and practice,* ed 7, vol 2, Philadelphia, 2008, Mosby.)

EPIDEMIOLOGY & DEMOGRAPHICS

INCIDENCE (IN U.S.): 1.6% to 12% in *newborns*
PREVALENCE (IN U.S.):
- Allergic conjunctivitis (Fig. 1), the most common form of ocular allergy, is usually associated with allergic rhinitis and may be seasonal or perennial.
- Bacterial or viral conjunctivitis is often seasonal and can be extremely contagious.

PREDOMINANT AGE: Occurs at *any* age. Most cases in adults are due to viral infection. Children are more prone to develop bacterial conjunctivitis than viral forms.
PEAK INCIDENCE: More common in the spring and fall, when *viral* infections and pollens increase.

PHYSICAL FINDINGS & CLINICAL PRESENTATION

- Infection and chemosis of conjunctivae with discharge. Gluing of the eyelids and no itching is more indicative of a bacterial cause (Fig. 2).
- Cornea is clear or can be involved.
- Vision is often normal but can be blurred.

ETIOLOGY

- Bacterial: *Haemophilus influenzae, Streptococcus pneumoniae,* and *Moraxella catarrhalis* in children; *Staphylococcus* species in adults. Gram-negative infections are more common in contact lens wearers. *Gonococcal ophthalmia neonatorum* is caused by *Neisseria gonorrhoeae* acquired by exposure of the neonatal conjunctivae to infected cervicovaginal secretions during delivery.
- Viral: most common overall cause of infectious conjunctivitis.
- Chlamydial.
- Allergic.
- Traumatic (chemical or toxin exposure).
- Chronic eyelid inflammation (blepharitis).

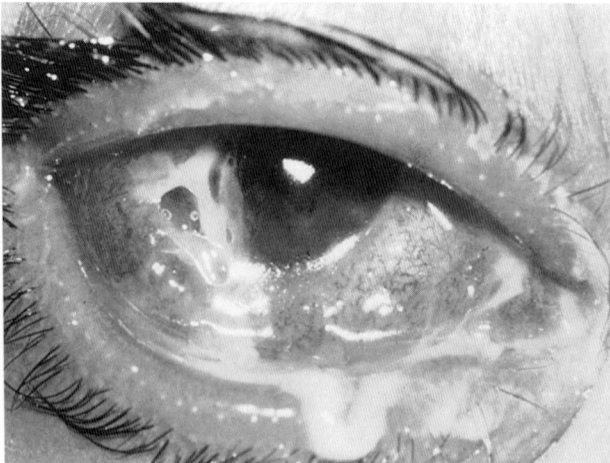

FIG. 2 Bacterial conjunctivitis. Purulent discharge and conjunctiva hyperemia suggest bacterial conjunctivitis. Viral conjunctivitis produces watery discharge, foreign body sensation, preauricular lymphadenopathy, and conjunctival follicles seen on slit lamp examination. (Reproduced with permission from the American Academy of Ophthalmology. From Goldman L, Schafer AI: *Goldman's Cecil medicine,* ed 24, Philadelphia, 2012, Saunders.)

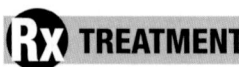 **DIAGNOSIS**

DIFFERENTIAL DIAGNOSIS

- Acute glaucoma (fixed pupil with headache may indicate acute angle closure).
- Corneal lesions.
- Acute iritis.
- Episcleritis.
- Scleritis.
- Canalicular obstruction.
- Table 1 compares allergic diseases of the eye. Histologic and laboratory manifestations of allergic ocular disease are described in Table 2.

WORKUP

- History and physical examination
- Visual acuity and eye examination
- Reports of itching, pain, and visual changes

LABORATORY TESTS

Cultures are useful if not *successfully* treated with antibiotics; initial culture is usually not necessary, since normal conjunctival flora interferes with helpful culture results.

Rx TREATMENT

NONPHARMACOLOGIC THERAPY

- Warm compresses if infective conjunctivitis.
- Cold compresses if irritative or allergic conjunctivitis.
- Contact lenses should be taken out until an infection is completely resolved. Nondisposable lenses should be cleaned thoroughly as recommended by the manufacturer, and a new lens case should be used. Disposable contact lenses should be thrown away.

ACUTE GENERAL Rx

- The majority of cases of bacterial conjunctivitis are self-limiting, and no treatment is necessary in uncomplicated cases.[1] Antibiotic drops (e.g., levofloxacin, ofloxacin, ciprofloxacin, tobramycin, gentamicin ophthalmic solution, 1 or 2 drops q2 to 4h) are indicated for complicated bacterial conjunctivitis, in conjunctivitis caused by gonorrhea or chlamydia, and in bacterial conjunctivitis in contact lens wearers.
- Caution: be careful with ophthalmic corticosteroid treatment and avoid unless sure of diagnosis; corticosteroids can exacerbate infections and have been associated with increased intraocular pressure and cataract formation.
- An oral antihistamine (e.g., cetirizine, loratadine, desloratadine, or fexofenadine) is effective in relieving itching.
- Mast cell stabilizers (e.g., ketotifen, olopatadine, azelastine bid) are effective for allergic conjunctivitis. Others include Elestat, Optivar, and Patanol.

[1]Azari AA, Barney NP: Conjunctivitis, a systematic review of diagnosis and treatment, *JAMA* 310(16):1721-1729, 2013.

TABLE 1 Allergic Diseases of the Eye

Disease	Clinical Parameters	Signs and Symptoms	Differential Diagnosis
Seasonal allergic conjunctivitis (SAC)	Occurs in sensitized individuals Both females and males affected Bilateral involvement Seasonal allergens Self-limiting	Ocular itching Tearing (watery discharge) Chemosis, redness Often associated with rhinitis Not sight threatening	Infective conjunctivitis Preservative toxicity (any eye drop with preservative) Medicamentosa Dry eye PAC/AKC/VKC
Perennial allergic conjunctivitis (PAC)	Occurs in sensitized individuals Both females and males affected Bilateral involvement Year-round allergens Self-limiting	Ocular itching Tearing (watery discharge) Chemosis, redness Often associated with rhinitis Not sight-threatening	Infective conjunctivitis Preservative toxicity Dry eye SAC/AKC/VKC
Atopic keratoconjunctivitis (AKC)	Occurs in sensitized individuals Peak incidence: 20-50 yr of age Both females and males affected Bilateral involvement Seasonal or perennial allergens Atopic dermatitis Chronic symptoms	Severe ocular itching Red, flaking periocular skin Mucoid discharge, photophobia Corneal erosions Scarring of conjunctiva Cataract (anterior subcapsular) Sight threatening	Contact dermatitis Infective conjunctivitis Blepharitis Pemphigoid VKC/SAC/PAC/GPC
Vernal keratoconjunctivitis (VKC)	Occurs in some sensitized individuals Peak incidence: 3-20 yr of age Males predominate (in 3:1 ratio) Bilateral involvement Warm, dry climate Seasonal/perennial allergens Chronic symptoms	Severe ocular itching Severe photophobia Thick, ropy discharge Cobblestone papillae Corneal ulceration and scarring Sight threatening	Infective conjunctivitis Blepharitis AKC/SAC/PAC/GPC
Giant papillary conjunctivitis (GPC)	Sensitization not necessary Both females and males affected Bilateral involvement Prosthetic exposure Occurs anytime Chronic symptoms Nonseasonal occurrence	Mild ocular itching Mild mucoid discharge Giant papillae Contact lens intolerance Foreign body sensation Protein buildup on contact lens Not sight threatening	Infective conjunctivitis Preservative toxicity SAC/PAC/AKC/VKC

From Adkinson NF, et al: *Middleton's allergy principles and practice*, ed 8, Philadelphia, 2014, Saunders.

TABLE 2 Histopathologic and Laboratory Manifestations of Allergic Ocular Disease

Disease	Histopathologic Features	Laboratory Manifestations
Seasonal/perennial allergic conjunctivitis	Mast cell/eosinophil infiltration in conjunctival epithelium and substantia propria Mast cell activation Upregulation of ICAM-1 on epithelial cells	Increased in tears: Specific IgE antibody Histamine Tryptase TNF-α
Atopic keratoconjunctivitis	Increased mast cells, eosinophils in conjunctival epithelium and substantia propria Epithelial cell/goblet cell hypertrophy Increased CD4/CD8 ratio in conjunctival epithelium and substantia propria Increased collagen	Increased specific IgE antibody in tears Depressed cell-mediated immunity Increased IgE antibody and eosinophils in blood Eosinophils found in conjunctival scrapings
Vernal keratoconjunctivitis	Increased mast cells, eosinophils in conjunctival epithelium and substantia propria Eosinophil major basic protein deposition in conjunctiva CD4+ clones from conjunctiva found to have helper function for local production of IgE antibody Increased collagen Increased ICAM-1 on corneal epithelium	Increased specific IgE/IgG antibody in tears Elevated histamine and tryptase in tears Reduced serum histaminase activity Increased serum levels of nerve growth factor and substance P
Giant papillary conjunctivitis	Giant papillae Conjunctival thickening Mast cells in epithelium	No increased histamine in tears Increased tryptase in tears

ICAM-1, Intercellular adhesion molecule 1; *IgE, IgG*, immunoglobulins E and G; *TNF-α*, tumor necrosis factor-α.
From Adkinson NF, et al: *Middleton's allergy principles and practice*, ed 8, Philadelphia, 2014, Saunders.

TABLE 3 Topical Ophthalmic Medications for Allergic Conjunctivitis

Generic Drug Name (Trade Name)	Mechanism of Action and Dosing	Cautions and Adverse Events
Azelastine hydrochloride 0.05% (Optivar)	Antihistamine Children ≥3 yr: 1 gtt bid	Not for treatment of contact lens–related irritation; the preservative may be absorbed by soft contact lenses. Wait at least 10 min after administration before inserting soft contact lenses.
Emedastine difumarate 0.05% (Emadine)	Antihistamine Children ≥3 yr: 1 gtt qid	Soft contact lenses should not be worn if the eye is red. Wait at least 10 min after administration before inserting soft contact lenses.
Levocabastine hydrochloride 0.05% (Livostin)	Antihistamine Children ≥12 yr: 1 gtt bid-qid up to 2 wk	Not for use in patients wearing soft contact lenses during treatment.
Pheniramine maleate 0.3% or 0.025% Naphazoline hydrochloride (Naphcon-A, Opcon-A)	Antihistamine/vasoconstrictor Children >6 yr: 1 to 2 gtt qid	Avoid prolonged use (>3 to 4 days) to avoid rebound symptoms. Not for use with contact lenses.
Cromolyn sodium 4% (Crolom, Opticrom)	Mast cell stabilizer Children >4 yr: 1 to 2 gtt q4-6h	Can be used to treat giant papillary conjunctivitis and vernal keratitis. Not for use with contact lenses.
Lodoxamide tromethamine 0.1% (Alomide)	Mast cell stabilizer Children ≥2 yr: 1 to 2 gtt qid up to 3 mo	Can be used to treat vernal keratoconjunctivitis. Not for use in patients wearing soft contact lenses during treatment.
Nedocromil sodium 2% (Alocril)	Mast cell stabilizer Children ≥3 yr: 1 to 2 gtt bid	Avoid wearing contact lenses while exhibiting the signs and symptoms of allergic conjunctivitis.
Pemirolast potassium 0.1% (Alamast)	Mast cell stabilizer Children >3 yr: 1 to 2 gtt qid	Not for treatment of contact lens–related irritation; the preservative may be absorbed by soft contact lenses. Wait at least 10 min after administration before inserting soft contact lenses.
Epinastine hydrochloride 0.05% (Elestat)	Antihistamine/mast cell stabilizer Children ≥3 yr: 1 gtt bid	Contact lenses should be removed before use. Wait at least 15 min after administration before inserting soft contact lenses. Not for the treatment of contact lens irritation.
Ketotifen fumarate 0.025% (Zaditor)	Antihistamine/mast cell stabilizer Children ≥3 yr: 1 gtt bid q8-12h	Not for treatment of contact lens–related irritation; the preservative may be absorbed by soft contact lenses. Wait at least 10 min after administration before inserting soft contact lenses.
Olopatadine hydrochloride 0.1%, 0.2% (Patanol, Pataday)	Antihistamine/mast cell stabilizer Children ≥3 yr: 1 gtt bid (8 hr apart), 1 gtt qid	Not for treatment of contact lens–related irritation; the preservative may be absorbed by soft contact lenses. Wait at least 10 min after administration before inserting soft contact lenses.
Ketorolac tromethamine 0.5% (Acular)	NSAID Children ≥3 yr: 1 gtt qid	Avoid with aspirin or NSAID sensitivity. Use ocular product with caution in patients with complicated ocular surgeries, corneal denervation or epithelial defects, ocular surface diseases (e.g., dry eye syndrome), repeated ocular surgeries within a short period of time, diabetes mellitus, or rheumatoid arthritis; these patients may be at risk for corneal adverse events that may be sight threatening. Do not use while wearing contact lenses.

NSAID, Nonsteroidal antiinflammatory drug.
Modified from Kliegman RM et al: *Nelson textbook of pediatrics,* ed 19, Philadelphia, 2011, Saunders.

- Bepotastine, alcaftadine, azelastine, epinastine, and ketotifen are H1-antihistamines and mast cell stabilizers effective for topical treatment of itching associated with allergic conjunctivitis. The topical NSAID ketorolac (0.5%, 1 drop qd) is also useful in allergic conjunctivitis. Table 3 describes topical ophthalmic medications for allergic conjunctivitis.
- Antihistamine/decongestant combinations such as pheniramine/naphazoline (Visine A), available over the counter, are more effective than either agent alone but have a short duration and can result in rebound vasodilatation with prolonged use. Others include Naphcon-A, Albalon-A, and Opcon-A.

CHRONIC Rx
- Depends on cause.
- If allergic, nonsteroidals such as ketorolac, and bromfenac ophthalmic solution; mast

cell stabilizers such as Patanol and Zaditor are useful for improving ocular itching in patients with allergic conjunctivitis.
- If an infection, use antibiotic drops (see "Acute General Rx").
- Dry eyes need artificial tears (Restasis) or lacrimal duct plugs when indicated.

DISPOSITION
Follow carefully for the first 2 wk to ensure secondary complications do not occur. Otitis media can develop in 25% of children with *H. influenzae* conjunctivitis. Bacterial keratitis occurs in 30/1000 contact lens wearers.

REFERRAL
To ophthalmologist if symptoms are refractory to initial treatment. Indications for urgent referral are severe eye pain or headache, photophobia, decreased vision, and contact lens use.

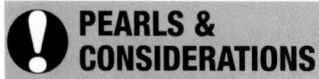

PEARLS & CONSIDERATIONS

COMMENTS
- Red eyes are not simply conjunctivitis when the patient has significant pain or loss of sight. However, it is usually safe to treat pain-free eyes and the normal-seeing red eye with lid hygiene and topical treatment.
- Use caution with patients wearing soft contact lenses, infants, and the elderly.
- Do not use steroids indiscriminately; use only when the diagnosis is certain.
- Bacterial conjunctivitis is generally self-limiting. More than 60% of persons will improve with placebo within 2 to 5 days.

RELATED CONTENT
Conjunctivitis (Patient Information)

AUTHOR: **R. SCOTT HOFFMAN, M.D.**

BASIC INFORMATION

DEFINITION

Contact dermatitis is an acute or chronic skin inflammation resulting from exposure to substances in the environment. It can be subdivided into "irritant" contact dermatitis (nonimmunologic physical and chemical alteration of the epidermis) and "allergic" contact dermatitis (delayed hypersensitivity reaction).

SYNONYMS

Irritant contact dermatitis
Allergic contact dermatitis

ICD-10CM CODES
L23   Allergic contact dermatitis
L23.0 Allergic contact dermatitis due to metals
L23.1 Allergic contact dermatitis due to adhesives
L23.2 Allergic contact dermatitis due to cosmetics
L23.3 Allergic contact dermatitis due to drugs in contact with skin
L23.4 Allergic contact dermatitis due to dyes
L23.5 Allergic contact dermatitis due to other chemical products
L25.9 Unspecified contact dermatitis, unspecified cause

EPIDEMIOLOGY & DEMOGRAPHICS

- 20% of all cases of dermatitis in children are caused by allergic contact dermatitis.
- Rhus dermatitis (poison ivy, poison oak, and poison sumac) is responsible for most cases of contact dermatitis.
- Frequent causes of irritant contact dermatitis are soaps, detergents, eye drops (Fig. E1) and organic solvents.
- Chemical irritants (e.g., cutting fluids used in machining, solvents) account for most cases of irritant contact dermatitis. Occupational skin diseases are second only to traumatic injuries as the most common types of occupational disease.

PHYSICAL FINDINGS & CLINICAL PRESENTATION

Clinical presentation varies with the responsible agent and affected area of skin.

IRRITANT CONTACT DERMATITIS:
- Mild exposure may result in dryness, erythema, and fissuring of the affected area (e.g., hand involvement in irritant dermatitis caused by exposure to soap (Fig. E2), genital area involvement in irritant dermatitis caused by prolonged exposure to wet diapers).
- Eczematous inflammation may result from chronic exposure.

ALLERGIC CONTACT DERMATITIS:
- Poison ivy dermatitis can present with vesicles and blisters; linear lesions (as a result of dragging of the resins over the surface of the skin by scratching) are a classic presentation.

- The pattern of lesions is asymmetric; itching, burning, and stinging may be present.
- The involved areas are erythematous, warm to touch, swollen, and may be confused with cellulitis.

ETIOLOGY

- Irritant contact dermatitis: cement (construction workers), rubber, ragweed, malathion (farmers), orange and lemon peels (chefs, bartenders), hair tints, shampoos (beauticians), rubber gloves (medical, surgical personnel)
- Allergic contact dermatitis: poison ivy, poison oak, poison sumac, rubber (shoe dermatitis), nickel (jewelry), balsam of Peru (hand and face dermatitis), neomycin, formaldehyde (cosmetics)

DIAGNOSIS

DIFFERENTIAL DIAGNOSIS

- Impetigo
- Lichen simplex chronicus
- Atopic dermatitis
- Nummular eczema, dyshidrotic eczema
- Seborrheic dermatitis
- Inverse psoriasis, palmoplantar psoriasis
- Scabies
- Tinea pedis

WORKUP

- Medical history: gradual onset versus rapid onset, number of exposures, clinical presentation, occupational history.
- Physical examination: contact dermatitis in the neck may be caused by necklaces, perfumes (Fig. E3), after-shave lotion. Involvement of the axillae is often secondary to deodorants, clothing. Face involvement can occur with cosmetics, airborne allergens, aftershave lotion.

LABORATORY TESTS

- Patch testing has a sensitivity and specificity of 70% to 80%. It is useful to confirm the diagnosis of contact dermatitis; it is indicated only when inflammation persists despite appropriate topical therapy and avoidance of suspected causative agent; patch testing should not be used for irritant contact dermatitis because this is a nonimmunologic-mediated inflammatory reaction.
- Dermoscopy and microscopy when suspecting scabies and mites.
- A potassium hydroxide (KOH) preparation may be useful if suspecting tinea or Candida infection.

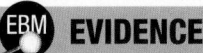 TREATMENT

NONPHARMACOLOGIC THERAPY

Avoidance of suspected allergens

ACUTE GENERAL Rx

- Removal of the irritant substance by washing the skin with plain water or mild soap within

15 min of exposure is helpful in patients with poison ivy, poison oak, or poison sumac dermatitis.
- Cold or cool water compresses for 20 to 30 min 5 to 6 times a day for the initial 72 hr are effective during the acute blistering stage.
- Topical steroids (clobetasol 0.05%, triamcinolone 0.1%) are effective for acute localized allergic contact dermatitis lesions. Lower-potency topical steroids are preferred on face, anogenital regions, and flexural surfaces to minimize risk of skin atrophy. Oral corticosteroids (e.g., prednisone 20 mg bid for 6 to 10 days) are generally reserved for severe, widespread dermatitis.
- IM steroids (e.g., Kenalog) are used for severe reactions and in patients requiring oral corticosteroids but unable to tolerate PO.
- Oral antihistamines (e.g., hydroxyzine 25 mg q6h) will control pruritus, especially at night; calamine lotion is also useful for pruritus; however, it can lead to excessive drying.
- Colloidal oatmeal (Aveeno) baths can also provide symptomatic relief.
- Patients with mild to moderate erythema may respond to topical steroid gels or creams.
- Patients with shoe allergy should change their socks at least once a day; use of aluminum chloride hexahydrate in a 20% solution (Drysol) qhs will also help control perspiration.
- Use hypoallergenic surgical gloves in patients with rubber and surgical glove allergy.

DISPOSITION

Allergic contact dermatitis generally resolves within 2 to 4 wk if re-exposure to allergen is prevented.

REFERRAL

For patch testing in selected patients, see "Laboratory Tests."

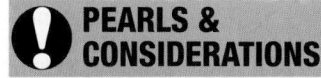 PEARLS & CONSIDERATIONS

COMMENTS

Commercially available corticosteroid dose packs should be avoided, because they generally provide an inadequate amount of medication.

EVIDENCE

Available at www.expertconsult.com

SUGGESTED READINGS
Available at www.expertconsult.com

RELATED CONTENT
Contact Dermatitis (Patient Information)
Poison Ivy Dermatitis (Related Key Topic)

AUTHOR: **FRED F. FERRI, M.D.**

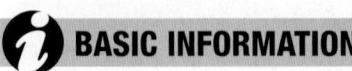

BASIC INFORMATION

DEFINITION

Contraception refers to the various modalities that a sexually active couple use to prevent pregnancy. These options can be either medical or nonmedical and used by men or women or both. The options are as follows:

- No contraception (unprotected intercourse) failure rate 85% both typical use and perfect use
- Abstinence
  1. 12.4% of unmarried men
  2. 13.2% of unmarried women
  3. More frequently practiced before age 17 yr
  4. No intercourse experienced by 13% of women ages 30 to 34 yr
  5. Failure rate 0%
- Withdrawal
  1. Used in only 2% of sexually active women
  2. Failure rate with perfect use, 4%; with typical use, 19%
- Rhythm method (natural family planning)
  1. Failure rate with perfect use, 1% to 9%; with typical use, 20%
  2. Symptothermal type: mucus method and ovulation pain combined with basal body temperature
  3. Ovulation (Billings' method): takes into account mucus quality
  4. Basal body temperature method: uses biphasic temperature chart
  5. Lactation amenorrhea method: effective in fully breastfeeding women, especially 70 to 100 days after delivery; depends on number of feedings per day
- Barriers
  1. Diaphragm and cervical cap: failure rate 5% to 9% in nulliparous women, 20% in multiparous women
  2. Female condom: failure rate with perfect use, 5.1%; with typical use, 12.4%; FDA labeling states 25% failure rate
  3. Male condom: failure rate with perfect use, 3%; with typical use, 12%
  4. Spermicides (aerosols, foam, jellies, creams, tabs): failure rate with perfect use, 3%; with typical use, 21%
- Oral contraceptives
  1. Failure rate with perfect use, <<1%; with typical use, 3%
  2. Come in combinations of estrogen/progestin or as progestin only
- Hormonal implants and injectables
  1. Implanon (etonogestrel) implant 2-yr cumulative pregnancy rate 0.05%. Nexplanon is essentially the same as Implanon but with a barium sulfate core for easier radiologic detection and a preloaded applicator to facilitate insertion.
  2. Depo-Provera: failure rate 0.3% in first year of use.
  3. Nestorone-releasing single implant: not yet available.
  4. Jadelle implant: Successor to the Norplant implant, which has been discontinued in the U.S. The Jadelle implant is not available in the U.S.

- Mini pill (progesterone only pill)
  1. Failure rate with typical use, 1.1% to 13.2%
  2. With perfect use, 5 pregnancies per 1000 women
     - Requires precise timing of daily use for effectiveness
- Emergency postcoital contraception
  1. Decreases pregnancy rate by 75% or more with women treated within 72 hrs of coitus
  2. Progestin-only method: 1.5 mg levonorgestrel single dose or 0.75 mg given 12 hrs apart
  3. Selective progesterone receptor modulator: 30 mg Ulipristal single dose is more effective than levonorgestrel
  4. Copper IUD: can be inserted up to 5 days after ovulation and results in the lowest pregnancy rate (0.1%)
- IUD (available over the counter in some states)
  1. Progestasert: failure rate with perfect use, 2%; with typical use, 3%
  2. Copper T (30-A): failure rate with perfect use, 0.6%; with typical use, 0.8%
  3. Levonorgestrel Intrauterine System (Mirena)
     1. 1-yr failure rate, 0.2%
     2. 5-yr cumulative failure rate, 0.7%
- Skyla, a smaller version of the Mirena, which also releases Levonorgestrel, and is targeted for younger users, was released in 2014. In 2015, the FDA approved Liletta, which also releases levonorgestrel. Liletta is marketed by Medicine 360, a nonprofit pharmaceutical firm, and is intended for use by women with fewer economic resources. Cost, which limits access to long-acting reversible contraceptives for many women, has been cited as a public health problem. Although Liletta has been approved for a 3-yr lifespan, the lower initial cost may allow many more women access to affordable contraception. Kyleena was FDA approved in 2016 for nulliparous and parous women, releases lower dose of levonorgestrel than Mirena, and was approved for 5 years.
- Female sterilization (tubal ligation): failure rate with perfect use, 0.2%; with typical use, 3%.
- Male sterilization (vasectomy): failure rate of 0.1% in first year.
- Vaginal ring (NuvaRring): failure rate pearl index 0.77.
- Contraceptive patch (Ortho Evra): failure rate 0.4% to 0.7%.

SYNONYMS

Birth control
Family planning

ICD-10CM CODES

Z30.011 Encounter for initial prescription of contraceptive pills
Z30.018 Encounter for initial prescription of other contraceptives
Z30.09 Encounter for other general counseling and advice on contraception
Z30.430 Encounter for insertion of intrauterine contraceptive device
Z30.2 Encounter for sterilization

DIAGNOSIS

WORKUP

- Thorough medical history
- Thorough surgical history
- Obstetric history (was fertility desired with conception?)
- Gynecologic history, including:
  1. History of previous sexually transmitted diseases
  2. Number of partners
  3. Previous difficulties with contraception
  4. Frequency of intercourse
- Family history
- Table E1 summarizes when to start using contraceptive methods.
- Examinations and tests needed before initiation of contraceptive methods are described in Table 2.
- Recommendations for routine follow-up after contraceptive initiation are summarized in Table E3.

LABORATORY TESTS

- Pap smear
- *Chlamydia* and *Gonorrhea* screening when appropriate
- Pregnancy test if suspected pregnancy
- Lipid profile if family history of premature vascular event

TREATMENT

NONPHARMACOLOGIC THERAPY

- Male condoms
  - 95% latex (rubber), 5% polyurethane, or natural membrane (lamb's intestine does not block transmission of sexually transmitted infections.
  - Proper use: place on an erect penis and leave ½-inch empty space at the tip of the condom; use with non–oil-based lubricants.
  - Effectiveness increased when used with spermicides.
  - Main advantage: condoms are the only method shown to reduce HIV transmission.
- Female condoms
  - Composed of polyurethane, with one end open and one end closed.
  - Proper use: place closed end over cervix, open end hanging out of vagina to cover penis and scrotum.
  - Highly effective against HIV.
- Spermicides
  - Types: nonoxynol, octoxynol.
  - Forms: jellies, creams, foams, suppositories, tablets, soluble films.
  - Proper use: put in immediately before intercourse; may be used with other barrier methods.

TABLE 2 Examinations and Tests Needed before Initiation of Contraceptive Methods

Examination or Test	Contraceptive Method and Class							
	Cu-IUD and LNG-IUD	Implant	Injectable	CHC	POP	Condom	Diaphragm or Cervical Cap	Spermicide
Examination								
Blood pressure	C	C	C	A*	C	C	C	C
Weight (BMI) (weight [kg]/ height [m]²)	—†	—†	—†	—†	—†	C	C	C
Clinical breast examination	C	C	C	C	C	C	C	C
Bimanual examination and cervical inspection	A	C	C	C	C	C	A§	C
Laboratory Test								
Glucose	C	C	C	C	C	C	C	C
Lipids	C	C	C	C	C	C	C	C
Liver enzymes	C	C	C	C	C	C	C	C
Hemoglobin	C	C	C	C	C	C	C	C
Thrombogenic mutations	C	C	C	C	C	C	C	C
Cervical cytology (Papanicolaou test)	C	C	C	C	C	C	C	C
STD screening with laboratory tests	—¶	C	C	C	C	C	C	C
HIV screening with laboratory tests	C	C	C	C	C	C	C	C

BMI, body mass index; CHC, combined hormonal contraceptive; Cu-IUD, copper-containing intrauterine device; HIV, human immunodeficiency virus; LNG-IUD, levonorgestrel-releasing intrauterine device; POP, progestin-only pill; STD, sexually transmitted disease; U.S. MEC, U.S. Medical Eligibility Criteria for Contraceptive Use.

*In instances in which blood pressure cannot be measured by a provider, blood pressure measured in other settings can be reported by the woman to her provider.

†Weight (BMI) measurement is not needed to determine medical eligibility for any methods of contraception because all methods can be used (U.S. MEC 1) or generally can be used (U.S. MEC 2) among obese women. However, measuring weight and calculating BMI at baseline might be helpful for monitoring any changes and counseling women who might be concerned about weight change perceived to be associated with their contraceptive method.

§A bimanual examination (not cervical inspection) is needed for diaphragm fitting.

¶Most women do not require additional STD screening at the time of IUD insertion. If a woman with risk factors for STDs has not been screened for gonorrhea and chlamydia according to CDC's STD Treatment Guidelines (http://www.cdc.gov/std/treatment), screening can be performed at the time of IUD insertion, and insertion should not be delayed. Women with current purulent cervicitis or chlamydial infection or gonococcal infection should not undergo IUD insertion (U.S. MEC 4).

From Curtis KM et al: U.S. selected practice recommendations for contraceptive use, 2016, MMWR Recomm Rep 65(4):1-66, 2016.

- Diaphragm and cervical cap
  - Must be fitted by practitioner, used with contraceptive gels, and refitted with weight gain or loss of 4.5 kg. Must also be refitted after pregnancy.
  - Diaphragm sizes: 50 to 105 mm; cervical cap sizes 26, 28, and 30 mm.
  - The correct fit allows the woman to remain ambulatory without feeling the device.
  - Proper use of diaphragm: put in immediately before intercourse and keep in for 6 hr after intercourse; must not remain in the vagina for longer than 24 hr.
  - Proper use of cervical cap: fit over the cervix exactly; must not remain in place for longer than 48 hr.
- Lactation amenorrhea method
  - Depends on number of feedings per day; effective as birth control for 6 mo if 15 or more feedings, lasting 10 min each, are accomplished daily. If woman meets criteria (e.g., breastfeeding only source of infant feeding) 0.5%-2.0% failure rate in the first 6 months after delivery.
- Not a common practice in the U.S.
- Withdrawal
  - Withdrawal of the penis from the vagina before ejaculation.
  - Depends on self-control, but there is a high typical use failure rate.
- Rhythm method
  - Depends on awareness of physiology of male and female reproductive tracts.
  - Sperm viable in vagina for 2 to 7 days.
  - Ovum life span 24 hr.
- Sterilization
  1. Male:
     - Vasectomy to interrupt vas deferens and block passage of sperm to seminal ejaculate.
     - Scalpel and nonscalpel techniques available.
     - More easily performed procedure than female sterilization and does not require general anesthesia.
  2. Female:
     - Leading method of birth control in U.S. in women older than 30 yr.

- Interrupts fallopian tubes, blocking passage of ovum proximally and sperm distally through tube.
- Several types; modified Pomeroy done during cesarean section or interval laparoscopic using clips (Filshie, Hulka) or banding.
- Essure-tubal occlusion through hysteroscopic placement of micro-inserts into the fallopian tubes; current controversy regarding safety and efficacy.

ACUTE GENERAL Rx

- Combination oral contraceptives
  - Standard administration: taken daily for 21 days, pill-free interval of 7 days.
  - Alternative regimen: extended or continuous administration of active pills.
  - Less than 50 mcg ethinyl estradiol in most common combination oral contraceptives; progestins most commonly used in combination pills are norethindrone, levonorgestrel, norgestrel, norethindrone acetate, ethynodiol diacetate, norgestimate,

or desogestrel; triphasic combination oral contraceptives (give varying doses of progestin and estrogens throughout cycle); monophasic oral contraceptives: offer same dose of progestin and estrogen throughout cycle, taken daily at same time; estrophasic pill (constant progesterone with variation of estrogen throughout the cycle).

- If pill taken with antibiotics, efficacy affected by inadequate gastrointestinal absorption in most cases; only rifampin truly reduces pill's effectiveness.
- Increased body weight decreases effectiveness.
- Table E4 describes oral contraceptive formulations available in the U.S. Guidelines for use of combination estrogen-progestin contraceptives in women 35 yr of age and older are described in Table E5.
- Fig. E1 describes recommended actions after late or missed combined oral contraceptives.
- Recommended actions after vomiting or diarrhea while using combined oral contraceptives are described in Fig. E2
- Mini pill
  - Progestin only; taken without a break.
  - May cause irregular bleeding because of the lack of estrogen effect on the lining of the uterus.
  - Table E6 provides a summary and recommendations for progestin-only oral contraceptive use.
- Hormonal implants and injectables
  1. Implanon/Nexplanon.
     - Single etonogestrel-secreting device that is inserted underneath the skin.
     - Among the most effective contraceptive available.
     - Approved by FDA in 2006 and effective over 3-yr period.
  2. Depo-Provera
     - Medroxyprogesterone acetate given every 3 mo in IM injection form.
     - Major side effect: irregular bleeding.
     - Fertility return possibly delayed up to 1 year or longer after last injection.
     - Table E7 provides a summary and recommendations for depot medroxyprogesterone acetate (DMPA) use.
- Postcoital contraception
  - Done on emergency basis, usually as a result of noncompliance with birth control or failure of birth control (e.g., condom breakage) at the time of ovulation.
  - Methods:
    - Hormonal methods:
      - Levonorgestrel is available either as two 0.75 mg tablets taken 12 hr apart

(next choice) or as a 1.5 mg tablet taken once (Plan B, one step). It is indicated for emergency contraception to be used within 72 hr after unexpected intercourse. It can be obtained OTC by women >15 yr of age and by prescription by younger patients.
      - Ulipristal (ELLA) is a progesterone-receptor agonist/antagonist available by prescription only. It is a 30-mg, single-dose tablet and can be taken up to 5 days after unexpected intercourse.
      - Copper IUD insertion within 5 days of coitus.
- IUD
  - Device inserted into uterus to prevent sperm and ovum from uniting in fallopian tube.
  - Types available in the U.S.:
    - ParaGard (Copper T/30-A): a polyethylene T wrapped with a fine copper wire effective for 10 yr.
    - Mirena Levonorgestrel Intrauterine System: a T-shaped system with a chamber that contains levonorgestrel. Releases 20 mcg/day; is effective for 5 yr.
    - Skyla: smaller and lowest dose of levonorgestrel, approved for 3 yr.
    - Liletta: cheaper levonorgestrel secreting system, approved for 3 yr.
    - Kyleena: another 5-yr levonorgestrel system.
- Vaginal ring (NuvaRing)
  - Provides daily dose of 120 mcg of etonogestrel and 15 mcg ethinyl estradiol.
  - Stays in vagina 3 wk and is removed the fourth for a contraceptive-free interval analogous to the placebo pills in oral contraceptive pills.
  - Increased body weight decreases effectiveness.
  - Delivers lower total dose of estrogen than the combination oral contraceptive, but may have higher risk of DVT.
  - Recommended actions after delayed insertion or reinsertion with combined vaginal ring are described in Fig. E3.
- Contraceptive patch
  - Releases a progestin and estrogen (ethinyl estradiol)
  - Each patch contains 6 mg norelgestromin and delivers an estimated continuous systemic dose of 150 mcg norelgestromin and 15 mcg of ethinyl estradiol daily
  - Worn 3 out of 4 wk
  - Increased body weight decreases effectiveness

- Concern for increased risk of thromboembolic events
- Ortha Evra brand discontinued; Xulane (generic) available in the U.S.
- Recommended actions after delayed application or detachment with combined hormonal patch are described in Fig. E4

CHRONIC Rx

- With all the previously mentioned types of birth control, patient is followed up at least yearly, or as necessary, if problems arise.
- Full history, physical examination, and Pap smear, including cultures when needed, are performed yearly.
- Patients with medical problems are followed up approximately every 6 mo when taking hormonal therapy.

DISPOSITION

- Follow yearly or more frequently according to patient's side effects.
- Tailor birth control to patient according to different needs or side effects present at different times in life. Effective counseling also requires an understanding of a woman's preference and medical risks, benefits, side effects, and contraindications of each contraceptive method.

COMMENTS

- With hormonal contraception, if neurologic or cardiac symptoms arise, stop method immediately, evaluate, and refer to internist when appropriate.
- The effectiveness of long-acting reversible contraception (IUDs and implants) is superior to that of contraceptive pills, patch, or ring and is not altered in adolescents and young women.
- Management of women with bleeding irregularities while using contraception is described in Fig. E5.

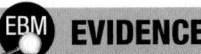 **EVIDENCE**

Available at www.expertconsult.com

SUGGESTED READINGS
Available at www.expertconsult.com

RELATED CONTENT

Contraception (Patient Information)
Emergency Contraception (Related Key Topic)

AUTHOR: **RUBEN ALVERO, M.D.,** and **GEORGE KOVALESKY, M.D.**

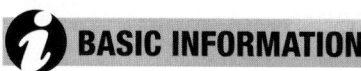

DEFINITION

A rise in serum creatinine of 0.5 mg/dl or >25% elevation from baseline 48 hours after iodinated contrast media exposure (Table 1).

SYNONYMS

Contrast-induced nephropathy (CIN)
Contrast nephropathy
Radiocontrast-induced nephropathy
CI-AKI

ICD-10CM CODES
N14.1 Nephropathy induced by other drugs, medicaments, and biological substances

EPIDEMIOLOGY & DEMOGRAPHICS

INCIDENCE: Overall incidence of CI-AKI is approximately 7% and is responsible for 11% of acquired AKI cases during hospitalization.
PEAK INCIDENCE: Incidence rates vary widely depending on the presence of known risk factors. In one risk prediction model of CI-AKI, the risk in patients undergoing percutaneous coronary intervention (PCI) ranged from 7.5% (lowest risk score group) to 57.1% (highest risk score group).
PREDOMINANT SEX AND AGE: Risk of CI-AKI increases with age. There is no gender predilection.
RISK FACTORS: Patient-related factors include chronic kidney disease, age >75 years, diabetes mellitus if CKD, severe anemia, nonnormovolemic states such as heart failure and volume depletion, and hemodynamic instability. Nonpatient-related factors include contrast osmolality, use of ionic contrast (rarely used), contrast total dose and sequential doses, and requirement for intraaortic balloon pump. Although initially thought to be higher, the risk of CI-AKI is <u>not</u> higher with intraarterial contrast administration (e.g., cardiac catheterization) than with intravenous contrast dosing (e.g., CT scans). Inpatients have a higher risk of developing CI-AKI than outpatients (Boxes 1 and 2).

PHYSICAL FINDINGS & CLINICAL PRESENTATION

- Elevation in serum creatinine generally occurs 24-48 hours after administration of contrast. Typically, there are no accompanying symptoms or exam findings. Acute kidney injury usually resolves within 10 days of radiocontrast exposure. Less than 1% of patients with CI-AKI will require dialysis, typically patients with a history of advanced renal disease.

ETIOLOGY

- Nephrotoxicity occurs due to renal medullary ischemia, a result of vasoconstrictive effects of the contrast medium on the large and small renal arteries.
- Contrast also exerts a direct cytotoxic effect on the vascular endothelium and renal tubular cells, leading to cell injury and death due to generation of damaging reactive oxygen species.

DX DIAGNOSIS

DIFFERENTIAL DIAGNOSIS

- Acute tubular necrosis, atheroembolic renal disease (i.e., postcardiac catheterization), acute interstitial nephritis, prerenal azotemia

WORKUP

- Diagnosis is dependent primarily on history and laboratory values. A search for clinical findings more suggestive of other etiologies of AKI should be conducted (e.g., livedo reticularis or dusky lower-extremity digits in the presence of atheroembolic disease, evidence of systemic infection accompanied by hypotension in the case of sepsis-mediated ATN).
- Urinalysis often reveals a fractional excretion of sodium (FE_{Na}) of <1% despite acute tubular necrosis. A high urine specific gravity may reflect the filtration of hyperosmolar contrast medium. Markers of renal tubular damage including muddy brown granular casts or renal epithelial cells may be seen on urinalysis.

- A renal biopsy is not recommended for diagnostic confirmation since biopsy findings are nonspecific for acute tubular necrosis.

LABORATORY TESTS

- Creatinine, urinalysis, and urine microscopy
- Urine and plasma sodium and creatinine concentrations for determination of FE_{Na}

IMAGING STUDIES

- No radiologic tests aid in the diagnosis of CI-AKI. A renal ultrasound should be obtained if postrenal obstruction is in the differential diagnosis.

Rx TREATMENT

Treatment for CI-AKI is supportive. Prevention has been the focus of research efforts.
Recommended strategies for CI-AKI prophylaxis:
- Avoidance of studies and procedures using intravenous contrast, if not emergent. Consider an alternative imaging modality, if available, for patients at high risk for developing CIN.
- Use low-osmolar nonionic contrast media.
- Minimize contrast volume (dose).
- Volume expansion with intravenous isotonic fluid. Normal saline and sodium bicarbonate solutions are both effective in reducing the risk of CIN, and normal saline is more effective than 0.45% saline. Although sodium bicarbonate solutions were initially thought to be superior to saline, current evidence reveals that neither solution is superior.

Preventive measures for CI-AKI that have NOT shown significant benefit include:
- Oral hydration solutions
- Prophylactic hemodialysis or hemofiltration
- Diuresis from diuretic medications or by osmotic diuretics (e.g., mannitol)
- Vasodilators (e.g., fenoldopam, nifedipine, theophylline)
- Ascorbic acid

Preventive measures for CI-AKI that may provide modest additional benefit include *N*-acetylcysteine (given at high dose with intravenous fluids), HMG Co-A reductase inhibitors, and repeat ischemia-reperfusion injury techniques.

GENERAL PROPHYLAXIS: INTRAVENOUS HYDRATION

- Outpatients with glomerular filtration rate (GFR) <60 ml/min: withhold medications that reduce GFR (e.g., nonsteroidal antiinflammatory drugs and, possibly, angiotensin converting enzyme inhibitors and angiotensin receptor blockers) or reduce extracellular fluid volume (e.g., thiazide or loop diuretics). An outpatient hydration protocol with either normal saline or sodium bicarbonate may be considered, particularly with GFR <45 ml/min. Notably, outpatient hydration protocols have not been rigorously evaluated. Sodium bicarbonate infused at 3 ml/kg/hr for 1 hour preprocedure and 1.5 mg/kg/hr 4-6 hours intra- and postprocedure can be performed in the outpatient setting.

TABLE 1 Classification of Iodinated Contrast Media

Ionicity	Relative Osmolality	Contrast Agent	Osmolality (mOsm/kg H_2O)
Ionic	High osmolality	Diatrizoate Ioxithalamate Ioxithalamate	1500-1860
Ionic	Low osmolality	Ioxaglate	600
Nonionic	Low osmolality	Iobitridol Iohexol Iomeprol Iopamidol Iopromide Ioversol	521-695
Nonionic	Iso-osmolal	Ioxaglate Iotrolan	290-320

From Vincent JL et al: *Textbook of critical care*, ed 6, Philadelphia, 2011, Saunders.

BOX 1 Recommedations to Reduce the Risk of Contrast-Induced Nephropathy

1. Identify patients at risk for contrast-induced nephropathy (CIN) and calculate their total risk score.
2. Assess risk/benefit of the proposed contrast-requiring intervention and consider alternative not requiring contrast intervention.
3. Assess kidney function by estimated glomerular filtration rate (eGFR) or calculated creatinine clearance prior to contrast, especially in patients at risk for CIN.
4. Modify correctable risk factors and hold medications that may act as co-nephrotoxins.
5. In high-risk patients receiving intraarterial contrast, consider either a low-osmolar contrast medium (other than iohexol) or an iso-osmolar contrast agent.
6. Use the lowest dose of appropriate contrast medium.
7. In high-risk patients, correct hypovolemia. Stop diuretics and consider IV fluid if there is no contraindication. The optimal fluid type and quantity are not clear. Data support the use of either 0.9% saline or isotonic sodium bicarbonate, beginning at least 1 hour prior to contrast injection and continuing for at least 6 hours postinjection. Initial rates of 3 ml/kg/hr, followed by 1 ml/kg/hr are commonly recommended. The patient should be monitored for signs and symptoms of hypervolemia or pulmonary edema.
8. In high-risk patients, consider *N*-acetylcysteine, particularly if higher doses of contrast media or intraarterial administration is necessary. A total of 4 doses of *N*-acetylcysteine, 1200 mg orally twice a day starting the day prior to contrast injection, is an acceptable regimen. For emergent procedures, may consider 1200 mg IV as an initial dose, followed by above 4 doses.
9. In patients with advanced kidney disease, prophylactic hemofiltration before and after contrast was associated with reduced mortality in one study.
10. In high-risk patients, serum creatinine should be rechecked within 24-72 hours post contrast injection.

Vincent JL et al: *Textbook of critical care*, ed 6, Philadelphia, 2011, Saunders.

BOX 2 Patient Risk Factors for Contrast-Induced Acute Kidney Injury

Chronic kidney disease (GFR <60 ml/min)
Diabetes
Age >75 years
Congestive heart failure
Hypotension
Intraaortic balloon pump placement
Anemia (Hct <36% in women, <39% in men)

Adapted from Mehran R, et al.: A simple risk score for prediction of contrast-induced nephropathy after percutaneous coronary intervention: development and initial validation, *J Am Coll Cardiol* 44(7):1393-1399, 2004.

- Inpatients with GFR <60 ml/min: intravenous normal saline or D5W with 3 amps sodium bicarbonate at 1 ml/kg/hr for 6-12 hours pre-procedure, during the procedure, and 6-12 hours postprocedure. If there are contraindications to intravenous fluid administration (e.g., congestive heart failure with pulmonary edema), consider postponement of studies involving contrast medium, if not emergently indicated. If the procedure is unavoidable, fluid management should be tailored to the individual patient.

DISPOSITION

- CI-AKI is usually self-limited. Patients with severe renal functional impairment may require hospitalization for supportive care and, potentially, dialysis.

REFERRAL

- Patients at high risk for CI-AKI or who develop significant CI-AKI should be referred to nephrology.

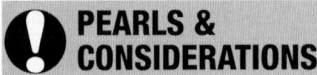 **PEARLS & CONSIDERATIONS**

- A diagnosis of CI-AKI should be considered in patients who develop acute kidney injury 24-72 hours after contrast exposure. Urine sediment may be bland or show signs of tubular injury. FE_{Na} is often <1% due to vasoconstriction.
- Administration of isotonic intravenous fluids as a preventive measure is indicated for patients with GFR <60 ml/min or who otherwise are at high risk for CI-AKI.
- NSAIDs and other potential nephrotoxic drugs should be avoided in patients receiving intravenous contrast media.
- Diabetic patients should have metformin held before receiving intravenous contrast due to an increased risk of metformin-related lactic acidosis in the setting of CI-AKI.

SUGGESTED READINGS
Available at www.expertconsult.com

RELATED CONTENT
Acute Kidney Injury (Related Key Topic)

AUTHOR: **LISA COHEN, M.D.**

BASIC INFORMATION

DEFINITION

Cor pulmonale is an alteration in the structure and function of the right ventricle (RV) from pulmonary hypertension caused by diseases of the upper or lower airways, lungs, or pulmonary vasculature. It is a state of cardiopulmonary dysfunction that may result from multiple etiologies rather than a specific disease state. Right-sided heart failure resulting from primary disease of the left heart and congenital heart disease are not considered in this disorder.

SYNONYMS

Acute cor pulmonale
Chronic cor pulmonale

ICD-10CM CODES
I26.0 Pulmonary embolism with acute cor pulmonale
I27.81 Cor pulmonale (chronic)
I26.01 Septic pulmonary embolism with acute cor pulmonale
I26.02 Saddle embolus of pulmonary artery with acute cor pulmonale
I26.09 Other pulmonary embolism with acute cor pulmonale
I26.90 Septic pulmonary embolism without acute cor pulmonale
I26.92 Saddle embolus of pulmonary artery without acute cor pulmonale
I26.99 Other pulmonary embolism without acute cor pulmonale

ETIOLOGY

Acute cor pulmonale is a disorder in which the right ventricle (RV) is dilated and the muscular wall is stretched thin, usually as a result of acute pulmonary embolism or acute respiratory distress syndrome (ARDS). This may present with often life-threatening cardiogenic shock, or death, but if the patient survives the initial event, then the RV often recovers and cor pulmonale no longer exists after several weeks. After its development, critical care echocardiography is the gold standard and defines acute cor pulmonale as the presence of RV dilatation along with a paradoxical interventricular septal motion at end systole, suggesting both RV systolic and diastolic overload.

Chronic cor pulmonale is hypertrophy of the right ventricle caused by increased afterload in the pulmonary circuit, i.e., pulmonary hypertension, resulting in either acute or chronic right ventricular failure depending on the time course of the elevation in pulmonary vascular resistance. Pulmonary hypertension associated with lung disease is defined as resting mean positive airway pressure (PAP) greater than 20 mm Hg, which is different from the definition of primary pulmonary arterial hypertension (mPAP >25 mm Hg). Mechanisms leading to pulmonary hypertension and thus predisposing to the development of cor pulmonale include:

- Pulmonary vasoconstriction leading to increased RV afterload, often resulting from conditions causing alveolar hypoxia and/ or respiratory acidosis (e.g., high altitude/hypobaric hypoxia, obstructive sleep apnea/obesity-hypoventilation syndrome, chronic obstructive pulmonary disease). In pulmonary arterial hypertension (PAH), pulmonary vasoconstriction may occur in the absence of a primary cause of hypoxemia, due to imbalances between vasoconstrictor and vasodilator expression in the pulmonary circulation.
- Anatomic reduction or remodeling of the pulmonary vascular bed leading to increased RV afterload (e.g., emphysema, interstitial lung disease, pulmonary emboli, pulmonary arterial hypertension).
- Increased blood viscosity leading to increased RV afterload (e.g., polycythemia related to chronic hypoxemia, polycythemia vera, Waldenström's macroglobulinemia).
- Chronic thrombotic and/or embolic disease.
- Pulmonary vascular endothelial dysfunction also plays a major role in the development of pulmonary hypertension. There is reduction in the production of nitric oxide as well as prostacyclins, resulting in an imbalance of vasoconstriction opposed to dilation.

PHYSICAL FINDINGS & CLINICAL PRESENTATION

No symptoms are specific for cor pulmonale. Typically, the symptoms depend on the underlying disease process. The symptoms are most often a result of right ventricular failure:

- Dyspnea, fatigue, chest pain, or syncope with exertion (from pulmonary hypertension, RV ischemia, and impaired cardiac output)
- Right upper quadrant abdominal pain and anorexia (from passive hepatic congestion)
- Hoarseness (caused by compression of the left recurrent laryngeal nerve by dilation of the main pulmonary artery; known as *Ortner's syndrome*)
- Signs of right ventricular failure: jugular venous distention, peripheral edema, hepatic congestion, ascites, and a right ventricular third heart sound
- Signs of associated tricuspid regurgitation: holosystolic murmur heard best along the left parasternal border (augments during inspiration), prominent V-wave on jugular venous pulse, and pulsatile hepatomegaly (in severe tricuspid regurgitation)
- Pulmonary hypertension will increase the intensity of the pulmonic component of S2, which may be narrowly split
- Rarely, cough and hemoptysis

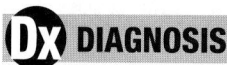

DIAGNOSIS

WORKUP

Search for an underlying pulmonary process resulting in pulmonary hypertension:

- Left ventricular dysfunction should be excluded in initial assessment with an echocardiogram.
- Worldwide, chronic mountain sickness is an important cause of cor pulmonale.
- 80% to 90% of cor pulmonale cases are attributable to chronic obstructive pulmonary disease (COPD) and should include complete pulmonary function tests (PFTs).
- Consideration of obstructive sleep apnea, chronic thromboembolic disease, pulmonary arterial hypertension, and musculoskeletal disease should be given in the absence of parenchymal lung disease.
- A MUGA RVEF <40% to 45% is considered abnormal, but RVEF is not a good marker of RV function because it is afterload dependent. Raised PAP and PVR will decrease the measured RVEF.

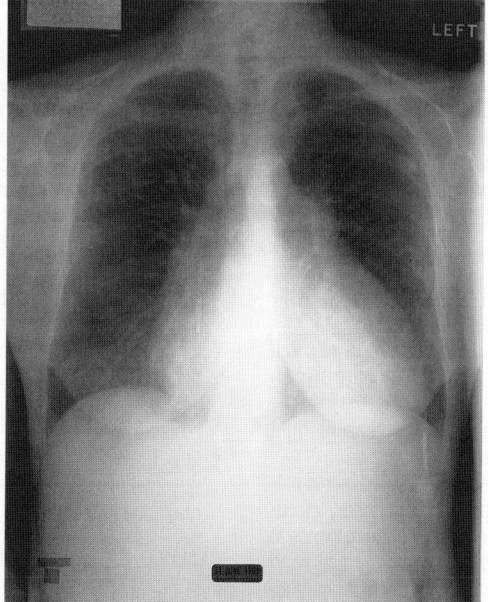

FIG. 1 Chest radiography in a patient with severe intrinsic pulmonary vascular disease demonstrating enlargement of the main pulmonary artery, right ventricle, and right atrium. (From Crawford MH et al [eds]: *Cardiology,* ed 2, St Louis, 2004, Mosby.)

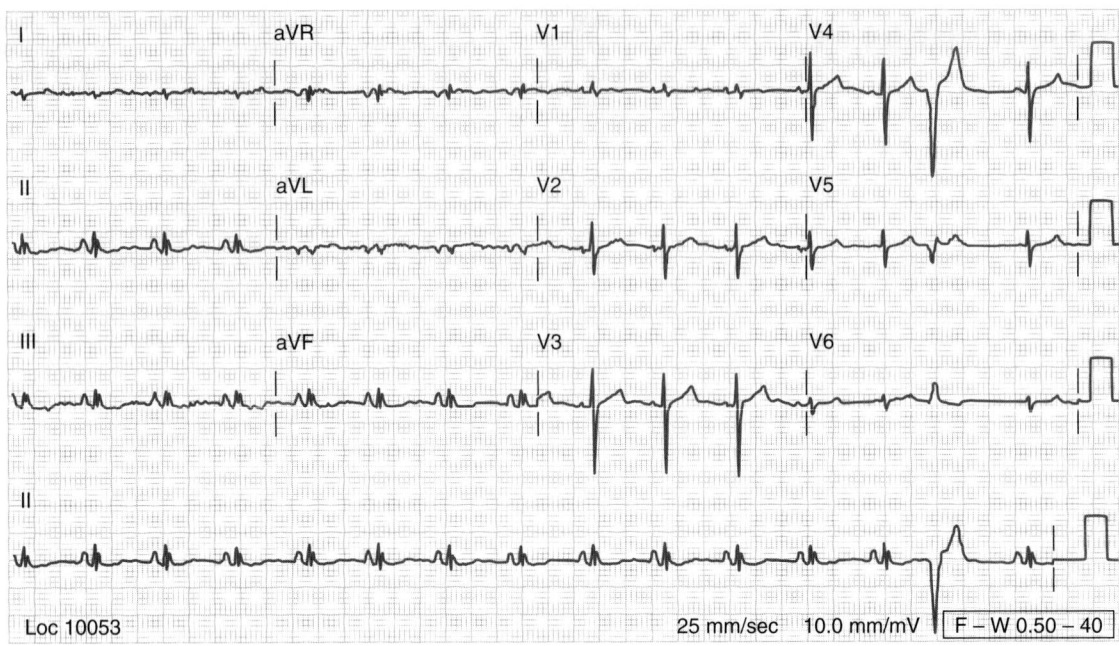

FIG. 2 An electrocardiogram in a patient with chronic cor pulmonale reveals prominent "p pulmonale" and other characteristic features (see text). (From Mason RJ: *Murray & Nadel's textbook of respiratory medicine,* ed 5, Philadelphia, 2010, Saunders.)

LABORATORY TESTS

- Complete blood count may show erythrocytosis from chronic hypoxia.
- Arterial blood gas levels confirm hypoxemia and acidosis or hypercapnia.
- BNP may be elevated from RV dilation and/or hypoxia.
- Connective tissue disorder workup to exclude scleroderma, lupus, rheumatoid arthritis
- HIV testing

IMAGING STUDIES

- Chest radiograph may show underlying pulmonary disease and evidence of pulmonary hypertension (e.g., enlargement of the pulmonary arteries or right atrium and right ventricular dilation or "pruning" of the peripheral vasculature) (Fig. 1).
- ECG (Fig. 2) may reveal right ventricular hypertrophy with R/S ratio >1 in leads V_1 and R/S ratio <1 in leads V_5, V_6, right atrial enlargement (P-pulmonale), right-axis deviation, or the triad of $S_1Q_3T_3$ indicative of RV strain.
- Echocardiogram to detect right ventricular enlargement and/or hypertrophy and estimate pulmonary artery pressure.
- Perfusion scintigraphy (VQ scan) to rule out chronic thromboembolic pulmonary hypertension (CTEPH)
- Cardiac MRI can accurately measure right ventricular dimensions and function.
- Right-sided heart catheterization measures pulmonary artery pressures and pulmonary vascular resistance. It can also determine response to oxygen or vasodilators. Importantly, right heart catheterization allows assessment of pulmonary capillary wedge pressure, allowing right heart failure from pulmonary venous hypertension due to left heart disease to be ruled out.

- Chest CT can assess for pulmonary parenchymal disease and embolus in the pulmonary vasculature.

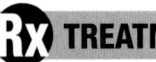 **TREATMENT**

The treatment of cor pulmonale is directed toward the underlying etiology while also reversing hypoxemia, improving right ventricular contractility, decreasing pulmonary artery vascular resistance, and improving pulmonary hypertension. Table 1 summarizes therapeutic strategies for cor pulmonale.

NONPHARMACOLOGIC THERAPY

Supplemental oxygen to correct hypoxemia is an important management step in the treatment of cor pulmonale related to hypoxemia. Goal O_2 sat of more than 90% is recommended.

- Continuous positive airway pressure is used in patients with obstructive sleep apnea.
- Sodium and fluid restriction in setting of edema from RV failure
- Phlebotomy is reserved as adjunctive therapy in patients with polycythemia (hematocrit >55%) who have acute decompensation of cor pulmonale or remain polycythemic despite long-term oxygen therapy. Phlebotomy has been shown to decrease mean pulmonary artery pressure and pulmonary vascular resistance.
- Low-level aerobic exercise, avoiding heavy physical exercise or isometric exercises that may cause syncope

ACUTE GENERAL Rx

- Pulmonary embolism is the most common cause of acute cor pulmonale (see "Pulmonary Embolism"). The treatment is anticoagulation, hemodynamic support, and

consideration of thrombolytics. Catheter-based thrombectomy or surgical embolectomy are potential salvage therapies in patients who cannot receive anticoagulation or thrombolysis, or whose condition continues to deteriorate despite thrombolytics and anticoagulation.

- Acute cor pulmonale may also be seen in cases of ARDS, related to hypercapnia/acidosis, hypoxic pulmonary vasoconstriction, and the effects of mechanical ventilation. The treatment is supportive care for ARDS with low tidal volume ventilation. Extracorporeal membrane oxygen support (ECMO) while awaiting lung recovery from ARDS may also be helpful in maintaining blood oxygenation. Venoarterial ECMO can provide hemodynamic support as well as blood oxygenation.
- In patients with preexisting cor pulmonale, acute pulmonary illnesses or hypoxia can increase pulmonary hypertension and worsen right ventricular function. The underlying exacerbating conditions should be treated.
- Careful attention to fluid balance is important in the management of acute decompensated right heart failure. Both overhydration and overdiuresis should be avoided, with careful monitoring of intake and output, electrolytes and creatinine, and hemodynamics.
- Intravenous inotropes may be employed to support right heart contractility in decompensated right heart failure.
- In acutely decompensated right heart failure due to pulmonary arterial hypertension, IV prostanoid medications are the treatment of choice. Oral pulmonary vasodilators may also be added to the IV prostanoids, but should not be initiated as monotherapy in patients with advanced right heart failure from PAH.

TABLE 1   Therapeutic Strategies for Cor Pulmonale

Diet and Lifestyle

Smoking cessation
Weight loss
Sodium restriction
Judicious exercise training
Structured rehabilitation and breathing training programs
Avoidance of overexertion
Avoidance of pregnancy
Avoidance of high altitudes

Interventions

Treatment of underlying condition
    COPD (bronchodilators, corticosteroids, antibiotics, oxygen)
    Interstitial lung disease (immunosuppression, oxygen, interferon gamma [investigational])
    Sleep-disordered breathing and alveolar hypoventilation disorders (CPAP, BiPAP, surgery)
    Chronic exposure to high altitudes (return to sea level)
    Chronic thromboembolic disease (anticoagulation, inferior vena cava filters, thromboendarterectomy)
Supplemental oxygen
Pulmonary vasodilators
Anticoagulation
Diuretics
Digitalis glycosides (chronic therapy)
Nonglycoside inotropes (low-dose dobutamine or dopamine in acute severe right heart decompensation with hypoperfusion)
Lung volume-reduction surgery
Lung transplantation
Heart-lung transplantation (PAH secondary to complex congenital heart disease)
Percutaneous blade-balloon atrial septostomy (investigational)
    Severe right-sided heart failure
    Recurrent syncope

BiPAP, bilevel positive airway pressure; *CPAP*, continuous positive airway pressure; *PAH*, pulmonary arterial hypertension.
From Mason RJ: *Murray & Nadel's textbook of respiratory medicine,* ed 5, Philadelphia, 2010, Saunders.

CHRONIC Rx

The long-term use of oxygen therapy results in decreased clinical right heart failure and improved pulmonary hemodynamics in hypoxic patients.

Indications for oxygen in COPD patients include the following:

1. Resting PaO_2 ≤55 mm Hg on arterial blood gas
2. Resting PaO 56–59 mm Hg if clinical presence of right heart failure with dependent edema, P pulmonale on EKG
3. Desaturation to SpO_2 ≤88% on oximetry with activity or at night
   - Right ventricular volume overload should be treated with loop diuretics (e.g., furosemide) and potassium-sparing diuretics such as spironolactone.
   - Anticoagulation with warfarin has been shown to have some benefit in patients with idiopathic pulmonary arterial hypertension with a target international normalized ratio (INR) of 1.5-2.5, unlike the target for thromboembolic disease, provided there are no obvious contraindications to long-term anticoagulation. Digoxin, though controversial, may be employed as an oral inotropic agent to improve right heart contractility and control atrial arrhythmias.
   - Selective oral or parenteral pulmonary vasodilators such as oral calcium channel blockers (CCBs), prostanoids, and endothelin receptor blockers may be used after a right heart catheterization that establishes pulmonary hypertension.

If vasoreactivity to calcium channel blockers is established, CCBs may be used to combat pulmonary hypertension. However, if there is no vasoreactivity, prostanoids such as epoprostenol or treprostinil or endothelin receptor blockers such as bosentan may be tried. However, such agents have been shown to be beneficial in the treatment of idiopathic PAH, PAH related to connective tissue disease, and PAH due to congenital heart disease. Pulmonary vasodilators are sometimes considered in other forms of PAH when primary disease management strategies have failed to improve right heart failure.

- Phosphodiesterase inhibitors such as sildenafil and tadalafil are newer vasodilators that improve symptoms, functional class, and mean pulmonary artery pressures as alternatives or in addition to prostanoids.
- Pulmonary thromboendarterectomy may be curative in the special case of cor pulmonale due to chronic thromboembolic pulmonary hypertension.
- Atrial septostomy is a salvage option for patients with ongoing decompensated right heart failure from PAH despite pulmonary vasodilators. Such patients should undergo rapid assessment for possible transplantation.
- Lung transplantation or heart-lung transplantation should be considered in the setting of cor pulmonale from lung diseases or from pulmonary vascular disease.

DISPOSITION

Patients with cor pulmonale should have regular assessment of their functional class (e.g., NYHA or WHO functional class); worse functional class indicates a poorer prognosis. Other poor prognostic features include high right atrial pressure, impaired cardiac output, presence of hyponatremia, elevated BNP levels, low systemic blood pressure, and poor exercise tolerance as demonstrated by a 6-minute walk test.

REFERRAL

Patients with pulmonary disease who have progressed to cor pulmonale should be followed up by a pulmonologist and a tertiary care center that specializes in treatment of advanced pulmonary hypertension.

! PEARLS & CONSIDERATIONS

- Identification and treatment of the underlying cause of cor pulmonale is key.
- Prognosis and treatment are related to the underlying cause, whereas the presence of cor pulmonale is merely a marker of the underlying disease severity.
- Right heart catheterization is the gold standard to establish diagnosis and to determine treatment, including response to calcium channel blockers, prostanoids, and endothelin receptor blockers.

COMMENTS

There is increasing interest in selective pulmonary vasodilators to improve right ventricular heart function in patients with cor pulmonale outside of the setting of idiopathic PAH, PAH related to connective tissue disease, and PAH related to congenital heart disease. However, more data on the safety and efficacy of these agents, especially in the setting of hypoxemic lung disease, is needed.

The importance of maintaining or improving right heart function, rather than solely lowering pulmonary pressures, is becoming increasingly apparent in the therapeutic management of patients with pulmonary hypertension and right heart failure.

Long-term survival is related to improved pulmonary artery hemodynamics (lower PAP). Improved pulmonary hemodynamics are apparent within the first 6 months of oxygen therapy. Twenty-four-hour oxygen therapy improves pulmonary hemodynamics more than 12 hr/day therapy.

SUGGESTED READINGS

Available at www.expertconsult.com

RELATED CONTENT

Pulmonary Embolism (Related Key Topic)
Pulmonary Hypertension (Related Key Topic)

AUTHOR: **WAJIH A. SYED, M.D.**

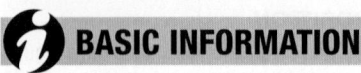

DEFINITION

A corneal abrasion is a loss of surface epithelial tissue of the cornea caused by trauma.

SYNONYMS

Corneal erosion
Corneal contusion
Corneal epithelial defect

ICD-10CM CODES

S05.00XA Injury of conjunctiva and corneal abrasion without foreign body, unspecified eye, initial encounter
S05.01XA Injury of conjunctiva and corneal abrasion without foreign body, right eye, initial encounter
S05.02XA Injury of conjunctiva and corneal abrasion without foreign body, left eye, initial encounter

EPIDEMIOLOGY & DEMOGRAPHICS

INCIDENCE (IN U.S.): A universal problem. Corneal abrasions comprise 8% of all eye presentations in primary care.
PEAK INCIDENCE: Childhood through active adulthood and older and debilitated patients
PREDOMINANT AGE: Any age

PHYSICAL FINDINGS & CLINICAL PRESENTATION

- Haziness of the cornea
- Disruption of the corneal surface (Fig. 1)
- Redness and injection of the conjunctiva
- Pain
- Light sensitivity
- Tearing
- Gritty or foreign-body feeling
- Pain on opening or closing eyes

ETIOLOGY

- Trauma (direct mechanical event)
- Foreign body
- Contact lenses
- Chemical or flash ultraviolet burns

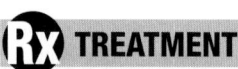

DIAGNOSIS

DIFFERENTIAL DIAGNOSIS

- Acute-angle closure glaucoma (pupil may be fixed, supraorbital headache)
- Herpes ulcers and other corneal ulcers
- Foreign body in the cornea (be certain it is not a keratitis)
- Infective keratitis (be cautious in contact lens wearers; bacterial infections are common, and symptoms are similar)

WORKUP

- Fluorescein staining, slit lamp evaluation. After fluorescein staining of the cornea, an abrasion will appear yellow under normal light and green in cobalt blue light.
- Assessment of visual acuity. Vision loss requires referral.
- Intraocular pressure.
- Rule out corneal laceration (flattened anterior chamber with perforation; refer urgently).
- Rule out other eye pathology. Inspect anterior chamber for blood (hyphema) or pus (hypopyon). If present, refer immediately to ophthalmologist.
- Examine for foreign bodies and remove them if present. (Evert upper eyelid to locate foreign body on the palpebral conjunctiva.)
- Confirm red reflex to rule out significant globe injury.

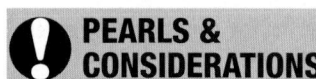

TREATMENT

NONPHARMACOLOGIC THERAPY

- Bandage contact lens can help to speed healing for large epithelial abrasions.
- Warm compresses.
- Pressure dressing (patching) is controversial. Although eye patching traditionally has been recommended in the treatment of corneal abrasions, several studies show that patching does not help and may hinder healing.
- Removal of any foreign particles if present.

ACUTE GENERAL Rx

- Topical antibiotics such as 10% sulfacetamide or ofloxacin 0.3% solution 2 drops qid are commonly prescribed to prevent bacterial superinfection, but evidence for their use is lacking. Ointment forms are often used (e.g., erythromycin, bacitracin ophthalmic QID) to also improve corneal surface lubrication. Antipseudomonal topical antibiotics are, however, recommended for contact lens–related abrasions.
- Pressure patching of eye with eyelid closed is no longer recommended because it can result in decreased oxygen delivery, increased moisture, and a higher chance of infection.
- Cycloplegics such as 5% homatropine are often prescribed to relieve ciliary muscle spasm; however, their benefit has been questioned and they are no longer routinely recommended.
- Topical nonsteroidal antiinflammatory drugs (NSAIDs) (e.g., diclofenac 0.1% or ketorolac 0.5%) 1 drop qid may be used for pain relief.
- Topical anesthetic drops immediately improve comfort for purposes of examination, but repeated use can lead to severe problems, delayed or arrested healing, infections, perforations, and loss of the eye.
- Oral NSAIDs may be used for severe pain.

DISPOSITION

Follow-up in 24 hr and then every 3 days until abrasion has cleared and vision has returned to normal. Less frequent follow-up is appropriate for abrasions ≤4 mm or for uncomplicated abrasions.

REFERRAL

To ophthalmologist if patient has no relief within 24 hr or for patients with deep eye injuries, foreign bodies that cannot be removed, or suspected recurrent corneal erosion or infections.

PEARLS & CONSIDERATIONS

COMMENTS

- Never give the patient topical anesthetic to use at home because these can cause decompensation of the cornea, severe delay of epithelial healing, and permanent damage.
- Corticosteroid drops (e.g., dexamethasone, prednisolone) should be avoided, since they can delay healing and exacerbate some corneal infections (herpes viral keratitis, pseudomonas, and fungal ulcers)
- Most corneal abrasions heal in 24 to 48 hr and rarely progress to corneal erosion or infection.
- Improvement in pain is a good indication of corneal epithelial healing. Severe worsening of pain could indicate corneal bacterial infection (keratitis) and should be evaluated urgently.

SUGGESTED READINGS

Available at www.expertconsult.com

RELATED CONTENT

Corneal Foreign Body or Abrasion (Patient Information)

AUTHOR: **R. SCOTT HOFFMAN, M.D.**

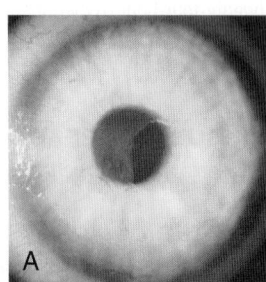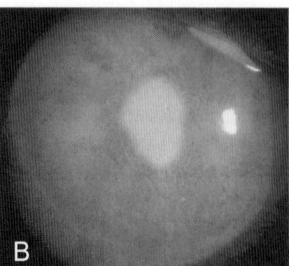

FIG. 1 Corneal epithelial abrasion. A, Epithelial defect without fluorescein highlighting the defect. An irregularity in the otherwise smooth corneal surface is the key to identifying the defect if no fluorescein is available. **B,** Classic fluorescein staining of an epithelial defect. (From Palay D [ed]: *Ophthalmology for the primary care physician,* St Louis, 1997, Mosby.)

BASIC INFORMATION

DEFINITION

Coronary artery disease (CAD) is a clinical syndrome that suggests limitation of coronary blood flow to the myocardium as a result of flow-limiting atherosclerotic lesions. It is silent in the early stages and characterized by exertional symptoms in later stages as described in the following.

This topic addresses only stable CAD. Acute coronary syndromes (ACS), angina pectoris, and myocardial infarction are addressed as separate topics elsewhere.

SYNONYMS

Atherosclerotic heart disease
CAD
Chronic stable angina
Stable ischemic heart disease
Coronary arteriosclerosis

ICD-10CM CODES
I25.1	Atherosclerotic heart disease
I25.0	Atherosclerotic cardiovascular disease
I25.10	Atherosclerotic heart disease of native coronary artery without angina pectoris
I25.110	Atherosclerotic heart disease of native coronary artery with unstable angina pectoris
I25.111	Atherosclerotic heart disease of native coronary artery with angina pectoris with documented spasm
I25.118	Atherosclerotic heart disease of native coronary artery with other forms of angina pectoris
I25.119	Atherosclerotic heart disease of native coronary artery with unspecified angina pectoris

EPIDEMIOLOGY & DEMOGRAPHICS

INCIDENCE: Increases with age.
PEAK INCIDENCE: Increases in age in women but peaks in men between the ages of 55 and 65 years.
PREVALENCE: 15.4 million Americans ≥20 years of age have CAD, and this includes 6.4% of US adults ≥20 years of age. CAD prevalence is 7.9% for men and 5.1% for women.
PREDOMINANT SEX AND AGE: Male predominance, no predominant age.
RISK FACTORS: Age, male sex, hypertension, hyperlipidemia, diabetes mellitus, obesity, tobacco use, family history, peripheral vascular disease. Coronary plaque, especially noncalcified plaque, is more prevalent and extensive in HIV-infected men, independent of CAD risk factors.

PHYSICAL FINDINGS & CLINICAL PRESENTATION

- Left anterior chest discomfort often described as squeezing, choking, heavy, and occasionally hot or cold sensations.
- Associated symptoms include fatigue, dyspnea, weakness, lightheadedness, nausea, diaphoresis, altered mental status, and syncope.
- Angina typically lasts 3 to 5 minutes but usually does not last more than 30 minutes.
- Women and diabetics may not present with classic symptoms, but may manifest more frequently with dyspnea.
- Elicited by physical exertion, emotional stress, cold exposure, consumption of heavy meal, smoking.
- Early coronary disease is asymptomatic.
- Stigmata of atherosclerosis may include xanthelasma, tendon xanthomata, and evidence of peripheral vascular disease such as claudication and diminished peripheral pulses.

ETIOLOGY

- Myocardial ischemia caused by the impairment of coronary blood flow secondary to coronary atherosclerosis that has built up over decades or nonatheromatous coronary artery disease, including Prinzmetal angina and congenital abnormalities of the coronary arteries in their origin or distribution.

DIAGNOSIS

DIFFERENTIAL DIAGNOSIS OF ACUTE CHEST PAIN
- Cardiovascular causes
  1. Aortic dissection.
  2. Pericarditis.
  3. Coronary arterial vasospasm.
- Pulmonary causes
  1. Pneumothorax.
  2. Pneumonia.
  3. Pleuritis.
  4. Pulmonary embolism.
- Gastrointestinal causes
  1. Esophageal spasm.
  2. Esophagitis.
  3. GERD.
  4. Cholecystitis.
  5. Choledocholithiasis.
  6. Cholangitis.
  7. Peptic ulcer.
  8. Pancreatitis.
- Chest wall causes
  1. Rib fracture.
  2. Sternoclavicular arthritis.
  3. Herpes zoster.
  4. Costochondritis.
- Psychiatric causes
  1. Anxiety disorders.

WORKUP
- See Fig. 1

LABORATORY TESTS
- Focused metabolic studies to rule out noncardiac causes.
- Complete blood count can help rule out anemia-related chest discomfort.
- Fasting cholesterol panel is important in assessment of control of lipid-related risk factors.
- Hemoglobin A1c is important to follow glycemic control.
- High-sensitivity C-reactive protein.

IMAGING STUDIES
- Electrocardiography (ECG) is important for assessing for prior cardiac injury or ischemia.
- Exercise treadmill test (ETT) is the gold standard to assess physiologic cardiac stress response if the patient is able to exercise and has a normal baseline ECG.
- Stress tests combined with imaging is the next best option if ETT cannot be performed due to physical limitation or if baseline ECG is abnormal.
- Echocardiogram to assess left ventricular ejection fraction (LVEF).
- Coronary artery calcium (CAC) score: can be used to improve CVD risk classification. The CAC is estimated from noncontrast CT (Fig. E2) images (radiation exposure 0.9 to 1.1 mSv of radiation, digital mammogram radiation is 0.44 mSv). Normal coronary arteries do not have plaques or calcium, and the normal score is 0. A CAC score of 300 or higher or 75th percentile or higher for age, sex, and ethnicity is considered a high risk. According to the recent ACC/AHA guidelines, CAC is most appropriate among adults with an estimated 10-year ASCVD risk <7.5% in whom questions remain about whether statin therapy is indicated. A CAC score >75th percentile for age, sex, and ethnicity is considered high risk and would justify revising a patient's risk upward.
- Those with high-risk features (Box 1) should undergo coronary angiography to assess coronary anatomy for revascularization.
- Cardiac computed tomography angiography is an emerging imaging modality that can be considered as an alternative to stress testing.
- Coronary angiography is useful for both diagnostic and therapeutic interventions if there is evidence of significant ischemia by noninvasive assessment or progressive symptoms despite optimal medical therapy (as in the following).

TREATMENT

- See Fig. 3.
- Successful treatment of CAD entails minimizing the likelihood of major adverse cardiac events (MACE), which include death, myocardial infarction, need for emergent coronary artery bypass grafting, or target lesion revascularization, while maximizing health and function.

NONPHARMACOLOGIC THERAPY
LIFESTYLE MODIFICATION:
- ≥150 min/wk of moderate-intensity activity or ≥75 min/wk of vigorous-intensity activity or a combination thereof (for adults) as 1 of the 7 components of ideal cardiovascular health.
- Mediterranean diet with a focus on vegetables, fruit, fish, whole grains, and olive oil has proven to reduce cardiovascular events to a degree greater than low-fat diets and equal to or greater than the benefit observed in statin trials.

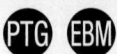

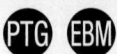

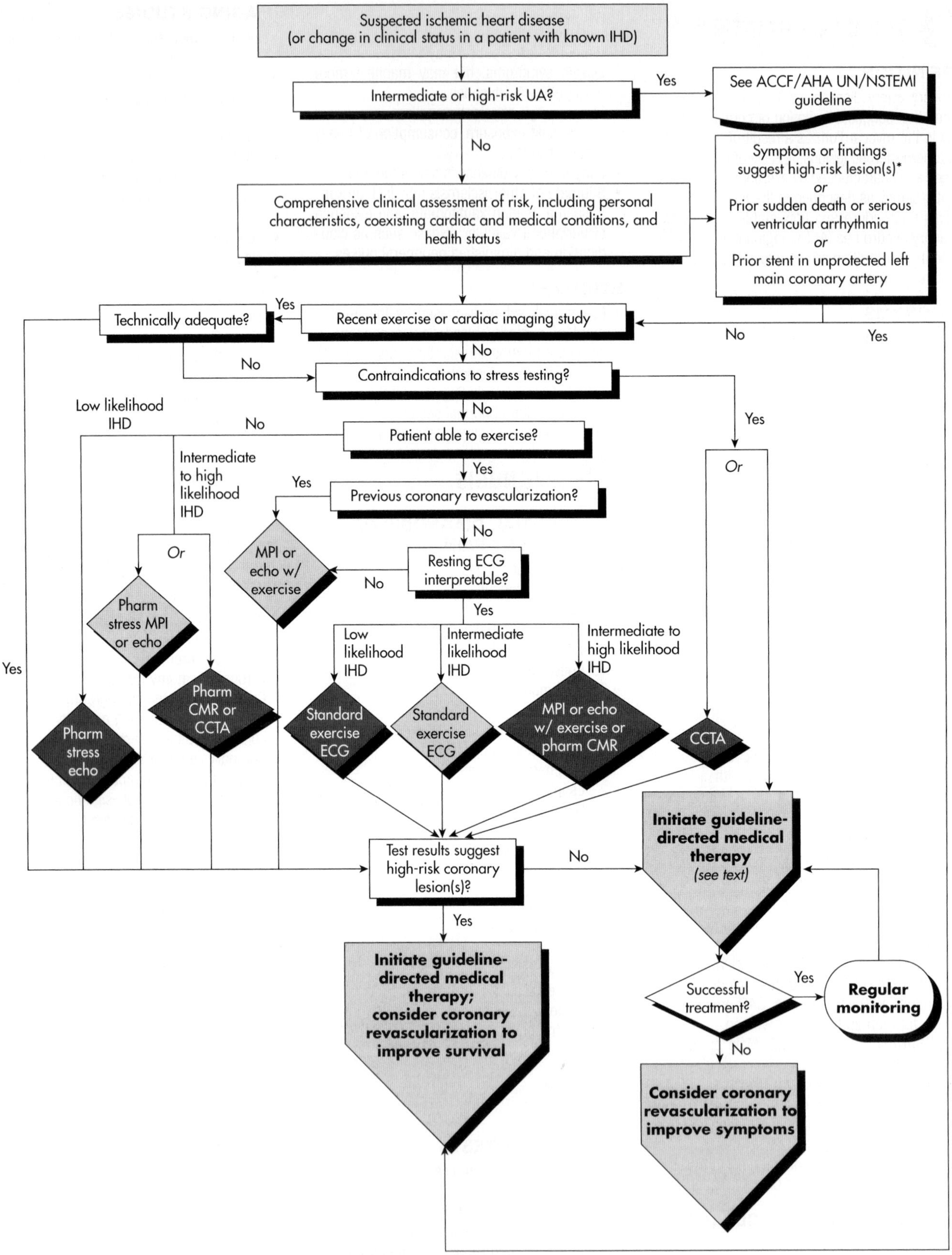

FIG. 1 Diagnosis of patients with suspected ischemic heart disease.

*CCTA is reasonable only for patients with intermediate probability of IHD. *CCTA*, Computed coronary tomography angiography; *CMR*, cardiac magnetic resonance; *ECG*, electrocardiogram; *Echo*, echocardiography; *IHD*, ischemic heart disease; *MI*, myocardial infarction; *MPI*, myocardial perfusion imaging; *Pharm*, pharmacologic; *UA*, unstable angina; *UA/NSTEMI*, unstable angina/non–ST-elevation myocardial infarction. (From 2012 ACCF/AHA/ACP/AATS/PCNA/SCAI/STS Guideline for the Diagnosis and Management of Patients With Stable Ischemic Heart Disease: A report of the American College of Cardiology Foundation/American Heart Association Task Force on Practice Guidelines, and the American College of Physicians, American Association for Thoracic Surgery, Preventive Cardiovascular Nurses Association, Society for Cardiovascular Angiography and Interventions, and Society of Thoracic Surgeons, *J Am Coll Cardiol* 60:e44-e164, 2012.)

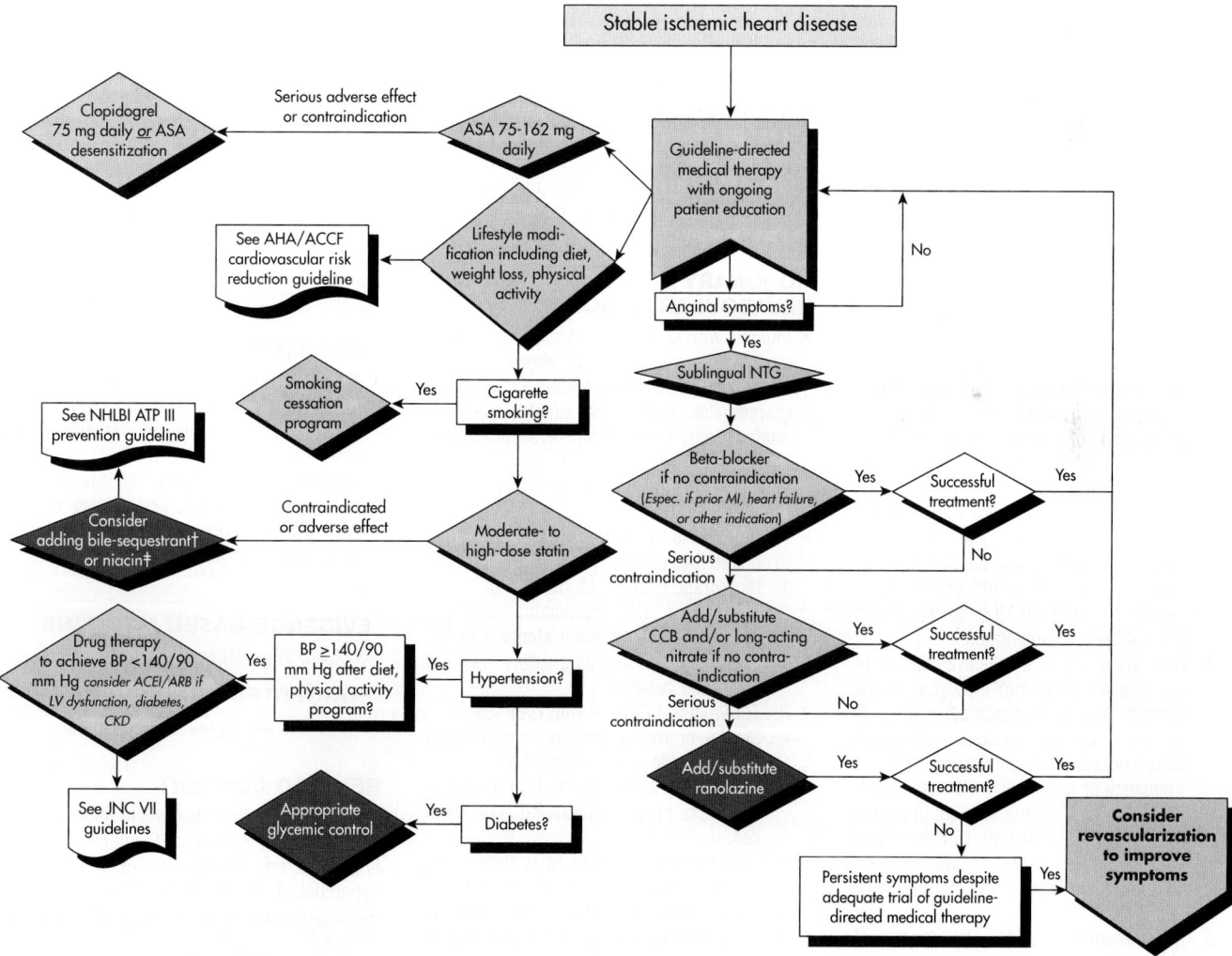

FIG. 3 Algorithm for guideline-directed medical therapy for patients with SIHD.*

*The algorithms do not represent a comprehensive list of recommendations (see text for all recommendations). †The use of bile acid sequestrant is relatively contraindicated when triglycerides are ≥200 mg/dl and is contraindicated when triglycerides are ≥500 mg/dl. ‡Dietary supplement niacin must not be used as a substitute for prescription niacin. *ACCF,* American College of Cardiology Foundation; *ACEI,* angiotensin-converting enzyme inhibitor; *AHA,* American Heart Association; *ARB,* angiotensin-receptor blocker; *ASA,* aspirin; *ATP III,* Adult Treatment Panel 3; *BP,* blood pressure; *CCB,* calcium channel blocker; *CKD,* chronic kidney disease; *HDL-C,* high-density lipoprotein cholesterol; *JNC VII,* Seventh Report of the Joint National Committee on Prevention, Detection, Evaluation, and Treatment of High Blood Pressure; *LDL-C,* low-density lipoprotein cholesterol; *LV,* left ventricular; *MI,* myocardial infarction; *NHLBI,* National Heart, Lung, and Blood Institute; *NTG,* nitroglycerin. (From 2012 ACCF/AHA/ACP/AATS/PCNA/SCAI/STS Guideline for the Diagnosis and Management of Patients With Stable Ischemic Heart Disease: A report of the American College of Cardiology Foundation/American Heart Association Task Force on Practice Guidelines, and the American College of Physicians, American Association for Thoracic Surgery, Preventive Cardiovascular Nurses Association, Society for Cardiovascular Angiography and Interventions, and Society of Thoracic Surgeons, *J Am Coll Cardiol* 60:e44-e164, 2012.)

- Smoking cessation.
- Weight reduction can reduce various risk factors with improved lipid and glycemic control.

THERAPEUTIC INTERVENTIONS:

- Enhanced external counterpulsation is used for refractory cases.
- Coronary angiography with PCI or CABG for patients on optimal medical therapy with persistent symptoms.

ACUTE GENERAL Rx FOR STABLE ANGINA

- Rest.
- Sublingual nitroglycerin if rest does not provide adequate relief.

CHRONIC Rx

- Antianginal therapy
  1. Nitrates (isosorbide mononitrate and isosorbide dinitrate). These medications treat ischemia by venodilation to decrease preload, dilate epicardial coronary arteries, and recruit coronary collaterals. Furthermore, they attenuate platelet aggregation. Although they do not influence survival or decrease cardiovascular death in patients with chronic CAD, they do lower the rate of angina frequency and increase time to ischemic ECG findings on treadmill testing.
  2. Beta-adrenergic antagonists (metoprolol, atenolol, carvedilol, or any other beta-blockers with the exception of those with intrinsic sympathomimetic activity). These medications work to relieve angina by decreasing myocardial oxygen demand by reducing heart rate, blood pressure, and contractility. Drugs should be titrated to a heart rate of 50 to 60 beats/min at rest and ≤100 beats/min with exercise
  3. Calcium channel blockers (CCBs; amlodipine or verapamil). The antianginal efficacy of CCBs is comparable to beta-blockers; however, the efficacy of monotherapy for reducing MI or cardiac death has not been demonstrated.
  4. Ranolazine. This is a selective inhibitor of late sodium influx into myocytes, which leads to decreased myocardial contractility. It can be used in combination with beta-blockers and significantly reduces frequency of angina and increases exercise duration and time to onset of angina (CARISA trial). Although it rarely may cause QT prolongation, it has not been linked to any clinically important arrhythmias.
  5. May benefit from combination therapy of the above.
- Antiplatelet therapy
  1. Aspirin therapy (81-162 mg/day).
  2. Clopidogrel for those intolerant to aspirin therapy.
  3. Combination of aspirin and clopidogrel does not reduce cardiovascular events (CHARISMA trial).

  4. Newer antiplatelet drugs such as prasugrel and ticagrelor have been studied in ACS but not in stable CAD.
- Statins
  1. HMG-CoA reductase inhibitors (statins) (atorvastatin, rosuvastatin) with high-intensity therapy for a target LDL reduction of >50% if safely achieved in high-risk patients; if not a candidate for high-intensity therapy, patient should receive at least moderate-intensity statin therapy that lowers LDL by 30% to 50% as advised by the new ATP IV cholesterol guidelines from the 2013 ACC/AHA expert panel.
- PCSK9 Inhibitors
  1. This is a novel class of monoclonal antibodies that inhibit proprotein convertase subtilisin/kexin type 9. In the recent OSLER trial, PCSK9 inhibition in addition to standard therapy reduced LDL cholesterol by 61%. The rate of cardiovascular events at 1 yr reduced to 0.98% with therapy versus 2.18% in the standard therapy group.
- ACE-inhibitors (captopril, enalapril, lisinopril) are a class I recommendation for patients with chronic CAD with LV dysfunction LVEF < 40% or diabetes and a class II recommendation for CAD patients without these features.

CORONARY ARTERY REVASCULARIZATION

- Patients with symptoms refractory to optimal medical therapy (OMT) as above or those with high clinical, stress testing, or an angiographic risk profile and suitable coronary anatomy may benefit from revascularization with either PCI (percutaneous coronary intervention) or CABG (coronary artery bypass graft) surgery.
- ACC/AHA class I indications for CABG surgery in chronic CAD patients include the following:
  1. High grade (>50%) left main CAD.
  2. Left main CAD-equivalent anatomy including >70% luminal stenosis in the left anterior descending artery and left circumflex arteries.
  3. Three-vessel disease with LVEF <50%.
  4. Single- or two-vessel CAD with a large area of viable myocardium at risk.
  5. Severe angina despite medical therapy if CABG can be performed with acceptable risk.
- PCI has not been shown to reduce long-term rates of MI and death in patients with stable chronic CAD and therefore has no class I indications in this group. PCI is suitable in patients with suitable anatomy with refractory or lifestyle-limiting angina who have failed optimal medical therapy (OMT). Recent trials such as the COURAGE Trial have demonstrated no significant difference between OMT and PCI in overall survival, MI, and ACS over 5 years in patients with chronic stable CAD. A recent

meta-analysis demonstrated no objective reduction in death, nonfatal MI, unplanned revascularization, or angina versus medical therapy alone.
- The SYNTAX trial, which used a numerical score based on qualitative plaque features on angiography, showed that surgical revascularization was associated with a lesser risk of stroke and major cardiac events if the SYNTAX score was high (>33).
- The FREEDOM trial showed that in diabetic patients with multivessel disease, CABG is superior to PCI with drug-eluting stents in chronic CAD and should remain the revascularization strategy of choice in this patient population. CABG resulted in lower rates of death and MI but a higher risk of stroke. This is true for patients with either insulin-dependent or non–insulin-dependent DM.

DISPOSITION

- Coronary artery disease is a common chronic condition with which many patients can live for years with good symptom control on optimal medical therapy.

REFERRAL

- Cardiovascular disease specialist.

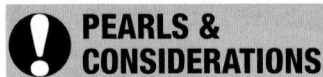

! PEARLS & CONSIDERATIONS

COMMENTS

- The transition from stable coronary artery disease to unstable angina must be carefully monitored. Symptoms of concern include more frequent episodes of chest pain, exertional dyspnea, chest pain that is less responsive to nitroglycerin, or first episode of chest pain. Regarding unstable angina, please refer to section on acute coronary syndromes.

EVIDENCE-BASED MEDICINE
Available at www.expertconsult.com

SUGGESTED READINGS
Available at www.expertconsult.com

RELATED CONTENT
Coronary Artery Disease (Patient Information)
Acute Coronary Syndrome (Related Key Topic)
Angina Pectoris (Related Key Topic)
Hypercholesterolemia (Related Key Topic)
Hyperlipoproteinemia, Primary (Related Key Topic)
Myocardial Infarction (Related Key Topic)

AUTHORS: **SYED R. LATIF, M.D., LILY CHEN, M.D.,** and **THOMAS SMITH, M.D.**

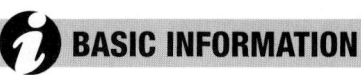

BASIC INFORMATION

DEFINITION
Clinical condition characterized by pain and tenderness at costochondral or chondrosternal joints of the anterior chest wall without obvious swelling or induration.

SYNONYMS
Anterior chest wall syndrome
Chest wall pain syndrome
Costosternal syndrome
Parasternal chondrodynia

ICD-10CM CODES
M94.0 Chondrocostal junction syndrome

EPIDEMIOLOGY & DEMOGRAPHICS
PREVALENCE: Fairly common, comprises approximately 28% of undifferentiated noncardiac chest pain patients.
PREDOMINANT SEX: Women more than men.
PREDOMINANT AGE: >40 years of age.

PHYSICAL FINDINGS & CLINICAL PRESENTATION
SYMPTOMS:
- Anterior chest wall pain, usually described as sharp, aching, or pressure-like. Pain is usually aggravated by coughing, sneezing, deep inspiration, or any chest wall movement.
- Pain is usually self-limited.
- May radiate to arms and shoulders mimicking cardiac pain.

SIGNS:
- Reproducible tenderness of costochondral (mostly second through fifth) or costosternal junction without localized swelling or induration.
- Pain on crossed-chest adduction of arm and backward extension of arm from 90 degrees of abduction signifies pain of musculoskeletal origin. Reproduction of symptoms during dry needling also suggests pain from musculoskeletal origin.

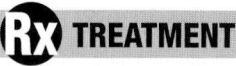

DIAGNOSIS

DIFFERENTIAL DIAGNOSIS
Usually self-limited and benign; however, it needs to be distinguished from other potentially serious conditions.
- Cardiac pain: primary concern; ischemic chest pain, acute pericarditis, aortic dissection.
- Gastrointestinal: gastroesophageal reflux disease.
- Pulmonary embolism, pneumonia, pneumothorax.
- Musculoskeletal (Table 1): Tietze's syndrome, cervical or thoracic spine disease, fibromyalgia, arthritis.
- Involvement of ribs by trauma, infections *(Candida albicans)* or neoplasms (breast cancer, prostate cancer, sarcoma, plasma cell cytoma, non-Hodgkin's lymphoma).
- Miscellaneous: fibromyalgia syndrome, panic attack.

WORKUP
- A diagnosis of exclusion for chest pain after ruling out more serious conditions including cardiac chest pain. Keys to diagnosis are a detailed history, a meticulous physical examination, and a few rationally selected diagnostic studies, including electrocardiogram and chest x-ray to rule out cardiopulmonary causes. Usefulness of nuclear scanning with technetium-99m scintigraphy, gallium, or bone scanning to assist diagnosis of costochondritis is not clear.

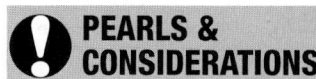

TREATMENT

ACUTE GENERAL Rx
- Often self-limiting, so reassurance is important.
- Symptomatic treatment includes local application of heat, minimizing of activities that aggravate symptoms, stretching exercises for chest wall muscles, and nonsteroidal anti-inflammatory drugs or acetaminophen.
- Refractory cases can be treated with local injections of combined lidocaine and corticosteroid (may be a useful diagnostic and therapeutic tool). Dry needling by a trained physical therapist may be helpful.
- Recurrent costochondritis may respond to sulfasalazine; however, there are no clinical trials of pharmacologic therapy for costochondritis.

PEARLS & CONSIDERATIONS

Presence of costochondritis in a patient with chest pain does not exclude more serious problems including cardiac pain. Further testing is required as clinically indicated.

SUGGESTED READINGS
Available at www.expertconsult.com

RELATED CONTENT
Costochondritis (Patient Information)

AUTHOR: **ASHA SHRESTHA, M.D.**

TABLE 1 Musculoskeletal Chest Pain		
Disorder	**Clinical Features**	**Comments**
Tietze's syndrome	Painful swelling of usually 2nd or 3rd costochondral junctions.	Less common than costochondritis; commonly affects young people of either sex. Exact cause is unknown, but a traumatic pathogenesis has been associated. The disease course is mostly self-limited. Non-Hodgkin's lymphoma of medial clavicular head has been reported to mimic Tietze's syndrome.
Costochondritis	Pain and tenderness at the costochondral or chondrosternal junctions without a notable swelling. The 2nd-5th costal cartilages are most commonly involved.	Certain maneuvers like "crowing rooster" maneuver (extension of the cervical spine and traction on the posteriorly extended arm) and traction on the adducted arm with head rotated to ipsilateral side may reproduce the pain.
Slipping rib syndrome	Pain at the lower costal cartilages, associated with increased mobility of the anterior end of a costal cartilage. Most commonly affects 10th rib and occasionally 8th and 9th ribs.	Maneuver such as hooking the fingers under the anterior costal margin and pulling the rib cage anteriorly may produce a palpable click of the cartilages slipping over one another.
Cervical, thoracic disc disease	Referred regional pain from affected areas. Often aggravated by spine motion and may be accompanied by radicular pain into arm if cervical origin or along intercostal nerve if thoracic origin. Symptoms reproduced by Spurling's maneuver (steady pressure to head causing increased axial loading on the nerve root).	May mimic chest disease if spinal complaints are minimal and referred or radicular symptoms predominate.
Fibromyalgia	Widespread pain with multiple other peripheral tender points.	Female/male ratio of 9:1. Prevalent age 30-50 yr. Frequently associated with tension headache, irritable bowel syndrome, and psychiatric symptoms.
Sternoclavicular or manubriosternal joint involvement in osteoarthritis, inflammatory conditions (rheumatoid arthritis, ankylosing spondylitis, psoriatic arthritis), and infection	Dull, aching local pain with tenderness. Occasional bony joint enlargement with soft tissue swelling.	Crepitus may rarely be present.

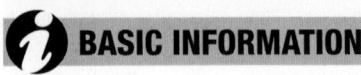

BASIC INFORMATION

DEFINITION

Crohn's disease is an inflammatory disease of the bowel of unknown etiology, most commonly involving the terminal ileum and manifesting primarily with diarrhea, abdominal pain, fatigue, and weight loss.

SYNONYMS

Regional enteritis
Inflammatory bowel disease (IBD)

ICD-10CM CODES

K50.00	Crohn's disease of small intestine without complications
K50.011	Crohn's disease of small intestine with rectal bleeding
K50.012	Crohn's disease of small intestine with intestinal obstruction
K50.013	Crohn's disease of small intestine with fistula
K50.014	Crohn's disease of small intestine with abscess
K50.018	Crohn's disease of small intestine with other complication
K50.019	Crohn's disease of small intestine with unspecified complications
K50.10	Crohn's disease of large intestine without complications
K50.111	Crohn's disease of large intestine with rectal bleeding
K50.112	Crohn's disease of large intestine with intestinal obstruction
K50.113	Crohn's disease of large intestine with fistula
K50.114	Crohn's disease of large intestine with abscess
K50.118	Crohn's disease of large intestine with other complication
K50.119	Crohn's disease of large intestine with unspecified complications
K50.80	Crohn's disease of both small and large intestine without complications
K50.811	Crohn's disease of both small and large intestine with rectal bleeding
K50.812	Crohn's disease of both small and large intestine with intestinal obstruction
K50.813	Crohn's disease of both small and large intestine with fistula
K50.814	Crohn's disease of both small and large intestine with abscess
K50.818	Crohn's disease of both small and large intestine with other complication
K50.819	Crohn's disease of both small and large intestine with unspecified complications
K50.90	Crohn's disease, unspecified, without complications
K50.911	Crohn's disease, unspecified, with rectal bleeding
K50.912	Crohn's disease, unspecified, with intestinal obstruction
K50.913	Crohn's disease, unspecified, with fistula
K50.914	Crohn's disease, unspecified, with abscess
K50.918	Crohn's disease, unspecified, with other complication
K50.919	Crohn's disease, unspecified, with unspecified complications

EPIDEMIOLOGY & DEMOGRAPHICS

PREVALENCE:

- One case per 1000 persons; most common in whites and Jews.
- Crohn's disease affects approximately 380,000 to 480,000 persons in the United States.
- Incidence: bimodal with a peak in the third decade of life and another in the fifth decade.

PHYSICAL FINDINGS & CLINICAL PRESENTATION

- Physical exam findings vary depending on disease location and severity.
- Abdominal tenderness, mass, or distention.
- Chronic or nocturnal diarrhea.
- Weight loss, fever, night sweats.
- Hyperactive bowel sounds in patients with partial obstruction, bloody diarrhea.
- Delayed growth and failure of normal development in children.
- Perianal and rectal abscesses, multiple sinuses and scarring (Fig. E1), mouth ulcers, cobblestone appearance of oral mucosa (Fig. E2), and atrophic glossitis.
- Extraintestinal manifestations (Table E1): joint swelling and tenderness, hepatosplenomegaly, erythema nodosum, clubbing, tenderness to palpation of the sacroiliac joints.
- Symptoms may be intermittent with varying periods of remission.
- Overall 40% of patients have ileocolonic inflammation, 30% have isolated small bowel disease, 25% have isolated colonic disease, and 5% have isolated upper GI or perianal manifestations.

ETIOLOGY

Unknown. Pathophysiologically, Crohn's disease involves an immune system dysfunction.

DIAGNOSIS

DIFFERENTIAL DIAGNOSIS

- Ulcerative colitis (see Table 2).
- Infectious diseases (tuberculosis, *Yersinia, Salmonella, Shigella, Campylobacter*).
- Parasitic infections (amebic infection).
- Pseudomembranous colitis.
- Ischemic colitis in elderly patients.
- Lymphoma.
- Colon carcinoma.
- Diverticulitis.
- Radiation enteritis.
- Collagenous colitis.
- Fungal infections (*Histoplasma, Actinomyces*).
- Gay bowel syndrome (in homosexual patient).
- Carcinoid tumors.
- Celiac sprue.
- Mesenteric adenitis.

LABORATORY TESTS

- Decreased hemoglobin and hematocrit from chronic blood loss, effect of inflammation on bone marrow, and malabsorption of vitamin B_{12}.
- Hypokalemia, hypomagnesemia, hypocalcemia, and low albumin in patients with chronic diarrhea.
- Vitamin B_{12} and folate deficiency.
- Elevated erythrocyte sedimentation rate and CRP.
- Positive anti–*Saccharomyces cerevisiae* antibodies.
- Elevated INR (due to vitamin K malabsorption).
- Fecal calprotectin has been reported as useful in screening of patients with suspected IBD. Based on a pretest probability of 32% in adults, an abnormal calprotectin test result increases the posttest probability to 91%, and a normal result reduces the probability of IBD to 3%. False elevations may occur with other gastrointestinal diseases such as bacterial, viral, and protozoal causes of infective diarrhea.

TABLE 2 Differentiating Features

	Ulcerative Colitis	Crohn's Disease
Site of involvement	Only involves colon Rectum almost always involved	Any area of the gastrointestinal tract Rectum usually spared
Pattern of involvement	Continuous	Skip lesions
Diarrhea	Bloody	Usually nonbloody
Severe abdominal pain	Rare	Frequent
Perianal disease	No	In 30% of patients
Fistula	No	Yes
Endoscopic findings	Erythematous and friable Superficial ulceration	Aphthoid and deep ulcers Cobblestoning
Radiologic findings	Tubular appearance resulting from loss of haustral folds	String sign of terminal ileum RLQ mass, fistulas, abscesses
Histologic features	Mucosa only Crypt abscesses	Transmural Crypt abscesses, granulomas (about 30%)
Smoking	Protective	Worsens course
Serology	p-ANCA more common	ASCA more common

ASCA, Anti–*Saccharomyces cerevisiae* antibodies; *p-ANCA,* perinuclear antineutrophil cytoplasmic antibody; *RLQ,* right lower quadrant.
From Andreoli TE et al: *Andreoli and Carpenter's Cecil essentials of medicine,* ed 8, Philadelphia, 2010, Saunders.

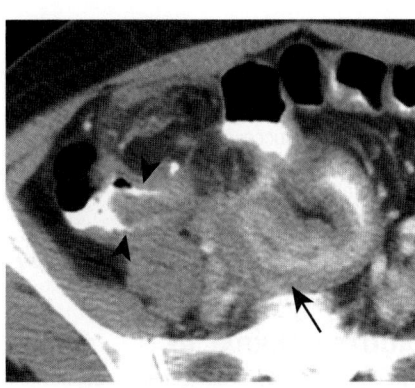

FIG. 3 Crohn's disease: fistulas. The ileum (*arrow*) in the right lower quadrant exhibits marked wall thickening and matting of bowel loops caused by inflammation of the mesentery. A double-tract bowel lumen (*arrowheads*) is seen, indicating the formation of an ileo–ileal fistula. (From Webb WR, Brant WE, Major NM: *Fundamentals of body CT*, ed 4, Philadelphia, 2015, Saunders.)

ENDOSCOPIC EVALUATION

Endoscopic features of Crohn's disease include asymmetric and discontinued disease, deep longitudinal fissures, cobblestone appearance, and presence of strictures. Crypt distortion and inflammation are also present. Granulomas may be present.

IMAGING STUDIES

- CT of abdomen may show thickening of the terminal ileum and is helpful in identifying abscesses, fistulas (Fig. 3), and other complications.
- Magnetic resonance enterography (MRe) is superior to other imaging modalities in its ability to distinguish active from chronic fibrotic disease. It is, however, more expensive.
- In 10% to 15% of patients with IBD, a clear distinction between ulcerative colitis and Crohn's disease cannot be made. In general, Crohn's disease can be distinguished from ulcerative colitis by the presence of transmural involvement and the frequent presence of noncaseating granulomas and lymphoid aggregates on biopsy.

Rx TREATMENT

The medical management of Crohn's disease is based on disease activity. According to Hanauer and Sanborn, disease activity can be defined as follows:

- Mild to moderate disease: The patient is ambulatory and able to take oral alimentation. There is no dehydration, high fever, abdominal tenderness, painful mass, obstruction, or weight loss of >10%.
- Moderate to severe disease: Either the patient has not responded to treatment for mild to moderate disease or has more pronounced symptoms, including fever, significant weight loss, abdominal pain or tenderness, intermittent nausea and vomiting, or significant anemia.
- Severe fulminant disease: Either the patient has persistent symptoms despite outpatient steroid therapy or has high fever, persistent vomiting, evidence of intestinal obstruction,

rebound tenderness, cachexia, or evidence of an abscess.
- Remission: The patient is asymptomatic or without inflammatory sequelae, including patients responding to acute medical intervention.

NONPHARMACOLOGIC THERAPY

- Nutritional supplementation is needed in patients with advanced disease. Total parenteral nutrition may be necessary in selected patients.
- Low-residue diet is necessary when obstructive symptoms are present.
- If diarrhea is prominent, increased dietary fiber and decreased fat in the diet are sometimes helpful.
- Psychotherapy is useful for situational adjustment crises. A trusting and mutually understanding relationship and referral to self-help groups are very important because of the chronicity of the disease and the relatively young age of the patients.
- Avoid oral feedings during acute exacerbation to decrease colonic activity: a low-roughage diet may be helpful in early relapse.

ACUTE GENERAL Rx

- Corticosteroids are used to induce remission. They have been the mainstay for treating moderate to severe active Crohn's disease. Prednisone 40 to 60 mg/day is useful for acute exacerbation. Steroids are usually tapered over approximately 2 to 3 mo. Some patients require a low dose for a prolonged period of maintenance.
- Steroid analogues are locally active corticosteroids that target specific areas of inflammation in the gastrointestinal tract. Budesonide is available as a controlled-release formulation and is approved for mild to moderate active Crohn's disease involving the ileum and/or ascending colon. The adult dose is 9 mg qd for a maximum of 8 wk.
- Patients responding to glucocorticoids are transitioned to immunomodulators as their glucocorticoid is tapered.
- Immunosuppressants such as azathioprine or mercaptopurine are used for maintenance of remission. Methotrexate is an alternative agent.
- Metronidazole 500 mg qid may be useful for colonic fistulas and treatment of mild to moderate active Crohn's disease. Ciprofloxacin 1 g qd has also been found to be effective in decreasing disease activity.
- TNF inhibitors are agents useful to induce remission and maintain remission in patients with moderate to severe Crohn's disease. Infliximab, a chimeric monoclonal antibody targeting tumor necrosis factor-α, is effective in the treatment of enterocutaneous fistulas. This medication can induce clinical improvement in 80% of patients with Crohn's disease refractory to other agents. It can be used in combination with other medications such as azathioprine in patients with severe Crohn's disease. A PPD test should be done before using this medication. Adalimumab and certolizumab are other TNF inhibitors also effective in inducing remissions and may be useful in adult patients with Crohn's disease who cannot tolerate infliximab or have symptoms despite receiving infliximab

therapy. Efficacy is better when an anti-TNF is used together with an immunomodulator.
- Natalizumab, a selective adhesion-molecule inhibitor, has been reported to be effective in increasing the rate of remission and response in patients with active Crohn's disease. It is effective for patients in whom anti-TNF therapy has been unsuccessful. Prior to using natalizumab, serologic testing should be done for JC virus, which causes multifocal leukoencephalopathy (PML), and if the patient is seronegative, the risk of PML from natalizumab is low. Vedolizumab is another IV integrin receptor antagonist recently FDA approved for moderate to severe Crohn's disease patients who have not responded to or cannot tolerate standard treatment. Vedolizumab use is not associated with high risk of PML. Ustekinumab, a monoclonal antibody to the P_40 subunit of interleukin-12 and interleukin-23, has shown efficacy for induction and maintenance therapy for Crohn's disease. It has been FDA-approved for moderate to severely active Crohn's disease unresponsive to immunomodulators or corticosteroids or a tumor necrosis factor inhibitor.
- Hydrocortisone enema bid or tid is useful for proctitis.
- Most patients who have anemia associated with Crohn's disease respond to iron supplementation. Erythropoietin is useful in patients with anemia refractory to treatment with iron and vitamins.

CHRONIC Rx

- Monitor disease activity with symptom review and laboratory evaluation (complete blood count and sedimentation rate).
- Liver tests and vitamin B_{12} levels monitored on a yearly basis.

DISPOSITION

One tenth of patients have prolonged remission, three quarters have a chronic intermittent disease course, and one eighth have an unremitting course. Patients with IBD are at increased risk of colon cancer.

REFERRAL

- Surgical referral is needed for complications such as abscess formation, obstruction, fistulas, toxic megacolon, refractory disease, or severe hemorrhage. Approximately 40% to 50% of patients will require some type of bowel surgery within the first 5 years of Crohn's disease. A conservative surgical approach is necessary because surgery is not curative. Multiple surgeries may also result in short bowel syndrome.

EBM EVIDENCE

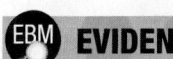

Available at www.expertconsult.com

SUGGESTED READINGS
Available at www.expertconsult.com

RELATED CONTENT
Crohn's Disease (Patient Information)

AUTHOR: **FRED F. FERRI, M.D.**

BASIC INFORMATION

DEFINITION

Cryoglobulins are serum immunoglobulins that precipitate when cooled and redissolve when heated. A classification of cryoglobulins is described in Table E1. Cryoglobulinemia is a clinical syndrome that results from systemic inflammation caused by cryoglobulin-containing immune complexes. Mixed cryoglobulinemia is a vasculitis of small and medium-sized arteries and veins due to the deposition of complexes of antigen, cryoglobulin, and complement in the vessel walls.

SYNONYMS

Cryoglobulinemic vasculitis
Cryoproteinemia
Mixed cryoglobulinemia
Essential cryoglobulinemia

ICD-10CM CODES
D89.1 Cryoglobulinemia

EPIDEMIOLOGY & DEMOGRAPHICS

PREVALENCE:
- Prevalence of mixed cryoglobulinemia is approximately 1:100,000.
- Approximately 50% of patients with HCV are found to have mixed cryoglobulinemia; only 5% to 10% develop vasculitis.
- Three types: I (monoclonal), II (IgM monoclonal and IgG polyclonal), and III (polyclonal).

PREDOMINANT SEX AND AGE: Female:male ratio of 3:1.

PREDOMINANT AGE: Mean age reported is 42 to 52 yr.

RISK FACTORS:
- Hepatitis C virus (HCV) infection
- Connective tissue disorders
- Lymphoproliferative disorders

PHYSICAL FINDINGS & CLINICAL PRESENTATION

- **Meltzer triad** of purpura, arthralgias/myalgia, and weakness.
- Other symptoms include dyspnea, cough, numbness, abdominal pain, acrocyanosis.
- Hypertension, hepatosplenomegaly, Raynaud's phenomenon, and in severe cases, distal necrosis and ulcerations of lower limbs (Fig. 1).

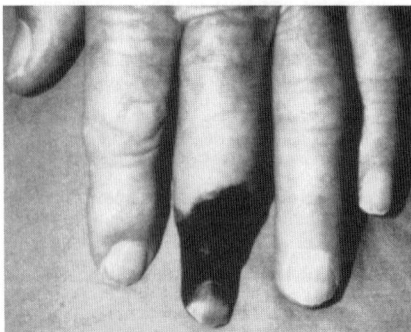

FIG. 1 Cryoglobulinemia. (From Hoffman R et al: *Hematology, basic principles and practice*, ed 6, New York, 2013, Elsevier.)

ETIOLOGY

- Intravascular deposition of cryoglobulins leading to ischemic insults in territory supplied by vasa nervorum
- Necrotizing vasculitis caused by cryoglobulin precipitation
- Infections: HCV, mycosis fungoides, HBV, HIV, Epstein-Barr virus, cytomegalovirus, *Treponema pallidum*, Mycobacterium leprae, and in post-streptococcal glomerulonephritis
- Lymphoproliferative disorders: chronic lymphocytic leukemia, Waldenström's macroglobulinemia, multiple myeloma
- Connective tissue disorders: rheumatoid arthritis, systemic lupus erythematosus (SLE), scleroderma, Sjögren's syndrome, vasculitis
- Renal diseases including proliferative glomerulonephritis

DIAGNOSIS

DIFFERENTIAL DIAGNOSIS

- Antiphospholipid syndrome
- SLE
- Churg-Strauss syndrome
- Cirrhosis
- Glomerulonephritis
- Goodpasture syndrome
- Hemolytic uremic syndrome
- Hepatitis
- Lymphoma
- Sarcoidosis
- Waldenström's hypergammaglobulinemia

WORKUP

History and physical examination; laboratory tests; imaging tests depending on patients' presentation.

LABORATORY TESTS

- Serum cryoglobulins, rheumatoid factor, serum complement, hepatitis C titer, urinalysis, CBC, ALT, AST, BUN, creatinine.
- Electromyogram/nerve conduction studies may demonstrate axonal changes and distal muscle denervation.
- Sural nerve and skin biopsy.

IMAGING STUDIES

Chest x-ray for pulmonary involvement, CT scan to evaluate for malignancy, and angiography for vasculitis.

TREATMENT

- Immunosuppressive therapies such as corticosteroids are the mainstay treatment for mixed cryoglobulinemia.
- In patients with HCV, IFN-α can be added. The treatment of HCV-related mixed cryoglobulinemia is difficult due to the multifactorial origin and polymorphism of the syndrome. Therapy is aimed at eradicating the HCV infection, suppressing B-cell clonal expansion and cryoglobulin production, and ameliorating symptoms.
- Combination of pegylated IFN-α with ribavirin results in 77% remission. Sofosbuvir-based regimens also result in high levels of clinical response.
- A variable success rate has been observed with plasma exchange, intravenous immunoglobulin, and anti-CD20 (rituximab) treatments.

NONPHARMACOLOGIC THERAPY

Avoidance of cold exposure

ACUTE GENERAL Rx

NSAIDs in those with general fatigue and arthralgia; see "Treatment" for further management.

DISPOSITION

Overall prognosis is worse with concomitant renal disease. Mean survival rate is ~50% at 10 yr.

REFERRAL

Consider referring to a
1. Nephrologist if there is renal involvement
2. Hematologist in patients with lymphoproliferative disorders
3. Gastroenterologist/hepatologist in patients with hepatitis
4. Rheumatologist in patients with connective tissue disease cases
5. Clinical immunologist in severe cases

PEARLS & CONSIDERATIONS

COMMENTS

Always look for underlying causes of cryoglobulinemia.

PREVENTION

Avoidance of cold exposure, avoidance of late complications.

PATIENT/FAMILY EDUCATION

Inform patients about early signs/symptoms of cryoglobulinemia so that treatment can be rendered before the development of complications.

SUGGESTED READINGS
Available at www.expertconsult.com

AUTHOR: **REBECCA SOINSKI, M.D.**

ℹ️ BASIC INFORMATION

DEFINITION

Cryptococcosis is an infection caused by the encapsulated yeast *Cryptococcus spp.*

SYNONYMS

C. neoformans infection
C. gattii infection
C. albidus infection
C. laurentii infection

ICD-10CM CODES
B45.9 Pulmonary cryptococcosis
B45.1 Cerebral cryptococcosis
B45.2 Cutaneous cryptococcosis
B45.3 Osseous cryptococcosis
B45.7 Disseminated cryptococcosis
B45.9 Cryptococcosis, unspecified

EPIDEMIOLOGY & DEMOGRAPHICS

INCIDENCE (IN U.S.):
- 0.8 cases/million persons/year; *C. neoformans* is an important opportunistic infection in patients with deficits in cell-mediated immunity.
- 6% to 7% in HIV-infected persons with AIDS.
PEAK INCIDENCE: 20 to 40 years (parallel to HIV/AIDS epidemic).
PREDOMINANT SEX: Equal sex distribution when adjusted for HIV status.
PREDOMINANT AGE: Less than 2 years of age; 20 to 40 years of age.
NEONATAL INFECTION: Very uncommon.

PHYSICAL FINDINGS & CLINICAL PRESENTATION

- More than 90% present with meningitis (generally subacute); almost all have fever and headache.
- Meningismus, photophobia, mental status changes are seen in approximately 25%.
- Increased intracranial pressure may be present.
- Most common infections outside the CNS:
  1. In the lungs (fever, cough, dyspnea, and typically with lobar consolidation).
  2. In the skin (cellulitis, papular eruption).
  3. In the lymph nodes (lymphadenitis).
  4. Potential involvement of virtually any organ (e.g., prostate and bone).

ETIOLOGY

- There are four *Cryptococcus spp.* that cause disease in humans, although most laboratories are not able to differentiate between species. *C. neoformans* is the cause of a majority of global disease burden, primarily in immunocompromised patients. *C. gattii* infections occur more often in normal hosts, are much less common, and have been associated with outbreaks in the Pacific Northwest. *C. albidus* and *C. laurentii* are rarer causes of disease.
- Infection originates by inhalation into the respiratory tract followed by dissemination to the CNS in most cases, usually without recognizable lung involvement.
- Almost always in the setting of AIDS (most with CD4 counts <100) or other disorders of cellular immune function, such as organ transplantation.
- Neutropenia alone poses a much lower risk of significant cryptococcal infection.

🅳🆇 DIAGNOSIS

DIFFERENTIAL DIAGNOSIS

- Subacute meningitis (caused by *Listeria monocytogenes,* Mycobacterium tuberculosis, *Histoplasma capsulatum,* viruses).
- Intracranial mass lesion (neoplasms, toxoplasmosis, TB).
- Pulmonary involvement confused with *Pneumocystis jiroveci* pneumonia when diffuse or confused with TB or bacterial pneumonia when focal or involving the pleura.
- Skin lesions confused with bacterial cellulitis or molluscum contagiosum.

WORKUP

- Lumbar puncture to exclude cryptococcal meningitis. In cryptococcal meningitis, CSF reveals lymphocytic pleocytosis (although a paucity of WBCs may be found in CSF of HIV patients).
- CT scan of the head when focal lesion or increased intracranial pressure is suspected.
- Biopsy of enlarged lymph nodes and skin lesions if feasible.

LABORATORY TESTS

- Culture and India ink stain (60% to 80% sensitive in culture-proven cases [Fig. 1]); examination of the CSF in all cases when CNS involvement is suspected.
- Blood and serum cryptococcal antigen assay (>90% sensitivity and specificity in immunocompromised patients; lower sensitivity in immunocompetent patients).
- Culture and histologic examination of biopsy material.
- HIV antibody testing.

IMAGING STUDIES

- CT scan or MRI of the head if focal neurologic involvement or cryptococcoma is suspected.
- Chest x-ray examination to exclude pulmonary involvement.

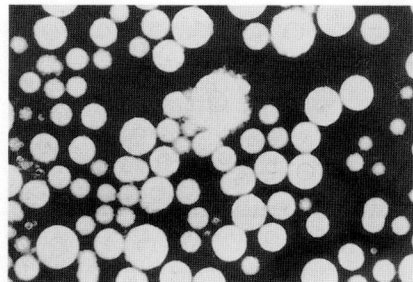

FIG. 1 India ink preparation of cerebrospinal fluid revealing encapsulated cryptococci. Note the large capsules surrounding the smaller organisms. (From Andreoli TE [ed]: *Cecil essentials of medicine,* ed 4, Philadelphia, 1997, Saunders.)

🆁🆇 TREATMENT

ACUTE GENERAL Rx

- Treatment of cryptococcosis consists of three stages: induction, consolidation, and maintenance. Induction therapy for CNS disease (meningitis) was historically initiated with IV amphotericin B deoxycholate (0.7 to 1.0 mg/kg/day) with flucytosine 100 mg/kg/day PO in 4 divided doses; however, there is growing clinical evidence for liposomal amphotericin B (3 to 6 mg/kg/day) plus flucytosine, especially in HIV-infected patients and in those with renal dysfunction. Induction therapy is generally recommended for 2 to 4 weeks and repeat CSF cultures negative, at which point one would transition to consolidation therapy with fluconazole 400 mg PO q24h for 8 weeks, followed by ongoing fluconazole 200 mg PO q24h maintenance therapy (up to 2 years) to reduce relapse rate. Maintenance therapy is indicated in patients with AIDS until these patients have been receiving antifungal therapy for at least 1 year and they have responded to antiretroviral therapy (CD4 cell count ≥100/microliter for ≥3 months). In patients without HIV, the duration of maintenance therapy is 6 to 12 months. Lifelong antifungal therapy is needed in organ transplant patients.
- Alternative: IV fluconazole combined with flucytosine for initial therapy in patients unable to tolerate amphotericin B.
- If symptomatic increased intracranial pressure, consider multiple therapeutic lumbar taps or intraventricular shunt.
- Data support increased mortality with early initiation of antiretroviral therapy in the setting of cryptococcal meningitis due to immune reconstitution syndrome; therefore, it is generally recommended to wait 2 to 10 weeks after starting cryptococcal therapy prior to starting antiretroviral therapy.

CHRONIC Rx

- Fluconazole (200-400 mg PO qd) is highly effective in preventing a relapse in HIV-infected patients; development of resistance may occur. Itraconazole is an alternative agent, along with growing evidence for voriconazole and posaconazole use.

DISPOSITION

Without maintenance therapy, relapse rate is >50% among AIDS patients.

REFERRAL

- For consultation with infectious diseases specialist in all cases.
- For neurologic consultation if level of consciousness is depressed or focal lesion is present.

SUGGESTED READINGS
Available at www.expertconsult.com

RELATED CONTENT
Cryptococcosis (Patient Information)

AUTHORS: **PHILIP A. CHAN, M.D., M.S.,** and **TARA C. BOUTON, M.D., M.P.H. & T.M.**

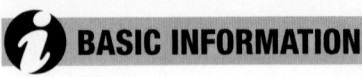

BASIC INFORMATION

DEFINITION

The intracellular protozoan parasite *Cryptosporidium parvum* is associated with gastrointestinal disease and diarrhea, especially in patients with AIDS or other immunocompromised hosts. It is also associated with sporadic infections and waterborne outbreaks in immunocompetent hosts. Cryptosporidiosis is a notifiable disease in the U.S.

Other species, including *C. hominis*, *C. felis*, *C. muris*, and *C. meleagridis*, are now described to be pathogens as well.

SYNONYMS

Cryptosporidiosis

ICD-10CM CODES
A07.2 Cryptosporidiosis

EPIDEMIOLOGY & DEMOGRAPHICS

INCIDENCE:
- Approximately 2% in industrial countries, 5% to 10% in developing countries.
- Immunocompromised patients, especially those with HIV/AIDS, are particularly susceptible to infection. 10% to 20% of HIV patients in the United States may excrete cyst.
- Cryptosporidiosis is a leading cause of all waterborne outbreaks in the U.S. An estimated 748,000 cryptosporidiosis cases occur annually, although fewer than 2% are reported. In 2011, more than 9000 cases of cryptosporidiosis were reported in the country. The highest overall reporting rates were observed in the Midwest.[1]

PREVALENCE: Worldwide, especially third world countries; associated with poor hygiene as a waterborne pathogen.

PREDOMINANT SEX: Male = female.

TRANSMISSION:
- Person-to-person (day care, family members).
- Animal to person (pets, farm animals). Fig. E1 describes the life cycle of *Cryptosporidium*.
- Environmental (water-associated outbreaks, including travel associated with swimming in or drinking contaminated water or eating contaminated food).
- May be significant pathogen causing diarrhea in patients with AIDS.

PHYSICAL FINDINGS & CLINICAL PRESENTATION

- Spectrum of illness ranging from asymptomatic to severe enteritis. Typical cases in immunocompetent hosts result in self-limited diarrhea, whereas immunocompromised hosts are characterized by profuse, watery, nonbloody diarrhea that may lead to dehydration and weight loss.
- Usually limited to the gastrointestinal tract; however, in individuals with AIDS, the disease may be fulminant and life-threatening (CD4 counts <50).
- Diarrhea, severe abdominal pain (2-28 days).
- Impaired digestion, dehydration.
- Fever, malaise, fatigue, nausea, vomiting.
- Pneumonia if aspirated.

ETIOLOGY

C. hominis, C. parvum, C. felis, C. muris, C. meleagridis.

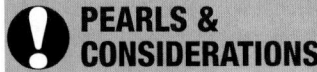

DIAGNOSIS

Clinical presentation of acute gastrointestinal illness, especially associated with HIV/AIDS or with travel and waterborne outbreaks.

DIFFERENTIAL DIAGNOSIS

- *Campylobacter*
- *Clostridium difficile*
- *Entamoeba histolytica*
- *Giardia lamblia*
- *Salmonella*
- *Shigella*
- Microsporidia
- Cytomegalovirus
- *Mycobacterium avium*

Disease may cause cholecystitis, reactive arthritis, hepatitis, urethritis, pancreatitis, or pneumonia in immunocompromised or HIV-infected patients.

WORKUP

- Stool evaluation looking for characteristic oocyst by modified acid-fast stain (Fig. 2).
- Direct immunofluorescence using monoclonal antibodies is the gold standard for stool exams.
- Rapid antigen detection.
- PCR.
- HIV antibody testing.

TREATMENT

- Handwashing and appropriate decontamination of drinking and recreational water sources.
- May be self-limited in normal host over several weeks. Antidiarrheal agents Pepto-Bismol, Kaopectate, or loperamide may give symptomatic relief.
- Pharmacologic treatment with antibiotics has been largely unsatisfactory in patients with AIDS. Antiviral therapy is the treatment of choice to restore the immune system. Oocyst excretion reduction has been shown with nitazoxanide 500 mg PO bid for three days in immunocompetent patients. If treatment fails,

consider a trial of paromomycin, metronidazole, azithromycin, or trimethoprim/sulfamethoxazole. However, these medications have not been approved for treatment of *Cryptosporidium*.
- Nitazoxanide elixir has been approved for the treatment of cryptosporidiosis in children ages 1 to 11 years.
- Biliary cryptosporidiosis can be treated with antiretroviral therapy in the HIV setting.

DISPOSITION

- A self-limited disease in immunocompetent patients with complete recovery over 2 to 3 weeks.
- In patients with AIDS, chronic infection often clears with initiation and maintenance of antiretroviral therapy.
- Chronic arthralgia, headache, malaise, and weakness may persist after infection, even in immunologically normal people.
- If severe and prolonged disease (>30 days), testing for HIV and other immunocompromised states is appropriate, along with a referral to an infectious diseases specialist or gastroenterologist.

REFERRAL

- To an infectious diseases specialist if symptoms persist and/or HIV infection is found.
- To a gastroenterologist if chronic malabsorption, or biliary or pancreatic complications occur.

PEARLS & CONSIDERATIONS

- Chronic cryptosporidiosis (>30 days of diarrhea from *Cryptosporidium* spp. infection) in a patient with HIV is an AIDS-qualifying opportunistic infection.
- *Cryptosporidium hominis* has a limited host range (humans), whereas *Cryptosporidium parvum* has a wide host range including humans, horses, cattle, other domesticated animals, and wild animals; both species present similarly in humans.

SUGGESTED READINGS
Available at www.expertconsult.com

AUTHORS: **SARA W.F. GEFFERT, M.D., M.S.,** and **PHILIP A. CHAN, M.D., M.S.**

[1]Cryptosporidiosis surveillance, United States, 2011-2012. MMWR 64 3 (2015).

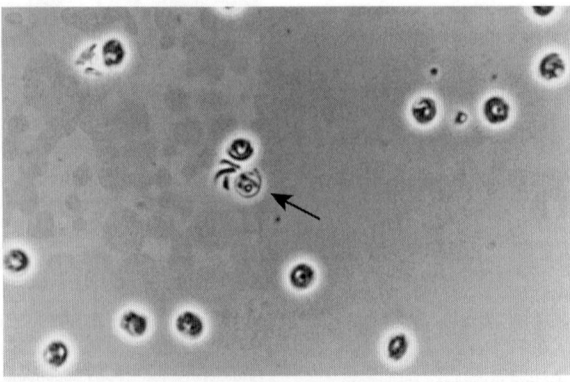

FIG. 2 Human stool-derived Cryptosporidium oocysts. Excysting oocyst (arrow) is releasing three of its four sporozoites. (Phase-control microscopy ×630.) (From Gorbach SL: *Infectious diseases*, ed 2, Philadelphia, 1998, Saunders.)

C

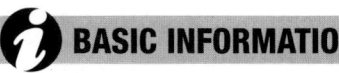

DEFINITION

- Cushing's syndrome is the occurrence of clinical abnormalities associated with glucocorticoid excess as a result of exaggerated adrenal cortisol production or long-term glucocorticoid therapy.
- Cushing's disease is Cushing's syndrome caused by pituitary adrenocorticotropic hormone (ACTH) excess.

ICD-10CM CODES
E24	Cushing syndrome
E24.2	Drug-induced Cushing syndrome
E24.3	Ectopic ACTH syndrome
E24.8	Other Cushing syndrome
E24.9	Cushing syndrome, unspecified
E24.9	Pituitary-dependent Cushing's disease

PHYSICAL FINDINGS & CLINICAL PRESENTATION

- Hypertension.
- Central obesity with rounding of the facies (moon facies); thin extremities.
- Hirsutism, menstrual irregularities, hypogonadism.
- Skin fragility, ecchymoses, red-purple abdominal striae (Fig. E1), acne, poor wound healing, hair loss, facial plethora, hyperpigmentation (with ACTH excess).
- Psychosis, emotional lability, paranoia.
- Muscle wasting with proximal myopathy.

NOTE: The previous characteristics are not commonly present in Cushing's syndrome caused by ectopic ACTH production. Many of these tumors secrete a biologically inactive ACTH that does not activate adrenal steroid synthesis. These patients may have only weight loss and weakness.

ETIOLOGY

- Iatrogenic from long-term glucocorticoid therapy (common).
- Pituitary ACTH excess (Cushing's disease; 60%).
- Adrenal neoplasms (30%).
- Ectopic ACTH production (neoplasms of lung, pancreas, kidney, thyroid, thymus; 10%).
- Table E1 summarizes the incidence of tumors associated with the ectopic adrenocorticotropic hormone syndrome.
- A classification of causes of Cushing's syndrome is described in Table E2.

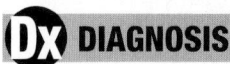 **DIAGNOSIS**

DIFFERENTIAL DIAGNOSIS

- Alcoholic pseudo-Cushing's syndrome (endogenous cortisol overproduction).
- Obesity associated with diabetes mellitus.
- Adrenogenital syndrome.

WORKUP (TABLE E3)

- Initial tests include the overnight low-dose dexamethasone suppression test (LDST), 24-hour urine free cortisol (UFC), and late-night (LN) salivary cortisol. The LN and UFC tend to be more convenient.

- In patients with a clinical diagnosis of Cushing's syndrome the initial screening test is the overnight dexamethasone suppression test:
  1. Dexamethasone 1 mg PO given at 11 PM.
  2. Plasma cortisol level measured 9 hr later (8 AM).
  3. Plasma cortisol level <5 mcg/100 ml excludes Cushing's syndrome.
- Late-night (LN) salivary cortisol: a single midnight serum cortisol level (normal diurnal variation leads to a nadir around midnight) >7.5 mcg/dl has been reported as 96% sensitive and 100% specific for the diagnosis of Cushing's syndrome.
- Serial measurements (two or three consecutive measurements) of 24-hr urinary free cortisol and creatinine (to ensure adequacy of collection) are undertaken if overnight dexamethasone test is suggestive of Cushing's syndrome. Persistent elevated cortisol excretion (>300 mcg/24 hr) indicates Cushing's syndrome.
- The low-dose (2 mg) dexamethasone suppression test is useful to exclude pseudo-Cushing's syndrome if the previous results are equivocal. Corticotropic-releasing hormone (CRH) stimulation after low-dose dexamethasone administration (dexamethasone-CRH test) is also used to distinguish patients with suspected Cushing's syndrome from those who have mildly elevated urinary free cortisol level and equivocal findings.
- The high-dose (8 mg) dexamethasone test and measurement of ACTH by radioimmunoassay are useful to determine the etiology of Cushing's syndrome.
  1. ACTH undetectable or decreased and lack of suppression indicate adrenal cause of Cushing's syndrome.
  2. ACTH normal or increased and lack of suppression indicate ectopic ACTH production.
  3. ACTH normal or increased and partial suppression suggest pituitary excess (Cushing's disease).

Bilateral inferior petrosal sinus sampling (BIPSS) can be used to distinguish pituitary Cushing's disease from the ectopic ACTH syndrome (Fig. 2).

LABORATORY TESTS

- Hypokalemia, hypochloremia, metabolic alkalosis, hyperglycemia, hypercholesterolemia.
- Increased 24-hr urinary free cortisol (>100 mcg/24 hr).
- Table 4 describes the differential diagnosis of hormonal values seen in Cushing's syndrome.

IMAGING STUDIES

- CT scan or MRI of adrenal glands in suspected adrenal Cushing's syndrome (Fig. E3).
- MRI of pituitary gland with gadolinium is the preferred procedure for localizing a pituitary edema in suspected pituitary Cushing's syndrome.
- Additional imaging studies to localize neoplasms of the lung, pancreas, kidney, thyroid, or thymus in patients with ectopic ACTH production.

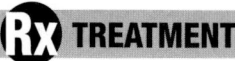 **TREATMENT**

GENERAL Rx

The definitive treatment of Cushing's syndrome is surgical removal of the tumor causing excessive production of cortisol:

- Pituitary adenoma: transsphenoidal microadenomectomy is the therapy of choice in adults. Pituitary irradiation is reserved for patients not cured by transsphenoidal surgery. In children, pituitary irradiation may be considered as initial therapy because 85% of children are cured by radiation. Stereotactic radiotherapy (photon knife or gamma knife) is effective and exposes the surrounding neuronal tissues to less irradiation than conventional radiotherapy. Total bilateral adrenalectomy is reserved for patients not cured by transsphenoidal surgery or pituitary irradiation.
- Adrenal neoplasm:
  1. Surgical resection of the affected adrenal.
  2. Glucocorticoid replacement for approximately 9 to 12 mo after the surgery to allow time for the contralateral adrenal gland to recover from its prolonged suppression.
  3. In nonsurgical candidates, suppression of adrenal steroid production can be accomplished with ketoconazole. Mifepristone, an antiprogestin, can also be used for control of hyperglycemia secondary to hypercortisolism in adults with endogenous Cushing's syndrome. It should be avoided in women who are or who could become pregnant.
- Bilateral micronodular or macronodular adrenal hyperplasia: bilateral total adrenalectomy.
- Ectopic ACTH:
  1. Surgical resection of the ACTH-secreting neoplasm.
  2. Control of cortisol excess with metyrapone, aminoglutethimide, mifepristone, or ketoconazole.
  3. Control of the mineralocorticoid effects of cortisol and 11-deoxycorticosteroid with spironolactone.
  4. Bilateral adrenalectomy: a rational approach to patients with indolent, unresectable tumors.

DISPOSITION

Prognosis is favorable in patients with surgically amenable disease.

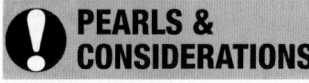 **PEARLS & CONSIDERATIONS**

COMMENTS

- Screening for multiple endocrine neoplasia type I should be considered in patients with Cushing's disease.

SUGGESTED READINGS

Available at www.expertconsult.com

RELATED CONTENT

Cushing's Syndrome (Patient Information)

AUTHOR: **FRED F. FERRI, M.D.**

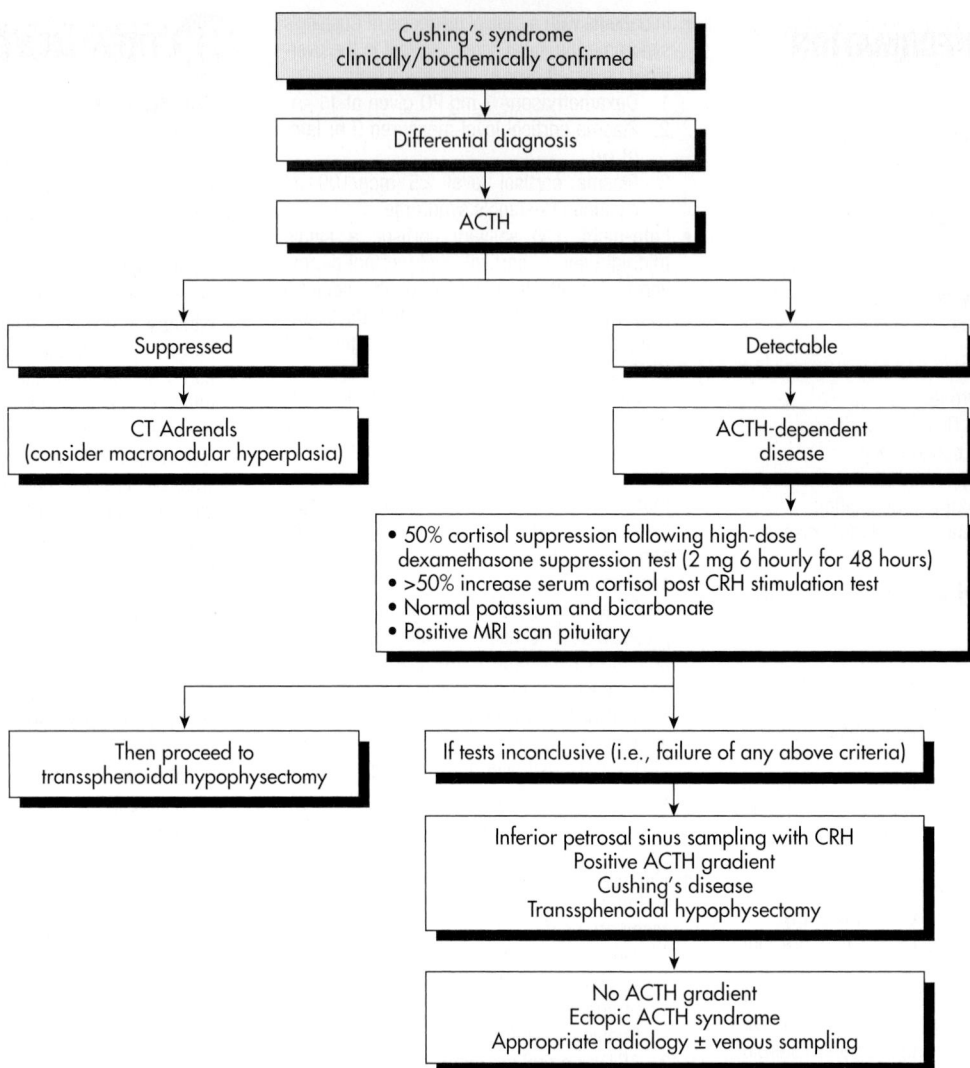

FIG. 2 The tests to uncover the cause of Cushing's syndrome are debatable and differ in any given center depending on many factors, including familiarity and turnaround time of hormone assays and local expertise in techniques such as inferior petrosal sinus sampling. Depicted here is an algorithm in use within many endocrine units based on the reported sensitivity and specificity of each endocrine test. *ACTH,* Adrenocorticotropin; *CT,* computed tomography; *MRI,* magnetic resonance imaging. (From Melmed S, Polonsky KS, Larsen PR, Kronenberg HM: *Williams textbook of endocrinology,* ed 12, Philadelphia, 2011, Saunders.)

TABLE 4 Differential Diagnosis of Hormonal Values Seen in Cushing's Syndrome

Cause	Plasma ACTH	Plasma Cortisol (PM)	High-Dose or Overnight Dexamethasone Suppression
Pituitary-dependent	N—slightly ↑	↑	Yes
Adrenal disease	↓—undetectable	↑	No
Ectopic Cushing's*	↑↑↑	↑↑	Usually no
Pseudo-Cushing's	N—slightly ↑	N–↑	Usually yes

ACTH, Adrenocorticotropin; *N,* normal.
*ACTH levels may overlap with values seen in pituitary-dependent disease.
From McPherson RA, Pincus MR (eds): *Henry's clinical diagnosis and management by laboratory methods,* ed 23, St Louis, 2017, Elsevier.

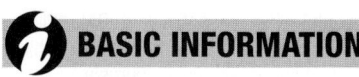 BASIC INFORMATION

DEFINITION

Cystic fibrosis (CF) is an autosomal recessive disorder characterized by dysfunction of exocrine glands.

ICD-10CM CODES
E84.0	Cystic fibrosis with pulmonary manifestations
E84.11	Meconium ileus in cystic fibrosis
E84.19	Cystic fibrosis with other intestinal manifestations
E84.8	Cystic fibrosis with other manifestations
E84.9	Cystic fibrosis, unspecified

EPIDEMIOLOGY & DEMOGRAPHICS

- CF is the most common fatal hereditary disorder amongst Caucasians in the U.S. (one case per approximately 2500) and the second most common life-shortening childhood-onset inherited disorder in the U.S., behind sickle cell disease.
- Median age at diagnosis is 5.3 mo. Median survival is 37 yr.
- Carrier screening is associated with a decrease in incidence of CF.

PHYSICAL FINDINGS & CLINICAL PRESENTATION

- Failure to thrive in children
- Increased anterior/posterior chest diameter
- Basilar crackles and hyperresonance to percussion
- Digital clubbing
- Chronic cough
- Abdominal distention
- Greasy, foul-smelling feces

ETIOLOGY

Caused by mutations to *CFTR* gene on chromosome 7. Over 1000 gene mutations have been associated with CF. About half of patients in the U.S. with CF are homozygous for the Phe508del mutation in *CFTR*, and more than 90% have at least one Phe508del allele. These mutations

result in abnormalities in chloride transport and thus water flux across the surface of epithelial cells; the resulting abnormally viscous secretions cause obstruction of glands and ducts in various organs and subsequent damage to exocrine tissue (recurrent pneumonia, atelectasis, bronchiectasis, diabetes mellitus, biliary cirrhosis, cholelithiasis, intestinal obstruction, increased risk of gastrointestinal malignancies).

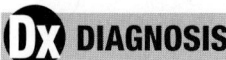 DIAGNOSIS

DIFFERENTIAL DIAGNOSIS

- Immunodeficiency states
- Celiac disease
- Asthma
- Recurrent pneumonia
- Primary ciliary dyskinesia

WORKUP

A diagnosis of CF requires proof of both CFTR dysfunction (i.e., elevated sweat chloride ≥60 mmol/L measured twice, two disease-causing mutations in CFTR from each parental allele, or abnormal nasal potential difference) and one or more phenotypic features consistent with CF (e.g., chronic suppurative obstructive lung disease, pancreatic insufficiency). Table 1 describes diagnostic criteria for CF. Conditions suggesting the diagnosis of CF in adults and recommended diagnostic studies are described in Table 2.

LABORATORY TESTS

- Pilocarpine iontophoresis (sweat chloride test): diagnostic of CF in children if sweat chloride is >60 mmol/L (>80 mmol/L in adults) on two separate tests on consecutive days. Repeat testing may be necessary because not all infants have sufficient quantities of sweat for reliable testing. Table 3 describes conditions associated with false-positive and false-negative sweat test results.
- DNA testing may be useful for confirming the diagnosis and providing genetic information for family members.

- Sputum culture and sensitivity and Gram stain (frequent bacterial infections with *Staphylococcus aureus*, *Pseudomonas aeruginosa* [most common virulent respiratory pathogen], *Haemophilus influenzae* and *Burkholderia cenocepacia*). Bronchoalveolar lavage (BAL) is used at times to aid in the early diagnosis of pulmonary infection in non-expectorating patients. However, evidence for its clinical benefit is lacking. Trials have shown that among infants diagnosed with CF, BAL-directed therapy did not result in a lower prevalence of *P. aeruginosa* infection or lower total CF-CT score when compared with standard therapy at age 5 years.
- Low albumin level, increased 72-hr fecal fat excretion.
- Pulse oximetry or arterial blood gases: hypoxemia.
- Pulmonary function studies: decreased total lung capacity, forced vital capacity, pulmonary diffusing capacity.

IMAGING STUDIES

- Chest x-ray (Fig. 1): may reveal focal atelectasis, peribronchial cuffing, bronchiectasis, increased interstitial markings, hyperinflation
- High-resolution chest CT scan: bronchial wall thickening, cystic lesions, ring shadows (bronchiectasis)

TABLE 1 Diagnostic Criteria for Cystic Fibrosis (CF)

Presence of typical clinical features (respiratory, gastrointestinal, or genitourinary)

OR

A history of CF in a sibling

OR

A positive newborn screening test

PLUS

Laboratory evidence for CFTR (CF transmembrane regulator) dysfunction:

Two elevated sweat chloride concentrations obtained on separate days

OR

Identification of two CF mutations

OR

An abnormal nasal potential difference measurement

From Kliegman RM et al: *Nelson textbook of pediatrics*, ed 19, Philadelphia, 2011, Saunders.

TABLE 2 Approach to Diagnosis of Cystic Fibrosis in Adult Patients

Conditions Suggesting the Diagnosis of Cystic Fibrosis in Adults

Recurrent pancreatitis
Male infertility
Chronic sinusitis
Nasal polyposis
Nontuberculous mycobacterial infection
Allergic bronchopulmonary mycosis
Bronchiectasis

Recommended Diagnostic Studies

Sweat electrolyte determination
Extended CFTR mutation analysis
Nasal potential difference
High-resolution CT scan to identify bronchiectasis
CT scan of sinuses for polyposis
Sputum induction or bronchoalveolar lavage to identify bacterial and fungal pathogens

CFTR, Cystic fibrosis transmembrane conductance regulator; *CT*, computed tomography.

From Goldman L, Schafer AI: *Goldman's Cecil medicine*, ed 24, Philadelphia, 2012, Saunders.

TABLE 3 Conditions Associated with False-Positive and False-Negative Sweat Test Results

With False-Positive Results

Eczema (atopic dermatitis)
Ectodermal dysplasia
Malnutrition/failure to thrive/deprivation
Anorexia nervosa
Congenital adrenal hyperplasia
Adrenal insufficiency
Glucose-6-phosphatase deficiency
Mauriac syndrome
Fucosidosis
Familial hypoparathyroidism
Hypothyroidism
Nephrogenic diabetes insipidus
Pseudohypoaldosteronism
Klinefelter's syndrome
Familial cholestasis syndrome
Autonomic dysfunction
Prostaglandin E infusions
Munchausen syndrome by proxy

With false-negative results

Dilution
Malnutrition
Edema
Insufficient sweat quantity
Hyponatremia
Cystic fibrosis transmembrane conductance regulator (CFTR) mutations with preserved sweat duct function

From Kliegman RM et al: *Nelson textbook of pediatrics*, ed 19, Philadelphia, 2011, Saunders.

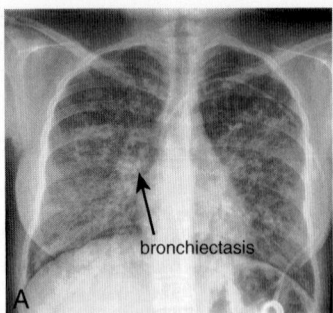
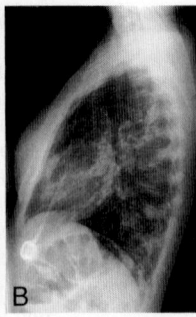
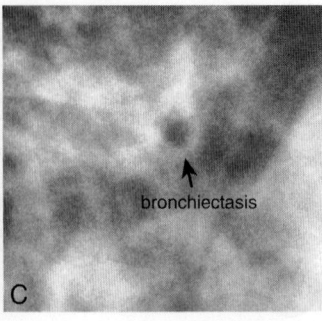
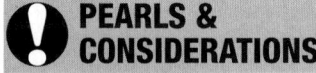

FIG. 1 Cystic fibrosis. Cystic fibrosis is aptly named. Chest x-ray findings include increased interstitial density of fibrosis and cystic changes of lung parenchyma similar to chronic obstructive pulmonary disease. Bronchiectasis (dilation of bronchi, potentially eroding into bronchial arteries and presenting with hemoptysis) may be visible on chest x-ray as large and thickened bronchioles particularly when viewed in short axis (when bronchioles are oriented perpendicular to the frontal plane). This I5-year-old with cystic fibrosis presented with cough and dyspnea. Does she have pneumonia? Comparison with prior x-rays showed no changes. **A,** Posterior-anterior chest x-ray. **B,** Lateral chest x-ray. **C,** Close-up from A showing bronchiectasis. (From Broder JS: *Diagnostic imaging for the emergency physician,* Philadelphia, 2011, Saunders.)

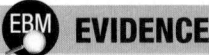 TREATMENT

NONPHARMACOLOGIC THERAPY

- Mucus clearance (i.e., using postural drainage techniques, chest percussion, pneumatic vest, acapella).
- Encouragement of regular exercise and proper nutrition (daily caloric intake of 120%-200% of healthy population).
- Psychosocial evaluation and counseling of patient and family members.

ACUTE GENERAL Rx

- Antibiotic therapy is based on the results of sputum gram stain and culture and sensitivity. *S. aureus* infections are treated with either cefazolin 1.5 g q6h or nafcillin 2 g 4-6h. MRSA should be treated with vancomycin 45-60 mg/kg/day in 3 divided doses or with linezolid 600 mg q12h. *P. aeruginosa* infections can be treated with piperacillin-tazobactam 4.5 g q6h plus ciprofloxacin 750 mg PO q12h. Treatment of CF exacerbations should be aimed at least at mucoid *P. aeruginosa* and *S. aureus* (i.e., piperacillin-tazobactam and ciprofloxacin). A recent study using azithromycin maintenance in children with CF for 6 mo found less use of additional antibiotics and improvement in some aspects of pulmonary function. Additional studies will be necessary to determine if azithromycin should be used as a primary therapy or rescue treatment. Inhaled antibiotics (aztreonam or tobramycin) can also be used and can achieve high airway concentration with lower systemic side effects. Intermittent administration of inhaled tobramycin has been reported to be beneficial in CF.
- Bronchodilators for patients with airflow obstruction.
- Long-term pancreatic enzyme replacement.
- Alternate-day prednisone (2 mg/kg) possibly beneficial in children with CF (decreased hospitalization rate, improved pulmonary function). Routine use of corticosteroids not recommended in adults. Boys with CF who have received alternate-day treatment with prednisone have shown persistent growth impairment after treatment is discontinued.
- Proper nutrition and vitamin supplementation (including fat-soluble vitamins A, D, E, and K).
- The mucolytic recombinant human deoxyribonuclease (DNase [dornase alfa]) 2.5 mg qd or bid given by aerosol for patients with viscid sputum. It lowers the viscosity of sputum. It is useful to improve mucociliary clearance by liquefying difficult-to-clear pulmonary secretions. It is, however, very expensive. It is most beneficial in patients with forced vital capacity values >40% of predicted. Its cost can be decreased by using alternate-day rhDNase therapy. Newer treatment modalities involve increasing the activity of CF transmembrane conductance regulator (CFTR) protein. Ivacaftor (a CFTR potentiator) is FDA approved for oral treatment of CF in patients 6 years and older with the G551D mutation (5% of patients with CF). It can decrease the frequency of pulmonary exacerbations and improve lung function. Dose is 150 mg PO BID. Cost is a significant limiting factor. A new oral combination treatment of Lumacaftor 400 mg (CFTR-corrector)-Ivacaftor 250 mg every 12 hr has been FDA approved in patients ages 12 yr and older who are homozygous for the F508del mutation in the *CFTR* gene. If the patient's genotype is unknown, an FDA-cleared CF mutation test should be used to detect the presence of the F508del mutation on both alleles of the *CFTR* gene.
  Limitations of use: Efficacy and safety have not been established in patients with CF other than those homozygous for the F508del mutation.
- Treatment of impaired glucose tolerance and diabetes mellitus.

CHRONIC Rx

Pneumococcal and influenza vaccination

DISPOSITION

- Bronchiectasis develops early in the course of cystic fibrosis, being detectable in infants as young as 10 wk of age, and is persistent and progressive. Recent data[1] reveal that

[1]Sly PD et al: Risk factors for bronchiectasis in children with cystic fibrosis, *N Engl J Med* 368:1963-1970, 2013.

neutrophil elastase activity in BAL fluid in early life is associated with early bronchiectasis in children with cystic fibrosis.

- More than 50% of children with CF live beyond age 20 yr. During the past 2 decades, survival among patients with late-stage CF has lengthened substantially. Survival has improved at the rate of 1.8% annually during the past decade. This is believed due to increased use of NBH DNase.
- Lung transplantation is the only definitive treatment; 3-yr survival after transplantation exceeds 50%.
- Obstructive azoospermia is present in >98% of postpubertal males.
- The SERPINA Z allele is a risk factor for liver disease in CF. Patients who carry the Z allele are at a greater risk of developing severe liver disease with portal hypertension.

REFERRAL

- For lung transplantation in selected patients. Indications for lung transplantation are FEV$_1$ <30% of predicted, rapidly progressive respiratory deterioration, increasing number of hospital admissions, massive hemoptysis, recurrent pneumothorax, arterial partial pressure of oxygen <55 mm Hg, arterial partial pressure of carbon dioxide >50 mm Hg, multiresistant organisms, wasting. Young female patients should be referred earlier because of overall poor prognosis.
- For screening of family members with DNA analysis.

! PEARLS & CONSIDERATIONS

COMMENTS

- Clinicians should think of CF in any patient with bronchiectasis plus any of the following: male infertility, recurrent idiopathic pancreatitis, recurrent nasal polyposis.
- Genetic testing for CF should be offered to adults with a positive family history of CF, couples currently planning a pregnancy, and couples seeking prenatal care.
- Inhalation of hypertonic saline (5 mL of 7% sodium chloride qid) has been reported to produce a sustained acceleration of mucus clearance and improved lung function.
- The prevalence of MRSA in the respiratory tract of individuals with CF has increased dramatically over the past decade and is associated with worse survival.

EBM EVIDENCE

Available at www.expertconsult.com
SUGGESTED READINGS
Available at www.expertconsult.com

RELATED CONTENT

Cystic Fibrosis (Patient Information)
Bronchiectasis (Related Key Topic)

AUTHORS: **FREDERIC CELESTIN, M.D.,** and **SAMAAN RAFEQ, M.D.**

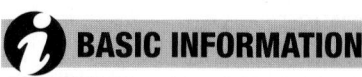 BASIC INFORMATION

DEFINITION

Cysticercosis is an infection caused by the tissue deposition of larval forms of the pork tapeworm *Taenia solium*. *T. solium* cysts, or cysticerci, may accumulate in any human tissue, including the eyes, spinal cord, skin, muscle, heart, and brain. Central nervous system (CNS) involvement is common and is known as neurocysticercosis. Humans most commonly acquire cysticercosis via fecal-oral transmission from human tapeworm carriers or via ingestion of larval cysts in infected pork or tapeworm eggs in contaminated water or soil. Larvae in the gastrointestinal tract migrate hematogenously to tissues, where they encyst, forming cysticerci.

SYNONYMS

Cysticerciasis
Taeniasis
Pork tapeworm

ICD-10CM CODES
B69	Cysticercosis
B69.0	Cysticercosis of central nervous system
B69.1	Cysticercosis of eye
B69.81	Myositis in cysticercosis
B69.89	Cysticercosis of other sites
B69.9	Cysticercosis, unspecified

EPIDEMIOLOGY & DEMOGRAPHICS

- *T. solium* infection is worldwide in distribution. Tapeworm infection and cysticercosis are endemic in developing countries where pigs are raised as a food source, including developing countries of Central America, South America, and parts of Africa and Asia.
- Serologic studies from endemic areas of Latin America have demonstrated seroprevalence rates of 4% to 24% in native populations.
- Neurocysticercosis is most common in the United States in states with large immigrant populations from countries where the disease is endemic.

PHYSICAL FINDINGS & CLINICAL PRESENTATION

- After ingestion of *T. solium* eggs or cysts, humans may remain asymptomatic for years.
- Cysticerci in muscles and skin may form asymptomatic "cold" nodules without erythema or tenderness that may calcify and be seen on radiographs. Any muscle may be involved, including the masseter.
- Neurocysticercosis, the presence of cysts within the brain parenchyma, is usually asymptomatic. Symptoms develop due to the inflammatory response to degeneration of cysts, which can result in focal encephalitis, vasculitis, chronic meningitis, and cranial nerve palsies.
- Seizures are the most common manifestation of neurocysticercosis, occurring in 70% to 90%

of symptomatic cases. Headache and focal neurologic deficits can also occur.
- Up to 40% of patients with epilepsy in endemic areas have neurocysticercosis.
- In 10% to 20% of cases of neurocysticercosis, cysts lodge within the ventricular system and result in obstructive hydrocephalus, causing acute intracranial hypertension. Symptoms are caused by the presence of the parasite itself, ependymal inflammation, and/or fibrosis, each of which blocks the circulation of cerebrospinal fluid (CSF). Death may occur from progressive hydrocephalus, cerebral edema, or intractable seizures.
- Ocular cysticercosis occurs in less than 5% of infections and is generally asymptomatic. Inflammation in response to degenerating cysticerci may result in chorioretinitis, vasculitis, or retinal detachment, threatening vision.

ETIOLOGY

- *T. solium* has a complex two-host life cycle.
- Humans are the only definitive host and harbor the adult worm in the intestine (taeniasis). However, both humans and pigs can serve as intermediate hosts and harbor the larvae or cysticerci.

Dx DIAGNOSIS

DIFFERENTIAL DIAGNOSIS

- Epilepsy of unknown etiology
- Migraine
- CNS vasculitis
- Primary neoplasia of CNS
- Chronic CNS infections, including toxoplasmosis, coccidioidomycosis, tuberculosis, and cryptococcosis
- Brain abscess
- CNS involvement with sarcoidosis or systemic lupus erythematosus

WORKUP

Comprehensive clinical history: obtain information on current and previous travel and residence, including geographic area, sanitary conditions, and consumption of undercooked pork.

LABORATORY TESTS

- Serum antibody detection by enzyme-linked immunoelectrotransfer blot (EITB) assay has a sensitivity of 98% and a specificity of 100% in patients with more than one cyst but has less predictive value in patients with a single cyst, in which up to 38% can be falsely negative. The same assay can be performed in CSF, with lower sensitivity. Antibodies detected by EITB can persist for years after successful therapy, limiting the usefulness of this assay in following patients after treatment. In endemic regions, a negative test result is useful in ruling out disease but a positive result is a marker of exposure, not necessarily symptomatic infection.
- Circulating cysticercus antigens can be detected in blood and CSF, providing a marker of viable organisms, even when CNS

lesions are calcified and presumed to be inactive. This method may be particularly useful in monitoring patients after therapy. Antigen levels usually fall within 3 months of successful treatment.
- Polymerase chain reaction (PCR) detection of *T. solium* DNA has been developed, with a reported sensitivity of 96.7%, but it is not widely available.
- Definitive diagnosis is based on the histopathologic demonstration of cysticerci in the tissue involved. Fine-needle aspiration cytology may be useful in diagnosing infection.
- Peripheral eosinophilia is usually absent.
- Stool examination for ova and proglottids of *T. solium* is insensitive and not specific for the diagnosis of cysticercosis.
- CSF examination in neurocysticercosis is usually unremarkable, but may demonstrate pleocytosis, with lymphocytic or eosinophilic predominance, low glucose, and elevated protein.

IMAGING STUDIES

- Plain radiographs of the extremities may reveal calcified cysts in patients with soft tissue or muscle involvement.
- For diagnosis of neurocysticercosis, CT and MRI are most commonly used.
- Brain CT (Fig. 1) has a sensitivity and specificity of 95% and can identify living cysticerci, which appear as hypodense lesions, as well as degenerating cysts, which appear as isodense or hyperdense lesions with surrounding edema. CT is the best method for detecting calcification associated with prior infection, which suggests inactivity.
- Brain MRI is the most accurate technique to assess the extent of infection, location, and evolutionary stage of the parasites. MRI provides detailed images of living and degenerating cysts, perilesional edema, as well as small cysts or those located in the ventricles, brainstem, and cerebellum. However, MRI has a low sensitivity for detecting calcified lesions, which are the most common neuroimaging finding in endemic populations.

Rx TREATMENT

ACUTE GENERAL Rx

Asymptomatic cysticercosis:
- There is no evidence that administering antiparasitic therapy is beneficial.

Symptomatic neurocysticercosis:
The goals of treatment are to control seizures and mass effect from cysticercal lesions, control intracranial hypertension, and reduce the size of active cysts.
- Treatment decisions in neurocysticercosis should be individualized. Initial measures should focus on the symptomatic management, considering antiparasitic therapy when appropriate.
- Patients with active lesions, with evidence of surrounding edema and/or inflammation, generally warrant treatment with antiparasitics, corticosteroids, and anticonvulsants.
  1. Patients who have seizures or are considered at risk for recurrent seizures based

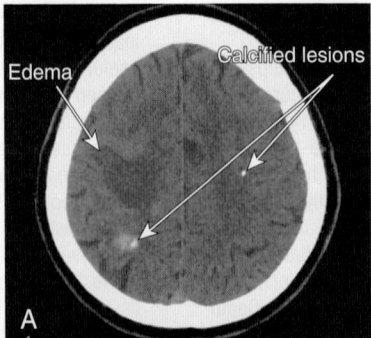

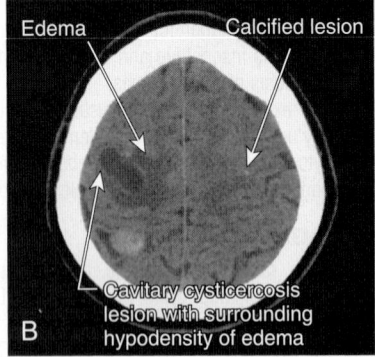

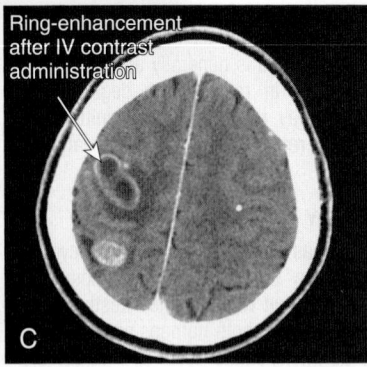

FIG. 1 Neurocysticercosis. This 40-year-old Bolivian man presented with left-hand weakness. **A, B,** Noncontrast head computed tomography (CT) scan, brain windows. **C,** CT scan with contrast moments later; compare this with (**B**). A slice through the same level of the brain before contrast administration. Hypodense lesions are present, with surrounding hypodensity (*dark gray*) representing edema. Scattered calcifications are also seen, which are a common feature of old neurocysticercosis lesions. Administration of intravenous contrast leads to ring enhancement, a feature of many infectious and inflammatory conditions, including neurocysticercosis, brain abscess, and toxoplasmosis. (From Broder JS: *Diagnostic imaging for the emergency physician,* Philadelphia, 2011, Saunders.)

on imaging should be treated with anticonvulsants.

2. Corticosteroids may decrease inflammation and edema, and should be given whenever antiparasitic therapy is given.
3. Antiparasitic therapy is indicated in the treatment of symptomatic patients with multiple viable brain parenchymal cysticerci. Despite treatment, only 30% to 50% of lesions resolve within 6 months.
4. Calcified cysticerci are generally inactive and do not warrant antiparasitic treatment.
5. Antiparasitic therapy is often unnecessary in patients with single cysts, which are usually self-limited and resolve spontaneously within 6 months.

Antiparasitic therapy:

1. Patients with viable parenchymal or subarachnoid cysts should be treated with albendazole 15 mg/kg/day PO divided twice daily for 7 days or praziquantel 50 mg/kg/day divided three times daily for 28 days. Albendazole is preferred since praziquantel management is more complicated due to an interaction with anticonvulsants such as phenytoin. Patients should receive prednisolone (2 mg/kg/day) or dexamethasone (0.15 mg/kg/day) orally before initiation of antiparasitic therapy. Antiparasitics should be used cautiously in patients with massive cysticercal infection of the brain parenchyma (≥50 cysts) or cysticercal encephalitis. These

patients should be managed initially with corticosteroids, and perhaps mannitol, to control intracranial hypertension. Once the inflammation and edema have resolved by MRI, antiparasitics can be administered.

2. Albendazole is considered to be the drug of choice due to slightly better efficacy, greater availability, fewer drug interactions, and lower cost.
3. Combination therapy with praziquantel (50 mg/kg/day) and albendazole (15 mg/kg/day) with dexamethasone (0.1 mg/kg/day) has been demonstrated to be more efficacious than albendazole and steroids alone for cyst resolution; seizures persisted despite treatment in many cases, so antiepileptic therapy is indicated.

Surgical therapy:

1. Surgery may be indicated in patients with obstructive hydrocephalus or giant cysts with associated intracranial hypertension.
2. Minimally invasive neurosurgery (neuroendoscopy) for cyst removal and ventricular shunt formation has greatly improved the management of intraventricular neurocysticercosis.
3. Extraparenchymal neurocysticercosis, including ocular, subarachnoid, and intraventricular disease, carries a poor prognosis and requires a more aggressive approach. When feasible, complete surgical excision of lesions remains the definitive therapy.

CHRONIC Rx

- Prolonged antiparasitic therapy does not improve outcomes in neurocysticercosis and may delay calcification of lesions. Antiepileptic medications should be continued for 2 years or 6 to 12 months after CT/MRI resolution of viable cysts, before tapering. In some cases, antiepileptic therapy needs to be continued indefinitely.
- Rare patients with neurocysticercosis develop chronic or recurrent perilesional inflammation, requiring long-term, high-dose steroid therapy. Methotrexate has been reported to be of use as a steroid-sparing agent in this setting.

DISPOSITION

- In seizure-free, stable neurocysticercosis, outpatient management is appropriate.
- Patients with seizures should be restricted from driving.

REFERRAL

- Infectious diseases consultation.
- Neurology consultation in patients with seizures.
- Neurosurgical consultation if extraparenchymal neurocysticercosis or obstructive hydrocephalus is present.

PREVENTION

- Eradication of taeniasis/cysticercosis is possible with implementation of meat inspection, improvement of pig husbandry, and improvement of socioeconomic conditions in endemic areas.
- A porcine vaccine against *T. solium* has been developed and successfully implemented in Peru, Mexico, and Australia.
- There is currently no human vaccine to prevent tapeworm infection or cysticercosis.

PATIENT & FAMILY EDUCATION

- Pork should be inspected for the presence of cysticerci, which are visible in raw meat.
- Pork must be well cooked.
- Proper disposal of human excreta and handwashing are of utmost importance to break the transmission cycle in households.

RELATED CONTENT

Cysticercosis (Patient Information)

AUTHOR: **STACI A. FISCHER, M.D.**

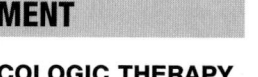

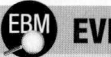 BASIC INFORMATION

DEFINITION

Infection with cytomegalovirus (CMV), a herpes virus, is common in the general population, with multiple mechanisms for transmission, often during childhood and adolescence. CMV is associated with pregnancy and can be a congenital disease. CMV is also associated with immunocompromised states and may be life-threatening.

SYNONYMS

CMV
Heterophil-negative mononucleosis
Cytomegalic inclusion disease virus

ICD-10CM CODES
B25.9	Cytomegaloviral disease, unspecified
P35.1	Congenital cytomegalovirus infection
Z20.820	Contact with and (suspected) exposure to varicella

EPIDEMIOLOGY & DEMOGRAPHICS

- Seroprevalence is widespread: 40% to 100% antibody positivity in adults.
- Increased infection develops perinatally, in day care exposure, and then during reproductive age, related to sexual activity.

ROUTES OF TRANSMISSION

- Blood transfusions.
- Sexually (STDs) via uterus, cervix, and semen.
- Perinatally via breast milk.
- Transplant of organs—bone marrow, kidneys, liver, heart, or lung.
- Saliva.

PHYSICAL FINDINGS & CLINICAL PRESENTATION

CHILDREN: Congenital—25% of infected children with symptoms if congenital:
- Petechial rash.
- Jaundice and/or hepatosplenomegaly.
- Lethargy.
- Respiratory distress.
- CNS involvement, seizures.
Postnatal acquisition:
- CMV mononucleosis.
- Pharyngitis, croup, bronchitis, pneumonia.
HEALTHY ADULTS: Common
- May be asymptomatic.
- CMV mononucleosis similar to EBV mononucleosis.
- Fever—lasting 9 to 30 days—mean of 19 days.
Less common
- Exudative pharyngitis.
- Lymphadenopathy, hepatitis, splenomegaly.
- Interstitial pneumonia (rare).
- Nonspecific rash.
- Thrombocytopenia/hemolytic anemia.
Rare
- Guillain-Barré syndrome.
- Meningoencephalitis.
- Myocarditis.

IMMUNOSUPPRESSED PATIENTS:
- Febrile mononucleosis.
- GI ulcerations, hepatitis, pneumonitis, retinitis, encephalopathy, meningoencephalopathy.
- HIV associated—dementia, demyelination, retinitis, acalculous cholecystitis, adrenalitis, diarrhea, enterocolitis, esophagitis.
- Diabetes associated with pancreatitis.
- Adrenalitis associated with HIV.

ETIOLOGY

CMV infection can remain latent, reactive with immunosuppression.

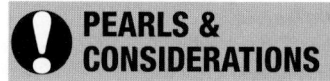 DIAGNOSIS

DIFFERENTIAL DIAGNOSIS

Congenital:
- Acute viral, bacterial, parasitic infections including other congenitally transmitted agents (toxoplasmosis, rubella, syphilis, pertussis, croup, bronchitis).
Acquired:
- EBV mononucleosis.
- Viral hepatitis—A, B, C.
- Cryptosporidiosis.
- Toxoplasmosis.
- *Mycobacterium avium* infections.
- Human herpesvirus 6.
- Acute HIV infection.

WORKUP

- Laboratory confirmation combined with clinical findings often with leukopenia, thrombocytopenia, lymphocytosis. Diagnostic modalities include serologic assays, PCR, detection of CMV PP25 antigen in leukocytes, isolation of virus from body fluids and urine, and cytopathic demonstration of "owl eye" intracellular inclusions.
- Serology:
  1. Detection of CMV-IgM antibodies suggests recent infection. CMV-IgG antibodies usually appear 2 to 3 weeks after infection.
  2. Molecular assays (PCR viral loads): on plasma.
  3. CMV antigenemia assays: detects antibodies to the pp65 protein of the virus in peripheral blood leukocytes. These tests and the PCR tests are used in immunocompromised, AIDS, and transplant patients.
- Cultures: using human fibroblast cultures of blood, CSF, urine, BAL, and biopsy specimens but can take 1 to 6 weeks.
- Funduscopic—necrotic patches with white granular component of retina.
- Biopsy—"owl's eye" inclusion bodies on tissue sample.
- HIV.

IMAGING STUDIES

- Chest radiograph—if pneumonitis suspected, consider bronchoscopy.
- Endoscopy—if GI involvement.
- CT scan/MRI—if CNS involvement.

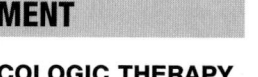 TREATMENT

NONPHARMACOLOGIC THERAPY

- Strict hand washing and standard precautions limit CMV transmission in health care facilities.
- Antiretroviral therapy (ART) in patients with CD4 count <50/mm^3 for the goal of CD4 >100/mm^3 for a 3- to 6-mo period.

ACUTE GENERAL Rx

For compromised hosts with CMV retinitis or pneumonitis:
- Ganciclovir 5 mg/kg q12h IV x 14 to 21 days, then valganciclovir: 900 mg PO q24h or alternative regimen.
- Ganciclovir intraocular implant plus valganciclovir 900 mg PO q24h or alternative regimen.
- Foscarnet 90 mg/kg q12h x 14 to 21 days, then 90 mg to 120 mg/kg IV q24h or alternative regimen.
- Cidofovir 5 mg/kg IV q day x 14 days, then 5 mg/kg IV q 2 weeks.
- Fomivirsen-salvage therapy for CMV retinitis 300 μg injected into vitreous.

DISPOSITION

- CMV infection in patients who are immunocompromised (especially those with AIDS, bone marrow and solid organ transplant recipients, and disorders of cell-mediated immune function) will need expert, long-term follow-up by an infectious disease specialist or immunologist familiar with the care of such patients.
- CMV mononucleosis, hepatitis, pharyngitis, etc. in immunologically normal hosts are usually self-limiting infections requiring no special follow-up plans.

REFERRAL

- To an ophthalmologist if CMV retinitis is present.
- To an infectious disease specialist or AIDS specialist for patients who are HIV-positive with CMV disease.
- To a cellular immunologist or transplant specialist in the case of CMV infection in a transplant recipient.
- To a pediatric infectious disease specialist for congenital CMV infection.

PEARLS & CONSIDERATIONS

CMV is ubiquitous in the environment and is asymptomatically shed by latently infected persons with CMV infection, making it difficult to protect patients who are immunocompromised from acquiring this infection.

EVIDENCE

Available at www.expertconsult.com

SUGGESTED READINGS

Available at www.expertconsult.com

AUTHOR: **GLENN G. FORT, M.D., M.P.H.**

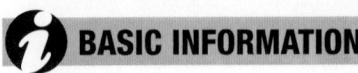

BASIC INFORMATION

DEFINITION

De Quervain's tenosynovitis is a stenosing tenosynovitis of the wrist's first dorsal extensor compartment, containing the abductor pollicis longus and extensor pollicis brevis tendons.

SYNONYMS

Stenosing tenosynovitis of the radial styloid process
Stenosing tenovaginitis of the first dorsal compartment
Radial styloid tenosynovitis
Tenosynovitis of radial styloid
De Quervain's disease
De Quervain's stenosing tenosynovitis
De Quervain's tendinitis
Washerwoman's sprain/strain
Tendinosis
Styloid tenovaginitis

ICD-10CM CODES

M65.4	Radial styloid tenosynovitis [de Quervain]
M65.9	Synovitis and tenosynovitis, unspecified
M65.849	Other synovitis and tenosynovitis, unspecified hand

EPIDEMIOLOGY & DEMOGRAPHICS

- More common in women than in men (10:1)
- Usually occurs between the ages of 30 and 50
- May be associated with systemic inflammatory diseases (rheumatoid arthritis)
- Often seen in new mothers or day care providers due to holding the babies with an extended and abducted thumb
- Seen more frequently in certain occupations involving repetitive wrist motion (e.g., clerical, assembly, and manual labor)

PHYSICAL FINDINGS & CLINICAL PRESENTATION

- Pain over the styloid process of the radius with grasping and resisted thumb abduction
- Tenderness with palpation over the radial styloid and first dorsal extensor compartment
- Pain may radiate up to the volar aspect of the wrist or to the thumb
- Swelling on the radial styloid
- Positive Finkelstein's test (Fig. 1)
- Crepitance
- Rarely, numbness of dorsum of thumb
- Absence of local heat on examination

ETIOLOGY

- Repetitive use or overuse of the hand and thumb involving pinching with the thumb while moving wrist in radial and ulnar directions (e.g., typing, writing, nailing, golfing, fly-fishing)
- Acute trauma to the first dorsal extensor compartment
- Anatomic abnormality or variation
- Increased volume states, such as occurring during pregnancy

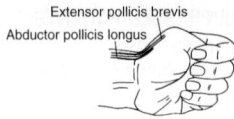
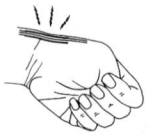

Extensor pollicis brevis
Abductor pollicis longus

FIG. 1 Finkelstein's test is positive in de Quervain's stenosing synovitis. Ulnar flexion of the wrist produces pain over the dorsal compartment containing the extensor pollicis brevis and abductor pollicis longus. (From Noble J [ed]: *Textbook of primary care medicine*, ed 2, St Louis, 1996, Mosby.)

DIAGNOSIS

- The diagnosis of de Quervain's tenosynovitis is based on the clinical triad of:
  1. Tenderness over the radial styloid
  2. Pain over the first dorsal extensor compartment on resisted thumb abduction or extension
  3. Pain on ulnar movement of the wrist with the thumb adducted and flexed (Finkelstein's test; see Fig. 1)
- Consideration can be given to injecting 1.5 mL of 1% Xylocaine into the tenosynovial sac, and if all three physical signs resolve, the diagnosis is confirmed, allowing for differentiation from carpometacarpal (CMC) osteoarthritis (OA).
- Finkelstein maneuver can also be present in first CMC joint OA.

DIFFERENTIAL DIAGNOSIS

- Carpal tunnel syndrome
- Radiocarpal arthritis (OA or RA)
- Gout
- Infiltrative tenosynovitis
- Thumb carpometacarpal arthritis (OA or RA)
- Compression neuropathy (e.g., superficial branch of the radial nerve "bracelet syndrome")
- Ganglion cysts
- Infection (e.g., tuberculosis, bacterial)
- Radial styloid fracture

IMAGING STUDIES

- Imaging of the wrist and thumb is not necessary unless fracture or arthritis is suspected.
- Radiographs (three views) of the wrist should be obtained if fracture is suspected.

TREATMENT

NONPHARMACOLOGIC THERAPY

- Avoiding repetitive movements of hand or thumb
- Thumb spica splinting
- Icing (4 to 6 times a day for 15 min)
- Physiotherapy

ACUTE GENERAL Rx

- Corticosteroid injection using 20 to 40 mg triamcinolone acetonide and 1% xylocaine is often diagnostic and therapeutic.
- Oral NSAIDs (ibuprofen 800 mg tid or naproxen 500 mg bid).

- Topical NSAIDs (Voltaren gel) or hydrocortisone.

CHRONIC Rx

- Once signs of active inflammation have resolved after 3 to 4 weeks, gentle stretching exercises involving abductor and extensor tendons usually help recovery.
- Maximum trial of three corticosteroid injections at minimum 3-month intervals (1 every 3 months or more).
- Surgical intervention is generally reserved for those patients not responding to NSAIDs and corticosteroid injection therapy.
- Surgery includes first dorsal extensor compartment and subcompartment releases with or without tenosynovectomy.

DISPOSITION

- ~82% of patients have initial relief of symptoms with corticosteroid injection.
- ~52% of patients remain symptom-free at 12 months after corticosteroid injection.
- Rarely, steroid injection use can cause infection, skin hypopigmentation, and tendon rupture.
- Diabetics may experience mild temporary hyperglycemia after corticosteroid injection.
- Accidental injection of the corticosteroid in the subcutaneous tissue instead of the sheath of the first dorsal extensor compartment should be avoided to prevent fat and dermal atrophy.
- If left untreated, can lead to fibrosis and decrease in mobility (stenosing tenosynovitis).
- Surgical resolution of symptoms achieved in 90% of referred cases.
- Complications of surgery include:
  1. Superficial branch of the radial nerve injury
  2. Paresthesia (10%)
  3. Neuroma formation
  4. Hypertrophic or painful scar
  5. Chronic regional pain syndrome
- Recovery rates with early treatment are higher to ~80% after 6 weeks but <40% after 4 years.

PEARLS & CONSIDERATIONS

- Steroid injection is generally recommended after failure of 2 to 6 weeks of conservative treatment.
- Pain relief usually noted within 48 hours, with patient becoming asymptomatic 1 to 2 weeks after corticosteroid injection.
- If no improvement 6 weeks after second corticosteroid injection, consider referral to an orthopedic hand surgeon.
- Condition can recur if triggering activity continues.

SUGGESTED READINGS

Available at www.expertconsult.com

RELATED CONTENT

De Quervain's Tenosynovitis (Patient Information)

AUTHOR: **ANDREW PAUL HARRIS, M.D.**

BASIC INFORMATION

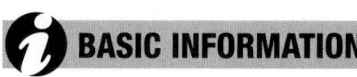

DEFINITION

Venous thromboembolism is any thromboembolic event occurring within the venous system. Deep vein thrombosis (DVT) is the development of thrombi in the deep veins of the extremities or pelvis.

SYNONYMS

DVT
Venous thromboembolism (VTE) (VTE includes DVT and pulmonary embolism [PE])
Deep venous thrombosis
VTE

ICD-10CM CODES

I82.401 Acute embolism and thrombosis of unspecified deep veins of right lower extremity
I82.402 Acute embolism and thrombosis of unspecified deep veins of left lower extremity
I82.403 Acute embolism and thrombosis of unspecified deep veins of lower extremity, bilateral
I82.621 Acute embolism and thrombosis of deep veins of right upper extremity
I82.622 Acute embolism and thrombosis of deep veins of left upper extremity
I82.623 Acute embolism and thrombosis of deep veins of upper extremity, bilateral

EPIDEMIOLOGY & DEMOGRAPHICS

- Annual incidence of VTE is 0.1% to 0.27%, affecting up to 5% of the population during their lifetimes.
- The risk of recurrent thromboembolism is higher among men than women.
- In the U.S., there are approximately 900,000 DVT events annually. About 5% to 15% of persons with untreated DVT die from pulmonary embolism.
- Venous thromboembolism occurs in nearly 2 cases per 1000 pregnancies and is a leading cause of maternal mortality and morbidity

PHYSICAL FINDINGS & CLINICAL PRESENTATION

- Pain and swelling of the affected extremity
- In lower extremity DVT: leg pain on dorsiflexion of the foot (*Homans' sign*)
- Physical examination may be unremarkable in early DVT

ETIOLOGY

The etiology is often multifactorial (prolonged stasis, coagulation abnormalities, vessel wall trauma). The following are risk factors for DVT:
- Prolonged immobilization (>3 days)
- Postoperative state
- Trauma to pelvis and lower extremities for lower extremity DVT; central line placement for upper extremity DVT
- Birth control pills, high-dose estrogen therapy; conjugated equine estrogen but not esterified estrogen is associated with increased risk of

DVT; estrogen plus progestin is associated with doubling the risk of venous thrombosis. The use of bevacizumab is also significantly associated with an increased risk of developing DVT in cancer patients receiving this drug.
- Visceral cancer (lung, pancreas, alimentary tract, genitourinary tract)
- Age >60 yr
- History of thromboembolic disease
- Hematologic disorders (e.g., factor V Leiden mutation [FVL], antithrombin III deficiency, protein C deficiency, protein S deficiency, heparin cofactor II deficiency, sticky platelet syndrome, G20210A prothrombin mutation, lupus anticoagulant, dysfibrinogenemias, anticardiolipin antibody, hyperhomocysteinemia, concurrent homocystinuria, high levels of factors VIII, XI, and single nucleotide polymorphisms [SNPs] such as CYP4V2)
- Pregnancy and early puerperium
- Obesity (BMI >30)
- Congestive heart failure
- Surgery, fracture, or injury involving lower leg or pelvis
- Plaster cast immobilization
- Surgery requiring >30 min of anesthesia
- Gynecologic surgery (particularly gynecologic cancer surgery)
- Recent travel (within 2 wk, lasting ≥2 hr). Every 2 hr spent traveling increases VTE risk by 18%.
- Smoking and abdominal obesity
- Central venous catheter or pacemaker insertion
- Superficial vein thrombosis (10% risk of DVT within 3 mo), varicose veins
- Collagen vascular disease
- Nephrotic syndrome
- Myeloproliferative disorders
- Long-term exposure to particulate air pollution is also associated with altered coagulation function and DVT risk.

DIAGNOSIS

DIFFERENTIAL DIAGNOSIS

- Postphlebitic syndrome
- Superficial thrombophlebitis
- Ruptured Baker's cyst
- Cellulitis, lymphangitis, Achilles tendinitis
- Hematoma
- Muscle or soft tissue injury, stress fracture
- Varicose veins, lymphedema
- Arterial insufficiency
- Abscess
- Claudication
- Venous stasis

WORKUP

- The clinical diagnosis of DVT is inaccurate. Pain, tenderness, swelling, or color changes are not specific for DVT.
- Clinical prediction rules can be used to establish pretest probability of DVT. The Wells prediction rules for DVT and for pulmonary embolism are described in Box 1. These rules perform better in younger patients without a history of DVT and in those without comorbidities. In younger patients without associated comorbidities and a low pretest probability using Wells criteria and a negative high-sensitivity D-dimer test, the diagnosis of DVT can be reasonably excluded.
- Compression ultrasonography (CUS; Fig. E1) is preferred as the initial study to diagnose DVT in patients with intermediate to high pretest probability. An initial negative test limited to the proximal leg should be repeated after 5 days (if the clinical suspicion of DVT persists) to exclude DVT that is propagating proximally from the calf. Comprehensive ultrasonography (whole-leg CUS) is a more extensive test that examines the deep veins from the inguinal ligament to the level of the malleolus. Literature reports indicate that it may be safe to withhold anticoagulation after negative results on comprehensive duplex ultrasonography in nonpregnant patients with a suspected first episode of symptomatic DVT of the leg.

LABORATORY TESTS

- Laboratory tests are not specific for DVT. Baseline prothrombin time (INR), partial thromboplastin time, and platelet count should be obtained on all patients before

---

BOX 1 Wells Prediction Rule for Diagnosing Deep Venous Thrombosis: Clinical Evaluation Table for Predicting Pretest Probability of Deep Venous Thrombosis*

Clinical Characteristic	Score
Active cancer (treatment ongoing, within previous 6 mo, or palliative)	1
Paralysis, paresis, or recent plaster immobilization of the lower extremities	1
Recently bedridden >3 days or major surgery within 12 wk requiring general or regional anesthesia	1
Localized tenderness along the distribution of the deep venous system	1
Entire leg swollen	1
Calf swelling 3 cm larger than asymptomatic side (measured 10 cm below tibial tuberosity)	1
Pitting edema confined to the symptomatic leg	1
Collateral superficial veins (nonvaricose)	1
Alternative diagnosis at least as likely as deep venous thrombosis	22

*Clinical probability: low, ≤0; intermediate, 1-2; high, ≥3. In patients with symptoms in both legs, the more symptomatic leg is used.
Reprinted from Wells PS et al: Value assessment of pretest probability of deep-vein thrombosis in clinical management, *Lancet* 351:1795-1798, 1997.

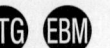

starting anticoagulation. D-dimer testing is sensitive but not specific for DVT. A negative result (D-dimer <0.5 mcg/ml) can exclude the diagnosis in a patient with low probability of DVT, but a positive result (≥0.5 mcg/ml) mandates additional testing with venous ultrasonography.

- Use of D-dimer assay by ELISA is useful in the management of suspected DVT. The combination of a normal D-dimer study on presentation together with a normal compression venous ultrasound is useful to exclude DVT. DVT can be ruled out in patients who are clinically unlikely to have DVT and who have a negative D-dimer test. Compressive ultrasonography can be safely omitted in such patients. Fig. 2 is an algorithm for the diagnosis of DVT.

- Laboratory evaluation of young patients with DVT, patients with recurrent thrombosis without obvious causes, and those with a family history of thrombosis should include protein S (both total and free PS), protein C, fibrinogen, antithrombin III level, lupus anticoagulant, anticardiolipin antibodies, anti-b2 glycoprotein1, factor V Leiden, factor VIII, factor IX, and fasting plasma homocysteine levels. HIT antibody may also be useful in the correct context (heparin exposure and abrupt onset of unexplained decrease in platelet count, whether thrombocytopenic or not). It is important to remember that the lupus anticoagulant assay and antithrombin, protein C, protein S, and dysfibrinogenemia testing cannot be properly interpreted if the patient is already on warfarin, whereas anticardiolipin antibody test, prothrombin G20210A factor

VII:C, factor V Leiden, and PT polymorphism can be performed when the patient is on warfarin.

IMAGING STUDIES

- Compression ultrasonography (CUS) is generally preferred as the initial study because it is noninvasive and can be repeated serially (useful to monitor suspected acute DVT); it offers good sensitivity for detecting proximal vein thrombosis (in the popliteal or femoral vein) (see Fig. E3). Its disadvantages are poor visualization of deep iliac and pelvic veins and poor sensitivity in isolated or nonocclusive calf vein thrombi. Whole-leg compression ultrasound can generally exclude proximal and distal DVT in a single evaluation. Withholding anticoagulation following a single negative whole-leg

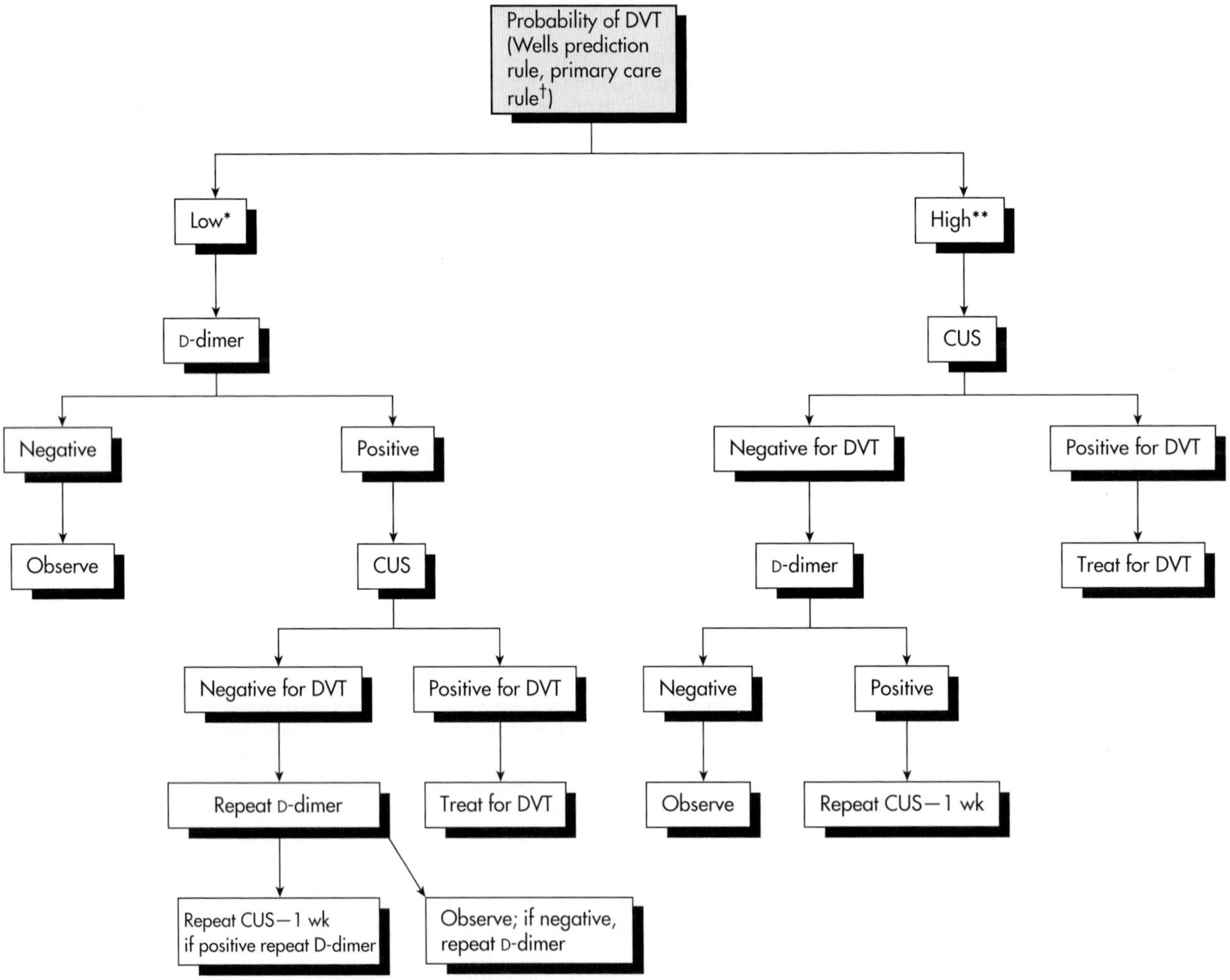

FIG. 2 Diagnostic approach to deep vein thrombosis. *Low probability: none of features of high probability and an alternative diagnosis likely. **High probability: (1) history of active cancer, (2) history of prolonged immobilization, (3) history of recent surgery, (4) history of recent leg trauma, (5) history of thromboembolic disease, (6) family history of thromboembolic disease, (7) birth control pill (BCP) use, (8) history of recent long travel, (9) exam positive for swelling and tenderness compared to other extremity. †The primary rule[1] assigns 1 point each to: male, use of hormonal contraceptives, active cancer in past 6 mo, surgery in previous mo, absence of leg trauma, distinction of collateral leg veins. It assigns 2 points to the presence of difference in calf circumference ≥3 cm and 6 points to abnormal D-dimer assay. A very low risk score is ≤3, and increased risk score is ≥4. *CUS,* Compressive ultrasound; *DVT,* deep vein thrombosis. [1]Toll DB, et al: A new diagnostic rule for deep vein thrombosis: safety and efficiency in clinically relevant subgroups, *Fam Pract* 25:3–8, 2008.

CUS is associated with a relatively low risk of venous thromboembolism (3.5% of inpatients will develop DVT) during a 3-mo follow-up.

- Contrast venography is the gold standard for evaluation of DVT of the lower extremity. It is, however, invasive and painful. Additional disadvantages are the increased risk of phlebitis, new thrombosis, renal failure, and hypersensitivity reaction to contrast media; it also gives poor visualization of the deep femoral vein in the thigh and the internal iliac vein and its tributaries.
- Magnetic resonance direct thrombus imaging (MRDTI) is an accurate noninvasive test for diagnosis of DVT. It is particularly useful in suspected DVT patients with leg casts, which prevent CUS, and in pregnant patients with positive D-dimer and negative CUS (Fig. E3). Current limitations are its cost and lack of widespread availability.

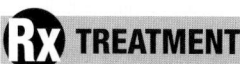 **TREATMENT**

NONPHARMACOLOGIC THERAPY

- Gradual resumption of normal activity. Immobility promotes stasis and propagation of DVT. Patients should get up and walk as tolerated. The theoretical risk that ambulation may dislodge thrombi in the legs, precipitating PE, is unfounded.
- Patient education on anticoagulant therapy and associated risks.

ACUTE GENERAL Rx

- Initial treatment of DVT requires therapeutic doses of heparin (low-molecular-weight heparin [LMWH] or unfractionated). LMWH is preferred due to ease of administration, less hemorrhage, and significantly fewer deaths. Unfractionated heparin is recommended in patients with renal insufficiency because LMWH is predominantly excreted in the urine.
- LMWH is generally administered for 5 to 7 days. Recommended dose of enoxaparin is 1 mg/kg q12h SC. Once-daily fondaparinux, a synthetic analogue of heparin, is also as effective and safe as twice-daily enoxaparin in the initial treatment of patients with symptomatic DVT. Once systemic anticoagulation is initiated, vitamin K antagonist warfarin or oral factor V inhibitors are initiated. When using warfarin, it is normally started on the same day as heparin and is titrated to maintain an INR between 2 and 3. Warfarin therapy at 10 mg daily for 2 days may be initiated in healthy patients with acute DVT. This higher dose helps to achieve therapeutic INR sooner and decreases LMWH doses needed as compared to the 5 mg/day dose. After ≥5 days, heparin is stopped and warfarin is continued as monotherapy. Long-term LMWH may be preferable to warfarin in patients with cancer or those whose INR is difficult to control. Alternatives to warfarin may include the oral factor Xa inhibitors rivaroxaban, apixaban, or edoxaban, or dabigatran, a direct oral thrombin inhibitor. These new

anticoagulants are noninferior to warfarin, do not require periodic lab monitoring, and have a relatively low bleeding risk. They are preferred agents for extended treatment of venous thromboembolism if cost is not a significant issue.

- Outpatient treatment of DVT is appropriate for patients without thrombophilic conditions or substantial comorbidity. Exclusions from outpatient treatment of DVT include patients with potential high complication risk (e.g., hemoglobin <7, platelet count <75,000, guaiac-positive stool, recent cerebrovascular accident or noncutaneous surgery, noncompliance).
- Compression stockings are effective in reducing the incidence of postthrombotic syndrome and should be used starting within 1 mo of proximal DVT and continued for at least 1 yr after diagnosis.
- Insertion of an inferior vena cava filter to prevent pulmonary embolism is recommended in patients with contraindications to anticoagulation (e.g., hemorrhagic stroke, active internal bleeding, pregnancy), HIT in a patient with an active VTE/PE, recurrent PE despite adequate anticoagulant therapy, emergent surgery in patient with DVT, presence of free-floating iliofemoral thrombus, lower IVC thrombosis (incipient embolization), and chronic pulmonary (thromboembolic) hypertension with limited pulmonary reserve.
- Thrombolytic therapy (streptokinase) can be used in rare cases (unless contraindicated) in patients with extensive iliofemoral venous thrombosis and a low risk of bleeding. There are concerns about hemorrhagic complications related to the large doses of thrombolytics required in systemic thrombolysis for DVT (2% to 10% risk of major hemorrhagic complications).
- Other treatment modalities for DVT include surgical thrombectomy and catheter-directed thrombolysis (CDT). Thromboreduction by surgical thrombectomy is effective but invasive and expensive. CDT is also invasive, carries a bleeding risk, and will generally require ICU admission.

CHRONIC Rx

- The optimal duration of anticoagulant therapy varies with the cause of DVT and the patient's risk factors. The risk of recurrence is low if VTE is provoked by surgery, intermediate if provoked by a nonsurgical risk factor, and high if unprovoked. These risks should determine whether patients with VTE should undergo short-term vs. indefinite treatment.
- Therapy for 3 mo is generally satisfactory in patients with reversible risk factors (low-risk group). A high D-dimer level measured after 3 mo of anticoagulation in patients with unprovoked DVT should favor a longer duration of therapy. The American College of Chest Physicians Guidelines suggests that patients with first unprovoked VTE receive indefinite anticoagulation unless their bleeding risk is high.
- The risk of recurrence in patients with a first unprovoked VTE who have negative D-dimer results is not low enough to justify stopping

anticoagulant therapy in men but may be low enough in some cases to justify stopping therapy in women who were taking estrogen at the time of initial VTE.[1]

- Anticoagulation for 6 mo is recommended for patients with idiopathic venous thrombosis or medical risk factors for DVT (intermediate-risk group). About 20% of patients with unprovoked venous thromboembolism have a recurrence within 2 yr after the withdrawal of oral anticoagulant therapy. Use of daily low-dose aspirin after discontinuation of anticoagulant treatment may provide a modest reduction in DVT risk.
- Indefinite anticoagulation is necessary in patients with DVT associated with active cancer; long-term anticoagulation is also indicated in patients with inherited thrombophilia (e.g., deficiency of antithrombin III, protein C or S antibody), high factor VIII levels, antiphospholipid antibody, and those with recurrent episodes of idiopathic DVT (high-risk group). Long-term anticoagulation should also be considered in the presence of comorbidities such as paroxysmal nocturnal hemoglobinuria (PNH), SLE (especially with nephrotic syndrome), some myeloproliferative disorders, IBD, and Cushing's syndrome.
- Measurement of D-dimer after withdrawal of oral anticoagulation may be useful to estimate the risk of recurrence in selected patients. In patients with a first unprovoked DVT, positive D-dimer test results after cessation of anticoagulation predict recurrence, regardless of test timing or patient's age. Patients with a first spontaneous DVT and a D-dimer level <250 mg/ml after withdrawal of oral anticoagulation have a low risk of DVT recurrence. Risk is lower in women than in men. In patients who have completed at least 3 mo of anticoagulation for a first episode of unprovoked DVT and after approximately 2 yr of follow-up, a negative D-dimer result is associated with a 3.5% annual risk of recurrent disease, whereas a positive D-dimer result is associated with an 8.9% annual risk for recurrence. Hence, elevated D-dimer levels would be an indication for prolonged therapy (for 1 or 2 more yr at a minimum).
- The presence of residual thrombosis on ultrasonography when warfarin therapy is discontinued is also associated with an increased risk for subsequent recurrent DVT; a recent trial showed that tailoring the duration of anticoagulation on the basis of the persistence of residual thrombi on ultrasonography may reduce the rate of recurrent DVT. Additional trials are needed before this approach can be adapted for all patients.
- Patients with DVT and pulmonary embolism are at high risk of recurrence whenever anticoagulation is discontinued; therefore, many experts recommend prolonged anticoagulation in this population group, especially if other risk factors for recurrence are present.

[1]Kearon C, et al: D-Dimer testing to select patients with a first unprovoked venous thromboembolism who can stop anticoagulant therapy: A cohort study. *Ann Intern Med* 162:27–34, 2015.

D

Diseases and Disorders

I

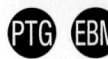

PEARLS & CONSIDERATIONS

COMMENTS

- The prevalence of occult cancer is low among patients with a first unprovoked venous embolism. Routine screening with CT of the abdomen and pelvis does not provide a clinically significant benefit.[2]
- When using heparin, there is a risk of heparin-induced thrombocytopenia (HIT) (with unfractionated more so than with LMWH). Platelet count should be obtained initially and repeated every 3 days while on heparin.
- **ISOLATED DEEP VEIN THROMBOSIS OF THE CALF:** The American College of Chest Physicians Guidelines suggest (1) anticoagulation in patients with severe symptoms or risk factors for proximal extension, and (2) repeat sonogram in 2 weeks in lower risk patients and anticoagulation only in those patients whose DVTs extend proximally.
- **PROPHYLAXIS OF DVT** Recommended in all patients at risk (e.g., low-molecular-weight heparin [enoxaparin 30 mg SC bid or fondaparinux 2.5 mg SC daily] after major trauma, postsurgery of hip and knee; enoxaparin 40 mg SC qd post-abdominal surgery in patients with moderate to high DVT risk; gradient elastic stockings alone or in combination with intermittent pneumatic compression [IPC] boots following neurosurgery). Graduated compression stockings (GCSs) are effective for preventing air-travel-related DVT and in reducing the risk of DVT in patients hospitalized for conditions other than stroke. The type of GCSs is also important because proximal DVT occurs more often in patients with stroke who wear below-knee stockings than in those who wear high-length stockings. The new oral anticoagulants (rivaroxaban, apixaban, etc.) are effective for thromboprophylaxis after THR and TKR. However, their clinical benefits over LMWH are marginal, they are more expensive, and they lack antidotes for timely reversal in case of bleeding.
- **RECURRENT THROMBOEMBOLISM:** The risk of recurrent venous thromboembolism in heterozygous carriers of factor V Leiden and a first spontaneous venous thromboembolism is similar to that of non-carriers of factor V Leiden; therefore, heterozygous patients should receive secondary thromboprophylaxis for a similar length of time as patients without factor V Leiden.
- **POSTTHROMBOTIC SYNDROME:**
  Approximately 20% to 50% of patients with DVT develop postthrombotic syndrome characterized by leg edema, pain, venous ectasia, skin induration, and ulceration. Patients with extensive DVT and those with more severe postthrombotic manifestations 1 month after DVT have poorer long-term outcomes. Recent trials have shown that compression

stockings after DVT do not prevent postthrombotic syndrome.

- Exercise following DVT is reasonable because it improves flexibility of the affected leg and does not increase symptoms in patients with postthrombotic syndrome.
- Previously undiagnosed cancer is frequent in patients with newly diagnosed DVT. A cancer screening strategy should be considered in all patients with unprovoked venous thromboembolism.
- **UPPER EXTREMITY DVT:** It is less common than lower extremity DVT and is seen more frequently in patients requiring central venous catheters or wires. It confers risk for mortality, recurrent thromboembolic events, and postthrombotic syndrome similar to that of lower extremity DVT. It is classified as primary upper extremity DVT **(Paget-Schroetter syndrome)**, defined as a thrombus in the axillary and subclavian veins in absence of identifiable thrombosis risk factors. It accounts for 20% of upper extremity DVT cases and may be due to an underlying anatomic abnormality at the thoracic outlet in combination with local hypercoagulability due to venous stretching or perivascular fibrosis from recurrent venous compression. Secondary upper extremity DVT is defined as any DVT related to a predisposing factor (e.g., insertion of central venous catheter, wires, or other devices, malignancy). In patients with secondary upper extremity DVT removal of the catheter is not routinely recommended but is warranted if there is a catheter malfunction or infection, if anticoagulation therapy is contraindicated or has failed, or if the catheter is no longer needed. Anticoagulation therapy in upper extremity DVT consists of use of vitamin K antagonists except in patients with cancer, for whom low-molecular-weight heparin is preferred. Optimal duration of anticoagulation treatment in upper extremity DVT is 3 to 6 mo (including in those in whom a central catheter has been removed).
- **DVT THERAPY IN PREGNANCY**
  Vitamin K antagonists such as warfarin are contraindicated in pregnancy. Low-molecular-weight heparins are safe and effective. Typical agents used in pregnancy include dalteparin (200 IU per kilogram of body weight daily or 100 IU per kilogram twice daily) or enoxaparin (1.5 mg per kilogram daily or 1 mg per kilogram twice daily).
- **REVERSAL OF ANTICOAGULATION:-**
  Vitamin K (1 mg PO or 2 mg IV) can be used to reverse elevated INR (3 to 6) from warfarin when elective or urgent procedures are needed. The administration of vitamin K can take more than 24 hr to fully restore vitamin K dependent coagulation factors II, VII, IX, and X. The American College of Chest Physicians recommends the following guidelines for managing elevated INRs or bleeding in patients receiving vitamin A antagonist therapy:
  1. INR between 4.5 and 10 and no significant bleeding: omit dose and monitor the

next day, routine use of vitamin K is not recommended
  2. INR >10 and no significant bleeding: hold vitamin K antagonist, give 5 to 10 mg orally of vitamin K. Monitor the next day and use additional vitamin K if necessary. Resume therapy at lower dose when INR therapeutic.
  3. Serious bleeding at any elevation of INR: hold vitamin K antagonist and supplement with prothrombin complex concentrates (PCC). Give vitamin K (10 mg by slow IV infusion over 30 min to reduce the risk of anaphylaxis). Vitamin K1 can be repeated every 12 hr. PCC composition in the United States (3-factor PCC) includes clotting factors II, IX, and X but minimal amounts of factor VII (unlike PCC products available outside of the United States [4-factor PCC], which have a significant amount of factor VII). In order to replace the low factor VII some clinicians in the United States will also give fresh frozen plasma (FFP) in addition to vitamin K and PCC in patients with life-threatening warfarin-related bleeding.
- **SPECIFIC REVERSAL AGENTS FOR NON–VITAMIN K ANTAGONIST ANTICOAGULANTS**
  - Idarucizumab, an antibody fragment given at a dose of 5 g IV, has been shown to completely reverse the anticoagulant effect of dabigatran within minutes.[3]
  - The anticoagulant activity of factor Xa inhibitors apixaban, rivaroxaban, and edoxaban can be rapidly reversed with IV administration of andexanet alfa.[4]

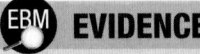 **EVIDENCE**

Available at www.expertconsult.com

SUGGESTED READINGS

Available at www.expertconsult.com

RELATED CONTENT

Deep Vein Thrombosis (DVT) (Patient Information)
Antiphospholipid Antibody Syndrome (Related Key Topic)
Hypercoagulable State (Related Key Topic)
Postthrombotic Syndrome (Related Key Topic)
Pulmonary Embolism (Related Key Topic)
Upper Extremity Deep Vein Thrombosis (Related Key Topic)

AUTHOR: **FRED F. FERRI, M.D.**

[2]Carrier M, Lazo-Langner A, Shivakumar S et al: Screening for occult cancer in unprovoked venous thromboembolism, N Engl J Med 373:697-704, 2015

[3]Pollack CV, Reilly PA, Eikleboom J et al: Idarucizumab for dabigatran reversal, N Engl J Med 373:511-20, 2015
[4]Siegal DM, et al.: Andexanet Alfa for the Reversal of Factor Xa Inhibitor Activity, N Engl J Med 373:2413-2424, 2015.

BASIC INFORMATION

DEFINITION

Delayed puberty is clinically defined as the absence of or incomplete development of secondary sexual characteristics by an age at which 95% of the population begins to mature sexually. For girls, a delay is defined as an absence of breast development by age 13 or primary amenorrhea by age 16. For boys, a delay is classified as an absence of testicular enlargement by age 14.

SYNONYMS

Pubertal delay

ICD-10CM CODES
E30.0 Delayed puberty

EPIDEMIOLOGY & DEMOGRAPHICS

PREVALENCE: The actual prevalence and incidence for children presenting with delayed puberty is unknown. Delayed puberty is more common in boys.
GENETICS: Constitutional pubertal delay (CPD) often runs in families. Although specific gene mutations have yet to be identified, studies have shown that 50% to 75% of patients with CPD have at least one parent who experienced a delay in puberty. The inheritance pattern for CPD is thought to be autosomal dominant.

PHYSICAL FINDINGS & CLINICAL PRESENTATION

- Girls with pubertal delay have an absence of breast development by age 13, absence of menarche by age 16, or absence of menarche within 3 years of thelarche. Boys with pubertal delay show no evidence of testicular enlargement, further defined as testes <2.5 cm, by age 14. Absence of pubic and/or axillary hair is common, as is lack of growth spurt.
- Patients with a constitutional delay in puberty are short in stature with a normal growth rate and otherwise good health.
- Boys often fall below the 10th percentile on a height chart with normal rate of growth between 4 and 6 cm per yr.

ETIOLOGY

Causes for pubertal delay (Fig. 1) can be separated into four categories (from most to least common):
1. Constitutional delay, which is a temporary delay in puberty that is seen mostly in boys and is genetic. Patients are typically short in stature with normal growth rate and appropriate skeletal age.
2. Functional hypogonadotropic hypogonadism secondary to malnutrition or chronic disease. Celiac sprue, inflammatory bowel disease (IBD), hypothyroidism, diabetes mellitus, cystic fibrosis, and eating disorders such as anorexia nervosa are examples of illnesses that may cause a temporary, reversible delay

in puberty. Clinical suspicion is warranted when underweight children present with pubertal delay.
3. Hypergonadotropic hypogonadism caused by primary gonadal failure. Congenital disorders such as cryptorchidism; chromosomal disorders such as gonadal dysgenesis, Klinefelter's syndrome, and Turner's syndrome; and acquired causes secondary to chemotherapy, pelvic radiation, and gonadal surgery are organic dysfunctions that result in gonadal failure despite adequate hypothalamic-pituitary function. In this group of disorders, luteinizing hormone (LH) and follicle-stimulating hormone (FSH) levels are elevated yet cannot stimulate ovaries and testicles to produce estrogen and testosterone, respectively, leading to hypogonadism and absence of secondary sex characteristics.
4. Permanent hypogonadotropic hypogonadism secondary to genetic or acquired defects along the hypothalamic-pituitary-gonadal (HPG) axis. Kallmann's syndrome is a genetic mutation in *KAL1* on the X chromosome and is responsible for the migration of gonadotropin-releasing hormone and olfactory neurons into the hypothalamus. Children with Kallmann's syndrome typically present with pubertal delay and anosmia. Other mutations

such as *FGFR1* and *DAX1* have been linked to congenital gonadotropin deficiencies and pubertal delay. Acquired defects such as hemochromatosis, sickle cell anemia, and pituitary tumors can cause delayed puberty and other hypothalamic syndromes, including Prader-Willi. Table E1 provides a classification of puberty and sexual infantilism.

DIAGNOSIS

DIFFERENTIAL DIAGNOSIS

Normal or low serum LH and FSH
- Constitutional pubertal delay
- Functional hypogonadotropic hypogonadism
  1. Malnutrition or eating disorder
  2. Strenuous exercise
  3. Chronic illness (e.g., hypothyroidism, celiac disease, IBD, cystic fibrosis)
- Hypopituitarism
  1. Panhypopituitarism
  2. Isolated gonadotropin deficiency
  3. Kallmann's syndrome (associated with anosmia)
  4. Prader-Willi syndrome
- Hyperprolactinemia
  1. Pituitary adenoma
  2. Drug-associated (e.g., cannabis, cocaine)

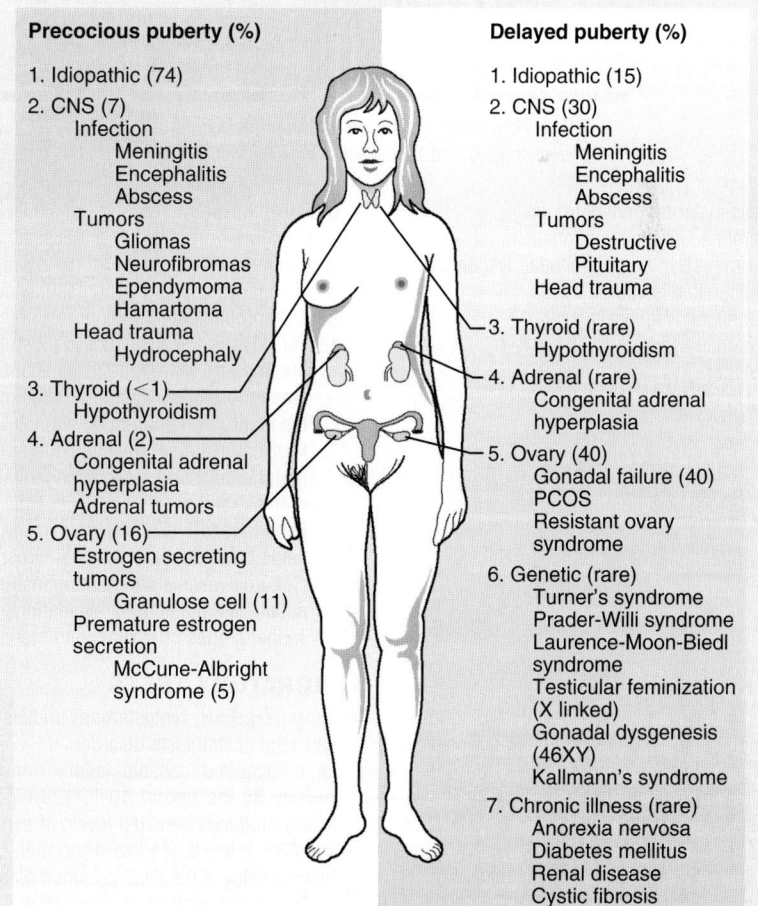

Precocious puberty (%)	Delayed puberty (%)
1. Idiopathic (74)	1. Idiopathic (15)

2. CNS (7)
Infection
  Meningitis
  Encephalitis
  Abscess
Tumors
  Gliomas
  Neurofibromas
  Ependymoma
  Hamartoma
Head trauma
Hydrocephaly
	2. CNS (30)
	Infection
	  Meningitis
	  Encephalitis
	  Abscess
	Tumors
	  Destructive
	  Pituitary
	Head trauma

3. Thyroid (<1) Hypothyroidism	3. Thyroid (rare) Hypothyroidism
4. Adrenal (2) Congenital adrenal hyperplasia Adrenal tumors	4. Adrenal (rare) Congenital adrenal hyperplasia

5. Ovary (16)
Estrogen secreting
tumors
  Granulose cell (11)
Premature estrogen
secretion
  McCune-Albright
  syndrome (5)
	5. Ovary (40)
	Gonadal failure (40)
	PCOS
	Resistant ovary
	syndrome

	6. Genetic (rare) Turner's syndrome Prader-Willi syndrome Laurence-Moon-Biedl syndrome Testicular feminization (X linked) Gonadal dysgenesis (46XY) Kallmann's syndrome
	7. Chronic illness (rare) Anorexia nervosa Diabetes mellitus Renal disease Cystic fibrosis

FIG. 1 Causes of precocious puberty and delayed puberty. (From Pariseai M: Gynaecological endocrinology. In *Obstetrics and gynaecology*, St. Louis, 2008, Mosby.)

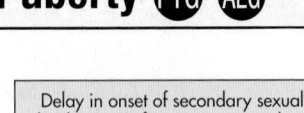

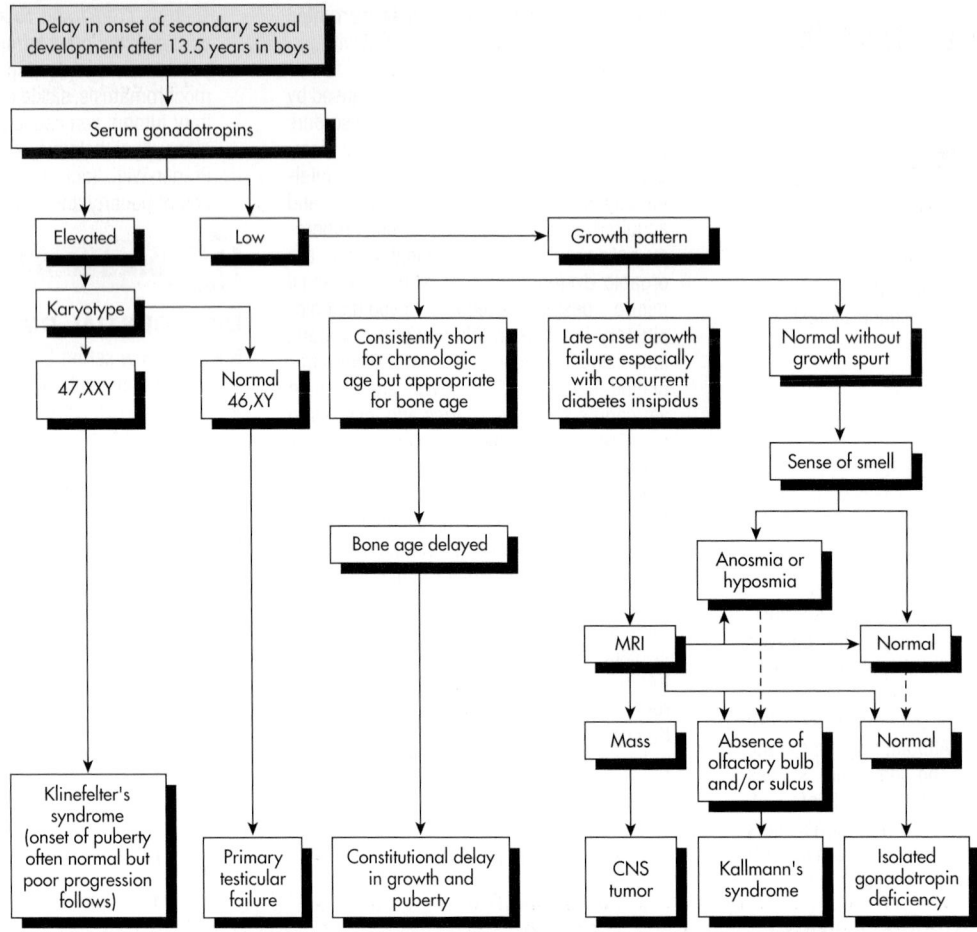

FIG. 2 Flow chart for the evaluation of delayed puberty in boys. (From Melmed S et al: *Williams textbook of endocrinology*, ed 12, Philadelphia, 2011, Saunders.)

Increased serum gonadotropins
- Hypergonadotropic hypogonadism
  1. Turner's syndrome (gonadal dysgenesis)
  2. Klinefelter's syndrome
  3. Gonadal dysgenesis
  4. Noonan syndrome
  5. Bilateral gonadal failure
     1. Primary testicular failure
     2. Anorchia
     3. Premature ovarian failure
     4. Resistant ovary syndrome
     5. Radiation, chemotherapy
     6. Trauma
     7. Infections (e.g., mumps, orchitis)
  Other conditions
- Androgen sensitivity syndrome
- Steroidogenic enzyme defects

WORKUP

- Given the extensive differential diagnosis for pubertal delay, a systematic and focused approach is necessary. Table E2 describes differential diagnostic features of delayed puberty and sexual infantilism. A careful history, including family and social history, can identify eating, exercise habits, chronic illnesses, weight loss, poor weight gain, changes in bowel habits, and parental history of pubertal delay. Figs. 2 and 3 describe an algorithm for the evaluation of delayed puberty in males and females.

- Growth measurement should include height and weight, a growth chart to assess rate of growth, and calculation of the sex-adjusted midparental height that represents the statistically probable adult height for the child.
  1. For boys, add 2.5 inches (6.5 cm) from the mean of the parents' heights. For girls, subtract 2.5 inches (6.5 cm) from the mean of the parents' heights.
  2. Physical exam can reveal signs of sexual maturation, stigmata of congenital syndromes, and nutritional deficiencies. It is important to include a neurologic (visual fields, ophthalmologic), thyroid, respiratory, cardiovascular, and abdominal examination, in addition to evaluation of the Tanner stages of sexual characteristics.

LABORATORY TESTS

- Serum LH, FSH, testosterone, and estradiol can help distinguish disorders of congenital or acquired gonadal failure from other causes. By the age of 10 to 12 yr gonadal failure produces elevated levels of serum LH and FSH. If levels are low or normal, constitutional delay is the most common diagnosis.
- Chromosomal analysis is indicated if there is a suspicion of gonadal dysgenesis or Klinefelter's syndrome.
- Screening studies include complete blood count, erythrocyte sedimentation rate, prolactin, thyroid-stimulating hormone, and free thyroxine level.
- Endocrinologist may incorporate further studies such as IGF-1 to screen for growth hormone disorders and GnRH stimulation testing.

IMAGING STUDIES

Bone age skeletal radiograph of the left hand and wrist determines skeletal age, which is delayed in constitutional delay and GnRH deficiency. MRI of the head should be considered if there is high clinical suspicion for tumors of pituitary or hypothalamic origin. Pelvic ultrasound can be helpful in detecting intraabdominal testes and evaluating müllerian anatomy.

Rx TREATMENT

- Treat underlying cause.
- Constitutional delay can be managed with reassurance that the delay will have no effect on the final adult height or overall development. Short-term hormonal therapy can be used to hasten puberty if the delay is causing severe psychosocial difficulties. Oxandrolone orally can be given daily or IM depot testosterone q6wk for 3-6 mo for boys to improve velocity of growth. Girls can receive oral estradiol once daily for 3-6 mo.

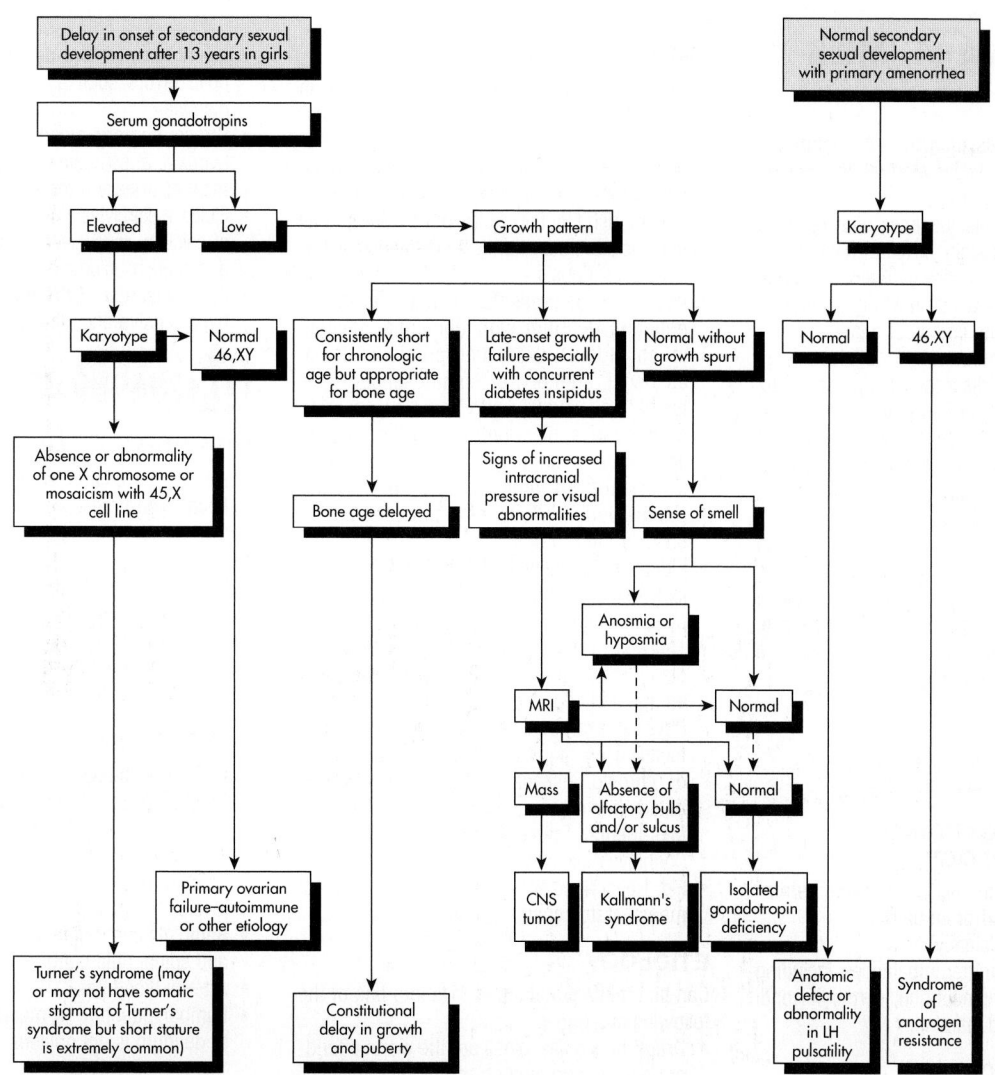

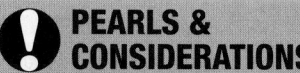

FIG. 3 Flow chart for the evaluation of delayed puberty in girls. (From Melmed S et al: *Williams textbook of endocrinology*, ed 12, Philadelphia, 2011, Saunders.)

- Malnutrition and chronic disease can best be treated by correcting the underlying etiology. A short (3-6 mo) treatment course, as described above, may be indicated for children with psychosocial difficulties.
- Permanent causes of pubertal delay can be treated by inducing puberty with testosterone for boys and estrogen plus progesterone for girls.
- Patients with Turner's syndrome will need adjunct growth hormone with or without oxandrolone.
- Gonadotropin deficiency or hypogonadism may require lifelong sex steroid replacement.
- Psychosocial evaluation, support, and treatment as needed.
- Table E3 summarizes the management and treatment of delayed puberty.

REFERRAL

Pediatric endocrinology

❗ PEARLS & CONSIDERATIONS

COMMENTS

- Constitutional delay is the most common cause of pubertal delay and is often associated with a positive family history in parents and/or siblings, but it is a diagnosis of exclusion, so other causes, such as Turner's syndrome and systemic disorders, need to be ruled out first.
- Bone age demonstrates more clearly than chronologic age how far an individual has progressed toward maturity and predicts the potential for further growth.
- No studies reliably differentiate constitutional delay from gonadotropin deficiency.

PATIENT & FAMILY EDUCATION

- The Magic Foundation, a support group for patients and their families (http://www.magicfoundation.org)

- The American Academy of Family Physicians (http://www.aafp.org)
- American Academy of Pediatrics (http://www.aap.org)
- Pediatric Endocrine Society (http://www.lwpes.org)
- Nemours Foundation (kiddshealth.rog/teen/sexual_health/changing_body/puberty)
- www.noonansyndrome.org

SUGGESTED READINGS

Available at www.expertconsult.com

RELATED CONTENT

Delayed Puberty (Patient Information)

AUTHORS: **STEPHANIE A. CURRY, M.D.,** and **RACHAEL M. BIANCUZZO, D.O.**

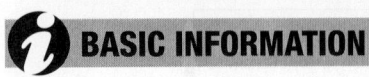

BASIC INFORMATION

DEFINITION

The American Psychiatric Association's *Diagnostic and Statistical Manual*, 5th edition (DSM-5) defines delirium as:
- Disturbance of consciousness with reduced ability to focus, sustain, or shift attention.
- The disturbance develops over a short period of time (usually hours to days) and tends to fluctuate during the course of a day.
- An additional disturbance in cognition (e.g., memory deficit, disorganization, language, visuospatial ability, or perception).
- A change in cognition or development of a perceptual disturbance that is not better accounted for by a preexisting, established, or evolving dementia.
- There is evidence from history, physical exam, or lab findings that the disturbance is caused by medical condition, substance intoxication or withdrawal (i.e., due to a drug of abuse or to a medication), or exposure to a toxin, or is due to multiple etiologies.

SYNONYMS

Acute confusional state
Toxic or metabolic encephalopathy

THEORIES REGARDING PATHOPHYSIOLOGY

- Neuroinflammation, with increased permeability of the blood-brain barrier.
- Acetylcholine deficiency.
- Other neurotransmitter imbalances, including excesses of norepinephrine, serotonin, and, most important, dopamine.

CLASSIFICATION

Hyperactive, hypoactive, and mixed subtype.

ICD-10CM CODES
F05	Delirium, not induced by alcohol and other psychoactive substances
F05.9	Delirium, unspecified
F06.0	Organic hallucinosis
F05.8	Other delirium
F05.0	Delirium not superimposed on dementia
F05.1	Delirium superimposed on dementia

EPIDEMIOLOGY & DEMOGRAPHICS

Nearly 30% of older patients experience delirium at some time during the hospital course. In old surgical patients, the risk varies from 10% to 50%. Hypoactive is more common. Delirium is the most common mental disorder in patients with medical illness. Any age, race, or gender can be affected. Pediatric delirium is often missed but remains important because delirium is associated with longer hospital stays, decreased cognitive performance, and increased mortality. Risk factors include extremes of age, severe pain, illicit substance use, surgery, dementia, and kidney or liver failure (Tables E1 and 2).

PHYSICAL FINDINGS & CLINICAL PRESENTATION

- One of the earliest symptoms is change in level of awareness and ability to focus, sustain, or shift attention. Symptoms may differ both among patients and within one patient. Family members or caregivers report that the patient "isn't acting quite right." Symptoms may include poor attention, sleepiness, agitation, or psychosis.
- Acuteness of presentation helps in differentiating delirium with dementia. Change in cognition, perceptual problems (such as visual, auditory, or somatosensory hallucination usually with lack of insight), memory loss, disorientation, difficulty with speech and language. It is important to ascertain from family member or caregivers the patient's level of functioning before onset of delirium.
- Elderly patients with delirium often do not look sick, but patients with delirium are sick by definition.
- There is often a prodrome phase that later blends into hypoactive delirium or erupts into an agitated confusional state.
- Physical examination should be performed, focusing on signs of infection, dehydration, or chronic disease that may be exacerbated. Vital signs are key. Consider using the Mini-Mental Status Exam or the Montreal Cognitive Assessment.
- Fig. 1 describes an algorithm for evaluation of mental status changes in an older patient.

ETIOLOGY

Can be multifactorial; often falls into one of the following categories:
- Drugs: benzodiazepines are the worst offenders, but other drugs such as narcotics, anticholinergics, beta-blockers, steroids, nonsteroidal antiinflammatory drugs, digoxin, cimetidine can cause delirium; also, withdrawal states such as alcohol withdrawal or benzodiazepine withdrawal can cause delirium.
- Infection or inflammation.
- Metabolic: kidney or liver failure, thyroid, adrenal, or glucose dysregulation, anemia, vitamin deficiency such as Wernicke's encephalopathy or vitamin B_{12} deficiency, inborn metabolic errors such as porphyrias or Wilson's disease.
- Stress: surgery, sleep problems, pain, fever, hypoxia, anesthesia, environmental changes, fecal or urinary retention, burns.
- Fluids, electrolytes, nutrition (FEN): dysregulation of calcium, magnesium, potassium, or sodium; dehydration; volume overload; altered pH.
- Brain disorder: CNS infection, head injury, hypertensive encephalopathy.

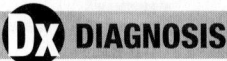

DIAGNOSIS

DIFFERENTIAL DIAGNOSIS

- Primary psychiatric illness.
- Focal syndromes.
- Dementia.
- Sundowning.
- Nonconvulsive status epilepticus.

Remember, delirium may coexist with any of the above. Table 3 describes clinical factors that help differentiate delirium and dementia from psychiatric disease.

LABORATORY TESTS

- Complete blood count, electrolytes, liver function tests, ammonia, drug levels (digoxin, lithium).
- Toxicology screen, urinalysis, urine culture.
- Thyroid function tests, vitamin B_{12}, and folate levels.
- Rapid plasma reagin for syphilis, blood, urine, and spinal fluid culture.
- Arterial blood gas.
- Lumbar puncture is mandatory when cause of delirium is not obvious.

IMAGING STUDIES

- Consider head CT (to look for bleed, trauma, tumor, atrophy, dementia, stroke)
- Chest radiograph (to look for tumor, infection).

ELECTROENCEPHALOGRAM

- To exclude seizure, confirm diagnosis of metabolic encephalopathy.

TABLE 2 Mnemonic for Risk Factors for Delirium and Agitation

Iwatchdeath	Delirium
Infection	**D**rugs
Withdrawal	**E**lectrolyte and physiologic abnormalities
Acute metabolic	**L**ack of drugs (withdrawal)
Trauma/pain	**I**nfection
Central nervous system pathology	**R**educed sensory input (blindness, deafness)
Hypoxia	**I**ntracranial problems (CVA, meningitis, seizure)
Deficiencies (vitamin B_{12}, thiamine)	**U**rinary retention and fecal impaction
Endocrinopathies (thyroid, adrenal)	**M**yocardial problems (MI, arrhythmia, CHF)
Acute vascular (hypertension, shock)	
Toxins/drugs	
Heavy metals	

CHF, Congestive heart failure; *CVA,* cerebrovascular accident; *MI,* myocardial infarction.
From Vincent JL et al: *Textbook of critical care,* ed 6, Philadelphia, 2011, Saunders.

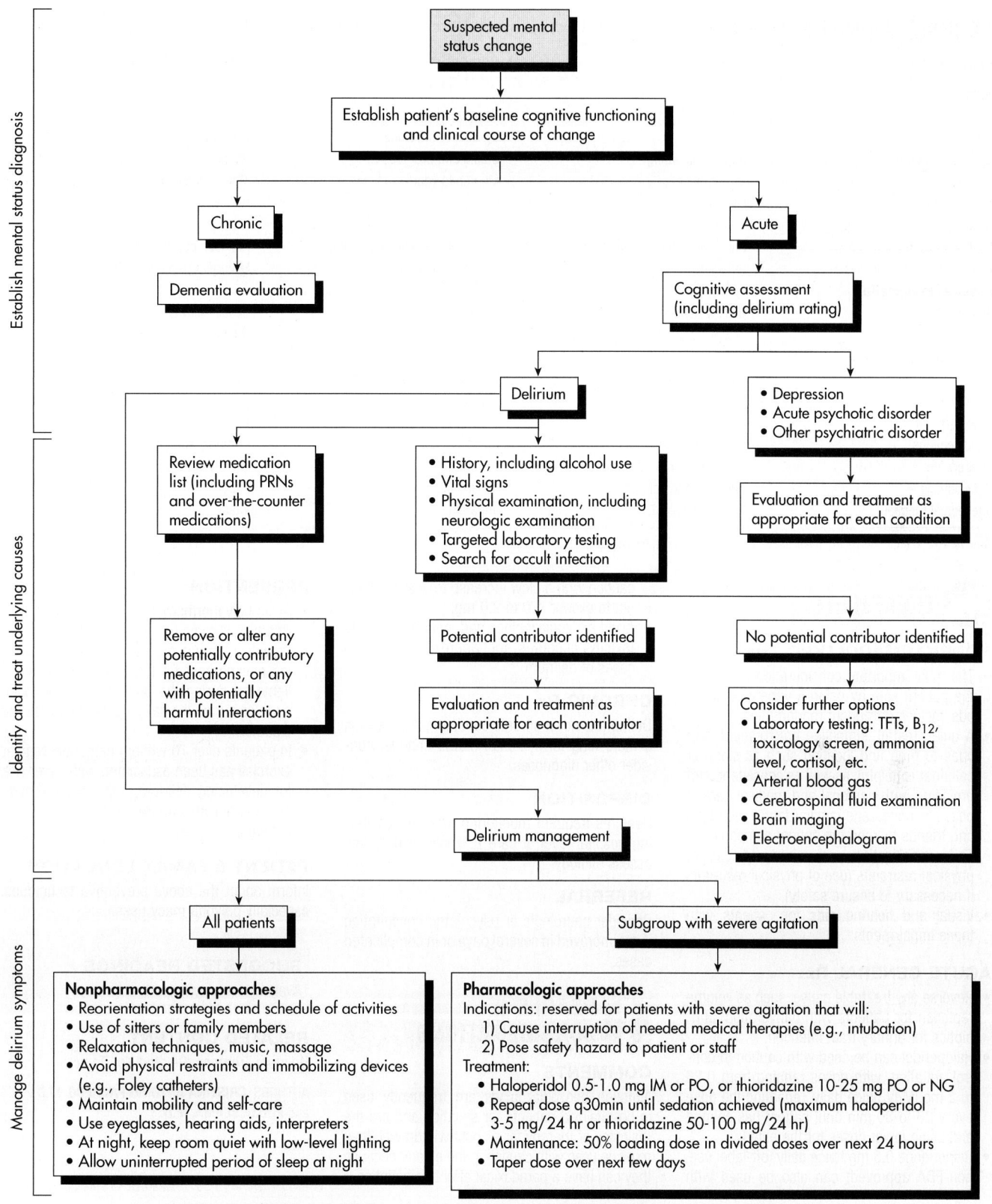

FIG. 1 Algorithm for evaluation of suspected mental status change in an older patient. *IM*, Intramuscular; *NG*, nasogastric; *PO*, by mouth; *PRN*, as needed; *TFTs*, thyroid function tests. (From Goldman L, Ausiello D [eds]: *Cecil textbook of medicine*, ed 24, Philadelphia, 2012, Saunders.)

TABLE 3 Clinical Factors That Help Differentiate Delirium and Dementia from Psychiatric Disease

Characteristic	Delirium	Dementia	Psychiatric Illness
Symptoms			
Age at onset	<12 or >40 yr	Usually elderly, >50 yr	13-40 yr
Onset	Acute	Gradual or insidious	Gradual
Symptom course	Rapid, fluctuating	Stable and progressive	Stable
Duration	Days to weeks	Months to years	Months to years
Reversibility	Usually	Rarely	Rarely
History			
Past medical history	Substance abuse, medical illness	Comorbid conditions of aging	Previous psychiatric history
Family history	Unusual	History of dementia	History of psychiatric illness
Physical Examination			
Vital signs	Usually abnormal	Usually normal	Usually normal
Involuntary activity	May have tremors, asterixis, etc.	None unless coexistent disease	None
Mental Status			
Affect	Emotional lability	Flat affect with advanced disease	Flat affect
Orientation	Usually impaired	Impaired with advanced disease	Rarely impaired
Attention	Impaired	Slow to focus	Disorganized
Hallucinations	Primarily visual	Rare	Primarily auditory
Speech	Slow, incoherent, dysarthric	Usually coherent	Usually coherent
Consciousness	Decreased to impaired	Normal (clear)	Alert
Intellectual function	Usually impaired	Impaired	Intact

From Adams JG et al: *Emergency medicine, clinical essentials*, ed 2, Philadelphia, 2013, Elsevier.

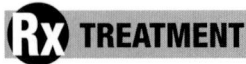 **TREATMENT**

NONPHARMACOLOGIC THERAPY

- The most important consideration is to keep the patient safe by using a variety of methods, including frequent reorientation.
- A quiet, restful, simplified environment with cues to time and location such as clock or calendar is helpful, as well as consistent staff providing both personal and medical care. If possible, encourage familiar family members and friends to keep the patient company.
- Early mobilization and minimized use of physical restraints (use of physical restraints if necessary to ensure safety).
- Visual and hearing aids for patients with these impairments.

ACUTE GENERAL Rx

- Reverse any treatable cause, such as volume repletion for patients with dehydration, antibiotics for urinary tract infection.
- Haloperidol can be used with caution to control agitation, with doses ranging from 0.25 to 2 mg IM/IV twice daily, repeating the dose every 20 to 30 min until patient has calmed and using lower doses for the elderly.
- Risperidone 0.5 mg twice daily (off-label use, non-FDA approved) can also be used with caution with a slow increase to desired dose, not to exceed 1.0 to 2.0 mg.
- Avoid benzodiazepines and meperidine. Drug toxicity accounts for approximately 30% cases of delirium.

CHRONIC Rx

Delirium is not a chronic condition; if assessing a more long-term mental status change, consider other diagnoses.

DISPOSITION

Requires frequent monitoring often necessitating hospital level of care to ensure safety and assess etiology.

REFERRAL

Consider neurologic or psychiatric consultation if not improved in several days or in complicated cases.

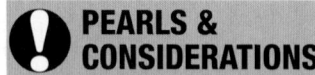 **PEARLS & CONSIDERATIONS**

COMMENTS

Although benzodiazepines are frequently used in hospitalized patients for sedation and are the mainstay of therapy for alcohol withdrawal, they must be used with caution in the elderly because they can have a paradoxical effect on agitation.

PREVENTION

- Avoid polypharmacy as much as possible.
- Optimize chronic medical conditions.
- Provide frequent reorientation and a soothing environment for high-risk patients (e.g., lights on during the day, off at night; open curtains during the day so patient can see the weather).
- In patients over 70 without dementia, regular exercise has been associated with lower risk for developing delirium, and early return to physical activity can improve outcomes in ill patients.

PATIENT & FAMILY EDUCATION

Inform about the above preventive techniques, especially polypharmacy risks.

SUGGESTED READINGS

Available at www.expertconsult.com

RELATED CONTENT

Delirium Tremens (Related Key Topic)

AUTHORS: **CRISTINA ANTONIO PACHECO, M.D.,** and **POOJA VERMA, M.D.**

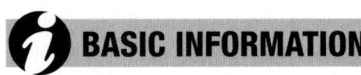

BASIC INFORMATION

DEFINITION

Delirium tremens, also known as withdrawal delirium, is overactivity of the central nervous system after cessation of alcohol intake. The time interval is variable; it usually occurs within 1 wk after reduction or cessation of heavy alcohol intake and persists for 1 to 3 days.

SYNONYMS

Withdrawal delirium
Alcohol withdrawal syndrome
DTs
Alcoholic delirium

ICD-10CM CODES
F10.231 Alcohol dependence with
withdrawal delirium

EPIDEMIOLOGY & DEMOGRAPHICS

INCIDENCE (IN U.S.): Up to 500,000 cases annually, 3% to 5% of patients who are hospitalized for alcohol withdrawal meet the criteria for withdrawal delirium
PEAK INCIDENCE: 30 yr and older
PREDOMINANT SEX: Male
PEAK AGE: Teenage years and older
GENETICS: More common with patients who have relatives who are alcoholics

PHYSICAL FINDINGS & CLINICAL PRESENTATION

- Ethanol withdrawal symptoms usually begin within 8 hours after blood alcohol levels decrease, peak at about 72 hours, and are markedly reduced by days 5 to 7 of abstinence.
- Initially: anxiety, insomnia, tremulousness
- Early: tachycardia, sweating, anorexia, agitation, headache, gastrointestinal distress
- Late: seizures, visual hallucinations, delirium

ETIOLOGY

Alcoholism

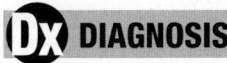

DIAGNOSIS

DIFFERENTIAL DIAGNOSIS

- Coexisting illness.
- Trauma.
- Drug use.

WORKUP

- Frequent rating of symptoms (hallucinations, tremor, sweating, agitation, orientation).
- The Clinical Institute Withdrawal Assessment-Alcohol (CIWA-A) scale can be used to measure the severity of alcohol withdrawal. It consists of the 10 following items:
  1. Nausea.
  2. Tremor.
  3. Autonomic hyperactivity.
  4. Anxiety.
  5. Agitation.
  6. Tactile disturbances.
  7. Visual disturbances.
  8. Auditory disturbances.
  9. Headache.
  10. Disorientation.

The maximum score is 67. Scores <8 indicate mild symptoms; scores 8-15 indicate moderate withdrawal symptoms; and scores >15 indicate severe withdrawal symptoms.

LABORATORY TESTS

- Electrolytes (including magnesium, phosphate).
- Close monitoring of glucose levels.
- Drug screen (blood and urine).

IMAGING STUDIES

CT scan of head if there is a history of head trauma.

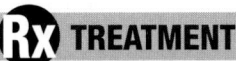

TREATMENT

NONPHARMACOLOGIC THERAPY

Refer to drug rehabilitation program after patient recovers.

ACUTE GENERAL Rx

- Admission to a detoxification unit where patient can be observed closely.
- Vital signs q30min initially (neurologic signs, if necessary).
- Use of lateral decubitus or prone position if restraints are necessary.
- Nothing by mouth: nasogastric tube for abdominal distention may be necessary but should not be routinely used.
- Vigorous hydration (4 to 6 L/day): IV with glucose (Na^+, K^+, PO_4^{-3}, and Mg^{2+} replacement). May be necessary in some patients but commonly there is little support for routine administration of magnesium. Use vigorous hydration with caution in patients with CHF.
- Vitamins: thiamine 500 mg infused IV over the course of 30 minutes daily for 3 days. The initial dose of thiamine should precede the administration of IV dextrose; multivitamins (may be added to the hydrating solution).
- Sedation (sedation can be achieved using fixed-dose regimen or individualized benzodiazepine administration [see CIWA-Ar score] in "Alcohol-Related Disorders"):
  1. Initially: lorazepam 8 mg IM/IV every 15 minutes as needed, after the patient has received 16 mg. If delirium is still severe, administer an 8 mg bolus IV, then administer 10-30 mg/hr.[1]
  2. Maintenance (individualized dosage): chlordiazepoxide, 50 to 100 mg PO q4 to 6h, lorazepam 2 mg PO q4h, or diazepam 5 to 10 mg PO tid; withhold doses or decrease subsequent doses if signs of oversedation are apparent.

---

[1]Schuckit MA: Recognition and management of withdrawal delirium (delirium tremens). *N Engl J Med* 371:2109-2113, 2014.

3. Midazolam is also effective for managing DTs. Its rapid onset (sedation within 2 to 4 min of IV injection) and short duration of action (approximately 30 min) make it an ideal agent for titration in continuous infusion.

- In addition to benzodiazepines, administer medications such as the antipsychotic agent haloperidol for uncontrolled agitation or hallucinations (0.5-5 mg IV/IM every 30-60 minutes as needed for severe agitation or hallucinations, not to exceed 20 mg).
- Treatment of seizures: diazepam 2.5 mg/min IV until seizure is controlled (check for respiratory depression or hypotension) may be beneficial for prolonged seizure activity; IV lorazepam 1 to 2 mg q2h can be used in place of diazepam. In general, withdrawal seizures are self-limited and treatment is not required; the use of phenytoin or other anticonvulsants for short-term treatment of alcohol withdrawal seizures is not recommended.
- Diagnosis and treatment of concomitant medical, surgical, or psychiatric conditions.

CHRONIC Rx

Alcoholics Anonymous has the best record in breaking addiction, but the results are still disappointing.

DISPOSITION

Refer to drug rehabilitation program.

REFERRAL

If cardiac arrhythmias are prominent or respiratory distress develops.

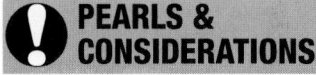

PEARLS & CONSIDERATIONS

COMMENTS

- This is a potentially lethal disease if not carefully treated. Mortality rate is 15% in untreated patients, and approximately 1% to 6% of hospitalized patients who have withdrawal delirium die.

SUGGESTED READINGS

Available at www.expertconsult.com

RELATED CONTENT

Delirium Tremens (Patient Information)
Alcohol Abuse (Related Key Topic)
Delirium (Related Key Topic)
Wernicke's Syndrome (Related Key Topic)

AUTHOR: **FRED F. FERRI, M.D.**

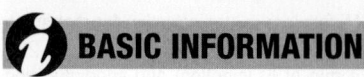

DEFINITION

Dementia with Lewy bodies (DLB) is a neurodegenerative dementia occurring concurrently with or within 1 year (either before or after) of the onset of parkinsonism. DLB also has other core features including fluctuations in attention and alertness and recurrent vivid visual hallucinations. Diagnostic criteria for dementia syndrome associated with Lewy body pathology are described in Box 1. Patients generally respond to cholinesterase inhibitors, are very sensitive to the adverse effects of neuroleptics, and compared with Parkinson's disease patients, are relatively unresponsive to L-dopa.

SYNONYMS

DLB
Lewy body dementia
Diffuse Lewy body disease
Lewy body type senile dementia
Cortical Lewy body disease

ICD-10CM CODES
G31.83 Dementia with Lewy bodies

EPIDEMIOLOGY & DEMOGRAPHICS

INCIDENCE: Accounts for 10% to 15% of all dementias. DLB is the second most common neurodegenerative cause of dementia after Alzheimer's disease.

PEAK INCIDENCE: Affects individuals in their sixth decade or older.

PREVALENCE: Estimated 0.7% of individuals older than age 65.

PREDOMINANT SEX AND AGE:
- Sex: Male predominance
- Mean age of onset: 75 years. On average, 10 years greater for dementia with Lewy bodies (DLB) than Parkinson's disease (PD).

GENETICS:
- Most cases are sporadic with a discordance among monozygotic twins, suggesting that either environmental or other epigenetic factors may play a major role in the incidence of DLB.
- Copy number variation of the alpha-synuclein gene (*SNCA*) has been reported in families with DLB. Rare autosomal dominant variants in *LRRK2* have also been reported. These genes are associated with Parkinson's disease and Parkinson's disease dementia in addition to DLB, suggesting a common molecular etiology with a spectrum of clinical phenotypes.
- The *APOE* ε4 allele has a higher prevalence in DLB than in control individuals, suggesting heightened disease risk conferred by the allele. Conversely, the *APOE* ε2 allele is enriched in control individuals, suggesting a neuroprotective role, or at least the lack of a deleterious effect, for the allele.
- Other factors include glucocerebrosidase genetic mutations, high prevalence of Lewy bodies with presenilin-1 mutations, and polymorphisms of the coding region for the synuclein genes.

RISK FACTORS:
- Male sex
- Advanced age

PHYSICAL FINDINGS & CLINICAL PRESENTATION
- Importance of recognizing DLB relates to its pharmacologic management, including responsiveness to cholinesterase inhibitors, sensitivity to the adverse effects of neuroleptics, and relative unresponsiveness to L-dopa.
- Onset of dementia is insidious, with core features of fluctuations in cognition, attention, and alertness; recurrent vivid visual hallucinations; and extrapyramidal motor symptoms, along with other features either suggestive or supportive of the clinical diagnosis. Refer to "Revised Criteria for the Clinical Diagnosis of Dementia with Lewy Bodies" (McKeith I et al, *Neurology*, 2005).
- Detailed neuropsychological assessment demonstrates a characteristic profile of impairments in visuoperceptual, attentional, and executive functions, with relative sparing of episodic memory (in contradistinction to Alzheimer's diseases, in which impairment in episodic memory is a hallmark), reflecting a combination of cortical and subcortical damage.

ETIOLOGY
- *SNCA* encodes for a protein normally found at the synapse with a role in vesicle production. In its insoluble form, SNCA aggregates into Lewy bodies found at the cortical and subcortical levels.

- Lewy bodies (Fig. 1) are round, eosinophilic, intracytoplasmic inclusions in the nuclei of neurons.
- Cortical Lewy bodies are found in deep cortical layers of the anterior frontal and temporal lobes, the cingulate gyrus, and insula.
- As in Parkinson's disease, Lewy bodies aggregate in the following structures: substantia nigra, locus coeruleus, raphe nuclei, nucleus basalis of Meynert, and brainstem nuclei.
- Fig. 2 shows the relationships among the subtypes of dementia.

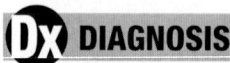

DIAGNOSIS

DIFFERENTIAL DIAGNOSIS
- Diagnosis of DLB when dementia occurs before or concurrently with extrapyramidal features—arbitrarily set as the "1-year rule" vs. Parkinson's disease with dementia, which occurs in the setting of well-established Parkinson's disease.
- Dementia: Alzheimer's disease (AD), vascular dementia.
- Parkinsonian features: Parkinson's disease dementia, progressive supranuclear palsy (PSP), multisystem atrophy (MSA), corticobasal syndrome (CBS).
- Rapidly progressive form: Creutzfeldt-Jakob disease (CJD). Lack of cerebellar signs and lack of typical MRI may help distinguish DLB from classic CJD (but not variant form of CJD).
- Psychiatric features: late-onset psychosis or depression with psychotic features.
- Hallucinations with fluctuations in consciousness: temporal lobe epilepsy (TLE) or delirium due to metabolic derangement.

BOX 1 Diagnostic Criteria for the Dementia Syndrome Associated With Lewy Body Pathology

The cognitive disturbance is of insidious onset and is progressive, based on evidence from the history or serial cognitive examination
The presence of at least two of the following:
    Parkinsonism (rigidity, resting tremor, bradykinesia, postural instability, parkinsonian gait disorder)
    Prominent, fully formed visual hallucinations
    Substantial fluctuations in alertness or cognition
    Rapid eye movement sleep behavior disorder
    Severe worsening of parkinsonism by antipsychotic drugs
    The disturbance is not better accounted for by a systemic disease or another brain disease

From Goldman L, Schafer AI: *Goldman's Cecil medicine,* ed 24, Philadelphia, 2012, Saunders.

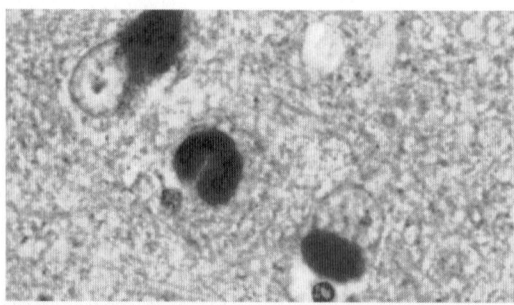

FIG. 1 Cortical Lewy bodies present in cerebral cortex, as opposed to Parkinson's disease without dementia, in which Lewy bodies are found in the substantia nigra. Immunostain for Alpha synuclein is characteristic for Lewy body immunohistological profile. (From MacDonald AB: Spirochetal cyst forms in neurodegenerative disorders, hiding in plain sight, *Medical Hypotheses* 67(4) 819–832, 2006.)

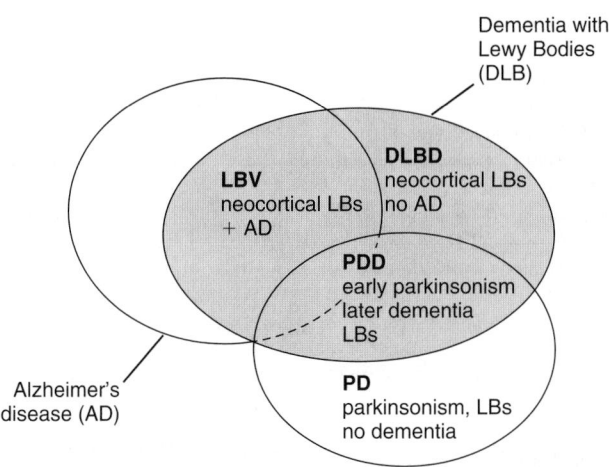

FIG. 2 Relationships among Alzheimer's disease (AD), the three subtypes of dementia with Lewy bodies (DLB), and Parkinson's disease (PD). Parkinsonism refers to the clinical symptoms of PD (hypokinesia, tremor, and muscular rigidity). *LBV*, Lewy body variant of Alzheimer's disease; *DLBD*, diffuse Lewy body disease; *PD*, Parkinson's disease; *PDD*, Parkinson's disease dementia; *LBs*, Lewy bodies. (From Lewis KA et al: Abnormal neurites containing C-terminally truncated α-synuclein are present in Alzheimer's disease without conventional Lewy body pathology. *Am J Pathol* 177(6) 3037–3050, 2010.)

WORKUP

- Lumbar puncture to rule out underlying chronic infections. Protein 14-3-3 may be present in both DLB and CJD.
- EEG to rule out potential TLE. However, either DLB or TLE may show nonspecific slowing or periodic complexes.
- MRI of the brain to evaluate for structural causes of dementia and to exclude MRI features of CJD.

LABORATORY TESTS

- Rule out other potential reversible causes for dementia including:
  1. Hormonal dysregulation: thyroid stimulating hormone, free thyroxine
  2. Vitamin deficiency: thiamine, cyanocobalamin, folate
  3. Vascular risk factors: lipid profile, Hgb A_{1c}, homocysteine, syphilis (FTA-ABS), or ApoE genotype

IMAGING STUDIES

- MRI typically shows a relative preservation of the hippocampi and medial temporal lobe volumes (as found in AD) but generalized atrophy and white matter changes.
- Functional imaging including single photon emission computed tomography (SPECT) may demonstrate hypoperfusion of the occipital region (specific finding but not sensitive).

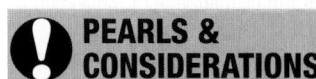 **TREATMENT**

Patient and caregiver education on benefits, side effects, and limitations of treatment is very important. Based on the preference of the patient and caregiver, a fine balance between psychosis and parkinsonism features confounds the treatment choices. Caregivers may be encouraged not to avoid neuroleptics unless the psychotic features either trouble or endanger the patient.

NONPHARMACOLOGIC THERAPY

- Social interaction and environmental novelty may improve cognitive dysfunction and psychiatric features often exacerbated by low levels of arousal and attention.
- Behavioral methods, such as avoiding previously exposed environmental triggers known to cause anxiety, agitation, or aggression.
- Physical therapy, mobility aids, and daily exercise.

ACUTE GENERAL Rx

Atypical neuroleptic for disabling, persistent, bothersome (to the patient) psychotic features despite initiation of a cholinesterase inhibitor. A very low dose of an atypical antipsychotic (quetiapine 12.5 mg daily) may be started after patient/caregiver education regarding the sensitivity to neuroleptics.

CHRONIC Rx

- Cholinesterase inhibitors for cognitive and behavioral symptoms. Rivastigmine (6 to 12 mg per day orally or 9.5 mg per day by transdermal patch) has shown in RCT a significant reduction in anxiety, delusions, and hallucinations, as well as significantly improved performance on neuropsychological testing.
- Antiparkinson medications for disabling parkinsonian features. L-dopa is reported to be more effective with fewer side effects than dopamine agonists. Begin at a low dose of L-dopa (25/100 mg tid), and slowly titrate over several weeks as tolerated and according to response.
- Selective serotonin reuptake inhibitors are commonly used for depression.
- If REM sleep disorder remains disabling (or patient has not responded to an atypical antipsychotic initiated for psychosis), a trial of low-dose clonazepam (0.25 to 0.5 mg) or melatonin (3 mg) at bedtime remains an option.
- Orthostatic hypotension may be aided by nonpharmacologic therapy such as supportive stockings or pharmacologically by midodrine and/or fludrocortisone.
- Memantine demonstrated an improvement in clinical global measure and remains well tolerated but may worsen hallucinations or delusions.
- Avoid anticholinergics (including tricyclic antidepressants) and benzodiazepines, as they can trigger delirium and worsen symptoms.

DISPOSITION

- Survival resembles the progression of AD, but a minority of cases may have a rapid disease course.
- Progression in cognitive decline, similar to AD, by approximately 10% per year on cognitive testing.

REFERRAL

DLB requires a multidisciplinary approach including the general practitioner, neurologist, neuropsychologist, and/or neuropsychiatrist.

! **PEARLS & CONSIDERATIONS**

COMMENTS

- Clinical presentation helps differentiate DLB from AD. AD presents with early signs of anterograde episodic memory loss without the benefit of cues on neuropsychological testing due to cortical atrophy at the medial temporal lobe region.
- Vascular dementia may also present with evidence of frontal-subcortical features but typically without the core features listed in the criteria above.
- Bed partners may report that individuals with DLB "act out their dreams," sometimes violently, leading to sleeping in separate beds. This history may indicate REM sleep behavior disorder. A history of REM sleep behavior may precede the diagnosis by many years. However, REM sleep behavior does not necessarily lead to DLB.

PATIENT/FAMILY EDUCATION

- Visual hallucinations (VH) typically consist of innocuous, well-formed, detailed images of animate figures. These are classically labeled Lilliputian, as the hallucinatory images are often relatively small. Unless VH lead to a potential threat to self or others, avoid antipsychotics due to the sensitivity of neuroleptics. Family/friends are often more alarmed by the VH than the patient with DLB.
- Apathy is a common clinical feature of DLB and mimics changes in mood, including depression, or excessive daytime somnolence. These features are often noticed by family/friends.

SUGGESTED READINGS

Available at www.expertconsult.com

AUTHORS: **ANGAD JOLLY,** and
JOSEPH S. KASS, M.D., J.D.

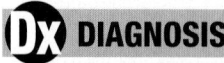 **BASIC INFORMATION**

DEFINITION

Dependent personality disorder (DPD) is characterized by a pervasive and excessive need to be taken care of that leads to submissive and clinging behavior and fears of separation. DPD begins by early adulthood and causes significant distress or impairment in multiple domains of functioning. Individuals must meet five or more of the following criteria:

1. Difficulty making routine decisions without an excessive amount of advice and reassurance from others
2. Need others to assume responsibility for most major areas of their lives
3. Difficulty expressing disagreement with others because of fear of loss of support or approval
4. Difficulty initiating or completing projects on own because of a lack of self-confidence in abilities rather than lack of motivation or energy
5. Excessive attempts to obtain nurturance and support from others
6. Feeling uncomfortable or helpless when alone because of exaggerated fears of being unable to care for self
7. Urgently seeking another relationship when a close relationship ends
8. Unrealistically preoccupied with being left to take care of self

SYNONYMS

None

ICD-10CM CODES
F60.7 Dependent personality disorder

EPIDEMIOLOGY & DEMOGRAPHICS

PREVALENCE: 0.5% in general population. Dependent traits, as opposed to the disorder itself, are among the most frequently reported in outpatient mental health clinics.
PREDOMINANT SEX: Female (2:1) in clinical settings

CLINICAL PRESENTATION

- Early onset and chronic course. Impairment is frequently mild.
- On interview, will defer excessively to partner or parent.
- Indecision in routine decisions.
- Depend on a parent or spouse to decide where they should live, work, and recreate and who they should befriend.
- Need for others to function for them goes beyond age-appropriate and situation-appropriate requests for assistance.

- Will agree with objectionable opinions, submit to unreasonable requests, and not express appropriate anger or disappointment for fear of alienating the person without whom they believe they cannot function.
- Convinced that they are not capable of independent function and present themselves as inept.
- Often do not develop independent living skills, perpetuating their dependency.
- Social relations tend to be limited to the few people on whom the person depends.

ETIOLOGY

Chronic physical illness or separation anxiety disorder may predispose for DPD.

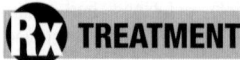 **DIAGNOSIS**

DIFFERENTIAL DIAGNOSIS

- Dependency and personality changes arising as a consequence of an Axis I disorder.
- Dependency arising as a consequence of a general medical condition.
- Most common comorbid Axis I conditions are major depressive and other mood disorders and anxiety disorders, including social phobia, and adjustment disorder.
- Most common comorbid personality disorders are histrionic, avoidant, and borderline. Each of these disorders is characterized by dependent features. DPD is distinguished by its predominantly submissive, reactive, and clinging behavior.

WORKUP

- History: Collateral information is essential to establishing the presence of longstanding interpersonal pattern in multiple domains of the patient's life.
- Physical examination.
- Mental status examination.

LABORATORY TESTS

Tests necessary to rule out medical causes of personality changes

IMAGING STUDIES

Tests necessary to rule out medical causes of personality changes

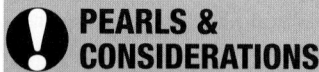 **TREATMENT**

NONPHARMACOLOGIC THERAPY

- Cognitive-behavioral and psychodynamic psychotherapy to diminish and better contain anxiety and to help patients develop sense of self as competent and requisite assertiveness skills.
- Psychodynamic psychotherapy to help develop improved self-concept and interpersonal functioning.

ACUTE GENERAL Rx

Benzodiazepines to control highly anxious states

CHRONIC Rx

Selective serotonin reuptake inhibitors (SSRIs) and selective serotonin-norepinephrine reuptake inhibitors (SNRIs) for comorbid depression, social phobia, other anxiety disorders, and agoraphobia

DISPOSITION

- Chronic course; severity is variable
- Impairments often mild
- At increased risk for major depression, social phobia, and other anxiety disorders, including panic and agoraphobia

REFERRAL

- If pharmacotherapy or psychotherapy is contemplated
- If patient's functioning is impaired

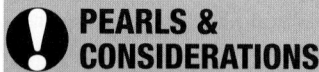 **PEARLS & CONSIDERATIONS**

COMMENTS

- Patients with DPD fear illness will lead to abandonment by others.
- This fear of simultaneous helplessness and abandonment intensifies neediness and may lead to dramatic demands for urgent medical attention.
- When physicians do not respond as wanted, angry outbursts may ensue.
- Medical care can also become a means by which dependency needs are met. As a result, some of these patients may unconsciously or consciously prolong their illnesses for primary gain.
- Physicians often react to the extreme neediness with avoidance or overengagement, leading to burnout.
- Management guidelines:
  1. Overall strategy is to provide reassurance and allay fear of abandonment.
  2. Specific strategies include scheduling frequent visits, noncontingent care (i.e., scheduling visits regardless of whether ill or not).
  3. Establish firm and realistic limits to availability as early as possible in treatment.
  4. Enlist other members of health care team for support.
  5. Encourage patient to develop additional "outside" support systems.

SUGGESTED READINGS
Available at www.expertconsult.com

AUTHOR: **JOHN Q. YOUNG, M.D., M.P.P.**

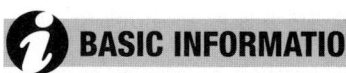

BASIC INFORMATION

DEFINITION

Major depression is an episodic, frequently recurring syndrome. The diagnosis requires that five of nine criteria be present for 2 wk. One of these nine criteria must be either a persistent depressed mood or pervasive anhedonia (loss of interest or pleasure in all, or almost all, usual interests or activities). Other symptoms include sleep disturbance (insomnia or hypersomnia), appetite loss/gain or weight loss/gain, fatigue, psychomotor retardation or agitation, difficulty concentrating or indecisiveness, feelings of guilt or worthlessness, and recurrent thoughts of death or suicidal ideation.

SYNONYMS

Unipolar affective disorder
Clinical depression
Melancholia
Manic-depressive illness, depressed type
Depressive episode
  Codes depend on whether the episode is single or recurrent, and also on clinical severity.

ICD-10CM CODES
F32.9 Depressive episode, unspecified
F33.0 Recurrent depressive episode, current episode mild
F33.1 Recurrent depressive disorder, current episode moderate
F33.2 Recurrent depressive disorder, current episode severe without psychotic symptoms
F33.3 Recurrent depressive disorder, current episode severe with psychotic symptoms
F33.4 Recurrent depressive disorder, currently in remission
F33.9 Recurrent depressive disorder, unspecified

EPIDEMIOLOGY & DEMOGRAPHICS

LIFETIME RISK (IN U.S.): 10% of men, 20% of women
PREVALENCE (IN U.S.): Point prevalence in a community sample is 3% of men, 4.5% to 9.3% of women, and 1% of children. Prevalence of 20% to 40% in patients with comorbid medical conditions.
PREDOMINANT SEX: Female/male ratio 2:1
PREDOMINANT AGE: 25 to 44 yr; 5% of adolescents
PEAK INCIDENCE: 30 to 40 yr; 13% of postpartum women
GENETICS:
- Clear evidence of familial predominance.
- Prevalence is 2 to 3 times greater among first-degree relatives.
- Concordance among monozygotic twins approximately 50%.
- No established pattern of inheritance.

PHYSICAL FINDINGS & CLINICAL PRESENTATION

- Clinical evaluation facilitated by organizing the major symptoms into four hallmarks:

(1) depressed mood, (2) anhedonia, (3) physical symptoms (sleep disturbance, appetite problem, fatigue, psychomotor changes), and (4) psychological symptoms (difficulty concentrating or indecisiveness, guilt or worthlessness, and suicidal ideation).
- A stressful life event, typically a serious loss, may trigger a depressive episode. DSM-5 recommends that clinical judgment be used to determine if depression in the context of a loss should be diagnosed as a major depressive episode.
- Patients often present with somatic complaints such as pain, fatigue, insomnia, dizziness, headache, or gastrointestinal problems. Somatic complaints may be reported more frequently among certain ethnic groups than depressed mood, increasing risk for under-detection in these groups.
- May be associated with mood-congruent delusional thinking (paranoid and melancholic themes).
- May be associated with active or passive suicidal ideation.
- Serious misconduct may appear in adolescents.
- May be underdiagnosed in elderly patients, with signs and symptoms attributed to normal aging.
- May be underdiagnosed in medically ill patients, with signs and symptoms attributed to medical illness or considered appropriate reaction to medical condition.

ETIOLOGY

- A heterogeneous group of disorders probably arising from various etiologies.
- Genetic and environmental experiences, and their interaction, each contribute.
- Significant psychosocial stressors, especially loss, often trigger depression, particularly for first episodes.
- Numerous biologic correlates have been identified, though none is considered causative or diagnostic. Genes that influence the production and reuptake of serotonin, norepinephrine, dopamine, and glutamate, as well as nerve cell growth in brain regions underlying memory and emotional processing, are of greatest interest. Abnormalities in brain regions underlying executive functioning, emotion regulation, and reward processing, as well as irregularities in cortisol responding and inflammation, appear to play a role.
- Cognitive risk factors include a pessimistic style of explaining negative events, a tendency to ruminate, and biases in processing emotional information and events.

DIAGNOSIS

DIFFERENTIAL DIAGNOSIS

- Anxiety disorders (e.g., social phobia, PTSD, obsessive compulsive disorder), substance abuse, and personality disorders often present with depressive symptoms.

- Important to determine if a depressive episode is part of major depression or part of bipolar disorder.
- Important to distinguish from adjustment disorder. Depression in the context of a stressful life event is diagnosed as major depressive disorder if the symptom criteria are met and adjustment disorder if the symptom criteria are not met. There is no evidence that medication is effective for adjustment disorder.
- Approximately 10% to 15% of depression caused by general medical illnesses, such as Alzheimer's disease, Parkinson's disease, stroke, end-stage renal failure, cardiac disease, HIV infection, and cancer.
- Some medical conditions present as depression (e.g., hypothyroidism, hyperthyroidism or neurosyphilis).
- Premenstrual dysphoric disorder.
- In elderly, depression often coexists with dementia.

WORKUP

- Careful medical history is required
- Physical examination reveals no specific diagnostic signs of depression
- Mental status examination
- Self-report scales can assist in screening.
- Commonly used validated screening tools include the 15-item Geriatric Depression Scale in the elderly and the Patient Health Questionnaire (PHQ)-2 and PHQ-9. The PHQ-2 has a 97% sensitivity and 67% specificity in adults. If it is positive for depression, the PHQ-9 should be administered. The PHQ-9 has a 61% sensitivity and 94% specificity for depression in adults.

LABORATORY TESTS

- No laboratory studies are diagnostic.
- The following can assist in ruling out other confounding issues:
  1. Routine blood chemistry evaluation
  2. CBC with differential
  3. Thyroid function studies
  4. Vitamin B_{12} levels

IMAGING STUDIES

With unusual presentations (e.g., associated with new-onset severe headache, focal neurologic signs, a cognitive or sensory disturbance), the following may be performed:
- EEG (diffuse slowing indicates metabolic encephalopathy)
- Anatomic brain imaging (CT scan or MRI)

TREATMENT

NONPHARMACOLOGIC THERAPY

- Good evidence that cognitive-behavioral therapy is as effective as antidepressant medication in achieving significant reduction or remission (Table 1).
- Problem solving and interpersonal psychotherapies are comparably efficacious.
- "New wave" cognitive-behavioral therapies (e.g., acceptance and commitment therapy, mindfulness-based CBT) have demonstrated

efficacy in numerous studies. It is unclear as of yet whether new-wave versus traditional behavioral therapies differ in mechanisms of action. Individuals not responding adequately to traditional behavioral therapies may benefit.

- Growing evidence indicates that Internet-based CBT and brief therapy interventions integrated into primary care to expand access to therapy are efficacious, but further research is needed.
- By 12 wk or earlier, psychotherapy and medication approaches are equally effective.
- Augmentation of standard depression treatment with CBT to address insomnia (CBT-I) was found to significantly improve response rates.
- Patients with severe symptoms should generally not be treated by psychotherapy alone.
- Evidence, although mixed, indicates that combined psychotherapy and medication may be more effective than either treatment alone. Various types of evidence-based psychotherapy or augmentation with psychotherapy appear to reduce the risk for future recurrences compared to medication alone, particularly when medication is discontinued after symptomatic remission.
- Factors, including history of childhood maltreatment, presence of precipitant stressful life events, family psychiatric history, the presence of anhedonia, and depression severity, may affect treatment response and risk of recurrence. Numerous genetic and neurobiologic variables that predict treatment response have been identified, particularly in combination with one another or with clinical characteristics. However, as of yet there are no universally accepted markers that can aid clinicians in matching individuals to particular medications or interventions.

ACUTE GENERAL Rx

- Concurrent medical or psychiatric illnesses, history of prior response, cost, patient preference, and side effects should be considered when selecting initial treatment.
- Antidepressants are helpful in approximately 60% to 70% of cases, though sustained remission rates are lower.
- Selective serotonin reuptake inhibitors (SSRIs) generally are first-line. According to the STAR-D trial, approximately 30% achieve remission with the first prescribed medication after 3 months of treatment. Another 25% to 30% respond to treatment, but do not achieve

remission. Treatment-refractory patients should be switched to another SSRI or to another class of medication, offered adjunctive medication such as bupropion, or referred for evidence-based counseling. Approximately 25% more patients will achieve remission with this secondary intervention.

- Response to antidepressants for many patients is seen as early as 2 wk, and among patients showing little to no response, the odds of later response decrease the longer patients remain unimproved.
- To date no benefit of combining antidepressants as first-line treatment. Also no clear advantage has been identified for switching medications within vs. across different classes, or to switching vs. augmentation.
- Therapy should be continued for 4 to 9 mo after the full remission of symptoms.
- Electroconvulsive therapy is the most effective means available for the treatment of severe, refractory depression. Transcranial magnetic stimulation has also shown evidence of efficacy though the magnitude of effects is more variable. To date electroconvulsive therapy has shown superior efficacy; research is underway to investigate whether higher-intensity TMS may enhance its efficacy.
- Antipsychotic medication should be added for psychotic depression. Antipsychotic medication has also been shown to be helpful in augmenting antidepressants for nonpsychotic depression, and it may be beneficial for individuals with mixed features, although more research is needed.
- Ketamine found to be rapidly effective in treatment-resistant depression. However, treatment remains experimental, and effects usually do not persist.

CHRONIC Rx

Long-term treatment, in some cases, lifelong recommended for multiple depressive episodes, an episode duration longer than 2 yr, a severe episode or significant suicidality, or a strong family history of severe depression or bipolar disorder.

DISPOSITION

- Major depression is often a relapsing and remitting illness.
- Physical symptoms predict a favorable response to biologic intervention.
- Additional episodes experienced by >50% after one episode, with each additional

episode linked to increased risk for subsequent episodes.

- Without treatment, episodes last an average of 6 to 12 mo; risk of recurrence higher without treatment.
- For many depressed individuals, subthreshold residual symptoms are present between episodes and define the majority of an individual's course of depression. Such symptoms may lead to impairment and warrant prolonged treatment.

REFERRAL

- If treatment refractory
- If patient suicidal or psychotic
- For suspected bipolar depression

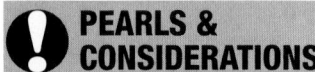 **PEARLS & CONSIDERATIONS**

COMMENTS

- All threats of suicide should be taken very seriously. Clinicians can use the mnemonic SAL: Is the method specific? Is it available? Is it lethal?
- Rule out bipolar affective disorder before initiating antidepressant medication. Screening scales for bipolar disorder can be helpful in primary care settings to identify patients at increased risk for bipolar disorder, although unclear benefit in mental health settings.
- Many patients and families reluctant to acknowledge depression because of stigma.
- A two-question screener is as effective as longer instruments. A positive answer to either question warrants a full assessment.
  1. Over the past 2 weeks, have you ever felt down, depressed, or hopeless?
  2. Over the past 2 weeks, have you felt little interest or pleasure in doing things?
- Depression screening programs without treatment programs are unlikely to improve depression outcomes.
- Strict monitoring of patients who initiate antidepressant therapy is necessary both for safety and to ensure optimal treatment. Use of self-report scales to measure symptom severity is helpful in monitoring outcome and may result in improved outcomes.

SUGGESTED READINGS

Available at www.expertconsult.com

RELATED CONTENT

Depression (Patient Information)
Bipolar Disorder (Related Key Topic)

AUTHORS: **MARK ZIMMERMAN, M.D.,** and **CATHERINE D'AVANZATO, PH.D.**

TABLE 1 Treatments of Depression

Name of Psychotherapy	Approach
Cognitive psychotherapy	Identify and correct negativistic patterns of thinking.
Interpersonal psychotherapy	Identify and work through role transitions or interpersonal losses, conflicts, or deficits.
Problem-solving therapy	Identify and prioritize situational problems; plan and implement strategies to deal with top-priority problems.
Psychodynamic psychotherapy	Use therapeutic relationship to maximize use of the healthiest defense mechanisms and coping strategies.

From Goldman L et al: *Goldman's Cecil medicine*, ed 24, Philadelphia, 2012, Saunders.

BASIC INFORMATION

DEFINITION

Dermatitis herpetiformis (DH) is an autoimmune blistering disease that is considered to be a cutaneous manifestation of celiac disease (CD). It is associated with gluten-sensitive enteropathy in nearly all cases, although only 20% of patients have gastrointestinal symptoms. 15% to 25% of patients with CD will have DH.

SYNONYMS

DH
Duhring disease

ICD-10CM CODES
L13.0 Dermatitis herpetiformis

EPIDEMIOLOGY & DEMOGRAPHICS

PREVALENCE (IN U.S.): 112 cases per 100,000 persons; prevalence for CD is one in 133 adults
PREDOMINANT SEX: Male predominance (2:1); however, female predominance in children
PREDOMINANT AGE: Fourth decade of life, but can occur at any age
PREDOMINANT RACE: Most common in Caucasians of Northern European ancestry
GENETICS: Both CD and DH have a strong genetic component. 10% to 15% of patients with DH have a first-degree relative with either DH or CD. Specific HLA genes (involved in processing gliadin antigen in genetically susceptible individuals) have also been shown to predispose to developing DH (HLA-DQ2 in 90%, DQ8 in the remaining 10%). However, less than 50% of genetic predisposition is attributed to HLA genes.

PHYSICAL FINDINGS & CLINICAL PRESENTATION

- Classically, the lesions of DH are small, grouped, "herpetiform" vesicles that are distributed symmetrically on extensor surfaces (elbows, knees, scalp, back, and buttocks) (Fig. 1). However, due to intense pruritus and scratching, pinpoint erosions and excoriations in the above distribution are often the most prominent findings on examination, with intact vesicles rarely seen.
- Spontaneous improvement with cyclic exacerbations is common.
- Celiac-type enamel defects to permanent teeth, oral vesicles, or palmoplantar purpura have been reported as potential associated findings.

PATHOGENESIS

CD and DH are both autoimmune-mediated by IgA class autoantibodies. Dietary gluten is central to the pathogenesis in both. In genetically predisposed individuals, it is hypothesized that the gluten byproduct, gliadin, complexes with tissue transglutaminase (tTG) in the gut, binding as an antigen to HLA-DQ2 on T-cells, creating an immune response that results in anti-tTG IgA antibodies (i.e., antiendomysial antibodies) in the blood. tTG cross-reacts with epidermal TG (eTG). The blood of CD patients with and without skin disease is found to have both skin and gut anti-TG IgA antibodies. Yet, it is thought that the high-affinity IgA against eTG form complexes that are responsible for DH. The deposition of IgA-eTG complexes in the papillary dermis triggers an immunologic cascade resulting in neutrophil recruitment and complement activation.

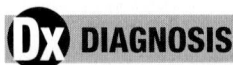 DIAGNOSIS

Physical examination and routine histopathology are often suggestive of DH; however, direct immunofluorescence (DIF) of a perilesional skin biopsy has pathognomonic findings and is the gold standard for diagnosis. Fig. 2 describes an approach to the patient with suspected dermatitis herpetiformis.

DIFFERENTIAL DIAGNOSIS

- Clinically and histologically, the differential diagnosis includes linear IgA dermatosis, bullous pemphigoid, and bullous lupus. These diagnoses can be differentiated by DIF on perilesional skin biopsy.
- Other clinical diagnoses to consider:
  1. Scabies (check for interdigital burrows and involvement of genitalia)
  2. Arthropod bite (papular urticaria over exposed areas)
  3. Eczematous dermatitis (ill-defined, weeping erythematous plaques)
  4. Herpes simplex or zoster infection (painful, not symmetric)
  5. Generalized pruritus (no blister history)

WORKUP, LABORATORY TESTS

- Evaluation for gastrointestinal symptoms, family history of DH or CD and pruritus should be sought in patients with suspected DH.
- **Lesional skin biopsy**: will demonstrate a neutrophil-rich subepidermal bulla and rule out many conditions.
- **DIF of normal-appearing perilesional skin biopsy**: will demonstrate pathognomonic IgA deposits localized to the dermal papillae and dermal-epidermal junction in a granular pattern.
- Checking for circulating antibodies in the blood (antigliadin, antiendomysial, or antireticulin IgA antibodies) is not recommended as part of the diagnostic workup for DH (as many as 10%-37% of DH patients have negative antiendomysial antibodies; a high false-positive rate for anti-tTG is found among patients with autoimmune diseases). However, they can be helpful in suggesting the diagnosis of DH in cases where linear IgA cannot be excluded on DIF.

TREATMENT

A gluten-free diet (GFD) and dapsone are considered first-line therapy and are often started in conjunction.

1. GFD improves symptoms of both GI and skin disease, with GI responding quicker (skin responds after 2 months). A retrospective study showed remission (2 years without symptoms) in 12%.
2. Dapsone results in improvement of skin manifestations within days but does not treat GI manifestations. Dapsone is typically tapered over time, while lifelong gluten avoidance is often necessary.
   A recent small study demonstrated that a GFD alone was comparable to a GFD plus dapsone in the treatment of DH; hence GFD is an essential component in the treatment of DH.

NONPHARMACOLOGIC THERAPY

- First line: GFD
  1. Avoid barley, rye, wheat (can consume rice, corn, and oats).
  2. Consultation with a dietitian is recommended.
  3. Most patients need to follow diet indefinitely; however, cases of spontaneous remission have been reported.
- Second line: elemental diet (controversial)
  1. Can consider elemental diet (avoidance of whole proteins) in those patients who do not adequately respond to a strict GFD; however, data are limited.

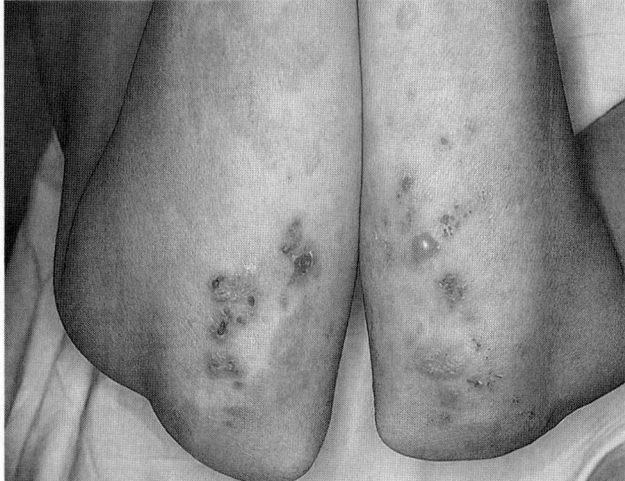

FIG. 1 Dermatitis herpetiformis is an immunologically mediated blistering disease. There is a strong association of dermatitis herpetiformis with HLA-B8, DR3. Gluten-sensitive enteropathy is a common associated finding. The lesions are grouped (herpetiform) and extremely pruritic. (From Callen JP [ed]: *Color atlas of dermatology,* ed 2, Philadelphia, 2000, Saunders.)

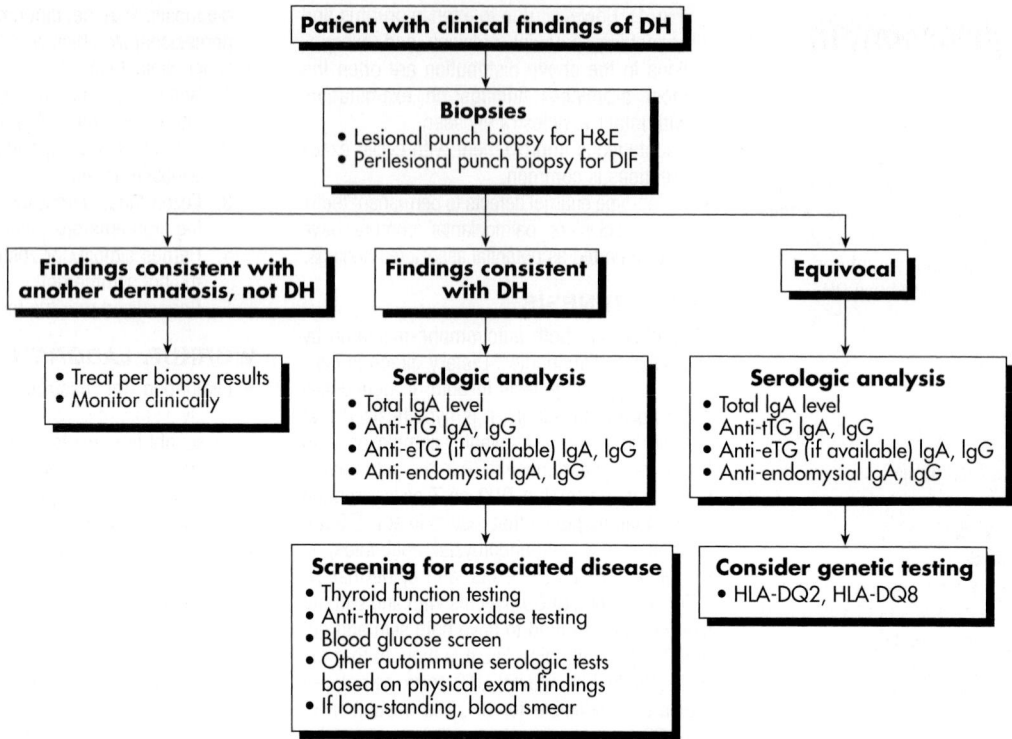

FIG. 2 Approach to the patient with suspected dermatitis herpetiformis. (From Bolotin D, Petronic-Rosic V: Dermatitis herpetiformis: Part II. Diagnosis, management, and prognosis. *J Am Acad Dermatol* 64(6):1027-1033, 2011.)

ACUTE GENERAL Rx

- First line: dapsone
  1. Initial dose 25-50 mg PO daily with gradual increase to an average maintenance dose of 0.5-1 mg/kg daily (often maintenance dose of 100 mg daily).
  2. Clinical monitoring weekly is recommended to optimize dose (optimal dose is when 1-2 new lesions/wk).
  3. Caution: dapsone may produce hemolysis (especially if G6PD deficiency), agranulocytosis, methemoglobinemia, systemic drug hypersensitivity reaction (DRESS), and a peripheral neuropathy.
  4. Baseline labs: CBC, LFTs, G6PD levels. After the initiation of therapy, monitor CBC every week ×1 month, then every other week ×2 months, monthly ×3 months, then every 3-4 months. Monitor LFTs every 3-4 months.
- Second-line alternatives
  1. Sulfapyridine (500-1500 mg/day) or sulfasalazine (500-1000 mg bid) may be substituted in cases of dapsone intolerance or in the rare case that neuropathy develops.
  2. Case reports of efficacy using topical dapsone 5% twice daily in patients who do not tolerate oral dapsone; also reported to be efficacious as an adjuvant to oral dapsone.
  3. Reported efficacy in uncontrolled studies and case reports have suggested efficacy with tetracyclines, nicotinamide, cyclosporine, colchicine, and heparin
- Symptomatic relief for pruritus
  1. Potent and superpotent topical corticosteroids (atrophy with prolonged use, limit to 14 days per month), nonsedating antihistamines twice daily, sedating antihistamines at bedtime, mentholated lotion

CHRONIC Rx

- As DH is considered to represent the cutaneous manifestations of CD, lifelong avoidance of gluten is typically recommended. Information about educational resources, such as national and local support groups, should be provided (www.celiac.org).
- Patients with DH and CD have an increased risk of developing Hashimoto's thyroiditis (50% with thyroid disease), non-Hodgkin's lymphoma, and GI lymphomas. An increased incidence of other autoimmune disorders (type 1 diabetes mellitus, pernicious anemia, Addison's disease, vitiligo, systemic lupus erythematosus, rheumatoid arthritis, and Sjögren's syndrome) and osteoporosis have also been reported.
  1. Screening for thyroid disease (TSH, antithyroid peroxidase antibody titers) is typically recommended
  2. Screening for autoimmune connective tissue diseases should be considered if suspicious signs or symptoms
  3. Routine screening for GI lymphomas is controversial

REFERRAL

- Dermatologist for skin biopsy and management of cutaneous disease
- Gastroenterologist for evaluation of CD
- Nutritionist to educate patients about gluten-free diet
- National support groups (www.celiac.org) and local support groups

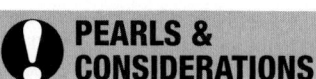

PEARLS & CONSIDERATIONS

- Classic areas involved are those that are exposed if in a "fetal position."
- Lesions may be worsened by iodides and certain NSAIDs; systemic steroids ineffective.
- Location of biopsies is IMPORTANT: False-negative DIF can result if biopsies are taken from lesional skin (should be taken from normal-appearing skin adjacent to lesion) as diagnostic IgA deposits are usually destroyed by the blistering process.
- GFD results in reduced IgA in skin on DIF (with eventual disappearance) and reduced antiendomysial antibodies in the blood. Hence, serologies (e.g., antiendomysial antibodies) can be used to monitor degree of compliance to dietary gluten restriction.
- Some studies have suggested a possible protective effect of GFD against intestinal lymphoma. First-degree relatives do not appear to be at increased risk for GI or systemic lymphomas in the absence of DH or CD.

SUGGESTED READINGS

Available at www.expertconsult.com

RELATED CONTENT

Celiac Disease (Related Key Topic)

AUTHOR: **LISA K. PAPPAS-TAFFER, M.D.**

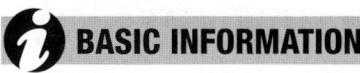 BASIC INFORMATION

DEFINITION

Diabetes insipidus is a polyuric disorder resulting from insufficient production of vasopressin (pituitary [neurogenic] diabetes insipidus) or unresponsiveness of the renal tubules to vasopressin (nephrogenic diabetes insipidus).

ICD-10CM CODES
E23.2 Diabetes insipidus

EPIDEMIOLOGY & DEMOGRAPHICS
GENETICS:
- Nephrogenic diabetes insipidus can be inherited as a sex-linked recessive trait.
- There is also a rare autosomal-dominant form of neurogenic diabetes insipidus.

PHYSICAL FINDINGS & CLINICAL PRESENTATION
- Central diabetes insipidus is usually abrupt in onset whereas in compulsive water drinking there is a more vague history of onset
- Nocturia is unusual in compulsive water drinkers and more common in central diabetes insipidus
- Polyuria: urinary volumes ranging from 2.5 to 6 L/day
- Polydipsia (predilection for cold or iced drinks)
- Neurologic manifestations (seizures, headaches, visual field defects)
- Evidence of volume contractions
  NOTE: The physical findings and clinical manifestations are generally not evident until vasopressin secretory capacity is reduced to <20% of normal.

ETIOLOGY
Neurogenic diabetes insipidus:
- Idiopathic (Autoimmune hypophysitis)
- Malignancy: Neoplasms of brain or pituitary fossa (craniopharyngiomas, metastatic neoplasms from breast or lung)
- Posttherapeutic neurosurgical procedures (e.g., hypophysectomy)
- Head trauma (e.g., basal skull fracture)
- Granulomatous disorders (sarcoidosis, granulomatosis with polyangiitis, or tuberculosis)
- Histiocytosis (Hand-Schüller-Christian disease, eosinophilic granuloma)
- Familial (autosomal dominant); some cases autosomal recessive
- Other: interventricular hemorrhage, aneurysms, meningitis, postencephalitis, multiple sclerosis, Guillain-Barré syndrome, IgG4-related disease, lymphocytic hypophysitis
Nephrogenic diabetes insipidus:
- Drugs: lithium, aminoglycosides, antivirals (foscarnet, didanosine), amphotericin B, demeclocycline, ifosfamide, methoxyflurane anesthesia
- Familial: X-linked
- Metabolic: hypercalcemia or hypokalemia
- Other: sarcoidosis, urinary tract infection, amyloidosis, Sjögren syndrome, pyelonephritis, nephronophthisis, polycystic disease, sickle cell nephropathy, postobstructive, low-protein diets (protein malnourishment)

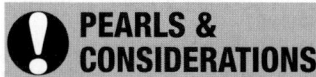 DIAGNOSIS

DIFFERENTIAL DIAGNOSIS
- Diabetes mellitus, nephropathies
- Primary polydipsia, medications (e.g., chlorpromazine)
- Osmotic diuresis (glucose, mannitol, anticholinergics)
- Psychogenic polydipsia, electrolyte disturbances

WORKUP
- The diagnostic workup is aimed at showing that polyuria is caused by the inability to concentrate urine and determining whether the problem is the result of decreased vasopressin or insensitivity to vasopressin. This is done with the water deprivation test (Table E1):
  1. After baseline measurement of weight, vasopressin, plasma sodium, and urine and plasma osmolarity, the patient is deprived of fluids under strict medical supervision.
  2. Frequent (q2h) monitoring of plasma and urine osmolarity follows.
  3. The test is generally terminated when plasma osmolarity is >295 mOsm/kg or the patient loses ≥3.5% of initial body weight.
  4. Diabetes insipidus is confirmed if the plasma osmolarity is >295 mOsm/kg and the urine osmolarity is <500 mOsm/kg.
  5. To distinguish nephrogenic from neurogenic diabetes insipidus, the patient is given 5 U of vasopressin and the change in urine osmolarity is measured. A significant increase (>50%) in urine osmolarity after administration of vasopressin is indicative of neurogenic diabetes insipidus.
- A diagnostic algorithm for diabetes insipidus is described in Fig. E1.

LABORATORY TESTS
- Decreased urinary specific gravity (≤1.005)
- Baseline plasma osmolality >295 mOsm/kg is suggestive of central diabetes mellitus whereas values below 270 mOsm/kg favor compulsive water drinking. Decreased urinary osmolarity (usually <200 mOsm/kg) even in the presence of high plasma osmolality
- Hypernatremia, increased plasma osmolarity, hypercalcemia, hypokalemia

IMAGING STUDIES
MRI of the pituitary if neurogenic diabetes insipidus is confirmed

(Rx) TREATMENT

NONPHARMACOLOGIC THERAPY
- Patient education regarding control of fluid balance and prevention of dehydration with adequate fluid intake or IV D_5W
- Daily weight

ACUTE GENERAL Rx
Therapy varies with the degree and type of diabetes insipidus (Table E2).

- Neurogenic diabetes insipidus:
  1. Desmopressin acetate (DDAVP) 20-40 mcg qd intranasally in 1 to 3 divided doses or in tablet form 0.1 to 1.2 mg. Usual oral dose is 0.1 to 1.2 mg/day in 2 to 3 divided doses. Desmopressin is also available in injectable form given as 2 to 4 mcg/day SC or IV in 2 divided doses.
  2. Vasopressin tannate in oil: 2.5 to 5 U IM q24 to 72h; useful for long-term management because of its long half-life.
  3. In mild cases of neurogenic diabetes insipidus, polyuria may be controlled with HCTZ 50 mg qd (decreases urine volume by increasing proximal tubular reabsorption of glomerular infiltrate).
- Nephrogenic diabetes insipidus:
  1. Removal of the underlying cause. However, prolonged lithium therapy can lead to irreversible nephrogenic diabetes insipidus even after lithium therapy is withdrawn.
  2. Amiloride 5 mg/day for lithium-related disease
  3. Low-sodium diet and chlorothiazide to induce mild sodium depletion

CHRONIC Rx
Patients should be aware of the danger of dehydration and the need for liberal water intake.

REFERRAL
Endocrinology consultation for diagnostic testing

(!) PEARLS & CONSIDERATIONS

COMMENTS
- Patients should be instructed to wear a medical identification tag or bracelet identifying their medical illness.
- In central diabetes insipidus, the use of DDAVP has become the standard of care. Extensive clinical experience has shown it to be both safe and effective in the treatment of this disorder.
- The treatment of nephrogenic diabetes insipidus is more complicated than the central form, and opinion varies among experts in the field. Consultation with a specialist is always recommended in this setting.

SUGGESTED READINGS
Available at www.expertconsult.com

RELATED CONTENT
Diabetes Insipidus (Patient Information)

AUTHOR: **FRED F. FERRI, M.D.**

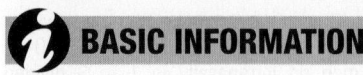

BASIC INFORMATION

DEFINITION

- Diabetes mellitus (DM) refers to a syndrome of hyperglycemia resulting from many different causes (see "Etiology"). It is broadly classified into type 1 (T1DM) and type 2 DM (T2DM). The terms "insulin-dependent" and "non–insulin-dependent" diabetes are obsolete because when a person with type 2 diabetes needs insulin, he or she remains labeled as type 2 and is not reclassified as type 1. Table 1 provides a general comparison of the two types of DM.
- The American Diabetes Association (ADA) defines DM as follows:
  1. A fasting plasma glucose (FPG) ≥126 mg/dl, which should be confirmed with repeat testing on a different day. Fasting is defined as no caloric intake for at least 8 hr.
  2. Symptoms of hyperglycemia and a casual (random) plasma glucose ≥200 mg/dl. Classic symptoms of hyperglycemia include polyuria, polydipsia, and unexplained weight loss.
  3. An oral glucose tolerance test (OGTT) with a plasma glucose ≥200 mg/dl 2 hr after a 75 g (100 g for pregnant women) glucose load.
  4. A hemoglobin A_{1c} (HbA_{1c}) value ≥6.5%.
- Individuals with glucose levels higher than normal but not high enough to meet the criteria for diagnosis of DM are considered to have "prediabetes," the diagnosis of which is made as follows:
  1. A fasting plasma glucose 100 to 125 mg/dl; this is referred to as **impaired fasting glucose**.
  2. After OGTT, a 2-hr plasma glucose 140 to 199; this is referred to as **impaired glucose tolerance**.
  3. A hemoglobin A_{1c} value 5.7% to 6.4%.

- Table 2 describes diagnostic categories for DM and at-risk states.

SYNONYMS

IDDM (insulin-dependent diabetes mellitus)
NIDDM (non–insulin-dependent diabetes mellitus)
Type 1 diabetes mellitus (insulin-dependent diabetes mellitus)
Type 2 diabetes mellitus (non–insulin-dependent diabetes mellitus)

ICD-10CM CODES

E11.5	Type 2 diabetes mellitus with peripheral circulatory complications
E11.7	Type 2 diabetes mellitus with multiple complications
E11.8	Type 2 diabetes mellitus with unspecified complications
E11.9	Type 2 diabetes mellitus without complications
E10.69	Type 1 diabetes mellitus with other specified complication
E10.8	Type 1 diabetes mellitus with unspecified complications
E10.9	Type 1 diabetes mellitus without complications
E11.69	Type 2 diabetes mellitus with other specified complication
E11.8	Type 2 diabetes mellitus with unspecified complications
E11.9	Type 2 diabetes mellitus without complications

EPIDEMIOLOGY & DEMOGRAPHICS

- DM affects 9% to 10% of the U.S. population. Prevalence rates vary considerably by race/ethnicity. T1DM accounts for approximately 5% of diagnosed diabetes cases and is defined by the presence of one or more autoimmune markers.
- Incidence rate increases with age, varying from 2% in persons age 20 to 44 yr to 18% in persons 65 to 74 yr. T2DM can have a long presymptomatic phase, leading to a 4- to 7-yr delay in diagnosis.
- Diabetes accounts for 8% of all legal blindness in the United States and is the leading cause of end-stage renal disease (ESRD).
- Patients with diabetes are 2-4 times more likely than nondiabetic patients to experience development of cardiovascular disease.

PHYSICAL FINDINGS & CLINICAL PRESENTATION

1. Physical examination varies with the presence of complications and may be normal in early stages
2. Diabetic retinopathy:
   a. Nonproliferative (background diabetic retinopathy):
      (1) Initially: microaneurysms, capillary dilation, waxy or hard exudates, dot and flame hemorrhages, arteriovenous shunts
      (2) Advanced stage: microinfarcts with cotton wool exudates, macular edema
   b. Proliferative retinopathy: characterized by formation of new vessels, vitreous hemorrhages, fibrous scarring, and retinal detachment
3. Cataracts and glaucoma occur with increased frequency in patients with diabetes
4. Diabetic neuropathy
   a. Distal sensorimotor polyneuropathy
      (1) Symptoms include paresthesia, hyperesthesia, or burning pain involving bilateral distal extremities, in a "stocking-glove" distribution. This can progress to motor weakness and ataxia.
      (2) Physical examination may reveal decreased pinprick sensation, sensation to light touch, vibration sense, and loss of proprioception. Motor disturbances such as decreased deep tendon reflexes and atrophy of interossei muscles can also be seen.

TABLE 1 General Comparison of the Two Types of Diabetes Mellitus

	Type 1	Type 2
Previous terminology	Insulin-dependent diabetes mellitus (IDDM), type I, juvenile-onset diabetes	Non–insulin-dependent diabetes mellitus, type II, adult-onset diabetes
Age of onset	Usually <30 yr, particularly childhood and adolescence, but any age	Usually >40 yr, but any age
Genetic predisposition	Moderate; environmental factors required for expression; 35%-50% concordance in monozygotic twins; several candidate genes proposed	Strong; 60%-90% concordance in monozygotic twins; many candidate genes proposed; some genes identified in maturity-onset diabetes of the young
Human leukocyte antigen associations	Linkage to DQA and DQB, influenced by DRB (3 and 4) (DR2 protective)	None known
Other associations	Autoimmune; Graves' disease, Hashimoto's thyroiditis, vitiligo, Addison's disease, pernicious anemia	Heterogenous group, ongoing subclassification based on identification of specific pathogenic processes and genetic defects
Precipitating and risk factors	Largely unknown; microbial, chemical, dietary, other	Age, obesity (central), sedentary lifestyle, previous gestational diabetes
Findings at diagnosis	85%-90% of patients have one and usually more autoantibodies to ICA512/IA-2/IA-2b, GAD$_{65}$, insulin (IAA)	Possibly complications (microvascular and macrovascular) caused by significant preceding asymptomatic period
Endogenous insulin levels	Low or absent	Usually present (relative deficiency), early hyperinsulinemia
Insulin resistance	Only with hyperglycemia	Mostly present
Prolonged fast	Hyperglycemia, ketoacidosis	Euglycemia
Stress, withdrawal of insulin	Ketoacidosis	Nonketotic hyperglycemia, occasionally ketoacidosis

GAD, Glutamic acid decarboxylase; *IA-2/IA-2b,* tyrosine phosphatases; *IAA,* insulin autoantibodies; *ICA,* islet cell antibody; *ICA512,* islet cell autoantigen 512 (fragment of IA-2).
From Andreoli TE (ed): *Cecil essentials of medicine,* ed 6, Philadelphia, 2005, Saunders.

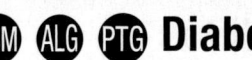
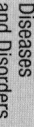

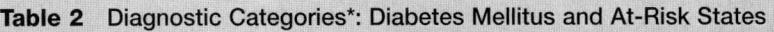

Table 2 Diagnostic Categories*: Diabetes Mellitus and At-Risk States

Fasting Plasma Glucose Level	2-Hour (75-g) OGTT Result		
	<140 mg/dl	140-199 mg/dl	≥200 mg/dl
<100 mg/dl	Normal	IGT†	DM
100-125 mg/dl	IFG†	IGT† and IFG†	DM
≥126 mg/dl	DM	DM	DM
HbA₁c Level	**<5.7%**	**5.7-6.4%**	**≥6.5%**
	Normal	High-risk†	DM

DM, Diabetes mellitus; *IFG*, impaired fasting glucose; *IGT*. impaired glucose tolerance.
*These diagnostic categories are based on the combined fasting plasma glucose level and a 2-hour, 75-g oral glucose tolerance test (OGTT) result. Note that a confirmed random plasma glucose level of 200 mg/dl or higher in the appropriate clinical setting is diagnostic of diabetes and precludes the need for further testing.
†May be referred to as prediabetes.
From Goldman L, Schafer AI: *Goldman's Cecil medicine*, ed 24, Philadelphia, 2012, Saunders.

b. Autonomic neuropathy:
   (1) GI disturbances: esophageal motility abnormalities, gastroparesis, diarrhea (usually nocturnal)
   (2) Genitourinary (GU) disturbances: neurogenic bladder (hesitancy, weak stream, and dribbling), impotence
   (3) Cardiovascular (CV) disturbances: orthostatic hypotension, tachycardia, decreased heart rate variability (HRV). Decreased heart rate variability is associated with increased cardiac mortality, independent of ejection fraction.
c. Polyradiculopathy: painful weakness and atrophy in the distribution of ≥1 contiguous nerve roots.
d. Mononeuropathy involving cranial nerves III, IV, or VI or peripheral nerves can also occur.
5. Diabetic nephropathy: pedal edema, pallor, weakness, uremic appearance
6. Foot ulcers: occur in 15% of individuals with diabetes (annual incidence rate 2%) and are the leading causes of hospitalization; they are usually secondary to a combination of factors, including peripheral vascular insufficiency, repeated trauma (unrecognized because of sensory loss), and superimposed infection.
   a. Patient symptoms are usually less than would be expected from clinical findings, due to loss of sensation related to peripheral neuropathy.
   b. Comprehensive foot exams include visual inspection, assessment of pedal pulses, and assessment of protective sensation using a 10-g monofilament to test sensation.
   c. Prevention of foot ulcers in an individual with diabetes includes strict glucose control, patient education, prescription footwear, intensive podiatric care, and evaluation for surgical interventions
7. Neuropathic arthropathy (Charcot's joints): bone or joint deformities from repeated trauma (secondary to peripheral neuropathy; Fig. E1).
8. Necrobiosis lipoidica diabeticorum: plaque-like reddened areas with a central area that fades to white-yellow found on the anterior surfaces of the legs (Fig. E2); in these areas, the skin becomes very thin and can ulcerate easily.

ETIOLOGY

IDIOPATHIC DIABETES: Type 1 DM: results from autoimmune beta-cell destruction, usually leading to absolute insulin deficiency
- Hereditary factors:
   1. Islet cell antibodies (found in 90% of patients within the first yr of diagnosis)
   2. Higher incidence of human leukocyte antigen (HLA) types DR3, DR4
   3. 50% concordance rate in identical twins
- Environmental factors: viral infection (possibly Coxsackie virus, mumps virus)
   Type 2 DM: results from insulin resistance and a progressive defect in insulin secretion.
- Hereditary factors: 90% concordance rate in identical twins
- Environmental factors: obesity, sedentary lifestyle, high carbohydrate content in food

DIABETES SECONDARY TO OTHER FACTORS:
- Hormonal excess: Cushing's syndrome, acromegaly, glucagonoma, pheochromocytoma
- Drugs: glucocorticoids, diuretics, oral contraceptives
- Insulin receptor unavailability (with or without circulating antibodies)
- Pancreatic disease: pancreatitis, pancreatectomy, hemochromatosis, cystic fibrosis
- Genetic syndromes: maturity onset diabetes of the young (MODY, monogenetic diabetes accounting for 2% to 5% of diabetes), familial hyperlipidemias, myotonic dystrophy, lipoatrophy
- Gestational diabetes (GDM): diabetes diagnosed during pregnancy that is due to pregnancy-related insulin resistance

(Dx) DIAGNOSIS

DIFFERENTIAL DIAGNOSIS
- Diabetes insipidus
- Stress hyperglycemia
- Diabetes secondary to hormonal excess, drugs, pancreatic disease

LABORATORY TESTS
- Diagnosis of DM is made on the basis of the following tests:
   1. Fasting glucose ≥126 mg/dl on two occasions.
   2. Non-FPG ≥200 mg/dl and symptoms of DM.

3. OGTT (75 g glucose load for nonpregnant individuals) with 2-hr value >200 mg/dl.
4. Glycosylated hemoglobin (HbA₁c) ≥6.5%. HbA₁c level reflects average glycemia over previous 3 months or longer. In known diabetics, this test should be performed at least twice yearly in stable patients and more frequently when therapy changes or patients are not meeting glycemic goals. HBA₁c alone does not provide a measure of glycemic variability or hypoglycemia and is affected by the presence of hemoglobin variants, hemolysis, or blood loss.
- Screening for prediabetes and diabetes in asymptomatic patients (see Table 3):
   1. Should be considered in adults of any age who are overweight (body mass index [BMI] >25 kg/m²) or obese (BMI >30) and who have one or more additional risk factors for diabetes.
   2. In those who are without these risk factors, testing should begin at age 45 yr.
   3. If screen is normal, repeat testing should be carried out at least at 3-yr intervals.
- Detection and diagnosis of gestational diabetes mellitus (GDM)
   1. Screen for GDM using risk factor analysis and use of an OGTT. Pregnant women who are not known to have diabetes should be screened for gestational diabetes at 24 to 28 weeks' gestation with a "1-step" strategy with 75 g oral glucose tolerance test or a "2-step" approach with a 50-g (nonfasting) screen followed by a 100-g oral glucose tolerance test for those who screen positive. A diagnosis of GDM is made if any of the following levels of plasma glucose are exceeded: ≥92 mg/dl (5.1 mmol/L) when fasting, ≥80 mg/dl (10 mmol/L) at 1 hour, or ≥153 mg/dl (8.5 mmol/L) at 2 hours.
   2. Women with GDM should be screened for diabetes 6 to 12 wk postpartum and should be followed with subsequent screening for the development of diabetes or prediabetes at least every 3 yr
- Screening for diabetic nephropathy (Fig. E3)
   1. Screening should be done at diagnosis and then yearly for type 2 diabetes and 5 yr after diagnosis then yearly in type 2 diabetics.
   2. Screening can be performed using a albumin:creatinine ratio (microalbumin) in a random spot urine collection or by measurement of a 24-hr urine collection for albumin, and creatinine clearance. The urine albumin to creatinine ratio (ACR) is independently associated with mortality at all levels of estimated glomerular filtration rate (eGFR) in older adults with diabetes.
   3. The diagnosis of microalbuminuria (ACR 30-299 mg/24 hr) should be based on 2 to 3 elevated levels within a 3- to 6-mo period because there is a marked variability in day-to-day albumin excretion. Patients with overt macroalbuminuria (>300 mg albumin/24 hr or albumin: creatinine ratio >300) should be followed by urine protein:creatinine ratio.

Table 3 Criteria for Diabetes Screening in Asymptomatic Individuals

1. Testing should be considered in all adults who are overweight (BMI >25 kg/m2*) and have additional risk factors:
   - Physical inactivity
   - A first-degree relative with diabetes
   - High-risk ethnic population (e.g., African American, Hispanic American, Native American, Asian American, Pacific Islander)
   - Delivered a baby weighing more than 9 lb or diagnosed with gestational diabetes mellitus
   - Systemic hypertension (blood pressure >140/90 mm Hg or on antihypertensive therapy)
   - High-density lipoprotein cholesterol level <35 mg/dl or triglyceride level >250 mg/dl
   - Polycystic ovary syndrome
   - Hemoglobin A1c ≥5.7%, impaired glucose tolerance or impaired fasting glucose on prior testing
   - Other clinical conditions associated with insulin resistance (e.g., severe obesity, acanthosis nigricans)
   - History of cardiovascular disease
2. If none of the above criteria are present, screening for diabetes should begin at age 45 yr.
3. If the results are normal, screening should be repeated at least every 3 yr. Depending on initial results and risk status, more frequent testing may need to be considered.

*In some ethnic groups, such as Asians, at-risk body mass index (BMI) may be lower.
Modified from American Diabetes Association, Diagnosis and classification of diabetes mellitus *Diabetes Care* 33(Suppl. 1):S14, 2010. Borrowed from Goldman L, Schafer AI: *Goldman's Cecil medicine,* ed 24, Philadelphia, 2012, Saunders.

- A fasting serum lipid panel, serum creatinine, and electrolytes should be obtained yearly on all adult patients with diabetes.
- Self-monitoring of blood glucose (SMBG) is crucial for assessing the effectiveness of the management plan. The frequency and timing of SMBG varies with the needs and goals of each patient. In most patients with type 1 DM and pregnant women taking insulin, SMBG is recommended at least 3 times/day. In patients with type 2 DM not on insulin, recommendations are unclear for SMBG, but testing once or twice/day is acceptable in most patients. Glycemic control is best evaluated when SMBG is combined with HbA_{1c} testing.
- Screening for thyroid dysfunction (TSH level), Vitamin B_{12} deficiency, and celiac disease should be considered in type 1 diabetes due to the increased frequency of other autoimmune diseases in these individuals.

℞ TREATMENT

- Type 1 diabetes requires immediate initiation of insulin therapy.
- In Type 1 diabetes, intensive glycemic control (HbA_{1c} <7) has been shown in randomized controlled trials (RCT) to reduce the risk of microvascular (neuropathy, retinopathy, nephropathy) and macrovascular (cardiovascular events) complications.
- Type 2 DM: The ADA and European Association for the Study of Diabetes recommend lifestyle intervention (diet and exercise) and metformin initiation (unless contraindication exist such as serum creatinine levels ≥1.5 mg/dl in males or ≥1.4 mg/dl in females or patients ≥30 years of age with reduced renal function as measured by creatinine clearance) at the time of diagnosis of type 2 diabetes. Therapy should then be augmented with additional agents (including early initiation of insulin therapy) to achieve adequate glycemic control.
- In Type 2 diabetes, intensive glycemic control (HbA_{1c} <7) has been shown in RCT to reduce the risk of microvascular complications. While intensive glucose control reduced the risk of some cardiovascular disease outcomes (such as nonfatal MI), it did not reduce the risk of cardiovascular death or all-cause mortality and increased the risk of severe hypoglycemia.
- It is important to remember that tight glycemic control may burden patients with complex treatment programs, hypoglycemia, weight gain, and costs. Clinicians should individualize HbA_{1c} targets so that they are reasonable and reflect patients' personal and clinical contexts and their informed values and preferences. A target HbA_{1c} <7 is reasonable for motivated new diabetic patients with long life expectancies, whereas less stringent controls (HbA_{1c} 7.5 or higher) may be reasonable in elderly patients with limited life expectancy and elevated risk of hypoglycemia. The American Geriatrics Society recommends a general goal for glycated hemoglobin in older adults of 7.5% to 8.0%. Higher HbA_{1c} targets (8%-9%) are appropriate for older adults with multiple comorbidities, poor health, and limited life expectancy.[1]

NONPHARMACOLOGIC THERAPY

1. Diet: Newly diagnosed diabetics who are overweight or obese should be counseled to lose at least 5% of their body weight.
   a. Calories
      (1) The patient with diabetes can be started on 15 calories/lb of ideal body weight; this number can be increased to 20 calories/lb for an active person and 25 calories/lb if the patient does heavy physical labor.
      (2) The calories should be distributed as 45% to 65% carbohydrates, <30% fat, with saturated fat limited to <7% of total calories, and 10% to 30% protein. Daily cholesterol intake should not exceed 300 mg.

      (3) The emphasis should be on complex carbohydrates rather than simple and refined starches, and on polyunsaturated instead of saturated fats in a ratio of 2:1.
   b. Seven food groups
      (1) The exchange diet of the ADA includes bread or starches, meat or proteins, vegetables, fruits, fats, milk, and free foods (e.g., black tea, sugar-free gelatin).
      (2) The name of each exchange is meant to be all-inclusive (e.g., cereal, muffins, spaghetti, potatoes, rice are in the bread group; meats, fish, eggs, cheese, peanut butter are in the protein group).
      (3) The glycemic index compares the increase in blood sugar after the ingestion of simple sugars and complex carbohydrates with the increase that occurs after the absorption of glucose; equal amounts of starches do not give the same increase in plasma glucose (pasta equal in calories to a baked potato causes less of an increase than the potato); thus, it is helpful to know the glycemic index of a particular food product.
      (4) Fiber: Insoluble fiber (bran, celery) and soluble globular fiber (pectin in fruit) delay glucose absorption and attenuate the postprandial serum glucose peak; they also appear to reduce the increased triglyceride level often present in patients with uncontrolled diabetes. A diet high in fiber should be emphasized (20 to 35 g/day of soluble and insoluble fiber).
   c. Other principles
      (1) Modest sodium restriction to 2400 to 3000 mg/day. If hypertension is present, restrict to <2400 mg/day; if nephropathy and hypertension are present, restrict to <2000 mg/day.
      (2) Moderation of alcohol intake recommended (≤2 drinks/day in men, ≤1 drink/day in women).
      (3) Non-nutritive artificial sweeteners are acceptable in moderate amounts.
2. Exercise: increases the cellular glucose uptake by increasing the number of insulin receptors. The following points must be considered:
   a. Exercise program must be individualized and built up slowly. Consider beginning with 15 min of low-impact aerobic exercise 3 times per wk and increasing the frequency and duration to 30 to 45 min of moderate aerobic activity (50% to 70% of maximum age predicted heart rate) to 3 to 5 days/wk.
      (1) In the absence of contraindications, resistance training three times per wk should be encouraged.
   b. Insulin is more rapidly absorbed when injected into a limb that is then exercised, and this can result in hypoglycemia.
   c. Physical activity can result in hypoglycemia if medication dose or carbohydrate consumption is not modified. Ingestion of additional carbohydrates is recommended if pre-exercise glucose levels are <100 mg/dl.
3. Weight loss: to ideal body weight if the patient is overweight. Recent trials have shown

[1]Huang ES, Davis AM: Glycemic control in older adults with diabetes mellitus, *JAMA* 314:1509-1510, 2015.

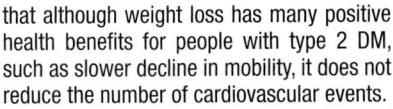

D

that although weight loss has many positive health benefits for people with type 2 DM, such as slower decline in mobility, it does not reduce the number of cardiovascular events.

4. Screening for nephropathy, neuropathy, and retinopathy: annual serum creatinine and urine albumin excretion; initial comprehensive eye examination and at least annually thereafter

5. Diabetes self-management education: could also address psychosocial issues

6. Self-monitoring of blood glucose should occur three to four times per day for patients using multiple insulin injections or on insulin pump therapy

7. Perform HbA1c at least two times a year in patients who are meeting treatment goals and who have stable glycemic control
   a. HbA1c quarterly in patients whose therapy has changed or who are not meeting glycemic goals
   b. The HbA1c goal for nonpregnant adults in general is <7%
   c. In the elderly, those with comorbidities, or those at risk for complications from hypoglycemia, a more moderate glycemic target (HbA1c 7-8) may be appropriate

GENERAL Rx

- When the previous measures fail to normalize the serum glucose, oral hypoglycemic agents should be added to the regimen in T2DM. Tables 4 and 5 compare therapies for T2DM and classes of antihyperglycemic agents.
- The primary mechanism of metformin is to decrease hepatic glucose production and improve insulin sensitivity. Because metformin does not produce hypoglycemia when used as a monotherapy, it is preferred initially for most patients. Metformin reduces mean HbA1c level by 1.1%. It is contraindicated in patients with severe renal insufficiency with an estimated glomerular filtrate rate <30 ml/min, serum creatinine level of 1.5 per dl or greater in men or 1.4 per dl or greater in women, heart failure, or other clinical states of hypoperfusion, and in patients with significant liver disease. Starting metformin in patients with GFR between 30 and 45 ml/min is also not recommended.
- When the HBA1c level is 9% or greater, initial dual-regimen combination therapy should be considered. Clinicians should consider adding either a DPP-4 inhibitor, an SGLT-2

inhibitor, a thiazolidinedione, or sulfonylurea to metformin to improve glycemic control when a dual regimen is considered.
- Sitagliptin, saxagliptin, vildagliptin, alogliptin, and linagliptin inhibit the enzyme DPP-4, responsible for inactivation and degradation of glucagon-like peptide-1 (GLP-1) and glucose-dependent insulinotropic polypeptide (GIP). These drugs, known as "DPP-4 inhibitors" or "gliptins," raise blood incretin levels, thereby inhibiting glucagon release and lowering blood glucose levels. When used with metformin they do not cause hypoglycemia and are preferred over sulfonylureas as second line agents. Linagliptin does not require a dosage adjustment in renal insufficiency. Cost is a major barrier to their use.
- Exenatide, dulaglutide, albiglutide, lixisenatide, and liraglutide are glucagon-like peptide-1 (GLP-1) agonists. They are incretin mimetics that stimulate release of insulin from pancreatic beta cells and can be used as adjunctive therapy for patients with T2DM. GLP-1 agonists are not indicated in T1DM and are contraindicated in patients with severe renal impairment. Cost is a barrier to their use.

Diseases and Disorders

I

Table 4 Comparison of Therapies for Type 2 Diabetes

Property	Lifestyle	Insulins	Sulfonylureas	Metformin	α-Glucosidase Inhibitors	Glitazones	Glinides	Exenatide	Pramlintide
Target tissue	Muscle or fat	Beta cell supplement	Beta cell	Liver	Gut	Muscle	Beta cell	Various	Brain
ΔHbA1c (%) as (monotherapy)	Variable	1->2	1-2	1-2	0.5-1	0.5-2	Re: 1-2 N: 0.5-1	~1	~0.5
Fasting effect	Good	Excellent	Good	Good	Poor	Good	Re: Moderate N: Poor	Poor	Poor
Postprandial effect	Good	Excellent	Good	Good	Excellent	Good	Re: Good N: Excellent	Excellent	Excellent
Severe hypoglycemia	No	Yes	Yes	No	No	No	Re: Yes N: No	No	No
Dosing interval	Continuous	qd to continuous	qd to tid	bid or tid	bid to qid	P: qd Ro: qd or bid	tid to qid with meals	bid	tid
ΔWeight (lb/yr)	+1	+3	+1 to 3	0 to −6	0 to −10	+1 to 13	+1 to 3	−6 to −12	−3 to −6
ΔInsulin	Variable	Increase	Increase	Modest decrease	Modest decrease	Decrease	Increase	Increase	None
ΔLDL	Minimal decrease	Minimal decrease	None	Decrease	Minimal decrease	Increase	None	None	None
ΔHDL	Minimal increase	None	None	Increase	None	Increase	None	Decrease	None
ΔTG	Minimal decrease	Decrease	None	Decrease	Minimal decrease	P: Decrease Ro: None	None	Decrease	None
Common problem	Recidivism, injury	Hypoglycemia, weight gain	Hypoglycemia, weight gain	Transient GI	Flatulence	Weight gain, edema, anemia	Hypoglycemia	GI	GI
Rare problem	—	—	—	Lactic acidosis	—	Hepatotoxicity?	—	—	—
Contraindications	None	None	Allergy	Renal failure, Liver failure, CHF (>80 yr old)	Intestinal disease	Hepatocellular disease	—	None	None
Cost ($/mo)	0-200	30-450	10-15	30-60	40-80	75-180	70-110	170-200	200-400
Maximum effective dose	—	1-2 U/kg per day	maximum or double starting	1000 mg bid	50 mg tid	P: 45 mg qd Ro: 4 mg bid	Re: 2 mg tid N: 120 mg tid	10 μg bid	120 μg ac

Δ, Change; *ac*, before food; *CHF*, congestive heart failure; *GI*, gastrointestinal disturbance; *HbA1c*, glycosylated hemoglobin; *HDL*, high-density lipoprotein; *LDL*, low-density lipoprotein; *N*, nateglinide; *P*, pioglitazone; *Re*, repaglinide; *Ro*, rosiglitazone; *TG*, triglycerides.

From Melmed S, Polonsky KS, Larsen PR, Kronenberg HM: *Williams textbook of endocrinology*, ed 12, Philadelphia, 2011, Saunders.

Table 5 Classes of Antihyperglycemic Therapy

Class	Representative Agents	Major Action	HbA$_{1c}$ Lowering (%)	Fasting or Prandial Effect	Usual Dosing Frequency (Doses/Day)	Route	Hypoglycemia	Weight Effect	CVD Risk Factor Benefits	Important Contraindications	Daily Cost ($)
Lifestyle	—	Broad	>1	Both	—	—	No	Loss	Yes	—	—
Biguanide	Metformin	Liver sensitizer	>1	Fasting	1-2	Oral	No	Neutral	Modest	Renal or hepatic failure	<$1
Sulfonylurea	Glimepiride, glipizide	Insulin secretagogue	>1	Fasting	1-2	Oral	Yes	Gain	Negligible	—	<<$1
Meglitinide	Repaglinide	Insulin secretagogue	>1	Both	With meals	Oral	Yes	Gain	Negligible	—	~$5
Benzoic acid–derived	Nateglinide	Insulin secretagogue	<1	Prandial	With meals	Oral	Minimal	Minimal	Negligible	—	~$5
Basal insulin	NPH, glargine, detemir	Insulin supplement/substitute	>1	Fasting	1	SQ	Yes++	Gain++	Lowers TG	—	~$5
Bolus insulin	R, lispro, aspart, glulisine	Insulin supplement/substitute	>1	Prandial	With meals	SQ	Yes++	Gain++	Lowers TG	—	~$5
Thiazolidinediones	Pioglitazone, rosiglitazone	Peripheral sensitizer	>1	Fasting	1	Oral	No	Gain++	Variable (see text)	Heart or liver failure	~$5
α-Glucosidase inhibitors	Acarbose, miglitol	Slow carbohydrate absorption	<1	Prandial	With meals	Oral	No	Neutral	Negligible	—	~$3
Amylinomimetics	Pramlintide	Broad	<1	Prandial	With meals	SQ	No	Loss	Negligible	—	~$10
GLP1 receptor agonists	Exenatide	Broad	~1	Prandial	2	SQ	No	Loss	Modest with weight loss	Pancreatitis, renal failure	~$9
Long-acting GLP1 receptor agonists	Liraglutide, albiglutide, dulaglutide	Broad	>1	Both	1	SQ	No	Loss	Lowers BP	Pancreatitis, medullary thyroid cancer	~$13
DPP4 inhibitors	Sitagliptin, saxagliptin	Improved insulin/glucagon secretion	<1	Both	1	Oral	No	Neutral	Negligible	Pancreatitis	~$7
Bile acid sequestrants	Colesevelam	Uncertain	<1	Prandial	1-2	Oral	No	Neutral	Lowers LDL	Hypertriglyceridemia	~$9
SGLT$_2$ inhibitor	Canagliflozin, dapagliflozin, empagliflozin	Decrease renal glucose reabsorption, increase urinary glucose excretion	<1	Both	1	Oral	No	Loss	Negligible	Volume dilution	~$10

BP, Blood pressure; CVD, cardiovascular disease; LDL, low-density lipoprotein; SGLT$_2$, sodium-glucose co-transporter 2; SQ, subcutaneous; TG, triglyceride.

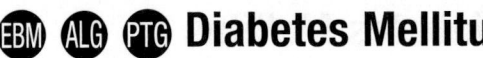

- Sodium-glucose co-transporter 2 (SGLT$_2$) inhibitors (e.g., canagliflozin [Invokana], dapagliflozin [Farxiga], empagliflozin [Jardiance]) are useful for oral treatment of type 2 DM. By inhibiting SGLT$_2$, these medications decrease glucose reabsorption, increase urinary glucose excretion, and lower blood glucose levels (decrease HbA$_{1c}$ by 0.7%). Empagliflozin has been shown to slow progression of renal disease in type 2 diabetics with cardiovascular disease. Side effects include increased risk of genital mycotic infections, UTIs, and volume depletion. Renal function should be evaluated before starting SGLT$_2$ inhibitors and periodically thereafter. Temporary discontinuation of these meds is recommended in cases of reduced oral intake or fluid loss. Higher cost and limited drug formulary availability are limiting factors.
- Sulfonylureas increase insulin secretion and work best when given before meals. All sulfonylureas are contraindicated in patients who are allergic to sulfa. Use of sulfonylureas confers a greater risk of hypoglycemia than the other agents.
- Acarbose and miglitol inhibit pancreatic amylase and small intestinal glucosidases, thereby delaying carbohydrate absorption in the gut and reducing associated postprandial hyperglycemia. The major side effects are flatulence, diarrhea, and abdominal cramps.
- The meglitinides nateglinide and repaglinide and the bile acid sequestrant colesevelam can also be used to lower glucose levels but are expensive and generally poorly tolerated.
- Pramlintide is a synthetic analog of human amylin, which is synthesized by pancreatic beta cells and cosecreted with insulin in response to food intake. It suppresses glucagon secretion and slows stomach emptying and can be used as an adjunctive treatment for patients with T1DM or T2DM who inject insulin at mealtime. Nausea is its major side effect.
- Thiazolidinediones (pioglitazone and rosiglitazone) increase insulin sensitivity and have been used in the therapy of type 2 diabetes. Serum transaminase levels should be obtained before starting therapy and monitored periodically. Thiazolidinediones, in general, result in moderate weight gain and increase the risk for heart failure and osteoporosis/fractures. Rosiglitazone has an FDA black box warning for heart failure exacerbations and myocardial ischemia. Pioglitazone and rosiglitazone cause increased incidence of bladder cancer.
- Combination therapy of various hypoglycemic agents is commonly used when dual therapy results in inadequate glycemic control.
- Insulin is indicated for the treatment of all T1DM and for T2DM patients whose condition cannot be adequately controlled with diet and oral agents. The American College of Endocrinology and the American Association of Clinical Endocrinologists recommend initiation of insulin therapy in patients with type 2 diabetes and an initial HbA$_{1c}$ level >9%, or if the diabetes is uncontrolled despite optimal oral glycemic therapy. Insulin therapy may be initiated as augmentation, starting at 0.1 to

Table 6 Types of Insulin[a]

Preparation	Brand	Onset (hr)[b]	Peak (hr)	Duration (hr)[c]	Route
Insulin Aspart	NovoLog[d]	<0.25	1-3	3-5	SC, IV, CSII
Insulin Aspart Protamine/Insulin Aspart	NovoLog Mix 70/30[d]	<0.25	1-4	24	SC
Insulin Detemir	Levemir	1-4	None	24	SC
Insulin Glargine	Lantus[d]	1-4	None	≥24	SC
Insulin Degludec	Tresiba	1-9	None	>42	SC
Insulin Glulisine	Apidra[d]	≤0.25	1	2-4	SC, IV
Insulin Lispro	Humalog[d]	<0.25	1	3.5-4.5	SC
Insulin Lispro Protamine/Insulin Lispro	Humalog Mix 75/25[d]	≤0.25	0.5-1.5	24	SC
	Humalog Mix 50/50[d]	≤0.25	1	16	SC
Insulin Injection Regular (R)	Humulin R[f]	0.5	2-4	6-8	SC, IM, IV
	Novolin N[e]	0.5	2.5-5	8	SC, IM, IV
Insulin Isophane Suspension (NPH)/ Regular Insulin (R)	Humulin 70/30[f]	0.5	2-12	24	SC
	Humulin 50/50[f]	0.5	3-5	24	SC
	Novolin 70/30[e]	0.5	2-12	24	SC
Insulin Isophane Suspension (NPH)	Humulin N[f]	1-2	6-12	18-24	SC
	Novolin N[e]	1.5	4-12	24	SC

CSII, Continuous subcutaneous infusion; *IM,* intramuscularly; *IV,* intravenously.
[a]Injectable insulins listed are available in a concentration of 100 U/ml; Humulin R, in a concentration of 500 U/ml for SC injection. SC injection only is available by prescription from Lilly for insulin-resistant patients who are hospitalized or in need of medical supervision.
[b]Onset for injectable formulations is always for the subcutaneous (SC) route. All times are approximate.
[c]Maximum effect occurs between these times; actual effect may last longer.
[d]Recombinant human insulin analogue (using *E. coli*).
[e]Recombinant (using *S. cerevisiae*).
[f]Recombinant (using *E. coli*).
Modified from Melmed S, Polonsky KS, Larsen PR, Kronenberg HM: *Williams textbook of endocrinology,* ed 12, Philadelphia, 2011, Saunders.

0.2 unit/kg of body weight, or as replacement, starting at 0.6 to 1.0 unit/kg. Table 6 describes commonly used types of insulin.
1. The risks of insulin therapy include weight gain, hypoglycemia, and in rare cases, allergic or cutaneous reactions.
2. Replacement insulin therapy should mimic normal release patterns.
    a. Approximately 50% to 60% of daily insulin can be given as a long-acting insulin (NPH, Ultralente, glargine, detemir) injected once or twice daily
    b. The remaining 40% to 50% can be short-acting (regular) or rapid-acting (lispro, aspart, glulisine) to cover mealtime carbohydrates and correct increased current glucose levels.
- Continuous subcutaneous insulin infusion (CSII, or insulin pump) provides comparable or slightly better control than multiple daily injections. It should be considered for diabetes presenting in childhood or adolescence and during pregnancy. The guidelines for insulin pump therapy from the American Association of Diabetes Educators include "frequent and unpredictable fluctuations in blood glucose" and "patient perceptions that diabetes management impedes the pursuit of personal or professional goals."
- Antiplatelet therapy: Low-dose aspirin (ASA; 81 mg/day) has been proven to lower the risk of subsequent myocardial infarction, stroke, or vascular death in secondary prevention studies. The ADA recommends low-dose aspirin for primary prevention in diabetic patients with one additional cardiovascular risk factor, including

age older than 40 yr, cigarette smoking, hypertension, obesity, albuminuria, hyperlipidemia, and family history of coronary artery disease. Clopidogrel can be used in patients with atherosclerotic cardiovascular disease (ASCVD) and a documented aspirin allergy.
- Lipid management: Measure fasting lipid profile at least annually in adults.
1. All patients with diabetes with one or more additional risk factors for cardiovascular disease should be on statin therapy together with lifestyle modification regardless of baseline lipid levels.
2. Diabetic patients aged 40 to 75 with LDL cholesterol of 70 to 189 mg/dl and without clinical ASCVD should receive at least moderate-intensity statin therapy and consider high-intensity statin therapy if 10-year ASCVD risk is ≥7.5%.
3. Ezetimibe can be added to moderate-intensity statin therapy in those who cannot tolerate high-intensity statin therapy.
4. Combination therapy with statin and fenofibrate is not recommended but may be considered in those with triglyceride levels equal or greater than 204 mg/dl.
- Hypertension: Antihypertensive therapy is recommended to keep systolic blood pressure (BP) <140 and diastolic BP <90 mm Hg. Use of angiotensin-converting enzyme (ACE) inhibitors or angiotensin receptor blockers (ARBs) to decrease albuminuria and for prevention of progression of kidney disease should be considered regardless of presence of hypertension. Combination therapy with an ACE inhibitor and

---

BOX 1 Sick Day Management Protocol for Diabetic Patients

Examples of "Sick Day" Scenarios
- Feeling sick or presence of fever for 2 days or longer without getting better
- Vomiting or diarrhea for more than 6 hours

Management
General Measures
- Check blood sugar levels at least every 4 hours, but when values are changing quickly, check more often.
- Check urine or blood ketones.
- Modify usual insulin regimen according to a plan developed by the diabetes physician or team.
- Maintain adequate food and fluid intake. If your appetite is poor, aim for consumption of 50 g of carbohydrate every 3-4 hours. If you are nauseous, high-carbohydrate liquids, such as regular (not diet) soft drinks or juice, or frozen juice bars, sherbet, pudding, creamed soups, or fruit-flavored yogurt usually are tolerated. Broth also is a good alternative.

Taking Medications When You Are Sick
- If you are eating: Continue taking your pills for diabetes or your insulin. Your blood sugar may continue to rise because of your illness.
- If you are nauseous or vomiting or otherwise cannot take your medicines:
  - Continue to take your long-acting insulin (Lantus, Levemir, NPH).
  - Call your doctor and discuss whether you need to adjust your short- or rapid-acting insulin dose (regular, lispro [Humalog], aspart [Novolog], glulisine [Apidra]) or your other diabetes medicines.

Examples of When to Call Physician or Diabetes Team
- If glucose levels are higher than 240 mg/dl despite taking extra insulin according to a sick day plan
- If you take diabetes pills and blood sugar is still above 240 mg/dl before meals and remains there for more than 24 hours
- If symptoms/signs develop that might signal DKA or dehydration, such as dizziness, trouble breathing, fruity breath, or dry and cracked lips or tongue

DKA, diabetic ketoacidosis.

Parrillo JE, Dellinger RP: *Critical care medicine: principles of diagnosis and management in the adult*, ed 4, Philadelphia, 2014, Mosby.

---

an ARB should be avoided due to increased risk of adverse effects among patients with diabetic nephropathy. In older adults a treatment goal of <130/70 mm Hg is not recommended due to higher mortality and morbidity.
- Bariatric surgery should be considered in adults with BMI >35 kg/m^2 and type 2 diabetes, especially if the diabetes is difficult to control with lifestyle and pharmacologic therapy. Five-year outcome data showed that, among patients with type 2 DM and a BMR of 27 to 43, bariatric surgery plus intensive medical therapy was more effective than intensive medical therapy alone in decreasing, or in some cases resolving, hyperglycemia.[2]
- Treat hypoglycemia in a conscious person with glucose tab or gel 15 to 20 g, and intramuscular injection of glucagon if unconscious. Patient and family members should be instructed on the administration of glucagon for individuals at significant risk for severe hypoglycemia. A sick day management protocol for diabetic patients is described in Box 1.

DISPOSITION
- Diabetic retinopathy occurs in nearly 15% of patients with diabetes after 15 yr of diagnosis and increases 1%/yr after diagnosis.

Glycemic, lipid, and blood pressure controls are essential to reduce the risk and progression of diabetic retinopathy. An annual comprehensive eye exam by an ophthalmologist or optometrist should begin at the time of diagnosis for those with T2DM and after 5 years in those with T1DM. Retinal laser photocoagulation and vitrectomy are effective treatment modalities. Prevention is best accomplished by strict glucose and BP control. Early blockade of the renin-angiotensin system has been shown to slow progression of retinopathy in patients with type 1 diabetes.
- The frequency of neuropathy in patients with type 2 diabetes approaches 70% to 80%. It can be subdivided into sensorimotor neuropathy and autonomic neuropathy. Duloxetine, a selective serotonin and norepinephrine reuptake inhibitor, is effective and FDA approved for relief of diabetic peripheral neuropathy. Pregabalin and gabapentin (900 to 3600 mg/day) are also effective for the symptomatic treatment of peripheral neuropathic pain. Topical capsaicin, 5% lidocaine transdermal patches, amitriptyline, and carbamazepine are also modestly effective.
- Diabetic gastroparesis is most often seen in patients who have had diabetes for at least 10 yr and typically have retinopathy, neuropathy, and nephropathy. Major manifestations are postprandial fullness, nausea, vomiting, and bloating. Pharmacologic therapy involves

prokinetic agents (metoclopramide). Endoscopic injection of botulinum toxin into the pylorus and gastric electrical stimulation (using f electrodes placed laparoscopically in the muscle wall of the stomach antrum and connected to a neurostimulator) represent newer approaches to nonpharmacologic therapy.
- Nephropathy: The first sign of renal involvement in patients with DM is most often microalbuminuria, which is classified as incipient nephropathy. Before the current period of intensive glycemic control and blood pressure with ACE inhibitors and angiotensin receptor blockade, it was suggested that 25% to 45% of diabetic patients would develop clinically evident renal disease (proteinuria) and 4% to 17% would progress to end-stage renal disease. In the current era of intensive glycemic and blood pressure control and ACE/ARB use, clinically evident diabetic nephropathy has declined to 9% and end-stage renal disease 2% to 7%.
- Infections are generally more common in patients with diabetes because of multiple factors, such as impaired leukocyte function, decreased tissue perfusion secondary to vascular disease, repeated trauma because of loss of sensation, and urinary retention secondary to neuropathy.
- Prevention/delay of type 2 diabetes: Patients with prediabetes should achieve weight loss of 5% to 10% of body weight and increase physical activity to at least 150 min/wk of moderate activity such as walking. Metformin therapy may be considered in those at high risk, especially if they have hyperglycemia (HbA$_{1c}$ ≥6) despite lifestyle interventions.

REFERRAL
- Patients with diabetes should be advised to have annual ophthalmologic examinations. In T1DM, ophthalmologic visits should usually begin 5 yr after diagnosis, whereas T2DM patients should be seen from disease onset.
- Podiatric care can significantly reduce the rate of foot infections and amputations in patients with DM. Noninfected neuropathic foot ulcers require debridement and reduction of pressure.
- Nephrology consultation in all cases of proteinuria, hyperkalemia, uncontrolled BP, and when GFR has decreased to <30 mL/min/1.73 m^2.

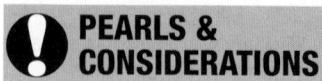 **PEARLS & CONSIDERATIONS**

COMMENTS
- Because normalization of serum glucose level is the ultimate goal, every patient with diabetes should measure his or her blood glucose with commercially available glucometers unless contraindicated by senility or blindness.
- Underinsured children and those with psychiatric illness are at greater risk for acute complications in T1DM and require frequent monitoring and aggressive risk management with diet, exercise, and periodic laboratory evaluation.

[2]Schauer PR, et al.: Bariatric surgery versus intensive medical therapy for diabetes—5-year outcomes, *N Engl J Med* 376(7):641–651, 2017.

- Significant sustained weight loss using bariatric surgery has been reported as effective in achieving remission of type 2 diabetes in morbidly obese patients. Bariatric surgery may be considered for adults with BMI >35 kg/m^2 and T2DM, especially if diabetes or associated comorbidities are difficult to control with lifestyle and pharmacologic therapy.
- Cigarette smoking predicts incident type 2 diabetes. For a smoker at risk for diabetes, smoking cessation should be coupled with strategies for diabetes prevention and early detection.
- Glycemic control in hospitalized patients: The American College of Physicians (ACP) recommends against using intensive insulin therapy to strictly control blood glucose in non-surgical intensive care unit (SICU)/medical intensive care unit (MICU) in patients with or without DM. The ACP recommends a target blood glucose level of 140 to 200 mg/dl if insulin therapy is used.

SUGGESTED READINGS

Available at www.expertconsult.com

RELATED CONTENT

Diabetes Mellitus Type 1(Patient Information)
Diabetes Mellitus Type 2 (Patient Information)
Diabetic Ketoacidosis (Related Key Topic)
Diabetic Foot (Related Key Topic)
Diabetic Polyneuropathy (Related Key Topic)
Diabetic Retinopathy (Related Key Topic)
Gestational Diabetes Mellitus (Related Key Topic)
Hyperosmolar Hyperglycemic Syndrome (Related Key Topic)

AUTHORS: **HILARY B. WHITLATCH, M.D.,
SAINATH GADDAM, M.D.,** and **FRED F. FERRI, M.D.**

D

Diseases and Disorders

I

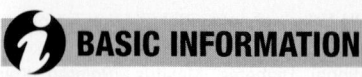
DEFINITION

Diabetic foot infections (DFIs) are a common and potentially serious problem in persons with diabetes. They usually arise from either a skin ulceration that occurs secondarily to peripheral neuropathy or in a wound caused by some form of trauma. The infection usually involves one or more bacteria and can spread to contiguous tissues including bone, causing an osteomyelitis.

SYNONYMS

Diabetic foot ulcer
Diabetic foot infection
DFI

ICD-10CM CODES	
E10.5	Diabetes mellitus with peripheral circulatory complications
E10.6	Diabetes mellitus with other specific complications
E11.621	Type 2 diabetes mellitus with foot ulcer

EPIDEMIOLOGY & DEMOGRAPHICS

INCIDENCE: DFIs are the most common cause of hospitalizations for diabetic patients. They account for 20% of all hospital admissions. Nearly one in six patients will die within a year of their infection.

PEAK INCIDENCE: More common in Hispanics, African Americans, and Native Americans due to increased rates of diabetes in those populations

PREVALENCE: 25 million people in the United States have diabetes, of which 15% to 25% will develop a foot ulcer in their lifetime and more than 50% of these will become infected.

PREDOMINANT SEX AND AGE: Females greater than males

RISK FACTORS:

- Diabetes greater than 10 years
- Poor glucose control
- Peripheral neuropathy: altered protective sensation and altered pain response
- Diabetic angiopathy: atherosclerotic obstruction of larger vessels leading to peripheral vascular disease
- Evidence of increased local pressure: callus or erythema

PHYSICAL FINDINGS & CLINICAL PRESENTATION

A. Based on guidelines by Infectious Diseases Society of America, infection is present if obvious purulent drainage and/or the presence of two or more signs of inflammation
  1. Erythema
  2. Pain
  3. Tenderness
  4. Warmth
  5. Induration
B. Systemic signs of infection include:
  1. Anorexia, nausea/vomiting
  2. Fever, chills, night sweats
  3. Change in mental status and recent worsening of glycemic control

An earlier and commonly used classification system was originally proposed by Wagner.

An update to the Wagner system was introduced at the University of Texas (UT), San Antonio, in the U.S. While similar to Wagner in its first three categories, this later system eliminated grades 4 and 5 and added stages A-D for each of the grades. The UT system was the first diabetic foot ulcer classification to be validated.
University of Texas system
  Grade:
- Grade 0: Pre- or postulcerative (Stages A-D)
- Grade 1: Full-thickness ulcer not involving tendon, capsule, or bone (Stage A-D)
- Grade 2: Tendon or capsular involvement without bone palpable (Stage A-D)
- Grade 3: Probes to bone (Stage A-D)
  Stage:
- A: Noninfected
- B: Infected
- C: Ischemic
- D: Infected and ischemic
C. Etiology: most diabetic foot infections are polymicrobial (can involve 5-7 different bacteria) and depend on the extent of involvement
  1. Superficial infections are likely due to gram-positive skin bacteria:
    a. *Staphylococcus aureus*, includes methicillin-resistant *S. aureus* (MRSA)
    b. *Streptococcus agalactiae* (group B streptococcus) and *Streptococcus pyogenes* (group A streptococcus)
    c. Coagulase-negative *Staphylococcus*
  2. Infections that are deep, chronically infected, or previously treated are likely to be polymicrobial:
    a. Include above bacteria plus enterococci, gram-negative rods including
    b. *Pseudomonas aeruginosa* and anaerobes
    c. With gangrene can expect more anaerobic bacteria such as *Clostridia* and *Bacteroides* species
    d. Patients with multiple admissions can have more resistant bacteria such as ESBL-type resistant gram-negative rod bacteria, MRSA, and *Acinetobacter*

DIAGNOSIS

DIFFERENTIAL DIAGNOSIS

Other inflammatory conditions that can mimic diabetic foot infections include:
- Crystal-associated arthritis such as gout
- Trauma
- Acute Charcot arthropathy from long-standing diabetes
- Venous stasis ulcers
- Deep vein thrombosis

WORKUP

Evaluation of a patient with a DFI involves determining the extent and severity of the infection, identifying the underlying factors that predispose to the infection, and determining the microbiologic etiology.

PHYSICAL EXAMINATION:

- Vital signs: fever, chills, hypotension, tachycardia can be present.
- Detailed wound description: length, width, and depth of wound, consistency of drainage, character of wound base: granular fibrous necrotic
- Determination of osteomyelitis: highly likely if bone visible. A positive probe test to bone has a sensitivity of 66% and specificity of 85% in diagnosing bone infection.
- Necrotizing infections may present with cutaneous bullae, soft tissue gas, foul odor, and skin discoloration (Fig. 1).
- Severe infections may present with gangrene, tissue necrosis, and evidence of tissue ischemia, all of which may be limb threatening.

LABORATORY TESTS

Important to obtain at baseline and to assess response to therapy
- Fewer than 50% of patients have an elevated WBC.
- Determine BUN/Cr, acidosis, hemoglobin A_{1C}, and blood sugar.
- Acute phase reactants: Sed rate and CRP are markers for inflammation.
  1. Sed rate >70 increases probability of bone infection.
- Serum prealbumin and albumin are markers for nutritional status and ability to heal.
- An ulcer size larger than 2 cm^2 is indicative of osteomyelitis.
- Gram stains and cultures: superficial cultures should not be obtained as they may contain colonizing bacteria and instead deep tissue cultures (aerobic and anaerobic) should be obtained.

IMAGING STUDIES

- Plain film x-ray evaluates bones and soft issues and can detect presence of tissue gas, which would represent an emergent situation (Fig. 2).

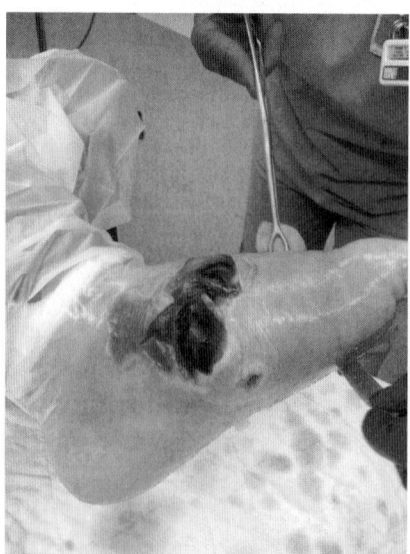

FIG. 1 Foot: Severe diabetic foot infection with significant tissue swelling and necrosis.

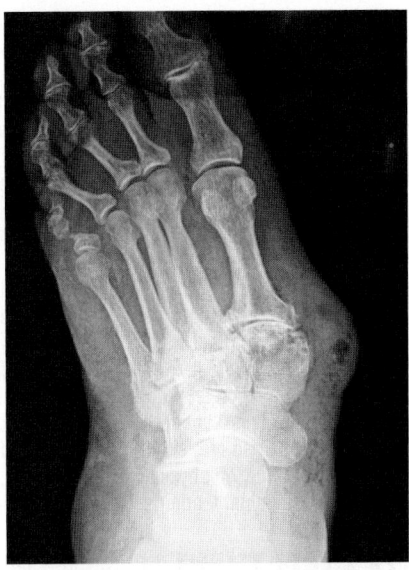

FIG. 2 X-ray: Significant soft tissue swelling in midfoot with numerous gas bubbles seen in the soft tissues.

- Osteomyelitis appears as radiolucencies, periosteal reaction, and destructive changes. Plain films are 67% specific and 60% sensitive for osteomyelitis.
- Bone scan: Indium-111 or technetium-99 can distinguish acute and chronic infections.
- CT and MRI: MRI is the most sensitive and specific test to detect osteomyelitis and abscess formation.

OTHER DIAGNOSTIC TESTS

- Noninvasive vascular studies: Ankle brachial index (ABI): <0.90 or >1.30 indicates peripheral arterial disease
- Transcutaneous oxygen (TcPO2) tension measurements: predictive of wound healing failure at levels below 25 mm Hg

Rx TREATMENT

Empiric antibiotic regimen should be started based on likely pathogens suspected and severity of disease. Wound management and debridement including surgical consultation are important as well.

NONPHARMACOLOGIC THERAPY

- Good nutrition will promote wound healing.
- Glycemic control will promote healing.
- Fluid and electrolyte balance will improve healing.

ACUTE GENERAL TREATMENT
WOUND MANAGEMENT:

- Debridement of callus and necrotic tissues by wound care specialist or surgeon and at times may require multiple debridements.
- Wound dressing: to absorb exudates and promote healing. Many products are available but none has been proven superior and include:
  1. Enzymes
  2. Gels
  3. Hydrocolloids
  4. Antiseptics containing iodine or silver salts
  5. Honey
- Relieve pressure on the foot: casts or special shoes.
- Amputation or revascularization procedures such as angioplasty or bypass grafting may be necessary.

Antibiotic management
- Prior to receiving culture results an empiric antibiotic regimen should be started as soon as possible to cover skin bacteria, gram-negative rods, and anaerobes. Options for intravenous therapy include:
- Piperacillin-tazobactam: 3.375 g IV q6h with normal kidney function. Will cover gram-negative rods including *Pseudomonas aeruginosa*, streptococci, anaerobes, and *Staphylococcus aureus.* Adjust dose based on CrCl.
- Meropenem: 1 g IV q8h with normal kidney function has comparable coverage as piperacillin-tazobactam. Similar agents include imipenem and doripenem.
- Third-generation cephalosporin such as cefepime, 2 g IV q8h, or ceftriaxone, 2 g IV qd, have excellent gram-negative coverage and for anaerobic coverage add metronidazole, 500 mg IV q8h, or clindamycin 900 mg IV q8h. Cefepime will cover *Pseudomonas aeruginosa* but ceftriaxone will not.
- For penicillin-allergic patients a combination of ciprofloxacin, 400 mg IV q12h, plus metronidazole or clindamycin is an option. Aztreonam is another option for gram-negative rod coverage, 2 g IV q8h.
- If MRSA suspected need to add IV vancomycin, 15-20 mg/kg IV q8-12h, depending on age and CrCL and follow trough levels to keep above 15. Other options include daptomycin, 4 mg/kg IV qd, which does not have to be adjusted for CrCL or linezolid, 400-600 mg IV q12h.
- If VRE suspected options include tigecycline, 100-mg IV load dose, then 50 mg IV q12h, which also covers MRSA and gram-negative rods but not *Pseudomonas aeruginosa,* or can use daptomycin or linezolid.
- If ESBL gram-negative bacteria are suspected then options include meropenem or ertapenem, 1 g IV qd, or tigecycline.
- Once culture results are known can tailor antibiotics to more specific agent.
- Oral antibiotics used for milder infections include: amoxicillin-clavulanate, 875 mg PO q12h, will cover gram-negative rods, streptococci, and anaerobes, or ciprofloxacin plus metronidazole or clindamycin. Bactrim will cover MRSA and MSSA and some gram-negative rods.

The expert panel on diabetic foot infection (DFI) of the International Working Group on the Diabetic Foot conducted a systematic review. Results of comparisons of different antibiotic regimens generally demonstrated that newly introduced antibiotic regimens appeared to be as effective as conventional therapy.

CHRONIC TREATMENT

- Length of therapy: highly variable depending on the severity of the infection. In general 2 to 4 weeks of antibiotics is sufficient. If bone infection suspected or documented may need 4-8 weeks of antibiotics preferably intravenous via a peripherally inserted central line (PICC line).
- Surgical debridement may also be necessary for several weeks.

COMPLEMENTARY MEDICINE

- Hyperbaric oxygen (HBO): Used as an adjunct to antibiotics, debridement, and revascularization in the therapy of chronic, nonhealing wounds associated with diabetes. HBO acts by:
  1. Inducing vasoconstriction and reducing vasogenic edema
  2. Facilitating fibroblast activity, angiogenesis, and wound healing
  3. Killing anaerobic bacteria and augmenting neutrophil bactericidal activity
- Negative pressure wound therapy (wound vac): controlled, subatmospheric pressure applied to an open wound can accelerate healing and closure.
  1. An open cell foam insert is cut to fit the open wound and then secured under a clear, vapor-permeable, plastic dressing.
  2. Tubing extends from the sponge to a disposable collection canister.
  3. A portable pump applies 125 mm Hg of controlled suction to the system. The subatmospheric pressure (suction) is equally distributed across the open wound and evacuates stagnant fluid from the wound.

DISPOSITION

- Following up on sed rates, CRP, BUN/CR, and levels of vancomycin if that antibiotic used.
- Surgical or wound center care follow-up.
- HBO usually involves multiple sessions over several weeks.
- Wound vac is applied for weeks and requires periodic nursing follow-up.

REFERRAL

- Infectious disease consultant for antibiotic management.
- Surgeon or wound care center for surgical treatments.
- Endocrinologist for good diabetes care.
- Vascular surgeon for angioplasty or bypass procedures.

❶ PEARLS & CONSIDERATIONS

- In a meta-analysis of randomized controlled trials on the outcome of DFIs, there was a 22.7% treatment failure rate.
- Patients should be advised to seek prompt medical attention as these infections can progress rapidly to gangrene.

AUTHOR: **GLENN G. FORT, M.D., M.P.H.**

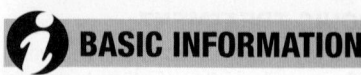

BASIC INFORMATION

DEFINITION

Diabetic ketoacidosis (DKA) is a life-threatening complication of diabetes mellitus resulting from absolute insulin deficiency or insulin resistance with relative insulin deficiency. It is characterized by the presence of an anion gap metabolic acidosis, ketonemia, and hyperglycemia. Patients often present with severe dehydration and altered sensorium.

SYNONYMS

DKA

ICD-10CM CODES
E10.10 Type 2 diabetes mellitus with other specified complication
E08.10 Diabetes mellitus due to underlying condition with ketoacidosis without coma
E08.11 Diabetes mellitus due to underlying condition with ketoacidosis with coma

EPIDEMIOLOGY & DEMOGRAPHICS

INCIDENCE/PREVALENCE: 6 episodes per 10,000 individuals with diabetes; it accounts for 8% to 29% of all hospital admissions of patients with diabetes
PREDOMINANT AGE: 36% in persons younger than age 30, 27% in persons 30 to 60 years of age, 23% in persons 51 to 70 years of age, and 14% occurring in persons older than 70 years.

PHYSICAL FINDINGS & CLINICAL PRESENTATION

- Evidence of dehydration (tachycardia, hypotension, dry mucous membranes, sunken eyeballs, poor skin turgor)
- Altered mental status
- Tachypnea with air hunger (Kussmaul's respiration)
- Fruity breath odor (caused by acetone)
- Lipemia retinalis in some patients
- Possible evidence of precipitating factors (infected wound, pneumonia)
- Abdominal tenderness in some patients

ETIOLOGY

- Metabolic decompensation in individuals with diabetes is frequently precipitated by an infectious process (up to 40%).
- Poor compliance with insulin therapy and severe medical illness (e.g., pancreatitis, cardiovascular events) are other common causes.
- There is a subgroup of type 2 diabetics who have ketosis-prone diabetes. These persons are often black or Latino, overweight, middle aged, males with a family history of diabetes or newly diagnosed diabetes. This subgroup represents 20% to 50% of persons with DKA.
- Cocaine abuse has been reported as a risk factor for DKA in adult and teenage

patients, particularly in patients with multiple admissions.
- Lack of education of primary caregiver (mother, sibling), as well as deficiencies in proper monitoring of blood glucose, correct administration of insulin, supervision of insulin pump maintenance, and monitoring of diabetic caloric restraints are causes of recurrent episodes of DKA.
- Use of sodium glucose co-transporter 2 inhibitors (SGLT2) increases risk of DKA.

DIAGNOSIS

DIFFERENTIAL DIAGNOSIS

- Hyperosmolar nonketotic state
- Alcoholic ketoacidosis
- Uremic acidosis
- Metabolic acidosis caused by methyl alcohol or ethylene glycol
- Salicylate poisoning

WORKUP

- Laboratory evaluation (see "Laboratory Tests") to confirm diagnosis and evaluate precipitating factors
- Identification of "trigger," such as infection (blood cultures, urine cultures, chest radiographs), pancreatitis (pancreatic enzymes), or myocardial ischemia (ECG, cardiac enzymes)

LABORATORY TESTS

- Glucose level demonstrates severe hyperglycemia (serum glucose generally >250 mg/dl)
- Arterial blood gases demonstrate metabolic acidosis: arterial pH usually <7.30 with Pco_2 <40 mm Hg
- Serum ketonemia (b-hydroxybutyrate >300 mmol/L), ketonuria, and glycosuria
- Serum electrolytes:
  1. Serum bicarbonate is usually <15 mEq/L.
  2. Serum potassium (K^+) may be low, normal, or elevated. There is always significant total body potassium depletion regardless of the initial potassium level.
  3. Serum sodium is usually decreased as a result of hyperglycemia, dehydration, and lipemia. Assume 1.6-mEq/L decrease in extracellular sodium for each 100-mg/dl increase in glucose concentration.
  4. Calculate the anion gap (AG): $AG = Na^+ - (Cl^- + HCO_3^-)$
  5. In DKA, the anion gap is increased (<12) because of high levels of ketones.
  6. Mixed metabolic disturbances demonstrating anion gap metabolic acidosis overlapping with metabolic alkalosis may be present; this is common in patients with DKA with persistent vomiting.
- CBC with differential, urinalysis, and urine and blood cultures to rule out infectious precipitating factor
- Serum calcium, magnesium, and phosphorus; the plasma phosphate and magnesium levels may be significantly depressed and should be rechecked within 12 hr because they may decrease further with correction of DKA

- Blood urea nitrogen and creatinine generally reveal significant dehydration and acute kidney injury.
- A pregnancy test should be performed in all female patients of child-bearing years who present with DKA.
- Amylase, lipase, and liver enzymes should be checked in patients with abdominal pain.

IMAGING STUDIES

- Chest radiographs are helpful to rule out pneumonia. The initial chest film may be negative if the patient has significant dehydration. Repeat chest x-ray after 24 hr if pulmonary infection is strongly suspected.
- Additional imaging, such as CT scanning or abdominal ultrasound, should be considered in the presence of physical exam findings, such as abdominal tenderness.

TREATMENT

NONPHARMACOLOGIC THERAPY

- Monitor mental status, vital signs, and urine output hourly until improved, then monitor every 2 to 4 hours.
- Fingersticks should be checked every 1 to 2 hours while patient is on an insulin drip.
- Basic metabolic panel should be checked every 2 to 4 hours to monitor for anion gap closure (see "Acute General Rx").

ACUTE GENERAL Rx (FIG. 1)

Fluid replacement (usual deficit is 6 to 8 L):
1. Do not delay fluid replacement until laboratory results have been received. Fluid deficits are typically 100 ml/kg of body weight. The total fluid administered should not exceed 4 L/m^2/24 hours for fear of causing cerebral edema (CE). One rule of thumb is to deliver fluids (deficit and maintenance) over a period of 48 hours if serum osmolality is >360 mOsm/L.
2. The initial fluid replacement should be with 0.9% normal saline (NS) to expand vascular volume and ensure blood pressure stabilization and organ perfusion. In patients with severe hypernatremia (serum sodium >160 mEq/L), 0.45% normal saline infusion can be used. Careful monitoring for fluid overload is necessary in elderly patients and those with a history of congestive heart failure.
3. The rate of fluid replacement varies with the age of the patient and the presence of significant cardiac or renal disease.
   1. The usual rate of infusion is 1 L of 0.9% NS over the first hour, followed by 15 ml/kg/hr 0.9% NS during the second hour. Then change to 0.45% NS at 15 ml/kg/hr to replenish free water.
   2. Switch to dextrose D5 0.45% NS when serum glucose is <250 to prevent hypoglycemia and introduce additional glucose substrate (necessary to suppress lipolysis and ketogenesis).

Insulin administration:
1. The patient should be given an initial loading IV bolus of 0.1 U/kg regular insulin followed by

Adult patient with DKA or HHS

Complete initial evaluation, including (but not limited to):

Medical history and physical
examination
Complete blood count with
differential
Fingerstick blood glucose
Serum chemistries ("Chem-10"
plus serum ketones)

Urine for urinalysis and ketones
Cultures as indicated (wound,
blood, urine, etc.)
Chest ± abdominal x-ray
12-lead electrocardiogram

Concurrently, begin empiric fluid
resuscitation with 0.9% NaCl at
1000 ml/hr
Consider volume expanders if hypovolemic
shock is present
Continue fluid resuscitation until volume
status and cardiovascular parameters
(pulse, blood pressure) have been
restored

IV fluids

Based on corrected serum sodium*
If high/normal, use 0.45% NaCl
If low/normal, use 0.9% NaCl
Continue IV fluids at 250-1000 ml/hr, depending
on volume status, cardiovascular history, and
cardiovascular status (pulse, BP)

Insulin therapy

Regular insulin bolus,
0.15 U/kg
IV infusion, 0.10 U/kg/hr
Check serum glucose
hourly—should fall by
50-80 mg/dl/hr

If serum glucose falling too
rapidly, back off on insulin
infusion
If serum glucose rising or falling
too slowly, increase insulin
infusion rate by 50%-100%

Continuing management:

Follow and replete serum electrolytes
(including divalent cations) q2-4h
until stable
After resolution of hyperglycemic
state, follow blood glucose q4h and
initiate sliding scale regular insulin
coverage
Convert IV insulin to subcutaneous
injections (or resumption of prior
therapy), ensuring adequate
overlap if treating patients without
endogenous insulin secretion

Begin clear liquid diet and advance as
tolerated. Encourage resumption of
ambulation and activity
Review and update diabetes
education, with special attention to
prevention of further hyperglycemic
crises

When serum glucose reaches 250-300 mg/dl:

Add dextrose to IV fluids. Continue IV fluids at
150-250 ml/hr, and adjust insulin infusion to
maintain serum glucose of 200-250 mg/dl until
metabolic control is achieved:
For DKA, continue until anion gap has closed and
acidosis has resolved
For HHS, continue until plasma osmolality drops
below 310 mOsm/kg
Begin more exhaustive search for
precipitant of metabolic
decompensation

Potassium (K⁺) repletion

Obtain baseline serum potassium
Obtain 12-lead ECG
[K⁺] ≥5.5 mEq/L

Hold K⁺ therapy

Treat hyperkalemia if
ECG changes present

Recheck [K⁺] in 2 hr

[K⁺] <5.5 mEq/L and
adequate urine output

Add K⁺ to IV fluids
(Use KCl and/or KPhos)

[K⁺] = 4.5-5.4: add 20 mEq/L IVF
[K⁺] = 3.5-4.4: add 30 mEq/L IVF
[K⁺] <3.5: add 40 mEq/L IVF

Follow serum [K⁺] every 2-4 hours until stable: anticipate rapid drop
of serum [K⁺] during therapy, due to dilution and intracellular shifting
Ensure adequate urine output to avoid over-repletion and hyperkalemia
Continue K⁺ repletion until serum [K⁺] is stable at between 4-5 mEq/L
If refractory hypokalemia, ensure concurrent magnesium repletion
Repletion may need to be continued for several days, as total body
losses may reach up to 500 mEq

Bicarbonate therapy

Obtain ABG
Obtain baseline serum bicarbonate

pH <6.9	6.9 ≤pH < 7.0	pH ≥7.0
88 mEq/L	44 mEq/L	Assess need
(2 amps)	(1 amp)	for bicarbonate
NaHCO₃	NaHCO₃	
over 2 hr	over 1 hr	

Repeat ABG after bicarbonate administration
Repeat NaHCO₃ therapy until pH ≥7.0, then discontinue therapy
Follow serum bicarbonate q4h until stable

*Sodium correction: Serum sodium should be corrected for
hyperglycemia. For every 100 mg/dl of glucose elevation
above 100 mg/dl, add 1.6 mEq/L to the measured sodium
value; this will yield the correction serum sodium concentration.

FIG. 1 Management of diabetic ketoacidosis (DKA) and hyperosmolar hyperglycemic state (HHS). *ABG,* Arterial blood gas; *ECG,* electrocardiograph. (From
Goldman L, Ausiello D [eds]: *Cecil textbook of medicine,* ed 23, Philadelphia, 2008, Saunders.)

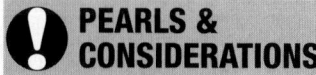
a constant infusion at a rate of 0.1 U/kg/hour. Insulin replacement should generally not be started until serum potassium is >3.3 mEq/L to prevent life-threatening hypokalemia.

2. Monitor serum glucose every 1 to 2 hr while patient is on insulin drip, then every 2 to 4 hr.

3. The goal is to decrease serum glucose level by 80 mg/dl/hour (after an initial decline because of rehydration); if the serum glucose level is not decreasing at the expected rate, double the rate of insulin infusion.

4. When the serum glucose level approaches 250 mg/dl, decrease the rate of insulin infusion to 2 to 3 U/hour and continue this rate until the patient has received adequate fluid replacement, HCO_3- is close to normal, and ketones have cleared. After target glucose levels are achieved, it usually takes 5 to 7 hr for ketosis to clear. Young children and adolescents have greater levels of human growth hormone, resulting in a prolonged time lag for plasma glucose to reach above levels. Patients with infection and fever have higher metabolic requirements and may need 15% to 20% more insulin than the usual starting dose.

5. Prior to stopping the IV insulin infusion, administer an SC dose of insulin (dose varies with the patient's demonstrated insulin sensitivity). Short (regular) or rapid-acting (aspart, lispro, glulisine) insulins should be administered SC 1 to 2 hr before stopping IV insulin infusion. Intermediate (NPH) or long-acting (glargine, detemir) insulins should be administered 2 to 4 hr before stopping IV insulin infusion.

6. In individuals with newly diagnosed diabetes, the total daily insulin dose to maintain metabolic control ranges from 0.5 to 0.8 U/kg/day. Approximately half of this dose should be given as intermediate or long-acting insulin, and half of this dose should be given as mealtime or prandial insulin, provided the patient is eating.

Electrolyte replacement:
- Potassium replacement: the average total potassium loss in DKA is 300 to 500 mEq.
- K^+ can be supplemented as chloride- and phosphate-containing solutions.
  1. The rate of replacement varies with the patient's serum potassium level, degree of acidosis (decreased pH, increased potassium level), and renal function (potassium replacement should be used with caution in patients with renal failure).
  2. As a rule of thumb, potassium replacement can be guided by presenting serum K level. If K is <3.3, give KCl 20 to 30 mEq/L of intravenous fluid (IVF) until K is >3.3. If K is 3.3 to 5.3, give KCl at 10 to

30 mEq/L IVF to maintain a K of >4. If K is >5.3, hold potassium supplementation until K is <5.3.
  3. Monitor serum potassium level hourly for the first 2 hours, then monitor q2 to 4h.

- Phosphate replacement: If the serum PO_4 is <1.5 mEq/L, give 2.5 mg/kg IV over 6 hours of elemental phosphate. Routine replacement of phosphate (in the absence of laboratory evidence of significant hypophosphatemia) is not indicated. Rapid IV phosphate administration can cause hypocalcemia.

- Magnesium replacement: Replacement is indicated only in the presence of significant hypomagnesemia or refractory hypokalemia/hypocalcemia.

Bicarbonate therapy:
- Routine use of bicarbonate in DKA is contraindicated because it can worsen hypokalemia and can cause cerebral edema. Bicarbonate therapy should be considered only if the arterial pH is <6.9 and HCO_3- is <5.

- In these patients, 44 to 88 mEq sodium bicarbonate can be added to 1 L of 0.45% NS q2-4h until pH increases to >7.

- Use of bicarbonate therapy is particularly dangerous in the pediatric population. Children with DKA are at increased risk for cerebral edema. Bicarbonate therapy in children with DKA should be limited to those with severe circulatory failure and a high risk for cardiac decompensation resulting from profound acidosis.

PREVENTION
- Provide information/education for teachers, parents, school staff, and caregivers on how to recognize children with undiagnosed diabetes.
- Review sick day management; increase home blood glucose monitoring, education on how to measure urinary or fingerstick ketones, compliance with insulin; and maintain adequate hydration and nutrition.

DISPOSITION
- Average mortality rate in DKA is 5% to 10%.
- In children <10 yr, DKA causes 70% of diabetes-related deaths.
- Cerebral edema (CE) occurs in 1% of episodes of DKA in children and is associated with a mortality rate of 40% to 90%.

REFERRAL
In general, patients with DKA should be admitted to the intensive care unit on an insulin drip. Alert patients who are able to take fluids orally and have mild DKA occasionally can be treated with short-acting insulin analogues under observation and sent home. The American Diabetes Association admission guidelines are

a plasma glucose level >250 mg/dl with arterial pH <7.30, serum bicarbonate level <15 mEq/L, and a moderate or greater level of ketones in the serum or urine.

! PEARLS & CONSIDERATIONS

COMMENTS
- Although DKA occurs more commonly in type 1 diabetes mellitus, a significant proportion (>20%) occurs in patients with type 2 diabetes, particularly under conditions of extreme stress, severe infection or surgery, and marked hyperglycemia (results in glucose toxicity).
- 30% to 40% of DKA admissions involve patients with newly diagnosed diabetes.
- Potential complications of DKA therapy include hypoglycemia, cerebral edema, cardiac arrhythmias, shock, myocardial infarction, and acute pancreatitis.
- Risk factors for cerebral edema include age <5 yr, high initial BUN, hyperventilation to a $Paco_2$ of <22 mm Hg, and presenting arterial pH of <7.00. It presents 4 to 8 hours after start of rehydration therapy. Presentation may be abrupt with sudden severe headache, vomiting, sudden hypertension, and obtunded sensorium. First management response to CE is to elevate head of the patient to 30-degree angle, IV mannitol, intubation and hyperventilation, and, finally, cutting back of the maintenance fluid to 75%.
- Underinsured children and those with psychiatric illness are at greater risk for DKA.
- Subcutaneous administration of rapid-acting insulin analogues may be reasonable alternatives to IV regular insulin infusion for treating uncomplicated DKA.
- DKA can occur with blood glucose <350 mg/dl in the setting of poor oral intake or pregnancy.
- Ketones can be positive in starvation or with heavy alcohol intake; DKA can coexist with other causes of metabolic acidosis such as lactic acidosis.

SUGGESTED READINGS
Available at www.expertconsult.com

RELATED CONTENT
Diabetes Mellitus (Related Key Topic)
Hyperosmolar Hyperglycemic Syndrome (Related Key Topic)

AUTHORS: **HILARY B. WHITLATCH, M.D.,**
SAINATH GADDAM, M.D., and
FRED F. FERRI, M.D.

BASIC INFORMATION

DEFINITION

Diabetic polyneuropathy is a distal symmetric polyneuropathy (DSPN) characterized by numbness, tingling, pain, or weakness that affects the nerves in a stocking-and-glove pattern, beginning in the distal extremities. DSPN leads to substantial pain, morbidity, and impaired quality of life.

SYNONYMS

Distal symmetric polyneuropathy (DSPN)
Diabetic peripheral neuropathy

ICD-10CM CODES
E11.40 Type 2 diabetes mellitus with neurological complications
E11.40 Type 2 diabetes mellitus with diabetic neuropathy, unspecified
E11.41 Type 2 diabetes mellitus with diabetic mononeuropathy
E11.42 Type 2 diabetes mellitus with diabetic polyneuropathy
E11.43 Type 2 diabetes mellitus with diabetic autonomic (poly)neuropathy
E11.44 Type 2 diabetes mellitus with diabetic amyotrophy
E11.49 Type 2 diabetes mellitus with other diabetic neurological complication

EPIDEMIOLOGY & DEMOGRAPHICS

PREVALENCE: The prevalence of diabetic polyneuropathy varies from 10% to 100% in patients with diabetes mellitus in population-based studies. It is the most common form of peripheral neuropathy in the western world.
RISK FACTORS: Patients with poor glycemic control, diabetic nephropathy, or retinopathy are at increased risk.

PHYSICAL FINDINGS & CLINICAL PRESENTATION

- Patients most commonly experience numbness and tingling, but they may also experience either feelings of tightness or a sensation of heat or cold.
- Pain is common, is often worst at night, and can be burning, aching, shooting, or lancinating in nature.
- Sensory symptoms begin in the feet and may slowly ascend over months to years. Symptoms in the hands do not generally occur until symptoms in the lower extremities have reached the level of the knees. In more severe cases, the symptoms can spread to the trunk and head.
- Neurologic examination reveals early loss of small-fiber modalities resulting in decreased pinprick and temperature sensation and later involvement of large-fiber modalities leading to a reduction in vibratory and proprioceptive sensation. Ankle reflexes are usually reduced or absent, and more proximal reflexes may

also become involved as the neuropathy progresses. Strength is usually normal, but there can be some motor involvement leading to mild weakness and atrophy, which is usually limited to intrinsic foot muscles and ankle dorsiflexors.

ETIOLOGY

The precise etiology is unknown but most likely involves a complex interaction of metabolic derangements and microvascular insults occurring in the setting of diabetes.

DIAGNOSIS

DIFFERENTIAL DIAGNOSIS

Although diabetes is the leading cause of peripheral neuropathy in developed countries, there are numerous other causes requiring further investigation(s).

WORKUP

- A thorough history and neurologic examination are essential to confirm features consistent with a diabetic polyneuropathy and exclude other features suggesting alternative diagnoses.
- For some patients, neuropathy may be the presenting feature of previously undiagnosed diabetes.
- Electrodiagnostic evaluation to include nerve conduction studies and electromyography can be helpful in confirming the presence, extent, and severity of a neuropathy.
- Patients with DSPN typically have a reduction of amplitudes and slowing of conduction velocities involving sensory and possibly motor nerves in a length-dependent and symmetric fashion.
- Electromyographic examination of distal muscles may reveal fibrillation potentials, positive sharp waves, and large motor unit action potentials, all suggestive of denervation and reinnervation.
- Neither skin biopsy nor nerve biopsy is necessary in the vast majority of cases.
- Fig. 1 describes a diagnosis and treatment algorithm of diabetic autonomic neuropathy.

LABORATORY TESTS

- Fasting blood sugar, hemoglobin A1c, and 2-hour oral glucose tolerance test should all be considered in patients with peripheral neuropathy without a known history of diabetes.
- A focused laboratory evaluation for other common or potentially treatable causes of neuropathy is also indicated: complete blood cell count, complete metabolic panel to include electrolytes and liver function tests, erythrocyte sedimentation rate, vitamin B12 and folate levels, thyroid function tests, serum protein electrophoresis with immunofixation electrophoresis.
- Additional laboratory tests can be considered, based on either history or exam findings suggesting other underlying diagnoses,

such as antinuclear antibodies, extractable nuclear antigens, ANCAs, rheumatoid factor, HIV, hepatitis B and C, and cryoglobulins.

IMAGING STUDIES

- Imaging is not necessary unless there is concern for an alternate or coexisting process based on the history and examination.

TREATMENT

CHRONIC Rx

- Table 1 summarizes clinical features, diagnosis, and treatment of diabetic autonomic neuropathy.
- Glycemic control: The primary treatment for diabetic polyneuropathy is effective glycemic control, as this may either improve or at least slow progression of the neuropathy.
- Symptomatic management: Another aspect of treatment is the symptomatic management of pain and paresthesias. The American Academy of Neurology, the American Association of Neuromuscular and Electrodiagnostic Medicine, and the American Academy of Physical Medicine and Rehabilitation have together developed an evidence-based guideline for the treatment of painful diabetic neuropathy. Pregabalin, an anticonvulsant, is the only agent in the guideline that has been established as effective for painful diabetic neuropathy. Other probably effective agents are listed in the following:
  1. Topical agents: Lidocaine 5% patch can be applied to painful areas for 12 hours a day, capsaicin 0.075% applied qid.
  2. Anticonvulsants: gabapentin (100 to 1200 mg tid) and pregabalin (50 to 100 mg tid).
  3. Antidepressants: amitriptyline (10 to 100 mg qhs), nortriptyline (25 to 150 mg qhs), duloxetine (60 to 120 mg daily), and venlafaxine (75 to 225 mg/day).
  4. Tramadol (50 mg qid as needed) can be a useful adjunctive analgesic.
- Fig. 2 describes a treatment algorithm for neuropathic pain after exclusion of nondiabetic etiologies and stabilization of glycemic control.

DISPOSITION

The distal sensory loss of diabetic polyneuropathy places patients at increased risk of trauma to the extremities, with the potential for ulceration and infection that could ultimately require amputation if not attended to in a timely fashion.

REFERRAL

- A neurologist can assist in the diagnosis and management of diabetic polyneuropathy.
- Patients with diabetic polyneuropathy should also be evaluated at least annually by a podiatrist and ophthalmologist
- Progression of diabetic polyneuropathy can be minimized by paying close attention to strict glycemic control as well as other risk factors such as hypertension and obesity.

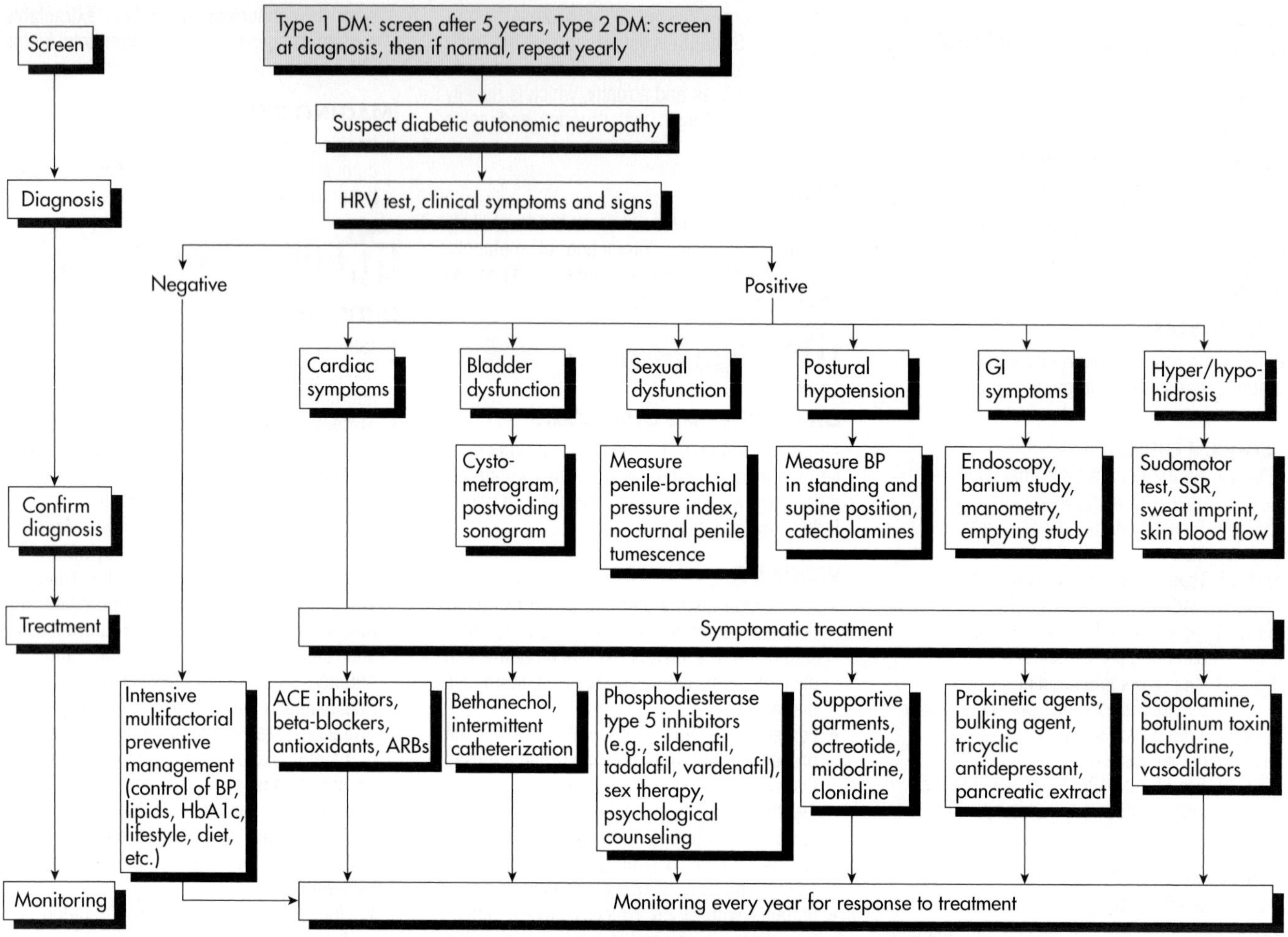

| Screen | Type 1 DM: screen after 5 years, Type 2 DM: screen at diagnosis, then if normal, repeat yearly |

Suspect diabetic autonomic neuropathy

| Diagnosis | HRV test, clinical symptoms and signs |

Negative — Positive

| Cardiac symptoms | Bladder dysfunction | Sexual dysfunction | Postural hypotension | GI symptoms | Hyper/hypo-hidrosis |

| | Cysto-metrogram, postvoiding sonogram | Measure penile-brachial pressure index, nocturnal penile tumescence | Measure BP in standing and supine position, catecholamines | Endoscopy, barium study, manometry, emptying study | Sudomotor test, SSR, sweat imprint, skin blood flow |

| Confirm diagnosis |

| Treatment | Symptomatic treatment |

| Intensive multifactorial preventive management (control of BP, lipids, HbA1c, lifestyle, diet, etc.) | ACE inhibitors, beta-blockers, antioxidants, ARBs | Bethanechol, intermittent catheterization | Phosphodiesterase type 5 inhibitors (e.g., sildenafil, tadalafil, vardenafil), sex therapy, psychological counseling | Supportive garments, octreotide, midodrine, clonidine | Prokinetic agents, bulking agent, tricyclic antidepressant, pancreatic extract | Scopolamine, botulinum toxin lachydrine, vasodilators |

| Monitoring | Monitoring every year for response to treatment |

FIG. 1 Diagnosis and treatment algorithm of diabetic autonomic neuropathy. *ACE,* Angiotensin-converting enzyme; *ARBs,* angiotensin receptor blockers; *BP,* blood pressure; *DM,* diabetes mellitus; *GI,* gastrointestinal; *HRV,* heart rate variability; *SSR,* sympathetic skin response. (Modified from Larsen PR et al [eds]: *Williams textbook of endocrinology,* ed 11, Philadelphia, 2008, Saunders.)

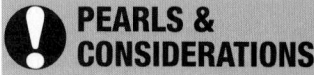

❗ PEARLS & CONSIDERATIONS

COMMENTS

- For many patients, either DSPN or another form of diabetic neuropathy may be the initial presentation of previously undiagnosed diabetes.
- In addition to regular visits with podiatry, patients with diabetic polyneuropathy should be educated on aggressive foot hygiene and the importance of examining their own feet

PATIENT/FAMILY EDUCATION

The following websites are recommended:
   http://patienteducationcenter.org/articles/diabetic-neuropathies/
   http://www.mayoclinic.com/health/diabetic-neuropathy/DS01045

AUTHOR: **DIVYA SINGHAL, M.D.**

TABLE 1 Clinical Features, Diagnosis, and Treatment of Diabetic Autonomic Neuropathy

Symptoms	Tests	Treatments
Cardiac		
Resting tachycardia, exercise intolerance	HRV, MUGA thallium scan, MIBG scan	Graded supervised exercise, ACE inhibitors, β-blockers
Postural hypotension, dizziness, weakness, fatigue, syncope	HRV, supine and standing BP, catecholamines	Mechanical measures, clonidine, midodrine, octreotide, erythropoietin
Gastrointestinal		
Gastroparesis, erratic glucose control	Gastric emptying study, barium study	Frequent small meals, prokinetic agents (metoclopramide, domperidone, erythromycin)
Abdominal pain, early satiety, nausea, vomiting, bloating, belching	Endoscopy, manometry, electrogastrogram	Antibiotics, antiemetics, bulking agents, tricyclic antidepressants, pyloric botulinum toxin, gastric pacing
Constipation	Endoscopy	High-fiber diet, bulking agents, osmotic laxatives, lubricating agents
Diarrhea (often nocturnal alternating with constipation)		Soluble fiber, gluten and lactose restriction, anticholinergic agents, cholestyramine, antibiotics, somatostatin, pancreatic enzyme supplements
Sexual Dysfunction		
Erectile dysfunction	H&P, HRV, penile-brachial pressure index, nocturnal penile tumescence	Sex therapy, psychological counseling, phosphodiesterase inhibitors, PGE$_1$ injections, devices or prostheses
Vaginal dryness		Vaginal lubricants
Bladder Dysfunction		
Frequency, urgency, nocturia, urinary retention, incontinence	Cystometrogram, postvoid sonography	Bethanechol, intermittent catheterization
Sudomotor Dysfunction		
Anhidrosis, heat intolerance, dry skin, hyperhidrosis	Quantitative sudomotor axon reflex, sweat test, skin blood flow	Emollients and skin lubricants, scopolamine, glycopyrrolate, botulinum toxin, vasodilators
Pupillomotor and Visceral Dysfunction		
Blurred vision, impaired adaptation to ambient light, Argyll-Robertson pupil	Pupillometry, HRV	Care with driving at night
Impaired visceral sensation: silent MI, hypoglycemia unawareness		Recognition of unusual presentation of MI, control of risk factors, control of plasma glucose levels

ACE, acetylcholinesterase; *BP*, blood pressure; *H&P*, history and physical examination; *HRV*, heart rate variability; *MI*, myocardial infarction; *MIBG*, metaiodobenzylguanidine; *MUGA*, multigated angiography; *PGE$_1$*, prostaglandin E$_1$.
From Melmed S, Polonsky KS, Larsen PR, Kronenberg HM: *Williams textbook of endocrinology*, ed 12, Philadelphia, 2011, Saunders.

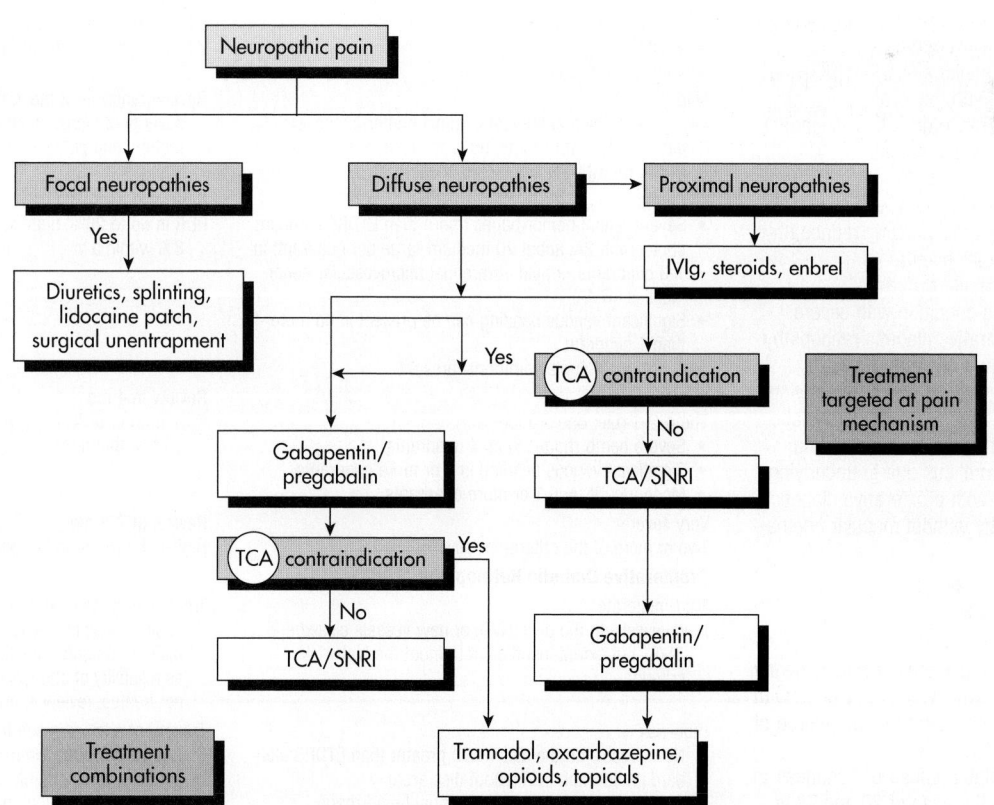

FIG. 2 Treatment algorithm for neuropathic pain after exclusion of nondiabetic etiologies and stabilization of glycemic control. *IVIg*, intravenous immune globulin; *SNRI*, serotonin-norepinephrine reuptake inhibitors; *TCA*, tricyclic antidepressants. (From Melmed S, Polonsky KS, Larsen PR, Kronenberg HM: *Williams textbook of endocrinology*, ed 12, Philadelphia, 2011, Saunders.)

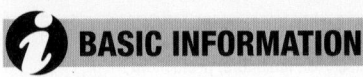

DEFINITION

Diabetic retinopathy is a microvascular abnormality of the retina resulting in microaneurysms, retinal hemorrhages, lipid exudates, macular edema, and neovascular vessel growth and can ultimately end in blindness. Diabetic retinopathy can be classified into two stages: nonproliferative (mild, moderate, and severe) and proliferative (Fig. E1 and Table 1).

SYNONYMS

Nonproliferative diabetic retinopathy (NPDR)
Proliferative diabetic retinopathy (PDR)
Diabetic macular edema (DME)

ICD-10CM CODES

E08.311 Diabetes mellitus due to underlying condition with unspecified diabetic retinopathy with macular edema
E08.319 Diabetes mellitus due to underlying condition with unspecified diabetic retinopathy without macular edema
E08.321 Diabetes mellitus due to underlying condition with mild nonproliferative diabetic retinopathy with macular edema
E08.329 Diabetes mellitus due to underlying condition with mild nonproliferative diabetic retinopathy without macular edema
E08.331 Diabetes mellitus due to underlying condition with moderate nonproliferative diabetic retinopathy with macular edema
E08.339 Diabetes mellitus due to underlying condition with moderate nonproliferative diabetic retinopathy without macular edema
E08.341 Diabetes mellitus due to underlying condition with severe nonproliferative diabetic retinopathy with macular edema
E08.349 Diabetes mellitus due to underlying condition with severe nonproliferative diabetic retinopathy without macular edema
E08.351 Diabetes mellitus due to underlying condition with proliferative diabetic retinopathy with macular edema
E08.359 Diabetes mellitus due to underlying condition with proliferative diabetic retinopathy without macular edema

EPIDEMIOLOGY & DEMOGRAPHICS

INCIDENCE (IN U.S.):

- After 20 years of diabetes mellitus, nearly 99% of patients with type 1 and 60% with type 2 disease demonstrate some degree of diabetic retinopathy.
- A leading preventable cause of blindness in the U.S. between the ages of 20 and 74 yr.
- There are approximately 8000 new cases of diabetic retinopathy–induced blindness each year in the U.S.

PEAK INCIDENCE: Begins 10 yr after onset of diabetes

PREVALENCE (IN U.S.):

- Prevalence of retinopathy increases with duration of diabetes. Found in 18% of people diagnosed with diabetes for 3- to 4-yr duration and in up to 80% of diabetics with a diagnosis of ≥15 yr.
- In the U.S., 700,000 people have proliferative retinopathy, and 500,000 have macular edema.
- CDC data reveal that 4 million Americans were visually impaired due to diabetic retinopathy in 2011.
- The number of Americans with diabetic retinopathy is expected to nearly double, from 7.7 million to 14.6 million between 2010 and 2050. Expected to triple in the Hispanic population.

PREDOMINANT SEX: Males and females affected equally
PREDOMINANT AGE: ≥30 yr

GENETICS:

- The development of diabetes involves the interaction of genetic and nongenetic factors.
- Type 1 has an autoimmune basis, resulting in destruction of beta islet cells and has strong HLA associations.

- Type 2 has genetic predisposition, but the specific genes are not yet well characterized.

PHYSICAL FINDINGS & CLINICAL PRESENTATION (FIG. 2)

- Microaneurysms.
- Hemorrhages.
- Cotton-wool spots.
- Lipid exudates.
- Macular edema.
- Neovascularization.
- Retinal detachment (in advanced cases).
- Vitreous hemorrhage.
- In early cases, patient may not report a visual disturbance.
- Figure E3 describes an initial ophthalmic examination flow chart.

ETIOLOGY

Prolonged hyperglycemia results in basement membrane thickening in retinal capillaries with subsequent loss of pericytes and endothelial decompensation resulting in breakdown of the blood–retina barrier and capillary occlusion, ischemia, and serum leakage. This leads to the clinical findings of dot hemorrhages, microaneurysms, lipid exudate, and edema. Upregulation of vascular endothelial growth

---

TABLE 1 Abbreviated Early Treatment Diabetic Retinopathy Study Classification of Diabetic Retinopathy

Category/Description	Management
Nonproliferative Diabetic Retinopathy (NPDR)	
No DR	Review in 12 mo
Very mild Microaneurysms only	Review most patients in 12 mo
Mild Any or all of: microaneurysms, retinal hemorrhages, exudates, cotton wool spots, up to the level of moderate NPDR. No IRMA or significant beading	Review range 6-12 mo, depending on severity of signs, stability, systemic factors, and patient's personal circumstances
Moderate • Severe retinal hemorrhages (more than ETDRS standard photograph 2A: about 20 medium-large per quadrant) in 1-3 quadrants *or* mild intraretinal microvascular abnormalities (IRMA) • Significant venous beading can be present in no more than 1 quadrant • Cotton-wool spots commonly present	Review in approximately 6 mo PDR in up to 26%, high-risk PDR in up to 8% within a yr
Severe The 4-2-1 rule; one or more of: • Severe hemorrhages in all 4 quadrants • Significant venous beading in 2 or more quadrants • Moderate IRMA in 1 or more quadrants	Review in 4 mo PDR in up to 50%, high-risk PDR in up to 15% within a yr
Very severe Two or more of the criteria for severe	Review in 2-3 mo High-risk PDR in up to 45% within a yr
Proliferative Diabetic Retinopathy (PDR)	
Mild-moderate New vessels on the disc (NVD) or new vessels elsewhere (NVE), but extent insufficient to meet the high-risk criteria	Treatment considered according to severity of signs, stability, systemic factors, and patient's personal circumstances such as reliability of attendance for review. If not treated, review in up to 2 mo
High-risk • New vessels on the disc (NVD) greater than ETDRS standard photograph 10A (about disc area) • Any NVD with vitreous or preretinal hemorrhage • NVE greater than disc area with vitreous or preretinal hemorrhage (or hemorrhage with presumed obscured NVD/E)	Treatment advised—see text Should be performed immediately when possible, and certainly same day if symptomatic presentation with good retinal view

From Kanski JJ, Bowling B: *Clinical ophthalmology, a systematic approach*, ed 7, Philadelphia, 2010, Saunders.

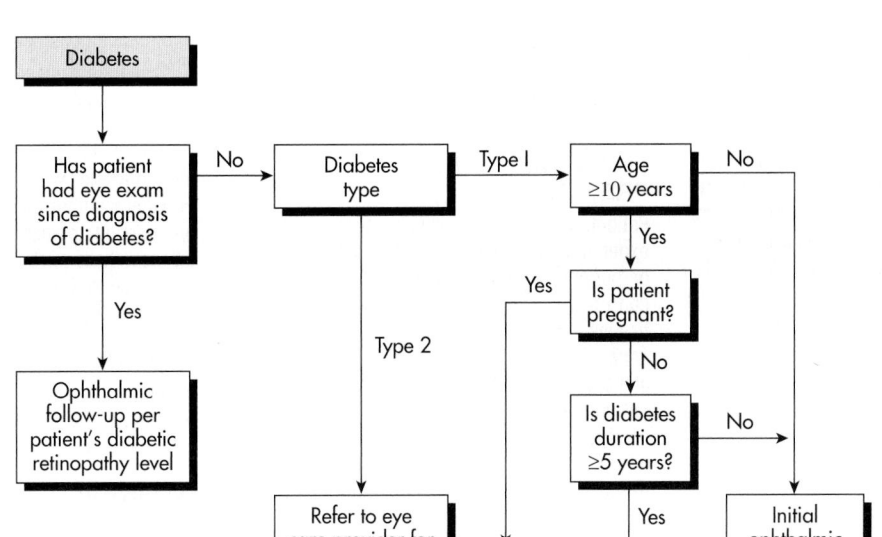

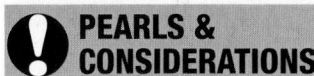

FIG. 2 Initial ophthalmic examination flow chart. Schematic flow chart of major principles involved in determining the timing of initial ophthalmic examination after a diagnosis of diabetes mellitus. These are minimal recommended times. Ocular symptoms, complaints, or other associated medical issues can necessitate earlier evaluation. Guidelines are regularly reevaluated based on new study results. (From Melmed S, Polonsky KS, Larsen PR, Kronenberg HM: *Williams textbook of endocrinology,* ed 12, Philadelphia, 2011, Saunders.)

factor (VEGF) and other cytokines contributes to vascular incompetence and promotes growth of neovascular tissue. Fig. E4 describes a diabetic retinopathy pathogenesis flow chart.

Dx DIAGNOSIS

DIFFERENTIAL DIAGNOSIS

- Branch or central retinal vein occlusion
- Hypertensive retinopathy
- Ocular ischemic syndrome (carotid occlusion)
- Radiation retinopathy
- Retinal macroaneurysm
- Sickle cell retinopathy
- Valsalva retinopathy
- Lupus
- Retinal vasculitis

WORKUP

- Fundus photography
- Optical coherence tomography
- Fluorescein angiogram
- Laboratory workup if indicated based on DDx

Rx TREATMENT

NONPHARMACOLOGIC THERAPY

- Tight glycemic control remains the cornerstone in the primary prevention of diabetic retinopathy, particularly in type 1 as seen in the Diabetes Control and Complications Trial (DCCT) and less so in type 2 as seen in the United Kingdom Prospective Diabetes Study (UKPDS) and more recently in the Action to Control Cardiovascular Risk in Diabetes Trial (ACCORD). ADA guidelines recommend A1c <7.0.

- Intensive lowering of blood pressure was shown in UKPDS but not ACCORD to reduce progression of diabetic retinopathy. ADA guidelines recommend BP target of <140/90 mm Hg.
- Lipid lowering results in reduction of retinopathy progression (ACCORD Trial).
- Laser treatment (photocoagulation) for proliferative disease or macular edema.

ACUTE GENERAL Rx

- Intravitreal pharmacotherapy with anti-VEGF agents (e.g., bevacizumab, ranibizumab, aflibercept) and/or corticosteroids is the standard of care for patients with center-involved diabetic macular edema.
- Laser therapy: Panretinal laser photocoagulation reduces the risk of severe visual loss in patients with proliferative retinopathy.
- Focal laser reduces risk of moderate visual loss by 50% in patients with clinically significant macular edema.
- Vitrectomy for traction retinal detachment or vitreous hemorrhage.

CHRONIC Rx

- Monthly anti-VEGF injections until macular edema has resolved with surveillance at regular intervals for additional treatment
- Repeated laser treatments may be necessary
- Diet and exercise; good medical control of disease, blood pressure, and cholesterol

DISPOSITION

- Retinal examination should be performed on all routine medical visits. Referral if abnormality seen.

- Routine annual eye examination in all patients with diabetes.
- Prognosis is improved with early diagnosis and treatment.

REFERRAL

Refer to ophthalmologist immediately on finding retinal abnormality to institute early treatment.

! PEARLS & CONSIDERATIONS

COMMENTS

- Early treatment of severe nonproliferative, and proliferative retinopathy may minimize complications and visual loss.
- Tight blood sugar control in type 1 patients significantly reduces the probability of developing new-onset retinopathy as well as progression of existing retinopathy.
- Retinopathy is an independent risk marker for cardiovascular disease in patients with type 2 DM.

SUGGESTED READINGS

Available at www.expertconsult.com

RELATED CONTENT

Diabetic Retinopathy (Patient Information)
Diabetes Mellitus (Related Key Topic)

AUTHOR: **ROBERT H. JANIGIAN, M.D.**

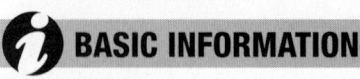

DEFINITION

Diffuse idiopathic skeletal hyperostosis (DISH) is a systemic disorder primarily involving the axial skeleton. DISH is characterized by widespread bone proliferation as well as calcification and ossification of soft tissues, including ligaments and their sites of insertion. DISH is known to be associated with certain metabolic abnormalities.

SYNONYMS

- Ankylosing hyperostosis
- Forestier disease
- DISH

ICD-10CM CODES
M48.10 Ankylosing hyperostosis, site unspecified
M48.11 Ankylosing hyperostosis, occipito-atlanto-axial region
M48.12 Ankylosing hyperostosis, cervical region
M48.13 Ankylosing hyperostosis, cervicothoracic region
M48.14 Ankylosing hyperostosis, thoracic region
M48.15 Ankylosing hyperostosis, thoracolumbar region
M48.16 Ankylosing hyperostosis, lumbar region
M48.17 Ankylosing hyperostosis, lumbosacral region
M48.18 Ankylosing hyperostosis, sacral and sacrococcygeal region
M48.19 Ankylosing hyperostosis, multiple sites in spine

EPIDEMIOLOGY & DEMOGRAPHICS

PREVALENCE: The prevalence of DISH varies in different populations. Factors such as age, ethnicity, geography, and clinical setting affect the prevalence of the disease. Studies have shown DISH is more common in developed nations, although this may be secondary to more frequent use of radiologic imaging in these countries. Higher prevalence rates are seen in men, 10% to 25% versus 5% to 15% in women over the age of 50 years. Rates increase with age, with prevalence reported as high as 35% in men and 26% in women over the age of 70 years.
PREDOMINANT SEX AND AGE:
- Male predominance with a ratio of 2:1
- Mostly seen in elderly patients, usually after the age of 50 years
GENETICS:
- Association with *COL6A1* gene in some populations, which causes ossification of the posterior longitudinal ligament, a condition that is related to DISH
RISK FACTORS:
- Obesity
- Type II diabetes mellitus
- Hyperuricemia
- Dyslipidemia
- Hypertension

- Hyperinsulinemia
- Elevated growth hormone levels
- Elevated insulin-like growth factor (IGF-1)
- Chronic vitamin A toxicity/retinoid use

PHYSICAL FINDINGS & CLINICAL PRESENTATION

Patients with DISH are usually asymptomatic or experience only increased stiffness in the spine or peripheral joints. In the spine, osteophytes can obstruct or impinge on other structures or tissues, causing dysphagia (DISH affecting the cervical spine), myelopathy, quadriplegia, spinal stenosis and ossification of posterior longitudinal ligament. Spinal ligament calcification and ossification leads to decreased range of motion and a stooped posture as well as an increase in the risk for fractures. Peripheral enthesopathies are usually asymptomatic, but mechanical stresses can injure the entheses and cause pain. In patients with DISH pronounced hypertrophic changes can be seen affecting certain peripheral joints that are not typically associated with OA, such as the metacarpophalangeal joints, elbows, shoulders, and ankles. Thoracic spinal involvement is common in DISH and not usually seen in OA. Patients with DISH are at increased risk for heterotopic ossification after orthopedic surgery (i.e., hip arthroplasty).

ETIOLOGY

Etiology of DISH is unknown and the cause of excess bone formation is unclear. Chondrocytes located in entheseal areas become activated and cause changes in the adjacent matrix leading to ossification. Local vascular infiltration in these areas promotes ossification as well.

Dx DIAGNOSIS

Diagnosis of DISH is made by radiographic imaging. Bone formation is typically seen in the thoracic spine, and less frequently in the cervical and lumbar spines. Coarse osteophytes that seem to "flow" between adjacent vertebrae are seen on the right side of the thoracic spine, thought to be subsequent to the pressure effect of the left-sided aorta (Figs. 1 and 2). Ossification occurs within the overlying anterior longitudinal ligament, preserving the original bone cortex. The intervertebral disc height is preserved in the involved segments. Peripheral bone formation is seen in entheseal areas, especially around the heels (Achilles tendon and plantar fascia), knees (peripatellar ligaments) and elbows (olecranon). Peripheral new bone formation can be seen as well, with increased distal finger tuft thickening, increased sesamoid bone size, and increased cortical bone thickness. There is no evidence of apophyseal joint ankylosis or sacroiliac involvement.

Resnick and Niwayama criteria: most frequently used and is based on radiographic findings in the spine
- Findings of new bone formation/osteophytes bridging four adjoining vertebral bodies or ossification of the anterolateral longitudinal ligament

- Preserved intervertebral disc height
- Absence of degenerative disc disease, sacroiliac joint or facet joint involvement or changes

Others have proposed different criteria for diagnosis, which include the presence of peripheral enthesopathy. New diagnostic criteria are needed to recognize milder forms of the disease, those affecting other parts of the spine, and those that manifest initially with peripheral enthesopathy.

DIFFERENTIAL DIAGNOSIS

- Ankylosing spondylitis
- Degenerative disc disease
- Acromegaly

WORK-UP

Diagnosis of DISH is made with radiologic imaging. Patients with the above risk factors (increased weight, BMI, waist circumference

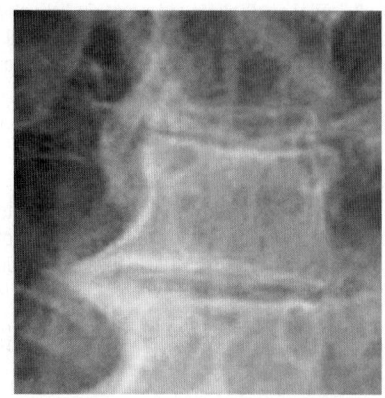

FIG. 1 Large, flowing, right-sided osteophytes of the thoracic spine (**A**). Note the translucent area between the vertebral body and the ossified ligamentous tissue (**B**). (Firestein GS, Budd RC, Gabriel SE, McInnes IB, O'Dell JR: Proliferative bone diseases. *In* Firestein G et al (eds): *Firestein: Kelley's textbook of rheumatology,* ed 9, Philadelphia, 2013, Elsevier, pp 1680-1691.)

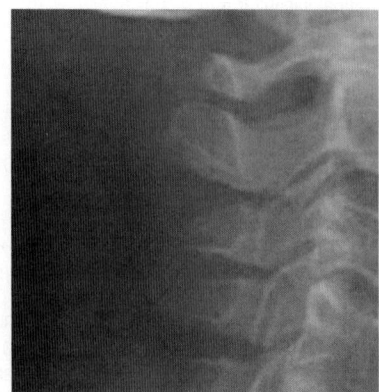

FIG. 2 Severe bulky ossification of the anterior longitudinal ligament of the cervical spine. (Firestein GS, Budd RC, Gabriel SE, McInnes IB, O'Dell JR: Proliferative bone diseases. *In* Firestein G et al (eds): *Firestein: Kelley's textbook of rheumatology,* ed 9, Philadelphia, 2013, Elsevier, pp 1680-1691.)

and systolic blood pressure) are at risk for cardiovascular disease and evaluation for this should be pursued.

LABORATORY TESTS

- Routine biochemical tests and erythrocyte sedimentation rate (ESR) are normal
- Laboratory testing should include evaluation for metabolic syndrome, i.e., fasting glucose or HgbA1c, cholesterol panel, etc.
- Uric acid

IMAGING STUDIES

- Posteroanterior and lateral (Fig. 3) X-ray views of the spine
- Computed tomography (CT) (Fig. 4) or magnetic resonance imaging (MRI) of the spine (not routinely needed unless evaluating for other possible conditions such as spinal stenosis)
- Plain radiographs of symptomatic peripheral joints

Rx TREATMENT

There is no specific treatment available for DISH
- Weight management
- Treatment and control of components of metabolic syndrome
- Treat cardiovascular risk factors

NONPHARMACOLOGIC THERAPY

- Physical therapy, light exercise
- Heat
- For peripheral enthesopathy pain, local soft applications such as insoles for plantar spurs or orthotics can be used as well as protective bandages at other sites.
- Surgical intervention rarely necessary, unless complications such as dysphagia from cervical osteophytes or spinal stenosis occurs

ACUTE GENERAL Rx

- Analgesics and nonsteroidal antiinflammatory medications (NSAIDs)
- Local corticosteroid injections

CHRONIC Rx

- Pain management as above
- Prevention of heterotopic ossification after orthopedic surgical procedures: NSAIDs, antivitamin K, and irradiation.

SUGGESTED READINGS

Available at www.expertconsult.com

RELATED CONTENT

Ankylosing Spondylitis (Related Key Topic)
Osteoarthritis (Related Key Topic)

AUTHOR: **JOANNE SZCZYGIEL CUNHA, M.D.**

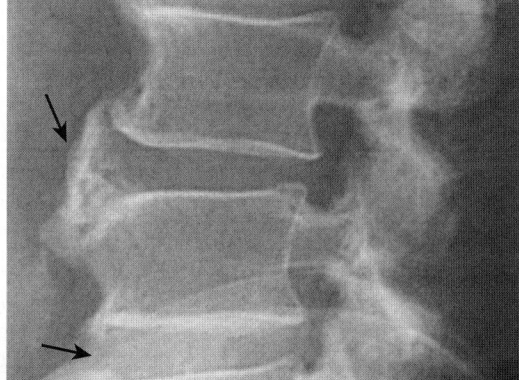

FIG. 3 Diffuse idiopathic skeletal hyperostosis (DISH): lumbar spine. This lateral radiograph of the lumbar spine shows early changes of DISH. Calcifications of the anterior longitudinal spinal ligament *(arrows)* are evident and will eventually evolve into flowing osteophytes extending across multiple spinal levels. (From Firestein GS: *Kelley's textbook of rheumatology*, ed 9, Philadelphia, 2013, Saunders.)

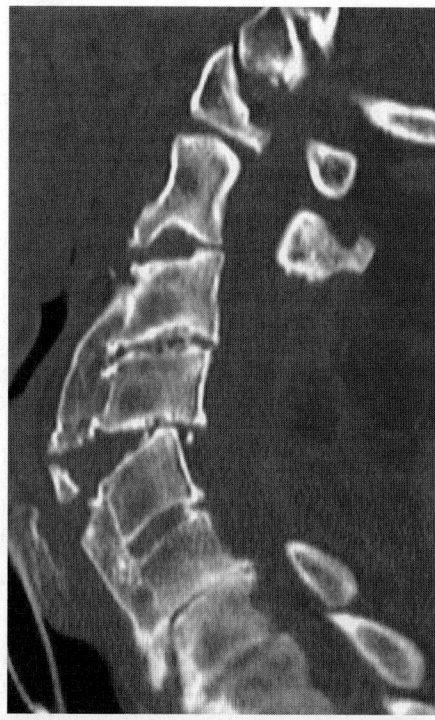

FIG. 4 Sagittal reformatted multidetector computed tomography image showing hyperextension fracture with subluxation through C4 and C5 levels in a patient with massive diffuse idiopathic skeletal hyperostosis. Such injuries may occur after relatively trivial trauma in such patients. (Pope TL, Bloem HL, Beltran J, Morrison WB, Wilson DJ: *Musculoskeletal imaging*, ed 2, Philadelphia, 2014, Saunders.)

BASIC INFORMATION

DEFINITION

Discoid lupus erythematosus (DLE) is a chronic inflammatory autoimmune cutaneous disorder that can lead to significant disfiguration and scarring. It can be associated with or occur independently of systemic lupus erythematosus (SLE).

SYNONYMS

Chronic cutaneous lupus erythematosus
CCLE

ICD-10CM CODES
L93.0 Discoid lupus erythematosus
L93.2 Other local lupus erythematosus

EPIDEMIOLOGY & DEMOGRAPHICS

- Slightly more common in African Americans than in Asians or whites
- DLE is two to three times more likely in women than in men.
- DLE most commonly occurs on the face, scalp, and ears, but can also appear on mucosal surfaces such as the conjunctiva, nasal mucosa, and lips.
- Approximately 5% to 10% of patients presenting with DLE will develop SLE; those with widespread, numerous lesions are more likely to progress.
- Highest prevalence of SLE occurs in persons ages 40 to 60, with SLE onset most often occurring in patients in their 20s and 30s.

PHYSICAL FINDINGS & CLINICAL PRESENTATION

General:
- Early lesions: single or multiple erythematous or violaceous, discrete papules or plaques with scale, often extending into dilated hair follicles. Intense inflammatory nature results in an indurated feel on palpation (Fig. 1)
- Older lesions: peripheral hyperpigmentation with scarring, central hypopigmentation (Fig. E2), and telangiectasia

Anatomic distribution:
- Commonly involves the scalp, face, ears (conchal bowls), and extensor surface of the arms (photodistributed pattern).
- Mucosal and nail involvement is also possible.

Lesion configuration:
- Irregularly grouped, confluent and disfiguring plaques.

Lesion morphology:
- Erythematous plaque with scale
- Rarely, hypertrophic plaques with thick scale
- Follicular plugging
- Atrophy
- Irreversible, scarring alopecia (34%)
- May be associated with other clinical findings of SLE (e.g., oral ulcers, arthritis, pleuritis, pericarditis)

ETIOLOGY

Unknown, but thought to be an autoimmune-mediated disorder and due to interaction between environmental and genetic factors

DIAGNOSIS

Clinical findings and skin biopsy are used to establish the diagnosis of DLE.

DIFFERENTIAL DIAGNOSIS

- Table 1 compares various cutaneous connective tissue diseases.
- Burn scar
- Dermotophyte infection
- Granuloma annulare
- Granuloma faciale
- Lichen planus
- Lichen planopilaris
- Psoriasis
- Radiation dermatitis
- Rosacea
- Sarcoidosis
- Scarring alopecia
- Subacute cutaneous lupus erythematosis
- Syphilis
- Vitiligo

LABORATORY TESTS

- Complete blood count is usually normal in isolated DLE.
- Blood urea nitrogen and creatinine are normal in isolated DLE.
- Erythrocyte sedimentation rate is elevated in active disease.
- Urinalysis may show proteinuria.
- Antinuclear antibody is positive in 20% of patients with isolated DLE.
- Anti-Ro (SS-A) and anti-La (SS-B) autoantibodies are present in 1% to 3% of patients.
- Histology of skin reveals hyperkeratosis with follicular plugging; interface dermatitis with Civatte bodies; melanophages at dermal-epidermal junction; a thickened basement membrane; and a perivascular, interstitial, and perifollicular lymphocytic infiltrate.

TREATMENT

NONPHARMACOLOGIC THERAPY

Avoid sun exposure by using protective clothing and a broad-spectrum sunscreen of SPF >30 that blocks UVB and UVA light (e.g., avobenzone with octocrylene, titanium dioxide, zinc oxide). Avoid exposure to sunlight during peak hours. Use sun-protective clothing.

ACUTE GENERAL Rx

1. Topical steroids: intermediate- to high-potency steroids are needed; use caution when applying to the face.
2. Intralesional triamcinolone acetonide (3-10 mg/cc)
3. Topical calcineurin inhibitors: pimecrolimus 1% cream and tacrolimus 0.1% ointment.
4. Systemic antimalarials: hydroxychloroquine sulfate 200 mg PO bid alone or in combination with quinacrine 100 mg PO daily.
5. Avoid use of systemic glucocorticoids in patients with isolated DLE because of risks of side effects.

CHRONIC Rx

1. Antimalarials remain the cornerstone of treatment: hydroxychloroquine 6 mg/kg of ideal body weight per day or chloroquine 4 mg/kg of ideal body weight per day. Combination therapy with quinacrine can also be used.
2. Second-line agents are methotrexate, acitretin, isotretinoin, and dapsone. Labs should be followed regularly on these medications.
3. Third-line agents are azathioprine, thalidomide, mycophenolate mofetil, sulfasalazine, and oral gold.
4. Oral corticosteroids can be considered in resistant cases with associated symptoms refractory to other measures.

DISPOSITION

If untreated, DLE can lead to significant and permanent atrophy and scarring of the skin.

REFERRAL

Dermatology, rheumatology, nephrology, internal medicine, ophthalmology

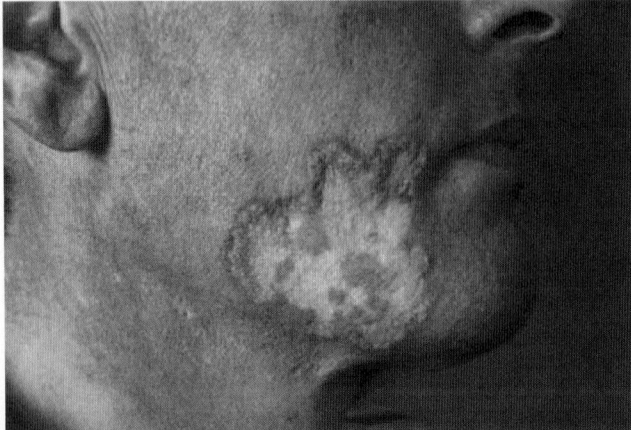

FIG. 1 Classic discoid lupus erythematosus of the face. Note central scarring and erythematous hyperkeratotic borders. (From Hochberg MC et al: *Rheumatology*, ed 5, St Louis, 2011, Mosby.)

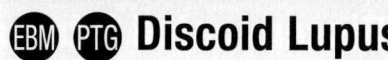
TABLE 1 Autoimmune Cutaneous Connective Tissue Diseases

Autoimmune Disease	Indirect Immunofluorescence Pattern of Antinuclear Antibody Staining in Serum*	Nuclear Antigens to Which Autoantibodies Are Directed	Direct Immunofluorescence of Tissue
Lupus Erythematosus			
Systemic LE	Peripheral (rim), homogeneous, nucleolar, speckled	nDNA or double-stranded DNA, single-stranded DNA, histones, nucleolar RNA, various ribonucleoproteins, cardiolipin, Sm (Smith), U1-snRNP, HMG-17	Two or more granular immunoglobulin and complement deposits at BMZ, IgG, IgM, and/or IgA with C3 in involved and uninvolved skin (lupus band); lichenoid changes with numerous cytoids and shaggy fibrinogen staining of BMZ also found
Discoid LE	Usually no circulating antibodies	Usually none detected	Two or more granular immunoglobulin and complement deposits at BMZ, IgG, IgM, and/or IgA with C3 in involved skin; lichenoid changes with numerous cytoids and shaggy fibrinogen staining of BMZ also found
Subacute cutaneous LE	Fine speckled or speckled, may be negative	SS-A/Ro, SS-B/La	Particulate intercellular staining with or without granular immune deposits at BMZ or lichenoid changes
Neonatal LE	Fine speckled or speckled, may be negative	SS-A/Ro, SS-B/La	Granular IgG (transplacental) at BMZ
Drug-induced LE	Peripheral, homogeneous	Histones	Granular immune deposits at the BMZ
Scleroderma			
Cutaneous scleroderma (localized and generalized morphea)	Peripheral	SCL-70, SS-A/Ro, SS-B/La	No characteristic changes; vascular staining may be observed
Limited disease (acrosclerosis, CREST)	Centromere	Centromere, SCL-70, U1-snRNP, HMG-17	No characteristic changes; vascular staining may be observed
Diffuse disease (systemic sclerosis)	Nucleolar, speckled	SCL-70, U1- and U3-snRNP, RNA pol I, II, and III	No characteristic changes; vascular staining may be observed
Dermatomyositis, polymyositis	Speckled, nucleolar	Jo-1, PM-Scl, Mi-2, U1-snRNP, SS-A/Ro	No characteristic changes; lichenoid features and vascular staining may be observed
Sjögren syndrome	Fine speckled, nucleolar	SS-A/Ro, SS-B/La, histones, U1-snRNP	No characteristic changes; vascular staining may be observed
Mixed connective tissue disease	Speckled	U1-snRNP, PM-Scl	No characteristic changes; granular immune deposits at the BMZ lichenoid features and vascular staining may be observed
Overlap and undifferentiated connective tissue disease	Any single or combination pattern	Any one or multiple	
PM-Scl	May show granular immune complex deposition at BMZ (lupus band), vascular staining, or lichenoid changes		

LE, Lupus erythematosus.
From Adkinson NF et al: *Middleton's allergy principles and practice*, ed 8, Philadelphia, 2014, Saunders.

! PEARLS & CONSIDERATIONS

- Discoid rash is one of 11 diagnostic criteria for SLE.
- Rarely, patients with DLE may develop cutaneous squamous cell carcinoma in areas of disease.
- It is unusual to see DLE involving areas below the neck if there is no disease above the neck. Biopsy for definitive diagnosis in these cases.

SUGGESTED READINGS

Available at www.expertconsult.com

RELATED CONTENT

Discoid Lupus Erythematosus (Patient Information)
Systemic Lupus Erythematosus (Related Key Topic)

AUTHORS: **KACHIU C. LEE, M.D., M.P.H.,** and **SARA CAPOBIANCO, B.S.**

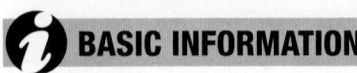

BASIC INFORMATION

DEFINITION

Disseminated intravascular coagulation (DIC) is an acquired thromboembolic disorder characterized by generalized activation of the clotting mechanism, which results in the intravascular formation of fibrin and ultimately thrombotic occlusion of small and midsize vessels.

SYNONYMS

Consumptive coagulopathy
DIC
Defibrination syndrome

ICD-10CM CODES
D65   Disseminated intravascular coagulation [defibrination syndrome]

EPIDEMIOLOGY & DEMOGRAPHICS

DIC can be found in up to 1% of hospitalized patients. There is no predilection for age or gender. More than 50% of cases are associated with gram-negative sepsis or other septicemic infections.

PHYSICAL FINDINGS & CLINICAL PRESENTATION

Both acute and chronic DIC can present with bleeding or thrombosis. Bleeding manifestations are more commonly seen in acute DIC. Sudden exposure to procoagulants may extensively activate a coagulation cascade and platelet consumption. Platelet regeneration from bone marrow and also replacement of coagulation factors from liver synthesis might not be able to keep up with this acute consumptive process. In contrast, chronic DIC more frequently causes thrombotic complications, although PT and PTT values may be normal. With DIC, multiple organs may be involved, as follows:

Central nervous system: altered mental status, transient neurological deficits
Cardiovascular: hypotension, tachycardia
Respiratory: hypoxia, dyspnea, localized rales, and acute respiratory syndrome
Gastrointestinal: intestinal bleeding, bowel infarction
Genitourinary: oliguria, anuria, uremia, acidosis, metrorrhagia
Skin: wound site bleeding, epistaxis, gingival bleeding, hemorrhagic bullae, petechiae, ecchymosis, purpura (Fig. E1)

ETIOLOGY

- Infections (e.g., gram-negative sepsis, Rocky Mountain spotted fever, malaria, viral or fungal infection).
- Obstetric complications (e.g., dead fetus, amniotic fluid embolism, toxemia, abruptio placentae, septic abortion, eclampsia, placenta previa, uterine atony).
- Tissue trauma (e.g., burns, hypothermia rewarming).
- Neoplasms (e.g., adenocarcinomas [gastrointestinal, prostate, lung, breast], acute promyelocytic leukemia).
- Quinine, cocaine-induced rhabdomyolysis.
- Liver failure.
- Acute pancreatitis.
- Transfusion reactions.
- Respiratory distress syndrome.
- Toxins (snake bites, amphetamine overdose).
- Other: systemic lupus erythematosus (SLE), vasculitis, aneurysms, polyarteritis, cavernous hemangiomas.
- Box E1 describes underlying conditions associated with DIC.

DIAGNOSIS

DIFFERENTIAL DIAGNOSIS

- Hepatic necrosis: normal or elevated factor VIII concentrations
- Vitamin K deficiency: normal platelet count
- Hemolytic uremic syndrome: coagulation assays are usually normal
- Thrombotic thrombocytopenic purpura: low ADAMTS13 activity
- Renal failure, SLE, sickle cell crisis, dysfibrinogenemias
- HELLP syndrome (**h**emolysis, **e**levated **l**iver function tests, and **l**ow **p**latelets)

WORKUP

Diagnostic workup includes laboratory screening to confirm the diagnosis and exclude conditions noted in the differential diagnosis (Figs. 2 and 3). Workup is also aimed at distinguishing DIC progression (acute vs. chronic), chief manifestations (thrombotic or hemorrhagic), and extent (localized or systemic). The International Society on Thrombosis and Haemostasis scoring system for DIC is described in Box E2.

LABORATORY TESTS

- Peripheral blood smear generally shows red blood cell fragments (schistocytes) and low platelet count.
- Coagulation factors are consumed at a rate in excess of the capacity of the liver to synthesize them, and platelets are consumed in excess of the capacity of the bone marrow megakaryocytes to release them. Diagnostic characteristics of DIC are decreased fibrinogen level; thrombocytopenia; and increased prothrombin time (PT), partial thromboplastin time (PTT), TT, fibrin split products, bleeding time, and D-dimer.
- Coagulopathy secondary to DIC must be differentiated from that secondary to liver disease or vitamin K deficiency.
  1. Vitamin K deficiency manifests with prolonged PT and normal PTT, TT, platelet, and fibrinogen level; PTT may be elevated in severe cases.
  2. Patients with liver disease have abnormal PT and PTT; TT and fibrinogen are usually normal unless severe disease is present; platelets are usually normal unless splenomegaly is present.
  3. Factor VIII is low in DIC but is normal in liver disease with coagulopathy.

IMAGING STUDIES

Imaging studies are generally not useful. Chest radiographs may be helpful to exclude infectious processes in patients with pulmonary symptoms such as dyspnea, cough, or hemoptysis.

TREATMENT

NONPHARMACOLOGIC THERAPY

No specific precautions regarding activity level are necessary unless thrombocytopenia is severe.

ACUTE GENERAL Rx

- Correct and eliminate underlying cause (e.g., antimicrobial therapy for infection, removal of necrotic bowel, evacuation of uterus in obstetric emergencies).
- Give replacement therapy with fresh frozen plasma (FFP) and platelets in patients with significant hemorrhage:
  1. FFP 10 to 15 ml/kg can be given with a goal of normalizing international normalized ratio.
  2. Platelet transfusions are given when platelet count is <10,000 (or higher if major bleeding is present).
  3. Cryoprecipitate 1 U/5 kg is reserved for fibrinogen level <100 mg/dl.
  4. Antithrombin treatment may be considered as a supportive therapeutic option in patients with severe DIC. Its modest results and substantial cost are limiting factors.
- Heparin therapy at a dose lower than that used in venous thrombosis (300 to 500 U/hr) may be useful in selected cases to increase neutralization of thrombin (e.g., DIC associated with acute promyelocytic leukemia, purpura fulminans, acral ischemia).

CHRONIC Rx

Follow-up management includes coagulation screening to assess factor replacement therapy. Laboratory abnormalities generally correct with treatment of the underlying disorder. Long-term laboratory monitoring is not required.

DISPOSITION

Mortality rate in severe DIC exceeds 75%. Death generally results from progression of the underlying disease and complications such as acute renal failure, intracerebral hematoma, shock, or cardiac tamponade.

REFERRAL

Hematology consultation is recommended in all cases of DIC.

PEARLS & CONSIDERATIONS

COMMENTS

The treatment of chronic DIC is controversial. Low-dose SC heparin and/or combination antiplatelet agents such as aspirin and dipyridamole may be useful.

SUGGESTED READINGS
Available at www.expertconsult.com

RELATED CONTENT

Disseminated Intravascular Coagulation (Patient Information)

AUTHORS: **PATAN GULTAWATVICHAI, M.D.,** and **BHARTI RATHORE, M.D.**

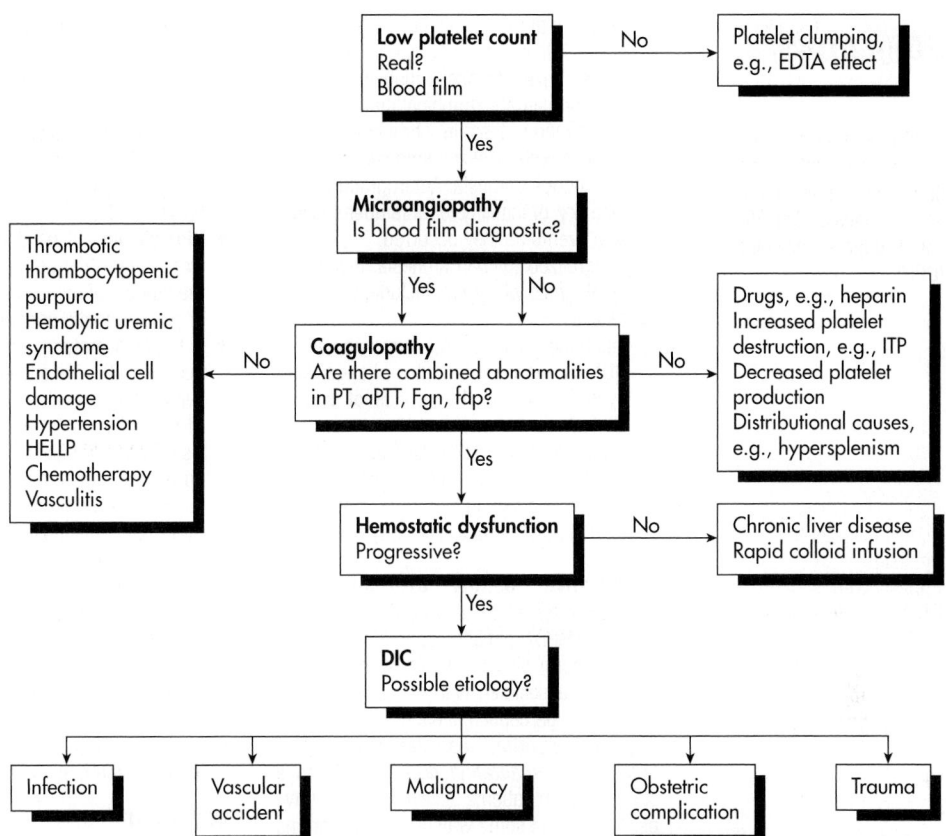

FIG. 2 Differential diagnostic algorithm for disseminated intravascular coagulation (DIC). *aPTT, Activated partial thromboplastin time; EDTA, ethylenediaminetetraacetic acid; ITP,* idiopathic thrombocytopenic purpura; *PT, prothrombin time.* (From Young NS et al [eds]: *Clinical hematology,* St Louis, 2006, Mosby.)

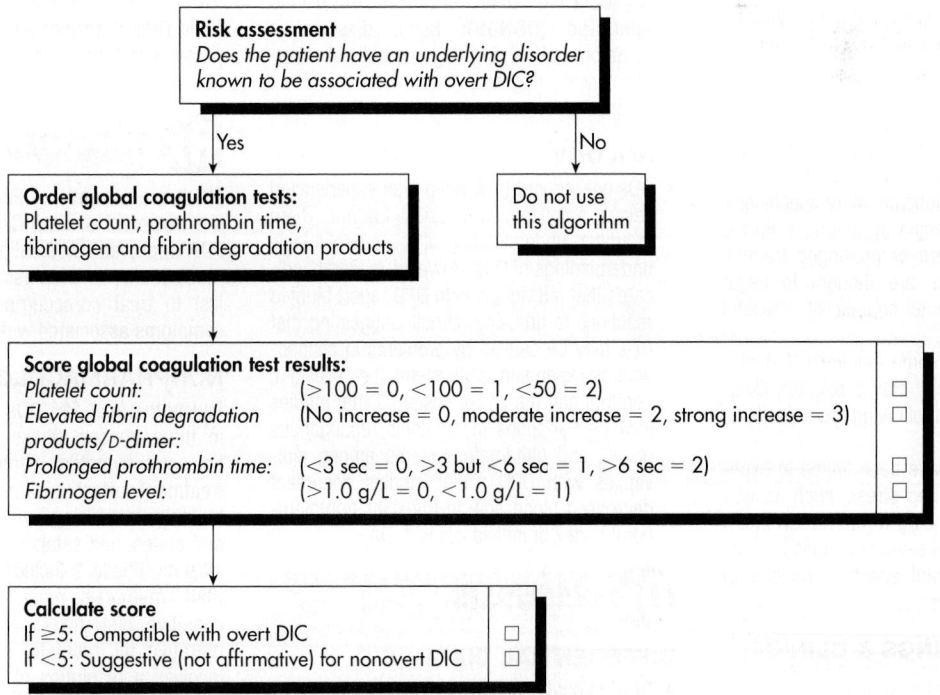

FIG. 3 Laboratory testing and diagnosis of overt disseminated intravascular coagulation (DIC). (From Young NS et al [eds]: *Clinical hematology,* St Louis, 2006, Mosby.)

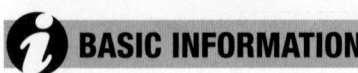

DEFINITION

Dissociative disorders (DDs) feature a disturbance in identity, memory, perception, and consciousness and include dissociative identity disorder (DID), dissociative amnesia (DA), dissociative fugue (DF), and depersonalization/derealization disorder (DPD).

SYNONYMS

DD
DID
DA
DF
DPD

ICD-10 CM CODES
300.14 Dissociative identity disorder
300.12 Dissociative amnesia
300.13 Dissociative amnesia with dissociative fugue
300.6 Depersonalization/derealization disorder
300.15 Other specified dissociative disorder
300.15 Dissociative disorder, unspecified

EPIDEMIOLOGY & DEMOGRAPHICS

- Incidence: Limited research documents incidence of DDs, and estimates vary based on the instrument utilized and the sample studied.
- Peak incidence: Age of peak incidence varies by the type of DD.
- Prevalence: The prevalence of DDs is thought to be between 0.1% and 1.0% of the general population.
- Predominant sex and age: Females are diagnosed with DDs more frequently than males. Diagnoses may be made among individuals of all ages; however, the age of onset is thought to vary by subtype. More specifically, DID is thought to begin in childhood during the course of severe or prolonged trauma, whereas other DDs are thought to begin within the immediate context of stressful events at any age.
- Genetics: There is some evidence that biologic differences may play a role the likelihood of dissociation following the experience of trauma.
- Risk factors: DDs have been linked to experiencing overwhelming stress, such as witnessing or experiencing traumatic events. A greater frequency of severe childhood sexual abuse is a significant specific predictor of dissociative disorders.

PHYSICAL FINDINGS & CLINICAL PRESENTATION

- **Dissociative amnesia (DA)**: Loss of autobiographic memory for previous experiences or before a certain point in time. Types of DA include:
  1. Localized amnesia: Inability to recall a specific (traumatic) period of time.
  2. Selective amnesia: Inability to recall parts, but not all, of a specific period of time.
  3. Systematized amnesia: Inability to recall categoric autobiographical memories, but not memory loss in chronologic order such as with localized amnesia.
  4. Continuous amnesia: Anterograde loss of memory, or inability to remember successive events as they occurred.
  5. Generalized (global) amnesia: Inability to recall one's whole life, including personal details.
  6. Thematic amnesia (as seen in DID & DDNOS): As identity states change, ability to recall specific periods of time is altered.
- **Dissociative fugue (DF):** DF carries all the same characteristics and features as DA, with the distinguishing feature of sudden and unplanned purposeful travel away from one's home.
- **Dissociative identity disorder (DID):** Formerly referred to as *multiple personality disorder* (MPD), patients appear to possess two (or more) distinct identities or personality states, associated with the patient's consciousness, perception, thoughts, and actions.
- **Depersonalization disorder (DPD):** Also known as *derealization disorder,* DPD is a state in which patients believe that they have been altered in some way or that they are no longer real. Features include persistent and recurring experiences of feeling detached from one's own body and mental processes (i.e., one observing oneself as an outsider). Reality testing remains intact.
- **Dissociative disorders not otherwise specified (DDNOS):** Some dissociative symptoms of varying degrees but not meeting clinical diagnostic criteria for a distinct diagnosis.

ETIOLOGY

- DDs are thought to develop after experiencing severe emotional or physical trauma. There is limited understanding of the neurobiologic underpinnings of DDs. However, research indicates that individuals with DPD report blunted reactions to arousing stimuli, suggesting that DDs may be caused by problems in connections between sensory systems (i.e., eyesight, hearing) and the limbic system. Other studies indicate variations in serotonin, endogenous opioid, and glutamate systems among individuals with DPD. Other studies document decreased blood flow in the right frontotemporal cortex of individuals with DA.

Dx DIAGNOSIS

DIFFERENTIAL DIAGNOSIS

- DDs should be distinguished from acute substance intoxication, withdrawal, or substance-induced persisting amnestic disorder.
- Symptoms due to the physiologic consequences of a medical condition should be diagnosed as a mental disorder NOS due to a general medical condition.
- DA should be distinguished from amnestic disorder due to a brain injury, seizure disorders, delirium, dementia, age-related cognitive decline, and nonpathologic forms of amnesia (i.e., amnesia for sleep, memory loss).
- DA and DPD should not be diagnosed separately if symptoms occur only during the course of DF.
- DPD should not be diagnosed when symptoms occur only during a panic attack or in the context of panic disorder, specific phobia, or posttraumatic or acute stress disorders.
- If fugue symptoms occur only in the context of DID, DF should not be diagnosed separately.
- DID diagnoses take precedence over diagnosis of other DDs (i.e., DA, DF, DPD).
- Purposeful travel that occurs during a manic episode should be distinguished from a DF.
- Differential diagnosis should also consider schizophrenia and other psychotic disorders, bipolar disorder with rapid cycling, anxiety disorders, somatization disorders, and personality disorders.
- Amnesia for trauma may also occur in posttraumatic stress disorder and acute stress disorder
- Clinicians may also consider malingered amnesia and malingered fugue states

WORKUP

Diagnosis is made based on structured clinical interviews such as Dissociative Disorders Interview Schedule (DDIS) or the Structured Clinical Interview for Dissociative Disorders (SCID-D). The Dissociative Experiences Scale (DES) is a self-questionnaire diagnostically useful in DDs. Diagnosis also includes a review of personal history and symptoms as well as ruling out any physical injury (i.e., head trauma).

Rx TREATMENT

There are currently no FDA-approved drugs for the treatment of DDs. Clinicians may consider FDA-approved medications (i.e., antianxiety medications, antidepressants, or antipsychotics) to treat co-occurring mood and anxiety symptoms associated with DDs.

NONPHARMACOLOGIC THERAPY

Psychotherapy for DDs generally proceeds in three phases. Phase 1 includes stabilization and symptom control, education about treatment, affect and impulse regulation skill building, increasing awareness of dissociated self-states, and establishment of a therapeutic alliance. Phase 2 includes processing of traumatic memories, resolution of trauma-related cognitive distortions, and development of a narrative of traumatic experiences. Phase 3 involves a resolution of dissociated self-state and a focus on current and future life issues.

- Therapists may be able to provide more effective treatment if trained in the importance of continuous and frequent assessments of the therapeutic alliance and methods for enhancing it.

- Experts treating dissociative disorders advise only occasionally processing traumatic material. During the trauma-processing stage, experts frequently stabilize safety and augment trauma processing by using containment and grounding modalities.

ACUTE GENERAL Rx

It is believed that a critical component of early treatment is the provision of a safe therapeutic environment. Identification of triggers associated with the onset of dissociation is useful. Controversy exists regarding the use of hypnosis for the purpose of recovering memories.

CHRONIC Rx

All stages of treatment may include psycho-education, skill building, alliance building, processing of reactions to therapy, emotion regulation, management of relationships, and stabilization. Grounding techniques, containment (i.e., imagery aimed at decreasing the intrusiveness of a memory), skill building (i.e., relaxation training and self-affirmation), and cognitive behavioral interventions (i.e., addressing irrational beliefs) are also used.

COMPLEMENTARY AND ALTERNATIVE MEDICINE

Research is lacking on complementary and alternative medicine for DDs.

DISPOSITION

Treatment should be delivered in the least restrictive environment possible to ensure patient safety. Patients who have comorbid psychiatric or medical diagnoses; who are experiencing suicidal or homicidal ideation, plans, or intention; or who are severely ill may require partial or inpatient hospitalization for the purpose of stabilization.

REFERRAL

Patients are treated by a mental health clinician.

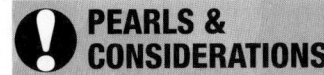

PEARLS & CONSIDERATIONS

COMMENTS

- Symptoms of DDs (i.e., derealization, dissociation) are seen in many other psychiatric disorders (e.g., panic disorder, PTSD). Incidence of dissociative symptoms following severe trauma is high. However, for most individuals, dissociative symptoms subside on their own within a few weeks following a traumatic event.
- Treatment approach may vary by the specific type of DD. Rigorous empiric studies assessing the treatment of specific DDs are lacking. For example, no randomized treatment studies have investigated the effectiveness of hypnosis in treating acute DA. Additionally, for chronic DA, pharmacologic facilitated intervention for the retrieval of memories (i.e., utilization of sodium pentobarbital or administration of intravenous lorazepam) is not well researched.

PREVENTION

Data are lacking on the prevention of DDs, but the prevention of child maltreatment may be useful in this regard.

PATIENT/FAMILY EDUCATION

International Society for the Study of Trauma and Dissociation (http://www.isst-d.org)

SUGGESTED READINGS

Available at www.expertconsult.com

RELATED TOPICS

Acute Stress Disorder (Related Key Topic)
Posttraumatic Stress Disorder (Related Key Topic)

AUTHORS: **LINDSAY M. ORCHOWSKI, Ph.D.,** and **DANIEL W. OESTERLE, B.S.**

D

Diseases and Disorders

I

ℹ️ BASIC INFORMATION

DEFINITION

- Colonic diverticula are herniations of mucosa and submucosa (Figs. 1 and 2) through the muscularis (Fig. 3). They are generally found along the colon's mesenteric border at the site where the vasa recta penetrates the muscle wall (anatomic weak point).
- *Diverticulosis* is the asymptomatic presence of multiple colonic diverticula.
- *Diverticulitis* is an inflammatory process or localized perforation of diverticulum.

ICD-10CM CODES
K57.30 Diverticulosis of large intestine without perforation or abscess without bleeding
K57.32 Diverticulitis of large intestine without perforation or abscess without bleeding
K57.31 Diverticulosis of large intestine without perforation or abscess with bleeding

EPIDEMIOLOGY & DEMOGRAPHICS

- Incidence of diverticulosis in the general population is 35% to 50%. Prevalence of diverticulosis increases with ages (<10% under age 40 to 80% in those >85).
- Diverticulosis is more common in Western countries, affecting >30% of people >40 yr and >50% of people >70 yr.
- Approximately 20% of patients with diverticula have an episode of diverticulitis.

PHYSICAL FINDINGS & CLINICAL PRESENTATION

- Physical examination in patients with diverticulosis is generally normal.
- Painful diverticular disease can present with left lower quadrant (LLQ) pain, often relieved by defecation; location of pain may be anywhere in the lower abdomen because of the redundancy of the sigmoid colon.
- Diverticulitis can cause muscle spasm, guarding, and rebound tenderness predominantly affecting the LLQ.

ETIOLOGY

- Diverticular disease is believed to be secondary to low intake of dietary fiber.
- Recent studies indicate a pathogenetic role for inflammation in diverticulitis that may be similar to that of IBS, IBD, or both, based on common histologic findings such as granulomas, infiltrating lymphocytes, TNF, histamine, and matrix metalloproteinases.[1]

🄳🅇 DIAGNOSIS

DIFFERENTIAL DIAGNOSIS

- Irritable bowel syndrome

[1]Morris AM et al: Sigmoid diverticulitis: a systematic review, *JAMA* 311(3):287-297, 2014.

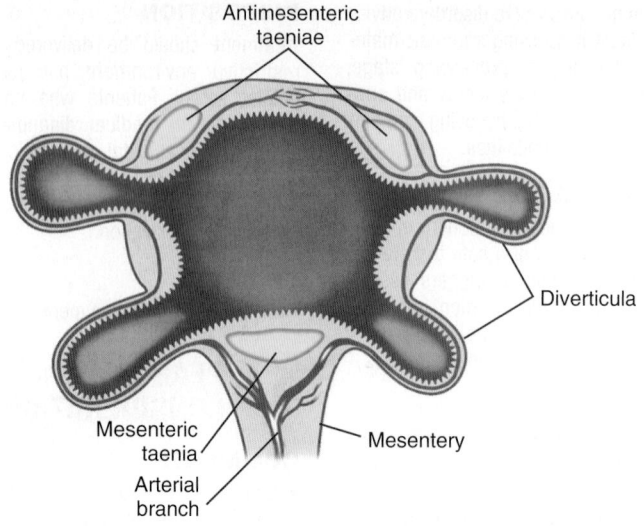

FIG. 1 Diagram showing colonic diverticula and their relationship to the taeniae coli. (From Feldman M et al (eds): *Sleisenger and Fordtran's gastrointestinal and liver disease*, ed 10, Philadelphia, 2016, Saunders.)

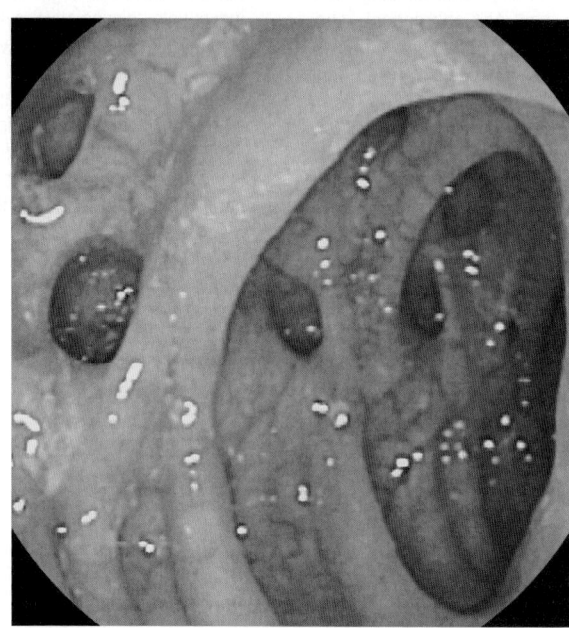

FIG. 2 Colonoscopic view of sigmoid diverticulosis. (From Feldman M et al (eds): *Sleisenger and Fordtran's gastrointestinal and liver disease*, ed 10, Philadelphia, 2016, Saunders.)

- IBD
- Carcinoma of colon
- Endometriosis
- Ischemic colitis
- Infections (pseudomembranous colitis, appendicitis, pyelonephritis, PID)
- Lactose intolerance
- Celiac disease

LABORATORY TESTS

- WBC count in diverticulitis reveals leukocytosis with left shift.
- Microcytic anemia can be present in patients with chronic bleeding from diverticular disease. MCV may be elevated in acute bleeding secondary to reticulocytosis.

PROCEDURES: Colonoscopy should be avoided during acute diverticulitis due to the risk of

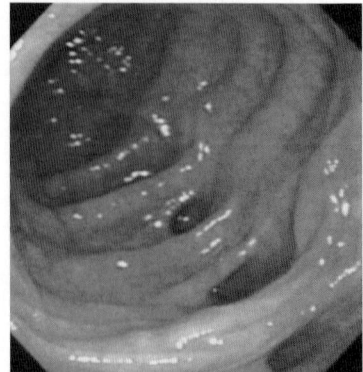

FIG. 3 Colonoscopic appearance of diverticular disease affecting the sigmoid colon. (From Forbes A et al: *Atlas of clinical gastroenterology*, ed 3, Edinburgh, 2005, Elsevier.)

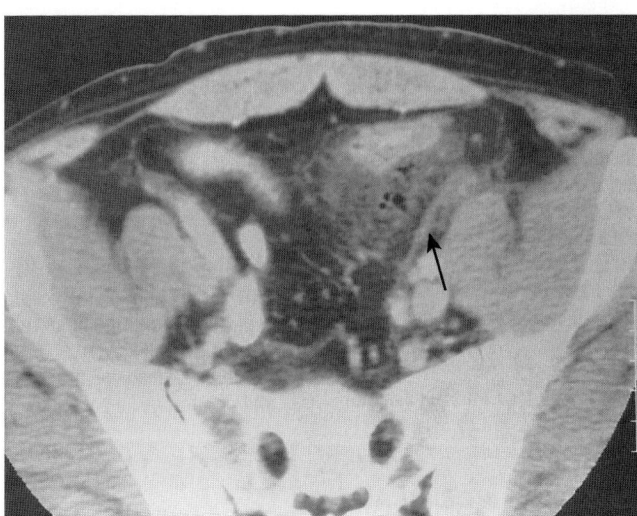

FIG. 4 Sigmoid diverticulitis. Enhanced CT shows haziness associated with extraluminal air in the sigmoid mesocolon due to perforated diverticulitis, also manifested as a thickened sigmoid wall. Thickening at the root of the sigmoid mesocolon is also present *(arrow).* (From Grainger RG et al [eds.]: *Grainger and Allison's diagnostic radiology,* ed 4, Philadelphia, 2001, Churchill Livingstone.)

perforation. It can generally be performed after 6 wk to rule out the presence of cancer and IBD.

IMAGING STUDIES

- If clinical features are highly suggestive of diverticulitis, imaging studies are generally not necessary.
- A CT scan of the abdomen (Fig. 4) is the preferred radiologic examination to diagnose acute diverticulitis. It can also diagnose diverticulosis. It has a sensitivity of 93% to 97% and a specificity approaching 100% for diverticulitis. Typical findings are thickening of the bowel wall, fistulas, or abscess formation. CT may also reveal other disease processes (e.g., appendicitis, tuboovarian abscess, Crohn's disease) accounting for lower abdominal pain
- Evaluation of suspected diverticular bleeding:
  1. Arteriography if the bleeding is faster than 1 ml/min (advantage: the possible infusion of vasopressin directly into the arteries supplying the bleeding, as well as selective arterial embolization; disadvantages: its cost and invasive nature)
  2. Technetium-99m sulfa colloid
  3. Technetium-99m labeled RBC (can detect bleeding rates as low as 0.12 to 5 ml/min)

Rx TREATMENT

NONPHARMACOLOGIC THERAPY

- Increase in dietary fiber intake and regular exercise to improve bowel function. However, recent studies have challenged the common view that fiber intake protects against diverticulosis
- NPO and IV hydration in severe diverticulitis; NG suction if ileus or small bowel obstruction is present
- Emergent surgery is required for perforation, peritonitis, or uncontrolled sepsis.

ACUTE GENERAL Rx
TREATMENT OF DIVERTICULITIS:

- Mild case: broad-spectrum PO antibiotics (e.g., ciprofloxacin 750 mg bid or levofloxacin 750 mg bid or trimethoprim/sulfamethoxazole DS bid to cover aerobic component of colonic flora *and* metronidazole 500 mg q6h for anaerobes) and liquid diet for 7 to 10 days are commonly prescribed. However, randomized trials and cohort studies have shown that antibiotics are not as beneficial or necessary as previously thought in cases of mild diverticulitis. Other modalities such as 5-aminosalicylate products and probiotics remain controversial and of unclear benefit. Severe case: NPO and aggressive IV antibiotic therapy
  a. Ampicillin-sulbactam 3 g IV q6h *or*
  b. Piperacillin-tazobactam 4.5 g IV q8h *or*
  c. Ciprofloxacin 400 mg IV q12h plus metronidazole 500 mg IV q6h *or*
  d. Ticarcillin-clavulanate 3.1 g IV q6h
- Life-threatening case: imipenem 500 mg IV q6h *or* meropenem 1 g IV q8h
- Surgical treatment (laparoscopic preferred over open colectomy) consisting of resection of involved areas and reanastomosis (if feasible); otherwise, a diverting colostomy with reanastomosis is performed when infection has been controlled. The need for surgery as well as its optimal timing is unclear, and surgery is no longer considered necessary after a couple of episodes of diverticulitis. Surgery may be considered in patients with:
  1. Repeated episodes of diverticulitis
  2. Poor response to appropriate medical therapy (failure of conservative management)
  3. Abscess or fistula formation
  4. Obstruction
  5. Peritonitis
  6. Immunocompromised patients, first episode in young patient (<40 yr old)

  7. Inability to exclude carcinoma (10% to 20% of patients diagnosed with diverticulosis on clinical grounds are subsequently found to have carcinoma of the colon)

DIVERTICULAR HEMORRHAGE:
1. Bleeding is painless and stops spontaneously in the majority of patients (60%); it is usually caused by erosion of a blood vessel by a fecalith present within the diverticular sac.
2. Medical therapy consists of blood replacement and correction of volume and any clotting abnormalities.
3. Colonoscopic treatment with epinephrine injections, bipolar coagulation, or both may prevent recurrent bleeding and decrease the need for surgery.
4. Surgical resection is necessary if bleeding does not stop spontaneously after administration of 4 to 5 U of PRBCs or recurs with severity within a few days; if attempts at localization are unsuccessful, total abdominal colectomy with ileoproctostomy may be indicated (high incidence of rebleeding if segmental resection is performed without adequate localization).

DISPOSITION
- The risk of recurrence among patients with uncomplicated diverticulitis is 32% to 36%. Most patients with diverticulitis respond well to antibiotic management and bowel rest. Up to 30% of patients with diverticulitis will eventually require surgical management.
- Diverticular bleeding can recur in 15% to 20% of patients within 5 yr.

REFERRAL
- GI referral for colonoscopy 4-6 wk after resolution of symptoms. In patients who have complications from diverticulitis, colonoscopy is generally not necessary after radiologically proven uncomplicated diverticulitis.
- Surgical referral when considering resection.

SUGGESTED READINGS
Available at www.expertconsult.com

RELATED CONTENT
Diverticular Disease (Patient Information)
Diverticulitis (Patient Information)
Diverticulosis (Patient Information)

AUTHOR: **FRED F. FERRI, M.D.**

BASIC INFORMATION

- Drowning aftereffects should be classified as death, morbidity, and absence of morbidity.
- The previously used terms *wet, dry, active, passive, silent,* and *secondary drowning* should no longer be used when considering statistical analysis; however, they remain in common use.

DEFINITION

Drowning is the process of experiencing respiratory impairment from submersion/immersion in liquid.

SYNONYMS

Suffocation
Asphyxiation

ICD-10CM CODES
W65 Accidental nontransport drowning and submersion
W67 Accidental drowning and submersion while in swimming pool
W69 Accidental drowning and submersion while in natural water
W74 Unspecified cause of accidental drowning and submersion

EPIDEMIOLOGY & DEMOGRAPHICS

- The fifth-leading cause of unintentional-injury death in the U.S.; 10 people die each day from drowning.
- Drowning is the most common injury-related cause of death in children 1 to 4 years of age.
- Nearly 6000 persons are treated in U.S. emergency departments each year for submersion or drowning injuries, with 50% of these patients requiring hospital admission.
- Between 2000 and 2007, the rate of fatal accidental drowning for African Americans was 130% that of whites; for Native Americans and Alaskan Natives, this rate was 170% that of whites.

INCIDENCE:
- From 2005 to 2014, an average of 3536 fatal unintentional drownings (nonboating related) occurred annually in the U.S. In California, Arizona, and Florida, drowning is the number one cause of injury-related death.
- Internationally the incidence is likely underestimated due to lack of reporting.

PEAK INCIDENCE:
- Ages 14 years of age or younger account for 25%. High-risk groups are in the toddler age group and in young males. Fifteen percent of children admitted for drowning die in the hospital.
- Highest occurrence on weekends (~40%) in the summertime months (May through August), and more commonly in the rural southern and western U.S. (62%).[3]

PREDOMINANT SEX AND AGE:
- Males are 400% more likely to suffer a drowning due to increased risk-taking behavior.
- Age distribution is bimodal with the very young and elderly showing higher rates of submersion injury.

RISK FACTORS:
- Alcohol abuse
- Male
- Youth, elderly
- Seizure disorder
- Mental illness
- Cardiac disease
- Neuromuscular disorder, musculoskeletal disorder
- Frigid liquid temperature

PHYSICAL FINDINGS & CLINICAL PRESENTATION

- Presentation varies; it most commonly is an unobserved individual found unconscious.
- Swimmers can suffer blackouts from hypocapnia when hyperventilating, and ascending divers may experience shallow water blackouts.
- A drowning classification system is used to classify victims at the rescue scene based on the following clinical parameters: pulse, respirations, pulmonary auscultation, and blood pressure.

ETIOLOGY

- The primary factor is hypoxemia with subsequent multiorgan damage.
- The initiation of breath holding is complicated by laryngospasm if liquid is detected in the posterior pharynx/larynx, which impedes immediate inhalation. Once serum oxygen levels decrease, involuntary larynx relaxation occurs, and the victim aspirates liquid.
- If hypoxemia ensues and progresses to acidosis, myocardial ischemia and CNS ischemia are the predominant threats.
- A minority of drownings are considered "dry," with laryngospasm persisting until death.

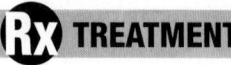

DIAGNOSIS

DIFFERENTIAL DIAGNOSIS

- Suicide
- Homicide
- Abuse
- Cranial/cervical trauma
- Seizure
- Cardiac arrhythmia
- Hypoglycemia

WORKUP

- Initiation of basic life support/advanced cardiac life support (BLS/ACLS)
- Cardiopulmonary monitoring
- Pulse oximetry
- EKG
- Assess for trauma
- Glasgow Coma Scale assessment

LABORATORY TESTS

- ABG
- Chemistry panel 7
- Toxicology screen
- Troponin
- Liver function tests
- Lactate
- Urinalysis

IMAGING STUDIES

- CXR for evaluation of pulmonary edema, aspiration, endotracheal tube placement, foreign body (Fig. E1)
- CT cervical/head for assessment of trauma and/or intracranial pathology

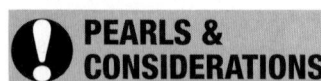

TREATMENT

- The foundation is management of basic cardiopulmonary functions of oxygenation, ventilation, respiration, and cardiac output as well as thermoregulation.

NONPHARMACOLOGIC THERAPY

- Supplemental oxygen.
- CPAP or intubation with mechanical ventilation for respiratory failure.
- Permissive therapeutic hypothermia may benefit comatose patients.
- Extracorporeal membrane oxygenation is beneficial under specific circumstances.
- Bronchoscopy to remove foreign aspirated bodies.
- Treat secondary causes such as seizure, trauma, hypoglycemia.

DISPOSITION

- Mental and cardiopulmonary status are core measures.
- ABG normalization.
- Correction of potential secondary etiologies.

REFERRAL

- Once the patient is stabilized, transfer to a tertiary care facility is ideal with comatose patients or those requiring a specialist.

PEARLS & CONSIDERATIONS

- Early resuscitation is key.
- All guardians should have BLS training.

PREVENTION

Unattended access to bodies of water and poor rescue/safety training are key.

PATIENT/FAMILY EDUCATION

All guardians should have BLS training.

SUGGESTED READINGS
Available at www.expertconsult.com

AUTHOR: **KEVIN V. PLUMLEY, M.D., M.P.H.**

BASIC INFORMATION

DEFINITION

Drug abuse is a recurring pattern of harmful use of a substance despite adverse consequences to work, school, relationships, the legal system, or physical health. This may occur concurrently with or independently from *substance dependence,* in which the impairment or distress is more pervasive and often (though not necessarily) includes physical dependence and withdrawal symptoms (Table 1).

SYNONYMS

Substance use disorder
Substance abuse
Addiction

ICD-10CM CODES
F19.129	Other psychoactive substance abuse, unspecified
F10-F19	Defined by specific substance
Z71.51	Drug abuse counseling and surveillance of drug abuser
Z71.51	Drug abuse counseling and surveillance of drug abuser

The new term *substance use disorder* in the fifth edition of the *Diagnostic and Statistical Manual of Mental Disorders* (DSM-5) combines the categories of substance abuse and substance dependence into a single disorder measured on a continuum from mild to severe.

EPIDEMIOLOGY & DEMOGRAPHICS

INCIDENCE (IN U.S.): Alcohol or drug dependence: 5% to 10% of population
PREVALENCE (IN U.S.): Approximately 15% of patients in primary care practice have an at-risk pattern of drug and/or alcohol use; lifetime prevalence of any alcohol use disorder: 30%; prescription drug misuse is on the rise with 5% past-year prevalence.
PREDOMINANT SEX: Males > females
PREDOMINANT AGE:
- Problematic use of substances may begin in early life (8 to 10 yr).
- Mean age of onset of problem drinking is approximately 25 yr for men and 30 yr for women.

PEAK INCIDENCE: For most substances: age 15 to 30 yr
DURATION OF CONDITION:
- Men: average >20 yr of heavy drinking
- Women: average 15 yr of heavy drinking
- In general, substance use disorders are chronic and relapsing and often progressive
GENETICS: There is evidence of nonspecific genetic factors. Addiction may result in part from underlying, inherited abnormalities in brain structure that impair behavior control and encourage impulsive behavior.

PHYSICAL FINDINGS & CLINICAL PRESENTATION

- Polysubstance use and comorbidity with psychiatric disorders are common.
- History often reveals recurring behavioral problems, such as relationship, work, or legal problems; violence and traumatic injuries; and anxiety, depression, insomnia, and cognitive and memory dysfunction.
- Repeated requests for early refills of controlled substances and obtaining prescriptions from multiple providers should raise concern for prescription drug abuse (Table 2).
- Physical findings may include injection marks (Fig. 1), nasal lesions or recurrent epistaxis, poor dentition, scars or bruises from falls or trauma, and poor nutritional status; signs/symptoms of intoxication or withdrawal are highly suggestive of substance use disorder.

ETIOLOGY

Several models of addiction have been proposed:
1. Disease model: Addiction is a mental illness, which occurs as a result of the impairment of healthy neurochemical or behavioral processes.
2. Genetic model: Genetic predisposition is often a factor in dependency and certain addictive behaviors.
3. Social model: Person–environment interactions (i.e., socialization, imitation of observable behavior, and the influence of modeling) shape addictive behavior.

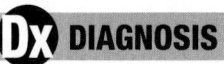

DIAGNOSIS

DIFFERENTIAL DIAGNOSIS

- Psychiatric disorders such as depression, mania, psychosis, and anxiety disorders may coexist or occur as a consequence of substance use.
- Rule out seizure disorder and underlying illness.

WORKUP

- A thorough history is crucial for diagnosis.
- The physician's history-taking style and techniques strongly affect patient's willingness to report use and participate in future treatment activities.
- A structured, nonjudgmental approach is generally preferable:
  1. Ask about quantity and frequency of alcohol or drug use. For example, the National Institute on Alcohol Abuse and Alcoholism (NIAAA) declares that *problem drinking* is defined as more than 2 drinks per day for men and more than 1 drink per day for women or anyone older than 65 yr.
  2. Use a short screening instrument such as the CAGE questionnaire ("1. Have you ever felt you need to Cut down on your alcohol or drug use? 2. Have people Annoyed you by criticizing your alcohol or drug use? 3. Have you ever felt Guilty about alcohol or drug use? 4. Have you ever felt you need to drink first thing in the morning [Eye opener] to stop shakiness?").
- Problematic behavior during intoxication or withdrawal is diagnostic.
- Because self-report of substance use and its consequences can be unreliable, obtaining corroborating information, such as from family members, past detoxifications, or drug rehabilitations, is often helpful.

TABLE 1   Key Features of Substance Abuse

1. The substance is often taken in larger amounts over a longer period than intended
2. Unsuccessful efforts to cut down
3. A great deal of time spent obtaining the substance or recovering from its effects
4. Craving
5. Social, occupational, or recreational
6. Recurrent despite hazards
7. Tolerance or withdrawal

Reprinted from Goldman L, Bennett JC (eds): *Cecil textbook of medicine,* ed 22, Philadelphia, 2004, Saunders.

TABLE 2   "Red Flags" for Abuse Behavior and Opioid Addiction

Potential Abuse/Addiction Behaviors*

1. Patient displays an overwhelming focus on opioid issues during clinic visits that occupies a significant proportion of the clinic visit and impedes progress with other pain issues or medical problems.
2. Patient has a pattern of early refills (three or more) or escalating drug use in the absence of acute change or progression of his or her medical condition.
3. Patient generates multiple telephone calls or unscheduled visits to request more opioids, early refills, or problems associated with the opioid prescription that often creates a disturbance of the clinic staff.
4. There is a pattern of prescription problems with reports of medications lost, spilled, or stolen.
5. Patient has supplemental sources of opioids from multiple providers, emergency departments, or illegal sources.

Additional "Red Flag" Abuse Behavior

1. Selling prescribed medications
2. Prescription forgery
3. Stealing another patient's medications
4. Injecting or snorting oral medication
5. Concurrent use of illicit drug(s)
6. Appears intoxicated or oversedated
7. Insists on obtaining a specific opioid medication

*Adapted from Chabal criteria for opioid abuse.
From Hochberg MC et al: *Rheumatology,* ed 5, St Louis, 2011, Mosby.

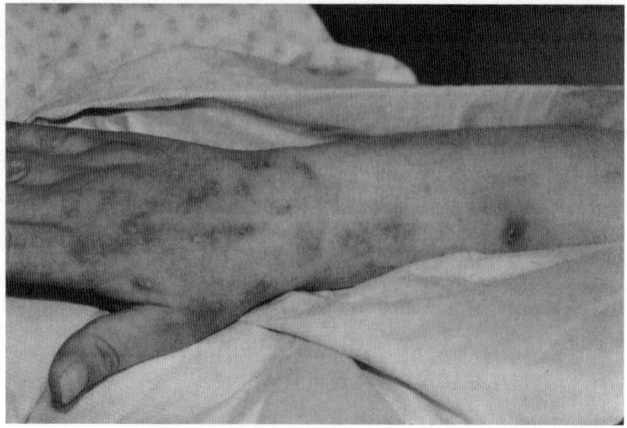

FIG. 1 Tracks secondary to intravenous heroin abuse. (Marx JA et al: *Rosen's emergency medicine*, ed 8, Philadelphia, 2014, Saunders.)

- Adolescent drug abuse detection and treatment is extremely challenging. Stages of adolescent substance use are described in Table 3. An assessment for evaluating the seriousness of adolescent drug abuse is described in Table 4.

TABLE 3 Stages of Adolescent Substance Abuse

Stage	Description
1	Potential for abuse Decreased impulse control Need for immediate gratification Available drugs, alcohol, inhalants Need for peer acceptance
2	Experimentation: learning the euphoria Use of inhalants, tobacco, marijuana, and alcohol with friends Few, if any, consequences Use may increase to weekends regularly Little change in behavior
3	Regular use: seeking the euphoria Use of other drugs, e.g., stimulants, LSD, sedatives Behavioral changes and some consequences Increased frequency of use; use alone Buying or stealing drugs
4	Regular use: preoccupation with the "high" Daily use of drugs Loss of control Multiple consequences and risk-taking Estrangement from family and "straight" friends
5	Burnout: use of drugs to feel normal Polysubstance use/cross-addiction Guilt, withdrawal, shame, remorse, depression Physical and mental deterioration Increased risk-taking, self-destructive, suicidal

From Kliegman RM et al: *Nelson textbook of pediatrics*, ed 19, Philadelphia, 2011, Saunders.

LABORATORY TESTS

- Blood alcohol content (BAC) measured on the breath is practical to define intoxication and provides a rough measure of impairment. In general, two standard drinks may cause BAC 0.08% or higher, which is considered legally impaired.
- Obtain toxicology screen in urine or blood samples.
- Biologic markers such as elevated mean corpuscular volume (MCV), γ-glutamyltransferase (GGT), liver function tests (AST and ALT), and carbohydrate deficient transferrin (CDT) may also be used to diagnose and monitor.

IMAGING STUDIES

Not helpful in routine diagnosis and management of substance abuse, but possibly useful in the management of sequelae of substance abuse (e.g., brain imaging to evaluate the alcohol abuse–associated increased risk of subdural hematomas or increased evidence of cerebral atrophy).

🆁🆇 TREATMENT

NONPHARMACOLOGIC THERAPY

- First assess readiness for change; if precontemplative or contemplative, counsel about risks of use and benefits of abstinence; a motivational interviewing approach has been shown to be effective.
- Nonpharmacologic strategies have the greatest documented efficacy: advice, feedback, goal setting, problem solving, and additional contacts for further assistance.
- Opiate contracts, prohibiting a patient from getting early refills or obtaining opiates from multiple prescribers, should be considered for all patients with chronic pain receiving opioid painkillers, especially for patients with a history of substance abuse or medication abuse.
- Relapse prevention facilitated by avoidance of trigger stimuli or by uncoupling trigger stimuli from substance ingestion.
- Self-help and support groups such as Alcoholics Anonymous and Narcotics Anonymous are helpful in achieving and maintaining sobriety.
- Residential or inpatient treatment programs should be a consideration for any individual with continued or escalating use despite outpatient treatment.

ACUTE GENERAL Rx

- Detoxification is an important first step. Its goals are to facilitate withdrawal and reduce

TABLE 4 Assessing the Seriousness of Adolescent Drug Abuse

Variable	0	+1	+2
Age (yr)	>15	<15	
Sex	Male	Female	
Family history of drug abuse		Yes	
Setting of drug use	In group		Alone
Affect before drug use	Happy	Always poor	Sad
School performance	Good, improving		Recently poor
Use before driving	None		Yes
History of accidents	None		Yes
Time of week	Weekend	Weekdays	
Time of day		After school	Before or during school
Type of drug	Marijuana, beer, wine	Hallucinogens, amphetamines	Whiskey, opiates, cocaine, barbiturates

Total score: 0-3, less worrisome; 3-8, serious; 8-18, very serious.
From Kliegman RM et al: *Nelson textbook of pediatrics*, ed 19, Philadelphia, 2011, Saunders.

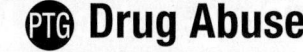
symptoms, initiate abstinence, and refer the patient to ongoing treatment.

- Benzodiazepines are effective in acute alcohol withdrawal for the management of symptoms as well as the prevention of seizures. One strategy is to give the patient a loading dose of a long-acting benzodiazepine (e.g., 20 mg of diazepam) and then continue the benzodiazepine as scheduled while tapering down the dose gradually. An alternative "symptom-driven" strategy is to follow the patient closely with serial assessments, such as the Clinical Institute Withdrawal Assessment for Alcohol (CIWA) scale, and to dose with 1 to 2 mg of lorazepam as needed to treat withdrawal symptoms.
- The prophylactic administration of thiamine and folic acid (first intravenously or intramuscularly followed by supplemental oral doses) in alcohol withdrawal is recommended before starting any carbohydrate-containing fluids or food to prevent Wernicke-Korsakoff syndrome (alcoholic encephalopathy and psychosis). Magnesium appears to be effective in the treatment of alcohol withdrawal–related cardiac arrhythmias, but not other symptoms of alcohol withdrawal.
- Beta-blockers and clonidine generally should be avoided in alcohol withdrawal; they may mask markers of the severity of the withdrawal (blood pressure and pulse rate).
- Unlike withdrawal from alcohol or benzodiazepines, opioid withdrawal is not life threatening.
- Clonidine alleviates the discomfort of opiate withdrawal. Clonidine tablets, 0.1 mg q4-6h as needed, can be used while monitoring patient's blood pressure. Clonidine transdermal patch, 0.1 mg/24 hr, can be used to treat autonomic hyperactivity symptoms; however, it has a very slow onset and may take 2-3 days to achieve therapeutic levels. Antidiarrheals, ibuprofen, and dicyclomine can be used as adjuncts to treat opiate withdrawal symptoms.
- Methadone taper is an effective approach for detoxification in opioid dependence.
- Buprenorphine is a partial μ-opioid receptor agonist that may be used for detoxification and maintenance in treatment of opioid dependence (see dosing in next section).

LONG-TERM Rx

- Naltrexone helps reduce craving for alcohol. Naltrexone 50 mg once daily for 12 wk can be a useful adjunct to substance abuse counseling or rehabilitation programs. Randomized treatment studies are equivocal for long-term outcomes. Naltrexone reduces relapse and the intensity or frequency of any drinking that does occur. It can be hepatotoxic and is contraindicated in opiate users. Intramuscular naltrexone (380 mg monthly) may be considered if adherence is an issue.
- Acamprosate also helps reduce craving for alcohol. Acamprosate 666 mg three times daily may be an effective adjunct to counseling. A recent meta-analysis showed overall benefit with increase in the number of abstinent days.
- Disulfiram provokes acetaldehyde accumulation after alcohol ingestion, producing a toxic state manifested by nausea, headache, flushing, and respiratory distress. Studies have shown limited efficacy mostly due to noncompliance.
- Topiramate may be an alternative treatment for alcoholism. In a 12-wk randomized trial topiramate up to 300 mg daily significantly reduced the number of heavy drinking days.
- Methadone maintenance for opiate addiction is effective and involves once-daily dosing of methadone in a controlled setting via methadone clinics.
- Buprenorphine is as effective as low-dose methadone and may be prescribed by physicians who have completed approved training. For induction, initiate 12 to 24 hr after short-acting opioid use and 24 to 48 hr after long-acting opioid use. Use buprenorphine/naloxone tablets in most patients, since buprenorphine-only tablets have risk of abuse. Maximum first-day dosage is 4 to 8 mg of buprenorphine. Titrate buprenorphine dose up to 12 mg on day 2 for signs of withdrawal. Then adjust dosage in frequent outpatient visits (weekly) to minimum needed for maintenance (up to 32 mg daily).
- Naltrexone (oral or injectable) may also be used for maintenance in opioid dependence treatment, though evidence of effectiveness is limited.
- Always combine pharmacotherapy with counseling.
- Treatment of comorbid psychiatric disorders improves outcomes.

- Intervention may be used to break through **denial** of a person with a serious addictive disorder to help the person acknowledge that he or she suffers from a disorder and agree to treatment.

DISPOSITION

- Substance abuse is a chronic relapsing illness, so relapses are best approached as part of the course of the illness, as opposed to as treatment failure.
- The goal of treatment is always abstinence, but success of treatment is measured by return of function, increasing duration between relapses, and prevention of sequelae of use.

REFERRAL

Physicians should refer patients who do not make progress on changing substance use patterns to addiction specialists and/or specialized substance abuse programs. Patients with comorbid psychiatric illness should be referred for mental health care.

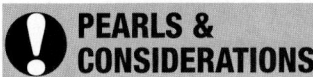

PEARLS & CONSIDERATIONS

- Acute withdrawal from alcohol can become life threatening.
- Withdrawal from opioids can resemble a severe case of the flu.
- A brief intervention (providing information and advising the patient to reduce consumption of alcohol) by the primary care doctor has been demonstrated in randomized trials to reduce drinking in at-risk patients.
- Treatment rates for alcohol use disorders remain low despite available effective treatments.

SUGGESTED READINGS
Available at www.expertconsult.com

RELATED CONTENT
Drug Abuse (Patient Information)
Alcohol Abuse (Related Key Topic)
Opioid Dependence (Related Key Topic)

AUTHOR: **TAHIR TELLIOGLU, M.D.**

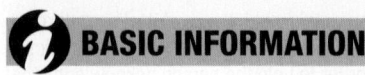

DEFINITION

Drug-induced liver injury (DILI) is defined as any injury to the liver by any medication such as a prescription medication, an over-the-counter medication, or an herbal/dietary supplement. It can present as asymptomatic liver test elevations or as acute liver failure.

SYNONYMS

Toxic liver disease
DILI

ICD-10CM CODES
K71.0	Toxic liver disease with cholestasis
K71.1	Toxic liver disease with hepatic necrosis
K71.10	Toxic liver disease with hepatic necrosis without coma
K71.11	Toxic liver disease with hepatic necrosis with coma
K71.2	Toxic liver disease with acute hepatitis
K71.3	Toxic liver disease with chronic persistent hepatitis
K71.4	Toxic liver disease with chronic lobular hepatitis
K71.5	Toxic liver disease with chronic active hepatitis
K71.50	Toxic liver disease with chronic active hepatitis without ascites
K71.51	Toxic liver disease with chronic active hepatitis with ascites
K71.6	Toxic liver disease with hepatitis, not elsewhere classified
K71.7	Toxic liver disease with hepatitis with fibrosis and cirrhosis of the liver
K71.8	Toxic liver disease with hepatitis, not elsewhere classified
K71.8	Toxic liver disease, unspecified

EPIDEMIOLOGY & DEMOGRAPHICS

INCIDENCE: Estimated annual incidence between 10 and 15 per 10,000 to 100,000 has been reported.

PEAK INCIDENCE: N/A
PREVALENCE: N/A
PREDOMINANT SEX AND AGE: Incidence increases with age and is more common in females.
GENETICS: Genetic polymorphisms can lead to altered expressions of various liver cytochrome p450 enzymes. Table 1 summarizes factors influencing the risk of liver diseases caused by drugs.
RISK FACTORS:
- Predisposing factors: female gender, race, and older age
- Acquired risk factors: chronic alcohol use, extrahepatic disease (i.e., hyperthyroidism, HIV, etc.)
- A patient's nutritional status can influence their ability to metabolize medications.

PHYSICAL FINDINGS & CLINICAL PRESENTATION

- The physical findings and presentation depend on the classification of hepatic injury incited by the drug.
- These are usually divided into hepatocellular, cholestatic, or a mixed picture of hepatocellular and cholestatic injury. Table 2 describes a clinicopathologic classification of drug-induced liver disease
- Some patients are asymptomatic, and DILI is detected only because of abnormal labs.
- Symptomatic patients present with fever, nausea, vomiting, malaise, anorexia, right upper quadrant pain, jaundice, acholic stools, or dark urine.
- Patients may also present with pruritus and hepatomegaly on physical examination.
- Patients may have muscular symptoms such as myalgia, stiffness, weakness, and elevated creatinine kinase level.

ETIOLOGY

- Drug-induced liver injury can result due to toxicity of over-the-counter drugs, prescription medications, anesthetics (Table E3), or herbal remedies/supplements (Table E4).

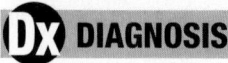

DIFFERENTIAL DIAGNOSIS

- Hepatitis (Tables E5 and E6): viral hepatitis, alcoholic liver disease, nonalcoholic fatty liver disease, autoimmune hepatitis, and Wilson's disease
- Cholestasis: biliary obstruction, primary biliary cirrhosis, primary sclerosing cholangitis, and intrahepatic cholestasis of pregnancy
- Steatosis: nonalcoholic fatty liver disease, nonalcoholic steatohepatitis, and acute fatty liver of pregnancy.
- Granulomatous hepatitis (Table E7): sarcoidosis, infection, and primary biliary cirrhosis.
- Peliosis hepatitis: infections, hematologic disorders, and organ transplantation

WORKUP

- A thorough history and blood tests to evaluate other possible causes of hepatic injury helps make the diagnosis.
- Liver function tests
- Hepatitis A, B, and C serologies, antinuclear antibody, anti-smooth muscle antibody, anti-liver kidney microsomal antibody, alpha 1 antitrypsin, ceruloplasmin, fasting glucose, triglycerides, and hemoglobin A1c

LABORATORY TESTS

- Hepatocellular findings:
  - Abnormal elevations in serum aminotransferases when compared to alkaline phosphatase (ALP)
  - Alanine aminotransferase (ALT)/ALP ratio greater than 5
- Cholestatic findings:
  - Abnormal elevations in the alkaline phosphatase compared to the serum aminotransferases
  - ALP >2 times the upper limit of normal and/or ALT to ALP ratio <2

TABLE 1 Factors Influencing the Risk of Liver Diseases Caused by Drugs

Factor	Examples of Drugs Affected	Influence
Genetic factors	Halothane, phenytoin, sulfonamides	Multiple cases in families
	Amoxicillin-clavulanic acid, flucloxacillin, abacavir	Strong HLA association
	Valproic acid	Familial cases; association with mitochondrial enzyme deficiencies
Age	Isoniazid, nitrofurantoin, halothane, troglitazone	Age >60 years: increased frequency, increased severity
	Valproic acid, salicylates	More common in children
Gender	Halothane, minocycline, nitrofurantoin	More common in women, especially in cases with chronic hepatitis
	Amoxicillin-clavulanic acid, azathioprine	More common in men
Dose	Acetaminophen, aspirin, some herbal medicines	Blood levels are directly related to the risk of hepatotoxicity
	Tetracycline, tacrine, oxypenicillins	Idiosyncratic reactions, with partial relationship to dose
	Methotrexate, vitamin A	Total dose, dosing frequency, and duration of exposure are related to the risk of hepatic fibrosis
Other drugs	Acetaminophen	Isoniazid, zidovudine, and phenytoin lower the dose threshold and increase the severity of hepatotoxicity
	Valproic acid	Other antiepileptic drugs increase the risk of hepatotoxicity
	Anticancer drugs	Interactive vascular toxicity

Continued

TABLE 1 Factors Influencing the Risk of Liver Diseases Caused by Drugs—cont'd

Factor	Examples of Drugs Affected	Influence
History of other drug reactions	Isoflurane, halothane, enflurane Erythromycins Diclofenac, ibuprofen, tiaprofenic acid Sulfonamides, COX-2 inhibitors	Instances of cross-sensitivity have been reported among members of each drug class but are rare
Excessive alcohol use	Acetaminophen	Lowered dose threshold, poorer outcome
	Isoniazid, methotrexate	Increased risk of liver injury, hepatic fibrosis
Nutritional status:		
Obesity	Halothane, troglitazone, tamoxifen, methotrexate	Increased risk of liver injury, hepatic fibrosis
Fasting	Acetaminophen	Increased risk of hepatotoxicity
Preexisting liver disease	Hycanthone, pemoline	Increased risk of liver injury
	Antituberculosis drugs, ibuprofen	Increased risk of liver injury with chronic hepatitis B and C
Other diseases/conditions:		
Diabetes mellitus	Methotrexate	Increased risk of hepatic fibrosis
HIV/AIDS	Sulfonamides	Increased risk of hypersensitivity
Renal failure	Tetracycline, methotrexate	Increased risk of liver injury, hepatic fibrosis
Organ transplantation	Azathioprine, thioguanine, busulfan	Increased risk of vascular toxicity

From Feldman M et al (eds): *Sleisenger and Fordtran's gastrointestinal and liver disease*, ed 10, Philadelphia, 2016, Elsevier.

Diseases and Disorders

I

TABLE 2 Clinicopathologic Classification of Drug-Induced Liver Disease

Category	Description	Implicated Drugs: Examples
Hepatic adaptation	No symptoms; raised serum GGTP and AP levels (occasionally raised ALT)	Phenytoin, warfarin, heparins
	Hyperbilirubinemia	Rifampin, HIV protease inhibitors
Dose-dependent hepatotoxicity	Symptoms of hepatitis; zonal, bridging, and massive necrosis; serum ALT level >5-fold increased, often >2000 U/L	Acetaminophen, nicotinic acid, amodiaquine, hycanthone
Other cytopathic toxicity, acute steatosis	Microvesicular steatosis, diffuse or zonal; partially dose dependent, severe liver injury, features of mitochondrial toxicity (lactic acidosis)	Valproic acid, didanosine, HAART agents, fialuridine, L-asparaginase, some herbal medicines
Acute hepatitis	Symptoms of hepatitis; focal, bridging, and massive necrosis; serum ALT level >5-fold increased; extrahepatic features of drug allergy in some cases	Isoniazid, dantrolene, nitrofurantoin, halothane, sulfonamides, phenytoin, disulfiram, acebutolol, etretinate, ketoconazole, terbinafine, troglitazone
Chronic hepatitis	Duration >3 months; interface hepatitis, bridging necrosis, fibrosis, cirrhosis; clinical and laboratory features of chronic liver disease; autoantibodies with some types of reaction	Nitrofurantoin, etretinate, diclofenac, minocycline, nefazodone
Granulomatous hepatitis	Hepatic granulomas with varying hepatitis and cholestasis; raised serum ALT, AP, GGTP levels	Allopurinol, carbamazepine, hydralazine, quinidine, quinine
Cholestasis without hepatitis	Cholestasis, no inflammation; serum AP levels > twice normal	Oral contraceptives, androgens
Cholestatic hepatitis	Cholestasis with inflammation; symptoms of hepatitis; raised serum ALT and AP levels	Chlorpromazine, tricyclic antidepressants, erythromycins, amoxicillin–clavulanic acid, cyproterone acetate
Cholestasis with bile duct injury	Bile duct lesions and cholestatic hepatitis; clinical features of cholangitis	Chlorpromazine, flucloxacillin, dextropropoxyphene
Chronic cholestasis	Duration >3 months	
Vanishing bile duct syndrome (VBDS)	Paucity of small bile ducts; resembles PBC but AMA negative	Chlorpromazine, flucloxacillin, trimethoprim/sulfamethoxazole
Sclerosing cholangitis	Strictures of large bile ducts	Intraarterial floxuridine, intralesional scolicidals
Steatohepatitis	Steatosis, focal necrosis, Mallory's hyaline, pericellular fibrosis, cirrhosis; chronic liver disease, portal hypertension	Perhexiline, amiodarone, tamoxifen
Fibrosis and cirrhosis	Fibrosis, nodular regeneration (Other features [e.g., interface hepatitis, steatohepatitis, paucity of bile ducts, cholestasis] depend on etiology.)	Methotrexate, cyproterone acetate; also see VBDS, chronic hepatitis, steatohepatitis
Vascular disorders	Sinusoidal obstruction syndrome, nodular regenerative hyperplasia, others	Many
Tumors	Hepatocellular carcinoma, adenoma, angiosarcoma, others	Many

AMA, antimitochondrial antibodies; *AP*, alkaline phosphatase.
From Feldman M et al (eds): *Sleisenger and Fordtran's gastrointestinal and liver disease*, ed 10, Philadelphia, 2016, Elsevier.

- Mixed hepatocellular/cholestatic findings:
  ○ ALT/ALP ratio >2 but <5
- In either of these types of DILI, the serum bilirubin may or may not be elevated.

IMAGING STUDIES

- Imaging studies such as right upper quadrant ultrasound or MRCP to rule out biliary obstruction may be needed if there is evidence of cholestasis
- Typically there is no need to do a liver biopsy unless the diagnosis is uncertain.

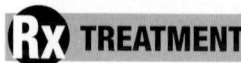 **TREATMENT**

NONPHARMACOLOGIC THERAPY

- Avoiding certain drugs and herbal supplements with underlying liver disease is very important.

ACUTE GENERAL Rx

- The mainstay of treatment is to avoid the offending agent.
- N-acetylcysteine is used for acetaminophen toxicity.
- L-carnitine is used for valproic acid toxicity.
- Glucocorticoids do not have proven benefit but are sometimes given for hypersensitivity reactions of the liver in which there is progressive cholestasis or in which biopsy reveals features similar to that of autoimmune hepatitis.
- For patients who present with pruritus in the setting of cholestatic liver disease, a bile acid sequestrant can be given.

CHRONIC Rx

- There is insufficient evidence to support the use of any medication, vitamin, or nutritional supplement for long-term treatment of DILI.

COMPLEMENTARY & ALTERNATIVE MEDICINE

- There are some studies on complementary and alternative medicine to help with prevention of drug-induced liver disease with certain medications. For instance, Haoqin Qingdan decoction has been used to prevent cyclophosphamide-induced hepatotoxicity.
- Alternative medicine such as herbal supplements can have adverse effects on the liver if they have not been well-tested for use in the general population. Table E4 summarizes hepatotoxic herbal remedies, dietary supplements, and weight loss products

DISPOSITION

- Hy's rule, which is known as a combination of high aminotransferases and jaundice, has been associated with mortality rate of 10% to 50% for various drugs.
- The mortality rate in hepatocellular injury depends on the drug involved.

REFERRAL

- Referral to a hepatologist may be needed if the patient develops signs of acute liver failure or chronic liver disease.

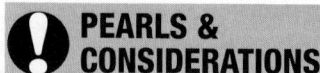 **PEARLS & CONSIDERATIONS**

COMMENTS

- Liver injury can occur due to many different drugs. The NIH has a searchable database of drugs that cause drug-induced liver injury.
- Taking a thorough history and ruling out other causes of liver injury is important.
- Withdrawal of the offending agent is the first and best form of management of the patient.
- Liver enzyme tests need to be carefully monitored with DILI.

PREVENTION

Educating patients about potential hepatotoxic medications and possible drug-to-drug interactions can prevent DILI.

PATIENT/FAMILY EDUCATION

http://livertox.nih.gov/

SUGGESTED READINGS

Available at www.expertconsult.com

RELATED CONTENT

Acute Liver Failure (Related Key Topic)
Acetaminophen Poisoning (Related Key Topic)

AUTHORS: **VICKY H. BHAGAT, M.D., M.P.H.**, and **MARIAM FAYEK, M.D.**

BASIC INFORMATION

DEFINITION

Damage to lung parenchyma caused by toxic effects of drugs. It is a diagnosis of exclusion.

SYNONYMS

Drug-induced interstitial lung disease
Drug-induced lung toxicity
DILD

ICD 10CM CODES
J70.2 Acute drug induced interstitial lung disorders

EPIDEMIOLOGY & DEMOGRAPHICS

INCIDENCE: Global incidence is not known but likely accounts for 2.5% to 3% of interstitial lung disease (ILD) cases. In the U.S., there are more than 2 million cases of adverse drug reactions annually, including 100,000 deaths. In the U.S., up to 10% of patients who receive chemotherapeutic agents develop lung toxicity.
PEAK INCIDENCE: Unknown
PREVALENCE: Not reported
PREDOMINANT SEX AND AGE: Extreme ends of ages are prone to develop severe drug-induced side effects. Some studies have shown severe side effects in individuals >40 years of age. Gender is not an independent risk factor.
GENETICS: Limited studies have shown that there may be a racial difference in the incidence of DILD.
RISK FACTORS: Age, sex, ethnicity, drug dose, oxygen, drug interaction, radiation, presence of underlying lung disease.

PHYSICAL FINDINGS & CLINICAL PRESENTATION

- Presentation is similar to other parenchymal lung diseases including shortness of breath, cough, fever, general malaise, and fatigue.
- No pathognomonic clinical, laboratory, physical, radiographic, or histologic findings. DILD is considered a diagnosis of exclusion.
- Significant exam findings include crackles. In advanced stages one can find clubbing.

ETIOLOGY

- Mechanism is not fully understood. Both cytotoxic and immune mechanisms of action may be involved independently or in combination.
- Two possible routes of exposure have been identified: inhalation vs. vasculature system.
- Initial exposure leading to acute toxicity may progress to chronic inflammation and fibrotic changes, which interfere with gas exchange.
- Amiodarone is a well-known cause of DILD and is usually associated with DILD at higher doses of administration (≥400 mg daily) in 5% to 15% of patients. The mechanism of lung damage is unknown. Chronic interstitial pneumonitis is the most common manifestation of amiodarone pulmonary toxicity, but there are reports of confluent lesions occurring as a result of amiodarone pneumonitis. Many of these lesions are bronchiolitis obliterans. CT scan of the lung (Fig. E1) can further define these lesions.

- Lung toxicity can occur after months to weeks of both low- and high-dose methotrexate administration. Hypersensitivity pneumonitis is its most common manifestation of lung toxicity. The mechanism by which it occurs is unknown.

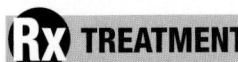 DIAGNOSIS

DIFFERENTIAL DIAGNOSIS

- Acute respiratory distress syndrome
- Alveolar proteinosis
- Congestive heart failure
- Diffuse lung diseases
- Hypersensitivity pneumonitis
- Lung malignancy
- Pulmonary infections
- Pulmonary vasculitis syndromes
- Radiation pneumonitis
- Respiratory failure secondary to hypoxia
- Occupational lung diseases:
  - Asbestosis
  - Berylliosis
  - Chemical worker's lung
  - Coal worker's pneumoconiosis
  - Farmer's lung
  - Silicosis
  - Nitrous dioxide toxicity (i.e., silo filler's disease)
  - Tobacco worker's lung

WORK-UP

- DILD is suspected after exclusion of other etiologies in patients with recent exposure to offending drug.
- Tables 1 and 2 list medications associated with pulmonary toxicities.
- Fig. 2 illustrates various radiographic presentations of DILD.

LABORATORY TESTS

- CBC may show increased eosinophils.
- Antinuclear antibody (ANA) and antihistone antibody labs. Complement levels are usually normal.
- Arterial blood gas (ABG) may show hypoxemia.

IMAGING STUDIES

- Chest x-ray (Fig. E3).
- CT scan (Fig. E4).
- Other studies include PTFs, flexible bronchoscopy with bronchoalveolar lavage (BAL), open lung biopsy.

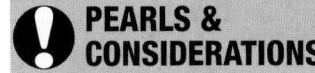 TREATMENT

There is no specific recognized treatment of DILD other than removal of offending agent.

NONPHARMACOLOGIC THERAPY

- Removal of offending agent. Supportive measures including smoking cessation, control of underlying lung disease, and prompt treatment of concomitant respiratory infection.

ACUTE GENERAL Rx

- Glucocorticoids have been used with rapid improvement in gas exchange and reversal in radiographic abnormalities.

CHRONIC Rx

- None

COMPLEMENTARY & ALTERNATIVE MEDICINE

- Lung transplantation in cases of severe irreversible fibrosis

DISPOSITION

- Most patients can be treated in the community setting. Transfer to a tertiary center is indicated when diagnosis is doubted.

REFERRAL

- For workup and diagnosis, early involvement of pulmonary specialist is advised.

! PEARLS & CONSIDERATIONS

COMMENTS

- DILD can manifest as noncardiogenic pulmonary edema (NCPE)/capillary leak syndrome, hypersensitivity reaction, cryptogenic pulmonary edema, or interstitial pneumonitis. Almost all histopathological subtypes of ILD may be observed.
- PFT findings are usually consistent with restrictive lung disease, demonstrating reduced TLC as well as reduced DLCO.
- BAL findings are nonspecific but may be helpful in the right context. Low $CD4^+$ to $CD8^+$ ratio suggests DILD. Elevated eosinophils (>40%) can be seen in patients with DILD.

PREVENTION

- When prescribing drugs known to cause DILD, close observation is in order.
- Avoidance of unnecessary drug administration.

SUGGESTED READING
Available at www.expertconsult.com

RELATED CONTENT

Acute Respiratory Distress Syndrome (ARDS) (Related Key Content)
Interstitial Lung Disease (Related Key Content)

AUTHORS: **FREDERIC CELESTIN, M.D.,** **FAHAD FAROOQ, M.D.,** and **SAMAAN RAFEQ, M.D.**

TABLE 1 Drugs Associated with the Development of Interstitial Lung Disease

Antimicrobial Agents
- Amphotericin B
- Isoniazid
- Nitrofurantoin
- Sulfasalazine

Anti-Inflammatory Agents
- Aspirin
- Etanercept
- Gold
- Infliximab
- Methotrexate
- Nonsteroidal Anti-Inflammatory Drugs
- Penicillamine

Biological Agents
- Adalimumab
- Alemtuzumab
- Bevacizumab
- Cetuximab
- Rituximab
- Trastuzumab
- Tumor necrosis factor (TNF)-a blockers

Cardiovascular Agents
- ACE inhibitors
- Amiodarone
- Anticoagulants

- ß-Blockers
- Flecainide
- Hydrochlorothiazide
- Procainamide
- Statins
- Tocainide

Chemotherapeutic Agents
- Azathioprine
- BCNU

Chemotherapeutic Agents
- Bleomycin
- Bortezomib
- Busulfan
- Carmustine
- Chlorambucil
- Colony-stimulating factors
- Cyclophosphamide
- Cytarabine
- Deferoxamine
- Docetaxel
- Doxorubicin
- Erlotinib
- Etoposide
- Fludarabine
- Flutamide

- Gefitinib
- Gemcitabine
- Hydroxyurea
- Imatinib
- Interferons
- Lomustine
- Melphalan
- Methotrexate
- Methyl-CCNU
- Mitomycin-C
- Nitrosoureas
- Paclitaxel
- Procarbazine
- Thalidomide
- Vinblastine
- Zinostatin

Miscellaneous
- Bromocriptine
- Carbamazepine
- Cabergoline
- Methysergide
- Penicillamine
- Phenytoin
- Sirolimus
- Talc

From Schwaiblmair M, et al.: Drug induced interstitial lung disease, *Open Respir Med J* 6:63-74, 2012.

TABLE 2 Pharmacologic Action of Selected Chemotherapeutic Agents with Associated Pulmonary Toxicities.

Antibiotic-Derived Agents
- Bleomycin
- Mitomycin C

Alkylating Agents
- Busulfan
- Cyclophosphamide
- Chlorambucil
- Melphalan

Antimetabolites
- Methotrexate
- 6-Mercaptopurine
- Azathioprine
- Cytosine arabinoside
- Gemcitabine
- Fludarabine

Nitrosoureas
- Bischloroethyl nitrosourea (BCNU)
- Chloroethyl cyclohexyl nitrosourea (CCNU)
- Methyl-CCNU

Podophyllotoxins
- Etoposide
- Paclitaxel
- Docetaxel

Novel Antitumor Agents
- All-*trans* retinoic acid (ATRA)
- Gefitinib
- Imatinib mesylate
- Irinotecan

Immune Modulatory Agents Used in Malignancy
- Interferons
- Interleukin-2
- Tumor necrosis factorα

Other Miscellaneous Chemotherapy Agents
- Procarbazine
- Zinostatin
- Vinblastine

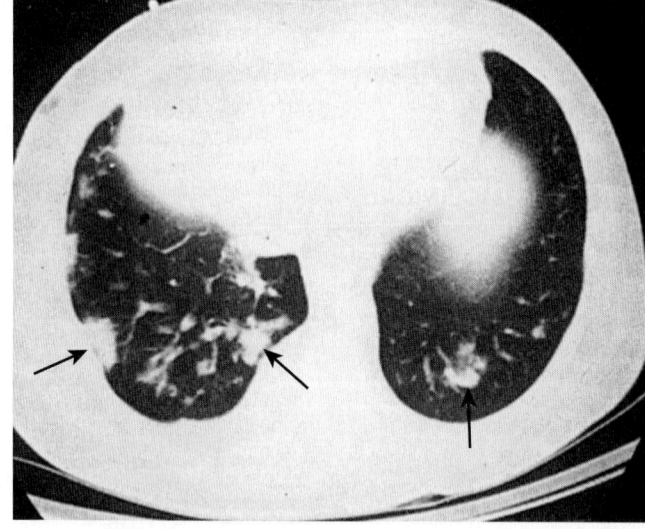

FIG. 2 Radiologic examples of DILD. A, Cryptogenic organizing pneumonia. **B,** Nonspecific interstitial pneumonia. **C,** Usual interstitial pneumonia. (From Schwaiblmair MM et al: Drug induced interstitial lung disease, *Open Respir Med J*, 6:63-74, 2012.)

Mason RJ, Broaddus CV et al: *Murray & Nadel's textbook of respiratory medicine*, ed 5, Philadelphia, 2010, Saunders.

BASIC INFORMATION

DEFINITION

Dysfunctional uterine bleeding (DUB) describes abnormal uterine bleeding in the absence of identified causative disease in the pelvis, pregnancy, or medical illness. Parameters of normal menstrual function are described in Box 1. Specific types of abnormal bleeding include the following:

- Menorrhagia: regular normal intervals, excessive flow and duration
- Metrorrhagia: irregular intervals
- Menometrorrhagia: irregular and excessive bleeding during menstruation and between periods
- Oligomenorrhea: intervals greater than 35 days
- Polymenorrhea: intervals less than 21 days
These terms, while commonly used in practice, increasingly are felt to be confusing. The term *dysfunctional uterine bleeding* was initially used in 1935 but has never been clearly defined and has been used as both a diagnosis and a symptom. It is generally understood to be a term of exclusion when no other cause of bleeding has been established. In 2011, the FIGO Working Group on Menstrual Disorders released a classification system intended to simplify these definitions. FIGO recommends that the three classifications typically comprising DUB—endometrial dysfunction, ovulatory dysfunction, and coagulopathy—be grouped under the nonstructural causes of abnormal uterine bleeding. However, these new FIGO terms have not yet made their way into common usage.

SYNONYMS

DUB

ICD-10CM CODES	
N92.5	Other specified irregular menstruation
N92.0	Excessive and frequent menstruation with regular cycle
N91.5	Oligomenorrhea, unspecified
N92.1	Excessive and frequent menstruation with irregular cycle
N94.6	Dysmenorrhea, unspecified

EPIDEMIOLOGY & DEMOGRAPHICS

- Most cases of DUB occur in postmenarchal and perimenopausal age groups.
- During reproductive age, <20% of abnormal bleeding results from anovulatory DUB.

PHYSICAL FINDINGS & CLINICAL PRESENTATION

- A clinical diagnosis of exclusion
- Thorough physical and pelvic examination to exclude the other causes of abnormal bleeding
  1. Includes thyroid, breast, liver, presence or absence of ecchymotic lesions
  2. Patient possibly obese and hirsute (polycystic ovarian disease)

3. No evidence of any vulvar, vaginal, cervical lesions, uterine (fibroid) or ovarian tumor, urethral caruncle, urethral diverticula, hemorrhoids, anal fissure, colorectal lesions
4. Bimanual pelvic examination: normal-sized or slightly enlarged uterus, regular or irregular contour

ETIOLOGY

- 90% is caused by anovulation.
- 10% is ovulatory in origin; can be caused by dysfunction of corpus luteum or midcycle (estrogen withdrawal) bleeding.
- Section II describes the various causes of abnormal uterine bleeding.

DIAGNOSIS

DIFFERENTIAL DIAGNOSIS

- Pregnancy-related cause
- Anatomic uterine causes:
  1. Leiomyomas
  2. Adenomyosis
  3. Polyps—endometrial or cervical
  4. Endometrial hyperplasia
  5. Cancer—uterine, cervical, vulvar, vaginal
  6. Sexually transmitted diseases
  7. Intrauterine contraceptive devices
- Anatomic nonuterine causes:
  1. Cervical neoplasia, cervicitis
  2. Vaginal neoplasia, adhesions, trauma, foreign body, atrophic vaginitis, infections, condyloma
  3. Vulvar trauma, infections, neoplasia, condyloma, dystrophy, varices
  4. Urinary tract: urethral caruncle, diverticulum, hematuria
  5. Gastrointestinal tract: hemorrhoids, anal fissure, colorectal lesions
- Systemic diseases/effects:
  1. Exogenous hormone intake
  2. Medications
  3. Coagulopathies: von Willebrand's disease, thrombocytopenia, hepatic failure
  4. Endocrinopathies: thyroid disorder, hypothyroidism and hyperthyroidism, diabetes mellitus
  5. Renal diseases
- Section II describes a differential diagnosis of vaginal bleeding abnormalities.

WORKUP

- A detailed history and thorough physical examination, including a pelvic examination to exclude causes mentioned above.
- Clinical algorithms for the evaluation of vaginal bleeding are described in Section III, "Bleeding, Vaginal."

BOX 1   Parameters of Normal Menstrual Function

Cycle interval (days)	21-35
Duration of flow (days)	2-8
Blood loss/cycle (ml)	30-80

From Carlson KJ et al: *Primary care of women,* ed 2, St Louis, 2002, Mosby.

LABORATORY TESTS

- Complete blood count with platelets to evaluate for possible iron-deficiency anemia or thrombocytopenia
- Prothrombin/INR; partial thromboplastin and bleeding time (or PFA-100 assay) if coagulopathy is suspected
- von Willebrand's panel, particularly in women with heavy bleeding since menarche
- Serum or urine human chorionic gonadotropin
- Chemistry profile, including liver function tests
- Thyroid profile
- Pap smear
- Cultures for gonorrhea and *Chlamydia*
- Serum gonadotropins and prolactin
- Serum androgens
- Endometrial biopsy or dilation and curettage in women, especially if there exists a long-standing history of anovulatory bleeding with fewer than three menstrual cycles per year or a high risk of endometrial neoplasia in women with prolonged unopposed estrogen exposure
- Stool testing for occult blood if source of bleeding is unclear
- Urinalysis for hematuria if source of bleeding is unclear

IMAGING STUDIES

- Pelvic ultrasound, including measurement of endometrial thickness and assessment of myometrial or endometrial defects
- Fluid contrast ultrasound (also called saline sonogram, sonohysterogram, saline infusion sonogram, etc.). Distends the uterine cavity so that "filling defects" of the endometrium can be assessed for possible endometrial polyp, uterine fibroid, or neoplasm.
- Hysteroscopy

TREATMENT

NONPHARMACOLOGIC THERAPY

Increase iron intake in the form of pills and a diet rich in iron to combat anemia.

ACUTE GENERAL Rx

- Progestational agents (see Box 2)
  1. Progesterone in oil, 100 to 200 mg
  2. Medroxyprogesterone acetate, 20 to 40 mg qd for 15 days
  3. Megestrol acetate, 40 to 120 mg daily in divided doses for 15 days
  4. Oral contraceptives: any oral contraceptive pill, 1 tablet tid for 5 to 7 days, followed by 1 tablet low-dose estrogen qd for 21 days; causes withdrawal bleeding; should then be on cyclical medroxyprogesterone or continue on oral contraceptives
- Estrogens
  1. Conjugated estrogen 25 mg IV q4h until bleeding is under control (in cases of severe or life-threatening bleeding); maximum 24 hr
  2. For prolonged bleeding that is not life threatening: Premarin 1.25 mg (Estrace 2 mg) q4h for 24 hr, followed by Provera

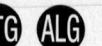

BOX 2 Equivalent Daily Doses of Oral Progestins for the Treatment of Dysfunctional Uterine Bleeding

Medroxyprogesterone acetate (Provera, Cycrin)	10 mg
Micronized progesterone (Prometrium)	400 mg
Norgestrel (Ovrette)	150 µg
Norethindrone acetate (Micronor, Nor-QD)	0.7 to 1.0 mg

From Carlson KJ et al: *Primary care of women*, ed 2, St Louis, 2002, Mosby.

to bring on withdrawal bleeding; then sequential regimen of estrogen and progestin (Premarin 1.25 mg qd for 24 days, Provera 10 mg for last 10 days) or oral contraceptives

CHRONIC Rx

- Progestational agents
  1. Medroxyprogesterone acetate 10 mg qd for 12 days, then cyclically to induce monthly withdrawal bleeding
  2. Norethindrone 2.5 to 10 mg qd for 12 days
  3. Depo-Provera 150 mg IM every 3 mo
  4. Oral contraceptives, 1 tablet qd either cyclically or continuously using only active pills

5. Levonorgestrel-releasing intrauterine device (Mirena, currently has an FDA indication for heavy menstrual bleeding)
- Letrozole or clomiphene citrate: patients with anovulatory bleeding who want to become pregnant. Progesterone withdrawal may be counterproductive in patients wishing to start an ovulation induction regimen. Pregnancy rates are lower when patients undergo withdrawal compared to when random ovulation induction start is used. Letrozole is superior to clomiphene citrate in ovulation induction in women with PCOS. Human menopausal gonadotropin (HMG) can be used for women who do not ovulate with oral agents or who have hypothalamic dysfunction.
- Others.
  1. Antiprostaglandins
  2. Danazol (rarely used due to side-effect profile).
  3. Gonadotropin-releasing hormone analogues (GnRH); often used to reduce bleeding and ameliorate anemia and in preparation for a surgical procedure.
  4. Tranexamic acid (Lysteda) is an antifibrinolytic agent FDA approved for cyclic heavy menstrual bleeding. Dosage in normal renal function is 3900 mg daily (650 mg tablets, 2 tablets tid) for up to 5 days during menses.
  5. Endometrial tamponade with Foley catheter

- Surgical treatment
  1. D&C and hysteroscopy
  2. Endometrial ablation
  3. Hysterectomy

DISPOSITION

Cyclical treatment on birth control pills or Provera for several cycles, then discontinue pill and watch patient for onset of regular menses. If the patient does not want to conceive, continued cycle management with oral contraceptives is commonly used.

REFERRAL

To gynecologist in case of failure of treatment

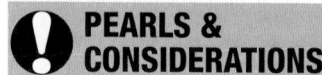

PEARLS & CONSIDERATIONS

COMMENTS

- Table 1 describes management options for DUB.
- Patient education material may be obtained from the American College of Obstetricians and Gynecologists, 409 12th Street SW, Washington, DC 20024-2188; phone 202-638-5577.

SUGGESTED READING

Available at www.expertconsult.com

RELATED CONTENT

Evaluation of ovulatory bleeding (Algorithm, Section III)
Evaluation of anovulatory bleeding (Algorithm, Section III)
Dysfunctional Uterine Bleeding (Patient Information)
Endometrial Cancer (Related Key Topic)
Menorrhagia (Related Key Topic)
Uterine Fibroids (Related Key Topic)

AUTHOR: **RUBEN ALVERO, M.D.,** and **NICOLE A. ROBERTS, M.D.**

TABLE 1 Management of Dysfunctional Uterine Bleeding (DUB)

Bleeding Pattern	Cause	Treatment
Ovulatory DUB		
Heavy menstrual bleeding	Imbalance in endometrial prostacyclins and prostaglandins	Nonsteroidal antiinflammatory drugs Combination oral contraceptive pill Progestin intrauterine device Endometrial ablation
Midcycle spotting	Periovulatory estrogen decline	None
Delayed menses	Persistent corpus luteum	None (rule out pregnancy)
Anovulatory DUB		
Irregular menses	Unopposed estrogen stimulation of endometrium	Combination oral contraceptive pill Cyclic progestins Endometrial ablation
Postmenopausal bleeding	Endometrial atrophy	Hormone replacement therapy Endometrial ablation

From Carlson KJ, Eisenstat SA, et al: *Primary care of women*, ed 2, St Louis, 2002, Mosby.

BASIC INFORMATION

DEFINITION

Dysmenorrhea is painful menstrual cramps of uterine origin. Prevalence is estimated to vary between 45% and 95%. Dysmenorrhea is the most common gynecologic condition in women, regardless of age and nationality.

Types of Dysmenorrhea

Primary dysmenorrhea is menstrual pain without organic disease.

Secondary dysmenorrhea is menstrual pain associated with an identifiable disease.

SYNONYMS

Menstrual cramps
Painful periods

ICD-10CM CODES
N94.3 Primary dysmenorrhea
N94.5 Secondary dysmenorrhea
N94.6 Dysmenorrhea, unspecified

EPIDEMIOLOGY & DEMOGRAPHICS

- Approximately 50% of menstruating women are affected by dysmenorrhea, with approximately 10% of them having severe dysmenorrhea with incapacitation for 1 to 3 days/mo.
- Dysmenorrhea is most common in the age group from 20 to 24 yr.
- Primary dysmenorrhea may appear 6 to 12 months after ovulatory menstrual cycles begin.
- Secondary dysmenorrhea may occur at any time after menarche, but it may arise in a woman's 30s to 40s due to a causative underlying condition. The woman may also complain of dyspareunia, menorrhagia, intermenstrual bleeding, or postcoital bleeding.

PHYSICAL FINDINGS & CLINICAL PRESENTATION

- Sharp, crampy, midline, lower abdominal pain without a lower quadrant or adnexal component but possible radiation to the lower back and upper thighs
- Unremarkable pelvic examination in nonmenstruating patient
- Accompanying symptoms: nausea, vomiting, headaches, anxiety, fatigue, diarrhea, fainting, and abdominal bloating
- Cramps usually lasting <24 hr and seldom lasting >2 to 3 days
- Secondary dysmenorrhea: dyspareunia is a common complaint, and bimanual pelvic-abdominal examination may demonstrate uterine or adnexal tenderness, fixed uterine retroflexion, uterosacral nodularity, a pelvic mass, or an enlarged, irregular uterus

ETIOLOGY

Prostaglandin $F_2\alpha$ is the agent responsible for dysmenorrhea. It stimulates uterine contractions and cervical stenosis (narrowing) and increases vasopressin release. Behavior and psychological factors have also been implicated in the etiology of primary dysmenorrhea. Primary dysmenorrhea only occurs in ovulatory cycles. Secondary dysmenorrhea is usually caused by endometriosis, adenomyosis, leiomyomas and, less commonly, intrauterine device (IUD) use, or congenital or acquired outflow tract obstruction, including cervical stenosis.

DIAGNOSIS

DIFFERENTIAL DIAGNOSIS: SECONDARY DYSMENORRHEA

- Adenomyosis
- Adhesions
- Cervical structures or stenosis
- Congenital malformation of müllerian system
- Ectopic pregnancy
- Endometriosis
- Imperforate hymen
- IUD use
- Leiomyomas
- Ovarian cysts
- Pelvic congestion syndrome
- Pelvic inflammatory disease
- Polyps
- Transverse vaginal septum

WORKUP AND EVALUATION

- Primary dysmenorrhea: characteristic history, physical examination and ultrasound normal with the absence of an identifiable cause of pelvic pain
- Secondary dysmenorrhea: physical examination and ultrasound may reveal vaginal/uterine abnormalities, fibroids, adenomyosis, polyps, endometriomas

LABORATORY TESTS

- No specific tests diagnostic for dysmenorrhea
- Elevated white blood cell count in the presence of infection
- Human chorionic gonadotropin to rule out ectopic pregnancy

IMAGING STUDIES

- Ultrasound scan of the pelvis to evaluate the presence of leiomyomas, adenomyosis, ovarian cysts
- Saline ultrasonography to assess the uterine cavity to rule out endometrial polyps or submucosal or intraluminal leiomyomas

TREATMENT

NONPHARMACOLOGIC THERAPY

- Applying heat to the lower abdomen with hot compresses, heating pads, or hot water bottles seems to offer some relief.
- Offer reassurance that this is a treatable condition.

ACUTE GENERAL Rx

- Nonsteroidal antiinflammatory drugs such as ibuprofen 400 to 600 mg q4 to 6h or naproxen sodium 500 mg q12h.

- Oral contraceptives cyclically or continuously (taking only active pills), primarily in women with primary dysmenorrhea.
- The levonorgestrel-containing IUD is increasingly being used to ameliorate symptoms of dysmenorrhea. Pain improvement has been shown in many cases to be even better than oral contraceptive pills.
- Magnesium supplements (research ongoing)
- Thiamine supplements (research ongoing)
- Fish oil supplements (research ongoing)
- Secondary dysmenorrhea: treatment directed to the specific underlying condition.

CHRONIC Rx

Acupuncture and transcutaneous electrical nerve stimulation may be tried. However, there is not enough evidence to support the use of yoga, acupuncture, or massage. In cases in which medical therapy has not worked, laparoscopy or other surgical treatments should be considered depending on the secondary cause of the dysmenorrhea. A directed physical examination, looking for gynecologic masses or nodularity should be performed. Nontraditional approaches such as acupuncture have been tried with relief in some patients. The levonorgestrel IUD has been shown to effectively reduce pain in women with primary dysmenorrhea.

DISPOSITION

The majority of patients are satisfactorily treated with good outcomes. Possible chronic complications with primary dysmenorrhea that has not been adequately treated can lead to anxiety and depression. With certain causes of secondary dysmenorrhea, infertility can become a problem.

REFERRAL

If a secondary cause of dysmenorrhea is revealed, refer to the appropriate specialist for further medical or surgical treatment (e.g., gynecologist, urogynecologist, reproductive endocrinologist, pain management center).

SUGGESTED READINGS
Available online at www.expertconsult.com

RELATED CONTENT

Dysmenorrhea (Patient Information)
Dyspareunia (Related Key Topic)
Endometriosis (Related Key Topic)
Premenstrual Dysphoric Disorder (Related Key Topic)
Premenstrual Syndrome (Related Key Topic)

AUTHOR: RUBEN ALVERO, M.D., and BARBARA MCGUIRK, M.D.

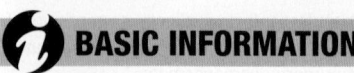

BASIC INFORMATION

DEFINITION

Persistent and/or recurrent pain associated with sexual activity that causes marked distress or interpersonal conflict.

SYNONYMS

Painful intercourse

ICD-10CM CODES
N94.1 Dyspareunia
F52.6 Dyspareunia not due to a substance or known physiological condition

EPIDEMIOLOGY & DEMOGRAPHICS

PREVALENCE (IN U.S.): Affects 10% to 20% of women
PREDOMINANT SEX: Female
AT-RISK POPULATION: No consistent findings regarding:
- Age
- Parity
- Educational status
- Race
- Income
- Marital status
- However, postmenopausal status is significant: Up to 50% of postmenopausal women note that sex can be painful

RISK FACTORS: Dyspareunia can lower:
- Frequency of intercourse
- Levels of desire and arousal
- Orgasmic response
- Physical and emotional satisfaction
- General happiness
- Relationship quality

HISTORICAL FACTORS—ASSESSMENT:
- Pain parameters
  1. Character (dryness, tightness, pain, burning, soreness)
  2. Location (introital, middle, deep)
  3. Onset
  4. Duration
  5. Timing (during sex or anticipation before sex, for example)
  6. Chronicity (worsening over the years)
  7. Cyclicity (related to menstrual cycle, other recurrent life events)
  8. Recurrence (one particular partner, positional, more/less frequent)
- Gynecologic history
  1. History of sexually transmitted disease
  2. History of herpes simplex virus (HSV) or human papillomavirus (HPV)
  3. Other sexual dysfunctions
  4. Prior abdominal or gynecologic surgery
  5. Prior pelvic or abdominal radiation
  6. History of endometriosis, adenomyosis, leiomyomata, pelvic mass/ovarian cyst
  7. History of genital or uterine prolapse
  8. History of gynecologic infection
  9. History of pelvic pain
  10. History of menopausal symptoms/genitourinary syndrome of menopause—most common cause of dyspareunia in women over 50 years old

  11. Diminished lubrication
  12. Sexual misinformation
  13. History of abuse
  14. Primary vs. secondary dyspareunia
      1. Secondary dyspareunia—prior history of pain-free coitus
- Obstetric history
  1. Lacerations
  2. Episiotomy
  3. Operative vaginal birth
  4. Prolonged labor
  5. Difficult vaginal birth
- General medical causes
  1. History of chronic diseases
  2. Gastrointestinal or genitourinary symptoms
  3. Medications
  4. History of psychological disorders
  5. History of dermatologic condition
  6. Religious beliefs
  7. Generalized anxiety
  8. Stress

PHYSICAL FINDINGS & CLINICAL PRESENTATION

- Visual inspection of lower genital tract
  1. Discoloration—consider hypopigmented lichen sclerosis
  2. Ulcerations
  3. Discharge
  4. Prolapse
  5. Dysplastic changes
  6. Infestations
  7. Dry/pale/thin vaginal walls
- Physical examination
  1. Sensitivity to light touch—single or multiple points
  2. Tenderness to palpation—single or multiple points
  3. Genital prolapse
     a. Uterus
     b. Bladder
     c. Cervix
     d. Vagina
     e. Adnexa
     f. Rectum
     g. Bowel
  4. Longitudinal or transverse vaginal septum
  5. Levator muscle tone
  6. Evidence of previous surgery
  7. Vaginal length, depth, caliber constrictions: assess for shortened or absent vagina
  8. Vaginismus—vaginal muscle tightening

ETIOLOGY—GENERAL CATEGORIES

- Pathology or alteration of genital-associated tissue
- Psychosocial factors
- Marital or relationship discord
- History of sexual or generalized physical/emotional abuse
- Menopause/aging
- Medication side effect
- Infection

Dx DIAGNOSIS

DIFFERENTIAL DIAGNOSIS

- Congenital deformities (septa/agenesis)

- Imperforate hymen
- Menopausal changes
- Atrophic/aging tissue
- Impaired lubrication
- Aromatase inhibitor usage/low estrogen levels
- Psychogenic
- Vaginismus
- Inadequate foreplay
- Virginity/hymenal factors
- Endometriosis/adenomyosis
- Levator ani myalgia
- Chronic pelvic pain
- Previous surgery (anterior/posterior colporrhaphy, perineorrhaphy, pelvic floor reconstruction, hysterectomy, episiotomy repair, labiaplasty, vaginoplasty)
  1. Alteration in vaginal length, depth, caliber, architecture, shape, elasticity
  2. Adhesions
- Infectious
  1. HPV
  2. HSV
  3. Candidiasis
  4. *Tinea cruris*
  5. Acute or chronic salpingitis or endometritis
  6. Sexually transmitted infections
- Pelvic carcinoma
- Previous radiation
- Adnexal attachment or tubal prolapse
- Pelvic tumor/leiomyoma/ovarian cyst or torsion
- Uterine prolapse, malposition, enlargement, or retroversion
- Genital prolapse
- Cystourethrocele, rectocele, enterocele
- Urethral or bladder pathology (interstitial cystitis, for example)
- Pelvic congestion (controversial)
- Vulvar vestibulitis
- Postcoital cystitis
- Broad ligament pathology
- Neuroma at the site of previous episiotomy
- Previous sexual/physical/emotional abuse
- Marital/relationship discord
- Vulvodynia
- Lichen sclerosus
- Contact or allergic dermatitis
- Vitamin A, B, or C deficiency
- Equestrian dyspareunia
- Pudendal neuralgia
- Myofascial pain syndrome
- Rectal/colon pathology
- Structural abnormalities or alterations
  1. Muscle
  2. Bone
  3. Ligament
  4. Nerve
  5. Adjacent tissues/structures

WORKUP

- History and physical examination are key and most likely all that is needed.
- If needed (unlikely, however):
  1. Colposcopy
  2. Cystoscopy
  3. Ultrasonography
  4. MRI
  5. Consider laparoscopy for unexplained deep dyspareunia

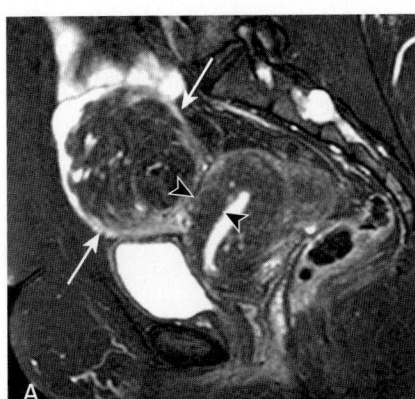

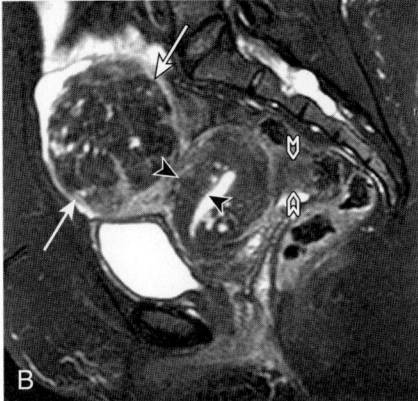

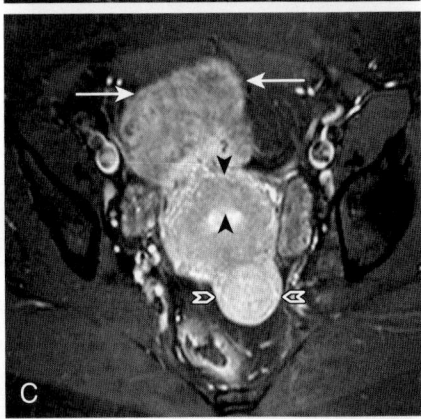

FIG. 1 Adenomyosis and leiomyomata in a 41-year-old woman with pelvic pain, irregular menses, menorrhagia, and dyspareunia. A and **B,** Sagittal T2-weighted fat-suppressed images show a large anterior subserosal fibroid with mixed but predominantly low signal *(arrows)* and a smaller posterior subserosal fibroid with low to intermediate signal *(chevrons)*. There is also widening of the junctional zone *(black arrowheads)* with areas of increased T2 signal, indicative of adenomyosis. **C,** Axial three-dimensional gradient echo postcontrast image with fat suppression shows enhancement of the leiomyomata *(white arrowheads and chevrons)* and the thickened junctional zone *(black arrowheads)*. (From Fielding JR et al: *Gynecologic imaging,* Philadelphia, 2011, Saunders.)

LABORATORY TESTS—USE JUDICIOUSLY

- Erythrocyte sedimentation rate
- White blood cell count
- Wet mount
  - ○ Trichomoniasis
  - ○ Candidiasis
  - ○ Bacterial vaginosis
- Cultures
  1. Cervical
     a. Gonorrhea
     b. *Chlamydia*
  2. Vaginal
  3. Lesions
  4. Urine
- Vulva, vaginal, or cervical biopsy
- Pap smear
- HSV antibodies
- Gonadotropin levels

IMAGING STUDIES

Pelvic or abdominal ultrasonography. Transvaginal ultrasonography provides for greater resolution of the uterus and adnexa (tubes/ovaries) due to proximity to pelvic organs. Consider an MRI when the diagnosis is unclear with other diagnostic modalities (Fig. 1).

Rx TREATMENT

NONPHARMACOLOGIC THERAPY

- Patient education
- Discontinue exacerbating activity, irritants, medications
- Lubrication with coitus
- Coital position changes
- Avoid deep thrusting
- Warm or cool soaks
- Reassurance to patient of nonmalignant/other worrisome conditions
- Psychosocial interventions
  1. Systemic desensitization techniques
  2. Behavior modification
  3. General counseling
  4. Marital/relationship counseling
- Vaginal dilators
- Vaginal muscle exercises and relaxation techniques
- Excision of pathologic tissue
- Surgical correction of altered, reduced, or deformed tissues

ACUTE GENERAL Rx

- Topical lidocaine, nonhormonal moisturizers and lubricants.
- Corticosteroids—for lichen sclerosus, for example.
- Antiinfective agents if vaginitis/cervicitis/adnexal abscess is found.
- Trigger point injections.
- Massage or physical therapy.
- Acupuncture.
- Transcutaneous electrical nerve stimulation.
- Stress reduction techniques.

- Safe sexual practices.
- Menopausal hormone (estrogen) therapy
  - ○ Local/intravaginal (pill/ring/cream)
  - ○ Systemic (pill/patch/gel/spray/cream/injection)
- Ospemifene (Osphena), an oral estrogen agonist/antagonist for treatment of moderate to severe dyspareunia in postmenopausal women with suspected vaginal atrophy. Dosage is 60 mg tablet daily.
- Antiviral agents.
- Intralesional interferon.
- Mild analgesics.
- Antidepressants.

CHRONIC Rx

All the previous plus:
- Set supportive visits as needed
- Oral contraceptives
- Regular sexual activity
- Balanced diet
- Vitamin supplementation
- Proper hygiene

DISPOSITION

Most patients will have a reduction and/or resolution of their symptoms by using the appropriate therapeutic approaches.

REFERRAL

As with other pain conditions, a multidisciplinary approach using the expertise of psychologists, dermatologists, gynecologic surgeons, infectious disease specialists, urologists, and others may be helpful.

! PEARLS & CONSIDERATIONS

- Dyspareunia is a symptom complex resulting from a multitude of etiologies, some of which act simultaneously.
- Uncovering the etiology of dyspareunia is predominantly based on a comprehensive history and physical examination.
- Ask about dyspareunia as part of your routine patient assessment. Don't wait for the patient to initiate the conversation.
- Sorting the differential diagnosis into superficial, intermediate, and deep dyspareunia categories is immensely helpful.
- As with the physical evaluation of any painful condition, attempt—by precise touching (moistened cotton swab), palpation, or applied pressure—to reproduce the patient's chief complaint.
- Performing a one-finger pelvic examination without concurrent abdominal palpation allows a more precise assessment as to the source of genital pain.
- Individualize therapy.
- Initiate and maintain an honest diagnosis and compassionate demeanor with the patient and her partner.

- Be open minded, approachable, nonjudgmental, and diligent in your search for a solution to help these often silently suffering patients.

PATIENT/FAMILY EDUCATION

www.menopause.org

SUGGESTED READING

Available at www.expertconsult.com

RELATED CONTENT

Painful Intercourse (Patient Information)
Dysmenorrhea (Related Key Topic)

Endometriosis (Related Key Topic)
Vaginitis, Estrogen Deficient (Related Key Topic)
Sexual Dysfunction in Women (Related Key Topic)
Menopause (Related Key Topic)

AUTHORS: **DAVID I. KURSS, M.D.,** and **RUBEN ALVERO, M.D.**

BASIC INFORMATION

DEFINITION

Dyspepsia is a constellation of symptoms referable to the gastroduodenal region of the upper GI tract. *Nonulcerative dyspepsia* is a term used to describe signs and symptoms of persistent or recurrent dyspepsia that have no identifiable organic cause.

SYNONYMS

Nonulcer dyspepsia
Functional dyspepsia
Idiopathic dyspepsia

ICD-10CM CODES
K30 Functional dyspepsia

EPIDEMIOLOGY & DEMOGRAPHICS

- Up to 25% of the general population will experience dyspepsia each year. Of these, 75% will have no evident causative agent.

PHYSICAL FINDINGS & CLINICAL PRESENTATION

Typical clinical presentation is dyspepsia without findings on physical examination to explain the symptoms

ETIOLOGY

The etiology and pathophysiology are still unclear. Research is focused on abnormalities of gastric motor function and visceral hypersensitivity, as well as
- *Helicobacter pylori* infection
- Psychosocial factors—associated with anxiety and depression

RISK FACTORS

Risk factors include:
- Genetic predisposition: homozygous *GNB3* gene.
- Dietary habits such as caffeine, alcohol, or smoking.
- Medications such as NSAIDs, calcium channel blockers, methylxanthines, alendronate, orlistat, acarbose, and potassium supplements.
- Psychological disorders such as anxiety, depression, somatization, or personal history of childhood sexual or physical abuse.

(Dx) DIAGNOSIS

DIFFERENTIAL DIAGNOSIS

Nonulcerative dyspepsia is diagnosed when all other organic causes have been excluded, including:
- PUD
- Gastroesophageal reflux
- Gastric/esophageal/other abdominal cancers
- Biliary tract disease
- Gastroparesis, including diabetic gastroparesis
- Pancreatitis
- Medications (i.e., NSAIDs, erythromycin)
- Metabolic disturbances (i.e., hypercalcemia, heavy metals, or hyperkalemia)
- Ischemic bowel disease

- Systemic disorders (i.e., eosinophilic gastritis, Crohn's disease, sarcoidosis, celiac disease, thyroid disorders)

DIAGNOSIS

Developed in 2006 in conjunction with the American Gastroenterological Association, the Rome III criteria lists the following factors, which must be present at least 3 months and first noticed within 6 months of diagnosis:
- At least one of the following:
  1. Postprandial fullness, *or*
  2. Early satiety, *or*
  3. Epigastric pain, *or*
  4. Epigastric burning
- *and* no evidence of structural disease likely to explain the symptoms

WORKUP

The American Gastroenterological Association, as well as the Maastricht III and the IV European consensus, suggest the following:
- The pattern of symptoms overlaps considerably for all types of dyspepsia; therefore, the history and physical should focus on finding specific symptoms that help exclude other causes of dyspepsia.
- Endoscopy should be performed only in patients >55 years old and in younger patients with alarming symptoms (e.g., weight loss, progressive dysphagia, recurrent vomiting, evidence of gastrointestinal bleeding, or family history of cancer) presenting with new-onset dyspepsia. Findings consistent with diagnosis of nonulcerative dyspepsia are not conclusive, no presence of *H. pylori*, no signs of gastroesophageal reflux disease, no mucosal inflammation. NOTE: Patients <55 years old and without any alarming symptoms can be treated without endoscopy.

LABORATORY TESTS

H. pylori: Laboratory methods include serologic tests[1], monoclonal stool antigen, or urea breath test.

(Rx) TREATMENT

ACUTE GENERAL Rx

PHARMACOLOGIC THERAPY: Primary treatment is usually initiated with proton pump inhibitors (PPIs), which can be started without performing endoscopy, especially if the patient comes from a population with low prevalence of *H. pylori* infection. If symptoms persist, a trial of antidepressants can be started.

Treatment of accompanying symptoms includes:

Predominant Symptom	Possible Etiology	Medication Recommended
Nausea	Motility dysfunction	Prokinetic agent
Bloating	Motility dysfunction	Simethicone and/or prokinetic agent

[1]Serologic testing for *H. pylori* has a low predictive value because colonization is lifelong; it can therefore determine prevalence better than incidence.

Predominant Symptom	Possible Etiology	Medication Recommended
Pain	Mucosal disease or *H. pylori* infection	Antibiotic trial
Somatic complaints	Psychosocial	Psychotropic medication trial

Medication categories:
- Antacids (i.e., aluminum hydroxide, calcium carbonate)
- Gas-reducing agents, such as those containing simethicone
- H_2-receptor antagonists (i.e., cimetidine)
- PPIs (i.e., omeprazole)
- Prokinetic agents (i.e., metoclopramide, domperidone)
- Antidepressants (i.e., selective serotonin receptor inhibitors, tricyclics)
- *H. pylori* therapy/antibiotic therapy (various antibiotic regimens, usually 1 PPI) if *H. pylori* present

CHRONIC Rx

Controversy currently exists around the long-term use of PPIs. Due to the high association with psychological factors, patients with functional dyspepsia should undergo psychological intervention, even if there is good response to pharmacotherapeutic approaches.

COMPLEMENTARY & ALTERNATIVE THERAPIES

Peppermint and caraway oil may be helpful, as well as acupuncture; however, no definitive trials have been performed.

REFERRAL

- Referral to gastroenterology if patient has alarming symptoms (such as GI bleeding, dysphagia, odynophagia, unexplained anemia, change in appetite, and weight loss) or when endoscopy is indicated—although controversy exists about the workup of younger patients.
- Referral to cardiology if cardiac etiology suspected.

(!) PEARLS & CONSIDERATIONS

PREVENTION

Avoid excessive amounts of caffeine, alcohol, smoking, or long-term use of steroids and NSAIDs.

PATIENT AND FAMILY EDUCATION

http://www.mayoclinic.com/health/stomach-pain/DS00524

SUGGESTED READINGS
Available at www.expertconsult.com

RELATED CONTENT

Approach to the patient with dyspepsia (Algorithm, Section III)

AUTHORS: **ALVARO M. RIVERA, M.D.,** and **NADINE MBUYI, M.D.**

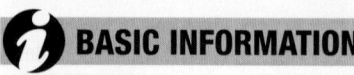
DEFINITION

The term "dysphagia" is derived from the Greek words *dys* (with difficulty) and *phagia* (to eat). It is characterized by abnormal transfer of food from mouth to the stomach, which may involve the oral, pharyngeal, or esophageal stages of swallowing.

ICD-10CM CODES
R13.10 Dysphagia, unspecified
D50.1   Sideropenic dysphagia
I69.091 Dysphagia following nontraumatic subarachnoid hemorrhage
I69.191 Dysphagia following nontraumatic intracerebral hemorrhage
I69.291 Dysphagia following other nontraumatic intracranial hemorrhage
I69.391 Dysphagia following cerebral infarction
I69.891 Dysphagia following other cerebrovascular disease
I69.991 Dysphagia following unspecified cerebrovascular disease
R13.11 Dysphagia, oral phase
R13.12 Dysphagia, oropharyngeal phase
R13.13 Dysphagia, pharyngeal phase
R13.14 Dysphagia, pharyngoesophageal phase
R13.19 Other dysphagia

EPIDEMIOLOGY & DEMOGRAPHICS

- This is seen in 10% of individuals above the age of 50 yr. Its prevalence increases with advancing age.
- Nearly 12% of hospitalized patients have symptoms of dysphagia.
- Up to 30% to 60% of nursing home patients have some form of dysphagia.
- Special populations, including patients with head injury, stroke, or Parkinson's disease, have 30% to 50% prevalence of oropharyngeal dysphagia.

ETIOLOGY

- Oropharyngeal
  1. Neuromuscular causes
     - Stroke.
     - Parkinson's disease.
     - Multiple sclerosis.
     - Myasthenia gravis.
     - Amyotrophic lateral sclerosis.
     - CNS tumors.
     - Muscular dystrophy.
     - Thyroid dysfunction.
     - Polymyositis and dermatomyositis.
     - Sarcoidosis.
     - Cerebral palsy.
     - Head trauma.
     - Metabolic encephalopathy.
     - Dementia.
     - Bell's palsy.
  2. Structural causes
     - Oropharyngeal tumors.
     - Zenker's diverticulum.
     - Infection of pharynx or neck (mucositis from *Candida*, herpes, and CMV).
     - Thyromegaly.
     - Prior surgery or radiotherapy.
     - Osteophytes and other spinal disorders.
     - Proximal esophageal webs.
     - Congenital anomalies (e.g., cleft palate).
     - Poor dentition.
- Esophageal
  1. Neuromuscular disorders
     - Achalasia.
     - Diffuse esophageal spasm.
     - Nutcracker esophagus.
     - Hypertensive lower esophageal sphincter.
     - Ineffective esophageal motility.
     - Scleroderma.
     - Reflex-associated dysmotility.
  2. Structural disorder
     - Peptic stricture.
     - Esophageal rings and webs.
     - Diverticuli.
     - Carcinoma and benign tumors.
     - Foreign bodies.
     - Vascular compression.
     - Mediastinal masses.
     - Spinal osteophytes.
     - Mucosal injury (from pills, infection, gastroesophageal reflux disease [GERD], etc.).

PATHOGENESIS

The inability to swallow is caused either by a problem in strength or coordination of the muscles required to move material from the mouth to stomach or by a fixed obstruction somewhere between the mouth and the stomach.

CLINICAL FEATURES

Oropharyngeal dysphagia
- Problem arises within 2 seconds of initiating the voluntary phase of swallowing.
- Typical symptoms include drooling, spillage of food, postnasal regurgitation, difficulty in initiation of swallowing, sialorrhea, sensation of food stuck in the neck, coughing or choking during swallowing, the need to swallow repeatedly to clear food or fluid from the pharynx, dysphonia, nasal speech, hoarseness of voice, and dysarthria.
- A thorough physical examination including that of the nervous system, oral cavity, and the head/neck is very important in patients with oropharyngeal dysphagia.

Esophageal dysphagia
- Problem usually arises several seconds after swallowing.
- Patients often complain of food being stuck in lower substernal area.
- Dysphagia to solids suggests mechanical obstruction.
- Neuromuscular causes result in dysphagia to both solids and liquids. Particularly, patients with achalasia tend to drink a lot of fluids while eating or apply maneuvers such as straightening the back, raising their arms over their heads, or standing to increase intraesophageal pressure to facilitate the emptying of food into the stomach.
- Oftentimes, ingestion of very cold or very hot foods precipitates the dysphagia associated with neuromuscular disorder.
- Delayed regurgitation of food, heartburn, and chest pain are usually present.
- Weight loss is usually associated with malignancy or achalasia.
- Symptoms are intermittent in patients with esophageal dysphagia from benign causes of structural obstruction or diffuse esophageal spasm. However, it is progressive in patients with peptic stricture, esophageal carcinoma, scleroderma, and achalasia.
- In patients with structural obstruction, when the luminal diameter is more than 18 to 20 mm, they are rarely symptomatic, whereas those with a diameter of less than 13 mm are nearly always symptomatic.
- These patients with esophageal dysphagia usually do not have any characteristic physical findings.

Laboratory evaluation
- CBC.
- Thyroid studies.
- Nutritional assessment by checking serum protein and albumin levels.
- Other studies based on specific clinical conditions.
Special studies
- Oropharyngeal dysphagia
  1. Videofluoroscopy is the first test often ordered in evaluation of patients with oropharyngeal dysphagia.
  2. Double contrast modified barium swallow study (Fig. E1).
  3. Fiberoptic flexible nasopharyngeal laryngoscopy is mandatory in all cases when a structural lesion, particularly malignancy, is suspected.
  4. Pharyngeal and upper esophageal manometry (Fig. E2) is occasionally of value to predict which patients will have a favorable outcome from cricopharyngeal myotomy or dilation.
  5. Radiography of head and neck when indicated.
- Esophageal dysphagia
  1. Barium esophagography should precede upper endoscopies to identify patients at risk from potential perforation with an endoscopy and to help plan fluoroscopically guided dilation. It is often the first step in evaluating patients with dysphagia, especially if an obstructive lesion is suspected.
  2. EGD.
  3. Esophageal manometry is indicated if no abnormality is identified by barium study or EGD.
  4. Esophageal pH monitoring in patients with suspected reflux disease.
  5. Endoscopic ultrasonography.
  6. Radiograph, CT, and MRI of chest.

DIFFERENTIAL DIAGNOSIS (FIG. 3)

- Globus pharyngeus.
- Odynophagia.
- Phagophobia.
- GERD.

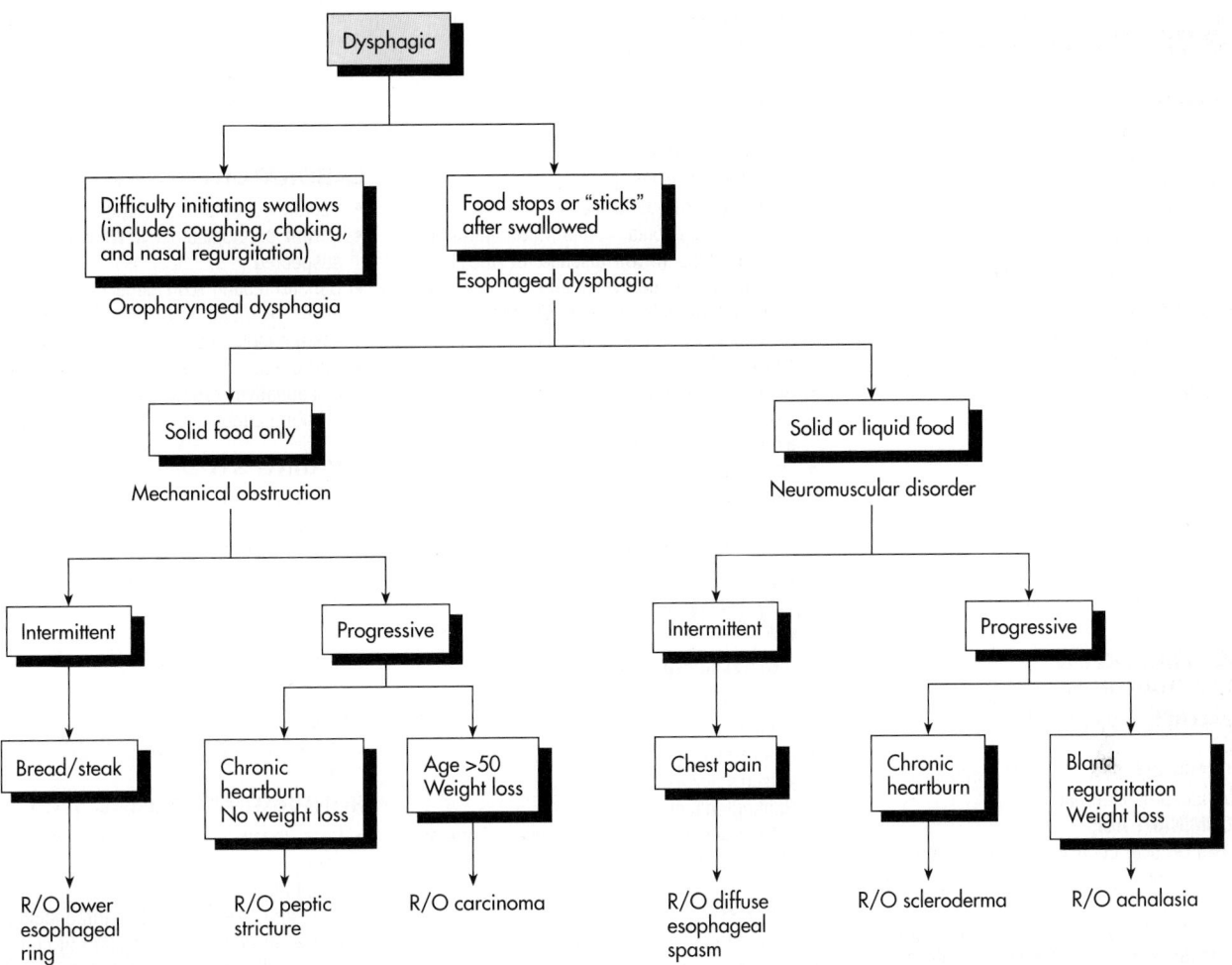

FIG. 3 Differential diagnosis of dysphagia. *RO,* Rule out. (Modified from Andreoli TE [ed]: *Cecil essentials of medicine,* ed 7, Philadelphia, 2008, Saunders.)

Rx TREATMENT

- Treatment should be approached with the help of specialists of multiple disciplines (ENT, head and neck surgeon, radiologist, speech pathologist, physical therapist, dietitian, gastroenterologist, physical medicine and rehabilitation specialist, dentist, neurologist, etc.).
- Goal of therapy is airway protection and maintenance of nutrition.
- Alteration of food consistency, volume, and delivery rate plays a major role.
- The goal of direct therapy is to change swallowing physiology with medical treatment of primary disease, maxillofacial prosthesis, and cricopharyngeal myotomy.
- Indirect therapies include exercise programs for tongue coordination and chewing under the guidance of a speech therapist.
- Maintenance of oral feeding often requires compensatory techniques such as chin-tuck position, rotation of head to the affected side, tilting of head to the strong side, and lying on one's back or on one's side during swallowing.
- Some of the voluntary maneuvers applied include supraglottic swallow, effortful swallow, Mendelson maneuver, Shaker exercise, and the Heimlich maneuver.
- Placement of nasogastric tube, jejunostomy tube, or percutaneous endoscopic gastrotomy

(PEG) tube is considered for enteral feeding when other measures fail and the patient remains at significant risk for aspiration or nutrition becomes compromised.
- Treatment of associated GERD should not be forgotten.
- Surgery for chronic aspiration may involve tracheostomy, medialization, laryngeal suspension, laryngeal closure, and/or laryngotracheal separation-diversion.
- Other measures include esophageal dilation removal of foreign body, esophageal resection, chemotherapy, radiotherapy, endoscopic ablation of tumor, photodynamic therapy, esophageal prosthesis/stents, diverticulectomy, intrasphincteric injection of botulinum toxin, surgical myotomy, and others. Smooth muscle relaxants such as nitrates and calcium channel blockers have been used to effectively treat patients with diffuse esophageal spasm and nutcracker esophagus.
- Several scales have been suggested to determine patients' functional outcome. One of them is the "Swallowing Rating Scale."

COMPLICATIONS

- Dehydration.
- Malnutrition.
- Aspiration pneumonia.
- Airway obstruction.
- Death resulting from pulmonary complications.

PROGNOSIS

- Depends on the etiology.
- Nursing home patients with oropharyngeal dysphagia and a history of aspiration have an approximately 45% mortality rate over 1 yr.
- All patients, especially the elderly, should take their medications with a full glass of water while in upright position well before bedtime.
- Dysphagia should be considered an alarm symptom, indicating the need for immediate evaluation.

PATIENT EDUCATION

Elderly patients with dysphagia should not attribute their symptoms to aging.

SUGGESTED READINGS

Available at www.expertconsult.com

RELATED CONTENT

Achalasia (Related Key Topic)
Dyspepsia, Nonulcerative (Related Key Topic)
Esophageal Tumors (Related Key Topic)
Gastroesophageal Reflux Disease (Related Key Topic)

AUTHOR: **HEMANT K. SATPATHY, M.D.,** and **FRED F. FERRI, M.D.**

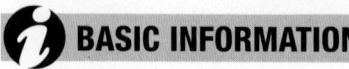

DEFINITION

Dystonia refers to a group of disorders characterized by involuntary muscle contractions (sustained or spasmodic) that lead to abnormal body movements or postures. Dystonia can be generalized or focal, of early (<20 yr) or late onset, and primary or secondary.

SYNONYMS

Blepharospasm
Oromandibular (orofacial) dystonia
Spasmodic (limb or axial) dystonia
Torticollis
Writer's cramp

ICD-10CM CODES
G24   Dystonia
G24.1 Idiopathic familial dystonia
G24.0 Drug induced dystonia
G24.3 Spasmodic torticollis

EPIDEMIOLOGY & DEMOGRAPHICS

PREVALENCE: Estimated at one in 3000 persons.
PREDOMINANT SEX: Cervical dystonia has a 3:2 female preponderance.
PREDOMINANT AGE:
- Onset of focal cervical dystonia is usually in the fifth decade.
- Hereditary forms may have an onset in childhood or adulthood and tend to be more severe.
GENETICS: Autosomal-dominant, autosomal-recessive, and X-linked forms of dystonia have been identified. Ashkenazi Jews are particularly susceptible to primary early-onset dystonia. Metabolic conditions in which dystonia is a feature can be inherited or, more frequently, caused by sporadic mutations.

CLINICAL PRESENTATION

Focal dystonias produce abnormal sustained muscle contractions in a single region of the body:
- Neck (**torticollis**): most commonly affected site with a tendency for the head to turn to one side.
- Eyelids (**blepharospasm**): involuntary closure of the eyelids that leads to excessive eye blinking, sometimes with persistent eye closure and functional blindness.
- Mouth (**oromandibular dystonia**): involuntary contraction of muscles of the mouth, tongue, or face.
- Hand (**writer's cramp**) (Fig. 1).
Generalized dystonia affects multiple areas of the body and can lead to marked joint deformities.
- Isolated foot dystonia is very rare and may suggest an underlying parkinsonian disorder or brain structural abnormality.

ETIOLOGY
- Exact pathophysiology of primary dystonia is unknown but believed to involve abnormalities of basal ganglia. Specifically, reduced and abnormal patterns of neuronal activity in the basal ganglia result in disinhibition of the motor thalamus and cortex, leading to abnormal movement.
- Fifteen hereditary forms have been described, including the severe progressive form, dystonia musculorum deformans.
- Secondary dystonia results from central nervous system (CNS) disease of the basal ganglia (stroke, demyelination, hypoxia, trauma), Huntington's disease, Wilson's disease, Parkinson syndromes, and lysosomal storage diseases.
- Acute dystonia can occur with drugs that block dopamine receptors, such as phenothiazines or butyrophenones.
- Tardive dyskinesia can result from long-term treatment with antiemetics (e.g., phenothiazines), antipsychotics (e.g., haloperidol), levodopa, anticonvulsants, or ergots.

DIFFERENTIAL DIAGNOSIS
- Drug effects.
- Parkinson's disease.
- Progressive supranuclear palsy.
- Wilson's disease.
- Huntington's disease.
- Table 1 describes selected causes of primary and secondary dystonia in childhood.

WORKUP

History (family history, birth history, trauma, medication use, age of onset, and temporal pattern), physical examination to determine associated features (weakness, myoclonus, tremor) and to determine pattern of dystonia—focal (single body region), segmental (two or more body contiguous body regions),

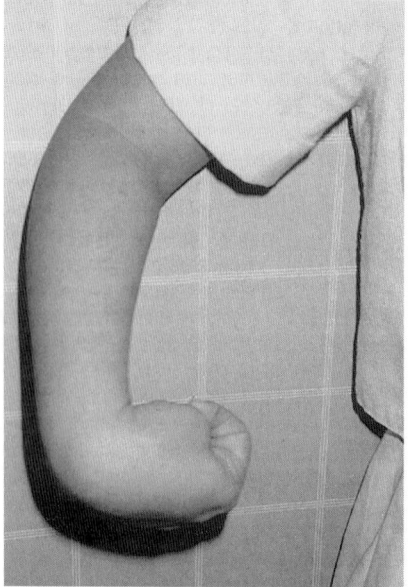

FIG. 1 Focal dystonia of the distal right arm.
(From Goldman L, Ausiello D [eds]: *Cecil textbook of medicine,* ed 22, Philadelphia, 2004, Saunders.)

multifocal (two or more noncontiguous body regions), generalized (involving the trunk and at least two other sites), or hemidystonia (involving more regions but restricted to one body side).

LABORATORY TESTS
- Usually not helpful for diagnosis
- Serum ceruloplasmin if Wilson's disease is suspected
- Genetic testing (*DYT* gene mutations, inborn errors of metabolism, or mitochondrial disease) if indicated
- Comprehensive toxicology screen indicated if causative drugs suspected (dopamine-blocking agents) and history unavailable

IMAGING STUDIES
- Primary dystonias are generally not associated with structural CNS abnormalities. CT scan or MRI of brain if a CNS lesion is suspected as a cause of secondary dystonia.
- Electrophysiologic testing can provide diagnostic support for the diagnosis, but dystonia is a clinical diagnosis.

NONPHARMACOLOGIC THERAPY
- Heat, massage, physical therapy to relieve pain
- Splints to prevent contractures.
- "Sensory trick" (geste antagoniste) can relieve discomfort: Application of light touch to the affected body part can abolish the dystonia; this also aids in diagnosis.

ACUTE GENERAL Rx
- For acute dystonic reactions to phenothiazines/butyrophenones, use diphenhydramine 50 mg IV or benztropine 2 mg IV.
- For patients presenting with subacute or chronic dystonia, a trial of L-dopa can be useful in distinguishing dopa-responsive dystonia from other causes.

CHRONIC Rx
- For treatment of drug-induced dystonia, slowly withdraw offending agents (antiemetics, antipsychotics most commonly).
- For generalized dystonia, a trial of carbidopa/levodopa may be beneficial and diagnostic of dopa-responsive dystonia.
- Trihexyphenidyl or benztropine may be helpful in up to 50% of tardive dystonias; these are the mainstay of treatment for generalized dystonias not responsive to dopa.
- Diazepam, clonazepam, or baclofen may be helpful.
- Injections of botulinum toxin into the affected muscles are the standard treatment for focal dystonias. Both type A and type B toxins produced by *Clostridium botulinum* block cholinergic transmission at the neuromuscular junction by inhibiting release of acetylcholine.

- Surgical procedures, including denervation, myectomy, rhizotomy, thalamotomy (pallidotomy), or deep brain stimulation, may be helpful for severe, refractory cases, depending on the etiology.
- Intrathecal baclofen can be useful for spastic or truncal dystonia.

DISPOSITION

Spontaneous remission of focal cervical dystonia can occur, but dystonia is generally progressive and pharmacologic therapy is often ineffective.

REFERRAL

Neurology (movement disorders) and/or neurosurgery for severe or refractory cases.
Physical therapy for maintaining flexibility.

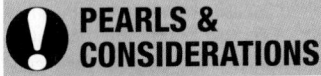

PEARLS & CONSIDERATIONS

COMMENTS

- Avoid triggers/exacerbating factors.
- Early physical therapy and splinting to prevent contractures.

- Consider botulism injections.
- Consider deep brain stimulation surgery for severe or refractory dystonia and for focal dystonias.

SUGGESTED READINGS

Available at www.expertconsult.com

AUTHOR: **JULIE L. ROTH, M.D.**

TABLE 1 Selected Causes of Primary and Secondary Dystonia in Childhood

Diagnosis	Additional Clinical Features	Diagnosis	Additional Clinical Features
Aicardi-Goutieres syndrome	Encephalopathy, developmental regression Acquired microcephaly Sterile pyrexias Lesions on the digits, ears (chilblain) Epilepsy CT: calcification of the basal ganglia	Leigh syndrome	Motor delays, weakness, hypotonia Ataxia, tremor Elevated lactate MRI: bilateral symmetric hyperintense lesions in the basal ganglia or thalamus
Alternating hemiplegia of childhood	Episodic hemiplegia/quadriplegia Abnormal ocular movements Autonomic symptoms Epilepsy Global developmental impairment Environmental triggers for spells	Lesch-Nyhan syndrome (X-linked)	Male Self-injurious behavior Hypotonia Oromandibular dystonia, inspiratory stridor Oculomotor apraxia Cognitive impairment Elevated uric acid
Aromatic amino acid decarboxylase deficiency (AADC)	Developmental delay Oculogyric crises Autonomic dysfunction Hypotonia	Myoclonus dystonia	Myoclonus Head, upper limb involvement
ARX gene mutation (X-linked)	Male Cognitive impairment Infantile spasms, epilepsy Brain malformation	Niemann-Pick type C	Hepatosplenomegaly Hypotonia Supranuclear gaze palsy Ataxia, dysarthria Epilepsy Psychiatric symptoms
Benign paroxysmal torticollis of infancy	Episodic Cervical dystonia only Family history of migraine	Neuroacanthocytosis	Oromandibular and lingual dystonia
Complex regional pain syndrome	Lower limb involvement Prominent pain	Neurodegeneration with brain iron accumulation	Cognitive impairment Retinal pigmentary degeneration, optic atrophy
Dopa-responsive dystonia (DRD)	Diurnal variation	Rapid onset dystonia parkinsonism (DYT12)	Acute onset Distribution face>arm>leg Prominent bulbar signs
Drug-induced dystonia		Rett syndrome	Female Developmental regression following a period of normal development Stereotypic hand movements Acquired microcephaly Epilepsy
Dystonia-deafness optic neuropathy syndrome	Sensorineural hearing loss in early childhood Psychosis Optic atrophy in adolescence		
DYT1 dystonia	Lower limb onset followed by generalization	Spinocerebellar ataxia 17 (SCA17)	Ataxia Dementia, psychiatric symptoms Parkinsonism
Glutaric aciduria type 1	Macrocephaly Encephalopathic crises MRI: striatal necrosis	Tics	Stereotyped movements Premonitory urge, suppressible
GM1 gangliosidosis type 3	Short stature, skeletal dysplasia Orofacial dystonia Speech/swallowing disturbance Parkinsonism MRI: putaminal hyperintensity	Tyrosine hydroxylase deficiency	Infantile encephalopathy, hypotonia Oculogyric crises, ptosis Autonomic symptoms Less diurnal fluctuation than DRD
Huntington disease (HD)	Parkinsonism Epilepsy Family history of HD		
Kernicterus	Jaundice in infancy Hearing loss Impaired upgaze Enamel dysplasia MRI: hyperintense lesions in the globus pallidus		

From Kliegman RM et al: *Nelson textbook of pediatrics,* ed 19, Philadelphia, 2011, Saunders.

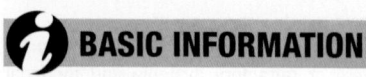
DEFINITION

An early repolarization pattern (ERP) in a QRS complex with a duration <120 ms, a peak J point elevation of ≥0.1 mV in two or more contiguous leads **excluding** leads V_1-V_3, with a notch or slur noted in the end of the QRS complex at the downslope of a prominent R wave (Fig. 1). This notch must be above the baseline T-P segment (Fig. 2). Previously thought to be benign, the pattern has been noted in higher prevalence in patients with idiopathic ventricular fibrillation (VF).

SYNONYM

1. Early repolarization syndrome—sudden cardiac arrest in a patient with ERP.
2. J point elevation
3. Persistent juvenile pattern

ICD-10CM CODES

R94.310	Abnormalities ECG—Abnormalities of ST segment
R00.9	Unspecified abnormalities of heart beat
I49.9	Cardiac arrhythmia unspecified

EPIDEMIOLOGY & DEMOGRAPHICS

INCIDENCE: The clinical entity "early repolarization pattern" is commonly asymptomatic; therefore, the true incidence of the pattern is difficult to definitively establish. In one comparison of patients with idiopathic ventricular fibrillation (VF) vs. young athletes vs. age-matched controls, the presence of ERP, defined as J point elevation >1.0 mm, in idiopathic VF patients was 31.1% in any lead, 17.8% in inferior leads, 11.1% in leads I and aVL, and 6.7% in leads V_4 to V_6. For comparison, the incidence in age-matched controls was 8.9% in any lead, 6.5% in inferior leads, 0% in leads I and aVL, and 4.9% in leads V_4 to V_6.

PREDOMINANT SEX: J point elevation >1 mm was documented significantly higher in males vs. females.

GENETICS: The mode of transmission and the genetic basis of the syndrome are unclear. An autosomal dominant pattern of inheritance of the *KCNJ8* gene, which has been associated with sporadic cases, has been shown. The prognostic value of the inheritance pattern is not known.

RISK FACTORS: Male sex, younger age, lower systolic blood pressure, higher Sokolow-Lyon index, and lower Cornell voltage have been shown to be associated with the presence of the early repolarization pattern. The early repolarization pattern carries an increased risk for future arrhythmic death. This is considered to be higher in the setting of a downsloping ST segment.

PHYSICAL FINDINGS & CLINICAL PRESENTATION

The physical exam will not show any findings specific for early repolarization. Rather, the clinical presentation is well documented in patients resuscitated from cardiac arrest. This is particularly shown in a pattern in which the early repolarization is seen in the inferior and/or the lateral leads but not in the precordial leads. The pattern has been shown to have an intermittent pattern of expression.[4]

ETIOLOGY

J point elevation is considered to be the electrocardiographic representation of a voltage gradient between different layers from the epicardium to the endocardium. The epicardium has a relatively higher density of transient outward potassium current (I_{TO}), when compared to the endocardium, resulting in a prominent notch in phase I of the action

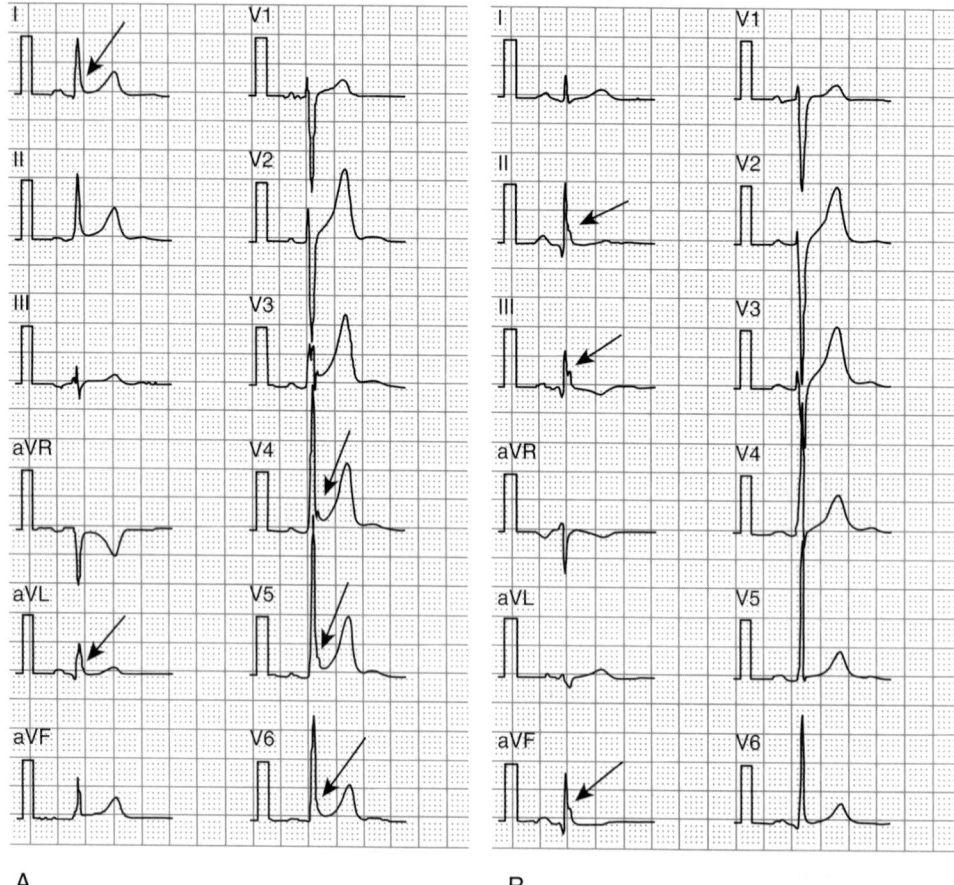

A   B

FIG. 1 A, Notching in lead V_6 progressing to slurring in V_6, I, aVL. **B,** Notching in lead III, aVF and slurring in lead II. (Macfarlane PW et al: The early repolarization pattern: a consensus pattern, *J Am Coll Cardiol* 66:470-477, 2015.)

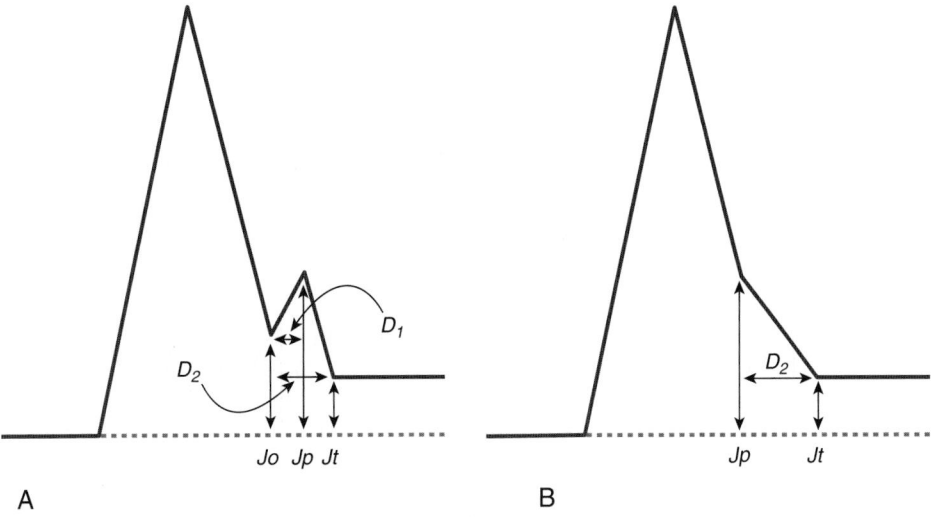

FIG. 2 A, Illustration of the amplitudes J onset (Jo), J peak (Jp), and J termination (Jt) as well as durations D1 and D2 in relation to an end QRS notch, as defined previously. **B,** Illustration of Jp and Jt as well as D2 in relation to an end QRS slur. (Macfarlane PW et al: The early repolarization pattern: a consensus pattern, *J Am Coll Cardiol* 66:470-477, 2015.)

potential. The Brugada syndrome is considered an extreme version of this phenomenon, where a loss of function mutation in the *SCN5A* gene results in loss of phase II in the action potential, causing marked J point and ST segment elevation, allowing for polymorphic ventricular tachycardia.

Dx DIAGNOSIS

Differential Diagnosis:
- Benign vs. malignant early repolarization
- Brugada syndrome
- Persistent juvenile pattern

WORK-UP
- Primarily guided by the clinical scenario. In a patient where the early repolarization pattern is an incidental finding (Figs. 3 and 4), detailed family history for sudden cardiac death is indicated.
- However, should the pattern be identified in the setting of a cardiac arrest, then the work-up would be directed to identification of potentially reversible causes.
  - Basic metabolic panel
  - Echocardiogram
  - Ischemic evaluation—noninvasive stress testing vs. left heart catheterization
  - Electrophysiology testing
  - ICD implant for secondary prevention of sudden cardiac death if no reversible cause is identified

LABORATORY TEST
- BMP
- Thyroid function studies

IMAGING STUDIES
Echocardiogram

Rx TREATMENT

No treatment is indicated in the case of the early repolarization pattern. In the setting of early repolarization syndrome with sudden cardiac death, the treatment would be that of sudden cardiac death as detailed under "Work-up."

REFERRALS
Cardiology referral should be obtained, particularly in the setting of syncope, nonsustained ventricular tachycardia, or cardiac arrest.

! PEARLS & CONSIDERATIONS

COMMENTS
The early repolarization pattern has previously been considered a benign pattern; however, the body of evidence suggests it to be a risk factor for sudden cardiac death. Therefore, all patients with early repolarization, particularly with risk factors or an isolated pattern in the inferior leads, merit a detailed evaluation.

PREVENTION
None

SUGGESTED READINGS
Available at www.expertconsult.com

RELATED CONTENT
Brugada Syndrome (Related Key Topic)
Ventricular Fibrillation (Related Key Topic)
Ventricular Tachycardia (Related Key Topic)

AUTHOR: **ALEEM MUGHAL, M.D.**

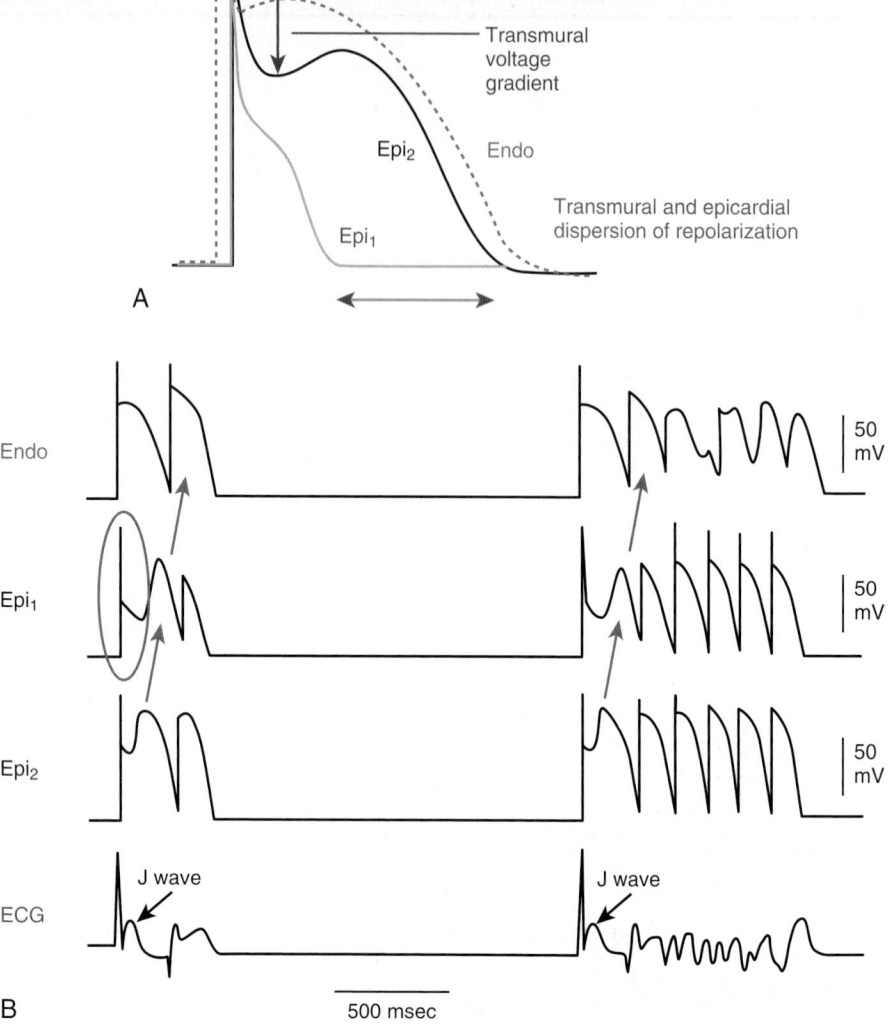

FIG. 3 Potential mechanism for arrhythmogenesis in the Brugada and early repolarization syndromes. **A,** With enhanced repolarization in regions with prominent transient outward current (I_{to}), all-or-none repolarization can occur, creating a substrate for arrhythmias. **B,** Simultaneous action potentials from two epicardial sites (Epi$_1$ and Epi$_2$) and one endocardial site (Endo), and surface ECG. A loss of the action potential dome in Epi$_1$, but not in Epi$_2$, leads to apparent propagation of the dome from Epi$_2$ to Epi$_1$, inducing reentry. (From Issa ZF, Miller JM: *Clinical arrhythmology and electrophysiology: a companion to Braunwald's heart disease*, ed 2, Philadelphia, 2012, Saunders.)

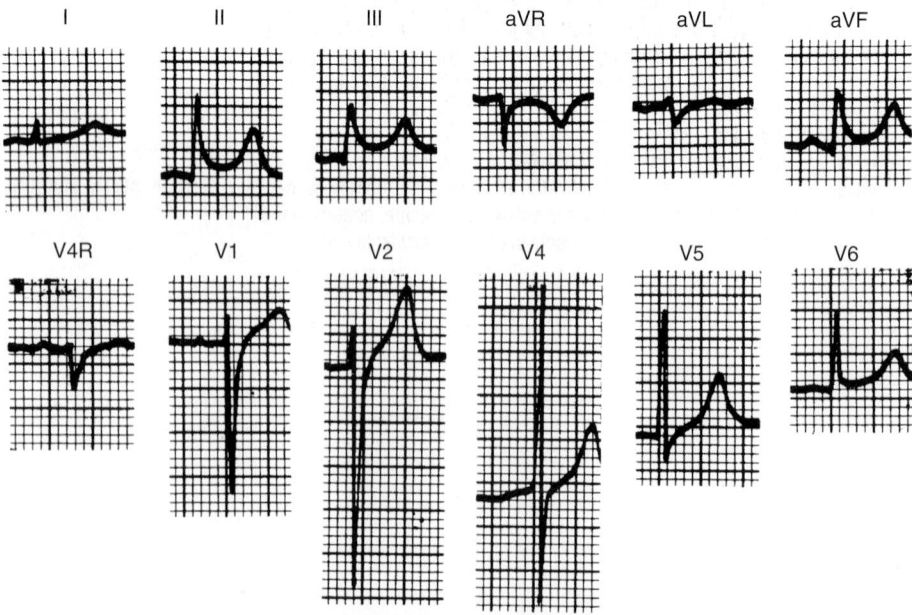

FIG. 4 Tracing from a healthy 16-year-old boy that exhibits early repolarization and J-depression. The ST segment is shifted toward the direction of the T wave and is most marked in II, III, and aVF. J-depression is seen in most of the precordial leads. (Park MK: *Park's Pediatric cardiology for practitioners*, ed 6, Philadelphia, 2014, Saunders.)

BASIC INFORMATION

DEFINITION

Echinococcosis is a chronic infection caused by the larval stage of several animal cestodes (tapeworms) of the genus *Echinococcus*.

SYNONYMS

Hydatid disease, hydatidosis, cystic echinococcosis (CE)
Alveolar echinococcosis (AE)
Polycystic echinococcosis

ICD-10CM CODES

B67.8   Echinococcosis, unspecified, of liver
B67.90 Echinococcosis, unspecified
B67.99 Other echinococcosis

EPIDEMIOLOGY & DEMOGRAPHICS

INCIDENCE (IN U.S.): Seen primarily in foreign-born patients, but local transmission of CE can occur in southwestern U.S., California, and Alaska. Found in areas where humans live in close proximity to dogs and livestock slaughtering. AE is found where humans have contact with wild foxes or coyotes, predominantly in the north central region of the U.S.
PEAK INCIDENCE: Presumed to be acquired in childhood or early adulthood in most cases, although prevalence increases with age.
PREVALENCE (IN U.S.): Prevalence in the U.S. is unknown.
PREDOMINANT SEX: Globally, women are more often affected by cystic echinococcosis than men. This higher prevalence in women is felt to be related to domestic activities that bring them in closer contact with dogs.
PREDOMINANT AGE: 0 to 50 years of age

PHYSICAL FINDINGS & CLINICAL PRESENTATION

- There are two predominant forms: cystic echinococcosis caused primarily by *E. granulosus* and alveolar echinococcosis caused by *E. multilocularis*. Rarely, polycystic echinococcus occurs in humans caused by *E. vogeli* and *E. oligarthrus*.
- Uncomplicated cystic echinococcosis is generally asymptomatic but may cause mass effect with signs of an enlarging mass lesion in a visceral site such as the liver, lungs, kidneys, bone, or CNS.
- Occasional cyst rupture may cause allergic manifestations such as urticaria, angioedema, or anaphylaxis that bring the patient to medical attention. Additionally, in the case of rupture, secondary bacterial infection may occur, or fistulas may develop (for example, cystobiliary).
- Incidental discovery of cysts by abdominal or thoracic imaging studies performed for other reasons
- Alveolar echinococcosis may mimic cirrhosis or liver cancer with upper abdominal discomfort, weight loss, and weakness. Rarely, it can spread to other tissues, including the brain.

ETIOLOGY

- There are currently nine recognized species of *Echinococcus*, of which seven cause human disease: *E. granulosus sensu stricto*, *E. equinus*, *E. ortleppi*, *E. Canadensis*, *E. multilocularis*, *E. oligarthrus*, and *E. vogeli*.
  1. Predominantly *E. granulosus* is the cause of cystic echinococcosis.
  2. *E. multilocularis* is the cause of alveolar echinococcosis.
- The disease is transmitted to humans by infected canines (domestic or wild dogs, wolves, foxes), which are the definitive hosts, and is seen most commonly in livestock-producing areas of the Middle East, Africa, Australia, New Zealand, Europe, and the Americas, including the southwestern U.S., whereby sheep, goats, camels, or cattle serve as intermediate hosts to humans. Humans are incidental hosts and do not play a role in the transmission cycle.
- The adult tapeworm resides in the small intestine of the canine definitive hosts. Eggs are then shed in the feces of infected canines; human infection occurs by ingestion of viable eggs in contaminated food from intermediate hosts or direct fecal-oral transmission.
- After ingestion of the eggs by intermediate hosts or humans, eggs hatch and release onchospheres, which migrate through intestinal mucosa to definitive organs and develop into enlarging fluid-filled cysts known as hydatid cysts (metacestode) (Fig. 1). The cyst is acellular and is surrounded by fibroblasts and lymphocytic infiltrate (Fig. E2).
- It is common in many areas of the world, especially the Middle East.

DIAGNOSIS

DIFFERENTIAL DIAGNOSIS

- Cystic neoplasms (see Table 1)
- Abscess (amebic or bacterial)
- Congenital polycystic disease

WORKUP

- Antibody assay (with limitations in sensitivity and specificity).
- Imaging study (CT scan [Fig. 3], ultrasonography).
- Classification (Fig. 4): Table 2 describes the World Health Organization Informal Working Group on Echinococcosis classification of hepatic echinococcal cysts.
- Histologic examination of cyst or contents obtained by aspiration or resection (if possible) to confirm diagnosis, although this is rarely indicated.

LABORATORY TESTS

Antibody assays (ELISA or Western blot) available through CDC: 80% to 100% sensitive and 88% to 96% specific for liver cysts, but less accurate for cysts in other sites, such as lung. A PCR assay is now available for problematic cases. Eosinophilia is not consistently seen and thus is not a reliable indicator.

IMAGING STUDIES

Ultrasonography, CT, and MRI:
- All are extremely sensitive for the detection of cysts, especially in the liver.
- All lack specificity and are inadequate to establish the diagnosis of echinococcosis with certainty.

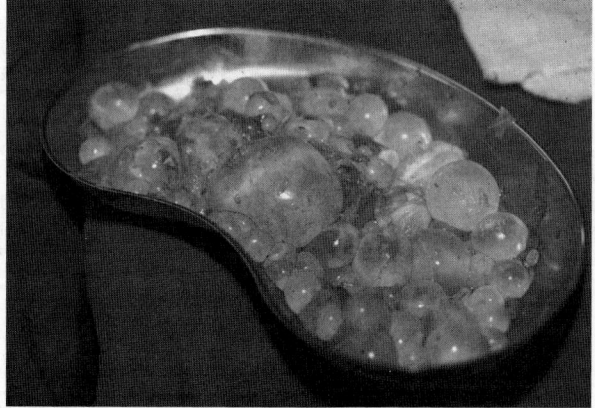

FIG. 1 Hydatid cysts removed surgically. (From Marx JA et al: *Rosen's emergency medicine*, ed 8, Philadelphia, 2014, Saunders.)

Table 1   Hepatic Cyst Disease: Differential Features on Imaging Studies

Characteristics	Hydatid Cyst	Congenital Cyst	Cystadenoma
Configuration	Cyst within cyst	Single or multiple ± septations	Single ± septations
Wall character	Thick, uniform ± calcification	Thin, uniform	Mural nodules
Cyst contents	Daughter cysts Hydatid sand	Low density	Low density

From Cameron JL, Cameron AM: *Current surgical therapy*, ed 10, Philadelphia, 2011, Saunders.

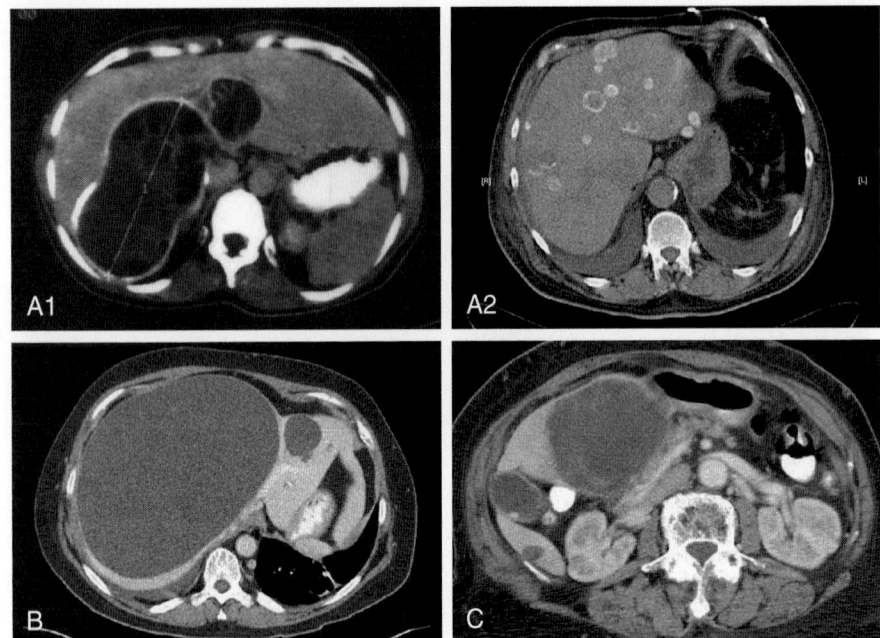

FIG. 3 A comparison of computed tomography scans. A, Hepatic echinococcal cysts. **B,** Congenital cyst. **C,** Cystadenoma. For echinococcal cyst. **A1** demonstrates a single cyst with calcification and daughter cyst caused by *E. granulosa*. **A2** shows multiple small cysts characteristic of *E. multilocularis* infection. (Courtesy Barbara M. Kadell, MD, Professor of Radiology, David Geffen School of Medicine at University of California, Los Angeles. From Cameron JL, Cameron AM: *Current surgical therapy,* ed 10, Philadelphia, 2011, Saunders.)

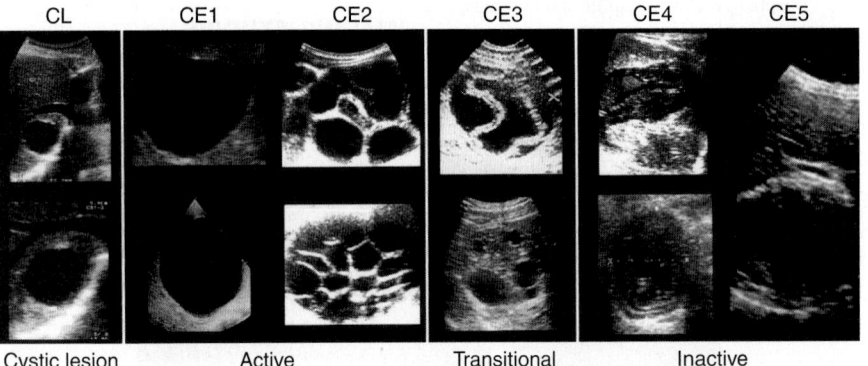

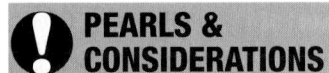

FIG. 4 WHO Informal Working Group on Echinococcosis standardized ultrasound classification of cystic echinococcosis. CL lesions are cystic lesions lacking a distinct wall and may have other diagnoses. CE1 lesions are cystic lesions with a visible wall that may demonstrate protoscolices ("hydatid sand"). CE2 lesions include internal septation. CE3 lesions may be detached from the wall or have daughter cysts with internal thickening. CE4 lesions are heterogeneous lesions with degeneration. CE5 lesions show thick calcification. (From Goldman L, Schafer AI: *Goldman's Cecil medicine,* ed 24, Philadelphia, 2012, Saunders.)

Rx TREATMENT

ACUTE GENERAL Rx

- There are four treatment modalities: percutaneous intervention, surgery, chemotherapy, and observation. Expert consultation is recommended.
- Albendazole 400 mg PO bid followed by percutaneous aspiration-injection-reaspiration (PAIR) for uncomplicated larval cysts. It consists of puncture (P) and needle aspirate (A) of cyst content followed by inspiration (I) of hypertonic saline (15%-30%) or absolute alcohol, waiting 20 to 30 minutes, then reaspirating (R) with final irrigation. Albendazole is continued for 28 days. Cure rate is 96%.
- Surgical resection: cure rate 90%.
- Alternatives to albendazole include mebendazole and praziquantel alone or in combination with mebendazole.

DISPOSITION

- Long-term follow-up is necessary following surgical or medical therapy because of the potential for late relapse.
- Antibody assays and imaging studies are repeated every 6 to 12 months for several years following successful surgical or medical therapy.

REFERRAL

All patients for evaluation for possible surgical resection of cysts versus PAIR

! PEARLS & CONSIDERATIONS

COMMENTS

Cyst resection, if indicated, should be performed by surgeons experienced with this procedure.

SUGGESTED READINGS

Available at www.expertconsult.com

RELATED CONTENT

Echinococcosis(Patient Information)

AUTHORS: **TARA C. BOUTON, M.D., M.P.H.&T.M.,** and **PHILIP A. CHAN, M.D., M.S.**

Table 2 WHO-IWGE Classification of Hepatic Echinococcal Cysts

Type of Cyst	Status	Ultrasound Features	Remarks
CL	Active	Signs not pathognomonic, unilocular, no cyst wall	Usually early stage, not fertile; differential diagnosis necessary
CE 1	Active	Cyst wall, hydatid sand	Usually fertile
CE 2	Active	Multivesicular, cyst wall, rosette-like	Usually fertile
CE 3	Transitional	Detached laminated membrane, "water lily" sign, less round, decreased intracystic pressure	Starting to degenerate, may produce daughter cyst
CE 4	Inactive	Heterogeneous hypoechogenic or hyperechogenic degenerative contents; no daughter cyst	Usually no living protoscolices; differential diagnosis necessary
CE 5	Inactive	Thick, calcified wall, calcification partial to complete; not pathognomonic but highly suggestive of diagnosis	Usually no living protoscolices

WHO-IWGE, World Health Organization Informal Working Group on Echinococcosis.
From Cameron JL, Cameron AM: *Current surgical therapy,* ed 10, Philadelphia, 2011, Saunders.

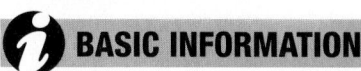 BASIC INFORMATION

DEFINITION

Eclampsia is the occurrence of seizures or coma in a woman with signs or symptoms of preeclampsia, occurring at >20 wk of gestation or <48 hr postpartum. Atypical eclampsia occurs at <20 wk of gestation or as much as 23 days postpartum.

SYNONYMS

Toxemia
Seizures of pregnancy

ICD-10CM CODES
015.00	Eclampsia in pregnancy, unspecified trimester
015.02	Eclampsia in pregnancy, second trimester
015.03	Eclampsia in pregnancy, third trimester
015.1	Eclampsia in labor
015.2	Eclampsia in the puerperium
015.9	Eclampsia, unspecified as to time period

EPIDEMIOLOGY & DEMOGRAPHICS

INCIDENCE: One case per 1500 to 3000 pregnancies; 2% to 4% of those with preeclampsia; one large Australian series found 8.6 cases per 10,000 live births.
GENETICS: Increased incidence with a first-degree relative (sister or mother) having had eclampsia.
RISK FACTORS: Multifetal gestation (3.6% in twin gestation), molar pregnancy, nonimmune hydrops fetalis, uncontrolled hypertension, preexisting hypertension, renal disease, systemic lupus, and existing heart disease.

PHYSICAL FINDINGS & CLINICAL PRESENTATION

- Seizure begins as facial twitching, then spreads to generalized tonic-clonic state, with cessation of respiration followed by a postictal period of amnesia, agitation, and confusion.
- The most common symptoms preceding eclampsia are headache (80%), visual disturbance (45%), and epigastric pain (20%). 50% will have proteinuria. 17% are completely asymptomatic prior to seizure.
- 40% have severe hypertension, 40% have mild to moderate hypertension, and 20% are normotensive.
- Generalized edema with rapid weight gain (>2 lb/wk) may precede eclampsia.
- Persistent occipital headache and hyperreflexia with clonus occur in 80% of patients with eclampsia; epigastric pain occurs in 20% of these patients.

ETIOLOGY

- Common pathway relates to abnormalities in autoregulation of cerebral blood flow. This may involve transient vasospasm, ischemia, cerebral hemorrhage, and edema occurring by a mechanism involving hypertensive encephalopathy, decreased colloid osmotic pressure, and prostaglandin imbalance.

Dx DIAGNOSIS

DIFFERENTIAL DIAGNOSIS

- Preexisting seizure disorder
- Metabolic abnormalities (hypoglycemia, hyponatremia, hypocalcemia)
- Substance abuse
- Head trauma, infection (meningitis, encephalitis)
- Intracerebral bleeding or thrombosis
- Amniotic fluid embolism
- Space-occupying brain lesions or neoplasms
- Pseudoseizure
- Hypertensive encephalopathy
- Venous or arterial thrombosis, arterial embolism
- Posterior reversible encephalopathy syndrome
- Vasculitis, angiopathy
- Thrombotic thrombocytopenic purpura

WORKUP

- Rule out other causes of seizures during pregnancy.
- Atypical presentations such as prolonged postictal state; status epilepticus; gestational age <20 wk or >48 hr postpartum; or signs of meningitis, substance abuse, or severe uncontrolled hypertension should prompt a search for other seizure etiologies.

LABORATORY TESTS

- Proteinuria: severe (49%), mild to moderate (29%), absent (22%).
- HCT: elevated as a result of hemoconcentration.
- Platelet count: decreased; LFTs elevated in HELLP syndrome (hemolysis, elevated liver enzymes, and low platelet count).
- BUN and creatinine: elevated with renal involvement.
- Serum electrolytes, glucose, calcium, toxicology profile: Rule out other causes of seizures.
- ABG: maternal acidemia and hypoxia.

IMAGING STUDIES

- CT scan or MRI indicated in atypical presentation, suspected intracerebral bleeding, or focal neurologic deficit.
- Over 90% of patients will have findings consistent with posterior reversible encephalopathy syndrome on MRI.
- There are abnormal findings, including cerebral edema, hemorrhage, and infarction, in 50% of patients.

Rx TREATMENT

ACUTE GENERAL Rx

- Maintain airway, adequate oxygenation, and IV access.
- Fetal resuscitation, involving maternal oxygenation, left lateral positioning, and continuous fetal heart rate monitoring, is needed.
- Magnesium sulfate is the drug of choice. Give magnesium sulfate 6 g IV load over 20 min, then 2 g/hr maintenance, for recurrent seizure prophylaxis. If repeated convulsions, may give an additional 2 g IV over 3 to 5 min. Approximately 10% to 15% of patients will have a second seizure after initial loading dose. Check magnesium level 1 hr after loading dose, then q6h (therapeutic range 4 to 7 mEq/L). Clinical signs of progressive Mg^{2+} toxicity, such as loss of reflexes, should also be followed. Respiratory and cardiac arrest occur at extremely high levels. Antidote for toxicity is calcium gluconate 10 ml of 10% solution. Phenytoin has been used as an alternative in patients in whom magnesium sulfate is contraindicated (renal insufficiency, heart block, myasthenia gravis, hypoparathyroidism).
- Give sodium amobarbital 250 mg IV over 3 min for persistent seizures.
- Treat blood pressure if >160 mm Hg/110 mm Hg with labetalol 20- to 40-mg IV bolus, hydralazine 10 mg IV, or nifedipine 10 to 20 mg sublingual q20 min.
- Evaluate patient for delivery.

CHRONIC Rx

- The first priority is stabilization of the mother in terms of adequate oxygenation, hemodynamics, and laboratory abnormalities, such as associated coagulopathies.
- Cervical status and gestational age should be assessed. If unfavorable cervix and <30 wk of gestation, consider C-section; otherwise consider induction.
- Give antenatal corticosteroids if 24 to 34-weeks' gestation. Consider antenatal corticosteroids if 34 to 36-6/7 weeks' gestation or 23-0/7 to 24 weeks' gestation.
- Controlled epidural is the anesthesia of choice for labor or C-section.
- Avoid general anesthesia in uncontrolled hypertension to minimize risk of catastrophic cerebral events.
- Continue magnesium sulfate through delivery process and for 24 hr postpartum or for at least 24 hr after the last convulsion.

DISPOSITION

The maternal mortality rate for eclampsia averages 5% to 6%. Morbidity rate is 25%, including placental abruption (10%), disseminated intravascular coagulation, maternal apnea with fetal asphyxia, aspiration pneumonia, pulmonary edema (4%), renal failure, cardiopulmonary arrest, and coma.

There is an increased risk of fetal death, neonatal death, preterm birth, and small-for-gestational-age birth.

REFERRAL

Because of the potential for serious permanent maternal and fetal sequelae, all cases should be managed by a team approach of obstetrician, neonatologist, and intensivist.

SUGGESTED READINGS
Available at www.expertconsult.com

RELATED CONTENT
Eclampsia (Patient Information)
HELLP Syndrome (Related Key Topic)
Preeclampsia (Related Key Topic)

AUTHOR: **RUBEN ALVERO, M.D.**, and **PHILIP A. SHLOSSMAN, M.D.**

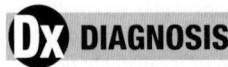

BASIC INFORMATION

DEFINITION

An ectopic pregnancy (EP) occurs when a fertilized ovum implants outside the endometrial cavity.

SYNONYMS

Tubal pregnancy (97%)
Interstitial (cornual) pregnancy (1%-2%)
Ovarian pregnancy (1%)
Abdominal pregnancy (0.03%-1%)
Cervical pregnancy (0.5%)

ICD-10CM CODES
O00.0 Abdominal pregnancy
O00.1 Tubal ectopic pregnancy
O00.2 Ovarian ectopic pregnancy
O00.8 Other ectopic pregnancy
O00.9 Ectopic pregnancy, unspecified

EPIDEMIOLOGY & DEMOGRAPHICS

- 1.5% to 2% of pregnancies
- 6% of maternal deaths

PREVALENCE (IN U.S.): Increasing number of EPs: 17,800 reported cases in 1970 and currently over 100,000 reported cases/year.

RISK FACTORS: Previous EP, previous pelvic infection (pelvic inflammatory disease, tubo-ovarian abscess, salpingitis), previous tubal ligation, previous tuboplasty, intrauterine device use, assisted reproductive techniques, cigarette use, age >35 years, multiple lifetime sexual partners

PHYSICAL FINDINGS & CLINICAL PRESENTATION:

- Abdominal tenderness: 95%
- Adnexal tenderness: 87% to 99%
- Peritoneal signs: 71% to 76%
- Amenorrhea or abnormal vaginal bleeding: 75%
- Adnexal mass: 33% to 53%
- Enlarged uterus: 6% to 30%
- Shock: 2% to 17%
- Shoulder pain: 10%
- Tissue passage: 6% to 7%

ETIOLOGY

- Anatomic obstruction to zygote passage
- Abnormalities in tubal motility
- Transperitoneal migration of the zygote

DIAGNOSIS

DIFFERENTIAL DIAGNOSIS

- Corpus luteum cyst
- Rupture or torsion of ovarian cyst
- Threatened or incomplete abortion

- Pelvic inflammatory disease
- Appendicitis
- Gastroenteritis
- Dysfunctional uterine bleeding
- Degenerating uterine fibroids
- Endometriosis

WORKUP

1. The classic presentation of EP includes the triad of abnormal vaginal bleeding, pelvic pain, and an adnexal mass. Fig. 1 describes a diagnostic approach to suspected EP. Fig. E2 *(top)* describes potential sites of ectopic implantations. Consider in all women with abdomino-pelvic pain and a positive pregnancy test.
2. Transvaginal ultrasound.
3. Quantitative serum human chorionic gonadotropin level.
4. Type and screen if presents with vaginal bleeding; give Rhogam if Rh-negative status on initial presentation of vaginal bleeding with positive pregnancy test.
5. Laparoscopy in equivocal situations and possibly for treatment.

LABORATORY TESTS

- Quantitative human chorionic gonadotropin (qhCG): Check on initial presentation. qhCG allows one to interpret initial ultrasound. If

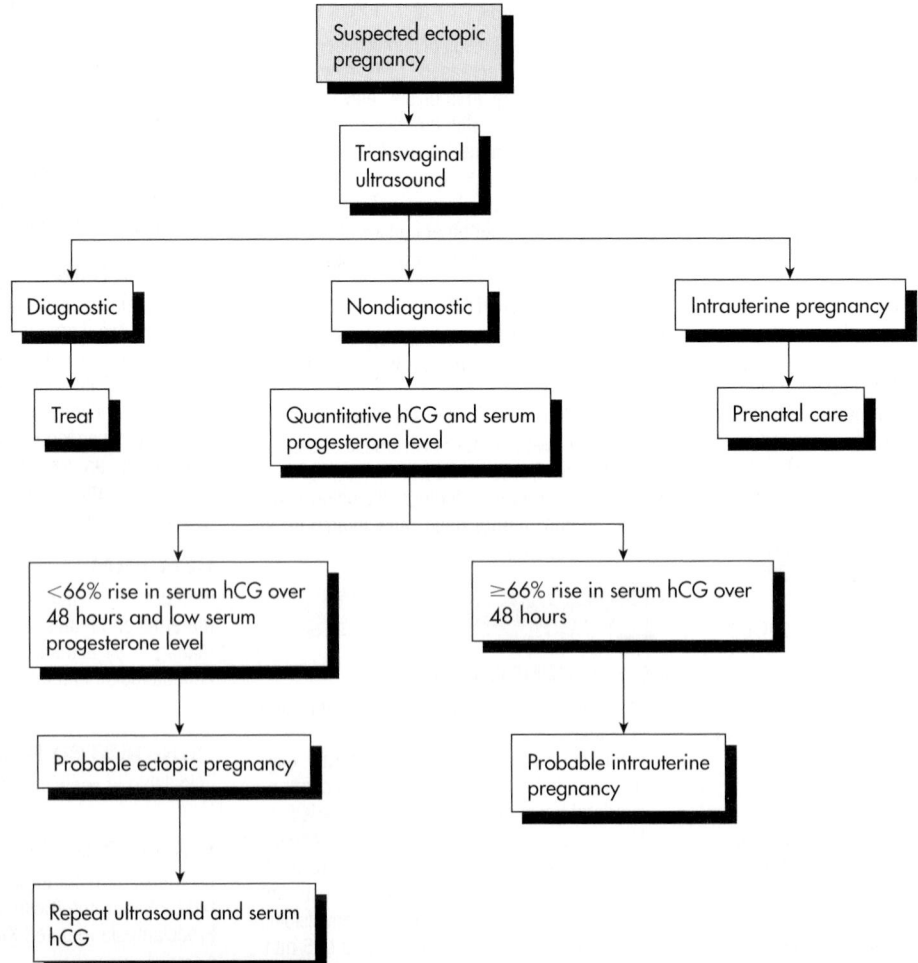

FIG. 1 Ectopic pregnancy. *hCG*, Human chorionic gonadotropin.

qhCG >6000 mIU/mL, should see intrauterine pregnancy (IUP) on abdominal scan; qhCG >1500 mIU/mL for transvaginal scan. The ability to visualize an early pregnancy is dependent on the gestational age and expertise of the ultrasonographer; therefore, some may use up to qhCG >3000 mIU/mL as the discriminatory threshold for transvaginal ultrasonography.

- Approximately 25% to 50% of women with an EP present with a pregnancy of unknown location, meaning that the initial ultrasound does not show a pregnancy in the uterus or the fallopian tube. Therefore, serial measurement of qhCG, typically obtained every 2 days, can help distinguish between an IUP, resolving miscarriage, or EP.
- 99% of normal IUP will have an increase of qhCG >53% within 2 days. However, 13% of ectopic pregnancies have a normal doubling time.
- Dropping hematocrit is associated with tubal rupture or possible abnormal intrauterine pregnancy.

IMAGING STUDIES

- Ultrasound: presence of an intrauterine yolk sac makes EP extremely unlikely. However, if the patient used assisted reproductive technologies, a heterotopic pregnancy (an EP with concurrent IUP) is much more likely to occur. A repeat ultrasonographic examination within 7 days after presentation may identify the location of a pregnancy that was not identified on initial ultrasonographic examination.
- Findings on ultrasound in EP include:
  1. Empty uterus (i.e., no yolk sac or fetal pole; a pseudosac in uterus may appear similar to a gestational sac).
  2. Adnexal mass (typically separate from adjacent ovary, commonly seen with "ring of fire" appearance).
  3. Fluid in cul-de-sac.
  4. Yolk sac and/or fetal pole in tube.
  5. Fetal cardiac activity in adnexa.

Rx TREATMENT

NONPHARMACOLOGIC THERAPY

Surgery performed via laparoscopy is preferred; however, laparotomy is appropriate if patient is very unstable or if visualization of the pelvis is poor at the time of laparoscopy.

- Salpingostomy, or resecting EP with conservation of tube, has the potential benefit of higher rates of subsequent IUP; however, recent randomized controlled trials suggest there is no difference in fecundity rate between salpingostomy and salpingectomy. The procedure requires postoperative serial monitoring of qhCG.
- Salpingectomy, or removal of affected fallopian tube, is considered the standard surgical procedure and is preferred in the following circumstances:
  1. Ruptured tube
  2. Future fertility not desired
  3. Recurrent EP in the same tube
  4. Uncontrolled hemorrhage
- Salpingiosis is the direct injection of chemotherapy into the EP by laparoscopy, transvaginal ultrasound, or hysteroscopy. Direct injection of methotrexate, and possibly KCl if there is active cardiac activity, may be performed when the pregnancy is in a location where there is high morbidity, such as the cervix, cesarean section scar, or cornu.

ACUTE GENERAL Rx

- Medical management with methotrexate, a folic acid antagonist, is a safe alternative if the patient is stable. Check the methotrexate safety labs prior to administration (CBC, creatinine, LFTs).
- Contraindications:
  1. Hemodynamically unstable; ruptured EP
  2. Patient unable to comply with follow-up
  3. Medical contraindication to methotrexate including the following: hepatic or renal disease, thrombocytopenia, leukopenia, or significant anemia
  4. Breastfeeding, preexisting blood dyscrasias, known sensitivity to methotrexate, active pulmonary disease, chronic liver disease, alcoholism, laboratory evidence of immunodeficiency, renal disease, and peptic ulcer disease
  5. Intrauterine gestation
- Relative contraindications
  1. EP >3.5 cm mass

  2. qhCG >5000 mIU/mL (more likely to require multidose regimen)
  3. Presence of cardiac activity in the fetus
- Most common regimen is methotrexate 50 mg/m^2 of body surface area and is administered on day 1. May require second dose or surgical intervention if qhCG increases or plateaus (<15% drop) when comparing values from day 4 and 7.
- Success rate of single-dose protocol approximately 88.1%. Rupture during methotrexate treatment ranges from 7% to 14%.
- Other methotrexate regimens include multidose protocol ± leucovorin rescue.
- Methotrexate side effects include nausea, vomiting, stomatitis, diarrhea, elevated LFTs, abdominal pain, and nephrotoxicity.

CHRONIC Rx

Persistent EP results from residual trophoblastic tissue or secondary implantation after conservative surgery. There is a 5% incidence of persistent EP with conservative treatment.

DISPOSITION

If diagnosed and treated early (before rupture), prognosis is excellent for good recovery. Monitor qhCG weekly until negative. Use reliable contraception until qhCG is negative. With subsequent pregnancies, follow qhCG and perform early ultrasound to confirm IUP. There is a 12% to 15% recurrence rate for EP.

REFERRAL

Should obtain gynecologic consultation if EP is suspected.

SUGGESTED READING
Available at www.expertconsult.com

RELATED CONTENT

Ectopic Pregnancy (Patient Information)
Spontaneous Miscarriage (Related Key Topic)
Vaginal Bleeding During Pregnancy (Related Key Topic)

AUTHORS: **TERRI Q. HUYNH, M.D.,** and **NIMA R. PATEL, M.D., M.S.**

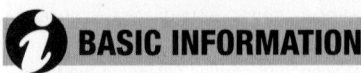

DEFINITION

Human monocytic ehrlichiosis (HME) and human granulocytic anaplasmosis (HGA) are tick-borne rickettsial diseases. Table 1 describes the agent, vector, and geographic prevalence of these diseases.

SYNONYMS

Human granulocytic ehrlichiosis (HGE)
Ehrlichiosis
Human monocytic ehrlichiosis (HME)
Human monocytotropic ehrlichiosis
Human granulocytic anaplasmosis (HGA)
Human granulocytotropic ehrlichiosis
Anaplasmosis
Ehrlichia phagocytophila
Anaplasma phagocytophilum

ICD-10CM CODES

A77.40 Ehrlichiosis, unspecified
A77.41 Ehrlichiosis chaffeensis [E. chaffeensis]
A77.49 Other ehrlichiosis

EPIDEMIOLOGY & DEMOGRAPHICS

INCIDENCE (IN U.S.): Highest overall incidence in Rhode Island (36.5 per 1 million), New York, New Jersey, Connecticut, Wisconsin, Minnesota, and northern California; >3000 cases identified in the United States since 2006.
PREDOMINANT SEX: Males outnumber females by 2 to 1.
PREDOMINANT AGE: Most severe disease 50 to 70 yr
PEAK INCIDENCE: Occurs throughout the year, with peak incidence between May and July and again in November.

PHYSICAL FINDINGS & CLINICAL PRESENTATION

- Symptoms of *E. chaffeensis* ehrlichiosis typically appear after a median of 9 days (range 5-14 days)
- Most common initial symptoms
  1. Fever (96%)
  2. Chills, rigor
  3. Headache (72%)
  4. Myalgia
- Subsequent symptoms
  1. Anorexia, nausea
  2. Arthralgia
  3. Cough
  4. Confusion (meningoencephalitis in 20% of patients with HME)
  5. Abdominal pain
  6. Rash (erythematous to pustular) <30% in HME, uncommon in HGA
- Complications
  1. Hepatitis
  2. Interstitial pneumonitis; acute respiratory distress syndrome
  3. Renal and respiratory failure
  4. Demyelinating polyneuropathy
  5. Toxic shock–like syndrome
  6. Life-threatening opportunistic infections

ETIOLOGY

- The causative agents are *Ehrlichia chaffeensis* and *Anaplasma phagocytophilum*
- Vector
  1. Almost certainly tick-borne, recently confirmed to be rarely transmitted by infected blood (including nosocomial infection).
  2. Transmitted by *Ixodes scapularis* in the northeastern states and *Amblyomma americanum* in the south central, southeastern, and mid-Atlantic states. Fig. 1 illustrates the life cycles of human monocytic ehrlichiosis (HME, with *Ehrlichia chaffeensis*) and human granulocytic ehrlichiosis (anaplasmosis).
  3. Tick exposure reported in >90% of patients, with ~60% reporting tick bite.
- Mammalian host: deer, horses, dogs, white-footed mice, cattle, sheep, goats, bison
- Host inflammatory and immune responses define final spectrum of disease beyond granulocytes, including hepatitis, interstitial pneumonitis, and nephritis with mild azotemia
- Between 6% and 21% of patients with HGE also have serologic evidence of other *Ixodes* spp. tick-borne diseases: Lyme disease or babesiosis
- Recovery is usual outcome; fatality rate of HGE is about 1%
- ICU care required: 7%

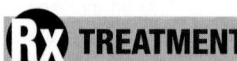

DIAGNOSIS

DIFFERENTIAL DIAGNOSIS

- Rocky Mountain spotted fever, Colorado tick fever, Q fever, relapsing fever
- Babesiosis
- Leptospirosis
- Lyme disease
- Tularemia
- Typhoid fever, paratyphoid fever
- Brucellosis
- Viral hepatitis
- Meningococcemia
- Infectious mononucleosis
- Hematologic malignancy
- TTP (thrombotic thrombocytopenic purpura)
- Table 2 describes clinical clues suggesting a diagnosis of a tick-borne illness manifesting as a nonspecific febrile illness

WORKUP

- Acute blood samples for Giemsa-stained smears
- CBC (leukopenia, thrombocytopenia), liver function (elevated), BUN/creatinine
- Acute serum samples for serology. Antibodies are seldom detected at time of acute infection (they usually appear 2-4 weeks following clinical illness).
- Chest radiograph examination
- Bone marrow rarely needed

LABORATORY TESTS

- Polymerase chain reaction (PCR) to facilitate early diagnosis: detection of *Ehrlichia* DNA in blood or CSF by PCR (Table E3)
- Giemsa-stained smear demonstrating morulae of the organism within granulocytes (sensitivity 20% to 75%) (Fig. E2)
- CBC: progressive leukopenia and thrombocytopenia with nadir near day 7

- C-reactive protein concentration is generally elevated
- Liver function tests (LFTs): increase in hepatic transaminases, lactate dehydrogenase, and alkaline phosphatase
- Elevated plasma creatinine concentration may be seen
- Serologic titer (IFA) >80 or fourfold increase in titer to *E. equi* antigen
- Culture on the first 7 days of illness; not readily available in most clinical laboratories

IMAGING STUDIES

- Chest radiograph examination to show interstitial pneumonitis (unusual)
- MRI of the brain

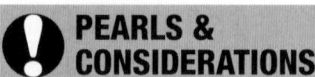

TREATMENT

ACUTE GENERAL Rx

- Immediate therapy to limit extent of acute illness and complication
- Doxycycline: 100 mg twice a day for 7 to 14 days is therapy of choice for adults and children >8 yr (4 mg/kg/day in 2 divided doses).
- Rifampin: 300 mg twice a day for 7 to 10 days can be used in pregnancy and for children <8 yr at 10 mg/kg twice per day
- Most patients defervesce within 24 to 48 hr given appropriate treatment.

PROGNOSIS

Poor prognostic indicators include:
- Advanced age
- Concomitant chronic illness (such as diabetes mellitus, collagen-vascular disease)
- Lack of diagnosis recognition
- Delayed onset of specific antibiotic therapy
- Concomitant HIV or organ transplant status

DISPOSITION

- Repeat CBC every 2 to 4 wk until normal.
- A new pathogenic *Ehrlichia* species, close relative of *E. muris* has been identified in Minnesota and Wisconsin. Organism-specific PCR and serologic testing can be used for identification.

REFERRAL

For consultation with infectious diseases specialist in suspected cases

! PEARLS & CONSIDERATIONS

COMMENTS

- Duration of time tick must be attached to produce illness as few as 4 hr
- Delay in antibiotic treatment results in poorer outcome. Antibiotic treatment should be initiated as soon as infection is suspected.

SUGGESTED READINGS

Available at www.expertconsult.com

RELATED CONTENT

Anaplasmosis (Patient Information)

AUTHOR: **PATRICIA CRISTOFARO, M.D.**

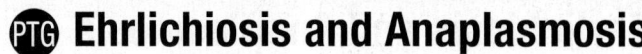

TABLE 1 Human Ehrlichioses and Anaplasmosis

	Human Monocytotropic Ehrlichiosis	Human Granulocytotropic Ehrlichiosis	Human Granulocytotropic Anaplasmosis
Former disease nomenclature	Human monocytic ehrlichiosis	Human granulocytic ehrlichiosis	Human granulocytic ehrlichiosis
Causative agent(s)	*Ehrlichia chaffeensis*	*Ehrlichia ewingii, Ehrlichia cani*—one asymptomatic human case reported in Venezuela	*Anaplasma phagocytophilum*
Leukocyte targets	Monocytic cell phagosomes	Neutrophil phagosomes	Granulocyte-neutrophil phagosomes
Tick vectors	*Amblyomma americanum* (lone star ticks)	*Amblyomma americanum* (lone star ticks), *Dermacentor variabilis* (American dog ticks)	*Ixodes persulcatus* complex (American deer ticks)—*I. scapularis, I. ricinus, I. pacificus*
Animal reservoirs	White-tailed deer, coyotes, dogs	White-tailed deer, dogs	Rodents, deer, ruminants, horses
U.S. regional distribution	Southeastern and south central United States	South central United States	Northeastern United States, upper Midwest, northern California
U.S. regional prevalence	2-5 cases/100,000	≤10% of presumed HME cases have *E. ewingii* infections in south central United States	50-60 cases/100,000; high seroprevalence rates in children (>20%) who have had subclinical infections
Seasonal occurrences	April-September, peaking in July	Spring-fall	May-July
Incubation periods (wk)	1-4	1-4	1-4
Modes of transmission	Tick bite, blood product transfusion	Tick bite, blood product transfusion	Tick bite, blood product transfusion, nosocomial
Frequently presenting clinical manifestations	Fever, malaise, headache, myalgias, rash in <40%	Same initial manifestations, but much milder, except in immunocompromised individuals	Fever, malaise, headache, myalgias; rarely rash
Laboratory abnormalities	Leukopenia, thrombocytopenia, transaminitis	Leukopenia, thrombocytopenia, transaminitis	More pronounced and prolonged leukopenia, thrombocytopenia, transaminitis
Potential complications, especially in immunocompromised individuals	Meningoencephalitis, acute renal and respiratory failure, hepatitis, myocarditis	Milder and less likely, except in patients immunocompromised by HIV/AIDS, organ transplantation, prolonged corticosteroid therapy	May be significant in immunocompromised patients with high fevers, seizures, confusion, hemorrhagic diathesis, rhabdomyolysis, shock, acute tubular necrosis, adult respiratory distress syndrome; some specific CNS complications may include eighth nerve palsy, brachial plexopathy, demyelinating polyneuropathy
Case-fatality rate (CFR)	3%, higher in immunocompromised individuals	No deaths reported	0.5%, higher CFR in immunocompromised individuals
Recommended confirmatory diagnostic tests	Wright-stained peripheral blood smears with characteristic intracytoplasmic morulae in monocytes, DNA detection by PCR assay, culture	Wright-stained peripheral blood smears with characteristic intracytoplasmic morulae in neutrophils, DNA detection by PCR	Wright-stained peripheral blood smears with characteristic intracytoplasmic aggregates in neutrophils, DNA detection by PCR assay, increased immunofluorescent antibodies in initial and paired serum samples
Current antibiotic resistance	Fluoroquinolones	Fluoroquinolones	Fluoroquinolones
Currently recommended antibiotic therapy, adults	Doxycycline, 100 mg PO bid, or tetracycline, 250-500 mg PO qid, for minimum of 3 days after defervescence to maximum of 14-21 days	Doxycycline, 100 mg PO bid, or tetracycline, 250-500 mg PO qid, for minimum of 3 days after defervescence to maximum of 14-21 days	Doxycycline, 100 mg PO bid, or tetracycline, 250-500 mg PO qid for minimum of 3 days after defervescence to maximum of 14-21 days
Currently recommended antibiotic therapy, children	Doxycycline, 4.4 mg/kg PO bid, or tetracycline, 25-50 mg/kg PO qid, for minimum of 3 days after defervescence to maximum of 14-21 days	Doxycycline, 4.4 mg/kg PO bid, or tetracycline, 25-50 mg/kg PO qid, for minimum of 3 days after defervescence to maximum of 14-21 days	Doxycycline, 4.4 mg/kg PO bid, or tetracycline, 25-50 mg/kg PO qid, for minimum of 3 days after defervescence to maximum of 14-21 days

CNS, Central nervous system; *HIV/AIDS,* human immunodeficiency virus infection/acquired immunodeficiency syndrome; *PCR,* polymerase chain reaction.
From Bennett JE , Dolin R, Blaser MJ: *Mandell, Douglas, and Bennett's principles and practice of infectious diseases,* ed 8, Philadelphia, 2015, Saunders.

E

Diseases and Disorders

I

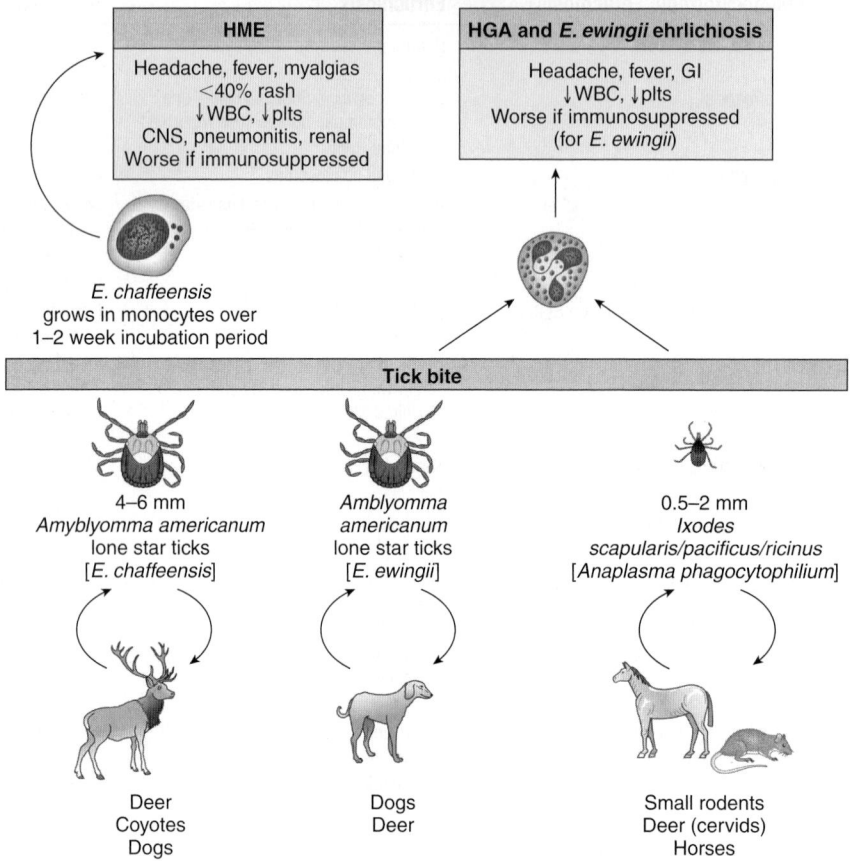

FIG. 1 Life cycles of human monocytic ehrlichiosis (HME, with *Ehrlichia chaffeensis*) and human granulocytic ehrlichiosis (anaplasmosis, HGA with *Anaplasma phagocytophilum*) or infection with *E. ewingii*. *CNS*, Central nervous system; *GI*, gastrointestinal; *WBC*, white blood cell count. (From Dumler JS: Ehrlichioses and anaplasmosis. In Guerrant RL, Walker DH, Weller PF (eds) *Tropical infectious diseases: principles, pathogens and practice*, 3rd ed, Philadelphia, 2011, Elsevier, pp. 339-343.)

TABLE 2 Clinical Clues (History, Physical Examination, or Laboratory) Suggesting the Diagnosis of a Tick-Borne Illness Manifesting as a Nonspecific Febrile Illness*

Disease	Clues
Anaplasmosis	Faint rash possible Low white blood cell or platelet count Elevated hepatic transaminases
Babesiosis	Findings of hemolysis History of splenectomy Presence of faint rash, hepatomegaly, or splenomegaly
Lyme disease	Careful skin examination for any rash consistent with erythema migrans Bradycardia from heart block Associated seventh nerve palsy or lymphocytic meningitis
Colorado tick fever	Saddle-back fever curve
Rocky Mountain spotted fever	Maculopapular or petechial rash Normal white blood cell count or low platelet count Hyponatremia Peripheral edema
Relapsing fever	Recurring episodes of fever with afebrile intervals
Tularemia	Acrally located ulcer Regional lymphadenopathy Possible associated pneumonia

*Apart from an epidemiologic context suggesting a tick-borne disease.

ⓘ BASIC INFORMATION

DEFINITION

Clinically significant disorders of ejaculation include failure of emission, retrograde ejaculation, premature ejaculation, delayed ejaculation, painful ejaculation, hematospermia, and anorgasmia. Failure of emission occurs when semen is not propulsed into the urethra during orgasm, resulting in a dry ejaculate. Retrograde ejaculation is a backward flow of semen into the bladder. Anejaculation refers to the absence of an antegrade and retrograde ejaculate, while aspermia refers to the absence of a visible antegrade ejaculate. Premature ejaculation refers to ejaculation that occurs sooner than desired, either before or shortly after penetration, causing distress to either one or both partners. Hematospermia is the appearance of blood in the ejaculate. Anorgasmia is the inability to achieve orgasm in a timely manner.

SYNONYMS

Ejaculatory dysfunction
Anejaculation
Dry ejaculate

ICD-10CM CODES
R36.1   Hematospermia; Bloody ejaculation
F52.4   Premature ejaculation
F52.32   Male orgasmic disorder; Inhibited male orgasm; Anorgasmia
N53.11   Delayed ejaculation; Retarded ejaculation
N53.12   Painful ejaculation
N53.13   Anejaculatory orgasm; Anejaculation
N53.14   Retrograde ejaculation
N53.19   Other ejaculatory dysfunction

EPIDEMIOLOGY & DEMOGRAPHICS

INCIDENCE: Not well understood, due to variability in definitions and reporting.
PEAK INCIDENCE: Not well understood.
PREVALENCE: Premature ejaculation is the most prevalent male sexual complaint, affecting 20% to 30% of men, and may be primary (lifelong) or acquired. Retarded or delayed ejaculation is the least common, least studied, and least understood of the male sexual dysfunctions.
PREDOMINANT SEX AND AGE: These disorders have been reported among men aged 18-70 years.
GENETICS: No known genetic predisposition.
RISK FACTORS: Men with ejaculatory dysfunction of any type usually indicate higher levels of relationship stress, sexual dissatisfaction, anxiety about sexual performance, and general health issues, compared to sexually functional men.

PHYSICAL FINDINGS & CLINICAL PRESENTATION

- Failure of emission: no ejaculate is produced during orgasm. Physical findings may reveal nervous system dysfunction (e.g., spinal cord injury); present with infertility.
- Retrograde ejaculation: little or no ejaculate is expelled out of the urethra at orgasm. Patients may report cloudy postcoital urine. Physical examination is usually normal; may present with infertility.
- Premature ejaculation: ejaculation occurs sooner than desired, often within 1 minute of penetration. Physical examination is normal. Up to 30% of patients may report concomitant erectile dysfunction.
- Delayed ejaculation: ejaculation requires prolonged sexual stimulation, often 30 minutes or longer. Physical examination is normal.
- Painful ejaculation: perineal, scrotal, or testicular pain during or shortly after ejaculation. Physical examination may demonstrate pain on examination of external genitalia, or with digital rectal examination; may present with infertility.
- Hematospermia: reddish-brown ejaculate, usually painless. Physical findings are usually unremarkable; not associated with malignancy.
- Anorgasmia: patient is not able to achieve orgasm despite appropriate stimulation.

ETIOLOGY

- Failure of emission may result from pelvic surgery, trauma, or radiation; from neurologic diseases such as Parkinson's disease, multiple sclerosis, spinal cord injury, or diabetes mellitus; from bilateral ejaculatory duct obstruction; or from psychological stress and anxiety.
- Retrograde ejaculation is most commonly caused by the use of medications (e.g., alpha-blockers) or surgical procedures (e.g., transurethral resection of prostate) that relax the bladder neck, but it can also be the result of retroperitoneal surgery and the previously mentioned neurologic diseases.
- Premature and delayed ejaculation represent opposite ends of the spectrum of ejaculatory disorders. The underlying etiology is complex and multifactorial, and includes organic and psychogenic contributions.
- Causes of painful ejaculation may be infectious (e.g., epididymo-orchitis, urethritis, prostatitis), obstructive (e.g., vasectomy, prostatectomy, hernia repair), or psychological.
- Hematospermia may be idiopathic, secondary to prolonged abstinence, or due to infection or inflammation of the genitourinary tract.
- Anorgasmia may be caused by spinal cord injury, psychological factors, dysfunctional sexual techniques, or medications, particularly serotonin reuptake inhibitors.

ⒹⓍ DIAGNOSIS

DIFFERENTIAL DIAGNOSIS

- Erectile dysfunction
- Hypogonadism
- Ejaculatory duct obstruction
- Urethral stricture disease
- Urethritis or sexually transmitted infection

LABORATORY TESTS

- Fig. 1 describes an algorithm for the evaluation of the patient with low-volume or absent (aspermia) ejaculate.
- For a low-volume ejaculate, post-ejaculate urine should be evaluated for the presence of spermatozoa to differentiate failure of emission from retrograde ejaculation.
- Hematuria, in the setting of hematospermia or painful ejaculation, may signal an underlying inflammatory disorder or a malignancy, and it should prompt a complete evaluation.
- A fasting blood glucose test may be considered if diabetes is suspected as a cause of lack of emission or retrograde ejaculation.
- Urinalysis, urine culture, and screening for sexually transmitted diseases, when indicated, can rule out an infectious etiology of painful ejaculation.

IMAGING STUDIES

Transrectal ultrasonography or pelvic MRI can rule out ejaculatory duct obstruction or absence of the seminal vesicles.

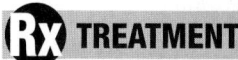 TREATMENT

NONPHARMACOLOGIC THERAPY

- Retrograde ejaculation and failure of emission do not require treatment unless fertility is desired.
- In the setting of retrograde ejaculation, viable sperm can be recovered from the post-ejaculate urine and used for intrauterine insemination or in vitro fertilization.
- Premature ejaculation can improve with psychotherapy and behavioral interventions (e.g., "coronal squeeze" or "start-and-stop" technique) and effective partner communication. These approaches may be more effective when combined with pharmacologic therapy.
- Idiopathic hematospermia may be followed expectantly and is usually self-limited to 10 or 15 ejaculations.
- Anorgasmia caused by serotonin reuptake inhibitors usually improves with withdrawal of the medication. Sexual therapy and counseling can improve anorgasmia caused by dysfunctional sexual techniques or psychological issues. Vibratory or electrical stimulation of emission is helpful in selected cases.

ACUTE GENERAL Rx

- Retrograde ejaculation: pharmacologic therapy is only effective in patients without an anatomic disturbance of the bladder neck. Sympathomimetic medications (phenylpropanolamine, ephedrine, pseudoephedrine) and imipramine may be useful in converting retrograde ejaculation to antegrade ejaculation.
- Premature ejaculation: selective serotonin reuptake inhibitors (SSRI) (e.g., sertraline, fluoxetine) and the tricyclic antidepressant clomipramine can successfully delay ejaculation when taken daily. Dapoxetine, a short-acting SSRI, may be used as an "on-demand" treatment for

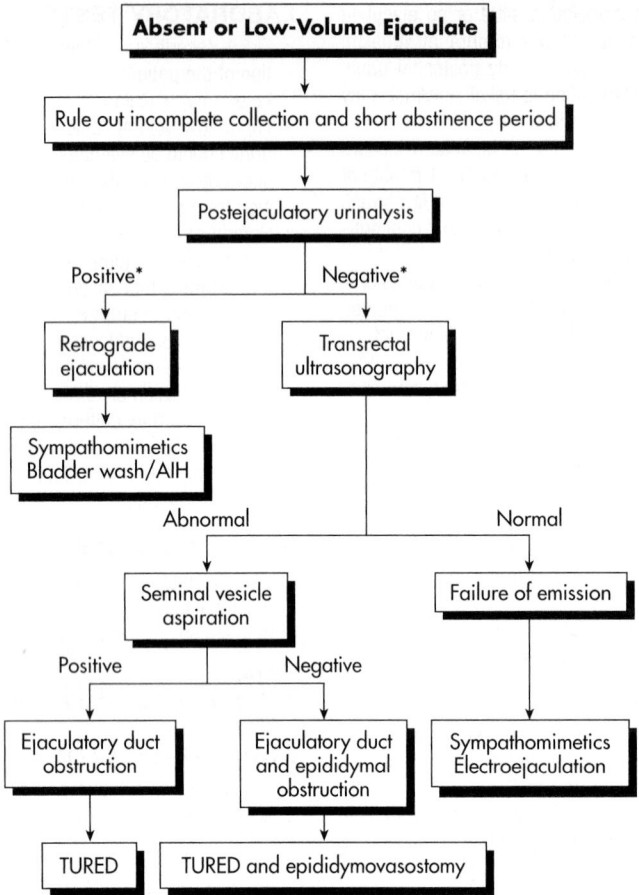

FIG. 1 Algorithm for the evaluation of the patient with low-volume or absent (aspermia) ejaculate. *AIH*, Artificial insemination using husband's sperm; *TURED*, transurethral resection of the ejaculatory ducts. *See text. (From Wein AJ; Male infertility. In Wein AJ et al (eds): *Campbell-Walsh urology*, Philadelphia, 2007, Elsevier.)

premature ejaculation (not available in the U.S.). Topical anesthetics such as lidocaine cream and topical sprays have been used with variable success. The use of phosphodiesterase inhibitors (PDE5i) (e.g., sildenafil, vardenafil, tadalafil) with SSRIs may be beneficial in men with concomitant erectile dysfunction and premature ejaculation.

- Antimicrobial treatment (if indicated), NSAIDs, and muscle relaxants may help decrease discomfort associated with painful ejaculation.
- The use of the pharmacologic therapies listed above for the treatment of various disorders of ejaculation is strictly off label and does not carry FDA approval.

CHRONIC Rx

Rarely, painful ejaculation due to long-standing obstructive causes may show improvement with surgical intervention (e.g., vasectomy reversal). The pharmacologic therapies listed previously can also be used for the chronic treatment of disorders of ejaculation and orgasm.

COMPLEMENTARY AND ALTERNATIVE MEDICINE

- A variety of nutritional supplements and herbs have been used for the treatment of erectile dysfunction, but their benefit for the specific treatment of ejaculation and orgasm disorders is unknown.
- Acupuncture and traditional Chinese medicine may be helpful in treating underlying hormonal imbalances.
- Yoga and meditation can reduce the effects of stress and relieve anxiety about sexual dysfunction.
- Therapeutic massage can decrease stress.

DISPOSITION

Prognosis varies with etiology. Ejaculatory dysfunction attributable to sexual techniques or psychological issues can improve with psychotherapy. Pharmacologic treatment is helpful in treating premature, retrograde, or painful ejaculation.

REFERRAL

All fertility issues and suspected anatomic problems should be referred to a urologist. Professional psychotherapy should be considered for appropriate patients.

ⓘ PEARLS AND CONSIDERATIONS

COMMENTS

Ejaculatory and orgasmic disorders are common male sexual dysfunctions and include failure of emission, retrograde ejaculation, premature ejaculation, delayed ejaculation, painful ejaculation, hematospermia, and anorgasmia.

PREVENTION

Preventing sexually transmitted infections and treating other inflammatory disorders of the genitourinary tract may be of some benefit in reducing the incidence of these sexual disorders.

PATIENT/FAMILY EDUCATION

These sexual disorders can exert a significant psychological burden on affected men and their partners. A combination of pharmacologic and nonpharmacologic therapies, including a urologic and psychologic evaluation, when indicated, may be helpful in the treatment of these complaints.

SUGGESTED READINGS
Available at www.expertconsult.com

RELATED CONTENT
Erectile Dysfunction (Patient Information)
Premature Ejaculation (Patient Information)
Erectile Dysfunction (Related Key Topic)

AUTHORS: **AKANKSHA MEHTA, M.D., M.S.,** and **MARK SIGMAN, M.D.**

BASIC INFORMATION

DEFINITION

Elder abuse includes abuse committed by someone in a trust relationship whether in the community or institutional setting.

- Physical abuse: inflicting physical pain or injury
- Sexual abuse: inflicting nonconsensual sexual activity
- Psychological abuse: inflicting mental anguish, including intimidation, humiliation, or threats
- Financial abuse: improper use of resources, property, or assets without the person's consent
- Neglect: abandonment, failure to fulfill a care-taking obligation, including provision of food, safe shelter, physical health and mental health care, or basic custodial care

SYNONYMS

Battered elder syndrome
Elder mistreatment
Domestic violence in the elderly
Diogenes syndrome
Intimate partner violence
IPV

Adult maltreatment and neglect problems cover a range of diagnostic codes depending on whether the issue is confirmed or suspected and whether the problem is physical, psychological, or sexual
Core Codes:
ICD-10CM CODES
T74   Maltreatment syndrome
T74.0 Neglect or abandonment
T74.1 Physical abuse
T74.2 Sexual abuse
T74.3 Psychological abuse
T74.8 Other maltreatment syndromes
T74.9 Maltreatment syndromes, unspecified

EPIDEMIOLOGY & DEMOGRAPHICS

INCIDENCE: 2013 CDC report estimates 500,000 adults 60 and older are subject to elder maltreatment yearly in the U.S.
PEAK INCIDENCE: >75 yr; more recent studies now suggest <75 yr
PREVALENCE:

- About 7.6% to 11% of those 60 yr or older.
- Emotional followed by financial abuse are the most common forms.
- 12-month U.S. prevalence rates: emotional abuse 9.0% and 4.6%; physical abuse 0.2% and 1.6%; sexual abuse 0.6%; neglect 0.5%; and financial abuse 3.5% and 5.2%.
- Family members reported 21% of nursing home residents were neglected on one or more occasion in the past 12 months, and over 24% had been subjected to physical abuse during their entire stay.

- Among caregivers of patients with dementia in the U.K., one half reported behaving abusively at least some of the time, and one third reported "important" levels of abuse. Verbal abuse was common and physical abuse was rare.
- Elder abuse is associated with increased risk of mortality, with the highest for caregiver neglect, functional impairment, and greater emotional distress, including depression, anxiety, and posttraumatic stress.
- Adult intimate partner violence perpetrators are significantly more likely to have witnessed intimate partner violence as a child than nonperpetrators.
- Older women are more likely than older men to be victims of abuse.

RISK FACTORS (VICTIM):

- Impaired cognition
- Behavioral problems
- Psychiatric illness or psychological problems
- Mental or physical dependence
- Poor physical health or frailty
- Trauma or past abuse
- Shared living situation and premorbid relationship with abuser
- Social isolation and poor social support
- Low household income

RISK FACTORS (PERPETRATOR):

- Relationship conflict with the victim
- Substance abuse, mental illness, particularly depression
- Caregiver burden or stress, being an involuntary caregiver, overwhelmed or resentful

PHYSICAL FINDINGS & CLINICAL PRESENTATION

- Physical abuse with multiple injuries at various stages with implausible descriptions of their origins.
- Fear, hypervigilance, or withdrawal.
- Evidence of poor nutrition, dehydration, poor hygiene, multiple or neglected pressure ulcers, genital or anal pain, neglected medical conditions, or evidence of restraint use (bruises around wrists or ankles).
- Toxicologic evidence of unprescribed medications.
- Poor adherence, frequent no-shows, or little contact with health care system.
- Caregiver not allowing interviewing the patient alone.

DIAGNOSIS

DIFFERENTIAL DIAGNOSIS

- Dementia
- Depression, substance misuse, or other psychiatric disorder
- Malnutrition from intrinsic causes
- Nonadherence to medical treatment
- Relationship distress
- Falling

WORKUP

1. Ask direct specific questions such as:

- "Has anyone close to you called you names or put you down recently?"
- "Are you afraid of anyone who lives with you or cares for you?"
- "Has anyone at home ever hurt you?"
- "Has anyone touched you without your consent?"
- "Has anyone forced you to do things you didn't want to do?"
- "Has anyone taken things or money that belong to you without your OK?"
- "Have you signed any documents that you don't understand?"
- "Are you often alone?"
- "When you need help has anyone ever failed to help you take care of yourself?"
- If appropriate, ask, "Have you been abused?"

2. Interview patient and alleged perpetrator separately.
3. Pelvic examination if sexual abuse suspected.
4. Take photographs of physical injuries as legal evidence.

LABORATORY TESTS & IMAGING STUDIES

- Screen for dehydration, malnutrition, and rhabdomyolysis.
- Toxicology screens and therapeutic drug monitoring are sometimes helpful.
- Other tests and radiology according to presentation.

TREATMENT

NONPHARMACOLOGIC THERAPY

- Separate patient and abuser.
- Patient and caregiver may benefit from psychiatric evaluation and treatment for substance abuse, mental illness, or cognitive impairment.
- If appropriate, assess the patient's capacity.
- Fig. 1 describes a management algorithm for elder abuse.

ACUTE GENERAL Rx

- As indicated for injury or pain relief
- As indicated for mental disorders, dementia, or delirium

DISPOSITION

If the patient's level of disability does not allow independent living, institutionalization may be required. Guidelines vary at the state and county levels regarding guardianship and conservatorship requirements.

REFERRAL

- For outpatients, report to local adult protective services agency. Reporting is mandatory in most states.
- Resident-to-resident elder mistreatment (R-REM) in nursing homes is highly prevalent. For nursing home patients, report to regional long-term care ombudsman. Reporting is mandatory under federal law.
- Mental health services may be needed.

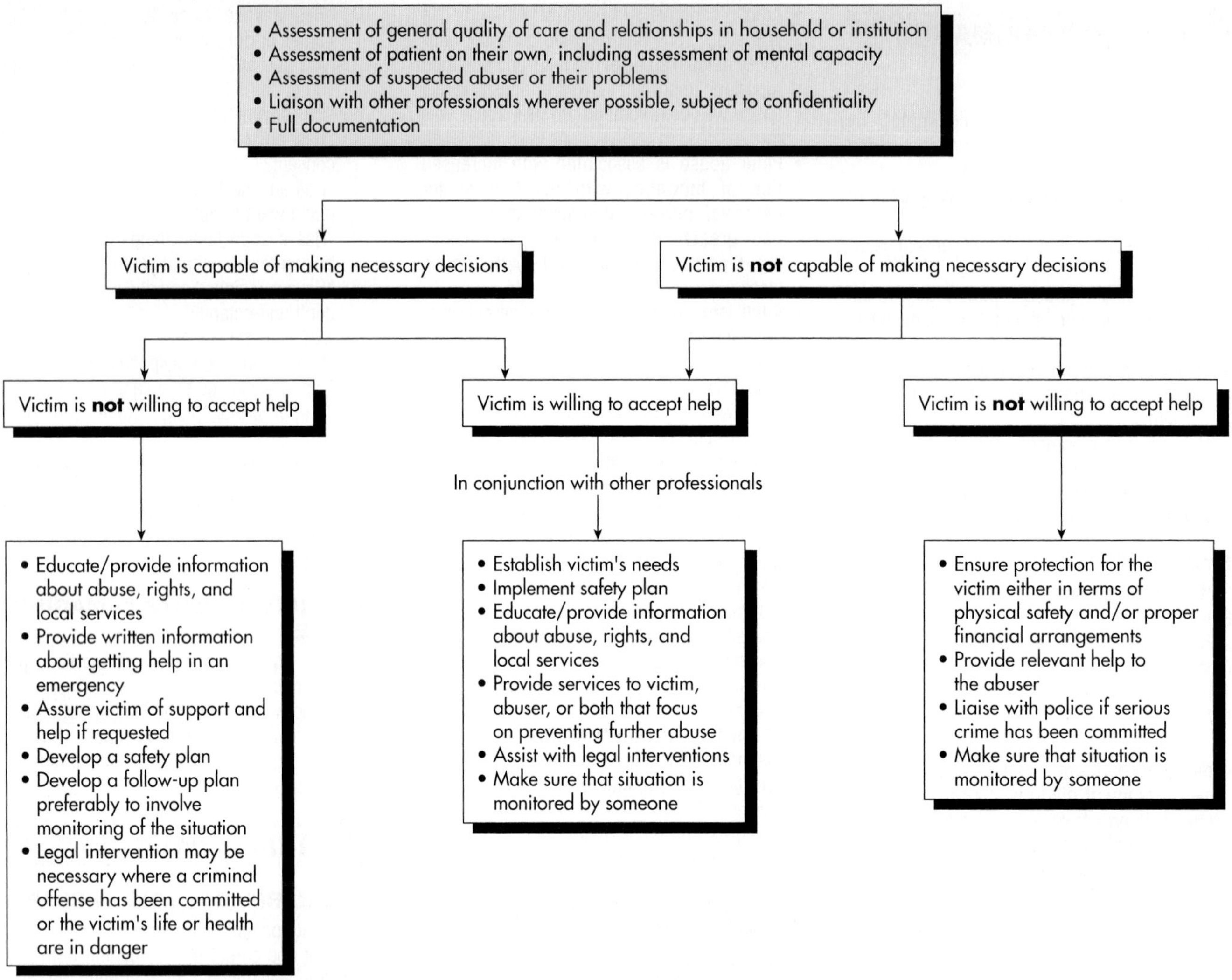

- Assessment of general quality of care and relationships in household or institution
- Assessment of patient on their own, including assessment of mental capacity
- Assessment of suspected abuser or their problems
- Liaison with other professionals wherever possible, subject to confidentiality
- Full documentation

| Victim is capable of making necessary decisions | Victim is **not** capable of making necessary decisions |

Victim is not willing to accept help

Victim is willing to accept help

In conjunction with other professionals

Victim is not willing to accept help

- Educate/provide information about abuse, rights, and local services
- Provide written information about getting help in an emergency
- Assure victim of support and help if requested
- Develop a safety plan
- Develop a follow-up plan preferably to involve monitoring of the situation
- Legal intervention may be necessary where a criminal offense has been committed or the victim's life or health are in danger

- Establish victim's needs
- Implement safety plan
- Educate/provide information about abuse, rights, and local services
- Provide services to victim, abuser, or both that focus on preventing further abuse
- Assist with legal interventions
- Make sure that situation is monitored by someone

- Ensure protection for the victim either in terms of physical safety and/or proper financial arrangements
- Provide relevant help to the abuser
- Liaise with police if serious crime has been committed
- Make sure that situation is monitored by someone

FIG. 1 Management of elder abuse. (From Tallis RC, Fillit HM [eds]: *Brocklehurst's textbook of geriatric medicine and gerontology,* ed 6, London, 2003, Churchill Livingstone.)

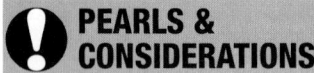

PEARLS & CONSIDERATIONS

COMMENTS
Care should be taken in interacting with the alleged abuser so that access to the victim is not lost.

PREVENTION
- Offer social services (e.g., respite care or homecare) for stressed caregivers.

- Make financial arrangements and arrange durable power of attorney for health care and finances while patient is still cognitively intact.

PATIENT & FAMILY EDUCATION
In the U.S., the elder care help line is 1-800-677-1116.
National Center on Elder Abuse: http://www.ncea.aoa.gov
JAMA Patient Page: Hildreth CJ et al: JAMA patient page. Elder abuse, *JAMA* 302(5):588, 2009

SUGGESTED READINGS
Available at www.expertconsult.com

RELATED CONTENT
Elder Abuse (Patient Information)

AUTHOR: **ROBERT KOHN, M.D.**

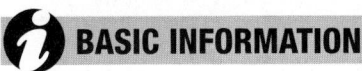

BASIC INFORMATION

DEFINITION

Injuries or wounds that occur as a result of contact with an electrical current or lightning.

ICD-10CM CODES
W87	Exposure to unspecified electric current
W86	Exposure to other specified electric current
W85	Exposure to electric transmission lines
X33	Victim of lightning
T75.4XXA	Electrocution, initial encounter

EPIDEMIOLOGY & DEMOGRAPHICS

- Causes approximately 1000 deaths annually, with two thirds occurring in persons between ages 15 and 40 yr.
- Most electrical injuries in children occur at home (e.g., oral burns from electrical appliances).
- Most electrical injuries in adults are occupationally related. They rank fifth as a cause of occupational death.
- Account for 4% to 6.5% of all admissions to burn units.
- Lightning strikes kill on average 100 people annually.
  1. Eight of every 10 lightning strike victims are male; 75% of lightning deaths in the U.S. occur in the South and Midwest.
  2. 25% of lightning deaths are work related.
- Electronic weapons (stun gun and Taser) are capable of causing fatal cardiac arrhythmias.
- Table 1 compares lightning injuries with high-voltage electrical injuries.

PHYSICAL FINDINGS & CLINICAL PRESENTATION

- Cognitive changes: depending on the extent of injury, the patient may be unconscious, seizing, or confused and unable to present a history.

TABLE 1 Lightning Injuries Compared with High-Voltage Electrical Injuries

Factor	Lightning	High Voltage
Energy level	30 million volts, 50,000 Å	Usually much lower*
Time of exposure	Brief, instantaneous	Seconds
Pathway	Flashover, orifice	Deep, internal
Burns	Superficial, minor	Deep, major injury
Renal	Rare myoglobinuria or hemoglobinuria	Myoglobinuric renal failure common
Fasciotomy	Rarely if ever necessary	Common, early, and extensive
Blunt injury	Explosive thunder effect	Falls, being thrown

*Range is 500 V up to millions of volts in transmission lines.
From Auerbach P: *Wilderness medicine, expert consult* Premium Edition—Enhanced Online Features and Print, Philadelphia, 2012, Saunders.

- Extensive skin burns (>10% of the body surface).
  1. Located over the entry and exit sites (Fig. 1).
  2. Most common entry sites are the hands and skull.
  3. Most common exit sites are the heels.
  4. "Kissing burns" over the flexor creases.
  5. Oral burns are common in children; bleeding from the labial artery may present 7 to 10 days after the injury.
  6. Charring at the contact site (Fig. E2).
- Asystole or ventricular fibrillation may be the initial cardiac rhythm.
- Bone fractures and periosteal burns.
- Compartment syndrome from severe muscle tissue damage.
- Headaches, memory disturbances.
- Weakness and paresthesias.
- Otologic injury, conductive hearing loss from tympanic membrane rupture or ossicular disruption.
- Rhabdomyolysis and myoglobin-induced acute tubular necrosis.
- Vascular injury from coagulation of small vessels or compartment syndrome.
- Box E1 summarizes the immediate and delayed effects of lightning injuries.

ETIOLOGY

- Electricity causes tissue injury by converting electrical energy into heat or by blunt trauma from being thrown from the electrical source or from continuous muscle contraction (tetany).
- The effects of electricity are determined by seven factors: (1) type of current, (2) amount of current, (3) pathway of current, (4) duration, (5) area of contact, (6) resistance of the body, and (7) voltage.
- Tissue damage is greater with higher voltage and longer duration of contact.
- Direct current (DC) contact causes a single muscle contraction, throwing the patient away from the source. Alternating current (AC) contact precipitates a tetanic contraction, not allowing the patient to withdraw from the source and prolonging the duration of contact. AC contact is more ominous than DC contact.
- Electrical injuries are arbitrarily divided into high-voltage (>1000 volts) and low-voltage (<1000 volts) burns. Low-voltage burns involve almost exclusively either the hands or oral cavity. High-voltage injuries have a wide variety of systemic manifestations.
- The entry and exit path of the electrical current determines which tissues are affected.
- Box 2 describes the mechanisms of lightning injury.

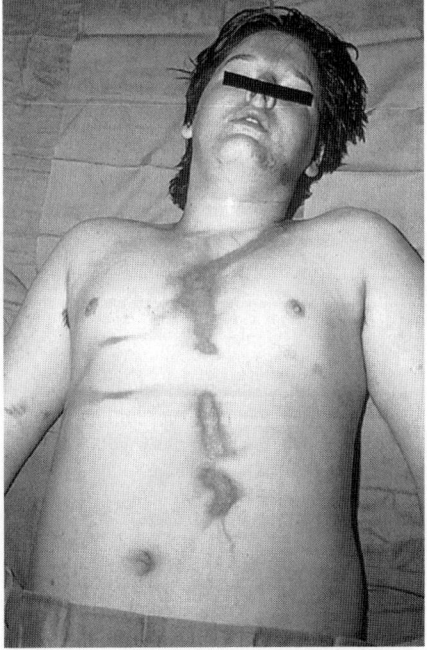

FIG. 1 The arborescent current markings on the face, neck, and anterior trunk of this young patient, which are characteristic of lightning injury, healed without the need for grafting. Note the focal lesions on the right arm, indicating the spread of the current that produced the marks on the right anterolateral aspect of the chest wall. (From Goldman L, Schafer AI: *Goldman's Cecil medicine,* ed 24, Philadelphia, 2012, Saunders.)

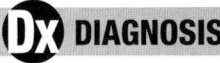

DIAGNOSIS

WORKUP

Physical examination may not reveal the extent of damage that has occurred. Detailed testing to determine the extent of internal organ damage is indicated. In lightning injuries, male victims may have scrotal (on the undersurface of the scrotum) and penile burns, which may often be overlooked. Hemorrhage behind the eardrum with or without perforation is not uncommon. An otoscopic examination is indicated in all lightning-strike victims.

LABORATORY TESTS

- Complete blood count
- Blood chemistry profile including electrolytes
- Blood urea nitrogen and creatinine
- Arterial blood gas analysis
- Myoglobin
- Creatinine kinase with isoenzyme fractionation
- Urinalysis, including screening for myoglobinuria
- Liver function tests
- Type and cross-match
- ECG

IMAGING STUDIES

- Radiographs: any suspicious area for bone fractures
- CT scan of the head and cervical spine in patients with suspected head injury, coma, or neurologic deficit

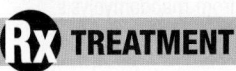

TREATMENT

NONPHARMACOLOGIC THERAPY

- At the scene: ensure the electrical power source of injury is turned off before approaching patients.
- Basic and advanced cardiac life support with cervical spine precautions. Prolonged cardiopulmonary resuscitation should be undertaken regardless of the initial cardiac rhythm.
- Cardiac monitoring.
- Oxygen.
- Tetanus prophylaxis.

BOX 2 Mechanisms of Lightning Injury

Electrothermal Effects
1. Direct strike
2. Contact potential
3. Side flash, sometimes called "splash" (1 to 3 may include surface arcs over the body surface)
4. Step voltage (also termed "Earth potential rise" or "ground current")
   a. Transmitted through the ground
   b. Surface arcing
5. Upward streamer current (also called "fifth mechanism")

Blunt Force Trauma Effects
1. Barotrauma
2. Concussive injury
3. Musculoskeletal injury from muscle contraction, falls

From Auerbach P: *Wilderness medicine, expert consult* Premium Edition—Enhanced Online Features and Print, Philadelphia, 2012, Saunders, Elsevier.

ACUTE GENERAL Rx

- IV fluids to maintain urine output of 50 to 100 ml/hr (IV hydration should be reassessed with central nervous system expert in patients at risk of developing cerebral edema).
- Alkalinization of the urine (sodium bicarbonate 50 mEq in 1 L of normal saline) in patients with or at risk of myoglobinuria.
- Furosemide 20 to 40 mg PO or IV and/or mannitol 12.5 g/kg/hr may be used to force diuresis.
- Seizures are treated in the standard fashion.
- Treat burns with sulfadiazine silver dressings.

CHRONIC Rx

- Hospitalization is indicated in patients with high-voltage injuries, extensive burns, central nervous system symptoms, myonecrosis (creatine kinase level more than twice normal, high serum myoglobin levels, or myoglobinuria), new cardiac arrhythmia or ECG changes, or any internal organ damage.
- Ophthalmology consultation at the follow-up to screen for cataract formation (occurs within 1 to 24 mo of a high-voltage electrical injury in 5% to 20% of patients).

DISPOSITION

- Patients with severe burns should be transferred to the regional burn center.
- Complications of electrical injuries include:
  1. Infection
  2. Renal failure from rhabdomyolysis
  3. Seizure disorder
  4. Fasciotomies
  5. Amputation
- Delayed neurologic damage may present as ascending paralysis, amyotrophic lateral sclerosis, or transverse myelitis weeks to years after the injury.
- Vascular damage may also present in a delayed fashion.

REFERRAL

- Referrals to general surgery, burn surgery, trauma surgery, orthopedic surgery, and/or

BOX 3 Myths Commonly Cited as Facts in Litigation

These apply to electrical injury as well as lightning injury.

Behavior of Current in the Body
- Current seeks earth.
- Current seeks the path of lowest resistance.
- Nerve tissue is a good conductor, or alternatively, current is preferentially conducted by nerve tissue.
- When a person touches a source of potential, current flows through the skin to other parts of the skin in contact with the same conductor (i.e., current passage is local only).

The Severity of Electric Shock
Myth: If the following are absent, the shock cannot be severe and no deleterious effect can result:
- Being thrown (i.e., if a person is not thrown, the shock is not severe).
- Burns (i.e., if burns are not present, the shock is not severe).
- If the only surface change is a blister, the shock was not severe.
- Entry and exit wounds:
  ○ Must be present.
  ○ Demonstrate the current path.
  ○ If not present, indicate no shock occurred.
- Fuses being blown (i.e., if a fuse does not blow, the shock is not severe enough to harm a victim).
- Low voltage cannot harm.
- Electroconvulsive therapy does not give long-term post–electric-shock symptoms (also false), so any other electric shock cannot be harmful.

Investigations
- If computed tomography (CT) and magnetic resonance imaging (MRI) scans are normal, there are no injuries.
- Negative investigations (e.g., nerve conduction study, electroencephalogram, CT, MRI) mean a victim has not sustained an electric shock.
- Neuropsychological testing is objective and easily interpreted.
- Burns of electrical origin can be distinguished on histologic examination.

Remote Symptoms
- Remote symptoms do not exist.
- Remote symptoms are proportional to the size of the shock.
- Symptoms of the shock that are not present immediately after the shock are not related to it.
- A person getting remote symptoms was psychologically vulnerable all the time.

Miscellaneous
- Litigation increases the potency of the claimed symptoms. Corollary: Resolving litigation terminates symptoms.
- Medical specialists understand electricity or lightning.
- Electrical experts can predict lightning or electrical injury.
- A diagnosis of depression, posttraumatic stress disorder, adjustment disorder, and so on negate an electrical injury causation.
- Residual current devices (RCDs) eliminate the possibility of all shocks. Corollary: A shock occurring when an RCD breaks the circuit cannot be severe.

From Auerbach P: *Wilderness medicine, expert consult* Premium Edition—Enhanced Online Features and Print, Philadelphia, 2012, Saunders, Elsevier.

critical care specialists as appropriate in any patient that meets hospitalization criteria. Ophthalmology and ear-nose-throat specialist referral may be indicated.
- Plastic surgery is recommended in children with oral burns.

(!) PEARLS & CONSIDERATIONS

COMMENTS

- The size of external skin burns can often underestimate the degree of internal injury.
- Lightning Strike and Electric Shock Survivors International is a support group that serves people from around the world who have sustained an electric injury (http://www.lightning-strike.org).

- Home safety education provided one-to-one in a clinical setting or at home, especially with the provision of safety equipment, is effective in increasing the range of safety practices.
- Box 3 describes myths regarding electrical and lightning injury commonly cited as facts in litigation.

RELATED CONTENT

Electrical Injury (Patient Information)

AUTHORS: **ROBERT M. KIRCHNER, M.D.,** and **PAUL GORDON, M.D.**

BASIC INFORMATION

DEFINITION

An accumulation of pus in the pleural space, most often caused by bacterial infection.

SYNONYMS

Infected pleuritis
Infected pleural effusion
Purulent pleural effusion

EPIDEMIOLOGY & DEMOGRAPHICS

- Empyema is most commonly a complication of bacterial pneumonia, especially in association with pneumococcal or anaerobic infection (40% to 60% of cases of empyema).
- Occurs as a complication of thoracic surgery (<20% of cases).
- Penetrating chest trauma (4% to 10% of cases).
- Bronchopleural fistulae resulting from malignancy or lung biopsy.

PHYSICAL FINDINGS & CLINICAL PRESENTATION

- May be abrupt or chronic and insidious depending on the etiologic agent and host factors.
- Typically presents as progressive pleuritic chest pain, persistent fever, and other sustained signs and symptoms of infection.
- In anaerobic empyema, particularly that caused by the actinomycetes, the clinical picture is dominated by systemic symptoms and signs: weight loss, malaise, and low-grade fever.
- A slowly enlarging chest wall mass.
- As a complication of thoracic trauma or surgery, empyema typically results from contamination of blood within the pleural space several days following the event.
- The physical findings of empyema are those of pleural effusion. Decreased breath sounds and dullness to percussion over the involved part of the thorax is typical. Systemic signs include fever, tachycardia, leukocytosis, and warmth and erythema over the involved area.

ETIOLOGY

Infection of the lung parenchyma spreading to pleural space caused by

- *Streptococcus pneumoniae.*
- *Haemophilus influenzae.*
- *Staphylococcus aureus.*
- *Legionella* species.
- *Mycobacterium tuberculosis.*
- *Actinomyces* spp.
- A variety of oral anaerobic bacteria have been cultured in 36% to 37% of empyemas: *Bacteroides fragilis, Prevotella* species, *Fusobacterium nucleatum,* and *Peptostreptococcus* are the most common.

DIAGNOSIS

DIFFERENTIAL DIAGNOSIS

- Uninfected parapneumonic effusion.
- Lung abscess (see Fig. 1)
- Congestive heart failure.
- Malignancy involving the pleura.
- Tuberculous pleurisy.
- Collagen vascular disease (particularly rheumatoid lung and systemic lupus erythematosus).

LABORATORY TESTS

- Complete blood count; arterial blood gas.
- Blood cultures.
- Pleural fluid analysis in empyema has the characteristics of an exudate with a ratio of pleural fluid to serum protein >0.5 or pleural fluid to serum LDH >0.6. Characteristically, empyema fluid is grossly purulent with visible organisms on Gram stain with glucose <50 mg/dl and pH <7. These findings justify immediate drainage by chest tube or surgery because of the high risk of loculation and progressive systemic infection.

IMAGING STUDIES

- Chest x-ray (Fig. E2*A*).
- Lateral decubitus view to establish the presence of free fluid in the pleural space.
- Computed tomography (Fig. E2*B*) to establish the presence of fluid loculation, underlying mass lesions, and other intrathoracic pathology.

TREATMENT

NONPHARMACOLOGIC THERAPY

Prompt drainage by thoracostomy (chest tube) or open thoracotomy. Video-assisted thorascopic surgery (VATS) has greatly improved surgical management of empyemas.

ACUTE GENERAL Rx

- Maintenance of drainage until infection controlled.
- Antibiotics directed at suspected or proven bacterial or fungal pathogens. Initial regimens include cefotaxime or ceftriaxone

for suspected *S. pneumoniae* or group A *Streptococcus*, nafcillin or oxacillin for suspected methicillin-sensitive *S. aureus*, vancomycin or linezolid for suspected MRSA, ceftriaxone for suspected *H. influenzae*, and clindamycin plus ceftriaxone when suspecting anaerobes. Other agents with excellent anaerobic coverage include carbapenem antibiotics such as meropenem and ertapenem and piperacillin/tazobactam (Zosyn). These agents also have excellent Gram-negative coverage.
- Thoracoscopy or instillation of thrombolytic agents (streptokinase or urokinase) may be considered in refractory, loculated empyema.

CHRONIC Rx

- If thorough drainage cannot be accomplished, open thoracotomy with pleural decortication may be required.
- Lung function should be monitored following completion of therapy.

DISPOSITION

Hospitalization with supplemental oxygen with ventilatory support if necessary

REFERRAL

Consultation by infectious diseases, pulmonary, or thoracic surgery specialists as needed.

PEARLS & CONSIDERATIONS

COMMENTS

- Empyema caused by actinomycetes may present with erosion through the chest wall and formation of a fistulous tract.
- Nosocomial infection caused by relatively resistant bacterial or fungal pathogens may result in empyema in patients with indwelling thoracostomy tubes.

SUGGESTED READINGS

Available at www.expertconsult.com

AUTHOR: **GLENN G. FORT, M.D., M.P.H.**

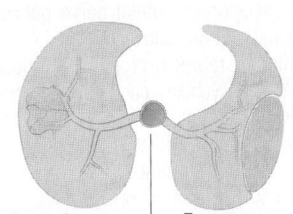

Lung abscess	Empyema
Poorly defined	Well defined
Irregular wall	Smooth, uniform wall
Spherical	Elliptical
Multiple cavities	"Split pleura"
Acute angles	Acute or obtuse angles
Vessels not displaced	Vessels displaced

FIG. 1 Empyema versus lung abscess. (From Webb WR, Brant WE, Major NM: *Fundamentals of body CT,* ed 4, Philadelphia, 2015, Saunders.)

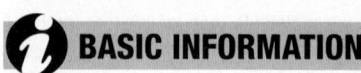

BASIC INFORMATION

DEFINITION

Acute viral encephalitis is an acute febrile syndrome with evidence of meningeal involvement and of derangement of the function of the cerebrum, cerebellum, or brain stem.

SYNONYMS

Arboviral encephalitis
Brain stem encephalitis
Acute necrotizing encephalitis
Rasmussen encephalitis
Encephalitis lethargica

ICD-10CM CODES
A86	Unspecified viral encephalitis
A83.0	Japanese encephalitis
A83.1	Western equine encephalitis
A83.2	Eastern equine encephalitis
A83.3	St Louis encephalitis
A83.4	Australian encephalitis
A83.5	California encephalitis
A83.8	Other mosquito-borne viral encephalitis
A83.9	Mosquito-borne viral encephalitis, unspecified
A84.8	Other tick-borne viral encephalitis
A84.9	Tick-borne viral encephalitis, unspecified
A85.0	Enteroviral encephalitis
A85.1	Adenoviral encephalitis
A85.2	Arthropod-borne viral encephalitis, unspecified
A85.8	Other specified viral encephalitis
A92.31	West Nile virus infection with encephalitis
B00.4	Herpesviral encephalitis
B01.11	Varicella encephalitis and encephalomyelitis
B02.0	Zoster encephalitis
B05.0	Measles complicated by encephalitis
B06.01	Rubella encephalitis
B10.01	Human herpesvirus 6 encephalitis
B10.09	Other human herpesvirus encephalitis
B26.2	Mumps encephalitis
B94.1	Sequelae of viral encephalitis
G04.00	Acute disseminated encephalitis and encephalomyelitis, unspecified
G04.81	Other encephalitis and encephalomyelitis
G04.90	Encephalitis and encephalomyelitis, unspecified
G05.3	Encephalitis and encephalomyelitis in diseases classified elsewhere

EPIDEMIOLOGY & DEMOGRAPHICS

INCIDENCE (IN U.S.):
- About 20,000 cases/yr are reported to the CDC. In 2014, there were 2205 cases of West Nile Virus with 97 deaths.

PEAK INCIDENCE: Any age, but children and older adults are more likely to have significant morbidity

PREVALENCE (IN U.S.):
- Arbovirus infections are transmitted by mosquitoes and thus cause infection when mosquitoes are active, especially summer and fall. Herpes simplex infections can occur at any time.
- Geography also plays a role: Whereas eastern equine encephalitis is more likely on the East Coast of U.S., West Nile Virus has spread to 48 states. Powassan virus is more common in northern New England and Canada. La Crosse virus is more common in the upper Midwestern and mid-Atlantic and southeastern states. There was a recent outbreak of enterovirus type 71 in Colorado.

PREDOMINANT SEX: Male = female
PREDOMINANT AGE: Any age
GENETICS: No specific genetic or congenital predisposition

ETIOLOGY

- Can be caused by a host of viruses, with herpes simplex the most common virus identified.
- Arboviruses transmitted by mosquitoes include Eastern equine encephalitis, Western equine encephalitis, St. Louis encephalitis, Venezuelan equine encephalitis, California virus encephalitis, Japanese B encephalitis, La Crosse encephalitis, Murray Valley and West Nile encephalitis. Tick-borne diseases include Russian spring-summer encephalitis, Powassan encephalitis, and other lesser known agents.
- Also implicated: rabies-causing agents, CMV, Epstein-Barr, varicella-zoster, echo virus, mumps, adenovirus, coxsackie, rubeola, and herpes viruses.
- Meningoencephalitis: acute retroviral infection from HIV.
- In the U.S., the most commonly identified etiologies are herpes simplex virus, West Nile virus, and the enteroviruses.

PHYSICAL FINDINGS & CLINICAL PRESENTATION

- Initially, fever and evidence of meningeal irritation
- Headache and stiff neck
- Later, development of signs of cortical dysfunction: lethargy, coma, stupor, weakness, seizures, facial weakness, as well as brain-stem findings
- Cerebellar findings: ataxia, nystagmus, hypotonia, myoclonus, cranial nerve palsies, and abnormal tendon reflexes
- Patients with rabies: hydrophobia, anxiety, facial numbness, psychosis, coma, or dysarthria
- Rarely, movement disorders, such as chorea, hemiballismus, or dystonia
- Recall of a prodromal viral-like illness (this finding is not at all uniform)

DIAGNOSIS

DIFFERENTIAL DIAGNOSIS

- Bacterial infections: brain abscess, toxic encephalopathies, TB
- Protozoal infections
- Behçet's disease

- Lupus encephalitis
- Sjögren's syndrome
- Multiple sclerosis
- Syphilis
- Cryptococcus
- Toxoplasmosis
- Brucellosis
- Leukemic or lymphomatous meningitis
- Other metastatic tumors
- Lyme disease
- Cat-scratch disease
- Vogt-Koyanagi-Harada syndrome
- Mollaret's meningitis

WORKUP

- Lumbar puncture to reveal pleocytosis, usually lymphocytic, although neutrophils may be seen early on
- Usually, elevated CSF protein
- Normal or low CSF glucose
- In herpes simplex encephalitis: RBCs and xanthochromia
- Selected tests on CSF fluid in viral encephalitis are described in Table 1
- EEG changes showing periodic high-voltage sharp waves in the temporal regions and slow wave complexes suggestive of herpes encephalitis (Fig. E1).
- CT scan and MRI to reveal edema and hemorrhage in the frontal and temporal lobes
- Temporal lobe involvement suggests herpes simplex encephalitis
- Basal ganglia and thalami are areas involved as generally seen in Eastern equine encephalitis
- With West Nile infection, MRI changes have shown changes in basal ganglia, thalami, mesial temporal structures, brain stem, and cerebellum
- Arboviral infections suspected during outbreaks in specific areas
- Rising titers of neutralizing antibodies from the acute to the convalescent stage demonstrated but often not helpful in the acutely ill patient
- Polymerase chain reaction (PCR) that amplifies DNA from the CSF for herpes simplex encephalitis
- Rarely, brain biopsy to assist in the diagnosis; viral culture of cerebral tissue obtained if biopsy done
- Classic herpetic skin lesions suggestive of herpes encephalitis
- In diagnosing arboviral encephalitis:
  1. Presence of antiviral IgM within the first few days of symptomatic disease; detected and quantified by ELISA
  2. Unusual to recover an arbovirus from the blood or CSF

LABORATORY TESTS

- Aside from the lumbar puncture, most other laboratory studies are nonspecific.
- Skin lesions and urine may be cultured for herpes simplex and CMV.

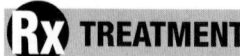 TREATMENT

ACUTE GENERAL Rx

- Supportive care, frequent evaluation, and neurologic examination

TABLE 1 Selected Tests for Viral Encephalitis

Organism/Syndrome	Test	Comment
West Nile Virus		
West Nile encephalitis	IgM in CSF	Diagnostic of CNS invasive disease or acute flaccid paralysis
Herpes Simplex Virus Type 1		
Herpes simplex encephalitis	PCR in CSF	Sensitive and specific in the acute phase
	CSF–serum antibody ratio	Useful 2 weeks to 3 months after onset
Herpes Simplex Virus Type 2		
Neonatal encephalitis	PCR in CSF	Confirmatory, high sensitivity
Relapsing meningitis	PCR in CSF	Sensitive and specific in first 3 days of illness
Varicella-Zoster Virus		
Meningoencephalitis	PCR in CSF	Confirmatory when used with clinical and spinal fluid findings; sensitivity unclear
Epstein-Barr Virus		
EBV encephalitis	PCR in CSF	Suggests CNS invasion by virus
JC Virus		
Progressive multifocal leukoencephalopathy	PCR in CSF	Diagnostic but incompletely (70%) sensitive
Cytomegalovirus		
CMV ventriculitis	PCR in CSF	Sensitive and specific

CMV, Cytomegalovirus; *CNS,* central nervous system; *CSF,* cerebrospinal fluid; *EBV,* Epstein-Barr virus; *PCR,* polymerase chain reaction.
From Goldman L, Schafer AI: *Goldman's Cecil medicine,* ed 24, Philadelphia, 2011, Saunders.

- Ventilatory assistance for patients who are moribund or at risk for aspiration
- Avoidance of infusion of hypotonic fluids to minimize the risk of hyponatremia
- For patients who develop seizures: anticonvulsant therapy and follow-up in a critical care setting
- For comatose patients:
  1. Aggressive care to avoid decubitus ulcers, contractures, and DVT
  2. Close attention to weights, input/output, and serum electrolytes
- Acyclovir 30 mg/kg/day IV total dose divided in q8 hour intervals for 14 days for herpes simplex encephalitis
- Short courses of corticosteroids to control brain edema and prevent herniation
- In patients with suspected rabies:
  1. Human rabies immune globulin (HRIG) should be given at a dose of 20 U/kg.
  2. Active immunization may be stimulated by rabies vaccine, which is grown on a human diploid cell line (HDCV) and has reduced the number of doses needed to five.

3. If suspect animal is a dog or cat and can be found, observe closely for 10 days to detect rabid behavior; any significant illness in the animal should promptly initiate humane sacrifice of the animal with the brain submitted to local or state health departments for pathology and immunologic testing for rabies. Any wild animal suspected of rabies should be humanely sacrificed, if possible, and submitted for rabies testing immediately.
4. If signs are seen, animal should be euthanized and its brain examined for signs of rabies.
- No specific pharmacologic therapy for most other viral pathogens

CHRONIC Rx

Some patients may develop permanent neurologic sequelae; these patients will benefit from intensive rehabilitation programs, including physical, occupational, and speech therapy.

DISPOSITION

- Patients with suspected encephalitis of any cause should generally be admitted for initial diagnostic workup and specific treatment (if available).
- Long-term management of patients with significant neurologic sequelae from encephalitis (e.g., memory defects, depression, difficulty with organization of thoughts, movement disorders) may benefit from rehabilitation services, home care, or nursing home placement.

REFERRAL

- To a neurologist for initial workup and management
- To an infectious disease specialist for diagnostic and therapeutic plan
- To a rehabilitation service for long-term evaluation and convalescent services

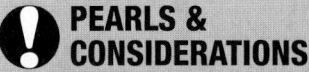 **PEARLS & CONSIDERATIONS**

- West Nile virus encephalitis occurs primarily in elderly patients >65 years of age.
- Rabies may occur months after contact with the rabid animal, and the exposure (especially bat rabies) may have been seemingly insignificant and even inapparent.
- Experimental therapies are worthy of consideration for some forms of viral encephalitis (e.g., immune plasma, ribavirin, interferons), and expert consultation should be obtained early on for possible treatment interventions with promising experimental therapies (e.g., Milwaukee protocol for rabies).

SUGGESTED READINGS

Available at www.expertconsult.com

RELATED CONTENT

Herpes Encephalitis (Patient Information)
Rabies (Related Key Topic)
West Nile Virus Infection (Related Key Topic)

AUTHOR: **GLENN G. FORT, M.D., M.P.H.**

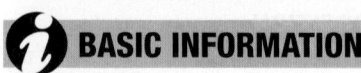

BASIC INFORMATION

DEFINITION

Encephalopathy is a clinical syndrome of global cognitive impairment characterized by impaired arousal, inattention, and disorientation.

SYNONYMS

Delirium, acute confusional state

ICD-10CM CODES

G93.40 Encephalopathy, unspecified
G93.41 Metabolic encephalopathy
G93.49 Other encephalopathy
G92 Toxic encephalopathy
E51.2 Wernicke's encephalopathy
G04.30 Acute necrotizing hemorrhagic encephalopathy, unspecified
G04.31 Postinfectious acute necrotizing hemorrhagic encephalopathy
G04.32 Postimmunization acute necrotizing hemorrhagic encephalopathy
G04.39 Other acute necrotizing hemorrhagic encephalopathy
G93.49 Other encephalopathy
I67.4 Hypertensive encephalopathy
I67.83 Posterior reversible encephalopathy syndrome
J10.81 Influenza due to other identified influenza virus with encephalopathy
J11.81 Influenza due to unidentified influenza virus with encephalopathy
P91.60 Hypoxic ischemic encephalopathy [HIE], unspecified
P91.61 Mild hypoxic ischemic encephalopathy [HIE]
P91.62 Moderate hypoxic ischemic encephalopathy [HIE]
P91.63 Severe hypoxic ischemic encephalopathy [HIE]

EPIDEMIOLOGY & DEMOGRAPHICS

POINT PREVALENCE: 1.1% of adults in the general population >55 yr, 10% to 40% of hospitalized elderly, and 60% of nursing home patients >75 yr; 100,000 to 200,000 cases annually with anoxic encephalopathy
RISK FACTORS: Age, cancer, AIDS, terminal illness, bone marrow transplant, surgery

PHYSICAL FINDINGS & CLINICAL PRESENTATION

- Common to all encephalopathies is a fluctuating level of arousal, poor attention, and disorientation.
- Some patients may appear agitated and others lethargic.
- Delusions (fixed false beliefs) and hallucinations are common.
- Asterixis (negative myoclonus) is common.
- Other physical findings, such as fever, ascites, jaundice, or tachycardia, may vary depending on the underlying cause of encephalopathy.
- Because toxins and metabolic disturbances are common causes of encephalopathy, the history should focus on exposure to toxins, especially medications, and symptoms suggesting a concurrent illness such as a urinary tract infection, pneumonia, sepsis, meningitis, or encephalitis.

ETIOLOGY

The final common pathway of all causes of encephalopathy is widespread neuronal dysfunction from either a structural or functional cause. Many conditions are reversible and carry a good prognosis if treated in a timely manner.
- Organ failure (e.g., hepatic encephalopathy [Fig. 1], hypoxia, hypercapnia, uremia).
- Infection: systemic (e.g., urinary tract, pneumonia, sepsis) or involving the central nervous system (e.g., meningitis, encephalitis).
- Toxin ingestion or withdrawal. Special consideration should be paid to alcohol, benzodiazepines, anticholinergics, neuroleptics, antibiotics (such as fluoroquinolones), and recreational drugs.
- Metabolic disturbance: hyperosmolar states, hypernatremia, hyponatremia, hyperglycemia, hypoglycemia, hypercalcemia, hypophosphatemia, acidosis, alkalosis, inborn errors of metabolism.
- Endocrinopathy: hyperthyroidism, hypothyroidism, Cushing's syndrome, adrenal insufficiency, pituitary failure.
- Neoplasm: tumors of the central nervous system, primary or metastatic; effects of distant tumors (e.g., paraneoplastic limbic encephalitis).
- Nutritional deficiency, mostly in alcoholics and chronically ill patients, such as vitamin B_1 deficiency (Wernicke's encephalopathy).
- Seizures: postictal state, nonconvulsive status epilepticus, complex partial seizures, absence seizures.
- Trauma: concussion, contusion, subdural hematoma, epidural hematoma, diffuse axonal injury.
- Vascular: ischemic and hemorrhagic strokes, vasculitis, venous thrombosis.
- Postanoxic encephalopathy.
- Psychiatric disease: acute psychosis, depression with psychiatric features.
- Acute demyelinating disease: acute disseminating encephalomyelitis, tumefactive multiple sclerosis.
- Other autoimmune diseases: autoimmune encephalitis (associated with antibodies such as anti-NMDA), lupus cerebritis, cerebral vasculitis (primary angiitis of the central nervous system [CNS] of a secondary cerebral vasculitis).
- Other: hypertensive encephalopathy, postoperative status, sleep deprivation.

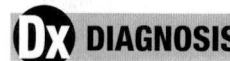 DIAGNOSIS

DIFFERENTIAL DIAGNOSIS

Differential diagnosis for encephalopathy is broad. It is typically helpful to distinguish toxic metabolic causes from primary neurologic causes.
- Dementia: distinguished from encephalopathy by a history of slowly progressive cognitive decline over time (fluctuating cognitive function is rare except in diffuse Lewy body disease).
- Hypersomnia
- Aphasia: distinguished from encephalopathy by virtue of it representing a specific disorder of language rather than a global disturbance of cognitive function.
- Depression

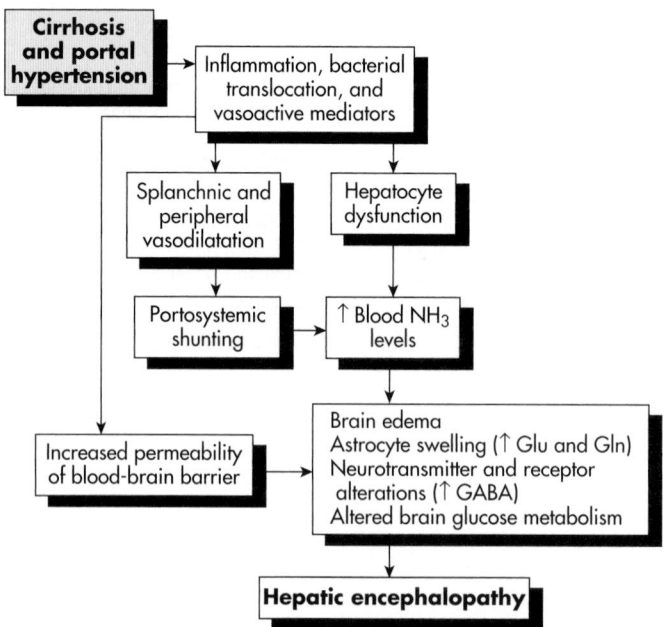

FIG. 1 Proposed pathophysiology of hepatic encephalopathy. *GABA*, gamma-aminobutyric acid; *Gln*, glutamine; *Glu*, glutamate; *NH₃*, ammonia. (From Feldman M et al (eds): *Sleisenger and Fordtran's gastrointestinal and liver disease*, ed 10, Philadelphia, 2016, Saunders.)

- Psychosis: some overlap with encephalopathy because delusions and hallucinations may be common to both.
- Mania
- Vegetative state from cerebral injury; these patients appear awake (eyes are open) but there is no content to their consciousness.
- Akinetic mutism: these patients do not talk and do not move; there is little fluctuation in their state and there is no asterixis or other focal deficit.
- Locked-in syndrome: may be distinguished from encephalopathy by the presence of fixed neurologic deficits (e.g., paralysis of all four limbs); however, the patient is aware of his or her environment.

WORKUP

The best tool in the evaluation of encephalopathy is a good history and physical exam, which will help tailor the remainder of the diagnostic workup. Interview family members and other providers to identify preceding events, medication changes, and medical history. Evaluate focal deficits.

LABORATORY TESTS

- General chemistry: electrolytes, glucose, creatinine, ammonia, blood urea nitrogen, transaminases, amylase, lipase
- Complete blood count
- Drug screen and alcohol level (must order ethylene glycol separately if suspected)
- Lumbar puncture if meningitis, encephalitis, autoimmune process, or subarachnoid hemorrhage with negative imaging is suspected
- HIV testing

- Endocrine testing: cortisol level, thyroid function test
- Urinalysis and microscopy, urine culture, blood cultures
- Arterial blood gases

IMAGING STUDIES

The following imaging and diagnostic studies may be indicated depending on history and physical examination:

- Chest radiograph to rule out pneumonia
- Head CT to rule out intracranial hemorrhage, hydrocephalus, tumors
- Brain MRI with and without contrast and with diffusion-weighted images for suspected encephalitis, tumors, acute strokes, or acute autoimmune processes
- Magnetic resonance angiography/venography for strokes, arterial dissection, venous thrombosis
- Conventional angiography for CNS vasculitis and aneurysms
- EEG: evaluate for subclinical status epilepticus

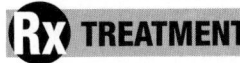 **TREATMENT**

The encephalopathy itself is a symptom of these underlying problems. In general, it is best to avoid treating the symptom of encephalopathy with antipsychotics or sedatives. The best approach is to treat the underlying toxic or metabolic disturbance.

- Thiamine supplementation.
- Glucose for hypoglycemia.
- Antibiotics in cases of infections (choose an agent with good CNS penetration in cases of primary CNS infections; to prevent exacerbation of underlying problem, ensure also that the agent is not associated with causing encephalopathy, if possible).
- Insulin in hyperglycemic conditions (e.g., diabetic ketoacidosis, hyperosmolar nonketosis, and sepsis).
- Correct electrolyte disturbances properly.
- Treat organ failure and its sequelae; for example, implement appropriate therapy for hyperammonemia and uremia.
- Ensure hemodynamic stability (blood pressure and heart rate).

SUGGESTED READINGS
Available at www.expertconsult.com

RELATED CONTENT
Delirium (Related Key Topic)
Encephalitis, Acute Viral (Related Key Topic)
Hepatic Encephalopathy (Related Key Topic)

AUTHORS: **CHLOE MANDER NUNNELEY, M.D., JOSEPH S. KASS, M.D., J.D.,** and **JOSHUA CHALKELY, M.S., D.O.**

E

Diseases and Disorders

I

DEFINITION

Infective endocarditis is an infection of the endocardial surface of the heart or mural endocardium. Box 1 describes the modified Duke criteria for the diagnosis of infective endocarditis.

ACUTE ENDOCARDITIS: Usually caused by *Staphylococcus aureus, Streptococcus pyogenes, S. pneumoniae,* and *Neisseria* organisms; classic clinical presentation of high fever, positive blood cultures, vascular and immunologic phenomenon

SUBACUTE ENDOCARDITIS: Usually caused by viridans streptococci in the presence of valvular pathology; less toxic, often indolent presentation with lower fevers, night sweats, fatigue

ENDOCARDITIS IN INJECTION DRUG USERS: Often involving *S. aureus* or *Pseudomonas aeruginosa* with variation that may be geographically influenced; tricuspid (Fig. 1) or multiple valvular involvement; high mortality rate of 50% to 60%

PROSTHETIC VALVE ENDOCARDITIS (EARLY): Usually caused by *S. aureus* (leading cause of PVE) within 2 mo of valve replacement; other organisms include *S. epidermidis,* gram-negative bacilli, diphtheroids, *Candida* organisms

PROSTHETIC VALVE ENDOCARDITIS (LATE): Typically develops >60 days after valvular replacement; involved organisms similar to early prosthetic valve endocarditis, including viridans streptococci, enterococci, and group D streptococci

NOSOCOMIAL ENDOCARDITIS: Secondary to intravenous catheters, TPN lines, pacemakers; coagulase-negative staphylococci, *S. aureus,* and streptococci most common

Non-HACEK gram-negative bacillus endocarditis is not primarily a disease of injection drug users. More than half of all cases are associated with health care contact

SYNONYMS

Bacterial endocarditis
Subacute bacterial endocarditis (SBE)
Endocarditis

ICD-10CM CODES

I33.0 Acute and subacute infective endocarditis
I33.9 Acute endocarditis, unspecified

EPIDEMIOLOGY & DEMOGRAPHICS

INCIDENCE (IN U.S.): 5 to 7.9 cases/100,000 persons/yr.
PEAK INCIDENCE: Females: often <35 yr old; males: 45 to 65 yr old.
NOSOCOMIAL ENDOCARDITIS: 14% to 28% of cases.
PREVALENCE (IN U.S.): 0.3 to 3 cases/1000 hospital admissions.
PREDOMINANT SEX: Male < female.
PREDOMINANT AGE: 45 to 65 yr.

PHYSICAL FINDINGS & CLINICAL PRESENTATION

- Clinical manifestations of infective endocarditis are described in Table 1.
- Fever may be variable in presentation; may be high, hectic, or absent.
- Fever, chills, fatigue, and rigors occur in 25% to 80% of patients.
- Heart murmur may be absent in right-sided endocarditis.
- Embolic phenomenon with peripheral manifestations is found in 50% of patients.
- Skin manifestations include petechiae, Osler nodes (Fig. E2), splinter hemorrhages, Janeway lesions (Fig. E3).
- Splenomegaly is more common with subacute course.

ETIOLOGY

Staphylococcal infection is now the leading cause of native or prosthetic valve infection.

Variation in incidence may occur that is influenced by the patient's risk for developing infection. Risk factors include hemodialysis (8%), IV drug use (10%), mitral regurgitation (43%), aortic regurgitation (26%), and rheumatic heart disease (3.3%).

ACUTE ENDOCARDITIS:
- *Staphylococcus aureus* (MSSA and MRSA)
- *Staphylococcus lugdunensis*
- *Streptococcus pneumoniae*
- Streptococcal species and groups A through G
- *Haemophilus influenzae*

SUBACUTE ENDOCARDITIS:
- Viridans streptococci (alpha-hemolytic).
- *S. bovis.*
- Enterococci.
- *S. aureus.*

ENDOCARDITIS IN INJECTION DRUG USERS:
- *S. aureus.*
- *P. aeruginosa.*
- *Candida* spp.

BOX 1 Modified Duke Criteria for the Diagnosis of Infective Endocarditis[1]

Major Criteria
Positive blood cultures for infective endocarditis.
Typical microorganism for infective endocarditis from two separate blood cultures in the absence of a primary focus: *Streptococcus viridans, Streptococcus bovis.*
HACEK group: *Haemophilus* species, *Actinobacillus actinomycetemcomitans, Cardiobacterium hominis, Eikenella corrodens,* and *Kingella kingae*
Community-acquired *Staphylococcus aureus* or enterococci
Persistently positive blood cultures, defined as recovery of a microorganism consistent with infective endocarditis from blood cultures drawn more than 12 hr apart or all of three or the majority of four or more separate blood cultures, with first and last drawn at least 1 hr apart
Single positive blood culture for *Coxiella burnetii* or antiphase IgG antibody titer >1:800
Evidence for endocardial involvement
TTE (TEE in prosthetic valve) showing oscillating intracardiac mass on a valve or supporting structures, in the path of regurgitant jet or on implanted material, in the absence of an alternative anatomic explanation, *or*
Abscess, *or*
New partial dehiscence of prosthetic valve.

Minor Criteria
Predisposition (e.g., prosthetic valve, intravenous drug use).
Fever: 38° C.
Vascular phenomena.
Immunologic phenomena.
Microbiologic evidence: positive blood culture but not meeting major criteria.

TEE, Transesophageal echocardiogram; *TTE,* transthoracic echocardiogram.
[1]Adapted from Li JS et al: Proposed modifications to the Duke criteria for the diagnosis of infective endocarditis, *Clin Infect Dis* 30:633-638, 2000.
From Ballinger A: *Kumar & Clark's essentials of clinical medicine,* ed 6, Edinburgh, 2012, Saunders.

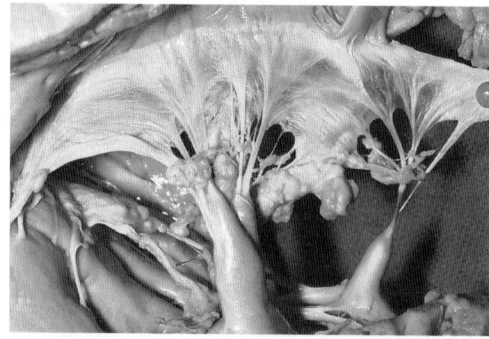

FIG. 1 Tricuspid valve endocarditis. There are large vegetations on the leaflets and the chordae tendineae. (From Crawford MH et al [eds]: *Cardiology,* ed 2, St Louis, 2004, Mosby.)

E

Diseases and Disorders

I

TABLE 1 Clinical Manifestations of Infective Endocarditis Myalgia/Arthralgia

Symptoms	Patients Affected (%)	Signs	Patients (%)
Fever	80	Fever	90
Chills	40	Heart murmur	85
Weakness	40	Changing murmur	5-10
Dyspnea	40	New murmur	3-5
Sweats	25	Embolic phenomenon	>50
Anorexia	25	Skin manifestations	18-50
Weight loss	25	Osler nodes	10-23
Malaise	25	Splinter hemorrhages	15
Cough	25	Petechiae	20-40
Skin lesions	20	Janeway lesion	<10
Stroke	20	Splenomegaly	20-57
Nausea/vomiting	20	Septic complications	20
Headache	20	(e.g., pneumonia, meningitis)	
Myalgia/arthralgia	15	Mycotic aneurysms	20
Edema	15	Clubbing	12-52
Chest pain	15	Retinal lesion	2-10
Abdominal pain and delirium/coma	15	Signs of renal failure	10-25
Delirium/coma	10-15		
Hemoptysis	10		
Back pain	10		

From Mandell GL et al: *Principles and practice of infectious diseases*, ed 6, Philadelphia, 2005, Churchill Livingstone.

- Enterococci.

PROSTHETIC VALVE ENDOCARDITIS (EARLY):
- *S. epidermidis.*
- *S. aureus.*
- Gram-negative bacilli.
- Group D streptococci.

PROSTHETIC VALVE ENDOCARDITIS (LATE):
- *S. epidermidis.*
- Viridans streptococci.
- *S. aureus.*
- Enterococci and group D streptococci.

NOSOCOMIAL ENDOCARDITIS:
- Coagulase-negative staphylococci
- *S. aureus*
- Streptococci: viridans, group B, enterococcus

HACEK ORGANISMS:
- Fastidious gram-negative bacilli.
- *H. parainfluenzae.*
- *H. aphrophilus.*
- *A. actinomycetemcomitans.*
- *Cardiobacterium hominis.*
- *Eikenella corrodens.*
- *Kingella kingae.*

RISK FACTORS
- Poor dental hygiene.
- Long-term hemodialysis.
- Diabetes mellitus.
- HIV infection.
- Mitral valve prolapse.

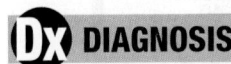 **DIAGNOSIS**

DIFFERENTIAL DIAGNOSIS
- Brain abscess.
- FUO.
- Pericarditis.
- Meningitis.

- Rheumatic fever.
- Osteomyelitis.
- *Salmonella.*
- TB.
- Bacteremia.
- Pericarditis.
- Glomerulonephritis.

WORKUP

Physical examination to evaluate for the previous physical findings followed by laboratory testing (see "Laboratory Tests"). Fig. 4 describes a diagnostic evaluation of suspected endocarditis. The modified Duke criteria for diagnosis of endocarditis defines "major criteria" as persistently positive blood cultures of organisms typical of endocarditis or endocardial involvement (new valvular regurgitation or positive echocardiogram). "Minor criteria" are defined as presence of predisposing condition or injection drug use, fever, embolic vascular pneumonia (e.g., glomerulonephritis, rheumatoid factor), or positive blood cultures not meeting major criteria. Definite endocarditis is 2 major criteria or 1 major criteria and 3 minor criteria or 5 minor criteria or presence of organisms by culture or histologic examination of a vegetation.

LABORATORY TESTS
- Blood cultures: three sets in first 24 hr. Table 2 describes causes of culture-negative endocarditis.
- More culturing if patient has received prior antibiotic.
- CBC (anemia possibly present, subacute).
- WBC (leukocytosis is higher in acute endocarditis).
- ESR and C-reactive protein (elevated).

- Positive rheumatoid factor (subacute endocarditis).
- Proteinuria, hematuria, RBC casts.

IMAGING STUDIES
- Echocardiogram: two-dimensional. Transthoracic echocardiography (TTE) (Fig. E5) is noninvasive and more easily available but has less-than-optimal sensitivity (50%-80%) for endocarditis.
- Transesophageal echocardiography (TEE): more sensitive in detecting vegetations and preferred diagnostic modality. It is especially helpful with prosthetic valves or in detecting perivalvular disease.
- Electrocardiogram: look for cardiac conduction abnormalities, injury pattern, or evidence of pericarditis—any such new findings are suggestive of myocardial abscess.

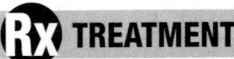 **TREATMENT**

Initial IV antibiotic therapy (before culture results) is aimed at the most likely organism. The American Heart Association has developed guidelines based on the most frequently encountered bacteria.

- **Native valve endocarditis** caused by penicillin-susceptible *S. viridians, S. bovis,* and other streptococci (MIC of penicillin ≤0.12 mcg/ml): Pen G 12-18 million U IV q24h continuous or divided q4h for 4 weeks **or** ceftriaxone 2 g IV or IM q day for 4 weeks for penicillin-allergic patients. Vancomycin at 30 mg/kg per 24 hr in 2 equally divided doses assuming normal kidney function, for 4 weeks.
- **Native valve endocarditis** caused by strains of viridians streptococci and *S. bovis* relatively resistant to penicillin (MIC >0.12 mcg/ml): Pen G: 24 million units per 24 hr IV either continuously or in 4 or 6 equally divided doses for 4 weeks **or** ceftriaxone 2 g per 24 hr IV or IM for 4 weeks **plus** gentamicin 3 mg/kg per 24 hr IV or IM in one dose or in 2 to 3 equally divided doses for two weeks or monotherapy with vancomycin 30 mg/kg per 24 hr IV in 2 equally divided doses for 4 weeks not to exceed 2 g per 24 hr unless concentrations in serum too low.
- **Native valve endocarditis** due to *Staphylococcus:*
  1. **MSSA:** nafcillin (or oxacillin) 12 per 24 hr IV in 4 or 6 equally divided doses for 6 weeks **plus** optional addition of gentamicin 3 mg/kg per 24 hr IV or IM in 2 or 3 equally divided doses for 3 to 5 days **or** cefazolin 6 g per 24 hr IV in 3 equally divided doses for 6 weeks, **plus** optional addition of gentamicin 3 mg/kg per 24 hr IV or IM in 2 or 3 equally divided doses for 3 to 5 days. A newer antibiotic daptomycin has an indication for right-sided endocarditis with MSSA at 6 mg/kg IV q24h.
  2. **MRSA:** vancomycin 30 mg/kg per 24 hr in 2 equally divided doses for 6 weeks; not to exceed 2 g per 24 hr unless concentrations in serum are low.

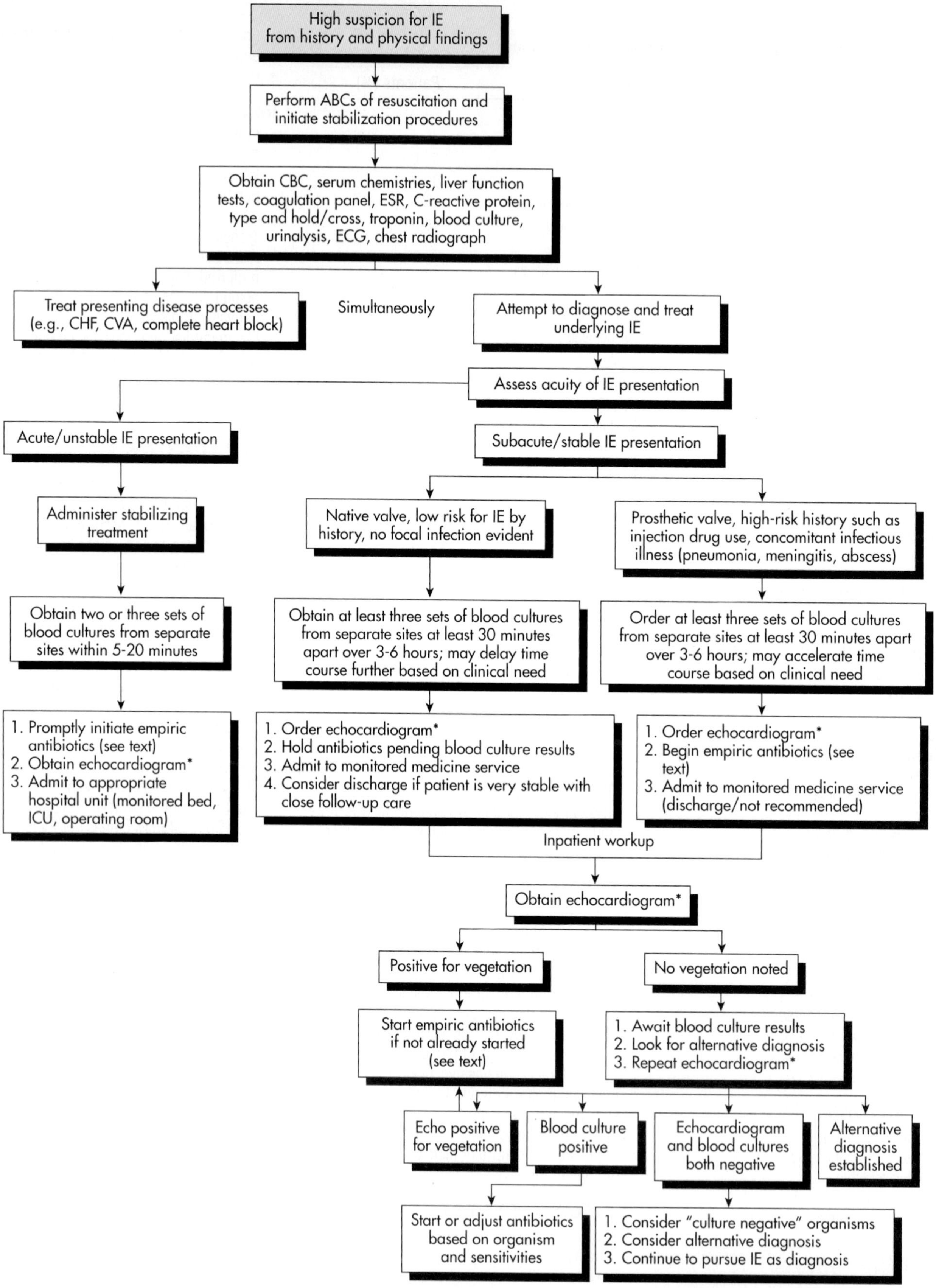

High suspicion for IE
from history and physical findings

↓

Perform ABCs of resuscitation and
initiate stabilization procedures

↓

Obtain CBC, serum chemistries, liver function
tests, coagulation panel, ESR, C-reactive protein,
type and hold/cross, troponin, blood culture,
urinalysis, ECG, chest radiograph

↓

Treat presenting disease processes
(e.g., CHF, CVA, complete heart block) ← Simultaneously → Attempt to diagnose and treat
underlying IE

↓

Assess acuity of IE presentation

↓   ↓

Acute/unstable IE presentation   Subacute/stable IE presentation

↓   ↓   ↓

Administer stabilizing   Native valve, low risk for IE by   Prosthetic valve, high-risk history such as
treatment   history, no focal infection evident   injection drug use, concomitant infectious
                                                                     illness (pneumonia, meningitis, abscess)

↓   ↓   ↓

Obtain two or three sets of   Obtain at least three sets of blood cultures   Order at least three sets of blood cultures
blood cultures from separate   from separate sites at least 30 minutes   from separate sites at least 30 minutes apart
sites within 5-20 minutes   apart over 3-6 hours; may delay time   over 3-6 hours; may accelerate time
                               course further based on clinical need   course based on clinical need

↓   ↓   ↓

1. Promptly initiate empiric   1. Order echocardiogram*   1. Order echocardiogram*
   antibiotics (see text)   2. Hold antibiotics pending blood   2. Begin empiric antibiotics (see
2. Obtain echocardiogram*   culture results   text)
3. Admit to appropriate   3. Admit to monitored medicine service 3. Admit to monitored medicine service
   hospital unit (monitored bed, 4. Consider discharge if patient is very   (discharge/not recommended)
   ICU, operating room)   stable with close follow-up care

Inpatient workup

↓

Obtain echocardiogram*

↓   ↓

Positive for vegetation   No vegetation noted

↓   ↓

Start empiric antibiotics   1. Await blood culture results
if not already started   2. Look for alternative diagnosis
(see text)   3. Repeat echocardiogram*

↓   ↓   ↓   ↓

Echo positive   Blood culture   Echocardiogram   Alternative
for vegetation positive   and blood cultures diagnosis
                                 both negative   established

↓   ↓

Start or adjust antibiotics   1. Consider "culture negative" organisms
based on organism   2. Consider alternative diagnosis
and sensitivities   3. Continue to pursue IE as diagnosis

FIG. 4 Diagnostic algorithm for the emergency department management of patients in whom infective endocarditis (IE) is suspected. *Echocardiography can be performed via either the transthoracic (TTE) or transesophageal (TEE) technique. TEE is more invasive but is more sensitive for detecting vegetations and complications of IE, such as perivalvular abscesses; it is recommended for prosthetic valves; for situations in which optimal visualization by TTE will be difficult, such as emphysema and morbid obesity; for high suspicion of IE but normal TTE findings; and for high suspicion of a complication of IE, such as perivalvular abscess. Normal findings with either technique do not exclude IE if clinical suspicion is high. Echocardiograms can be repeated in an attempt to identify problems such as vegetations and abscesses that may not be noted initially. *ABCs*, Airway, breathing, and circulation; *CBC*, complete blood count; *CHF*, congestive heart failure; *CVA*, cerebrovascular accident; *ECG*, electrocardiogram; *ESR*, erythrocyte sedimentation rate; *ICU*, intensive care unit. (From Adams JG et al: *Emergency medicine, clinical essentials*, ed 2, Philadelphia, 2013, Elsevier.)

TABLE 2   Causes of Culture-Negative Endocarditis

Organism	Epidemiology and Exposures	Diagnostic Approaches
Aspergillus and other noncandidal fungi	Prosthetic valve	Lysis-centrifugation technique; also culture and histopathologic examination of any emboli
Bartonella spp.	*B. henselae:* exposure to cats or cat fleas *B. quintana:* louse infestation; homelessness, alcohol abuse	Most common cause of culture-negative IE in United States; serologic testing (may cross-react with *Chlamydia* spp.); PCR assay of valve or emboli is best test; lysis-centrifugation technique may be useful
Brucella spp.	Ingestion of unpasteurized milk or dairy products; livestock contact	Blood cultures ultimately become positive in 80% of cases with extended incubation time of 4-6 wk; lysis-centrifugation technique may expedite growth; serologic tests are available
Chlamydia psittaci	Bird exposure	Serologic tests available but exhibit cross-reactivity with *Bartonella;* monoclonal antibody direct stains on tissue may be useful; PCR assay now available
Coxiella burnetii (Q fever)	Global distribution; exposure to unpasteurized milk or agricultural areas	Serologic tests (high titers of antibody to both phase 1 and phase 2 antigens); also PCR assay on blood or valve tissue
HACEK spp.	Periodontal disease or preceding dental work	Although traditionally a cause of culture-negative IE, HACEK species are now routinely isolated from most liquid broth continuous monitoring blood culture systems without prolonged incubation times
Legionella spp.	Contaminated water distribution systems; prosthetic valves	Serology available; periodic subcultures onto buffered charcoal yeast extract medium; lysis-centrifugation technique; PCR assay available
Nutritionally variant streptococci	Slow and indolent course	Supplemented culture media or growth as satellite colonies around *Staphylococcus aureus* streak; antimicrobial susceptibility testing often requires processing specialized microbiology laboratory
Tropheryma whipplei (Whipple's disease)	Typical signs and symptoms include diarrhea, weight loss, arthralgias, abdominal pain, lymphadenopathy, central nervous system involvement; IE may be present without systemic symptoms	Histologic examination of valve with periodic acid–Schiff stain; valve cultures may be done using fibroblast cell lines; PCR assay on vegetation material

HACEK, *Haemophilus* spp., *Aggregatibacter* spp., *Cardiobacterium hominis, Eikenella corrodens,* and *Kingella* spp.; IE, infective endocarditis; PCR, polymerase chain reaction.
From Bennett JE, Dolin R, Blaser MJ: *Mandell, Douglas, and Bennett's principles and practice of infectious diseases,* ed 8, Philadelphia, 2015, Saunders.

- For culture-negative native valve endocarditis one of the following regimens is suggested: ampicillin-sulbactam: 12 g per 24 hr IV in 4 equally divided doses for 4 to 6 weeks **plus** gentamicin 3 mg/kg per 24 hr IV or IM in 3 equally divided doses for 4 to 6 weeks **or** vancomycin 30 mg/kg per 24 hr IV in 2 equally divided doses for 4 to 6 weeks; not to exceed 2 g per 24 hr unless concentrations in serum low **plus** gentamicin 3 mg/kg per 24 hr IV or IM in 3 equally divided doses for 4 to 6 weeks **plus** ciprofloxacin 1000 mg per 24 hr orally or 800 mg per 24 hr IV in 2 equally divided doses for 4 to 6 weeks.
- For treatment of native valve endocarditis due to HACEK organisms: ceftriaxone 2 g per 24 hr IV or IM in 1 dose for 4 weeks **or** ampicillin-sulbactam 12 g per 24 hr IV in 4 equally divided doses for 4 weeks **or** ciprofloxacin 1000 mg per 24 hr orally or 800 mg per 24 hr IV in 2 equally divided doses for 4 weeks.
- **Patients with prosthetic valves** endocarditis:
- Methicillin-susceptible strains: nafcillin or oxacillin 12 g per 24 hr IV in 6 equally divided doses for at least 6 weeks **plus** rifampin 900 mg per 24 hr IV or orally in 3 equally divided doses for at least 6 weeks **plus** gentamicin 3 mg/kg IV or IM in 2 or 3 equally divided doses for 2 weeks.
- Methicillin-resistant strains: vancomycin 30 mg/kg per 24 hr in 2 equally divided doses

for at least 6 weeks **plus** rifampin 900 mg per 24 hr IV or orally in 3 equally divided doses for at least 6 weeks **plus** gentamicin 3 mg/kg per 24 hr IV or IM in 2 or 3 equally divided doses for 2 weeks.

Antibiotic therapy after identification of the organism should be guided by susceptibility testing, preferably by formal testing by MIC (minimum inhibitory concentration).

DISPOSITION

- The patient may need outpatient IV antibiotic therapy, and arrangements need to be made to ensure safe vascular access and continuity of care with outpatient IV therapy team.
- Long-term follow-up is essential after therapy has ended; relapse of endocarditis may occur.
- Prophylaxis with antibiotics will be needed before dental procedures as a previous episode of endocarditis increases the risk of recurrent endocarditis associated with transient bacteremia from dental procedures.

REFERRAL

- To an infectious disease specialist.
- To a cardiologist or a cardiac surgeon if evidence of heart failure, refractory infection, myocardial abscess, valve disruption, or major embolic events occur.
- The timing and indications for surgical intervention to prevent systemic embolism in infective endocarditis remain controversial.

Trials have shown that early surgery in patients with infective endocarditis and large vegetations significantly reduced death and embolic events by decreasing the risk of systemic embolism.

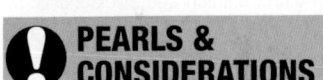

PEARLS & CONSIDERATIONS

COMMENTS

For endocarditis prophylaxis refer to Section V.
Streptococcus viridians are a large group of commensal bacteria that are either alpha hemolytic on blood agar plates or nonhemolytic. Common members of this family include *S. mutans, S. anginosus, S. mitis, S. sanguis,* and *S. salivarius.* These tend to be oral/dental flora.

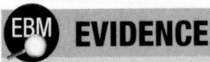 **EVIDENCE**

Available at www.expertconsult.com

SUGGESTED READINGS
Available at www.expertconsult.com

RELATED CONTENT
Endocarditis (Patient Information)

AUTHOR: **GLENN G. FORT, M.D., M.P.H.**

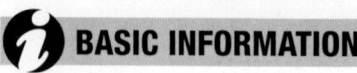

BASIC INFORMATION

DEFINITION

Endometrial carcinoma (EC) is the malignant transformation of endometrial glands with stromal invasion. The changes are typified by irregular nuclear membranes, nuclear atypia, mitotic activity, loss of glandular pattern, loss of intervening stroma, and irregular cell size. The two main histologic subcategories of EC, low-grade endometrioid (Type 1) and high-grade endometrioid and nonendometrioid EC (Type 2), show unique molecular aberrations and differing clinical behaviors.

SYNONYMS

Uterine cancer (some forms)
Carcinoma of the endometrium
EC

ICD-10CM CODES
C54.1 Malignant neoplasm of endometrium
C55 Malignant neoplasm of uterus, part unspecified
C54.9 Malignant neoplasm of corpus uteri, unspecified

EPIDEMIOLOGY & DEMOGRAPHICS

INCIDENCE: 25.4 cases per 100,000 persons; approximately 60,000 new cases annually. It is the most common gynecologic malignancy in the U.S. 2.8% of women will be diagnosed in their lifetime

PREDOMINANCE: Median age at diagnosis: 62 yr; only 5% occur in women <40 yr; 5-year survival >80%

RISK FACTORS: Obesity, diabetes, nulliparity, early menarche and late menopause, unopposed estrogen therapy, tamoxifen use, oligoovulation with chronic unopposed estrogen exposure such as with polycystic ovary syndrome (PCOS), endometrial atypical hyperplasia,

endometrial polyps (malignancy is found in 3.6% of endometrial polyps), family history

PHYSICAL FINDINGS & CLINICAL PRESENTATION

- Abnormal uterine bleeding or postmenopausal bleeding in 90%
- Pyometra or hematometra
- Abnormal Pap smear
- Incidental finding at hysterectomy

ETIOLOGY

Endogenous or exogenous chronic unopposed estrogen stimulation of the endometrium

DIAGNOSIS

DIFFERENTIAL DIAGNOSIS

- Endometrial atypical hyperplasia
- Transvaginal sonography
- Other genital tract malignancy
- Uterine polyps
- Atrophic vaginitis
- Granulosa cell tumor
- Fibroid uterus
- Adenomyosis

WORKUP

- Complete history and physical examination
- Endometrial biopsy or dilation and curettage
- Assessment of operative risk
- Staging (Tables 1 and 2)

LABORATORY TESTS

- Complete blood count
- Prothrombin time and partial thromboplastin time if bleeding is heavy
- Chemistry profile including liver function tests
- Consider CA-125 level

IMAGING STUDIES

- Chest x-ray
- CT scan if concern for metastatic disease, and/or pelvic ultrasound (Fig. 1)

- Transvaginal ultrasound (Fig. 2) in postmenopausal women with vaginal bleeding

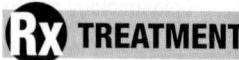

TREATMENT

NONPHARMACOLOGIC THERAPY

- Surgery is the mainstay of treatment, with or without adjuvant radiation and/or chemotherapy, depending on tumor histology, stage, and grade. Laparoscopic surgery for early-stage EC is as safe and effective as laparotomy. Robotic laparoscopy procedures have increased significantly in recent years for this indication.
- Surgery generally consists of pelvic washings, total abdominal hysterectomy and bilateral salpingo-oophorectomy, selective pelvic and periaortic lymphadenectomy, and omental biopsy depending on stage, grade, and histology.
- Brachytherapy and/or teletherapy are added in an advanced stage.
- Chemotherapy (carboplatin, paclitaxel) or hormonal therapy (tamoxifen, progestational agents, aromatase inhibitors) may also be used, especially for advanced or recurrent endometrial cancers.
- Hormonal therapy is an option for some young women with early-stage, low-grade EC who wish to preserve fertility. This choice should be discussed with a gynecologic oncologist.

ACUTE GENERAL Rx

- A thorough workup should be completed before any therapy for EC.
- Surgery hysterectomy with bilateral salpingo-oophorectomy is the treatment of choice.

CHRONIC Rx

- Physical and pelvic examination every 3 mo for 2 yr, then every 6 mo for 2 yr, and annually thereafter with imaging as clinically indicated
- Hormone replacement (combination) a consideration in low-risk patients (stage I or early stage II)

DISPOSITION

- Survival is generally defined by the stage of the disease and histology.
- The majority of cases present early, and the 5-yr survival is generally good (Fig. 3).

TABLE 1 Revised FIGO Staging for Endometrial Cancer (Adopted 2009)

Stages*	Characteristic
I	Tumor confined to the corpus uteri
IA	No or less than half myometrial invasion
IB	Invasion equal to or more than half of the myometrium
II	Tumor invades cervical stroma but does not extend beyond the uterus†
III	Local or regional spread of the tumor
IIIA	Tumor invades serosa of the corpus uteri or the adnexa‡
IIIB	Vaginal or parametrial involvement‡
IIIC	Metastases to pelvic or paraaortic lymph nodes‡
IIIC1	Positive pelvic nodes
IIIC2	Positive paraaortic lymph nodes with or without positive pelvic lymph nodes
IV	Tumor invades bladder or bowel mucosa, or distant metastasis
IVA*	Tumor invasion of bladder or bowel mucosa
IVB	Distant metastases, including intraabdominal or inguinal lymph nodes

*G1, G2, or G3.
†Endocervical glandular involvement only should be considered as stage I and no longer as stage II.
‡Positive cytology has to be reported separately without changing the stage.
From Lobo RA et al: *Comprehensive gynecology*, ed 7, Philadelphia, 2017, Elsevier.

TABLE 2 Carcinoma of the Corpus Uteri: Patients Treated in 1990-1992: Survival by 1988 FIGO Surgical Stage, *N* = 5562

Stage	5-Year Survival Rate
IA	90.9%
IB	88.2%
IC	81.0%
II	71.6%
III	51.4%
IV	8.9%

From Lobo RA et al: *Comprehensive gynecology*, ed 7, Philadelphia, 2017, Elsevier.

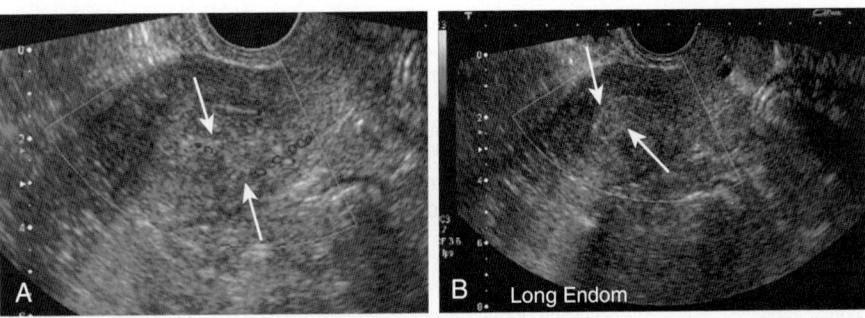

FIG. 1 A 48-year-old woman with endometrial carcinoma. A, Endovaginal ultrasound (US) showing thickened, heterogeneous, cystic, and vascular hyperechoic tissue filling the endometrial cavity *(arrows).* **B,** Second, sagittal US image showing the same. (From Fielding JR et al: *Gynecologic imaging,* Philadelphia, 2011, Saunders.)

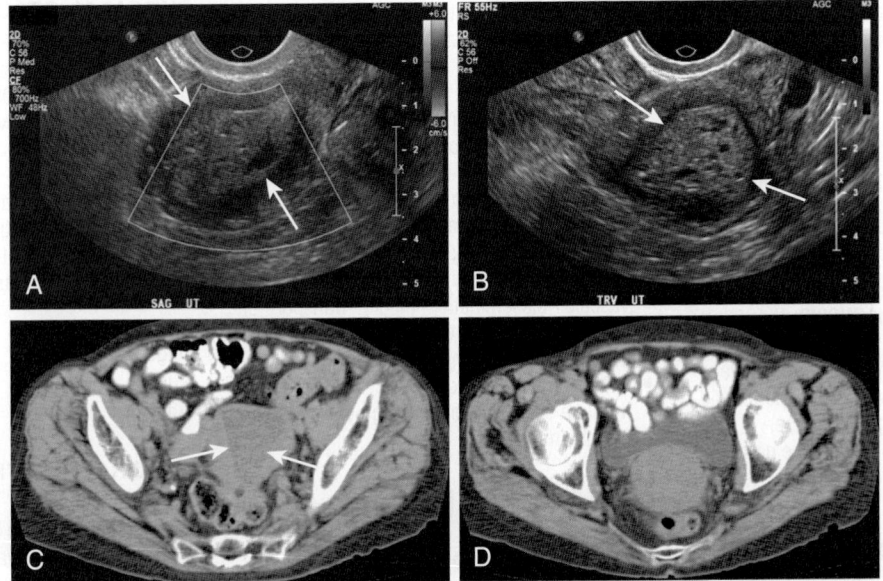

FIG. 2 A 56-year-old woman with endometrial carcinoma. A, Sagittal ultrasound (US) image showing thickened cystic echogenic soft tissue filling the endometrial cavity *(arrows).* **B,** Axial US image showing thickened cystic echogenic soft tissue filling the endometrial cavity *(arrows).* **C,** Non–contrast-enhanced axial computed tomographic (CT) image showing low-attenuation tissue filling the endometrial canal *(arrows)* in a postmenopausal patient. Note fundal thinning. **D,** Non–contrast-enhanced axial CT image showing cervical soft tissue fullness. (From Fielding JR et al: *Gynecologic imaging,* Philadelphia, 2011, Saunders.)

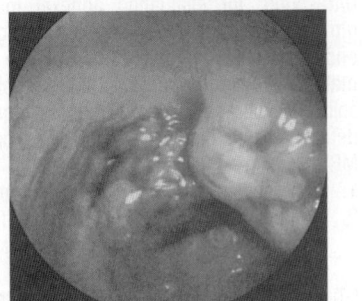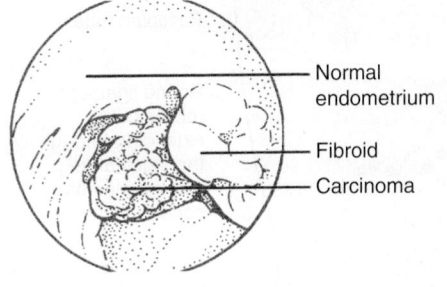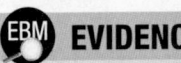

Normal endometrium

Fibroid

Carcinoma

FIG. 3 Stage I endometrial carcinoma. A small carcinoma can be seen adjacent to a uterine fibroid in this hysteroscopy photograph. Occasionally, a tumor this small may be missed on curettage. (From Skarin AT: *Atlas of diagnostic oncology,* ed 4, St Louis, 2010, Mosby.)

- Some histologic types (clear cell, papillary serous) have worse survival rates, as they tend to be more aggressive with higher rates of metastatic disease at the time of diagnosis.

⚠ **PEARLS & CONSIDERATIONS**

Any woman with postmenopausal bleeding or abnormal uterine bleeding with risk factors for endometrial cancer needs evaluation by a gynecologist and either endometrial biopsy and/or pelvic ultrasound. When endometrial cancer is diagnosed, the patient should be cared for by a gynecologic oncologist and undergo surgical staging in a minimally invasive procedure when possible.

EBM **EVIDENCE**

Available at www.expertconsult.com

SUGGESTED READINGS

Available at www.expertconsult.com

RELATED CONTENT

Endometrial Cancer (Patient Information)
Dysfunctional Uterine Bleeding (Related Key Topic)
Uterine Malignancy (Related Key Topic)

AUTHORS: **TONI PICERNO, D.O.,** and **MARK ELIOT BOROWSKY, M.D.**

BASIC INFORMATION

DEFINITION

Endometriosis is defined as the presence of functioning endometrial glands and stroma outside the uterine cavity (Fig. 1).

ICD-10CM CODES
N80.0 Endometriosis of uterus
N80.1 Endometriosis of ovary
N80.2 Endometriosis of fallopian tube
N80.3 Endometriosis of pelvic peritoneum
N80.4 Endometriosis of rectovaginal septum and vagina
N80.5 Endometriosis of intestine
N80.6 Endometriosis in cutaneous scar
N80.8 Other endometriosis
N80.9 Endometriosis, unspecified

EPIDEMIOLOGY & DEMOGRAPHICS
PREVALENCE:
- Endometriosis affects 10% of reproductive-aged women.
- Women with dysmenorrhea: 40% to 60%.
- Subfertile women: 28% to 50%.
- Incidence peaks at approximately 40 yr.

MOST COMMON AGE AT DIAGNOSIS: 25 to 29 yr.

GENETICS:
- Familial association: If first-degree relative is affected, the patient has a seven- to tenfold increased risk of having the disease.
- Polygenic-multifactorial inheritance pattern.
- 6.9% occurrence rate in first-degree female relatives.

PHYSICAL FINDINGS & CLINICAL PRESENTATION
- Classic triad is dysmenorrhea, dyspareunia, and infertility.

- Presence of pelvic pain does not correlate with the total area of endometriosis (stage of disease), type of lesion, or volume of disease but is correlated with the depth of infiltration.
- Other symptoms include abnormal bleeding (premenstrual spotting, menorrhagia), cyclic abdominal pain, intermittent constipation/diarrhea, dyschezia, dysuria, hematuria, and urinary frequency.
- Rare manifestations: catamenial hemothorax, bloody pleural effusion, massive ascites occurring during menses.
- Most severe discomfort is associated with lesions >1 cm in depth.
- Bimanual examination may reveal tender uterosacral ligaments, cul-de-sac nodularity, induration of the rectovaginal septum, fixed retroversion of the uterus, adnexal mass, and generalized or localized tenderness.

ETIOLOGY
- Reflux and direct implantation theory: retrograde menstruation with implantation of viable endometrial cells to surrounding pelvic structures (Sampson's theory).
- Coelomic metaplasia theory: transformation of multipotential cells of the coelomic epithelium into endometrium-like cells.
- Vascular dissemination theory: transport of endometrial cells to distant sites by the uterine vascular and lymphatic systems.
- Autoimmune disease theory: disorder of immune surveillance allows growth of endometrial implants.

DIAGNOSIS

DIFFERENTIAL DIAGNOSIS
- Ectopic pregnancy
- Acute appendicitis
- Chronic appendicitis

- Pelvic inflammatory disease (PID)
- Pelvic adhesions
- Hemorrhagic cyst
- Hernia
- Irritable bowel syndrome
- Uterine leiomyomata
- Adenomyosis
- Nerve entrapment syndrome
- Interstitial cystitis

WORKUP
- Thorough history and physical examination including ultrasound.
- Definitive diagnosis of endometriosis can be made only by histologic confirmation during surgery (gold standard).

SURGICAL STAGING
- American Society for Reproductive Medicine classification system for endometriosis (ASRM revised 1996) is the most widely accepted staging system.
- Value: uniform recording of operative findings.
- Limitations
  ○ Not a good predictor of successful pregnancy after treatment.
  ○ Does not correlate well with the symptoms of pain, dyspareunia, or infertility.

Stage I	Minimal
Stage II	Mild
Stage III	Moderate
Stage IV	Severe

LABORATORY TESTS
Cancer antigen 125 (CA125): limited overall value in the diagnosis of endometriosis
- Also elevated in ovarian epithelial neoplasm, myomas, adenomyosis, acute PID, ovarian cysts, pancreatitis, chronic liver disease, menstruation, and pregnancy.
- CA125 value >35 U/ml: positive predictive value of 0.58 and a negative predictive value of 0.96 for the presence of endometriosis.

IMAGING STUDIES
- Ultrasound: for evaluating adnexal mass; ultrasound characteristics may suggest endometriomas versus other benign or malignant ovarian conditions but persistent solid or cystic-solid ovarian masses require definitive tissue diagnosis with laparoscopy.
- MRI:
  1. Highly accurate in detecting endometriomas.
  2. Limited sensitivity in detecting diffuse pelvic endometriosis, especially if sessile lesions.
- CT scan may show adnexal masses of varying density (Fig. 2).

TREATMENT

NONPHARMACOLOGIC THERAPY
Expectant management (observation for 5 to 12 months) for stage I or stage II endometriosis-associated infertility. Evaluation should take place if the couple meet the diagnostic criteria for infertility.

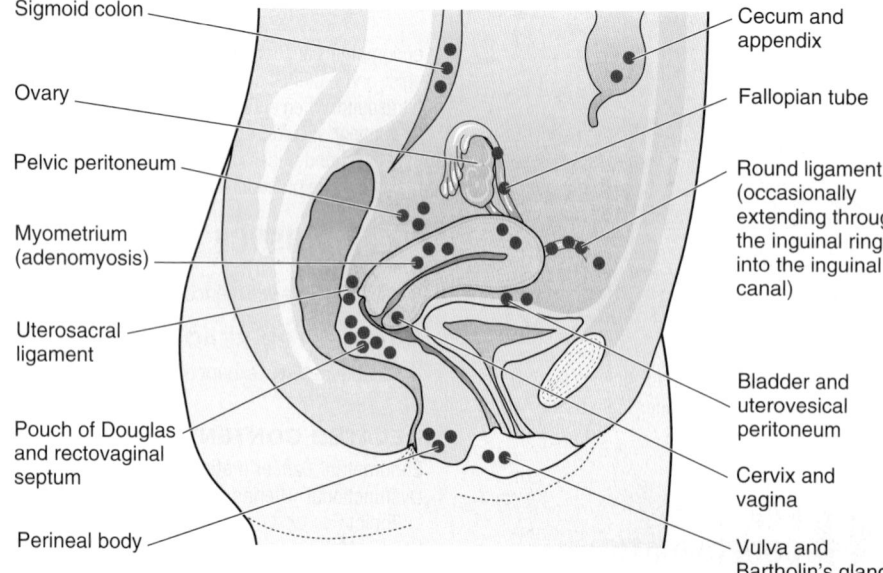

Sigmoid colon
Ovary
Pelvic peritoneum
Myometrium (adenomyosis)
Uterosacral ligament
Pouch of Douglas and rectovaginal septum
Perineal body

Cecum and appendix
Fallopian tube
Round ligament (occasionally extending through the inguinal ring into the inguinal canal)
Bladder and uterovesical peritoneum
Cervix and vagina
Vulva and Bartholin's gland

FIG. 1 Common sites for endometriotic deposits in the pelvis. (From Drife J, Magowan B: *Clinical obstetrics and gynecology,* Philadelphia, 2004, Saunders.)

ACUTE GENERAL Rx

Nonsteroidal antiinflammatory drugs for symptomatic relief of dysmenorrhea.

CHRONIC Rx

PHARMACOLOGIC MANAGEMENT: Estrogen-progesterone:
- State of "pseudopregnancy" created by continuous (discarding pill pack when placebo pills remaining and starting active pills from new pill pack) use of combination oral contraceptives for minimum of 6 months and continuing indefinitely.

Progestins:
- Medroxyprogesterone acetate 10 to 30 mg orally qd and occasionally up to 100 mg orally qd.
- Alternatively, 100 mg IM q2wk for four doses, followed by 200 mg IM monthly for 4 mo.
- Comparison with danazol: progestins cost less, have a more tolerable side-effect profile, and have comparable efficacy with regard to pain relief and so are often the first-line drug. Very little justification for the use of danazol.

Gonadotropin-releasing hormone (GnRH) agonists:
- Induces medical menopause
- Use usually limited to 6-12 months due to hypoestrogenic effects such as osteopenia or osteoporosis but can be given longer in certain circumstances, particularly when paired with estrogen add-back therapy. Referral to specialist strongly advised.
- Leuprolide acetate depot 3.75 mg IM monthly or 11.25 mg IM q3mo or nafarelin 400 mcg nasal puffs bid or goserelin 3.6 mg SC monthly.
- Add-back therapy for protection against vasomotor symptoms and bone loss: norethindrone acetate 5 mg PO qd alone or in combination with conjugated estrogen 0.625 mg orally qd.

- Add-back therapy allows gonadotropin-releasing hormone (GnRH) agonist use to be extended to 1 yr based on limited studies available.

Alternative therapies for inhibition of estrogen action currently under investigation are:
- Aromatase inhibitors: anastrozole, letrozole
- SERM: raloxifene
- Agents enhancing cell-mediated immunity are cytokines (interleukin-12 and interferon-α2b)
- Immunomodulators (loxoribine, levamisole)
- Antiinflammatory: pentoxifylline

SURGICAL MANAGEMENT: Conservative:
- Directed at enhancing fertility or treating pain unresponsive to first-line medical treatment.
- Usually accomplished through laparoscopy.
- Removal or destruction of endometriotic implants by excision, electrocautery, or laser.
- Cystectomy for endometrioma; must remove cyst wall to be effective long-term.
- Laparoscopic uterosacral nerve ablation (LUNA) for midline pain such as dysmenorrhea or dyspareunia (evidence does not support its use).
- Unless pregnancy is desired, patient is usually started on GnRH agonist therapy or continuous OCP immediately after surgery.
- For those desiring pregnancy, surgery alone results in significant increase in fertility.

Definitive:
- Directed at relieving endometriosis-associated pain.
- Total abdominal hysterectomy with bilateral salpingo-oophorectomy and complete excision or ablation of endometriosis.
- Thorough abdominal exploration to ensure removal of all disease.
- Must be prepared to manage possible gastrointestinal and urinary tract endometriosis.
- 90% effective in pain relief; patient must be counseled that pain relief is not guaranteed.
- Estrogen replacement therapy (ERT) to be considered in all women undergoing definitive surgical management; after ERT, recurrence rate is 0% to 5% in women with endometriosis confined to the pelvis but 18% in women with bowel involvement.
- Concern for malignant degeneration exists in implants if unopposed estrogen is used after definitive surgical therapy.

MANAGEMENT OF ENDOMETRIOSIS-ASSOCIATED INFERTILITY:
Conservative surgery:
- Yields significantly higher pregnancy rate than does expectant management, in part because of correction of mechanical factors such as adhesions.

Assisted reproductive technologies:
- Can be used to circumvent unknown mechanism of endometriosis-associated infertility.
- Superovulation with clomiphene citrate or human menopausal gonadotropins; clomiphene citrate results in threefold pregnancy rate over expectant management.
- Further improvement with intrauterine insemination combined with superovulation.
- In vitro fertilization if above procedures are unsuccessful.

DISPOSITION

Tends to recur unless definitive surgery is performed, and should be considered a chronic condition.

REFERRAL

To a reproductive endocrinologist for advanced surgical management or infertility management.

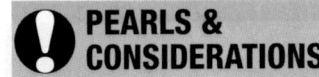

PEARLS & CONSIDERATIONS

COMMENTS

Patient information can be obtained through the following organizations: Endometriosis Association, 8585 North 76th Place, Milwaukee, WI 53223, 414-355-2200 or 800-992-ENDO; Women's Reproductive Health Network, P.O. Box 30167, Portland, OR 97230-9067 or 503-667-7757.

SUGGESTED READINGS
Available at www.expertconsult.com

RELATED CONTENT

Endometriosis (Patient Information)
Dysmenorrhea (Related Key Topic)
Dyspareunia (Related Key Topic)

AUTHOR: **RUBEN ALVERO, M.D.,** and **BARBARA MCGUIRK, M.D.**

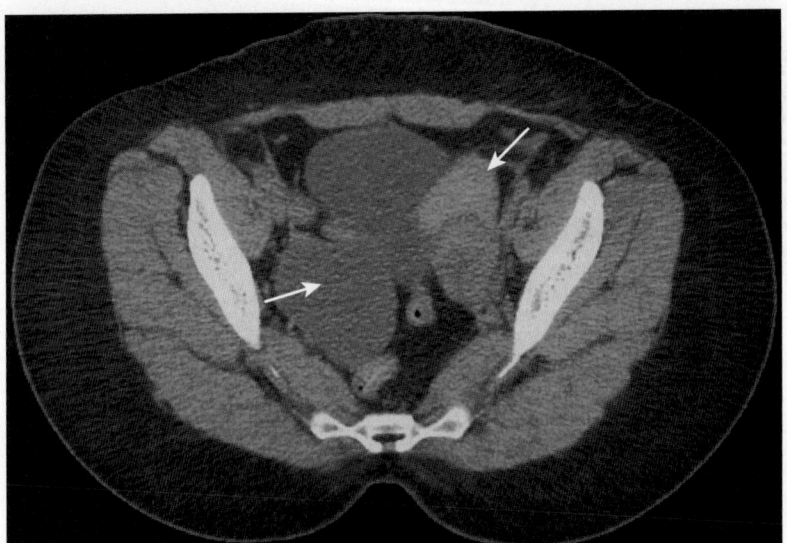

FIG. 2 Computed tomographic scan demonstrates adnexal masses of varying density, subsequently proven to be endometriomas. (From Fielding JR et al: *Gynecologic imaging,* Philadelphia, 2011, Saunders.)

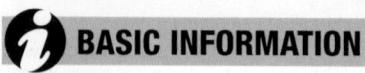 **BASIC INFORMATION**

DEFINITION

Endometritis is defined as a uterine infection after delivery or abortion.

SYNONYMS

Endomyometritis
Metritis

ICD-10CM CODES
O85	Puerperal sepsis
O86	Other puerperal infections
O86.1	Other infection of genital tract following delivery
O86.8	Other specified puerperal infections

EPIDEMIOLOGY & DEMOGRAPHICS

- Overall rate of postpartum infection: estimated between 1% and 8%
- Most common genital tract infection after delivery
- Usually presents early in postpartum period; more commonly seen after cesarean section than vaginal delivery; also seen with an incomplete abortion (spontaneous abortion, legal abortion, or illegal abortion)
- More common in preterm deliveries
- Possible after any uterine manipulation in the presence of undiagnosed cervicitis or vaginitis

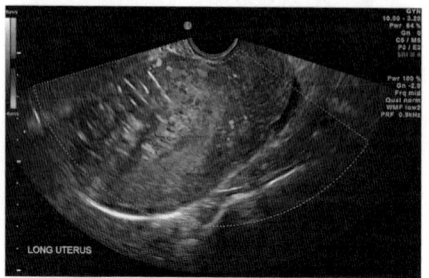

FIG. 1 Endometritis. Patient with uterine tenderness and fever 7 days after classic cesarean section for premature rupture of membranes, chorioamnionitis, and fundic presentation at 27 weeks' gestational age. Sagittal transvaginal ultrasound shows increased vascularity within the endometrium, which can be seen with endometritis. Linear echogenic foci within the anterior myometrium likely represent air and suture material in the vertical uterine incision. Patient's symptoms resolved with antibiotics. (From Fielding JR et al: *Gynecologic imaging*, Philadelphia, 2011, Saunders.)

PHYSICAL FINDINGS & CLINICAL PRESENTATION

- Postpartum oral temperature >37.8° C
- Localized uterine tenderness, purulent or foul lochia; physical examination revealing uterine or parametrial tenderness
- Nonspecific signs and symptoms such as malaise, abdominal pain, chills, and tachycardia

ETIOLOGY

Endometritis is usually associated with multiple organisms: group A or B streptococci, *Staphylococcus aureus* and *Bacteroides* species, *Neisseria gonorrhoeae*, *Chlamydia trachomatis*, enterococci, *Gardnerella vaginalis*, *Escherichia coli*, and *Mycoplasma*.

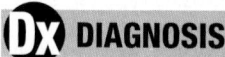 **DIAGNOSIS**

DIFFERENTIAL DIAGNOSIS

Causes of postoperative or postprocedural infections

WORKUP

Diagnosis based on symptoms of fever, malaise, abdominal pain, uterine tenderness, and purulent, foul vaginal discharge.

LABORATORY TESTS

Complete blood count, blood cultures, and uterine culture

IMAGING STUDIES

Ultrasound (Fig. 1) may be useful if retained products are considered a possible source of infection.

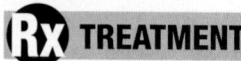 **TREATMENT**

ACUTE GENERAL Rx

Treatment options include doxycycline plus one of the following:
1. Cefoxitin.
2. Ticarcillin-clavulanate.
3. Ertapenem.
4. Imipenem-cilastatin.
5. Meropenem.
6. Ampicillin-sulbactam.
7. Piperacillin-tazobactam.

An alternative regimen is clindamycin plus aminoglycoside or ceftriaxone.

Regimen should be continued for at least 48 hr after substantial clinical improvement. If response is not adequate (Table 1), check cultures and treat with appropriate antibiotics.

CHRONIC Rx

Watch for recurrent infection.

DISPOSITION

With appropriate antibiotic therapy, 95% to 98% cure rate.

REFERRAL

For patients who do not respond within 48 to 72 hr of appropriate antibiotic therapy, obtain an infectious disease consultation or gynecologic consultation.

AUTHOR: **ANTHONY SCISCIONE, D.O.**

TABLE 1 Identified Causes of Poor Response to Antibiotic Therapy in Patients with Endometritis

Cause	Approximate Prevalence (%)
Infected mass, including abscess, hematoma, septic pelvic thrombophlebitis, pelvic cellulitis, retained placenta	40-50
Resistant organisms, commonly enterococci, in a patient receiving clindamycin-aminoglycoside or a cephalosporin	20
Additional cause, including catheter phlebitis, inadequate dose of antibiotics	10
No cause evident but response to empirical change in antibiotic therapy	20-30

From Gorbach SL: *Infectious diseases*, ed 2, Philadelphia, 1998, Saunders.

ⓘ BASIC INFORMATION

DEFINITION

Enteropathic arthritis (EA) is a spondyloarthritis that occurs in patients with inflammatory bowel diseases such as Crohn's disease (CD) and ulcerative colitis (UC). It also includes inflammatory arthritis seen in other gastrointestinal diseases such as Whipple's disease, celiac disease, and after intestinal bypass surgery. Arthritis is the most common extraintestinal manifestation of inflammatory bowel disease (IBD). Spondyloarthritis or spondyloarthropathy (SpA) is a collective term to describe peripheral arthritis, periarticular disease, and axial involvement such as spondylitis or sacroiliitis.

SYNONYM(S)

IBD-related spondyloarthropathy
Enteroarthritis
Arthritis associated with gastrointestinal disease
EA

ICD 10-CM CODE(S)

M.07.60 Enteropathic arthropathies, unspecified sites
M.07.69 Enteropathic arthropathies, multiple sites
M.07.68 Enteropathic arthropathies, vertebra
M07.611 Enteropathic arthropathies, right shoulder
M07.612 Enteropathic arthropathies, left shoulder
M07.619 Enteropathic arthropathies, unspecified shoulder
M07.621 Enteropathic arthropathies, right elbow
M07.622 Enteropathic arthropathies, left elbow
M07.629 Enteropathic arthropathies, unspecified elbow
M07.631 Enteropathic arthropathies, right wrist
M07.632 Enteropathic arthropathies, left wrist
M07.639 Enteropathic arthropathies, unspecified wrist
M07.641 Enteropathic arthropathies, right hand
M07.642 Enteropathic arthropathies, left hand
M07.649 Enteropathic arthropathies, unspecified hand
M07.651 Enteropathic arthropathies, right hip
M07.652 Enteropathic arthropathies, left hip
M07.659 Enteropathic arthropathies, unspecified hip
M07.661 Enteropathic arthropathies, right knee
M07.662 Enteropathic arthropathies, left knee
M07.669 Enteropathic arthropathies, unspecified knee
M07.671 Enteropathic arthropathies, right ankle and foot
M07.672 Enteropathic arthropathies, left ankle and foot
M07.679 Enteropathic arthropathies, unspecified ankle and foot
M07.68 Enteropathic arthropathies, vertebrae
M07.69 Enteropathic arthropathies, multiple sites

EPIDEMIOLOGY AND DEMOGRAPHICS

Arthritis occurs in 6% to 46% of patients with IBD. Inflammatory back pain usually presents before the age of 45 yr. Onset of peripheral arthritis is usually between 25 and 45 years of age.

PREDOMINANT SEX AND AGE: Males and females equally affected. Whereas women more frequently have a peripheral joint involvement, men tend to have an axial involvement (sacroiliac and/or spine joint arthritis).

GENETICS: The presence of HLA-B27 is the strongest association with spondyloarthropathies.

RISK FACTORS:
- Active large bowel disease
- Family history of IBD
- Appendectomy
- Cigarette smoking
- Other extraintestinal manifestations such as erythema nodosum, pyoderma gangrenosum, uveitis, and complicating intestinal manifestations such as abscesses and perianal disease

PHYSICAL FINDINGS & CLINICAL PRESENTATION

- Axial: affects the spine in the form of sacroiliitis with or without spondylitis; can be similar to ankylosing spondylitis or other idiopathic SpA (e.g., psoriatic arthritis, reactive arthritis, undifferentiated SpA).
- Peripheral: affects peripheral joints, predominantly lower limb joints.

- Axial involvement is found more commonly in CD than in UC. Axial disease is independent of IBD activity.
- Peripheral arthritis is the most frequent finding in both CD and UC, equally affecting both sexes (Table 1).
- Periarticular and other extraintestinal manifestations include enthesitis (inflammation of tendon insertion sites into bone such as Achilles or plantar fascia), dactylitis (flexor tenosynovitis of a finger or toe causing sausage-like swelling of digit), uveitis, and psoriasis.
- Main complaints are inflammatory back pain, buttock pain, joint pain (with prolonged morning stiffness and fatigue); symptoms worse with rest or inactivity and improve with exercise.
- Examination reveals evidence of synovitis, progressive limitation of spinal mobility.
- Type 1 arthropathy or pauciarticular (less than five joints): usually acute and self-limited asymmetric inflammatory arthritis; commonly affects large joints of legs such as the knee; occurs early in the course of IBD and commonly parallels the disease activity or flares of IBD.
- Type 2 arthropathy or polyarticular (five or more joints): affects mainly the metacarpophalangeal (MCP) joints; bilateral and symmetric; may be migratory. Symptoms may take a more chronic course, independent of IBD activity.
- Type 3 includes patients with both axial and peripheral forms.

ETIOLOGY

- Theorized that in genetically predisposed individuals with bacterial gut infections, the occurrence of joint inflammation provides important evidence for a possible relationship between inflammation of the gut mucosa and arthritis.

TABLE 1 Enteropathic Arthritis

Feature	Peripheral Arthritis	Sacroiliitis, Spondylitis
Crohn's Disease		
Frequency in CD	10%-20%	2%-7%
HLA-B27 associated	No	Yes
Pattern	Transient, symmetrical	Chronic
Course	Related to activity of CD	Unrelated to activity of CD
Effect of surgery	Remission of arthritis uncommon	No effect
Effect of anti-TNF therapy	Effective	Effective
Ulcerative Colitis		
Frequency in UC	5%-10%	2%-7%
HLA-B27 associated	No	Yes
Pattern	Transient	Chronic
Course	More common in pancolitis than proctitis; related to activity of UC	Unrelated
Effect of surgery	Remission of arthritis	No effect

CD, Crohn's disease; HLA, human leukocyte antigen; TNF, tumor necrosis factor; UC, ulcerative colitis.
From Goldman L, Schafer AI: *Goldman's Cecil Medicine*, ed 24, Philadelphia, 2012, Saunders.

DIAGNOSIS

DIFFERENTIAL DIAGNOSIS

- Hypertrophic osteoarthropathy
- Osteonecrosis (avascular necrosis)
- Septic arthritis
- Erythema nodosum
- Other idiopathic seronegative spondyloarthropathies
- Behçet's disease
- Rheumatoid arthritis

WORK-UP

- Diagnosis mainly relies on clinical evidence and imaging data. There is no gold standard for diagnosis

LABORATORY TEST(S)

- Laboratory testing: Markers of inflammation such as sedimentation rate and CRP may reflect underlying disease activity of bowel disease and thus may not be useful to track for EA activity. CBC can reveal leukocytosis, anemia, thrombocytosis; suggestive of inflammatory response.
- Synovial fluid is nonspecific; shows mild to marked inflammation: WBC 1500-50,000/mm^3.
- Serologic tests are negative for rheumatoid factor, and antinuclear antibodies (ANA) are absent.

IMAGING STUDIES

- Plain x-ray of the spine and pelvis may appear normal in early disease but with progression may show evidence of sacroiliitis, spondylitis, or ankyloses.
- X-ray of peripheral joints may show soft tissue swelling, periostitis, or joint effusion.
- MRI may be used to assess early changes of spondyloarthritis when plain x-rays are negative. MRI is the most sensitive method of detecting sacroiliitis in IBD patients.
- Musculoskeletal ultrasonography is a noninvasive, safe, and easily reproducible means of detecting early pathologic changes in SpA patients. It can identify characteristic features of enthesitis, bone erosions, synovitis, bursitis, and tenosynovitis.

TREATMENT

- Effective treatment of underlying IBD is helpful in controlling the peripheral arthritis. The goal of treatment of EA is reducing inflammation to relieve suffering and prevent joint deformity and disability.
- When IBD and SpA coexist, treatment strategy should also address extraintestinal features such as enthesitis, dactylitis, and uveitis.

NONPHARMACOLOGIC THERAPY

- Rest, physical therapy, and exercise such as swimming

ACUTE GENERAL Rx

- Axial and peripheral arthritis symptoms respond to NSAIDs and physical therapy.
- There has been concern that NSAIDs exacerbate IBD and that NSAID-related adverse events such as ulcers and GI bleeding may mimic IBD flares. COX-2 inhibitors may be preferred to traditional NSAIDs, but similar concerns and cautions apply.
- Intraarticular steroid injections may help treat joint synovitis.
- Systemic steroids can help reduce polyarticular joint and IBD activity but should be used at the lowest effective dose and ideally for only short courses.

CHRONIC Rx

- Immunomodulatory agents such as sulfasalazine, azathioprine, 6-mercaptopurine, methotrexate, and cyclosporine can be used to treat active IBD and peripheral arthritis. Peripheral joint disease responds better to these agents than axial disease. TNF inhibitors, particularly infliximab, adalimumab, and certolizumab, are useful to treat both arthritis (axial or peripheral) and severe, refractory IBD. Golimumab is also in use for refractory IBD and is used for arthritis. Etanercept is effective only to control the arthritis but not the IBD.
- The axial disease associated with IBD is treated as is any SpA. Newer medications approved for other SpAs such as psoriatic arthritis may be promising treatments for EA; these medications include ustekinumab (anti-IL12/23) and secukinumab (anti-IL17A), although their effectiveness for IBD treatment is not clear.
- The choice of biologic requires the consideration of extraintestinal features such as uveitis. This condition can be treated with infliximab or adalimumab, both of which also treat the IBD.
- For highly active IBD, particularly UC, colectomy has been found to ameliorate peripheral joint inflammatory disease but does not influence axial involvement.

REFERRAL

Rheumatology and gastroenterology

PEARLS & CONSIDERATIONS

- When a single joint is affected, consider joint aspiration to rule out septic arthritis. Signs of infection may be atypical in those receiving antiinflammatory or immunosuppressive medications.
- Other extraintestinal manifestations of enteropathic arthritis include skin and mucous membrane involvement, anterior uveitis, Hashimoto's thyroiditis, genitourinary involvement (nephrolithiasis), aortic insufficiency, and cardiac conduction abnormalities. These are often seen in patients with prolonged disease activity and with positive HLA-B 27.
- Pyoderma gangrenosum is the most severe skin manifestation in IBD.

RELATED TOPICS

Ankylosing Spondylitis (Related Key Topic)
Crohn's Disease (Related Key Topic)
Psoriatic Arthritis (Related Key Topic)
Ulcerative Colitis (Related Key Topic)

AUTHOR: **CANDICE YUVIENCO, M.D., RH.M.S.U.S.**

BASIC INFORMATION

DEFINITION

Enuresis refers to the voiding of urine into clothes or in bed that is either voluntary or involuntary in individuals who are expected to be continent (>5 yr of age). The diagnosis is made if voiding occurs at least twice a week for 3 months. Primary enuresis refers to enuresis without a period of continence, whereas secondary enuresis occurs after a 6-month period of normal bladder control.

SYNONYMS

Urinary incontinence
Bedwetting
Nocturia

ICD-10CM CODES
N39.44 Nocturnal enuresis
F98.0 Enuresis not due to a substance or known physiological condition

EPIDEMIOLOGY & DEMOGRAPHICS

PEAK INCIDENCE: Ages 5 to 10 yr. 5 to 7 million children in the U.S. have enuresis.
PREVALENCE (IN U.S.):
- Age 5 yr: 7% of males and 3% of females.
- Age 10 yr: 3% of males and 2% of females.
- Ages 15 and older: 1% of males and females.
PREDOMINANT SEX: Twice as many males as females at all ages
PREDOMINANT AGE: Highest prevalence at age 5 with a steady decrease thereafter at a rate of approximately 12% to 15% per year
GENETICS:
- Approximately 75% of children with enuresis have a first-degree relative with enuresis.
- Almost twice as common in monozygotic than dizygotic twins.
RISK FACTORS:
- Developmental delays
- Behavior problems and ADHD
- Younger age
- Male
- Positive family history

PHYSICAL FINDINGS & CLINICAL PRESENTATION

Three enuresis subtypes are defined in DSM-5:
- Nocturnal only (also known as monosymptomatic enuresis): occurs in each sleep stage in proportion to the time spent in the particular stage. May occur during transition from deep sleep to REM and is without other lower urinary tract symptoms.
- Diurnal only (also referred to as non-monosymptomatic or urinary incontinence): more frequent in girls and rarely after age 9 yr; voiding occurs in early afternoon on school days. Within this subtype, individuals have "urge incontinence" with sudden symptoms of urgency and detrusor instability or "voiding postponement" where individuals ignore urges until the point of incontinence.
- Combined nocturnal and diurnal.

ETIOLOGY

- Enuresis often correlates with other maturational delays, particularly language, motor skills, and social development.
- May be related to toilet training issues, stress (secondary enuresis), inability to concentrate urine, altered smooth muscle physiology, small bladder capacity, or dysfunction of the arousal system.
- Diurnal enuresis associated with a higher rate of urinary tract infections.

DIAGNOSIS

DIFFERENTIAL DIAGNOSIS

- The pathophysiology of primary enuresis involves the inability to awaken from sleep in response to full bladder, or a decreased functional capacity of the bladder with possible excessive nighttime urine production.
- May be associated with encopresis and sleep disorders such as sleep terrors; much less likely to be a primary psychological disorder.
- Organic causes of enuresis include diabetes mellitus, diabetes insipidus, bladder outlet obstruction, small bladder capacity, detrusor instability, urethral valves, meatal stenosis, cerebral palsy, spina bifida, pelvic mass, impacted stool, sedating medications, nocturnal seizures, urinary tract infections, kidney disease, hyperthyroidism, pinworms, and obstructive sleep apnea.

WORKUP

- History and physical examination to rule out anatomic abnormalities, look for signs of obstructive sleep apnea. Fluid intake, voiding diaries, and stooling histories may be useful. Family history of enuresis, particularly for nocturnal enuresis.
- Children frequently experience shame, so gentleness and care must be exercised when questioning or examining the child.
- Observation of voiding is useful to assess for weak stream.

LABORATORY TESTS

- Urinalysis with specific gravity and urine culture if white cells or nitrites to rule out infection.
- Serum studies to rule out diabetes, electrolyte abnormalities, or renal dysfunction.

IMAGING STUDIES

- In complicated cases, or if there is evidence of obstructive sleep apnea, sleep studies may be useful.
- If an anatomic abnormality is suspected, urologic imaging, including voiding cystourethrogram and renal sonogram is possibly indicated: an abdominal x-ray may demonstrate stool retention; MRI of the spine if evidence of abnormalities of lower spine or perineum is found on examination.

TREATMENT

NONPHARMACOLOGIC THERAPY

Behavioral treatment:
- Scheduled voiding to reduce the frequency of enuretic episodes.
- Motivational therapy including sticker or star charts to reward child for dry nights.
- Alarm and pad technique: 66% response rate (compared with 4% of control participants), although about half relapse.
- Punishment for enuresis is not effective.

ACUTE GENERAL Rx

- Desmopressin (DDAVP) administered orally at bedtime significantly reduces the incidence of bedwetting with complete response in 30% of patients and another 40% with dramatic reduction in symptoms. Relapse rate is as high as 70% after discontinuation. Of note, the intranasal preparation is associated with a greater risk for water intoxication and is not recommended.
- Tricyclic antidepressants (imipramine): efficacy supported by randomized control trials. Use with care in children, given the side effect profile.
- Serotonin reuptake inhibitors: lack of adequate trials is notable.
- Indomethacin suppositories may reduce normal prostaglandin inhibitory effects on antidiuretic hormone.
- Table 1 summarizes medications commonly used for treatment of monosymptomatic nocturnal enuresis. Fig. 1 describes an algorithm for management of pediatric enuresis and voiding dysfunction.

DISPOSITION

- After age 5 yr, the rate of spontaneous remissions is approximately 12% to 15% per year.
- The disorder usually resolves by adolescence. However, effective treatment spares considerable misery.
- Fewer than 1% will have enuresis as adults.

REFERRAL

- If coexisting, a psychiatric condition complicates the course of treatment.
- Referral to a pediatric urologist is indicated for primary enuresis refractory to therapy and for selected secondary causes (e.g., urinary tract malformations, neurologic disorders).

PEARLS & CONSIDERATIONS

Illness, hospitalization, and family stressors may precipitate recurrent enuresis after a period of dryness.

PATIENT & FAMILY EDUCATION

American Academy of Pediatrics www.healthychildren.org/English/ages-stages/toddler/toilet-training/Pages/default.aspx

Kidshealth http://kidshealth.org/parent/general/sleep/enuresis.html

SUGGESTED READINGS
Available at www.expertconsult.com

RELATED CONTENT

Bedwetting (Patient Information)

AUTHOR: **MARTA MAJCZAK, M.D.**

TABLE 1 Medications for Treatment of Monosymptomatic Nocturnal Enuresis

Generic Name (Trade Name)	Dosage Formulation	Dosage Regimen	Mechanisms of Action	Comments
Desmopressin acetate (DDAVP)	Tablets: 0.1 mg, 0.2 mg	0.2 mg PO qhs, increasing up to 0.4 mg	Decreased urine volume Possible effect on sleep arousal through its action as a central nervous system neurotransmitter	Risk of water intoxication (headache, seizures); hence, limit fluids 1 hr before and 3 hours after the dose Stop treatment during illness or conditions necessitating increased fluid intake
Imipramine hydrochloride (Tofranil)	Tablets: 10 mg, 25 mg, 50 mg; Tofranil PM capsule 75, 100, 125, 150 mg	1.5-2 mg/kg 2 hr before bedtime, not to exceed 50 mg in children less than 12 yr and 75 mg in older children	Anticholinergic effect on bladder Increased resistance of bladder outlet Possible central inhibition of micturition reflex Possible effect on sleep arousal by central noradrenergic facilitation	Can cause sleep disturbance, mood alteration, decreased appetite Risk of cardiac arrhythmia with overdose

Modified from Chandra MM: Enuresis and voiding dysfunction. In Burg FD et al (eds): *Current pediatric therapy*, ed 18, Philadelphia, 2006, Saunders.

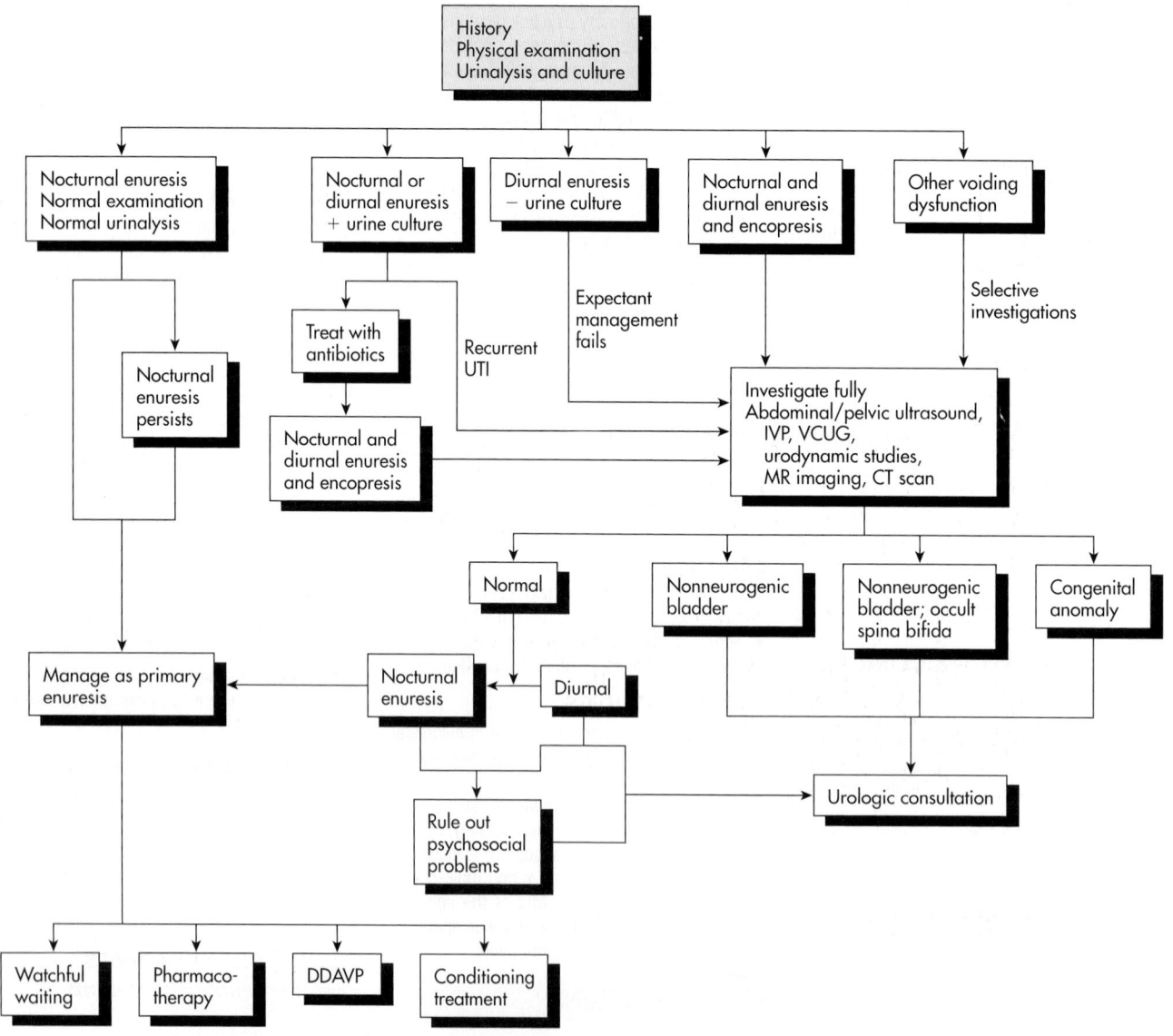

FIG. 1 Algorithm of management of pediatric enuresis and voiding dysfunction. *CT,* Computed tomography; *DDAVP,* desmopressin acetate; *IVP,* intravenous pyelogram; *MR,* magnetic resonance; *UTI,* urinary tract infection; *VCUG,* voiding cystourethrogram. (From Nseyo UO [ed]: *Urology for primary care physicians,* Philadelphia, 1999, Saunders.)

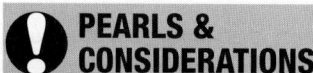

BASIC INFORMATION

DEFINITION

- Epididymitis is an inflammatory reaction of the epididymis caused by either an infectious agent or local trauma. In most cases of acute epididymitis, the testis is also involved (orchitis).
- Epididymitis is considered chronic if lasting ≥6 wk. Chronic epididymitis has been subcategorized into inflammatory chronic epididymitis, obstructive chronic epididymitis, and chronic epididymalgia.

SYNONYMS

Nonspecific bacterial epididymitis
Sexually transmitted epididymitis

ICD-10CM CODES
N45.1   Epididymitis
A54.00 Gonococcal infection of lower
        genitourinary tract, unspecified

EPIDEMIOLOGY & DEMOGRAPHICS

INCIDENCE (IN U.S.): Cause of >600,000 visits to physicians per year
PEAK INCIDENCE: Sexually active years
PREDOMINANT SEX: Exclusive to males
PREDOMINANT AGE: All ages affected but usually in sexually active men or older males
CONGENITAL: Congenital urologic structural disorders possibly predisposing to infections

PHYSICAL FINDINGS & CLINICAL PRESENTATION

- Tender swelling of the scrotum with erythema, usually unilateral testicular pain and tenderness
- Dysuria and/or urethral discharge
- Fever and signs of systemic illness (less common)
- Pain and redness on scrotal examination
- Hydrocele or even epididymoorchitis, especially late
- Chronic draining scrotal sinuses with a "beadlike" enlargement of the vas deferens in tuberculous disease

ETIOLOGY

- In young, sexually active men (<35 years of age), the most common infectious agents isolated are *Neisseria gonorrhoeae* and *Chlamydia trachomatis.*
- In older men (>35 years of age) or with underlying urologic disease:
  1. Gram-negative aerobic rods are predominant (i.e., *Escherichia coli*).
  2. Similar organisms are found in men following invasive urologic procedures.
  3. Gram-positive cocci are rarely seen in these groups.
  4. Mycobacteria may also be a cause of epididymitis.
- Acute epididymitis caused by sexually transmitted enteric organisms (e.g., *Escherichia coli*) also occurs among men who are the insertive partner during anal intercourse.
- Young, prepubertal boys may present with epididymitis caused by coliform bacteria;

almost always a complication of underlying urologic disease such as reflux.
- In AIDS patients, CMV and *Salmonella* epididymitis have been described. CMV may have a negative urine culture. Toxoplasmosis and *Cryptococcus* should also be considered as a cause of epididymitis in AIDS patients.
- Chronic infectious epididymitis is mostly frequently seen in conditions associated with granulomatous reaction; mycobacterium tuberculosis is the most common granulomatous disease affecting the epididymis.

DIAGNOSIS

DIFFERENTIAL DIAGNOSIS

- Orchitis
- Testicular torsion, trauma, or tumor
- Epididymal cyst
- Hydrocele
- Varicocele
- Spermatocele
- Testicular torsion should be considered in all cases (Table E1).

WORKUP

- Consideration of a full assessment of the urologic tract in patients with bacterial infection, especially if recurrent
- If discharge is present, cultures and Gram stain smear of urethral exudate. Gram stain will demonstrate ≥5 WBC per oil immersion field.
- In sexually active men: gonococcal cultures of the throat and rectum possibly of value
- If testicular torsion a consideration: radionuclear imaging
- Examination of first void uncentrifuged urine for leukocytes if the urethral Gram stain is negative. Positive leukocyte esterase test on first-void urine or microscopic examination of first-void urine sediment will demonstrate ≥10 WBC per high power field. A culture and Gram-stained smear of this urine specimen should be obtained along with nucleic acid amplification studies (ligase chain reaction [LCR]) from urine samples for gonorrhea and *Chlamydia* spp.
- Imaging with sonogram

LABORATORY TESTS

- All suspected cases of acute epididymitis should be tested for *C. trachomatis* and for *N. gonorrhoeae* by NAAT. Urine is the preferred specimen for NAAT testing.
- Urinalysis and urine culture if dysuria is present or if urinary tract infection is suspected
- HIV testing and counseling
- PPD placed and chest x-ray viewed if TB suspected (rare cases)
- Rarely, biopsy to ensure the diagnosis of tuberculous epididymitis

TREATMENT

ACUTE GENERAL Rx

- Ice packs and scrotal elevation for relief of pain
- Analgesia with acetaminophen with or without codeine or NSAIDs

- Antibiotics to cover suspected pathogens. Empiric therapy is indicated before laboratory test results are available.
- Recommended regimens are ceftriaxone 250 mg IM in a single dose plus doxycycline 100 mg bid for 10 days. For acute epididymitis most likely caused by enteric organisms, treatment options are levofloxacin 500 mg qd × 10 days or ofloxacin 300 mg bid × 10 days. Add ceftriaxone 250 mg IM single dose to levofloxacin or ofloxacin in men who practice insertive anal sex and are suspected to have chlamydia and gonorrhea and enteric organisms.
- Best treatment for older men with gram-negative bacteriuria: ofloxacin 300 mg PO bid for 10 days or levofloxacin 500 mg PO qd for 10 days
- *Pseudomonas* covered by ciprofloxacin PO or IV or cefepime (2 g IV q12h)
- Consider ampicillin-sulbactam, 3rd-generation cephalosporin, ticarcillin-clavulanate, or piperacillin-tazobactam in toxic-appearing patients.
- Surgical aspiration of local abscesses or even open surgical drainage
- Diabetics: especially prone to develop more extensive scrotal infections, including Fournier's gangrene
- Reinforcement of compliance with antibiotics to avoid partial treatment

CHRONIC Rx

- Repair of underlying structural defects is considered especially if infections are severe or recur.
- Surgical repair of reflux in young boys should be undertaken promptly and at a young age when possible.
- Sex partners of patient should be referred for evaluation and treatment.

REFERRAL

- If abscess or chronic structural problems suspected
- If another diagnosis, such as testicular torsion, is suspected

PEARLS & CONSIDERATIONS

- Recurrent epididymitis in sexually active men is usually related to failure to simultaneously treat sexual partners for STDs.
- Recurrent epididymitis in non-sexually active men is generally related to structural-anatomic defects in the genitourinary system or relapsing disease from inadequate initial treatment or antimicrobial resistance.
- Tuberculous epididymitis fails to respond to seemingly adequate antimicrobial therapy even without characteristic radiographic changes on chest films.

SUGGESTED READINGS

Available at www.expertconsult.com

RELATED CONTENT

Epididymitis (Patient Information)
Orchidis (Related Key Topic)
Testicular Torsion (Related Key Topic)

AUTHOR: **PHILIP A. CHAN, M.D., M.S.**

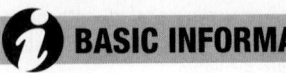 **BASIC INFORMATION**

DEFINITION

Epidural abscess is a suppurative infection of the central nervous system localized between the dura mater and the overlying skull or vertebral column. There are two types of epidural abscess: spinal epidural abscess (SEA) and intracranial epidural abscess (IEA), depending on the location within the central nervous system.

SYNONYMS

Spinal epidural abscess
Intraspinal abscess

ICD-10CM CODES
G06.2 Extradural and subdural abscess, unspecified

EPIDEMIOLOGY & DEMOGRAPHICS

INCIDENCE: Spinal epidural abscess: 2 to 25 patients per 100,000 admissions; spinal epidural abscess is 9 times more common than intracranial abscess
PEAK INCIDENCE: Median age at onset of spinal epidural abscess: 50 years old
PREVALENCE: Greatest between 50 and 70 years of age
PREDOMINANT SEX: More common in men
RISK FACTORS: Bacteremia, secondary to distant infection; epidural catheter placement (0.5% to 3% risk), paraspinal injections of glucocorticoids or for pain management, contiguous bone or soft tissue infection, intravenous drug abuse, diabetes, immunosuppressive therapy, HIV

PHYSICAL FINDINGS & CLINICAL PRESENTATION

- Initially nonspecific, such as fever and malaise
- Classic triad: fever, spinal pain, and neurologic deficits are not common
- More commonly:
  1. Localized and significant back pain is present.
  2. Nerve root pain is present ("shooting" or "electrical" from involved nerve root).
  3. Motor weakness, sensory changes, and even paralysis can occur.
  4. Fever may not be a prominent sign.

ETIOLOGY

- Bacteria enter the epidural space most often secondary to hematogenous spread from foci elsewhere in the body (25% to 50% of cases) or by direct extension from nearby infected tissues such as vertebral body or psoas muscle. A local intervention such as injection can also cause infection.
- Hematogenous foci include furuncles, cellulitis, urinary tract infection, pharyngitis, and pneumonia.
- Microbiology:
  1. *Staphylococcus aureus*, including methicillin-resistant S. *aureus* (MRSA), accounts for 50% to 90% of cases.
  2. Aerobic and anaerobic streptococci account for 8% to 17% of cases.
  3. Aerobic gram-negative rods (*Escherichia coli* and *Pseudomonas*) account for 10% to 17% of cases.
  4. Coagulase-negative staphylococci can be seen with spinal procedures.

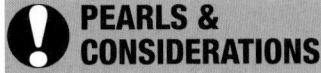 **DIAGNOSIS**

DIFFERENTIAL DIAGNOSIS

- Disc and degenerative bone disease
- Metastatic tumors
- Vertebral discitis and osteomyelitis

WORKUP

Includes a combination of physical exam with neurologic evaluation, blood work, and radiographic studies

LABORATORY TESTS

- Blood cultures
- Culture of fluid or pus by CT-guided aspiration if possible
- Erythrocyte sedimentation rate and/or C-reactive protein
- CBC with differential

IMAGING STUDIES

- MRI with gadolinium is the diagnostic test of choice and imperative if diagnosis is considered.
- CT is an alternative but not as good as MRI for visualizing spinal cord and epidural space.
- CT myelography can be performed if MRI is not available.

TREATMENT

NONPHARMACOLOGIC THERAPY

- Immediate surgery is required if neurologic deficits occur or the patient worsens with medical therapy.
- CT-guided aspiration of abscess with antimicrobial therapy is an alternative treatment to surgery for patients without neurologic deficits.

ACUTE GENERAL Rx

- Empiric antibiotic regimen should include antibiotics effective against staphylococci (including MRSA), streptococci, and gram-negative rods.
- Examples are vancomycin (30 to 60 mg/kg daily divided in q12h doses adjusted for creatinine clearance *plus* metronidazole (500 mg IV q8h) *plus* ceftriaxone (2 g IV q12h) or ceftazidime (2 g IV q8h) if *Pseudomonas* is suspected.
- If cultures reveal methicillin-sensitive S. *aureus*, use nafcillin 2 g IV q4h.

CHRONIC Rx

Antimicrobial therapy tailored to culture results may have to be continued for 4 to 6 weeks depending on whether or not there was surgical or CT-guided drainage. If osteomyelitis is suspected, treat for 6 to 8 weeks.

DISPOSITION

- Mortality rates vary from 5% to 32%. Irreversible paralysis can affect 4% to 22% of patients.
- Complete recovery is more likely if neurologic signs are present less than 24 hours before the start of treatment.
- Final functional capacity may continue to improve for up to 1 year after the end of treatment.

REFERRAL

- Neurosurgery should be involved early when this diagnosis is considered.
- Refer to an interventional radiologist for possible aspiration.
- An infectious diseases evaluation is needed for antimicrobial therapy.

PEARLS & CONSIDERATIONS

COMMENTS

It is important to think of spinal epidural abscess early to permit early treatment and prevent permanent neurologic deficits.

SUGGESTED READINGS
Available at www.expertconsult.com

RELATED CONTENT
Abscess, Brain (Related Key Topic)

AUTHOR: **GLENN G. FORT, M.D., M.P.H.**

BASIC INFORMATION

DEFINITION

Epidural hematoma (EDH) is the accumulation of blood in the potential space surrounding the brain, between the dura mater and the inner surface of the skull.

SYNONYMS

Extradural hematoma/hemorrhage
EDH

ICD-10CM CODES

S06.4	Epidural hemorrhage
I62.1	Non-traumatic extradural hemorrhage
S06.4X0A	Epidural hemorrhage without loss of consciousness, initial encounter
S06.4X1A	Epidural hemorrhage with loss of consciousness of 30 minutes or less, initial encounter
S06.4X9A	Epidural hemorrhage with loss of consciousness of unspecified duration, initial encounter

EPIDEMIOLOGY & DEMOGRAPHICS

INCIDENCE: Exact incidence is unknown; however, it is found in 1% to 4% of traumatic head injury cases and 5% to 15% of autopsy series.
PREDOMINANT SEX AND AGE: Male > female
PEAK INCIDENCE: Peak incidence is among adolescents and young adults. It is rarely found in patients older than 50-60 years old.
GENETICS: There is a role for genetics in spontaneous (nontraumatic) EDH caused by coagulopathies and vascular malformations.
RISK FACTORS: Head trauma, especially in cases involving skull fracture.

PHYSICAL FINDINGS & CLINICAL PRESENTATION

- History of head trauma is present.
- Signs and symptoms vary depending on severity.
- Symptoms: altered mental status, nuchal rigidity, headache, drowsiness, confusion, aphasia, photophobia, and paralysis
- Signs: transient loss of consciousness, followed by a "lucid interval" in 47% of cases, in which the patient is free of any neurologic signs or symptoms. This is followed by clinical deterioration including vomiting, lethargy, confusion, or seizures. Other signs may include focal neurologic deficits such as paralysis of limbs, unequal pupils, and coma. Signs of increased intracranial pressure could be found including the Cushing reflex of hypertension, bradycardia, and respiratory distress. External signs of skull fracture—lacerations, ecchymoses, cerebrospinal fluid (CSF) rhinorrhea or otorrhea—may be observed. Skull fractures can be found in 75% to 95% of EDH patients.

ETIOLOGY

- Traumatic: commonly caused by arterial injury (the middle meningeal artery) (Fig. 1) but may also be injury of the anterior meningeal artery, a dural arteriovenous (AV) fistula at the vertex, or from venous bleeding
- Nontraumatic: caused by an infection/eroding abscess, coagulopathy, hemorrhagic tumors, vascular malformations, postsurgical procedures, and in special populations (e.g., pregnant women, patients receiving hemodialysis)

DIAGNOSIS

DIFFERENTIAL DIAGNOSIS

In the setting of head trauma: subdural hematoma, subarachnoid hemorrhage, cerebral contusion, brain laceration, diffuse brain swelling

WORKUP

- Imaging is the mainstay of diagnosis.
- Serial head CT is the test most commonly used due to its simplicity, widespread use, and availability. Typical appearance is a "lens shaped," or "lentiform" hyperdensity (Fig. 2). Box 1 describes CT findings of EDH.
- Note: Head CT is not conclusive in 8% of cases possibly due to severe anemia, early scanning (before blood has time to accumulate), and severe hypotension.
- Brain MRI: more sensitive. Indicated in situations in which there is a strong clinical suspicion but no evidence of EDH on head CT (Fig. 3).
- Angiography: rarely necessary but may be used to evaluate an underlying vascular lesion.
- NOTE: lumbar puncture (LP) is contraindicated in EDH due to risk of brain stem herniation.

LABORATORY TESTS

- Laboratory tests are helpful as adjunct to diagnosis but are not the mainstay of diagnosis or treatment.

- CBC may be helpful to evaluate for anemia, although in an acute onset of bleeding hemoglobin levels can be normal.
- Other tests: renal functions, electrolytes, liver functions, INR may be helpful depending on the case scenario.

TREATMENT

Acute symptomatic EDH is a neurologic emergency that requires surgical treatment to prevent permanent brain injury.

NONPHARMACOLOGIC THERAPY

- Immediate surgical decompression, ideally within 1-2 hr after traumatic event

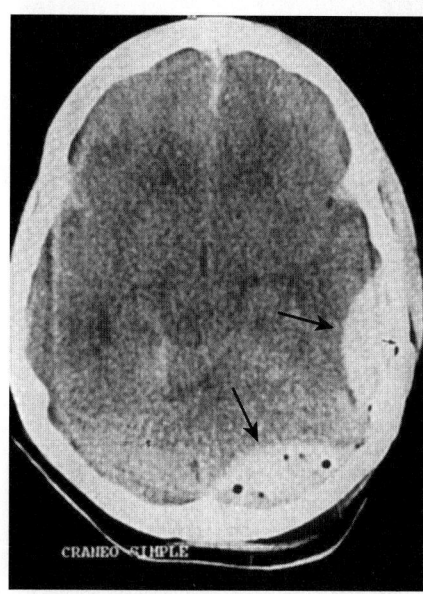

FIG. 2 Head CT showing two epidural hematomas in a 23-year-old involved in a motor vehicle accident. Note air bubbles that are a result of linear fracture in the left temporal bone *(short arrow)*.

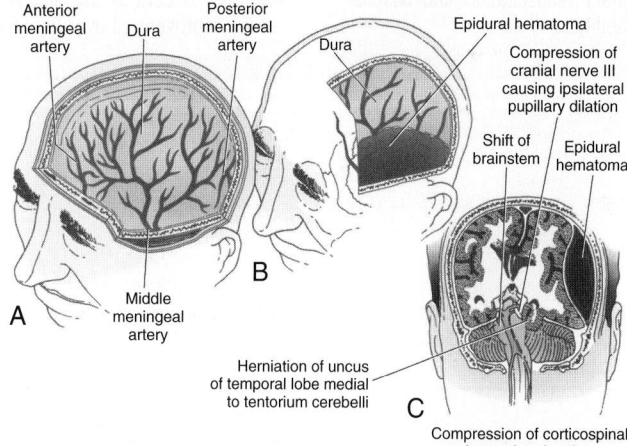

FIG. 1 Epidural hematoma is typically caused by trauma resulting in laceration of the middle meningeal artery. **A,** The middle meningeal artery. The typical traumatic epidural hematoma is caused by a laceration of this vessel. **B** and **C,** A linear fracture of the squamous portion of the temporal bone has torn the middle meningeal artery, which has resulted in an epidural hematoma. (From Rothrock, JC: Neurosurgery. In Rothrock, JC (ed): *Alexander's care of the patient in surgery*, 13th edition, Philadelphia, 2007, Elsevier.)

BOX 1 CT Findings of Epidural Hematoma

- CT appearance: variable white to gray on brain windows
- Location: peripheral to brain, variable but usually temporal region
- Shape: biconvex disc or lens
- Pearl: does not cross suture lines
- White swirl sign means active bleeding

- Significance: may cause mass effect and herniation
- Look for midline shift
- Look for effacement of ventricles and sulci
- Surgical indications: 15-mm thickness or 5-mm midline shift

From Broder JS: *Diagnostic imaging for the emergency physician*, Philadelphia, 2011, Saunders.

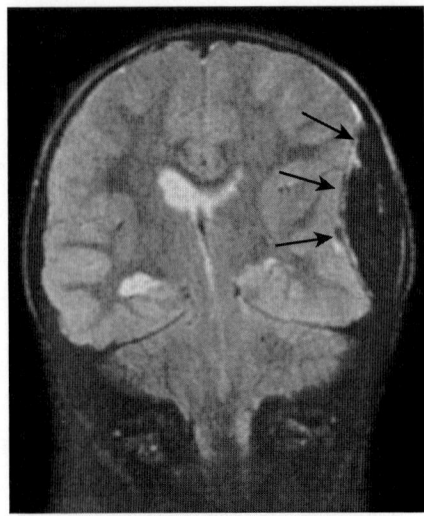

FIG. 3 Epidural hematoma on MRI. Coronal T2-weighted images show hypointense biconvex extraaxial collection in the left temporal region.

- Craniotomy and hematoma evacuation is the treatment of choice. When indicated, identify and ligate the bleeding vessel.
- Burr hole evacuation: this involves drilling a hole in the skull to evacuate the hematoma. It is a lifesaving procedure that is indicated if surgical expertise is limited.

ACUTE GENERAL Rx

- Cardiopulmonary resuscitation and assessment for disability.

- Medical resuscitation maneuvers: head elevation, hyperventilation, monitoring of vital signs and avoidance of hypotension and hyperthermia, sedation if necessary.
- Medications: osmotic diuresis with IV mannitol, cerebrosedating medications, antiepileptics may be used to treat or, in some situations, prevent seizures. The patient should also be started on a proton pump inhibitor to decrease risks of developing an upper gastrointestinal bleed.
- Reversing anticoagulation should be weighed in terms of advantages versus disadvantages.
- NOTE: glucocorticoid therapy is *not* indicated following head injury and may be related to increased mortality.
- Evaluation for surgery: the best available evidence points toward advantages of decompression procedures. Nonoperative treatment may only be indicated if the patient has no symptoms, no focal neurologic deficit, no coma (Glasgow coma score >8), and EDH volume is less than 30 ml by CT scan, with clot thickness <15 mm and midline shift of less than 5 mm.
- Nonoperative treatment involves close monitoring, hourly neurologic checks, and serial head CT scans.

CHRONIC Rx

- There is a risk of permanent brain damage whether the disorder is treated or not. Most recovery occurs in the first 6 months with some improvement over 2 years.

- Children have a tendency to recover more quickly.
- Patients should be educated on rehabilitative exercises and to alert medical professionals in the event of new neurologic symptoms.
- Support and encouragement to patient and family should always be provided.

REFERRAL

Neurosurgery should be the first service consulted. If not available, then general surgery needs to be called. Clinical nurse practitioners, pastoral care staff, and social workers to help patients and families are also appropriate.

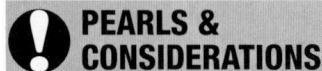

PEARLS & CONSIDERATIONS

- Acute symptomatic EDH is a neurologic emergency.
- EDH should be suspected in any patient with a history of blow to the head leading to a period of loss of consciousness.
- Initial resuscitation is extremely important, but surgery is the mainstay of treatment for acute symptomatic EDH.

PREVENTION

Should be directed toward preventing head trauma: use of appropriate safety equipment (e.g., helmets, hard hats, safe driving, avoiding diving into unknown depths)

PATIENT/FAMILY EDUCATION

Online head injury support groups are helpful: www.headinjury.com/linktbisup.htm, www.headinjury.com/, www.dailystrengthorg/c/Brain-Injury/support-group.

SUGGESTED READINGS

Available at www.expertconsult.com

AUTHOR: **SCOTT M. SOUTHER, M.D.**

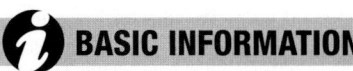

BASIC INFORMATION

DEFINITION

Epiglottitis is a rapidly progressive cellulitis of the epiglottis and adjacent soft tissue structures with the potential to cause abrupt airway obstruction, which can be life-threatening.

SYNONYMS

Supraglottitis
Cherry-red epiglottitis

ICD-10CM CODES
J05.1 Acute epiglottitis

EPIDEMIOLOGY

INCIDENCE (IN U.S.): Due to vaccination against *Haemophilus influenzae* type B, this is a rare infection in children estimated at between 0.6 to 0.8 per 100,000 in one study and for adults at 1.6 per 100,000.
PEAK INCIDENCE: Now highest in children ages 6 to 12
PREDOMINANT SEX: Males

PHYSICAL FINDINGS & CLINICAL PRESENTATION

- Irritability, fever, dysphonia, and dysphagia.
- Respiratory distress, with child tending to lean up and forward.
- Often, drooling or oral secretions.
- Often, presence of tachycardia and tachypnea.
- On visualization, edematous and cherry-red epiglottis.
- Often, no classic barking cough as seen in croup.
- Possibly fulminant course (especially in children), leading to complete airway obstruction.

ETIOLOGY

- In children, *Haemophilus influenzae* type b, still most common cause but now rare due to vaccination *Streptococcus pyogenes,* (group A Streptococcus) *Streptococcus pneumoniae, Staphylococcus aureus* (includes MRSA).

- In adults, *Streptococcus pyogenes* (group A Streptococcus), *H. influenzae* (can be isolated from blood and/or epiglottis [about 26% of cases]).
- Pneumococci, streptococci, and staphylococci are also implicated.
- Role of viruses in epiglottitis unclear.

DIAGNOSIS

DIFFERENTIAL DIAGNOSIS

- Croup (Table E1)
- Angioedema
- Retropharyngeal or peritonsillar abscess
- Diphtheria
- Foreign body aspiration
- Lingual tonsillitis
- Bacterial tracheitis

WORKUP

- Cultures of blood and urine.
- Lateral neck radiograph to show an enlarged epiglottis, ballooning of the hypopharynx, and normal subglottic structures (Fig. 1).
  1. Radiographs are of only moderate sensitivity and specificity and take time to perform.
  2. Visualization of the epiglottis may be safer in adults than in children.
- Cultures of the epiglottis.

LABORATORY TESTS

- CBC: may reveal a leukocytosis with a shift to the left.
- Chest radiograph examination: may reveal evidence of pneumonia in close to 25% of cases.
- Cultures of blood, urine, and the epiglottis, as noted previously.

TREATMENT

ACUTE GENERAL Rx

- Maintenance of adequate airway is critical. Fig. E2 describes the optimal assessment and management of upper airway

obstruction caused by epiglottitis or severe croup. It is crucial to have a tracheostomy set "at bedside."
- Early placement of an endotracheal or naso-tracheal tube in a child is advised.
- Closely follow the adult patient, if no signs of airway obstruction, and defer intubation.
- In children, visualization and intubation are best done in the most controlled environment.
- *H. influenzae* in children is much less common in large part due to the HIB vaccine. Empiric antibiotics:
1. **In children:** use cefotaxime 50 mg/kg IV q8h or ceftriaxone 50 mg/kg IV q24h *plus* vancomycin for its coverage of MRSA. If penicillin allergy, use levofloxacin 10 mg/kg IV q24h *plus* clindamycin 7.5 mg/kg IV q6h.
2. **In adults:** ceftriaxone 2 g IV q24h or cefotaxime *plus* vancomycin.
3. If possible, obtain cultures before initiating antibiotics.
4. If there is an unvaccinated child for *H. influenzae* at home (or in a day care center) who is >4 yr and living with an index case, give close family contacts of the patient (including adults) rifampin 20 mg/kg/day for 4 days (up to 600 mg/day) for prophylaxis.
5. Role of epinephrine or corticosteroids in the management of epiglottitis is not firmly established.

DISPOSITION

Invasive *H. influenzae* infections and epiglottitis are reportable illnesses; this may be particularly important in recognizing an outbreak in a day care center with unvaccinated children.

REFERRAL

- Close cooperation between the pediatrician or internist, anesthesiologist, and otorhinolaryngologist, especially when epiglottis is visualized and when the patient requires endotracheal intubation.
- Best managed in a critical care setting or ICU.

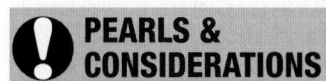

PEARLS & CONSIDERATIONS

The incidence of epiglottitis has diminished markedly since the introduction of the conjugate vaccine against *H. influenzae* serotype B into routine childhood immunization.

SUGGESTED READINGS
Available at www.expertconsult.com

RELATED CONTENT
Epiglottitis (Patient Information)

AUTHOR: **GLENN G. FORT, M.D., M.P.H.**

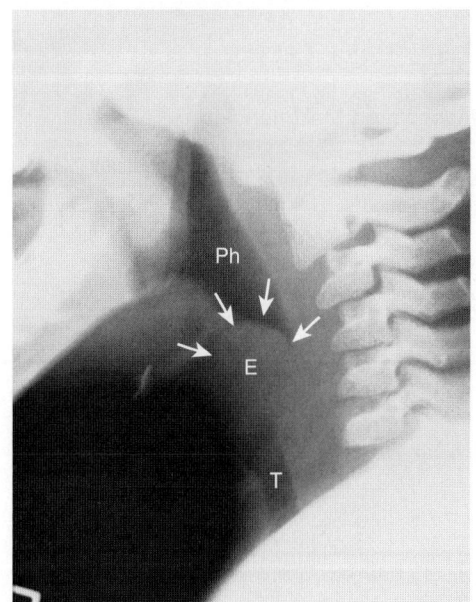

FIG. 1 Epiglottitis. A lateral soft tissue view of the neck shows a ballooned pharynx *(Ph)* with swollen epiglottis *(E)* in the shape of a large thumbprint *(arrows)*. T, Trachea. (From Mettler FA [ed]: *Primary care radiology,* Philadelphia, 2000, Saunders.)

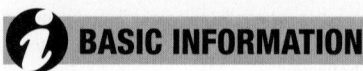

DEFINITION

Epstein-Barr virus infection refers to a disease caused by Epstein-Barr virus (EBV), a human herpesvirus.

SYNONYMS

Infectious mononucleosis (IM)
Kissing disease

ICD-10CM CODES

B27.80 Other infectious mononucleosis without complication
B27.81 Other infectious mononucleosis with polyneuropathy
B27.82 Other infectious mononucleosis with meningitis
B27.89 Other infectious mononucleosis with other complication
B27.90 Infectious mononucleosis, unspecified without complication
B27.91 Infectious mononucleosis, unspecified with polyneuropathy
B27.92 Infectious mononucleosis, unspecified with meningitis
B27.99 Infectious mononucleosis, unspecified with other complication

EPIDEMIOLOGY & DEMOGRAPHICS

INCIDENCE (IN U.S.): 5 cases/100,000 persons per yr of IM.
PREDOMINANT SEX: Neither, although peak incidence occurs about 2 yr earlier in women.
PREDOMINANT AGE:
- Clinical evidence of IM: occurs most commonly at ages 15 to 24 yr.
- EBV infection: occurs earlier in life in lower socioeconomic groups.

PHYSICAL FINDINGS & CLINICAL PRESENTATION

- Most EBV infections either are asymptomatic or cause a nonspecific viral illness.
- Incubation period is 1 to 2 mo, possibly followed by a prodrome of anorexia, low-grade fever, malaise, headache, and chills; after several days, clinical triad of pharyngitis, moderate to high fever, and adenopathy may appear, accompanied by fatigue and malaise.
- Pharyngitis is usually the most severe symptom; white or necrotic exudates are common.
- Symmetrical lymphadenopathy is most prominent in the posterior more than anterior cervical region but may be diffuse.
- Splenomegaly (50% of cases) is possible, most commonly during the second week of illness.
- Maculopapular or morbilliform rash is uncommon but will often occur in patients who receive ampicillin (Fig. 1). Patients may have palatal petechiae, periorbital, or palpebral edema. Mucocutaneous oral hairy leukoplakia (OHL), which is associated with intense EBV replication and the action of EBV-encoded proteins such as latent membrane protein-1, may occur.

- Possible IM presentation: fever and adenopathy without pharyngitis.
- Nausea, vomiting, and anorexia are frequent in patients with IM, probably reflecting mild hepatitis encountered in 90% of infected individuals.
- Although complications such as spleen rupture, airway obstruction, and malignancy may be severe and fatal, they are uncommon and tend to resolve completely.
- Hematologic involvement includes hemolytic or aplastic anemia, thrombocytopenia, thrombotic thrombocytopenic purpura/hemolytic-uremic syndrome, and disseminated intravascular coagulation (DIC). Pneumonia, myocarditis, pancreatitis, mesenteric adenitis, myositis, and glomerulonephritis may occur as well. Nervous system involvement includes Guillain-Barré syndrome, facial nerve palsy, meningoencephalitis, aseptic meningitis, transfer myelitis, peripheral neuritis, and optic neuritis.
- IM is usually a self-limited illness. Acute symptoms resolve in 1 to 2 wk, but symptoms of malaise and fatigue often persist for months.
- EBV is related to lymphoproliferative syndromes in transplant recipients and in AIDS patients.
- Increasing evidence showing an association between EBV infection and African Burkitt's, B-cell, T-cell lymphoma, and nasopharyngeal carcinoma. Table 1 describes EBV-associated malignancies.

ETIOLOGY

- EBV is a ubiquitous virus.
- Infection during childhood is much less likely to cause significant illness.
- Frequency of IM in late adolescence is attributed to the onset of social contact between the sexes.
- Close personal contact is usually necessary for transmission, although EBV is occasionally transmitted by blood transfusion; transfer via saliva while kissing may be responsible for many cases.

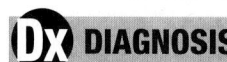
DIAGNOSIS

DIFFERENTIAL DIAGNOSIS

- Heterophile-negative IM caused by cytomegalovirus (CMV).
- Although clinical presentation similar, CMV more frequently follows transfusion.
- Bacterial and viral causes of pharyngitis.
- Toxoplasmosis.
- Acute retroviral syndrome of HIV.
- Lymphoma.
- Lyme disease.

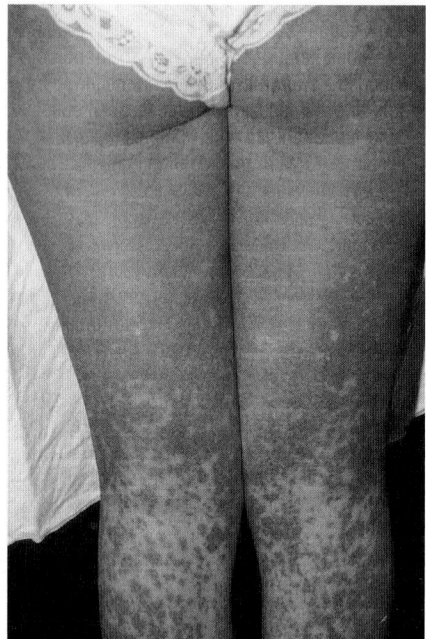

FIG. 1 Patient with infectious mononucleosis and ampicillin-induced rash. Maculopapular rash extends over the trunk and extremities. Rash frequently has a violaceous hue and is often accompanied by pruritus. (Bennett JE et al: *Mandell, Douglas, and Bennett's principles and practice of infectious diseases,* ed 8, Philadelphia, 2015, Saunders.)

TABLE 1 Epstein-Barr Virus (EBV)–Associated Malignancies

Malignancy	EBV Frequency (%)
Hodgkin disease	~40
Non-Hodgkin lymphomas	
Burkitt's lymphoma	20-95
Diffuse large B-cell lymphoma and CD30+ Ki-1+ anaplastic large cell lymphoma	10-35
Lymphomatoid granulomatosis	80-95
T-cell–rich B-cell lymphoma	20
Angioimmunoblastic lymphoma	>80
T-cell, NK-cell, and T/NK-cell lymphomas	30-90
Nasopharyngeal carcinoma	>95
Gastric adenocarcinoma	5-10
Pyothorax-associated lymphoma	>95
Leiomyosarcoma in immunocompromised patients	>95

From Hoffman R et al: *Hematology: basic principles and practice,* ed 5, Philadelphia, 2009, Churchill Livingstone.

TABLE 2 Frequently Determined EBV-Specific Antibodies

Antibody Specificity	Positive in IM (%)	Time of Appearance in IM	Persistence	Comments
Viral Capsid Antigen				
VCA-IgM	100	At clinical presentation	4-8 weeks	Highly sensitive and specific; of major diagnostic utility
VCA-IgG	100	At clinical presentation	Lifelong	Useful for documentation of past EBV infection
Early Antigen				
Anti-D	70	Peaks 3-4 weeks after onset	3-6 months	Correlates with disease severity; seen in NPC patients
Anti-R	Low	2 weeks to several months after onset	2 months to >3 years	Occasionally seen with unusually severe cases; seen in African Burkitt's lymphoma patients
EBNA	100	3-4 weeks after onset	Lifelong	Presence excludes primary EBV infection

EBNA, EBV nuclear antigen; *EBV*, Epstein-Barr virus; *IM*, infectious mononucleosis; *NPC*, nasopharyngeal carcinoma; *VCA*, viral capsid antigen.
Adapted from Schooley RT: Epstein-Barr virus (infectious mononucleosis). In Mandell GL et al (eds): *Principles and practice of infectious diseases*, Philadelphia, 2010, Churchill Livingstone.

WORKUP

Heterophile antibody and CBC with blood smear. Table 2 describes frequently determined EBV-specific antibodies.

LABORATORY TESTS

- Increased WBC common, with a relative lymphocytosis of more than 50% and neutropenia identified.
- Hallmark of IM: atypical lymphocytes of more than 10% (not pathognomonic) are found.
- Mild thrombocytopenia is present.
- Falling hematocrit signals the possibility of splenic rupture or immune hemolytic anemia.
- Elevated hepatocellular enzymes and cryoglobulins are found in most cases.
- Heterophile antibody:
  1. As measured by the monospot test, may be positive at presentation or may appear later in the course of illness.
  2. Negative test is repeated in 1 wk if clinical suspicion is high.
  3. A positive test has been reported with primary HIV infection.
- Viral capsid antigen (VCA) IgG and IgM are rarely used for diagnosis, but better value in children because heterophile antibody is negative in most children younger than 8 years.
- PCR DNA for CMV is the test of choice in transplant recipients who develop lymphoproliferative syndromes.

IMAGING STUDIES

Chest radiograph examination:
- May rarely show infiltrates.
- Possible elevated left hemidiaphragm with splenic rupture.

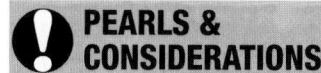 **TREATMENT**

NONPHARMACOLOGIC THERAPY

- Supportive including rest.
- Splenectomy if rupture occurs.
- Transfusions for severe anemia or thrombocytopenia.

ACUTE GENERAL Rx

- Pharmacologic therapy is not indicated in uncomplicated illness.
- Avoid aspirin due to the risk of Reye's syndrome.
- Avoid ampicillin and amoxicillin as their use can frequently precipitate a nonallergic rash.
- Use of steroids is suggested in patients who have severe thrombocytopenia, hemolytic anemia, impending airway obstruction resulting from enlarged tonsils, or fulminant liver failure. Prednisone 60 to 80 mg PO qd for 3 days, then tapered over 1 to 2 wk.
- Although it may reduce initial viral shedding, there is little evidence to support the use of antiviral agents such as acyclovir in the management of IM.

CHRONIC Rx

An extremely rare, chronic form of IM with persistent fevers and fatigue has been described and should be differentiated from chronic fatigue syndrome, which is not related to EBV.

DISPOSITION

Eventual resolution of all symptoms.

REFERRAL

If more than mild illness.

PEARLS & CONSIDERATIONS

COMMENTS

Avoidance of contact sports during the first month of illness because splenic rupture can occur even in the absence of clinically detectable splenomegaly.

RELATED CONTENT

Epstein-Barr Virus Infection (Patient Information)
Mononucleosis (Related Key Topic)

AUTHOR: **MONZR M. AL MALKI, M.D.**

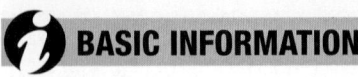

DEFINITION

Erectile dysfunction (ED) is the persistent inability to achieve or sustain a penile erection of adequate rigidity to make sexual penetration possible or satisfactory.

SYNONYMS

ED
Impotence
Male erectile disorder
Sexual dysfunction (a nonspecific term)

ICD-10CM CODES

N48.4	Impotence of organic origin
F52.2	Failure of genital response
F52.9	Unspecified sexual dysfunction, not caused by organic disorder or disease
N52.01	Erectile dysfunction due to arterial insufficiency
N52.02	Corporo-venous occlusive erectile dysfunction
N52.03	Combined arterial insufficiency and corporo-venous occlusive erectile dysfunction
N52.1	Erectile dysfunction due to diseases classified elsewhere
N52.2	Drug-induced erectile dysfunction
N52.31	Erectile dysfunction following radical prostatectomy
N52.32	Erectile dysfunction following radical cystectomy
N52.33	Erectile dysfunction following urethral surgery
N52.34	Erectile dysfunction following simple prostatectomy
N52.39	Other post-surgical erectile dysfunction
N52.8	Other male erectile dysfunction
N52.9	Male erectile dysfunction, unspecified

EPIDEMIOLOGY & DEMOGRAPHICS

PREVALENCE (IN U.S.):
- Increases with age and presence of specific medical comorbidities.
- Approximately 8% in the 20s to 30s, 18% in the 50s, 25% in the 60s, 37% in the 70s, 80% in the 80s.

PREDOMINANT SEX: By definition, only in males

PREDOMINANT AGE: Increases with age

RISK FACTORS: Age, coronary artery disease, peripheral vascular disease, hypertension, hypogonadism, diabetes mellitus, hypercholesterolemia, prostate surgery, neurologic injury, numerous medications, alcohol, smoking or drug abuse, obesity, obstructive sleep apnea, systemic sclerosis

ETIOLOGY

- Most cases involving men older than 50 yr are caused by organic problems related to neurologic, hormonal, or vascular abnormalities or prescription or recreational drugs. In organic ED, nocturnal penile tumescence is generally abnormal, and ED is also experienced during private masturbation and across partners.
- Psychogenic ED results from mental stress, depression, a stressful partner relationship, a partner's sexual and mental health problems, and performance anxiety. Performance anxiety is extremely common and is characterized by a focus on the performance outcome of sex (i.e., obtaining and maintaining an erection) rather than a focus on the process and enjoyment of sex. Psychogenic ED is characterized by normal nocturnal penile tumescence and/or erections associated with erotic material or other partners, and by otherwise negative medical test results.
- Vascular disease: history of hypertension (HTN), peripheral vascular disease, ischemic heart disease, diabetes, smoking. In approximately 40% of men >50 yr, the primary cause of ED is related to atherosclerotic disease, diabetes mellitus (DM), neuropathy, or vascular disease.
- Medication side effects: antihypertensives such as thiazides and clonidine, guanethidine or methyldopa (consider change to ACE inhibitors and calcium channel blockers with lower reported incidence of ED); antiandrogens such as spironolactone, finasteride, ketoconazole; cimetidine (but not ranitidine or famotidine); antidepressants such as selective serotonin reuptake inhibitors [SSRIs]; and antipsychotics.
- Excessive alcohol and nicotine use.
- Recreational drugs, including cocaine, heroin, amphetamines, and marijuana. These may increase libido but impair performance.
- Hormonal dysfunction such as testosterone deficiency (decreases libido and erection), hypothyroidism or hyperthyroidism, hyperprolactinemia, and adrenal insufficiency.
- Neurogenic causes including spinal cord lesions, cortical lesions, and peripheral neuropathies.
- Trauma or pelvic surgeries such as radical prostatectomy or cystectomy.

Dx DIAGNOSIS

DIFFERENTIAL DIAGNOSIS

- A useful tool to diagnose/evaluate ED severity is the Sexual Health Inventory for Men.
- Distinguish psychogenic from organic ED.
- Evaluate for underlying etiology of organic ED and comorbid psychiatric condition.

WORKUP

- Clinical history should include time course (abrupt onset may correlate with reversible cause such as medications, psychosocial stress, psychiatric complaint, trauma. Nonsustained erection may be secondary to anxiety or vascular steal syndrome), cause (psychogenic vs. organic), and change in libido.
- Report of spontaneous nocturnal or morning erections indicate intact neurologic reflexes and penile blood flow.
- Decreased libido may indicate endocrinologic or psychogenic cause.
- If possible, interview partner regarding sexual function, relationship satisfaction, and mental health history.
- Medical and social history should address cardiac disease symptoms and risk factors (HTN, DM, hyperlipidemia, smoking, and substance abuse), pelvic surgery, medications, and mental health.
- Physical examination to check blood pressure, visual field defects to evaluate for pituitary tumors; femoral and peripheral pulses, femoral bruits; gynecomastia; neuronal damage (genital sensation, cremasteric reflex); direct penile damage (e.g., plaque formation such as Peyronie's disease); prostate examination; or testicular atrophy and other secondary sexual characteristics.

LABORATORY TESTS

Screen for diabetes mellitus with fasting glucose. Consider lipid panel, thyroid-stimulating hormone, morning serum testosterone (free and total). If decreased testosterone, check prolactin, follicle-stimulating hormone, and luteinizing hormone.

IMAGING STUDIES

Imaging studies are rarely performed except in situations of pelvic trauma or surgery.

OTHER STUDIES

- Nocturnal penile tumescence testing very specific for distinguishing psychogenic versus organic causes.
- Neurogenic etiologies examined by the cremasteric reflex (inner-thigh touch elicits scrotal contraction), the bulbocavernosus reflex, or the pudendal-evoked response.
- Intracorporeal injection of prostaglandin E_1 to distinguish vascular and nonvascular etiologies (erection is achieved in patients with normal vascular systems). If no erection with direct injection of vasoactive substance, consider duplex ultrasound of penile vasculature.
- In patients without an obvious cause of ED, consider screening for cardiovascular disease prior to starting treatment.

Rx TREATMENT (FIG. 1)

NON-PHARMACOLOGIC THERAPY

- Various psychotherapeutic approaches: cognitive-behavioral therapy preferred; success rates decrease with advancing age and duration of symptoms.
- Psychosexual therapy is first line for psychogenic ED. Psychosexual therapy may be used as for adjunctive therapy in ED from any cause to address contributing, performance anxiety, social, and relationship issues.
- Performance anxiety is best addressed by sensate focus in which a couple is asked to refrain from sexual penetration but enjoy erotic touching.
- Mechanical vacuum devices (function by drawing blood into corpus cavernosum) are 70% to 90% effective but are difficult to use.
- Incorporate vascular risk factor reduction including counsel on diet, exercise, smoking cessation, ETOH intake and screening/treatment for HTN, insulin resistance, and hypercholesterolemia as appropriate. Trials

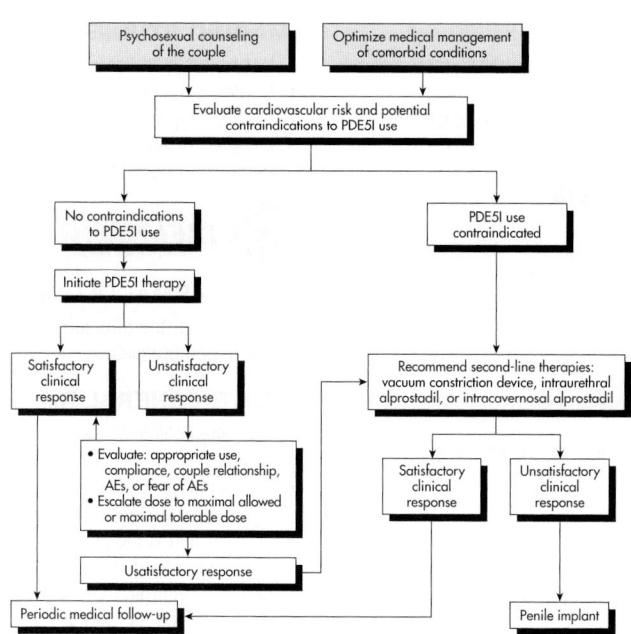

FIG. 1 An algorithmic approach to the treatment of erectile dysfunction in men. *AE,* Adverse effects; *PDE5I,* phosphodiesterase 5 inhibitor. (From Melmed S, Polonsky KS, Larsen PR, Kronenberg HM: *Williams textbook of endocrinology,* ed 12, Philadelphia, 2011, Saunders.)

have shown that lifestyle modification and pharmacotherapy for cardiovascular risk factors are effective in improving sexual function in men with ED.

ACUTE GENERAL Rx

- First-line treatment: In setting of sexual stimulation, four selective phosphodiesterase type 5 (PDE5) inhibitors prolong nitric oxide–induced vasodilation by increase of intracavernosal cyclic guanosine monophosphate levels. Sildenafil (Viagra) and vardenafil (Levitra, Staxyn) can be taken 30 to 60 min before sexual activity, and both are effective for about 4 hr. Avanafil (Stendra) can be taken 15 to 30 min before sexual activity and is effective for about 6 hr. Tadalafil (Cialis) can be taken several hours before sexual activity (although 50% respond within 30 min) and lasts up to 36 hr. All four PDE5 inhibitors have similar efficacy and tolerability, but tadalafil has a longer duration of action and is less affected by high-fat meals and alcohol. Counsel patients to avoid high-fat meals and excessive alcohol when taking PDE5 inhibitors, as they may impede effectiveness.
- With PDE5 inhibitors, avoid concomitant use of nitrates (absolute contraindication), drugs that inhibit or induce cytochrome P450 CYP3A4, and drugs that prolong the QT interval. Caution in men on alpha-adrenergic blocker therapy because of concern for hypotension; start the lowest dose of PDE5 inhibitor. Caution in men who have had myocardial infarction in the past 6 mo, resting hypotension or uncontrolled hypertension,

unstable angina, positive exercise stress test or poor exercise tolerance. Counsel on side effects of headache, flushing, dyspepsia, nasal congestion, changes in color perception (including blue vision for sildenafil and vardenafil but not tadalafil), sudden hearing loss, and priapism (rare). Nonarteritic anterior ischemic optic neuropathy is also a rare association with sildenafil and tadalafil. Consider counseling on safe sexual practices when prescribing PDE5 inhibitors.

- Second-line treatment if PDE5 inhibitors fail: self-injection with intraurethral alprostadil (prostaglandin E_1 [medicated urethral suppository]) applied into meatus of penis before intercourse; or intracavernosal injections of vasodilators (e.g., papaverine or prostaglandin E_1). Consider combining intraurethral alprostadil with PDE5 inhibitor. Relatively high success with self-injection, but attrition is high (Table E1).
- Second-line treatment alternative: vacuum constriction pump; has variable satisfaction rate.

CHRONIC Rx

- Psychosexual therapy is helpful as an adjunctive treatment.
- Psychogenic impotence: PDE5 inhibitors are effective in patients with depression because tissues, nerves, hormones, and vasculature are normal. PDE5 inhibitors are also effective as a way of providing positive experiences and building sexual confidence. Full psychological evaluation is recommended before starting treatment.

- For men not responding to other approaches: surgical implantation of penile prosthesis may be considered. Full psychological evaluation is recommended to evaluate the possibility of unrealistic expectations or partner problems contributing to ED.
- Testosterone therapy in men with low testosterone (i.e., hypogonadal); evaluate for prostate cancer before prescribing testosterone.
- Aerobic exercise may improve ED along with pharmacologic treatment.

DISPOSITION

- Psychogenic-acquired ED will remit spontaneously in 15% to 30% of cases.
- Lifelong ED is usually a chronic and unremitting condition.
- Situational ED may remit with changes in social environment and reducing performance anxiety.

REFERRAL

- Refer if psychotherapy, sex therapy, or invasive organic treatment required
- Refer to urology if PDE5 inhibitors fail or sudden onset occurs after penile trauma

PEARLS & CONSIDERATIONS

- ED is commonly evaluated and treated by primary care physician; refer to urologist if oral therapy fails or surgery is required.
- PDE5 inhibitors are treatment of choice for most causes of ED. Main contraindications are nitrate use and decompensated cardiac disease. Caution in patients on alpha-adrenergic blockers and with blood pressures at extreme ends (significant hypotension or hypertension).
- For optimal response, patients should be appropriately informed of proper use, precautions, and adverse effects of PDE5 inhibitors. Try six to eight times at optimal doses before declaring PDE5 inhibitors a failure. Consider switching among the four PDE5 inhibitors if one fails.
- Men with ED are at increased risk of coronary, cerebrovascular, and peripheral vascular diseases. Screen for cardiovascular risk factors in these patients.

SUGGESTED READINGS

Available at www.expertconsult.com

RELATED CONTENT

Erectile Dysfunction (Patient Information)
Ejaculation and Orgasm Disorders (Related Key Topic)

AUTHOR: **JOHN P. WINCZE, PH.D.**

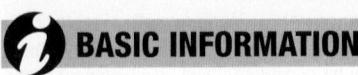

DEFINITION

Erysipelas is a type of cellulitis caused by infection of the superficial layers of the skin and cutaneous lymphatics. Erysipelas is characterized by redness, induration, and a sharply demarcated, raised border.

SYNONYMS

St. Anthony's fire

ICD-10CM CODES
A46 Erysipelas

EPIDEMIOLOGY & DEMOGRAPHICS

PREDOMINANT AGE: Occurs most often in the young or old
RISK FACTORS: Patients with impaired lymphatic or venous drainage (mastectomy, saphenous vein harvesting) and immunocompromised patients. Athlete's foot is a common portal of entry.
RECURRENCE RATE: Relatively common

PHYSICAL FINDINGS & CLINICAL PRESENTATION

- Distinctive red, warm, tender skin lesion with induration and a sharply defined, advancing, raised border (Fig. 1).
- Most common sites are lower extremities and face.
- Systemic signs of infection (fever) are often present.
- Vesicles or bullae may develop.
- After several days lesions may appear ecchymotic.
- After 7 to 10 days, desquamation of affected area may occur.

ETIOLOGY

- Usually group A β-hemolytic streptococci (GABHS)
- Less often group B, C, or G streptococci
- Rarely *Staphylococcus aureus*

COMPLICATIONS

- Abscess
- Necrotizing fasciitis
- Thrombophlebitis
- Gangrene
- Metastatic infection

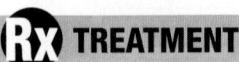 **DIAGNOSIS**

DIFFERENTIAL DIAGNOSIS

- Other types of cellulitis
- Necrotizing fasciitis
- Deep vein thrombosis
- Contact dermatitis
- Erythema migrans (Lyme disease)
- Insect bite
- Herpes zoster
- Erysipeloid
- Acute gout
- Pseudogout

WORKUP

History, physical examination, and laboratory evaluation

LABORATORY TESTS

Diagnosis is usually made by characteristic clinical setting and appearance.
- Complete blood count; white blood cell count often elevated
- Blood cultures positive in 5% of patients
- Gram stain and culture of any drainage from skin lesions
- Culture of aspirated fluid from leading edge of skin lesion has low yield

IMAGING STUDIES

- Not routinely indicated
- Duplex ultrasound for patients suspected of having deep vein thrombosis
- CT scan or MRI for patients with suspected necrotizing fasciitis

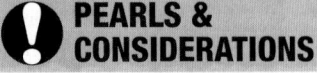 **TREATMENT**

NONPHARMACOLOGIC THERAPY

- Elevation of the affected limb
- Warm compresses

ACUTE GENERAL Rx

Typical erysipelas of extremity in nondiabetic patient:
- PO: penicillin V 500 mg q6h. Use azithromycin in patients who are allergic to penicillin.
- IV: penicillin G (aqueous) 1 to 2 million units q6h. Use vancomycin 15 mg/kg IV q12h in penicillin-allergic patients.

Facial erysipelas (include coverage for *Staphylococcus aureus*):
- PO dicloxacillin 500 mg q6h
- IV nafcillin or oxacillin 2 g q4h
- IV vancomycin 1 g q12h
- Daptomycin 4 mg/kg IV q24h
- Linezolid 600 mg IV q12h

DISPOSITION

Prognosis is good with antibiotic treatment but recurrence is common.

REFERRAL

For surgical debridement for patients with necrotizing fasciitis or for drainage of abscess

! **PEARLS & CONSIDERATIONS**

- Consider early surgical referral when necrotizing fasciitis suspected. Consider skin biopsy when not responding to appropriate antibiotics.
- Look for tinea pedis as portal of entry in erysipelas of lower extremities. Treat if present.

RELATED CONTENT

Erysipelas (Patient Information)
Cellulitis (Related Key Topic)

AUTHOR: **GAIL M. O'BRIEN, M.D.**

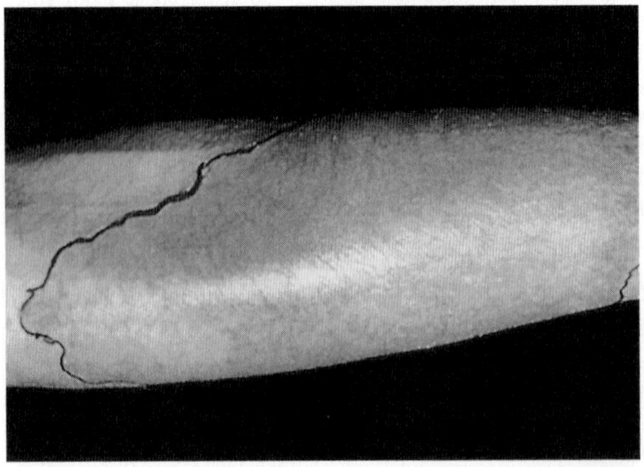

FIG. 1 Erysipelas. Note well-demarcated erythematous plaque on arm. (From Goldstein B [ed]: *Practical dermatology,* ed 2, St Louis, 1997, Mosby. Courtesy Department of Dermatology, University of North Carolina at Chapel Hill.)

BASIC INFORMATION

DEFINITION

Erythema elevatum diutinum (EED) is a chronic form of leukocytoclastic vasculitis consisting of violaceous, red-brown, or yellowish papules, plaques, or nodules that favor the extensor surfaces.

EED may occur in association with infections, hematologic abnormalities, autoimmune diseases, or other conditions.

SYNONYM

EED

ICD 10CM CODES

L951 Erythema elevatum diutinum

EPIDEMIOLOGY & DEMOGRAPHICS

- EED is a rare disease.
- It most frequently affects young and middle-aged adults between the ages of 30 and 60 years.
- There is no known sex or racial predilection.

ASSOCIATED FACTORS

- Infections: human immunodeficiency virus (HIV) infection, beta-hemolytic streptococcal infections, hepatitis, and tuberculosis.
- Hematologic disorders: plasma cell dyscrasias (particularly IgA monoclonal gammopathies), myelodysplasia, myeloproliferative disorders, B-cell lymphoma, and hairy cell leukemia. EED may appear years after the diagnosis of the hematologic disease.
- Autoimmune disease: inflammatory bowel disease, rheumatoid arthritis, celiac disease, relapsing polychondritis, lupus erythematosus, granulomatous polyangiitis, and dermatomyositis.
- Other sporadic reports of disease associations include breast carcinoma and dermatitis herpetiformis.

PHYSICAL FINDINGS & CLINICAL PRESENTATION

- EED most commonly manifests as a bilateral eruption of violaceous, red-brown, or yellowish papules, plaques, or nodules.
- Early EED tends to be soft and erythematous.
- Older lesions are often more firm secondary to fibrosis.
- EED is most frequently found on acral skin and periarticular skin.
- The extensor surfaces of the elbows (Fig. 1), knees, ankles, hands, and fingers are commonly involved.
- Less frequently involved sites include the face, retroauricular area, trunk, axillae, buttocks, and genitalia.
- Nodular lesions progressing to bulky masses appear to be more common in patients with EED associated with human immunodeficiency virus (HIV) infection.
- Additional reported presentations of EED include annular plaques with raised borders, verrucous plaques on the soles, and vesicobullous presentations.

- The cutaneous manifestations of EED may be asymptomatic or associated with a burning or stinging sensation or pruritus (especially in early stages).
- Extracutaneous symptoms include arthralgia, fever, or other constitutional symptoms.
- Ocular abnormalities such as peripheral keratitis, nodular scleritis, panuveitis, and blindness also have been reported.

ETIOLOGY

- The pathogenesis of EED is not well understood.
- It appears to be a form of immune complex–mediated vasculitis.
- The cutaneous findings may result from the deposition of immune complexes in small blood vessels in the skin, leading to complement activation, neutrophilic infiltration, and the release of destructive enzymes.
- Direct immunofluorescence studies reveal perivascular deposition of complement, IgG, IgM, IgA, and fibrin in EED.
- In vitro studies suggest that activation of cytokines such as interleukin-8 contributes to selective recruitment of leukocytes to affected skin.
- Antineutrophil cytoplasmic antibodies (ANCA) may also be pathogenic in EED.

DIAGNOSIS

DIFFERENTIAL DIAGNOSIS

- Granuloma faciale
- Sweet syndrome
- Rheumatoid neutrophilic dermatitis
- Palisaded neutrophilic and granulomatous dermatitis
- Rheumatoid nodules
- Multicentric reticulohistiocytosis
- Sarcoidosis
- Leprosy

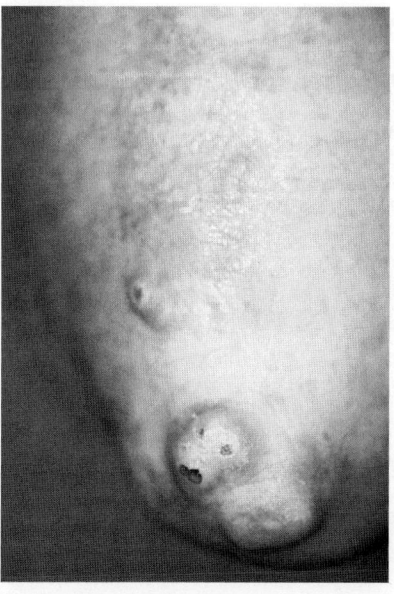

FIG. 1 Erythema elevatum diutinum. Nodules typically form over the extensor surfaces of the knuckles and other joints. (Firestein GS et al: *Kelley's textbook of rheumatology*, Philadelphia, 2013, Saunders.)

WORKUP/LABORATORY TESTS/ IMAGING STUDIES

- Complete blood count, comprehensive metabolic panel
- Human immunodeficiency virus (HIV) test
- Immunofixation electrophoresis
- Streptozyme test
- Hepatitis B and C serology
- Antinuclear antibody (ANA)
- Antineutrophil cytoplasmic antibodies
- Anti-nDNA antibody, antiphospholipid antibodies
- Chest radiograph, urinalysis
- Specific testing for other infections or autoimmune diseases should be based upon the presence of suggestive signs, symptoms, or patient history.

Rx TREATMENT

NONPHARMACOLOGIC THERAPY

Local surgical excision can be beneficial for localized fibrotic nodules of EED.

ACUTE GENERAL Rx

Dapsone (with or without glucocorticoids) is the medical treatment of choice for EED.

CHRONIC Rx

Dapsone, colchicine, methotrexate, tetracycline

DISPOSITION

- EED usually has a prolonged course, characterized by fluctuating periods of exacerbation and stability.
- The disease may resolve spontaneously after 5 to 10 years; however, persistence up to 40 years has occurred.
- EED does not progress to systemic vasculitis.
- Recurrence is common after cessation of dapsone.

SUMMARY & RECOMMENDATIONS

- EED is a rare form of leukocytoclastic vasculitis consisting of violaceous, red-brown, or yellowish papules, plaques, or nodules that favor the extensor surfaces.
- It may occur in association with infections, hematologic disorders, or autoimmune diseases.
- The diagnosis of EED is made based upon correlation of the clinical and histologic findings.
- Treatments for EED have included local medications, systemic medications, and surgery.
- In addition, the associated underlying disease (when present) should be treated.
- Erythema elevatum diutinum exhibits a prolonged relapsing-remitting course.

REFERRAL

- Ophthalmology, dermatology, rheumatology

SUGGESTED READINGS

Available at www.expertconsult.com

AUTHOR: **CATHERINE E. NAJEM, M.D.**

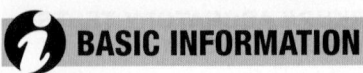

DEFINITION

Erythema multiforme is an inflammatory disease characterized by eruption of annular, maculopapular lesions with dark raised, erythematous, or vesiculobullous center surrounded by a pale zone. It is believed to be caused by immune complex formation and subsequent deposition in the skin and mucous membranes. It is considered a hypersensitivity reaction to infection or drugs.

SYNONYMS

EM

ICD-10CM CODES
L51.9 Erythema multiforme, unspecified
L51.0 Nonbullous erythema multiforme
L51.8 Other erythema multiforme

EPIDEMIOLOGY & DEMOGRAPHICS

PREDOMINANT AGE: 20 to 40 yr.
RISK FACTORS: Often associated with herpes simplex and other infectious agents, drugs, or connective tissue diseases.

PHYSICAL FINDINGS & CLINICAL PRESENTATION

- Prodromal symptoms are mild or absent. Itching or burning at the site of eruption may occur.
- Symmetric skin lesions with a classic "target" appearance (caused by the centrifugal spread of red maculopapules to circumference of 1 to 3 cm with a purpuric, cyanotic, or vesicular center) are present (Fig. 1). The papules may enlarge into plaques measuring a few centimeters in diameter with a dark or red central portion. Target lesions may not be apparent for several days.
- Lesions are most common on the back of the hands and feet and extensor aspect of the forearms and legs. Trunk involvement can occur in severe cases.
- Urticarial papules, vesicles, and bullae may also be present and generally indicate a more severe form of the disease.
- Individual lesions heal in 1 to 2 wk without scarring.
- Bullae and erosions may also be present in the oral cavity. The most common sites are the lips and buccal mucosa.

ETIOLOGY

- Immune complex formation and subsequent deposition in the cutaneous microvasculature may play a role in the pathogenesis of erythema multiforme.
- The majority of cases follow outbreaks of herpes simplex virus 1 and 2.
- *Mycoplasma pneumoniae,* fungal infections, medications (bupropion, sulfonamides, penicillins, nonsteroidal antiinflammatory drugs, barbiturates, phenothiazines, hydantoins).
- In >50% of patients no specific cause is identified.

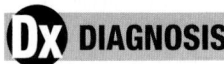 DIAGNOSIS

DIFFERENTIAL DIAGNOSIS

- Chronic urticaria.
- Pityriasis rosea.
- Contact dermatitis.
- Pemphigus vulgaris.
- Lichen planus.
- Serum sickness.
- Drug eruption.
- Granuloma annulare.
- Polymorphic light eruption.
- Viral exanthema.
- Stevens-Johnson syndrome (SJS).
- Toxic epidermal necrolysis (TEN).
- Bullous pemphigoid.
- Viral exanthems.
- Leukocytoclastic vasculitis.
- Lupus erythematosus.
- Secondary syphilis.

WORKUP

- Medical history with emphasis on drug ingestion.
- Laboratory evaluation in patients with suspected collagen-vascular diseases.
- Skin biopsy when diagnosis is unclear.

LABORATORY TESTS

- Complete blood count with differential elevated ESR.
- Antinuclear antibody.
- Serology for *Mycoplasma pneumoniae,* HSV-1, HSV-2.
- Biopsy for atypical cases.
- Direct immunofluorescence if suspecting bullous diseases.

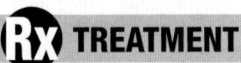 TREATMENT

NONPHARMACOLOGIC THERAPY

- Mild cases generally do not require treatment; lesions resolve spontaneously within 1 mo.
- Potential drug precipitants should be removed.

ACUTE GENERAL Rx

- Treatment of associated diseases (e.g., valacyclovir or famciclovir for herpes simplex, erythromycin for *Mycoplasma* infection).
- Dapsone, antimalarials or azathioprine for severe or resistant cases.
- Prednisone 40 to 80 mg/day for 1 to 3 wk may be tried in patients with many target lesions; however, the role of systemic steroids remains controversial.
- Levamisole, an immunomodulator, may be effective in the treatment of patients with chronic or recurrent oral lesions (dose is 150 mg/day for 3 consecutive days used alone or in combination with prednisone).
- IV immunoglobulins in severe cases.

DISPOSITION

The rash generally evolves over a 2-wk period and resolves within 3 to 4 wk without scarring. A severe bullous form can occur (see entry for "Stevens-Johnson Syndrome").

REFERRAL

Hospital admission in patients with suspected Stevens-Johnson syndrome

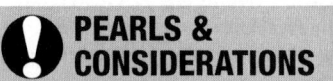 PEARLS & CONSIDERATIONS

COMMENTS

The risk of recurrence of erythema multiforme exceeds 30%. Recurrence may be treated with valacyclovir 500 to 1000 mg/day, famciclovir 125 to 250 mg/day, or acyclovir 400 mg bid. Dapsone, antimalarials, azathioprine, or cyclosporine use is reserved for cases resistant to antivirals.

RELATED CONTENT

Erythema Multiforme (Patient Information)
Stevens-Johnson Syndrome (Related Key Topic)

AUTHOR: **FRED F. FERRI, M.D.**

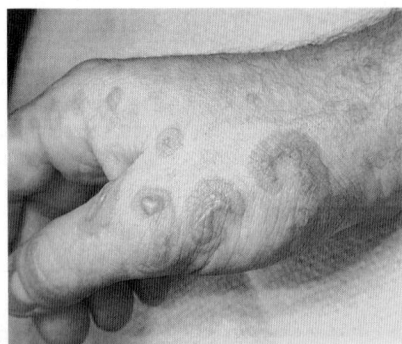

FIG. 1 Iris and arcuate lesions of erythema multiforme. Note erythematous lesions with multiform configurations: target, arcuate, and vesicles. (From Noble J et al: *Textbook of primary care medicine,* ed 2, St Louis, 1995, Mosby.)

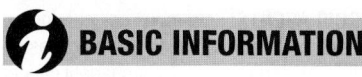

BASIC INFORMATION

DEFINITION

Erythema nodosum (EN) is an acute, tender, erythematous, nodular skin eruption resulting from inflammation of subcutaneous fat, often associated with bruising. It is the most common form of panniculitis.

SYNONYMS

EN

ICD-10CM CODES
L52 Erythema nodosum

EPIDEMIOLOGY & DEMOGRAPHICS

INCIDENCE: Two to three cases/100,000 persons per yr.
PREDOMINANT SEX: Female/male ratio of 3 to 4:1.
PREDOMINANT AGE: 25 to 40 yr.

PHYSICAL FINDINGS & CLINICAL PRESENTATION

- Prodromal symptoms of fatigue, malaise, upper respiratory infection symptoms may precede eruption by 1 to 2 weeks.
- Acute onset of tender nodules typically located on the shins (Fig. 1) and occasionally seen on the thighs and forearms.
- The nodules are usually 1/8 to 1 inch in diameter but can be as large as 4 inches; they begin as light red lesions, then become darker and often ecchymotic. The nodules heal within 8 wk without ulceration.
- Associated findings:
  1. Fever (60%).

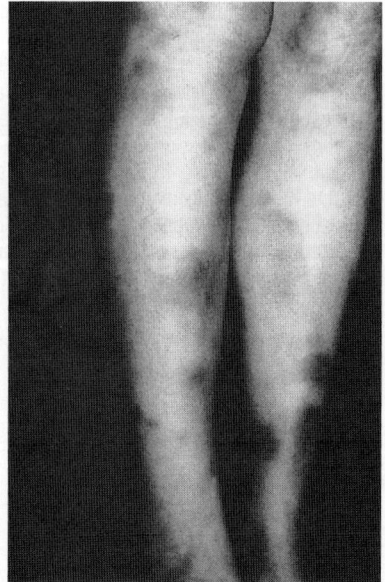

FIG. 1 Erythema nodosum. (From Arndt KA et al: *Cutaneous medicine and surgery, vol 1,* Philadelphia, 1997, Saunders.)

2. Lymphadenopathy (<50%).
3. Arthralgia (64%).
4. Signs of the underlying illness.

ETIOLOGY

Cell-mediated hypersensitivity reaction is seen more frequently in persons with human leukocyte antigen (HLA) B8. The lesion results from an exaggerated interaction between an antigen and cell-mediated immune mechanisms leading to granuloma formation. Up to 55% of cases of EN are idiopathic.
Infections:
- Bacteria
  Campylobacter.
  Streptococcal pharyngitis (28% to 48%).
  Salmonella enteritis.
  Yersinia enteritis.
  Psittacosis.
  Chlamydia pneumoniae infection.
  Mycoplasma pneumonia.
  Meningococcal infection.
  Gonorrhea.
  Syphilis.
  Lymphogranuloma venereum.
  Tularemia.
  Cat-scratch disease.
  Leprosy.
  Tuberculosis.
- Fungi
  Histoplasmosis.
  Coccidioidomycosis.
  Blastomycosis.
  Trichophyton verrucosum.
- Viruses
  Cytomegalovirus.
  Hepatitis B.
  Epstein-Barr virus.
- Drugs (3% to 10%)
  Sulfonylureas.
  Sulfonamides.
  Penicillins.
  Oral contraceptives.
  Gold salts.
  Prazosin.
  Aspirin.
  Bromides.
- Sarcoidosis (11% to 25%).
- Inflammatory bowel disease.
- Hodgkin's disease, non-Hodgkin's lymphoma.
- Ankylosing spondylosis and reactive arthropathies (e.g., associated with inflammatory bowel disease)
- Behçet's disease.
- Lofgren's syndrome.
- Acute myelogenous leukemia.

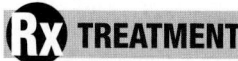

DIAGNOSIS

DIFFERENTIAL DIAGNOSIS

- Insect bites.
- Posttraumatic ecchymoses.
- Vasculitis.
- Weber-Christian disease.
- Fat necrosis associated with pancreatitis.

- Necrobiosis lipoidica.
- Scleroderma.
- Lupus panniculitis.
- Subcutaneous granuloma.

WORKUP

- Physical examination.
- Diagnosis of underlying illness by history, physical examination, and laboratory tests as indicated.

LABORATORY TESTS

- Erythrocyte sedimentation rate.
- Throat culture and antistreptolysin O titer.
- PPD.
- Others depending on index of suspicion (e.g., stool culture and evaluation for ova and parasites in patients with diarrhea and gastrointestinal symptoms).
- Skin biopsy in doubtful cases:
  1. Early lesion: inflammation and hemorrhage in subcutaneous tissue.
  2. Late lesion: giant cells and granulomata.

IMAGING STUDIES

Chest radiograph to rule out sarcoidosis and tuberculosis.

TREATMENT

- The disease is self-limited and treatment is symptomatic. EN nodules develop in pretibial locations and resolve spontaneously over several weeks without scarring or ulceration.
- Treatment of underlying disorders.
- Avoidance of contact irritation of affected areas.
- Nonsteroidal antiinflammatory drugs for pain.
- Systemic steroids (prednisone 1 mg/kg of body weight/day, tapered over several days) may be useful in severe cases if underlying risk of sepsis and malignancy have been excluded.
- Potassium iodide given as tablet 300 mg tid or as a supersaturated solution (5 drops 3 times/day in orange juice) has been reported as effective for symptom control.
- Intralesional corticosteroid injections for persistent lesions.

PROGNOSIS

Typical case:
- Pain for 2 wk.
- Resolution within 8 wk.

RELATED CONTENT

Erythema Nodosum (Patient Information)
Sarcoidosis (Related Key Topic)

AUTHOR: **FRED F. FERRI, M.D.**

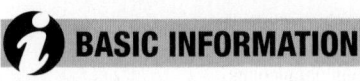

BASIC INFORMATION

DEFINITION

Esophageal tumors include benign and malignant neoplasms of the esophageal mucosa and wall. Carcinomas of the esophageal epithelium, both squamous cell and adenocarcinoma, are by far the most common tumors of the esophagus (see Table 1). Rare esophageal tumors include both malignant (spindle cell, small cell, sarcoma, lymphoma) and benign neoplasms (leiomyoma, papilloma, and fibrovascular polyps). Approximately 15% of esophageal tumors arise in the proximal esophagus, 50% in the middle third of the esophagus, and 35% in the lower third. Tumors in the upper two thirds are usually squamous cell cancers, and tumors in the lower third are usually adenocarcinomas.

SYNONYMS

Cancer of esophagus
Esophageal cancer
Neoplasm of the esophagus.
Malignancy of the esophagus.

ICD-10CM CODES
C15.X   Malignant neoplasm of the esophagus (X defines location)
C15.3   Malignant neoplasm of upper third of esophagus
C15.4   Malignant neoplasm of middle third of esophagus
C15.5   Malignant neoplasm of lower third of esophagus
D00.2   Carcinoma of esophagus, in situ

EPIDEMIOLOGY & DEMOGRAPHICS

INCIDENCE: It is the eighth most common cancer and the seventh leading cause of cancer deaths worldwide. Rates are increasing every decade and are highest in the Asian esophageal cancer belt, extending from the Caspian Sea to northern China, with certain high-incidence pockets in Finland, Ireland, southeast Africa, and northwest France. Incidence has increased six-fold since 1975. Rates of squamous cell

TABLE 1   Classification of Esophageal Cancer

Epithelial

Squamous cell
   Ordinary squamous cell
   Verrucous squamous cell
   Spindle cell (carcinosarcoma)
Adenocarcinoma
   Ordinary
   Adenoacanthoma
   Mucoepidermoid
   Adenoid cystic
Small cell
Melanoma
Choriocarcinoma

Metastatic Disease

Lymphoma
Sarcoma

From Abeloff MD: *Clinical oncology*, ed 3, Philadelphia, 2004, Churchill Livingstone.

carcinoma are decreasing while those of adeno-carcinomas are dramatically increasing.

PREVALENCE: In the United States, there will be an estimated 17,000 new cases and 15,600 deaths in 2015, making it the seventh leading cause of death by cancer among men. The majority of cases are diagnosed at an advanced stage (unresectable or metastatic disease).

RACE, AGE, & SEX PREDOMINANCE: In the United States, squamous cell esophageal cancer is more common among blacks than whites, whereas adenocarcinoma is more common in whites than blacks. The overall male/female ratio is 3 to 4:1; the highest male/female ratio is in the Hispanic population. It usually develops in the seventh and eighth decades and is associated with lower socio-economic status.

GENETICS: Increasing evidence shows that genetics may play a role by increasing susceptibility to esophageal cancer. One well-identified disease associated with esophageal cancer is tylosis (focal non-epidermolytic palmoplantar keratoderma), linked to loss of heterozygosity on chromosome 17q. Familiar clustering of Barrett's esophagus and the recent identification of germ-line mutations in affected sibling pairs support a genetic link to esophageal adenocarcinoma.

CLINICAL PRESENTATION

Symptoms and signs:
- Dysphagia (74%): initially with solid foods, gradually progresses to semisolids and liquids; the latter signs usually indicate incurable disease with tumor involving more than 60% of the esophageal circumference. It may be felt as chest pain.
- Unintentional weight loss: usually of short duration. Losing >10% of body mass predicts poor outcome.
- Hoarseness: suggests recurrent laryngeal nerve involvement.
- Odynophagia and halitosis: unusual symptoms.
- Cervical adenopathy: usually involving supra-clavicular lymph nodes.
- Dry cough: suggests tracheal involvement.
- Aspiration pneumonia: caused by fistula between the esophagus and trachea.
- Iron deficiency anemia: related to chronic GI blood loss.
- Massive hemoptysis or hematemesis from the invasion of vascular structures.
- Advanced disease spreads to lymph nodes, liver, lungs, peritoneum, and pleura.
- Hypercalcemia: associated with squamous cell carcinoma from secretion of a parathyroid-like tumor peptide.
Clinical findings:
- 50% to 60% of patients present with the inoperable stage of their disease (locally advanced, regional, or metastatic).

ETIOLOGY

The pathogenesis of esophageal cancers is attributable to chronic recurrent oxidative damage from any of the following etiologic agents, which cause inflammation, and esophagitis, increased cell turnover, and, ultimately, initiation of the carcinogenic process.

ETIOLOGIC AGENTS: Squamous cell carcinoma
- Excess alcohol consumption is strongly associated with squamous cell esophageal cancer in the United States; hard liquor is associated with a higher incidence than wine or beer.
- Tobacco and alcohol synergistically increase risk for squamous cell cancer.
- Other ingested carcinogens:
  1. Nitrates (converted to nitrites): South Asia, China.
  2. Smoked opiates: Northern Iran.
  3. Fungal toxins in pickled vegetables.
  4. Betel nut chewing.
- Mucosal damage:
  1. Long-term exposure to extremely hot tea (>70° C).
  2. Lye ingestion.
- Radiation-induced strictures.
- Achalasia: incidence of esophageal cancer is seven times greater in this population.
- Host susceptibility as a result of precancerous lesions:
  1. Plummer-Vinson syndrome (Paterson-Kelly): glossitis with iron deficiency.
  2. Congenital hyperkeratosis and pitting of palms and soles (tylosis).
- Human papillomavirus infection (particularly types 16 and 18) has been variably detected in squamous cell carcinoma of the esophagus, sometimes associated with p53 tumor suppressor gene mutations.
- Questionable relationship with prolonged bisphosphonate use (≥10 prescriptions, or use >3 years).
- Possible association with celiac sprue or dietary deficiencies of molybdenum, selenium, zinc, vitamin A.

ADENOCARCINOMA: The incidence of adeno-carcinoma is continually rising, whereas that of squamous cell carcinoma is unchanged.
- Smoking increases the risk of developing adenocarcinoma, particularly in patients with Barrett's.
- Obesity, hiatal hernia, and diets lacking in fresh fruit and vegetables and high in fat (particularly from red meat and processed foods).
- Chronic GERD leading to Barrett's metaplasia and adenocarcinoma via immune cell infiltration and production of inflammatory mediators and reactive oxygen species. The annual rate of transformation from Barrett's to adenocarcinoma is <0.5%.
- *H. pylori* infection may reduce the risk of adenocarcinoma.

DIAGNOSIS

DIFFERENTIAL DIAGNOSIS

- Achalasia.
- Scleroderma of the esophagus.
- Diffuse esophageal spasm.
- Esophageal rings and webs.

LABORATORY TESTS

Complete blood cell count, blood chemistry, liver enzymes. No biomarkers are available currently to diagnose, monitor, or predict outcomes.

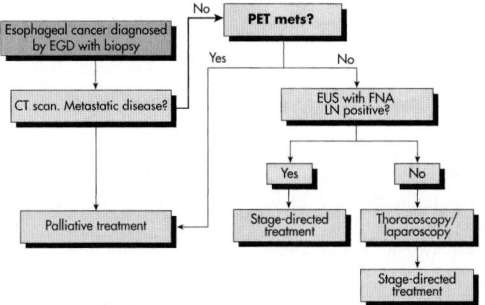

FIG. 1 Algorithm for staging esophageal cancer. *CT,* Computed tomography; *EGD,* esophagogastroduo-denoscopy; *mets,* metastases; *PET,* positron emission tomography. (From Cameron JL, Cameron AM: *Current surgical therapy,* ed 10, Philadelphia, 2011, Saunders.)

IMAGING STUDIES

Imaging studies are important not only for diagnosis but for accurate staging (Fig. 1):

- Esophagogastroduodenoscopy (EGD) (Fig. E2) should be performed initially to visualize smaller tumors, which may be missed by esophagogram, and to allow histopathologic confirmation.
- Endoscopic inspection of the larynx, trachea, and bronchi may identify concomitant cancers of head, neck, and lung ("triple endoscopy").
- Endoscopic ultrasound (EUS) (Fig. E2) is the most accurate method for locoregional staging: to determine the depth of tumor invasion and to assess for and possibly obtain fine needle aspiration biopsies of suspicious lymph nodes.
- Double-contrast esophagogram effectively identifies large esophageal lesions (Fig. E3).
  1. In contrast to benign esophageal leiomyomata, which cause narrowing with preservation of normal mucosal pattern, esophageal carcinomas cause ragged ulcerating mucosal changes in association with deeper infiltration.
- PET CT has become the standard of care, along with EUS, for the most accurate staging. These modalities can determine tumor spread for preoperative staging. CT scans of the chest and abdomen are more useful for restaging patients after initial therapy.
- Staging laparoscopy may alter treatment plans in 20% to 30% of cases by more accurately staging regional lymph nodes and detecting occult peritoneal metastases.

STAGING

Table 2 describes the TNM staging system for cancer of the esophagus from the American Joint Committee on Cancer Criteria.

Rx TREATMENT

TREATMENT OF ALL STAGES OF ESOPHAGEAL CANCER
SURGICAL RESECTION:
- Surgical resection of squamous cell carcinoma and adenocarcinoma of the middle esophagus and lower third of the esophagus is an acceptable initial modality for local and resectable disease in the absence of

widespread metastases detected by CT-PET and transesophageal ultrasound (T1 and T2 tumors). Gastric pull-through or colonic interposition typically is used to provide luminal continuity.
- Endoscopic mucosal resection may replace radical surgical resection in patients with dysplasia and some small early tumors with no lymph node involvement (Tis or T1a), but a recent Cochrane review found no studies comparing endoscopic treatment vs. surgery. Endoscopic mucosal resection may be beneficial for patients who are poor surgical candidates. It may be performed in conjunction with ablative therapies, including radiofrequency ablation, thermal ablation techniques, laser ablation, argon plasma coagulation, or photodynamic therapy. Electrocoagulation (electrofulguration) is also being used and may aid in the relief of esophageal blockage.
- Complications of surgery:
  1. Anatomic fistula (usually with colon interposition, subphrenic abscesses).
  2. Respiratory complications.
  3. Cardiovascular complications are most common, including MI, CVA, and PE.
  4. Mortality is lower and clinical outcomes are better at high-volume hospitals and with minimally invasive surgery.

Despite adequate preoperative staging, 25% of patients initially treated with surgical resection will have microscopically positive resection margins and are upstaged at the time of surgery. This has led to the majority of patients receiving neoadjuvant chemoradiotherapy as demonstrated in the CROSS Trial. The median disease-free survival for this group of patients was significantly prolonged as compared with the surgery-alone group. Death from recurrent cancer was decreased by 9% in the neoadjuvant group as well. The benefit of neoadjuvant therapy on survival was consistent regardless of histologic subtype.

PRE-TREATMENT PATIENT PREPARATION

The patient needs to stop smoking and drinking alcohol if at all possible. Before neoadjuvant or definitive chemoradiotherapy, the patient should have placement of an intravenous access device and a feeding tube (J-tube is preferable before surgical resection).

TABLE 2 TNM Staging System for Cancer of the Esophagus (American Joint Committee on Cancer Criteria)

Primary Tumor (T)*

TX	Primary tumor cannot be assessed
T0	No evidence of primary tumor
Tis	High-grade dysplasia†
T1	Tumor invades lamina propria, muscularis mucosae, or submucosa
T1a	Tumor invades lamina propria or muscularis mucosae
T1b	Tumor invades submucosa
T2	Tumor invades muscularis propria
T3	Tumor invades adventitia
T4	Tumor invades adjacent structures
T4a	Resectable tumor invading pleura, pericardium, or diaphragm
T4b	Unresectable tumor invading other adjacent structures, such as aorta, vertebral body, trachea, etc.

Lymph Node (N)‡

NX	Regional lymph nodes cannot be assessed
N0	No regional lymph node metastasis
N1	Metastasis in 1-2 regional lymph nodes
N2	Metastasis in 3-6 regional lymph nodes
N3	Metastasis in 7 or more regional lymph nodes

Distant Metastasis (M)

MX	Metastasis cannot be assessed
M0	No distant metastasis
M1	Distant metastasis

*(1) At least maximal dimension of the tumor must be recorded and (2) multiple tumors require the T(m) suffix.
†High-grade dysplasia includes all noninvasive neoplastic epithelia that was formerly called carcinoma in situ.
‡Number must be recorded for total number of regional nodes sampled and total number of reported nodes with metastasis.

RADIATION THERAPY:
- Squamous cell carcinomas are more radiosensitive. Radiotherapy achieves good local control but is generally only used as monotherapy in a palliative mode for obstructive symptoms in patients with unresectable or advanced cancer or those with multiple comorbidities that limit treatment. It is best used for cervical esophageal tumors, but response rates are best when combined with chemotherapy.
- Radiotherapy in the preoperative/neoadjuvant setting is taken to a total dose of 40-50 Gy. For definitive therapy, the dose range is 50-55 Gy.
- Palliative radiotherapy for bone metastasis is also effective.
- Complications of radiotherapy: can best be avoided by 3D conformal therapy.
  1. Esophageal stricture, fistula formation, radiation-induced pulmonary fibrosis, and transverse myelitis are the most common.
  2. Radiotherapy-induced cardiomyopathy and skin changes are rare.

COMBINATION CHEMOTHERAPY, RADIOTHERAPY RX, & SURGICAL RX:

- Chemotherapy is most often given with concurrent radiotherapy. Chemotherapy acts as a radiosensitizer and makes tumor cells more vulnerable to the effects of ionizing radiation, thus improving tumoricidal effects on cancer. Neoadjuvant chemoradiotherapy followed by surgery is the most common approach for patients with resectable disease but is employed primarily for patients with stage IIA or higher disease. Five-year survival is improved with neoadjuvant approach (39%) vs. surgery alone (16%). Several trials have now shown that preoperative therapy improves survival among patients with potentially curable esophageal or esophagogastric junction cancer. Neoadjuvant chemotherapy alone is another option for locally advanced disease, but results are not as good as with neoadjuvant chemoradiotherapy.
- Chemoradiotherapy followed by surgery should be offered to late stage I (T1bN0 or higher), stage II, and stage III esophageal cancer patients as the current standard of care. In several studies, this approach significantly improved local control, reduced recurrence, and reduced mortality compared with surgery alone in patients with resectable esophageal cancer. Trimodality therapy is the preferred treatment for most esophageal cancers.
- Chemoradiotherapy alone may be offered as the definitive treatment for patients who are not surgical candidates, and some of these patients may be cured.
- Combination chemotherapy utilizing a platinum doublet (platinum agent plus second agent) can achieve significant tumor reduction in 30% to 60% of patients. Cisplatin, oxaliplatin or carboplatin is usually given with 5-FU (5-fluorouracil) or paclitaxel to obtain the desired tumoricidal effects.
- Capecitabine in combination with either cisplatin or oxaliplatin is as effective as 5FU in the neoadjuvant or definitive treatment setting.
- Complications of chemotherapy primarily include mucositis, nausea, vomiting, diarrhea, myelosuppression, nephrotoxicity, ototoxicity, and neurotoxicity. These can occur to varying degrees and are certainly more significant in the elderly and otherwise infirmed.
- Postoperative adjuvant chemotherapy with or without radiation therapy may be offered to node-positive patients who underwent initial surgery alone.

TREATMENT OF UNRESECTABLE, LOCALLY ADVANCED, OR METASTATIC DISEASE

- Combination chemotherapy regimens as a rule have a higher response rate than single-agent therapy. Response rates can be as high as 50% but that does not always translate into prolonged survival.
- Neoadjuvant chemotherapy regimens can also be utilized in locally advanced or metastatic settings. Cisplatin is probably the most active agent, and this combined with 5FU can yield response rates shown in several studies of 20% to 50%. If a taxane is added to this regimen in the metastatic setting, the triple drug regimen can lead to a prolongation in disease progression by about 2 months, which may translate into prolonged survival. However, the patients have to be carefully chosen for this triple drug regimen because of increased toxicity. Other active double regimens can combine cisplatin with irinotecan, etoposide, or gemcitabine. Again, capecitabine can be substituted for 5FU in these regimens.

TARGETED MOLECULAR THERAPY

- Ramucirumab is a recombinant monoclonal IgG1 antibody that is a vascular endothelial growth factor receptor 2 (VEGFR-2) antagonist. It inhibits ligand proliferation and migration of endothelial cells and ultimately inhibits angiogenesis. It is indicated for second-line therapy in conjunction with paclitaxel or as third line as monotherapy.
- Trastuzumab, in combination with cisplatin and 5FU, can be used as first-line therapy for metastatic esophageal cancer in patients with HER-2 overexpressing adenocarcinoma. Approximately 22% of adenocarcinomas will overexpress the type II epidermal growth factor receptor HER2. The overall response rate is 47%.

FOLLOW-UP CARE

The majority of recurrences develop within 12 months. Clinical monitoring, lab tests, imaging, and endoscopic evaluation where appropriate (particularly Barrett's), are performed for postoperative surveillance, without clear benefit in earlier detection or decreased mortality. For patients who have undergone definitive therapy, it is recommended that endoscopic surveillance be performed every 3 months for the first year, and then annually. Palliative procedures such as repeated endoscopic dilation, endoscopic ablation, endoscopic mucosal resection, photodynamic therapy, brachytherapy, feeding tube insertion, or placement of expandable metal stents or polyvinyl prostheses to bypass tumors have been used for unresectable patients. The morbidity and mortality associated with resection in patients with advanced disease and/or for palliation argues against offering this modality to most of these patients.

SURVIVORSHIP

- Overall 5-yr survival for all stages at presentation is 15% (39% for localized disease, 21% for regional disease, and 4% for distant disease).
- Endoscopic therapy for highly selected stage 0 or stage I patients with disease limited to the submucosa may have 5-year survival rates of 70% to 90%.
- Surgical resection without neoadjuvant treatment: 5-yr survival rate is 5% to 30%, with higher survival (up to 45%-50%) in early-stage cancers.
- Radiation therapy without chemotherapy or surgery: 5-yr survival rate of 6% to 20%.
- Chemoradiotherapy without surgery: 5-year survival up to 30%.
- Combined trimodality treatment: up to 45% to 50% 5-year survival rates (all stages of disease treated).
- Patients with metastatic disease have median survivals of less than 1 year with palliative chemotherapy.

REFERRAL

- To gastroenterologist for endoscopy for patients with dysphagia, odynophagia, or unexplained weight loss, or for palliative care.
- To medical oncologist for evaluation of preoperative chemotherapy and care of the metastatic patient.
- To radiation oncologist for palliative therapy if tumor is unresectable or obstruction is present.
- To hospice if appropriate.

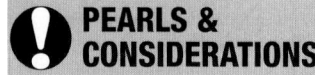 **PEARLS & CONSIDERATIONS**

COMMENTS

More than 50% of patients with esophageal cancer are diagnosed when the disease is metastatic or unresectable.

PREVENTION

- A diet high in fruits, vegetables, and antioxidants may be associated with lower risk of esophageal cancer.
- Avoid tobacco and excessive alcohol use.
- Avoid ingested toxins known to cause esophageal cancers.
- Aspirin may have a chemopreventive role in Barrett's but is only currently recommended for patients with other (e.g., cardiac) indications.
- There is no evidence that vitamins, Chinese herbal regimens, or green tea prevent esophageal cancer.
- Screening the general population is not recommended. If Barrett esophagus is detected, regularly scheduled surveillance endoscopies are necessary, with consideration for radiofrequency or other ablation therapy if dysplasia is detected.

PATIENT/FAMILY EDUCATION

Provide education and support about the likely prognosis because most esophageal cancers are diagnosed at an advanced stage.

SUGGESTED READINGS

Available at www.expertconsult.com

RELATED CONTENT

Esophageal Cancer (Patient Information)
Barrett Esophagus (Related Key Topic)

AUTHOR: **ANTHONY G. THOMAS, D.O.**

BASIC INFORMATION

DEFINITION
Esophageal varices are dilated submucosal veins that occur in patients with underlying portal hypertension, function as a shunt between the portal venous and systemic venous circulation, and can result in severe upper GI hemorrhage.

ICD-10CM CODES
I85.00 Esophageal varices without bleeding
I85.01 Esophageal varices with bleeding

EPIDEMIOLOGY & DEMOGRAPHICS
INCIDENCE:
- Esophageal varices: 5% to 15% per year in patients with cirrhosis
- Hemorrhage:
  1. One third of all patients with varices will develop hemorrhage.
  2. Variceal hemorrhage occurs in 25% to 40% of patients with cirrhosis
  3. The risk of bleeding from varices is approximately 15% at 1 year.
  4. Survivors of an episode of active bleeding have a 70% risk of recurrent hemorrhage within 1 year.

PREVALENCE: Approximately 50% of patients with cirrhosis have varices at the time of diagnosis.
RISK FACTORS: Cirrhosis, low platelet count and advanced Child-Pugh class, hepatitis C with advanced fibrosis

PHYSICAL FINDINGS & CLINICAL PRESENTATION
- Often asymptomatic until acute upper GI hemorrhage: hematemesis, hypovolemia
- No physical findings specific for esophageal varices
- Stigmata of cirrhosis and portal hypertension may be evident: palmar erythema, telangiectasias, gynecomastia, testicular atrophy, jaundice, caput medusae, lower extremity edema, ascites, splenomegaly, hemorrhoids, asterixis

ETIOLOGY
- Portal hypertension results from obstruction to portal venous outflow, and varices subsequently develop in order to decompress the hypertensive portal vein and return blood to the systemic circulation.
- Varices may appear when portal vein pressures rise above 10 to 12 mm Hg.
- Cirrhosis is the most common cause of portal hypertension.

DIAGNOSIS

DIFFERENTIAL DIAGNOSIS
- Budd-Chiari syndrome, cirrhosis, portal vein thrombosis, schistosomiasis, Wilson's disease
- Other causes of upper GI bleeding: duodenal or gastric ulcers, gastric cancer, Mallory-Weiss tear

WORKUP
Upper endoscopy, laboratory tests, and imaging

LABORATORY TESTS
- CBC
  1. Anemia (blood loss, nutritional deficiencies, alcohol myelosuppression)
  2. Thrombocytopenia (hypersplenism, alcohol myelosuppression)
- Renal function panel
  1. BUN: often increased in setting of upper GI bleeding
  2. Creatinine: often elevated by hypovolemia, monitor for hepatorenal syndrome
  3. Sodium: dilutional hyponatremia
- Heme-positive stools
- Type and Crossmatch: in preparation for blood transfusion
- INR/PT and PTT: coagulation factors produced in liver and may be prolonged in liver disease or impairment
- Liver function tests: ALT/AST may be normal in cirrhotic patients due to longstanding fibrosis; elevated alkaline phosphatase and a direct hyperbilirubinemia may be present if cholestatic liver disease is present
- Serum albumin: severe liver disease results in hypoalbuminemia

IMAGING STUDIES (FIG. E1)
Invasive:
- Esophagogastroduodenoscopy (EGD) (upper endoscopy):
  1. In all patients with cirrhosis, screen for the presence or absence of varices and determine subsequent risk for variceal hemorrhage.
  2. In patients with compensated cirrhosis who do not have varices, screening is repeated every 2 to 3 years.
  3. In patients with decompensated cirrhosis (ascites, hepatic encephalopathy, variceal hemorrhage, or jaundice), it is repeated every year or at the time of first decompensation.
  4. Emergently performed if there is evidence of acute upper GI bleeding to diagnose and treat variceal hemorrhage.

Noninvasive:
- Esophagography with barium can diagnose esophageal varices (Fig. E1).
- Capsule endoscopy can also diagnose esophageal varices, although sensitivity is not yet established.
- CT scan (Figs. E1 and E2).

TREATMENT

NONPHARMACOLOGIC THERAPY
- Endoscopic variceal ligation (Fig. E3) is an alternative to nonselective beta-blockers for primary prophylaxis against variceal hemorrhage.
  1. Typically for patients with medium or large varices at highest risk for hemorrhage (Child-Pugh B/C or red wale markings viewed on endoscopy)
  2. Usually 2 to 4 sessions

  3. May not be a permanent solution because varices can recur after initial eradication
  4. Associated with significant complications, including hemorrhage from banding-induced ulcerations
     1. Therefore should be performed by endoscopists with expertise in prophylactic banding
     2. First surveillance endoscopy 1-3 months after obliteration, then every 6 to 12 months indefinitely

ACUTE GENERAL Rx
- Variceal hemorrhage: acute hemodynamic resuscitation with packed red blood cell transfusion, correct coagulopathy and thrombocytopenia, airway protection and intubation as necessary, antibiotics (ceftriaxone or norfloxacin) for SBP prophylaxis, octreotide maintained for 2 to 5 days in conjunction with endoscopic therapy
- EGD to treat bleeding esophageal varices by esophageal band ligation or sclerotherapy

CHRONIC Rx
Primary prophylaxis:
- Nonselective beta-blockers such as propranolol (20 mg twice daily) and nadolol (40 mg once daily)
  1. Increase as tolerated for goal heart rate of approximately 55 beats/min
  2. Blocks the adrenergic dilatory tone in mesenteric arterioles, resulting in unopposed alpha-adrenergic mediated vasoconstriction and therefore a decrease in portal inflow

Secondary prophylaxis:
- All patients with compensated cirrhosis who have bled from esophageal varices should receive esophageal band ligation and beta-blockers, unless beta-blockers are contraindicated.
  1. Transjugular intrahepatic portosystemic shunt or surgical shunt may be performed if bleeding from esophageal varices continues or recurs despite this dual therapy.
- For patients with decompensated cirrhosis there is evidence, although limited, against the use of prophylactic beta-blockers due to the risk for increased mortality.

REFERRAL: Consultation with a gastroenterologist is recommended in all patients with cirrhosis or portal hypertension in order to screen for esophageal varices.

PEARLS & CONSIDERATIONS

Besides variceal size, risk factors for variceal hemorrhage include Child-Pugh class B/C or variceal red wale markings on endoscopy.

RELATED CONTENT
Cirrhosis (Related Key Topic)
Portal Hypertension (Related Key Topic)

AUTHOR: **ADAM J. WEINBERG, M.D.**

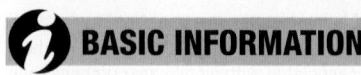

BASIC INFORMATION

DEFINITION

A predominantly postural and action tremor that is bilateral and tends to progress slowly over the years in the absence of other neurologic abnormalities.

SYNONYMS

Benign essential tremor
Familial tremor

ICD-10CM CODES

G25.0 Essential tremor

EPIDEMIOLOGY & DEMOGRAPHICS

Essential tremor is one of the most prevalent neurologic diseases. It affects nearly 7 million persons in the United States.
PREDOMINANT AGE: Can begin at any age, but incidence increases after age 40 years. Prevalence is 6% to 9% for those >60 years of age.
GENETICS: No gender or racial predominance.

PHYSICAL FINDINGS & CLINICAL PRESENTATION

- Tremor, 4 to 12 Hz, bilateral postural and action tremor of the upper extremities (90%-95%), head (30%), legs (10%-15%), and voice (20%). Typically, it is the same amplitude throughout the action, such as bringing a cup to the mouth.
- No other neurologic abnormalities on examination except difficulty with tandem gait.
- Symptoms worsen under emotional distress and improve with intake of small amounts of alcohol.

ETIOLOGY

Often an inherited disease in an autosomal dominant pattern. Sporadic cases without a family history can occur.

DIAGNOSIS

DIFFERENTIAL DIAGNOSIS (SEE TABLE 1)

- Parkinson's disease: The tremor is usually asymmetric, especially early on in the disease, and is predominantly a resting tremor. Patients with Parkinson's disease will often also have increased tone, decreased facial expression, slowness of movement, and shuffling gait.
- Cerebellar tremor: This is an intention tremor that increases at the end of a goal-directed movement (such as finger to nose testing). Other associated neurologic abnormalities include ataxia, dysarthria, and difficulty with tandem gait.
- Drug-induced: Many drugs enhance normal, physiologic tremor. These include caffeine, nicotine, lithium, levothyroxine, β-adrenergic bronchodilators, amiodarone, valproate, and SSRIs.
- Wilson's disease: This is often characterized by a wing-beating tremor that is most pronounced with shoulders abducted, elbows flexed, and fingers pointing toward each other. Usually there are other neurologic abnormalities including dysarthria, dystonia, and Kayser-Fleischer rings on ophthalmologic examination.
- Physiologic tremor.

WORKUP

- Essential tremor is a clinical diagnosis.
- All imaging studies (MRI, CT) are unnecessary unless other neurologic abnormalities are present.
- Obtain TSH to rule out hyperthyroidism.
- In patients younger than 40 years old with other neurologic abnormalities, send ceruloplasmin, serum copper, and 24-hr urine copper to evaluate for Wilson's disease.

TREATMENT

Treat essential tremor when it is functionally impairing. Treatments are up to 75% effective.

NONPHARMACOLOGIC THERAPY

- Stress management
- Minimization of caffeine use if consumption is correlated with worsened symptoms
- Consumption of small quantities of alcohol at social functions, although relief may be short in duration and may be followed by tremor rebound
- A recent trial using MRI-guided focus ultrasound thalamotomy found it effective in reducing hand tremor in patents with essential tremor. Side effects included sensory and gait disturbances.[1]

---

[1]Elias WJ, et al.: A randomized trial of focused ultrasound thalamotomy for essential tremor, *N Engl J Med* 375:730-739, 2016.

ACUTE GENERAL Rx

Propranolol (20-40 mg) may be used in preparation for specific event.

CHRONIC Rx

First-line agents:
- Propranolol/Inderal LA: Typical starting dose is 30 mg. The usual therapeutic dose is 160 to 320 mg. Although not contraindicated, this medication may be used with caution in those with asthma, depression, cardiac disease, and diabetes.
- Primidone: Typical starting dose is 12.5 to 25 mg qhs. Usual therapeutic dose is between 62.5 and 750 mg daily (assuming side effects are tolerated). Sedation and nausea are common at treatment initiation.
- Topiramate: 25 mg qhs, may titrate up to about 400 mg
Other (second-line) agents:
- Gabapentin: Typical starting dose is 300 mg tid. Usual therapeutic dose is 1200 to 3600 mg daily.
- Pregabalin: Typical starting dose is 50 mg twice a day. Usual therapeutic dose is 150 to 600 mg per day.
- Benzodiazepines (i.e., alprazolam): 0.125 to 3 mg daily.
- Focal botulinum toxin injections.

SURGICAL Rx

Thalamic deep brain stimulation (or possibly thalamotomy) contralateral to side of tremor is reserved for resistant tremor or for patients who do not tolerate drug therapy.

DISPOSITION

Patients should be reassured that the condition is not associated with other neurologic disabilities; however, it can become quite functionally disabling over time.

REFERRAL

This is a condition that usually can be treated by the primary care physician; however, if patient fails first-line therapies, the patient should be referred to a neurologist for other drug trials and discussion of possible surgical options.

PEARLS & CONSIDERATIONS

- Essential tremor is the most common of all movement disorders.
- In addition to motor dysfunction, essential tremor can cause significant psychological impact on patients in social situations.

SUGGESTED READINGS

Available at www.expertconsult.com

RELATED CONTENT

Essential Tremor (Patient Information)

AUTHORS: **CHLOE MANDER NUNNELEY, M.D.,**
JOSEPH S. KASS, M.D., J.D., and
U. SHIVRAJ SOHUR, M.D., PH.D.

TABLE 1 Overlapping Features of Various Types of Tremor

Feature	Parkinson's Syndrome	Cerebellar Tremor	Essential Tremor
Present at rest	Yes	No	Yes
Increased tone	Yes	No	No
Decreased tone	No	Yes	No
Postural abnormality	Yes	Yes	No
Head involvement	Yes	Yes	Yes
Intentional component	No	Yes	Yes
Incoordination	No	Yes	No

From Remmel KS et al: *Handbook of symptom-oriented neurology,* ed 3, St Louis, 2002, Mosby.

Diseases
and Disorders

I

BASIC INFORMATION

DEFINITION

Factitious disorder, according to the DSM-5, occurs when an individual feigns physical or psychological signs or symptoms or induces injury or disease with identified deception. Individuals present to others as ill, impaired, or injured and create signs or symptoms by lying, simulating (e.g., putting drops of blood into a urine sample), or actually creating disease (e.g., injecting bacteria or taking medications). The primary aim is to achieve the patient role, and the behavior persists even in the absence of apparent external rewards such as monetary gain or obtaining narcotics. More is known about factitious physical disorder.

The individual may seek examination and treatment to include invasive diagnostic testing or surgery. The term *Munchausen syndrome* is reserved for the most severe variant of factitious physical disorder and is characterized by exaggerated lying (pseudologia fantastica), sociopathy, geographic wandering (peregrinating) from hospital to hospital, and seeking to be in the patient role.

SYNONYMS

Munchausen syndrome (severe form of factitious disorder).
Munchausen by proxy (factitious disorder created in another person, usually a child).
Hospital addiction syndrome.
Surreptitious illness.

ICD-10CM CODES
F68.10 Intentional production or feigning of symptoms or disabilities, either physical or psychological (factitious disorder)

EPIDEMIOLOGY & DEMOGRAPHICS

INCIDENCE (IN U.S.): Unknown
PEAK INCIDENCE: Approximately 30 to 40 yr of age
PREVALENCE (IN U.S.): Likely underdiagnosed because of the role of deception, but estimates range between 0.5% and 2%.
PREDOMINANT SEX: Variable. With psychological subtype M > F; with predominant physical symptoms F > M by a ratio of 3:1. Munchausen syndrome M > F, and Munchausen by proxy mostly younger females.
PREDOMINANT AGE: 30 to 40 yr of age.
GENETICS: No genetic predisposition known

PHYSICAL FINDINGS & CLINICAL PRESENTATION

- Patient is inconsistent or intentionally misleading and resistant to allowing providers to obtain outside records.
- Clinical picture is atypical for the natural history of disease (e.g., an infection that does not respond to multiple courses of appropriate antibiotics).
- Tests, consultations, and medical and surgical treatments done to no avail and often contradicting history provided by the patient.

- Presentation may be acute and dramatic and in excess of what might be expected.
- The patient may predict deterioration or report exacerbation just before scheduled discharge.
- Opposition to psychiatric consultation.

ETIOLOGY

- A history of significant childhood illness; traumatic experiences such as having witnessed violence and physical, emotional, or sexual abuse can predispose.
- Personality disorders and psychodynamic factors often play a significant role in the development and maintenance of this problem.

DIAGNOSIS

This is a diagnosis of exclusion. It requires demonstrating that the individual is taking surreptitious actions to misinterpret, simulate, or cause signs or symptoms of illness or injury in the absence of any obvious external reward. Early diagnosis is helpful to prevent extensive and unnecessary testing.

There may be direct observation of fabrication, the presence of signs or symptoms that contradict laboratory testing, nonphysiologic response to treatment, physical evidence of fabrication (e.g., syringes at the bedside), recurrent patterns of illness exacerbation, or failure to follow the expected natural history of disease.

DIFFERENTIAL DIAGNOSIS

- Primary medical condition.
- Somatic symptoms disorder: not intentionally produced.
- Conversion disorder.
- Conditions in which self-injurious behavior is common such as borderline personality disorder. The goal is self-injury and not to attain the sick role.
- Malingering: clear secondary gain (e.g., financial gain or avoidance of unwanted duties).

WORKUP

- Dictated by the presenting complaints. A reasonable index of suspicion when presentation is not consistent with known pathology.

LABORATORY TESTS

- Laboratory testing often reveals inconsistencies.
- Laboratory abnormalities may reflect the underlying factitious behavior (e.g., hypokalemia in an individual surreptitiously taking furosemide or a clean urine sample obtained by straight catheterization in someone complaining of hematuria).

TREATMENT

NONPHARMACOLOGIC THERAPY

Two approaches may be considered:
- Nonpunitive constructive confrontation by the primary physician and a psychiatrist in collaboration. A supportive stance should be maintained and an offer for ongoing support and follow-up made.

- Avoid overt confrontation with patient but provide him or her with a face-saving way to recover. For example, a therapeutic double bind would involve saying, "There are two possibilities here: one is that you have a medical problem that should respond to the next intervention we do, or two, you have a factitious disorder. The outcome will give us the answer."
- Munchausen's syndrome is the most severe variant and may be virtually impossible to treat except to avoid further invasive and iatrogenic intervention.

ACUTE GENERAL Rx

- Treatment of comorbid psychiatric disorders may be helpful with medications and/or psychotherapy, which may ameliorate the factitious behavior.
- Multidisciplinary staff meetings can be useful to ventilate feelings and develop cohesive treatment plans.

CHRONIC Rx

- Attempt to engage the patient in some form of psychotherapy or at least a harm-reduction strategy.
- Establishment of a central reporting register has been proposed to aid development of evidence-based guidelines.

DISPOSITION

- After being confronted with their behavior, patients may cease factitious behavior, but they may also seek other physicians or hospitals, as in the Munchausen variant.
- Some patients may enter psychotherapy, particularly when they have been given a face-saving approach with avoidance of a humiliating confrontation.

REFERRAL

Always obtain psychiatric referral. Risk management attorneys and hospital ethicists may contribute to challenging decision making in these patients.

PEARLS & CONSIDERATIONS

- Think of factitious disorders whenever there is an unexplained medical course that continues to repeat itself despite appropriate treatment.
- Patients may have a history of working in the healthcare field.
- Gratuitous, self-aggrandizing lying may be noted.

SUGGESTED READINGS
Available at www.expertconsult.com

AUTHOR: **DWAYNE R. HEITMILLER, M.D.**

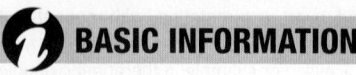

BASIC INFORMATION

DEFINITION

Failure to thrive (FTT) describes a delay in growth and development among children. FTT is a cluster of symptoms rather than a specific disease.

CLINICALLY

The term (FTT) is often used for infants and children with weight below the 5th percentile for sex and corrected age.

SYNONYMS

Pediatric undernutrition
Faltering growth
Weight faltering
Growth failure
FTT

ICD-10CM CODES

R62.51 Failure to thrive (child)

EPIDEMIOLOGY & DEMOGRAPHICS

INCIDENCE: FTT is a common problem, though its incidence in the community is unclear. A total of 1% to 5% of inpatient pediatric admissions are for evaluation of FTT.

PREDOMINANT SEX AND AGE: FTT most commonly occurs among children ages 6 to 12 months, with 80% presenting before 18 months of age. Most FTT patients present before 3 years of age. Males and females are equally affected.

RISK FACTORS: Poverty is the single greatest risk factor. Nonmedical: poverty, food insecurity, social isolation, neglect, and physical or emotional abuse. Medical: Intrauterine growth restriction (IUGR), prematurity, medical conditions leading to inadequate food intake, food malabsorption, or increased metabolic demand.

PHYSICAL FINDINGS & CLINICAL PRESENTATION

Children have blunted growth in height, weight, head circumference, or any combination of these. Children may have pallid, dry, or cracked skin, sparse hair growth, poorly developed musculature, lack of subcutaneous fat, swollen abdomen, or evidence of vitamin deficiencies.

ETIOLOGY

FTT is the result of inadequate nutrition, which may be due to a wide range of medical or psychosocial causes. FTT can be thought of as stemming from inadequate nutritional intake, malabsorption of nutrients, or increased caloric expenditure, though the actual cause is commonly multifactorial.

DIAGNOSIS

DIFFERENTIAL DIAGNOSIS

- Inadequate nutritional intake: food insecurity, poor parent knowledge of child's needs, formula dilution, excessive juice, breastfeeding difficulties, neglect, behavioral feeding problem, oromotor dysfunction, developmental delay, emesis, gastroesophageal reflux, volvulus, increased intracranial pressure, genetic disease (trisomy 13, 18, 21), and psychiatric conditions
- Malabsorption: cystic fibrosis, celiac disease, eosinophilic esophagitis, food protein insensitivity or intolerance, and inflammatory bowel disease
- Increased metabolic demand: insulin resistance, congenital infection, other infection, genetic syndrome, hyperthyroidism, chronic disease, and malignancy

WORKUP

- Evaluation should include the child's eating habits, caloric intake, parent-child interactions, psychosocial history, past medical history, medications, family history to include parent stature and weight, review of systems, and physical exam. Fig. 1 illustrates an algorithm for management of a child with failure to thrive (FTT).
- Height, weight, and weight-to-length measurements are most sensitive, whereas head circumference and body mass index (BMI) may be useful. Common FTT criteria for children younger than 2 years are below, but clinical judgment should be used because normal causes and biologic variants may exist.
  1. Length, weight, or BMI below the 3rd or 5th percentile on more than one consecutive visit
  2. Weight that drops below two major percentile lines
  3. Weight less than 80% of the ideal weight for age
  4. Weight-to-length below the 5th percentile or weight-for-length less than 70% to 79% of the median
  5. Weight velocity below the 3rd or 5th percentile
  6. Weight less than 70% of the 50th percentile; may require hospitalization
- Obtain caliper measurements of skinfold thickness and midarm muscle circumference.
- Observation of a meal being taken to assess potential feeding difficulties.
- A 3-day food diary is helpful, as well as consultation by a nutritionist, to calculate the child's intake of energy, protein, vitamins, and minerals.
- Assess stool frequency, consistency, quantity, as well as fat, blood, or mucus content.
- Routine hospitalization for FTT evaluation is not recommended. Rarely, hospitalization for observed feedings and further workup is warranted.

LABORATORY TESTS

- Laboratory tests should be based on medical history and physical exam findings and should consider the risk for refeeding syndrome and other medical complications.
- Consider CBC with red blood cell indices, complete chemistry panel including phosphorus, thyroid function, urinalysis, HIV testing, C-reactive protein or erythrocyte sedimentation rate, celiac screening, stool examination for fats or reducing substances,

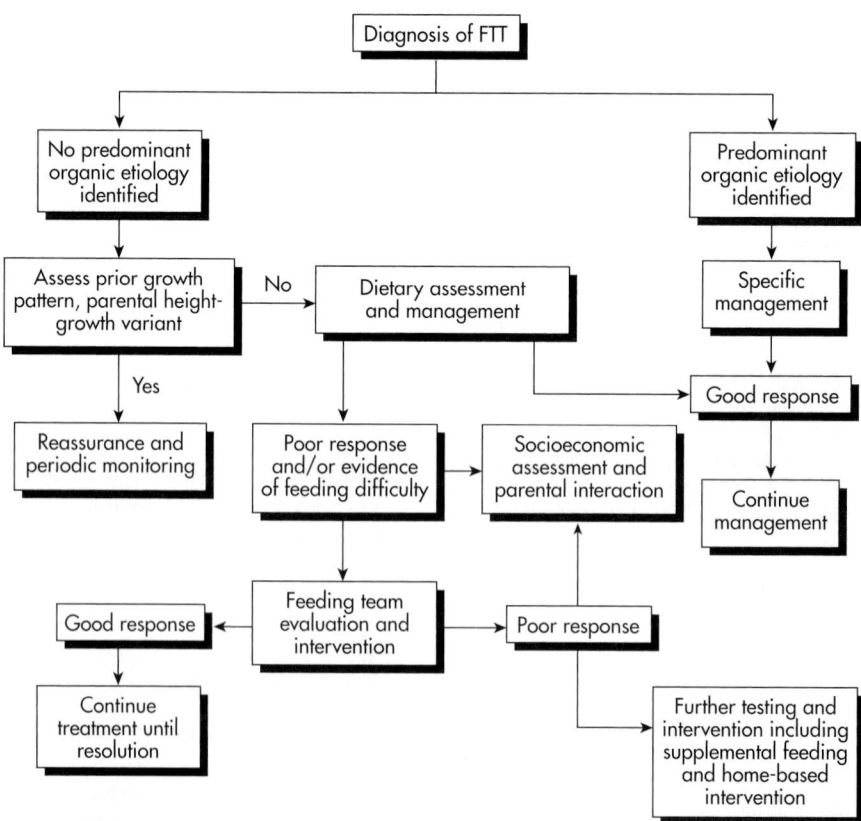

FIG. 1 Algorithm for management of a child with failure to thrive (FTT). (Shashidhar H, Tolia V: Failure to Thrive. *In* Wyllie R, Hyams, JS (eds): *Pediatric gastrointestinal and liver disease*, 4th ed, Philadelphia, 2011, Elsevier, pp. 136–145.e3.)

or sweat chloride testing. If clinically indicated, growth hormone level and genetic sequencing can be checked.

IMAGING STUDIES

Imaging tests are not routinely performed but may be warranted depending on underlying medical cause.

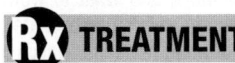

TREATMENT

Identification and management of underlying causes should be implemented. In cases in which there is no underlying medical condition, providing nutrition repletion will, by definition, correct FTT. A multidisciplinary team (including, but not limited to, social workers, occupational/ speech therapists, nutritionists/dietitians, nurses, advanced practice nurses, and pediatricians) should be used.

NONPHARMACOLOGIC THERAPY

- Add calorie-dense foods or increase the number of feedings.
- Enteral feeding, percutaneous endoscopic gastrostomy (PEG), and nasogastric feeding tubes can be used to accelerate weight gain, and results should be seen within 2 to 7 days. Caloric intake should be titrated up to goal over 5 to 7 days. Caloric goals by age group: 0 to 6 months: 108 kcal/kg/day, 6 to 12 months: 98 kcal/kg/day, and 1 to 3 years: 102 kcal/kg/day.
- Swift restoration of nutrition can lead to life-threatening refeeding syndrome, where shifts in electrolyte balance (low phosphate, magnesium, potassium), fluid balance (edema), hypoglycemia, gastroparesis or ileus, impaired heart function or arrhythmia,

and sudden death can occur. Calories must therefore be titrated slowly to goal with close monitoring.
- Treat underlying medical conditions, including mental health disorders.
- Assist with family psychosocial stressors.
- Follow up closely, including home nursing visits.
- In cases where economic, psychosocial, or parental issues are suspected and the child's growth is not maintained, state and federal legislation regarding reporting to child protection services must be followed.

ACUTE GENERAL Rx

Multivitamins including iron and zinc

CHRONIC Rx

Nutrient repletion with the goal of accelerated growth should be continued for 4 to 9 months

DISPOSITION

Children with FTT commonly remain small in height and weight. Studies consistently find that children with FTT are more prone to long-term cognitive, learning, and behavioral abnormalities.

REFERRAL

- Indicated based on the cause of FTT
- Hospitalization should be considered in cases of FTT in which a child is less than 70% of predicted weight for length, where outpatient management has failed, when a suspicion of abuse or neglect exists, where signs of traumatic injury are present, where serious impairment of the child's caregiver is evident, or for close observation and treatment for refeeding syndrome.

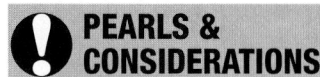

PEARLS & CONSIDERATIONS

COMMENTS

- FTT is a common childhood symptom encountered in the outpatient and inpatient pediatric populations, is caused by undernutrition, and is associated with inadequate nutritional intake, malabsorption, or increased metabolic demand.
- A thorough multidisciplinary approach to assessment, diagnosis, and management should be used to manage nutrient status and any underlying cause(s).
- Child height/length, weight, and weight-for-length measurements with comparison to standard growth curves are useful in the identification of potential cases of FTT.
- FTT treatment should include restoration of nutrition along with treatment of the underlying cause(s), including psychosocial factors.
- Although FTT can usually be managed effectively in the outpatient setting, specific indications for inpatient treatment should be considered.

PREVENTION

Nutritional counseling and anticipatory guidance should be provided at each well-child visit. Growth parameters should be measured during serial clinical assessments and compared with growth standards. Enlist dietitians and visiting nurses to provide support to families with children at high risk of FTT.

SUGGESTED READINGS

Available at www.expertconsult.com

AUTHOR: GRAYSON W. ARMSTRONG, M.D., M.P.H.

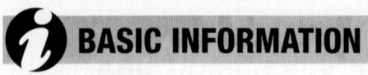

BASIC INFORMATION

DEFINITION

A fall is an "event which results in a person coming to rest inadvertently on the ground and other than a consequence of the following: loss of consciousness, sudden onset of paralysis, or epileptic seizure" (Kellogg International Work Group, *Danish Medical Bulletin*, 34, 1-24).

SYNONYMS

Syncope
Collapse

ICD-10CM CODES
E880-E888.9   Accidental fall
R29.6   Repeated falls

EPIDEMIOLOGY & DEMOGRAPHICS

INCIDENCE:

- Trauma is the fifth leading cause of death in persons >65 years of age, and falls are responsible for 70% of accidental deaths in persons ≥75 yr.
- The incidence of falls among community-dwelling older adults is 30% to 40%. Two thirds of falls in the community are preventable; 6% to 7% of these falls result in fracture.
- The incidence of falls for nursing home and hospitalized older adults is three times the rate of community-dwelling older adults. Over 50% of nursing home residents fall during their stay.
- 20% to 30% of older adults who fall suffer significant injury leading to immobility, dependence, and an increased risk of early death.

HEALTH CARE COST:

- In 2006, patients ≥65 had over 2.1 million visits to the ED for injurious falls, which was 10.5% of all ED visits among the elderly and 29.6% of these visits required hospital admission. In those that were admitted, the mean length of stay was 5.5 days with a mean cost of $10,800. The aggregate hospital cost for those requiring admission in 2006 was $6.8 billion. (Source: Healthcare Cost and Utilization Project).

PREDOMINANT SEX & AGE:

- Fall-related mortality is highest among older white men followed by white women, black men, and black women.
- The incidence rates of falls increase with advancing age.
- Older adults ≥85 years are 10 to 15 times more likely to have a fracture compared with those aged 60 to 65 years.

RISK FACTORS: Four groups of risk factors for falls have been identified (Table 1):

1. Intrinsic factors inherent in the older adult who falls.
2. Extrinsic factors circumstantial to the older adult who falls.
3. Falls in nursing homes.
4. Situational or the activity in which the older adult is engaged in when a fall occurs.

CLINICAL PRESENTATION

- Older adults who fall may present with minor soft tissue injuries, such as lacerations or bruising, hip fracture, or head trauma; however, most falls are not reported unless an injury has occurred.
- If an older adult presents for medical attention for a fall or reports recurrent falls in the past year or difficulties in walking or balance, a multifactorial fall risk assessment should be completed.
- The multifactorial fall risk assessment should include:
  1. Focused history: A detailed history of events and circumstances surrounding fall, relevant risk factors including review of medications, acute and chronic medical problems (e.g., osteoporosis, urinary incontinence, and cardiovascular disease), and whether the fall was witnessed.
  2. Physical examination
     1. Vital signs including orthostatics.
     2. Cardiovascular examination assessing for arrhythmias, carotid bruits, or new murmurs.
     3. Neurologic examination including vision assessment, evaluation of lower-extremity strength, peripheral nerves, proprioception, and testing of cortical, extrapyramidal, and cerebellar function.
     4. Gait and balance assessment: "Get up and go test" is a rapid assessment that will quickly tell you if the patient needs rehabilitation and what to work on. (Ask patient to stand from a seated position without use of hands, walk 10 feet forward, turn around, and return to chair and sit).
     5. Musculoskeletal exam with attention to joints of lower extremity, feet, and footwear.
  2. Functional assessment including the older adult's activities of daily living skills, use of adaptive equipment, and fear of falling
  3. Environmental assessment of home safety

ETIOLOGY

- Falls are a multifactorial syndrome resulting from the cumulative effects of impaired gait

---

TABLE 1   Risk Factors for Falls in the Elderly

Intrinsic

Aging

Age-related decline in vestibular function might lead to loss of balance, dizziness, and falls. Aging of the vision system (e.g., glaucoma, cataracts, retinopathy) may result in decreased visual acuity, inability to discriminate dark/light, and decreased spatial perception.

Cardiac

Cardiac arrhythmias, carotid sinus hypersensitivity, neurocardiogenic syncope

Neurologic

Parkinson's disease, normal pressure hydrocephalus (NPH), sensory neuropathy, dementia/impaired cognition, cervical myelopathy, senile gait disorder, prior stroke (One third of the elderly have abnormal position sense)

Musculoskeletal

Lower extremity weakness, impaired knee extension and ankle plantar flexion strength contribute to abnormalities in gait velocity and step length, deconditioning, arthritis, foot abnormalities (such as bunions, calluses, or nail abnormalities)

Vascular

Vertebrobasilar insufficiency, postural hypotension, postprandial hypotension

Metabolic

Hypoglycemia, hypothyroidism, hyponatremia

Psychiatric

Depression

Medications

Use of more than four medications may be associated with an increased risk of falls. Medications that may increase fall risk include benzodiazepines, sleeping medications, neuroleptics, antidepressants, anticonvulsants, class I antiarrhythmics, and antihypertensives (Rao, 2005).

Extrinsic

Environmental

Environmental hazards cause >50% of falls in the elderly (cords, furniture, small objects, ill-fitting shoes, slippery surfaces, loose rugs, uneven steps, optical patterns on escalators). Majority occurs with mild-moderate activity (walking, stepping up/down, changing position); 70% occur at home and 10% on stairs (descending > ascending).

Nursing Home Falls

20% have a cardiovascular cause (hypotension: drug induced, postprandial, postural, or bradycardia)
5% are the result of an acute illness such as PNA, febrile illness, UTI, CHF.
3% are from an overwhelming intrinsic event such as syncope, seizure, stroke, psychoactive drugs.

Situational

Tripping over obstacles, carrying heavy items, descending/ascending stairs, rapid turning, reaching overhead, climbing ladders, ill-fitting shoes, lack of assistive devices and balance, aging, polypharmacy, depression, cognitive impairment, acute medical illness, or environmental factors (Fig. E1).

- Most falls among community-dwelling older adults are due to environmental factors, whereas falls among nursing home residents are a result of confusion, gait impairment, or postural hypotension.

Dx DIAGNOSIS

DIFFERENTIAL DIAGNOSIS

Falls are often a nonspecific symptom of an acute illness (such as delirium, urinary tract infection, acute anemia, or pneumonia) or an exacerbation of a chronic disease (chronic heart failure [CHF] or chronic obstructive pulmonary disease [COPD]). The mnemonic "DELIRIUMS" can be used to assess the differential diagnosis in acute delirium. (**D**rugs, **E**motional [depression], **L**ow PaO_2 [CHF, COPD], **I**nfection, **R**etention [urinary, fecal], **I**ctal status, **U**nder nutrition/hydration, **M**etabolic, **S**ubdural/Sensory [all neurologic causes] workup).

WORKUP

- Older adults presenting with a noninjurious fall need a detailed history and physical exam to identify acute medical illnesses and potential modifiable risk factors. Laboratory and neuroimaging studies may be necessary if the history and physical exam indicate a specific problem. ECG and Holter monitoring may be considered if cardiac arrhythmia is suspected.
- See Fig. E1.

LABORATORY TESTS

CBC, stool guaiac, blood chemistries, thyroid function, liver function, vitamin B_{12} level, folate level, erythrocyte sedimentation rate, vitamin D level, drug levels, and urinalysis depending on physical/historical findings.

IMAGING STUDIES

- CT or MRI of the brain or cervical spine films in the presence of neurologic or gait impairment.
- Chest x-ray if pulmonary pathology (pneumonia, pulmonary edema) is suspected.
- Consider ECG, echocardiography, or Holter monitor if suspicious for structural cardiac abnormality or syncope.

Rx TREATMENT

NONPHARMACOLOGIC THERAPY

- Physical therapy evaluation for gait and balance training, evaluation of appropriate assisted devices (e.g., cane, walker), the use of fall prevention equipment (e.g., low beds, bed alarms).
- Home safety assessment: studies show that 50% of recurrent fallers fell doing the same

activity that caused them to fall the first time. This can be prevented by creating a home safety evaluation checklist (preferably done by family member to improve compliance) or arranging for a home safety inspection by a visiting nurse or occupational therapist.

- Minimization or discontinuation of certain medications associated with falls (psychotropics).
- Customized exercise program to improve strength, gait, and balance
- Evaluation of proper footwear, hard sole, and low heel height.

ACUTE GENERAL Rx

Hospitalization may be necessary for treatment of hip fracture, subdural hematoma, lacerations, or trauma as well as the treatment of underlying cause of the fall such as infection, metabolic disturbances, cardiovascular (e.g., carotid sinus hypersensitivity, vasovagal syndrome, bradyarrhythmias, and tachyarrhythmias) or neurologic abnormality.

CHRONIC Rx

- Screen and treat for osteoporosis as low bone density increases the risk of hip or other fractures.
- Optimize treatment of chronic illnesses such as CHF, COPD, osteoarthritis, Parkinson's disease, dementia, postural hypotension, and visual problems.
- Vitamin D supplementation of at least 800 IU per day. Epidemiological studies reveal that compared with usual care, short-term intervention with oral nutritional supplementation and dietetic counseling significantly decrease falls in malnourished older adults.

COMPLEMENTARY & ALTERNATIVE MEDICINE

T'ai chi has been shown to reduce the risk of falls in community-dwelling study participants.

DISPOSITION

Falls increase the older adult's risk of hospitalization, institutionalization, and mortality.

REFERRAL

- Referral may be appropriate to cardiologist, ophthalmologist, neurologist, or podiatrist depending on the presence of a specific condition.
- Consider referral to physical therapist for gait and balance training, evaluation for assisted device, or strengthening program.

! PEARLS & CONSIDERATIONS

COMMENTS

- Fear of falling may lead to restriction of activities, social isolation, and dependence.
- Older adults with four or more risk factors have a 78% chance of falling.

- Mortality from falls has increased by 42% over the past decade.

PREVENTION

The U.S. Preventive Services Task Force recommends exercise or physical therapy and vitamin D supplementation to prevent falls in community-dwelling adults aged ≥65 who are at increased risk for falls. It does not recommend automatically performing an in-depth multifactorial risk assessment in conjunction with comprehensive management of identified risks to prevent falls in community-dwelling adults aged 65 or older because the likelihood of benefit is small. In determining whether this service is appropriate in individual cases, patients and clinicians should consider the balance of benefits and harms on the basis of the circumstances of prior falls, comorbid medical conditions, and patient values.

SCREENING

The "get up and go test" is a quick assessment of balance and gait. A more in-depth screening tool for falls is the Tinetti gait and balance assessment, which evaluates normal and adaptive ability to maintain balance when rising from a chair, standing with eyes closed, turning, and receiving a sternal nudge. It also evaluates several components of gait (step height, postural sway, path deviation). The test is scored on the patient's ability to perform specific tasks. Scoring is done on a 3-point scale with a range of 0 to 2. Individual scores are combined to form three measures: an overall gait assessment score (maximum score = 12), an overall balance assessment score (maximum score = 16), and a gait and balance score (maximum score = 28). In general, patients who score below 19 are at high risk for falls, and those who score 19-24 are at risk for falls.

PATIENT/FAMILY EDUCATION

Providing education and information for the patient and caregiver regarding fall prevention strategies in addition to multifactorial risk reduction strategies

EBM EVIDENCE

Available at www.expertconsult.com

SUGGESTED READINGS

Available at www.expertconsult.com

AUTHORS: **SEAN H. UITERWYK, M.D., ALICIA J. CURTIN, PH.D.,** and **KEITH BRENNAN, M.D.**

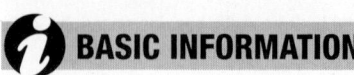

BASIC INFORMATION

DEFINITION

Familial adenomatous polyposis (FAP) is a highly penetrant autosomal-dominant condition characterized by hundreds of colorectal adenomatous polyps that inevitably progress to cancer (Fig. 1). *Gardner's syndrome* is a subset of FAP, with prominent extraintestinal manifestations including dental abnormalities, soft tissue lesions, desmoid tumors, and osteomas.

SYNONYMS

Familial adenomatous polyposis
FAP
Gardner's syndrome

ICD-10CM CODES
D12.5 Benign neoplasm of sigmoid colon
D12.4 Benign neoplasm of descending colon
D12.3 Benign neoplasm of transverse colon
D12.2 Benign neoplasm of ascending colon
D12.6 Benign neoplasm of colon, unspecified

EPIDEMIOLOGY & DEMOGRAPHICS

- FAP occurs in approximately 1 in 10,000 births.
- FAP accounts for <1% of all colorectal cancers.
- Individuals develop hundreds to thousands of adenomatous colorectal polyps.
- Polyps usually present in adolescence.
- 100% lifetime risk for colorectal cancer; most diagnosed by 40 yr of age.
- Gastric, duodenal, periampullary, and small bowel polyps occur but have lower malignant potential.
- Increased risk for other tumors: desmoid (15%), duodenal/periampullary (7%), thyroid (2%), brain (1%), childhood hepatoblastoma (1%), nasopharyngeal angiofibroma (benign), pancreatic (2%), adrenal adenoma (10%), and gastric (1%).

PHYSICAL FINDINGS & CLINICAL PRESENTATION

Phenotypic variability is seen in individuals and families with the same mutation. Soft tissue and bone abnormalities may precede intestinal disease. These findings are reported in at least 20% of individuals with FAP.

- Congenital hypertrophy of the retinal pigment epithelium (CHRPE): benign fundus lesions, usually present at birth
- Dental abnormalities: supernumerary or unerupted teeth
- Soft tissue lesions: epidermal or sebaceous cysts, fibromas, lipomas, desmoid tumors (benign, locally invasive, aggressive connective tissue tumor)
- Osteomas (benign bone growths): skull, mandible, long bone
- Anemia, occult blood in stool, bowel obstruction, weight loss

ETIOLOGY

- FAP is caused by mutations of the tumor suppressor gene adenomatous polyposis coli *(APC)* on chromosome 5q21-q22; more than 1000 disease-causing mutations identified. The site of the mutation may explain the prominent extraintestinal lesions found in Gardner's syndrome.
- De novo mutations are responsible for approximately 20% of FAP cases. These may be due to germline mutations or somatic cell mosaicism, which is seen when a new mutation occurs in the APC gene post-fertilization and is present in only a subset of cell types or tissues.

DIAGNOSIS

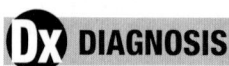

In individuals with a family history, more than 100 adenomatous colorectal polyps, CHRPE lesions, or genetic testing confirms diagnosis. In those without a family history, more than 100 adenomatous colorectal polyps suggest the diagnosis, and genetic testing confirms it.

DIFFERENTIAL DIAGNOSIS

- Turcot's syndrome.
- Attenuated FAP.
- MUTYH-associated polyposis.
- Peutz-Jeghers syndrome.
- Juvenile polyposis syndrome.
- Cowden Disease.
- Lynch syndrome.
- Hereditary mixed polyposis syndrome.
- POLE or POLD1 polyposis.
- Hyperplastic polyposis.
- Table 1 compares various adenomatous polyposis syndromes.

WORKUP

History, physical examination, laboratory tests, imaging studies

DIAGNOSTIC SCREENING OPTIONS

GENETIC TESTING: NOTE: Genetic counseling should be performed, and written informed consent obtained before testing. Refer to a specialized center for counseling and evaluation.

- Should be offered to first-degree relatives of affected individuals (with an identified mutation) at age 10 to 12 yr and clinically suspected individuals.
- Able to identify a mutation in approximately 80% of families. To ensure that the family has a detectable mutation, test an affected family member first.
- If positive in the affected individual, the test can differentiate with 100% accuracy affected and unaffected family members. If negative in the affected individual, screening family members will not be useful in determining disease status.
- If no known family history exists, screening the clinically suspected individual is reasonable. A positive test rules in FAP but a negative test does not rule it out.
- Numerous testing techniques available; may require multiple tests to identify the mutation.

SIGMOIDOSCOPY:

- Individuals with a positive genetic test, untested at-risk family members, or patients from families with an unidentified *APC* mutation: annual flexible sigmoidoscopy or colonoscopy beginning at 10 to 12 yr of age.
- Once adenomatous polyps are detected, patients should undergo colonoscopy and evaluation for colectomy.
- Negative genetic test in patients from families with an identified mutation: average risk screening.

CHRPE: Lesions occur in up to 80% of families and are a reliable indicator of affected status in these families.

TREATMENT

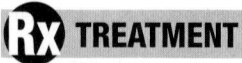

- Prophylactic colectomy or proctocolectomy: timing determined by polyp number, size, and degree of dysplasia. Postsurgical endoscopic surveillance annually.

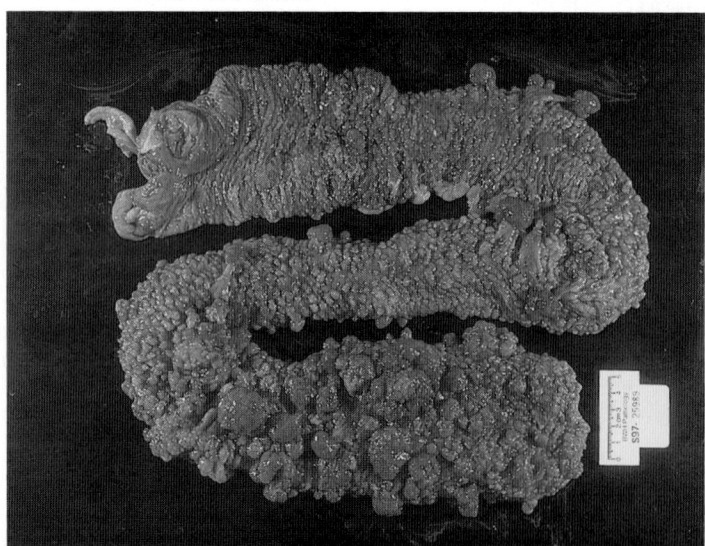

FIG. 1 Familial adenomatous polyposis with innumerable adenomatous polyps, increasing in size and density from proximal *(upper left)* to distal *(lower right)*. (From Skarin AT: Atlas of diagnostic oncology, ed 4, St. Louis, 2010, Mosby.)

TABLE 1   Adenomatous Polyposis Syndromes

Syndrome	Gene Mutation	Polyps	Extraintestinal Abnormalities
Classic FAP	*APC* (usually truncated protein)	Colonic adenomas (thousands) Duodenal, periampullary adenomas Gastric fundic gland polyps Jejunal and ileal adenomas Ileal lymphoid polyps	Mandibular osteomas Dental abnormalities
Gardner variant of FAP	*APC*	Same as FAP	Osteomas (mandible, skull, long bones) CHRPE Desmoid tumors Epidermoid and sebaceous cysts Fibromas, lipomas Thyroid, adrenal tumors
Turcot variant of FAP	*APC* DNA MMR*	Colonic adenomas (sometimes fewer than in classic FAP)	Medulloblastoma Glioblastoma multiforme CHRPE
Attenuated FAP	*APC* 5′ and 3′ regions	Colonic adenomas (<100; proximal colon) Duodenal, periampullary adenomas Gastric fundic gland polyps	Mandibular osteomas (rare)
Familial tooth agenesis	*Axin2* (APC pathway)	Colonic adenomas Hyperplastic polyps	Agenesis of teeth
Bloom's syndrome	*BLM*	Colonic adenomas	Small stature Facial erythema/telangiectasia Male sterility Adenocarcinomas, leukemia, lymphoma
MUTYH polyposis	*MUTYH (MYH)*	Colonic adenomas (5-100) Duodenal polyposis Gastric cancer	CHRPE Osteomas

*May be more appropriately classified under hereditary nonpolyposis colon cancer.
APC, adenomatous polyposis coli; *CHRPE,* congenital hypertrophy of the retinal pigment epithelium; *FAP,* familial adenomatous polyposis; *MMR,* mismatch repair; *MUTYH* (mutY homolog [*E. coli*]).
From Feldman M et al (eds): *Sleisenger and Fordtran's gastrointestinal and liver disease,* ed 10, Philadelphia, 2016, Saunders.

- Screening of remaining GI tract and screening for extraintestinal manifestations continues after colectomy
  1. Annual physical examination: history, examination (including thyroid), and blood tests
  2. Upper endoscopy to screen for gastric/duodenal polyps: baseline at age 25 yr (earlier if colon polyps detected) and repeated every 0.5 to 4 yr based on findings
  3. Some recommend annual thyroid ultrasound
  4. Other possible cancer sites imaged if symptoms occur or if these cancers have occurred in relatives
- Treat soft tissue lesions and osteomas for symptoms or cosmetic concerns. Treat desmoid tumors if they pose a risk to adjacent structures.

DISPOSITION

- 100% chance of colorectal cancer in untreated individuals. Many other neoplasms occur at higher rates.
- Metastatic colorectal cancer is the leading cause of death (58%), followed by desmoid tumors (11%), and duodenal/periampullary adenocarcinoma (8%).

REFERRAL

- Patients should be managed at centers with expertise in FAP, including a gastroenterologist, medical geneticist, and surgeon.
- Genetic counselors can be found at www.nsgc.org.
- Genetic testing sites can be found at www.genetests.org.

ⓘ PEARLS & CONSIDERATIONS

- Management should be individualized based on genotype, phenotype, and individual preferences.
- Sulindac (NSAID) and celecoxib (COX-2 inhibitor) can cause colorectal polyp regression in individuals with FAP. Cancer risk remains; neither replaces colon resection for cancer prevention.
- Preliminary study suggests that combination therapy with sulindac and erlotinib may decrease duodenal polyp burden.

- Desmoid tumors usually present in the 30s, frequently occur in the abdomen, and are difficult to treat with high rates of recurrence. Growth and recurrence are stimulated by surgery.
- Screen children of affected parents (from infancy to age 7 yr) biannually with alpha-fetoprotein level and liver ultrasound to rule out hepatoblastoma.
- Preimplantation and prenatal genetic testing is available.

SUGGESTED READINGS

Available at www.expertconsult.com

RELATED CONTENT

Familial Adenomatous Polyposis and Polyposis Syndromes (Patient Information)
Colorectal Cancer (Related Key Topic)
Peutz-Jeghers Syndrome (Related Key Topic)
Lynch Syndrome (Related Key Topic)

AUTHOR: **SUDEEP K. AULAKH, M.D.**

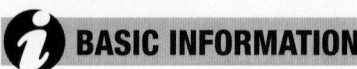

BASIC INFORMATION

DEFINITION

Familial Mediterranean fever (FMF) is a hereditary periodic fever syndrome. FMF type 1 is characterized by recurrent short episodes of inflammation and serositis, while FMF type 2 is characterized by amyloidosis as the first clinical manifestation.

SYNONYMS

Non-neuropathic heredofamilial amyloidosis
Benign paroxysmal peritonitis
Familial paroxysmal polyserositis
Recurrent polyserositis
Periodic fever
FMF

ICD-10CM CODES
E85.0 Non-neuropathic heredofamilial amyloidosis

EPIDEMIOLOGY & DEMOGRAPHICS

PREVALENCE: Varies depending on the ethnic background of the population. FMF affects primarily eastern Mediterranean populations (e.g., Armenians, Arabs, Turks, Sephardic Jews). In Armenians, the prevalence is 1 case per 500, and in Turks, estimates are 1 case per 1000. As many as 1 in 5 people of these ethnic backgrounds is a carrier of FMF.

PREDOMINANT SEX AND AGE: Male:female ratio of 1.5-2:1. Disease onset is typically before age 20, with about 50% of cases before age 10. Very rare to have onset after age 40.

GENETICS: Pattern of inheritance is primarily autosomal recessive. Mutations in the *MEFV* gene, which encodes the pyrin protein, causes the disease in many cases; there are more than 80 known mutations, and 30% have only one or no mutations found.

RISK FACTORS: Affected first-degree relatives, consider offering genetic testing

PHYSICAL FINDINGS & CLINICAL PRESENTATION

- Sporadic, recurrent attacks of fever and severe pain, abrupt in onset, usually lasting 1 to 3 days, with spontaneous resolution.
- Almost all patients have episodic abdominal pain. On exam may have tenderness, guarding, rebound and rigidity; may be mistaken for an acute surgical abdomen.
- Attacks localized to chest in up to half of patients due to pleural inflammation or referred from subdiaphragmatic inflammation.
- Arthritis is usually mono- or oligoarticular, involving large joints (e.g., knee, ankle, hip). Pain is out of proportion to swelling.
- Up to 50% of patients can have an erysipelas-like rash, usually on lower extremities (Fig. E1).
- Rarer manifestations include prolonged febrile myalgias, orchitis, aseptic meningitis, polyarthritis, Henoch-Schönlein purpura, sacroiliitis, infertility.

ETIOLOGY

MEFV is the only gene in which pathogenic variants are known to cause FMF, and it encodes pyrin, a protein that plays a role in the innate immune system and helps regulate the inflammasome. The exact mechanism that triggers acute FMF attacks remains unclear.

DIAGNOSIS

DIFFERENTIAL DIAGNOSIS

- Other periodic fever syndromes (e.g., TRAPS, hyperimmunoglobulin D)
- Systemic rheumatic diseases (e.g., rheumatoid arthritis, systemic lupus erythematosus, adult Still's disease)

WORKUP

- The diagnosis is based on a detailed history with suggestive clinical symptoms and is supported by ethnic origin and positive family history; the diagnosis is not excluded by negative genetic testing.
- In patients who have abdominal surgery, a negative laparotomy or removal of a normal appendix is expected, as is a favorable response to colchicine.

LABORATORY TESTS

- CBC: leukocytosis with neutrophil predominance
- Elevated acute phase reactants: ESR, CRP, fibrinogen, serum amyloid A protein
- Inflammatory synovial fluid if aspirated
- Urinalysis with proteinuria should raise concern for possible amyloidosis
- *MEFV* with gene mutations

IMAGING STUDIES

- During an acute attack, depending on manifestations such as peritonitis, pleuritis, or arthritis, may see air-fluid levels, pleural effusions, and/or synovial effusions.

TREATMENT

The main goals of treatment are to: (1) prevent acute attacks and (2) prevent the development of amyloidosis.

ACUTE GENERAL AND CHRONIC Rx

- Supportive care during acute episodes with IVF, NSAIDs, pain control.
- To prevent attacks first-line Rx is colchicine, 0.6 to 1.8 mg daily.
  1. If colchicine unresponsive, possibility of noncompliance, or reconsider diagnosis.
  2. Recommended to continue colchicine in pregnant patients with FMF.
- If truly colchicine unresponsive, therapeutic strategy less clear, but successful reports of using interferon-alfa, thalidomide, etanercept, infliximab, anakinra, and rilonacept.

DISPOSITION

- Since the usage of colchicine, most treated patients are asymptomatic and do not commonly see previous complication of AA amyloidosis.

REFERRAL

- Rheumatology

PEARLS & CONSIDERATIONS

COMMENTS

Most patients have disease onset before age 20, and attacks typically last 1 to 3 days. Colchicine is the standard of care for prophylaxis of attacks and prevention of amyloidosis. Should continue treatment with colchicine during pregnancy. Should question diagnosis if there is no response to colchicine. Type AA amyloidosis is the most frequent complication of FMF, with the kidneys being the most affected organ.

PREVENTION

Should consider referring all first-degree relatives of FMF patients for genetic testing, whether or not they have symptoms.

PATIENT/FAMILY EDUCATION

https://rarediseases.info.nih.gov/diseases/6421/disease

SUGGESTED READINGS
Available at www.expertconsult.com

AUTHOR: **DAPHNE SCARAMANGAS-PLUMLEY, M.D.**

BASIC INFORMATION

DEFINITION

Acute fatty liver of pregnancy (AFLP) is characterized histologically by microvesicular fatty cytoplasmic infiltration of hepatocytes with minimal hepatocellular necrosis.

SYNONYMS

Acute fatty metamorphosis
Acute yellow atrophy
AFLP
Fatty liver of pregnancy

ICD-10CM CODES
O26.611 Liver and biliary tract disorders in pregnancy, first trimester
O26.612 Liver and biliary tract disorders in pregnancy, second trimester
O26.613 Liver and biliary tract disorders in pregnancy, third trimester
O26.619 Liver and biliary tract disorders in pregnancy, unspecified trimester

EPIDEMIOLOGY & DEMOGRAPHICS

INCIDENCE:
- Rare: 1 in 10,000 to 1 in 20,000 pregnancies
- Equal frequencies in all races and at all maternal ages

AVERAGE GESTATIONAL AGE: 37 wk (range 28 to 42 wk)
20% present postnatally

RISK FACTORS:
- Primiparity
- Multiple gestation
- Male fetus

GENETICS: Some with a familial deficiency of long-chain 3-hydroxyacyl-coenzyme A dehydrogenase (LCHAD)

PHYSICAL FINDINGS & CLINICAL PRESENTATION

- Initial manifestations:
  1. Nausea and vomiting (70%)
  2. Pain in right upper quadrant or epigastrium (50% to 80%)
  3. Malaise and anorexia
- Jaundice often in 1 to 2 wk
- Hypoglycemia
- Late manifestations:
  1. Fulminant hepatic failure
  2. Encephalopathy
  3. Renal failure
  4. Pancreatitis
  5. Gastrointestinal and uterine bleeding
  6. Disseminated intravascular coagulation (10%)
  7. Seizures
  8. Coma
- Liver:
  1. Usually small
  2. Normal or enlarged in preeclampsia, eclampsia, HELLP syndrome (hemolysis, elevated liver enzymes, and low platelets), and acute hepatitis

  3. Coexistent preeclampsia in up to 46% of patients

ETIOLOGY

- Fetal LCHAD deficiency results in transplacental passage of excess fetal fatty acids and subsequent accumulation in the maternal liver.
- Postulated that inhibition of mitochondrial oxidation of fatty acids may lead to microvesicular fatty infiltration of liver.
- Fatty metamorphosis of preeclamptic liver disease believed to be of different etiology.

DIAGNOSIS

DIFFERENTIAL DIAGNOSIS

- Acute gastroenteritis
- Preeclampsia or eclampsia with liver involvement
- HELLP syndrome
- Acute viral hepatitis
- Fulminant hepatitis
- Drug-induced hepatitis caused by halothane, phenytoin, methyldopa, isoniazid, hydrochlorothiazide, or tetracycline
- Intrahepatic cholestasis of pregnancy
- Gallbladder disease
- Reye's syndrome
- Hemolytic-uremic syndrome
- Budd-Chiari syndrome
- Systemic lupus erythematosus

WORKUP

- A clinical diagnosis is based predominantly on physical and laboratory findings (Swansea criteria).
- Most definitive diagnosis is through liver biopsy with oil red O staining and electron microscopy.
- Liver biopsy is reserved for atypical cases only and only after any existing coagulopathy is corrected with fresh frozen plasma because of concerns for excessive bleeding.

LABORATORY TESTS

Tests to determine the following:
- Hypoglycemia (often profound <60 mg/dl).
- Hyperammonemia.
- Elevated aminotransferases (usually <500 U/mL).
- Thrombocytopenia.
- Leukocytosis (white blood cell count >15,000).
- Hyperbilirubinemia (usually <10 mg/dl).
- Low albumin.
- Hypofibrinogenemia (<300 mg/dl).
- Disseminated intravascular coagulation (DIC) (in 75%).

IMAGING STUDIES

- Ultrasound: best used to rule out other diseases in the differential diagnosis such as gallbladder disease
- CT scan: plays minimal role because of a high false-negative rate

TREATMENT

NONPHARMACOLOGIC THERAPY

- Patient is admitted to intensive care unit for stabilization.
- Fetus is delivered; spontaneous resolution usually follows delivery.
- Mode of delivery is based on obstetric indications and clinical assessment of disease severity.

ACUTE GENERAL Rx

- Decrease in endogenous ammonia through dietary protein restriction; neomycin 6 to 12 g/day PO to decrease presence of ammonia-producing bacteria; magnesium citrate 30 to 50 mL PO or enema to evacuate nitrogenous wastes from colon.
- Administration of IV fluids with glucose to keep glucose levels >60 mg/dl.
- Coagulopathy corrected with fresh frozen plasma.
- Avoidance of drugs metabolized by liver.
- Aggressive avoidance and treatment for nosocomial infections; consideration of prophylactic antibiotics.
- Monitor closely for development of complications such as hepatic encephalopathy, pulmonary edema, DIC, and respiratory arrest.
- Plasma exchange after delivery may result in a lower maternal mortality.

CHRONIC Rx

Orthotopic liver transplantation is the only treatment for irreversible liver failure.

DISPOSITION

- Before 1980, both maternal and fetal mortality rates were approximately 85%.
- Since 2008, maternal mortality rates have been less than 10%.
- Usually rapid return of liver function to normal after delivery.
- Minimal risk of recurrence with future pregnancies.

REFERRAL

- To tertiary health care facility as soon as diagnosis is suspected.
- 20% of infants born to mothers with AFLP have LCHAD; after birth, all infants should be evaluated for the deficiency.

SUGGESTED READINGS
Available at www.expertconsult.com

RELATED CONTENT
Eclampsia (Related Key Topic).
Preeclampsia (Related Key Topic).

AUTHOR: **RUBEN ALVERO, M.D.,** and **KELLY RUHSTALLER, M.D.**

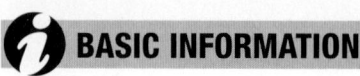

DEFINITION

- Adverse effects of alcohol on developing humans represent spectrum of structural anomalies and behavioral and neurocognitive disabilities, most accurately termed fetal alcohol spectrum disorder (FASD) (Table 1).
- Children at severe end of spectrum defined as having fetal alcohol syndrome (FAS).

SYNONYMS

Fetal alcohol spectrum disorder
FAS

ICD-10CM CODES
Q86.0 Fetal alcohol syndrome (dysmorphic)
P04.3 Newborn (suspected to be) affected by maternal use of alcohol

EPIDEMIOLOGY & DEMOGRAPHICS

- Alcohol considered to be most common teratogen to which the fetus is liable to be exposed.
- 10% report drinking alcohol during pregnancy and 2% to 4% admit to binge drinking.
- Most common form of mental retardation in the United States.
- Prevalence is 1 to 2/1000 live births across the United States.
- Each year 40,000 babies are born with FASD.

RISK FACTORS

- Advanced maternal age (>30 yr).
- High parity.
- African-American, Alaskan Natives, and Native Indian race.
- Binge drinking (>4 drinks per occasion).
- History of prior affected child.
- Genetic susceptibility.
- Undernutrition.
- Low socioeconomic group.

PHYSICAL FINDINGS & CLINICAL PRESENTATION

Typical features:
- Growth retardation.
  1. Prenatal or postnatal.
  2. Height and/or weight <10%.
- Facial dysmorphia
  1. Smooth philtrum.
  2. Thin vermilion border.
  3. Small palpebral fissure (<10%).
  4. Others: epicanthic folds, ptosis of eyelids, flat nasal bridge and midface, upturned nose, railroad track ears, and so forth.
- CNS abnormalities
  1. Structural
     ○ Head circumference, 10%.
     ○ Clinically significant brain abnormalities observable through imaging.
  2. Neurologic
     ○ Neurologic problems not due to a postnatal insult or fever.
  3. Functional
     ○ Intellectual deficit.
     ○ Cognitive or developmental deficits.
     ○ Executive function deficits.
     ○ Motor function delays.
     ○ Problem with attention and hyperactivity.
     ○ Social skills.
     ○ Other problems such as sensory, pragmatic language, and memory.
Rare birth defects:
- Cardiac
  1. Ventricular septal defect (VSD).
  2. Atrial septal defect (ASD).
  3. Tetralogy of Fallot.
  4. Aberrant great vessels.
- Skeletal
  1. Radioulnar synostosis.
  2. Hypoplastic nails.
  3. Clinodactyly.
  4. Shortened fifth digit.
  5. Pectus excavatum and carinatum.
  6. Klippel-Feil syndrome.
  7. Hemivertebrae.
  8. Camptodactyly.
  9. Scoliosis.
- Renal
  1. Aplastic kidneys.
  2. Dysplastic kidneys.
  3. Ureteral duplication.
  4. Hypoplastic kidneys.
  5. Hydronephrosis.
  6. Horseshoe kidneys.
- Ocular
  1. Strabismus.
  2. Refractive problems.
  3. Retinal vascular abnormalities.
- Auditory
  1. Conductive hearing loss.
  2. Neurosensory hearing loss.
- Others
  1. Hockey stick–like palmar crease.

ETIOLOGY

- Prenatal damage comes about primarily by direct action of ethanol or its metabolites (e.g., acetaldehyde) on the fetus.
- Exact damaging mechanism is unclear.
- Although the damaging effect of alcohol is different in the various phases of pregnancy, it is by no means limited to first trimester.
- No exact dose-response relationship between alcohol consumed during prenatal period and extent of damage inflicted on infant.
- An occasional drink during pregnancy carries no risk to the fetus, but no level of drinking is known to be safe during pregnancy.
- The least significant effect recognized at 2 drinks/day is smaller birth weight (160 g less than average).
- Until 4 to 6 drinks/day are consumed, no additional subtle clinical features are evident.
- Most children who have FAS have been born to frankly alcoholic mothers whose intake is ≥8 to 10 drinks/day, and those who engage in binge drinking.
- The risk of serious problem in the offspring of a chronically alcoholic woman is ~30% to 50%; the greatest risk is mental retardation.

SECONDARY DISABILITIES

- Mental health problems.
- Dependent living.
- Employment problems.
- Disruptive school problems.
- Trouble with law.
- Confinement.
- Inappropriate sexual behavior.
- Alcohol or drug problems.

DX DIAGNOSIS

- It is a diagnosis of exclusion.
- Diagnosis is difficult prenatally and at birth. Most cases are not diagnosed until school age.
- As the characteristic facial features tend to become decreasingly recognizable as the child reaches adolescence, the diagnosis

---

TABLE 1 Institute of Medicine's Diagnostic Criteria for Fetal Alcohol–Related Abnormalities

Category 1		
FAS with confirmed maternal alcohol exposure	Presence of classic triad of growth retardation, characteristic facial dysmorphology, and neurodevelopmental abnormalities. This is often defined as full-blown FAS.	
Category 2		
FAS without confirmed maternal alcohol exposure	Triad in category 1 is present without confirmed maternal drinking	
Category 3		
Partial FAS with confirmed maternal alcohol exposure	Presence of some of the characteristic facial anomalies plus growth retardation or CNS neurodevelopmental abnormalities or behavioral/cognitive abnormalities	
Category 4		
FAS with confirmed maternal alcohol exposure and alcohol-related birth defects	Some congenital anomalies as a result of alcohol toxicity	
Category 5		
FAS with confirmed maternal alcohol exposure and alcohol-related neurodevelopmental disorder	Evidence of CNS neurodevelopmental abnormalities, a complex pattern of behavioral/cognitive abnormalities, or both, but not necessarily any obvious physical changes	

CNS, Central nervous system; *FAS*, fetal alcohol syndrome.

becomes increasingly difficult with advancing age.

- Prenatal exposure to alcohol is not sufficient to warrant a diagnosis. According to the CDC, diagnosis of FAS requires 3 specific findings and history of prenatal alcohol exposure:
  1. Growth restriction (intrauterine or postnatal)
  2. CNS involvement
  3. Documentation of all three facial abnormalities (smooth philtrum, thin vermilion border, and short palpebral fissure)
- Imaging recommendation during pregnancy with alcohol exposure:
  1. High-risk anatomy scan.
  2. Serial growth scan.
  3. Fetal echocardiogram at 22 to 24 weeks' intrauterine pregnancy.
- Measurement of the ethyl esters of fatty acids in the meconium and hair of the newborn can substantiate maternal alcohol exposure.
- In school-aged children, the diagnostic process should include a thorough psychological evaluation that assesses multiple domains. Also, supplement the observation by obtaining standardized testing through early intervention programs, public schools, and psychologists in private practice.

DIFFERENTIAL DIAGNOSIS

- Other causes of symmetric growth retardation including intrauterine infection and aneuploidy.
- Aneuploidy (T21, T18, T13).
- Syndromes with overlapping features of FAS:
  1. Fetal anticonvulsant syndrome.
  2. Maternal phenylketonuria.
  3. Toluene embryopathy.
  4. Velocardiofacial syndrome (deletion 22q11).
  5. Williams syndrome.
  6. Dubowitz syndrome.
  7. Cornelia de Lange syndrome.

(Rx) TREATMENT

- As there is no cure for FAS, we need to emphasize prevention.
- For women who are planning pregnancy or who could become pregnant, the United States Surgeon General recommends the safest course: to avoid alcohol entirely during pregnancy.
- Women of childbearing age who are not pregnant should drink ≤7 alcoholic drinks/wk and ≤3 drinks on any one occasion.
- Preconception counseling should be offered to women of childbearing age who are at risk for an alcohol-exposed pregnancy.
- Screen all pregnant women for alcohol use.
- The National Institute on Alcohol Abuse and Alcoholism recommends that any woman who reports drinking >7 drinks/wk or >3 drinks on a given day be further assessed for alcohol-related problems.
- The T-ACE (Table 2) and TWEAK (Table 3) questionnaires are used to identify women drinking enough to potentially damage the fetus. The CAGE questionnaire is less sensitive for screening pregnant women.

- Effective treatment alternatives for women who screen positive for hazardous alcohol use include brief interventions to promote reductions in alcohol use and that facilitate referral to specialized treatment programs.
- Discontinuation or reduction of alcohol consumption at any point in pregnancy may be beneficial.
- The use of alcohol-containing tonics and medications should be avoided. This applies to medications with an alcohol base when the concentration exceeds 10%.
- Alcoholism is one of the few situations in which pregnancy interruption may be discussed with the patient as it may result in FAS.
- Early diagnosis and appropriate treatment may decrease secondary disabilities and recurrence in future pregnancies.
- A child should be referred for full FAS evaluation when substantial prenatal alcohol use by the mother has been confirmed (>7 drinks/wk, >3 drinks on multiple occasions, or both).
- If substantial prenatal exposure is known, with no other positive criteria, the physician should document exposure and closely monitor the child's growth and development.
- When information about prenatal exposure is unknown, a child should be referred for

TABLE 2   T-ACE Questions*

T (tolerance)	How many drinks does it take to make you feel high? (3 or more drinks = 2 points)
A (annoyed)	Have people annoyed you by criticizing your drinking? (Yes = 1 point)
C (cut down)	Have you felt you ought to cut down on your drinking? (Yes = 1 point)
E (eye opener)	Have you ever had to drink first thing in the morning to steady your nerves or to get rid of a hangover? (Yes = 1 point)

*A score of 2 or more indicates heavy or problem drinker. Its sensitivity is 70% and specificity is 85%.

TABLE 3   TWEAK*

T (tolerance)	How many drinks does it take before you begin to feel the first effects of alcohol? (3 or more drinks = 2 points)
W (worried)	Have close friends or relatives worried about your drinking in the past year? (Yes = 2 points)
E (eye opener)	Do you sometimes take a drink in the morning when you first get up? (Yes = 1 point)
A (amnesia)	Has a friend or family member ever told you about things you said or did while you were drinking that you could not remember? (Yes = 1 point)
K (kut down)	Do you sometimes feel the need to cut down on your drinking? (Yes = 1 point)

*A total of 3 or more points indicates the woman is likely to be a heavy or problem drinker. Its sensitivity is 79% and specificity is 83%.

full FAS if any of the following conditions are present: (1) all three dysmorphic facial features (smooth philtrum, thin vermilion border, and small palpebral fissure), (2) one or more of these facial features with growth deficit, (3) one or more facial features with one or more CNS abnormalities, (4) one or more dysmorphic facial features with growth deficit and one or more CNS abnormalities, or (5) any report of concern by a caregiver or parent that a child has or may have FAS.

- Infants and children who are diagnosed with FAS should be evaluated by a physician who is knowledgeable and competent in the evaluation of neurodevelopment and psychosocial problems associated with the diagnosis.
- A multidisciplinary team including a clinical geneticist, developmental pediatrician, mental health professional, social worker, and education specialist is often necessary for management.
- Treatment options include:
  1. Medications to help with symptoms
  2. Behavior and education therapy
     a) Friendship training
     b) Specialized math training
     c) Executive function training
     d) Parent-child interaction training
     e) Parenting and behavior management training
  3. Parenting training
     a) Concentrate on child's strengths and talents.
     b) Accept child's limitations.
     c) Be consistent with everything.
     d) Use concrete language and examples.
     e) Use stable routine that does not change daily.
     f) Keep everything simple.
     g) Be specific (i.e., say exactly what you mean).
     h) Structure your child's world to provide a foundation for daily living.
     i) Use visualized aids, music, and hands-on activities to help your child learn.
     j) Use positive reinforcement often.
     k) Supervise.
     l) Repeat, repeat, and repeat.
  4. Emphasis on the following protective factors helps reduce the effects and also assists people with this condition to reach their full potential:
     a) Diagnosing before 6 yr
     b) Living in stable nurturing home environment in school years
     c) Absence of violence
     d) Involvement in special education and social services
  5. Alternative approaches such as biofeedback, auditory training, relaxation therapy, visual imagery, yoga/exercise, acupuncture/acupressure, massage, Reiki, energy healing, animal-assisted therapy, and so forth may play a role.

AUTHOR: **HEMANT K. SATPATHY, M.D.**

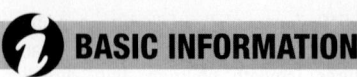
BASIC INFORMATION

DEFINITION

Fever of undetermined origin (FUO) was defined by Petersdorf and Beeson in 1961 as an illness characterized by temperatures >38.3° C (101° F) on several occasions for >3 weeks with no known cause despite extensive workup.

- Persistence for >2 weeks separates an FUO from an insignificant viral illness.
- Traditionally, diagnosis was made only after a 1-week inpatient workup. In contemporary practice, much of the workup is performed as an outpatient.

  FUO can be classified into classic, nosocomial (health-care associated), neutropenic (immune deficient), and HIV-associated. Table 1 provides a summary of definitions and major features of subtypes of FUO.

SYNONYMS

Fever of unknown origin

ICD-10CM CODES
R50.9 Fever, unspecified

EPIDEMIOLOGY & DEMOGRAPHICS

- The incidence of undiagnosed FUO dropped to <10% in the 1950s but has steadily increased since then.

- True FUOs are uncommon.

CLINICAL PRESENTATION

Fever 38.3° C (101° F or higher) on several occasions >3 weeks.

ETIOLOGY

- Infection (16%-23%).
  1. Abscess: abdominal, pelvic
  2. Tuberculosis
  3. HIV infection
  4. Nosocomial: urinary tract infection, pneumonia, line-related bacteremia, *Clostridium difficile* colitis, sinusitis
  5. Bacterial endocarditis (especially caused by difficult-to-isolate organisms)
  6. Biliary tract infection
  7. Osteomyelitis, vertebral and mandibular
  8. Less common infections: Q fever, leptospirosis, psittacosis, tularemia, secondary syphilis, gonococcemia, chronic meningococcemia, Whipple's disease, yersiniosis, fungal infections
- Malignancy (7%-10%): lymphoma (especially non-Hodgkin's lymphoma), leukemia, renal cell carcinoma, hepatocellular carcinomas, other tumors metastatic to liver
- Noninfectious inflammatory disease (22%-31%)
  1. Adult Still's disease (young to middle-aged patients)
  2. Temporal arteritis (elderly patients)

3. Other vasculitis: polyarteritis nodosa, Takayasu's arteritis, Wegener's granulomatosis, mixed cryoglobulinemia
- Other
  1. Drug-induced fever
  2. Inflammatory bowel disease
  3. Sarcoidosis
  4. Pulmonary embolism
  5. Alcoholic hepatitis
- No diagnosis

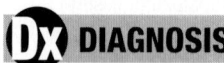
DIAGNOSIS

DIFFERENTIAL DIAGNOSIS

Factitious fever

WORKUP

- Accurate history and careful physical examination are essential. Fig. E1 describes an approach to the patient with FUO.
- Laboratory tests and imaging dependent on medical history clues and physical findings.
- When in doubt, perform another complete history and physical examination. Examples of subtle physical findings in patients with FUO are described in Table 2.

MEDICAL HISTORY CLUES

- Fever duration, tempo; inciting factors
- Rash, myalgia, weight loss, pain
- Sick contacts

TABLE 1 Summary of Definitions and Major Features of the Four Subtypes of Fever of Undetermined Origin

Feature	Classic FUO	Health Care–Associated FUO	Immune-Deficient FUO	HIV-Related FUO
Definition	>38.0° C, >3 wk, >2 visits or 1 wk in hospital	≥38.0° C, >1 wk, not present or incubating on admission	≥38.0° C, >1 wk, negative cultures after 48 hr	≥38.0° C, >3 wk for outpatients, >1 wk for inpatients, HIV infection confirmed
Patient location	Community, clinic, or hospital	Acute care hospital	Hospital or clinic	Community, clinic, or hospital
Leading causes	Cancer, infections, inflammatory conditions, undiagnosed, habitual hyperthermia	Health care–associated infections, postoperative complications, drug fever	Majority due to infections, but cause documented in only 40%-60%	HIV (primary infection), typical and atypical mycobacteria, CMV, lymphomas, toxoplasmosis, cryptococcosis, immune reconstitution inflammatory syndrome (IRIS)
History emphasis	Travel, contacts, animal and insect exposure, medications, immunizations, family history, cardiac valve disorder	Operations and procedures, devices, anatomic considerations, drug treatment	Stage of chemotherapy, drugs administered, underlying immunosuppressive disorder	Drugs, exposures, risk factors, travel, contacts, stage of HIV infection
Examination emphasis	Fundi, oropharynx, temporal artery, abdomen, lymph nodes, spleen, joints, skin, nails, genitalia, rectum or prostate, lower limb deep veins	Wounds, drains, devices, sinuses, urine	Skinfolds, IV sites, lungs, perianal area	Mouth, sinuses, skin, lymph nodes, eyes, lungs, perianal area
Investigation emphasis	Imaging, biopsies, sedimentation rate, skin tests	Imaging, bacterial cultures	CXR, bacterial cultures	Blood and lymphocyte count; serologic tests; CXR; stool examination; biopsies of lung, bone marrow, and liver for cultures and cytologic tests; brain imaging
Management	Observation, outpatient temperature chart, investigations, avoidance of empirical drug treatments	Depends on situation	Antimicrobial treatment protocols	Antiviral and antimicrobial protocols, vaccines, revision of treatment regimens, good nutrition
Time course of disease	Months	Weeks	Days	Weeks to months
Tempo of investigation	Weeks	Days	Hours	Days to weeks

CMV, Cytomegalovirus; *CXR,* chest radiograph; *FUO,* fever of undetermined origin.
Adapted from Mandell GL, Bennett JE, Dolin R (eds): *Mandell, Douglas, and Bennett's principles and practice of infectious diseases,* ed 7, Philadelphia, 2010, Churchill Livingstone. Borrowed from Kliegman RM et al: *Nelson textbook of pediatrics,* ed 19, Philadelphia, 2011, Saunders.

- Past medical history: tuberculosis, HIV, malignancies, surgeries
- Medications
- Family history: tuberculosis, malignancies, familial Mediterranean fever
- Social history: daily routine, rural versus urban, pets and animal contacts, arthropod bites, recent and remote travel, socioeconomic status, occupation, military service, sexual history

PHYSICAL FINDINGS

- HEENT (head, ears, eyes, nose, throat): sinus tenderness, dental abscesses, funduscopic lesions
- Neck: adenopathy, palpable thyroid
- Lungs: auscultate for rales
- Heart: murmur
- Abdomen: organomegaly
- Rectal: prostate tenderness
- Pelvic: cervical motion tenderness, fundal or adnexal masses or pain, inguinal adenopathy
- Extremities: clubbing, splinter hemorrhages, tenderness or fluctuance at IV access site
- Musculoskeletal: joint effusions
- Skin: rashes, wounds

LABORATORY TESTS

- Most FUO workups include:
  1. Blood cultures (three sets from different sites)
  2. Complete blood count with differential
  3. Erythrocyte sedimentation rate or C-reactive protein
  4. Urinalysis with microscopic exam and culture
  5. Transaminases
  6. Serum lactate dehydrogenase
  7. PPD testing
- Consider
  1. HIV antibody testing
  2. Creatinine phosphokinase
  3. Rheumatoid factor
  4. Serum protein electrophoresis
  5. Lumbar puncture
  6. Thyroid function testing
  7. Stool culture and *C. difficile* assay
  8. Biopsy (bone marrow, skin, liver lymph nodes, pleural, etc., based on clinical and laboratory findings)
  9. Antinuclear antibody testing

May need to repeat tests at regular intervals until diagnosis is established.

IMAGING STUDIES

- Most workups eventually include chest radiograph and abdominal CT scan.
- Further imaging is based on medical history clues and physical findings.
- FDG-PET is very sensitive to detect anatomic sites of inflammation or malignancy. It may help to identify sites requiring further investigation.

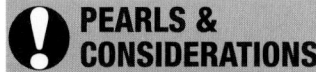 **TREATMENT**

ACUTE GENERAL Rx

Antibiotics and other treatment indicated only after definitive or highly probable diagnosis is established unless patient is neutropenic, severely ill, or septic.

DISPOSITION

In some cases a diagnosis is not made for years. At 5-yr follow-up, mortality rate among patients with undiagnosed FUO was only 3.2% in one study.

REFERRAL

To an infectious disease specialist, hematologist, or rheumatologist if no diagnosis after thoughtful workup.

! PEARLS & CONSIDERATIONS

COMMENTS

Because of improvements in imaging and laboratory tests, fewer cases of FUO are attributed to infectious causes and more are attributable to tumors and collagen-vascular diseases.

SUGGESTED READING

Available at www.expertconsult.com

RELATED CONTENT

Fever of Unknown Origin (Patient Information).

AUTHOR: **ETSUKO AOKI, M.D., PH.D.**

F

Diseases and Disorders

I

TABLE 2 Examples of Subtle Physical Findings Having Special Significance in Patients with Fever of Undetermined Origin

Body Site	Physical Finding	Diagnosis
Head	Sinus tenderness	Sinusitis
Temporal artery	Nodules, reduced pulsations	Temporal arteritis
Oropharynx	Ulceration	Disseminated histoplasmosis
	Tender tooth	Periapical abscess
Fundi or conjunctivae	Choroid tubercle	Disseminated granulomatosis*
	Petechiae, Roth's spot	Endocarditis
Thyroid	Enlargement, tenderness	Thyroiditis
Heart	Murmur	Infective or marantic endocarditis
Abdomen	Enlarged iliac crest lymph nodes, splenomegaly	Lymphoma, endocarditis, disseminated granulomatosis*
Rectum	Perirectal fluctuance, tenderness	Abscess
	Prostatic tenderness, fluctuance	Abscess
Genitalia	Testicular nodule	Periarteritis nodosa
	Epididymal nodule	Disseminated granulomatosis
Lower extremities	Deep venous tenderness	Thrombosis or thrombophlebitis
Skin and nails	Petechiae, splinter hemorrhages, subcutaneous nodules, clubbing	Vasculitis, endocarditis

*Includes tuberculosis, histoplasmosis, coccidioidomycosis, sarcoidosis, and syphilis.
From Mandell GL et al (eds): *Mandell, Douglas, and Bennett's principles and practice of infectious diseases*, ed 7, Philadelphia, 2010, Churchill Livingstone.

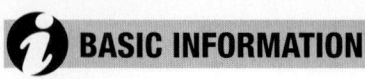

DEFINITION

Fibrocystic breast disease (FCD), now called "fibrocystic breast changes" (FBC), includes nonmalignant breast lesions including:
- Microcystic and macrocystic changes
- Fibrosis
- Mild and moderate hyperplasia
- Sclerosing adenosis
- Apocrine metaplasia
- Fibroadenoma
- Papilloma
- Papillomatosis
- Radial scar

SYNONYMS

Cystic changes
Chronic cystic mastitis
Fibrocystic breast changes
FBC
Mammary dysplasia
FCD
Fibrocystic mastopathy
Diffuse cystic mastopathy

ICD-10CM CODES

N60.01 Solitary cyst of right breast
N60.02 Solitary cyst of left breast
N60.09 Solitary cyst of unspecified breast
N60.11 Diffuse cystic mastopathy of right breast
N60.12 Diffuse cystic mastopathy of left breast
N60.19 Diffuse cystic mastopathy of unspecified breast
N60.3 Fibrosclerosis

EPIDEMIOLOGY & DEMOGRAPHICS

- FBC affects 30% to 60% of reproductive-age women.
- Most commonly seen in women ages 30 to 50 years

PHYSICAL FINDINGS & CLINICAL PRESENTATION

- Lumpy or ropey breast texture.
- Nodular areas
- Tenderness of breasts and/or nipples.
- Dominant mass more often in the upper outer quadrants.
- Symptoms tend to be affected with changes in the menstrual cycle.
- Symptoms can be aggravated in postmenopausal women who initiate hormone therapy.
- Nipple discharge.

ETIOLOGY

- Because it is found in the majority of healthy breasts, it is regarded as a nonpathologic process.
- The relationship of FBC to the menstrual cycle suggests hormonal influence.

DIAGNOSIS

DIFFERENTIAL DIAGNOSIS

Table 1 differentiates breast masses. Characteristics of breast masses suspect for cancer (90% sensitivity, 40%-60% specificity) are:
- Fixed mass
- Poorly defined mass
- Hard (scirrhous) mass.

WORKUP

- Rule out breast carcinoma if breast mass, thickening, discharge, and/or pain are present.
- Perform biopsy of suspected area for histologic confirmation.

IMAGING STUDIES

Mammography and ultrasound studies required:
- For mammographic changes (suspicious densities, microcalcifications, architectural distortion): careful evaluation, including possibly biopsy to exclude breast cancer.
- Ultrasound study: to evaluate the presence of a solid vs. cystic mass.

TREATMENT

NONPHARMACOLOGIC THERAPY

Treatment is symptomatic:
- Reassurance.
- Supportive bra.
- OTC pain medications including NSAIDs and Tylenol.
- Reduced intake of methylxanthines (coffee, chocolate), although this is not as effective as previously thought.
- Decreasing vitamin E or salt has not proved to be effective.
- Periodic physician examination to monitor patients with FCD who have pronounced nodular features.
- Aspiration for palpable or symptomatic cysts (NOTE: Cysts often recur; repeat aspiration is not always required unless pain is a problem).

PHARMACOLOGIC TREATMENT

For breast pain:
- Danocrine (Danazol): This is the only FDA-approved drug for breast pain. Moderate success has been reported, but the side effect profile is significant due to androgenic effects.
- Bromocriptine: The medication inhibits prolactin, and its effects are better than a placebo, but side effects such as lightheadedness and gastrointestinal symptoms limit its use.
- Tamoxifen: This has been found to reduce breast pain in 70% of affected women with cyclic breast pain, but the side effects of hot flashes and vaginal dryness interfere with compliance.
- Pharmacology therapy is usually tapered down after 3 to 6 months of treatment.

FOLLOW-UP

- Evaluate carefully to exclude breast cancer; then offer reassurance and periodic reevaluation as required.
- Regular self-examination, annual physician examination.

REFERRAL TO BREAST SURGEON

- For further evaluation and/or biopsy if suspicious changes are associated with FBC (including progression of dominant mass or thickening, persistent or spontaneous nipple discharge, or suspicious mammographic changes or lesions)
- To alleviate anxiety associated with breast symptoms or changes

RELATED CONTENT

Fibrocystic Breast Changes (Patient Information)
Breast Cancer (Related Key Topic)
Mastodynia (Related Key Topic)
Mastitis (Related Key Topic)

AUTHOR: **RUBEN ALVERO, M.D.,** and **ESTELLE H. WHITNEY, M.D.**

TABLE 1 Differentiation of Breast Masses

Characteristic	Cystic Disease	Benign Adenoma	Malignant Tumor
Patient age	25-60 yr	10-55 yr	25-85 yr
Number	One or more	One	One
Shape	Round	Round	Irregular
Consistency	Elastic, soft to hard	Firm	Stony hard
Delimitation	Well delimited	Well delimited	Poorly delimited
Mobility	Mobile	Mobile	Fixed
Tenderness	Present	Absent	Absent
Skin retraction	Absent	Absent	Present

From Swartz, MH: *Textbook of physical diagnosis*, ed 7, Philadelphia, 2014, Saunders.

BASIC INFORMATION

DEFINITION

Fibromyalgia (FM) is a syndrome characterized by chronic, widespread musculoskeletal pain without evidence of soft tissue inflammation. Key features include fatigue, sleep disruption, cognitive disturbance, and psychiatric and somatic symptoms. Research suggests that FM is a disorder of pain regulation, which is often classified as a form of central sensitization.

SYNONYMS

- "Fibrositis" is a term that is no longer used because there is no evidence of connective tissue inflammation in FM
- FM

ICD-10CM CODES
M79.7 Fibromyalgia

EPIDEMIOLOGY & DEMOGRAPHICS

Worldwide, the prevalence of FM is believed to be 2% to 8%, and it increases with age. In the U.S., FM is the most common cause of musculoskeletal pain in women ages 20 to 55 yr. Using the 2010 American College of Rheumatology (ACR) diagnostic criteria for FM, the female-to-male ratio is approximately 2:1.

PHYSICAL FINDINGS & CLINICAL PRESENTATION

Patients with FM often report the following symptoms:
- Chronic (>3 months) widespread (affecting both sides of the body, above and below the waist, and involving the axial spine) musculoskeletal pain
- Cognitive disturbances
- Fatigue and sleep disturbances (e.g., unrefreshed sleep, easy fatigability)
- Psychiatric symptoms (e.g., anxiety, depression)
- Headache (present in more than half of patients with FM; this includes migraine and tension-type headaches)
- Paresthesias

- Associated disorders: irritable bowel syndrome, interstitial cystitis/painful bladder syndrome

On physical examination, patients with FM may have tenderness in particular soft tissue locations called tender points (Fig. 1). Examination of tender points requires that the examiner be familiar with the areas to palpate and that they apply enough pressure (4 kg/cm^2 or enough pressure to whiten the nail bed of the fingertips of the examiner).

ETIOLOGY

Although the exact cause of FM is unknown, many factors are believed to contribute to the development of this disorder:
- Genetic and environmental factors predispose individuals to FM. Evidence suggests that both the ascending and descending pain pathways operate abnormally, resulting in central amplification of pain signals. Familial associations of FM provide strongest evidence that reflect both these factors.
- In those predisposed, FM may be precipitated by stressful events such as abuse, injury from accidents, illnesses (including autoimmune disorders), infections, surgical procedures, and psychological stressors.
- Psychosocial, neuroendocrine, hormonal, and sociocultural factors also influence symptom expression.

PATHOGENESIS

Much remains to be discovered about the pathogenesis of FM, even though significant advances have been made in our understanding of this syndrome over the past few decades. Researchers have shown that biochemical, metabolic, and immunoregulatory abnormalities exist in patients with FM. Hence, this condition is now believed to be neurosensory in nature.
- Augmented pain and sensory processing is a hallmark, resulting in diffuse pain, allodynia (pain brought on by nonpainful stimuli), and hyperalgesia (more intense and prolonged pain perception).
- Afflicted persons show altered physiologic responses to painful stimulation at spinal and supraspinal levels.

- Brain neuroimaging studies found differences in brain structure, neurochemical concentrations, and functional brain networks in FM compared with control subjects.
- Pain augmentation may also result from a loss of tonic inhibition by descending inhibitory pathways from the brain to the spinal cord.

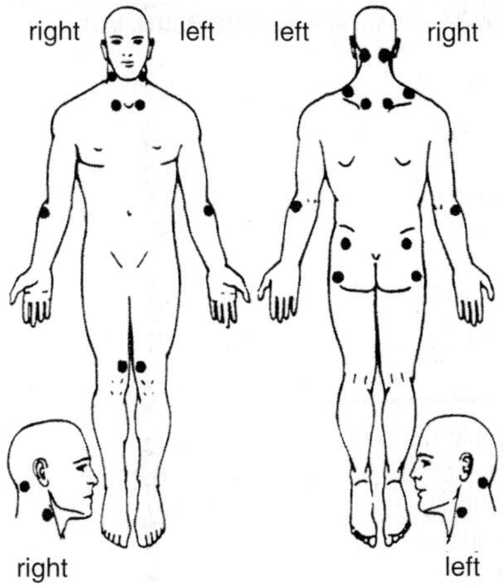

DIAGNOSIS

DIFFERENTIAL DIAGNOSIS

The presence of any of the disorders mentioned below does not necessarily exclude a diagnosis of FM because it may coexist with many conditions:
- Other functional somatic or "central sensitivity" syndromes: myofascial pain, chronic fatigue syndrome, irritable bowel syndrome, headache/migraines, chronic pelvic and bladder pain disorders, and temporomandibular disorder.
- Disorders that can mimic FM and must be ruled out include metabolic (e.g., hypothyroidism), infectious, and neurologic disorders. Arthritis and rheumatic diseases (e.g., rheumatoid arthritis, systemic lupus erythematosus, osteoarthritis, Sjögren's syndrome)
- Myalgias and other muscle disease (e.g., inflammatory and metabolic myopathies).
- Mood and anxiety disorders.
- Sleep disorders (e.g., sleep apnea, restless leg syndrome).
- Neurologic disorders.
- Medications: statin-induced muscle pain, opioid-induced hyperalgesia.

WORKUP

A thorough history, physical examination, and appropriately selected laboratory or imaging studies can usually differentiate FM from connective tissue or other systemic diseases.
- Chronic (>3 months), widespread pain is the hallmark symptom of FM, but fatigue, tenderness, depression/anxiety, nonrestorative sleep, cognitive difficulties (the so-called "fibrofog"), and functional impairment are other key symptoms.
- The 1990 American College of Rheumatology (ACR) FM Classification Criteria was used for clinical studies:
  1. Chronic, widespread pain in all four quadrants of the body and the axial skeleton.
  2. Pain on digital palpation of at least 11 of 18 tender points (see Fig. 1).
- The 2010 ACR diagnostic criteria for FM do not require a tender point examination; it requires the exclusion of other disorders that would otherwise explain the pain (Table 1)
- A diagnostic screening tool (Fibromyalgia Diagnostic Screen) developed by Arnold and colleagues was found to accurately screen for FM. This tool includes a patient self-reported questionnaire and an abbreviated physical examination with targeted lab tests.

right · left · left · right

1. Occiput
2. Low cervical
3. Trapezius
4. Supraspinatus
5. Second rib
6. Lateral epicondyle
7. Gluteal
8. Greater trochanter
9. Knees

right · left

FIG. 1 The sites of the 18 tender points of the 1990 American College of Rheumatology criteria for the classification of fibromyalgia. (From Conn R: *Current diagnosis*, ed 9, Philadelphia, 1997, Saunders.)

TABLE 1   2010 Fibromyalgia Diagnostic Criteria

Criteria

A patient satisfies diagnostic criteria for fibromyalgia if the following three conditions are met:
1. Widespread pain index (WPI) 7 and symptom severity (SS) scale score of 5 or WPI 3-6 and SS scale score of 9.
2. Symptoms have been present at a similar level for at least 3 months.
3. The patient does not have a disorder that would otherwise explain the pain.

Ascertainment

1. WPI: Note the number of areas in which the patient has had pain over the past week. In how many areas has the patient had pain?
Score will be between 0 and 19

Shoulder girdle, left	Hip (buttock, trochanter), left	Jaw, left	Upper back
Shoulder girdle, right	Hip (buttock, trochanter), right	Jaw, right	Lower back
Upper arm, left	Upper leg, left	Chest	Neck
Upper arm, right	Upper leg, right	Abdomen	
Lower arm, left	Lower leg, left		
Lower arm, right	Lower leg, right		

2. SS scale score:
   - Fatigue
   - Waking unrefreshed
   - Cognitive symptoms

For the each of the three symptoms above, indicate the level of severity over the past week using the following scale:

0 No problem
1 Slight or mild problems, generally mild or intermittent
2 Moderate, considerable problems, often present at a moderate level
3 Severe: pervasive, continuous, life-disturbing problems
Considering somatic symptoms in general, indicate whether the patient has:*
0 no symptoms
1 Few symptoms
2 A moderate number of symptoms
3 A great deal of symptoms
The SS scale score is the sum of the severity of the three symptoms (fatigue, waking unrefreshed, cognitive symptoms) plus the extent (severity) of somatic symptoms in general. The final score is between 0 and 12.

*Somatic symptoms that might be considered include muscle pain, irritable bowel syndrome, fatigue or tiredness, thinking or remembering problem, muscle weakness, headache, pain or cramps in the abdomen, numbness or tingling, dizziness, insomnia, depression, constipation, pain in the upper abdomen, nausea, nervousness, chest pain, blurred vision, fever, diarrhea, dry mouth, itching, wheezing, Raynaud's phenomenon, hives or welts, ringing in ears, vomiting, heartburn, oral ulcers, loss of or change in taste, seizures, dry eyes, shortness of breath, loss of appetite, rash, sun sensitivity, hearing difficulties, easy bruising, hair loss, frequent urination, painful urination, and bladder spasms.
Table adapted from Wolfe et al, 2010.

LABORATORY TESTS

- Selective use of ancillary tests complements the history and physical examination in the diagnosis of FM. Testing should be highly focused on the exclusion of FM mimickers or suspected concurrent diseases.
- Complete blood cell count, routine chemistries, thyroid-stimulating hormone (TSH), 25-hydroxy vitamin D level (low levels can cause muscle pain), vitamin B_{12} level (low levels can cause fatigue and pain), iron studies (low levels can cause fatigue and depressive symptoms), and magnesium levels (low levels can cause muscle spasms).
- Erythrocyte sedimentation rate (ESR), and C-reactive protein (CRP) are normal in FM.
- Routine testing for antinuclear antibody (ANA) and/or rheumatoid factor should be avoided unless history and physical examination suggest an autoimmune disease.

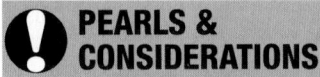 **TREATMENT**

GENERAL Rx (FIG. E2)

The goal in treating patients with fibromyalgia is to reduce the main symptoms of the syndrome (musculoskeletal pain, fatigue, depression, anxiety, poor sleep).

- Best approach may be combination of drug and nondrug therapies.
- FM can be due to abnormalities in many different neurotransmitter systems, thus, approaches and treatment responses may vary.
- Best evidence for tricyclics (low-dose amitriptyline and cyclobenzaprine), serotonin-norepinephrine reuptake inhibitors (milnacipran and duloxetine), and gabapentinoids (gabapentin and pregabalin).
- Second-tier drug classes include SSRIs.
- "Start low, go slow" approach is best to avoid side effects from medications.
- The only analgesic that has demonstrated efficacy in FM has been tramadol, either alone or in combination with acetaminophen.
- There is no evidence that NSAIDs or corticosteroids are effective in FM.
- Avoid narcotic use. There is concern that opioid use and abuse may aggravate chronic widespread pain.
- Nonpharmacologic: strong evidence to support exercise (aerobic, strengthening, and stretching exercises), cognitive behavioral therapy, physical therapy, and patient education (e.g., regarding the disease, importance of good sleep hygiene)

DISPOSITION

- The pain and symptoms of FM can wax and wane, vary in physical location and in intensity day to day; many patients continue to have chronic pain and fatigue regardless of therapy.
- Disability rates vary from 10% to 30%.

REFERRAL

Referral to rheumatology, neurology, mental health professionals, physical medicine and rehabilitation, including physical therapy, may be helpful for a multidisciplinary team approach.

! PEARLS & CONSIDERATIONS

- Fibromyalgia is a neurosensory disorder whereby affected individuals have abnormal central nociceptive processing.
- Diagnosis is based on the presence of chronic musculoskeletal pain in the absence of physical or laboratory evidence of inflammation and in the absence of any other condition that would explain the symptoms.
- Treatment options are varied, but a combination of drug and nondrug options is likely to provide optimal results.
- Myofascial pain syndrome may represent a localized form of FM. It is associated with trigger points (rather than tender points as seen in FM). Some patients with myofascial pain syndrome may progress to FM.

COMMENTS

FM occurs frequently in patients with some rheumatic diseases such as rheumatoid arthritis, ankylosing spondylitis, and systemic lupus erythematosus, in which prevalence of FM may reach 20%.

SUGGESTED READINGS

Available at www.expertconsult.com

RELATED CONTENT

Fibromyalgia (Patient Information)

AUTHOR: **NADINE MBUYI, M.D.**

BASIC INFORMATION

DEFINITION

Parvovirus B19 is a small, non-enveloped ssDNA virus that belongs to the *Erythrovirus* genus of the *Parvoviridae* family. It was first discovered in 1975 when units of blood were being screened for hepatitis B and was read as a false-positive result (sample 19 in panel B). It causes a spectrum of human disease, from asymptomatic to fatal, depending on the underlying host. Classically, it has been associated with erythema infectiosum (EI), or "fifth disease," the fifth in a series of six viral exanthems that commonly affect school-aged children and are named in order of the dates they were first described. In addition, parvovirus B19 causes a variety of diseases in fetuses, adults, and the immunocompromised.

SYNONYMS

Parvovirus B19
Erythema infectiosum
Fifth disease

ICD-10CM CODES
B08.3 Erythema infectiosum [fifth disease]

EPIDEMIOLOGY & DEMOGRAPHICS

INCIDENCE: Between 1% and 9% of pregnancies are affected by B19 infection. Up to 1 in 200 units of blood are contaminated by B19, and 16% of schoolteachers and 9% of daycare workers and homemakers are infected with B19 during epidemics. The infection rate of household contacts may be as high as 50%.
PEAK INCIDENCE: Temperate climates between late winter and early summer, often in cycles of local epidemics that peak every 3 to 10 yr.
PREVALENCE: 15% of school-aged children, and 30% to 85% of adults have demonstrated protective IgG antibodies to parvovirus B19.
PREDOMINANT AGE: 5 to 18 yr
RISK FACTORS:
- Exposure to school-aged children
- Immunosuppression
- Congenital or acquired hematologic abnormalities,
- Blood transfusion
- Tissue transplantation

PHYSICAL FINDINGS & CLINICAL PRESENTATION

- Approximately 25% of those infected are asymptomatic, 50% have nonspecific flu-like symptoms, and 25% have the classic symptoms of B19 infection, including rash and/or arthralgias.
- Parvovirus B19 is the most common viral agent associated with rashes in school-aged children. EI is characterized by a bright red, non-tender rash most prominent on the cheeks with a circumoral pallor producing the classic "slapped face" appearance (Fig. 1), which is often followed by a reticular, lacelike rash on the trunk and extremities. This is typically a transient, self-limited illness that begins with a prodrome of flu-like symptoms, such as fever, malaise, myalgias, coryza, headache, nausea, and diarrhea, and ends with the malar rash once viremia has resolved and antibody production has occurred.
- Polyarthralgias and polyarthritis are more commonly seen in adults (especially women) and typically involve symmetric small joints of the extremities. The arthritis is nonerosive. Joint symptoms usually resolve within 3 weeks but may rarely become persistent or recurrent. A rash develops in 75% of infected adults, but less than 20% have the classic "slapped face" rash seen in EI. The rash may be exacerbated by changes in temperature, sunlight, exercise, or emotional stress.
- B19 infection during pregnancy can result in fetal anemia, nonimmune hydrops fetalis, miscarriage, or fetal loss. Pregnant women with B19 infection have a 30% chance of fetal transmission. The risk of fetal loss is 5% to 10% and greatest when fetal infection occurs in the first 20 weeks of gestation.
- In patients with congenital or acquired hematologic abnormalities, B19 infection can cause severe anemia or transient aplastic crisis, which is usually manifested as pure red cell aplasia and may be fatal. Chronic infection and anemia have been described in patients with leukemia and other cancers, HIV, or congenital immunodeficiency and in recipients of tissue transplantation.
- B19 has also been associated with immune thrombocytopenic purpura, vasculitis, nephritis, lymphadenitis, meningitis, encephalitis, and fulminant liver disease and is the most prevalent pathogen responsible for acute myocarditis, which progresses to dilated cardiomyopathy in 21% of cases.

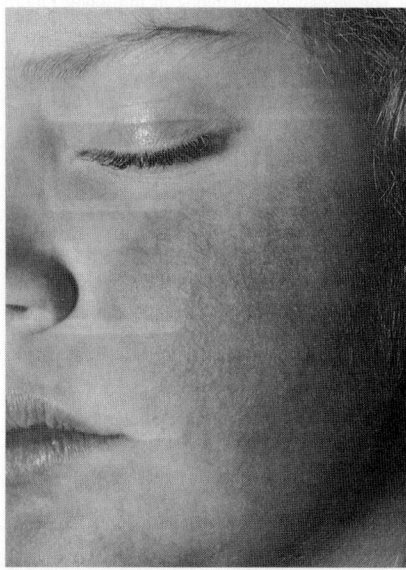

FIG. 1 Fifth disease (erythema infectiosum). Facial erythema "slapped face." The red plaque covers the cheek and spares the nasolabial and the circumoral region. (From Habif TP: *Clinical dermatology: a color guide to diagnosis and therapy*, ed 3, St Louis, 1996, Mosby.)

- B19 can cause a severe acute myocarditis in children. Patients with fulminant myocarditis, ST segment changes, or a short prodrome have the worst outcome. Transplantation may be considered but is rarely required in the acute period if mechanical circulatory support is utilized. If the initial presentation is survived, recovery of the myocardium can occur even in those who had fulminant myocarditis.
- B19 has now been shown to play a role in the pathogenesis of autoimmunity and autoimmune disease.
- It has been suggested that parvovirus B19 infection may precipitate the development of rheumatoid arthritis, systemic lupus erythematosus, or juvenile rheumatoid arthritis.
- As many as 15% of new cases of inflammatory arthritis may be caused by parvovirus infection.

ETIOLOGY, INFECTIVITY, & TRANSMISSION

B19 preferentially infects, replicates in, and is directly cytotoxic to erythroid progenitor cells, which may result in profound anemia or pure red cell aplasia. Viremia and the period of greatest infectivity occur 7 to 10 days after exposure and last about 1 week in immunocompetent individuals, after which time antibody production begins and typical symptoms of rash and arthralgias manifest. Transmission is thought to occur primarily through droplet exposure, as well as person-to-person contact, fomites, vertical transmission, and hematogenous transmission. Because of its non-enveloped capsid, parvovirus B19 is heat stable and difficult to inactivate with solvent detergents, often leading to contamination of blood products.

DIAGNOSIS

DIFFERENTIAL DIAGNOSIS

- Juvenile rheumatoid arthritis (Still's disease)
- Rubella, measles (rubeola), and other childhood viral exanthems
- Mononucleosis
- Lyme disease
- Acute HIV infection
- Drug eruption

WORKUP

Diagnosis can be made by typical clinical presentation in well children. Laboratory tests may be required for confirmation in immunosuppressed populations, those with severe anemia or transient aplastic crisis (TAC), and pregnant women.

LABORATORY TESTS

- About half of adults are immune to parvovirus infection, most likely because of a previous, unnoticed childhood infection. People who are at risk of severe parvovirus complications might benefit from serum antibody testing to determine whether they are immune to parvovirus or whether there is recent infection.
- Complete blood count (CBC) and reticulocyte count: CBC evaluation ranges from mild to profound classically normocytic normochromic anemia. Reticulocytes are markedly

decreased or absent in pure red blood cell aplasia. White blood cell and platelet counts are typically unchanged.

- Parvovirus B19 IgM and IgG: Parvovirus B19 IgM enzyme immunoassay is widely available and the preferred method of diagnosis in immunocompetent individuals. IgM can be found within 7 to 10 days of exposure and may persist for several months. IgG antibodies are detectable about 15 days after exposure and persist long term.
- Parvovirus B19 viral DNA polymerase chain reaction (PCR): Nucleic acid antigen testing (NAAT) of B19 DNA by PCR is the most sensitive method of infection detection and the preferred method for diagnosis in immunocompromised individuals, fetuses, immunocompetent patients with suspected persistent infection, and blood products.
- Bone marrow biopsy: Bone marrow examination in patients with pure red cell aplasia demonstrates complete or near-complete absence of red cell precursors. Characteristic giant proerythroblasts containing large eosinophilic nuclear inclusions can be seen.
- Fig. 2 illustrates investigations for parvovirus B19 infection in pregnancy.

Prenatal testing: Fetal nuchal translucency measurement and ductus venosus Doppler velocimetry may indicate the presence of severe fetal anemia. Ultrasound may show fetal edema, ascites, pleural effusions, and cardiomegaly in hydrops fetalis.

Rx TREATMENT

NONPHARMACOLOGIC THERAPY

- Treatment for Fifth disease is generally supportive because the majority of B19 infections are asymptomatic or mild and self-limited. Nonsteroidal antiinflammatory drugs may be used for relief of joint symptoms, antipyretics for fever, and adequate hydration.

- Use caution when giving aspirin to children or teenagers. Although aspirin is approved for use in children older than age 3, children and teenagers recovering from chickenpox or flulike symptoms should never take aspirin. This is because aspirin has been linked to Reye's syndrome, a rare but potentially life-threatening condition, in such children.
- Reye's (Ryes) syndrome is a rare but serious condition that causes swelling in the liver and brain in children who have had a recent viral infection and take aspirin. Reye's syndrome is rarely fatal. However, it can cause varying degrees of permanent brain damage.

ACUTE GENERAL TREATMENT

- No antiviral drug is available.
- Blood transfusion is often required in cases of severe anemia and pure red cell aplasia until red blood cell (RBC) production returns; intrauterine transfusion may be required in fetal infection.
- Initiation of antiretroviral therapy (ART) has been associated with resolution of B19-induced anemia in HIV-infected patients.
- Bone marrow transplantation has been used in individuals with nonresolving aplastic crisis.
- The mainstay of fetal therapy is delivery, which may be followed by resuscitation and ventilation in cases of severe hydrops.

CHRONIC GENERAL TREATMENT

- IV immunoglobulin (IVIG) treatment may be considered for immunocompromised patients with chronic B19 infection and chronic anemia.

DISPOSITION

- B19 infection is typically self-limited, with symptoms usually resolving within a few weeks and most often only requiring supportive care.
- The illness is contagious in the week before the rash appears. Once the rash appears, the person with the illness is no longer considered contagious and does not require isolation.
- Patients in whom persistent arthritis with or without joint erosion develops should be evaluated by a rheumatologist.
- In immunocompetent patients, anemia is typically transient with spontaneous resolution and return of RBC production in days to weeks. In patients with hematologic abnormalities, however, anemia may be severe and may be the result of transient aplastic crisis or pure red cell aplasia, which warrants immediate hematologic evaluation and transfusion.
- Patients with TAC or chronic parvovirus B19 infection pose a risk for nosocomial spread and, when hospitalized, should be isolated with droplet precautions.
- Patients with chronic infection and anemia may require evaluation for possible IVIG treatment.
- Pregnant women with B19 infection have a 30% risk of fetal transmission; they should undergo close monitoring of fetal health and development and may require fetal transfusion or referral to a tertiary care center for delivery in the case of hydrops fetalis.
- Vaccines have not progressed beyond phase I/II clinical trials.

REFERRAL

- To hematologist if signs of marrow suppression
- To rheumatologist if signs of severe or erosive arthritis
- To cardiologist if suspicion of myocarditis

! PEARLS & CONSIDERATIONS

- Generally self-limited disease lasting up to 3 weeks in immunocompetent individuals.
- Symmetric arthritis involving small joints is common in adults, whereas facial rash is common in children.
- Can cause severe anemia with or without transient aplastic crisis that may become chronic in patients with hematologic abnormalities, immunocompromise, malignancy, or a history of organ transplantation.
- Infection during pregnancy can cause fetal anemia, hydrops fetalis, or fetal loss.

PREVENTION

- Hand-washing and not sharing food or drinks during epidemics.
- Testing of plasma pools and blood products for B19 contamination.
- Once you've become infected with parvovirus, you have acquired lifelong immunity.

SUGGESTED READINGS

Available at www.expertconsult.com.

RELATED CONTENT

Fifth Disease (Patient Information)

AUTHORS: **LINDSEY CILIA, M.D.,** and **DOMINICK TAMMARO, M.D.**

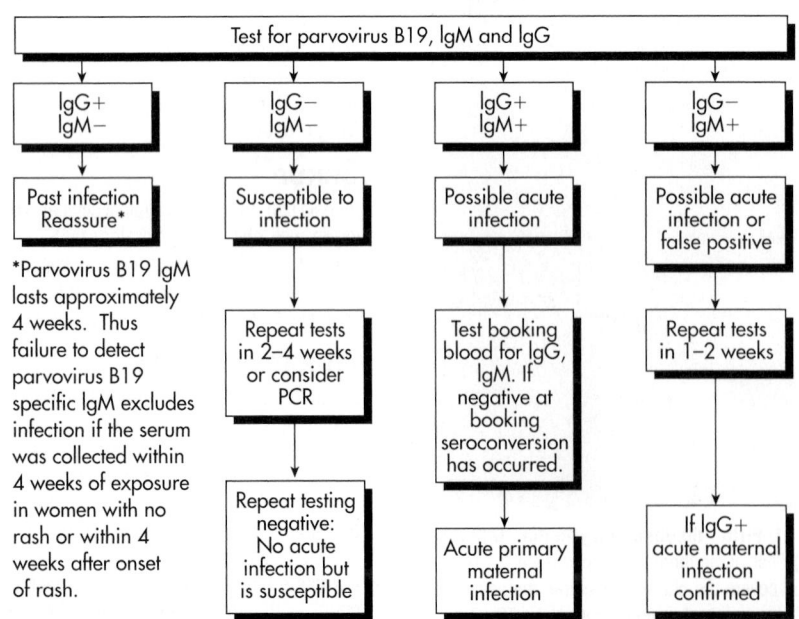

FIG. 2 Investigations for parvovirus B19 infection. (From Stephen G, Gillham J: Fetal infection: a pragmatic approach to recognition and management. *Obstet Gynecol Reprod Med* 22(10): 299–303, 2012.)

ⓘ BASIC INFORMATION

DEFINITION

Folliculitis is inflammation of the hair follicle as a result of infection, physical injury, or chemical irritation.

SYNONYMS

Sycosis barbae

ICD-10CM CODES
L72.9 Follicular cyst of skin and subcutaneous tissue, unspecified
L73.1 Pseudofolliculitis barbae
L73.8 Other specified follicular disorders
L66.2 Folliculitis decalvans
L66.4 Folliculitis ulerythematosa reticulata
L66.3 Perifolliculitis capitis abscedens

EPIDEMIOLOGY & DEMOGRAPHICS

PREVALENCE: Staphylococcal folliculitis is the most common form of infectious folliculitis; it occurs most commonly in persons with diabetes. Gram-negative folliculitis occurs in patients who have had moderately inflammatory acne for long periods and have been treated with long-term antibiotics such as tetracycline.

PREDOMINANT SEX: Sycosis barbae occurs most frequently in men who have commenced shaving.

PHYSICAL FINDINGS & CLINICAL PRESENTATION

- The lesions generally consist of painful yellow pustules surrounded by erythema; a central hair is present in the pustules. Furuncles with pus may be present (Fig. 1).
- Patients with sycosis barbae may initially present with small follicular papules or pustules that increase in size with continued shaving; deep follicular pustules may occur surrounded by erythema and swelling; the upper lip is frequently involved.

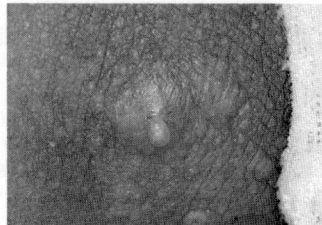

FIG. 1 Rupture and discharge of pus in a furuncle. (From Kliegman RM et al: *Nelson textbook of pediatrics,* ed 19, Philadelphia, 2011, Saunders.)

- "Hot tub" folliculitis occurs within 1 to 4 days after the use of a hot tub with poor chlorination. It is characterized by papules and pustules (Fig. 2) with surrounding erythema generally affecting the torso, buttocks, and limbs.

ETIOLOGY

- Staphylococcus infection (e.g., sycosis barbae), *Pseudomonas aeruginosa* ("hot tub" folliculitis)
- Gram-negative folliculitis *(Klebsiella, Enterobacter, Proteus)* associated with antibiotic treatment of acne
- Chronic irritation of the hair follicle (use of cocoa butter or coconut oil, chronic irritation from workplace)
- Initial use of systemic corticosteroid therapy (steroid acne), eosinophilic folliculitis (AIDS patients), *Candida albicans* (immunocompromised patients)
- *Pityrosporum orbiculare*

Ⓓˣ DIAGNOSIS

DIFFERENTIAL DIAGNOSIS

- Pseudofolliculitis barbae (ingrown hairs)
- Acne vulgaris
- Dermatophyte fungal infections
- Keratosis pilaris
- Cutaneous candidiasis
- Superficial fungal infections
- Miliaris

WORKUP

- Physical examination and medical history (e.g., use of hot tub: "hot tub" folliculitis; adolescent patients who have started shaving: sycosis barbae; use of occlusive topical steroid therapy: *Staphylococcus* folliculitis).
- Gram-negative folliculitis in acne patients on prolonged antibiotic treatment manifests with superficial pustules 3 to 6 mm in diameter flaring out from anterior nares or fluctuant, deep-seated nodules.

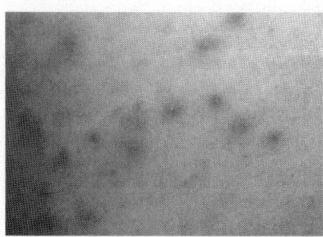

FIG. 2 Papules and pustules in hot tub folliculitis. (From Kliegman RM et al: *Nelson textbook of pediatrics,* ed 19, Philadelphia, 2011, Saunders.)

LABORATORY TESTS

- Generally not necessary.
- Gram stain is useful to identify the infective organisms in infectious folliculitis and to differentiate infectious folliculitis from noninfectious.

℞ TREATMENT

NONPHARMACOLOGIC THERAPY

- Prevention of chemical or mechanical skin irritation
- Glycemic control in diabetics
- Proper chlorination of hot tubs and spas
- Shaving with a clean razor

ACUTE GENERAL

- Cleansing of the area with chlorhexidine and application of saline compresses to involved area.
- Application of 2% mupirocin ointment or 1% retapamulin ointment for bacterial folliculitis affecting a limited area (e.g., sycosis barbae).
- Treatment of severe cases of *Pseudomonas* folliculitis with ciprofloxacin.
- Treatment of *S. aureus* folliculitis with dicloxacillin 250 mg qd for 10 days.
- Isotretinoin is the treatment of choice in gram-negative folliculitis. Amoxicillin or TMS-SMX can be used when isotretinoin is contraindicated or cannot be tolerated.

CHRONIC Rx

- Chronic nasal or perineal *S. aureus* carriers with frequent folliculitis can be treated with rifampin 300 mg bid for 5 days.
- Mupirocin or retapamulin ointment applied to nares bid is also effective for nasal carriers.

DISPOSITION:
- Most cases of bacterial folliculitis resolve completely with proper treatment.
- Steroid folliculitis responds to discontinuation of steroids.

❗ PEARLS & CONSIDERATIONS

COMMENTS

Patients should be instructed in good personal hygiene and avoidance of sharing razors, towels, and washcloths.

RELATED CONTENT

Folliculitis (Patient Information)

AUTHOR: **FRED F. FERRI, M.D.**

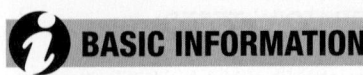

BASIC INFORMATION

DEFINITION

Food allergies are divided into IgE-mediated and immunologically mediated non-IgE reactions. They include a spectrum of disorders that involve adverse immunologic responses to dietary antigens.

ICD-10CM CODES

T78.0	Adverse food reaction (including anaphylactic shock)
T78.1	Other adverse food reactions, not elsewhere classified
L27.2	Dermatitis due to ingested food
Z91.010	Allergy to peanuts
Z91.011	Allergy to milk products
Z91.012	Allergy to eggs
Z91.013	Allergy to seafood
Z91.018	Allergy to other foods
Z91.02	Food additives allergy status

EPIDEMIOLOGY & DEMOGRAPHICS

INCIDENCE: Food allergies have a cumulative incidence of 6% to 8% for the first 3 yr of life.
PREVALENCE:
- Overall prevalence is 1% to 2% in general population, ~3.9% to 8% in children.
- Patient self-reported food allergies have a prevalence of 12% to 13%, demonstrating the importance of objective measures in assessing food allergies.
- Nearly 40% of children with food allergy have a history of severe reactions that, if not treated immediately with proper medication, can lead to hospitalization or even death.[1]
- There is insufficient evidence to conclude a racial predilection (Greenhawt, 2013).

PREDOMINANT SEX: Males are more affected than females among children, and among adults, females are more frequently affected.
GENETICS: Children with parents or close relatives with allergies may have a tendency to become allergic to foods.

PHYSICAL FINDINGS & CLINICAL PRESENTATION

- IgE-mediated reactions: (within minutes to a few hours) pruritus, urticaria or angioedema, atopic dermatitis, GI symptoms, conjunctival injection, sneezing, nasal congestion, rhinorrhea, bronchospasm, and anaphylaxis
- Non–IgE-mediated reactions: food-induced enterocolitis, celiac disease, Crohn's disease, dermatitis herpetiformis, and pulmonary reactions such as Heiner syndrome. These illnesses are discussed separately.
- Signs, symptoms, and presentation reflect specific allergic manifestation, but in food allergies there is a reproducible temporal relationship to ingested food allergens.

[1]Gupta RS et al: The prevalence, severity, and distribution of childhood food allergy in the United States, *Pediatrics* 128(l):e9-e17, 2011.

ETIOLOGY

Failure to establish tolerance to food antigens. IL-33 mediated epithelial permeability and Th2 skewing result in sensitization to food proteins which are presented to primed T cells. Food processing conditions that may affect allergenic activity are described in Table 1.

DIAGNOSIS

- Thorough history and physical exam should be performed.
- The temporal relationship and reproducibility of the symptoms are most important to establishing the diagnosis.
- A review of ingredient labels may be helpful.
- Confirmatory testing can include skin testing or in vitro testing.
- Skin prick testing (SPT): positive predictive value <50%, but negative predictive value >95%. Thus a negative skin test effectively rules out an IgE-mediated process.
- In vitro testing: RAST testing: Historically it is less sensitive than skin testing, but sensitivity has improved with cut off points indicating a positive predictive value of 95% for allergies to eggs, milk, peanuts, wheat, and fish.
- Atopy patch test: used in conjunction with RAST and skin testing in multiallergic children to plan widening the elimination diet. However, it is not recommended in the routine evaluation of food allergies.
- Double-blind, placebo-controlled food challenges are the gold standard test for determining food allergies. These need to be done in a supervised and controlled setting.
- In summary, if the history and lab tests are suggestive of a specific food allergy, that food should be confirmed by SPT, RAST, or food challenge and, once confirmed, eliminated from the diet.

DIFFERENTIAL DIAGNOSIS

- Gastrointestinal disorders
- Irritable bowel syndrome
- Carcinoid syndrome
- Giardiasis
- Structural abnormalities like hiatal hernia, pyloric stenosis, Hirschsprung's disease, tracheoesophageal fistula
- Disaccharidase deficiencies: lactase, sucrase-isomaltase complex, glucose-galactose complex
- Pancreatic insufficiency: cystic fibrosis
- Gallbladder disease
- Peptic ulcer disease
- Malignancy
- Metabolic disorders
- Galactosemia
- Phenylketonuria
- Pharmacologic-related conditions
- Gustatory rhinitis
- Auriculotemporal syndrome (facial flush from tart food)

TREATMENT

NONPHARMACOLOGIC THERAPY

- Elimination diet should be used in conjunction with nutritional counseling. Fig. 1 illustrates an algorithm for the management of food allergy

- Formula-fed infants: brief trial of hydrolyzed milk formula as most children with milk allergy–induced skin symptoms will respond to the change of formula. Nonresponders may require amino acid–based formula.
- In older children: elimination of one to two suspected foods is appropriate for 2 wk or longer and then reintroducing the foods to determine if symptoms recur.

ACUTE GENERAL Rx

- Antihistamines (both H_1 and H_2 antihistamines), albuterol if wheezing, epinephrine and glucocorticoids in patients with anaphylaxis.
- Patients with documented IgE-mediated reactions should receive and be counseled on the use of epinephrine autoinjector.

NEW TREATMENTS FOR FOOD ALLERGIES

- Oral and sublingual immunotherapy may play a role in management of food allergies, but this is currently under investigation.
- Recombinant vaccines and other immuno-modulatory strategies are under development, although monoclonal anti-IgE antibody has shown benefit in adults with peanut allergy.

PEARLS & CONSIDERATIONS

- Eczema that develops in first 6 to 12 mo of life is usually the first manifestation of atopy.
- Egg allergy or sensitization is the strongest recognized predictor of respiratory allergies in children and asthma in adults.
- Neither the size of the wheal in skin prick testing nor the IgE antibody level correlates with severity. However, there may be increased positive predictive value with larger wheals and higher titers.
- Consultation with trained dietitian is critical to avoid potentially adverse nutritional consequences in children with multiple food allergies.
- Skin testing is the preferred method for identifying food-specific IgE. RAST is useful if there is chance of severe food reaction causing risk to the patient.
- American Academy of Pediatrics recommends avoiding influenza vaccine in patients with severe systemic allergic reactions to egg. Skin prick testing using influenza vaccine containing egg is recommended before vaccination in children with egg allergy and asthma. Skin prick testing not required before MMR vaccine in children with egg allergy.

COMMENTS

- Milk allergy usually resolves by age 5. Risk factors for persistence are early cutaneous manifestations following milk ingestion, development of other atopic conditions, and persistence of milk-specific high IgE titers. Soy milk is recommended for these children, keeping in mind that about 15% of these children can develop soy allergy.
- Egg allergy has been thought to resolve in 66% of children by 5 yr of age and in 75% of children by 7 yr of age. Trials have shown

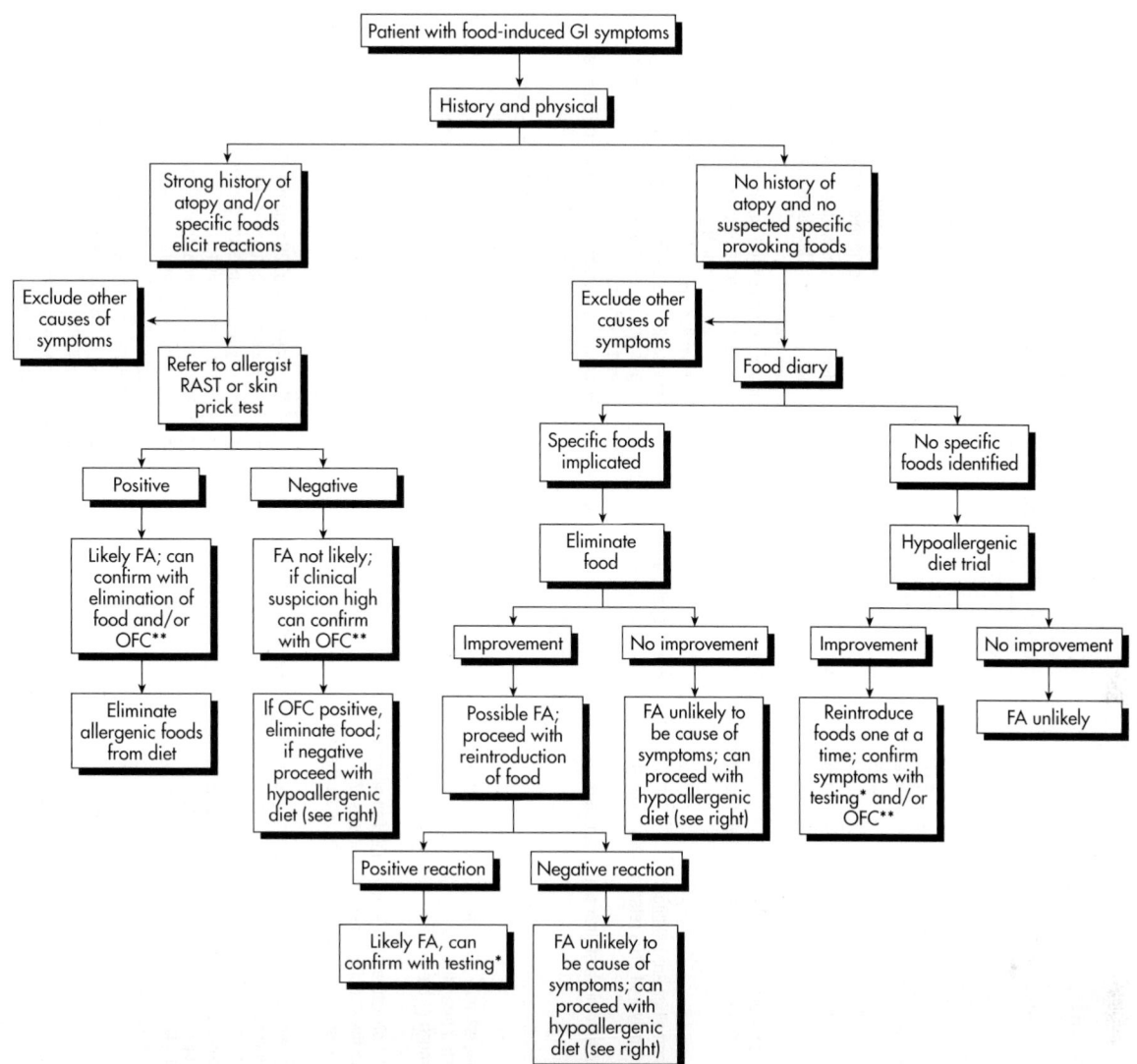

FIG. 1 Algorithm for the management of food allergy. *Testing indicates skin-prick testing, radioallergosorbent tests (RAST), IgG₄ assay, and/or patch testing. Note that clinical symptoms must be associated with the food(s) that test positive before the food(s) should be eliminated from the diet. **Oral food challenge (OFC) involves reintroducing the food and observing for signs/symptoms of food allergy (FA). Treatment of food allergy involves elimination of the causative food(s) from the diet. (From Stephen G, Gillham J: Fetal infection: a pragmatic approach to recognition and management. *Obstetr Gynaecol Rep Med* 22(10) 299–303, 2012.)

that oral immunotherapy can desensitize a high proportion of children with egg allergy and induce sustained unresponsiveness in a clinically significant subset.
- Wheat allergy found to resolve by 5 yr of age and soybean allergy by 2 yr of age.

PREVENTION
- There is conflicting evidence regarding the protective effect of breastfeeding on food allergies.
- There is no evidence to suggest that exclusive breastfeeding for 6 mo or more is superior to exclusive breastfeeding for 4 to 6 mo in terms of developing food allergies.
- In high-risk infants who are not exclusively breast fed, there is limited evidence to suggest that feeding with hydrolyzed formula compared to cow's milk formula reduces allergies.

- Currently, there is no evidence to support the use of prebiotics, probiotics, or synbiotics for the prevention of allergic diseases.
- No current evidence exists to support delaying the introduction of solid foods beyond 4 to 6 mo.
- The early introduction of peanuts significantly decreases the frequency of the development of peanut allergy among children at high risk for this allergy and modulated immune responses to peanuts.[2] Early peanut introduction (ages 4-11 months) lowers the risk of developing peanut allergy by 80% compared with peanut introduction after age 5 years.

PATIENT/FAMILY EDUCATION
Information can be found on American Academy of Allergy, Asthma and Immunology

[2]DuToit G et al.: Randomized trial of peanut consumption in infants at risk for peanut allergy, *N Engl J Med* 372:803-13, 2015

(www.aaaai.org), the Food Allergy and Anaphylaxis Network (www.foodallergy.org), and the Anaphylaxis Campaign (www.anaphylaxis.org.uk).

REFERRAL
Patients may be referred to an allergy/immunology specialist when the diagnosis is uncertain or if avoidance measures are not successful.

SUGGESTED READINGS
Available at www.expertconsult.com

RELATED CONTENT
Food Allergies (Patient Information)

AUTHOR: **LUKE BARRÉ, M.D.**

TABLE 1 Food Processing Conditions That May Affect Allergenic Activity

Processing Stage	Nature of Processing	Impact of Processing on Allergens	Food-Level Evidence	Clinical Implications
Post-harvest treatments	Modified atmosphere for storage of fruit and vegetables	Expression of Bet v 1 homologs is upregulated during storage; levels are higher in fruit stored for 4–5 mo compared with fresh fruit. Expression of LTP allergens is downregulated during storage; levels are higher in fresh fruit and decrease during storage.	Apple	Individuals with birch pollen–related fruit allergies may tolerate freshly picked but not stored fruit. LTP-allergic individuals may experience reverse symptoms, although severity of LTP allergies may completely preclude consumption of problem fruit.
Primary processing	Removal of outer layers by physical or chemical peeling	Loss of allergens such as LTPs located in the outer layers	Peach	Peeling fruits can make them safe for consumption by certain individuals with LTP allergies.
Secondary processing	Fruit purees and fresh juices	Labile Bet v 1 homologs are modified. Prolamin superfamily fruit LTPs retain a native-like structure.	Peach, apple	Individuals with Bet v 1–related fruit allergies usually can consume pureed fruit products. These foods can still trigger reactions in individuals with LTP fruit allergies.
	Preparation of pasteurized, UHT fruit juices and milk	Labile Bet v 1 homologs are modified. Prolamin superfamily fruit LTPs retain a native-like structure. Milk allergens retain much of their native structure.	Peach, apple, milk	Individuals with Bet v 1–related fruit allergies usually can consume UHT-processed fruit products. Processing is insufficient to make UHT juices safe for individuals with LTP fruit allergies. The allergenic potential of UHT milk resembles that of pasteurized and raw milk.
	Boiling	The prolamin superfamily LTPs and 2S albumin retain a native-like structure after boiling, although when seeds are boiled, much of the protein is lost into cooking water. Boiling alters the structure of milk, egg, and fish allergens. Boiling alters the structure of cupin allergens (7S and 11S seed storage proteins) and can render them insoluble.	Maize, wheat, peanut, lentil, fish, milk, egg	Boiling seeds (e.g., peanuts) and milk reduces their allergenicity but does not abolish it. For some foods (e.g., polenta), the extent of cooking affects the residual level of allergenic activity.
	Roasting and frying	Thermostable allergens, notably the prolamin superfamily 2S albumin allergens, retain their native structure and solubility after roasting and frying. Some cupin allergens (7S and 11S seed storage proteins) are altered by roasting and become insoluble. Maillard modification of allergens may take place under these processing conditions	Peanut	The major peanut 2S albumin allergens retain their allergenic activity, explaining why roasted peanuts possess significant allergenic activity. Allergenic activity of the 7S and 11S globulins is retained to some extent after roasting. Maillard modifications may further contribute to the allergenic activity of roasted peanuts.
	Preparation of powdered ingredients, such as celery spice, skimmed milk, and pasteurized egg white powder	Major allergens retain their three-dimensional structure and activity in dry-processed goods. Maillard modifications take place under these processing conditions when residual sugars are present (e.g., lactose in skimmed milk powder).	Celery spice, milk	Powdered food ingredients have allergenic activity similar to unprocessed foods and can promote trigger reactions when included in recipes or through cross-contact in other foods (e.g., residual milk powder in foods otherwise free from milk).

Deamidation	Gluten	Acidic conditions are used to treat food ingredients (notably gluten) to improve their food functional properties through deamidation. Induces formation of novel IgE epitopes through glutamine deamidation, which results in individuals reacting to foods prepared with deamidated gluten ingredients who can otherwise safely consume wheat flour–containing foods.
Hydrolyzed food ingredients	Milk, egg, gluten	Enzymatic (usually microbial proteases) and chemical treatments are used to hydrolyze protein ingredients to change their functional properties. Ingredients may originate from soy, milk (e.g., caseinates, whey protein), gluten, and other sources. Hydrolysis reduces IgE reactivity but does not abolish it completely, which may in part result from the presence of residual intact protein. Evidence is largely limited to in vitro IgE binding studies and animal models with little direct, in vivo evidence for allergic humans.
Oil refining	Soybean, peanut	Proteins are removed during the refining process, and residual protein levels in highly refined oils are very low. In the EU, highly refined soybean oils are considered safe for consumption by individuals with soy allergies. Highly refined peanut oils do not appear to cause adverse reactions in peanut-allergic individuals, but these oils do not have an EU labeling derogation.
Complex foods		
Fining agents added to alcoholic beverages	Beer, wine, and spirits	Certain beverages contain residual levels of fining agents based on isinglass, fish gelatin, milk casein, egg albumin, or lysozyme. Fining agents and their residues in beverages usually are highly modified compared with the raw, unprocessed foods. Individuals with allergies to fish triggered by collagen or egg can react to alcoholic beverages when they are used as fining agents, although this depends on the nature of the individual's allergy and whether fining agents are used in conjunction with other agents, such as bentonite. Reactions to fining agents are rare, and many individuals with egg, milk, or fish allergy can safely consume these beverages.
Fermented foods	Milk, soybean	Lactic acid fermentations can cause proteins to unfold and precipitate or form gelled networks due to the reduced pH. Fermentative organisms secrete proteases that can hydrolyze proteins. Although fermented milk and yogurt may retain some allergenic activity, other highly modified foods, such as soy sauce, may have substantially reduced allergenic activity and may not present a hazard to certain allergic patients.
Baked foods	Milk	Food ingredients may be included that are raw or have already been processed (e.g., skimmed milk powder, pasteurized egg white). Complex interactions between different food ingredients coupled with further cooking modify allergens and result in their becoming part of the insoluble food matrix, but data are limited because of the poor solubility of allergens in physiologic buffers. Evidence from oral food challenge studies indicates that baking reduces the allergenic activity of milk, and foods with baked milk may be given to children whose infantile cow's milk allergy is beginning to resolve.

EU, European Union; *LTP,* lipid transfer protein; *UHT,* ultrahigh temperature.
From Adkinson NF et al: *Middleton's allergy principles and practice,* ed 8, Philadelphia, 2014, Saunders.

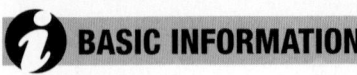

BASIC INFORMATION

DEFINITION

Food poisoning is an illness caused by ingestion of food contaminated by bacteria and/or bacterial toxins. Table 1 describes pathogenic mechanisms in bacterial foodborne disease.

SYNONYMS

Enterotoxin-poisoning
Epidemic vomiting disease

ICD-10CM CODES
A05.9 Bacterial foodborne intoxication, unspecified

EPIDEMIOLOGY & DEMOGRAPHICS

INCIDENCE (IN U.S.):

- CDC estimates that each year one in six Americans will experience a foodborne illness.
- CDC reported 13,405 foodborne disease outbreaks from 1998 to 2008 in the United States.
- Majority of identifiable causes are bacterial, although more than 250 known diseases can be transmitted through food.

PEAK INCIDENCE: Varies with specific organism.

- Summer: *Staphylococcus aureus, Salmonella, Shigella* spp.
- Summer and fall: *Clostridium botulinum, Vibrio parahaemolyticus.*
- Spring and fall: *Campylobacter jejuni.*
- Winter: *Clostridium perfringens, Yersinia enterocolitica.*

PREDOMINANT AGE: Varies with specific agent.

NEONATAL INFECTION: Rare but severe with *Shigella* and *Salmonella* spp.

PHYSICAL FINDINGS & CLINICAL PRESENTATION

- Any combination of GI symptoms and fever. Orthostatic pulse and blood pressure changes should be noted.
- Specific organisms suspected on the basis of the incubation period and predominant symptoms (Table E2), although a great deal of overlap exists.
  1. Short incubation period (1 to 6 hr): involve the ingestion of preformed toxin; noninvasive.
     a. *S. aureus:* nausea, profuse vomiting, and abdominal cramps common; diarrhea possible, but fever uncommon; usually resolves within 24 hr; foods implicated in outbreaks include meats, mayonnaise, and cream pastries.
     b. *B. cereus:* two forms, a short incubation (emetic) form (characterized by vomiting and abdominal cramps in virtually all patients, diarrhea in one third of patients, fever uncommon) and a long incubation (diarrheal) form; illness usually mild, resolves within 12 hr; unrefrigerated rice most often implicated as vehicle. Other sources include gravy, meats, stews, vanilla, and sauces.
  2. Moderate incubation period (8 to 16 hr): involves the in vivo production of toxin; noninvasive.
     a. *C. perfringens:* severe crampy abdominal pain and watery diarrhea common; fever and vomiting unlikely; symptoms usually resolving within 24 hr; outbreaks invariably related to cooked meat or poultry that is allowed to cool without refrigeration; most cases in the fall and winter months. *C. perfringens* is the third most common cause of foodborne illness in the United States.
     b. *B. cereus:* diarrheal (or long incubation) form most commonly beginning with diarrhea, abdominal cramps, and occasionally vomiting; fever uncommon; usually resolves within 24 hr; the responsible food is usually fried rice.
  3. Long incubation period (>16 hr): some toxin-mediated, some invasive.
- Toxin-producing organisms include:
  1. *C. botulinum:* should be considered when a diarrheal illness coincides with or precedes paralysis; severity of illness related to the quantity of toxin ingested; characteristic cranial nerve palsies progressing to a descending paralysis; fever usually absent; usually associated with home-canned foods.
  2. Enterotoxigenic *E. coli* (ETEC): most common cause of travelers' diarrhea; after 1- to 2-day incubation period, abdominal cramps and copious diarrhea occur; vomiting and fever uncommon; usually resolves after 3 to 4 days; vehicle usually unbottled water or contaminated salad or ice.
  3. Enterohemorrhagic *E. coli* (EHEC): can cause severe abdominal cramps and watery diarrhea, which may eventually become bloody; bacteria (strain O157:H7) are noninvasive; no fever; illness may be complicated by hemolytic-uremic syndrome; associated with contaminated beef (especially hamburger), unpasteurized milk or juice.
  4. *V. cholerae:* varies from a mild, self-limited illness to life-threatening cholera; diarrhea, nausea, and vomiting, abdominal cramps, and muscle cramps; no fever; severe cases may progress to shock and death within hours of onset; survivors usually have resolution of symptoms in 1 wk; U.S. cases are either imported or result from ingestion of imported food.
- Invasive organisms include:
  (1) *Salmonella:* associated most often with nontyphoidal strains; incubation period generally 12 to 48 hr; nausea, vomiting, diarrhea, and abdominal cramps typical; fever possible; outbreaks of gastroenteritis related to contaminated poultry, meat, and dairy products.
  (2) *Shigella:* asymptomatic infection possible, but some with fever and watery diarrhea that may progress to bloody diarrhea and dysentery; with mild illness, usually self-limited, resolves in a few days; with severe illness, may develop complications; transmission usually from person to person but can occur via contaminated food or water.
  (3) *C. jejuni:* the most common foodborne bacterial pathogen; incubation period is about 1 day, then a prodrome of fever, headache, and myalgias; intestinal phase marked by diarrhea associated with fever, malaise, and abdominal pain; diarrhea mild to profuse and bloody; usually resolves in about 7 days, but relapse is possible; associated with undercooked meats and poultry, unpasteurized dairy products, and drinking from freshwater streams.
  (4) *Y. enterocolitica* and *Y. pseudotuberculosis:* infrequent causes of enteritis in the United States; children affected more often than adults; fever, diarrhea, and abdominal pain lasting 1 to 3 wk; some with mesenteric adenitis that mimics acute appendicitis; contaminated food or water is usually responsible.
  (5) *V. parahaemolyticus:* In the United States, most outbreaks in coastal states or on cruise ships during the summer months; incubation period usually >1 day, followed by explosive watery diarrhea in

---

TABLE 1 Pathogenic Mechanisms in Bacterial Foodborne Disease

Preformed Toxin	Toxin Production in Vivo	Tissue Invasion	Toxin Production and/or Tissue Invasion
Staphylococcus aureus	*Clostridium perfringens*	*Campylobacter jejuni*	*Vibrio parahaemolyticus*
Bacillus cereus (short incubation)	*B. cereus* (long incubation)	*Salmonella*	*Yersinia enterocolitica*
Clostridium botulinum	*C. botulinum* (infant botulism)	*Shigella*	
	Enterotoxigenic *Escherichia coli*	Invasive *E. coli*	
	Vibrio cholerae 01 or 0139		
	V. cholerae non-01		
	Shiga toxin–producing *E. coli*		

From Mandell GL et al: *Principles and practice of infectious diseases*, ed 6, Philadelphia, 2005, Churchill Livingstone.

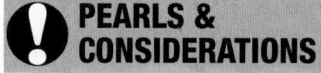

the majority of cases; nausea, vomiting, abdominal cramps, and headache also common; fever less common; usually resolves by 1 wk; related to ingestion of seafood.

(6) Enteroinvasive *E. coli* (EIEC): a rare cause of disease in the United States; high incidence of fever and bloody diarrhea; may resemble bacillary dysentery.

(7) *V. vulnificus:* may cause serious, often fatal illness in persons with chronic liver disease; GI symptoms usually absent, but fever, chills, hypotension, and hemorrhagic skin lesions possible; patients with liver disease or at increased risk of developing liver disease should avoid eating raw oysters.

ETIOLOGY

Classically categorized as either inflammatory (invasive) or noninflammatory:

- Noninflammatory: *B. cereus, S. aureus, C. botulinum, C. perfringens, V. cholerae,* enterotoxigenic *E. coli* (ETEC), and enterohemorrhagic *E. coli* (EHEC); toxin-producing organisms that are noninvasive; fecal leukocytes are not seen.
- Inflammatory: *Campylobacter,* enteroinvasive *E. coli* (EIEC), *Salmonella, Shigella, V. parahaemolyticus,* and *Yersinia;* cause disease by invasion of intestinal tissue; fecal leukocytes are seen.

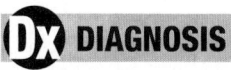 **DIAGNOSIS**

DIFFERENTIAL DIAGNOSIS

Gastroenteritis caused by viruses (Norwalk, Noro, or rotavirus), parasites *(Amoeba histolytica, Giardia lamblia),* or toxins (ciguatoxins, mushrooms, heavy metals).

LABORATORY TESTS

- Watchful waiting is often the most appropriate option and ancillary testing is usually not necessary.
- In severe or persistent cases stool test for fecal leukocytes may help narrow the differential diagnosis:
  1. Send stool for culture and for ova and parasites.
  2. Send stool for *C. difficile* toxin in patients with current or recent antibiotic use.
  3. Note: Some pathogens are not identified on routine stool culture; laboratory should be advised if *Yersinia, C. botulinum, Vibrio,* or enterohemorrhagic *E. coli* (O157:H7) are suspected.

4. Finding *B. cereus, C. perfringens,* or *E. coli* in stool is of little value, because these may be part of the normal bowel flora.
5. Stool cultures are positive in less than 40% of cases.
6. Newer techniques such as polymerase chain reaction (PCR) testing provide a more rapid and reliable determination of specific pathogens.
- If botulism suspected, send food, serum, and stool for toxin assay.
- Blood cultures should be considered for all febrile patients.
- Consider toxic megacolon (identified on plain abdominal sonography).
- Consider sigmoidoscopy to obtain tissue and histology in hospitalized patients with bloody diarrhea.
- Consider lactoferrin measurement if an inflammatory etiology is suspected.

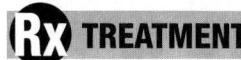 **TREATMENT**

NONPHARMACOLOGIC THERAPY

Adequate rehydration is the mainstay of therapy.

ACUTE GENERAL Rx

- Most cases of acute infectious diarrhea are viral and antibiotics are not indicated.
- Gastroenteritis caused by the following bacterial organisms requires no antimicrobial treatment: *B. cereus, S. aureus, C. perfringens, V. parahaemolyticus, Yersinia,* and enterohemorrhagic and enteroinvasive *E. coli.*
- The usual cause of traveler's diarrhea is enterotoxigenic *E. coli.* Although usually a self-limited illness, antibiotics can shorten the course in patients with fever or dysentery.
  1. Azithromycin 1000 mg in a single oral dose or
  2. SMX/TMP one DS tab bid for 3 days or
  3. Ciprofloxacin 500 mg PO bid for 3 days.
- The mainstay of therapy for cholera is fluid replacement. Antibiotics should be given to decrease shedding and duration of illness.
  1. Doxycycline 300 mg in a single dose or 100 mg PO bid for 3 days.
  2. SMX/TMP one DS tab bid for 3 days.
- Treatment is not indicated for *Salmonella* gastroenteritis. Patients who are at high risk of developing bacteremia may be treated for 48 to 72 hr (see "Salmonellosis").
- Although shigellosis tends to be a self-limited illness, antibiotics shorten the course of illness and may limit transmission of the illness (see "Shigellosis").

- Those with moderate or severe *Campylobacter* diarrhea may benefit from treatment.
  1. Azithromycin 500 mg qd for 3 days or
  2. Erythromycin 500 mg PO qid for 5 days or
  3. Ciprofloxacin 500 mg PO bid for 5 days.
- *V. vulnificus* sepsis should be treated with:
  1. Doxycycline 100 mg IV bid for 2 wk.
  2. Ceftazidime 2 g IV q8h for 2 wk.
- For suspected botulism, antitoxin should be administered early (see "Botulism").

CHRONIC Rx

Patients with *Salmonella* infections may become carriers and may require treatment (see "Salmonellosis").

DISPOSITION

- Most infections are self-limited and do not require therapy.
- In immunocompromised host or patient with underlying disease, serious complications are possible.
- Postinfectious syndromes are important with some infections:
  1. Reiter's syndrome: *Salmonella, Shigella, Campylobacter, Yersinia* spp.; more common in genetically susceptible host (HLA-B27+).
  2. Guillain-Barré syndrome: *Campylobacter* spp.

REFERRAL

If more than a mild illness.

PEARLS & CONSIDERATIONS

COMMENTS

- Grossly underreported and undiagnosed.
- All cases to be reported to the local health department.
- Table E3 summarizes control and prevention measures of foodborne diseases.

SUGGESTED READINGS

Available at www.expertconsult.com

RELATED CONTENT

Bacterial Food Poisoning (Patient Information)
Salmonellosis (Related Key Topic)

AUTHOR: **GLENN G. FORT, M.D., M.P.H.**

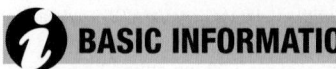

DEFINITION

Frostbite represents tissue injury (or death) from freezing and vasoconstriction induced by severe environmental cold exposure.

SYNONYMS

Cold-induced tissue injury.

ICD-10CM CODES
T35.0 Superficial frostbite involving multiple body regions
T34 Frostbite with tissue necrosis
T345 Frostbite with tissue necrosis of wrist and hand
T34.8 Frostbite with tissue necrosis of ankle and foot
T34.9 Frostbite with tissue necrosis of other and unspecified sites
T35.4 Superficial frostbite involving multiple body regions
T33.9 Superficial frostbite of unspecified sites, initial encounter

EPIDEMIOLOGY & DEMOGRAPHICS

- Environmental factors include windchill factor, temperature, duration of exposure, altitude, and degree of wetness. Hands and feet account for 90% of injuries; nose, cheeks, ears, and male genitalia are also more susceptible.
- Host factors include psychiatric illness and neuroleptic and sedative drugs (especially alcohol, which, in addition to impairing judgment, inhibit shivering and cause cutaneous vasodilation). Other risk factors include immobility, previous frostbite, malnutrition, tobacco use, peripheral neuropathy, peripheral vascular disease, diabetes, exhaustion, and constricting clothing and footwear.

  Patients at the extremes of age are at greatest risk, but frostbite is more common in adults ages 30 to 49 yr, and African Americans may be more susceptible than whites.

PHYSICAL FINDINGS & CLINICAL PRESENTATION

- Frostbite may be classified into four degrees of injury severity or, more practically, into *superficial* (corresponding to first and second degree) and *deep* (corresponding to third and fourth degree) groups. In both cases, the degree of frostbite can only be accurately determined after rewarming as initially most frostbite injuries appear similar.
- *Superficial* frostbite involves the skin and subcutaneous tissue. The frozen part is waxy, white (or mottled), and firm but soft and resilient below the surface when gently depressed. After rewarming, there is an initial hyperemia that may be followed by swelling and formation of superficial blisters with clear or milky fluid within 6 to 24 hr (Fig. 1). There is no ultimate tissue loss.

- *Deep* frostbite extends into the dermis and may involve muscles, nerves, tendons, or bones. The skin may be hard or wooden, without tissue resilience. Nonblanching cyanosis, hemorrhagic blisters, tissue necrosis (Fig. 2), and gangrene may develop. Affected tissue has a poor prognosis and debridement or amputation is generally required.
- Patients initially feel numbness, prickling, and itching. More severe injury can produce paresthesias and stiffness, with burning or throbbing pain upon thawing.

PATHOPHYSIOLOGY

Two phases of tissue injury:
1. The actual freezing of the tissues, during which cellular damage is caused by the formation of extracellular ice crystals, which cause osmotic shifts, cellular dehydration, cell membrane lysis, and cell death.
2. The reperfusion injury, during which the thawing of damaged endothelial cells releases a cascade of inflammatory mediators (e.g., prostaglandin F, thromboxane A2, bradykinins, histamine), resulting in capillary compression, vascular stasis, progressive ischemic injury, and thrombus formation. These conditions ultimately lead to the destruction of the microcirculation and to cell death.

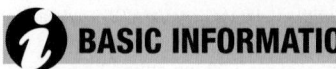 **DIAGNOSIS**

DIFFERENTIAL DIAGNOSIS

- Frostnip: a superficial nonfreezing cold injury associated with intense vasoconstriction and characterized by frost forming on the surface of the skin. Transient numbness, tingling, and pallor resolve quickly with warming
- Pernio (chilblains): self-limited, cold-induced vasculitis associated with purple plaques or nodules, often affecting dorsum of hands and feet; seen with prolonged cold exposure to above-freezing temperatures
- Cold immersion (trench foot): caused by ischemic injury resulting from sustained, severe vasoconstriction in appendages exposed to wet cold at temperatures above freezing

WORKUP

- Laboratory workup is not indicated unless the patient has systemic hypothermia.

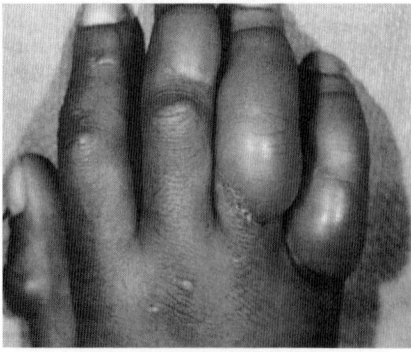

FIG. 1 Large, clear frostbite blisters on the right hand. (From Rosen P [ed]: *Emergency medicine*, ed 4, St Louis, 1998, Mosby.)

- Early presentation (<24 hr from thawing): If there is deep frostbite with potential significant morbidity, angiography should be done emergently in anticipation of potential thrombolysis treatment.
- Late presentation (>24 hr from thawing): Noninvasive imaging with MRA or multiphase bone scintigraphy (ideally with SPECT/CT) can be used to predict the likely levels of tissue viability for future reconstruction after amputation.

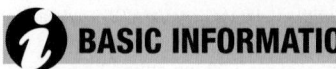 **TREATMENT (3 PHASES)**

1. FIELD MANAGEMENT

- Prioritize treatment of hypothermia (core body temperature <35° C) with systemic and adjunctive rewarming measures if available (e.g., warmed, humidified oxygen, heated IV saline [45° C], and warming blankets) before thawing frostbitten extremities.
  - Shelter patient out of wind and give warm fluids.
- Remove constricting or wet clothing and jewelry from affected digits.
  - Place cold extremity in a companion's axilla or groin for 10 minutes, then replace dry gloves/boots.
- Insulate, splint, and elevate affected areas if practical to do so.
  - Never rub or massage the affected area. Avoid dry heat (e.g., fires and heaters).
- Avoid thawing if there is any risk of refreezing and if possible avoid ambulation on thawed lower extremities (unless only distal toes affected).
- Administer pain medication and topical aloe if available.
- Box 1 describes the Alaska State Guidelines for prehospital treatment of frostbite.

2. REWARMING

- Rapid rewarming (with warm water) limits the freezing injury and yields better outcomes than slow rewarming (e.g., moving to a warmer location).
- Rapid rewarming is achieved by immersing the affected area in a circulating warm water bath with or without a mild

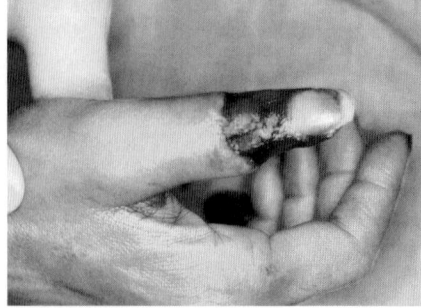

FIG. 2 Third- and fourth-degree frostbite with tissue death. Note demarcation beyond the interphalangeal joint. (From Cameron, JL, Cameron AM: *Current surgical therapy*, ed 10, Philadelphia, 2011, Saunders.)

F

BOX 1 Alaska State Guidelines for Prehospital Treatment of Frostbite

First Responder/Emergency Medical Technician—I, II, III/Paramedic/Small Bush Clinic
Evaluation and Treatment

A Anticipate, assess, and treat the patient for hypothermia, if present.
B Assess the frostbitten area carefully because the loss of sensation may cause the patient to be unaware of soft tissue injuries in that area.
C Obtain a complete set of vital signs and the patient's temperature.
D Remove jewelry and clothing, if present, from the affected area.
E Obtain a patient history, including the date of the patient's last tetanus immunization.
F If there is frostbite distal to a fracture, attempt to align the limb unless there is resistance. Splint the fracture in a manner that does not compromise distal circulation.
G Determine whether rewarming the frostbitten tissue can be accomplished in a medical facility. If it can, transport the patient while protecting the tissue from further injury from cold or impacts.
H If the decision is made to rewarm frostbitten tissue in the field, you should prepare a warm water bath in a container large enough to accommodate the frostbitten tissues without them touching the sides or bottom of the container. The temperature of the water bath should be 99° to 102° F (37° to 39° C).
  ○ Generally, patients with frostbite do not require opiates for pain relief; they occasionally need non-opiate pain medication or anxiolytics. If possible, consult a physician regarding the administration of oral analgesics, such as acetaminophen, ibuprofen or aspirin. Aspirin or ibuprofen may help improve outcomes by blocking the arachidonic acid pathway.
  ○ Immersion injury or frostbite with other associated injuries may produce significant edema and high pain levels. These patients may need opiate pain medications for initial treatment. In this case, advanced life support personnel should administer morphine or other analgesics in accordance with physician-signed standing orders or online medical control.
I A source of additional warm water must be available.
J Water should be maintained at approximately at 99° to 102° F (37° to 39° C) and gently circulated around the frostbitten tissue until the distal tip of the frostbitten part becomes flushed.
K Pain after rewarming usually indicates that viable tissue has been successfully rewarmed.
L After rewarming, let the frostbitten tissues dry in the warm air. Do **not** towel dry.
M After thawing, tissues that were deeply frostbitten may develop blisters or appear cyanotic. Blisters should not be broken and must be protected from injury.
N Pad between affected digits and bandage affected tissues loosely with a soft, sterile dressing. Avoid putting undue pressure on the affected parts.
O Rewarmed extremities should be kept at a level above the heart, if possible.
P Protect the rewarmed area from refreezing and other trauma during transport. A frame around the frostbitten area should be constructed to prevent blankets from pressing directly on the injured area.
Q Do not allow an individual who has frostbitten feet to walk except when the life of the patient or rescuer is in danger. Once frostbitten feet are rewarmed, the patient becomes nonambulatory.

antibacterial agent (e.g., chlorhexidine or povidone-iodine) maintained at 37° to 39° C for at least 15 to 30 min up to 1 hour, until all tissues are thoroughly rewarmed and pliable with a red-purple color. Active motion during rewarming is advisable; massage is not.
- Administer analgesics during rewarming (ibuprofen and possibly narcotics).

3. POST-THAW TREATMENT

- Tetanus prophylaxis and topical antibiotics if potentially contaminated skin wound.
- Consider systemic antibiotics for patients with significant trauma or signs of infection.
- Debride broken clear vesicles and avoid disrupting intact blisters (especially hemorrhagic ones) unless they interfere with mobility.
- Topical aloe vera (a potent anti-prostaglandin agent) q6h and ibuprofen (a thromboxane inhibitor) 400 to 600 mg bid to tid (or daily aspirin) can be given until wounds are healed or surgery occurs.

- Thrombolytic therapy: If <24 hr from thawing in a patient with severe frostbite and poor prognostic indicators (e.g., cool skin after rewarming, numb, dusky or blue digits, hemorrhagic blisters). First, angiography (or possibly MRA) is performed to assess for arterial compromise followed by intraarterial (or intravenous) tPA if perfusion defects are demonstrated and there is no contraindication to thrombolysis. The use of early thrombolytic therapy appears to limit reperfusion injury considerably and to reduce subsequent digit amputation significantly. The tissue salvage rate correlates with elapsed time to treatment from time of rewarming.
- Heparin is recommended in addition to tPA to prevent recurrent local thrombosis.
- Vasodilator therapy: Various vasodilators (NTG, pentoxifylline, phenoxybenzamine, nifedipine, reserpine, and buflomedil) have been tried, with the best evidence favoring prostacyclin (or iloprost, which is available in Europe). If iloprost is available, at least one study shows superior efficacy to tPA, and it

is easier to administer, has a better safety profile, has fewer contraindications, and can be managed on a general ward with benefit seen up to 48 hours after frostbite thawing.
- Daily dressing changes with dry, sterile, noncompressive, and nonadherent dressings. Splint and elevate hands and feet to reduce edema and separate digits with cotton gauze. Avoid any abrasion to limit risk of infection.
- Whirlpool hydrotherapy: 1 to 2 times per day for 30 minutes with warm water (37°-39° C), +/- an antiseptic solution if severe edema is present, until there is a clear demarcation of necrotic tissues or evidence of tissue healing.
- Gentle, progressive physical therapy after edema resolves.
- Keep site warm, and avoid all vasoconstrictors, including nicotine.
- Dextran, warfarin, sympathectomy, and hyperbaric oxygen are of potential but unproven benefit. In patients treated with thrombolysis, an oral anticoagulant or antiplatelet therapy upon discharge is included in some treatment protocols.

DISPOSITION

A majority of patients have long-term residual symptoms, including cold hypersensitivity, neuropathic pain, sensory deficits, hyperhidrosis, secondary Raynaud's disease, localized osteoporosis, edema, hair or nail deformities, and (rarely) arthritis. Treatment with tricyclics, gabapentin, calcium channel blockers, and careful protection from further cold exposure may be helpful.

REFERRAL

- Hospitalize for hypothermia or deep frostbite; a burn unit is best.
- Surgical decisions regarding amputation should be deferred until demarcation of viable tissue is clear (6 to 12 weeks), unless refractory pain, sepsis, or gangrene occurs.

SUGGESTED READINGS
Available at www.expertconsult.com

RELATED CONTENT
Frostbite (Patient Information)

AUTHOR: **MICHAEL P. JOHNSON, M.D.**

BASIC INFORMATION

DEFINITION

Biliary pain caused by gallbladder dysmotility in the absence of gallstones, sludge, or microlithiasis. It is a diagnosis of exclusion with no evidence of structural disease seen with normal hepatobiliary and pancreatic laboratory and diagnostic imaging modalities.

SYNONYM(S)

Biliary dyskinesia
Gallbladder dyskinesia
Gallbladder spasm
Acalculous biliary disease
Chronic acalculous cholecystitis
Chronic acalculous
Gallbladder dysfunction
Cystic duct syndrome

ICD-10CM CODES
K82.9 Disease of gallbladder, unspecified

EPIDEMIOLOGY & DEMOGRAPHICS

INCIDENCE: Biliary dyspepsia has an incidence rate of 1% to 6%.
PREVALENCE: 10% to 45% of total population report dyspepsia.
PREDOMINANT SEX AND AGE: There is a 3:1 female-to-male predominance.

RISK FACTORS

There is no consistent relationship to meals or fatty meal intake.

PHYSICAL FINDINGS & CLINICAL PRESENTATION

These patients present with typical biliary pain that fulfills the Rome III criteria:
- Patients present with sporadic epigastric or right upper quadrant pain lasting for 30 minutes but less than 6 hours.
- Episodes are recurrent and occur in sporadic intervals (but not daily).
- The pain is not relieved by bowel movements.
- The pain is not relieved by postural movements.
- The pain is not relieved by antacids.
- The pain builds up to a steady level.
- The pain is severe enough it impedes daily activities and may even require an emergency department visit.

DIAGNOSIS

DIFFERENTIAL DIAGNOSIS

- Primary gallbladder disorders: gallstones, cholecystitis
- Pancreatobiliary disorders: cholelithiasis, choledocholithiasis, pancreatitis, pancreatic neoplasm
- Gastrointestinal disorders: gastroesophageal reflux disorder, peptic ulcer disease, inflammatory bowel disease, irritable bowel syndrome, gastric or esophageal neoplasm
- Metabolic disorders: obesity, diabetes mellitus
- Cholecystokinin deficiency: celiac disease

WORKUP

- This is a diagnosis of exclusion in a patient with biliary pain. Patients will have normal blood test results and hepatobiliary and pancreatic enzymes, including AST, ALT, ALP, bilirubin, amylase, and lipase. Imaging, including abdominal ultrasound, is essentially normal without evidence of gallstone or gallbladder sludge pathology.

LABORATORY TESTS

- Laboratory tests, including serum AST, ALT, ALP, bilirubin, GGT, amylase, and lipase, are within normal limits.

IMAGING STUDIES

- To exclude gallstone pathology, a transabdominal ultrasound is initial choice for imaging. Transabdominal ultrasound is capable of detecting gallstones up to 3 to 5 mm in size. Patients should fast for at least 8 hours before ultrasound to optimize visualization of the gallbladder.
- If gallstones or gallbladder is not found on ultrasound but still suspected, endoscopic ultrasound (EUS) may be used to detect microlithiasis or gallstones smaller than 3 mm.
- Assessing gallbladder emptying through cholecystokinin (CCK)–stimulated cholescintigraphy is essential in the diagnosis. CCK-stimulated cholescintigraphy allows for the calculation of gallbladder ejection fraction (GBEF). Normal GBEF is >38%. Patients with a GBEF <35% to 40% with reproducible pain on CCK stimulation is suggestive of functional gallbladder disorder.

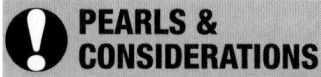 TREATMENT

In patients with appropriate evaluation for suspected functional gallbladder disorder, surgical management with cholecystectomy is the preferred method of treatment.

NONPHARMACOLOGIC THERAPY

- Surgical cholecystectomy is the preferred method of treatment. Studies have shown symptomatic relief in up to 98% of patients postcholecystectomy.

ACUTE GENERAL Rx

- Initial management should include adequate analgesic control for abdominal pain.
- Opioid analgesics should be avoided because they may exacerbate symptoms involved in a hypofunctioning gallbladder.

COMPLEMENTARY AND ALTERNATIVE MEDICINE

- Turmeric (Curcuma) has been known to alleviate biliary dyspepsia by stimulating gallbladder contractions.

DISPOSITION

- Patients with functional gallbladder disorder are often misdiagnosed. These patients require appropriate evaluation to exclude other hepatobiliary etiology. After they are properly diagnosed, these patients have a favorable prognosis after surgical intervention.

REFERRAL

- Gastroenterology consultation may be considered to rule out microlithiasis via EUS.
- Surgical consultation should be considered for possible cholecystectomy in select patients.

PEARLS & CONSIDERATIONS

COMMENTS

Functional gallbladder disorder is a diagnosis of exclusion. It is essential that other hepatobiliary pathology be ruled out first. CCK-stimulation scintigraphy showing a reduced GBEF without any other pathology is suggestive of this disorder. Patients fare well with surgical intervention.

SUGGESTED READINGS
Available at www.expertconsult.com

RELATED TOPICS

Cholangiocarcinoma (Related Key Topic)
Cholecystitis (Related Key Topic)
Choledocholithiasis (Related Key Topic)
Cholelithiasis (Related Key Topic)

AUTHOR: **GEORGE CHOLANKERIL, M.D.**

BASIC INFORMATION

DEFINITION

Galactorrhea can be defined as inappropriate lactation (in the absence of pregnancy or postpartum state) as a result of nonphysiologic augmentation of prolactin release.

ICD-10CM CODES
N64.3 Galactorrhea not associated with childbirth
O92.6 Galactorrhea

PHYSICAL FINDINGS & CLINICAL PRESENTATION

- Milky discharge from nipples (Fig. 1), usually occurring bilaterally.
- Evidence of chest wall irritation from ill-fitting clothing, herpes zoster, or atopic dermatitis may be present.
- Visual field defects (bitemporal hemianopsia) may be present with prolactinomas, particularly if large, such as macroadenomas.
- Headaches may also occur in cases of large pituitary adenomas.
- Evidence of acromegaly, Cushing's disease, or hypothyroidism when galactorrhea is caused by these disorders.

ETIOLOGY

- Medications (phenothiazines, metoclopramide, selective serotonin reuptake inhibitors, anxiolytics, buspirone, risperidone, atenolol, valproic acid, conjugated estrogen and medroxyprogesterone, methyldopa, verapamil, H_2 receptor blockers [cimetidine], octreotide, danazol, tricyclic antidepressants, isoniazid, amphetamine, reserpine, opiates, sumatriptan, rimantadine, oral contraceptive formulations), cocaine; after infancy, galactorrhea is often medication induced
- Breast stimulation (prolonged suckling), sexual intercourse
- Pituitary tumors (prolactinomas, craniopharyngiomas)
- Chest wall irritation from ill-fitting clothing, herpes zoster, atopic dermatitis, burns

- Hypothyroidism (diminished feedback inhibition increases thyroid-releasing hormone [TRH], which increases prolactin)
- Increased stress, major trauma
- Chronic renal failure (decreased prolactin clearance)
- Cushing's disease
- Herbs (e.g., fennel, red clover, anise, red raspberry, marshmallow)
- Cannabis
- Spinal cord surgery or injury, or tumors
- Severe gastroesophageal reflux disease, esophagitis (stimulation of thoracic nerves by the cervical and thoracic ganglia)
- Breast surgery
- Idiopathic
- Neonatal ("witch's milk" produced by 2%-5% of neonates because of precipitous drop in maternal estrogen and progesterone postdelivery)
- Lymphomas, Hodgkin's disease, bronchogenic carcinoma, renal adenocarcinomas
- Sarcoidosis and other infiltrative disorders
- Tuberculosis affecting pituitary gland
- Pituitary stalk resection
- Multiple sclerosis
- Empty sella syndrome
- Acromegaly
- Exercise

DIAGNOSIS

DIFFERENTIAL DIAGNOSIS

- Intraductal papilloma
- Breast cancer
- Paget's disease of breast
- Breast abscess

WORKUP

- Complete history focusing on menstrual irregularity, infertility, previous pregnancies, duration of galactorrhea, medications, visual complaints, fatigue. Age of onset is also significant (e.g., prolactinoma most common between ages 20 and 35 yr; neonatal galactorrhea is usually secondary to transplacental transfer of maternal estrogen).

- Physical examination: hirsutism, acne, obesity, visual field defects, goiter.
- Breast examination for presence of nodules, evaluation of discharge (milky versus serosanguineous versus purulent).
- Laboratory testing and imaging studies (see "Laboratory Tests")

LABORATORY TESTS

- Prolactin level (elevated, often >200 ng/ml in prolactinoma but may occur at any prolactin level)
- Human chorionic gonadotropin level (positive in pregnancy)
- Thyroid-stimulating hormone (TSH) (elevated in hypothyroidism)
- Blood urea nitrogen, creatinine (elevated in renal failure), glucose (elevated in Cushing's syndrome)
- Urinalysis (hematuria in renal cell carcinoma)
- Microscopic examination of nipple discharge (scant cellular material, numerous fat globules, can be seen without specific staining)

IMAGING STUDIES

- MRI of brain if prolactin level is elevated, amenorrhea is present, or visual field defects are detected on physical examination.
- High-resolution CT of brain with special coronal cuts through the pituitary region may be helpful in patients with contraindications to MRI; however, it may miss small lesions.

TREATMENT

- Discontinuation of potential offending agents.
- Avoidance of excessive breast stimulation.
- Galactorrhea resulting from prolactinoma can be managed medically or with careful surveillance depending on size and growth of tumor, associated symptoms, and prolactin level. Surgical treatment of prolactinomas is usually reserved for medication failures. Please refer to the topic "Prolactinoma" in Section I for additional information.
- No treatment is necessary for normoprolactinemic patients with idiopathic nonbothersome galactorrhea.
- Normoprolactinemic patients with bothersome galactorrhea may respond to low dose dopamine agonist (e.g., cabergoline 0.25 mg twice weekly).

REFERRAL

Endocrine and surgical consultation if prolactinoma is detected

SUGGESTED READING
Available at www.expertconsult.com

RELATED CONTENT
Galactorrhea (Patient Information)
Pituitary Adenoma (Related Key Topic)
Prolactinoma (Related Key Topic)

AUTHOR: **FRED F. FERRI, M.D.**

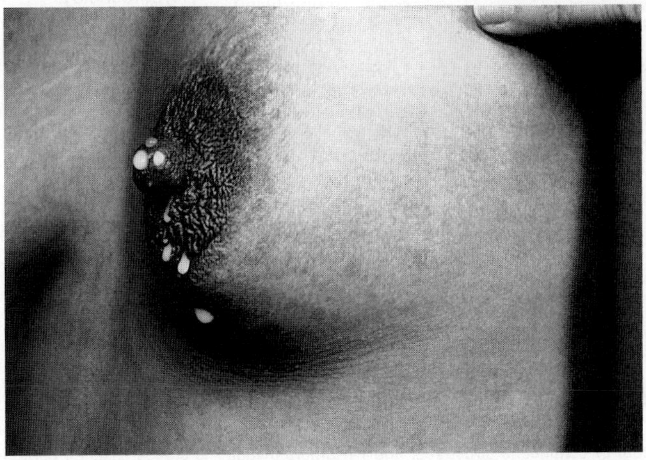

FIG. 1 Galactorrhea. Milk production in a nonpregnant woman resulting from a prolactinoma. (From Haines DE: *Fundamental neuroscience for basic and clinical applications,* ed 3, Philadelphia, 2006, Churchill Livingstone.)

BASIC INFORMATION

DEFINITION

Gastric cancer is an adenocarcinoma arising from the stomach. Cancers in the cardia arising within 5 cm of the gastroesophageal junction (GEJ) are typically classified as GEJ cancers. It is subdivided into intestinal and diffuse histology. The diffuse form of gastric cancer is more common in women and young patients, whereas the intestinal type is predominantly related to environmental factors. The classification of gastric adenocarcinoma by depth of invasion is illustrated in Fig. 1.

SYNONYMS

Gastric adenocarcinoma
Stomach cancer
Linitis plastica

ICD-10CM CODESs
C16   Malignant neoplasm of stomach
C16.0 Malignant neoplasm of cardia of stomach
C16.1 Malignant neoplasm of stomach
C16.2 Malignant neoplasm of body of stomach
C16.3 Malignant neoplasm of pyloric antrum
C16.5 Malignant neoplasm of lesser curvature of stomach, unspecified
C16.6 Malignant neoplasm of greater curvature of stomach, unspecified
C16.8 Malignant neoplasm of overlapping sites of stomach

EPIDEMIOLOGY & DEMOGRAPHICS

- Gastric cancer is the fourth commonest cancer in the world, with an annual incidence of approximately 950,000 cases annually; of these, 70% occur in developing countries. The highest incidence is in Asia (80 cases per 100,000 persons in Japan) and the lowest in North America. Annual estimated deaths due to gastric cancer are 723,000 worldwide.
- In the U.S., an estimated 26,370 new cases and 10,730 deaths were expected for 2016.
- The incidence of distal stomach tumors has greatly declined, whereas that of proximal tumors of the cardia and fundus is on the rise.
- Gastric cancer occurs most commonly in male patients >65 yr (70% of patients are >50 yr).
- Incidence of gastric cancer has been declining over the past 30 yr.
- Male/female ratio is 3:2.
- Familial diffuse gastric cancer is a disease with autosomal-dominant inheritance in which gastric cancer develops at a young age. Germ-line truncating mutations in the E-cadherin gene *(CDH1)* are found in these families. It is associated with an 80% lifetime risk of gastric cancer. Increased risk of gastric cancer is also seen with Lynch syndrome, FAP, Peutz-Jeghers, juvenile polyposis syndrome, and hyperplastic gastric polyps.

PHYSICAL FINDINGS & CLINICAL PRESENTATION

- Medical history may reveal complaints of postprandial fullness with significant weight loss (70%-80%), nausea/emesis (20%-40%), dysphagia (20%), and dyspepsia, usually unrelieved by antacids; epigastric discomfort, usually lessened by fasting and exacerbated by food intake, is also common.
- Epigastric or abdominal mass (30%-50%), epigastric pain.
- Anemia from tumor bleeding and hemoccult-positive stools.
- Hard, nodular liver: generally indicates metastatic disease to the liver.
- Ascites, lymphadenopathy, or pleural effusions: may indicate metastases.

ETIOLOGY

RISK FACTORS:

- Chronic *Helicobacter pylori* gastritis. Gastric cancer develops in persons infected with *H. pylori* but not in uninfected persons. Those with histologic findings of severe gastric atrophy, corpus-predominant gastritis, or intestinal metaplasia are at increased risk. Persons with *H. pylori* infection and duodenal ulcer are not at risk, whereas those with gastric ulcers, nonulcer dyspepsia, and gastric hyperplastic polyps are. Eradication of *H. pylori* reduces gastric cancer risk.
- Tobacco abuse, alcohol consumption.
- Food additives (nitrosamines), smoked foods, occupational exposure to heavy metals, rubber, asbestos.
- Chronic atrophic gastritis with intestinal metaplasia, hypertrophic gastritis, and pernicious anemia.
- Box 1 summarizes risk factors for gastric adenocarcinoma.

DIAGNOSIS

DIFFERENTIAL DIAGNOSIS

- Gastric lymphoma (5% of gastric malignancies).
- Hypertrophic gastritis.
- Peptic ulcer.
- Reflux esophagitis.

WORKUP

Upper endoscopy (Fig. E2) with biopsy will confirm diagnosis. Endoscopic ultrasonography in combination with CT scanning and operative lymph node dissection can be used in staging of the tumor. Table 1 and Fig. 1 describe staging systems for gastric carcinoma.

LABORATORY TESTS

- Microcytic anemia.
- Hemoccult-positive stools.
- Hypoalbuminemia.
- Abnormal liver enzymes in patients with metastasis to the liver.
- Up to 20% of gastric cancers overexpress the HER2 growth factor receptor.

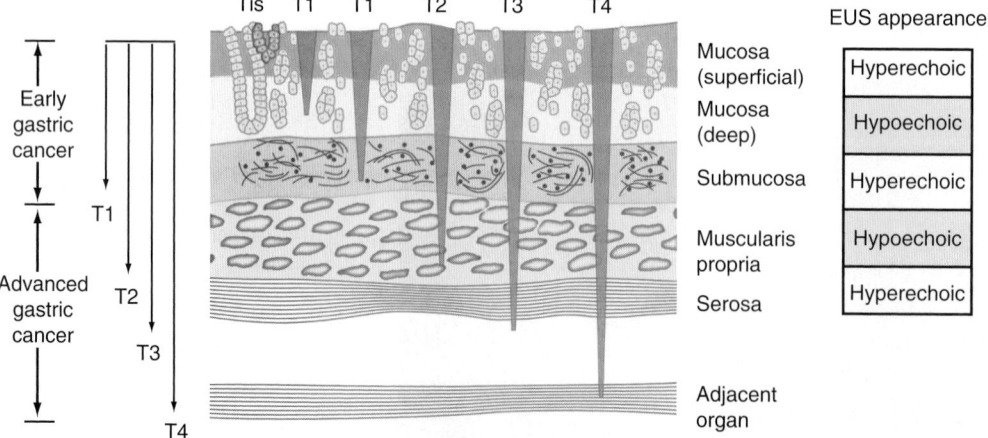

FIG. 1 Classification of gastric adenocarcinoma by depth of invasion (T classification). In the TNM classification, T denotes depth of invasion: Tis designates carcinoma in situ; T1 tumors are confined to the mucosa (T1a) and submucosa (T1b); T2 tumors invade the muscularis propria but not the serosa; T3 tumors penetrate the subserosal connective tissue without involving the visceral peritoneum or contiguous structures; and T4 tumors invade the serosa (visceral peritoneum) and may involve adjacent organs and tissues. In early gastric cancer, the disease is confined to the mucosa and submucosa (T1), regardless of nodal involvement. (From Feldman M et al [eds]: *Sleisenger and Fordtran's gastrointestinal and liver disease*, ed 10, Philadelphia, 2016, Saunders.)

G

BOX 1 Risk Factors for Gastric Adenocarcinoma

Definite
Hp infection
Chronic atrophic gastritis
Intestinal metaplasia
Dysplasia*
Adenomatous gastric polyps*
Cigarette smoking
History of gastric surgery (esp. Billroth II)*
Genetic factors:
   Family history of gastric cancer (first-degree relative)*
   Familial adenomatous polyposis (with fundic gland polyps)*
   Hereditary nonpolyposis colorectal cancer*
   Peutz-Jeghers syndrome*
   Juvenile polyposis*

Probable
High salt intake
Obesity (adenocarcinoma of the cardia only)
Snuff tobacco use
History of gastric ulcer
Pernicious anemia*
Regular aspirin or other NSAID use (protective)

Possible
Statin use (protective)
Heavy alcohol use
Low socioeconomic status
Ménétrier's disease
High intake of fresh fruits and vegetables (protective)
High ascorbate intake (protective)

Questionable
Hyperplastic and fundic gland polyps
Diet high in nitrates
High green tea consumption (protective)

* Surveillance for cancer is recommended in patients with this risk factor. From Feldman M et al [eds]: *Sleisenger and Fordtran's gastrointestinal and liver disease*, ed 10, Philadelphia, 2016, Saunders.

- Mutation-specific predictive genetic testing by polymerase chain reaction amplification followed by restriction: enzyme digestion and DNA sequencing for truncating mutations in *CDH1* is recommended in families of patients with familial diffuse cancer because gastric cancer develops in three of every four carriers of a mutant *CDH1* gene. Genetic abnormalities in gastric adenocarcinoma are summarized in Table E2.

IMAGING STUDIES
Chest and abdomen CT scan (Fig. E3) to evaluate for metastases.

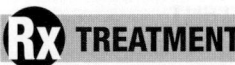 **TREATMENT**

ACUTE GENERAL Rx
- Gastrectomy with regional lymphadenectomy is performed in patients who have early cancers with curative potential (<30% of patients at time of diagnosis).

TABLE 1 Staging Systems for Gastric Carcinoma*

Modified Astler-Coller	TNM	Characteristics
A	TisN0	Nodes negative; lesion limited to mucosa
B1	T1–2N0	Nodes negative; extension of lesion beyond mucosa but still within gastric wall
B2	T3N0	Nodes negative; extension beyond the entire wall (including serosa if present) without adherence to or invasion of surrounding organs or structures
B3	T4N0	Nodes negative; beyond wall with adherence to or invasion of surrounding organs or structures
C1	Tis–2N1–3	Nodes positive; lesion limited to wall
C2	T3N1–3	Nodes positive; extension of lesion through the entire wall (including serosa)
C3	T4N1–3	Nodes positive; beyond wall with adherence to or invasion of surrounding organs or structures

*Comparison of TNM system with a modification of the Astler-Coller rectal system by Gunderson and Sosin.
From Abeloff MD: *Clinical oncology,* ed 3, Philadelphia, 2004, Elsevier.

- In patients with operable gastric cancer, a perioperative regimen of epirubicin, cisplatin, and infused fluorouracil decreases tumor size and stage and significantly improves progression-free and overall survival.
- Postoperative adjuvant chemoradiotherapy using 5-fluorouracil (5-FU) and leucovorin improves overall survival and is now the standard of care for stage II-III patients able to tolerate such treatment. When surgical cure is not possible, palliative resection may prolong duration and quality of life, especially in the case of major bleeding.
- Chemotherapy with triplet or doublet regimens is associated with improvement in overall survival. The addition of trastuzumab to cisplatin plus 5-FU or capecitabine may prolong survival in gastric cancer patients expressing HER2-2/neu oncogene (20%-25% of patients). Patients progressing after first-line chemotherapy can derive a survival benefit with the use of chemotherapy in combination with antivascular endothelial growth factor receptor-2 antibody ramucirumab.

DISPOSITION
- Median survival rate of metastatic or recurrent gastric carcinoma is 10-15 months overall.
- The 5-yr survival for early gastric cancers is >35%.

⚠ PEARLS & CONSIDERATIONS

COMMENTS
- Gastrectomy patients will need vitamin B_{12} replacement. They are also at risk for dumping syndrome and should be advised to ingest frequent, small meals.
- Prophylactic gastrectomy should be considered in young, asymptomatic carriers of germ-line truncating *CDH1* mutations who belong to families with highly penetrant heredity diffuse gastric cancer.

- Gastric cancer screening for average-risk patients is not recommended in the U.S.

SUGGESTED READINGS
Available at www.expertconsult.com

RELATED CONTENT
Stomach Cancer (Patient Information)

AUTHOR: **RITESH RATHORE, M.D.**

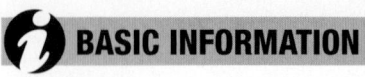

BASIC INFORMATION

DEFINITION

Histologically, *gastritis* refers to inflammation in the stomach. Endoscopically, gastritis refers to a number of abnormal features such as erythema, erosions, and subepithelial hemorrhages. Gastritis can also be subdivided into erosive, nonerosive, and specific types of gastritis with distinctive features both endoscopically and histologically.

SYNONYMS

Erosive gastritis
Hemorrhagic gastritis
Helicobacter pylori gastritis

ICD-10CM CODES
K29.00	Acute gastritis without bleeding
K29.01	Acute gastritis with bleeding
K29.20	Alcoholic gastritis without bleeding
K29.21	Alcoholic gastritis with bleeding
K29.30	Chronic superficial gastritis without bleeding
K29.31	Chronic superficial gastritis with bleeding
K29.40	Chronic atrophic gastritis without bleeding
K29.41	Chronic atrophic gastritis with bleeding
K29.50	Unspecified chronic gastritis without bleeding
K29.51	Unspecified chronic gastritis with bleeding
K29.60	Other gastritis without bleeding
K29.61	Other gastritis with bleeding
K29.70	Gastritis, unspecified, without bleeding
K29.71	Gastritis, unspecified, with bleeding
K52.81	Eosinophilic gastritis or gastroenteritis

EPIDEMIOLOGY & DEMOGRAPHICS

- Erosive and hemorrhagic gastritis is most commonly seen in patients taking nonsteroidal antiinflammatory drugs (NSAIDs), alcoholics, and critically ill patients (usually on ventilator support).
- *H. pylori* infection with gastritis is believed to be present in 30% to 50% of the population; however, the majority are asymptomatic.
- The prevalence of *H. pylori* infection increases with age from <10% in whites <40 yr to >50% in patients >50 yr.

PHYSICAL FINDINGS & CLINICAL PRESENTATION

- Patients with gastritis generally present with nonspecific clinical signs and symptoms (e.g., epigastric pain, abdominal tenderness, bloating, anorexia, nausea [with or without vomiting]). Symptoms may be aggravated by eating.
- Epigastric tenderness in acute alcoholic gastritis (may be absent in chronic gastritis).
- Foul-smelling breath.
- Hematemesis ("coffee grounds" emesis).

ETIOLOGY

- Alcohol, NSAIDs, stress (critically ill patients usually on mechanical respiration), hepatic or renal failure, multiorgan failure.
- *H. pylori* infection.
- Bile reflux, pancreatic enzyme reflux.
- Gastric mucosal atrophy, portal hypertension gastropathy.
- Irradiation.

DIAGNOSIS

DIFFERENTIAL DIAGNOSIS

- Peptic ulcer disease.
- Gastroesophageal reflux disease.
- Nonulcer dyspepsia.
- Gastric lymphoma or carcinoma.
- Pancreatitis.
- Gastroparesis.

WORKUP

Diagnostic workup includes a comprehensive history and endoscopy with biopsy.

LABORATORY TESTS

- *H. pylori* testing by urea breath test, stool antigen test (*H. pylori* stool antigen), endoscopic biopsy, or specific antibody test is recommended.
  1. The urea breath test documents active infection (sensitivity and specificity >90%). It uses a flat breath card read by a small analyzer.
  2. The stool antigen test is an enzymatic immunoassay (ELISA) that identifies *H. pylori* antigen in a stool specimen with a polyclonal anti–*H. pylori* antibody. It is as accurate as the urea breath test for diagnosis of active infection and follow-up evaluation of patients treated for *H. pylori*. A negative result on the stool antigen test 8 wk after completion of therapy identifies patients in whom eradication of *H. pylori* was successful.
  3. Histologic evaluation of endoscopic biopsy samples is considered by many the gold standard for accurate diagnosis of *H. pylori* infection. However, detection of *H. pylori* depends on the site and number of biopsy samples, the method of staining, and experience of the pathologist.
  4. Serologic testing for antibodies to *H. pylori* is easy and inexpensive; however, the presence of antibodies demonstrates previous but not necessarily current infection. Antibodies to *H. pylori* can remain elevated for months to years after infection has cleared; therefore antibody levels must be interpreted in light of patient's symptoms and other test results (e.g., peptic ulcer disease [PUD] seen on upper gastrointestinal series).
- Vitamin B_{12} level in patients with atrophic gastritis.
- Hematocrit (low if significant bleeding has occurred).

TREATMENT

NONPHARMACOLOGIC THERAPY

- Avoidance of mucosal irritants such as alcohol and NSAIDs
- Lifestyle modifications with avoidance of tobacco and foods that trigger symptoms

ACUTE GENERAL Rx

Eradication of *H. pylori,* when present, can be accomplished with various regimens:
1. Proton pump inhibitor (PPI) (omeprazole 20 mg, lansoprazole 30 mg, pantoprazole 40 mg, rabeprazole 20 mg) bid *plus* amoxicillin 1000 mg bid *plus* metronidazole 500 mg BID for 10 to 14 days.
2. PPI bid *plus* clarithromycin 500 mg bid *and* metronidazole 500 mg bid for 10 to 14 days. This regimen is useful in those with penicillin allergy.
3. Ranitidine 150 mg bid plus bismuth subsalicylate 525 mg qid plus metronidazole 250 mg qid plus doxycycline 100 mg bid.
4. A combination of levofloxacin 250 mg bid, amoxicillin 1000 mg bid, and a PPI bid for 10 to 14 days can be used as salvage therapy after unsuccessful attempts to eradicate *H. pylori* using other regimens.
   - A 10-day sequential therapy has been reported to be superior to standard triple therapy for eradication of *H. pylori*. It consists of 5 days of treatment with a PPI and one antibiotic (usually amoxicillin) followed by 5-day treatment with the PPI and two other antibiotics (usually clarithromycin and metronidazole).
   - Prophylaxis and treatment of stress gastritis with sucralfate suspension 1 g orally q4-6h, H_2-receptor antagonists, or PPIs in patients on ventilator support.

CHRONIC Rx

- Omeprazole, H2RB, or sucralfate in patients receiving long-term NSAIDs.
- Avoidance of alcohol, tobacco, and prolonged NSAID or corticosteroid use.

DISPOSITION

- Undetectable stool antigen tested at least 4 wk after therapy accurately confirms cure of *H. pylori* infection in initially seropositive healthy subjects with reasonable sensitivity. PPI therapy should be stopped at least 2 weeks prior to testing.
- Surveillance gastroscopy in patients with atrophic gastritis (increased risk of gastric cancer).

RELATED CONTENT

Gastritis (Patient Information)
Helicobacter pylori Infection (Related Key Topic)
Peptic Ulcer Disease (Related Key Topic)

AUTHOR: **FRED F. FERRI, M.D.**

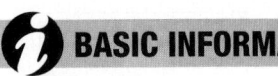 BASIC INFORMATION

DEFINITION

- Gastroenteritis is a broad term used for various gastrointestinal pathologic states. The main manifestation is diarrhea, defined as daily stool of at least 200 g, often accompanied by nausea, vomiting, malaise, anorexia, fever, abdominal pain, and dehydration. Gastroenteritis is usually self-limited, but if it is not managed properly, it can lead to a prolonged course.
- Gastroenteritis is a common cause of morbidity/mortality around the world. In the developing world, it is a leading cause of death.

ICD-10CM CODES
K52.9 Non-infective gastroenteritis and colitis
558.3 Allergic gastroenteritis and colitis
K52.1 Infectious gastroenteritis and colitis
K52.0 Gastroenteritis and colitis due to radiation

EPIDEMIOLOGY & DEMOGRAPHICS

- Frequency is difficult to determine. Gastroenteritis is underreported in adults.
- Statistics on sporadic cases of adult viral gastroenteritis are not known. Norovirus is the leading cause of medically attended acute gastroenteritis in U.S. children and is associated with nearly 1 million health care visits annually.
- It is estimated that there are 1.5 billion cases a year worldwide.
- It is the leading cause of death in many developing countries. Children under the age of 5 yr are most vulnerable.
- Traveler's diarrhea affects 20% to 50% of residents of industrialized countries who travel to developing countries.

SEX: Higher mortality seen in women.
Females have a higher incidence of *Campylobacter* infections.

AGE:
- May occur at any age
- High morbidity and mortality in the very young (younger than 5 yr), the elderly (people aged 65 or older), and the immunosuppressed.

PHYSICAL FINDINGS & CLINICAL PRESENTATION

- A well-taken history is important. The onset, duration, and frequency of diarrhea should be noted. The aim of the physical examination is to assess the patient's degree of hydration. This helps to identify the cause of diarrhea and identify patients at risk of complications.
Viral gastroenteritis has a short prodome with vomiting, mild fever, nonbloody and watery diarrhea, usually for 1 to 4 days.
- Bacterial gastroenteritis presents with high fever, bloody diarrhea, severe abdominal pain, and at least 6 stools in a 24-hour period.
- Patients usually present with:
  1. Diarrhea: usually more than 6 stools a day indicates bacterial cause of gastroenteritis
  2. Vomiting

  3. Abdominal pain
  4. Mucus and/or blood in stool: indicating bacterial or parasitic infection
  5. Fever
  6. Dehydration: this is the main cause of morbidity and mortality. Check for lethargy, dry mucous membrane, poor skin turgor, sunken eyes as signs of dehydration.
  7. Malnutrition: this occurs when diarrhea is chronic. There is reduced muscle and fat mass.
  8. Abdominal pain: this is a very common symptom in gastroenteritis.
  9. Borborygmi: there is significantly increased peristaltic activity, which may cause audible or palpable bowel activity.
  10. Perianal erythema: secondary to constantly wet area. Wet buttock and perianal area may result in redness and skin breakdown.

ETIOLOGY

- Bacterial gastroenteritis: The top three leading cause of bacterial diarrhea worldwide are *Salmonella*, *Shigella*, and *Campylobacter* spp.
  1. *Salmonella*
  2. *Shigella*
  3. *Campylobacter*
  4. *Aeromonas species*
  5. *Yersinia*
  6. Enterohemorrhagic *Escherichia coli*
  7. *E. coli*
  8. *Clostridium perfringens*
- Viral gastroenteritis (in adults)
  1. The caliciviruses such as *Norovirus* genogroup I (e.g., Norwalk), *Norovirus* genogroup II (e.g., South Hampton), *Sapovirus* (e.g., Sapporo).
  2. Non-group A *Rotavirus*
  3. *Astrovirus*
  4. Adenovirus

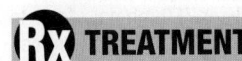 DIAGNOSIS

DIFFERENTIAL DIAGNOSIS

- Amebiasis
- Appendicitis
- Celiac disease
- Inflammatory bowel disease
- Colon cancer
- Bowel obstruction
- Botulism
- Hemolytic uremic syndrome
- Food poisoning
- Intraabdominal abscess
- Crohn's disease

WORKUP

- In most cases laboratory tests are not indicated.
- Further workup is indicated in patients who:
  1. Have persistent diarrhea
  2. Are extremely dehydrated
  3. Appear seriously ill
  4. Have high fever
  5. Present with severe abdominal pain
  6. Have bloody diarrhea
  7. Have persistent nausea

LABORATORY TESTS

- Routine laboratory tests
  1. Tests such as CBC and BMP may not be indicated in making a diagnosis. However, electrolytes and BUN are indicated in patients with severe diarrhea or dehydration.
  2. CBC is indicated with severe diarrhea or toxicity. WBC is increased in *Salmonella* infection; eosinophilia is present in parasitic infections.
- Stool studies
  1. Presence of blood/leukocytes in stool may indicate inflammatory diarrhea.
  2. In *Salmonella* or *Shigella* infections there is an increased fecal leukocyte.
  3. Stool leukocytes are absent in viral diarrhea.
- Stool culture
  1. Are only useful when positive
  2. Usually not necessary in most cases of diarrhea
  3. Indications for stool cultures include: bloody stools; prolonged, untreated diarrhea; fever; leukocytes in stool; immunosuppressed patients; immunocompromised patients; and patients who have traveled to remote, exotic, or developing nations. It should also be considered in patients with concurrent or very recent use of antibiotics to rule out *Clostridium difficile* infection as a cause of the diarrhea.
- Examination for ova and parasites (O&P) is indicated in immunosuppressed patients, immunocompromised patients, and patients who have traveled to remote, exotic, or developing nations

IMAGING STUDIES

- In patients with suspected bowel obstruction, perforation, or toxic megacolon, abdominal series is warranted.
- Consider CT scan of the abdomen in older patients with severe abdominal pain.

Rx TREATMENT

GENERAL CONSIDERATIONS

- Most infectious diarrhea is self-limited. Medical care is mainly supportive. Fig. 1 describes an approach to the management of gastroenteritis.
- It is important to assess the degree of dehydration by checking BP, pulse, HR, skin turgor, mucous membrane, thirst, urine output, and mental status change.
- Oral rehydration therapy is very important in diarrhea treatment.
- Consider intravenous rehydration when oral rehydration fails. Watch out for potassium depletion.
- Early re-feeding decreases recovery time. Principles of treatment include:
- Rehydration: orally or intravenously, PRN
- Treatment of symptoms such as fever, abdominal pain, nausea, vomiting as needed
- Identify and treat complications

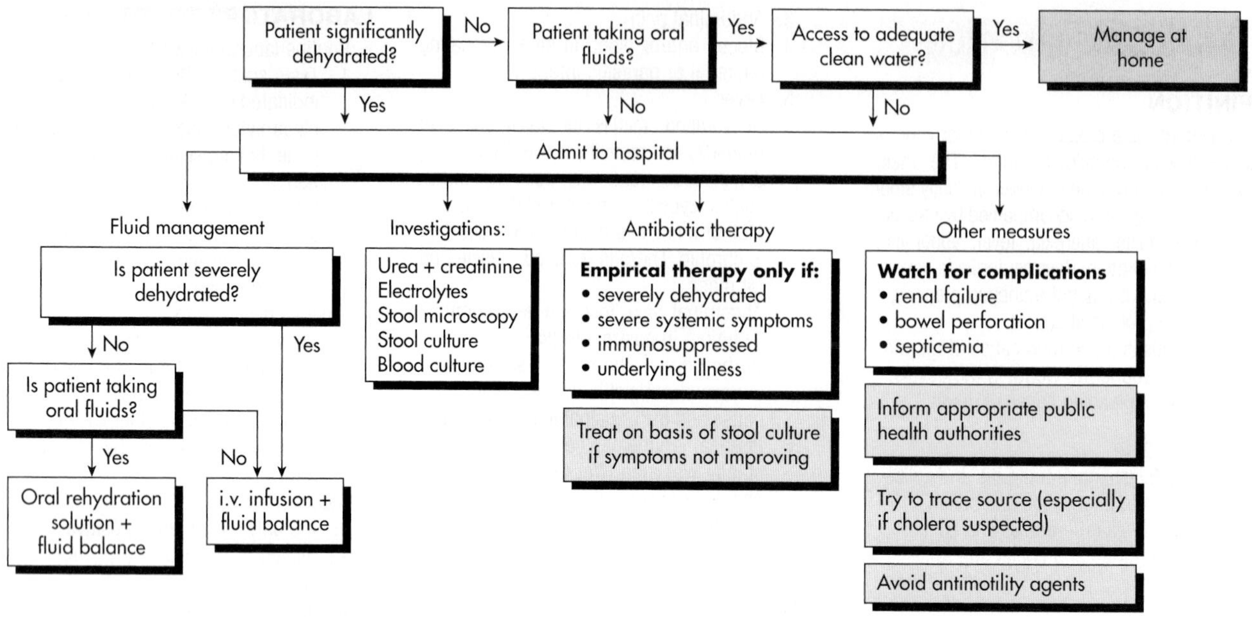

FIG. 1 Management of gastroenteritis. (From Currie G, Douglas G: *Flesh and bones of medicine*, St. Louis, 2011, Mosby, pp 8-9.)

REHYDRATION:
- Oral hydration products include Naturalyte, Rehydralyte.
- Intravenous solutions used include dextrose 5% in 0.5 isotonic NaCl with 50 mEq NaHCO$_3$ and 10-20 mEq KCl.
  1. Indications for IV hydration include intractable vomiting, severe dehydration, change in mental status or consciousness, and ileus.
  2. Oral hydration is not appropriate due to environmental conditions

TREATMENT OF SYMPTOMS:
- Infectious diarrhea sometimes requires empiric treatment with antibiotics. Food-borne toxigenic diarrhea usually does not.
- Traveler's diarrhea: patients without fever or dysentery may be treated with rifaximin 200 mg thrice daily for 3 days, or ciprofloxacin 500 mg twice daily or 750 mg daily for 1 to 3 days; patients with fever or dysentery can be treated with azithromycin 1000 mg in a single dose.
- *C. difficile* diarrhea and parasitic infestations with *Giardia* or *Entamoeba* are treated with metronidazole or vancomycin. For *C. difficile*, it is important to discontinue the causative antibiotic.
- Treat severe nausea and vomiting with antiemetics.
- Antidiarrheal agents may be useful for systemic relief in mild to moderate diarrhea.
- Loperamide (Imodium) or bismuth subsalicylate (Pepto-Bismol) may provide limited relief in traveler's or non-bloody diarrhea.

Dietary measures may include:
- Start with banana, rice, applesauce, toast diet (BRAT diet)
- As early as possible introduce lean meats and clear liquid

In recent years the use of probiotics (nonpathogenic live microorganism) has increased. They are known to provide beneficial effects on the host's health. Beneficial effects have been noted with *Lactobacillus casei GG* and *S. boulardii*.

REFERRAL

Referral to infectious disease or gastroenterologist specialist may be indicated in patients:
- With chronic diarrhea
- In whom a parasitic etiology is suspected
- With *C. difficile* resistant to treatment with metronidazole and vancomycin
- With HIV/AIDS
- Who relapse

⚠ PEARLS AND CONSIDERATIONS

PREVENTION
- Perform proper hand washing before and after eating and after each bowel movement to prevent spread to family members.
- Avoid (raw) shellfish served in certain unregulated places.
- Avoid raw or undercooked eggs and/or poultry.
- Wash all produce before consumption.

- For travelers to high-risk areas:
  1. Eat only cooked foods.
  2. Drink hot or carbonated beverages.
  3. Avoid water, raw peeled fruits/vegetables, green leafy vegetables, and street food sold by street vendors.
  4. Vaccines are available for *Salmonella typhi* and *Vibrio cholerae* (the latter provides about 50% protection for 3-6 months).

PATIENT EDUCATION
- Stress the importance of oral rehydration.
- Stress the need for early appropriate feeding.
- Relapse occurs due to dietary noncompliance.
- Travelers to developing areas should be educated on proper avoidance measures and treatment.
- Also stress the importance of good hygiene, hand washing, safe food preparation, and access to clean water as key in preventing gastroenteritis.

SUGGESTED READINGS
Available at www.expertconsult.com

RELATED CONTENT
Gastroenteritis (Patient Information)

AUTHOR: **DANIEL K. ASIEDU, M.D., PH.D.**

BASIC INFORMATION

DEFINITION

Gastroesophageal reflux disease (GERD) is a motility disorder characterized primarily by heartburn and caused by the reflux of gastric contents into the esophagus. A current definition is a condition that develops when the reflux of stomach contents causes at least two heartburn episodes per week and/or complications.

SYNONYMS

Peptic esophagitis
Reflux esophagitis
GERD

ICD-10CM CODES
K21.9 Gastroesophageal reflux disease
without esophagitis
R12   Heartburn

EPIDEMIOLOGY & DEMOGRAPHICS

- GERD is one of the most prevalent gastrointestinal disorders. It is the most common GI diagnosis recorded during visits to outpatient clinics. From 14% to 20% of adults are affected.
- Nearly 7% of persons in the United States have heartburn daily, 20% have it monthly, and 60% have it intermittently. Incidence in pregnant women exceeds 80%.
- Nearly 20% of adults use antacids or over-the-counter H_2 blockers at least once a week for relief of heartburn.

PHYSICAL FINDINGS & CLINICAL PRESENTATION

- Physical examination: generally unremarkable.

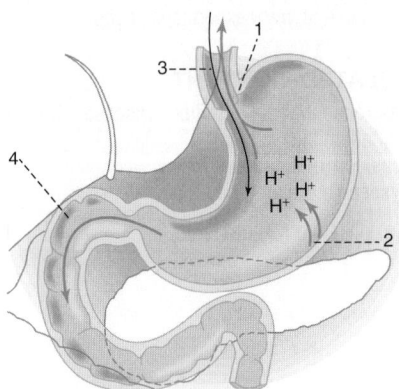

FIG. 1 Pathogenesis of gastroesophageal reflux disease: *(1)* impaired lower esophageal sphincter—low pressures or frequent transient lower esophageal sphincter relaxation; *(2)* hypersecretion of acid; *(3)* decreased acid clearance resulting from impaired peristalsis or abnormal saliva production; *(4)* delayed gastric emptying or duodenogastric reflux of bile salts and pancreatic enzymes. (From Andreoli TE et al: *Andreoli and Carpenter's Cecil essentials of medicine,* ed 8, Philadelphia, 2010, Saunders.)

- Clinical signs and symptoms: heartburn, dysphagia, sour taste, regurgitation of gastric contents into the mouth.
- Chronic cough and bronchospasm.
- Chest pain, laryngitis, early satiety, abdominal fullness, and bloating with belching.
- Dental erosions in children.

ETIOLOGY

- Incompetent lower esophageal sphincter (LES) (see Fig. 1).
- Medications that lower LES pressure (calcium channel blockers, alpha-adrenergic antagonists, nitrates, theophylline, anticholinergics, sedatives, prostaglandins).
- Foods that lower LES pressure (chocolate, yellow onions, peppermint).
- Tobacco abuse, alcohol, coffee.
- Pregnancy.
- Gastric acid hypersecretion.
- Hiatal hernia (controversial) present in >70% of patients with GERD; however, most patients with hiatal hernia are asymptomatic.
- Obesity is associated with a statistically significant increase in the risk for GERD symptoms, erosive esophagitis, and esophageal carcinoma.

DIAGNOSIS

DIFFERENTIAL DIAGNOSIS

- Peptic ulcer disease.
- Unstable angina.
- Esophagitis (from infections such as herpes, *Candida*), medication induced (doxycycline, potassium chloride).
- Esophageal spasm (nutcracker esophagus).
- Cancer of esophagus.

WORKUP

- Aimed at eliminating the conditions noted in the differential diagnosis and documenting the type and extent of tissue damage. Generally, when symptoms of GERD are typical and the patient responds to therapy, there is no need for further diagnostic tests to verify the diagnosis.
- Upper GI endoscopy is useful to document the type and extent of tissue damage in persistent GERD and to exclude potentially malignant conditions such as Barrett esophagus. The American College of Physicians recommends endoscopy in the setting of GERD in people with heartburn and alarm symptoms (dysphagia, bleeding, anemia, weight loss, and recurrent vomiting). It is also indicated in people with GERD symptoms that persist despite a therapeutic trial of 4 to 8 weeks of bid proton pump inhibitor (PPI) therapy in patients with severe erosive esophagus after a 2-month course of PPI therapy to assess healing and rule out Barrett esophagus.
- Fig. E2 describes an approach to patients with heartburn.

LABORATORY TESTS

- 24-hr esophageal pH monitoring and Bernstein test are sensitive diagnostic tests;

however, they are not practical and generally not done. They are useful in patients with atypical manifestations of GERD, such as chest pain or chronic cough.
- Esophageal manometry is indicated in patients with refractory reflux in whom surgical therapy is planned.
- *Helicobacter pylori* testing is not indicated in GERD.

IMAGING STUDIES

An upper GI series is useful in patients unwilling to have endoscopy or with medical contraindications to the procedure. It can identify ulcerations and strictures; however, it may miss mucosal abnormalities. Only one third of patients with GERD have radiographic signs of esophagitis on an upper GI series.

TREATMENT

NONPHARMACOLOGIC THERAPY

- Lifestyle modifications with avoidance of foods (e.g., citrus- and tomato-based products, onions, spicy foods, carbonated beverages, mint, chocolate, fried foods) and drugs that exacerbate reflux (e.g., caffeine, β-blockers, calcium channel blockers, α-adrenergic agonists, theophylline).
- Avoidance of tobacco and alcohol use.
- Elevation of head of bed (4 to 8 in) with blocks.
- Avoidance of lying down directly after late or large evening meals, consumption of smaller and more frequent meals.
- Weight reduction to BMI <25, decreased fat intake.
- Avoidance of clothing that is tight around the waist.

GENERAL Rx

- PPIs (esomeprazole 40 mg qd, omeprazole 20 mg qd, lansoprazole 30 mg qd, rabeprazole 20 mg qd, or pantoprazole 40 mg qd, or dexlansoprazole 30 mg) are generally safe, tolerated, and highly effective in most patients when used on a short-term basis (Table 1). Omeprazole and esomeprazole are inhibitors of CYP2C19 and can increase serum concentrations of phenytoin and diazepam. Concomitant use of clopidogrel should also be avoided with omeprazole and esomeprazole. Increased risk of pneumonia has been documented in hospitalized patients. Long-term use of PPIs has been associated with increased risk of osteoporosis. Use of PPIs in patients with cirrhosis increases risk of spontaneous bacterial peritonitis and hepatic encephalopathy.
- H_2 blockers (nizatidine 300 mg qhs, famotidine 40 mg qhs, ranitidine 300 mg qhs, or cimetidine 800 mg qhs) can be used but are generally much less effective than PPIs.
- Antacids (may be useful for relief of mild symptoms; however, they are generally ineffective in severe cases of reflux).
- Prokinetic agents (metoclopramide) are indicated only when PPIs are not fully effective. They can be used in combination therapy; however, side effects limit their use.

TABLE 1 Drug Therapy for Esophageal Disorders

Agent	Dose
Antacids: Liquid (to Buffer Acid and Increase LESP)	
For example, Mylanta II/Maalox TC (acid-neutralizing capacity, 25 mEq/5 mL)*	15 mL qid 1 hr after meals and at bedtime or as needed
Gaviscon (to Decrease Reflux via a Viscous Mechanical Barrier and Buffer Acid)	
Al(OH)$_3$, NaHCO$_3$, Mg trisilicate, alginic acid	2-4 tablets qid at bedtime or as needed
H$_2$-Receptor Antagonists (to Decrease Acid Secretion)	
Cimetidine	800 mg bid, 400 mg qid, ≈13 mL bid
Ranitidine	150 mg qid or 10 mL qid; maintenance dose, 150 mg bid, 10 mL bid
Famotidine	20-40 mg bid or 2.5-5 mL bid
Nizatidine	150 mg bid
Proton Pump Inhibitors (to Decrease Acid Secretion and Gastric Volume)†	
Omeprazole	20 mg/day; maintenance dose, 20 mg/day
Lansoprazole	30 mg/day; maintenance dose, 15 mg/day
Pantoprazole	40 mg/day; maintenance dose, 40 mg/day
Rabeprazole	20 mg/day; maintenance dose, 20 mg/day
Esomeprazole	20-40 mg/day; maintenance dose, 20 mg/day
Dexlansoprazole	30-60 mg/day; maintenance dose, 30 mg/day

LESP, Lower esophageal sphincter pressure.

*Patients with reflux are not generally hypersecretors of gastric acid, so the therapeutic doses of antacids are based on their capacity to buffer (normal) basal acid secretion rates of approximately 1 to 7 mEq/hr (mean, 2 mEq/hr) and peak meal-stimulated acid secretion rates of about 10 to 60 mEq/hr (mean, 30 mEq/hr).

†High-dose therapy is a twice-daily administration of the usual daily dose.

From Goldman L, Schafer AI: *Goldman's Cecil medicine,* ed 24, Philadelphia, 2012, Saunders.

- For refractory cases: surgery with Nissen fundoplication. Potential surgical candidates should have reflux esophagitis documented by esophagogastroduodenoscopy and normal esophageal motility as evaluated by manometry. Surgery generally consists of reduction of hiatal hernia when present and placement of a gastric wrap around the gastroesophageal (GE) junction (fundoplication). Although laparoscopic fundoplication is now widely used, long-term medical therapy is a better choice for most patients who are willing to remain on daily acid-reduction medication. In patients preferring surgical intervention, surgery should not be advised with the expectation that patients with GERD will no longer need to take antisecretory medications or that the procedure will prevent esophageal cancer among those with GERD and Barrett esophagus.
- Endoscopic radiofrequency heating of the GE junction (Stretta procedure) is a newer treatment modality for GERD patients unresponsive to traditional therapy. Its mechanism of action remains unclear. Endoscopy gastroplasty (EndoCinch procedure) is also aimed at treating GERD. Initial results appear encouraging; however, long-term studies are needed before recommending these procedures.

- Lifestyle modification must be followed for life because this is generally an irreversible condition.

DISPOSITION

- Recurrence of reflux is common if treatment is discontinued. Preliminary trials have shown that in patients with severe reflux esophagitis successfully treated with PPI therapy, stopping PPI medication was associated with T lymphocyte–predominant esophageal inflammation and basal cell and papillary hyperplasia without loss of surface cells. If replicated, these findings suggest that the pathogenesis of reflux esophagitis may be cytokine mediated rather than the result of chemical injury.[1]
- The majority of patients respond well to therapy. In patients with chronic GERD, long-term outcomes are similar between medical therapy with PPIs and anti-reflux surgery. Prolonged use of PPIs is associated with increased risk of fractures of hip, wrist, and spine; increased risk of diarrhea

[1]Dunbar KB, et al.: Association of acute gastroesophageal reflux disease with esophageal histologic changes. *JAMA* 315(19):2104–2112, 2016.

from *Clostridium difficile;* pneumonia; and possible iron deficiency from impaired iron absorption. PPIs also block the effects of clopidogrel by inhibiting cytochrome P450 2C19 isozyme. Therefore all PPIs (other than pantoprazole) should be avoided in patients using clopidogrel. H$_2$ blockers (e.g., ranitidine) can be used for patients with GERD taking clopidogrel.

- Postsurgical complications occur in nearly 20% of patients (dysphagia, gas, bloating, diarrhea, nausea). Long-term follow-up studies also reveal that within 3 to 5 yr, 52% of patients who had undergone antireflux surgery are taking antireflux medications again.

REFERRAL

- There is a strong and probably causal relation between symptomatic prolonged and untreated GERD, Barrett esophagus, and esophageal adenocarcinoma. GI referral for upper endoscopy is needed when there are concerns about associated peptic ulcer disease, Barrett esophagus, or esophageal cancer.
- Patients with Barrett esophagus should undergo surveillance endoscopy with mucosal biopsy every 2 yr or less because the risk of developing adenocarcinoma of esophagus is at least 30 times greater than that of the general population.
- Testing and treating for *Helicobacter pylori* in patients with GERD has not been shown to improve symptoms.
- All children with dental erosions should be evaluated for GERD.

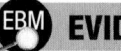 **EVIDENCE**

Available at www.expertconsult.com

SUGGESTED READINGS

Available at www.expertconsult.com

RELATED CONTENT

Gastroesophageal Reflux Disease (GERD) (Patient Information)
Achalasia (Related Key Topic)
Dysphagia (Related Key Topic)

AUTHOR: **FRED F. FERRI, M.D.**

BASIC INFORMATION

DEFINITION

- Glucose intolerance that occurs during pregnancy and resolves postpartum.
- In the U.S., a "two-step approach is commonly used and is currently endorsed by the American College of Obstetricians and Gynecologists (ACOG) and the National Institutes of Health (NIH). Women are initially screened with a 1-hr, nonfasting 50-g oral glucose tolerance test. If the result is abnormal, ≥130 mg/dl as defined by Carpenter and Coustan, a 3-hr, 100-g oral glucose tolerance test is performed. The diagnosis of gestational diabetes (GDM) is made if two or more of the following glucose values are met or exceeded:
  Fasting: 95 mg/dl
  1-hr: 180 mg/dl
  2-hr: 155 mg/dl
  3-hr: 140 mg/dl
- The International Association of Diabetes in Pregnancy Study Group has recommended a simplified "one-step" approach to screening and diagnosing GDM, which involves a 2-hr fasting 75-g oral glucose tolerance test. A diagnosis of GDM is made according to the following: plasma glucose ≥92 mg/dl when fasting, ≥180 mg/dl at 1 hr, or ≥153 mg/dl at 2 hr. Although this approach is endorsed by the American Diabetes Association, the NIH Consensus on GDM did not endorse these guidelines in 2013 because of increases in the prevalence of GDM, along with corresponding costs and interventions related to treatment, without clear evidence of improvement in obstetrical outcomes.
- Pregnant women with diabetes mellitus (DM) (gestational or preexisting) are classified according to White's classification (Table E1).

SYNONYMS

Gestational diabetes
Diet-controlled gestational diabetes (A1)
Medication-treated gestational diabetes (A2)

ICD-10CM CODES
O24.410 Gestational diabetes mellitus in pregnancy, diet controlled
O24.414 Gestational diabetes mellitus in pregnancy, insulin controlled
O24.419 Gestational diabetes mellitus in pregnancy, unspecified control
O99.810 Abnormal glucose complicating pregnancy

EPIDEMIOLOGY & DEMOGRAPHICS

INCIDENCE: Approximately 5% to 6% of pregnant women will be diagnosed with GDM using the two-step approach and 15% to 20% using the one-step approach.
PREDOMINANT SEX AND AGE: Women of childbearing age.
GENETICS: Higher rate in women with family history of GDM or type 2 diabetes; specific HLA alleles (DR3 or DR4) predispose to the development of DM type 2 after pregnancy.

RISK FACTORS

- Obesity.
- Family history of GDM or type 2 diabetes, particularly in first-degree relatives.
- Polycystic ovarian syndrome.
- Multiple gestation.
- Hypertensive disorder of pregnancy or chronic hypertension.
- Chronic systemic steroid use.
- Previous infant weighing >9 lb or history of shoulder dystocia.
- Unexplained perinatal loss or malformation in previous or current pregnancy.
- Personal history of abnormal glucose tolerance or GDM in previous pregnancy.
- Hispanic, Native American, African American, Asian, or Pacific Islander ethnicity.
- Advanced maternal age.

PHYSICAL FINDINGS & CLINICAL PRESENTATION

Suspect GDM if:
- Fetal size greater than dates, especially if significantly enlarged abdominal circumference on fetal ultrasound.
- Macrosomia or polyhydramnios on ultrasound.
- Marked maternal obesity or weight gain above expected range.

ETIOLOGY

- During normal pregnancy there is increased insulin resistance because of placental secretion of diabetogenic hormones in the late second and third trimesters. Maternal pancreatic beta-cells secrete more insulin to compensate for the increased insulin resistance. GDM occurs when maternal insulin secretion cannot meet the increased demand.
- Insulin resistance is also exacerbated by an increase in maternal adipose deposition, decreased exercise, and increased caloric intake.

DIAGNOSIS

DIFFERENTIAL DIAGNOSIS

Preexisting type 1 or 2 DM not previously diagnosed.

WORKUP

- History with focus on personal medical history, prior pregnancy history, and family history.
- Routine prenatal examination.
- Laboratory evaluation (see the following).

LABORATORY TESTS

- "Two-step" approach.
  1. For screening without risk factors, order a 1-hr glucose tolerance test (Nonfasting; 50-g oral glucose load) at 24 to 28 weeks.
  2. For screening with risk factors, order a 1-hr glucose tolerance test at the first prenatal visit, then repeat at 24 to 28 weeks if initial screen was normal. If abnormal at intake, consider possibility of undiagnosed preexisting DM and check hemoglobin A1c.
- If 1-hr test result is abnormal (≥130 mg/dl), order 3-hr glucose tolerance test (Fasting: 100-g oral glucose load).

1. Performed after 3 days of unrestricted diet (carbohydrate load is probably not necessary).
2. Carpenter and Coustan Criteria (see previous page for cutoff values).
3. GDM is diagnosed if two or more of the glucose values are met or exceeded.
- If one of four values on 3-hr glucose tolerance test is abnormal, consider repeat testing in 1 month and recommend a diabetic diet immediately.
- "One-step" approach
  1. Rule out overt diabetes at the initial prenatal visit. A diagnosis of diabetes is made if a woman meets any of the following criteria: fasting plasma glucose >126 mg/dl, A1c >6.5%, random plasma glucose >200 mg/dl.
  2. Perform a one-step screening at 24 to 28 weeks on all pregnant patients who have not already been diagnosed with diabetes. This is a 2-hr, 75-g oral glucose tolerance test performed after an overnight fast. A diagnosis of GDM is made if one or more of the following values are met or exceeded:
  Fasting: ≥92 mg/dl
  1-hr plasma glucose ≥180 mg/dl
  2-hr plasma glucose ≥153 mg/dl
- The U.S. Preventive Services Task Force (USPSTF) recommends screening for gestational diabetes in all pregnant women after 24 weeks' gestation. The current evidence is insufficient to assess the balance between the benefits and harms of screening women for GDM in asymptomatic women before 24 weeks' gestation. Clinicians should discuss early screening for GDM with their patients and make case-by-case decisions after considering patient risk factors. The discussion should include information about the potential benefits and harms of screening as well as the uncertain meaning of a positive screening test result.
- Women with GDM have an increased risk of developing diabetes during their lifetime. Women with GDM should be screened at or after 6 weeks postpartum with a 75-g 2-hour GTT to diagnose impaired glucose tolerance or type 2 diabetes. Up to 12 weeks' gestation, the HgA1c test is also a reasonable method to use to screen for preexisting insulin resistance or type 2 DM.

IMAGING STUDIES

Ultrasound for fetal size is performed at least once at 36 to 37 weeks; it may be initiated at an earlier gestational age and repeated every 3 to 4 weeks if macrosomia is suspected.

TREATMENT

NONPHARMACOLOGIC THERAPY

- Glucose monitoring:
  1. Four times daily: fasting and 2-hr postprandial (defined as 2 hr after the start of each meal).
  2. Goals: fasting <95 mg/dl; 2-hr postprandial <120 mg/dl.
  3. Can also use 1-hr postprandial goal of <140 mg/dl.

- Dietary modifications aimed at glycemic control:
  1. Follow a low-fat, high-fiber diet; avoid sugar and concentrated sweets; and eat small, frequent meals.
  2. Ongoing nutrition counseling; diet should adequately meet the needs of pregnancy (below) while restricting carbohydrates to 35% to 40% of daily calories.
  3. Prepregnancy BMI: 30 kcal/kg/day; BMI above 30: 25 kcal/kg/day; and BMI >40: 12 to 14 kcal/kg/day.
- Regular moderate exercise.

PHARMACOLOGIC Rx

Initiate if >20% of fasting, postprandial, or a combination of glucose values are elevated after trial of diet control:

- Oral hypoglycemics:
  1. According to recent studies, oral hypoglycemics show equivalent efficacy to insulin and can be appropriate first-line agents. There is no consistent evidence from randomized trials showing any increase in short-term adverse maternal or neonatal outcomes with oral medications vs. insulin. There are no long-term trials available, and both metformin and glyburide may cross the placenta.
  2. Glyburide: begin at 2.5 mg qd and titrate up to a maximum of 20 mg qd (10 mg bid). Increase dose as needed by 2.5 to 5 mg/wk.
  3. Metformin: begin at 500 mg PO qd or bid and titrate up to a max of 2000 mg daily.
- Insulin: considered gold standard in GDM management.
  - There are no randomized controlled trials on insulin regimens, and therapy is largely guided by expert opinion.
  - Insulin may be started first line or added when oral medications have failed to achieve glycemic control. The authors consider factors such as the degree of hyperglycemia, obstacles to medication adherence, and gestational age at time of diagnosis (with early-onset diagnosis more likely to progress and require insulin) when initiating therapy.
  1. One commonly used regimen:
     1. Insulin 0.7 to 1.0 U/kg/day SQ (based on current pregnant weight), with two thirds of the total daily dose given in the morning and one third of the total daily dose given in the evening
     2. One third of each dose is given as short-acting (regular, lispro, or aspart) insulin and the remaining two thirds as NPH insulin
  2. Another option:
     1. If fasting values are elevated, use NPH at bedtime with initial dose of 0.2 U/kg
     2. If postprandial values are elevated, use rapid-acting insulin before meals with initial dose 1.5 U/10 g carbohydrate at breakfast and 1 U/10 g carbohydrate at lunch and dinner
     3. Long-acting insulin such as glargine (Lantus) does not have sufficient data to determine whether it crosses the placenta; it may be continued in persons with preexisting diabetes who are well controlled but is not recommended in patients with newly diagnosed GDM.

ANTENATAL TESTING

Antepartum testing is recommended for women with pre-gestational diabetes. There is no consensus regarding antepartum testing in gestational diabetes, and this should be guided by local standards.

ONE COMMONLY USED REGIMEN

- Class A1: NST/AFI at 40 wk.
- Class A2: weekly NST/AFI beginning at 32 wk or when medications are initiated.
- Poorly controlled diabetes, vascular complications, or hypertension: biweekly NST/AFI beginning at 28 wk. and consider admission for initial glycemic control.

TIMING AND ROUTE OF DELIVERY

- Women with preexisting diabetes should be induced at 39 weeks.
- Women with GDM may also be induced at 39 weeks, with decisions regarding induction guided by local standards of care.
  ACOG states that there is no single evidence-based recommendation that can be made regarding timing of delivery in women with GDM.
- Counseling regarding elective cesarean section at or after 39 weeks if estimated fetal weight is over 4500 g.
- Consider delivery earlier than 39 weeks if poor control or other medical indications such as growth restriction or preeclampsia.

INTRAPARTUM MANAGEMENT

- Goal is normoglycemia (80 to 120 mg/dl) using insulin and D5 lactated Ringer's IV fluid if needed.
- Monitor glucose every 1 to 2 hours in active labor.
- Preparation for shoulder dystocia.
- If on glyburide, discontinue in labor or 12 hr before a scheduled induction.
- If on insulin consider decreased long-acting insulin by one third to one half before scheduled induction. Most experts recommend holding insulin entirely the morning of a scheduled cesarean delivery.

NEONATAL MANAGEMENT

- Check 30- and 60-min glucose at a minimum. Most institutions have their own protocol regarding glucose management for the neonate.
- Watch for signs of hypoglycemia, hypocalcemia, hyperbilirubinemia, and polycythemia.

POSTPARTUM MANAGEMENT

- Class A2: check fasting level before discharge; if abnormal, continue checking at home and early follow-up with primary care physician to confirm diagnosis of DM.
- 6-wk postpartum visit: screen for impaired glucose tolerance and diabetes in A1 and A2 women with a 75 g, 2-hr glucose tolerance test
- If no evidence of DM, screen annually for DM and counsel on risk factor modification

REFERRAL

- Nutritionist.
- High-risk obstetrician.
- Maternal-fetal medicine.
- Diabetes educator.
- Nurse care manager, when available.

COMPLICATIONS

- Maternal: preeclampsia, future type 2 DM or GDM, operative delivery.
- Fetal: polyhydramnios, macrosomia, shoulder dystocia, birth trauma, congenital malformations.
- Neonatal: hypoglycemia, hypocalcemia, hyperbilirubinemia, polycythemia, perinatal death, impaired glucose homeostasis at birth, respiratory distress, future obesity and DM, increased rates of inattention and hyperactivity in childhood.

❗ PEARLS & CONSIDERATIONS

- Trials have shown that although treatment of mild gestational DM did not significantly reduce the frequency of a composite outcome that included stillbirth or perinatal death and several neonatal complications, it did reduce the risks of fetal overgrowth, shoulder dystocia, cesarean delivery, and hypertensive disorders.
- Lactation improves maternal glucose metabolism and may prevent or delay the development of type 2 DM following GDM. Higher lactation intensity and longer duration are independently associated with lower 2-year incidences of DM after a GDM-affected pregnancy.[1]

PREVENTION

Regular exercise, maintenance of ideal body weight, and high-fiber low-glycemic diet.

SUGGESTED READINGS

Available at www.expertconsult.com

RELATED CONTENT

Gestational Diabetes (Patient Information)
Diabetes Mellitus (Related Key Topic)

AUTHORS: **SUSANNA R. MAGEE, M.D., M.P.H., MARY BETH SUTTER, M.D., HAYLEY RYAN, D.O., HEIDI RADLINSKI, M.D., M.P.H.,** and **ASHLEY LAKIN, D.O., M.A.**

[1]Gunderson EP, et al.: Lactation and progression to type 2 diabetes mellitus after gestational diabetes mellitus: a prospective cohort study, *Ann Intern Med* 163:889-898, 2015.

BASIC INFORMATION

DEFINITION

Giant cell arteritis (GCA) is a segmental systemic granulomatous arteritis affecting medium and large arteries in individuals >50 yr. Inflammation primarily targets branches of the extracranial head and neck blood vessels (external carotids, temporal arteries, ciliary and ophthalmic arteries). The aorta and subclavian and brachial arteries can also be affected. Intracranial arteritis is rare.

SYNONYMS

Temporal arteritis
Cranial arteritis
GCA
Horton's disease

ICD-10CM CODES
M31.5 Giant cell arteritis with polymyalgia
        rheumatica
M31.6 Other giant cell arteritis

EPIDEMIOLOGY & DEMOGRAPHICS

INCIDENCE: Approximately 20 new cases per 100,000 persons >50 yr; peak incidence is in patients ages 60 to 80 yr.
PREVALENCE: 200 cases per 100,000 persons; it is the most common primary vasculitis; female/male predominance of twofold to fourfold; more common in Caucasians.

PHYSICAL FINDINGS & CLINICAL PRESENTATION

GCA can present with the following clinical manifestations:

TABLE 1 Atypical Manifestations of Giant Cell Arteritis

Fever of unknown origin
Respiratory symptoms (especially cough)
Otolaryngeal manifestations
    Glossitis
    Lingual infarction
    Throat pain
    Hearing loss
Large-artery disease
    Aortic aneurysm
    Aortic dissection
    Limb claudication
    Raynaud's phenomenon
Neurologic manifestations
    Peripheral neuropathy
    Transient ischemic attack (TIA) or stroke
    Dementia
    Delirium
Myocardial infarction
Tumorlike lesions
    Breast mass
    Ovarian and uterine mass
Syndrome of inappropriate antidiuretic hormone
    secretion (SIADH)
Microangiopathic hemolytic anemia

From Harris ED et al: *Kelly's textbook of rheumatology,* ed 7, Philadelphia, 2005, Saunders.

- Headache, often associated with marked scalp tenderness—noticed while brushing hair (hair comb allodynia).
- Constitutional symptoms (fever, weight loss, anorexia, fatigue).
- Polymyalgia rheumatica (aching and stiffness of the trunk and proximal muscle groups).
- Visual disturbances (transient or permanent monocular or binocular visual loss).
- Intermittent claudication of jaw and tongue on mastication that is especially prominent when solid food such as steak is chewed.
- Table 1 describes atypical manifestations of GCA.
  Important physical findings in GCA:
- Vascular examination: The temporal artery demonstrates tenderness, decreased pulsation, and nodularity (ropy) (Fig. 1); diminished or absent pulses in upper extremities may be seen.

ETIOLOGY

Vasculitis of unknown etiology. Recent demonstration of varicella zoster virus virion, antigen, and DNA within the vessel walls of the temporal arteries on histopathologic specimens of giant cell arteritis suggest an association.

Dx DIAGNOSIS

Clinical history and vascular examination remain cornerstones of diagnosis. An algorithm for diagnosing GCA is described in Fig. 2. The American College of Rheumatology has proposed classification criteria to aid in the diagnosis of GCA. Presence of three or more of these criteria in a patient with suspected vasculitis is considered to be suggestive of GCA.

- Age of onset of symptoms >50 yr.
- New-onset of or new type of localized headache.
- Temporal artery abnormalities including tenderness or decreased pulsation.
- Westergren erythrocyte sedimentation rate (ESR) elevated (typically >50 mm/hr).
- Temporal artery biopsy with vasculitis and mononuclear cell infiltrate or granulomatous changes.

DIFFERENTIAL DIAGNOSIS

- Other vasculitic syndromes.
- Nonarteritic anterior ischemic optic neuropathy (NAION).
- Pituitary apoplexy.
- Primary amyloidosis.
- Transient ischemic attack, stroke.
- Infections.
- Occult neoplasm, multiple myeloma.

LABORATORY TESTS

- ESR elevated although up to 22% of patients with GCA have normal ESR before treatment.

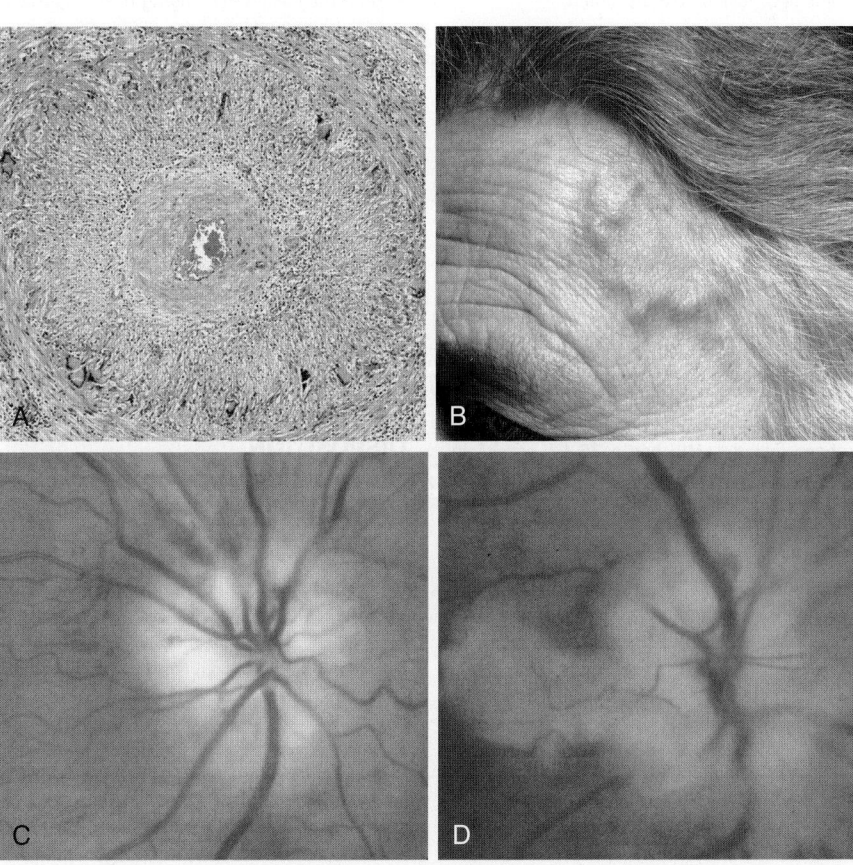

FIG. 1 **Giant cell arteritis. A,** Histology shows transmural granulomatous inflammation, disruption of the internal elastic lamina, proliferation of the intima, and gross narrowing of the lumen. **B,** The superficial temporal artery is pulseless, nodular, and thickened. **C,** Ischemic optic neuropathy. **D,** Ischemic optic neuropathy and cilioretinal artery occlusion. (From Kanski JJ, Bowling B: *Clinical ophthalmology, a systematic approach,* ed 7, Philadelphia, 2010, Saunders.)

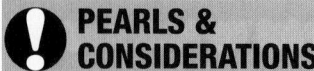
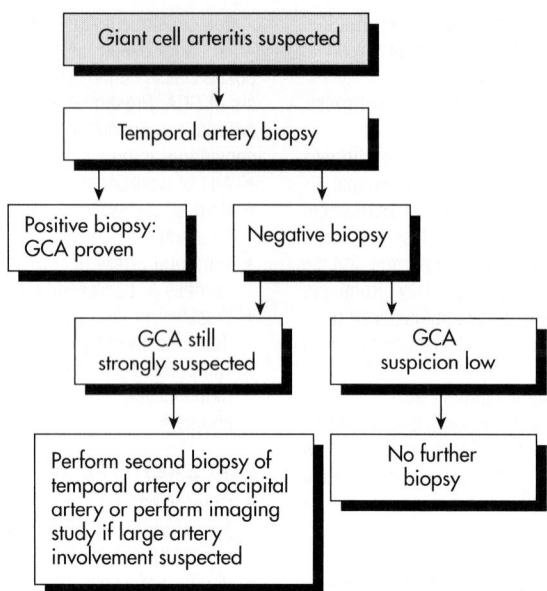

FIG. 2 Algorithm for diagnosing giant cell arteritis (GCA). (From Firestein GS et al: *Kelly's textbook of rheumatology,* ed 9, Philadelphia, 2013, Saunders.)

- C-reactive protein (CRP) is typically included in laboratory investigation; it may have greater sensitivity than ESR. CRP typically rises before the ESR.
- Mild to moderate normochromic normocytic anemia, elevated platelet count.

IMAGING STUDIES

- Color duplex ultrasonography (CDUS) of temporal artery produces three characteristic features—periluminal "halo" over the temporal artery involved, segmental arterial stenosis, and arterial luminal occlusion in severe cases. CDUS of the temporal artery has 40% to 75% sensitivity and 79% to 83% specificity for diagnosis of GCA. Clinical utility is not superior to clinical examination with biopsy.
- Contrasted MRI of temporal artery may be performed in patients with contraindications to surgical biopsy of the superficial temporal artery, if treatment with steroids has not been initiated. MRI has a 78.4% sensitivity and 90.4% specificity in detecting temporal artery involvement in patients with a clinical diagnosis of GCA.
- Angiography of the arms is indicated in patients with peripheral vascular insufficiency.
- FDG-PET imaging may be used to detect large-vessel inflammation in GCA.

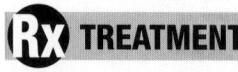 **TREATMENT**

ACUTE GENERAL Rx

- If there is clinical suspicion of GCA, treatment should be initiated without waiting for results of laboratory or imaging studies.

- IV methylprednisolone (250-1000 mg for 1-3 days) is considered standard of care in patients with severe clinical manifestations such as visual loss from ischemic optic neuropathy.
- Oral prednisone (1 mg/kg/day): high-dose oral regimen should be continued at least until symptoms resolve and ESR returns to normal; usually 3 to 4 weeks after treatment initiation. Steroid taper is very slow (10%-20% per month) with monitoring of clinical features as well as ESR and CRP. When dose <10 mg/day, taper by 1 mg/month. Treatment may last up to 2 yr or more.
  Corticosteroids are the treatment of choice. There is no evidence for the role of steroid-sparing agents. Methotrexate, tocilizumab, and cyclophosphamide may be considered in cases of contraindications to or failure of corticosteroid therapy. Evidence for their efficacy is limited.

DISPOSITION

With steroid therapy there is a dramatic improvement of systemic symptoms, but not vision in patients with ischemic optic neuropathy. In one study only 4% of eyes improved in both visual acuity and central visual field.

Management of flares: Repeat prednisone induction if patient experiences severe flare. If mild flare, increase prednisone by 10% to 20%.

REFERRAL

- Surgical or ophthalmologic referral for biopsy of temporal artery.
- Rheumatology referral for long-term immunosuppressive treatment management.

⚠ PEARLS & CONSIDERATIONS

- Treatment of GCA should be started if there is clinical suspicion of the disease. This usually includes patients above the age of 50 presenting with a severe headache and systemic features that suggest GCA as well. Physicians should not wait for laboratory or pathologic confirmation before starting treatment as the risk of visual loss increases.
- Temporal artery biopsy should be performed as soon as possible, but within 2 weeks of initiating treatment with steroids. The biopsy may remain positive for two to six weeks after initiation of corticosteroids.
- Treatment should not be withheld pending temporal artery biopsy.
- Temporal artery biopsy may not be required in patients with typical disease features accompanied by characteristic ultrasound or MRI findings.

COMMENTS

- The relation between polymyalgia rheumatica and GCA is unclear, but the two frequently coexist. They are considered to be different points along the gradient or spectrum of the same disease.
- Clinical picture rather than ESR should be the prime yardstick for continuing prednisone therapy. A rising ESR in a clinically asymptomatic patient with normal hematocrit should raise suspicion for alternate explanations (e.g., infections, neoplasms).
- GCA is associated with a markedly increased risk for the development of aortic aneurysm, which is often a late complication and may cause death. Annual chest radiograph in chronic CGA patients has been suggested, as well as emergent chest CT or MRI for clinical suspicion.
- GCA is also associated with increased risk of myocardial infarction, stroke, and peripheral vascular disease.
- Coadministration of low dose aspirin (81 mg/day) has been reported by some as effective for further reduction of risk of blindness. Additional trials may be needed before it can be recommended as standard therapy.

SUGGESTED READINGS

Available at www.expertconsult.com.

RELATED CONTENT

Giant Cell Arteritis (Patient Information)
Temporal Arteritis (Patient Information)

AUTHORS: **ARUN SWAMINATHAN, M.B.B.S.,** and **SACHIN KEDAR, M.B.B.S., M.D.**

BASIC INFORMATION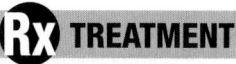

DEFINITION
Giardiasis is an intestinal and/or biliary tract infection caused by the protozoal parasite *Giardia intestinalis* (also known as *G. lamblia* or *G. duodenalis*). The organism is a widespread zoonotic parasite and frequently contaminates fresh water sources worldwide.

SYNONYMS
Giardiasis
Giardia duodenalis
Giardia intestinalis

ICD-10CM CODES
A07.1 Giardiasis [lambliasis]

EPIDEMIOLOGY & DEMOGRAPHICS
INCIDENCE (IN U.S.):
- Exact incidence unknown. CDC estimates 20,000 cases a year in the U.S.
- Frequently occurs as waterborne outbreaks in international adoptees, travelers, immunocompromised patients, and those with cystic fibrosis.
- *G. lamblia* has been demonstrated in 4% to 7% of submitted stool specimens, making it the most commonly identified intestinal parasite.

PREVALENCE (IN U.S.): 4%
PREDOMINANT SEX: Male = female
PREDOMINANT AGE:
- Preschool children, especially if in day care
- 20 to 40 yr of age, especially among sexually active homosexual men

PEAK INCIDENCE:
- Varies with risk factors, outbreaks, but peak onset from early summer through early fall
- All age groups affected

GENETICS: Familial disposition: Patients with common variable immunodeficiency or X-linked agammaglobulinemia are at increased risk of infection.

PHYSICAL FINDINGS & CLINICAL PRESENTATION
- More than 70% with one or more intestinal symptoms (diarrhea, flatulence, cramps, bloating, nausea). Table 1 summarizes clinical signs and symptoms of giardiasis
- Incubation period averages 7 to 14 days but can be longer
- Fever in <30%
- Chronic diarrhea, malabsorption, and weight loss, which can be up to 10% of body weight, are common
- GI bleeding is unusual
- Continuous or intermittent symptoms, lasting for 2 to 4 weeks
- Of infected patients, 20% to 25% are asymptomatic and can shed cysts for months

ETIOLOGY
Infection is acquired by ingestion of viable cysts of the organism (Fig. 1), typically in contaminated water or food or by fecal-oral contact. *Giardia* cysts are resistant to chlorination and survive well in cold mountain streams.

DIAGNOSIS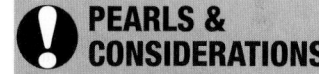

DIFFERENTIAL DIAGNOSIS
- Other agents of infective diarrhea (amebae, *Salmonella* sp., *Shigella* sp., *Staphylococcus aureus, Cryptosporidium,* etc.)
- Noninfectious causes of malabsorption

WORKUP
- Stool specimen (three specimens yield 90% sensitivity) as a saline suspension or duodenal aspirate for microscopic examination to establish diagnosis and exclude other pathogens
- Immunoassays for *Giardia* sp. Antigens in stool samples such as the DFA or ELISA are now routinely used in most clinical laboratories. These assays are 85% to 98% sensitive and 90% to 100% specific. They also have a faster turnaround time.

LABORATORY TESTS
Serum albumin, vitamin B_{12} levels, and stool fat test to exclude malabsorption

IMAGING STUDIES
- Not necessary unless biliary obstruction is suspected
- In detection of organism, possible interference by barium in stool from radiographic studies

TREATMENT

NONPHARMACOLOGIC THERAPY
Avoidance of milk products to reduce symptoms of transient lactase deficiency that occur in many patients and can last for weeks to months

GENERAL Rx
Adult and pediatric:
- Tinidazole: 2 g single dose (50 mg/kg in children over 3 years of age).
- Metronidazole 250 mg PO three times daily for 5 to 7 days. Pediatric dose: 5 mg/kg tid × 7 days (metronidazole should be avoided in pregnancy).
- Nitazoxanide: aged 12 to 47 mo: 100 mg bid × 3 days. Aged 4 to 11 yr: 200 mg bid × 3 days
- Albendazole 400 mg PO qd x 5 days
- Paromomycin 25 to 35 mg/kg/day in three doses for 5 to 10 days
- Can be used in pregnancy

DISPOSITION
Reinfection is possible.

PEARLS & CONSIDERATIONS

COMMENTS
Travelers to endemic areas (developing world, wilderness areas) should be cautioned to boil drinking water or use water purification tablets (for iodine-containing products, chlorination is not effective). Chronic giardiasis as seen in developing nations can cause delays in growth and development in children due to malabsorption and diarrhea.

SUGGESTED READINGS
Available at www.expertconsult.com

RELATED CONTENT
Giardiasis (Patient Information)

AUTHOR: **GLENN G. FORT, M.D., M.P.H.**

TABLE 1 Clinical Signs and Symptoms of Giardiasis

Symptom	Frequency (%)
Diarrhea	64-100
Malaise, weakness	72-97
Abdominal distention	42-97
Flatulence	35-97
Abdominal cramps	44-81
Nausea	14-79
Foul-smelling, greasy stools	15-79
Anorexia	41-73
Weight loss	53-73
Vomiting	14-35
Fever	0-28
Constipation	0-27

From Kliegman RM et al: *Nelson textbook of pediatrics,* ed 19, Philadelphia, 2011, Saunders.

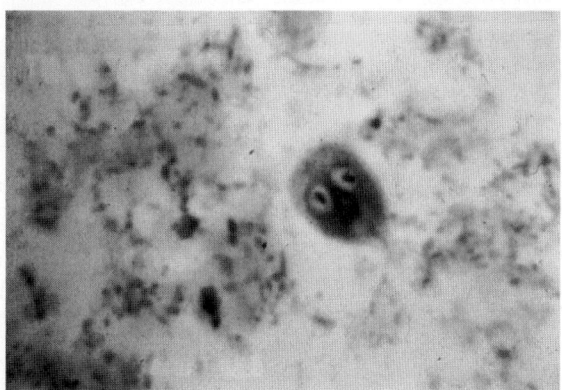

FIG. 1 *Giardia lamblia* trophozoite is demonstrated in a trichrome stain of fecal material. Note the prominent nuclei in the trophozoite. (Bennett JE, Dolin R, Blaser MJ: Mandell, Douglas, and Bennett *'s principles and practice of infectious diseases,* ed 8, Philadelphia, 2015, Saunders.)

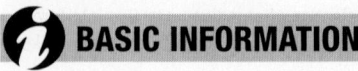

BASIC INFORMATION

DEFINITION

Gilbert's syndrome is an autosomal-dominant disorder characterized by indirect hyperbilirubinemia caused by impaired glucuronyl transferase activity.

SYNONYMS

Gilbert's disease

ICD-10CM CODES
E80.4 Gilbert's syndrome

EPIDEMIOLOGY & DEMOGRAPHICS

INCIDENCE (IN U.S.): Probable autosomal-dominant disease affecting >5% of the U.S. population
PREDOMINANT SEX: Male/female ratio of 3:1
GENETICS: Most common hereditary hyperbilirubinemia (genotypic prevalence 12%)

PHYSICAL FINDINGS & CLINICAL PRESENTATION

- No abnormalities on physical examination other than mild jaundice when bilirubin exceeds 3 mg/dl.
- A family history of unconjugated hyperbilirubinemia may be present.

ETIOLOGY

- Decreased elimination of bilirubin in bile is caused by inadequate conjugation of bilirubin.
- Alcohol consumption and starvation diet can increase bilirubin level.
- The pathogenesis of Gilbert's syndrome has been linked to a reduction in the bilirubin UGT-1 gene *(HUG-Brl)* transcription, resulting from a mutation in the promoter region.

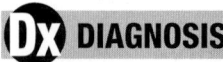

DIAGNOSIS

DIFFERENTIAL DIAGNOSIS

- Hemolytic anemia.
- Liver disease (chronic hepatitis, cirrhosis).
- Crigler-Najjar syndrome.

WORKUP

- Most patients are diagnosed during or after adolescence, when isolated hyperbilirubinemia is detected as an incidental finding on routine biochemical testing.
- Laboratory evaluation to exclude hemolysis and liver diseases as a cause of the elevated bilirubin level (Table 1 and Fig. 1).

LABORATORY TESTS

Elevated indirect (unconjugated) bilirubin (rarely exceeds 5 mg/dl).

TABLE 1 Characteristic Patterns of Liver Function Tests

Disorder	Bilirubin	Alkaline Phosphatase	AST	ALT	Prothrombin Time	Albumin
Gilbert's syndrome (abnormal bilirubin metabolism)	↑	NL	NL	NL	NL	NL
Bile duct obstruction (pancreatic cancer)	↑↑↑	↑↑↑	↑	↑	↑-↑↑	NL
Acute hepatocellular damage (toxic, viral hepatitis)	↑-↑↑↑	↑-↑↑	↑↑↑	↑↑↑	NL-↑↑↑	NL-↓↓
Cirrhosis	NL-↑	NL-↑	NL-↑	NL-↑	NL-↑↑	NL-↓↓

ALT, Alanine aminotransferase; *AST,* aspartate aminotransferase; *NL,* normal; ↑ increase; ↓, decrease (arrows indicate extent of change: ↑-↑↑↑, slight to large).
From Andreoli TE (ed): *Cecil essentials of medicine,* ed 6, Philadelphia, 2005, Saunders.

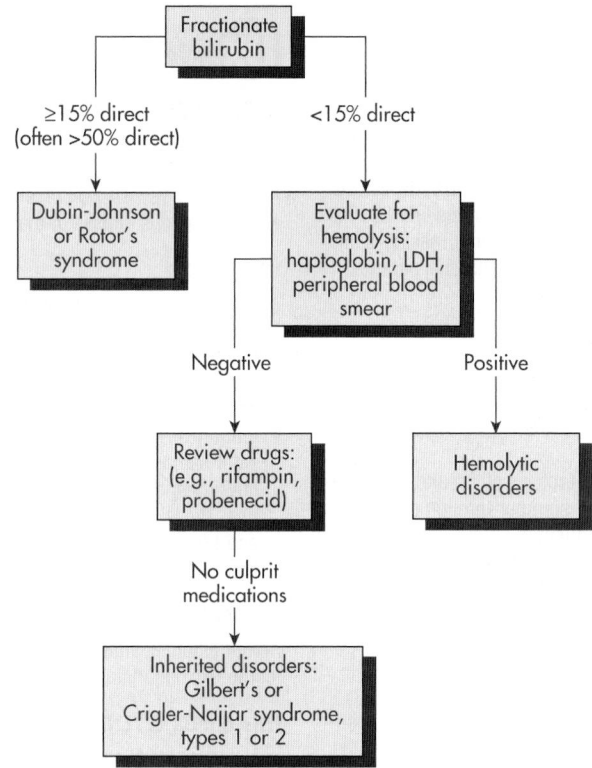

FIG. 1 Evaluation of an isolated elevation of the serum bilirubin level. (From Feldman M et al [eds]: *Sleisenger and Fordtran's gastrointestinal and liver disease,* ed 10, Philadelphia, 2016, Saunders.)

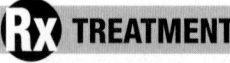

TREATMENT

ACUTE GENERAL Rx

Treatment is generally unnecessary. Phenobarbital (if clinical jaundice is present) can rapidly decrease serum indirect bilirubin level.

DISPOSITION

Prognosis is excellent. Treatment is generally unnecessary.

REFERRAL

Referral is generally not necessary.

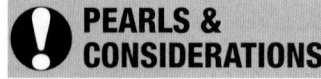

PEARLS & CONSIDERATIONS

COMMENTS

- Patients should be reassured about the benign nature of the condition.
- Fasting for 2 days or significant dehydration may raise the bilirubin level and result in the clinical recognition of jaundice.

AUTHOR: **FRED F. FERRI, M.D.**

BASIC INFORMATION

DEFINITION

Glaucoma is a chronic degenerative optic neuropathy (or the high potential for such degeneration due to risk factors) in which the neuro-retinal rim of the optic nerve becomes progressively thinner, thereby enlarging the optic-nerve cup. The classification of glaucoma is based on the appearance of the iridocorneal angle (open angle vs. closed angle) and is further subdivided into primary and secondary types. Primary open-angle glaucoma can occur with or without elevated intraocular pressure (IOP). Normal tension glaucoma refers to primary open-angle glaucoma without elevated intraocular pressure.

SYNONYMS

Primary open-angle glaucoma (POAG)
Open-angle glaucoma (OAG)
Secondary open-angle glaucoma (e.g., pseudoexfoliation, pigment dispersion, trauma, inflammatory)
Chronic open-angle glaucoma

ICD-10CM CODES
H40.10X0	Unspecified open-angle glaucoma, stage unspecified
H40.10X1	Unspecified open-angle glaucoma, mild stage
H40.10X2	Unspecified open-angle glaucoma, moderate stage
H40.10X3	Unspecified open-angle glaucoma, severe stage
H40.10X4	Unspecified open-angle glaucoma, indeterminate stage
H40.11X0	Primary open-angle glaucoma, stage unspecified
H40.11X1	Primary open-angle glaucoma, mild stage
H40.11X2	Primary open-angle glaucoma, moderate stage
H40.11X3	Primary open-angle glaucoma, severe stage
H40.11X4	Primary open-angle glaucoma, indeterminate stage

EPIDEMIOLOGY & DEMOGRAPHICS

INCIDENCE (IN U.S.): Third most common cause of vision loss (75% to 95% of all forms of glaucoma are open angle)
PEAK INCIDENCE:
- Increases after age 40 yr
- Three million cases expected by 2020 because of the rapid increase in aging population

PREVALENCE (IN U.S.):
- Overall prevalence in U.S. population aged >40 yr is estimated to be 1.86%, with 1.57 million white and 398,000 black patients affected. By 2020, we may expect more than 3 million cases in the U.S.
- 150,000 patients have bilateral blindness.
- Prevalence is higher in diabetics, those with high myopia, and older persons.
- More common in African-American population (three times the age-adjusted prevalence

than whites). There is a genetic tendency to OAG; multiple genes have been isolated that are associated with development of high IOP and optic nerve damage.

PREDOMINANT AGE:
- Persons >50 yr
- Can occur in 30s and 40s, and juvenile forms are rare

PHYSICAL FINDINGS & CLINICAL PRESENTATION

- High intraocular pressures and/or large optic nerve cup (Ocular Hypertension Treatment Study results help to delineate important risk factors).
- Abnormal visual fields (with advanced glaucoma damage to the optic nerve).
- Open anterior chamber angle—evaluated with gonioscopy.
- Since early treatable stages of OAG normally have no symptoms, it's important to have routine eye exams, especially patients with family history and patients over 60 yr.
- Secondary forms of OAG may exhibit ocular findings such as pseudo-exfoliation, pigment dispersion, blood in anterior chamber, inflammation.

ETIOLOGY

- Uncertain hereditary tendency (multifactorial genetics).
- Topical steroids can induce high IOP and cause glaucoma.
- Trauma.
- Inflammatory (e.g., history of uveitis).
- High-dose oral corticosteroids taken for prolonged periods.

DIAGNOSIS

DIFFERENTIAL DIAGNOSIS

- Other optic neuropathies (previous retinal vascular disorders, optic nerve pits, or coloboma).
- Physiologic cupping of the optic nerve: The optic nerve may appear similar to glaucoma damage but does not progress. This is followed for any signs of progression.
- Ocular hypertension: IOP is chronically elevated, but not causing optic nerve damage, must monitor closely.
- Secondary glaucoma from inflammation and steroid therapy.
- Trauma.

WORKUP

- Comprehensive eye examination
- Intraocular pressure
- Slit lamp examination
- Visual fields
- Gonioscopy: to determine the type of glaucoma
- Nerve fiber analysis (e.g., GDx, OCT, and HRT)
- Corneal thickness (thick central cornea will result in possible overestimation of the true physiologic IOP, and vice versa, so this is important information in diagnosis and treatment of OAG)

LABORATORY TESTS

Blood sugar

IMAGING STUDIES

- Optic nerve photography—stereo photographs (Fig. E1).
- Visual field testing.
- Laser scan of nerve fiber layer, OCT, HRT. Rarely, MRI of orbits if the glaucoma findings are atypical or suspicious of other causes of optic nerve atrophy (Fig. E1).

TREATMENT

ACUTE GENERAL Rx

- β-blockers (e.g., timolol) qd to bid depending on individual response to drug.
- Carbonic anhydrase inhibitors (e.g., Diamox 250 mg qid or 500 mg bid).
- Prostaglandin analogues (latanoprost, bimatoprost, travoprost, tafluprost) are commonly used as first-line treatment. They lower intraocular pressure by 25% to 30% by increasing uveoscleral outflow and reducing aqueous production.
- Alpha-2 agonists and cholinergic agonists.
- Hyperosmotic agents (mannitol) in acute treatment (IV).
- Selective laser trabeculoplasty (SLT) may delay or forestall need for second eyedrop. The effect may be temporary but the laser can be repeated.

CHRONIC Rx

- At least biannual checks of intraocular pressure and adjustment of medication.
- Surgical trabeculectomy and filter valve surgeries can be considered for glaucoma that progresses (optic nerve changes or visual field progression) despite maximal tolerated medical therapies. Recently, minimally invasive glaucoma surgeries (MIGS) have been advocated for IOP control. Some are performed at the time of cataract procedures and some are independent procedures. The effort is to reduce the risks associated with traditional trabeculectomy.

DISPOSITION

Must be followed by ophthalmologist.

REFERRAL

Immediately to ophthalmologist.

PEARLS & CONSIDERATIONS

COMMENTS

- Glaucoma is a serious blinding disease that must be monitored professionally by an ophthalmologist. It is mostly asymptomatic until late in the disease when visual problems arise. Even in developed countries half of glaucoma cases are undiagnosed.
- Risk factors that should prompt referral to an ophthalmologist for evaluation of glaucoma are high intraocular pressure, family history of glaucoma, use of systemic or topical corticosteroids, older age, and black race.

- Vision loss from glaucoma cannot be recovered. Early diagnosis and treatment may minimize visual loss.
- Glaucoma is not solely caused by increased intraocular pressure because approximately 20% of patients with glaucoma have normal intraocular pressure. However, high pressure is definitely a risk factor to be considered.

Potential sites of increased resistance to aqueous flow are described in Fig. 2.

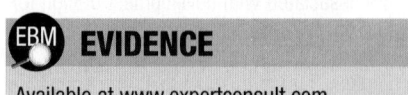

Available at www.expertconsult.com

SUGGESTED READINGS

Available at www.expertconsult.com

RELATED CONTENT

Glaucoma (Patient Information)

AUTHOR: **R. SCOTT HOFFMAN, M.D.**

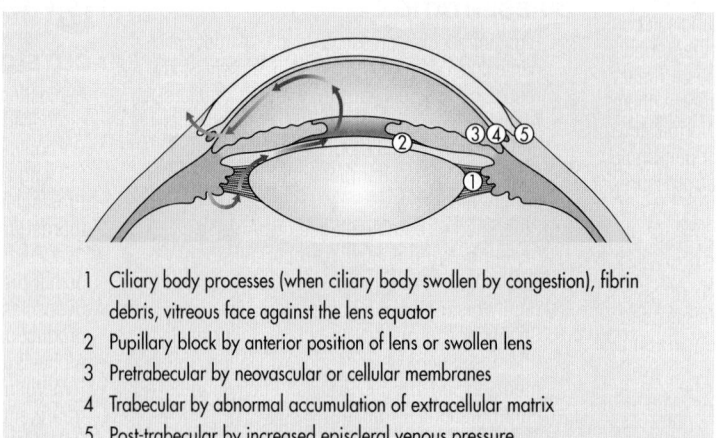

1 Ciliary body processes (when ciliary body swollen by congestion), fibrin debris, vitreous face against the lens equator
2 Pupillary block by anterior position of lens or swollen lens
3 Pretrabecular by neovascular or cellular membranes
4 Trabecular by abnormal accumulation of extracellular matrix
5 Post-trabecular by increased episcleral venous pressure

FIG. 2 Potential sites of increased resistance to aqueous flow. (From Yanoff M, Duker JS: *Ophthalmology,* ed 2, St Louis, 2004, Mosby.)

BASIC INFORMATION

DEFINITION

Primary angle-closure glaucoma occurs when elevated intraocular pressure is associated with closure of the filtration angle or obstruction in the circulating pathway of the aqueous humor.

SYNONYMS

Acute glaucoma, angle-closure glaucoma (ACG)
Pupillary block glaucoma
Narrow-angle glaucoma
Angle-closure glaucoma

ICD-10CM CODES
H40.061 Primary angle closure without glaucoma damage, right eye
H40.062 Primary angle closure without glaucoma damage, left eye
H40.063 Primary angle closure without glaucoma damage, bilateral
H40.069 Primary angle closure without glaucoma damage, unspecified eye

EPIDEMIOLOGY & DEMOGRAPHICS

INCIDENCE (IN U.S.):
- 2% to 8% of all patients with glaucoma.
- Higher incidence among those with hyperopia, small eyes, dense cataracts, shallow anterior chambers.

PEAK INCIDENCE: Greater >50 yr; high association with hyperopia, cataracts, and eye trauma
PREDOMINANT SEX: Females are affected more often than males.
PREDOMINANT AGE: 50 to 60 yr.
GENETICS: Family history is not particularly helpful; far-sighted (hyperopes) individuals with thickening lenses (i.e., cataracts) are often those with angle-closure attacks

PHYSICAL FINDINGS & CLINICAL PRESENTATION

- Although angle-closure glaucoma can present with an acute painful crisis associated with blurred vision, more than 75% of patients present with an asymptomatic course with progressive loss of the visual field (similar to that in patients with primary open-angle glaucoma; referred to as intermittent, subacute, or chronic angle closure).
- Hazy cornea.
- Narrow angle (Fig. E1).
- Red eyes.
- Pain may be present (supraorbital headache is typical.)
- Injection of conjunctiva.
- Shallow anterior chamber.
- Thick cataract.
- Pupil may be mid-dilated and nonreactive to light.

ETIOLOGY

- Narrow angles with acute closure: blockage of circulatory path of the aqueous humor

causing increase in intraocular pressure (IOP). ACG occurs more commonly in eyes with shorter axial length (farsightedness), shallower anterior chamber, and a relatively larger lens (enlarging cataract).
- Secondary angle-closure glaucoma resulting from neovascularization of iris, iris tumors, lens induced, iris scarring, trauma, chronic inflammation with scarring, malignant glaucoma with aqueous misdirection

DIAGNOSIS

DIFFERENTIAL DIAGNOSIS

- Open-angle glaucoma: Angle-closure glaucoma is distinguished from open-angle glaucoma by the closure of the angle between the iris and cornea, obstructing outflow of aqueous humor.
- High intraocular pressure.
- Optic nerve cupping.
- Shallow chamber.
- Open-angle glaucoma.
- Conjunctivitis.
- Corneal disease, keratitis.
- Uveitis.
- Scleritis.
- Allergies.
- Contact lens wearing with irritation.

WORKUP

Comprehensive eye examination: if one suspects narrow angle or angle closure, avoid pupil dilation since this may exacerbate the attack
- Intraocular pressure.
- Gonioscopy.
- Slit lamp examination.
- Visual field examination.
- GDx examination (laser scan of nerve fiber layer), OCT.
- Optic nerve evaluation.
- Anterior chamber depth.

LABORATORY TESTS

- Blood sugar and complete blood count (if diabetes or inflammatory disease is suspected).
- Visual field.
- GDx nerve fiber analysis, OCT, Heidelberg retinal tomography.

IMAGING STUDIES

- Fundus photography (optic nerve photos).
- Fluorescein angiography for neovascular disease such as diabetic retinopathy, retinal vein occlusions.
- Ultrasound biomicroscopy and anterior OCT can show relationships of anterior eye structures.

TREATMENT

The goal of treatment is to acutely lower pressure on the eye and keep it down.

NONPHARMACOLOGIC THERAPY

Laser iridotomy early in disease process.

ACUTE GENERAL Rx

- IV mannitol.
- Pilocarpine.
- β-blockers.
- Diamox.
- Laser iridotomy.
- Anterior chamber paracentesis (as emergency treatment).

CHRONIC Rx

- Iridotomy: When there is an adequate peripheral hole in the iris, the chance for future angle closure is usually eliminated.
- Lens removal (cataract extraction) can also eliminate the possibility of ACG.
- Trabeculectomy and filter valve procedures for non-responsive cases.
- Other laser procedures, such as gonioplasty for atypical angle closures.

DISPOSITION

Refer to ophthalmologist immediately.

REFERRAL

If acute angle-closure episode is suspected, should refer emergently to ophthalmologist.

PEARLS & CONSIDERATIONS

COMMENTS

- Do not use antihistamines or vasodilators with narrow-angle glaucoma.
- After iridotomy, the majority of patients will be totally cured and will need no further medication and have no visual loss.
- Lower socioeconomic status and higher levels of social deprivation are risk factors for delayed detection and probable worse outcomes in glaucoma.
- Risk factors that should prompt referral to an ophthalmologist for evaluation of glaucoma are high intraocular pressure, family history of glaucoma, use of systemic or topical corticosteroids, older age, and black race.
- Glaucoma is undiagnosed in 9 out of 10 affected people worldwide and is undiagnosed in 50% of those in developed countries.
- Angle closure has become rarer because most people have cataract extractions at an earlier stage than in the past.

EVIDENCE

Available at www.expertconsult.com

SUGGESTED READINGS

Available at www.expertconsult.com

RELATED CONTENT

Glaucoma (Patient Information).
Glaucoma, Open Angle(Related Key Topic)

AUTHOR: **R. SCOTT HOFFMAN, M.D.**

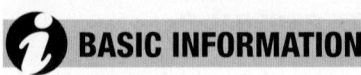

BASIC INFORMATION

DEFINITION

Acute glomerulonephritis is an immunologically mediated inflammation of the filtering units of the nephron, the glomeruli. The inflammation may result in damage to the glomerular basement membrane (GBM), mesangium, and/or capillary endothelium.

SYNONYMS

Acute nephritic syndrome

ICD-10CM CODES

N00.0 Acute nephritic syndrome with minor glomerular abnormality
N00.1 Acute nephritic syndrome with focal and segmental glomerular lesions
N00.2 Acute nephritic syndrome with diffuse membranous glomerulonephritis
N00.3 Acute nephritic syndrome with diffuse mesangial proliferative glomerulonephritis
N00.4 Acute nephritic syndrome with diffuse endocapillary proliferative glomerulonephritis
N00.5 Acute nephritic syndrome with diffuse mesangiocapillary glomerulonephritis
N00.6 Acute nephritic syndrome with dense deposit disease
N00.7 Acute nephritic syndrome with diffuse crescentic glomerulonephritis
N00.8 Acute nephritic syndrome with other morphologic changes
N00.9 Acute nephritic syndrome with unspecified morphologic changes

EPIDEMIOLOGY & DEMOGRAPHICS

- Incidence rates of primary glomerulonephritis vary between 0.2/100,000 per year and 2.5/100,000 per year.
- Immunoglobulin A (IgA) nephropathy (Berger's disease) is the most common glomerulonephritis worldwide.
- Glomerulonephritis accounts for 23% of end-stage renal disease cases.
- Glomerulonephritis affects adults and children.

PHYSICAL FINDINGS & CLINICAL PRESENTATION

- Acute onset of hypertension.
- Dark, "tea-colored" urine.
- Edema (peripheral, periorbital, or pulmonary).
- Fatigue.
- Concurrent pulmonary hemorrhage and kidney disease may indicate anti-neutrophil cytoplasmic antibody (ANCA) vasculitis or anti-GBM disease.
- Joint pains, oral ulcers, and malar rash are frequently seen with systemic lupus erythematosus.
- Palpable purpura may be found in patients with systemic vasculitis such as Henoch-Schönlein purpura, ANCA-associated vasculitis, or cryoglobulinemia.
- Recent history of endocarditis or cellulitis or preceding pharyngitis may indicate infection-related glomerulonephritis.

- Hepatitis C infection may cause membrano-proliferative glomerulonephritis (MPGN) with or without cryoglobulinemia.
- Concurrent upper respiratory tract infection "synpharyngitic" is commonly associated with flares of IgA nephropathy.
- Nonspecific flulike symptoms, fatigue, and myalgias are frequent with ANCA-associated vasculitis.

ETIOLOGY

Acute glomerulonephritis may occur as a kidney-limited disease or a systemic disease. The 3 mechanisms of primary glomerulonephritis are immune-complex deposition, anti-glomerular basement membrane disease antibodies, and vasculitis with minimal immune staining ("pauci-immune" glomerulonephritis)

Immune Complex	Pauci-Immune	Anti-Glomerular Basement Membrane
IgA nephropathy/Henoch-Schönlein purpura (IgA Vasculitis)	Myeloperoxidase (MPO)–associated vasculitis	Goodpasture disease
Lupus nephritis	Proteinase 3–associated vasculitis	
Infection-related glomerulonephritis, including poststreptococcal GN and endocarditis-associated GN	Eosinophilic vasculitis	
Membranoproliferative GN		
Cryoglobulinemic vasculitis		

Table 1 summarizes primary renal diseases that present as acute glomerulonephritis (GN). Diseases associated with rapidly progressive glomerulonephritis and pertinent laboratory findings are described in Table 2.

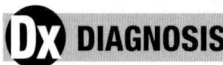

DIAGNOSIS

DIFFERENTIAL DIAGNOSIS

- Cirrhosis with edema and ascites.
- Congestive heart failure.
- Acute interstitial nephritis.
- Acute tubular necrosis.
- Thrombotic microangiopathy.
- Nephrotic syndrome.
- Hereditary nephritis.
- Nephrolithiasis.

WORKUP

Initial evaluation of suspected glomerulonephritis consists of laboratory testing.

LABORATORY TESTS

- Urinalysis (hematuria [dysmorphic erythrocytes and red cell casts], proteinuria).
- Blood urea nitrogen and serum creatinine (to estimate glomerular filtration rate [GFR]).
- 24-hr urine for protein excretion and creatinine clearance (to document degree of renal dysfunction and amount of proteinuria). Random urine (spot specimen) protein-to-creatinine ratio is also acceptable in place of a 24-hour collection. Proteinuria in acute glomerulonephritis typically ranges from 500 mg per day to 3 g per day, but nephrotic-range proteinuria (>3.5 g per day) may be present.

- Streptococcal tests (Streptozyme), antistreptolysin O (ASO) quantitative titer (highest in 3 to 5 weeks); ASO titer, however, is not related to severity of renal disease, duration, or prognosis.
- Additional serologic testing: anti-DNA antibodies (rule out SLE), C3, C4, cryoglobulins, rheumatoid factor, hepatitis B and C serologies, antineutrophil cytoplasmic antibodies (MPO and PR3), and anti–glomerular basement membrane antibodies, serum and urine protein electrophoresis, and serum kappa and lambda free light chains.
- Hematocrit and platelet count (decreased in thrombotic microangiopathy).
- Blood cultures are indicated in all febrile patients.
- Antigens identified in glomerulonephritis are described in Table 3.

IMAGING STUDIES

- Chest x-ray: Pulmonary involvement may be seen in ANCA-associated vasculitis and Goodpasture syndrome.
- Renal ultrasound to evaluate renal size. A kidney size of <9 cm is suggestive of extensive scarring and low likelihood of reversibility.
- Echocardiogram in patients with new cardiac murmurs or positive blood cultures to rule out endocarditis and pericardial effusion.
- Renal biopsy with light, electron, and immunofluorescence microscopy to confirm diagnosis.
- Biopsy of other affected organs if systemic vasculitis is suspected.

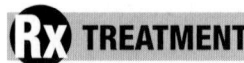

NONPHARMACOLOGIC THERAPY

- Low-salt diet if edema or hypertension is present
- Avoidance of high-potassium foods if patient is hyperkalemic

ACUTE GENERAL Rx

- Diuretics in patients with significant edema or hypertension.
- Correction of electrolyte abnormalities (hypocalcemia, hyperkalemia) and acidosis.
- High-dose steroids for rapidly progressive glomerulonephritis.
- Additional immunosuppressive treatment with alkylating agents, calcineurin inhibitors, or biologic agents (e.g., rituximab) may be necessary depending on the underlying disease.

TABLE 1 Summary of Primary Renal Diseases That Manifest as Acute Glomerulonephritis

Diseases	Poststreptococcal Glomerulonephritis	IgA Nephropathy	Goodpasture Syndrome	Idiopathic Rapidly Progressive Glomerulonephritis
Clinical Manifestations				
Age and sex	All ages, mean 7 yr, 2:1 male	10-35 yr, 2:1 male	15-30 yr, 6:1 male	Adults, 2:1 male
Acute nephritic syndrome	90%	50%	90%	90%
Asymptomatic hematuria	Occasionally	50%	Rare	Rare
Nephrotic syndrome	10%-20%	Rare	Rare	10%-20%
Hypertension	70%	30%-50%	Rare	25%
Acute renal failure	50% (transient)	Very rare	50%	60%
Other	Latent period of 1-3 wk	Follows viral syndromes	Pulmonary hemorrhage; iron deficiency anemia	None
Laboratory findings	↑ ASO titers (70%) Positive Streptozyme (95%)↓ C3-C9; normal C1, C4	↑ Serum IgA (50%) IgA in dermal capillaries	Positive anti-GBM antibody	Positive ANCA in some
Immunogenetics	HLA-B12, D "EN" (9)*	HLA-Bw 35, DR4 (4)*	HLA-DR2 (16)*	None established
Renal Pathology				
Light microscopy	Diffuse proliferation	Focal proliferation	Focal → diffuse proliferation with crescents	Crescentic GN
Immunofluorescence	Granular IgG, C3	Diffuse mesangial IgA	Linear IgG, C3	No immune deposits
Electron microscopy	Subepithelial humps	Mesangial deposits	No deposits	No deposits
Prognosis	95% resolve spontaneously 5% RPGN or slowly progressive	Slow progression in 25%-50%	75% stabilize or improve if treated early	75% stabilize or improve if treated early
Treatment	Supportive	Uncertain (options include steroids, fish oil, and ACE inhibitors)	Plasma exchange, steroids, cyclophosphamide	Steroid pulse therapy

ACE, Angiotensin-converting enzyme; *ANCA,* antineutrophil cytoplasmic antibody; *ASO,* anti–streptolysin O; *GBM,* glomerular basement membrane; *GN,* glomerulonephritis; *HLA,* human leukocyte antigen; *Ig,* immunoglobulin; *RPGN,* rapidly progressive glomerulonephritis.
*Relative risk.
From Kliegman RM et al: *Practical strategies in pediatric diagnosis and therapy,* ed 2, Philadelphia, 2004, Saunders.

TABLE 2 Diseases Associated with Rapidly Progressive Glomerulonephritis and Pertinent Laboratory Studies

Disease	Studies
Renal Limited	
IgA nephropathy	
Infection-related glomerulonephritis	Low complement, streptococcal serologies, Bacterial cultures Echocardiography
ANCA-associated glomerulonephritis (pauci-immune glomerulonephritis)	ANCA titers
Anti-GBM disease (Goodpasture syndrome)	Anti-GBM antibodies
Systemic Disorders	
Lupus nephritis	Low complement, ANA, dsDNA antibodies
ANCA-associated small-vessel vasculitis	ANCA titers
Goodpasture disease	Anti-GBM antibodies
Henoch-Schönlein purpura	None
Cryoglobulinemic vasculitis	Low complement, cryoglobulins, rheumatoid factor, hepatitis C serologies

ANCA, Antineutrophil cytoplasmic antibody; *ANA,* antinuclear antibodies; *dsDNA,* double-stranded DNA; *GBM,* glomerular basement membrane; *IgA,* immunoglobulin A.
From Vincent JL et al: *Textbook of critical care,* ed 6, Philadelphia, 2011, Saunders.

- Treatment of streptococcal infection with penicillin (or erythromycin in penicillin-allergic patients). Hemodialysis in patients with diuretic-resistant volume overload, hyperkalemia, uremic symptoms, and encephalopathy. Plasma exchange therapy for concurrent diffuse alveolar hemorrhage or rapidly progressive glomerulonephritis with a low GFR.
- Treatment of hepatitis C–associated glomerulonephritis is rapidly changing due to the introduction of direct-acting antiviral agents.
- Table 4 summarizes suggested management of idiopathic MPGN.

CHRONIC Rx

- Frequent monitoring of blood pressure, urinalysis, serum creatinine, serum albumin, and random urine for protein-to-creatinine ratio
- Angiotensin-converting enzyme (ACE) inhibitors or angiotensin receptor II blockers (ARBs) are used in patients with persistent proteinuria
- Lipid management with statins and fibrates as indicated
- Monitoring for side effects related to immunosuppression, such as infections, leukopenia and anemia, osteoporosis or osteopenia, gastrointestinal ulcers, high blood pressure, and tumors.

- Routine health maintenance with vaccinations for influenza and pneumococcal pneumonia, age-appropriate vaccinations, as well as age-appropriate malignancy screening. Live-vaccines are contraindicated in patients on immunosuppression.

DISPOSITION

- Prognosis is generally related to the initial serum creatinine and degree of fibrosis on biopsy.
- In general, prognosis is worse in patients with heavy proteinuria, low GFR at presentation, severe hypertension, and crescentic glomerulonephritis.
- Recovery of renal function occurs within 8 to 12 wk in 95% of patients with poststreptococcal glomerulonephritis.

REFERRAL

- Nephrology consultation for all patients with suspected glomerulonephritis. Urgent consultation is recommended if GFR is significantly abnormal or rapidly deteriorating or if the patient has systemic symptoms.

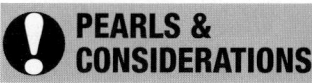
PEARLS & CONSIDERATIONS

COMMENTS

- Diagnosis of glomerulonephritis is made on kidney biopsy. Kidney biopsy is necessary when the histologic diagnosis will alter the treatment plan; this is usually the case in patients with systemic illnesses, significant proteinuria (>500 mg to 1 g per day),

TABLE 3 Antigens Identified in Glomerulonephritis

Poststreptococcal GN	Streptococcal pyrogenic exotoxin B, plasmin receptor
Anti-GBM disease	α3 type IV collagen (likely induced by molecular mimicry)
IgA nephropathy	Possibly no antigen but rather polymerized polyclonal IgA (?superantigen driven)
Membranous nephropathy	Phospholipase A_2 receptor (idiopathic), neutral endopeptidase in podocyte (congenital), HBeAg (hepatitis associated)
Staphylococcus aureus–associated GN	*Staphylococcus* superantigens induce polyclonal response; not necessarily antigen in glomeruli
Membranoproliferative GN	HCV and HBsAg in hepatitis-associated MPGN
ANCA-associated vasculitis	Proteinase 3 (c-ANCA) and myeloperoxidase (p-ANCA) in neutrophils; antibodies to lysosome-associated membrane protein 2 on endothelial cells (likely induced by molecular mimicry to fimbriated bacterial antigens)

ANCA, Antineutrophil cytoplasmic antibody; *GBM,* glomerular basement membrane; *GN,* glomerulonephritis; *HBeAg,* hepatitis B virus early antigen; *HBsAg,* hepatitis B surface antigen; *HCV,* hepatitis C virus; *IgA,* immunoglobulin A; *MPGN,* membranoproliferative glomerulonephritis.
From Floege J et al: *Comprehensive clinical nephrology,* ed 4, Philadelphia, 2010, Saunders.

TABLE 4 Suggested Management of Membranoproliferative Glomerulonephritis

Type	Treatment
All types	Supportive therapy following the recommendations discussed in text
Idiopathic MPGN in children	Non-nephrotic proteinuria, normal renal function: follow with 3-month visits Normal renal function and moderate proteinuria (>3 g/day): prednisone 40 mg/m² on alternate days for 3 months Nephrotic or impaired renal function: prednisone 40 mg/m² on alternate days (80 mg maximum) for 2 years, tapering to 20 mg on alternate days for 3-10 years
Idiopathic MPGN in adults	Non-nephrotic, normal renal function: follow with 3-month visits Nephrotic or impaired renal function: 6-month course of corticosteroid with/without cytotoxic agents (cyclophosphamide) or other drugs used: cyclosporine, tacrolimus, mycophenolate mofetil Rapidly progressive renal failure with diffuse crescents: treat as for idiopathic rapidly progressive glomerulonephritis In the presence of chronic renal failure or nephrotic proteinuria: angiotensin-converting enzyme inhibitors

MPGN, Membranoproliferative glomerulonephritis.
From Floege J et al: *Comprehensive clinical nephrology,* ed 4, Philadelphia, 2010, Saunders.

or rising serum creatinine. Not all patients with suspected glomerulonephritis require a kidney biopsy because of success with supportive therapies (e.g., infection-related GN). A search for systemic illness, including infections, autoimmune disease, and malignancy is needed with careful history, physical examination, and serologic tests.

- Nephrology consultation is necessary before initiation of immunosuppressive therapy. In the absence of contraindications to their use, ACE inhibitor or ARB therapy is essential for proteinuria reduction. Aldosterone receptor antagonists may be used for additional reduction in proteinuria.
- Monitoring of lipids and aggressive treatment of hyperlipidemia is recommended when persistent disease is present.
- Close monitoring of side effects of immunosuppressive drugs and complications of corticosteroids is necessary.

SUGGESTED READINGS
Available at www.expertconsult.com

RELATED CONTENT
Glomerulonephritis (Patient Information)
Acute Kidney Injury (Related Key Topic)

AUTHOR: **RUPALI AVASARE, M.D.**

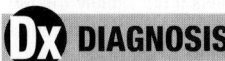 BASIC INFORMATION

DEFINITION

Glossitis is an inflammation of the tongue that can lead to loss of filiform papillae.

ICD-10CM CODES
K14.0 Glossitis
K14.2 Median rhomboid glossitis

EPIDEMIOLOGY & DEMOGRAPHICS

Glossitis is seen more frequently in patients of lower socioeconomic status, malnourished patients, alcoholics, smokers, elderly patients, immunocompromised patients, and patients with dentures.

PHYSICAL FINDINGS & CLINICAL PRESENTATION

- The appearance of the tongue varies depending on the etiology of the glossitis (Fig. E1). Loss of filiform papillae results in a red, smooth-surfaced tongue.
- The tongue may appear pale in patients with significant anemia.
- Pain and swelling of the tongue may be present when glossitis is associated with infections, trauma, or lichen planus.
- Ulcerations may be present in patients with herpetic glossitis, pemphigus, or streptococcal infection.
- Excessive use of mouthwash may result in a "hairy" appearance of the tongue (Fig. E2)

ETIOLOGY

- Nutritional deficiencies (vitamin E, riboflavin, niacin, vitamin B_{12}, iron).
- Infections (viral, candidiasis, tuberculosis, syphilis).
- Trauma (generally caused by poorly fitting dentures).
- Irritation of the tongue from toothpaste, medications, alcohol, tobacco, citrus.
- Lichen planus, pemphigus vulgaris, erythema multiforme.
- Neoplasms.

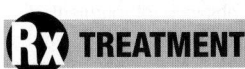 DIAGNOSIS

DIFFERENTIAL DIAGNOSIS

- Infections.
- Use of chemical irritants.
- Neoplasms.
- Skin disorders (e.g., Behçet's syndrome, erythema multiforme).

WORKUP

- Laboratory evaluation to exclude infectious processes, vitamin deficiencies, and systemic disorders,
- Biopsy of lesion only when there is no response to treatment,

LABORATORY TESTS

- Complete blood count: decreased hemoglobin and hematocrit, low mean corpuscular volume (MCV) (iron-deficiency anemia), elevated MCV (vitamin B_{12} deficiency).
- Vitamin B_{12} level.
- 10% KOH scrapings in patients with white patches suspect for candidiasis.

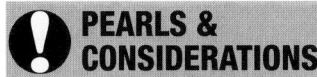 TREATMENT

NONPHARMACOLOGIC THERAPY

Avoidance of primary irritants such as hot foods, spices, tobacco, and alcohol.

ACUTE GENERAL Rx

Treatment varies with the etiology of the glossitis.
- Malnutrition with avitaminosis: multivitamins.
- Candidiasis: fluconazole 200 mg on day 1, then 100 mg/day for at least 2 wk or nystatin 400,000 U suspension qid for 10 days or 200,000 pastilles dissolved slowly in the mouth four to five times qd for 10 to 14 days.
- Painful oral lesions: rinsing of the mouth with 2% lidocaine viscous, 1 to 2 tablespoons q4h prn; triamcinolone 0.1% applied to painful ulcers prn for symptomatic relief.

CHRONIC Rx

- Lifestyle changes with elimination of tobacco, alcohol, and other primary irritants.
- Dental evaluation for correction of ill-fitting dentures.
- Correction of associated metabolic abnormalities such as hyperglycemia from diabetes mellitus.

DISPOSITION

Most patients experience prompt improvement with identification and treatment of the cause of the glossitis.

REFERRAL

Surgical referral for biopsy of solitary lesions unresponsive to treatment to rule out neoplasm.

PEARLS & CONSIDERATIONS

COMMENTS

If the primary cause of glossitis is not identified or cannot be corrected, enteric nutritional replacement therapy should be considered in malnourished patients.

RELATED CONTENT

Glossitis (Patient Information)

AUTHOR: **FRED F. FERRI, M.D.**

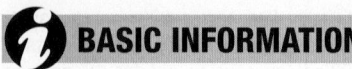

BASIC INFORMATION

DEFINITION

Gonorrhea is a sexually transmitted bacterial infection with a predilection for columnar and transitional epithelial cells. It commonly manifests as urethritis, cervicitis, or salpingitis. Infection may be asymptomatic. It differs between males and females in course, severity, and ease of recognition.

SYNONYMS

Gonococcal urethritis
Gonococcal vulvovaginitis
Gonococcal cervicitis
Gonococcal bartholinitis
GC

ICD-10CM CODES

A54.9	Gonococcal infection, unspecified
O98.211	Gonorrhea complicating pregnancy, first trimester
O98.212	Gonorrhea complicating pregnancy, second trimester
O98.213	Gonorrhea complicating pregnancy, third trimester
O98.219	Gonorrhea complicating pregnancy, unspecified trimester
O98.22	Gonorrhea complicating childbirth
O98.23	Gonorrhea complicating the puerperium
A54.03	Gonococcal cervicitis, unspecified
A54.00	Gonococcal infection of lower genitourinary tract, unspecified

EPIDEMIOLOGY & DEMOGRAPHICS

- The disease is common worldwide, affects both sexes and all ages, especially younger adults; highest incidence is in inner-city areas, with an estimated 820,000 new cases annually. Gonorrhea is the second most commonly reported communicable disease.
- Asymptomatic anterior urethral carriage may occur in 12% to 50% of cases in men.
- Asymptomatic in 50% to 80% of cases in women. Most common dissemination by mucosal passage to fallopian tubes, resulting in pelvic inflammatory disease (PID) in 10% to 15% of infected women. Hematogenous spread may result in septic arthritis and skin lesions. Conjunctivitis rarely occurs but may result in blindness if not rapidly treated. Infection can occur in both men and women in oropharynx and anorectally.
- 700,000 new infections per year (second most commonly reported bacterial STD).

PHYSICAL FINDINGS & CLINICAL PRESENTATION

- Males: purulent discharge from anterior urethra (Fig. 1, with dysuria appearing 2 to 7 days after infecting exposure. May have rectal infection causing pruritus, tenesmus, and discharge or may be asymptomatic.
- Females: initial urethritis or cervicitis may occur a few days after exposure, frequently mild. Infections may be asymptomatic or may not produce recognizable symptoms until complications have occurred. In approximately 20% of cases uterine invasion occurs after menstrual period with signs and symptoms of endometritis, salpingitis, or pelvic peritonitis. The patient may have purulent discharge or inflamed Skene or Bartholin glands.
- Classic presentation of acute gonococcal PID is fever, abdominal and adnexal tenderness, and often absence of purulent discharge. Physical examination may be normal if asymptomatic. Disseminated gonococcal infection (DGI) may manifest with petechial or pustular acral skin lesions (Fig. 2), asymmetric polyarthralgia, tenosynovitis, or oligoarticular septic arthritis. The infection is complicated occasionally by perihepatitis and rarely endocarditis or meningitis.

ETIOLOGY

- *Neisseria gonorrhoeae* is the gonococcus. Plasmids coding for β-lactamase render some strains resistant to penicillin or tetracycline. There is an increasing frequency of chromosomally mediated resistance to penicillin, tetracycline, fluoroquinolones, and cefoxitin. In the Far East, high-level resistance to spectinomycin is endemic.
- There are a rising number of cases of quinolone-resistant *N. gonorrhoeae* worldwide, with the expected number to rise in the U.S. from importation.
- Men who have sex with men are vulnerable to the emerging threat of antimicrobial-resistant *N. gonorrhoeae.*

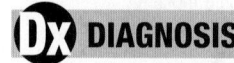 DIAGNOSIS

DIFFERENTIAL DIAGNOSIS

- Nongonococcal urethritis (NGU)
- Nongonococcal mucopurulent cervicitis
- *Chlamydia trachomatis*

WORKUP

Diagnosis depends on bacteriologic investigation. Culture and nucleic acid amplification tests (NAAT) are available for the detection of genitourinary infection with *N. gonorrhoeae.*

- NAATs are preferred testing modalities for the detection of genitourinary infection with *N. gonorrhoeae.* The performance of NAATs with respect to overall sensitivity, specificity, and ease of specimen transport is better than that of any of the other tests available for the diagnosis of gonococcal infections. NAATs should be used to detect gonorrhea except in cases of child sexual assault involving boys and rectal and oropharyngeal infections in prepubescent girls and when evaluating a potential gonorrhea treatment failure, in which case culture and susceptibility testing might be required. NAATs allow testing of the widest variety of specimen types, including endocervical swabs, vaginal swabs, urethral swabs (men), and urine (from both men and women).
- Culture: Gonorrhea culture on Thayer-Martin medium (organism is fastidious; requires aerobic conditions with increased carbon dioxide atmosphere; incubate ASAP). Culture has a sensitivity of 95% or more for urethral specimens from men with symptomatic urethritis and 80% to 90% for endocervical infection in women. Gram-negative intracellular diplococci are diagnostic in male urethral smears (Fig. 3). There is a false-negative rate of 60% to 70% in female cervical or urethral smears.
  - Concomitant serologic testing for syphilis for all patients
  - Concomitant *Chlamydia* testing for all patients
  - Offer of HIV testing and counseling to all patients

LABORATORY TESTS

- Gonorrhea culture on Thayer-Martin medium (organism is fastidious; requires aerobic conditions with increased carbon dioxide atmosphere; incubate ASAP). Culture has a sensitivity of 95% or more for urethral specimens from men with symptomatic urethritis and 80% to 90% for endocervical infection in women.

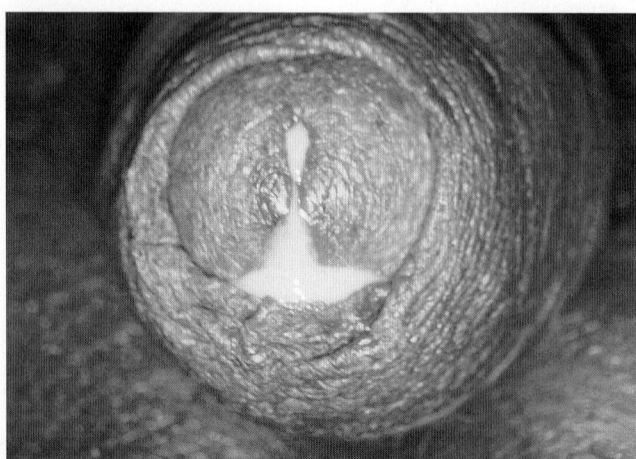

FIG. 1 Purulent urethral discharge from a man with gonococcal urethritis. (From Mandell GL et al: *Principles and practice of infectious diseases,* ed 6, Philadelphia, 2005, Churchill Livingstone.)

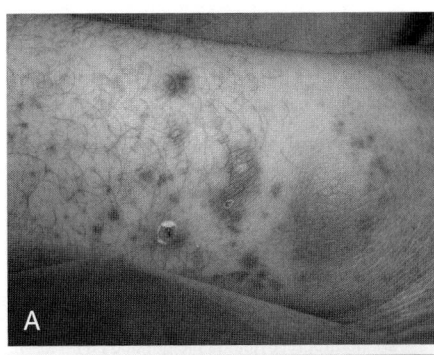
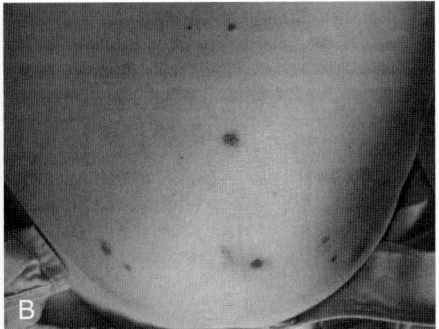
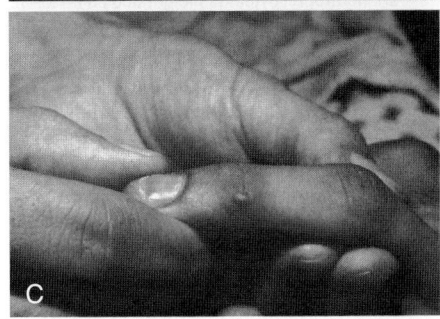

Diseases and Disorders

I

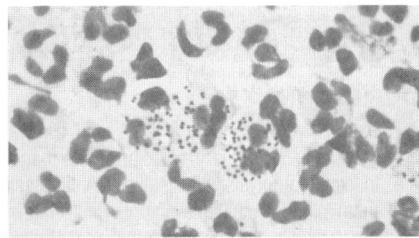

FIG. 3 _Neisseria gonorrhoeae._ Gram stain of urethral exudate in gonorrhea, showing intracellular gram-negative reniform diplococci. (Courtesy of Dr. S.E. Thompson. From Hochberg MC et al: _Rheumatology,_ ed 5, St Louis, 2011, Mosby.)

FIG. 2 Disseminated gonococcal infection: skin lesions. A, Macules, papules, and pustules over an ankle. **B,** Hemorrhagic papules localized in trunk. **C,** Hemorrhagic vessel over a distal interphalangeal joint. (**C** Courtesy of Dr. Peter Schlessinger. From Hochberg MC et al: _Rheumatology,_ ed 5, St Louis, 2011, Mosby.)

- NAATs: These tests have largely replaced culture in many settings where persons are screened for asymptomatic genital infection. They are not more sensitive than culture for detecting _N. gonorrhoeae_ in cervical or urethral specimen; however, they have specificities >99% and retain sensitivity when used to test voided urine or self-collected vaginal swabs.
- Nonamplified DNA probe tests are less sensitive than culture or NAATs and are not useful in the diagnosis of rectal or pharyngeal infection or for testing urine; however, they are inexpensive, readily available and offered in many laboratories in combination assays for _C. trachomatis._
- Concomitant serologic testing for syphilis on all patients.
- Concomitant _Chlamydia_ testing on all patients.
- Offer of HIV testing and counseling to all patients.

Rx TREATMENT

ACUTE GENERAL Rx

Uncomplicated infections of the cervix, urethra, and rectum. Critical for the practitioner to know local resistance characteristics to best treat the patient:
- Ceftriaxone 250 mg IM × 1 dose _plus_ azithromycin 1 g PO single dose. Doxycycline 100 mg PO bid for 7 days can be substituted for azithromycin in patients with azithromycin allergy.

Alternative regimens if ceftriaxone is not available:
- Ceftizoxime (500 mg IM), cefoxitin (2 gm IM with probenecid 1 gm orally), and cefotaxime (500 mg IM). None of these injectable cephalosporins offer any advantage over ceftriaxone.
- Cefixime 400 mg PO × 1 dose _plus_ azithromycin 1 g orally single dose. Doxycycline 100 mg PO bid for 7 days can be substituted for azithromycin in patients with azithromycin allergy.

- If the patient has severe cephalosporin allergy, then azithromycin 2 g PO single dose _plus_ single-dose gemifloxacin 320 mg PO or gentamicin 240 mg IM.
- A test-of-cure is not needed for persons who receive a diagnosis of uncomplicated urogenital or rectal gonorrhea who are treated with any of the recommended or alternative regimens.

Uncomplicated gonococcal infections of the pharynx:
- Ceftriaxone 250 mg IM × 1 dose _plus_ azithromycin 1 g PO single dose. Doxycycline 100 mg PO bid for 7 days can be substituted for azithromycin in patients with azithromycin allergy.
- Treatment of the cephalosporin-allergic patient: oral azithromycin 2 g _plus_ single dose gemifloxacin 320 mg PO _or_ 240 mg IM of gentamicin is effective.
- Any person with pharyngeal gonorrhea who is treated with an alternative regimen should return 14 days after treatment for a test-of-cure using either culture or NAAT.

Treatment of arthritis and arthritis-dermatitis syndrome:
- Recommended regimen: Ceftriaxone 1 g IM or IV every 24 hours plus azithromycin 1 g orally as a single dose.
- Alternative regimens: Cefotaxime 1 g IV every 8 hours or ceftizoxime 1 g IV every 8 hours _plus_ azithromycin 1 g orally in a single dose.

DISPOSITION

- Pregnant women infected with _N. gonorrhoeae_ should be treated with dual therapy consisting of ceftriaxone 250 mg in a single IM dose or azithromycin 1 g PO as a single dose. When cephalosporin allergy or other considerations preclude treatment and

spectinomycin is not available, consultation with an ID specialist is recommended.
- To reduce development of drug resistance, reculture should be done for patients who show continued symptoms despite treatment. These patients should be tested with a culture-based gonorrhea test that can detect antibiotic resistance.
- All sexual partners should be identified, examined, tested, and receive presumptive treatment.

REFERRAL

PID requiring hospitalization, disseminated gonococcal infection

❗ PEARLS & CONSIDERATIONS

COMMENTS

- This is a reportable disease.
- The proportion of gonorrhea cases in heterosexual men who are fluoroquinolone resistant (QRNG) has reached 6.7%, an 11-fold increase from 0.6% in 2001. Fluoroquinolone antibiotics are no longer recommended to treat gonorrhea in the U.S.
- The use of azithromycin as the second antimicrobial is preferred over doxycycline due to the high prevalence of tetracycline resistance.
- The U.S. Preventive Services Task Force (USPSTF) recommends screening for gonorrhea in sexually active females 24 years or younger and in older women who are at increased risk for infection. The USPSTF also concludes that the current evidence is insufficient to assess the balance of benefits and harms of screening for gonorrhea in men.
- High-intensity counseling on sexual risk reduction has been shown to reduce sexually transmitted infections (STIs) in primary care and related settings.

SUGGESTED READINGS

Available at www.expertconsult.com

RELATED CONTENT

Gonorrhea (Patient Information)
Cervicitis (Related Key Topic)
Chlamydia Genital Infections (Related Key Topic)
Pelvic Inflammatory Disease (Related Key Topic)

AUTHOR: **RUBEN ALVERO, M.D.**

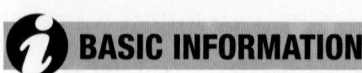

DEFINITION

A pulmonary-renal syndrome is defined as the coexistence of pulmonary alveolar hemorrhage (i.e., triad of hemoptysis, diffuse alveolar infiltrates, and anemia) and acute kidney injury, usually manifesting as rapidly progressive glomerulonephritis. Goodpasture *disease* refers specifically to alveolar hemorrhage and rapidly progressive glomerulonephritis (RPGN) caused by an anti–glomerular basement membrane (anti–GBM) antibody.

SYNONYMS

Anti–glomerular basement membrane disease
Goodpasture syndrome

ICD-10CM CODES
N01.7 Rapidly progressive nephritic syndrome with diffuse crescentic glomerulonephritis
N00.7 Acute nephritic syndrome with diffuse crescentic glomerulonephritis

EPIDEMIOLOGY & DEMOGRAPHICS

- Goodpasture disease affects predominantly young, white, male smokers
- Male-to-female ratio is 6:1
- Goodpasture disease accounts for 5% of all cases of RPGN
- HLA-BR2 positive is positive in 80% of patients
- Goodpasture disease may occur in up to 5% of syndrome patients with Alport disease who undergo kidney transplantation.

PHYSICAL FINDINGS & CLINICAL PRESENTATION

- Dyspnea, cough, hemoptysis
- Skin pallor, fever, arthralgias (may be mild or absent at the time of initial presentation)

ETIOLOGY

Goodpasture disease is caused by autoantibodies directed against type IV collagen, a primary component of the GBM. Antibody deposition leads to immune cell- and complement-mediated tissue damage that results in pulmonary hemorrhage and glomerulonephritis.

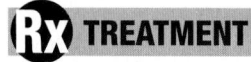 DIAGNOSIS

DIFFERENTIAL DIAGNOSIS

- Granulomatosis with polyangiitis
- Systemic lupus erythematosus
- Churg-Strauss syndrome
- Essential mixed cryoglobulinemia
- Idiopathic rapidly progressive glomerulonephritis
- Drug-induced renal pulmonary disease (e.g., penicillamine)

WORKUP

Laboratory evaluation, diagnostic imaging, and kidney biopsy

LABORATORY TESTS

- Serum anti-GBM antibodies.
- Absence of circulating immune complexes, antineutrophil cytoplasmic antibodies (ANCAs), and cryoglobulins.
- Urinalysis with microscopic hematuria, proteinuria, and red blood cell casts.
- Elevated blood urea nitrogen and creatinine.
- Immunofluorescence studies of kidney biopsy material demonstrates linear deposition of anti-GBM antibody, often with C3 deposition.
- Complete blood count and serum iron studies demonstrate anemia and iron deficiency from blood loss and iron sequestration in the lungs.

IMAGING STUDIES

Chest radiograph with airspace disease composed of alveolar infiltrates or evidence of pulmonary hemorrhage (Fig. 1)

TREATMENT

ACUTE GENERAL Rx

- Apheresis with albumin replacement for 1 to 2 weeks with ongoing immunosuppressive and medical therapy consisting of prednisone (1 mg/kg/day) and oral cyclophosphamide (2 mg/kg/day).
- Hemodialysis support in patients with renal failure.
- Factors influencing the decision to treat or not to treat aggressively in Goodpasture disease are described in Table 1.

DISPOSITION

Life-threatening pulmonary hemorrhage and irreversible glomerular damage are the major causes of death.

REFERRAL

- Referral for kidney biopsy to guide the management.
- Consider kidney transplantation in patients with end-stage renal disease.

SUGGESTED READING

Available at www.expertconsult.com

RELATED CONTENT

Goodpasture Syndrome (Patient Information)

AUTHOR: **KAUSIK UMANATH, M.D., M.S.**

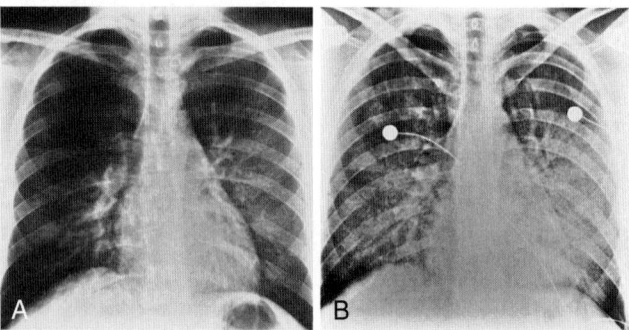

FIG. 1 Lung hemorrhage. A, Patient with early pulmonary hemorrhage. The chest radiograph still appears normal. **B,** Radiograph taken 4 days later shows the evolution of alveolar shadowing caused by lung hemorrhage. (From Floege J et al: *Comprehensive clinical nephrology,* ed 4, Philadelphia, 2010, Saunders, p. 285.)

TABLE 1 Factors Influencing Decision to Treat Aggressively in Goodpasture Disease

	Factors Favoring Aggressive Treatment	Factors Against Aggressive Treatment
Pulmonary hemorrhage	Present	Absent
Oliguria	Absent	Present
Creatinine	<5.5 mg/dl (~500 μmol/L)	>5.5–6.5 mg/dl (~500–600 μmol/L) and ANCA negative Severe damage on kidney biopsy No desire for early kidney transplantation
Other factors	Creatinine >5.5–6.5 mg/dl (~500–600 μmol/L) Rapid and recent progression ANCA-positive status Glomerular damage less severe than expected Crescents recent, nonfibrous Early renal transplantation desired	
Associated disease	Absent	Unusually high risk from immunosuppression

ANCA, Antineutrophil cytoplasmic antibody.
From Floege J et al: *Comprehensive clinical nephrology,* ed 4, Philadelphia, 2010, Saunders.

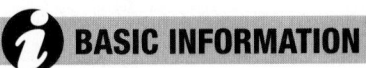

BASIC INFORMATION

DEFINITION

Gout is a term used to refer to a group of disease states caused by tissue deposition of monosodium urate due to prolonged hyperuricemia. Clinical manifestations of gout include acute and chronic arthritis, soft tissue inflammation, tophus formation, gouty nephropathy, and nephrolithiasis. Untreated hyperuricemia in patients with gout may lead to chronic destructive deforming arthritis.

ICD-10CM CODES
M10	Gout
M10.0	Idiopathic gout
M10.2	Drug-induced gout
M10.3	Gout due to impairment of renal function
M10.4	Other secondary gout
M10.9	Gout, unspecified
M10.1	Lead-induced gout

EPIDEMIOLOGY & DEMOGRAPHICS

PREVALENCE: 5 cases per 1000 persons in the U.S. Globally 8 cases per 10,000. Incidence is rising.
PREDOMINANT SEX: Male:female ratio ~4:1.
PREDOMINANT AGE: 30 to 50 years in men. Older than 60 years in women.

ETIOLOGY

- Gout is induced by inflammation from monosodium urate (MSU) crystal deposition. The primary risk factor for MSU deposition is hyperuricemia, though local factors such as temperature, pH, and mechanical stress may play a role.
- Hyperuricemia and gout develop from excessive uric acid production, a decrease in the renal excretion of uric acid, or both.
- Primary hyperuricemia results from an inborn error of metabolism and may be attributed to several biochemical defects.
- Secondary hyperuricemia may develop as a complication of acquired disorders (e.g., leukemia) or as a result of the use of certain drugs (e.g., diuretics). Consumption of alcohol, especially beer, increases the risk of gout, and fructose-rich beverage intake is associated with hyperuricemia.

PHYSICAL FINDINGS & CLINICAL PRESENTATION

ACUTE GOUT:
- Rapid onset of pain and swelling and erythema of a distal joint and/or periarticular soft tissue. Table 1 summarizes key components of gout flares.
- May present as monoarthritis of any joint. Acute gout of the first metatarsophalangeal (MTP) joint (Fig. E1) is known as *podagra*.
- 10% to 15% of attacks are polyarticular.
- Spontaneous resolution occurs over days to weeks.

CHRONIC TOPHACEOUS GOUT (FIG. E2):
- Insidious onset of painless arthritis and soft tissue swelling
- Distal small joints characteristic
- May be confused with nodal osteoarthritis

TABLE 1   Key Components of Gout Flares

- Marked tenderness and swelling of affected joint
- Acute onset with maximum pain in 4-12 hr
- Recurrent pattern of similar attacks
- Marked impairment of physical function
- Resolution of symptoms within 3-14 days

From Hochberg MC et al: *Rheumatology*, ed 5, St Louis, 2011, Mosby.

DIAGNOSIS

DIFFERENTIAL DIAGNOSIS OF ACUTE GOUT
- Infectious arthritis cellulitis
- Pseudogout
- Trauma

DIFFERENTIAL DIAGNOSIS OF CHRONIC GOUT
- Osteoarthritis (especially nodal OA in women)
- Rheumatoid arthritis
- Psoriatic arthritis
  Section II describes the differential diagnosis of acute monoarticular and oligoarticular arthritis.

WORKUP
Arthrocentesis and examination of synovial fluid

LABORATORY TESTS
- Uric acid: All patients with gout are hyperuricemic at some time, but during an acute attack the serum uric acid may be normal or low.
- Synovial aspirate: usually cloudy and markedly inflammatory in nature. Urate crystals in fluid are needle-shaped and strongly negatively birefringent under polarized microscopy (Fig. E3).
- CBC: mild leukocytosis often present.
- Inflammatory markers: ESR and CRP often elevated.

IMAGING STUDIES
- Plain radiography for diagnosis and evaluation. Not generally indicated in typical gout presentation.
- No typical findings in early gouty arthritis, but late disease is associated with characteristic punched-out marginal erosions and overhanging edges.
- Musculoskeletal ultrasound has been shown to be an effective means of detecting monosodium urate crystal deposition. Ultrasound can differentiate urate crystals that are found on the surface of articular cartilage from CPPD crystals that are seen within the substance of the cartilage (Fig. 4).

TREATMENT OPTIONS FOR ACUTE GOUT

- Nonsteroidal antiinflammatory medication (see Table 2).
  ○ Indomethacin 75 mg bid
  ○ Ibuprofen 800 mg tid

  ○ Naproxen 500 mg bid
  ○ Celecoxib 800 mg, then 400 mg/day
- Low-dose colchicine (less toxic and as effective as traditional high-dose colchicine): 1.2 mg colchicine PO, followed by 0.6 mg PO 1 hr later.
- Intraarticular corticosteroid injection (treatment of choice for monoarticular large joint attack): triamcinolone acetonide 40 mg or equivalent for knee.
- Systemic corticosteroid therapy: prednisone 40 mg PO for 3 days, then taper over 10 days (effective and safe, but evidence is lacking).

NONPHARMACOLOGIC THERAPY

Lifestyle and dietary modification may be effective in highly motivated patients. Recommendations include reducing ingestion of red meat, kidney, liver, yeast extract, shellfish, and overall protein along with restricting alcohol intake. These recommendations should be attempted only in patients with modestly elevated uric acid, as dietary modification can only lower uric acid 1 mg/dl. Discontinuation of diuretic therapy may help.

PHARMACOLOGIC TREATMENT OF SYMPTOMATIC HYPERURICEMIA

ALLOPURINOL: Allopurinol is very effective and safe when used properly. Correct dosing and patient compliance are essential elements in the prevention of erosive and tophaceous gout. Patients with renal insufficiency are at increased risk for allopurinol hypersensitivity, which manifests as fever, rash, and hepatitis occurring most commonly in the first 3 mo of therapy. The rash may progress to life-threatening toxic epidermal necrolysis if not recognized early.

Traditionally, therapy with allopurinol is initiated several weeks after the acute attack has resolved. However, initiation of allopurinol at presentation may improve long-term compliance without reducing the efficacy of acute treatment. The initial dose should be low (≤100 mg/day depending on creatinine clearance) in patients with renal insufficiency and those with very high uric acid levels. High initial doses are associated with increased incidence of allopurinol hypersensitivity. The serum uric acid should be reevaluated after 4 to 6 wk of therapy, and the allopurinol dose adjusted to reduce the serum uric acid to less than 6 mg/dl. The most common therapeutic dosage of allopurinol is 300 mg/day, but dose may be increased by 50 to 100 mg every 2 to 3 wk until the target serum uric acid level is achieved. There is evidence that increasing allopurinol doses in patients with renal insufficiency does not result in significant toxicity, but concurrent use with statins and colchicine is associated with a higher incidence of adverse effects. Some authors have reported using doses as high as 800 mg daily without excess toxicity. It is recommended that patients of Han Chinese, Thai, and Korean ancestry be tested for HLA-B*5801 before initiating allopurinol as these individuals are at high risk of allopurinol hypersensitivity if this antigen is present.

TABLE 2 Treatment of Gout

Acute Gout	Interval Gout	Treatment of Hyperuricemia
NSAIDs (preferred): Indomethacin 50 mg qid or ibuprofen 800 mg tid (or other NSAID in full doses). Contraindicated in patients with renal insufficiency and gastrointestinal disorders. *Or* **Colchicine, oral:** 1.2 mg followed by a second dose of 0.6 mg 1 hr later. Contraindicated in patients with renal insufficiency and gastrointestinal disorders *Or* **Intraarticular steroids** (Treatment of choice for large joint monoarthritis): Triamcinolone 40 mg or equivalent for knee *Or* Systemic steroid therapy (for patients in whom NSAIDs and colchicine are contraindicated) Prednisone 30-50 mg PO daily or in divided doses. May use lower dose in diabetic or postsurgical patients.	**Colchicine, oral:** 0.6-1.2 mg/day as prophylaxis against recurrent attacks. **NSAIDs may also be used for prophylaxis.** **Hypouricemic agent:** Indicated for patients with recurrent attacks despite prophylaxis, severe hyperuricemia, presence of tophi, urolithiasis, or gouty arthritis **Other:** Weight loss, reduce alcohol (especially beer), diet low in seafood, red meat, organ meat, and fructose	**Colchicine, oral:** 0.6-1.2 mg/day for 4-6 wk before initiating hypouricemic therapy and for several months afterward to prevent recurrent attacks during initiation of hypouricemic therapy. *And* **Allopurinol:** Initial dose 100 mg/day in patients with renal insufficiency or very high uric acid levels. Increase dose as needed to attain uric acid less than 6 mg/dl. *Or* **Uricosuric agent** (Use only in patients with good renal function and <600 mg uric acid in a 24-hr collection): probenecid, 0.5-1 g bid, or sulfinpyrazone 100 mg tid or qid **Other:** Consider febuxostat for patients allergic to allopurinol. Pegloticase may be useful for selected patients with severe tophaceous gout.

NSAIDs, Nonsteroidal antiinflammatory drugs.

FEBUXOSTAT: Febuxostat is a xanthine oxidase inhibitor that has been shown to be more potent than allopurinol 300 mg daily for reducing serum uric acid. The chemical structure of febuxostat is different from allopurinol, making cross-reactive allergy unlikely. The metabolism of febuxostat is primarily hepatic, which obviates the need for dose adjustments due to renal insufficiency. Some cases of hepatic toxicity have been reported, and it is recommended that liver function tests be monitored periodically. Febuxostat may help preserve renal function in patients with chronic kidney disease (CKD) but has not been tested in patients with severe renal failure.

The primary indication for febuxostat is demonstrated allergy to allopurinol. The cost of febuxostat may be as much as 40 times that of allopurinol.

PROBENECID: Uricosuric agents may be used in patients with good renal function and urinary uric acid less than 600 mg in a 24-hr collection. Probenecid can be used in patients with intolerance to xanthene-oxidase inhibitors. Compliance is poor due to the necessity of taking the drug more often than once daily. In December 2015, the U.S. Food and Drug Administration (FDA) approved lesinurad, which is an inhibitor of the URAT1 transport enzyme, for treatment of hyperuricemia in patients with gout who have not achieved target serum acid

levels with xanthine oxidase inhibitors alone. The approved dose is 200 mg PO qd, and lesinurad must be taken in combination with a xanthene oxidase inhibitor.

LESINURAD: Uric acid transporter 1 (URAT 1) inhibitor recently FDA-approved for gout-associated hyperuricemia unresponsive to xanthine oxidase inhibitor monotherapy. It prevents reuptake of uric acid at the proximal renal tubule. Dosage is 200 mg once daily taken with allopurinol or febuxostat. Increased fluid intake (at least 2 L of liquid per day) and frequent monitoring of renal function is necessary. This drug should not be used in patients with CrCl <45 ml/min.

PEGLOTICASE: Intravenous PEGylated uricase is FDA-approved for treatment of severe refractory tophaceous gout. It is a PEGylated recombinant mammalian uricase that rapidly degrades urate when given intravenously. Use is limited by very high cost and significant toxicities, including frequent gout flares and anaphylaxis.

PATIENT/FAMILY EDUCATION

It is essential that patients, families, physicians, and other members of the health care team appreciate the importance of compliance with a daily allopurinol regimen if recurrent flares and progression to chronic arthritis and tophi are to be avoided. Allopurinol should be

discontinued only for symptoms suggesting the hypersensitivity syndrome. It should be continued during flares, medical illnesses, and surgical procedures.

REFERRAL

- Rheumatologist if diagnosis is not clear or therapy is complicated
- Podiatrist for management of pedal complications

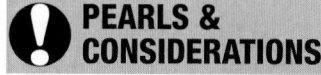
PEARLS & CONSIDERATIONS

Do not stop allopurinol during hospitalizations, surgery, or acute attacks unless there is evidence of drug allergy.

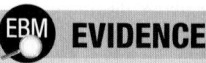
EVIDENCE

Available at www.expertconsult.com

SUGGESTED READINGS

Available at www.expertconsult.com

RELATED CONTENT

Gout (Patient Information)
Hyperuricemia (Related Key Topic)

AUTHOR: **BERNARD ZIMMERMANN, M.D**

BASIC INFORMATION

DEFINITION

Granuloma annulare (GA) is a chronic, usually self-limited, inflammatory disorder of the dermis that classically presents as arciform to annular plaques located on the extremities.

SYNONYMS

Pseudorheumatoid nodule—subcutaneous granuloma annulare
GA

ICD-10CM CODES
L92.0 Granuloma annulare

EPIDEMIOLOGY & DEMOGRAPHICS

- Most common in children and young adults; most cases of localized GA are diagnosed in patients <30 yr.
- Female predominance (2:1).
- Disseminated form associated with diabetes mellitus.
- Recurrent in 40% of affected individuals.
- A generalized form of GA can occur in up to 15% of patients.

PHYSICAL FINDINGS & CLINICAL PRESENTATION

- The main clinical variants of GA are localized (75%), disseminated (>10 lesions), subcutaneous (occurring primarily in children aged 2 to 5 yr), patch-type or macular GA, and perforating (rare form manifesting with 1- to 4-mm papules with a central crust usually appearing on the dorsal hands).
- Localized GA starts as a small ring of colored skin or pale erythematous papules. More common in children and young to middle-age adults. Usually, only one or a few lesions occur at any one time.
- Lesions coalesce and evolve into annular plaques over several weeks.
- Plaques undergo central involution and increase in diameter over several months (0.5 to 5 cm) (Fig. 1).
- Most frequently found on the lateral and dorsal surfaces of the hands and feet.
- Most lesions resolve spontaneously after several months.
- The generalized form of GA is characterized by hundreds of small (lesions rarely exceed 5 cm in diameter), flesh-colored papules in a symmetric distribution on the trunk and extremities. It most commonly affects women in the fifth or sixth decades but can also be seen in adolescents and children. Some patients are completely asymptomatic, whereas others complain of severe pruritus.
- Macular GA is more common in women between ages 30 to 70 and manifests with flat or slightly palpable erythematous or red-brown lesions on upper medial thighs and in bathing-trunk distribution.
- Deep dermal GA (subcutaneous GA) presents as large, painless, skin-colored nodules that are frequently mistaken for rheumatoid nodules.

ETIOLOGY

Unknown, but may be related to vasculitis, trauma, monocyte activation, or delayed hypersensitivity.

DIAGNOSIS

DIFFERENTIAL DIAGNOSIS

- Tinea corporis.
- Lichen planus.
- Necrobiosis lipoidica diabeticorum.
- Sarcoidosis.
- Rheumatoid nodules.
- Late secondary or tertiary syphilis.
- Arcuate and annular plaques of mycosis fungoides.
- Papular GA can simulate insect bites, secondary syphilis, xanthoma.
- Annular elastolytic giant cell granuloma.

WORKUP

- Diagnosis based on clinical appearance and presentation.
- Biopsy when diagnosis is unclear.

LABORATORY TESTS

- No laboratory tests will help confirm the diagnosis.
- Biopsy shows focal degeneration of collagen and elastic fibers, mucin deposition, and perivascular and interstitial lymphohistiocytic infiltrate in the upper and middle dermis.

TREATMENT

NONPHARMACOLOGIC THERAPY

Reassurance, given the self-limited and benign nature of GA

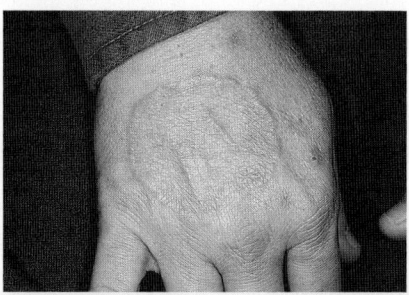
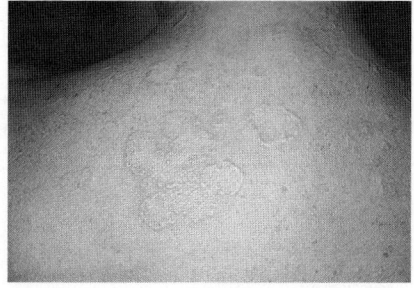

FIG. 1 Granuloma annulare. (From Callen JP [ed]: *Color atlas of dermatology,* ed 2, Philadelphia, 2000, Saunders.)

CHRONIC Rx

High-potency topical corticosteroids with or without occlusion and intralesional steroid injection into elevated border with triamcinolone 2.5 to 10 mg/ml are useful first-line local therapies.

- Cryosurgery, psoralen ultraviolet-A (UVA) range or UVA-1 therapy, and carbon dioxide laser treatment can also be used.
- Systemic agents (e.g., niacinamide, hydroxychloroquine, chloroquine, cyclosporine, dapsone) are generally reserved for severe cases. Recent case reports indicate positive outcomes with tacrolimus and pimecrolimus and the tumor necrosis factor infliximab.

DISPOSITION

Most lesions resolve spontaneously within 2 yr.

REFERRAL

Dermatology referral recommended for symptomatic, disseminated disease

PEARLS & CONSIDERATIONS

COMMENTS

GA has been described as a paraneoplastic granulomatous reaction to Hodgkin's disease, non-Hodgkin's lymphoma, solid organ tumors, and mycosis fungoides.

RELATED CONTENT

Granuloma Annulare (Patient Information)

AUTHOR: **FRED F. FERRI, M.D.**

BASIC INFORMATION

DEFINITION

Granulomatosis with polyangiitis (GPA), formerly known as "Wegener's granulomatosis," is a multisystem necrotizing vasculitis that generally affects the upper and lower respiratory tracts and the kidneys. It is characterized as an ANCA-associated granulomatous small-vessel vasculitis. Clinical manifestations depend on the tropism of blood vessel involvement and organ systems commonly affected beyond the respiratory tract and kidneys and include neurologic involvement and involvement of the skin and the musculoskeletal systems as well as the gastrointestinal tract.

The disease can also present in a limited form that is generally confined to the upper respiratory tract and can be managed less aggressively than the more diffuse systemic form.

SYNONYMS

GPA
Wegener's granulomatosis (WG)

ICD-10CM CODES
M31.3 Wegener's granulomatosis

EPIDEMIOLOGY & DEMOGRAPHICS

INCIDENCE: 3/100,000 in recent U.S. epidemiologic studies, equal in men and women, more common in whites.
MEAN AGE AT ONSET: 41 yr.

PHYSICAL FINDINGS & CLINICAL PRESENTATION

- Clinical manifestations often vary with the stage of the disease and degree of organ involvement; localized disease often has upper respiratory tract involvement without systemic vasculitis, whereas systemic disease stages include early systemic, generalized, and severe disease.
- Frequent manifestations are:
  1. Upper respiratory tract: chronic sinusitis, chronic otitis media, mastoiditis, nasal crusting, obstruction and epistaxis, nasal septal perforation, nasal lacrimal duct stenosis, saddle nose deformities (Fig. 1), and tracheal and subglottic stenosis. Up to 90% of patients with GPA have one or more nasal manifestations.
  2. Eyes: conjunctivitis, ulcerative keratosis, episcleritis or scleritis, optic neuropathy, nasolacrimal duct obstruction, retinal vasculitis, uveitis, proptosis.
  3. Ears: sensorineural and conductive hearing loss, otorrhea, and polychondritis.
  4. Mouth: chronic ulcerative lesions of the oral mucosa, "mulberry" gingivitis.
  5. Lung: nodules, pulmonary infiltrates or effusions, cavitary lesions, and frank hemoptysis (6%-85%).
  6. Kidney: rapidly progressive glomerulonephritis (38%-70%), microscopic hematuria with or without red cell casts, and proteinuria.
  7. Skin: cutaneous nodules over extensor surfaces of joints, necrotizing skin lesions, palpable purpura (30%-46%), urticaria, and livedo reticularis.
  8. Nervous system: mononeuritis multiplex and peripheral neuropathies (15%-40%), meningeal inflammation (pachymeningitis), headaches, and CNS involvement (7%-11%).
  9. Musculoskeletal: monoarthritis or polyarthritis (nondeforming), usually affecting large joints (60%).
  10. Constitutional: fever (23%-30%), weight loss (50%), and fatigue (61%).

ETIOLOGY

Unknown; believed to begin with granulomatous inflammation that progresses to systemic vasculitis

DIAGNOSIS

DIFFERENTIAL DIAGNOSIS

- Other granulomatous lung diseases (e.g., sarcoidosis, lymphomatoid granulomatosis, eosinophilic granulomatosis with polyangiitis [Churg-Strauss syndrome]), and necrotizing bronchocentric granulomatosis). The differential diagnosis of granulomatous lung disease is described in Section II. Table 1 describes differential diagnostic features of ANCA-associated vasculitis.
- Other ANCA-associated vasculitides, including microscopic polyangiitis.
- Goodpasture's disease and other causes of glomerulonephritis (e.g., poststreptococcal nephritis).
- Neoplasms (especially lymphoproliferative disease).
- Bacterial or fungal sinusitis.
- Viral infections.
- Cocaine-induced midline destructive lesions and levamisole-induced vasculitis.
- Other causes of glomerulonephritis (e.g., poststreptococcal nephritis).

WORKUP

- Granulomatosis with polyangiitis should be suspected in a patient presenting with sinus disease that is unresponsive to conventional treatment and/or pulmonary hemorrhage, glomerulonephritis, mononeuritis multiplex resulting in wrist drop or foot drop or progressive migratory arthralgias or arthritis.
- Chest x-ray, laboratory evaluation, PFTs, and tissue biopsy for granulomatous lesions (Fig. 2).

LABORATORY TESTS

- ANCA serology: Most patients with GPA have a positive test result for cytoplasmic pattern of ANCA (c-ANCA). In GPA, ANCAs are

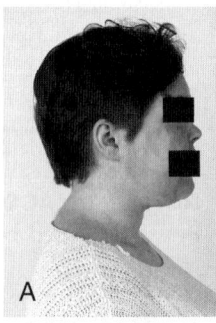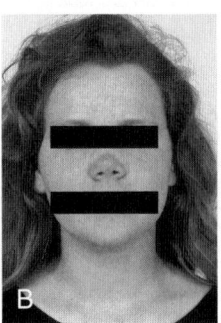

FIG. 1 Saddle-nose deformity in a patient with Wegener's granulomatosis. (From *Kelley's textbook of rheumatology,* ed 8, Philadelphia, 2009, Elsevier.)

TABLE 1 Differential Diagnostic Features of the Antineutrophil Cytoplasm Antibody–Associated Vasculitides

Feature	Microscopic Polyangiitis	GPA	AGPA	Comments
Glomerulonephritis	+++	+++	+	Progressive renal failure uncommon in AGPA
Pulmonary infiltrates or nodules	++	+++	+++	Asthma and eosinophilia in AGPA
Alveolar hemorrhage	++	++	+	
Upper airway disease	+	+++	++	Ear, nose, and throat disease usually favors GPA
Skin, purpura	+++	+	++	
Peripheral nerve involvement	+	++	+++	Often a prominent feature of AGPA
Central nervous system involvement	+	+	+	

+++, Very commonly seen; ++, seen often; +, uncommon finding; *AGPA,* allergic granulomatosis with polyangiitis; *GPA,* granulomatosis with polyangiitis.
From Firestein GS et al: *Kelly's textbook of rheumatology,* ed 9, Philadelphia, 2013, Saunders.

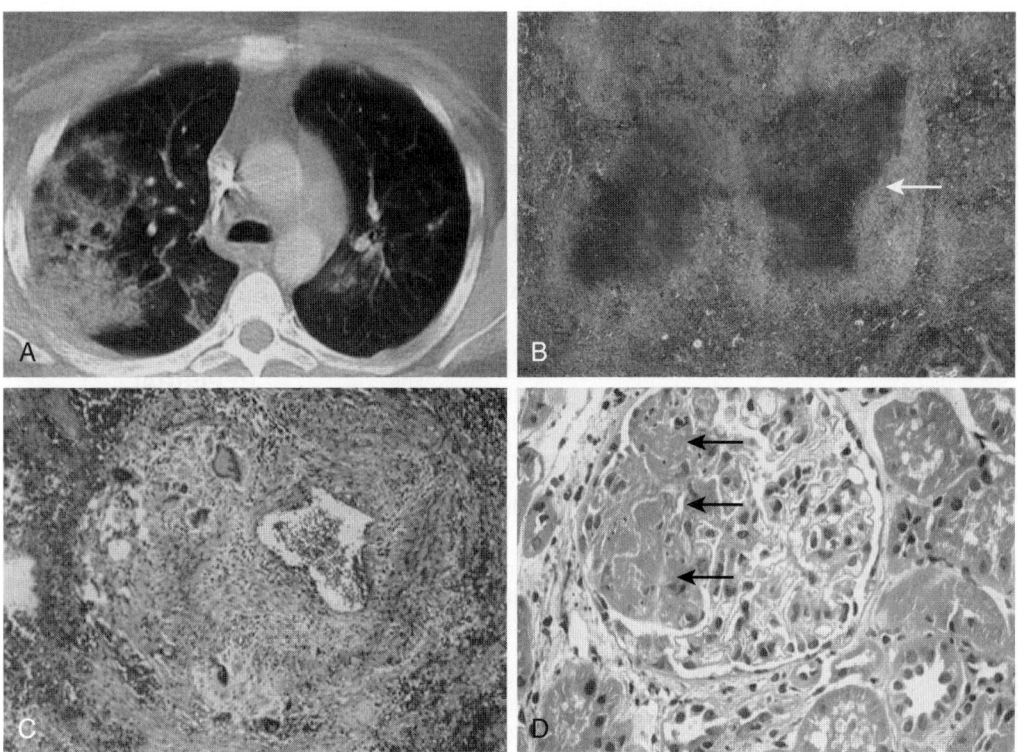

FIG. 2 A, Chest computed tomographic scan of a patient with granulomatosis with polyangiitis (GPA) shows typical nodular lung infiltrate with cavitation. **B,** Low-power view of granulomatous inflammation and geographic necrosis (*arrow*) in a lung biopsy from a patient with GPA. **C,** Granulomatous vasculitis involving a small pulmonary artery in the lung of a patient with GPA. The vessel wall is markedly thickened with an inflammatory infiltrate that includes multinucleated giant cells. **D,** Glomeruli showing segmental necrosis with early crescent formation (*arrows*). (Adkinson NF, et al: *Middleton's allergy principles and practice*, ed 8, Philadelphia, 2014, Saunders.)

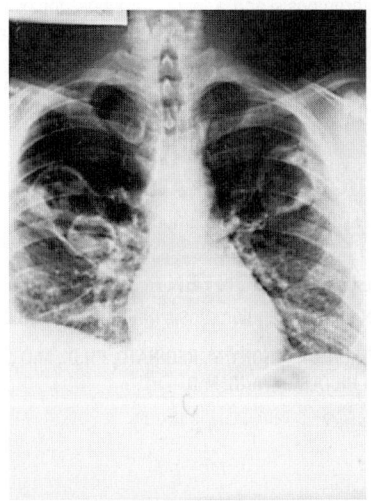

FIG. 3 Chest radiograph shows multiple cavitary pulmonary nodules in patient with Wegener's granulomatosis. (From Weinberg SE, et al: *Principles of pulmonary medicine*, ed 5, Philadelphia, 2008, Saunders.)

predominantly directed against proteinase 3 (anti-PR3), which is the confirmatory laboratory test in a patient with positive ANCA staining on immunofluorescence. However, between 10% and 15% of patients with GPA are positive for p-ANCA (usually MPO), and up to 10% are ANCA negative.

- CBC: anemia, leukocytosis, thrombocytosis (>400,000/μL).
- Chemistry: elevated serum creatinine, decreased creatinine clearance.
- Urinalysis: may reveal hematuria, RBC casts, and proteinuria.
- Inflammatory markers: increased ESR, positive rheumatoid factor, and elevated C-reactive protein may be found.
- Liver function, hepatitis serologies, cryoglobulins, HIV screens, ANA, C3-C4, and cultures to exclude other processes with similar constitutional symptoms.

IMAGING STUDIES

- Chest x-ray: may reveal bilateral multiple nodules, cavitary mass lesions, pleural effusion (20%). Up to one third of patients without pulmonary signs or symptoms have an abnormal chest x-ray (Fig. 3).
- Computed tomography (Fig. 4) or MRI (Fig. E5).
- PFTs: useful in detecting stenosis of the airways.
- Fiberoptic bronchoscopy and endoscopic ENT examination: nasal crusting ("golden crusts") are typical on evaluation (Fig. 6).
- Biopsy of one or more affected organs should be attempted; the most reliable source for tissue diagnosis is the lung. Lesions in the nasopharynx can be easily biopsied but biopsy is positive in only 20%. Biopsy of radiographically abnormal pulmonary parenchyma provides the highest yield (>90%).

Rx TREATMENT

NONPHARMACOLOGIC THERAPY

- Ensure proper airway drainage.
- Give nutritional counseling.

ACUTE GENERAL Rx

- Immunosuppressive therapy should be considered in all patients with GPA.
- Induction therapy in GPA consists of glucocorticoid with either cyclophosphamide or rituximab. Selected patients with severe disease may benefit from the addition of plasma exchange to this regimen.
- Historically, the gold standard for treatment is pulse methylprednisolone followed by prednisone 60 to 80 mg/day and pulse cyclophosphamide (1 g/m² every 4 weeks) or daily oral cyclophosphamide (2 mg/kg/day) was generally effective and used to control clinical manifestation. MESNA is required in intermittent pulses of cyclophosphamide for the prevention of cyclophosphamide-induced hemorrhagic cystitis.
- Based on the RAVE trial, rituximab (375 mg/m²/wk ×4 wk) appears to be more effective than traditional therapy in treating GPA that presents with disease flares and is at least as effective as traditional therapy for the induction of remission. The RITUXVAS trial concluded that a combined cyclophosphamide-rituximab regimen was not inferior to

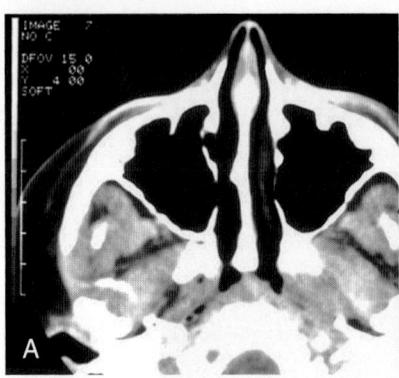
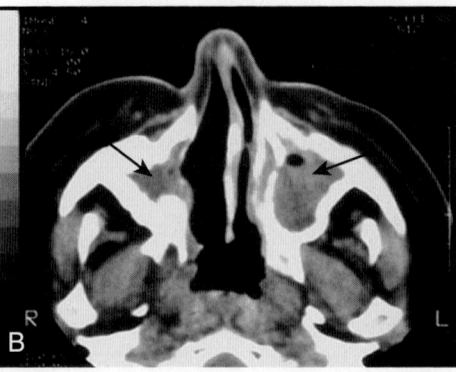

FIG. 4 Computed tomography (CT) scans of the sinuses. A, Normal maxillary sinuses in a recently diagnosed Wegener's granulomatosis (WG) patient. **B,** Sinus CT scan of a patient with long-standing WG: nasal septal deviation to the left, destruction of the medial walls of the right maxillary sinus, opacification of both sinuses with soft tissue densities *(arrows),* and neo-ossification of all maxillary bony structures due to chronic inflammation. (From Hochberg MC, et al: *Rheumatology,* ed 5, St Louis, 2011, Mosby.)

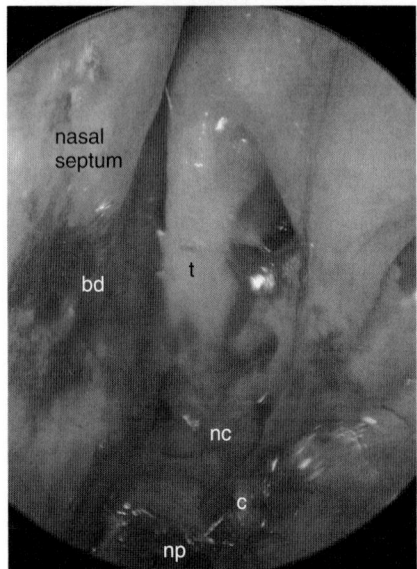

FIG. 6 Endoscopic view of nasal cavity of GPA patient showing crusting and bloody discharge. (From Holle, et al: *Rheum Dis Clin North Am* 36(3):507-526, 2010).

pulse cyclophosphamide alone. Both of these studies used concurrent methylprednisone followed by prednisone.
- Methotrexate and glucocorticoids alone may be used with mild extrarenal disease or little to no renal involvement.

- For severe active renal disease, the MEPEX trial demonstrated that plasma exchange in addition to cyclophosphamide and glucocorticoids may enhance renal function recovery.
- Potentially useful agents for maintenance therapy include rituximab, methotrexate, azathioprine, and mycophenolate mofetil. The MAINRITSAN trial showed that rituximab may be preferable for maintenance therapy, and the CYCAZAREM (for azathioprine) and LEM (for leflunomide) trials showed that these agents can also be used. The WEGENT study showed oral methotrexate and azathioprine were also noninferior for maintenance than intravenous cyclophosphamide.
- Maintenance therapy should generally be continued for 18 to 24 months, and, if ANCA positivity remains, even as long as 5 years.
- TMP-SMX therapy has a limited role in patients with lesions confined to the upper or lower respiratory tracts in absence of vasculitis or nephritis. Treatment with TMP-SMX (160 mg/800 mg bid) may reduce the incidence of relapses in patients with granulomatosis with polyangiitis in remission. It is also useful in preventing *Pneumocystis jirovecii* pneumonia (PJP), which occurs in 10% of patients receiving induction therapy. When used for prophylaxis, dose of TMP-SMX (160 mg/800 mg) is 1 tablet three times/week.
- In patients unable to tolerate TMP-SMX, often because of rash or allergy, PJP prophylaxis can also be achieved with dapsone, atovaquone, or inhaled pentamidine.

DISPOSITION
- Five-year survival with aggressive treatment is approximately 80%; without treatment 2-yr survival is 20%.
- Age >50 yr, impaired renal function, pulmonary involvement at diagnosis, and lack of ENT changes at diagnosis are all associated with worse outcomes and increased mortality rate.
- With standard therapy, remission is achieved by 90% to 94% of patients, but relapse is frequent (from 18% to 40% at 24 months.).

REFERRAL
- Rheumatology referral for continued treatment.
- ENT, surgical referral for biopsy

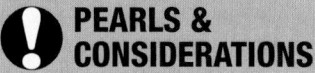
PEARLS & CONSIDERATIONS

COMMENTS
- Granulomatosis with polyangiitis is characterized by granulomatous lesions and vasculitis involving the respiratory tract, lung, and kidneys.
- C-ANCA levels should not dictate changes in therapy, because they correlate erratically with disease activity.
- The incidence of venous thrombotic events in patients with granulomatosis with polyangiitis is significantly higher than in the general population. Clinicians should maintain a heightened awareness of the risks of venous thrombosis and a lower threshold for evaluating patients for possible DVT or pulmonary embolism.
- Disease relapse remains a major problem in the course of the disease.

SUGGESTED READINGS
Available at www.expertconsult.com

RELATED CONTENT
Wegener's Granulomatosis (Patient Information).

AUTHORS: **ANTHONY M. REGINATO, PH.D., M.D.,** and **NICOLE B. YANG, M.D.**

BASIC INFORMATION

DEFINITION

Graves' disease is a hypermetabolic state caused by circulating IgG antibodies that bind to and activate the G-protein–coupled thyrotropin receptor. This activation stimulates follicular hypertrophy and hyperplasia, causing thyroid enlargement as well as increases in thyroid hormone production. It is characterized by thyrotoxicosis, diffuse goiter, and infiltrative ophthalmopathy (edema and inflammation of the extraocular muscles and an increase in orbital connective tissue and fat); infiltrative dermopathy characterized by lymphocytic infiltration of the dermis; accumulation of glycosaminoglycans; and occasionally edema.

SYNONYMS

Thyrotoxicosis

ICD-10CM CODES
E05.00	Thyrotoxicosis with diffuse goiter without thyrotoxic crisis or storm
E05.01	Thyrotoxicosis with diffuse goiter with thyrotoxic crisis or storm

EPIDEMIOLOGY & DEMOGRAPHICS

INCIDENCE/PREVALENCE: Graves' disease is the most common cause of hyperthyroidism. It affects 3% of women and 0.5% of men during their lifetime. There is a slight increased incidence among young African Americans. The annual incidence of Graves' disease-associated ophthalmopathy is 16 cases per 100,000 women and 3 cases per 100,000 men. It is more common in whites than Asians.
PREDOMINANT AGE: Peak incidence is between 30 and 60 yr.
GENETICS: Patients often report a family history of Hashimoto thyroiditis, Graves' disease, or other autoimmune conditions. Increased prevalence of HLA-B8 and HLA-DR3 in whites with Graves' disease. Concordance rate is 20% among monozygotic twins.

PHYSICAL FINDINGS & CLINICAL PRESENTATION

- Elevated systolic blood pressure with a widened pulse pressure.
- Diffusely enlarged thyroid. Thyroid bruit may be present.
- Tachycardia, palpitations, tremor, hyperreflexia.
- Exophthalmos (50% of patients), lid retraction (lid lag), in which contraction of the levator palpebrae muscles of the eyelids shows immobility of the upper eyelid with downward rotation of the eye.
- Nervousness, weight loss (weight gain in 10% of patients), heat intolerance, pruritus, muscle weakness, atrial fibrillation.
- Increased sweating, brittle nails, clubbing of fingers.
- Localized infiltrative dermopathy (1% to 2% of patients) is most frequent over the anterolateral aspects of the legs, commonly over the pretibial area (pretibial myxedema) (Fig. 1) but can be found at other sites (especially after trauma). It is typically patchy with a peau d'orange appearance to the skin.
- Men may have gynecomastia, reduced libido, and erectile dysfunction. Women often have irregular menses.

ETIOLOGY

Autoimmune etiology: the activity of the thyroid gland is stimulated by the action of T cells, which induce specific B cells to synthesize antibodies against thyroid-stimulating hormone (TSH) receptors in the follicular cell membrane.

DIAGNOSIS

DIFFERENTIAL DIAGNOSIS

- Anxiety disorder.
- Premenopausal state.
- Thyroiditis.
- Other causes of hyperthyroidism (e.g., toxic multinodular goiter, toxic adenoma).
- Other: metastatic neoplasm, diabetes mellitus, pheochromocytoma.

WORKUP

- The diagnosis is made clinically on most instances.
- The diagnostic workup includes a detailed medical history followed by laboratory and imaging studies and ECG. Patients often present with anxiety, heat intolerance, menstrual dysfunction, increased appetite, and weight loss. Elderly patients can have an atypical presentation (apathetic hyperparathyroidism). For additional information, refer to the topic "Hyperthyroidism."
- Table 1 describes the clinical assessment of the patient with Graves' ophthalmopathy.

LABORATORY TESTS

- Increased free thyroxine (T_4) and free triiodothyronine (T_3).
- Decreased TSH.
- Measurement of thyroid-stimulating antibodies (TSI) is generally reserved for patients without classic presentation of thyrotoxicity (see "Clinical Findings") to differentiate Graves' disease from toxic nodular goiter.

IMAGING STUDIES

- 24-hr radioactive iodine uptake (RAIU): increased homogeneous uptake.
- CT or MRI of the orbits (Fig. 2) is useful if there is uncertainty about the cause of ophthalmopathy.

TREATMENT

NONPHARMACOLOGIC THERAPY

- Patient education and discussion of therapeutic options.
- Smoking cessation: smoking is associated with an increased risk of progression of Graves' ophthalmopathy.

ACUTE GENERAL Rx

- Antithyroid drugs (ATDs) to inhibit thyroid hormone synthesis or peripheral conversion of T_4 to T_3:
  1. Methimazole or propylthiouracil (PTU) are available. Methimazole is generally preferred because it has a longer half-life, allowing for once-daily dosing. PTU is preferred during pregnancy.
  2. Side effects: skin rash (3% to 5%), arthralgias, myalgias, granulocytopenia (0.5%); rare side effects: aplastic anemia, hepatic necrosis (PTU), cholestatic jaundice.
  3. Thionamide antithyroid drug therapy results in a remission in 40% to 50% of patients treated for 12 to 18 months.
- Radioactive iodine (RAI):
  1. Treatment of choice for patients >21 yr and younger patients who have not achieved remission after 1 yr of ATD therapy
  2. Contraindicated during pregnancy and lactation
  3. Following radioactive therapy there may be an acute elevation of thyroid antibody titers and exacerbation of ocular symptoms in 15% to 20% of patients.
- Surgery: near-total thyroidectomy. Indications: obstructing goiters despite RAI and ATD therapy, patients who refuse RAI and cannot be adequately managed with ATDs, and pregnant women inadequately managed with ATDs. Complications of surgery include hypoparathyroidism (4%) and vocal cord paralysis (1%).
- Adjunctive therapy: Beta-adrenergic receptor blockers (e.g., atenolol 50 to 100 mg/day) to alleviate the beta-adrenergic symptoms of hyperthyroidism (tachycardia, tremor); contraindicated in patients with bronchospasm.
- Graves' ophthalmopathy: methylcellulose eye drops to protect against excessive dryness, sunglasses to decrease photophobia, intraocular and systemic high-dose corticosteroids for severe exophthalmos. Worsening of ophthalmopathy after RAI therapy is often transient and can be prevented by the administration of prednisone. Other treatment options include antiinflammatory and immunosuppressive agents, radiation, and corrective surgical procedures. The administration of the antioxidant selenium (100 μg PO bid) has been recently reported as effective in improving quality of

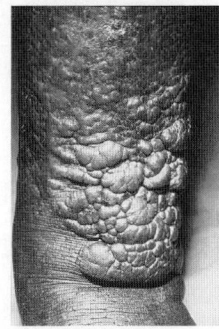

FIG. 1 Chronic pretibial myxedema in a patient with Graves' disease and orbitopathy. The lesions are firm and nonpitting, with a clear edge to feel. (Courtesy of Dr. Andrew Werner, New York, NY.)

life, reducing ocular involvement, and slowing progression of the disease in patients with mild Graves' orbitopathy. Its mechanism of action is believed to be an effect on the oxygen free radicals and cytokines that play a pathogenic role in Graves' orbitopathy.

- Dermopathy and acropachy: topical corticosteroids are often used but are generally ineffective. Trials using rituximab infusion for dermopathy have shown striking improvement.

CHRONIC Rx

Patients undergoing treatment with ATDs should be seen every 1 to 3 mo until euthyroidism is achieved and every 3 to 4 mo while they are receiving ATDs.

DISPOSITION

- ATDs induce sustained remission in <60% of cases.
- The incidence of hypothyroidism after RAI is >50% within the first year and 2% per year thereafter.
- Complications of surgery include hypothyroidism (28% to 43% after 10 yr), hypoparathyroidism (4%), and vocal cord paralysis (1%).
- Successful treatment of hyperthyroidism requires lifelong monitoring for the onset of hypothyroidism or the recurrence of thyrotoxicosis.

- RAI therapy is followed by the appearance or worsening of ophthalmopathy more often than is therapy with methimazole, particularly in patients who are cigarette smokers. It can be prevented with the administration of prednisone 0.5 mg/kg body weight per day starting 2 to 3 days after RAI, continued for 1 mo, then tapered off over 2 mo.
- Mild to moderate ophthalmopathy often improves spontaneously. Severe cases can be treated with high-dose glucocorticoids, orbital irradiation, or both. Orbital decompression may be used in patients with optic neuropathy and exophthalmos (see "Hyperthyroidism").

TABLE 1 Clinical Assessment of the Patient with Graves' Ophthalmopathy

Activity Measures*

Spontaneous retrobulbar pain

Pain on attempted up or down gaze

Redness of the eyelids

Redness of the conjunctiva

Swelling of the eyelids

Inflammation of the caruncle and/or plica

Conjunctival edema

Severity Measures

Lid aperture: distance between lid margins in millimeters with the patient looking in the primary position, sitting relaxed, and with distant fixation

Swelling of the eyelids (absent/equivocal, moderate, severe)

Redness of the eyelids (absent/present)

Redness of the conjunctivae (absent/present)

Conjunctival edema (absent, present)

Inflammation of the caruncle or plica (absent, present)

Exophthalmos: measured in millimeters using the same Hertel exophthalmometer and the same intercanthal distance for an individual patient

Subjective diplopia score†

Eye muscle involvement (ductions in degrees)

Corneal involvement (absent/punctate keratopathy/ulcer)

Optic nerve involvement: best-corrected visual acuity, color vision, optic disk, relative afferent pupillary defect (absent/present), plus visual fields if optic nerve compression is suspected

*Based on the seven classic features of inflammation in Graves' ophthalmopathy. The clinical activity score (CAS) is the total number of items present; a CAS ≥3 indicates active ophthalmopathy.
†Subjective diplopia score: 0 = no diplopia; 1 = intermittent (i.e., diplopia in primary position of gaze, when tired, or when first awakening); 2 = inconstant (i.e., diplopia at extremes of gaze); 3 = constant (i.e., continuous diplopia in primary or reading position).
From Melmed S, Polonsky KS, Larsen PR, Kronenberg HM: *Williams textbook of endocrinology,* ed 12, Philadelphia, 2011, Saunders.

ⓔⓑⓜ **EVIDENCE**

Available at www.expertconsult.com

SUGGESTED READINGS

Available at www.expertconsult.com

RELATED CONTENT

Graves' Disease (Patient Information)
Hyperthyroidism (Related Key Topic)

AUTHOR: **FRED F. FERRI, M.D.**

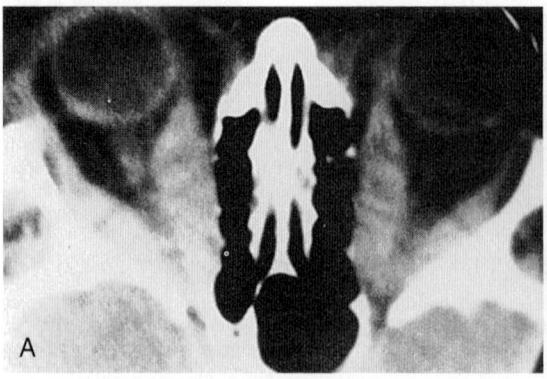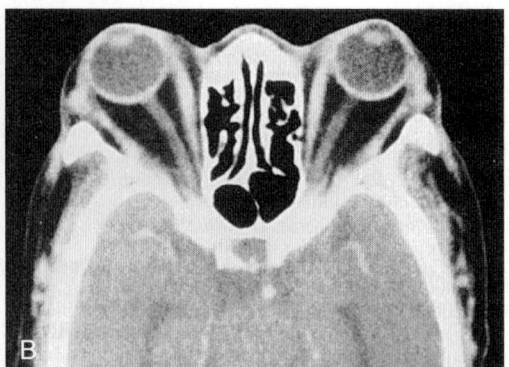

FIG. 2 Computed tomographic scans of orbits in two patients with Graves' orbitopathy. A, Notice the obviously grossly swollen medial rectus extraocular muscles in both orbits and the resulting proptosis. **B,** The patient shows considerable proptosis with only minimal muscle enlargement, suggesting the presence of a large amount of retroorbital fat. (Courtesy of Dr. Peter Som, New York, NY.)

BASIC INFORMATION

DEFINITION

Guillain-Barré syndrome (GBS) is an acute immune-mediated polyradiculoneuropathy (affects nerve roots and peripheral nerves), with predominant motor involvement. It is the most common cause of acute flaccid paralysis in the Western hemisphere and probably worldwide. By definition, maximal clinical weakness, the clinical nadir, occurs within 4 weeks of disease onset.

SYNONYMS

AIDP (acute inflammatory demyelinating polyradiculoneuropathy)
Acute polyneuropathy
Ascending paralysis
GBS
Postinfectious polyneuritis

ICD-10CM CODES
G61.0 Guillain-Barré syndrome

EPIDEMIOLOGY & DEMOGRAPHICS

INCIDENCE: 0.6 to 1.9 cases/100,000 persons annually without geographic variation. Incidence increases with age. A slight peak in incidence occurs between late adolescence and early adulthood. A slight male preponderance (1.25:1) also exists.

PREDISPOSING FACTORS: Viral (HIV, CMV, EBV, influenza) and bacterial (*Campylobacter jejuni, Mycoplasma pneumoniae*) infections; systemic illness (Hodgkin's lymphoma, immunizations). Major antecedents of GBS are described in Box 1.

ETIOLOGY

- Unknown, but believed to be caused by infection-induced aberrant immune response.
- Preceding infectious illness 1 to 4 weeks before disease onset has been noted. The most frequent antecedent infection is *C. jejuni* infection (associated with 30% of cases of GBS and 20% of cases of Miller-Fisher syndrome).
- Humoral and cell-mediated immune attack of peripheral nerve myelin, Schwann cells; sometimes with primary axonal involvement.

PHYSICAL FINDINGS & CLINICAL PRESENTATION

- Symmetric weakness, most commonly involving proximal muscles initially, subsequently involving both proximal and distal muscles; difficulty in ambulating, getting up from a chair, or climbing stairs (Box 2).
- Depressed or absent reflexes bilaterally.
- Minimal to moderate glove and stocking paresthesias/dysesthesia/anesthesia or back pain.
- Pain (caused by involvement of posterior nerve roots) may be prominent.
- Autonomic abnormalities (bradyarrhythmias or tachyarrhythmias, hypotension or hypertension).
- Respiratory insufficiency (caused by weakness of bulbar/intercostal muscles).
- Facial paresis, ophthalmoparesis, dysphagia (secondary to cranial nerve involvement).

BOX 1 Major Antecedents of Guillain-Barré Syndrome

Frequent
Upper respiratory tract infections
Campylobacter jejuni enteritis
Cytomegalovirus infection
Epstein-Barr virus infection
Hepatitis A infection
Hepatitis B infection
Hepatitis C infection
HIV infection

Infrequent
Mycoplasma pneumoniae infection
Haemophilus influenzae infection
Leptospira icterohaemorrhagiae infection
Salmonellosis
Rabies vaccine
Tetanus toxoid
Bacille Calmette-Guérin immunization
Sarcoidosis
Systemic lupus erythematosus
Lymphoma
Trauma
Surgery

Questionable
Hepatitis B vaccine
Influenza vaccine
Hyperthermia
Epidural anesthesia

From Vincent JL et al: *Textbook of critical care*, ed 6, Philadelphia, 2011, Saunders.

BOX 2 Findings Suggesting Guillain-Barré Syndrome

Relative symmetry of symptoms
Mild sensory signs and symptoms
Cranial nerve involvement
Autonomic dysfunction
Absence of fever at onset
Cytoalbuminologic dissociation of cerebrospinal fluid
Typical electrodiagnostic findings
Progression over days to weeks
Recovery beginning 2 to 4 weeks after cessation of progression

From Adams JG: *Emergency medicine: clinical essentials*, Philadelphia, 2013, Saunders.

- GBS consists of several clinical variants based on the pattern of clinical involvement and electrophysiologic findings. These include:
  1. AIDP (most common form in Europe and North America)
  2. Acute motor axonal neuropathy (AMAN; most prevalent form in China and Japan)
  3. Acute motor and sensory axonal neuropathy (AMSAN; has more severe sensory involvement and is associated with more severe clinical course and poorer prognosis)
  4. **Miller Fisher syndrome** (MFS; triad of ophthalmoplegia, ataxia, and areflexia)
  5. Acute pandysautonomia (rapid onset of parasympathetic and sympathetic failure without motor or sensory involvement)
  6. Regional variants (e.g., pharyngeal-cervical-brachial GBS, pure ataxic GBS)

DIAGNOSIS

DIFFERENTIAL DIAGNOSIS

- Toxic peripheral neuropathies: heavy metal poisoning (lead [microcytic anemia], thallium [alopecia], arsenic [typically accompanied by acute GI illness]), medications (vincristine, disulfiram), organophosphate poisoning, hexacarbon (glue sniffer's neuropathy)
- Nontoxic peripheral neuropathies: acute intermittent porphyria, fulminant vasculitic polyneuropathy, infectious (poliomyelitis, diphtheria, Lyme disease, West Nile virus); tick paralysis
- Neuromuscular junction disorders: myasthenia gravis, botulism, snake envenomation
- Myopathies such as polymyositis and acute necrotizing myopathies caused by drugs
- Metabolic derangements such as hypermagnesemia, hypokalemia, hypophosphatemia
- Acute CNS disorders such as basilar artery thrombosis with brainstem infarction, brainstem encephalomyelitis, transverse myelitis, or spinal cord compression
- Hysterical paralysis or malingering

WORKUP

1. Exclude other causes based on clinical history, examination, and laboratory tests.
2. Lumbar puncture (may be normal in the first 1 to 2 weeks of the illness). Typical findings include elevated CSF protein with few mononuclear leukocytes (albuminocytologic dissociation) in 80% to 90% of patients. Elevated CSF cell counts is an expected feature in cases associated with HIV seroconversion.
3. EMG/nerve conduction study (NCS) may be normal in the first 10 to 14 days of the disease. The earliest electrodiagnostic abnormality is prolongation or absence of H-reflexes. NCS evidence of demyelination (prolonged distal latency, conduction velocity slowing, conduction block, temporal dispersion, and prolonged F-waves) in two or more motor nerves confirms diagnosis of AIDP in the appropriate clinical context.

LABORATORY TESTS

- CBC may reveal early leukocytosis with left shift. Electrolytes are tested to exclude metabolic causes of weakness.
- Heavy metal testing; urine porphyria screen; creatine kinase; HIV testing, including tests for HIV seroconversion, especially if CSF demonstrates lymphocytic pleocytosis. MRI brain and spinal cord with and without contrast may be indicated if diagnosis is uncertain. In GBS, a gadolinium-enhanced MRI of the lumbosacral spine may reveal nerve root enhancement.
- Antibodies against ganglioside GQ1b may be present in up to 90% of patients with MFS. IgG antibodies against ganglioside GM1 may be associated with AMAN. There are no antiganglioside antibodies commonly associated with AIDP.
- In equivocal cases, especially if peripheral nerve vasculitis is a concern, nerve biopsy may aid in confirming a diagnosis of GBS. Sensory

nerve biopsy demonstrates segmental demyelination with infiltration of monocytes and T cells into the endoneurium. Axonal loss is commonly seen in sensory nerve biopsy specimens in GBS.

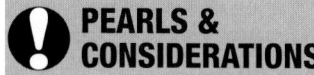

TREATMENT

NONPHARMACOLOGIC THERAPY

- Close monitoring of respiratory function (frequent measurements of vital capacity, negative inspiratory force, and tidal volume) and pulmonary toilet should be done because respiratory failure is the major complication in GBS (Fig. E1).
- Frequent repositioning of patient to minimize formation of pressure sores.
- Prevention of venous thromboembolism with antithrombotic stockings as a supplement to pharmacologic venous thromboembolism prevention.
- Emotional support and social counseling for patient and family.
- Physical and occupational therapy once patient is medically stable and able to participate.

ACUTE GENERAL Rx

- Option 1: Infusion of IV immunoglobulins (IVIG; 0.4 g/kg/day for 5 days). Always check serum IgA levels before infusion to prevent anaphylaxis in IgA-deficient patients.
- Option 2: Early therapeutic plasma exchange (TPE or plasmapheresis: 200 to 250 ml/kg over five sessions every other day), started within 7 days of onset of symptoms, is beneficial in reducing the need for mechanical ventilation in patients with rapidly progressive disease and results in improved rate of recovery. It is contraindicated in patients with cardiovascular disease (recent MI, unstable angina), active sepsis, and autonomic dysfunction.
- Both therapies are equally effective and may shorten recovery time by 50%. There is no proven benefit from combining IVIG and plasma exchange. Glucocorticoids are contraindicated.
- Mechanical ventilation may be needed if FVC is <12 to 15 mL/kg, vital capacity is rapidly decreasing or is <1000 ml, negative inspiratory force is <20 cm H_2O, PaO_2 is <70, or the patient is having significant difficulty clearing secretions or is aspirating.

CHRONIC Rx

- Ventilatory support may be necessary in 10% to 20% of patients. Adequate fluid/electrolyte support and nutrition are necessary, especially in patients with dysautonomia or bulbar dysfunction.
- Aggressive nursing care to prevent decubitus, infections, fecal impactions, and pressure nerve palsies.
- Monitoring and treatment of autonomic dysfunction (bradyarrhythmias or tachyarrhythmias, orthostatic hypotension, systemic hypertension).
- Treatment of back pain and dysesthesia with low-dose tricyclics, gabapentin, and so on. Opiate narcotics can be used cautiously in the short term but may compound dysautonomia.
- Pharmacologic venous thromboembolism prevention with agents such as heparin (5000 U SC q12h) or enoxaparin (40 mg SC daily) in poorly ambulating and nonambulatory patients.
- Stress ulcer prevention in patients receiving ventilator support.
- Physical and occupational therapy rehabilitation, including supportive devices.

DISPOSITION

- Mortality rate is approximately 5% to 10% worldwide. Causes of death include cardiac arrest, pulmonary embolism, and fulminant infections. A recent study showed 62% complete motor recovery, 14% mild weakness, 9% moderate weakness, 4% bed-bound or ventilated, and 8% dead at 1 year. Another study suggested that about 33% of patients were free from sensory symptoms at 1 year, with residual sensory loss present in the lower extremities in 67% and 36% in the upper extremities. About 32% had to change their work, 30% were unable to function at home as well as they could before the disease, and 52% had to alter their leisure activities 1 year after GBS onset. Excessive fatigue is a common complaint in patients during the recovery phase of GBS. This may be treated with exercise therapy (e.g., bicycle exercise training).
- Predictors for poor recovery (inability to walk independently at 1 year): age >60 years, preceding diarrheal illness, recent CMV infection, fulminant or rapidly progressing course, ventilatory dependence, reduced motor amplitudes (<20% normal), or unexcitable nerves on NCS. Outcomes may also be influenced by complications of medical therapy.
- GBS is typically a monophasic illness. Recurrence may occur in <5% of patients following full recovery.

REFERRAL

- Neurology to aid in diagnosis and direct treatment
- Pulmonary/critical care for ICU management
- Otolaryngology or general surgery for tracheostomy in patients requiring prolonged ventilatory support
- Gastroenterology for percutaneous endoscopic gastrostomy for patients with prolonged inability to obtain nutrition orally

ⓘ PEARLS & CONSIDERATIONS

- GBS is the most common cause of acute flaccid paralysis.
- Close monitoring of ventilatory function with respiratory mechanics (FVC and NIF) is of paramount importance in all patients with suspected GBS.
- Glucocorticoids are not indicated in GBS and may even slow recovery.

PATIENT/FAMILY EDUCATION

Patient education information may be obtained from the Guillain-Barré Foundation International, The Holly Building, 104 1/2 Forrest Avenue, Narberth, PA 19072; phone: (610) 667-0131; fax: (610) 667-7036; toll-free: (866) 224-3301; E-mail: info@gbs-cidp.org

SUGGESTED READINGS
Available at www.expertconsult.com

RELATED CONTENT
Guillain-Barre Syndrome (Patient Information)

AUTHOR: **DIVYA SINGHAL, M.D.**

BASIC INFORMATION

DEFINITION
Gynecomastia is a benign enlargement of male breast, resulting from proliferation of glandular breast tissue.

ICD-10CM CODES
N62 Hypertrophy of breast

EPIDEMIOLOGY
- Most common reason for male breast evaluation.
- Seen in patients of all age groups.
- 60% to 90% of infants have transient gynecomastia due to high estrogenic state of pregnancy.
- Prevalence during adolescence ranges from 4% to 69%. It results from transient increase of estradiol concentration at the onset of puberty.
- Higher incidence in body builders due to use of anabolic steroids.
- 24% to 65% of older men have gynecomastia. It is secondary to decreased testosterone production with advanced age, increased peripheral conversion of testosterone to estrogen, and at times from side effects of medications.

PATHOPHYSIOLOGY
Altered estrogen-androgen balance, in favor of estrogen.

ETIOLOGY
- Physiologic
  Infancy
  Puberty
  Persistent pubertal gynecomastia seen in 25% of cases
  Elderly
- Pathologic
  Idiopathic (25%)
  Increased estrogen production or action
  Testicular tumors (3%)
  Chronic liver disease
  Malnutrition
  Hyperthyroidism
  Adrenal tumors
  Familial gynecomastia
  Decreased testosterone production or action (10%)
  Testicular trauma
  Testicular torsion
  Viral orchitis
  Congenital anorchia
  Renal failure (1%)
  Hyperthyroidism (1.5%)
  Malnutrition
  Androgen insensitivity syndrome
  Five-alpha reductase deficiency
  Pituitary tumors
  Kallmann syndrome
  Klinefelter's syndrome
  Medications (10% to 25%)

Estrogen, gonadotropins, clomiphene, phenytoin, ketoconazole, metronidazole, metoclopramide, alkylating agents, busulfan, methotrexate, cisplatin, cimetidine, ranitidine, omeprazole, flutamide, finasteride, etomidate, HAART therapy, INH, tricyclic antidepressants, phenothiazines, diazepam, haloperidol, calcium channel blocker, ACE inhibitors, spironolactone, digoxin, amiodarone, methyldopa, alcohol, marijuana, heroin, methadone, amphetamine, anabolic steroids. Table E1 summarizes the various causes of gynecomastia.

CLINICAL FEATURES
- Although gynecomastia is usually bilateral, it could be unilateral.
- Characterized by concentric rubbery to firm disk of tissue, which is often mobile and located directly beneath the areola (Fig. 1).
- Pain is usually not severe. Varying degree of tenderness and nipple sensitivity are more common than pain, usually in the first 6 mo.

DIAGNOSIS

- Good history and physical examination including review of all medications the patient is taking is helpful.
- Mammogram is recommended for suspected breast cancer.
- Serum concentration of hCG, LH, testosterone, and estradiol should be measured, preferably in the morning, unless the cause is clearly apparent. There is no uniformity of opinion regarding what biochemical evaluation, if any, should be performed in patients

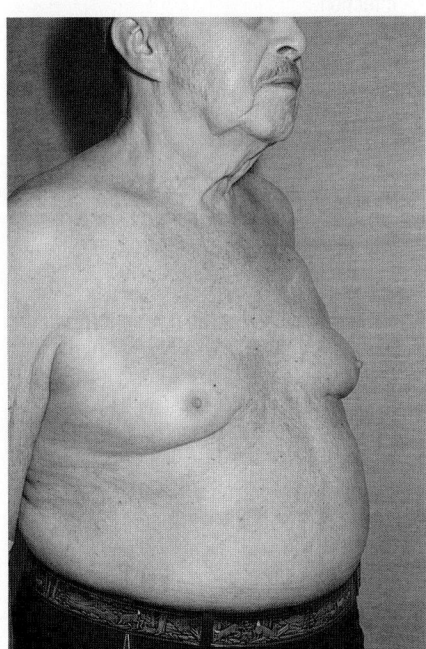

FIG. 1 Gynecomastia. (From Swartz, MH: *Textbook of physical diagnosis*, ed 7, Philadelphia, 2014, Saunders.)

with asymptomatic gynecomastia. Fig. E2 describes an algorithm for evaluation of gynecomastia.

DIFFERENTIAL DIAGNOSIS
- Breast cancer
  1. Mass is usually firm to hard
  2. Unilateral
  3. Eccentric in location
  4. Could be associated with nipple discharge and retraction, lymphadenopathy, and skin dimpling
- Pseudogynecomastia or lipomastia
  1. Characterized by fat deposition without glandular proliferation
  2. Seen in obese men
  3. Bilateral
  4. Remain unchanged over time

TREATMENT

- Observation is recommended for most patients with physiologic gynecomastia. They often regress spontaneously. Reassurance and follow-up examination in 3 to 6 mo usually suffice.
- Treat the underlying cause, and stop the offending medications.
- Treatment is most effective in the early stages (first 6 mo). Medical therapy often fails when given for longstanding (>12 mo) cases because of the presence of fibrosis.
- Potential indications of early therapy include severe breast enlargement, pain, tenderness, and psychological embarrassment. Consider giving tamoxifen 10 mg orally twice a day to these patients for up to 3 mo. It is not FDA-approved for this purpose. It results in regression of gynecomastia in approximately 80% of patients and, of which, only 60% had complete regression. As far as breast symptoms, such as pain and tenderness, some improvement is usually seen within a month of therapy.
- Surgery is offered for symptomatic gynecomastia that does not respond to medical therapy. However, for adolescents, surgery is deferred until puberty is completed. The different surgical options include subcutaneous mastectomy, ultrasound-guided liposuction, and suction-assisted lipectomy.
- For prevention of gynecomastia in patients with prostate cancer using antiandrogen therapy, one could offer tamoxifen or radiotherapy.

SUGGESTED READING
Available at www.expertconsult.com

RELATED CONTENT
Gynecomastia (Patient Information)

AUTHOR: **HEMANT K. SATPATHY, M.D.**

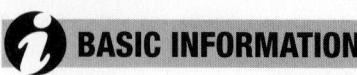

DEFINITION

Hand-foot-mouth disease (HFMD) is a viral illness characterized by superficial lesions of the oral mucosa and skin of the extremities. HFMD is primarily caused by coxsackie or enterovirus infection and can be transmitted by either respiratory droplet contact or fecal-oral contact. Although young children are predominantly affected, adults are also at risk. This disease is usually self-limited and benign, although outbreaks in the Asia Pacific region have been increasingly complicated by neurologic and cardiopulmonary sequelae.

SYNONYMS

HFMD
Vesicular stomatitis with exanthema
Coxsackie virus infection
Enterovirus infection

ICD-10CM CODES
B08.4 Enteroviral vesicular stomatitis with exanthem

EPIDEMIOLOGY & DEMOGRAPHICS

- HFMD most often affects children <10 yr.
  - Children <5 yr are at the highest risk of infection and have the most severe cases.
- HFMD is contagious. Close contacts of affected children, including family members and health care workers, are the most commonly infected adults. Outbreaks can also occur in clustered populations of young adults (a recent outbreak at a military base affected 4.7% of the exposed population).
- Infection is spread from person to person by direct contact with saliva, respiratory secretions, fluid in vesicles, or stool.
- A person is most contagious during the first week of illness.
- Outbreaks tend to occur during the summer.
- Infection leads to immunity, but a subsequent episode may occur after infection with a different etiologic virus or type.

PHYSICAL FINDINGS & CLINICAL PRESENTATION

Symptoms:
- After a 4- to 6-day incubation period, patients may report odynophagia, sore throat, malaise, and fever (38.3° to 40° C).
- 1 to 2 days later, the characteristic oral lesions appear (small red spots that blister and may ulcerate). The fluid from these lesions is infectious, and disease can be transmitted through contact with the fluid.
- In 75% of cases, skin lesions on the extremities accompany these oral manifestations (small flat or raised red bumps, sometimes with blisters), but the lesions may be absent.
- Only 11% of adults have cutaneous findings.
- Lesions appear over the course of 1 or 2 days.
Physical findings:
- Oral lesions are common and are usually found on the tongue, buccal mucosa, gingivae, and hard palate.

- Oral lesions initially start as 1- to 3-mm erythematous macules and evolve into gray vesicles on an erythematous base.
- Vesicles are frequently broken by the time of presentation and appear as superficial, gray ulcers with surrounding erythema.
- Skin lesions of the palms of the hands and soles of the feet are common and start as linear erythematous papules (3 to 10 mm in diameter) that evolve into gray vesicles that may be mildly painful (Fig. E1). These vesicles are usually intact at presentation and remain so until they desquamate within 2 wk.
- Involvement of the buttocks and genital area is also common (present in 31% of cases).
- Although rare, atypical findings such as fingernail or toenail loss (nail separation from the nail matrix, otherwise known as onychomadesis) after HFMD (notably with the A6 strain of coxsackie virus) has been reported in children. The nail loss is temporary, and nails grow back without intervention.
- Another atypical skin manifestation is that of "eczema coxsackium," which is described as the typical skin lesions of coxsackie virus but with a more extensive distribution involving the trunk and extremities, localized to areas of active or past atopic dermatitis.
- In rare cases, encephalitis, meningitis, myocarditis, poliomyelitis-like paralysis, and pulmonary edema may develop. Sporadic acute paralysis and long-term neurologic sequelae have been reported with enterovirus 71.
- Although information is limited, there is no clear evidence that pregnancy outcomes are affected in the setting of maternal infection.

ETIOLOGY

- Coxsackie virus group A, type 16, was the first and is the most common cause of HFMD.
- Enterovirus 71 is the second leading cause of HFMD. Enterovirus 71 is neurotropic and has a predilection for the brainstem, leading to more severe cases of the disease. Infection rates have been rising in the Asia Pacific region with clusters of severe disease.
- Coxsackie viruses A5, A6, A7, A9, A10, B1, B2, B3, and B5 have also been implicated.
- Coxsackie A6 has been known to cause a severe skin rash and self-limited nail abnormalities (onychomadesis). Patients with this strain may lack oral lesions.
- Epidemic outbreaks have been reported with coxsackie A16 and enterovirus 71.

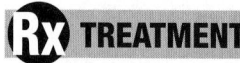 DIAGNOSIS

DIFFERENTIAL DIAGNOSIS

- Aphthous stomatitis
- Herpes simplex infection
- Herpangina
- Behçet's disease
- Erythema multiforme
- Pemphigus
- Gonorrhea

- Acute leukemia
- Lymphoma
- Allergic contact dermatitis

WORKUP

The diagnosis is made on the basis of typical history and characteristic physical examination.

LABORATORY TESTS

- Not indicated unless the diagnosis is in doubt such as for a suspected case with an atypical presentation.
  - Oropharyngeal specimen, stool specimen, or vesicular fluid may be obtained to identify the presence of enterovirus or coxsackie virus by polymerase chain reaction (PCR), but may take from 2 to 4 weeks for results.
    - Identification of a certain strain is only available in public health laboratories.

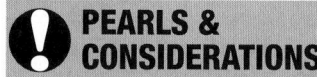 TREATMENT

ACUTE GENERAL Rx

- Symptomatic therapy is given for this usually self-limited disease.
- There are currently no available approved therapies for more severe cases. Antivirals and IV immunoglobulin have been evaluated for enterovirus 71 infections, but these treatments have not been evaluated in randomized, placebo-controlled studies.
- Systemic steroids should be avoided because they have been associated with more severe disease and higher viral loads.

DISPOSITION

Prognosis is excellent except in rare cases of central nervous system or cardiac involvement. Most are managed as outpatients.

REFERRAL

Not usually needed

PEARLS & CONSIDERATIONS

- Frequent handwashing, disinfection of contaminated surfaces, and washing of soiled articles of clothing can help reduce transmission.
- HFMD has no relation to hoof and mouth disease in cattle.

SUGGESTED READINGS
Available at www.expertconsult.com

RELATED CONTENT

Hand, Foot, and Mouth Disease (Patient Information)

AUTHOR: **ERICA HARDY, M.D., M.M.S.**

BASIC INFORMATION

DEFINITION

Head and neck squamous cell carcinoma is a malignant disease entity that arises from the epithelium of the mucosal surfaces of the upper aerodigestive tract and accounts for about 90% of head and neck cancers. This disease results from exposure to carcinogens and from the accumulation of genetic alterations. The workup and management of these patients depends upon the specific subsite of the aerodigestive tract in the head and neck from which the primary tumor arises. These subsites are the oral cavity, oropharynx, nasopharynx, hypopharynx, and larynx. Cutaneous malignancies, thyroid neoplasms, and salivary gland neoplasms also occur in the head and neck but are beyond the scope of this chapter.

SYNONYMS

HNC
Head and neck cancer
HNSCC
Head and neck squamous cell carcinoma

ICD 10-CM CODES
C77.0	Secondary and unspecified malignant neoplasm of lymph nodes of head, face, and neck
C00-C14	Malignant neoplasms of lip, oral cavity, and pharynx
C30	Malignant neoplasm of nasal cavities, middle ear, and accessory sinuses
C32	Malignant neoplasm of larynx

EPIDEMIOLOGY & DEMOGRAPHICS

INCIDENCE:

- U.S. annual incidence of head and neck cancer (90% of which is squamous cell carcinoma) is approximately 62,000 persons per year.
- Annual mortality is approximately 13,000 persons per year.
- Accounts for approximately 3% of all cancers in the U.S.
- Human papilloma virus (HPV)-associated squamous cell carcinoma of the head and neck accounts for 5% to 20% of all HNSCCs, and 40% to 90% of those arise in oropharynx.
- Incidence of all forms of HNSCC is on the decline, except oropharyngeal squamous cell carcinoma, which is increasing in incidence, likely related to the rise in human papilloma virus (HPV) associated HNSCC.

PEAK INCIDENCE: Sixth decade of life.
PREDOMINANT SEX AND AGE: Male:female ratio is about 3:1. Risk increases significantly over the age of 40.
GENETICS: Research is ongoing in genetic factors that lead to the development and progression of HNSCC. Tumor suppressor genes including *p53*, *NOTCH1*, and *CDKN2A*, among others, have been shown to harbor mutations in patients with HNSCC.

RISK FACTORS: The two most strongly implicated risk factors associated with HNSCC are tobacco and alcohol use. These carcinogens place the entire epithelium of the upper respiratory tract at risk for multiple primary tumors via a process known as field cancerization. More recently, a new subset of HNSCC caused by the HPV has been increasing in prevalence. HPV 16 is the most common genotype detected. Patients are more likely to be white middle-aged men, nonsmokers, with minimal alcohol use and higher socioeconomic status.

PHYSICAL FINDINGS & CLINICAL PRESENTATION

- Presenting signs and symptoms are related to local effects of the primary tumor, regional spread, metastatic disease, or paraneoplastic phenomena.
  - Oral cavity, oropharynx, hypopharynx: painful mass or ulceration (Fig. 1), dysphagia, odynophagia, weight loss.
  - Larynx: hoarseness, voice change, shortness of breath, stridor.
  - Nasal cavity, paranasal sinus, nasopharynx—referred otalgia, conductive hearing loss from middle ear effusion, epistaxis, cranial nerve palsies.
  - All sites: cranial nerve palsies, painless neck mass from regional metastases to cervical lymph nodes. Most common site of distant metastases is the lung, with bone and liver being much less common.
- Physical exam: A thorough examination of the head and neck including cranial nerve exam, otoscopy, inspection and palpation of oral cavity, oropharynx, and neck, and general physical exam.
  - Concerning exam findings: Unilateral middle ear effusion, ulcerated mass of the oral cavity (Fig. E2) or oropharynx, trismus, painless neck mass.

ETIOLOGY

- Exposure to carcinogens including tobacco and alcohol causes genetic alterations in the epithelium of mucosal surfaces lining the upper aerodigestive tract, leading to malignant transformation of epithelial cells.

HPV-associated HNSCC is a direct result of the carcinogenic effects of the virus and is not related to alcohol and tobacco use. Primary nasopharyngeal carcinoma has a weak association with tobacco and alcohol and is endemic to southern China, Southeast Asia, and northern Africa. There is a strong association between Epstein-Barr virus infection and primary nasopharyngeal carcinoma.

DIAGNOSIS

DIFFERENTIAL DIAGNOSIS

Lymphoma, primary salivary gland malignancy, thyroid malignancy, benign tumors of the upper aerodigestive tract, metastases.

WORKUP

- Initial workup includes incudes a full physical examination, indirect and/or direct laryngoscopy, imaging studies of the head and neck as well as the chest and/or body to assess for metastases, laboratory tests as indicated, and referral to a head and neck cancer specialist.
- Additional workup by head and neck cancer specialist:
  - Flexible fiber-optic laryngoscopy or mirror laryngoscopy
  - Biopsy of the tumor in office or under anesthesia
  - Fine-needle aspiration (FNA) and biopsy for patient who presents with a suspicious neck mass
  - Panendoscopy with biopsy under anesthesia, which may include direct laryngoscopy, esophagoscopy, and/or bronchoscopy

LABORATORY TESTS

- Complete blood count (CBC), coagulation studies, electrolytes, ECG, liver function tests (albumin, transaminases, alkaline phosphatase)

IMAGING STUDIES

- CT scan of the neck with contrast: necessary to evaluate extent of primary tumor and nodal metastases in neck (Fig. 3).

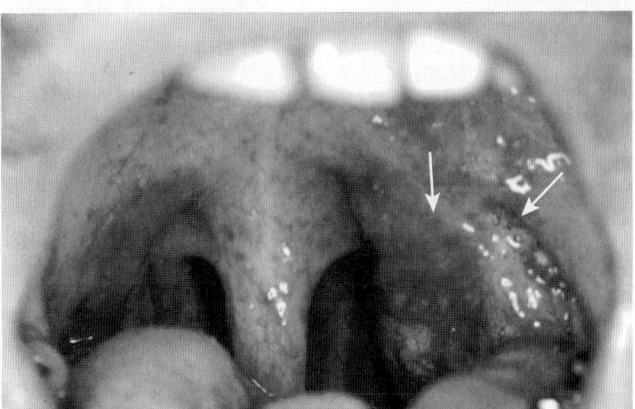

FIG. 1 Squamous cell carcinoma of the left tonsil *(arrows)*. (From Richardson MA et al: *Cummings otolaryngology–head and neck surgery*, ed 5, Philadelphia, 2010, Mosby, pp. 1358-1374, Figure 100-8 (978-0323052832).)

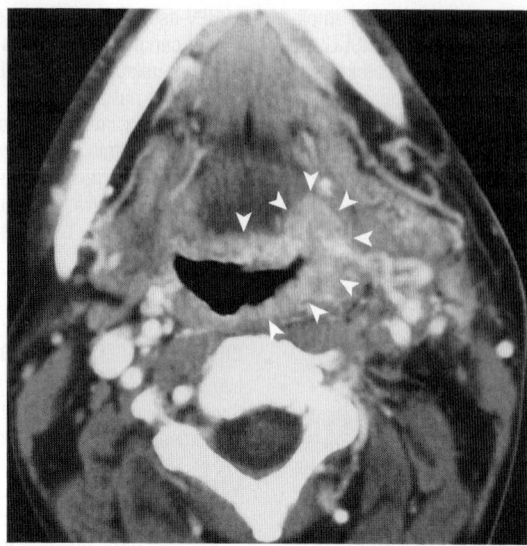

FIG. 3 CT scan with contrast showing tumor of the base of the left oropharynx *(arrowheads)*. (From Richardson MA et al: *Cummings otolaryngology–head and neck surgery*, ed 5, Philadelphia, 2010, Mosby, pp. 1393-1420, Figure 102-47 (978-0323052832).)

- MRI of head and neck (optional): Useful for nasopharyngeal, infratemporal fossa, temporal bone, parotid, parapharyngeal, skull base, or intracranial involvement.
- Chest x-ray or CT chest with contrast: To evaluate for lung metastases.
- PET/CT: Highlights areas in the body with increased metabolic uptake. Useful initially to assess extent of primary tumor, location of unknown primary tumor, cervical metastases, distant metastases, and second primary tumors. Can be used to monitor for recurrence in the posttreatment setting.

STAGING

- Staging is based on the tumor, node, metastasis (TNM) staging system provided by the AJCC. Staging varies depending on the head and neck subsite that is involved. Any nodal metastasis in the neck automatically classifies as advanced disease (Stage III or IV). Distant metastases place patients at Stage IVC.

TREATMENT

- Treatment consists of surgery, radiation, chemotherapy, or a combination of any or all of the three modalities. The goal is to use as few modalities as possible to minimize side effects of treatment.
  - Surgery: Complete surgical resection of the primary tumor along with unilateral or bilateral neck dissections to remove involved or potentially involved lymph nodes as clinically indicated.
  - Radiation: Allows for easier access to poorly exposed tumors such as those of the larynx, oropharynx, nasopharynx, or hypopharynx. Disadvantages include lengthy, time-intensive treatment course, xerostomia, pain, and higher surgical morbidity if salvage surgery is needed.

- Chemotherapy: Useful only as an adjuvant to radiation therapy or for palliation. Single-agent cisplatin therapy is widely accepted in the U.S. as a standard for chemoradiation regimens for head and neck cancers of any site. Major toxicities include nausea, vomiting, renal toxicity, ototoxicity, and myelosuppression.
  - Reconstruction: Performed with the goal of optimizing functional and cosmetic outcomes. Options include primary closure, local flaps, regional flaps, skin grafts, and microvascular free flaps from other parts of the body (e.g., radial forearm, fibula, anterolateral thigh, latissimus, etc.).

ACUTE GENERAL Rx

- Early-stage disease (Stage I or II)
  - Single-modality treatment with surgery or radiation alone may be appropriate for early-stage head and neck cancer. The choice between one or the other depends on the specific subsite of the head and neck that is involved and the side effects profile for each modality.
  - Treatment of the potentially involved lymph nodes in the neck with either neck dissection or radiation is controversial and depends on the clinical scenario and the judgment of the treatment team.
- Locoregionally advanced disease (Stage III or IV)
  - In general, these patients have large tumors >4 cm and/or cervical nodal metastases. Treatment typically involves multimodality therapy with either surgery followed by radiation therapy or upfront chemoradiation alone. Depending on the presence of certain adverse pathologic features of the surgical specimen, adjuvant chemoradiation may be necessary. If chemoradiation is the initial treatment modality, surgery may be needed in the adjuvant setting for residual or recurrent disease.

- Laryngeal cancers are the exception where select advanced disease with T3 or N1 tumors can be managed with single-modality therapy with surgery or radiation alone.
- Nasopharyngeal cancer is also an exception. This is not a surgical disease. Managed primarily by radiation to primary site and neck for early-stage disease. Chemoradiation is primary treatment for advanced disease. Surgery is reserved for recurrent or residual disease of primary site or neck following radiation therapy.
- Metastatic disease (Stage IVC)
  - Palliation of symptoms is the primary goal of treatment.
- All patients should be counseled on smoking cessation and avoidance of alcohol.

DISPOSITION

- Prognosis depends on the specific subsite of the head and neck that is involved. Overall 5-year survival rate for head and neck squamous cell carcinoma is about 55%. This varies with 5-year survival rates for carcinoma of the lip as high as 89.7% and carcinomas of the hypopharynx as low as approximately 30%.
- Patients are followed on a regular basis multiple times a year by a head and neck cancer specialist. After a 5-year disease-free survival, patients are followed on a yearly basis.

REFERRAL

- Referral should be made to an otolaryngologist or oral surgeon who specializes in head and neck cancer.

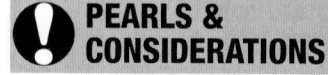

PEARLS & CONSIDERATIONS

PREVENTION

- Encourage all patients to cease using tobacco and to limit alcohol consumption.
- Examine the oral cavity and palpate the neck during the annual physical examination. Work up any suspicious masses or lesions.

PATIENT/FAMILY EDUCATION

http://www.entnet.org/content/head-and-neck-cancer
http://www.cancer.gov/types/head-and-neck

SUGGESTED READINGS

Available at www.expertconsult.com

RELATED CONTENT

Laryngeal Carcinoma (Related Key Topic)
Oral Cancer (Related Key Topic)

AUTHOR: **LOUIS INSALACO, M.D.**

BASIC INFORMATION

DEFINITION

The term *cluster headache* refers to attacks of severe, unilateral pain that is orbital, supraorbital, temporal, or any combination of these sites, lasting 15 to 180 minutes, and occurring from once every other day to eight times a day. The attacks are associated with ipsilateral signs and symptoms including one or more of the following: conjunctival injection, lacrimation, nasal congestion, rhinorrhea, forehead and facial sweating, miosis, ptosis, and eyelid edema. Most patients are restless or agitated during an attack.

SYNONYMS

Cluster headache
Ciliary neuralgia
Erythromelalgia of the head
Erythroprosopalgia of Bing
Horton's headache

ICD-10CM CODES

G44.001 Cluster headache syndrome, unspecified, intractable
G44.009 Cluster headache syndrome, unspecified, not intractable
G44.011 Episodic cluster headache, intractable
G44.019 Episodic cluster headache, not intractable
G44.021 Chronic cluster headache, intractable
G44.029 Chronic cluster headache, not intractable

EPIDEMIOLOGY & DEMOGRAPHICS

INCIDENCE: Estimated to occur in 0.05% to 1% of the population
PREDOMINANT SEX: Occurs in males at least five times more commonly than in females
PREDOMINANT AGE: Peak age of onset between 20 and 40 yr
GENETICS: May be inherited in up to 20% of cases, although uncertainty exists over the mode or modes of inheritance.

PHYSICAL FINDINGS & CLINICAL PRESENTATION

- During attack: conjunctival injection, lacrimation, nasal congestion, rhinorrhea, facial sweating, Horner's syndrome.
- In contrast to migraine sufferers, patients are agitated and active during an attack.
- Symptoms associated with an attack remain ipsilateral during the attack but may switch sides from one attack to the next.
- Permanent partial Horner's syndrome in 5% of patients; otherwise examination is normal.

ETIOLOGY

Activation of the posterior hypothalamic gray matter resulting in trigeminal activation coupled with parasympathetic activation. The pathophysiology remains controversial.

DIAGNOSIS

Per the *International Classification of Headache Disorders, 3rd edition,* the diagnosis of cluster headache requires all of the following:

- At least five attacks of severe or very severe unilateral orbital, supraorbital, and/or temporal pain lasting 15 to 180 minutes.
- Frequency of every other day to eight per day; they may cluster seasonally or at a certain time in a patient's life.
- Headache is accompanied by a sense of restlessness or agitation and/or at least one of the following (ipsilateral):
  1. Conjunctival injection and/or lacrimation
  2. Nasal congestion and/or rhinorrhea
  3. Eyelid edema
  4. Forehead and facial sweating
  5. Forehead and facial flushing
  6. Miosis and/or ptosis
  7. Sensation of fullness in the ear
  8. Restlessness or agitation

A diagnosis of episodic cluster headache requires the above criteria plus attacks that occur in bouts, also called cluster periods. These periods last 1 week to 1 year and are separated by attack-free intervals lasting at least 1 month.

A diagnosis of chronic cluster headache requires meeting the criteria for cluster headache plus at least 1 year of attacks without a pain-free interval of at least 1 month.

DIFFERENTIAL DIAGNOSIS

- Migraine
- Trigeminal neuralgia
- Primary stabbing headache
- Temporal arteritis
- Post-herpetic neuralgia
- Venous sinus thrombosis
- Carotid-cavernous fistula or other cavernous sinus lesions
- Other trigeminal autonomic cephalalgias
- Section II describes the differential diagnosis of headaches

WORKUP

Diagnosis is made clinically.

IMAGING STUDIES

- None, unless history or examination suggests focal neurologic deficit or headaches change in character or are of new onset.
- MRI of the brain along with vascular imaging may be necessary to exclude secondary headaches at the time of initial diagnosis.

TREATMENT

NONPHARMACOLOGIC THERAPY

Avoidance of alcohol, histamine, nitroglycerin, and tobacco during clusters

ABORTIVE Rx

- Inhalation of 100% oxygen by face mask at a flow rate of 12 L/min or greater for 15 min aborts the attack in 60% to 80% of patients.

- About 75% of users of triptans (sumatriptan, zolmitriptan) will be pain free within 20 minutes. Only injectable and nasal formulations achieve a response that is rapid enough to be efficacious.
- Cafergot, octreotide, intranasal lidocaine, or dihydroergotamine may abort an attack or prevent one if given just before a predictable episode. An attack typically resolves before oral analgesics can take effect, although indomethacin and other NSAIDs may be effective in prolonged attacks.

PROPHYLAXIS Rx

For patients with episodic cluster headache, prophylactic treatment should be started at the onset of the cluster period and tapered at its end. Patients with chronic cluster headache should be started on prophylactic treatment at increasing doses until good control is achieved. Preventative therapy should begin with verapamil. Alternative treatment options are also listed below.

- Verapamil: Start at 240 mg/day; increase up to 960 mg/day as tolerated. Dosing three times per day may be more effective than extended release. First-degree AV block may develop with escalating doses, so ECG should be checked.
- Topiramate: up to 50 mg bid; can be used as add-on to verapamil.
- Lithium: 200 mg tid with frequent monitoring and adjustment to maintain therapeutic serum level of 0.4 to 1 mEq/L. Equally effective as verapamil, but with more side effects.
- Methysergide: 1 to 2 mg tid; requires familiarity with the potential adverse effects and use of "drug holidays" to decrease risk of fibrosis.
- Ergotamine tartrate: 3 to 4 mg/day during clusters.
- Prednisone: 60 mg PO daily for 1 wk followed by taper; headaches can return during taper.
- Greater and lesser occipital nerve blocks, with the use of local anesthetics including lidocaine and bupivacaine along with steroids like Depo-Medrol, dexamethasone, or triamcinolone, may be used to shorten the duration of the cluster period. Consensus guidelines from the American Headache Society have been published recently.
- There is emerging evidence for benefit of a sphenopalatine ganglion block that may be available at some centers for both treatment and prophylaxis of cluster attacks.

DISPOSITION

Headache-free periods tend to increase with increasing age.

REFERRAL

Refractory cluster headaches may require referral to a headache specialist.

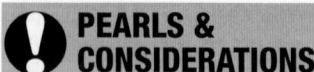
PEARLS & CONSIDERATIONS

COMMENTS

- Cluster headaches are divided into episodic (attacks lasting up to 1 year with more than 1 month pain-free periods) and chronic (>1 year without remission). Episodic cluster headache is six times more common than the chronic form.
- Home oxygen therapy is reasonable for cluster headache sufferers.

SUGGESTED READING

Available at www.expertconsult.com

RELATED CONTENT

Cluster Headaches (Patient Information)

AUTHORS: **MICHAEL POHLEN, M.D.,**
JOSEPH S. KASS, M.D., J.D., and
SIDDHARTH KAPOOR, M.D.

BASIC INFORMATION

DEFINITION

Migraine headaches are recurrent headaches that are either preceded by a focal neurologic symptom (migraine with aura), occur independently without preceding focal neurologic symptoms (migraine without aura), or have atypical presentations (migraine variants). The migraine aura typically is characterized by visual or sensory symptoms that develop over 5 to 60 min. If aura includes motor weakness, the migraine is referred to as hemiplegic. In migraine with and without aura, the headache is typically moderate to severe, unilateral, pulsatile, made worse with head movement, and associated with nausea and vomiting, photophobia, and phonophobia. Migraines that occur ≥15 days every month for ≥3 months are known as chronic; otherwise, they are referred to as episodic.

ICD-10CM CODES
G43.909 Migraine, unspecified, not intractable, without status migrainosus
G43.1 Migraine with aura (classical migraine)
G43.0 Migraine without aura (common migraine)
G43.2 Status migrainosus
G43.3 Complicated migraine

EPIDEMIOLOGY & DEMOGRAPHICS

INCIDENCE: Increases from infancy, peaks during the third decade of life, then decreases
PREVALENCE (IN U.S.): Females: 18%; males: 6%. More than 50% of persons affected by migraine headaches report reduced work or school productivity.
AGE: Peak prevalence between ages of 18 and 49
PREDOMINANT SEX: Female/male ratio of 3:1
GENETICS:
- Familial predisposition: more than 50% of migraine sufferers have an affected family member
- Autosomal-dominant transmission for some rare migraine variants (familial hemiplegic migraine, cerebral autosomal-dominant arteriopathy with subcortical infarcts and leukoencephalopathy [CADASIL]); familial hemiplegic migraines have been associated with calcium channelopathy, sodium channelopathy, and Na^+/K^+-ATPase dysfunction.

PHYSICAL FINDINGS & CLINICAL PRESENTATION

- Normal between episodes
- Normal for migraine without aura.
- Focal motor or sensory abnormalities possible for migraine with aura or migraine variants.
- Common aura types include scintillating scotoma, bright zigzags, homonymous visual disturbance such as paresthesia, speech disturbances, or hemiparesis (familial or sporadic hemiplegic migraine). Other visual phenomena include image distortion or "Alice in Wonderland" effect.

ETIOLOGY

The pathophysiology of migraines is not clearly understood, although the primary neuronal event results in a trigeminovascular reflex causing neurogenic inflammation. Serotonin, substance P, nitric oxide, and calcitonin gene-related peptide also play a role, but the exact mechanism is unknown. Cortical spreading depression is likely responsible for the aura.

DIAGNOSIS

Migraine without aura:
- Five attacks fulfilling criteria
- Headache attacks lasting 4 to 72 hr
- Headache has at least two of the following characteristics:
  1. Unilateral location
  2. Pulsating quality
  3. Moderate or severe pain intensity
  4. Aggravation or causing avoidance of routine physical activity
- At least one of the following during headache:
  1. Nausea and/or vomiting
  2. Photophobia and phonophobia
Migraine with typical aura:
- At least two attacks
- Aura consisting of at least one of the following, but no motor weakness:
  1. Fully reversible visual symptoms, including positive and/or negative features
  2. Fully reversible sensory symptoms, including positive and/or negative features
  3. Fully reversible dysphasic speech disturbance
- At least two of the following:
  1. Homonymous visual symptoms and/or unilateral sensory symptoms
  2. At least one aura symptom develops gradually over >5 min and/or different aura symptoms occur in succession over >5 min
  3. Each symptom lasts between 5 and 60 min
- A migraine occurring during or within 60 min of the aura

DIFFERENTIAL DIAGNOSIS

- A diagnosis of migraine is possible only after five recurrent episodes.
- The first or the worst headache should always be investigated and the differential includes headaches from all secondary causes.
- Headache red flags can be remembered by the mnemonic SSNOOP5:
  1. S: systemic symptoms of fever, weight loss
  2. S: secondary risk factors of immunosuppression from any cause, cancer
  3. N: neurologic deficits, altered consciousness
  4. O: onset is sudden, abrupt, split second thunderclap
  5. O: older, age >50 for new-onset headache should be worked up for giant cell arteritis
  6. P: pattern: change in headache pattern
  7. P: pregnancy
  8. P: positional or postural
  9. P: papilledema
  10. P: precipitation with Valsalva maneuver or exertion
- Section II describes the differential diagnosis of headaches

WORKUP

- In general, no additional investigation is needed with recurrent, typical attacks with usual age of onset, family history, and a normal physical examination.
- If there is an unusual presentation and/or unexpected findings on examination, investigation for other causes is required.

LABORATORY TESTS

Lumbar puncture for history of abrupt-onset headaches and uncertain diagnosis of migraine

IMAGING STUDIES

- Imaging should be done in patients with any of the red flags for secondary headache such as described by the SSNOOP5 mnemonic (see differential diagnosis section above).
- MRI brain with and without contrast is the imaging modality of choice for almost all headache types, although CT head without contrast may be used in the acute setting to evaluate for subarachnoid hemorrhage or other causes of acute intracranial hemorrhage.

TREATMENT

Consider the use of a headache log/diary to identify triggers of headaches, record efficacy of treatments, and track history of headaches.

NONPHARMACOLOGIC THERAPY

- Avoid any identifiable provoking factors: caffeine, tobacco, and alcohol may trigger attacks, as may dietary or other environmental precipitants (less common).
- Avoid emotional stressors and minimize variations in daily routine with regular sleep, meals, and exercise.
- Relaxation training, behavioral therapy, and biofeedback. Trials have shown that among young persons with chronic migraine, the use of cognitive behavior therapy (CBT) plus amitriptyline results in greater reductions in days with headaches and migraine-related disability compared with use of headache education plus amitriptyline.[1]

ACUTE ANALGESIC Rx

- Many oral agents are ineffective because of poor absorption from migraine-induced gastric stasis. Non-oral route of administration should be selected in patients with severe nausea or vomiting.

[1]Powers SW et al: Cognitive behavioral therapy plus amitriptyline for chronic migraine in children and adolescents, *JAMA* 310(24):2622-2630, 2013.

TABLE 1	Abortive and Analgesic Therapy for Migraine*	
Drug	**Route**	**Dose**
Triptans (Serotonin Agonists)		
Sumatriptan	Subcutaneous	6 mg, repeat in 2 hr (max 2 doses/day)
Sumatriptan	Oral	25 mg, 50 mg, 100 mg, repeat in 2 hr (max 200 mg/day)
Sumatriptan	Nasal spray	5 mg, 20 mg, repeat in 2 hr (max 40 mg/day)
Zolmitriptan	Oral	1.25, 2.5 mg, 5 mg, repeat in 2 hr (max 10 mg/day)
Zolmitriptan	Nasal spray	5 mg, repeat in 2 hr (max 10 mg/day)
Zolmitriptan	Orally disintegrating tab	2.5, 5 mg, repeat in 2 hr (max 10 mg/day)
Naratriptan	Oral	1 mg, 2.5 mg, repeat in 4 hr (max 5 mg/day)
Rizatriptan	Oral	5 mg, 10 mg, repeat in 2 hr (max 30 mg/day)
Almotriptan	Oral	6.25 mg, 12.5 mg, may repeat in 2 hr (max 25 mg/day)
Eletriptan	Oral	20 mg, 40 mg, may repeat in 2 hr (max 80 mg/day)
Frovatriptan	Oral	2.5 mg, may repeat in 2 hr (max 7.5 mg/day); may also be used for mini prophylaxis
Ergotamine Preparations		
Ergotamine and caffeine	Oral	2 tablets, may repeat 1 tab q30 min (max 6/day)
Ergotamine and caffeine	Rectal	1 suppository, repeat in 1 hr (max 2/day)
Ergotamine	Sublingual	1 tablet, repeat in 1 hr (max 2/day)
Dihydroergotamine	Intramuscular	0.5-1.0 mg, repeat twice at 1-hr intervals (max 3 mg/attack)
	Subcutaneous	
	Intravenous	
	Nasal spray	
Isometheptene+ dichloralphenazone+ acetaminophen	Oral	1 to 2 capsules, repeat in 4 hr (max 8/day)
Nonsteroidal Antiinflammatory Drugs		
Acetaminophen+ (should not be used alone)	Oral	2 tablets, repeat in 6 hr (max 8/day aspirin+caffeine)
Naproxen	Oral	550-750 mg, repeat in 1 hr (max 3 times/wk)
Meclofenamate	Oral	100-200 mg, repeat in 1 hr (max 3 times/wk)
Flurbiprofen	Oral	50-100 mg, repeat in 1 hr (max 3 times/wk)
Ibuprofen	Oral	200-300 mg, repeat in 1 hr (max 3 times/wk)
Antiemetics		
Promethazine	Oral	50-125 mg
	Intramuscular	No clear benefit in migraine, may be used
Prochlorperazine	Oral	1-25 mg
	Rectal	2.5-25 mg (suppository)
	Intramuscular/IV	5-10 mg, good evidence for strong benefit
Chlorpromazine	Oral	10-25 mg
	Rectal	50-100 mg (suppository)
	Intravenous	Up to 35 mg, use with monitoring, some evidence for good benefit
Trimethobenzamide	Oral	250 mg
	Rectal	200 mg
Metoclopramide	Oral	5-10 mg
	Intramuscular	10 mg
	Intravenous	5-10 mg
Dimenhydrinate	Oral	50 mg

*For side effects and contraindications, consult the manufacturer's drug insert before prescribing any of these drugs.
Modified from Wiederholt WC: *Neurology for non-neurologists*, ed 4, Philadelphia, 2000, Saunders.

- NSAIDs such as ketorolac, ibuprofen, and naproxen, or combination analgesics, may be used first line for mild migraine headaches. Barbiturate-containing compounds are potentially addictive and promote medication overuse headaches.

ACUTE ABORTIVE Rx

- Triptans (SC, PO, and intranasal) are now considered the drug class of choice for abortive therapy. Meta-analysis suggests that 10 mg rizatriptan, 40 mg eletriptan, and 12.5 mg almotriptan are most effective. Sumatriptan may also be given, especially in combination with naproxen. Early administration improves effectiveness.
- IV antiemetics (prochlorperazine, metoclopramide, chlorpromazine) may be used in addition to triptans. Acute dystonic reactions, QT prolongation, and akathisia are rare side effects. These are generally not used as monotherapy.
- Ergotamine, ergotamine combinations (PO/PR), and dihydroergotamine (DHE 45) (SC, IV, IM, intranasal) have well-documented efficacy against migraines. DHE is usually administered in combination with an antiemetic drug (Table 1).
- IV dexamethasone may be used to prevent recurrence but should not be used frequently due to risk for toxicity.
- Greater and lesser occipital nerve blocks may also be performed to alleviate pain in the acute setting. This may be combined with auriculotemporal, supraorbital, and supratrochlear nerve block to achieve anesthesia in the area of perceived pain. Steroids should generally be avoided with these nerve blocks because of lack of benefit.

PROPHYLAXIS Rx

- Prophylactic treatment is generally indicated when headaches occur more than once a week or when symptomatic treatments are contraindicated or not effective. They are most effective when initiated during a headache-free period. All prophylaxis should be maintained for at least 3 months before deeming the medication a failure.
- Well-established options for prophylactic treatment include β-blockers (propranolol, timolol, atenolol, metoprolol), tricyclic antidepressants (amitriptyline), and the antiepileptic drugs topiramate and sodium divalproate (valproic acid).
- Less-established options include calcium channel blockers and selective norepinephrine serotonin reuptake inhibitors.
- Supraorbital transcutaneous electrical stimulation has been approved by the FDA for prophylaxis of episodic migraine and is widely available with a prescription in Europe and North America.
- The FDA has approved injection of onabotulinum toxin A (Botox) for prevention of headaches in adult patients with chronic migraines only (≥15 headache days/mo for ≥3 mo).
- Surgical treatment for migraine using nerve decompression has been recently advocated but remains highly controversial, with poorly established results. This should be pursued only in collaboration with a headache specialist.

DISPOSITION

With advancing age, many patients will have sustained reduction in frequency of migraine headaches.

REFERRAL

To neurologist if uncertain about diagnosis or treatment not effective

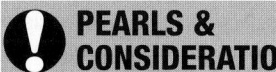

PEARLS & CONSIDERATIONS

- Avoid use of narcotics, barbiturates, and benzodiazepines because they are habit-forming. Narcotics and barbiturates also promote medical overuse headaches.
- Long-term use of analgesic medications can result in medication overuse or rebound headaches.
- Useful mnemonic for migraine is POUND: *P*ulsatile, *O*ne-day in duration, *U*nilateral, *N*ausea/vomiting, *D*isabling.
- Migraine with aura is a significant contributor to stroke risk in women and a contraindication to the use of combined oral contraceptives.

SUGGESTED READINGS

Available at www.expertconsult.com

RELATED CONTENT

Migraine Headache (Patient Information)

AUTHORS: **MICHAEL POHLEN, M.D., JOSEPH S. KASS, M.D., J.D.,** and **SIDDHARTH KAPOOR, M.D.**

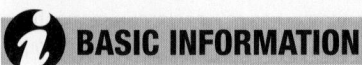

BASIC INFORMATION

Tension-type headache (TTH) is a highly prevalent primary headache disorder that is not associated with nausea or vomiting. Although previously thought to be caused by psychological factors and muscle contraction, current thinking implicates neurobiological mechanisms.

ICD-10CM CODES
G44.209 Tension-type headache, unspecified, not intractable
G44.201 Tension-type headache, unspecified, intractable

EPIDEMIOLOGY & DEMOGRAPHICS

Most common type of headache, representing 70% of all headaches presenting to primary care physicians. Women are affected more often than men.

PHYSICAL FINDINGS & CLINICAL PRESENTATION

Headaches have an insidious progression, ranging from infrequent (<1 day per month) to chronic. Although considered a "featureless" headache disorder, either the symptom photophobia or phonophobia may still be present. Concurrent problems, such as anxiety, depression, and analgesic overuse, may aggravate the headaches. Patients may have pericranial tenderness to palpation on exam. The rest of the examination should be normal.

PATHOPHYSIOLOGY

- TTH is no longer thought to be due to either a psychological problem or abnormal muscle contraction. Similar to migraine, TTH is likely a heterogeneous disorder with several possible pathophysiologic mechanisms.
- In episodic TTH, peripheral mechanisms may predominate, whereas in chronic TTH central mechanisms are involved.

DIAGNOSIS

Tension-type headache:
- At least 10 headaches
- Lasting from 30 minutes to 7 days
- Having at least two of the following features:
  1. Bilateral
  2. Pressure or tightening (non-pulsating) quality
  3. Mild or moderate intensity
  4. Not aggravated by routine physical activity such as walking or climbing stairs

- Both of the following:
  1. No nausea or vomiting
  2. No more than one of either photophobia or phonophobia
- Not better accounted for by another diagnosis

DIFFERENTIAL DIAGNOSIS

- Migraine (would expect associated symptoms [i.e., nausea]; see topic "Headache, Migraine").
- Cervical spine disease.
- Intracranial mass (may present with focal neurologic signs, seizures, or headache awakening patient from sleep).
- Idiopathic intracranial hypertension (found more often in obese women of childbearing age).
- Medication overuse headache.
- Secondary headache (e.g., obstructive sleep apnea, temporomandibular joint syndrome, hypo- or hyperthyroidism, drug side effects).
- Section II describes the differential diagnosis of headaches.

WORKUP

- Routine testing is not needed; the diagnosis may be established clinically.
- Thorough history to identify any red flag features (see topic "Headache, Migraine," SSNOOP5 mnemonic in differential diagnosis) and physical examination (looking for papilledema) for all patients being evaluated for headache.
- Neuroimaging, preferably with contrast-enhanced MRI, should be performed when red flag features are identified by history or unexplained neurologic findings are present on examination.
- Erythrocyte sedimentation rate and C-reactive protein in patients 50 years of age and older to screen for giant cell arteritis.

TREATMENT

Current evidence supports synergistic benefits of combined nonpharmacologic and pharmacologic interventions. Nonpharmacologic therapy may include behavioral sleep modification, acupuncture, cognitive-behavioral therapy, relaxation training, and biofeedback.

ACUTE Rx

- Simple analgesics (i.e., NSAID, acetaminophen).
- Combination analgesics containing caffeine may be used as second-line treatment, although use on more than 10 days per month may lead to medication overuse headache.
- As with migraine headaches, narcotic- and barbiturate-containing analgesics should be avoided in tension-type headaches.

PREVENTIVE Rx

- Tricyclic antidepressants (e.g., amitriptyline 10-50 mg qhs) (first choice)
  Other options: mirtazapine, venlafaxine, and tizanidine

DISPOSITION

The headache prognosis is generally favorable. Some patients will not respond to treatment.

REFERRAL

If red flags are present on history or exam or if the patient is not improving with treatment

PEARLS & CONSIDERATIONS

It is imperative to avoid overuse of caffeine-, narcotic-, and barbiturate-containing medications because of the risk of rebound headaches.

SUGGESTED READINGS
Available at www.expertconsult.com

RELATED CONTENT
Tension Headache (Patient Information)

AUTHOR: **JONATHAN H. SMITH, M.D.**

BASIC INFORMATION

DEFINITION

Complete heart block (CHB) is the absence of electrical impulse transmission from the atria to the ventricles when atrioventricular (AV) junction is not physiologically refractory, due to a functional or anatomical impairment of the conduction system, resulting in a bradycardia characterized by AV dissociation. It may be acquired or congenital. CHB can be permanent or reversible.

SYNONYMS

Third-degree AV block
CHB
Complete AV block

ICD-10CM CODES
I44.2 Atrioventricular block, complete

EPIDEMIOLOGY & DEMOGRAPHICS

- The prevalence of CHB is 0.04%.
- The prevalence of CHB increases with age.

PHYSICAL FINDINGS & CLINICAL PRESENTATION

Physical examination may be normal. Cannon A waves may appear in the jugular vein periodically due to the right atrium contracting during ventricular systole. Patients may present with the following clinical manifestations:
- Dizziness, palpitations
- Syncope or presyncope (due to reduced cardiac output)
- Fatigue, impaired exercise tolerance
- Mental status changes
- Congestive heart failure
- Angina pectoris
- Some patients may be asymptomatic (e.g., congenital CHB)

ETIOLOGY

- Fibrosis or sclerosis of the conduction system, Lenegre and Lev disease
- Acute myocardial infarction—inferior (14%) or anterior (2%) wall of patients, usually within 24 hours
- Drug effect (digitalis, calcium channel blockers, beta-blockers, amiodarone)
- Cardiomyopathy and myocarditis
- Infiltrative processes of the myocardium (amyloidosis, sarcoidosis, scleroderma, tumor)

- Metabolic abnormalities (hyperkalemia, hypoxia, hypothyroidism)
- Lyme carditis, rheumatoid nodules, polymyositis, Chagas' disease
- Neuromuscular disorders (Becker muscular dystrophy, myotonic muscular dystrophy)
- Congenital (birth from mothers with systemic lupus)
- Hyperkalemia
- Familial: SCN5 sodium channel mutations have been associated with CHB
- Iatrogenic (cardiac surgery, catheter ablation of arrhythmias, percutaneous coronary intervention). Transcatheter aortic valve implantation (TAVI) is shown to be frequently associated with new conduction abnormalities; patients with preexisting right bundle-branch block are at increased risk of CHB (resolves over time in most patients).
- Paroxysmal due to phase 4 block of the His-Purkinje system

DIAGNOSIS

DIFFERENTIAL DIAGNOSIS

- The differential diagnosis includes lesser degree of AV block, automatic accelerated junctional rhythms, and nonconducted premature atrial contractions.
- The atrial rate must be faster than the ventricular rate (more As than Vs) and the junctional or ventricular rate is regular. Episodes of AV dissociation with an accelerated ventricular or junctional pacemaker overtaking the sinus node can often look like heart block on a single electrocardiogram.

WORKUP

- Workup such as routine labs, cardiac biomarkers, and cardiac imaging should be dictated by the clinical circumstances.
- ECG: diagnostic of the disease (Figs. 1 and 2):
  1. P waves are present with a regular atrial rate that is faster than the ventricular rate.
  2. P waves are not related to the QRS complexes. The PR intervals are variable.
  3. RR intervals are regular.
  4. QRS complexes may be narrow with rate of 40 to 60 beats/min (block proximal to His bundle) or wide with a rate of <40 beats/min (block distal to His bundle)—depending on the location of the block in the conduction system.
  5. Complete AV block can result from block at the level of AV node, within the His bundle, or distal to it, in the Purkinje system.

TREATMENT

ACUTE GENERAL Rx

- Initial treatment should focus on the hemodynamic stability and symptoms of the patient.
- Consider temporary pacemaker insertion if ventricular escape rate is slow (<40 beats/

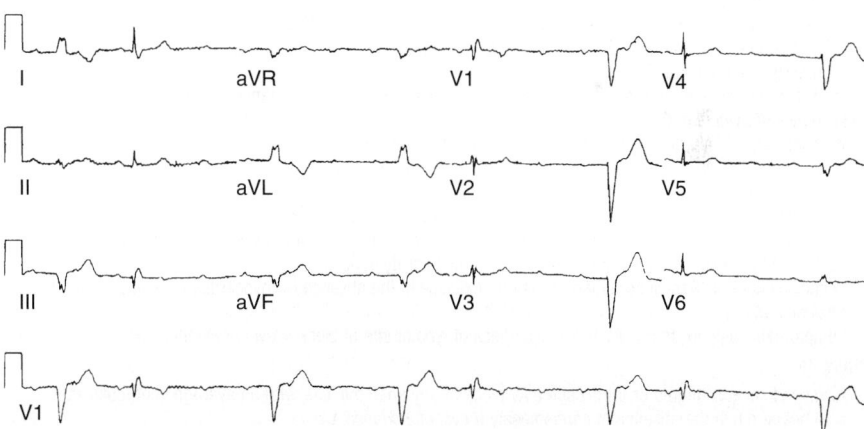

FIG. 2 High-grade atrioventricular block. Note that only three P waves conducted to the ventricle in the whole tracing. Conducted P waves were associated with normal PR intervals and right bundle branch block, a finding suggesting infranodal block. All other P waves were blocked, and ventricular escape rhythm with a left bundle branch block pattern is observed. Note that the block is not caused by retrograde concealment in the atrioventricular node or His-Purkinje system from the ventricular escape complexes because the conducted P waves occurred at a short cycle following the escape complexes. (From Issa Z, et al.: *Clinical arrhythmology and electrophysiology,* ed 2, Philadelphia, 2012, Saunders.)

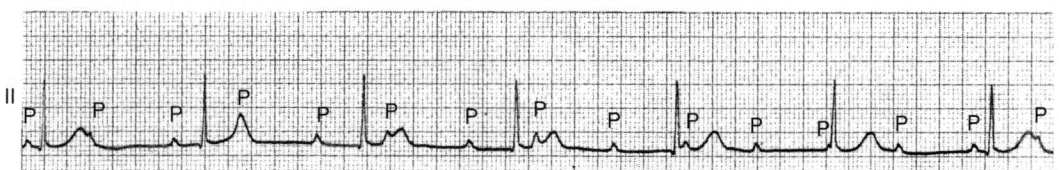

FIG. 1 Third-degree (complete) atrioventricular heart block is characterized by independent atrial (P) and ventricular (QRS) activity. The atrial rate is always faster than the ventricular rate. The PR intervals are completely variable. Some P waves fall on the T wave, distorting its shape. Others may fall in the QRS complex and be "lost." Notice that the QRS complexes are of normal width, indicating that the ventricles are being paced from the atrioventricular junction. (From Goldberger AL, editor: *Clinical electrocardiography,* ed 5, St Louis, 1994, Mosby.)

min) and associated with symptoms or hemodynamic compromise as well as wide QRS escape rhythms, which can be unstable, and QT prolongation above 500 ms, increasing the risk of torsade de pointes ventricular tachycardias.

- CHB as a complication of inferior MI usually only requires temporary pacing; however, a CHB as a result of anterior MI often requires permanent pacing (Table 1).
- Acquired CHB usually requires pacing, but patients with congenital CHB often have sufficiently rapid escape rhythm to prevent symptoms and avoid permanent pacemaker implantation.
- Withdraw AV-nodal blocking agents if any.
- Short-term therapy (until adequate pacing therapy is established)
  1. Vagolytic agents such as atropine may be used to increase the rate of the escape rhythm (for AV nodal level blocks)
  2. Catecholamines such as isoproterenol transiently used for a CHB at any site (use with extreme caution or not at all in patients with coronary artery disease or in patients with digitalis toxicity).

3. Percutaneous external cardiac pacing (uncomfortable for patients and not always reliably capturing the ventricle).
- Drugs cannot be relied on to increase HR for more than several hours or days without side effects; therefore, temporary or permanent pacemaker insertion is indicated.
- Symptomatic CHB in the absence of a condition that is likely to resolve is an ACC/AHA/HRS Class I indication for permanent pacemaker (PPM) placement.
- Class 1 indications for PPM placement in asymptomatic patients according to the ACC/AHA guidelines include:
  1. Patients in sinus rhythm, with documented asystolic pauses greater than or equal to 3.0 sec or an escape rate <40 beats/min, or with an escape rhythm that is below the AV node
  2. Patients with atrial fibrillation and bradycardia with one or more pauses of at least 5 sec or longer
  3. After catheter ablation of the AV junction
  4. If cardiomegaly or LV dysfunction is present with ventricular rates of 40 beats/min or faster

5. Postoperative CHB that is not expected to resolve
6. When it is associated with neuromuscular diseases, such as Erb dystrophy (limb-girdle muscular dystrophy), Kearns-Sayre syndrome, myotonic muscular dystrophy, and peroneal muscular atrophy
7. CHB present during exercise in the absence of myocardial ischemia
- Therapy is directed toward the underlying etiology if there is a reversible source (i.e., IV antibiotics for Lyme disease).

CHRONIC Rx

Dual-chamber pacemaker implantation. Patients with PPM need regular follow-up and pacemaker monitoring to ensure proper device functioning.

DISPOSITION

- Mortality is highest in the neonatal period in congenital CHB.
- Prognosis is favorable after insertion of pacemaker and related to the underlying etiology of complete AV block (e.g., myocardial infarction, cardiomyopathy).
- Nonrandomized studies have shown that PPM insertion improves survival in patients with CHB.

REFERRAL

All patients with CHB should be referred to a cardiologist for consideration of temporary and/or PPM implantation.

❗ PEARLS & CONSIDERATIONS

COMMENTS

- Patients should be instructed to avoid activities that may damage the pacemaker (e.g., contact sports).
- Pacemaker manufacturers do not recommend any special restrictions regarding proximity to typical household items.
- The presence of a permanent pacemaker is a strong relative contraindication to MRI, although now many MRI-compatible pacemakers are available.
- Some medical procedures, such as lithotripsy, hyperbaric chamber, and electrocautery used during surgery, may require pacemaker programming and testing perioperatively.
- Table E2 describes the five-letter pacemaker code, and Table E3 summarizes common permanent pacemakers.

RELATED CONTENT

Complete Heart Block (Patient Information)

AUTHORS: **BARRY FINE, M.D., Ph.D.,** and **HEIKO SCHMITT, M.D., PH.D.**

TABLE 1 Indications for Pacing in AV Block

Class I

1. Third-degree or advanced second-degree AV block at any anatomic level associated with any one of the following conditions:
   a Symptoms (including heart failure) attributable to AV block (*Level of Evidence: C*)
   b Arrhythmias and other medical conditions that require drugs that result in symptomatic bradycardia (*Level of Evidence: C*)
   c Documented periods of asystole >3.0 seconds, any escape rate <40 beats/min, or any escape rhythm below the AV junction (e.g., a wide QRS morphology) in awake, asymptomatic patients in sinus rhythm (*Level of Evidence: C*)
   d A documented period of asystole >5 seconds in awake, asymptomatic patients in atrial fibrillation (*Level of Evidence: C*)
   e After catheter ablation of the AV junction (*Level of Evidence: C*)
   f Postoperative AV block that is not expected to resolve after cardiac surgery (*Level of Evidence: C*)
   g Neuromuscular diseases, such as myotonic muscular dystrophy, Kearns–Sayre syndrome, Erb (limb-girdle) dystrophy, and peroneal muscular atrophy, with or without symptoms of bradycardia (*Level of Evidence: B*)
2. Asymptomatic third-degree AV block at any anatomic site with an average awake ventricular rate >40 beats/min in patients with cardiomegaly or left ventricular dysfunction
3. Second-degree or third-degree AV block during exercise in the absence of myocardial ischemia (*Level of Evidence: C*)
4. Symptomatic second-degree AV block regardless of type or site of block (*Level of Evidence: B*)

Class IIa

1. Advanced second-degree or third-degree AV block at any anatomic site with an average ventricular rate >40 beats/min in the absence of cardiomegaly (*Level of Evidence: C*)
2. Asymptomatic second-degree AV block at intra- or infra-His levels found at electrophysiologic study (*Level of Evidence: B*)
3. First-degree or second-degree AV block with symptoms similar to those of pacemaker syndrome (*Level of Evidence: B*)
4. Asymptomatic type II second-degree AV block with a narrow QRS. When type II second-degree AV block occurs with a wide QRS, including isolated right bundle branch block, pacing becomes a Class I recommendation. (*Level of Evidence: B*)

Class IIb

1. AV block due to drug use or toxicity when the block is expected to recur even after withdrawal of the drug (*Level of Evidence: B*)
2. Neuromuscular diseases, such as myotonic muscular dystrophy, Kearns–Sayre syndrome, Erb (limb-girdle) dystrophy, and peroneal muscular atrophy with any degree of AV block (including first-degree AV block), with or without symptoms of bradycardia (*Level of Evidence: B*)

Class III

1. Asymptomatic first-degree AV block (*Level of Evidence: B*)
2. Asymptomatic type I second-degree AV block at a site above the His (i.e., the AV node) level or not known to be intra- or infra-Hisian by electrophysiologic study (*Level of Evidence: B*)
3. AV block expected to resolve and unlikely to recur (e.g., drug toxicity, Lyme disease, nocturnally in sleep apnea, early postoperative status, transient increases in vagal tone) (*Level of Evidence: B*)

From Bonow RO, et al.: Braunwald's heart disease: a textbook of cardiovascular medicine, ed 9, Philadelphia, 2012, Saunders.

BASIC INFORMATION

DEFINITION

Second-degree heart block or second-degree atrioventricular (AV) heart block is characterized by a failure of one or more, but not all, atrial impulses to conduct to the ventricles. The block may be at any level of AV conduction system. In both types of second-degree heart block, the sinus rate will continue at regular intervals resulting in a constant sinus rate. When more than one atrial impulse is present for each ventricular complex, the rhythm may be described as a ratio of the number of atrial impulses to the number of ventricular complexes. Electrocardiographically there are three types of second-degree block:

- Mobitz type I (Wenckebach):
  1. Characterized by a progressive prolongation of the PR interval prior to a blocked nonconducted beat and a shorter PR interval after that blocked beat; the conducted impulse will generally be narrow. The cycle may repeat periodically, leading to "grouped beating."
  2. Site of block is usually AV node (proximal to the His bundle).
- Mobitz type II:
  1. Characterized by fixed PR intervals before and after blocked beats and may be associated with a wide QRS morphology (right bundle branch block [RBBB] or left bundle branch block [LBBB] patterns).
  2. Site of block is usually infranodal, especially when QRS is wide.
  3. It has a greater propensity for progressing to third-degree AV block.
- Pure 2:1 conduction patterns cannot be reliably classified as Mobitz type I or type II because there are not enough P waves to characterize prolongation of the PR interval.

SYNONYMS

Wenckebach block (Mobitz type I block)
Mobitz type II block
AV block

ICD-10CM CODES
I44.1 Atrioventricular block, second degree
I45.5 Other specified heart block
Q24.6 Congenital heart block

EPIDEMIOLOGY & DEMOGRAPHICS

Mobitz type I block is more common and may occur in individuals with heightened vagal tone or as a side effect of medications, such as β-blockers or calcium channel blockers.

PHYSICAL FINDINGS & CLINICAL PRESENTATION

- Patients with Mobitz type I are usually asymptomatic. Patients with either type may feel palpitations or the feeling of "missing a beat." Sudden loss of consciousness without warning (Adams-Stokes attack) can occur in patients with Mobitz type II; however, it is much more common in patients with complete heart block.
- Type I block: there is gradual decrease in the intensity of the first heart sound with widening of the a-c interval in the central venous waveform, ending in a pause, and an a wave not followed by a v wave in the neck along with an irregular pulse.
- Type II block: the first heart sound retains a constant intensity, with intermittent ventricular pauses and a waves not followed by v waves in the neck. There is an irregular pulse for most times with intermittent pauses.

ETIOLOGY

- High vagal tone (young patients, athletes at rest)
- Degenerative changes in the AV conduction system
- Ischemia at the AV nodes (type I with inferior wall myocardial infarction [MI] and type II with anterior wall MI)
- Drugs (digitalis, quinidine, procainamide, adenosine, calcium channel blockers [nondihydropyridines], β-blockers)
- Cardiomyopathies, collagen vascular diseases, infiltrative diseases (amyloidosis, sarcoidosis, hematochromatosis)
- Myocarditis/endocarditis (infectious, e.g., Lyme disease, Chagas disease; and noninfectious, e.g., systemic lupus erythematosus)
- Hyperkalemia, hypermagnesemia
- Hypothyroidism
- Prior cardiac valve surgery
- Catheter trauma, catheter ablation for arrhythmias

(DX) DIAGNOSIS

DIFFERENTIAL DIAGNOSIS

The ECG easily and reliably distinguishes Mobitz type I from Mobitz type II block and from other conduction abnormalities. It should be distinguished from the less common phenomenon of second-degree sinoatrial node exit block.

Mobitz type I block with a normal QRS complex tends to be benign and usually does not progress to more advanced forms of AV conduction within a short period of time because the disease is mostly confined to within the AV node. Mobitz type II block often precedes the development of Adams-Stokes syncope, symptoms are frequent, prognosis is compromised, and progression to third-degree AV block is common and sudden. Thus, type II second-degree AV block with a wide QRS typically indicates diffuse conduction system disease involving even the infranodal His-Purkinje system.

WORKUP

ECG, ambulatory monitoring (Holter or external loop recorders) in selected patients

- Mobitz type I (Fig. 1) ECG shows:
  1. Sequential and gradual prolongation of PR interval leading to a nonconducted P wave
  2. Shortened PR interval following the pause as compared to the pre-pause PR interval
  3. Progressive shortening of the R-R interval prior to nonconducted atrial impulse
  4. Usually see "grouped beating" pattern.
- Mobitz type II ECG shows (Fig. 2):
  1. Fixed duration of PR interval with constant P-P and R-R intervals
  2. Sudden nonconducted P wave
  3. Abnormal QRS duration or fascicular blocks are common.
- In 2:1 AV block (Fig. 3), it cannot be determined based on the 12-lead ECG whether there is Mobitz type I or type II AV block, although a wide QRS complex is suggestive of Mobitz type II.
  1. Administering atropine can improve AV conduction if the AV block is type I or within the AV node; however, if it is infranodal (i.e., type II), the increased sinus rate caused by atropine may worsen the ratio of AV conduction, resulting in worsening bradycardia.
  2. Exercise stress testing may function in the same way as atropine above. If the disease is confined to the AV node, it may improve with exercise, but in cases of Mobitz type II AV block, the degree of AV block will worsen.
  3. Carotid sinus stimulation and other vagal maneuvers may worsen the AV block if it is at the level of the AV node (i.e., Mobitz type I) but will paradoxically improve the ratio of AV conduction by slowing down the sinus rate if it is a Mobitz type II or infranodal AV block.

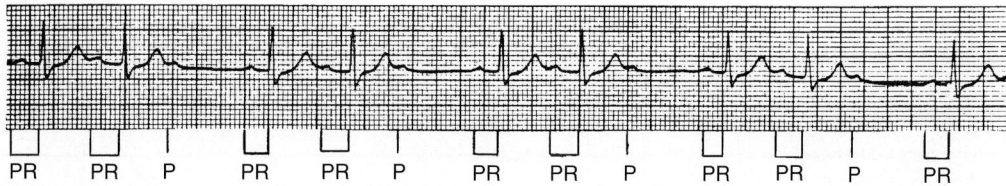

FIG. 1 Wenckebach (Mobitz type I) second-degree atrioventricular block. Notice the progressive increase in PR intervals, with the third P wave in each sequence not followed by a QRS. Wenckebach block produces a characteristically syncopated rhythm with grouping of the QRS complexes (group beating). (From Goldberger AL [ed]: *Clinical electrocardiography,* ed 5, St Louis, 1994, Mosby.)

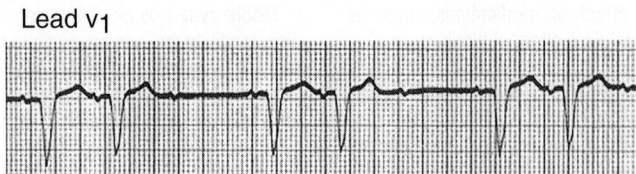
Lead v₁

2nd degree AV block (type II) with LBBB

FIG. 2 Mobitz type II AV block with left bundle branch block (LBBB). Note the fixed P-P intervals with no change in PR intervals followed by a sudden nonconducted P wave. The LBBB indicates infranodal disease in the His-Purkinje system that is suggestive of Mobitz type II block.

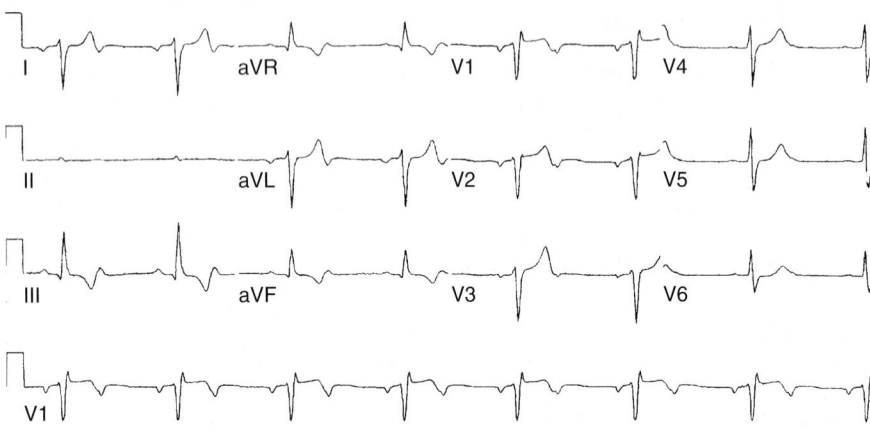

I   aVR   V1   V4

II   aVL   V2   V5

III   aVF   V3   V6

V1

FIG. 3 Second-degree 2:1 atrioventricular block. Notice the short PR interval during conducted complexes and the wide QRS complexes, suggesting block in the His-Purkinje system. (From Issa Z, et al.: *Clinical arrhythmology and electrophysiology,* ed 2, Philadelphia, 2012, Saunders.)

℞ TREATMENT

NONPHARMACOLOGIC THERAPY

Elimination of drugs that may induce AV block such as digoxin, beta-blockers, and calcium channel blockers

ACUTE GENERAL Rx

- Treatment is usually not necessary unless the resting heart rate is <40 beats per min (bpm) while awake.
- If symptomatic (e.g., dizziness), atropine 1 mg (may repeat once after 5 min) may be tried to increase AV conduction; if no response, trial of dobutamine or isoproterenol may be helpful prior to insertion of a pacemaker.

- Atropine
  1. Reduces heart block due to hypervagotonia but not due to AV node ischemia
  2. Does not increase infranodal conduction (third-degree and second-degree AV block that is below the AV node)
  3. Should be used with caution in Mobitz type II AV block due to possible paradoxical decrease in heart rate (as atrial rate increases, AV conduction decreases)
  4. Is ineffective in heart transplantation patients
- If associated with anterior wall MI and wide QRS complex, consider insertion of a temporary pacemaker.
- Indications for permanent pacemaker (PPM) implantation by ACC/AHA/HRS 2008 guidelines:
  1. Second-degree AV block with associated symptomatic bradycardia regardless of the type or site of the block (class I; level of evidence: B).
  2. Second-degree AV block provoked by exercise in the absence of myocardial ischemia (class I; level of evidence: C).
  3. Asymptomatic second-degree AV block at intra- or infra-His levels found at electrophysiologic study (class IIa; level of evidence: B).
  4. First- or second-degree AV block with symptoms similar to those of pacemaker syndrome or hemodynamic compromise (class IIa; level of evidence: B).
  5. Asymptomatic type II second-degree AV block with a wide QRS, including isolated right bundle-branch block (class I; level of evidence: B).
  6. PPM is not indicated for asymptomatic type I second-degree AV block at supra-His (AV node) level or that which is not known to be intra- or infra-Hisian (class III; level of evidence: C)

DISPOSITION

Prognosis is good with insertion of a pacemaker.

REFERRAL

Referral for pacemaker insertion (see "Acute General Rx")

❗ PEARLS & CONSIDERATIONS

COMMENTS

Patients with symptomatic Mobitz type II should be referred for a pacemaker. Asymptomatic patients should be referred if the AV block worsens with exercise and should be followed up routinely for potential development of high-grade AV block.

RELATED CONTENT

Second-Degree Heart Block (Patient Information)

AUTHORS: **ALEEM MUGHAL, M.D.,** and **JOHN WYLIE, M.D.**

BASIC INFORMATION

DEFINITION

Heart failure (HF) is a complex clinical syndrome that can result from any structural or functional cardiac disorder that impairs the ability of the ventricle to fill with or eject blood. The cardinal manifestations of heart failure are dyspnea and fatigue that can limit exercise tolerance. The pathophysiology of HF is related to progressive activation of the neuroendocrine system to compensate for decreased effective circulating volume (Table 1), leading to total body volume overload and circulatory insufficiency. These events culminate in the development of pulmonary congestion as well as peripheral edema. Specifically, the renin-angiotensin-aldosterone system (RAAS) is implicated as being activated in HF, leading to volume expansion (sodium retention) and cardiac fibrosis (mediated through angiotensin II). Disordered adrenergic stimulation has also been recognized as a key component of progression of disease. The term "congestive heart failure" (CHF) usually denotes a volume-overloaded status as a result of HF. Given that not all patients have volume overload at the time of the evaluation, "congestive heart failure" should be distinguished from the broader term "heart failure."

CLASSIFICATION: The American College of Cardiology/American Heart Association (ACC/AHA) describes the following four stages of HF. This staging model was designed to emphasize the evolution and progression of HF over a continuum and the preventability of HF in at-risk patients.

Stage A: Patients at high risk (e.g., with hypertension, atherosclerotic disease, diabetes mellitus, metabolic syndrome, cytotoxin, family history) for HF but without structural heart disease or symptoms of HF

Stage B: Patients with structural heart disease (e.g., left ventricular [LV] dysfunction) but without symptoms of HF

Stage C: Patients with structural heart disease with prior or current symptoms of HF

Stage D: Patients with refractory HF requiring specialized interventions

In addition to the ACC/AHA stages described above, the New York Heart Association (NYHA) defines four functional classes of HF designed to describe the symptoms of stage C and D HF. The functional classes are intended to assess the symptoms of HF and may fluctuate with therapy. It should be noted that current guidelines employ the functional classes to aid in determination of appropriate treatment.

I. Asymptomatic or symptomatic only at activity levels that would limit normal individuals

II. Symptomatic with ordinary exertion (e.g., 2 city blocks or 1 flight of stairs in a faster than usual pace)

III. Symptomatic with less than ordinary exertion (e.g., less than 2 city blocks or 1 flight of stairs)

IV. Symptomatic at rest

TERMINOLOGY: HF has been traditionally dichotomized as systolic vs. diastolic (see Table 2), which has now been replaced with the terms "HF with reduced ejection fraction" (HFrEF) and "HF with preserved ejection fraction" (HFpEF), respectively. Other common classifications include right-sided vs. left-sided and high-output vs. low-output. Systolic HF or HFrEF is defined by the presence of impaired contractility of the LV, as measured by ejection fraction (EF) less than 40% with clinical signs or symptoms of HF. In contrast, HFpEF has been described as evidence (clinical) of HF with an EF above 50% with or without evidence of diastolic dysfunction. The term "HF with preserved EF" is preferred over the term "diastolic HF," given that many of the physiologic derangements in this subset of HF are not solely restricted to diastolic

function of the heart. Right-sided HF denotes peripheral signs and symptoms of HF without evidence of pulmonary congestion, as opposed to left-sided HF, which typically manifests with pulmonary congestion and subsequent signs and symptoms of right-sided HF. The most common cause of right-sided HF is left-sided HF. High-output HF involves signs and symptoms of HF but features an elevated cardiac output unable to meet the abnormally high metabolic demands of peripheral tissues and is the result of myriad systemic disorders (e.g., systemic arteriovenous fistulas, hyperthyroidism, anemia). The term "acute decompensated HF" (ADHF) refers to worsening of signs or symptoms of HF due to a wide range of causes. Of note, HF is not equivalent to cardiomyopathy or LV dysfunction. These latter terms describe the possible structural or functional reasons for the development of HF, whereas HF is a clinical syndrome characterized by specific symptoms and signs.

SYNONYMS

HF
Congestive heart failure
CHF
Cardiac failure
Cardiogenic shock
Cardiogenic pulmonary edema

ICD-10CM CODES
I50.20 Unspecified systolic (congestive) heart failure
I50.21 Acute systolic (congestive) heart failure
I50.22 Chronic systolic (congestive) heart failure
I50.23 Acute on chronic systolic (congestive) heart failure
I50.30 Unspecified diastolic (congestive) heart failure

Continued

TABLE 1 Compensatory Mechanisms in Heart Failure

Compensatory Response	Stimuli	Beneficial Effects	Adverse Effects	Potential Pharmacologic Interventions
Renin-angiotensin system activation	↓CO/BP ↓Renal blood flow ↑β-adrenergic activity	Maintain vital organ perfusion through vasoconstriction and sodium retention	↑Afterload → worsened LV function Adverse LV remodeling (apoptosis, myocyte hypertrophy)	ACE inhibitors ARBs
Adrenergic activation	↓CO/BP	↑CO through ↑ in heart rate and contractility ↑BP	↑Ischemia ↑Afterload → worsened LV function ↑LVEDP → pulmonary congestion Adverse LV remodeling (apoptosis, myocyte hypertrophy)	β-adrenergic blocking agents
Renal salt and water retention	↑Antidiuretic hormone ↑Norepinephrine ↑Angiotensin II ↑Aldosterone ↓Renal blood flow	↑Preload → ↑stroke volume and CO	Pulmonary and systemic congestion Adverse LV remodeling	Diuretics Aldosterone inhibitors ACE inhibitors, ARBs β-adrenergic blocking agents
↑Natriuretic peptide secretion	Volume expansion (atrial stretch)	Diuresis Natriuresis Partial inhibition of renin-angiotensin system and norepinephrine	None known	Natriuretic peptides

ACE, Angiotensin-converting enzyme; *ARB*, angiotensin receptor blocker; *BP*, blood pressure; *CO*, cardiac output; *LV*, left ventricular; *LVEDP*, left ventricular end-diastolic pressure.
From Sellke FW et al: *Sabiston & Spencer surgery of the chest*, ed 9, 2016, Elsevier.

I50.31	Acute diastolic (congestive) heart failure
I50.32	Chronic diastolic (congestive) heart failure
I50.33	Acute on chronic diastolic (congestive) heart failure
I50.40	Unspecified combined systolic (congestive) and diastolic (congestive) heart failure
I50.41	Acute combined systolic (congestive) and diastolic (congestive) heart failure
I50.42	Chronic combined systolic (congestive) and diastolic (congestive) heart failure
I50.43	Acute on chronic combined systolic (congestive) and diastolic (congestive) heart failure
I50.9	Heart failure, unspecified

EPIDEMIOLOGY & DEMOGRAPHICS

- There is variability in the reported demographics of HF due to heterogeneous definitions and classifications of HF. African Americans have the highest risk for HF of the demographic groups. Incidence rate is lowest among white women and highest among black men, with blacks having a higher 5-yr mortality rate than whites.
- The lifetime risk of developing HF is 20% for Americans ≥40 years of age.
  1. In the United States, HF incidence has largely remained stable over the past several decades, with >650,000 new HF cases diagnosed annually.
- HF is primarily a condition of the elderly. Approximately 80% of patients hospitalized with HF are older than 65 yr. HF is the most common inpatient diagnosis in the U.S. for patients aged >65 yr.
- HF incidence increases with age, rising from approximately 20 per 1,000 individuals 65 to 69 yr to >80 per 1,000 individuals among those >85 yr. Before age 75, the incidence of HF is higher in males, but both sexes are equally affected after this age cutoff.
- In the U.S., 1.1 million hospital discharges and 3.2 million hospitalizations/ambulatory care visits were associated with HF in 2007.
- Prevalence: 5.1 million persons in the U.S. and an estimated 23 million persons worldwide. The prevalence of HF is rising, especially in the elderly, particularly due to aging of the population and improved survival from other conditions.
- The estimated (direct and indirect) cost of HF in the U.S. was >$40 billion in 2012, with over half of these costs spent on hospitalizations. The mean cost of HF-related hospitalizations is $23,077 per patient and is higher when HF was a secondary rather than the primary diagnosis.
- HFrEF and HFpEF each make up about half of the overall HF burden.
- Among patients with HF in one large population study, hospitalizations were common after HF diagnosis, with 83% of patients hospitalized at least once and 43% hospitalized at least 4 times. More than half of the hospitalizations were related to non-cardiovascular causes.

TABLE 2 Systolic vs. Diastolic Heart Failure*

Parameters	Systolic (HFrEF)	Diastolic (HFpEF)
History		
Coronary artery disease	+++†	++
Hypertension	++	++++
Diabetes	++	++
Valvular heart disease	++++	+
Paroxysmal dyspnea	++	+++
Physical Examination		
Cardiomegaly	+++	+
Soft heart sounds	++++	+
S3 gallop	+++	+
S4 gallop	+	+++
Hypertension	++	++++
Mitral regurgitation	+++	+
Rales	++	+
Edema	+++	+
Jugular venous distention	+++	+
Chest Radiograph		
Cardiomegaly	+++	+
Pulmonary congestion	+++	+++
Electrocardiogram		
Left ventricular hypertrophy	++	++++
Q waves	++	+
Low voltage	+++	-
Echocardiogram		
Left ventricular hypertrophy	++	++++
Left ventricular dilation	++	-
Left atrial enlargement	++	++
Reduced ejection fraction	++++	-

*Certain aspects of the history and physical examination, along with clinical measurements, may help to distinguish diastolic from systolic heart failure. For example, patients with hypertensive heart disease and severe left ventricular hypertrophy often experience heart failure because of diastolic dysfunction.
†Plus signs indicate "suggestive" (the number reflects relative weight). Minus signs indicate "not very suggestive." HFpEF, Heart failure with preserved ejection fraction; HFrEF, heart failure with reduced ejection fraction.
From Zipes DP et al (eds): Braunwald's heart disease, ed 7, Philadelphia, 2005, Saunders.

PHYSICAL FINDINGS & CLINICAL PRESENTATION

The clinical and physical exam findings should be given the highest priority when determining the diagnosis of HF. These signs and symptoms are dependent on the severity of disease, precipitant factors, comorbid conditions, and whether the HF symptoms are predominantly right-sided or left-sided.

- Common clinical manifestations are:
  1. Dyspnea on exertion, that can progress to dyspnea at rest, caused by increasing pulmonary vascular congestion
  2. Orthopnea, caused by increased venous return in the recumbent position and further elevated pulmonary venous pressure
  3. Paroxysmal nocturnal dyspnea (PND) resulting from multiple factors including increased venous return in the recumbent position, decreased PaO_2 and decreased adrenergic stimulation of myocardial function during sleep
  4. Nocturnal angina resulting from increased myocardial oxygen demand (secondary to increased venous return in the recumbent position causing increased preload) in patients with concomitant coronary artery disease (CAD)
  5. *Cheyne-Stokes respiration* (alternating phases of apnea and hyperventilation) caused by prolonged circulation time from lungs to brain as a result of impaired cardiac output
  6. Fatigue, lethargy, and decreased functional capacity resulting from low cardiac output and hypoperfusion of peripheral tissues
- Physical examination:
  1. Fine pulmonary crackles, wheezes, tachypnea, hypoxia (due to elevated pulmonary pressures). Crackles may be absent in chronic and longstanding high pulmonary venous pressure because it allows for lymphatic drainage in the lungs to increase.
  2. Tachycardia and narrowed pulse pressure (due to increased sympathetic tone)
  3. S3 gallop, paradoxical splitting of S2, jugular venous distention, peripheral edema in dependent tissues, congestive hepatomegaly, ascites, and hepatojugular reflux (due to volume overload)
  4. Perioral and peripheral cyanosis, decreased capillary refill, pulsus alternans, and cool extremities (due to decreased cardiac output)

- Six common clinical presentations identified by European Society of Cardiology of Acute Heart Failure Syndromes:
  1. ADHF presenting with hypertension (SBP >160): the hypertension leads to increased afterload causing pulmonary vascular congestion.
  2. Worsening or decompensation of chronic HF
  3. Flash pulmonary edema
  4. Cardiogenic shock
  5. Acute coronary syndrome (ACS) and ADHF
  6. Isolated RV failure
- Each of these scenarios may require different therapies to effectively stabilize and treat the patient.

Acute precipitants of HF decompensation include noncompliance with salt restriction or medications (most common cause), infection, arrhythmias (e.g., atrial fibrillation), ischemia or infarction, uncontrolled hypertension, new medications (e.g., negative inotropic agents such as calcium channel blockers/antiarrhythmic agents), nonsteroidal antiinflammatory drugs (NSAIDs), renal dysfunction, toxins (e.g., ethanol and anthracyclines), cardiac surgery, or valvular catastrophe.

ETIOLOGY

LEFT VENTRICULAR FAILURE: The dichotomy of whether HF occurs in the setting of preserved or reduced LV systolic function plays an important role in treatment strategies. Patients with HFpEF may have significant abnormalities in active relaxation and passive stiffness of the LV as well as valvular disease. HFrEF denotes poor pump function.
- Abnormal LV systolic function
  1. CAD (acute or chronic ischemia, myocardial infarction [MI], LV aneurysm), the most common cause of cardiomyopathy in the U.S., comprising 50% to 75% HF patients.
  2. Increased afterload or pressure overload (severe hypertension, aortic stenosis)
  3. Increased preload or volume overload (mitral regurgitation, aortic regurgitation)
  4. Cardiomyopathy: Idiopathic, infiltrative (non-ischemic)
  5. Infectious (Chagas, myocarditis)
  6. Infiltrative (amyloidosis, sarcoidosis, hemochromatosis)
  7. Toxins (ethanol, cocaine, anthracyclines)
  8. Tachycardia induced (e.g., with atrial fibrillation)
- Preserved LV systolic function
  1. Impaired relaxation (myocardial ischemia, diabetes mellitus, metabolic syndrome)
  2. Tachyarrhythmia (featuring reduced diastolic filling time)
  3. Restrictive cardiomyopathy (myocardial stiffness, such as hypereosinophilic syndrome, amyloidosis, hemochromatosis)
  4. High cardiac output (thiamine deficiency, anemia, thyrotoxicosis, arteriovenous malformations)
  5. Increased afterload (uncontrolled hypertension, aortic stenosis, hypertrophic obstructive cardiomyopathy)
  6. Hypervolemia (oliguric renal failure, iatrogenic)

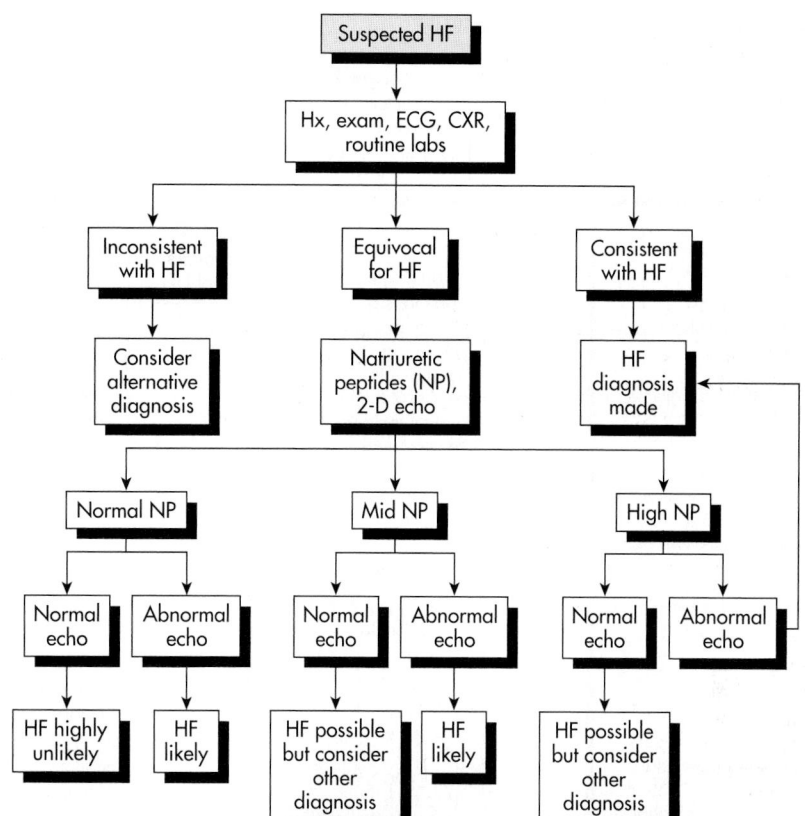

FIG. 1 Flow chart for the evaluation of patients with heart failure. *CXR,* Chest radiograph; *ECG,* electrocardiograph; *echo,* echocardiograph; *HF,* heart failure; *Hx,* history; *NP,* natriuretic peptides. (From Bonow RO et al: Braunwald*'s heart disease: a textbook of cardiovascular medicine,* ed 9, Philadelphia, 2012, Saunders.)

RIGHT VENTRICULAR FAILURE:
- Left-sided HF
- Chronic hypoxemic pulmonary disease
- Valvular heart disease (mitral stenosis or regurgitation)
- Pulmonary embolism
- Primary pulmonary hypertension
- Right-to-left shunts that cause systemic hypoxemia (e.g., large patent foramen ovale and tetralogy of Fallot)
- Left-to-right shunts that cause volume overload (e.g., atrial and ventricular septal defects)
- Bacterial endocarditis (right-sided)
- Right ventricular infarction

DX DIAGNOSIS

DIFFERENTIAL DIAGNOSIS
- COPD, asthma
- Cirrhosis
- Nephrotic syndrome
- Venous insufficiency
- Pulmonary embolism
- ARDS (adult respiratory distress syndrome)
- Pneumonia
- Heroin overdose

WORKUP
- A flow chart for the evaluation of patients with heart failure is outlined in Fig. 1. Fig. 2 describes the stages and treatment options for HF.

- Blood work (to diagnose potentially reversible causes, identify comorbidities, and assess disease severity)
  1. CBC (to evaluate for anemia, infections), urinalysis, blood urea nitrogen (BUN), creatinine, electrolytes (worsening hyponatremia is a marker of disease severity and is associated with higher mortality rates), liver enzymes (hepatic congestion), thyroid function (especially in the elderly or patients with comorbid atrial fibrillation or known thyroid disease)
  2. B-type natriuretic peptide (BNP) is a cardiac neurohormone secreted from the ventricles in response to elevated LV end-diastolic pressure. The sensitivity is low in asymptomatic patients (but elevated BNP levels have been shown to have a negative predictive value up to 90% in symptomatic patients), and BNP elevation generally correlates with severity of disease and parallels closely morbidity and mortality outcome measures. The cleavage remnant N-terminal-pro-BNP (NT-pro-BNP) has a longer half-life and is cleared through the kidneys, making it susceptible to alterations in renal function. A level of <300 pg/mL has an age-independent 98% negative predictive value.
  3. Cardiac biomarkers may be elevated if ischemia is the precipitant factor. However, slight elevations are very common and may not always be due to obstructive

AT RISK FOR HEART FAILURE

HEART FAILURE

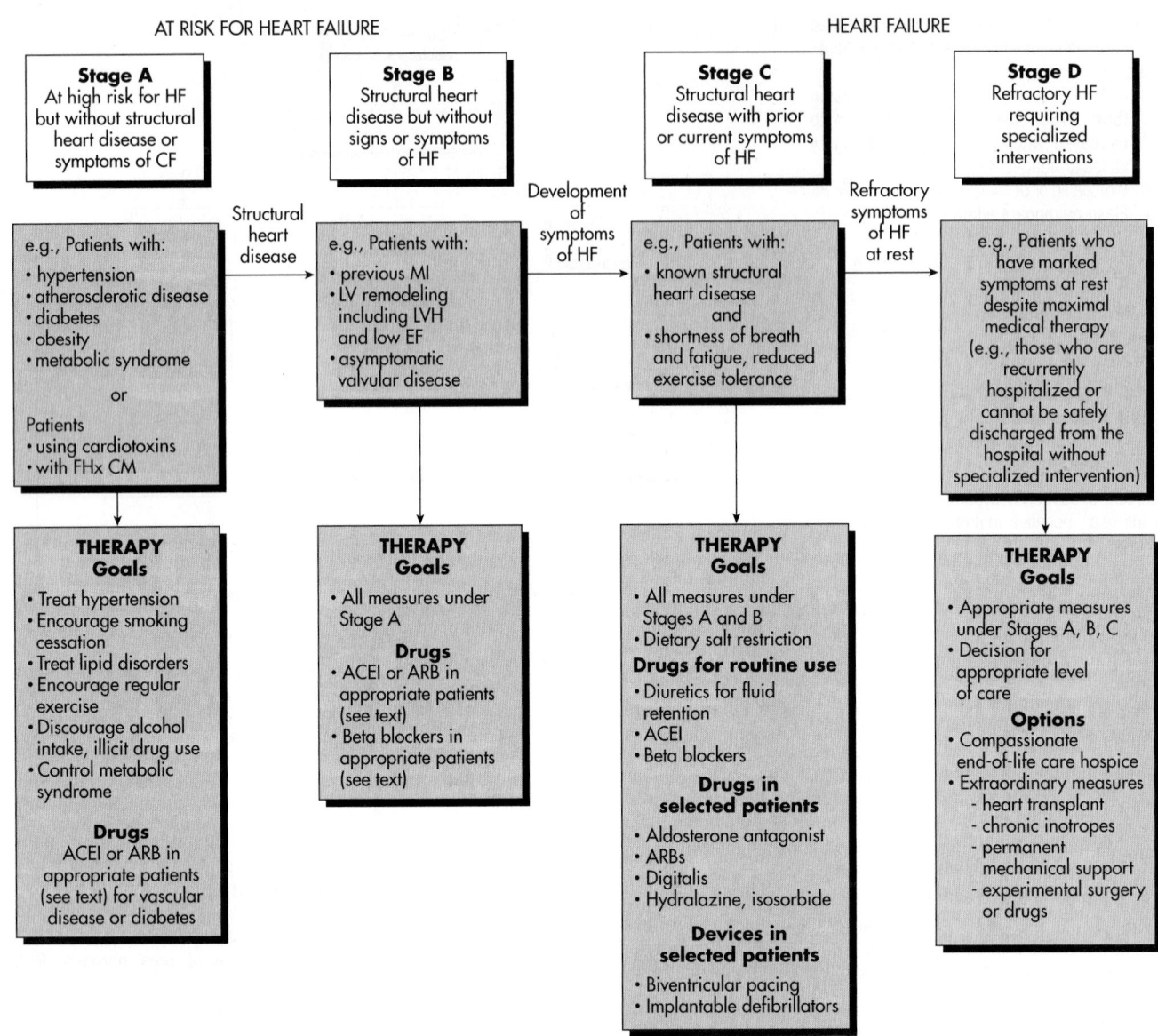

FIG. 2 Stages in the evolution of heart failure (HF) and recommended therapy by stage. *ACEI,* Angiotensin-converting enzyme inhibitor; *ARB,* angiotensin receptor blocker; *EF,* ejection fraction; *FHx CM,* family history of cardiomyopathy; *IV,* intravenous; *LV,* left ventricular; *LVH,* left ventricular hypertrophy; *MI,* myocardial infarction. (From Hunt SA, Baker DW, Chin MH, et al: ACC/AHA guidelines for the evaluation and management of chronic heart failure in the adult: Executive summary. A report of the American College of Cardiology/American Heart Association Task Force on Practice Guidelines [Committee to Revise the 1995 Guidelines for the Evaluation and Management of Heart Failure]. *J Am Coll Cardiol* 104:2996, 2001.)

coronary artery disease. These elevations could be due to subendocardial ischemia (due to increased end-diastolic pressure resulting in decreased perfusion) and necrosis, or cardiomyocyte damage from the inflammatory cytokines or oxidative stress. Impaired renal function is very common, and decreased clearance of the biomarkers can contribute to their elevation. Therefore these elevations should be interpreted in the context of the clinical setting. Despite that, in patients with acute decompensated heart failure (ADHF), a positive cardiac troponin test (from whatever mechanism) is associated with worse prognosis.

4. Screening for dyslipidemia and glucose intolerance, which are risk factors for CAD.

5. If hemochromatosis is suspected (specifically in Northern European patients), consider checking a transferrin saturation and ferritin level.

6. Consider HIV testing in high-risk patients.

- Electrocardiogram (ECG)
  1. Look for signs of prior MI, chamber enlargement, hypertrophy, heart block, arrhythmia, and evidence of pericardial effusion.
  2. More than 25% of patients with HF have some form of intraventricular conduction abnormality that manifests as an increased QRS duration. The most common pattern seen is left bundle-branch block.
- Chest x-ray (Fig. 3)
  1. Evaluate for pulmonary venous congestion, pulmonary edema, pleural effusion,

cardiomegaly, chamber dilation, and Kerley B lines.

- Echocardiography
  1. Plays a critical diagnostic role in patients with HF and is useful in assessment of systolic, diastolic function in addition to assessment of valvular structure and function
- Exercise stress testing
  1. May be useful in evaluating concomitant ischemic etiologies and assessment of degree of disability in stable compensated patients.
- Cardiac catheterization
  1. Left heart catheterization can help to identify coronary artery disease as a cause of HF. Right heart catheterization can help to evaluate intracardiac filling

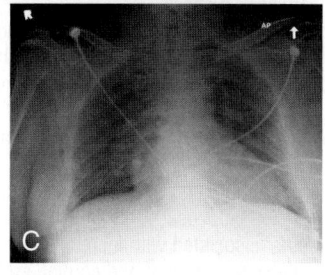

FIG. 3 Congestive heart failure. Mild left ventricular hypertrophy with restricted filling, ejection fraction >55%, and no pericardial effusion. This 63-year-old man with coronary artery disease, chronic renal insufficiency, and diastolic heart failure (ejection fraction >55%) presented multiple times for dyspnea (**A, B,** and **C,** first through third clinical presentations). Each of these three radiographs shows signs of moderate pulmonary edema. The diaphragms and costophrenic angles are clear, suggesting no pleural effusion. The right heart border in all three images is indistinct because of interstitial edema in these locations. Portions of the left heart border are also indistinct. The upper lung fields have a hazy appearance indicating mild edema. Fluid is visible in the minor fissure on all three images. Does the similarity of these radiographs mean that edema is not the cause of the patient's dyspnea? No, he simply presented with pulmonary edema on all three occasions. (From Broder JS: *Diagnostic imaging for the emergency physician,* Philadelphia, 2011, Saunders.)

pressures, estimates of valvular areas, presence of intracardiac shunts, and calculation of hemodynamic properties such as cardiac output, systemic vascular resistance, and pulmonary artery wedge pressure to further guide management.
- Cardiac MRI
  1. Useful modality in accurately estimating EF (with less variability than conventional 2D echocardiography). MRI is also useful in excluding pericardial disease, identifying infiltrative disease, and assessing viability in cases of HF caused by underlying ischemic heart disease.

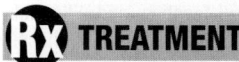 **TREATMENT**

NONPHARMACOLOGIC GENERAL MEASURES
- Assess the etiology and severity of disease. Educate the patient and family about the nature of the disorder. Assess the home setting and if patient has social support to ensure compliance, especially for patients with dementia.
- Identify and correct precipitating factors (e.g., increased sodium load, medication noncompliance, ischemia, infections, anemia, thyrotoxicosis) and address lifestyle modification (e.g., smoking and alcohol cessation, weight reduction, avoiding use of nonsteroidal antiinflammatory drugs [NSAIDs]). Anemia is common in patients with HF. However,

treatments with erythropoiesis-stimulating agents (ESAs) have not shown improved clinical outcomes in patients with systolic HF and mild-to-moderate anemia and are thus not recommended.
- Review list of medications and discontinue the ones that can contribute to HF (e.g., NSAIDs, antiarrhythmic drugs, calcium channel blockers, thiazolidinediones)
- Dietary sodium restriction of <2 g/day is commonly recommended to patients with HF and is endorsed by many guidelines.
- Restrict fluid intake to <2 L/day in patients with hyponatremia.
- Caloric supplementation should be provided to patients with advanced HF with weight loss and muscle wasting due to cardiac cachexia. Weight loss may reflect cachexia caused by the higher total energy expenditure associated with HF compared with that of healthy sedentary subjects. The diagnosis of cardiac cachexia independently predicts a worse prognosis.
- For patients with coexisting obstructive sleep apnea, continuous positive airway pressure (CPAP) is often recommended after polysomnography, thereby reducing systolic blood pressure and improving LV function (class IIa recommendation).
- Exercise training (or regular physical activity) is recommended as safe and effective for patients with class I to III HF who are able to participate to improve functional status (class I recommendation). Cardiac rehabilitation is unfortunately an underused

preventive measure, although it has been shown to reduce morbidity and mortality. Cardiac rehabilitation can be useful in clinically stable patients with HF to improve functional capacity, exercise duration, health-related quality of life, and mortality (class IIa recommendation).
- Pneumococcal vaccination and annual influenza vaccination.

TREATMENT OF ADHF
- Four phases in treatment of ADHF (Fig. 2):
  1st phase: initial stabilization and management
  2nd phase: inpatient hospital care
  3rd phase: early discharge planning and care
  4th phase: early post-discharge care
- 1st phase: Initial stabilization and management
  Short-term goals: hemodynamic stabilization, stabilization of respiratory status, symptom relief, optimization of tissue perfusion, and recognition of more immediately life-threatening conditions (e.g., arrhythmias, valvular catastrophe, MI, cardiac tamponade). Initial therapy of ADHF is contingent on appropriate determination of clinical scenario.

  Management as per clinical scenario:
  1. ADHF-associated hypertension: goal is afterload reduction and decrease of systemic hypervolemia. Mode of treatment: diuresis (IV loop diuretics) and vasodilators (acutely nitrates and morphine followed by treatment with ACE inhibitors or angiotensin receptor blockers [ARBs])

2. Worsening or decompensation of chronic HF (HFrEF or HFpEF): goal is control of volume status. Treatment is accomplished with vasodilators and diuretics.

3. Flash pulmonary edema: goal is afterload reduction (vasodilators such as nitrates acutely), respiratory status stabilization, and diuresis (IV loop diuretics). Rate control can be initiated in patients with atrial fibrillation or tachyarrhythmias as it may improve cardiac filling and function.

4. Cardiogenic shock: goal is hemodynamic stabilization. Treatment consists of inotropes + vasopressors ± mechanical circulatory support ± emergent revascularization if indicated.

5. ACS and ADHF: goal is hemodynamic stabilization + emergent restoration of coronary perfusion. See "Acute Coronary Syndromes."

6. Isolated RV failure: goals are identification of etiology: (1) valvular, (2) pulmonary hypertension, and (3) primary RV failure secondary to ischemia. Treatment: depends on etiology, either corrective surgery vs. treatment of pulmonary hypertension (endothelin antagonists, calcium channel blockers, phosphodiesterase inhibitors) vs. coronary reperfusion therapies.

ACUTE PHARMACOLOGIC TREATMENTS:

- Vasodilators are appropriate in most patients with ADHF (contraindicated in cardiogenic shock and severe aortic stenosis)

  1. Nitroglycerin (0.4 to 0.8 mg sublingually every 3 to 5 min, or by intravenous infusion starting at 0.2 to 0.4 mcg/kg/min with subsequent up titration) may be administered in the emergency setting until relative hypotension ensues. Nitrates are contraindicated after use of phosphodiesterase inhibitors such as sildenafil due to risk of hypotension.

  2. Sodium nitroprusside (0.1 to 0.2 mcg/kg/min as an intravenous infusion) is a potent vasodilator with balanced venous and arteriolar effects that usually requires hemodynamic monitoring with an arterial line and may precipitate coronary steal and thiocyanate toxicity (elevated risk in renal failure).

  3. When given intravenously, loop diuretics have an immediate vasodilator effect that provides clinical relief of symptoms before diuresis begins. Due to gut edema and unpredictable patterns of absorption, oral formulation may become less effective. Therefore intravenous formulation should be used in the acute setting. Studies showed no difference in outcome when using bolus dosing vs. continuous IV infusion. Administration of smaller doses of short-acting loop diuretics multiple times daily is preferable to a single large dose because the kidneys can avidly reabsorb sodium after the initial diuresis. However, if a certain dose is not adequate to force diuresis, the dose, rather than the frequency, should be increased until a single effective dose is reached; more frequent doses can be added as needed.

Therefore monitoring of urine output, renal function, and electrolytes is key. The addition of a distal tubule inhibitor such as metolazone 30 min prior to loop diuretic dosing has a synergistic effect and often enhances diuresis because it inhibits sodium reabsorption in the distal segment in the face of increased sodium delivery from the loop. Diuretics should be used with caution in patients with aortic stenosis and are contraindicated in patients with severe hypotension or cardiogenic shock.

- Inotropic agents are used for temporary hemodynamic support in cardiogenic shock, but have not been shown to improve survival. Many of these agents have serious associated adverse events including myocardial necrosis and malignant arrhythmias.

  1. Dobutamine (starting at 2.5 to 5 mcg/kg/min) can be used for inotropic support but is associated with increased myocardial oxygen demand and cardiac arrhythmias and may result in hypotension from decreased systemic vascular resistance.

  2. Milrinone (37.5 to 75 mcg/kg loading dose, followed by 0.375 to 0.75 mcg/kg/min) can be used as a vasodilator and inotropic agent, but is associated with increased oxygen demand and cardiac arrhythmias, and may result in hypotension from decreased systemic vascular resistance.

- Renal replacement therapy or ultrafiltration (can be used as an alternative to pharmacologic diuresis in ADHF when renal function is significantly compromised).

- ACE inhibitors or ARBs, if part of a patient's chronic medication regimen, should be continued in the absence of hypotension, acute renal failure, or hyperkalemia.

- Beta-blockers, if part of a patient's chronic medication regimen, may be continued or reduced in dosage in mild exacerbations of HF but should be discontinued in patients with hypotension or those requiring inotropic support. Beta-blockers should not be initiated in patients who are not on chronic beta-blocker therapy until euvolemia is achieved unless used for rate control.

- Morphine sulfate can cause venodilation and thus reduce cardiac preload. It may be used to reduce patient work of breathing and anxiety, but recent retrospective studies have suggested increased incidence of mechanical ventilation and in-hospital mortality in patients who received morphine.

- If ADHF with preserved EF is suspected, therapy is usually aimed at relief of symptoms and correction of any potential precipitating etiologies (e.g., tachycardia, hypertension, ischemia). Treatment generally involves diuretics to reduce pulmonary congestion with caution to not overdiurese given the need for elevated filling pressures in these patients to ensure adequate stroke volume and cardiac output. Nitrates may be useful in providing symptomatic relief but may precipitate hypotension. Ventricular rate

should be controlled in the presence of atrial fibrillation, which, at rapid rates, is poorly tolerated in patients with impaired diastolic filling. Negative inotropic agents such as beta-blockers and calcium channel blockers can be used with caution.

- Nesiritide (recombinant brain natriuretic protein) does not reduce morbidity or mortality (ASCEND-HF trial)

- 2nd phase: Inpatient hospital care

  This phase of treatment includes further diuresis and stabilization of volume status. The patient should be carefully brought to euvolemia with daily volume status and electrolyte monitoring. The patient should also be transitioned to oral diuretics when stabilized. Whilst inpatient, the patient should have his/her medical and device management optimized with the therapies discussed later.

3rd phase: Early discharge planning and care

The patient should be transitioned to oral diuretics and be placed on optimum outpatient maintenance therapy. If the patient was on IV inotropic therapy, oral regimens should be adjusted while these infusions are tapered off. Prolonged physiologic effects of these IV inotropic agents after their discontinuation before discharge may mask the inadequate diuretic regimen and intolerance to the vasodilator doses. This can result in readmission, especially with milrinone due to its long half-life that can be further prolonged by the common coexisting impaired renal function. Therefore it may be recommended that patients who received inotropic infusions remain hospitalized for at least 48 hours after inotropic agents are discontinued, and optimize the oral regimen.

4th phase: Early post-discharge care

The patient will require reevaluation and constant monitoring in order to avoid another episode of ADHF. Emphasis should be placed on importance of compliance with instructions regarding dietary restrictions and daily body weight monitoring. Early follow-up should be scheduled as well as outpatient electrolyte monitoring if required after medication adjustments.

CHRONIC TREATMENT OF HFrEF: The goals of HF therapy are clinical improvement followed by stabilizing, slowing, or even reversing deterioration in myocardial function, and ultimately a reduction in risk of morbidity (including hospitalization rates) and mortality.

- ACE inhibitors

  1. Reduce morbidity and mortality.

  2. Produce both venous and arterial vasodilation acutely, thereby reducing both preload and afterload.

  3. Potential mechanism of long-term benefit is attenuation of RAAS activation and decreased myocardial remodeling and fibrosis.

  4. Used as first-line therapy for asymptomatic LV dysfunction (LVEF <40%) and symptomatic systolic HF (ACC/AHA grades A-D).

  5. Therapy should be initiated at low doses to prevent hypotension and rapidly titrated to higher doses as tolerated.

6. Contraindications to the use of ACE inhibitors are renal insufficiency (creatinine clearance <30 ml/min), bilateral renal artery stenosis, hyperkalemia, hypotension, or adverse reactions (e.g., angioedema).

- ARBs
  1. Receptor antagonists to the angiotensin II receptor.
  2. Clinical trials have not shown any superiority compared to ACE inhibitors in patients with systolic HF (LVEF <40%).
  3. Reserved for patients who are ACE inhibitor intolerant.
  4. Combination therapy with ARBs and ACE inhibitors is generally not recommended.
  5. Have a similar contraindication profile to ACE inhibitors. Routine combined use of an ACE inhibitor, ARB, and aldosterone antagonist is potentially harmful for patients with HFrEF.

- Angiotensin receptor–neprilysin inhibitor (ARNI) (valsartan/sacubitril or Entresto)
  1. Neprilysin is an enzyme that degrades natriuretic peptides, bradykinin, adrenomedullin, and other vasoactive peptides.
  2. Reduces morbidity and mortality. In a randomized controlled trial (PARADIGM-HF) that compared valsartan/sacubitril with enalapril in symptomatic patients with HFrEF tolerating an adequate dose of either ACE inhibitor or ARB, the ARNI reduced the composite end point of cardiovascular death or HF hospitalization significantly, by 20%.
  3. In patients with chronic symptomatic HFrEF NYHA class II or III who tolerate an ACE inhibitor or ARB, replacement by an ARNI is recommended to further reduce morbidity and mortality (class I).
  4. ARNI should not be administered concomitantly with ACE inhibitors or within 36 hours of the last dose of an ACE inhibitor (class III: Harm).
  5. ARNI should not be administered to patients with a history of angioedema (class III: Harm).

- Beta-adrenergic blockers (beta-blockers)
  1. Reduce morbidity and mortality. Such benefits observed with bisoprolol (CIBIS II trial), metoprolol succinate (MERIT-HF trial), and carvedilol (COPERNICUS trial).
  2. Benefit is believed to be conferred by blockade of sympathetic effects of neurohormonal stimulation due to HF.
  3. Are considered first-line therapy for symptomatic patients with systolic HF (NYHA class ≥II and LVEF <35%).
  4. Only carvedilol, bisoprolol, and metoprolol succinate (long acting) have been approved for the medical treatment of chronic HF; these agents are generally started in patients judged to be euvolemic and dosage is to be slowly uptitrated as tolerated.
  5. Adverse effects include worsening HF (due to negative inotropic effects), fatigue, dizziness, bradycardia, hypotension, and bronchospasm.

- Aldosterone receptor antagonists

1. Reduce morbidity and mortality
2. Indicated in patients with NYHA class II-IV HF, with LVEF ≤35%, already treated with ACE inhibitors and beta-blockers without significant renal insufficiency or hyperkalemia. Patients with NYHA class II should have a history of prior cardiovascular hospitalization or elevated plasma natriuretic peptide levels to be considered for aldosterone receptor antagonists. Creatinine should be ≤2.5 mg/dL in men or ≤2.0 mg/dL in women (or estimated glomerular filtration rate >30 mL/min/1.73 m2), and potassium should be <5.0 mEq/L. They are also indicated for post-MI patients with EF ≤40% who have either symptomatic HF or diabetes mellitus.
3. Spironolactone may cause gynecomastia, galactorrhea, and hyperkalemia (especially in patients with baseline renal insufficiency or type 4 renal tubular acidosis).It has been best studied in chronic HF with NYHA class III to IV symptoms (RALES study).
4. Eplerenone is associated with fewer endocrine side effects and has especially been studied in postmyocardial infarction left ventricular dysfunction (EPHESUS trial) and in chronic systolic HF with only class II symptoms (EMPHASIS-HF trial).
5. Inappropriate use of aldosterone receptor antagonists is potentially harmful because of life-threatening hyperkalemia or renal insufficiency when serum creatinine is >2.5 mg/dL in men or >2.0 mg/dL in women (or estimated glomerular filtration rate <30 mL/min/1.73 m2), and/or potassium >5.0 mEq/L.

- Diuretics
  1. Are used to maintain euvolemia and to improve symptoms as discussed previously.
  2. Although data on diuretic efficacy are limited, a meta-analysis of a few small trials found that they were associated with reduction in mortality as well as reduced hospitalization for HF.
  3. Of note, loop diuretics with better bioavailability, such as torsemide and bumetanide, may be used in diuretic-resistant patients but are generally more expensive.

- Combination of isosorbide dinitrate and hydralazine
  1. Cause venous (nitrates) and arteriolar (hydralazine) vasodilation resulting in decreased preload and afterload.
  2. The combination of hydralazine and isosorbide dinitrate is recommended to reduce morbidity and mortality for patients self-described as African Americans with NYHA class III–IV HFrEF receiving optimal therapy with ACE inhibitors and beta-blockers, unless contraindicated.
  3. A combination of hydralazine and isosorbide dinitrate can be useful to reduce morbidity or mortality in patients with current or prior symptomatic HFrEF who cannot be given an ACE inhibitor or ARB

because of drug intolerance, hypotension, or renal insufficiency, unless contraindicated.
4. Adverse effects of nitrates include hypotension, headaches, and tolerance as well as reflex tachycardia and lupus-like syndrome with hydralazine.

- Digoxin
  1. Positive inotropic and negative chronotropic drug that works by inhibition of the sodium-potassium transmembrane exchange pump and through its vagomimetic action
  2. Commonly used in patients with concomitant atrial fibrillation
  3. Has been shown to reduce HF-related hospitalizations but does NOT confer any mortality benefit (DIG trial). However, there is evidence suggesting that digoxin may actually have an effect on survival that varies with the serum digoxin level; survival was improved when the level was between 0.5 and 0.8 ng/ml (most often in men) and significantly worsened when it was ≥1.2 ng/ml and >0.9 ng/ml in women.
  4. Caution must be used in patients with abnormal renal function to avoid digoxin toxicity and life-threatening arrhythmia. Avoid hypokalemia because potassium competes with digoxin on the same site of the Na^+-K^+-ATPase pump.

- I_f channel inhibitor (ivabradine)
  1. Ivabradine is a new therapeutic agent that selectively inhibits the I_f current in the sinoatrial node, providing heart rate reduction.
  2. Ivabradine can be beneficial to reduce HF hospitalization for patients with symptomatic (NYHA class II-III) stable chronic HFrEF (LVEF ≤35%) who are receiving guideline-directed therapy, including a beta-blocker at maximum tolerated dose, and who are in sinus rhythm with a heart rate of 70 bpm or greater at rest (class II).

- Cardiac resynchronization therapy (CRT)
  1. Improves morbidity and mortality rates in selected patients.
  2. The presence of a bundle-branch block or other intraventricular conduction delay (IVCD) can cause ventricular dyssynchrony, which induces regional loading disparities and reduces the efficiency of ventricular contraction, thereby further impairing the systolic function of a failing ventricle.
  3. CRT is indicated for patients who have LVEF ≤35%, sinus rhythm, left bundle-branch block with a QRS duration of 150 ms or greater, and NYHA class II, III, or ambulatory IV symptoms on guideline-directed medical therapy. CRT is NOT indicated in patients whose functional status and life expectancy are limited predominantly by chronic noncardiac conditions. Life expectancy should be >1 yr.

H

Diseases and Disorders

I

4. In the appropriate subset of patients, CRT in addition to optimal medical therapy has been shown in numerous clinical trials to improve symptoms by at least one NYHA class, improve 6-min walk distance and quality of life, reduce rate of HF-related hospitalization, and reduce rate of all-cause and cardiovascular mortality.

5. Detailed guidelines for CRT are beyond the scope of this chapter. Consultation with cardiology service may be indicated.

- Implantable cardioverter-defibrillators (ICDs)

1. Sudden cardiac death (SCD) is a common cause of death in patients with HF in both ischemic and nonischemic cardiomyopathies. Ventricular tachycardia (VT) degenerating into ventricular fibrillation (VF) is the culprit in the majority of patients with SCD, although bradyarrhythmias do also occur with less frequency.

2. ICD therapy is recommended for primary prevention of SCD to reduce total mortality in selected patients with nonischemic dilated cardiomyopathy or ischemic heart disease at least 40 days post-MI with LVEF ≤35% and NYHA class II or III symptoms on chronic guideline-directed medical therapy, who have reasonable expectation of meaningful survival for >1 year.

3. Patients with HF who survive an episode of sudden cardiac arrest or experience sustained VT in the presence of LVEF <35% are at high risk for future arrhythmic events and SCD and obtain a mortality benefit from ICD placement for secondary prevention, with or without adjunctive therapies such as antiarrhythmic drugs, radiofrequency ablation, surgery, or transplant.

- In the absence of an indication (e.g., atrial fibrillation), routine use of anticoagulation is currently not recommended in patients with HF. Even with the increased risk for LV thrombus formation in dilated cardiomyopathy and subsequent thromboembolization, data are conflicting about benefits of antithrombotic (antiplatelet or anticoagulant) therapy for primary prevention to reduce thromboembolic events or mortality in patients with systolic HF who are in sinus rhythm (SOLVD, V-HeFT, SAVE, HELAS, and WASH trials). It may be reasonable to consider anticoagulation for secondary prevention in patients with HF who had a prior thromboembolic event; however, risks and benefits should be carefully assessed.

- Antiplatelet agents are recommended for patients with concomitant CAD.

- Statins are not beneficial as adjunctive therapy when prescribed solely for the diagnosis of HF in the absence of other indications for their use.

- Calcium channel blocking drugs are not recommended as routine treatment for patients with HFrEF.

- Omega-3 polyunsaturated fatty acid supplementation is reasonable to use as adjunctive therapy in patients with NYHA class II-IV symptoms and HFrEF or HFpEF, unless contraindicated, to reduce mortality and cardiovascular hospitalizations.

- Percutaneous coronary intervention (PCI) or surgical revascularization should be considered in patients with HF and significant CAD who are revascularization candidates.

- In general, the following sequence of drugs is recommended:

1. Loop diuretics to provide symptom relief and achieve a euvolemic state.

2. ACE inhibitor or ARB started at low doses, then increased to a moderate dose in 1-2 weeks. Replace with ARNI in those tolerating ACE inhibitor or ARB.

3. Beta-blockers after the patient is stable on ACE/ARB treatment. Start a low dose, then uptitrate to goal based on trial data or maximal dose tolerated. Once achieved, uptitration of ACE or ARB to goal doses can be completed.

- The following drugs can be added in selected patients in the absence of contraindications:

1. Aldosterone antagonists improve survival in NYHA class II with LVEF <30% or NYHA class III-IV with EF <35%. Kidney function should be stable with eGFR ≥30 ml/min and potassium <5 mEq/L.

2. Combination of hydralazine with a nitrate in patients (particularly African Americans) with a reduced EF.

3. Digoxin reduces hospitalizations for HF and controls HR rate in atrial fibrillation. It can also help control symptoms.

CHRONIC TREATMENT OF HFpEF:

- To date, there is a relative dearth of clinical trials examining effective chronic treatment strategies in this subset of patients with HFpEF. Current therapies are mainly for symptomatic relief.

- Therapy centers on relief of volume overload with judicious diuretic use, treatment of ischemia via coronary revascularization, management of atrial fibrillation, controlling heart rate and blood pressure to prevent acute decompensation, and restriction of sodium and fluid to prevent volume overload.

- Diuretics should be used for relief of symptoms due to volume overload in patients with HFpEF.

- The use of beta-blocking agents, ACE inhibitors, and ARBs in patients with hypertension is reasonable to control blood pressure in patients with HFpEF.

- The use of ARBs might be considered to decrease hospitalizations for patients with HFpEF.

- HF hospitalization was less frequent in the spironolactone group compared with the

placebo group (TOPCAT trial); therefore, spironolactone may be considered in HPpEF patients who can be reliably and carefully monitored for changes in potassium and creatinine, and they should have potassium levels <5 meq/L and glomerular filtration rate <30 mL/min per 1.73m^2 at baseline.

- Omega-3 polyunsaturated fatty acid supplementation is reasonable, unless contraindicated, to reduce mortality and cardiovascular hospitalizations.

- There is no evidence to support routine use of nutritional supplements and they are not recommended for patients with HFpEF.

- Surgical options for contributing critical aortic stenosis, constrictive pericarditis, and hypertrophic cardiomyopathy (HCM) should be entertained in appropriate patients.

DISPOSITION

- Annual mortality of systolic HF ranges from 10% in stable patients with mild symptoms to 50% in patients with NYHA class IV disease (a mortality rate rivaling some malignancies). The Seattle Heart Failure Model provides an accurate estimate of 1-, 2-, and 3-year survival before and after different therapies. This model can be useful to assess the need for LV assist device implantation or urgent transplantation. The calculator is available online at http://depts.washington.edu/shfm/.

- Cardiac transplantation has a 5-yr survival rate of ~70% and represents a viable option in selected patients.

- The use of an LV assist device (LVAD) in patients with advanced HF can result in a clinically meaningful survival benefit and improve quality of life in patients who are not candidates for cardiac transplantation. There are two approved uses of LVADs specifically as a bridge to transplant and as destination therapy. There are two major categories of LVAD pulsatile flow devices vs. continuous flow devices. Continuous flow devices are associated with increased survival as destination therapy as compared to medically managed controls (REMATCH trial).

EBM EVIDENCE

Available at www.expertconsult.com

SUGGESTED READINGS

Available at www.expertconsult.com

RELATED CONTENT

Heart Failure (Patient Information)

AUTHORS: **DHAVAL KOLTE, M.D., PH.D.,** and **ARAVIND RAO KOKKIRALA, M.D.**

BASIC INFORMATION

DEFINITION

Heat exhaustion and heat stroke are part of a continuum of heat-related illness, and unless factors leading to heat exhaustion are corrected swiftly, affected patients can progress to heat stroke.

- **Heat exhaustion:** an illness resulting from prolonged, heavy activity in a hot environment with subsequent dehydration, electrolyte depletion, and rectal temperature >37.8° C but ≤40° C.
- **Heat stroke:** a life-threatening heat illness characterized by extreme hyperthermia (core temperature >40° C [104.0° F]), dehydration, and neurologic manifestations. Heat stroke can be further subdivided into "exertional heat stroke" occurring in generally healthy individuals undergoing strenuous physical activity in warm conditions and "non-exertional heat stroke" often seen in elderly and/or debilitated patients with impaired thermal regulations due to illness or medications (see Etiology).

SYNONYMS

Heat illness
Hyperthermia

ICD-10CM CODES
T67.5   Heat exhaustion, unspecified
T67.0   Heatstroke and sunstroke
T67.1   Heat syncope
T67.2   Heat cramp
T67.3   Heat exhaustion, anhydrotic
T67.6   Heat fatigue, transient

EPIDEMIOLOGY & DEMOGRAPHICS

INCIDENCE (IN U.S.): Incidence of heat stroke is approximately 20 cases/100,000 population.
PREDOMINANT AGE: Heat exhaustion and stroke occur more frequently in elderly patients, especially those taking diuretics or medications that impair heat dissipation (e.g., phenothiazines, anticholinergics, antihistamines, beta-blockers). Table 1 describes factors predisposing to serious heat illness.

PHYSICAL FINDINGS & CLINICAL PRESENTATION

Heat exhaustion:
- Generalized malaise, weakness, headache, muscle and abdominal cramps, nausea, vomiting, hypotension, tachycardia.
- Rectal temperature is usually normal.
- Sweating is usually present.
Heat stroke:
- Neurologic manifestations (seizures, tremor, hemiplegia, coma, psychosis, other bizarre behavior).
- Evidence of dehydration (poor skin turgor, sunken eyeballs).
- Tachycardia, hyperventilation.
- Skin is hot, red, and flushed.
- Sweating is often (not always) absent, particularly in elderly patients.
- Classic heat stroke generally develops slowly over days and occurs predominantly in older

persons and in those with chronic illness. Exertional heat stroke is more common in young, healthy persons, has a more rapid onset, and is associated with higher core temperatures. Table 2 compares classic and exertional heat stroke. Box 1 summarizes organ dysfunction seen in patients with heat stroke.

ETIOLOGY

- Exogenous heat gain (increased ambient temperature).
- Increased heat production (exercise, infection, hyperthyroidism, drugs).
- Impaired heat dissipation (high humidity, heavy clothing, neonatal or elderly patients, drugs [phenothiazines, anticholinergics, antihistamines, butyrophenones, amphetamines, cocaine, alcohol, β-blockers]).
- Diuretics, laxatives.
- Fig. E1 describes an algorithm of the pathophysiology of heat stroke.

TABLE 1   Factors Predisposing to Serious Heat Illness

Individual Factors

Lack of acclimatization
Low physical fitness
Excessive body weight
Dehydration
Advanced age
Young age

Health Conditions

Inflammation and fever
Viral infection
Cardiovascular disease
Diabetes mellitus
Gastroenteritis
Rash, sunburn, and previous burns to large
   areas of skin
Seizures
Thyroid storm
Neuroleptic malignant syndrome
Malignant hyperthermia
Sickle cell trait
Cystic fibrosis
Spinal cord injury

Drugs

Anticholinergic properties (atropine)
Antiepileptic (topiramate)
Antihistamines
Glutethimide (Doriden)
Phenothiazines
Tricyclic antidepressants
Amphetamines, cocaine, "Ecstasy"
Ergogenic stimulants (e.g., ephedrine, ephedra)
Lithium
Diuretics
β-Blockers
Ethanol

Environmental Factors

High temperature
High humidity
Little air motion
Lack of shade
Heat wave
Physical exercise
Heavy clothing
Air pollution (nitrogen dioxide)

From Goldman L, Schafer AI: *Goldman's Cecil medicine*, ed 24, Philadelphia, 2012, Saunders.

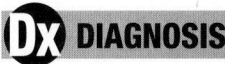

DIAGNOSIS

DIFFERENTIAL DIAGNOSIS

- Infections (meningitis, encephalitis, sepsis).
- Head trauma.
- Epilepsy.
- Thyroid storm.
- Acute cocaine intoxication.
- Malignant hyperthermia.
- Heat exhaustion can be differentiated from heat stroke by the following:
  1. Essentially intact mental function and lack of significant fever in heat exhaustion.
  2. Mild or absent increases in creatine phosphokinase (CPK), aspartate aminotransferase (AST), lactate dehydrogenase (LDH), and alanine aminotransferase (ALT) in heat exhaustion.

WORKUP

- Heat stroke: comprehensive history, physical examination, and laboratory evaluation.
- Heat exhaustion: in most cases, laboratory tests are not necessary for diagnosis.

LABORATORY TESTS

Laboratory abnormalities may include the following:
- Elevated BUN, creatinine, hematocrit.
- Hyponatremia or hypernatremia, hyperkalemia or hypokalemia.
- Elevated LDH, AST, ALT, CPK, bilirubin.
- Lactic acidosis, respiratory alkalosis (from hyperventilation).
- Myoglobinuria, hypofibrinogenemia, fibrinolysis, hypocalcemia.

TREATMENT

- Treatment of heat exhaustion consists primarily of placing the patient in a cool, shaded area and providing rapid hydration and salt replacement.
  1. Fluid intake should be at least 2 L q4h in patients without history of CHF.
  2. Salt replacement can be accomplished by using one-quarter teaspoon of salt or two 10-grain salt tablets dissolved in 1 L of water.
  3. If IV fluid replacement is necessary, young athletes can be given normal saline IV (3 to 4 L over 6 to 8 hr); in elderly patients, consider using D5½NS IV with the rate titrated to cardiovascular status.
- Patients with heat stroke should undergo rapid cooling.
  1. Remove the patient's clothes and place the patient in a cool and well-ventilated room.
  2. If patient is unconscious, position on his or her side and clear the airway. Protect airway and augment oxygenation (e.g., nasal O_2 at 4 L/min to keep oxygen saturation >90%).
  3. Monitor body temperature every 5 min. Measurement of the patient's core temperature with a rectal probe is recommended. The goal is to reduce the body temperature to 39° C (102.2° F) in 30 to

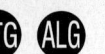

TABLE 2 Comparison of Classic and Exertional Heat Stroke

Patient Characteristics	Classic	Exertional
Age	Young children or elderly	15-55 yr
Health	Chronic illness	Usually healthy
Fever	Unusual	Common
Prevailing weather	Frequent in heat waves	Variable
Activity	Sedentary	Strenuous exercise
Drug use	Diuretics, antidepressants, anticholinergics, phenothiazines	Ergogenic stimulants or cocaine
Sweating	Often absent	Common
Acid-base disturbances	Respiratory alkalosis	Lactic acidosis
Acute renal failure	Uncommon	Common ($\approx$15%)
Rhabdomyolysis	Uncommon	Common ($\approx$25%)
CK	Mildly elevated	Markedly elevated (500-1000 U/L)
ALT, AST	Mildly elevated	Markedly elevated
Hyperkalemia	Uncommon	Common
Hypocalcemia	Uncommon	Common
DIC	Mild	Marked
Hypoglycemia	Uncommon	Common

ALT, Alanine aminotransferase; *AST,* aspartate aminotransferase; *CK,* creatine kinase; *DIC,* disseminated intravascular coagulation.
From Goldman L, Schafer AI: *Goldman's Cecil medicine,* ed 24, Philadelphia, 2012, Saunders.

BOX 1 Organ Dysfunction Seen in Patients with Heat Stroke

Encephalopathy
Rhabdomyolysis
Acute renal failure
Acute respiratory distress syndrome
Myocardial injury
Hepatocellular injury
Intestinal ischemia and infarction
Pancreatic injury
Hemorrhagic complication (e.g., disseminated intravascular coagulation)

From Adams JG, et al.: *Emergency medicine, clinical essentials,* ed 2, Philadelphia, 2013, Elsevier.

60 min. Advantages, disadvantages, and efficacy of various cooling methods are described in Table E3.

4. Spray the patient with a cool mist and use fans to enhance airflow over the body (rapid evaporation method).
5. Immersion of the patient in ice water, stomach lavage with iced saline solution, intravenous administration of cooled fluids, and inhalation of cold air are advisable only when the means for rapid evaporation are not available. Immersion in tepid water (15° C, 59° F) is preferred over ice water immersion to minimize risk of shivering.
6. Use of ice packs on axillae, neck, and groin is controversial because they increase peripheral vasoconstriction and may induce shivering.

7. Antipyretics are ineffective because the hypothalamic set point during heat stroke is normal despite the increased body temperature.
8. Intubate a comatose patient, insert a Foley catheter, and start nasal O_2. Continuous ECG monitoring is recommended.
9. Insert at least two large-bore IV lines and begin IV hydration with NS or Ringer's lactate.
10. Draw initial laboratory studies: electrolytes, complete blood count, blood urea nitrogen, creatinine, AST, ALT, CPK, LDH, glucose, PT (INR), PTT, platelet count, Ca^{2+}, lactic acid, and arterial blood gases.
11. Treat complications as follows:
    a. Hypotension: vigorous hydration with normal saline or Ringer's lactate.
    b. Convulsions: diazepam 5 to 10 mg IV (slowly).
    c. Shivering: chlorpromazine 10 to 50 mg IV.
    d. Acidosis: use bicarbonate judiciously (only in severe acidosis).
- Observe for evidence of rhabdomyolysis and hepatic, renal, or cardiac failure and treat accordingly.

DISPOSITION

Most patients recover completely within 48 hr. Central nervous system injury is permanent in 20% of cases. Mortality rate can exceed 30% in patients with prolonged and severe hyperthermia. Delayed access to cooling is the leading cause of morbidity and mortality in persons with heat stroke.

SUGGESTED READINGS

Available at www.expertconsult.com

RELATED CONTENT

Heat Exhaustion and Heat Stroke (Patient Information)

AUTHOR: **FRED F. FERRI, M.D.**

BASIC INFORMATION

DEFINITION

Infection of the human gastric mucosa with the organism *Helicobacter pylori,* a spiral-shaped gram-negative organism with unique features that allow it to survive in the hostile gastric environment.

SYNONYMS

Previously known as *Campylobacter pylori*

ICD-10CM CODES
B96.81 *Helicobacter pylori (H. pylori)* as the cause of diseases classified elsewhere

EPIDEMIOLOGY & DEMOGRAPHICS

H. pylori is the most common chronic bacterial infection in human beings, probably affecting 50% of the earth's population in all age groups and probably 30% to 40% of the U.S. population. In developing nations, infection is acquired at an earlier age and occurs more frequently.

CLINICAL PRESENTATION

- *H. pylori* causes histologic gastritis in all affected individuals. The majority of cases are asymptomatic and unlikely to proceed to serious consequences.
- *H. pylori* is a causative agent in peptic ulcer disease (PUD), gastric adenocarcinoma, and gastric mucosa-associated lymphoid tissue lymphoma, and may be a risk factor for iron-deficiency anemia and chronic idiopathic thrombocytopenic purpura. It may present with the signs and symptoms of these disorders, including abdominal pain, bloating, anorexia, and early satiety. Fig. 1 describes association of *H. pylori* infection and disease states.
- "Alarm symptoms" that should prompt more immediate and aggressive workup include weight loss, dysphagia, protracted nausea or vomiting, anemia, melena, and palpable abdominal mass.

ETIOLOGY

- Route of acquisition is unknown but is presumed to be person to person by oral-oral or fecal-oral exposure.
- The majority of cases are acquired in childhood. Socioeconomic status and living conditions in childhood affect risk of acquisition of infection. These factors include housing density, number of siblings, overcrowding, sharing a bed, and lack of running water.
- *H. pylori* does not invade gastroduodenal tissue, but disrupts the mucous layer, causing the underlying mucosa to be more vulnerable to acid peptic damage.
- What differentiates the subset of patients with *H. pylori* who go on to develop ulcers or cancer remains unclear.

DIAGNOSIS

DIFFERENTIAL DIAGNOSIS

- Infection with *H. pylori* should be considered in the face of PUD, gastric cancer, gastritis, and gastric MALT lymphoma.
- *H. pylori* should be considered in the differential diagnosis of upper gastrointestinal (GI) tract disease, along with non-ulcer dyspepsia, reflux esophagitis, biliary tract disease, gastroparesis, pancreatitis, and ischemic bowel.

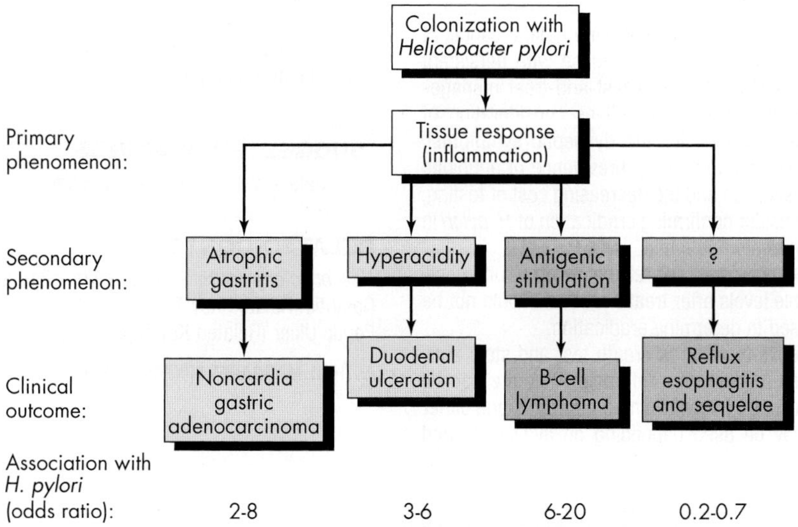

FIG. 1 Association of *Helicobacter pylori* colonization and disease states. After *H. pylori* acquisition, virtually all persons develop persistent colonization that lasts for life. Colonization induces tissue responses termed *chronic gastritis.* This process affects gastric physiology, including glandular structure, acid secretion, and antigen processing, which in turn affect disease risk. Colonization with *H. pylori* increases the risk for certain diseases (duodenal ulcer, gastric ulcer, noncardia gastric adenocarcinoma, and B-cell lymphomas) but appears to decrease the risk for gastroesophageal reflux disease and its complications, including Barrett's esophagus, and adenocarcinoma of the esophagus or gastric cardia. (From Mandell GL, et al.: *Principles and practice of infectious diseases,* ed 7, Philadelphia, 2010, Churchill Livingstone.)

WORKUP

- Workup is indicated in patients with active PUD, a past history of documented peptic ulcer, or gastric MALT lymphoma. The role of routine screening in high-risk populations is not clear. However, numerous studies suggest that *H. pylori* eradication is protective against progression of premalignant lesions. Consider testing for *H. pylori* in patients with idiopathic thrombocytopenic purpura, with otherwise unexplained iron deficiency anemia or unexplained B12 deficiency, as well as patients facing long-term NSAID or PPI therapy. Consider a test-and-treat approach in asymptomatic first-degree relatives of gastric cancer patients.
- Routine identification and treatment of *H. pylori* in cases of non-ulcer dyspepsia, gastroesophageal reflux disease (GERD), nonsteroidal antiinflammatory drug (NSAID) use, and in asymptomatic individuals in populations at high risk for gastric cancer is considered controversial, although it may be indicated in specific cases. A test-and-treat strategy may be used in patients younger than 55 with uncomplicated dyspepsia who have no alarm symptoms.
- Results of testing must be interpreted in relation to the individual patient's likelihood of *H. pylori* infection based on demographic risk factors. In the U.S. population, increased probability of infection exists in African Americans, Hispanics/Latinos, immigrants from developing nations, patients with poor socioeconomic status, Native Americans from Alaska, and persons >50 yr.
- Routine screening for *H. pylori* is not indicated in asymptomatic patients who are at low risk of infection.
- Infected patients with functional dyspepsia often benefit from treatment and should be evaluated for *H. pylori.*

LABORATORY TESTS

- Testing may be invasive or noninvasive depending on the need for endoscopy for other indications. There is no indication for endoscopy solely to diagnose *H. pylori.*
- Tests for *H. pylori* are differentiated as active or passive. Active tests provide direct evidence that *H. pylori* infection is currently present and include urea breath testing and stool antigen testing. Passive testing, which includes all serologic testing for *H. pylori,* gives indirect evidence of its presence by detecting the presence of antibodies to the organism. Serologic testing is limited by its inability to distinguish between active current infection and prior infection that has resolved.
- Tests that use urease as a marker (urea breath and stool antigen tests and biopsy for urease activity) may result in false-negative results in patients taking antibiotics, bismuth, or antisecretory therapy, as well as those with active ulcer bleeding. Patients should be off antibiotics for 4 wk and off protein pump inhibitors for 2 wk before urea breath or stool antigen testing.
- When diagnostic endoscopy is indicated (for suspicion or follow-up of PUD or gastric

MALT), antral biopsy should be tested for urease activity. If urease testing is likely to show a false-negative result because of recent proton pump inhibitor (PPI), bismuth, or antibiotic use or active ulcer bleeding, the sample should undergo histologic examination.

- In cases in which biopsy is not indicated, urea breath testing or stool antigen testing is indicated to evaluate for active infection. The sensitivities and specificities of these two tests are similar (>90%). Urea breath testing is slightly more expensive than stool antigen testing, but both costs are in the modest range. Choice can be made based on patient preference and availability.
- In cases in which biopsy is not indicated, consider using serologic testing as the initial approach. However, in individuals with a low pretest probability of infection, positive results should be confirmed with another testing method.

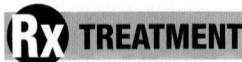 **TREATMENT**

ACUTE GENERAL Rx

- Test only patients whom you intend to treat if positive (see "Workup"). At this time, the value of eradicating *H. pylori* infection is proven in patients with PUD or gastric MALT lymphoma.
- The optimal antibiotic regimen has not been defined. In addition to efficacy, side effects, cost, and ease of administration must be considered.
- Due to increasing resistance to clarithromycin, decisions regarding appropriate regimens should take into account local rates of clarithromycin resistance.
- The following regimens may be considered for first-line therapy:
  1. PPI twice daily, with twice-daily clarithromycin (500 mg) and amoxicillin (1 g) may be used in areas of low clarithromycin resistance.
  2. In cases of penicillin allergy, metronidazole (500 mg bid) may be substituted for amoxicillin.
  3. PPI twice daily, combined with bismuth four times daily, as well as tetracycline (500 mg) and metronidazole (250 mg), both four times daily, is now recommended as first-line therapy in areas of high clarithromycin resistance. Sequential therapy, consisting of 5 days of treatment with a PPI and one antibiotic (usually amoxicillin) followed by 5-day treatment with the PPI and two other antibiotics (usually

clarithromycin and metronidazole), may be used in areas of high clarithromycin resistance when bismuth-based therapy is not available.
- Duration of treatment remains controversial. Extending therapy to 10 to 14 days may improve eradication rates. Use of combination capsules may improve compliance but is likely to be more expensive.
- Prior exposure to a macrolide or metronidazole, for any reason, is associated with increased resistance. A preferable regimen would include medications to which the patient has not been previously exposed.
- Diarrhea and abdominal cramping are commonly observed with many of the regimens. (Probiotics may diminish this effect.) Other side effects may include a metallic taste with metronidazole or clarithromycin, neuropathy, seizures, and disulfiram-like reaction with metronidazole, diarrhea with amoxicillin, photosensitivity with tetracycline, and *Clostridium difficile* infection with any antibiotic exposure. Bismuth may cause black stool and constipation. Tetracycline is contraindicated in pregnant patients.
- 20% of patients may not respond to initial therapy. Optimal retreatment regimens are under investigation. It is important to reinforce compliance. Second-line therapy should be either bismuth-containing quadruple therapy or levofloxacin-containing triple therapy (regardless of local clarithromycin resistance patterns). When possible, management of those who do not respond to two courses of therapy should be guided by antimicrobial sensitivity testing (although this is not indicated before initial treatment).

CHRONIC Rx

- Accepted indications for confirming eradication include *H. pylori*–associated ulcers, MALT lymphoma, and early gastric cancer. It may be considered in those with persistent dyspepsia despite a test-and-treat management strategy (as well as consideration of other causes for the dyspeptic symptoms). Given the increasing prevalence of antibiotic resistance and the decreasing cost of testing, consider confirming eradication of *H. pylori* in all treated patients.
- Serology does not reliably revert to undetectable levels after treatment and should not be used to determine eradication.
- Active tests (urea breath test and stool antigen testing) are preferable. They are equally accurate in confirming eradication, and either may be used depending on availability and

patient preference. To reduce the likelihood of false-negative results, testing should be performed at least 4 wk after eradication therapy with PPI and antibiotics or at least 2 wk after the cessation of PPI therapy alone.

DISPOSITION

Consider further evaluation in patients with recurrent symptoms after appropriate treatment.

REFERRAL

- Patients with gastric MALT lymphoma should be followed by a gastroenterologist and oncologist with expertise in the care of lymphoid neoplasms.
- Patients with dyspepsia who have tested positive for *H. pylori* and been treated without resolution should be referred for endoscopy.
- Consider referral for biopsy for culture and sensitivity in patients who have not responded to two attempts at treatment.

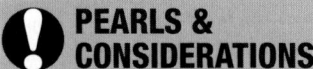 **PEARLS & CONSIDERATIONS**

- Whether *H. pylori* eradication reduces the risk of gastric cancer is unclear.
- Outcomes in PUD and gastric MALT lymphoma are improved with treatment of associated *H. pylori* infection.
- Tests that provide direct evidence of active *H. pylori* infection (urea breath and stool antigen testing) are preferred but may result in false-negative results in patients taking antibiotics, bismuth, or antisecretory agents.
- Serologic testing does not differentiate active from prior infection. It may be useful when active tests are not indicated, particularly in high-risk patients.
- Be aware of high-risk populations in low-prevalence settings, including immigrants from Mexico, South America, Southeast Asia, and Eastern Europe.

SUGGESTED READINGS

Available at www.expertconsult.com

RELATED CONTENT

Helicobacter pylori Infection (Patient Information)
Gastritis (Related Key Topic)
Peptic Ulcer (Related Key Topic)

AUTHOR: **MARGARET TRYFOROS, M.D.**

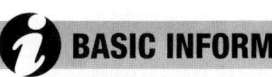

BASIC INFORMATION

DEFINITION

Hemochromatosis is an autosomal-recessive disorder that disrupts the body's regulation of iron and is characterized by increased accumulation of iron in various organs (adrenals, liver, pancreas, heart, testes, kidneys, pituitary) and eventual dysfunction of these organs if not treated appropriately.

SYNONYMS

Bronze diabetes

ICD-10CM CODES
E83.110 Hereditary hemochromatosis
E83.111 Hemochromatosis due to repeated red blood cell transfusions
E83.118 Other hemochromatosis
E83.119 Hemochromatosis, unspecified

EPIDEMIOLOGY & DEMOGRAPHICS

INCIDENCE: In whites, approximately 1 in 385 persons.
PREDOMINANT SEX AND AGE: Generally diagnosed in males in their fifth decade. Diagnosis in females is generally not made until 10 to 20 yr after menopause.
GENETICS: Most common genetic disorder in North European ancestry. Homozygosity for the *C282Y* mutation is now found in approximately 5 of every 1000 persons of European descent.

PHYSICAL FINDINGS & CLINICAL PRESENTATION

- In earlier stages patients completely asymptomatic and diagnosed due to abnormal laboratory tests.
- Hepatic dysfunction leading to hepatomegaly, fibrosis, and eventually cirrhosis.
- Arthritis.
- Gonadal insufficiency leading to loss of libido and testicular atrophy.
- Diabetes mellitus: risk greater in patients with family history.
- Iron-induced cardiac disease resulting in cardiomyopathy, heart failure, and arrhythmias.
- Skin pigmentation.

ETIOLOGY

- The majority of the patients diagnosed with hemochromatosis have mutation in the *HFE* gene and are either homozygous for the *C282Y* mutation *(C282Y/C282Y)* or compound heterozygote for the *C282Y* mutation and either the mutation *H63D (C282Y/H63D)* or less commonly the *S65C (C282Y/S65C)*.
- The remainder of the patients are classified as non–*HFE*-associated hemochromatosis.

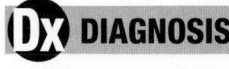 DIAGNOSIS

DIFFERENTIAL DIAGNOSIS

- Hereditary anemias with defect of erythropoiesis.
- Cirrhosis, chronic liver disease, porphyria cutanea tarda.
- Repeated blood transfusions.
- African dietary iron overload.

WORKUP

Medical history, physical examination, and laboratory evaluation should be focused on affected organ systems (see "Physical Findings & Clinical Presentation"). Fig. 1 outlines evaluation for possible hereditary hemochromatosis in an individual with negative family history. Liver biopsy is the gold standard for diagnosis; it reveals iron deposition in hepatocytes, bile ducts, and supporting tissues.

LABORATORY TESTS

- Transferrin saturation is the best screening test. Values >45% are an indication for further testing.
- Elevated serum ferritin is good evidence of iron overload, but other causes like chronic inflammatory conditions, malignancy, and so forth need to be ruled out as ferritin is also an acute phase reactant.
- Genotypical screening for *C282Y* and *H63D* mutation in *HFE* gene should be done in patients with high transferrin saturation, elevated ferritin, or both.

- Liver biopsy (Fig. 2) is the gold standard but is not needed in somebody who has a persistently elevated transferrin saturation, elevated ferritin, or both.
- Hepatic iron index can help differentiate between various causes of iron overload.
- Elevated aspartate aminotransferase, alanine aminotransferase, and alkaline phosphatase are seen.
- Hyperglycemia is found.
- Endocrine abnormalities (decreased testosterone, luteinizing hormone, follicle-stimulating hormone) are noted.
- Table 1 describes laboratory findings in patients with hereditary hemochromatosis.

IMAGING STUDIES

Routine radiologic imaging is not needed.

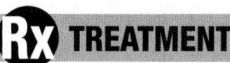 TREATMENT

The goal of therapy is the removal of excess iron and maintaining it at a normal or near-normal level.

NONPHARMACOLOGIC THERAPY

Phlebotomy is the treatment of choice.

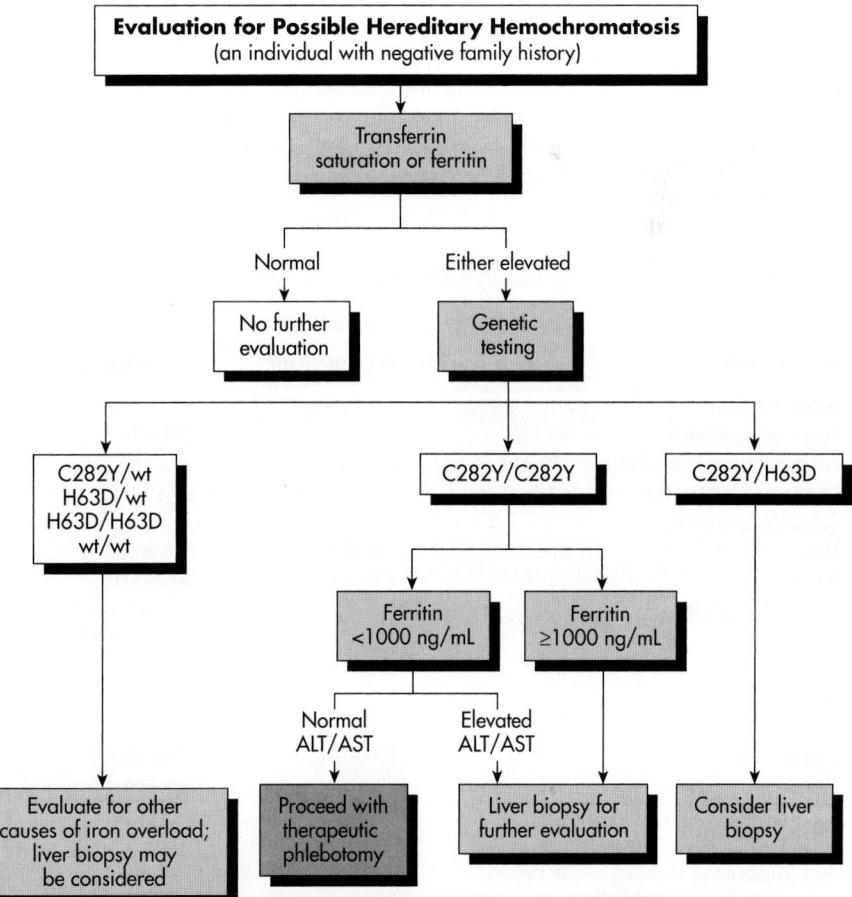

FIG. 1 Algorithm for evaluation of possible hereditary hemochromatosis in a person with a negative family history. *ALT,* Alanine transminase; *AST,* aspartate transminase. (From Goldman L, Schafer AI: *Goldman's Cecil medicine,* ed 24, Philadelphia, 2012, Saunders.)

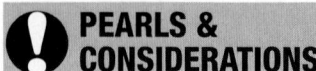

ACUTE GENERAL Rx

- The timing and frequency of phlebotomy needs to be individualized for each patient.
- For patients with heavy iron overload twice-weekly phlebotomies should be started. In most patients, weekly phlebotomy is adequate.
- The effectiveness of treatment is monitored by periodic ferritin measurement. The goal is to bring ferritin level below 50 ng/mL.
- Patients with iron overload due to transfusion-dependent anemias may not tolerate phlebotomy. For these patients iron chelation may be needed.
- The chelating agent deferoxamine has to be given daily as a 9- to 12-hr IV or SC infusion and compliance is difficult.
- The oral chelating agent deferasirox (Exjade) is effective, but should not be used in patients with high-risk myelodysplastic syndrome because it can cause renal impairment, hepatic impairment, or gastrointestinal hemorrhage, which can be fatal.

CHRONIC Rx

After the ferritin has been brought to less than 50 ng/mL, phlebotomy is needed on an as-needed basis to keep the ferritin at that level.

DISPOSITION

- Serum ferritin measurement is the most useful prognostic indicator of disease severity.
- Prognosis is good if phlebotomy is started early (before onset of cirrhosis or diabetes mellitus); women can have the full phenotypic expression of the disease, including cirrhosis, and should also be aggressively treated.

REFERRAL

For liver biopsy if diagnosis is uncertain.

PEARLS & CONSIDERATIONS

COMMENTS

- Persons who are homozygous for the HFE gene mutation *C282Y* comprise 85% to 90% of phenotypically affected individuals.
- Patients with hemochromatosis and serum ferritin levels <1000 ng/mL are unlikely to have cirrhosis. Liver biopsy to screen for cirrhosis may be unnecessary in such patients.
- Cirrhotic patients must be periodically monitored (ultrasound or CT scan) because of their increased risk of hepatocellular carcinoma.
- *HFE* gene testing for *C282Y* mutation is a cost-effective method of screening relatives of patients with hereditary hemochromatosis. The American College of Gastroenterology recommends genotyping persons who have abnormal iron screening tests and first-degree relatives of those identified with *C282Y* homozygosity.
- Established cirrhosis, hypogonadism, destructive arthritis, and insulin-dependent diabetes mellitus secondary to hemochromatosis cannot be reversed with repeated phlebotomy, but their progress can be slowed.
- In patients who are heterozygotes for *C282Y* or *H63D* mutation, clinically meaningful iron overload does not develop.
- Screening for hepatocellular carcinoma is reserved for those with hereditary hemochromatosis and cirrhosis.

SUGGESTED READINGS

Available at www.expertconsult.com

RELATED CONTENT

Hemochromatosis (Patient Information)

AUTHOR: **FRED F. FERRI, M.D.**

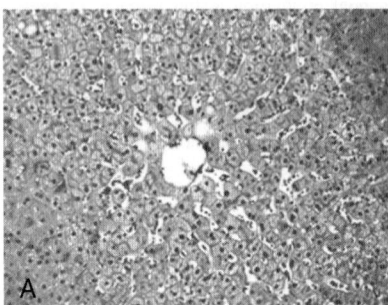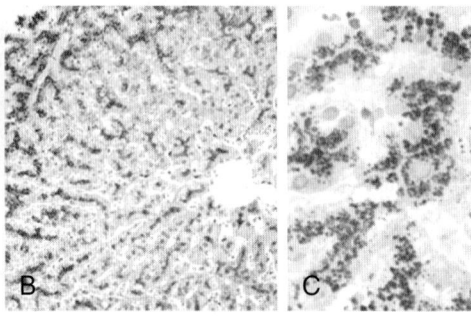

FIG. 2 Hemochromatosis. Liver biopsy sample from a 46-year-old man with homozygous hemochromatosis. Hematoxylin and eosin stain of the liver **(A)** shows intact hepatic architecture. Iron stain **(B, C)** shows marked diffuse iron deposits in the hepatocytes throughout the lobules. A normal liver would show essentially no iron in the hepatocytes. (From Hoffman R et al: *Hematology, basic principles and practice,* ed 5, Philadelphia, 2009, Churchill Livingstone.)

Table 1 Laboratory Findings in Patients with Hereditary Hemochromatosis

		Patients With Hereditary Hemochromatosis	
Measurements	Normal Subjects	Asymptomatic	Symptomatic
Blood (Fasting)			
Serum iron level (µg/dl)	60-180	150-280	180-300
Serum transferrin level (mg/dl)	220-410	200-280	200-300
Transferrin saturation (%)	20-45	45-100	80-100
Serum ferritin level (ng/ml)			
Men	20-200	150-1000	500-6000
Women	15-150	120-1000	500-6000
Genetic (*HFE* Mutation Analysis)			
C282Y/C282Y	wt/wt‡	*C282Y/C282Y*	*C282Y/C282Y*
*C282Y/H63D**	wt/wt	*C282Y/H63D*	*C282Y/H63D*
Liver			
Hepatic iron concentration			
µg/g dry weight	300-1500	2000-10,000	8000-30,000
µmol/g dry weight	5-27	36-179	140-550
Hepatic iron index†	<1	1 to >1.9	>1.9
Liver histology			
Perls' Prussian blue stain	0, 1+	2+ to 4+	3+, 4+

*Compound heterozygote.
†Calculated by dividing the hepatic iron concentration (in µmol/g dry weight) by the age of the patient (in yr). With the increased use of genetic testing in patients with iron overload, the specificity of the hepatic iron index has diminished.
‡wt/wt: wild type (normal).
From Goldman L, Schafer AI: *Goldman's Cecil medicine,* ed 24, Philadelphia, 2012, Saunders.

BASIC INFORMATION

DEFINITION

Thrombotic microangiopathy (TMA) is characterized by microvascular injury and occlusion resulting in microangiopathic hemolytic anemia, thrombocytopenia, and ischemic injury to multiple organs. Hemolytic-uremic syndrome (HUS) is a life-threatening form of thrombotic microangiopathy usually caused by bacterial infections such as those secondary to Shiga toxin–producing E. coli (STEC). In 5% to 10% of patients presenting with TMA resembling HUS, a preceding bacterial infection is not identified (so-called atypical HUS [aHUS]). Accumulating evidence indicates that uncontrolled complement activation can lead to aHUS in genetically susceptible individuals.

SYNONYMS

HUS

ICD-10CM CODES
D59.3 Hemolytic-uremic syndrome

EPIDEMIOLOGY & DEMOGRAPHICS

HUS affects mainly young children less than 5 years of age and has an incidence of 1 to 2 cases per 100,000 in the U.S. At times, HUS clusters in rural populations during the summer months. aHUS can occur at any age. The prevalence of aHUS is estimated to be 1 to 9 cases per million.

PHYSICAL FINDINGS AND CLINICAL PRESENTATION

HUS is usually preceded by an infection such as STEC-induced gastroenteritis, in which case HUS occurs 2 to 10 days following the onset of diarrhea. Diarrhea is bloody in approximately three fourths of cases and is accompanied by abdominal pain, vomiting, and fever. Oligoanuric acute kidney injury and hypertension are common manifestations of HUS. Neurologic manifestations occur in ~20% of cases and include altered mental status, seizure, and stroke. Stroke and coma are associated with increased mortality. Hepatomegaly and abnormal liver function tests may be present.

aHUS occurs in sporadic and familial forms. While aHUS is usually abrupt in onset, it can be insidious in ~20% of cases. aHUS often leads to severe acute kidney injury that requires therapy. Hypertension, proteinuria, and hematuria are frequently noted. C3 hypocomplementemia is present in ~20% of cases. Extrarenal involvement is increasingly being recognized and includes neurologic, gastrointestinal, and cardiovascular manifestations.

ETIOLOGY

Endothelial injury and microvascular thrombosis are the common denominators of HUS and aHUS. Endothelial injury in HUS is usually secondary to toxins produced by pathogenic bacteria such as STEC (especially E. coli serotype 0157:H7). However, endothelial injury in aHUS is secondary to complement activation via the alternative pathway. Complement activity is normally regulated by several soluble and membrane-bound proteins. Unrestrained complement activity and amplification produce and sustain endothelial injury. Loss-of-function genetic mutations affecting complement regulators are found in 40% to 60% of patients with aHUS. Conditions that amplify complement activity may precipitate aHUS. Complement-amplifying conditions include inflammatory diseases such as systemic lupus erythematosus, infections, pregnancy-related complications such as preeclampsia and HELLP, and transplantation. In up to two thirds of cases of aHUS, a complement-amplifying condition can be identified.

DIAGNOSIS

The first step in making a diagnosis of HUS/aHUS is establishing the presence of TMA. Most cases of HUS occur following a bacterial infection such as acute gastroenteritis due to STEC. aHUS remains a diagnosis of exclusion.

DIFFERENTIAL DIAGNOSIS

TMA also can be associated with thrombotic thrombocytopenic purpura (TTP), malignant hypertension, scleroderma renal crisis, and antiphospholipid antibody syndrome. TMAs are also associated with certain drugs (cyclosporine, tacrolimus, clopidogrel, quinine, mitomycin, gemcitabine), pregnancy, malignancy, bone marrow transplantation, HIV infection, and systemic lupus erythematosus.

WORKUP

The workup for suspected HUS/aHUS includes blood and stool tests.

LABORATORY TESTS

Anemia in HUS/aHUS is primarily secondary to microangiopathic hemolysis characterized by low-to-undetectable haptoglobin and increased LDH levels. The peripheral blood smear reveals fragmented erythrocytes (schistocytes) and increased numbers of reticulocytes. Indirect (unconjugated) bilirubin may be elevated. Platelet consumption secondary to microvascular thrombosis leads to relative (>25% reduction) or absolute (<150,000/mm^3) thrombocytopenia. In the absence of blood transfusion or autoimmunity, the direct Coombs test is typically negative. Increased blood urea nitrogen and creatinine levels are indicative of reduced kidney function. Urinalysis may show proteinuria and hematuria. Stool culture using special agar plates may detect STEC, especially during the first week of diarrhea. Specific immunoassays and genetic tests are available for detection of Shiga toxin from a stool specimen. TTP is suspected when the plasma activity of von Willebrand factor–cleaving protease ADAMTS-13 (*a disintegrin and metalloproteinase with a thrombospondin type 1 motif, member 13*) is <5%.

IMAGING STUDIES

Imaging studies are not very helpful in the diagnosis of HUS/aHUS.

TREATMENT

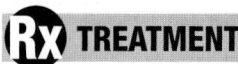

While the treatment of HUS is primarily supportive, pharmacologic complement inhibition is the mainstay of therapy for aHUS.

NONPHARMACOLOGIC THERAPY

Careful attention must be paid to volume status and electrolyte derangements. Severe anemia may require blood transfusion. Platelet transfusion is reserved for patients with clinically significant bleeding and those who require invasive procedures.

ACUTE GENERAL Rx

The treatment of HUS is supportive. Antibiotics and antimotility agents are avoided. Corticosteroids and therapeutic plasma exchange have no proven benefit in HUS. Therapeutic plasma exchange is considered as first- or second-line therapy for aHUS, either as stand-alone treatment or in conjunction with other treatment modalities. Eculizumab has been successfully used for the treatment of aHUS. Eculizumab is a humanized monoclonal antibody that binds to complement C5 and blocks its activation, thereby inhibiting terminal complement activation.

CHRONIC Rx

Renal replacement therapy (e.g., dialysis or kidney transplantation) may be required for renal failure in HUS/aHUS. Long-term therapeutic plasma exchange or eculizumab may be required for aHUS.

DISPOSITION

HUS has a mortality rate of <5%. The prognosis in adults is less favorable than in children. aHUS has a grave prognosis. While aHUS mortality approaches 25% during the acute phase, end-stage renal disease develops in nearly half of patients within a year. aHUS has a high recurrence rate after renal transplantation, and recurrent disease often leads to graft loss.

REFERRAL

The local health department is to be notified if STEC is isolated in a stool sample. Large foodborne outbreaks of STEC-HUS have occurred as a result of contaminated commercial beef products and asparagus.

Hematology and nephrology consultation are recommended.

PEARLS & CONSIDERATIONS

- STEC is transmissible from person to person. Therefore, universal precautions including handwashing are recommended. Children testing positive for STEC should not return

to the school or day care facility until two consecutive stool specimens test negative.
- The clinical presentation of HUS overlaps with TTP. As a rule of thumb, HUS is more common in children and is associated with more severe renal injury and milder neurologic manifestations than TTP.

SUGGESTED READINGS
Available at www.expertconsult.com

RELATED CONTENT
Hemolytic-Uremic Syndrome (Patient Information)

Thrombotic Thrombocytopenic Purpura (Related Key Topic)

AUTHORS: **ALI NAYER, M.D.,** and **ARIF ASIF, M.D.**

BASIC INFORMATION

DEFINITION

Hemophilia is a hereditary bleeding disorder caused by low factor VIII coagulant activity (hemophilia A) or low levels of factor IX coagulant activity (hemophilia B).

SYNONYMS

Hemophilia A: Classic hemophilia, factor VIII deficiency hemophilia

Hemophilia B: Christmas disease, factor IX hemophilia

ICD-10CM CODES
D66	Hereditary factor VIII deficiency
D67	Hereditary factor IX deficiency
D68.311	Acquired hemophilia
Z14.01	Asymptomatic hemophilia A carrier
Z14.02	Symptomatic hemophilia A carrier

EPIDEMIOLOGY & DEMOGRAPHICS

INCIDENCE/PREVALENCE (IN U.S.): Hemophilia A: 100 cases per 1 million males; hemophilia B: 20 cases per 1 million males. Approximately 400,000 patients have severe hemophilia worldwide.

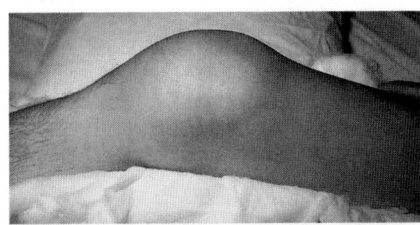

FIG. 1 Acute hemarthrosis of the knee is a common complication of hemophilia. It may be confused with acute infection unless the patient's coagulation disorder is known because the knee is hot, red, swollen, and painful. (From Forbes CD, Jackson WF: *Color atlas and text of clinical medicine*, ed 3, London, 2003, Mosby.)

GENETIC: Both hemophilias have an X-linked recessive pattern of inheritance with only males affected.

PHYSICAL FINDINGS & CLINICAL PRESENTATION

- The clinical features of hemophilia A and B are generally indistinguishable from each other. The clinical symptoms are determined by the baseline factor activity in each patient. Spontaneous bleeding can occur with those with severe hemophilia (<1% factor VIII or IX activity). Trauma-induced bleeding can occur in those with moderate hemophilia (factor levels 1%-5%) and mild disease (factor levels >5%).
- Bleeding is most commonly seen in joints (knees, ankles, elbows), resulting in hot, swollen, painful joints (Fig. 1) and subsequent crippling joint deformity (Fig. 2).
- Bleeding can also occur into the muscles and the gastrointestinal tract.
- Compartment syndrome can occur from large hematomas.
- Hematuria may be present.

ETIOLOGY

- Both disorders are congenital. X-linked recessive disorders of hemostasis.
- Hemophilia A: low factor VIII coagulant (VIII:C) activity; can be classified as mild if factor VIII:C levels are >5%, moderate if levels are 1% to 5%, and severe if levels are <1%.
- Hemophilia B: low levels of factor IX coagulant activity.
- Spontaneous acquisition of factor VIII inhibitors (acquired hemophilia) is rare.

DIAGNOSIS

DIFFERENTIAL DIAGNOSIS

- Other clotting factor deficiencies.
- Platelet function disorders.
- Vitamin K deficiency.

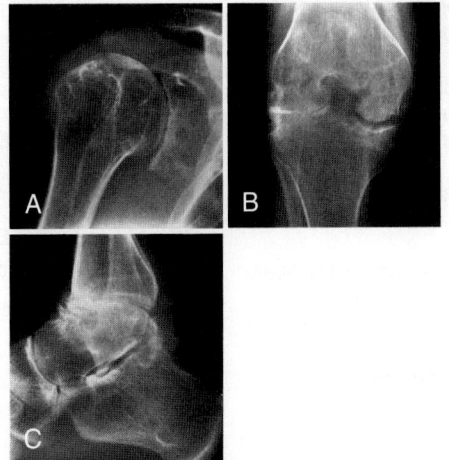

FIG. 2 Radiographic changes associated with hemophilic arthropathy. A, Radiograph of the shoulder showing multiple subchondral cysts in the head of the humerus, an early finding in hemophilic arthropathy. The glenohumeral joint space is fairly well preserved, and range of motion is normal. **B,** Widening of the intercondylar notch and near fusion of the femur and medial tibial condyle in the knee joint affected by hemophilic arthropathy. **C,** Narrowing and fusion of the tibiotalar joint in the ankle. (From Hoffman R et al: *Hematology, basic principles and practice*, ed 5, Philadelphia, 2009, Churchill Livingstone.)

WORKUP

Patients with mild hemophilia bleed only in response to major trauma or surgery and may not be diagnosed until young adulthood. Diagnostic workup includes laboratory evaluation (see "Laboratory Tests").

LABORATORY TESTS

- Partial thromboplastin time (aPTT) is prolonged. Prothrombin time (PT) is normal, and the aPTT mixing study will fully correct.
- Reduced factor VIII: C level distinguishes hemophilia A from other causes of prolonged PTT.
- Factor VIII antigen, fibrinogen level, and bleeding time are normal.
- Factor IX coagulant activity levels are reduced in patients with hemophilia B.
- Coagulation factor activity measurement is useful to correlate with disease severity. Normal range is 50 to 150 U/dl; 5 to 20 U/dl indicates mild disease, 2 to 5 U/dl indicates moderate disease, and <2 U/dl indicates severe disease with spontaneous bleeding episodes.

TREATMENT

NONPHARMACOLOGIC THERAPY

- Avoidance of contact sports.
- Patient education regarding the disease; promotion of exercises such as swimming.
- Avoidance of aspirin or other NSAIDs.
- Orthopedic evaluation and physical therapy evaluation in patients with joint involvement.
- Hepatitis vaccination.

ACUTE GENERAL Rx

(See Table 1).
HEMOPHILIA A:

- Reversal and prevention of acute bleeding in hemophilia A and B are based on adequate replacement of deficient or missing factor protein.
- The choice of the product for replacement therapy is guided by availability, capacity, concerns, and cost. Recombinant factors cost two to three times as much as plasma-derived factors, and the limited capacity to produce recombinant factors often results in periods of shortage. In the United States 60% of patients with severe hemophilia use recombinant products.
- Factor VIII concentrates are effective in controlling spontaneous and traumatic hemorrhage in severe hemophilia. The new recombinant factor VIII is stable without added human serum albumin (decreased risk of transmission of infectious agents).
- Alloantibodies (inhibitors) that neutralize factor VIII clotting function occur in nearly 30% of patients with severe hemophilia A after exposure to factor VIII. In these patients, bypassing agents (anti-inhibitor coagulant complex [AICC] and recombinant activated factor VII [rFVIIa]) can be used to treat bleeding. AICC can also be used prophylactically to decrease the frequency of joint and other bleeding events in patients with severe hemophilia A and factor VIII inhibitors.

TABLE 1 Treatment of Hemophilia

Type of Hemorrhage	Hemophilia A	Hemophilia B
Hemarthrosis*	50 IU/kg factor VIII concentrate[†] on day 1; then 20 IU/kg on days 2, 3, 5 until joint function is normal or back to baseline. Consider additional treatment every other day for 7-10 days. Consider prophylaxis.	80-100 IU/kg on day 1; then 40 IU/kg on days 2, 4. Consider additional treatment every other day for 7-10 days. Consider prophylaxis.
Muscle or significant subcutaneous hematoma	50 IU/kg factor VIII concentrate; 20 IU/kg every-other-day treatment may be needed until resolved.	80 IU/kg factor IX concentrate[‡]; treatment every 2-3 days may be needed until resolved.
Mouth, deciduous tooth, or tooth extraction	20 IU/kg factor VIII concentrate; antifibrinolytic therapy; remove loose deciduous tooth.	40 IU/kg factor IX concentrate[‡]; antifibrinolytic therapy[§]; remove loose deciduous tooth.
Epistaxis	Apply pressure for 15-20 min; pack with petrolatum gauze; give antifibrinolytic therapy; 20 IU/kg factor VIII concentrate if this treatment fails.[ǁ]	Apply pressure for 15-20 min; pack with petrolatum gauze; antifibrinolytic therapy; 30 IU/kg factor IX concentrate[‡] if this treatment fails.
Major surgery, life-threatening hemorrhage	50-75 IU/kg factor VIII concentrate, then initiate continuous infusion of 2-4 IU/kg/hr to maintain factor VIII >100 IU/dl for 24 hr[ǁ] then give 2-3 IU/kg/hr continuously for 5-7 days to maintain the level at >50 IU/dl and an additional 5-7 days to maintain the level at >30 IU/dl.[¶]	120 IU/kg factor IX concentrate[‡], then 50-60 IU/kg every 12-24 hr to maintain factor IX at >40 IU/dl for 5-7 days, and then at >30 IU/dl for 7 days.
Iliopsoas hemorrhage	50 IU/kg factor VIII concentrate, then 25 IU/kg every 12 hr until asymptomatic, then 20 IU/kg every other day for a total of 10-14 days.**	120 IU/kg factor IX concentrate[‡]; then 50-60 IU/kg every 12-24 hr to maintain factor IX at >40 IU/dl until patient is asymptomatic; then 40-50 IU every other day for a total of 10-14 days.[#].**
Hematuria	Bed rest; 1½ × maintenance fluids; if not controlled in 1-2 days, 20 IU/kg factor VIII concentrate; if not controlled, give prednisone (unless patient is HIV-infected).	Bed rest; 1½ × maintenance fluids; if not controlled in 1-2 days, 40 IU/kg factor IX concentrate[‡]; if not controlled, give prednisone (unless patient is HIV-infected).
Prophylaxis	20-40 IU/kg factor VIII concentrate every other day to achieve a trough level ≥1%.	30-50 IU/kg factor IX concentrate[‡] every 2-3 days to achieve a trough level ≥1%.

*For hip hemarthrosis, orthopedic evaluation tor possible aspiration is advisable to prevent avascular necrosis of the femoral head.

[†]For mild or moderate hemophilia, desmopressin, 0.3 µg/kg, should be used instead of factor VIII concentrate, if the patient is known to respond with a hemostatic level of factor VIII; if repeated doses are given, monitor factor VIII levels for tachyphylaxis.

[‡]Stated doses apply for recombinant factor IX concentrate; for plasma-derived factor IX concentrate, use 70% of the stated dose.

[§]Do not give antifibrinolytic therapy until 4 to 6 hr after a dose of prothrombin complex concentrate.

[ǁ]Over-the-counter coagulation-promoting products may be helpful.

[¶]Alternatively, give 25 IU/kg every 12 hr to maintain a trough level >50% for 5 to 7 days followed by 25-30 IU/kg for an additional 5 to 7 days to maintain trough >25%.

[#]Repeat radiologic assessment should be performed before discontinuation of therapy.

**If repeated doses of factor IX concentrate are required, use highly purified, specific factor IX concentrate.

Adapted from Montgomery RR et al: Hemophilia and von Willebrand disease. In Nathan DG, Orkin SH (eds): *Nathan and Oski's hematology at infancy and childhood*, ed 5, Philadelphia, 1998, Saunders.

- Recombinant activated factor VII is useful to stop spontaneous hemorrhages and prevent excessive bleeding during surgery in 75% of patients with inhibitors. Recommended dose is 90 µg/mg of body weight every 2 to 3 hr for treatment of life-threatening hemorrhage. It is, however, very expensive ($1 per µg).
- Desmopressin acetate 0.3 µg/kg q24h (causes release of factor VIII:C) may be used in preparation for minor surgical procedures in mild hemophiliacs.
- Aminocaproic acid (EACA, Amicar) 4 g PO q4h can be given for persistent bleeding that is unresponsive to factor VIII concentrate or desmopressin.

HEMOPHILIA B:
- Infuse factor IX concentrates. It is important to remember that factor IX concentrates contain other proteins that may increase the risk of thrombosis with recurrent use. Therefore factor IX concentrates must be used only when clearly indicated.
- Daily administration of oral cyclophosphamide and prednisone without empirical factor VIII therapy is an effective and well-tolerated treatment for acquired hemophilia.

CHRONIC Rx
- The aim of chronic treatment is to prevent spontaneous bleeding and excessive bleeding during any surgical intervention. Monitoring and treatment of patients with hemophilia at comprehensive hemophilia treatment centers is cost-effective and decreases morbidity and mortality.
- Prophylaxis with recombinant factor VIII can prevent joint damage and decrease the frequency of joint and other hemorrhages in young boys with severe hemophilia A. The estimated annual cost for treatment of one patient with recombinant factor VIII is $300,000.
- Implantation of genetically altered fibroblasts that produce factor VIII is safe and well tolerated. This form is feasible in patients with severe hemophilia. Hemophilia will likely be the first common, severe genetic disease to be cured by gene therapy.

DISPOSITION
- Despite the advent of virally safe blood products and blood treatment programs, nearly 70% of hemophiliacs are HIV seropositive. Survival is of normal expectancy in HIV-negative patients with mild disease.
- Intracranial bleeds are the second most common cause of death in hemophiliacs after AIDS. They are fatal in 30% of patients, occur in 10% of patients, and are generally the result of trauma.

SUGGESTED READINGS
Available at www.expertconsult.com

RELATED CONTENT
Hemophilia (Patient Information)

AUTHOR: **BHARTI RATHORE, M.D.**

i BASIC INFORMATION

DEFINITION

Hemoptysis is coughing up of blood originating from the lower respiratory tract, ranging from blood-streaked sputum to gross blood. If greater than 400 to 600 ml in 24 hours or if the bleeding rate is >100 ml/hr, it is considered massive hemoptysis.

ICD-10CM CODES
R04.2 Hemoptysis

EPIDEMIOLOGY & DEMOGRAPHICS

INCIDENCE: Unknown, varies based on underlying pathology
RISK FACTORS: Tobacco smoking predisposes to lung cancer, a common cause of hemoptysis. Systemic processes (rheumatologic, renal, hematologic) may contribute to alveolar hemorrhage or vasculitis. Anticoagulation can worsen bleeding.

PHYSICAL FINDINGS & CLINICAL PRESENTATION

- Presentation of hemoptysis is variable and can range from minimal blood-tinged sputum to more than 500 mL of gross blood in 24 hr. Other symptoms depend on the underlying etiology and can include cough, sputum production, fever, shortness of breath, weight loss, night sweats, wheezing, and chest pain.
- There are no specific exam findings, but clues to the etiology may be present, for example, focal wheezing, rhonchi or rales on pulmonary exam, murmur of mitral stenosis on cardiac exam.

ETIOLOGY

- There are many potential causes of hemoptysis including airway disease (bronchitis, bronchiectasis, lung neoplasm), infection (necrotizing pneumonia, lung abscess, tuberculosis, fungal infection), inflammatory diseases (granulomatosis with polyangiitis, Goodpasture's syndrome, lupus), cardiac disease (mitral stenosis after rheumatic heart disease, congenital heart diseases), and others (pulmonary embolism, cocaine use, foreign body, airway trauma, iatrogenic and cryptogenic).
- Acute respiratory tract infections, asthma, COPD, malignancy, and bronchiectasis are the most common diagnoses in outpatient primary care.
- Worldwide tuberculosis accounts for 7% to 85% of cases of massive hemoptysis. Highest incidence is in South Africa; lowest incidence in the U.S.

Dx DIAGNOSIS

DIFFERENTIAL DIAGNOSIS

- Various potential causes of lower respiratory tract bleeding.
  1. Airway disease (bronchitis, bronchiectasis, lung neoplasm).
  2. Infection (necrotizing pneumonia, lung abscess, tuberculosis, fungal infection).
  3. Inflammatory diseases (granulomatosis with polyangiitis, Goodpasture's syndrome, lupus).
  4. Cardiac disease (mitral stenosis after rheumatic heart disease, congenital heart diseases).
  5. Pulmonary embolism.
  6. Cocaine use.
  7. Foreign body.
- Bleeding from upper respiratory tract.
- Hematemesis or epistaxis
- Coagulopathy.

WORKUP

- The initial history should focus on determining the anatomic origin of the bleeding and on quantifying the volume of the hemoptysis in order to triage appropriately.
- Complete history and physical exam may suggest a particular etiology; important to ask about duration and quantity of hemoptysis and smoking history.

LABORATORY TESTS

- Complete blood count.
- Coagulation profile.
- Serum chemistries including creatinine, urinalysis.
- If indicated, consider vasculitis serologies (i.e., ANA, ANCA, anti-GBM).
- Arterial blood gas to assess oxygenation.
- Sputum for cultures and cytologic studies.
- PPD

IMAGING STUDIES

- Chest x-ray: all patients with hemoptysis should have a chest x-ray but will likely need additional studies to localize site of bleeding.
- Chest CT: chest CT scan combined with flexible bronchoscopy has the highest yield for localizing the site of bleeding.

Rx TREATMENT

Varies based on underlying etiology and non-massive versus massive hemoptysis

NONPHARMACOLOGIC THERAPY

Massive hemoptysis:

- Arteriographic embolization of bronchial arteries and/or collateral systemic vessels.
- Surgical resection of affected lung.

ACUTE GENERAL Rx

Massive hemoptysis (Fig. 1):
- Stabilize hemodynamic status and oxygenation.
- Reverse any coagulopathy.
- Bronchoscopy can be used to identify cause of hemoptysis (e.g., neoplasm), as well as to help isolate a site/segment of bleeding.
- If site of bleeding is known, place patient with bleeding lung in dependent position to prevent blood from spilling into non-affected lung and consider selective intubation with large-bore single-lumen endotracheal tube or double-lumen endotracheal tube.
- Bronchoscopic lavage with iced saline or topical application of epinephrine can be tried as a temporizing measure.
- Bronchoscopic balloon tamponade of bleeding site can be used as temporizing measure.
- Early consultation with interventional radiology, interventional pulmonology, and/or thoracic surgery for definitive intervention is recommended.

Submassive hemoptysis:
For submassive hemoptysis, identify and treat underlying condition. Refer to pulmonologist or hematologist if indicated.

CHRONIC Rx

For patients requiring anticoagulation or antiplatelet therapy for another disorder, consider risks/benefits of continued anticoagulation or antiplatelet therapy.

DISPOSITION

Generally, patients have a good prognosis after an episode of hemoptysis, but those with massive bleeding and/or malignancy tend to have a poorer prognosis.

SUGGESTED READING
Available at www.expertconsult.com

RELATED CONTENT

Evaluation of hemoptysis (Algorithm, Section III)

AUTHOR: **GAETANE MICHAUD, M.D.**

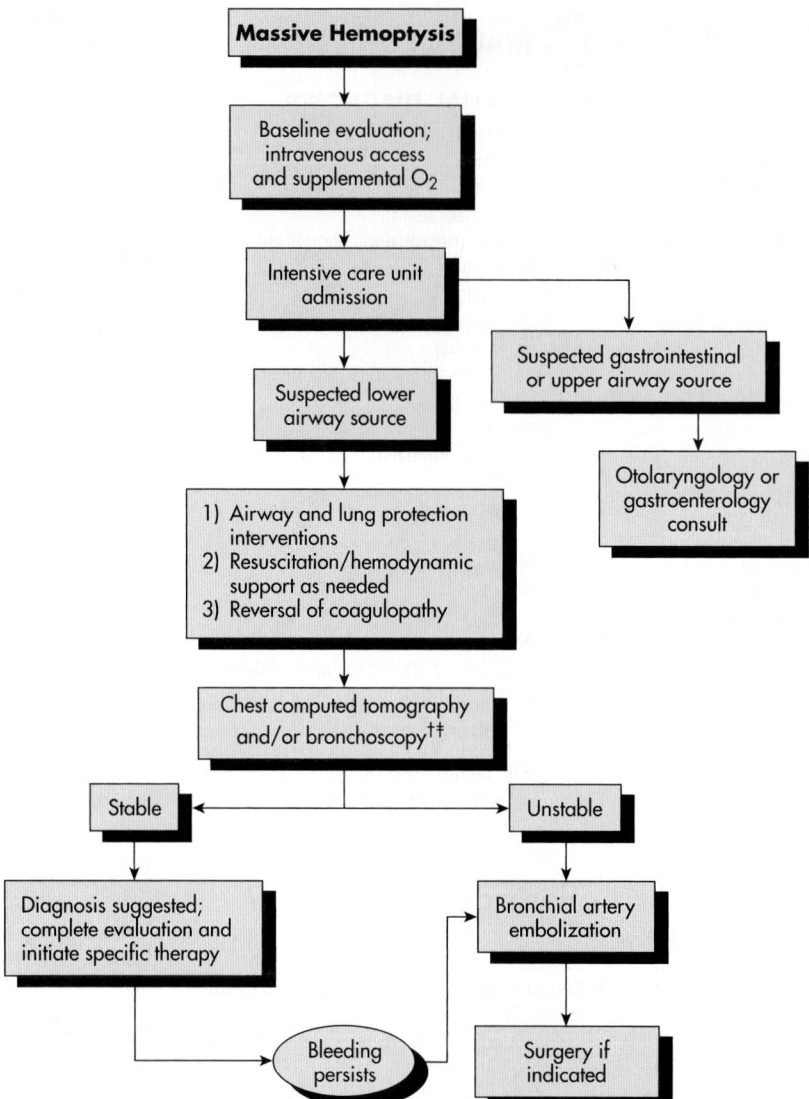

FIG. 1 Massive hemoptysis. *History and physical examination, complete blood count, coagulation studies, type and cross-match, chest radiograph, and arterial blood gas. †Local availability and patient stability should guide choice; computed tomography is preferred for the initial evaluation of a stable patient. ‡Local measures including topical vasoconstrictors, bronchial blockers, laser photocoagulation, electrocautery, and hemostatic agents can be used endobronchially. (From Parrillo JE, Dellinger RP: *Critical care medicine: principles of diagnosis and management in the adult*, ed 4, Philadelphia, 2014, Saunders.)

BASIC INFORMATION

DEFINITION

Henoch-Schönlein purpura (HSP) is a systemic, small-vessel, IgA immune complex–mediated leukocytoclastic vasculitis characterized by a tetrad of palpable purpura (without thrombocytopenia), abdominal pain, renal disease, and arthritis/arthralgias. It may also present with gastrointestinal (GI) bleeding.

SYNONYMS

Anaphylactoid purpura
Allergic purpura
HSP

ICD-10CM CODES
D69.0 Allergic purpura

EPIDEMIOLOGY & DEMOGRAPHICS

INCIDENCE: Annual incidence of 20 cases/100,000 population in children. Approximately 1/100,000 in adults
PEAK INCIDENCE: Late autumn to early spring, rarely in summer. Seasonal variation is not seen in adults.
PREVALENCE: Most common vasculitis seen in children and younger age groups; seen in white and Asian populations 3 to 4 times more commonly than in black patients.
PREDOMINANT SEX AND AGE: 2:1 male/female ratio. Seen mostly from ages 3 to 12, although can be seen in older adolescents and young adults; 90% of all patients <10 years old.
GENETICS: Recent studies have identified genetic susceptibility factors, but familial recurrence is very rare. An association has been seen with the "Mediterranean fever" (*MEFV*) gene; HSP seen in up to 7% of gene carriers.

RISK FACTORS

No formally identified risk factors

PHYSICAL FINDINGS & CLINICAL PRESENTATION

- Palpable purpura (Fig. 1) of dependent areas, especially lower extremities (palms and soles) and areas subjected to pressure, such as the beltline in adults or buttocks in toddlers.
- GI symptoms are seen in up to two thirds of patients. Common findings are abdominal pain, nausea, vomiting, diarrhea, cramping, hematochezia, and melena. Complications include GI bleeding (20% to 30%), bowel ischemia, intussusception (1%-5%), and bowel perforation (<1%).
- Subcutaneous edema.
- Arthralgias and arthritis in 60% to 85%. Typically oligoarticular, affecting lower extremity and large joints. Periarticular swelling and tenderness also noted.
- Renal involvement is seen in as many as 80% of older children, usually within the first month of illness. Fewer than 5% progress to end-stage renal failure, a major cause of morbidity. Renal manifestations may range from isolated hematuria or proteinuria to acute nephropathy with renal insufficiency.
- 10% to 20% of male children can present with pain and swelling of the scrotum that can mimic testicular torsion.

ETIOLOGY

- Presumptive etiology is exposure to a trigger antigen that causes antibody formation.
- Antigen-antibody (immune) complex deposition then occurs in arteriole and capillary walls of skin, renal mesangium, and GI tract. Immunoglobulin A (IgA) deposition is most common.
- Antigen triggers postulated include drugs, foods, immunization, and upper respiratory and other viral illnesses. Group A streptococcal infection is the most common precipitant in children, seen in up to one third of cases. A recent adult case triggered by pantoprazole has also been reported.
- 30% to 65% of cases reviewed in children were preceded by an unspecified upper respiratory infection.
- Serologic and pathologic evidence suggests an association between parvovirus B19 and HSP, which may explain observed cases of HSP that do not respond to corticosteroids or other immunosuppressive therapy.
- Case reports have been published describing development of HSP after treatment with a variety of medications including immunosuppressive agents (e.g., etanercept) and more widely used medications such as pantoprazole.
- In a meta-analysis of 749 HSP children and 560 controls, 49.27% of HSP children had evidence of *Helicobacter pylori* infection compared to 23.39% of controls. The pooled odds ratio of *H. pylori* infection in HSP children was 3.80 (95% CI 2.54-5.68). Case reports suggest that eradication of *H. pylori* improves symptoms of HSP. Though causation between *H. pylori* and HSP has not been established, there appears to be a strong correlation.

DIAGNOSIS

- Diagnosis is based on the finding of IgA in the affected vessels. Nonthrombocytopenic purpura (see Fig. 2) is essential to the diagnosis.
- Skin manifestations are most common. See Table 1 for common clinical manifestations of HSP.
- Skin biopsy shows leukocytoclastic vasculitis. Renal biopsy shows mesangial IgA deposition.
- The presence of two of the following four American College of Rheumatology criteria yields a diagnostic sensitivity of 87.1% and specificity of 87.7%:
  1. Palpable purpura unrelated to thrombocytopenia
  2. Age <20 yr at onset of first symptoms
  3. Bowel angina or ischemia
  4. Granulocytic infiltration of arteriole or venule walls on biopsy
- In 2010, a European consortium published a set of validated diagnostic criteria that showed 100% sensitivity and 87% specificity. Their

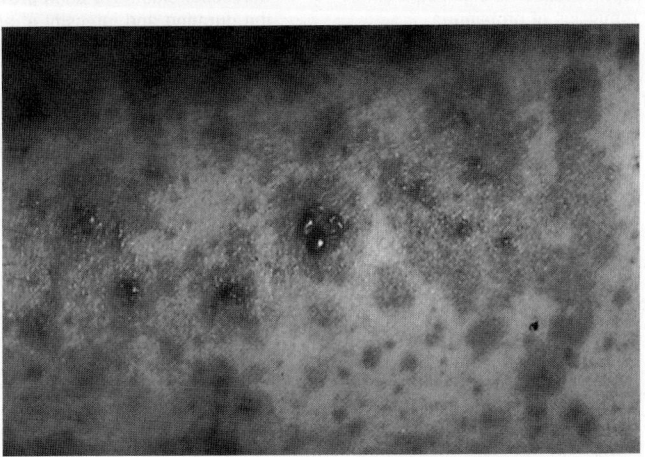

FIG. 1 Palpable purpura in a patient with Henoch-Schönlein purpura. (From Hoffman R et al [eds]: *Hematology: basic principles and practice,* ed 4, Philadelphia, 2005, Saunders.)

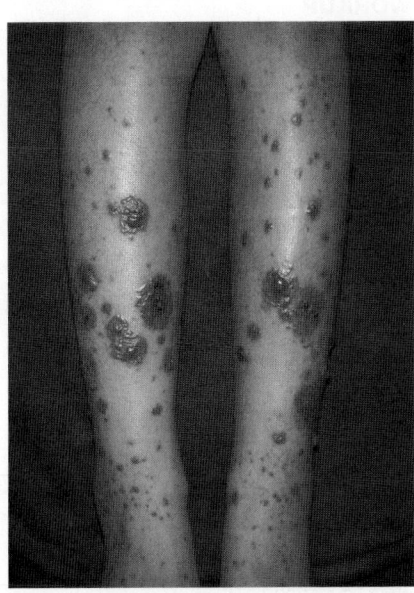

FIG. 2 Extensive palpable purpura over the lower extremities in a 7-yr-old girl with Henoch-Schönlein purpura. (From Hochberg MC et al: *Rheumatology,* ed 5, St Louis, 2011, Mosby.)

TABLE 1 Clinical Manifestations of Henoch-Schönlein Purpura

	% at Onset	% during Course
Purpura (nl platelet count)	50	100
Subcutaneous edema	10-20	20-50
Arthritis (large joints)	25	60-85
Gastrointestinal	30	85
Renal	?	10-50
Genitourinary (ddx torsion)	?	2-35
Pulmonary (T_LCO)	?	95
Pulmonary hemorrhage	?	Rare, may be fatal
Central nervous system (headache, organic brain syndrome, seizures)	?	Rare, may be fatal

From Hochberg MC et al: *Rheumatology*, ed 5, St Louis, 2011, Mosby.

criteria described purpura with lower limb predominance and one or more of the following:
○ Abdominal pain
○ Predominant IgA deposits of histopathology
○ Arthritis or arthralgia
○ Renal involvement

DIFFERENTIAL DIAGNOSIS

- Polyarteritis nodosa
- Acute abdomen
- Meningococcemia
- Thrombocytopenic purpura
- Hypersensitivity vasculitis
- Microscopic polyangiitis
- Granulomatosis with polyangiitis (Wegener granulomatosis)

WORKUP

History, physical examination, laboratory testing, skin or renal biopsy

LABORATORY TESTS

- Electrolytes, blood urea nitrogen, and creatinine
- Urinalysis
- Complete blood count
- Prothrombin time, fibrinogen, and fibrin degradation products
- Blood cultures
  Laboratory abnormalities are not specific for HSP but may help identify complications and rule out other diseases. Leukocytosis and eosinophilia may be seen. IgA levels are elevated in approximately 50% of patients. Glomerulonephritis may be present (microscopic hematuria, proteinuria, and red blood cell casts).

IMAGING STUDIES

Imaging studies are generally not useful in the diagnosis of HSP. Arteriography or magnetic resonance angiography may be helpful in distinguishing from polyarteritis nodosa. Abdominal ultrasound is recommended for patients with severe abdominal pain to detect increased bowel wall thickness, peritoneal fluid, or intussusception.

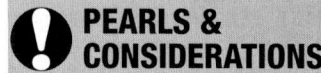

TREATMENT

NONPHARMACOLOGIC THERAPY

- Supportive care with pain management, adequate hydration, and nutrition is the primary intervention as up to 94% of cases in children and 87% cases in adults will resolve spontaneously.

ACUTE GENERAL Rx

Prednisone 1 to 2 mg/kg PO daily for 2 weeks is typically given for severe arthritis and/or abdominal pain. An equivalent dose of methylprednisolone can be used with same efficacy.
- A double-blind, randomized, controlled trial (RCT) found that early treatment with prednisone reduced abdominal pain and joint symptoms but did not prevent development of renal disease. It was effective in the treatment of renal disease once it was established.
- Another recent trial showed no evidence that treatment with prednisolone at diagnosis reduces the prevalence of proteinuria 12 mo after disease onset in children with HSP.
- Corticosteroids are the first-line therapy for inducing remission of HSP-induced kidney disease; cyclosporine, azathioprine, and mycophenolate mofetil are used to maintain remission.
- A retrospective review of 29 patients showed successful induction of remission with cyclosporine. However, two subsequent RCTs with a total of 110 patients did not show that cyclosporine was superior to placebo in achieving remission.
- An observational study of 12 patients with HSP nephritis who failed steroids showed normalization of renal function with mycophenolate mofetil.
- Azathioprine may be beneficial if rapidly progressive glomerulonephritis is present.
- A study comparing mycophenolate mofetil to azathioprine found no significant difference in remission of proteinuria.
- Not all patients with HSP nephritis or nephrotic-range proteinuria respond to these treatments.
- Recent case series and case reports on a total of 12 patients with biopsy-proven renal involvement who failed steroids +/- immunosuppressives had improvement in kidney function or proteinuria or hematuria with rituximab therapy. More systematic studies are needed to examine renal outcomes with rituximab.
- Severe gastrointestinal involvement (defined by intense pain, GI bleeding, and protein-losing enteropathy) improved with intravenous immunoglobulin in eight pediatric patients with HSP.

CHRONIC Rx

- Even if renal involvement is not present after initial episode, urinalysis and blood pressure should be checked every 2 to 4 weeks for first 6 months to detect development and progression of kidney disease.

COMPLEMENTARY AND ALTERNATIVE MEDICINE:

- No complementary or alternative treatment modalities proven to be effective for HSP.

DISPOSITION

- Prognosis excellent, with spontaneous recovery within 4 weeks in most patients.
- Hospitalization is recommended for significant GI or renal involvement.
- Increased age of onset generally correlates with morbidity. While end-stage renal disease (ESRD) occurs in 10% to 30% of adult patients with HSP at 15 years, chronic renal insufficiency is the most common long-term morbidity and affects adults more than children.
- Recurrences in up to one third of patients, especially within first 4 to 6 mo after initial episode and most commonly in patients with renal involvement. Recurrences are characteristically less severe than initial episode.

REFERRAL

Rheumatologist, nephrology, or general surgery consultation based on clinical manifestations

PEARLS & CONSIDERATIONS

- HSP is an IgA-related vasculitis.
- Organ systems involved are skin, joints, GI tract, and kidneys.
- Palpable purpura without thrombocytopenia more common in adults; GI symptoms more common in children.
- GI symptoms and arthritis may precede rash. Skin and renal manifestations occur at same time.
- Most with spontaneous recovery within 4 weeks of onset of symptoms.
- End-stage renal disease occurs in only 5% of patients.
- Corticosteroids have been proven to shorten the duration and intensity of arthritis and GI symptoms but do not prevent nephritis or recurrences.

SUGGESTED READINGS

Available at www.expertconsult.com

RELATED CONTENT

Henoch-Schönlein Purpura (Patient Information)

AUTHORS: **CANTING GUO, M.D.,** and **DOMINICK TAMMARO, M.D.**

BASIC INFORMATION
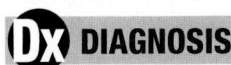

DEFINITION

There are two forms of heparin-induced thrombocytopenia (HIT). Type 1 HIT is a mild, transient decrease in platelet count that occurs during the first few days of heparin exposure due to platelet agglutination. This form is a benign, non–immune-mediated reaction, and the platelet count will return to normal while heparin is continued. This chapter will refer to Type 2 HIT, an antibody-mediated thrombocytopenia that is associated with thrombosis.

SYNONYMS

Type II heparin-induced thrombocytopenia

Heparin-induced thrombocytopenia and thrombosis (HITT)

Heparin-associated immune thrombocytopenia

ICD-10CM CODES
D75.82 Heparin-induced thrombocytopenia (HIT)

EPIDEMIOLOGY & DEMOGRAPHICS

INCIDENCE: Occurs in 0.2% to 5% of patients exposed to heparin. Unfractionated heparin is associated with a 5 to 10 times higher risk of HIT compared with low-molecular-weight heparin. Initially, there was an overwhelming underdiagnosis of HIT; however, since the introduction of HIT antibody ELISA test, there is a propensity to overdiagnose HIT irrespective of the clinical scenario.

PREDOMINANT SEX AND AGE: Females are at slightly higher risk than males. More common in adults but may also occur in children.

RISK FACTORS: Longer duration of exposure to heparin, type of heparin (unfractionated heparin has a greater risk), type of patient (surgical patients, especially cardiac and orthopedic surgery, are at higher risk than medical patients).

PHYSICAL FINDINGS & CLINICAL PRESENTATION

Suspect in a patient with:
- Exposure to heparin for 4 to 14 days OR who was exposed to heparin in the prior 3 mo.
- Unexplained platelet count decrease to 50% below pretreatment baseline.
- Onset of thrombocytopenia 5 to 10 days after heparin initiation.
- Evidence of acute venous or arterial thrombosis.
- Phlegmasia cerulea dolens
- Skin lesions or necrosis at heparin injection sites.
- Acute anaphylaxis during administration of heparin bolus.
- Adrenal hemorrhage.

ETIOLOGY

Occurs due to the formation of IgG antibodies, directed against heparin in complex with platelet factor 4, which bind to and activate platelets. Activated platelets release platelet factor 4 (leading to more antibody production) and undergo aggregation and premature removal from the circulation (resulting in thrombocytopenia). This platelet activation and antibody formation also can lead to thrombosis. Fig. E1 illustrates the mechanism of HIT.

DIAGNOSIS

DIFFERENTIAL DIAGNOSIS

Thrombocytopenia due to other causes including:
- Sepsis
- Disseminated intravascular coagulation
- Thrombocytopenic thrombotic purpura
- Hemolytic uremic syndrome
- Drug-induced thrombocytopenia (other than heparin)
- Antiphospholipid antibody syndrome
- Liver failure
- Splenic sequestration
- Digital or distal limb ischemia from embolism or shock

WORKUP

HIT is first and foremost a clinical diagnosis that is confirmed with laboratory testing. See Table 1 for workup based on pretest probability. If the patient has a low pretest probability score, heparin can be safely continued, and there is no need to send for further testing for HIT. If the

Table 1 A Diagnostic and Treatment Approach to Heparin-Induced Thrombocytopenia

Suspicion of HIT Based upon the "4 T's"	Score	Pre-Test Probability Score Criteria 2	1	0
Thrombocytopenia	☐	nadir 20-100, or >50% platelet fall	nadir 10-19, or 30%-50% platelet fall	nadir <10, or <30% platelet fall
Timing of onset of platelet fall	☐	day 5-10, or ≤day 1 with recent heparin*	>day 10 or timing unclear (but fits with HIT)	≤day 1 (no recent heparin)
Thrombosis or other sequelae	☐	proven thrombosis, skin necrosis, or ASR†	progressive, recurrent, or silent thrombosis; erythematous skin lesions	none
Other cause of platelet fall	☐	none evident	possible	definite
Total Pre-Test Probability Score	☐	periodic reassessment as new information can change pre-test probability (e.g., positive blood cultures)		

Total Pre-Test Probability Score

High			Moderate		Low			
8	7	6	5	4	3	2	1	0
Stop heparin‡, give alternative non-heparin anticoagulant argatroban¶ or lepirudin# or danaparoid** (or bivalirudin†† or fondaparinux‡‡)			Physician judgment		Continue (LMW) heparin			

Positive test for HIT antibodies ← **HIT Test** → **Negative** test for HIT antibodies
Continue non-heparin anticoagulant until platelet count recovery
Consider continuing or switching back to (LMW) heparin ##

Thrombosis* ← **Imaging studies for lower-limb DVT†††** → **No Thrombosis**
If HIT, continue non-heparin anticoagulant until platelet count recovery, then **cautious coumarin overlap¶¶**
If HIT, consider anticoagulating until platelet count recovery, even if no thrombosis apparent (± coumarin¶¶)

---

*recent heparin indicates exposure within the past 30 days (2 points) or past 30-100 days (1 point)
†ASR, acute systemic reaction following i.v. heparin bolus
‡stop all heparin, including catheter "flushes" and, possibly, heparin-coated catheters
¶argatroban: approved (U.S., Canada) for isolated HIT and HIT complicated by thrombosis (2 μg/kg/min i.v., adjusted to 1.5-3.0X patient's baseline aPTT or the mean of the laboratory normal range); reduce dose for hepatobiliary compromise: may increase INR more than the other direct thrombin inhibitors, thus requiring care in managing coumarin overlap (see ¶¶ below)
#lepirudin: approved (U.S., Canada, E.U., elsewhere) for treatment of thrombosis complicating HIT (±0.4 mg/kg i.v. bolus, then 0.15 mg/kg/h adjusted to 1.5-2.5X patient's baseline aPTT or mean of the laboratory normal range); used (off-label) also to treat isolated HIT (0.1 mg/kg/h, adjusted by aPTT); to avoid overdosing and anaphylaxis, it may be preferable to omit the bolus, and begin as i.v. infusion (except when facing life- or limb-threatening thrombosis); reduce dose for renal insufficiency
**danaparoid: usual i.v. bolus, 2250 U (body weight 60-75 kg) followed by infusion (400 U/h for 4 h, then 300 U/h for 4 h, then 200 U/h, adjusted by anti-factor Xa levels); this therapeutic-dose regimen is appropriate both for isolated HIT and for HIT complicated by thrombosis (though higher than approved dose in some jurisdictions); withdrawn from U.S. market (2002)
††bivalirudin: no bolus, i.v. infusion 0.15 mg/kg/h adjusted by aPTT; limited experience (off-label)
‡‡fondaparinux: dosing for HIT not established; limited experience (off-label)
¶¶delay coumadin pending substantial platelet count recovery (at least >100, preferably >150); begin coumadin in low doses, with at least 4-5 day overlap, stopping alternative anticoagulant when INR therapeutic for 2 days and platelets recovered
##depending on physician confidence in the laboratory's ability to rule out HIT antibodies (usually, negative PF4-dependent enzyme-immunoassay and/or washed platelet activation assay performed by an experienced laboratory)
***some thrombi may require special treatment, e.g., thrombectomy for large limb artery thrombosis
†††routine ultrasound of lower-limb veins recommended, since many HIT patients have subclinical deep-vein thrombosis (DVT)

From Warkentin TE et al: Platelet-endothelial interactions: sepsis, HIT, and antiphospholipid syndrome. *Hematology Am Soc Hematol Educ Program* 497-519, 2003.

patient has a moderate to high pretest probability, HIT testing (Table E2), imaging studies for lower-extremity deep venous thrombosis (also consider imaging of upper extremities if swelling is present or venous catheters are in place), cessation of heparin products, and alternative anticoagulation should all be performed. Patients with intermediate and high pretest probability but no HIT antibodies or intermediate pretest probability and only weakly positive HIT antibodies (based on optical density, see below) can resume heparin use as HIT is unlikely in these scenarios. Patients with high pretest probability and weakly positive antibodies or intermediate/high pretest probability and moderate to strongly positive antibodies likely have HIT and should be treated as such.

LABORATORY TESTS

These can be broadly divided into immunoassays (high sensitivity) and functional assays (high specificity).

In the appropriate clinical setting, testing for HIT antibodies with an enzyme-linked immunosorbent assay, or ELISA, can be useful. This test is very sensitive, but not specific. The majority of patients with positive testing for HIT antibodies will not develop clinical HIT. Thus, HIT antibody testing is more effective for ruling out rather than confirming the diagnosis of HIT.

More recently, use of the HIT antibody optical density as well as the immunoglobulin subtypes of the HIT antibody have entered the diagnostic realm. Higher optical density levels are associated with increased likelihood of a positive functional assay, higher pretest probability score, and increased risk of thrombosis. Weakly positive optical densities (0.4 to 1.0) are only rarely associated with functional assay positivity. In contrast, optical densities >2.0 almost always show heparin-dependent platelet activation. Optical densities are thus defined as weakly positive (0.4-1.0), moderately positive (1.0-2.0), or strongly positive (>2.0). The HIT antibody IgG subtype is the pathologic antibody for HIT. Hence, use of IgG-specific ELISA kits increases the test specificity over the polyspecific (IgA/M/G) antibody. Patients with low pretest probability via the 4T clinical prediction score should not have HIT antibody testing performed because it has a more than 99% negative predictive value, while all patients with intermediate and high pretest probability of HIT benefit from HIT antibody testing.

The gold standard test for HIT is to measure heparin-dependent platelet activation via the functional serotonin release assay (14C-SRA). This is both a highly sensitive and specific test. Donor platelets are incubated with radiolabeled serotonin. The platelets internalize the serotonin and are then exposed to the patient's serum and heparin at a therapeutic concentration. If antibodies to the platelet factor 4-heparin complex are present in the patient's serum, the platelets react and released radioactive serotonin is then measured. Availability and turnaround time of this test is dependent on the institution, which can influence the test's clinical utility. Cases where there is intermediate pretest probability, but only a weakly positive HIT antibody optical density, benefit the most from confirmatory SRA testing.

IMAGING STUDIES

Doppler ultrasonography of the extremities in the correct clinical setting.

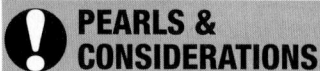

TREATMENT

- For patients with a moderate or high pretest probability, discontinue all heparin exposure. Even if the patient does not have a clinically evident thrombosis, there is a 50% risk of developing an incident clot within the subsequent 30 days. Thus, the patient must be started on an alternate anticoagulant.
- Two agents, both direct thrombin inhibitors, are approved for this indication:
  1. Argatroban (preferred agent in renal failure; avoid in liver dysfunction).
  2. Bivalirudin (approved only for patients with HIT or at risk of HIT who are undergoing PCI; dose adjustment is required in renal failure). Note: Lepirudin is no longer available.
- The safety and efficacy of the oral direct thrombin inhibitor dabigatran in HIT has yet to be shown in clinical trials.
- Platelet transfusion in the absence of life-threatening hemorrhage or extreme thrombocytopenia should be avoided. Platelet recovery should occur with discontinuation of heparin and initiation of a direct thrombin inhibitor.
- These drugs should be continued as a single agent until the platelet count returns to baseline (generally a platelet count of 150 × 109/L but it is important to consider the individual patient's baseline), then warfarin can be added at a maximum dose of 5 mg/day. This overlap therapy should continue until the platelet count has reached a stable plateau, the INR has reached the intended target (remember that argatroban artificially elevates the INR), and after a minimum overlap of 5 days of both the direct thrombin inhibitor and warfarin. The length of treatment is controversial, but most clinicians agree that 1 month of alternate anticoagulation is sufficient in the absence of thrombosis, while 3 to 6 months of treatment are required in the presence of thrombosis.
- Argatroban has been safely used in hemodialysis patients with HIT.
- Care should be taken when initiating warfarin in HIT because the risk of warfarin-induced skin and limb necrosis is increased in this setting. Risk is increased with higher loading doses of warfarin.

- There are emerging data showing similar efficacy and lower bleeding risk in HIT for fondaparinux when compared with the direct thrombin inhibitors. Fondaparinux is a synthetic pentasaccharide that binds antithrombin, causing long-acting inhibition of activated factor X, but not thrombin. It is not FDA approved for HIT, but its use in HIT has been reported. Rare cases of fondaparinux-induced HIT have been reported, however.
- The use of novel oral anticoagulants (e.g., rivaroxaban, dabigatran, apixaban) is being studied.
- Outside of the U.S., the factor Xa inhibitor danaparoid may be used.

NONPHARMACOLOGIC THERAPY

All nonpharmacologic therapies including surgical procedures.

REFERRAL

Request a hematology consultation.

PEARLS & CONSIDERATIONS

COMMENTS

HIT paradoxically causes thrombocytopenia and *clotting*, not bleeding.

It is unclear whether patients who have had HIT should be considered heparin allergic lifelong. Risk of recurrent HIT with heparin rechallenge years later is relatively low, about 5% in one small study (though recurrence risk is higher perioperatively). If such a patient requires surgery with heparin (e.g., on-pump cardiac bypass), consider perioperative argatroban.

Consult the coagulation laboratory and/or hematology when bridging patients on argatroban to warfarin, as argatroban concomitantly raises the INR in most assays. Some clinicians will use a higher target than 2-3 during the bridging period for this reason.

Beware heparin exposure in the absence of anticoagulation or DVT prophylaxis: hospitalized patients are often exposed to heparin lock flushes, heparin-coated catheters, or heparin-coated guidewires—any of which could precipitate HIT.

PREVENTION

Strongly consider the use of low-molecular-weight heparin instead of unfractionated heparin in hospitalized patients with a stable creatinine clearance (CrCl) of 30 mL/min or greater. Such a preventive strategy can reduce the risk of HIT by over 90%, as well as yield cost savings in testing and treatment.

SUGGESTED READINGS

Available at www.expertconsult.com

AUTHORS: **WILLIAM M. RAFELSON, M.D., M.B.A.,** and **JOHN L. REAGAN, M.D.**

BASIC INFORMATION

DEFINITION

Hepatic encephalopathy is a neuropsychiatric syndrome occurring in patients with severe impairment of liver function and consequent accumulation of toxic products not metabolized by the liver. It is characterized by gradual impairment of the ability to perform mental tasks and to react to external stimuli. *Minimal hepatic encephalopathy* refers to patients with hepatic cirrhosis and mild cognitive impairment, but no history of overt encephalopathy.

SYNONYMS

Hepatic coma
Portal systemic encephalopathy
HE

ICD-10CM CODES

K72.0	Acute and subacute hepatic failure
K72.1	Chronic hepatic failure
K72.9	Hepatic failure, unspecified
G92	Toxic encephalopathy
G93.40	Encephalopathy, unspecified
G93.41	Metabolic encephalopathy
K70.40	Alcoholic hepatic failure without coma
K70.41	Alcoholic hepatic failure with coma
K72.00	Acute and subacute hepatic failure without coma
K72.01	Acute and subacute hepatic failure with coma
K72.10	Chronic hepatic failure without coma
K72.11	Chronic hepatic failure with coma
K72.90	Hepatic failure, unspecified without coma
K72.91	Hepatic failure, unspecified with coma
K91.82	Postprocedural hepatic failure

EPIDEMIOLOGY & DEMOGRAPHICS

INCIDENCE/PREVALENCE: Hepatic encephalopathy occurs in >40% of all cases of cirrhosis.

PHYSICAL FINDINGS & CLINICAL PRESENTATION

Hepatic encephalopathy can be classified by clinical stages described in Table 1. Other widely used scales are the four score criteria and the West Haven criteria. The West Haven criteria for grading hepatic encephalopathy is as follows:

- Grade (0): No abnormalities noted
- Grade (1): Unawareness (mild), euphoria or anxiety, shortened attention span, impairment of calculation ability, lethargy or apathy
- Grade (2): Disorientation to time, obvious personal change, inappropriate behavior
- Grade (3): Somnolence to stupor, responsiveness to stimuli, gross disorientation, bizarre behavior
- Grade (4): Coma

The physical examination in hepatic encephalopathy varies with the stage and may reveal the following abnormalities:

- Skin: jaundice, palmar erythema, spider angiomata, ecchymosis, dilated superficial periumbilical veins (caput medusae) in patients with cirrhosis.
- Eyes: scleral icterus, Kayser-Fleischer rings (Wilson's disease).
- Breath: fetor hepaticus.
- Chest: gynecomastia in men with chronic liver disease.
- Abdomen: ascites, small nodular liver (cirrhosis), tender hepatomegaly (congestive hepatomegaly).
- Rectal examination: hemorrhoids (portal hypertension), guaiac-positive stool (alcoholic gastritis, bleeding esophageal varices, peptic ulcer disease, bleeding hemorrhoids).
- Genitalia: testicular atrophy in males with chronic liver disease.
- Extremities: pedal edema from hypoalbuminemia.
- Neurologic: flapping tremor (asterixis), obtundation, coma with or without decerebrate posturing.

ETIOLOGY

- Hepatic encephalopathy is thought to be caused mainly by accumulation of unmetabolized ammonia. The shunting of ammonia into the systemic circulation results in neuronal dysfunction leading to hepatic encephalopathy.
- Precipitating factors in patients with underlying cirrhosis (upper gastrointestinal bleeding, hypokalemia, hypomagnesemia, analgesic and sedative drugs, sepsis, alkalosis, increased dietary protein).
- Acute fulminant viral hepatitis.
- Drugs and toxins (e.g., isoniazid, acetaminophen, diclofenac and other NSAIDs, statins, methyldopa, loratadine, propylthiouracil, lisinopril, labetalol, halothane, carbon tetrachloride, erythromycin, nitrofurantoin, troglitazone, herbal products, flavocoxid).
- Reye's syndrome.
- Shock and/or sepsis.
- Fatty liver of pregnancy.
- Metastatic carcinoma, hepatocellular carcinoma.
- Other: autoimmune hepatitis, ischemic veno-occlusive disease, sclerosing cholangitis, heat stroke, amebic abscesses.

DIAGNOSIS

DIFFERENTIAL DIAGNOSIS

- Delirium caused by medications or illicit drugs.
- Cerebrovascular accident, subdural hematoma.
- Meningitis, encephalitis.
- Hypoglycemia.
- Uremia.
- Cerebral anoxia.
- Hypercalcemia.
- Metastatic neoplasm to brain.
- Alcohol withdrawal syndrome/Wernicke-Vorsakoff syndrome.
- Hyponatremia
- Postictal state

WORKUP

Hepatic encephalopathy should be considered in any patient with cirrhosis who presents with neuropsychiatric manifestations. Exclude other etiologies with comprehensive history (obtained from patient, relatives, and others), physical examination, and laboratory and imaging studies. A pertinent history should include exposure to hepatitis, ethanol intake, drug history, exposure to toxins, IV drug abuse, measles or influenza with aspirin use (Reye's syndrome), and history of carcinoma (primary or metastatic). Minimal hepatic encephalopathy may not be obvious on clinical examination, but can be detected with neurophysiologic and neuropsychiatric testing.

LABORATORY TESTS

- Alanine aminotransferase, aspartate aminotransferase, bilirubin, alkaline phosphatase, glucose, calcium, electrolytes, blood urea nitrogen, creatinine, albumin.
- Complete blood count, platelet count, prothrombin time, partial thromboplastin time.
- Serum and urine toxicology screen in suspected medication or illegal drug use.
- Blood and urine cultures, urinalysis.
- Venous ammonia level. Measurement of serum ammonia level is useful in the evaluation of acute liver failure because levels correlate with the severity of encephalopathy and elevated levels are predictive of severe encephalopathy and cerebral edema. It is not useful for the evaluation or screening

TABLE 1 Clinical Stages of Hepatic Encephalopathy

Stage	Asterixis	EEG Changes	Clinical Manifestations
I (prodrome)	Slight	Minimal	Mild intellectual impairment, disturbed sleep-wake cycle
II (impending)	Easily elicited	Usually generalized	Drowsiness, confusion, coma/inappropriate behavior, disorientation, mood swings
III (stupor)	Present if patient cooperative	Grossly abnormal slowing of rhythm	Drowsy, unresponsive to verbal commands, markedly confused, delirious, hyperreflexia, positive Babinski sign
IV (coma)	Usually absent	Appearance of delta waves, decreased amplitudes	Unconscious, decerebrate or decorticate response to pain present (stage IVA) or absent (stage IVB)

EEG, Electroencephalogram.
From Fuhrman BP et al: *Pediatric critical care,* ed 4, Philadelphia, 2011, Saunders.

of hepatic encephalopathy in patients with chronic liver disease because it can neither rule in nor rule out hepatic encephalopathy, and levels do not correlate with the degree of encephalopathy.

- Arterial blood gases.

IMAGING STUDIES

CT scan or MRI of the brain may be useful in selected patients to exclude other etiologies when diagnosis is unclear.

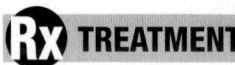 TREATMENT

NONPHARMACOLOGIC THERAPY

- Identification and treatment of precipitating factors.
- Restriction of protein intake is ill-advised and not necessary, since normal protein intake does not appear to exacerbate hepatic encephalopathy.

ACUTE GENERAL Rx

Fig. 1 illustrates the initial management of patients with high grade hepatic encephalopathy. Table 2 summarizes the management of fulminant hepatic failure.

Reduction of colonic ammonia production:

- Lactulose 25 ml twice daily initially; dose is subsequently adjusted depending on clinical response to achieve production of 3 bowel movements daily. IV ornithine aspartate should be considered for those not responding to lactulose.
- The oral antibiotic rifaximin (550 mg PO bid) is effective in reducing the risk of recurrent hepatic encephalopathy in patients with cirrhosis. It can be taken with lactulose, and the combination of lactulose and rifaximin is superior to lactulose alone in reversing hepatic encephalopathy. Rifamaxin has also been shown to be effective in improving psychometric performance and health-related quality of life in patients with minimal hepatic encephalopathy. It is well tolerated but expensive.
- Probiotics (e.g., 1 capsule containing 112.5 billion viable lyophilized bacteria tid) might also be beneficial in altering gut flora to reduce ammonia production.

Treatment of cerebral edema:

- Cerebral edema is often present in patients with acute liver failure, and it accounts for nearly 50% of deaths. Monitoring intracranial pressure by epidural, intraparenchymal, or subdural transducers and treatment of cerebral edema with mannitol (100 to 200 ml of 20% solution [0.3 to 0.4 g/kg of body weight]) given by rapid IV infusion are helpful in selected patients (e.g., potential transplantation patients).
- Dexamethasone and hyperventilation (useful in head injury) are of little value in treating cerebral edema from liver failure.

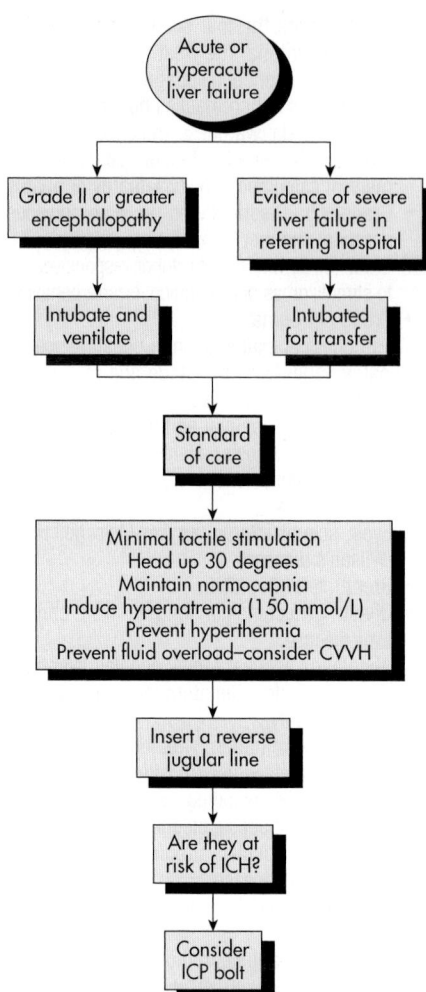

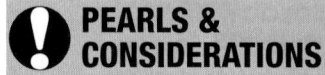

FIG. 1 Initial management of patient with high-grade encephalopathy. *CVVH*, continuous venovenous hemofiltration; *ICH*, intracranial hypertension; *ICP*, intracranial pressure. (From Parrillo JE, Dellinger RP: *Critical care medicine: principles of diagnosis and management in the adult*, ed 4, Philadelphia, 2014, Saunders.)

CHRONIC Rx

- Avoidance of any precipitating factors (e.g., high-protein diet, medications).
- Consideration of liver transplantation in selected patients with progressive or recurrent encephalopathy (Box 1). Liver transplantation remains the only curative therapeutic option.

DISPOSITION

Prognosis varies with the underlying etiology of the liver failure and the grade of encephalopathy (generally good for grades 1 or 2; poor for grades 3 or 4). Without proper therapy, the survival rate at 1 yr is 42% and decreases to 23% at 3 yr.

REFERRAL

The early stages of hepatic encephalopathy can be managed in the outpatient setting, whereas stages 3 or 4 require hospital admission.

TABLE 2 Management of Fulminant Hepatic Failure

No sedation except for procedures
Minimal handling
Enteric precautions until infection ruled out
Monitor:
- ○ Heart and respiratory rate
- ○ Arterial BP, CVP
- ○ Core/toe temperature
- ○ Neurologic observations
- ○ Gastric pH (>5.0)
- ○ Blood glucose (>4 mmol/L)
- ○ Acid-base
- ○ Electrolytes
- ○ PT, PTT
Fluid balance
- ○ 75% maintenance
- ○ Dextrose 10%-50% (provide 6-10 mg/kg/min)
- ○ Sodium (0.5-1 mmol/L)
- ○ Potassium (2-4 mmol/L)
Maintain circulating volume with colloid/FFP
Coagulation support only if required
Drugs
- ○ Vitamin K
- ○ H_2 antagonist
- ○ Antacids
- ○ Lactulose
- ○ *N*-acetylcysteine for acetaminophen toxicity
- ○ Broad-spectrum antibiotics
- ○ Antifungals
Nutrition
- ○ Enteral feeding (1-2 g protein/kg/day)
- ○ PN if ventilated

BP, Blood pressure; *CVP*, central venous pressure; *FFP*, fresh frozen plasma; *PN*, parenteral nutrition; *PT*, prothrombin time; *PTT*, partial thromboplastin time.
From Fuhrman BP et al: *Pediatric critical care*, ed 4, Philadelphia, 2011, Saunders.

⚠ PEARLS & CONSIDERATIONS

COMMENTS

- Trials have shown that adding IV albumin to lactulose may improve outcomes in severe hepatic encephalopathy by reducing oxidative stress through reduction of levels of circulating cytokines and endotoxins.
- Long-acting benzodiazepines should not be used to treat anxiety and sleep disorders in patients with cirrhosis, as they may precipitate encephalopathy.
- Patients not responding to supportive therapy should be evaluated for liver transplantation.
- Not all patients with cirrhosis develop hepatic encephalopathy. It has been shown that 40% of persons with cirrhosis and minimal hepatic encephalopathy do not develop overt hepatic encephalopathy in long-term follow-up. There are genetic factors associated with development of hepatic encephalopathy in patients with cirrhosis. Genetic analyses have shown that glutaminase TACC and CACC haplotypes are linked to the risk for overt hepatic encephalopathy.

BOX 1 Various Prognostic Criteria Used for Liver Transplantation in Patients with Fulminant Hepatic Failure

King's College Criteria
Acetaminophen overdose:
- Arterial pH <7.3 (irrespective of grade of encephalopathy) or
- PT >100 sec (INR >6.5)
- Serum creatinine >3.4 mg/dl (>300 μmol/L)
- Patients with grade III and IV hepatic encephalopathy

Nonacetaminophen liver injury:
- PT >100 sec (INR >6.5) (irrespective of grade of encephalopathy) or any three of the following variables:
  1. Age <10 or >40 years
  2. Non-A, non-B hepatitis, halothane hepatitis, idiosyncratic drug reactions
  3. Jaundice >7 days before onset of encephalopathy
  4. Serum bilirubin 17.4 mg/dl (300 μmol/L)
  5. PT >50 sec

Cliché Criteria
Factor V <20% in persons <30 years or both of the following:
- Factor V <30% in patients >30 years
- Grade III or IV encephalopathy

Serum Gc Globulin Levels
- Decreasing Gc levels due to dying hepatocytes

Serum α-Fetoprotein Level
- Serial increase from day 1 to day 3 has shown correlation with survival

Liver Biopsy[32]
70% necrosis is discriminant of 90% mortality

Gc, Plasma group-specific component protein; *INR,* international normalized ratio; *PT,* prothrombin time.
From Vincent JL et al: *Textbook of critical care,* ed 6, Philadelphia, 2011, Saunders.

EBM **EVIDENCE**
Available at www.expertconsult.com

SUGGESTED READINGS
Available at www.expertconsult.com

RELATED CONTENT
Hepatic Encephalopathy (Patient Information)
Cirrhosis (Related Key Topic)
Encephalopathy (Related Key Topic)

AUTHOR: **FRED F. FERRI, M.D.**

H

Diseases
and Disorders

I

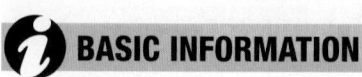

DEFINITION

Hepatitis A is generally an acute self-limiting infection of the liver by an enterically transmitted picornavirus, hepatitis A virus (HAV). Infection may range from asymptomatic to fulminant hepatitis.

SYNONYMS

Infectious hepatitis
Short incubation hepatitis
Type A hepatitis
HAV (hepatitis A virus)

ICD-10CM CODES
B15.9 Hepatitis A without hepatic coma
B15.0 Hepatitis A with hepatic coma

EPIDEMIOLOGY & DEMOGRAPHICS

INCIDENCE:
- Hepatitis A occurs worldwide, affecting 1.4 million people annually and accounting for 20% to 40% of cases of viral hepatitis in the United States.
- The seroprevalence increases with age, ranging from 10% in individuals aged <5 yr to 74% in those aged >50 yr.
- In the United States, average disease rate was ~15 cases/100,000 persons/yr before routine vaccination of all children in certain states. The incidence after 2005 is about 1 case/100,000.
- The incidence is relatively higher in some regions in the United States, including Arizona, Alaska, California, Idaho, Nevada, New Mexico, Oklahoma, Oregon, South Dakota, and Washington.
- At-risk groups include:
  1. Residents and staff of group homes.
  2. Children and employees of day care centers.
  3. People who engage in oral-anal contact, regardless of sexual orientation.
  4. IV drug abusers.
  5. Travel to endemic areas.
  6. Areas of overcrowding, poor sanitation, inadequate sewage treatment.

PREVALENCE:
- Approximately three fourths of the U.S. population has serologic evidence of prior infection.
- Anti-HAV prevalence has an inverse relation to income and household size.

PREDOMINANT SEX: None, except higher infection rates seen in homosexual males who engage in oral-anal contact.

PREDOMINANT AGE/PEAK INCIDENCE:
- In areas of high rates of hepatitis A, virtually all children are infected while younger than 10 yr, but disease is rare.
- In areas of moderate rates of hepatitis A, disease occurs in late childhood and young adults.
- In areas of low rates of hepatitis A, most cases occur in young adults.

INCUBATION PERIOD: Averages 30 days (15 to 50)

PHYSICAL FINDINGS & CLINICAL PRESENTATION

- Infection with HAV may have acute or subacute presentation, icteric or anicteric. Severity of illness seems to increase with age (90% of infection in children aged <5 yr may be subclinical).
- The incubation period of HAV is 2 to 6 weeks.
- A preicteric, prodromal phase of approximately 1 to 14 days; 15% no apparent prodrome. Symptoms are usually abrupt in onset and may include anorexia, fatigue, malaise, nausea, vomiting, fever, headache, and mild abdominal pain.
- Less common symptoms are chills, myalgias, arthralgias, upper respiratory symptoms, constipation, diarrhea, pruritus, urticaria.
- Jaundice occurs in >70% of patients. Patients older than 30 years are more likely than younger individuals to have jaundice.
- The icteric phase is preceded by dark urine.
- Bilirubinuria is typically followed a few days later by clay-colored stools and icterus.

PHYSICAL EXAMINATION

- Jaundice: Peaks in severity 2 wk after onset.
- Hepatomegaly.
- Splenomegaly.
- Cervical lymphadenopathy.
- Evanescent rash.
- Petechiae.
- Cardiac arrhythmias.

COMPLICATIONS

- Cholestasis.
- Fulminant hepatitis.
- Arthritis.
- Myocarditis.
- Optic neuritis.
- Transverse myelitis.
- Thrombocytopenic purpura.
- Aplastic anemia.
- Red cell aplasia.
- Henoch-Schönlein purpura.
- IgA dominant glomerulonephritis.

ETIOLOGY

- Caused by HAV, a 27-nm, nonenveloped, icosahedral, positive-stranded RNA virus.
- Transmission is fecal-oral route, from person to person. Transmission occurs with close contact or with food- or water-borne outbreaks with inadequately purified water or cooked foods. Recent outbreaks have involved green onions and tomatoes.
- Parenteral transmission is considered rare.
- Vertical transmission has also been reported.

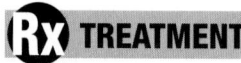
DIAGNOSIS

DIFFERENTIAL DIAGNOSIS

- Other hepatitis virus (B, C, D, E).
- Infectious mononucleosis.
- Cytomegalovirus infection.
- Herpes simplex virus infection.
- Leptospirosis.
- Brucellosis.
- Drug-induced liver disease.
- Ischemic hepatitis.
- Autoimmune hepatitis.

WORKUP

- IgM antibody specific for HAV.
- Liver function tests; ALT and AST elevations are sensitive for liver damage but not specific for HAV.
- Elevated ESR.
- CBC; may find mild lymphocytosis.

LABORATORY TESTS

- Diagnosis confirmed by IgM anti-HAV; it is detectable in almost all infected patients at presentation and remains positive for 3 to 6 mo.
- A fourfold rise in titer of total antibody (IgM and IgG) to HAV confirms acute infection.
- HAV detection in stool and body fluids by electron microscopy.
- HAV RNA detection in stool, body fluids, serum, and liver tissue.
- ALT and AST usually more than 8 times normal in acute infection.
- Bilirubin usually 5 to 15 times normal.
- Alkaline phosphatase minimally elevated but higher level in cholestasis.
- Albumin and prothrombin time are generally normal; if elevated, they may herald hepatic necrosis.
- Fig. 1 illustrates the typical course of hepatis A.

IMAGING STUDIES

- Rarely useful.
- Sonogram (fulminant hepatitis).

TREATMENT

- Usually self-limited.
- Supportive care.
- Those with fulminant hepatitis may require hospitalization and treatment of associated complications.
- Activity as tolerated.
- Advise to avoid alcohol and hepatotoxic drugs.
- Patients with fulminant hepatitis should be assessed for liver transplantation.

CHRONIC Rx

No chronic HAV and no chronic carrier state. The majority of patients have resolution of symptoms and liver abnormalities within 3 months.

DISPOSITION

- Follow-up as outpatient.
- Most patients recover within 3 months of infection, although 5% to 10% of patients will experience a relapse in the first 6 months.
- HAV is a self-limited infection and does not cause chronic hepatitis.

REFERRAL

- To a hepatologist if severe, fulminant hepatitis develops
- To a transplant surgeon if liver transplant becomes a consideration for fulminant hepatitis and liver failure

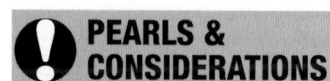
PEARLS & CONSIDERATIONS

- All cases of hepatitis A should be reported to the public health authorities because food-borne or

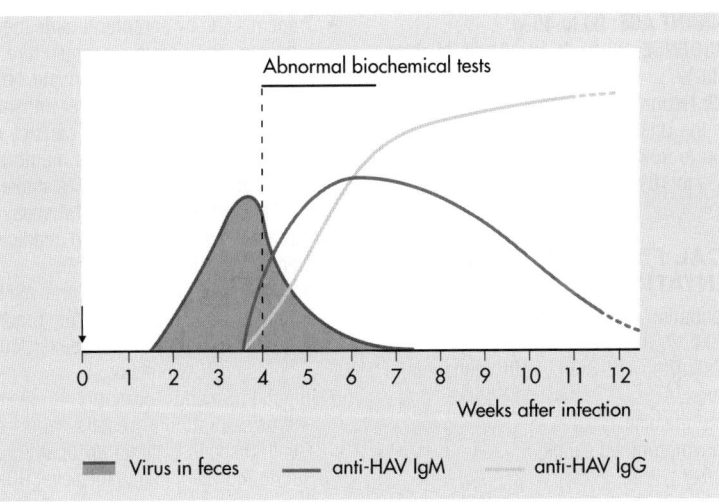

FIG. 1 Course of acute hepatitis A. (From Cohen J, Powderly WG: *Infectious diseases,* ed 2, St Louis, 2004, Mosby.)

Table 1 Recommendations for Routine Preexposure Use of Hepatitis A Virus Vaccine

GROUP	COMMENTS
Children	Vaccine should be given to all children at age 1 yr (12-23 mo).* Vaccination of children 2-18 yr may also be warranted.[†]
International travelers[‡]	IG may be given in addition to or instead of vaccine; children <12 mo should receive IG.
Close contacts of newly arriving international adoptees	All persons who anticipate close personal contact (e.g., household contact or regular babysitter) during the first 60 days after arrival
Men who have sex with men	Includes adolescents
Illicit drug users	Includes adolescents
Persons with chronic liver disease, such as those with hepatitis B or C	Increased risk of fulminant hepatitis A with HAV infection
Persons receiving clotting factor concentrates	
Persons who work with HAV in research laboratory settings	

HAV, hepatitis A virus; *IG,* immunoglobulin.
*Hepatitis A vaccine is not licensed for children <12 months.
[†]States and communities with existing vaccination programs for children ages 2 to 18 years are encouraged to maintain these programs. Catch-up vaccination for this age group may be warranted elsewhere in the context of ongoing outbreaks among children.
[‡]Persons traveling to Canada, Western Europe, Japan, Australia, or New Zealand are at no greater risk than in the U.S.
From Bennett JE et al: *Mandell, Douglas, and Bennett's principles and practice of infectious diseases,* ed 8, Philadelphia, 2015, Saunders.

water-borne outbreaks may occur, and public health efforts (mass vaccination or immunoglobulin therapy) may prevent secondary cases.

- Hepatitis A is a common illness in internationally traveled and developing countries. Pretravel vaccination is strongly recommended for travelers who are HAV susceptible. Table 1 summarizes recommendations for preexposure use of hepatitis A virus vaccine.

- Handwashing is important, as the hepatitis A virus may survive for up to 4 hours on the fingertips.

PREVENTION

- Improvement in hygiene and sanitation.
- Heating food.
- Avoidance of water and foods from endemic area.

PASSIVE IMMUNIZATION

- Immunoglobulin provides protection against HAV through passive transfer of antibody.
- Preexposure prophylaxis indicated for people traveling to endemic areas (Ig 0.02 or 0.06 ml/kg given IM) who have not received or cannot receive the hepatitis A vaccine before departure. The lower dose is effective for up to 3 mo, and the higher dose is effective for up to 5 mo.
- Postexposure prophylaxis: For individuals with a recent exposure to hepatitis A who have not received the vaccine, post-exposure prophylaxis is warranted with either immune globulin (Ig 0.02 ml/kg given IM) or a single dose of the hepatitis A vaccine within 2 weeks of the exposure. For healthy persons ages 12 months to 40 years of age, a single dose of the hepatitis A vaccine should be given. Children <12 months, adults >40 years of age, and persons who have chronic liver disease and who are immunocompromised should receive immunoglobulin.

ACTIVE IMMUNIZATION

- There are several inactivated and attenuated hepatitis vaccines; only the inactivated vaccines are currently available for use and they have been found to be safe and highly immunogenic: HAVRIX or VAQTA. These can be used in adults and children older than 12 mo. They are given as a two-dose regimen 6 mo to 1 yr apart. A combined hepatitis A and hepatitis B vaccine called TWINRX is also available.
- Protective antibody levels were reached in 94% to 100% of adults 1 mo after the first dose; similar results have been found for children and adolescents.
- Theoretic analyses of antibody levels estimate duration of immunity to be 10 to 20 yr.
- Vaccine should be considered for persons who are at risk: those traveling to or working in endemic areas, homosexual men, illegal drug users, persons with chronic liver disease, children in areas with high rates of hepatitis A infection.
- The Advisory Committee on Immunization Practices recommends routine hepatitis A vaccination for all children beginning at 12 to 23 mo of age.

SUGGESTED READINGS
Available at www.expertconsult.com

RELATED CONTENT
Hepatitis A (Patient Information)

AUTHOR: **GLENN G. FORT, M.D., M.P.H.**

H

Diseases and Disorders

I

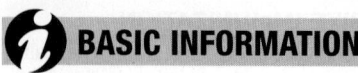
DEFINITION

Hepatitis B is an acute infection of the liver parenchymal cells caused by the hepatitis B virus (HBV).

SYNONYMS

Serum hepatitis
Long incubation (30 to 180 days) hepatitis HBV
HBV

EPIDEMIOLOGY & DEMOGRAPHICS

INCIDENCE (IN U.S.):

- ~200,000 to 300,000 infections annually in the United States.
- Much higher incidence in Europe (~1 million new cases annually) and in areas of high endemicity.
- In the United States, transmission is mainly horizontal (percutaneous and mucous membrane exposure to infectious blood and other body fluids [e.g., sexual transmission, either homosexual or heterosexual]); also from needle sharing among drug abusers; occupational exposure to contaminated blood and blood products; persons receiving transfusions of blood and blood products; and hemodialysis patients.

NOTE: Improved screening of blood and blood products has greatly reduced, although not eliminated, the risk of posttransfusion HBV infection.

- In areas of high endemicity, transmission is largely vertical (perinatal): HBV exists in the blood and body fluids. Perinatal transmission from HBsAg-positive mothers is as high as 90% unless immunoprophylaxis is given.

PREVALENCE (IN U.S.):

- The WHO estimates that 400 million people worldwide (6% of the population) are chronic HBV carriers. North America, Western Europe, and Australia are areas of low prevalence, <2%. In the United States an estimated 800,000 to 1.4 million people have chronic HBV infection.
- Africa, Asia, and the Western Pacific region are areas of high prevalence, ≥8%.
- Southern and Eastern Europe have intermediate rates, 2% to 7%.
- Chronically infected persons, those with positive HBsAg for >6 mo, represent the major source of infection.
- As many as 95% of infants and children aged <5, who typically have subclinical acute infection, will become chronic HBV carriers.
- Adults are more likely to have clinically evident acute infection, but only 1% to 5% will develop chronic infection.
- ~0.1% of patients with acute infection will develop fulminant acute hepatitis resulting in death.

PREDOMINANT SEX:

- Predominant in males because of increased IV drug abuse, homosexuality.
- Females more commonly terminate in chronic carrier state.

PREDOMINANT AGE: 20 to 45 yr.
PEAK INCIDENCE: 30 to 45 yr of age, at rates of 5% to 20%.
GENETICS: Neonatal infection:

- Rare in the United States.
- High (up to 90%) in areas of high endemicity (only 5% to 10% of perinatal infections occur in utero).

PHYSICAL FINDINGS & CLINICAL PRESENTATION (FIG. 1)

- The incubation period of HBV infection is 4 to 24 weeks.
- Patients often present with nonspecific symptoms.
- Profound malaise.
- Many asymptomatic cases.
- Prodrome:
  1. 15% to 20% serum sickness (urticaria, rash, arthralgia) during early HBsAg.
  2. HBsAg-Ab complex disease (polyarteritis nodosa–arthritis, arteritis, glomerulonephritis).
- Hepatomegaly (87%) with right upper quadrant (RUQ) tenderness.
  1. Hepatic punch tenderness.
  2. Splenomegaly: rare (10% to 15%).
- Jaundice, dark urine, with occasional pruritus.
- Variable fever (when present, generally precedes jaundice and rapidly declines following onset of icteric phase).
- Spider angiomata: rare; resolves during recovery.
- Rare polyarteritis nodosa, cryoglobulinemia.

ETIOLOGY

- Caused by HBV (42-nm hepadnavirus with an outer surface coat [HBsAg], inner nucleocapsid core [HBcAg; HBeAg]; DNA polymerase; and partially double-stranded DNA genome). There are eight genotypes (A to H) based on nucleotide sequence. The prevalence of each genotype varies widely.

- Transmission by parenteral route (needle use, tattooing, ear piercing, acupuncture, transfusion of blood and blood products, hemodialysis, sexual contact), perinatal transmission.
- Infection may result from contact of infectious material with mucous membranes and open skin breaks (e.g., HBV is stable and can be transmitted from toothbrushes, utensils, razors, baby toys, assorted medical equipment [respirators, endoscopes]).
- Oral intake of infectious material may result in infection through breaks in the oral mucosa.
- Food or water are virtually never found to be sources of HBV infection.
- Infection occurs primarily in liver, where necrosis probably results from cytotoxic T-cell response, direct cytopathic effect of HBcAg (core antigen), high-level HBsAg (surface antigen) expression, or coinfection with delta (D) hepatitis virus (RNA delta core within HBsAg envelope).
- Recovery (>90%):
  1. Fulminant hepatitis occurring in <1% (especially if coinfected with hepatitis D); 80% fatal.
  2. Unusual (5%) prolonged acute disease for 4 to 12 mo, with recovery.
  3. Overall fatality increases with age and viral inoculation (e.g., transfusions).
- Chronic hepatitis B (CHB) infection (1% to 2%), four phases:
  1. Immune-tolerant phase: A highly replicative/low-inflammatory phase where HBV DNA levels are high (typically >1 million IU/ml), ALT levels are normal, and biopsies have minimal signs of significant inflammation or fibrosis.
     a) This phase can persist for years, especially in those infected prenatally.
     b) With age there is a likely transformation to an HBeAg-positive immune-active phase.
  2. HBeAg-positive immune-active phase: elevated ALT and HBV DNA levels in conjunction with liver injury (≥ 20,000 IU/ml).

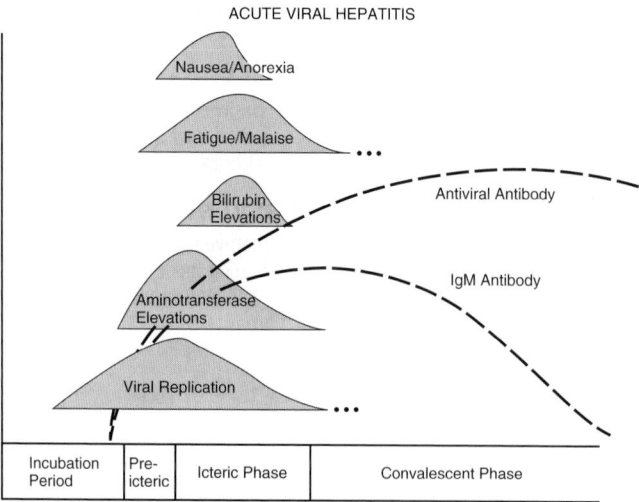

ACUTE VIRAL HEPATITIS

Nausea/Anorexia

Fatigue/Malaise

Bilirubin Elevations

Antiviral Antibody

IgM Antibody

Aminotransferase Elevations

Viral Replication

| Incubation Period | Pre-icteric | Icteric Phase | Convalescent Phase |

Time after Exposure

FIG. 1 The typical course of acute viral hepatitis. (From Goldman L, Ausiello D [eds]: *Cecil textbook of medicine,* ed 22, Philadelphia, 2004, Saunders.)

Median age of onset is 30 years in those infected at a young age. Biopsy will show moderate to severe inflammation or fibrosis.
3. Inactive CHB phase: HBV DNA levels are low or undetectable (<2000 IU/ml), ALT levels are normal, and anti-HBe is present. Biopsy shows minimal necroinflammation but variable fibrosis.
4. HBeAg-negative immune reactivation phase: elevated ALT and elevated HBV DNA (≥2000 IU/ml). Biopsy will show moderate to severe necroinflammation and fibrosis.
• Table 1 summarizes causes of hepatitis flares in patients with CHB.
• The most feared complications of CHB are cirrhosis and hepatocellular carcinoma (HCC), which kill more than 300,000 people a year globally. One quarter to one third of patients will go on to develop these complications. The risk of developing HCC appears to be greatest among individuals with the highest serum levels of HBV DNA.

Dx DIAGNOSIS

DIFFERENTIAL DIAGNOSIS

• Acute disease confused with other viral hepatitis infections (A, C, D, E).
• Any viral illness producing systemic disease and hepatitis (e.g., yellow fever, EBV, CMV, HIV, rubella, rubeola, coxsackie B, adenovirus, herpes simplex or zoster).
• Nonviral causes of hepatitis (e.g., leptospirosis, toxoplasmosis, alcoholic hepatitis, drug-induced [e.g., acetaminophen, INH], toxic hepatitis [carbon tetrachloride, benzene]).

WORKUP

• Acute serum specimen for hepatitis B serology (HBsAg, HBsAb, HBcAb, HBeAg, HBeAb), HBDNA by PCR.
• LFTs.

• CBC.
• Liver biopsy: rarely indicated for diagnosis of fulminant viral hepatitis, chronic hepatitis, cirrhosis, carcinoma.

LABORATORY TESTS

• Diagnosis of acute HBV infection is best confirmed by IgM HBcAb in acute or early convalescent serum or by HBDNA by PCR.
  1. Generally, IgM present during onset of jaundice.
  2. Coexisting HBsAg.
• HBsAg and IgG-HBcAb during acute jaundice are strongly suggestive of remote HBV infection and another cause for current illness (Fig. 2).
• HBsAb alone is suggestive of immunization response.
• With recovery, HBeAg is rapidly replaced by HBeAb in 2 to 3 mo, and HBsAg is replaced by HBsAb in 5 to 6 mo.
• In chronic HBV hepatitis, HBsAg and HBeAg are persistent without corresponding Ab.

TABLE 1 Causes of Hepatitis Flares in Patients with Chronic Hepatitis B

Cause of Flare	Comment
Spontaneous	Factors that precipitate viral replication are unclear
Immunosuppressive therapy	Flares are often observed during withdrawal of the agent; preemptive antiviral therapy is required
Antiviral therapy for HBV	
Interferon	Flares are often observed during the second to third month of therapy in 30% of patients; may herald virologic response
Nucleoside analog	
During treatment	Flares are no more common than with placebo
Drug-resistant HBV	Severe consequences can occur in patients with advanced liver disease
On withdrawal	Flares are caused by the rapid reemergence of wild-type HBV; severe consequences can occur in patients with advanced liver disease
HIV treatment	Flares can occur as a result of the direct toxicity of HAART or with immune reconstitution; HBV increases the risk of antiretroviral drug hepatotoxicity
Genotypic variation	
Precore and core promoter mutants	Fluctuations in serum ALT levels are common with precore mutants
Superinfection with other hepatitis viruses	May be associated with suppression of HBV replication

HAART, highly active antiretroviral therapy; *HBV,* hepatitis B virus.
From Feldman M et al [eds]: *Sleisenger and Fordtran's gastrointestinal and liver disease,* ed 10, Philadelphia, 2016, Saunders.

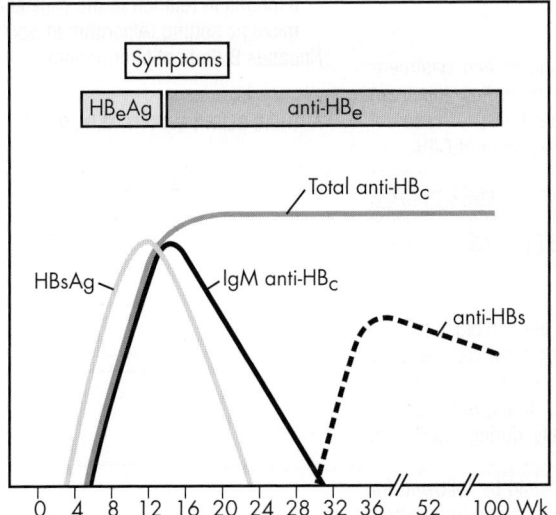 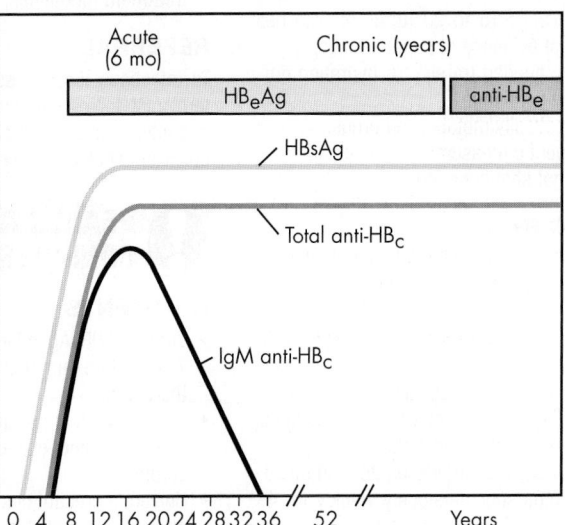

FIG. 2 Typical course of hepatitis B. *Left,* Typical course of acute hepatitis B. *Right,* Chronic hepatitis B. *HBc,* Hepatitis B core; *HBe,* hepatitis B early; *HBsAg,* hepatitis B surface antigen; *IgM,* immunoglobulin M. (From Mandell GL et al: *Principles and practice of infectious diseases,* ed 7, Philadelphia, 2010, Saunders.)

- In chronic carrier state, HBsAg is persistent, but HBeAg is replaced by HBeAb.
- HBcAb develops in all outcomes.
- HBeAg correlation with highest infectivity; appearance of HBeAb heralds recovery.
- LFTs:
  1. ALT and AST: usually more than eight times normal (often 1000 U/L) at onset of jaundice (minimal acute ALT/AST rises often followed by chronic hepatitis or hepatocellular carcinoma).
  2. Bilirubin: variably elevated in icteric viral hepatitis.
  3. Alkaline phosphatase: minimally elevated (one to three times normal) acutely.
- Albumin and prothrombin time:
  1. Generally normal.
  2. If abnormal, possible harbinger of impending hepatic necrosis (fulminant hepatitis).
- WBC and ESR: generally normal.

IMAGING STUDIES

- Sonogram to document rapid reduction in liver size during fulminant hepatitis or mass in hepatocellular carcinoma.
- Fibroscan (transient elastography): A noninvasive test to quantify liver fibrosis without liver biopsy.

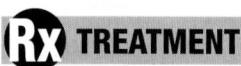 **TREATMENT**

NONPHARMACOLOGIC THERAPY

- Symptomatic treatment as necessary.
- Activity as tolerated.
- High-calorie diet preferred; often best tolerated in morning.

ACUTE GENERAL Rx

- In most cases of acute HBV infection no treatment necessary; >90% of adults will spontaneously clear infection.
- Hospitalization advisable for any patient in danger from dehydration caused by poor oral intake, whose PT is prolonged, who has rising bilirubin level >15 to 20 μg/dl, or who has any clinical evidence of hepatic failure.
- IV therapy needed (rarely) for hydration during severe vomiting.
- Avoid hepatically metabolized drugs.
- No therapeutic measures are beneficial.
- Steroids not shown helpful.

CHRONIC Rx

- Treatment of chronic HBV infection is dependent on which phase the patient is found to be in:
  1. Therapy is warranted for patients in immune-active CHB stage (HBeAg negative or HBeAg positive) to decrease the risk of liver-related complications. Treatment options include:
     a. a. Pegylated interferon 2a: 180 micrograms subcutaneously weekly for 48 weeks. This will lead to seroconversion rates of 20% to 30% (HBeAg to anti-HBe), and 65% of patients

will have HBV DNA <2000 IU/ml off therapy.
     b. Entecavir: 0.5 to 1 mg daily
     c. Tenofovir: 300 mg daily
     d. Other agents: Lamivudine, telbivudine, and adefovir are less frequently used.
  2. Therapy is not warranted in adults with immune-tolerant CHB. LFTs should be checked every 6 months to look for conversion to immune-active or inactive status.
     a. Therapy may be warranted for select adults >40 with normal ALT and elevated HBV DNA (≥1 million IU/ml) with liver biopsy showing significant necroinflammation or fibrosis.
  3. HBeAg-positive adults without cirrhosis who seroconvert to anti-HBe on therapy with entecavir or tenofovir can discontinue treatment after a period of treatment consolidation.
  4. It is recommended that patients receive indefinite therapy with entecavir or tenofovir if HBeAg-negative immune-active CHB is present, unless there is a competing rationale for treatment discontinuation.
  5. Adults with compensated cirrhosis and low levels of viremia (<2000 IU/ml) should be treated with entecavir or tenofovir to reduce the risk of decompensation, regardless of ALT level.

DISPOSITION

- Follow-up as outpatient.
- Acute disease: infection will resolve (defined as clearance of hepatitis B surface antigen within 6 months) in 90% of adult patients.
- Rare fatalities (fulminant hepatitis).
- Possible chronic carrier state, cirrhosis, hepatocellular carcinoma.
- Cure of HBV is an unrealistic goal for most patients with chronic infection since only a few patients will become HBsAb with current treatment modalities.

REFERRAL

To infectious disease specialist and gastroenterologist for consultation regarding fulminant hepatitis or prolonged cholestasis, for cases of uncertain etiology, or for treatment of CAH.

PEARLS & CONSIDERATIONS

COMMENTS

- Virus and HBsAg in high titers in blood for 1 to 7 wk before jaundice and for a variable time thereafter.
- Transmission is possible during entire period of HBsAg (and especially during HBeAg) in serum.
- Universal precautions should be followed for all contacts with blood or secretions/excretions contaminated with blood.
- Antiviral therapy is recommended in pregnancy to reduce perinatal transmission if

HBsAg positive and HBV DNA >200,00 IU/ml. Can use tenofovir, lamivudine, or telbivudine. Fig. 3 describes an algorithm for the treatment of hepatitis B surface antigen (HBsAg)–positive mothers during pregnancy.

- Preventing before exposure:
  1. Lifestyle changes
  2. Meticulous testing of blood supply (although some chronically infected, infectious donors are HBsAg negative).
  3. Sterilization via steam or hypochlorite.
  4. Hepatitis B vaccine for high-risk groups given IM in deltoid to induce HBsAb (response should be confirmed) is protective (>90% effective).
  5. Recommendation for universal childhood immunization with doses at birth, 1 mo, and 6 mo.
- Prevention after exposure:
  1. HBV hyperimmune globulin (HBIG) (0.06 ml/kg IM) given immediately after needlestick, within 14 days of sexual exposure, or at birth, followed by HBV vaccination. A second dose of HBIG is given in 28 days for those refusing vaccine or vaccine nonresponders.
  2. Standard immune globulin: nearly as effective as HBIG
- Preventive therapy with entecavir or tenofovir for patients who test positive for HBsAg and are undergoing chemotherapy may reduce the risk for HBV reactivation and HBV-associated morbidity and mortality,
- Hepatitis B prophylaxis is described in Section V.
- Table 2 summarizes interpretation of serologic markers and serum DNA in hepatitis B.

SUGGESTED READINGS
Available at www.expertconsult.com

RELATED CONTENT

A flow diagram showing the use of specific serologic tests for the diagnosis of acute viral hepatitis in relation to the clinical and epidemiologic setting (Algorithm in Section III)
Hepatitis B (Patient Information)

AUTHOR: **GLENN G. FORT, M.D., M.P.H.**

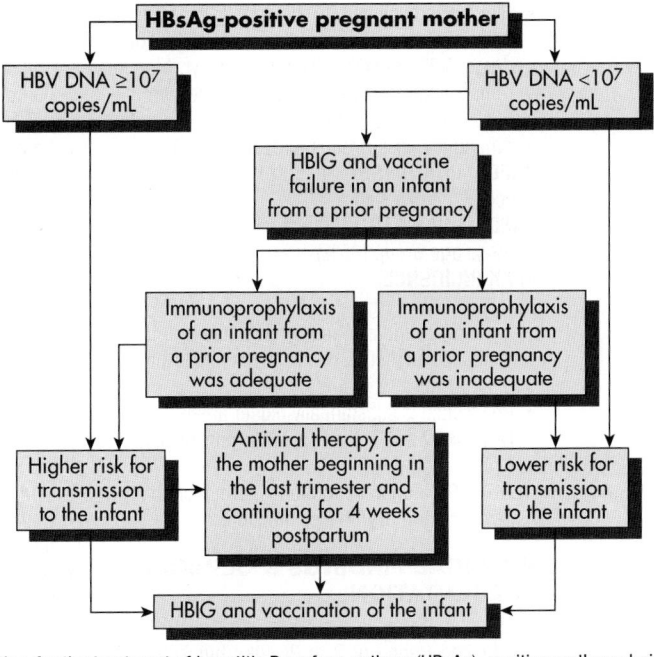

FIG. 3 Algorithm for the treatment of hepatitis B surface antigen (HBsAg)–positive mothers during pregnancy. The goal of treatment in highly viremic mothers is to lower the serum HBV DNA level by several log_{10} IU/ml by the time of delivery to minimize the chance of newborn infection. The choice of antiviral agent is less important if treatment of the mother is not needed long term. In the event that the treatment needs to be continued after delivery, the patient should be started on a high-genetic-barrier drug initially or switched to one immediately after delivery. See text for further details about drug selection. *HBIG,* hepatitis B immune globulin. (From Feldman M et al [eds]: *Sleisenger and Fordtran's gastrointestinal and liver disease,* ed 10, Philadelphia, 2016, Saunders.)

TABLE 2 Interpretation of Serologic Markers and Serum DNA in Hepatitis B

	HBsAg	HbeAg	Anti-HBc IgM	Anti-HBc IgG	Anti-HBs	Anti-HBe	HBV DNA*
Acute hepatitis	+	+/–	+				+
Acute hepatitis, window period			+				
Recovery from acute hepatitis			+	+	+	+/–	
Chronic hepatitis	+	+					+
Chronic hepatitis (precore mutant)	+					+	+
Inactive carrier	+					+/–	
Vaccinated					+		

HBsAg, Hepatitis B surface antigen; *HBeAg,* hepatitis Be antigen; *anti-HBc IgM,* hepatitis B core antibody (IgM type); *anti-HBc IgG,* hepatitis B core antibody (IgG type); *anti-HBs,* hepatitis B surface antibody; *anti-HBe,* hepatitis Be antibody; *HBV DNA,* hepatitis B viral DNA.
*HBV DNA >10^5 copies/mL.
From Andreoli TE et al: *Andreoli and Carpenter's Cecil essentials of medicine,* ed 8, Philadelphia, 2010, Saunders.

Diseases and Disorders

I

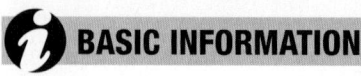

BASIC INFORMATION

DEFINITION

Hepatitis C is an acute liver parenchymal infection caused by hepatitis C virus (HCV).

SYNONYMS

Transfusion-related non-A, non-B hepatitis (incubation period averages 6 wk, intermediate between hepatitis A and B)

ICD-10CM CODES
B17.1   Acute hepatitis C
B18.2   Chronic viral hepatitis C
B17.10 Acute hepatitis C without hepatic coma
B17.11 Acute hepatitis C with hepatic coma
B19.20 Unspecified viral hepatitis C without hepatic coma
B19.21 Unspecified viral hepatitis C with hepatic coma

EPIDEMIOLOGY & DEMOGRAPHICS

Hepatitis C infection is the most common chronic blood-borne infection in the United States. About 3% of baby boomers test positive for the virus. The CDC now recommends testing for hepatitis C for anyone born from 1945 to 1965.

INCIDENCE (IN U.S.): HCV infects more than 185 million individuals worldwide. Approximately 20% of patients chronically infected with HCV progress to cirrhosis.

- 150,000 new cases/yr (37,500 symptomatic; 93,000 later chronic liver disease; 30,700 cirrhosis). The incidence of acute HCV has declined substantially over the past 30 yr (from 7.4/100,000 to 0.7/100,000).
- ~9000 of these ultimately die of HCV infection; most common (40%) cause of nonalcoholic liver disease in the United States

PREVALENCE (IN U.S.):
- Overall prevalence of anti-HCV antibody is 1% to 1.2% (an estimated 2.7 million persons nationwide).

- Highest prevalence in hemophiliacs transfused before 1987 and users of injection drugs, 72% to 90%. Over past 30 yr, blood transfusion as a risk factor declined from 15% of cases to 1.9%.
- Among low-risk groups, prevalence 0.6%.

PREDOMINANT SEX: Slight male predominance.

PREDOMINANT AGE: Highest prevalence in 30- to 49-yr age group (65%).

PEAK INCIDENCE:
- 20 to 39 yr of age.
- African Americans and whites have similar incidence of acute disease; Hispanics have higher rates.
- Prevalence is substantially higher among non-Hispanic blacks than among non-Hispanic whites.

GENETICS: Neonatal infection is rare; increased risk with maternal HIV-1 coinfection.

PHYSICAL FINDINGS & CLINICAL PRESENTATION

- Symptoms usually develop 7 to 8 wk after infection (range of 2 to 26 wk), but 70% to 80% of cases are subclinical.
- 10% to 20% report acute illness with jaundice and nonspecific symptoms (abdominal pain, anorexia, malaise).
- Fulminant hepatitis may rarely occur during this period.
- After acute infection, 15% to 25% have complete resolution (absence of HCV RNA in serum, normal ALT).
- Progression to chronic infection is common, 50% to 84%. 74% to 86% have persistent viremia; spontaneous clearance of viremia in chronic infection is rare. 60% to 70% of patients will have persistent or fluctuating ALT levels; 30% to 40% with chronic infection have normal ALT levels.
- 15% to 20% of those with chronic HCV will develop cirrhosis over a period of 20 to 30 yr; in most others, chronic infection leads to hepatitis and varying degrees of fibrosis. Table 1 summarizes factors associated with progression of hepatic fibrosis in patients with chronic HCV infection. Table 2 describes

factors associated with cirrhosis in persons with hepatitis C infection.
- 0.4% to 2.5% of patients with chronic infection develop hepatocellular carcinoma (HCC).
- 25% of patients with chronic infection continue to have an asymptomatic course with normal LFTs and benign histology.
- In chronic HCV infection, extrahepatic sequelae include a variety of immunologic and lymphoproliferative disorders (e.g., cryoglobulinemia, membranoproliferative glomerulonephritis, and possibly Sjögren's syndrome, autoimmune thyroiditis, polyarteritis nodosa, aplastic anemia, lichen planus, porphyria cutanea tarda, B-cell lymphoma, others).
- Fig. 1 illustrates the natural history of HCV infection.

ETIOLOGY

- Caused by HCV (single-stranded RNA flavivirus).
- Most HCV transmission is parenteral.
- In the United States, advances in screening of blood and blood products have made transfusion-related HCV infection rare (the risk is estimated to be 0.001% per unit transfused).
- Injecting-drug use accounts for most HCV transmission in the United States (60% of newly acquired cases, 20% to 50% of chronically infected persons).
- Occupational needlestick exposure from an HCV-positive source has a seroconversion rate of 1.8% (range 0% to 7%).
- Nosocomial transmission rates (from surgery and procedures such as colonoscopy and hemodialysis) are extremely low.
- Sexual transmission and maternal-fetal transmission are infrequent (estimated at 5%).
- No identifiable risk in 40% to 50% of community-acquired hepatitis C, but snorting of cocaine by shared use of straw or rolled-up paper has been identified as a risk factor because it causes microscopic bleeding of nasal mucosa.
- HCV infection may stimulate production of cytotoxic T lymphocytes and cytokines (INF-γ), which probably mediate hepatic necrosis.

TABLE 1   Factors Associated With Progression of Hepatic Fibrosis in Patients With Chronic Hepatitis C Virus Infection

Established	Possible	Not Associated
Age >40 years	Increased hepatic iron concentration	Viral genotype
Alcohol consumption	Male gender	Viral load
Hepatitis B virus coinfection	Serum ALT level	
HIV coinfection		
Immunosuppressed state		
Insulin resistance		
Marijuana use		
Obesity		
Schistosomiasis		
Severe hepatic necroinflammation		
Smoking		
White race		

From Feldman M et al [eds]: *Sleisenger and Fordtran's gastrointestinal and liver disease*, ed 10, Philadelphia, 2016, Saunders.

TABLE 2 Factors Associated With Cirrhosis in Persons With Hepatitis C Infection

Factor	Impact	Comment
Environmental		
Alcohol use	+4	The importance of minimal alcohol ingestion (<20 g/day) has not been established
Host		
HIV infection	+4	Increasingly important as HIV-related survival improves; may be masked by competing mortality
HBV infection	+3	Strong effect when HBsAg positive; relatively uncommon
Age	+4	Strong effect; increases as low as 40 yr. Hard to distinguish from infection duration
Body mass index	+2	Associated with metabolic syndrome
Duration of HCV infection	+3	Cirrhosis is rare before 10 yr
HLA type	+1?	HLA B54 is correlated with increased risk of cirrhosis; DRB1*0301 with lack of cirrhosis
Viral		
Quasispecies complexity	+1	Cross-sectional studies cannot assess causality and complexity may be confounded by duration of infection
HCV genotype 1	+1?	Genotype 1b in some, but not other studies, could be confounded by longer duration of 1b infections
Quantitative measures of viremia (serum or plasma HCV RNA level)	+2	Not always detected or lost in multivariate analysis of age or HIV

HCV, Hepatitis C virus; *HIV,* human immunodeficiency virus; *HLA,* human leukocyte antigen; *RNA,* ribonucleic acid.
From Bennett JE et al: Mandell, Douglas, and Bennett*'s principles and practice of infectious diseases,* ed 8, Philadelphia, 2015, Saunders.

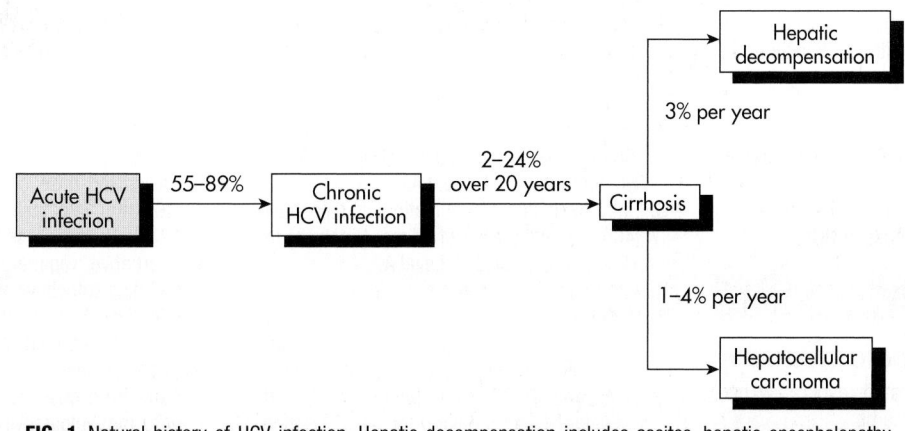

FIG. 1 Natural history of HCV infection. Hepatic decompensation includes ascites, hepatic encephalopathy, variceal hemorrhage, hepatorenal syndrome, or hepatic synthetic dysfunction. (From Feldman M et al [eds]: *Sleisenger and Fordtran's gastrointestinal and liver disease,* ed 10, Philadelphia, 2016, Saunders.)

Dx DIAGNOSIS

DIFFERENTIAL DIAGNOSIS

- Other hepatitis viruses (A, B, D, E).
- Other viral illnesses producing systemic disease (e.g., yellow fever, EBV, CMV, HIV, rubella, rubeola, coxsackie B, adenovirus, HSV, HZV).
- Nonviral hepatitis (e.g., leptospirosis, toxoplasmosis, alcoholic hepatitis, drug-induced hepatitis [acetaminophen, INH], toxic hepatitis).

WORKUP

- Acute hepatitis C antibody, viral genotyping, viral titers.
- LFTs; CBC.

NOTE: ALT is an easy and inexpensive test to monitor infection and efficacy of therapy. However, ALT levels may fluctuate or even be normal in active or chronic infection and even with cirrhosis, and ALT may remain elevated even after clearance of viremia.

- Liver biopsy with histologic staging is the gold standard for assessing the degree of disease activity and the likelihood of disease progression, and also to help rule out other causes of liver disease.
- Transient elastography (Fibroscan) is a noninvasive test to quantify liver fibrosis and is being increasingly used in place of liver biopsy in many institutions.

LABORATORY TESTS

- Diagnosis is often by exclusion, because it takes 6 wk to 12 mo to develop anti-HCV antibody (70% positive by 6 wk, 90% positive by 6 mo).
- Diagnostic tests include serologic assays for antibodies and molecular tests for viral particles.

1. Enzyme immunoassay is the test for anti-HCV antibody:
   The current version can detect antibody within 4 to 10 wk after infection.
   False-negative rate in low-risk populations is 0.5% to 1%.
   False negatives also occur in immune-compromised persons, HIV-1, renal failure, HCV-associated essential mixed cryoglobulinemia.
   False positives in autoimmune hepatitis, paraproteinemia, and persons with no risk factors.

- The recombinant immunoblot assay that was previously recommended as a follow-up to positive antibody test is no longer available. The CDC now recommends that anyone who tests positive for HCV antibodies receive a follow-up HCV RNA test.

- Qualitative and quantitative HCV RNA tests using PCR: Lower limit of detection is <43 IU/ml.
- Used to confirm viremia and to assess response to treatment.
- Qualitative polymerase chain reaction (PCR) useful in patients with negative enzyme immunoassay in whom infection is suspected.
- Quantitative tests use either branched-chain DNA or reverse transcription PCR; the latter is more sensitive.
- Viral genotyping can distinguish among genotypes 1, 2, 3, 4, 5, and 6, which is helpful in choosing therapy; most of these tests use PCR (genotypes 1, 2, 3, and 4 predominate in the United States and Europe [genotype 1 is especially common in North America (60% to 75% of Hep C infections in the United States).
- LFTs: ALT and AST may be elevated to more than eight times normal in acute infection; in chronic infection ALT may be normal or fluctuate.
- Bilirubin may be five to 10 times normal.
- Albumin and prothrombin time generally normal; if abnormal, may be harbinger of impending hepatic necrosis.
- WBC and erythrocyte sedimentation rate (ESR) are generally normal.
- HIV testing. Infection with HCV is seen in 15% to 30% of individuals with HIV infection due to shared risk factors.

IMAGING STUDIES

- Transient elastography (Fibroscan) to quantify liver fibrosis.
- Sonogram: rapid liver size reduction during fulminant hepatitis or mass in HCC.

(Rx) TREATMENT

NONPHARMACOLOGIC THERAPY

Activity and diet as tolerated; avoid saw palmetto and green tea leaf herbs.

ACUTE GENERAL Rx

- Supportive care.
- Avoid hepatically metabolized drugs.

CHRONIC Rx

Response to therapy is influenced by HCV genotype. Recommendations for the treatment of hepatitis C in adults are changing constantly as new therapies come to the market. The advent of direct-acting antiviral agents (DAAs) has drastically changed treatment options and improved cure rates to greater than 95%. The most up-to-date guidance is available at the website www.hcvguidelines.org. The following is a brief summary of the guidelines based on genotype as of July 2016. Newer agents are expected to be FDA approved in the next few years. Currently, these treatment regimens are extremely expensive.

Genotype 1a: Options for treatment-naïve patients without cirrhosis, listed by level of evidence:

A. Daily fixed-dose combination of elbasvir (50 mg)/grazoprevir (100 mg) [Zepatier] for 12 wk and in those who do not have baseline NS5A RAVs (amino acid substitutions at 28, 30, 31, or 93 that confer resistance to elbasvir). Rating: Class I, Level A.

B. Daily fixed-dose combination of ledipasvir (90 mg)/sofosbuvir (400 mg) [Harvoni] for 12 wk. Rating: Class I, Level A.

C. Daily fixed-dose combination of paritaprevir (150 mg)/ritonavir (100 mg)/ombitasvir (25 mg) plus twice-daily dosed dasabuvir (250 mg) with weight-based ribavirin for 12 wk [Viekira Pak]. Rating: Class I, Level A.

D. Daily simeprevir (150 mg) plus sofosbuvir (400 mg) for 12 wk. Rating: Class I, Level A.

E. Daily fixed-dose combination of sofosbuvir (400 mg)/velpatasvir (100 mg) [Epclusa] for 12 wk.

F. Daily daclatasvir (60 mg) [Daklinza] plus sofosbuvir (400 mg) [Solvaldi] for 12 wk. Rating: Class I, Level B.

G. Alternative regimen: Daily fixed-dose combination of elbasvir (50 mg)/grazoprevir (100 mg) [Zepatier] with weight-based ribavirin for 16 wk and in those who do not have baseline NS5A RAVs for elbasvir. Rating: Class IIa, Level B.

Genotype 1a: Options for treatment-naïve patients with compensated cirrhosis:

A. Daily fixed-dose combination of elbasvir (50 mg)/grazoprevir (100 mg) [Zepatier] and in those in whom no baseline NS5A RAVs for elbasvir are detected. Rating: Class I, Level A.

B. Daily fixed-dose combination of ledipasvir (90 mg)/sofosbuvir (400 mg) [Harvoni] for 12 wk. Rating: Class I, Level A.

C. Daily fixed-dose combination of sofosbuvir (400 mg)/velpatasvir (100 mg) [Epclusa] for 12 wk. Rating: Class I, Level A.

D. Alternative Regimens:
1. Daily fixed-dose combination of paritaprevir (150 mg)/ritonavir (100 mg)/ombitasvir (25 mg) plus twice-daily dosed dasabuvir (250 mg) [Viekira Pak] with weight-based ribavirin for 24 wk. Rating: Class I, Level A.
2. Daily simeprevir (150 mg) plus sofosbuvir (400 mg) with or without weight-based ribavirin for 24 wk. Rating: Class II, Level B.
3. Daily daclatasvir (60 mg) plus sofosbuvir (400 mg) with or without weight-based ribavirin for 24 weeks. Rating: Class IIa, Level B.
4. Daily fixed-dose combination of elbasvir (50 mg)/grazoprevir (100 mg) [Zepatier] with weight-based ribavirin for 16 wk. Rating: Class IIa, Level B.

Genotype 1b: Treatment-naïve patients without cirrhosis:

A. Daily fixed-dose combination of elbasvir (50 mg)/grazoprevir (100 mg) [Zepatier] for 12 wk. Rating: Class I, Level A.

B. Daily fixed-dose combination of ledipasvir (90 mg)/sofosbuvir (400 mg) [Harvoni] for 12 wk. Rating: Class I, Level A.

C. Daily fixed combination of paritaprevir (150 mg)/ritonavir (100 mg)/ombitasvir (25 mg) plus twice-daily dosed dasabuvir (250 mg) [Viekira Pak] for 12 wk. Rating: Class I, Level A.

D. Daily simeprevir (150 mg) plus sofosbuvir (400 mg) for 12 wk. Rating: Class I, Level A.

E. Daily fixed combination of sofosbuvir (400 mg)/velpatasvir (100 mg) [Epclusa] for 12 wk. Rating: Class I, Level A.

F. Daily daclatasvir (60 mg) plus sofosbuvir (400 mg) for 12 wk. Rating: Class I, Level B.

Genotype 1b: Treatment-naïve patients with compensated cirrhosis:

A. Daily fixed-dose combination of elbasvir (50 mg)/grazoprevir (100 mg) [Zepatier] for 12 wk. Rating: Class I, Level A.

B. Daily fixed-dose combination of ledipasvir (90 mg)/sofosbuvir [Harvoni] for 12 wk. Rating: Class I, Level A.

C. Daily fixed-dose combination of paritaprevir (150 mg)/ritonavir (100 mg)/ombitasvir (25 mg) plus twice-daily dosed dasabuvir (250 mg) [Viekira Pak] for 12 wk. Rating: Class I, Level A.

D. Daily fixed combination of sofosbuvir (400 mg)/velpatasvir (100 mg) [Epclusa] for 12 wk. Rating: Class I, Level A.

E. Alternative regimens:
1. Daily daclatasvir (60 mg) plus sofosbuvir (400 mg) with or without weight-based ribavirin for 24 wk. Rating: Class IIa, Level B.
2. Daily simeprevir (150 mg) plus sofosbuvir (400 mg) with or without weight-based ribavirin for 24 wk. Rating: Class IIa, Level B.

Genotype 2: Treatment-naïve regimens without cirrhosis:

A. Daily fixed-dose combination of sofosbuvir (400 mg)/velpatasir (100 mg) [Epclusa] for 12 wk. Rating: Class I, Level A.

B. Alternative regimen: Daily daclatasvir (60 mg) plus sofosbuvir (400 mg) for 12 wk. Rating: Class IIa, Level B.

Genotype 2: Treatment-naïve patients with compensated cirrhosis:

A. Daily fixed-dose combination of sofosbuvir (400 mg)/velpatasvir (100 mg) [Epclusa] for 12 wk. Rating: Class I, Level A.

B. Alternative regimen: Daily daclatasvir (60 mg) plus sofosbuvir (400 mg) for 16 to 24 wk. Rating: Class IIa, Level B.

Genotype 3: Treatment-naïve patients without cirrhosis:

A. Daily daclatasvir (60 mg) and sofosbuvir (400 mg) for 12 wk. Rating: Class I, Level A.

B. Daily fixed-dose combination of sofosbuvir (400 mg)/velpatasvir (100 mg) [Epclusa] for 12 weeks. Rating: Class I, Level A.

Genotype 3: Treatment-naïve patients with compensated cirrhosis:

A. Daily fixed-dose combination of sofosbuvir (400 mg)/velpatasvir (100 mg) [Epclusa] for 12 wk. Rating: Class I, Level A.

B. Daily daclatasvir (60 mg) plus sofosbuvir (400 mg) for 24 wk with or without weight-based ribavirin. Rating: Class IIa, Level B.

Genotype 4: Treatment-naïve patients without cirrhosis:

A. Daily fixed-dose combination of paritaprevir (150 mg)/ritonavir (100 mg)/ombitasvir (25 mg) and weight-based ribavirin for 12 weeks. Rating: Class I, Level A.

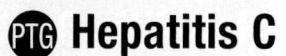 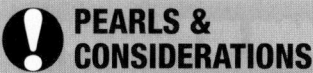

B. Daily fixed-dose combination of sofosbuvir (400 mg)/velpatasvir (100 mg) [Epclusa] for 12 weeks. Rating: Class I, Level A.

C. Daily fixed-dose combination of elbasvir (50 mg)/grazoprevir (100 mg) [Zepatier] for 12 weeks. Rating: Class IIa, Level B.

D. Daily fixed-dose combination of ledipasvir (90 mg)/sofosbuvir (400 mg) [Harvoni] for 12 weeks. Rating: Class IIa, Level B.

Genotype 4: Treatment-naïve patients with compensated cirrhosis:

A. Daily fixed-dose combination of paritaprevir (150 mg)/ritonavir (100 mg)/ombitasvir (25 mg) and weight-based ribavirin for 12 wk. Rating: Class I, Level A.

B. Daily fixed-dose combination of sofosbuvir (400 mg)/velpatasvir (100 mg) [Epclusa] for 12 wk. Rating: Class I, Level A.

C. Daily fixed-dose combination of elbasvir (50 mg)/grazoprevir (100 mg) [Zepatier] for 12 wk. Rating: Class IIa, Level B.

D. Daily fixed-dose combination of ledipasvir (90 mg)/sofosbuvir (400 mg) [Harvoni] for 12 wk. Rating: Class IIa, Level B.

Genotypes 5 and 6: Treatment-naïve patients with and without cirrhosis:

A. Daily fixed-dose combination of sofosbuvir (400 mg)/velpatasvir (100 mg) [Epclusa] for 12 wk. Rating: Class I, Level A. Daily fixed-dose combination of ledipasvir (90 mg)/sofosbuvir (400 mg for 12 weeks).

B. Daily fixed-dose combination of ledipasvir (90 mg)/sofosbuvir (400 mg) [Harvoni] for 12 wk. Rating: Class IIa, Level B.

Drug interactions can be significant with these regimens (http://www.hep-druginteractions.org). With DAA regimens, viral loads are measured at 4 wk into the therapy to monitor success and at the end of therapy. A final viral load is measured 12 wk after completing the treatment, and if undetectable, the patient is considered to have a sustained virologic response (SVR), which equates to a cure.

- Liver transplantation:
  1. Hepatitis C is the main indication for liver transplantation in the United States.
  2. It is the only option for patients with deteriorating HCV-related cirrhosis and for some patients with HCC.
  3. Recurrent infection occurs in almost all patients with progressive fibrosis and cirrhosis; as many as 20% progress to cirrhosis within 5 yrs posttransplant.

DISPOSITION

- SVR after treatment among HCV-infected persons at any stage of fibrosis is associated with reduced HCC.
- Periodic abdominal ultrasonography for HCC screening.
- Recent guidelines recommend against measurement of alpha-fetoprotein (AFP) to screen for HCC in patients with chronic hepatitis C due to lack of sensitivity, specificity, and predictive values.

REFERRAL

- To a hepatologist or infectious disease specialist for treatment for hepatitis C in patients who have been previously treated or for treatment failures with DAA agents.
- To a transplant surgeon for consideration of liver transplant if indicated.

PEARLS & CONSIDERATIONS

- More rapid progression of disease in persons who drink alcohol regularly, persons of advanced age at time of infection, and those coinfected with other viruses (HIV, hepatitis B). All persons with identified HCV infection should receive a brief alcohol screening and intervention as clinically indicated.
- Regression of cirrhosis has been demonstrated after antiviral therapy in some patients with chronic hepatitis C. Regression is associated with decreased disease-related morbidity and improved survival.
- The presence of interleukin (IL)-28B and HLA class II is independently associated with spontaneous resolution of HCV infection, and single nucleotide polymorphism IL-28B and DQB1*03:01 may explain approximately 15% of spontaneous resolution of HCV infection.

SUGGESTED READINGS

Available at www.expertconsult.com

RELATED CONTENT

Hepatitis C (Patient Information)

AUTHOR: **GLENN G. FORT, M.D., M.P.H.**

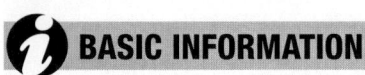 **BASIC INFORMATION**

DEFINITION

- A defective RNA virus
- Depends on hepatitis B virus (HBV) for its active viral replication
- Most severe form of viral hepatitis

SYNONYMS

HDV
Delta virus
Delta agent

ICD-10-CM CODES
B16.1	Acute hepatitis B with delta-agent without hepatic coma
B16.0	Acute hepatitis B with delta-agent with hepatic coma
B18. 0	Chronic viral hepatitis B with delta-agent

EPIDEMIOLOGY AND DEMOGRAPHICS

- The least common cause of chronic viral hepatitis worldwide.
- Endemic in many parts of the world in 1980s (Fig. E1).
- The rates of occurrence in the tropical and subtropical areas were higher compared with those in northern Europe or North America due to the increased HBV in those locations.
- Immigration from endemic areas to northern Europe and the U.S. has increased HDV in these areas.

INCIDENCE:
- Remains a major health concern in developing countries.

PEAK INCIDENCE:
- Peak incidence was in the 1980s.

PREVALENCE:
- 15 to 20 million people affected worldwide
- The highest prevalence is in the Middle East, Central Africa, northern parts of South America, and the Mediterranean basin (Fig. 2).

PREDOMINANT SEX AND AGE:
- Occurs in both sexes
- Age varies

GENETICS:
- There are eight identified genotypes of HDV.
- The genotype has no influence on management.
- It is unclear whether the genotypes carry substantial clinical or prognostic significance.
- Genotype does have an important role when studying epidemiology.
- Different HBV genotypes may interact with different genotypes of HDV.
- Table 1 illustrates the individual genotypes, their geographical distribution, and the few associated clinical observations.

RISK FACTORS

- Transmitted by parenteral routes.
- Shares the same risk factors as HBV.
- Highest rates of infection are in intravenous drug users.
- Sexual transmission through heterosexual contact can occur.
- Its spread among homosexual men has not been evident.
- Vertical transmission can also occur but is rare.
- Box 1 describes persons who should be clinically suspected of having HDV infection.

PHYSICAL FINDINGS & CLINICAL PRESENTATION

- Clinical manifestations can vary.
- Symptoms can include nausea, lethargy, and abdominal pain.
- The presentation depends on whether it occurs as a coinfection with HBV or as a superinfection in a chronic HBV carrier.
- HBV/HDV coinfection is usually a self-limited acute hepatitis.
- Superinfection can cause a severe acute hepatitis with a drastic clinical course.
- Severe infection can result in liver cirrhosis, liver cancer, liver failure, and even death.
- Coinfection with HBV, HCV, and HIV has increased risk of liver cirrhosis.

ETIOLOGY

- HDV requires the hepatitis B surface antigen (HBsAg) for hepatocyte adherence and virion assembly.
- HBsAg carriers serve as the main reservoirs for hepatitis D infection and often become chronic carriers of the virus.
- At least 5% of HBV carriers worldwide are infected with HDV.

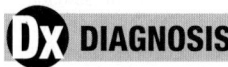 **DIAGNOSIS**

DIFFERENTIAL DIAGNOSIS

- Acute hepatitis B infection
- Recrudescence of HBV infection in a known HBV carrier

WORKUP

- The first step is to measure the immunoglobulin (Ig) G antibodies to HDV, also known as anti-HD.

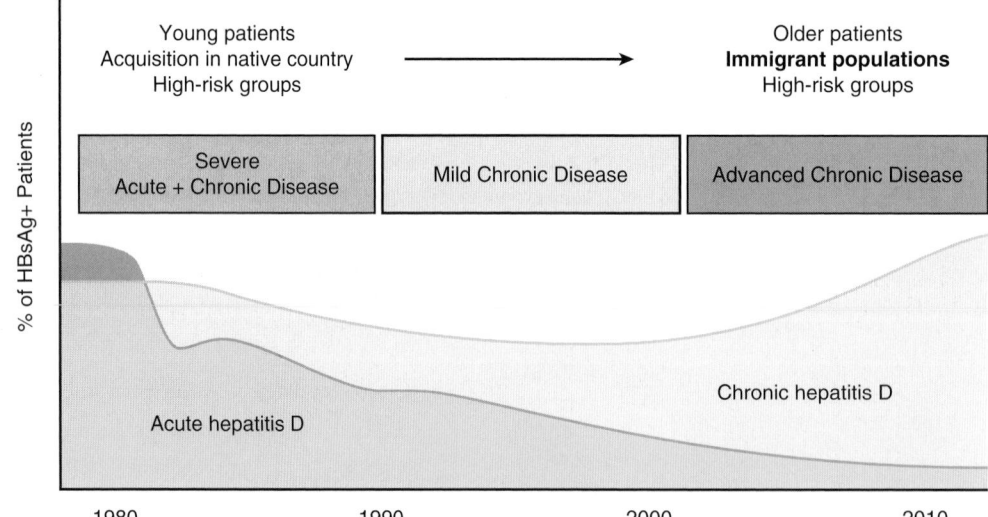

Young patients
Acquisition in native country
High-risk groups
→
Older patients
Immigrant populations
High-risk groups

% of HBsAg+ Patients

Severe Acute + Chronic Disease | Mild Chronic Disease | Advanced Chronic Disease

Chronic hepatitis D

Acute hepatitis D

1980   1990   2000   2010

FIG. 2 Timeline of the changing epidemiology of HDV infection since the late 1970s. HDV had a dramatic acute appearance in the early to mid-1980s, and many of the patients were young, from countries with a high prevalence of HDV infection, or identified as being in high-risk groups (e.g., people who inject drugs). Since that time, many of the patients with severe liver injury have died because of the infection, and many of those with initially mild hepatitis have developed advanced liver disease and its complications. With changing immigration patterns in Europe and the U.S. (see Fig. 1), more cases of chronic HDV infection are being seen in persons who have relocated from high-prevalence areas. *HBsAg,* hepatitis B surface antigen. (From Feldman M et al [eds]: *Sleisenger and Fordtran's gastrointestinal and liver disease*, ed 10, Philadelphia, 2016, Saunders.)

TABLE 1 Hepatitis D Virus Genotypes

Genotype	Geography	Clinical Observations
1 (Most common)	North America, Europe, Middle East, North Africa, Mediterranean, and Taiwan	Lower remission rates and more adverse events compared to genotype 2 in Taiwan
2	North and East Asia	Milder disease (in East Asia)
3	South America (Northern)	Fulminant hepatitis
4	Japan and Taiwan	Milder disease (in East Asia)
5-8	West and Central Africa	N/A

BOX 1 Persons Who Should Be Clinically Suspected of Having Hepatitis D Virus Infection*

HBsAg-positive immigrants from regions that are moderately to highly endemic for HDV
HBsAg carriers with a history of injection drug use
Persons with chronic hepatitis B and rapid evolution to cirrhosis or hepatocellular carcinoma
HBsAg carriers who are persistently HBV DNA negative but have active liver disease
Persons with an unexplained acute flare of chronic hepatitis B that is not due to acute hepatitis A or C or reactivation of hepatitis B

* Initial screening with anti-HDV is recommended.
Anti-HDV, antibody to HDV; *HBsAg,* hepatitis B surface antigen.
From Feldman M et al [eds]: *Sleisenger and Fordtran's gastrointestinal and liver disease,* ed 10, Philadelphia, 2016, Saunders.

- Antibody response may be diminished in immunocompromised individuals, such as those with HIV.
- The most sensitive and specific test is the HDV-RNA measured by polymerase chain reaction (PCR).
- Level of viremia does not correlate with the severity of disease.
- There are no distinct histological characteristics from biopsy when compared to findings from isolated HBV infection.

LABORATORY TESTS

- Patients with coinfection can experience a biphasic course with two peaks of alanine aminotransferase (ALT) elevations several weeks apart.
- The first peak occurs during HBV replication, and the second peak occurs during delayed HDV replication.
- Key serological markers in acute coinfection include HDV-RNA, HBV-DNA, HBsAg, immunoglobulin (Ig) M antibody to hepatitis B core antigen (HBcAb), and IgM anti-HDV.
- HDV-RNA and HBV-DNA titers decrease as the infection resolves.

- Antibody to hepatitis B surface antigen (HbSAb) is formed as HBsAg disappears.
- IgM anti-HDV can persist even after HbSAb appears and aminotransferases normalize.
- Superinfection with HDV is differentiated from an acute HBV flare by detecting the presence of HDV-RNA and IgM anti-HDV along with measuring HBV-DNA titers, which are elevated in acute HBV infection.
- The lack of IgM to HBcAb also suggests superinfection in a chronic HBV carrier, rather than acute HBV infection.
- See Fig. 3, *A* and *B*, which illustrates the natural course in coinfection and superinfection, respectively. Table 2 describes diagnostic markers for HDV infection, their importance, and potential weaknesses.

IMAGING STUDIES

- Imaging studies are not used in diagnosis.

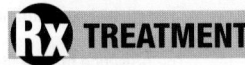 **TREATMENT**

NONPHARMACOLOGIC THERAPY

- Supportive care
- Management of symptoms

ACUTE GENERAL TREATMENT

- Interferon-alpha is the only therapeutic option.

CHRONIC TREATMENT

- Interferon-alpha should be continued as long as possible.
- Response is determined by the loss of HBsAg.
- Response is often delayed.
- Treatment should be given for at least 1 year before the individual is determined to be a nonresponder.
- Longer-term therapy is associated with a sustained disappearance of HDV-RNA and HBsAg along with regression of liver fibrosis.
- Investigations of other therapies, such as prenylation inhibitors, are currently ongoing.

DISPOSITION

- HBV/HDV coinfection is usually a self-limited illness that resolves after a few weeks.
- 2% of patients with coinfection progress to chronic HDV infection.
- Superinfection can cause a severe acute hepatitis but usually results in chronic infection.

REFERRAL

- Patients should be referred to a hepatologist or someone who is experienced in treating liver disease.

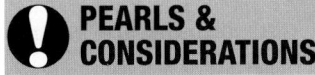 **PEARLS & CONSIDERATIONS**

COMMENTS

- Consider HDV infection in patients with underlying HBV and progressive liver disease.
- Investigational therapies are under way.

PREVENTION

- Aimed at modifying risk factors.
- No vaccine available for HDV.
- Vaccinating against HBV helps prevent HDV.
- High-risk populations, such as intravenous drug users, should be vaccinated against HBV.

RELATED CONTENT

Hepatitis B Virus (Related Key Topic)

AUTHOR: **HIRSH D. TRIVEDI, M.D.**

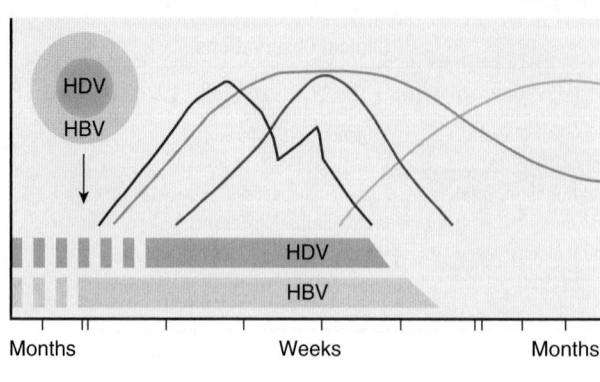

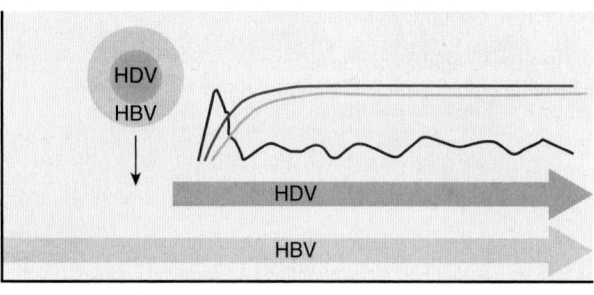

FIG. 3 A, Course of hepatitis B virus (HBV) and hepatitis D virus (HDV) coinfection. **B,** Course of hepatitis D virus superinfection in chronic hepatitis B carriers. *ALT,* alanine aminotransferase; *Ig,* immunoglobulin. (From Boyer TD et al: *Zakim & Boyer's hepatology: a textbook of liver disease*, ed 6, Philadelphia, 2012, Saunders.)

TABLE 2 Diagnostic Markers for Hepatitis D Virus Infection, Their Importance, and Potential Weaknesses

Diagnostic Markers and Their Importance	Potential Weaknesses
IgG anti-HDV	
Positive in all persons exposed to HDV; persists long term, even after viral clearance	May not be elevated in immunocompromised persons.
May indicate active or past infection; not a neutralizing antibody	
IgM anti-HDV	
Positive in acute infection; negative in past infection	Often persists in chronic infection, particularly with active liver disease.
May be used as a surrogate marker for HDV replication	Neither 100% sensitive nor specific for HDV replication.
Decrease in titers and subsequent clearance in chronic HDV infection is a predictor of spontaneous or therapy-induced remission	
HDAg	
Can be demonstrated in hepatocytes by immunohistochemical staining	The reliability of immunochemistry decreases as the disease becomes chronic.
	The presence of high titers of neutralizing antibodies (anti-HDV) interferes with detection of HDAg.
	Less sensitive than molecular assays.
HDV RNA (qualitative)	
Marker of HDV replication	Variability in the HDV genome and assay primers influences the sensitivity of HDV RNA detection.
Positive in all patients with chronic HDV infection	
Negative in spontaneous or treatment-induced viral clearance	No WHO standardized assay.
HDV RNA (quantitative)	
Used to measure the level of HDV RNA in serum	HDV RNA may be present at a lower titer than the limit of detection (as low as 10 copies/mL).
Useful method for predicting and monitoring treatment response	Levels do not reflect the grade or stage of liver disease.
	May be useful for monitoring patients during therapy with interferon, but there is no WHO standardized assay.
	Results may differ significantly among laboratories.
HBsAg (quantitative)	
May be useful for predicting or monitoring treatment response during therapy with interferon, because a falling titer heralds HBsAg loss and hence HDV RNA clearance	Confined to research laboratories in the U.S. but commercially licensed in Asia and Europe.

HBsAg, hepatitis B surface antigen; *HDAg,* hepatitis D antigen; *HDV,* hepatitis D virus; *IgG,* immunoglobulin G; *IgM,* immunoglobulin M.
From Feldman M et al [eds]: *Sleisenger and Fordtran's gastrointestinal and liver disease*, ed 10, Philadelphia, 2016, Saunders.

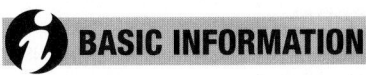
BASIC INFORMATION

DEFINITION

Hepatitis E is an RNA virus transmitted mostly by the fecal-oral route that is among the most frequent causes of acute hepatitis worldwide, with an estimated 20 million cases annually and 70,000 deaths.

SYNONYMS

Previously known as enterically transmitted non-A non-B hepatitis
HEV
Hepatitis E virus
Epidemic non-A, non-B hepatitis

ICD-10CM CODES
B17.2 Acute hepatitis E

EPIDEMIOLOGY & DEMOGRAPHICS

INCIDENCE:
- Considered hyperendemic in India, Bangladesh, China, and Mexico (Fig. 1). It is probably the most common cause of acute hepatitis and jaundice in the world
- In developed nations usually associated with travelers returning from endemic countries (Table 1)
- Large outbreaks can occur and are associated with fecal-contaminated water
- Person-to-person transmission is thought not to contribute to morbidity in epidemics

PEAK INCIDENCE:
- Some waterborne outbreaks are more common in summer months.
- Foodborne transmission through raw or undercooked meat of wild deer, boar and domestic pigs, and probably rabbit contribute to cases of hepatitis E in developed nations.

PREVALENCE:
- In endemic countries, HEV prevalence of 25% for all non-A and non-B acute hepatitis cases.
- In endemic countries among blood donors, IgG antibodies are found in as high as 45% of donors.
- In developing countries, prevalence of IgG antibodies is 1% to 4% among blood donors.

PREDOMINANT SEX AND AGE:
- High attack rates are found in adults 15 to 40 years of age.
- Fulminant hepatic failure occurs more frequently during pregnancy, with mortality rates of 15% to 25%.
- Vertical transmission commonly occurs via intrauterine and perinatal routes and can lead to severe liver disease and high mortality in fetuses and neonates.
- Men are more frequently affected than women.

PHYSICAL FINDINGS & CLINICAL PRESENTATION
- After an incubation period of 15 to 60 days, most cases are self-limited and asymptomatic (80%).
- Symptomatic patients will experience nonspecific findings:
  - Flu-like myalgia, arthralgia, anorexia
  - Hepatomegaly, fever, weakness, vomiting, diarrhea
  - Jaundice, pale stools, darkened urine can also occur as in other hepatitis infections
- Elevated liver function tests: total bilirubin, ALT, AST occur 1 to 6 weeks after onset of illness.
- Case fatality rate is very low: 0.5% to 4%, except in pregnancy: 15% to 25%.
- Rare complications include pancreatitis, encephalitis, proximal myopathy.

ETIOLOGY
- HEV is the sole member of the *Orthohepevirus* genus of the *Hepeviridae* family.
- HEV is an icosahedral, nonenveloped, single-stranded RNA virus about 27 to 34 nm in diameter.
- There are four genotypes, of which humans are the host for all four genotypes, and swine and other mammals may also be the hosts for genotypes 3 and 4. Box 1 summarizes features of HEV genotypes 1 and 2. Table 2 compares epidemiologic and clinical features associated with HEV genotypes 1 and 3.

DIAGNOSIS

DIFFERENTIAL DIAGNOSIS
- Hepatitis A: another fecal-oral hepatitis virus with low mortality and low chronic state rate
- Hepatitis B, hepatitis C, hepatitis D
- Drug-induced induced liver injury such as from isoniazid
- Dengue fever, malaria
- Typhoid fever

WORKUP
- Consists of tests on blood and feces on a clinical-compatible patient/travel to endemic areas
- Patients will shed detectable virus in stool 1 week prior to start of illness and persists for up to 2 weeks afterward

LABORATORY TESTS
- Anti-HEV IgM antibodies can be detected 4 days after onset of jaundice and persist for 5 months.
- Anti-HEV IgG antibodies are detectable shortly after appearance of the IgM antibodies.
- PCR on blood and feces.
- Fig. 2 illustrates the typical course of HEV infection.

PATHOLOGY
- On liver biopsy will demonstrate a cholestatic picture and classic types of acute viral hepatitis.
- In fulminant cases, there is massive hepatic necrosis.

TREATMENT

- Treatment is supportive, as most cases are self-limited in normal hosts.

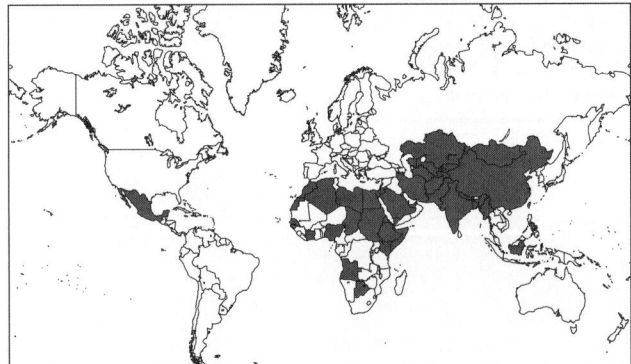

FIG. 1 Geographic distribution of areas where infection with HEV genotypes 1 and 2 is highly endemic *(red areas)*. (From Feldman M et al [eds]: *Sleisenger and Fordtran's gastrointestinal and liver disease*, ed 10, Philadelphia, 2016, Saunders.)

TABLE 1 HEV Genotypes and Their Geographic Distribution

Genotype	Human Cases	Animal Cases
1	South, Southeast and Central Asia, Africa	—
2	Mexico, Western Africa	—
3	U.S., South America, Europe (France, Spain, U.K., the Netherlands), Japan	U.S., China, Japan, Southeast Asia, Australia, New Zealand, South America
4	China, Taiwan, Japan, Vietnam	India, China, Taiwan, Japan

From Feldman M et al [eds]: *Sleisenger and Fordtran's gastrointestinal and liver disease*, ed 10, Philadelphia, 2016, Saunders.

BOX 1 Features of HEV Genotypes 1 and 2

Acute infection with no evidence of chronicity.
Large outbreaks involving up to several thousand persons in developing countries.
Frequent sporadic cases.
Disease is more common among young adults.
Fecal-oral transmission, usually through contaminated water.
Highest attack rates are among young adults aged 15 to 40 years, with relative sparing of children.
Infrequent person-to-person transmission.
No evidence of parenteral or sexual transmission.
Greater likelihood of severe disease (liver failure) with high mortality rates (15% to 25%) in pregnant women, especially in the third trimester.
Mother-to-newborn (transplacental) transmission is known to occur.

From Feldman M et al [eds]: *Sleisenger and Fordtran's gastrointestinal and liver disease*, ed 10, Philadelphia, 2016, Saunders.

TABLE 2 Comparison of Epidemiologic and Clinical Features Associated With HEV Genotypes 1 and 3

Characteristic	Genotype 1	Genotype 3
Epidemiologic patterns of human disease	Large epidemics, small outbreaks, and frequent sporadic cases	A small proportion of cases with sporadic acute hepatitis
Persons affected	Young, otherwise healthy persons; males > females	Mostly elderly, often with other comorbid conditions; males > females
Animal-to-human transmission	Not reported	Demonstrated; a likely mode of transmission through consumption of undercooked meat or close contact with animals
Water-borne transmission	Well known to occur; most common route	Unknown
Animal reservoir	No	Yes (pigs, wild boars, deer)
Severity	Variable severity, including fulminant hepatic failure; severe disease is particularly more common in pregnant women	Severity and poor outcome are related to comorbid conditions
Chronic infection	Not known to occur after acute infection	Immunosuppressed persons; transplant recipients receiving immunosuppressive drugs

From Feldman M et al [eds]: *Sleisenger and Fordtran's gastrointestinal and liver disease*, ed 10, Philadelphia, 2016, Saunders.

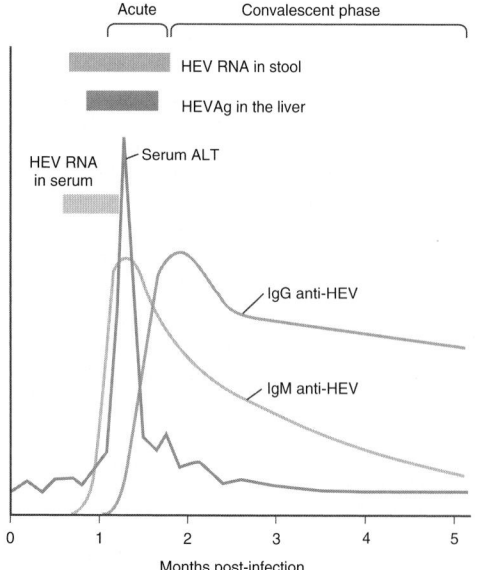

FIG. 2 Typical course of HEV infection (based on studies with human subjects and with experimentally infected primates). *anti-HEV,* antibody to HEV; *Ag,* antigen; *IgG,* immunoglobulin G; *IgM,* immunoglobulin M. (From Feldman M et al [eds]: *Sleisenger and Fordtran's gastrointestinal and liver disease*, ed 10, Philadelphia, 2016, Saunders.)

REFERRAL

- To gastroenterologist or infectious diseases for correct diagnosis

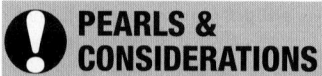

PEARLS & CONSIDERATIONS

COMMENTS

- HEV can become chronic in organ transplant patients on immunosuppressive therapy, and ribavirin appears to produce a sustained virologic response.

PREVENTION

- Hepatitis E vaccines are available and appear to be 96% effective.

PATIENT/FAMILY EDUCATION

- Travelers to endemic areas should take precautions and drink only potable water and not eat uncooked shellfish, fruits, and vegetables.

SUGGESTED READINGS

Available at www.expertconsult.com

RELATED CONTENT

Hepatitis A (Related Key Topic)

AUTHOR: **GLENN G. FORT, M.D., M.P.H.**

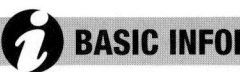

BASIC INFORMATION

DEFINITION

Autoimmune hepatitis is a chronic inflammatory condition of the liver characterized by elevated serum globulin levels (IgG), presence of circulating autoantibodies, interface hepatitis on histology, and plasma cell rich infiltrate. Two types have been described:

- Type 1, or "classic," autoimmune hepatitis is the most predominant form in the U.S. and worldwide (80%) and has a bimodal age distribution with peaks between 10 and 20 and 45 and 70 years of age. Patients are positive for antinuclear antibodies (ANA) and/or antismooth muscle antibodies (ASMA) and have specific associated HLA haplotypes: B8, DR3, DR4.
- Type 2 is rare in the U.S., primarily affects young children between 2 and 14 years of age, and is characterized by the presence of antibodies to liver/kidney microsomes (anti-LKM-1) or liver cytosol 1. Patients have associated HLA haplotypes: B14, DR. This form is generally more advanced at presentation and is more difficult to treat.

SYNONYMS

Autoimmune chronic active hepatitis
Chronic active hepatitis
Lupoid hepatitis
Plasma cell hepatitis

ICD-10CM CODES
K75.4 Autoimmune hepatitis
K73.2 Chronic active hepatitis, not elsewhere classified

EPIDEMIOLOGY & DEMOGRAPHICS

- Annual incidence (estimated): 0.2 to 2.0 cases per 100,000, similar to PBC, more common than PSC.
- Point prevalence (estimated): 16.9 per 100,000.
- Type 1: age of onset has a bimodal distribution with peaks between 10 and 20 and 45 and 70 years.
- Type 2: more common in young children 2-14 years of age.
- Female/male ratio is 3.6:1; type 1 has an 80% female predominance, whereas type 2 has a 90% female predominance.
- Approximately 100,000 to 200,000 persons affected in the U.S.
- Accounts for 4% to 6% of liver transplants in the U.S.
- Associated with HLA-DRB1*0301 and HLA-DRB1*0401 alleles.

CLINICAL PRESENTATION

- Varies from intermittent asymptomatic elevations of liver enzymes to advanced cirrhosis. Cirrhosis is often the presenting stage. AIH can also present initially as a fulminant hepatitis.
- Symptoms may include fatigue, anorexia, nausea, abdominal pain, pruritus, and arthralgia.

- Autoimmune findings may include arthritis, xerostomia, keratoconjunctivitis, cutaneous vasculitis, and erythema nodosum.
- Patients with advanced disease can show hepatosplenomegaly, ascites, peripheral edema, abnormal bleeding, and jaundice.

ETIOLOGY

- Exact etiology is unknown; liver histology demonstrates cell-mediated immune attack against hepatocytes.
- Presence of a variety of autoantibodies suggests an autoimmune mechanism.
- There are likely two components involved: genetic predisposition and an inciting environmental trigger.
- Potential triggering agents such as viruses (hepatitis A, B, C) or drugs (minocycline, nitrofurantoin) likely possess some homology similar to liver-specific antigens.

DIAGNOSIS

- A simplified diagnostic criteria for routine clinical practice has been developed by the International Autoimmune Hepatitis Group (see Table 1).
- Histology: lymphoplasmacytic infiltrate invading the hepatocyte boundary surrounding the portal triad (limiting plate). Also, a periportal infiltrate may be seen (interface hepatitis).
- The European Association for the Study of the Liver guidelines do require liver biopsy as part of the diagnostic evaluation.
- The American Association for the Study of Liver Disease (AASLD) approach is to obtain a liver biopsy if the diagnosis is unclear or to assess disease activity prior to initiating treatment.

DIFFERENTIAL DIAGNOSIS

- Acute viral hepatitis (A, B, C, D, E, cytomegalovirus, Epstein-Barr, herpes)
- Chronic viral hepatitis (B, C)
- Toxic hepatitis (alcohol, drugs)
- Primary biliary cirrhosis
- Primary sclerosing cholangitis
- Hemochromatosis
- Nonalcoholic steatohepatitis
- Systemic lupus erythematosus
- Wilson's disease
- Alpha-1 antitrypsin deficiency

WORKUP

- History and physical examination with attention to the presence of autoimmune

abnormalities such as autoimmune thyroiditis, Graves' disease, inflammatory bowel disease, celiac sprue, and rheumatoid arthritis.
- Liver function tests and serum gamma-globulins.
- Tests for autoantibodies: ANA, ASMA, anti-LKM.
- Liver biopsy for establishing diagnosis and disease severity.

LABORATORY TESTS

- Aminotransferases generally elevated and may fluctuate
- Bilirubin and alkaline phosphatase moderately elevated or normal
- Elevation of gamma globulin (>2.0 g/dl [20 g/L]) and immunoglobulin G
- Circulating autoantibodies often present:
  1. Rheumatoid factor
  2. ANAs
     a. Present in two thirds of patients
     b. Typical pattern is homogeneous or speckled
     c. Titer does not correlate with the stage, activity, or prognosis
  3. Anti-SMAs
     a. Present in 87% of patients
     b. Titer does not correlate with course or prognosis
  4. Anti-LKM antibodies
     a. Typically found in patients who are ANA negative and SMA negative
     b. Characterizes type 2 AIH
     c. Present in pediatric population and up to 20% of adults in Europe; also present in patients with drug-induced hepatitis
  5. Autoantibodies against soluble liver antigen and liver-pancreas antigen (anti-SLA/LP)
     a. Present in 10% to 30% of patients
     b. Associated with higher rate of relapse after corticosteroid therapy
     c. Several studies suggest that patients with anti-SLA/LP have a more severe course

  Serum p-ANCA levels are useful for diagnosis of the 10% to 15% of patients with negative ASMA, negative ANA, and low gamma globulin levels.
- Hypoalbuminemia and prolonged prothrombin time with advanced disease.
- There is a well-described overlap syndrome with primary biliary cirrhosis (7%), primary sclerosing cholangitis (6%), and autoimmune

TABLE 1 Simplified Diagnostic Criteria for Autoimmune Hepatitis

Variable	Cutoff	Points	Cutoff	Points
ANA or SMA	≥1:40	1	≥1:80	2
LKM			≥1:40	2
SLA			Positive	2
IgG	≥ULN	1	≥1.1 × ULN	2
Histology	Compatible with AIH	1	Typical of AIH	2
Absence of viral hepatitis			Yes	2

Maximum number of points for all antibodies = 2, total = 8. Probable AIH ≥6 points, definite AIH ≥7 points. 88% sensitivity and 97% specificity. *AIH,* Autoimmune hepatitis; *ANA,* antinuclear antibody; *IgG,* immunoglobulin G; *LKM,* liver/kidney microsomes; *SLA,* soluble liver antigen; *SMA,* smooth muscle antibody; *ULN,* upper limit of normal.

cholangitis (11%). In patients who do not respond to therapy after 3 months, consider cholangiographic studies to evaluate for primary sclerosing cholangitis.

IMAGING STUDIES

- Ultrasound of liver and biliary tree to rule out obstruction or hepatic mass.
- Cirrhosis secondary to AIH is a risk factor for development of hepatocellular carcinoma (although less so than viral hepatitis). Patients with cirrhosis should get ultrasonography and AFP every 6 months.

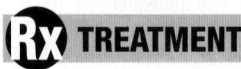

NONPHARMACOLOGIC THERAPY

- Avoid alcohol and hepatotoxic medications.
- Liver transplantation is an option for end-stage disease or fulminant hepatic failure.

PHARMACOLOGIC THERAPY

- Initial treatment:
  1. Prednisone or prednisolone 40 to 60 mg/day PO or combination treatment with prednisone 30 mg PO daily plus azathioprine 50 mg PO daily, with a gradual taper to prednisone 10 mg PO daily over 2 to 3 months as liver function test (LFT) results normalize. A combination of oral budesonide (6 to 9 mg/day) and azathioprine (1-2 mg/kg/day) can be used to induce and maintain remission in patients with non-cirrhotic AIH, with a lower rate of steroid-specific side effects. Steroids are contraindicated in brittle diabetes mellitus, uncontrolled hypertension, prior steroid intolerance, severe osteopenia, and psychosis. Azathioprine is contraindicated by thiopurine S-methyltransferase (TPMT) deficiency, leukopenia, or thrombocytopenia. Budesonide is contraindicated in cirrhosis because portal systemic shunting and abnormal hepatic metabolism prevent complete hepatic first-pass extraction, reducing therapeutic efficacy and causing systemic steroid side effects.
  2. Combination therapy allows lower prednisone doses, fewer steroid side effects, and faster normalization of LFTs.

  The primary goal of therapy in AIH is to achieve remission. The 2010 AASLD Practice Guideline (2010 PG) redefined remission to require: normal levels of AST, ALT (optimally <19 U/L in women and <30 U/L in men), total bilirubin, gamma-globulin or IgG and absence of inflammatory activity on liver biopsy. Secondary goals of therapy are the prevention of progression of fibrosis to cirrhosis and reversion of cirrhosis to a lower stage of fibrosis, which has been documented.
- Indications for treatment:
  1. Serum aminotransferases >10 times the upper limit of normal
  2. Serum aminotransferases >5 times the upper limit of normal, with serum gamma-globulin level twice the upper limit of normal

  3. Histologic features of bridging necrosis
  4. Symptomatic disease: incapacitating symptoms such as fatigue and arthralgia
- Relative indications:
  - Asymptomatic patients with elevated liver enzymes or limited histological activity
- Treatment not indicated:
  - Inactive cirrhosis
- Evaluation of treatment response:
  1. Goals are the absence of symptoms, normalization of liver function tests, and absence of inflammatory activity on liver biopsy. Generally, this is a steroid-responsive condition, but up to 20% do not respond.
  2. Patients whose transaminase levels normalize may continue to have ongoing active hepatitis involving inflammation and fibrosis.
  3. Histologic improvement may lag behind clinical and laboratory improvement by as much as 6 months. Because of this, repeat liver biopsy should be considered after normalization of transaminase levels. A review of AIH studies between 1972 and 2013 shows that hepatic fibrosis improves in 53% to 57% of cases and that progressive fibrosis slows or is prevented in 79% of patients.
  4. After initial remission is achieved, one may consider tapering medications. Steroid withdrawal should be done only if liver function tests normalize and histologic quiescence is achieved. About 50% to 86% of patients will relapse after this and require long-term maintenance medications.
  5. Complete normalization on biopsy is associated with a 15% to 20% risk of relapse, whereas persistent interface hepatitis is associated with a 90% risk of relapse. Do not attempt multiple treatment withdrawals. The risk of developing cirrhosis with single relapse is 9.5%, whereas multiple relapses are associated with 37.5% risk of developing cirrhosis. The patient with sustained remission has a risk of cirrhosis of 4.5%.

DISPOSITION

- Long-term treatment may be necessary for sustained remission in individuals who continuously relapse and in partial responders.
- Sixty-five percent of patients achieve remission by 18 months; 80% achieve remission by 3 years.
- Approximately 10% to 15% of patients do not respond to conventional therapy. The risk factors for nonresponse include presence of underlying cirrhosis, younger age, or longer duration of disease, HLA-B8 or DR3. High-dose therapy can achieve remission in 70%: prednisone 60 mg or dual therapy with prednisone 30 mg and AZA 150 mg. Other alternatives such as mycophenolate, the calcineurin inhibitors (CNIs), tacrolimus (TAC) and cyclosporine (CSA), sirolimus (SIR), everolimus (EVR), rituximab,

and infliximab, have been used successfully. However, none of the alternative therapies has been studied in multicenter, randomized, controlled trials.
- Orthotopic liver transplantation (OLT) is a life-saving option for AIH patients with acute liver failure, decompensated cirrhosis, or HCC. Allograft and patient survival are excellent; however, AIH recurs in the allograft in a minority (25% probability in first 5 years, 50% in 10 years).

REFERRAL

Patients with advanced cirrhosis or who progress to end-stage liver disease are candidates for liver transplantation and should be referred to appropriate medical centers that provide liver transplantation services.

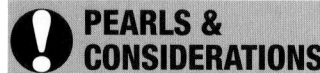

COMMENTS

- ANA and SMA are observed together in 60% of cases. Serum titers >1:40 suggest autoimmune hepatitis.
- A variety of autoimmune conditions can be seen in association with autoimmune hepatitis, including thyroiditis, Graves' disease, ulcerative colitis, rheumatoid arthritis, uveitis, pernicious anemia, Sjögren's syndrome, mixed connective tissue disease, CREST syndrome, and vitiligo.
- Variant forms of autoimmune hepatitis (overlap syndrome) have clinical and serologic findings of autoimmune hepatitis plus features of other forms of chronic liver disease such as primary biliary cirrhosis (PBC) or primary sclerosing cholangitis (PSC).

PREVENTION

None

PATIENT & FAMILY EDUCATION

- American Liver Foundation (ALF): Phone: 800-GO-LIVER (465-4837); Internet: www.liverfoundation.org
- National Digestive Diseases Information clearinghouse: http://digestive.niddk.nih.gov/ddiseases/pubs/autoimmunehep

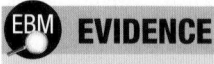

Available at www.expertconsult.com.

SUGGESTED READINGS

Available at www.expertconsult.com.

RELATED CONTENT

Autoimmune Hepatitis (Patient Information).

AUTHORS: **ANDREEA M. CATANA, M.D.,** and **KITTICHAI PROMRAT, M.D.**

BASIC INFORMATION

DEFINITION

Hepatocellular carcinoma (HCC) is a malignant neoplasm of the hepatocytes.

SYNONYMS

Hepatoma
HCC

ICD-10CM CODES
C22.0 Liver cell carcinoma

EPIDEMIOLOGY & DEMOGRAPHICS

HCC is the fifth most common cancer worldwide (~600,000 new cases/year) and third most common cause of cancer deaths. Incidence varies worldwide:

- Areas with high rates of hepatitis B and C (East Asia, sub-Saharan Africa) have highest incidence.
- Males more affected than females, with ratios between 2:1 and 4:1.
- Peak incidence: fifth and sixth decades in Western countries, earlier in areas with perinatal transmission of hepatitis B.
- Incidence is growing in the U.S. due to chronic hepatitis C, increasing obesity, and diabetes mellitus.
  1. During the past two decades, the incidence of HCC in the U.S. doubled. The greatest proportional increase has been among Hispanics and whites between 45 and 60 years of age.
  2. Mean age of diagnosis approximately 65 years.
  3. HCC is the fastest-rising cause of cancer-related deaths in the U.S.
- Risk factors:
  1. Chronic hepatitis B infection accounts for 50% of all cases and virtually all childhood cases.
  2. Chronic hepatitis C infection markers are found in 80% to 90% of patients with HCC in Japan and 30% to 50% in the U.S.
  3. Cirrhosis from other causes: alcoholic liver disease, nonalcoholic steatohepatitis, primary biliary cirrhosis, hemochromatosis, α1-antitrypsin deficiency, and autoimmune hepatitis.
  4. Hepatotoxins: aflatoxin B1.
  5. Systemic diseases affecting the liver: tyrosinemia.
  6. Obesity and diabetes mellitus.

PHYSICAL FINDINGS & CLINICAL PRESENTATION

- One third of patients are asymptomatic.
- Abdominal pain may be the initial presentation.
- Signs of underlying cirrhosis and portal hypertension are often present.
- Previously compensated cirrhosis with new ascites, encephalopathy, jaundice, or bleeding.
- Paraneoplastic syndromes (hypoglycemia, erythrocytosis, hypercalcemia, severe diarrhea, dermatomyositis) may be present.

DIAGNOSIS

DIFFERENTIAL DIAGNOSIS

- Metastatic cancers to liver
- Intrahepatic cholangiocarcinoma
- Benign liver neoplasms (adenomas, focal nodular hyperplasia, and hemangiomas)
- Focal fatty infiltration

WORKUP

- History regarding risk factors
- Physical examination with attention to signs of chronic liver disease
- Laboratory evaluation and imaging studies
- Imaging studies: ultrasound for initial testing; 3-phase CT scan or dynamic contrast-enhanced MRI

LABORATORY TESTS

- Liver function tests
- α-Fetoprotein (AFP) levels can be elevated in 70% of patients. An AFP level of 400 ng/mL or greater is highly suggestive of HCC; however, elevations may not be seen in up to 40% of patients with small lesions (1-2 cm).
- Paraneoplastic syndromes associated with HCC may cause hypercalcemia, hypoglycemia, and polycythemia
- Elevated serum HBV DNA level (≥10,000 copies/mL) is a strong risk predictor of HCC independent of HBeAg, serum aminotransferase level, and liver cirrhosis

IMAGING STUDIES

Ultrasound (US), CT scan (Fig. 1), or MRI. Ultrasound is most commonly used as a screening test for HCC in high-risk patients every 6 months. Fig. E2 shows a laparoscopic view of a cirrhotic liver with a nodular hepatoma.

The following imaging modalities are recommended based on US findings:

- Hepatic lesion <1 cm needs to be followed with a repeat US every 3 months to ensure the lesion does not change in size. If stable

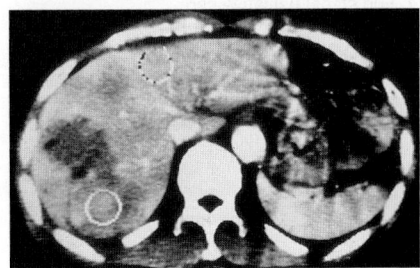

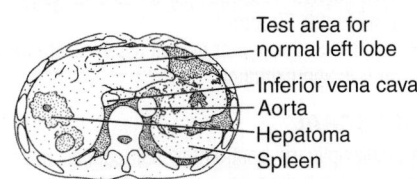

Test area for
normal left lobe
Inferior vena cava
Aorta
Hepatoma
Spleen

FIG. 1 Hepatoma. CT scan shows a diffuse lesion in the right lobe of an otherwise normal liver. (From Skarin AT: *Atlas of diagnostic oncology*, ed 3, St Louis, 2003, Mosby.)

for 24 months, the interval for US can be increased back to every 6 months.
- Hepatic lesion >1 cm needs further confirmatory imaging with either a CT scan or a MRI scan. If the chosen imaging modality shows characteristics typical of HCC (hypervascular in the arterial phase with washout in the portal venous or delayed phase) the diagnosis of HCC is confirmed with no need for additional diagnostic testing or biopsy. If the imaging modality is inconclusive or atypical for HCC then the alternate imaging test must be performed. If the second imaging modality is also inconclusive, an image-guided biopsy is recommended.

BIOPSY: Percutaneous biopsy under ultrasound or CT scan is obtained in the event that imaging studies are nondiagnostic or atypical for HCC, or if no cirrhosis is present. Negative biopsy results should be followed and the hepatic nodule reassessed every 3 to 6 months until it is no longer seen, enlarges, or shows diagnostic characteristics.

SCREENING: Screening high-risk patients with US every 6 months is currently recommended to identify early-stage HCC. The use of AFP in addition to US is debatable; though it does increase detection rate it also increases false-positive results. The use of AFP alone should be discouraged due to limited sensitivity and specificity. Patients on transplant waiting lists should be regularly screened for HCC because in the U.S. the development of HCC gives increased priority for liver transplantation. Screening for HCC is recommended in the following groups:

- Hepatitis B carriers (HBsAg positive): Asian males >40 years, Asian females >50 years, all cirrhotic hepatitis B carriers, family history of HCC and North American blacks/Africans older than age 20 years
- Cirrhosis (nonhepatitis B): hepatitis C, alcoholic cirrhosis, hemochromatosis, primary biliary cirrhosis, and possibly α1-antitrypsin deficiency, autoimmune hepatitis, and nonalcoholic steatohepatitis

STAGING: The commonly used Barcelona Clinic Liver Cancer (BCLC) staging system includes patient performance status, cancer symptoms, number and size of nodules, and liver function. Treatment is determined according to stage:

- Early stage (A): asymptomatic single tumor 5 cm or 3 nodules, each ≤3 cm
- Intermediate stage (B): patients with tumors that exceed early criteria but do not yet show cancer-related symptoms, vascular invasion, or metastases
- Advanced stage (C): patients with mild cancer-related symptoms and/or vascular invasion or extrahepatic spread
- End-stage (D): patients with advanced, symptomatic disease

TREATMENT

- Fig. 3 describes a treatment algorithm for HCC.
- Early stage: curative treatment (surgical resection or liver transplantation). Patients who have

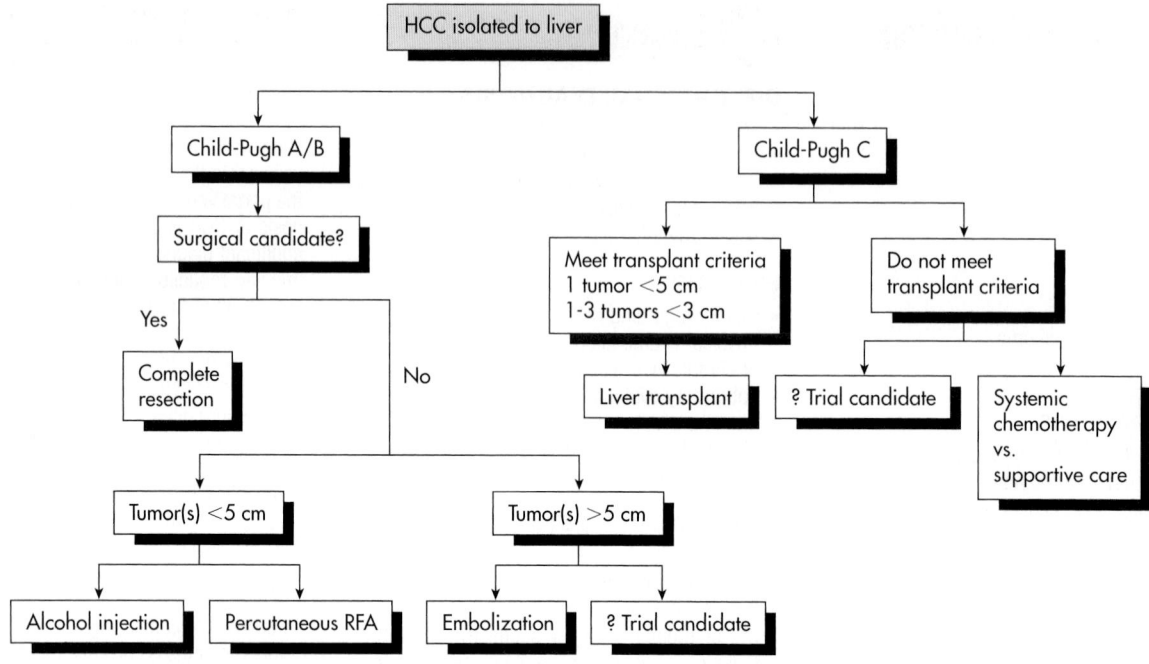

FIG. 3 Treatment algorithm for hepatocellular carcinoma (HCC). (From Bruix J, Sherman M. AASLD practice guideline. Management of hepatocellular carcinoma: an update. *Hepatology* 53(3):1020-1022, 2011.)

TABLE 1 Milan Criteria of Eligibility for Liver Transplantation

Presence of a tumor ≤5 cm in diameter in patients with single hepatocellular carcinomas
Or
≤3 tumor nodules, each 3 cm or less in diameter, in patients with multiple tumors

From Cameron JL, Cameron AM: *Current surgical therapy*, ed 10, Philadelphia, 2011, Saunders.

a single lesion can be offered surgical resection if they are non-cirrhotic or have cirrhosis with well-preserved liver function, normal bilirubin, and no significant portal hypertension. Liver transplantation is an effective option for patients with HCC corresponding to the Milan criteria (Table 1). Living donor transplantation can be offered for HCC if the waiting time is expected to be long. Local ablation is safe and effective therapy for patients who cannot undergo resection or as a bridge to transplantation. With these options, survival at 5 year ranges from 50% to 70%. Radiofrequency ablation (RFA) is used in patients with early HCC who are not surgical candidates, and very high local control rates at 2 years are obtained (>90%), but eventual recurrence rates can approach 70% at 5 years.
- Intermediate stage: Transarterial chemoembolization (TACE) is recommended as first-line, noncurative therapy for nonsurgical patients with large/multifocal HCC who do not have vascular invasion or extrahepatic spread. More recently, transarterial use of selective internal radiation therapy (SIRT) with yttrium-90 radio-labeled glass microspheres is an alternative to traditional TACE approaches in this setting. Median survivals exceed 2 years.
- Advanced stage: Palliative therapy or clinical trials are used in this stage. Sorafenib, an oral multikinase inhibitor, is the standard of care and has been shown to improve overall survival.

The effectiveness has been demonstrated in patients with Child-Pugh A cirrhosis and the greatest benefit is seen in patients with hepatitis C related HCC. A recent trial demonstrated a survival benefit with the use of regorafenib, an oral multikinase inhibitor, in patients who progressed after receiving sorafenib. Doxorubicin chemotherapy may be considered, although survival benefits are unclear.
- End stage: palliative care.

DISPOSITION
- For resectable HCC, the 5-year survival after liver transplantation is 50% to 70% and 30% to 50% with surgical resection. For unresectable HCC, the overall prognosis is poor.
- Tumor size is an independent prognostic factor for resected small HCC (≤50 mm in diameter). Patients with tumors of 0-35 mm diameter have a better 60-month HCC specific survival rate than do those with larger tumors (36-50 mm).[1]
- In the U.S. the 5-year overall survival rate for HCC is approximately 10%.

REFERRAL
Multidisciplinary gastrointestinal cancer team for treatment planning

[1]Zhang W, et al.: Effect of Tumor Size on Cancer-Specific Survival in Small Hepatocellular Carcinoma, *Mayo Clin Proc* 90(9):1187–1195, 2015.

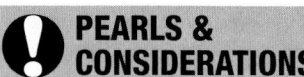 **PEARLS & CONSIDERATIONS**

PREVENTION
- Universal hepatitis B vaccination in children in endemic areas has been shown to decrease the incidence of HCC.
- Treatment of patients with chronic hepatitis B–associated cirrhosis with lamivudine reduces the incidence of HCC. Treatment with entecavir in chronic hepatitis B-HCC can improve hepatic function and MELD score.
- Treatment with interferon-based therapy in patients with noncirrhotic hepatitis C reduces risk of HCC in patients demonstrating a sustained viral response
- HCC screening is recommended in high-risk patients because curative therapies are available only for small and early HCC.
- Patients diagnosed with HCC with an AFP >1000 are at increased risk for recurrence after transplantation regardless of tumor size.
- There are numerous ongoing trials with tyrosine kinase inhibitors and monoclonal antibodies for advanced HCC in patients who are intolerant or resistant to sorafenib. The future of therapy for advanced HCC will likely lead to the personalized combination of multiple agents targeting different oncogenic pathways to optimize treatment success.

SUGGESTED READINGS
Available at www.expertconsult.com

RELATED CONTENT
Liver Cancer (Patient Information)

AUTHOR: **BHARTI RATHORE, M.D.**

BASIC INFORMATION

DEFINITION

Hepatopulmonary syndrome (HPS) is characterized by intrapulmonary vascular dilation in the setting of liver disease causing an increased alveolar-arterial (A-a) gradient.

SYNONYMS

HPS

ICD-10CM CODES
K76.81 Hepatopulmonary syndrome

EPIDEMIOLOGY & DEMOGRAPHICS

PREVALENCE: Between 5% and 30% of patients with cirrhosis; wide range due to lack of diagnostic criteria.
PREDOMINANT SEX AND AGE: There are no data on gender or age prevalence.
RISK FACTORS: Can occur with any degree or etiology of liver disease but is more common in patients with established cirrhosis and portal hypertension. There is no clear relationship between severity of hepatic dysfunction and level of hypoxemia. One recent study suggests that HPS is more common in patients with history of viral hepatitis than in patients with alcoholic cirrhosis.
GENETICS: There are new data suggesting that genes involved in the regulation of angiogenesis are associated with the risk of HPS.

PHYSICAL FINDINGS & CLINICAL PRESENTATION

- Dyspnea.
- Platypnea: worsened dyspnea when sitting upright compared with supine position due to further ventilation-perfusion mismatch.
- Orthodeoxia: decreased Pao_2 when the patient is sitting upright compared with supine position due to ventilation-perfusion mismatch.
- Spider angiomata seen in high number.
- Signs of severe hypoxemia (e.g., cyanosis and clubbing of the digits).

ETIOLOGY

Dilation of intrapulmonary arterioles and dilated vascular channels between pulmonary arteries and veins leading to a ventilation-perfusion mismatch and right-to-left shunting (Fig. E1). Research shows that nitric oxide plays a role in vasodilation. The relationship of vasodilation to liver disease is unclear. New areas of research include endothelin-1, which is produced by proliferating cholangiocytes, pulmonary angiogenesis, and opiate receptors' influence on NO production.

DIAGNOSIS

DIFFERENTIAL DIAGNOSIS

- Portopulmonary hypertension.
- Cavopulmonary anastomosis.
- Hereditary hemorrhagic telangiectasia (Rendu-Osler-Weber syndrome).
- Chronic lung disease (i.e., COPD or pulmonary fibrosis) with coexisting liver disease.

WORKUP

- Diagnosis should be suspected in patients with cirrhosis who develop hypoxemia in absence of other causes (e.g., COPD, thromboembolism).
- Workup includes lab testing and imaging studies (see following), but diagnosis is based on clinical findings.

LABORATORY TESTS

- Arterial blood gas at rest, both supine and erect; Pao_2 <80 mm Hg.
- Pulmonary function tests will show nonspecific reduction in DLco.

There is new evidence showing that blood testing for elevated von Willenbrand factor antigen is a good screening test for HPS because it is a surrogate marker for endothelial dysfunction.

IMAGING STUDIES

- The most effective screening tool is transthoracic echocardiogram with bubble study to rule out right-to-left cardiac shunt; microbubble opacification in left atrium shows vasodilation of pulmonary vascular bed.
- Chest x-ray may show nonspecific bibasilar interstitial pattern.
- Scintigraphic perfusion scanning: technetium-99m–labeled albumin found in brain or spleen indicates dilated pulmonary vasculature or cardiac right-to-left shunt.
- Pulmonary angiography rarely used unless there is potential to embolize arteriovenous malformation (AVM).

TREATMENT

Ideal treatment would be targeted against pulmonary vasodilation. Most medications have targeted NO production, the activity of NO synthase or endothelin-1, pulmonary angiogenesis, or even bacterial translocation, but no controlled trials exist. Liver transplantation is the only successful treatment, which leads to improvement in gas exchange or complete resolution in gas exchange in the majority of patients. However, severe hypoxemia with Pao_2 <50 has been associated with a high posttransplant mortality. Some studies have shown benefit of transjugular portosystemic shunting, although it is not currently established treatment. Coil embolization in the setting of pulmonary AVMs is another possible area of treatment.

NONPHARMACOLOGIC THERAPY

Oxygen to correct hypoxemia; Pao_2 will partially correct with administration of supplemental O_2.

ACUTE GENERAL Rx

Correct hypoxemia with supplemental O_2.

CHRONIC Rx

Liver transplantation is the only successful treatment; the majority of patients show improvement in oxygenation at 1 year post transplant. There are some data showing worse outcomes for patients with severe HPS (PaO_2 <50%), but mortality appears to be improving.

COMPLEMENTARY & ALTERNATIVE MEDICINE

One study suggested that garlic supplements might decrease A-a gradient in patients with HPS. Studies of diets containing low amount of L-arginine have not shown benefit.

DISPOSITION

The diagnosis of HPS confers a poor prognosis. Patients with HPS have high mortality and shorter median survival than other patients with liver disease, even after adjusting for severity of liver disease. According to one natural history study, compared with patients with similar severity of liver disease and comorbidities whose 5-yr survival was estimated at 63%, those patients with the diagnosis of HPS had a 5-yr survival rate of 23%.

REFERRAL

- Referral to pulmonologist to help in establishing diagnosis.
- Referral to a liver transplant center.

PEARLS & CONSIDERATIONS

COMMENTS

Consider the diagnosis of HPS in patients with cirrhosis who present with dyspnea without signs of pulmonary edema from fluid overload.

SUGGESTED READING

Available at www.expertconsult.com.

RELATED CONTENT

Cirrhosis (Related Key Topic)

AUTHOR: **SAMAAN RAFEQ, M.D.**

BASIC INFORMATION

DEFINITION

Hepatorenal syndrome (HRS) is a functional cause of acute kidney injury that occurs in patients with severe acute or chronic liver disease, most commonly with advanced cirrhosis and portal hypertension. In HRS, severe liver dysfunction leads to increased production or activity of vasodilators. Vasodilation is most pronounced in the splanchnic circulation, resulting in systemic hypotension that ultimately is unable to be reversed due to cardiac dysfunction. Homeostatic responses lead to intense renal vasoconstriction, renal cortical hypoperfusion, and a decline in kidney function (see Fig. 1).

There are two types of HRS (see Table 1):
1. Type 1: acute and rapid deterioration in kidney function (serum creatinine >2.5 mg/dl (220 μmol/L) in <2 weeks
2. Type 2: moderate stable kidney impairment (average serum creatinine 2 mg/dl [176 μmol/L])

SYNONYMS

Hepatorenal failure
Hepatic nephropathy
Oliguric renal failure of cirrhosis

ICD-10CM CODES
K76.7　Hepatorenal syndrome, hepatorenal failure
Z87.19　History of hepatorenal syndrome
Z84.1　Family history of hepatorenal syndrome

EPIDEMIOLOGY & DEMOGRAPHICS

The probability of HRS in cirrhotic patients is 18% at 1 year and 39% at 5 years. HRS is associated with poor prognosis. HRS type 1 is associated with >90% mortality in 3 months, and HRS type 2 is associated with 30% mortality in 3 months and 60% in 1 year. The cause of liver failure or the model for end-stage liver disease (MELD) score does not predict the development of HRS, although dilutional hyponatremia is an independent risk factor.

PHYSICAL FINDINGS & CLINICAL PRESENTATION

There are no specific physical findings associated with HRS, although it is usually associated with signs and symptoms of acute or chronic decompensated liver failure, such as hypotension, jaundice, spider angiomas, splenomegaly, ascites, fetor hepaticus, pedal edema, asterixis, encephalopathy, or coma. Usually, HRS is associated with oliguria and a bland urine sediment. However, a nonoliguric state or an active urine sediment (blood and/or protein) does not exclude the diagnosis of HRS.

PRECIPITANTS

Precipitating events are identified in 70% to 100% of cases of HRS. Contributory factors include bacterial infection, alcoholic hepatitis, gastrointestinal bleeding, or large-volume paracentesis without albumin administration. By definition, overdiuresis does not cause HRS, because HRS is a condition in which volume depletion is not present or has been treated appropriately (see "Treatment"). Unlike HRS, prerenal azotemia, irrespective of its etiology (diuresis or other fluid removal), improves with cessation of diuretic therapy and/or volume resuscitation. Nevertheless, HRS may present in the absence of a clear precipitating factor.

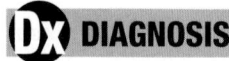 DIAGNOSIS

HRS is a diagnosis of exclusion. Tables 2 and 3 summarize the revised diagnostic criteria for HRS.

DIFFERENTIAL DIAGNOSIS

- Prerenal azotemia: must be excluded or treated appropriately before establishing a diagnosis of HRS. Prerenal azotemia typically responds to volume expansion and cessation of diuretic therapy. Both prerenal conditions and HRS are often associated with low fractional excretions of sodium (FENa) <1%.
- Acute tubular necrosis: urine sodium >30 mEq/L, FENa >1.5%, urine-to-plasma creatinine ratio <30, urine-to-plasma osmolality ratio = 1; urine sediment reveals brown casts and cellular debris, without significant response to sustained plasma expansion.
- Other: Renal artery or vein thrombosis, cardiorenal syndrome, urinary tract obstruction, glomerulonephritis, and toxicity from drugs, organic solvents, heavy metals, heme pigments, and intravenous contrast medium.

WORKUP

Acute azotemia and oliguria in the setting of liver disease requires laboratory evaluation to differentiate HRS from acute tubular necrosis.

TABLE 1　Definition of hepatorenal syndrome.

Type 1

Acute and rapid deterioration in kidney function (serum creatinine >2.5 mg/dl (220 μmol/l) in <2 weeks.

Occurs in parallel with the failure of other organs or systems (e.g., coagulopathy, hepatic encephalopathy).

In cirrhosis, is a form of acute-on-chronic liver failure.

Frequently follows a precipitating event, mainly bacterial infection; rapidly fatal without treatment: mean survival 2 to 3 weeks.

Type 2

Moderate stable renal impairment (average serum creatinine 2 mg/dl [176 μmol/l]).

Mainly causes refractory ascites.

Mean survival without treatment: 6 months.

From Fernández J, Arroyo V: Hepatorenal syndrome. *In* Johnson RJ et al (eds): *Comprehensive clinical nephrology*, ed 5, Philadelphia, 2015, Saunders, pp. 873-882.

TABLE 2　Revised diagnostic criteria for hepatorenal syndrome.

Cirrhosis with ascites.

Serum creatinine >1.5 mg/dl (133 μmol/L).

No improvement in serum creatinine (decrease to a level of 1.5 mg/dl) after at least 2 days with diuretic withdrawal and volume expansion with albumin. The recommended dose of albumin is 1 g/kg of body weight per day up to a maximum of 100 g/day.

Absence of shock.

No current or recent treatment with nephrotoxic drugs.

Absence of parenchymal kidney disease as indicated by proteinuria >500 mg/day, microhematuria (>50 red blood cells per high-power field), and/or abnormal kidney ultrasound.

From Fernández J, Arroyo V: Hepatorenal syndrome. *In* Johnson RJ et al (eds): *Comprehensive clinical nephrology*, ed 5, Philadelphia, 2015, Saunders, pp. 873-882.

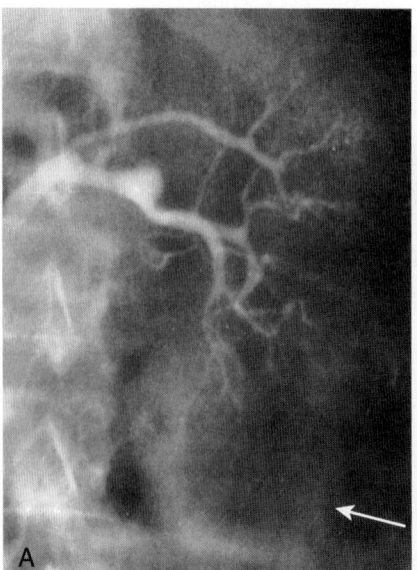 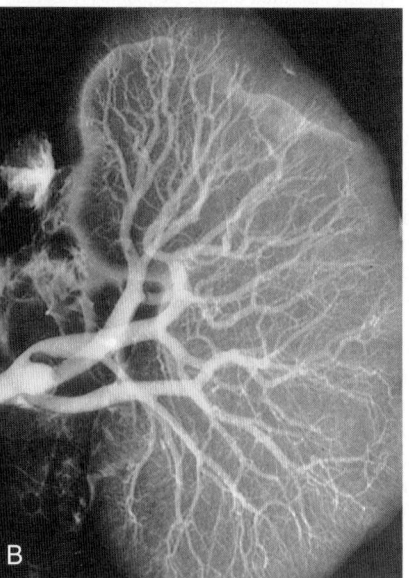

FIG. 1 Circulatory dysfunction in hepatorenal syndrome (HRS). **A,** Renal angiogram (the *arrow* marks edge of the kidney). **B,** The angiogram carried out in the same kidney at autopsy. Note complete filling of the renal arterial system throughout the vascular bed to the periphery of the cortex. The vascular attenuation and tortuosity seen previously (**A**) are no longer present. The vessels are also histologically normal. This indicates the functional nature of the vascular abnormality in HRS. (From Floege J et al: *Comprehensive clinical nephrology*, ed 4, St Louis, 2010, Saunders.)

TABLE 3 Pharmacologic options in the treatment of hepatorenal syndrome.

- **Terlipressin + albumin***: Terlipressin: 1 mg/4-6 h to start, increasing to a maximum of 2 mg/4-6 h if serum creatinine decreases <25% at day 3. Terlipressin can also be administered as continuous infusion. Treatment is maintained until serum creatinine has decreased below 1.5 mg/dl (133 μmol/L). Maximum duration of treatment: 14 days.
- **Norepinephrine + albumin***: Norepinephrine: IV infusion at 0.5 mg/h to start, increasing the dose by 0.25 to 0.5 mg/h every 4 hours up to a maximum of 3 mg/h to achieve an increase in mean arterial pressure (MAP) of at least 10 mm Hg. Maximum duration of treatment: 14 days.
- **Vasopressin + albumin***: Vasopressin: IV infusion at 0.01 units/min to start, increasing the dose upward to a maximum of 0.8 units/min to achieve an increase in MAP of at least 10 mm Hg. Maximum duration of treatment: 11 days.
- **Midodrine + octreotide + albumin***: Oral midodrine 2.5 to 7.5 mg/8 h + subcutaneous octreotide 100 μg/8 h to start, increasing midodrine dose to a maximum of 12.5-15 mg/8 h and octreotide dose to a maximum of 200 μg/8 h to achieve an increase in MAP of at least 15 mm Hg. Maximum duration is not defined.

*Albumin: 1 g/kg on day 1 (up to 100 g) followed by 20 to 40 g/day. Central venous pressure monitoring is advised (but not mandatory) to achieve a value of 10 to 15 mm Hg.
From Fernández J, Arroyo V: Hepatorenal syndrome. *In* Johnson RJ et al (eds): *Comprehensive clinical nephrology*, ed 5, Philadelphia, 2015, Saunders, pp. 873-882.

Extracellular fluid volume challenge may be required to differentiate HRS from prerenal azotemia. Rule out concurrent bacterial infection. Serum creatinine and BUN are poorly sensitive markers of kidney function in cirrhosis.

LABORATORY TESTS

- Serum electrolytes (serum sodium <135 mEq/L), blood urea nitrogen, creatinine, osmolality.
- Urinalysis, urine sodium, creatinine, osmolality.
- FENa will not adequately differentiate HRS from other common etiologies associated with acute kidney injury in liver dysfunction. Only a minority of patients with HRS have high urine sodium concentrations.
- Urine sodium <10 mEq/L, FENa <1%, urine-to-plasma creatinine ratio >30, urine plasma-to-urine osmolality ratio >1.5, bland urine sediment.

IMAGING STUDIES

Kidney, bladder, and ureter ultrasound may be indicated if obstructive uropathy is suspected. CT scan may be required to diagnose occult infection(s), and prophylaxis directed at preventing contrast-induced nephropathy is recommended.

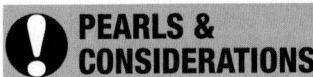 **TREATMENT**

ACUTE GENERAL Rx

- Avoidance of precipitating factors and their appropriate therapy are cornerstones of HRS management.
- Primary prophylaxis of spontaneous bacterial peritonitis with norfloxacin has recently been shown to prevent or delay the development of HRS.
- Improvement in liver function due to partial resolution of the primary disorder or successful liver transplantation is the optimal treatment. Liver transplantation leads to resolution of HRS type 1 in 76% of cases.
- Splanchnic vasoconstrictor agents (e.g., terlipressin, norepinephrine, midodrine).
- Ornipressin prevents further deterioration of kidney function in patients awaiting liver transplantation.
- Dopamine and prostaglandins are generally ineffective in treating patients with HRS.

PHARMACOLOGIC THERAPY

Most therapy is centered on the use of vasoconstrictor therapy and albumin resuscitation targeted at the reversal of splanchnic arterial vasodilation. Table 3 summarizes the commonly used regimens.

NONPHARMACOLOGIC THERAPY

- Liver transplantation
- Transjugular, intrahepatic, or portosystemic shunts
- Extracorporeal liver support therapy as a bridge to liver transplantation

REFERRAL

- Referral for hepatology, nephrology, and liver transplantation as indicated (see "Comments")

⚠ PEARLS & CONSIDERATIONS

COMMENTS

- Liver transplantation may be indicated in an otherwise healthy patient (age, preferably <65 years) with sclerosing cholangitis, chronic hepatitis with cirrhosis, or primary biliary cirrhosis. Contraindications to liver transplantation are AIDS, most metastatic malignancies, active alcohol and substance abuse, uncontrolled sepsis, and uncontrolled cardiac or pulmonary disease.
- Recurrence rates of HRS after successful treatment are variable and tend to be more common in type 2 (around 50%) than in type 1 HRS (20%).

SUGGESTED READINGS
Available at www.expertconsult.com

RELATED CONTENT
Hepatorenal Syndrome (Patient Information)

AUTHORS: **NAUSHABA ISHRATH KHALID, M.D.,** and **JAMES E. NOVAK, M.D., PH.D.**

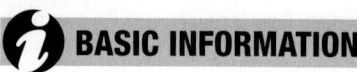

BASIC INFORMATION

DEFINITION

Hereditary breast and ovarian cancer syndrome patients carry a significant cancer-associated alteration in the *BRCA1* or *BRCA2* gene. These genetic mutations can confer a heightened risk of malignancy in the breast, ovary, fallopian tube, peritoneum, and endometrium of the uterus in women, and an elevated risk of prostate and breast cancer in men. Pancreatic cancer and skin cancer are elevated for both men and women. The risk for that particular cancer is significantly greater than the risk associated with the general population or with one's personal and/or family cancer history. Frequently, a cancer that is associated with a heritable genetic mutation presents at a younger age than that seen in the general population and/or affects multiple same-side family members. Identifying carriers can significantly reduce the morbidity and mortality of the patient and her/his close family members.

SYNONYMS

Hereditary breast and ovarian cancer syndrome (HBOC)
Lynch syndrome/hereditary nonpolyposis colorectal cancer (HNPCC)
Hereditary cancer syndrome

ICD-10CM CODES
Z84.81	Family history of carrier of genetic disease
Z80.3	Family history of malignant neoplasm of breast
Z80.41	Family history of malignant neoplasm of ovary
Z80.49	Family history of malignant neoplasm of other genital organs (uterus, vagina, for example)
Z15.01	Genetic susceptibility to malignant neoplasm of breast
Z15.02	Genetic susceptibility to malignant neoplasm of ovary

EPIDEMIOLOGY & DEMOGRAPHICS

INCIDENCE: Overall, an estimated 6% to 10% of gynecologic cancers are heritable. Approximately 7% to 10% of the estimated 235,000 new breast cancer cases are likely to be hereditary. Inherited *BRCA 1, 2* mutations account for an estimated 11% to 15% of ovarian cancer cases. Less than 1% of the general population has a mutation in the *BRCA 1* or *2* gene. Lynch syndrome–associated mutations increase ovarian and uterine cancer as well as colorectal cancer (up to 5% of colorectal cancers are considered heritable) and pancreatic and gastric cancers. This topic will, however, focus on gynecologic disease.

PREDOMINANT SEX AND AGE: Although predominantly females are affected, males who carry deleterious mutations in *BRCA 1, 2* are at a significantly higher risk for cancer. Both sexes can transmit the altered gene to their offspring.

GENETICS: Autosomal dominant transmission pattern. A child whose parent has a *BRCA* mutation has a 50% chance of inheriting that genetic mutation.

RISK FACTORS: BRCA 1 and 2 mutations can generate a greater risk of breast cancer than other such well-established factors as increased breast density, history of atypical ductal or lobular hyperplasia, nulliparity, obesity, and family history.

Up to 37% of breast cancer patients and 100% of ovarian/tubal/peritoneal cancer patients are at risk for hereditary breast and ovarian cancer syndrome.

Hereditary Breast and Ovarian Cancer Syndrome (HBOC):
- Individuals with *BRCA1, BRCA2* mutations (Fig. 1)
- Red flags for HBOC include personal or family history of (not an exhaustive list):
  ○ Personal breast cancer diagnosed at ≤45 years old
  ○ Triple-negative breast cancer (ER-, PR-, Her2-)
  ○ Ovarian cancer—very important factor (mostly papillary serous)
  ○ Male breast cancer
  ○ Two primary breast cancers
  ○ Ashkenazi Jewish ancestry
  ○ Breast cancer with ≥2 relatives with an HBOC-associated cancer (breast, ovary, prostate, pancreatic cancers)
  ○ A previously identified HBOC mutation
  ○ Two or more close relatives with breast cancer <50 years old
  ○ Three or more HBOC-associated cancers at any age

Note:
1. One half of *BRCA* carriers inherit the mutation from their father.
2. Early onset of cancer may be a more important red flag than the number of affected family members, especially if the number of family members is small to begin with.
3. Testing criteria, as per National Comprehensive Cancer Network (NCCN) guidelines, may differ from the red flags noted previously.
4. Family history extends to first-, second-, and third-degree relatives.
5. Consider Lynch syndrome–associated cancers (e.g., colorectal, gastric, brain, small bowel, skin, ureter, renal pelvis, GI polyps), as Lynch syndrome is associated also with ovarian and uterine (endometrial) cancer.
6. BRCA stands for BReast CAncer.
- The majority (84%) of the approximately 7% of breast cancers and 14% of ovarian cancers that result from a heritable mutation are due to a *BRCA1* (52%) and *BRCA2* (32%) gene mutation.
- By age 70, in comparison to the 7.3% risk of breast cancer in the general population, or approximately double that risk if one has an affected first-degree relative, *BRCA1* and *BRCA2* mutation carriers have up to an 87% reported risk of developing breast cancer. As opposed to a general-population risk of 2% for developing a second breast primary within 5 years of a first diagnosis, women with HBOC mutations have a 12% to 27% risk. This risk climbs to a reported 50% (*BRCA2*) and up to 64% (*BRCA1*) by age 70.
- By age 70, in contrast to the 0.7% risk of ovarian cancer in the general population, there is a reported risk of up to 27% to 44% for *BRCA2* and *BRCA1* mutation carriers, respectively. The risk for ovarian cancer within 10 years of a breast cancer diagnosis is 6.8% (*BRCA2*) to 12.7% (*BRCA1*) as opposed to a general-population risk of less than 1.0%.
- Men with HBOC have an up to tenfold increased risk for breast cancer and a more than twofold increase in prostate cancer in comparison to the general-population risk.

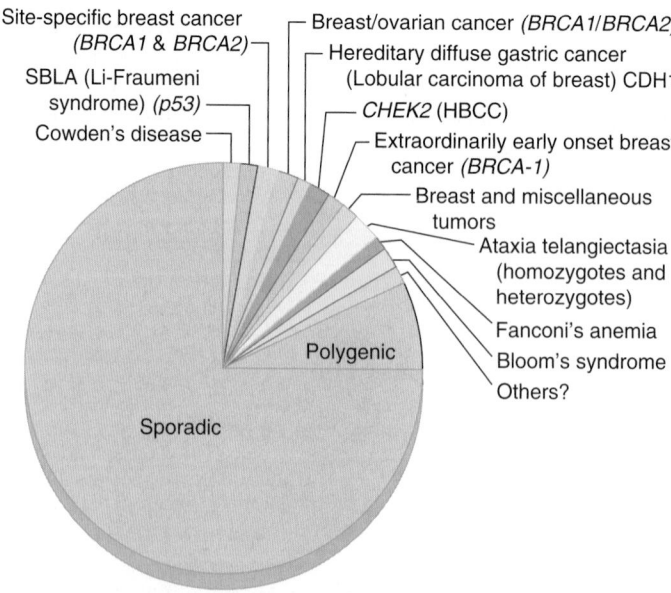

FIG 1 Schematic depicting heterogeneity in breast cancer. *HBCC*, hereditary breast and colorectal cancer; *SBLA*, sarcoma, breast and brain tumors, leukemia, laryngeal and lung cancer, and adrenal cortical carcinoma. (From Goldman L, Schafer AI: *Goldman's Cecil medicine*, ed 24, Philadelphia, 2012, Saunders.)

In men, the *BRCA2* mutation increases the cancer risk more than the *BRCA1* mutation. In fact, the breast cancer risk for a male with a *BRCA2* mutation is up to 80 times the risk seen in the general population.

- Both men and women have an elevated risk (up to sevenfold) for pancreatic cancer (*BRCA2* >1) and for melanoma (2.5-fold increase with *BRCA2*).
- Ashkenazi Jewish ancestry is associated with founder mutations 187delAG (*BRCA1*), 5382insC (*BRCA1*), and 6174delT (*BRCA2*), which confer a significantly elevated risk for breast and ovarian cancer. As opposed to the 1 in 300 risk in the general population, 1 in 40 individuals of Ashkenazi Jewish descent have a *BRCA 1* or *2* mutation.

Lynch Syndrome (Hereditary Nonpolyposis Colorectal Cancer)

- Individuals with *MLH1, MSH2, MSH6, PMS2, EPCAM* mutations
- By age 70, Lynch syndrome carriers have—in addition to an increased risk for colorectal, gastric, hepatobiliary, urinary tract, small bowel, brain, skin, and pancreatic cancers—up to an approximately twentyfold increase in ovarian cancer (4%-12% risk vs. the general-population risk of 0.7%) and up to an approximately fortyfold increase in uterine cancer (25%-60+% risk vs. the general-population risk of 1.6%).
- The previously listed genes and others (e.g., *PTEN, TP53, CDH1, STK11*) that are found less frequently and carry a lower lifetime risk of cancer are considered high-penetrance genes, as they can increase the relative risk of their respective syndromes by greater than four- to fivefold.
- Other, more moderate-penetrant genes (e.g., *CHEK2, ATM, PALB2, BRIP1, RAD51C, RAD51D*), that is, those that are associated with a two- to fourfold increase in the relative risk of cancer, should be considered when assessing risk and ordering genetic tests.
- More than 12 known gene mutations are associated with an elevated risk for breast cancer, and a similar number are associated with an elevated risk for ovarian cancer. As such, screening for *BRCA 1, 2* alone will miss these mutations.
- Deleterious mismatch repair gene mutations and those gene alterations that are categorized in the literature as emerging risk mutations are also associated with hereditary gynecologic and other cancers.

PHYSICAL FINDINGS & CLINICAL PRESENTATION

- Present at a younger age
- Bilaterality more likely
- Multiple primaries in one individual

ETIOLOGY

- Hereditary cancers are typically due to a genetic mutation in a tumor suppression gene that interferes with DNA repair and allows an otherwise potentially avoidable

cancer to develop. This is distinct from familial cancers in which there is no isolated gene mutation but, nonetheless, cancers appear in the family to a degree more than that which would be statistically seen in the general population. Nongenetic factors such as lifestyle habits and environmental influences contribute to cancer risk as well.

Dx DIAGNOSIS

DIFFERENTIAL DIAGNOSIS

- General (sporadic) population or familial basis for the cancer in question
- Hereditary cancer is more likely to present at a younger age, to span a number of generations, to affect more family members than would be expected (if a large enough family), especially in a suspicious pattern, and to include some rare (ovary, male breast cancer, for example) presentations.
- In addition to the more common syndromes listed previously, consider Cowden (*PTEN*), Peutz-Jeghers (*STK11*), Li-Fraumeni (*TP53*), and others.

WORKUP

- Family history questionnaire, patient and family interviews, genetic counseling/risk assessment (including tools such as Tyrer-Cuzick/Gail/Claus models), and tailored genetic testing.

LABORATORY TESTS

- A simple blood or saliva sample drawn in the office or a lab, after informed consent, is needed. This specimen should be sent to a reliable laboratory recognized nationally for its genetic cancer testing accuracy (technologic and interpretation), reporting format, and the support staff ability and availability for consultation and office counseling and testing integration. Look for a laboratory that has published peer-reviewed data and has an accurate classification methodology that relies on an extensive database. Realize that these labs are not FDA approved and that CLIA certification, while needed, relies on just in-house data. Remember also that most patients get tested only once in their lifetime.
- Options include:
  - Syndrome specific: for example, HBOC-BRCA testing (including large rearrangement detection); Lynch syndrome; founder mutation testing (187delAG, 5382insC, 6174delT); Ashkenazi Jewish population (often recommended as the first test for this population); single-site testing (if a previously identified gene mutation is known in the family); cancer specific, for example, breast cancer panel–*BRCA 1, 2* with/without reflex to broader panel (i.e., sequential testing).
  - Comprehensive panel testing (can include HBOC syndrome *BRCA1, BRCA2*), Lynch syndrome (*MLH1, MSH2, MSH6, PMS2, EPCAM*), Li-Fraumeni (*TP53*), Cowden (*PTEN*), Peutz-Jeghers (*STK11*), *PALB2*,

CHEK2, ATM, BRIP1, RAD51C, and others [upward of 25+ genes]).

- Choice of the test is generally based on personal/family history, although thoroughness of the risk assessment may be limited by attempting to choose a gene test based on history/phenotype alone.
- Comprehensive panel testing has been shown to increase mutation detection and to aid in test selection when patients qualify for more than one syndrome/cancer-specific test, or it can be used to capture a potentially broader view of risk. There is a concern, however, for detecting mutations that are not clinically actionable.
- Categories of results include positive or negative for a deleterious mutation or a genetic variant of uncertain significance, in which a cancer risk is not yet established or ruled out. It is critical that the classification of these variants is accurate.
- Markers such as CA-125 may be clinically helpful.

IMAGING STUDIES

- Screening transvaginal ultrasonography, annual mammography, annual MRI (when breast cancer risk is 20% or more based on Tyrer-Cuzick or other breast cancer screening models)

Rx TREATMENT/RISK REDUCTION

- Heightened surveillance, judicious chemoprevention, and prophylactic surgery have been associated with improved outcomes.
- Surveillance includes patient breast awareness, clinical breast exam, mammography, MRI, transvaginal ultrasonography, and CA-125 blood testing, for example.
- Chemopreventive approaches have been shown to reduce the risk of ovarian cancer by 60% (with an oral contraceptive) and risk of contralateral breast cancer by as much as 53% (with tamoxifen).
- In HBOC patients, prophylactic total mastectomy can reduce the risk for breast cancer by 90%, and a bilateral salpingo-oophorectomy, after childbearing or by age 40, can reduce the risk of ovarian cancer by up to 96% and the risk of breast cancer by up to 68%.
- Consider preimplantation genetic diagnosis in conjunction with in vitro fertilization.

REFERRAL

- If services are needed beyond one's practice or comfort level, consider consulting with genetic counselors, gynecologists, gynecologic oncologists, breast surgeons, and gastroenterology specialists, among others.

PEARLS & CONSIDERATIONS

- Be vigilant. Be motivated by the risks: Women with these mutations are approximately 10 times more likely to develop breast cancer and 20 to 30 times more likely to develop ovarian cancer. Look for red flags during every encounter, regardless of the patient's chief complaint or scheduled visit type, and inquire and update information about the patient's personal and family history of cancer. Consider that approximately 10% of general practice patients have a significant family history. Supply a printed family history questionnaire. Always consider your patient's cancer risk, especially when charting a new treatment course or planning a surgical procedure. Oftentimes, a more comprehensive approach may be taken if a patient proves to be a mutation carrier.

- Adjust the age at which screening/treatment is initiated and the frequency of the visits depending on the age of the youngest affected family member, the at-risk cancer site, and the carrier status of the patient.
- Encourage input from the patient during the screening, workup, follow-up, and treatment.
- Recommend that the patient verify any questionable family history, collect appropriate family documentation/testing, and involve her family in the process; this involvement can include advising counseling and testing for close relatives.
- Try to counsel and test (if appropriate) the family member(s) who, if tested, would render testing of progeny/other family members less necessary. Testing an affected family member is oftentimes the most appropriate, efficient, cost-effective, and informative approach.
- Genetic testing can more accurately predict risk and enable a more tailored management approach than relying on one's family history alone. Be mindful that there may be other, although as yet unidentified, mutations at the root of one's patient's personal or family cancer history.
- Refer to your professional societies and the NCCN for screening and surveillance/imaging/treatment guidelines. Don't hesitate to engage the assistance of a genetic counselor, gynecologist, oncologist, breast surgeon, and/or a gastroenterologist during this initial phase.

- Involve other appropriate specialists in the patient's short- and long-term care, depending on the at-risk anatomic systems.
- Remember that *BRCA1*- and *BRCA2*-positive men are at a significantly higher risk for breast and prostate cancer.
- Consider prophylactic bilateral mastectomy or bilateral salpingo-oophorectomy.
- Encourage high-risk patients to complete childbearing at a younger age and consider, as appropriate, subsequent prophylactic bilateral salpingo-oophorectomy and menopause hormone therapy options.
- Recommend prophylactic salpingectomy for at-risk patients during any other surgical procedure—once childbearing is complete. Consider such assistive reproductive options as preimplantation genetic diagnosis.
- Genetic information cannot be used as the basis for a "preexisting condition" with regard to health insurance or employment, according to federal and state laws. It may play a role in life insurance, disability insurance, and long-term care insurance.
- While insurance coverage generally is available, panel testing reimbursement may occasionally be challenged. Vocalize and document your support of the appropriate testing and management, with both your patient and her/his insurance company. Enlist the assistance of your local professional society, as needed.
- There may be a medical-legal risk if a failure to identify and/or genetically counsel or test a high-risk patient and/or her family results in a delay in the diagnosis of breast or ovarian cancer. The provider, laboratory, insurance company, and the employer may have legal exposure for failing to order testing, for providing inaccurate results, or for denial of coverage, respectively.
- Being aware of a patient's cancer risk facilitates initiation of those preventive screenings and management strategies that have been shown to reduce the likelihood of cancer and improve early cancer detection rates. This can be of tremendous benefit for the patient's family members as well as the patient.

PREVENTION

Consider appropriate screening and surveillance (awareness/physical exam by patient and health care provider, imaging studies, diagnostic procedures, counseling and genetic testing) as well as prophylactic surgery and chemopreventive measures.

PATIENT/FAMILY EDUCATION

Always encourage patients to revisit their personal and family history and to update this information with all of their health care providers and their family members. Recommend that patients initiate discussions with their family members and other health care providers in an ongoing effort to reduce their and their loved ones' risk of heritable cancer.

Refer to NCCN guidelines (www.nccn.org) and national specialty society recommendations.

SUGGESTED READINGS
Available at www.expertconsult.com

RELATED CONTENT
Breast Cancer (Related Key Topic)
Lynch Syndrome (Related Key Topic)
Ovarian Cancer (Related Key Topic)

AUTHOR: **DAVID I. KURSS, M.D.**

BASIC INFORMATION

DEFINITION

Herpes simplex is a viral infection caused by the herpes simplex virus (HSV). HSV-1 is associated primarily with oral infections, and HSV-2 causes mainly genital infections. However, either type can infect any site. After the primary infection, the virus enters the nerve endings in the skin directly below the lesions and ascends to the dorsal root ganglia, where it remains in a latent stage until it is reactivated.

SYNONYMS

Genital herpes
Herpes labialis
Herpes gladiatorum
Herpes digitalis
Oral herpes

ICD-10CM CODES
B00.1	Herpesvirus vesicular dermatitis
B00.0	Eczema herpeticum
A60.9	Anogenital herpesviral infection, unspecified
B00.9	Herpesviral infection, unspecified
B00.82	Herpes simplex myelitis
P35.2	Congenital herpesviral [herpes simplex] infection

EPIDEMIOLOGY & DEMOGRAPHICS

- More than 85% of adults have serologic evidence of HSV-1 infection. The seroprevalence of adults with HSV-2 in the United States is 25%; however, only approximately 20% of these persons recall having symptoms of HSV infection.
- Most cases of eye or digital herpetic infections are caused by HSV-1.
- Worldwide, more than 400 million persons have genital herpes caused by HSV-2. In the U.S., 1 in 5 adults is infected with HSV-2, and 1 million new infections occur yearly.
- Frequency of recurrence of HSV-2 genital herpes is higher than HSV-1 oral labial infection.
- The frequency of recurrence is lowest for oral labial HSV-2 infections.
- The incidence of complications from herpes simplex (e.g., herpes encephalitis) is highest in immunocompromised hosts.
- Male circumcision significantly reduces the incidence of HSV-2.

PHYSICAL FINDINGS & CLINICAL PRESENTATION

Primary infection
- Symptoms occur from 3 to 7 days after contact (respiratory droplets, direct contact).
- Constitutional symptoms include low-grade fever, headache and myalgias, regional lymphadenopathy, and localized pain.
- Pain, burning, itching, and tingling last several hours.
- Grouped vesicles (Fig. 1), usually with surrounding erythema, appear and generally ulcerate or crust within 48 hr.
- The vesicles are uniform in size (differentiating it from herpes zoster vesicles, which vary in size). Scattered erosions covered

with exudate may be noted on genitals (Fig. E2).
- During the acute eruption the patient is uncomfortable; involvement of lips and inside of mouth may make it unpleasant for the patient to eat; urinary retention may complicate involvement of the genital area.
- Lesions generally last from 2 to 6 wk and heal without scarring.

Recurrent infection:
- Generally caused by alteration in the immune system; fatigue, stress, menses, local skin trauma, and exposure to sunlight are contributing factors.
- The prodromal symptoms (fatigue, burning and tingling of the affected area) last 12 to 24 hr.
- A cluster of lesions generally evolves within 24 hr from a macule to a papule and then vesicles surrounded by erythema; the vesicles coalesce and subsequently rupture within 4 days, revealing erosions covered by crusts.
- The crusts are generally shed within 7 to 10 days, revealing a pink surface.
- The most frequent location of the lesions is on the vermilion border of the lips (HSV-1), the penile shaft or glans penis and the labia (HSV-2), buttocks (seen more frequently in women), fingertips (herpetic whitlow), and trunk (may be confused with herpes zoster).
- Rapid onset of diffuse cutaneous herpes simplex (eczema herpeticum) may occur in certain atopic infants and adults. It is a medical emergency, especially in young infants, and should be promptly treated with acyclovir.
- Herpes encephalitis, meningitis, and ocular herpes can occur in patients with immunocompromised status and occasionally in normal hosts.

ETIOLOGY

HSV-1 and HSV-2 are both DNA viruses.

DIAGNOSIS

DIFFERENTIAL DIAGNOSIS

- Impetigo.
- Behçet's syndrome.
- Coxsackie virus infection.
- Syphilis.

- Stevens-Johnson syndrome.
- Herpangina.
- Aphthous stomatitis.
- Varicella.
- Herpes zoster.

WORKUP

Diagnosis is based on clinical presentation. Laboratory evaluation confirms diagnosis.

LABORATORY TESTS

- Direct immunofluorescent antibody slide tests provide a rapid diagnosis.
- Viral culture is the most definitive method for diagnosis; results are generally available in 1 or 2 days. The lesions should be sampled during the vesicular or early ulcerative stage; cervical samples should be taken from the endocervix with a swab.
- Pap smear will detect HSV-infected cells in cervical tissue from women without symptoms.
- Serologic tests for HSV: immunoglobulin (Ig) G and IgM serum antibodies. Antibodies to HSV occur in 50% to 90% of adults. The presence of IgM or a fourfold or greater rise in IgG titers indicates a recent infection (convalescent sample should be drawn 2 to 3 wk after the acute specimen is drawn).
- Tzanck smear is a readily available test that will demonstrate multinucleated giant cells. However, it is not a highly sensitive test.

TREATMENT

- Table 1 summarizes antiviral chemotherapy for HSV infection.
- Topical acyclovir, penciclovir, and docosanol are optional treatments for recurrent herpes labialis, but they are less effective than oral treatments.

DISPOSITION

Most patients recover from the initial episode or recurrences without complications; immunocompromised hosts are at risk for complications (e.g., disseminated herpes simplex infection, herpes encephalitis).

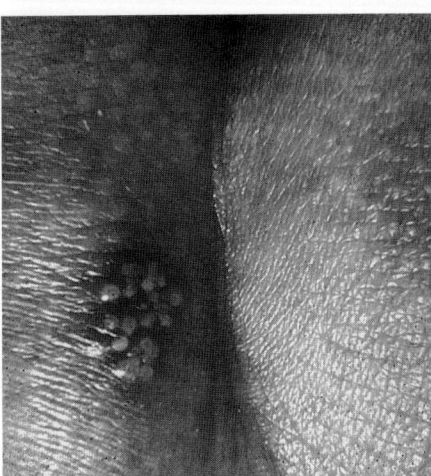
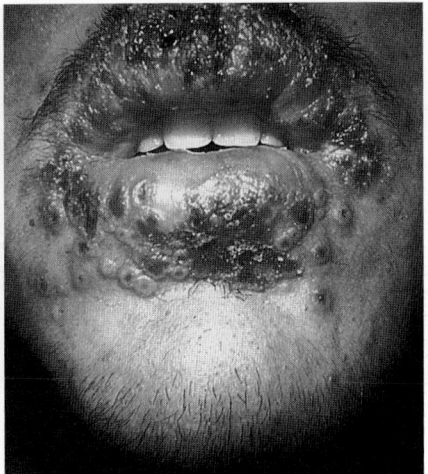

FIG. 1 Herpes simplex. (From Scuderi G [ed]: *Sports medicine: principles of primary care,* St Louis, 1997, Mosby.)

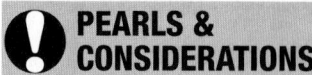

REFERRAL

- Hospital admission in patients with herpes encephalitis or herpes meningitis and in immunocompromised hosts with diffuse herpes simplex infection.
- Ophthalmology referral in patients with suspected ocular herpes.

ⓘ PEARLS & CONSIDERATIONS

COMMENTS

- Provide patient education regarding transmission of HSV.
- Condom use offers significant protection against HSV-1 infection in susceptible women.
- Patients should be instructed on the use of condoms for sexual intercourse and on avoiding kissing or sexual intercourse until lesions are crusted. Pericoital application of tenofovir gel, an antiretroviral vaginal gel, has also been shown to reduce the risk of HSV-2 in women. This may be useful in regions of the world where use of condoms is shunned.
- Patients should also avoid contact with immunocompromised hosts or neonates while lesions are present.
- Proper handwashing techniques should be explained.
- Patients with herpes gladiatorum (cutaneous herpes in athletes involved in contact sports) should be excluded from participation in active sports until lesions have resolved.
- Many new HSV-2 infections are asymptomatic. Since HSV-2 antibody tests have become commercially available, an increasing number of persons have learned that they have genital herpes through serologic testing. Persons with asymptomatic HSV-2 infection shed virus in the genital tract less frequently than persons with symptomatic infection, but much of the difference is attributable to less frequent genital lesions because generally lesions are accompanied by frequent viral shedding. The U.S. Preventive Services Task Force (USPSTF) recommends against routine serologic screening for genital HSV infection in asymptomatic adolescents and adults, including those that are pregnant.
- Suppressive treatment of HSV-2 infection lowers the incidence of genital lesions by 70% to 80%, but cuts the rate of HSV-2 transmission to uninfected partners by only 50%.
- Pregnancy: Antiviral prophylaxis with acyclovir is recommended from 36 weeks of gestation until delivery in women with a history of genital herpes. Elective cesarean delivery should be performed in laboring patients with active lesions to decrease the risk of neonatal herpes.
- Trials involving investigational herpes simplex vaccine have found it to be effective in preventing HSV-1 genital disease and infection, but not in preventing HSV-2 disease or infection.

RELATED CONTENT

Genital Herpes (Patient Information)
Oral Herpes (Patient Information)

AUTHOR: **FRED F. FERRI, M.D.**

TABLE 1 Antiviral Chemotherapy for Herpes Simplex Virus Infection

Mucocutaneous HSV Infections

Infections in Immunosuppressed Patients

Acute symptomatic first or recurrent episodes: IV acyclovir (5 mg/kg q8h) and oral acyclovir (400 mg qid), famciclovir (500 mg PO tid), or valacyclovir (500 mg PO bid) for 7-10 days are effective. Treatment duration may vary from 7-14 days.

Suppression of reactivation disease: IV acyclovir (5 mg/kg q8h), valacyclovir (500 mg PO bid), or oral acyclovir (400-800 mg 3-5 times per day) prevents recurrences during the immediate 30-day post-transplantation period. Longer-term suppression is often used for persons with continued immunosuppression. In bone marrow and renal transplant recipients, valacyclovir 2 g 4 times daily is also effective in preventing CMV infection. Valacyclovir 4 g 4 times daily has been associated with TTP after extended use in HIV-positive persons. In HIV-infected persons, oral famciclovir (500 mg bid) is effective in reducing clinical and subclinical reactivations of HSV-1 and -2.

Genital Herpes

First episodes: Oral acyclovir (200 mg five times per day or 400 mg tid), oral valacyclovir (1000 mg bid), or famciclovir (250 mg bid) for 10-14 days is effective. IV acyclovir (5 mg/kg q8h for 5 days) is given for severe disease or neurologic complications such as aseptic meningitis.

Symptomatic recurrent genital herpes: Oral acyclovir (200 mg 5 times per day for 5 days, 800 mg PO tid for 2 days), valacyclovir (500 mg bid for 3 or 5 days), or famciclovir (125 mg bid for 5 days). All these therapies are effective in shortening lesion duration.

Suppression of recurrent genital herpes: Oral acyclovir (200-mg capsules bid or tid, 400 mg bid, or 800 mg qd), famciclovir (250 mg bid), or valacyclovir (500 mg or 1000 mg qd or 500 mg bid) prevents symptomatic reactivation. Persons with frequent reactivation (<9 episodes/year) can take 500 mg daily; those with >9 episodes/year should take 1000 mg/daily or 500 mg bid.

Oral-Labial HSV Infections

First episode: Oral acyclovir (200 mg) is given 4 or 5 times per day. Famciclovir (250 mg bid) or valacyclovir (1000 mg bid) has been used clinically.

Recurrent episodes: Valacyclovir 1000 mg bid for 1 day or 500 mg bid for 3 days is effective in reducing pain and speeding healing. Self-initiated therapy with six times daily topical 1% penciclovir cream is effective in speeding the healing of oral-labial HSV; topical acyclovir cream has also been shown to speed healing.

Suppression of reactivation of oral-labial HSV: Oral acyclovir (400 mg bid), if started before exposure and continued for the duration of exposure (usually 5-10 days), prevents reactivation of recurrent oral-labial HSV infection associated with severe sun exposure.

Herpetic Whitlow

Oral acyclovir (200 mg) 5 times daily for 7-10 days.

HSV Proctitis

Oral acyclovir (400 mg five times per day) is useful in shortening the course of infection. In immunosuppressed patients or in patients with severe infection, IV acyclovir (5 mg/kg q8h) may be useful.

Herpetic Eye Infections

In acute keratitis, topical trifluorothymidine, vidarabine, idoxuridine, acyclovir, penciclovir, and interferon are all beneficial. Debridement may be required; topical steroids may worsen disease.

CNS HSV Infections

HSV encephalitis: Intravenous acyclovir (10 mg/kg q8h; 30 mg/kg per day) for 14-21 days is preferred.

HSV aseptic meningitis: No studies of systemic antiviral chemotherapy exist. If therapy is to be given, IV acyclovir (15-30 mg/kg/day) should be used.

Autonomic radiculopathy: No studies are available.

Neonatal HSV infections: Acyclovir (60 mg/kg/day, divided into three doses) is given. The recommended duration of treatment is 21 days. Monitoring for relapse should be undertaken, and some authorities recommend continued suppression with oral acyclovir suspension for 3 to 4 mo.

Visceral HSV Infections

HSV esophagitis: IV acyclovir (15 mg/kg per day). In some patients with milder forms of immunosuppression, oral therapy with valacyclovir or famciclovir is effective.

HSV pneumonitis: No controlled studies exist. IV acyclovir (15 mg/kg per day) should be considered.

Disseminated HSV infections: No controlled studies exist. Intravenous acyclovir (10 mg/kg q8h) nevertheless should be tried. No definite evidence indicates that therapy decreases the risk of death.

Erythema multiforme-associated HSV: Anecdotal observations suggest that oral acyclovir (400 mg bid or tid) or valacyclovir (500 mg bid) suppresses erythema multiforme.

Surgical prophylaxis: Several surgical procedures such as laser skin resurfacing, trigeminal nerve root decompression, and lumbar disk surgery have been associated with HSV reactivation. Intravenous acyclovir (3 mg/kg) and oral acyclovir 800 mg bid, valacyclovir 500 mg bid, or famciclovir 250 mg bid is effective in reducing reactivation. Therapy should be initiated 48 hours before surgery and continued for 3-7 days.

Infections with acyclovir-resistant HSV: Foscarnet (40 mg/kg IV q8h) should be given until lesions heal. The optimal duration of therapy and the usefulness of its continuation to suppress lesions are unclear. Some patients may benefit from cutaneous application of trifluorothymidine or 5% cidofovir gel.

CMV, Cytomegalovirus; *CNS,* central nervous system; *HIV,* human immunodeficiency virus; *HSV,* herpes simplex virus; *TTP,* thrombotic thrombocytopenic purpura.

From Mandell GL et al: *Principles and practice of infectious diseases,* ed 7, Philadelphia, 2010, Saunders.

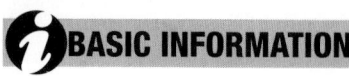

BASIC INFORMATION

DEFINITION

Herpes zoster is a disease caused by reactivation of the varicella-zoster virus, with spread of the virus alone from the sensory nerve to the dermatome. After the primary infection (chickenpox), the virus becomes latent in the dorsal root ganglia and reemerges when there is a weakening of the immune system (as a result of disease or advanced age).

SYNONYMS

Shingles
HZ

ICD-10CM CODES
B02	Herpes zoster
B02.7	Disseminated zoster
B02.8	Zoster with other complications
B02.9	Zoster without complications
B02.39	Other herpes zoster eye disease
B02.0	Zoster encephalitis
B02.1	Zoster meningitis
B02.30	Zoster ocular disease, unspecified
B02.31	Zoster conjunctivitis
B02.32	Zoster iridocyclitis
B02.33	Zoster keratitis
B02.34	Zoster scleritis
B02.39	Other herpes zoster eye disease

EPIDEMIOLOGY & DEMOGRAPHICS

- Herpes zoster occurs during the lifetime of 10% to 20% of the population.
- There is an increased incidence in immunocompromised patients (AIDS, malignancy), the elderly (Fig. 1), and children who acquired chickenpox when younger than 2 mo.

PHYSICAL FINDINGS & CLINICAL PRESENTATION

- Pain generally precedes skin manifestation by 3 to 5 days and is generally localized to the dermatome that will be affected by the skin lesions.
- Constitutional symptoms are often present (malaise, fever, headache).
- The initial rash consists of erythematous maculopapules generally affecting one dermatome (thoracic region in majority of cases [Fig. 2]). Typically the rash does not cross the midline. Some patients (<30%) may have scattered vesicles outside the affected dermatome. In rare cases the rash can be generalized (Fig. 3).
- The initial maculopapules evolve into vesicles and pustules by the third or the fourth day.
- The vesicles have an erythematous base (Fig. 4), are cloudy, and have various sizes (a distinguishing characteristic from herpes simplex, in which the vesicles are of uniform size) and may have a classic appearance of grouped vesicles (Fig. 5).
- The vesicles subsequently become umbilicated and then form crusts that generally fall off within 3 wk; scarring may occur.

- Pain during and after the rash is generally significant. Post-herpetic neuralgia occurs after herpes zoster in approximately one third of patients aged 60 years and older and can persist for months or years.
- Secondary bacterial infection with *Staphylococcus aureus* or *Streptococcus pyogenes* may occur.
- Regional lymphadenopathy may occur.
- Herpes zoster may involve the trigeminal nerve (most frequent cranial nerve involved); involvement of the geniculate ganglion can cause facial palsy and a painful ear, with the presence of vesicles on the pinna and external auditory canal (Ramsay Hunt syndrome).

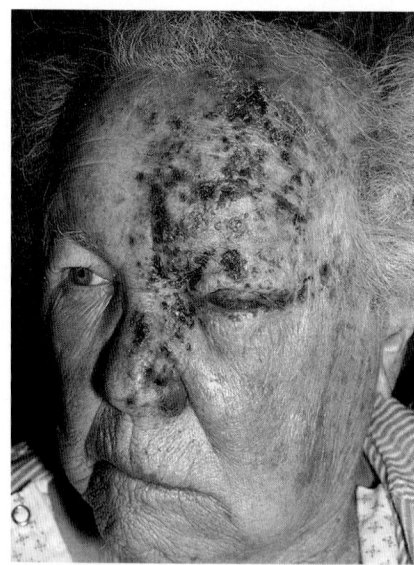

FIG. 1 Herpes zoster, involvement of the V1 dermatome. (From James WD et al: *Andrews' diseases of the skin: clinical dermatology*, ed 12, Philadelphia, 2016, Elsevier.)

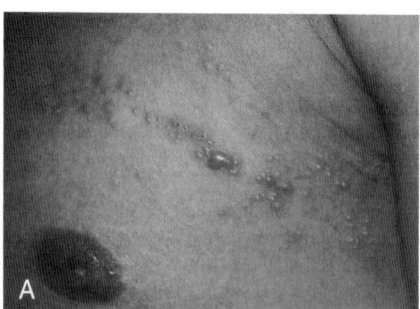

FIG. 2 A and **B,** Herpes zoster lesions in T3 distribution. (From Swartz, MH: *Textbook of physical diagnosis*, ed 7, Philadelphia, 2014, Saunders.)

ETIOLOGY

Reactivation of varicella virus (human herpes virus III)

DIAGNOSIS

DIFFERENTIAL DIAGNOSIS

- Rash: herpes simplex and other viral infections
- Pain from herpes zoster: may be confused with acute myocardial infarction, pulmonary embolism, pleuritis, pericarditis, renal colic

LABORATORY TESTS

Laboratory tests are generally not necessary (viral cultures and Tzanck smear will confirm diagnosis in patients with atypical presentation).

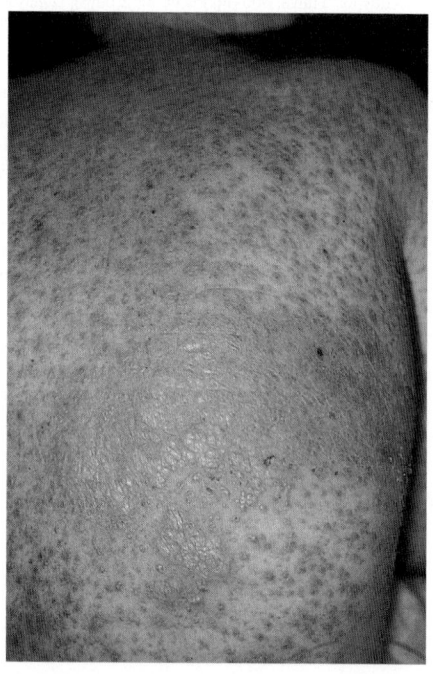

FIG. 3 Herpes zoster, generalized. (From Swartz, MH: *Textbook of physical diagnosis*, ed 7, Philadelphia, 2014, Saunders.)

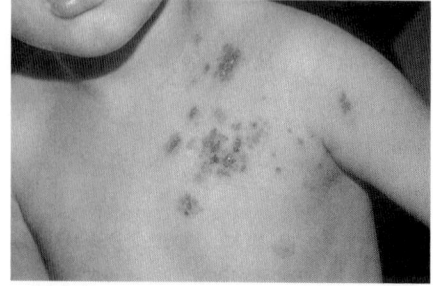

FIG. 4 Herpes zoster occurred in this 3-year-old. She had chickenpox at age 18 months. The varicella-zoster virus causes both conditions. Spontaneous resolution can be expected. (From White GM, Cox NH [eds]: *Diseases of the skin, a color atlas and text*, ed 2, St Louis, 2006, Mosby.)

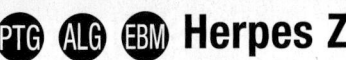

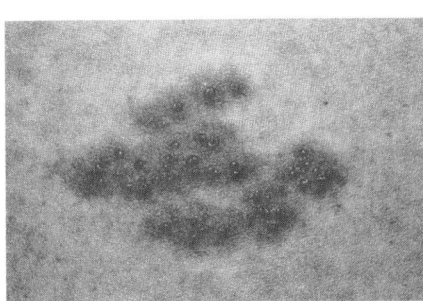

FIG. 5 Herpes zoster. Classic appearance of grouped vesicles. (From White GM, Cox NH [eds]: *Diseases of the skin, a color atlas and text,* ed 2, St Louis, 2006, Mosby.)

Rx TREATMENT

NONPHARMACOLOGIC THERAPY

- Wet compresses (using Burow's solution or cool tap water) applied for 15 to 30 min five to 10 times a day are useful to break vesicles and remove serum and crust.
- Care must be taken to prevent any secondary bacterial infection.

ACUTE GENERAL Rx

- Oral antiviral agents can decrease acute pain, inflammation, and vesicle formation when treatment is begun within 48 hr of onset of rash. Treatment options are:
  1. Valacyclovir 1000 mg tid for 7 days
  2. Famciclovir 500 mg tid for 7 days
  3. Acyclovir 800 mg 5 times daily for 7 to 10 days
- Corticosteroids should be considered in older patients within 72 hr of clinical presentation or if new lesions are still appearing if there are no contraindications. Initial dose is prednisone 40 mg/day decreased by 5 mg/day until finished. When used there is a decrease in the use of analgesics and time to resumption of usual activities, but there is no effect on the incidence and duration of postherpetic neuralgia.
- Immunocompromised patients should be treated with IV acyclovir 500 mg/m^2 or 10 mg/kg q8h in 1-hr infusions for 7 days, with close monitoring of renal function and adequate hydration; vidarabine (continuous 12-hr infusion of 10 mg/kg/day for 7 days) is also effective for treatment of disseminated herpes zoster in immunocompromised hosts.
- Patients with AIDS and transplant recipients may develop acyclovir-resistant varicella-zoster; these patients can be treated with foscarnet (40 mg/kg IV q8h) continued for at least 10 days or until lesions are completely healed.
- Postherpetic neuralgia
  1. Gabapentin 100 to 600 mg tid is effective in the treatment of pain and sleep interference associated with postherpetic neuralgia. Other effective agents are pregabalin, duloxetine, and tricyclic antidepressants.
  2. Lidocaine patch 5% is also effective in relieving postherpetic neuralgia. Patches are applied to intact skin after resolution of blisters and crusts to cover the most painful area for up to 12 hr within a 24-hr period.
  3. Capsaicin cream can be useful for treatment of postherpetic neuralgia. It is generally applied 3 to 5 times daily for several weeks after the crusts have fallen off. A topical 8% patch formulation of capsaicin is now available by prescription for post-herpetic neuralgia.
  4. Sympathetic blocks (stellate ganglion or epidural) with 0.25% bupivacaine and rhizotomy are reserved for severe cases unresponsive to conservative treatment.

DISPOSITION

- The incidence of postherpetic neuralgia (defined as pain that persists more than 90 days after onset of rash) increases with age (<30% by age 40 yr, >70% by age 70 yr); antivirals reduce the risk of postherpetic neuralgia.
- Incidence of disseminated herpes zoster is increased in immunocompromised hosts (e.g., 15% to 50% of patients with active Hodgkin's disease).
- Immunocompromised hosts are also more prone to neurologic complications (encephalitis, myelitis, cranial and peripheral nerve palsies, acute retinal necrosis). The mortality rate is 10% to 20% in immunocompromised hosts with disseminated zoster.
- Motor neuropathies occur in 5% of all cases of zoster; complete recovery occurs in >70% of patients.
- Rates of HZ recurrence are more frequent than previously reported and are comparable to rates of first HZ occurrence in immunocompetent individuals.

REFERRAL

- Hospitalization for IV acyclovir in patients with disseminated herpes zoster.
- Patients with herpes zoster ophthalmicus should be referred to an ophthalmologist.
- Vaccination: In the absence of the herpes zoster vaccine, persons who live to 85 yr of age have a 50% risk of herpes zoster. Immunocompetent adults ≥60 yr are appropriate candidates for a single dose of varicella-zoster vaccine (VZV) whether or not they have had a previous episode of herpes zoster. Immunization with VZV (Zostavax) boosts waning immunity in older adults and reduces the severity and duration of pain caused by herpes zoster by 61%. Adults who are VZV seronegative (never had varicella) should be immunized against varicella with two doses of varicella vaccine (Varivax). Despite its efficacy and safety, use of this vaccine remains low (<8% of potential recipients).

EBM EVIDENCE

Available at www.expertconsult.com

SUGGESTED READINGS

Available at www.expertconsult.com

RELATED CONTENT

Shingles (Patient Information)
Post-Herpetic Neuralgia (Related Key Topic)

AUTHOR: **FRED F. FERRI, M.D.**

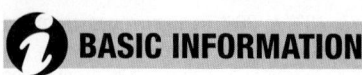

DEFINITION

Hidradenitis suppurativa (HS) is a chronic, relapsing suppurative cutaneous disease affecting skin that bears apocrine glands and is manifested by abscesses, fistulating sinus tracts, and chronic infection leading to scarring.

SYNONYMS

Acne inversa
Apocrinitis
Verneuil's disease
HS

ICD-10CM CODES
L73.2 Hidradenitis suppurativa

EPIDEMIOLOGY & DEMOGRAPHICS

Onset is postpubertal, with an average age of onset of 23 yr; rates decline after age 55 yr.
PREVALENCE: Overall prevalence in the United States is ~1% to 2%.
PREDOMINANT SEX: Female to male ratio is 3:1.
PREDOMINANT AGE: HS most often manifests after puberty, usually in the second or third decade of life. It is rare in the elderly.
RISK FACTORS:
- Obesity and metabolic syndrome.
- Family history (approximately 30%).
- Hyperandrogenism in women.
- Cigarette smoking.

PHYSICAL FINDINGS & CLINICAL PRESENTATION

The diagnosis is primarily clinical, based on the development of typical lesions in a characteristic distribution, with a relapsing nature. The course of HS is prolonged and marked by intermittent periods of activity and remission.
- Early symptoms include pain, itching, burning, erythema, and hyperhidrosis.
- Typical lesions include:
  1. Painful erythematous papules and nodules leading to painful abscesses with foul-smelling discharge.
  2. Dermal contractures and ropelike elevation of the skin.
  3. Comedones in the apocrine, gland-bearing skin.
- Classified into Hurley Stages
  1. Stage I: abscesses without sinus tracts or scarring.
  2. Stage II: multiple abscesses plus sinus tracts and scarring.
  3. Stage III: diffuse involvement of entire area with abscesses, sinus tracts, and scarring.
- The axilla is the most common site (Fig. 1).
- Less common sites include the inguinal region, the breasts (more often in women), and the perineal or perianal skin (more often in men).
- There is a strong tendency toward relapse and recurrence.

- There is often a poor response to conventional antibiotics and no pathogens isolated from cultures of lesions.
- The disease is often mistaken for a simple infection and a long delay in diagnosis is common.
- Three clinical subtypes of HS have been recently proposed[1]:
  1. A classic axillary-mammary HS subtype, representing 48% of cases and characterized by breast and axillary involvement and hypertrophic scarring.
  2. A follicular HS subtype, representing 26% of cases manifesting primarily in male smokers with a family history of HS and characterized by follicular lesions, including epidermal cysts, pilonidal sinus, comedones, and severe acne.
  3. A gluteal HS subtype, representing 26% of cases, most often seen in smokers with lower body mass index (BMI) and with a morphology characterized by follicular papules, folliculitis, and gluteal involvement.

ETIOLOGY

- Keratinous materials plug apocrine glands in hair follicles leading to stasis, dilation, rupture, and re-epithelialization. Fig. 2 illustrates the pathogenesis of hidradenitis suppurativa.
- Bacteria are trapped and multiply, leading to gland rupture with surrounding inflammation and local bacterial infection.
- Over time, repeated nodules and infections cause scarring, which can lead to deep tissue damage and sinus tracts.
- Infectious agents such as *Streptococcus, Staphylococcus,* and *Escherichia coli,* and enteric flora have been identified in cultures but are likely a secondary component of the disease.
- There is likely a significant genetic component to the disease. 35% to 40% of patients report a family history of HS. An HS spectrum of different phenotypes has been characterized involving genetic factors that are not yet well described but may be important for future therapy.
- HS has been associated with other endocrine and autoimmune disorders such as diabetes, Cushing's disease, acromegaly, Crohn's disease, and inflammatory arthritis.
- Metabolic syndrome affects as many as 50% of patients with HS and may exacerbate the associated inflammation.

DIAGNOSIS

DIFFERENTIAL DIAGNOSIS

- Follicular pyodermias such as folliculitis, furuncles, carbuncles, and pilonidal cysts.
- Noduloulcerative syphilis.
- Cat scratch disease.
- Granuloma inguinale.
- Perianal and vulvar manifestations of Crohn's disease.

[1]Woodruff CM, Charlie AM, Leslie KS: Hidradenitis suppurative: a guide for the practicing physician, *Mayo Clin Proc* 90(12):1679-1693, 2015.

- Actinomycosis.
- Lymphogranuloma venereum.
- Dermoid, epidermoid, or Bartholin's cysts.
- Tuberculous inflammation of the skin.
- Lymphadenitis.
- Erysipelas.

WORKUP

Primarily a clinical diagnosis based on typical lesion (see "Physical Findings & Clinical Presentation").

LABORATORY TESTS

- Patients with acute lesions may have an elevated erythrocyte sedimentation rate or WBC.
- Febrile and toxic-appearing patients should have complete blood count, chemistries, and blood cultures.
- Any pus should be sampled for bacterial culture and sensitivity.

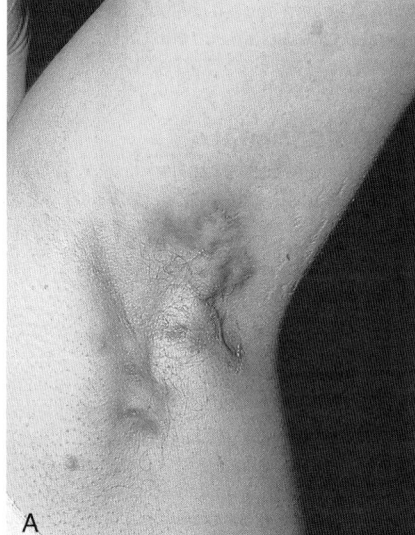

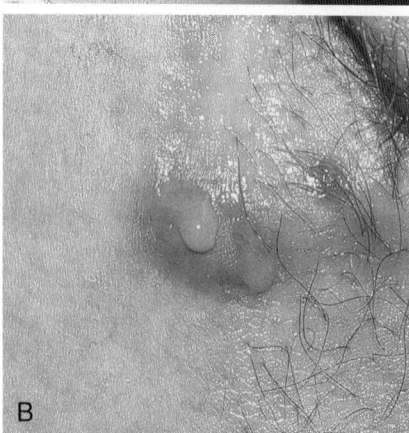

FIG. 1 Hidradenitis suppurativa (HS). *A,* HS of the axilla. This is the classic appearance with inflammatory nodules and scarred areas. This condition is commonly misdiagnosed as a bacterial infection. ***B,*** HS of the axilla, a close-up view of the draining pus. When intact, the lesions represent sterile abscesses. Once open, they may become secondarily infected. (From White GM, Cox NH [eds]: *Diseases of the skin: a color atlas and text,* ed 2, St Louis, 2006, Mosby.)

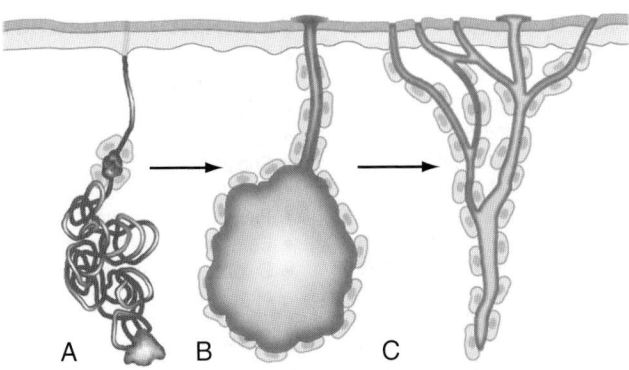

A   B   C

FIG. 2 Pathogenesis of hidradenitis suppurativa, an inflammatory disease of the apocrine sweat glands and adjacent connective tissue. *A*, The initiating event is occlusion of the apocrine duct by a keratinous plug. *B*, Bacteria are trapped beneath the keratinous plug and multiply to form an abscess, which can rupture into adjacent tissue. *C*, The end result is recurrent abscesses, chronic draining sinuses, and indurated scarred skin and subcutaneous tissues. Often, multiple tracts are interconnected and lead to the skin. (From Feldman M, et al.: *Sleisenger and Fortran's gastrointestinal and liver disease*, ed 10, Philadelphia, 2016, Elsevier.)

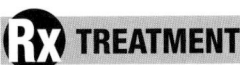

TREATMENT

There is no definitive cure for hidradenitis.

NONPHARMACOLOGIC THERAPY

- Weight loss and control of metabolic syndrome.
- Smoking cessation.
- Avoidance of shaving, depilatory creams, deodorants.
- Avoidance of tight-fitting clothing.
- Warm compresses.
- Incision and drainage of nonpurulent lesions is *not* recommended due to recurrence and scarring.
- Laser therapy, radiotherapy, and cryotherapy currently under study.
- Wide local excision for stage III disease with or without vacuum-assisted closure device.

ACUTE AND CHRONIC Rx

- NSAIDs for inflammation and pain, consider gabapentin, pregabalin, SSRIs for chronic pain management.
- Antibiotics never proven to be effective; however, they are a mainstay of treatment. Can base treatment on the basis of aspirate culture and sensitivities or empirically.
  1. Clindamycin is the only topical antibiotic proven to be effective in randomized controlled trial and is appropriate for stage I disease.
  2. For oral therapy in stage II: consider clindamycin and rifampin in combination. Cephalosporins, dicloxacillin, erythromycin, minocycline, and tetracycline have also been used.
  3. Severe, recurrent disease can require up to 3 to 6 mo of antibiotics.
- Oral contraceptives with low androgenic progesterone (norgestimate, desogestrel, or gestodene) for women show mixed effectiveness. They are especially advantageous for female patients of childbearing age who also require some form of birth control.
- Isotretinoin has been used with mixed effectiveness. They should be avoided in women of childbearing age.
- Metformin has mixed effectiveness, possibly due to related metabolic syndrome and hyperandrogenism.
- Trials using zinc gluconate 75 to 118 mg/day in patients with mild (grade 1) disease have shown mixed effectiveness.
- Corticosteroids and other immune suppressants such as cyclosporin, infliximab, and etanercept have been used for stage II disease, with mixed results.
- Adalimumab, an antitumor necrosis factor-α antibody given once per week (dose 40 mg/wk) has shown significantly higher clinical response as compared to placebo in phase 3 trials. Infliximab has also been used in trials with variable success rates, with most patients exhibiting clinical improvement within 8 wk.

COMPLICATIONS

- Squamous cell carcinoma.
- Scarring leading to restricted limb mobility or lymphedema.
- Rectal or urethral fistulas.
- Psychological effects related to disfiguring nature of disease.

REFERRAL

- Referral to dermatology during stage I to II disease.
- Referral to a surgeon is indicated for stage III disease.
- Surgical approaches include laser surgery and excisional surgery.

PEARLS & CONSIDERATIONS

COMMENTS

- Patients with hidradenitis are at risk for severe depression, social isolation, and negatively impacted sexuality as a result of their disease.
- There is an average delay in diagnosis of 12 years and most patients are diagnosed in stage II of the disease.
- It is important to maximize nonmedical treatment, start medical treatment, and refer to a surgeon early in the disease course to ensure the best quality of life for patients.
- The only definitive treatment for hidradenitis is wide excision of the involved skin.

SUGGESTED READINGS

Available at www.expertconsult.com

AUTHOR: **MARY BETH SUTTER, M.D.**

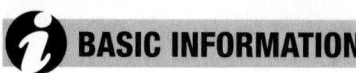

DEFINITION

High-altitude illness refers to a spectrum of cerebral and pulmonary syndromes related to hypoxemia occurring during rapid ascension to high altitudes. Common acute syndromes include high-altitude pulmonary edema (HAPE), acute mountain sickness (AMS), and high-altitude cerebral edema (HACE). The latter two are thought to represent different points of severity along the same pathophysiologic process in the brain.

SYNONYMS

Altitude sickness
High-altitude headache
Acute mountain sickness
High-altitude pulmonary edema
High-altitude cerebral edema

ICD-10CM CODES
W94   Exposure to high and low air pressure and changes in air pressure
T70.2 Other and unspecified effects of high altitude

EPIDEMIOLOGY & DEMOGRAPHICS

- More than 30 million people are at risk of developing altitude sickness.
- 80% of people who ascend to high altitudes have HAH_2.
- AMS is the most common of the altitude diseases. It affects approximately 40% to 50% of people ascending to 14,000 ft (4200 m) from lowland.
- The incidence of HACE is reported to be 0.1% to 2% at elevations in excess of 12,000 ft (3000 m). HACE is often complicated by concomitant HAPE.
- Men are five times more likely to develop HAPE than are women.
- AMS and HACE affect men and women equally.
- Some studies have suggested that climbers with a prior history of HAPE have a roughly 60% chance of recurrence if they ascend to the same elevation at the same rate.

PHYSICAL FINDINGS & CLINICAL PRESENTATION (TABLE E1)

HAH_1
- Headache that develops within 24 hr of ascent.
- Bilateral, frontal or frontotemporal, dull or pressing quality.
- Mild to moderate intensity and aggravated by exertion, movement, straining, coughing, or bending.
- Headache resolves within 8 hr of descent.
- HAH should resolve with analgesics and/or 10 to 15 min of supplementary oxygen.
- Difficult to distinguish from headaches secondary to dehydration.

AMS
- AMS is thought to be a progression of HAH_2.

- Occurs within 6 to 12 hours after rapid ascent to 8000 ft (2500 m) in 10% to 25% of unacclimatized persons.
- Headache is the most common symptom.
- Dizziness and lightheadedness.
- Nausea, vomiting, and loss of appetite.
- Fatigue.
- Sleep disturbance from an exaggerated hyperventilatory phase of Cheyne-Stokes respiration in response to hypoxemia and alkalosis.
- AMS can evolve into HAPE and HACE.
- Retinal hemorrhages can be present from increased blood flow or breakdown in the blood-retina barrier.
- Supplemental oxygen may be used to support the clinical diagnosis.

HACE
- Usually presents several days after AMS.
- Confusion, irritability, drowsiness, stupor, hallucinations, mild fever.
- Headache, nausea, vomiting.
- Truncal ataxia, paralysis, and seizures.
- The sixth cranial nerve is the nerve most commonly affected from the compression of the trunk adjacent to brain swelling.
- Coma and death from brain herniation may develop within hours of the first symptoms.

HAPE (Fig. E1)
- Typically occurs 2 to 4 days after ascent more than 8000 ft (2500 m).
- It can occur at a lower elevation in patients with pulmonary hypertension.
- Dyspnea out of proportion to the level of exertion, loss of stamina.
- Dry cough or cough with frothy rust- or pink-tinged sputum.
- Chest tightness.
- Tachycardia, tachypnea, rales, cyanosis.

ETIOLOGY

- During ascent to altitudes above sea level, the atmospheric pressure decreases. Although the percentage of oxygen in the air remains the same, the partial pressure of oxygen decreases with increased altitude, and can cause hypoxemia. Fig. E2 illustrates the effect of altitude on alveolar Pao_2 and oxygen saturation.
- Increased cerebral blood flow and the loss of autoregulation of intracranial pressure may contribute to increased cerebral vascular permeability and subsequent brain edema (HACE).
- Hypobaric hypoxia can trigger elevated pulmonary pressures, resulting in protein-rich, hemorrhagic exudates into the lung alveoli due to a breakdown in the pulmonary blood-gas barrier (HAPE).
- The body responds to low oxygen partial pressures through a process of acclimatization (see "Comments").

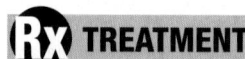 DIAGNOSIS

Made by clinical presentation and physical findings.

DIFFERENTIAL DIAGNOSIS

- Dehydration.
- Carbon monoxide poisoning.
- Hypothermia.
- Infection.
- Substance abuse.
- Congestive heart failure.
- Pulmonary embolism.
- Cerebrovascular accident.
- Box E1 summarizes the differential diagnosis of high-altitude illnesses.

WORKUP

Typically the diagnosis is self-evident after history and physical examination. Laboratory tests and imaging studies help monitor cardiopulmonary and central nervous system status in patients admitted to the intensive care unit for pulmonary and/or cerebral edema. In patients with HAPE occurring at lower altitudes (<8000 ft), an evaluation of preexisting pulmonary hypertension or a left-to-right shunt should be considered.

LABORATORY TESTS

Not useful, unless to rule out an alternative diagnosis.

IMAGING STUDIES

- Chest x-ray showing Kerley B-lines and patchy edema (see Fig. E1).
- CT scan of the head showing diffuse or patchy edema.
- MRI of the head showing characteristic intense T2 signal in the white matter.

【Rx】 TREATMENT

NONPHARMACOLOGIC THERAPY

- Stop the ascent to allow acclimatization or start to descend until symptoms have resolved.
- Patient with AMS can stay at the same height and may ascend once symptoms resolve but should strongly consider using acetazolamide for the remainder of the trip.
- If the symptoms recur or fail to resolve after 2 to 3 days, descent is indicated.
- Descent is the definitive treatment and should begin immediately at the first suspicion of HACE.
- Oxygen 4 to 6 L/min is used for severe AMS, HAPE, and HACE.
- Portable hyperbaric bags are useful if available at the site.
- Altitude can cause diuresis that may be mediated by enhanced release of atrial natriuretic peptide. When coupled with the increased fluid loss through increased ventilation, there is a higher risk for dehydration, and adequate hydration should be maintained.

ACUTE PHARMACOLOGIC Rx

- Nonsteroidal antiinflammatory drugs (e.g., ibuprofen 600 mg every 6 hours, beginning 6 hours before ascending) are effective prophylaxis of traditional altitude sickness and in treating headaches in AMS.
- Acetazolamide 125 to 250 mg PO bid is the preferred agent and has been effective for

both prevention and acute therapy in patients with AMS and HACE. Dexamethasone should also be added in patients with HACE.

- Nifedipine 10 mg sublingual followed by long-acting nifedipine 30 mg bid is used for patients with HAPE who cannot descend immediately.
- Dexamethasone 4 mg PO every 6 hr is used in patients with severe AMS, HAPE, or HACE.

CHRONIC Rx

Prevention is the most prudent therapy.

1. Slow, staged ascent to avoid altitude sickness.
2. Start the ascent below 8000 feet.
3. Ascend 1000 feet/day (300 m/day).
4. Spend two nights at the same altitude every 3 days.
5. Sleep at lower heights than the altitude climbed ("climb high, sleep low").
6. Prophylactic therapy with NSAIDs (ibuprofen 600 mg every 6 hours, beginning 6 hours before ascending) or acetazolamide up to 750 mg daily and/or dexamethasone 8 to 16 mg daily decreases the risk of developing AMS (combination may have additive benefit). The drugs should be used until acclimatization occurs.
7. Prophylactic inhalation of a β-adrenergic agonist, salmeterol 125 mcg q12h, or the use of slow-release nifedipine 20 mg bid have both been shown to reduce the risk of HAPE in susceptible individuals.
8. Tadalafil, a long-acting phosphodiesterase inhibitor, has recently been shown to decrease the incidence of HAPE in susceptible individuals.

9. Box 2 summarizes field treatment of high-altitude illness.

DISPOSITION

- AMS improves over a period of 2 to 3 days.
- HAPE is the most common cause of death among patients with altitude illnesses.
- More than 60% of patients with HAPE will have recurrence of symptoms on subsequent climbs.
- In HACE, neurologic deficits may persist for weeks but eventually resolve. If coma occurs, prognosis is poor.

REFERRAL

Cardiology and neurology referrals are made in patients with pulmonary edema and central nervous system findings, respectively.

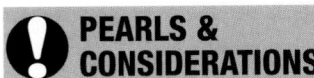

PEARLS & CONSIDERATIONS

COMMENTS

- Acclimatization is the process in which an individual who normally resides at low altitude adapts to hypobaric hypoxia to improve tolerance and performance at higher altitude. These mechanisms include:
  1. An increase in respiratory rates and tidal volume. This hyperventilation allows lowering of arterial carbon dioxide to preserve oxygen delivery, even at extreme altitudes.
  2. An early increase in heart rate and stroke volume to improve oxygen delivery. After 1 week, both parameters decrease

because of diuresis and lower catecholamine levels.
  3. Pulmonary hypertension develops in response to hypoxemia, resulting in improvement of the ventilation-perfusion mismatch but may be maladaptive and lead to the development of HAPE.
  4. Cerebral vasodilation to increase blood flow to the brain.
  5. Rise in hemoglobin and hematocrit. This is a long-term process that takes up to 1 week to occur in response to the need for improved oxygen delivery.
- Adaptation to altitude is different from acclimatization and refers to physiologic differences in permanent residents at high altitude (e.g., an increased oxygen diffusion capacity).
- High altitude illness can generally be prevented by ascending to 300 to 500 meters per day at altitudes above 3000 meters and including a rest day every 3 to 4 days.
- Risk factors for the development of altitude sicknesses are:
  1. Rapid ascent.
  2. Previous history of altitude sickness.
  3. Strenuous exertion on arrival.
  4. Obesity.
  5. Male gender.
- Physical fitness is not protective against high-altitude illness.
- Both dexamethasone and tadalafil decrease systolic pulmonary artery pressure and may reduce the incidence of HAPE in adults with a history of HAPE. Dexamethasone prophylaxis may also reduce the incidence of AMS in these adults.
- Descent is mandatory for all persons with HACE or HAPE.
- The American College of Chest Physicians has released a primer on caring for passengers with a variety of health conditions who are traveling to high-altitude places or areas (http://www.accpstorage.org/newOrganization/patients/TravelingwithOxygen.pdf). Specific indications for supplemental oxygen are provided in the document.

SUGGESTED READINGS

Available at www.expertconsult.com

RELATED CONTENT

Altitude Sickness (Patient Information)

AUTHORS: **FAHAD FAROOQ, M.D.,** and **SAMAAN RAFEQ, M.D.**

BOX 2   Field Treatment of High-Altitude Illness

High-Altitude Headache and Mild Acute Mountain Sickness
- Stop ascent, rest, acclimatize at same altitude.
- Symptomatic treatment as necessary with analgesics and antiemetics.
- Consider acetazolamide, 125 to 250 mg bid, to speed acclimatization.
- OR descend 500 m (1640 feet) or more.

Moderate to Severe Acute Mountain Sickness
- Low-flow oxygen, if available.
- Acetazolamide, 125 to 250 mg bid, with or without dexamethasone, 4 mg PO, IM, or IV q6h.
- Hyperbaric therapy.
- OR immediate descent.

High-Altitude Cerebral Edema
- Immediate descent or evacuation.
- Oxygen, 2 to 4 L/min.
- Dexamethasone, 8 mg PO, IM, or IV, then 4 mg q6h.
- Hyperbaric therapy.

High-Altitude Pulmonary Edema
- Minimize exertion and keep warm.
- Immediate descent or hyperbaric therapy.
- Oxygen, 4 to 6 L/min until improving, then 2 to 4 L/min.
  If above unavailable, one of the following:
- Nifedipine, 30 mg extended release q12h.
- Sildenafil 50 mg q8h.
- Tadalafil 10 mg q12h.
- Consider inhaled β-agonist.

Periodic Breathing
- Acetazolamide, 62.5 to 125 mg at bedtime as needed.

IM, Intramuscularly; *IV,* intravenously; *PO,* orally.
From Auerbach P: *Wilderness medicine, expert consult* Premium Edition—Enhanced Online Features and Print, Philadelphia, 2012, Saunders.

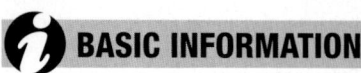

DEFINITION

Hip fractures are fractures of the proximal part of the femur and typically are classified as intracapsular or extracapsular. Intracapsular fractures include femoral head and femoral neck fractures (Fig. 1, Table 1). Extracapsular fractures include intertrochanteric fractures, subtrochanteric fractures and, less commonly, greater or lesser trochanteric fractures. These fractures can be further categorized by the fracture pattern and the fracture stability.

SYNONYMS

Hip fracture
Proximal femur fracture
Intracapsular fracture
Femoral neck fractures (subcapital vs. transcervical vs. basicervical)
Extracapsular fracture
Intertrochanteric fracture

ICD-10CM CODES: Code x Y (Y = encounter type: A [initial], D [subsequent with routine healing], G [subsequent with delayed healing], K [subsequent with nonunion], P [subsequent with malunion], S [sequelae]).

S72.0	Fracture of neck of femur
S72.1	Pertrochanteric fracture
S72.2	Subtrochanteric fracture
S72.3	Fracture of shaft of femur
S72.4	Fracture of lower end of femur
S72.7	Multiple fractures of femur
S72.8	Fractures of other parts of femur
S72.009	fracture of unspecified part of neck of unspecified femur
M84.359xY	Stress fracture hip, unspecified
M84.459xY	Pathologic fracture of the hip, unspecified
M85.353xY	Stress fracture unspecified femur

EPIDEMIOLOGY & DEMOGRAPHICS

PREVALENCE: Lifetime risk in women ~16%.
INCIDENCE: 350,000 hip fractures annually in the U.S.
EPIDEMIOLOGY: Female > male
Caucasian > African American
90% >65 yr
Mean age, 80 years old
MORTALITY: 20%-25% mortality within a year following the fracture

PHYSICAL FINDINGS & CLINICAL PRESENTATION

- Hip or groin pain.
- Displaced fractures: affected extremity may be shortened and externally rotated (less often internally rotated).
- Impacted/stressed/nondisplaced fracture: pain with motion or ambulation; often without obvious deformity.
- Ecchymosis or bruising about the hip.
- Inability to bear weight and tenderness to palpation.

RISK FACTORS

- Osteoporosis.
- Age >75.
- Gait instability, foot deformities, and muscular weakness.
- Sensory impairment such as neuropathy.
- Polypharmacy.
- Impaired cognition, depression.
- Use of alcohol or benzodiazepines.
- Orthostatic hypotension.
- Environmental hazards at home (e.g., loose rugs, loose cords).
- Subclinical hyperthyroidism.

ETIOLOGY

- Trauma.
- Age-related bone fragility usually caused by osteoporosis or decreased bone mineral density.
- Increased risk of fractures in elderly (decline in muscle function, reduced bone quality, use of psychotropic medication, etc.).

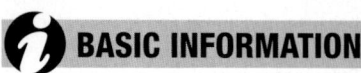

DIFFERENTIAL DIAGNOSIS

- Osteoarthritis/rheumatoid arthritis of the hip
- Hip dislocation
- Pathologic fracture
- Muscle strain or tendonitis
- Lumbar disk syndrome with radicular pain
- Insufficiency fracture of pelvis or pubic ramus fracture
- Trochanteric bursitis
- Septic hip joint
- Pelvic fracture
- Lateral femoral cutaneous nerve entrapment (meralgia paresthetica)
- Labral tear or pathology
- Paget's disease
- Neoplasm

WORKUP

In most cases, the diagnosis is based on clinical presentation and plain radiographs (Figs. 2 and 3). Fig. E4 illustrates the Garden classification of femoral neck fractures, which classifies the fracture based on the amount of displacement or gapping between the fracture fragments. Additional imaging may be required to aid in the diagnosis of

fractures not evident on plain radiographs (e.g., stress or occult fractures).

IMAGING STUDIES

- Standard radiographs should include an anteroposterior view of the pelvis and hip, and a cross-table lateral view of the hip to confirm the diagnosis. Full-length femur and knee films should also be obtained.
- If initial radiographs are negative, then computed tomography (CT) or magnetic resonance imaging (MRI) may be indicated. Stress fractures can be diagnosed with CT scan; however, occult fractures may require an MRI. Bone scanning may also be used to identify fractures.

TREATMENT

- Orthopedic consultation.
- Preoperative workup in elderly patient: CBC, BMP, type and screen, coagulation panel, CXR, ECG, and urinalysis.
- Surgery is indicated in most cases, usually within 24-48 hr. Treatment depends on fracture pattern and stability:

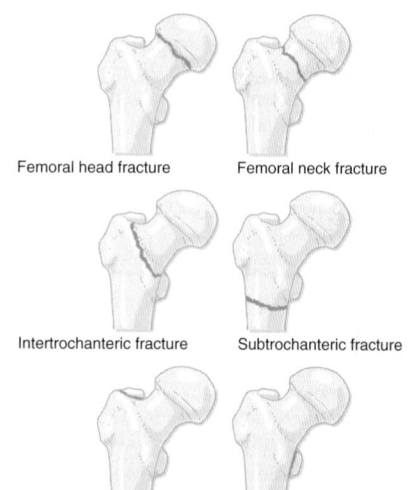

Femoral head fracture

Femoral neck fracture

Intertrochanteric fracture

Subtrochanteric fracture

Greater trochanter fracture

Lesser trochanter fracture

FIG. 1 Types of hip fractures. (From Adams JG.; et al. *Emergency medicine, clinical essentials*, ed 2, Philadelphia, 2013, Elsevier.)

TABLE 1	Garden's Classification of Femoral Neck Fractures
Type I	Nondisplaced, slightly impacted, incomplete fracture line The medial trabeculae of the femoral head and neck form an angle of 180 degrees The femoral head is tilted into valgus The distal fragment lies in external rotation
Type II	Nondisplaced, complete fracture line The medial trabeculae of the femoral head and neck form an angle of 160 degrees Nondisplaced femoral head Normal distal alignment
Type III	Complete fracture line, with displacement <50% The femoral head trabeculae are not in alignment with those of the pelvis The femoral head is tilted into varus and medially rotated The distal fragment lies in external rotation
Type IV	Complete fracture line, with displacement >50% and dissociation The femoral head trabeculae lie in alignment with those of the pelvis The femoral head is detached and frequently realigns with the acetabulum The distal fragment is proximally displaced and lies in external rotation

From Pope TL, Bloem HL, Beltran J, Morrison WB, Wilson DJ: *Musculoskeletal imaging*, ed 2, Philadelphia, 2014, Saunders.

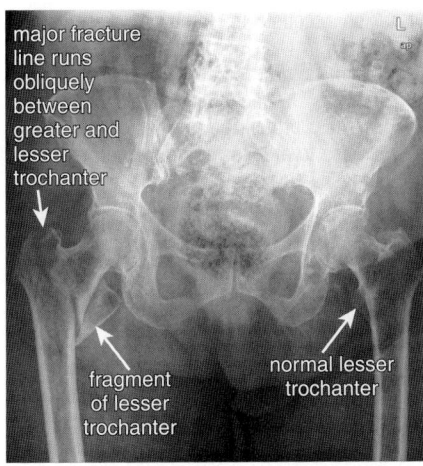

FIG. 2 Intertrochanteric femur fracture: three parts (proximal, distal, and one trochanter).

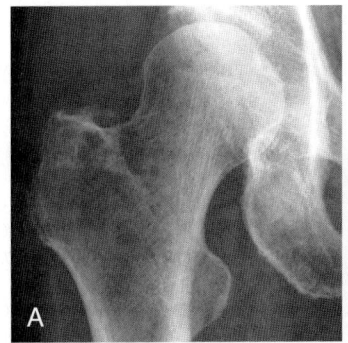
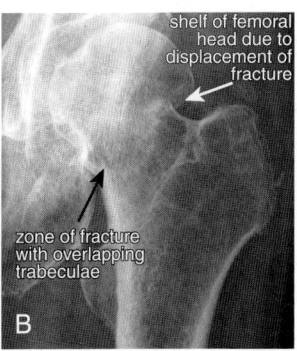

FIG. 3 **Femoral neck fracture.** This 84-year-old female had an unwitnessed fall. **A,** Normal right hip, osteoporotic. **B,** Left hip, another relatively subtle femoral neck fracture. Note the smudging of the trabeculae of the femoral neck. In addition, the distal fragment has shifted medially, creating an overhanging ledge of the femoral head not seen on the opposite normal side. Some femoral neck fractures are more obvious. (From Broder JS: *Diagnostic imaging for the emergency physician*, Philadelphia, 2011, Saunders.)

FIG. 2 Intertrochanteric femur fracture: three parts (proximal, distal, and one trochanter). Intertrochanteric femur fractures are common, with the mechanism often being a fall from standing in an elderly patient. The major fracture line usually runs obliquely between the greater and the lesser trochanters. These fractures may have two, three, or four parts classically, although badly comminuted combinations are also possible. Two-part fractures consist of the proximal and distal fragments. Three-part fractures also include a fragment of one trochanter. Four-part fractures include fragments of both trochanters. This 86-year-old female had an unwitnessed fall. She has a typical 3-part fracture, with a fragment of the lesser trochanter visible. Note her generalized severe osteopenia. (From Broder JS: *Diagnostic imaging for the emergency physician,* Philadelphia, 2011, Saunders.)

1. Femoral neck, nondisplaced/valgus impacted: internal fixation with 3 cannulated screws.
2. Displaced femoral neck: <65 years: urgent anatomic reduction, cannulated screws; >65 years: 3 cannulated screws vs. dynamic hip screw (DHS) vs. intramedullary nail (IMN) vs. hemiarthroplasty vs. total hip arthroplasty.
3. Intertrochanteric: DHS vs. IMN.
4. Unstable intertrochanteric/reverse obliquity: IMN, blade plate, dynamic condylar screw (not DHS).
- Deep vein thrombosis (DVT) prophylaxis (enoxaparin, fondaparinux, heparin). Mechanical DVT prophylaxis in the nonaffected limb. Pharmacologic DVT prophylaxis is usually continued for 14 to 30 days postop.
- Pain management: effective pain management is a primary goal in hip fracture. Opioid analgesics have a high incidence of delirium and constipation. Nerve blockade is effective in reducing acute pain following a hip fracture. A bowel regimen and adequate hydration are recommended in patients taking narcotics.
- Prophylactic antibiotics should be administered before surgery and continued for 24 hours after surgical repair.
- Rehabilitation is a major component of hip fracture treatment and should be initiated on the first postoperative day.

- Conservative therapy and pain control should be considered in patients who are not surgical candidates (e.g., significant medical risk or bed-/wheelchair-bound).

DISPOSITION
- Mortality associated with surgery is 2% to 4%. Older adults have a 5- to 8-fold increased risk for all-cause mortality during the first 3 months after a hip fracture.
- Mortality rate within 1 year in elderly patients is 20% to 30%.
- Increased annual mortality persists over time for both women and men, but at any given age, the annual mortality following a hip fracture is higher in men than in women.
- Dementia is a particularly poor prognostic sign.

REFERRAL
To orthopaedic surgeon for surgical consideration when the diagnosis is made.

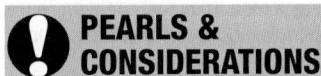 **PEARLS & CONSIDERATIONS**

COMMENTS
- Complications: nonunion, malunion, infection, avascular necrosis, DVT, delirium, decubitus ulcers, persistent pain, loosening of prosthesis, and periprosthetic fractures.
- Nonoperative management:
  1. Should be considered for nonambulatory patients, patients with severe dementia or cognitive impairment, or patients who are at high risk of complications associated with surgery (e.g., severe cardiac or pulmonary disease).
  2. Early bed-to-chair mobilization and vigilant nursing care to avoid skin breakdown and decubitus ulcers.
  3. Patients may experience pain relief prior to physiologic union of the fracture.
- Severe groin pain or inability to ambulate may be the only finding associated with an occult fracture of the femoral neck. If suspected, MRI can be obtained.

- The rate of hip fracture could be reduced by:
  1. Elimination of environmental hazards (e.g., poor lighting, loose rugs, low sitting furniture).
  2. Regular exercise for balance and strength.
  3. Patient education about fall prevention.
  4. Medication review to minimize side effects and reduce polypharmacy.
  5. Prevention and treatment of osteoporosis (e.g., calcium/vitamin D, resistance exercise, reversal of underlying pathology).
- In the U.S., hip fracture rates and subsequent mortality among persons aged 65 years and older are declining, and comorbidities among patients with hip fractures are very expensive ($40,000 in the first year following hip fracture for direct medical costs and $5000 in subsequent years). The estimated cost related to hip fractures was >$20 billion in 2007.
- Fragility (or low-energy) hip fractures are common in elderly patients with reduced bone quality. These types of fractures are associated with a 1-year mortality of 26% with 58% of patients requiring long-term care in a nursing facility. Diagnosis of a fragility fracture of the hip is associated with a second fragility fracture within the next 5 years.
- Concurrent prolonged use of proton-pump inhibitors (≥1 yr) is associated with reduced effectiveness of alendronate for preventing hip fractures in older adults.

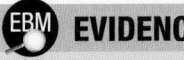 **EVIDENCE**

Available at www.expertconsult.com

SUGGESTED READINGS
Available at www.expertconsult.com

RELATED CONTENT
Hip Fracture (Patient Information)

AUTHOR: **MICHAEL C. MARIORENZI, M.S., M.D.**

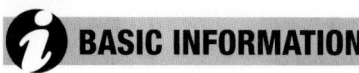

BASIC INFORMATION

DEFINITION

Hirsutism is the development of stiff, pigmented (terminal) facial and body hair (male distribution) in women as a result of excess androgen production.

SYNONYMS

Excessive hair growth

ICD-10CM CODES
L68.0 Hirsutism

EPIDEMIOLOGY & DEMOGRAPHICS

- Overall prevalence unknown, estimated 5% to 10% in reproductive age women.
- Race and genetics should be considered. Some distinct ethnic populations have minimal body hair and others (Mediterranean, Middle Eastern, South Asian) have moderate to large amounts of body hair while serum androgen levels are similar.
- Social norms and culture also determine how much body hair is cosmetically acceptable.
- Half of all cases of mild hirsutism do not have hyperandrogenemia. "Patient-important hirsutism" refers to hirsutism causing woman sufficient distress to seek care.
- Incidence and presentation of hirsutism is dependent on underlying cause of androgen excess (see "Differential Diagnosis").
- Most women with hirsutism have polycystic ovary syndrome.

PHYSICAL FINDINGS & CLINICAL PRESENTATION

- Timing of symptoms: abrupt onset, short duration, rapid progression, progressive worsening, more severe signs of virilization (Fig. 1), or later age of onset suggest androgen-producing tumor, late-onset congenital adrenal hyperplasia, or Cushing's syndrome.

- Weight increases may produce increased androgen production.
- Menstrual history: menarche, cycle regularity and symptoms of ovulation, fertility, and contraception use. Anovulatory cycles are the most common underlying cause of androgen excess.
- Medication use history: some drugs cause hirsutism or produce androgenic effects (danazol, phenytoin, valproic acid, androgenic progestins [e.g., norgestrel], cyclosporin, minoxidil, metoclopramide, phenothiazines, methyldopa, diazoxide, and penicillamine).
- Family history: known or suspected family history of hirsutism, congenital adrenal hyperplasia, insulin resistance, polycystic ovary syndrome (PCOS), infertility, obesity, menstrual irregularity may be found.
- Physical exam reveals deepening voice, body habitus, increased muscle mass, galactorrhea; abdominal and pelvic exam.
- Associated cutaneous manifestations (Fig. 2) are acne, acanthosis nigricans, striae, hair distribution, location and quantity, frontotemporal balding, muscle mass, clitoromegaly.
- Ferriman-Gallwey scale, a simple, pictorial system of scoring nine body areas, is the most common tool used to quantify hirsutism. It may be unreliable in non-Caucasian women of other ethnicities.

ETIOLOGY

- Presence of hirsutism indicates androgen excess. Total testosterone may be normal, but free testosterone is elevated.
- Androgens induce vellus hair follicles (soft, unpigmented hair) in sex-specific areas (upper lip, chin, midsternum, upper abdomen, back, buttocks) to develop into thicker, more heavily pigmented terminal hairs.
- Anovulatory ovaries are usual source of excess androgens through thecal cell steroidogenesis and conversion of androstenedione to testosterone. The most common cause of hirsutism is polycystic ovary syndrome,

which accounts for three out of every four cases.
- Conditions that decrease hepatic production of sex hormone binding globulin (SHBG) decrease protein-bound testosterone and increase free testosterone fraction (e.g., low estrogen, high androgen, and hyperinsulinemic states).
- Late-onset, congenital adrenal hyperplasia enzyme deficiency (most commonly 21-hydroxylase deficiency) produces excess 17 hydroxyprogesterone (17-OHP) and overproduction of androstenedione.
- Rare ovarian tumors primarily derived from Sertoli-Leydig cells, granulosa theca cells, or hilus cells produce excess androgens.
- Rare adrenal tumors produce excess androgens.
- Rare pituitary or hypothalamic tumors produce excess prolactin and can lead to anovulation.
- Box 1 summarizes causes of androgen excess in women of reproductive age.

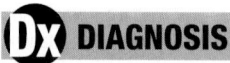 DIAGNOSIS

DIFFERENTIAL DIAGNOSIS

- Androgen-independent vellus hair: soft, unpigmented hair that covers entire body
- Hypertrichosis: diffusely increased total body hair (vellus or lanugo-type) not restricted to androgen-dependent areas often an adverse response to a medication or systemic illness (e.g., anorexia nervosa, porphyria, malnutrition, hypothyroidism)
- PCOS 75%
- Idiopathic 5% to 15%
- Congenital adrenal hyperplasia 1% to 8%
- Insulin resistance syndrome 3% to 4%
- Cushing's syndrome <1%
- Drug induced <1%
- Ovarian tumor <1%
- Adrenal tumor <1%
- Hyperthecosis <1%
- Hyperprolactinemia <1%

WORKUP

- Hirsutism is a clinical diagnosis.
- Management of hirsutism is largely independent of the etiology.
- Workup in selected hirsute women is directed to determine underlying cause of androgen excess.
- See specific conditions for more detailed workup of individual diagnoses.

LABORATORY TESTS

Establishing laboratory evidence of excess androgens in women with moderate or severe hirsutism, sudden onset, rapid progression, or associated menstrual dysfunction, central obesity, clitoromegaly, or acanthosis nigricans is an approach consistent with guidelines from the Endocrine Society, the American College of Obstetricians and Gynecologists, the Androgen Excess and Polycystic Ovary Syndrome Society and the American Association of Clinical Endocrinologists.

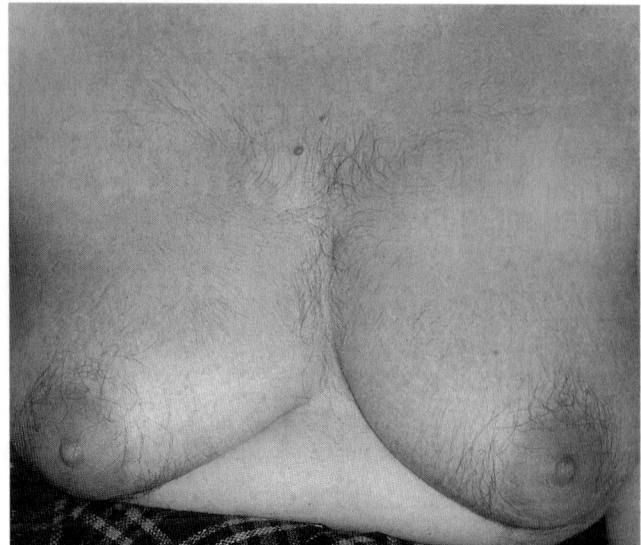

FIG. 1 Hirsutism. (From James WD et al: *Andrews' diseases of the skin*, ed 12, Philadelphia, 2016, Saunders.)

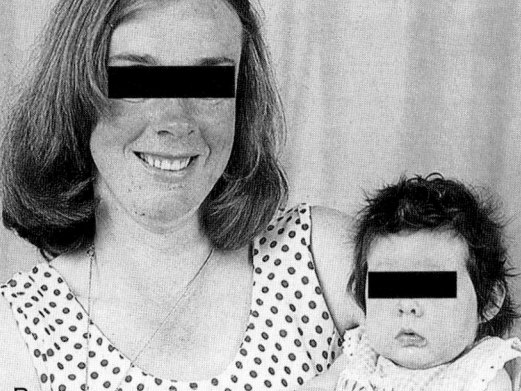

FIG. 2 A patient with an arrhenoblastoma with associated polycystic ovaries before and after treatment. **A,** Before treatment, the patient had marked facial hirsutism. **B,** The patient is shown successfully treated. The tumor was resected and ovulation ensued with clomiphene and human chorionic gonadotropin therapy. (From Besser CM, Thorner MO: *Comprehensive clinical endocrinology,* ed 3, St Louis, 2002, Mosby.)

BOX 1 Causes of Androgen Excess in Women of Reproductive Age

Ovarian
Polycystic ovary syndrome (PCOS)
Hyperthecosis (a severe PCOS variant)
Ovarian tumor (e.g., Sertoli-Leydig cell tumor)

Adrenal
Nonclassic adrenal hyperplasia
Cushing's syndrome
Glucocorticoid resistance
Adrenal tumor (e.g., adenoma, carcinoma)

Specific Conditions of Pregnancy
Luteoma of pregnancy
Hyperreaction luteinalis
Aromatase deficiency in fetus

Other
Hyperprolactinemia, hypothyroidism
Medications (danazol, testosterone, anabolizing agents)
Idiopathic hirsutism (normal serum testosterone in an ovulatory woman)
Idiopathic hyperandrogenism (patients who do not fall into any of the other categories listed)

From Melmed S et al: *Williams textbook of endocrinology,* ed 12, Philadelphia, 2011, Saunders.

- Total plasma testosterone (normal range 20-60 ng/dl [0.69-2.1 nmol/L]) or free testosterone: early morning on day 4 to 10 of menstrual cycle to screen for testosterone-secreting tumors. If moderately or markedly elevated (total testosterone >150 ng/dl [5.2 nmol/L], free testosterone >2 ng/dl [0.07 nmol/L]) may image adrenals and ovaries for androgen-secreting tumors.
  Other laboratory test considerations if appropriate:
- Prolactin: moderately elevated values should prompt imaging of pituitary-hypothalamic region
- 17-OHP (17 α-hydroxyprogesterone): screen for adrenal enzyme deficiencies. Morning value >200 ng/dl in early follicular phase suggests nonclassic (late onset) congenital adrenal hyperplasia due to 21-hydroxylase deficiency and may be confirmed with high-dose (250 mcg) ACTH stimulation test.
- Thyroid-stimulating hormone (TSH): rule out hypothyroidism

- Dehydroepiandrosterone sulfate (DHEA-S): screen for adrenal androgen production as almost entirely produced by adrenals. Levels >700 mcg/dl (13.6 nmol/L) raise suspicion for adrenal androgen-secreting tumor.
  Additional laboratory test considerations if appropriate:
- Follicle-stimulating hormone: (FSH): rule out hypoestrogenic state (perimenopausal).
- Luteinizing hormone: (LH): typically elevated in PCOS with low or normal FSH.
- 24-hour urinary free cortisol: rule out Cushing's syndrome and overproduction of cortisol.
- Overnight single-dose dexamethasone suppression test: rule out Cushing's syndrome and adrenal hyperfunction.
- Fasting blood sugar (FBS), 2-hr 75-g oral glucose tolerance test, fasting insulin levels: rule out insulin resistance syndrome.
- Table 1 summarizes laboratory tests for the differential diagnosis of androgen excess

IMAGING STUDIES

Imaging study considerations if appropriate:
- Pelvic ultrasound (high resolution, transvaginal): rule out ovarian tumor if total testosterone is elevated.
- Abdominal CT/MRI: rule out adrenal tumor if elevated DHEAS.
- Pituitary-hypothalamic region CT/MRI: rule out pituitary tumor if prolactin elevated.
- Laparoscopy/laparotomy: rule out small ovarian tumor in cases of elevated testosterone levels without radiologic evidence of adrenal or ovarian pathology.

Rx TREATMENT

NONPHARMACOLOGIC THERAPY

- Weight reduction: can reduce androgen production indirectly by reducing insulin-stimulated theca cell androgen production and improve menstrual function, and slow hair growth in obese women.
- Cosmetic: temporary.
  1. Shaving: does not stimulate hair growth; lasts days, leaves stubble.
  2. Epilation: electronic plucking.
  3. Bleaching: removes hair pigment. May cause skin irritation.
  4. Mechanical waxing/plucking.
  5. Depilatories: gels, lotions, or creams that chemically disrupt sulfide bonds of hair causing dissolution of hair shaft. No stubble.
  6. Photoepilation (laser and intense pulsed light [IPL]): hair follicles destroyed by wavelengths of light absorbed by melanin. Good for pigmented hair; laser treatment is more effective than shaving, waxing, and electrolysis. It lasts 3 to 6 months as vellus follicles remain and can be converted to terminal pigmented hair under excess androgens.
- Cosmetic: permanent. Electrolysis: destroys individual hair follicles. May be expensive and time consuming.

ACUTE GENERAL Rx

See "Pharmacologic Therapy."

CHRONIC Rx

See "Pharmacologic Therapy."

PHARMACOLOGIC THERAPY

- Usually second-line treatment following non-pharmacologic, physical methods of hair control, and in consideration of patient's comorbidities and risk factors, patient preferences, area of excess hair amenable to treatment, and access and affordability of treatments.
- Pharmacologic treatments categorized as topical, oral contraceptive pills (OCPs), anti-androgens (potential adverse effects on a developing male fetus, so use with reliable contraception), other treatments directed at specific underlying etiology.
- Topical: Eflornithine topical cream 13.9%: unclear mechanism of action; may inhibit

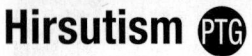
TABLE 1 Laboratory Tests for the Differential Diagnosis of Androgen Excess

Initial Testing

Total testosterone
Prolactin
Thyroid-stimulating hormone

Further Testing Based on Clinical Presentation

17-Hydroxyprogesterone (8:00 a.m.)
17-Hydroxyprogesterone 60 min after IV ACTH
Cortisol (8:00 a.m.) after 1 mg dexamethasone at midnight
DHEAS
Androstenedione
Imaging of ovaries (transvaginal ultrasonography)
Imaging of adrenals (abdominal ultrasonography, CT, MRI)
Nuclear imaging after IV administration of radiolabeled cholesterol

ACTH, Adrenocorticotropic hormone; *DHEAS,* dehydroepiandrosterone sulfate.
From Melmed S et al.: *Williams textbook of endocrinology,* ed12, Philadelphia, 2011, Saunders.

ornithine decarboxylase, retarding hair growth. Temporary cosmetic treatment for facial hair. Applied directly to unwanted facial hair bid with at least 8 hr spaced applications. Does not remove hair, rather slows growth. Slow response over 4 to 8 wk. Hair growth returns upon discontinuation of treatment.

- OCPs: Suppress ovarian steroidogenesis and LH through low-dose estrogen and low androgenic progestational agents. Slow response to treatment. Suppresses new hair growth. Established hair unaffected. Low-dose OCPs with low androgenic progestational agents, for example, desogestrel, drospirenone, norgestimate. Avoid norgestrel and levonorgestrel (higher androgenic progestational agents).
- Antiandrogens: Spironolactone: when OCPs unacceptable or may be added for disappointing results after 6 mo of OCP treatment.
  1. Aldosterone-antagonist diuretic inhibits adrenal and ovarian biosynthesis of androgens. May result in ovulation, so consider contraception needs.
  2. Slow response usually 6 mo or more.
  3. 200 mg PO qd, then decrease to 25 to 50 mg qd maintenance.
  4. May cause hyperkalemia.
  5. Anovulatory, unopposed estrogen states require progestin management.

REFERRAL

- To endocrinologist if difficulty in determining diagnosis, achieving therapeutic goals, or resistant to first-line therapies. Prepubertal and postmenopausal hirsutism is suspicious for neoplastic or secondary endocrine causes and should be referred for further evaluation.
- Consider referral or consultation for following therapies:
  1. Finasteride: antiandrogen, in hair follicle blocks 5α-reductase conversion of testosterone to intranuclearly active 5α-dihydrotestosterone (DHT).
     1. Use only with reliable contraception because DHT necessary for normal male fetus urogenital development.
     2. Not FDA approved for treatment of hirsutism.
     3. 1 to 5 mg PO qd.
  2. Flutamide: inhibits androgen uptake and receptor binding
     1. Not recommended by Endocrine Society Clinical Practice Guidelines and not FDA approved for treatment of hirsutism, but used by some European endocrinologists.
     2. Use only with reliable contraception.
     3. Reserved for women with severe, resistant hirsutism because of risk of hepatic dysfunction.
     4. 250 mg PO bid.

3. Cyproterone acetate (not available in the United States): antiandrogen that competes with DHT for binding androgen receptors. Used as progestin component of OCPs outside the United States.

- Other treatments directed at specific underlying etiology:
  1. Metformin/thiazolidinediones: therapy reserved for documented insulin-resistant states.
  2. GnRH agonists: recommended only in women with severe hyperandrogenemia (e.g., ovarian hyperthecosis) with suboptimal response to combination low-dose estrogen/progestin pills and antiandrogen treatment. Inhibits gonadotropin and consequently ovarian androgen and estrogen secretion.
  3. Dexamethasone: adrenal glucocorticoid suppression is reserved for diagnosis of adrenal enzyme deficiency.
  4. Total abdominal hysterectomy/bilateral salpingo-oophorectomy reserved for recalcitrant hirsutism in older female with hyperthecosis and undesired fertility.

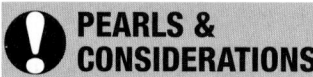

PEARLS & CONSIDERATIONS

COMMENTS

- Hirsutism is both an endocrine and cosmetic problem for patients.
- Ovulation induction therapy is indicated in women desiring pregnancy.
- Delay checking serum androgens until oral contraceptives have been discontinued for 2 to 3 mo.
- Evaluation of incidental adrenal mass is always warranted.

SUGGESTED READINGS

Available at www.expertconsult.com

RELATED CONTENT

Hirsutism (Patient Information)

AUTHOR: **RICHARD LONG, M.D.**

BASIC INFORMATION

DEFINITION

Histoplasmosis is caused by the fungus *Histoplasma capsulatum* and characterized by a primary pulmonary focus with occasional progression to chronic pulmonary histoplasmosis (CPH) or various forms of dissemination. Progressive disseminated histoplasmosis (PDH) may present with a diverse clinical spectrum, including adrenal necrosis, pulmonary and mediastinal fibrosis, and ulcerations of the oropharynx and GI tract. In those patients coinfected with HIV, it is a defining disease for AIDS.

SYNONYMS

North American histoplasmosis
Ohio Valley fever
Vanderbilt disease

ICD-10CM CODES
B39.0 Acute pulmonary histoplasmosis capsulati
B39.1 Chronic pulmonary histoplasmosis capsulati
B39.2 Pulmonary histoplasmosis capsulati, unspecified
B39.3 Disseminated histoplasmosis capsulati
B39.4 Histoplasmosis capsulati, unspecified
B39.5 Histoplasmosis duboisii
B39.9 Histoplasmosis, unspecified

EPIDEMIOLOGY & DEMOGRAPHICS

INCIDENCE (IN U.S.):
- Unknown for acute pulmonary disease
- For CPH, estimated at 1/100,000 cases in endemic areas
- For PDH in immunocompetent adults, estimated at 1/2000 cases of histoplasmosis

PREVALENCE: Unknown

PREDOMINANT SEX: Clinically evident disease is most common in males; male/female ratio of 4:1

PREDOMINANT AGE:
- CPH is most often seen in males >50 yr old with an associated history of COPD.
- Presumed ocular histoplasmosis syndrome (POHS) is seen between ages of 20 and 40 yr.

PEAK INCIDENCE: Unknown

PHYSICAL FINDINGS & CLINICAL PRESENTATION

- Conidia are deposited in alveoli then converted to yeast forms where they spread to regional lymph nodes and other organs, especially liver and spleen.
- 1 to 2 wk later, a granulomatous inflammatory response begins to contain the yeast in the form of discrete granulomas.
- Delayed-type hypersensitivity to *Histoplasma* antigens occurs 3 to 6 wk after exposure.
- Clinical disease manifests in various forms, depending on host cellular immunity and inoculum size:
  1. **Acute primary pulmonary histoplasmosis**
     a. An overwhelming number of patients are asymptomatic.
     b. Most clinically apparent infections manifest by complaints of fever, headache, malaise, pleuritic chest pain, nonproductive cough, and weight loss.
     c. Less than 10%, mainly women, complain of arthralgias, myalgias, and skin manifestations such as erythema multiforme or erythema nodosum.
     d. Acute pericarditis presents in a smaller percentage of patients.
     e. Hepatosplenomegaly is most commonly observed in children.
     f. With particularly heavy exposure, there is severe dyspnea, marked hypoxemia, impending respiratory failure.
     g. Most patients are asymptomatic within 6 wk.
  2. **CPH**
     a. Presents insidiously with low-grade fever, malaise, weight loss, cough, sometimes with blood-streaked sputum or frank hemoptysis.
     b. Most patients with cavitary lesions present with associated COPD or chronic bronchitis, masking underlying fungal disease.
     c. Tends to worsen preexisting pulmonary disease and further contribute to eventual respiratory insufficiency.
  3. **PDH**
     a. In both acute and subacute forms, constitutional symptoms of fever, fatigue, malaise, and weight loss are common.
     b. Acute form (seen in infants and children) presents with respiratory symptoms, fever ≥101° F (38.3° C), generalized lymphadenopathy, marked hepatosplenomegaly, and fulminant course resembling septic shock associated with a high fatality rate.
     c. Subacute form is more common in adults and associated with lower temperatures, hepatosplenomegaly, oropharyngeal ulceration, focal organ involvement (including adrenal destruction, endocarditis, chronic meningitis, and intracerebral mass lesions).
     d. Course of subacute form is relentless, with untreated patients dying within 2 yr.
     e. Chronic PDH is found in adults and marked by gradual symptoms of weight loss, weakness, easy fatigability; low-grade fever when present; oropharyngeal ulcerations and hepatomegaly and/or splenomegaly in one third of patients.
     f. Less clinical evidence of focal organ involvement in chronic form than in subacute form.
     g. Natural history of chronic form is protracted and intermittent, spanning months to years.
- **Histoplasmoma**
  1. A healed area of caseation necrosis surrounded by a fibrous capsule
  2. Usually asymptomatic
- **Mediastinal fibrosis**
  1. A rare consequence of a fibroblastic process that encases caseating mediastinal lymph nodes producing severe retraction, compression, and distortion of mediastinal structures
  2. Constriction of the bronchi resulting in bronchiectasis, also esophageal stenosis associated with dysphagia, and superior vena cava syndrome
- **POHS**
  1. Diagnosis characterized by distinct clinical features, including atrophic choroidal scars and maculopathy in patients with histories suggestive of exposure to the fungus (e.g., residence in an endemic area)
  2. Patient complains of distortion or loss of central vision without pain, redness, or photophobia
  3. Usually no evidence of infection except for a positive skin reaction to histoplasmin
- **In patients with AIDS**
  1. Possible presentation as overwhelming infection similar to acute PDH seen in children
  2. Constitutional symptoms: fever, weight loss, malaise, cough, dyspnea
  3. About 10% with cutaneous maculopapular, erythematous eruptions or purpuric lesions on face, trunk, and extremities
  4. Up to 20% with CNS involvement, manifesting as intracerebral mass lesions, chronic meningitis, or encephalopathy

ETIOLOGY

- *H. capsulatum* is a dimorphic fungus present in temperate zones and river valleys worldwide.
- In the U.S., it is highly endemic in southeastern, mid-Atlantic, and central states.
- Exists as mold at ambient temperature and favors soils enriched with bird or bat droppings.

DIAGNOSIS

DIFFERENTIAL DIAGNOSIS

- Acute pulmonary histoplasmosis
  1. Mycobacterium tuberculosis
  2. Community-acquired pneumonias caused by Mycoplasma and Chlamydia
  3. Other fungal diseases, such as Blastomyces dermatitidis and Coccidioides immitis
- Chronic cavitary pulmonary histoplasmosis: *M. tuberculosis*
- Histoplasmomas: true neoplasms

WORKUP

- Suspect diagnosis in patients who present with a history of residence or travel in an endemic area, especially if engaged in occupations (e.g., outside construction or street cleaning) or hobbies (e.g., cave exploring) that increase the likelihood of exposure to fungal spores.
- Suspect diagnosis in immunosuppressed patients with remote history of exposure, especially if associated with characteristic calcifications on chest x-ray.

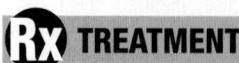
LABORATORY TESTS

- Demonstration of organism on culture from body fluid or tissues biopsy (Fig. E1) to make definitive diagnosis
  1. Especially high yield in patients with AIDS
  2. Characteristic oval yeast cells in neutrophils with Giemsa stain from peripheral smear
  3. Preparations of infected tissue with Gomori's silver methenamine for revealing yeast forms, especially in areas of caseation necrosis
- Serologic tests, including complement-fixing (CF) antibodies and immunodiffusion assays
- Detection of *Histoplasma* antigen in serum and urine. Urine antigen is 75% accurate in normal hosts and 95% in immunocompromised patients with disseminated disease. The serum test is close to 100% accurate, but with *Blastomyces* and *Coccidioides,* tests may cross-react with infections.
- In PDH
  1. Pancytopenia
  2. Marked elevations in alkaline phosphatase and alanine aminotransferase (ALT) common
- In chronic meningitis (majority of cases)
  1. CSF pleocytosis with either lymphocytes or neutrophils predominating
  2. Elevated CSF protein levels
  3. Hypoglycorrhachia

IMAGING STUDIES

- Chest x-ray in acute pulmonary histoplasmosis
  1. Singular or multiple patchy infiltrates, especially in the lower lung fields
  2. Hilar or mediastinal lymphadenopathy with or without pneumonitis
  3. Diffuse nodular or confluent bilateral miliary infiltrates characteristic of heavier exposure
  4. Infrequent pleural effusions, except when associated with pericarditis
- Chest x-ray in histoplasmoma: coin lesion displaying central calcification, ranging from 1 to 4 cm in diameter, predominantly located in the subpleural regions
- Chest x-ray in CPH (Fig. E2):
  1. Upper lobe disease frequently associated with cavities
  2. Preexisting calcifications in the hilum associated with peribronchial streaking extending to the parenchyma
- Chest x-ray in acute PDH: hilar adenopathy and/or diffuse nodular infiltrates

- CT scan of adrenals to reveal bilateral enlargement and low-attenuation centers

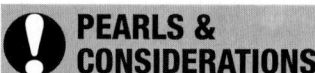

NONPHARMACOLOGIC THERAPY

For life-threatening disease seen in acute disseminated disease or infection in patients with AIDS: supportive therapy with IV fluids

ACUTE GENERAL Rx

- No drug therapy is required for asymptomatic pulmonary disease.
- A course of therapy with itraconazole 200 mg PO tid for 3 days, then 200 mg/day PO for 6-12 wk may be beneficial in some patients with acute pulmonary distress. Avoid fluconazole because it is not as active.
- Same therapy appropriate for immunocompetent, mild to moderately symptomatic patients with CPH and subacute and chronic forms of PDH, but duration for 6 to 12 mo.
- Use amphotericin B 0.7 to 1 mg/kg IV q day for initial therapy in moderate to severe disease and then transition to oral itraconazole within 1 to 2 wk. Lipid formulations of amphotericin can be used to avoid nephrotoxicity of amphotericin B, and they produce better outcomes in terms of mortality, rates of culture conversion, and side effects.
- (Liposomal amphotericin: 3 mg/kg/day IV or amphotericin B lipid complex: 5 mg/kg/day)
- Posaconazole is highly effective as well, but voriconazole is less active in vitro than itraconazole and posaconazole. Isavuconazole is also active in vitro, but echinocandins such as micafungin are not effective.
- Chronic cavitary pulmonary histoplasmosis: itraconazole 200 mg PO tid for 3 days, then once or twice daily for at least 12 mo.
- CNS histoplasmosis: liposomal amphotericin B, 5 mg/kg/day for a total of 175 mg/kg over 4 to 6 wk, then itraconazole 200 mg 2 to 3×/day for at least 12 mo.
- Endocarditis: surgical treatment with excision of infected valve or graft combined with amphotericin for a total dose of 35 mg/kg or 2.5 g.
- For pericardial disease:
  1. Antifungal therapy: no apparent benefit
  2. Best managed with NSAIDs
- For POHS:
  1. Antifungal therapy: no apparent benefit
  2. May respond to laser therapy

CHRONIC Rx

- In patients with AIDS: lifelong suppressive therapy with either itraconazole, given 200 mg PO q day, or IV amphotericin B at a dose of 50 mg once weekly; a triazole compound posaconazole (400 mg PO bid) may be useful in refractory cases, but clinical experience is limited at this point.
- Prophylaxis in HIV-infected patients with <150 CD4 cells/mm³: itraconazole 200 mg PO qd

DISPOSITION

For those with chronic or progressive disease, especially if immunocompromised, prognosis is dependent on prompt recognition and timely administration of appropriate antifungal drugs.

REFERRAL

- To an infectious disease specialist in suspected cases of disseminated disease, especially if immunocompromised
- To a pulmonologist for patients with CPH form because of progressive respiratory compromise
- To a thoracic surgeon for decompression procedures for progressive mediastinal fibrosis

PEARLS & CONSIDERATIONS

- *H. capsulatum,* variety *duboisii,* also known as African histoplasmosis, is restricted to Senegal, Nigeria, Zaire, and Uganda.
- Unlike *H. capsulatum,* pulmonary forms of *duboisii* are not seen, and the disease is limited to the skin, soft tissues, and bone.

COMMENTS

- Patients living in endemic areas, especially if immunocompromised, should take appropriate respiratory precautions when disposing of bird waste from rooftop or home aviaries.
- Appropriate respiratory precautions should also be taken when leisure traveling to areas that act as a natural haven for the fungus, such as bat caves.

SUGGESTED READINGS

Available at www.expertconsult.com

RELATED CONTENT

Histoplasmosis (Patient Information)

AUTHOR: **GLENN G. FORT, M.D., M.P.H.**

BASIC INFORMATION

- HIV-associated cognitive dysfunction (HAND) covers a spectrum of disorders ranging from asymptomatic to clinically severe (including AIDS dementia complex or HIV encephalopathy).
- Cognitive, motor, and behavioral abnormalities

SYNONYMS

HAD
HAND
HIV-associated neurocognitive disorder
HIV dementia
HIV-associated dementia
Mild neurocognitive disorder
AIDS dementia complex
HIV-1 encephalopathy

ICD-10CM CODES
B20   Human immunodeficiency virus [HIV] disease
R41.8 Other and unspecified symptoms and signs involving cognitive functions and awareness
B97.35 Human immunodeficiency virus, type 2 [HIV 2] as the cause of diseases classified elsewhere

EPIDEMIOLOGY

- According to the CHARTER study, approximately 52% of HIV-infected individuals have HAND. The largest group has asymptomatic neurocognitive impairment (approximately 33%), followed by minor neurocognitive disorder (12%) and HIV-associated dementia (2%).
- The epidemiology has changed in the era of antiretroviral therapy (ART), with the number of cases of HIV-associated dementia (HAD) falling from 15% in the pre-ART era to 2% now, but the proportion of mildly affected patients is increasing.
- As HIV-infected patients live longer, the prevalence of HAND may be increasing.

CLINICAL FEATURES

- The 2007 Frascati Criteria for HAND require assessment of five cognitive domains when evaluating a patient for the presence of HAND: verbal/language ability, attention and working memory, abstraction and executive function, speed of information processing, sensory perceptual skills, and motor skills. The criteria define three levels of HAND:
  ○ Asymptomatic neurocognitive disorder: an acquired impairment in at least two cognitive domains as defined by a performance on neuropsychological testing of more than 1 SD below expected age and education-adjusted norms. This impairment does not impact daily functioning, and the patient may be unaware of its existence.
  ○ Mild neurocognitive disorder: an acquired impairment in at least two cognitive domains as defined by a performance on neuropsychological testing of more than 1 SD below expected age and education-adjusted norms. This impairment does

impact daily functioning to a mild degree. For example, work efficiency is decreased, but the patient can compensate for the deficits.
  ○ HIV-associated dementia: an acquired impairment in at least two cognitive domains as defined by a performance on neuropsychological testing of more than 2 SD below expected age and education-adjusted norms. This impairment does impact daily functioning to a significant degree.
- Cognitive changes: forgetfulness, poor attention and concentration, increased difficulty performing complex tasks, slowed psycho-motor speed.
- Behavioral changes: apathy, lack of initiative, social withdrawal, irritability, occasionally agitation, psychosis or obsessive-compulsive disorder.
- Motor problems: clumsiness, unsteady gait, poor balance, tremor, leg weakness.
- Progressive/later stages: bedbound, severe dementia, bowel/bladder incontinence.
- Classically HIV-associated dementia was described as a classic subcortical dementia (attention, concentration, working memory, and executive function difficulties being prominent features). However, in the ART era, more patients are developing cortical features.
- Results from inflammation triggered by HIV itself (not related to opportunistic infection) and immune activation of microglia and brain macrophages.
- In children: developmental delay, microcephaly, and spasticity are common.

- Table 1 summarizes features of HIV-associated neurocognitive disorder.

RISK FACTORS

- Low CD4 count (less than 200 cells/mm³)
- High viral load
- Anemia
- Injection drug use
- Hepatitis C
- Female gender
- Older age

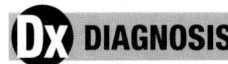 DIAGNOSIS

DIAGNOSTIC EVALUATION

- Diagnosis is based on clinical examination and neuropsychologic tests and exclusion of opportunistic processes.
- CT of brain may show subcortical hypodensities, enlarged ventricles, and cortical atrophy greater than expected for age.
- MRI head (Fig. 1): diffuse, confluent, periventricular white matter lesions on T2-weighted images with cortical atrophy and enlarged ventricles. The white matter hypointensities are not mandatory for the diagnosis.
- Lumbar puncture: CSF analysis helps to rule out opportunistic infections. In HIV-related cognitive dysfunction the CSF may show a nonspecific increase in cell count and protein.
- Subtle electrophysiologic abnormalities can be found in early HIV-1 infection (on electro-encephalography, evoked potentials, nerve conduction studies), but they do not seem to have a predictive value for the later onset of

TABLE 1 Clinical Triad in Human Immunodeficiency Virus Type 1–Associated Neurocognitive Disorder

Cognition	Behavioral	Motor
Forgetfulness	Apathy	Gait instability
Mental slowing	Social withdrawal	Poor coordination
Decreased concentration	Lack of spontaneity	Leg weakness

From Bennett JE et al: *Mandell, Douglas, and Bennett's principles and practice of infectious diseases,* ed 8, Philadelphia, 2015, Saunders.

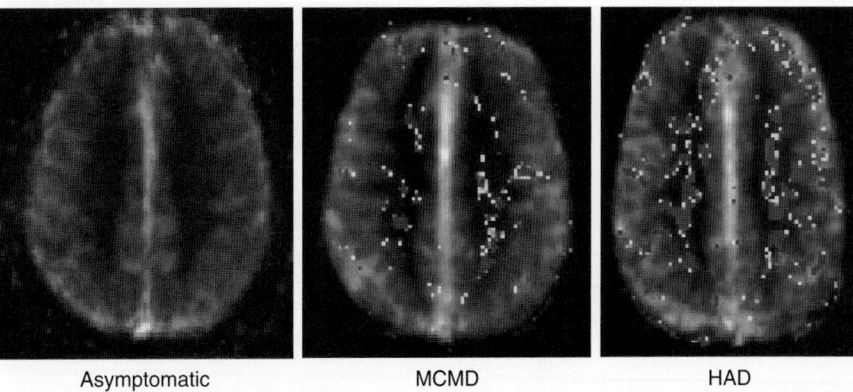

Asymptomatic   MCMD   HAD

FIG. 1 Perfusion MRI (pMRI) maps showing regions of increasing cerebral blood volume (CBV) with advancing HIV groups: asymptomatic, minor cognitive–motor disorder (MCMD), and HIV-associated dementia (HAD). Areas of red indicate >2 standard deviations elevation in CBV. (Tucker KA et al: Neuroimaging in human immunodeficiency virus infection, *J Neuroimmunol* 157(1-2):153-162, 2004.)

AIDS dementia, which generally occurs when the CD4+ T-lymphocyte counts are less than 200 cells/microliter.[1]

- Potential causes for cognitive impairment that must be ruled out include:
  1. Opportunistic central nervous system (CNS) processes (toxoplasmosis, CNS lymphoma, progressive multifocal leukoencephalopathy, cytomegalovirus encephalitis)
  2. General paresis of the insane due to syphilis
  3. Vitamin B_{12} deficiency
  4. Substance use
  5. Alcoholism
  6. Psychiatric disorders such as depression, anxiety, bipolar disorder
  7. Side effects of prescribed medications

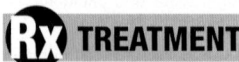 **TREATMENT**

Early treatment with antiretroviral therapy (ART) may lead to clinical improvement in some patients, but in most cases, cognitive dysfunction persists despite ART.

Maintaining high CD4 count and not allowing CD4 count to nadir below 200 cells/microliter may protect against the development of HAND.

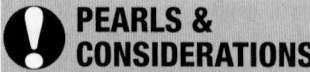 **PEARLS & CONSIDERATIONS**

- Initiation of ART can lead to rapid improvement in cognitive function in early stages (untreated, life span of patient with HIV-associated dementia is typically 4-6 mo)
- Most common presenting complaint in children infected with HIV
- Usually cognitive symptoms precede motor abnormalities
- Five HIV-related opportunistic infections that commonly cause cognitive impairment are: toxoplasmosis, cryptococcal meningitis, progressive multifocal leukoencephalopathy, primary CNS lymphoma, and cytomegalovirus encephalitis

REFERRALS

- Upon diagnosis/clinical suspicion for HIV-associated cognitive dysfunction, referral to neurology is recommended
- Referral to neuropsychology may be considered
- Referral to infectious disease specialist to manage HIV infection

SUGGESTED READINGS

Available at www.expertconsult.com

AUTHORS: **JOSEPH S. KASS, M.D., J.D.,** and **DIVYA SINGHAL, M.D.**

BASIC INFORMATION

DEFINITION

Hodgkin lymphoma is a malignant disorder arising from germinal center B cells and characterized histologically by the presence of multinucleated giant cells (Reed-Sternberg cells) in a mixed inflammatory background.

ICD-10CM CODES

C81.90 Hodgkin lymphoma, unspecified, unspecified site
C81.00 Nodular lymphocyte predominant Hodgkin lymphoma, unspecified site
C81.10 Nodular sclerosis classical Hodgkin lymphoma, unspecified site
C81.20 Mixed cellularity classical Hodgkin lymphoma, unspecified site
C81.30 Lymphocyte depleted classical Hodgkin lymphoma, unspecified site
C81.79 Other classical Hodgkin lymphoma, extranodal and solid organ sites
C81.90 Hodgkin lymphoma, unspecified, unspecified site
C81.91 Hodgkin lymphoma, unspecified, lymph nodes of head, face, and neck
C81.92 Hodgkin lymphoma, unspecified, intrathoracic lymph nodes
C81.93 Hodgkin lymphoma, unspecified, intra-abdominal lymph nodes
C81.94 Hodgkin lymphoma, unspecified, lymph nodes of axilla and upper limb
C81.95 Hodgkin lymphoma, unspecified, lymph nodes of inguinal region and lower limb
C81.96 Hodgkin lymphoma, unspecified, intrapelvic lymph nodes
C81.97 Hodgkin lymphoma, unspecified, spleen
C81.98 Hodgkin lymphoma, unspecified, lymph nodes of multiple sites
C81.99 Hodgkin lymphoma, unspecified, extranodal and solid organ sites

EPIDEMIOLOGY & DEMOGRAPHICS

- There is a bimodal age distribution (15-34 yr and >50 yr).
- Incidence is 4 in 100,000 cases; >8000 new cases of Hodgkin lymphoma diagnosed annually in the U.S.
- Concordance for Hodgkin lymphoma in identical twins suggests that a genetic susceptibility underlies Hodgkin lymphoma in young adulthood.
- There is association between certain HLA haplotypes, especially HLA-A1.
- The disease is more common in males (in childhood Hodgkin lymphoma, >80% occur in males), whites, and higher socioeconomic groups.
- There is an increased risk in smokers and HIV-infected individuals.

PHYSICAL FINDINGS & CLINICAL PRESENTATION

- Painless palpable lymphadenopathy is the most common presenting symptom.
- The most common site of involvement is the neck region.
- Fever and night sweats: fever in a cyclical pattern (days or weeks of fever alternating with afebrile periods) is known as Pel-Ebstein fever.
- Unexplained weight loss, generalized malaise.
- Persistent, nonproductive cough.
- Lymph node pain associated with alcohol ingestion often because of heavy eosinophil infiltration of the tumor sites is relatively uncommon.
- Generalized pruritus.
- Hepatosplenomegaly.
- Other: superior vena cava syndrome, spinal cord compression (rare), erythema nodosum (very rare), ichthyosis (very rare).

ETIOLOGY

Evidence implicating Epstein-Barr virus remains controversial.

DIAGNOSIS

DIFFERENTIAL DIAGNOSIS

- Non-Hodgkin lymphoma.
- Sarcoidosis.
- Infections (e.g., cytomegalovirus, Epstein-Barr virus, toxoplasmosis, HIV, tuberculosis).
- Drug reaction.

WORKUP

Diagnosis is confirmed by lymph node biopsy. The World Health Organization classifies Hodgkin lymphoma into two groups: classical Hodgkin lymphoma (92%-97%) and nodular lymphocyte-predominant Hodgkin lymphoma (3%-8%). Classical Hodgkin lymphoma has four main histologic subtypes based on the number of lymphocytes, Reed-Sternberg cells, and the presence of fibrous tissue:
1. Nodular sclerosis (60%-80%) (Fig. E1).
2. Mixed cellularity (15%-30%) (Fig. E2).
3. Lymphocyte rich (2%-7%).
4. Lymphocyte depleted (1%-6%).

Nodular sclerosis occurs mainly in young adulthood, whereas the mixed cellularity type is more prevalent after age 50 yr. Table 1 summarizes key features of Hodgkin lymphomas.

Staging: Table 2 describes the Cotswolds staging classification.

Proper staging requires the following:
- Detailed history (with documentation of "B symptoms" and physical examination).
- Excisional biopsy with histologic, immunophenotypic and immunohistochemical analysis.
- Laboratory evaluation (complete blood count, erythrocyte sedimentation rate (ESR), blood

---

TABLE 1 Key Features of Hodgkin Lymphomas

Lymphoma	Demographics, Clinical Presentation	Morphology	Cell Surface Markers	Prognosis
Nodular, lymphocyte predominant (NLPHL)	M > F, 30-50 years, with peripheral lymphadenopathy	Mononuclear cells with convoluted nuclei (popcorn or L&H cells) loosely aggregated in nodules of small B cells	CD45, CD20, bcl-6, J-chain, Oct-2, BOB.1, EBV absent in LP cells	Excellent for stages I, II
Nodular sclerosis	M = F, <30 years with mediastinal mass, occasional spleen or lung involvement; 40% have B symptoms; most patients present with stage II disease	Broad bands of collagen, nodules of lymphoid tissue with aggregates of HRS cells and lacunar cells, multi-nucleated variants	CD15, CD30, CD45-EBV in 1%-40%	Good with systemic therapy
Mixed cellularity	M > F; median age, 38 years; peripheral lymphadenopathy common, spleen, BM; B symptoms common; patients often stage III or IV	Classic HRS cells in mixture of lymphocytes, plasma cells, eosinophils, histiocytes	CD15, CD30, CD45-EBV in 75%	Good with systemic therapy
Lymphocyte depletion	M > F; median age, 30-37 years; B symptoms, advanced stage common; associated with HIV	Classic HRS cells common with paucity of background lymphocytes; pleomorphic HRS cells mimic sarcoma	CD15, CD30, CD45-EBV positive in HIV-affected patients	Associated with advanced stage
Lymphocyte-rich classical	M > F, older age; peripheral lymphadenopathy; B symptoms rare; most patients with stage I or II disease	Scattered classic HRS cells among numerous small lymphocytes; nodular growth pattern	CD15, CD30; Oct2 and BOB.1 vary; J-chain absent; EBV in 40%-75%	Good, similar to NLPHL

BM, Bone marrow; *CHL*, classical Hodgkin lymphoma; *EBV*, Epstein-Barr virus; *F*, female; *HIV*, human immunodeficiency virus; *HRS*, Hodgkin Reed-Sternberg; *L&H*, lymphocytic and histiocytic; *LP*, lymphoplasmacytic; *M*, male.
From McPherson RA, Pincus MR: *Henry's clinical diagnosis and management by laboratory methods*, ed 23, St Louis, 2017, Elsevier.

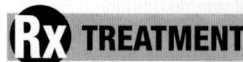

urea nitrogen, creatinine, liver function tests, albumin, lactate dehydrogenase, HIV test), immunophenotypic markers (see Table 3).
- Positron emission tomography (PET)/computed tomography (CT) scan of the chest, abdomen, and pelvis.
- Unilateral bone marrow biopsy in selected patients.

Box 1 summarizes recommended staging procedures for Hodgkin lymphoma.

Rx TREATMENT

ACUTE GENERAL Rx

The main therapeutic modality includes chemotherapy with or without radiotherapy depending on stage and other risk factors. In general, chemotherapy plus involved-site radiotherapy is standard treatment for Hodgkin lymphoma in the early stages; however, recent data suggest that chemotherapy alone is appropriate for a significant proportion of patients. Chemotherapy is used for advanced stage disease with radiotherapy in selected patients, such as those with bulky disease.

Most oncologists prefer the combination of adriamycin (doxorubicin), bleomycin, vinblastine, and dacarbazine (ABVD). ABVD does not cause infertility or stem cell damage and has also shown to be effective in patients with HIV infection and Hodgkin lymphoma. Table 4 describes characteristics of the ABVD regimen.

Recent trials have shown that in patients with early-stage Hodgkin lymphoma and favorable prognosis, defined by fewer than three nodal sites without bulky or extranodal disease in the absence of ESR >50 without symptoms or 30 with symptoms, treatment with two cycles of ABVD followed by 20 Gy of involved-field radiation therapy may be as effective as, and less toxic than, four cycles of ABVD followed by 30 Gy of involved-field radiation therapy. For patients with early stage disease who do not meet these criteria, options include three or four cycles of ABVD plus involved site radiotherapy to 30 Gy. In addition, chemotherapy alone, in the absence of bulky disease, is an alternative approach, especially in women younger than 30 years, given the increased risk of including breast cancer, as well as cardiac and thyroid disease. Although the risk of disease recurrence is slightly higher in patients who receive chemotherapy alone, there is no difference in overall survival.

BEACOPP, an intensified regimen consisting of bleomycin, etoposide, doxorubicin, cyclophosphamide, vincristine, procarbazine, and prednisone, has been advocated by some as the new standard for treatment of advanced Hodgkin lymphoma in place of ABVD. Recent trials have shown that treatment with BEACOPP, as compared with ABVD, results in better initial tumor control, but the long-term clinical outcome does not differ significantly between the two regimens. In addition, with the use of the escalated BEACOPP regimen, the rate of complications is higher (3% treatment-related death, 20% rate of hospitalization, and 3% rate of secondary leukemia, and near-universal infertility). Thus, if the goal is cure with the least overall toxic effects, it is best to favor ABVD therapy, reserving rescue therapy with high-dose chemotherapy and autologous hematopoietic stem-cell transplantation for the small number of patients in whom the primary treatment fails.
- Definitions of treatment groups are described in Table 5.
- Recommendations for the primary treatment of Hodgkin lymphoma outside of clinical trials are described in Table 6.
- In 2011, the FDA approved the use of the anti-CD30 antibody drug conjugate brentuximab vedotin for the treatment of patients with Hodgkin lymphoma who have relapsed after autologous stem cell transplant and for patients with Hodgkin lymphoma who have

TABLE 2 Cotswolds Staging Classification for Hodgkin Lymphoma

Classification	Description
Stage I	Involvement of a single lymph node region or lymphoid structure (e.g., spleen, thymus, Waldeyer ring) or involvement of a single extralymphatic site (IE)
Stage II	Involvement of two or more lymph node regions on the same side of the diaphragm (hilar nodes, when involved on both sides, constitute stage II disease); localized contiguous involvement of only one extranodal organ or site and lymph node regions on the same side of the diaphragm (IIE). The number of anatomic regions involved should be indicated by a subscript (e.g., II$_3$)
III$_1$	With or without involvement of splenic, hilar, celiac, or portal nodes
III$_2$	With involvement of paraaortic, iliac, and mesenteric nodes
Stage IV	Diffuse or disseminated involvement of one or more extranodal organs or tissues, with or without associated lymph node involvement Designations applicable to any disease stage
A	No symptoms
B	Fever (temperature, >38° C [100.4° F]), drenching night sweats, unexplained loss of >10% of body weight within the preceding 6 mo
X	Bulky disease (a widening of the mediastinum by more than one third of the maximal intrathoracic diameter, or presence of a nodal mass with a maximal dimension >10 cm)
E	Involvement of a single extranodal site that is contiguous or proximal to the known nodal site

From Hoffman R et al: *Hematology: basic principles and practice*, ed 5, Philadelphia, 2009, Churchill Livingstone.

TABLE 3 Selected Immunophenotypic Markers and Histologic Characteristics of Use in the Differential Diagnosis of Hodgkin Lymphoma and Other Lymphoid Neoplasms

Marker	Classical HL	Nodular Lymphocyte Predominant HL	TCRBCL	ALCL
CD30	+	−	−	+
CD15	+	−	−	−
CD20	−/+*	+	+	−
CD45	−	+	+	+/−
CD79a	−	+	+	−
ALK	−	−	−	+/−
EMA	−	+	+	+
Nodular growth protein	+/−†	+	−	−

+, >90% of cases positive; +/−, majority of cases positive; −/+, minority of cases positive; −, <10% of cases positive; *ALCL*, anaplastic large cell lymphoma; *HL*, Hodgkin lymphoma; *TCRBCL*, T-cell rich B-cell lymphoma.
*CD20 positivity in classical Hodgkin lymphoma is quite heterogeneous, with a wide range in brightness of staining.
†In classical Hodgkin lymphoma, a nodular growth pattern is confined to the nodular sclerosing subtype.
From Abeloff MD: *Clinical oncology*, ed 3, Philadelphia, 2004, Saunders.

BOX 1 Recommended Staging Procedures for Hodgkin Lymphoma

The following staging procedures are recommended for the initial workup of Hodgkin lymphoma:
1. Adequate surgical biopsy reviewed by an experienced hematopathologist
2. Cytologic examination of any effusion in selected cases
3. Detailed history, with attention to the presence or absence of systemic symptoms, and a careful physical examination, emphasizing node chains, size of the liver and spleen, and inspection of Waldeyer ring
4. Routine laboratory tests: complete blood cell count, erythrocyte sedimentation rate, and liver function tests
5. Neck, chest, and abdominal CT imaging fused with 18-FDG PET scan (Fig. 3)

From Hoffman R. et al. *Hematology: basic principles and practice*, ed 5, Philadelphia, 2009, Churchill Livingstone.

relapsed but are not candidates for transplant. Brentuximab vedotin is associated with an overall response rate of 75% in patients with HL who have relapsed after autologous stem cell transplantation. Brentuximab vedotin is approved as consolidation therapy after autologous transplant in patients at high risk for relapse.

- In May 2016, the FDA granted accelerated approval to the anti-PD-1 monoclonal antibody nivolumab for patients with Hodgkin lymphoma who relapse after autologous stem cell transplant and posttransplant brentuximab vedotin. In this setting, nivolumab was associated with an overall response rate of 65%. Continued approval will be contingent upon verification of clinical benefit in a randomized phase III study.

DISPOSITION

- Cure rates as high as 85% to 90% in early stage patients and 75% in stage III/IV disease are now possible with appropriate initial therapy.
- Poor prognostic features (Table 7) include presence of B symptoms, advanced age, advanced stage at initial presentation, male sex, low albumin, high ESR, lymphocyte depletion histology, and increased number of tumor-associated macrophages.
- Unlike escalated BEACOPP, ABVD is not associated with a risk of leukemia.
- Mediastinal irradiation increases the risk of subsequent cardiac disease, including valvular and pericardial disease, accelerated coronary artery disease, and conduction abnormalities.
- Radiation therapy increases the risk of developing secondary solid tumors, especially breast cancer in women younger than age 30 years (Table 8).
- Table 9 describes potential late complications of Hodgkin lymphoma treatment and appropriate clinical responses and preventive strategies.

REFERRAL

- To surgery for lymph node biopsy
- Fertility clinic for sperm banking
- Hematology/oncology
- Radiation oncology, in selected cases

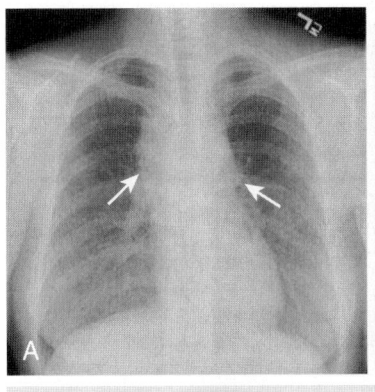
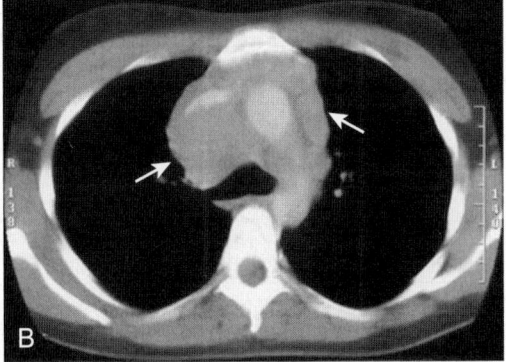
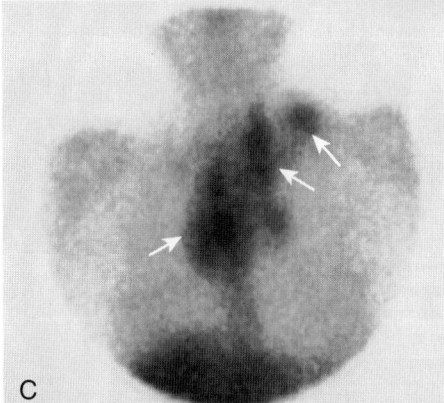
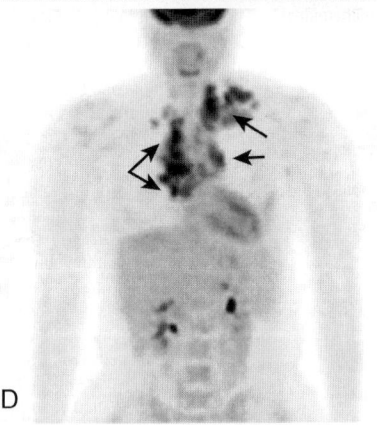

FIG. 3 Imaging of Hodgkin lymphoma. Bulky Hodgkin disease as seen on chest radiograph (**A**), computed tomography (CT) of the chest (**B**), gallium scan (**C**), and positron emission tomography (PET) (**D**). The *arrows* indicate sites of disease. Note that the PET and CT scans provide more detailed information than the chest radiograph and gallium scan. (From Goldman L., Schafer AI. *Goldman's Cecil medicine*, ed 24, Philadelphia, 2012, Saunders.)

TABLE 4   Characteristics of the ABVD Regimen

Agents: doxorubicin, bleomycin, vinblastine, dacarbazine

All intravenous, total compliance

80% complete response rate

10% primary refractory disease

60%-65% overall disease-free survival

Most relapses occur within the first 4 yr; however, about 10% of all relapses occur beyond 5 yr

Major side effects are nausea, phlebitis, myelosuppression, less cumulative myelotoxicity than MOPP

No infertility

No leukemia

ABVD, Adriamycin (doxorubicin), bleomycin, vinblastine, dacarbazine; *MOPP*, mechlorethamine, Oncovin (vincristine), procarbazine, prednisone.
From Abeloff MD: *Clinical oncology*, ed 3, Philadelphia, 2004, Saunders.

TABLE 5   Definition of Treatment Groups According to the EORTC/GELA and GHSG

Treatment Group	EORTC/GELA	GHSG	NCIC/ECOG
Early-stage favorable	CS I-II without risk factors (supradiaphragmatic)	CS I-II without risk factors	Standard risk group: favorable CSD I-II (without risk factors)
Early-stage unfavorable (intermediate)	CS I-II with ≥1 risk factors (supradiaphragmatic)	CS I, CSIIA ≥1 risk factors; CS IIB with C/D but without A/B	Standard risk group: unfavorable CS I-II (at least one risk factor)
Advanced stage	CS III-IV	CS IIB with A/B;CS III-IV	High-risk group: CS I or II with bulky disease; intraabdominal disease; CS III, IV
Risk factors (RF)	A large mediastinal mass B age ≥50 yr C elevated ESR* D ≥4 involved regions	A large mediastinal mass B extranodal disease C elevated ESR* D ≥3 involved areas	A ≥40 years B not NLPHL or NS histology C ESR ≥50 mm/h D ≥4 involved nodal regions

CS, Clinical stage; *ECOG*, Eastern Cooperative Oncology Group; *EORTC*, European Organization for Research and Treatment of Cancer; *GELA*, Groupe d'Etude des Lymphomes de l'Adulte; *GHSG*, German Hodgkin Study Group; *NCIC*, National Cancer Institute of Canada.
*Erythrocyte sedimentation rate (ESR) (≥50 mm/h without or ≥30 mm/h with B-symptoms).
From Hoffman R et al: *Hematology, basic principles and practice*, ed 5, New York, 2009, Churchill Livingstone.

H

Diseases and Disorders

I

TABLE 6 Recommendations for the Primary Treatment of Hodgkin Lymphoma Outside of Clinical Trials

Group	Stage	Recommendation
Early stages (favorable)	CS I-II A/B, no RFs	2 cycles ABVD + ISRT (20 Gy)
	Early stages (unfavorable, intermediate)	4-6 cycles ABVD ±30 Gy for nonbulky disease
	CS I-II A/B + RFs	4-6 cycles ABVD + 30 Gy for bulky disease
Advanced stages	CS IIB + RFs, CS III A/B, CS IV A/B	6 cycles ABVD; BEACOPP-escalated or BEACOPP-14 ± RT, 20-30 Gy for residual tumor (PET positive) and/ or bulky disease

ABVD regimen, Adriamycin (doxorubicin), vinblastine, bleomycin, and dacarbazine; *BEACOPP-baseline* regimen, bleomycin, etoposide, Adriamycin (doxorubicin), cyclophosphamide, Oncovin (vincristine), procarbazine, and prednisone; *BEACOPP-escalated* regimen, bleomycin, etoposide, Adriamycin (doxorubicin), cyclophosphamide, Oncovin (vincristine), procarbazine, prednisone, and G-CSF; *BEACOPP-14* regimen, bleomycin, etoposide, Adriamycin (doxorubicin), cyclophosphamide, Oncovin (vincristine), procarbazine, prednisone, and G-CSF; *CS,* clinical stage; *IF,* involved field; *MOPP* regimen, mechlorethamine, Oncovin (vincristine), procarbazine, and prednisone; *PET,* positron emission tomography; *RF,* risk factors; *RT,* radiation therapy; *Stanford V* regimen, nitrogen mustard, doxorubicin, vinblastine, bleomycin, vincristine, etoposide, and prednisone.
From Hoffman R et al: *Hematology, basic principles and practice,* ed 5, New York, 2009, Churchill Livingstone.

TABLE 7 Prognostic Factors of Importance in Advanced Hodgkin Lymphoma*

Gender	Male
Age	>45 years
Stage	IV
Hemoglobin	<10.5 g/dl
White blood cell count	>15 × 10⁹/L
Lymphocyte count	<0.6 × 10⁹/L or <8% of the white cell differential
Serum albumin	<4 g/dl

*Identified by the International Prognostic Factors Project on Advanced Hodgkin Disease.
From Abeloff MD: *Clinical oncology,* ed 3, Philadelphia, 2004, Saunders.

TABLE 8 Second Neoplasms Seen with Increased Frequency After Successful Hodgkin Lymphoma Treatment

Acute myelogenous leukemia/myelodysplasia (BEACOPP)
Non-Hodgkin lymphoma
Melanoma
Soft tissue sarcoma
Adenocarcinoma
  Breast
  Thyroid
  Lung
Stomach and esophagus
  Squamous cell carcinoma
  Skin
  Uterine cervix
  Head and neck

From Abeloff MD: *Clinical oncology,* ed 3, Philadelphia, 2004, Saunders.

❗ PEARLS & CONSIDERATIONS

COMMENTS

- Young male patients should consider sperm banking before the initiation of therapy even though the risk of infertility with ABVD is low. Symptomatic males, particularly with advanced stage Hodgkin lymphoma, may have disease-related oligospermia at diagnosis.
- Chemotherapy with or without involved-field radiotherapy should be the standard treatment for Hodgkin lymphoma with early stage disease. Chemotherapy with radiation in selected cases should be the standard of care for advanced stage.
- After failure of ABVD therapy, more than 60% of patients who have had a relapse and about 30% of patients with initially refractory lymphoma can be reliably cured with high-dose

chemotherapy and autologous hematopoietic stem-cell transplantation.

SUGGESTED READINGS

Available at www.expertconsult.com

TABLE 9 Potential Late Complications of Hodgkin Lymphoma Treatment and Appropriate Clinical Responses and Preventive Strategies

Risk/Problem	Incidence/Response
Dental caries	Neck or oropharyngeal irradiation can cause decreased salivation. Patients should have careful dental care follow-up and should make their dentist aware of the previous irradiation.
Hypothyroidism	After external beam irradiation that encompasses the thyroid with doses sufficient to cure Hodgkin lymphoma, at least 50% of patients will eventually become hypothyroid. All patients whose TSH level becomes elevated should be treated with lifelong thyroxine replacement in doses sufficient to suppress TSH levels to low normal. This is also necessary to ensure that the radiation-damaged thyroid is not subjected to long-term stimulation by thyroid-stimulating hormone, which can increase the risk of thyroid neoplasm.
Infertility	ABVD is not known to cause any permanent gonadal toxicity, although oligospermia for 1-2 yr after treatment is common. Direct or scatter radiation to gonadal tissue can cause infertility, amenorrhea, or premature menopause, but this seldom occurs with the current fields used for the treatment of Hodgkin lymphoma. Thus, with the current chemotherapy regimens and radiation fields used, most patients will not develop these problems. In general, after treatment, women who continue menstruating are fertile, but men require semen analysis to provide a specific answer. High-dose chemoradiotherapy and hematopoietic stem cell transplantation almost always cause permanent infertility in both genders, although some young women occasionally recover fertility.
Impaired immunity to infections	Hodgkin lymphoma and its treatment can lead to lifelong impairment of full immunity to infection. All patients should be given annual influenza immunization and pneumococcal immunization every 5 years. Patients whose spleen has been irradiated or removed should also be immunized against meningococcal types A and C and *Haemophilus influenza* type B. As for all adults, diphtheria and tetanus immunizations should be kept up-to-date.
Secondary neoplasms	Although uncommon, certain secondary neoplasms occur with increased frequency in patients who have been treated for Hodgkin lymphoma. These include acute myelogenous leukemia, thyroid, breast, lung, and upper gastrointestinal carcinoma and melanoma, and cervical carcinoma in situ. It is appropriate to screen for these neoplasms for the rest of the patient's life because they might have lengthy induction periods.

ABVD, Adriamycin, bleomycin, vinblastine, dacarbazine; *TSH,* thyroid-stimulating hormone.
From Abeloff MD: *Clinical oncology,* ed 3, Philadelphia, 2004, Saunders.

RELATED CONTENT

Hodgkin Lymphoma (Patient Information)

AUTHORS: **JORGE J. CASTILLO, M.D.,** and **ANN S. LACASCE, M.D., M.M.SC.**

BASIC INFORMATION

DEFINITION
Hookworm is a parasitic infection of the intestine caused by the soil helminths *Necator americanus* and *Ancylostoma duodenale*.

SYNONYMS
Ground itch
Ancylostoma duodenale infection
Necator americanus infection

ICD-10CM CODES
B76.9 Hookworm disease, unspecified
B76.8 Other hookworm diseases

EPIDEMIOLOGY & DEMOGRAPHICS
INCIDENCE (IN U.S.):
- Varies greatly in different areas of the United States.
- Most common in rural areas of southeastern United States.
- Poor sanitation and increased rainfall increase incidence.

PREVALENCE (IN U.S.): Varies from 10% to 90% in regions where it is found.
PREDOMINANT AGE: Schoolchildren.

PHYSICAL FINDINGS & CLINICAL PRESENTATION
- Nonspecific abdominal complaints.
- Symptoms related to iron deficiency anemia depending on the amount of iron in the diet and worm burden (these organisms consume host's RBCs).
- Fatigue, tachycardia, dyspnea, and high-output failure.

- Hypoproteinemia and edema from loss of proteins into the intestinal tract.
- Unusual for pulmonary manifestations to occur when the larvae migrate through the lungs.
- Skin rash at sites of larval penetration in some individuals without prior exposure: ground itch.

ETIOLOGY
Two species can cause this disease: *N. americanus* and *A. duodenale*. *N. americanus* is the predominant cause of hookworm in the United States. They are soil nematodes (geohelminthic infections) that are acquired by skin contact (i.e., bare feet) with contaminated soils in moist, warm climate. Worldwide, over 700 million people are infected.
- Infection occurs via penetration of the skin by the larval form, with subsequent migration via the bloodstream to the alveoli, up the respiratory tract, then into the GI tract (Fig. 1).
- *Ancylostoma* spp. infection can also occur via the oral route through ingestion of contaminated water supplies.
- Sharp mouth parts allow for attachment to intestinal mucosa.
- *Ancylostoma* spp. are more likely to cause iron deficiency anemia because they are larger and remove more blood daily from the bowel wall than the other hookworm species, *N. americanus*.

DIAGNOSIS

DIFFERENTIAL DIAGNOSIS
- Strongyloidiasis.
- Ascariasis.
- Other causes of iron deficiency anemia and malabsorption.

WORKUP
Examine stool for hookworm eggs. Shedding of eggs starts around 8 weeks after skin penetration in *N. americanum* infections and longer with *A. duodenale,* but eggs are indistinguishable between the two species.

LABORATORY TESTS
CBC to show hypochromic, microcytic anemia; possible mild eosinophilia and hypoalbuminemia.

IMAGING STUDIES
Chest x-ray: generally not helpful, occasionally shows opacities.

TREATMENT

NONPHARMACOLOGIC THERAPY
- Prevention of disease by not walking barefoot and by improving sanitary conditions.
- Vaccines are in development.

ACUTE GENERAL Rx
- Albendazole 400 mg once PO has become preferred treatment.
- Mebendazole 100 mg PO bid for 3 days is more effective than as a 500-mg single dose.
- Pyrantel pamoate 11 mg/kg (to max dose of 1 g) PO qd × 3 days.
- Iron supplementation may be helpful in patients with iron deficiency.

DISPOSITION
Easily treated.

REFERRAL
To gastroenterologist and infectious disease specialist if diagnosis uncertain.

PEARLS & CONSIDERATIONS

COMMENTS
- Appropriate disposal of human waste is important in controlling the disease in areas with a high prevalence of hookworm infestation.
- Wearing shoes will avoid contact with contaminated soil, and the provision of safe water and sanitation for disposing human excreta is important in control of hookworm.

EVIDENCE

Available at www.expertconsult.com

SUGGESTED READING
Available at www.expertconsult.com

RELATED CONTENT
Hookworm Infection (Patient Information)

AUTHOR: **GLENN G. FORT, M.D., M.P.H.**

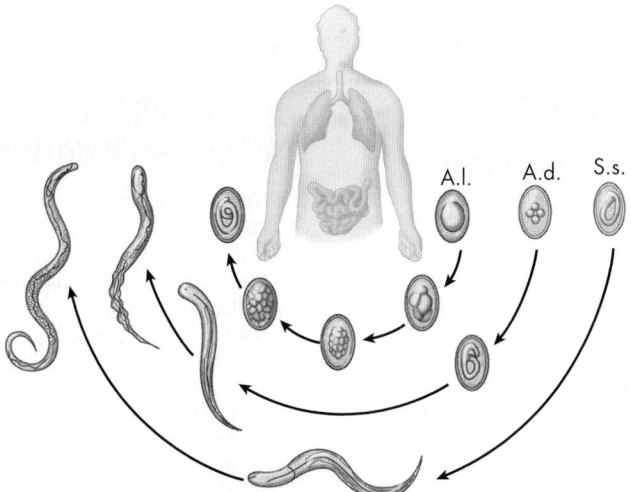

FIG. 1 Life cycle of intestinal nematodes with a migratory phase through the lungs. Eggs are passed with stools in *Ascaris lumbricoides (A.l.), Necator americanus,* or *Ancylostoma duodenale (A.d.),* or they hatch on their way out in *Strongyloides stercoralis (S.s.).* Ascaris eggs mature in soil, and humans are infected upon ingestion of these eggs. With hookworm and strongyloidiasis, humans are infected via skin penetration by filariform larvae. In all three infections, larvae pass through a migratory phase via the lungs before reaching maturity at their final habitat in the small intestine. (From Mandell GL et al: *Principles and practice of infectious diseases,* ed 7, Philadelphia, 2010, Churchill Livingstone.)

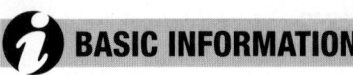

DEFINITION

Horner's syndrome is the clinical triad of ipsilateral ptosis, miosis, and sometimes facial anhidrosis. Disruption of any of the three neurons in the oculosympathetic pathway (first-order, second-order, or third-order) can cause Horner's syndrome.

SYNONYMS

Oculosympathetic paresis
Raeder's paratrigeminal syndrome: Horner's syndrome of the third-order neuron associated with pain in the trigeminal nerve distribution

ICD-10CM CODES
G90.2 Horner's Syndrome

EPIDEMIOLOGY & DEMOGRAPHICS

Congenital or acquired.

PHYSICAL FINDINGS & CLINICAL PRESENTATION

- Ptosis is usually mild. It results from loss of sympathetic tone to Müller's muscle, which contributes approximately 2 mm of upper eyelid elevation. Weakness of the corresponding muscle in the lower eyelid causes it to elevate slightly. This combination causes narrowing of the palpebral fissure. Levator function of the eyelid is preserved.
- Miosis results from loss of sympathetic innervation to the iris dilator muscle (Fig. 1). The affected pupil reacts normally to bright light and accommodation. Anisocoria is greater in dim light.
  1. Dilation lag: Horner's pupil dilates more slowly than the normal pupil when lights are dimmed (20 versus 5 sec) because it dilates passively as a result of relaxation of the iris sphincter.
- Presence of facial anhidrosis is variable and depends on the site of injury. It occurs with lesions affecting first-order or second-order neurons.
- Congenital Horner's syndrome may result in heterochromia. The affected eye has a lighter-colored iris.
- Acute cases may also present with conjunctival injection from the loss of sympathetic vasoconstriction.

ETIOLOGY

Disruption of the ipsilateral sympathetic innervation to the eye and face. Lesions can damage any of the three neurons in the oculosympathetic

FIG. 1 Horner's syndrome. The mild ptosis (1 to 2 mm) and the smaller pupil (in room light) can be seen on the affected right side. (From Palay D [ed]: *Ophthalmology for the primary care physician,* St Louis, 1997, Mosby.)

pathway (Fig. E2). First order neuron lesions are least common but are usually caused by pathology in the hypothalamus, brainstem, or cervicothoracic spinal cord. Second order neuron lesions are often caused by disease involving the cervicothoracic spinal cord, lung apex, or anterior neck. Third order neuron lesions are usually seen with disease in the internal carotid artery, skull base, cavernous sinus, or orbital apex. Location is often suggested by the presence of associated findings. Vascular disease and neoplasm must be considered.

Mechanical:
- Syringomyelia
- Trauma
- Tumors: benign, malignant head and neck cancers (thyroid, apical lung, mediastinal)
- Cervical rib

Vascular (ischemia, hemorrhage or arteriovenous malformation):
- Brainstem lesion: commonly occlusion of the posterior inferior cerebellar artery but other arteries may be responsible (vertebral; superior, middle or inferior lateral medullary arteries; superior or anterior inferior cerebellar arteries).
- Carotid artery aneurysm, dissection, arteritis: can also be from injury to other major vessels (internal carotid artery, subclavian artery, ascending aorta).
- Jugular venous ectasia.
- Cavernous sinus thrombosis.
- Cluster headache, migraine.

Miscellaneous:
- Idiopathic
- Congenital
- Demyelination (multiple sclerosis)
- Infection (apical tuberculosis, herpes zoster, Lyme disease)
- Myelitis
- Pneumothorax
- Iatrogenic (angiography, internal jugular/subclavian catheter, chest tube, neck or upper thoracic surgery, epidural spinal anesthesia)

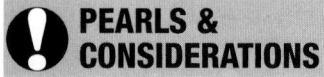 DIAGNOSIS

DIFFERENTIAL DIAGNOSIS

Causes of anisocoria (unequal pupils):
- Normal variant
- Mydriatic use
- Prosthetic eye
- Prior eye surgery
- Unilateral cataract
- Iritis
  Causes of ptosis are described in Section II.

WORKUP

History, physical examination, pharmacologic testing, imaging.

PHARMACOLOGIC TESTING

These medications may not be readily available. Pharmacologic testing should not delay evaluation in acute, painful, or traumatic cases or in patients with a history of malignancy.
- Topical cocaine test: confirms diagnosis (drops increase anisocoria by dilating normal pupil but not Horner's pupil).

- Topical apraclonidine test: confirms diagnosis (drops reverse anisocoria by causing dilation of Horner's pupil and slight constriction of normal pupil).
- Topical hydroxyamphetamine test: distinguishes first- and second-order neuron lesions from third-order sympathetic lesions (drops dilate normal pupil and first- or second-order Horner's pupil, but not third-order Horner's pupil). Testing must be delayed >48 hr after topical cocaine or apraclonidine testing. Topical phenylephrine may be used as an alternative (causes dilatation of pupil due to third-order neuron lesions).

IMAGING STUDIES

Results of pharmacologic testing as well as accompanying signs and symptoms should guide imaging:
- MRI brain: brainstem (diplopia, vertigo, ataxia, lateral medullary syndrome); cavernous sinus (eye movement abnormalities, sixth nerve palsy).
- MRI cervical and upper thoracic spinal cord: sensory changes/weakness of extremities, bowel/bladder dysfunction.
- MR or CT angiography (ultrasound is less sensitive): internal carotid artery dissection (acute Horner's syndrome with face or neck pain).
- CT chest and neck: evaluate lung apex, perivertebral areas, mediastinum if symptoms do not localize to the central nervous system; brachial plexus lesion (arm/hand pain or weakness).

Rx TREATMENT

- Treatment depends on underlying cause.
- Ptosis can be surgically corrected or treated with medication (phenylephrine drops).

REFERRAL

Ophthalmologist for pharmacologic testing to confirm diagnosis and localize lesion.

! PEARLS & CONSIDERATIONS

- May be the presentation of a life-threatening condition. Horner's syndrome presenting acutely or associated with head/neck pain, trauma, or history of malignancy should be evaluated urgently.
- Normal variant anisocoria:
  1. Occurs in 20% of people
  2. Usually <1 mm difference between pupils
  3. Pupils are round and display a normal, brisk constriction and dilation response to light

SUGGESTED READING
Available at www.expertconsult.com

RELATED CONTENT
Horner's Syndrome (Patient Information)
Lung Neoplasms, Primary (Related Key Topic)

AUTHOR: **SUDEEP K. AULAKH, M.D.**

BASIC INFORMATION

DEFINITION

Hot flashes are sudden onset of intense warmth that begins in the neck or face, or in the chest and progresses to the neck and face; often associated with profuse sweating, anxiety, and palpitations.

SYNONYMS

HFs
Vasomotor symptoms (VMSs)

ICD-10CM CODES
N95.1 Menopausal and female climacteric states
R23.2 Flushing

EPIDEMIOLOGY & DEMOGRAPHICS

- Hot flashes affect 75% of postmenopausal women.
- Most hot flashes begin 1 to 2 yr before menopause and may resolve after 2 yr. Average duration is 5 yr.
- 15% of women report duration of hot flashes >15 yr.
- Complementary therapies for hot flashes account for $34 billion in out-of-pocket spending in the U.S. annually.

PHYSICAL FINDINGS & CLINICAL PRESENTATION

- Profuse sweating and red blotching of skin may be noted during the vasomotor event.
- Palpitations and hyperreflexia may be present during the hot flash.
- Hot flashes typically last 1 to 5 min.
- Each hot flash is associated with increase in temperature, increased pulse rate, and increased blood flow into the hands and face.
- Hot flashes during sleep are common and are referred to as *night sweats.*
- There is considerable variation in the frequency of hot flashes. One third of women report more than 10 flashes per day.

ETIOLOGY

- Dysfunction of central thermoregulatory centers caused by changes in estrogen level at the time of menopause
- Tamoxifen use
- Chemotherapy-induced ovarian failure
- Androgen ablation therapy for prostate carcinoma

DIAGNOSIS

DIFFERENTIAL DIAGNOSIS

- Carcinoid syndrome
- Anxiety disorder.
- Idiopathic flushing
- Lymphoma (night sweats)
- Hyperthyroidism
- Hyperhidrosis

WORKUP

Evaluation of hot flashes is aimed at excluding the conditions listed in the differential diagnosis.

LABORATORY TESTS

- Follicle-stimulating hormone (FSH), luteinizing hormone, estradiol level. The serum FSH levels rather than estradiol levels are associated with greater severity of hot flashes in older postmenopausal women, suggesting that nonestrogen feedback systems may be important in modulating the severity of hot flashes. It is not necessary to obtain an FSH to make the diagnosis of menopausal status, however. An amenorrheic woman over age 50 with vasomotor symptoms is assumed to have made the menopausal transition and serum markers of menopause are not required to complete the diagnosis.
- Thyroid-stimulating hormone (TSH).

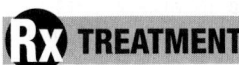 TREATMENT

NONPHARMACOLOGIC THERAPY

- Behavioral interventions such as relaxation training and paced respiration have been reported effective in reducing symptoms in some women.
- Avoidance of caffeine, alcohol, tobacco, and spicy foods may be beneficial.

GENERAL Rx

- Estrogen replacement therapy reduces hot flashes by 80% to 90%. Estrogen therapy, however, is contraindicated in many women, and others are fearful of its use. Potential risks and side effects should be considered before using estrogen in any patient. When using estrogen, it is best to use low dose (e.g., Prempro [conjugated equine estrogen 0.45 mg or 0.3 mg plus medroxyprogesterone 1.5 mg]). Femring is an intravaginal ring that is changed every 3 mo and approved to treat vasomotor symptoms in women who have had a hysterectomy. It provides both local and systemic estrogen.
- Megestrol acetate, a progestational agent, is a safer alternative to estrogen in women with a history of receptor-positive breast or uterine cancer and in men receiving androgen ablation therapy for prostate cancer. Usual dose is 20 mg bid.
- The antidepressant venlafaxine has been reported to be 60% effective in reducing hot flashes and represents an alternative treatment modality in women unable or unwilling to use estrogens. Starting dose is 37.5 mg qd, increased as tolerated up to a maximum of 300 mg/day. Other antidepressants such as desvenlafaxine and escitalopram have

also been shown to be effective in reducing the number and severity of menopausal hot flashes. Trials have shown that paroxetine is also an effective agent for diminishing hot flashes in postmenopausal women and men receiving androgen ablation therapy.

- Duavee is a new FDA-approved treatment of moderate to severe vasomotor menopausal symptoms. It consists of a combination of conjugated estrogens and bazedoxifene, a new selective estrogen receptor modulator (SERM).
- The anticonvulsant gabapentin (300-1200 mg/day) represents another nonhormonal alternative in the treatment of hot flashes and can be used alone or in combination with venlafaxine.
- The antihypertensive clonidine is also somewhat effective in reducing the frequency of hot flashes in mild cases. Adverse effects include dry mouth, sedation, and dizziness.
- Vitamin E (800 IU/day) may be effective in patients with mild symptoms that do not interfere with sleep or daily function.
- Soy protein (use of soy extracts that contain plant-derived estrogens [phytoestrogens]) is often used; however, clinical trials have not shown clear efficacy.
- Several classes of herbal remedies are available to patients and are commonly used, generally without significant benefit. Frequently used agents are *Cimicifuga racemosa* (black cohosh, snakeroot, bugbane), *Angelica sinensis,* and evening primrose (evening star). Recent trials using the isopropanolic extract of black cohosh rootstock (Remefemin) did show some improvement in controlling menopausal symptoms. Such alternative medications may be used to treat mild to moderate symptoms, but it is possible that symptomatic improvements may derive in part from a placebo effect. Acupuncturists are the second most consulted therapists by menopausal women. Evidence of acupuncture efficacy as an HF treatment is conflicting. A recent randomized trial[1] revealed that Chinese medicine acupuncture was not superior to noninsertive sham acupuncture for women with moderately severe menopausal HFs.

SUGGESTED READING

Available at www.expertconsult.com

RELATED CONTENT

Hot Flashes (Patient Information)
Menopause (Related Key Topic)

AUTHOR: **FRED F. FERRI, M.D.**

[1]Ee C, et al.: Acupuncture for Menopausal Hot Flashes: A Randomized Trial, Ann Intern Med 164:146-154, 2016.

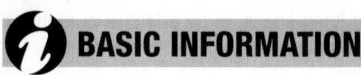

BASIC INFORMATION

DEFINITION

The human immunodeficiency virus (HIV) is a retrovirus that is responsible for causing acquired immunodeficiency syndrome (AIDS). HIV infection does not necessarily mean a person has AIDS.

SYNONYMS

HIV

AIDS: The result of progressive HIV infection in which a person has a weakened immune system and meets specific diagnostic criteria (See "Acquired Immunodeficiency Syndrome" in Section I.)

ICD-10CM CODES
B20 Human immunodeficiency virus [HIV]

EPIDEMIOLOGY & DEMOGRAPHICS (IN U.S.)

- There are an estimated 1.2 million people infected with HIV in the U.S., with approximately 1 out of 8 (13%) who do not know they are infected.
- In 2014, there were an estimated 44,073 new HIV infections, according to the CDC.
- Greatest incidence is in gay, bisexual, and other men who have sex with men (MSM) and in minority racial and ethnic populations.

PREDOMINANT RISK GROUPS:

- Gay, bisexual, and other MSM are the groups most affected by HIV.
- In 2014, MSM accounted for 67% of all new infections, according to the CDC.
- HIV disproportionately affects MSM of younger age and black/African American and Hispanic/Latino background.
- Heterosexual transmission and injection drug use accounted for 24% and 9%, respectively, of new HIV infections in 2014.

- Table 1 summarizes risk factors associated with sexual transmission of HIV.

RACIAL DATA:

- In 2014, blacks/African Americans accounted for 44% of new HIV infections despite being 12% of the U.S. population.
- In 2014, Hispanics/Latinos accounted for 23% of new HIV infections despite being 17% of the U.S. population.

GENETICS

Familial Disposition:

Individuals with deletions in the *CCR5* gene are immune from infection with macrophage tropic virus (the predominant virus in sexual transmission). Other genetic variants may contribute to rapid progression or long-term control of the virus once infected. One in 300 individuals infected with HIV is an "elite controller," which means they are able to maintain a normal CD4 count and undetectable viral load through immune control.

Congenital Infection:

- 73% of HIV cases diagnosed in children younger than age 13 years in 2014 were caused by peripartum infection, which may occur in utero, during delivery, or after delivery via breastfeeding.
- No specific congenital abnormalities are associated with HIV infection, although there is a higher risk of spontaneous abortion and low birth weight.

Neonatal Infection:

- May occur during delivery or via breastfeeding.
- Typically asymptomatic.

PHYSICAL FINDINGS & CLINICAL PRESENTATION

- Signs and symptoms are variable with stage of disease. "Stage 0" indicates very early infection diagnosed when antibody tests are converting from negative to positive.

- Acute HIV infection (0 to 3 months, usually within several weeks):
  1. Causes a self-limited mononucleosis-like illness in 50% to 80% of individuals, characterized by fever, sore throat, lymphadenopathy, headache, and a rash resembling roseola. Individuals may also be asymptomatic.
  2. In a minority of acute cases, aseptic meningitis, Bell's palsy, or peripheral neuropathy may occur.
  3. Rarely, opportunistic infections such as thrush or *Pneumocystis jiroveci* pneumonia (PJP) may occur.
- Chronic HIV infection is usually characterized by a prolonged asymptomatic phase followed by nonspecific symptoms of lymphadenopathy, fatigue, weight loss, diarrhea, and skin changes including seborrheic dermatitis, localized herpes zoster, and/or fungal infection.
- Advanced disease is characterized by AIDS-associated diseases, including infections and malignancies (see specific disorders).
- HIV infection in women may be associated with lower levels of viral load at comparable degrees of immunosuppression when compared with men. Furthermore, women may, on average, have higher CD4 counts at the time of HIV diagnosis.
- Another special consideration in women infected with HIV is the high incidence of human papillomavirus (HPV) co-infection and risk for cervical cancer. HIV-positive women should be screened for cervical cancer twice in the first year and then annually thereafter if pap smears are normal.
- Co-infection with HIV and hepatitis C is common because of similar transmission risk. Hepatitis C is most commonly transmitted by contaminated needles or blood exposure. Hepatitis C can be transmitted sexually, but the risk is low. Patients with HIV and hepatitis C progress faster to cirrhosis. Patients may already have signs of advanced liver disease at the time of diagnosis.

ETIOLOGY

- HIV is a single-stranded RNA retrovirus (Fig. 1) that is categorized as type 1 or 2.
- HIV-1 was derived from transmission of a simian immunodeficiency virus (SIV) from chimpanzees in Central Africa; HIV-2 was derived from an SIV found in sooty mangabey monkeys from West Africa.
- HIV-1 is the predominant pathogenic retrovirus in human populations; HIV-2 has limited distribution (primarily West Africa) and tends to progress less rapidly than HIV-1. HIV-2 should be considered in individuals from West Africa or whose sexual partners are from West Africa.
- HIV-1/2 are transmitted by sexual contact, shared needles, blood transfusion, or from mother to child during pregnancy, delivery, or breastfeeding.
- Primary target of infection: CD4 lymphocytes.

TABLE 1 Risk Factors Associated with Sexual Transmission of HIV

Sexually transmitted infections
    Ulcerative or nonulcerative diseases
Genital tract inflammation
HIV disease
    Higher viral loads
    Lower CD4+ levels
    Acute HIV infection
    Lack of effective antiretroviral therapy
    Lack of heterozygosity or homozygosity for the inactivating 32-base pair deletion in the chemokine receptor gene *(CCR5)*
Anatomic factors
    Lack of circumcision
    Cervical ectopy
    Leukocytospermia
    ?Hormonal contraception
Sexual practices
    Receptive anal intercourse
    Sexual activity during menses
    Bleeding during intercourse (disruption of vaginal mucosa through trauma)
    Lack of barrier protection
HIV viral features
    Syncytium formation
    Certain viral clades

HIV, Human immunodeficiency virus.
From Bennett JE, Dolin R, Blaser MJ: *Mandell, Douglas, and Bennett's principles and practice of infectious diseases,* ed 8, Philadelphia, 2015, Saunders.

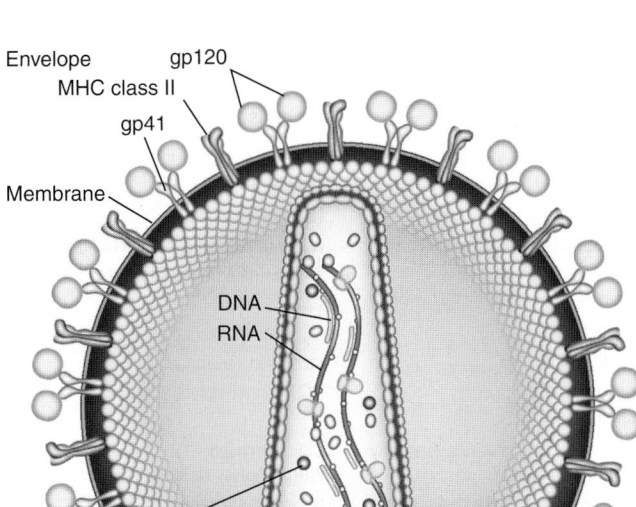

FIG. 1 Structure of the HIV-1 virion. The viral envelope is formed from the host cell membrane, into which the HIV-1 envelope proteins gp41 and gp120 have been inserted and may include several host cell proteins, most significantly the major histocompatibility complex class II proteins. The matrix between the envelope and the core is formed predominantly from gag protein p17. The core contains the viral RNA, closely associated with gag protein p7, in addition to RT and integrase. It has also been proven that virions contain complementary DNA, as shown, synthesized by the RT. The major structural proteins of the core are gag proteins p24 and p6. Also present within the virion are the protease and two cleavage products from the gag precursor protein (p1 and p2, not shown) of undetermined position within the virion. Viral protein R (Vpr) is also packaged in the virion and is thought to be localized within the core, as shown. (From Mandell GL et al: *Principles and practice of infectious diseases*, ed 7, Philadelphia, 2010, Saunders.)

Dx DIAGNOSIS

DIFFERENTIAL DIAGNOSIS

- Acute HIV infection: often diagnosed or confused with mononucleosis or other respiratory viral infections
- Late symptoms: similar to those produced by other wasting/chronic illnesses such as neoplasms, tuberculosis (TB), disseminated fungal infection (such as *Candida*), malabsorption, or depression
- HIV-related encephalopathy: confused with Alzheimer's disease or other causes of chronic dementia (cognitive impairment in HIV infection is described in another chapter in Section I); myelopathy and neuropathy possibly resembling other demyelinating diseases such as multiple sclerosis.
- Direct central nervous system (CNS) involvement: manifests as encephalopathy, myelopathy, or neuropathy in advanced cases. Table 2 summarizes neuromuscular syndromes in HIV infection.
- Renal failure, rheumatologic disorders, thrombocytopenia, or cardiac abnormalities may be seen in association with HIV-1.

WORKUP

Diagnosis is established by testing for antibodies to the virus in the blood. The CDC recommends routine testing for patients in all health care settings unless the patient declines (opt-out screening). This includes routine testing of pregnant women. It is also recommended that separate written consent should no longer be required, although by law this is being addressed on a state-by-state basis. Generally, all persons aged 13 to 64 years should undergo HIV testing at least once, and more frequently (at least once a year) if sexually active.

- An FDA-approved at-home rapid HIV screening test is available. It uses swabs of oral fluids from upper and lower gums. A positive test requires confirmatory testing in the office.

LABORATORY TESTS

HIV antibodies are detected by a two-step technique:
- ELISA (enzyme-linked immunosorbent assay), which is a sensitive screening test.
- Confirmation of positive ELISA tests with more specific assays. The classic confirmatory test is the Western blot, but this is not commonly used anymore.
- Screening ELISA antibody tests will measure HIV-1 and HIV-2 antibodies. Confirmatory tests will generally differentiate between HIV-1 and HIV-2 as well. However, the viral load assays (HIV RNA PCR) are specific only for HIV-1.
- Fourth-generation antibody/antigen tests can detect the "p20" antigen, which is present early in HIV infection and can be used to diagnose HIV earlier than previous generations. An HIV RNA PCR should still be sent if acute HIV is suspected.
- Baseline viral resistance testing (e.g., genotype) is recommended for all newly diagnosed patients with HIV to guide choice of antiretroviral therapy (ART).
- The CD4 count and HIV viral load (e.g., HIV RNA PCR) should be measured in all patients.
- The CD4 count is a marker of current immune status. Table 3 describes the World Health Organization (WHO) immunologic classification for established HIV infection.
- The HIV RNA PCR (viral load) is predictive of disease progression.
- Rapid serologic tests have been increasingly used and are useful in specific settings: occupational exposures, pregnant women in labor without previous testing, and patients in high seroprevalence areas (for immediate results). Specimens are either blood or saliva and results are given within 1 to 20 min. Although sensitivity is high (99%), false-positive tests are more common in low seroprevalence populations. Thus, all positive results must be confirmed with standard serology.
- Early during infection (i.e., acute HIV infection), standard antibody tests may be negative ("window period"). The standard for

TABLE 2 Neuromuscular Syndromes in Human Immunodeficiency Virus Type–1 Infection

Diagnosis	Disease Stage	Clinical Features	Diagnostic Studies	Treatment
AIDP CIDP	Early > late	Weakness more than sensory loss	CSF: ↑ WBCs ↑↑ Protein NCSs: demyelination	Early: IVIG, steroids, plasmapheresis Late: consider ganciclovir/foscarnet
MM	Early or late	Multiple painful mononeuropathies	NCSs: multifocal axonal neuropathy Biopsy: inflammation/vasculitis CMV	Early: none Late: steroids/cyclophosphamide Ganciclovir/foscarnet
Nucleoside Neuropathy	Any stage	Distal sensory loss Neuropathic pain	NCSs: distal axonopathy Increased serum lactate	Nucleoside withdrawal
DSPN	Late	Distal sensory loss Neuropathic pain	NCSs: distal axonopathy	NSAIDs, capsaicin AED, tricyclics
PP	Late	Progressive flaccid paraparesis, urinary dysfunction, LS pain	CSF: increased WBCs (PMNs), CMV PCR+	Ganciclovir/foscarnet Cidofovir
DILS	Late	Sjögren's syndrome, distal motor and sensory loss, pain	NCSs: axonal neuropathy Biopsy: CD8+ T cells, HIV-1	Zidovudine/ART Steroids
Zidovudine Myopathy	Any stage	Proximal weakness Myalgias	EMG: ± irritative Biopsy: ragged red fibers	Zidovudine withdrawal
Polymyositis	Any stage	Proximal weakness Myalgias	EMG: ± irritative Biopsy: inflammatory infiltrates	Steroids, IVIG Immunosuppressants
ALS-like	Late	Weakness, dysphagia	EMG: neurogenic	ART

AED, Antiepileptic drug; *AIDP,* acute inflammatory demyelinating polyneuropathy; *ALS,* amyotrophic lateral sclerosis; *ART,* antiretroviral therapy; *CIDP,* chronic inflammatory demyelinating polyneuropathy; *CMV,* cytomegalovirus; *CSF,* cerebrospinal fluid; *DILS,* diffuse infiltrative lymphocytosis syndrome; *DSPN,* distal sensory polyneuropathy; *EMG,* electromyography; *HIV,* human immunodeficiency virus; *IVIG,* intravenous immunoglobulin; *LS,* lumbosacral; *MM,* mononeuritis multiplex; *NCS,* nerve conduction studies; *NSAID,* nonsteroidal anti-inflammatory drug; *PCR,* polymerase chain reaction; *PMNs,* polymorphonuclear leukocytes; *PP,* progressive polyradiculopathy; *WBCs,* white blood cells.
From Bennett JE, Dolin R, Blaser MJ: *Mandell, Douglas, and Bennett's principles and practice of infectious diseases,* ed 8, Philadelphia, 2015, Saunders.

TABLE 3 World Health Organization Immunologic Classification for Established HIV Infection

HIV-Associated Immunodeficiency	Age-Related CD4 Values			
	<11 mo (% CD4+)	12-35 mo (% CD4+)	36-59 mo (% CD4+)	>5 yr (Absolute No./mm³ or % CD4+)
None or not significant	>35	>30	>25	>500
Mild	30-35	25-30	20-25	350-500
Advanced	25-29	20-24	15-19	200-349
Severe	<25	<20	<15	<200 or <15%

From Bennett JE, Dolin R, Blaser MJ: *Mandell, Douglas, and Bennett's principles and practice of infectious diseases,* ed 8, Philadelphia, 2015, Saunders.

diagnosing HIV during acute HIV infection is by testing for HIV RNA (viral load).

- In 2014, the CDC released a revised surveillance case definition for HIV infection. This information has been added in the EBM section of this topic. Table 4 describes the WHO clinical staging of HIV/AIDS for adults and adolescents with confirmed HIV infection. Table 5 compares the WHO and CDC staging systems.

Fig. 2 describes the immunologic response to HIV infection.

Rx TREATMENT

NONPHARMACOLOGIC THERAPY
Maintenance of adequate nutrition

ACUTE GENERAL Rx
Acute management of opportunistic infections and malignancies (see AIDS-associated disorders, "*Pneumocystis jiroveci* Pneumonia," "Cryptococcosis," "Tuberculosis," "Cryptosporidiosis," "Toxoplasmosis," etc., elsewhere in this text).

CHRONIC Rx
All HIV-infected patients should be considered for ART regardless of CD4 cell count. The benefit of ART is well established in preventing progression to AIDS and associated comorbidities.

- Therapy is strongly recommended for all patients with symptomatic established HIV disease regardless of the CD4 count. Symptomatic HIV disease is defined as the presence of any of the following: thrush, vaginal candidiasis, herpes zoster, peripheral neuropathy, bacillary angiomatosis, cervical dysplasia in situ, constitutional symptoms such as fever or diarrhea for more than 1 month, ITP, PID, or listeriosis.
- In asymptomatic individuals, ART is now recommended regardless of CD4 cell counts. The updated recommendations are due to the safety and benefit of newer antivirals in preventing AIDS and decreasing both morbidity and mortality. Earlier treatment may also help reduce transmission of the virus to others due to reductions in viral loads.

- ART generally consists of using a 3-drug regimen to treat HIV infection. Classes of antiretrovirals include:
  1. Nucleoside/nucleotide reverse transcriptase inhibitor (NRTI): zidovudine (AZT), lamivudine (3TC), emtricitabine (FTC), tenofovir disoproxil fumarate (TDF), tenofovir alafenamide (TAF), abacavir (ABC), stavudine (D4T), or didanosine (DDI).
  2. Protease inhibitors (PI): lopinavir/ritonavir, atazanavir, fosamprenavir, darunavir, saquinavir, amprenavir, tipranavir, nelfinavir, and indinavir. These PIs may be "boosted" by ritonavir or cobicistat to increase levels.
  3. Non-nucleoside reverse transcriptase inhibitors (NNRTI): Nevirapine, efavirenz, etravirine, delavirdine, or rilpivirine.
  4. Integrase Inhibitors (II): Raltegravir, elvitegravir, and dolutegravir.
  5. Fusion Inhibitors: Enfuvirtide (T-20). This drug is administered through subcutaneous

TABLE 4 World Health Organization Clinical Staging of HIV/AIDS for Adults and Adolescents With Confirmed HIV Infection

Clinical Stage 1
Asymptomatic
Persistent generalized lymphadenopathy

Clinical Stage 2
Moderate unexplained weight loss (<10% of presumed or measured body weight)*
Recurrent respiratory tract infections (e.g., sinusitis, tonsillitis, otitis media, pharyngitis)
Herpes zoster
Angular cheilitis
Recurrent oral ulceration
Papular pruritic eruptions
Seborrheic dermatitis
Fungal nail infections

Clinical Stage 3
Unexplained* severe weight loss (>10% of presumed or measured body weight)
Unexplained chronic diarrhea for longer than 1 month
Unexplained persistent fever (>37.6°C [99.7°F]), intermittent or constant, for longer than 1 month
Persistent oral candidiasis
Oral hairy leukoplakia
Pulmonary tuberculosis (current)
Severe bacterial infections (e.g., pneumonia, empyema, pyomyositis, bone or joint infection, meningitis, or bacteremia)
Acute necrotizing ulcerative stomatitis, gingivitis, or periodontitis
Unexplained anemia (<8 g/dL), neutropenia (<0.5 × 10^9/L), or chronic thrombocytopenia (<50 × 10^9/L)

Clinical Stage 4†
HIV wasting syndrome
Pneumocystis jirovecii
Recurrent severe bacterial pneumonia
Chronic herpes simplex infection (orolabial, genital or anorectal, longer than 1 month's duration, or visceral at any site)
Esophageal candidiasis (or candidiasis of trachea, bronchi, or lungs)
Extrapulmonary tuberculosis
Kaposi sarcoma
Cytomegalovirus infection (retinitis or infection of other organs)
Central nervous system toxoplasmosis
HIV encephalopathy
Extrapulmonary cryptococcosis, including meningitis
Disseminated nontuberculous mycobacterial infection
Progressive multifocal leukoencephalopathy
Chronic cryptosporidiosis (with diarrhea)
Chronic isosporiasis
Disseminated mycosis (coccidioidomycosis or histoplasmosis)
Recurrent nontyphoidal *Salmonella* bacteremia
Lymphoma (cerebral or B-cell non-Hodgkin's) or other solid HIV-associated tumors
Invasive cervical carcinoma
Atypical disseminated leishmaniasis
Symptomatic HIV-associated nephropathy or symptomatic HIV-associated cardiomyopathy

*Unexplained refers to when the condition is not explained by other causes.
†Some additional specific conditions can also be included in regional classifications (e.g., reactivation of American trypanosomiasis [meningoencephalitis or myocarditis]) in the World Health Organization region of the Americas and disseminated penicilliosis in Asia.
From Bennett JE, Dolin R, Blaser MJ: *Mandell, Douglas, and Bennett's principles and practice of infectious diseases,* ed 8, Philadelphia, 2015, Saunders.

injections and is only used as part of a salvage regimen for individuals who have failed multiple other regimens.
6. CCR5 Inhibitors: Maraviroc. Before using this drug, a viral trophism assay should be checked to determine if the virus uses the CCR5 co-receptor to infect cells. If the virus uses the CXCR4 co-receptor, this drug will not be effective.
• Adding a fourth drug to the three-drug regimen does not improve viral suppression or outcomes and is not recommended.

Treatment interruptions based upon CD4 responses appear harmful in recent comparative studies versus standard continuous treatment protocols and should be avoided. Antiretroviral regimens for initial therapy are summarized in Table 6.
• Typical dosing regimen consists of two NRTIs and either a NNRTI, PI, or II. IIs are now the preferred third drug because of tolerability. Data support inclusion of lamivudine or emtricitabine as one of the two NRTIs.

Standard NRTIs include:
• Truvada (tenofovir disoproxil fumarate/emtricitabine) 1 tablet once daily. Individuals with underlying renal dysfunction or requiring other nephrotoxic agents may be at increased risk of renal toxicity while taking tenofovir. TDF may also be associated with reductions in bone mineral density.
• Descovy (tenofovir alafenamide/emtricitabine) 1 tablet once daily. TAF is a newer formulation of TDF with less nephrotoxicity and bone mineral density effects. Both TDF/

TABLE 5 Comparison of WHO and CDC Staging Systems*

WHO Stage†	WHO T-Lymphocyte Count and Percentage‡	CDC Stage§	CDC T-Lymphocyte Count and Percentage
Stage 1 (HIV infection)	CD4+ T-lymphocyte count of ≥500 cells/mm³	Stage 1 (HIV infection)	CD4+ T-lymphocyte count of ≥500 cells/mm³ or CD4+ T-lymphocyte percentage of ≥29
Stage 2 (HIV infection)	CD4+ T-lymphocyte count of 350-499 cells/mm³	Stage 2 (HIV infection)	CD4+ T-lymphocyte count of 200-499 cells/mm³ or CD4+ T-lymphocyte percentage of 14-28
Stage 3 (advanced HIV disease [AHD])	CD4+ T-lymphocyte count of 200-349 cells/mm³	Stage 2 (HIV infection)	CD4+ T-lymphocyte count of 200-499 cells/mm³ or CD4+ T-lymphocyte percentage of 14-28
Stage 4 (acquired immunodeficiency syndrome [AIDS])	CD4+ T-lymphocyte count of <200 cells/mm³ or CD4+ T-lymphocyte percentage of <15	Stage 3 (AIDS)	CD4+ T-lymphocyte count of <200 cells/mm³ or CD4+ T-lymphocyte percentage of <14

CDC, Centers for Disease Control and Prevention; *WHO,* World Health Organization.
*For reporting purposes only.
†Among adults and children aged ≥5 years.
‡Percentage applicable for stage 4 only.
§Among adults and adolescents (ages ≥13 years). CDC also includes a fourth stage, stage unknown; laboratory confirmation of HIV infection but no information on CD4+ T-lymphocyte count or percentage and no information on AIDS-defining conditions.
From Bennett JE, Dolin R, Blaser MJ: *Mandell, Douglas, and Bennett's Principles and Practice of Infectious Diseases,* ed 8, Philadelphia, 2015, Saunders.

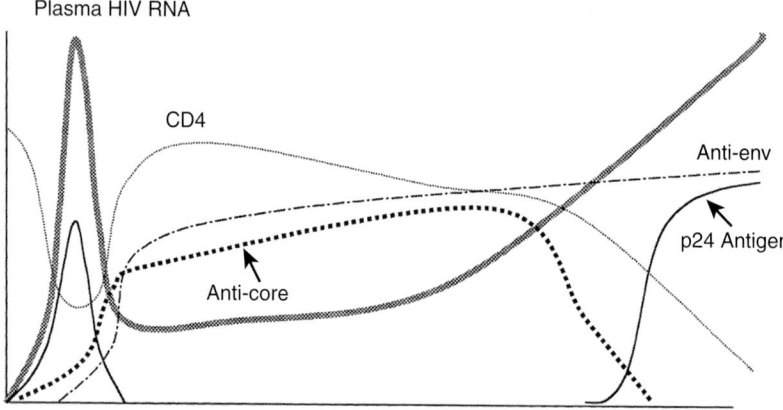

FIG. 2 Course of human immunodeficiency virus infection. (From Mandell GL [ed]: *Mandell, Douglas, and Bennett's principles and practice of infectious diseases,* ed 6, New York, 2005, Churchill Livingstone.)

FTC, and TAF/FTC are recommended components of the initial regimen (with a "backbone" medication). TDF should be avoided in patients with a creatinine clearance (CrCl) <60 ml/min. TAF should be avoided in patients with a CrCl <30 ml/min.

- Epzicom (abacavir/lamivudine) 1 tablet once daily. Abacavir may be associated with increased risk of myocardial infarction. Before using this drug, individuals should be checked for HLA-B*5701. Individuals with this allele are at higher risk of serious hypersensitivity reactions, and this drug should be avoided.
- Combivir (zidovudine/lamivudine) 1 tablet twice daily. Once widely prescribed; now rarely used due to lower efficacy compared with tenofovir-emtricitabine; zidovudine is associated with lipoatrophy and anemia, as well as GI and CNS side effects.

Standard Backbone Regimens include:

- IIs (These are now considered first line)
  1. Dolutegravir (50 mg once daily): The FDA has approved Triumeq, a fixed-dose combination of the integrase strand inhibitor dolutegravir and the NRTIs abacavir and lamivudine, for once-daily treatment of HIV-1 infection.
  2. Elvitegravir: Given with cobicistat (booster) and tenofovir/emtricitabine in a fixed-dose combination called Stribild.
  3. Raltegravir (400 mg twice a day).
- NNRTIs
  1. Efavirenz 600 mg daily: not recommended for women in the first trimester or those who are contemplating pregnancy.
  2. Rilpivirine: given with tenofovir and emtricitabine as part of a fixed-dose combination called Complera.
  3. Nevirapine 200 mg two times a day: avoid with CD4 count >250 in men and >350 cells per cubic millimeter in women because of the risk of hepatitis. The newer agent rilpivirine had higher virologic failures and should be considered an alternative agent.
  4. Etravirine 200 mg two times a day: This drug is generally used in patients for whom other regimens have failed. Etravirine retains activity in many patients who have developed resistance against efavirenz and nevirapine.
- PIs (ritonavir boosted)
  1. Lopinavir and ritonavir (200 mg/50 mg) 2 tablets twice a day (or 4 tablets once a day): most likely to cause diarrhea and has the greatest negative effect on triglyceride levels.
  2. Atazanavir and ritonavir (300 mg and 100 mg) 2 tablets a day: lower pill burden but use with caution with acid-reducing agents—can alter absorption.
  3. Fosamprenavir and ritonavir (700 mg and 100 mg) 2 tablets twice a day (or 4 tablets once a day): cannot take fosamprenavir with sulfa allergy.
  4. Darunavir and ritonavir (800 mg and 100 mg a day). This is considered a preferred PI regimen within the DHHS guidelines.
  5. Saquinavir and ritonavir: Saquinavir is no longer recommended for initial treatment of any patient and should be prescribed only in consultation with a specialist.
- All these drugs have their own unique, as well as class-specific, side effects and require careful follow-up to achieve optimal antiviral effects. Compliance with the drug regimen and tolerance of common side effects are critically important to maintain drug efficacy. Antiviral response should be monitored by baseline HIV viral load and CD4 count and repeat measurement at 2 and 4 weeks into

TABLE 6 What Antiretroviral Regimen to Choose for Initial Therapy

Preferred Regimens	Comments
Integrase inhibitor-based regimen	
RAL + TDF/FTC	
Dolutegravir + TDF/FTC	
Dolutegravir/ABC/3TC	
Elvitegravir/cobicistat/TDF/FTC	
PI-based regimen	
DRV/r (once daily) + TDF/FTC	
Preferred regimen for pregnant women	
LPV/r (twice daily) + ZDV/3TC	

Alternative Regimens	**Comments**
NNRTI-based regimens (in alphabetical order)	These regimens are now preferred.
EFV/TDF/FTC	EFV should not be used during the first trimester of pregnancy or in women trying
EFV + ABC/3TC	to conceive.
RPV/TDF/FTC	NVP should not be used in patients with moderate to severe hepatic impairment
RPV + ABC/3TC	(Child-Pugh B or C) Should not be used in women with pre-treatment CD4
	>250 cells/mm^3 or men with CD4 >400 cells/mm^3
PI-based regimens (in alphabetical order)	ABC should not be used in patients who test positive for HLA-B*5701
ATV/r + ABC/3TC	Use with caution in patients with high risk of cardiovascular disease or with
ATV/r + TDF/FTC	pretreatment HIV
DRV + ABC/3TC FPV/r (once or twice daily) + either ABC/3TC or TDF/FTC	RNA >100,000 copies/mL
LPV/r (once or twice daily) + either [(ABC or ZDV)/3TC] or TDF/FTC	Once-daily LPV/r is not recommended in pregnant women.
Integrase inhibitor-based regimens RAL + ABC/3TC	

Acceptable Regimens	
EFV + AZT/3TC	
NVP + TDF/FTC or ABC/3TC or AZT/3TC	
RPV + AZT/3TC	
ATV + ABC/3TC or AZT/3TC	
ATV/r + AZT/3TC	
DRV/r + AZT/3TC	
FPV/r + AZT/3TC	
LPV/r + AZT/3TC	
RAL + AZT/3TC	
MVC + AZT/3TC or TDF/FTC or ABC/3TC	

3TC, Lamivudine; *ABC*, abacavir; *ATV*, atazanavir; *ddI*, didanosine; *DRV*, darunavir; *EFV*, efavirenz; *FPV*, fosamprenavir; *FTC*, emtricitabine; *INSTI*, integrase strand transfer inhibitor; *LPV*, lopinavir; *MRV*, maraviroc; *NNRTI*, nonnucleoside reverse transcriptase inhibitor; *NRTI*, nucleos(t)ide reverse transcriptase inhibitor; *NVP*, nevirapine; *PI*, protease inhibitor; *r*, low dose ritonavir; *RAL*, raltegravir; *RVP*, rilpivirine; *SQV*, saquinavir; *TDF*, tenofovir; *ZDV*, zidovudine. The following combinations in the recommended list are available as fixed-dose combination formulations: ABC/3TC, EFV/TDF/FTC, LPV/r, TDF/FTC, RPV/TDF/FTC, and ZDV/3TC.
Modified from Panel on Antiretroviral Guidelines for Adults and Adolescents. Guidelines for the use of antiretroviral agents in HIV-1–infected adults and adolescents. Department of Health and Human Services 1-161, 2012. http://www.aidsinfo.nih.gov/ContentFiles/AdultandAdolescentGL.pdf.

treatment and then periodically (every 3-6 months) to ensure viral suppression.

- All patients should have genotypic resistance testing upon entry into medical care and before initiation of ART.
- In experienced patients, an antiretroviral regimen should be constructed based on past antiretroviral use and the results of genotypic or phenotypic testing.
- Patients with a CD4 count <200/mm^3 should be given preventive therapy for PJP (see "*Pneumocystis jiroveci [P. carinii]* Pneumonia").
- Evaluation of chronic diarrhea in patients with HIV is described in the AIDS topic in Section I.
- Criteria for discontinuing and restarting opportunistic infection prophylaxis for adults and adolescents with HIV infection is described in Table 7.
- HIV infection in a pregnant woman poses special challenges and considerations. Appropriate and timely ART given to mother and newborn has been shown to dramatically reduce the risk of perinatal transmission of HIV. The goal of therapy is to achieve an undetectable viral load. For HIV-infected pregnant women who are already receiving

ART: (1) Continue therapy if suppressing viral replication, but avoid use of efavirenz in the first trimester (substitution is recommended in the first trimester); (2) If viremia on therapy, genotypic testing is recommended; (3) Nevirapine should be continued, regardless of CD4 count, if there is viral suppression. For HIV-infected pregnant women who have never received ART: (1) Women who require ART for their own health should start on ART in the first trimester. Most antiretrovirals are safe in pregnancy, however, efavirenz should be avoided because of teratogenicity (Class D), DDI and D4T should be avoided (potential of lactic acidosis), and some protease inhibitors may be dose-altered in pregnancy. Nevirapine should not be initiated in an antiretroviral-naive pregnant patient with CD4 counts >250 cells/mm^3 because of the risk of hepatotoxicity. (2) Women who do not need ART for their own health should also initiate three-drug therapy, but may do so at the end of the first trimester.

- Therapy should continue through the baby's birth. Zidovudine is given intravenously at the time of labor, regardless of whether it is an existing component of her three-drug regimen.

In women with viral loads persistently >1000 copies/ml despite appropriate ART, cesarean section may further lower risk of transmission. Zidovudine (AZT) should also be given to the newborn for the first six weeks of life, and mothers should completely avoid nursing.

DISPOSITION

- Ongoing care consisting of frequent medical evaluations and monitoring of CD4 counts and HIV viral loads.
- Long-term care focused on providing up-to-date ART and prophylaxis of PJP and other opportunistic infections, as well as early detection of complications.
- Ongoing assessment for cardiovascular risk and other primary prevention interventions.
- Screening for hepatitis A, B, and C. Treatment when indicated. Drugs such as TDF and lamivudine have activity against both HIV and hepatitis B and may be used in patients with co-infection.
- Vaccinations including hepatitis A and B (when susceptible), Pneumovax, tetanus/diphtheria/pertussis, and influenza. Box 1H-9 summarizes vaccinations in HIV-positive adults.

TABLE 7 Criteria for Discontinuing and Restarting Opportunistic Infection Prophylaxis for Adults and Adolescents with Human Immunodeficiency Virus Infection

Opportunistic Infection	Criteria for Discontinuing Primary Prophylaxis	Criteria for Restarting Primary Prophylaxis	Criteria for Discontinuing Secondary Prophylaxis/Chronic Maintenance Therapy	Criteria for Restarting Secondary Prophylaxis/Chronic Maintenance Therapy
Pneumocystis pneumonia (PJP)	CD4+ count >200 cells/mm³ for >3 mo in response to ART	CD4+ count <200 cells/mm³	CD4+ count increased from <200 cells/mm³ to >200 cells/mm³ for ≥3 mo in response to ART. If PJP is diagnosed when CD4+ count >200 cells/mm³, prophylaxis should probably be continued for life regardless of CD4+ count rise in response to ART.	CD4+ count <200 cells/mm³, or if PCP recurred at a CD4+ count >200 cells/mm³
Toxoplasma gondii encephalitis (TE)	CD4+ count >200 cells/mm³ for >3 mo in response to ART	CD4+ count <100-200 cells/mm³	Successfully completed initial therapy, remain asymptomatic of signs and symptoms of TE, and CD4+ count >200 cells/mm³ for >6 mo in response to ART	CD4+ count <200 cells/mm³
Microsporidiosis	Not applicable	Not applicable	No signs and symptoms of non-ocular microsporidiosis and CD4+ count >200 cells/mm³ for >6 mo in response to ART. Patients with ocular microsporidiosis should be on therapy indefinitely regardless of CD4+ count.	No recommendation
Disseminated *Mycobacterium avium* complex (MAC) disease	CD4+ count >100 cells/mm³ for ≥3 mo in response to ART	CD4+ count <50 cells/mm³	If fulfill the following criteria: Completed ≥12 mo therapy, and No signs and symptoms of MAC, and Have sustained (≥6 mo) CD4+ count >100 cells/mm³ in response to ART	CD4+ count <100 cells/mm³
Bartonellosis	Not applicable	Not applicable	If fulfill the following criteria: Received 3-4 mo of treatment, CD4+ count >200 cells/mm³ for ≥6 mo. Certain specialists would discontinue therapy only if *Bartonella* titers have also decreased by fourfold.	No recommendation
Mucosal candidiasis	Not applicable	Not applicable	If used, reasonable to discontinue when CD4+ count >200 cells/mm³	No recommendation
Cryptococcal meningitis	Not applicable	Not applicable	If fulfill the following criteria: Completed course of initial therapy, Remain asymptomatic of cryptococcosis, CD4+ count ≥200 cells/mm³ for >6 mo in response to ART. Certain specialists would perform a lumbar puncture to determine if cerebrospinal fluid is culture and antigen negative before stopping therapy.	CD4+ count <200 cells/mm³
Histoplasma capsulatum infection	If used, CD4+ count >150 cells/mm³ for 6 mo on ART	For patients at high risk for acquiring histoplasmosis, restart at CD4+ count ≤150 cells/mm³.	If fulfill the following criteria: Received itraconazole for ≥1 yr, Negative blood cultures, CD4+ count >150 cells/mm³ for ≥6 mo in response to ART, Serum *Histoplasma* antigen <2 units	CD4+ count ≤150 cells/mm³
Coccidioidomycosis	If used, CD4+ count ≥250 cells/mm³ for ≥6 mo	If used, restart at CD4+ count <250 cells/mm³	**Only for patients with focal coccidioidal pneumonia:** Clinically responded to ≥12 mo of antifungal therapy, CD4+ count >250 cells/mm³, Receiving ART. Suppressive therapy should be continued indefinitely, even with increase in CD4+ count on ART for patients with diffuse pulmonary, disseminated, or meningeal diseases.	No recommendation
Cytomegalovirus retinitis	Not applicable	Not applicable	CD4+ count >100 cells/mm³ for >3-6 mo in response to ART. Therapy should be discontinued only after consultation with an ophthalmologist, taking into account magnitude and duration of CD4+ count increase, anatomic location of the lesions, vision in the contralateral eye, and the feasibility of regular ophthalmologic monitoring. Routine (every 3 mo) ophthalmologic follow-up is recommended for early detection of relapse or immune restoration uveitis.	CD4+ count <100 cells/mm³
Isospora belli infection	Not applicable	Not applicable	Sustained increase in CD4+ count to >200 cells/mm³ for >6 mo in response to ART and without evidence of *I. belli* infection	No recommendation

Modified from Centers for Disease Control and Prevention. Guidelines for prevention and treatment of opportunistic infections in HIV-infected adults and adolescents. Recommendations from CDC, the National Institutes of Health, and the HIV Medicine Association of the Infectious Disease Society of America. *MMWR Morb Mortal Wkly Rep* 58(RR-4), 2009.

BOX 1 Vaccination in HIV-Positive Adults

Generally Avoid
- VZV
- BCG
- Oral polio
- Oral typhoid

Avoid if CD4+ Cells <200
- Yellow fever
- Measles

Give Routinely
- Tetanus/diphtheria (or Tdap)
- Hepatitis B
- *Streptococcus pneumoniae*
- Hib
- Influenza, yearly
- Hepatitis A

Give if Indicated for Travel
- Typhoid Vi
- Meningococcal
- Polio, IPV
- Rabies
- Japanese encephalitis
- Tick-borne encephalitis

From Auerbach P: *Wilderness medicine, expert consult* Premium Edition—Enhanced Online Features and Print, Philadelphia, 2012, Saunders.

- Yearly screening for other sexually transmitted infections (chlamydia, gonorrhea, syphilis).
- Consideration of AIDS (lymphomas, HPV) and non-AIDS related (screening for general population, age-specific cancers).

REFERRAL

To a physician knowledgeable and experienced in the management of HIV infection and its complications.

PREVENTION:

- TDF/FTC may be used as pre-exposure prophylaxis (PrEP). Individuals who are HIV negative may take TDF/FTC once a day to prevent HIV infection. PrEP has been demonstrated to be effective in MSM, heterosexuals, and injection drug users. Individuals on PrEP should be monitored every three months for renal dysfunction, HIV status, and adherence.
- Post-exposure prophylaxis (PEP) is an effective prevention intervention for individuals exposed to HIV infection, either occupationally or through a sexual exposure (Table 8). PEP should be taken within 72 hours of an exposure and continued for 28 days. Baseline HIV status, renal function, hepatitis B/C, and liver function should be assessed. The recommended first-line regimen is raltegravir and FTC/TDF.

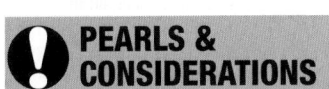 **PEARLS & CONSIDERATIONS**

COMMENTS

- HIV chemoprophylaxis after occupational exposure is described in Section V.
- ART should be initiated in all HIV-infected individuals regardless of CD4 cell counts.

- Trials involving antiretroviral chemoprophylaxis before exposure for the prevention of HIV acquisition in MSM have shown that oral tenofovir disoproxil fumarate (FTC-TDF) provides protection against acquisition of HIV infection. This is known as *pre-exposure prophylaxis (PrEP)*. Detected blood levels strongly correlated with the prophylactic effect.
- ART in combination with avoidance of breast-feeding and elective cesarean section in women with viremia reduces risk for mother-to-child transmission.
- Use of a monthly vaginal ring containing dapivirine has been shown effective in reducing the risk of HIV-1 infection.

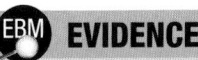 **EVIDENCE**

Available at www.expertconsult.com

SUGGESTED READINGS

Available at www.expertconsult.com

RELATED CONTENT

Human Immunodeficiency Virus (HIV) Infection (Patient Information)
Acquired Immunodeficiency Syndrome (Related Key Topic)

AUTHOR: **PHILIP A. CHAN, M.D., M.S.**

TABLE 8 Prophylaxis to Prevent First Episode of HIV-related Opportunistic Disease

Pathogen	Indication	First Choice	Alternative
Pneumocystis jiroveci pneumonia (PJP, previously referred to as *Pneumocystis carinii*, PCP)	CD4+ count <200 cells/mm³ or oropharyngeal candidiasis CD4+ <14% or history of AIDS-defining illness CD4+ count >200 but <250 cells/mm³ if monitoring CD4+ count every 1-3 mo is not possible	Trimethoprim-sulfamethoxazole (TMP-SMX) double-strength PO daily; *or* single-strength daily	TMP-SMX 1 double-strength PO 3 times weekly; *or* Dapsone 100 mg PO daily or 50 mg PO bid; *or* Aerosolized pentamidine 300 mg via Respirgard II nebulizer every month; *or* Atovaquone 1500 mg PO daily
Toxoplasma gondii encephalitis	*Toxoplasma* IgG–positive patients with CD4+ count <100 cells/mm³ Seronegative patients receiving PCP prophylaxis not active against toxoplasmosis should have *Toxoplasma* serology retested if CD4+ count declines to <100 cells/mm³. Prophylaxis should be initiated if seroconversion occurred.	TMP-SMX, 1 double-strength PO daily	TMP-SMX 1 double-strength PO 3 times weekly; *or* TMP-SMX 1 single-strength PO daily; *or* Dapsone 50 mg PO daily + pyrimethamine 50 mg PO weekly + leucovorin 25 mg PO weekly; *or* Dapsone 200 mg PO weekly + pyrimethamine 75 mg PO weekly + leucovorin 25 mg PO weekly
Mycobacterium tuberculosis infection (TB) (treatment of latent TB infection or LTBI)	(1) Diagnostic test for LTBI, no evidence of active TB, and no prior history of treatment for active or latent TB (2) Diagnostic test for LTBI, but close contact with a person with infectious pulmonary TB and no evidence of active TB (3) A history of untreated or inadequately treated healed TB (i.e., old fibrotic lesions) regardless of diagnostic tests for LTBI and no evidence of active TB	Isoniazid (INH) 300 mg PO daily or 900 mg PO twice weekly for 9 mo—both plus pyridoxine 50 mg PO daily; *or* For persons exposed to drug-resistant TB, selection of drugs after consultation with public health authorities	Rifampin (RIF) 600 mg PO daily × 3-4 mo; *or* Rifabutin (RFB) 300 mg once daily for 4 mo. Be careful of drug interactions with these medications (PIs and NNRTIs).
Disseminated *Mycobacterium avium* complex (MAC) disease	CD4+ count <50 cells/mm³—after ruling out active MAC infection	Azithromycin 1200 mg PO once weekly; *or* Clarithromycin 500 mg PO bid; *or* Azithromycin 600 mg PO twice weekly	RFB 300 mg PO daily (dosage adjustment based on drug-drug interactions with antiretroviral therapy); rule out active TB before starting RFB

Continued

TABLE 8 Prophylaxis to Prevent First Episode of HIV-related Opportunistic Disease—cont'd

Pathogen	Indication	First Choice	Alternative
Streptococcus pneumoniae infection	CD4$^+$ count >200 cells/mm^3 and no receipt of pneumococcal vaccine in the past 5 yr CD4$^+$ count <200 cells/mm^3—vaccination can be offered In patients who received polysaccharide pneumococcal vaccination (PPV) when CD4$^+$ count <200 cells/mm^3 but has increased to >200 cells/mm^3 in response to antiretroviral therapy	23-valent PPV 0.5 mL IM × 1 Revaccination every 5 yr may be considered	
Influenza A and B virus infection	All HIV-infected patients	Inactivated influenza vaccine 0.5 mL IM annually	
Histoplasma capsulatum infection	CD4$^+$ count ≤150 cells/mm^3 and at high risk because of occupational exposure or live in a community with a hyperendemic rate of histoplasmosis (>10 cases/100 patient-yr)	Itraconazole 200 mg PO daily	
Coccidioidomycosis	Positive IgM or IgG serologic test result in a patient from a disease-endemic area; and CD4$^+$ count <250 cells/mm^3	Fluconazole 400 mg PO daily Itraconazole 200 mg PO bid	
Varicella-zoster virus (VZV) infection	*Pre-exposure prevention:* Patients with CD4$^+$ count ≥200 cells/mm^3 who have not been vaccinated, have no history of varicella or herpes zoster, or who are seronegative for VZV Note: Routine VZV serologic testing in HIV-infected adults is not recommended. *Postexposure—close contact with a person who has active varicella or herpes zoster* For susceptible patients (those who have no history of vaccination or of either condition, or are known to be VZV seronegative)	*Pre-exposure prevention:* Primary varicella vaccination (Varivax), 2 doses (0.5 mL SC) administered 3 mo apart. If vaccination results in disease because of vaccine virus, treatment with acyclovir is recommended. *Postexposure therapy:* Varicella-zoster immune globulin (VariZIG) 125 IU per 10 kg (maximum of 625 IU) IM, administered within 96 hr after exposure to a person with active varicella or herpes zoster Note: As of June 2007, VariZIG can be obtained only under a treatment IND (1-800-843-7477, FFF Enterprises).	VZV-susceptible household contacts of susceptible HIV-infected persons should be vaccinated to prevent potential transmission of VZV to their HIV-infected contacts. Alternative postexposure therapy: Postexposure varicella vaccine (Varivax) 0.5 ml SC × 2 doses, 3 mo apart if CD4$^+$ count >200 cells/mm^3; *or* Preemptive acyclovir 800 mg PO 3×/day for 5 days These two alternatives have not been studied in the HIV population.
Human papillomavirus (HPV) infection	Women aged 11-26 yr. Men aged 11-21 yr	HPV quadrivalent vaccine 0.5 ml IM mo 0, 2, and 6	
Hepatitis A virus (HAV) infection	HAV-susceptible patients with chronic liver disease or who are injection-drug users, or men who have sex with men. Certain specialists might delay vaccination until CD4$^+$ count >200 cells/mm^3.	Hepatitis A vaccine 1 ml IM × 2 doses—at 0 and 6-12 mo IgG antibody response should be assessed 1 mo after vaccination; nonresponders should be revaccinated	
Hepatitis B virus (HBV) infection	All HIV patients without evidence of prior exposure to HBV should be vaccinated with HBV vaccine, including patients with CD4$^+$ count <200 cells/mm^3. *Patients with isolated anti-HBc:* consider screening for HBV DNA before vaccination to rule out occult chronic HBV infection	Hepatitis B vaccine IM (Engerix-B 20 μg/mL or Recombivax HB 10 μg/ml) at 0, 1, and 6 mo Anti-HBs should be obtained 1 mo after completion of the vaccine series.	Some experts recommend vaccinating with 40-μg doses of either vaccine.
	Vaccine nonresponders: Defined as anti-HBs <10 IU/mL 1 mo after a vaccination series For patients with low CD4$^+$ count at the time of first vaccination series, certain specialists might delay revaccination until after a sustained increase in CD4$^+$ count with antiretroviral therapy.	Revaccinate with a second vaccine series.	Some experts recommend revaccinating with 40-μg doses of either vaccine.

Modified from Centers for Disease Control and Prevention. Guidelines for prevention and treatment of opportunistic infections in HIV-infected adults and adolescents: Recommendations from CDC, the National Institutes of Health, and the HIV Medicine Association of the Infectious Disease Society of America, *MMWR Morb Mortal Wkly Rep* 58(RR-4), 2009.

BASIC INFORMATION

DEFINITION

Huntington's disease (HD) is a trinucleotide repeat autosomal dominant neurodegenerative disorder characterized by involuntary movements, psychiatric disturbance, and cognitive decline. The disease exhibits the genetic phenomenon of anticipation, such that subsequent generations have longer repeats and a younger age of onset (Table 1).

SYNONYMS

Huntington's chorea
HD

ICD-10CM CODES
G10 Huntington's disease

EPIDEMIOLOGY & DEMOGRAPHICS

PEAK INCIDENCE: Late 30s and 40s, with onsets from ages 2 to 70 yr.

Age of onset, but not necessarily disease severity, correlates with CAG repeat numbers.
PREVALENCE (IN U.S.): 4.1 to 8.4 cases/100,000 persons. Most common neurodegenerative cause of generalized chorea
PREDOMINANT SEX: Female = male
PREDOMINANT AGE: Adulthood
GENETICS: Autosomal dominant

PHYSICAL FINDINGS & CLINICAL PRESENTATION

- Chorea: irregular, rapid, flowing, nonstereotyped involuntary movements. When there is a writhing quality, it is referred to as choreoathetosis. Chorea is present early on and tends to decrease in end stages of disease.
- Dancelike, lurching gait, often caused by chorea.
- Westphal variant: cognitive dysfunction, bradykinesia, and rigidity. This variant is more commonly seen in juvenile-onset Huntington's.
- Oculomotor abnormalities are common early on and include increased latency of response and insuppressible eye blinking.
- Psychiatric disorders (can be present early on): depression is commonly seen as well as obsessive-compulsive behaviors and aggression associated with impaired impulse control.

ETIOLOGY

- Trinucleotide repeat disorder; repeat of CAG, which codes for glutamine
- The responsible gene is the *huntingtin* gene (*HTT*), located on chromosome 4. Its function is not known.

DIAGNOSIS

DIFFERENTIAL DIAGNOSIS

- Drug-induced chorea: dopamine, stimulants, anticonvulsants, antidepressants, and oral contraceptives have all been known to cause chorea.
- Sydenham's chorea: decreased incidence with decline of rheumatic fever.
- Benign hereditary chorea: autosomal dominant with onset in childhood; nonprogressive and without associated dementia or behavioral problems.
- Senile chorea: possibly vascular in origin.
- Wilson's disease: autosomal recessive; tremor, dysarthria, and dystonia are more common presentations than chorea. A total of 95% of patients with neurologic manifestations will have Kayser-Fleischer rings.
- Postinfectious.
- Systemic lupus erythematosus: can be the presenting feature of lupus (rare).
- Chorea gravidarum: presents during first 4 to 5 mo of pregnancy and resolves after delivery.
- Paraneoplastic: seen most commonly in small-cell lung cancer and lymphoma.

WORKUP

Onset of symptoms in an individual with an established family history requires no additional investigation.

LABORATORY TESTS

- Genetic testing for CAG repeat numbers
- If genetic tests are normal, obtain complete blood count with smear, erythrocyte sedimentation rate, electrolytes, serum ceruloplasmin, 24-hr urinary copper excretion, TFTs, antinuclear antibody, liver function tests, HIV, and ASO titer. Consider paraneoplastic markers.

IMAGING STUDIES

CT scan or MRI scan will show atrophy, most notably in the caudate and putamen. In some cases, the striatal atrophy causes a characteristic appearance of the lateral ventricles on imaging termed "boxcar ventricles." The cortex is involved to a lesser extent. A normal scan does not exclude the diagnosis.

TREATMENT

NONPHARMACOLOGIC THERAPY

- Supportive counseling
- Physical and occupational therapy
- Home health care
- Genetic counseling

CHRONIC Rx

- Chorea does not need to be treated unless it is disabling.
- Tetrabenazine (TBZ) is approved by the FDA for the symptomatic treatment of chorea seen in Huntington's disease. It is a reversible inhibitor of the vesicle monoamine transporter type 2 (VMAT-2). It inhibits primarily dopamine and to a lesser degree serotonin and norepinephrine. Side effects include parkinsonism and severe depression.
- Neuroleptics, typical or atypical, can be used for symptomatic management of neuropsychiatric issues and chorea at low doses (e.g., haloperidol 1 to 10 mg/day).
- Amantadine (up to 300 to 400 mg divided tid).
- Depression with suicidal ideation is common; may improve with tricyclic antidepressants or SSRI

DISPOSITION

Relentless course of variable duration leading to progressive disability and death

REFERRAL

- Should refer to psychiatry and neurology for treatment of mood disorders and movement disorders
- Genetic counseling

PEARLS & CONSIDERATIONS

- Suicide rate is fivefold that of the general population.
- Generational transmission is often associated with the phenomenon of "anticipation" with disease starting at an earlier age in a child because of increased repeat length compared with that of the parent.
- The number of repeats does correlate with age of onset but does not clearly correlate with disease severity. Interpretation of number of repeats is still difficult at this time; therefore it is debatable whether to disclose this information to patients.

SUGGESTED READING

Available at www.expertconsult.com

RELATED CONTENT

Huntington's Disease (Patient Information)

AUTHORS: **ANGAD JOLLY,**
JOSEPH S. KASS, M.D., J.D., and
FARIHA ZAHEER, M.D.

TABLE 1 CAG Repeats and Disease Risk

CAG Repeat #	Allele Classification	Disease Risk	Risk to Offspring
≤26	Normal	No symptoms	None
27-35	Intermediate	No symptoms	Low
36-39	Disease	At risk for HD	Moderate
≥40	Disease	HD imminent	High

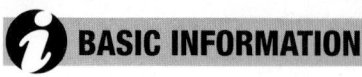

BASIC INFORMATION

DEFINITION

A hydrocele is a fluid collection in a serous scrotal space, usually between the layers of the tunica vaginalis (Fig. 1). A hydrocele that fills with fluid from the peritoneum is termed *communicating*. This is distinguished from a *noncommunicating* hydrocele by history of variation in size throughout the day and palpation of a thickened cord above the testicle on the affected side. A communicating hydrocele is a small inguinal hernia in which fluid, but not peritoneal structures, traverses the processus vaginalis. In noncommunicating hydrocele, the processus vaginalis was obliterated during development. An abdominoscrotal hydrocele is a rare variant of a hydrocele in which there is a large, tense hydrocele that extends into the lower abdominal cavity.

ICD-10CM CODES
N43.3 Hydrocele, unspecified
N43 Hydrocele and spermatocele
N43.0 Encysted hydrocele
N43.1 Infected hydrocele
N43.2 Other hydrocele
P83.5 Congenital hydrocele

PHYSICAL FINDINGS & CLINICAL PRESENTATION

Symptoms:
- Scrotal enlargement
- Scrotal heaviness or discomfort radiating to the inguinal area
- Back pain

Physical findings:
- Most hydroceles are smooth and nontender. Scrotal distention may make it difficult to palpate the testis, but it is important to palpate the testis because some young men develop a hydrocele in association with a testis tumor
- Transillumination of the scrotum confirms the fluid-filled nature of the mass

ETIOLOGY

Hydroceles may occur as a congenital abnormality in which the processus vaginalis fails to close. In this case an inguinal hernia is virtually always associated with the malformation. Congenital hydroceles are most common in infants (1%-2% of neonates have hydroceles) and children. In adults, hydroceles are more frequently caused by infection, tumor, or trauma. Infection of the epididymis often results in the development of a secondary hydrocele. Tropical infections such as filariasis may produce hydroceles.

DIAGNOSIS

DIFFERENTIAL DIAGNOSIS

- Spermatocele
- Inguinoscrotal hernia
- Testicular tumor
- Varicocele
- Epididymitis

IMAGING STUDIES

Scrotal ultrasound is useful to rule out a testicular tumor as the cause of the hydrocele (Fig. 2). The acute development of a hydrocele might be associated with the onset of epididymitis, testicular tumor, trauma, and torsion of a testicular appendage. An ultrasound of the scrotum may provide important diagnostic information.

TREATMENT

- No treatment if asymptomatic and testis is believed to be normal. Most congenital hydroceles resolve by 12 months of age following reabsorption of the hydrocele fluid.
- Surgical repair should be considered if the hydrocele is tense and large. Communicating hydroceles should be repaired in the same manner as an indirect hernia. The indications for repair of a noncommunicating hydrocele include failure to resolve and increase in size to one that is large and tense.
- Surgical correction is similar to a herniorrhaphy: an inguinal incision is made, the spermatic cord is identified, the hydrocele fluid is drained, and a high ligation of the processus vaginalis is performed.

PEARLS & CONSIDERATIONS

- The long-term risk of a communicating hydrocele is the development of an inguinal hernia.
- An inguinal hernia/hydrocele is likely if compression of the fluid-filled mass completely reduces the hydrocele.

RELATED CONTENT

Hydrocele (Patient Information)

AUTHOR: **FRED F. FERRI, M.D.**

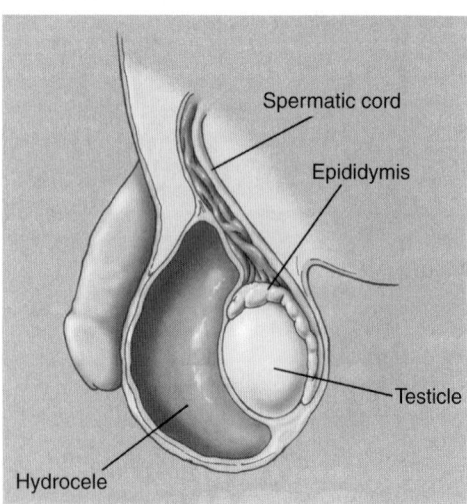

FIG. 1 Schematic representation of the testicle, epididymis, spermatic cord, and a hydrocele. (From Lipshultz LI et al: *Urology and the primary care practitioner,* ed 3, Philadelphia, 2008, Elsevier.)

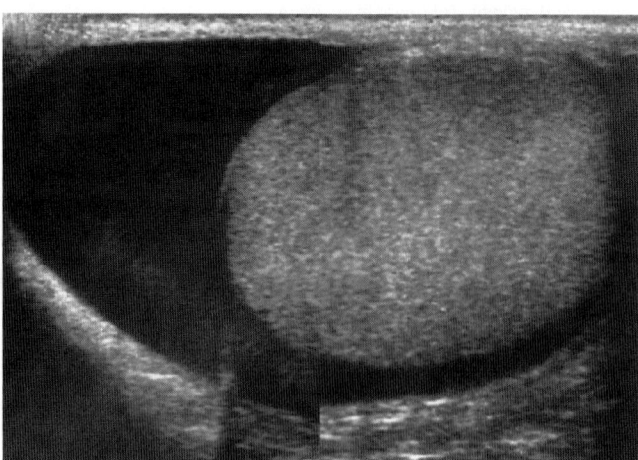

FIG. 2 Longitudinal ultrasound view of normal testis and moderate hydrocele. (From Grainger RG et al [eds.]: *Grainger & Allison's diagnostic radiology,* ed 4, London, 2001, Harcourt.)

BASIC INFORMATION

DEFINITION

Normal pressure hydrocephalus (NPH) is a syndrome of symptomatic hydrocephalus in the setting of normal cerebrospinal fluid (CSF) pressure. The classic clinical triad of NPH includes gait disturbance, cognitive decline, and incontinence.

SYNONYMS

Occult hydrocephalus
Extraventricular obstructive hydrocephalus
Chronic hydrocephalus

ICD-10CM CODES
G91.2 Normal pressure hydrocephalus
G91.8 Other hydrocephalus

EPIDEMIOLOGY & DEMOGRAPHICS

INCIDENCE: The exact incidence is not known. In one study the incidence was found to be 5.5 per 100,000, but it may account for up to 5% of dementia in the U.S. Hospital discharge data suggest approximately 11,500 new cases diagnosed annually (may be overestimated). The prevalence of NPH may be as high as 14% among extended care facility patients.
PREDOMINANT SEX: Males = females
PREDOMINANT AGE: NPH is more common with increasing age. In one study of 1238 patients who had undergone a head CT and neuropsychiatric evaluation, 0.2% of patients between 70 and 79 had probable NPH, and 5.9% of those 80 years old and older had probable NPH.

PHYSICAL FINDINGS & CLINICAL PRESENTATION

- Gait difficulty: patients often have difficulty initiating ambulation, and the gait may be broad based and shuffling, with the appearance that the feet are stuck to the floor
- ("magnetic gait" or "frontal gait disorder").
- Cognitive decline: mental slowing, forgetfulness, and inattention, typically without agnosia, aphasia, or other cortical disturbances.
- Incontinence: initially may have urinary urgency; incontinence later develops. Fecal incontinence also occasionally occurs. In one prospective study of 55 consecutive patients with idiopathic NPH, nocturia was the most common symptom, urge incontinence was the most bothersome, and 100% had detrusor overactivity on urodynamic studies.
- *Gegenhalten* (paratonia or involuntary resistance with passive movement) or other frontal lobe signs may be seen.

ETIOLOGY

- Approximately 50% of cases are idiopathic; the remaining cases have a variety of causes, including prior subarachnoid hemorrhage, meningitis, head trauma, or intracranial surgery.
- Symptoms are presumed to result from stretching of sacral motor and limbic fibers that lie near the ventricles as dilation occurs.

DX DIAGNOSIS

DIFFERENTIAL DIAGNOSIS

- Alzheimer's disease with extrapyramidal features
- Cognitive impairment in the setting of Parkinson's disease or parkinsonism-plus syndromes
- Dementia with Lewy bodies
- Frontotemporal dementia
- Cervical spondylosis with cord compromise in the setting of degenerative dementia
- Multi-infarct dementia
- HIV-associated dementia

WORKUP

- Large-volume lumbar puncture:
  1. Mental status testing (e.g., MOCA, www.moca.org/) and time to walk a prespecified distance (usually 25 feet) are measured, followed by removal of 40 to 50 ml of CSF.
  2. Retest of mental status and timed walking are done later (sometimes at 1 and 4 hr). Patients who have significant improvement in gait or mental status may have a better surgical outcome; those with mild or negative response can have variable outcomes.
  3. Opening and closing pressure are measured; if pressure is elevated, alternative causes must be considered. Higher *normal* pressure may predict a good outcome from CSF shunting (normal CSF pressure: 8-15 mm Hg or 10-18 cm H_2O).
- Measurement of CSF outflow resistance by an infusion test or CSF pressure monitoring is sometimes used to help predict surgical outcome. External lumbar drainage (ELD) is being used more commonly.

LABORATORY TESTS

- CSF should be sent for routine fluid analysis to exclude other pathologies.
- CSF biomarkers may be useful in excluding Alzheimer's disease (e.g., Tau/A beta 42).

IMAGING STUDIES

- CT scan or MRI can be used to document ventriculomegaly. The distinguishing feature of NPH is ventricular enlargement out of proportion to sulcal atrophy (Fig. E1), and typically the frontal horn ratio (Evans ratio) exceeds 0.40. An algorithm for evaluation of patients with enlarged ventricles is described in Fig. 2.

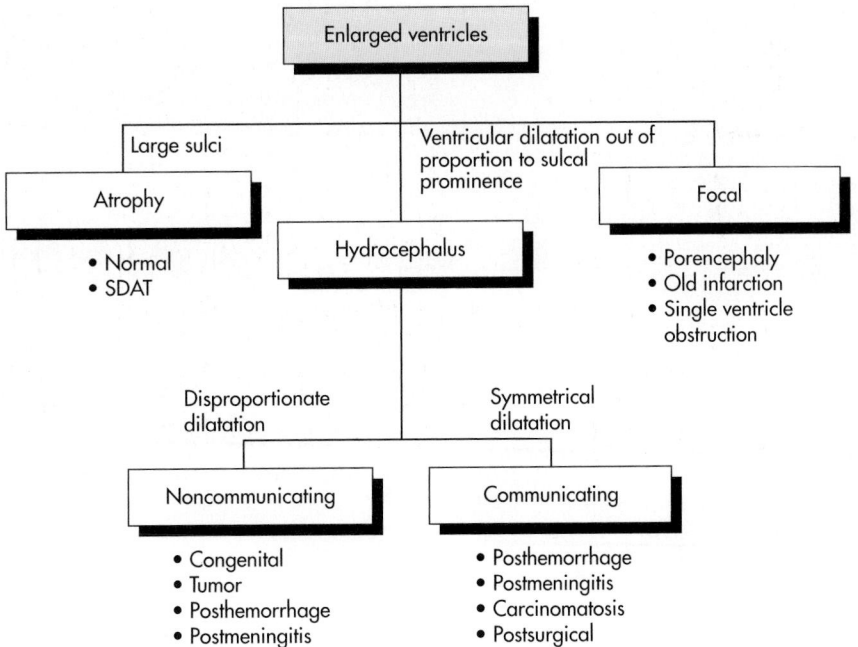

FIG. 2 Radiographic differential diagnosis of enlarged ventricles. (From Weissleder R et al: *Primer of diagnostic imaging*, ed 5, St. Louis, 2011, Mosby.)

- MRI has advantages over CT, including better ability to visualize structures in the posterior fossa, visualize transependymal CSF flow (seen as periventricular hyperintensity), and document extent of white matter lesions. On MRI a flow void in the aqueduct and third ventricle ("jet sign"), thinning and elevation of the corpus callosum on sagittal images, rounding of the frontal horns, and a narrow CSF space at the high convexity/midline areas relative to Sylvian fissure size may be seen. MRI time-resolved 2D phase contrast imaging with velocity encoding can also be used to visualize CSF flow.
- Isotope cisternography and dynamic MRI studies have not been shown to be superior in predicting shunt outcome.

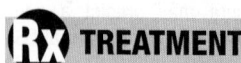 **TREATMENT**

There is no evidence that NPH can be effectively treated with medications.

NONPHARMACOLOGIC THERAPY

Response to ventriculoperitoneal shunting is variable. Some patients (variable depending on series reported) show significant improvement from shunting; however, effectiveness of shunting has never been demonstrated in a randomized-controlled trial. Gait is most likely to improve.

Factors that may predict positive outcome with surgery:
- NPH caused by prior trauma, subarachnoid hemorrhage, or meningitis

- History of mild impairment in cognition <2 yr duration
- Onset of gait abnormality before cognitive decline
- Imaging demonstrates hydrocephalus without sulcal enlargement, including normal-sized sylvian fissures and cortical sulci, and absent or mild white matter lesions.
- Transependymal CSF flow visualized on MRI
- Large-volume tap or ELD produces dramatic but temporary relief of symptoms
- High *normal* opening pressure
Factors that may predict negative outcome with surgery:
- Extensive white matter lesions or diffuse cerebral atrophy on MRI
- Moderate to severe cognitive impairment
- Onset of cognitive impairment before gait disorder
- History of alcohol abuse

ACUTE GENERAL Rx

Shunting in selected patients

DISPOSITION

Symptoms of NPH may progress over time. Prompt diagnosis may improve chances for treatment success.

REFERRAL

To neurologist for initial evaluation, including lumbar puncture, followed by neurosurgeon for shunting in appropriate patients

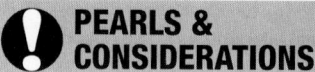 **PEARLS & CONSIDERATIONS**

Each of the cardinal symptoms of NPH is commonly seen in the elderly and occurs in multiple disease processes; therefore, differential diagnoses should always be considered carefully.

CAUTION

Shunt complications, including subdural or intracerebral hematoma, may occur in 30% to 40% of patients. In one retrospective study spanning 10 years, which included patients with idiopathic as well as other forms of adult hydrocephalus, the shunt failure rate was 32%.

SUGGESTED READINGS

Available at www.expertconsult.com

RELATED CONTENT

Normal Pressure Hydrocephalus (Patient Information)

AUTHORS: **TAMARA G. FONG, M.D., PH.D.,** and **IRINA A. SKYLAR-SCOTT, M.D.**

BASIC INFORMATION

DEFINITION

Hydronephrosis, which literally means "water inside the kidney," is an anatomic dilation of the collecting system of the kidneys (renal pelvis and/or calyces). When combined with dilation of the ureters, this is known as hydroureteronephrosis. This finding is *not* synonymous with obstruction and can occur with or without obstruction of the urine flow.

SYNONYMS

Pelviectasis
Caliectasis
Pelvocaliectasis
Pyelocaliectasis

ICD-10-CM CODES

N13.1 Hydronephrosis with ureteral stricture, not elsewhere classified
N13.2 Hydronephrosis with renal and ureteral calculous obstruction
N13.30 Unspecified hydronephrosis
N13.39 Other hydronephrosis
Q62.0 Congenital hydronephrosis

EPIDEMIOLOGY & DEMOGRAPHICS

Prevalence from multiple autopsy series ranges from 2% to 4% (subjects ranging in age from neonates to geriatric patients). Antenatal hydronephrosis is one of the most common findings in prenatal ultrasound scans, affecting up to 5% of pregnancies, with 30% to 40% persisting postnatally and, of these, 40% resolving spontaneously. Hydronephrosis in children is often caused by congenital and structural abnormalities of the kidneys and ureters, such as ureteropelvic junction obstruction (UPJO) and vesicoureteral reflux (VUR). Hydronephrosis in adults is often a result of obstruction of one or both kidneys, usually caused by stones, tumors, infections, and trauma. In young adults, obstruction from renal calculi is common, while in young females, gynecologic causes predominate. During pregnancy, physiologic hydronephrosis (more commonly on the right since the uterus dextrorotates) can occur in up to 90% and is often asymptomatic. In older patients, obstructions from prostate enlargement (in males) or malignancy are the most common causes.

CLINICAL PRESENTATION

This may present as an asymptomatic incidental finding during imaging performed for another purpose. Symptoms often indicate an element of obstruction, and the presentation will depend on the *degree* of obstruction (complete or partial), the *chronicity* of obstruction (acute or chronic), and *anatomic* factors (unilateral, bilateral, and whether intrinsic or extrinsic in the ureter).

HISTORY:

• Pain: Pain is usually present along the flank with radiation toward the ipsilateral groin or lower abdominal quadrant. If very sudden and severe in onset, consider a ureteral stone. If the pain is induced by diuresis (e.g., following consumption of alcohol), consider UPJO (known as "Dietl's crisis"). When obstruction is subacute to chronic, symptoms may be vague, less intense, or absent, and they may wax and wane in severity (colic). Extrinsic compression (e.g., malignant compression of the ureters) usually has a more insidious onset compared to intrinsic obstruction (e.g., from a ureteral stone or blood clot).

• Nausea and vomiting.

• Oliguria/anuria: can occur with complete bilateral obstruction or with an obstructed solitary kidney.

• Urinary symptoms: often absent unless there is an associated condition, for example, a distal ureteral calculus. Irritative urinary symptoms may be present, along with bladder outflow obstruction preceding obstructive urinary symptoms, obstruction in the setting of a urinary tract infection, dysuria, flank pain, and fevers.

• Hematuria: may indicate a stone or malignancy.

PHYSICAL EXAMINATION: A complete physical examination is warranted but is typically is not helpful in the assessment of hydronephrosis. Areas to pay special attention to include:

• Blood pressure measurement

• Abdominal exam: Palpable abdominal masses are rare, except in children with massive hydronephrosis. Costovertebral angle tenderness is not a particularly helpful finding. Palpate and percuss for an enlarged bladder.

• Complete genitourinary and pelvic exams: Digital rectal exam in men will assess for prostatic abnormality or rectal mass, and pelvic exam in women will assess for any pelvic masses.

• Residual urine volume: If incomplete emptying of the bladder is a concern, residual urine volume can be evaluated indirectly by bedside ultrasonography or directly by catheterization.

ETIOLOGY

Hydronephrosis can be caused by extrinsic or intrinsic factors relative to the urinary tract. Causes can also be grouped as congenital or acquired (Table 1).

DIAGNOSIS

Diagnostic workup will depend upon the age of the patient, whether the hydronephrosis was diagnosed incidentally, and which associated symptoms are present.

DIFFERENTIAL DIAGNOSIS

• Extrarenal pelvis: not obstructed and often confused for obstruction
• Urinary stones
• Neoplastic disease: kidney, ureter, bladder, urethra
• Prostatic hyperplasia
• Neurologic disease
• Urinary reflux
• Urinary tract infection
• Medication effects
• Trauma
• Congenital abnormality of urinary tract
• Urinary retention
• Retroperitoneal fibrosis

• Urinary trauma
• Iatrogenic injuries

LABORATORY TESTS

• **Evaluation of kidney function** by blood urea nitrogen and creatinine (if impaired, usually implies bilateral obstruction or unilateral obstruction of a solitary/functionally solitary kidney).

• **Evaluation of electrolyte abnormalities** including hypo- or hypernatremia, hyperkalemia, or distal renal tubular acidosis.

• **Urinalysis and sediment examination** may reveal white blood cells, red blood cells, or bacteria in the appropriate setting (e.g., infection, stones). Often the sediment is normal in obstructive renal disease. Urine culture should be sent if urinary tract infection is a concern.

IMAGING STUDIES

• Ultrasound is an excellent initial test, especially for children and pregnant women and for screening purposes, permitting evaluation of kidneys and bladder volume as well as the contour of the collecting system and ureters (Fig. 1). Ultrasound is >90% sensitive

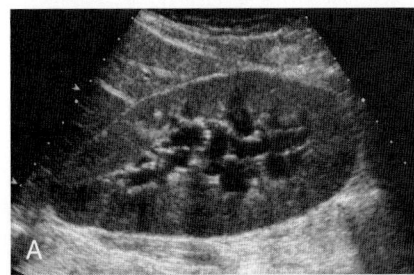

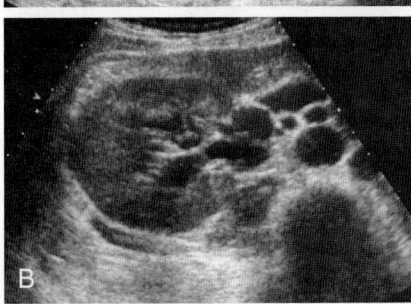

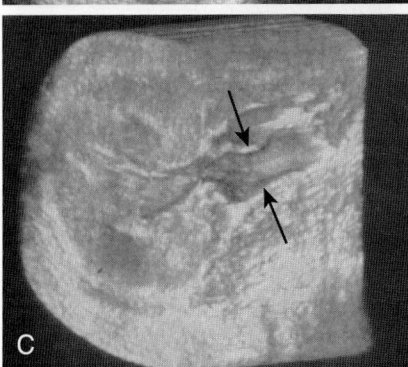

FIG. 1 Renal ultrasound study demonstrating hydronephrosis. A, Sagittal image. **B,** Transverse image. **C,** Transverse three-dimensional surface-rendered image; *arrows* indicate the dilated proximal ureter. (From Floege J et al: *Comprehensive clinical nephrology,* ed 4, Philadelphia, 2010, Saunders.)

Table 1 Causes of Hydronephrosis

Obstructive

Intrinsic to the Urinary Tract	Ureter: ureteropelvic junction obstruction, ureterovesical junction obstruction, stricture, tumor, ureterocele, stone, blood clot, sloughed papilla, infection
	Bladder: malignancy, stone, bladder neck obstruction, urine retention
	Prostate: benign prostatic enlargement, calculus, abscess, malignancy
	Urethra: stricture, stone, diverticulum, malignancy, posterior urethral valves, phimosis

Extrinsic to the Urinary Tract	Reproductive System:
	  Uterus: pregnancy, prolapse, fibroids, malignancy
	  Ovary: malignancy, cyst, abscess
	Vascular System:
	  Aneurysm: Abdominal aorta, iliac vessel
	  Aberrant vessels: ureteropelvic junction
	  Venous: retrocaval ureter, ovarian vein syndrome
	Gastrointestinal System:
	  Inflammatory bowel disease, GI malignancy, abscesses, cysts
	Diseases of the Retroperitoneum
	  Retroperitoneal fibrosis
	  Retroperitoneal malignancy (primary or metastatic deposits)
	  Hematoma
	  Lymphocele
	Iatrogenic injury

Nonobstructive

Vesicoureteral reflux
Extrarenal pelvis
Megaureter/megacalycosis
Pyelonephritis

and specific for hydronephrosis. Absence of ureteral jets may be an indirect sign of obstruction but is not definitive.

- Abdominal CT scan without intravenous contrast medium provides excellent localization of the site of obstruction (Fig. E2), especially if a ureteral calculus is the cause of obstruction. If kidney function is normal, CT urography (without and then with contrast, with delayed images of the ureters, provides excellent anatomic information). This is the modality of choice for assessment of possible upper tract tumors or for workup of incidental hydronephrosis.
- MRI is an alternative to CT. MRI provides good detail but cannot directly detect a stone and is cumbersome, time-consuming, and expensive. Impaired renal function may preclude gadolinium administration. MRI is considered after other tests are inconclusive or contraindicated.
- Antegrade or retrograde ureterograms can be used additionally if there are contraindications to CT or MRI scans with contrast (e.g., contrast allergy, renal impairment).
- Voiding cystourethrogram can diagnose vesicoureteral reflux and bladder neck or urethral obstruction.
- Diuretic renography (MAG3 renogram) is a functional radioisotopic test, providing differential function of each kidney and also indicating whether obstruction is present.

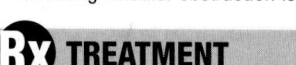

TREATMENT

ACUTE GENERAL Rx

Analgesics, antiemetics, and fluids for treatment of pain, nausea, and vomiting

Antibiotics for urinary tract infection/pyelonephritis

Definitive management:
- This will depend upon the presence of obstruction, the etiology, and the location of the hydronephrosis. Prompt treatment of infection and rapid relief of obstruction prevent long-term loss of kidney function. Chronic bilateral obstruction, such as from benign prostatic hypertrophy or neurogenic bladder, may cause chronic kidney disease.
- General principles include:
- Observation and outpatient workup for asymptomatic or minimally symptomatic patients with no infection concerns and no severe electrolyte derangements or acute kidney injury.
- Surgical treatment aimed at relieving the obstruction is indicated in the setting of acute obstruction associated with urinary tract infection, acute kidney injury, or uncontrollable pain.

- Urinary catheter or suprapubic catheter placement is indicated for bladder outlet obstruction.
- Ureteral stenting for internal decompression of one or both kidneys.
- Percutaneous nephrostomy tubes may be required in the setting of extrinsic ureteral compression or when ureteral stenting is not possible or fails.

REFERRAL

Prompt emergent referral is paramount in the setting of severe symptoms, infection, or impaired renal function.
- Urology for timely diagnostic and/or therapeutic procedures (pediatric urologist for antenatal or postnatal hydronephrosis)
- Oncology if a neoplasm is diagnosed
- Gynecology if pregnancy or female pelvic anatomy is involved

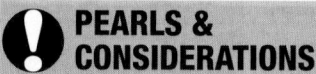

PEARLS & CONSIDERATIONS

COMMENTS

- Hydronephrosis is not a primary disorder; an underlying etiology must be sought.
- Children often have congenital causes; adults usually have acquired intrinsic or extrinsic causes.
- There are obstructive and nonobstructive causes of hydronephrosis. Further evaluation can be diagnosed without specialty consultation by a diuretic renogram, CT urogram, or MR urogram.
- Prompt renal decompression is paramount when hydronephrosis is associated with infection, severe kidney injury, and/or severe electrolyte abnormalities.

PREVENTION

Timely and appropriate management of acute kidney obstruction prevents long-term kidney damage. Hydronephrosis may persist after relief of the obstructing cause.

SUGGESTED READINGS

Available at www.expertconsult.com

RELATED CONTENT

Hydronephrosis (Patient Information)

AUTHORS: **NAVEEN KACHROO, M.D., PH.D.,** and **DAVID A. LEAVITT, M.D.**

BASIC INFORMATION

DEFINITION

Hypercholesterolemia refers to a blood cholesterol measurement ≥200 mg/dl.

SYNONYMS

Hypercholesteremia
Dyslipidemia
Type II familial hyperlipoproteinemia

ICD-10CM CODES
E78.0 Pure hypercholesterolemia

EPIDEMIOLOGY & DEMOGRAPHICS

- Over 105 million (37%) adults in the U.S. have total blood cholesterol levels higher than 200 mg/dl. Of this group, more than 36 million adults have extremely high-risk cholesterol levels over 240 mg/dl (13%).
- For men over the age of 20 years, approximately 48% of white men, 45% of black men, and 50% of Hispanic men have high blood cholesterol.
- For women over the age of 20, approximately 50% of white women, 42% of black women, and 50% of Hispanic women have hypercholesterolemia.
- Prevalence of hypercholesterolemia increases with increasing age.
- According to NHANES data for 2009-2010, about 47% of adults had at least one of three risk factors for cardiovascular disease—uncontrolled high blood pressure, uncontrolled high levels of low-density lipoproteins (LDL) cholesterol, or current smoking.

PHYSICAL FINDINGS & CLINICAL PRESENTATION

- A detailed medication history should be performed because some medications may affect lipid levels (e.g., thiazides, corticosteroids, beta-blockers, and estrogens).
- The physical examination should include measurements of BMI and BP, thyroid and liver assessments, and examining peripheral pulses including carotids for bruits.
- Physical findings, particularly in the familial forms may include
  1. Tendon xanthomas
  2. Xanthelasma
  3. Arcus corneae
  4. Arterial bruits (young adulthood)

ETIOLOGY

Primary:
- Genetics
- Obesity
- Dietary intake
Secondary:
- Hypothyroidism
- Diabetes mellitus
- Nephrotic syndrome
- Obstructive liver disease: Hepatoma, extrahepatic biliary obstruction, primary biliary cirrhosis
- Alcohol or tobacco use
- Dysgammaglobulinemia (multiple myeloma, SLE)
- Drugs: Oral contraceptives, progesterone, corticosteroids, thiazide diuretics, β-blockers, androgenic steroids, retinoic acid derivatives, protease inhibitors

DIAGNOSIS

DIFFERENTIAL DIAGNOSIS

- Always consider underlying secondary causes for the elevated cholesterol.
- Patients with very high LDL cholesterol usually have genetic forms of hypercholesterolemia (see "Hyperlipoproteinemia, Primary"). Early detection of these cases and family testing to identify similarly affected relatives is important.
- Metabolic syndrome:
  1. A constellation of lipid and nonlipid risk factors of a metabolic origin
  2. Diagnosed when three or more of the following are present: abdominal obesity (waist circumference >40 in in men and >35 in in women); fasting triglycerides >150 mg/dl; HDL <40 mg/dl in males and <50 mg/dl in females; systolic BP >130 mmHg and diastolic BP >85 mmHg; fasting glucose >110 mg/dl

WHO SHOULD BE SCREENED:

- AACE recommends screening of patients >20 yr of age for elevated cholesterol every 5 yr, males >45 yr and females >55 yr of age every 1-2 yr, and >65 yr of age every yr up to 75 yr of age regardless of CAD risk status. Patients above 75 yr of age with multiple CAD risk factors should still continue to get screened annually.
- The USPSTF supports routine screening for men aged >35 yr and women aged >45 yr by measurement of nonfasting total and HDL cholesterol alone.
- In 2010, the USPSTF recommended routine screening for overweight and obesity in persons aged <20 yr.
- In 2011, ACC/AHA recommended screening for hypertriglyceridemia by a nonfasting measurement. A nonfasting level of <200 mg/dl is commensurate with an optimal level of <100 mg/dl and no further testing is required. However, a nonfasting level of >200 mg/dl warrants further testing with a fasting lipid profile.

LABORATORY TESTS

- Obtain a fasting lipid profile.
- Perform a workup for secondary causes if clinically indicated such as TSH, metabolic profile, LFTs, and fasting glucose.

TREATMENT

NONPHARMACOLOGIC THERAPY

- First line of treatment: dietary therapy can result in 5% to 15% reduction in LDL cholesterol level.
- Composition of the **TLC diet:**
  1. Total fat 25% to 30% of total calories
  2. Polyunsaturated fat up to 10% of total calories
  3. Monounsaturated fat up to 20% of total calories

TABLE 1 Risk Factors for Heart Disease

1. Cigarette smoking
2. Hypertension (BP ≤140/90 mm Hg or on medications)
3. Low HDL cholesterol (<40 mg/dl)*
4. Family history of premature CHD (<55 yr in first-degree male relative or <65 yr in first-degree female relative)
5. Age (men ≥45 yr, women ≥55 yr)

*HDL cholesterol >60 mg/dl counts as a negative risk factor; its presence removes one risk factor from the total count.

4. Saturated fats <7% of total calories
5. Carbohydrate 50% to 60% of total calories
6. Protein 15% of total calories
7. No more than 200 mg/day of cholesterol
8. Fiber 20 to 30 g/day

- Increased physical activity: encourage 30 min of moderately intense physical activity, four to six times a week (e.g., brisk walking, riding stationary bike, water aerobics)
- Maintenance of a healthy weight
- Avoidance of tobacco products
- Counseling on CAD risk factors (Table 1)
- Plant-based diets (including stanol-containing margarines, oat bran, and nuts) have shown effectiveness in controlling lipids.

ACUTE GENERAL Rx

No acute treatment needed

CHRONIC Rx

- Box 1 summarizes the key recommendations for the treatment of blood cholesterol to reduce ASCVD (atherosclerotic cardiovascular disease) risk in adults.
- The current guidelines represent a substantial departure from previous recommendations, which were based on LDL levels.
- The new guidelines identify four high-risk groups that benefit from statin therapy:
- Patients with clinical ASCVD (Table 2)
  LDL ≥190 mg/dl
  DM aged 40-75 years and LDL 70-189 mg/dl
  Ten-year risk for ASCVD ≥7.5% and LDL 70-189 mg/dl
- The 10-year risk of ASCVD is calculated with the risk calculator available at http://my.americanheart.org/cvriskcalculator
- ASCVD events are reduced by using the maximum tolerated statin intensity in the above groups shown to benefit the most (Tables 3 and 4).
- Additional factors such as CRP >2 mg/L, primary LDL >160, genetic hyperlipidemias, family history of premature CHD, ABI <0.9, and CAD score >300 Agatston units may be used in patients who are not in one of four statin benefit groups and for whom a decision to initiate statin therapy is otherwise unclear.
- Percent reduction in LDL cholesterol is used as a guide to compliance and adherence to therapy but is not considered a treatment goal.
- Moderate-intensity statin therapy should be continued for individuals >75 years of age for secondary prevention. However, factors such

BOX 1   2013 ACC/AHA Summary of Key Recommendations for the Treatment of Blood Cholesterol to Reduce ASCVD Risk in Adults

A. Heart-healthy lifestyle habits should be encouraged for all individuals.
B. The appropriate intensity of statin therapy should be initiated or continued:
  1. Clinical ASCVD*
    a. Age 75 years or less and no safety concerns: high-intensity statin (class I, level A)
    b. Age 75 years or safety concerns: moderate-intensity statin (class I, level A)
  2. Primary prevention: primary LDL-C 190 mg/dl or greater
    a. Rule out secondary causes of hyperlipidemia (class I, level B)
    b. Age 21 years or older: high-intensity statin (class I, level B)
    c. Achieve at least a 50% reduction in LDL-C (class IIa, level B)
    d. LDL-C lowering nonstatin therapy may be considered to further reduce LDL-C (class IIb, level C)
  3. Primary prevention: diabetes 40 to 75 years of age and LDL-C 70 to 189 mg/dl
    a. Moderate-intensity statin (class I, level A)
    b. Consider high-intensity statin when 7.5% or greater 10-year ASCVD risk using the Pooled Cohort Equations† (class IIa, level B)
  4. Primary prevention: no diabetes 40 to 75 years of age and LDL-C 70 to 189 mg/dl
    a. Estimate 10-year ASCVD risk using the Risk Calculator based on the Pooled Cohort Equations† in those *not* receiving a statin; estimate risk every 4 to 6 years (class I, level B)
    b. To determine whether to initiate a statin, engage in a clinician-patient discussion of the potential for ASCVD risk reduction, adverse effects, drug-drug interactions, and patient preferences
    c. Reemphasize heart-healthy lifestyle habits and address other risk factors (class IIa, level C)
      i. 7.5% or greater 10-year ASCVD risk: moderate- or high-intensity statin (class I, level A)
      ii. 5% to 7.5% 10-year ASCVD risk: consider moderate-intensity statin (class IIa, level B)
      iii. Other factors may be considered‡: LDL-C 160 mg/dl or greater, family history of premature ASCVD, hs-CRP 2.0 mg/L or greater, CAC score 300 Agatston units or greater, ABI less than 0.9, or lifetime ASCVD risk (class IIb, level C)
  5. Primary prevention when LDL-C is less than 190 mg/dl and age is less than 40 or more than 75 years, or less than 5% 10-year ASCVD risk
    a. Statin therapy may be considered in selected individuals‡ (class IIb, level C)
  6. Statin therapy is not routinely recommended for individuals with NYHA class II-IV heart failure or who are receiving maintenance hemodialysis
C. Regularly monitor adherence to lifestyle and drug therapy with lipid and safety assessments
  1. Assess adherence, response to therapy, and adverse effects within 4 to 12 weeks following statin initiation or change in therapy (class I, level A)
    a. Measure a fasting lipid panel (class I, level A)
    b. Do not routinely monitor ALT or CK unless symptomatic (class IIa, level C)
    c. Screen and treat type 2 diabetes according to current practice guidelines. Heart-healthy lifestyle habits should be encouraged to prevent progression to diabetes (class I, level B)
    d. Anticipated therapeutic response: approximately 50% or greater reduction in LDL-C from baseline for high-intensity statin and 30% to 50% for moderate-intensity statin (class IIa, level B)
      i. Insufficient evidence for LDL-C or non–HDL-C treatment targets from RCTs
      ii. For those with unknown baseline LDL-C, an LDL-C less than 100 mg/dl was observed in RCTs of high-intensity statin therapy
    e. Less than anticipated therapeutic response:
      i. Reinforce improved adherence to lifestyle and drug therapy (class I, level A)
      ii. Evaluate for secondary causes of hyperlipidemia if indicated (class I, level A)
      iii. Increase statin intensity, or if on maximally tolerated statin intensity, consider addition of nonstatin therapy in selected high-risk individuals§ (class IIb, level C)
    f. Regularly monitor adherence to lifestyle and drug therapy every 3 to 12 months once adherence has been established. Continue assessment of adherence for optimal ASCVD risk reduction and safety (class I, level A)
D. In individuals intolerant of the recommended intensity of statin therapy, use the maximally tolerated intensity of statin (class I, level B)
  If there are muscle or other symptoms, establish that they are related to the statin (class IIa, level B)

ABI, ankle-brachial index; *ACC*, American College of Cardiology; *AHA*, American Heart Association; *ALT*, alanine aminotransferase, a test of hepatic function; *ASCVD*, atherosclerotic cardiovascular disease; *CAC*, coronary artery calcium; *CHD*, coronary heart disease; *CK*, creatine kinase, a test of muscle injury; *HDL-C*, high-density lipoprotein cholesterol; *hs-CRP*, high-sensitivity C-reactive protein; *LDL-C*, low-density lipoprotein cholesterol; *NHLBI*, National Heart, Lung, and Blood Institute; *NYHA*, New York Heart Association; *RCTs*, randomized controlled trials; and *TIA*, transient ischemic attack.

* Clinical ASCVD includes acute coronary syndromes, history of MI, stable or unstable angina, coronary or other arterial revascularization, stroke, TIA, or peripheral arterial disease presumed to be of atherosclerotic origin.

† Estimated 10-year or "hard" ASCVD risk includes first occurrence of nonfatal MI, CHD death, and nonfatal and fatal stroke as used by the Risk Assessment Work Group in developing the Pooled Cohort Equations on the basis of age, sex, smoking status, total cholesterol level, HDL-C level, systolic blood pressure, and the use of antihypertensive therapy.

‡ These factors may include primary LDL-C of 160 mg/dl or greater or other evidence of genetic hyperlipidemias; family history of premature ASCVD with onset at less than 55 years of age in a first-degree male relative or at less than 65 years of age in a first-degree female relative; hs-CRP 2 mg/L or greater; CAC score 300 Agatston units or greater or 75th percentile or greater for age, sex, and ethnicity; ABI less than 0.9; or lifetime risk of ASCVD. Additional factors that might aid in individual risk assessment could be identified in the future.

§ High-risk individuals include those with clinical ASCVD, an untreated LDL-C 190 mg/dl or greater, suggesting genetic hypercholesterolemia, or individuals with diabetes 40 to 75 years of age and LDL-C 70 to 189 mg/dl.

From 2013 ACC/AHA guideline on the treatment of blood cholesterol to reduce atherosclerotic cardiovascular risk in adults: a report of the American College of Cardiology/American Heart Association Task Force on Practice Guidelines, *J Am Coll Cardiol* 63(25 Pt B):2889-2934, 2014.

- as comorbidities, safety, and priorities of care should be considered before initiating statins for primary prevention of ASCVD.
- Adherence to lifestyle and to statin therapy should be reiterated with patients before the addition of a nonstatin drug.
- Nonstatin therapies do not provide acceptable ASCVD risk reduction benefits compared with their potential adverse effects in ASCVD prevention. (Table 5) summarizes oral drugs affecting lipoprotein metabolism.
- PCSK9 (proprotein convertase subtilisin/kexin type 9) inhibitors (alirocumab [Praluent], evolocumab [Repatha]) are indicated as adjunct to diet and maximally tolerated statin therapy for the treatment of adults with heterozygous familial hypercholesterolemia or clinical atherosclerotic cardiovascular disease, who require additional lowering of LDL cholesterol. These medications are administered by subcutaneous injection and are expensive.

- High-risk patients with a suboptimal response to statins who are unable to tolerate a recommended intensity or who are completely statin intolerant may benefit from the addition of a nonstatin cholesterol-lowering agent.
- The management of metabolic syndrome includes weight reduction, increased physical activity, and treatment of hypertension, elevated triglycerides, and low HDL cholesterol.
- According to recent studies, each 40 mg/dl reduction in LDL cholesterol by statin therapy confers a 20% reduction in ASCVD. In other words, a relative risk reduction of 30% in ASCVD by moderate-intensity therapy and 45% by high-intensity therapy has been approximated.

DISPOSITION AND FOLLOW-UP

- Baseline LFT testing should be done before initiation of statin therapy and as clinically indicated thereafter.
- CK level monitoring is not recommended unless a patient reports muscle weakness or myalgias.
- Statin therapy should be monitored by repeating a lipid profile within 4 to 12 weeks after initiation of therapy.
- Counseling about behavioral lifestyle changes and risk factors for CHD should be provided at every follow-up visit.
- Adverse effects of statin-associated diabetes varies by statin intensity: 1 excess case of diabetes per 1000 treated individuals

with moderate-intensity statin and 3 excess cases of diabetes per 1000 treated individuals with high-intensity statin per year has been reported. Myopathy and hemorrhagic stroke incidence is around 1 excess case per 10,000 treated individuals.
- Per new guidelines, those who develop diabetes during statin therapy should be advised to continue it to reduce their risk of ASCVD events and should adhere to a heart-healthy diet, engage in physical activity, cease tobacco use, and maintain a healthy body weight (Table E5).

REFERRAL

Patients with rare lipid disorders, hyperlipoproteinemias, patients resistant to treatment, on complex regimens, and with evidence of disease progression despite treatment should be referred to a lipid specialist.

❗ PEARLS & CONSIDERATIONS

COMMENTS

- Familial hypercholesterolemia (FH) is characterized by elevated cholesterol concentrations early in life. Untreated FH is associated with premature cardiovascular disease in adulthood. Screening can detect FH in children, and lipid-lowering treatment in childhood can reduce lipid concentrations in the short term, with little evidence of harm.
- The American Academy of Pediatrics (AAP) guideline (*Pediatrics* 122:198, 2008) recommends consideration toward pharmacologic treatment for children with LDL >190 mg/dl or >160 mg/dl if other risk factors are present.
- *HDL cholesterol efflux capacity* refers to the ability of HDL to accept cholesterol from macrophages, which is a key step in reverse cholesterol transport. It is inversely associated with the incidence of cardiovascular events and may be a useful biomarker when added to traditional risk factors.

TABLE 2 Atherosclerotic Cardiovascular Disease

1. Coronary heart disease: acute coronary syndromes, history of myocardial infarction, stable or unstable angina, coronary or other arterial revascularization
2. Stroke or transient ischemic attack
3. Peripheral arterial disease

TABLE 3 Statin Intensity Therapies

High Intensity (Decrease LDL-C ≥50%)	Moderate Intensity (Decrease LDL-C 30%-49%)
Atorvastatin 40-80 mg	Atorvastatin 10-20 mg
Rosuvastatin 20-40 mg	Rosuvastatin 5-10 mg
—	Simvastatin 20-40 mg
—	Pravastatin 40-80 mg
—	Lovastatin 40 mg
—	Fluvastatin XL 80 mg
—	Fluvastatin 40 mg bid
—	Pitavastatin 2-4 mg

LDL-C, Low-density lipoprotein cholesterol.
From Stone N et al: 2013 ACC/AHA guideline on the treatment of blood cholesterol to reduce atherosclerotic cardiovascular risk in adults: a report of the American College of Cardiology/American Heart Association Task Force on Practice Guidelines, *J Am Coll Cardiol* 63(25 Pt. B):2889, 2014.

TABLE 4 Statin Benefit Groups and Recommended Therapy

Statin Benefit Group	High Intensity	Moderate Intensity	Additional Testing
Clinical ASCVD	Yes	Consider[†]	None
Primary LDL-C >190 mg/dl	Yes	Consider[†]	None
Diabetes without ASCVD and 10-year risk ≥7.5%*	Yes	Consider[†]	None
Diabetes without ASCVD and 10-year risk <7.5%*	Consider[‡]	Yes	Case-by-case
Primary prevention and 10-year risk ≥7.5%*	Consider[‡]	Yes	Case-by-case
Primary prevention and 10-year risk <7.5%*	Consider[‡]	Consider[‡]	Case-by-case

ASCVD, Atherosclerotic cardiovascular disease; LDL-C, low-density lipoprotein cholesterol.
*Based on Pooled Cohort Risk Equations.
[†]If age >75 years or not candidate for high intensity.
[‡]If abnormal high-sensitivity C-reactive protein, coronary artery calcium, ankle-brachial index, lifetime risk.
From Boyden TF et al: Implementing new guidelines in the management of blood cholesterol, *Am J Med* 127:705, 2014.

EBM EVIDENCE

Available at www.expertconsult.com

SUGGESTED READINGS

Available at www.expertconsult.com

RELATED CONTENT

High Cholesterol (Patient Information)
Hyperlipoproteinemia, Primary (Related Key Topic)
Statin Induced Muscle Syndrome (Related Key Topic)

AUTHORS: **PRIYA BANSAL, M.D., M.P.H.,** and **FRED F. FERRI, M.D.**

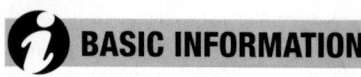

BASIC INFORMATION

DEFINITION

Hypercoagulable state is an inherited or acquired condition associated with an increased risk of thrombosis.

SYNONYMS

Thrombophilia

ICD-10CM CODES
D68.5 Primary thrombophilia
D68.6 Other thrombophilia
D68.8 Other specified coagulation defects
D68.9 Coagulation defect, unspecified

EPIDEMIOLOGY & DEMOGRAPHICS

INCIDENCE: See Table 1.
PREVALENCE, PREDOMINANT SEX, AND AGE:
Significant variations in the prevalence rates and thrombotic risks for thrombophilia are reported. This may reflect geographic variation in the prevalence of genetic defects, different populations, or the presence of other unidentified thrombophilic risk factors. When thrombosis occurs, it is often associated with an acquired risk factor (e.g., surgery, pregnancy, oral contraceptive [OC] use).
GENETICS:
- Most people with a genetic defect will not have thrombotic disease.
- Multiple genetic defects are not uncommon (1% to 2% prevalence in patients with idiopathic venous thromboembolism [VTE]); a strong synergistic effect occurs when multiple defects are present. Low risk of recurrent thrombosis in patients with a single genetic defect. Approximately half of patients with unprovoked thrombosis have an identifiable inherited thrombophilia.
RISK FACTORS: Family history of thrombosis, increasing age, tobacco use, immobility, surgery, prior history of DVT, pregnancy, hormone replacement therapy, trauma, connective tissue disease, underlying malignancy, medications (megestrol acetate, tamoxifen, oral contraceptives)

PHYSICAL FINDINGS & CLINICAL PRESENTATION

- Inherited thrombophilia is usually associated with VTE, most commonly deep vein thrombosis (DVT)

- Some acquired thrombophilias are associated with arterial thrombosis. Table E2 describes sites of thrombosis according to coagulation defect.
- Pregnancy complications
- Medical conditions associated with increased risk of thrombosis

ETIOLOGY

See Table 3. The differential diagnosis of the patient presenting with thrombosis or thrombotic diathesis is described in Section II. Fig. E1 describes components of thrombus formation and actions of various antithrombotic and thrombolytic agents.
- Thrombosis is often a multifactorial process with genetic, environmental, and acquired factors. Table 4 describes causes of acquired deficiencies in antithrombin, protein S, or protein C.
- Thrombotic risk increases with use of OCs or hormone replacement therapy (HRT) and during the pregnancy/postpartum period.
- Adverse pregnancy outcomes may be caused by thrombosis of the uteroplacental circulation.

DIAGNOSIS

DIFFERENTIAL DIAGNOSIS

INHERITED: Factor V Leiden (FVL) mutation:
- Autosomal-dominant mutation with low penetrance.
- Causes activated protein C resistance (APCR); 90% of APCR is caused by FVL mutation.
- Most common inherited thrombophilia; accounts for 40% to 50% of cases.
- OC use in heterozygous carriers is associated with an eightfold increased risk of VTE compared with noncarriers and a thirty-fivefold increased risk of VTE compared with noncarriers not using OCs.
- May be associated with cardiovascular disease in select high-risk subgroups.
Prothrombin G20210A mutation:
- Autosomal-dominant mutation with low penetrance.
- OC use in heterozygous carriers is associated with a sixteenfold increased risk of VTE compared with noncarriers not using OCs.
- May be associated with cardiovascular disease in select high-risk subgroups and young patients with ischemic stroke.

- Causes increased mRNA accumulation and protein synthesis, leading to elevated prothrombin plasma concentrations.
Protein C, protein S, antithrombin (AT) deficiency:
- Autosomal-dominant inheritance; many mutations identified for each of these conditions.
- Decreased level (type I deficiency) or abnormal function (type II deficiency).
- First episode of thrombosis is usually in young adults.
Protein C and protein S:
- Homozygous condition is very rare; usually associated with lethal thrombosis in infancy.
- Associated with warfarin-induced skin necrosis, which occurs secondary to depletion of

TABLE 3 Potential Prothrombotic States

Congenital

Deficiency of anticoagulants
AT-III, protein C or protein S, plasminogen
Resistance to cofactor proteolysis
Factor V Leiden
High levels of procoagulants
Prothrombin 20210 mutation
Damage to endothelium

Acquired

Obstruction to flow
Indwelling lines
Pregnancy
Polycythemia/dehydration
Immobilization
Injury
Trauma, surgery, exercise
Inflammation
IBD, vasculitis, infection, Behçet's syndrome
Hypercoagulability
Pregnancy
Malignancy
Antiphospholipid syndrome
Nephrotic syndrome
Oral contraceptives
L-Asparaginase

Rare Other Entities

Congenital
Dysfibrinogenemia
Acquired
Paroxysmal nocturnal hemoglobinuria
Thrombocythemia
Vascular grafts

AT-III, Antithrombin III; *IBD,* inflammatory bowel disease.
From Kliegman RM et al: *Nelson textbook of pediatrics,* ed 19, Philadelphia, 2011, Saunders.

TABLE 1 Hypercoagulable Conditions

	Prevalence in General Population (%)	Prevalence in Population with Thrombosis (%)	A/V Events	Relative Risk of Thrombosis
FVL mutation	5% of whites; rare in nonwhites	12-40%	V	Heterozygous: 3-7; homozygous: 80
Prothrombin G20210A mutation	3% of whites; rare in nonwhites	6-18%	V	3
AT deficiency	0.02%	1-3%	V	20-50
PC deficiency	0.2-0.4%	3-5%	V	7-15
PS deficiency	0.03-0.1%	1-5%	V	5-11
Antiphospholipid antibody syndrome	1-2%	5-21%	V + A	2-11

A, Arterial; *AT,* antithrombin; *FVL,* factor V Leiden; *PC,* protein C; *PS,* protein S; *V,* venous.

TABLE 4 Causes of Acquired Deficiencies in Antithrombin III, Protein C, or Protein S

Antithrombin III	Protein C	Protein S
Neonatal period	Neonatal period	Neonatal period
Pregnancy	Liver disease	Pregnancy
Liver disease	DIC	Liver disease
DIC	Chemotherapy (CMF)	DIC
Nephrotic syndrome	Acute thrombosis	Inflammatory states
Major surgery		Acute thrombosis
Acute thrombosis		
Treatment with:		
Heparin	Warfarin	Warfarin
L-Asparaginase	L-Asparaginase	L-Asparaginase
Estrogens		Estrogens

CMF, Cyclophosphamide, methotrexate, 5-fluorouracil; *DIC,* disseminated intravascular coagulation.
From Hoffman R et al: *Hematology, basic principles and practice,* ed 5, Philadelphia, 2009, Churchill Livingstone.

vitamin K–dependent anticoagulant factors sooner than procoagulant factors in the first few days of therapy.
AT deficiency:
- Most thrombogenic of the inherited thrombophilias; 50% lifetime risk of thrombosis.
- Homozygous condition is very rare, probably not compatible with normal fetal development.
- Arterial thrombosis can occur rarely.
- Can cause heparin resistance.
Elevated factor VIII level:
- May be an important risk factor for thrombosis in African-American population.
- Increased risk of recurrent thrombosis.
- Genetic etiology is suspected but not yet identified.
Other possible causes: Non-O blood group, dysfibrinogenemia, elevated thrombin-activatable fibrinolysis inhibitor, elevated factor IX and factor XI levels
ACQUIRED: Antiphospholipid antibody syndrome (APS):
- Most common cause of acquired thrombophilia.
- Can present as arterial or venous thrombosis, recurrent pregnancy loss, and adverse pregnancy outcomes.
- Thromboembolic events occur in up to 30% of population; high risk of recurrent thrombosis (up to 70% reported).
- See "Antiphospholipid Antibody Syndrome" for more information.
Conditions associated with increased risk of thrombosis:
- Prior thrombosis
- Trauma
- Medical illness: heart failure, respiratory failure, infection, diabetes mellitus, obesity, nephrotic syndrome, inflammatory bowel disease
- Chronic hemolysis–paroxysmal nocturnal hemoglobinuria, atypical hemolytic uremic syndrome, sickle cell anemia
- Pregnancy (sixfold increased risk of VTE), postpartum, OC use (fourfold increased risk, higher risk with third-generation OCs), transdermal contraceptive patch, HRT (twofold increased risk), tamoxifen, raloxifene

- Immobilization, travel
- Surgery (especially orthopedic), central venous catheters
- Hyperviscosity syndromes
- Myeloproliferative disorders
- Malignancy: disease or treatment related
- Heparin-induced thrombocytopenia and thrombosis
- Smoking

WORKUP
- History (presence of conditions or use of medications predisposing to thrombosis, family history of thrombosis), physical examination, laboratory tests, imaging studies.
- Age-appropriate cancer screening.
- No consensus exists regarding screening for thrombophilia; few cost-effectiveness or outcomes data are available. Screening laboratory evaluation for patients suspected of having a biologic defect predisposing to thrombosis is described in Box E1. Thrombophilia screening is probably overused, as results usually don't change management.
- Thrombophilia screening is not recommended for primary prevention of VTE; some advocate testing prior to OC use or pregnancy in women with a strong family history of thrombosis or thrombophilia.
- Screening not recommended if VTE was associated with an identified risk factor. A possible exception is thrombosis associated with pregnancy, the postpartum period, or with OC use.
- Unprovoked VTE:
  1. Screen individuals for APCR, prothrombin G20210A mutation, protein C, protein S, AT deficiency, and APS if any of the following are present: <50 yr of age at first episode of thrombosis, family history of thrombosis, recurrent thrombosis, thrombosis in unusual anatomic location, life-threatening thrombotic event, warfarin-induced skin necrosis or thrombosis in pregnancy/postpartum
  2. Screen all others for APS.
- Arterial thrombosis: Screen for APS.
- Note: Routine screening for factor VIII level or hyperhomocysteinemia is not recommended.

TIMING OF WORKUP:
- Ideally >3 wk after discontinuation of anticoagulation (except for APS, which requires prolonged anticoagulation).
- Note: Acute thrombosis, anticoagulation, pregnancy, and many medical conditions can affect the results and must be considered in the timing and interpretation of the workup.

LABORATORY TESTS
- CBC with peripheral smear, electrolytes, calcium, creatinine, BUN and liver function tests, prothrombin time/partial thromboplastin time, prostate-specific antigen (in men aged >50 years), urinalysis.
- Note: Genetic counseling and written informed consent should be obtained before genetic testing. Abnormal nongenetic tests should be repeated after 6 wk to decrease false-positive results.
- APCR: APC-resistance assay (using factor V–deficient plasma). Presence of lupus anticoagulant causes false positives. Follow-up positive APCR assay with genetic test for FVL.
- Prothrombin G20210A mutation testing.
- AT, protein C, and protein S deficiency: functional assays; if decreased perform antigenic assay to determine type of deficiency. Antigenic assays for protein S should measure free and total levels. In protein C and protein S deficiency, the functional assay may be falsely low in the presence of APCR or elevated factor VIII level and falsely high if lupus anticoagulant is present.
- APS: any one of the following found on two occasions at least 12 weeks apart: lupus anticoagulant, anticardiolipin antibodies, or anti–B$_2$-glycoprotein-I antibodies.

IMAGING STUDIES
Chest radiograph and other tests as appropriate to diagnose thrombosis and rule out associated conditions

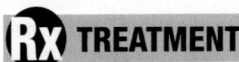 **TREATMENT**

NONPHARMACOLOGIC THERAPY
OC/HRT use and smoking should be avoided.

PROPHYLAXIS
- Prophylactic anticoagulation in high-risk situations.
- Patients with AT deficiency may benefit from antithrombin concentrates in high-risk situations.
- Pregnancy prophylaxis: timing and intensity of therapy is based on the patient's risk (genetic or acquired defect and clinical history). Women with thrombophilia and recurrent adverse pregnancy outcomes may benefit from prophylaxis with heparin (low-molecular-weight heparin most commonly used) and low-dose aspirin.

ACUTE GENERAL Rx
Initial therapy is the same as for individuals with and without thrombophilia, with exceptions for

protein C and AT deficiency as detailed in the following.

Venous thrombosis:
- Begin low-molecular-weight heparin (LMWH) and warfarin simultaneously. Continue heparin for at least 5 days and until international normalized ratio (INR) is therapeutic for 2 consecutive days; continue warfarin for at least 3 months. Aim for INR of 2 to 3. Unfractionated heparin (UH) or fondaparinux (factor Xa inhibitor) may be used as alternatives to LMWH. LMWH is preferred over UH (except in patients with massive pulmonary embolism, increased risk of bleeding or renal failure) because of equivalent or superior effectiveness and a better safety profile.
- Direct oral anticoagulants (DOACs) such as direct thrombin inhibitor (dabigatran) and the direct Xa inhibitors (rivaroxaban, edoxaban, apixaban) have been FDA approved for treatment in acute DVT. They have been found to be noninferior to warfarin, appear easier to use with fewer drug interactions, and have a trend toward less major bleeding. Prothrombin concentrates (three-factor or four-factor concentrates) are currently utilized in instances of bleeding associated with DOACs. Andexanet alpha is a recombinant protein effective against Xa inhibitors that is undergoing phase III clinical testing.
- Thrombophilia is not associated with a higher risk of recurrent VTE during warfarin therapy, with the exception of cancer patients in whom LMWH for 3 to 6 mo is associated with lower rates of recurrence than warfarin therapy.
- In pregnancy, anticoagulate with heparin throughout pregnancy and for at least 6 wk postpartum. Minimum duration of anticoagulation should be 6 mo. LMWH is preferred over UH. Warfarin may be used postpartum.
- Consider thrombolysis or thrombectomy in patients with massive pulmonary embolism or large proximal lower extremity DVT.

Protein C deficiency:
- Warfarin-induced skin necrosis: Discontinue warfarin, give vitamin K, and start heparin anticoagulation. Consider protein C replacement with protein C concentrate or fresh frozen plasma. Warfarin may be restarted at a low dose (2 mg daily for 3 days and increase by 2 to 3 mg daily until target INR is reached). Continue heparin for at least 5 days and until warfarin-induced anticoagulation is achieved.

AT deficiency:
- AT concentrates may be used if difficulty achieving anticoagulation (heparin resistance), severe thrombosis, or recurrent thrombosis despite adequate anticoagulation.

Arterial thrombosis:
- Anticoagulation and evaluation for thrombolysis or surgery.

CHRONIC Rx

- Optimal duration of anticoagulation remains unknown. Length of therapy may be individualized by assessing the risk of recurrence. Residual thrombosis (on ultrasonography) or elevated D-dimer levels after completion of anticoagulation are associated with an increased risk of recurrence. With these findings, consider prolonging anticoagulation.
- Must consider risk and benefit; risk of major bleeding 2% to 3% annually in general population on anticoagulation but higher in the elderly (7% to 9% per year). Long-term anticoagulation is usually not indicated given the low risk of recurrent thrombosis for most conditions and the bleeding risk associated with anticoagulation.
- Indefinite anticoagulation considered if ≥2 spontaneous thromboses or spontaneous thrombosis associated with any of the following:
  1. Life-threatening thrombosis or thrombosis at an unusual site
  2. More than a single genetic defect
  3. Presence of AT deficiency or APS
- Patients with active cancer may benefit from indefinite anticoagulation.

DISPOSITION

Depends on underlying condition

REFERRAL

Hematology, maternal-fetal medicine, obstetric medicine

(!) PEARLS & CONSIDERATIONS

COMMENTS

- Warfarin therapy effectively reduces the risk of recurrent VTE; when therapy is discontinued VTE risk increases.
- Previous episode of VTE is a major risk factor for recurrence regardless of the presence of thrombophilia. Risk is greatest in the first 2 yr after thrombosis. 20% of all patients with unprovoked VTE have recurrence within 5 yr.
- Genetic risk factors for thrombosis in nonwhites remain largely unknown.
- Interpreting workup: many medical conditions cause acquired abnormalities.
  1. Acute thrombosis may be associated with lupus anticoagulant, increased anticardiolipin antibodies, and elevated factor VIII levels

  2. Heparin therapy: antithrombin levels decrease by up to 30%; can affect lupus anticoagulant testing
  3. Warfarin therapy: cannot measure protein C and protein S (levels and function decrease); antithrombin levels may increase; can affect lupus anticoagulant testing
  4. Protein C, protein S, and antithrombin levels decrease with acute thrombosis (<2 wk), surgery, liver disease, disseminated intravascular coagulation, and chemotherapy. Protein C level also decreases with severe infection but levels increase with age and hyperlipidemia. Protein S and antithrombin levels also decrease with nephrotic syndrome, pregnancy, and estrogen therapy (HRT, OC).
  5. APCR is increased with pregnancy, estrogen therapy (HRT, OCs), and certain cancers; elevated factor VIII level and antiphospholipid antibodies can cause APCR

PREVENTION

Risk of post-thrombotic syndrome decreases if compression stockings are worn for at least 1 year, starting in the first month after the DVT.

PATIENT & FAMILY EDUCATION

National Blood Clot Alliance
120 White Plains Road, Suite 100
Tarrytown, NY 10591
http://www.stoptheclot.org/contact.htm

National Collaborative Outreach Project of the Blood Clot Outreach Program at the Hemophilia and Thrombosis Center University of North Carolina at Chapel Hill
http://www.clotconnect.org/about-clot-connect/about

Factor V Leiden Resources
http://www.fvleiden.org/resources/index.html

APS Foundation of America, Inc.
P. O. Box 801
LaCrosse, WI 54602-0801
http://www.apsfa.org/

SUGGESTED READINGS

Available at www.expertconsult.com

RELATED CONTENT

Thrombophilia (Patient Information)
Antiphospholipid Syndrome (Related Key Topic)
Deep Vein Thrombosis (Related Key Topic)
Pulmonary Embolism (Related Key Topic)

AUTHOR: **JOHN L. REAGAN, M.D.**

BASIC INFORMATION

DEFINITION

Hyperemesis gravidarum is a severe and persistent form of nausea and vomiting resulting in at least a 5% weight loss, dehydration, ketonuria, and electrolyte imbalance, with typical onset at 4 to 8 wk of pregnancy continuing through 14 to 16 wk of pregnancy.

ICD-10CM CODES
O21.0 Mild hyperemesis gravidarum
O21.1 Hyperemesis gravidarum with metabolic disturbance

EPIDEMIOLOGY & DEMOGRAPHICS

INCIDENCE: 0.5% to 2% of pregnancies
GENETICS: No genetic disposition
RISK FACTORS: Women with increased placental mass, including molar pregnancy or multiple gestation, family history or personal history of hyperemesis gravidarum, prior miscarriage, nulliparity, preexisting diabetes, hyperthyroid disorder, peptic ulceration or other gastrointestinal disorders, depression, and asthma. Female fetus increases the risk by 1.5-fold.

PHYSICAL FINDINGS & CLINICAL PRESENTATION

- Weight loss of more than 5% from pregravid weight
- Symptoms—nausea, vomiting, spitting, enhanced olfactory senses, food and/or fluid intolerance, lethargy
- Signs—dehydration, poor skin turgor, dry mucous membranes, ketonuria, anemia, tachycardia, hypotension
- Complications include inadequate caloric intake, nutritional deficiencies, dehydration, and electrolyte abnormalities including hyponatremia, hypocalcemia, hypokalemia, and in severe cases hypochloremic metabolic acidosis or Wernicke's encephalopathy from thiamine deficiency

ETIOLOGY

Unknown but likely multifactorial. Theories include gestational hyperestrogenemia, gastric dysrhythmias, and hyperthyroidism.

DIAGNOSIS

DIFFERENTIAL DIAGNOSIS

- Gastrointestinal conditions—gastroenteritis, gastroparesis, achalasia, biliary tract disease, hepatitis, intestinal obstruction, peptic ulcer disease, appendicitis
- Genitourinary tract conditions—pyelonephritis, uremia, ovarian torsion, kidney stones, degenerating uterine leiomyoma
- Metabolic disease—diabetic ketoacidosis, porphyria, Addison's disease, hyperthyroidism

- Neurologic conditions—pseudotumor cerebri, vestibular lesions, migraines, tumors of the central nervous system
- Miscellaneous—drug toxicity or intolerance, psychologic
- Pregnancy-related conditions—acute fatty liver of pregnancy, preeclampsia

WORKUP

Diagnosis is one of exclusion. History and physical examination along with laboratory tests to rule out other causes of vomiting should be performed.

LABORATORY TESTS

- Urinalysis may show elevated specific gravity, ketonuria, or proteinuria
- Liver enzymes (elevated but usually <300 U/L)
- Serum bilirubin (<4 mg/dl)
- Serum amylase or lipase (up to 5× greater than normal)
- BMP, may reveal hyponatremia, hypokalemia, low serum urea
- CBC
- Calcium
- TSH and free T4 (transient hyperthyroidism occurs in 2/3 of women with hyperemesis gravidarum; this is biochemical hyperthyroidism that usually resolves by 18 wk gestation; treatment should not be undertaken without evidence of intrinsic thyroid disease)

IMAGING STUDIES

- Ultrasound to evaluate for multiple gestation or molar pregnancy
- Right upper quadrant ultrasound to evaluate for biliary tract disease

TREATMENT

NONPHARMACOLOGIC THERAPY

- Reassurance and support
- Avoidance of foods and smells that trigger nausea
- Oral ginger root
- Small frequent dry meals
- Eating prior to getting out of bed

ACUTE GENERAL Rx

- Nothing by mouth
- Intravenous fluid and electrolyte replacement with vitamin supplementation
- Thiamine administration prior to giving dextrose to avoid Wernicke's encephalopathy
- Pyridoxine (vitamin B$_6$)
- Doxylamine 25 mg qhs
- Antiemetics, including promethazine, phenothiazines, metoclopramide, and ondansetron, have been shown to be generally safe and effective in improving pregnancy outcome
- Restart oral intake gradually no less than 48 hr after vomiting has stopped

CHRONIC Rx

- Nasogastric feedings are useful alternatives in severe cases
- Total parenteral nutrition may be necessary in life-threatening cases

COMPLEMENTARY AND ALTERNATIVE MEDICINE

- Supportive psychotherapy
- Acupuncture
- Acupressure with use of a wrist band

DISPOSITION

- Infants born to pregnancies complicated by hyperemesis are more likely to be premature and small for gestational age.
- Lower rates of miscarriage have also been documented when comparing pregnancies complicated by hyperemesis gravidarum vs. controls.

PEARLS & CONSIDERATIONS

COMMENTS

Nausea and vomiting in early pregnancy are associated with psychosocial morbidity.

PREVENTION

Taking a multivitamin from time of conception

RELATED CONTENT

Hyperemesis Gravidarum (Patient Information)

AUTHORS: **ALISON PATTERSON, M.D.,** and **ANTHONY SCISCIONE, D.O.**

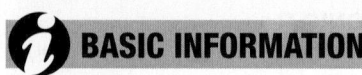

DEFINITION

Hyperglycemic hyperosmolar syndrome (HHS) is a life-threatening complication of diabetes mellitus characterized by marked hyperglycemia, dehydration, and hyperosmolality with or without mental obtundation, in the absence of significant ketoacidosis.

SYNONYMS

HHS
Hyperosmolar hyperglycemic syndrome
Diabetic hyperosmolar syndrome
Hyperglycemic hyperosmolar nonketotic syndrome
Hyperglycemic hyperosmolar nonketotic coma
Hyperosmolar hyperglycemic state
Nonketotic hyperosmolar syndrome

ICD-10CM CODES
E08.00	Diabetes mellitus due to underlying condition with hyperosmolarity without nonketotic hyperglycemic-hyperosmolar coma (NKHHC)
E08.01	Diabetes mellitus due to underlying condition with hyperosmolarity with coma
E09.00	Drug or chemical induced diabetes mellitus with hyperosmolarity without nonketotic hyperglycemic-hyperosmolar coma (NKHHC)
E09.01	Drug or chemical induced diabetes mellitus with hyperosmolarity with coma
E11.00	Type 2 diabetes mellitus with hyperosmolarity without nonketotic hyperglycemic-hyperosmolar coma (NKHHC)
E11.01	Type 2 diabetes mellitus with hyperosmolarity with coma
E13.00	Other specified diabetes mellitus with hyperosmolarity without nonketotic hyperglycemic-hyperosmolar coma (NKHHC)
E13.01	Other specified diabetes mellitus with hyperosmolarity with coma

EPIDEMIOLOGY AND DEMOGRAPHICS

HHS is a rare condition that most commonly affects patients with type 2 diabetes mellitus. Approximately 20% of the patients may have no prior history of diabetes. Elderly individuals with new-onset diabetes or those with poorly controlled type 2 diabetes who are predisposed to dehydration are at increased risk for HHS. Mortality from HHS is estimated to be 5% to 20%, which is higher than the mortality with diabetic ketoacidosis.

PHYSICAL FINDINGS & CLINICAL PRESENTATION

- Polyuria, polydipsia, weight loss, weakness
- Mental obtundation (can range from full alertness to coma)
- Focal neurologic signs (e.g., hemiplegia, hemianopsia) or seizures (focal or generalized), aphasia, visual hallucinations
- Symptoms of coexisting illnesses or comorbidities that may have precipitated the event
- Signs of dehydration such as dry mucous membranes, poor skin turgor, sunken eyes, hypotension, tachycardia
- Normo- or hypothermia even in the presence of infection, due to peripheral vasodilation

ETIOLOGY

HHS can be precipitated by various conditions:
- Infection (most common precipitant)
- Insulin deficiency (undiagnosed diabetes, inadequate insulin, or medication noncompliance)
- Inflammatory conditions (e.g., acute pancreatitis, acute cholecystitis)
- Ischemia/infarction (e.g., myocardial infarction, stroke, bowel ischemia)
- Renal failure
- Severe dehydration (e.g., burns, heatstroke)
- Drugs (e.g., steroids, thiazides, atypical antipsychotics, sympathomimetics including cocaine, alcohol, pentamidine)

A relative insulin deficiency provides enough insulin to inhibit ketogenesis but not enough to inhibit hepatic gluconeogenesis, glycogenolysis, or peripheral glucose uptake, thereby resulting in hyperglycemia. With underlying illness, counter-regulatory hormone excess leads to further blood glucose rise. The resultant extreme hyperglycemia leads to osmotic diuresis. If adequate hydration is not maintained, dehydration and worsening renal function ensue. Diminished renal filtration further impairs glucose excretion, thus exacerbating the hyperglycemia, dehydration, and hyperosmolality.

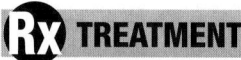 **DIAGNOSIS**

DIFFERENTIAL DIAGNOSIS

- Diabetic ketoacidosis
- Stroke (especially in the elderly with neurologic abnormalities)
- Hypovolemic or septic shock
- Encephalopathy

WORKUP

After the initial history is obtained, a physical examination should be performed that includes immediate evaluation of airway, breathing, circulation, mental status, volume status, and signs suggestive of precipitating event including infection, myocardial infarction, or stroke.

LABORATORY TESTS

- Hyperglycemia: blood glucose >600 mg/dl (Box 1).
- Serum osmolality: typically >320 mOsm/kg.
- Complete metabolic panel including serum creatinine, blood urea nitrogen (BUN), electrolytes, glucose.
- Serum sodium: may be low, normal, or high. Hyperglycemia causes increase in plasma osmolality, which causes movement of water from intracellular to the extracellular compartment, thereby decreasing the serum sodium concentration. Serum sodium can be corrected by adding 1.6 mg/dl to the measured serum sodium for every 100 mg/dl rise in serum glucose above 100 mg/dl. Marked osmotic diuresis induced by hyperglycemia may sometimes cause the serum sodium level to be normal or high.
- Serum potassium and phosphate: There is typically a total body potassium and phosphate deficit due to urinary losses from osmotic diuresis. However, the levels may acutely be normal or high due to extracellular shift secondary to insulin deficiency and hyperosmolality.
- Anion gap and serum lactate: Anion gap may be normal or elevated in the setting of lactic acidosis.
- Arterial blood gas: pH >7.3.
- Serum and urine ketones: negative or small.
- Serum bicarbonate: >15 mEq/L.
- Hemoglobin A1c.
- Complete blood count with differential (may indicate presence of underlying infection, inflammatory condition, hemoconcentration, or simply the stress of illness).
- Urine analysis, urine/sputum/blood cultures as indicated based on the physical exam findings to evaluate the precipitating illness and other comorbidities.

IMAGING STUDIES

- ECG, chest x-ray, and other imaging studies as indicated to evaluate the precipitating causes

TREATMENT

ACUTE GENERAL Rx

- Aggressive fluid resuscitation, IV insulin, and electrolyte correction are the mainstays of treatment. Patients with HHS are very ill, and many are elderly; therefore, slower correction of osmolality may be required to limit cerebral edema.

Aggressive IV fluid replacement
- Due to trivial ketonemia and the insulin sensitivity of most HHS patients, initial treatment

---

BOX 1 Diagnostic Testing Criteria for Patients with Hyperglycemic Hyperosmolar State

Glucose higher than 600 mg/dl
Normal pH (classically, however, patients are often mildly acidotic)
No significant ketosis*
Serum osmolarity
- >320 mOsm/L with any mental status changes, *or*
- >350 mOsm/L

*Acetoacetate is often present, typically with no to low β-hydroxybutyrate.
From Adams JG, et al., editors: *Emergency medicine: clinical essentials*, ed 2, Philadelphia, 2013, Saunders.

is IV fluid alone without insulin. Insulin used prior to IV hydration or early in resuscitation risks a precipitous drop in serum osmolality. In the absence of cardiac compromise, 0.9% normal saline (NS) should be infused at an initial rate of 1000 ml/hour. A lower rate of 250 to 500 ml/hr may be adequate in the absence of severe dehydration. If the serum sodium is high, 0.45% NS may be infused instead. Reassess sodium needs by frequent measurement. Ideal decline is 0.5 mEq/L/hr and must not surpass 10 to 12 mEq/L per day. Use measured or calculated osmolality to guide rate of fluid resuscitation for gradual normalization of osmolality. Once serum glucose decreases to 300 mg/dl, change the IV fluid to 5% dextrose with 0.45% NS at 150 to 250 ml/hr.

Insulin

- Once glucose is no longer significantly improving with fluids alone, reassess patient's fluid status and initiate IV insulin. Administer initial bolus of IV regular insulin 0.1 units/kg followed by 0.1 units/kg/hr infusion or a continuous infusion of 0.14 units/kg/hr without initial bolus. If the decline in serum glucose is less than 50 to 75 mg/dl in the first hour, the insulin infusion rate should be increased. Once the serum glucose reaches 300 mg/dl, the insulin infusion rate should be decreased to 0.02 to 0.05 units/kg/hr to maintain the serum glucose between 200 and 300 mg/dl until resolution of HHS.

Potassium replacement

- Insulin therapy shifts potassium intracellularly, frequently causing hypokalemia. If the serum potassium at presentation is between 3.3 and 5.2 mEq/L, infuse 20 to 30 mEq of potassium chloride with each liter of IV fluid to maintain serum potassium between 4 to 5 mEq/L. If the serum potassium at presentation is <3.3 mEq/L, replace potassium by administering potassium chloride infusion at 20 to 30 mEq/hr and hold insulin until serum potassium is >3.3 mEq/L. If serum potassium at presentation is >5.2 mEq/L, monitor serum potassium level every 2 hr without potassium replacement.

Phosphate and magnesium replacement

- Phosphate and magnesium replacement are not routinely recommended. There are no studies on phosphate use in the treatment of HHS. Very low phosphorus levels may limit ATP generation, thus limiting adequate diaphragm function. In patients with cardiac dysfunction, respiratory depression, or anemia and serum phosphate <1 mg/dl, 20 to 30 mEq/L of potassium phosphate may be added to the IV fluids.
- Monitor serum glucose every 1 hr and serum electrolytes, BUN, and creatinine every 2-4 hr until resolution of HHS.

Transition to subcutaneous insulin

- Normalization of serum osmolality and mental status indicates resolution of HHS. At this point, one can transition to subcutaneous insulin. One must overlap the initiation of subcutaneous long- or intermediate-acting insulin and discontinuation of IV insulin by 1 to 2 hr to ensure adequate insulin levels and to prevent rebound hyperglycemia. In patients with a known history of diabetes, their home insulin regimen may be initiated if it was adequate prior to presentation. In patients with a history of poorly controlled diabetes, the subcutaneous insulin dose can be determined on the basis of their regular insulin drip requirement when stable. Insulin-naïve patients may be started on basal-bolus insulin therapy, starting with a total daily dose of 0.5 to 0.8 units/kg (split as half-basal and half-bolus: administer 1/3 total bolus for each meal). Their stable insulin drip requirement will also help guide initial doses of subcutaneous insulin. Further subcutaneous insulin dose titration will be based on resultant blood glucoses. Resolution of glucotoxicity and the inciting condition(s) will decrease insulin requirements. The underlying infection/inflammatory condition or precipitating event must be adequately treated.

Chronic therapy

- Most patients will need insulin at discharge, at least short-term. Patients whose diabetes was previously well controlled on oral agents may resume oral therapy after stabilization of blood glucoses with the use of insulin.

Disposition

- Most patients will need to be managed in an emergency care setting such as the intensive care unit or in a step-up facility where close supervision and monitoring are feasible.

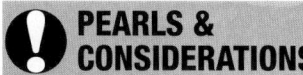

❗ PEARLS & CONSIDERATIONS

COMMENTS

- Educating the patient, family, and caregivers at chronic care facilities regarding optimal glycemic control, limiting modifiable risk factors for HHS, and prevention of dehydration are paramount.

SUGGESTED READINGS
Available at www.expertconsult.com

AUTHORS: **RESHMA RAMAKRISHNAN, M.D.,** and **JESSICA E. SHILL, M.D.**

H

Diseases and Disorders

I

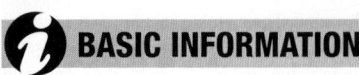

BASIC INFORMATION

DEFINITION

- Primary hyperlipoproteinemia is a group of genetic disorders of the lipid transport proteins in the blood that manifests as abnormally elevated levels of cholesterol, triglycerides, or both in the serum of affected patients.
- Usually defined as total cholesterol, LDL, triglycerides or lipoprotein A levels above 90th percentile or HDL or apo A-1 levels below the 10th percentile for the general population. Fig. E1 illustrates the structure of lipoproteins. Plasma lipoprotein composition is described in Table E1.

SYNONYMS

Hyperlipidemia

ICD-10CM CODES
E78.0 Pure hypercholesterolemia
E78.2 Mixed hyperlipidemia
E78.1 Pure hyperglyceridemia
E78.4 Other hyperlipidemia
E78.3 Hyperchylomicronemia

EPIDEMIOLOGY & DEMOGRAPHICS

INCIDENCE: The most common types are lipoprotein A excess, hypertriglyceridemia, and combined hyperlipidemia.
- Incidence of heterozygous familial hypercholesterolemia: 1:500.
- Incidence of homozygous familial hypercholesterolemia: 1:1 million.
- Familial hypercholesterolemia: autosomal-dominant disorder.
- Familial combined hyperlipidemia: possibly an autosomal-dominant disorder.
- Multifactorial predilection: apparent in majority of affected individuals.

GENETICS:
- Familial lipoprotein lipase deficiency: autosomal recessive, resulting in an elevation in the plasma chylomicrons and triglycerides
- Familial apoprotein CII deficiency: autosomal recessive, resulting in increased serum chylomicrons, very-low-density lipoprotein (VLDL), and hypertriglyceridemia
- Familial type 3 hyperlipoproteinemia: single-gene defect requiring contributory factors to manifest
- Familial hypercholesterolemia: autosomal-dominant defect of the LDL receptor, resulting in an elevated serum cholesterol level and normal triglycerides
- Familial hypertriglyceridemia: common, autosomal-dominant defect resulting in elevated VLDL and triglycerides
- Multiple lipoprotein–type hyperlipidemia: autosomal dominant, manifesting as isolated hypercholesterolemia, isolated hypertriglyceridemia, or hyperlipidemia
- Polygenic hypercholesterolemia: multifactorial
- Polygenic hyperalphalipoproteinemia: autosomal dominant or polygenic, causing an elevated high-density lipoprotein
- A classification of lipoprotein disorders is described in Table E2.

PHYSICAL FINDINGS & CLINICAL PRESENTATION

- Familial lipoprotein lipase deficiency: recurrent bouts of abdominal pain in infancy, eruptive xanthomas, hepatomegaly, splenomegaly, lipemia retinalis
- Familial apoprotein CII deficiency: occasional eruptive xanthomas
- Familial type 3 hyperlipoproteinemia: xanthoma striata palmaris or tuberoeruptive xanthomas, xanthelasmas, arterial bruits at a young age, gangrene of the lower extremities at a young age
- Familial hypercholesterolemia: tendon xanthomas, arcus corneae, xanthelasma
- Familial hypertriglyceridemia: associated obesity; eruptive xanthomas can develop with exacerbations

ETIOLOGY

- Genetic defects causing lipid abnormalities
- Environmental influences including diet, drugs, and alcohol intake

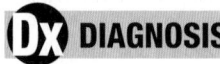

DIAGNOSIS

DIFFERENTIAL DIAGNOSIS

Secondary causes of hyperlipoproteinemias:
- Hypothyroidism
- Diabetes mellitus
- Pancreatitis
- Autoimmune hyperlipoproteinemia
- Nephrotic syndrome
- Biliary obstruction. Table E3 describes the differential diagnosis of hyperlipidemia and dyslipidemia.

WORKUP

- Family history for premature cardiac disease
- Personal history of recurrent pancreatitis
- Detailed physical examination

LABORATORY TESTS

- Standard lipid profile
- If normal, further testing with measurement of lipoprotein A, apo B, and apo A-1
- Lipoprotein electrophoresis and ultracentrifugation (for phenotypic classification)
- Workup for secondary causes: TSH, fasting glucose, liver function, renal function, urinary protein

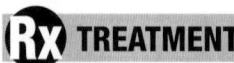

TREATMENT

NONPHARMACOLOGIC THERAPY

- Cornerstone of treatment: dietary therapy
  1. TLC diet (therapeutic lifestyle changes): see "Hypercholesterolemia" topic
- Risk factor reduction includes smoking cessation, treatment of hypertension, exercise
- Familial lipoprotein lipase deficiency and familial apoprotein CII deficiency: fat-free diet
- Remainder of cases, except those with polygenic hyperalphalipoproteinemia: fat- and cholesterol-restricted diets
- Interventions to improve adherence are described in Table E4

ACUTE GENERAL Rx

No acute treatment needed.

CHRONIC Rx

- Familial lipoprotein lipase deficiency, polygenic hyperalphalipoproteinemia, or familial apoprotein CII deficiency: no chronic drug therapy
- Familial type 3 hyperlipoproteinemia: usually responds well to secondary causes being treated and diet therapy; if not, fibric acids may be tried
- Familial hypercholesterolemia: HMG-CoA reductase inhibitors, bile acid sequestrants, or niacin. Alirocumab and evolocumab are subcutaneously injected PCSK9 (protein convertase subtilisin kexin type 9) inhibitors available as an adjunct diet and maximally tolerated statin therapy for adults with heterozygous familial hypercholesterolemia (HeFH).
- Familial hypertriglyceridemia: fibric acids (fenofibrate), niacin, omega-3 PUFA-containing fish oil capsules
- Multiple lipoprotein–type hyperlipidemia: drug therapy aimed at the predominant lipid abnormality noted
- Recent data suggest in patients with lipoprotein abnormalities that treatment goals should be based on non-HDL cholesterol rather than LDL cholesterol
- The FDA has approved mipomersen and lomitapide in patients with homozygous familial hypercholesterolemia already taking maximum doses of other lipid-lowering drugs. Both medicines are hepatotoxic and very expensive.
- Table E5 describes the various medications used to treat hyperlipidemia.

DISPOSITION

- Those with polygenic hyperalphalipoproteinemia: excellent prognosis for longevity
- Those with familial hypercholesterolemia, familial type 3 hypercholesterolemia, or multiple lipoprotein–type hyperlipidemia: even with aggressive treatment, at high risk for accelerated atherosclerosis and coronary artery disease

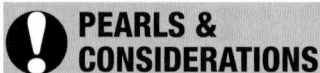

PEARLS & CONSIDERATIONS

COMMENTS

- Patient information is available through the American Heart Association.
- Lipid-lowering drug therapy is recommended for children ≥10 yr whose LDL-C levels remain extremely elevated after 6 mo to 1 yr of dietary modification. Drug therapy also can be considered for children with LDL-C levels of ≥190 mg/dl.

SUGGESTED READINGS

Available at www.expertconsult.com

RELATED CONTENT

Hypercholesterolemia (Related Key Topic)

AUTHOR: **PRIYA BANSAL, M.D., M.P.H.**

BASIC INFORMATION

DEFINITION

Hyperparathyroidism is an endocrine disorder caused by excessive secretion of parathyroid hormone (PTH) from the parathyroid glands. Autonomous production of PTH resulting in hypercalcemia defines primary hyperparathyroidism. Secondary hyperparathyroidism occurs when the parathyroid glands appropriately increase PTH production in response to low calcium or vitamin D states. Primary hyperparathyroidism is the focus of this section.

ICD-10CM CODES
E21.0	Primary hyperparathyroidism
E21.1	Secondary hyperparathyroidism, not elsewhere classified
E21.2	Other hyperparathyroidism
E21.3	Hyperparathyroidism, unspecified
N25.81	Secondary hyperparathyroidism of renal origin

EPIDEMIOLOGY & DEMOGRAPHICS

INCIDENCE: 4 cases per 100,000 persons per year. Although malignancy is the most common cause of hypercalcemia in hospitalized patients, primary hyperparathyroidism is the most common cause of hypercalcemia in the outpatient setting.
PREVALENCE: 3 cases/1000 persons
PREDOMINANT SEX AND AGE: Higher prevalence in women (female:male ratio 2:1) and older age (peaks in the seventh decade of life).

PHYSICAL FINDINGS & CLINICAL PRESENTATION

The majority of patients with primary hyperparathyroidism are asymptomatic. Diagnosis is usually considered in patients after an incidental discovery of hypercalcemia or during the evaluation for decreased bone mass. The development of symptoms varies with severity and rapidity of disease progression and reflects both the hypercalcemic and hyperparathyroid components of the disease process.
- Cardiovascular: hypertension, shortened QT interval, bradycardia, arrhythmia, valvular calcification, left ventricular hypertrophy, increased mean carotid intima-media thickness.
- GI: anorexia, nausea, vomiting, constipation, abdominal pain, peptic ulcer disease, pancreatitis
- GU: nephrolithiasis, nephrocalcinosis, renal insufficiency, polyuria, nocturia, nephrogenic diabetes insipidus, renal tubular acidosis
- Musculoskeletal: weakness, myopathy, bone pain, osteopenia, osteoporosis, gout, pseudogout, chondrocalcinosis, osteitis fibrosa cystica, subperiosteal bone resorption (Fig. E1)
- CNS: confusion, anxiety, fatigue, lethargy, obtundation, depression, coma
- Other: pruritus, metastatic calcifications, band keratopathy

ETIOLOGY
- Most cases of primary hyperparathyroidism are sporadic, but hyperparathyroidism can be associated with rare familial conditions such as multiple endocrine neoplasia (MEN-1 and MEN-2). Mutations in certain genes have been linked to tumor development in both sporadic and familial cases such as hyperparathyroidism-jaw tumor syndrome. Higher prevalence of hyperparathyroidism is noted with head and neck irradiation, chronic low calcium or vitamin D status, and lithium therapy.
- Pathologic characteristics include adenoma (80%-85%), hyperplasia (10%-15%), or carcinomas (<1%-2%).

DIAGNOSIS

DIFFERENTIAL DIAGNOSIS
- Primary hyperparathyroidism
  1. Adenoma (80%-85%)
  2. Hyperplasia (10%-15%)
  3. Carcinomas (<1%-2%)
- Secondary hyperparathyroidism precipitated by conditions that result in hypocalcemia
  1. Renal calcium loss (i.e., medication: loop diuretics and hypercalcuria)
  2. Calcium deficiency
  3. Vitamin D deficiency
  4. Malabsorption
  5. Chronic kidney disease (most common)
  6. Pseudohypoparathyroidism (PTH resistance)
  7. Inhibition of bone resorption (i.e., bisphosphonates)
- Other causes of hypercalcemia include:
  1. Medications: thiazide diuretics, lithium therapy
  2. Vitamin D intoxication, milk-alkali syndrome
  3. Familial hypocalciuric hypercalcemia (FHH)
  4. Renal failure (tertiary hyperparathyroidism)
  5. Granulomatous disorders (e.g., sarcoidosis)
  6. Malignancy (e.g., lung cancer, lymphoma, multiple myeloma, bone metastasis)
  7. Prolonged immobilization

WORK-UP
- Typically, primary hyperparathyroidism is confirmed with an elevated serum calcium and PTH level.
  1. Two measurements of serum calcium are required for the confirmation of hypercalcemia. Total calcium should be corrected for low albumin utilizing the formula: Corrected Calcium = Serum Calcium + 0.8 × 4 − serum albumin). If a reliable laboratory is available, ionized calcium should be considered, especially in conditions associated with acid-base disturbances or low albumin states. Patients with primary hyperparathyroidism can also present with normal calcium levels. The most common reason for this finding is concomitant vitamin D deficiency and primary hyperparathyroidism.
  2. The serum intact PTH (iPTH) level is the single best test to evaluate the etiology of hypercalcemia. PTH is elevated or in the high normal range (i.e., inappropriately normal for an elevated calcium state) in primary hyperparathyroidism. PTH is decreased in most other conditions associated with elevated calcium.
- Other causes of hypercalcemia should be ruled out. These are typically associated with low PTH levels. Exceptions include lithium use and FHH.
  1. Review medication history to determine lithium, thiazide, vitamin D, or calcium intake.
  2. Check 24-hr urine calcium:creatinine to rule out FHH. Urine calcium is usually low in FHH. PTH can be normal or high in FHH.
  3. Consider PTH-related peptide (PTHrP) to evaluate hypercalcemia related to malignancies and vitamin D 1,25 to assess hypercalcemia secondary to granulomatous diseases or lymphomas.
  4. Multiple myeloma and bone metastasis can also result in a high calcium state and therefore must be appropriately evaluated.
- Rule out other causes of elevated PTH (i.e., secondary hyperparathyroidism). Serum calcium is typically low or low-normal in secondary hyperparathyroidism.
  1. Check calcium and 25 OH-vitamin D to rule out deficiency states.
  2. Check serum creatinine to assess renal function and 24-hr urine calcium and creatinine to evaluate renal loss.

LABORATORY TESTS
- Serum calcium (ionized or corrected calcium): normal or elevated in primary hyperparathyroidism
- Serum phosphorus: low or low-normal in primary hyperparathyroidism
- PTH: elevated or high normal in primary hyperparathyroidism
- Serum creatinine and estimated glomerular filtration rate (eGFR)
- 24-hr urine calcium and creatinine
- PTHrP and 1,25 OH-vitamin D levels 25 OH-vitamin D level
- ECG may reveal shortening of the QT interval secondary to severe hypercalcemia (>12 mg/dl)

IMAGING STUDIES
- Parathyroid localization with technetium-99m sestamibi can identify potential adenomas to help with surgical planning.
- Parathyroid ultrasound is also used to localize the parathyroid adenoma.
- Bone mineral density (BMD) of the spine, hip, and forearm (distal third) is recommended for all patients with hyperparathyroidism in order to assess the risk for osteoporosis and fragility fractures. Cortical bone loss (i.e., forearm or hip) is greater than trabecular bone loss (i.e., spine) in hyperparathyroidism.
- Renal ultrasound can be considered to assess asymptomatic renal stones.

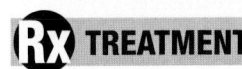 TREATMENT

Modality of treatment depends on disease progression and which patients are more likely to suffer end-organ effects of hyperparathyroidism or benefit the most from surgery.

- Surgery is the only definitive treatment for symptomatic primary hyperparathyroidism. Surgery can normalize calcium levels, decrease the risk for kidney stones, improve bone mineral density and fracture risk, and enhance quality of life measures.
  1. Indications for parathyroidectomy
     1. All patients younger than 50 yr
     2. Hypercalcemia (Ca >1 mg/dl above upper limit normal)
     3. Creatinine clearance <60 mL/min
     4. 24-h urine for calcium >400 mg/dL (>10 mmol/dl)
     5. Presence of nephrolithiasis or nephrocalcinosis by x-ray, ultrasound, or CT
     6. Osteoporosis
        a. BMD by dual-energy x-ray absorptiometry (DXA): T-score ≤2.5 at lumbar spine, total hip, femoral neck, or distal 1/3 radius
        b. Vertebral fracture by x-ray, CT, MRI, or vertebral fracture assessment (VFA) by DXA
  2. Surgical approaches include:
     1. Minimally invasive parathyroidectomy has increased in popularity. The surgeon will identify and remove the abnormal gland that was identified on preoperative imaging. This technique has limited dissection and has improved recovery time. Intraoperative monitoring of PTH level is done to ensure the removal of the abnormal gland. Fall of PTH level by 50%, into the normal range, is expected within 10 to 15 minutes after removal of the abnormal gland.
     2. Bilateral neck exploration under general anesthesia is the traditional surgical approach. All parathyroid glands are identified and compared. An experienced endocrine surgeon cures >95% of patients undergoing bilateral neck exploration. Potential complications include transient and permanent hypocalcemia secondary to hypoparathyroidism and recurrent laryngeal nerve injury.
- Ablation therapy (e.g., ethanol, angiographic, radiofrequency) can be considered in patients who are not surgical candidates. Limited data are available on efficacy and side effects. Repeat ablations may be required if hypercalcemia persists.
- Medical management
  1. Avoid medications that precipitate hypercalcemia (e.g., thiazide or lithium)

2. Because inadequate calcium and vitamin D status stimulates PTH, it is not necessary to restrict calcium and vitamin D intake. Vitamin D replacement safely improves vitamin D level and decreases PTH level without significantly increasing serum calcium level and urinary calcium excretion. Calcium intake is based on the recommendations established for the general population.
3. Encourage physical activity since immobilization increases bone resorption.
4. Recommend adequate hydration (at least 2 L) to minimize the risk of nephrolithiasis.
   1. For patients who are not surgical candidates or who refuse surgery, pharmacologic options are available. The choice of pharmacologic agents is dependent on the desired goal. Cinacalcet (Sensipar) is an oral calcimimetic agent that activates the calcium sensing receptor in the parathyroid gland. It decreases PTH production and subsequently normalizes or decreases serum calcium levels, without significant BMD changes. It is indicated for the treatment of severe hypercalcemia in patients with primary hyperparathyroidism who are unable to undergo surgery. It is also indicated for the treatment of secondary hyperparathyroidism associated with chronic kidney disease and for hypercalcemia associated with parathyroid carcinoma.
   2. Agents such as bisphosphonates (e.g., alendronate, zoledronate) that inhibit bone resorption and increase BMD should be considered when improvement in BMD is the primary goal in patients with hyperparathyroidism.
- Medical monitoring is recommended for asymptomatic primary hyperparathyroidism. The majority of patients do not manifest disease progression during observation. However, approximately 25% of asymptomatic patients require surgery over a 10-yr follow-up period.
  1. Indications for medical monitoring
     1. Clinically asymptomatic and >50 yr old
     2. Serum calcium level only mildly elevated (<1 mg/dl above upper limit normal)
     3. GFR >60 mL/min and no nephrolithiasis or nephrocalcinosis
     4. No evidence of osteoporosis
     5. Medically unfit for surgery or refusing surgery
- Symptoms should be assessed regularly. Serum calcium, creatinine, and eGFR should be checked yearly. DXA performed at three

sites every 1 to 2 years or VFA of the spine is clinically indicated (e.g., height loss, back pain).

ACUTE GENERAL Rx

Severe and/or symptomatic hypercalcemia may require hospitalization especially if serum calcium >12 mg/dl. Acute management of hypercalcemia includes:

- Vigorous hydration with IV normal saline (2-4 L/day). Fluid status must be monitored in patients with cardiac dysfunction or renal insufficiency in order to avoid fluid overload.
- Bisphosphonates can effectively decrease calcium levels. Zoledronate (4 mg IV over 15 min) or pamidronate (60-90 mg IV over 4 hr) are both effective. Onset of action is 24 to 48 hr.
- Calcitonin (4 units/kg IM/SC every 12 hr) may be used with bisphosphonates to achieve a more rapid reduction of calcium levels. Onset of action is within hours.

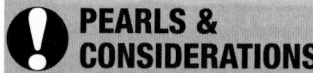

PEARLS & CONSIDERATIONS

COMMENTS

- Parathyroidectomy should be considered for all patients with symptomatic hyperparathyroidism. If surgery is contraindicated or not desired, cinacalcet and bisphosphonates can be used.
- Asymptomatic patients can be monitored with serial calcium, creatinine, eGFR, and bone mineral density measurements. Disease progression may result in surgery.
- Most patients can be managed medically by limiting factors that result in hypercalcemia (e.g., dehydration, immobilization, thiazide diuretics) and maintaining normal calcium and vitamin D intake.
- Patients with osteopenia and high fracture risk may require antiresorptive therapy such as bisphosphonates.

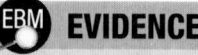 **EVIDENCE**

Available at www.expertconsult.com

SUGGESTED READINGS

Available at www.expertconsult.com

RELATED CONTENT

Hyperparathyroidism (Patient Information)

AUTHOR: **VICKY CHENG, M.D.**

BASIC INFORMATION

DEFINITION

Hypersensitivity pneumonitis (HP) is a group of immunologically mediated pulmonary diseases, with or without systemic manifestations (e.g., fever, weight loss), caused by the inhalation of an antigen to which the patient is sensitized and hyperresponsive. Sensitization and exposure alone in the absence of symptoms do not define the disease.

SYNONYMS

HP - Extrinsic allergic alveolitis (EAA)
Some specific examples:
- ○ Bird fancier's lung
- ○ Farmer's lung
- ○ Malt worker's lung
- ○ "Ventilation" pneumonitis
- ○ Maple bark-stripper's lung
- ○ Sauna taker's lung
- ○ Hot tub lung

ICD-10CM CODES
J67.8 Hypersensitivity pneumonitis due to other organic dusts
J67.9 Hypersensitivity pneumonitis due to unspecified organic dust

EPIDEMIOLOGY & DEMOGRAPHICS

- Prevalence and incidence of HP vary considerably.
- Depend on definition and methods to establish diagnosis, intensity of exposure, environmental conditions, and genetic risk factors that remain poorly understood.
- More than 300 causative agents have been identified, and the number continues to grow.
- Causative agents in residential and occupational exposures include birds, mold, humidifiers, fountains, steam irons, dry sausage molds, moldy cheese, contaminated wood, biofilm contained within wind instruments (e.g., trombone, saxophone), and organic and inorganic chemicals, including metalworking fluids. It is likely that genetic factors are involved that cause an exaggerated lung response to an offending agent. The major histocompatibility complex is the most studied thus far.

PHYSICAL FINDINGS & CLINICAL PRESENTATION

Vary depending on frequency and intensity of antigen exposure.
- Acute: fever, cough, malaise, and dyspnea 4 to 6 hr after an intense exposure, lasting 18 to 24 hr
- Often misdiagnosed initially as a viral illness or asthma
- Subacute: insidious onset of productive cough, dyspnea on exertion, anorexia, and weight loss, usually from a heavy, sustained exposure
- Chronic: gradually progressive cough, dyspnea, malaise, and weight loss, usually from low-grade or recurrent exposure
- Physical examination: hypoxemia, cyanosis, rales, possible fever

ETIOLOGY

- Numerous environmental agents, often encountered in occupational settings.
- Common sources of antigens: "moldy" hay, silage, grain, or vegetables; bird droppings or feathers (including those found commonly in down pillows, blankets, and upholstered furniture); low-molecular-weight chemicals (e.g., isocyanates); pharmaceutical products.
- Fig. E1 illustrates the pathogenesis of hypersensitivity pneumonitis.

DIAGNOSIS

- Accurate diagnosis is important for differentiating HP from other interstitial lung diseases because the prognosis and treatment may differ.
- The clinical syndrome of acute HP is indistinguishable from an acute respiratory infection with a history of illness occurring within hours of exposure to an antigen.
- Need high index of suspicion.
- Detailed occupational and home exposure history is required.
- Lung biopsy is often necessary for diagnosis.

DIFFERENTIAL DIAGNOSIS

Acute Stages	Chronic Stages
Allergic bronchopulmonary aspergillosis	Idiopathic pulmonary fibrosis (IPF)
Pulmonary embolism	
Asthma	
Aspiration pneumonia	Bronchiectasis
Bacterial pneumonia	Chronic bronchitis
Fungal or mycobacterial pneumonia	
Bronchiolitis obliterans–organizing pneumonia	Nonspecific interstitial pneumonia (NSIP)
Eosinophilic pneumonia	Connective tissue–related lung disease
Churg-Strauss syndrome	
Wegener granulomatosis	Sarcoidosis

WORKUP

No single radiologic, physiologic, or immunologic test is specific for the diagnosis of HP. HP must be suspected in any patient presenting with cough, dyspnea, fever, and malaise. A thorough history focusing on potential exposures is essential. Table 1 describes examples of occupational causes of HP.

Environmental and occupational history questions should ask about grain dusts, animal handling, food processing, cooling towers, fountains, metalworking fluids, symptom improvement away from exposure, pets (particularly birds), hobbies involving chemicals, feathers, or fur, organic dusts, presence of humidifiers, dehumidifiers, or hot tubs/saunas, leaking or flooding indoors, visible fungal growth in living or working environment, feather pillows, bedding, or upholstered furniture.

Major criteria:
- History of symptoms compatible with HP that appear to worsen within hours after antigen exposure
- Confirmation of exposure to the offending agent by history, investigation of the environment, serum precipitin tests to potential agents (often referred to as a "hypersensitivity panel" by many labs), or bronchoalveolar lavage (BAL) antibody
- Compatible clinical symptoms, physical exam, and changes on chest radiograph or high-resolution CT (HRCT) of the chest
- BAL fluid lymphocytosis (if performed)
- Compatible histologic changes by lung biopsy (if performed): poorly formed granulomas or mononuclear cell infiltrate
- Positive natural challenge (reproduction of symptoms and laboratory abnormalities after exposure to the suspected environment) or controlled inhalation challenge

Minor criteria:
- Basilar crackles
- Decreased diffusion capacity
- Arterial hypoxemia (either at rest or with exercise)

LABORATORY TESTS

- Routine laboratory tests do not make the diagnosis, but typically the erythrocyte sedimentation rate, C-reactive protein, lactate dehydrogenase, and leukocyte count are increased; elevated immunoglobulins IgG and IgM are nonspecific; rheumatoid factor (RF) and immune complexes are often positive; peripheral eosinophil count and serum IgE are generally normal.
- Lactate dehydrogenase (LDH) is increased and tends to decrease with improvement.
- Pulmonary function tests: restrictive ventilatory pattern is typically seen. Decreased FEV_1, decreased forced vital capacity, decreased total lung capacity, decreased diffusion capacity, and decreased static compliance.
- Arterial blood gases show mild hypoxemia (worsens with exercise).
- A-a gradient shows slight increase.
- Serum precipitin test for IgG antibodies against offending antigen detected in serum. It is sensitive but not specific for HP (asymptomatic patients may have IgG antibodies in serum). HP may also be present without a positive precipitin test.
- Skin testing: unclear if helpful. However, some believe it to be a safe, effective, and rapid procedure in the diagnosis and follow-up of patients with HP. Sensitivity is similar to that of the precipitin test but the specificity is higher.

IMAGING STUDIES

Chest x-ray: nonspecific; may be normal in early stage.
- Acute/subacute: bilateral interstitial and alveolar nodular infiltrates in a patchy or homogeneous distribution. Apices are often spared.
- Chronic: diffuse reticulonodular infiltrates and fibrosis.

TABLE 1 Examples of Occupational Causes of Hypersensitivity Pneumonitis

Occupation	Cause
Farmer	Thermophilic actinomycetes in moldy hay
Metal worker	Contamination of metal-working fluids with microorganisms such as Mycobacteria immunogens or fungi
Worker exposed to humidifiers	Contamination with microorganisms such as protozoa or fungi
Sugarcane worker	Moldy sugarcane (bagassosis)
Maple bark stripper	Fungi
Chicken or turkey worker	Avian proteins
Pharmaceutical worker	Penicillin
Food handler	Soybeans
Office worker	Microorganisms contaminating air conditioners or humidifiers
Swimming pool attendant	Fungal contamination in sprays around pool area
Animal worker	Rat proteins
Mushroom worker	Fungi
Wheat farmer or handler	Weevil-infested flour
Greenhouse worker	Fungi
Workers spraying urethane paint or adhesives/sealants (or less often, other workers using diisocyanate)	Methylene diphenyl diisocyanate, hexamethylene diisocyanate, toluene diisocyanates
Chemical worker using plastics, resins, paints	Trimellitic anhydride

From Goldman L, Schafer AI: *Goldman's Cecil medicine,* ed 24, Philadelphia, 2012, Saunders.

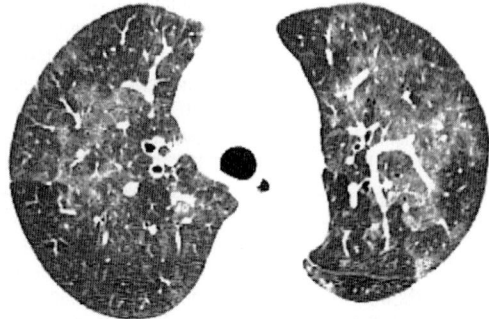

FIG. 2 In this patient with hypersensitivity pneumonitis, patchy ground-glass opacity is visible bilaterally. (From Mason RJ: *Murray & Nadel's textbook of respiratory medicine,* ed 5, Philadelphia, 2010, Saunders.)

High-resolution chest CT scan (Fig. 2): no pathognomonic features but demonstrates air-space and interstitial patterns in the acute and subacute stage. The chronic stage reveals honeycombing and bronchiectasis.

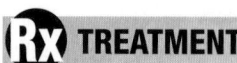 **TREATMENT**

NON-PHARMACOLOGIC THERAPY

Early recognition and avoidance of the causative antigen

ACUTE GENERAL Rx

- Glucocorticoids accelerate initial lung recovery but may have no effect long term (from a controlled study in farmer's lung). No prospective, randomized, placebo-controlled trials for other types of HP or subacute and chronic stages.
- Prednisone 0.5 to 1 mg/kg usually over 1 to 2 wk then tapered over 4 wk. Some patients, particularly those with subacute or chronic presentation, may require a longer course of therapy.

DISPOSITION/PROGNOSIS

Prognosis is generally better in patients with acute or subacute HP. Prognosis is worse in those with older age, desaturation during exercise, and findings of severe fibrosis by lung biopsy.

Acute: 4 to 48 hr
- Clinical: fever, chills, cough, hypoxia, malaise
- HRCT: ground-glass infiltrates
- Immunopathology: poorly formed, noncaseating granulomas or mononuclear cell infiltration in a peribronchial distribution, frequently with giant cells
- Prognosis: good
Subacute: weeks to 4 mo
- Clinical: dyspnea, cough, episodic flares
- HRCT: micronodules, air trapping
- Immunopathology: more well-formed, noncaseating granulomas, bronchiolitis, organizing pneumonia, and interstitial fibrosis
- Prognosis: good
Chronic: 4 mo to years
- Clinical: dyspnea, cough, fatigue, weight loss
- HRCT: fibrosis (possible), honeycombing, emphysema
- Immunopathology: granulomatous inflammation may be seen in addition to bronchiolitis obliterans (with or without organizing pneumonia) and honeycombing and fibrosis, lymphocytic infiltration, centrilobular and bridging fibrosis, neutrophil-mediated air space destruction, giant cells

REFERRAL

- Bronchoscopy: BAL provides useful supportive data in the diagnosis of HP. Usually reveals intense lymphocytosis (typically T cells >50%) of predominantly CD8+ suppressor cells. In the acute stage neutrophils predominate, but as the disease progresses to chronic form the ratio of CD4+ to CD8+ cells increases. When fibrosis is present the number of neutrophils increases.
- Lung biopsy: the histopathologic features of HP are distinctive but not pathognomonic. Bronchiolitis and interstitial pneumonitis with granuloma formation typically is seen. Variable degrees of interstitial fibrosis are seen in the chronic form. Chronic HP may be difficult to distinguish from IPF or NSIP pathologically.
- Laboratory inhalation challenge: testing to prove a direct relation between a suspected antigen and disease; extract of antigen is inhaled by nebulizer.

ⓘ PEARLS & CONSIDERATIONS

A clinical prediction rule using six features has high specificity and sensitivity for the diagnosis of acute and subacute HP:
- Exposure to a known offending agent
- Positive specific precipitating antibody
- Recurrent episodes of symptoms
- Inspiratory crackles
- Symptoms occurring 4 to 8 hr after exposure
- Weight loss
HP occurs more frequently in smokers than nonsmokers (likely from an immunosuppressive effect).

SUGGESTED READINGS

Available at www.expertconsult.com

RELATED CONTENT

Hypersensitivity Pneumonitis (Patient Information)

AUTHOR: **MELISSA H. TUKEY, M.D., M.SC.**

BASIC INFORMATION

DEFINITION

Hypersplenism is a syndrome characterized by splenomegaly, cytopenias (one or more of the following: anemia, thrombocytopenia, or leukopenia), and compensatory hyperplastic bone marrow. These cytopenias are correctable with splenectomy.

ICD-10CM CODES
D73.1 Hypersplenism

EPIDEMIOLOGY & DEMOGRAPHICS

Most often seen in patients with liver disease, hematologic malignancy, and infection

PHYSICAL FINDINGS & CLINICAL PRESENTATION

- Symptoms depend on the size of the spleen, rate of growth, and underlying disease.
- History: early satiety, abdominal discomfort or fullness, acute left upper quadrant (LUQ) pain (infarction, sequestration crisis), referred pain to left shoulder
- Physical examination: splenomegaly (normal spleen usually not palpable), LUQ tenderness, presence of a rub in LUQ (suggestive of splenic infarct), stigmata of cytopenias

ETIOLOGY

- The spleen is an important component of the hematologic and immune systems (antigen processing and antibody synthesis). The spleen is responsible for the modification (removal of particles and parasites) and clearance of senescent or poorly deformable red blood cells (RBCs). It also filters blood, removing foreign particles (microorganisms) and other particulates (e.g., complement- or antibody-coated cells) from the circulation. The spleen is a platelet reservoir, storing 30% of platelet mass. It can become the site of hematopoiesis in certain disease states. The spleen's normal activities are augmented when enlarged.
- Splenomegaly increases the proportion of blood channeled through the red pulp, causing inappropriate splenic pooling of both normal and abnormal blood cells. The size of the spleen determines the amount of cell sequestration. Up to 90% of platelets may be pooled in an enlarged spleen. Prolonged sequestration leads to increased destruction of RBCs. Platelets and white blood cells (WBCs) have about normal survival time even when sequestered and may be available if needed.
- Splenomegaly exacerbates cytopenias by dilution, possibly due to plasma volume expansion.

DIAGNOSIS

DIFFERENTIAL DIAGNOSIS

Hypersplenism can be caused by splenomegaly of almost any cause.

- Splenic congestion: cirrhosis (portal hypertension); congestive heart failure; portal, splenic, or hepatic vein thrombosis

- Hematologic causes: hemolytic anemia, spherocytosis, elliptocytosis, sickle cell anemia, thalassemia, extramedullary hematopoiesis, chronic transfusions, following use of granulocyte colony-stimulating factor
- Infections: viral (hepatitis, infectious mononucleosis, cytomegalovirus, HIV/AIDS), bacterial (endocarditis, sepsis, tuberculosis, salmonella, brucella), parasitic (babesiosis, malaria, leishmaniasis, schistosomiasis, toxoplasmosis), fungal
- Malignancy: acute or chronic leukemia, lymphoma, histiocytosis, myeloproliferative diseases (polycythemia vera, essential thrombocythemia, myelofibrosis), splenic or metastatic tumors
- Inflammatory diseases: rheumatic fever, rheumatoid arthritis (Felty's syndrome), systemic lupus erythematosus, sarcoid, serum sickness
- Infiltrative diseases: amyloidosis, Gaucher's disease, Niemann-Pick disease, glycogen storage disease

WORKUP

History (including travel), physical examination, laboratory tests, imaging studies

LABORATORY TESTS

- CBC with differential: cytopenias, neutrophilia (infection)
- Peripheral smear: RBC and WBC morphology (abnormal cells may suggest infection, malignancy, bone marrow disease, rheumatologic disease), organisms (bacteria, malaria, babesiosis)
- Bone marrow aspiration/biopsy: hyperplasia of cytopenic cell lines; hematologic, infiltrative, or infectious disorders
- Tests to diagnose suspected cause of splenomegaly: liver function, hepatitis serology, HIV, rheumatoid factor, antinuclear antibody, tissue biopsy
- Note: red cell mass (^{51}Cr assay) may be used to assess severity of anemia. RBC mass measurement will differentiate true anemia (decrease in RBCs) from dilutional anemia (plasma volume expansion).

IMAGING STUDIES

- Ultrasound: splenic size, presence of cyst or abscess
- CT: estimate volume, obtain structural information: cyst, abscess, malignancy
- MRI: most useful for assessing vascular lesions and infections
- Nuclear medicine: liver-spleen scan: assess anatomy and function; may suggest presence of portal hypertension
- Consider other studies as suggested by history and examination: chest radiograph, echocardiogram, PET scan

TREATMENT

ACUTE GENERAL Rx

- Treat underlying disease
- Splenectomy is considered if:
  1. Indicated for the management of the underlying cause

  2. Persistent symptomatic disease (severe cytopenia) not responding to therapy
  3. Necessary for diagnosis
  Risks:
- Infections (especially encapsulated organisms): risk greatest in the first 2 yr after splenectomy. Mortality rate from sepsis is fiftyfold greater in asplenic patients. Attempts to decrease risk include:
  1. Immunization with pneumococcal (PCV13 and PPSV23), meningococcal (MenACWY and MenB), and *Haemophilus influenza* type b (Hib) vaccines (if not previously vaccinated) at least 2 wk before splenectomy. Preferred: PCV13 vaccination followed by PPSV23 vaccination at least 8 wk later. If already immunized with PPSV23, PCV13 vaccine should be given at least 1 year later. Revaccination with PPSV23 in 5 yr and again after age 65 yr (and 5 yr after most recent dose). Revaccination for meningococcal (MenACWY) every 5 yr. Annual inactivated influenza vaccination.
  2. Prophylactic antibiotics after splenectomy in highest-risk patients.
  3. Patient education regarding the importance of rapid initiation of antibiotics at the first sign of infection.
- Thromboembolic complications, especially high risk of portal vein thrombosis.
- Possible increased risk of atherosclerotic heart disease and cancer.
- Splenectomy should not be performed if the spleen is the main site of hematopoiesis as a result of bone marrow failure (e.g., myelofibrosis).
- Other options include partial splenectomy, partial splenic embolization, radiofrequency ablation, portosystemic shunting (for congestive splenomegaly).

DISPOSITION

- Cytopenias are usually correctable with splenectomy; normal cell counts result in a few weeks.
- Splenectomy may alleviate portal hypertension.
- Prognosis depends on the underlying disease.

REFERRAL

Hematology

PEARLS & CONSIDERATIONS

- Thrombocytopenia in hypersplenism is usually moderately severe (>50 × 10⁹/L) and asymptomatic; severe thrombocytopenia (<20 × 10⁹/L) suggests another diagnosis.

SUGGESTED READINGS

Available at www.expertconsult.com

RELATED CONTENT

Hypersplenism (Patient Information)
Felty's Syndrome (Related Key Topic)

AUTHOR: **SUDEEP K. AULAKH, M.D.**

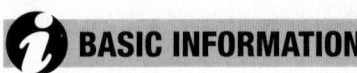

BASIC INFORMATION

DEFINITION

Normal blood pressure (BP) in adults can be defined as systolic BP <120 mm Hg and diastolic BP <80 mm Hg. Prehypertension is defined as systolic BP between 120 and 139 mm Hg or diastolic between 80 and 89 mm Hg. Hypertension can be divided into stage 1: systolic BP from 140 to 159 mmHg or diastolic BP from 90 to 99 mm Hg and stage 2: systolic BP ≥160 mm Hg or diastolic BP ≥100 mm Hg. Measurements should be appropriately taken as described below.

SYNONYMS

Essential hypertension
Idiopathic hypertension
High BP

ICD-10CM CODES
I10	Essential (primary) hypertension
I15.0	Renovascular hypertension
I15.1	Hypertension secondary to other renal disorders
I15.2	Hypertension secondary to endocrine disorders
I15.8	Other secondary hypertension
I15.9	Secondary hypertension, unspecified
O10.919	Unspecified pre-existing hypertension complicating pregnancy, unspecified trimester
I67.4	Hypertensive encephalopathy

EPIDEMIOLOGY & DEMOGRAPHICS

- In the U.S., 50% of people age 60 to 69 yr and approximately 75% of people >70 yr of age are affected, Worldwide, it is estimated that 41% of people ages 35 to 70 yr have hypertension, and only 46.5% of them are aware of it.
- Peak prevalence increases with age and was highest among non-Hispanic black adults in the U.S.
- Hypertension is linked with a higher risk of heart attack, stroke, heart failure, and kidney disease.

PHYSICAL FINDINGS & CLINICAL PRESENTATION

Physical examination may be entirely within normal limits except for the presence of elevated BP. A proper initial physical examination on a hypertensive patient should include the following:
- The BP should be measured with an appropriately sized cuff (bladder of the cuff should cover at least two thirds of the circumference of the arm) and in both arms (the higher of the readings being used).
- The BP should be measured twice on each visit, and separated by at least 1 to 2 min to allow the return of trapped blood.
- The patient should be seated in a calm environment for at least 5 minutes with the arm in which BP is measured rested on support level with the heart.

- Postural BP change should always be recorded in the elderly to diagnose postural hypotension. This is assessed by taking BP in supine (after 5 minute rest) and standing (after 2 minutes) positions. A drop of ≥20 mm Hg in systolic, a drop of ≥10 mm Hg diastolic BP, or symptoms of cerebral hypoperfusion is suggestive of postural (orthostatic) hypotension.
- A diagnosis of HTN may be established if the BP is markedly elevated (>180/110 mm Hg) or has evidence of end organ damage; otherwise such a diagnosis should wait until BP is found elevated on at least 3 visits, spaced over a period of weeks to months.
- Measure heart rate, height, weight, body mass index, and waist circumference.
- Physical examination should include searching for secondary causes, and sequelae of hypertension.
- Examine skin for the presence of café-au-lait spots (neurofibromatosis), uremic appearance (renal failure), and violaceous striae (Cushing's syndrome).
- Perform careful funduscopic examination; check for papilledema, retinal exudates, hemorrhages, arterial narrowing, arteriovenous compression.
- Examine neck for carotid bruits, distended neck veins, and enlarged thyroid gland.
- Perform extensive cardiopulmonary examination: check for a laterally displaced point of maximal intensity, an S3 or S4, and valvular murmurs.
- Palpate abdomen for renal masses (pheochromocytoma, polycystic kidneys), and auscultate for bruit over the aorta and renal arteries.

- Examine arterial pulses (dilated or absent femoral pulses and BP greater in upper extremities than lower extremities suggest aortic coarctation).
- Look for truncal obesity (Cushing's syndrome) and pedal edema (congestive heart failure [CHF]).
- Table 1 provides a guide to evaluation of identifiable causes of HTN.
- Fig. E1 and Box E1 describe the investigation of suspected endocrine causes of HTN.
- Table 2 summarizes clinical clues to guide the investigation in young patients with hypertension that has a potentially hereditary cause.

ETIOLOGY

- Essential (primary) HTN (85%)
- Drug induced or drug related (5%)
  1. NSAIDs
  2. Oral contraceptives
  3. Corticosteroids
- Renal HTN (5%)
  1. Renal parenchymal disease (3%)
  2. Renovascular HTN (RVH) (<2%)
- Endocrine (<2%)
  1. Primary aldosteronism (at least 5%)
  2. Pheochromocytoma (0.2%)
  3. Cushing's syndrome and long-term steroid therapy (0.2%)
  4. Hyperparathyroidism or thyroid disease (0.2%)
- Coarctation of the aorta (0.2%)

TABLE 1 Guide to Evaluation of Identifiable Causes of Hypertension

Suspected Diagnosis	Clinical Clues	Diagnostic Testing
Chronic kidney disease	Estimated GFR <60 ml/min/1.73 m² Urine albumin-to-creatinine ratio ≥30 mg/g	Renal sonography
Renovascular disease	New elevation in serum creatinine, marked elevation in serum creatinine with ACEI or ARB, drug-resistant hypertension, flash pulmonary edema, abdominal, or flank bruit	Renal sonography (atrophic kidney), CT or MR angiography, invasive angiography
Coarctation of the aorta	Arm pulses > leg pulses, arm BP > leg BP, chest bruits, rib notching on chest radiography	MR angiography, TEE, invasive angiography
Primary aldosteronism	Hypokalemia, drug-resistant hypertension	Plasma renin and aldosterone, 24-hr urine aldosterone and potassium after oral salt loading, adrenal vein sampling
Cushing's syndrome	Truncal obesity, wide and blanching purple striae, muscle weakness	1 mg dexamethasone-suppression test, urinary cortisol after dexamethasone, adrenal CT
Pheochromocytoma	Paroxysms of hypertension, palpitations, perspiration, and pallor; diabetes	Plasma metanephrines, 24-hr urinary metanephrines and catecholamines, abdominal CT or MR imaging
Obstructive sleep apnea	Loud snoring, large neck, obesity, somnolence	Polysomnography

ACEI, Angiotensin-converting enzyme inhibitor; *ARB*, angiotensin receptor blocker; *BP*, blood pressure; *CT*, computed tomography; *GFR*, glomerular filtration rate; *MR*, magnetic resonance; *TEE*, transesophageal echocardiography.
From Goldman L, Schafer AI: *Goldman's Cecil medicine*, ed 24, Philadelphia, 2012, Saunders.

TABLE 2 Clinical Clues to Guide the Investigation in Young Patients with Hypertension That Has a Potentially Hereditary Cause

Specific Conditions	Possible Causes of Familial Hypertension	Clinical Clues
Catecholamine-Producing Tumors		
Pheochromocytoma/paraganglioma	Familial cases are responsible for <30% of cases, including MEN2A and MEN2B, von Hippel-Lindau disease, neurofibromatosis, and familial paraganglioma syndromes (SDH complex mutations)	Paroxysmal palpitations, headaches, diaphoresis, pale flushing; syndromic features of any of the associated disorders
Neuroblastomas (adrenal)	1%-2% of neuroblastomas are familial	
Aortic or renovascular lesions		
Coarctation of the aorta	Overrepresented in families but no familial distribution	Asymmetry between upper- and lower-extremity BP, radial-formal pulse delay; associated with Turner syndrome, Williams syndrome, and bicuspid aortic valve
Renal artery stenosis caused by fibromuscular dysplasia or inherited arterial wall lesions	<10% familial with AD pattern	Abnormal renal vascular imaging results; vascular disease in the carotid territory at an early age; common in neurofibromatosis and Williams syndrome; also present in tuberous sclerosis, Ehlers-Danlos syndrome, and Marfan syndrome
Parenchymal kidney disease GN	Alport disease (X-linked, AR, or AD), familial IgA nephropathy (AD with incomplete penetrance)	Proteinuria, hematuria, low eGFR
PKD	ADPKD type 1 or 2, ARPKD	Multiple renal cysts (as few as 3 in patients under 30 yr)
Adrenocortical disease		
Glucocorticoid-remediable aldosteronism (familial hyperaldosteronism type I)	AD chimeric fusion of the 11β-hydroxylase and aldosterone synthase genes	Cerebral hemorrhages at young age, cerebral aneurysms; mild hypokalemia; high plasma aldosterone, low renin
Familial hyperaldosteronism	AD; unknown defect	Severe type 2 hypertension in early adulthood; high plasma aldosterone, low renin; no response to glucocorticoid treatment
Familial hyperaldosteronism type III	AD; unknown defect	Severe hypertension in childhood with extensive target-organ damage; high plasma aldosterone, low renin; marked bilateral adrenal enlargement
Congenital adrenal hyperplasia	AR mutations in 11β-hydroxylase or 21-hydroxylase	Hirsutism, virilization; hypokalemia and metabolic alkalosis; low plasma aldosterone and renin
Monogenic Primary Renal Tubular Defects		
Gordon syndrome	AD mutations of *KLHL3*, *CUL3*, *WNK1*, and *WNK4*; AR mutations of *KLHL3*	Hyperkalemia and metabolic acidosis with normal renal function
Liddle syndrome	AD mutations of the epithelial sodium channel	Hypokalemia and metabolic alkalosis; low plasma aldosterone and renin
Apparent mineralocorticoid excess	AD mutation in 11β-hydroxysteroid dehydrogenase type 2	Hypokalemia and metabolic alkalosis; low plasma aldosterone and renin
Geller syndrome	AD mutation in the mineralocorticoid receptor	Hypokalemia and metabolic alkalosis; low plasma aldosterone and renin; increased BP during pregnancy or exposure to spironolactone
Hypertension-brachydactyly syndrome	AD mutations in the phosphodiesterase E3A enzyme	
Unknown Mechanisms		
Hypertension-brachydactyly syndrome	AD	Short fingers (small phalanges) and short stature; brainstem compression from vascular tortuosity in the posterior fossa
Essential Hypertension		
	Polygenic	When obesity or metabolic syndrome is present, the likelihood of essential hypertension is higher

AD, Autosomal dominant; *ADPKD,* autosomal dominant polycystic kidney disease; *AR,* autosomal recessive; *ARPKD,* autosomal recessive polycystic kidney disease; *BP,* blood pressure; *eGFR,* estimated glomerular filtration rate; *GN,* glomerulonephritis; *IgA,* immunoglobulin A; *MEN,* multiple endocrine neoplasia; *PKD,* polycystic kidney disease; *SDH,* succinate dehydrogenase.
(From Skorecki K et al: *Brenner and Rector's the kidney,* ed 10, Philadelphia, 2016, Elsevier.)

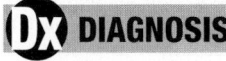 **DIAGNOSIS**

WORKUP

- The objective for the initial evaluation of HTN is to establish the diagnosis and stage of HTN. Table 3 summarizes initial laboratory evaluation of the hypertensive patient.
- Gather office and nonoffice BP readings, assess presence of target organ damage (TOD), assess the level of global cardiovascular disease risk and produce a plan for individualized monitoring and therapy.

- Patient counseling and education should be prominent features of the initial evaluation.
- Pertinent history:
  1. Age of onset of HTN, previous antihypertensive therapy
  2. Family history of HTN, stroke, cardiovascular disease
- Diet, salt intake, caffeine, alcohol, drugs (e.g., oral contraceptives, NSAIDs, decongestants, steroids)
- Occupation, lifestyle, pain, socioeconomic status, psychologic factors

- Other cardiovascular risk factors: hyperlipidemia, obesity, diabetes mellitus
- Symptoms of secondary HTN:
  1. Headache, palpitations, excessive perspiration (possible pheochromocytoma)
  2. Weakness, polyuria (consider hyperaldosteronism)
  3. Claudication of lower extremities (seen with coarctation of aorta)
  4. Loud snoring, day-time somnolence, morning confusion (may warrant evaluation for sleep apnea)

Diseases and Disorders

I

TABLE 3 Initial Laboratory Evaluation of the Hypertensive Patient to Investigate the Presence of Comorbid Conditions, Secondary Causes, or Established Target-Organ Damage

Test	Clinical Usefulness
Serum creatinine (and estimated glomerular filtration rate)	Assessment of renal function. Identifies parenchymal kidney disease as a possible secondary cause as well as established TOD.
Serum potassium	Low potassium (of renal origin) suggests mineralocorticoid excess (primary or secondary), glucocorticoid excess, Liddle syndrome. High potassium with normal renal function suggests Gordon syndrome. Low levels raise caution about the use of thiazides and loop diuretics. High levels preclude the use of ACEIs, ARBs, renin inhibitors, and potassium-sparing diuretics.
Serum sodium	If high, suggests primary aldosteronism. If low, alerts to the need to avoid thiazide diuretics.
Serum bicarbonate	If high, suggests aldosterone excess (primary or secondary). If low with normal renal function, suggests Gordon syndrome (with high potassium) or primary hyperparathyroidism (with high calcium).
Serum calcium	If high, suggests primary hyperparathyroidism.
Serum glucose	Identifies prediabetes or diabetes. In the appropriate setting, suggests glucocorticoid excess, pheochromocytoma, or acromegaly.
Lipid profile	Identifies hyperlipidemia.
Hemoglobin/hematocrit	If high, in the absence of other hematologic abnormalities or underlying lung disease, suggests sleep apnea.
Urinalysis*	Proteinuria and hematuria identify a possible secondary cause (glomerulonephritis). Proteinuria can also be a marker of TOD.
Electrocardiogram	Identifies left ventricular hypertrophy, old myocardial infarction, or other ischemic changes. Identifies conduction abnormalities that may preclude the use of β-blockers or nondihydropyridine CCBs.

The most recent guidelines do not recommend BUN measurement alone.
ACEI, angiotensin-converting enzyme inhibitor; *ARB,* angiotensin receptor blocker. *CCB,* calcium channel blocker; *TOD,* target-organ damage.
*Some organizations recommend screening microalbuminuria as a more sensitive tool to identify early renal injury.
From Skorecki K et al: *Brenner and Rector's the kidney,* ed 10, Philadelphia, 2016, Elsevier.

LABORATORY TESTS
- Routine laboratory tests recommended before initiating therapy include:
  1. Urinalysis with microscopic evaluation; for signs of glomerulopathy
  2. Basic metabolic panel and calcium; for signs of kidney damage, hypokalemia (primary aldosteronism and Cushing's syndrome), hypercalcemia (hyperparathyroid).
  3. Complete blood count.
  4. Screening for coexisting diseases that may adversely affect prognosis; hemoglobin a1c or fasting glucose level, serum lipid panel.
  5. Optional tests include measurement of urinary albumin or albumin/creatinine ratio.
- Nonoffice (home, workplace, 24-hr ambulatory) BP determination to establish the pattern of HTN (sustained, "white coat," or "masked" HTN) in selected patients.
- Some general clinical clues for when to screen for secondary HTN include:
  1. Severe or resistant HTN.
  2. An acute rise in BP developing in a patient with previous stable BP.
  3. Age less than 30 yr, non-obese, non-black with no family history of HTN.
  4. Sudden onset or accelerated hypertension.
  5. Age of onset before puberty. If above is suspected, additional tests for secondary

HTN should be done including renin, aldosterone, cortisol levels, 24-hr urine metanephrines, and serum catecholamines

IMAGING STUDIES
- ECG: check for presence of left ventricular hypertrophy (LVH) with strain pattern.
- Renal duplex ultrasonography, CT angiography or magnetic resonance angiography of the renal arteries in suspected renovascular hypertension (renal artery stenosis) may be considered.

(Rx) TREATMENT

NONPHARMACOLOGIC THERAPY
Lifestyle modifications (the initial treatment of hypertension should focus on lifestyle modifications):
- Weight loss if overweight (target BMI <25).
- Limit alcohol intake to 1 oz of ethanol per day (<2 drinks/day) in men or 0.5 oz (<1 drink/day) in women.
- Regular aerobic exercise (at least 30 min/day on most days).
- Reduce sodium intake to <100 mmol/day (<1.5 g of sodium/day).
- Maintain adequate dietary potassium (>3500 mg/day) intake in patients with normal kidney function.
- Smoking cessation.

- The BP reduction seen ranges from 2 to 20 mm Hg, most significant with substantial weight loss and the implementation of the Dietary Approaches to Stop Hypertension (DASH) eating plan, which relies on a diet high in fruits and vegetables, moderate in low-fat dairy products, and low in animal protein but with substantial amount of plant protein from legumes and nuts.

ACUTE GENERAL Rx
- Multiple recent consensus documents regarding blood pressure goals and when to initiate treatment have been published.
- According to AHA/ACC/CDC advisory algorithm, American Society of Hypertension/International Society of Hypertension (ASH/ISH), European Society of Hypertension and European Society of Cardiology (ESH/ESC), Canadian Hypertension Education Program (CHEP)[1]:
  ○ In patients age <80 yr old without diabetes or chronic kidney disease (CKD) or all ages with CKD, initiate therapy for BP ≥140/90 mm Hg (≥130/90 mm Hg in ESH/ESC). For patients ≥80 yr old without diabetes or CKD, initiate therapy for BP ≥150/90 mm Hg. For patients of all ages with diabetes, initiate therapy for BP ≥140/90 mm Hg (ASH/ISH), ≥140/85 mm Hg (ESH/ESC), and ≥130/80 mm Hg (CHEP).
- According to the writing group for JNC 8[2]:
  - In all patients, initiate pharmacologic treatment if diastolic BP is ≥90 mm Hg. In patients <60 years old, in diabetics, and in those with CKD, pharmacologic treatment should be initiated for systolic BP ≥140 mm Hg, whereas in patients ≥60 years, the threshold for pharmacologic treatment for systolic BP has been raised to ≥150 mm Hg.
  - In the general non-black population, preferred initial agents are thiazide-type diuretics, angiotensin-converting enzyme inhibitors (ACEi), calcium channel blockers (CCBs), or angiotensin receptor blockers (ARBs). ACEi or ARBs are preferred initial agents in diabetics and those with CKD in this population.
- Preferred initial agents in the black population (including diabetics) are thiazide-type diuretics or CCBs.
- When selecting drugs, try to give once per day dosages to improve compliance. Also consider the cost of the medication, metabolic and subjective side effects, and drug-drug interactions.
- All consensus guidelines agree that for patients <60 yr old without diabetes or CKD, target BP is <140/90 mm Hg, and

[1]Salvo M et al: Reconciling multiple hypertension guidelines to promote effective clinical practice. *Ann Pharmacother* 48:1242-8, 2014.
[2]James PA et al: 2014 Evidence-based guidelines for the management of high blood pressure in adults. Report from the panel members appointed to the eighth Joint National Committee (JNC8), *JAMA* 311(5):507-520, 2014.

for patients >80 yr old without diabetes or CKD, target BP is <150/90 mm Hg.

○ The major advantages and limitations of each class of drugs are described as follows:

1. Thiazide diuretics:
   a. Advantages: inexpensive, once-daily dosing. Useful in edematous states, CHF, chronic renal disease, elderly patients (decreased incidence of hip fractures in elderly patients)
   b. Disadvantages: significant adverse metabolic effects (hypokalemia), increased risk of cardiac arrhythmias, sexual dysfunction, gout flares, possible adverse effects on lipids and glucose levels

2. Beta-blockers:
   a. Advantages: ideal in hypertensive patients with ischemic heart disease or status post MI. Favored in hyperkinetic, young patients (resting tachycardia, wide pulse pressure, hyperdynamic heart) and stable CHF patients.
   b. Disadvantages: adverse effect on quality of life (increased incidence of fatigue, depression, impotence), bronchospasm, hypoglycemia, peripheral vascular disease, adverse effects on lipids, masking of signs and symptoms of hypoglycemia in diabetics.

3. Calcium antagonists:
   a. Advantages: helpful in hypertensive patients with ischemic heart disease. Generally favorable effect on quality of life; can be used in patients with bronchospastic disorders, renal disease, peripheral vascular disease, metabolic disorders, and salt sensitivity. CCBs BP-lowering effect is independent of Na^+ intake.
   b. Disadvantages: diltiazem and verapamil should be avoided in patients with CHF due to systolic dysfunction because of their negative inotropic effects; pedal edema may occur with nifedipine and amlodipine; constipation can be severe in elderly patients receiving verapamil. CCB-related edema is positional in nature, it improves with lying position; additional strategies include switching CCB classes, reducing dosage, giving the medication later in the day, and adding a venodilator (nitrates, an ACE, or an ARB); diuretics may improve edema, but at the expense of a reduction in plasma volume.

4. ACE inhibitors:
   a. Advantages: first-line therapy for patients with left ventricular dysfunction, helpful in prevention of diabetic renal disease; effective in decreasing LVH, and remodeling.
   b. Disadvantages: dry cough is a frequent side effect (5% to 20% of patients); hyperkalemia may occur in patients with diabetes or severe renal insufficiency; hypotension may occur in volume-depleted patients; increased risk of renal failure in patients with renal artery stenosis; contraindicated in pregnancy.

5. ARBs:
   a. Advantages: well tolerated, favorable impact on quality of life; useful in patients unable to tolerate ACE inhibitors because of persistent cough and in CHF and diabetic patients; single daily dose. An episode of renal insufficiency with ACE inhibitors does not rule out future therapy with an ARB unless high-grade bilateral renal artery stenosis exists.
   b. Disadvantages: hypotension may occur in volume-depleted patients; hyperkalemia; risk of renal failure in renal artery stenosis; contraindicated in pregnancy.

6. Alpha-adrenergic blockers:
   a. Advantages: no adverse effect on blood lipids or insulin sensitivity; helpful in benign prostatic hypertrophy.
   b. Disadvantages: postural hypotension, sedation; syncope can be avoided by giving an initial low dose at bedtime. Generally considered third- or fourth-line agent.

7. Central alpha-antagonists:
   a. Oral clonidine mainstay of therapy for hypertensive urgencies because of the ease of administration and relative safety.
   b. Transdermal clonidine; useful in management of labile HTN, the hospitalized patient who cannot take medications by mouth, and patients subject to early-morning BP surges. At equivalent doses, transdermal clonidine is more apt to precipitate salt and water retention than is the case with oral clonidine.
   c. Dose beyond 0.4 mg causes fatigue, sedation, dry mouth, salt and water retention, and rebound HTN upon abrupt termination of the medication.

8. Combined alpha- and beta-adrenergic receptor blockers:
   a. Labetalol, nebivolol, and carvedilol: Use is reserved to treat complicated hypertensive patient when an antihypertensive effect beyond beta-blockade is sought. IV labetalol is used for hypertensive emergencies. Carvedilol is shown to have less adverse effect on glycemic control than metoprolol and to reduce urinary protein excretion in hypertensive diabetic patients.

9. Direct-acting smooth muscle relaxant: Hydralazine
   a. Advantages: beneficial in black patients when used with isosorbide dinitrate.
   b. Disadvantages: may lead to reflex tachycardia, worsening ischemia (best used with nitrates), at higher doses or with renal failure can lead to a reversible drug-induced lupus.

10. Renin inhibitors: newest class of antihypertensives (Aliskiren):
    a. Advantages: generally well tolerated; once-daily dosing; can be used alone or in combination with other antihypertensive agents (avoid combining with ACEI or ARBs given increase of hyperkalemia)
    b. Disadvantages: contraindicated in pregnancy; should not be used in patients with impaired renal function; excessive cost; paucity of cardiovascular outcomes data showing benefit.

TREATMENT OF RENOVASCULAR HYPERTENSION: The therapeutic approach varies with the cause of the renovascular hypertension (RVH) (refer to "Renal Artery Stenosis" for additional information).

1. Young patients with fibromuscular dysplasia refractory to medical therapy can be treated with percutaneous transluminal renal angioplasty (PTRA).

2. Medical therapy is advisable in elderly patients with atheromatous RVH; useful agents are:
   a. Beta-blockers: highly effective in patients with elevated plasma renin
   b. ACE inhibitors: highly effective; however, should be avoided in patients with bilateral renal artery stenosis or with a solitary kidney and renal artery stenosis
   c. Diuretics: often used in combination with ACE inhibitors

3. Surgical revascularization: A recent trial revealed that renal-artery stenting does not confer a significant benefit with respect to the prevention of clinical events when added to comprehensive, multifactorial medical therapy in people with atherosclerotic renal-artery stenosis and hypertension or CKD.[3]

HTN DURING PREGNANCY:

1. HTN complicates 5% to 12% of all pregnancies.

2. The American Obstetrical Committee defines BP of 130/80 mm Hg as the upper limit of normal at any time during pregnancy.

3. A rise of 30 mm Hg systolic or 15 mm Hg diastolic is also considered abnormal regardless of the absolute values obtained.

4. Hypertension during pregnancy can be from chronic HTN, gestational HTN, preeclampsia or preeclampsia superimposed on chronic HTN. It is important to distinguish the etiology because the risk to mother and fetus is much greater in preeclampsia.

[3]Cooper CJ et al: Stenting and medical therapy for atherosclerotic renal-artery stenosis, *N Engl J Med* 370:13-22, 2014.

5. Treatment of chronic HTN during pregnancy is as follows:
   a. Initial treatment with conservative measures (proper nutrition, limited physical activity).
   b. When drug therapy is necessary, initiation of methyldopa, hydralazine, labetalol, or atenolol is preferred. Table 4 summarizes drugs used to treat hypertension in pregnancy.
   c. ACE inhibitors can cause fetal and neonatal complications; their use should be avoided in pregnancy.
   d. The safety of CCBs remains unclear.
   e. Diuretics should be used only if there is a specific reason for initiating and maintaining their use (e.g., HTN associated with severe fluid overload or left ventricular dysfunction).

MALIGNANT HTN, HYPERTENSIVE EMERGENCIES, AND HYPERTENSIVE URGENCIES: Definitions:
1. Malignant HTN occurs with HTN when there are grades III and IV retinopathy (exudates, hemorrhages and papilledema).
   a. The rate of BP rise is a critical factor in the development of malignant HTN.
   b. Complications and mortality rates are much higher in malignant HTN compared to essential HTN.
   c. Requires immediate BP reduction (not necessarily into normal ranges) to prevent or limit target organ disease.
2. Hypertensive emergencies is when the BP elevation causes evidence of impending or progressive organ dysfunction. It requires rapid lowering of BP to prevent end-organ damage.
3. Hypertensive urgencies are significant BP elevations without end-organ damage that should be corrected within 24 hrs of presentation.
   a. Patients are usually treated with oral antihypertensive medications.
   b. Most clinicians suggest lowering the BP to <160 mm Hg/<100 mm Hg or to a level no more than 30% lower than the patient's baseline BP.

Therapy: The choice of therapeutic agents varies with the cause. IV medications are preferred in hypertensive emergencies.
1. Nitroprusside is the drug of choice in hypertensive encephalopathy, HTN and intracranial bleeding, malignant HTN, HTN and heart failure, dissecting aortic aneurysm (used in combination with propranolol); its onset of action is immediate. Because it is metabolized to cyanide, patients should be carefully monitored for toxicity (mental status changes, acidemia).
2. Fenoldopam is a vasodilator agent useful for the short-term (up to 48 hr) management of severe HTN when rapid but quickly reversible reduction of BP is required. It should be avoided in patients with glaucoma.
3. Other commonly used agents are the IV CCBs nicardipine and clevidipine (useful for urgent treatment of HTN in the intensive care unit or operating room), the beta-blocker esmolol (useful in aortic dissection or postoperative HTN), labetalol (combined β-adrenergic and α-blocker useful in patients with coronary disease), phentolamine (useful for catechol-

amine-related emergencies), IV nitroglycerin (used in patients with cardiac ischemia and hypertensive crisis), and hydralazine (used for hypertensive emergencies in pregnancy).

4. Table 5 describes parenteral agents for management of hypertensive emergencies. *The following are important points to remember when treating hypertensive emergencies:*

TABLE 4 Drugs Used to Treat Hypertension in Pregnancy

Drug	Starting Dose	Maximum Dose	Comments
Acute Treatment of Severe Hypertension			
Hydralazine	5-10 mg IV every 20 min	20 mg*	Avoid in cases of tachycardia and persistent headaches
Labetalol	20-40 mg IV every 10-15 min	220 mg*	Avoid in women with asthma or congestive heart failure
Nifedipine	10-20 mg oral every 30 min	50 mg*	Avoid in case of tachycardia and palpitations
Long-Term Treatment of Hypertension			
Methyldopa	250 mg bid	4 g/day	
Labetalol	100 mg bid	2400 mg/day	
Nifedipine	10 mg bid	120 mg/day	
Thiazide diuretic	12.5 mg bid	50 mg/day	

*If desired blood pressure levels are not achieved, switch to another drug.
From Gabbe SG: *Obstetrics*, ed 6, Philadelphia, 2012, Saunders.

TABLE 5 Parenteral Agents for Management of Hypertensive Emergencies

Agent	Dose	Onset of Action	Precautions
Parenteral Vasodilators			
Sodium nitroprusside	0.25-10 mcg/kg/min IV infusion	Immediate	Thiocyanate toxicity with prolonged use
Nitroglycerin	5-100 mcg/min IV infusion	2-5 min	Headache, tachycardia, tolerance
Nicardipine	5-15 mg/hr IV infusion	1-5 min	Protracted hypotension after prolonged use
Fenoldopam mesylate	0.1-0.3 mcg/kg/min IV infusion	1-5 min	Headache, tachycardia, increased intraocular pressure
Hydralazine	5-10 mg as IV bolus or 10-40 mg IM; repeat every 4-6 hr	10 min IV 20 min IM	Unpredictable and excessive falls in blood pressure; tachycardia, angina exacerbation
Enalaprilat	0.625-1.25 mg every 6 hr IV bolus	15-60 min	Unpredictable and excessive falls in blood pressure; acute renal failure in patients with bilateral renal artery stenosis
Parenteral Adrenergic Inhibitors			
Labetalol	20-80 mg as slow IV injection every 10 min, or 0.5-2.0 mg/min IV as infusion	5-10 min	Bronchospasm, heart block, orthostatic hypotension
Metoprolol	5 mg IV every 10 min for three doses	5-10 min	Bronchospasm, heart block, heart failure, exacerbation of cocaine-induced myocardial ischemia
Esmolol	500 mcg/kg IV over 3 min; then 25-100 mg/kg/min as IV infusion	1-5 min	Bronchospasm, heart block, heart failure
Phentolamine	5-10 mg IV bolus every 5-15 min	1-2 min	Tachycardia, orthostatic hypotension

IM, Intramuscular; *IV*, intravenous.
From Andreoli TE et al: *Andreoli and Carpenter's Cecil essentials of medicine*, ed 8, Philadelphia, 2010, Saunders.

a. Introduce a plan for long-term therapy at the time of the initial emergency treatment.

b. Agents that reduce arterial pressure can cause the kidney to retain sodium and water; therefore the judicious administration of diuretics should accompany their use.

c. The initial goal of antihypertensive therapy is not to achieve a normal BP, but rather to gradually reduce the BP; cerebral hypoperfusion may occur if the mean BP is hypertension in patients with CKD.

Fig. 2 illustrates an evidence-based approach to blood pressure management in stage 3 or higher CKD.

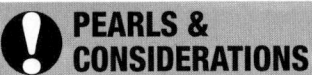 **PEARLS & CONSIDERATIONS**

COMMENTS

- For patients with prehypertension, every 20/10 mm Hg increase in BP doubles the risk of cardiovascular events.
- Most patients will require at least two medications for BP control.
- If BP is greater than 20/10 mm Hg above goal, therapy should be initiated with two drugs.

- Resistant HTN: HTN is considered resistant if the BP cannot be reduced below target levels in patients who are compliant with an optimal triple-drug regimen that includes a diuretic. Terms *refractory* and *resistant* are used interchangeably. Causes include pseudohypertension, measurement artifact, medication nonadherence, volume overload, and secondary HTN.
  1. Pseudohypertension in elderly: hardened and sclerotic artery is not compressible hence falsely elevates BP measurement artifact
  2. Measurement artifact: BP taken incorrectly (small cuff, improper support).

Fig. E3 describes an approach to patients with resistant HTN.

- Renal sympathetic denervation: A recent blinded trial did not show a significant reduction of systolic blood pressure in patients with resistant hypertension 6 mo after renal artery denervation as compared with a sham control.[4]

---

[4]Bhatt DL et al: A controlled trial of renal denervation for resistant hypertension, *N Engl J Med* 370:1393-1401, 2014.

- Fig. E4 describes an algorithm for evaluation of secondary causes of HTN.
- Barriers to BP control: system issues, provider issues; patient issues, and behavior issues. The rate at which physicians adopt recommended changes based on evidence-based findings can be quite slow and has been properly described as "clinical inertia."
- Indications for specialist referral for patients with HTN are described in Table E6.

SUGGESTED READINGS
Available at www.expertconsult.com

RELATED CONTENT
High Blood Pressure (Patient Information)
High Blood Pressure—Child (Patient Information)
Eclampsia (Related Key Topic)
Pre-Eclampsia (Related Key Topic)
Renal Artery Stenosis (Related Key Topic)

AUTHORS: **TANIA B. BABAR, M.D.,** and **CRAIG L. BASMAN, M.D.**

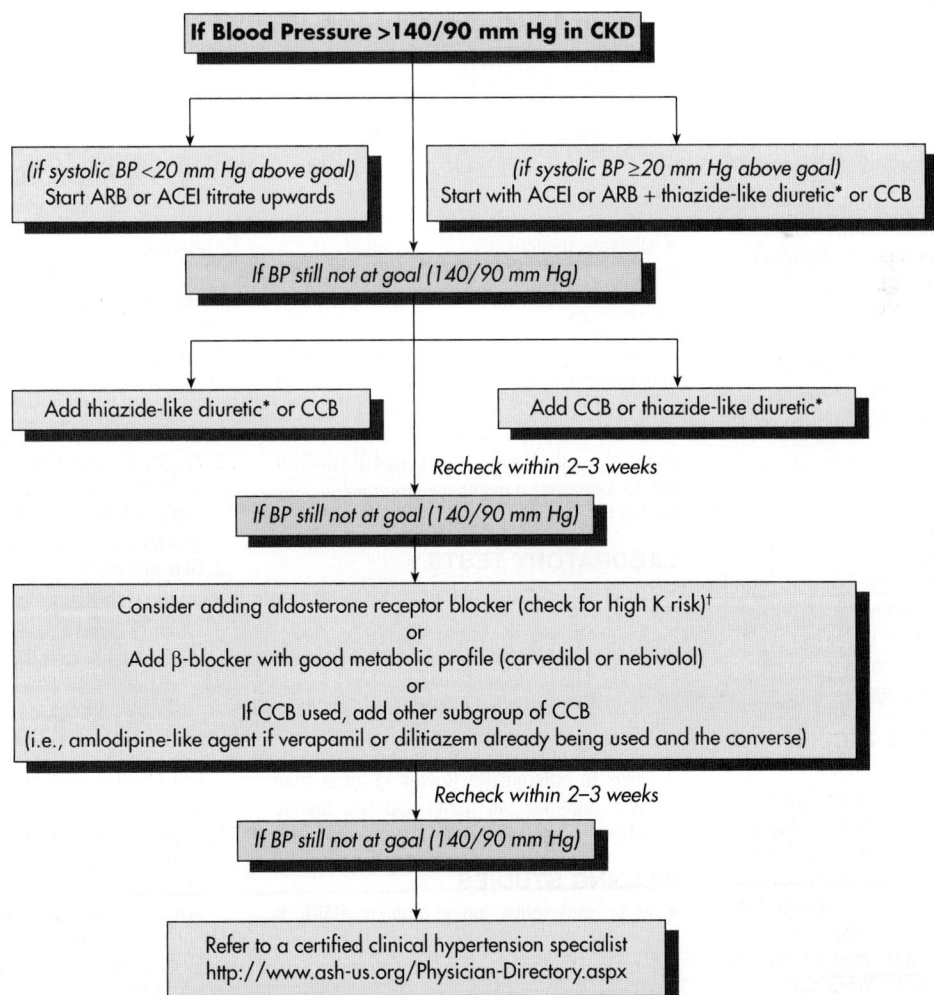

FIG. 2 An evidence-based approach to blood pressure management in stage 3 or higher chronic kidney disease, updated from the National Kidney Foundation consensus report. *Chlorthalidone or indapamide are preferred diuretics, as they work to achieve estimated glomerular filtration rate (eGFR) 30 ml/min. Below this GFR, torsemide, the long-acting loop diuretic, is preferred. †Risk for hyperkalemia—if on diuretic, eGFR <45 ml/min/1.73 m² or [K⁺]ₛ >4.5 mEq/L. *ACE,* angiotensin-converting enzyme; *ACEI,* angiotensin-converting enzyme inhibitor; *ARB,* angiotensin receptor blocker; *CCB,* calcium channel blocker. (From Skorecki K et al: *Brenner and Rector's the kidney,* ed 10, Philadelphia, 2016, Elsevier.)

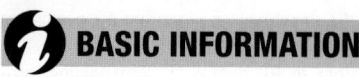

BASIC INFORMATION

DEFINITION

Hyperthyroidism is a hypermetabolic state resulting from excess thyroid hormone.

SYNONYMS

Thyrotoxicosis

ICD-10CM CODES

E05.00 Thyrotoxicosis with diffuse goiter without thyrotoxic crisis or storm
E05.01 Thyrotoxicosis with diffuse goiter with thyrotoxic crisis or storm
E05.10 Thyrotoxicosis with toxic single thyroid nodule without thyrotoxic crisis or storm
E05.11 Thyrotoxicosis with toxic single thyroid nodule with thyrotoxic crisis or storm
E05.20 Thyrotoxicosis with toxic multinodular goiter without thyrotoxic crisis or storm
E05.21 Thyrotoxicosis with toxic multinodular goiter with thyrotoxic crisis or storm
E05.30 Thyrotoxicosis from ectopic thyroid tissue without thyrotoxic crisis or storm
E05.31 Thyrotoxicosis from ectopic thyroid tissue with thyrotoxic crisis or storm
E05.40 Thyrotoxicosis factitia without thyrotoxic crisis or storm
E05.41 Thyrotoxicosis factitia with thyrotoxic crisis or storm
E05.80 Other thyrotoxicosis without thyrotoxic crisis or storm
E05.81 Other thyrotoxicosis with thyrotoxic crisis or storm
E05.90 Thyrotoxicosis, unspecified without thyrotoxic crisis or storm
E05.91 Thyrotoxicosis, unspecified with thyrotoxic crisis or storm
E06.2   Chronic thyroiditis with transient thyrotoxicosis

EPIDEMIOLOGY & DEMOGRAPHICS

INCIDENCE/PREVALENCE:

- Hyperthyroidism affects 2% of women and 0.2% of men in their lifetimes.
- Toxic multinodular goiter usually occurs in women >55 yr and is more common than Graves' disease in the elderly.

PHYSICAL FINDINGS & CLINICAL PRESENTATION

- Patients with hyperthyroidism generally present with tachycardia, tremor, hyperreflexia, anxiety, irritability, emotional lability, panic attacks, heat intolerance, sweating, increased appetite, diarrhea, weight loss, menstrual dysfunction (oligomenorrhea, amenorrhea). Presentation may be different in elderly patients (see the following).
- Patients with Graves' disease may present with exophthalmos, lid retraction, and lid lag (Graves' ophthalmopathy). The following signs and symptoms of ophthalmopathy may be present: blurring of vision, photophobia, increased lacrimation, double vision, and deep orbital pressure. Clubbing of fingers associated with periosteal new bone formation in other skeletal areas (Graves' acropachy) and pretibial myxedema may also be noted.
- Clinical signs of hyperthyroidism in the elderly may be masked by manifestations of coexisting disease (e.g., new-onset atrial fibrillation, exacerbation of congestive heart failure).

ETIOLOGY

- Graves' disease (diffuse toxic goiter): 80% to 90% of all cases of hyperthyroidism
- Toxic multinodular goiter (Plummer's disease)
- Toxic adenoma
- Iatrogenic and factitious
- Transient hyperthyroidism (subacute thyroiditis, Hashimoto's thyroiditis)
- Rare causes: hypersecretion of thyroid-stimulating hormone (TSH) (e.g., pituitary neoplasms), struma ovarii, ingestion of large amount of iodine in a patient with preexisting thyroid hyperplasia or adenoma (Jod-Basedow phenomenon), hydatidiform mole, carcinoma of thyroid, amiodarone therapy

DIAGNOSIS

DIFFERENTIAL DIAGNOSIS

- Anxiety disorder
- Pheochromocytoma
- Metastatic neoplasm
- Diabetes mellitus
- Premenopausal state

WORKUP

Suspected hyperthyroidism requires laboratory confirmation and identification of its etiology because treatment varies with cause. A detailed medical history will often provide clues to the diagnosis and etiology of the hyperthyroidism. Fig. E1 describes a diagnostic approach to suspected hyperthyroidism.

LABORATORY TESTS

- Elevated free thyroxine (T_4)
- Elevated free triiodothyronine (T_3): generally not necessary for diagnosis
- Low TSH (unless hyperthyroidism is a result of the rare hypersecretion of TSH from a pituitary adenoma)
- Thyroid autoantibodies useful in selected cases to differentiate Graves' disease from toxic multinodular goiter (absent thyroid antibodies)

IMAGING STUDIES

- 24-hr radioactive iodine uptake (RAIU) is useful to distinguish hyperthyroidism from iatrogenic thyroid hormone synthesis (thyrotoxicosis factitia) and from thyroiditis.
- An overactive thyroid shows increased uptake, whereas a normal underactive thyroid (iatrogenic thyroid ingestion, painless or subacute thyroiditis) shows normal or decreased uptake.
- The RAIU results also vary with the etiology of the hyperthyroidism:
  1. Graves' disease: increased homogeneous uptake
  2. Multinodular goiter: increased heterogeneous uptake
  3. Hot nodule: single focus of increased uptake
- RAIU is also generally performed before the therapeutic administration of radioactive iodine to determine the appropriate dose.

TREATMENT

NONPHARMACOLOGIC THERAPY

Patient education regarding thyroid disease and discussion of the therapeutic options. Patients should be informed that radioiodine, antithyroid drugs, and surgery are all reasonable treatment options for hyperthyroidism. It is crucial for the physician to have a detailed discussion with the patient about the benefits and risks relative to lifestyle, patients' values, and coexisting conditions.

ACUTE GENERAL Rx

ANTITHYROID DRUGS (THIONAMIDES): Propylthiouracil (PTU) and methimazole inhibit thyroid hormone synthesis by blocking production of thyroid peroxidase (PTU and methimazole) or inhibit peripheral conversion of T_4 to T_3 (PTU). Methimazole is favored by most endocrinologists because of the potential for hepatic failure with PTU. PTU is preferred in pregnant women during the first trimester because methimazole has been associated with aplasia cutis and with choanal and esophageal atresia. Complete blood count and differential should be obtained before their use.

1. Dosage: methimazole 15 to 30 mg/day given as a single dose; PTU 50 to 100 mg PO q8h.
2. Antithyroid drugs can be used as the primary form of treatment or as adjunctive therapy before radioactive therapy or surgery or afterward if the hyperthyroidism recurs.
3. Side effects: skin rash (3% to 5% of patients), arthralgias, myalgias, granulocytopenia (0.5%). Rare side effects are aplastic anemia, hepatic necrosis from PTU, cholestatic jaundice from methimazole.
4. When antithyroid drugs are used as primary therapy, they are usually given for 6 to 18 mo; prolonged therapy may cause hypothyroidism. Monitor thyroid function every 2 mo for 6 mo, then less frequently.
5. The use of antithyroid drugs before radioiodine therapy is best reserved for patients in whom exacerbation of hyperthyroidism after radioactive iodine therapy is hazardous (e.g., elderly patients with coronary artery disease or significant coexisting morbidity). In these patients the antithyroid drug can be stopped 2 days before radioactive iodine therapy, resumed 2 days later, and continued for 4 to 6 wk.

H

RADIOIODINE THERAPY (RADIOACTIVE IODINE [RAI; ^{131}I]):

1. RAI is the treatment of choice for patients aged >21 yr and younger patients who have not achieved remission after 1 yr of antithyroid drug therapy. RAI is also used in hyperthyroidism caused by toxic adenoma or toxic multinodular goiter.
2. Contraindicated during pregnancy (can cause fetal hypothyroidism) and lactation. Pregnancy should be excluded in women of childbearing age before RAI is administered.
3. A single dose of RAI is effective in inducing a euthyroid state in nearly 80% of patients.
4. There is a high incidence of post-RAI hypothyroidism (>50% within first year and 2%/yr thereafter); these patients should be frequently evaluated for the onset of hypothyroidism (see "Chronic Rx").

SURGICAL THERAPY (SUBTOTAL THYROIDECTOMY):

1. Indicated in obstructing goiters, in any patient who refuses RAI and cannot be adequately managed with antithyroid medications (e.g., patients with toxic adenoma or toxic multinodular goiter), and in pregnant patients who cannot be adequately managed with antithyroid medication or develop side effects to them. Thyroidectomy can also be considered as primary therapy in refractory cases of amiodarone-induced hyperthyroidism. Thyroidectomy is not indicated for low RAIU hyperthyroidism.
2. Patients should be rendered euthyroid with antithyroid drugs before surgery.
3. Complications of surgery include hypothyroidism (28% to 43% after 10 yr), hypoparathyroidism, and vocal cord paralysis (1%).
4. Most patients should be started on replacement doses of levothyroxine (1.7 mcg/kg/day) before discharge from hospital.
5. Hyperthyroidism recurs after surgery in 10% to 15% of patients.

ADJUNCTIVE THERAPY: Propranolol alleviates the beta-adrenergic symptoms of hyperthyroidism; initial dose is 20 to 40 mg PO q6h; dosage is gradually increased until symptoms are controlled. Major contraindications to propranolol are congestive heart failure and bronchospasm. Diagnosis and treatment of thyrotoxic storm are also discussed in Section I.

CHRONIC Rx

- Patients undergoing treatment with antithyroid drugs should be seen every 1 to 3 mo until euthyroidism is achieved and every 3 to 4 mo while they remain on antithyroid therapy. After treatment is stopped, periodic monitoring of thyroid function tests with TSH is recommended every 3 mo for 1 yr, then every 6 mo for 1 yr, then annually.
- Orbital decompression surgery can be used to correct Graves' orbitopathy (Fig. E2). The administration of the antioxidant selenium (100 mcg PO bid) has been recently reported as effective in improving quality of life, reducing ocular involvement, and slowing progression of the disease in patients with mild Graves' orbitopathy. Its mechanism of action is believed to be an effect on the oxygen free radicals and cytokines that play a pathogenic role in Graves' orbitopathy.

DISPOSITION

Successful treatment of hyperthyroidism requires lifelong monitoring for the onset of hypothyroidism or the recurrence of thyrotoxicosis.

REFERRAL

- Endocrinology referral is recommended at the time of initial diagnosis and during treatment.
- Surgical referral in selected patients (see "Surgical Therapy").
- Hospitalization of all patients with thyroid storm.

⊘ PEARLS & CONSIDERATIONS

COMMENTS

- Elderly hyperthyroid patients may have only subtle signs (weight loss, tachycardia, fine skin, brittle nails). This form is known as **apathetic hyperthyroidism** and manifests with lethargy rather than hyperkinetic activity. An enlarged thyroid gland may be absent. Coexisting medical disorders (most commonly cardiac disease) may also mask the symptoms. These patients often have unexplained congestive heart failure, worsening of angina, or new-onset atrial fibrillation resistant to treatment. See the topic "Graves' Disease" for additional information on diagnosis and treatment.
- Subclinical hyperthyroidism is defined as a normal serum-free thyroxine and free triiodothyronine levels with a TSH level suppressed below the normal range and usually undetectable. These patients usually do not present with signs or symptoms of overt hyperthyroidism. Treatment options include observation or a therapeutic trial of low-dose antithyroid agents for 6 mo to attempt to induce remission.
- ***Thyrotoxic periodic paralysis (TPP)*** is a hyperthyroidism-related hypokalemia and muscle-weakening condition resulting from a sudden shift of potassium into cells. Many patients do not have other symptoms of hyperthyroidism. Typical presentation involves an Asian adult male with acute fatigue and muscle weakness initially presenting in the lower extremities. Physical examination reveals decreased deep tendon reflexes, hypertension, and tachycardia. ECG often reveals U waves, high QRS voltage, and first-degree atrioventricular block. Additional laboratory testing reveals normal acid-base state, hypokalemia with low urinary potassium excretion (spot urinary potassium concentration <20 mEq/L from potassium shift into cells), hypophosphatemia, hypophostaturia, and hypercalciuria. Electromyography during attacks shows low-amplitude compound muscle action potential of the tested muscle. Therapy consists of cautious potassium supplementation (increased risk of rebound hyperkalemia). Use of nonselective beta-blockers (e.g., propranolol) to counteract hyperadrenergic activity, which may be causing TPP, may also be useful.

SUGGESTED READINGS

Available at www.expertconsult.com

RELATED CONTENT

Hyperthyroidism (Patient Information)
Graves' Disease (Related Key Topic)
Thyrotoxic Storm (Related Key Topic)

AUTHOR: **FRED F. FERRI, M.D.**

BASIC INFORMATION

DEFINITION

Hypertrophic osteoarthropathy (HOA) is a syndrome of clubbing of the digits, periostosis of long bones, abnormal proliferation of skin, and arthritis. Periostosis is usually involved with pain on palpation of the involved area. HOA may be primary or secondary to other underlying disease processes.

SYNONYMS

- Primary hypertrophic osteoarthropathy:
  1. Pachydermoperiostosis
  2. Idiopathic clubbing
  3. Touraine-Solente-Golé syndrome
- Secondary hypertrophic osteoarthropathy
- HOA

ICD-10CM CODES
M89.3	Hypertrophy of bone
M89.40	Other hypertrophic osteoarthropathy, unspecified site
M89.411	Other hypertrophic osteoarthropathy, right shoulder
M89.412	Other hypertrophic osteoarthropathy, left shoulder
M89.419	Other hypertrophic osteoarthropathy, unspecified shoulder
M89.421	Other hypertrophic osteoarthropathy, right upper arm
M89.422	Other hypertrophic osteoarthropathy, left upper arm
M89.429	Other hypertrophic osteoarthropathy, unspecified upper arm
M89.431	Other hypertrophic osteoarthropathy, right forearm
M89.432	Other hypertrophic osteoarthropathy, left forearm
M89.439	Other hypertrophic osteoarthropathy, unspecified forearm
M89.441	Other hypertrophic osteoarthropathy, right hand
M89.442	Other hypertrophic osteoarthropathy, left hand
M89.449	Other hypertrophic osteoarthropathy, unspecified hand
M89.451	Other hypertrophic osteoarthropathy, right thigh
M89.452	Other hypertrophic osteoarthropathy, left thigh
M89.459	Other hypertrophic osteoarthropathy, unspecified thigh
M89.461	Other hypertrophic osteoarthropathy, right lower leg
M89.462	Other hypertrophic osteoarthropathy, left lower leg
M89.469	Other hypertrophic osteoarthropathy, unspecified lower leg
M89.471	Other hypertrophic osteoarthropathy, right ankle and foot
M89.472	Other hypertrophic osteoarthropathy, left ankle and foot
M89.479	Other hypertrophic osteoarthropathy, unspecified ankle and foot
M89.48	Other hypertrophic osteoarthropathy, other site
M89.49	Other hypertrophic osteoarthropathy, multiple sites

EPIDEMIOLOGY & DEMOGRAPHICS

- Fig. 1 provides a classification of HOA.
- Primary HOA is a familial autosomal-dominant disease affecting the age group between 1 and 20 years and is rare.
- There is a male/female ratio of 9:1 in occurrence.
- Secondary HOA is more common, typically occurs in adults 55 to 75 years of age. 80% to 90% of secondary HOA is associated with non–small cell lung cancer, most frequently adenocarcinoma; other associated illnesses include:
  1. Pulmonary: mesothelioma, bronchogenic carcinoma, lung abscesses, empyema, bronchiectasis, cystic fibrosis, pulmonary fibrosis, sarcoidosis, arteriovenous malformations
  2. Gastrointestinal: Carcinoma of esophagus or colon, biliary atresia, peptic ulcer disease, inflammatory bowel disease, hepatocellular carcinoma, liver cirrhosis, amebiasis, laxative abuse, achalasia.
  3. Cardiac: infective endocarditis, right-to-left cardiac shunts, aortic aneurysms, infected aortic bypass graft
  4. Hematologic: thalassemia, myelofibrosis, Hodgkin lymphoma
  5. Endocrine: thyroid acropachy, POEMS syndrome (polyneuropathy, organomegaly, endocrinopathy, M component, and skin changes)
  6. Connective tissue diseases
  7. Thymoma
  8. HIV infection
  9. Osteosarcoma
  10. Nasopharyngeal sarcoma

PHYSICAL FINDINGS & CLINICAL PRESENTATION

- Primary HOA typically presents with the insidious onset of clubbing of the hands (Fig. 2) and feet, described as "spade-like." Finger clubbing is diagnosed by measurement of the digital index (Fig. 3). Other signs and symptoms of HOA include:
  1. Joint pain and swelling
  2. Sensation of warmth or burning in the hands and feet

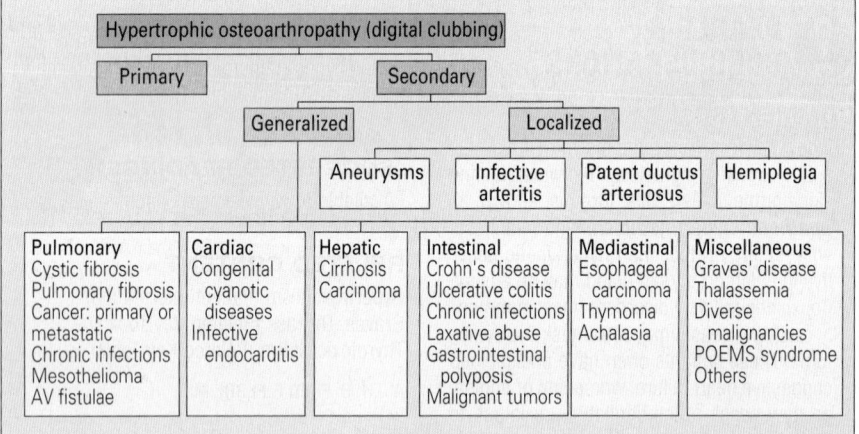

FIG. 1 Classification of hypertrophic osteoarthropathy. *AV,* Arteriovenous; *POEMS,* polyneuropathy, organomegaly, endocrinopathy, monoclonal proteins, and skin changes. (From Hochberg MC, et al.: *Rheumatology,* ed 5, St Louis, 2011, Mosby.)

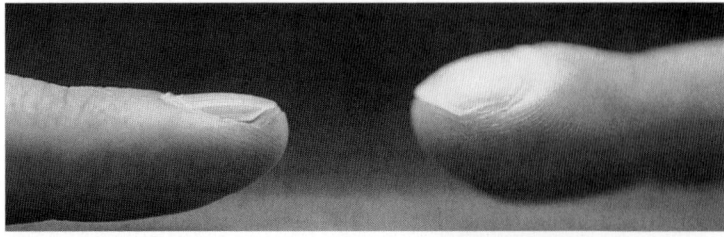

FIG. 2 Clubbing deformity. The finger on the right is clubbed compared with the normal finger shape on the left. (From Hochberg MC, et al.: *Rheumatology,* ed 5, St Louis, 2011, Mosby.)

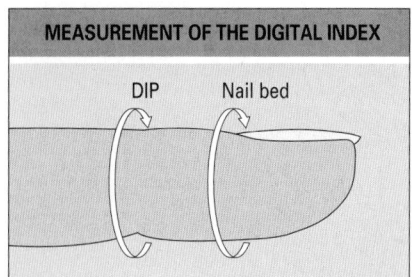

FIG. 3 The digital index. The perimeter of each of the 10 fingers is measured at the nail bed (NB) and at the distal interphalangeal joint (DIP). If the sum of the 10 NB:DIP ratios is more than 10, clubbing is probably present. (From Hochberg MC, et al.: *Rheumatology,* ed 5, St Louis, 2011, Mosby.)

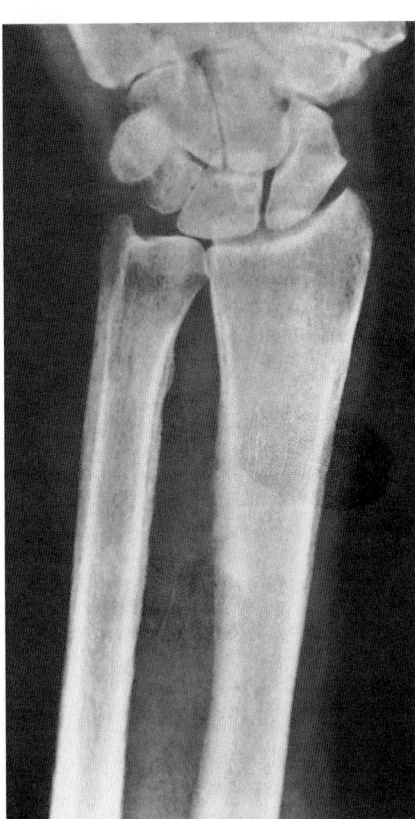

FIG. 4 Hypertrophic osteoarthropathy. Wrist radiograph showing periostosis at the distal ends of the radius and ulna. The coarse, layered appearance is most evident along the diaphyses. The relative sparing of the radial epiphyses is characteristic. (From Hochberg MC, et al.: *Rheumatology*, ed 5, St Louis, 2011, Mosby.)

3. Coarsening of facial features with grooves or depressions in the scalp, ptosis of the lids
4. Thickening of the arms and legs
5. Oily skin, diaphoresis, gynecomastia, and acne
6. Thin and shiny appearance of the skin around the nail bed
7. Nail convexity with nail "floating" sensation within the soft tissue is noticed on palpation of the base of the nail bed
8. Elephant legs: nonpitting soft tissue swelling with tenderness can be seen

- Secondary HOA patients may present with clinical symptoms before the underlying disorder can be detected. Signs and symptoms are similar to the previous symptoms in addition to findings related to the underlying disease (e.g., bronchogenic carcinoma, infective endocarditis).
- Patients presenting with painful joints prior to developing clubbing can be misdiagnosed as having inflammatory arthritis.

ETIOLOGY

The pathogenesis of HOA is not fully understood; current knowledge suggests that HOA results from the activation of one or more growth fac-

tors, such as vascular endothelial growth factor (VEGF) and platelet-derived growth factor, which are normally inactivated in the lungs and systemic circulation.

DX DIAGNOSIS

Diagnosis is primarily clinical; radiographs and bone scans can help confirm the diagnosis.

DIFFERENTIAL DIAGNOSIS

Paget's disease, reactive arthritis, psoriatic arthritis, syphilitic periostosis, osteoarthritis, rheumatoid arthritis, osteomyelitis, scleromyxedema, and acromegaly.

WORKUP

HOA warrants an investigation into any associated illnesses.

LABORATORY TESTS

- Routine laboratory studies such as blood count, electrolytes, and urine studies are typically normal in primary and secondary HOA.
- Erythrocyte sedimentation rate is elevated in secondary HOA.
- Liver function tests may be abnormal in patients with secondary HOA from gastrointestinal pathology.
- Alkaline phosphatase may be elevated as a result of periostosis of long bones.
- Analysis of the synovial fluid from joint effusions reveals a low white blood cell count with normal viscosity, color, and complement levels.

IMAGING STUDIES

- Radiographs of the long bones show periosteal new bone formation (Fig. 4).
- A chest radiograph should be obtained to rule out underlying lung cancer.
- Bone scan with technetium-99m reveals cortical uptake; SPECT/CT can increase specificity by excluding bony metastasis.
- Angiography findings may demonstrate hypervascularization of the finger pads.

RX TREATMENT

ACUTE GENERAL Rx

- Treatment of primary HOA is symptomatic. Nonsteroidal antiinflammatory medications, corticosteroids, tamoxifen citrate, or retinoids can be used.
- Colchicine can be helpful for the pain due to subperiosteal new bone formation.
- Reconstructive surgery is indicated for correction of gross disfigurement.
- Case reports of infliximab use and arthroscopic synovectomy with some relief in primary HOA are present.
- Treatment of secondary HOA is to eradicate the underlying disease (e.g., antibiotics for infective endocarditis, surgery for bronchogenic carcinoma). Correction of heart

malformation or removal of an underlying tumor is rapidly followed by regression of HOA.

CHRONIC Rx

In patients with secondary HOA refractory to NSAIDs and aspirin, octreotide (100 mcg subcutaneously twice daily) and bisphosphonates, including pamidronate (1 mg/kg intravenously to a maximum of 60 mg) and zoledronic acid, which inhibit VEGF expression, have significantly reduced pain.

Vagotomy has been tried with some success. However, the definitive treatment is to treat the underlying disease.

DISPOSITION

- Patients with primary HOA typically have symptoms of joint pain and swelling for the early part of their life. However, the disease becomes quiescent thereafter.
- Prognosis and disease course in patients with secondary HOA will depend on the underlying cause. The insidious development of clubbing suggests an infectious process, whereas the rapid progression of clubbing may suggest underlying malignancy.

REFERRAL

Referral should be made to rheumatology when the diagnosis of HOA is suspected and the cause remains unclear.

! PEARLS & CONSIDERATIONS

Some cases of primary HOA may later be found to be associated with an underlying disease such as patent ductus arteriosus, Crohn's disease, or myelofibrosis, in which case they become secondary.

COMMENTS

- Infections and intrathoracic malignancies are the most common causes of secondary HOA.
- The periostosis and the extent of involvement do not depend on the form of the disease (primary or secondary), but rather on its duration.
- HOA secondary to infection of an arterial graft has been reported.

SUGGESTED READINGS

Available at www.expertconsult.com

AUTHOR: **DURKHANI MAHBOOB, M.D.**

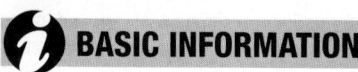

BASIC INFORMATION

DEFINITION

Hyperuricemia may be defined as serum uric acid >7.0 mg/dl in males or >6.0 mg/dl in females. Some persons who are not hyperuricemic by this definition will have levels of uric acid that exceed the limit of solubility of uric acid in tissue. Data from the Framingham study indicate that hyperuricemia increased from 4.8% of the population in the early 1970s to 9.3% in the mid-1980s. Age is an important risk factor in the increasing incidence of hyperuricemia and gout. Women become hyperuricemic at an older age than men due to the uricosuric effect of estrogen. Most people with hyperuricemia are asymptomatic and will remain so; however, 20% of those with serum uric acid >9 mg/dl will develop gout in 5 yr. Hyperuricemia is strongly associated with gout, obesity, diabetes, hypertension, and cardiovascular disease but has not been proven to cause any of these conditions.

ASYMPTOMATIC HYPERURICEMIA

Definition: laboratory evidence of elevated serum uric acid without clinical disease known to be caused by hyperuricemia

ETIOLOGY

Overproduction of uric acid accounts for a minority of cases of hyperuricemia. Most cases are due to decreased renal clearance of uric acid and high dietary purine consumption. Fig. E1 describes factors affecting urate balance. Table 1 describes a classification of hyperuricemia and gout.

ICD-10CM CODES
E79.0 Hyperuricemia without signs of inflammatory arthritis and tophaceous disease

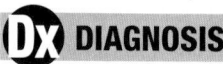 DIAGNOSIS

EVALUATION

The finding of hyperuricemia should prompt a thorough evaluation of potential causes and related diseases. Fig. 2 describes the evaluation of patients with hyperuricemia. If there is no clinical evidence of gout, nephrolithiasis, or acute kidney injury, the patient may be said to have asymptomatic hyperuricemia. Potential causes of elevated uric acid include malignancy, renal insufficiency, toxins, lead toxicity, and dietary indiscretion. If a careful history and physical exam does not reveal an evident cause of persistent hyperuricemia, a

---

TABLE 1 Classification of Hyperuricemia and Gout

Impaired Uric Acid Excretion
Primary gout with decreased uric acid clearance
Secondary gout
Clinical conditions
Reduced glomerular filtration rate
Hypertension
Obesity
Systemic acidosis
Familial juvenile hyperuricemic nephropathy
Medullary cystic kidney disease
Lead nephropathy
Drugs
Diuretics
Ethanol
Low-dose salicylates (0.3-3.0 g/day)
Cyclosporine
Tacrolimus
Levodopa

Excessive Urate Production
Primary metabolic disorders
HPRT deficiency
PRPP synthetase overactivity
Glucose-6-phosphatase deficiency
Fructose-1-phosphate aldolase deficiency
Secondary causes
Clinical conditions
Myelo- and lymphoproliferative disorders
Obesity
Psoriasis
Glycogenoses III, V, VII
Drugs and dietary components
Nicotinic acid
Pancreatic extract
Cytotoxic drugs
Red meat, organ meat, shellfish
Alcoholic beverages (especially beer)
Fructose

HPRT, Hypoxanthine-guanine phosphoribosyltransferase; *PRPP*, phosphoribosyl pyrophosphate.
From Goldman L, Schafer AI: *Goldman's Cecil medicine*, ed 24, Philadelphia, 2012, Saunders.

24-hr urine collection for uric acid and creatinine may be considered. Patients with urinary excretion of uric acid >800 mg/24 hr are likely to be overproducers of uric acid and should be investigated more thoroughly for the underlying cause of their hyperuricemia.

LABORATORY TESTS
- CBC with differential.

- BUN/creatinine.
- Urinalysis.
- Lipid profile.
- Consider 24-hr urine collection for uric acid.

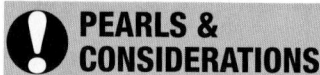 TREATMENT

No specific therapy is indicated for most patients with asymptomatic hyperuricemia. Lifestyle and dietary modification are often advisable.

NONPHARMACOLOGIC THERAPY
- Weight loss
- Reduce alcohol intake, especially beer
- Reduce consumption of foods known to be high in purines such as red meat, organ meat, and high-fructose soft drinks.

PEARLS & CONSIDERATIONS

- Research suggests there may be a causal relationship between hyperuricemia and early hypertension.
- Very high levels of serum uric acid may warrant treatment even if asymptomatic.
- Patients with hyperuricemia and a family history of gout should be followed closely for the development of gouty arthritis.
- Hyperuricemia in patients with gout (Fig. E3) should almost always be treated with urate-lowering medication (see "Gout").
- The presence of gouty tophi or arthritis due to gout are absolute indications for urate-lowering therapy.

There is evidence from several sources suggesting that treatment of hyperuricemia slows the progression of chronic kidney disease in patients without gout. Recent studies have suggested that allopurinol use is associated with a reduced risk of myocardial infarction and reduction in all-cause mortality. These preliminary studies have sparked renewed interest in research to evaluate the effects of treatment of asymptomatic hyperuricemia in hopes of improving the many disease states associated with high levels of serum uric acid.

SUGGESTED READINGS
Available at www.expertconsult.com

RELATED CONTENT
Gout (Related Key Topic)

AUTHOR: **BERNARD ZIMMERMANN, M.D.**

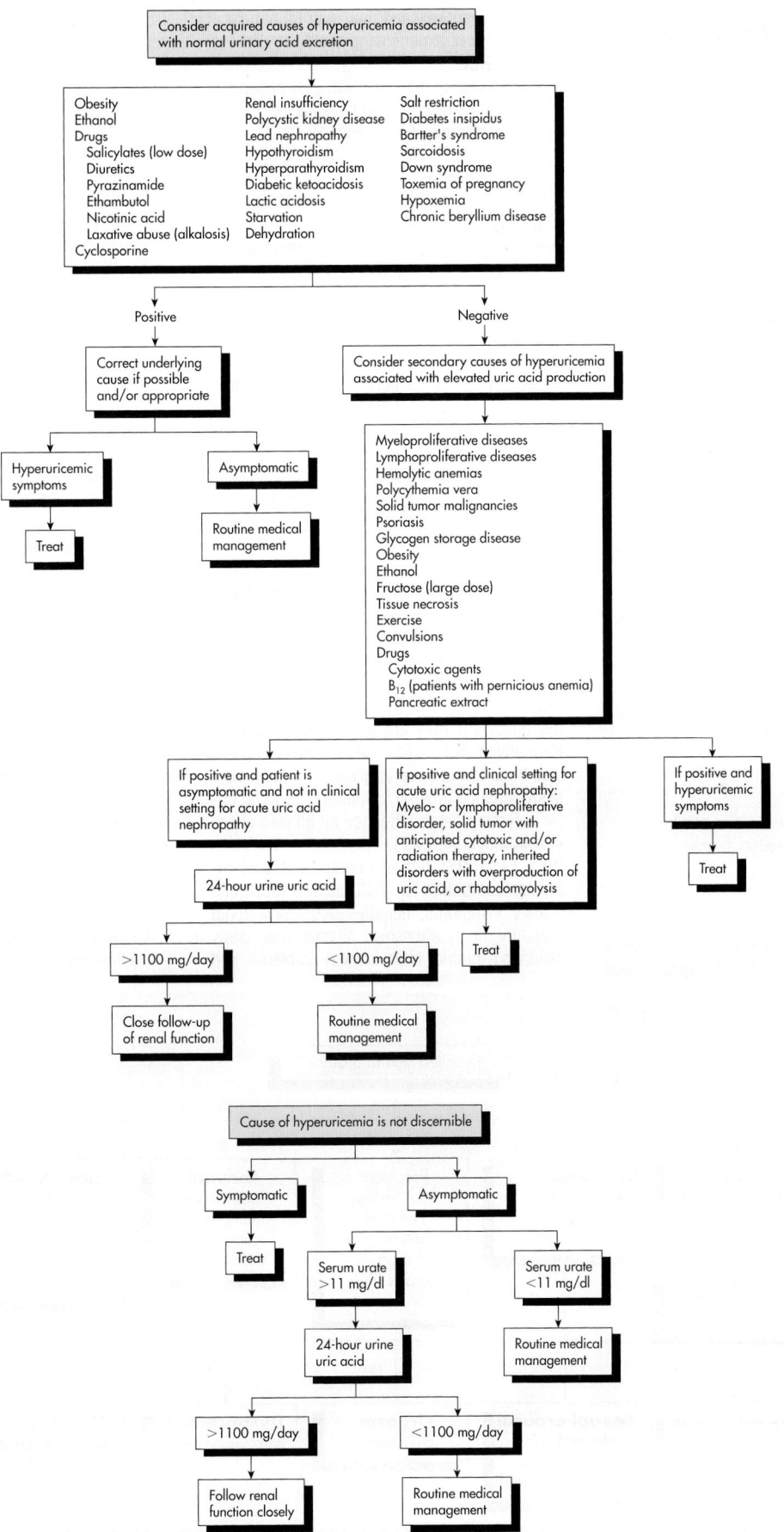

FIG. 2 Evaluation of patients with hyperuricemia. (From Harris ED et al, eds: *Kelley's textbook of rheumatology,* ed 7, Philadelphia, 2005, Saunders.)

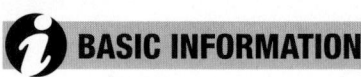

BASIC INFORMATION

DEFINITION

- Persistently or recurrently diminished or absent sexual/erotic thoughts or fantasies and desire for sexual activity.
- The judgment of deficiency is made by the clinician taking into account factors related to age, social context, and general contexts of the individual's life.
- Symptoms must have been present for a minimum of 6 months, the majority of the time, and be distressing to the individual.
- The lack of desire must not be better explained by a nonsexual mental disorder or by a severe relationship distress or other significant stressor.
- Must also not be better attributable to substance/medication or another medical condition.

SYNONYMS

Subsumed in female sexual interest/arousal disorder
Hypoactive sexual desire disorder, situational
Psychosexual desire disorder, situational hypoactive
Psychosexual dysfunction associated with inhibited libido
Psychosexual dysfunction with inhibited libido
Situational hypoactive sexual desire disorder
HSDD

ICD-10CM CODES
F52.0   Hyperactive sexual desire disorder
F52.22 Female sexual arousal disorder

EPIDEMIOLOGY & DEMOGRAPHICS

PEAK INCIDENCE: Prevalence of low sexual desire increases with age. Middle-aged women (45 to 65 years old) and men over 60 appear at greatest risk of experiencing qualifying distress.

PREVALENCE:
- Among males, rates of HSDD vary depending on country of origin and means of assessment. Generally, 6% of men 18-24 and 41% of men 66-74 report problems with sexual desire. Persistent lack of sexual interest that lasts longer than 6 months is seen in approximately 1.8% of men 16-44.
- For women, rates of HSDD are more uncertain, especially given the new inclusion of HSDD into female sexual interest/arousal disorder. Prior studies with less stringent criteria suggest approximately 36% of women endorse low sexual desire, but roughly only 8% report experiencing clinical levels of related distress. These rates also vary by country of origin and method of assessment (Fig. 1).

PREDOMINANT SEX AND AGE: HSDD appears to be more prevalent in women; however, men are more likely to be underdiagnosed or misdiagnosed with another sexual dysfunction.

GENETICS: There appears to be a strong influence of genetics in the vulnerability of women to sexual dysfunction. Specifically, women with the ll genotype for the SCL6A4 promoter region (5HTTLPR) appear to be eight times more likely to have selective serotonin reuptake inhibitor (SSRI) associated sexual dysfunction if they are also taking oral contraceptives. Men with the ll genotype have also been found to be at greater risk of sexual dysfunction. Similarly, dopamine (D4) receptor polymorphisms influence all phases of the sexual response cycle.

RISK FACTORS: Temperamental and environmental risk factors for HSDD include mood and anxiety symptoms, negative cognitions about sexuality or relationship, alcohol use, early childhood trauma, interpersonal problems, and lack of adequate sex education. Physiological risk factors include age, medical conditions such as diabetes mellitus, thyroid dysfunction, hyperprolactinemia, coronary disease, renal failure, and androgen deficiency, as well as other neuroendocrine changes.

PHYSICAL FINDINGS & CLINICAL PRESENTATION

- HSDD can be lifelong or acquired as well as generalized or situational.
- Men appear more likely to present with the acquired, situational subtype.
- For women, lack of pleasure is a common presenting clinical complaint.
- Consideration of initiation of sexual activity and receptivity to sexual activity initiated by the partner should be assessed. Men are often more likely to initiate sexual encounters, and noninitiation may be a signifier of a possible problem, but any shift in pattern of initiation should be investigated further.
- Other sexual activities such as masturbation or partnered sexual activity may still occur even in the context of low sexual desire.
- The interpersonal context of HSDD should be taken into account, as often a desire discrepancy between partners leads to discussions of possible HSDD, but this is not sufficient for diagnosis.
- Symptoms should be present for approximately 6 months, but clinical judgment can be used if symptoms are of lesser duration.

ETIOLOGY

- Best evidence suggests a multifactorial etiology, including factors along the biopsychosocial continuum including genetic vulnerability, interpersonal distress, cultural factors, mental health, medical conditions, and medical treatments.

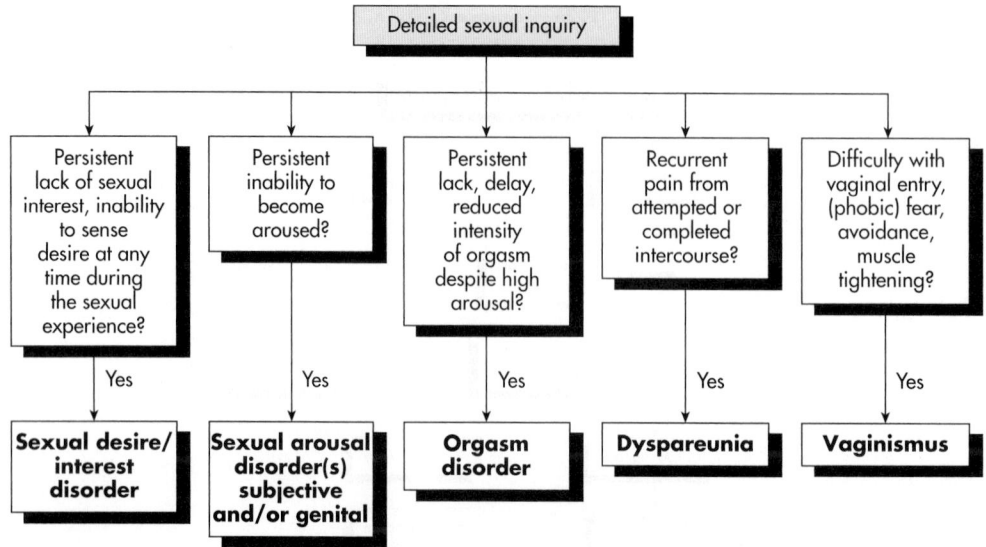

FIG. 1 Currently recommended definitions for women's sexual dysfunction. Comorbidity is usual, especially sexual desire/interest disorder with one of the sexual arousal disorders. (From Melmed S et al: *Williams textbook of endocrinology*, ed 12, Philadelphia, 2011, Saunders.)

Dx DIAGNOSIS

DIFFERENTIAL DIAGNOSIS

If low sexual desire can be attributed largely to one of these factors, HSDD should not be diagnosed, and the underlying factor should be addressed.

- Nonsexual mental disorder: depression, anxiety, posttraumatic stress disorder, and schizophrenia
- Substance/medication use: drugs of abuse (e.g., alcohol), anticonvulsants (e.g., carbamazepine), cardiovascular and antihypertensive agents (e.g., clonidine), hormonal medications (e.g., oral contraceptives), and psychotropic medications (e.g., SSRIs).
- Another medical condition: endocrine disorders (e.g., diabetes mellitus), coronary artery disease, cancer, central nervous system disease, hypertension, and arthritis.
- Interpersonal factors: relationship discord, partner sexual problems, dissatisfaction with partner or relationship, communication deficits, and intimate partner violence.
- Other sexual dysfunctions: erectile disorder, female orgasmic disorder, and genitopelvic pain/penetration disorder.

WORKUP

- Clinical interview should include a sexual history, medical history, and psychosocial history. The sexual history should include questions about prior sexual issues, sexual behavior and practices, and patient's treatment goals.
- A physical examination may be warranted for some female patients to identify possible contributing factors to low desire such as vulvovaginal atrophy, genital sensory changes, and pelvic floor prolapse.
- Symptom of depression and anxiety should be assessed. This can be done with brief screeners such as the PHQ-9 and GAD-7.
- Adequate endocrine functioning can be assessed through a combination of history taking (e.g., menstrual patterns) and laboratory tests when warranted by history.
- Self-rating scales and standardized symptom-specific checklist may be helpful in diagnosis and determining treatment. Example screeners include The Brief Sexual Symptom Checklist (BSSC), The Decreased Sexual Desire Screener (DSDS), and Female Sexual Function Index (FSFI).

LABORATORY TESTS

- Laboratory tests should be undertaken if indicated by history or physical exam.
- Common tests include
  - Thyroid function, serum total testosterone, prolactin, follicle-stimulating hormone (FSH), and luteinizing hormone (LH).

Rx TREATMENT

NONPHARMACOLOGIC THERAPY

- Multimodal interventions are often needed to address the complex etiology of HSDD.
- Basic sex education can be a valuable in-office intervention that can alleviate distress that arises from unrealistic norms or misunderstandings related to basic reproductive anatomy and physiology.
- Simple suggestions related to reducing stress, increasing communication with partner, and leading a healthy lifestyle can help to improve sexual function for some.
- Patients should be referred for psychological intervention when medical rule-outs have been completed. Therapist should have experience with treating sexual problems.
- The number of controlled trials studying the efficacy of psychological treatment for HSDD is limited; however, available evidence suggests significant improvements with the use of cognitive behavioral therapy, traditional sex therapy, or both.
- There is support for both individual- and couple-based treatments.

ACUTE GENERAL Rx

- Currently, only one FDA-approved treatment exists for HSDD: flibanserin (Addyi). Addyi is a multifunctional serotonin agonist/antagonist that passes through the blood-brain barrier and selectively affects the prefrontal cortex. Addyi has been shown to increase the number of satisfying sexual events per month.
- Addyi is contraindicated for use with moderate and strong CYP3A4 inhibitors, with alcohol, and in patients with hepatic impairments. Side effects include dizziness, somnolence, fatigue, and nausea.
- Bupropion hydrochloride is a mild dopamine and norepinephrine reuptake inhibitor and nicotinic acetylcholine receptor antagonist that is used as an antidepressant and smoking cessation aid. There is some empirical evidence for off-label use suggesting that bupropion significantly increases sexual desire in nondepressed women. It has also been shown to be effective in reversing SSRI-induced sexual dysfunction.
- Testosterone is widely prescribed off-label for postmenopausal women, with substantial evidence suggesting testosterone therapy improves sexual well-being among postmenopausal women. There is limited evidence for similar effects among premenopausal women.
- Testosterone is a well-established treatment for men with HSDD secondary to low testosterone.

COMPLEMENTARY & ALTERNATIVE MEDICINE

- Recent studies have shown good preliminary efficacy of treating both sexual arousal and desire disorders with mindfulness, yoga, and meditation as a complement to psychotherapy.

DISPOSITION

- HSDD is a common sexual dysfunction that affects both men and women across the life span. With appropriate identification and treatment, many patients will experience improvement in sexual desire; however, finding appropriate referrals and support for patients may be challenging.
- Specific types of HSDD can resolve in time untreated if a patient's contextual factors change (e.g., new partner), but for others HSDD will persist or worsen without treatment.
- Patients may be at higher risk for relationship discord and other psychiatric disorders such as depression and anxiety.

REFERRAL

- Most patients presenting with HSDD would benefit from referral to a therapist skilled in treating sexual problems.
- Patients with unresolved physical or sexual trauma should be promptly referred to a specialist.
- Establishing a referral network of specialists in sexual medicine and therapy is important.

! PEARLS & CONSIDERATIONS

- Biological and psychological factors often co-mingle and contribute to the individual picture of HSDD.
- Linguistic and cultural variations can heavily impact the presentation of HSDD and the associated distress as well as treatment.
- New FDA-approved medication Addyi is highly controversial among sexual medicine specialists.
- Discussions of potential sexual side effects of medications and of general sexual health with all patients will allow for more open conversations when problems do arise.

SUGGESTED READINGS

Available at www.expertconsult.com

RELATED CONTENT

Ejaculation and Orgasm Disorders (Related Key Topic)
Sexual Dysfunction in Women (Related Key Topic)

AUTHOR: **KARLENE CUNNINGHAM, PH.D.**

Diseases and Disorders

H

I

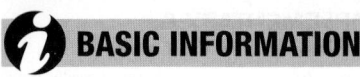

BASIC INFORMATION

DEFINITION

Hypoaldosteronism is defined as an aldosterone deficiency or impaired aldosterone function.

ICD-10CM CODES
E27.40 Unspecified adrenocortical insufficiency
E27.3 Drug-induced adrenocortical insufficiency
E27.9 Disorder of adrenal gland, unspecified
E27.1 Primary adrenocortical insufficiency
E27.40 Unspecified adrenocortical insufficiency
E27.49 Other adrenocortical insufficiency

EPIDEMIOLOGY & DEMOGRAPHICS

Selective hypoaldosteronism accounts for as many as 10% of cases of unexplained hyperkalemia.

PHYSICAL FINDINGS & CLINICAL PRESENTATION

- Physical examination may be entirely within normal limits.
- Hypertension may be present in some patients.
- Profound muscle weakness and cardiac arrhythmias may be present.

ETIOLOGY

- Hyporeninemic hypoaldosteronism (renin-angiotensin dependent): decreased aldosterone production as a result of decreased renin production; the typical patient has renal disease attributable to various factors (e.g., diabetes mellitus, interstitial nephritis, multiple myeloma, HIV infection, urinary tract obstruction, aging) and medications (NSAIDs, COX-2 inhibitors, ACEI/ARBs).
- Hyperreninemic hypoaldosteronism (renin-angiotensin independent): renin production by the kidneys is intact; the defect is in aldosterone biosynthesis or in the action of angiotensin II. Common causes of this form of hypoaldosteronism are medications (ketoconazole, heparin), lead poisoning, aldosterone enzyme defects, and severe illness.

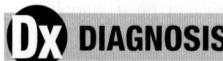

DIAGNOSIS

DIFFERENTIAL DIAGNOSIS

Pseudohypoaldosteronism: renal unresponsiveness to aldosterone. In this condition both renin and aldosterone levels are elevated. Pseudohypoaldosteronism can be caused by medications (spironolactone), chronic interstitial nephritis, systemic disorders (systemic lupus erythematosus, amyloidosis), or primary mineralocorticoid resistance.

WORKUP

Measurement of plasma renin activity after 4 hr of upright posture can differentiate hyporeninemic from hyperreninemic causes. Renin levels in the normal or low range identify cases that are renin-angiotensin dependent, whereas high renin levels identify cases that are renin-angiotensin independent. The diagnosis and etiology of hypoaldosteronism can be confirmed with the renin-aldosterone stimulation test:
- Hyporeninemic hypoaldosteronism: low stimulated renin and aldosterone levels
- End-organ refractoriness to aldosterone action: high stimulated renin and aldosterone levels
- Adrenal gland abnormality: high stimulated renin and low aldosterone levels

LABORATORY TESTS

- Increased potassium, normal or decreased sodium
- Hyperchloremic metabolic acidosis (caused by the absence of hydrogen-secreting action of aldosterone)
- Increased BUN and creatinine (secondary to renal disease)
- Hyperglycemia (diabetes mellitus is common in these patients)

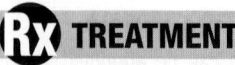

TREATMENT

NONPHARMACOLOGIC THERAPY

- Low-potassium diet with liberal sodium intake (at least 4 g of sodium chloride per day)
- Avoidance of ACE inhibitors and potassium-sparing diuretics

ACUTE GENERAL Rx

- Judicious use of fludrocortisone (0.05 to 0.1 mg PO every morning) in patients with aldosterone deficiency associated with deficiency of adrenal glucocorticoid hormones
- Furosemide 20 to 40 mg qd to correct hyperkalemia of hyporeninemic hypoaldosteronism

DISPOSITION

Prognosis varies with the etiology of hypoaldosteronism and presence of associated disorders.

REFERRAL

Endocrinology referral for renin-aldosterone stimulation test

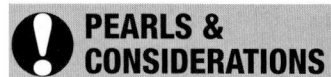

PEARLS & CONSIDERATIONS

COMMENTS

Treatment of pseudohypoaldosteronism is the same as for hypoaldosteronism; however, effect is limited because of impaired renal sensitivity.

AUTHOR: **FRED F. FERRI, M.D.**

BASIC INFORMATION

DEFINITION

- Hypocomplementemic urticarial vasculitis (HUV) is the term used to describe patients with urticarial vasculitis and hypocomplementemia who do not meet diagnostic criteria for hypocomplementemic urticarial vasculitis syndrome.
- In general, patients with HUV have cutaneous disease and few or no systemic manifestations.

SYNONYMS

Urticarial vasculitis
Hypocomplementemic urticarial vasculitis syndrome
HUV

ICD 10CM CODES
M31.8 Hypocomplementeric vasculitis

EPIDEMIOLOGY & DEMOGRAPHICS

INCIDENCE:
- Urticarial vasculitis (UV) is a rare diagnosis.
- The incidence and prevalence of the disorder are uncertain.

PEAK INCIDENCE:
- The peak reported incidence is in the fourth decade of life.

PREVALENCE:
- The prevalence of UV in patients with chronic urticaria varies from 5% to 20%.

PREDOMINANT SEX AND AGE:
- Women comprise 60% to 80% of reported patients.
- UV has also been described in children; the youngest reported case occurred in a patient 1 year of age.

GENETICS:
- A study including two families with autosomal-recessive HUVS found that mutations in DNASE1L3 were associated with a familial form of HUVS and HUVS associated with SLE.

RISK FACTORS:
- The association with some disorders in which the antigen-antibody complexes are well defined (e.g., hepatitis B, hepatitis C), and the observation that removal of immune complexes by plasmapheresis is temporally associated with the resolution of the urticarial lesions.
- Medications and viruses (particularly hepatitis B and C) have been implicated as the target antigen in some cases.
- There have also been reports demonstrating the development of UV in association with infliximab, glatiramer acetate, and the injection of hyaluronic acid.

PHYSICAL FINDINGS & CLINICAL PRESENTATION

- **Dermatologic**: The urticarial lesions (or wheals) of urticarial vasculitis (UV) can be found anywhere on the body. Urticarial lesions are typically more pruritic than painful and can be associated with angioedema, purpura, and livedo reticularis.
- **Musculoskeletal**: Arthralgias and arthritis are the most common systemic manifestation of UV. Joint pain is usually migratory and transient, frequently affecting the hands, elbows, feet, ankles, and knees.
- **Renal**: Renal disease is characterized by proteinuria and hematuria. The renal disease of UV includes proliferative glomerulonephritis, focal necrotizing vasculitis, crescentic glomerulonephritis, membranoproliferative glomerulonephritis, and tubulointerstitial nephritis. The renal involvement of UV tends to be more severe in children.
- **Pulmonary**: Pulmonary involvement is a leading cause of morbidity and mortality in UV and may include cough, dyspnea, hemoptysis, chronic obstructive pulmonary disease (COPD), asthma, pleuritis, and pleural effusions. The most common pulmonary manifestations are COPD and asthma.
- Smoking accelerates pulmonary parenchymal destruction by helping to recruit neutrophils. Thus, patients with UV should not smoke and should avoid secondhand smoke.
- **Gastrointestinal**: GI symptoms include substernal pain, abdominal pain, nausea, vomiting, and diarrhea. Hepatomegaly and splenomegaly have been reported.
- **Ophthalmologic**: Ophthalmologic symptoms include episcleritis, uveitis, and conjunctivitis. A rare case of serpiginous choroidopathy with subsequent blindness was reported; optic atrophy has been reported also.
- **Cardiovascular**: Symptoms include pericarditis, tamponade, valvular disease, and pericardial effusion.
- **Neurologic**: Central nervous system (CNS) involvement includes pseudotumor cerebri (the most common CNS manifestation), aseptic meningitis, cranial nerve palsies, peripheral neuropathy, and transverse myelitis.

ETIOLOGY

- HUV results from the formation of immune complexes in the blood that then deposit in vessel walls.
- In some patients with UV (particularly those with hypocomplementemic urticarial vasculitis), a collagen-like region on C1q has been implicated as the antigenic target.
- The autoantibody is referred to as a C1q precipitin.
- Once antigen-antibody complexes have formed, they can activate the classical complement pathway. This generates C3a and C5a, which cause mast cell degranulation resulting in urticarial eruptions. C3a and C5a also cause increased vessel permeability and chemotaxis of neutrophils.
- Infiltrating neutrophils release proteolytic enzymes, causing further tissue destruction and edema.
- IL-1 may play a role in the pathogenesis of UV.

DIAGNOSIS

DIFFERENTIAL DIAGNOSIS
- Common urticarial
- Erythema multiforme
- Neutrophilic urticarial dermatosis
- Acquired angioedema

WORKUP

LABORATORY TESTS: The most common abnormal laboratory results associated with urticarial vasculitis (UV) include:
- Elevated erythrocyte sedimentation rate (ESR)
- Hypocomplementemia (usually decreased C1q, C3, and C4)
- Circulating immune complexes by the C1q solid phase test and/or anti-C1q antibody assay
- Positive antinuclear antibodies (ANA)
- Anti-double stranded DNA (ds-DNA)
- Anti-Ro, -La, -Sm, and -RNP antibodies
- Anti-neutrophil cytoplasmic antibodies (ANCA), particularly enzyme immunoassays for antibodies to proteinase-3 and myeloperoxidase (PR3- and MPO-ANCA)
- Rheumatoid factor and/or anti-cyclic citrullinated peptides (anti-CCP)
- Immunofixation electrophoresis
- Cryoglobulins and cryofibrinogens
  Skin biopsy: Leukocytoclasis, or fragmentation of leukocytes with nuclear debris, and fibrinoid deposits are important histopathologic findings that represent direct signs of vessel damage. Immunofluorescence reveals deposits of immunoglobulins, complement, or fibrin around blood vessels in most patients.

TREATMENT

GENERAL Rx
- UV is often difficult to treat, and therapy is based upon case reports and small series.
- Systemic glucocorticoids are considered the mainstay of therapy for UV, and additional agents are typically added.
- Antihistamines are used to manage pruritus.
- Glucocorticoids in combination with either dapsone, colchicine, or hydroxychloroquine are typically used as initial therapy for patients with mild to moderate disease.
- For patients with refractory symptoms or those with organ- or life-threatening disease manifestations, other agents in combination with glucocorticoids are recommended: mycophenolate mofetil, methotrexate, azathioprine, and cyclosporine; rarely, cyclophosphamide, rituximab, anakinra, canakinumab, and omalizumab are used.
- The assistance of a rheumatologist with experience in the management of vasculitides is suggested for patients with evidence of significant systemic disease.

DISPOSITION

Patients with hypocomplementemia have severe disease and may experience significant morbidity and mortality; however, they rarely die as a direct result of the disease, even in the setting of multisystem involvement

Pulmonary involvement is a leading cause of morbidity and mortality, due largely to complications of COPD

REFERRAL

Rheumatology, dermatology, pulmonary critical care, cardiology, nephrology

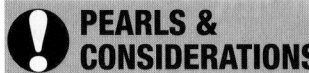

PEARLS & CONSIDERATIONS

- UV is a clinicopathologic entity consisting of urticaria and evidence of leukocytoclastic vasculitis on skin biopsy.
- UV predominantly involves the skin but may affect other organs, particularly the lungs, kidney, and gastrointestinal tract.

- Hypocomplementemia, when present, may be associated with extensive vasculitis and systemic features.
- The pathophysiology of UV is believed to involve the deposition of immune complexes in vessel walls, complement activation, and mast cell degranulation due to C3a and C5a with resultant urticaria
- The diagnosis of UV requires the presence of urticaria with leukocytoclastic vasculitis (LCV) on skin biopsy.
- If LCV is present, further testing is indicated to define the presence and extent of systemic disease and to evaluate for associated conditions.
- UV is a benign and self-limited disease for the majority of patients, although symptoms can last for decades in some individuals.

SUGGESTED READING

Available at www.expertconsult.com

AUTHOR: **CATHERINE E. NAJEM, M.D.**

BASIC INFORMATION

DEFINITION

Male hypogonadism is a clinical syndrome involving subnormal testosterone levels and/or impaired sperm production due to dysfunction at one or both levels of the hypothalamic-pituitary-testicular axis.

SYNONYMS

Testicular dysfunction

ICD-10CM CODES

E29	Testicular dysfunction
E29.1	Testicular hypofunction
E29.8	Other testicular dysfunction
E29.9	Testicular dysfunction, unspecified
E23.0	Hypopituitarism
E23.1	Drug-induced hypopituitarism
E89.3	Postprocedural hypopituitarism

EPIDEMIOLOGY & DEMOGRAPHICS

INCIDENCE: Hypogonadism is the most common clinical disorder of the testis. Incidence is unclear due to the many possible underlying factors, nonspecificity of symptoms, and questions relating to the adequacy of a diagnostic serum total testosterone threshold.

PREVALENCE: Prevalence of hypogonadism increases with aging, obesity, diabetes mellitus, and other comorbidities. The average decrease in serum total testosterone levels in aging men is 1% to 2% per year. Prevalence rises to 23% among men in their 70s. However, in population-based surveys of community-dwelling middle-aged and older males, prevalence of hypogonadism is approximately 6%.

GENETICS: Genetic abnormalities underlie a number of hypogonadal disorders including Klinefelter syndrome, Noonan syndrome, hemochromatosis, Kallmann syndrome, and Prader-Willi syndrome.

RISK FACTORS: These are many and include genetic abnormalities; the aging process; pituitary and testicular lesions and disorders; medications; drug abuse; HIV disease; acute illnesses; chronic cardiac, hepatic, renal, and pulmonary diseases; cancer; ionizing radiation; chemotherapy; obesity; and malnutrition.

PHYSICAL FINDINGS & CLINICAL PRESENTATION

Sexual (specific)
- Decrease in frequency of erections
- Erectile dysfunction
- Decrease in libido
- Decreased fertility
- Small or shrinking testes
- Gynecomastia
- Diminished sexual hair
- Hot flushes and sweats

Neuropsychologic (less specific)
- Depression
- Inability to concentrate
- Diminished motivation and vitality

- Decrease in self-confidence
- Diminished energy and stamina
- Sleep disturbances

Physical features and findings
- Diminished capacity for physical activity
- Decrease in physical endurance and performance
- Diminished muscle mass and strength
- Increase in body fat
- Decrease or loss of axillary and pubic hair and decrease in shaving frequency
- Fine wrinkling over the lateral aspects of the face
- Breast enlargement with or without tenderness
- Change in consistency and decrease in size of testes
- Fragility fractures
- Anemia

ETIOLOGY

- The importance of a careful history and examination cannot be overstated to determine the etiology of possible hypogonadism. Primary hypogonadism is a result of a decrease in testicular testosterone secretion and/or a decrease in spermatogenesis with an associated increase in gonadotropin levels as in Klinefelter syndrome, cryptorchidism, and following orchitis, testicular trauma, chemotherapy, and irradiation.
- Secondary hypogonadism is due to hypothalamic-pituitary dysfunction, which results in a decrease in testosterone levels and/or spermatogenesis with gonadotropin levels that are subnormal or inappropriately within the normal range.
- Combined primary and secondary hypogonadism is a result of deficits at both the level of the hypothalamic-pituitary axis and testes with variable gonadotropin levels depending upon the predominance of the level of the defect.

DIAGNOSIS (FIG. 1)

DIFFERENTIAL DIAGNOSIS

Hypogonadotropic or secondary hypogonadism
- Pituitary dysfunction—hypopituitarism, functioning or nonfunctioning pituitary tumor, lymphocytic hypophysitis, infiltrative disease as with sarcoidosis, hemochromatosis, and histiocytosis X
- Hyperprolactinemia—prolactinoma, medication-related, chronic kidney disease
- Genetic—Kallmann syndrome with anosmia, Prader-Willi syndrome with morbid obesity
- Acute and chronic illnesses, malnutrition, emotional disorders, HIV, sleep apnea, aging, malignancies, obesity, and renal, hepatic, pulmonary, and cardiac diseases
- Opioids, CNS—active medications, glucocorticoid excess, and GnRH analogues (androgen deprivation therapy)
Hypergonadotropic or primary hypogonadism
- Genetic—Klinefelter syndrome, Noonan syndrome, myotonic dystrophy
- Gonadal damage due to drugs, alcohol, radiation, chemotherapy, trauma

- Congenital anorchia (vanishing testis syndrome)
- Cryptorchidism
- Mumps orchitis, HIV orchitis
- Diabetes mellitus
- Hodgkin's disease
- Aging
Combined primary and secondary hypogonadism
- Hemochromatosis, sickle cell disease, thalassemia
- Alcoholism, glucocorticoid therapy, aging
- Chronic cardiac, hepatic, renal, pulmonary diseases, and HIV disease

WORKUP

- Determine the presence or absence of male hypogonadism on the basis of history, clinical manifestations and findings, and documentation of consistently low serum total testosterone levels and/or abnormal seminal fluid analysis.
- Morning serum total testosterone levels should be measured on at least 2 or 3 occasions for confirmation of diagnosis and when necessary followed by measurement of serum free or bioavailable testosterone.
- Serum FSH and LH levels are measured to determine whether hypogonadism is primary, secondary, or a result of combined defects of the hypothalamic-pituitary axis and testis. The case of testosterone deficiency should be definitively determined before initiation of testosterone replacement therapy.
- Hormonal assessment of gonadal status should not be done during an acute or subacute illness.

LABORATORY TESTS

- Serum total testosterone is tightly bound to sex hormone binding globulin (SHBG) and weakly bound to circulating albumin. 0.5% to 3% of serum total testosterone is unbound or free.
- Liquid chromatography tandem mass spectrometry assays for total serum testosterone are more accurate than immunoassays.
- Bioavailable testosterone refers to unbound testosterone plus the testosterone that is loosely bound to albumin.
- Free testosterone, if necessary, is best measured by equilibrium dialysis or centrifugal ultrafiltration.
- An SHBG measurement is helpful in determining the adequacy or normality of a serum total testosterone measurement. Conditions that lower SHBG include obesity, protein-losing states, androgens, hypothyroidism, and familial SHBG deficiency. Increases in SHBG occur in those with hyperthyroidism, hepatitis, cirrhosis, and HIV disease, aging, and by estrogens.
- The lower limit of normal for serum total testosterone in a healthy young male is approximately 240 to 280 ng/dl and a low-normal serum free testosterone in a young normal male is 9 pg/ml.
- Serum total testosterone levels can vary from day-to-day and there is a diurnal rhythm in

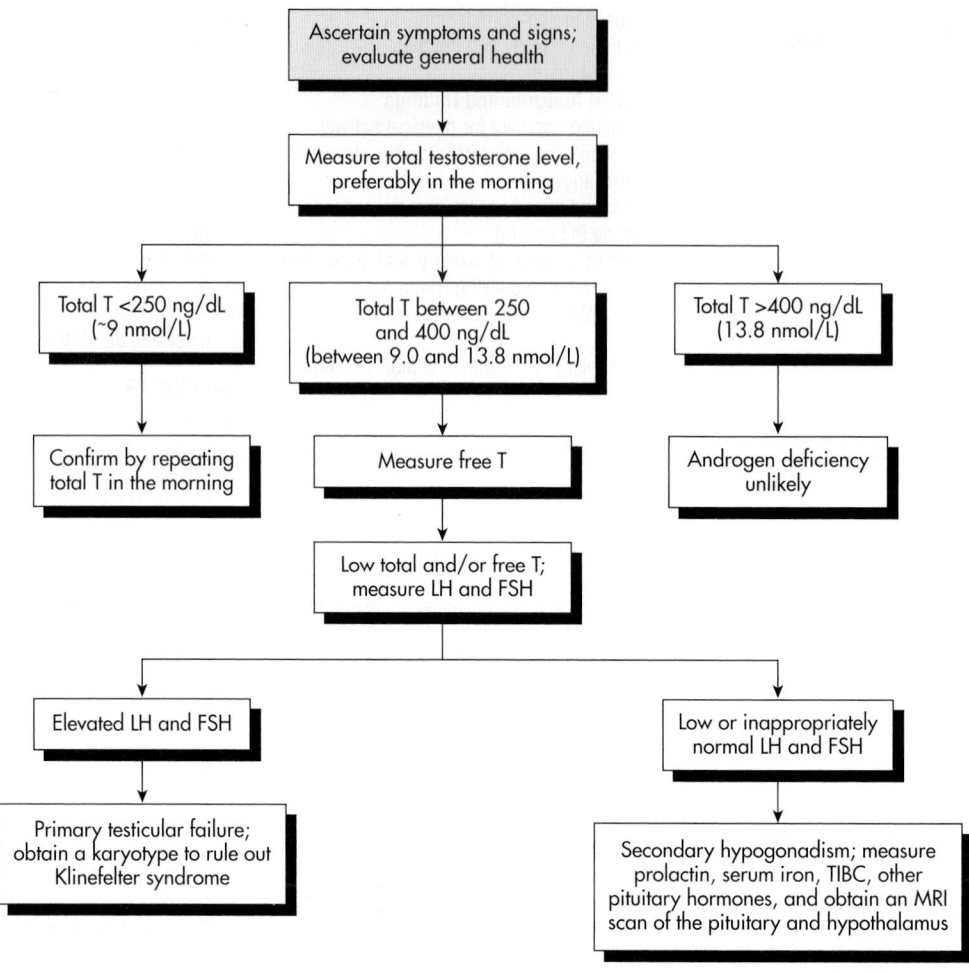

FIG. 1 Algorithm showing an approach for the diagnostic evaluation of adult men suspected of having androgen deficiency. (From Shalender B, Shehzad B: Diagnosis and treatment of hypogonadism in men, *Best Pract Res Clin Endocrin* 25(2):251-270, 2011.)

young normal males with morning levels that are higher by approximately 20% to 25% as compared with levels in the afternoon.

- In elderly males, the diurnal rhythm is diminished with levels approximately 10% lower in the afternoon as compared with morning levels.
- Serum FSH and LH measurements are important in delineating primary, secondary, and combined hypogonadism.
- Hypogonadal symptoms are more likely to be seen in those with total serum testosterone level below the lower limit of values for young normal males. Serum total testosterone levels of <150 ng/dl are unequivocally low.
- Transient suppression of total serum testosterone may occur during acute illness, in males that are being treated with glucocorticoid, in those taking opiates or CNS-active medications, in those with malnutrition or poor eating habits, and during excessive physical exercise.
- Quantity and quality of sperm counts and activity can vary in a significant way for a variety of reasons. Therefore, in assessing fertility, seminal fluid analysis should be done on two or more occasions each separated by two or more weeks and on semen collected within an hour of ejaculation after more than two days of abstinence.

- Depending on the clinical picture and examination, other studies may be necessary including a karyotype analysis, for example, for Klinefelter syndrome, or serum prolactin measurement for patients with possible hyperprolactinemia which may be drug-induced, related to a prolactinoma, or to chronic renal disease.

IMAGING STUDIES

- In males with severe androgen deficiency with low serum gonadotropin levels, increased serum prolactin levels, hypopituitarism, severe headaches, and visual defects, an MRI of the pituitary would be appropriate. In males with hypogonadism and a history of fractures, DXA measurements of spine and hip should be obtained to further delineate the status of the skeletal system.

Ⓡⓧ TREATMENT

- Testosterone replacement therapy is indicated when patients have symptoms and signs of hypogonadism and serum testosterone levels that are consistently subnormal with levels of <250 ng/dl. The goal of replacement therapy is to restore serum testosterone levels to within the normal range of values

and to have a positive effect on the constellation of hypogonadal symptoms and signs. Subnormal spermatogenesis, if present in such patients, is not affected by testosterone therapy. In patients with hypogonadotropic or secondary hypogonadism, chorionic gonadotropin and/or GnRH therapy can optimize spermatogenesis, whereas, generally in patients with primary hypogonadism, subnormal spermatogenesis and infertility are irreversible.

NONPHARMACOLOGIC THERAPY

- Weight reduction, especially when it appears to be a major factor underlying male hypogonadism.
- Discontinuation of anabolic steroids, CNS-active medications, and narcotic abuse.
- Surgery or radiation therapy for patients with a pituitary functioning or nonfunctioning tumor with visual field abnormality and headaches who are not candidates for further medical therapy or have been unsuccessfully treated with medication.
- Surgery indicated for chronic gynecomastia and, occasionally, in cases with recent-onset gynecomastia that has not responded to testosterone replacement therapy.

CHRONIC THERAPY

Testosterone formulations:

- Parenteral testosterone preparations:
  1. Testosterone enanthate (generic) and testosterone cypionate (Depo-Testosterone and generic) 150 to 200 mg are injected intramuscularly every 2 weeks. Following injections, there are appreciable fluctuations in serum testosterone, with levels rising within the first several days and a subsequent decrease to normal and in some cases to below normal at the end of the two weeks. As a result of the varying levels of testosterone, patients may have related symptoms. Adjustments in dose and dosing interval may help to alleviate the serum fluctuations and clinical symptoms. Testosterone undecanoate (AUEFD-ENDO) is an injectable depot formulation FDA-approved for male hypogonadism. The recommended dosage is 750 mg injected IM at 0 and 4 wk, and then every 10 wk thereafter.
- Topical testosterone preparations:
  1. Testosterone adhesive patch (Androderm) delivers 2.5 or 5 mg of testosterone when applied nightly to the back, abdomen, upper arms, or thighs. Serum testosterone levels rise to within normal range in a few hours after application and, thereafter, are relatively stable. Daily doses of up to 10 mg may be necessary.
  2. Testosterone 1% gels (AndroGel and Testim). Androgel is available in 2.5 g and 5 g gel units that deliver 2.5 mg and 5 mg of testosterone, respectively. The gel is applied daily in the morning by hand over the shoulder, upper arms, or abdomen. Adjustments in dose to 7.5 g or 10 g of gel may be necessary to optimize serum testosterone levels. AndroGel (1.62%) pump is also available for daily application. Testim is available in 5 g and 10 g tubes and with morning applications over the shoulders or arms delivers 5 mg and 10 mg of testosterone, respectively. Both AndroGel and Testim provide relatively stable serum testosterone levels. Two new transdermal formulations, Fortesta and Axiron, are now available and are applied daily by metered dose pumps. With these preparations, care is necessary to avoid skin-to-skin contact exposure with others.
- Testosterone pellets:
  1. 3 to 6 pellets of testosterone each containing 75 mg of testosterone are surgically inserted subcutaneously every 3 to 6 months and provide relatively stable serum testosterone levels.

RISKS AND ADVERSE EFFECTS

- Contraindications to testosterone therapy include prostate cancer and breast cancer. Relative contraindications include severe benign prostatic hyperplasia, hematocrit ≥50% at baseline, sleep apnea, and severe congestive heart failure.
- Patients on chronic testosterone therapy need to be followed carefully with prostate and PSA assessments and hematocrit measurements for possible excessive induction of erythrocytosis, initially at 3 to 6 months and at regular intervals thereafter.

REFERRAL

Endocrinology for full endocrine and metabolic assessment and therapy. Urology for further assessment and follow-up of the prostate and for evaluation and therapy of erectile dysfunction. Neurosurgery for evaluation and possible surgery for a pituitary lesion. Plastic surgery for chronic gynecomastia. Reproductive endocrinology for those with an infertility problem.

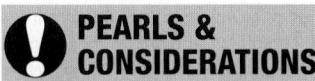

PEARLS & CONSIDERATIONS

COMMENTS

- Male hypogonadism is an important and frequently encountered problem that requires a complete medical history, examination, and hormonal assessment to determine whether a patient has hypogonadism and requires testosterone replacement therapy. Treated patients need to be seen on a regular basis to avoid possible testosterone adverse effects. Patients requiring testosterone replacement should have testosterone, prostate specific antigen, and hematocrit levels monitored.
- A recent trial to evaluate the effects of testosterone treatment in older men revealed that in symptomatic men 65 years of age or older, raising testosterone concentrations for 1 year from moderately low to the mid-normal range had a moderate benefit with respect to sexual function and some benefit with respect to mood and depressive symptoms but no benefit with respect to vitality or walking distance.[1]
- Controversy exists regarding the safety of testosterone replacement therapy following reports of increased risk of cardiovascular events. However, a recent trial among men with androgen deficiency dispensed testosterone prescriptions revealed lower risk of cardiovascular outcomes over a median follow-up of 3.4 years.[2]
- Clinical trials have also demonstrated that testosterone replacement in men with low testosterone increases volumetric bone mineral density (vBMD) and estimated bone strength more in trabecular than peripheral bone and more in the spine than the hip.[3]

AUTHOR: **JOSEPH R. TUCCI, M.D.**

[1]Snyder PJ, et al.: Effects of testosterone treatment in older men, *N Engl J Med* 374:611–624, 2016.
[2]Cheetham TC, et al.: Association of testosterone replacement with cardiovascular outcomes among men with androgen deficiency, *JAMA Int Med* 177(4):491–499, 2017.
[3]Synder PJ, et al.: Effect of testosterone treatment on volumetric bone density and strength in older men with low testosterone, *JAMA Int Med* 177(4):471–479, 2017.

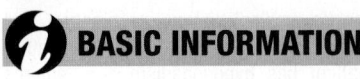

DEFINITION

In its broadest sense, hyponatremia is defined as a measured serum sodium concentration (S_{Na}) less than the lower limit of normal, that is, less than 135 mEq/L in most clinical labs. Since the clinical manifestations of hyponatremia are actually due to hypotonicity, appropriate clinical management depends on correctly distinguishing between the majority of patients with hypotonic hyponatremia from patients who are either hypertonic or who have pseudohyponatremia (low measured S_{Na} due solely to laboratory artifact). For the remainder of this chapter, hyponatremia will be used synonymously with hypotonic hyponatremia. Pseudohyponatremia and hypertonic hyponatremia will be identified specifically by those names.

SYNONYMS

Low serum sodium concentration
Hypo-osmolality

ICD-10CM CODES
E87.1 Hypo-osmolality and hyponatremia

EPIDEMIOLOGY & DEMOGRAPHICS

PREVALENCE: The prevalence of hyponatremia varies widely according to setting and population age. In the general US population captured by the NHANES data base there was an overall prevalence of 1.72%. One study of patients coming to an Emergency Department reported a prevalence of 2.3% in patients 16 to 21 years and 16.9% in patients >80 years of age. The point prevalence in stable older outpatient adults has been reported as around 8%, and as much as 18% to 20% in sicker or frailer populations. The overall incidence (at or subsequent to hospital admission) is similar, with even higher rates in patients admitted for CHF or cirrhosis, or in elderly patients admitted for fragility fracture or hip fracture.
PREDOMINANT SEX AND AGE: Prevalence of hyponatremia was significantly higher in NHANES women (2.09%; P = 0.004) and increased with age.
GENETICS: While rare, a familial gain-of-function mutation of the AVP V2 receptor in the renal collecting duct resulting in hyponatremia has been reported
RISK FACTORS: In NHANES, hyponatremia was more common in subjects with hypertension, diabetes, coronary artery disease, stroke, chronic obstructive pulmonary disease, cancer, and psychiatric disorders, and less common in those with no comorbidities (1.04%, P <0.001). There was a significant risk of death associated with hyponatremia in unadjusted (hazard ratio [HR], 3.61; P <0.001) and adjusted Cox models controlling for demographics, smoking, comorbidities, and insurance status (HR, 2.43; P <0.001). The incidence in outpatients using thiazide diuretics was 15.1%, a HR of 4.95 (95% CI,

4.12-5.96). Reported incidences in outpatients using selective serotonin reuptake inhibitors (SSRIs) or selective norepinephrine reuptake inhibitors (SNRIs) has varied widely between 0.5% and 32%.

PHYSICAL FINDINGS & CLINICAL PRESENTATION

- Critical historical information that the health care provider needs to obtain includes detailed documentation of fluid consumption and diet, GI and insensible losses of fluid and electrolytes, urine outputs, and changes in weight; medication use, changes in behavior or cognition, and presence of comorbid conditions that increase the risk of hyponatremia including malignancies, CNS or pulmonary diseases, adrenal or thyroid diseases, CHF, liver disease, or nephrotic syndrome. In the appropriate setting participation in marathons or other strenuous endurance exercise or attendance at "rave" parties where the use of 3,4-methylenedioxy-methamphetamine [MDMA, "Ecstasy"] is common should be noted.
- The clinical presentation and physical findings are determined primarily by the acuity and severity of the hyponatremia as well as the underlying etiology. The etiology of hyponatremia may affect the clinical presentation both directly and/or by its effect on the extracellular fluid volume (ECFV). Hypovolemia and hypervolemia (decreased or increased ECFV respectively) are identified by the usual clinical criteria, although if available vector bioimpedance analysis has been shown to further increase accuracy. Specific manifestations of the precipitating cause or underlying diseases may be evident (e.g., fever and delirium following the use of MDMA, stigmata of alcoholism or malnutrition, fever and/or localizing symptoms related to pneumonia or other pulmonary disease, or headaches and visual field defects from an intracranial mass).
- Neurologic symptoms predominate as the direct clinical manifestations of hyponatremia due to cerebrocyte swelling. Compensatory processes that reduce cerebral edema by extrusion of electrolytes, amino acids, and carbohydrates from brain cells take 24 hours to fully engage and up to 7 days to reach completion. Therefore, patients who develop hyponatremia over less than 24 to 48 hours have the highest degree of brain swelling, the most severe neurologic symptoms, and the highest risk of permanent or fatal brain injury. Postpubertal, premenopausal women appear to undergo cerebral compensation more slowly, placing them at greater risk from acute hyponatremia.
- Acute hyponatremia may result in nausea and malaise as S_{Na} reaches 130 mEq/L or less, and headache, lethargy, obtundation, neurogenic pulmonary edema, and/or seizures in cases of S_{Na} less than 120 mEq/L. In the most severe cases death from brain stem herniation can occur.
- Chronic hyponatremia almost never presents with life-threatening clinical manifestations.

However, more subtle neurologic disturbances such as ataxia, short-term memory deficits, fatigue, lethargy and nausea have been commonly reported. Muscular weakness and elevated creatine kinase and even rhabdomyolysis have been reported. Chronic hyponatremia has also been associated with increased risk of falls, fractures, and osteoporosis in elderly patients. In addition, hyponatremia has been associated with increased risk of cardiovascular complications and mortality in a diverse group including elderly outpatients, general hospital admissions, and patients admitted for stroke, subarachnoid hemorrhage, CHF, cirrhosis, pneumonia, hip fracture and liver transplantation.

ETIOLOGY

- In patients with hypotonic hyponatremia, S_{Na} is closely approximated by the ratio ($TBNa_e$ + TBK_e)/TBW, where $TBNa_e$ and TBK_e represent exchangeable total body sodium and potassium, respectively, and TBW represents total body water. Hypotonic hyponatremia results from decreases in this numerator of total body cations, increases in this denominator, or both. TBNa is the main determinant of extracellular fluid volume (ECFV).
- ECFV depletion (with proportionately greater decrease in TBNa and possibly TBK than in TBW)
  ○ GI losses with intake of hypotonic fluids
  ○ Renal losses (diuresis, tubulopathies) with intake of hypotonic fluid
  ○ Cerebral salt wasting
- Euvolemic (normal ECFV)
  ○ Syndrome of inappropriate antidiuresis (SIAD, see "Syndrome of Inappropriate Antidiuresis")
  ○ Medications (thiazide diuretics, selective serotonin reuptake inhibitors (SSRIs) and serotonin-norepinephrine reuptake inhibitors (SNRIs), narcotics, "ecstasy" (MDMA), carbamazepine, cyclophosphamide, nicotine, DDAVP, phenothiazines, terlipressin)
  ○ Pain, nausea, stress
  ○ Marathon running or other endurance exercise
  ○ Primary polydipsia
  ○ Solute-limited water excretion (tea-and-toast diet, beer potomania)
  ○ Severe potassium deficiency with normal total body sodium
  ○ Adrenal insufficiency or hypothyroidism
  ○ Reset osmostat
- Increased ECFV (with decreased effective arterial blood volume, EABV). Hyponatremia results from proportionately greater increase in TBW than in TBNa and TBK
  ○ Congestive heart failure (CHF)
  ○ Nephrotic syndrome
  ○ Cirrhosis

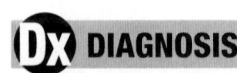 **DIAGNOSIS**

DIFFERENTIAL DIAGNOSIS

- *Pseudohyponatremia.* Clinical laboratories by convention report and to some extent measure the concentration of sodium (mEq)

TABLE 1 S_{Na} Corrected for Known Effective Osmoles (Including Glucose)

			S_{Na} Corrected for Known Effective Osmoles (Including Glucose)		
			Low	**Normal**	**High**
Osmolar Gap	**Elevated**	**Low S_{Na}**	Pseudohyponatremia ± hypotonic hyponatremia	Hypernatremia + Pseudohyponatremia	Hypernatremia ++ Hyperglycemia +++ Pseudohyponatremia
		Normal S_{Na}		Hypernatremia ++ Pseudohyponatremia	Hypernatremia ++ Hyperglycemia ++ Pseudohyponatremia
		High S_{Na}			Hypernatremia ++ Hyperglycemia + Pseudohyponatremia
	Normal	**Low S_{Na}**	Hypotonic hyponatremia	Hyperglycemia ++	Hypernatremia + Hyperglycemia +++
		Normal S_{Na}		Normal	Hypernatremia + Hyperglycemia ++
		High S_{Na}			Hypernatremia + Hyperglycemia +

This table outlines the relationship between the serum osmolar gap (see text) and the serum sodium concentration (S_{Na}) corrected for known effective osmoles such as glucose. Hypernatremia and hypotonic hyponatremia refer to elevation and depression, respectively, of S_{Na} in the absence of hyperglycemia or pseudohyponatremia. Pseudohyponatremia increases the osmolar gap because it decreases measured S_{Na} and calculated S_{osm} without altering measured S_{osm}. Hyperglycemia decreases S_{Na} while increasing S_{osm}.
S_{Na}, serum sodium; S_{osm}, serum osmolality; +, ++, and +++ indicate mild, moderate, and severe alterations of S_{Na}.
From Parrillo JE, Dellinger RP: *Critical care medicine: principles of diagnosis and management in the adult*, ed 4, Philadelphia, 2014, Saunders.

per liter of plasma, not plasma water. As a result, conditions (severe hypertriglyceridemia and hyperproteinemia) that significantly reduce the aqueous fraction of plasma (~0.93) lead to a decrease in the reported S_{Na} despite the presence of serum normal osmolality (S_{osm}, mOsm/kg H_2O). However, since the condition can coexist with preexisting hypernatremia or hypotonic hyponatremia, a more reliable method for identifying the disorder is the presence of an increased osmolal gap (i.e., a difference between laboratory-measured serum osmolality and the calculated S_{osm} of >10 mOsm/L) and a low S_{Na}. Calculated S_{osm} = 2 × (S_{Na}) + serum glucose (mg/dL)/18 + BUN (mg/dL)/2.8.

- *Hypertonic hyponatremia.* Small solutes such as glucose (in the absence of insulin), mannitol, sorbitol, and glycine that accumulate in higher concentrations in ECF than ICF induce a shift of water from ICF to ECF compartments. Since ICF is virtually sodium free, this dilutes the ECF sodium concentration and results in hyponatremia. In the case of glucose, a decrease in S_{Na} of 1.6 mEq/L occurs for each increment of serum glucose of 100 mg/dL up to 400 mg/dL, using a baseline serum glucose of 100 mg/dL; for serum glucose levels > 400 mg/dL, the increment is 4 mEq/L per 100 mg/dL increment in serum glucose. The tendency of a solute in vivo to shift fluid from ICF to ECF is known as tonicity, and is of clinical importance because increases and decreases in tonicity also result in brain cell shrinkage and edema respectively. In contrast, solutes such as urea or ethanol that equilibrate across cell membranes affect in vitro osmolality (measured by freezing point depression) but not tonicity or S_{Na}.
- The relationships between S_{Na}, measured and calculated S_{osm}, osmolar gap, and serum glucose are shown in Table 1 to aid in differential diagnosis and interpretation of laboratory values.

WORK-UP

- Comprehensive history including medication and drug abuse history, psychiatric history, exercise history, prior serum sodium measurements, dietary history, history of external fluid losses, volume and composition of oral and IV fluid intake, and history of (or suggestive of) disorders associated with hyponatremia (e.g., disorders of lungs, CNS, heart, kidney, liver, adrenal gland, or thyroid; malignancies; diabetes mellitus; nausea; vomiting; pain; or stress)
- Comprehensive physical examination including careful review of vital signs, weights, intake and outputs; evidence of increased extracellular fluid volume (ECFV) manifested by edema, ascites, or pleural effusions, or ECFV depletion; and evidence of comorbid diseases listed above (e.g., abnormal pulmonary, neurological or cardiovascular exam, hepatomegaly, thyromegaly or nodular thyroid)

LABORATORY TESTS

- S_{osm} to detect pseudohyponatremia or hypertonic hypernatremia due to solutes other than glucose, in the appropriate clinical circumstances (see Table 1)
- Serum triglycerides and total protein, if pseudohyponatremia is suspected
- Serum glucose to adjust for influence on serum sodium (see previously)
- Serum potassium: Since S_{Na} = (TBNa$_e$ + TBK$_e$)/TBW, decreases in TBK lower both S_K and S_{Na}
- Random urine osmolality and 24-hour urine volume. U_{osm} <100 mOsm/kg H_2O usually indicates appropriate suppression of ADH, suggesting the diagnoses of solute-limited water excretion, primary polydipsia, or a reset osmostat. U_{osm} ≥100 mOsm/kg H_2O usually implies effective ADH bioactivity. However, large quantities of isosmotic urine (U_{osm} ~290 mOsm/kg H_2O with total urine osmolar excretion >900 mOsm/day) are indicative of osmotic diuresis (with accompanying intake of hypotonic fluids).

- Random urine sodium (U_{Na}), and urine potassium (U_K). U_{Na} <20–40 mEq/L suggests either decreased ECFV or decreased EABV. U_K has to be taken into consideration when prescribing and monitoring therapy (see the following) because urine potassium losses may substantially increase with increased urine output.
- Specific testing for comorbid diseases listed previously as clinically indicated (e.g., AM or cosyntropin-stimulated serum cortisol level, BNP, TSH)

IMAGING STUDIES

- Not routinely required but may be indicated to diagnose associated etiologies, or to evaluate associated delirium that may be present in acute hyponatremia

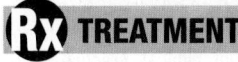 **TREATMENT**

NONPHARMACOLOGIC THERAPY

- By definition, hyponatremic patients excrete less free water than they take in. In most cases their capacity to excrete free water insufficient to match even conventional quantities of (hypotonic) fluid intake. Moderate fluid restriction (10-15 ml/kg) is indicated while patients are hyponatremic, especially if free water excretion capacity remains impaired. Diets that are high in protein, sodium, and potassium (including the use of NaCl tablets) increase osmolar generation and can increase free water excretion modestly.

ACUTE GENERAL Rx

- Acute (hypotonic) hyponatremia is defined as developing over <24 hours. Acute hyponatremia results in larger increases in brain water than equivalent changes in S_{Na} developing over longer durations. As a result, correction of acute hyponatremia is a medical emergency mandating an increase in S_{Na} of 4 to 6 mEq/L in the first 1 to 3 hours depending on the severity of symptoms and the acuity of the increase. Iatrogenic cases (classically children or premenopausal women receiving perioperative hypotonic fluids), fortunately rare now, can present with headache or nausea prior to severe symptoms but still require emergent correction. Acute hyponatremia is rare in patients with high ECFV because the increased TBNa partially offsets the decreased $(TBNa_e + TBK_e)/TBW$ ratio driven by high TBW.

- Controlled increases in S_{Na} at this rapid rate almost always require the use of hypertonic (3%) saline. A useful rule-of-thumb is that 2 ml/kg of 3% saline can be expected to increase S_{Na} by 1.6 to 2 mEq/L. The recommended rate of correction in severe acute hyponatremia is an increase in S_{Na} of 4 to 6 mEq/L in the first hour. In euvolemic patients (i.e., having normal TBNa), furosemide 20 to 40 mg IV has been used in conjunction with hypertonic saline to lessen the expansion of ECFV while maintaining the rapid increase in S_{Na} by increasing free water excretion.
- Regardless of the therapies employed, patients with acute hyponatremia require monitoring in an ICU setting with frequent measurements of S_{Na}, urine volume, and U_{osm} until patients are neurologically stable and the S_{Na} is near normal.

CHRONIC Rx

- Chronic hyponatremia develops over >24 to 48 hours, which allows brain cells to adapt by extrusion of electrolytes and other osmoles such as amino acids. As a result, brain edema in minimized while the risks of rapid correction increase. Precipitous increases in S_{Na} in this setting have been associated with serious demyelinating brain injuries. The appropriate target for correction of hyponatremia in this setting is 6 to 8 mEq/L/day
- In hypovolemic patients with chronic hyponatremia the usual clinical practice is to administer 0.9% saline until patients are euvolemic. 0.9% saline results in very little direct change in S_{Na} because it proportionately increases $(TBNa_e + TBK_e)$ and TBW, but indirectly can trigger a rapid increase in S_{Na} when hypovolemia-induced (non-osmotic) stimulation of ADH is turned off. The simultaneous use of DDAVP (1–2 mcg IV every 6-12 hours) is a recommended adjuvant to therapy in these patients to prevent unanticipated and unwanted increases in free water loss than can result in unpredictably high rates of change. Once the patient is euvolemic IV fluids can be stopped and the patient monitored. If the rate or magnitude of S_{Na} correction starts to exceed prudent targets, DDAVP may be redosed as needed. Since decreased ECFV may not always be recognized, DDAVP administration may also be

judiciously administered in some apparently euvolemic patients with chronic hyponatremia treated with 0.9% or 3% saline.

- The treatment of euvolemic patients is covered in detail in the Section I topic "Syndrome of Inappropriate Antidiuresis" and will be only briefly reviewed here. The goals of therapy in these patients are to restore TBW to normal while keeping TBNa and TBK normal, correcting S_{Na} at safe rate. Some patients with chronic euvolemic hyponatremia (especially those with drug-induced etiologies or primary polydipsia) have self-limited abnormalities and primarily require monitoring to prevent excessively rapid correction, although active therapy as described below can be started to avoid delays. If needed, DDAVP can be administered intermittently to temporarily block further losses of free water to slow the overall rate of correction. If overcorrection has occurred oral and/or IV hypotonic fluids can be quantitatively given to lower the serum sodium actively in addition. Other disorders may only slowly resolve if at all, and will require more active therapy as outlined in "Syndrome of Inappropriate Antidiuresis," consisting of either a direct AVP V2 receptor antagonist or a loop diuretic combined with replacement of electrolytes lost during diuresis.

DISPOSITION

- Patients with symptomatic or severe hyponatremia require monitoring in an ICU setting until the S_{Na} has stabilized at a safe level. Frequent monitoring of serum sodium, urine volume, and urine osmolality and electrolytes is required, with adjustments in therapy as outlined previously as needed.
- All potential contributing causes should be evaluated and treated appropriately. In addition to obvious disorders, less apparent conditions such as adrenal insufficiency and hypothyroidism should be ruled out.
- The risk of recurrence depends primarily on the nature of the underlying disorders present. Hypovolemic hyponatremia (e.g., diarrheal or diuretic-induced electrolyte and water losses) or drug-induced SIAD may have little chance of recurrence if the offending medication is discontinued or if the gastrointestinal losses are not chronic. Elderly patients with solute limited diuresis due to low electrolyte and protein intake may be resistant to major changes in diet, but may agree to NaCl tablets and/or protein supplements. In addition to disease-specific management, incurable conditions (e.g., chronic CNS or pulmonary disease, CHF, or

cirrhosis) may require life-long fluid restriction (10-15 ml/kg/day), high protein and electrolyte diets as tolerated, and periodic monitoring of the S_{Na} to reduce the risk of recurrence.

REFERRAL

- Referral to specialists in nephrology, endocrinology, and/or critical care medicine are recommended in cases of severe or symptomatic hyponatremia to aid in setting appropriate rates of correction and to recommend, monitor, and adjust therapeutic regimens to achieve those target rates.
- Outpatient referral to nephrology or endocrinology may be indicated to help manage patients with recurrent hyponatremia or mild hyponatremia that does not warrant hospitalization

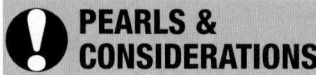 **PEARLS & CONSIDERATIONS**

COMMENTS

PREVENTION: Well-meaning family members, friends, news media, and even health care providers often tell patients who have chronic kidney disease or are taking diuretics to drink large amounts of water. When this causes patients to consume more free water than they can excrete, this can lead to hyponatremia. Similarly, participants in marathons or other high-intensity endurance activities may ingest so much water that in place of TBW depletion they develop high TBW and hyponatremia. Patients at risk for hyponatremia should receive a specific fluid prescription that avoids both extremes. On the other hand patients with diarrheal losses or who actually develop decreased ECFV from loop or combination diuretics need to be counseled that intake of water or other hypotonic fluids alone will lead to hyponatremia but not effectively restore ECFV. Safe outpatient correction of ECFV requires the consumption of electrolyte-containing solutions such as those marketed for infants. Standard sports drinks have high sugar content but relatively low quantities of electrolytes.

SUGGESTED READINGS
Available at www.expertconsult.com

RELATED CONTENT
Syndrome of Inappropriate Antidiuresis (Related Key Topic)

AUTHORS: **MARK D. FABER, M.D.,** and **JERRY YEE, M.D.**

BASIC INFORMATION

DEFINITION

A decrease in parathyroid hormone (PTH) secretion or function results in hypoparathyroidism. In primary hypoparathyroidism, absence or dysfunction of the parathyroid gland results in inadequate PTH secretion and subsequent hypocalcemia and hyperphosphatemia. Surgical hypoparathyroidism is the most common etiology, followed by autoimmune disorders. Individuals with autoimmune polyglandular syndrome 1 typically present in childhood/adolescence with candidiasis, hypoparathyroidism, and adrenal insufficiency. Impaired function of PTH (i.e., PTH resistance) can also cause hypocalcemia and hyperphosphatemia, but the measured PTH level is elevated in this circumstance. A maternally transmitted mutation in the GNAS1 gene results in PTH resistance (i.e., pseudohypoparathyroidism). It is associated with characteristic features that include developmental delay, short stature, round facies, and short 4th metacarpal known as Albright's hereditary osteodystrophy (AHO). Paternal transmission manifests with AHO without PTH resistance (i.e., pseudopseudohypoparathyroidism; Table 1). Secondary hypoparathyroidism, a condition in which PTH levels are low in response to hypercalcemic states, is discussed in Section IV (see hypercalcemia discussion in the "Calcium" topic).

ICD-10CM CODES
E20.0 Idiopathic hypoparathyroidism
E20.1 Pseudohypoparathyroidism
E20.8 Other hypoparathyroidism
E20.9 Hypoparathyroidism, unspecified
E89.2 Postprocedural hypoparathyroidism
P71.4 Transitory neonatal hypoparathyroidism

EPIDEMIOLOGY & DEMOGRAPHICS

The incidence and prevalence of primary hypoparathyroidism depends on the etiology of the condition. Postoperative hypoparathyroidism is the most common etiology (75%). This occurs in the setting of thyroid or parathyroid surgery as a result of removal of, or vascular compromise of, the parathyroid glands during surgery. Transient hypoparathyroidism (<6 months) can be as high as 20% postoperatively, but permanent dysfunction (>6 months) is less common (3%). Autoimmune disorders are the second most common cause of hypoparathyroidism in adults (female/male ratio of 1.4:1.0). Autoimmune polyglandular syndrome type I is reported to have

an incidence worldwide of 1:1,000,000. Other etiologies of hypoparathyroidism are very rare.

PHYSICAL FINDINGS & CLINICAL PRESENTATION

The symptoms of hypoparathyroidism are primarily related to hypocalcemia. The presentation of symptoms varies with the severity and duration of illness.
- Cardiovascular: prolonged QT intervals, QRS and ST segment changes, ventricular arrhythmias
- Musculoskeletal: muscle cramps, laryngospasm, osteomalacia (adults), rickets (children), weakened tooth enamel, osteosclerosis
- CNS: tetany (Chvostek's sign and Trousseau's sign), seizures, paresthesias, visual impairment from cataract formation, altered mental status, papilledema, and basal ganglia calcifications with longstanding disease
- GI: abdominal pain
- Renal: hypercalciuria and nephrolithiasis
- Other: dry scaly skin, brittle nails, dry hair
  In addition to the hypocalcemia-related symptoms, syndromes associated with hypoparathyroidism can have distinct clinical findings. Conditions associated with hypoparathyroidism include:
- Autoimmune polyglandular syndrome type 1: mucocutaneous candidiasis and adrenal insufficiency
- DiGeorge syndrome: dysmorphic facies, cleft palate
- Pseudohypoparathyroidism: developmental delay, short stature, round face, short 4th metacarpal (Albright's hereditary osteodystrophy)
- Hypoparathyroidism-retardation-dysmorphism syndrome: short stature, microcephaly, microphthalmia, small hands and feet, abnormal teeth
- Hypoparathyroidism-deafness-renal dysplasia syndrome: sensorineural deafness

ETIOLOGY

There are several etiologies of hypoparathyroidism:
- Postoperative hypoparathyroidism
- Destruction of the parathyroids
  1. Autoimmune polyglandular syndrome type 1
  2. Radiation to the neck
  3. Infiltrative disease (e.g., metastatic carcinoma, Wilson's disease, hemochromatosis, thalassemia, granulomatous disease)
- Developmental defects of the parathyroids:
  1. Isolated hypoparathyroidism
  2. Branchial dysembryogenesis (DiGeorge syndrome)

3. Hypoparathyroidism-retardation-dysmorphism syndrome
4. Hypoparathyroidism-deafness-renal dysplasia syndrome
5. Mitochondrial dysfunction associated with hypoparathyroidism
- Functional and secretory defects of the parathyroid glands:
  1. Activating mutation of the calcium-sensing receptor alters the set point of the receptor and decreases PTH secretion
  2. Activating antibodies to calcium-sensing receptor alters the set point of the receptor and decreases PTH secretion
  3. PTH resistance (i.e., target organs unresponsive to PTH action)
     1. Pseudohypoparathyroidism (PHP): heterogeneous disorder presenting in childhood characterized by hypocalcemia, hyperphosphatemia, and elevated PTH levels. Table 2 summarizes the various types of PHP.
     2. Hypermagnesemia and hypomagnesemia

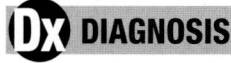 DIAGNOSIS

DIFFERENTIAL DIAGNOSIS
- Secondary hypoparathyroidism as a result of hypercalcemia (discussed in the "Hypercalcemia" section)
- Other conditions associated with hypocalcemia. These conditions are usually associated with an elevated PTH hormone level.

WORKUP
- Hypoparathyroidism is characterized by hypocalcemia and hyperphosphatemia as a result of inadequate PTH secretion.
  1. Two measurements of serum calcium are required for the confirmation of hypocalcemia. Total calcium should be corrected for low albumin utilizing the formula: Corrected calcium = measured calcium + [(4 − albumin) × 0.8]. If a reliable laboratory is available, ionized calcium should be considered especially in conditions associated with acid-base disturbances or low albumin states.
  2. Serum phosphorus is usually high-normal or elevated in primary hypoparathyroidism.
  3. Serum intact PTH (iPTH) level is the single best test to evaluate the etiology of hypocalcemia. Typically, PTH is decreased in primary hypoparathyroidism and elevated in most other conditions associated with low calcium levels. However, PTH is also elevated in disorders associated with impaired PTH function (i.e., pseudohypoparathyroidism). Genetic studies as indicated if medical or family history is suggestive.

LABORATORY TESTS
- Total and ionized calcium: low in hypoparathyroidism
- PTH: low in hypoparathyroidism and high in PTH resistance states like pseudohypoparathyroidism

TABLE 1 Types of Hypoparathyroidism

Type	Calcium	PO$_4$	PTH	Comments
Hypoparathyroidism	↓	↑	↓	Surgical removal (most common cause)
Pseudohypoparathyroidism	↓	↑	Ø↑	End-organ resistance to parathyroid hormone and Albright's hereditary osteodystrophy
Pseudo-pseudohypoparathyroidism	Normal	Normal	Normal	Only Albright's hereditary osteodystrophy

Adapted from Weissleder R et al: *Primer of diagnostic imaging*, ed 5, St Louis, 2011, Mosby.

TABLE 2   Types of Pseudohypoparathyroidism (PHP)

Disorder	Urinary cAMP Response to PTH	Urinary PO$_4$ Response to PTH	Other Hormonal Resistance	AHO	Pathophysiology
PHP type 1A	Decreased	Decreased	Yes	Yes	G$_s$α mutation
Pseudo-PHP	Normal	Normal	No	Yes	G$_s$α mutation
PHP type 1B	Decreased	Decreased	No	No	*GNAS1* imprinting mutations
PHP type 1C	Decreased	Decreased	Yes	Yes	G$_s$α activity normal
PHP type 2	Normal	Decreased	No	No	Vitamin D deficiency or myotonic dystrophy in some cases

AHO, Albright's hereditary osteodystrophy; *cAMP*, cyclic adenosine monophosphate; *GNAS1*, portion of the *GNAS* complex locus encoding G$_s$α; *G$_s$α*, α-subunit of the stimulatory G protein; *PO$_4$*, phosphate; *PTH*, parathyroid hormone.
From Melmed: *Williams textbook of endocrinology*, ed 12, Philadelphia, 2011, Saunders.

- Phosphorus: high-normal or high in hypoparathyroidism
- Magnesium: both hypomagnesemia and hypermagnesemia can cause hypoparathyroidism
- 24-hr urine for calcium to evaluate the risk for renal stones
- ECG should be considered. Hypocalcemia associated with prolonged QT interval, rarely ST-segment elevations

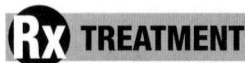 **TREATMENT**

NONPHARMACOLOGIC THERAPY

Parathyroid autotransplantation:

Hypoparathyroidism and subsequent hypocalcemia are common problems after neck exploration for total or near-total thyroidectomy or parathyroidectomy. In cases where there is concern for postoperative hypoparathyroidism, parathyroid autotransplantation of one or two parathyroid glands into the forearm or sternocleidomastoid muscle should be performed to prevent postoperative hypoparathyroidism.

PHARMACOLOGIC THERAPY

The mainstay of treatment for primary hypoparathyroidism is pharmacologic therapy with calcium and vitamin D supplementation. The goals of therapy are to control symptoms and minimize complications of therapy. The aim should be to achieve low-normal serum calcium level (8.0-8.5 mg/dl), high-normal serum phosphorus level, 24-hr urinary calcium <300 mg/day, and a calcium-phosphorus product <55 mg^2/dL^2.

- Vitamin D:
  1. There are several vitamin D preparations available on the market but the treatment of choice for patients with primary hypoparathyroidism is calcitriol. It is an active metabolite that does not require hydroxylation in the liver or kidney and therefore bypasses the PTH-mediated 1-α hydroxylation defect that occurs with hypoparathyroidism.
  2. Dose of 0.25 to 1 μg once or twice daily is usually required to correct hypocalcemia and improve symptoms. Its maximal effect is seen after 10 hours and it lasts for 2 to 3 days.
  3. Vitamin D$_2$ (ergocalciferol) or vitamin D$_3$ (cholecalciferol) may also be supplemented if levels are found to be low.
- Calcium:
  1. Calcium carbonate or calcium citrates are common oral agents used for treatment of hypocalcemia associated with hypoparathyroidism. Calcium carbonate contains 40% elemental calcium, and calcium citrate contains 21% elemental calcium. Calcium carbonate requires an acidic environment for effective absorption, and as a result, it must be taken with food. Its effectiveness is decreased with concomitant use of H$_2$ blockers or proton pump inhibitors. Calcium citrate does not require an acidic environment for effective absorption.
  2. Start with a dose of 500 to 1000 mg of elemental calcium two to three times daily and adjust the dose for a desired calcium in the low-normal range.
- Magnesium:
  1. Hypocalcemia is difficult to correct without normalizing magnesium levels.
  2. Magnesium sulfate IV 2 g over 20 min followed by 1 g/hr infusion can be considered in severe deficiency states. Milder deficiencies can be managed with oral magnesium 100 mg tid.
- Thiazide diuretics:
  1. Thiazide diuretics (25 to 100 mg daily) decrease urine calcium excretion and decrease kidney stones. They should be considered in individuals with urine calcium >250 mg/day.
- PTH replacement:
  1. Injectable synthetic human PTH (1-84) decreases urinary calcium excretion and maintains serum calcium in the normal range with reduced requirements for calcium and vitamin D supplementation.
  2. PTH (1-84, Natpara, an 84 amino acid single-chain polypeptide identical to native parathyroid hormone) is the first FDA approved for use in the treatment of hypoparathyroidism. The cost for a 4-week supply of Natpara exceeds $7000.
  3. PTH (1-84) is recommended for patients who cannot be well controlled on conventional therapy alone.

ACUTE GENERAL Rx

Severe and/or symptomatic hypocalcemia requires hospitalization. Acute management of hypocalcemia includes:

- Telemetry monitoring for arrhythmias associated with severe hypocalcemia
- IV infusion of calcium gluconate 10 mL of 10% solution to receive a bolus of 90 mg of elemental calcium followed by an infusion of 0.5 to 2 mg/kg/hr until calcium levels are in the low-normal range.

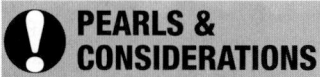 **PEARLS & CONSIDERATIONS**

COMMENTS

- The mainstay of treatment for primary hypoparathyroidism is calcitriol and calcium supplementation to maintain a goal serum calcium level in the low-normal range. IV calcium should be considered if calcium <7.0 mg/dl. Magnesium levels should be assessed and appropriately replaced in all patients with hypocalcemia. Clinical trials are under way to evaluate the role of recombinant PTH for the treatment of primary hypoparathyroidism.
- In patients undergoing neck exploration, consideration should be given to the parathyroid glands. Autotransplantation of one or more parathyroid glands should be considered when appropriate to prevent postoperative hypoparathyroidism.

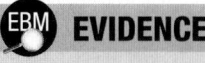 **EVIDENCE**

Available at www.expertconsult.com

SUGGESTED READINGS

Available at www.expertconsult.com

AUTHOR: **VICKY CHENG, M.D.**

BASIC INFORMATION

DEFINITION

Hypopituitarism (from the Latin *pituita,* meaning "phlegm") is the deficiency of one or more of the hormones of the anterior or posterior pituitary gland resulting from diseases of the hypothalamus or pituitary gland. Panhypopituitarism indicates the loss of all the pituitary hormones but is often used in clinical practice to describe patients deficient in growth hormone (GH), gonadotropins, corticotropin, or thyrotropin in whom posterior pituitary function remains intact.

SYNONYMS

Panhypopituitarism
Pituitary insufficiency

ICD-10CM CODES
E23.0 Hypopituitarism
E23.0 Hypopituitarism
E23.1 Drug-induced hypopituitarism
E89.3 Postprocedural hypopituitarism

EPIDEMIOLOGY & DEMOGRAPHICS

Incidence of 4.2 cases per 100,000 persons

PHYSICAL FINDINGS & CLINICAL PRESENTATION

Symptoms depend on type of onset, number and severity of hormone deficiencies, their target organs, and age of onset.
- Mass effect of a pituitary tumor can cause headaches and visual disturbances (typically as bitemporal hemianopsia).
- Rhinorrhea.
- Corticotropin deficiency:
  1. Fatigue and weakness, no appetite, abdominal pain, nausea, vomiting, failure to thrive in children, and hyponatremia. If the onset is abrupt, hypotension and shock
- Thyrotropin deficiency:
  1. Fatigue and weakness, weight gain, cold intolerance, anemia, constipation
  2. Bradycardia, hung-up reflexes, pretibial edema, change in voice, and hair loss
- Gonadotropin deficiency:
  1. Loss of libido, erectile dysfunction, amenorrhea, hot flashes, dyspareunia, infertility, gynecomastia, decreased muscle mass, and anemia
- GH deficiency:
  1. Growth retardation in children
  2. Easy fatigue, hypoglycemia
  3. Lean mass is reduced and fat mass is increased, leading to obesity
  4. Decreased bone mineral density, increased low-density lipoprotein cholesterol, obesity, increased inflammatory cardiovascular markers (interleukin-6 and C-reactive protein)
- Hyperprolactinemia:
  1. Galactorrhea, hypogonadism, inability to lactate after delivery

2. Posterior pituitary (vasopressin; antidiuretic hormone [ADH] deficiency): diabetes insipidus with polyuria, polydipsia, nocturia, hypotension, and dehydration

ETIOLOGY

It can be congenital or acquired:
- Congenital: mutations in transcription factors produce multiple hormonal deficiencies. Mutations in genes produce single hormonal deficiency.
- Acquired: the result of destruction of pituitary cells caused by:
  1. Pituitary apoplexy: hemorrhage or infarction of the pituitary gland. Predisposing factors include diabetes mellitus, anticoagulation therapy, head trauma, and radiation therapy. Sheehan's syndrome: postpartum necrosis, a rare complication after pregnancy.
  2. Infiltrative disease, including sarcoidosis, hemachromatosis, histiocytosis X, Wegener's granulomatosis, lymphocytic hypophysitis, and infection of the pituitary (tuberculosis, mycosis, syphilis).
  3. Primary empty sella syndrome: flattening of the pituitary gland caused by extension of the subarachnoid space and filling of cerebrospinal fluid into the sella turcica.
  4. Pituitary tumors: classified by size (microadenomas, <10 mm; macroadenomas, >10 mm) and function. Prolactin-secreting tumors and nonfunctioning tumors account for the majority of pituitary adenomas.
  5. Suprasellar tumors: craniopharyngiomas are the most common.

DIAGNOSIS

The diagnosis of hypopituitarism is suspected by clinical history and physical findings and is established by blood tests to confirm the presence of hormone deficiency.

DIFFERENTIAL DIAGNOSIS

The differential diagnosis is as outlined under "Etiology."

WORKUP

Includes baseline determination of each anterior pituitary hormone followed by dynamic provocative stimulation tests, radiograph imaging, and formal visual field testing. Table 1 summarizes testing for assessment of anterior pituitary function.

LABORATORY TESTS

- Corticotropin deficiency:
  1. The presence of a 9:00 am cortisol level >20 mcg/dl or <4 mcg/dl usually confirms sufficiency or deficiency, respectively.
  2. Corticotropin stimulation test using 250 mcg of corticotropin given IV and measuring serum cortisol before and 30 and 60 min after administration. A normal

response is an increase in serum cortisol level >20 mcg/dl.
  3. With pituitary disease these test results may be indeterminate, and more dynamic testing such as an insulin-tolerance or metyrapone test may be necessary.
- Thyrotropin deficiency:
  1. Thyroid-stimulating hormone (TSH) and free T_4 measurements
  2. Primary hypothyroidism shows elevated TSH with low free T_4. Secondary hypothyroidism shows normal or low TSH with low free T_4 and low T_3 resin uptake.
- Gonadotropin deficiency:
  1. Follicle-stimulating hormone (FSH), luteinizing hormone (LH), estrogen, and testosterone measurements.
  2. In men, hypogonadotropic hypogonadism is seen with low testosterone levels and normal or low FSH and LH levels (ideally measured at 9:00 AM because of diurnal rhythm). Check free testosterone if patient is obese.
  3. In premenopausal women with amenorrhea, low estrogen with normal or low FSH and LH levels is typically seen.
- GH deficiency:
  1. Insulin-induced hypoglycemia stimulation test using 0.1 to 0.15 unit/kg regular insulin given IV and measuring GH 30, 60, and 120 min after administration. A normal response is a GH level >3 mcg/dl. This test is contraindicated in seizure disorder or ischemic heart disease.
  2. Combination of GH-releasing hormone plus arginine is an alternative test, with a diagnostic threshold of 9 mcg/L.
  3. Because the relation between serum insulinlike growth factor (IGF)-1 and GH levels blurs with age, a normal serum IGF-1 does not exclude the diagnosis in older adults.
- Hyperprolactinemia: prolactin levels may be elevated in prolactin-secreting pituitary adenomas.
- Vasopressin deficiency:
  1. Urinalysis shows low specific gravity.
  2. Urine osmolality is low.
  3. Serum osmolality is high.
  4. Fluid deprivation test over 18 hr with inability to concentrate the urine.
  5. Serum vasopressin level is low.
  6. Electrolytes may show hyponatremia and exclude hyperglycemia.

IMAGING STUDIES

- Imaging is the first step in identifying an underlying cause.
- MRI (Fig. 1) is more sensitive than CT in visualizing the pituitary fossa, sella turcica, optic chiasm, pituitary stalk, and cavernous sinuses. It is also more sensitive in detecting pituitary microadenomas. CT with contrast can be used if MRI is not available.
- Surveillance scan at baseline and 12 mo thereafter depending on protocol and clinical symptoms.

TABLE 1 Assessment of Anterior Pituitary Function

Test	Dose	Normal Response	Side Effects
ACTH			
Insulin tolerance	0.1-0.15 U/kg IV	Peak cortisol response >18 µg/dl, or ≥5 µg/dl	Sweating, palpitation, tremor
Metyrapone	30 mg/kg PO at 11 P.M.	Peak 11-DOC ≥=7 µg/dl Peak cortisol ≤7 µg/dl Peak ACTH >75 pg/ml	Nausea, insomnia, adrenal crisis
CRH stimulation	100 µg IV	Peak ACTH ≥2-4-fold Peak cortisol ≥20 µg/dl or ↑ ≥=7 µg/dl	Flushing
ACTH stimulation	250 µg IV or IM, or 1 µg IV	Peak cortisol ≥20 µg/dl	Rare
TSH			
Serum T$_4$ (free T$_4$) Total T$_3$ TSH—third-generation TRH stimulation	200-500 µg IV	Peak TSH ≥2.5-fold, or ↑ ≥5-6 mU/L (females) or ≥2-3 mU/L (males)	Flushing, nausea, urge to micturate
PRL			
Serum PRL TRH stimulation	200-500 µg IV	PRL ↑ ≥2.5-fold	Flushing, nausea, urge to micturate
LH/FSH			
Serum LH and FSH Serum testosterone GnRH stimulation	100 µg IV	Elevated in menopause and in men with primary testicular failure (otherwise normal) 300-900 ng/ml LH ≥2-3-fold, or ↑ by 10 IU/L FSH ≥1.5-2-fold, or ↑ ≥2 IU/L	Rare
GH			
Insulin tolerance	0.1-0.15 U/kg	GH peak >5 µg/L	Sweating, palpitation, tremor
L-Arginine	Arginine 0.5 g/kg (maximum, 30 g) IV over 30-120 min	GH peak >0.4 µg/L	Nausea
Plus			
GHRH	GHRH 1-5 µg/kg	GH peak >4 µg/L	Flushing

ACTH, Adrenocorticotropic hormone; *CRH,* corticotropin-releasing hormone; *11-DOC,* 11-deoxycorticosterone; *FSH,* follicle-stimulating hormone; *GH,* growth hormone; *GHRH,* growth hormone–releasing hormone; *GnRH,* gonadotropin-releasing hormone; *LH,* luteinizing hormone; *PRL,* prolactin; *T$_3$,* triiodothyronine; *T$_4$,* thyroxine; *TSH,* thyroid-stimulating hormone; *TRH,* thyrotropin-releasing hormone.
From Melmed S, Polonsky KS, Larsen PR, Kronenberg HM: *Williams textbook of endocrinology,* ed 12, Philadelphia, 2011, Saunders, Elsevier Inc.

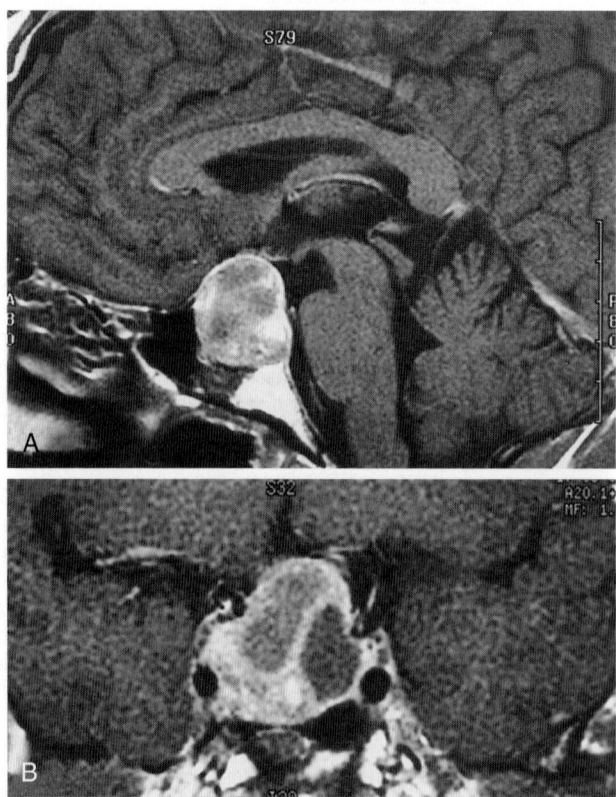

FIG. 1 T1-weighted gadolinium-enhanced MR of a pituitary adenoma. **(A)** Sagittal and **(B)** coronal images. (Courtesy of D. Thomas. From Bowling B: *Kanski's clinical ophthalmology,* ed 8, Philadelphia, 2016, Elsevier.)

Rx TREATMENT

Threefold: removing underlying cause (surgery or radiation), treating hormonal deficiencies, and addressing any other repercussions from deficiency. Table 2 summarizes replacement therapy for adult hypopituitarism.

NONPHARMACOLOGIC THERAPY

- IV fluid resuscitation, correction of electrolyte and metabolic abnormalities with potassium bicarbonate, and oxygen therapy.
- Transsphenoidal surgery for tumors causing specific symptoms.
- Radiation or stereotactic radiosurgery ("gamma knife") for medically unresponsive, surgically unresectable tumors and tumors for which other modalities are contraindicated. It is both safe and effective for recurrent or residual pituitary adenomas.

TABLE 2 Replacement Therapy for Adult Hypopituitarism*

Deficient Hormone

Treatment

Remarks

ACTH

Hydrocortisone: 10-20 mg/day in divided doses
Cortisone acetate: 15-25 mg/day in divided doses

TSH

L-Thyroxine: 0.05-0.2 mg/day according to T_4 levels

FSH/LH (in males)

Testosterone enanthate: 200 mg IM q2-3 wk
Testosterone skin patch: 2.5-5.0 mg/day (or up to 7.5 mg/day)
Testosterone gel: 3-6 g/day
For fertility: hCG three times weekly, or hCG + either FSH or menopausal gonadotropin or GnRH

FSH/LH (in females)

Conjugated estrogen: 0.3-0.625 mg/day
Micronized estradiol: 1 mg/day
Estradiol valerate: 2 mg
Piperazine estrone sulfate: 1.25 mg
Estradiol skin patch: 4-8 mg twice weekly
All of the estrogens are administered with progesterone or progestin sequentially or in combination if uterus is present
For fertility: Menopausal gonadotropin, and hCG, or GnRH

Growth hormone

Somatotropin (in adults): 0.2-1.0 mg/day SC
Somatotropin (in children): 0.02-0.05 mg/kg per day

Vasopressin

Intranasal desmopressin: 10-20 μg bid
Oral DDAVP: 300-600 μg/day, usually in divided doses

ACTH, Adrenocorticotropic hormone; *DDAVP,* desmopressin acetate; *FSH,* follicle-stimulating hormone; *GnRH,* gonad-otropin-releasing hormone; *hCG,* human chorionic go-nadotropin; *LH,* luteinizing hormone; *T4,* thyroxine; *TSH,* thyroid-stimulating hormone.
From Melmed S, Polonsky KS, Larsen PR, Kronenberg HM: *Williams textbook of endocrinology,* ed 12, Philadelphia, 2011, Saunders, Elsevier Inc.

ACUTE GENERAL Rx

Acute situations such as adrenal crisis or myxedema coma can occur in untreated hypopituitarism and should be treated accordingly with IV corticosteroids (e.g., hydrocortisone 100 to 250 mg bolus followed by hydrocortisone 100 mg IV q6h for 24 hr) and levothyroxine (e.g., 5 to 8 mcg/kg IV over 15 min, then 100 mcg IV q24h).

CHRONIC Rx

Treatment is lifelong:
- Adrenocorticotropic hormone (ACTH) deficiency: hydrocortisone 10 mg PO every morning and 5 mg PO every evening or prednisone 5 mg PO every morning and 2.5 mg PO every evening. Dexamethasone or prednisone is often preferred because of longer duration of action.
- LH and FSH deficiency:
  1. In men, testosterone enanthate or propionate 200 to 300 mg IM every 2 to 3 wk, or transdermal testosterone scrotal patches can be tried.
  2. In women who are not interested in fertility, conjugated estrogen 0.3 to 1.25 mg/day and held the last 5 to 7 days of each month with the addition of medroxyprogesterone 10 mg/day given during days 15 to 25 of the normal menstrual cycle. In those who have secondary hypogonadism and wish to become pregnant, pulsatile gonadotropic-releasing hormone may be of benefit.
- TSH deficiency: levothyroxine 0.05 to 0.15 mg/day.
- GH deficiency:
  1. GH replacement in children is universally accepted.
  2. GH replacement in adults is not generally recommended and requires careful consideration of each individual case. It may have effects on quality of life, body composition, bone density, and cardiovascular risk factors.
  3. Side effects of replacement include peripheral edema, arthralgia, and headaches.
  4. Usual GH dose is between 0.2 and 0.4 mg, determined by the age and gender of a patient and increments of 0.1 mg every 2 to 4 wk until serum IGF-1 is in the upper part of the normal range. Young adults and women taking estrogen require a higher dose.
- ADH deficiency:
  1. Desmopressin (DDAVP) 10 to 20 mcg by intranasal spray or 0.05 to 0.1 mg PO bid is used in patients with diabetes insipidus.
  2. Vasopressin: 5-10 U given IM or SC q6h.

DISPOSITION

- Hormone replacement therapy is adjusted according to serum hormone monitoring.
- If untreated can lead to adrenal crisis, severe hyponatremia and hypothyroidism, metabolic abnormalities, and death.
- Complications: visual deficit, adrenal crisis, susceptibility to infection and other stressors.

- Prognosis: stable patients have a favorable prognosis with replacement hormone therapy. Patients with acute decompensation are in critical condition with a high mortality rate.

REFERRAL

Consultation with an endocrinologist and neurosurgeon for surgical treatment

! PEARLS & CONSIDERATIONS

- All patients sustaining moderate to severe head injury should undergo assessment of anterior pituitary function during the acute phase and at 6 mo.
- IGF-1 can be used as a marker of GH deficiency.
- All tests of GH secretion are more likely to give false-positive results in obese patients.
- The GH axis is the most vulnerable to the effects of radiotherapy; doses as low as 18 Gy in children have caused GH deficiency.
- Sequence of hormonal disruption: GH secretion then gonadotropin secretion. TSH and adrenocorticotropic hormone secretion are somewhat resistant.
- Thyroxine supplementation increases the rate of cortisol metabolism and can lead to adrenal crisis, so corticosteroids should be replaced first.
- All patients receiving glucocorticoid replacement therapy should wear proper identification stating the need for this therapy.
- Stress doses of corticosteroids are indicated before surgery or for any medical emergency (e.g., sepsis, acute myocardial infarction).
- Antidiuretic hormone deficiency may be masked if there is ACTH deficiency with symptoms only appearing when cortisol has been replaced.

COMMENTS

- Mineralocorticoid replacement is not necessary in secondary adrenal insufficiency because the renin-angiotensin-aldosterone system is unaffected by pituitary failure.
- Patients with adult-acquired GH deficiency must meet at least two criteria before replacement therapy: a poor GH response to at least two standard stimuli and hypopituitarism from pituitary or hypothalamic damage. The criteria are different in children in whom GH is required for normal growth.
- Prevention of acute decompensation can be accomplished by reminding patients to increase the dose of hydrocortisone in response to stress.
- Medical therapy should precede surgical therapy.

RELATED CONTENT

Hypopituitarism (Patient Information)

AUTHOR: **SHAHNAZ PUNJANI, M.D.**

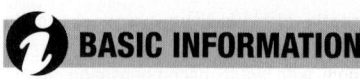

BASIC INFORMATION

DEFINITION

Hypothermia is a rectal temperature <35° C (95.8° F). Accidental hypothermia is an unintentionally induced decrease in core temperature in the absence of preoptic anterior hypothalamic conditions.

ICD-10CM CODES
T68   Hypothermia
R68.0 Hypothermia, not associated with low environmental temperature

EPIDEMIOLOGY & DEMOGRAPHICS

- Hypothermia occurs most frequently in the following groups: alcoholics; homeless; learning-impaired; patients with cardiovascular, cerebrovascular, or pituitary disorders; those using sedatives or tranquilizers; and elderly patients.
- >700 persons in the United States die from hypothermia annually.

PHYSICAL FINDINGS & CLINICAL PRESENTATION

The clinical presentation varies with the severity of hypothermia. Shivering may be absent if body temperature is <33.3° C (92° F) or in patients taking phenothiazines.

Hypothermia may masquerade as cerebrovascular accident, ataxia, or slurred speech, or the patient may appear comatose or clinically dead. Signs of hypothermia are summarized in Box E1.
Physiologic stages of hypothermia:

1. Stage HT I: Mild hypothermia (typical core temperature 32.2° to 35° C [90° to 95° F]): arrhythmias, ataxia
2. Stage HT II: Moderate hypothermia (core temperature 28° to 32.2° C [82.4° to 90° F]):
   a. Progressive decrease of level of consciousness, pulse, cardiac output, and respiration
   b. Fibrillation, dysrhythmias (increased susceptibility to ventricular tachycardia)
   c. Elimination of shivering mechanism for thermogenesis
3. Stage HT III: Severe hypothermia (core temperature ≤28° C to 24° C [82.4° F to 75° F]):
   a. Absence of reflexes or response to pain
   b. Decreased cerebral blood flow, decreased CO_2
   c. Increased risk of ventricular fibrillation or asystole
   d. Vital signs present
4. Stage IV: No vital signs (core temperature <24° C [75° F])

ETIOLOGY

Exposure to cold temperatures for a prolonged period. Contributing factors include:
1. Drugs: ethanol, phenothiazines, sedative-hypnotics
2. Skin disorders: extensive burns, severe psoriasis, exfoliative dermatitis
3. Metabolic disorders: hypopituitarism, hypothyroidism, hypoadrenalism

4. Neurologic abnormalities: stroke, head trauma, acute spinal cord transection, impaired shivering
5. Other: lack of acclimatization, aggressive fluid resuscitation, sepsis, heat stroke treatment
6. Box E2 summarizes factors predisposing to hypothermia

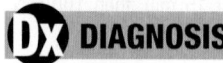

DIAGNOSIS

DIFFERENTIAL DIAGNOSIS

- It is crucial to determine an accurate core temperature measurement. Advantages and considerations of various methods to determine core temperature are summarized in Table 1.
- Cerebrovascular accident
- Myxedema coma
- Drug intoxication
- Hypoglycemia

LABORATORY TESTS

1. Metabolic and respiratory acidosis are usually present.
   a. When blood cools, the arterial pH increases, oxygen tension (Po_2) increases, and the Pco_2 falls:
   (1) pH increases 0.008 U/° F (or 0.015 U/° C), causing a decrease in temperature.
   (2) Pao_2 increases 3.3%/° F, causing a decrease in temperature. Oxygenation considerations during hypothermia are described in Box 3.
   (3) $Paco_2$ decreases 2.4%/° F, causing a decrease in temperature.
   b. Blood gas analyzers warm the blood to 37° C, increasing the partial pressure of dissolved gases, resulting in higher oxygen and carbon dioxide levels and a lower pH than the patient's actual values. Correction of arterial blood gases for temperature is unnecessary as a guide to therapy. The use of uncorrected values also permits reference to the standard acid–base nomograms.
2. A decrease in K^+ initially, then an increase in K^+ with increasing hypothermia; extreme hyperkalemia indicates a poor prognosis.
3. Hematocrit increases (caused by hemoconcentration), decreasing leukocytes and platelets (caused by splenic sequestration).
4. Blood viscosity, increased clotting time

TABLE 1 Core Temperature Measurements

Type	Advantages	Considerations
Rectal	Convenient	Insert 15 cm (6 inches)
	Continuous monitoring	Lags during transition from cooling to rewarming
		Falsely elevated with peritoneal lavage
		Falsely low if probe is in cold feces or when lower extremities are frozen
Esophageal	Convenient	Insert 24 cm (9.5 inches) below larynx
	Continuous monitoring	Tracheal misplacement
		Aspiration
		Falsely elevated with heated inhalation
Tympanic	Approximates hypothalamic temperature via internal carotid artery	Probe: tympanic membrane perforation; canal hemorrhage Infrared: unreliable; cerumen effect
Bladder	Convenient	Unreliable
	Continuous monitoring	Falsely elevated with peritoneal lavage
		Falsely low with cold diuresis

From Auerbach P: *Wilderness medicine, expert consult* Premium Edition—Enhanced Online Features and Print, Philadelphia, 2012, Saunders.

BOX 3 Oxygenation Considerations During Hypothermia

Detrimental Factors
Oxygen consumption increases with rise in temperature; caution if rapid rewarming; shivering also increases demand
Decreased temperature shifts oxyhemoglobin dissociation curve to the left
Ventilation-perfusion mismatch; atelectasis; decreased respiratory minute volume; bronchorrhea; decreased protective airway reflexes
Decreased tissue perfusion from vasoconstriction; increased viscosity
"Functional hemoglobin" concept: capability of hemoglobin to unload oxygen is lowered
Decreased thoracic elasticity and pulmonary compliance

Protective Factors
Reduction of oxygen consumption: 50% at 28° C (82.4° F); 75% at 22° C (71.6° F); 92% at 10° C (50° F)
Increased oxygen solubility in plasma
Decreased pH and increased $Paco_2$ shift oxyhemoglobin dissociation curve to right

From Auerbach P: *Wilderness medicine*, ed 4, St Louis, 2001, Mosby.

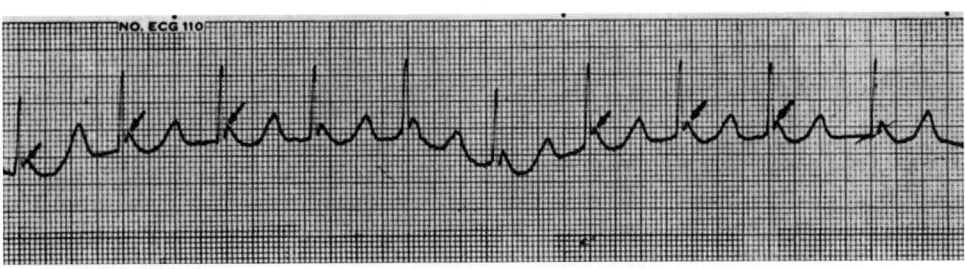

FIG. 1 Hypothermic J waves (Osborne waves) *(arrows)* **in an 80-year-old man with core temperature of 86° F (30° C)**.These waves disappeared with rewarming. (From Morse CD, Rial WY: Emergency medicine. In Rakel RE [ed]: *Textbook of family practice*, ed 4, Philadelphia, 1990, Saunders.)

BOX 4   Preparing Hypothermic Patients for Transport

1. The patient must be dry. Gently remove or cut off wet clothing, and replace it with dry clothing or a dry insulation system. Keep the patient horizontal, and do not allow exertion or massage of the extremities.
2. Stabilize injuries (i.e., the spine; place fractures in the correct anatomic position). Open wounds should be covered before packaging.
3. Initiate heated intravenous infusions (IVs) if feasible; bags can be placed under the patient's buttocks or in a compressor system. Administer a fluid challenge.
4. Active rewarming should be limited to heated inhalation and truncal heat. Insulate hot water bottles in stockings or mittens, and then place them in the patient's axillae and groin.
5. The patient should be wrapped. Begin building the wrap by placing a large plastic sheet on the available surface (floor, ground), and on it place an insulated sleeping pad. A layer of blankets, a sleeping bag, or bubble wrap insulating material is laid over the sleeping pad. The patient is then placed on the insulation. Heating bottles are put in place along with IVs, and the entire package is wrapped layer over layer, with the plastic as the final closure. The patient's face should be partially covered, but a tunnel should be created to allow access for breathing and monitoring.

From Auerbach P: *Wilderness medicine, Expert Consult premium edition—enhanced online features and print*, Philadelphia, 2012, Elsevier.

IMAGING STUDIES

- Chest x-ray: generally not helpful; may reveal evidence of aspiration (e.g., intoxicated patient with aspiration pneumonia)
- ECG: prolonged PR, QT, and QRS segments, depressed ST segments, inverted T waves, atrioventricular block, and hypothermic J waves (Osborne waves) may appear at temperatures less than 33.0° C (91.4° F); characterized by notching of the junction of the QRS complex and ST segments (Fig. 1).

Rx TREATMENT

NONPHARMACOLOGIC THERAPY

- The first critical step in management of accidental hypothermia is initiating passive external rewarming by removing wet clothing and covering the patient with insulating material.
- Specific treatment of hypothermia varies with the following:
  1. Degree of hypothermia
  2. Existence of concomitant diseases (e.g., cardiovascular insufficiency)
  3. Patient's age and medical condition (e.g., elderly, debilitated patients vs. young, healthy patients)
- General measures:
  1. Secure an airway before warming all unconscious patients; precede endotracheal intubation with oxygenation (if pos-

sible) to minimize the risk of arrhythmias during the procedure.
  2. Peripheral vasoconstriction may impede placement of a peripheral intravenous catheter; consider femoral venous access as an alternative to the jugular or subclavian sites to avoid ventricular stimulation.
  3. A Foley catheter should be inserted, and urinary output should be monitored and maintained >0.5 to 1 ml/kg/hr with intravascular volume replacement.
  4. Box 4 summarizes measures for preparing hypothermic patients for transport.

ACUTE GENERAL Rx

- Continuous ECG monitoring of patients is recommended. Ventricular arrhythmias can be treated with bretylium; lidocaine is generally ineffective, and procainamide is associated with an increased incidence of ventricular fibrillation in hypothermic patients.
- Correct severe acidosis and electrolyte abnormalities.
- Hypothyroidism, if present, should be promptly treated (see "Myxedema Coma").
- If clinical evidence suggests adrenal insufficiency, administer IV methylprednisolone.

In patients unresponsive to verbal or noxious stimuli or with altered mental status, 100 mg of thiamine, 0.4 mg of naloxone, and 1 ampule of 50% dextrose may be given.

Warm (104° to 113° F [40° to 45° C]), humidified oxygen should also be given if available. Specific treatment:
1. Mild hypothermia (rectal temperature <32.3° C [90° F]): passive external rewarming is indicated. Place the patient in a warm room (temperature >21° C [69.8° F]), and cover with insulating material after gently removing wet clothing; recommended rewarming rates vary between 0.5° and 20° C/hr but should not exceed 0.55° C/hr in elderly persons.
2. Moderate to severe hypothermia:
   a. Active core rewarming
      (1) Delivery of heat by way of fluids: warm gastrointestinal irrigation (with saline enemas and by nasogastric tube); IV fluids (usually D_5NS without potassium) warmed to 104° to 107.6° F (40° to 42° C), peritoneal dialysis with dialysate heated to 40.5° to 42.5° C.
      (2) Inhalation of heated, humidified oxygen (warmed to 40° C [104° F]) increases core temperature by 1° C (1.8° F) per hr and decreases evaporative heat loss from respiration.
3. Active external rewarming: immersion in a bath of warm water (40° to 41° C); active external rewarming may produce shock because of excessive peripheral vasodilation. Ideal candidates are previously healthy, young patients with acute immersion hypothermia.
4. Extracorporeal blood warming with cardiopulmonary bypass appears to be an efficacious rewarming technique in young, otherwise healthy persons.
5. Patients with cardiac instability and those in cardiac arrest should be transported to a center capable of providing extracorporeal membrane oxygenation (ECMO) unless other conditions (e.g., trauma) require transport to a closer facility.

SUGGESTED READING
Available at www.expertconsult.com

RELATED CONTENT
Hypothermia (Patient Information)

AUTHOR: **FRED F. FERRI, M.D.**

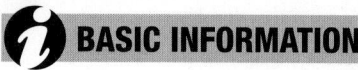

BASIC INFORMATION

DEFINITION

Hypothyroidism is a disorder caused by the inadequate secretion of thyroid hormone.

SYNONYMS

Myxedema

ICD-10CM CODES

E03.9 Hypothyroidism, unspecified
E00.9 Congenital iodine-deficiency syndrome, unspecified
E89.0 Postprocedural hypothyroidism
E03.2 Hypothyroidism due to medicaments and other exogenous substances
E02 Subclinical iodine-deficiency hypothyroidism
E03.0 Congenital hypothyroidism with diffuse goiter
E03.1 Congenital hypothyroidism without goiter
E03.3 Postinfectious hypothyroidism
E03.8 Other specified hypothyroidism

EPIDEMIOLOGY & DEMOGRAPHICS

INCIDENCE/PREVALENCE: 1.5% to 2% of women and 0.2% of men. Overall, about 1 in 300 persons in the United States has hypothyroidism.
PREDOMINANT AGE: Incidence of hypothyroidism increases with age; among persons older than 60 yr, 6% of women and 2.5% of men have laboratory evidence of hypothyroidism (thyroid-stimulating hormone [TSH] more than twice normal level).

PHYSICAL FINDINGS & CLINICAL PRESENTATION

- Hypothyroid patients generally present with the following signs and symptoms: fatigue, lethargy, weakness, constipation, weight gain, cold intolerance, muscle weakness, slow speech, slow cerebration with poor memory.
- Skin: dry, coarse, thick, cool, sallow (yellow color caused by carotenemia); nonpitting edema in skin of eyelids and hands (myxedema) secondary to infiltration of subcutaneous tissues by a hydrophilic mucopolysaccharide substance. (Fig. E1, *A* and *B*)
- Hair: brittle and coarse; loss of outer third of eyebrows.
- Facies: dulled expression, thickened tongue, thick and slow-moving lips.
- Thyroid gland: may or may not be palpable (depending on the cause of the hypothyroidism).
- Heart sounds: distant, possible pericardial effusion.
- Pulse: bradycardia.
- Neurologic: delayed relaxation phase of the deep tendon reflexes, cerebellar ataxia, hearing impairment, poor memory, peripheral neuropathies with paresthesia.
- Musculoskeletal: carpal tunnel syndrome, muscular stiffness, weakness.

ETIOLOGY

1. Primary hypothyroidism (thyroid gland dysfunction): the cause of >90% of the cases of hypothyroidism

  o Hashimoto's thyroiditis is the most common cause of hypothyroidism after age 8 yr
  o Idiopathic myxedema (nongoitrous form of Hashimoto's thyroiditis)
  o Previous treatment of hyperthyroidism (radioiodine therapy, subtotal thyroidectomy)
  o Subacute thyroiditis
  o Radiation therapy to the neck (usually for malignant disease)
  o Iodine deficiency or excess
  o Drugs (lithium, para-aminosalicylate, sulfonamides, phenylbutazone, amiodarone, thiourea)
  o Congenital (approximately one case per 4000 live births)
  o Prolonged treatment with iodides
2. Secondary hypothyroidism: pituitary dysfunction, postpartum necrosis, neoplasm, infiltrative disease causing deficiency of TSH
3. Tertiary hypothyroidism: hypothalamic disease (granuloma, neoplasm, or irradiation causing deficiency of thyrotropin-releasing hormone)
4. Tissue resistance to thyroid hormone: rare

DIAGNOSIS

DIFFERENTIAL DIAGNOSIS

- Depression
- Dementia from other causes
- Systemic disorders (e.g., nephrotic syndrome, congestive heart failure, amyloidosis)

LABORATORY TESTS

- Increased TSH: TSH may be normal if patient has secondary or tertiary hypothyroidism, is receiving dopamine or corticosteroids, or the level is obtained after severe illness
- Decreased free T_4
- Other common laboratory abnormalities: hyperlipidemia, hyponatremia, and anemia
- Increased antimicrosomal and antithyroglobulin antibody titers: useful when autoimmune thyroiditis is suspected as the cause of the hypothyroidism. The American Thyroid Association recommends treatment of pregnant patients with subclinical hypothyroidism and thyroid peroxidase antibody (anti-TPO) positivity.
- Fig. E1, *C* describes a strategy for the laboratory evaluation of patients with suspected hypothyroidism

TREATMENT

NONPHARMACOLOGIC THERAPY

Patients should be educated regarding hypothyroidism and its possible complications. Patients should also be instructed about the need for lifelong treatment and monitoring of their thyroid abnormality.

ACUTE GENERAL Rx

Start replacement therapy with levothyroxine (L-thyroxine) 25 to 100 μg/day, depending on the patient's age and the severity of the disease. Physiologic combinations of L-thyroxine plus liothyronine do not offer any objective advantage over L-thyroxine alone. The levothyroxine dose may be increased every 6 to 8 wk, depending on the clinical response and serum TSH level. Elderly patients and patients with coronary

artery disease should be started with 12.5 to 25 μg/day (higher doses may precipitate angina). The average maintenance dose of levothyroxine is 1.7 μg/kg/day (100 to 150 μg/day in adults). The elderly may require <1 μg/kg/day, whereas children generally require higher doses (up to 3 to 4 μg/kg/day). Pregnant patients also have increased requirements. Estrogen therapy may also increase the need for thyroxine. Women with hypothyroidism should increase their levothyroxine dose by approximately 30% as soon as pregnancy is confirmed. Close monitoring of serum thyrotropin levels and adjustment of levothyroxine dose to maintain a TSH level of 4.0 mU per liter as upper limit is recommended throughout pregnancy. Table E1 summarizes conditions that alter levothyroxine requirements.

CHRONIC Rx

- Periodic monitoring of TSH level is an essential part of treatment. Patients should be evaluated initially with office visit and TSH levels every 6 to 8 wk until the patient is clinically euthyroid and the TSH level is normalized. The frequency of subsequent visits and TSH measurement can then be decreased to every 6 to 12 mo. Pregnant patients should be checked every trimester.
- For monitoring therapy in patients with central hypothyroidism, measurement of serum free thyroxine (free T_4 level) is appropriate and should be maintained in the upper half of the normal range.

REFERRAL

Admission to the hospital intensive care unit is recommended in all patients with myxedema coma. Additional information on the diagnosis and treatment of this life-threatening complication of hypothyroidism is available under "Myxedema Coma" in Section I.

PEARLS & CONSIDERATIONS

COMMENTS

Subclinical hypothyroidism occurs in as many as 15% of elderly patients and is characterized by an elevated serum TSH and a normal free T_4 level. Subclinical hypothyroidism is associated with an increased risk of coronary heart disease events and mortality, particularly in those with a TSH concentration of 10 mU/L or greater. Treatment is individualized. In general, replacement therapy is recommended for all patients with serum TSH >10 mU/L and with presence of goiter or thyroid autoantibodies.

EVIDENCE

Available at www.expertconsult.com

SUGGESTED READINGS

Available at www.expertconsult.com

RELATED CONTENT

Hypothyroidism (Patient Information)
Myxedema Coma (Related Key Topic)

AUTHOR: **FRED F. FERRI, M.D.**

ⓘ BASIC INFORMATION

DEFINITION

Idiopathic pulmonary fibrosis (IPF) is a specific form of chronic fibrosing interstitial pneumonia with histopathologic characteristics of usual interstitial pneumonia (UIP) occurring in the absence of an identifiable cause of lung injury. Clinically, it is characterized by progressive parenchymal scarring and loss of pulmonary function.

SYNONYMS

Cryptogenic fibrosing alveolitis
IPF
Pulmonary fibrosis
Usual interstitial pneumonia

ICD-10CM CODES
J84.112 Idiopathic pulmonary fibrosis

EPIDEMIOLOGY & DEMOGRAPHICS

- Incidence: 7-16 cases/100,000 persons worldwide. Clinically IPF affects >50,000 people in the U.S. and accounts for 20%-30% of interstitial lung diseases. It is the most common idiopathic interstitial pneumonia.
- Most commonly presents in 6th and 7th decades
- More common in men than women
- More common in current and past smokers
- Familial forms account for 3% to 25% of cases. Genetic variants: include mutations in surfactant protein C and telomerase as well as polymorphisms of the *MUC5B* gene.
- No distinct geographic distribution; no clear racial predilection

PHYSICAL FINDINGS & CLINICAL PRESENTATION

- Most present with gradual onset (>6 mo) of exertional dyspnea and nonproductive cough. Progressive dyspnea is usually the most prominent symptom. Cough affects up to 80% of patients with IPF, is frequently disabling, and lacks effective therapy.
- Fine bibasilar inspiratory crackles in >80% of patients, with progression upward as the disease advances.
- Clubbing is found in 25% to 50% of patients.
- Cyanosis and right heart failure (cor pulmonale) may occur late in the disease course.
- There are no extrapulmonary manifestations beyond clubbing and complications of right heart failure. Fever and wheezing are rare and suggest alternative diagnosis.
- Fig. 1 is a chest radiograph showing diffuse bilateral lower lung predominant reticular opacities in a patient with IPF.

ETIOLOGY

- Unknown
- Cigarette smoking, environmental exposure, and microaspiration have been associated with IPF.
- Aberrant tissue repair and fibrosis are believed to play a greater role in the pathogenesis than generalized inflammation. Immune system activation and increased vascular permeability contribute to the underlying pathology.

⑁ DIAGNOSIS

DIFFERENTIAL DIAGNOSIS

- Sarcoidosis
- Drug-induced interstitial lung disease
- Pulmonary manifestations of collagen vascular diseases (e.g., rheumatoid arthritis [RA], systemic sclerosis)
- Hypersensitivity pneumonitis (HP)
- Occupational exposures (e.g., asbestos, silica) may cause pneumoconiosis that mimics IPF
- Other idiopathic interstitial pneumonias:
  1. Desquamative interstitial pneumonia (DIP)
  2. Respiratory bronchitis–interstitial lung disease (RB-ILD)
  3. Acute interstitial pneumonia (AIP)
  4. Nonspecific interstitial pneumonia (NSIP)
  5. Cryptogenic organizing pneumonia (COP)

WORKUP

- Almost all patients have abnormal chest radiograph at presentation, with bilateral reticular opacities most prominent in the periphery and lower lobes. Peripheral honeycombing may be seen.
- High-resolution CT scan (Fig. 2) shows patchy peripheral reticular abnormalities with intralobular linear opacities, irregular septal thickening, subpleural honeycombing, and minimal, if any, ground-glass opacities.
- Pulmonary function testing shows restrictive pattern and reduced carbon monoxide diffusion into the lung.
- Six-minute walk test may show reduced exercise tolerance and/or exertional hypoxia.
- Laboratory abnormalities (nondiagnostic): mild anemia; increases in erythrocyte sedimentation rate, lactate dehydrogenase, C-reactive protein; low titer antinuclear antibody seen in up to 30% of patients.
- There is a limited role for bronchoalveolar lavage either in diagnosis or monitoring IPF.
- Gold standard for diagnosis is lung biopsy (open thoracotomy or video-assisted thoracoscopy). Hallmark features: heterogeneous distribution of parenchymal fibrosis against background of mild inflammation (UIP). In patients with characteristic chest CTs, lung biopsies can be avoided.
- When there is uncertainty, lung biopsy is critical to distinguish IPF from diseases with better prognosis and different treatment options.
- Table 1 summarizes histologic findings for immunologic diseases.

⑀ TREATMENT

- Two FDA-approved oral therapies have proven efficacy in slowing disease progression.
- Pirfenidone is an antifibrotic medication without a known mechanism of action. It is taken three times a day. Its major side effects are nausea, abdominal discomfort, and photosensitivity. LFTs require periodic surveillance.

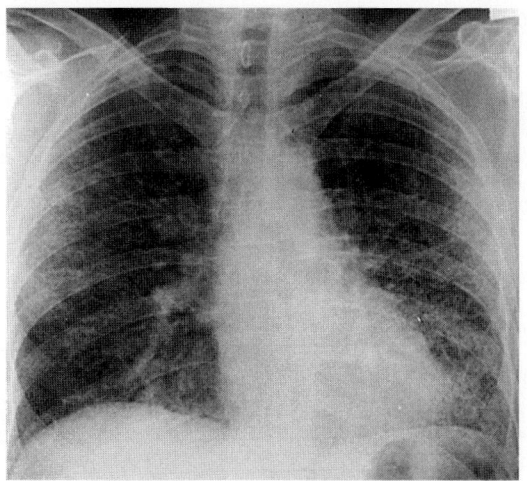

FIG. 1 Chest radiograph shows diffuse bilateral lower lung predominant reticular opacities in a patient with idiopathic pulmonary fibrosis (IPF). (From Mason RJ: *Murray & Nadel's textbook of respiratory medicine,* ed 5, Philadelphia, 2010, Saunders.)

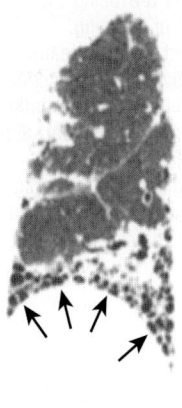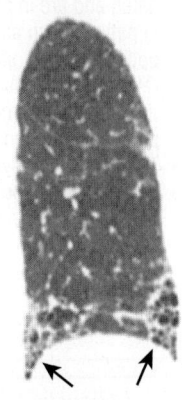

FIG. 2 **Pulmonary fibrosis, honeycombing, and a usual interstitial pneumonia (UIP) pattern in idiopathic pulmonary fibrosis (IPF).** Coronal high-resolution computed tomography reconstruction shows honeycombing (*arrows*) with a basal and subpleural predominance. This is typical of a UIP pattern. (Webb WR, Brant WE, Major NM: *Fundamentals of body CT,* ed 4, Philadelphia, 2015, Saunders.)

TABLE 1 Summary of Histologic Findings for Immunologic Lung Diseases

Disease	Histology
Granulomatous	
Foreign body, inorganic dust	Simple granuloma
Hypersensitivity pneumonitis	Granulomas with CD4+/CD8+ T cells; interstitial edema; fibrosis in later stages
Infections	
Tuberculosis	Caseating granulomas
Sarcoidosis	Noncaseating granulomas
Granulomatous Vasculitides	
Wegener granulomatosis	Necrotizing granulomas involving vasculature
Churg-Strauss syndrome	Necrotizing granulomas involving vasculature
Eosinophilic pneumonias	Granulomas with eosinophilic predominance; interstitial edema
Histiocytosis X	Granulomas with Langerhans cells
Alveolitic	
Drug-associated injury	Interstitial edema with inflammatory cells
Goodpasture syndrome	Linear staining of basement membrane with anti-IgG antibodies typically seen on renal biopsy; interstitial edema with inflammatory cells
Idiopathic Interstitial Pneumonias	
Idiopathic pulmonary fibrosis	Interstitial edema and/or fibrosis with inflammatory cells; patchy fibrotic change
Desquamative interstitial pneumonia	Interstitial edema with sparse inflammatory cells; mild diffuse fibrotic change
Idiopathic nonspecific interstitial pneumonia	Thickened interstitium with inflammatory cells; some patchy fibrosis
Acute interstitial pneumonia	Diffuse alveolar damage with thickened fibrotic interstitium; proliferating fibroblasts
Respiratory bronchiolitis–associated interstitial lung disease	Macrophages infiltrating distal bronchioles
Cryptogenic organizing pneumonia	Chronically inflamed alveoli with granulation tissue in bronchioles and macrophages in alveoli
Lymphocytic interstitial pneumonia	Diffuse lymphocytic and plasma cell infiltration; minimal alveolar injury
Idiopathic pleuroparenchymal fibroelastosis	Diffuse alveolar damage with fibrosis

From Sellke FW et al: *Sabiston & Spencer Surgery of the Chest*, ed 9, 2016, Elsevier.

- Nintedanib is a tyrosine kinase inhibitor taken twice daily. Its major side effect is diarrhea, which often resolves. LFTs also need to be followed.
- Additional new therapies are being investigated and are in phase I or II testing.
- In patients with advanced disease, treatment options include supportive care (pulmonary rehabilitation, supplemental oxygen, influenza and pneumococcal vaccination) and potential lung transplantation.
- Treatment of asymptomatic gastroesophageal reflux may be reasonable given association between pulmonary fibrosis and reflux or microaspiration.

- Lung transplantation is the only therapy shown to prolong survival in IPF. Posttransplant 5-yr survival for IPF patients is approximately 50% to 60%. Median survival time is longer after bilateral lung transplantation than single lung transplantation but is associated with more complications during the first year.
- Acute exacerbation of IPF, defined as worsening dyspnea (<1 mo), the presence of new opacities on radiograph, and the lack of evidence of infection, has a yearly incidence of 10% to 20%. Progressive respiratory failure may require mechanical ventilation. Treatment often includes high-dose corticosteroids and broad-spectrum antibiotics,

although the efficacy of this approach is unproven and questionable.

DISPOSITION

- Spontaneous remissions do not occur.
- Natural history includes progressive loss of pulmonary function.
- There is an increased risk of lung cancer.
- Mean survival after the diagnosis of biopsy-confirmed IPF is 4 to 5 yr, although with new therapies available, survival is less defined.
- Respiratory failure is the most common cause of death.

REFERRAL

- To pulmonologist for review of abnormal chest imaging and establishing diagnosis.
- Encouraging participation in clinical trials is a priority.
- Early referral for lung transplant.

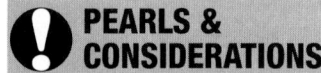

- The course is progressive, with a high mortality rate. The most common cause of death in IPF is respiratory failure.
- Critical to differentiate IPF from other interstitial lung diseases because prognosis and response to treatment differ.
- Two new oral therapies shown to slow disease progression were recently approved. Additional novel treatments are being investigated.[1]

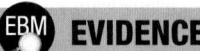 **EVIDENCE**

Available at www.expertconsult.com

SUGGESTED READINGS

Available at www.expertconsult.com

RELATED CONTENT

Idiopathic Pulmonary Fibrosis (Patient Information)

AUTHOR: **PETER LACAMERA, M.D.**

[1]Peljto AL, et al.: Association between the MUC5B promoter polymorphism and survival in patients with idiopathic pulmonary fibrosis, *JAMA* 309(21):2232-2239, 2013.

BASIC INFORMATION

DEFINITION

Immunoglobulin A (IgA) nephropathy is a proliferative glomerulonephritis associated with predominant deposition of IgA in the mesangium. The diagnostic hallmark of IgA nephropathy is the predominance of IgA deposits, either alone or with IgG, IgM, or both, and typically with C3 complement in the glomerular mesangium.

SYNONYM

Berger's disease
IgAN

ICD-10CM CODES
N02.8 IgA nephropathy
N02.1 IgA nephropathy with glomerular lesion, focal and segmental hyalinosis or sclerosis
N02.3 IgA nephropathy with glomerular lesion, mesangial proliferative (diffuse)
N02.5 IgA nephropathy with glomerular lesion, membrane proliferative (diffuse)

EPIDEMIOLOGY & DEMOGRAPHICS

INCIDENCE: IgA nephropathy is the most common primary glomerulonephropathy worldwide. The annual incidence of IgA nephropathy in the U.S. is about 1 to 4 cases per 100,000 person-years. There is a west-to-east increase in incidence and prevalence, with a very low incidence in Africa relative to the U.S. and a higher incidence in East Asia. In Japan, the incidence is 10 times as high as in the U.S. In Europe, there is a south-to-north increase in incidence, with Nordic populations having more than a twofold greater risk than southern Europeans.

PREVALENCE: Prevalence data ranges from 1.3% to 16% in the general population based on necropsy studies demonstrating IgA deposits. In most reports, prevalence rates are expressed as a percentage of cases of primary glomerulonephritis or as a percentage of total series of renal biopsies. Prevalence rate in kidney biopsies is lowest in the Middle East (5%), 10% to 35% in Europe, 20% in the U.S., and 32% to 54% in Japan and China, reflecting the west-to-east increase in incidence and prevalence. Lower rates may be biased by a more conservative approach by nephrologists in the U.S., who are reluctant to perform renal biopsies in asymptomatic patients with minimal renal abnormalities.

PREDOMINANT SEX AND AGE: IgA nephropathy is most prevalent in the second and third decades of life with a male:female ratio of 2:1 in the U.S. and 3:1 in Europe. In East Asia, the male:female ratio is closer to 1:1.

GENETICS: Galactose-deficient IgA1 in the serum is a known heritable trait in diverse racial and ethnic groups. The disease is characterized by galactose-deficient IgA1 deposits in the mesangium, and the genetic predisposition is demonstrated by the fact that 75% of patients with IgA nephropathy have elevated galactose-deficient IgA1 serum levels.

Although it is considered a sporadic disease in more than 90% of cases, recent genome-wide association studies have identified 6% to 8% of cases with at least 15 susceptibility loci, with the strongest signal from the MHC region of chromosome 6. Certain loci are more prevalent in Asia than in the U.S. and Europe. Geospatial analysis of the genetic risk in 85 worldwide populations mirrors the west-to-east worldwide pattern and south-to-north European distribution of the disease. In addition, Asian Americans have a fourfold higher end-stage renal disease incidence than European Americans and a sevenfold higher end-stage renal disease incidence than African Americans, reflecting the genetic basis for this disease. One interesting theory is that the greater prevalence of risk alleles in East Asia may have been selected for to protect against intestinal helminthic infestation.

RISK FACTORS: Disease development: higher association in Asians, whites, and Native Americans and rarely seen in African Americans. IgA nephropathy is more common in males outside of East Asia.

Renal outcomes: The most robust risk factors and predictors of poor renal outcomes include older age, hypertension, proteinuria >1 g/day, and decreased glomerular filtration rate (GFR) at diagnosis. Lower hemoglobin and albumin have recently been shown as robust, poor outcome risk factors. Pathologic risk factors for poor renal outcomes include increased mesangial cellularity, segmental glomerulosclerosis, and tubular atrophy and interstitial fibrosis (see Box 1).

PHYSICAL FINDINGS & CLINICAL PRESENTATION

- 75% of children and young adults present with macroscopic hematuria often associated with upper respiratory infection or gastrointestinal illness. Older adults present with microscopic hematuria, proteinuria, and hypertension.
- Loin pain may be associated with macroscopic hematuria, not to be confused with the much rarer disorder termed "loin pain hematuria syndrome."
- Physical findings are usually unremarkable, except hypertension seen in 20% to 30% of patients with chronic kidney disease and edema in the uncommon (5%) number of patients with nephrotic-range proteinuria.
- IgA nephropathy presents as acute kidney injury due to hemoglobin toxicity from macroscopic hematuria in 5% of patients and as chronic kidney disease in 10% to 20% of patients.

ETIOLOGY

- Most cases are idiopathic/primary. Henoch-Schönlein purpura may represent a vasculitic, more systemic form of IgA nephropathy.
- Secondary causes of IgA nephropathy (Table E1) include hepatitis B; alcoholic cirrhosis; celiac disease; inflammatory bowel disease; psoriasis; sarcoidosis; cystic fibrosis; cancer of the lungs, larynx, or pancreas; HIV infection; systemic lupus erythematosus; rheumatoid arthritis; diabetic nephropathy; Sjögren's syndrome; and Reiter's syndrome.
- There is currently a four-hit pathogenesis model, as demonstrated in Fig. 1. The first hit with high heritability is abnormal glycosylation resulting in the production of galactose-deficient IgA1 (Gd-IgA1). The second hit is production of anti-glycan antibodies that recognize epitopes on the Gd-IgA1, forming immune complexes that deposit in the mesangium as the third hit. The activation of complement and release of inflammatory cytokines from activated leukocytes represent the fourth and final hit.

DIAGNOSIS

DIFFERENTIAL DIAGNOSIS

The differential diagnosis is the group of glomerular, hematuric diseases.
- Henoch-Schönlein purpura.
- Hereditary nephritis.
- Thin glomerular basement membrane disease.
- Lupus nephritis.
- Vasculitis.
- Poststreptococcal nephritis.
- Secondary causes associated with IgA nephropathy are mentioned above.

WORKUP

- The diagnosis of IgA nephropathy is suspected on the basis of clinical history and laboratory data. Episodes of gross hematuria with upper respiratory infections and urinalysis demonstrating worsening hematuria and RBC casts with negative serologies for other glomerulonephritides (e.g., lupus and vasculitis) strongly point to the diagnosis. Although serum IgA levels are elevated in

---

Box 1 Prognostic Markers in IgA Nephropathy

Clinical
Poor prognosis
- Increasing age
- Severity of proteinuria
- Hypertension (increased systolic blood pressure)
- Renal impairment (decreased GFR)
- Decreased serum albumin
- Decreased hemoglobin
- Persistent microscopic hematuria

Good prognosis
- Recurrent macroscopic hematuria

Histopathologic (Oxford Classification)
Poor prognosis
- Increased mesangial cellularity
- Segmental glomerulosclerosis
- Tubular atrophy/interstitial fibrosis
- Crescents

No impact on prognosis
- Endocapillary hypercellularity

From Cancetta PA, et al.: *Clin J Am Soc Nephrol* 9:617, 2014; and Jicheng L, et al.: *Am J Kidney Dis* 62(5):891, 2013.

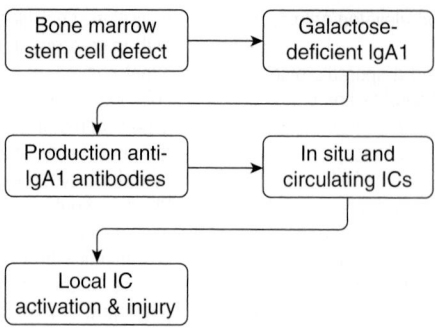

FIG. 1 Pathogenesis of IgA nephropathy.

50% of patients, their sensitivity and specificity is low, and the diagnosis is confirmed by kidney biopsy showing IgA deposits in the mesangium. To standardize diagnosis and provide prognostication, the pathology is scored via the Oxford IgAN MEST classification that evaluates *m*esangial hypercellularity, *e*ndocapillary hypercellularity, *s*egmental glomerulosclerosis, and *t*ubular atrophy/interstitial fibrosis.

- Prognosis is excellent with normal function and low proteinuria; accordingly, kidney biopsy is restricted to patients with sustained proteinuria >1 g/day or worsening kidney function.

LABORATORY TESTS

- Urinalysis variably shows protein, red blood cells, and red blood cell casts.
- Serum creatinine may be elevated.
- Urine protein:creatinine ratio shows mild increases in proteinuria.
- Serum IgA is elevated in only 50% of patients and supports the diagnosis, but it has little clinical utility.

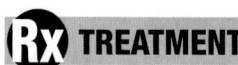 **TREATMENT**

Although initially considered a benign disease, IgA nephropathy is now recognized as a common cause of kidney failure. Currently there is no cure.

NONPHARMACOLOGIC THERAPY

- Moderate dietary protein restriction.
- Discourage smoking.

ACUTE AND CHRONIC GENERAL Rx

- Aggressive therapy for hypertension, preferably with angiotensin-converting enzyme (ACE) inhibitors or angiotensin receptor blockers (ARBs). The goal blood pressure is <125/75 mm Hg if proteinuria is >1 g/day and <130/80 if <1 g/day per international guidelines.
- Patients with recurrent gross hematuria or isolated microscopic hematuria, no or minimal proteinuria (<1 g/day), normal blood pressure, and normal kidney function should be monitored every 6 to 12 months to evaluate disease progression. Fish oil should be considered.

- If bouts of recurrent macroscopic hematuria are associated with tonsillitis, tonsillectomy may benefit these patients, but this treatment is controversial.
- Patients with persistent proteinuria >1 g/day with or without hypertension are treated with ACE inhibitors and/or ARBs. Based on three prior randomized, controlled trials, a 6-month regimen of glucocorticoid steroids is advocated for patients with good kidney function but persistent proteinuria >1 g/day despite ACE and/or ARB administration and fish oil after 6 months. However, a recent prospective randomized, controlled trial showed no benefit of corticosteroids in subnephrotic patients followed for 3 years. Patients with nephrotic syndrome, preserved kidney function, and minimal change in disease are treated with steroids for a 6-month course.
- Based primarily on treatment of crescentic glomerulonephritis with other diseases, patients with crescentic, rapidly progressive glomerulonephritis, in the absence of changes of chronic kidney disease by kidney biopsy, are treated with pulse steroids followed by oral steroids, combined with cyclophosphamide for the first 2 to 3 months. This initial regimen is followed by oral steroids and azathioprine for 2 years as maintenance treatment.
- Patients with acute kidney injury require a renal biopsy to differentiate acute tubular necrosis from pigment nephropathy that requires only supportive therapy from crescentic IgA nephropathy that is treated with aggressive medical management.
- Kidney transplantation is the treatment of choice for end-stage kidney disease. Although the recurrence rate of IgA nephropathy in the transplant is 50%, allograft loss from recurrent IgA nephropathy is only 5%.
- Statins are indicated for all IgA nephropathy patients with dyslipidemia, hypertension, and other cardiovascular risks.
- The roles of mycophenolate, rituximab, and plasmapheresis are not clearly defined given lack of evidence.

COMPLEMENTARY & ALTERNATIVE MEDICINE

The role of fish oil is controversial. One large randomized, placebo-controlled study showed benefit, although many small randomized studies showed no benefit. The recommendation for mild disease is to leave fish oil as optional for patients. International consensus guidelines recommend fish oil along with ACE inhibitors/ARBs if proteinuria is >1 g/day.

DISPOSITION/PROGNOSIS

- Complete remission occurs in <10% of patients.
- End-stage renal failure develops in 12% of patients followed for 5 years, in 15% to 20% within 10 years, and in 20% to 40% within 20 years. Prognostic markers in IgA nephropathy are described in Box 1.
- Poor prognostic indicators include hypertension, extent of renal insufficiency, extent of proteinuria (and certain histologic changes seen in renal biopsy, such as crescents, increased mesangial cells, glomerulosclerosis, and tubulointerstitial fibrosis or atrophy).
- Although not in commercial use, increased serum levels of glycan-specific IgG antibodies predict progression to end-stage kidney disease or death, and increased serum levels of galactose-deficient IgA1 are correlated with risk of deterioration of kidney function.

REFERRAL

Patients with suspected IgA nephropathy are commonly referred to nephrologists for diagnosis and treatment, typically presenting with gross hematuria and urinalysis with blood and proteinuria.

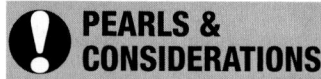 **PEARLS & CONSIDERATIONS**

COMMENTS

- Gross hematuria (red urine) is uncommon with intrinsic kidney diseases but is commonly encountered in IgA nephropathy and cyst rupture in autosomal dominant polycystic kidney disease.
- IgA nephropathy is not an entirely benign condition, even when microhematuria is the only clinical presentation: Nearly 40% of patients reach end-stage kidney disease after 20 years.
- Episodic gross hematuria that occurs during upper respiratory infections is a classic presentation for IgA nephropathy.

SUGGESTED READINGS

Available at www.expertconsult.com

AUTHOR: **PAUL S. KELLERMAN, M.D.**

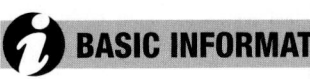

BASIC INFORMATION

DEFINITION

Immune thrombocytopenic purpura (ITP) is an autoimmune disorder in which antibody-coated or immune complex–coated platelets are destroyed prematurely, resulting in peripheral thrombocytopenia. In primary ITP the thrombocytopenia is isolated, whereas in secondary ITP the condition is associated with other disorders (e.g., SLE, HIV, CLL, lymphomas).

ICD-10CM CODES
D69.3 Immune thrombocytopenic purpura

EPIDEMIOLOGY & DEMOGRAPHICS

INCIDENCE: Primary ITP incidence is 10 in 100,000 adults, 5 in 100,000 children.
PREVALENCE: Five to 10 cases per 100,000 persons.
PREDOMINANT SEX: 72% of patients >10 years are female; in children, males are more commonly affected than females.
PREDOMINANT AGE: Children ages 1 to 6 years and young women (70% are <40 yr). New onset of ITP after age 60 years is uncommon; comprehensive workup may be required.

PHYSICAL FINDINGS & CLINICAL PRESENTATION

The presentation of ITP is different in children and adults:

- Children generally present with sudden onset of bruising and petechiae from severe thrombocytopenia.
- In adults the presentation is insidious; a history of prolonged purpura may be present; many patients are diagnosed incidentally on the basis of automated laboratory tests that now routinely include platelet counts.
- The physical examination may be entirely normal.
- Patients with severe thrombocytopenia may have petechiae, purpura, epistaxis, or heme-positive stool from gastrointestinal bleeding. Life-threatening bleeding is uncommon and generally confined to patients with platelets <10,000/m^l.
- Splenomegaly is unusual; its presence should alert to the possibility of other etiologies of thrombocytopenia.
- The presence of dysmorphic features (skeletal anomalies, auditory abnormalities) may indicate a congenital disorder as the cause of the thrombocytopenia.

ETIOLOGY

Increased platelet destruction is caused by autoantibody targets to platelet-membrane antigens, in particular, antibodies against platelet GPIIb/IIIa or GPIb/IX. The spleen has a major role in ITP by producing autoantibodies in the white pulp and removing autoantibody-coated platelets in the red pulp. Production of antibodies could be triggered either by immunogenicity of membrane glycoproteins (GPs) on the platelet surface or by external factors such as infections or medications.

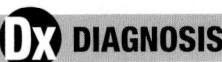

DIAGNOSIS

DIFFERENTIAL DIAGNOSIS

- Falsely low platelet count (resulting from EDTA-dependent or cold-dependent agglutinins).
- Viral infections (e.g., HIV, hepatitis C, mononucleosis, rubella).
- Drugs commonly implicated are quinidine, heparin, antibiotics (linezolid, vancomycin, sulfonamides, rifampin), platelet inhibitors (tirofiban, abciximab, eptifibatide), cimetidine, NSAIDs, thiazide diuretics, antirheumatic agents (gold salts, penicillamine), and chemotherapeutic agents (cyclosporine, fludarabine, oxaliplatin).
- Hypersplenism resulting from liver disease.
- Myelodysplastic and lymphoproliferative disorders.
- Pregnancy, hypothyroidism.
- SLE, TTP, hemolytic-uremic syndrome.
- Congenital thrombocytopenia (e.g., Fanconi's syndrome, May-Hegglin anomaly, Bernard-Soulier syndrome).

LABORATORY TESTS

- Complete blood count, platelet count, and peripheral smear: platelets are decreased. The peripheral smear should show large platelets and no schistocytes (Fig. E1). Red blood cells and white blood cells have a normal morphology. Unless the patient has been bleeding, the hemoglobin level and leukocyte count should be normal.
- Additional tests may be ordered to exclude other causes of the thrombocytopenia when clinically indicated (e.g., HIV, ANA, TSH [hypothyroidism and hyperthyroidism can cause thrombocytopenia], liver enzymes, Hep C ab).
- The direct assay for the measurement of platelet-bound antibodies has an estimated positive predictive value of 80% to 83%. A negative test cannot be used to rule out the diagnosis.
- Bone marrow aspiration and biopsy are recommended in adults older than 60 yr; evidence of immature cells on peripheral smear, or persistent neutropenia.

IMAGING STUDIES

CT scan of abdomen/pelvis in patients with splenomegaly to exclude other disorders causing thrombocytopenia

TREATMENT

NONPHARMACOLOGIC THERAPY

- Minimize activity to prevent injury or bruising (e.g., contact sports should be avoided).
- Stop any potentially offending drugs (see "Etiology"). Avoid medications that increase the risk of bleeding (e.g., aspirin and other NSAIDs).

ACUTE GENERAL Rx

- Treatment varies with the platelet count, patient's age, and bleeding status (Fig. 2).

- Observation and frequent monitoring of platelet count are needed in asymptomatic patients with platelet counts >30,000/mm^3.
- Oral prednisone 1 mg/kg/day in a tapering dose generally for 4 to 6 wk is the most common initial regimen. Methylprednisolone 30 mg/kg/day IV infused over a period of 20 to 30 min (maximum dose of 1 g/day for 2 or 3 days) plus IV immunoglobulin (1 g/kg/day for 2 or 3 days) and infusion of platelets should be given to patients with neurologic symptoms, internal bleeding, or those undergoing emergency surgery.
- Prednisone continued until the platelet count is normalized then slowly tapered off is indicated in adults with platelet counts <20,000/mm^3 and those who have counts <50,000/mm^3 and significant mucous membrane bleeding. Response rates range from 50% to 75%, and most responses occur within the first 3 wk. Oral dexamethasone at a dosage of 40 mg/day for 4 consecutive days has also been reported to induce a high response rate (85%). Continuation of corticosteroids is limited by long-term complications associated with its use (osteoporosis, weight gain, opportunistic infections, emotional lability)
- IV immunoglobulin (0.8 to 1.0 g/kg) is used in patients who have not responded to corticosteroids and often in pregnant patients. It rapidly increases platelet count in nearly 80% of patients, but its effect is transient. Anti-D immunoglobulin, a pooled IgG product derived from the plasma of Rh(D)-negative donors, is also effective. It can be given only to patients who are Rh(D) positive with hemoglobin >8 mg/dl with a usual dose of 50 to 75 mcg/kg.
- Rituximab, a monoclonal antibody directed against the CD20 antigen, is used as a second-line agent. Usual dose is 375 mg/m^2 weekly × 4 wk.
- Splenectomy is considered second-line treatment and should be considered in adults with platelet count <20,000/mm^3 after 6 wk of medical treatment or after 6 mo if more than 10 to 20 mg of prednisone per day is required to maintain a platelet count >30,000/mm^3. In children, splenectomy is generally reserved for persistent thrombocytopenia (>1 yr) and clinically significant bleeding. Appropriate immunizations (pneumococcal vaccine in adults and children, *Haemophilus influenzae* vaccine, meningococcal vaccine in children) should be administered before splenectomy.
- Additional second-line agents are thrombopoietin receptor agonists, azathioprine, cyclosporin A, cyclophosphamide, danazol, dapsone, mycophenolate mofetil, and *Vinca* alkaloids. Romiplostim, a recombinant fusion protein, and the oral thrombopoietin-receptor agonist eltrombopag are effective in increasing platelet count in adult patients with chronic ITP refractory to corticosteroids and/or splenectomy. The American Society of Hematology guidelines revised in 2011 recommend the use of thrombopoietin-receptor agonists for adult patients with ITP at risk for bleeding, who have a contraindication to

splenectomy, or do not have a response to at least one other therapy.
- Platelet transfusion is needed only in case of life-threatening hemorrhage.
- Third-line therapy for ITP consists of combination chemotherapy and hematopoietic stem cell transplantation.

PREGNANCY Rx
- No treatment is required when platelet count is >30,000/mm^3 or higher until 36 weeks' gestation, except anticipating premature labor.

- Oral corticosteroids and intravenous immunoglobulin (IVIG) are first-line treatments.
- Refractory ITP may require splenectomy in the second trimester.

DISPOSITION
- More than 80% of children have a complete remission within 8 wk.
- In adults, the course of the disease is chronic; only 5% of adults have spontaneous remission.

- The principal cause of death from ITP is intracranial hemorrhage (1% of children, 5% of adults).

SUGGESTED READINGS
Available at www.expertconsult.com

Immune Thrombocytopenic Purpura (Patient Information).

AUTHORS: **PATAN GULTAWATVICHAI, M.D.,** and **BHARTI RATHORE, M.D.**

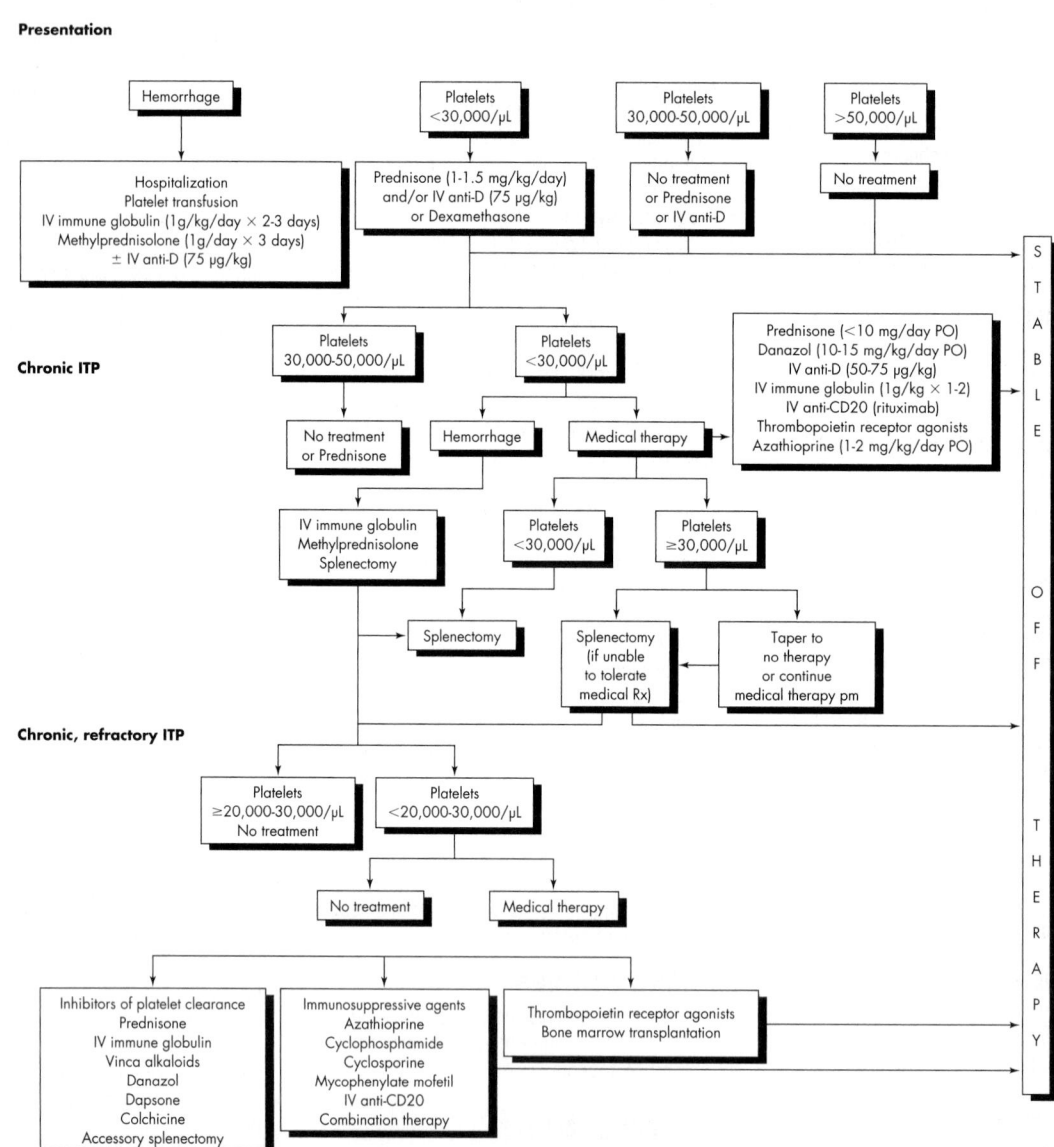

FIG. 2 Treatment algorithm for management of adult-onset immune thrombocytopenic purpura. Some advocate the use of 20,000/mcL as a guideline for therapy. The decision to treat patients with platelet counts lower than 50,000/mcL is based in part on evidence of bleeding, a history of bleeding, comorbid risk factors, lifestyle, and tolerance of therapy. There is no consensus as to duration of steroid therapy. The use of anti-D as initial therapy is appropriate only for Rh(D)-positive individuals who are not markedly anemic or hemolyzing. The goal of medical therapy is to attain a hemostatic platelet count, generally >20,000 to 30,000/mcL. The threshold for treatment depends on comorbid risk factors for bleeding and risk of trauma. Higher platelet counts may be appropriate for surgery or after trauma. Medications can be used individually, but combinations of azathioprine and danazol (or corticosteroids) may provide added benefit and allow lower doses to be used. IVIG and anti-D are generally reserved for severe thrombocytopenia unresponsive to oral agents. The decision to proceed to splenectomy depends on intensity of therapy required, tolerance to side effects, risk of surgery, and patient preference. IVIG and/or methylprednisolone may help to increase the platelet count immediately before splenectomy. Laparoscopic and open splenectomy have comparable outcomes. The decision to treat patients who have platelet counts lower than 20,000 to 30,000/mcL after splenectomy involves an assessment of the risk of hemorrhage versus the side effects of each form of therapy. (Modified from Hoffman R, et al.: *Hematology, basic principles and practice,* ed 5, Philadelphia, 2009, Churchill Livingstone.)

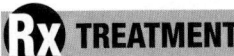

BASIC INFORMATION

DEFINITION

Impetigo is a superficial skin infection generally caused by *Staphylococcus aureus* and/or *Streptococcus* spp.

Common presentations are bullous impetigo (generally caused by staphylococcal disease) and nonbullous impetigo (from streptococcal infection and possible staphylococcal infection); the bullous form is caused by an epidermolytic toxin produced at the site of infection.

SYNONYMS

Impetigo vulgaris
Pyoderma
Impetigo contagiosa
Bullous impetigo

ICD-10CM CODES
L01.00 Impetigo, unspecified
L01.01 Non-bullous impetigo
L01.02 Bockhart's impetigo
L01.03 Bullous impetigo
L01.09 Other impetigo

EPIDEMIOLOGY & DEMOGRAPHICS

Impetigo is the most common bacterial skin infection in children 2 to 5 yr of age. Bullous impetigo accounts for 30% of cases and nonbullous for 70% of cases. Impetigo is most common in temperate zones, mostly during the summer in hot, humid weather. Common sources for children are dirty fingers, pets, and other children in school or day care centers. Impetigo often complicates insect bites, pediculosis, scabies, eczema, and poison ivy.

- Bullous impetigo is most common in infants and children. The nonbullous form is most common in children ages 2 to 5 yr with poor hygiene in warm climates.
- The overall incidence of acute nephritis with impetigo varies between 2% and 5%.

PHYSICAL FINDINGS & CLINICAL PRESENTATION

- Nonbullous impetigo begins as a single red macule or papule that quickly becomes a vesicle. Rupture of the vesicle produces an

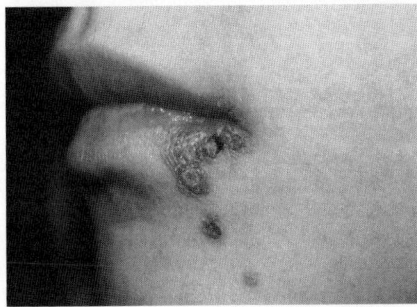

FIG. 1 Multiple crusted and oozing lesions of impetigo. (From Kliegman RM et al: *Nelson textbook of pediatrics,* ed 19, Philadelphia, 2011, Saunders.)

erosion of which the contents dry to form honey-colored crusts. Multiple lesions with golden yellow crusts and weeping areas are often found on the skin around the nose, mouth (Fig. 1), and limbs.
- Bullous impetigo is manifested by the presence of vesicles that enlarge rapidly to form bullae with contents that vary from clear to cloudy. There is subsequent collapse of the center of the bullae; the peripheral areas may retain fluid, and a honey-colored crust may appear in the center. As the lesions enlarge and become contiguous with the others, a scaling border replaces the fluid-filled rim; there is minimal erythema surrounding the lesions.
- Regional lymphadenopathy is most common with nonbullous impetigo.
- Constitutional symptoms are generally absent.

ETIOLOGY

- *S. aureus* coagulase positive is the dominant microorganism (50%–70% of cases).
- *S. pyogenes* (group A β-hemolytic streptococci): M-T serotypes of this organism associated with acute nephritis are 2, 49, 55, 57, and 60. Group B streptococci are associated with newborn impetigo.

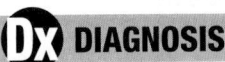 DIAGNOSIS

DIFFERENTIAL DIAGNOSIS

- Atopic dermatitis
- Herpes simplex infection
- Ecthyma
- Folliculitis
- Dermatitis herpetiformis
- Insect bites
- Scabies, pediculosis
- Tinea corporis, cutaneous candidiasis
- Pemphigus vulgaris and bullous pemphigoid
- Chickenpox
- Thermal burns
- Contact dermatitis
- Stevens-Johnson syndrome, Sweet syndrome

WORKUP

Diagnosis is clinical.

LABORATORY TESTS

- Generally not necessary.
- Gram stain and culture and sensitivity to confirm the diagnosis when the clinical presentation is unclear.
- Sedimentation rate parallel to activity of the disease.
- Increased anti-DNAse B and antihyaluronidase.
- Urinalysis revealing hematuria with erythrocyte casts and proteinuria in patients with acute nephritis (most frequently occurring in children between ages 2 and 4 yr in the southern part of the United States).
- If recurrent staphylococcal impetigo develops, a culture of the anterior nares should be done to rule out a carrier state.

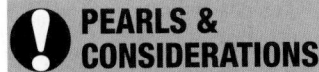 TREATMENT

NONPHARMACOLOGIC THERAPY

Remove crusts by soaking with wet cloth compresses (crusts block the penetration of antibacterial creams).

GENERAL Rx

- Application of 2% mupirocin ointment tid for 10 days or retapamulin 1% applied bid for 5 days to the affected area or until all lesions have cleared.
- Oral antibiotics are used in severe cases: commonly used agents are dicloxacillin 250 mg qid for 7 to 10 days, cephalexin 250 mg qid for 7 to 10 days, azithromycin 500 mg on day 1, 250 mg on days 2 through 5, amoxicillin/clavulanate 500 mg q8h.
- Impetigo can be prevented by prompt application of mupirocin or triple-antibiotic ointment (bacitracin, Polysporin, and neomycin) to sites of skin trauma.
- Patients who are carriers of *S. aureus* in their nares should be treated with mupirocin ointment applied to their nares bid for 5 days or a 10-day course of rifampin, 600 mg/day, combined with dicloxacillin (for MSSA) or TMP-SMX (for MRSA).
- Fingernails should be kept short, and patients should be advised not to scratch any lesions to avoid spread of infection.

DISPOSITION

Most cases of impetigo resolve promptly with appropriate treatment. Both bullous and nonbullous forms of impetigo heal without scarring.

REFERRAL

Nephrology referral in patients with acute nephritis

PEARLS & CONSIDERATIONS

COMMENTS

- Patients should be instructed on use of antibacterial soaps and avoidance of sharing of towels and washcloths because impetigo is extremely contagious.
- Children attending day care should be removed until 48 to 72 hr after initiation of antibiotic treatment.
- Bullous impetigo may be an early manifestation of HIV infection.

SUGGESTED READINGS

Available online at www.expertconsult.com

RELATED CONTENT

Impetigo (Patient Information)

AUTHOR: **FRED F. FERRI, M.D.**

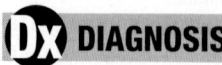

BASIC INFORMATION

DEFINITION

Inclusion body myositis (IBM) is the most common acquired idiopathic myopathy with onset after the age of 50. The idiopathic inflammatory myopathies include polymyositis (PM), dermatomyositis (DM), and inclusion body myositis. They are associated with inflammatory movement of muscle fibers and recurrent weakness. Although IBM is classified among the inflammatory myopathies, its underlying pathophysiology has not yet been delineated, and antiinflammatory medications do not improve weakness.

SYNONYMS

IBM

ICD-10CM CODES
G72.41 Inclusion body myositis [IBM]

EPIDEMIOLOGY & DEMOGRAPHICS

INCIDENCE: 0.22 to 0.79 cases/100,000 persons; uncommon in Asians and African Americans
PREVALENCE: 0.5 to 7.1 cases/100,000 persons
PREDOMINANT SEX: Male/female ratio 1.3:1
PREDOMINANT AGE: 87% older than 50 yr; mean age of 60 yr
PEAK INCIDENCE: Seventh decade
RISK FACTORS: None known
GENETICS: Less than 10% of cases familial

PHYSICAL FINDINGS & CLINICAL PRESENTATION

- Insidious onset of slowly progressive proximal leg and distal arm weakness.
- Time to diagnosis from symptom onset often lags by years to a decade.
- Functional loss of strength in the legs most often precedes arm weakness.
- The cardinal clinical features include early weakness and atrophy of quadriceps muscles (difficulty climbing stairs, rising from chairs, and getting out of cars) along with wrist and finger flexor muscles (difficulty grasping, opening jars, and turning doorknobs). Ankle dorsiflexion weakness may also be prominent leading to foot drop and tripping.
- When examining strength, side-to-side asymmetries are seen in one or more muscle groups in the majority of patients. This stands in contrast to the symmetrical, proximal involvement of polymyositis and most muscular dystrophies.
- Dysphagia and/or mild facial weakness are present in about one third to one half of cases. Dysphagia may be the presenting symptom.
- Although sensory symptoms are usually lacking, one third have evidence of peripheral neuropathy on physical examination and/or electrodiagnostic testing.
- 10% to 15% of patients have concomitant autoimmune disorders such as systemic lupus erythematosus, Sjögren's syndrome, scleroderma, sarcoidosis, or thrombocytopenia. However, unlike polymyositis and dermatomyositis, IBM does not portend an increased risk of heart disease, lung disease, or cancer.

ETIOLOGY

The pathogenesis of IBM is not known. Inflammatory, degenerative, viral, and prion etiologies have been postulated, but none substantiated.

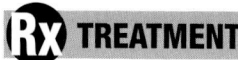

DIAGNOSIS

DIFFERENTIAL DIAGNOSIS

- Polymyositis (Table E1)
- Dermatomyositis
- Amyotrophic lateral sclerosis
- Late-onset muscular dystrophies
- Acid maltase deficiency

WORKUP

- Thorough neurologic examination with emphasis on the motor exam.
- Nerve conduction studies should be performed to exclude other causes and EMG to document a myopathy.
- The diagnosis of definite IBM requires the following features on muscle biopsy (Fig. E1): (1) inflammation, (2) inflammatory cells invading healthy muscle fibers, (3) vacuoles, and (4) amyloid deposits by Congo red staining, TDP-43 sarcoplasmic staining, or tubulofilaments on electron microscopy.

LABORATORY TESTS

- Creatine kinase level (mildly elevated early in disease but less than 10× normal levels; creatine kinase levels may normalize as the disease progresses).
- Complete blood count and coagulation studies should be drawn in anticipation of the muscle biopsy.

IMAGING STUDIES

MRI may reveal atrophy and signal abnormalities in volar forearm muscle groups and quadriceps atrophy with relative preservation of the rectus femoris muscle.

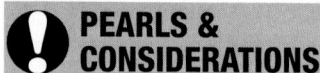

TREATMENT

NONPHARMACOLOGIC THERAPY

- Physical therapy and occupational therapy with the use of assistive mobility devices such as canes, walkers, and wheelchairs are the mainstay of therapy.
- Occasionally knee orthoses or ankle-foot orthoses may improve and prolong ambulation.

ACUTE GENERAL Rx
None

CHRONIC Rx

- Experts have not found clinically significant improvement in functional strength with any pharmacologic therapy. Clinical trials of corticosteroids, methotrexate, intravenous immunoglobulin, anti-T lymphocyte globulin, etanercept, interferon β-1a, and oxandrolone have all failed to demonstrate functional improvements in limb strength.
- A short, small trial of a home exercise program demonstrated mild improvements in strength.
- IBM is generally refractory to therapy.

COMPLEMENTARY & ALTERNATIVE MEDICINE

Some patients choose to self-treat with creatine supplementation, coenzyme Q10, or lithium. There is no evidence supporting these treatments.

REFERRAL

- Patients with suspected IBM should be referred to a neurologist with subspecialty expertise in neuromuscular medicine.
- Physical therapy and occupational therapy consultations help the patient optimize ambulation and fine motor tasks, respectively.
- Speech therapy consultations can assist with symptomatic dysphagia.

PROGNOSIS

Life expectancy is not significantly altered in this late-onset, slowly progressive disorder. Some patients require wheelchair use 10 to 20 years after disease onset.

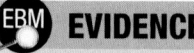

PEARLS & CONSIDERATIONS

COMMENTS

- In contrast to PM and DM, muscle weakness in IBM generally affects both distal and proximal muscles.
- A key to diagnosis rests in finding weakness of wrist and/or finger flexors (especially the deep finger flexors at the DIP joints) on examination.

PREVENTION

None known

PATIENT/FAMILY EDUCATION

Patient information and support groups can be found at: www.ninds.nih.gov/disorders/inclusion_body_myositis and http://www.myositis.org.

EVIDENCE

Available at www.expertconsult.com

SUGGESTED READING

Available at www.expertconsult.com

RELATED CONTENT

Inflammatory Myopathies (Related Key Topic)

AUTHORS: **EMMA H. WEISS, B.B.A., MATTHEW P. WICKLUND, M.D.,** and **JOSEPH S. KASS, M.D., J.D.**

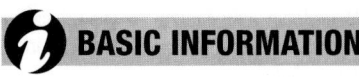

BASIC INFORMATION

DEFINITION

Fecal incontinence is defined as the involuntary loss of gas or liquid stool (minor incontinence) or the involuntary loss of solid stool (major incontinence).

SYNONYMS

Anal or bowel incontinence
Accidental bowel leakage

ICD-10CM CODES
R15.9 Full incontinence of feces
F98.1 Encopresis not due to a substance or known physiological condition

EPIDEMIOLOGY & DEMOGRAPHICS

INCIDENCE: Affects 0.5% to 1.5% of the population younger than age 65, but >10% older than 65. More common in institutionalized patients.
PREVALENCE: Varies widely depending on definition used and population studied; often underreported. In community-based studies, ranges from 1% to 24%. Increases with age and BMI in women.
PREDOMINANT SEX AND AGE: Slightly more common in females versus males and age >65
RISK FACTORS:
- Cognitive or behavioral dysfunction.
- Structural anorectal abnormalities (e.g., rectal prolapse).
- Neurologic disorders, comorbidities (e.g., diabetes mellitus), inflammatory bowel disease (IBD).
- Poor mobility in female gender, advanced age.
- Anal sphincter trauma (surgery, obstetrical injury).
- Fecal impaction from constipation or diarrhea.

PHYSICAL FINDINGS & CLINICAL PRESENTATION

- Should inspect perianal area and perform an internal digital rectal exam to evaluate for the presence of fecal material, prolapsing hemorrhoids, chemical dermatitis, scars, fistula or rectal prolapse.
- Assess for anocutaneous reflex. This may be elicited by stroking skin in each perianal quadrant (normal response is a brisk anal wink). Absent reflex is suggestive of nerve damage. Assess resting to squeezing anal tone by asking the patient to bear down.
- Ask patient to bear down to assess for rectal prolapse or excessive perianal descent.

ETIOLOGY

- Usually multifactorial
- Overflow due to fecal impaction
- Anal sphincter weakness
  - Trauma (e.g., anorectal surgery, childbirth).
  - Nontraumatic (e.g., neurologic, spinal cord lesions, diabetes, scleroderma).
- Anorectal inflammation
  - Radiation, IBD
- CNS disorders (e.g., dementia, multiple sclerosis, stroke)
- Anatomic disturbance of pelvic floor
  - Fistula, prolapse
- Idiopathic

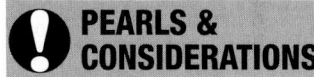 DIAGNOSIS

DIFFERENTIAL DIAGNOSIS

- Fecal encopresis.
- Irritable bowel syndrome or IBD.

WORKUP

- Requires detailed history taking that includes the onset and precipitating events, duration and severity, stool consistency and urgency. Important to evaluate for history of urinary incontinence, anorectal surgery or radiation, neurologic disorders, or prior vaginal deliveries and complete a thorough physical exam. Box E1 describes a structured clinical approach to focal incontinence in older adults.
- Diagnostic workup may include anorectal manometry, endorectal ultrasound (simple and economical), MRI, proctosigmoidoscopy, defecography, pudendal nerve terminal latency, and anal electromyography (EMG).

TREATMENT

- Therapy is focused on supportive care, medications, biofeedback, and surgery.
- Medications focus on decreasing stool frequency and improving consistency.
  - Fiber supplements
  - Antidiarrheals: loperamide, diphenoxylate/atropine sulfate, cholestyramine.
  - Topical phenylephrine, oral valproate sodium: increases smooth muscle tone.
  - Solesta: dextrananomer-hyaluronic gel that is FDA approved for the treatment of fecal incontinence in adults who have failed conservative therapy. It consists of four 1-ml injections into the deep submucosal layer of the anal canal. It is hypothesized that Solesta may narrow the anal canal and allow for better sphincter control.

NONPHARMACOLOGIC THERAPY

- Supportive therapy:
  1. Education, behavioral training, pelvic floor exercises.
  2. Dietary modifications (e.g., increased fiber/fluid intake, less caffeine), keeping food diary.
  3. Incontinence pads, barrier cream.
- Biofeedback therapy
- Electrical stimulation
  - Anal electrodes
  - Sacral nerve stimulation
  - Tibial nerve stimulation
- Surgery:
  1. Overlapping sphincteroplasty (most common).
  2. Implanted devices (e.g., artificial anal sphincter).
  3. Colostomy (if intractable symptoms and/or failed all other therapies).

REFERRAL

Colorectal surgery

PEARLS & CONSIDERATIONS

COMMENTS

The shame, embarrassment, and stigma associated with fecal and urinary incontinence pose significant barriers to seeking professional treatment, resulting in many people suffering from these conditions without help. Therefore, during routine office visits, asking all patients older than 70 about incontinence may be helpful.

PREVENTION

- Reduce constipation and avoid straining during bowel movements.
- Routine episiotomy is the most easily preventable risk factor for fecal incontinence in females.

PATIENT/FAMILY EDUCATION

http://digestive.niddk.nih.gov/ddiseases/pubs/fecalincontinence/index.aspx

SUGGESTED READINGS
Available at www.expertconsult.com

AUTHOR: **DAPHNE SCARAMANGAS-PLUMLEY, M.D.**

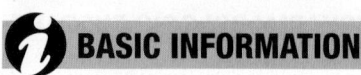

BASIC INFORMATION

DEFINITION

Urinary incontinence is the involuntary loss of urine.

ICD-10CM CODES	
R32	Unspecified urinary incontinence
N39.3	Stress incontinence (female) (male)
N39.41	Urgency urinary incontinence
N39.46	Mixed incontinence
N39.49	Disorder of urinary system, unspecified
R39.81	Functional urinary incontinence

EPIDEMIOLOGY & DEMOGRAPHICS

INCIDENCE/PREVALENCE: In the general population between the ages of 15 and 64 years, 1.5% to 5% of men and 25% to 57% of women have urinary incontinence. In the nursing home population, 75% of the population has some degree of incontinence. Nearly 20% of children through the mid-teenage years have episodes of urinary incontinence.

CLINICAL, PSYCHOLOGICAL, & SOCIAL IMPACT

Fewer than 50% of women living with incontinence in the U.S. consult health care professionals for care, resulting in significant physical and psychological limitations. Many women choose to turn to home remedies, commercially available absorbent materials, and supportive aids. As the incontinence worsens, many women become depressed, limit social interaction, refrain from sexual intimacy, and become homebound. It is estimated that $19.5 billion in direct costs is spent annually on incontinence in the U.S. Urinary incontinence contributes to approximately 6% of nursing home admissions in the older population, leading to a cost of $3 billion per year. With aging populations around the world, this cost is dramatically increasing every year.

MAJOR TYPES OF INCONTINENCE

- **Stress Urinary Incontinence (SUI)** (Table E1) is the complaint of involuntary loss of urine on effort or physical exertion (sporting activities), or on sneezing or coughing (any activity that increases intraabdominal pressure). SUI may be demonstrated in the office with a simple cough stress test during examination and further characterized with degree of urethral mobility (cotton swab test).
- **Urgency Urinary Incontinence (UUI)** is the complaint of involuntary loss of urine associated with urgency, a sudden compelling desire to pass urine that is difficult to defer. The diagnosis is often made clinically based on patient's report of symptoms but may also be associated with involuntary detrusor contractions on urodynamic investigation. May be idiopathic or neurogenic.
- **Overactive Bladder (OAB)** is described as a constellation of symptoms including urgency, with or without urgency urinary incontinence, usually with urinary frequency and nocturia. It should be distinguished from excessive fluid intake and must exclude urinary tract infection. Can occur in up to 27% of men and up to 43% of women.
- **Mixed Urinary Incontinence** is the complaint of involuntary leakage of urine associated with urgency and also with exertion, effort, sneezing or coughing (see Fig. E1).
- **Overflow Incontinence** is the leakage of urine resulting from urinary retention with resultant overflow or spilling of the urine. Causes include hypotonic bladder resulting from age, neurologic conditions such as diabetes or spinal cord injury, prior surgery, drug effects, or fecal impaction. It may also be caused by obstruction at the bladder neck and urethra, such as from prior anti-incontinence surgery, pelvic organ prolapse, urethral stenosis, or detrusor-sphincter dyssynergia.
- **Functional Urinary Incontinence** is the complaint of involuntary leakage of urine resulting from chronic impairments of physical and/or cognitive functioning. This is a diagnosis of exclusion and may be cured by improving the patient's functional status, treating comorbidities, changing medications, and reducing environmental barriers.
- **Extraurethral Urinary Incontinence** is leakage that bypasses the urethral meatus (i.e., vesicovaginal fistula or ectopic ureter).

DIAGNOSIS

HISTORY

- Since many women are hesitant to bring up symptoms of incontinence, these symptoms should be elicited through simple screening.
- History of present illness, psychosocial factors, congenital disorders, access issues for the physically challenged, neurologic disorders, and medication use are coexistent disorders that may affect the urinary tract.
- Urinary incontinence may be characterized by frequency of incontinence episodes, severity, and extent of bother.
- Voiding diary to assess total voided volume, frequency of micturition, mean volume voided, largest single volume, diurnal distribution, nature and severity of incontinence.
- Assessments of the severity of symptoms and goals for treatment are important parts of the history.

WORKUP

- General physical examination
  - Confounding conditions including mobility issues
  - Neuromuscular deficits (gait of the patient)
- Pelvic exam
  - Concurrent pelvic organ prolapse
  - Vaginal discharge
  - Estrogen status
  - Pelvic floor strength assessment
  - Neurologic examination to assess sacral nerves with anal wink and bulbocavernosus reflex
- Rectal examination to assess sphincter tone and stool impaction
- Simple cough stress test
- Urethral hypermobility
- Postvoid residual check with bladder scan or catheter to exclude retention
- 3-day bladder diary to assess frequency, timing, and volume of voids

LABORATORY TESTS

- It is important to rule out urinary tract infection and microscopic hematuria with urinalysis and/or culture prior to more invasive testing for other causes for incontinence.

SPECIALIZED STUDIES

- **Urodynamic testing**: measures different facets of urine storage and evacuation; usually necessary only if basic office evaluation does not elicit the cause of incontinence, or if incontinence is persistent despite treatments.
  - Simple cystometrogram: graph of bladder and abdominal pressures related to fluid volume during filling/storage/voiding to assess sensation and capacity; also assesses presence of detrusor contractions, whether voluntary or involuntary.
  - Uroflowmetry and pressure-flow studies: measure the mechanism of bladder emptying and rate of urine flow.
  - Urethral mechanism and pressure studies.
  - Electromyography: studies the neuromuscular activity of pelvic muscles and striated urethral sphincter during filling and micturition.
- **Cystourethroscopy**: procedure that can be done in the office or the operating room in which an endoscope is inserted into the urethra to view the inside of the bladder and urethra. This procedure is not routinely used to evaluate incontinence unless hematuria is present or prior pelvic surgery is noted on history.

IMAGING STUDIES

- These are usually ordered only if history and/or physical findings suggest other, less common causes of incontinence (i.e., genitourinary fistula) or if microscopic hematuria is present.
- Renal ultrasound may be used to assess for hydronephrosis.
- CT urogram may be used to assess upper tract abnormalities, congenital anomalies, genitourinary fistula, and microscopic hematuria etiologies.

TREATMENT

- The recommended approach to urinary incontinence is a stepped care plan first offering noninvasive behavioral modifications such as bladder training, weight loss, and fluid management.

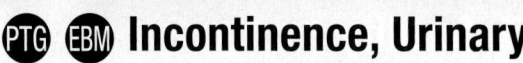

- **Pelvic floor muscle training,** including Kegel exercises and often augmented with biofeedback or electrical stimulation, is an important component of first-line therapy for stress, urge, and mixed incontinence.
- **Pharmacotherapy** is usually reserved for urgency urinary incontinence.
  - ○ Antimuscarinic (anticholinergic) medications: block parasympathetic muscarinic receptors (detrusor M2/M3 receptors) to inhibit involuntary detrusor contractions.
    - ■ Agents available: darifenacin, fesoterodine, oxybutynin (available orally and as a transdermal patch), solifenacin, tolterodine, and trospium.
    - ■ Efficacy: shown to improve symptoms and continence but only modestly compared with placebo.
    - ■ Side effects: high rates of discontinuation due to side effects, most often dry mouth and constipation. May also exacerbate urinary retention, blurred vision, dyspepsia, and impaired cognitive function; contraindicated in narrow-angle glaucoma.
  - ○ Beta-agonists: stimulate β3-adrenergic receptor in the detrusor muscle to cause relaxation and increase bladder capacity.
    - ■ Agent available: mirabegron
    - ■ Efficacy: significant reductions in urgency incontinence in randomized trials
    - ■ Side effects: tachycardia, headache, and diarrhea (similar to placebo); not recommended in uncontrolled hypertension
  - ○ OnabotulinumtoxinA (Botox A): inhibits the presynaptic release of acetylcholine from motor neurons at the neuromuscular junction to paralyze the muscle; given by cystoscopic injection.
    - ■ Efficacy: Similar rates of improvement seen when compared with antimuscarinic medications, but more women reporting complete resolution of urgency urinary incontinence with Botox A; third-line treatment due to adverse effects
    - ■ Adverse effects: urinary retention or incomplete bladder emptying (5% requiring catheterization) and urinary tract infections (33%)
- **Peripheral tibial nerve stimulation**: 30-minute session of tibial nerve stimulation once per week for 12 weeks followed by a customized maintenance plan to treat OAB. Compared to placebo, pooled success rate was 60% in a guideline published by American Urological Association; fewer adverse events noted when compared to antimuscarinic medication.
- **Sacral neuromodulation**: stimulation of bladder and pelvic floor nerves to treat OAB, UUI, and idiopathic urinary retention. The mechanism is unknown. The procedure occurs in a two-stage process: First the electrode is placed near S3 to determine if symptoms are improved; if so, then next the pulse generator is implanted. Evidence suggests 70% of women experience significant improvement in their symptoms with sacral neuromodulation.
- **Surgery**: indicated for women with SUI without symptom control after conservative management or as first-line treatment in appropriately counseled women who decline more conservative treatment.
  - ○ Synthetic slings are the most common primary surgical treatment for SUI.
    - ■ Cure rates of 62% to 98% in a recent systematic review.
- Transvaginal/retropubic: Trocars are passed through the retropubic space from the midurethra to the abdomen (or vice versa). Cure rates range from 81% to 84% at all time points with de novo urgency in approximately 6% of patients.
- Transobturator: Trocars are passed from the vagina behind the ischium (or vice versa).
- Single-incision slings: Only one vaginal incision is needed beneath the urethra; ends of the sling are secured in the internal obturator muscle.
  - ○ Autologous fascial slings: usually considered second line after the failure of synthetic slings due to length and morbidity of the operation. Cure rates estimated to be 90% at 12 to 23 months and 82% at 48 months or greater.
  - ○ Cadaveric slings: usually second line; use has declined more recently due to concerns with early failure and declining success rate over time. Cure rates of 74% at 12 to 23 months and 80% at 48 months or greater.
  - ○ Retropubic urethropexy, i.e., Burch procedure (open abdominal or laparoscopic): a large meta-analysis estimated cure rates to be 82% at 12 to 23 months and 73% at 48 months or longer for open procedures.
- **Bulking Agents**: for treatment of stress incontinence without hypermobility or in poor surgical candidates.
  - ○ Available agents: pyrolytic carbon-coated beads, calcium hydroxylapatite
  - ○ Effectiveness: relatively noninvasive but less effective than surgical intervention; cure rate at 63% to 80% at 1 year
- Treatment for urinary retention and overflow incontinence focuses on reversal of modifiable factors and drainage of urine from the bladder
  - ○ Clean intermittent self-catheterization
  - ○ Sacral neuromodulation

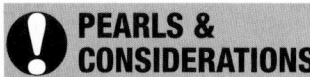

TABLE 2 Transient Causes of Urinary Incontinence (DIAPPERS)

D	Delirium/confusional state
I	Infection—urinary (symptomatic)
A	Atrophic urethritis/vaginitis
P	Pharmaceuticals (diuretics, and so on)
P	Psychological, especially depression
E	Endocrine (hypercalcemia, hypokalemia, glycosuria)
R	Restricted mobility
S	Stool impaction

From Floege J et al. *Comprehensive clinical nephrology,* ed 4, Philadelphia, 2010, Saunders.

! PEARLS & CONSIDERATIONS

COMMENTS

- Weight loss and exercise are helpful for urinary incontinence in obese women. Overweight and obese women with urinary incontinence also have a high prevalence of monthly fecal incontinence (16% found to be associated with low dietary fiber intake after adjustment for other known risk factors for fecal incontinence).
- Transient causes of urinary incontinence in the elderly are described in Table 2.
- Other forms of incontinence:
  1. Nocturnal enuresis: loss of urine occurring during sleep; can occur as idiopathic or neurogenic.
  2. Postvoid dribble: a postsphincteric collection of urine seen with urethral diverticulum; can be idiopathic.
  3. Extraurethral incontinence: enterovesical, urethral; also known as *fistula.*
- Conditions that predispose to surgical failure: advanced age, prior failed incontinence surgery, concurrent detrusor instability, abnormal perineal electromyography, pelvic radiation

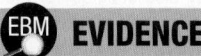 EVIDENCE

Available at www.expertconsult.com

SUGGESTED READINGS

Available at www.expertconsult.com

RELATED CONTENT

Urinary Incontinence (Patient Information)
Pelvic Organ Prolapse (Related Key Topic)

AUTHORS: **MEAGAN CRAMER, M.D.,** **EMILY K. SAKS, M.D., M.S.C.E.,** and **RUBEN ALVERO, M.D.**

Diseases and Disorders

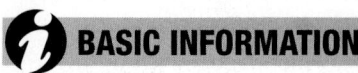

DEFINITION

Infertility in a reproductive-age couple is the inability to conceive after unprotected intercourse for ≥1 year. When a female is greater than 35 years of age, an evaluation is justified after 6 months without successful pregnancy. Earlier evaluation at any age is warranted with known symptoms or medical conditions.

SYNONYM

Sterility

ICD-10CM CODES
N46	Male infertility
N46.8	Other male infertility
N46.9	Male infertility, unspecified
N97.0	Female infertility associated with anovulation
N97.1	Female infertility of tubal origin
N97.2	Female infertility of uterine origin
N97.8	Female infertility of other origin
N97.9	Female infertility, unspecified
O09.00	Supervision of pregnancy with history of infertility, unspecified trimester
O09.01	Supervision of pregnancy with history of infertility, first trimester
O09.02	Supervision of pregnancy with history of infertility, second trimester
O09.03	Supervision of pregnancy with history of infertility, third trimester
Z31.81	Encounter for male factor infertility in female patient

EPIDEMIOLOGY & DEMOGRAPHICS

PEAK INCIDENCE: The incidence of infertility increases with age. Subtle decreases in female fertility start as early as age 30. The rate of infertility increases dramatically after age 37, and unassisted pregnancies become extremely uncommon as women reach the mid-40s. There is also a subtle, but still detectable, decrease in male fertility that may also start as early as age 30.

PREVALENCE: One in eight reproductive age couples experience infertility. This prevalence is consistent in all developed countries and there is evidence that it is historically stable.

PREDOMINANT SEX AND AGE: By definition this is a diagnosis of reproductive age couples. Infertility increases with aging in both males and females, but more dramatically in women. Male factor is responsible in ~40% of couples and the female factor is responsible in ~40% of couples. The remainder of the cases are either combined male and female or unexplained infertility, meaning a clear cause is not identified.

RISK FACTORS: Aging is among the most common of risk factors, predominantly among females. Women are increasingly deferring pregnancy as a result of careers, which is likely associated with the increasing prevalence in certain sectors of the population. Sexually transmitted disease with chlamydia and gonorrhea is associated with pelvic inflammatory disease, which frequently results in tubal factor infertility. Extremes of weight, particularly obesity, are associated with ovulatory dysfunction. Male factor infertility may be idiopathic or due to trauma, infection, varicocele, and exposure to environmental toxins. Smoking is the most common lifestyle choice that impairs fertility.

PHYSICAL FINDINGS & CLINICAL PRESENTATION

- Age
- Previous fertility, particularly if no pregnancy has occurred in another relationship despite absence of contraception
- Absence of secondary sexual characteristics
- Abnormal uterine bleeding or absent menstruation
- Clinical signs of androgen excess: hirsutism, acne, alopecia
- Abnormal pelvic exam: enlarged uterus, adnexal masses, pelvic/abdominal tenderness
- History of urological surgery in male or trauma to testes

ETIOLOGY

- Female factor
  ○ Advanced age
  ○ Tubal factor: pelvic inflammatory disease, endometriosis, prior pelvic surgery, history of ruptured appendicitis, prior elective sterilization
  ○ Anatomic: uterine fibroids, polyps, intrauterine adhesions, uterine anomalies
  ○ Oligo-/anovulation: most frequently due to polycystic ovarian syndrome (PCOS) but also due to thyroid abnormalities, hyperprolactinemia, nonclassic congenital adrenal hyperplasia, hypothalamic amenorrhea
- Male factor
  ○ Abnormal semen analysis
  ○ Elective sterilization
- Idiopathic: both male and female

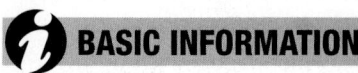

WORKUP

- Confirmation of ovulation: history of regular menstrual cycles, mid-luteal serum progesterone, basal body temperature testing, urinary luteinizing hormone predictor kits (Box E1, Fig. E1)
- Complete transvaginal pelvic ultrasound
- Ovarian reserve testing: anti-müllerian hormone, FSH, and estradiol obtained on cycle day 2-4 and antral follicle count
- Fallopian tube evaluation: hysterosalpingogram (HSG) (Fig. 2)
- Uterine cavity evaluation: HSG, saline infusion sonohysterography, hysteroscopy, or 3D ultrasound of uterus
- Male factor: semen analysis

LABORATORY TESTS

- Semen analysis, using Kruger strict morphology. Abstain 2 to 5 days prior to test.
- FSH and estradiol collected cycle day 2, 3, or 4 and anti-müllerian hormone as a measure of ovarian reserve.
- Mid-luteal progesterone (ideally 7 days prior to expected menses). Given variability of serum progesterone measurements throughout the day and absence of a reliable threshold, most practitioners use clinical criteria to diagnose ovulatory dysfunction.
- Urinary luteinizing hormone measurement
- TSH
- In patients with oligo- or anovulation: prolactin, testosterone, 17-hydroxyprogesterone

IMAGING STUDIES

- Day 2 or 3 transvaginal pelvic ultrasound to assess uterine or adnexal abnormalities and to count the number of small antral follicles (2-9 mm) as a measure of ovarian reserve. If oligo- or anovulatory, to assess for polycystic-appearing ovary.

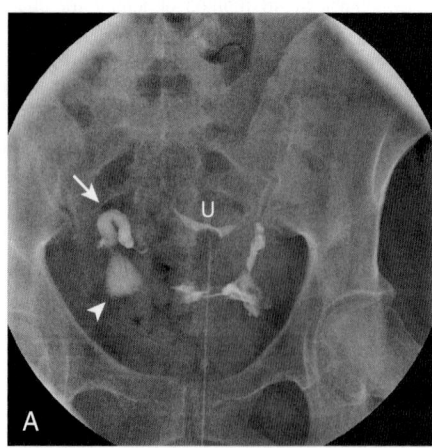 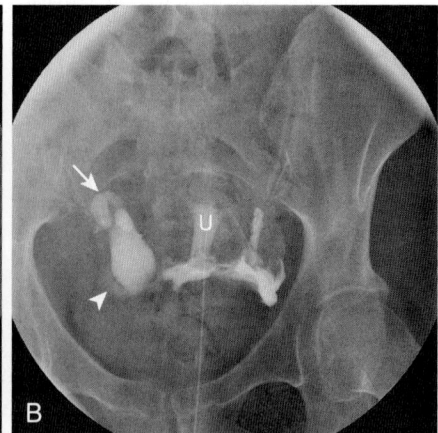

FIG. 2 Hysterosalpingogram spot radiographs early **(A)** and late **(B)** demonstrate a rounded collection of contrast material *(arrowhead)* adjacent to the dilated ampullary portion of the right fallopian tube *(arrow)*, caused by peritubal pelvic adhesions related to previous pelvic inflammatory disease. Normal patient left fallopian tube. *U,* Uterus. (From Fielding JR et al: *Gynecologic imaging,* Philadelphia, 2011, Saunders.)

Diseases
and Disorders

I

- Hysterosalpingogram (early follicular phase after menses complete but before ovulation, typically between days 5 and 12 of the menstrual cycle).
- Also used for imaging of uterine cavity: saline infusion sonohysterography, 3D ultrasound of uterus, hysteroscopy.

Rx TREATMENT

Once the patient presents for evaluation, testing should be completed as quickly as possible, ideally within one menstrual cycle. The couple should follow up with the evaluating provider once all testing is completed and treatment initiated as abnormalities are found.

ACUTE GENERAL Rx

- Oligo- or anovulation should be treated with ovulation induction agents, such as clomiphene citrate or aromatase inhibitors. A recent multicenter trial found that aromatase inhibitors achieved higher live birth rates than clomiphene citrate.[1] Historically, clomiphene citrate has been used, but a very well done randomized controlled trial convincingly demonstrated that letrozole is superior. Far less commonly, ovulatory dysfunction is the result of hypothalamic dysfunction. In these patients, once hypothalamic or pituitary abnormalities are excluded with MRI, ovulation can be achieved using injected gonadotropins.
- Tubal factor infertility may be treated surgically if mild and if the female patient is young and can afford the time to attempt pregnancy over multiple menstrual cycles. If the patient is older or if the tubal pathology is moderate to severe, in vitro fertilization (IVF) is recommended.
- Uterine anatomic abnormalities such as submucosal fibroids, polyps, intrauterine adhesions, or septate uterus should be corrected if they are identified. Fibroids that do not impact the uterine cavity probably do not interfere with fertility. Removal of intramural or subserosal fibroids is reserved for situations in which these cause excessive vaginal bleeding, pain, or pressure.
- Male infertility: referral to urologist for complete evaluation. If semen analysis is severely abnormal, the following laboratory testing is recommended: testosterone, FSH, estradiol, luteinizing hormone, TSH and prolactin, karyotype and Y-chromosome microdeletion.
  - Mild male factor infertility may be treated with intrauterine insemination (IUI), but severe male factor will usually require assisted reproductive technologies (ART) with intracytoplasmic sperm injection (ICSI) in the laboratory, where sperm is injected directly into the oocyte. ICSI use has increased from 36.4% in 1996 to 76.2% in 2012 with the largest increase among cycles without male factor infertility. Donor sperm may be necessary in cases of azoospermia due to testicular failure, if male

partner has a genetic disorder, or if couple is unable to proceed with IVF/ICSI.
- Unexplained infertility can be treated empirically using superovulation with clomiphene citrate or gonadotropins combined with intrauterine insemination with partner's or donor sperm. Most providers recommend using clomiphene citrate with insemination as a first-line superovulatory agent because it is inexpensive. After 3 to 4 such cycles, few pregnancies occur and the couple should be advised to become more aggressive. Controversy exists as to whether gonadotropins with insemination or IVF should be used after clomiphene citrate superovulation induction. There is evidence suggesting that moving to IVF after 3 months of clomiphene citrate and insemination shortens the time interval to achieving pregnancy.[2] A randomized trial in women with unexplained infertility revealed ovarian stimulation with letrozole resulted in a significantly lower frequency of multiple gestation but also a lower frequency of live birth, as compared with gonadotropin but not as compared with clomiphene.
- Donor egg or embryo may be required in cases of premature ovarian insufficiency or due to age. Some couples may elect to pursue adoption.
- For LGBT couples, many family building options are available, including IUI or IVF utilizing donor sperm, donor oocytes, and/or gestational carrier, depending on the needs of the couple.

COMPLEMENTARY & ALTERNATIVE MEDICINE

Acupuncture is widely used by women being treated for infertility. Limited data suggest some benefit, with possible mechanisms of action including increasing blood flow to the uterus and/or ovaries. Despite these studies, it is unproven whether acupuncture definitely improves IVF outcomes. Patients may additionally benefit from the stress relief that acupuncture provides.

DISPOSITION

- Most couples will achieve a pregnancy, provided that they are willing to proceed with treatment including ovulation induction, superovulation, IUI, IVF, or gamete donation.
- Adoption is also a worthwhile and viable possibility for couples unable to conceive.

REFERRAL

Couples should be referred to a reproductive endocrinologist once the complexity of treatment exceeds the comfort level of the provider, whether a family physician, internist, or general gynecologist. Complex ovulation and superovulation induction and ART are best managed by a board-certified reproductive endocrinologist.

[1]Legro RS, et al.: Letrozole versus clomiphene for infertility in the polycystic ovary syndrome, *N Engl J Med* 371:119-129, 2014.11

[2]Reindollar RH, et al.: A randomized clinical trial to evaluate optimal treatment for unexplained infertility: the fast track and standard treatment (FASTT) trial, *Fertil Steril* 94:888-899, 2010.

⚠ PEARLS & CONSIDERATIONS

COMMENTS

- The incidence of heterotopic pregnancy in patients who have undergone IVF is relatively common; identification of a patient with ultrasound-proved intrauterine pregnancy who used ART to conceive should NOT necessarily exclude the possibility of an ectopic gestation.
- Single-embryo transfer is becoming more common in IVF cycles to reduce the rate of multiple gestation.
- Preimplantation genetic diagnosis is used in selected IVF cycles when one or both parents has one or more known genetic abnormalities to test embryos for these specific genetic abnormalities prior to implantation.
- Preimplantation genetic screening is used in IVF cycles to screen embryos for aneuploidy prior to implantation.

PREVENTION

- Techniques that reduce the incidence of pelvic inflammatory disease, such as condom use, can reduce pelvic adhesions that are associated with tubal factor infertility.
- Women should be made aware of the fact that delaying pregnancy into the later reproductive years reduces the likelihood for successful pregnancy. Many women are electing to cryopreserve oocytes or embryos for future use.
- Oocyte, embryo, or sperm cryopreservation is recommended for patients undergoing gonadotoxic chemotherapy or radiation treatment as a means of fertility preservation. Ovarian or testicular tissue cryopreservation may also be performed under a research protocol. All patients should be referred to a reproductive endocrinologist before planned treatment to discuss fertility preservation options.

PATIENT & FAMILY EDUCATION

Patient support groups such as *Resolve* (www.resolve.org) are available to help couples during evaluation and treatment of infertility, which can be extraordinarily stressful.

EBM EVIDENCE

Available at www.expertconsult.com

SUGGESTED READINGS

Available at www.expertconsult.com

RELATED CONTENT

Infertility (Patient Information)
Amenorrhea (Related Key Topic)
Pelvic Inflammatory Disease (Related Key Topic)
Polycystic Ovary Syndrome (Related Key Topic)

AUTHOR: **EMELIA ARGYROPOULOS BACHMAN, M.D.**

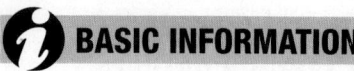

BASIC INFORMATION

DEFINITION

Inflammatory myopathies are idiopathic diseases of muscle characterized clinically by muscle weakness and pathologically by inflammation and muscle fiber breakdown. The four most common are dermatomyositis (DM), necrotizing autoimmune myositis, polymyositis (PM), and inclusion body myositis (IBM). See separate topic on "Inclusion Body Myositis" for details regarding the latter.

SYNONYMS

Idiopathic inflammatory myopathies
Myositis syndromes
Polymyositis
Dermatomyositis

ICD-10CM CODES
M33.90 Dermatopolymyositis, unspecified, organ involvement unspecified
M33.20 Polymyositis, organ involvement unspecified
M33.02 Juvenile dermatopolymyositis with myopathy
M33.12 Other dermatopolymyositis with myopathy
M33.22 Polymyositis with myopathy
M33.92 Dermatopolymyositis, unspecified with myopathy

EPIDEMIOLOGY & DEMOGRAPHICS

Inflammatory myopathies are the largest group of potentially treatable myopathies in children and adults.
DM:
- Occurs in children and in adults (bimodal age peak)
- Average age at diagnosis is 40 years in adults. Age range in children: 5 to 14 years
- More common in females than in males (2:1)
- Incidence 1:100,000
- Prevalence 1 to 10 cases/million in adults and 1 to 3.2 cases/million in children
- Up to one third of patients older than 50 with DM have an associated malignancy
PM:
- Occurs mostly in adults, very rare in children
- Average age at diagnosis >20 years
- More common in females
- Least common inflammatory myopathy
- Exact incidence unknown

PHYSICAL FINDINGS & CLINICAL PRESENTATION

DM and PM:
- Most patients have a subacute onset over weeks to months.
- Pattern is typically symmetric proximal muscle weakness involving the proximal limbs (shoulder and pelvic girdles).
- Weakness of neck flexion and extension is common.
- Difficulty getting up from a chair, climbing stairs, reaching for objects above head, or combing hair.

- Distal muscle and ocular involvement is uncommon.
- Sensation is preserved.
- Reflexes may be preserved or diminished.
- Dysphagia and dysphonia result from involvement of striated muscle of the pharynx and proximal esophagus.
- Esophageal dysmotility is common in DM.
- Respiratory failure from associated pulmonary fibrosis.
- Cardiac conduction abnormalities can be seen with DM.
- Systemic autoimmune disease occurs frequently in PM, and rarely in DM.
- Skin findings in DM:
  1. Heliotrope rash on the upper eyelids (Fig. E1)
  2. Erythematous rash on the face (see Fig. E1)
  3. May also involve the back and shoulders (shawl sign), neck and chest (V-shape), knees (Fig. E2), and elbows
  4. Photosensitivity
  5. Gottron's papules (violaceous papules overlying dorsal interphalangeal or metacarpophalangeal areas, elbow or knee joints—Fig. E3)
  6. Nail cracking, thickening, and irregularity (Fig. E4) with periungual telangiectasia
  7. Mechanic's hand: fissured, hyperpigmented, scaly, and hyperkeratotic; also associated with increased risk of interstitial lung disease

ETIOLOGY

DM: complex, immune-mediated microangiopathy. Adaptive immune response via humorally mediated complement attack
PM: unknown:
- Cell-mediated immune major histocompatibility-I (MHC-1) process directed against muscle fibers is likely, given biopsy features.
- A viral etiology has been proposed secondary to the presence of autoantibodies to histidyl transferase, anti-Jo-1, and signal recognition particle.

DIAGNOSIS

- The diagnosis of each subtype of inflammatory myopathy is based on clinical history, pattern of muscle involvement, electromyographic findings, muscle biopsy, and presence of certain antibodies.
- Myopathic pattern of muscle weakness
- Characteristic rash in DM
- EMG shows myopathic (small-amplitude, short-duration, polyphasic) motor potentials with early recruitment
- Majority of patients have "irritable" features (fibrillations and positive sharp waves) on EMG
- See "Laboratory Tests."
- Biopsy is required for diagnosis and should confirm inflammation before treatment is started. Table 1 describes histologic features of idiopathic inflammatory myopathies. In idiopathic inflammatory myopathies, myopathic features (variation in fiber size, fiber splitting, fatty replacement of muscle tissue, and increased endomysial connective

tissue) should be seen in addition to the following:
1. DM: perifascicular atrophy, MAC deposition along capillaries
2. PM: endomysial infiltrates composed of CD8+ T cells and macrophages invading nonnecrotic muscle fibers that express MHC-I antigen

DIFFERENTIAL DIAGNOSIS

- IBM
- Muscular dystrophies
- Amyloid myoneuropathy
- Amyotrophic lateral sclerosis
- Myasthenia gravis
- Eaton-Lambert syndrome
- Drug-induced myopathies (e.g., quinidine, NSAIDs, penicillamine, HMG CoA-reductase inhibitors)
- Diabetic amyotrophy
- Guillain-Barré syndrome
- Hyperthyroidism or hypothyroidism
- Lichen planus
- Amyopathic DM (rash without weakness)
- DM sine rash (weakness with characteristic biopsy, but no rash)
- Systemic lupus erythematosus (SLE)
- Contact atopic or seborrheic dermatitis
- Psoriasis

LABORATORY TESTS

- Creatine kinase (CK) is the most sensitive muscle enzyme test for muscle breakdown. It should be checked at onset, and serially monitored several times during treatment.
- CK is typically elevated (5-50x normal) in active PM.
- CK may be normal or only slightly elevated in DM.
- Aldolase, AST, ALT, alkaline phosphatase, and LDH may be elevated.
- Anti-Jo-1 antibodies are seen in myositis with associated interstitial lung disease but are not specific for either DM or PM.
- DM: Anti-MDA-5, anti-Mi-2, anti-TIF-1, and anti-NXP2 (implicated in cancer-associated dermatomyositis).
- PM: Antisynthetase antibodies (often seen in overlap myositis) associated with interstitial lung disease, arthritis, fever, and "mechanic's hands."
- Electrolytes, thyroid-stimulating hormone (TSH), Ca, and Mg should be evaluated to exclude other causes of weakness.
- Check ECG for cardiac involvement.

IMAGING STUDIES

- Chest x-ray is used to rule out pulmonary involvement. If suspicious for pulmonary interstitial disease, a high-resolution CT scan of the chest may be helpful.
- Radiography is an efficient means of identifying and characterizing soft-tissue calcinosis (Fig. E5).
- Although MRI arguably has greater diagnostic value than electromyography or serum enzyme measurements in cases of suspected idiopathic inflammatory myopathy, MRI findings have not been formalized as a diagnostic

TABLE 1 Histologic Features of Idiopathic Inflammatory Myopathies

Feature	Dermatomyositis	Polymyositis	Inclusion Body Myositis
Necrosis of muscle fibers	+	+	+
Variation in fiber diameter	+	+	+
Regeneration of muscle fibers	+	+	+
Proliferation of connective tissue	+	+	+
Infiltration of mononuclear cells*	+	+	+
Perivascular and perimysial inflammation	+	–/+	–/+
Endomysial inflammation	–/+	+	+
Perifascicular atrophy	+	–	–
Abnormally dilated capillaries	+	–/+	–
Reduced capillary density	+	–/+	–
Deposition of complement on vessel walls	+	–/+	–
Microinfarcts	+	–	–
Invasion of non-necrotic fibers by cytotoxic T lymphocytes and macrophages	–	+	+
Expression of major histocompatibility complex class I on muscle fibers	–/+	+	+
Rimmed vacuoles with amyloid deposits and tubulofilaments†	–	–	+
Angulated or atrophic and hypertrophic fibers	–	–	+
Ragged red or cytochrome oxidase–negative fibers	–	–	+

*Inflammation is absent in a small proportion of polymyositis and dermatomyositis biopsies.
†Also seen in chronic neurogenic conditions and distal myopathies.
From Firestein GS et al: *Kelly's textbook of rheumatology*, ed 9, Philadelphia, 2013, Saunders, Elsevier.

criterion for idiopathic inflammatory myopathy. The acceptance of MRI as a diagnostic tool in myositis may be inhibited by the high cost and the need for more reliable and validated methods of summarizing the findings of MRI. MRI evaluation before biopsy, however, has become routine at many tertiary care centers. Fascial disease is manifested on MRI by fascial or perifascial hyperintensity on fluid-sensitive sequences. The edema-like signal in the deep subcutis may accompany fasciitis and can indicate associated panniculitis (Fig. E6).
- Video fluoroscopy or barium swallow study to look for upper esophageal dysfunction in patients with dysphagia and DM.

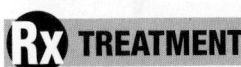 **TREATMENT**

Goal: maintain function, minimize disease/iatrogenic sequelae

NONPHARMACOLOGIC THERAPY
- Sun-blocking agents with SPF 15 or greater for skin protection in patients with DM
- Physical therapy beneficial for gait training and increasing muscle tone and strength
- Occupational therapy assists with activities of daily living
- Speech therapy to monitor patients with swallowing dysfunction

ACUTE GENERAL Rx
- Corticosteroids are the mainstay of therapy. Start prednisone 1 to 2 mg/kg per day, up to a maximum dose of 100 mg/day. Continue until muscle strength improves or muscle enzymes have normalized for at least 4 wk. Begin tapering by 10 mg/month until 60 mg/day, then slowly taper by 5 mg/month. Consider every-other-day prednisone treatment at same dose (may decrease side effects).
- Consider IV immunoglobulin (IVIG) if patient fails to improve on prednisone, or muscle enzymes begin rising when tapering off prednisone. See "Chronic Rx" for specific dosage.
- Hydroxychloroquine can be used to treat the cutaneous lesions of DM.
- A treatment algorithm for adult patients with PM and DM is described in Fig. 7.

CHRONIC Rx
- Chronic prednisone therapy may be needed for years, but other immunosuppressive ("steroid-sparing") agents may be added early to decrease long-term steroid side effects.
- Azathioprine 2 to 3 mg/kg per day tapered to 1 mg/kg per day once steroid is tapered to 15 mg/day. Reduce dosage monthly by 25-mg intervals. Maintenance dosage is 50 mg/day.
- Methotrexate 7.5 to 10 mg PO/wk, increased by 2.5 mg/wk to total of 25 mg/wk; consider IM dosing if PO is ineffective.
- IV immunoglobulin 2 g/kg total dose over 2 to 5 days.
- IV cyclophosphamide 1 g/M^2 monthly for 6 mo is preferred to oral dosing for refractory cases. However, oral dosing of cyclophosphamide is 1 to 3 mg/kg per day PO or 2 to 4 mg/kg per day in conjunction with prednisone.

- Cyclosporine A: initial dose 2.0 to 2.5 mg/kg bid; long-term maintenance is lowest effective dose.
- Mycophenolate mofetil 500 mg PO bid, titrate to 1500 mg PO bid over 1 to 2 months.
- Hydroxychloroquine 200 mg PO daily; monitor for visual changes.

DISPOSITION
- 30% to 40% of patients achieve clinical remission with treatment.
- In patients with residual weakness, deficits typically remain stable over long-term follow-up.
- 10% experience recurrent disease.
- Serum CK often returns to normal before symptoms improve.
- During exacerbations, enzymes may rise before clinical symptoms appear.
- Poor prognostic indicators include delay in diagnosis, older age, recalcitrant disease, malignancy, interstitial pulmonary fibrosis, dysphagia, leukocytosis, fever, and anorexia.
- Infection, malignancy, and cardiac and pulmonary dysfunction are the most common causes of death.
- With early treatment, 5- and 8-yr survival rates of 80% and 73%, respectively, have been reported.

REFERRAL
Neurology or rheumatology referral should be made to help establish the diagnosis and implement treatment.

! PEARLS & CONSIDERATIONS

- Do not implement treatment before muscle biopsy.
- When assessing response to treatment, clinical muscle strength is more important than muscle enzyme tests.
- The concern for malignancies (ovary, lung, breast, GI) associated with DM is legitimate and merits screening in patients older than age 40 at time of diagnosis and every 2 to 3 yr thereafter.
- There does not appear to be any association between juvenile DM and malignancy.
- Overlap syndrome refers to patients with DM who also meet criteria for a connective tissue disorder (e.g., rheumatoid arthritis, scleroderma, SLE).
- In any patient taking steroids, closely monitor for:
  1. Diabetes or glucose intolerance (2-hour oral glucose tolerance test)
  2. Osteopenia/osteoporosis (DEXA scan q6mo)
  3. Cataracts (yearly ophthalmologic appointment)
  4. Hypertension
  5. Psychiatric side effects including depression or psychosis
  6. Poor sleep
  7. Peptic ulcer disease (prescribe H$_2$ antagonist or proton pump inhibitor)

- Clinical and immune response features can be used for categorizing heterogeneous myositis syndromes and mutually exclusive and stable phenotypes and are useful for predicting clinical signs and symptoms, associated environmental and genetic risk factors, and responses to therapy and prognosis.

EBM EVIDENCE

Available at www.expertconsult.com

SUGGESTED READING

Available at www.expertconsult.com

RELATED CONTENT

Dermatomyositis and Polymyositis (Patient Information)
Inclusion Body Myositis (Related Key Topic)

AUTHOR: **JOSEPH S. KASS, M.D., J.D.,** and **GAVIN BROWN, M.D.**

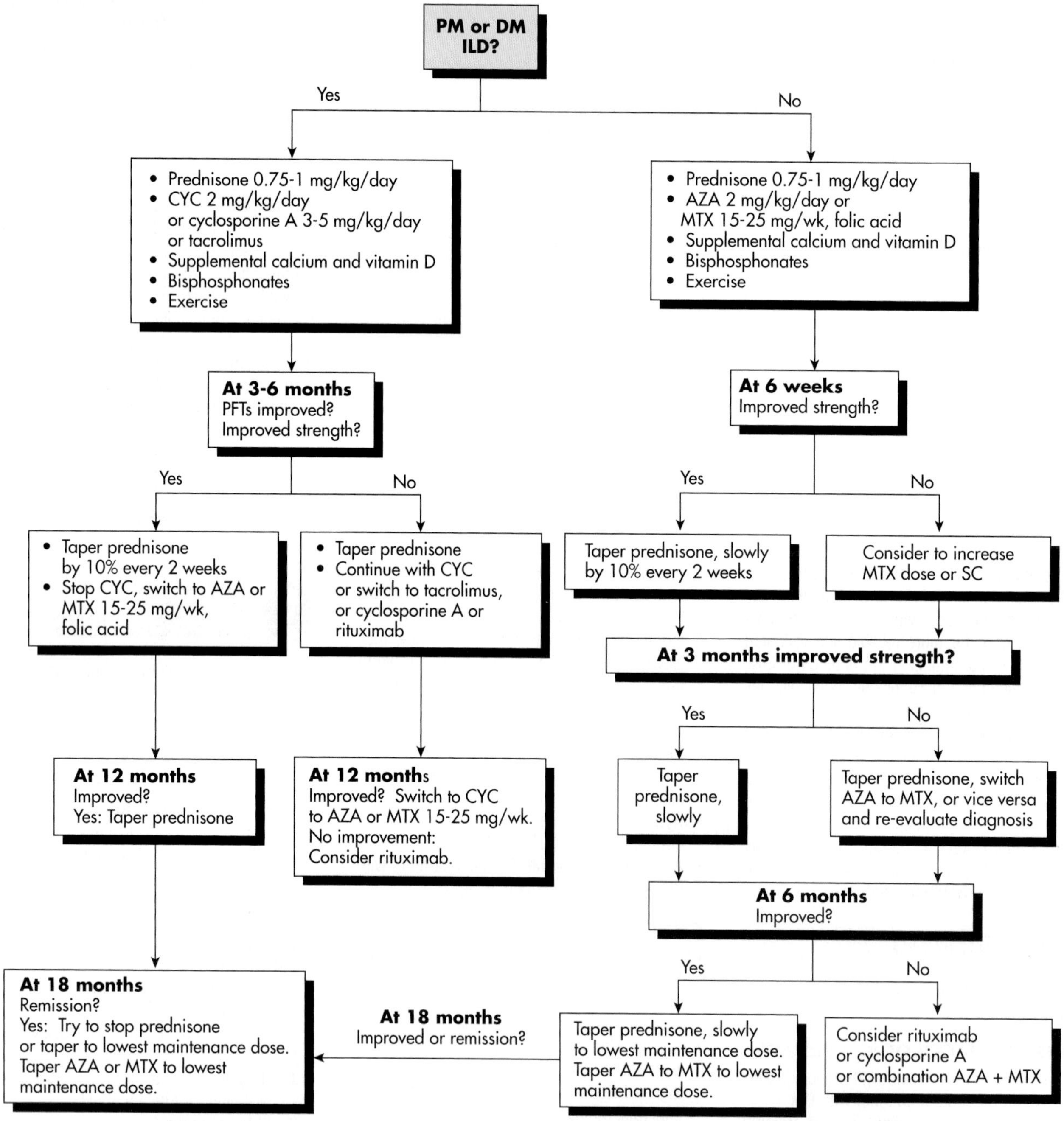

PM or DM ILD?

Yes

- Prednisone 0.75-1 mg/kg/day
- CYC 2 mg/kg/day or cyclosporine A 3-5 mg/kg/day or tacrolimus
- Supplemental calcium and vitamin D
- Bisphosphonates
- Exercise

At 3-6 months
PFTs improved?
Improved strength?

Yes

- Taper prednisone by 10% every 2 weeks
- Stop CYC, switch to AZA or MTX 15-25 mg/wk, folic acid

No

- Taper prednisone
- Continue with CYC or switch to tacrolimus, or cyclosporine A or rituximab

At 12 months
Improved?
Yes: Taper prednisone

At 12 months
Improved? Switch to CYC to AZA or MTX 15-25 mg/wk. No improvement: Consider rituximab.

No

- Prednisone 0.75-1 mg/kg/day
- AZA 2 mg/kg/day or MTX 15-25 mg/wk, folic acid
- Supplemental calcium and vitamin D
- Bisphosphonates
- Exercise

At 6 weeks
Improved strength?

Yes
Taper prednisone, slowly by 10% every 2 weeks

No
Consider to increase MTX dose or SC

At 3 months improved strength?

Yes
Taper prednisone, slowly

No
Taper prednisone, switch AZA to MTX, or vice versa and re-evaluate diagnosis

At 6 months
Improved?

Yes
Taper prednisone, slowly to lowest maintenance dose. Taper AZA to MTX to lowest maintenance dose.

No
Consider rituximab or cyclosporine A or combination AZA + MTX

At 18 months
Improved or remission?

At 18 months
Remission?
Yes: Try to stop prednisone or taper to lowest maintenance dose. Taper AZA or MTX to lowest maintenance dose.

FIG. 7 Treatment algorithm for adult patients with polymyositis (PM) or dermatomyositis (DM).
AZA, Azathioprine; *CYC,* cyclophosphamide; *ILD,* interstitial lung disease; *MTX,* methotrexate; *PFT,* pulmonary function test; *SC,* subcutaneous. (From Firestein GS et al: *Kelly's textbook of rheumatology,* ed 9, Philadelphia, 2013, Saunders, Elsevier.)

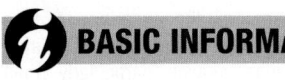

BASIC INFORMATION

DEFINITION

Influenza is an acute febrile illness caused by infection with influenza type A or B virus. Seasonal influenza can include the H1N1 virus. A similar respiratory illness is severe acute respiratory syndrome (SARS) caused by a coronavirus called SARS-associated coronavirus (SARS-CoV). A new novel coronavirus was recognized in two patients in September 2012. This is a very different virus from the SARS agent; the two patients exhibited acute respiratory distress syndrome, renal failure, consumptive coagulopathy, and/or pericarditis. Now called the Middle East respiratory syndrome (MERS-CoV) virus, it has affected more than 1700 persons in 27 countries since 2012. Patients have fever and pneumonia requiring hospitalization. Transmission spread in 2015 from the Middle East to Korea and China, resulting in more than 185 cases. There were 558 cases in Saudi Arabia from January 2015 through early June 2016. Dromedary camels and their milk are documented to harbor MERS-CoV.

SYNONYMS

Flu
Influenza-like illness (ILI)

ICD-10CM CODES
J11.00 Influenza due to other unidentified influenza virus with unspecified type of pneumonia
J12.9 Viral pneumonia, unspecified
J11.1 Influenza due to unidentified influenza virus with other respiratory manifestations

INFLUENZA EPIDEMIOLOGY & DEMOGRAPHICS

PEAK INCIDENCE: Winter outbreaks lasting 5 to 6 wk.
PREDOMINANT SEX: Male =female.
PREDOMINANT AGE: Attack rates are higher among children than adults, although children are less prone to develop pulmonary complications. During the 2014-2015 flu season, the highest hospitalization rate occurred with people 65 years and older (323/100,000)
INCIDENCE (IN U.S.): Annual incidence of influenza-related deaths is ~36,000 deaths/yr.

PHYSICAL FINDINGS & CLINICAL PRESENTATION

- "Classic flu" is characterized by abrupt onset of fever, headache, myalgias, anorexia, and malaise after a 1- to 2-day incubation period.
- Clinical syndromes are similar to those produced by other respiratory viruses, including pharyngitis, common colds, tracheobronchitis, bronchiolitis, and croup.
- Respiratory symptoms such as cough, sore throat, and nasal discharge are usually present at the onset of illness, but systemic symptoms predominate.
- Elderly patients may experience fever, weakness, and confusion without any respiratory complaints.

- Acute deterioration to status asthmaticus may occur in patients with asthma.
- Influenza pneumonia: rapidly progressive cough, dyspnea, and cyanosis may occur after typical flu onset. This may be caused by primary influenza pneumonia or secondary bacterial pneumonia (often pneumococcal or staphylococcal co-infection).
- For influenza A (H3N2v), children younger than 10 years lack immunity. People ≥65 years and those with morbid obesity are at high risk.

ETIOLOGY

- Variation in the surface antigens of the influenza virus, hemagglutinin (HA) and neuraminidase (NA), leading to infection with variants to which immunity is inadequate in the population at risk.
- Droplet transmission by small-particle aerosols and deposited on the respiratory tract epithelium.

DIAGNOSIS

DIFFERENTIAL DIAGNOSIS

- Respiratory syncytial virus, adenovirus, parainfluenza virus infection.
- Secondary bacterial pneumonia or mixed bacterial-viral pneumonia.

WORKUP

- The accuracy of clinical diagnosis of influenza on the basis of symptoms alone is limited because symptoms from illness caused by other pathogens can overlap considerably with influenza. Diagnostic tests available for influenza include viral cultures, serology, rapid influenza diagnostic tests (RIDTs), reverse transcription-polymerase chain reaction (RT-PCR), and immunofluorescence assays.
- Virus isolation from nasal or throat swab or sputum specimens is the most rapid diagnostic method in the setting of acute illness.
- Specimens are placed into virus transport medium and processed by a reference laboratory.
- For serologic diagnosis:
  1. Paired serum specimens, acute and convalescent, the latter obtained 10 to 20 days later
  2. Fourfold rises or falls in the titer of antibodies (various techniques) considered diagnostic of recent infection
  3. Commercial rapid influenza diagnostic tests (RIDTs) are available. They can detect influenza virus antigens within 15 minutes of testing. Rapid flu test should be collected as early as possible, ideally within 4 days of onset. False-negative results are common during the flu season. A negative test result does NOT exclude diagnosis of influenza.
  4. Commercial RIDTs cannot determine if an H3N2 is a variant virus; when suspect H3N2v virus infection, send nasopharyngeal swab or aspirate in viral transport

medium to state public health laboratory for rRT-PCR testing using Centers for Disease Control and Prevention (CDC) FLU rRT-PCR diagnostic panel assay.

LABORATORY TESTS

Septic syndrome presentation: CBC, ABG analysis, blood cultures

IMAGING STUDIES

- Chest x-ray examination when suspecting viral pneumonia: peribronchial and patchy interstitial infiltrates in multiple lobes with atelectasis. Table 1 describes x-ray pulmonary findings based on virus type.
- Possible progression to diffuse interstitial pneumonitis.

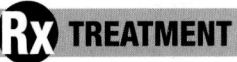 TREATMENT

NONPHARMACOLOGIC THERAPY

- Bed rest.
- Hydration.

ACUTE GENERAL Rx

- Supportive care: antipyretics; avoid use of aspirin in children because of the association with Reye's syndrome.
- Antibiotics if bacterial pneumonia is proved or suspected.
- Amantadine is NOT recommended due to resistant isolates.
- Neuraminidase inhibitors block release of virions from infected cells, resulting in shortened duration of symptoms and decrease in complications; effective against both influenza A and B, including A (H3N2v) for all hospitalized patients, those with severe and progressive illness, and high-risk patients with suspected or confirmed H3N2v.
  1. Zanamivir, administered via inhaler:
     For treatment, 10 mg (2 inhalations of 5 mg each) twice daily for 5 days.
     For prevention in households, 10 mg (2 inhalations of 5 mg each) once daily for 17 days. Not recommended in persons with underlying airways disease such as asthma or chronic obstructive pulmonary disease.
  2. Oseltamivir, administered orally:
     For treatment, 75 mg PO twice daily for 5 days.
     For prevention, 75 mg PO once daily for a minimum of 2 wk in an outbreak setting or 7 days after exposure for an adult.
  3. Emergency use authorization by the CDC for intravenous peramivir during the H1N1 pandemic was terminated in June 2010. Intravenous zanamivir is available in clinical trials or as an emergency investigational new drug.
- Placebo-controlled studies have suggested that antiviral therapy with any of the previously mentioned agents must ideally be initiated within 1 to 2 days of the onset of symptoms and reduces the duration of illness by ~1 day.

- Oseltamivir resistance developed on therapy in individuals with avian flu (H5N1) in Asia, and this is associated with poor outcome.
- Amantadine and rimantadine resistance are documented for novel (H1N1) influenza and H3N2 influenza virus.
- Systemic corticosteroids should not be routinely administered to patients with suspected or confirmed influenza, including H3N2v virus infection, except for patients on chronic corticosteroid therapy for COPD, asthma.

DISPOSITION

Patients are hospitalized if signs of pneumonia are present.

REFERRAL

Infectious disease and/or pulmonary consultation when influenza pneumonia is suspected.

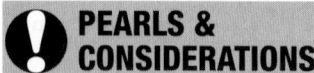

PEARLS & CONSIDERATIONS

COMMENTS

- Prevention of influenza in patients at high risk is an important goal of primary care.
- Vaccines reduce the risk of infection and the severity of illness.
  1. Antigenic composition of the vaccine is updated annually. The northern hemisphere's 2016 to 2017 season trivalent vaccine includes an A/California/7/2009 (H1N1) pdm09-like virus, an A/HongKong/4801/2014 (H3N2)–like virus, and a B/Brisbane/60/2008–like virus (B/Victoria lineage).
  2. Quadrivalent vaccines contain these three antigens, plus an antigen from a second influenza B vaccine virus strain called B/Phuket/3073/2013-like virus (B/Yamagata lineage).
  3. Revaccination is recommended annually before onset of influenza activity in the community, even for those who received the vaccine in the previous season.
  4. Delaying vaccination to ensure persistence of vaccine-induced protection during flu season could result in missed opportunities to vaccinate.
  5. Seasonal influenza vaccine does not provide protection against the influenza

A (H3N2v) virus that is associated with agricultural fairs.
  6. Vaccination should be given at the start of the flu season (September-October) for all persons aged ≥6 mo. Vaccination is particularly important for persons who are at increased risk for severe complications from influenza. When vaccine supply is limited, vaccination efforts should focus on the following groups:
     a. All children aged 6 mo to 4 yr (59 mo).
     b. People 50 years and older.
     c. Adults and children with chronic cardiac (except hypertension) or pulmonary (including asthma), renal, hepatic, neurologic, hematologic or metabolic disease (including diabetes mellitus).
     d. Immunocompromised patients (including HIV-infected persons or patients immunosuppressed due to medications).
     e. Women who are or will be pregnant during the influenza season.
     f. Children aged 6 mo to 18 yr who are receiving long-term aspirin therapy.
     g. Residents of nursing homes and other long-term care facilities.
     h. American Indians/Alaska Natives.
     i. Persons who are morbidly obese (BMI ≥40).
     j. Health care workers (HCWs).
     k. Household contacts and caregivers of persons in the previous groups.
  7. Vaccination should be delayed for persons with moderate to severe acute febrile illness. Precautions include:
     a. Guillain-Barré syndrome within 6 wk following a previous dose of influenza vaccine.
     b. Moderate or severe acute illness with or without fever (for trivalent inactivated influenza vaccine).
  8. Contraindication to receiving vaccine is a previous severe allergic reaction to influenza vaccine.
  9. Special efforts should be made to vaccinate high-risk patients <65 yr, only 10% to 15% of whom are vaccinated each year.
  10. HCW vaccination minimizes transmission to patients and coworkers. Some states mandate vaccination of HCWs; some healthcare facilities and other

states require the wearing of face masks by unvaccinated HCWs during the influenza season, particularly when there is widespread flu.
  11. Vaccine efficacy varies by age and by type of circulating virus. Efficacy varies each year and has ranged from 23% to 60% overall efficacy during the past 5 seasons. The 2015-2016 season overall vaccine efficacy was 47%.
  12. Alternate vaccine formulations.
     a. Intradermal vaccine is available for injection into skin instead of muscle. This uses a smaller needle than the regular flu vaccine and might be preferred by adults aged 18 to 64 yr who do not like shots.
     b. Nasal spray, live-attenuated influenza vaccine (LAIV) is not recommended during the 2016-2017 flu season. The CDC's Advisory Committee on Immunization Practices (ACIP) found no measurable protective benefit during the 2015-2016 flu season.
     c. Give TIV if recipient has egg allergy or asthma or cares for immunosuppressed persons who require a protective environment.
     d. A new adjuvanted seasonal vaccine is available for the 2016-2017 flu season for adults >65 yr. This is designed to create a stronger immune response.
     e. Thimerosal-free vaccine is available.
     f. IIV can be trivalent or quadrivalent, and egg-based or non-egg-based (cell culture or recombinant hemagglutinin).
     g. There is no preference for standard dose IIV, high dose IIV (age 65 or over) or intradermal IIV (ages 18-64).
     h. ACIP guidance for egg allergies:
        - If a person with egg allergy experiences only hives, then administer trivalent recombinant hemagglutinin influenza vaccine (RIV3) if ages 18 to 49, or IIV and observe for at least 30 minutes for reaction following vaccine.
        - If a person with egg allergy experiences other symptoms such as cardiovascular (e.g., hypotension), respiratory distress (e.g., wheezing), gastrointestinal (e.g., nausea/

TABLE 1 Pulmonary Radiographic Findings Based on Virus Type					
Virus	**Centrilobular Nodules**	**Lobar Ground-Glass**	**Diffuse Ground-Glass**	**Thickened Interlobular Septa**	**Consolidation**
Influenza	+++	+++	+		+
Epstein-Barr	+	+	+		+
Cytomegalovirus	++	++	++	+	+
Varicella-zoster	+++	+	+		
Herpes simplex	+	+++	+		+++
Measles	++	+	+		+
Hantavirus			+++	+	++
Adenovirus	++	+			+++

From Weissleder R et al: *Primer of diagnostic imaging*, ed 5, St Louis, 2011, Mosby.

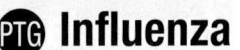

vomiting), reaction requiring epinephrine or emergency medical attention, administer RIV3 if age 18 to 49, or refer to a physician with expertise in management of allergic conditions.
- If there is no known history of exposure to egg, but the person is suspected of having egg allergy, consult with a physician who has expertise in the management of allergies before vaccinating, or give RIV3 (if ages 18 to 49).
- Chemoprophylaxis:
1. Table 2 describes antiviral agents for influenza. Oseltamivir and zanamivir are recommended in the United States during the influenza season.
2. Consider (after the current circulating strain of influenza has been shown to be sensitive):
   a. For high-risk patients in whom vaccination is contraindicated.
   b. When the available vaccine is known not to include the circulating strain.
   c. To provide added protection to immunosuppressed patients likely to have a diminished response to vaccination.
   d. In the setting of an outbreak, when immediate protection of unvaccinated

or recently vaccinated patients at high risk of complications is desired.
3. Chemoprophylaxis with antiviral drugs is not recommended for healthy persons exposed to seasonal influenza.
4. Give for 2 wk in the case of late vaccination and for the duration of the flu season in all other patients.
5. Treatment should not wait for laboratory confirmation of influenza.
6. Do not give aspirin or aspirin-containing products to children with influenza-like illness due to the risk of Reye's syndrome.
- Other prevention strategies:
1. Hand hygiene, cough etiquette (cover your cough), respiratory hygiene (use of tissues, facemasks for the ill and proper disposal).
2. Seasonal flu personal protective equipment (PPE)—wear gloves and gowns as per universal/standard precautions. Per the CDC, wear a facemask, adhering to Droplet Precautions for 7 days after illness onset or until 24 hr after fever and respiratory symptoms are resolved, whichever is longer. Patient placement in a negative pressure room and N95 respirator for health care workers are recommended when conducting aerosol-generating procedures.

3. For HPAI (H5N1, H7N9, H5N2, H5N8) per the CDC, wear eye protection, N95 respirator, gown, and gloves as for airborne and contact precautions.
4. Management of ill health care workers—exclude from work until at least 24 hr after they no longer have a fever (without the use of fever-reducing medication). Extended exclusion time period when caring for severely immunocompromised patients.
5. Standard cleaning and disinfection procedures.
- The Centers for Medicare and Medicaid Services links healthcare worker vaccine acceptance with payment for performance.

SUGGESTED READINGS
Available at www.expertconsult.com

RELATED CONTENT
Influenza (Flu) (Patient Information)

AUTHOR: **MARLENE FISHMAN WOLPERT, M.P.H.**

TABLE 2 Antiviral Agents for Influenza

	Amantadine	Rimantadine	Zanamivir	Oseltamivir
Protein target	M2	M2	Neuraminidase	Neuraminidase
Activity	A only (H1N1 and H3N2 are resistant)	A only (H1N1 and H3N2 are resistant)	A and B	A and B
Side effects	CNS (13%) GI (3%)	GI (6%)	? Bronchospasm	GI (9%)
Metabolism	None	Multiple (hepatic)	None	Hepatic
Excretion	Renal	Renal,+ others	Renal	Renal (tubular secretion)
Drug interactions	Antihistamines, anticholinergics	None	None	Probenecid (increased levels of oseltamivir)
Dose adjustments needed	≥65 yr old CrCl <50 ml/min	≥65 yr old CrCl <10 ml/min	None	CrCl <30 ml/min Severe liver dysfunction
Contraindications	Acute-angle glaucoma	Severe liver dysfunction	Underlying airway disease, asthma	
FDA-Approved Indications				
Therapy	Adults and children ≥1 yr old	Adults only	Adults and children ≥7 yr old	Adults and children ≥1 yr old*
Prophylaxis	Yes	Yes	Adults and children ≥5 yr old	Adults and children ≥13 yr old†

CrCl, Creatinine clearance; *FDA*, U.S. Food and Drug Administration; *GI*, gastrointestinal.
*FDA has authorized treatment of S-OIV (novel H1N1) virus with oseltamivir in children ≥3 mo of age.
†FDA has authorized prophylaxis for S-OIV (novel H1N1) virus with oseltamivir in children ≥1 yr.
From Mandell GL et al: *Principles and practice of infectious diseases*, ed 7, Philadelphia, 2010, Churchill Livingstone.

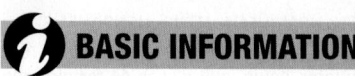

DEFINITION

Insomnia is a disturbance of initiating or maintaining sleep. Restless, nonrestorative sleep may also be described as another specified insomnia. The disturbance occurs despite adequate circumstances and opportunity for sleep and is accompanied by significant distress or impairment in daytime functioning. In the new DSM-5, the diagnosis of primary insomnia has been replaced with **insomnia disorder** in order to avoid the distinction between primary and secondary forms of the disorder. This paradigm shift relates to widely accepted research in the field suggesting that there is a bidirectional and interactive relationship between insomnia and any coexisting medical and/or mental disorders. As such it suggests that insomnia is deserving of direct clinical attention that may be expected to have beneficial impact on both the insomnia and comorbid disorder as well.

SYNONYMS

Sleeplessness
Sleep disorder, sleep disturbance, dyssomnia (NOTE: The terms *sleep disorder, sleep disturbance,* and *dyssomnia* are generic and can refer to disorders of wakefulness [hypersomnia] or sleep-related behavior disorders [parasomnias])
Insomnia disorder

ICD-10CM CODES
F51.01 Primary insomnia
F51.02 Adjustment insomnia
F51.03 Paradoxical insomnia
F51.04 Psychophysiologic insomnia
F51.05 Insomnia due to other mental disorder
F51.09 Other insomnia not due to a substance or known physiological condition
G47.00 Insomnia, unspecified
G47.01 Insomnia due to medical condition
G47.09 Other insomnia
Z73.810 Behavioral insomnia of childhood, sleep-onset association type
Z73.811 Behavioral insomnia of childhood, limit setting type
Z73.812 Behavioral insomnia of childhood, combined type
Z73.819 Behavioral insomnia of childhood, unspecified type

EPIDEMIOLOGY & DEMOGRAPHICS

INCIDENCE (IN U.S.): 30% to 45% of adults experience insomnia per year.
PREVALENCE (IN U.S.): 1% to 15% of all adults and 25% of older adults develop persistent insomnia.
PREDOMINANT SEX: More common in women.
PREDOMINANT AGE: Transient insomnia can occur at any age; persistent insomnia can also occur at any age but is more common after age 60 yr.
GENETICS: Can run in families and may be genetically influenced. Circadian rhythm disorders and narcolepsy have been traced to specific genes.

PHYSICAL FINDINGS & CLINICAL PRESENTATION

- Difficulty falling asleep, difficulty staying asleep, or early morning awakening.
- Significant distress or impairment in daytime functioning such as fatigue or low energy, sleepiness, cognitive impairments, mood disturbances, or behavioral problems.
- Difficulty occurs despite adequate opportunity for sleep.
- Symptoms may be acute and self-limited, chronic but intermittent, or chronic and frequent.

ETIOLOGY

- Transient insomnia:
  1. Any stressful biopsychosocial change in life circumstance (e.g., marriage, divorce, birth of a child, loss of a loved one, illness, retirement, etc.).
  2. Travel (across time zones).
  3. Environmental disruptions (noise, heat, cold, poor bedding, bed partners, unfamiliar surroundings, etc.).
- Persistent insomnia (Fig. 1):
  1. Mood and anxiety disorders (depression, hypomania/mania, PTSD).
  2. Psychophysiologic insomnia (conditioned arousal, extended sleep opportunity, sleep effort, poor sleep hygiene).
  3. Sleep-related breathing disorders (e.g., obstructive apnea and hypopnea, increased upper airway resistance).
  4. Chronobiologic (also known as circadian rhythm) disorder (delayed sleep phase, advanced sleep phase, shift work, non-24-hr sleep wake disorder secondary to blindness).
  5. Drug and alcohol abuse.
  6. Restless legs syndrome and periodic leg movements.
  7. Neurodegenerative (Alzheimer's disease, Parkinson's disease, etc.).
  8. Medical (pain, GERD, nocturia, orthopnea, menopause, medications, etc.).

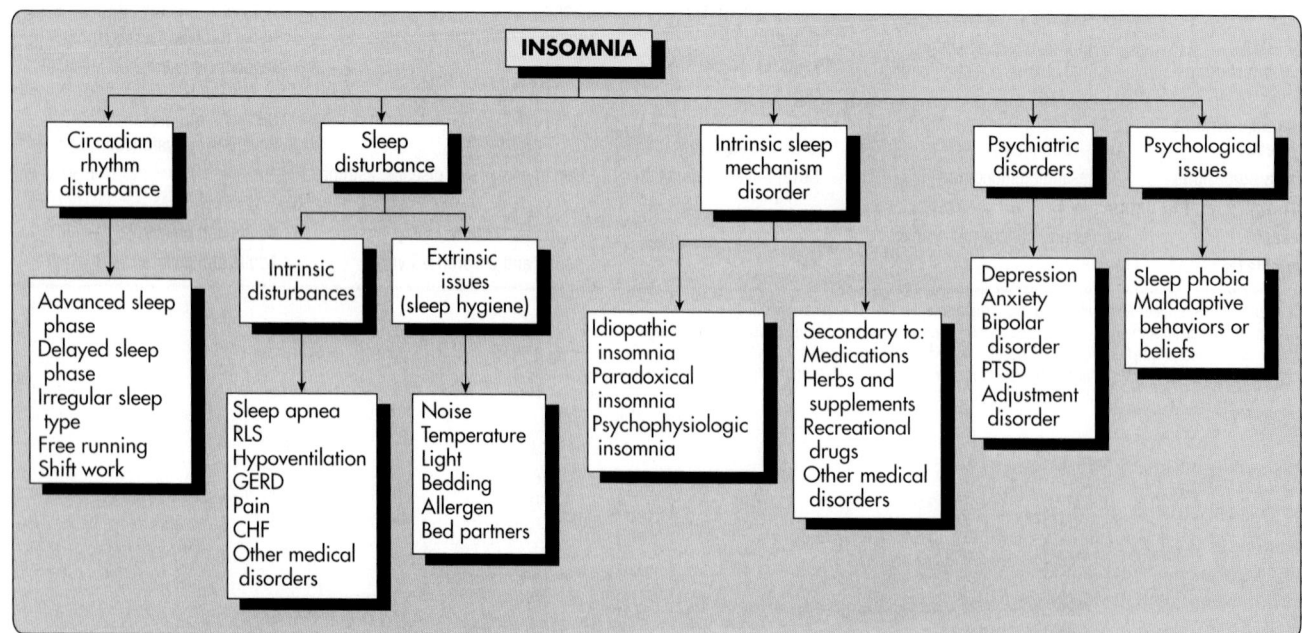

FIG. 1 Diagnostic flow chart to approach insomnia. *CHF,* congestive heart failure; *GERD,* gastroesophageal reflux disease; *PTSD,* posttraumatic stress disorder; *RLS,* restless legs syndrome. (From Kryger MH et al: *Principles and practice of sleep medicine,* ed 6, Philadelphia, 2017, Elsevier.)

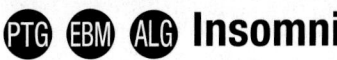

BOX 1 Sleep Habits (Sleep Hygiene Measures) That May Improve Sleep

1. Reduce caffeine, alcohol, or tobacco late in the day or especially evening.
2. Avoid heavy meals at night, but consider a light snack before bed such as toast or a handful of nuts.
3. Increase daytime activity, but avoid exercise within 3-5 hours of bedtime.
4. Increase daytime exposure to natural light.
5. Reduce liquids in the last 4 hours before bedtime.
6. Consider white noise as background sound for the sleep environment.
7. Maintain regular bed and wake times.
8. Go to bed with calm mind; resolve arguments or set a time earlier in the day to review problems and perhaps write down plans, solutions, or things to do.
9. Keep light exposure in the middle of the night to a minimum when awake and attenuate morning light in the bedroom.
10. Avoid pets in the bed.

Dx DIAGNOSIS

Diagnostic and Statistical Manual of Mental Disorders (DSM-5) criteria for the diagnosis of insomnia disorder is as follows:[1]

- Dissatisfaction with sleep quantity or quality, with one or more of the following symptoms:
- Difficulty initiating sleep
- Difficulty maintaining sleep, characterized by frequent awakenings or trouble returning to sleep after awakenings
- Early-morning awakening with inability to return to sleep
- The sleep disturbance causes clinically significant distress or impairment in daytime functioning, as evidenced by at least one of the following:
  - Fatigue or low energy
  - Daytime sleepiness
  - Impaired attention, concentration, or memory
  - Mood disturbance
  - Behavioral difficulties
  - Impaired occupational or academic function
  - Impaired interpersonal or social function
  - Negative effect on caregiver or family functioning
- The sleep difficulty occurs at least 3 nights per week, is present for at least 3 months, and occurs despite adequate opportunity for sleep

DIFFERENTIAL DIAGNOSIS

Insomnia disorder is only ruled out when the disorder is seen exclusively during other etiologies (see "Etiology"). It can be precipitated by a "primary" medical, mental health, or other sleep-wake disorder, but continues as a comorbid condition even after the "primary disorder" has been treated.

WORKUP

- History (with bed partner interview, if possible).
- Sleep diary for 2 wk (Consider the Consensus Sleep Diary [Carney CE, et al. in Suggested Readings]).

[1]American Psychiatric Association: *Diagnostic and statistical manual of mental disorders*, 5th ed, American Psychiatric Publishing, Arlington, VA, 2013.

- Wrist actigraphy (detects gross limb movements and can distinguish wake from sleep states) and as an adjunct to a diary—provides some objective verification of the diary data.
- Validated sleep-quality rating scale (optional).
  1. Insomnia Severity Index.
  2. Pittsburgh Sleep Quality Index.
  3. Epworth Sleepiness Scale (see Daytime Sleepiness Test at http://www.sleepfoundation.org).

LABORATORY TESTS

- Evaluate for anemia (especially low ferritin level), uremia (for restless legs), thyroid function (if other signs present).
- Polysomnography (in home or in sleep laboratory) is not standard for insomnia but should be reserved for patients whose history suggests specific sleep-related breathing or movement disorders. It is indicated for symptoms suggestive of daytime sleepiness (obstructive sleep apnea, narcolepsy), nonrestorative sleep (periodic leg movements, chronic pain conditions), or sleep behavior suggesting parasomnia (somnambulism, REM sleep behavior).

IMAGING STUDIES

- Not generally helpful.
- Brain CT or MRI for severe daytime sleepiness or acute onset.

Rx TREATMENT

NONPHARMACOLOGIC THERAPY

- Sleep hygiene measures (Box 1) as a monotherapy are not very effective in cases of persistent insomnia. More useful if combined with procedures described next.
- Cognitive-behavioral therapy (CBT-I) has been shown to reduce time to fall asleep and time awake during the night, can reduce reliance on sleep medications, and has shown lasting effects after treatment has been discontinued.
- The standard components that comprise CBT-I are as follows:
  1. Stimulus control, which addresses the conditioned cues that create arousal when attempting to sleep by restricting activity in bed to sleep and sex and not permitting sleep effort, worrying, watching TV, reading, etc., in bed (reconditioning of this type can take several days or weeks—patients should not come to expect positive changes on the first night)
  2. Sleep restriction therapy restricts sleep opportunity to the average amount of total sleep time the patient is getting as determined by baseline sleep diary data. Sleep time is increased incrementally, based on improving sleep efficiency. Note that restricted time in bed should never be <5 hr. For the elderly and infirm, average total sleep time plus 30 min is sometimes considered. For patients whose estimated average total sleep time is <4 hr, a diagnosis of paradoxical insomnia should be considered and CBT-I would be contraindicated.
  3. Cognitive therapy targets unhelpful beliefs and worries about sleep, negative and unwanted thoughts, selective attention bias and monitoring, misperception of sleep and daytime deficits, and counterproductive safety behaviors that are thought to maintain insomnia.
  4. Sleep hygiene is aimed at improving sleep habits (e.g., initiating or maintaining exercise, avoiding heavy meals at night, and altering the timing of or eliminating caffeine, nicotine, and alcohol intake). Environmental factors can also be addressed (e.g., using white noise and/or light attenuating bedroom). Caffeine sometimes can prove useful when used judiciously in the morning and early afternoon to combat the increased fatigue and somnolence that are produced early in therapy with sleep restriction and stimulus control. In addition, exercise contingently applied to daytime fatigue can also help to improve alertness during the day and increase sleep pressure at bedtime.
  5. Relaxation exercises (e.g., progressive muscle relaxation, diaphragmatic breathing) may be good adjunctive therapy, especially in highly anxious patients, but are not thought to be essential in CBT-I. Increasingly, mindfulness-based practices are being effectively utilized alone and in combination with other elements of CBT-I. Mindfulness may help patients to adopt a more flexible and accepting stance toward insomnia.
- Circadian rhythm disturbances, such as in shift workers, many blind individuals who lack light-dark cycle to synchronize body clock, adolescents and young adults with delayed sleep phase syndrome, and jet lag can be treated with chronobiologic therapies such as chronotherapy, bright light exposure, melatonin, or melatonin agonists. However, the timing of these interventions can be critical to outcome and constitutes therapies that are very different from standard medical and/or behavioral treatment for insomnia.

ACUTE GENERAL Rx

- Benzodiazepine receptor agonists zolpidem 5 mg and zaleplon 5 mg for sleep-onset insomnia, and zolpidem continuous-release formulation 6.25 to 12.5 mg and eszopiclone 1 to 3 mg for maintenance insomnia.
- Suvorexant is an orexin receptor antagonist FDA approved for insomnia. Signaling of orexin neuropeptides sustains wakefulness. Suvorexant promotes sleep by blocking orexin neuropeptides from binding to their receptors. The initial dose is 10 mg once daily within 30 minutes of bedtime. Most common side effect (10%) is next-day somnolence.
- Benzodiazepine sedative-hypnotics (e.g., temazepam 7.5 to 30 mg, triazolam 0.125 to 0.25 mg).
- A low-dose formulation (6 mg) of the tricyclic antidepressant doxepin, brand name Silenor, is also FDA approved for treatment of insomnia associated with sleep maintenance. This dose retains the hypnotic effect of doxepin without the typical tricyclic effects. A generic 10 mg/ml liquid formulation of doxepin is also available.
- In critical care: lorazepam 0.25 to 0.5 mg PO, SL, or IV as needed for sleep. In patients with acute delirium, haloperidol 0.25 to 0.5 mg IV as needed up to 2 mg/day may be less likely to worsen confusion.
- Melatonin agonist ramelteon 8 mg for sleep-onset insomnia when a mild agent without benzodiazepine side effects is desired.
- Avoid antihistamines except for occasional use.
- Optimize treatment of medical symptoms, especially pain.
- Most prescription and over-the-counter medications carry significant risk of adverse events and drug interactions, especially in the geriatric patient. Preferred pharmacotherapeutic agents in the elderly are zolpidem, zaleplon, eszopiclone, and ramelteon.

CHRONIC Rx

- Considerable research supports the efficacy of CBT-I, with acute treatment outcomes equivalent to pharmacotherapy, and better long-term outcomes and maintenance of treatment gains. Although there is limited availability of CBT-I specialists, especially in certain geographic areas, there are now online interactive evidence-based self-help programs that can serve as an effective base for a stepped model of care. Patients who fail these attempts should still be encouraged to seek more tailored treatment with a specialist, especially when the insomnia is comorbid with other conditions.
- Note that the American College of Physicians recently published clinical guidelines for the management of chronic insomnia disorder suggesting that CBT-I be the first-line treatment for insomnia and recommending that it be attempted before pharmacologic approaches when possible.

- Three sedative-hypnotics—zolpidem continuous release, eszopiclone, and ramelteon—FDA approved for long-term use.
- Some evidence shows that benzodiazepines and benzodiazepine receptor agonists can be used for chronic insomnia on either intermittent or nightly use with moderate risk of tolerance and dependence but low risk of addiction.
- Sedating antidepressants (e.g., trazodone 25 to 150 mg, mirtazapine 7.5 to 30 mg, amitriptyline 25 to 50 mg, doxepin 10 mg) are in widespread use, with limited data on safety and efficacy. Amitriptyline should be avoided in older adults.
- Sedating antipsychotics (e.g., quetiapine 25 to 200 mg, olanzapine 2.5 to 10 mg at night) considered for severe mood or psychotic disorders associated with insomnia.

COMPLEMENTARY & ALTERNATIVE MEDICINE

Melatonin may shorten sleep-onset latency in some individuals. It may have more clinical utility in the management of circadian rhythm disorders. Timing of administration in these types of cases requires careful consideration and would not be often administered at bedtime.

DISPOSITION

- Transient (acute) insomnia: usually self-limited. May require follow-up if stress-related or illness-related because of risk of depression or persistence. Prophylactic education regarding maladaptive sleep practices such as extending time in bed, and/or remaining in bed when unable to sleep, might be helpful in avoiding a more protracted course of insomnia.

  Persistent insomnia: Patients who respond well to CBT-I often continue to maintain gains at 1-and 2-yr follow-ups. Patients may need periodic follow-up to reinforce good sleep hygiene and stimulus control and for reevaluation of pharmacologic therapies. There is now a compelling amount of evidence that insomnia, if left untreated, is associated with significant negative mental and health effects over time.

REFERRAL

- A referral to a behavioral medicine specialist may be required for CBT-I or for circadian rhythm disturbances (find a directory at http://www.behavioralsleep.org/findspecialist.aspx).
- Excessive daytime sleepiness not obviously caused by insomnia (e.g., narcolepsy, sleep-related breathing disorder).
- Nighttime behavior suggestive of a parasomnia (e.g., somnambulism, REM behavior disorder).
- Severe insomnia not responsive to basic interventions.

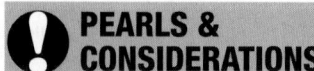

PEARLS & CONSIDERATIONS

COMMENTS

CBT-I often results in worse sleep and more fatigue in the short run. Patients often respond to initial worsening of symptoms as a sign of failure; however, they should be encouraged to see this as an important piece of the therapy and to stay the course as new conditioned patterns begin to emerge, sleep efficiency improves, and total sleep time gradually increases. Patients should avoid compensating for lost sleep by extending sleep opportunity in the form of sleeping in or napping. Therefore, early treatment should focus on helping patients to manage daytime fatigue and sleepiness by engaging in activities that help patients stay awake and maintain set bed and wake times.

PREVENTION

It is estimated that 50% to 70% of individuals demonstrating the syndrome of insomnia (e.g., insomnia symptoms more than 3 days per week for a month along with deleterious daytime sequelae) are still syndromic 1 to 5 years later. Therefore, early intervention with medication or education to prevent the development of maladaptive compensatory behaviors (e.g., napping, sleeping late, tossing and turning in bed, avoiding or decreasing daytime activity) may help to reduce the risk of developing persistent insomnia.

PATIENT & FAMILY EDUCATION

The National Sleep Foundation (http://www.sleepfoundation.org) is a comprehensive resource for health care providers and patients.

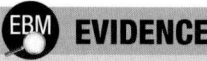 **EVIDENCE**

Available at www.expertconsult.com

SUGGESTED READINGS

Available at www.expertconsult.com

RELATED CONTENT

Sleep disorders (Algorithm in Section III)
Insomnia (Patient Information)

AUTHOR: **DONN POSNER, PH.D.**

BASIC INFORMATION

DEFINITION

The International Continence Society defines interstitial cystitis (IC), otherwise known as painful bladder syndrome, as a clinical syndrome consisting of suprapubic pain related to bladder filling and accompanied by other symptoms such as increased daytime and nighttime frequency in the absence of proven infection or other obvious pathology. The American Urological Association defines interstitial cystitis/bladder pain syndrome (IC/BPS) as an unpleasant sensation perceived to be related to the urinary bladder that is associated with lower urinary tract symptoms >6 weeks' duration, in the absence of infection or other unidentifiable causes.

SYNONYMS

Interstitial cystitis/bladder pain syndrome (IC/BPS)
Painful bladder syndrome
Tic douloureux of bladder

ICD-10CM CODES
N30.1 Interstitial cystitis (chronic)
N30.9 Cystitis, unspecified
N30.10 Interstitial cystitis (chronic) without hematuria
N30.11 Interstitial cystitis (chronic) with hematuria

EPIDEMIOLOGY & DEMOGRAPHICS

INCIDENCE: 21 cases per 100,000 women and four cases per 100,000 men annually
PREVALENCE:
- 197 per 100,000 women and 41 per 100,000 men in the U.S.
- Because the disease is substantially under-diagnosed, it may actually affect one in five women and one in 20 men.
- More than 81% of women diagnosed with chronic pelvic pain and up to 84% of men initially diagnosed with chronic prostatitis actually have IC.
- More than 90% of patients diagnosed with overactive bladder who do not respond to anticholinergics are subsequently diagnosed with IC.

PREDOMINANT SEX AND AGE:
- White women constitute 95% of patients with IC.
- Female/male ratio of 5 to 10:1.
- Most prevalent in fourth and fifth decades of life.

PHYSICAL FINDINGS & CLINICAL PRESENTATION

- Urinary urgency, frequency (>8 in daytime), nocturia (>2 at night), and suprapubic pain are the most common symptoms.
- Suprapubic pain is worse with bladder filling or urinating and relieved after emptying.
- Dyspareunia.
- Symptoms lasting longer than 6 mo.
- Intensity of symptoms waxes and wanes.

- Insidious onset and worsens to the final stage within 5 to 15 yr.
- Exercise, stress, sexual activity, ejaculation, certain foods with high potassium and acids (beer, spices, bananas, tomatoes, chocolate, strawberries, artificial sweeteners, oranges, cranberries, caffeine), menstruation, prolonged sitting, and activation of allergies exacerbate the symptoms.
- Often associated with irritable bowel syndrome, migraine, endometriosis, skin sensitivities, multiple drug allergies, other allergies, vulvodynia, fibromyalgia, chronic fatigue syndrome, systemic lupus erythematosus, and mood disorders.
- Dysphoric mood.
- Lower abdominal tenderness.
- Tender prostate in digital rectal examination.
- Levator ani tenderness in female.
- Tenderness of anterior vaginal wall/bladder neck in female.

ETIOLOGY

Unknown. Fig. 1 illustrates a hypothesis for etiologic cascade of painful bladder syndrome/interstitial cystitis.

Dx DIAGNOSIS

DIFFERENTIAL DIAGNOSIS

- Chronic pelvic pain
- Overactive bladder
- Recurrent urinary tract infection
- Endometriosis
- Pelvic adhesions
- Vulvar vestibulitis
- Vulvodynia
- Urethral pain syndrome
- Chronic nonbacterial prostatitis
- Frequent vaginitis
- Benign prostatic hyperplasia

WORKUP

- IC can be considered a diagnosis of exclusion when no known cause of painful bladder can be identified.
- There is no definite diagnostic test.
- Validated questionnaires such as Pelvic Pain and Urgency/Frequency scale (PUF), O'Leary-Sant symptoms and problem index, and Wisconsin IC scale. PUF is the most commonly used.

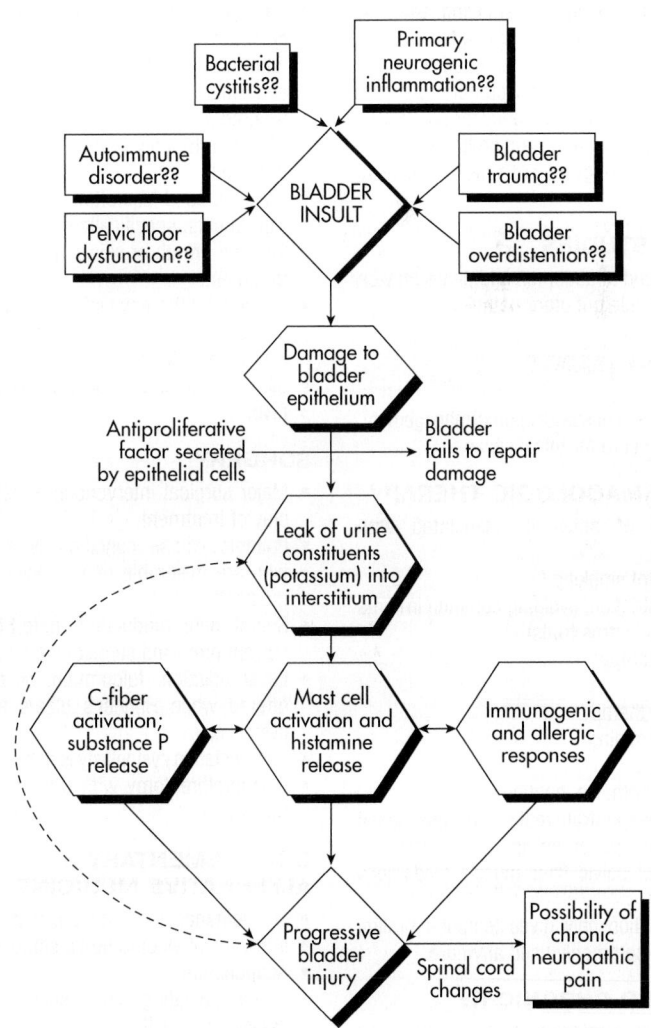

FIG. 1 Hypothesis for etiologic cascade of painful bladder syndrome/interstitial cystitis. (From Wein AJ: Painful bladder syndrome/interstitial cystitis and related disorders. In Wein AJ, et al., editors: *Campbell-Walsh urology*, ed 11, Philadelphia, 2007, Elsevier.)

- Voiding diary shows low-volume (<100 ml) and high-frequency voiding pattern.
- National Institute of Diabetes and Diseases of the Kidney diagnostic criteria misses 60% of IC patients and is not clinically used anymore.
- Anesthetic bladder challenge: with this test the symptoms dissipate on instillation of an anesthetic cocktail into the bladder.
- Cystoscopy and hydrodistention under general anesthesia may show terminal hematuria, glomerulation, Hunner's ulcers, and small bladder capacity of less than 350 ml. Cystoscopy and/or urodynamic testing should be considered when the diagnosis is in doubt, but the tests are not necessary to confirm an IC/BPS diagnosis in uncomplicated cases.
- Bladder biopsy is not essential for diagnosis of IC.
- Parson's potassium sensitivity test (PST).
- Urodynamics are unnecessary in diagnosis of IC.

LABORATORY TESTS

- Urine analysis and culture.
- Urine cytology should be performed if microscopic or gross hematuria is present, or with other risk factors such as smoking, age >40 yr, and other bladder cancer risk factors.
- Culture of sexually transmitted diseases if clinically indicated. Nonbacteriuric patients with pyuria should be screened for *Chlamydia*.
- Urine biomarkers (e.g., antiproliferative factor) are promising but not ready for clinical use.

IMAGING STUDIES

CT or ultrasound of abdomen and pelvis may be considered to rule out other pathology.

Rx TREATMENT

- There is no consensus for optimal management.
- There is no cure for this disease.

NONPHARMACOLOGIC THERAPY

- Avoidance of activities associated with flare-ups
- Avoidance of smoking
- Dietary restriction, avoiding common irritants (e.g., coffee, citrus fruits)
- Physical therapy
- Exercise
- Behavioral therapy
- Bladder retraining
- Biofeedback
- Warm sitz bath, ice, heating pad
- Thiele massage (transrectal and transvaginal manual therapy of pelvic floor muscle) in presence of pelvic floor muscle tenderness and spasm
- Hydrodistention only gives temporary relief, so it is not commonly used anymore

ACUTE AND CHRONIC Rx

- A course of empiric antibiotics if not tried yet. Long-term oral antibiotics are not recommended.

- Oral therapy is tried first.
- Pentosan polysulfate sodium (Elmiron) is the only FDA-approved and most effective oral therapy.
- Most treatment takes 3 to 6 mo before maximum benefit is seen.
- Adjunct oral therapy includes tricyclic antidepressants (amitriptyline), cimetidine, antihistaminics (hydroxyzine, montelukast), neuroleptics (gabapentin, topiramate), analgesics (NSAIDs, opioid analgesics), and occasionally antimuscarinics.
- Oral therapies can be used in combination.
- Antihistaminics are preferred for patients with an allergy history or those who show mast cells in bladder biopsy.
- Oral prednisone is used in presence of Hunner's ulcers.
- Other drugs rarely used for IC are cyclosporin A, interleukin-10, imatinib, methotrexate, suplatast, misoprostol, and quercetin.
- Growth factor inhibitors, gene therapy, RDP 58, and vitamin B_3 analogue (BXL 628) may represent future therapies.
- Intravesical treatment is used when oral medications fail, for acute flare-ups, or before the oral medications take full effect.
- Dimethyl sulfoxide (DMSO), heparin, lidocaine, hyaluronic acid, capsaicin, botulinum toxin A, chondroitin sulfate, steroids, and Elmiron are drugs used for intravesical treatment.
- DMSO is the only FDA-approved intravesical treatment.
- DMSO is used less often now because of its side effects, specifically a garlic-like odor or taste on breath or skin that lasts 72 hr after treatment.
- Intravesical therapy typically involves mixture of heparin or Elmiron with lidocaine and sodium bicarbonate.
- Silver nitrate and clorpactin have fallen out of favor.

SURGERY

- Major surgical intervention is not the mainstay of treatment.
- Patients whose condition is extreme and who are miserable may consider surgery if medications fail.
- Sacral neuromodulation (InterStim) is the current preferred surgical intervention.
- Laser ablation, fulguration, or resection is offered when Hunner's ulcers are seen in cystoscopy.
- Augmentation cystoplasty is not recommended.
- Cystourethrectomy with urinary diversion is rarely done.

COMPLEMENTARY & ALTERNATIVE MEDICINE

- Transcutaneous electric nerve stimulation
- Intravaginal electric nerve stimulation
- Acupuncture
- Urinary chelating agents such as Polycitra-K crystals, Urocit-K
- Prelief, an over-the-counter food additive
- Herbal remedies such as Algnot Plus, CystoProtek, Cysta-Q, aloe vera

DISPOSITION

- Close follow-up every month for 3 mo and every 3 mo thereafter.
- Voiding diary and symptom questionnaire are helpful to monitor response to treatment.

REFERRAL

- Urologist
- Pain specialist
- Physical therapist

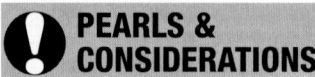 **PEARLS & CONSIDERATIONS**

COMMENTS

- On average these patients see five physicians and endure irritating voiding symptoms for 5 yr before the disease is identified.
- Besides symptom questionnaire and urine analysis, all other diagnostic tests are optional.
- PST is well tolerated.
- Negative cystoscopy does not rule out IC.

PREVENTION

Early identification and timely intervention improve patient outcome.

PATIENT & FAMILY EDUCATION

- IC support groups
- Interstitial Cystitis Association
- Interstitial Cystitis Network

SUGGESTED READINGS

Available at www.expertconsult.com

AUTHOR: **HEMANT K. SATPATHY, M.D.**

BASIC INFORMATION

DEFINITION

The interstitial lung diseases (ILDs) include more than 150 nonmalignant disorders, characterized by varying degrees of damage to the lung parenchyma or interstitium via inflammation and fibrosis. The term "ILD" can be confusing as processes affecting the alveolar space (e.g., pulmonary alveolar proteinosis) are also lumped under the title. A clinical classification of the interstitial lung diseases is summarized in Table 1. The diseases can generally divided into three subgroups—those that are caused by an identifiable or suspected trigger, those that are associated with an underlying, more systemic disorder, and those that are idiopathic.

SYNONYMS

Interstitial pulmonary disease
ILD
Diffuse parenchymal lung disease (DPLD)
Interstitial pneumonia

ICD-10CM CODES
J84.17	Other interstitial pulmonary diseases with fibrosis in diseases classified elsewhere
J84.89	Other specified interstitial pulmonary diseases
J84.9	Interstitial pulmonary disease, unspecified
J84.115	Respiratory bronchiolitis interstitial lung disease
J84.848	Other interstitial lung diseases of childhood

EPIDEMIOLOGY & DEMOGRAPHICS

INCIDENCE AND PREVALENCE: Varies widely with type of ILD. The most common ILDs are sarcoidosis, cryptogenic organizing pneumonia, and idiopathic pulmonary fibrosis. The prevalence of these syndromes varies widely across different populations as defined by age, gender, and race.

PREDOMINANT SEX & AGE: Some ILDs are more common in women, such as those resulting from connective tissue disorders. Lymphangiomyomatosis occurs exclusively in premenopausal women. ILD caused by occupational exposures are more common in men. Most ILDs occur in people >50 yr; however, sarcoidosis most often presents in younger populations.

RISK FACTORS: Although many ILDs are categorized as idiopathic, the most common identifiable risk factors include environmental exposures such as silicone, asbestos, or bird droppings; reactions to drugs such as chemotherapeutic agents, radiation therapy, cardiac medications, and finally some history of connective tissue disease such as rheumatoid arthritis or scleroderma.

PHYSICAL FINDINGS & CLINICAL PRESENTATION

- Shortness of breath (especially with exertion)
- Cough (dry)

- Tachypnea
- Bibasilar end-inspiratory dry crackles
- Pulmonary hypertension
- Cyanosis, clubbing

Hallmarks of ILD include a restrictive pattern and decreased diffusing capacity for carbon monoxide (DLCO) as demonstrated by pulmonary

---

function testing. The restrictive process can be the result of a number of factors depending on the type of ILD. Different types of ILD are characterized by varying degrees of acute inflammatory changes, which are potentially reversible, and fibrosis, which is largely irreversible.

- Specific changes may be seen:
  1. Granulomatous: accumulation of T lymphocytes, macrophages, and epithelioid cells into granulomas in lung parenchyma
  2. Inflammation and fibrosis: injury to epithelium causes inflammation; if chronic, inflammation spreads to interstitium and vascular areas

  Etiology

There is a wide range of environmental and workplace exposures that can directly result in an ILD. The mechanism by which underlying autoimmunity can lead to an associated ILD is not clear.

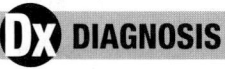

DIAGNOSIS

DIFFERENTIAL DIAGNOSIS

- Congestive heart failure
- Pneumonia: viral, bacterial, mycobacterial, fungal
- Pulmonary embolism
- COPD
- Pulmonary hypertension
- Vasculitis
- Metastatic malignancy manifesting as lymphangitic carcinomatosis

WORKUP

- Well-defined patterns in pulmonary function tests are usually consistent with restrictive defect (decreased FVC, FRC, RV, and TLC) owing to decreased lung compliance caused by alveolar wall thickening as a result of inflammation and fibrosis. Diffusion capacity is usually reduced also because of inflammation and thickening of alveolar walls, though nonspecific. FEV_1/FVC is usually normal or increased because lung stiffness keeps small airways open, although some conditions (e.g., sarcoidosis) may result in air trapping.
- Bronchoscopy and bronchoalveolar lavage (BAL) may help identify type of ILD. However, their role in defining stage of disease and response to therapy is controversial. Histologic patterns in the interstitial lung diseases and their disease associations are summarized in Table 2.
- If laboratory studies and imaging including HRCT fail in yielding a diagnosis, a surgical biopsy may be required.
- Fig. 1 describes a diagnostic approach to occupational ILD.

LABORATORY TESTS

- ABGs may be normal or show respiratory alkalosis and widened Aa gradient.
- Blood tests for connective tissue diseases, such as antinuclear antibodies, anti-immunoglobulin antibodies (rheumatoid factors), LDH. Laboratory findings in the interstitial lung diseases are summarized in Table 3.

TABLE 2 Histologic Patterns in the Interstitial Lung Diseases and Their Disease Associations

Histologic Patterns	Clinical Associations
Usual interstitial pneumonia	Idiopathic pulmonary fibrosis; connective tissue diseases (uncommon); asbestosis; chronic hypersensitivity pneumonitis; chronic aspiration pneumonia; chronic radiation pneumonitis; Hermansky-Pudlak syndrome
Nonspecific interstitial pneumonia	Idiopathic; connective tissue diseases; drugs; AIDS
Diffuse alveolar damage	Acute interstitial pneumonia (Hamman-Rich syndrome); acute respiratory distress syndrome (ARDS); drugs (cytotoxic agents, heroin, paraquat, ethchlorvynol, aspirin); toxic gas inhalation; radiation therapy; oxygen toxicity; connective tissue disease; infections
Organizing pneumonia	Cryptogenic organizing pneumonia; organizing stage of diffuse alveolar damage; drugs (amiodarone, cocaine); infections; connective tissue diseases
Desquamative interstitial pneumonia/respiratory bronchiolitis	Cigarette smoking; idiopathic DIP of childhood
Lymphocytic interstitial pneumonia	Idiopathic; hypogammaglobulinemia; autoimmune diseases, including Hashimoto's thyroiditis, lupus erythematosus, primary biliary cirrhosis, Sjögren's syndrome, myasthenia gravis, chronic active hepatitis; AIDS; allogeneic bone marrow transplantation
Eosinophilic pneumonia	Idiopathic acute and chronic; tropical filarial eosinophilia; parasitic infections; allergic bronchopulmonary aspergillosis; allergic granulomatosis of Churg and Strauss; hypereosinophilic syndrome; AIDS
Alveolar proteinosis	Pulmonary alveolar proteinosis; acute silicosis; aluminum dust; AIDS; myeloproliferative disorder
Diffuse alveolar hemorrhage	
With capillaritis	Wegener's granulomatosis; microscopic polyangiitis; systemic lupus erythematosus; polymyositis; scleroderma; rheumatoid arthritis; mixed connective tissue disease; lung transplantation; drugs (retinoic acid, propylthiouracil, Dilantin); Behçet's disease; cryoglobulinemia; Henoch-Schönlein purpura; pauci-immune glomerulonephritis; immune complex glomerulonephritis
Without capillaritis	Idiopathic pulmonary hemosiderosis; systemic lupus erythematosus; Goodpasture's syndrome; diffuse alveolar damage; pulmonary venoocclusive disease; mitral stenosis; lymphangioleiomyomatosis
Amyloid deposition	Primary amyloidosis; multiple myeloma; lymphocytic interstitial pneumonia
Granuloma	Sarcoidosis; hypersensitivity pneumonitis; pulmonary Langerhans cell histiocytosis; silicosis; intravenous talcosis; berylliosis; lymphocytic interstitial pneumonia; infections

AIDS, Acquired immunodeficiency syndrome.
Modified from Mason RJ: *Murray & Nadel's textbook of respiratory medicine,* 5th ed, Philadelphia, 2010, Saunders.

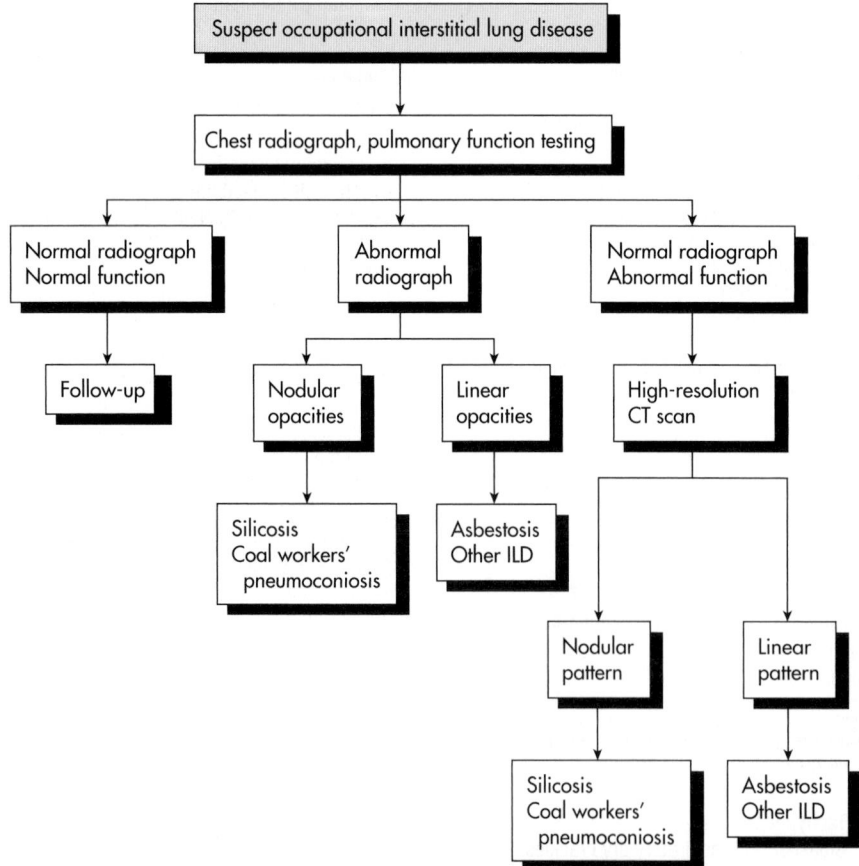

FIG. 1 Diagnostic approach to occupational interstitial lung disease (ILD). *CT,* Computed tomography. (From Goldman L, Ausiello D, editors: *Goldman's Cecil textbook of medicine,* ed 23, Philadelphia, 2008, Saunders.)

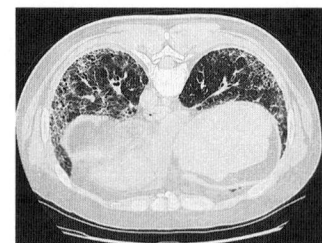

FIG. 2 High-resolution computed tomography scan of the chest shows fibrotic changes in a subpleural distribution with honeycombing consistent with usual interstitial pneumonia. (From Hochberg MC, et al.: *Rheumatology,* ed 5, St Louis, 2011, Mosby.)

- Serum precipitins confirm exposure if hypersensitivity pneumonitis is suspected.
- Antineutrophil cytoplasmic antibodies or antibasement membrane antibodies if vasculitis is suspected.
- Angiotensin-converting enzyme testing (ACE levels) in sarcoidosis is of unclear value.

IMAGING STUDIES

- Chest x-ray may be normal but commonly shows a bibasilar reticular pattern. Table 4 summarizes radiographic features of the interstitial lung diseases.
- High-resolution CT (HRCT) (Fig. 2) is the gold standard for evaluating parenchymal opacities seen on chest x-ray; it is also useful for determining potential biopsy sites.
- Echocardiography may be useful to evaluate cardiac function/dilation or to evaluate for pulmonary hypertension, which can complicate advanced ILDs.

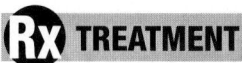
TABLE 3 Radiographic Features of the Interstitial Lung Diseases

Feature	Diseases
Upper zone–predominant disease	Radiation pneumonitis; neurofibromatosis; chronic sarcoidosis; pulmonary Langerhans cell histiocytosis; silicosis; chronic hypersensitivity pneumonitis; chronic eosinophilic pneumonia; ankylosing spondylitis; nodular rheumatoid arthritis; berylliosis; drug-induced (amiodarone, gold, BCNU [carmustine]); radiation
Increased lung volumes	Lymphangioleiomyomatosis; chronic sarcoidosis; chronic pulmonary Langerhans cell histiocytosis; tuberous sclerosis; neurofibromatosis
Radiographic honeycomb lung	Idiopathic pulmonary fibrosis; connective tissue disease; asbestosis; drug-induced; lymphocytic interstitial pneumonia; chronic aspiration pneumonia; hemosiderosis; Hermansky-Pudlak syndrome; alveolar proteinosis
Pneumothorax	Pulmonary Langerhans cell histiocytosis; lymphangioleiomyomatosis; tuberous sclerosis; neurofibromatosis, IPF
Kerley's B lines	Lymphangitic carcinomatosis; lymphangioleiomyomatosis; left atrial hypertension (mitral valve disease, venoocclusive disease); lymphoma; amyloidosis
Lymphadenopathy	Sarcoidosis; lymphoma; lymphangitic carcinomatosis; lymphoid interstitial pneumonia; berylliosis; amyloidosis; Gaucher's disease
Pleural disease	Lymphangitic carcinomatosis; connective tissue disease; asbestosis (pleural calcification); lymphangioleiomyomatosis (chylous effusion); drug-induced (nitrofurantoin, radiation); sarcoidosis
Eggshell calcification of lymph nodes	Silicosis; sarcoidosis; radiation

From Mason RJ: *Murray & Nadel's textbook of respiratory medicine*, 5th ed, Philadelphia, 2010, Saunders.

TABLE 4 Laboratory Findings in the Interstitial Lung Diseases

Finding	Diseases
Leukopenia	Sarcoidosis; connective tissue disease; lymphoma; drug-induced
Leukocytosis	Systemic vasculitis; hypersensitivity pneumonitis; lymphoma
Eosinophilia	Eosinophilic pneumonia; sarcoidosis; systemic vasculitis; drug-induced (sulfa, methotrexate)
Thrombocytopenia	Sarcoidosis; connective tissue disease; drug-induced; Gaucher's disease; idiopathic pulmonary fibrosis
Hemolytic anemia	Connective tissue disease; sarcoidosis; lymphoma; drug-induced; idiopathic pulmonary fibrosis
Normocytic anemia	Diffuse alveolar hemorrhage syndromes; connective tissue disease; lymphangitic carcinomatosis
Urinary sediment abnormalities	Connective tissue disease; systemic vasculitis; drug-induced
Hypogammaglobulinemia	Lymphocytic interstitial pneumonia
Hypergammaglobulinemia	Connective tissue disease; sarcoidosis; systemic vasculitis; idiopathic pulmonary fibrosis; asbestosis; silicosis; lymphocytic interstitial pneumonia; lymphoma
Serum autoantibodies	Connective tissue disease; systemic vasculitis; sarcoidosis; idiopathic pulmonary fibrosis; silicosis; asbestosis; lymphocytic interstitial pneumonia
Serum immune complexes	Idiopathic pulmonary fibrosis; lymphocytic interstitial pneumonia; systemic vasculitis; connective tissue disease; pulmonary Langerhans cell histiocytosis
Serum angiotensin-converting enzyme	Sarcoidosis; hypersensitivity pneumonitis; silicosis; acute respiratory distress syndrome; Gaucher's disease
Antibasement membrane antibody	Goodpasture's syndrome
Antineutrophil cytoplasmic antibody	Systemic vasculitis

From Mason, RJ: *Murray & Nadel's textbook of respiratory medicine*, 5th ed, Philadelphia, 2010, Saunders.

TREATMENT

NONPHARMACOLOGIC THERAPY
Avoidance of tobacco and occupational exposures

ACUTE GENERAL Rx
- Supplemental oxygen in patients with hypoxemia is helpful short and long term.
- Glucocorticoids are the mainstay of therapy for many of the ILDs. Patients should be continuously reevaluated after the initiation of treatment to gauge the response. If they are improved or stable, steroids may be tapered. If not, the same course may be maintained 4 additional wk. If patient's condition is unresponsive to steroids or declines as the steroids are tapered, may consider adding second agent (cyclophosphamide, azathioprine, mycophenolate, among other options).

CHRONIC GENERAL Rx
- Outpatient pulmonary rehabilitation may be of value.
- Lung transplantation may be considered in appropriate patients in severe stages of the disease.

DISPOSITION
The prognosis is highly variable and depends on the cause, severity of illness, and initial response to treatment.

REFERRAL
- Pulmonary referral for workup and management
- Surgical referral for biopsy

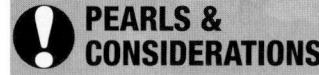 **PEARLS & CONSIDERATIONS**

COMMENTS
It is very important when working up an ILD to take a thorough history of prior medications, workplace and environmental exposures and pets, as well as a review of systems, including signs and symptoms that might suggest an underlying connective tissue disease.

PREVENTION
Proper industrial hygiene from a respiratory perspective is important as well as close surveillance when patients are given medications with known pulmonary toxicity. Symptoms of an ILD in the setting of an autoimmune condition need to be evaluated thoroughly.

SUGGESTED READINGS
Available at www.expertconsult.com

RELATED CONTENT
Interstitial Pulmonary Disease (Patient Information)

AUTHOR: **PETER LACAMERA, M.D.**

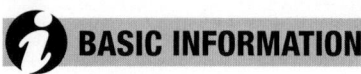
DEFINITION

Can be classified into two broad categories:
1. Acute interstitial nephritis (AIN):
   - Decrease in renal function resulting from delayed hypersensitivity immune-mediated injury, most often drug-induced
   - Characterized on renal biopsy by edema and leukocyte infiltration of the renal interstitium and tubules, classically sparing glomeruli and blood vessels
2. Chronic interstitial nephritis:
   - Final common pathway of many chronic kidney diseases including unresolved AIN, chronic obstruction, high-grade vesicoureteral reflux, and chronic bacterial infections
   - Characterized on renal biopsy by interstitial fibrosis with mononuclear leukocyte infiltration and tubular atrophy

SYNONYMS

AIN
Acute tubulo-interstitial nephritis
Contracted kidney
Cirrhosis of the kidney
Granular kidney
Gouty kidney
Renal sclerosis
Chronic productive nephritis without exudation

ICD-10CM CODES
N05.9 Unspecified nephritic syndrome with unspecified morphologic changes
N17.2 Acute kidney failure with medullary necrosis
N05.8 Unspecified nephritic syndrome with other morphologic changes
N10 Acute tubulo-interstitial nephritis
N11.8 Other chronic tubulo-interstitial nephritis
N11.9 Chronic tubulo-interstitial nephritis, unspecified
N12 Tubulo-interstitial nephritis, not specified as acute or chronic

EPIDEMIOLOGY & DEMOGRAPHICS

PREVALENCE:
- Prevalence is significantly underestimated.
- AIN is found in 11% to 15% of patients biopsied with acute kidney injury (AKI) and may comprise 10% to 27% of all AKI cases.

DEMOGRAPHICS:
- Increasing incidence in the elderly, thought to be due to reduced glomerular filtration rate and comorbidities
- Median age at presentation is 65 yr

RISK FACTORS:
- Advanced age (>65 yr)
- Volume depletion
- Underlying kidney disease
- Congestive heart failure
- Diabetes
- HIV infection

PHYSICAL FINDINGS & CLINICAL PRESENTATION

Signs and Symptoms
- Most common presentation is an elevation of serum creatinine and BUN that is asymptomatic or associated with nonspecific symptoms of acute renal failure due to any cause, including:
  - Malaise
  - Anorexia
  - Nausea and vomiting
  - Oliguria or polyuria
  - Hematuria
  - Flank pain
- Classic triad (fever, maculopapular rash, and arthralgias) is present in only 5% of cases:
  - When present, the rash is usually a truncal maculopapular morbilliform eruption,
  - Triad was characteristic of methicillin-related AIN; methicillin is no longer used clinically in the U.S.
- A small minority present with tubulo-interstitial nephritis and uveitis (TINU) syndrome. The uveitis may be symptomatic or subclinical and may develop before, during, or after the renal injury. Adolescent females are most often affected by TINU.

Etiology
Acute Interstitial Nephritis
- **Drug-induced** (70%). More than 150 agents have been implicated. AKI usually develops 10 to 14 days after exposure to the drug but may develop sooner if there was a previous exposure.
- Antibiotics (beta-lactams, sulfonamides, rifampin, fluoroquinolones)
- NSAIDs (including selective COX-2 inhibitors)
- Proton pump inhibitors and H2 antagonists
- Anti-neoplastic agents
- Anticonvulsants
- Allopurinol (particularly common cause of drug reaction or rash with eosinophilia and systemic symptoms [DRESS] with AIN)
- **Infection** (10%-15%). May be systemic or localized to genitourinary system.
- Bacterial: staphylococci, streptococci, *Corynebacterium diphtheria, Legionellae, Yersiniae, Mycobacteria, Mycoplasmas, Rickettsiae*
- Viral: cytomegalovirus, Epstein-Barr virus, hantaviruses, hepatitis C virus, herpes simplex virus, HIV, mumps, polyomavirus, influenza A virus
- Other: *Treponema pallidum, Toxoplasma gondii*, Babesia
- **Other Causes** (15%-20%)
- Idiopathic (10%)
- Immune disorders: systemic lupus erythematosus, Sjögren's syndrome, small-vessel vasculitides, autoimmune pancreatitis
- Neoplastic disorders (multiple myeloma)
- DRESS syndrome
- IgG4-related tubulo-interstitial nephritis
- Hypocomplementemic tubulo-interstitial nephritis

Chronic Interstitial Nephritis
- Metabolic diseases (urate nephropathy, hypercalcemic nephropathy, hypokalemic nephropathy, oxalate nephropathy)
- Sarcoidosis
- Heavy metals
- Chronic urinary tract obstruction
- Aristolochia
- Diabetes mellitus
  Overlap of Acute and Chronic Interstitial Nephritis
Some metabolic processes and autoimmune disorders can present either as acute or chronic interstitial nephritis. For example, oxalate nephropathy can present with acute interstitial nephropathy in the setting of ethylene glycol ingestion, or with chronic interstitial nephritis in patients with prior bariatric surgery and a high oxalate-containing diet.

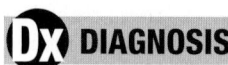 **DIAGNOSIS**

DIFFERENTIAL DIAGNOSIS

Other causes of AKI or chronic kidney disease, including acute tubular necrosis, glomerulonephritis, hypertensive nephrosclerosis, prerenal azotemia, obstructive nephropathy, renal vascular disease

WORKUP

- Diagnosis is most often made by defining the temporal relationship between onset and resolution of an AKI episode with use and discontinuation of a known culprit drug.
- Gold standard for diagnosis is renal biopsy, but biopsy is performed only when diagnosis is unclear, removal of offending agent does not result in improvement, removal of offending agent may impact medical care, or steroid initiation is being considered.

LABORATORY TESTS

- There is no single laboratory test with significant positive or negative predictive value.
- Diagnosis may be made based on clinical history, constellation of urine and serum abnormalities, and clinical course.

URINE TESTS

- Urine eosinophils were historically thought to be a marker of AIN, but they are neither sensitive nor specific for AIN and have a low positive and negative predictive value. They do not help diagnose or rule out AIN and should not be used in diagnosis.
- Urinalysis findings may include sterile pyuria, microhematuria, glucosuria, and proteinuria.
- Urine sediment analysis may include WBCs, WBC casts, possible red cells, and possible tubular epithelial cells (Fig. 1).

BLOOD TESTS

- Serum chemistry profile: elevated BUN and creatinine, low serum phosphorus, low serum urate
- Complete blood count with differential may show the following:
- Eosinophilia (not sensitive, but if present greatly increases clinical suspicion for a

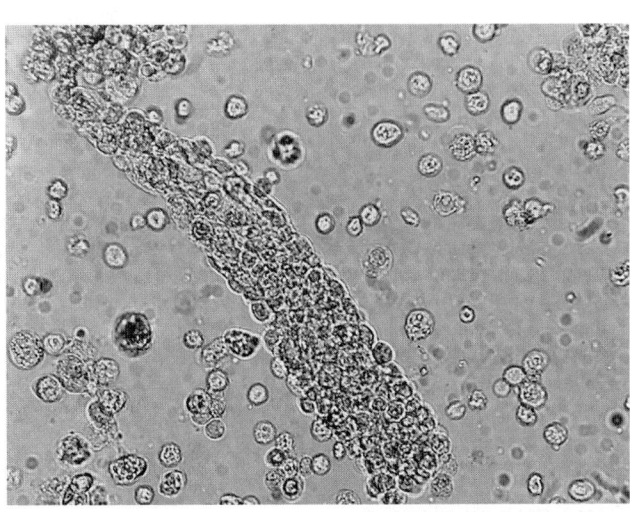

FIG. 1 Urinary sediment showing white blood cells and white blood cell cast. (Courtesy Randy L. Luciano, M.D.)

systemic drug reaction; may also occur in other causes of AKI including cholesterol emboli, vasculitis, and hematologic or solid organ malignancy).
- Anemia (may be out of proportion to degree of AKI since erythropoietin-producing cells reside within the interstitium and may be decreased by inflammation in this kidney compartment).
- If drug-related AIN is not suspected, laboratory workup for infection, vasculitis, and autoimmune disorders may be warranted depending on the clinical context.

IMAGING STUDIES
- Gallium scintigraphy and PET/CT have both been used to evaluate AIN in patients. May distinguish between AIN and other forms of AKI in patients who may be too unstable for a renal biopsy.

KIDNEY BIOPSY
Critical in diagnosis of interstitial nephritis in patients in whom the differential of AKI is broad. Biopsy findings include (Fig. E2):
- Predominant lymphocytic and monocytic infiltrate (Fig. E2B).
- Presence of eosinophils is suggestive of drug-induced AIN (Fig. E2C).
- Tubulitis (renal tubular invasion by inflammatory cells) is suggestive of AIN.
- Early on, inflammation is associated with edema, but a transition to fibrosis with underlying tubular atrophy occurs with chronicity (Fig. E2D).

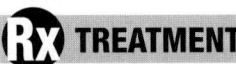

TREATMENT

NONPHARMACOLOGIC THERAPY
Largely supportive; removal of offending agent, if known, will resolve 60% of all cases

ACUTE GENERAL Rx
- Maintain adequate hydration and urine output but avoid volume overload.
- Identify and treat infection if present.
- Avoid nephrotoxins and medications that impair renal blood flow.
- Uveitis in the tubulo-interstitial nephritis and uveitis syndrome may be asymptomatic; therefore, ophthalmologic exam is required in idiopathic AIN.
- Initiation of steroids is controversial, but retrospective studies and anecdotal literature have shown that steroid treatment, started within 7 days of diagnosis, may reduce need for chronic dialysis in patients with drug-induced AIN who have not responded to drug withdrawal alone. Steroids are the basis of treatment in idiopathic AIN, AIN associated with systemic disease, and TINU. Dosing is typically pulsed steroids with IV methylprednisolone (250 mg daily ×3 days) followed by 0.5 to 1 mg/kg/day tapering over 4 to 6 weeks.
- Cyclophosphamide, cyclosporine, and mycophenolate mofetil have all been used anecdotally in steroid-resistant disease. Additionally, mycophenolate mofetil has been used as a steroid-sparing agent if AKI recurs when steroids are tapered or discontinued.

CHRONIC Rx
- Limit exposure to known nephrotoxic agents.
- Adjust dosages of all medications as indicated by glomerular filtration rate.
- Tight control of blood pressure, diabetes, and cholesterol.
- Relieve any sources of chronic obstruction (treat benign prostatic hyperplasia).

DISPOSITION
With AIN:
- Complete recovery with return to baseline creatinine occurs in 60% to 65% of cases
- Partial recovery is seen in 10% to 20%
- Irreversible damage in 5% to 10%
- Relapse is common with reexposure to offending agents

REFERRAL
Renal consultation is often necessary, especially if the diagnosis is unclear, biopsy is required, or there is treatment-resistant disease.

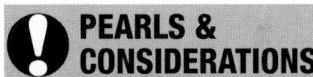

PEARLS & CONSIDERATIONS

COMMENTS
Acute interstitial nephritis is most often due to drugs started in the preceding 30 days. The most common drug classes are beta-lactam antibiotics, NSAIDs, and proton pump inhibitors. In contrast to acute tubular necrosis, which is often associated with oliguria, early AIN may be associated with polyuria; therefore, a high index of suspicion in this clinical setting is essential for early diagnosis.

PREVENTION
Use known offending agents with care, especially in the elderly and those with known underlying kidney disease.

PATIENT/FAMILY EDUCATION
http://www.nlm.nih.gov/medlineplus/ency/article/000464.htm

SUGGESTED READINGS
Available at www.expertconsult.com

RELATED CONTENT
Interstitial Nephritis (Patient Information)

AUTHORS: **RANDY L. LUCIANO, M.D., PH.D.,** and **SAMANTHA L. GELFAND, M.D.**

Diseases and Disorders

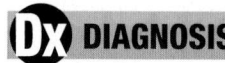

i BASIC INFORMATION

DEFINITION

Intraventricular conduction delay (IVCD) is a common clinical abnormality related to a conduction disturbance that occurs at various levels in the His-Purkinje system. This defect does not meet criteria for right bundle branch (RBBB), left bundle branch (LBBB), or hemifascicular block (Fig. 1). It can be caused by anatomic abnormalities and the physiologic properties of cardiac tissue. It may occur between ventricles (interventricular), within Purkinje fibers or ventricular myocardium (intraventricular), or between layers of the myocardium (intramural). Parietal block occurs in the terminal Purkinje system and presents with prolonged QRS in leads V1 to V3 that exceeds significantly the QRS width from V4 to V6. This particular type of IVCD is associated with right ventricular arrhythmogenic dysplasia.

IVCD is defined by a QRS duration of >110 ms in adults, in children 8 to 16 yr of age >90 ms, and in children younger than 8 yr of age >80 ms in the ECG provided there is no criteria for either LBBB or RBBB. The conduction delay causing the prolonged QRS is considered to take place beyond the Purkinje's myocardial gates and arises from a slowing down in the cell-to-cell conduction.

SYNONYMS

IVCD
Nonspecific intraventricular conduction disturbance
Unspecified intraventricular conduction disturbance
Intraventricular conduction delay
Intraventricular block
Intraventricular conduction defect
Fragmented QRS complex

ICD-10CM CODES
145.4 Non-specific intraventricular block
145.8 Other specified conduction disorders
145.9 Conduction disorder, unspecified

EPIDEMIOLOGY

- A Finnish Social Security Study, which consisted of 10,899 subjects with baseline ECGs, showed a prevalence of IVCD in 0.6% of the total population. 45.6% of subjects with a QRS duration ≥110 ms without evidence of cardiac disease or bundle branch block, had an increased risk of all-cause mortality (relative risk [RR] 1.75, 95% CI, cardiac mortality (RR 1.87, 95% CI), and mortality due to arrhythmias (RR 2.90, 95% CI). The P values were .002, .04, and .007, respectively.
- IVCD has a consensus prevalence of 30% in patients with heart failure (HF) ranging between 14% and 47% in various studies.
- The reported prevalence in military aviators was similar to RBBB at 2:1000.

ETIOLOGY

Patients with IVCD are not a homogeneous group of patients and cannot be classified as such. A patient with IVCD secondary to dilated cardiomyopathy cannot be compared with a patient with IVCD secondary to LVH caused by hypertension or with patients with myocardial scarring secondary to myocardial infarction and other conditions. Therefore, the treatment for each patient has to be individualized and tailored to the underlying cause of the conduction defect.

The most common clinical conditions associated with IVCD are as follows:
- Coronary artery disease
- Infiltrative cardiomyopathy (CMO): amyloidosis, sarcoidosis, hemosiderosis, and so on
- Cardiomyopathies of other etiologies
- Left ventricular hypertrophy
- Endocarditis of the aortic valve
- Myocarditis
- Chagas disease (parasitic)
- Primary conduction diseases: Lenegre's disease, Lev disease
- Congenital anomalies
- Progressive systemic scleroderma
- Pulmonary embolism
- Cyclic antidepressants
- Hyperkalemia
- Hypothermia
- Intracardiac catheter manipulation

It constitutes a prognostic marker for cardiac events in CAD, hypertrophic cardiomyopathy, structural heart disease with implanted cardiac defibrillators, Chagas' disease, arrhythmogenic right ventricular dysplasia, Brugada's syndrome, and acquired long QT syndrome. It is associated with heart failure hospitalization in patients with hypertrophic cardiomyopathy.

Antiarrhythmic drugs, class IA (e.g., procainamide, disopyramide, quinidine), and class IC (e.g., flecainide, encainide, and propafenone), amantadine, carbamazepine, cocaine, diphenhydramine, mesoridazine, and thioridazine. In addition, propoxyphene and propranolol can also cause IVCD by sodium channel blockade in older adults due to myocardial fibrosis caused by apoptosis.

Etiology can also be unknown in many cases.

PHYSICAL FINDINGS & CLINICAL PRESENTATION

IVCD per se is asymptomatic and is recognizable only with a 12-lead ECG.

Dx DIAGNOSIS

Intraventricular conduction delay (IVCD) is usually an incidental ECG finding. This defect does not meet criteria for RBBB, LBBB, or hemifascicular block.

DIFFERENTIAL DIAGNOSIS

- Unifascicular block
- Bifascicular block
- Wolff-Parkinson-White (WPW) pattern and variants
- LBBB
- RBBB

EVALUATION

The evaluation of the patient with IVCD should be oriented to discovering the cause of the ECG abnormality to implement appropriate therapy and counseling. Thorough history and physical exams must be performed to implement adequate laboratory and imaging testing based on the level of suspicion for the causes of IVCD listed earlier. Such tests could include but are not limited to:
- Standard laboratory testing appropriate for age, gender, and metabolic abnormalities
- Resting ECG
- Exercise ECG, with or without imaging
- Ambulatory ECG
- Echocardiogram
- Specialized studies based on known comorbidities and risk assessment or suspicion of them such as heart failure, myocardial infarction, cardiomyopathies, and so on

Rx TREATMENT

The management goal of patients with IVCD should be the optimization of treatment for the underlying contributing conditions to the conduction defect. In selected patients at risk for sudden cardiac death (SCD) due to significant CAD or arrhythmogenic right ventricular dysplasia, appropriate referral should be made without delay.

Although cardiac resynchronization therapy (CRT) has been effective in reducing clinical events in patients with LBBB (LBBB and RBBB are independent predictors of increased risk of

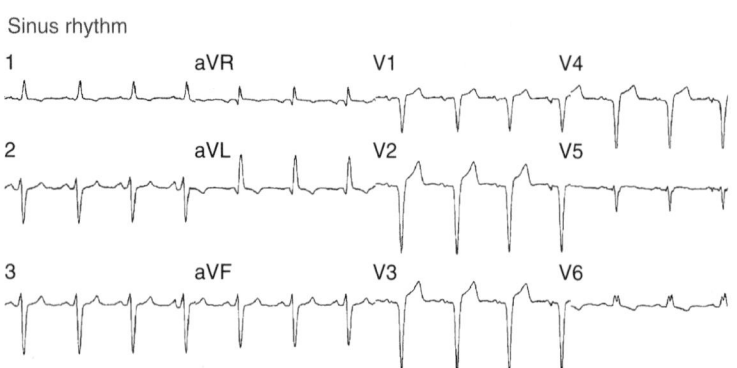

Sinus rhythm

FIG 1 Normal sinus rhythm baseline with intraventricular conduction delay resembling left bundle branch block (LBBB). (From Issa ZF: *Clinical arrhythmology and electrophysiology: a companion to Braunwald's heart disease*, ed 2, Philadelphia, 2012, Saunders.)

cardiac death in patients with HF), patients with IVCDs do not correlate with worsened prognosis nor clinical improvement of heart failure.

CRT offers no benefit for the management of patients with IVCD and in fact there may be an increased risk of ventricular tachycardia for this group of patients when receiving CRT or intracardiac defibrillator (ICD) devices.

However, intraventricular dyssynchrony has been found to be directly related to IVCD and to have major implications in the identification of adequate electronic pacing sites in patients who require device implantation therapy.

Strauss et al. have recently proposed that criteria for LBBB be changed to >140 ms in the male population and >130 ms in the female population for better guidance of device therapy.

PROGNOSIS

Different studies have shown that IVCD is associated with increased all-cause mortality with relative risk of (RR): 1.75-2.01, increased cardiac mortality with RR:1.87-2.53, and a markedly elevated risk of sudden arrhythmic death with RR: 2.9-3.11. Nevertheless, clinical correlation is needed because prognosis depends on underlying associated clinical conditions.

An area of increasing clinical and research interest is the presence of intra- and interatrial conduction delay as it relates to the generation of atrial fibrillation and as a more reliable parameter than left atrial volume and dimension in the prediction of atrial fibrillation and ischemic stroke. It has been found to have a direct correlation with aortic strain in patients with hypertension, and it correlates also with an increase in symptoms and mortality in patients with systolic heart failure.

REFERRAL

Refer to a cardiologist if there is history of palpitations, dizziness, heart failure, myocardial infarction, or an abnormal cardiac exam.

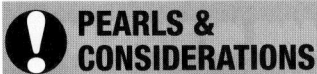

PEARLS & CONSIDERATIONS

IVCD can be due to drugs such as Class I antiarrhythmic drugs.

IVCD can be a normal variant and is not always associated with cardiac pathology.

Clinical correlation (history and physical exam) is needed to identify associated cardiac abnormalities.

In patients with heart failure, cardiac resynchronization for IVCD does not influence prognosis or clinical improvement unless it is associated with LBBB.

SUGGESTED READINGS
Available at www.expertconsult.com

AUTHORS: **JUAN A. ESCARFULLER, M.D.,** and **CLAUDIA SERRANO, M.D.**

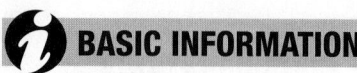

BASIC INFORMATION

DEFINITION

Irritable bowel syndrome (IBS) is a chronic functional disorder manifested by alteration in bowel habits and recurrent abdominal pain and bloating. IBS is a symptom complex influenced by a variety of physiologic determinants from gut to brain and back. The ROME III criteria for diagnosis of IBS are:

- Recurrent abdominal pain or discomfort at least 3 days per month in the past 3 mo associated with ≥ two of the following:
  1. Pain is relieved or improved with defecation.
  2. Its onset is associated with a change in the frequency of bowel movement.
  3. Its onset is associated with a change in the form or appearance of the stool.
- The criteria must be fulfilled for at least the past 3 mo with symptom onset at least 6 mo before the diagnosis.

SYNONYMS

Irritable colon
Spastic colon
IBS

ICD-10CM CODES
K58   Irritable bowel syndrome
K58.9 Irritable bowel syndrome without
      diarrhea
K58.0 Irritable bowel syndrome with diarrhea

EPIDEMIOLOGY & DEMOGRAPHICS

- IBS is the most common functional bowel disorder. An estimated 15 million people in the United States have IBS.
- IBS occurs in 7% to 21% of the general population of industrialized countries and is responsible for >50% of gastrointestinal (GI) referrals. Worldwide adult prevalence is 12%. Incidence increases during adolescence and peaks in third and fourth decades of life.
- Female/male ratio is 2:1. Peak prevalence is from 20 to 39 years of age.
- Nearly 50% of patients have psychiatric abnormalities, with anxiety disorders being most common.

PHYSICAL FINDINGS & CLINICAL PRESENTATION

- The clinical presentation of IBS consists of abdominal pain and abnormalities of defecation, which may include loose stools, usually after meals and in the morning, alternating with episodes of constipation.
- Physical examination is generally normal.
- Nonspecific abdominal tenderness and distention may be present.

ETIOLOGY

- Unknown, believed to be multifactorial. Fig. 1 illustrates a biopsychological model of IBS pathophysiology.
- Associated pathophysiology includes altered GI motility, alteration in gut flora, and increased gut sensitivity
- Risk factors: anxiety, depression, personality disorders, history of childhood sexual abuse, and domestic abuse in women

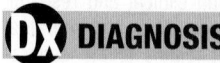

DIAGNOSIS

Table 1 summarizes the diagnostic criteria for IBS and Table 2 subtypes IBS by predominant stool pattern.

DIFFERENTIAL DIAGNOSIS

- Inflammatory bowel disease (IBD)
- Diverticulitis
- Colon malignancy
- Endometriosis
- Peptic ulcer disease
- Biliary liver disease
- Chronic pancreatitis
- Constipation caused by medications (opiates, calcium channel blockers, anticholinergics)
- Diarrhea caused by medications (metformin, colchicine, proton pump inhibitors, antacids, antibiotics)
- Small-bowel overgrowth
- Celiac disease
- Parasites
- Lymphoma of GI tract

WORKUP

Diagnostic workup (Table 3) is aimed primarily at excluding the conditions listed in the differential diagnoses. A step-wise approach is critical. It is important to identify red flags of other diseases, such as weight loss, rectal bleeding, onset in patients >50 yr, fever, nocturnal pain, and family history of malignancy or IBD. Additional red flags include abnormal examination (e.g., mass, enlarged lymph nodes, stool positive for occult blood, muscle wasting) and abnormal laboratory values (anemia, leukocytosis, abnormal chemistry).

Common clinical criteria for diagnosis of IBS are >3 mo of symptoms, including abdominal pain that is relieved by a bowel movement, or pain accompanied by a change in bowel pattern, and abnormality in bowel movement 25% of the time, characterized by two of the following features:

- Abdominal distention
- Abnormal consistency
- Abnormal defecation (e.g., straining, sense of incomplete evacuation)
- Abnormal frequency
- Mucus with bowel movement

LABORATORY TESTS

- Blood work is generally normal. CBC is reasonable to evaluate for anemia. The presence of anemia should alert to the possibility of a colonic malignancy or IBD.
- Testing of stool for ova and parasites should be considered only in patients with chronic diarrhea. Evaluation of stool for *Clostridium difficile* may be helpful in patients with predominant diarrhea symptoms who have recently taken antibiotics.

IMAGING STUDIES

Imaging studies (e.g., flat and upright abdominal radiograph, small-bowel series, sonogram or CT of abdomen and pelvis) are normal and not necessary for diagnosis.

Lower endoscopy is generally normal except for the presence of some spasms. Colonoscopic imaging should be performed only in persons who have alarm features to rule out organic disease and in persons older than 50 yr to screen for colorectal cancer.

TREATMENT

NONPHARMACOLOGIC THERAPY

- Fig. 2 illustrates the management of irritable bowel syndrome. The patient should be encouraged to maintain an adequate fiber intake and to eliminate foods that aggravate symptoms. Avoidance of caffeine, dairy products, fatty foods, and dietary excesses is also helpful. Several clinical trials have shown that a diet low in fermentable oligosaccharides, disaccharides, monosaccharides, and polyols (FODMAPs) improves symptoms in nearly 70% of patients with IBS.
- Cognitive-behavioral therapy is also recommended, particularly in younger patients because psychosocial stressors are important triggers of IBS. Reassurance and education about trigger avoidance and stress management are important.
- Importance of regular exercise and adequate fluid intake should be stressed.

GENERAL Rx

- The mainstay of treatment of IBS is a high-fiber diet. Fiber is helpful for relief of constipation but not for relief of pain. Because symptoms are chronic, the use of laxatives should generally be avoided.
- Soluble fiber (psyllium) is more effective in symptom relief than insoluble fiber (bran). Fiber supplementation with psyllium 1 tbsp bid or calcium polycarbophil (FiberCon) 2 tablets one to four times daily followed by 8 oz of water may be necessary in some patients.
- Patients should be instructed that there might be some increased bloating on initiation of fiber supplementation, which should resolve within 2 to 3 wk. It is important that patients take these fiber products on a regular basis and not only as needed. Fiber is not effective in patients with diarrhea-predominant IBS and may worsen symptoms in these patients.
- Patients who appear anxious can benefit from use of sedatives or selective serotonin reuptake inhibitors (SSRIs). Tricyclic antidepressants in low doses are also effective in some patients with diarrhea-predominant IBS.
- C-2 chloride channel activators: Lubiprostone (Amitiza) is a chloride channel activator that stimulates chloride-rich intestinal fluid secretion and accelerates small intestine

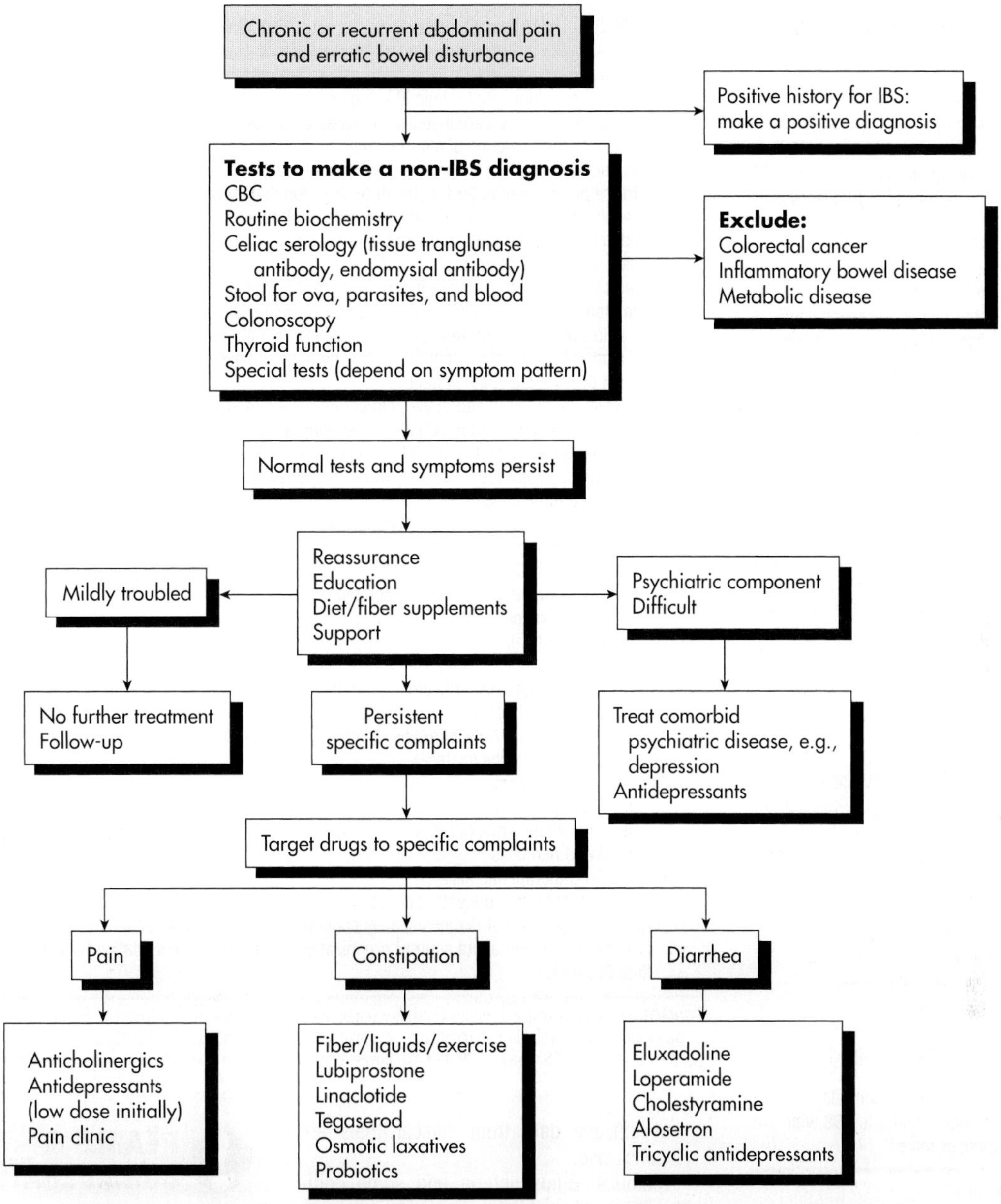

Chronic or recurrent abdominal pain
and erratic bowel disturbance

Positive history for IBS:
make a positive diagnosis

Tests to make a non-IBS diagnosis
CBC
Routine biochemistry
Celiac serology (tissue tranglunase
    antibody, endomysial antibody)
Stool for ova, parasites, and blood
Colonoscopy
Thyroid function
Special tests (depend on symptom pattern)

Exclude:
Colorectal cancer
Inflammatory bowel disease
Metabolic disease

Normal tests and symptoms persist

Reassurance
Education
Diet/fiber supplements
Support

Mildly troubled

Psychiatric component
Difficult

No further treatment
Follow-up

Persistent
specific complaints

Treat comorbid
psychiatric disease, e.g.,
depression
Antidepressants

Target drugs to specific complaints

Pain

Constipation

Diarrhea

Anticholinergics
Antidepressants
(low dose initially)
Pain clinic

Fiber/liquids/exercise
Lubiprostone
Linaclotide
Tegaserod
Osmotic laxatives
Probiotics

Eluxadoline
Loperamide
Cholestyramine
Alosetron
Tricyclic antidepressants

FIG. 1 A biopsychosocial model of irritable bowel syndrome pathophysiology. Irritable bowel syndrome is thought to be a multifactorial disorder, deriving from a potential multitude of etiopathogenic factors, including environmental, psychological, and physiologic factors. This model highlights the complex, often bidirectional interplay of these factors in the experience of irritable bowel syndrome symptoms. *cGMP,* cyclic guanosine monophosphate; *5-HT3,*serotonin type 3; *5-HT4,*serotonin type 4; *FODMAPS,* fermentable oligosaccharides, disaccharides, monosaccharides, and polyols; *HRQOL,* health-related quality of life; *IBS,* irritable bowel syndrome. (Adapted from Sayuk GS, Gyawali CP: Irritable bowel syndrome: modern concepts and management options, *Am J Med* 128(8), 817-827, 2015.)

and colonic transmit time. It may be effective in chronic constipation-predominant IBS unresponsive to conventional treatment. Usual dose is 8 to 24 mcg bid with food. Side effects include headache and nausea.

- Linaclotide (Linzess) is a guanylate cyclase-C (GC-C) agonist FDA approved for IBS with constipation. It stimulates secretion of chloride and bicarbonate into the intestinal lumen, mainly through activation of the CFTR ion channel, resulting in increased intestinal fluid and accelerated transit. Usual dose for

IBS is 290 mcg 30 min before eating. The most common adverse effects are diarrhea, abdominal pain, flatulence, and abdominal distension.

- Eluxadoline (Viberzi) is a μ-opioid receptor agonist and Δ-opioid receptor antagonist FDA approved for IBS with diarrhea. It decreases muscle contractility, inhibits water and electrolyte secretion, and increases rectal sphincter tone. Usual dose is 100 mg PO bid taken with food.
- Loperamide is effective for diarrhea. Alosetron, a serotonin type-3 receptor

antagonist previously withdrawn because of severe constipation and ischemic colitis, has been reintroduced with limited availability. It is indicated only for women with severe chronic diarrhea-predominant IBS unresponsive to conventional therapy and not caused by anatomic or metabolic abnormality. Starting dose is 1 mg qd.

- Alterations in gut flora have been identified as potentially contributing to IBS (84% of IBS patients have an abnormal lactulose breath test, suggesting small-intestinal bacterial overgrowth). Rifaximin,

TABLE 1 Diagnostic Criteria* for Irritable Bowel Syndrome

Recurrent abdominal pain or discomfort† at least 3 d/mo in the previous 3 mo associated with ≥2 of the following:

1. Improvement with defecation
2. Onset associated with a change in frequency of stool
3. Onset associated with a change in form (appearance) of stool
4. Supporting symptoms (not required for diagnosis but helpful in confirming IBS presentation): (1) abnormal stool frequency (<3 bowel movements per week or >3 bowel movements per day), (2) abnormal stool form, (3) defecation straining, (4) urgency (feeling of incomplete evacuation), (5) passage of mucus, and (6) bloating.

IBS, Irritable bowel syndrome.
*Criteria fulfilled for the previous 3 mo with symptom onset at least 6 mo before diagnosis.
†Discomfort means an uncomfortable sensation not described as pain. In pathophysiology research and clinical trials, a pain or discomfort frequency of at least 2 d/wk during screening evaluation for subject eligibility.
Adapted from Sayuk GS, Gyawali CP: Irritable bowel syndrome: modern concepts and management options. *Am J Med* 128(8), 817-827, 2015.

TABLE 2 Subtyping Irritable Bowel Syndrome by Predominant Stool Pattern

1. IBS with constipation—hard or lumpy stools* ≥25% and loose (mushy) or watery stools† ≥25% of bowel movements‡
2. IBS with diarrhea—loose (mushy) or watery stools† ≥25% and hard or lumpy stool* ≥25% of bowel movements‡
3. Mixed IBS—hard or lumpy stools* ≥25% and loose (mushy) or watery stools† ≥25% of bowel movements‡
4. Unsubtyped IBS—insufficient abnormality of stool consistency to meet criteria for IBS with constipation, diarrhea, or mixed‡

IBS, Irritable bowel syndrome.
*Bristol Stool Form Scale 1-2 (separate hard lumps like nuts [difficult to pass] or sausage-shaped but lumpy).
†Bristol Stool Form Scale 6-7 (fluffy pieces with ragged edges, a mushy stool or watery, no solid pieces, entirely liquid).
‡In the absence of use of antidiarrheals or laxatives.
Adapted from Sayuk GS, Gyawali CP: Irritable bowel syndrome: modern concepts and management options. *Am J Med* 128(8), 817-827, 2015.

TABLE 3 Irritable Bowel Syndrome Treatment Strategy: A Way Forward

1. Evaluation
   a. Consider conditions that mimic IBS (e.g., celiac disease, microscopic colitis, bile acid diarrhea, pancreatic insufficiency, carbohydrate intolerances, medication side effects, postsurgical neoanatomy)
   b. Assess for the presence of alarm symptoms
   c. Evaluate for symptom triggers (e.g., stressors, diet)
   d. Explore presence of other functional GI (e.g., functional dyspepsia) and non-GI disorders (e.g., fibromyalgia), psychiatric comorbidity, and drug intolerances
   e. Understand previous IBS treatment experiences
2. Selection of treatment approach
   a. Predicated on symptom severity and dominant symptoms
   b. Symptom severity (intensity, bother, effects on quality of life)
      i. Mild symptoms, intermittent symptoms, low symptom burden: symptomatic or peripheral therapy
      ii. Moderate symptoms: centrally acting neuromodulators, especially if symptomatic therapy does not provide adequate benefit
      iii. Severe symptoms and those with comorbidities (non-GI functional disorders, psychiatric): both centrally acting neuromodulators and peripheral therapy
         a. Concurrent affective disorders need to be managed.
         b. Other central therapies (cognitive and behavioral therapy, hypnosis, stress reduction) may need to be considered.
   b. Dominant symptoms (diarrhea, constipation, pain, other GI symptoms)
      i. Constipation predominant
         a. Laxatives, fiber
         b. Novel agents (linaclotide, lubiprostone)
      ii. Diarrhea predominant
         a. Antidiarrheals
         b. Alosetron
         c. Address dysbiosis (rifaximin, probiotics)
         d. Diet (low FODMAP)
         e. Bile binders (cholestyramine, colesevelam)
         f. Disaccharidases (lactase)
      iii. Pain predominant
         a. Antidepressants (TCAs and SNRIs preferred)
         b. Linaclotide when constipation present
         c. Avoid narcotics
3. Education and therapeutic alliance
   a. Inform patient about etiopathogenesis.
   b. Reaffirm legitimacy of diagnosis; allay concerns about organic disease.
   c. Provide information about support organizations (International Foundation for Functional Gastrointestinal Disorders).

FODMAP, fermentable oligosaccharides, disaccharides, monosaccharides, and polyols; *GI,* gastrointestinal; *IBS,* irritable bowel syndrome; *SNRI,* serotonin-norepinephrine reuptake inhibitor; *TCA,* tricyclic antidepressant.
Adapted from Sayuk GS, Gyawali CP: Irritable bowel syndrome: modern concepts and management options. *Am J Med* 128(8), 817-827, 2015.

a gut-selective antibiotic, has been used in recent trials to eradicate bacterial overgrowth (70% eradication rate). A dose of 400 mg tid for 10 days was reported effective in improving IBS symptoms up to 10 wk after discontinuation of therapy. Until additional evidence is available, use of rifaximin or other antibiotics in IBS should be reserved for patients with proven bacterial overgrowth.

- Antispasmodics-anticholinergics (e.g., dicyclomine, hyoscyamine) are often used, but efficacy data from clinical trials are inconclusive.
- Probiotics: Bifidobacteria and some combinations of probiotics have shown some limited efficacy. Lactobacilli do not appear to be effective for the treatment of IBS. Additional data showing efficacy is needed before probiotics can be endorsed for treatment of IBS.
- Antidepressants: SSRIs are more effective than placebo for relief of global IBS symptoms.

DISPOSITION

More than 60% of patients respond successfully to treatment over the initial 12 mo; however, IBS is a chronic, relapsing condition and requires prolonged therapy.

REFERRAL

GI referral is recommended in patients with rectal bleeding, fever, nocturnal diarrhea, anemia, weight loss, or onset of symptoms >40 yr. Consultation is also necessary if specialized diagnostic procedures such as endoscopy are necessary.

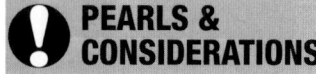

PEARLS & CONSIDERATIONS

COMMENTS

- Patients should be educated regarding maintenance of a high-fiber diet and elimination of stressors, which can precipitate attacks of IBS. They should be reassured that their condition does not lead to cancer.
- Recent drug efforts (alosetron, tegaserod) are aimed at serotonergic receptors in the gut because most of the serotonin in the body is found in the GI tract and is believed to be involved in the mediation of visceral sensation and motility.
- Cognitive-behavioral therapy is effective in the treatment of patients with IBS and should be considered as part of the armamentarium against this disorder.
- Some patients with IBS but without celiac disease show symptom improvement on a wheat-free diet. A 2- to 3-week trial of wheat avoidance may be reasonable in patients with treatment-resistant IBS.

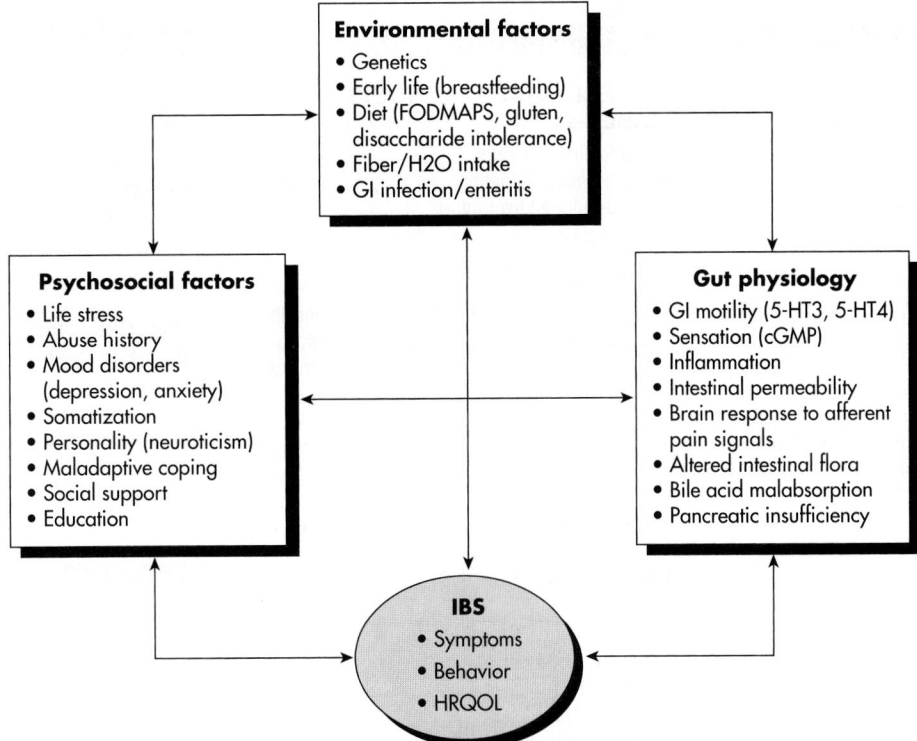

FIG. 2 Management of irritable bowel syndrome. (Modified from Palmer K.R., Penman I.D.: 22 Alimentary tract and pancreatic disease. In Colledge N.R., Walker B.R., Ralston S.H.: *Davidson's principles and practice of medicine*, Philadelphia, 2010, Elsevier.)

EBM **EVIDENCE**

Available at www.expertconsult.com

SUGGESTED READINGS
Available at www.expertconsult.com

RELATED CONTENT

Irritable Bowel Syndrome (Patient Information)

AUTHOR: **FRED F. FERRI, M.D.**

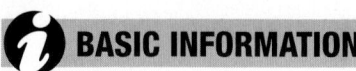 BASIC INFORMATION

DEFINITION

- A common form of vascular liver disease
- Occurs when a severe systemic disturbance leads to decreased perfusion to the liver resulting in tissue hypoxia.

SYNONYMS

- Hypoxic hepatitis
- Shock liver
- Ischemic hepatopathy
- Hepatic necrosis

ICD10-CM
K76.2   Central hemorrhagic necrosis of liver
K75.89 Other specified inflammatory liver disease

EPIDEMIOLOGY & DEMOGRAPHICS

- Occurs worldwide

INCIDENCE:
- Less than 1% on the inpatient medical wards
- Incidence is higher (2.5%) in intensive care unit.

PEAK INCIDENCE:
- Highest in the cardiac care units

PREVALENCE:
- Recognized as most frequent cause of acute liver injury
- 57% of patients with liver enzymes >1000 IU/L have ischemic hepatitis
- Prevalence up to 10% in the intensive care setting

PREDOMINANT AGE AND SEX:
- Can occur in all ages
- Most common in elderly

GENETICS:
- No genetic predisposition

RISK FACTORS:
- Most common is cardiovascular disease
- Chronic heart failure
- Cirrhosis

PHYSICAL FINDINGS & CLINICAL PRESENTATION

- Altered mental status may be present due to decreased cerebral perfusion.
- Other symptoms are often masked by the overall disease state.
- Hepatic synthetic function is usually preserved in ischemic hepatitis

ETIOLOGY

- Cardiac disease in the most common (Fig. E1).
- This includes myocardial infarction, arrhythmias, cardiac tamponade, and cardiogenic shock.
- Respiratory failure and sepsis are the second and third most common.
- Hypovolemic shock from hemorrhage, dehydration, and heat stroke.
- Hypotension.
- See Table 1 for a brief summary of the different causes of ischemic hepatitis.

Dx DIAGNOSIS

DIFFERENTIAL DIAGNOSIS (TABLE 2)

- Acute viral hepatitis
- Autoimmune hepatitis
- Drug-induced liver injury
- Other toxins and medications

WORKUP

- Diagnosed by laboratory parameters and the clinical context of a hospitalized patient.
- Workup is directed at identifying the predisposing cause.
- Liver biopsy is not required.
- Histology shows centrilobular (zone 3) necrosis with preservation of the hepatic architecture.
- Necrosis can extend to the midzonal hepatocytes in the setting of prolonged ischemia.

LABORATORY TESTS

- Extremely elevated aminotransferase levels, often exceeding 200 times the upper limit of normal.
- Aspartate aminotransferase (AST) and alanine aminotransferase (ALT) rapidly rise after the ischemic insult.
- They peak within 1 to 3 days.
- They usually return to normal within 7 to 10 days if the initial ischemic insult is resolved.
- Lactate dehydrogenase (LDH) level is extremely elevated.
- ALT/LDH ratio of less than 1.5 is suggestive.
- Prothrombin time can be slightly prolonged.
- The serum bilirubin can be mildly increased.
- Serum bilirubin peaks after the aminotransferases peak.
- Increased blood urea nitrogen and creatinine levels from acute tubular necrosis and renal dysfunction.

IMAGING STUDIES

- Imaging is not required for the diagnosis.

Rx TREATMENT

NONPHARMACOLOGIC THERAPY

- Management is directed at treating the underlying illness causing the systemic disturbance.

ACUTE GENERAL TREATMENT

- Hemodynamic resuscitation
- Inotropic agents for cardiogenic shock
- Intravenous fluid resuscitation with or without vasoconstrictors for septic or hypovolemic shock
- Blood transfusions if hypovolemic shock from blood loss
- These measures optimize hepatic perfusion and resolve tissue hypoxia

CHRONIC TREATMENT

- Ensure stability of underlying illness
- No specific liver-directed therapy

TABLE 1   Causes of Ischemic Hepatitis

Cardiovascular disease (most common): cardiogenic shock
Respiratory Failure
Sepsis/Septic Shock
Hypovolemic Shock: hemorrhage, volume depletion
Hypotension

TABLE 2   Common Differentials of Ischemic Hepatitis

Acute Viral Hepatitis (e.g., hepatitis A, hepatitis B)
Autoimmune hepatitis
Toxins (e.g., herbal supplements)
Medications (e.g., acetaminophen)

DISPOSITION

- Most commonly self-limited and benign condition.
- Occasionally associated with significant mortality.
- Prognosis is determined by the severity of the underlying illness. In-hospital mortality associated with ischemic hepatitis is roughly 50%.
- Patients with underlying chronic heart failure or cirrhosis have worse outcomes.
- Other poor prognostic factors include persistently elevated aminotransferase and multiorgan failure.

REFERRAL

- Referral to a hepatologist is not required once illness is resolved.
- Referral is appropriate if patient has underlying cirrhosis.

! PEARLS AND CONSIDERATIONS

COMMENTS

- Have a high index of suspicion for this diagnosis in a hospitalized patient with severe systemic illness and significantly elevated AST and ALT
- Do not be alarmed if bilirubin continues to rise after AST and ALT peak

PREVENTION

- Ensure stability of comorbidities (e.g., cardiac disease)

AUTHOR: **HIRSH D. TRIVEDI, M.D.**

DEFINITION

Ischemic optic neuropathy (ION) is a general term for dysfunction of the optic nerve due to decreased blood supply and subsequent neuronal death.
Subclassifications
Arteritic anterior ischemic optic neuropathy (AAION)
Non-arteritic anterior ischemic optic neuropathy (NAION)
Posterior ischemic optic neuropathy (PION)

SYNONYMS

ION
AAION
NAION
PION

ICD-10CM CODES
H47.01 Ischemic Optic Neuropathy

EPIDEMIOLOGY AND DEMOGRAPHICS
INCIDENCE:
- 2.3-10 cases of anterior ischemic optic neuropathy per 100,000 per year (15% AAION, 85% NAION)
- PION is much less common than anterior ischemic optic neuropathy (AION).

AGE, RACE, AND SEX:
- Age >50, though may occur at any age
- White women are at particular risk of AAION due to giant cell arteritis (GCA).
- 95% of NAION patients are white.

RISK FACTORS:
- NAION: Diabetes mellitus, hypertension, episodic hypotension, obstructive sleep apnea, hypercholesterolemia. Emboli can be refractile yellow-white cholesterol (Hollenhorst) plaques (Fig. 1*A*), grayish elongated fibrin-platelet aggregates (Fig. 1*B*), or nonscintillating white calcific particles (Fig. 1*C*).
- PION: Surgery (hemodilution, prolonged hypotension, orbital edema, and orbital compression), or factors associated with AAION and NAION.

CLINICAL PRESENTATION

- AAION: Sudden, unilateral, often painless vision loss. Will commonly have systemic symptoms of GCA including headache, jaw claudication, scalp tenderness, fever, and weight loss, but vision loss may be the only presenting sign/symptom.
- NAION: Sudden, unilateral, painless vision loss, often upon awakening.
- PION: Sudden, painless loss of vision that is either unilateral or bilateral. Typically bilateral if following surgery or unilateral

in its arteritic or non-arteritic form with symptoms similar to AAION and NAION, respectively.

PHYSICAL FINDINGS

- All types of ION may result in a relative afferent pupillary defect and/or dyschromatopsia in the affected eye.
- AAION: Severe vision loss with visual acuity worse than 20/200 in a majority of patients. Fundoscopic view of the optic nerve head in the affected eye will show pallid edema ("chalky white" disc).
- NAION: Blurring/cloudiness of vision with relatively preserved central visual acuity (>20/64 in 31%-52% of patients). Fundoscopic view of the optic nerve head during the acute phase will show edema and surface capillary dilation with peripapillary splinter hemorrhages. The unaffected eye will likely reveal a small cup-to-disc ratio.
- PION: Vision loss is worst in surgical PION, otherwise similar to AAION and NAION. Fundoscopic exam typically normal in acute setting, but may show pallor weeks later.

ETIOLOGY

- AAION: Sudden occlusion of the short posterior ciliary arteries that supply the optic nerve head as a result of vasculitis. The

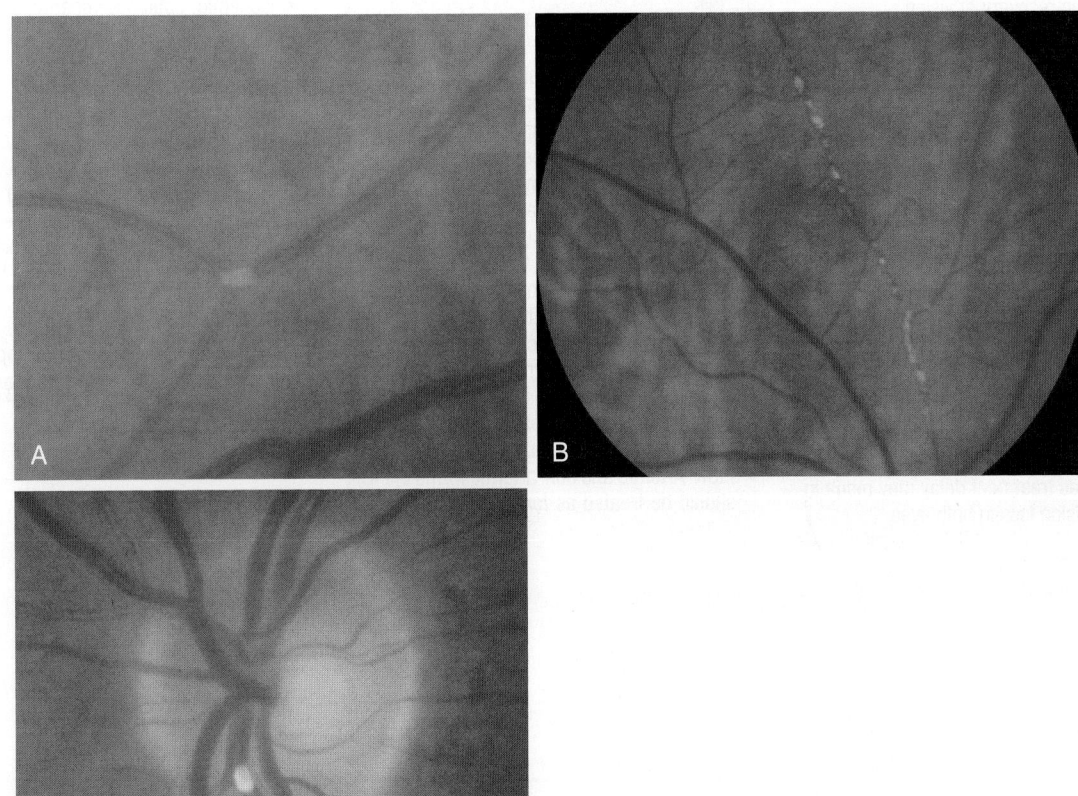

FIG. 1 Retinal emboli. A, Hollenhorst plaque; **B,** fibrin-platelet emboli; **C,** calcific embolus at the disc. (From Bowling B: Kanski's clinical ophthalmology: a systemic approach, ed 8, 2016, Elsevier.)

most common vasculitis is GCA, but others include eosinophilic granulomatosis with angiitis (previously Churg-Strauss syndrome), polyarteritis nodosa, or rheumatoid arthritis
- NAION: It is hypothesized that hypoxia of the optic nerve head results in slight edema of the axons of the optic nerve. As the edema increases, a compartment syndrome develops resulting in the occlusion of the short posterior ciliary arteries in the optic nerve head.
- PION: Ischemia in the retrobulbar optic nerve due to hypoperfusion of the pial plexus. This may be secondary to either surgery or arteritic/non-arteritic causes as discussed previously.

DIAGNOSIS

DIFFERENTIAL DIAGNOSIS

- Optic neuritis: Typically associated with painful vision loss and may be the presenting sign of multiple sclerosis or neuromyelitis optica.
- Toxic/nutritional optic meuropathy: Typically bilateral, symmetric, painless, and slowly progressive, although may be acute (such as with methanol or ethylene glycol poisoning).
- Radiation-induced optic neuropathy: Typically develops within 3 years of radiation to structures near the optic nerve. Progresses within weeks with no recovery of vision.
- Infectious optic neuropathy: Optic neuropathy can develop as a result of a number of infections including bacterial (*B. henselae, M. tuberculosis*), spirochetes (*B. burgdorferi, T. pallidum*), fungi (cryptococcus *sp.,* aspergillus *sp.*), or viruses (cytomegalovirus, Epstein-Barr virus, or varicella-zoster virus in immunocompromised patients).
- Compressive optic neuropathy (e.g., from tumor): Typically progressive vision loss but may present acutely.

WORKUP

- Complete history focused on pertinent symptoms and risk factors.
- Workup should focus on excluding GCA (headache, jaw claudication, scalp tenderness, fever), as treatment delay may result in permanent vision loss in both eyes.

- Careful examination of optic disc, look for "chalky white" pallor suggestive of AAION or edema and peripapillary hemorrhages suggestive of NAION.
- The unaffected eye should also be examined and compared.

LABORATORY TESTS

- Complete blood count with C-reactive protein (level above 2.45 mg/dL highly suggestive of GCA) and erythrocyte sedimentation rate.
- Tests to rule out infectious optic neuropathy as appropriate.

IMAGING STUDIES

- Visual Field Testing: May detect any visual field defects associated with optic nerve injury (including altitudinal, arcuate, and central visual field defects). PION in particular is associated with central visual field defects.
- Optical Coherence tomography: May show swelling of the optic disc.
- Fluorescein angiography: May show generalized choroidal filling delay (AAION) or delayed filling in the optic disc prelaminar layers (NAION). PION will show no abnormalities.

SURGICAL WORKUP

- Temporal artery biopsy if high suspicion for GCA.

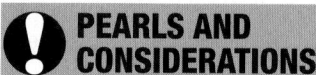 TREATMENT

- AAION: Treatment should begin as soon as GCA is suspected. Corticosteroids are the mainstay of treatment. Recommendations include either oral prednisone (80-120 mg daily) or intravenous methylprednisolone (1 gram daily) for 3 to 5 days followed by 1 to 2 mg/kg/day oral prednisone for 4 to 6 weeks and tapered gradually to 10 to 15 mg/day and maintained for 12 or more months.
- NAION: There is currently no effective treatment for NAION. Proposed treatments that have not been shown to be efficacious include corticosteroids, intravitreal anti-VEGF injections, aspirin, hyperbaric oxygen, and surgical decompression.
- PION: Arteritic and non-arteritic forms of PION should be treated as for AAION, and there is

currently not an effective treatment for surgical PION.

DISPOSITION

- AAION: If not treated, the second eye is similarly affected in 50% to 95% of patients. With treatment, contralateral eye involvement is generally prevented and some patients have slight improvement in affected eye.
- NAION: Approximately 20% to 25% will spontaneously recover some vision, and the same amount may have some worsening. Although recurrent NAION in the same eye is not likely (3%-8%), up to 30% to 40% of patients experience contralateral eye involvement in their lifetime.
- PION: Arteritic/non-arteritic forms as mentioned previously, patients with surgical PION generally have little change following vision loss.

REFERRAL

- Recommend referral to an ophthalmologist or neuro-ophthalmologist for evaluation and workup. Again, if GCA is suspected, begin treatment immediately.

PEARLS AND CONSIDERATIONS

- Ischemic optic neuropathy can be classified as either anterior or posterior, and may be due to arteritic, non-arteritic, or surgical causes.
- Correct identification of the underlying etiology is key to preventing further vision loss, especially in patients with GCA.
- Patients suspected of having GCA should be treated with corticosteroids immediately and undergo temporal artery biopsy within a week of starting corticosteroid treatment.

RELATED CONTENT

Giant Cell Arteritis (Related Key Topic)

AUTHORS: **PAUL D. CHAMBERLAIN, B.S.,** and **JOSEPH S. KASS, M.D., J.D.**

BASIC INFORMATION

DEFINITION

Jaundice is a yellowish discoloration of the sclera (Fig. E1), skin, and mucous membranes caused by an excessive amount of bilirubin in the bloodstream. Clinically detectable jaundice in adults is a serum bilirubin of 2.5 to 3 mg/dl.

SYNONYMS

Icterus

ICD-10CM CODES
R17 Unspecified jaundice

EPIDEMIOLOGY & DEMOGRAPHICS

The prevalent causes of jaundice by age and sex:
- Young adulthood (for either sex): viral hepatitis, Gilbert's disease
- Middle adulthood (for either sex): drug-induced hepatitis and cirrhosis
- Middle-aged and older men: alcoholic liver disease, pancreatic cancer, hepatoma, primary hemochromatosis
- Women: primary biliary cirrhosis, chronic active hepatitis, choledocholithiasis, carcinoma of the gallbladder

PHYSICAL FINDINGS & CLINICAL PRESENTATION

Presentation can vary from an incidental finding to acute and life threatening. History and physical examination give important clues to the underlying condition.
Key history of present illness findings:
- Duration of jaundice
- Associated symptoms: abdominal pain, fever, nausea, malaise, pruritus, chills, changes in urine and stool color, anorexia and/or weight loss
Key social history/exposure findings:
- Alcohol use, injection of illicit drugs, use of hepatotoxic medication or herbal products, blood transfusions, unprotected sex, ingestion of shellfish, travel, occupational exposure to toxins
Key medical history findings:
- Prior abdominal/biliary surgery, prior episodes of jaundice, prior diagnosis of hepatitis B or C, inflammatory bowel disease
Key physical findings:
- Vital sign abnormalities: fever, hypotension, tachycardia
- Signs of acute disease: abdominal tenderness, splenomegaly, abdominal mass, encephalopathy, Murphy's sign
- Signs of chronic liver disease: palmar erythema, spider angiomas, bruising, gynecomastia, testicular atrophy, ascites, weight loss, Kayser-Fleischer rings (Wilson's), caput medusa, internal hemorrhoids, scleral icterus

ETIOLOGY

Disruption in any of the three phases of bilirubin metabolism can lead to jaundice:

- Prehepatic phase: an increase in heme degradation products from red blood cell catabolism, ineffective erythropoiesis, or breakdown of muscle myoglobin and cytochromes; leads to indirect (unconjugated) hyperbilirubinemia
- Intrahepatic phase: destruction of the hepatocytes or disruption of either of the two separate biochemical processes that conjugate bilirubin in the hepatocyte; may lead to indirect (unconjugated) or direct (conjugated) hyperbilirubinemia
- Posthepatic phase: blockage of the release of water-soluble bilirubin from the hepatobiliary system, preventing excretion into the stool or urine or recycling within the gut flora; leads to direct (conjugated) hyperbilirubinemia

DIAGNOSIS

DIFFERENTIAL DIAGNOSIS

Prehepatic causes:
- Hemolytic processes (e.g., sickle cell disease, spherocytosis, thalassemia, G6PD, immune hemolysis, HUS), ineffective erythropoiesis (e.g., thalassemia, folate, severe iron deficiency), or large hematoma reabsorption.
Intrahepatic causes:
- If unconjugated hyperbilirubinemia: enzyme metabolism disorders (Gilbert's disease, Crigler-Najjar syndrome), drugs that alter the enzymatic pathways such as rifampin, isoniazid, and probenecid.
- If conjugated hyperbilirubinemia: intrahepatic cholestasis caused by:
  1. Viruses: hepatitis A, B, and C; Epstein-Barr, hemorrhagic viruses (yellow fever, Ebola)
  2. Other infections: bacteria (leptospirosis, MAI), parasites (schistosomiasis, malaria, amebiasis), fungal (blastomyces, histoplasma)
  3. Alcohol: alcoholic hepatitis, alcoholic cirrhosis
  4. Autoimmune: primary biliary cirrhosis, primary sclerosing cholangitis, autoimmune hepatitis
  5. Hepatotoxic drug-induced: acetaminophen (most common), penicillins (most commonly Augmentin), chlorpromazine, steroids (estrogenic or anabolic), NSAIDs, valproic acid, some herbals such as kava, ma huang, and off-market weight-loss supplements
  6. Hereditary/metabolic: sickle cell disease and other RBC dyscrasias, hemochromatosis, Wilson's disease, Dubin-Johnson and Rotor's syndromes, α-antitrypsin deficiency, glycogen storage disease, NASH (non-alcoholic steatohepatitis), porphyria, benign recurrent intrahepatic cholestasis
  7. Systemic disease: invading liver: sarcoidosis, amyloidosis, hemochromatosis, tuberculosis, *Mycobacterium avium intracellulare*
  8. Other: cirrhosis, sepsis, total parenteral nutrition, intrahepatic cholestasis of pregnancy, graft-versus-host disease, environmental toxins, benign postoperative state

Posthepatic causes:
- Intrinsic or extrinsic obstruction of the biliary system
  1. Blockage within hepatobiliary tree: strictures, cholangiocarcinoma, gallbladder cancer, carcinoma of ampulla of Vater, infection (e.g., cytomegalovirus, *Cryptosporidium* in patients with AIDS, parasites), choledocholithiasis
  2. Blockage outside of hepatobiliary tree: pancreatitis, pancreatic carcinoma, pancreatic pseudocyst, lymphoma
- Pseudojaundice: not related to bilirubin but rather resulting from excessive ingestion of foods containing beta carotene (e.g., carrots, melons, squash)

WORKUP

- History, physical examination, and first-line lab tests can often clarify diagnosis. Fig. 2 describes a clinical approach to jaundice.
- Table 1 summarizes the differential diagnosis of critical and emergent diagnoses in patients with jaundice.

LABORATORY TESTS

- First-line tests:
  - Serum total and direct bilirubin
  - Urinalysis
  - Liver function tests (AST, ALT, GGTP, alkaline phosphatase), CBC, liver synthetic function (albumin, PT, PTT), pancreatic function (amylase, lipase)

If serum total bilirubin and direct bilirubin are elevated and urine is positive for bilirubin, consider intrahepatic or posthepatic process. If serum total bilirubin is elevated but direct bilirubin is normal (unconjugated hyperbilirubinemia) and urine is negative for bilirubin, consider prehepatic or intrahepatic processes.
Additional tests if diagnosis unclear:
- Screen for hepatitis A, B, and C; if still unclear, then consider following options based on H&P.
- Other viruses: EBV, CMV.
- Autoimmune disorders: antimitochondrial antibody (elevated in primary biliary cirrhosis); antismooth muscle antibody, ANA (elevated in autoimmune hepatitis); antinuclear cytoplasmic antibody (elevated in primary sclerosing cholangitis).
- Ceruloplasmin (elevated in Wilson's disease).
- Alpha-1 antitrypsin deficiency (elevated in cirrhosis and emphysema).
- Ferritin, Fe saturation (elevated in hemochromatosis).
- Blood smear (RBC dyscrasias).
- Diagnosis of exclusion: Gilbert's syndrome
- Liver biopsy: essential in diagnosis of chronic hepatitis. Can be used for diagnosis of liver masses but carries a substantial risk.

IMAGING STUDIES

- Abdominal ultrasound: first-line study (Figs. E3 and E4) may be completed bedside, most sensitive for proximal biliary tract disease; presence of dilated ducts hints at an extrahepatic process.

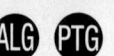

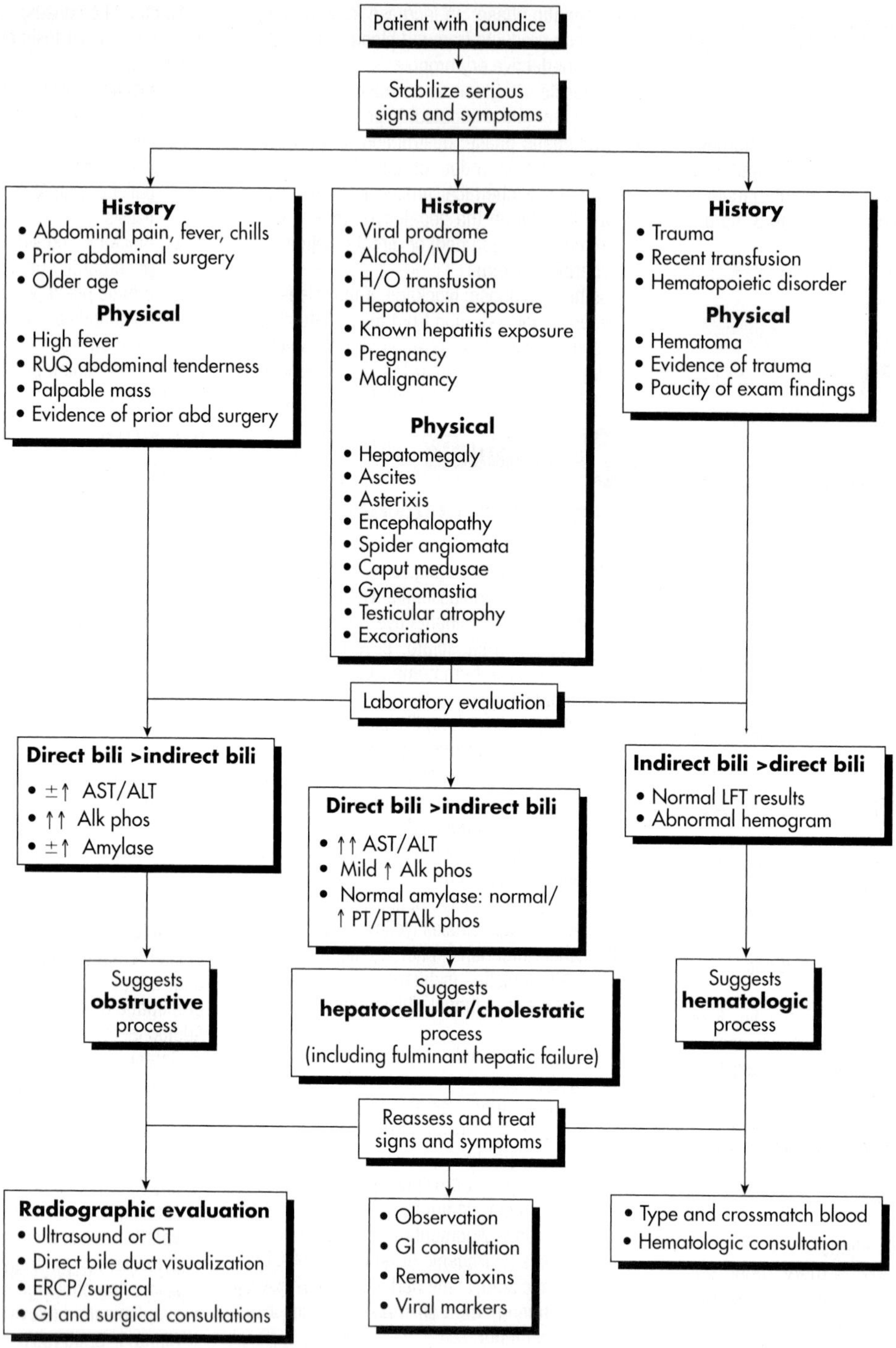

Patient with jaundice

Stabilize serious
signs and symptoms

History
- Abdominal pain, fever, chills
- Prior abdominal surgery
- Older age

Physical
- High fever
- RUQ abdominal tenderness
- Palpable mass
- Evidence of prior abd surgery

History
- Viral prodrome
- Alcohol/IVDU
- H/O transfusion
- Hepatotoxin exposure
- Known hepatitis exposure
- Pregnancy
- Malignancy

Physical
- Hepatomegaly
- Ascites
- Asterixis
- Encephalopathy
- Spider angiomata
- Caput medusae
- Gynecomastia
- Testicular atrophy
- Excoriations

History
- Trauma
- Recent transfusion
- Hematopoietic disorder

Physical
- Hematoma
- Evidence of trauma
- Paucity of exam findings

Laboratory evaluation

Direct bili >indirect bili
- ±↑ AST/ALT
- ↑↑ Alk phos
- ±↑ Amylase

Direct bili >indirect bili
- ↑↑ AST/ALT
- Mild ↑ Alk phos
- Normal amylase: normal/
  ↑ PT/PTTAlk phos

Indirect bili >direct bili
- Normal LFT results
- Abnormal hemogram

Suggests
obstructive
process

Suggests
hepatocellular/cholestatic
process
(including fulminant hepatic failure)

Suggests
hematologic
process

Reassess and treat
signs and symptoms

Radiographic evaluation
- Ultrasound or CT
- Direct bile duct visualization
- ERCP/surgical
- GI and surgical consultations

- Observation
- GI consultation
- Remove toxins
- Viral markers

- Type and crossmatch blood
- Hematologic consultation

FIG. 2 Management of the patient with jaundice. *Alk phos,* Alkaline phosphatase; *ALT,* alanine aminotransferase; *AST,* aspartate aminotransferase; *bili,* bilirubin; *CT,* computed tomography; *ERCP,* endoscopic retrograde cholangiopancreatography; *GI,* gastrointestinal; *H/O,* history of; *IVDU,* intravenous drug use; *LFT,* liver function test; *PT,* prothrombin time; *PTT,* partial thromboplastin time; *RUQ,* right upper quadrant. (From Marx AJ et al: *Rosen's emergency medicine: concepts and clinical practice,* ed 7, Philadelphia, 2010, Elsevier)

- Abdominal CT: often necessary to elucidate more information on liver, pancreas, and distal biliary system.
- Endoscopic retrograde cholangiopancreatography: rarely necessary for diagnostics. Refer to GI consultant.
- Percutaneous transhepatic cholangiography: rarely necessary for diagnostics. Refer to GI or surgical consultant.

- Magnetic resonance cholangiopancreatography: noninvasive visualization of bile and pancreatic ducts. Refer to GI consultant.
- Endoscopic ultrasound: used for characterization and, if needed, biopsy of any focal lesions found within biliary tree and/or pancreas. Refer to GI consultant.

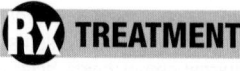 **TREATMENT**

NONPHARMACOLOGIC THERAPY

Depends on underlying cause of the jaundice and clinical stability of the patient. Generally, obstructive causes require surgical treatment, while nonobstructive causes require medical treatment.

TABLE 1 Jaundice: Differential Diagnosis of Critical and Emergent Diagnoses

System	Critical	Emergent	Nonemergent
Hepatic	Fulminant hepatic failure	Hepatitis of any cause with confusion, bleeding, or coagulopathy	Hepatitis with normal mental status, normal vital signs, and no active bleeding
	Toxin	Wilson's disease	
	Virus	Primary biliary cirrhosis	
	Alcohol	Autoimmune hepatitis	
	Ischemic insult	Liver transplant rejection	
	Reye's syndrome	Infiltrative liver disease	
		Drug induced (isoniazid, phenytoin, acetaminophen, ritonavir, halothane, sulfonamides)	
		Toxin ingestion or exposure	
Biliary	Cholangitis	Bile duct obstruction (stone, inflammation, stricture, neoplasm)	
Systemic	Sepsis	Sarcoidosis	Posttraumatic hematoma resorption
	Heatstroke	Amyloidosis	Total parenteral nutrition
		Graft-versus-host disease	
Cardiovascular	Obstructing AAA	Right-sided congestive heart failure	
	Budd-Chiari syndrome	Veno-occlusive disease	
	Severe congestive heart failure		
Hematologic-oncologic	Transfusion reaction	Hemolytic anemia	Gilbert's syndrome
		Massive malignant infiltration	Physiologic neonatal jaundice
		Inborn error of metabolism	
		Pancreatic head tumor	
		Metastatic disease	
Reproductive	Preeclampsia or HELLP syndrome	Hyperemesis gravidarum	
	Acute fatty liver of pregnancy		Cholestasis of pregnancy

AAA, Abdominal aortic aneurysm; *HELLP*, hemolysis, elevated liver enzymes, low platelets.
From Marx JA, et al: *Rosen's emergency medicine*, ed 8, Philadelphia, 2014, Saunders.

ACUTE GENERAL Rx

Acute, life-threatening illness (e.g., cholecystitis or ascending cholangitis) requires prompt diagnosis with basic labs and bedside diagnostics, with early surgical and GI consultation in conjunction. Suspicious medications should be stopped. Initiate medical management of symptoms with analgesia, IV fluids, correction of coagulopathies, and consideration of antibiotics. *N*-Acetylcysteine can be given for acetaminophen overdose.

CHRONIC Rx

Reversible causes must be ruled out first—suspicious medications and EtOH must be discontinued. Consider GI consult for management of many intrahepatic diseases, such as treatment of hepatitis B or C, Wilson's disease with penicillamine, hemochromatosis with phlebotomy, or for stent insertion with ERCP for posthepatic obstruction. Consider surgical consult for resection of pancreatic masses, cholecystectomy, etc.

Symptomatic pruritus may be treated with cholestyramine for bilirubin binding or with antihistamines to decrease the itch reflex. Ursodiol to treat primary biliary cirrhosis and for gallstone prevention/dissolution.

(!) PEARLS & CONSIDERATIONS

COMMENTS

- Heed the warning signs of unstable vital signs to diagnose life-threatening illness; early collaboration with surgical and gastroenterology colleagues is helpful in complex patient care scenarios.

- Careful history and physical examination, basic labs, and prompt bedside imaging frequently lead to accurate diagnosis.
- Very high serum bilirubin (>15 mg/dl) is most likely to be seen in cirrhosis. Watch for hepatorenal syndrome in these patients.

SUGGESTED READINGS
Available at www.expertconsult.com

RELATED CONTENT
Jaundice (Patient Information)

AUTHORS: **ALLA GOLDBURT, M.D.,** and **PAOLO G. PACE, M.A.SC., M.D**

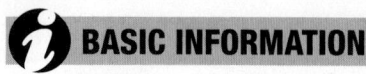
DEFINITION

Juvenile idiopathic arthritis (JIA), previously referred to as juvenile rheumatoid arthritis (JRA), is a diverse spectrum of chronic arthritides, involving ≥1 joints for at least 6 weeks in a patient ≤16 yr of age. Other causes of arthritis must be excluded.

SYNONYMS

JIA
Juvenile rheumatoid arthritis
Still's disease (specifically systemic JIA)
JRA

ICD-10CM CODES

M08.00 Unspecified juvenile rheumatoid arthritis of unspecified site
M08.29 Juvenile rheumatoid arthritis with systemic onset, multiple sites
M08.40 Pauciarticular juvenile rheumatoid arthritis, unspecified site
M08.09 Unspecified juvenile rheumatoid arthritis, multiple sites
M08.20 Juvenile rheumatoid arthritis with systemic onset, unspecified site

EPIDEMIOLOGY & DEMOGRAPHICS

PREVALENCE: About 1 per 1000 children in the U.S.; more common in children of European ancestry

PHYSICAL FINDINGS & CLINICAL PRESENTATION

JIA is subdivided into seven categories based on the International League of Associations for Rheumatology (ILAR) classification criteria (summarized in Table 1).
Systemic onset JIA (4%-17%)
Arthritis in ≥1 joints with or preceded by fever of at least 2-wk duration that is quotidian (once daily) for at least 3 days and associated with at least one of the following: (1) evanescent erythematous rash (Fig. E1); (2) generalized lymphadenopathy; (3) hepatomegaly, splenomegaly, or both; and (4) serositis.
Oligoarticular JIA (Fig. 2) (27%-56%)
Arthritis in <4 joints in the first 6 mo of disease. There are two subtypes:
Persistent: ≤4 joints throughout the disease course.
Extended: ≤4 joints during the first 6 mo extending to >4 joints after 6 mo.
Polyarthritis, rheumatoid factor (RF) negative (11%-28%)
Arthritis in >5 joints during first 6 mo of the disease with negative RF.
Polyarthritis, RF positive (2%-7%)
Arthritis involves ≥5 joints during first 6 mo of the disease with positive RF on at least two tests run 3 mo apart.
Anti–cyclic citrullinated (CCP) antibodies may also be present.

Most similar to adult rheumatoid arthritis; most likely to progress.
Psoriatic arthritis (2%-11%)
Psoriasis and arthritis or psoriasis and ≥2 of the following:
Dactylitis, nail pitting, onycholysis, and psoriasis in a first-degree relative.
Enthesitis-related arthritis (3%-11%)
Arthritis or enthesitis and ≥2 of the following:
Sacroiliac tenderness, positive HLA-B27, male age >6 yr, acute anterior uveitis, or first-degree relative with HLA-B27-associated disease.
Undifferentiated arthritis (11%-21%)
Fulfills criteria in ≥2 categories above, or none of them

ETIOLOGY

Influenced by both genetic and environmental factors. Childhood antibiotic use may increase the risk of JIA due to disruption of the microbiome.

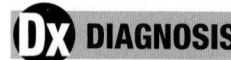 **DIAGNOSIS**

DIFFERENTIAL DIAGNOSIS

- Infection: viral (parvovirus, toxic synovitis) or bacterial (Lyme, osteomyelitis, septic joints)
- Inflammation: lupus, serum sickness, inflammatory bowel disease
- Reactive: post-streptococcal, rheumatic fever
- Malignancy: leukemia, bone tumors

TABLE 1 Overview of the Main Features of the Subtypes of Juvenile Idiopathic Arthritis

ILAR Subtype	Peak Age of Onset (yr)	Female: Male; % of All JIA	Arthritis Pattern	Extraarticular Features	Investigations	Notes on Therapy
Systemic arthritis	2-4	1:1; ~10% of JIA cases	Polyarticular, often knees, wrists, and ankles; also fingers, neck, and hips	Daily fever; evanescent rash; pericarditis; pleuritis	Anemia; WBC↑↑; ESR↑↑; CRP↑↑; ferritin;↑ platelets↑↑ (normal or ↑ in MAS)	Less responsive to standard treatment with MTX and anti-TNF agents; consider IL-1Ra in resistant cases
Oligoarthritis	>6	4:1; 50%-60% of JIA (but ethnic variation)	Knees ++; ankles, fingers +	Uveitis in ~30%	ANA positive in 60%; other tests usually normal; may have mildly ↑ ESR/CRP	NSAIDs and intraarticular steroids; occasionally require MTX
Polyarthritis, RF negative	6-7	3:1; 30% of JIA cases	Symmetric or asymmetric; small and large joints; cervical spine; TMJ	Uveitis in ~10%	ANA positive in 40%; RF negative; ESR ↑ or; ↑↑ CRP↑/normal; mild anemia	Standard therapy with MTX and NSAIDs, then if nonresponsive, anti-TNF agents or other biologics
Polyarthritis, RF positive	9-12	9:1; >10% of JIA cases	Aggressive symmetric polyarthritis	Rheumatoid nodules in 10%; low-grade fever	RF positive; ESR ↑↑; CRP ↑/normal; mild anemia	Long-term remission unlikely; early aggressive therapy is warranted
Psoriatic arthritis	7-10	2:1; >10% of JIA cases	Asymmetric arthritis of small or medium sized joints	Uveitis in 10%; psoriasis in 50%	ANA positive in 50%; ESR ↑; CRP ↑/normal; mild anemia	NSAIDs and intraarticular steroids; second-line agents less commonly
Enthesitis-related arthritis	9-12	1:7; 10% of JIA cases	Predominantly lower limb joints affected; sometimes axial skeleton (but less than adult AS)	Acute anterior uveitis; association with reactive arthritis and IBD	80% HLA-B27[1]	NSAIDs and intraarticular steroids; consider sulfasalazine as alternative to MTX

ANA, Antinuclear antibody; *AS,* ankylosing spondylitis; *CRP,* C-reactive protein; *ESR,* erythrocyte sedimentation rate; *IBD,* inflammatory bowel disease; *ILAR,* International League of Associations for Rheumatology; *IL-1Ra,* interleukin-1 receptor antagonist; *JIA,* juvenile idiopathic arthritis; *MAS,* macrophage activation syndrome; *MTX,* methotrexate; *NSAID,* nonsteroidal anti-inflammatory drug; *RF,* rheumatoid factor; *TMJ,* temporomandibular joint; *TNF,* tumor necrosis factor; *WBC,* white blood cell count.
From Firestein G et al: *Kelley's textbook of rheumatology,* ed 9, Philadelphia, 2013, Saunders.

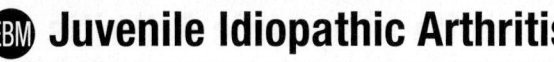

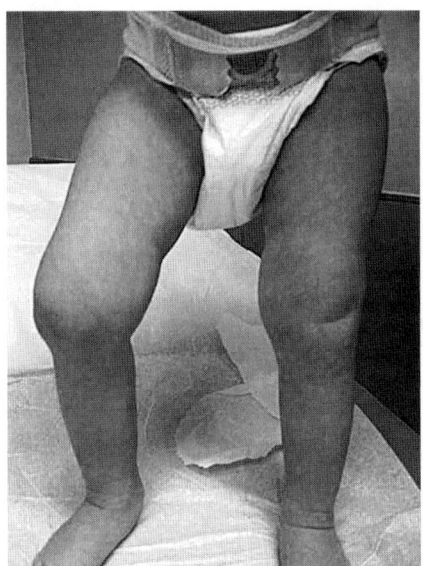

FIG. 2 Oligoarticular juvenile idiopathic arthritis with swelling and flexion contracture of the right knee. (From Kliegman RM et al: *Nelson textbook of pediatrics,* ed 19, Philadelphia, 2011, Saunders.)

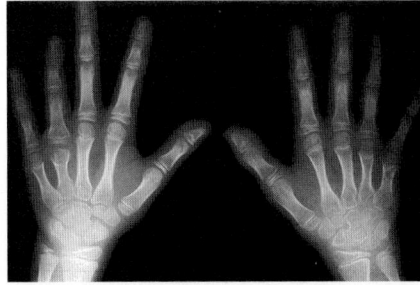

FIG. 3 Juvenile idiopathic arthritis (JIA). Oligoarticular-onset JIA in an 8-year-old. Epiphyseal destruction and undergrowth of the third metacarpophalangeal joint of the left hand are seen, as well as overgrowth of the carpal bones of the right wrist compared with the left wrist. Also note the widened appearance of the third phalanges caused by periosteal new bone formation. (From Hochberg MC et al: *Rheumatology,* ed 5, St Louis, 2011, Mosby.)

LABORATORY TESTS

- No single diagnostic test. Other causes of arthritis must be excluded.
- Elevated sedimentation rate and C-reactive protein
- Mild anemia, leukocytosis
- Rheumatoid factor: rarely positive in children
- Antinuclear antibodies: elevation associated with ocular complications

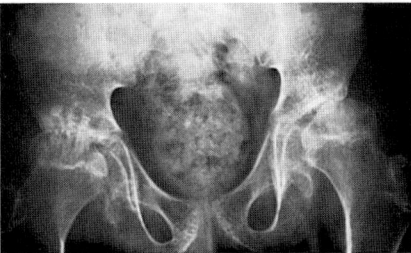

FIG. 4 Severe hip disease in a 13-yr-old boy with active, systemic-onset juvenile idiopathic arthritis. Radiograph shows destruction of the femoral head and acetabula, joint space narrowing, and subluxation of left hip. The patient had received corticosteroids systemically for 9 yr. (From Kliegman RM et al: *Nelson textbook of pediatrics,* ed 19, Philadelphia, 2011, Saunders.)

- Pancytopenia, lab results consistent with a consumptive coagulopathy, and elevated liver enzymes are indicative of macrophage activation syndrome in systemic JIA. Bone marrow biopsy is needed to confirm diagnosis.

IMAGING STUDIES

- Radiographs show soft tissue swelling and periarticular osteopenia early in the disease (Fig. 3).
- Joint destruction (Fig. 4) is less frequent, but bony erosion and cyst formation may be present.

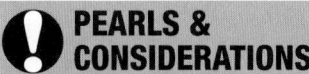 **TREATMENT**

NONPHARMACOLOGIC THERAPY

Collaboration among the patient's pediatrician, pediatric rheumatologist, orthopedist, and physical therapist yields the best outcome. The goal is complete remission.
- Physical and occupational therapy.
- Education regarding diet and weight management (Fig. 5).

CHRONIC GENERAL Rx

- NSAIDs, used as monotherapy or in conjunction with intraarticular steroids
- DMARDs: methotrexate, leflunomide, sulfasalazine
  - Required by two-thirds of children
  - Axial involvement is less responsive to methotrexate.
- Biologics: improve morbidity associated with JIA
  1. Tumor necrosis factor antagonists such as etanercept and adalimumab.
  2. T-cell modulator, abatacept, is approved for patients with polyarticular JIA who have not responded to anti-TNF therapy.

3. IL-1 and IL-6 antagonists, anakinra and tocilizumab, respectively, offer promising results in patients with systemic JIA.
- Systemic corticosteroids should be limited when possible.

DISPOSITION

- 50% continue to have active disease into adulthood.
- 70% to 85% regain normal function.
- Macrophage activation syndrome is a life-threatening complication in systemic JIA.
- Oligoarticular JIA patients with positive ANA are at the highest risk for blindness due to chronic iridocyclitis and require frequent ophthalmologic monitoring.
- Systemic and localized growth disturbance can lead to growth failure and leg length discrepancies.

REFERRAL

- Early rheumatology consultation.
- Ophthalmology consultation at diagnosis and at least annually.
- Children age <7 years, with + ANA are at the highest risk for iritis, and require screening every 3 to 4 months.

 PEARLS & CONSIDERATIONS

COMMENTS

Research has shown that systemic JIA is an acquired autoinflammatory disease. Thus, the development of IL-1 and IL-6 antagonists has improved therapy in refractory disease. Increasingly, many pediatric rheumatologists are opting to use these biologics as first-line therapy, with the hope that normalization of the immune response early in the disease can limit disease progression. More research into this strategy for management is in process. The long-term effect of using biologic agents in children is unclear.

EVIDENCE

Available at www.expertconsult.com

SUGGESTED READINGS

Available at www.expertconsult.com

RELATED CONTENT

Juvenile Rheumatoid Arthritis (Patient Information)

AUTHOR: **MICHELLE C. MACIAG, M.D.**

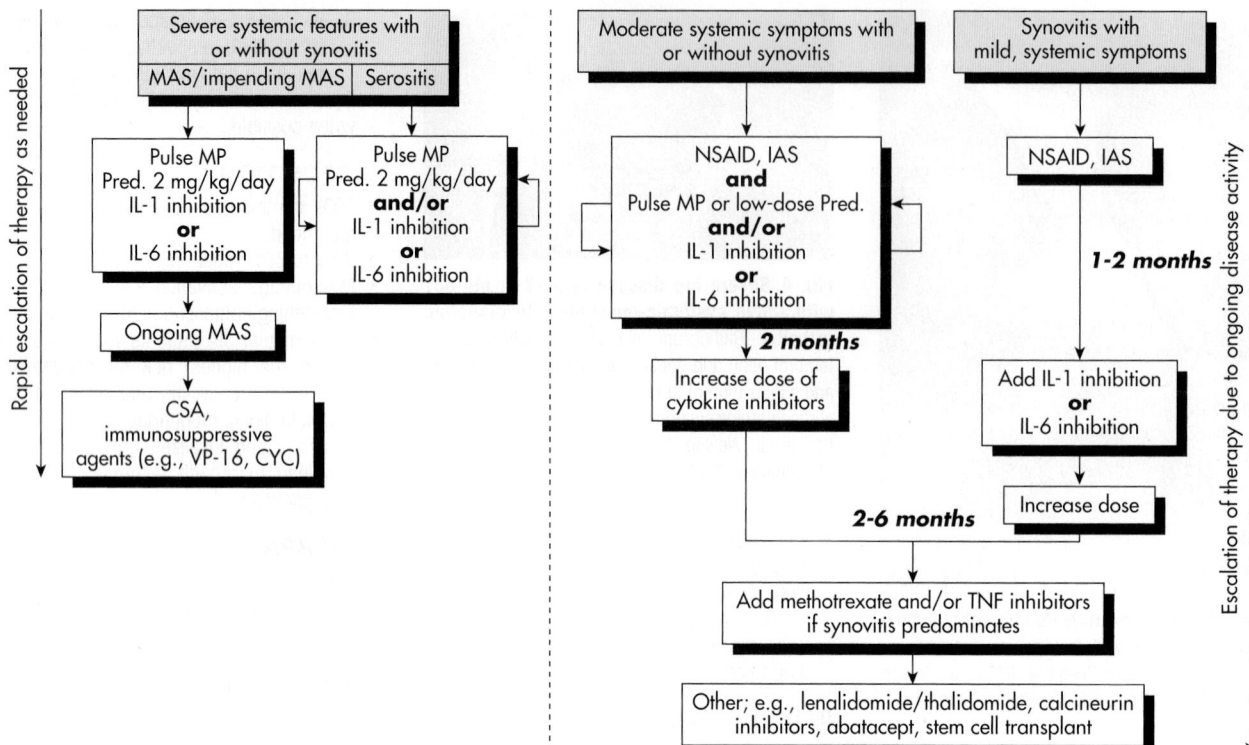

FIG. 5 Systemic juvenile idiopathic arthritis treatment algorithm. The treatment goal is remission of disease activity, both systemic and articular, and is stratified by severity of disease. Algorithm is divided into severe systemic disease manifestations (macrophage activation syndrome [MAS], serositis) or synovitis with milder systemic disease. Currently there is significant variability in practice regarding using corticosteroid as initial systemic therapy or moving directly to inflammatory cytokine inhibitors. At the time of this writing, interleukin (IL)-1 inhibition and IL-6 inhibition are currently in trials, and more information is likely to be available in the future. *CSA*, cyclosporine A; *CYC*, cyclophosphamide; *IAS*, intraarticular steroid; *MP*, methylprednisolone; *NSAID*, nonsteroidal antiinflammatory drug; *Pred.*, prednisone; *TNF*, tumor necrosis factor. (From Firestein GS et al: *Kelly's textbook of rheumatology*, ed 9, Philadelphia, 2013, Saunders.)

BASIC INFORMATION

DEFINITION

Kaposi's sarcoma (KS) is a vascular neoplasm most frequently occurring in AIDS patients. It can be divided into the following four subsets:
1. Classic KS: most frequently found in elderly Eastern European and Mediterranean males. It consists initially of violaceous macules and papules with subsequent development of plaques and red-purple nodules. Growth is slow, and most of the patients die of unrelated causes.
2. Epidemic or AIDS-related KS: most frequently occurs in homosexual men. Lesions are generally multifocal and widespread (Fig. E1). Lymphadenopathy may be associated.
3. Endemic KS: usually affects African children and adults. An aggressive lymphadenopathic form affects African children in particular.
4. Immunosuppression-associated, or transplantation-associated, KS: usually associated with chemotherapy.

SYNONYM

KS

ICD-10CM CODES

C46.0	Kaposi's sarcoma of skin
C46.1	Kaposi's sarcoma of soft tissue
C46.2	Kaposi's sarcoma of palate
C46.3	Kaposi's sarcoma of lymph nodes
C46.4	Kaposi's sarcoma of gastrointestinal sites
C46.50	Kaposi's sarcoma of unspecified lung
C46.51	Kaposi's sarcoma of right lung
C46.52	Kaposi's sarcoma of left lung
C46.7	Kaposi's sarcoma of other sites
C46.9	Kaposi's sarcoma, unspecified

EPIDEMIOLOGY & DEMOGRAPHICS

- AIDS-related KS affects >35% of AIDS cases.
- Highest incidence is in homosexual men.

PHYSICAL FINDINGS & CLINICAL PRESENTATION

- AIDS-related KS: multifocal and widespread red-purple (Fig. 1) or dark plaques (Fig. E2) and/or nodules on cutaneous or mucosal surfaces (Fig. E3).
- Generalized lymphadenopathy at the time of diagnosis is present in >50% of patients with AIDS-related KS; the initial lesions have a rust-colored appearance; subsequent progression to red or purple nodules or plaques occurs (Fig. E4).
- Most frequently affected areas are the face, trunk, oral cavity, and upper and lower extremities.
- The GI tract is the most frequent site of internal involvement in classic KS.
- In AIDS-associated KS, 25% of patients have cutaneous involvement alone, whereas 29% have visceral lesions only (lymph nodes 50%, GI tract 50%, lungs 37%).

ETIOLOGY

A herpesvirus (HHV-8, KS-associated herpesvirus KSHV) has been isolated from patients with most forms of KS and is believed to be the causative agent. It can be transmitted sexually (homosexual or heterosexual activities) and by other forms of nonsexual contact such as maternal-infant transmission (common in African countries).

DIAGNOSIS

DIFFERENTIAL DIAGNOSIS

- Stasis dermatitis.
- Pyogenic granuloma.
- Capillary hemangiomas.
- Granulation tissue.
- Postinflammatory hyperpigmentation.
- Cutaneous lymphoma.
- Melanoma.
- Dermatofibroma.
- Hematoma.
- Prurigo nodularis.

The differential diagnosis of cutaneous lesions in patients with HIV infection is described in Section II.

WORKUP

Diagnosis can generally be made on clinical appearance; tissue biopsy will confirm diagnosis.

LABORATORY TESTS

HIV in patients suspected of AIDS.

TREATMENT

NONPHARMACOLOGIC THERAPY

Observation is a reasonable option in patients with slowly progressive disease.

GENERAL Rx

- All types of KS are radiosensitive. Radiation therapy is effective in non-AIDS KS and for large tumor masses that interfere with normal function.
- Excisional biopsy often provides adequate treatment for single lesions and resected recurrences in classic KS.

- Liquid nitrogen cryotherapy can result in complete response in 80% of lesions.
- Interlesional chemotherapy with vinblastine is useful for nodular lesions >1 cm in diameter. Intralesional injection of interferon alfa-2b has also been reported as effective and well tolerated.
- HIV treatment is patients with HIV-related KS.
- Liposomal anthracyclines and paclitaxel are FDA approved as first-line and second-line monotherapy for advanced KS.
- Sirolimus (rapamycin), an immunosuppressive drug, is effective in inhibiting the progression of dermal KS in kidney transplant recipients.
- Alitretinoin gel (Panretin) for local lesions.

PEARLS & CONSIDERATIONS

COMMENTS

- Immunosuppression-associated KS usually regresses with the cessation, reduction, or modification of immunosuppression therapy in most patients. Similarly, in HIV patients KS responds concurrently with the decrease in serum HIV RNA and increase in the CD4 count.
- Kaposi sarcoma is associated with an increased risk of developing secondary malignancies (lymphomas, leukemia, myeloma).

SUGGESTED READINGS

Available at www.expertconsult.com

RELATED CONTENT

Kaposi's Sarcoma (Patient Information)
Acquired Immunodeficiency Syndrome (Related Key Topic)

AUTHOR: **BHARTI RATHORE, M.D.**

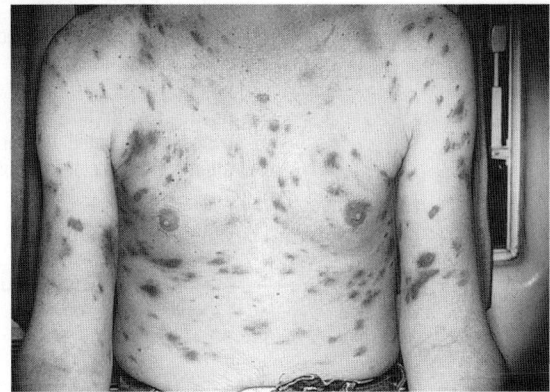

FIG. 4 Kaposi's sarcoma. More advanced lesions. Note widespread hemorrhagic plaques and nodules. (From Noble J [ed]: *Textbook of primary care medicine,* ed 2, St Louis, 1995, Mosby.)

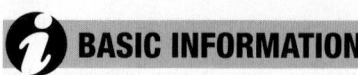

BASIC INFORMATION

DEFINITION

Labyrinthitis is a peripheral vestibulopathy characterized by acute onset of vertigo usually associated with nausea and vomiting. It can be associated with hearing loss and gait abnormalities and may be either serous or purulent.

SYNONYMS

Acute labyrinthitis
Acute vestibular neuronopathy
Vestibular neuronitis
Viral neurolabyrinthitis

ICD-10CM CODES
H81.23 Vestibular neuronitis, bilateral
H83.09 Labyrinthitis, unspecified ear
H83.01 Labyrinthitis, right ear
H83.02 Labyrinthitis, left ear
H83.03 Labyrinthitis, bilateral

EPIDEMIOLOGY & DEMOGRAPHICS

INCIDENCE (IN U.S.): Most common cause of prolonged spontaneous vertigo associated with nausea at any age
PREDOMINANT AGE: Any

CLINICAL PRESENTATION

- Vertigo, nausea, and vomiting with onset over several hours
- Symptoms usually peak within 24 hours, then resolve gradually over several weeks
- During the first day, the patient usually has difficulty focusing the eyes because of spontaneous nystagmus
- Usually has benign course with complete recovery within 1 to 3 months, though older patients may have intractable dizziness that persists for many months

PHYSICAL FINDINGS

- Nystagmus
- Nausea
- Vomiting
- Vertigo worsening with head movement
- Abnormal caloric ENG tests
- May have hearing loss in the affected ear or ears
- Normal otoscopic exam typically
- Normal neurologic exam; may have signs of vestibular loss, such as a positive head thrust test

ETIOLOGY

Symptoms often preceded for 1 to 2 weeks by a viral-like illness. Labyrinthitis may be either bacterial or viral and may be either tympanogenic (i.e., resulting from spread of infection into the inner ear from the middle ear, antrum, or petrous apex), meningogenic, or hematogenic from encephalitis or brain abscess. The round window membrane is considered the most likely pathway of inflammatory mediators from the middle to the inner ear that subsequently give rise to labyrinthitis.

DIAGNOSIS

DIFFERENTIAL DIAGNOSIS

- Acute labyrinthine ischemia (ischemic stroke of the labyrinthine artery)
- Labyrinthine fistula
- Benign paroxysmal positional vertigo
- Meniere's disease
- Cholesteatoma
- Drug-induced vestibulocochlear nerve damage
- Vestibulocochlear nerve (cranial nerve VIII) tumor
- Head trauma
- Vertebrobasilar stroke
- Dehiscence of the superior semicircular canal

WORKUP

- Otoscopic examination
- Neurologic examination, with close attention to cranial nerves
- Bedside test of vestibular function, specifically head thrust or head heave test
- Audiogram if symptoms accompanied by hearing loss
- Caloric test if presentation is atypical

LABORATORY TESTS

- Routine laboratory tests are generally not helpful.
- If there is a history of significant emesis, check electrolytes, BUN, and creatinine.

IMAGING STUDIES

- Imaging studies are usually not necessary.
- Gadolinium-enhanced MRI may show enhancement of bony labyrinth. MRI of the brain with and without contrast with fine cuts through the internal auditory canal is indicated if there is an abnormal cranial nerve exam, headache, concern for stroke, or suspicion of cranial nerve VIII nerve tumor.
- Head CT with fine cuts through temporal bones is indicated if there is a history of trauma or suspicion of cholesteatoma.

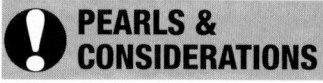

TREATMENT

NONPHARMACOLOGIC THERAPY

- Reassurance.
- Initial bed rest, then encourage increase in activity as tolerated.

ACUTE GENERAL Rx

- Phenergan or other antiemetics are typically effective.
- Vestibular suppressant: meclizine 12.5 to 25 mg qid is often used. Scopolamine patch is also effective.
- Methylprednisolone 100 mg per day for 3 days, with slow taper over 3 wk.
- Valacyclovir has not been shown to be helpful.

CHRONIC Rx

No specific chronic therapy

DISPOSITION

Usually does not require hospital admission unless the patient is unable to tolerate oral intake of liquids.

REFERRAL

- Refer if symptoms persist or neurologic abnormalities are present.
- Consider vestibular rehabilitation, particularly in the elderly.

PEARLS & CONSIDERATIONS

COMMENTS

Labyrinthitis is a term that usually implies peripheral vestibulopathy associated with hearing loss. The term *vestibular neuronitis* is typically used when hearing is not affected. Despite this technical distinction, many physicians use these terms interchangeably.

RELATED CONTENT

Labyrinthitis (Patient Information)
Benign Paroxysmal Positional Vertigo (Related Key Topic)
Vestibular Neuronitis (Related Key Topic)

AUTHORS: **MICHAEL POHLEN, M.D.,**
JOSEPH S. KASS, M.D., J.D., and
SHARON S. HARTMAN POLENSEK, M.D., PH.D.

BASIC INFORMATION

DEFINITION

Lactic acidosis (LA) is a life-threatening condition characterized by accumulation of lactate, especially L-lactate, in the body. It represents an imbalance of lactate overproduction or underutilization usually resulting from tissue hypoperfusion and hypoxia (type A LA), or caused by toxins or medication-induced cellular toxicity (type B LA).

SYNONYMS

Lactic acidosis
Hyperlactatemia
LA

ICD-10CM CODES
E87.2 Acidosis

RISK FACTORS

- Sepsis
- Liver disease
- Severe anemia
- Severe trauma
- Advanced heart failure
- Cardiogenic shock
- Hypovolemic shock
- Diabetes mellitus
- Seizures
- Vigorous exercise
- Cocaine
- Medications (metformin, salicylates, beta-2 agonists, propofol, nucleoside reverse-transcriptase inhibitors)
- Thiamine deficiency
- Pheochromocytoma

PHYSICAL FINDINGS & CLINICAL PRESENTATION

- Shock, dehydration (tachycardia, decreased skin turgor, decreased urine output, hypotension, dry mucous membranes)
- Possible clues or precipitating factors (sepsis, bleeding, intoxication)
- Altered mental status
- Nausea, vomiting, abdominal pain
- Weakness, lethargy
- Tachypnea, rapid shallow breathing caused by acidosis (Kussmaul's breathing)

ETIOLOGY

- Type A, related to tissue hypoperfusion or hypoxia, is probably the most common cause of LA.
  - Sepsis leading to systemic hypotension and microcirculation dysfunction leading to decreased extraction of oxygen and lactate clearance by the peripheral tissues
  - Shock: cardiogenic, hemorrhagic and obstructive shock; LA in those conditions is believed to be related to decreased clearance
  - Regional ischemia, such as acute mesenteric ischemia
  - Burns
- Type B: related to toxins, medications and liver dysfunction, alcoholism, malignancy
  - Metformin: patients who are at increased risk of LA are those who are taking metformin and have renal or hepatic dysfunction, cardiac dysfunction, or those who overdose on the medication
  - Cyanide poisoning, beta^2 agonist excessive use, thiamine deficiency
  - Seizure

D-lactic acidosis is a rare type of LA that is associated with short bowel syndrome and bacterial overgrowth.

DIAGNOSIS

DIFFERENTIAL DIAGNOSIS

- Alcoholic ketoacidosis
- Uremic acidosis
- Diabetic ketoacidosis
- Fulminant hepatic failure

WORKUP

- Laboratory measurement of lactic acid to confirm diagnosis and assess for precipitating factors
- Identification of triggering conditions such as infections (blood cultures, urine cultures, chest radiographs), blood drug and toxins level (alcohol, metformin, cyanide); liver and kidney function tests (hepatitis, acute kidney insufficiency)

LABORATORY TESTS

- Normal lactate level is 2.0 to 2.5 mEq/l.
- LA is defined by serum lactate concentration >4 mEq/L. An elevated blood lactate level is essential for confirmation of the diagnosis.
- Arterial blood gas analysis demonstrates metabolic acidosis usually with PH <7.3 and PCO_2 <40.
- Serum chemistries:
  - Low serum bicarbonate <15 mEq/L
  - Large anion gap (AG) metabolic acidosis: AG >12 usually caused by lactate accumulation. A normal AG does not rule out lactic acidosis. Correction of the AG for the effect of serum albumin can improve its sensitivity.
  - Calculate AG: $AG = NA^+ - (Cl^- + HCO_3^-)$.
  - Mixed metabolic disturbances might demonstrate more than only AG acidosis, especially in patients with vomiting, diarrhea, and acute kidney injury.

IMAGING STUDIES

- Chest radiography is helpful if chest infection is suspected as a cause of sepsis or cardiogenic or obstructive shock is suspected.
- Abdominal CT scan or ultrasound might aid in the diagnosis if abdominal pain, regional ischemia, or liver failure is suspected as a cause of the lactic acidosis.

TREATMENT

NONPHARMACOLOGIC THERAPY

- The cornerstone of L.A treatment is reversing the causative condition.
- Continuous monitoring for patients with LA is warranted, including monitoring of mental status, urine output, and vital signs.
- Lactate levels should be checked every 2 to 6 hr.
- Surgery in the case of regional tissue ischemia or trauma with shock.
- Cardiac assist devices in the case of cardiogenic shock.
- Hemodialysis for drugs or toxins removal (i.e., metformin-induced LA).

ACUTE GENERAL Rx

Pharmacologic treatment consists of:
- Resuscitating the intravascular component with IV crystalloid or colloid solution fluids in cases of shock.
- Sodium bicarbonate IV infusion should be considered only if pH <7.1 and serum bicarbonate level is less than 6 mEq/L. Infusion of 1-2 mEq/L of sodium bicarbonate in a bolus form repeated every 30-60 min if the pH is less than 7.1.
- Vasopressor therapy is cases of shock might be required; increasing doses of vasopressor might be needed as the acidosis can blunt the effect of catecholamines. Norepinephrine is generally preferred over dopamine as the initial vasopressor in most types of shock.
- Optimize oxygen delivery: When an inotrope is indicated to improve cardiac output, dobutamine is usually the preferred agent.

DISPOSITION

- Septic shock and lactic acid level >4 mEq/L is associated with a 28% mortality rate.
- There is a clear correlation with increasing lactate level and increased mortality.

REFERRAL

- In general, patients with LA should be admitted to the intensive care unit for close monitoring, frequent lactate, chemistries, and arterial blood gas analysis.

PEARLS & CONSIDERATIONS

COMMENTS

- Hemodialysis is not an effective way of clearing lactate or reversing LA, especially in cases of overproduction and tissue hypoxemia; it could be of value in cases of drug- and toxin-induced LA for removal of the offending agent.

PREVENTION

- Aggressive treatment of shock
- Avoidance of metformin in high-risk populations such as patients older than 85 yr and patients with kidney or liver impairment
- Early use of antibiotics in patients with sepsis

RELATED CONTENT

Diabetic Ketoacidosis (Related Key Topic)

SUGGESTED READINGS
Available at www.expertconsult.com

AUTHOR: **AHMAD M. ISMAIL, M.D.**

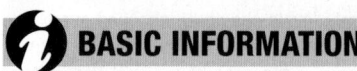

BASIC INFORMATION

DEFINITION

Lactose intolerance is the insufficient concentration of lactase enzyme, leading to fermentation of malabsorbed lactose by intestinal bacteria with subsequent production of intestinal gas and various organic acids, manifesting clinically with diarrhea, abdominal pain, flatulence, or bloating after lactose intake. *Lactose malabsorption* occurs when a substantial amount of lactose is not absorbed in the intestine. *Lactase deficiency* is defined as brush-border lactase activity that is markedly reduced relative to the activity observed in infants.

SYNONYMS

Lactase deficiency
Milk intolerance Carbohydrate malabsorption

ICD-10CM CODES
E73.9 Lactose intolerance, unspecified
E73.8 Other lactose intolerance

EPIDEMIOLOGY & DEMOGRAPHICS

- Nearly 50 million people in the United States have partial or complete lactose intolerance. There are racial differences, with <25% of white adults being lactose intolerant but >85% of Asian Americans and >60% of African Americans having some form of lactose intolerance.
- There are geographic variations: highest in Asians (up to 90%), lowest in northern Europeans (approximately 10%), intermediate in southern Europeans and Middle Eastern populations (up to 40%).

PHYSICAL FINDINGS & CLINICAL PRESENTATION

- Abdominal tenderness and cramping, bloating, flatulence.
- Diarrhea.
- Symptoms are directly related to the osmotic pressure of substrate in the colon and occur approximately 2 hr after ingestion of lactose.
- Physical examination: may be entirely within normal limits.

ETIOLOGY

- Before it can be absorbed, lactose is cleared to glucose and galactose by the enzyme lactase in the brush border of the small intestine. If the amount of lactase is marginal or its expression is left, lactose intolerance will results.
- Congenital lactase deficiency: common in premature infants; rare in term infants and generally inherited as a chromosomal recessive trait.
- Secondary lactose intolerance: usually a result of injury of the intestinal mucosa (Crohn's disease, viral gastroenteritis, AIDS enteropathy, cryptosporidiosis, Whipple's disease, sprue)

DIAGNOSIS

DIFFERENTIAL DIAGNOSIS

- Inflammatory bowel disease.
- Irritable bowel syndrome.
- Pancreatic insufficiency.
- Nontropical and tropical sprue.
- Cystic fibrosis.
- Diverticular disease.
- Bowel neoplasm.
- Laxative abuse.
- Celiac disease.
- Parasitic disease (e.g., giardiasis).
- Viral or bacterial infections.

WORKUP

- A detailed dietary history is essential in the evaluation of patients with suspected carbohydrate malabsorption.
- The diagnosis can usually be made on the basis of the history and improvement with dietary manipulation.
- Diagnostic workup may include confirming the diagnosis with hydrogen breath test and excluding other conditions listed in the differential diagnosis that may also coexist with lactase deficiency.

LABORATORY TESTS

- Lactose breath hydrogen test: a rise in breath hydrogen >20 ppm within 90 min of ingestion of 50 g of lactose is positive for lactase deficiency. This test is positive in 90% of patients with lactose malabsorption. Common causes of false-negative results are recent use of oral antibiotics or recent high colonic enema.
- The lactose tolerance test is an older and less accurate testing modality (20% rate of false-positive and false-negative results). The patient is administered an oral dose of 1 to 1.5 g of lactose/kg body weight. Serial measurement of blood glucose level on an hourly basis for 3 hr is then performed. The test is considered positive if the patient develops intestinal symptoms and the blood glucose level rises <20 mg/dl above the fasting baseline level.
- Diarrhea associated with lactase deficiency is osmotic in nature with an osmotic gap and a pH <6.5.

IMAGING STUDIES

Imaging studies are generally not indicated. A small bowel series may be useful in patients with significant malabsorption.

TREATMENT

NONPHARMACOLOGIC THERAPY

Management consists of reducing lactose exposure by avoiding milk and milk-containing products or using milk in which the lactose has been prehydrolyzed with lactase. A lactose-free diet generally results in prompt resolution of symptoms. Lactose is primarily found in dairy products but may be present as an ingredient or component of common foods and beverages. Possible sources of lactose include breads, candies, cold cuts, dessert mixes, cream soups, bologna, commercial sauces and gravies, chocolate, drink mixes, salad dressings, and medications. Labels should be read carefully to identify sources of lactose.

ACUTE GENERAL Rx

- Addition of lactase enzyme supplement (Lactaid tablets, Dairy Ease) before the ingestion of milk products may prevent symptoms in some patients. However, it is not effective for all lactose-intolerant patients.
- Lactose-intolerant patients must ensure adequate calcium intake. Calcium supplementation is recommended to prevent osteoporosis.

CHRONIC Rx

Patient education regarding foods high in lactose, such as milk, cottage cheese, or ice cream, is recommended.

DISPOSITION

Clinical improvement with restriction or elimination of milk products.

REFERRAL

GI referral for endoscopic procedures if concomitant GI disorders are suspected.

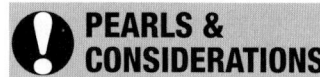

PEARLS & CONSIDERATIONS

COMMENTS

- There is great variability in signs and symptoms in patients with lactose intolerance depending on the degree of lactase deficiency. Most individuals with presumed lactose malabsorption can tolerate 12 to 15 g of lactose or up to 12 oz of milk daily without symptoms.
- Nondairy synthetic drinks (e.g., Coffee-Mate) and use of rice milk are well tolerated.

SUGGESTED READINGS

Available at www.expertconsult.com

RELATED CONTENT

Lactose Intolerance (Patient Information)

AUTHOR: **FRED F. FERRI, M.D.**

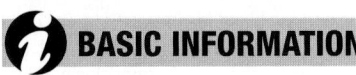 **BASIC INFORMATION**

DEFINITION

Laryngitis is an acute or chronic inflammation of the laryngeal mucous membranes.

SYNONYMS

Lower respiratory tract infection

ICD-10CM CODES
J04.0 Acute laryngitis
J37.0 Chronic laryngitis

EPIDEMIOLOGY & DEMOGRAPHICS

It is a common illness worldwide in both genders and all age groups, but the diagnosis is imprecise and, therefore, statistics are not readily available with respect to incidence and prevalence.

PHYSICAL FINDINGS & CLINICAL PRESENTATION

ACUTE LARYNGITIS:
- Clinical syndrome characterized by the onset of hoarseness, voice breaks, or episodes of aphonia; may also have accompanying sore throat, cough, nasal congestion, and rhinorrhea.
- Usually associated with viral upper respiratory infection.
- Larynx with diffuse erythema, edema, and vascular engorgement of the vocal folds, and occasionally mucosal ulceration.
- In young children subglottis is often affected, resulting in airway narrowing with marked hoarseness, inspiratory stridor, dyspnea, and restlessness.
- Respiratory compromise rare in adults.

CHRONIC LARYNGITIS: Characterized by hoarseness or dysphonia persisting for longer than 2 wk.

ETIOLOGY

ACUTE LARYNGITIS:
- Most often caused by viruses so treatment consists of supportive measures as outlined in "Nonpharmacologic Therapy" section.
- Studies evaluating the use of antibiotics (erythromycin, penicillin) in acute laryngitis failed to show objective clinical benefit over placebo so they are not routinely recommended. Antibiotics and other antimicrobials may be indicated in cases in which specific treatable pathogens are identified.
- Avoid decongestants because of their drying effect.
- Guaifenesin may be a useful adjunct as a mucolytic agent.

- In gastroesophageal reflux disease (GERD)-associated laryngitis use acid-suppressive therapy (H_2 blockers, proton pump inhibitors) and nocturnal antireflux precautions.

CHRONIC LARYNGITIS:
- Results from any of the following: tuberculosis, usually through bronchogenic spread; leprosy, from nasopharyngeal or oropharyngeal spread; syphilis, in secondary and tertiary stages; rhinoscleroma, extending from the nose and nasopharynx; actinomycosis; cryptococcosis; histoplasmosis; blastomycosis; paracoccidioidomycosis; coccidiosis; candidiasis; aspergillosis; sporotrichosis; rhinosporidiosis; parasitic infections including leishmaniasis and *Clinostomum* infection following raw fresh-water fish ingestion.
- Noninfectious causes of both acute and chronic laryngitis include malignancy, voice abuse (singers), GERD, and chemical or environmental irritants such as cigarettes and allergens. Other causes of inflammatory or granulomatous lesions of the larynx include relapsing polychondritis, Wegener's granulomatosis, and sarcoidosis.

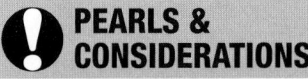 **DIAGNOSIS**

DIFFERENTIAL DIAGNOSIS

- Young children with signs of airway obstruction:
  1. Supraglottitis (epiglottitis).
  2. Laryngotracheobronchitis.
  3. Tracheitis.
  4. Foreign body aspiration.
- Adults with persistent hoarseness, consider noninfectious causes of laryngitis as listed previously.

WORKUP

- History and physical examination: diagnosis is usually apparent.
- Laryngoscopy for severe or persistent cases.
- Laryngeal cultures should be performed if a cause other than acute viral infection is suspected.
- Imaging not indicated unless there is evidence of airway compromise. Obtain plain radiographs of neck, anteroposterior and lateral views, to differentiate laryngitis from acute laryngotracheobronchitis or supraglottitis.

TREATMENT

NONPHARMACOLOGIC THERAPY

- Rest the voice.
- Use an air humidifier.
- Ensure adequate hydration. Avoid alcohol and caffeine because of diuretic effect.

ACUTE GENERAL Rx
- Antibiotics and other antimicrobials should generally not be used. They are indicated only when a specific pathogen is isolated; commonly employed antibacterial agents are macrolides; clarithromycin 500 mg by mouth bid for 5 to 7 days or azithromycin 500 mg followed by 250 mg once daily for 4 to 5 days if the cause of laryngitis is found to be *Mycoplasma pneumoniae* or *Chlamydophila pneumoniae* (the new name for what was formerly known as *Chlamydia pneumoniae*).
- Avoid decongestants because of their drying effect.
- Guaifenesin may be a useful adjunct as a mucolytic agent.
- In GERD-associated laryngitis use acid-suppressive therapy (H_2 blockers, proton pump inhibitors) and nocturnal antireflux precautions.

DISPOSITION

Uncomplicated laryngitis is usually benign, with gradual resolution of symptoms.

REFERRAL

- If symptoms persist for >2 wk, refer to otolaryngologist for laryngoscopy.
- Consider referral to gastroenterologist if GERD is suspected.

⬤ PEARLS & CONSIDERATIONS

- Most cases of uncomplicated acute laryngitis are viral in origin, and antibacterial agents should not be routinely administered.
- A recent Cochrane analysis in 2013 found no evidence for the use of empiric antibiotics in adults with laryngitis.
- The most difficult clinical challenge is often convincing patients with acute laryngitis that they do not need and will not benefit from antibacterial agents.

SUGGESTED READING
Available at www.expertconsult.com

RELATED CONTENT
Laryngitis (Patient Information)

AUTHOR: **GLENN G. FORT, M.D., M.P.H.**

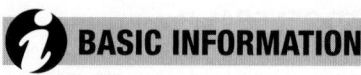

BASIC INFORMATION

DEFINITION

Lead is a potent, pervasive neurotoxicant. Lead poisoning refers to multisystem abnormalities resulting from excessive lead exposure.

SYNONYM

Plumbism

ICD-10CM CODES

T56.0 X1A	Toxic effect of lead and its compounds, accidental (unintentional), initial encounter
T56.0X1D	Toxic effect of lead and its compounds, accidental (unintentional), subsequent encounter
T56.0X1S	Toxic effect of lead and its compounds, accidental (unintentional), sequela
T56.0X2A	Toxic effect of lead and its compounds, intentional self-harm, initial encounter
T56.0X2D	Toxic effect of lead and its compounds, intentional self-harm, subsequent encounter
T56.0X2S	Toxic effect of lead and its compounds, intentional self-harm, sequela
T56.0X3A	Toxic effect of lead and its compounds, assault, initial encounter
T56.0X3D	Toxic effect of lead and its compounds, assault, subsequent encounter
T56.0X3S	Toxic effect of lead and its compounds, assault, sequela
T56.0X4A	Toxic effect of lead and its compounds, undetermined, initial encounter
T56.0X4D	Toxic effect of lead and its compounds, undetermined, subsequent encounter
T56.0X4S	Toxic effect of lead and its compounds, undetermined, sequela

EPIDEMIOLOGY & DEMOGRAPHICS

- Lead poisoning is most common in children ages 1 to 5 yr (17,000 cases/100,000 persons). The highest rates are among blacks, those with low income, and urban children.
- In 1991 the Centers for Disease Control and Prevention (CDC) lowered the definition of a safe blood lead level to <10 mcg/dl of whole blood (a blood lead level of 25 mcg/dl was considered acceptable before 1991).
- It is estimated that >15% of preschoolers in the United States have a blood lead level >15 mcg/dl.

PHYSICAL FINDINGS & CLINICAL PRESENTATION

- Findings vary with the degree of toxicity (Table 1). Examination may be normal in patients with mild toxicity.

- Myalgias, irritability, headache, and general fatigue may be present initially.
- Abdominal cramping, constipation, weight loss, tremor, paresthesias and peripheral neuritis, seizures, and coma may occur with severe toxicity.
- Motor neuropathy is common in children with lead poisoning; learning disorders are also frequent.

ETIOLOGY

Chronic, repeated exposure to paint containing lead, plumbing, storage of batteries, pottery, or lead soldering. Concentration of lead is generally highest in lead-based paint on exterior surfaces. Among interior surfaces, windows are most likely to have the highest lead content.

DIAGNOSIS

DIFFERENTIAL DIAGNOSIS

- Polyneuropathies from other sources.
- Anxiety disorder, attention deficit disorder.
- Malabsorption, acute abdomen.
- Iron-deficiency anemia.

WORKUP

Laboratory screening: all U.S. children should be considered to be at risk for lead poisoning and should be screened routinely starting at age 1 yr for low-risk children and age 6 mo for high-risk children.

LABORATORY TESTS

- Venous blood lead level: normal level, <5 mcg/dl; levels of 50 to 70 mcg/dl, indicative of moderate toxicity; levels >70 mcg/dl, associated with severe poisoning.
- Mild anemia with basophilic stippling on peripheral smear.
- Elevated zinc protoporphyrin levels or free erythrocyte protoporphyrin level.
- An increased body burden of lead with previous high-level exposure in patients with occupational lead poisoning can be demonstrated by measuring the excretion of lead in urine after premedication with calcium ethylenediamine tetraacetic acid (EDTA) or another chelating agent.

IMAGING STUDIES

- Imaging studies are generally not necessary.
- A plain abdominal film can visualize lead particles in the gut.
- "Lead lines" may be noted on x-ray films of long bones.

TREATMENT

NONPHARMACOLOGIC THERAPY

- Provide adequate amounts of calcium, iron, zinc, and protein in patient's diet.
- Family education on sources of lead exposure and potential adverse health effects.

ACUTE GENERAL Rx

- The use of chelation in cases of acute lead poisoning is guided by the patient's clinical status and the blood lead level (BLL). For children with blood levels of 10 to 19 mcg/dl, the CDC recommends nonpharmacologic interventions (see "Nonpharmacologic Therapy").
- For children with blood levels between 20 and 44 mcg/dl, the CDC recommendations include case management by a qualified social worker, clinical management, environmental assessment, and lead hazard control. Chelation therapy should be considered in children with refractory blood lead levels. Chelation therapy (Table 2) is indicated in children with blood lead levels >45 mcg/dl:
- Succimer (DMSA) 10 mg/kg PO q8h for 5 days then q12h for 2 wk can be used in patients with levels between 45 and 70 mcg/dl.
- Edetate calcium disodium (EDTA) and dimercaprol (BAL) are effective in patients with severe toxicity.
- Use of both EDTA and DMSA is indicated in children with blood levels >70 mcg/dl.
- d-Penicillamine (Cuprimine) can also be used for lead poisoning, but it is not FDA approved for this condition.

CHRONIC Rx

- Reduce exposure, remove any potential lead sources.
- Correct iron deficiency and any other nutritional deficiencies.
- Recheck blood lead level 7 to 21 days after chelation therapy.

DISPOSITION

Patients with mild to moderate toxicity generally improve without any residual deficits. The presence of encephalopathy at diagnosis is a poor prognostic sign. Residual neurologic deficits may persist in these patients. Chelation therapy seems to slow the progression of renal insufficiency in patients with mildly elevated body lead burden.

REFERRAL

If exposure to lead is work related, it should be reported to the Office of the United States Occupational Safety and Health Administration (OSHA). Follow-up testing is mandatory in all patients after an abnormal screening blood lead level.

PEARLS & CONSIDERATIONS

COMMENTS

- Even blood lead concentrations as low as 5-10 mcg/dl are inversely associated with children's IQ scores at age 3 and 5 yr.
- Screening of household members of affected individuals is recommended.
- In children with blood lead levels of >45 mg/dl, treatment with succimer does not improve scores on tests of cognition, behavior, or neuropsychological function.
- Lead toxicity may delay growth and pubertal development in girls.
- Low-level environmental lead exposure may accelerate progressive renal insufficiency in

patients without diabetes who have chronic renal disease. Repeated chelation therapy may improve renal function and slow the progression of renal failure.

RELATED CONTENT

Lead Poisoning (Patient Information)

AUTHOR: **FRED F. FERRI, M.D.**

TABLE 1 Serum Lead Levels and Symptoms

Level (µg/dL)	Symptoms	
	Adults	**Children**
10	None	Decreased IQ
		Decreased hearing
		Decreased growth
20	Increased protoporphyrin	Decreased nerve conduction velocity
	No symptoms	Increased protoporphyrin
30	Increased blood pressure	Decreased vitamin D metabolism
	Decreased hearing	
40	Peripheral neuropathies	Decreased hemoglobin synthesis
	Nephropathy	
	Infertility (men)	
50	Decreased hemoglobin synthesis	Lead colic
70	Anemia	Anemia
		Encephalopathy
		Nephropathy
100	Encephalopathy	Death

From Marx JA, et al.: *Rosen's emergency medicine*, ed 8, Philadelphia, 2014, Saunders.

TABLE 2 Chelators*

Chelator	Dose	Indications	Contraindications
Deferoxamine	15 mg/kg/hr up to 24 hr (titrate up slowly because of hypotension)	Iron level >500 g/dL or systemic symptoms	
Dimercaprol (British anti-Lewisite [BAL])	Lead encephalopathy: 75 mg/m^2 deep IM injection every 4 hr for 5 days in children or 4 mg/kg every 4 hr for adults Arsenic (severe): no established regimen; consider 3 mg/kg IM every 4 hr for 48 hr; then twice daily for 7-10 days Mercury: 5 mg/kg IM first; then 2.5 mg/kg every 12-24 hr	Lead level >70 g/dL or encephalopathy Arsenic: symptomatic patient with known exposure Mercury: inorganic	Peanut allergy Organic mercury poisoning
CaNa$_2$EDTA	1500 mg/m^2/day continuous IV infusion 50 mg/kg/day or 1000 mg/m^2/day in 2-4 divided doses for up to 5 days if less severe symptoms	Lead: given after first dose of BAL for blood lead level above 70 g/dL or encephalopathy	
Succimer (DMSA)	10 mg/kg q8h × 5 days; then q12h for 14 days	Lead level of 45-69 g/dL Arsenic: if tolerated orally for subacute and chronic toxicity Mercury: acute and chronic	
D-Penicillamine	25 mg/kg q6h × 5 days	Lead level of 45-69 g/dL, succimer not tolerated Arsenic: only if BAL and DMSA are unavailable Mercury: if BAL and DMSA are unavailable or not tolerated	Penicillin allergy
DMPS (investigational)	5 mg/kg/dose IM q6-8h day 1, q8-12h day 2, q12-24h day 3 and until 24-hr urine is <50 µg/L	Lead (chronic) Arsenic Mercury	

IM, Intramuscular; *IV*, intravenous.
*Indications for chelation and dosing regimens may change. Consult with a toxicologist or poison control center for the most up-to-date recommendations.
From Marx JA, et al.: *Rosen's emergency medicine*, ed 8, Philadelphia, 2014, Saunders.

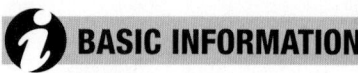

DEFINITION

Legg-Calvé-Perthes disease (LCPD) is characterized by vascular compromise to the immature proximal femoral head leading to avascular necrosis of the femoral head. The classification of LCPD is outlined in Fig. 1.

SYNONYMS

Perthes disease
Coxa plana
Capital femoral osteochondrosis
Osteonecrosis of the proximal femoral epiphysis
LCPD

ICD-10CM CODES

M91.10 Juvenile osteochondrosis of head of femur [Legg-Calvé-Perthes], unspecified leg

EPIDEMIOLOGY & DEMOGRAPHICS

PREVALENCE: One case in 1300 children. More common in Caucasians.
INCIDENCE: One in 1200 children younger than 15 years of age.
PREDOMINANT SEX: Male/female ratio of 4:1.
PREDOMINANT AGE: 4 to 10 years old

PHYSICAL FINDINGS & CLINICAL PRESENTATION

- Initial symptom: usually a mildly painful limp.
- Pain may be referred down the medial aspect of the thigh to the knee.
- Positive roll test: with the patient in the supine position, rolling of the affected extremity into internal and external rotation elicits guarding, with limited range of motion.
- Pain at the extremes of motion and tenderness over the anterior aspect of the hip joint.
- No history of trauma.
- Condition is bilateral in 10% to 20% of patients.

ETIOLOGY

Unknown. Increased association with ADHD, delayed bone age.

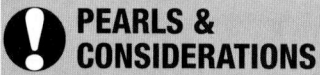 DIAGNOSIS

DIFFERENTIAL DIAGNOSIS

Unilateral Disease
- Transient synovitis
- Sickle cell disease
- Septic arthritis
- Neoplastic process
- Spondyloepiphyseal dysplasia tarda
- Slipped capital femoral epiphysis

BILATERAL DISEASE

- Multiple epiphyseal dysplasia.
- Sickle cell disease.
- Juvenile idiopathic arthritis.

WORKUP

Diagnosis is usually based on physical examination findings and radiographic evaluation.

IMAGING STUDIES

- MRI is most sensitive for early LCPD.
- Plain x-ray (AP and frog-leg lateral x-rays) (Fig. 2) will show late changes.
- Technetium bone scan may help confirm the diagnosis in early cases.

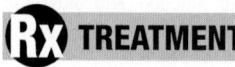 TREATMENT

ACUTE GENERAL Rx

- Non-weight bearing followed by bracing
- Bracing may be required for 2 to 3 years in a small subset of patients.
- NSAIDs for pain control.
- Range-of-motion physical therapy exercises.
- Surgery may be required in refractory cases, usually femoral or pelvic osteotomies.

DISPOSITION

- Prognosis depends on the age of patient and the degree of involvement of the femoral head at onset.
- In patients younger than 6 years, outcome is generally favorable, regardless of treatment.
- Patients over the age of 8 years at onset often have less favorable outcomes. Females tend to do worse than males in this age group.
- A subset of patients may go on to develop degenerative arthritis.

REFERRAL

Referral to pediatric orthopedist when diagnosis is suspected.

PEARLS & CONSIDERATIONS

Both the etiology and treatment of LCPD remain controversial. Treatment recommendations vary widely and continue to evolve. Children over the age of 8 years at onset may benefit from early surgical intervention.

SUGGESTED READINGS

Available at www.expertconsult.com

RELATED CONTENT

Legg-Calvé-Perthes Disease (Patient Information)

AUTHOR: **ANDREW P. THOME, JR., M.D.**

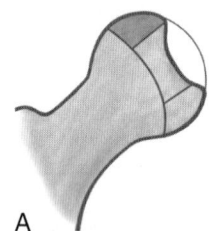 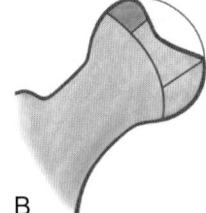 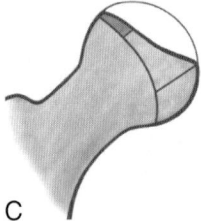

FIG. 1 Lateral pillar classification for Legg-Calvé-Perthes disease. A, There is no involvement of the lateral pillar. **B,** >50% of the lateral pillar height is maintained. **C,** <50% of the lateral pillar height is maintained. (From Kliegman RM et al: *Nelson textbook of pediatrics,* ed 19, Philadelphia, 2011, Saunders.)

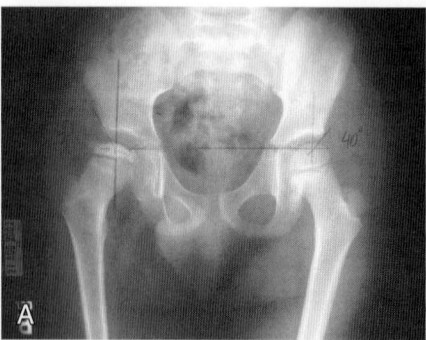 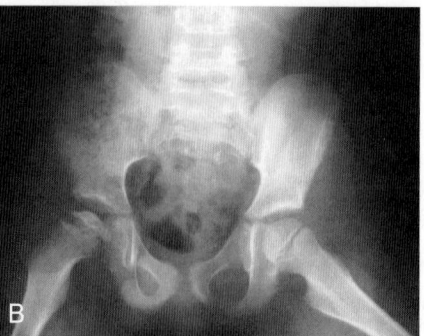

FIG. 2 A, Anteroposterior radiograph of the pelvis shows epiphyseal fragmentation in the right hip, characteristic of the fragmentation phase of Legg-Calvé-Perthes disease. **B,** The frog-leg lateral view demonstrates subchondral fracture, increased density of the femoral head, and some collapse. (From Kliegman RM et al: *Nelson textbook of pediatrics,* ed 19, Philadelphia, 2011, Saunders.)

BASIC INFORMATION

DEFINITION

Acute lymphoblastic leukemia (ALL) is a malignancy of precursor B or T lymphocytes (lymphoblasts) characterized by uncontrolled proliferation of malignant lymphocytic cells with replacement of normal bone marrow elements and bone marrow failure. Lymphoblastic lymphoma is diagnosed when the disease presents in extramedullary sites (most commonly as mediastinal mass in T cell disease) *and* less than 25% of the bone marrow is involved.

SYNONYMS

Acute lymphocytic leukemia
Acute lymphoblastic leukemia
ALL

ICD-10CM CODES

C91.00 Acute lymphoblastic leukemia not having achieved remission
C91.01 Acute lymphoblastic leukemia, in remission
C91.02 Acute lymphoblastic leukemia, in relapse

EPIDEMIOLOGY & DEMOGRAPHICS

- ALL is primarily a disease of children (peak incidence occurring at 3-5 years of age).
- Overall incidence is 4.5 cases per 100,000 persons per year; 60% are under age 20. It is the most common malignancy of childhood. (SEER database accessed 11/26/15)
- Incidence varies according to race and ethnic group: 14.8 cases per million for blacks, 35.6 cases per million for whites, and 40.9 cases per million for Hispanics.
- Male:female ratio is 55% to 45%.

PHYSICAL FINDINGS & CLINICAL PRESENTATION

- Findings consistent with bone marrow failure and peripheral cytopenias—pallor, bruising, petechiae.
- Lymphadenopathy or hepatosplenomegaly.
- Fever (disease related or infectious), bone pain, weakness, weight loss, mental status changes, and neurologic findings associated with central nervous system (CNS) involvement (if present).
- T cell lymphoblastic lymphoma is usually associated with a mediastinal mass.
- Table 1 summarizes the clinical presentation of acute lymphoblastic leukemia.

ETIOLOGY

- Most cases are sporadic without established risk factors.
- Ionizing radiation exposure appears to be a risk factor.
- Down's syndrome (trisomy 21) is associated with an approximately 3% risk of developing leukemia by age 30, predominantly ALL. ALL may be seen with other hereditary premalignancy syndromes (e.g., ataxia-telangiectasia)

DIAGNOSIS

DIFFERENTIAL DIAGNOSIS

Disorders associated with lymphocytosis (lymphocytes >5000/mcl):

- Adults: Chronic lymphocytic leukemia, mantle cell lymphoma, marginal zone lymphoma, hairy cell leukemia.
- Adolescents/young adults: Infectious mononucleosis syndromes due to Epstein-Barr virus or cytomegalovirus, among others, may present with lymphocyte abnormalities with appearance suggestive of leukemic blasts.
- Disorders associated with circulating blasts or blastlike cells such as acute myeloid leukemia, prolymphocytic leukemia, blastoid mantle cell lymphoma, and Burkitt's lymphoma (mature B cell leukemia/lymphoma).
- Lymphoblastic lymphoma.
- Aplastic anemia; ALL may present without circulating leukemia cells and with only manifestations of bone marrow failure.

WORKUP

- Identification of circulating abnormal cell population by flow cytometry. CD19 identifies most precursor B cells. Immature leukemic blasts should have *absence* of surface immunoglobulin and will usually express CD34 and stain positive for terminal deoxynucleotidyltransferase (TdT). Cytoplasmic CD3 and CD7 establish immature T cell lineage in most cases. Aberrant myeloid markers (CD13, CD33) can be seen.
- Cytochemical stains are sometimes easier to perform and may be available sooner but are less specific. ALL blasts should be negative for myeloperoxidase and esterase stains.
- Bone marrow examination (Fig. E1).
- Genetic studies define important treatment categories, of which the most important is Philadelphia chromosome positive (Ph+) vs. Philadelphia chromosome negative (Ph−) disease, as these are treated differently. Ph status can be determined rapidly by polymerase chain reaction (PCR) or fluorescence *in situ* hybridization (FISH) and should be available within 24 to 48 hours of diagnosis. The WHO classification recognizes genetic variants of ALL as distinct syndromes (Table 2), and the clinical significance of common abnormalities is outlined in Table 3.

- Genetic profiling for "Ph-like" ALL (genetic profile similar to Ph+ disease, but no BCR/ABL abnormality) or IKZF1 (IKAROS) mutations may provide additional prognostic information, but may not be uniformly available. Ph-like ALL may respond to tyrosine kinase inhibitor therapy and may behave more like Ph+ ALL.
- Lumbar puncture is usually done at diagnosis, if practical, to assess for CNS involvement and to initiate CNS prophylactic therapy.

LABORATORY TESTS

- Complete blood count reveals normochromic, normocytic anemia, thrombocytopenia.
- Peripheral smear will usually reveal lymphoblasts, but in some cases only the marrow is involved.
- Initial blood work should also include assessment for basic organ function (creatinine, bilirubin), blood glucose (glucocorticoids are part of therapy) and spontaneous tumor lysis syndrome (K^+, Ca^{++}, PO_4^{++}, uric acid).
- Coagulation studies (full disseminated intravascular coagulation [DIC] screen) prior to lumbar puncture.
- Studies appropriate to identifying and risk-stratifying leukemia as outlined previously.

IMAGING STUDIES

- Chest x-ray to evaluate fever and for the presence of mediastinal mass.
- CT for symptomatic complaints. Be cautious about contrast dye exposure in patients with evidence of spontaneous tumor lysis syndrome to avoid further renal injury.

TREATMENT
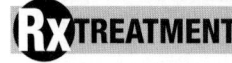

ACUTE GENERAL Rx

- Survival of children with ALL has improved from 10% to 90% in the last 40 years and is a major success story of modern medical science and research. Adults have fared less

---

TABLE 1 Clinical Presentation of Acute Lymphoblastic Leukemia

Symptoms and Signs	Etiology	Management
Fever	Disease or infection	Fever workup with blood, urine cultures, and chest x-ray. Broad-spectrum antimicrobial coverage with attention to localizing symptoms (i.e., cough, abdominal pain).
Fatigue, pallor	Anemia (bone marrow failure, bleeding)	RBC transfusion. Transfuse with caution if hyperleukocytosis is present.
Petechiae, bruising, bleeding	Thrombocytopenia, DIC (bone marrow failure, tumor lysis)	Transfuse with platelets, coagulation protein support if indicated (uncommon).
Pain	Leukemia infiltrating bones or joints or expanding BM cavity	Establish diagnosis and start chemotherapy.
Respiratory distress, superior vena cava syndrome	Mediastinal mass	Avoid sedation in the presence of tracheal compression; establish diagnosis as soon as possible and start chemotherapy.

ALL, Acute lymphoblastic leukemia; *BM,* bone marrow; *RBC,* red blood cell.
Adapted from Hoffman R: *Hematology, basic principles and practice,* 6th ed, Philadelphia, 2013, Saunders.

TABLE 2 WHO Classification of Precursor Lymphoid Neoplasms

B-lymphoblastic leukemia/lymphoma, not otherwise specified.
B-lymphoblastic leukemia/lymphoma with recurrent cytogenetic abnormalities
    B-lymphoblastic leukemia/lymphoma with t(9;22)(q34;q11.2); *BCR-ABL1*
    B-lymphoblastic leukemia/lymphoma with t(v*;11q23) *MLL* rearranged.
    B-lymphoblastic leukemia/lymphoma with t(12;21)(p13;q22); *TEL-AML1 (ETV6-RUNX1)*
    B-lymphoblastic leukemia/lymphoma with hyperdiploidy
    B-lymphoblastic leukemia/lymphoma with hypodiploidy
    B-lymphoblastic leukemia/lymphoma with t(5;14)(q32;q32); *IL3-IGH*
    B-lymphoblastic leukemia/lymphoma with t(1;19)(q23;p13.3); *EZA-PBX1 (TCF3-PBX-1)*
T-lymphoblastic leukemia/lymphoma.
Provisional entities:
B-lymphoblastic leukemia/lymphoma BCR/ABL1 like
B lymphoblastic leukemia/lymphoma with iAMP21
Early T cell precursor lymphoblastic leukemia/lymphoma

v*, Variable gene partners.
From Arber DA et al: The 2016 revision to the World Health Organization classification of myeloid neoplasms and acute leukemia, *Blood* 127:2391-2405, 2016.

TABLE 3 More Common Recurrent Cytogenetic Abnormalities in B-Lymphoblastic Leukemia/Lymphoma

Abnormality	Clinical Relevance
t(9;22)(q34;q11.2); *BCR-ABL1*	Incidence approximately 3% in children, 25% in adults, rising with age; requires therapy with tyrosine kinase inhibitors.
t(v*;11q23) *MLL* rearranged.	Most common variant is t(4;11); often presents with very high WBC; confers worse prognosis; rare in adults; common in infant leukemia.
t(12;21)(p13;q22); *TEL-AML1*	Common in children (20%-30%); rare in adults; confers improved prognosis.
Hyperdiploidy	Seen in about 25% of children, less in adults; confers favorable prognosis.
Hypodiploidy	Uncommon; confers worse prognosis.
t(5;14)(q32;q32); *IL3-IGH*	Rare; commonly associated with eosinophilia; T cell disease, ? neutral prognostically
t(1;19)(q23;p13.3);	Incidence approximately 5%; intermediate/favorable in children, intermediate/poor in adults.

v*, Variable gene partners. Many of these disorders also have distinct immunophenotypes by flow cytometry. Additional molecular abnormalities of recently defined relevance include mutations of IKZF1, which encodes a lymphoid transcription factor IKAROS, is associated with high relapse rates and gene expression profile similar to BCR-ABL1 translocated disease. Gene expression profiling has identified a subgroup of "Philadelphia chromosome-like" ALL with a gene expression similar to BCR-ABL1 translocation associated disease, which confers worse prognosis, but which may identify new opportunities for targeted therapies.

well, but cure rates have also improved to about 60% to 70% in standard-risk patients in recent trials. Adults in particular have benefited from tyrosine kinase inhibitor therapy for Ph+ ALL, since this disease is more common in adults and may represent 50% or more of disease in patients over 50.

- **Hyperleukocytic leukemia** (WBC >100,000/mcl) is uncommon in ALL and lymphocyte counts of 100,000 may be well tolerated. Prednisone and vincristine usually offer rapid cytoreduction and leukapheresis is rarely (but sometimes) required.
- **Tumor lysis syndrome** is common in ALL and was seen in 23% of patients in one large series. It is sometimes spontaneous—i.e., present before therapy is given—and is a potential cause of early death. Tumor lysis syndrome is caused by release of intracellular potassium, phosphate, and nucleic acids. The nucleic acids adenosine and guanosine are eventually metabolized to uric acid. Elevated potassium may cause cardiac dysrhythmia and death. Elevated uric acid may cause renal failure through renal urate crystal deposition and possibly other mechanisms. Elevated

phosphates cause renal calcium phosphate deposition and kidney injury while also lowering serum calcium, which can cause cardiac dysrhythmia and spasms. Therapy is directed mainly at maintaining renal function through vigorous hydration (3 liters normal saline per day if practical, alkalinization *not* recommended); "forced diuresis" if necessary to maintain urine output at 2 ml/kg/h; and dialysis if necessary to control K$^+$, phosphates, or fluid balance. Allopurinol, up to 800 mg/day for adults, 300 to 450 mg/m^2/day for children is given routinely. Rasburicase is a recombinant urate oxidase that rapidly lowers uric acid levels. The dose is 0.2 mg/kg, and one dose is usually enough. Rasburicase should be avoided in patients with G6PD deficiency. Phosphate binders are of uncertain value but are usually given. Asymptomatic hypocalcemia is not treated to avoid increasing calcium phosphate deposition. Definitions of laboratory and clinical tumor lysis and defined risk categories are outlined in Table 4.

- Numerous protocols have been used in North America, Europe, and Asia for Ph-ALL, and the specific protocol is likely to be determined by

institution/physician familiarity and access to clinical trials (participation is strongly recommended), among other factors.

- In the 1990s and early 2000s, it was noted that adolescents and young adult (AYA) patients had better outcomes on pediatric trials than on adult trials. Consequently, this group (currently defined as ages 15-39) is now often (especially younger AYAs) treated on pediatric protocols by pediatric services or on adult "pediatric inspired" protocols.
- Therapy for Ph- negative ALL generally has four components:
  1. Induction therapy, typically with corticosteroids, cyclophosphamide (some regimens), vincristine, an anthracycline (doxorubicin or daunorubicin usually), and asparaginase. The CD20 directed antibody rituximab has shown benefit in patients with greater than 20% CD20 expression on their blast cells.
  2. Consolidation therapy is high-dose therapy aimed at preventing relapse after remission has been obtained and varies by protocol, commonly consisting of cytarabine and methotrexate in combination with other agents.
  3. Maintenance therapy is low-intensity outpatient therapy that is continued for 2-3 years after completion of consolidation. Prednisone, monthly vincristine ("Oncovin"), methotrexate, and oral 6-mercaptopurine (POMP) are commonly used.
  4. CNS prophylaxis is required since roughly two thirds of patients relapsed in the CNS in early trials. This is usually done with intrathecal therapy (methotrexate at a minimum, commonly with cytarabine and hydrocortisone) administered by lumbar puncture or sometimes Ommaya reservoir. Because of increased toxicity, cranial radiation is reserved for patients with high-risk features, such as active CNS disease at diagnosis.
- The use of allogeneic bone marrow transplant in first remission of ALL is controversial because of improving results with current nontransplant therapies. It is usually recommended for patients in whom the likelihood of cure is considered less than 50% to 60% with chemotherapy alone, if practical by age and donor availability. Autologous bone marrow transplant is rarely used in Ph- ALL.
- Risk factors for treatment failure in recent protocols are outlined in Table 5.
- Therapy of Ph+ ALL consists of a tyrosine kinase inhibitor—imatinib, dasatinib, nilotinib, ponatinib have been used—with chemotherapy.
  - 2-year survival has been reported as 50% to 65%, with various regimens.
  - Low-intensity induction (i.e., without myelosuppressive chemotherapy) with dasatinib and prednisone or imatinib, vincristine and prednisone have resulted in remission rates of 100% and 98% and may allow for less toxicity and hospitalization at diagnosis.

TABLE 4 Tumor Lysis Syndrome

Laboratory Tumor Lysis Syndrome[a]
Uric acid: ≥8 mg/dl or 476 μmol/L
Potassium: ≥6.0 mmol/L
Phosphorus: ≥4.5 mg/dl or 1.5 mmol/L (adults), ≥6.5 mg/dl or 2.1 mmol (children)
- Calcium: Corrected[b] Ca^{++} <7.0 mg/dl or 1.75 mmol/L or ionized Ca^{++} <1.12 mg/dl or 0.3 mmol/L, or 25% increase from baseline uric acid, potassium, phosphorus; 25% decrease for calcium.

Clinical Tumor Lysis Syndrome
Acute kidney injury
- Rise in serum creatinine ≥0.3 mg/dl (26.5 μmol/L).
- Any creatinine >1.5 age-appropriate upper limit normal if no baseline available.
- Oliguria defined as urine output <0.5 ml/kg/hr for 6 hours.

Cardiac arrhythmia
Seizure
Symptomatic hypocalcemia (e.g., neuromuscular irritability such as tetany)

[a]Laboratory tumor lysis syndrome present if two or more abnormalities are present within 3 days before or 7 days after therapy.
[b]Corrected calcium is measured calcium (mg/dl) + 0.8 x (4 − measured albumin g/dl).
Adapted from Howard SC et al: The tumor lysis syndrome, *N Engl J Med* 364:1844-1854, 2011 and Coiffier B et al: Guidelines for the management of pediatric and adult tumor lysis syndrome: an evidence based review, *J Clin Oncol* 26:2767-2778, 2008.

TABLE 5 Risk Factors for Treatment Failure in Recent ALL trials

t(v*;11q23) *MLL* rearranged.

Hypodiploidy

Minimal residual disease after remission or consolidation*

Philadelphia chromosome like genomic signature (in Ph- ALL)†

Early precursor T (ETP) ALL (absent CD1a, CD8, weak CD5, myeloid or stem cell antigen expression).

*Measured variously after induction or consolidation therapy.
†Standardized testing for this is still in development, but it may have important treatment implications. Note also that many historic risk factors (e.g., T cell vs B cell disease) have not been independent risk factors in current trials.
Roberts KG et al: Targetable kinase-activating lesions in Ph-like acute lymphoblastic leukemia, *N Engl J Med* 371(11):1005-1015, 2014.

- Allogeneic bone marrow transplant is commonly used as consolidative therapy if available but has become more controversial. Maintenance therapy with tyrosine kinase inhibitor is usually given after BMT or non-BMT therapy.
- Therapy of relapsed disease
  - Allogeneic bone marrow transplant is offered for relapsed disease, but relapse after BMT is common, and long-term cure rates have been low at about 20%.
  - Blinatumomab is a bispecific antibody that binds CD19 and CD3, redirecting T cells to leukemia cells, with approximately 40% of relapsed patients having remission.
- Chimeric antigen receptor T cell (CAR-T) therapy, a form of targeted immunotherapy, has yielded remission rates of 70% to 90% in relapsed patients. Availability of this therapy is slowly expanding.

- Survivorship
  - Survivors of childhood and adult ALL are increasingly been seen in primary care practices; as of 2006 there were estimated > 50,000 survivors, likely increasing by about 2000+ per year.
  - Long-term complications of ALL therapy include secondary malignancy from chemotherapy (usually in first 5-10 years) or from radiation (if given, no plateau in risk, congestive heart failure from anthracycline therapy (often manifesting 20-30 years after treatment), osteopenia and avascular necrosis from glucocorticoid therapy, obesity and neurocognitive defects. Key recommendations include the following:
  - Echocardiography every 3 to 5 years for asymptomatic congestive heart failure, more often if anthracycline exposure was >250 to 300 mg/m^2, since asymptomatic congestive heart failure may warrant therapy. This may show up decades after therapy.
  - Screening for malignancy and endocrinopathies in pertinent radiation fields.
  - Attention to the increased risk of obesity and metabolic derangement in survivors.
  - Recent reviews (see references) summarizing current recommendations and guidelines are accessible online (http://www.survivorshipguidelines.org/pdf/LTFUGuidelines_40.pdf, http://www.sign.ac.uk/pdf/sign132.pdf).

SUGGESTED READINGS
Available at www.expertconsult.com

RELATED CONTENT
Acute Lymphocytic Leukemia (ALL) (Patient Information)
Tumor Lysis Syndrome (Related Key Topic)

AUTHOR: **PETER RINTELS, M.D.**

BASIC INFORMATION

DEFINITION

Acute myelogenous leukemia (AML) is a malignancy of hematopoietic progenitor cells that would normally give rise to mature granulocytes. Strictly speaking, AML is a subset of acute nonlymphocytic leukemia (ANLL), a designation that broadly distinguishes these diseases from the biologically distinct leukemias of lymphocytic origin. ANLL includes leukemias involving the spectrum of myeloid stem cells, including precursors of granulocytes, monocytes, erythrocytes, and megakaryocytes. Acute promyelocytic leukemia is a distinct leukemia syndrome that is part of the ANLL spectrum, but which has very different treatment implications. ANLL is characterized by maturation failure of myeloid progenitors, excessive numbers of immature progenitors ("blasts"), and various degrees of bone marrow failure (neutropenia, thrombocytopenia, anemia).

SYNONYMS

Acute nonlymphocytic leukemia (ANLL)
Acute myeloid leukemia (AML)

ICD-10CM CODES

C92.60	Acute myeloid leukemia with 11q23-abnormality not having achieved remission
C92.61	Acute myeloid leukemia with 11q23-abnormality in remission
C92.62	Acute myeloid leukemia with 11q23-abnormality in relapse
C92.90	Myeloid leukemia, unspecified, not having achieved remission
C92.91	Myeloid leukemia, unspecified in remission
C92.92	Myeloid leukemia, unspecified in relapse
C92.A0	Acute myeloid leukemia with multilineage dysplasia, not having achieved remission
C92.A1	Acute myeloid leukemia with multilineage dysplasia, in remission
C92.A2	Acute myeloid leukemia with multilineage dysplasia, in relapse
C92.Z0	Other myeloid leukemia not having achieved remission
C92.Z1	Other myeloid leukemia, in remission
C92.Z2	Other myeloid leukemia, in relapse
C92.00	Acute myeloblastic leukemia, not having achieved remission
C92.01	Acute myeloblastic leukemia, in remission
C92.02	Acute myeloblastic leukemia, in relapse

EPIDEMIOLOGY & DEMOGRAPHICS

- AML incidence rises with age:
  - Incidence 20 to 55 years old: 1 to 3/100,000 persons/year.
  - Incidence 65 to 80 years old: 11 to 20/100,000 persons/year.
- Annual incidence is 4 cases/100,000 persons/year.
- Males slightly > females; European ancestry slightly > African ancestry.

PHYSICAL FINDINGS & CLINICAL PRESENTATION

Symptoms/Exam Findings:
- Complications of bone marrow failure:
  - Thrombocytopenia associated bleeding.
  - Fatigue and shortness of breath associated with anemia.
  - Infection associated with neutropenia.
- Complications of leukocytosis (hyperleukocytic leukemia, WBC >100,000/mcl)
  - Retinal hemorrhage with visual symptoms.
  - Headache and intracranial bleeding.
  - Respiratory symptoms from pulmonary involvement.
- Systemic symptoms
  - Fatigue, fever (usually infectious, rarely tumor), bone pain (more common in ALL).
- Hemorrhagic complications of disseminated intravascular coagulation (DIC), especially with APML)
- Physical exam will reflect consequences of cytopenias (bruising from thrombocytopenia, pallor from anemia). Enlarged lymph nodes and enlarged liver and spleen are rare. Exam is often normal.
- Rarely disease will present as skin lesions (leukemia cutis) or mass lesions (granulocytic sarcoma).
- Gum hypertrophy and organ/skin involvement is more common in monocytic leukemia.

ETIOLOGY

- Environmental/exposure related: Benzene (best documented), organic solvents (including gasoline), cigarettes smoking (≥20 pack-year 1.34 relative risk), obesity, best documented in women.
- Hereditary disorders: Numerous, including Fanconi anemia, Bloom syndrome, Schwachman Diamond syndrome, Diamond Blackfan anemia, among others.
- Therapy related:
  - Alkylator (e.g. melphalan, busulfan, cisplatin) related: typical latency 5 to 7 years, associated with chromosome 5 and 7 abnormalities.
  - Topoisomerase II inhibitor (e.g. etoposide, doxorubicin): typical latency 1-3 years, associated with 11q23 (mixed lineage leukemia (MLL) gene) rearrangements.
- Radiation exposures (therapeutic—generally low risk), occupational.
- Antecedent hematologic disorders: Myelodysplasia, myeloproliferative disorders, aplastic anemia.

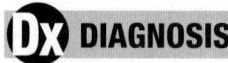 DIAGNOSIS

DIFFERENTIAL DIAGNOSIS

- Disorders that can present with circulating blasts or cells with blast like appearance:
  - Acute myeloid leukemia/acute lymphocytic leukemia.
  - Myelodysplasia (up to 20% circulating blasts, if ≥20% = AML).
  - Primary myelofibrosis.
  - Chronic myeloid leukemia
  - Blastoid variant of mantle cell lymphoma.
  - Prolymphocytic leukemia
  - Blastic plasmacytoid dendritic cell neoplasm.
  - Atypical lymphocytes of Epstein-Barr and cytomegalovirus infection may have blast-like appearance.

LABORATORY TESTS

- Complete blood counts and blood smear evaluation. Note that morphologic evaluation of blasts may suggest myeloid or lymphoid origin, but flow cytometry or cytochemistries (often faster) are needed to confirm. Auer rods are seen in blasts of myeloid origin.
- LDH is commonly elevated. Other biochemistries to assess organ function (creatinine, liver enzymes) and spontaneous tumor lysis syndrome (uric acid, potassium, phosphate, calcium).
- Coagulation studies to assess DIC. DIC is always present in APML, but can be present in **all** forms of acute leukemia, especially acute monocytic leukemia.
- HLA typing for possible bone marrow transplant and platelet support.
- Cytochemical stains –
  - Myeloperoxidase can be performed in minutes, + in myeloid origin leukemia.
  - Alpha naphthyl acetate esterase ("nonspecific esterase") stains mainly monocytic cells.
- Flow cytometry on blood and/or bone marrow (see Table 1)
- Cytogenetic studies, ideally on bone marrow, but can be done on peripheral blood. Fluorescence in situ hybridization (FISH) is often used as an adjunct to conventional chromosome analysis.
- Molecular studies to further stratify risk and prognosis, which may affect treatment choices (see Tables 2 and 3). Directing this workup

---

TABLE 1 Flow Cytometry Markers Used For Diagnosis of ANLL

Precursor stage	CD34, CD38, CD117, CD133, HLA-DR
Granulocytic (myeloid) markers	CD13, CD15 CD16, CD33, CD65, cytoplasmic myeloperoxidase
Monocytic markers	CD11c, CD14, CD64, CD4, CD11b, CD36, NG2 homologue
Megakaryocytic markers	CD41 (glycoprotein IIb/IIIa), CD61 (glycoprotein IIIa), CD42 glycoprotein 1b
Erythroid markers	CD235 (glycophorin A)

Adapted from Doehner H et al, Diagnosis and management of acute myeloid leukemia in adults, recommendations from an international expert panel, on behalf of the European LeukemiaNet, *Blood* 115: 453-474, 2010.

TABLE 2 Significance of Molecular Abnormalities in Cytogenetically Normal Patients With AML

Molecular profile	Patients	4-year overall survival
Mutant CEBPA	67	62%
Mutant NPM, without FLT-3 ITD	150	60%
FLT-3 ITD present	164	24%
FLT-3 ITD absent, wild type NPM, wild type CEBPA (triple negative leukemia)	69	33%

CEBPA, CCAAT/enhancer binding protein α gene; *FLT-3 ITD*, fms-related tyrosine kinase gene internal tandem duplication; *NPM*, nucleophosmin gene. Improved prognosis in patients with CEBPA mutations is limited to patients who lack FLT-3 ITD and have biallelic mutations. CEBPA mutations are seen in approximately 6% to 10% of AML cases, NPM mutations in 25% to 35% (more common in cytogenetically normal cases) and FLT-3 ITD in approximately 20% to 30% of cases.
Data from Schlenk RF et al: *N Engl J Med* 358: 1909-18, 2008, and Green CL et al: *J Clin Oncol* 28: 2739-47, 2010.

TABLE 3 European LeukemiaNet Defined Cytogenetic and Molecular Abnormalities Relevant to Prognosis in AML

Favorable	t(8;21)(q22;q22)* inv (16)(p13.1;q22) or t(16;16) (p13.1;q22)* Normal karyotype with mutated NPM1 and absent FLT-3 ITD Normal karyotype and mutated CEBPA
Intermediate-1†	Normal karyotype and mutated NPM1 and FLT3-ITD Normal karyotype with wild type NPM1 and FLT3-ITD Normal karyotype without FLT3-ITD
Intermediate-2	t(9;11)(p22;q23) Cytogenetic abnormalities not classified as favorable or adverse
Adverse	Complex (3 or more abnormalities, unless associated with a known favorable abnormality), inv(3)(q21;q26.2) or t(3;3)(q21;q26.2); t(6;9)(p23;q34) t(variable;11)(variable;q23) (MLL gene rearrangement), -5 or del (5q); -7; abnormal (17p)

ITD,
*AML associated with t(8;21)(q22;q22), inv (16)(p13.1;q22) or t(16;16) (p13.1;q22) are referred to core binding factor (CBF) leukemias. CBF is a modulator of DNA transcription that is affected by these mutations. Favorable risk groups have had 5-year survivals of about 60%, intermediate risk of approximately 25% to 30%, and unfavorable risk of less than 5% in clinical trials from the 1990s.
†The updated 2016 NCCN guidelines place patients with normal karyotype and FLT3-ITD mutations in the unfavorable risk group. A second FLT3 mutation that is commonly seen involving the tyrosine kinase domain (FLT3-TKD) has either no prognostic significance or is potentially favorable.
Adapted from Doehner H et al, Diagnosis and management of acute myeloid leukemia in adults, recommendations from an international expert panel, on behalf of the European LeukemiaNet, *Blood* 115: 453-474, 2010.

should be done with combined hematology and laboratory expertise and typically will consist of studies for fms-related tyrosine kinase gene (*FLT3*) mutations, nucleophosmin gene (*NPM*) mutations, and CCAAT/enhancer binding protein α gene (CEBPA) mutations. Wider molecular panels are increasingly common because of the increasing numbers of potential markers and the potential availability of targeted therapies for *FLT3* mutated disease and those with isocitrate dehydrogenase mutations, among others.

- Formal diagnosis of acute nonlymphocytic leukemia is established if the marrow blast percentage is ≥20%, unless t(8;21), inv(16), t(16;16) or t(15;17) are present, in which case the percentage of blasts may be lower.
  - Myeloperoxidase (MPO) staining of 3% of blasts establishes myeloid lineage, but MPO may be negative in some AML cases diagnosed by flow cytometry.
  - Specific criteria exist for diagnosing other forms of ANLL, mainly to distinguish from myelodysplasia. The WHO AML classification is outlined in Table 4.

- Cytogenetic risk categories in AML are described in Table 3. Bone marrow findings are described in Fig. E1.

IMAGING STUDIES

- Imaging studies are typically directed to evaluating specific complaints.
- Echocardiogram or MUGA is usually performed to verify that cardiac function is adequate to tolerate anthracycline (usually daunorubicin) therapy, with left ventricular ejection fraction (LVEF) of >50% typically considered acceptable.

Rx TREATMENT

ACUTE GENERAL Rx

- Therapy of AML typically has three components:
  - Immediate therapy to correct metabolic, infectious, or hyperleukocytic emergencies (if needed).
  - Induction therapy, which is therapy of active disease intended to obtain remission

and restore normal bone marrow function. Remission is defined as blasts <5% in the bone marrow, absolute neutrophils (ANC) of >1000/mcl, platelets >100,000/mcl and transfusion independence.
- Consolidation therapy, typically some form of intensive chemotherapy or stem cell transplant therapy intended to prevent relapse.
- Hyperleukocytic symptoms are typically seen with WBC >100,000/ml. Leukapheresis requires catheter placement and pheresis but spares tumor lysis. Rapid cytoreduction with chemotherapy (hydroxyurea 3 to 6 g orally or cytarabine) is often adequate and easier but risks tumor lysis. Optimal management is therefore individualized.
- Tumor lysis syndrome is associated with a rise in uric acid, potassium, and serum phosphate, the last causing a reciprocal fall in calcium. The metabolic changes may result in renal failure, cardiac dysrhythmias, muscle spasms (due to low calcium), seizures, and death (a more detailed discussion is in the section on acute lymphocytic leukemia).
- Induction chemotherapy typically consists of daunorubicin 60 or 90 mg/m^2 IV for 3 days and cytarabine (Ara-C) 100 or 200 mg/m^2/day as continuous infusion for 7 days ("7+3").
- Success rates are 60% to 80% and have been better in recent trials. Other agents used have included etoposide, idarubicin, and fludarabine, among others. Bone marrow examination is commonly performed at day 14 to assess adequacy of response with additional therapy given for large amounts of persisting disease.
- For patients with FLT-3 (fms-like tyrosine receptor kinase) internal tandem duplication or tyrosine kinase domain mutations, the addition of midostaurin, an oral FLT-3 inhibitor, significantly prolonged survival when added to induction and consolidation therapy as compared to placebo. As of this writing, it is available from the manufacturer but not commercially in the U.S. Sorafenib is another FLT-3 inhibitor that has shown activity in FLT-3 mutated AML.
- Consolidation therapy is controversial. Suggested consolidation strategy by risk group is outlined in Table 5. For patients managed with chemotherapy, cytarabine 3 g/m^2 for six doses is commonly used (day 1, 3, 5), but intermediate doses (1000-1500 mg/m^2) for six doses appear equally effective and less toxic. Doses above 1000 mg/m^2 are poorly tolerated in patients over 60 yr because of cerebellar toxicity. Renal insufficiency also increases the risk of cerebellar toxicity from Ara-C, which can be severe.
- The role of autologous bone marrow transplant is controversial, with some evidence of decreased relapse rates after chemotherapy but no clear benefit in overall survival.

TABLE 4 Classification of Acute Myeloid Leukemia According to the Revised World Health Organization Classification (2016)

Category	Subtype/Definition*
AML with recurrent cytogenetic abnormalities	t(8;21)(q22;q22); RUNX1-RUNX1T1[†]
	inv(16)(p13.1q22); CBFB-MYH11[†]
	t(16;16)(p13.1q22); CBFB-MYH11[†]
	t(15;17)(q22;q12); PML-RARA[†] (= acute promyelocytic leukemia)
	t(9;11)(p22;q23); MLLT3-KMT2A
	t(6;9)(p23;q34); DEK-NUP214
	inv(3)(q21q26.2); GATA2, MECOM
	t(3;3)(q21;q26.2); RPN1-EVI1
	t(1;22)(p13q13); RBM15-MKL1 (megakaryoblastic)
	with mutated NPM1
	with biallelic mutations of CEBPA
AML with MDS-related changes	Morphologic features of MDS, or
	Prior history of MDS or MDS/MPN, or
	MDS-related karyotype, and
	None of the recurrent genetic abnormalities above
Therapy-related myeloid neoplasms	Late complications of cytotoxic chemotherapy (alkylating agents, topoisomerase II inhibitors) and/or ionizing radiation therapy[†]
AML, not otherwise specified	AML with minimal differentiation
	AML without maturation
	AML with maturation
	Acute myelomonocytic leukemia
	Acute monoblastic/monocytic leukemia
	Pure erythroid leukemia
	Acute megakaryoblastic leukemia
	Acute basophilic leukemia
	Acute panmyelosis with myelofibrosis
Myeloid sarcoma	
Myeloid proliferations related to Down syndrome	Transient abnormal myelopoiesis
	Myeloid leukemia associated with Down syndrome
Blastic plasmacytoid dendritic cell neoplasm	
Acute leukemia of ambiguous lineage	Acute undifferentiated leukemia
	Mixed-phenotype acute leukemia with:
	t(9;22)(q34;q11.2); BCR-ABL1
	t(v;11q23); KMT2A rearranged
	Mixed-phenotype acute leukemia, B/myeloid, NOS
	Mixed-phenotype acute leukemia, T/myeloid, NOS
Provisional entities	AML with mutated NPM1
	AML with mutated CEBPA
	NK-cell lymphoblastic leukemia/lymphoma

AML, Acute myeloid leukemia; *MDS,* myelodysplastic syndrome; *MPN,* myeloproliferative neoplasm; *NK,* natural killer.
*Diagnosis of AML regardless of percentage of blasts.
[†]Excluded are patients with AML who have transformed from MPN.
For AML with recurrent genetic abnormalities, specific genes rearranged follow the chromosome rearrangement. In 2016, the *MLL* gene has been renamed *KMT2A.*

TABLE 5 Recommendations for Consolidation Therapy for Acute Myelogenous Leukemia in First Remission by Risk Category

Risk Group	Typical Consolidation
Favorable	Chemotherapy with high-dose cytarabine. Allo-BMT usually offered in second remission; may be considered in first remission in selected high-risk situations: high presenting WBC, c-KIT mutations, persisting minimal residual disease.
Intermediate-1	Chemotherapy with high-dose cytarabine *or* first remission allo-BMT. For patients with FLT3-ITD, allo-BMT is often recommended.
Intermediate-2	Chemotherapy with high-dose cytarabine or allo-BMT.
Adverse	Allo-BMT in first remission if a donor is available.

High-dose cytarabine is usually 3 g/m^2 every 12 hr on days 1, 3, and 5 (6 doses) for 3 to 4 cycles, but other doses and schedules have been used. The cytarabine dose is usually lowered to 1 g/m^2 in patients over 60, and high-dose cytarabine should be used with caution in patients with renal failure due to high risk of cerebellar toxicity. *Allo-BMT,* allogeneic bone marrow transplant.

- Allogeneic bone marrow transplant is offered to patients with relapsed disease if a second remission can be obtained. It is offered to high-risk patients in first remission if a donor is available.
- Relapses after bone marrow transplant can sometimes be managed with donor lymphocyte infusions, adjustment of immune suppression, and chemotherapy (often low intensity). In general, outcomes are poor with posttransplant relapses.
- Treatment of older patients (>60 yr) is problematic, with cure rates of 10% to 15%. Older patients do worse because they are more likely to have high-risk features and less likely to tolerate therapy. Options for these patients include:
  - Standard induction therapy is reasonable for patients likely to tolerate it. Even in the absence of cure, quality of life is often excellent in remission. More recent studies suggest that the early death rate (within 30 days of diagnosis) was lower for patients in their 70s and 80s receiving standard induction. A study of induction therapy in patients ages 80 to 89 identified a complete remission rate of 30%, with 37% in remission at 1 yr and 13% at 3 yr. There is no standardized approach to evaluating fitness for therapy; one algorithm is at http://www.aml-score.org/.
  - Hypomethylating agents—decitabine and azacytidine—may be considered in patients unlikely to tolerate induction therapy. Azacytidine 75 mg/m^2 daily for 7 days resulted in a median survival rate of 10.4 months and 1-year survival of 46.5% in one recent multinational study. Decitabine at 20 mg/m^2 for 5 days yielded a median survival of 7.7 months and a remission rate of 17.8% in one trial large trial. Decitabine in particular is well tolerated in older patients who are not considered appropriate for induction chemotherapy.
  - Low-dose cytarabine (20 mg/m^2 twice daily or 40 mg/m^2 daily for 10 days subcutaneously) has shown survival benefit over hydroxyurea in low-/intermediate-risk patients.
  - Oral hydroxyurea dosed to counts and cytopenias.
  - Best supportive care.
  - Reduced-intensity allogeneic stem cell transplant (RIT) is an option for patients in remission after standard therapy. A recent meta-analysis of studies including 749 patients over 60 receiving RIT identified a 3-year relapse-free survival of 35%.
- **Acute Promyelocytic Leukemia** (APML)
  APML is a distinct leukemia syndrome with very different treatment implications. Cure rates greater than 95% have been seen in current protocols in the absence of high-risk features. It is associated with t(15;17), which translocates the PML gene to retinoic acid receptor α (PML-RARα). Uncommon variants are t(11;17) and t(5;17).

- Risk groups in APML receiving anthracycline and retinoic acid therapy:
- Patients in low- and intermediate-risk groups (WBC ≤10,000) had a 2-year event-free survival of 97% using all transretinoic acid (ATRA) and arsenic trioxide (AsO₃) therapy in a recent trial.
- Patients in the high-risk group had approximately 75% 5-year survival using anthracycline (idarubicin) and ATRA therapy.
- APML is a medical emergency because of the high risk of bleeding complications.
  - All patients with APML have DIC, caused by overexpression of annexin II, (which increases generation of plasmin, degrading fibrin), elastases (which degrade fibrinogen and fibrinolytic inhibitors), and increased endothelial tissue plasminogen activator release.
  - Early death due to hemorrhage is seen in 5% to 17% of newly diagnosed APML patients, usually intracranial or pulmonary. Risk factors include elevated WBC, increased age, and elevated creatinine.
  - Retinoic acid rapidly stabilizes the coagulopathy of APML; consideration should be given to starting this immediately for suspected cases.
  - Cryoprecipitate (usual dose 10 bags) to raise the fibrinogen level to 150 mg/dl and platelet transfusion to raise the count to >50,000//mcl should be given as needed.
  - Unfractionated heparin may paradoxically stop bleeding in APML by inhibiting DIC, but is rarely used in the retinoic acid treatment era.
- Diagnosis of APML
  - Rapid diagnosis is essential due to treatment implications.

- Diagnosis by classic APML blast morphology and clinical syndrome (especially DIC with low fibrinogen) is sufficient to justify starting treatment with retinoic acid pending confirmation with molecular studies. Immediate therapy with retinoic acid will rapidly stabilize the coagulopathy and help prevent catastrophic bleeding.
- Polymerase chain reaction for PML/RARa
- FISH for t(15;17) or variants
- Flow cytometry is typically distinct with lack of HLA-DR and CD34; CD13, CD33 and CD64 are usually positive
- Therapy of APML
  - Emergency measures to stabilize coagulopathy as outlined previously.
  - Patients with WBC ≤10,000 (low/intermediate risk) are treated with retinoic acid and arsenic trioxide ("differentiation therapy").
  - Optimal therapy of higher-risk patients is less well defined and may include anthracyclines (commonly idarubicin, also daunorubicin) to lower WBC and decrease risk of differentiation syndrome as well as cytarabine.
  - Maintenance therapy for 2 years is given in some APML protocols.
  - Patients with high-risk disease receive central nervous system prophylaxis with intrathecal chemotherapy.
  - Treatment of relapsed disease typically consists of autologous bone marrow transplant after obtaining second remission.
- Differentiation syndrome (DS) is a potentially fatal complication of therapy with retinoic acid and arsenic trioxide. It is associated with fever, interstitial pulmonary infiltrates, peripheral edema, pleural and pericardial effusions and renal failure; it is commonly associated with rising WBC seen in patients on differentiation therapy.
- Therapy for suspected differentiation syndrome is dexamethasone 10 mg/m² every 12 hr. Stopping retinoic acid and arsenic is appropriate for inadequate response to dexamethasone.
- Prophylaxis for differentiation syndrome with dexamethasone 2.5 mg/m² every 12 hr has been suggested for WBC >5000 or creatinine >1.4 mg/dl. Hydroxyurea is used to keep the WBC below 10,000/mcl in some protocols.

⓵ PEARLS & CONSIDERATIONS

- The diagnosis of acute myeloid leukemia or variants is often, but not always, a medical emergency requiring rapid clinical and laboratory assessment by appropriate expertise.
- APML is a distinct clinical entity that has a high cure rate with current protocols, but which requires intensive supportive care at the time of diagnosis.

SUGGESTED READINGS
Available at www.expertconsult.com

RELATED CONTENT
Acute Myelogenous Leukemia (Patient Information)

AUTHOR: **PETER RINTELS, M.D.**

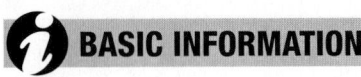

BASIC INFORMATION

DEFINITION

Chronic lymphocytic leukemia (CLL) is a lymphoproliferative disorder characterized by proliferation and accumulation of mature-appearing neoplastic B-cells.

SYNONYMS

CLL

ICD-10-CM CODES
C91.10 Chronic lymphocytic leukemia of B-cell type not having achieved remission
C91.11 Chronic lymphocytic leukemia of B-cell type in remission
C91.12 Chronic lymphocytic leukemia of B-cell type in relapse

EPIDEMIOLOGY & DEMOGRAPHICS

- Most frequent form of leukemia in Western countries (18,960 new cases and 4660 deaths annually in the U.S.). Incidence rate is 4.6 per 100,000 person-years, increasing to 17 cases per 100,000 at age 65. It is more common in Caucasians and in those with a family history of CLL or other lymphoid malignancy.
- Generally occurs in older patients (67% are >65 years of age). Median age at diagnosis in the U.S. is 71 years.
- Male/female ratio of 2:1.
- CLL accounts for 1.1% of all cancers and 11% of all hematologic neoplasms.
- May be preceded by monoclonal B-cell lymphocytosis—a premalignant, asymptomatic condition with less than 5000 /mm³ CLL-like cells circulating in the blood

PHYSICAL FINDINGS & CLINICAL PRESENTATION

- At presentation most patients are asymptomatic. Many cases are diagnosed on the basis of incidental laboratory results.
- Symptoms include fatigue, recurrent infections (pneumonia, herpes zoster), enlarging lymph nodes.
- B symptoms (fever, weight loss, and drenching night sweats) in 10% of patients at initial presentation.
- Small diffuse lymphadenopathy and splenomegaly are typical findings on clinical examination, but they are absent in a majority of patients at diagnosis.
- A minority of CLL patients (~1%-10%) may develop autoimmune hemolytic anemia or immune thrombocytopenia at diagnosis or during the course of the disease.
- At a rate of 1% per year, CLL patients may experience a transformation of their disease into an aggressive lymphoma (Richter's transformation), characterized by a rapidly growing nodal mass, elevated LDH, and constitutional symptoms.

ETIOLOGY

The etiology of CLL remains largely unknown, although accumulation of genetic defects causing resistance to apoptosis and chronic stimulation of the B-cell receptor by autoantigens or undefined microorganisms have been implicated.

DIAGNOSIS

- The diagnosis of CLL requires presence of >5000/mm³ clonal B-cells, for >3 months, with a characteristic immunophenotype on flow cytometry, which is essential for diagnosis
- CLL cells are typically positive for CD5, CD19, CD23 and weakly positive for CD20, while they are negative for CD10, Cyclin D1, and CD103. In some cases, molecular studies for CLL-specific chromosomal alterations (deletion of chromosome 13q, 11q, 17p or trisomy 12) may be helpful.
- Table 1 describes the evaluation of CLL patients at diagnosis.

DIFFERENTIAL DIAGNOSIS

- Few acute infections with lymphocytosis (mononucleosis, pertussis)
- Other lymphoproliferative disorders that involve blood (can be distinguished using flow cytometry): follicular lymphoma, mantle cell lymphoma, splenic marginal zone lymphoma, prolymphocytic leukemia, adult T-cell lymphoma/leukemia, hairy cell leukemia.
- Acute lymphocytic leukemia can be differentiated by presence of lymphoblasts rather than mature lymphocytes
- Persistent polyclonal B-cell lymphocytosis: a rare, benign condition affecting (predominantly female) middle-aged smokers

LABORATORY TESTS

- Complete blood count demonstrates lymphocytosis with mature lymphocytes and characteristic "smudge cells" on the peripheral smear (Fig. 1); anemia and thrombocytopenia may be present in more advanced cases.
- Bone marrow examination is **not** indicated in most cases, except when differentiation between autoimmune cytopenias and marrow infiltration by CLL is difficult.
- Hypogammaglobulinemia and elevated lactate dehydrogenase may be present at the time of diagnosis.
- Cytogenetic evaluation (using fluorescent *in-situ* hybridization, FISH) is essential for prognostic assessment and optimal treatment selection (Table 2).
- Other prognostic markers include: mutational status of the immunoglobulin heavy chain variable region (*IGHV*, unmutated gene with >98% homology indicates poor prognosis), presence of CD38 or ZAP-70 (also associated with poor prognosis). Additional mutation analysis is gaining importance for identifying patients with worse prognosis (mutations in *TP53, NOTCH1, SF3B1* and *BIRC3* genes).

TABLE 1 Evaluation of Chronic Lymphocytic Leukemia (CLL) Patients at Diagnosis

History

B-symptom and fatigue assessment
Infectious history assessment
Occupational assessment for chemical exposure
Familial history of CLL and lymphoproliferative disorders
Preventive interventions for infections and secondary cancers

Physical Exam with attention to lymph nodes, spleen, liver, and Waldeyer's ring

Laboratory Assessment—Essential

Complete blood count with differential
Morphology assessment of lymphocytes
Kidney and liver function tests, lactate dehydrogenase
Flow cytometry assessment to confirm immunophenotype of CLL
FISH analysis for del 17, del 11q, del 13, and trisomy 12
Hepatitis B screening prior to immunochemotherapy

Selected Tests Under Certain Circumstances

IGVH mutational analysis, CD38 or ZAP-70 expression
TP53 mutation status
Serum immunoglobulins
Serum beta-2-microglobulin levels
Direct antiglobulin test (direct Coombs test), reticulocyte count if anemia present
CT scan of chest, abdomen and pelvis if there is a clinical concern for symptomatic adenopathy, or prior to chemotherapy
PET scan and/or biopsy if large nodal mass with suspected Richter's transformation present
Bone marrow aspirate and biopsy if unexplained cytopenias present
Familial counseling if first-degree relative with CLL

Teaching

Varicella zoster identification instruction
Skin cancer identification
Disease education (Leukemia and Lymphoma Society, CLL Topics, ACOR)

Adapted from Hoffmann R et al: *Hematology: basic principles and practice*, ed 6, Philadelphia, 2013, Elsevier.

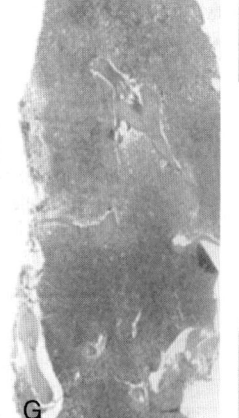
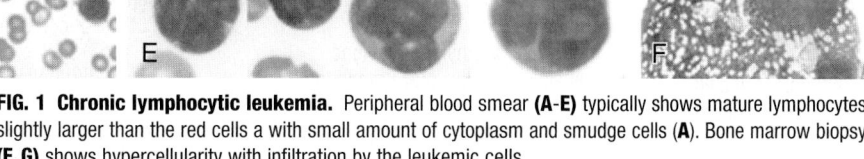

FIG. 1 Chronic lymphocytic leukemia. Peripheral blood smear **(A-E)** typically shows mature lymphocytes slightly larger than the red cells a with small amount of cytoplasm and smudge cells **(A)**. Bone marrow biopsy **(F, G)** shows hypercellularity with infiltration by the leukemic cells.

TABLE 2 Prognosis of Patients With CLL at the Time of Diagnosis, Stratified by Cytogenetic Risk Group

Cytogenetic alteration	Risk group	Percent of patients (some may overlap)	Median time to first chemotherapy	Median survival
Deletion 13q	Favorable	40%-60%	8 yr	11 yr
None	Intermediate	<20%	4 yr	9 yr
Trisomy 12	Intermediate	15%-30%	3 yr	9 yr
Deletion 11q	High	15%-20%	1 yr	7 yr
Deletion 17p	Ultra-high	~10%	<1 yr	3 yr

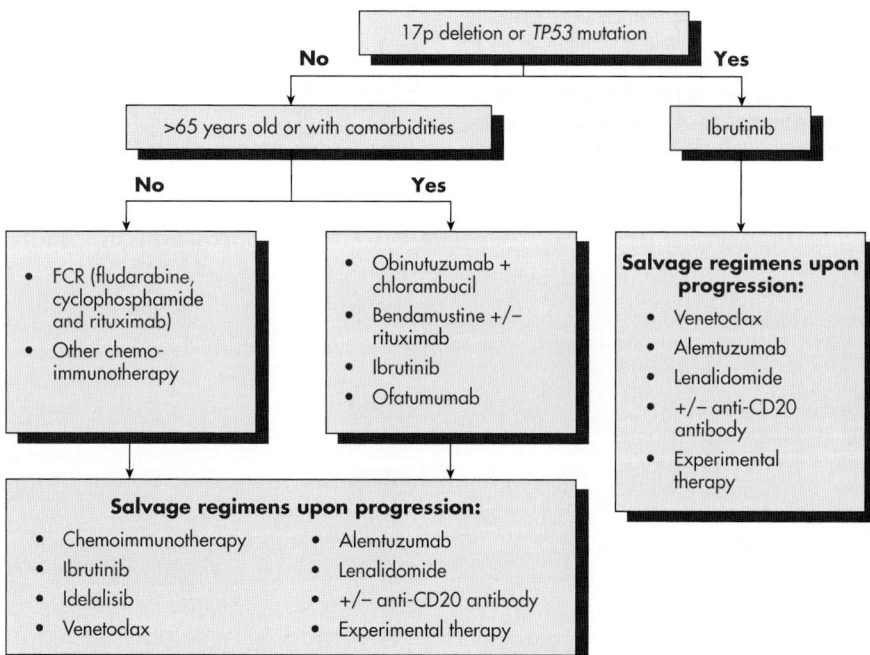

FIG. 2 Treatment approach in chronic lymphocytic leukemia. (Courtesy of **ADAM J. OLSZEWSKI, M.D.**)

STAGING: Staging reflects the clinical burden of disease and aids assessment of prognosis and treatment decision-making. The historical staging systems by Rai and Binet remain in clinical use. They use **only** physical examination and the CBC (i.e., no scans).

The modified Rai system distinguishes three risk groups:
• Low risk (lymphocytosis alone, or Stage 0)
• Intermediate risk (presence of lymphadenopathy, hepatomegaly or splenomegaly, formerly Stage I/II)

• High risk (presence of anemia with hemoglobin <11 g/dL, or thrombocytopenia with platelet count <100,000/mm³, formerly stage III/IV).

The Binet system divides CLL into three stages:
• Stage A: involvement of <3 nodal areas (counting separately cervical, axillary, or inguinal lymph nodes, spleen, and liver).
• Stage B: three or more areas involved.
• Stage C: presence of anemia (hemoglobin <10 g/dl) or thrombocytopenia (<100,000/mm³), independent of the areas involved.

Prognosis in CLL can be determined using the CLL-International Prognostic Index (CLL-IPI), which includes five factors: 17p/*TP53* status, *IGVH* mutational status, serum beta-2-microglobulin, Rai/Binet stage (0/A vs. I-IV/B-C), and age >65 years. Overall 5-year survival varies from 93% for the low-risk group to 23% for the very high risk group.

IMAGING STUDIES

Imaging studies (CT or PET/CT scans) are not necessary for asymptomatic patients at diagnosis. They are obtained in case of clinical concerns for bulky internal adenopathy, Richter's transformation, or prior to starting chemotherapy.

Rx TREATMENT

• At present, there is no standard curative therapy for CLL, so treatment is only instituted for progressive or symptomatic disease with a goal of symptom relief and prolongation of life.
• "Watchful waiting" (i.e., observation without therapy) is the optimal strategy for all early-stage, asymptomatic patients outside of clinical trials because early chemotherapy provides no survival or quality-of-life benefit.
• Immunochemotherapy is the standard of care for patients with symptoms related to disease, bulky adenopathy, rapidly increasing lymphocyte count, or progressive cytopenias (except for autoimmune cytopenias, which can be treated without chemotherapy).

ACUTE GENERAL Rx

- The initial chemotherapy is chosen depending on the patient's age, comorbidities, and CLL cytogenetics (Fig. 2).
- The combination of fludarabine, cyclophosphamide, and rituximab is considered the most active immunochemotherapy regimen; it results in complete remission in 72% of patients, while about 30% remain in remission after 12 years of follow-up. It is considered a standard of care for fit patients younger than 65 years and without *TP53* abnormalities.
- Although chlorambucil was the historical standard for therapy of older patients, randomized controlled trials have now demonstrated improved outcomes of alternative approaches: ibrutinib or combinations of chlorambucil with anti-CD20 antibodies (obinutuzumab or ofatumumab). Fit older patients are often treated with a combination of bendamustine with rituximab. With these regimens, a majority (>80%) of patients achieve at least a partial remission, with median progression-free survival of about 2 to 4 years.
- CLL with deletion 17p or *TP53* mutation does not respond well to standard immunochemotherapy, and alternative agents (B-cell receptor complex inhibitors ibrutinib or idelalisib, anti-CD52 monoclonal antibody alemtuzumab) are recommended. Venetoclax, an oral selective BCL-2 inhibitor, has been FDA-approved for treatment of CLL in patients with 17p deletion who have received at least one prior therapy.
- Recurrent CLL is often characterized by acquired deletion or mutation of the *TP53* gene and can also be treated with a variety of salvage regimens:
  - B-cell receptor complex inhibitors: ibrutinib and idelalisib. These oral agents are characterized by relatively good tolerance, a high rate of durable responses, occasional persistent lymphocytosis, and extremely high cost of therapy.
  - Venetoclax, an oral BCL2 inhibitor, is characterized by a high response rate (79%) and risk of tumor lysis.
  - Anti-CD20 monoclonal antibodies: ofatumumab, obinutuzumab, rituximab, alone or in combination with chemotherapy: purine analogues (fludarabine, pentostatin); alkylating agents (bendamustine, cyclophosphamide, CHOP-like combinations)
  - Alemtuzumab (anti-CD52 monoclonal antibody)
  - High-dose methylprednisolone
  - Lenalidomide (an oral immunomodulatory drug)
  - Palliative radiation therapy to bulky lymph nodes or spleen.
- Allogeneic bone marrow transplantation can be used for younger patients with recurrent, refractory, or ultra-high cytogenetic risk disease, but is associated with high rates of transplant-related mortality

CHRONIC Rx

Treatment of systemic complications:
- Tumor lysis syndrome may occur during initial or subsequent chemotherapy but is extremely unlikely without chemotherapy in CLL, even with high lymphocyte counts.
- CLL patients are at increased risk of solid tumors and should adhere to age-appropriate screening modalities; skin cancers, including melanoma, are particularly common.
- Hypogammaglobulinemia is frequent in CLL and may cause recurrent infections, particularly pneumonias. Immunoglobulin supplementation (250 mg/kg IV every 4 wk) may prevent infections but has no effect on the course of CLL.
- Patients after chemoimmunotherapy are at risk for, and often ultimately succumb to, opportunistic infections. Herpes zoster and *Pneumocystis jiroveci* prophylaxis is used during and after some chemoimmunotherapy regimens.
- Autoimmune hemolytic anemia, thrombocytopenia, and (rare) neutropenia may be treated with steroids, immunoglobulin, or immune suppression without cytotoxic chemotherapy
- Granulocyte colony stimulating factor is often used for older CLL patients to prevent neutropenia infections after chemotherapy.
- CLL is a contraindication to administration of live vaccines (varicella zoster, mumps/measles/rubella, yellow fever, intranasal influenza). Patients should adhere to the recommended schedule of immunization against *Pneumococcus* and influenza.

DISPOSITION

Most patients die due to infectious complications of therapy for refractory disease after several lines of treatment. Histologic transformation to an aggressive lymphoma is also associated with high mortality. Palliative treatment should be offered to patients who are no longer benefitting from aggressive therapy to avoid pervasive and futile treatment with distressing complications.

SUGGESTED READINGS
Available at www.expertconsult.com.

RELATED CONTENT
Chronic Lymphocytic Leukemia (Patient Information)

AUTHOR: **ADAM J. OLSZEWSKI, M.D.**

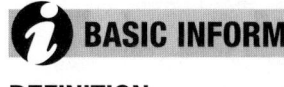

BASIC INFORMATION

DEFINITION

Chronic myelogenous leukemia (CML) is a malignant clonal stem disease. The hallmark of CML is the Philadelphia chromosome, an acquired cytogenetic abnormality arising out of the reciprocal translocation of long arms of the *ABL* and *BCR* genes on chromosomes 9 and 22, resulting in the *BCR:ABL* fusion oncogene. CML is characterized by abnormal myeloid proliferation and accumulation of immature granulocytes. CML manifests with a chronic phase (CP-CML) lasting months to years, which evolves into an advanced phase (AP-CML) characterized by poor response to therapy, worsening anemia, or thrombocytopenia; this phase then evolves into a terminal blast phase (BP) resulting in acute leukemia (70% myeloid and approximately 30% lymphoid subtype). The WHO criteria for accelerated and blast phases of CML are described in Table 1.

SYNONYMS

CML
Chronic granulocytic leukemia
Chronic myeloid leukemia

ICD-10CM CODES
C92.10 Chronic myeloid leukemia, BCR/ABL-positive, not having achieved remission
C92.11 Chronic myeloid leukemia, BCR/ABL-positive, in remission
C92.12 Chronic myeloid leukemia, BCR/ABL-positive, in relapse

EPIDEMIOLOGY & DEMOGRAPHICS

- The median age for CML presentation is usually in the mid-50 year range. It accounts for 15% to 20% of adult leukemias.
- Incidence is 1 to 2 cases per 100,000 people annually.
- In 2016, an estimated 8220 new cases and 1070 deaths will occur in the U.S.

PHYSICAL FINDINGS & CLINICAL PRESENTATION

- Up to 50% patients are asymptomatic, with diagnosis based on abnormal blood counts.
- In chronic phase, symptomatic patients can have fatigue, weight loss, early satiety, and left abdomen pain. Examination can reveal splenomegaly. Occasionally, a very high WBC count may lead to hyperviscosity-related symptoms.
- Patients in accelerated phase are usually symptomatic with fevers, sweats, weight loss, abdomen pain, and progressive splenomegaly.
- Patients in blast phase in addition can have bone pain; symptoms of anemia, infectious complications and bleeding are also present.

ETIOLOGY

The etiology of CML is unclear though radiation exposure has been linked in its development.

TABLE 1 WHO Criteria for Accelerated and Blast Phases of CML

Accelerated phase	Diagnosis can be made if one or more of the following is present: Blasts 10%-19% of peripheral blood white cells or bone marrow cells Peripheral blood basophils at least 20% Persistent thrombocytopenia (<100 × 10⁹/L) unrelated to therapy, or persistent thrombocytosis (>1000 × 10⁹/L) unresponsive to therapy Increasing spleen size and increasing WBC count unresponsive to therapy Cytogenetic evidence of clonal evolution (i.e., the appearance of an additional genetic abnormality that was not present in the initial specimen at the time of diagnosis of chronic phase CML) Megakaryocytic proliferation in sizable sheets and clusters, associated with marked reticulin or collagen fibrosis, and/or severe granulocytic dysplasia, should be considered as suggestive of CML-AP. (These findings have not yet been analyzed in large clinical studies; thus it is not clear whether they are independent criteria for accelerated phase. They often occur simultaneously with one or more of the other features listed.)
Blast crisis	Diagnosis can be made if one or more of following is present: Blasts 30% or more of peripheral blood white cells or bone marrow cells Extramedullary blast proliferation Large foci or clusters of blasts in bone marrow biopsy

From Hoffman R: *Hematology, basic principles and practice*, ed 6, Philadelphia, 2013, Saunders.

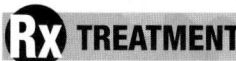

DIFFERENTIAL DIAGNOSIS

- Splenic lymphoma.
- Myeloproliferative syndrome.
- Chronic neutrophilic leukemia.
- Essential thrombocythemia.

LABORATORY TESTS

- CBC showing left-shifted myeloid cells, with broad spectrum and also can be accompanied by thrombocytosis.
- Median leukocyte count of 100,000/microliter with classic "myelocyte bulge" (more myelocytes than the more mature metamyelocytes seen on the blood smear.
- Bone marrow biopsy demonstrates hypercellularity with granulocytic hyperplasia, increased ratio of myeloid cells to erythroid cells, and increased megakaryocytes (Fig. 1).
- Bone marrow cytogenetics demonstrated the 9:22 translocation (Philadelphia chromosome) in >95% of patients (Fig. 2).
- Leukocyte alkaline phosphatase is markedly decreased (unlike other myeloproliferative disorders).
- *BCR-ABL* fusion transcripts can be measured using quantitative RT-PCR technology using either peripheral blood or bone marrow; serial peripheral blood monitoring of transcript level is utilized at 3-month intervals to determine molecular remission status.

RISK STRATIFICATION

- Chronic phase CML patients can be stratified into low-, intermediate-, or high-risk criteria using the Sokal or Hasford criteria; more recently, the EUTOS score has been validated as an effective tool used to stratify patients into low- or high-risk categories.
- Patients developing secondary mutations have variable response to second-line therapies; the T315I mutation is typically associated with resistance and is treated with allogeneic stem cell transplantation

IMAGING STUDIES

Ultrasound or CT scan of abdomen can be done.

TREATMENT

Treatment with a potential to either cure CML or prolong long-term survival should be used according to the phase of the disease.

- Chronic phase: the therapeutic approach involves the use of either a first-generation (imatinib) or second-generation (dasatinib, nilotinib) oral tyrosine kinase inhibitor (TKI). The large majority of patients obtain hematologic and cytogenetic remissions; major molecular remissions are observed in 25%-60% cases. Patients who lose their initial response, develop secondary mutations, or develop intolerance to therapy can be treated with newer third-generation drugs (bosutinib, ponatinib). Accelerated phase: patients are initially treated with second-generation TKIs but ultimately require allogeneic stem cell transplantation.
- Blast phase: patients are initially treated with conventional induction chemotherapy as per the type of evolved acute leukemia and then subsequently undergo allogeneic stem cell transplantation.
- Symptomatic hyperleukocytosis can be treated with leukapheresis and hydroxyurea; allopurinol should be started to prevent urate nephropathy after the rapid lysis of the leukemia cells.
- Interferon-alfa is active in early chronic phase patients but has been replaced by the oral TKIs.

DISPOSITION

- Median survival for patients with chronic phase CML undergoing therapy with current TKIs is estimated to last 25+ years.
- Median survivals for patients with accelerated and blast phase CML are 5 years and 7 to 11 months, respectively.
- Discontinuing oral TKI therapy in chronic phase CML patients who have achieved deep molecular remissions is associated with molecular relapses in up to half the cases; as such, indefinite therapy is preferred in all cases.

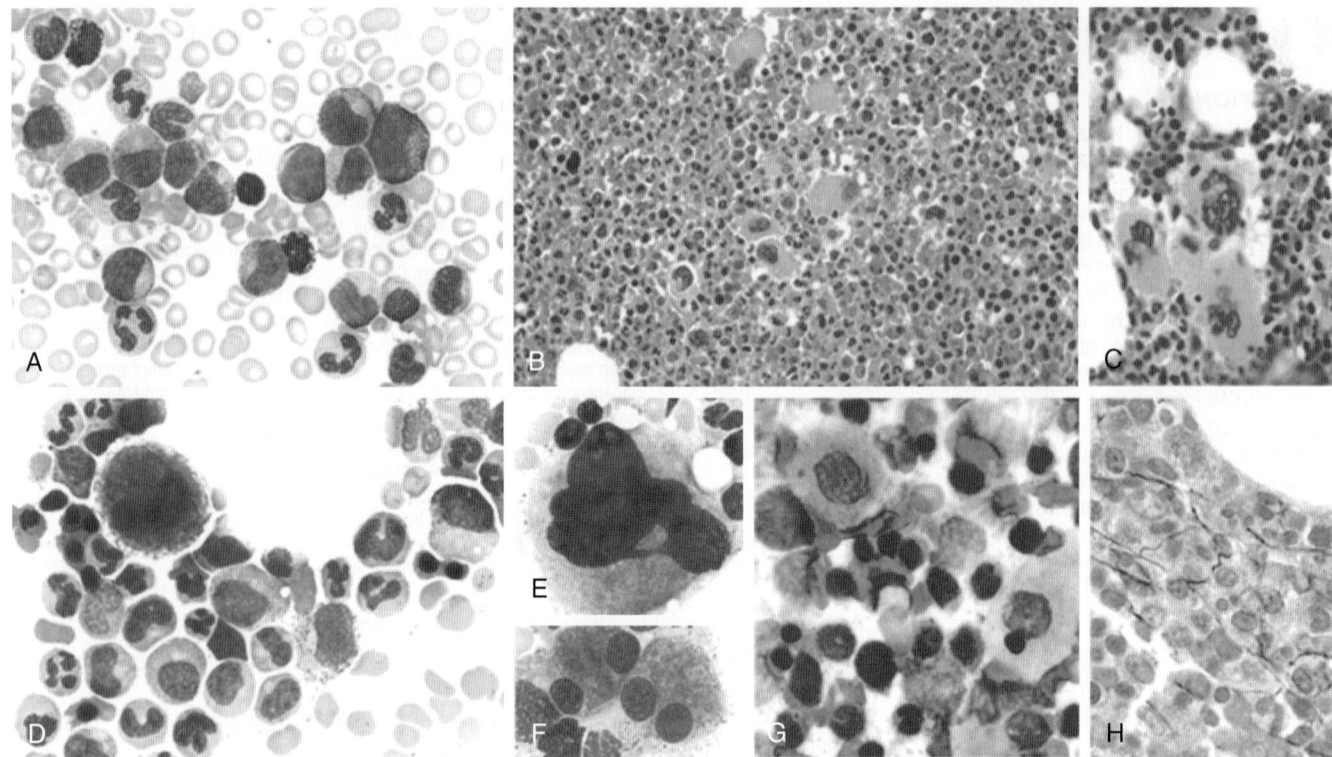

FIG. 1 Chronic myelogenous leukemia, chronic phase. Peripheral smear **(A)** showing marked leukocytosis due to a granulocytic proliferation of all stages with particularly increased myelocytes and absolute basophilia. Bone core biopsy **(B)** illustrating markedly hypercellular marrow due to granulocytic proliferation and increased small hypolobated megakaryocytes. Compare with large megakaryocytes **(C)** from a myeloproliferative disorder other than CML. Bone marrow aspirate **(D)** showing granulocytic proliferation and small, "dwarf" megakaryocyte, compared with large-sized megakaryocyte **(E)** and micro-megakaryocytes **(F)** typical of MDS. Pseudo-Gaucher cells **(G)** and mild fibrosis **(H)** as seen on reticulin stain. (From Hoffman R, et al.: *Hematology: basic principles and practice,* ed 5, Philadelphia, 2009, Churchill Livingstone.)

REFERRAL

- To hematology physician.

PEARLS

- Chronic phase CML patients should be risk-stratified at diagnosis to define prognosis upfront; patients achieving complete cytogenetic remission or major molecular remission by 12 months have consistently superior long-term outcomes.
- Regular monitoring of molecular response using peripheral blood RT-PCR for BCR:ABL transcript levels is done every 3 to 6 months for disease monitoring.
- Allogeneic stem cell transplantation is a useful modality for advanced CML patients and chronic phase CML patients who develop resistance to standard TKI therapy.

SUGGESTED READINGS

Available at www.expertconsult.com

RELATED CONTENT

Chronic Myelogenous Leukemia (Patient Information)

AUTHOR: **RITESH RATHORE, M.D.**

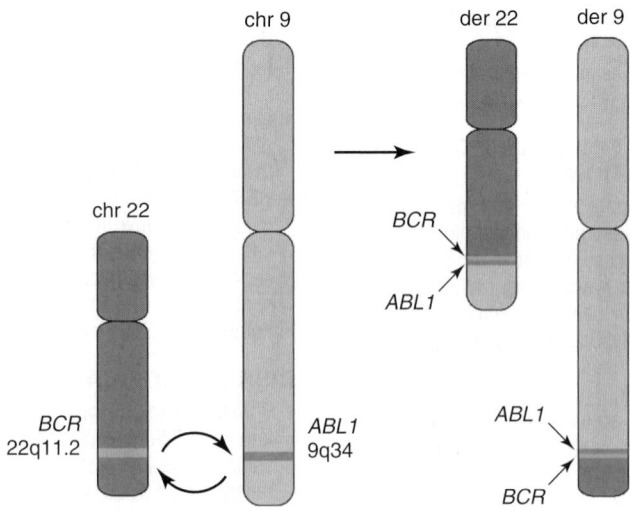

FIG. 2 The Philadelphia chromosome, der(22q), results from the reciprocal translocation of a portion of the *ABL1* gene on chromosome 9 at band q34 to the region of the *BCR* gene on chromosome 22 at band q11.2. In turn, a portion of *BCR* is translocated to chromosome 9 to the region of *ABL1*. In 5% to 10% of patients with chronic myelogenous leukemia, cryptic or complex rearrangements result in a *BCR-ABL1* fusion gene, even though no Philadelphia chromosome is detected cytogenetically. (From Jaffe ES, et al.: *Hematopathology,* Philadelphia, 2011, Saunders.)

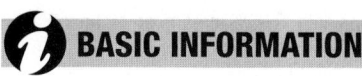 BASIC INFORMATION

DEFINITION

Oral hairy leukoplakia (OHL) is a painless, white, nonremovable, plaquelike lesion typically located on the lateral aspect of the tongue.

SYNONYMS

Oral hairy leukoplakia
OHL

ICD-10CM CODES
K13.3 Hairy leukoplakia

EPIDEMIOLOGY & DEMOGRAPHICS

INCIDENCE AND PREVALENCE: EBV is implicated in the etiology of OHL, and the incidence of Epstein-Barr virus (EBV) seroprevalence is high in individuals who are HIV seropositive. However, OHL occurs in only 25% of these cases.

RISK FACTORS: OHL is usually found in HIV-seropositive individuals (median CD4 count is 468/mL) but may also be identified in smokers and other immunocompromised patients such as transplant recipients (particularly renal) and patients taking steroids. Diagnosing OHL is an indication to institute a workup to evaluate and manage HIV disease.

PHYSICAL FINDINGS & CLINICAL PRESENTATION

- Varying morphology and appearance, which may change daily.
- May be unilateral or bilateral.
- White plaques can be small with fine, vertical corrugations on the lateral margin of the tongue (Fig. 1). The plaques from OHL are adherent to the tongue surface (in contrast to candidal plaques, which may be easily scraped off).
- Irregular surface; may have prominent folds or projection, occasionally markedly resembling hairs.

- May spread to cover the entire dorsal surface or spread onto the ventral surface of the tongue where the lesions usually appear flat.
- Rarely, lesions can manifest on the soft palate, buccal mucosa, or posterior oropharynx.
- Usually asymptomatic, but some patients have mouth pain, soreness, or a burning sensation; impaired taste; or difficulty eating; others complain of its unsightly appearance.
- OHL may rarely progress to oral squamous cell carcinoma particularly in smokers, which has a poor prognosis.

ETIOLOGY

EBV is implicated in its etiology, and OHL is a result of replication EBV in the epithelium of keratinized cells. OHL differs from most EBV-related diseases in that infection is predominantly lytic, with abundant virus production results in cell lysis, rather than latent.

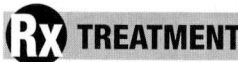 DIAGNOSIS

DIFFERENTIAL DIAGNOSIS

- *Candida albicans*
- Lichen planus
- Idiopathic leukoplakia
- White sponge nevus
- Dysplasia
- Squamous cell carcinoma

WORKUP

Requires physical examination and evaluation of HIV disease

LABORATORY TESTS

The *provisional* diagnosis is clinical and based on:
- Visual inspection
- Inability to scrape the lesion off the tongue with a blade
- Failure to respond to antifungal therapy

The *presumptive* diagnosis requires biopsy and histologic demonstration of:
- Epithelial hyperplasia with hairs
- Absence of inflammatory cell infiltrate

The *definitive* diagnosis requires:
- In situ hybridization of histologic or cytologic specimens revealing EBV DNA or
- Electron microscopy of specimens revealing herpes-like particles
- Measurement of the DNA content in cells of oral leukoplakia may be used to predict the risk of oral carcinoma

NOTE: Specimens obtained from lesions may demonstrate hyphae of *Candida albicans,* which may coexist and potentiate EBV-induced OHL.

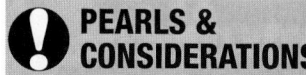 TREATMENT

NONPHARMACOLOGIC THERAPY

OHL is usually asymptomatic and requires no specific therapy. It may resolve spontaneously and is generally benign in HIV-seropositive patients.

ACUTE GENERAL Rx

- Antiretroviral therapy (ART) has considerably changed the frequency of oral lesions caused by opportunistic infections in HIV-seropositive individuals.
- Topical retinoids (0.1% vitamin A) may improve the appearance of OHL-affected oral surfaces through their dekeratinizing and immunomodulation effects; however, they are expensive and prolonged use may result in a burning sensation over the treated area.
- Topical podophyllin resin 25% solution has been reported to induce resolution.
- Surgical excision and cryotherapy may help, but the lesions may recur.
- High-dose acyclovir 800 mg five times per day, valacyclovir 1000 mg tid, famciclovir 500 mg tid, ganciclovir 1000 mg tid, or foscarnet 40 mg/kg IV tid will cause lesions to resolve but only temporarily.

⚠ PEARLS & CONSIDERATIONS

- OHL may be the presenting sign of patients infected with HIV who are unaware of their status.
- The incidence has decreased significantly in the era of ART.

RELATED CONTENT

Oral Hairy Leukoplakia (Patient Information)
Epstein-Barr Virus Infection (Related Key Topic)
Human Immunodeficiency Virus (Related Key Topic)

AUTHOR: **SAJEEV HANDA, M.D.**

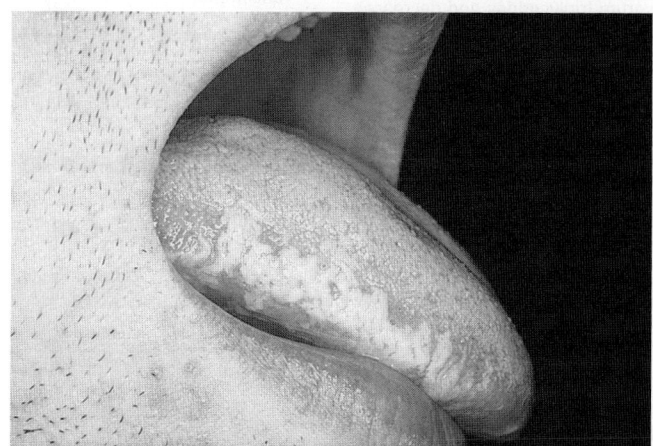

FIG. 1 Oral hairy leukoplakia. Note white verrucoid plaques on the lateral border of the tongue. (From Noble J: *Primary care medicine*, ed 3, St Louis, 2001, Mosby.)

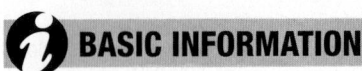

BASIC INFORMATION

DEFINITION

Lichen planus (LP) refers to an idiopathic inflammatory disease manifesting with a papular skin eruption characteristically found over the flexor surfaces of the extremities, genitalia, and mucous membranes.

SYNONYMS

Lichen
Lichen planus et atrophicus
LP

ICD-10CM CODES
L43 Lichen planus
L43.0 Hypertrophic lichen planus
L43.1 Bullous lichen planus
L43.9 Lichen planus, unspecified
L43.8 Other lichen planus

EPIDEMIOLOGY & DEMOGRAPHICS

INCIDENCE: One in every 100 new patients seen in dermatology clinics in the United States is diagnosed with LP.
PREVALENCE: 440 cases/100,000 persons
PREDOMINANT SEX: Found equally between males and females (1:1).
PREDOMINANT AGE: Usually found in people between the ages of 30 and 60 yr.
PREDISPOSING FACTORS:
- Associated with other autoimmune disorders (e.g., primary biliary cirrhosis, myasthenia gravis, ulcerative colitis, diabetes).
- Associated with hepatitis C infection.
- Drug-induced form affects any area of the body surface (e.g., beta-blocker, methyldopa, penicillamine, quinidine, nonsteroidal anti-inflammatory drugs, angiotensin-converting enzyme inhibitors, sulfonylurea agents).

PHYSICAL FINDINGS & CLINICAL PRESENTATION

The clinical presentation varies depending on the area involved.
History:
- Usually starts on an extremity and may remain localized or spread to involve other areas over a 1- to 4-mo period.
- Pruritic.
  Physical findings:
- Anatomic distribution:
  1. Flexor surface of wrists, forearms, shins, and upper thighs.
  2. Neck and back area.
  3. Nails (5%-10% of patients).
  4. Scalp (lichen planopilaris).
  5. Oral mucosa, buccal mucosa, tongue, gingiva, and lips; oral lichen planus can cause extensive desquamative gingivitis.
  6. Vulva, penis (Fig. E1).
  Genital mucosa:
- Lesion configuration:
  1. Linear.
  2. Annular (more common).

  3. Reticular pattern noted on oral mucosa and genital area.
- Lesion morphology:
  1. Papules most common presentation (flat, smooth, shiny) (Fig. E2)
  2. Hypertrophic
  3. Follicular
  4. Vesicular
- Color:
  1. Dark red, bluish red, purplish-violaceous color is noted in cutaneous LP.
  2. Individual lesions characteristically have white lines visible (Wickham's striae) (Fig. E3).
  3. Oral and genital LP has a reticular network of white lines that may be raised or annular in appearance.
- Scalp lesions may result in alopecia.

ETIOLOGY

Lichen planus is characterized by an immunologic reaction mediated by CD8+ T cells. These cells induce keratinocytes to undergo apoptosis. Although the inflammatory reaction is believed to be autoimmune, the antigen targeted by these effector T lymphocytes is unknown.

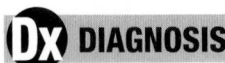 DIAGNOSIS

- Clinical history and physical findings usually establish the diagnosis of LP.
- Skin biopsy (deep shave or punch biopsy of the most developed lesion) can be performed to confirm the diagnosis.

DIFFERENTIAL DIAGNOSIS

- Drug eruption, psoriasis, Bowen's disease, leukoplakia, candidiasis, lupus rash, secondary syphilis, seborrheic dermatitis, chronic graft-versus-host disease

WORKUP

If the diagnosis is questionable, a skin biopsy is performed.

LABORATORY TESTS

Laboratory tests are not specific for the diagnosis of LP. Lipid panels screening is useful since increases in serum triglycerides and decreases in HDL cholesterol are common in patients with LP.

IMAGING STUDIES

Imaging studies are not helpful in diagnosing LP.

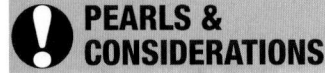 TREATMENT

NONPHARMACOLOGIC THERAPY

- Avoid scratching.
- Use mild soaps and emollients after bathing to prevent dryness.

GENERAL Rx

For cutaneous LP:
- Topical steroids (e.g., triamcinolone acetonide 0.1%, fluocinonide 0.05%, clobetasol propionate 0.05% cream or ointment) with occlusion used twice daily.
- Acitretin 30 mg/day PO for 8 wk.
- Systemic prednisone 30 to 60 mg/day as a starting dose and tapered to 15 to 20 mg/day maintenance for 6 wk can be used for widespread lesions.
- Intradermal steroid triamcinolone acetonide 5 mg/mL can be tried for thick hyperkeratotic lesions.
- Hydroxyzine 25 mg PO q6h can be used for pruritus.
- Phototherapy: PUVA or narrow-band ultraviolet B therapy: 2 or 3 times per week, for a total of 12 sessions (i.e., one cycle).

For oral LP:
- Topical steroid fluocinonide in an adhesive base used six times/day for 9 wk.
- Topical calcineurin in steroid-unresponsive cases.
- Topical or systemic retinoids 0.1% retinoic acid in an adhesive base or gel.
- Etretinate 75 mg/day for 2 mo.

DISPOSITION

- Spontaneous remissions of cutaneous LP occur in >65% of cases within the first year.
- Spontaneous remission of oral LP usually occurs by 5 yr.
- Approximately 10% to 20% of patients will have recurrence.

REFERRAL

To dermatologist if diagnosis is unclear

PEARLS & CONSIDERATIONS

COMMENTS

- LP can be remembered as purple, planar, pruritic, polygonal, papules, and plaques (six Ps).
- Lesions can develop at the site of prior skin injury (Koebner's phenomenon).
- Although there is an increased risk of squamous cell carcinoma in chronic lesions of mucosal LP, transformation to skin cancer is uncommon.

SUGGESTED READINGS

Available at www.expertconsult.com

RELATED CONTENT

Lichen Planus (Patient Information)

AUTHOR: **TANYA ALI, M.D.**

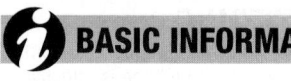 BASIC INFORMATION

DEFINITION

Lichen sclerosus (LS) is a chronic inflammatory condition of the skin usually affecting the vulva, penis, perianal area, and groin.

SYNONYMS

Lichen sclerosus et atrophicus
Kraurosis vulvae
Balanitis xerotica obliterans
LS

ICD-10CM CODES
L90.0 Lichen sclerosus et atrophicus

EPIDEMIOLOGY & DEMOGRAPHICS

- Most common in postmenopausal women and men between ages 40 and 60 yr.
- More common in females (female/male ratio of 5:1). It affects 1.7% of the general adult female population.
- Can occur in children (usually prepubertal girls with involvement of the vulva and perineum).

PHYSICAL FINDINGS & CLINICAL PRESENTATION

- Erythema may be the only initial sign. A characteristic finding is the presence of ivory-white atrophic lesions on the involved area.
- Close inspection of the affected area will reveal the presence of white-to-brown follicular plugs on the surface (dells).
- When the genitals are involved, the white, parchment-like skin assumes an hourglass configuration around the introital and perianal area ("keyhole" distribution; Fig. 1). Inflammation, subepithelial hemorrhages, and chronic ulceration may develop.
- In males, lesions are atrophic and may be hypopigmented or depigmented, resembling vitiligo. Phimosis and paraphimosis are common complications in uncircumcised males with LS.
- Lesions may be surrounded by an erythematous to violaceous halo.

- Dyspareunia, genital bleeding, and anal bleeding are common.
- Pruritus may be a prominent symptom.

ETIOLOGY

Unknown. There may be an autoimmune association and a genetic familial component.

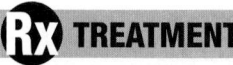 DIAGNOSIS

DIFFERENTIAL DIAGNOSIS

- Localized scleroderma (morphea).
- Cutaneous discoid lupus erythematosus.
- Atrophic lichen planus.
- Psoriasis.
- Lichen simplex chronicus.
- Vulvar intraepithelial neoplasm.
- Extramammary Paget's disease.

WORKUP

Diagnosis is based on close examination of the lesions for the presence of ivory-white atrophic lesions and typical location.

LABORATORY TESTS

- Punch or deep shave biopsy can be used to confirm the diagnosis.
- Autoantibodies to extracellular matrix protein 1 (ECM-1) are present in 80% of LS patients and the ECM-1 titer correlates with disease activity.

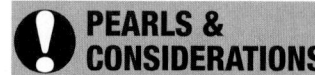 TREATMENT

NONPHARMACOLOGIC THERAPY

- Attention to hygiene and elimination of irritants or excessive bathing with harsh soaps.
- Cryotherapy and photodynamic therapy can be used in refractory cases.

GENERAL Rx

- Application of clobetasol propionate 0.05% topically bid for up to 4 wk is usually effective. Repeat courses of corticosteroids may be necessary because of the chronic nature of this disorder. Continual application of topical steroids may lead to atrophy of the vulva.

- There is no substantial evidence that use of topical sex hormones (e.g., topical testosterone [2%]) is effective in genital lichen sclerosus.
- Lubricants (e.g., Nutraplus cream) are useful to soothe dry tissues.
- Hydroxyzine 25 mg at bedtime is effective in decreasing nocturnal itching.
- Use of intralesional steroids, etretinate, and surgical management is usually reserved for refractory cases.

DISPOSITION

- The disease persists in approximately one third of patients.
- Most prepubertal girls improve spontaneously at menarche.
- Squamous cell carcinoma can develop within the lesions in 3% to 10% of older patients; therefore periodic examination and biopsy of suspicious areas are indicated.

! PEARLS & CONSIDERATIONS

COMMENTS

- Prepubertal lichen sclerosus may be confused with sexual abuse in prepubertal girls and may lead to false accusations and investigations.
- Pregnancy leads to improvement and often complete resolution of lesions, suggesting a hormonal component to etiology of lesions.
- Lichen sclerosus of the vulva (kraurosis vulvae) usually occurs after menopause and is generally chronic. It can be painful and interfere with sexual activity.
- Lichen sclerosus of the penis (balanitis xerotica obliterans) is seen more commonly in uncircumcised males. It affects the glans and prepuce and may lead to stricture if it encroaches into the urinary meatus.

SUGGESTED READING
Available at www.expertconsult.com

RELATED CONTENT
Lichen Sclerosus (Patient Information)

AUTHOR: **FRED F. FERRI, M.D.**

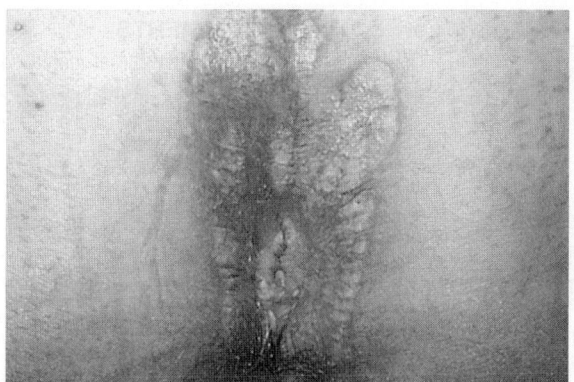

FIG. 1 Lichen sclerosus. Perianal area is thinned and chalk white (keyhole distribution). (Courtesy Department of Dermatology, University of North Carolina at Chapel Hill. From Goldstein BG, Goldstein AO: *Practical dermatology*, ed 2, St Louis, 1997, Mosby.)

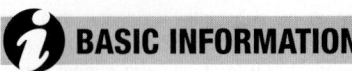

DEFINITION

Lichen simplex chronicus is neurodermatitis manifesting with localized areas of thickened, hyperplastic scaly skin due to prolonged and severe scratching in patients with no underlying dermatologic condition.

SYNONYMS

Neurodermatitis from rubbing
Circumscribed neurodermatitis

ICD-10CM CODES
L28.0 Lichen simplex chronicus

EPIDEMIOLOGY & DEMOGRAPHICS

PEAK INCIDENCE: Between 35 and 50 yr old
PREVALENCE: Increased in patients with underlying anxiety disorders
PREDOMINANT SEX AND AGE:
- Sex: Females > males (2:1)
- Age: Adults over 60

RISK FACTORS: Anxiety disorders, dry skin, insect bites

PHYSICAL FINDINGS & CLINICAL PRESENTATION

- Patients present with profound pruritus and localized scaly plaques with accentuated skin markings said to resemble tree bark (Fig. 1).
- Lichenified circumscribed plaques. Trauma from rubbing and scratching accounts for persistence of the plaque.
- Commonly involved areas include hands and wrists (Fig. 2), back and sides of neck, anterior tibias, anogenital areas, the scalp, the upper eyelid, the orifice of both ears, and ankles.

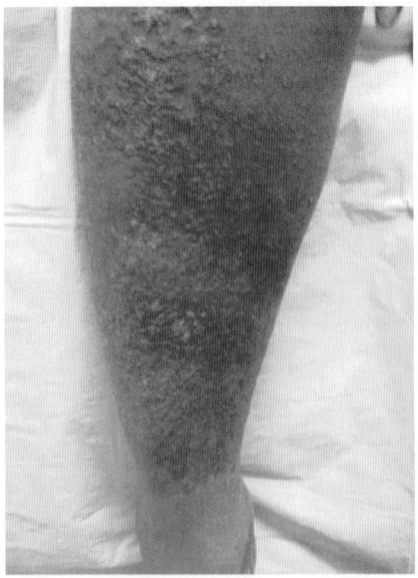

FIG. 1 Lichenified skin of the lower extremity caused by habitual rubbing. The confluence of multiple scaling papules has formed a large plaque of palpably thickened skin. (From Ferri FF et al: *Ferri's fast facts in dermatology,* Philadelphia, 2010, Saunders.)

ETIOLOGY

- Neurodermatitis due to long-term chronic rubbing and scratching more vigorously than a normal pain threshold would allow, resulting in thickened and leathery skin.
- Common triggers are excess dryness of skin, heat, sweat, and psychological stress. It can also accompany other conditions such as the fungal infections candidiasis or tinea cruris, or psoriasis, lichen sclerosus, and neoplasia, leading to squamous cell hyperplasia.
- Other causes include atrophic dermatitis and insect bites. Rare cases have shown links to lithium use, hair dye containing PPD, and long-term exposure to vehicle pollution.

Dx DIAGNOSIS

DIFFERENTIAL DIAGNOSIS

- Lichen planus
- Psoriasis
- Atopic dermatitis
- Insect bite
- Nummular eczema
- Contact dermatitis
- Stasis dermatitis

WORKUP

Patient history and skin examination. Skin biopsy when diagnosis is unclear or persistent symptoms.

LABORATORY TESTS

- Not generally necessary.
- Biopsy reveals hyperkeratosis, acanthosis, and mild to moderate lymphohistiocytic inflammatory infiltrate with prominent lichenification.

Rx TREATMENT

NONPHARMACOLOGIC THERAPY

- Patient education is essential to break the itch-scratch cycle and facilitate treatment of any underlying dermatitis.
- Psychotherapy.

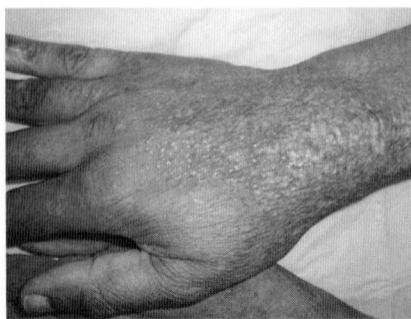

FIG. 2 Long-standing pruritus and scratching resulted in this thickened, hyperpigmented skin on the wrist consisting of numerous 1- to 2-mm papules. This "follicular" pattern is more common in African Americans. (From Ferri FF et al: *Ferri's fast facts in dermatology,* Philadelphia, 2010, Saunders.)

ACUTE GENERAL Rx

- Cessation of pruritus is the goal. Antihistamine hydroxyzine 25 mg at bedtime is effective in decreasing nocturnal itching.
- High-potency topical corticosteroids can be used initially but not indefinitely because of potential for steroid-induced atrophy.
- Steroid-containing tape may be effective in providing both occlusion and antiinflammatory effect.
- Intralesional corticosteroids.
- Anxiolytics, SSRIs.
- Oral doxepin (an antidepressant and anxiolytic).
- Mirtazapine.
- Tropical calcineurin inhibitor for vulvar lichenification.
- Cyclosporin A
- Topical tacrolimus, 0.1% ointment, can be used for sensitive skin, face.
- Botulinum intradermal injections.
- Alitretinoin, 30 mg daily for 3 mo, has shown some clinical improvement in case studies but needs further investigation as a potential Rx.

CHRONIC Rx

Constant irritation of the skin must be avoided. Keeping skin moisturized, covering to prevent scratching, or filing nails may be necessary.

DISPOSITION

Psychological intervention improves recovery. Regular follow-up visits facilitate long-term management.

REFERRAL

Refer to a psychologist for psychological evaluation and consultation, and a dermatologist in resistant cases.

! PEARLS & CONSIDERATIONS

- Significant scratching may occur during nocturnal hours.
- The involved area is always at a site that is easily reached for scratching.
- Chronic scratching can also cause keratinocyte necrosis and the development of amyloid in the papillary dermis, called lichen amyloidosis.

COMMENTS

Patients may be at increased risk for scarring of the skin, changes in skin pigmentation, and bacterial and fungal infections of the involved skin.

PREVENTION

Prevent future incidences by continued therapy, stress management, and avoidance of common triggers and accompanying conditions.

AUTHORS: **FRED F. FERRI, M.D.,** and **HEATHER FERRI, D.O.**

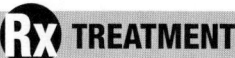

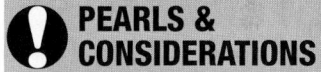 BASIC INFORMATION

DEFINITION

Listeriosis is a systemic infection caused by the gram-positive aerobic bacterium *Listeria monocytogenes*. The range of clinical syndromes varies from gastroenteritis to life-threatening meningitis and tends to be more severe in immunocompromised patients and in patients who are pregnant.

SYNONYMS

Listerial infection
Granulomatosis infantisepticum

ICD-10CM CODES
A32	Listeriosis
A32.0	Cutaneous listeriosis
A32.11	Listeria meningitis
A32.81	Oculoglandular listeriosis
A32.89	Other forms of listeriosis
P37.2	Neonatal (disseminated) listeriosis

EPIDEMIOLOGY & DEMOGRAPHICS

INCIDENCE (IN U.S.):
- *Listeria* meningitis: about 0.7 cases/100,000 persons (fourth most common cause of community-acquired bacterial meningitis in adults).
- In pregnant women: 3.0 cases per 100,000 population.
- In general population: 0.29 confirmed cases per 100,000 persons in 2009-2011 in the United States, but 1.3 per 100,000 cases in persons over the age of 65.

PREDOMINANT SEX: Pregnant women are more susceptible to *Listeria* bacteremia, accounting for up to one third of reported cases.

PREDOMINANT AGE:
- Pregnant women
- Immunocompromised patients of any age
- Elderly patients are susceptible even in the absence of recognized immunocompromised states

GENETICS: Congenital infection:
- With transplacental transmission, syndrome termed *granulomatosis infantisepticum* in neonate
- Characterized by disseminated abscesses in multiple organs, skin lesions, and conjunctivitis
- Mortality: 33% to 100%

Neonatal infection:
- Infant becoming ill after 3 days of age; mother invariably asymptomatic
- Clinical picture of sepsis of unknown origin

PHYSICAL FINDINGS & CLINICAL PRESENTATION

Infections in pregnancy
1. More common in third trimester
2. Usually present with fever and chills without localizing symptoms or signs of infection

Meningoencephalitis
1. More common in neonates and immunocompromised patients, but up to 30% of adults have no underlying condition

2. In neonates: poor appetite with or without fever possibly the only presenting signs
3. In adults: presentation often subacute, with low-grade fever and personality change as only signs
4. Focal neurologic signs seen without demonstrable brain abscess on CT scan

Cerebritis/rhombencephalitis
1. Headache and fever may be only presenting complaints
2. Progressive cranial nerve palsies, hemiparesis, seizures, depressed level of consciousness, cerebellar signs, respiratory insufficiency may also be seen

Focal infections
1. Ocular infections (purulent conjunctivitis) and skin lesions (granulomatosis infantisepticum) as a result of inadvertent inoculation by laboratory and veterinary personnel
2. Others: arthritis, prosthetic joint infections, peritonitis, osteomyelitis, organ abscesses, cholecystitis

ETIOLOGY

- Listeria is a gram-positive rod that acts as a facultative intracellular parasite that helps protect the cell from host innate and adaptive immune responses. The primary habitat for the bacterium is soil and decaying vegetable matter.
- Direct invasion of skin and eye has been documented, but mechanism of GI entry is unclear.
- Organism's intracellular life cycle explanatory of:
  1. Importance of cell-mediated immunity in host defense
  2. Increased infection in neonates, pregnant women, and immunocompromised hosts

DX DIAGNOSIS

DIFFERENTIAL DIAGNOSIS

- Meningitis caused by other bacteria, mycobacteria, or fungi
- CNS sarcoidosis
- Brain neoplasm or abscess
- Tuberculous and fungal (especially cryptococcal) meningitis
- Cerebral toxoplasmosis
- Lyme disease
- Sarcoidosis

LABORATORY TESTS

- Cultures of blood and other appropriate body fluids
- Variable CSF findings, but neutrophils usually predominate
- Organisms uncommonly seen on Gram stain and may be difficult to identify morphologically
- Monoclonal antibodies, polymerase chain reaction, and DNA probe techniques to detect *Listeria* in foods

IMAGING STUDIES

- If focal cerebral involvement suspected: CT scan or MRI
- MRI most sensitive for evaluation of brainstem and cerebellum

Rx TREATMENT

Empiric therapy should be administered when diagnosis is suspected because overall mortality is 23%.

ACUTE GENERAL Rx

- Drugs of choice:
  1. IV ampicillin 2 g IV q 4 hr for adults. Children: 300 mg/kg per day IV in 4 to 6 divided doses. Infants 8 days to 1 month: 150 to 200 mg/kg per day divided in four doses. For infants ≤7 days: 100 mg/kg per day divided in two doses for infants weighing <2000 g and 150 mg/kg per day divided in three doses for infants weighing more than 2000 g.
  2. IV penicillin 12 to 24 million U/day in divided doses.
- Continuation of therapy for 2 weeks for bacteremia; 2 to 4 weeks for meningitis.
- Alternative (if penicillin allergic): trimethoprim/sulfamethoxazole (10-20 mg/kg based on trimethoprim component) IV per day divided every 6-12 hr or vancomycin.
- Gentamicin IV added to provide synergy in meningitis or endocarditis patients of any age (adults: 3 mg/kg per day IV in three divided doses and for children and infants will depend on age and weight).

CHRONIC Rx

Relapses reported, especially in immunocompromised hosts, after 2 wk of therapy.

REFERRAL

Infectious disease consultation for all patients.

! PEARLS & CONSIDERATIONS

COMMENTS

- Foodborne cases have been linked to various products in recent years: coleslaw, soft cheeses, unpasteurized milk and milk products, vegetables, undercooked chicken, hot dogs, luncheon meats, refrigerated smoked seafood, caramel apples, cantaloupes, and so on.
- Complete decontamination of food products is difficult because *Listeria* is resistant to pasteurization and refrigeration.
- Immunocompromised states include glucocorticoid use, anti-TNF therapies, malignancies (hematologic and solid), AIDS, end-stage renal disease, iron overload, collagen vascular diseases, liver disease, and alcoholism.

SUGGESTED READINGS

Available at www.expertconsult.com

RELATED CONTENT

Listeriosis (Patient Information)

AUTHOR: **GLENN G. FORT, M.D., M.P.H.**

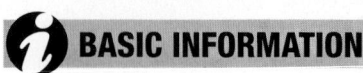

DEFINITION

Liver abscess is a necrotic infection of the liver usually classified as pyogenic or amebic.

SYNONYMS

Pyogenic hepatic abscess
Amebic hepatic abscess

ICD-10CM CODES
K75.0 Abscess of liver

EPIDEMIOLOGY & DEMOGRAPHICS

INCIDENCE: Incidence of pyogenic liver abscess is 2.3 cases per 100,000 population.
PREVALENCE (WORLDWIDE): Amebic liver abscess is more common than pyogenic liver abscess.
PREVALENCE (IN U.S.): Pyogenic liver abscess is more common than amebic liver abscess.
PREDOMINANT SEX AND AGE: More common in men than women; male/female ratio of 2:1; most common in fourth to sixth decades of life.

PHYSICAL FINDINGS & CLINICAL PRESENTATION

- Fever, chills, and sweats
- Weakness/malaise
- Anorexia with weight loss
- Nausea, vomiting, and diarrhea
- Cough with pleuritic chest pain
- Right upper quadrant abdominal pain
- Hepatomegaly
- Splenomegaly
- Jaundice
- Pleural effusions, rales, and friction rubs may be present
- Most abscesses occur on the right lobe of the liver

ETIOLOGY

- Pyogenic liver abscess is usually polymicrobial (*Klebsiella pneumoniae* [43%], *Escherichia coli* [33%], *Streptococcus* spp. [37%], *Pseudomonas aeruginosa*, *Proteus* spp., *Bacteroides* spp. [24%], *Fusobacterium* spp., *Actinomyces* spp., gram-positive anaerobes, and *Staphylococcus aureus*).
- Pyogenic liver abscess occurs from:
  1. Biliary disease with cholangitis (accounts for approximately 40%-60%).
  2. Gallbladder disease with contiguous spread to the liver.
  3. Diverticulitis or appendicitis with spread via the portal circulation.
  4. Hematogenous spread via the hepatic artery, though uncommon; if a solitary organism is isolated, a distant source of hematogenous seeding should be sought.
  5. Penetrating wounds.
  6. Cryptogenic.
  7. Infection by way of portal system (portal pyemia).
  8. No causes found in approximately half of cases.
  9. Incidence increased in patients with diabetes and metastatic cancer.
  10. Table 1 summarizes underlying etiology and bacteriology of liver abscesses.
- Amebic hepatic abscess is caused by the parasite *Entamoeba histolytica*. Amebiasis is usually due to fecal-oral contamination and invades the intestinal mucosa, gaining entry into the portal system to reach the liver. Amebic abscess occurs in 3% to 7% of patients with amebiasis.

Box 1 describes pearls for amebic liver abscesses. The abscess is usually solitary (85%) and in the right lobe (72%).

DIAGNOSIS

The diagnosis of liver abscess requires a high index of suspicion after a detailed history and physical examination. Imaging studies and microbiologic, serologic, and percutaneous techniques (e.g., aspiration) confirm the presence of a liver abscess.

DIFFERENTIAL DIAGNOSIS

- Cholangitis
- Cholecystitis
- Diverticulitis
- Appendicitis

TABLE 1 Underlying Etiology and Bacteriology

Etiology	Bacteriology
Biliary, benign	*Escherichia coli* *Klebsiella* spp. *Enterococcus*
Biliary, malignant	*Pseudomonas* spp. Multiply resistant GN aerobes VRE Yeast
Diverticulitis/ appendicitis	GN aerobes *Bacteroides fragilis*
Severe cholecystitis	See Biliary, benign *Clostridium perfringens* *Bacteroides* spp.
Subcutaneous abscess	*Staphylococcus* spp. MRSA
Endocarditis	*Enterococcus* spp. *Staphylococcus* spp.
Cryptogenic	Anaerobes

GN, Gram-negative.
From Cameron, JL, Cameron AM: *Current surgical therapy*, ed 10, Philadelphia, 2011, Saunders.

- Perforated viscus
- Mesentery ischemia
- Pulmonary embolism
- Pancreatitis

WORKUP

- The workup of a liver abscess should focus on differentiating between amebic and pyogenic causes.
- Features suggesting an amebic cause include travel to an endemic area, single abscess rather than multiple abscesses, subacute onset of symptoms, and absence of conditions predisposing to pyogenic liver abscess, as highlighted under "Etiology."
- Laboratory studies are not specific but are useful as adjunctive tests.
- Imaging studies cannot differentiate between the two, and bacteriologic cultures may be sterile in 50% of the cases.

LABORATORY TESTS

- Complete blood count: leukocytosis
- Liver function tests: alkaline phosphatase is most commonly elevated (95%-100%); aspartate transaminase (AST) and alanine transaminase (ALT) elevated in 50% of cases; elevated bilirubin (28%-30%); decreased albumin
- Prothrombin time (INR): prolonged (70%)
- Blood cultures: positive in 50% of cases
- Aspiration (50% sterile)
- Stool samples for *E. histolytica* trophozoites (positive in 10%-15% of amebic liver abscess cases)
- Serologic testing for *E. histolytica* should be done on all patients, but it is important to remember that it does not differentiate acute from old infections.

IMAGING STUDIES

- Ultrasound (80%-100% sensitivity in detecting abscesses) shows round or oval hypoechogenic mass (Fig. 1, *A*).
- CT scan is more sensitive in detecting hepatic abscesses and contiguous organ extension and is the imaging study of choice (Fig. 1, *B*, and Fig. 2).
- Chest x-ray: abnormal in 50% of the cases, may reveal elevated right hemidiaphragm, subdiaphragmatic air-fluid levels, pleural effusions, and consolidating infiltrates.
- Most liver abscesses are single; however, multiple liver abscesses can occur with systemic bacteremia.

BOX 1 Pearls for Amebic Liver Abscesses

- Only 10%-20% of patients with amebic liver abscess have a history of diarrhea.
- Treat the intestinal infection to prevent relapse of amebic liver abscess. Failure to use luminal amebicidal agents after metronidazole in cases of amebic abscess results in a 10% relapse rate.
- Failure to show response to antiamebic medication requires evaluation for polymicrobial infection with bacteria.
- Amebic abscess usually responds clinically to antimicrobial therapy in 3 to 7 days, although imaging takes several months to show resolution.
- Percutaneous drainage is rarely required.

From Cameron, JL, Cameron AM: *Current surgical therapy*, ed 10, Philadelphia, 2011, Saunders.

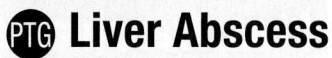

L

Diseases
and Disorders

I

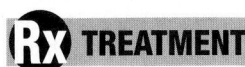 **TREATMENT**

NONPHARMACOLOGIC THERAPY

- The management of pyogenic liver abscess differs from that of amebic liver abscess.
- Medical management is the cornerstone of therapy in amebic liver abscess, whereas early intervention in the form of surgical therapy or catheter drainage and parenteral antibiotics is the rule in pyogenic liver abscess.

ACUTE GENERAL Rx

- Percutaneous drainage under CT or ultrasound guidance is essential in the treatment of pyogenic liver abscesses.
- Aspiration of hepatic amebic abscesses is not required unless there is no response to treatment or a pyogenic cause is being considered.
- Empiric broad-spectrum antibiotics are recommended initially until culture results are available. Common choices include:
  1. Metronidazole (500 mg IV q8h) plus ceftriaxone or levofloxacin.
  2. Monotherapy with a beta-lactam/beta-lactamase inhibitor, such as piperacillin/tazobactam (4.5 g q6h), ticarcillin-clavu-lanate (3.1 g q4h), or ampicillin-sulbactam (3 g q6h).
  3. Monotherapy with a carbapenem, such as imipenem (500 mg IV q6h), meropenem (1 g q8h), or ertapenem (1 g daily).
  4. Duration of antibiotic treatment is usually 4 to 6 wk with IV antibiotics used for the first 1 to 2 wk or until a favorable clinical response, followed thereafter with oral antibiotics (e.g., metronidazole 500 mg PO q8h plus ciprofloxacin 500 mg PO q12h).
  5. Third-generation cephalosporins should not be used as single agents for empiric therapy because of risk of the emergence of beta-lactamase-producing bacteria.
- Antibiotic coverage for amebic liver abscesses includes:
  1. Tissue agent: metronidazole 750 mg PO tid for 10 days
  2. Luminal agent: after therapy with tissue agent treatment with any luminal agent is required even if the stool is negative, such as paromomycin for 10 days or diiodohydroxyquin for 20 days.

CHRONIC Rx

- If fever persists for 2 wk despite percutaneous drainage and antibiotic therapy as outlined under "Acute General Rx," or if there is failure of aspiration or failure of percutaneous drainage, surgery is indicated.
- In patients not responding to intravenous antibiotics and percutaneous drainage, hepatic artery antibiotic infusion can be considered.
- In patients with evidence of metastatic disease that is causing biliary obstruction, a gastroenterology consultation for endoscopic retrograde cholangiopancreatography and stenting should be considered.

DISPOSITION

- Most patients with pyogenic liver abscesses defervesce within 2 wk of treatment with antibiotics and drainage.
- No randomized controlled studies have evaluated the optimal duration of antibiotic therapy for pyogenic liver abscess. Typical duration of antibiotic therapy is at least 4 to 6 wk.
- Pyogenic liver abscess cure rates using percutaneous drainage and antibiotics have been reported to be between 88% and 100%.
- Mortality rate of untreated pyogenic liver abscess is nearly 100%.
- Most patients with amebic liver abscesses defervesce within 4 to 5 days of treatment.
- Amebic liver abscess mortality rate is <1% unless complications occur (see "Comments").
- Follow-up imaging should be used to monitor response to therapy; continue treatment until CT scan shows complete or near-complete resolution of cavity.

REFERRAL

Infectious disease, gastroenterology, interventional radiology, and general surgical consultations are recommended in any patient with hepatic abscess.

PEARLS AND CONSIDERATIONS

COMMENTS

- Complications of pyogenic and amebic liver abscesses include:
  1. Pleuropulmonary extension, resulting in empyema, abscess, and fistula formation
  2. Peritonitis
  3. Purulent pericarditis
  4. Sepsis
- Amebic liver abscesses complicate amebic colitis in nearly 10% of cases.

RELATED CONTENT

Liver Abscess (Patient Information)

AUTHOR: **TANYA ALI, M.D.**

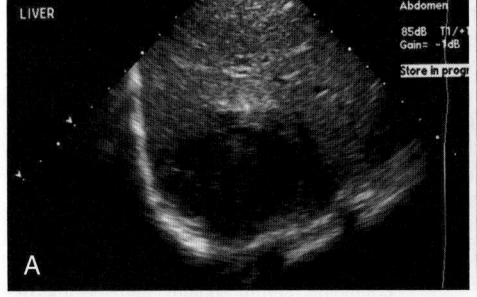 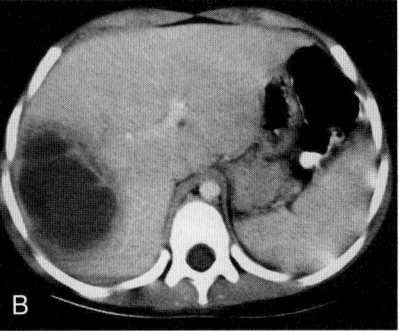

FIG. 1 A, Amebic abscess. Sonogram demonstrates a hypoechogenic mass in the right lobe of the liver with a more hypoechoic surrounding rim. **B,** CT scan demonstrates a low-attenuation mass in the right lobe of the liver with a prominent halo. (From Kuhn JP et al: *Caffrey's pediatric diagnostic imaging*, vol 2, ed 10, Philadelphia, 2004, Mosby.)

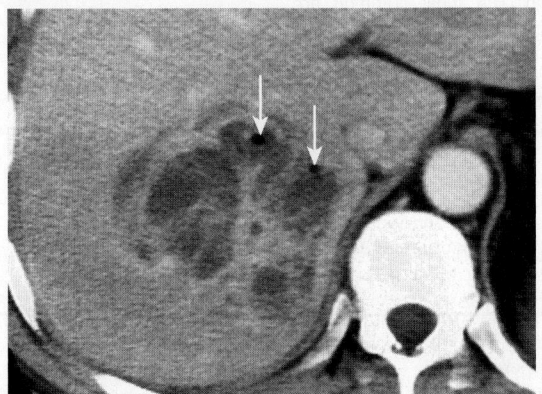

FIG. 2 Pyogenic liver abscess. A liver abscess containing *Escherichia coli* has irregular septations and contains a few bubbles of air (*arrows*). Because of the multiple loculations, this abscess did not respond to a percutaneous catheter for drainage and required surgical debridement. (Webb WR, Brant WE, Major NM: *Fundamentals of body CT*, ed 4, Philadelphia, 2015, Saunders.)

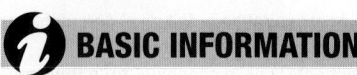

BASIC INFORMATION

DEFINITION

Liver transplantation is surgery to remove a diseased liver and replace it with a donated whole or partial healthy liver. Liver transplantation is a treatment option for acute liver failure, end-stage liver disease, and primary hepatic malignancy. Box 1 summarizes indications for liver transplantation.

ICD-10 CM CODES
Z94.4 Liver transplant status

EPIDEMIOLOGY & DEMOGRAPHICS

- Cirrhosis remains the twelfth-leading cause of death for adults in the U.S., with a death rate of 9.2 cases per 100,000 people.
- Accounts for 1.1% of total deaths in the U.S.
- Hepatocellular carcinoma is a primary cancer originating in the liver. Hepatocellular carcinoma is responsible for more than 12,000 deaths a year in the U.S. and is the highest rising malignancy in the U.S. It is more common in men than women and in African Americans than whites.

INCIDENCE: Number of patients on liver transplant list exceeds 15,000

PREVALENCE: 6000 liver transplants are performed annually in the U.S.

GENETICS: Genetic factors that may induce end-stage liver failure include hemachromatosis, Wilson's disease, alpha-1 antitrypsin deficiency, glycogen storage disease, tyrosinemia

RISK FACTORS

- Viral hepatitis (hepatitis B and hepatitis C [Hepatitis C is the leading indication for liver transplantation])
- Alcoholic liver disease or Laennec's cirrhosis (second most common cause of liver transplant)
- Nonalcoholic steatohepatitis (NASH)
- Autoimmune liver disease (autoimmune hepatitis, cholestatic liver disease, primary biliary cholangitis, primary sclerosing cholangitis, neonatal sclerosing cholangitis, biliary atresia, Caroli's disease, TPN-induced cholestasis)
- Genetics (hemachromatosis, Wilson's disease, alpha-1 antitrypsin deficiency, glycogen storage disease, tyrosinemia)
- Vascular liver disease (Budd-Chiari syndrome)
- Hepatocellular carcinoma
- Acute liver failure (drug-induced liver failure [paracetamol/acetaminophen or APAP, non-APAP acute viral hepatitis [acute hepatitis B], Epstein-Barr virus, cytomegalovirus, herpes simplex virus, human immunodeficiency virus) (Box 2)

PHYSICAL FINDINGS & CLINICAL PRESENTATION

- Cirrhosis alone does not warrant transplantation. Transplantation is considered when a patient presents with manifestations of compromised hepatic function such as portal hypertension or a manifestation of compromised hepatic function. Complications of portal hypertension include esophageal varices, hepatic encephalopathy, ascites, spontaneous bacterial peritonitis, hepatopulmonary syndrome.
- Physical findings and clinical presentation that warrant liver transplantation in patients with end-stage liver disease are recurrent variceal hemorrhage, intractable ascites, spontaneous bacterial peritonitis, refractory encephalopathy, severe jaundice, exacerbated synthetic dysfunction, sudden deterioration, fulminant hepatic failure.

ETIOLOGY

- The etiology of a liver transplant is from end-stage liver disease that has resulted in cirrhosis scarring. The most common are chronic hepatitis C virus (30%), alcoholic cirrhosis (18%), fatty liver disease including NASH, primary liver cancer, acute or chronic hepatitis B virus, bile duct disease, genetic disease, and autoimmune liver disease.

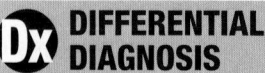

DIFFERENTIAL DIAGNOSIS

- Differential diagnosis of acute liver decompensation in patients diagnosed with end-stage liver disease include eclampsia, preeclampsia, and sepsis with multiorgan failure.

WORKUP

- Patients with end-stage liver disease requiring a transplant are accessed by using the MELD-Na score (Model for End-Stage Liver Disease-Na). The MELD-Na score measures the severity of chronic liver disease and can predict mortality within 3 months of surgery in patients who received a transjugular intrahepatic portosystemic shunt (TIPS) procedure. The score prioritizes who is in need of a transplant as soon as possible.
- MELD-Na score testing includes: serum bilirubin, serum creatinine, international normalization ratio for prothrombin time, and serum sodium
- MELD-Na = [[3.78×ln[serum bilirubin (mg/dL)] + 11.2×ln[INR] + 9.57×ln[serum creatinine (mg/dL)] + 6.43]]+1.59 (135-Na)
  - Maximum and minimum Na of 135 and 120 mmol/L, respectively
- 40 or more: 71.3% mortality
- 30-39: 52.6% mortality
- 20-29: 19.6% mortality
- 10-19: 6.0% mortality (MELD >15 warrants liver transplantation workup for waitlist)
- <9:1.9% mortality

LABORATORY TESTS

- MELD score testing: serum bilirubin, serum creatinine, serum sodium, and the international normalization ratio for prothrombin time.

IMAGING STUDIES

- Abdominal CT scanning or MRI to screen for hepatocellular carcinoma

---

BOX 1 Indications for Liver Transplantation

Acute liver failure
Complications of cirrhosis
  Ascites
  Chronic GI blood loss due to portal hypertensive gastropathy
  Encephalopathy
  Liver cancer
  Refractory variceal hemorrhage
  Synthetic dysfunction
Liver-based metabolic conditions with systemic manifestations
  α_1-antitrypsin deficiency
  Familial amyloidosis
  Glycogen storage disease
  Primary oxaluria
  Tyrosinemia
  Urea cycle enzyme deficiencies
  Wilson's disease
Systemic complications of chronic liver disease
  Hepatopulmonary syndrome
  Portopulmonary hypertension

From Feldman M et al [eds]: *Sleisenger and Fordtran's gastrointestinal and liver disease*, ed 10, Philadelphia, 2016, Saunders.

BOX 2 Absolute Contraindications to Liver Transplantation

AIDS
Active alcoholism or substance abuse
Advanced cardiac or pulmonary disease
Anatomic abnormality that precludes liver transplantation
Cholangiocarcinoma
Extrahepatic malignancy
Fulminant hepatic failure with sustained ICP >50 mm Hg or CPP <40 mm Hg
Hemangiosarcoma
Persistent nonadherence
Uncontrolled sepsis
ICP, intracranial pressure; *CPP,* cerebral perfusion pressure (CPP = mean arterial pressure minus ICP).

From Feldman M et al [eds]: *Sleisenger and Fordtran's gastrointestinal and liver disease,* ed 10, Philadelphia, 2016, Saunders.

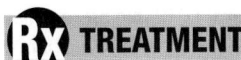

TREATMENT

Patients with decompensated liver disease, end-stage liver disease, hepatocellular carcinoma within Barcelona with a MELD >15 warrant evaluation at a liver transplant center for further workup and possible registration for the liver transplant waitlist. Allocation for liver transplantation is prioritized by a patient's acuity of illness determined by a patient's MELD score.

LIVING DONOR OR DECEASED DONOR LIVER TRANSPLANTATION

Living Donor:
- The scarcity of cadaveric organs has prompted some centers to use living donors, which guarantees transplantation but entails a risk to the donor. Donor compatibility is based on candidates who are family members or close friends of the recipient. The donor must be aged 18 to 60, have compatible blood type with the recipient, be the same physical size or larger, and in excellent health with no history of uncontrolled high blood pressure, liver disease, diabetes, or heart disease. Donor risk includes wound infections, hernia, abdominal bleeding, bile leakage, narrowing of the bile duct, intestinal problems including blockages and tears, organ impairment or failure that leads to the need for transplantation, and death.

Deceased Donor:
- Orthotopic liver transplantation is effective for nonresectable early hepatocellular carcinoma, acute liver failure, and end-stage liver disease.

HEPATOCELLULAR CARCINOMA PATIENTS EVALUATED BY THE UCSF CRITERIA

UCSF criteria
- Criteria for liver transplant are as follows: single tumor <6.5 cm, maximum of 3 total tumors with none >4.5 cm, and cumulative tumor size <8 cm, or exceeded UCSF criteria.

Acute Liver Failure

In the case of acute liver failure, the patient is evaluated for liver transplantation based on the "Kings Criteria," which is based on:
- pH <7.3

or, in a 24-hour period, all 3 of:
- INR >6 (PT >100s) + Cr >300 mmol/L + Grade III or IV encephalopathy

Pretransplant Care

Pretransplantation treatment is focused on testing the patients' ability to handle stress of the surgery, immunosuppression, and post-transplantation care. This is achieved by extensive cardiopulmonary evaluation, screening for occult infection or cancer, and psychosocial evaluation. Additional testing includes ABO-Rh blood typing; liver biochemical and function tests (alanine aminotransferase, aspartate aminotransferase, alkaline phosphatase, bilirubin, international normalized ratio [INR]); complete blood count with differential; creatinine clearance; serum alpha-fetoprotein; calcium and vitamin D levels; serologies for cytomegalovirus, Epstein-Barr virus, varicella, HIV, hepatitis A, hepatitis B, hepatitis C, rapid plasma regain; urinalysis; and urine drug screen.

Posttransplant Care

The primary goal is to prevent posttransplant rejection of the donated liver. This is accomplished with immunosuppression of the immune system with corticosteroids, calcineurin inhibitors such as tacrolimus (FK-506, Profraf), mycophenolate mofetil (Cellcept, Myfortic), mTOR inhibitors (Sirolimus; everolimus), antibodies that remove T cells from the circulation (Thymoglobulin, OKT-3).

REFERRAL

- Gastroenterologist and liver transplant team

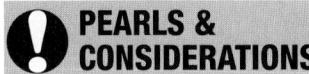

PEARLS & CONSIDERATIONS

COMMENTS

- Cirrhosis alone does not warrant transplantation. Liver transplantation is considered when a patient has suffered either an end-stage liver disease or a manifestation of compromised hepatic function.
- Liver transplantation is always a last option, as the overall determining factor is the number of donor livers available at any time.

PREVENTION

Nongenetic factors such as lifestyle modification and hepatitis B vaccination to avoid developing end-stage liver disease.

PATIENT/FAMILY EDUCATION

Patients who have a genetic predisposition to developing end- stage liver disease from having hemochromatosis, Wilson's disease, alpha-1 antitrypsin deficiency, glycogen storage disease, and tyrosinemia would be advised to have genetic screening of immediate family members.

SUGGESTED READINGS
Available at www.expertconsult.com

RELATED CONTENT
Acute Liver Failure (Related Key Topic)
Cirrhosis (Related Key Topic)

AUTHORS: **EDDIE L. COPELIN II, M.D., M.H.A, ROSANN CHOLANKERIL,** and **GEORGE CHOLANKERIL, M.D.**

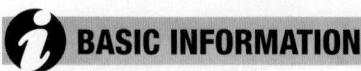

BASIC INFORMATION

DEFINITION

Long QT syndrome (LQTS) is a disorder of myocardial repolarization characterized by a prolongation of the QT interval on the ECG associated with an increased risk of developing life-threatening ventricular arrhythmias, most commonly torsades de pointes (a specific type of polymorphic ventricular tachycardia), which may lead to ventricular fibrillation and sudden cardiac death (SCD). This syndrome may be either genetic or acquired.

SYNONYMS

LQTS
Congenital forms:
    Jervell and Lange-Nielsen syndrome (associated with deafness)
    Romano-Ward syndrome (associated with normal hearing)

ICD-10CM CODES
I45.81 Long QT syndrome

EPIDEMIOLOGY & DEMOGRAPHICS

- Congenital LQTS is thought to account for >3000 deaths in childhood per year in the United States.
- Prevalence is felt to be 1:2000 of apparently healthy white young births. It may be higher because this is based on genetic testing of infants in whom the QTc was in excess of 470 and 460 milliseconds, respectively (Schwartz, 2009).
- Presence of LQTS has been shown in all racial groups. Review of data from the US portion of the international LQTS registry found a lower incidence but higher severity of QT prolongation among African Americans. These findings could be in part attributable to socioeconomic factors (Fugate 2010).
- Incidence of LQTS is thought to be between 1:2500 and 1:10,000 in the general population, although it has been difficult to estimate due to incomplete penetrance. Congenital form associated with deafness is autosomal recessive (Jervell and Lange Nielsen syndrome) and is less common than the autosomal dominant form as well as more severe.
- Congenital form associated with normal hearing (Romano-Ward syndrome) is autosomal dominant. Although inheritance of LQTS is autosomal dominant, female predominance has often been observed and has been attributed to an increased susceptibility to cardiac arrhythmias in women. LQTS is more likely to express itself before puberty in males and after puberty in females.
- At least 15 different LQTS genes have been identified to date. LQTS is more common in women than in men.
- Mortality rate is estimated to be about 1% per year.
- Genetic mutations in the congenital LQTS are described in Table 1. Common types of LQTS are described in Table 2.

PHYSICAL FINDINGS & CLINICAL PRESENTATION

- Many episodes are stress mediated.
- Palpitations, presyncope.
- Syncope caused by ventricular tachycardia.
- SCD.
- Seizure.
- Family history of LQTS, but a family history of SCD has not been proved to be a risk factor for SCD in patients with LQTS.
- Abnormal ECG (prolonged QT) in asymptomatic relatives of known case.
- Prolonged QTc interval on ECG (QTc should be >460 ms in women and >440 ms in men). Notably, 20% to 25% genotype positive LQTS may have normal QTc on resting ECG.
- In case of congenital LQTS, the presentation of syncope or SCD is typically triggered by exercise and swimming in LQT1 patients, in LQT2 patients by emotion, pregnancy, or noise, and patients with LQT3 are at highest risk of events when at rest or asleep.

ETIOLOGY

- Cardiac repolarization abnormality.
- Congenital cause (hundreds of mutations on more than 10 genes have been identified).
- Most of the gene mutations affect function of ion channels leading to prolonged repolarization (i.e., sodium and potassium channels resulting in either increased Na^+ influx or decreased K^+ efflux). These mutations

---

TABLE 1   Genetic Mutations in Congenital Long QT Syndrome

		Location	Gene	Current	Effect
Romano-Ward syndrome (autosomal-dominant inheritance)	LQT1	11p15.5	KCNQ1 (K+ channel)	I_{Ks}	↓ Function ↓ Repolarization
	LQT2	7q35-36	KCNH2 (K+ channel)	I_{Kr}	↓ Function ↓ Repolarization
	LQT3	3q21-24	SCN5A (Na+ channel)	I_{Na}	↑ Function ↑ Depolarization
	LQT4	4q25-27	ANK2	Unknown	Unknown
	LQT5	21q22	KCNE1 (K+ channel, subunit minK)	I_{Ks}	↓ Function ↓ Repolarization
Jervell and Lange-Nielsen syndrome (autosomal-recessive inheritance)		11p15.5	KvLQT1 (K+ channel)	I_{Ks}	↓ Function ↓ Repolarization
		21q22	KCNE 1 (K+ channel, subunit minK)	I_{Ks}	↓ Function ↓ Repolarization

From Crawford MH et al (eds): *Cardiology,* ed 2, St Louis, 2004, Mosby.

TABLE 2   Common Types of Long QT (LQT) Syndrome

	LQT1	LQT2	LQT3
Pathophysiology			
Gene	KCNQ1 (KvLQT1)	KCNH2 (HERG)	SCN5A
Protein	$K_v7.1$	$K_v11.1$	$Na_v1.5$
Ionic current	Decreased I_{Ks}	Decreased I_{Kr}	Increased late I_{Na}
Clinical Presentation			
Incidence of cardiac events	63%	46%	18%
Incidence of SCD	4%	4%	4%
Arrhythmia triggers	Emotional/physical stress (swimming, diving)	Emotional stress, arousal (alarm clock, telephone), rest	Sleep/rest
ECG	Broad-based T wave	Low-amplitude, bifid T wave	Long isoelectric ST segment
QT response to exercise	Attenuated QTc shortening and an exaggerated QTc prolongation during early and peak exercise	Normal QT during exercise but with exaggerated QT hysteresis	Supernormal QT shortening
Management			
Exercise restriction	+++	++	?
Response to beta blockers	+++	+++	?
Potassium supplement	+	++	+
Left cervicothoracic sympathectomy	++	++	++
Response to mexiletine	+	+	++

From Issa Z et al: *Clinical arrhythmology and electrophysiology,* ed 2, Philadelphia, 2012, Saunders.

prolong depolarization and predispose the patient to torsades de pointes.

- Acquired causes:
  1. Drugs: dofetilide, ibutilide, bepridil, quinidine, procainamide, sotalol, amiodarone, ranolazine, disopyramide, phenothiazines and antiemetic agents (droperidol, domperidone), tricyclic antidepressants, antipsychotics (quetiapine, ziprasidone, iloperidone), citalopram, antihistamines, quinolones, azithromycin, astemizole or cisapride given with ketoconazole or erythromycin, clarithromycin, and antimalarials, particularly among patients with asthma or those using potassium-lowering medications; also common in patients receiving methadone.
  2. Hypokalemia, hypomagnesemia, hypocalcemia (especially in patients with malabsorption syndrome).
  3. Liquid protein diet.
  4. Central nervous system lesions.
  5. Ischemia.
  6. Hypothyroidism.

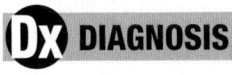 **DIAGNOSIS**

DIFFERENTIAL DIAGNOSIS

See "Syncope." Brugada's syndrome, arrhythmogenic right ventricular dysplasia, and LQTS are major causes of genetic sudden death syndromes (Fig. 1).

Diagnostic criteria for the congenital LQTS as per 2013 HRS Guidelines:
LQTS is diagnosed:

a. In the presence of an LQTS risk score ≥3.5 in the absence of a secondary cause for QT prolongation and/or

b. In the presence of an unequivocally pathogenic mutation in one of the LQTS genes or

c. In the presence of a QT interval corrected for heart rate using Bazett's formula (QTc) ≥500 ms in repeated 12-lead electrocardiogram (ECG) and in the absence of a secondary cause for QT prolongation.

d. LQTS can be diagnosed in the presence of a QTc between 480 and 499 ms in repeated 12-lead ECGs in a patient with unexplained syncope in the absence of a secondary cause for QT prolongation and in the absence of a pathogenic mutation.

LQTS Risk Score (Schwartz 2011):

ECG Criteria

QTc >480 ms	3 points
QTc 460-480 ms	2 points
QTc 450-460 ms (males)	1 point
QTc 4th minute of recovery from exercise stress test >480 ms	1 point
Torsades de pointes	2 points
T-wave alternans	1 point
Notched T wave in three leads	1 point
Bradycardia	0.5 point

History

Syncope with stress	2 points
Syncope without stress	1 point
Congenital deafness	0.5 point
Definite family history of long QT	1 point
Unexplained cardiac death in first-degree relative <30 yr	0.5 point

Total score: 1 point: low probability of LQTS. 1.5 to 3 points: intermediate probability of LQTS. ≥ 3.5 points high probability.

WORKUP

Cardiology referral is recommended for all cases.

Genetic analysis is an essential step for risk stratification of patients with congenital prolonged QT and is important for identification of potential mutation carriers within the proband family. There is evidence for gene-specific triggers of events and therapeutic efficacy. Molecular screening should become part of the routine clinical management of LQTS.

In relatives of known patients with LQTS or in young patients with syncope:

- Stress test may prolong the QT interval or cause T-wave alternans.
- Valsalva maneuver: may prolong the QT interval or cause T-wave alternans.
- Prolonged ECG monitoring with various stimulations aimed at increasing catecholamines and assess for QT prolongation (perform in a setting that can provide resuscitation with α- and β-antagonists readily available).
- Epinephrine-induced prolongation of the QT interval (epinephrine infusion QT stress test)
- Genetic analysis
  1. LQT1 locus of KCNQ1 potassium channel gene.
  2. LQT2 locus of KCNH2 potassium channel gene.
  3. LQT3 locus of SCN5A sodium channel gene.
  4. These three variants account for >90% of all genotyped LQTS patients, whereas the remaining genes are responsible for a minority of cases.
- Risk stratification for each genetic variant on the basis of gender and QTc: groups are defined on the basis of the probability of the first cardiac event (syncope, cardiac arrest, or sudden death) before the age of 40 years or before therapy. Specific mutations, depending on type, location, and degree, may confer a high risk even if the ECG abnormalities are mild. Clinically, QT interval duration was the strongest predictor of risk for cardiac events; a QTc exceeding 500 ms identifies patients with the highest risk.
  1. High risk (>50% of cardiac event): QTc ≥ 500 ms and LQT1 or LQT2, or male with LQT3.
  2. Moderate risk (30%-50%): QTc <500 ms in male with LQT3 or in female with LQT2 or LQT3, and female with LQT3 with QTc ≥500 ms.
  3. Low risk (<30%): QTc <500 ms and LQT1 or male LQT2 with QTc <500 ms.

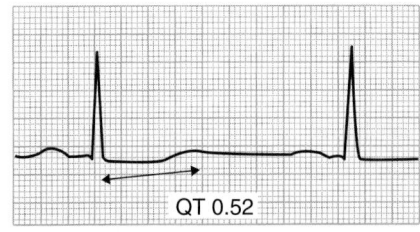

A

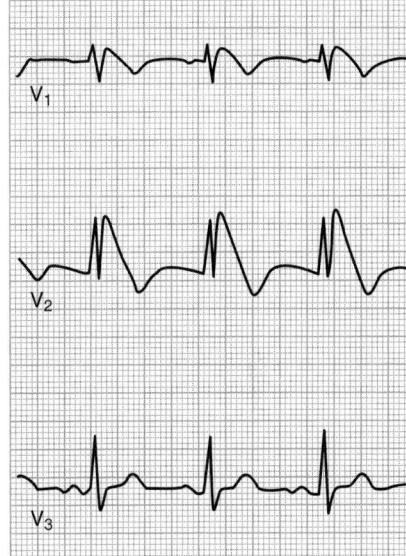

B

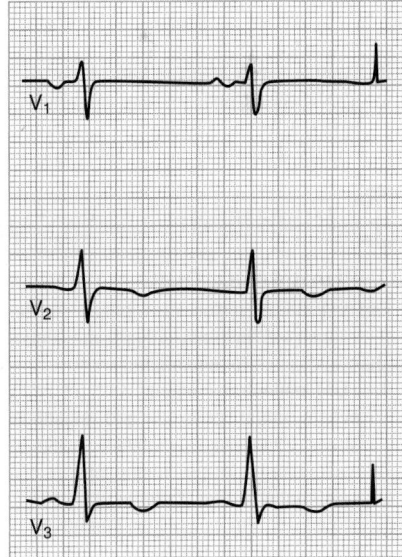

C

FIG. 1 Sinus rhythm electrocardiogram findings in three genetic sudden death syndromes. A, QT prolongation during sinus rhythm in a patient with long QT syndrome. **B,** ST elevation in V₁ and V₂ in a patient with Brugada's syndrome. **C,** T wave inversion in V₁-V₃ in a patient with arrhythmogenic right ventricular dysplasia. (From Goldman L, Schafer AI: *Goldman's Cecil medicine,* ed 24, Philadelphia, 2012, Saunders.)

TABLE 3 Cardiac Event Risk Stratification Scheme Based on Genes, Gender, and QTc

Genetic Subtype	QTc <500 ms		QTc ≥550 ms	
	Male	Female	Male	Female
LQT1	Low	Low	High	High
LQT2	Low	Intermediate	High	High
LQT3	Intermediate	Intermediate	High	Intermediate

Probability of the first cardiac event (syncope, cardiac arrest, or sudden death) before the age of 40 years or before therapy. High = >50%, Intermediate = 30%-50%, Low = <30%.

TABLE 4 Management of Patients with Long QT Syndrome

Type of Syndrome	Management	Indication
Congenital	Beta-blockers	Asymptomatic patients, symptomatic patients (who do not have bronchospasm)
	Cervicothoracic sympathectomy	Refractory symptoms, especially in pediatric patients
	Cardiac pacing	Refractory symptoms associated with bradycardia, pauses
	Implantable cardioverter-defibrillator	Cardiac arrest, refractory syncope, prophylaxis for moderate- to high-risk patients for cardiac events
Acquired	Elimination of causative drug or condition	All patients
	Magnesium sulfate	Nonsustained ventricular tachycardia, torsades de pointes (even with a normal serum magnesium concentration)
	Administration of potassium (to keep serum K+ >4.5 mEq/L)	Serum K+ <4.5 mEq/L
	Maneuvers to increase heart rate (cardiac pacing, isoproterenol)	Bradycardia, arrhythmias refractory to magnesium sulfate

K^+, Potassium.
Adapted from Crawford MH et al (eds): *Cardiology*, ed 2, St Louis, 2004, Mosby.

4. Prophylactic treatment should be considered in all patients with moderate or high risk for cardiac events based on the above risk stratification scheme (Table 3).

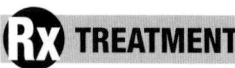 **TREATMENT**

NONPHARMACOLOGIC

- Focuses on exclusion of triggers of life-threatening arrhythmia—there are gene-specific triggers for symptoms:
  1. *LQT1* patients experience 90% of lethal events under physical and emotional stress. Swimming and diving should be avoided or performed under supervision.
  2. *LQT2* patients are at highest risk during arousal or emotions, also during sleep and at rest but not at all during exercise; avoid sudden or excessive acoustic stimuli, especially during sleep (e.g., avoid telephone and/or alarm clock in the proximity)—as opposed to *LQT3* patients, in whom 80% of the events occur at rest or while asleep.
- Previously, all patients with LQTS have been instructed to avoid competitive sports. More recently, low-risk, genetically confirmed LQTS with borderline QTc prolongation, without prior cardiac symptoms and no familial history of SCD are thought to be safe to participate in competitive sports where AED and BLS personnel is available.
- Implantation of an implantable cardioverter-defibrillator (ICD) is recommended according to the ACC/AHA guidelines for patients with a good functional status for more than 1 yr and the following conditions (Table 4):
  1. Survivors of cardiac arrest (class 1).
  2. Patients with syncope or ventricular tachycardia while receiving β-blockers (class IIa).
  3. Prophylaxis of SCD with use of β-blocker in patients with characteristics that suggest high risk (such as *LQT2* and *LQT3*, QTc >500 ms) (class IIb).

PHARMACOLOGIC

- With few exceptions (mostly borderline QTc and *LQT1* males aged >25 to 30 yr), all mutation carriers should be treated because of the risk of SCD during first cardiac event. All symptomatic patients should be treated as well.
- Beta-blockers an initial therapy of choice—there are differential responses to β-blocker therapy among different genetic variants; especially effective among LQT1 patients. Studies showed the efficacy of β-blockers with an overall mortality <2% over a mean follow-up exceeding 5 yr.
- In patients with LQT3, mexiletine shortens the QTc and can be given with a β-blocker.
- In the 20% to 30% of patients who continue to have symptoms on a β-blocker, the main options are either left cardiac sympathetic denervation (LCSD) or the prophylactic implantation of an ICD.
- In patients with frequent ICD shocks or in those with high risk for SCD where ICD placement cannot be performed, cardiac pacing and/or LCSD may be indicated.
- In patients with recurrent syncope and/or aborted cardiac arrest despite combined ICD and β-blocker, LCSD as adjunctive therapy can be performed.
- Correctable factors including electrolyte disorder—hypokalemia and hypomagnesemia—and avoidance of precipitating drugs that may further prolong the QT interval is mandatory. A complete list of drugs that can potentially prolong QT may be found at www.qtdrugs.org.
- For patients with acquired form and torsades de pointes, IV magnesium and atrial or ventricular pacing are initial choices.
- Table 4 summarizes management of patients with LQTS.

PROGNOSIS

In carefully treated patients, mortality is around 0.5% to 1% over 20 years.

The timing and frequency of syncope, QTc prolongation, and gender are predictive of risk for aborted cardiac arrest and SCD during adolescence. Higher risk is present in those with one or two or more episodes of syncope in the last 10 yr compared with those with no syncopal episodes, those with QTc >530 ms, and males aged 10 to 12 yr.

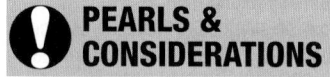 **PEARLS & CONSIDERATIONS**

COMMENTS

Family history should be assessed for a history of sudden death and other deaths that may have occurred as manifestations of LQTS (e.g., sudden infant death, drowning, and loss of consciousness while driving).

SUGGESTED READINGS

Available at www.expertconsult.com

RELATED CONTENT

Long QT Syndrome (Patient Information)
Torsades des Pointes (Related Key Topic)

AUTHOR: **SIMON GRINGUT, M.D.**

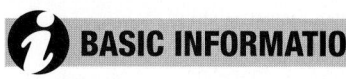

BASIC INFORMATION

DEFINITION
A lung abscess is an infection of the lung parenchyma resulting in a necrotic cavity containing pus.

SYNONYMS
Pulmonary abscess

ICD-10CM CODES
J85.1 Abscess of lung with pneumonia
J85.2 Abscess of lung without pneumonia
A06.5 Amebic lung abscess

EPIDEMIOLOGY & DEMOGRAPHICS
INCIDENCE: Has decreased over the last 30 years as a result of antibiotic therapy.
- Lung abscess in patients age 50 and over is associated with primary lung neoplasia in 30% of the cases.
- Lung abscesses commonly coexist with empyemas.

RISK FACTORS (SEE TABLE 1):
1. Alcohol-related problems
2. Seizure disorders
3. Cerebrovascular disorders with dysphagia
4. Drug abuse
5. Esophageal disorders (e.g., scleroderma, esophageal carcinoma, etc.)
6. Poor oral hygiene
7. Obstructive malignant lung disease
8. Bronchiectasis

PHYSICAL FINDINGS & CLINICAL PRESENTATION
- Symptoms are generally insidious and prolonged, occurring for weeks to months
- Fever, chills, and sweats
- Cough
- Sputum production (purulent with foul odor)
- Pleuritic chest pain
- Hemoptysis
- Dyspnea
- Malaise, fatigue, and weakness
- Tachycardia and tachypnea
- Dullness to percussion, whispered pectoriloquy, and bronchophony
- Amphoric breath sounds (low-pitched sound of air moving across a large open cavity)

ETIOLOGY
- The most important factor predisposing to lung abscess is aspiration.
- Following aspiration as a major predisposing factor is periodontal disease.
- Lung abscess is rare in an edentulous person.
- Approximately 90% of lung abscesses are caused by anaerobic microorganisms (peptostreptococci, microaerophilic streptococci such as *Streptococcus milleri*, *Bacteroides* species, *Fusobacterium nucleatum*, *Prevotella*). Pulmonary actinomycosis will also generate lung abscess.
- In most cases anaerobic infection is mixed with aerobic or facultative anaerobic organisms (*S. aureus*, *E. coli*, *K. pneumoniae*, *P. aeruginosa*).
- Parasitic organisms including *Paragonimus westermani* and *Entamoeba histolytica*.
- Fungi including *Aspergillus*, *Cryptococcus*, *Histoplasma*, *Blastomyces*, and *Coccidioides* spp.
- Immunocompromised hosts may become infected with *Aspergillus*, mycobacteria, *Nocardia*, *Legionella micdadei*, and *Rhodococcus equi*.
- Lung necrosis caused by community strains of MRSA (USA 300 strain) in young adults or adolescents after acute influenza was initially reported in 2002 and can be quite fulminant.

DIAGNOSIS

Lung abscess may be primary or secondary.
- *Primary lung abscess* refers to infection from normal host organisms within the lung (e.g., aspiration, pneumonia).
- Secondary lung abscess results from other preexisting conditions (e.g., endocarditis, underlying lung cancer, pulmonary emboli). Lung abscess may be acute or chronic.
- Acute lung abscess is present if symptoms are of less than 4 to 6 wk.
- Chronic lung abscess is present if symptoms last longer than 6 wk.

DIFFERENTIAL DIAGNOSIS
The differential diagnosis is similar to that for cavitary lung lesions:
- Bacterial (anaerobic, aerobic, infected bulla, empyema, actinomycosis, tuberculosis)

- Fungal (histoplasmosis, coccidioidomycosis, blastomycosis, aspergillosis, cryptococcosis, zygomycetes)
- Parasitic (amebiasis, echinococcosis)
- Malignancy (primary lung carcinoma, metastatic lung disease, lymphoma, Hodgkin's disease)
- Granulomatosis with polyangiitis, sarcoidosis, endocarditis, and septic pulmonary emboli

WORKUP
- The workup of a patient with lung abscess attempts to elicit a primary or a secondary cause.
- Blood tests are not specific in diagnosing lung abscesses.
- Most diagnoses are made from imaging studies; however, to diagnose a specific cause bacteriologic studies are needed.

LABORATORY TESTS
- CBC with leukocytosis
- Bacteriologic studies
  1. Sputum Gram stain and culture (commonly contaminated by oral flora)
  2. Percutaneous transtracheal aspiration
  3. Percutaneous transthoracic aspiration
  4. Fiberoptic bronchoscopy using bronchial brushings or bronchoalveolar lavage is the most widely used intervention when trying to obtain diagnostic bacteriologic cultures
- Blood cultures on some occasions (<30%) may be positive
- If an empyema is present, obtaining empyema fluid via thoracentesis may isolate the organism

IMAGING STUDIES
- Chest x-ray makes the diagnosis of lung abscess showing the cavitary lesion with an air-fluid level.
- Lung abscesses are most commonly found in the posterior segment of the right upper lobe.
- Chest CT scan can localize and size the lesion and assist in differentiating lung abscesses from other pathologic processes (e.g., tumor, empyema, infected bulla, etc.) (Fig. 1).

TREATMENT

NONPHARMACOLOGIC THERAPY
- Oxygen therapy
- Postural drainage
- Respiratory therapy maneuvers

ACUTE GENERAL Rx
- Piperacillin/tazobactam 3.375 g IV q6h in aspiration pneumonia with lung abscess.
- Ceftriaxone 1 to 2 g IV q24h plus metronidazole: 500 mg IV q8h.
- Clindamycin is more effective for anaerobic lung abscess than penicillin alone. Dose: 600 mg IV q8h until improved, then 300 to 600 mg PO q6h.
- Penicillin 1 to 2 million units IV q4h until improvement (afebrile, decreased phlegm production), followed by penicillin VK 500 mg PO q6h for 2 to 3 weeks but often up to 6 to

---

TABLE 1 Risk Factors for Aspiration Pneumonia and Lung Abscess

Increased bacterial inoculum	Periodontal disease, gingivitis, tonsillar or dental abscess, drugs that decrease gastric acidity
Impairment of consciousness	Drugs, alcohol, general anesthesia, metabolic encephalopathy, coma, shock, cerebrovascular accident, cardiopulmonary arrest, seizures, surgery, trauma
Impaired cough and gag reflexes	Vocal cord paralysis, intratracheal anesthesia, endotracheal tube, tracheostomy, myopathy, myelopathy, other neurologic disorders
Impairment of esophageal function	Diverticula, achalasia, strictures, disorders of gastrointestinal motility, neoplasm, tracheoesophageal fistula, pseudobulbar palsy
Emesis	Nasogastric tube, gastric dilation, ileus, intestinal obstruction

From Cohen J, Powderly WG: *Infectious diseases*, ed 2, St Louis, 2004, Mosby.

8 weeks) can be given with metronidazole doses of 7.5 mg/kg IV q6h followed by PO 500 mg bid to qid dosing as an alternative to clindamycin.

- Penicillin should not be used alone because many mouth flora anaerobes now produce penicillinase enzymes. Metronidazole should not be used alone because it is not active against microaerophilic streptococci and some anaerobic cocci.
- Other alternatives are ampicillin/sulbactam and carbapenems such as ertapenem and meropenem.

CHRONIC Rx

- Bronchoscopy to assist with drainage and/or diagnosis is indicated in patients who fail to respond to antibiotics or if there is suspected underlying malignancy.
- Surgery is indicated on rare occasions (<10%) in patients with complications of lung abscess (see "Comments").

DISPOSITION

- More than 95% of patients are cured with the use of antibiotics alone.

- Complications of lung abscesses include:
  1. Empyema
  2. Massive hemoptysis
  3. Pneumothorax
  4. Bronchopleural fistula
  5. Hepatobronchial fistula
  6. Brain abscess
  7. Bronchiectasis
- Mortality is low in community-acquired lung abscess (2.5%).
- Hospital-acquired lung abscess carries a high mortality rate (65%).

REFERRAL

If lung abscess is present, consultation with pulmonary and infectious disease specialist is recommended.

⚠ PEARLS & CONSIDERATIONS

COMMENTS

- Refractory cases are usually the result of:
  1. Large cavity size (>6 cm)
  2. Recurrent aspiration

  3. Thick-walled cavities
  4. Underlying lung carcinoma
  5. Empyema formation
- Necrotizing pneumonia is similar to a lung abscess but differs in size (<2 cm in diameter) and number (usually multiple suppurative cavitary lesions).

SUGGESTED READING

Available at www.expertconsult.com

RELATED CONTENT

Lung Abscess (Patient Information)

AUTHOR: **GLENN G. FORT, M.D., M.P.H.**

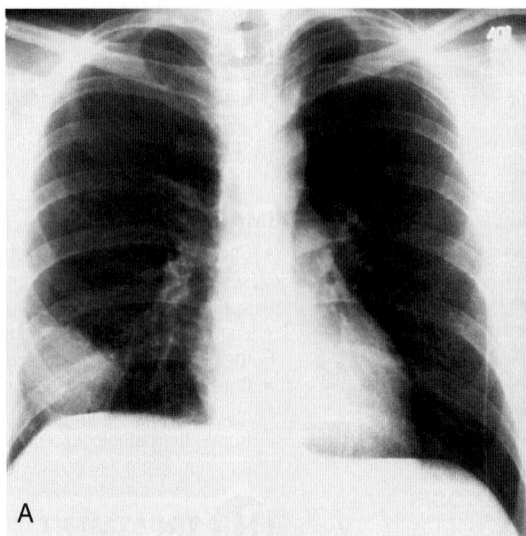 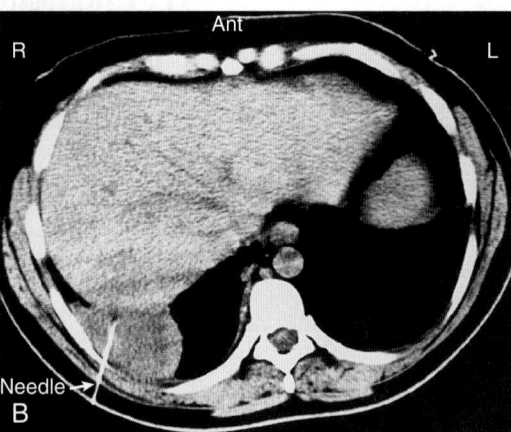

FIG. 1 Lung abscess. On a chest radiograph, a lung abscess may look to be a solid rounded lesion **(A),** or, if it has a connection with the bronchus, there may be an air-fluid level in a thick-walled cavitary lesion. CT scanning **(B)** can be used to localize the lesion and to place a needle for drainage and aspiration of contents for culture. (From Mettler FA [ed]: *Primary care radiology,* Philadelphia, 2000, Saunders.)

BASIC INFORMATION

DEFINITION

A primary lung neoplasm is a malignancy arising from lung tissue. The different types are non-small cell lung cancer (NSCLC; squamous cell carcinoma, adenocarcinoma, and large cell carcinoma) and small cell lung cancer (SCLC).

ADENOCARCINOMA: Represent 35% to 40% of lung carcinomas; frequently located in mid-lung and periphery; initial metastases are to lymphatics; frequently associated with peripheral scars; adenocarcinoma is described as preinvasive, minimally invasive, or invasive

SQUAMOUS CELL (EPIDERMOID): Represent 20% to 30% of lung cancers; central location; metastasis by local invasion; frequent cavitation and obstructive phenomena

SMALL CELL (OAT CELL): Represent 15% to 20% of lung carcinomas; central location; metastasis through lymphatics; associated with lesion of the short arm of chromosome 3; high cavitation rate

LARGE CELL: Represent 10% to 15% of lung carcinomas; frequently located in the periphery; metastasis to central nervous system and mediastinum; rapid growth rate with early metastasis

LEPIDIC-PREDOMINANT PATTERN (BRONCHOALVEOLAR): Represent 5% of lung carcinomas; frequently located in the periphery; may be bilateral; initial metastasis through lymphatic, hematogenous, and local invasion; no correlation with cigarette smoking; cavitation rare

SYNONYMS

Lung cancer

ICD-10CM CODES

C34.10 Malignant neoplasm of upper lobe, unspecified bronchus or lung
C34.11 Malignant neoplasm of upper lobe, right bronchus or lung
C34.12 Malignant neoplasm of upper lobe, left bronchus or lung
C34.2 Malignant neoplasm of middle lobe, bronchus or lung
C34.30 Malignant neoplasm of lower lobe, unspecified bronchus or lung
C34.31 Malignant neoplasm of lower lobe, right bronchus or lung
C34.32 Malignant neoplasm of lower lobe, left bronchus or lung
C34.80 Malignant neoplasm of overlapping sites of unspecified bronchus and lung
C34.81 Malignant neoplasm of overlapping sites of right bronchus and lung
C34.82 Malignant neoplasm of overlapping sites of left bronchus and lung
C34.90 Malignant neoplasm of unspecified part of unspecified bronchus or lung
C34.91 Malignant neoplasm of unspecified part of right bronchus or lung
C34.92 Malignant neoplasm of unspecified part of left bronchus or lung

EPIDEMIOLOGY & DEMOGRAPHICS

- Lung cancer is responsible for >30% of cancer deaths in males and >25% of cancer deaths in females. It has been the most common cancer in the world since 1985 and is the leading cause of cancer-related death in both sexes.
- Tobacco smoke is implicated in 90% of cases; of these, secondhand smoke is responsible for approximately 20% of cases.
- There will be an estimated 224,390 new cases of lung cancer and 158,080 deaths from lung cancer in 2016 in the U.S.
- Among women there has been a 600% increase in incidence of lung cancer during the past 80 years. The rates of death among women with lung cancer in the U.S. are the highest in the world.

PHYSICAL FINDINGS & CLINICAL PRESENTATION

- Weight loss, fatigue, fever, anorexia, dysphagia
- Cough, hemoptysis, dyspnea, wheezing
- Chest, shoulder, and bone pain
- Paraneoplastic syndromes (see Table 1):
  1. *Lambert-Eaton myasthenic syndrome:* myopathy involving proximal muscle groups
  2. Endocrine manifestations: hypercalcemia, ectopic adrenocorticotropic hormone secretion, syndrome of inappropriate excretion of adrenocorticotropic hormone (SIADH)
  3. Neurologic: subacute cerebellar degeneration, peripheral neuropathy, cortical degeneration
  4. Musculoskeletal: polymyositis, clubbing, hypertrophic pulmonary osteoarthropathy
  5. Hematologic or vascular: migratory thrombophlebitis, marantic thrombosis, anemia, thrombocytosis, or thrombocytopenia
  6. Cutaneous: acanthosis nigricans, dermatomyositis
- Pleural effusion (10% of patients), recurrent pneumonias (from obstruction), localized wheezing
- *Superior vena cava syndrome:*
  1. Obstruction of venous return of the superior vena cava is most commonly caused by bronchogenic carcinoma or metastasis to paratracheal nodes.
  2. The patient usually reports headache, nausea, dizziness, visual changes, syncope, and respiratory distress.
  3. Physical examination reveals distention of thoracic and neck veins, edema of face and upper extremities, facial plethora, and cyanosis.
- *Horner's syndrome:* constricted pupil, ptosis, facial anhidrosis caused by spinal cord damage between C8 and T1 as a result of a superior sulcus tumor (bronchogenic carcinoma of the extreme lung apex)
- *Pancoast tumor:* a superior sulcus tumor associated with ipsilateral Horner's syndrome and shoulder pain

ETIOLOGY

- Tobacco abuse; the chance of developing lung cancer for a 40-pack-year persistent smoker is 20 times that of someone who never smoked.
- Environmental agents (e.g., radon) and industrial agents (e.g., ionizing radiation, asbestos, nickel, uranium, vinyl chloride, chromium, arsenic, coal dust).
- Lung cancer susceptibility and risk increased in inherited cancer syndromes caused by germline mutations in p53, retinoblastoma, and epidermal growth factor receptor (*EGFR*) genes.

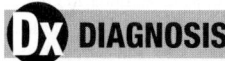

DIAGNOSIS

DIFFERENTIAL DIAGNOSIS

- Pneumonia
- Tuberculosis (TB)
- Metastatic carcinoma to the lung
- Lung abscess
- Granulomatous disease
- Carcinoid tumor
- Sarcoidosis
- Benign lesions that simulate thoracic malignancy:
  1. Lobar atelectasis: pneumonia, chronic inflammatory disease, allergic bronchopulmonary aspergillosis

TABLE 1 Paraneoplastic Syndromes Associated with Bronchogenic Carcinoma

Syndrome	Cell Type	Mechanism
Hypertrophic pulmonary osteoarthropathy and clubbing	All types	Unknown
Hyponatremia	SCLC most common; may be any type	SIADH, ectopic antidiuretic hormone production by tumor
Hypercalcemia	Usually squamous cell	Bone metastases, osteoclast-activating factor, parathyroid hormone–like hormone, prostaglandins
Cushing's syndrome	Usually SCLC	Ectopic ACTH production
Lambert-Eaton myasthenic syndrome	Usually SCLC	Voltage-sensitive calcium channel antibodies in >75%; affects presynaptic neuronal calcium channel activity
Other neuromyopathic disorders	SCLC most common; may be any type	Antineuronal nuclear antibodies, also known as anti-Hu; others unknown
Thrombophlebitis	All types	Unknown

ACTH, Adrenocorticotropic hormone; *SIADH,* syndrome of inappropriate secretion of antidiuretic hormone.
Adapted from Andreoli TE et al: *Andreoli and Carpenter's Cecil essentials of medicine,* ed 8, Philadelphia, 2010, Saunders.

2. Multiple pulmonary nodules: septic emboli, Wegener's granulomatosis, sarcoidosis, rheumatoid nodules, fungal disease, multiple pulmonary atrioventricular fistulas
3. Mediastinal adenopathy: sarcoidosis, lymphoma, primary TB, fungal disease, silicosis, pneumoconiosis, drug-induced (e.g., phenytoin, trimethadione)
4. Pleural effusion: congestive heart failure, pneumonia with parapneumonic effusion, TB, viral pneumonitis, ascites, pancreatitis, collagen-vascular disease

WORKUP

The workup generally includes chest CT, positron-emission tomographic (PET) scan, and tissue biopsy. Lab tests include CBC, serum chemistry studies. Diagnosis and staging of lung cancer should be performed simultaneously to minimize invasive testing.

LABORATORY TESTS

Various modalities are available to obtain a tissue diagnosis:
- Biopsy of any suspicious lymph nodes (e.g., supraclavicular or mediastinal node)
- Flexible fiberoptic bronchoscopy: brush and biopsy specimens are obtained from any visualized endobronchial lesions. The use of a gene-expression classifier has a high sensitivity across different lesion sizes, locations, stages, and cell type of lung cancer. The combination of the classifier plus bronchoscopy has a sensitivity of >85%. In intermediate-risk patients with a non-diagnostic bronchoscopic examination, a negative classifier score provides support for a more conservative diagnostic approach.[1]
- Transbronchial needle aspiration: done with a special needle passed through the bronchoscope; this technique is useful to sample mediastinal masses or paratracheal lymph nodes
- Transthoracic fine-needle aspiration biopsy with fluoroscopic or CT scan guidance to evaluate peripheral pulmonary nodules
- Endobronchial ultrasound (EBUS) guided biopsy and staging can be used to evaluate suspected mediastinal and hilar nodes
- Mediastinoscopy and anteromedial sternotomy in suspected tumor involvement of the mediastinum
- Pleural biopsy in patients with pleural effusion
- Thoracentesis of pleural effusion and cytologic evaluation of the obtained fluid may confirm diagnosis

IMAGING STUDIES

- Chest x-ray (Fig. E1): The radiographic presentation often varies with the cell type. Presence of pleural effusion, lobar atelectasis, and mediastinal adenopathy can occur in any cell type.
- CT scan of the chest (Fig. 2) can evaluate mediastinal and pleural extension. The chest

[1]Silvestri GA et al: A bronchial genomic classifier for the diagnostic evaluation of lung cancer, *N Engl J Med* 373:243-251, 2015.

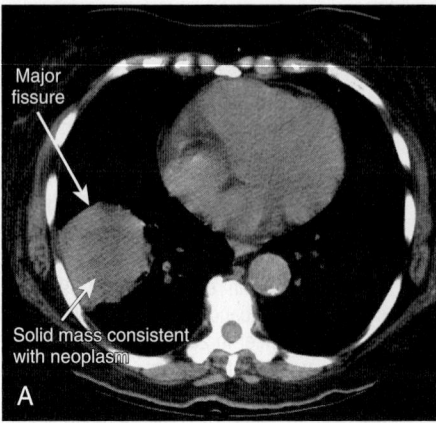
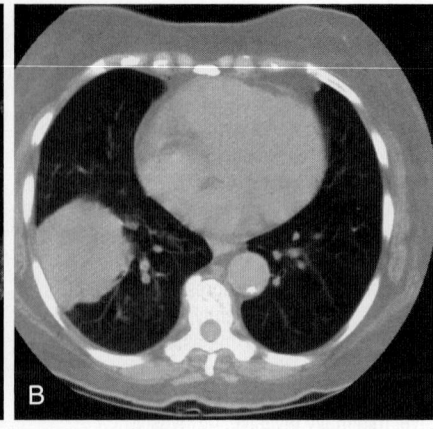

FIG. 2 Lung neoplasm, primary. Lung mass presenting with hemoptysis. Same patient as in Fig. 2. Noncontrast computed tomography was performed (contrast was withheld as a consequence of the patient's renal dysfunction) and shows a 6 by 6 cm round lesion abutting the oblique fissure (also called the major fissure) and lateral chest wall. **A,** Soft tissue windows. **B,** Lung windows. On soft tissue windows, the center appears slightly darker, indicating lower density that may represent central necrosis. If IV contrast had been given, an area of necrosis would have failed to enhance. Infection or infarction is technically possible, but a pulmonary neoplasm is the most likely explanation for this lesion. Biopsy showed this to be a moderately differentiated squamous cell carcinoma. (From Broder JS: *Diagnostic imaging for the emergency physician*, Philadelphia, 2011, Saunders.)

TABLE 2 Brief Description of the TNM Stage Groups for Lung Cancer

Stage 0	Carcinoma in situ					
Stage IA	T1a,b	N0	M0			
Stage IB	T2a	N0	M0			
Stage IIA	T1a,b, T2a	N1	M0	T2b N0 M0		
Stage IIB	T2b	N1	M0	T3	N0 M0	
Stage IIIA	T3	N1	M0	T1-3	N2 M0	T4 N0-1 M0
Stage IIIB	T4	N2	M0	Any T N3 M0		
Stage IV	Any T	Any N	M1a,b			

From Sellke FW et al: *Sabiston & Spencer surgery of the chest*, ed 9, 2016, Elsevier.

CT should include liver and adrenal glands (common sites of metastases). CT or MRI of brain should be considered in a patient presenting with neurologic symptoms (e.g., headaches, vision disturbances).
- PET with ^{18}F-fluorodeoxyglucose (^{18}FDG-PET) (Fig. E3) is superior to CT in detecting mediastinal and distant metastases in NSCLC. It is useful for preoperative staging of NSCLC.
- The use of PET-CT for preoperative staging of NSCLC reduces both the total number of thoracotomies and the number of futile thoracotomies.

STAGING

After confirmation of diagnosis, patients should undergo staging:
1. In NSCLC, the TNM staging system is used. Table 2 summarizes TNM stage groups. Stage I (N0; no lymph node involvement) and stage II (N1; spread to ipsilateral bronchopulmonary or hilar lymph nodes) include localized tumors for which surgical resection is the preferred treatment. Stage III is subdivided into IIIA (potentially resectable) and IIIB (unresectable). Stage IV indicates metastatic disease. In SCLC, the staging system developed by the

Veterans Administration Lung Cancer Study Group is used. It contains two stages:
   a. Limited-stage disease: confined to the regional lymph nodes and to one hemithorax (excluding pleural surfaces), which can be included in a single radiation portal
   b. Extensive-stage disease: spread beyond the confines of limited-stage disease
2. Pretreatment staging procedures for lung cancer patients, in addition to complete history and physical examination, generally include the following tests:
   a. Chest radiograph (posteroanterior and lateral), ECG.
   b. Laboratory evaluation: complete blood count, complete metabolic panel; arterial blood gases and pulse oximetry in selected cases.
   c. Pulmonary function studies.
   d. CT scan of chest and PET scan: trials have shown a reduction in futile thoracotomies for patients with suspected NSCLC who undergo preoperative assessment with PET in addition to conventional workup.
   e. Mediastinoscopy or anterior mediastinotomy in patients being considered for possible curative lung resection.
   f. Biopsy of any accessible suspect lesions.
   g. CT scan to include liver and brain.

TABLE 3 Summary of Multimodality Guidelines

Stage	Surgery	Adjuvant Therapy	Radiation	Chemotherapy	Level of Evidence
I	Yes	No	No	No	1B—Surgical resection 1B—Against postoperative chemotherapy 1A—Against postoperative radiation therapy
II	Yes	Yes	No	Yes	1B—Surgical resection 1A—Postoperative chemotherapy 2A—Against postoperative radiation therapy
IIIA					
(N2-occult)	Yes	Yes	May be considered	Yes	1A—Adjuvant chemo 2C—Adjuvant radiation
(N2-discrete)	Yes	No	Yes	Yes	1A—Definite or induction followed by surgery
			(Definitive or induction recommended)		1C—Against primary resection followed by adjuvant therapy
IIIB	No	No	Yes	Yes	1A—Definitive concurrent
(N2, N3)			(Definitive concurrent)		1A—Against induction followed by surgery

From Sellke FW et al: *Sabiston & Spencer surgery of the chest*, ed 9, 2016, Elsevier.

h. Bone marrow aspiration and biopsy only in selected patients with small cell carcinoma of the lung. In the absence of an increased lactate dehydrogenase or cytopenias, routine bone marrow examination is not recommended.

i. Newer technologies in preoperative staging include endoscopic bronchial ultrasonography and esophageal ultrasonography to guide biopsies; however, cervical mediastinoscopy is standard criterion in preoperative nodal staging (sensitivity >93%, specificity >95%).

Rx TREATMENT

NONPHARMACOLOGIC THERAPY

- Nutritional support
- Avoidance of tobacco and other substances toxic to the lungs
- Supplemental oxygen

ACUTE GENERAL Rx

NON–SMALL CELL CARCINOMA:

- Surgical resection is standard in patients with operable NSCLC (stage I or II) who are surgical candidates. Lobectomy is the best standard surgical approach. Lesser resections may be necessary in patients with marginal pulmonary reserve. Video-assisted thoracic surgery (VATS) is helpful in decreasing morbidity and shortening hospital stay.
  1. Surgical resection is indicated in patients with limited disease (not involving mediastinal nodes, ribs, pleura, or distant sites). This represents approximately 15% to 30% of diagnosed cases. Stereotactic ablative radiotherapy is a reasonable option for patients with localized NSCLC who are not surgical candidates. Multimodality treatment guidelines are summarized in Table 3.
  2. Preoperative evaluation includes cardiac status and pulmonary function assessment. Pneumonectomy is possible if the patient has a preoperative $FEV_1 = 2$ L or if the maximal voluntary ventilation is >50% of predicted capacity. Individuals with FEV_1 >1.5 L are suitable for lobectomy without further evaluation unless there is evidence of interstitial lung disease or undue dyspnea on exertion. In that case, carbon dioxide diffusion in the lung (DLCO) should be measured. If the DLCO is <80% predicted normal, the individual is not clearly operable.
  3. Conventional radiotherapy fails to durably control the primary lung tumor in nearly 70% of patients and 2-yr survival is less than 40%. Stereotactic body radiation (SBRT) uses several highly focused radiation beams to deliver high doses in 3 to 5 fractions and appears to be more effective than conventional radiotherapy, with a local control rate equivalent to that with surgery in inoperable early stage lung cancer.
  4. Preoperative chemotherapy should be considered in patients with more advanced disease (stage IIIA) who are being considered for surgery because it increases the median survival time in patients with NSCLC compared with the use of surgery alone.
  5. Postoperative adjuvant chemotherapy with cisplatin plus vinorelbine significantly increases 5-yr survival (69% vs. 54%) in patients with completely resected stage II-IIIA NSCLC.

- Treatment of unresectable NSCLC:
  1. Radiotherapy alone is used primarily for treatment of central nervous system and skeletal metastases, superior vena cava syndrome. Thoracic radiotherapy in combination with chemotherapy is standard therapy for unresectable stage 3 disease.
  2. Chemotherapy is the mainstay of treatment for advanced stage IIIB-IV NSCLC. Initial stratification is done based on pathology (squamous vs. non-squamous cancers) and presence of driver mutations (e.g. EGFR, ALK, and ROS1 mutations in adenocarcinomas). Table 4 summarizes selected NSCLC oncogenes and targeted therapy. A platinum-based double regimen is recommended for fit patients, and single agents are offered to elderly patients and those with poor performance status. Various combination regimens are available with platinum plus pemetrexed preferred for non-squamous cancers while other for squamous cancers other doublets such as paclitaxel plus carboplatin, cisplatin plus vinorelbine, gemcitabine plus cisplatin, and cisplatin plus docetaxel are utilized with none being clearly superior to the others. The addition of bevacizumab to paclitaxel plus carboplatin results in significant survival benefit in nonsquamous cancers.
  3. Upfront therapy with pembrolizumab, a PD-1 immune-checkpoint inhibitor antibody that disrupts PD-1 mediated signaling and restores antitumor immunity, has been recently shown to be superior to chemotherapy in patients with >50% PD-L1 expression. Both pembrolizumab and nivolumab (another PD-1 inhibitor antibody) have been shown to have superior survival benefit versus docetaxel in advanced squamous cell and nonsquamous cell NSCLC that had progressed during or after platinum-based chemotherapy.
  4. Tyrosine kinase inhibitors targeting activating mutations are of use in patients whose adenocarcinomas harbor the EGFR mutations. Gefitinib, erlotinib, and afatinib are oral EGFR inhibitors that have showed impressive responses and improvements in median overall survival to the range of 30 months. (These mutations are more common in adenocarcinomas found in patients who are never or light smokers and in Asian patients). Patients with EGFR mutations can acquire secondary T790M mutations that can be targeted with the oral inhibitor osimertinib.
  5. Oncogenic fusion genes consisting of EML4 and anaplastic lymphoma kinase (ALK) are present in 4% to 5% of adenocarcinomas and can be treated with inhibitors crizotinib or ceritinib. Approximately 2% of adenocarcinomas have genetic rearrangements involving the ROS1 proto-oncogenic receptor tyrosine kinase (ROS1). Recent trials have shown that the oral inhibitors crizotinib and ceritinib

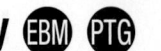

TABLE 4 Selected Non-Small Cell Lung Cancer Oncogenes and Targeted Therapy

Oncogene Alteration	Incidence (%)	Clinical Relevance	Treatment
BRAF			
Mutation	1-5	V600E mutation: most common, equal association with smokers and nonsmokers May be mechanism of acquired EGFR TKI resistance	V600E mutation: dabrafenib vemurafenib
EGFR (ErbB1, HER1)			
Mutation	13-50	Exon 19 deletion and Exon 21 point mutation are the most common Predominantly adenocarcinoma and nonsmokers Up to 50% frequency in Asian	TKI: gefitinib, erlotinib Monoclonal antibodies: cetuximab
EML4-ALK			
Fusion	3-13	Most frequent in adenocarcinomas, nonsmokers, men, and younger patients	Nonspecific TKI: crizotinib
Her2/neu (ErbB2)			Monoclonal antibodies: trastuzumab
Mutation	2-6	Mostly adenocarcinomas and nonsmokers	
Amplification	23	Mechanism of resistance to EGFR TKI	
KRAS			
Mutation	5-30	Mostly adenocarcinomas and smokers May contribute to resistance to ALF, BRAF, and PI3K inhibitors	No approved therapy Small-molecule inhibitors in preclinical trials
MET			Nonspecific TKI: crizotinib
Mutation	<5		
Amplification	21	Mechanism of resistance to EGFR TKI	
PIK3CA			Nonspecific TKI: crizotinib
Mutation	<10	Frequently occurs in association with other mutations; more common in squamous cell	
Amplification	5-43	Mechanism of resistance to EGFR TKI	
PTEN			Nonspecific TKI: crizotinib
Mutation	1.7-10	Associated with PI3K activation, resistance to EGFR TKI, and sensitivity to PI3K inhibitors More frequent in squamous cell	
Loss of function	4-21	Associated with PI3K activation, resistance to EGFR TKI, and sensitivity to PI3K inhibitors More frequent in squamous cell	
RET fusion gene	1-2	Mostly adenocarcinomas and nonsmokers	RET inhibitors: cabozantinib
ROS1 fusion gene	2	Mostly adenocarcinomas, nonsmokers, and younger patients	ALK inhibitor: crizotinib
VEGF			Monoclonal antibodies: bevacizumab VEGFR TKI

BRAF, v-raf murine sarcoma viral oncogene homolog B1; *EGFR,* epidermal growth factor receptor; *EML4-ALK,* echinoderm microtubule-associated protein-like 4 anaplastic lymphoma kinase; *ERBB,* avian erythroblastosis oncogene B; *Her2,* human epidermal growth factor receptor 2; *KRAS,* Kirsten Rat sarcoma viral oncogene homolog; *MET,* mesenchymal-epithelial transition; *PIK3CA,* phosphoinositide-3-kinase catalytic alpha polypeptide; *PTEH,* phosphatase and tensin homolog; *RET,* rearranged during transfection; *ROS1,* reactive oxygen species 1; *TKI,* tyrosine kinase inhibitor; *VEGF,* vascular endothelial growth factor; *VEGFR,* vascular endothelial growth factor receptor.
(From Sellke FW et al: *Sabiston & Spencer surgery of the chest,* ed 9, 2016, Elsevier.)

have marked antitumor activity in these patients.
6. The addition of chemotherapy to radiotherapy improves survival in patients with locally advanced, unresectable (stages IIIA-IIIB) NSCLC.
7. Early initiation of palliative care focusing on management of symptoms, psychosocial support, and assistance with decision making in patients with metastatic NSCLC leads to improved quality of life, longer survival, and less use of aggressive end-of-life care.

SMALL CELL LUNG CANCER:
- Limited-stage disease: standard treatments include thoracic radiotherapy and chemotherapy (cisplatin and etoposide).
- Extensive-stage disease: standard treatments include combination chemotherapy (platinum plus etoposide or platinum plus irinotecan).

- Prophylactic cranial irradiation for patients in complete remission to decrease the risk of central nervous system metastasis.
- Despite high initial response rates, most patients eventually relapse. Topotecan or irinotecan may be an option for these patients.
- The anti-PD-1 antibody, nivolumab, has demonstrated survival benefit in SCLC patients who have failed standard therapies.

DISPOSITION
- The 5-yr survival of patients with NSCLC when the disease is resectable is approximately 30%.
- Median survival time in patients with limited-stage disease SCLC is 15 mo; in patients with extensive-stage SCLC, it is 9 mo.
- Among patients with metastatic NSCLC, early palliative care results in longer survival and significant improvements in both quality of life and mood.

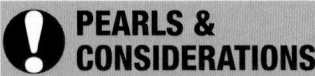 **PEARLS & CONSIDERATIONS**

- CT screening with use of low-dose computed tomography (LDCT) for detection of lung cancer among persons with a heavy history of smoking increases the percentage of lung cancer cases that are diagnosed in stage 1 and reduces mortality from lung cancer. The National Lung Screening Trial (NLST) showed that lung cancer screening with LDCT resulted in a 20% reduction in lung cancer mortality. New guidelines recommend annual LDCT for those who are current or former smokers aged 55 to 74. Screening should be discontinued once a person has not smoked for 15 years or develops a health problem that substantially limits life expectancy or the ability or willingness to have curative lung surgery.

RELATED CONTENT

Lung Cancer (Patient Information)
Lung Cancer Screening (Patient Information)
Horner's Syndrome (Related Key Topic)
Lambert-Eaton Myasthenic Syndrome (Related Key Topic)
Paraneoplastic Syndromes (Related Key Topic)
Superior Vena Cava Syndrome (Related Key Topic)

AUTHOR: **BHARTI RATHORE, M.D.**

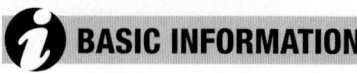

DEFINITION

Lyme disease is a multisystem inflammatory disorder caused by the transmission of a spirochete, *Borrelia burgdorferi*. Lyme disease is spread by the bite of infected *Ixodes* ticks, taking 36 to 48 hr for a tick to feed and transmit the infecting organism *B. burgdorferi* to the host.

SYNONYMS

Bannworth's syndrome (Europe)
Acrodermatitis chronica atrophicans

ICD-10CM CODES
A69.20 Lyme disease, unspecified
A69.21 Meningitis due to Lyme disease
A69.22 Other neurologic disorders in Lyme disease
A69.23 Arthritis due to Lyme disease
A69.29 Other conditions associated with Lyme disease

EPIDEMIOLOGY & DEMOGRAPHICS

INCIDENCE (IN U.S.): In the United States, 4.4 cases/100,000 persons; it is the most common vector-borne infection in the U.S., with more than 30,000 new cases reported each year. 90% of cases are found in: Massachusetts, Connecticut, Rhode Island, New York, New Jersey, Pennsylvania, Minnesota, Wisconsin, and California. The disease also occurs in Europe and Asia with a different *Ixodes* tick vector.
PEAK INCIDENCE: May to November.
PREDOMINANT SEX: Male = female.
PREDOMINANT AGE: Median age of 28 yr.

PHYSICAL FINDINGS & CLINICAL PRESENTATION

Lyme disease may present in the following stages:

- *Early localized stage (incubation period 3-30 days):* early Lyme disease, erythema migrans (EM); skin rash, often at site of tick bite (the CDC has defined EM rash as an expanding red macule or papule that must reach at least 5 cm in size, with or without central clearing); target lesions from ECM can be found in 60% to 80% of localized infections; possible fever, myalgias 3 to 32 days after tick bite.
- *Early disseminated stage (incubation period 3-6 weeks):* days to weeks later; multiorgan system involvement, including CNS with aseptic meningitis–type picture or Bell's palsy, joints (arthritis or arthralgias), cardiac including varying degrees of heart block; related to dissemination of spirochete
- *Late stage (incubation period months to years):* mo to yr after tick exposure; affects central and peripheral nervous system, cardiac, joints

Common presenting signs and symptoms include:

- EM (Fig. 1). Most patients with EM (about 80%) have a single lesion but the bacteria can disseminate hematogenously to other sites in the skin and result in often smaller erythema migrans lesions.
- Lymphadenopathy, neck pains, pharyngeal erythema, myalgias, hepatosplenomegaly.
- Patients will complain of malaise, fatigue, lethargy, headache, fever/chills, neck pain, myalgias, back pain.

ETIOLOGY

B. burgdorferi transmitted from bite of an *Ixodes* tick (mostly in the nymph stage, but can also be from adult ticks). Human infection occurs through inoculation of spirochetes in infected saliva and usually requires tick attachment for more than 36 hours.

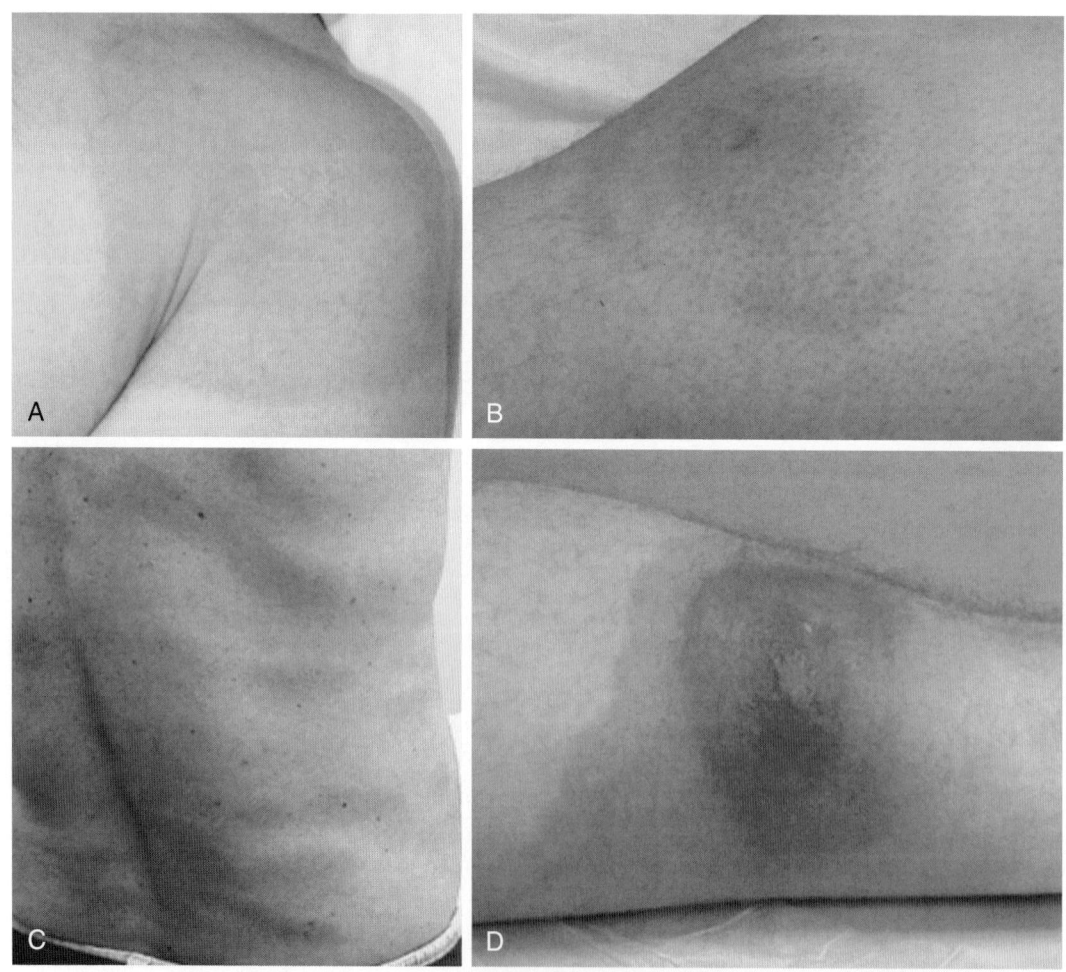

FIG. 1 Erythema migrans rash of Lyme disease. A, Typical macular lesion on left shoulder. **B,** Bull's eye lesion on lateral thigh with central punctum. **C,** Multiple lesions on back. **D,** Lesion with vesicular center on posterior thigh. (Courtesy Juan Salazar, MD, University of Connecticut Health Center.)

TABLE 1 Criteria for Western Blot Interpretation in the Serologic Confirmation of Lyme Disease

Duration of Disease	Isotype Tested	Criteria for Positive Test
First month of infection	IgM	2 of the following 3 bands are present: 23 kD (OspC), 39 kD (BmpA), and 41 kD (Fla)
After first month of infection	IgG	5 of 10 bands are present: 18 kD, 21 kD, 28 kD, 30 kD, 39 kD, 41 kD, 45 kD, 58 kD (not GroEL), 66 kD, and 93 kD

Modified from Centers for Disease Control and Prevention: Recommendations for test performance and interpretation from the Second National Conference on Serologic Diagnosis of Lyme Disease, *MMWR Morb Mortal Wkly Rep* 44:590–591, 1995.

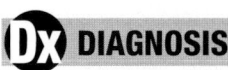 **DIAGNOSIS**

Clinical presentation, exposure to ticks in endemic area, and diagnostic testing for antibody response to *B. burgdorferi*. Serologic testing at early stages is usually negative; therefore, in early stage, documentation of erythema migrans lesion with a compatible epidemiologic history is sufficient for diagnosis, and laboratory testing is not indicated.

DIFFERENTIAL DIAGNOSIS

- Chronic fatigue/fibromyalgia.
- Acute viral illnesses.
- Babesiosis.
- Human granulocytic anaplasmosis

WORKUP

- ELISA testing and if positive or equivocal then followed by a Western blot IgM and IgG (Table 1). A Western blot IgM assay is positive if 2 of 3 bands present. The Western blot IgG is positive if 5 of 10 bands present.
- An alternative serologic test is the VlsE C6 ELISA, which detects an IgG response earlier.
- Early disease often difficult to diagnose serologically secondary to slow immune response
- Culturing of skin lesions (EM) and polymerase chain reaction (PCR) of synovial fluid or CSF can also give the diagnosis of active infection.

IMAGING STUDIES

- ECG
- Echocardiogram if conduction abnormalities are present with cardiac involvement.
- CT scan, MRI of head for CNS involvement.

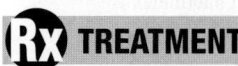 **TREATMENT**

Early localized Lyme disease:

- Doxycycline 100 mg bid in adults (children: 2 mg/kg twice daily if ≥8 yr) [doxycycline offers the advantage of treating possible coinfection with the bacterial agents of Ehrlichiosis] for 10 to 14 days or amoxicillin 500 mg tid for adults (children: 50 mg/kg per day in three divided doses) for 14 to 21 days.

- Alternative treatments for pregnancy and children ≤8 years: cefuroxime axetil 500 mg bid for 14 to 21 days (children: 30 mg/kg per day in two divided doses), azithromycin 500 mg PO for 7 to 10 days but should **not** be used as a first-line agent, as it is less effective than doxycycline and amoxicillin.
- A single dose of 200 mg doxycycline given within 72 hr of removing an engorged *Ixodes* tick can significantly reduce the risk of developing of Lyme disease in endemic areas and is reasonable prophylaxis in nonpregnant adults and children ≥8 years old.

Early disseminated and late persistent infection:

- 28 days of treatment is often prescribed, although recent evidence supports treating patients with a 14-day course of oral doxycycline for early neurologic Lyme disease in ambulatory patients.[1] Doxycycline and ceftriaxone appear equally effective for acute disseminated Lyme disease.
- Arthritis: 28 days of doxycycline or amoxicillin plus probenecid.
- Neurologic involvement requires parenteral antibiotics. Those who fail to respond should be treated with IV ceftriaxone or cefotaxime.
- Ceftriaxone 2 g/day IV for 21 to 28 days; alternative: cefotaxime 2 g q8h IV; alternative: penicillin G 5 million U qid.
- Cardiac involvement: IV ceftriaxone or cefotaxime plus cardiac monitoring.
- Prolonged treatment with IV or PO antibiotic therapy for up to 90 days did not improve symptoms more than placebo.

Post–Lyme disease syndrome:

- Presence of disabling symptoms such as fatigue, malaise, diffuse pains, and poor concentration, which may be due to an exuberant host inflammatory response
- Antibiotics are not indicated. Antibiotic treatment of patients with persistent unexplained

[1]Sanchez E, et al.: Diagnosis, treatment, and prevention of Lyme disease, human granulocytic anaplasmosis, and babesiosis: a review, *JAMA* 315(16):1767–1777, 2016.

symptoms despite previous antibiotic treatment of Lyme disease provides little, if any, benefit and carries significant risk.

- Supportive care

DISPOSITION

- The patient often needs careful follow-up and supportive care for the arthralgia-neuritis symptoms.
- 10% to 20% of treated patients may have lingering symptoms of fatigue, disrupted sleep, and musculoskeletal complaints. Repeat episodes of EM in appropriately treated patients are due to reinfection and not to relapse.

REFERRAL

- To a neurologist if significant neurologic complications (meningitis, myelitis, ophthalmoplegia, Bell's palsy).
- To a cardiologist if the patient develops evidence of cardiac conduction disturbances or pericarditis.

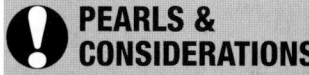 **PEARLS & CONSIDERATIONS**

- A physician diagnosis of classic EM in an endemic region of Lyme disease is sufficient to make a definitive diagnosis.
- In some patients with Lyme disease, nonspecific complaints such as headache, fatigue, and arthralgia may persist for months after appropriate (and ultimately successful) antibiotic treatment. Long-term antibiotic treatment does not provide additional beneficial effects.
- There is no evidence of current or previous *Borrelia burgdorferi* infection in most patients evaluated at university-based Lyme disease referral centers. Psychiatric comorbidity and other psychological factors are prominent in the presentation and outcome of some patients who inaccurately ascribe longstanding symptoms to "chronic Lyme disease."
- It is important to realize that one tick bite can transmit Lyme disease *and* the bacterial agents of either Ehrlichiosis or Babesiosis, or even both, and these latter agents require separate serologic testing and possibly therapy. *Ehrlichiosis* is treated with doxycycline, but *Babesia* would require a different therapy.

SUGGESTED READINGS

Available at www.expertconsult.com

RELATED CONTENT

Lyme Disease (Patient Information)

AUTHOR: **GLENN G. FORT, M.D., M.P.H.**

L

Diseases and Disorders

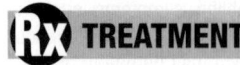

BASIC INFORMATION

DEFINITION

Lymphangitis refers to the inflammation of lymphatic vessels due to infectious or noninfectious causes. Infectious causes include bacteria, mycobacteria, viruses, fungi, and parasites.

SYNONYMS

Nodular lymphangitis
Sporotrichoid lymphangitis

ICD-10CM CODES

I89.1 Lymphangitis

EPIDEMIOLOGY & DEMOGRAPHICS

INCIDENCE (IN U.S.): Several hundred cases/yr of sporotrichoid lymphangitis; bacterial lymphangitis more common but not reported.

PHYSICAL FINDINGS & CLINICAL PRESENTATION

ACUTE LYMPHANGITIS:
- Commonly associated with a bacterial cellulitis.
- Usually develops after cutaneous inoculation of microorganisms into the lymphatic vessels through disrupted skin or as a result of spread from a distal infection.
- May or may not recognize a site of skin trauma (i.e., laceration, puncture, ulcer).
- In hours to days, distal appearance of erythema, edema, and tenderness, with linear erythematous streaks extending proximally to regional lymph nodes.
- Possible lymphadenitis and fever.
- Predisposition to group A streptococcal infection of the skin in those with uncontrolled diabetes mellitus, chronic lymphedema, and superficial fungal infections (e.g., tinea pedis).

SPOROTRICHOID OR NODULAR LYMPHANGITIS:
- Includes subcutaneous nodules that develop along the path of involved lymphatics.
- Most commonly results from inoculation of the skin of the hand.
- Usually preceded by well-defined episode of cutaneous inoculation or trauma.
- Lesions apparent from one to several weeks after inoculation.
- Initially, nodular or papular lesion; may ulcerate.
- May have frank pus or a serosanguineous discharge.
- Systemic complaints uncommon, but infection with certain microorganisms associated with fever, chills, myalgias, and headache.

ETIOLOGY

- Acute lymphangitis: usually associated with *Streptococcus pyogenes* (group A streptococcus), and to a lesser extent staphylococcus species, including community-acquired methicillin-resistant *S. aureus* (CA-MRSA).
- Nodular lymphangitis caused by one of several organisms.
  1. *Sporothrix schenckii* ("Rose gardener's disease").
     a. Most common recognized cause in the United States, usually in the Midwest.
     b. Found in soil and plant debris.
  2. *Nocardia brasiliensis:* found in soil.
  3. *Mycobacterium marinum:* associated with trauma related to water (e.g., aquariums, swimming pools, fish).
  4. *Leishmania brasiliensis.*
     a. Protozoal parasite transmitted to humans by sandflies, mostly to travelers in endemic areas.
     b. Small endemic focus in Texas.
  5. *Francisella tularensis.*
     a. Most often in Southern/Midwestern states (Arkansas, Missouri, Oklahoma).
     b. Associated with contact with infected mammals, (e.g., rabbits, squirrels) tick bites, and (rarely) water exposure.

DIAGNOSIS

DIFFERENTIAL DIAGNOSIS

- Nodular lymphangitis.
- Insect or snake bites.
- Filariasis.

WORKUP

- Acute lymphangitis: blood cultures.
- Nodular lymphangitis: various stains and cultures of drainage or biopsy specimens of inoculation sites to make definitive diagnosis.

LABORATORY TESTS

- WBCs possibly elevated with cellulitis.
- Eosinophilia common with helminthic infections.
- Skin biopsy and microbiologic cultures may be necessary to confirm diagnosis in nodular lymphangitis.

TREATMENT

NONPHARMACOLOGIC THERAPY

Limb elevation.

ACUTE GENERAL Rx

- Penicillin possibly sufficient, but 1 wk of dicloxacillin or cephalexin 500 mg PO qid commonly used to ensure antistaphylococcal coverage; if CA-MRSA suspected, then use oral Bactrim DS one PO bid or clindamycin 300 mg PO q6H. Reserve vancomycin 1 g IV every 12 hr for patients requiring IV therapy.
- If allergic to penicillin:
  1. Clindamycin 300 mg PO qid for 7 days *or*
  2. Erythromycin 500 mg PO qid for 7 days.
  3. Levofloxacin 500 mg PO daily or moxifloxacin 400 mg PO daily for 7 days.
- Nodular lymphangitis: specific therapy directed at etiologic agent.
- For superficial fungal infections: treatment may prevent recurrence of acute lymphangitis.

DISPOSITION

- Acute lymphangitis: usually resolves with therapy.
- Recurrent attacks: may lead to chronic lymphedema of limb, rarely resulting in elephantiasis nostras (nonfilarial elephantiasis).
- Nodular lymphangitis: usually responds to appropriate therapy.

REFERRAL

- If acute lymphangitis is more than a mild disease or if it involves the face.
- If nodular lymphangitis or filariasis is suspected.

PEARLS & CONSIDERATIONS

COMMENTS

- Outside of the United States, initial episodes of filariasis caused by *Brugia malayi* resemble acute lymphangitis.
- Chronic lymphedema or elephantiasis results from recurrent episodes.
- For chronic lymphedema, adherence to limb elevation, compression/support stockings, and adequate glycemic control (for patients with diabetes) all can reduce risk of acute lymphangitis.

RELATED CONTENT

Lymphangitis (Patient Information)

AUTHOR: **RUSSELL J. MCCULLOH, M.D.**

BASIC INFORMATION

DEFINITION
A primary role of the lymphatic system is to transport proteins from the interstitium to the heart. When the transport capacity of the lymphatic system is reduced, proteins accumulate in the interstitium. Accumulated proteins attract water, which creates a high protein swelling in the subcutaneous tissues called lymphedema.

SYNONYMS
Elephantiasis

ICD-10CM CODES
I97.2 Postmastectomy lymphedema syndrome
I89.0 Lymphedema, not elsewhere classified
Q82.0 Hereditary lymphedema

EPIDEMIOLOGY & DEMOGRAPHICS
PRIMARY LYMPHEDEMA:
- Found in 1.1/100,000 people aged <20 yr.
- Females outnumber males 3.5:1.
- Incidence peaks between ages 12 and 16 (puberty).

SECONDARY LYMPHEDEMA: See specific etiology in the following.

PHYSICAL FINDINGS & CLINICAL PRESENTATION
Lymphedema is a slow-onset, progressive disease characterized by an asymmetrical, inflammatory swelling, traveling distal to proximal, that can affect any body part including limbs, trunk, head/neck, and genitals (Fig. 1). Box 1 summarizes lymphedema staging from the International Society of Lymphology.

STAGE 0: LATENCY:
- Decreased lymphatic system transport capacity due to primary or secondary etiology.

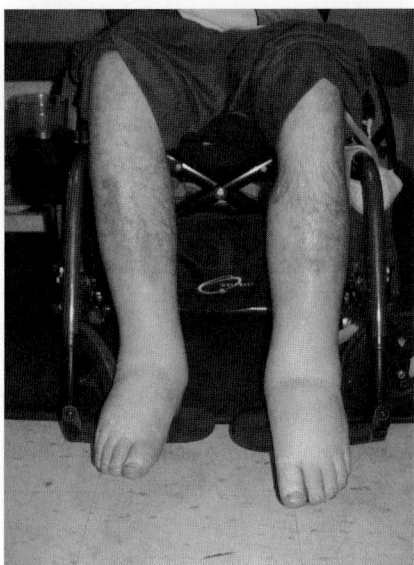

FIG. 1 Lymphedema before treatment.

- Subjective complaints of affected body part feeling heavy or achy.
- No objective findings, no apparent swelling.

STAGE I: REVERSIBLE:
- Edema is observable, soft, pitting and reversible with elevation.
- No secondary skin changes are present.

STAGE II: SPONTANEOUSLY IRREVERSIBLE:
- Skin becomes more firm/fibrotic, therefore less pitting.
- Edema does not reverse to normal with elevation.
- Possibility of infections (cellulitis), wounds, or weeping (lymphorrhea).

STAGE III: ELEPHANTIASIS:
- Skin becomes very firm/fibrotic, therefore nonpitting.
- Evidence of substantial skin changes (e.g., papillomas, lobules, *"peau d' orange"*).

ETIOLOGY: Lymphedema is caused by a reduction in lymphatic system transport and is classified into primary and secondary forms.

Primary Lymphedema.
- Occurs when the lymphatic system does not mature properly during fetal development.
  1. Aplasia.
  2. Hypoplasia.
  3. Hyperplasia.
- Can be familial, genetic, or hereditary.
- Lymphedema congenital: symptoms present at birth.
- Lymphedema praecox: symptoms onset before the age of 35 (commonly during puberty).
- Lymphedema tardum: symptoms onset at the age of 35 or after.

Secondary Lymphedema.
- Occurs secondary to a disruption or obstruction of the lymphatic system caused by:
  1. Filariasis (#1 cause worldwide).
  2. Lymph node surgery/radiation due to cancer (#1 cause in the United States).

BOX 1 Lymphedema Staging

Stage 0: Latent
- Impaired lymphatic function
- No evident edema; subclinical
- May last months or years before progression

Stage I: Spontaneously Reversible
- Early accumulation of protein-rich fluid
- Pitting edema
- Subsides with elevation

Stage II: Spontaneously Irreversible
- Accumulation of protein-rich fluid
- Pitting edema progresses to fibrosis
- Does not resolve with elevation alone

Stage III: Lymphostatic Elephantiasis
- Nonpitting
- Significant fibrosis
- Trophic skin changes

From International Society of Lymphology: The diagnosis and treatment of peripheral edema: 2009 consensus document of the International Society of Lymphology, *Lymphology* 42(2):51-60, 2009.

---

3. Other: chronic venous insufficiency (CVI), deep vein thrombosis (DVT), infection, surgery/trauma, lipedema, and obesity.

DIAGNOSIS

- Lymphedema is primarily a clinical diagnosis made on the basis of past medical history and objective findings that distinguish it from other causes of chronic edema.
- A Stemmer's sign is often used to identify lymphedema (inability to pick up or pinch a fold of skin at the base of the second toe or finger).
- When physical examination is inconclusive, other available imaging tests can help make the diagnosis (see "Imaging Studies").

DIFFERENTIAL DIAGNOSIS
Other causes of edema that should be ruled out before treatment for lymphedema include cardiac, renal, hepatic, and thyroid dysfunction.

WORKUP
A detailed history and physical examination should help exclude most of the differential diagnoses.

LABORATORY TESTS
- Blood urea nitrogen, creatinine, liver function tests, albumin, urine analysis, and thyroid function tests are obtained to exclude possible systemic causes of edema.
- Genetic testing may be practical in defining a specific hereditary syndrome with a discrete gene mutation such as lymphedema distichiasis (*FOXC2*), Milroy's disease (*VEGFR-3*), Meige's disease, or Klippel-Trenaunay-Weber syndrome.

IMAGING STUDIES
- Lymphoscintigraphy: diagnostic image of choice for lymphedema (if needed).
- Indocyanine green (ICG) fluorescent lymphography: can now be used to identify sentinel nodes, to demonstrate superficial lymph channels and functional lymphatics, to indicate treatment pathways, and to confirm the effectiveness of therapeutic techniques.
- Magnetic resonance imaging (MRI): primarily used in tumor diagnosis.
- Duplex ultrasound: determines venous involvement in the edema.
- Computed axial tomography (CAT): distinguishes between fatty tissue and accumulations of protein-rich fluids.
- Lymphography: phased out in favor of less invasive techniques.

TREATMENT

NONPHARMACOLOGIC THERAPY
- Complete decongestive therapy (CDT) is backed by longstanding research and experience as the primary treatment of choice for lymphedema in both children and adults (Fig. 2). It should be delivered by a certified

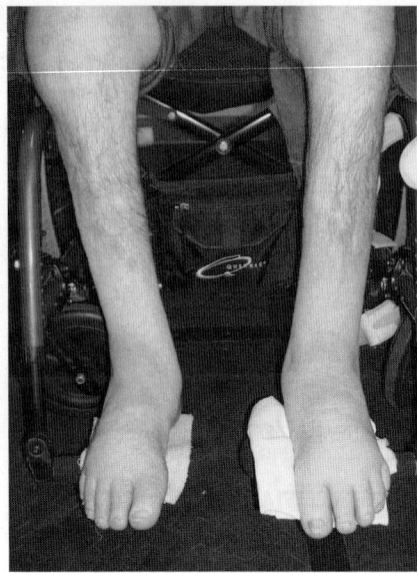

FIG. 2 Lymphedema after treatment.

lymphedema therapist (CLT). CDT involves a two-phase treatment program:

1. Phase 1—Reduce tissue congestion of affected body part with daily treatments:
   1. Manual lymph drainage.
   2. Skin care.
   3. Compression wrapping of limb.
   4. Decongestive exercises.
2. Phase 2—Maintain decongestion with Home Maintenance Program:
   1. Daily use of elastic and inelastic compression garments that are properly fitted according to circumference and length to prevent lymphedema from returning.
   2. Compression is graduated; most of the compression is distal with decreasing compression in the stocking proximally.
   3. Different knits and compression classes are available for different stages of lymphedema.
   4. Choices of garments include below-the-knee stockings, thigh-high stockings, pantyhose, sleeves, bras, and truncal garments.

- Massage (or any modality that increases blood flow) can have negative effects on lymphedema by increasing vasodilation. Therefore it is contraindicated on the lymphedematous quadrants.
- Compression pumps have not been found to be effective in removing proteins from lymphedematous quadrants.
- Nutritional therapy (reducing the amount of proteins ingested) is ineffective in the treatment of lymphedema.

PHARMACOLOGIC THERAPY

No drugs have been shown to be beneficial in the treatment of lymphedema. Diuretics, in particular, have not been found to be effective in removing proteins from lymphedematous quadrants and may promote the development of volume depletion.

SURGERY

Surgery for lymphedema has been proven largely unsuccessful and should not be considered before CDT. Surgical procedures are divided into two types:

- Physiologic procedures: those performed to improve lymph node drainage (e.g., anastomoses of the lymph system with the venous system, lymph node transplant).
- Excisional or debulking procedures: those performed to excise the subcutaneous tissue (e.g., Charles' procedure, Thompson's procedure, the modified Homans' procedure, and liposuction). Liposuction-circumferential suction-assisted lipectomy represents a newly proposed method to reduce morbidity involved in the traditional excisional techniques.

ⓘ PEARLS & CONSIDERATIONS

- Lymphedema is a chronic, generally incurable but very manageable condition that requires lifelong care and attention along with psychosocial support.
- Children and adolescents (along with parents and adults) should be encouraged to pursue a normal life, participating in school activities and sports (preferably noncontact, such as swimming).
- Infections such as cellulitis should be treated promptly.
- If the etiology is filariasis caused by the parasites *Wuchereria bancrofti* or *Brugia malayi*, treatment is diethylcarbamazine citrate 5 mg/kg in divided doses for 3 wk.
- Patients with lymphedema commonly manifest psychiatric comorbidities as a result of their disease, such as anxiety, depression, adjustment problems, and difficulty in vocational, domestic, or social domains.
- Lymphedema can be complicated in rare cases by development of lymphangiosarcomata or other cutaneous malignancies.
- Gene therapy to develop new lymphangioses in the affected body parts is a potential clinical remedy in the future.

SUGGESTED READING

Available at www.expertconsult.com

RELATED CONTENT

Lymphedema (Patient Information)

AUTHORS: **FRANK G. FORT, M.D.,** and **KATHRYN TAYLOR ANILOWSKI, M.S., P.T., C.L.T.-L.A.N.A.**

BASIC INFORMATION

DEFINITION

Non-Hodgkin's lymphoma (NHL) is a heterogeneous group of malignancies of the lymphoreticular system. There are approximately 40 different NHL subtypes.

SYNONYMS

NHL
Non-Hodgkin's lymphoma

ICD-10CM CODES
C85.90 Non-Hodgkin lymphoma, unspecified, unspecified site
C85.91 Non-Hodgkin lymphoma, unspecified, lymph nodes of head, face, and neck
C85.92 Non-Hodgkin lymphoma, unspecified, intrathoracic lymph nodes
C85.93 Non-Hodgkin lymphoma, unspecified, intra-abdominal lymph nodes
C85.94 Non-Hodgkin lymphoma, unspecified, lymph nodes of axilla and upper limb
C85.95 Non-Hodgkin lymphoma, unspecified, lymph nodes of inguinal region and lower limb
C85.96 Non-Hodgkin lymphoma, unspecified, intrapelvic lymph nodes
C85.97 Non-Hodgkin lymphoma, unspecified, spleen
C85.98 Non-Hodgkin lymphoma, unspecified, lymph nodes of multiple sites
C85.99 Non-Hodgkin lymphoma, unspecified, extranodal and solid organ sites

EPIDEMIOLOGY

- Sixth most common neoplasm in the U.S. (>70,000 new cases annually). Incidence increases with age; majority of patients are above 60 years of age.
- Diffuse large B-cell lymphoma (DLBCL) is the most common subtype (30% of the cases). Follicular lymphoma (FL) is the second most common subtype (25% of the cases).
- In patients with HIV, NHL is the most common tumor (followed by Kaposi sarcoma). DLBCL accounts for 80% to 90% of the cases of HIV-associated NHL.

PHYSICAL FINDINGS & CLINICAL PRESENTATION

- Patients often present with lymphadenopathy.
- Approximately one third of the NHL involve extranodal sites, which can result in unusual presentations (e.g., gastrointestinal tract involvement can simulate peptic ulcer disease).
- Presence of B symptoms like unexplained weight loss, fever, fatigue, and night sweats are seen typically in aggressive or highly aggressive lymphomas.
- Aggressive lymphomas have acute or subacute presentation with increasing size of the mass and B symptoms.
- Indolent lymphomas have a more chronic course, with asymptomatic lymphadenopathy and/or slowly progressive cytopenias.
- Hepatomegaly and splenomegaly may be present.
- Cough, dyspnea with bulky mediastinal involvement

DIAGNOSIS

DIFFERENTIAL DIAGNOSIS

- Hodgkin's lymphoma.
- Viral infections.
- Metastatic carcinoma.
- Autoimmune conditions.
- Sarcoidosis

A clinical algorithm for evaluation of lymphadenopathy is described in Section III. The differential diagnosis of lymphadenopathy is described in Section II.

WORKUP

Initial laboratory evaluation may be entirely normal. Elevated LDH may be seen in aggressive lymphoma or in indolent lymphoma with high disease bulk. In cases of highly aggressive NHL (e.g., Burkitt lymphoma), spontaneous tumor lysis syndrome (TLS) may be seen, but rarely; it is characterized by hyperkalemia, hyperuricemia, hypocalcemia, hyperphosphatemia, and acidosis. TLS can be life threatening, and is considered a medical emergency. Acute management includes aggressive IV fluid repletion and rasburicase. Proper staging of NHL includes the following:

- A thorough history and physical examination.
- Excisional or incisional surgical biopsy is preferred. Image-guided core needle biopsies may be acceptable in patients without peripheral adenopathy. Fine needle aspirates are not adequate for precise lymphoma subclassification. Laparoscopic lymph node biopsy or mediastinoscopy can be used on an outpatient basis for most patients with intraabdominal or mediastinal lymphoma, respectively.
- Tissue biopsy with histologic, immunophenotypic, and genetic studies interpretation.
- Routine laboratory evaluation (complete blood count, flow cytometry in selected circumstances, ESR, urinalysis, LDH, blood urea nitrogen, creatinine, serum calcium, uric acid, liver function tests, serum protein electrophoresis).
- HIV and hepatitis B testing.
- Bone marrow evaluation (aspirate and biopsy) (Fig. E1).
- CT scan of chest, abdomen and pelvis with IV contrast, if possible.
- Fluorine-18 fluorodeoxyglucose (FDG) positron emission tomography (PET) integrated with CT has emerged as a powerful tool for staging, response evaluation, and post-treatment surveillance in patients with aggressive subtypes of NHL.
- Depending on the histopathology (Table 1), the results of the previous studies and the planned therapy, some other tests may be performed.
- Lumbar puncture is needed in some patients with aggressive NHL, and most patients with HIV-associated NHL, to evaluate for CNS involvement by lymphoma.

CLASSIFICATION: For clinical approach, NHL is subdivided lymphomas into indolent, aggressive, and highly aggressive disease.

STAGING: The Ann Arbor staging system with Cotswold modification is described in Table 2. Histopathology has greater therapeutic implications in NHL than in Hodgkin's lymphoma. The frequency of indolent lymphomas among all lymphomas is described in Table 3. The classification of aggressive lymphomas is described in Table 4.

TREATMENT

ACUTE GENERAL Rx

The therapeutic regimen varies with specific lymphoma subtype and pathologic stage. Following are the commonly used therapeutic modalities:

INDOLENT NHL:
1. Deferment of therapy and careful observation in asymptomatic patients with low volume disease.
2. Local radiotherapy for stage I disease.
3. Rituximab, an anti-CD20 monoclonal antibody, with or without chemotherapy is used in patients with symptomatic or progressive disease.
4. The addition of rituximab to chemotherapy is generally well tolerated and has increased response and survival rates in these patients.
5. Patients who received rituximab, cyclophosphamide, doxorubicin, vincristine, and prednisone (R-CHOP) had higher response rates (96% vs. 90%) with a better 2-year overall survival rate (95% vs. 90%) than patients who received CHOP without rituximab.
6. Similarly, patients who received rituximab, cyclophosphamide, vincristine, and prednisone (R-CVP) had higher response rates (81% vs. 57%) and better overall survival at 4 years (83% vs. 77%) than patients who were treated with CVP without rituximab.
7. In a recent phase III noninferiority study, the combination of bendamustine and rituximab was associated with better progression-free survival rates than R-CHOP (70 vs. 31 months) with fewer toxic effects.
8. Maintenance rituximab after rituximab-containing regimens has been associated with a better progression-free survival at 3 years (75% vs. 58%) than observation alone without a difference in overall survival.
9. Second-line chemotherapy or novel agents such as lenalidomide, ibrutinib, idelalisib, or obinutuzumab are highly active in relapsed disease.
10. Stem cell transplantation (autologous or allogeneic) may confer long-term disease control in multiple relapsed or refractory disease.
11. *H. pylori*-associated gastric marginal zone lymphoma can be treated with a course of antibiotics. For persistent cases after eradication or *H. pylori*-negative cases, radiotherapy is highly effective.
12. Table 5 summarizes treatment strategies for indolent lymphomas.

AGGRESSIVE NHL: The most common aggressive NHL is DLBCL. The addition of rituximab against CD20 B-cell lymphoma to the CHOP regimen (R-CHOP) increases the complete response rate and prolongs overall survival in patients with DLBCL without clinically significant increase in toxicity. R-CHOP has shown to be safe and

TABLE 1 Histologic Features of Non-Hodgkin's Lymphomas Involving Bone Marrow

Type of Lymphoma	Incidence of Involvement (%)	Pattern of Involvement*	Cytology	Comments
Small lymphocytic	85	FR, I, D	Small, mature lymphocytes; proliferation centers may be present	CD5+, CD19+ cells; paratrabecular infiltrates essentially rule out this diagnosis
Lymphoplasmacytic	80-100	FR, I, D, FP	Spectrum of cells from lymphocytes to plasma cells; immunoblasts may be present; Dutcher bodies common	Unlike SLL/CLL, occasional paratrabecular infiltrates may be present
Mantle cell	55-95	FR, I, D, FP	Small irregular lymphocytes; may be blastoid; rare cells with prominent nucleoli	CD5+, cyclin D1 positive; paratrabecular infiltrates may be present
Follicular	50-60	FP, D, FR, I	Small cleaved lymphocytes usually predominate; large cleaved or noncleaved cells may be present	CD10+; characteristically paratrabecular; neoplastic follicles may be apparent
Splenic marginal zone	73-100	FR, I, D, IS	Small lymphocytes with slightly irregular nuclei, condensed chromatin, and abundant cytoplasm	Intrasinusoidal infiltrates often prominent; reactive germinal centers may be present
Low-grade extranodal marginal zone	44	FR, P, I, IS	Small cells with condensed chromatin and scant to moderate amounts of cytoplasm; rare large cells may be admixed	Extent of bone marrow infiltration usually minimal
Nodal marginal zone	30-40	FR, I, P, D	Small cells with condensed chromatin and scant to moderate amounts of cytoplasm	
Diffuse large B cell	15-30	FR, D	Large cells with prominent nucleoli	Prominent component of T lymphocytes with or without histiocytes may be present; immunohistochemistry for B-cell antigens and other markers is essential in these cases; rare cases of large cell lymphoma are intravascular
Burkitt	35-60	I, D	Medium-sized cells with reticular chromatin, multiple small nucleoli, and basophilic cytoplasm; cytoplasmic vacuoles common	CD10+, c-MYC+; necrosis common; "starry sky" pattern may be seen
Peripheral T cell (unspecified)	80	FR, D	Polymorphic lymphoid population—nuclei often hyperchromatic and irregular; large cells with nucleoli may be present; prominent reactive cell component often intermixed with lymphoma cells	Vascularity and reticulin fibrosis frequently prominent
Anaplastic large cell	4-40	FR, I (scattered cells), D	Large cells with lobulated nuclei, prominent nucleoli, and abundant cytoplasm	Detection rate is higher with immunostaining for CD30 or ALK-1
Hepatosplenic T cell	100	IS	Medium-sized lymphocytes with dispersed chromatin	Lesions may be subtle; immunohistochemistry is often helpful
Lymphoblastic	50-60	I, D	Blastic cells with high mitotic rate	Identical to acute lymphoblastic leukemia
NK/T cell	0-25	I (scattered cells)	Variable size with pleomorphic nuclei	Immunostains or in situ hybridization (EBER) may be necessary to identify lymphoma cells in bone marrow sections

D, Diffuse; EBER, Epstein-Barr virus–encoded RNA; FP, focal paratrabecular; FR, focal random; I, interstitial; IS, intrasinusoidal; NK, natural killer; P, paratrabecular.
*Patterns may be mixed; the most common patterns are listed.
From Jaffe ES, et al.: *Hematopathology*, Philadelphia, 2011, Saunders.

TABLE 2 Ann Arbor Staging System for Lymphomas

Stage*	Cotswold Modification of Ann Arbor Classification
I	Involvement of a single lymph node region or lymphoid structure
II	Involvement of two or more lymph node regions on the same side of the diaphragm (the mediastinum is considered a single site, whereas the hilar lymph nodes are considered bilaterally); the number of anatomic sites should be indicated by a subscript (e.g., II_3)
III	Involvement of lymph node regions on both sides of the diaphragm: III_1 (with or without involvement of splenic hilar, celiac, or portal nodes) and III_2 (with involvement of para-aortic, iliac, and mesenteric nodes)
IV	Involvement of one or more extranodal sites in addition to a site for which the designation E has been used

*All cases are subclassified to indicate the absence (A) or presence (B) of the systemic symptoms of significant fever (>38.0° C [100.4° F]), night sweats, and unexplained weight loss exceeding 10% of normal body weight within the previous 6 months. The clinical stage (CS) denotes the stage as determined by all diagnostic examinations and a single diagnostic biopsy only. In the Ann Arbor classification, the term pathologic stage (PS) is used if a second biopsy of any kind has been obtained, whether negative or positive. In the Cotswold modification, the PS is determined by laparotomy; X designates bulky disease (widening of the mediastinum by >one third or the presence of a nodal mass >10 cm), and E designates involvement of a single extranodal site that is contiguous or proximal to the known nodal site.
From Hoffmann R, et al.: *Hematology: basic principles and practice*, ed 5, Philadelphia, 2009, Churchill Livingstone.

TABLE 3 Frequency of Indolent Lymphomas Among All Lymphomas in the World Health Organization Classification

Follicular lymphoma	22.1%
Extranodal marginal zone lymphoma of mucosa-associated lymphoid tissue type	7.6%
Small lymphocytic lymphoma/chronic lymphocytic leukemia	6.7%
Mantle cell	6.0%
Splenic marginal zone lymphoma	1.8%
Lymphoplasmacytic lymphoma	1.2%
Nodal marginal zone B-cell lymphoma (±monocytoid B cells)	1.0%

From Hoffman R, et al.: *Hematology: basic principles and practice*, ed 5, Philadelphia, 2009, Churchill Livingstone.

TABLE 4 Classification of Aggressive Lymphomas

B-cell Neoplasms
Precursor B-cell lymphoma
Precursor B lymphoblastic leukemia/lymphoma
Mature B-cell lymphoma
Mantle cell lymphoma
Diffuse large B-cell lymphoma
Mediastinal (thymic) large B-cell lymphoma
Intravascular large B-cell lymphoma
Primary effusion lymphoma
Burkitt lymphoma
B-cell proliferations of uncertain malignant potential
Lymphomatoid granulomatosis
Posttransplant lymphoproliferative disorder, polymorphic

T-cell and NK-cell Neoplasms
Precursor T-cell
Precursor T lymphoblastic leukemia/lymphoma
Blastic NK cell lymphoma
Mature T-cell and NK-cell lymphoma
Adult T-cell leukemia/lymphoma
Extranodal NK/T cell lymphoma, nasal type
Hepatosplenic T-cell lymphoma
Peripheral T-cell lymphoma, unspecified
Angioimmunoblastic T-cell lymphoma
Anaplastic large cell lymphoma

NK, Natural killer.
From Hoffman R, et al.: *Hematology: basic principles and practice*, ed 5, Philadelphia, 2009, Churchill Livingstone.

TABLE 5 Treatment Strategies for Indolent Lymphomas

Advanced Stage Disease
Watchful waiting
Alkylating agents
Purine analogs (rarely used)
Combination chemotherapy (e.g., CVP, CHOP)
Single agent rituximab
Chemoimmunotherapy (e.g., R-CVP, R-CHOP, R-bendamustine)
Idelalisib +/– rituximab
Lenalidomide +/– rituximab
High dose chemotherapy plus autologous stem cell transplantation
Reduced intensity conditioning allogeneic transplantation
Palliative radiotherapy
Localized Disease
Radiotherapy
Single agent rituximab

Adapted from Hoffman R, et al.: *Hematology: basic principles and practice*, ed 5, Philadelphia, 2009, Churchill Livingstone.

effective in patients with HIV-associated NHL with CD4+ counts >50 cells/mm^3.

Most commonly regimens used in DLBCL include:
○ Three cycles of R-CHOP followed by involved-field radiotherapy or 6 cycles of R-CHOP

alone are appropriate approaches in patients with localized DLBCL.
○ 6 cycles of R-CHOP with or without radiotherapy are appropriate in patients with advanced-stage DLBCL.
○ For patients with double-hit lymphomas (defined as harboring rearrangement of MYC, BCL-2, and/or BCL-6), which are more aggressive and have poorer outcomes to R-CHOP than regular DLBCL, the use of R-EPOCH (infusional etoposide, doxorubicin, and vincristine, along with cyclophosphamide, prednisone, and rituximab) might be more effective.
○ In patients with HIV infection, the use of R-EPOCH might produce better results than R-CHOP.
○ Granulocyte-colony stimulating factor (e.g., filgrastim, MYC) may be effective in reducing the risk of febrile neutropenia in patients over 65 years with aggressive lymphoma undergoing chemotherapy.
○ Treatment with high-dose chemotherapy and autologous bone marrow transplant: compared with conventional chemotherapy, increases overall survival in patients with chemotherapy-sensitive relapsed DLBCL.
○ Combination chemotherapy regimens for NHL are described in Table 6.

HIGHLY AGGRESSIVE NHL: The most common high-grade NHL subtype is Burkitt lymphoma (BL). BL affects younger patients than DLBCL, and is common in HIV-infected individuals. Regimens more intensive than R-CHOP are needed to cure patients with high-grade NHL. The most commonly used multi-agent regimens include hyperCVAD or CODOX-M/IVAC, usually in combination with rituximab. The 5-year survival approximates 75%.

DISPOSITION

- Patients with indolent NHL in the rituximab era experience long survival despite the lack of curative potential of chemoimmunotherapy. Patients with aggressive NHL may achieve a cure with chemoimmunotherapy.
- Complete remission occurs in 35% to 50% of patients with aggressive NHL. Prognostic factors include the lymphoma subtype, age of patient, and extent of disease. Table E7 describes the International Prognostic Index for aggressive lymphomas.
- Patients who present with HIV-related NHL and low CD4+ cell count have a poor prognosis (median duration of survival is 15-34 mo). Despite therapeutic advances, the management of HIV-associated lymphomas is challenging due to potential pharmacologic interactions and increased risk of infectious complications. It is important to optimize the CD4 cell count during treatment. Referral to an HIV oncologist is recommended.

SUGGESTED READINGS
Available at www.expertconsult.com

RELATED CONTENT
Non-Hodgkin's Lymphoma (Patient Information)

AUTHORS: **JORGE J. CASTILLO, M.D.,** and **ANN S. LACASCE, M.D., M.M.SC.**

TABLE 6 Combination Chemotherapy Regimens for Non-Hodgkin's Lymphoma

Regimen	Dose	Days of Administration	Frequency
R-bendamustine			Every 28 days
Bendamustine	90 mg/m2 IV	1-2	
Rituximab	375 mg/m^2 IV	1	
R-CHOP			Every 21 days
Cyclophosphamide	750 mg/m^2 IV	1	
Doxorubicin	50 mg/m^2 IV	1	
Vincristine	1.4 mg/m^2 IV	1	
Prednisone, fixed dose	100 mg PO	1-5	
Rituximab	375 mg/m^2 IV	1	
R-CVP			Every 21 days
Cyclophosphamide	1000 mg/m^2 IV	1	
Vincristine	1.4 mg/m^2 IV	1	
Prednisone, fixed dose	100 mg PO	1-5	
Rituximab	375 mg/m^2 IV	1	

Adapted from Goldman L, Schafer AI: *Goldman's Cecil medicine*, ed 24, Philadelphia, 2012, Saunders.

BASIC INFORMATION

DEFINITION

Lynch syndrome is a hereditary predisposition to malignancy of the colon that is explained by a germline mutation in a DNA mismatch repair gene.

SYNONYMS

Hereditary non-polyposis colorectal cancer
HPNCC
Hereditary site-specific colon cancer

ICD-10CM CODES
C18.9 Malignant neoplasm of colon, unspecified

EPIDEMIOLOGY & DEMOGRAPHICS

The lifetime risk for developing colon cancer in the United States is approximately 6%. Up to 30% of colon cancer is inherited and 2% to 4% may be attributable to Lynch syndrome. The incidence of Lynch syndrome is estimated to be between 1:660 and 1:2000. Lynch syndrome is the most common form of hereditary colon cancer. The average age of diagnosis for Lynch syndrome is 45 years, although diagnosis can occur as early as the 20s or as late as the 70s.
RISK FACTORS: Family history of colon cancer or other hereditary non-polyposis colorectal cancer (HNPCC)-related cancers such as endometrial (up to 40% of women with Lynch syndrome may develop endometrial cancer), biliary tract, ovarian, stomach, upper urinary tract, or brain.
GENETICS: Autosomal-dominant inheritance pattern.

ETIOLOGY

Lynch syndrome is thought to be secondary to germline mutations in DNA mismatch repair genes. The predominant genes involved are *MSH2* and *MLH1*, which are tumor suppressor genes, although other genes have documented involvement (*PMS1*, *PMS2*, *MSH6*, and *EpCAM*). Mutations in these genes prevent repair of DNA mismatches during DNA replication. This is most prevalent in regions of DNA called microsatellites causing DNA microsatellite instability and leading to an increased risk for malignancy, especially colon cancer. *MSH6* mutations are associated with a markedly lower cancer risk than *MLH1* or *MSH2* mutations.

PHYSICAL FINDINGS & CLINICAL PRESENTATION

- Changes in bowel habits (prolonged constipation).
- Melena.
- Hematochezia.
- Abdominal pain.
- Unexplained weight loss.
- Decreased appetite.
- Right sided colon cancer (70%-85% of cases)

DX DIAGNOSIS

DIFFERENTIAL DIAGNOSIS

- Familial adenomatosis polyposis.
- Peutz-Jeghers syndrome.
- Juvenile polyposis.
- Nonhereditary colorectal cancer.
- Gardner syndrome.

WORKUP

If an individual presents with numerous adenomatous polyps or has multiple relatives with cancer at a young age, a family history complete with pedigree must be obtained. Clinical diagnosis of the Lynch syndrome can be made with the Amsterdam or Bethesda criteria.

- Revised Amsterdam (II) criteria (must meet all criteria):
  1. HNPCC-associated carrier diagnosis in at least three individuals in the family.
  2. One of the patients is a first-degree family member of two other patients.
  3. Involved patients occur in at least two successive generations with diagnosis of HNPCC.
  4. At least one diagnosis in family of HNPCC was made before age 50.
  5. The diagnoses are histologically confirmed.
  6. Familial adenomatous polyposis is excluded.
- Bethesda criteria (must meet all criteria):
  1. Colorectal cancer before age 50.
  2. Multiple colorectal cancers or other HNPCC-related cancers such as biliary tract, endometrial, stomach, or ovary.
  3. Colorectal cancer with microsatellite instability histology <60 years of age.
  4. Colorectal cancer or HNPCC-related cancer in first-degree relative <50 years of age.
  5. Colorectal cancer or HNPCC-related cancer in at least two first- or second-degree relatives, any age.
- If criteria for the Lynch syndrome are not met, no further analysis is necessary (although a genetic syndrome cannot be definitively excluded and genetic referral may be warranted).

LABORATORY TESTS

- If a patient meets criteria for Lynch syndrome, immunohistochemistry can be performed for the presence or absence of mismatch repair genes *MLH1*, *MSH2*, *MSH6*, and *PMS2*. Rarely, *MLH3* is identified.
- Microsatellite instability analysis should also be performed if criteria for Lynch syndrome are met.

Rx TREATMENT

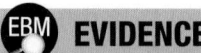

- If the mutation has been identified in a family member, screening for this mutation can be performed via genetic testing. Informed consent must be obtained after a thorough explanation has been provided to each individual.
- Surveillance using colonoscopy can be performed in individuals who screen positive, while those who screen negative can be discharged. The mismatch repair gene that is mutated guides screening.
- According to the Netherlands Surveillance Protocol, for example, individuals with mutations in *MLH1*, *MSH2*, or *MSH6* should have colonoscopies every 1 to 2 yr starting at age 20 to 25 yr; urine cytology every 1 to 2 yr starting at age 30 to 35 yr; esophagogastroduodenoscopy every 1 to 2 yr starting at age 30 to 35 yr; and, in females, ultrasound of endometrium and CA-125 every 1 to 2 yr starting at age 30 to 35 yr.
- Aspirin may be protective against colorectal cancer in Lynch syndrome patients.

REFERRALS

- To gastroenterology for surveillance colonoscopies.
- To genetic counselor if patient satisfies Bethesda criteria.
- To psychologist as necessary for psychological support.

! PEARLS & CONSIDERATIONS

- Before genetic testing is instituted, informed consent must be obtained because consequences of this testing include the necessity of lifelong screenings such as colonoscopies.
- The risk of pancreatic cancer is increased in families with Lynch syndrome compared with the U.S. population.
- **Familial Colorectal Cancer Type X** refers to patients who meet the Amsterdam criteria for HPNCC but have no molecular evidence of a MMR deficiency. These patients have a lower risk of colon cancer and no increased risk of extracolonic cancer compared to those with Lynch syndrome.

PATIENT & FAMILY EDUCATION

- For information on local genetic counselors, visit the National Society of Genetic Counselors Web site at www.nsgc.org.
- For information on Lynch syndrome, visit www.mayoclinic.com/health/lynch-syndrome/DS00669.

EBM EVIDENCE

Available at www.expertconsult.com

SUGGESTED READINGS

Available at www.expertconsult.com

RELATED CONTENT

Colorectal Cancer (Related Key Topic)
Familial Adenomatous Polyposis and Gardner's Syndrome (Related Key Topic)
Peutz-Jeghers Syndrome and other Polyposis Syndromes (Related Key Topic)

AUTHORS: **PAUL F. GEORGE, M.D., M.H.P.E.,** and **JOANNE M. SILVIA, M.D.**

BASIC INFORMATION

DEFINITION

Macular degeneration, usually referred to as *age-related macular degeneration* (ARMD), is an acquired degeneration of the retinal pigment epithelium and subsequently the neurosensory retina and choroid resulting in loss of central vision. The etiology is not known but a combination of genetic predisposition and certain risk factors plays an important role. Nonexudative (or "dry") AMD is the most common but exudative (or "wet") AMD is the most visually devastating.

SYNONYMS

AMD
ARMD

ICD-10CM CODES
H35.31 Nonexudative age-related macular degeneration
H35.32 Exudative age-related macular degeneration

EPIDEMIOLOGY & DEMOGRAPHICS

INCIDENCE (IN U.S.):
- Leading cause of irreversible blindness in people ≥50 yr in the developed world.
- Increases with age.
- In North America 15 million people currently have nonexudative AMD and 1.7 million have neovascular AMD. The overall prevalence is projected to increase by >50% by 2020.
- About 10% of patients with AMD have the neovascular form manifested by an often rapid decrease in central visual acuity caused by bleeding and scarring secondary to choroidal neovascularization.

PEAK INCIDENCE:
- Ages 75 to 80 yr
- Risk increases threefold in patients over the age of 75 as compared with younger age groups

PREVALENCE (IN U.S.):
- Varies, but ~5% of people >50 yr have some signs of macular degeneration.
- In the U.S., approximately 30% of people over the age of 75 have some form of macular degeneration.

PREDOMINANT SEX: Males and females are affected equally (15% of white women >80 yr have severe AMD)

PREDOMINANT AGE: >50 yr

RISK FACTORS:
- Advancing age, especially over 70
- Genetic factors
- History of smoking within past 20 yr
- Dietary factors (low intake of antioxidants, zinc, and omega-3 fatty acids; high fat intake)
- Obesity
- White race

PHYSICAL FINDINGS & CLINICAL PRESENTATION

- Decreased central vision, distortion of vision (metamorphopsia), poor night vision
- Drusen, atrophy, macular hemorrhage, pigmentation, macular edema, subretinal fluid
- The most common abnormality seen in AMD is the presence of drusen, or yellowish deposits deep to the retina
- Choroidal neovascular membrane (CNVM) develops with rapid change in vision due to leakage of exudative fluid and hemorrhage.

ETIOLOGY

- Oxidative and inflammatory changes in the retinal pigment epithelium due to a combination of environmental factors and genetic predisposition
- Genetics: 19 genes with mutations have been identified—dysregulation of the alternate complement system among other biochemical pathways
- Pigmentary and vascular changes with exudate, edema, and ultimately scar tissue development in exudative AMD
- Dry-type atrophy of the macula retinal pigment epithelium in nonexudative AMD
- The main mediator of neovascularization in wet AMD is vascular endothelial growth factor (VEGF). It induces angiogenesis and increases inflammation and vascular permeability

DIAGNOSIS

DIFFERENTIAL DIAGNOSIS

- Central serous chorioretinopathy
- Pattern dystrophy of the retinal pigment epithelium
- Drug toxicity (hydroxychloroquine, deferoxamine)
- Hypertensive retinopathy
- Histoplasmosis and high myopia (less common causes of CNVM)
- Angioid streaks
- Trauma with macular scar

WORKUP

- Careful history including family history of ocular disease.
- Complete eye examination including slit lamp biomicroscopy.
- Optical coherence tomography (OCT) is essential.

IMAGING STUDIES

- High-resolution OCT
- Fluorescein angiography
- Fundus autofluorescence
- Possibly indocyanine green angiography if other diseases are being considered

TREATMENT

NONPHARMACOLOGIC THERAPY

- There is no laser treatment for dry AMD.
- Photodynamic treatment with verteporfin can be used in the rare case of exudative AMD that does not respond to intravitreal pharmacotherapy.
- Thermal laser (argon) for certain classic membranes (CNVM) is rarely used in the era of biologics

ACUTE GENERAL Rx

- The introduction of therapies blocking VEGF has dramatically changed the management of AMD and is now the standard of care in the management of neovascular AMD. Intravitreal injections of anti-VEGF agents (ranibizumab, bevacizumab, and aflibercept) are first-line treatments for neovascular AMD. Intravitreal administration of ranibizumab, a humanized antibody fragment that neutralizes all active forms of VEGF A, was shown to stabilize or improve vision in 95% of patients compared to 65% of patients treated with verteporfin PDT. Aflibercept is a soluble protein that acts as a VEGF receptor decoy and is the most recently FDA-approved intravitreal therapy. Randomized controlled trials showed it to be non-inferior to ranibizumab. Bevacizumab, a full-length monoclonal antibody to VEGF, is used off-label as intravitreal therapy. Its cost per intravitreal dose is significantly lower than that of ranibizumab and aflibercept. However, several comparative effectiveness trials have shown bevacizumab to be non-inferior to ranibizumab.
- A major concern regarding anti-VEGF treatment is the potential increased risk of stroke and cardiovascular disease but no study to date has shown an increased incidence due to intravitreal therapy.
- Laser photocoagulation therapy may be useful in patients with extrafoveal lesions but is no longer routinely recommended for wet AMD.

CHRONIC Rx

- Age Related Eye Disease Study 1 and 2 (AREDS): a large randomized controlled trial showed that supplementation with the antioxidant vitamins C (500 mg) and E (400 IU), beta carotene (15 mg), and the micronutrient zinc (80 mg zinc oxide and 2 mg cupric oxide to prevent zinc-induced anemia) in patients with intermediate nonexudative AMD resulted in a 25% risk reduction of progression to advanced AMD at 5 years.
- AREDS 2 formula eliminates beta carotene and replaces it with 10 mg lutein and 2 mg zeaxanthin, thus avoiding the risk of lung cancer in former smokers.

DISPOSITION

- Follow closely by ophthalmologist, retinal specialist
- Frequency of follow-up determined by severity of disease
- Patients should self-monitor with Amsler grid daily and report changes immediately
- Smoking cessation, sunglasses with UV A and B protection, diet high in green leafy vegetables and fish
- Most anti-VEGF treatment failures are due to missed follow-up visits. Patients should be reminded repeatedly to call if their vision worsens

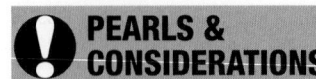

PEARLS & CONSIDERATIONS

COMMENTS

- Recent trials with embryonic stem cell transplants have shown promise in macular degeneration. Although stem cells represent new therapeutic strategies to repair and regenerate tissues damaged by disease or injury, much remains to be learned about how stem cells and their derivatives can be manufactured and delivered safely.[1] Recent reports show success with autologous-induced stem-cell–derived retinal cells for macular degeneration,[2] whereas others

performed outside of clinical trial settings have resulted in vision loss after intravitreal injection of autologous "stem cells" for AMD.[3] The International Society for Stem Cell Research has recently released guidelines for clinical translation of stem cells.[4]

- Statistically, the vision of only 1 of 10 affected persons can be saved, but the disease is so devastating that vigorous therapy should be considered in all patients.
- Vitamins with zinc and antioxidants may slow progression of AMD.
- Quitting smoking significantly reduces the risk of developing AMD.

[1]Daley GQ: Polar extremes in the clinical use of stem cells, *N Engl J Med* 376:1075–1077, 2017.

[2]Mandai M, et al.: Autologous induced stem-cell–derived retinal cells for macular degeneration, *N Engl J Med* 376:1038–1046, 2017.

[3]Kuriyan AE, et al.: Vision loss after intravitreal injection of autologous "stem cells" for AMD, *N Engl J Med* 376:1047–1053, 2017.

[4]Daley QC, et al.: Setting global standards for stem cell research and clinical translation: the 2016 ISSCR guidelines, *Stem Cell Reports* 6(6):787–797, 2016.

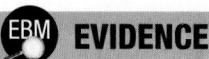 **EVIDENCE**

Available at www.expertconsult.com

SUGGESTED READINGS
Available at www.expertconsult.com

RELATED CONTENT

Macular Degeneration (Patient Information)

AUTHOR: **ROBERT H. JANIGIAN, M.D.**

BASIC INFORMATION

DEFINITION

Malabsorption is the diminished intestinal absorption of dietary nutrients. The majority of malabsorption is due to either congenital or acquired defects in the membrane transport system, absorption, and brush border processing in the intestinal epithelium.

SYNONYM

Maldigestion

ICD-10CM CODES

K90.9	Intestinal malabsorption, unspecified
K90.4	Malabsorption due to intolerance, not elsewhere classified
K90.89	Other intestinal malabsorption
K91.2	Postsurgical malabsorption, not elsewhere classified

EPIDEMIOLOGY & DEMOGRAPHICS

PREDOMINANT SEX AND AGE: More common in females with a mean age of 40
GENETICS:
- HLA-DQ2 present in 95% of celiac disease.

RISK FACTORS:
- Excessive alcohol consumption
- History of celiac disease
- History of IBD
- Intestinal surgery

PHYSICAL FINDINGS & CLINICAL PRESENTATION

- Most commonly nonspecific symptoms such as abdominal flatulence and distention are seen.
- Due to the osmotic load from maldigestion/malabsorption, watery diarrhea may be present. In the case of fat digestive disorder, steatorrhea ensues.
- Weight loss is very common but many patients are able to compensate by increased caloric load. Diffuse disease often has much more pronounced weight loss.
- Chronic protein malabsorption can cause hypoalbuminemia, leading to edema and ascites.
- Both microcytic and macrocytic anemia can result from micronutrient deficiency (iron/B12). These patient can be pale and present with fatigue.
- Bleeding disorders from vitamin K deficiency can lead to ecchymosis, melena, and hematuria.
- Vitamin D deficiency can lead to bone disorders. Secondary hyperparathyroidism can be a presenting feature.
- Electrolyte and vitamin deficiency can lead to neurologic disorders such as ataxia, weakness, and neuropathy, and may have positive Chvostek or trousseau sign.
- Disease-specific dermatologic findings such as alopecia, pellagra, erythema nodosum, pyoderma gangrenosum, cheilosis, glossitis, and aphthous ulcers may be present.

ETIOLOGY

- Can be congenital or acquired
- Disease-specific etiology

DIFFERENTIAL DIAGNOSIS

- Crohn's disease
- Celiac disease
- Hartnup disease
- Chronic pancreatitis
- Pancreatic insufficiency
- Cystic fibrosis
- Short bowel syndrome
- Neoplasm
- Abetalipoproteinemia
- Lactose intolerance
- Small intestine bacterial overgrowth
- Chronic atrophic gastritis
- Zollinger-Ellison syndrome
- Chronic cholestasis
- Cirrhosis

WORKUP

- A detailed history including alcohol consumption, surgical history as well as autoimmune disease can help diagnose the underlying disease. It is important to screen for anemia and electrolyte abnormalities due to malabsorption.

LABORATORY TESTS

- CBC, serum iron, Vitamin B12, and folate to detect for anemia.
- Prothrombin time: elevated PT can suggest vitamin K deficiency.
- **Fat malabsorption:** The gold standard is the 72-hour stool fat collection. More than 6/g day in the stool is pathologic. This test can be cumbersome so other options are available. Sudan III stain and acid steatocrit tests are qualitative measures of steatorrhea. Serologic testing for celiac disease should be considered as well.
- **Carbohydrate malabsorption:** Carbohydrate malabsorption leads to fermentation of the undigested carbohydrates by intestinal bacteria.
- The urinary D-xylose test for carbohydrate absorption in the small intestine. After loading with D-xylose, urinary D-xylose levels are measured. Low levels suggest intestinal malabsorption.
- Lactose intolerance can be tested by the lactose tolerance test or the breath test. The lactose tolerance test measures blood glucose after lactose administration. Development of symptoms or inadequate increase in blood sugar is indicative of lactose intolerance. H_2/CO_2 breath tests using specific forms of carbohydrates can detect malabsorption as well.
- **Protein malabsorption:** Protein malabsorption is likely due to small intestinal bacterial overgrowth or protein gastroenteropathies. Alpha-1 antitrypsin clearance or 99mTc-albumin gamma camera scintigraphy may aid in this diagnosis.
- **Pancreatic insufficiency:** Fecal elastase and chymotrypsin levels can distinguish from pancreatic and intestinal causes.

- **Vitamin deficiency:** It is important to assess serum vitamin B12 and methylmalonic acid levels. Schilling's test is rarely used but can be useful in some cases.
- **Bile acid malabsorption:** Quantitative stool bile acid measurement is the preferred method of diagnosis. SeHCAT test (selenium homocholic acid taurine test) is another option but less likely used.
- **Bacterial overgrowth:** This can be detected with endoscopic jejunal aspirate culture or a less invasive hydrogen breath test.
- Table 1 summarizes useful laboratory tests for evaluating patients with suspected malabsorption and for establishing possible nutrient deficiencies.

IMAGING STUDIES

- Abdominal US can identify thickened small bowel wall.
- Endoscopy for visualization and biopsy
- Small bowel follow through
- Abdominal CT/MRI
- ERCP/MRCP/EUS for identification of pancreatic abnormalities
- Capsule endoscopy

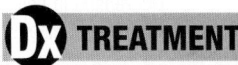 TREATMENT

Involves identification and treatment of the underlying illness, treatment of diarrhea, and nutritional repletion

NONPHARMACOLOGIC THERAPY

- A gluten-free diet in patients with celiac disease. Avoidance of lactose-containing product in lactose intolerance.
- Avoidance of caffeine and high sugar containing compounds has been found to decrease diarrhea in some cases.

ACUTE GENERAL Rx

- Control of the underlying disease should be primary goal
- It is also essential to control any volume and electrolyte abnormalities that might exist.

CHRONIC Rx

- Control of chronic diarrhea with loperamide or diphenoxylate with atropine should be one of the goals in a chronic malabsorptive state.
- Correction of volume and electrolyte disturbance with oral rehydration therapy should be made a priority.
- Bile acid conjugates can decrease steatorrhea in some cases.
- Pancreatic insufficiency is typically treated with a low-fat diet and exogenous pancreatic enzymes
- Teduglutide-homolog of GLP-2 has been shown to increase absorptive surface area in short bowel syndrome.
- Periodic DEXA scans are indicated in chronic malabsorption in the setting of vitamin D deficiency
- Oral supplementation with vitamins and minerals is important, sometimes requiring parenteral therapy

TABLE 1 Useful Laboratory Tests for Patients With Suspected Malabsorption and for Establishing Possible Nutrient Deficiencies

Test	Comment(s)
Blood Cell Count	
Hematocrit, hemoglobin	Decreased in iron, vitamin B_{12}, and folate malabsorption or with blood loss
Mean corpuscular hemoglobin or mean corpuscular volume	Decreased in iron malabsorption; increased in folate and vitamin B_{12} malabsorption
White blood cells, differential	Decreased in vitamin B_{12} and folate malabsorption; low lymphocyte count in lymphangiectasia
Biochemical Tests (Serum)	
TGs	Decreased in severe fat malabsorption
Cholesterol	Decreased in bile acid malabsorption or severe fat malabsorption
Albumin	Decreased in severe malnutrition, lymphangiectasia, protein-losing enteropathy
Alkaline phosphatase	Increased in calcium and vitamin D malabsorption (severe steatorrhea); decreased in zinc deficiency
Calcium, phosphorus, magnesium	Decreased in extensive small intestinal mucosal disease, after extensive intestinal resection, or in vitamin D deficiency
Zinc	Decreased in extensive small intestinal mucosal disease or intestinal resection
Iron, ferritin	Decreased in celiac disease, in other extensive small intestinal mucosal diseases, and with chronic blood loss
Other Serum Tests	
Prothrombin time	Prolonged in vitamin K malabsorption
β-Carotene	Decreased in fat malabsorption from hepatobiliary or intestinal diseases
Immunoglobulins	Decreased in lymphangiectasia, diffuse lymphoma
Folic acid	Decreased in extensive small intestinal mucosal diseases, with anticonvulsant use, in pregnancy; may be increased in SIBO
Vitamin B_{12}	Decreased after gastrectomy, in pernicious anemia, terminal ileal disease, SIBO, and infection with *Diphyllobothriumlatum*
Methylmalonic acid	Markedly elevated in vitamin B_{12} deficiency
Homocysteine	Markedly elevated in vitamin B_{12} or folate deficiency
Citrulline	May be decreased in destructive small intestinal mucosal disease or intestinal resection
Stool Tests	
Fat	Qualitative or quantitative increase in fat malabsorption
Elastase, chymotrypsin	Decreased concentrations and output in exocrine pancreatic insufficiency
pH	Less than 5.5 in carbohydrate malabsorption

From Feldman M et al [eds]: *Sleisenger and Fordtran's gastrointestinal and liver disease*, ed 10, Philadelphia, 2016, Saunders.

REFERRAL

- Gastroenterology consultation can help in diagnosis when initial laboratory testing is unclear.
- Nutrition consultation can help patients with diet modification to alleviate symptoms.

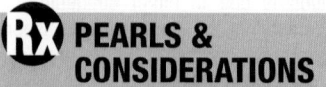 **PEARLS & CONSIDERATIONS**

COMMENTS

- Malabsorption should be considered a sign of an underlying disease.
- Treatment should focus on treating the underlying disorder.
- Nutrient and volume repletion should be priority in any treatment plan of malabsorption.

RELATED CONTENT

Section III Suspected Malabsorption (Algorithm)
Section III Table 34 Tests for the Evaluation of Malabsorption (Algorithm)
Celiac Disease(Related Key Topic)
Crohn's Disease (Related Key Topic)
Cystic Fibrosis (Related Key Topic)
Lactose Intolerance (Related Key Topic)
Pancreatitis, Chronic (Related Key Topic)
Short Bowel Syndrome (Related Key Topic)
Small Intestinal Bacterial Overgrowth (Related Key Topic)
Ulcerative Colitis (Related Key Topic)

AUTHORS: **GEORGE CHOLANKERIL, M.D.,**
DIMITRI GITELMAKER, M.D., and
ALAN EPSTEIN, M.D.

BASIC INFORMATION

DEFINITION

Malaria is a protozoan disease caused by intraerythrocytic protozoa of the genus *Plasmodium* and transmitted by female *Anopheles* spp. mosquitoes. It is endemic throughout most of the tropics and is characterized by hectic fever and often presents with classic malarial paroxysm. Five species of genus *Plasmodium* usually infect humans (Table 1):
- *P. falciparum*
- *P. vivax*
- *P. malariae*
- *P. ovale*
- *P. knowlesi*

SYNONYMS

Periodic fever
Tertian malaria
Quartan malaria
Tropical splenomegaly

ICD-10CM CODES
B54   Unspecified malaria
B50.9 *Plasmodium falciparum* malaria, unspecified
B51.9 *Plasmodium vivax* malaria without complications
B52.9 *Plasmodium malariae* malaria without complications
53.0   *Plasmodium ovale* malaria
B53.8 Other parasitologically confirmed malaria, not elsewhere classified

EPIDEMIOLOGY & DEMOGRAPHICS

Global:
- ~300 million cases a year in more than 100 countries
- Around 900,000 deaths per year, with more than 80% of the deaths occurring in children of sub-Saharan Africa
- 3 billion people live in malaria-endemic areas

U.S.:
- ~1500 cases reported to the CDC in the U.S. each year (Fig. 1). In the majority of reported cases, U.S. civilians who acquired infection abroad had not adhered to a chemoprophylaxis regimen that was appropriate for the country in which they acquired malaria.
- More than 50% of the reported cases in the U.S. are *P. falciparum*. On average, there are six deaths per year in the U.S.
- Most infections limited to:
  1. Immigrant population
  2. Returned travelers or troops from endemic area
- Occasionally, transmission through exposure to infected blood product or shared intravenous needles by users of injection drugs.
- Congenital transmission is possible.
- Local mosquito-borne transmission has been reported.
- Competent mosquito vectors are present.
  1. *A. albimanus* in eastern U.S.
  2. *A. freeborni* in western U.S.
  Geographic distribution:
- *P. falciparum:* Sub-Saharan Africa, Papua New Guinea, Solomon Islands, Haiti, Indian subcontinent
- *P. vivax:* Central America, South America, North Africa, Middle East, Indian subcontinent
- *P. ovale:* West Africa
- *P. malariae:* worldwide
  Parasite life cycle (Fig. 2):
- Human infection begins when a female anopheline mosquito bites (only female anopheline mosquito takes blood meal) and inoculates plasmodial sporozoites into bloodstream. The bite usually occurs between dusk and dawn.
- The sporozoites then travel to liver and invade to hepatocytes.
- In the hepatocytes, the sporozoites mature to tissue schizont or become dormant hypnozoites.
- The tissue schizonts amplify the infection by producing a large number of merozoites (10,000 to 30,000).

- Each merozoite is capable of invading an RBC and can establish the asexual cycle of replication in RBCs.
- Asexual cycles produce and release 24 to 32 merozoites at the end of 48- or 72-hr (*P. malariae*) cycles.
- The hypnozoites are only found in relapsing malaria *P. vivax* or *P. ovale* and may remain dormant for up to 5 yr.
- Eventually some intraerythrocytic parasites develop into gametocytes. Male and female gametocytes are taken up by a female anopheline mosquito with a blood meal where they fertilize in the mosquito gut to produce a diploid zygote that matures to an ookinete; haploid sporozoites are generated that migrate to the salivary gland of the mosquito to infect another human.

PHYSICAL FINDINGS & CLINICAL PRESENTATION

- Fever is the hallmark of malaria, known as malarial paroxysm, initially daily until synchronization of infection after several wk, when fever may occur every other day (tertian) in *P. vivax*, *P. ovale*, or *P. falciparum* malaria or every third day (quartan) in *P. malariae* malaria. Table 2 describes the WHO criteria for severe malaria.
- Classic malarial paroxysm characterized by
  1. Cold stage: abrupt onset of cold feeling associated with rigors, shakes.
  2. Hot stage: high fever (~40° C) associated with restlessness.
  3. Sweating stage: patient defervesces.
- Nonspecific symptoms are
  1. Headache.
  2. Cough.
  3. Myalgia.
  4. Vomiting.
  5. Diarrhea.
  6. Jaundice.
- *P. falciparum:*
  1. Most pathogenic of the four species.
  2. Rapidly progresses to high-level parasitemia.
  3. Important cause of the fatal malaria.

TABLE 1   Features of the Five Species of Malaria Known to Cause Disease in Humans

	Plasmodium falciparum	Plasmodium vivax	Plasmodium ovale	Plasmodium malariae	Plasmodium knowlesi
Incubation period (days)	6-25	8-27	8-27	16-40	12
Asexual cycle (hours)	48 (tertian)	48 (tertian)	48 (tertian)	72 (quartan)	24 (tertian)
Relapse	No	Yes*	Yes*	No†	No
Chloroquine resistance	Yes‡	Rare§	No	No‖	No
Characteristic on thin blood film	Rings predominate, multiply infected RBCs, high parasitemia, rings with thread-like cytoplasm, double nuclei, banana-shaped gametocytes	Enlarged RBCs, Schüffner's dots, trophozoite cytoplasm ameboid, 12-24 merozoites in mature schizont	Oval RBCs with fringed edges, Schüffner's dots, trophozoite cytoplasm compact, 6-16 merozoites in mature schizont	Trophozoite cytoplasm compact (band forms), 6-12 merozoites in mature schizont, RBC unchanged	Similar to *P. malariae*, 8-10 merozoites in mature schizont, often in rosette pattern with central clump of pigment

*Relapses may appear months to years after initial infection due to dormant hypnozoites in the liver.
†Although relapse does not occur, *P. malariae* can produce persistent infections that remain below detectable limits in the blood for 20 to 30 years or more.
‡*P. falciparum* resistance to sulfadoxine/pyrimethamine, mefloquine, halofantrine, and artemisinin have also been reported in some areas, along with partial resistance to quinine and quinidine.
§*P. vivax* resistance to chloroquine now reported in some areas of Southeast Asia, Oceania, and South America.
‖Chloroquine-resistant *P. malariae* has also been reported in south Sumatra, Indonesia.
From Vincent JL et al: *Textbook of critical care,* ed 6, Philadelphia, 2011, Saunders.

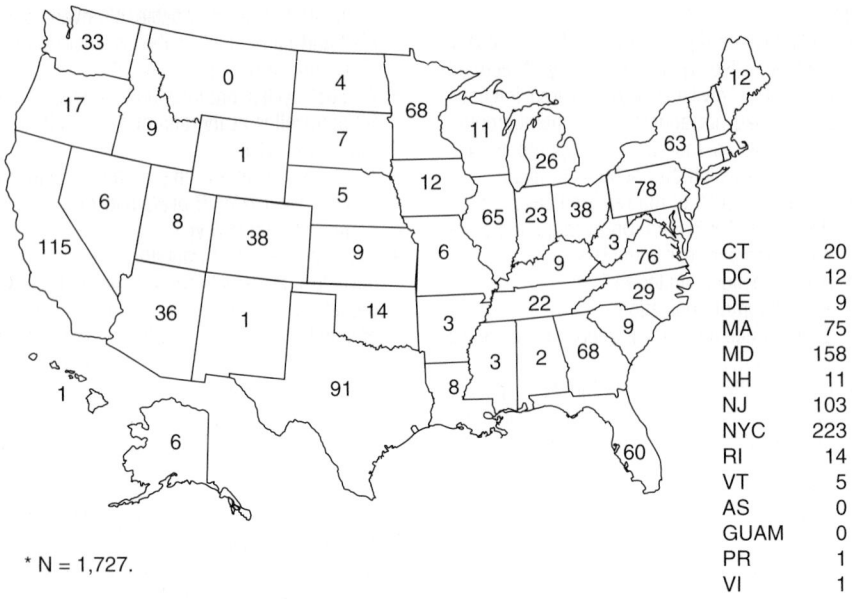

CT	20
DC	12
DE	9
MA	75
MD	158
NH	11
NJ	103
NYC	223
RI	14
VT	5
AS	0
GUAM	0
PR	1
VI	1

* N = 1,727.

FIG. 1 Number* of malaria cases, by state in which the disease was diagnosed—United States, 2013 (Cullen KA et al: Malaria surveillance—United States, 2013, *MMWR Surveill Summ* 65:1-22, 2016.)

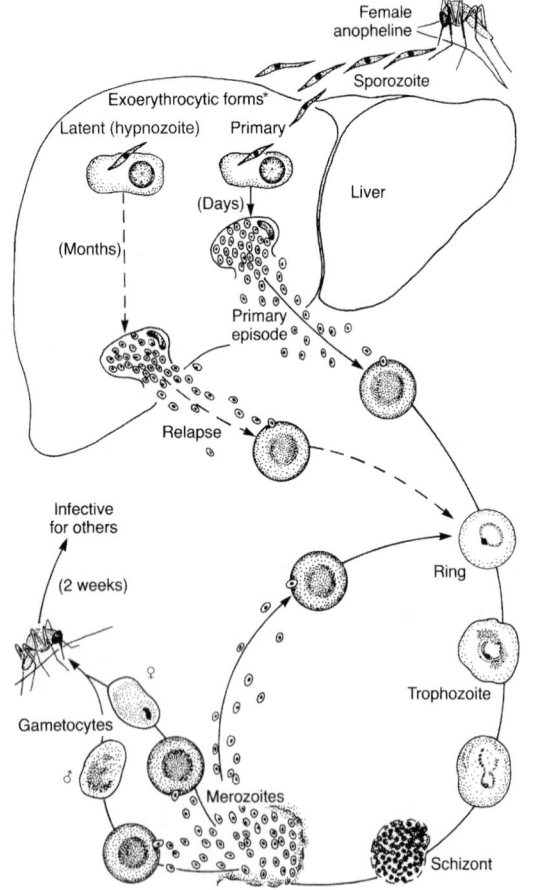

FIG. 2 Life cycle of plasmodia in humans. Exoerythrocytic forms are also called schizonts. (From Gorbach SL: *Infectious diseases*, ed 2, Philadelphia, 1998, Saunders.)

TABLE 2 World Health Organization Criteria for Severe Malaria, 2000
Impaired consciousness
Prostration
Respiratory distress
Multiple seizures
Jaundice
Hemoglobinuria
Abnormal bleeding
Severe anemia
Circulatory collapse
Pulmonary edema

From Kliegman RM et al: *Nelson textbook of pediatrics*, ed 19, Philadelphia, 2011, Saunders.

8. Cerebral malaria is a feared complication.
9. Invades erythrocytes of all ages.
10. Lacks hypnozoites (intrahepatic stage), does not relapse.
11. Blood smear usually shows ring form only.
12. Pigment color is black.
13. Banana-shaped gametocytes; if seen in blood, smear is diagnostic.
14. Chloroquine resistance is widely present.

- *P. vivax:*
  1. Known as tertian malaria: fever occurs every other day.
  2. Duffy blood-group antigen FYA- or FYB-related receptor is needed for attachment to RBC.
  3. FyFy phenotype (most West African) individuals are resistant to *P. vivax* malaria.
  4. Incubation period after exposure is 14 days (range: 8 to 27 days).
  5. Hypnozoites may cause relapse of infection after years.
  6. Infects mainly reticulocytes.
  7. Irregularly shaped large rings and trophozoites, enlarged RBCs, and Schüffner's dots are seen in peripheral blood smear (Fig. 2).
  8. Pigment color is yellow-brown.
  9. *P. vivax* from Papua New Guinea have reduced sensitivity to chloroquine.
  10. Primaquine is needed to eradicate the hypnozoites.

- *P. ovale:*
  1. Also known as tertian malaria; fever occurs every other day.
  2. Occurs mainly in tropical Africa.
  3. Incubation period after exposure is 14 days (range: 8-27 days).
  4. Hypnozoites may cause relapse of infection.
  5. Infects mainly reticulocytes.
  6. Infected RBC is seen as enlarged, oval shape containing large ring or trophozoites with Schüffner's dots.
  7. Pigment color is dark brown.
  8. Primaquine needed to eradicate the hypnozoites.
  9. No chloroquine resistance has been encountered.

4. Classic malarial paroxysm is usually absent.
5. Incubation period after exposure is 12 days (range: 9 to 60 days).
6. Cytoadherence and resetting of RBCs play central role in pathogenesis.
7. The sequestration of RBCs in vital organs leads to fatal complications.

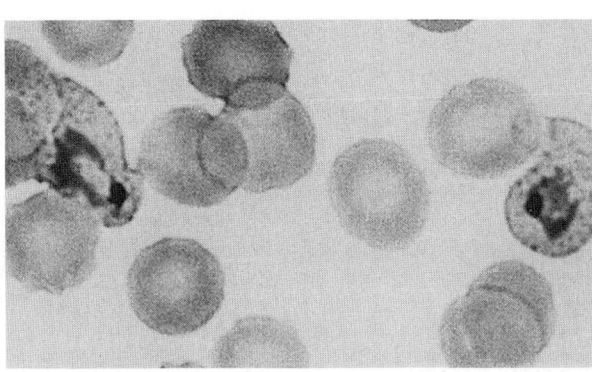

FIG. 3 Giemsa-stained blood smear in *Plasmodium vivax* malaria. Asexual parasites. Note that the parasites are large and ameboid; the infected erythrocytes are the largest cells in the field (because they are reticulocytes), and the erythrocytes contain numerous pink dots (Schüffner's dots) (×2000). (From Klippel JH et al [eds]: *Internal medicine*, ed 5, St Louis, 1998, Mosby.)

- *P. malariae:*
  1. Known as quartan malaria; fever occurs every third day.
  2. Common cause of chronic malarial infection.
  3. May persist for 20 to 30 yr after leaving the endemic area.
  4. Worldwide distribution.
  5. Incubation period after exposure is 30 days (range: 16-60 days).
  6. Lacks hypnozoites (intrahepatic stage).
  7. May persist in blood for many years if treated inadequately.
  8. Chronic infection may cause soluble immune-complex, resulting in nephritic syndrome.
  9. Infects mainly mature RBCs.
  10. Band or rectangular forms of trophozoites are commonly seen in peripheral blood smear.
  11. Pigment color is brown-black.
- Cerebral malaria:
  1. Feared complication of *P. falciparum* infection.
  2. Mortality is ~20%.
  3. Pathogenesis is poorly understood.
  4. Ischemia as a result of sequestration of parasites or cytokines induced by parasite toxin(s) is the key debate.
  5. Seizure and altered mental status leading to coma are cardinal manifestation.
  6. Hypoglycemia, lactic acidosis, and elevated circulating TNF-α may be present.
  7. CSF studies: no increase of WBC count or protein, raised lactate concentrate, and increased opening pressure, especially in children, may be present.

DX DIAGNOSIS

DIFFERENTIAL DIAGNOSIS
- Typhoid fever
- Dengue fever
- Yellow fever
- Viral hepatitis
- Influenza
- Brucellosis
- UTI
- Leishmaniasis

- Trypanosomiasis
- Rickettsial diseases
- Leptospirosis

WORKUP
- Clinical diagnosis is notoriously inaccurate.
- Demonstration of malarial parasites in blood smear is essential.
- Newer molecular diagnostic techniques (polymerase chain reaction, rapid diagnostic tests) are promising.

LABORATORY TESTS
- The thick and thin blood film is required to identify malarial parasites. A Giemsa-stained film of the patient's peripheral blood (Fig. 3) should be examined for parasites as soon as possible.
- The thick smears are more sensitive and primarily used to detect the presence of parasites.
- The thin smears are used for species differentiation and parasite density estimation.
- A patient who is suspected of having malaria but who has no parasite seen in blood smears should have blood smears repeated every 12 to 24 hr for 3 consecutive days.

PREPARATION OF BLOOD SMEAR:
- Must be prepared from fresh blood obtained by pricking the finger.
- The thin smear is fixed in methanol before staining.
- The thick smear is stained unfixed.
- The smear should be stained with a 3% Giemsa solution (pH of 7.2) for 30 to 45 min.
- The parasite density should be estimated by counting the percentage of RBCs infected, not the number of parasites, under an oil immersion lens on thin film.

COMMON ERRORS IN READING MALARIAL SMEARS:
- Platelets overlying an RBC
- Misreading artifacts as parasites
- Concern about missing a positive slide

MOLECULAR DIAGNOSIS OF MALARIA:
- Rapid diagnostic tests (RDT)
  1. Employ immunochromatographic lateral flow technology for antigen detection.
  2. Thus far only one RDT has been FDA approved: BinaxNOW Malaria test kit.

  3. This kit is based on antigens HRP-2 and aldolase.
  4. For *P. falciparum:* sensitivity 95% and specificity 94%.
  5. For *P. vivax:* sensitivity 69% and specificity 100%.
- Limitations of the BinaxNOW Malaria test:
  1. Not approved for mixed infections
  2. Should not be used for *P. malariae* and *P. ovale* as data are limited
  3. Positive test must be confirmed by microscopy
  4. Negative results require confirmation by thick and thin smears
  5. This test cannot be used to monitor therapy as antigen persists after the elimination of the parasite, causing false positives
- Other diagnostic tests available include:
  1. Tagged monoclonal antibodies for malaria antigen detection
  2. Nucleic acid amplification and detection: PCR can detect parasites down to a level of 1 to 5 parasites per microliter of blood. PCR can detect mixed species infection
  3. Fluorescence microscopy with acridine orange or other staining
  4. Dark field microscopy

RX TREATMENT

NONPHARMACOLOGIC THERAPY
ANTIMOSQUITO MEASURES:
1. Eradication of mosquito breeding places by chemical spray
2. Use of mosquito nets properly in the endemic areas
3. Use of protective clothing
4. Use of insect spray (permethrin), mosquito coils, or repellents such as diethyltoluamide (DEET). For adults, DEET (30%-50%) is generally protective for at least 4 hr. For smaller children, use DEET at ≤20% concentration.

ACUTE GENERAL Rx
A definitive diagnosis of malaria is essential for specific antimalarial chemotherapy.
NON-FALCIPARUM MALARIA:
- Chloroquine 600 mg base (1000 mg chloroquine phosphate) PO loading dose, 6 hr later 300 mg base (500 mg salt), then 300 mg base (500 mg salt) daily for 2 days.
- In the case of *P. vivax* and *P. ovale,* treatment with primaquine 15 mg daily for 14 days is needed to eradicate the exoerythrocytic forms, especially the hypnozoites responsible for relapses.
- G6PD should be measured before primaquine is given. Primaquine is not recommended for those who are glucose-6-phosphate dehydrogenase deficient, because primaquine can cause hemolysis and even death in G6PD-deficient persons. Normal G6PD levels must be documented before using primaquine for either chemoprophylaxis or treatment.
- Chloroquine-resistant *P. vivax* has been documented; in that case, quinine is given.

FALCIPARUM MALARIA:

- Chloroquine can be used cautiously for falciparum malaria acquired in chloroquine-sensitive areas (chloroquine is more rapidly effective than quinine).
- Mainstay of treatment is oral quinine sulfate 10 mg (salt)/kg (usually 650 mg) q8h for 3 to 7 days + doxycycline 100 mg PO bid both for 7 days for adults. Pediatrics: quinine sulfate: 10 mg/kg PO tid plus clindamycin: 20 mg/kg per day divided in tid dose both for 7 days.
- Atovaquone-proguanil (Malarone): 250 mg atovaquone/100 mg proguanil): 4 adult tabs PO once a day for 3 days with food in adults or for pediatrics: pediatric tablets (62.5 mg atovaquone/25 mg proguanil) are used based on weight:
- 5 to 8 kg: 2 pediatric tabs PO once daily for 3 days
- 9 to 10 kg: 3 pediatric tabs PO once daily for 3 days
- 11 to 20 kg: 1 adult tab PO once daily for 3 days
- 21 to 30 kg: 2 adult tabs PO once daily for 3 days
- 31 to 40 kg: 3 adult tabs PO once daily for 3 days
- >40 kg: 4 adult tabs PO once daily for 3 days artemether-lumefantrine (Coartem) tablets: 4 tabs PO (at time zero and 8 hr later) then bid × 2 days for a total of six doses. For pediatrics:
- 5 to <15 kg: 1 tablet per dose
- 15 to <25 kg: 2 tablets per dose
- 25 to <35 kg: 3 tablets per dose
- >35 kg: 4 tablets per dose. The child should receive initial dose based on weight, then followed by second dose 8 hr later, then 1 dose PO bid for following 2 days

ALTERNATIVES:

- Quinine sulfate plus clindamycin 900 mg tid for 7 days in adults, or
- Mefloquine 750 mg PO then 500 mg PO 6 to 12 hr later in adults

NOTE: Parasitemia may paradoxically rise in the first 24 to 36 hr and is not an indication of treatment failure.

SEVERE FALCIPARUM MALARIA:

- It is a medical emergency; intensive care is preferred.
- Measurement of blood glucose, lactate, ABG is important.
- IV quinidine gluconate 10 mg salt/kg loading dose (maximum 600 mg) in NS; infuse slowly over 1 to 2 hr, followed by continuous infusion of 0.02 mg/kg/min until patient can swallow.
- Need to monitor ECG for observation of QT interval as can prolong. Also need to monitor blood pressure and glucose to avoid hypoglycemia.
- Alternatively, IV artesunate: 2.4 mg/kg IV first dose then at 12 and 24 hr followed by 2.4 mg/kg once daily. One recent study showed the superiority of parenteral artesunate over parenteral quinine in adults and children who could not take an oral medication.
- Plasmapheresis is an option for parasitemia >30% or in pregnant women and in elderly with severe malaria.

NOTE: WHO recommends IV artesunate as the treatment of choice for severe malaria in adults and children in area of low transmission. Data on children in high-transmission regions are limited, and WHO recommends treatment with artesunate, artemether, or quinine.

MULTIDRUG-RESISTANT MALARIA:

- Mefloquine 1250 mg as a single dose, or
- Halofantrine 500 mg every 6 hr for 3 doses, repeat same course after 1 wk
- Combination therapy usually preferred

DISPOSITION

RISK FACTORS FOR FATAL MALARIA:

- Failure to take chemoprophylaxis
- Delay in seeking medical care
- Misdiagnosis

COMPLICATIONS OF MALARIA:

- Anemia
- Acidosis
- Hypoglycemia
- Respiratory distress
- DIC
- Blackwater fever
- Renal failure
- Shock

REFERRAL

- To an infectious disease specialist or travel medicine expert for severe malaria complications
- To an intensive care specialist if severe cerebral malaria or other major organ failure develops
- All malaria cases are mandated to be reported to local and state health departments by health care providers or laboratory staff

ⓘ PEARLS & CONSIDERATIONS

HOST RESPONSE

- The specific immune response to malaria confers protection from high-level parasitemia and disease, but not from infection.
- Asymptomatic parasitemia without illness (premunition) is common among adults in endemic areas.
- Immunity is specific for both the species and the strain of infecting malarial parasites.
- Immunity to all strains is never achieved.
- Normal spleen function is an important host factor because of immunologic as well as filtering functions of the spleen.
- Both humoral and cellular immunity is necessary for protection.
- Polyclonal increase in serum level of IgG, IgM, and IgA occurs in immune individuals.
- Antibody to antigenically variant protein PfEMP1 is important for protection in case of *P. falciparum* malaria.
- Passively transferred IgG from immune individuals has been shown to be protective.
- Maternal antibody confers relative protection of infants from severe disease.
- Genetic disorders (sickle cell disease, thalassemia, and G6PD deficiency) confer protection from death because parasites are unable to grow efficiently in low-oxygen tensions, thus preventing high-level parasitemias.
- Individuals deficient of Duffy factor in RBCs are resistant to infection by *P. vivax*.
- Nonspecific defense mechanisms, such as cytokines (TNF-α, IL-1, -6, -8), also play an important role in protection, causing fever (temperatures of 40° C damage mature parasites) and other pathologic effects.

PREVENTION OF MALARIA: Medications are available for the prophylaxis of malaria and will vary depending on level of chloroquine resistance in a given area.

Areas free of chloroquine-resistant Falciparum malaria

Chloroquine 300 mg base (500 mg chloroquine phosphate) PO/wk. Start 1 wk prior to arrival in malaria area, then weekly while there and for 4 wk on leaving malaria area. Pediatric dose: 8.3 mg/kg (5 mg/kg base). Alternatives for adults include atovaquone-proguanil (Malarone): 1 adult tablet per day starting 1 to 2 days prior to arriving in malaria area, then daily while there and then for 7 days daily on leaving malaria area. For children, atovaquone-proguanil pediatric tablets based on weight:

11 to 20 kg 1 pediatric tablet
21 to 30 kg 2 pediatric tablets
31 to 40 kg 3 pediatric tablets
>40 kg 1 adult tablet

Areas with chloroquine-resistant Falciparum malaria

- Atovaquone-proguanil (Malarone): dosing as previously
- Mefloquine 250 mg (228 mg base) PO/wk, starting 1 wk before arriving in malaria area, weekly while there and then weekly for 4 wk on return. In children, mefloquine dose is based on weight:
- <15 kg 5 mg/kg
- to 19 kg ¼ adult dose
- to 30 kg ½ adult dose
- to 45 kg ¾ adult dose
- >45 kg adult dose
- Doxycycline 100 mg PO/day for adults and children aged >8. Start 1 to 2 days before travel, daily while in malaria area, and then daily for 4 wk on return.

SPECIAL CONSIDERATIONS:

- Long-term visitors or travelers
- Children aged <12 yr
- Immunocompromised host
- Pregnant women: chloroquine and mefloquine are safe in pregnancy but not atovaquone-proguanil. A recent trial revealed that the burden of malaria in pregnancy was significantly lower among adolescent girls or women who received intermittent preventive treatment with dihydroartemisinin-piperaquine than among those who received sulfadoxine-pyrimethamine, and monthly treatment with dihydroartemisinin-piperaquine was superior to three-dose dihydroartemisinin-piperaquine with regards to several outcomes.[1] Avoid doxycycline and primaquine.

[1]Kakuru A, et al: Dihydroartemisinin-piperaquine for the prevention of malaria in pregnancy, *N Engl J Med* 374:928-939, 2016.

TABLE 3 Sources for Malaria Prophylaxis, Diagnosis, and Treatment Recommendations

Type of Information	Source	Availability	Telephone Number, Internet Address, or Electronic Mail Address
Prophylaxis	CDC's Traveler's Health Internet site (includes online access to Health Information for International Travel)	24 hours/day	http://www.nc.cdc.gov/travel
	(The Yellow Book)	Order from Oxford University Press, Inc. Order Fulfillment 198 Madison Avenue, New York, NY 10016-4314	800-451-7556 or http://www.oup.com/us/
	CDC's Malaria Branch Internet site with Malaria Information and Prophylaxis, By Country (Red Pages)	24 hours/day	http://www.cdc.gov/malaria/travelers/country_table/a.html
	CDC Malaria Map Application	24 hours/day	http://www.cdc.gov/malaria/map
Diagnosis	CDC's Division of Parasitic Diseases and Malaria diagnostic internet site (DPDx)	24 hours/day	http://www.dpd.cdc.gov/dpdx
	CDC's Division of Parasitic Diseases and Malaria diagnostic CD-ROM (DPDx)	Order by electronic mail from CDC Division of Parasitic Diseases and Malaria	dpdx@cdc.gov
Treatment	CDC Malaria Branch	9:00 A.M.–5:00 P.M. Eastern time, Monday–Friday	770-488-7788 or toll-free 855-856-4713*
	CDC Malaria Branch	5:00 P.M.–9:00 A.M. Eastern time on weekdays and all day weekends and holidays	770-488-7100* (This number is for the CDC's Emergency Operations Center. Ask staff member to page the person on call for the Malaria Branch.) http://www.cdc.gov/malaria/ diagnosis_treatment/treatment.html

*These numbers are intended for health care professionals only.
Cullen KA et al: Malaria surveillance—United States, 2013, *MMWR Surveill Summ* 65:1-22, 2016.

VACCINATION:
- In 2015, Mosquirix (RTS,S): a recombinant protein-based vaccine, was approved in Europe to prevent malaria in babies in Africa. It showed an efficacy of about 30% in babies 6 to 12 weeks old and about 46% in babies 5 to 17 months old.
- New DNA-based vaccines are in development

MALARIA INFORMATION:
- CDC Travelers' Health Hotline (877) 394-8747; CDC Travelers' Health Fax (888) 232-3299
- CDC Malaria Epidemiology (770) 488-7788; internet: www.cdc.gov
- Table 3 summarizes sources for malaria prophylaxis, diagnosis, and treatment recommendations.

SUGGESTED READINGS
Available at www.expertconsult.com

RELATED CONTENT
Malaria (Patient Information)

AUTHOR: **GLENN G. FORT, M.D., M.P.H.**

DEFINITION

Malignant hyperthermia (MH) is a rare and life-threatening subclinical myopathy that can occur in genetically susceptible individuals after exposure to triggering agents, most commonly halogenated anesthetic gases, such as halothane, isoflurane, sevoflurane, and desflurane, or the depolarizing agent succinylcholine. These agents, given to susceptible individuals, often those with a genetic anomaly in the ryanodine or dihydropyridine receptor, may lead to excessive skeletal muscle contraction. Initial signs include rising end tidal carbon dioxide (PET CO_2) levels, tachycardia, and skeletal muscle rigidity. Mortality has recently been reported to be 1.4% to 5%, down from 70% in the past, likely due to monitoring for changes in PET CO_2 and intraoperative temperature. Advanced age, muscularity, comorbidities, and disseminated intravascular coagulation (DIC) increase risk of death.

SYNONYMS

Malignant hyperthermia of anesthesia
Malignant hyperpyrexia
MH

ICD-10CM CODES
T88.3 Malignant hyperthermia due to anesthesia, initial encounter

EPIDEMIOLOGY & DEMOGRAPHICS

INCIDENCE: In the population as a whole undergoing general anesthesia, the incidence is approximately 1:100,000. It is widely believed that we fail to include a large number of unrecognized events, and that half of afflicted patients have had prior uneventful exposures to the same triggering agents. Children account for 42% to 52% of cases; however, any age may be affected.
GENETICS: Susceptibility to MH is due to mutation of the ryanodine receptor, less frequently the dihydropyridine (DHP) receptor, and sometimes both. Recently studied are four mutations in the RYR1 gene at the p.Arg2508, which were found to have a crucial effect on the pathological conditions related to malignant hyperthermia. *Mutations in the CACNA1S gene on chromosome 1q32 have been linked to MH as well.* Of note, however, in a patient with known genetic susceptibility to MH, a history of uneventful anesthesia while using known triggering agents does not exclude the possibility of a future MH crisis.
ETIOLOGY: Susceptibility to MH is inherited in an autosomal dominant fashion in 50% of cases, the rest presumed to be new mutations. At least 31 mutations on chromosome 19 are known to cause changes in the ryanodine receptor (RYR1) that result in the abnormalities of skeletal muscle calcium homeostasis and susceptibility to MH, with significant clinical variability due to incomplete penetrance and variable expressivity. In approximately 1% of cases, MH susceptibility is due to mutations of the gene on chromosome one coding for the dihydropyridine receptor.

PREVALENCE OF SUSCEPTIBILITY TO MALIGNANT HYPERTHERMIA: In the general population, 1:3000 are thought to carry a defective gene for the ryanodine receptor. However, the prevalence of susceptibility to MH (MHS) is estimated to be 1:2000. The difference is likely accounted for by other genetic abnormalities such as abnormalities of the DHP receptor and certain clinical risk factors (see risk factors). In family cohorts of patients who are susceptible, the prevalence of susceptibility ranges from 1:200 to 1:5000 due to incomplete penetrance and variable expressivity.

RISK FACTORS:
- Preoperatively, the patient and family history is used to evaluate the risk of MH crisis and the need for further testing. Patients with myopathies due to RYR1 abnormalities, such as central core myopathy, rather than true MH, should not receive succinylcholine or volatile anesthetics.
- Patients with dystrophinopathies such as Duchenne and Becker muscular dystrophy, enzymopathies of skeletal muscle such as McArdle's disease, or exercise- and heat-induced rhabdomyolysis, may develop rhabdomyolysis when exposed to these agents, and many authors deem it prudent to use only nontriggering agents. Other syndromes such as osteogenesis imperfecta, myotonia, and neuroleptic malignant syndrome are no longer felt to be associated with MHS.

PREDOMINANT AGE AND SEX: Male to female ratio of 2:1. Children account for up to half of cases.

PATHOPHYSIOLOGY

- In subjects genetically susceptible to dysregulated calcium release from the sarcoplasmic reticulum, administration of volatile anesthetic gases results in excessive release of sarcoplasmic Ca^{++}. Halothane will inhibit Ca^{++} reuptake resulting in unmitigated muscle contraction, increased aerobic and anaerobic metabolism, leading to CO_2 production, elevated PET CO_2, and tachycardia in patients unable to increase their alveolar minute volume.
- Hyperpyrexia results from hypermetabolism of skeletal muscle with an overwhelming amount of heat production resulting in the body's inability to dissipate this heat.
- L-cysteine/hydrogen sulfide pathway has been shown to have a role in the pathogenesis of MH, as hydrogen sulfide has the same effect on the sarcoplasmic reticulum as either halothane or caffeine.

PHYSICAL FINDINGS & CLINICAL PRESENTATION

- Within minutes to hours after the triggering anesthetic is administered, the patient develops muscle rigidity, resulting in tachypnea and tachycardia. In the operating room, however, MH may be difficult to recognize because the latter signs are often attributed to inadequate sedation.
- Masseter muscle rigidity is common after initial induction of anesthesia; however, when prolonged, it may suggest MH.
- Hyperthermia or a rapidly increasing temperature from an anesthesia-induced hypothermic state is present in more than 50% of MH events. Hyperthermia is not always present early in MH crisis, and thus core body temperature is not a definitive inclusion factor in diagnosing MH at an early stage. Higher core body temperature correlates with morbidity, and in the OR, skin temperature underestimates core body temperature.
- The skin may initially be erythematous, progressing to a mottled, cyanotic appearance.
- Due to increased skeletal muscle metabolism, CO_2 production is increased, leading to elevated mixed venous and arterial pCO_2, and an elevated PET CO_2. Muscle injury with an elevated creatine kinase (CK) may lead to rhabdomyolysis and subsequent acute renal failure. Disseminated intravascular coagulation (DIC) may develop.
- Box 1 summarizes the findings consistent with MH.

BOX 1   Positive Findings Consistent with Malignant Hyperthermia (MH)

History of recent exposure to trigger agent, including volatile anesthetic agents or succinylcholine
Family or personal history of MH susceptibility
Total body rigidity
Masseter spasm
Inappropriately elevated (38.8° C) or rapidly increasing temperature (>1.5° C over 5 min)
Inappropriate tachypnea
Profuse sweating
Mottled, cyanotic skin
Dark urine, urine dipstick testing shows a positive result from blood without red cells in the sediment and no hemolysis
Unexplained, excessive bleeding
Unexplained ventricular tachycardia or fibrillation
Inappropriate hypercarbia (venous $Paco_2$ >65 mm Hg, arterial $Paco_2$ >55 mm Hg) if the patient is receiving positive-pressure ventilation or is spontaneously breathing with greater than normal minute ventilation
Arterial base excess more negative than −8 mEq/L
Arterial pH <7.25
Potassium concentration >6 mEq/L
Creatine kinase >10,000 IU/L

From Fuhrman BP et al: *Pediatric critical care*, ed 4, Philadelphia, 2011, Saunders.

Dx DIAGNOSIS

DIFFERENTIAL DIAGNOSIS

- Exertional heatstroke
- Neuroleptic malignant syndrome
- Fever
- Thyrotoxicosis
- Pheochromocytoma
- Central nervous system infection or space-occupying lesion
- MDMA (Ecstasy), cocaine, alcohol withdrawal, or amphetamine use
- Serotonin syndrome
- Adverse reaction to MAOIs or anticholinergic drug
- Strychnine poisoning
- Sepsis
- Drug withdrawal
- Rhabdomyolysis
- Transfusion reactions

WORKUP

MH can often be distinguished from other causes of hyperthermia based on history.

LABORATORY TESTS

- If the cause of hyperthermia is uncertain, thyroid function studies, CBC, toxicology screen, and urine vanillylmandelic acid (VMA) may be useful.
- Once the diagnosis is established, it is important to monitor end organ function through serial lab data including electrolytes, especially potassium, calcium, and phosphorus; creatinine; blood urea nitrogen; liver transaminases; and creatinine kinase.
- Prothrombin time and partial thromboplastin time should be followed to evaluate for DIC.

IMAGING STUDIES

CT scan of the head to evaluate for space-occupying lesion if clinically indicated.

SUSCEPTIBILITY TESTING: Testing of MH susceptibility involves genetic evaluation or the in vitro muscle contracture test. The latter involves placing a muscle biopsy specimen in a bath of caffeine or halothane. Significant muscle contraction is 97% to 99% sensitive for MH susceptibility, with a specificity of 78% to 94% and a cost of $6 to $10,000. It is performed in only a few sites in the U.S. Genetic testing, while noninvasive, has a sensitivity of <50% and a cost of $1 to $4000. Generally, a positive contracture test leads to genetic testing, unless there is a positive family member, in which case the patient can go directly to genetic testing.

Testing for MHS can be performed preoperatively in patients at risk or those with personal or family history of anesthesia-induced complications suggestive of MH. In such patients, regardless of the test results, it is prudent to avoid volatile agents or succinylcholine, and thus this testing will only delay surgery and not change the anesthetic plan.

After an acute event, the patient should undergo susceptibility testing to confirm the diagnosis and the need for testing other immediate family members at risk.

Rx TREATMENT

After diagnosis of acute MH is made, MH protocol should be initiated. This begins with calling for assistance and in most institutions, obtaining access to the MH treatment cart. Potential triggering agents must be discontinued, substituting nontriggering agents in the setting of surgical intervention that cannot be terminated emergently. The patient should be hyperventilated on an FiO_2 of 100%. Dantrolene should be administered immediately and continued for a period of 24 to 48 hours. ABGs, serum electrolytes, clotting studies, CK, capnography, central venous pressure, and urine output should be followed closely. Sodium bicarbonate to mitigate metabolic acidosis, and dextrose and insulin to treat hyperkalemia may be warranted.

NONPHARMACOLOGIC THERAPY

- The patient should be cooled to 38°C. This can be accomplished with ice packs to the axillae and groin, a cooling blanket, a fan with cool mist, or chilled IV fluids. In extreme situations, partial extracorporeal bypass or iced peritoneal lavage have proven helpful.
- Frequent evaluation of core temperature, hemodynamics, and gas exchange are imperative.

ACUTE GENERAL Rx (SEE *BOX* 2)

- Dantrolene, which binds to ryanodine receptors and limits calcium release, is the only known antidote for MH. It has no effect on cardiac or smooth muscle but can cause weakness of the diaphragm and other skeletal muscles. After a loading dose of 2.5 mg/kg IV over 10 minutes, it should be administered at 1mg/kg IV every 5 minutes until elevated PET CO_2, rigidity, and fever abate. Patients with greater muscle mass may require an initial dose of up to 10 mg/kg.

ONGOING CARE

- Up to 25% of patients will have recrudescence of their symptoms, on average 13 hours after the initiation of MH. Dantrolene, 1mg/kg IV every 4 to 6 hours or by continuous infusion at 0.1 to 0.3 mg/kg/hr IV, is recommended for at least 24 to 48 hours. Additional boluses may be needed for breakthrough signs.
- Aggressive hydration with forced diuresis and alkalization of the urine should be instituted for rhabdomyolysis. Observe closely for the development of compartment syndrome.
- Beta-blockers and lidocaine may be useful for dysrhythmias. Use of calcium channel blockers should be avoided as in combination with dantrolene may produce profound hyperkalemia and significantly depress cardiac function.

BOX 2 Management of an Acute Malignant Hyperthermia Episode in the Intensive Care Unit

1. Administer high-flow 100% oxygen via a nonrebreathing mask, and consider endotracheal intubation.
2. For ventilated patients, administer an FiO_2 of 1.0 and increase minute ventilation to control $PaCO_2$.
3. Administer dantrolene (2.5 mg/kg intravenously) over 10 min, and repeat until acidosis and muscle rigidity have resolved. Repeat dantrolene (1 mg/kg) every 6 hr.
4. Initiate cooling with ice packs in the axillae and groin; decrease room temperature; use hypothermia blankets, iced intravenous saline solution (10 mL/kg over 10 min, repeated as needed), and lavage body cavities with cold saline solution if temperature is greater than 39° C. Stop cooling when core temperature falls to 38° C.
5. Correct metabolic acidosis with sodium bicarbonate (1-2 mEq/kg initially), and give subsequent doses based on base excess and body weight.
6. Administer calcium chloride (10 mg/kg) or calcium gluconate (100-200 mg/kg) for cardiotoxicity associated with hyperkalemia.
7. Give regular insulin (0.1 U/kg) and glucose (0.3-0.5 g/kg) to correct hyperkalemia.
8. Administer lidocaine (1 mg/kg) to treat ventricular arrhythmias. Consider amiodarone (5 mg/kg IV) for refractory, stable ventricular tachycardia. Do not delay defibrillation or cardiopulmonary resuscitation if indicated by cardiovascular instability.
9. Maintain urine output of 2 mL/kg/hr with aggressive cold fluid administration, furosemide (0.5-1 mg/kg), and additional mannitol (0.25-0.3 g/kg) if needed.
10. Consider quantitative end-tidal CO_2 monitoring.
11. Monitor core temperature (pulmonary artery, esophageal temperature probe, rectal probe).
12. Place arterial catheter for invasive blood pressure monitoring and frequent blood sampling. Consider central venous catheter and/or pulmonary artery catheter if indicated by cardiovascular instability.
13. Repeat venous blood gas and electrolytes analysis until these normalize. Repeat CK at least every 6 hr while the patient is in ICU and then daily until CK returns to normal. Assess glucose, clotting function, and hepatic and renal functions, and treat symptomatically. Repeat lactic acid measurement after each dantrolene administration.
14. Consider hemodialysis if indicated.
15. Consider intensive care monitoring for at least 24 hr after MH episode or after recrudescence of MH.
16. Refer the patient for muscle caffeine-halothane contracture testing and consider testing of RYR1. Pursue a pathologic diagnosis for other occult myopathies.

CK, Creatine kinase; *ICU,* intensive care unit; *MH,* malignant hyperthermia.

From Fuhrman BP et al: *Pediatric critical care,* ed 4, Philadelphia, 2011, Saunders.

BOX 3 Anesthetics Associated with the Development of Malignant Hyperthermia and Neuroleptic Malignant Syndrome

Malignant Hyperthermia
Volatile Anesthetics
Cyclopropane, diethyl ether, enflurane, ethylene, halothane, isoflurane, methoxyflurane, sevoflurane

Muscle Relaxants
Succinylcholine, decamethonium

Neuroleptic Malignant Syndrome
Phenothiazines
Fluphenazine, chlorpromazine, levomepromazine, thioridazine, trimeprazine, trifluoroperazine, prochlorperazine

Butyrophenones
Haloperidol, bromperidol, droperidol

Dibenzoxepine
Loxapine

Dopamine-Depleting Drugs
Alpha-methyltyrosine, tetrabenazine

Dopaminergic Agent Withdrawal
Levodopa-carbidopa, amantadine

From Parrillo JE, Dellinger RP: *Critical care medicine: principles of diagnosis and management in the adult*, ed 4, Philadelphia, 2014, Saunders.

CHRONIC Rx

- This is an acute disease, resolving in 24 to 48 hours with appropriate treatment.
- The patient should be aware that exercise in excessive heat and/or humidity could trigger an episode of MH.
- The patient as well as immediate family members should be advised to undergo susceptibility testing.

COMPLEMENTARY & ALTERNATIVE MEDICINE

None

DISPOSITION

After MH crisis, patients should be admitted to the intensive care unit for at least 24 hrs where close monitoring and supportive care can be maximized.

REFERRAL

Anesthesia, cardiology, renal, and hematologic consultation as appropriate.

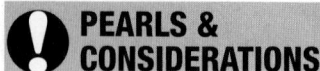 **PEARLS & CONSIDERATIONS**

COMMENTS

- MH is a life-threatening condition that requires prompt recognition to minimize illness and end-organ damage.
- Family or personal history of problems with general anesthesia in the past are clues to susceptibility and should prompt careful preoperative evaluation.
- Prophylactic dantrolene is no longer recommended for MH patients undergoing general anesthesia with nontriggering agents.
- Box 3 summarizes anesthetics associated with the development of malignant hyperthermia and neuroleptic malignant syndrome.

PATIENT & FAMILY EDUCATION

The patient and his/her family should be made aware of the diagnosis in order either to undergo susceptibility testing or to provide information to the anesthesiologist and other intraoperative caregivers if they are to be undergoing any type of surgery or procedure under sedation.

SUGGESTED READINGS

Available at www.expertconsult.com

AUTHORS: **JOSEPH MEHARG, M.D., SOMWAIL RASLA, M.D.,** and **MARINA GARAS, D.O.**

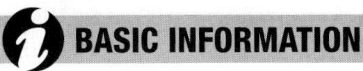

BASIC INFORMATION

DEFINITION

A Mallory-Weiss tear (MWT) is a longitudinal mucosal laceration in the region of the gastro-esophageal junction.

SYNONYMS

Mallory-Weiss syndrome

ICD-10CM CODES
K22.6 Mallory-Weiss syndrome

EPIDEMIOLOGY & DEMOGRAPHICS

- Accounts for 5% to 15% of cases of upper gastrointestinal (GI) bleeding
- Reported from early childhood to old age; the majority of patients are age 40 to 60 yr
- More common in males
- Alcohol use is present in 30% to 60%

PHYSICAL FINDINGS & CLINICAL PRESENTATION

- Vomiting, retching, or vigorous coughing will often, but not always, precede hematemesis.
- Patients may be clinically stable or present with tachycardia, hypotension, melena, hematochezia, epigastric pain, or back pain.
- Bleeding may be self-limited or severe. Rebleeding is more common in patients with advanced alcoholic liver disease.
- Tears may be seen in association with other upper GI tract lesions, including hiatal hernia (present in as many as 90% of patients), ulcers, and esophageal varices, particularly in alcoholics.

ETIOLOGY

- An acute increase in intragastric and intraabdominal pressure is transmitted to the gastroesophageal junction and esophagus, resulting in mucosal laceration.
- Vomiting may be associated with alcohol use, cannabinoid use, ketoacidosis, ulcer disease, uremia, pancreatitis, chemotherapy, cholecystitis, pregnancy (in particular associated with hyperemesis gravidarum), myocardial infarction, or the postoperative period.
- Infrequently reported causes include chest wall trauma (including CPR), hiccups, coughing, seizures, lifting/straining, blunt abdominal trauma, acute severe asthma, and labor and delivery.
- Tears may be iatrogenic, related to routine endoscopy (especially in struggling or retching patients, or in association with hiatal hernias), enteroscopy with or without overtubes, esophageal dilation, lower esophageal pneumatic disruption therapy for achalasia, endoscopic submucosal dissection, transesophageal echocardiography, or in association with polyethylene glycol electrolyte colonic lavage preparation. They are frequently found on the right lateral wall of the esophagus.

DIAGNOSIS

DIFFERENTIAL DIAGNOSIS

- Esophageal or gastric varices
- Esophagitis or esophageal ulcers (peptic or pill-induced)
- Gastric erosions
- Gastric or duodenal ulcer
- Dieulafoy lesion
- Arteriovenous malformations
- Neoplasms (usually gastric)
- Boerhaave's syndrome

WORKUP

Endoscopy is the diagnostic method of choice.

LABORATORY TESTS

- Complete blood count, prothrombin time, partial thromboplastin time
- Electrolytes, blood urea nitrogen, creatinine, liver function tests, pregnancy test, tests to evaluate for predisposing conditions

IMAGING STUDIES

Upper GI series is usually not sensitive. Patients with concurrent chest pain, dyspnea, shock, or physical examination findings of crepitus or pleural effusion should have a chest radiograph or CT to exclude Boerhaave's syndrome.

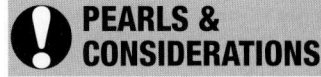 TREATMENT

NONPHARMACOLOGIC THERAPY

- Supportive care
- Avoidance of aspirin, nonsteroidal antiinflammatory drugs, and anticoagulants

ACUTE GENERAL Rx

- Patients with active bleeding or hemodynamic instability require large-bore IVs, fluid resuscitation, and transfusion of blood products (red blood cells, fresh frozen plasma, and platelets) as appropriate.
- Nasogastric decompression and antiemetics may be considered.
- Endoscopic therapy for patients with active or ongoing hemorrhage (Fig. 1). Therapeutic modalities include electrocoagulation, argon plasma photocoagulation, injection (e.g., 1:10,000 epinephrine, polidocanol), sclerotherapy (for bleeding associated with esophageal varices), band ligation, or endoscopic hemoclips (therapies may be used alone or in combination) (Fig. E2).

- Arterial embolization in patients with active bleeding who are poor surgical candidates.
- Laparotomy, with gastrotomy and oversewing of the tear, is required in a small percentage of patients with uncontrolled bleeding.

CHRONIC Rx

- Healing will usually occur without specific therapy.
- H_2 blockers or proton pump inhibitors may be given to help facilitate healing but should not be used long term unless appropriate indications are present.

DISPOSITION

- Prognosis is good, with spontaneous cessation of bleeding in upwards of 90% of patients. Endoscopic features can guide treatment. Blatchford score <6 suggests no need for transfusion or endoscopic intervention.
- Delayed rebleeding is described in patients with high-risk stigmata (shock at initial presentation, spurting or oozing at initial endoscopy).
- Death has been reported in 3% to 12%, often in association with severe bleeding and underlying comorbid conditions such as advanced age, coagulopathy, elevated transaminases, thrombocytopenia, alcohol use, presentation with a very low hemoglobin level or melena, and multi-system organ failure.

REFERRAL

- Gastrointestinal referral for endoscopy
- Surgical referral for bleeding unresponsive to endoscopic treatment or in the setting of coexistent perforation

PEARLS & CONSIDERATIONS

Conditions predisposing to retching or vomiting should be identified and treated at presentation.

SUGGESTED READINGS
Available at www.expertconsult.com

RELATED CONTENT

Mallory-Weiss Tear (Patient Information)

AUTHOR: **HARLAN G. RICH, M.D.**

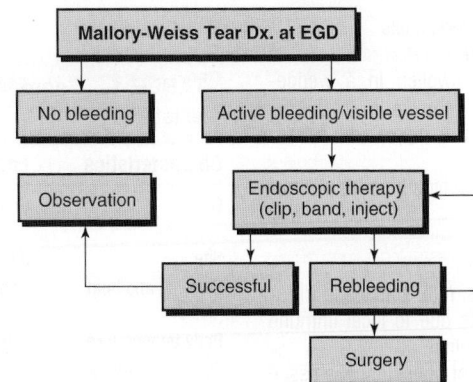

FIG. 1 Treatment algorithm for Mallory-Weiss tear. *EGD,* Esophagogastroduodenoscopy. (From Cameron JL, Cameron AM: *Current surgical therapy,* ed 10, Philadelphia, 2011, Saunders.)

M

Diseases and Disorders

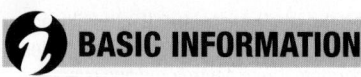

DEFINITION

Mastitis is local painful inflammation of the breast that may or may not be accompanied by infection, flulike symptoms, and abscess formation.

ICD-10CM CODES
N61 Inflammatory disorders of breast
O91.12 Abscess of breast associated with the puerperium
O91.22 Nonpurulent mastitis associated with the puerperium

EPIDEMIOLOGY & DEMOGRAPHICS

- In lactating mothers, typically occurs in first 3 mo postpartum (74%-95% of cases)
- When severe, mastitis can lead to a breast abscess (5%-11%) or septicemia
- Delayed diagnosis and treatment of lactational mastitis can lead to discontinuation of breastfeeding, breast tissue damage, recurrence
- In nonlactating women of childbearing age, often presents as granulomatous mastitis (GM)
- In older nonlactating women, often presents as periductal mastitis (PM) and is caused by inflamed milk ducts near the nipple
- Mastitis can also occur in infancy, when breast hypertrophy from maternal hormone leads to infection

PREVALENCE: Lactational mastitis occurs in up to 33% of mothers
PREDOMINANT SEX: Females
RISK FACTORS:
- Previous mastitis
- Milk stasis and missed feedings
- Cracked, fissured, or sore nipples
- Primiparity and infant attachment difficulties
- Cleft lip or palate or short frenulum in infant
- Use of manual breast pump
- Diabetes
- Breast implants
- Nipple piercings

PHYSICAL FINDINGS & CLINICAL PRESENTATION

- Warmth, redness, tenderness in breast
- Unilateral or bilateral
- Malaise, myalgias, fevers, chills
- Decreased milk output
- Breast is hard and swollen in a wedge-shaped area
- In PM, breast mass near nipple with retraction or discharge
- In GM, enlarged axillary lymph nodes or sinus tract formation

ETIOLOGY

- In lactational mastitis, milk stasis and irritation of the milk ducts due to local immune response to milk proteins.
  - Bacterial infection of subcutaneous tissue due to breaks in skin.

- Most commonly, *S. aureus;* less common, *S. epidermidis,* group A beta-hemolytic streptococci, *S. pneumoniae, E. coli, Candida albicans, M. tuberculosis.*
- GM results from inflammation with epithelioid histiocytes and multinucleated giant cells and can be caused by etiologies like tuberculosis, sarcoidosis, foreign body reaction, parasitic and mycotic infections, or idiopathic.
- Neonatal mastitis caused by *S. aureus* or gram-negative enteric bacteria.

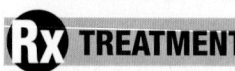 DIAGNOSIS

DIFFERENTIAL DIAGNOSIS

- Engorgement, plugged duct (see Table 1)
- Breast abscess
- Inflammatory or other breast cancer (3% of women diagnosed with breast cancer are lactating)
- Mastitis as a symptom of hyperprolactinemia or galactorrhea
- GM can be manifestation of systemic disease (sarcoidosis, Wegener granulomatosis, GCA, polyarteritis nodosa, TB, syphilis)

WORKUP

- History and clinical exam with thorough breast exam and assessment of axillary nodes and nipple discharge are sufficient for diagnosis
- Recurrent mastitis should include workup for underlying breast disease

LABORATORY TESTS

- Simple lactational mastitis requires no milk culture or laboratory studies
- Obtain midstream sample of milk for culture and sensitivities in refractory mastitis or in MRSA-suspected cases
- CBC and blood cultures in toxic patients
- In abscess formation, culture of drainage or aspirate fluid
- Gram stain and culture indicated in infant mastitis

IMAGING STUDIES

- Not necessary unless refractory mastitis or abscess suspected
- Consider US (Fig. 1) to evaluate for abscess or mammogram when appropriate to exclude carcinoma

- In GM, mammogram and US-guided FNA are standard

TREATMENT

NONPHARMACOLOGIC THERAPY

- Mainstay of therapy is effective milk removal through continued breastfeeding or pumping
- Consider referral to a certified lactation consultant to improve breastfeeding technique
- Warm compresses, increased fluid intake, good nutrition, and rest
- In abscess formation (10% of women who are treated for bacterial mastitis), surgical drainage or needle aspiration is necessary, followed by antibiotic therapy based on sensitivities of culture

ACUTE GENERAL Rx

- NSAIDs and analgesics (e.g., acetaminophen, ibuprofen). There is insufficient evidence to support or refute the effectiveness of antibiotic therapy. Common regimens include:
- No history of MRSA:
  1. Dicloxacillin 250 mg 4x/d for 7 d
  2. Cephalexin 500 mg 4x/d for 10-14 d
  3. Inpatient: nafcillin or oxacillin 2 g IV q4h
  4. Erythromycin may be used in patients allergic to penicillin
- Suspected MRSA or high-risk penicillin allergy:
  1. Trimethoprim/sulfamethoxazole 160 mg/800 mg 2x/d for 10 to 14 d; should not be used when breastfeeding healthy infants <2 mo or compromised infants
  2. Clindamycin 300 mg 4x/d for 10 to 14 d
  3. Inpatient: vancomycin 1 g IV q12h
- Oxytocin nasal spray if letdown reflex disturbed
- Consider treatment for candidal infection if bilateral symptoms and infant with thrush
  - Topical clotrimazole for mother and oral nystatin for infant, with careful washing of all pacifiers and nipples
  - If resistant to topical treatment, can consider oral fluconazole; however, data in breastfeeding are limited
- Infant mastitis typically treated in an inpatient setting with parenteral antibiotics based on results of Gram stain

---

TABLE 1 Comparison of Findings of Engorgement, Plugged Duct, and Mastitis

Characteristics	Engorgement	Plugged Duct	Mastitis
Onset	Gradual, immediately	Gradual, after feedings	Sudden, after 10 days postpartum
Site	Bilateral	Unilateral	Usually unilateral
Swelling and heat	Generalized	May shift/little or no heat	Localized red, hot, and swollen
Body temperature	<38.4° C	<38.4° C	>38.4° C
Systemic symptoms	Feels well	Feels well	Flulike symptoms

From Lawrence RA, Lawrence RM: *Breastfeeding: a guide for the medical profession,* ed 5, St Louis, 1999, Mosby.

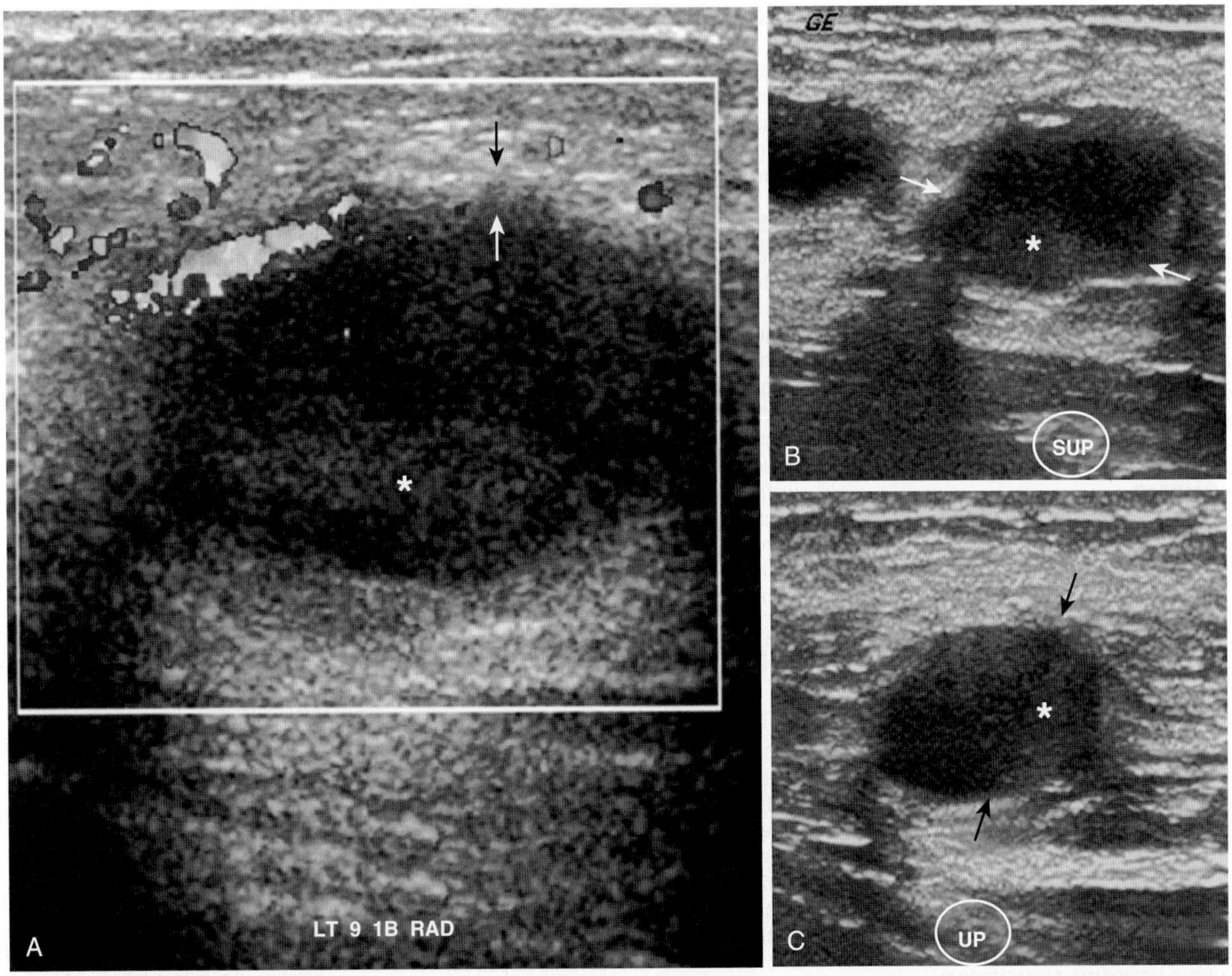

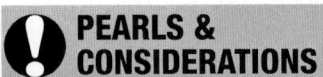

FIG. 1 Inflamed or infected cyst. A, Acutely inflamed or infected cysts demonstrate three findings: (1) abnormal uniform isoechoic wall thickening *(between arrows)*, (2) dependent debris *(asterisk)*, and (3) hyperemia of the thickened wall. **B,** Supine, and **C,** upright, images show the debris *(asterisk)*, resembling sludge within a gallbladder, shifting to the dependent part of the cyst when the position of the patient is changed from supine to upright or lateral decubitus positions. Note the change in the position of the interface between the nondependent fluid and the dependent debris or pus *(between arrows)*. (From Rumack CM et al: *Diagnostic ultrasound*, ed 4, Philadelphia, 2011, Mosby.)

CHRONIC Rx

- No evidence proving benefit of prophylactic antibiotics to prevent lactational mastitis
- In GM, systemic corticosteroids or wide surgical resection

COMPLEMENTARY & ALTERNATIVE MEDICINE

- Complementary therapies not assessed in prospective studies: *Belladonna, Phytolacca, Chamomilla,* sulfur, *Bellis perennis*
- Several strains of lactobacilli have shown promise as probiotic agents that might be useful in treating mastitis, including *L. fermentum* and *L. salivarius*. These results should be replicated before this approach is adopted widely.

REFERRAL

Refer to surgeon for severe PM or significant lactational abscess that does not resolve with conservative measures

⚠ PEARLS & CONSIDERATIONS

COMMENTS

- 25% of breastfeeding mothers with 1 episode of mastitis stop breastfeeding.
- Increasing incidence of MRSA mastitis.
- Lactational mastitis is risk factor for vertical transmission of infections (i.e., HIV-1, CMV, measles, hepatitis B and C).
- When reassessing refractory nonlactational mastitis, the most important consideration is the possibility of cancer.
- Nonlactational mastitis can be a manifestation of systemic disease.
- GM mimics breast cancer both clinically and radiologically (>50% of reported cases are initially mistaken for carcinoma). This includes fine needle aspiration, which is sometimes interpreted as malignant.

RELATED CONTENT

Lactational Mastitis (Patient Information)
Abscess, Breast (Related Key Topic)
Fibrocystic Breast Disease (Related Key Topic)
Mastitis (Related Key Topic)

SUGGESTED READINGS

Available at www.expertconsult.com

AUTHORS: **MARY BETH SUTTER, M.D.,** and **ANDRE LEVCHENKO, PH.D.**

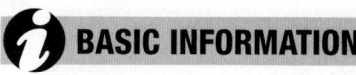

DEFINITION

Mastocytosis is a rare clonal disorder of hematopoiesis caused by the accumulation of an abnormal mast cell population primarily in skin and bone marrow, less commonly in liver and other tissues. Children usually have disease confined to the skin (urticaria pigmentosa) that resolves with adolescence. Adults typically have systemic disease of varying severity that is chronic. Indolent disease is typically defined by mast cell mediator related symptoms; advanced disease is associated with tissue injury from mast cell infiltrates and is less common.

SYNONYMS

Systemic mastocytosis
Urticaria pigmentosa (refers to skin disease only).
"Mastocytosis in the skin" (MIS, refers to skin disease only)

ICD-10CM CODES
Q82.2 Mastocytosis
D47.0 Indolent systemic
C96.2 Aggressive systemic
C96.2 Malignant
D47.0 Systemic, with an associated hematologic neoplasm (SM-AHM)

EPIDEMIOLOGY & DEMOGRAPHICS

INCIDENCE (SYSTEMIC MASTOCYTOSIS, EXCLUDING URTICARIA PIGMENTOSA):
0.4 per 1,000,000 persons per year (US)
0.45 cases per 100,000 persons per year (Denmark)
Male/female approximately equal.
Age at diagnosis typically 50-70, with wide range including teenager/young adult.
Approximately 2/3's of cases are indolent (excluding UP and SM-ASM).

PHYSICAL FINDINGS & CLINICAL PRESENTATION

Most symptoms are related to release of mast cell mediators, mainly histamine. Mast cells also contain serotonin, heparin, several proteases (most important tryptase, which is a diagnostic marker), leukotrienes and numerous cytokines (e.g. IL-6), among other mediators.

SYMPTOMS:

- Mast cell mediator symptoms:
  ○ Cutaneous: flushing (distinctive color change of face and skin), pruritus, urticaria, angioedema.
  ○ Extra-cutaneous: lightheadedness (due mediator related vasodilation), sometimes with syncope; palpitations; wheezing (less common).
- Gastrointestinal symptoms, due to mediator release, histamine related gastritis or ulcers or GI tract involvement with disease: nausea/vomiting, diarrhea, constipation, bloating.

- Musculoskeletal symptoms due to mastocytosis related osteopenia/osteoporosis or direct bone involvement with mast cells lesions: bone pain, less commonly myalgia/arthralgia.
- Severe anaphylactoid reactions, especially to Hymenoptera (bees, wasps, ants) venom.

PHYSICAL EXAM

- Urticaria pigmentosa is the hallmark lesion of systemic mastocytosis. In adults, the lesions are small, brown/red (Fig. E1), generally flat (maculopapular). Pediatric lesions are commonly larger and may be more nodular or plaque like. In adults, skin lesions are usually seen in indolent mast cell disease, less common in advanced disease.
- Darier's sign: wheal and reddening of lesions with stroking, persisting minutes to hours.
- Hepatomegaly and/or splenomegaly are common in advanced disease.
- Lymphadenopathy, by exam or imaging (about 20%).

DX DIAGNOSIS

DIFFERENTIAL DIAGNOSIS

- Mastocytosis is a rare disorder with a wide spectrum of symptoms and presentations. It should be considered in the evaluation of severe urticarial reactions to Hymenoptera venom exposures (i.e., bee stings mainly), unexplained angioedema, episodic hypotension and unexplained nausea or diarrhea. It should also be considered in premature osteopenia/osteoporosis, especially in males.
- Elevated tryptase levels may be seen with many myeloid hematologic malignancies, transiently with allergic reactions and helminth infections. Tryptase is elevated in renal failure and about 1%-3% of the normal population.
- Mast cell activation syndrome (MCAS) is a poorly understood disorder with mast cell mediator symptoms, possibly from hyperresponsive mast cells, but who lack pathologic findings of systemic mast cell disease.

WORKUP

- WHO diagnostic criteria for various forms of mastocytosis are outlined in Tables 1 through 3.
- Serum tryptase (mast cell protease). Approximately 20% of cases have serum tryptase less than WHO cut off of 20 ng/ml. Elevated levels have high specificity (98%). May be elevated after urticarial reactions; should not be elevated at baseline.
- Skin biopsy (Fig. E2) for urticarial pigmentosa/mastocytosis in the skin (MIS).
- Bone marrow examination should be performed in adults with MIS or elevated tryptase (> 25 ng/ml, or 15-25 ng/ml with high clinical suspicion).
- Flow cytometry/immune histochemistry for aberrant CD25 and/or CD2 expression, in addition to normal mast cell markers.

- Molecular studies (polymerase chain reaction, PCR) for *KIT* D816V mutation, preferably on tissue (marrow/skin); peripheral blood studies are less sensitive. If *KIT* D816V negative, consider evaluation for other KIT mutations.
- CBC and liver function studies; imaging of liver/spleen if appropriate.
- Bone density study for early osteoporosis in all patients; skeletal imaging if symptomatic (bone scan, plain x-rays).

Rx TREATMENT

Therapy of mastocytosis is primarily directed to blockade of histamine release symptoms with histamine receptor blockade and anti-inflammatory medications with cytoreductive therapy for organ injury or refractory histamine release symptoms. Cromolyn sulfate is a mast cell stabilizer that has been used for GI symptoms. Due to high incidence of anaphylaxis, epinephrine injectors are often recommended for mastocytosis patients. Triggers (e.g., alcohol, abrupt temperature changes e.g. with swimming) should be identified and avoided.

- Pruritus/flushing
  ○ H1 blockade: Cetirizine 5-10 mg/day, fexofenadine 60 mg BID, others. Doses sometimes adjusted upwards with caution. Use with caution in glaucoma, BPH; may cause dry mouth.
  ○ Leukotriene antagonist (second line): Montelukast 10 mg/day, zafirlukast 20 mg BID.
  ○ Aspirin (third line): Low doses sometimes helpful; use with caution with GI symptoms, or any other form of aspirin sensitivity
  ○ Psoralen and ultraviolet A light (PUVA) (third/fourth line)
- Abdominal pain/nausea/diarrhea/bloating
  ○ H2 blockade: Ranitidine 150 mg BID, famotidine 10 mg BID.
  ○ Proton pump inhibitors (second line): Omeprazole 20 mg/day, others.
  ○ Cromolyn sulfate (mast cell stabilizer, third line) 100-200 mg before meals and HS. This agent is expensive; availability may vary.
  ○ Corticosteroids for short courses (fourth line); doses vary.
- Recurrent hypotension
  ○ Epinephrine injector ("Epi-Pen")
  ○ H1/H2 receptor blockade.
  ○ Specific therapy for defined allergies (e.g., bee stings).
- Osteoporosis
  ○ Bisphosphonates: Alendronate 70 mg weekly, others.
  ○ Optimize vitamin D/calcium replacement.
- Cytoreductive therapy
  ○ Cladribine (2-CdA, 2-chlorodeoxyadenosine) 0.14 mg/kg x 5 days; a recent study found response rates of 72%, more durable in indolent disease (3.71 years for indolent, 2.47 for advanced). Increased infection risk was the main toxicity.

TABLE 1 WHO Diagnostic Criteria for Systemic Mastocytosis

Major Criterion
Multifocal dense infiltrates of mast cells (>15 mast cells in aggregates) detected in sections of bone marrow and/or in another extracutaneous organ.

Minor Criteria
1) In biopsy section of the BM or in other extracutaneous organ, >25% of the mast cells (MC) in the infiltrate are spindle-shaped or have atypical morphology, or, of all MC in the bone marrow aspirate smears, >25% are immature or atypical (mostly spindle-shaped).
2) Detection of an activating point mutation at codon 816 of *KIT* in bone marrow, peripheral blood or other extracutaneous organ.
3) Expression of CD2 and/or CD25 by MCs in bone marrow, peripheral blood or other extracutaneous organ.
4) Serum total tryptase persistently >20 ng/ml. The diagnosis of systemic mastocytosis (SM) can be made if at least one major and one minor criterion or at least three minor criteria are present.

Adapted from Arock, MD et al: *Eur J Hematol* 94(4), 474-490, 2015.

TABLE 2 Variants of Mastocytosis

Cutaneous mastocytosis	Cutaneous lesions present, but systemic mastocytosis (SM) criteria are not fulfilled.
Indolent systemic mastocytosis (ISM)	Meets criteria for SM but no "B" or "C" findings (Table 3 below), no mast cell leukemia and no associated hematologic neoplasm
Systemic mastocytosis with associated hematologic neoplasm (SM-AHN)	Criteria for SM met, with associated hematologic neoplasm*
Aggressive systemic mastocytosis (ASM)	SM with one or more "C" findings, but no evidence of mast cell leukemia.
Mast cell leukemia	Bone marrow (BM) shows diffuse and dense infiltration by atypical (mostly immature) mast cells. Bone aspirate smear is ≥20% mast cells; peripheral blood ≥10% mast cells.
Mast cell sarcoma (MCS)	Unifocal mast cell tumor with destructive growth pattern, but no evidence of SM.

*Usually myeloid–myelodysplasia, acute myeloid leukemia, or myeloproliferative neoplasms.
Adapted from Arock, MD et al: *Eur J Hematol* 94(4), 474-490, 2015; Arber DA; *Blood* 20(127):2391-2405, 2016.

TABLE 3 B and C Findings For Assessment of Mast Cell Burden and Aggressive Disease.

B ("Borderline benign") findings	1. Bone marrow biopsy with > 30% infiltration by mast cells and/or tryptase level > 200 ng/ml. 2. Signs of dysplasia or myeloproliferation in non-mast cell lineage but insufficient for diagnosis of associated hematologic neoplasm, with normal or slightly abnormal blood counts. 3. Hepatomegaly without impairment of liver function and or palpable splenomegaly without hypersplenism and/or lymphadenopathy by imaging or palpation.
C ("Consider cytoreduction") findings.	1. BM damage caused by infiltration of neoplastic mast cells with ANC <1000/mcl, Hgb <10.0 g/dl, platelets <100,000/mcl. 2. Palpable hepatomegaly with SM-related impairment of liver function, ascites, and/or portal hypertension. 3. Skeletal involvement with large osteolytic lesions and/or pathologic fractures caused by local mast cell infiltration. 4. Palpable splenomegaly with hypersplenism. 5. Malabsorption with weight loss due to gastrointestinal mast cell infiltrates

Adapted from Arock, MD et al: *Eur J Hematol* 94(4), 474-490, 2015.

○ Interferon alpha, 1-2 million units TIW, adjusted to response and tolerance.
○ Midostaurin is an oral multikinase inhibitor that had a response rate of 60% in a recent study; duration of response averaged 14.1 months. It is not commercially available, but has been used on a compassionate use basis.
○ Tyrosine kinase inhibitors such as imatinib mesylate have limited efficacy in *KIT* D816V mutated disease, but have use with other *KIT* mutations.

DISPOSITION

• Indolent mastocytosis patients had survivals that roughly parallel age-matched controls in a study 159 patients seen between 1976 and 2007 at Mayo Clinic. In the same era, advanced mastocytosis patients had median survival of 41 months. It is not known what impact changes in treatment standards in the current treatment era will have on survival.

SUGGESTED READINGS
Available at www.expertconsult.com

AUTHOR: **PETER RINTELS, M.D.**

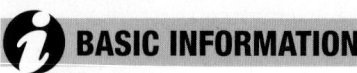

BASIC INFORMATION

DEFINITION

- Pain in the breast
- Usually cyclic condition but may be noncyclic or extramammary

SYNONYMS

Mastalgia

ICD-10CM CODES
N64.4 Mastodynia

EPIDEMIOLOGY & DEMOGRAPHICS

- Mastodynia affects up to 70% of women at some time in their reproductive lives.
- Severe cyclic mastodynia lasting more than 5 days/mo and of sufficient intensity to interfere with sexual, physical, social, and work-related activities is reported among 30% of premenopausal women.
- Underlying fear of breast cancer is the reason most of these women seek medical consultation.
- One tenth of women with mastodynia require pain-relieving therapy.

PHYSICAL FINDINGS & CLINICAL PRESENTATION

- Usually the breasts are normal bilaterally
- Full, tender breasts
- Generalized breast nodularity without discrete lumps
- Chest wall tenderness: extramammary breast pain
- Distinguishing mammary from extramammary pain can be difficult
- With the patient lying on her side so that the breast tissue falls away from the chest wall, tenderness can then be reproduced by direct pressure over the offending site
- Cyclic mastodynia presents in the luteal phase of the menstrual cycle
- Women with cyclic mastodynia tend to have abdominal bloating, leg swelling, and other symptoms of premenstrual syndrome
- Noncyclic mastodynia, on the other hand, is unrelated to the menstrual cycle
- Extramammary breast pain simulates noncyclic mastodynia

ETIOLOGY

- Hormonal imbalance
- Abnormal lipid metabolism
- Premenstrual syndrome (20%)
- Fibrocystic breast disease
- Emotional abuse and anxiety
- Excessive caffeine intake
- Breast cancer (10%)
- Tietze syndrome (idiopathic costochondritis)

DIAGNOSIS

DIFFERENTIAL DIAGNOSIS

- See "Etiology."

- The majority of women with mastodynia have no underlying abnormality.
- Breast fullness and tenderness associated with hormonal changes fluctuate with the menstrual cycle.
- Similarly, breast nodularity, which may or may not be the result of fibrocystic breast disease, also fluctuates with the menstrual cycle.
- Discrete breast lumps need full evaluation to rule out malignancy.
- Tietze syndrome is usually unilateral and may be associated with chest wall swelling.

LABORATORY TESTS

Although hormonal imbalance and abnormal lipid metabolism have been implicated in the etiopathogenesis of mastodynia, there is no good evidence to support any consistent pattern of serum hormonal or lipid profile in women with mastodynia. These tests are therefore not recommended.

IMAGING STUDIES

- Mammography should be part of the baseline investigation if the woman is >35 yr.
- Ultrasound can be performed as needed; it is particularly helpful in the assessment of cystic breast lesions.
- In women <35 yr, imaging investigations are not helpful unless a lump has been palpated clinically. Consideration of family history for breast disease is important.
- There are no radiologic features associated with mastodynia: rather, radiologic investigations are performed to exclude the rare presence of a subclinical carcinoma.

TREATMENT

NONPHARMACOLOGIC THERAPY

- 85% of the women with mastodynia can be reassured after full clinical evaluation. In fact, reassurance can be considered first-line therapy for mastodynia since many women who present are concerned about significant pathology, especially cancer.
- The remaining 15% require some form of therapy in addition to reassurance.
- A firm, supportive brassiere designed for postpartum use is particularly helpful if mastodynia is associated with breast swelling.
- Follow a low-fat, high-carbohydrate diet.
- Reduce caffeine intake.

ACUTE GENERAL Rx

- Evening primrose oil, which contains gamma-linolenic acid, has been shown to have some effectiveness and is an acceptable treatment for mastodynia.
- Topical NSAID preparations may confer some benefit and can be prescribed for these women.
- Hormonal therapy is the mainstay of treatment and may include progesterone-only oral contraceptives or cyclic Provera.
- Danazol is the only drug approved by the FDA for the treatment of mastodynia. Danazol has some androgenic and peripheral antiestrogenic effects. Its efficacy is well established, with significant relief of mastodynia in 70% to 93% of cases.

  ○ Widespread use of danazol is limited because of its adverse side effects. These include menstrual irregularities, depression, acne, hirsutism, and, in severe cases, voice deepening. Women taking danazol should be advised to use effective nonhormonal contraception because of the drug's potential adverse effects on the fetus.
  ○ The side effects of danazol can be significantly reduced by using a low dose (100 mg daily) and confining treatment to 2 wk preceding menstruation. However, alternatives should be explored.

- Tamoxifen, a synthetic antiestrogen, has also been shown to be effective in the treatment of mastodynia. Although effective in relieving symptoms, its use is extremely limited because of side effects. When used, it should be at a low dosage of 10 mg/day and duration should be limited to 6 mo at a time. In the U.S. this agent is not approved for use in women with mastodynia.
- Bromocriptine is a dopamine-receptor agonist whose primary action is inhibition of prolactin release. It has been used extensively in the treatment of severe cyclic mastodynia and is effective. Again, side effects such as headache and lightheadedness have limited its use.
- Lisuride maleate was recently found to be effective by one study.
- Other hormonal agents that have been reported to be effective in small studies cannot be recommended. Either they have unacceptable side effect profiles or their efficacy is not established. These agents include gestrinone, gonadotropin-releasing hormone analogues, progesterone, and hormone replacement therapy.

CHRONIC Rx

- Longstanding cases of mastodynia can be managed with intermittent low-dose danazol therapy to limit side effects. In between these courses of hormone, nonpharmacologic and nonhormonal therapy can be used.
- Severe, unremitting mastodynia that does not respond to medical treatment may require mastectomy; this is rare.

DISPOSITION

- Cyclic mastodynia resolves spontaneously in 20% to 30% of women.
- Up to 60% of women may develop recurrent symptoms 2 yr after treatment.
- Noncyclic mastodynia responds poorly to treatment but may resolve spontaneously in up to 50% of women.

RELATED CONTENT

Breast Pain (Patient Information)
Abscess, Breast (Related Key Topic)
Fibrocystic Breast Disease (Related Key Topic)
Mastitis (Related Key Topic)

AUTHORS: **ALEXANDER B. OLAWAIYE, M.D.,** and **RUBEN ALVERO, M.D.**

BASIC INFORMATION

DEFINITION

Mastoiditis is inflammation of the mastoid process and air cells, a complication of otitis media.

SYNONYMS

Mastoid abscess

ICD-10CM CODES
H70.0 Acute mastoiditis
H40.1 Chronic mastoiditis
H70.8 Other mastoiditis and related conditions
H70.9 Mastoiditis, unspecified

EPIDEMIOLOGY & DEMOGRAPHICS

INCIDENCE (IN U.S.): Since the introduction of antibiotic therapy and use of broad-spectrum antibiotics, there has been a marked decline in the incidence of acute mastoiditis.
PREDOMINANT SEX: More common in males
PREDOMINANT AGE: 2 mo to 18 yr
PEAK INCIDENCE: Early childhood

PHYSICAL FINDINGS & CLINICAL PRESENTATION

- Acute mastoiditis is usually a complication of acute otitis media.
- Most common presenting symptom is pain and tenderness in the postauricular region.
- Other signs or symptoms include:
  1. Fever
  2. Postauricular erythema and edema
  3. Protrusion of the pinna inferiorly and anteriorly
  4. Tympanic membrane usually intact with signs of acute otitis media
- Complications of acute mastoiditis include:
  1. Subperiosteal abscess (most common complication)
  2. Hearing loss
  3. Facial nerve palsy
  4. Labyrinthitis
  5. Intracranial complications such as hydrocephalus, meningitis, encephalitis, intracranial abscess, and lateral sinus thrombosis
- Chronic mastoiditis is characterized by chronic otorrhea and chronic tympanic membrane perforation.

ETIOLOGY

- Continuity exists between the middle air space and the mastoid cavity.
- Initial hyperemia and edema of the mucosal lining of the air cells result in accumulation of purulent exudate.
- Dissolution of calcium from bony septa and osteoclastic activity in the inflamed periosteum lead to bone necrosis and coalescence of air cells.
- Most common bacterial isolates are:
  1. *Streptococcus pneumoniae*
  2. *Streptococcus pyogenes*
  3. *Haemophilus influenzae*
  4. *Moraxella catarrhalis*
  5. *Staphylococcus aureus*
- Often, there are multiple organisms in chronic mastoiditis, with predominance of anaerobes and gram-negative bacteria.
- *Mycobacterium tuberculosis,* nontuberculous mycobacteria, *Aspergillus,* and *Rhodococcus equi* have been reported in cases of mastoiditis in severely immunocompromised individuals.

DIAGNOSIS

DIFFERENTIAL DIAGNOSIS

- Children
  1. Rhabdomyosarcoma
  2. Histiocytosis X
  3. Leukemia
  4. Kawasaki syndrome
- Adults
  1. Fulminant otitis externa
  2. Histiocytosis X
  3. Metastatic disease

WORKUP

A thorough history and physical examination are important in establishing diagnosis.

LABORATORY TESTS

- Fluid for Gram stain and culture may be obtained by myringotomy.
- If there is a perforation in the tympanic membrane with drainage, cultures of this may be taken after carefully cleaning the external canal.

IMAGING STUDIES

- Plain x-rays of the mastoid region may demonstrate clouding or opacification in areas of pneumatization.
- CT scan can demonstrate early involvement of bone (mastoiditis with bone destruction).
- MRI is more sensitive than CT scan in evaluating soft-tissue involvement and is useful in conjunction with CT scan to investigate other complications of mastoiditis.

TREATMENT

NONPHARMACOLOGIC THERAPY

Myringotomy, if the ear is not already draining

ACUTE GENERAL Rx

- Initiated with IV antibiotics directed against the common organisms *S. pneumoniae* and *H. influenzae.* Useful agents are amoxicillin/clavulanate, ceftriaxone, and cefotaxime. If the disease in the mastoid has had a prolonged course, coverage for *S. aureus* with gram-negative enteric bacilli may be considered for initial therapy until results of cultures become available. Add vancomycin if MRSA suspected or nafcillin/oxacillin if culture is positive for *S. aureus*, methicillin susceptible.
- Antibiotics continued until all signs of mastoiditis have resolved
- Directed against enteric gram-negative organisms and anaerobes in chronic mastoiditis
- Indications for mastoidectomy:
  1. Failure to improve after 72 hr of therapy
  2. Persistent fever
  3. Imminent or overt signs of intracranial complications
  4. Evidence of a subperiosteal abscess in the mastoid bone

DISPOSITION

Proceed with mastoidectomy when medical therapy fails.

REFERRAL

- To otorhinolaryngologist:
  1. If diagnosis is in doubt
  2. If aural complications present
  3. To evaluate for surgical intervention
- To neurosurgeon if intratemporal or intracranial extension of infection suspected
  1. Aural complications: bone destruction, subperiosteal abscess, petrositis, facial paralysis, labyrinthitis
  2. Intracranial complications: extradural abscess, lateral sinus thrombophlebitis or thrombosis, subdural abscess, meningitis, brain abscess, otitic hydrocephalus

PEARLS & CONSIDERATIONS

Mastoiditis is particularly difficult to eradicate because the mastoid air cells are poorly vascularized and difficult to drain.

SUGGESTED READING
Available at www.expertconsult.com

RELATED CONTENT
Mastoiditis (Patient Information)

AUTHOR: **GLENN G. FORT, M.D., M.P.H.**

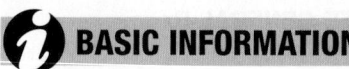

DEFINITION

Mediastinitis is an infection involving the connective mediastinal tissue that fills the interpleural spaces and surrounds the mediastinal organs. It can be acute or chronic.

SYNONYMS

Fibrosing mediastinitis
Sclerosing mediastinitis
Granulomatous mediastinitis

ICD-10CM CODES
J98.5 Mediastinitis

EPIDEMIOLOGY

Acute mediastinitis occurs most frequently as a postoperative infection after a median sternotomy and can be a life-threatening infection. Most infections are bacterial in nature.

Chronic mediastinitis is a chronic form of infection in the mediastinum characterized by an invasive and compressive inflammatory infiltrate. It is mostly caused by fungi and some bacteria.

INCIDENCE: Incidence of postoperative mediastinitis ranges from 0.4 to 5%.

RISK FACTORS: Mediastinal infections have four possible sources:
- Direct contamination as seen in trauma or surgery (e.g., open heart, esophageal)
- Hematogenous or lymphatic spread
- Extension of infection from the neck or retroperitoneum
- Extension from the lung, pleura, or chest wall

PHYSICAL FINDINGS & CLINICAL PRESENTATION

- Patients with acute mediastinitis present with acute onset of fever, tachycardia, chest pain, dysphagia, or respiratory distress. There may be signs of sternal wound infection or cellulitis and/or crepitus and edema of the chest wall.
- Patients with chronic mediastinitis are mostly asymptomatic until symptoms develop related to invasion or obstructions of structures within the mediastinum or adjacent to the mediastinum, such as cough, dyspnea, wheezing, chest pain, dysphagia, or hemoptysis. Complications of chronic or sclerosing mediastinitis include:
  - Superior vena cava syndrome. Histoplasma is the most common nonmalignant cause of this syndrome, marked by edema of face, neck and torso; neck vein distention; and headache.
  - Pulmonary venous or arterial obstruction.
  - Esophageal obstruction, cor pulmonale, constrictive pericarditis.
  - Thoracic duct obstruction.

ETIOLOGY (TABLE 1)

Acute mediastinitis:
- Related to head and neck infections or esophageal perforation

- Anaerobic bacteria: Peptostreptococci, Veillonella, Fusobacterium, Actinomyces, Prevotella, Eubacterium, Bacteroides
- Aerobic bacteria: Streptococcus, Staphylococcus, Corynebacterium, Moraxella, enteric gram-negative rods
- Fungi: Candida albicans
- Related to cardiothoracic surgery
- Gram-positive bacteria: Staphylococcus aureus, Staphylococcus epidermidis, Enterococcus, Streptococcus

---

TABLE 1 Microbiology of Mediastinitis

Organisms Frequently Recovered in Mediastinitis Secondary to Infection of the Head and Neck or Esophageal Perforation

Anaerobic

Gram-positive cocci—*Peptostreptococcus* spp.

Gram-positive bacilli—*Actinomyces, Eubacterium, Lactobacillus*

Gram-negative cocci—*Veillonella*

Gram-negative bacilli—*Bacteroides* spp., *Fusobacterium* spp., *Prevotella* spp., *Porphyromonas* spp.

Aerobic or Facultative

Gram-positive cocci—*Streptococcus* spp., *Staphylococcus* spp.

Gram-positive bacilli—*Corynebacterium*

Gram-negative cocci—*Moraxella*

Gram-negative bacilli—Enterobacteriaceae, *Pseudomonas* spp., *Eikenella corrodens*

Fungi—*Candida albicans*

Representative Organisms Recovered in Mediastinitis Secondary to Cardiothoracic Surgery, with Representative Rate and Range

Gram-Positive Cocci

Staphylococcus aureus, 25% (7.1%-66.7%)

Staphylococcus epidermidis, 30% (6%-45.5%)

Enterococcus spp., 10% (8%-18.8%)

Streptococcus spp., 2% (0%-18.2%)

Gram-Negative Bacilli

Escherichia coli, 5% (0%-12.5%)

Enterobacter spp., 10% (4%-21.4%)

Klebsiella spp., 3% (0%-21.1%)

Proteus spp., 2% (0%-7.1%)

Other Enterobacteriaceae, 2% (0%-20%)

Pseudomonas spp., 2% (0%-54%)

Fungi

C. albicans, <2 (0%-20.5%)

Polymicrobial, 10% (0%-40%)

Others Occasionally Reported

Acinetobacter, Salmonella spp., *Legionella* spp., *Bacteroides fragilis, Corynebacterium* spp., *Burkholderia cepacia, Mycoplasma hominis, Candida tropicalis, Aspergillus* spp., *Nocardia* spp., *Kluyvera, Gordonia sputi, Mycobacterium fortuitum, Mycobacterium chelonae, Rhodococcus bronchialis*

Other Unusual Causes of Mediastinitis

Anthrax, brucellosis, actinomycosis, paragonimiasis, *Streptococcus pneumonia*

From Bennett JE et al: *Mandell, Douglas, and Bennett's principles and practice of infectious diseases*, ed 8, Philadelphia, 2015, Saunders.

- Gram-negative bacteria: Escherichia coli, Enterobacter, Klebsiella, Proteus, Pseudomonas, other Enterobacteriaceae
- Fungi: Candida albicans

Chronic mediastinitis:
- *Histoplasma capsulatum,* a dimorphic fungus, is the most common and can cause mediastinal granuloma or fibrosing mediastinitis. A leakage of fungal antigens from lymph nodes into the mediastinal space is believed to cause a hypersensitivity reaction and subsequent exuberant fibrotic response.
- Other: *Mycobacterium tuberculosis, Nocardia,* actinomycosis, aspergillosis.

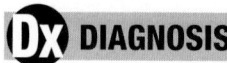 DIAGNOSIS

DIFFERENTIAL DIAGNOSIS

For chronic mediastinitis:
- Tumors that can also cause superior vena cava syndrome (e.g., Hodgkin's and non-Hodgkin's lymphomas, mesothelioma)
- Sarcoidosis
- Behçet's syndrome
- Mediastinal fibrosis associated with radiation
- Silicosis

LABORATORY TESTS

- CBC with differential, C-reactive protein, and procalcitonin can point to bacterial infection
- Obtain cultures: aerobic and anaerobic bacteria and fungi, intraoperatively or of any purulent drainage
- Pathologic examination: distinguish between cancer and infection for chronic mediastinitis and allow for specific fungal stains on tissues

IMAGING STUDIES

- Chest x-ray: can show diffuse mediastinal widening or evidence of mediastinal abscess, including gas bubbles or fluid level. Pneumomediastinum (Fig. 1) or pneumothorax can be seen with esophageal perforation (Table 2).
- Chest CT: can show the same as x-ray but is more sensitive in determining degree of mediastinal involvement and may guide drainage procedures for treatment or diagnosis.
- MRI may be superior to CT for sclerosing mediastinitis.

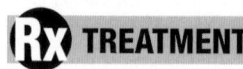 TREATMENT

NONPHARMACOLOGIC THERAPY

Surgery remains the gold standard treatment of mediastinitis for optimal drainage and debridement.

- Open techniques: debridement of infected tissue and open packing of the wound with delayed closure or use of vacuum-assisted closure for acute mediastinitis
- Closed techniques: debridement of infected tissues, closure of the sternum, and postoperative irrigation through drainage tubes for acute mediastinitis

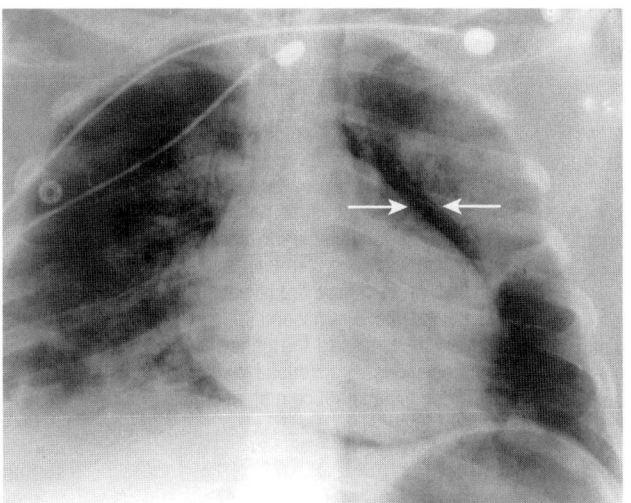

FIG. 1 Mediastinitis. Chest radiograph shows large pneumomediastinum and pneumopericardium *(arrows)* in a patient with mediastinitis. (From Bennett JE et al: *Mandell, Douglas, and Bennett's principles and practice of infectious diseases,* ed 8, Philadelphia, 2015, Saunders.)

TABLE 2   Risk Factors for Surgical Site Infection/Mediastinitis Post–cardiac Surgery

Preoperative Risk Factors	Operative Risk Factors	Postoperative Risk Factors
Increasing age	Emergent surgery	Need for reexploration
Diabetes	Heart transplant	Prolonged ICU stay
Staphylococcus aureus nasal colonization	Increasing complexity of surgery	Need for mechanical ventilation >48 hr
Previous sternotomy	Use of internal thoracic arteries in CABG	Lack of perioperative glucose control
COPD	Prolonged operative time	Placement of tracheostomy
Peripheral vascular disease	Hair removal by razor, not clippers	Postoperative myocardial infarction
Class 3-4 angina	Inappropriate timing of antibiotics	Receipt of multiple blood products
Renal failure requiring hemodialysis	Prolonged time on cardiopulmonary bypass	Postoperative low cardiac output state
History of endocarditis	High core temperature during bypass (>38°C)	
Cigarette smoking		
Low cardiac output		
Concurrent infection		
Prolonged preoperative hospitalization		
Preoperative use of a ventricular assist device		

CABG, Coronary artery bypass grafting; *COPD,* chronic obstructive pulmonary disease; *ICU,* intensive care unit.
From Bennett JE et al: *Mandell, Douglas, and Bennett's principles and practice of infectious diseases,* ed 8, Philadelphia, 2015, Saunders.

ACUTE GENERAL Rx

- Intravenous antibiotics: also a cornerstone of therapy but without surgery may fail. Broad-spectrum antibiotics should be used until cultures are finalized. Combination of piperacillin-tazobactam or meropenem plus vancomycin offers good initial coverage for acute mediastinitis. Other options include ciprofloxacin or cefepime for gram-negative rods, linezolid for gram-positive bacteria, metronidazole for anaerobic bacteria.
- Therapy is 2 to 3 weeks, but some cases may require 4 to 6 weeks.

CHRONIC Rx

- There is no definitive cure for chronic fibrosing or sclerosing mediastinitis. Antifungal agents and steroids generally do not work. The goal of therapy is to palliate symptoms by relieving airway, vascular, or esophageal obstruction. Surgery in patients with extensive fibrosis has high morbidity and mortality.

DISPOSITION

- Patients may need extensive wound care and possible vacuum-assisted closure and prolonged intravenous antibiotics.

REFERRAL

- Thoracic surgeon and/or head and neck surgeon for surgery and debridement
- Infectious diseases consultant for antibiotic selection and long-term management

! PEARLS & CONSIDERATIONS

COMMENTS

Histoplasma capsulatum is a dimorphic fungus found commonly in bird and bat fecal material and is most prevalent in the Ohio and Mississippi river valleys of the United States.

PREVENTION

Antibiotic prophylaxis should be given within 60 minutes before incision for surgeries requiring sternotomy. Options include cefazolin 1 g IV if <80 kg and 2 g if >80 kg, or cefuroxime 1.5 g IV. If the patient is penicillin allergic or has a history of methicillin-resistant *S. aureus* (MRSA) infection or surgery is to be done in a hospital where MRSA infection is common, use vancomycin 1 g IV.

SUGGESTED READINGS

Available online at www.expertconsult.com

AUTHOR: **GLENN G. FORT, M.D., M.P.H.**

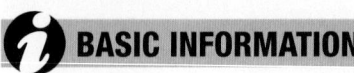

BASIC INFORMATION

DEFINITIONS

1. **Classic Meigs' syndrome:** a triad characterized by the presence of a benign fibroma or fibroma-like ovarian tumor (thecoma, granulosa cell tumor, or Brenner tumor) with ascites and pleural effusion (usually right-sided that resolves after resection of the tumor).
2. **Nonclassic Meigs' (Demons-Meigs') syndrome:** characterized by ascites and pleural effusion in conjunction with a benign ovarian, fallopian tube, or broad ligament tumor that is not included in the definition of classic Meigs' syndrome.
3. **Pseudo-Meigs' syndrome:** characterized by both ascites and pleural effusion but caused by a pelvic or abdominal tumor, either benign or malignant, not included in either classic Meigs' or nonclassic Meigs' syndrome.
4. **Pseudo-pseudo Meigs' (Tjalma) syndrome:** characterized by the triad of ascites, pleural effusion, and an elevated CA-125 (Cancer antigen 125) in a patient with systemic lupus erythematosus.

ICD-10CM CODES
C56.9 Malignant neoplasm of unspecified ovary
D27.9 Benign neoplasm of unspecified ovary
D28.2 Benign neoplasm of uterine tubes and ligaments
D28.7 Benign neoplasm of other specified female genital organs
J91.8 Pleural effusion in other conditions classified elsewhere
R18.0 Malignant ascites
R18.8 Other ascites

EPIDEMIOLOGY & DEMOGRAPHICS

- Occurs in 1% to 2% of ovarian fibromas (associated with approximately 0.004% of ovarian tumors).
- <1% progress to malignancy.
- Incidence begins to increase in the 30s. Most frequently encountered during middle age (average age, approximately 50 yr).

PHYSICAL FINDINGS & CLINICAL PRESENTATION

- Abdominal bloating/increased girth
- Intermittent pelvic pain (intermittent torsion)
- Weight gain or loss
- Pelvic mass on bimanual examination
- Acute pelvic/abdominal tenderness
- Fluid wave
- Shifting dullness
- "Puddle sign" (physical exam maneuver)
- Hyperresonance or flatness to chest percussion, absence of tactile and vocal fremitus
- Absent or loud bronchial breath sounds, rales, mediastinal displacement, tracheal shift

ETIOLOGY

- Unclear
- Often associated with "edematous" fibromas (or other benign ovarian solid tumor) in excess of 10 cm that may irritate the peritoneal lining, thereby stimulating production of peritoneal fluid
- Hypothesized that large fibroma with narrow stalk has inadequate lymphatic drainage; when coupled with intermittent torsion, results in backflow transudation into the peritoneal cavity; accumulated peritoneal ascites then pass to the right pleural cavity by the lymphatics (overloaded thoracic duct) or abdominal pleural commutation (i.e., foramen of Bochdalek)

DIAGNOSIS

DIFFERENTIAL DIAGNOSIS

- Ovarian malignancy
- Various gynecologic disorders:
  1. Uterus: endometrial tumor, sarcoma, leiomyoma ("pseudo-Meigs' syndrome")
  2. Fallopian tube: hydrosalpinx, granulomatous salpingitis, fallopian tube malignancy
  3. Ovary: benign, serous, mucinous, endometrioid, clear cell, Brenner tumor, granulosa, stromal, dysgerminoma, fibroma, metastatic tumor
- Nongynecologic causes of abdominopelvic ascites
  1. Portal vein obstruction
  2. Inferior vena cava obstruction
  3. Hypoproteinemia
  4. Thoracic duct obstruction
  5. Tuberculosis
  6. Amyloidosis
  7. Pancreatitis
  8. Gastrointestinal/genitourinary neoplasm
  9. Ovarian hyperstimulation
  10. Pleural effusion
  11. Congestive heart failure
  12. Collagen-vascular disease
  13. Cirrhosis

WORKUP

- Clinical condition characterized by ovarian mass, ascites, and predominantly right-sided pleural effusion
- History of early satiety, weight loss with increased abdominal girth, bloating, intermittent abdominal pain, dyspnea, and nonproductive cough

LABORATORY TESTS

- Complete blood count to rule out inflammatory process
- Tumor markers (CA-125, hCG, AFP, CEA, LDH) to evaluate gynecologic malignancy
- Chemical and liver function testing profile to evaluate metabolic or hepatic involvement
- Arterial blood gases if respiratory compromise

IMAGING STUDIES

- Pelvic sonography (color-flow Doppler evaluation of adnexal mass) initially to evaluate pelvic pathology (CT scan or MRI to further delineate neoplastic lesions [Fig. E1])
- Chest x-ray to confirm pleural effusion Procedures
- Paracentesis/thoracentesis will usually show a transudate.

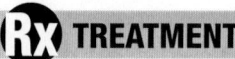

TREATMENT

NONPHARMACOLOGIC THERAPY

- Informed consent and proper preparation of patient for possible staging laparotomy (total abdominal hysterectomy and bilateral salpingo-oophorectomy, possible omentectomy, possible bowel resection, and possible pelvic/periaortic lymphadenectomy)
- Bowel prep if considering pelvic malignancy

ACUTE GENERAL TREATMENT

Depending on clinical presentation, size of pelvic mass, amount of ascites, and pleural effusion:

- If pelvic mass <10 cm with minimal ascites/pleural effusion: consider diagnostic laparoscopy (possible exploratory laparotomy) and salpingo-oophorectomy with removal of ovarian fibroma (tumor).
- If pelvic mass >10 cm with moderate/large amount ascites/pleural effusion: consider pleurocentesis if respiratory compromise (cytology: AFB) and exploratory laparotomy with salpingo-oophorectomy and removal of ovarian tumor.
- Treat pelvic malignancy, gastrointestinal or genitourinary tumor as indicated.

CHRONIC TREATMENT

- Resolution of ascites and pleural effusion after removal of ovarian tumor
- Routine gynecologic follow-up for benign ovarian tumor

DISPOSITION

Dramatic resolution of ascites and effusion within weeks of resection of pelvic mass is seen. Excellent progress and complete survival are expected. Recurrence rate is low.

REFERRAL

To gynecologic oncologist for evaluation and treatment, especially if malignancy considered or encountered

To pulmonologist for management of pleural effusion

SUGGESTED READING
Available at www.expertconsult.com

AUTHORS: **JORDAN KLEBANOFF, M.D.,** and **NIMA R. PATEL, M.D., M.S.**

 **BASIC INFORMATION**

DEFINITION

Melanoma is a skin neoplasm arising from the malignant degeneration of melanocytes. It is classically subdivided in four types:
1. Superficial spreading melanoma (70%) (Fig. 1, *A*)
2. Nodular melanoma (15%-20%) (Fig. 1, *B*)
3. Lentigo maligna melanoma (5%-10%) (Fig. 2)
4. Acral lentiginous melanoma (7%-10%)

SYNONYMS

Malignant melanoma
Cutaneous malignant melanoma

ICD-10CM CODES

C43.9	Malignant melanoma of skin, unspecified
C43.30	Malignant melanoma of unspecified part of face
C43.31	Malignant melanoma of nose
C43.4	Malignant melanoma of scalp and neck
C43.51	Malignant melanoma of anal skin
C43.52	Malignant melanoma of skin of breast
C43.59	Malignant melanoma of other part of trunk
C43.8	Malignant melanoma of overlapping sites of skin
D03.8	Melanoma in situ of other sites
D03.9	Melanoma in situ, unspecified

EPIDEMIOLOGY & DEMOGRAPHICS

- In 2016, an estimated 76,380 new cases and 10,130 deaths are expected in the U.S.; the estimated lifetime risk of development of melanoma is 1 in 50.
- Melanoma is much more common in whites (17.2 per 100,000 white men) than in African Americans (1 per 100,000 African American men). Increased risk of developing melanomas is found in patients with fair skin, red hair, light eyes, abundance of freckles, atypical moles or large amount of moles (>50). A personal history of any skin cancer or a family history of melanoma also increases the risk.

- Melanoma is the leading cause of death from skin cancer. Although it represents <10% of all skin-cancers, it accounts for at least 70% of deaths related to skin cancer.
- The median age at diagnosis is 53 years.
- Superficial spreading melanoma occurs most often in young adults on sun-exposed areas.
- Acral lentiginous melanoma is most often found in Asian Americans and African Americans and is unrelated to sun exposure.
- 8% to 10% of melanomas arise in people with a family history of the disease.

PHYSICAL FINDINGS & CLINICAL PRESENTATION

Variable depending on the subtype of melanoma:
- Superficial spreading melanoma is most often found on the lower legs, arms, and upper back. It may have a combination of many colors or may be uniformly brown or black.
- Nodular melanoma can be found anywhere on the body, but it most frequently occurs on the trunk on sun-exposed areas. It has a dark-brown or red-brown appearance and can be dome shaped or pedunculated. Lesions are frequently misdiagnosed because they may resemble a blood blister or hemangioma and may also be amelanotic.
- Lentigo maligna melanoma is generally found in older adults in areas continually exposed to the sun and frequently arising from lentigo maligna (Hutchinson's freckle) or melanoma in situ. It might have a complex pattern and variable shape; color is more uniform than in superficial spreading melanoma.
- Acral lentiginous melanoma frequently occurs on soles, subungual mucous membranes, and palms (sole of the foot is the most prevalent site). Unlike other types of melanoma, it has a similar incidence in all ethnic groups.
- The warning signs that the lesion may be a melanoma can be summarized with the ABCDE mnemonic:
  A: Asymmetry (e.g., lesion is bisected and halves are not identical)
  B: Border irregularity (uneven, ragged border)

C: Color variegation (presence of various shades of pigmentation)
D: Diameter enlargement (>6 mm)
E: Evolving (mole changing in size, shape, or color, or mole that differs visibly from surrounding moles ["ugly duckling" sign]) (Fig. 3)

ETIOLOGY

- Ultraviolet light is the most important cause of malignant melanoma.
- There is a modest increase in melanoma risk in patients with small nondysplastic nevi and a much greater risk in those with dysplastic lesions.
- The *CDKN2A* gene, residing at the *9p21* locus, is often deleted in patients with familial melanoma.
- A mutated signal transduction molecule, v-raf murine sarcoma viral oncogene homolog B_1 (BRAF), has been identified in 50% to 70% of patients with melanoma.

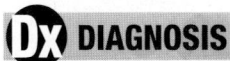 **DIAGNOSIS**

DIFFERENTIAL DIAGNOSIS

- Dysplastic nevi
- Solar lentigo
- Vascular lesions
- Blue nevus
- Basal cell carcinoma
- Seborrheic keratosis

WORKUP

- Dermoscopy (use of an instrument that shines polarized light on skin surfaces and magnifies skin lesions) can increase the accuracy in diagnosing melanoma by 10% to 27%.
- Any suspicious lesion (Fig. 4) should be biopsied. Perform excisional biopsy with elliptical excision that includes 1 to 2 mm of normal skin surrounding the lesion and extends to the subcutaneous tissue; incisional punch biopsy is sometimes necessary in surgically sensitive areas (e.g., digits, nose). It is essential that the size of the specimen be adequate to determine the histologic depth of penetration, which is known as the Breslow depth.

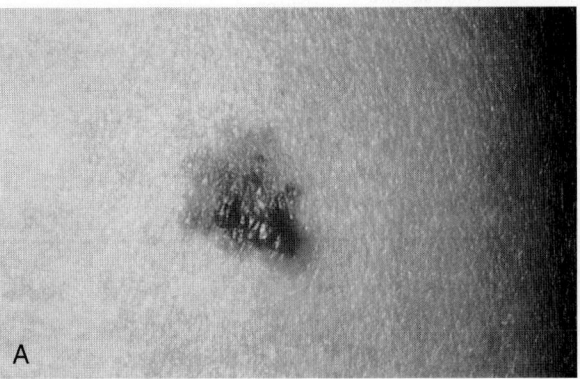
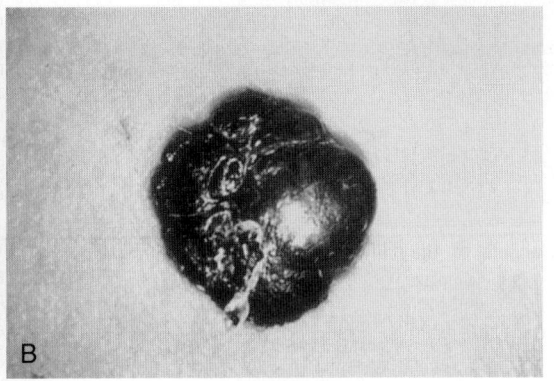

FIG. 1 A, Superficial spreading melanoma. **B,** Nodular melanoma. (From Abeloff MD [ed]: *Clinical oncology,* ed 3, New York, 2004, Churchill Livingstone.)

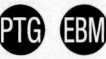

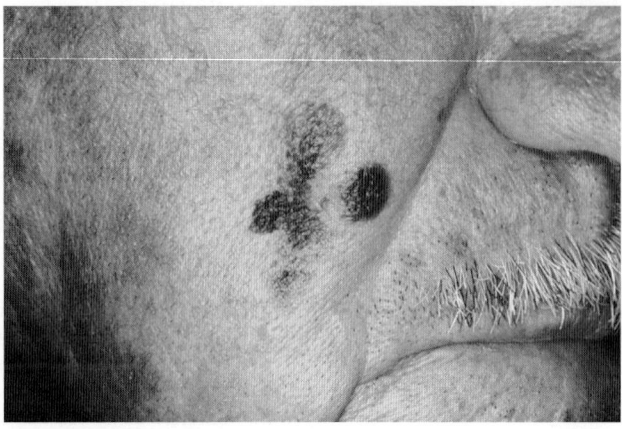

FIG. 2 Lentigo maligna melanoma. (From James WD et al: *Andrews' diseases of the skin: clinical dermatology*, ed 12, Philadelphia, 2016, Elsevier.)

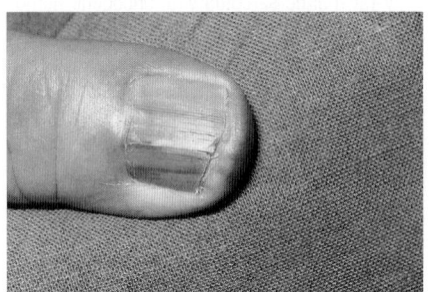

FIG. 3 Subungual melanoma with Hutchinson sign (pigment spreading from under the nail to involve the adjacent skin, usually of the proximal or lateral nail fold). These lesions are thought to emanate from the nail matrix. (From White GM, Cox NH [eds]: *Diseases of the skin, a color atlas and text,* ed 2, St Louis, 2006, Mosby.)

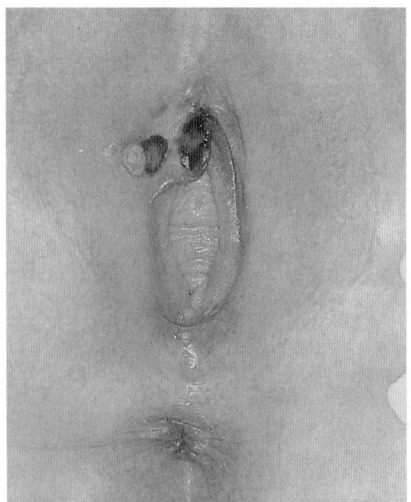

FIG. 4 Melanoma of the vulva. Benign nevi, vulva melanosis, and melanoma may occur in the vulvar region. Any suspicious pigmented lesion should be biopsied. The patient here is 75 years old. (Courtesy Paul Koonings, M.D. From White GM, Cox NH [eds]: *Diseases of the skin, a color atlas and text,* ed 2, St Louis, 2006, Mosby.)

- Sentinel lymph node excision (SLNE) is the most important staging and potentially therapeutic procedure for patients with melanoma. It should be considered in patients with intermediate (1 to 4 mm) melanomas or

TABLE 1 The Staging System for Melanoma Adapted by the American Joint Committee on Cancer (AJCC)

T classification	Thickness (mm)	Ulceration status/mitoses
Tis	-	-
T1	≤1.00	a: no ulceration and mitoses <1/mm^2 b: with ulceration or mitoses ≥1/mm^2
T2	1.01-2.00	a: no ulceration b: with ulceration
T3	2.01-4.00	a: no ulceration b: with ulceration
T4	≥4.00	a: no ulceration b: with ulceration
Regional nodes (N)	Number of nodes	Nodal metastatic mass
N0	0	None
N1	1	a: micrometastases b: macrometastases
N2	2-3	a: micrometastases b: macrometastases
N3	>4, or matted nodes, or in transit met(s)/ satellite(s) with metastatic nodes	a: micrometastases b: macrometastases c: in transit met(s)/ satellite(s) without metastatic nodes
Distant Metastases	M stage	
M0	No distant metastases	
M1a	Metastases to skin, subcutaneous tissue, distant nodes	
M1b	Metastases to lungs	
M1c	Metastases to any other visceral sites or to any site combined with elevated LDH	

Clinical Stage	TNM classification
Stage 0	TisN0M0
Stage I	A: T1aN0M0 B: T1b-T2aN0M0
Stage II	A: T2b-T3aN0M0 B: T3b-T4aN0M0 C: T4bN0M0
Stage III	A: T(1-4)aN(1-2)aM0 B: T(1-4)bN(1-2)aM0 or T(1-4) aN(1-2)bM0 C: T(1-4)bN1bM0 or T(1-4) bN2b-cM0 or any TN3M0
Stage IV	Any M1 disease

high-risk skin tumors to obtain information regarding a patient's subclinical lymph node status with minimal morbidity. The National Comprehensive Cancer Network (NCCN) recommends that SLNE be discussed with and offered to patients classified as stage IB or II, and should be considered for patients with stage IA melanoma and "adverse" features that might portend a higher risk of sentinel node involvement (e.g., Clark level IV or V, tumor thickness of 0.75 mm or more, lymphovascular invasion, positive deep margins). SLNE involves the use of radiologic lymphoscintigraphy to map lymphatic drainage from the site of the primary melanoma to the first sentinel lymph node in the region. When properly performed, if the sentinel node is negative the remaining lymph nodes in the region will not have metastases in more than 98% of cases. If the sentinel nodes are negative, no additional regional surgery is recommended. The staging of intermediate thickness (1.2-3.5 mm) primary melanomas, according to the results of sentinel node biopsy, provides important prognostic information and identifies patients with nodal metastases whose survival can be prolonged by immediate lymphadenectomy.
- The staging system for melanoma adapted by the American Joint Committee on Cancer (AJCC) can be found in Table 1.

LABORATORY TESTS

The pathology report should indicate the following:
- Tumor thickness (Breslow microstage).
- Tumor depth: the depth of invasion is the most important histologic prognostic parameter in evaluating the primary tumor.
- Mitotic rate: tabulated as mitoses per square millimeter in the dermal part of the tumor in which most mitoses are identified.
- Radial growth rates versus vertical growth rate: radial growth phase describes the growth of melanoma within the epidermis and along the dermal-epidermal junction.
- Tumor infiltrating lymphocytes have a strong predictive value in vertical growth phase melanomas and are defined as brisk, non-brisk, or absent.

- Histologic regression: characterized by the absence of melanoma in the epidermis and dermis flanked on one or both sides by melanoma.
- Reverse-transcription polymerase chain reaction assay for tyrosine messenger RNA is a useful marker for the presence of melanoma cells. It is performed on sentinel lymph node biopsy and is useful for detection of submicroscopic metastases.
- Identification of somatic mutations in the gene encoding the serine-threonine protein kinase B-RAF (*BRAF*) which is found in approximately 50% to 70% of melanomas.

Rx TREATMENT

- Initial excision of the melanoma
- Re-excision of the involved area after histologic diagnosis:
  1. The margins of re-excision depend on the Breslow depth. For melanoma in situ with Breslow depth ≤2.0 mm, recommended surgical margin is 1 cm. If Breslow depth is ≤2.0 mm, margin should be 2 cm. For melanoma in situ, margin should be 5 mm.
  2. Low-risk or intermediate-risk tumors require excision of 1 to 3 cm.
  3. Melanomas of moderate thickness (0.9-2.0 mm) can be excised safely with 2-cm margins.
  4. A 1-cm margin of excision for melanoma with a poor prognosis (as defined by a tumor thickness ≥2 mm) is associated with a significantly greater risk of regional recurrence than is a 3-cm margin, but with a similar overall survival rate. Randomized clinical trials have also shown that radical surgery with 2 cm excision margins did not differ from that with 4 cm margins for survival in patients with cutaneous melanoma >2 mm thick.
- Lymph node dissection: recommended in all patients with enlarged lymph nodes. Lymph node evaluation is important in patients with melanoma 1 mm in depth because it determines the overall prognosis and need

for therapeutic lymph node dissection or adjuvant treatment.
  1. Elective lymph node dissection remains controversial.
  2. It is indicated with positive sentinel node. It may be considered in those with a primary melanoma between 1 and 4 mm thick (especially in patients >60 yr).
- Adjuvant therapy with interferon alfa-2b is approved by the FDA for AJCC stages IIb-III melanoma; however, it has modest survival benefit. Peginterferon alfa-2b (which has a longer duration of action and can be given once a week) has also been FDA approved for adjuvant treatment of stage III melanoma.
- Ipilimumab, an immune checkpoint inhibitor that blocks cytotoxic T-lymphocyte–associated antigen 4 to potentiate an antitumor T cell response, has been demonstrated to improve survival in stage III high-risk resected melanoma.
- The use of immune checkpoint inhibitors has come to the forefront in the therapy of metastatic melanoma. Ipilimumab has shown improved overall survival in patients with previously treated or untreated metastatic melanoma. Impressive and durable long-term survival rates have been demonstrated in approximately 20% of patients beyond 7 years. More recently, inhibitors of program death receptor (PD-1) and /or their ligands (PDL1 have been found to provide impressive responses and improved survival in both relapsed and untreated patients with metastatic disease. The PD-1 inhibitors, nivolumab and pembrolizumab, have both been approved for the treatment of metastatic melanoma which has progressed or not responded after initial therapy with ipilimumab. Combined use of nivolumab and ipilimumab in previously untreated patients with BRAF V600 wild-type unresectable or metastatic melanoma has been shown more effective than ipilimumab alone and is a new option for first-line treatment of metastatic melanoma.
- In patients who carry the V600E *BRAF* mutation, the current approach involves the use of

oral BRAF-inhibitors, with resultant improved rates of overall and progression-free survival in patients with previously untreated melanoma. Vemurafenib is a selective BRAF inhibitor with a response rate of greater than 60% in patients with metastatic melanomas with V600 BRAF mutation. Oral selective MEK inhibitors (e.g., trametinib, cobimetinib) or combinations of these two receptor-inhibitors have showed improved survival outcomes when used together in this setting. Targeted therapy is useful in patients with rapidly growing melanoma with BRAF mutations, but resistance appears in almost all patients and median progression-free survival is 15 to 18 months.
- Patients with a history of melanoma should be followed up with skin examinations every 6 mo or sooner if patient detects any new lesions; the assessments usually consist of medical history, physical examination, laboratory values, and chest radiograph.

DISPOSITION

- Prognosis varies with the stage of the melanoma. The 5-yr survival related to thickness is as follows: <0.76 mm, 99% survival; 0.6 to 1.49 mm, 85%; 1.5 to 2.49 mm, 84%; 2.5 to 3.9 mm, 70%; >4 mm, 44%.
- The 5-yr survival in patients with distant metastasis is <10%.
- Treatment of advanced disease consists (in addition to surgical excision and lymph node dissection) of chemotherapy, immunotherapy, and radiation therapy.

SUGGESTED READINGS
Available at www.expertconsult.com

RELATED CONTENT
Melanoma (Patient Information)

AUTHOR: **BHARTI RATHORE, M.D.**

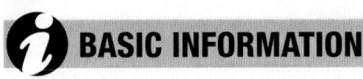

BASIC INFORMATION

DEFINITION

Ménière's disease is a syndrome characterized by recurrent vertigo with fluctuating hearing loss, tinnitus, and fullness in the ear.

SYNONYMS

Endolymphatic hydrops
Lermoyez's syndrome
Idiopathic endolymphatic hydrops

ICD-10CM CODES
H81.09 Ménière's disease, unspecified ear
H81.01 Meniere's disease, right ear
H81.02 Meniere's disease, left ear
H81.03 Meniere's disease, bilateral

EPIDEMIOLOGY & DEMOGRAPHICS

INCIDENCE (IN U.S.): Approximately 190/100,000 persons
PREDOMINANT SEX: Female:male ratio of 1.3:1
PEAK INCIDENCE: Fourth to sixth decade of life

PHYSICAL FINDINGS & CLINICAL PRESENTATION

- Hearing may be unilaterally decreased.
- Pallor, sweating, and nausea may occur during a severe attack.
- Usually the patient develops a sensation of fullness and pressure along with decreased hearing and tinnitus in a single ear.
- The patient typically experiences severe vertigo, which peaks within minutes, then slowly subsides over hours.
- May see spontaneous nystagmus on examination.
- Persistent sense of disequilibrium for days is typical after an acute episode
- May have vestibulopathy demonstrable with a positive head thrust test.

ETIOLOGY

- Unknown; viral, autoimmune, and genetic causes have been suggested.
- Endolymphatic hydrops is the postmortem histologic hallmark. Endolymphatic hydrops may create cytochemical changes that disturb endolymphatic fluid homeostasis, leading to spiral ganglion cell death.

DIAGNOSIS

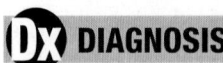

Proposed guidelines by the American Academy of Otolaryngology-Head and Neck Surgery (AAO-HNS) for diagnosis of Ménière's disease:

DIFFERENTIAL DIAGNOSIS

- Acoustic neuroma
- Migrainous vertigo
- Multiple sclerosis
- Autoimmune inner ear syndrome
- Otitis media
- Vertebrobasilar disease
- Labyrinthitis

WORKUP

- Diagnosis is primarily made by history, although further diagnostic tests may help support the diagnosis. Guidelines to define Ménière's disease are described in Table 1.
- Audiogram may show sensorineural hearing loss with lower frequencies primarily affected. Hearing loss may recover either partially or completely after an attack. Recurrent attacks may lead to a persistent and progressive sensorineural hearing loss.
- Electronystagmography may show peripheral vestibular deficit.
- Both vestibular-evoked myogenic potential (VEMP) studies and electrocochleography (ECoG) have low sensitivity and specificity for Ménière's disease and are not clinically useful.

LABORATORY TESTS

No laboratory serologic test is specific for Ménière's disease. A thyroid panel, glucose, hemoglobin A1C, antinuclear antibodies, urinalysis, chemistry panel, rapid plasma reagin, Lyme disease antibodies, and allergy testing can be ordered to screen for other disorders such as thyroid or autoimmune diseases, diabetes, otorenal syndrome, syphilis, Lyme disease, and allergy-mediated Ménière's disease.

IMAGING STUDIES

- MRI to rule out acoustic neuroma or other retrocochlear lesion, especially if cerebellar or CNS dysfunction is present.
- Recent efforts have shown a role for MRI with intratympanic gadolinium.

TREATMENT

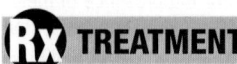

NONPHARMACOLOGIC THERAPY
Limit activity during attacks.

ACUTE GENERAL Rx

- Prochlorperazine 5 to 10 mg PO q6h or 25 mg PO bid
- Promethazine 12.5 to 25 mg PO q4 to 6h
- Diazepam 5 to 10 mg IV/PO for acute attack
- Meclizine 25 mg q6h
- Scopolamine patch

CHRONIC Rx

- Diuretics such as hydrochlorothiazide or acetazolamide.
- Lifestyle modification recommendations include salt restriction and avoidance of caffeine.
- For refractory cases, intratympanic gentamicin injections to the affected ear; endolymphatic sac surgery.

DISPOSITION

- Patients are usually followed by an otoneurologist or ENT specialist.
- Usual course of disease consists of alternating attacks and remissions.
- Majority of patients can be managed medically. Of all patients, 10% to 30% will undergo surgical intervention for persistent incapacitating vertigo.

REFERRAL

To an otolaryngologist for surgical intervention if attacks persist despite medical therapy

SUGGESTED READINGS
Available at www.expertconsult.com

RELATED CONTENT

Ménière's Disease (Patient Information)

AUTHORS: **KATHERINE KOSTROUN, B.S.,**
JOSEPH S. KASS, M.D., J.D., and
SHARON S. HARTMAN POLENSEK, M.D., PH.D.

TABLE 1 Guidelines to Define Ménière's Disease

Definition	Symptoms
Certain Ménière's disease	Histopathologic confirmation
Definite Ménière's disease	≥2 definitive spontaneous episodes of vertigo 20 min to 12 hours Audiometrically documented low- to medium-frequency sensorineural hearing loss in one ear, defining the affected ear on at least one occasion before, during, or after one of the episodes of vertigo Fluctuating aural symptoms (hearing, tinnitus, or fullness) in the affected ear Not better accounted for by another vestibular diagnosis
Probable Ménière's disease	One definite episode of vertigo Audiometrically documented hearing loss on at least one occasion Tinnitus or aural fullness in the treated ear Other causes excluded
Possible Ménière's disease	Episodic vertigo without documented hearing loss, or sensorineural hearing loss (SNHL) fluctuating or fixed, with disequilibrium but nonepisodic Other causes excluded

ⓘ BASIC INFORMATION

DEFINITION

Meningiomas are generally slow-growing tumors arising from arachnoid cells of the arachnoid villi; 90% are benign.

ICD-10CM CODES
D32.0 Benign neoplasm of cerebral meninges

EPIDEMIOLOGY & DEMOGRAPHICS

INCIDENCE: 6/100,000 persons/year; second most common brain tumor in adults, accounting for about one third of primary brain tumors; often underreported.

PREDOMINANT SEX AND AGE: Female/male ratio of almost 3:1 in the brain and up to 6:1 in the spinal cord; 1:1 in childhood

PEAK INCIDENCE: Males: sixth decade, females: seventh decade, incidence increases with age; rare in childhood

RISK FACTORS: Ionizing radiation results in increased incidence and a shorter latency period. Neurofibromatosis type 2 (NF2) is an autosomal dominant genetic disorder that predisposes to multiple intracranial tumors. Approximately half of all individuals with NF2 have meningiomas, most of which are intracranial. Studies have suggested a link between hormonal factors and development of meningioma. At present, there is no conclusive evidence to support a causal relationship with cell phone usage and subsequent development of meningioma.

GENETICS: Meningiomas may be isolated or found in association with other genetic diseases, such as NF2 and familial meningioma. Approximately half of meningiomas have allelic losses involving the *NF2* and *DAL-1* genes. Allelic losses of chromosomes 1p, 2p, 6q, 9q, 10q, 14q, 17p, and 18q may be associated with histologic progression.

TABLE 1 Locations and Presentations of Meningiomas

Location	Presenting Manifestation
Parasagittal	Urinary incontinence, dementia, gradual paraparesis, seizures
Lateral convexity	Variable depending on structures compressed, including slow hemiparesis, speech abnormalities
Olfactory groove	Anosmia, visual disturbance, dementia, Foster-Kennedy syndrome
Suprasellar	Hormonal failure, bitemporal hemianopsia, optic atrophy
Sphenoid ridge	Extraocular nerve paresis, exostoses, proptosis, seizures

From Goetz CG, Pappert EJ: *Textbook of clinical neurology,* Philadelphia, 1999, Saunders.

PHYSICAL FINDINGS & CLINICAL PRESENTATION

- Neurologic symptoms vary with location and size (see Table 1); meningiomas can arise from the dura at any site, although they most commonly occur within the skull and at sites of dural reflection (i.e., the cerebral convexities and the falx). Other less common locations include the sphenoid wing, olfactory groove, and optic nerve sheath.
- The presence of focal symptoms such as vision loss, hearing loss, or mental status change depend on the site of origin and the time course of growth.
- Most common presentation is with a focal or generalized seizure or gradually worsening neurologic deficit. Seizures are present preoperatively in 30% to 40%.
- Typically are slow growing and asymptomatic; many meningiomas are asymptomatic and/or discovered incidentally on a neuroimaging study or at autopsy.

ETIOLOGY

- Meningiomas are thought to arise from a multistep progression of genetic changes.
- Mutations of the *NF2* gene on chromosome 22 are found in patients with neurofibromatosis type 2 and >50% of sporadic meningiomas. This gene is thought to act as a tumor suppressor gene; the protein product, merlin, is also involved in cytoskeletal organization.
- *DAL-1* is another tumor suppressor gene, located on chromosome 18p, that has been identified in a subset of the approximately 40% of sporadic meningiomas with neither the *NF2* gene mutations nor allelic loss of chromosome 22q.
- Cranial radiation may be responsible for some cases following an appropriate latency period from 10 to 20 years. Meningiomas

---

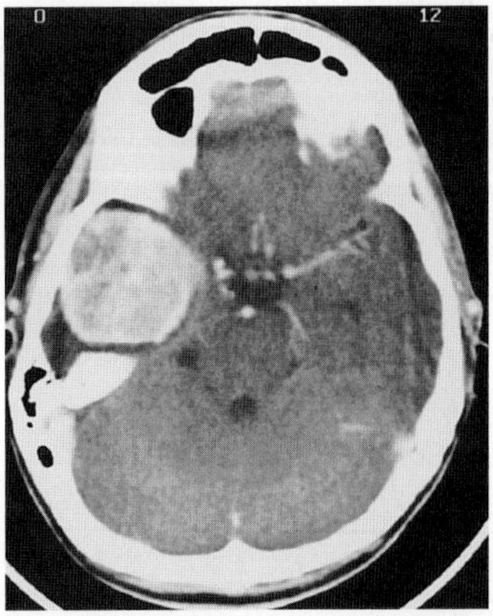

FIG. 1 Contrast-enhanced CT scan demonstrates a large contrast-enhancing right sphenoid wing meningioma. (From Specht N, editor: *Practical guide to diagnostic imaging,* St Louis, 1998, Mosby.)

---

that result from radiation are generally more aggressive.
- The link with steroid hormones and their receptors is suggested by the increase in growth rate and/or development of meningiomas during pregnancy, increased incidence in women who use postmenopausal hormones, and in association with breast carcinomas.

Ⓓⅹ DIAGNOSIS

DIFFERENTIAL DIAGNOSIS

Other well-circumscribed intracranial tumors that involve the dura or subdural space:
- Acoustic schwannoma (typically at the pontocerebellar junction)
- Ependymoma, lipoma, and metastases within spinal cord
- Metastatic disease from lymphoma/adenocarcinoma
- Inflammatory disease such as sarcoidosis and Wegener's granulomatosis
- Infections such as tuberculosis

WORKUP

Imaging studies with CT or MRI, followed by surgical removal with histologic confirmation

LABORATORY TESTS

According to the World Health Organization (WHO) classification, there are nine benign histologic variants (account for 90% of all meningiomas) and four variants associated with increased recurrence and rates of metastasis. Ninety percent of meningiomas are classified as benign meningiomas or WHO grade I.

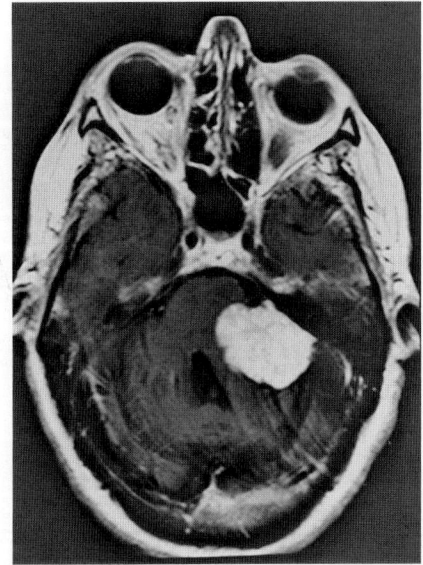

FIG. 2 MRI picture of a posterior fossa meningioma, demonstrated an extra-axial homogeneously contrast-enhanced mass arising from the tentorium and compressing the cerebellar hemisphere. (From Goetz CG, Pappert EJ: *Textbook of clinical neurology,* Philadelphia, 1999, Saunders.)

IMAGING STUDIES

- Cranial CT scanning or MRI can detect and determine the extent of meningiomas (Fig. 1). CT can show hyperostosis and/or intratumoral calcifications. MRI (Fig. 2) is the imaging modality of choice to demonstrate the dural origin of the tumor in most cases, with the characteristic "tail" sign.
- On nonenhanced scans, meningiomas are typically isodense or slightly hyperdense to brain and are homogeneous in appearance. They show homogeneous contrast enhancement; gadolinium can facilitate imaging of smaller additional lesions that are missed on unenhanced images.
- Indistinct margins, marked edema, mushroomlike projections from tumor, brain parenchymal infiltration, and heterogeneous enhancement are suggestive of more aggressive behavior.
- PET scan may help in predicting the aggressiveness of the tumor and the potential for recurrence, but it is not used routinely.

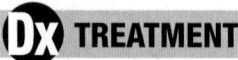 **TREATMENT**

Primary management depends on signs or symptoms, age of patient, and location and size of tumor. Observation may be appropriate if tumors are discovered incidentally and/or if growth is indolent and unlikely to cause symptoms.

PHARMACOLOGIC THERAPY

- Although a variety of chemotherapeutic agents have been studied, such as hydroxyurea, there is no established effective systemic therapy.
- Inhibition of hormone receptors, such as progesterone, estrogen, and androgen, has failed to demonstrate clinical benefit.
- Treatment with molecularly targeted approaches, such as angiogenesis inhibition, is currently under way.

NONPHARMACOLOGIC THERAPY

- The mainstay of treatment for meningiomas remains surgical removal. Complete resection is usually attempted, when feasible. After total excision, recurrence rates of 0% to 20% have been observed, while 20% to 50% of patients recur within 5 yr of a subtotal resection.
- Active surveillance to monitor for tumor recurrence is important.
- Radiation therapy is the only validated form of adjuvant therapy and may be beneficial in patients with incomplete resections or inoperable tumors. Stereotactic radiosurgery can provide local control with more limited toxicity.

ACUTE GENERAL Rx

- For lesions that cause significant mass effect, steroids are sometimes used to decrease brain edema.
- Anticonvulsants are used if the patient presents with seizures.

CHRONIC Rx

- Prophylactic use of anticonvulsants is not recommended in patients without a history of seizures.
- There is limited data on the efficacy of traditional chemotherapy, and the evidence is largely anecdotal. The most extensively evaluated agents are hydroxyurea, mifepristone (RU486), and interferon alfa-2b. Recently, somatostatin analogs have been evaluated in multicenter clinical trials.

DISPOSITION

- Estimated surgical mortality is 7%. Significant morbidity and mortality can be observed in meningiomas with otherwise favorable pathology secondary to unfavorable location (e.g., skull base).
- Long-term outcome varies based on pathology, tumor grade, location, and completeness of resection.
- Most incidentally discovered meningiomas remain asymptomatic and have a slow rate of growth. Calcified tumors may be less likely to progress than noncalcified ones.
- Meningiomas may recur after surgical resection or progress to a higher grade. Risk factors for recurrence include multiple allelic chromosomal losses, local brain invasion, high rate of mitosis, and highly anaplastic features.

REFERRAL

- Neurosurgical consultation for all cases.
- Neurology, radiation oncology, and oncology consults depending on presence of other sequelae or in the setting of recurrence.

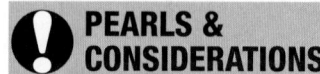 **PEARLS & CONSIDERATIONS**

COMMENTS

- Many meningiomas are discovered incidentally; most are benign and remain asymptomatic. A first follow-up MRI should be performed 3 to 6 months after the tumor is identified to rule out an atypical meningioma with rapid growth.
- "Dural tail," which is the thickening of the dura adjacent to the mass, is a classic finding on neuroimaging studies.
- Individuals with neurofibromatosis type 2 are at high risk to develop meningiomas.

PATIENT & FAMILY EDUCATION

Meningioma mommas: www.meningiomamo mmas.org

Meningioma Support and Patient Information Group

National Brain Tumor Society

Meningioma Online Support Group: http://www. brainstrust.org/meningioma.htm

SUGGESTED READINGS

Available at www.expertconsult.com

RELATED CONTENT

Meningioma (Patient Information)

AUTHORS: **DANYELLE EVANS, M.D.,**
JOSEPH S. KASS, M.D., J.D., and
NICOLE J. ULLRICH, M.D., PH.D.

BASIC INFORMATION

DEFINITION

Bacterial meningitis is an inflammation of meninges with increased intracranial pressure, and pleocytosis or increased WBCs in cerebrospinal fluid (CSF) secondary to bacteria in the pia-subarachnoid space and ventricles, leading to neurologic sequelae and abnormalities.

SYNONYMS

Spinal meningitis
Bacterial meningitis

ICD-10CM CODES
G00.9 Bacterial meningitis, unspecified
G00.8 Other bacterial meningitis
G01 Meningitis in bacterial diseases classified elsewhere

EPIDEMIOLOGY & DEMOGRAPHICS

INCIDENCE (IN U.S.): 1.3 to 2.0 cases/100,000 persons; 1.2 million cases per year in the world; 135,000 deaths annually worldwide. The rate of bacterial meningitis declined dramatically in the U.S. starting in the early 1990s with the introduction of the *Haemophilus influenzae* type b (Hib) vaccine and in 2000 with the introduction of the conjugate pneumococcal vaccine.
PREDOMINANT SEX: Male = female
PREDOMINANT AGE: All ages, neonate to geriatric

PHYSICAL FINDINGS & CLINICAL PRESENTATION

- Fever
- Headache
- Neck stiffness, nuchal rigidity, meningismus
- Altered mental state, lethargy
- Vomiting, nausea
- Photophobia
- Seizures
- Coma; lethargy, stupor
- Rash: petechial associated with meningococcal infection (Fig. 1), purpura fulminans (Fig. 2)
- Myalgia
- Cranial nerve abnormality (unilateral)
- Papilledema
- Dilated, nonreactive pupil(s)
- Posturing: decorticate/decerebrate
- Physical examination findings of Kernig's sign and Brudzinski sign in adults with meningitis are often not helpful in determining meningeal inflammation

ETIOLOGY

The bacterial etiology of meningitis depends on the age of the patient. *Neisseria meningitidis* is now more common than *Haemophilus influenzae* as a cause of bacterial meningitis in children as well as adults, and streptococci are still common causes of bacterial meningitis. *H. influenzae* is the cause of >30% of cases of meningitis (usually in infants and children <6 yr of age). It is associated with sinusitis, otitis media.

- Neonates: group B streptococcus, gram-negative rods such as *E. coli, Listeria monocytogenes*

- Infants ≥1 mo and <3 mo: group B streptococci (40%), gram-negative rods (30%), *Streptococcus pneumoniae* (14%), and *Neisseria meningitidis* (12%)
- Infants ≥3 mo and <3 yr:
  1. *S. pneumoniae* (45%)
  2. *N. meningitidis* (34%)
  3. *S. agalactiae* (group B streptococci) (11%)
  4. *H. influenzae*
  5. *E. coli*
- Ages ≥3 yr and <10 yr:
  1. *S. pneumoniae* (47%)
  2. *N. meningitidis* (32%)
- Ages ≥10 yr and <19 yr
  1. *N. meningitidis* (55%)
  2. *S. pneumoniae*
- Adults: *S. pneumoniae, N. meningitidis,* and *L. monocytogenes* (especially over age 50-60 or with cell-mediated immune deficiencies)
- People with HIV/AIDS are at increased risk for invasive meningococcal disease (IMD).

DIAGNOSIS

Diagnostic approach is based on patient presentation and physical examination (Fig. 3). Lumbar puncture should be performed as soon as possible. Key elements to diagnosis are CSF evaluation and CT scan or MRI if the patient is in a coma or has focal neurologic deficits, pupillary abnormalities, or papilledema. Table 1 describes tests of CSF in patients with suspected CNS infection.

DIFFERENTIAL DIAGNOSIS

- Endocarditis, bacteremia
- Intracranial tumor
- Lyme disease
- Brain abscess
- Partially treated bacterial meningitis
- Medications
- SLE
- Seizures
- Acute mononucleosis

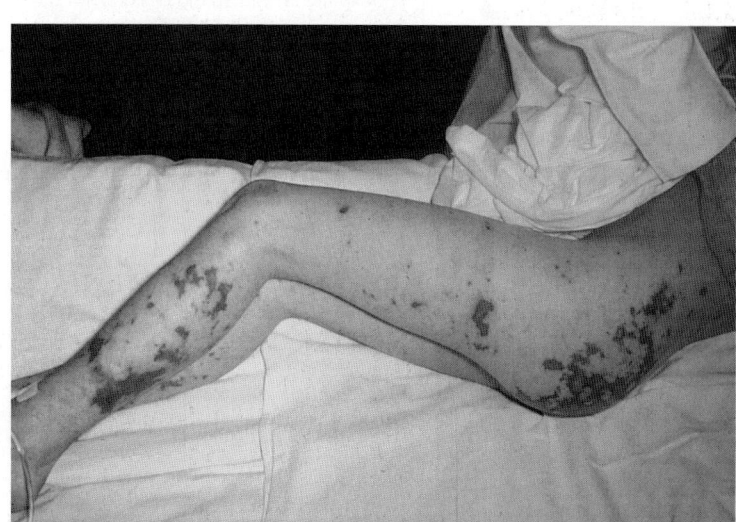

FIG. 1 Fully developed, almost pathognomonic hemorrhagic rash of meningococcal sepsis. (From Cohen J, Powderly WG: *Infectious diseases,* ed 2, St Louis, 2004, Mosby.)

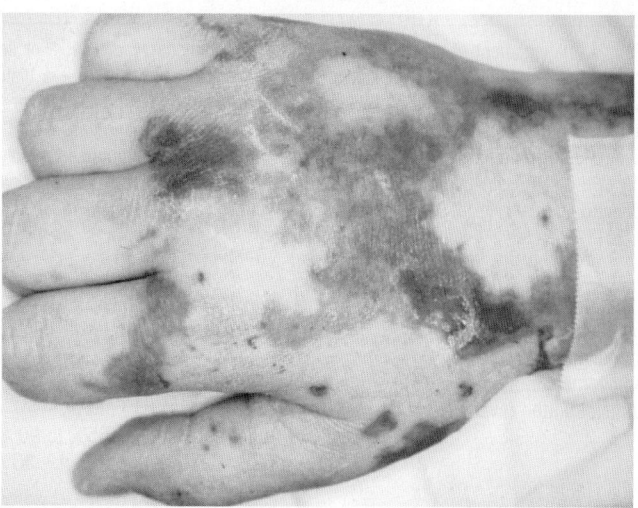

FIG. 2 Meningococcal purpura fulminans in overwhelming meningococcal meningitis. (From Adams JG et al: *Emergency medicine, clinical essentials,* ed 2, Philadelphia, 2013, Elsevier.)

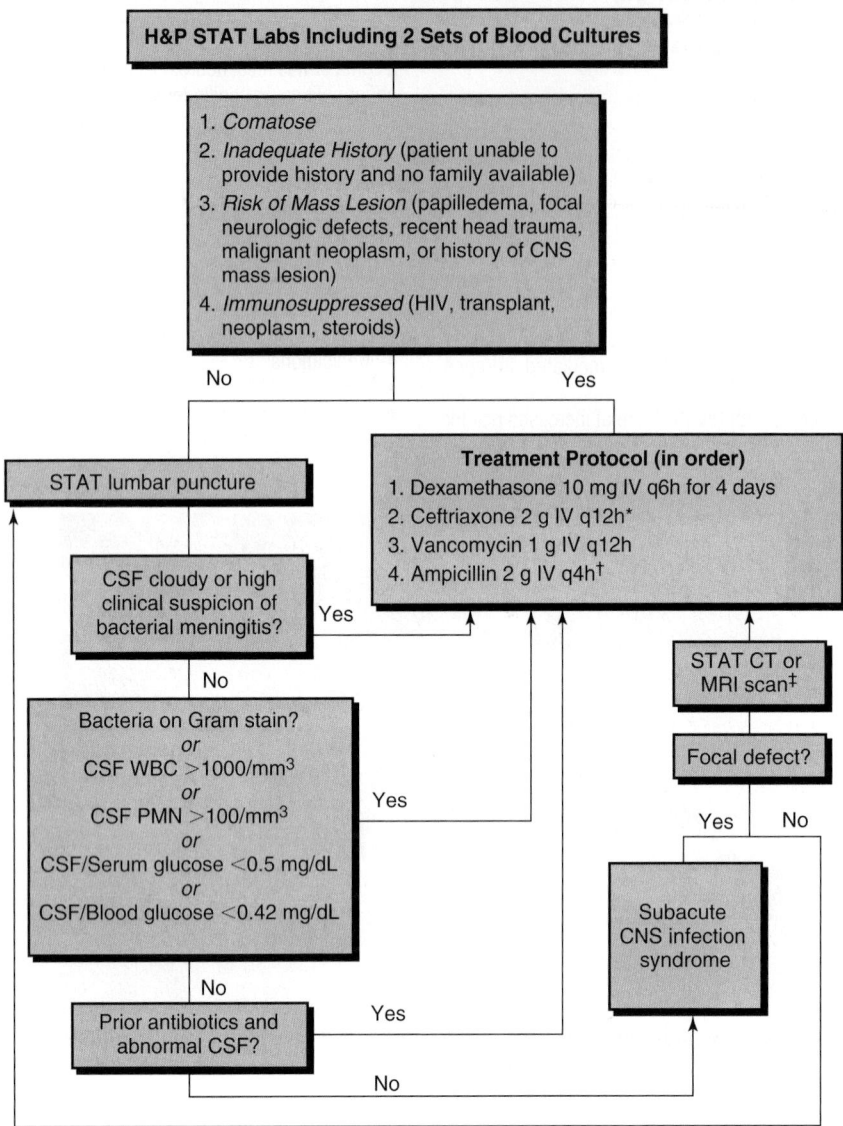

Management of Adults with Acute Meningitis Syndrome
(Fulminant course (<48 h) with fever, headache, usually with impaired sensorium and stiff neck. This protocol is not applicable if the dominant clinical impression is subarachnoid hemorrhage or acute psychosis.)

FIG. 3 Algorithm for management of adult patients with acute meningitis syndrome. *For severe cephalosporin allergy, consider meropenem or moxifloxacin. †Ampicillin is indicated if there is a history of alcoholism, organ transplant, malignancy, pregnancy, or age older than 50 years. For penicillin-allergic patients, an alternative is trimethoprim-sulfamethoxazole. ‡Consider magnetic resonance imaging *(MRI)* if the patient is known or suspected to have human immunodeficiency virus *(HIV)*, if it can be obtained rapidly. *CNS,* Central nervous system; *CSF,* cerebrospinal fluid; *CT,* computed tomography; *H&P,* history and physical examination; *PMN,* polymorphonuclear leukocyte; *WBC,* white blood cell. (From Vincent JL et al: *Textbook of critical care*, ed 6, Philadelphia, 2011, Saunders.)

- Other infectious meningitides
- Neuroleptic malignant syndrome
- Subdural empyema
- Rocky Mountain spotted fever

WORKUP
CSF examination (Table 2):
- Opening pressure >100 to 200 mm Hg
- WBC usually >1000 WBC/mm³
- Neutrophilic predominance: >80%

- Gram stain of CSF: positive in 60% to 90% of patients
- CSF protein: >50 mg/dl
- CSF glucose: <40 mg/dl
- Culture: positive in 65% to 90% of cases
- CSF bacterial antigen: 50% to 100% sensitivity
- E-test for susceptibility of pneumococcal isolates

TABLE 1 Tests of Cerebrospinal Fluid in Patients with Suspected Central Nervous System Infection

Routine Tests
White blood cell count with differential
Red blood cell count[a]
Glucose concentration[b]
Protein concentration
Gram stain
Bacterial culture

Selected Specific Tests Based on Clinical Suspicion
Viral culture[c]
Smears and culture for acid-fast bacilli
Venereal Disease Research Laboratory (VDRL)
India ink preparation
Cryptococcal polysaccharide antigen
Fungal culture
Antibody tests (IgM or IgG, or both)[d]
Nucleic acid amplification tests (e.g., polymerase chain reaction)[e]
Cytology[f]
Flow cytometry

[a]Should be checked in the first and last tubes; in patients with a traumatic tap, there should be a decrease in the number of red blood cells with continued flow of cerebrospinal fluid (CSF). See text for the formula for determining whether the numbers of CSF red blood cells and white blood cells are consistent with a traumatic tap.
[b]Compare with serum glucose drawn just before lumbar puncture.
[c]Yield of viral culture may be low.
[d]May be useful for specific causes of meningitis and encephalitis.
[e]Most useful for specific viral causes of encephalitis and causes of chronic meningitis.
[f]In patients with suspected malignancy.
From Bennett JE, Dolin R, Blaser MJ: *Mandell, Douglas, and Bennett's principles and practice of infectious diseases*, ed 8, Philadelphia, 2015, Saunders.)

LABORATORY TESTS
Blood culturing, WBC with differential, and CSF examination (see "Workup")

IMAGING STUDIES
- Guidelines from the Infectious Society of America recommend CT of brain before lumbar puncture in patients presenting with:
  - A high clinical suspicion for subarachnoid hemorrhage
  - New focal neurologic deficit
  - Pailledema
  - Seizures within a week
  - Altered mental status
  - History of central nervous system disease (e.g., tumor, stroke)
  - Immunodeficiency
  - Age 60 or older

(Rx) TREATMENT

Empiric therapy is necessary with IV antibiotic treatment if patient has purulent CSF fluid at time of lumbar puncture, is asplenic, or has signs of DIC/sepsis pending Gram stain and culture results. Try to obtain blood and CSF cultures before starting antimicrobial therapy, but do not

TABLE 2 Typical Cerebrospinal Fluid Findings in Patients With Selected Infectious Causes of Meningitis

Cause of Meningitis	White Blood Cell Count (cells/mm³)	Primary Cell Type	Glucose (mg/dL)	Protein (mg/dL)
Viral	50-1000	Mononuclear[a]	>45	<200
Bacterial	1000-5000[b]	Neutrophilic[c]	<40[d]	100-500
Tuberculous	50-300	Mononuclear[e]	<45	50-300
Cryptococcal	20-500[f]	Mononuclear	<40	>45

[a]May be neutrophilic early in presentation.
[b]Range from <100 to >10,000 cells/mm³.
[c]About 10% of patients have cerebrospinal fluid lymphocyte predominance.
[d]Should always be compared with a simultaneous serum glucose; ratio of CSF to serum glucose is ≤0.4 in most cases.
[e]May see a "therapeutic paradox," in which a mononuclear predominance becomes neutrophilic during antituberculous therapy.
[f]More than 75% of patients with acquired immunodeficiency syndrome have <20 cells/mm³.
From Bennett JE, Dolin R, Blaser MJ: *Mandell, Douglas, and Bennett's principles and practice of infectious diseases,* ed 8, Philadelphia, 2015, Saunders.

delay therapy if obtaining them is not possible. Therapy after Gram stain pending cultures is recommended for the following:

1. Neonates: ampicillin: 200 to 400 mg/kg per day divided q6 to 8 hr plus gentamicin: 7.5 mg/kg IV in 3 divided doses plus a third-generation cephalosporin: cefotaxime or ceftriaxone
2. 1-23 mo: vancomycin: 60 mg/kg per day IV (maximum up to 4 g/day) divided in 4 doses plus third-generation cephalosporin: ceftriaxone: 100 mg/kg (maximum dose 4 g/day) in 1 or 2 divided doses or cefotaxime: 300 mg/kg per day IV (maximum dose of 12 g/day) in 3 or 4 divided doses
3. Children: vancomycin: 60 mg/kg per day IV (maximum dose 4 g/day) in 4 divided doses plus third-generation cephalosporin: ceftriaxone 100 mg/kg per day IV (maximum 4 g/day) or cefotaxime: 300 mg/kg IV (maximum dose of 12 g/day) in 3 or 4 divided doses
4. Adults: vancomycin: 15-20 mg/kg IV every 8 to 12 hours plus third-generation cephalosporin: ceftriaxone: 2 g IV q12 hours or cefotaxime: 2 g IV q4 to 6 hr. For adults over 50 yr of age also add ampicillin 2 g IV every 4 hr to cover *Listeria*
5. Immunocompromised patients: vancomycin *plus* ampicillin *plus* either cefepime 2 g IV every 8 hr to cover *Pseudomonas* or meropenem 2 g IV q8 hr for adults, which also covers *Pseudomonas*

Use of corticosteroids in adults:
1. Dexamethasone 0.15 mg/kg q6h for first 4 days of therapy should be used for adults in developed countries with known or suspected bacterial meningitis. Decreased mortality and neurologic sequelae are seen with adjunct therapy. The benefit of dexamethasone is less clear in developing countries with high HIV prevalence and malnutrition or with delayed clinical presentations.
2. Dexamethasone also benefits children with Hib meningitis if given at the same time or before the first dose of the antibiotic: 0.15 mg/kg per dose q6 hr for 2 to 4 d. The use and benefit of corticosteroids in suspected or pneumococcal or meningococcal meningitis to prevent neurologic

sequelae is not as clear and should be individualized after analysis of risk and benefits.

DISPOSITION
Bacterial meningitis is a reportable disease that needs to be reported to local health authorities. Droplet precautions should be used for first 24 hr of therapy for suspected or confirmed *N. meningitidis* infection.

REFERRAL
- To a neurologist if persistent neurologic sequelae develop after bacterial meningitis
- To an infectious disease consultant if a patient has recurrent bacterial meningitis; such patients deserve a workup for an anatomic (CSF dural leak) or immunologic defect (complement defect, hyposplenism, immunoglobulin deficiency)

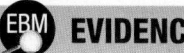

ⓘ PEARLS & CONSIDERATIONS

COMMENTS
- Nosocomial bacterial meningitis may result from invasive procedures (e.g., placement of ventricular catheters, lumbar puncture, craniotomy, spinal anesthesia). Treatment of this different spectrum of microorganisms requires empirical antimicrobial therapy with vancomycin plus either cefepime, ceftazidime, or meropenem. In cases of basilar skull fracture, effective empirical antimicrobial therapy consists of vancomycin plus a third-generation cephalosporin.
- False-positive elevations of CSF where blood cell counts can be found after traumatic lumbar puncture or in patients with intracerebral or subarachnoid hemorrhage in which RBCs and WBCs are introduced into the subarachnoid space. In those instances, the following formula should be used as a correction factor for the true WBC count in the presence of CSF RBCs:

$$\text{Adjusted WBC in CSF} = \frac{\text{Actual WBC in CSF} - \text{WBC in blood} \times \text{RBC in CSF blood}}{\text{RBC in blood}}$$

In the previous equation, the amount being subtracted is the predicted CSF WBC that would occur if all the CSF WBCs were the result of blood contamination.[1]
- Prevention of meningitis can be achieved through chemoprophylaxis of close contacts (household members and anyone exposed to oral secretions).
- Effective medications are rifampin 10 mg/kg PO bid for 2 days or ceftriaxone 250 mg IM single dose in patients older than age 12; 125 mg IM if age 12 or younger.
- Ciprofloxacin 500 mg for prevention of *Neisseria* meningitis can be given to patients older than 18 yr who cannot tolerate rifampin to eradicate pharyngeal colonization.
- Menactra: a protein-conjugate vaccine against serogroup A, C, Y, W-135 capsular polysaccharides is available for adults (up to 55 yr) and children older than 2 yr.

ⒺⒷⓂ EVIDENCE
Available at www.expertconsult.com

SUGGESTED READINGS
Available at www.expertconsult.com

RELATED CONTENT
Meningitis (Patient Information)
Meningitis, Viral (Related Key Topic)
Meningitis, Fungal (Related Key Topic)

AUTHOR: **GLENN G. FORT, M.D., M.P.H.**

[1]Bennett JE, et al: *Mandell, Douglas and Bennett's principles and practice of infectious diseases,* ed 8, Philadelphia, 2015, Saunders, p 1093.

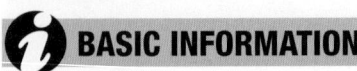

BASIC INFORMATION

DEFINITION

Viral meningitis is an acute febrile illness with signs and symptoms of meningeal irritation, usually with a lymphocytic pleocytosis of the cerebrospinal fluid (CSF) and negative CSF bacterial stains and cultures.

SYNONYMS

Aseptic meningitis
Viral meningitis

ICD-10CM CODES
A87.8 Other viral meningitis
A87.9 Viral meningitis, unspecified

EPIDEMIOLOGY & DEMOGRAPHICS (TABLE 1)

INCIDENCE (IN U.S.): 11 cases/100,000 persons. Leads to 26,000 to 42,000 hospitalizations a year.
PREDOMINANT SEX: Male = female
GENETICS: Those with abnormal humoral immunity and agammaglobulinemia have associated difficulty with viral clearance.

PHYSICAL FINDINGS & CLINICAL PRESENTATION

- Fever
- Headache
- Nuchal rigidity
- Photophobia
- Myalgias
- Vomiting
- Rash

ETIOLOGY

- Enterovirus: 85% to 95% of all cases. Most common are coxsackie viruses and echoviruses
- Parechoviruses

- Mumps virus
- Measles
- Arboviruses from mosquitoes: EEE, West Nile, St Louis
- Herpes: HSV-1, HSV-2, VZV, HHV-6, and HHV-7
- Acute HIV
- Lymphocytic choriomeningitis virus
- Adenovirus
- CMV and EBV
- Other arthropod-borne viruses: Powassan virus
- Influenza A and B virus

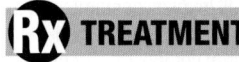

DIAGNOSIS

The diagnostic approach is similar to that for bacterial meningitis (see "Meningitis, Bacterial"); the foremost need is to rule out bacterial meningitis with CSF evaluation. Presentation may be similar to that of meningitis with bacterial involvement.

DIFFERENTIAL DIAGNOSIS

- Bacterial meningitis
- Meningitis secondary to Lyme disease, TB, syphilis, amebiasis, leptospirosis
- Rickettsial illnesses: Rocky Mountain spotted fever
- Migraine headache
- Medications
- SLE
- Acute mononucleosis/Epstein-Barr virus
- Seizures
- Carcinomatous meningitis

WORKUP

CSF examination:
- Usually shows pleocytosis
- Lymphocytic predominance (neutrophils in early stages)
- Opening pressure: 200 to 250 mm Hg H_2O (≤250 mm/H_2O)
- WBC: 100 to 1000 mm^3

- Increased CSF protein (<200 mg/dl)
- Slightly decreased or normal CSF glucose (>45 mg/dl)
- Negative Gram stain, cultures, CIE, latex agglutination
- Viral cultures or serologic testing may be diagnostic
- Polymerase chain reaction for HSV or enterovirus (which could shorten duration of antibiotic treatment and hospitalization if bacterial meningitis was suspected)
- Antibody detection in CSF for diagnosis of West Nile virus meningitis

LABORATORY TESTS

CBC with differential, blood culturing, and CSF examination (see "Workup")

IMAGING STUDIES

CT scan or MRI: if cerebral edema, focal neurologic findings develop

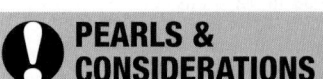

TREATMENT

- No specific antiviral therapy for most viruses. Treatment is supportive unless HSV is detected, which would be treated with IV acyclovir: 10 mg/kg q8h in adults for 14 to 21 days. Up to 20 mg/kg q8h in children >12 yr.
- Empiric antibiotics may be given until CSF cultures exclude bacterial meningitis.

DISPOSITION

Viral meningitis is almost always an uncomplicated illness that will resolve; however, relapsing headache, myalgia, and weakness may occur for 2 to 3 wk after onset of symptoms.

PEARLS & CONSIDERATIONS

- Enteroviruses are the most common cause of viral meningitis and are transmitted by fecal-oral route and less commonly by the respiratory route. They are more common in summer and fall months. From 2000 to 2005, the most common serotypes were coxsackie viruses A9, B5, and B1 and echoviruses 6, 9, 13, 18, and 30.
- Herpes simplex type 2 (HSV-2) can be a cause of a primary episode of meningitis and also be a cause of recurrent episodes of lymphocytic meningitis. HSV-2 meningitis presents most often without a history of genital herpes or genital symptoms. Recurrent aseptic meningitis, also known as Mollaret's disease, is predominantly caused by HSV-2 infection.

RELATED CONTENT

Meningitis (Patient Information)

AUTHOR: **GLENN G. FORT, M.D., M.P.H.**

TABLE 1 Epidemiology of Acute Viral Meningitis

| | | | Epidemiologic Factors* | |
Season	Patient's Age (yr)	Patient's Sex	Risk Factor	Suggested Viral Agent
Summer-fall	Infant	—	Infected mother	Coxsackievirus B
	1-15	—	Swimming pools, closed communities	Enteroviruses
			Geographic area: California, southeastern United States	California serogroup virus
Winter	1-15	—	School exposure	Varicella virus, measles virus
		Male/female 3:1		Mumps virus
	16-21	—	College exposure	Measles virus
		Male/female 3:1 —		Mumps virus
				Epstein-Barr virus (mononucleosis)
	Any	—	Mice, rats, hamsters	Lymphocytic choriomeningitis virus
	Adults	—	Varicella-zoster	Varicella-zoster virus
Any	Any	—	Immunocompromise	Adenovirus
		—	Acquired immunodeficiency syndrome	Human immunodeficiency virus

*Epidemiologic factors are suggestive but should not be used to exclude diagnoses in individual cases.
From Gorbach SI: *Infectious diseases*, ed 2, Philadelphia, 1998, Saunders.

BASIC INFORMATION

DEFINITION

Menopause is the permanent cessation of menstrual periods for 1 yr after age 40 yr or permanent cessation of ovulation after lost ovarian activity. It is the reproductive stage of life marked by waxing and waning estrogen levels followed by decreasing ovarian function. Primary ovarian insufficiency (previously also referred to as premature ovarian failure) and no menstrual periods may also occur because of depletion of ovarian follicles before the age of 40 yr.

SYNONYMS

Change of life
Climacteric ovarian failure

ICD-10CM CODES
Z78.0	Asymptomatic menopausal state
N95.1	Menopausal and female climacteric states
N95.8	Other specified menopausal and perimenopausal disorders
E28.310	Symptomatic premature menopause
E28.319	Asymptomatic premature menopause

EPIDEMIOLOGY & DEMOGRAPHICS

- Average age of menopause in the United States is 51 yr.
- Age at which menopause occurs is primarily genetically determined.
- Smokers experience menopause an average of 1.5 yr earlier than nonsmokers.
- More than one third of a woman's life may be spent after menopause.
- Onset of perimenopause is usually in a woman's mid- to late-40s.
- Approximately 4000 women begin menopause each day.

PHYSICAL FINDINGS & CLINICAL PRESENTATION

- Atrophic vaginitis, which can cause burning, itching, bleeding, dyspareunia
- Either complete cessation of menses or a period of irregular cycles and diminished or heavier bleeding
- Osteoporosis
- Osteopenia/psychological dysfunction:
  1. Anxiety
  2. Depression
  3. Insomnia
  4. Nervousness
  5. Irritability
  6. Inability to concentrate
- Sexual changes, decreased libido, dyspareunia
- Urinary incontinence
- Menopausal vasomotor symptoms (VMS, hot flashes, flushes), night sweats, cardiovascular disease, coronary artery disease, atherosclerosis, headaches, tiredness, and lethargy. A study from the University of Pennsylvania noted that the median duration of moderate-to-severe hot flashes is 10.2 yr but that the length of hot flashes was largely dictated by how early these began in the perimenopause.

ETIOLOGY

- The most common etiology: physiologic, caused by depleted granulosa and theca cells that fail to react to endogenous gonadotropins, producing less estrogen; decreased negative feedback in the hypothalamic pituitary access, increased follicle-stimulating hormone (FSH), and increased luteinizing hormone (LH), which leads to stromal cells that continue to produce androgens as a result of the LH stimulation
- Surgical castration
- Family history of early menopause, cigarette smoking, blindness, abnormal chromosomal karyotype (Turner's syndrome, gonadal dysgenesis), precocious puberty, and left-handedness

DIAGNOSIS

DIFFERENTIAL DIAGNOSIS

- Asherman's syndrome
- Hypothalamic dysfunction
- Hypothyroidism
- Pituitary tumors
- Adrenal abnormalities
- Ovarian abnormalities
- Polycystic ovarian syndrome
- Pregnancy
- Ovarian neoplasm
- Tuberculosis of the endometrium

WORKUP

- If the clinical picture is highly suggestive of menopause, estrogen can be prescribed. If all symptoms resolve, then a diagnosis essentially has been made. Before estrogen is prescribed, however, a complete history and physical examination are needed. If a patient has an estrogen-dependent malignancy, unexplained abnormal uterine bleeding, a history of thrombophlebitis, or acute liver disease, estrogen therapy is contraindicated.
- Progesterone challenge test: medroxyprogesterone 10 to 20 mg PO or progesterone 100 mg IM to induce withdrawal bleeding. If no withdrawal bleeding is obtained, a hypoestrogenic state is assumed to be present. This test is increasingly controversial, even if very commonly performed.
- Physical examination, height, weight, blood pressure, breast examination, and pelvic examination are needed.
- Assess risk for coronary artery disease, osteoporosis, cigarette smoking, personal history, history of breast cancer, liver disease, active coagulation disorder, or any unexplained vaginal bleeding.

LABORATORY TESTS

- FSH, LH, and estrogen levels: markedly elevated FSH and markedly depressed estrogen level constitute laboratory diagnosis of ovarian failure; LH only if polycystic ovarian disease is to be ruled out in a younger patient. It is not necessary to obtain an FSH if the patient fulfills the clinical criteria for menopause. Similarly, since estradiol levels vary during the menstrual cycle, estradiol levels are rarely necessary or informative.
- TSH to rule out thyroid dysfunction and prolactin level if patient has symptoms of galactorrhea and if suspicion of pituitary adenoma exists
- A general chemistry profile to check for any systemic diseases
- Pap smear per standard guidelines, endometrial biopsy, or dilation and curettage in patients who have had irregular periods or intermenstrual or postmenopausal bleeding
- Mammogram as recommended by American Congress of Obstetricians and Gynecologists.

IMAGING STUDIES

- Per standard protocols, CT scan or MRI of sella if pituitary tumor is suspected
- Bone density studies if high-risk condition for osteoporosis exists
- Pelvic ultrasound to check endometrial stripe

TREATMENT

NONPHARMACOLOGIC THERAPY

- A balanced diet: low in fat, with total fat intake being <30% of calories; total calories sufficient to maintain body weight or produce weight loss if that is desired
- Avoidance of smoking and excessive alcohol or caffeine intake
- Exercise: weight-bearing exercise for osteoporosis prevention
- Kegel exercises for strengthening the pelvic floor
- Adequate calcium intake: 1500 mg elemental calcium qd is necessary to maintain zero calcium balance in postmenopausal women
- Change in the ambient temperature (may ameliorate hot flashes and reduce night sweats)
- Vitamin E
- Avoidance of caffeine, alcohol, and spicy foods if they trigger hot flashes
- Vaginal lubricants to help with the dyspareunia attributable to vaginal dryness (e.g., Replens, K-Y Jelly, or Gyne-Moistrin cream)

ACUTE GENERAL Rx

Vasomotor symptoms are best managed with systemic hormone therapy given in the lowest dose and for the shortest period possible. Estrogen replacement in symptomatic patients can be administered in a variety of forms, including oral estrogen and transdermal estrogen patch. The lowest effective dose should be prescribed.

- Examples of oral estrogen include:
  1. Conjugated estrogens: start with 0.3 mg qd and increase to 1.25 mg qd depending on symptoms.
  2. Estradiol: start with 0.5 mg qd and increase to 2 mg qd.
  3. Esterified estrogens: start with 0.3 to 1.25 mg qd.

4. Estropipate: start with 0.625 to 2.5 mg qd.
5. Esterified estrogen/testosterone combination: give 1.25 mg and methyltestosterone 2.5 mg (Estratest) and esterified estrogen 0.625 mg and methyltestosterone 1.25 mg (Estratest HS [half-strength]). May improve sexual enjoyment and libido.

- If the patient has had a hysterectomy for benign disease, estrogen alone is sufficient. In patients who have an intact uterus, progestin is necessary to prevent endometrial hyperplasia associated with unopposed estrogen, which is protective against endometrial cancer. Progestins can be prescribed as continual daily dose or cyclic fashion. Most commonly prescribed progestins include medroxyprogesterone acetate 2.5 mg, 5 mg, and 10 mg; Prometrium 100 mg, 200 mg, and 400 mg; and Aygestin 5 mg. Continuous hormone replacement therapy is preferred because after time the patient should be amenorrheic. Patients should be counseled that they may experience some irregular spotting for the first 6 to 9 mo after starting hormone replacement therapy. Cyclic therapy will cause withdrawal bleeding.
- Combination oral preparations FemHRT, Prefest, Prempro, Activella, Premphase are commonly used. However, the U.S. Preventive Services Task Force recommends against the use of combined estrogen and progestin for the prevention of chronic conditions such as cardiovascular disease in postmenopausal women.
- Transdermal patches can be either estradiol (Estraderm, Vivelle, FemPatch) 0.025 to 0.1 mg applied twice weekly or Climara 0.025 to 0.1 mg used once a week. With these preparations, progesterone should be used in a similar fashion. Apply CombiPatch twice weekly (combination estrogen and progesterone) or Climara Pro once per week (one patch).
- Vaginal creams can be used; these should be reserved for local therapy of atrophic vaginitis. Minimal systemic absorption does occur; however, blood levels are unpredictable. Usual dose 0.5 to 2 g intravaginally daily, cyclically 3 wk on 1 wk off. When symptoms improve, once to twice weekly is adequate maintenance.
- Vagifem estradiol vaginal tablets. Initial dosage: one Vagifem tablet, inserted vaginally, qd for 2 wk. Maintenance dose: one Vagifem tablet, inserted vaginally, twice weekly.
- Femring vaginal ring delivering the equivalent of 0.5 mg/day inserted every 3 months or Estring 0.0075 mg/day.
- EstroGel 0.06% (estradiol gel) One Pump (1.25 g/day) applied to one arm from wrist to shoulder.
- The FDA contraindications to menopause hormone therapy include the following diseases and disorders: active liver disease; current, past, or suspected breast cancer; active or recent anterior thromboembolic disease (angina, myocardial infarction); known or suspected estrogen-sensitive malignant conditions; known hypersensitivity to the active substance of the therapy or to any of the excipients; porphyria cutanea tarda; previous idiopathic or current venous thromboembolism; undiagnosed genital bleeding; untreated hypertension; untreated endometrial hyperplasia.
- For women in whom estrogen is contraindicated or for those who do not wish to take estrogen, the following regimens can be used:
  1. Serotonin reuptake inhibitors
  2. Depo-Provera 150 mg IM every month (may be helpful in alleviating hot flashes)
  3. Clonidine 0.05 to 0.15 mg PO qd (questionable efficacy) or transdermal clonidine patch
  4. Bellergal-S (questionable efficacy)
- Tibolone significantly improves vasomotor symptoms, libido, and vaginal lubrication. Not available in the U.S.

CHRONIC Rx

Hormone replacement therapy should be used only for the short term unless benefits outweigh the risks of long-term use. As a result of the results of the Women's Health Initiative (WHI), the FDA has instituted a "black box" warning on postmenopausal hormone replacement products suggesting that the lowest dose should be used for the shortest period of time. This necessitates a considered and nuanced counseling session with patients contemplating hormone replacement prior to the initiation of therapy and then on a periodic basis after that, usually at least a yearly basis.

DISPOSITION

If treated, the patient should have resolution of her symptoms and reduced incidence of osteoporosis. Lifelong medical supervision is necessary to monitor adequacy of treatment and prevention of complications. This should include regular Pap smears in accordance with ASCCP guidelines until the age of 65, pelvic examinations, breast examinations, mammography, and endometrial sampling of any type of abnormal bleeding. If untreated, the vasomotor symptoms will eventually dissipate; however, this may take several years in a small percentage of women. Some women who are in their 80s have experienced hot flashes. Urogenital atrophy will continue to worsen. Osteoporosis and coronary artery disease risks will increase with every passing year.

REFERRAL

Most menopausal women are managed by their gynecologists. However, this condition can be managed adequately by the patient's primary care physician who has an interest in treating menopausal women.

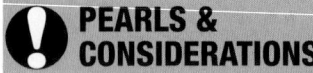

PEARLS & CONSIDERATIONS

COMMENTS

- Short-term risks of hormone replacement therapy (HT) include an eighteenfold increased rise for cholecystitis, three-and-a-half-fold risk of a thrombocardiac event in the first year, and possible increased risk of stroke and myocardial infarction.
- Results of the WHI study found that for every 10,000 women taking HT (combination of both estrogen and progesterone) for 1 yr (10,000 person-yr), seven more would have coronary events, eight would have more strokes, eight would have more pulmonary emboli, and eight would have earlier breast cancer than would 10,000 women taking placebo. Benefits of HT were six fewer cases of colorectal cancer and five fewer hip fractures per 10,000 women.
- HT should not be initiated or continued for the primary or secondary prevention of coronary heart disease.
- Estrogen-replacement therapy should only be prescribed for patients with sufficient menopausal symptoms that impact the patient's quality of life.
- Interestingly, women who start hormone therapy early in menopause may have cardiac and other benefits. A recent trial showed that oral estradiol therapy was associated with less progression of subclinical atherosclerosis (measured as change in carotid-artery intima media thickness [CIMT]) than with placebo when therapy was initiated within 6 years after menopause but not when it was initiated 10 or more years after menopause. Estradiol had no significant effect on cardiac CT measures of atherosclerosis in either postmenopause stratum.[1]

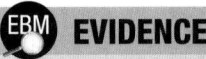 **EVIDENCE**

Available at www.expertconsult.com

SUGGESTED READINGS
Available at www.expertconsult.com

RELATED CONTENT

Menopause (Patient Information)
Hot Flashes (Related Key Topic)
Osteoporosis (Related Key Topic)

AUTHOR: **RUBEN ALVERO, M.D.,** and **ELIZABETH ZADZIELSKI, M.D., M.B.A.**

[1]Hodis HN, et al.: Vascular effects of early versus late postmenopausal treatment with estradiol, *N Engl J Med* 374:1221-1231, 2016.

BASIC INFORMATION

DEFINITION

Normal duration of menstrual flow is 5 days; normal menstrual cycle is 21 to 35 days.

Menorrhagia is menstrual blood loss greater than 80 ml.

Metrorrhagia is bleeding between menses.

Polymenorrhea is bleeding that occurs more often than every 21 days.

Oligomenorrhea is bleeding less than every 35 days.

PALM-COEIN classification of abnormal uterine bleeding was adopted in 2011 to standardize terminology: PALM-COEIN (Polyp, Adenomyosis, Leiomyoma, Malignancy or hyperplasia, Coagulopathy, Ovulatory dysfunction, Endometrial, Iatrogenic, or Not yet classified).

Abnormal bleeding termed as AUB with the addition of PALM-COEIN terminology (i.e., AUB-P for polyp).

SYNONYMS

Abnormal uterine bleeding
Menometrorrhagia
Dysfunctional uterine bleeding

ICD-10CM CODES
N92.0	Excessive and frequent menstruation with regular cycle
N92.1	Excessive and frequent menstruation with irregular cycle
N92.4	Excessive bleeding in the premenopausal period
N92.2	Excessive menstruation at puberty
N92.6	Irregular menstruation, unspecified

EPIDEMIOLOGY & DEMOGRAPHICS

INCIDENCE: 10% to 15% of reproductive-aged women; 30% of outpatient office visits; 70% of all gynecologic consults

PEAK INCIDENCE: Reproductive-aged women, ages 18 to 50

PREVALENCE: 53 per 1000 women annually

PREDOMINANT SEX AND AGE: Female; peak in adolescence and perimenopausal periods

GENETICS: Von Willebrand disease; hereditary platelet dysfunction disorders; 20% of women at any age have underlying bleeding disorder

RISK FACTORS: Genetic predisposition, anticoagulation treatment, obesity

PHYSICAL FINDINGS & CLINICAL PRESENTATION

- History: age, age at menarche or menopause, menstrual bleeding patterns, severity of bleeding, pain, underlying medical conditions, surgical history, use of medications, signs and symptoms of hemostatic disorder including history of heavy bleeding since menarche, postpartum hemorrhage, surgery-related bleeding, bleeding from dental work, easy bruising, epistaxis, and frequent gum bleeding, family history of bleeding disorder

- Physical exam: general findings including excessive weight, signs of polycystic ovarian syndrome (PCOS) (hirsutism and acne), signs of thyroid disease (nodule), signs of insulin resistance (acanthosis nigricans), signs of bleeding disorder including petechiae, ecchymoses, pallor, swollen joints, pelvic examination including external, speculum, and bimanual exam, Pap test if indicated

ETIOLOGY

- Pregnancy/miscarriage
- Endometrial polyps
- Adenomyosis
- Uterine leiomyoma
- Endometrial hyperplasia or carcinoma
- Coagulopathy, inherited or acquired
- Ovulatory dysfunction, most likely PCOS
- Endometrial
- Iatrogenic

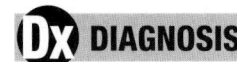 DIAGNOSIS

DIFFERENTIAL DIAGNOSIS

Pregnancy, sexually transmitted disease, polycystic ovary syndrome (PCOS), thyroid dysfunction, anovulation due to immature hypothalamic-pituitary-ovarian axis, perimenopausal transition, uterine pathology including endometrial hyperplasia or carcinoma, leiomyoma, adenomyosis, or endometrial polyp, von Willebrand's disease, platelet dysfunction disorder, iatrogenic due to medications including oral contraceptives or anticoagulants (warfarin)

WORK-UP

- History
- Physical exam to evaluate for uterine pathology
- Laboratory, pathology, and imaging studies to determine etiology

LABORATORY TESTS

- Pregnancy test
- Complete blood count (CBC)
- Thyroid-stimulating hormone (TSH)
- *Chlamydia trachomatis* testing if high risk
- Evaluation for cyclic menses for determination of ovulatory status
- Prothrombin time and partial thromboplastin time
- Testing for von Willebrand disease if clinically suspected (von Willebrand–ristocetin cofactor activity, von Willebrand factor antigen, and factor VIII)
- Endometrial sampling by endometrial biopsy or hysteroscopic sampling for women >45 yr or <45 yr with history of unopposed estrogen (PCOS, obesity), failed medical management, or persistent abnormal bleeding

IMAGING STUDIES

- Transvaginal ultrasound
- Sonohysterography or hysteroscopy if ultrasound is not adequate or further evaluation of the cavity is required
- Transabdominal ultrasound in adolescents
- MRI not indicated initially

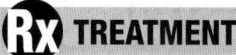 TREATMENT

NONPHARMACOLOGIC THERAPY

- Dilation and curettage
- Uterine artery embolization
- Hysteroscopic resection of uterine pathology including endometrial polyps and submucosal leiomyoma
- Endometrial ablation
- Hysterectomy

ACUTE GENERAL Rx

- Progestin
- Combined oral contraceptive methods
- Conjugated estrogens
- Tranexamic acid
- Surgical management if indicated including dilation and curettage, uterine artery embolization, or hysterectomy
- Hospitalization to maintain hemostasis and administer blood transfusion if severe menorrhagia

CHRONIC Rx

- Oral contraceptive pills: continuous preferred over cyclic regimens
- Levonorgestrel intrauterine device: high degree of efficacy
- Gonadotropin-releasing hormone agonist (goserelin)
- Nonsteroidal antiinflammatory drugs
- Tranexamic acid, aminocaproic acid
- Danazol (significant side-effect profile requires justification for use; this is rare)
- Surgery for anatomic causes including resection of leiomyoma and hysterectomy
Endometrial ablation if completed childbearing

REFERRAL

- If concern for uterine pathology as etiology for menorrhagia, referral to a gynecologist for surgical management is indicated.
- If endometrial sampling reveals endometrial hyperplasia or malignancy, referral to a gynecologist is indicated. Cyclic progestin therapy is necessary with resampling. If endometrial hyperplasia associated with complex glands or atypia, consultation with gynecologic oncologist due to high degree of progression to malignancy.

RELATED CONTENT

Menorrhagia (Patient Information)
Dysfunctional Uterine Bleeding (Related Key Topic)

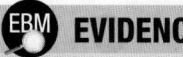 EVIDENCE

Available at www.expertconsult.com

SUGGESTED READINGS

Available at www.expertconsult.com

AUTHOR: **ERIN E. MEDLIN, M.D.**

BASIC INFORMATION

DEFINITION

Acute mesenteric lymphadenitis is a syndrome of acute right lower quadrant abdominal pain associated with mesenteric lymph node enlargement and a normal appendix.

SYNONYMS

Acute mesenteric lymphadenitis
Mesenteric lymphadenitis

ICD-10CM CODES

I88.0 Nonspecific mesenteric lymphadenitis

EPIDEMIOLOGY & DEMOGRAPHICS

- Incidence unknown
- Affects mostly children (<18 yr) with no sex preference
- When *Yersinia* enterocolitis is the cause, boys are more frequently involved

PHYSICAL FINDINGS & CLINICAL PRESENTATION

- Abdominal pain of variable severity (mild ache to severe colic) beginning in upper abdomen or right lower quadrant; eventually localizes in the right side but not in a precise location (unlike appendicitis)
- In *Yersinia* infection outbreaks (see Table E1. symptoms include abdominal pain (84%), diarrhea (78%), fever (43%), anorexia (22%), nausea (13%), and vomiting (8%)
- Physical findings:
  1. Other lymphadenopathy (20% of cases)
  2. Right lower quadrant tenderness (site of maximal tenderness may vary from one examination to the next)
  3. Guarding (rare)
  4. Mild fever

ETIOLOGY & PATHOGENESIS

- Reactive hyperplasia of lymph nodes that drain the ileocecal region, similar to that seen in inflammatory or allergic conditions. One study reported that approximately two thirds of cases are secondary (reactive) and one third are primary (no demonstrable associated inflammatory process).
- *Yersinia enterocolitica, Y. pseudotuberculosis, Salmonella* species, *Escherichia coli,* and streptococci have been implicated in mesenteric adenitis. Clinical manifestations of yersiniosis are described in Table E2.

DIAGNOSIS

In general, the diagnosis is made on exploration of the abdomen of a patient suspected of having acute appendicitis. On examination the appendix appears normal, and enlarged mesenteric lymph nodes are noted. Excision of an enlarged lymph node with culture and nodal histology may provide information regarding the etiology but is not routinely used.

DIFFERENTIAL DIAGNOSIS

- Acute appendicitis (5%-10% of patients admitted to hospitals with a diagnosis of appendicitis are discharged with a diagnosis of mesenteric adenitis)
- Crohn's disease
  Section II describes the differential diagnosis of right lower quadrant abdominal pain.

LABORATORY TESTS

- Complete blood count may show leukocytosis
- Abdominal sonography and CT scan with IV and oral contrast (Fig. 1) may be useful
- Laparotomy if appendicitis is suspected

PROGNOSIS

Recurrent bouts are common; therefore if laparotomy is performed and a normal appendix is found, it should be removed.

AUTHOR: **FRED F. FERRI, M.D.**

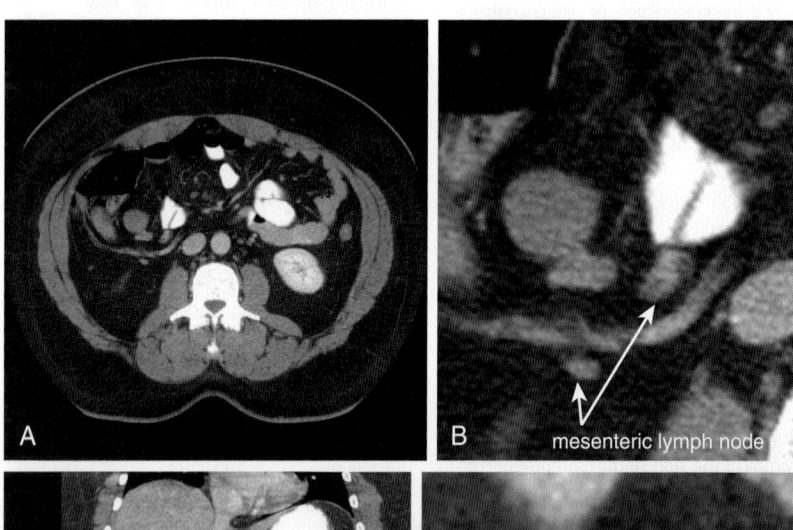

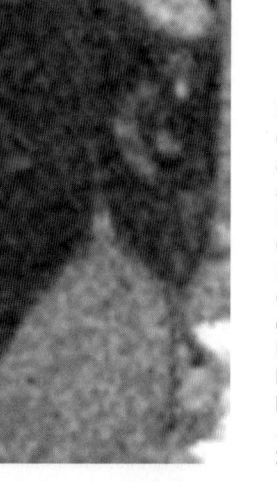

FIG. 1 Mesenteric adenitis, CT with IV and oral contrast, soft-tissue window. Mesenteric adenitis can mimic appendicitis in its clinical presentation. Enlarged lymph nodes are visible on CT. Lymph nodes have soft-tissue density and appear as discrete, rounded structures. On a single image they may appear similar to blood vessels or to the appendix, but on inspection of adjacent images it becomes clear that lymph nodes are rounded, not tubular like a blood vessel or the appendix. **A,** Axial image. **B,** Close-up from **A. C,** Coronal reconstruction. **D,** Close-up from **C.** (From Broder JS: *Diagnostic imaging for the emergency physician,* Philadelphia, 2011, Saunders.)

BASIC INFORMATION

DEFINITION

Acute mesenteric ischemia (AMI) is the sudden onset of intestinal hypoperfusion to all or part of the small bowel caused by emboli, arterial or venous thrombosis (Fig. E1), or vasoconstriction from low-flow states.

SYNONYMS

Acute mesenteric ischemia
AMI

ICD-10CM CODES
K55.0 Acute vascular disorders of intestine

EPIDEMIOLOGY & DEMOGRAPHICS

INCIDENCE:
- AMI accounts for 0.1% of hospital admissions.
- The incidence appears to be increasing. Factors for this include increased awareness among clinicians, the aging of the population, and improved intensive care, leading to longer survival of sicker patients. The mortality rate is 60% to 85%.

PREDOMINANT SEX AND AGE:
- AMI caused by arterial embolism or thrombosis occurs more frequently in the elderly.
- AMI due to mesenteric venous thrombosis often presents in younger age groups.

GENETICS: No specific genetic predisposition but may be related to underlying factors such as cardiac disease, atherosclerosis, and hypercoagulable states.

RISK FACTORS:
- Advanced age, atherosclerosis, low cardiac output (especially atrial fibrillation), severe cardiac valvular disease, intraabdominal malignancy.
- In the subgroup of cases caused by venous thrombosis, risk factors include hypercoagulable states, portal hypertension, abdominal infection, blunt trauma, pancreatitis, and portal malignancy.
- Additional risk factors for AMI caused by nonocclusive mesenteric ischemia include recent cardiac surgery, dialysis, and cocaine use.
- Table 1 summarizes risk factors for ischemic bowel disease.
- AMI may occur rarely in patients with no identifiable risk factors.

PHYSICAL FINDINGS & CLINICAL PRESENTATION

- The classic presentation is rapid onset of severe periumbilical pain "out of proportion to physical examination findings." An epigastric bruit may be present in some patients. Generally, patients with mesenteric venous thrombosis tend to present with a less abrupt onset of abdominal pain than those with acute arterial occlusion.
- Nausea and vomiting are commonly associated.
- Initial abdominal examination may be normal, with no rebound or guarding, or may include minimal distention or stool positive for occult blood.

- Later in the course the patient may present with gross distention, absence of bowel sounds, and peritoneal signs. In the elderly, mental status changes may occur.

ETIOLOGY

The pathophysiologic mechanisms that cause AMI include:
- Mesenteric arterial embolism (40% to 50% of cases of AMI): typically from the left atrium, left ventricle, or cardiac valves. The superior mesenteric artery is most commonly affected.
- Mesenteric arterial thrombosis: often in patients with prior progressive atherosclerotic stenoses, with superimposed abdominal trauma or infection. Thrombotic occlusion of previously stenotic mesenteric vessels accounts for 20% to 35% of cases of AMI.

- Mesenteric venous thrombosis may occur in the setting of hypercoagulable states (acquired or inherited), blunt trauma, abdominal infection, portal hypertension, pancreatitis, and portal malignancy.
- Nonocclusive mesenteric ischemia is caused by reduced intestinal perfusion, as seen with hypotension, hypovolemia, vasoconstricting drugs, and hemodialysis.
- Dissection or inflammation of the mesenteric artery accounts for less than 5% of cases of AMI.

DIAGNOSIS

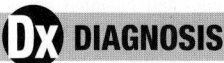

DIFFERENTIAL DIAGNOSIS

Initially include other causes of abdominal pain of acute onset, including perforated peptic ulcer and early appendicitis, as well as the varied causes of peritonitis.

TABLE 1 Risk Factors for Ischemic Bowel Diseases*

Risk Factor	Arterial Thrombosis	Embolus	Mesenteric Vein Thrombosis	Nonobstructive Mesenteric Ischemia
Advanced age	+	+	+	+
Atherosclerosis	+			
Aortic dissection	+			
Low cardiac output	+	+		+
Congestive heart failure				+
Shock				+
Severe dehydration	+		+	
Cardiac arrhythmias, especially atrial fibrillation		+		+
Severe cardiac valvular disease		+		
Recent myocardial infarction	+			+
Intraabdominal malignancy			+	
Abdominal trauma			+	
Intraabdominal infection			+	
Intraabdominal inflammatory conditions			+	
Parasitic infection (ascariasis)			+	
Hypercoagulable states (venous thrombosis)			+	
Sickle cell anemia			+	
Recent cardiac surgery	+	+		+
Recent abdominal surgery			+	
Vascular aortic prosthetic grafts proximal to the superior mesenteric artery		+		
Hemodialysis				+
Vasculitis	+		+	
Pregnancy			+	
Decompression sickness			+	
Blast lung caused by systemic air embolism		+		
Drugs that cause constriction				
• Digitalis				+
• Cocaine				+
• Amphetamines				+
• Pseudoephedrine				+
• Vasopressin			+†	+
Estrogen therapy			+	

*A plus sign (+) indicates that the factor is a risk for the disease subtype.
†Especially after sclerotherapy
From Adams JG et al: *Emergency medicine, clinical essentials*, ed 2, Philadelphia, 2013, Elsevier.

WORKUP

- Early diagnosis is key. Treatment success is related to the duration of symptoms prior to diagnosis.
- Consider early laparotomy for diagnosis in cases with a high index of suspicion when imaging is not readily available.

LABORATORY TESTS

- Laboratory test results are nonspecific, especially early in the course. Elevated lactic acid, leukocytosis, acidosis, and elevated hematocrit from hemoconcentration can occur later in the course, often after progression to bowel necrosis has occurred, hence are not useful for early diagnosis.
- When a hypercoagulable state is suspected, workup may include proteins C and S, antithrombin III, and factor V Leiden. This will likely not affect the diagnosis of AMI but may help guide long-term therapy.
- Normal D-dimer testing may help rule out AMI. Elevated levels are nonspecific.

IMAGING STUDIES

- Biphasic contrast-enhanced CT is the preferred diagnostic mode (Fig. E2). It is more easily available and has similar sensitivity to angiography, the prior gold standard test. Computed tomographic angiography (CTA) has 95% to 100% accuracy for the diagnosis of visceral ischemic syndromes and is also useful in detecting potential sources of emboli and other pathologic processes.
- Plain CT findings are nonspecific and more often found late in the course. Portal venous gas or intramural gas may be seen after the development of gangrene. In many cases, CT findings remain nonspecific even at advanced stages.
- MR angiography (MRA) may be more useful in cases of mesenteric vein thrombosis causing AMI. It has also been found useful in monitoring the progress of patients with superior mesenteric venous thrombosis who are treated nonsurgically. MRA, however, takes longer than CTA to perform and can overestimate the degree of stenosis.
- Angiography may be considered if the diagnosis remains unclear after CT or MR imaging.
- Plain films are normal 25% of the time in early stages. Suggestive findings may include ileus, bowel wall thickening, or intramural gas. Free air under the diaphragm may support early surgical intervention prior to further radiologic evaluation.
- Doppler ultrasound evaluation of intestinal blood flow is often limited by the presence of air-filled loops of bowel and is not an appropriate part of the diagnostic workup if AMI is the leading working diagnosis.

℞ TREATMENT

- The goal of treatment is to restore blood flow to ischemic bowel as rapidly as possible before the occurrence of infarction.
- Treatment varies depending on etiology.

ACUTE GENERAL Rx

- Initial management should include hemodynamic monitoring and support, correction of acidosis, administration of broad-spectrum antibiotics, and gastric decompression by nasogastric tube.
- Vasoconstricting agents should be avoided.
- In the absence of active bleeding, the use of systemic anticoagulation is usually indicated. The optimal timing of initiation is unclear.

NONPHARMACOLOGIC THERAPY

- Signs of peritonitis mandate early laparotomy and resection of infarcted bowel.
- Specific management will depend on patient status and most likely etiology of the ischemia.
- When workup is positive for major superior mesenteric artery (SMA) embolus, embolectomy is considered standard treatment in the absence of peritoneal signs. Depending on the location and degree of occlusion of the embolus, surgical revascularization, intraarterial infusion of thrombolytics or vasodilators, or systemic anticoagulation may be considered.
- In cases of SMA thrombosis, emergency surgical revascularization is the treatment of choice; stent placement may be a viable alternative.
- Angiography is needed to diagnose nonocclusive mesenteric ischemia before infarct and should be followed up by intraarterial vasodilator infusion. This approach has been shown to significantly reduce mortality rate. Underlying risk factors for reduced blood flow should be assessed and mitigated.
- In patients with mesenteric vein thrombosis, treatment depends on the presence or absence of peritoneal signs. Laparotomy and resection of infarcted bowel is indicated in more advanced cases. If there are no peritoneal signs, immediate anticoagulant therapy with heparin, and ultimately warfarin, may be adequate treatment.
- In general, percutaneous treatment with lytic therapy, balloon angioplasty, or stenting may be limited by the frequent presence of nonviable bowel, which would require laparotomy despite success with percutaneous treatment.
- A "second look" procedure is indicated in most patients, 24-48 hours after initial revascularization.

CHRONIC Rx

- In the subgroup of patients with mesenteric venous thrombosis, prevention of further thrombosis is indicated. The optimal duration of anticoagulation is unclear.
- Patients who receive endovascular treatment should be managed with 1-3 months of clopidogrel; additionally, periodic surveillance for restenosis with duplex ultrasound or CTA is indicated.

DISPOSITION

- Prognosis is best in AMI due to mesenteric venous thrombosis and after surgical treatment for acute arterial embolism. It remains poor in cases of arterial thrombosis and nonocclusive ischemia.
- With delayed diagnosis, intestinal infarction—resulting in perforation or gangrenous bowel, sepsis, shock, and death—is typical.

REFERRAL

- Early surgical consultation should be considered. There should be no delay with peritoneal signs.
- Surgery may be warranted for diagnostic purposes.

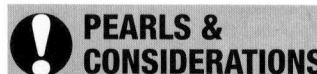

❗ PEARLS & CONSIDERATIONS

COMMENTS

- The diagnosis of AMI should be considered in any patient with acute onset of abdominal pain out of proportion to physical findings, particularly in at-risk patients.
- Early diagnosis, before intestinal infarction occurs, is critical and correlates with improved survival rates.
- The use of endovascular procedures for AMI is becoming more common and may be most appropriate for patients with ischemia that is not severe and for those who have severe coexisting conditions that place them at high risk for complications and death associated with open surgery.

PREVENTION

Prevention of underlying factors, most notably atherosclerotic disease (smoking cessation, management of hypertension, and use of statins) is indicated for primary prevention as well as prevention of recurrence.

SUGGESTED READINGS
Available at www.expertconsult.com

RELATED CONTENT
Mesenteric Venous Thrombosis (Related Key Topic)

AUTHOR: **MARGARET TRYFOROS, M.D.**

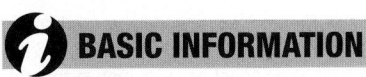

BASIC INFORMATION

DEFINITION

Mesenteric venous thrombosis (MVT) is a thrombotic occlusion of the mesenteric venous system involving major trunks or smaller branches and leading to intestinal infarction in its acute form.

SYNONYMS

MVT

ICD-10CM CODES
K55.0 Acute vascular disorders of intestine
K55.1 Chronic vascular disorders of intestine

EPIDEMIOLOGY & DEMOGRAPHICS

Between 5% and 15% of patients with acute mesenteric infarction have MVT. MVT is slightly more common in men than women. The typical age of occurrence is 50 to 60 yr. Table 1 summarizes the incidence of ischemic bowel disease.

PHYSICAL FINDINGS & CLINICAL PRESENTATION

Acute MVT:
- Symptoms: abdominal pain in 90% of patients, typically out of proportion to the physical findings. Nausea and vomiting occur in 50% and gastrointestinal (GI) bleeding occurs in 50% (occult) and 15% (gross).
- Physical findings:
  1. Early: abdominal tenderness, decreased bowel sounds, abdominal distention
  2. Later: guarding and rebound tenderness, fever, septic shock

Subacute MVT:
- Symptoms: nonspecific abdominal pain for weeks or months
- Physical findings: none

Chronic MVT:
- Symptoms: upper GI hemorrhage from bleeding varices
- Physical findings: none other than signs of blood loss if significant

ETIOLOGY & PATHOGENESIS

Hypercoagulable states:
- Peripheral deep venous thrombosis
- Neoplasms
- Antithrombin III, protein C, protein S deficiencies
- Lupus anticoagulant (antiphospholipid antibody)
- Oral contraceptive use, pregnancy
- Polycythemia vera
- Thrombocytosis
- Paroxysmal nocturnal hemoglobinuria

Portal hypertension:
- Cirrhosis
- Inflammation:
- Pancreatitis
- Peritonitis (e.g., appendicitis, diverticulitis, perforated viscus)
- Inflammatory bowel disease
- Pelvic or intraabdominal abscess
- Intraabdominal cancer
- Postoperative state or trauma:
- Blunt abdominal trauma

TABLE 1 Incidence of Ischemic Bowel Diseases

Disease	Incidence (%)*
Superior mesenteric artery (SMA) embolism: • The SMA is susceptible to embolism because of large vessel caliber and a narrow angle of departure from the aorta. • The proximal SMA is most commonly obstructed within 6-8 cm of the aorta	50
Nonocclusive ischemia	25
SMA thrombosis	20
Mesenteric venous thrombosis	5

*Percentage of all cases of acute mesenteric ischemia.
From Adams JG et al: *Emergency medicine, clinical essentials,* ed 2, Philadelphia, 2013, Elsevier.

BOX 1   Factors Associated with Mesenteric Venous Thrombosis

Hypercoagulable states
  Polycythemia vera
  Sickle cell disease
  Antithrombin III deficiency
  Protein C or S deficiency
  Malignancy
  Myeloproliferative disorders
  Estrogen therapy, oral contraceptive pills
  Pregnancy
Inflammatory conditions
  Pancreatitis
  Diverticulitis
  Appendicitis
  Cholangitis
Trauma
  Operative venous injury
  Postsplenectomy
  Blunt or abdominal trauma
Miscellaneous
  Congestive heart failure
  Renal failure
  Decompression sickness

Portal hypertension. From Marx JA et al: *Rosen's emergency medicine,* ed 8, Philadelphia, 2014, Saunders.

- Postoperative states (abdominal surgery)
- Box 1 summarizes factors associated with mesenteric venous thrombosis

Thrombosis may begin in small mesenteric branches (e.g., in hypercoagulable states) and propagate to the major venous mesenteric trunks or begin in large veins (e.g., in cirrhosis, intraabdominal cancer, surgery) and extend distally. If collateral drainage is inadequate, the intestine becomes congested, edematous, cyanotic, and hemorrhagic and eventually may infarct.

DIAGNOSIS

DIFFERENTIAL DIAGNOSIS

All other causes of abdominal pain (e.g., peritonitis, intestinal obstruction, pancreatitis, peptic ulcer disease, gastritis, inflammatory bowel disease, perforated viscus) are also to be considered in the differential diagnosis of GI hemorrhage.

WORKUP

Laboratory tests and imaging studies

LABORATORY TESTS
- Complete blood count: leukocytosis
- Electrolytes: metabolic acidosis (lactic) indicates bowel infarction
- Tests for hypercoagulable status

IMAGING STUDIES
- Computed tomographic angiography (CTA) is preferred imaging modality due to high accuracy (95%-100%). Use of two-phase imaging improves sensitivity for venous thrombosis
- Magnetic resonance angiography (MRA) can also be used; it avoids the risk of radiation and contrast material, but takes longer and may overestimate degree of stenosis
- Abdominal plain radiograph: ileus, ascites, bowel dilation, bowel wall thickening, loop separation, thumbprinting.

TREATMENT

- Anticoagulation with heparin or thrombolytic therapy. When medical treatment is unsuccessful, options include transhepatic and percutaneous mechanical thrombectomy, thrombolysis, and open intraarterial thrombolysis
- Laparotomy if intestinal infarction is suspected
- Short ischemic segment: resection
- Long ischemic segment:
  1. Nonviable: resection or close
  2. Viable: intraarterial papaverine and/or thrombectomy followed by "second look" intervention

PROGNOSIS
- Mortality rate of acute MVT: 20% to 50%
- Recurrence rate: 15% to 25%

SUGGESTED READING
Available at www.expertconsult.com

RELATED CONTENT
Mesenteric Ischemia, Acute (Related Key Topic)

AUTHOR: FRED F. FERRI, M.D.

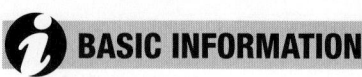
BASIC INFORMATION

DEFINITION

Malignant mesothelioma is a neoplasm that originates from the mesothelial surfaces of the pleural cavities (80%) or peritoneal cavities (20%).There are three major histologic subtypes: epithelial (most common), sarcomatous, and mixed (epithelial/sarcomatous).

SYNONYMS

Malignant mesothelioma

ICD-10CM CODES
C45.0 Mesothelioma of pleura
C45.1 Mesothelioma of peritoneum
C45.2 Mesothelioma of pericardium
C45.7 Mesothelioma of other sites
C45.9 Mesothelioma, unspecified

EPIDEMIOLOGY & DEMOGRAPHICS

- Associated with asbestos exposure (all fiber types)
- About 2000 to 3000 new cases are diagnosed in the U.S. annually
- More common in men as a result of workplace asbestos exposure
- Incidence in the U.S. has leveled off due to lack of asbestos use and mining.
- Incidence of mesothelioma increases with age; median age at presentation is >70 years
- More than 8 million persons in the U.S. are currently at risk for mesothelioma because of prior asbestos exposure.

PHYSICAL FINDINGS & CLINICAL PRESENTATION

- Dyspnea
- Nonpleuritic chest pain
- Fever, weight loss, sweats, fatigue, loss of appetite
- Dysphagia, superior vena cava syndrome, Horner's syndrome in advanced stages
- Auscultation may reveal unilateral loss of breath sounds
- Dullness on percussion may be present

ETIOLOGY

- Asbestos exposure (>70% of patients)
- Other reported potentially causal factors include prior radiation therapy and extravasated thorotrast, zeolite, and erionite fibers

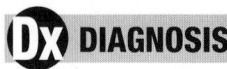
DIAGNOSIS

DIFFERENTIAL DIAGNOSIS

Metastatic adenocarcinomas (from lung, breast, ovary, kidney, stomach, prostate)

WORKUP

- Staging evaluation (Fig. 1) includes complete history (including occupational history), physical examination, and testing to determine potential operability (CT, bone scan, pulmonary function tests [PFTs])
- Thoracoscopy, pleuroscopy, and open-lung biopsy are useful in obtaining adequate tissue samples for diagnosis
- Pulmonary function tests
- PET-CT scan is performed only in patients considered candidates for surgery to determine resectability.
- Staging: the TNM system categories mesothelioma in stages I to IV similar to that used for non–small cell lung cancer

LABORATORY TESTS

- Diagnostic thoracentesis is generally insufficient for diagnosis because pleural effusions may only reveal atypical mesothelial cells.
- Immunohistochemistry is useful to distinguish adenocarcinoma from epithelial malignant mesothelioma (mesotheliomas are generally carcinoembryonic antigen negative and cytokeratin positive).
- Thrombocytosis and anemia may be found on initial laboratory evaluation.
- Serum osteopontin levels (when available) can also be used to distinguish persons with exposure to asbestos who do not have cancer from those with exposure to asbestos who have pleural mesothelioma.

IMAGING STUDIES

- Chest radiographs may reveal pleural plaques (Figs. 2 and E3) or calcifications in the diaphragm.
- CT scans of the chest and abdomen, bone scan, and PET scan are used to assess the stage of disease.

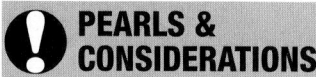
TREATMENT

GENERAL Rx

- Operable patient (epithelial type, no positive nodes, confined to pleura, adequate PFTs): the two surgical techniques for therapeutic intervention are decortication (pleurectomy) and extrapleural pneumonectomy. Postoperative chemotherapy with cisplatin and pemetrexed and subsequent external-beam radiation are used with limited success.
- Inoperable patient (elderly patient, extensive disease, sarcomatous or mixed histology type, poor PFTs): chemotherapy to improve survival, plus supportive care is a standard option. Combined modality therapies (radiation therapy, chemotherapy, and biologics) have also been used to reduce both local and distant recurrences. The combination of cisplatin and pemetrexed is used as front-line

chemotherapy. More recently, a randomized trial has revealed the survival benefit of adding antiangiogenic agent bevacizumab in this setting to the standard chemotherapy regimen.
- Patients with progressive cancer after initial chemotherapy can often be treated with single-agent chemotherapy such as gemcitabine or vinorelbine.
- Intrapleural instillation of cisplatin or biologics (e.g., interferons, interleukin-2) is generally limited to very early disease because it can only penetrate a very limited depth of the tumor and there is a propensity of the pleural space to become progressively obliterated with advancing disease.
- Radiation therapy is often used for palliation of local chest pain.
- Obliteration of the pleural space (pleurodesis) with instillation of talc or tetracycline into the pleural cavity is done in the treatment of recurrent symptomatic pleural effusions.

DISPOSITION

Median survival is from 6 to 21 months for patients undergoing pleurectomy and ranges from 4 to 21 mo for extrapleural pneumonectomy. Survival is better for patients with the epithelial form, although overall median survival is approximately still 1 year.

PEARLS & CONSIDERATIONS

- Patients with early disease should be referred to treatment centers specializing in multidisciplinary therapy before attempts are made to obliterate the pleural space with pleurodesis.
- Patients with advanced or resected disease should be treated with appropriate combination chemotherapy as listed previously.
- Fibulin-3 may be useful as a blood and effusion biomarker for pleural mesothelioma. Recent data reveal that plasma fibulin-3 levels can distinguish healthy persons with exposure to asbestos from patients with mesothelioma. In conjunction with effusion fibulin-3 levels, plasma fibulin-3 levels can further differentiate mesothelioma effusions from other malignant and benign effusions.

SUGGESTED READINGS
Available at www.expertconsult.com

RELATED CONTENT
Mesothelioma (Patient Information)
Asbestosis (Related Key Topic)

AUTHOR: **BHARTI RATHORE, M.D.**

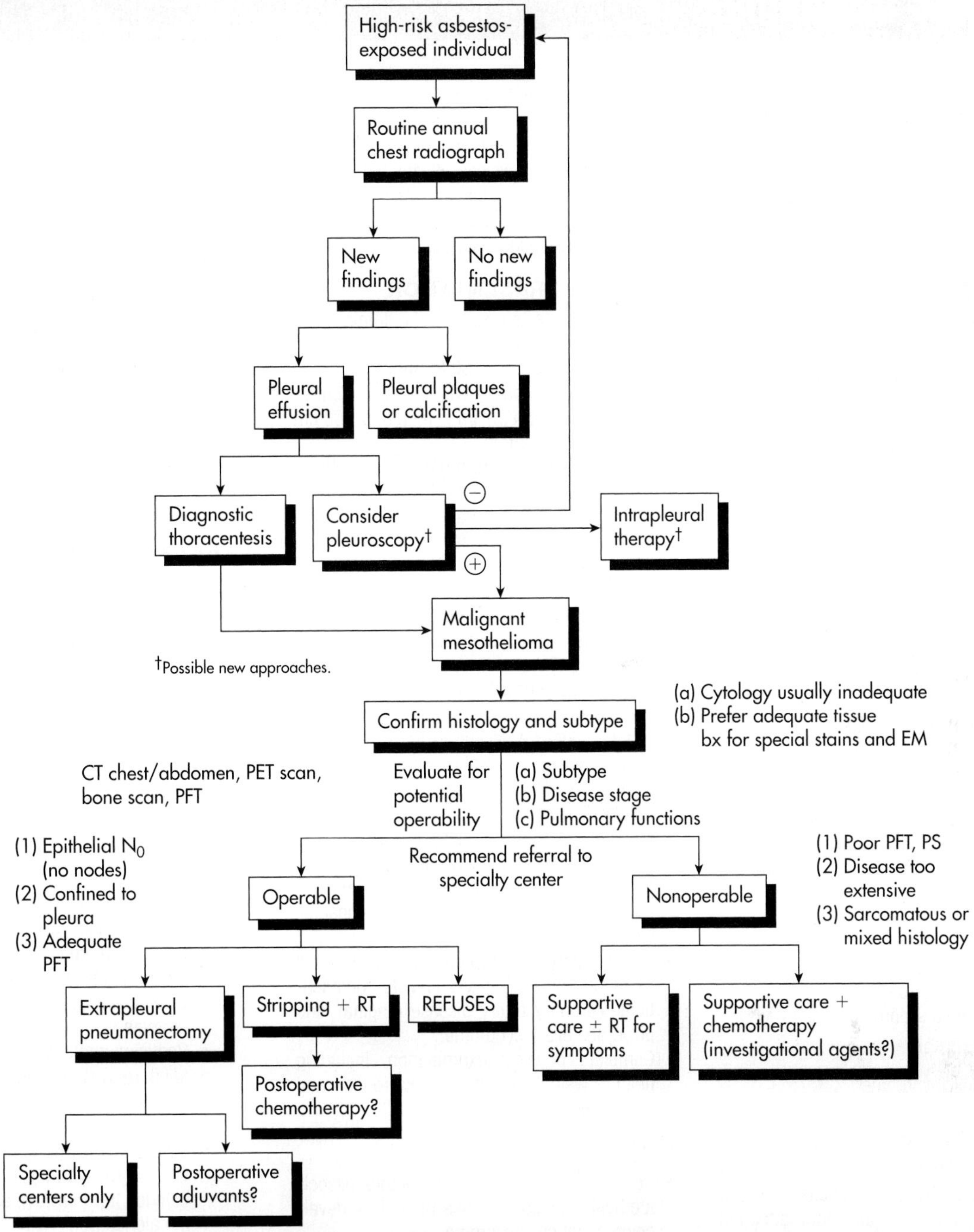

High-risk asbestos-exposed individual

Routine annual chest radiograph

New findings

No new findings

Pleural effusion

Pleural plaques or calcification

Diagnostic thoracentesis

Consider pleuroscopy†

⊖

Intrapleural therapy†

⊕

Malignant mesothelioma

†Possible new approaches.

Confirm histology and subtype

(a) Cytology usually inadequate
(b) Prefer adequate tissue bx for special stains and EM

CT chest/abdomen, PET scan, bone scan, PFT

Evaluate for potential operability

(a) Subtype
(b) Disease stage
(c) Pulmonary functions

(1) Epithelial N_0 (no nodes)
(2) Confined to pleura
(3) Adequate PFT

Recommend referral to specialty center

(1) Poor PFT, PS
(2) Disease too extensive
(3) Sarcomatous or mixed histology

Operable

Nonoperable

Extrapleural pneumonectomy

Stripping + RT

REFUSES

Supportive care ± RT for symptoms

Supportive care ± chemotherapy (investigational agents?)

Postoperative chemotherapy?

Specialty centers only

Postoperative adjuvants?

FIG. 1 Evaluation and treatment of mesothelioma. *bx,* Biopsy; *CT,* computed tomography; *EM,* electron microscopy; *PET,* positron emission tomography; *PFT,* pulmonary function test; *PS,* pleural sclerosis; *RT,* respiratory therapy. (From Abeloff MD: *Clinical oncology,* ed 3, New York, 2004, Churchill Livingstone.)

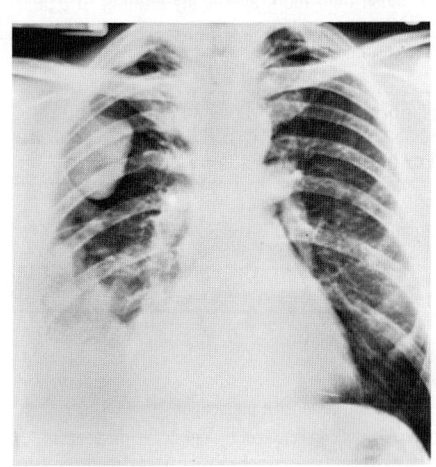

FIG. 2 Chest radiograph of patient with mesothelioma. Note several lobulated, pleural-based masses in right hemithorax accompanied by right pleural effusion. (From Weinberg SE et al: *Principles of pulmonary medicine,* ed 5, Philadelphia, 2008, Saunders.)

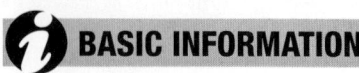

DEFINITION

Hyperglycemia, dyslipidemia, abdominal obesity, and hypertension are critical components of metabolic syndrome. Over the years, many definitions of the syndrome have been proposed and debated (see Table 1). In 2009, a consensus statement from several organizations including the International Diabetes Federation (IDF) and American Heart Association defined "metabolic syndrome" as the presence of any three of the following criteria:

- Abdominal waist circumference >94 cm (37 in) in men and >80 cm (31 in) in women (the use of population- and country-specific definitions is suggested; however, until better data are available, IDF recommends using these cutoffs)
- Serum hypertriglyceridemia ≥150 mg/dl (1.7 mmol/L) or drug treatment for elevated triglycerides
- Serum high-density lipoprotein (HDL) cholesterol <40 mg/dl (1 mmol/L) in men and <50 mg/dl (1.3 mmol/L) in women or drug treatment for low HDL-C
- Blood pressure ≥130/85 mm Hg or drug treatment for elevated blood pressure
- Fasting glucose ≥100 mg/dl (5.6 mmol/L) or drug treatment for elevated blood glucose

A new concept of the metabolic syndrome includes not only insulin resistance, visceral obesity, and hypertension but also obstructive sleep apnea (Fig. 1).

SYNONYMS

Syndrome X
Insulin resistance syndrome
Obesity dyslipidemia syndrome

ICD-10CM CODES
E88.81 Metabolic syndrome

EPIDEMIOLOGY & DEMOGRAPHICS

- Affects close to 25% of U.S. adults
- Prevalence increases with age, affecting more than 40% of individuals >60 yr.
- Increasing prevalence among women, especially in the African American and Mexican American populations.
- Prevalence increases with weight. Metabolic syndrome is noted in 5% of normal weight,

22% of overweight, and 60% of obese individuals.
- Other risk factors include low socioeconomic status, lack of physical activity, high-carbohydrate diet, alcohol intake, smoking, genetic predisposition, use of atypical antipsychotics, and postmenopausal status.

CLINICAL PRESENTATION

- Obesity, hypertension, dyslipidemia, and hyperglycemia as defined.
  1. Blood pressure: ≥130/85 mm Hg
  2. Abdominal obesity with waist circumference: >94 cm (37 in) in men and >80 cm (31 in) in women
  3. Triglycerides: ≥150 mg/dl (1.7 mmol/L)
  4. HDL: <40 mg/dl (1 mmol/L) in men and <50 mg/dl (1.3 mmol/L) in women
  5. High fasting glucose: ≥100 mg/dl (5.6 mmol/L)
- Patients with metabolic syndrome are at twice the risk of developing cardiovascular disease and have a sevenfold increase in risk for type 2 diabetes and a 1.5-fold increase in all-cause mortality compared to patients without the syndrome. Other complications include cognitive decline in the elderly, fatty liver disease, polycystic ovary syndrome, obstructive sleep apnea, gout, and chronic kidney disease.
- Metabolic syndrome is also associated with decreased sexual activity, desire, and satisfaction and with sexual dysfunction in most domains in sexually active postmenopausal women.
- Focus history on symptoms of diabetes and its complications, obesity and its complications, coronary artery disease (angina), and polycystic ovary syndrome.
- Complete physical examination, including height, weight, waist circumference, and blood pressure.

ETIOLOGY

- Genetic and environmental factors associated with obesity increase the risk of developing metabolic syndrome.
- Abdominal obesity is associated with insulin resistance and hyperinsulinemia.
- Insulin resistance results in ineffective glucose utilization, eventually leading to type 2 diabetes mellitus

- Hyperinsulinemia and inflammatory markers/cytokines play an important role in development of abnormal lipid profile, hypertension, and vascular endothelial dysfunction, which can lead to the development of atherosclerotic cardiovascular disease.

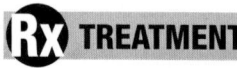 DIAGNOSIS

DIFFERENTIAL DIAGNOSIS

- Other causes of weight gain or obesity (Cushing's syndrome, hypothyroidism)
- Other causes of hyperlipidemia (familial hyperlipidemia, hypothyroidism)
- Other causes of hypertension (Cushing's syndrome, hyperaldosteronism)
- Other forms of diabetes (type 1)

LABORATORY TESTS

- Fasting lipid profile (total cholesterol, low-density lipoprotein [LDL] cholesterol, HDL cholesterol, and triglycerides)
- Fasting glucose

Rx TREATMENT

NONPHARMACOLOGIC THERAPY

- Lifestyle modification:
  1. Dietary modifications aimed at weight loss. The American Heart Association (AHA) recommendations include
     - Consuming vegetables and fruits
     - Eating whole grains and high-fiber foods (≥30 g/day)
     - Eating fish twice weekly
     - Consuming lean animal and vegetable proteins
     - Reducing intake of sugary beverages
     - Minimizing sugar and sodium intake
     - Maintaining moderate to no alcohol intake
     - Consuming 50% to 55% of calories from carbohydrates, 15% to 20% of calories from protein, and 30% to 35% of calories from fat
     - Limiting saturated fat to less than 7% of energy, trans fat to less than 1% of energy, and cholesterol to less than 300 mg/day
  2. Physical activity of moderate intensity (i.e., brisk walking): 30 min daily
  3. Smoking cessation
- Consider bariatric surgery in the management of obesity:
  1. Body mass index (BMI) ≥40 kg/m^2 in patients who have not responded to diet and exercise (with or without drug therapy).
  2. Individuals with BMI >35 kg/m^2 and comorbidities (hypertension, impaired glucose tolerance, diabetes mellitus, dyslipidemia, sleep apnea) are also potential surgical candidates.

ACUTE GENERAL Rx

- Treat obesity (see "Obesity"): Pharmacologic treatment: consider orlistat and other approved agents (e.g., liraglutide, topiramate/

TABLE 1 Common Definitions for Metabolic Syndrome

Criterion	NCEP ATP III (3 or more criteria)
Abdominal obesity	Waist circumference
Men	>40 inches (>102 cm)
Women	>35 inches (>88 cm)
Hypertriglyceridemia	>150 mg/dl (≥1.7 mmol/L)
Low HDL	
Men	<40 mg/dl (<1.03 mmol/L)
Women	<50 mg/dl (<1.30 mmol/L)
Hypertension	≥130/85 mm Hg or on antihypertensive medication
Impaired fasting glucose or diabetes	>100 mg/dl (5.6 mmol/L) or taking insulin or hypoglycemic medication

From Floege J et al: *Comprehensive clinical nephrology,* ed 4, Philadelphia, 2010, Saunders.

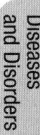

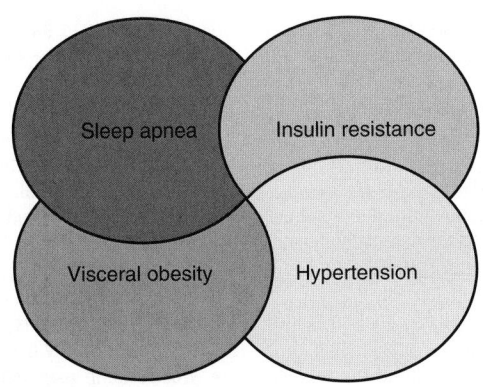

FIG. 1 A new concept of the metabolic syndrome. It includes not only insulin resistance, visceral obesity, and hypertension but also obstructive sleep apnea. (From Mason RJ et al: *Murray and Nadel's textbook of respiratory medicine*, Philadelphia, 2010, Saunders.)

phentermine) in patients who have not responded to diet and exercise if BMI >30 kg/m^2 or a BMI of 27 to 30 kg/m^2 with comorbid conditions. Drug therapy still needs to be in conjunction with diet and exercise.
- Treat hypertension (see "Hypertension"): Systolic blood pressures >130/85 mm Hg: consider angiotensin-converting enzyme inhibitors or angiotensin II receptor blocker as first-line therapy.
- Treat hyperlipidemia: In the 2013 guidelines from the American College of Cardiology and American Heart Association (ACC/AHA), treatment goals for LDL-C and non-HDL-C are no longer recommended, and there are no guidelines for treating high triglyceride levels. The new guidelines specify four groups that may require statin therapy[1] (potential statin side effects will need to be discussed with the patient prior to any initiation):
  1. People with clinical atherosclerotic cardiovascular disease (ASCVD)
  2. People with LDL-C levels of ≥190 mg/dl
  3. People with diabetes, age 40 to 75
  4. People without diabetes, age 40 to 75 with LDL-C levels 70-190 mg/dl, and a

10-year ASCVD risk of 7.5% or higher as determined by the new risk calculator.[2]
- Treat diabetes:
  1. Goal HgAlC <7.0%
  2. Metformin as first-line therapy to improve insulin sensitivity
- Treat cardiovascular risk factors:
  1. Consider aspirin. Aspirin should be started in patients with metabolic syndrome and an intermediate or elevated Framingham cardiovascular risk, if there are no contraindications.
  2. Risk can be lowered with weight loss, exercise, smoking cessation, blood pressure control, diabetes management, and treatment of hyperlipidemia.

CHRONIC Rx
- Encourage lifestyle modification as discussed previously.
- Pharmacologic and surgical management to maintain therapeutic goals described previously.

[1]Raymond C et al: New cholesterol guidelines: worth the wait? *Clev Clin J Med* 81:11-19, 2014.

[2]American Heart Association: *2013 Prevention Guideline Tools. CV risk calculator.* Available at http://my.americanheart.org/professional/statementsguidelines/preventionguidelines/preventionguidelines_VCM_subhomepage.jsp.

DISPOSITION
Weight loss can prevent disease progression. Appropriate treatment of obesity, hypertension, hyperlipidemia, and diabetes can improve morbidity and mortality rates.

REFERRAL
- To nutritionist for dietary counseling
- To weight loss and exercise programs
- To endocrinologist if difficulty reaching therapeutic goal and also to consider weight loss pharmacotherapy.
- To bariatric surgeon if patient meets surgical criteria (as noted previously)

PEARLS & CONSIDERATIONS

PREVENTION
- Weight loss is essential for the prevention and treatment of metabolic syndrome.
- Recommend dietary modifications and moderate physical activity.
- Consider pharmacologic and surgical options in select individuals (as noted previously).

PATIENT & FAMILY EDUCATION
- Weight reduction programs, including Weight Watchers, Curves, etc.
- American Diabetes Association: http://www.diabetes.org
- Polycystic Ovarian Syndrome Association: http://www.pcosupport.org
- The Hormone Foundation: http://www.hormone.org

SUGGESTED READINGS
Available at www.expertconsult.com

RELATED CONTENT
Obesity (Related Key Topic)
Metabolic Syndrome (Patient Information)

AUTHORS: **HARIKRASHNA B. BHATT, M.D.,** and **SHIVANG U. DANAK, M.D.**

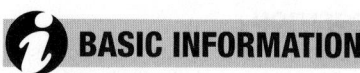

BASIC INFORMATION

DEFINITION

An accidental or intentional ingestion of 1 g per kg methanol or ethylene glycol is considered lethal, although even small amounts can be toxic. Inhalational and dermal exposures rarely cause toxicity.

SYNONYMS

Toxic alcohols
Moonshine
Wood alcohol
Antifreeze

ICD-10CM CODES
T51.8   Toxic effect of alcohols
T51.1X1 Toxic effect of methanol
T51.1X2 Toxic effect of methanol, intentional
        self-harm
T52.8X1 Ethylene glycol poisoning

EPIDEMIOLOGY & DEMOGRAPHICS

INCIDENCE:
- In 2014, the American Association of Poison Control Centers reported 6089 and 1747 single-exposure cases of ethylene glycol and methanol poisoning, respectively.
- Most cases are reported in adults and predominantly in men.
- Accidental exposure is common in children, while alcoholism, polysubstance abuse, depression, and suicide are seen in adults.
- Suicide attempts involving toxic alcohols frequently involve the ingestion of multiple substances.
- Outbreaks or epidemic poisoning with methanol is frequently the result of bootleg distillation or counterfeit alcohol.

PHYSICAL FINDINGS & CLINICAL PRESENTATION

- Clinical manifestations depend on the quantity of ingestion, duration of time since ingestion, and whether co-ingestion of other substances occurs.
- Early ingestion of either substance causes CNS depression, nausea, and vomiting; inebriation can mimic ethanol ingestion. Late effects include progressive CNS dysfunction, including seizure and coma, as well as respiratory and cardiopulmonary failure.
- Visual symptoms ranging from blurry or snowy vision to complete visual loss and findings of papillary edema and, later, optic atrophy, fixed and dilated pupils, retinal hyperemia, and a Parkinson-like syndrome are indicative of methanol poisoning. Other CNS effects are hemorrhage and white matter lesions in the putamen, subcortical structures, brainstem, and cerebellum.
- Oliguria, hematuria, calcium oxalate crystalluria, tetany, cranial nerve palsy, and acute kidney injury suggest ethylene glycol toxicity.
- Abdominal pain may result from exposure to either substance, while methanol can cause acute pancreatitis.
- Küssmaul respirations (rapid, labored breathing) may be evident with severe acidosis.

PATHOPHYSIOLOGY

- Toxicity of these alcohols is related to their metabolites rather than the parent compound.
- Lethal dose for methanol is >15 to 30 mL and >1 to 1.5 mL/kg for ethylene glycol.
- Sequential metabolism by alcohol and aldehyde dehydrogenases converts methanol to formaldehyde and then formic acid, while ethylene glycol is converted to glycoaldehyde, glycolic acid, and then oxalate.
- Fig. E1 depicts the pathways involved in methanol metabolism.
- While methanol metabolites primarily cause retinal injury, ethylene glycol metabolites produce renal tubular injury and calcium oxalate stones.
  1. Formaldehyde binds to tissue proteins and is likely the major toxin in methanol poisoning involving necrosis of retinal and optic neurons and the basal ganglia (putamen). Formic acid, the acid produced in the largest quantity, inhibits cytochrome oxidase, preventing oxygen utilization by mitochondria and causing further organ dysfunction.
  2. Glycoaldehyde may be the major nephrotoxin, while glycolic acid is the acid produced in the largest quantity in ethylene glycol poisoning, with a small quantity converted to oxalic acid by lactate dehydrogenase. Oxalate then forms calcium oxalate crystals, which are deposited in the renal parenchyma, cerebral blood vessels, and meninges, causing hypocalcemic tetany.

DIAGNOSIS

DIFFERENTIAL DIAGNOSIS

- Other causes of a high anion gap metabolic acidosis include lactic acidosis, diabetic and alcoholic ketoacidosis, kidney failure (acute and chronic), early toluene toxicity, and salicylate intoxication. Of note, L-lactate may be elevated in methanol toxicity due to cytochrome oxidase inhibition by formic acid and an increase of the NADH:NAD$^+$ ratio that is driven by methanol metabolism.
- Elevated plasma osmolal gap may be encountered in ethyl alcohol or isopropyl alcohol ingestion

EVALUATION AND WORKUP

- Diagnosis depends on history, clinical presentation, and laboratory abnormalities.
- High anion gap metabolic acidosis (AG >12 mEq/L) with elevated plasma osmolal gap (>10 mOsm/kg; usually >25 mOsm/Kg) in an appropriate clinical setting should raise the suspicion of methanol or ethylene glycol ingestion.
- In either intoxication, an osmolal gap will initially be positive, but as the parent compound is converted to its metabolites, the osmolal gap will normalize and the serum anion gap will increase.
- Serum methanol and ethylene glycol levels are elevated in their respective ingestions.
- Acute kidney injury, hypocalcemia with prolonged QT interval, and calcium oxalate crystalluria are seen with ethylene glycol toxicity.
- Metabolic acidosis in the absence of acute kidney injury suggests methanol toxicity; that is, ethylene glycol is more often associated with acute kidney injury.
- Wood's lamp uses ultraviolet light to detect urinary presence of fluorescein, which is contained in some ethylene glycol preparations. Fluorescence lacks sensitivity and specificity. Therefore, fluorescence is not considered a reliable clinical tool.

LABORATORY TESTS

- Calculation of the anion gap and serum osmolal gap
  1. Anion gap determination: electrolytes and albumin
  2. Osmolal gap determination: measured and calculated serum osmolalities (sodium, BUN, glucose, ± ethanol)
- Arterial blood gas analysis, lactate, calcium, and creatine kinase
- Creatinine and urinalysis to evaluate presence of tubular injury and calcium oxalate crystals
- ECG to evaluate QT interval
- Toxicology screen with quantification: acetaminophen, salicylate, ethanol, methanol, ethylene glycol, and isopropyl alcohol

TREATMENT

High index of suspicion and immediate recognition with early treatment remain crucial to reduce mortality. Box 1 describes common commercial products that may contain ethylene glycol.

NONPHARMACOLOGIC THERAPY

- Cardiorespiratory support as required
- Rapid (within 60 minutes) gastric decontamination (charcoal and/or gastric lavage)
- Induction of vomiting is contraindicated even in conscious patients given the risks

---

BOX 1   Common Commercial Products That May Contain Ethylene Glycol

Paints and lacquers
  Polishes and detergents
Inks
Cosmetics
  Hydraulic brake fluids
  Solar collector fluids
  Car wash fluids

Data from Kruse JA: Methanol, ethylene glycol, and related intoxications. In Carlson RW, Geheb MA (eds): *Principles and practice of medical intensive care*, Philadelphia, 1993, Saunders.

of development of central nervous system depression in these patients

ACUTE GENERAL Rx

- Principles of therapy include prevention of formation of toxic metabolites, correction of acidosis, and toxin removal.
- Ethanol, a competitive substrate, and fomepizole (4-methylpyrazole or 4-MP), a competitive inhibitor of alcohol dehydrogenase, prevent formation of toxic metabolites of ethylene glycol and methanol.
- Fomepizole is preferred over ethanol given the increased incidence of adverse events with ethanol administration, its greater inhibition of alcohol dehydrogenase, and easier administration. Cost and availability of fomepizole may influence the decision to administer this agent vs. ethanol.
- Intravenous isotonic fluids can facilitate urinary excretion of volatile alcohol and its metabolites; when acidosis is present (pH <7.3), isotonic bicarbonate should be utilized because reversal of acidosis helps prevent end-organ damage from toxic metabolites (target pH: 7.35-7.45).
- Treatment with medications and/or hemodialysis is continued until the methanol or ethylene glycol concentration is <20 mg/dl.
- Ethanol: dosing
  1. Target ethanol concentration is 100-200 mg/dl and requires close monitoring.
  2. Loading dose: 800 mg/kg in a 10% solution of 5% dextrose in water will raise serum ethanol by 100 mg/dl.
  3. Maintenance dose: infusion of 80-160 mg/kg/hr based on blood concentrations.
  4. Comment on dosing adjustment in patients receiving concomitant dialysis.
- Fomepizole: indications for use
  1. Plasma concentration of methanol or ethylene glycol >20 mg/dl OR
  2. Documented ingestion with an osmolal gap >10 mOsm/L OR
  3. Suspected ingestion with at least two of the following criteria:
     A. Arterial pH <7.3
     B. Serum bicarbonate <20 mEq/L
     C. Osmolal gap >10 mOsm/L
     D. Urinary oxalate crystals in the case of ethylene glycol toxicity
- Fomepizole (4-methylpyrazole): dosing
  1. Loading dose: 15 mg/kg body weight
  2. Maintenance dose: 10 mg/kg body weight every 12 hr for 4 doses, then 15 mg/kg every 12 hr (if blood levels do not reach goal by 48 hours)

  3. During hemodialysis: Add 1-1.5 mg/kg/hr, or repeat loading dose every 4 hr
- The half-lives of ethylene glycol and methanol increase with ethanol or fomepizole.
- Hemodialysis should be considered in patients with significant metabolic acidosis (pH <7.15), kidney failure, new visual abnormalities, electrolyte imbalances refractory to pharmacologic treatments, hemodynamic instability, seizures, coma, and serum concentrations as low as 20 mg/dl with acidosis or other end organ damage.
- The half-life of methanol metabolism is long (as much as 70 hr). Treatment with fomepizole alone is not recommended, and hemodialysis should be considered to prevent a prolonged requirement for intensive care. Duration of hemodialysis can be estimated using the formula: Time (hr) equals $-V \ln(5/A)/0.06k$, where V is the Watson total body water volume (L); A is the initial alcohol concentration (mmol/L); and k is 80% of the manufacturer's specified urea clearance (mL/min).
- Average duration of dialysis in studies was 8.4 ± 3.2 hr.
  1. Intermittent hemodialysis is the preferred modality of dialysis, as continuous renal replacement therapy (CRRT) alone is ineffective in achieving rapid clearance of methanol and ethylene glycol.
  2. CRRT is an acceptable alternative when intermittent hemodialysis is not available.
  3. If blood concentration levels are not available, start by conducting an 8-hr intermittent hemodialysis session followed by 18 hr of continuous renal replacement therapy; adjust therapy afterward as clinically indicated.
  4. Do not use heparin with dialysis, as heparin may increase the risk of cerebral hemorrhage.

ADJUNCTIVE Rx

- In ethylene glycol poisoning, thiamine (100 mg q6h) and pyridoxine (500 mg IM q6h) may decrease oxalic acid formation and direct metabolism to less toxic metabolites.
- In methanol poisoning, folinic acid doses of 1 mg/kg given IV every 4 to 6 hr may increase formic acid metabolism to CO_2 and H_2O. Correct electrolyte abnormalities (hypocalcemia, etc.).
- Treat seizures.

DISPOSITION

Transfer to a hospital with an intensive care unit and hemodialysis capabilities should be carried out early in the course of intoxication.

REFERRAL

- Regional poison center (toxicologist) and nephrology recommended to avoid treatment delays
- Ophthalmology for patients with visual symptoms
- Psychiatry if depression and suicidal ideation are present
- Detoxification centers for patients with substance abuse

PROGNOSIS

- Coma or seizures at presentation and prolonged severe acidosis correlate with increased mortality
- High osmolal gap and high anion gap acidosis associated with high mortality
- Hyperglycemia may correlate with worse prognosis in methanol poisoning

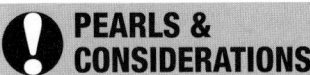

PEARLS & CONSIDERATIONS

- Profound plasma osmolal gap or anion gap metabolic acidosis should raise suspicion for ethylene glycol and/or methanol ingestion. A high index of suspicion and early treatment are crucial to reducing mortality. The metabolites of methanol and ethylene glycol produce the clinical toxidrome.
- Complaints of visual blurring, central scotomata, and blindness are consistent with methanol poisoning.
- Calcium oxalate crystalluria, oliguria, hematuria, and acute kidney injury are consistent with ethylene glycol poisoning.
- Fomepizole is preferred to ethanol due to complications associated with ethanol use.
- Emergent hemodialysis is indicated with end organ damage and/or severe metabolic acidosis.
- Elevated osmolal gap and anion gap metabolic acidosis may occur rarely with other toxic alcohols such as diethylene glycol and propylene glycol.

SUGGESTED READINGS
Available at www.expertconsult.com

RELATED CONTENT
Algorithm for the management of acute poisoning (Algorithm, Section III)

AUTHORS: **NIKOLAS HARBORD, M.D.,** and **JAMES F. WINCHESTER, M.D.**

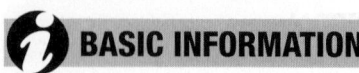

BASIC INFORMATION

DEFINITION

Methicillin-resistant *Staphylococcus aureus* (MRSA) is a common bacterial pathogen with resistance to many antibiotics. It is defined as a *S. aureus* that shows a minimum inhibitory concentration (MIC) of greater than or equal to 4 mcg/mL to oxacillin. There are two types of MRSA:

- HA-MRSA: hospital-acquired MRSA, usually multidrug resistant
- CA-MRSA: community-acquired MRSA; an emerging pathogen, usually acquired outside of the hospital setting; resistance may differ from HA-MRSA and is generally susceptible to more antibiotics than HA-MRSA

SYNONYMS

Multidrug-resistant *Staphylococcus aureus*
Oxacillin-resistant *Staphylococcus aureus*

ICD-10CM CODES

A41.02	Sepsis due to Methicillin resistant *Staphylococcus aureus*
A49.02	Methicillin resistant *Staphylococcus aureus* infection, unspecified site
B95.62	Methicillin resistant *Staphylococcus aureus* infection as the cause of diseases classified elsewhere
J15.212	Pneumonia due to Methicillin resistant *Staphylococcus aureus*
Z22.322	Carrier or suspected carrier of Methicillin resistant *Staphylococcus aureus*
Z86.14	Personal history of Methicillin resistant *Staphylococcus aureus* infection

EPIDEMIOLOGY & DEMOGRAPHICS

INCIDENCE: 1:3000
PEAK INCIDENCE: Occurs year round; may peak during summer and fall months for CA-MRSA
PREVALENCE: The national rate of MRSA colonization or infection is 46.3 per 10,000 inpatients. Hospital prevalence rate of MRSA is as high as 60% in hospitals, which means that 60% of *S. aureus* strains in that hospital will be MRSA.
PREDOMINANT SEX AND AGE: All ages and both sexes
RISK FACTORS:

- HA-MRSA: hospitalization; invasive medical device; residing in long-term nursing facility
- CA-MRSA: initially seen in young men engaged in athletic activities and in gyms, prisons, military barracks, etc., but has now spread to the entire age spectrum including neonates and the elderly.

PHYSICAL FINDINGS & CLINICAL PRESENTATION

- CA-MRSA: can present with skin infection, associated with opening in the skin; red bump, pustule, or boil; erythema, swelling; edema, often fluctuant and very painful
- HA-MRSA: bacteremia; infection associated with intravenous device

1. Catheters: pneumonia
2. Skin: cellulitis
3. Bone: osteomyelitis
4. Endocarditis
5. Abscesses: skin or organ
6. Pneumonia: nosocomial

ETIOLOGY

- CA-MRSA: the most prevalent strain in the US on pulse field electrophoresis (PFGE) is called USA 300
  1. CA-MRSA: common cause of skin and soft tissue infections seen in the emergency room. It can, however, also cause necrotizing pneumonia, sepsis, osteomyelitis, etc.
  2. Virulence factors particular to CA-MRSA: Panton-Valentine leukocidin (PVL) toxin, alpha-hemolysin toxin, phenol soluble modulins, etc., that enhance ability to cause infection
- HA-MRSA: most strains on PFGE are USA 100 or USA 200 and tend to have multidrug resistance. Patients with HA-MRSA infection have higher mortality and morbidity than patients with a methicillin-sensitive *S. aureus* (MSSA) infection.

DIAGNOSIS

WORKUP

- Culture of wound, abscess, blood, sputum; rule out colonization; culture of nares or axillae

LABORATORY TESTS

- See previously.
- PFGE: usually done only for epidemiologic or outbreak purposes.

IMAGING STUDIES

- Radiographs or computed tomography scan of suspected organ
- Echocardiogram: all adult patients with *S. aureus* bacteremia should undergo echocardiography

TREATMENT

- CA-MRSA: oral antibiotics that may be effective include trimethoprim-sulfamethoxazole, doxycycline, minocycline, or clindamycin; linezolid and tedizolid are other options but are very expensive.
- HA-MRSA: intravenous antibiotics, vancomycin, linezolid, tedizolid, daptomycin, tigecycline

NONPHARMACOLOGIC THERAPY

Abscess surgically drained

ACUTE GENERAL Rx

- Trimethoprim-sulfamethoxazole, one double-strength tablet PO bid, is useful in cases of CA-MRSA since 95% of community-acquired MRSA strains are susceptible to it in vitro. Other agents that can be used for CA-MRSA include:

1. Clindamycin: 300 to 450 mg q6 to 8h also inhibits toxin production. If strain tests sensitive to clindamycin but resistant to erythromycin, then a D test must be done to ensure there will not be inducible resistance while on therapy with the clindamycin.
2. Doxycycline: 100 mg PO q12h and minocycline also have some activity against MRSA.
3. Rifampin: never used alone but can be used with one of the other oral agents
- Vancomycin 15 to 20 mg/kg IV q8 to 12h is the mainstay of parenteral therapy for MRSA infections. There is an increasing concern of MRSA strains developing tolerance to vancomycin, requiring higher doses to achieve eradication. True vancomycin resistant strains (MIC ≥32 mg/L) remain rare. Vancomycin trough levels of at least 15 to 20 mcg/ml are recommended to treat MRSA infections.
- Linezolid 600 mg PO or IV bid is a synthetic oxazolidinone FDA-approved for MRSA skin and soft tissue infections and pneumonia. It has been shown to be more effective than vancomycin for MRSA pneumonia. A similar agent, tedizolid (200 mg IV or PO for 6 days), was recently approved for skin and soft tissue infections. These agents are much more expensive than vancomycin.
- Daptomycin: 4 mg/kg/day to 6 mg/kg/day IV is approved for skin and soft tissue infections, bacteremia and right-sided endocarditis but should not be used for pneumonia as it is inactivated by pulmonary surfactant.
- Tigecycline: 100 mg IV load, then 50 mg IV q12h, is approved for MRSA skin and soft tissue infections and intraabdominal abscess.
- Ceftaroline is a fifth-generation cephalosporin, also effective against MRSA but only skin and soft tissue infections, not pneumonia: 600 mg IV q12h.
- Newer glycopeptide agents: dalbavancin (1000 mg IV followed by 500 mg IV a week later for complicated skin and soft tissue infections) and telavancin (10 mg/kg IV daily for 7-14 days) to treat skin infections or pneumonia; these are expensive alternatives to vancomycin.

CHRONIC Rx

- Patients with MRSA colonization may have reexposure or may be unable to eradicate colonized state.
- Oral agents used to attempt eradication of colonization are rifampin, tetracycline, and minocycline.

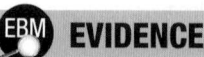 **EVIDENCE**

Available at www.expertconsult.com

SUGGESTED READINGS
Available at www.expertconsult.com

RELATED CONTENT

Methicillin-Resistant *Staphylococcus aureus* (Patient Information)

AUTHOR: **GLENN G. FORT, M.D., M.P.H.**

BASIC INFORMATION

DEFINITION

Microscopic polyangiitis (MPA) is an ANCA (anti-neutrophil cytoplasmic autoantibody)-associated small to medium vessel systemic vasculitis. It is characterized by necrotizing, pauci-immune, small-vessel vasculitis in the absence of granulomatous inflammation. Most patients present with both renal and pulmonary involvement that may cause severe organ dysfunction leading to renal and respiratory failure. However, MPA may affect any organ or tissue, including the skin, nervous system, and gastrointestinal (GI) tract. MPA belongs to the family of ANCA-associated vasculitides that also includes granulomatosis with polyangiitis (GPA, previously known as Wegener's granulomatosis) and eosinophilic granulomatosis with polyangiitis (EGPA, previously known as Churg-Strauss syndrome) (Table 1).

ICD-10CM CODES
M31.7 Microscopic polyangiitis

SYNONYMS

Microscopic polyarteritis
MPA

TABLE 1 Classification Scheme of Vasculitides According to Size of Predominant Blood Vessels Involved

Predominantly Large-Vessel Vasculitides

Takayasu's arteritis
Giant cell arteritis
Cogan's syndrome
Behçet's syndrome*
Predominantly Medium-Vessel Vasculitides
Classic polyarteritis nodosa
Cutaneous polyarteritis nodosa
Rheumatoid vasculitis†
Buerger's disease
Kawasaki disease
Primary angiitis of the central nervous system

Predominantly Small-Vessel Vasculitides

Immune complex mediated
- Cutaneous leukocytoclastic angiitis ("hypersensitivity" vasculitis)
- Henoch-Schönlein purpura
- Urticarial vasculitis
- Cryoglobulinemia†

"ANCA-associated" disorders
- Wegener's granulomatosis†
- Microscopic polyangiitis†
- Churg-Strauss syndrome†

Miscellaneous small-vessel vasculitides

- Connective tissue disorders†
- Paraneoplastic diseases
- Infection
- Inflammatory bowel disease

ANCA, Antineutrophil cytoplasmic antibody.
*May involve small, medium, and large blood vessels.
†Frequent overlap of involvement of small- and medium-sized blood vessels.
From Goldman L, Schafer AI: *Goldman's Cecil medicine,* ed 24, Philadelphia, 2012, Saunders.

EPIDEMIOLOGY & DEMOGRAPHICS

- Incidence is 5 to 10 per 1,000,000 adults annually in U.S.
- Prevalence is 20 to 50 cases per 1,000,000.
- More common in Caucasians than in African Americans.
- The male:female ratio is independent of age and is around or slightly above 1.

MPA occurs at all ages and even in young children; incidence rises with increasing age, peaking in the sixth and especially seventh decades.

PHYSICAL FINDINGS & CLINICAL PRESENTATION

- In 60% to 80% of cases, there is a protracted and indolent course over many weeks to months with nonspecific symptoms such as fatigue, fever, "flu-like" symptoms, weight loss, and anorexia.
- Many have migratory arthralgias with no or only mild signs of arthritis affecting a few joints at a time.
- Macroscopic hematuria, proteinuria, edema, decreased urinary output.
- Pulmonary symptoms including hemoptysis, cough, dyspnea, pulmonary hemorrhage, pleuritic pain.
- Palpable purpura (41%) is the most common cutaneous manifestation. Livedo reticularis (12%), skin ulcers, digital gangrene may also be present.
- Inflammation of visceral blood and gut vessels causes pain, bloody stools, and perforation.
- Peripheral nervous system involvement manifesting as mononeuritis multiplex (57%), CNS involvement manifesting as seizures (11%).
- Kidney involvement 90%.
- Weight loss >70%.
- Myalgias 50%, arthralgias (10%-50%).
- Chest pain, heart failure symptoms.
- Mild ENT symptoms including nasal congestion, sinusitis, and epistaxis can occur in up to 30% of cases.
- Severe or destructive disease of the upper airways is not compatible with MPA and suggests a diagnosis of GPA.
- Ophthalmic involvement: Episcleritis and ulcerative keratitis are the most common clinical manifestations, occurring in 10% to 20% of cases. Uveitis, conjunctivitis, and necrotizing scleritis have also been described.

ETIOLOGY

- Autoimmune process of unknown etiology. ANCA, most specifically those directed at cytoplasmic myeloperoxidase, are felt to contribute to the inflammatory process. Once bound to their cellular epitope, anti-myeloperoxidase (MPO) antibodies likely contribute to degranulation of the neutrophil, which presumably contributes to endothelial injury. Most recently, investigators have demonstrated that anti-MPO antibodies alone can cause necrotizing and crescentic glomerulonephritis.
- In addition to antibodies directed against PR3 and MPO, it has been demonstrated that patients with ANCA-associated necrotizing glomerulonephritis tend to have IgG antibodies against human lysosomal membrane protein 2 (hLAMP-2).
- Many hypotheses involve microbial agents in the development of disease activity.

DIAGNOSIS

DIFFERENTIAL DIAGNOSIS

- Polyarteritis nodosa
- Kawasaki's disease
- Infective endocarditis
- Lymphoma
- Amyloidosis
- Hypercoagulable states
- Systemic lupus erythematosus
- Paraproteinemias
- Cryoglobulinemia

MPA is distinguished from GPA by the absence of granuloma formation (Table 2) and from EGPA by absence of asthma and eosinophilia.

WORKUP

- Thorough medical history and physical examination to detect sites of organ involvement and to exclude other illnesses that may have a similar appearance, especially infections.

LABORATORY TESTS

- Laboratory testing may reveal elevated sedimentation rate (ESR), C-reactive protein, leukocytosis, thrombocytosis, and normocytic anemia.
- Elevated serum blood urea nitrogen and creatinine suggest renal impairment.
- Urinalysis to detect proteinuria, hematuria, erythrocyte casts, abnormal urine sediment.
- ANCA positive 82% to 94%.
- Perinuclear ANCA directed at myeloperoxidase (50%-70%).
- Cytoplasmic ANCA directed at proteinase 3 (25%-30%).
- Serum complement levels.
- Aspartate aminotransferase, alanine aminotransferase, and creatine phosphokinase to evaluate for liver or muscle involvement.
- Blood cultures to rule out bacterial endocarditis.
- Intestinal angina is often a result of mesenteric ischemia and can be assessed using mesenteric angiography when renal function permits.
- Tissue for pathology diagnosis is usually required to confirm the diagnosis.
- The characteristic histologic lesion in MPA is pauci-immune necrotizing small-vessel vasculitis.
- Biopsy of the skin reveals nonspecific leukocytoclastic vasculitis with little or no complement and immunoglobulin on immunofluorescence.
- Kidney biopsy usually reveals necrotizing crescentic glomerulonephritis that is usually pauci-immune on immunofluorescence and necrotizing vasculitis of microscopic vessels (small arteries, arterioles, capillaries, venules).

TABLE 2 Names and Definitions of Vasculitis Adopted by the Chapel Hill Consensus Conference on the Nomenclature of Systemic Vasculitis

Name	Large-Vessel Vasculitis*
Giant cell (temporal arteritis)	Granulomatous arteritis of the aorta and its major branches, with a predilection for the extracranial branches of the carotid artery. Often involves the temporal artery. Usually occurs in patients older than 50 yr and often is associated with polymyalgia rheumatica
Takayasu's arteritis	Granulomatous inflammation of the aorta and its major branches. Usually occurs in patients younger than 50 yr
	Medium-Sized Vessel Vasculitis*
Polyarteritis nodosa (classic polyarteritis nodosa)	Necrotizing inflammation of medium-sized or small arteries without glomerulonephritis or vasculitis in arterioles, capillaries, or venules. Kawasaki's disease arteritis involving large, medium-sized, and small arteries and associated with mucocutaneous lymph node syndrome. Coronary arteries are often involved. Aorta and veins may be involved. Usually occurs in children
	Small-Vessel Vasculitis*
Granulomatosis with polyangiitis[†,‡]	Granulomatous inflammation involving the respiratory tract and necrotizing vasculitis affecting small- to medium-sized vessels, e.g., capillaries, venules, arterioles, and arteries. Necrotizing glomerulonephritis is common
Churg-Strauss syndrome[†,‡]	Eosinophil-rich and granulomatous inflammation involving the respiratory tract and necrotizing vasculitis affecting small- to medium-sized vessels and associated with asthma and blood eosinophilia
Microscopic polyangiitis (microscopic polyarteritis)[†,‡]	Necrotizing vasculitis with few or no immune deposits affecting small vessels, e.g., capillaries, venules, or arterioles. Necrotizing arteritis involving small- and medium-sized arteries may be present. Necrotizing glomerulonephritis is very common. Pulmonary capillaritis often occurs
Henoch-Schönlein purpura[‡]	Vasculitis with immunoglobulin A–dominant immune deposits affecting small vessels, e.g., capillaries, venules, or arterioles. Typically involves the skin, gut, and glomeruli and is associated with arthralgias or arthritis
Essential cryoglobulinemic vasculitis[‡]	Vasculitis with cryoglobulin immune deposits affecting small vessels, e.g., capillaries, venules, or arterioles, and associated with cryoglobulins in serum. Skin and glomeruli are often involved
Cutaneous leukocytoclastic angiitis	Isolated cutaneous leukocytoclastic angiitis without systemic vasculitis or glomerulonephritis

*Large artery refers to the aorta and the largest branches directed toward major body regions (e.g., to the extremities and the head and neck); medium-sized artery refers to the main visceral arteries (e.g., renal, hepatic, coronary, and mesenteric arteries); and small artery refers to the distal arterial radicals that connect with arterioles (e.g., renal arcuate and interlobular arteries). Note that some small- and large-vessel vasculitides may involve medium-sized arteries; but large- and medium-sized vessel vasculitides do not involve vessels smaller than arteries.
[†]Strongly associated with antineutrophil cytoplasmic autoantibodies (ANCA).
[‡]May be accompanied by glomerulonephritis and can manifest as nephritis or pulmonary renal vasculitic syndrome.

IMAGING STUDIES

- Chest radiograph would show diffuse parenchymal infiltrates secondary to pulmonary alveolar hemorrhages (Fig. E1).
- Computed tomographic (CT) scanning may disclose previously undetected nodules, unsuspected cavitation in nodules, alveolar opacities, large-airway inflammation or stenotic lesions, and pleural-based lesions.
- An EMG may reveal a sensorimotor peripheral neuropathy in patients with mononeuritis multiplex.
- Electrocardiography is indicated in myocardial infection, pericarditis, and congestive heart failure.

- Gastrointestinal endoscopy and mesenteric angiography in cases of gastrointestinal involvement.

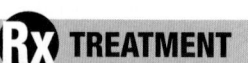 **TREATMENT**

ACUTE GENERAL Rx

Induction
- Corticosteroids combined with cyclophosphamide, followed by maintenance therapy with methotrexate, azathioprine, or mycophenolate mofetil.
- Rituximab is an effective alternative to cyclophosphamide for initial induction therapy as well as for relapse.

- Plasmapheresis is an option for patients with severe bleeding in the lungs or rapidly progressive kidney failure leading to dialysis.

CHRONIC Rx

Maintenance therapy
- Low-dose steroids, azathioprine, methotrexate, and rituximab have been demonstrated to be non-inferior to cyclophosphamide and can be used for maintenance therapy, although dosing intervals and duration of therapy are still being determined.

Prophylaxis for opportunistic infections like *Pneumocystis jirovecii (carinii)* pneumonia (PCP) is with low-dose sulfamethoxazole/trimethoprim given as one double-strength tablet three times weekly or as a single-strength tablet once daily. Atovaquone is preferred in patients who are allergic to sulfonamides or who do not tolerate trimethoprim-sulfamethoxazole.

Relapse therapy
- Mild or non-life-threatening relapses while on maintenance therapy can be treated by increasing glucocorticoid dose and/or by adding azathioprine or methotrexate.
- In severe cases, treatment is the same as in remission induction; however, rituximab is often preferred over cyclophosphamide.

DISPOSITION

- Poor prognosis if untreated.
- Prompt diagnosis is important to permit initiation of therapy that may be life-saving and organ sparing.
- Renal failure and pulmonary involvement are the major causes of morbidity and mortality.
- With treatment, 2- to 5-yr survival rates are 74%.

REFERRAL

Nephrology consultation is needed for the diagnosis and management of renal disease.

Multiple specialists may be consulted depending on other organ system involvement.

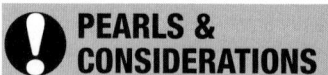 **PEARLS & CONSIDERATIONS**

Relapse occurs in one third of the cases.
PCP occurs in 6% of the patients as a complication of immunosuppressive therapy.

SUGGESTED READINGS

Available at www.expertconsult.com

AUTHOR: **CATHERINE E. NAJEM, M.D.**

M

Diseases
and Disorders

I

BASIC INFORMATION

DEFINITION

Microsporidiosis is an infection caused by single-celled protozoan intracellular spore-forming organisms called Microsporidia. Recent evidence suggests a relationship between microsporidia and fungi. Infections occur more commonly in patients with HIV/AIDS, travelers, children, organ transplant recipients, contact lens wearers, and the elderly.

SYNONYMS

Enterocytozoon bieneusi infection
Encephalitozoon species infections

ICD-10CM CODES
B60.8 Microsporidiosis
A07.8 Microsporidiosis, intestinal

EPIDEMIOLOGY & DEMOGRAPHICS

Microsporidia exist worldwide in the environment and can infect vertebrate and invertebrate hosts, entering via ingestion or inhalation of spores and by direct contact through broken skin or lesions in the eyes.
PREVALENCE: One European study showed a prevalence of 5% to 8% in immunocompetent persons.

In a study of asymptomatic HIV patients, 15% had evidence of microsporidia on small bowel biopsy. The advent of highly active antiretroviral therapy has effectively decreased the incidence of microsporidiosis in those with HIV.
RISK FACTORS: Infections such as a non-bloody watery diarrhea and keratoconjunctivitis in contact lens wearers can occur in normal hosts, but immunocompromised hosts such as AIDS patients, organ transplant recipients, and bone marrow graft recipients are at greater risk for more severe disease and other organ involvement.

ETIOLOGY

- There are 1200 species of Microsporidia, but only 14 infect humans. The four most common are:
  1) *Enterocytozoon bieneusi*
  2) *Encephalitozoon intestinalis*
  3) *Encephalitozoon cuniculi*
  4) *Encephalitozoon hellem*
- These genotypes that infect humans have been identified in domestic, farm, and wild animals and thus may be a form of zoonotic disease.

PHYSICAL FINDINGS & CLINICAL PRESENTATION

Each species of microsporidia has different reported infections:
1) *Enterocytozoon bieneusi* can cause diarrhea, wasting syndrome, cholangitis, rhinitis, or bronchitis.
2) *Encephalitozoon intestinalis* can cause diarrhea, intestinal perforation, cholangitis, nephritis, keratoconjunctivitis, and disseminated infection.
3) *Encephalitozoon cuniculi* can cause hepatitis, peritonitis, encephalitis, urethritis, prostatitis, nephritis, sinusitis, keratoconjunctivitis, cystitis, cellulitis, and disseminated infection.
4) *Encephalitozoon hellem* can cause keratoconjunctivitis, sinusitis, pneumonitis, nephritis, prostatitis, urethritis, cystitis, and disseminated infection.

DIAGNOSIS

DIFFERENTIAL DIAGNOSIS

- Other causes of watery non-bloody diarrhea: *Norovirus, Giardia, Cryptosporidia, Cyclospora,* and *Isospora belli*
- Other causes of keratoconjunctivitis: herpetic keratoconjunctivitis and acanthamoeba keratitis

WORKUP

Consists of the microscopic detection of microsporidia spores (1-2 mcm in diameter) in stool, body fluids, or tissue samples

LABORATORY TESTS

- Modified trichrome stain with light microscopy can be used on stool, urine, mucus, or tissues. Spores stain pink against a blue-green background.
- Fluorescent techniques: calcofluor white stain, Uvitex 2B, and Fungi-Fluor kit
- Indirect immunofluorescence
- Serology: detects IgM and IgG antibodies
- For exact speciation: PCR

TREATMENT

ACUTE GENERAL Rx

Treatment will depend on organism and site involved.
1) *Encephalitozoonidae* species:
   a) Intestinal or disseminated infection: albendazole 400 mg PO bid for 2 to 4 weeks depending on level of immunosuppression. Children: 15 mg/kg/day PO in divided doses.

   b) Keratoconjunctivitis: topical fumagillin 70 mcg/mL eye drops (2 drops every 2 hours for 4 days, then 2 drops 4 times a day). If associated with intestinal disease, add albendazole 400 mg PO bid for 2 to 4 weeks depending on degree of immunosuppression.
2) *Enterocytozoon bieneusi:* intestinal or disseminated disease—albendazole is not effective but can use fumagillin 20 mg PO tid (although this is not commercially available in the U.S.). Alternative: nitazoxanide 1 g PO bid for 60 days in patients with AIDS.

CHRONIC Rx

Antimotility agents are useful to control diarrhea.

REFERRAL

- Infectious diseases physician for antiretroviral therapy if positive for HIV/AIDS
- Ophthalmologist if keratoconjunctivitis is suspected

PEARLS & CONSIDERATIONS

COMMENTS

- Microsporidia infections occur particularly in HIV-positive patients with CD4+ cell counts <50/ml.
- Microsporidia spores can remain active in the environment for prolonged periods of time (e.g., months).

PREVENTION

The most effective prevention in HIV-positive patients is to start antiretroviral therapy to increase CD4+ count >100/ml; this will result in resolution of symptoms of enteric microsporidiosis (if already present) and serve as a prevention.

SUGGESTED READINGS
Available at www.expertconsult.com

AUTHORS: **SARA W.F. GEFFERT, M.D., M.S.,** and **PHILIP A. CHAN, M.D., M.S.**

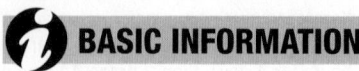

BASIC INFORMATION

DEFINITION

Significant cognitive impairment in the absence of dementia with preserved activities of daily living (ADLs). Mild cognitive impairment (MCI) is an intermediate state between normal cognitive function and dementia. The main distinctions between MCI and mild dementia are that in the latter, more than one cognitive domain is invariably involved and substantial interference with daily life is evident.[1]

SYNONYMS

Mild neurocognitive disorder
MCI

ICD-10CM CODES
G31.84 Mild cognitive impairment, so stated

EPIDEMIOLOGY & DEMOGRAPHICS

INCIDENCE:
- 12 to 15 cases per 1000 person-yr age ≥65
- 51 to 77 cases per 1000 person-yr age ≥75

PEAK INCIDENCE: In the elderly
PREVALENCE: 15% to 25% in those older than age 70.
PREDOMINANT SEX AND AGE: Male, age ≥75
GENETICS: *APOE4* genotype
- Various pathways result in amyloid accumulation and deposition in pre-Alzheimer's presenting as MCI.

RISK FACTORS: Male sex, age, lower socioeconomic status, lower educational level

CLINICAL PRESENTATION

- Subjective memory problems, preferably corroborated by another person.
- Preserved functional status (ADLs).
- Normal general thinking and reasoning skills.
- Subtypes of MCI include amnestic (mainly involves memory loss) vs. nonamnestic with involvement of other cognitive domains (single domain vs. multiple domains).
- Domains affected in MCI include memory, visuospatial skills, language, attention, and executive function.
- Olfactory dysfunction may be associated with amnestic MCI and progression to Alzheimer's dementia.

ETIOLOGY

Neurodegenerative, vascular, traumatic, depression, or due to underlying medical condition

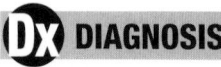 DIAGNOSIS

DIFFERENTIAL DIAGNOSIS

- Delirium
- Dementia

[1]Knopman Ds, Petersen RC: Mild cognitive impairment and mild dementia: a clinical perspective, *Mayo Clin Proc* 89:1452, 2014.

- Depression
- "Reversible" cognitive impairment:
  1. Medication related (anticholinergics)
  2. Hypothyroidism
  3. Vitamin B_{12} deficiency
- Reversible CNS conditions
  1. Subdural hematoma
  2. Normal pressure hydrocephalus
  3. Metastatic disease

WORKUP

History
- Focus on cognitive deficits and impairment.
- Review all medications that may impact cognition (i.e., anticholinergics).
- Rule out depression and delirium.
- Perform functional assessment.
- Additional history from family members or caregivers is important.
Physical exam
- Check blood pressure
- Neurologic exam to rule out reversible CNS causes of cognitive impairment
- Gait and balance assessment
Cognitive function testing:
  Brief mental status testing using MOCA (Montreal Cognitive Assessment) or SLUMS (Saint Louis University Mental Status) for office screening followed by neuropsychological testing if appropriate for specific deficits in cognitive domains. MOCA may be a better tool in identifying and following MCI with higher sensitivity to monitor cognitive decline in longitudinal monitoring.

LABORATORY TESTS

- Complete blood count
- Comprehensive metabolic profile
- TSH
- Vitamin B_{12}

IMAGING STUDIES

- CT imaging can detect most reversible CNS conditions leading to cognitive impairment.
- MRI further evaluates vascular, infectious, neoplastic, and inflammatory conditions.

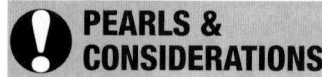 TREATMENT

- There is insufficient evidence to recommend use of cholinesterase inhibitors for MCI. They are not approved for treating MCI, have shown little efficacy in altering progression to dementia, and can have significant side effects.
- Consider treatment with these medications only if memory complaints appear to be affecting day-to-day quality of life in individual patients or in amnestic subtypes of MCI after risk-versus-benefit discussion with patient and family.

NONPHARMACOLOGIC THERAPY

- Role of cognitive rehabilitation to target specific deficits
- Caregiver education and counseling
- Physical and mental exercises to maintain cognition should be recommended

COMPLEMENTARY & ALTERNATIVE MEDICINE

No clear indications for antioxidants, and studies in humans are inconclusive.

DISPOSITION

- Progression to Alzheimer's at the rate of 5% to 15% per year
  1. Risk factors for progression to dementia include presence of vascular risk factors, significant cognitive impairment, depression, and presence of extrapyramidal signs.
- Mortality of those with MCI is twice that of those without MCI.
- Two- to threefold increase in risk of nursing home placement in those with MCI.

REFERRAL

Consider referral to a memory specialist if more than just memory is involved or for further evaluation of specific deficits.

PEARLS & CONSIDERATIONS

COMMENTS

Patients with MCI usually report short-term memory concerns such as misplacing things, not remembering names of people, word-finding difficulties, forgetting day-to-day tasks, not being able to read a book, or not being able to follow a conversation.

MCI becomes clinically relevant when quality of life is affected such as problems making financial decisions and problems with personal day-to-day interactions.

Depression should be ruled out prior to making a diagnosis of MCI since it is highly prevalent in the elderly.

Anticholinergic medication use should be evaluated carefully prior to making a diagnosis of MCI.

PREVENTION

Patients with MCI should be counseled on strategies to prevent progression to dementia. They should remain physically and mentally active, have a well-balanced diet, continue activities that are socially engaging, reduce stress in their lives, and aggressively pursue treatment of vascular risk factors.

PATIENT & FAMILY EDUCATION

- Patients with MCI typically have poor retention and rapid loss of newly learned information.
- For additional information for patients, families, and clinicians: Alzheimer's Association (www.alzheimers.org)

SUGGESTED READINGS
Available at www.expertconsult.com

AUTHORS: **BIRJU B. PATEL, M.D.**, and **N. WILSON HOLLAND, M.D.**

BASIC INFORMATION

DEFINITION

Mitral regurgitation (MR) is retrograde blood flow into the left atrium resulting from an incompetent mitral valve. This condition may cause left ventricular (LV) failure as well as increased left atrial and pulmonary pressures leading to pulmonary hypertension and right-sided heart failure.

SYNONYMS

Mitral insufficiency
MR

ICD-10CM CODES

I34.0 Nonrheumatic mitral (valve) insufficiency
I05.1 Rheumatic mitral insufficiency
I05.9 Mitral valve disease, unspecified
I05.2 Rheumatic mitral stenosis with insufficiency
Q23.3 Congenital mitral insufficiency

EPIDEMIOLOGY & DEMOGRAPHICS

The incidence of MR has increased over the past 30 yr; however, this may be due to increasing availability of echocardiography leading to MR diagnosis rather than to an actual increase in the prevalence of this condition.

PHYSICAL FINDINGS & CLINICAL PRESENTATION

- Holosystolic, high-pitched, "blowing" murmur at apex with radiation to base, left axilla, or back. There is a poor correlation between the intensity of the systolic murmur and the degree of regurgitation. However, an early diastolic to mid-diastolic rumble (pseudo-mitral stenosis) suggests severe MR.
- The murmur of acute MR (e.g., from papillary muscle rupture) can be very soft or inaudible due to a large regurgitant volume entering a noncompliant left atrium, causing an acute rise in left atrial pressure and thus a lack of significant gradient for an audible murmur.
- Hyperdynamic apex, sometimes with palpable LV lift and apical thrill.
- Diminished S1, reflecting failure of valve leaflets to coapt completely; widely split S2 (decreased LV ejection time results in early A2); and presence of an S3.
- Many patients with mild to moderate MR will remain asymptomatic and without evidence of hemodynamic compromise for years until LV remodeling occurs.
- Symptomatic patients with MR generally present with the following:
  1. Symptoms suggestive of heart failure (fatigue, dyspnea, orthopnea, paroxysmal nocturnal dyspnea, edema)
  2. Hemoptysis (caused by pulmonary hypertension)
  3. Atrial fibrillation

ETIOLOGY

Primary MR
- Idiopathic myxomatous degeneration of the mitral valve, mitral valve prolapse (most common cause of MR in industrialized countries)
- Papillary muscle dysfunction or rupture (typically as a result of an inferior wall myocardial infarction)
- Ruptured chordae tendineae
- Infective endocarditis
- Calcified mitral valve annulus
- Rheumatic valvulitis (may be combined with mitral stenosis; common in developing countries)
- Systemic lupus erythematosus (Libman-Sacks endocarditis)
- Drugs: fenfluramine, dexfenfluramine, pergolide, cabergoline
- Congenital cleft valve
- Ischemic mitral regurgitation due to papillary muscle dysfunction from multivessel CAD
Secondary MR
- Hypertrophic cardiomyopathy
- LV dilation (e.g., secondary to dilated cardiomyopathy)

DIAGNOSIS

DIFFERENTIAL DIAGNOSIS

- Hypertrophic cardiomyopathy
- Tricuspid regurgitation
- Aortic stenosis
- Aortic sclerosis
- Ventricular septal defect
- Atrial septal defect

WORKUP

- Diagnostic workup consists of echocardiography, ECG, and chest radiograph; cardiac catheterization is sometimes needed to confirm severity of the disease.
- Recent studies suggest that in patients with severe asymptomatic MR, normal LV function and elevations of brain natriuretic peptide (BNP) >105 pg/ml have an independent and additive prognostic value that may identify high-risk patients and aid in the selection of patients for early surgery.

IMAGING STUDIES

- Echocardiography (Fig. 1): dilated left atrium, hyperdynamic left ventricle (erratic motion of the leaflet is seen in patients with ruptured chordae tendineae); color flow Doppler will show evidence of MR. The most important aspect of the echocardiographic examination is the quantification of the severity of MR (Table 1); LV systolic performance, estimated right ventricular (RV) systolic pressure vena contracta width >0.6 cm, regurgitant volume >60 ml, regurgitant orifice area >0.40 cm^2 by PISA (proximal isovelocity surface area), and systolic pulmonary vein flow reversal are all echocardiographic criteria of severe MR.

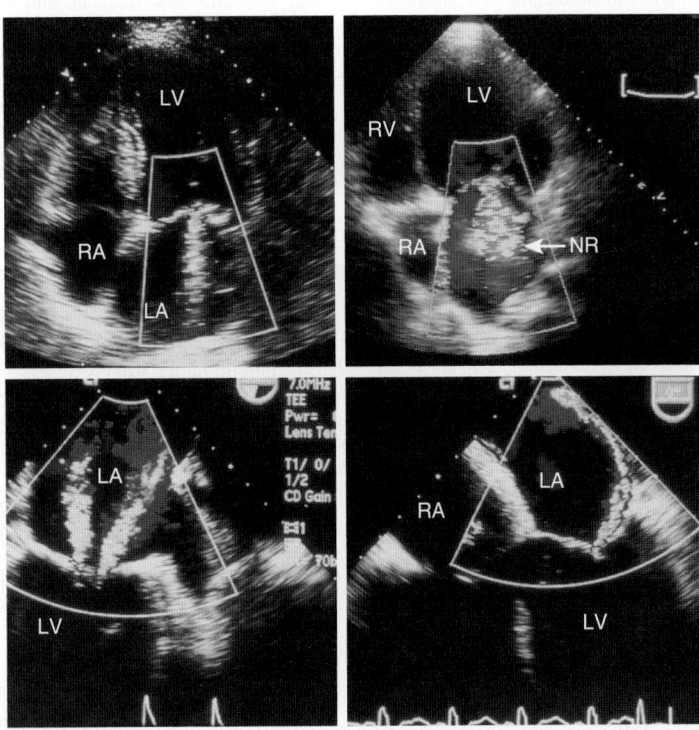

FIG. 1 Mitral regurgitation. Four panels depicting varying degrees of mitral regurgitation; the two *top panels* are apical four-chamber transthoracic views showing, on the *left*, mild mitral regurgitation and, on the *right*, moderate to severe mitral regurgitation. On the *left*, note the relatively narrow jet directed from the tips of the mitral valve toward the posterior left atrial wall. On the right, note the larger jet, filling approximately 40% of the left atrial cavity. The two *bottom panels* are transesophageal echocardiograms. On the *left*, note the mitral regurgitation occurring in two discrete jets and, on the *right*, the highly eccentric jet, which courses along the extreme lateral wall of the left atrium. *LA,* Left atrium; *LV,* left ventricle; *RA,* right atrium; *RV,* right ventricle. (From Zipes DP et al [eds]: *Braunwald's heart disease,* ed 7, Philadelphia, 2005, Saunders.)

TABLE 1 Mitral Regurgitation Severity*

	(Mild)	II	III	IV (Severe)
MR = jet (%LA)	<15	15-30	35-50	>50
Spectral Doppler	Faint	—	—	Dense
Vena contracta	<3 mm	—	—	>6 mm
Pulmonary vein flow	S > D	—	—	Systolic reversed
RV (ml)	<30	30-44	45-59	≥60
ERO (cm^2)	<0.2	0.2-0.29	0.3-0.39	≥0.40
PISA	Small	—	—	Large

D, Antegrade flow in diastole; *ERO*, effective regurgitant orifice; *%LA*, percentage of left atrial area encompassed by the *MR* jet with color flow Doppler; *MR*, mitral regurgitation; *PISA*, proximal iso-velocity surface area; *RV*, regurgitant volume; *S*, antegrade flow in systole.
*For some parameters, the observation is valid at the extremes of MR severity and there may be marked overlap in intermediate (grades II, III) MR. In these instances, no value is presented.
From Zipes DP et al (eds): *Braunwald's heart disease*, ed 7, Philadelphia, 2005, Saunders and the 2003 American Society of Echocardiography Guidelines.

- Chest x-ray:
  1. Left atrial enlargement, LV enlargement
  2. Possible pulmonary congestion, although most often normal
- ECG:
  1. Left atrial enlargement
  2. LV hypertrophy
  3. Atrial fibrillation
- Cardiac catheterization: to confirm severity of MR, or to rule out presence of coronary artery disease in patients being evaluated for surgical replacement
- Can consider cardiac MRI in cases where echocardiography is limited or LV function/dimensions are borderline, or when clinical condition and echocardiographic findings are discordant.

(Rx) TREATMENT

NONPHARMACOLOGIC THERAPY

- Salt restriction
- Surgical repair or replacement (see the following)

ACUTE GENERAL Rx

- Medical: medical therapy is primarily directed toward treatment of the source or its complications (e.g., atrial fibrillation, ischemic heart disease, infective endocarditis, hypertension, and heart failure).
  1. The utility of afterload reduction to decrease the regurgitant fraction and to increase cardiac output depends upon the etiology of MR. In acute MR, intravenous nitroprusside has shown some utility. Long-term use of oral afterload reducers (e.g., ACE inhibitors or angiotensin receptor blockers), while they do not slow the progression of mitral regurgitation, should be implemented when other indications such as hypertension and LV dysfunction are present.
  2. Control ventricular response in atrial fibrillation with rapid ventricular response when present. Use anticoagulants if atrial fibrillation occurs, which of note is not considered valvular, and novel anticoagulation agents may be used for stroke prophylaxis.

- Surgery: Surgery is the only definitive treatment for MR. Although no randomized trial of mitral valve repair vs. replacement exists, repair is favored over replacement in degenerative mitral valve disease due to its lower perioperative risk, improved event-free survival, freedom from complications of prosthetic valves, and better postoperative LV function. It is a class I indication in patients with (Fig. 2):
  1. Acute severe MR
  2. Symptomatic patients with severe primary MR despite optimal medical therapy and LVEF >30%, LV dilation, severe MR by echo criteria
  3. Asymptomatic patients with severe MR but with evidence of declining LV function (EF 30% to 60%) or progressive dilation (LV at end-systole >40 mm)
     1. Concomitant mitral valve repair or MVR is indicated in patients with chronic severe primary MR undergoing cardiac surgery for other indications
- Surgery is a class IIa (reasonable) recommendation in:
  1. Severe MR with new-onset atrial fibrillation, even if asymptomatic.
  2. Asymptomatic severe MR with pulmonary hypertension (≥50 mm Hg at rest or ≥60 mm Hg during exercise).
  3. Asymptomatic severe MR secondary to flail leaflet.
  4. A recent study of early surgical intervention for severe MR secondary to a flail leaflet in patients with asymptomatic disease shows greater long-term survival and reduced rates of heart failure when compared with medical therapy alone.
     a. Asymptomatic severe MR with preserved LVEF (>60%) and size (<40 mm in end-systole) in whom the likelihood of successful repair without residual MR is >95% and operative mortality is <1%.
- Surgery is a class IIb recommendation in symptomatic patients (NYHA class III-IV) with severe MR with severe LV dysfunction or dilation (LVEF <30% or LV at end-systole >55 mm, respectively) in whom LV dysfunction is not the primary cause for the MR as well

as functional MR where it is secondary to LV dysfunction.
- Quantitative grading of MR is a powerful predictor of the clinical outcome of asymptomatic MR. In general, patients with regurgitant orifice areas of ≥40 mm^2 should be considered for prompt surgery, whereas those with orifices between 20 and 39 mm^2 can be followed closely.
- Percutaneous mitral valve repair methods are currently being investigated. The MitraClip device is now FDA approved for use in patients with significant symptomatic degenerative MR (>3+) who are too high risk for surgery. The device is a catheter-delivered clip that grasps and approximates the edges of the mitral leaflets at the origin of the regurgitant jet. Early data have not demonstrated a significant efficacy in MR reduction compared with surgical replacement; however, it has been shown to improve NYHA functional class and quality of life measures.
- Ischemic MR has been a source of controversy as to whether moderate or greater MR should be fixed at the time of revascularization with CABG. Based on the new 2015 CT surgery guidelines, mitral valve repair can be considered at the time of CABG in moderate MR or for other cardiac surgery such as aortic valve replacement (class IIb); mitral valve repair is reasonable for severe MR (class IIa) in the presence of a basal aneurysm or dyskinesis, significant leaflet tethering due to wall motion abnormalities, and moderate to severe LV remodeling (LV end diastolic diameter >65 mm).

DISPOSITION

Prognosis is generally good unless there is significant impairment of left ventricular function or significantly elevated pulmonary artery pressures. Most patients remain asymptomatic for many years (average interval from diagnosis to onset of symptoms is 16 yr). In patients with chronic severe MR, MR is commonly progressive, with onset of other symptoms or left ventricular dysfunction within 6 to 10 yr. However surgery should be advised well before the onset of symptoms in case of worsening LVEF and LV systolic dimensions and presence of pulmonary

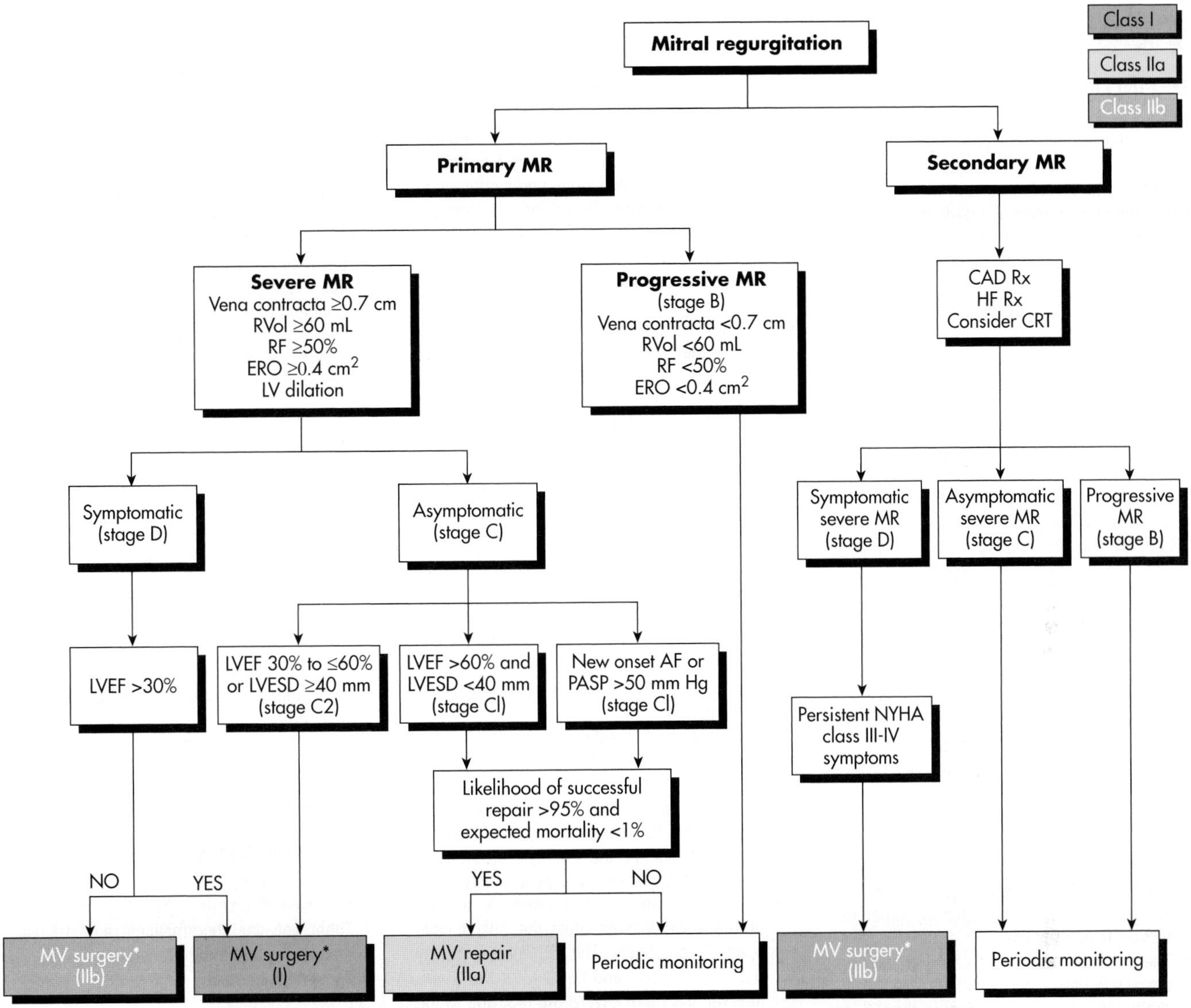

M

Class I
Class IIa
Class IIb

Mitral regurgitation

↓

Primary MR | **Secondary MR**

Primary MR:

Severe MR
Vena contracta ≥0.7 cm
RVol ≥60 mL
RF ≥50%
ERO ≥0.4 cm^2
LV dilation

Progressive MR
(stage B)
Vena contracta <0.7 cm
RVol <60 mL
RF <50%
ERO <0.4 cm^2

Secondary MR:
CAD Rx
HF Rx
Consider CRT

Severe MR →
- Symptomatic (stage D)
- Asymptomatic (stage C)

Symptomatic → LVEF >30%
- NO → MV surgery* (IIb)
- YES → MV surgery* (I)

Asymptomatic →
- LVEF 30% to ≤60% or LVESD ≥40 mm (stage C2) → MV surgery* (I)
- LVEF >60% and LVESD <40 mm (stage CI)
- New onset AF or PASP >50 mm Hg (stage CI)

LVEF >60% and New onset AF → **Likelihood of successful repair >95% and expected mortality <1%**
- YES → MV repair (IIa)
- NO → Periodic monitoring

Secondary MR branches:
- Symptomatic severe MR (stage D) → Persistent NYHA class III-IV symptoms → MV surgery* (IIb)
- Asymptomatic severe MR (stage C)
- Progressive MR (stage B) → Periodic monitoring

FIG. 2 Indications for surgery for MR. *Mitral valve repair is preferred over MVR when possible. *AF,* Atrial fibrillation; *CAD,* coronary artery disease; *CRT,* cardiac resynchronization therapy; *ERO,* effective regurgitant orifice; *HF,* heart failure; *LV,* left ventricular; *LVEF,* left ventricular ejection fraction; *LVESD,* left ventricular end-systolic dimension; *MR,* mitral regurgitation, *MV,* mitral valve; *MVR,* mitral valve replacement; *NYHA,* New York Heart Association; *PASP,* pulmonary artery systolic pressure; *RF,* regurgitant fraction; *RVol,* regurgitant volume; and *Rx,* therapy. (From Nishimura RA, et al. ACC/AHA guidelines for the management of patients with valvular heart disease. *J Am Coll Cardiol* 63(22):e57-e185, 2014.) http://dx.doi.org/10.1016/j.jacc.2014.02.536.)

hypertension or atrial fibrillation, all of which are poor prognostic signs.

REFERRAL

- Surgical referral in selected patients (see "Acute General Rx"). Emergency surgery is usually necessary in patients with acute MR caused by ruptured papillary muscle or chordae tendineae after myocardial infarction.
- Mitral valve repair can also be accomplished with percutaneous implantation of a MitraClip device in patients who are too high risk for surgery. The role of percutaneous repair of functional MR is still under active investigation.

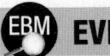

PEARLS & CONSIDERATIONS

COMMENTS

- Although vasodilators and other agents should be used to treat hypertension in patients with severe mitral regurgitation, there is no evidence that they will delay the need for eventual valve surgery, which is the definitive treatment for severe MR.
- In 2007, the AHA guidelines for prevention of infectious endocarditis were revised and routine antibiotic prophylaxis to undergo dental or other invasive procedures is no longer recommended, unless the patient has prior endocarditis.

EBM **EVIDENCE**

Available at www.expertconsult.com

SUGGESTED READINGS

Available at www.expertconsult.com

RELATED CONTENT

Mitral Regurgitation (Patient Information)

AUTHOR: **UYEN T. LAM, M.D.**

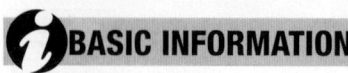

BASIC INFORMATION

DEFINITION

Mitral stenosis is a narrowing of the mitral valve orifice that prevents proper opening during diastole and obstruction of blood flow from the left atrium to the left ventricle. Due to thickening of the leaflets there is restricted movement. The cross section of a normal orifice measures 4 to 6 cm^2. Symptoms usually develop with exercise when the orifice measures <2.5 cm^2, and symptoms may develop at rest when the orifice is <1.5 cm^2.

SYNONYMS

MS

ICD-10CM CODES
I05.0	Rheumatic mitral stenosis
I05.2	Rheumatic mitral stenosis with insufficiency
I34.2	Nonrheumatic mitral (valve) stenosis
Q23.2	Congenital mitral stenosis

EPIDEMIOLOGY & DEMOGRAPHICS

- The predominant cause of mitral stenosis is rheumatic heart disease; however, the occurrence of mitral valve stenosis has decreased worldwide over the past 30 years (particularly in developed countries) as a result of declining incidence of rheumatic fever due to appropriate antibiotic use.
- Rheumatic heart disease has a predilection for the mitral valve, aortic valve, and to some extent the tricuspid valve.
- The incidence of MS is higher in women (2:1 female-to-male ratio).
- There is high prevalence of rheumatic heart disease in developing countries.
- Outbreaks of rheumatic fever in the U.S. are due to increased virulence of a streptococcal strain or enhanced immigration from where rheumatic heart disease is prevalent.

PHYSICAL FINDINGS & CLINICAL PRESENTATION

- Dyspnea is the most common symptom along with fatigue and decreased exercise capacity. These symptoms occur due to an inability to increase cardiac output, especially with exercise, and elevated pulmonary capillary wedge pressures, with resultant increase in pulmonary artery pressures.
- The left ventricle is unaffected in pure MS; however, MS often coexists with mitral regurgitation and occasionally with aortic valve dysfunction, both of which can cause left ventricular dysfunction.
- "Mitral facies" which are pinkish-purple patches on the cheek due to low cardiac output and vasoconstriction, usually indicate severe MS.
- Paroxysmal nocturnal dyspnea (PND) and orthopnea secondary to elevated left atrial pressure may occur.

- Acute pulmonary edema may occur after an increase in flow across the mitral valve secondary to an increase in cardiac output or heart rate (exertion, tachyarrhythmias, fever, anemia, etc.).
- Pulmonary hypertension that results from chronically elevated pulmonary capillary wedge pressures can lead to right ventricular (RV) dysfunction and signs and symptoms of right heart failure (hepatomegaly, pulsatile liver, peripheral edema, ascites).
- The left ventricle is typically "protected" in mitral stenosis and exists in a low-pressure state.
- Hemoptysis can be present secondary to rupture of thin-walled dilated bronchial veins due to an abrupt increase in left atrial pressure.
- Systemic embolic events are caused by left atrial thrombi. These are associated with atrial fibrillation 80% of the time, since mitral stenosis leads to left atrial enlargement, which is a predisposing factor for atrial arrhythmias.
- Atrial fibrillation is more prevalent in patients with more severe MS, increasing age, and other valvular abnormalities.
- Chest pain can be caused by RV pressure overload and/or concomitant coronary artery disease in up to 15% of patients.
- Irregularly irregular pulse caused by atrial fibrillation.
- Loud first heart sound (S$_1$) caused by delayed valve closure preceded by an opening snap and rapid rising left ventricular (LV) pressure.
- A low-pitched rumbling diastolic murmur is heard best at the apex. The intensity of the murmur is not related to the severity of the stenosis, but the duration is holodiastolic in severe MS.
- An opening snap (OS) caused by tensing of the valve leaflets after the cusps have opened completely. The OS follows S$_2$ by 0.03 to 0.14 sec, and the shorter the S$_2$-OS interval, the more severe the MS, due to the increasing left atrial pressures.
- Prominent A wave on the pulmonary capillary wedge pressure tracing. This is analogous to the prominent A wave seen in systemic venous pressure tracings with tricuspid stenosis.
- A diastolic thrill may be palpable at the apex, especially with the patient in the left lateral recumbent position.
- An RV lift may be palpable at the left sternal border secondary to RV hypertrophy and pulmonary hypertension.
- An accentuated P$_2$ and/or a soft, early diastolic decrescendo murmur *(Graham Steell murmur)* caused by pulmonary regurgitation may be present in patients with pulmonary hypertension (not specific for mitral stenosis).
- Hoarseness due to the enlargement of the left atrium compressing the recurrent laryngeal nerve.
- Straightening of the left heart border seen on chest radiography indicative of left atrial enlargement.
- Fig. 1 shows schematic representations of LV, aortic, and left atrial (LA) pressures, showing normal relationships and alterations with mild and severe MS.

ETIOLOGY

- Rheumatic fever (RF) is the predominant cause of MS. RF causes thickening of the leaflet tips, commissure fusion, and chordal shortening and fusion. This leads to the classic doming of the leaflets in diastole due to fusion of the leaflet tips at the commissures. Rheumatic fever involves the leaflet tips first with progression toward the annulus. This is opposite of mitral annular calcification, which typically starts in the annulus and proceeds out to the leaflet tips, leading to mitral stenosis in severe cases.
- Congenital defect (parachute valve) has the usual two mitral leaflets, but the chordae, instead of diverging to insert into two papillary muscles, converge into one major papillary muscle, which allows little mobility of the leaflets, as in cor triatriatum (heart with three atria), in which there is a thin membrane that obstructs the pulmonary vein flow and simulates mitral stenosis.
- Rare causes are severe mitral annular calcification usually seen in end-stage renal disease patients, endomyocardial fibroelastosis, malignant carcinoid syndrome, systemic lupus erythematosus, Whipple disease, Fabry disease, and rheumatoid arthritis.
- Atrial septal defect in association with rheumatic mitral stenosis is termed Lutembacher syndrome.
- Medications: methysergide

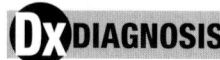

DIAGNOSIS

DIFFERENTIAL DIAGNOSIS

- Left atrial myxoma
- Ball valve thrombus
- Other valvular abnormalities (e.g., tricuspid stenosis, mitral regurgitation)
- Atrial septal defect

WORKUP

Physical examination and echocardiography

IMAGING STUDIES

- Echocardiography (Fig. 2):
  1. Two-dimensional echocardiogram can measure valve area by direct planimetry or calculate it by the Doppler pressure half-time method (this may be inaccurate in patients with concomitant diastolic dysfunction or aortic insufficiency and in patients who have recently undergone mitral valvuloplasty) or the continuity equation can be used to calculate the valve area. A valve area ≤1.5 cm^2 is consistent with severe MS (and ≤1.0 cm^2 with very severe MS). The transmitral gradient can also be calculated. A mean gradient of >10 mm Hg indicates severe MS, a gradient of 5 to 10 mm Hg is consistent with moderate MS, and 0 to 5 mm Hg is consistent with mild MS or no MS.
  2. Echocardiography will also show a markedly diminished E-to-F slope of the anterior mitral valve leaflet during diastole; there is also fusion of the commissures,

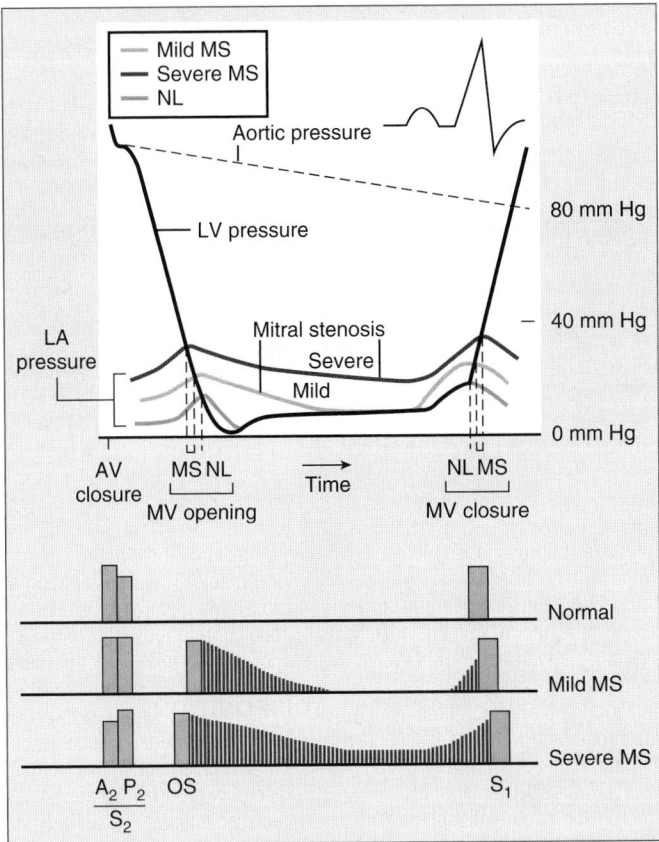

FIG. 1 Schematic representation of LV, aortic, and left atrial (LA) pressures, showing normal relationships and alterations with mild and severe MS. Corresponding classic auscultatory signs of MS are shown at the bottom. The higher left atrial v wave of severe MS causes earlier pressure crossover and earlier MV opening, leading to a shorter time interval between aortic valve (AV) closure and the opening snap (OS). The higher left atrial end-diastolic pressure with severe MS also results in later closure of the mitral valve. With severe MS, the diastolic rumble becomes longer and there is accentuation of the pulmonic component (P_2) of the second heart sound (S_2) in relation to the aortic component (A_2). (From Bonow R.O.: *Heart disease,* 9th ed, Philadelphia, 2012, Saunders.)

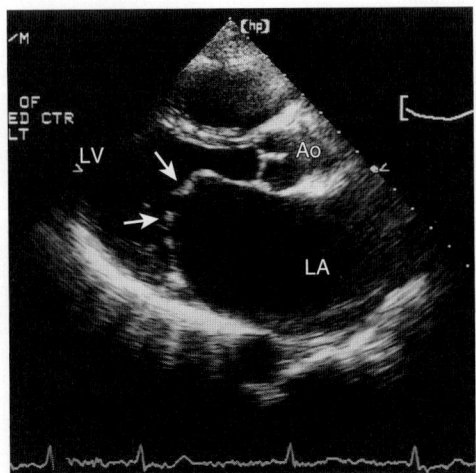

FIG. 2 Mitral stenosis. Parasternal long-axis view of a patient with mitral stenosis and a pliable non-calcified mitral valve leaflet. Note the "doming" motion of the mitral valve leaflets *(arrows)*. Valves with these morphologic features are excellent candidates for percutaneous balloon valvotomy. *Ao,* Aorta; *LA,* left atrium; *LV,* left ventricle. (From Zipes DP et al [eds]: *Braunwald's heart disease,* ed 7, Philadelphia, 2005, Saunders.)

resulting in "doming" of the leaflets during diastole.

3. Grading of leaflet thickness, mobility, calcification, and subvalvular thickening (Wilkins score) with a score of 0 to 4 for each characteristic can predict hemodynamic results and outcome of balloon mitral valvuloplasty (a low score of less than 8 is favorable for balloon valvuloplasty and a high score is unfavorable). A score above 8 would favor a surgical approach. In addition, mitral regurgitation that is greater than mild would preclude a balloon mitral valvuloplasty procedure.

4. Doppler echocardiography can be used to assess for pulmonary hypertension and to give an estimate of the pulmonary artery systolic pressure at rest and with exercise.

5. Patients with known mitral stenosis: a follow-up echocardiography is recommended to assess for pulmonary artery pressures and valve gradient (very severe MS with mitral valve area <1.0 cm² every year, severe MS with mitral valve area ≤1.5 cm² every 1 to 2 years, and progressive MS with mitral valve area >1.5 cm² every 3 to 5 years).

- Chest radiograph:
  1. Straightening of the left cardiac border caused by enlarged left atrium
  2. Left atrial enlargement on lateral chest radiograph
  3. Prominence of pulmonary arteries that indicates pulmonary hypertension
  4. Possible pulmonary congestion and edema (Kerley B lines)

- ECG:
  1. RV hypertrophy; right axis deviation caused by pulmonary hypertension
  2. Left atrial enlargement (broad, biphasic P waves in lead V1 and duration of P-waves >0.11 sec in lead II). This is termed "P-mitrale."
  3. Atrial fibrillation

- Cardiac catheterization:
  1. Allows the measurement of pulmonary artery pressure and transmitral pressure gradients at rest or with exercise (supine biking or raising weights with arms while lying supine).
  2. Allows the measurement of transmitral flow and calculation of the valve area.
  3. Is not routinely recommended for the evaluation of MS but is useful when the echocardiographic findings are nondiagnostic or discrepant with the clinical scenario.
  4. Cardiac catheterization in addition to echocardiography can be used to monitor the hemodynamics during a balloon mitral valvuloplasty procedure.

Rx TREATMENT

NONPHARMACOLOGIC THERAPY

Decrease level of activity in symptomatic patients and salt restriction if pulmonary congestion is present.

TABLE 1 Approaches to Mechanical Relief of Mitral Stenosis

Approach	Advantages	Disadvantages
Closed surgical valvotomy	Inexpensive Relatively simple Good hemodynamic results in selected patients Good long-term outcome	No direct visualization of valve Only feasible with flexible, noncalcified valves Contraindicated if MR >2+Surgical procedure with general anesthesia
Open surgical valvotomy	Visualization of valve allows directed valvotomy Concurrent annuloplasty for MR is feasible	Best results with flexible, noncalcified valves Surgical procedure with general anesthesia
Valve replacement	Feasible in all patients regardless of extent of valve calcification or severity of MR	Surgical procedure with general anesthesia Effect of loss of annular-papillary muscle continuity on LV function Prosthetic valve Chronic anticoagulation
Balloon mitral valvotomy	Percutaneous approach Local anesthesia Good hemodynamic results in selected patients Good long-term outcome	No direct visualization of valve Only feasible with flexible, noncalcified valves Contraindicated if MR >2+

LV, Left ventricular; *MR,* mitral regurgitation.
From Otto CM: *Valvular heart disease,* ed 2, Philadelphia, 2004, Saunders.

ACUTE GENERAL Rx
- Medical:
  1. Anticoagulation for the prevention of systemic embolic events in patients with MS and:
     1. Atrial fibrillation
     2. Prior embolic event
     3. Documented left atrial thrombus or left atrial appendage thrombus
  2. Ventricular rate control (to increase diastolic filling period) with beta-blockers, non-dihydropyridine calcium channel blockers, or digitalis and aggressive treatment of tachyarrhythmias.
  3. Treat congestive heart failure with loop diuretics and sodium restriction.
  4. Antibiotic prophylaxis to prevent recurrent rheumatic fever is usually not indicated unless presence of high-risk features such as prior endocarditis, prosthetic heart valves, valvulopathy of the transplanted heart, and certain cases of cyanotic congenital heart disease.
  5. Pregnancy in females with advanced MS may be poorly tolerated due to the hemodynamic changes such as increased cardiac output occurring in pregnancy. Mild to moderate MS may be tolerated in pregnancy with medical therapy alone.

- Table 1 summarizes approaches to mechanical relief of mitral stenosis.
- Percutaneous mitral balloon commissurotomy (PMBC) is the therapy of choice for symptomatic patients with severe MS (valve area ≤1.5 cm^2) with a favorable valvuloplasty score, minimal or no mitral regurgitation, and no left atrial thrombus. PMBC is reasonable for asymptomatic patients with very severe MS (mitral valve area ≤1.0 cm^2) and favorable valve morphology in the absence of left atrial thrombus or moderate to severe MR (class IIa indication). PMBC is also considered the procedure of choice in pregnant women with rheumatic MS and in NYHA class III to IV heart failure and/or unresponsive to adequate medical treatment. In addition, it may be considered for severely symptomatic (NYHA class III/IV) patients with very severe MS (mitral valve area ≤1.5 cm^2) who are not candidates for surgery or are at high risk for surgery, even if they have suboptimal valve anatomy (class IIb indication).
- Mitral valve surgery is indicated for patients with moderate to severe symptomatic MS when PMBC is not available or is contraindicated (valvuloplasty score greater than or equal to 8) or the valve is calcified, when MR is more than mild, when left atrial thrombus

is present, and when the surgical risk is acceptable. The surgical approaches include closed mitral valvotomy, open valvotomy and repair (preferred), and mitral valve replacement when repair is not possible.

DISPOSITION
- Prognosis is generally good except in patients with chronic pulmonary hypertension.
- Operative mortality rates for mitral valve replacement are 1% to 5% at most institutions.

SUGGESTED READING
Available at www.expertconsult.com

RELATED CONTENT
Mitral Stenosis (Patient Information)

AUTHORS: **DHAVAL KOLTE, M.D., PH.D.,** and **ARAVIND RAO KOKKIRALA, M.D.**

ⓘ BASIC INFORMATION

DEFINITION

Mitral valve prolapse (MVP) is the bulging of one or both of the mitral valve leaflets ≥2 mm above the annular plane into the left atrium during systole. MVP syndrome refers to a constellation of MVP and associated symptoms (e.g., autonomic dysfunction, palpitations) or other physical abnormalities (e.g., pectus excavatum). Table 1 describes a classification of mitral valve prolapse.

SYNONYMS

MVP
Mitral click murmur syndrome
Barlow's syndrome

ICD-10CM CODES
I34.1 Nonrheumatic mitral (valve) prolapse
I34.0 Nonrheumatic mitral (valve) insufficiency

EPIDEMIOLOGY & DEMOGRAPHICS

- MVP can be found by echocardiogram in 1% to 2.4% of the general population, with some studies suggesting that it is more common in women than in men.
- Increased incidence is seen with autoimmune thyroid disorders, Ehlers-Danlos syndrome, Marfan syndrome, osteogenesis imperfecta, pseudoxanthoma elasticum, pectus excavatum, anorexia nervosa, and bulimia.
- Compared to men, women with MVP have less posterior prolapse (22% vs. 31%), less flail (2% vs. 8%), more leaflet thickening (32% vs. 28%), and less frequent severe mitral regurgitation (MR) (10% vs. 23%).

TABLE 1   Classification of Mitral Valve Prolapse

Mitral Valve Prolapse Syndrome
- Younger age (20-50 yr)
- Predominantly female
- Click or click-murmur on physical examination
- Thin leaflets with systolic displacement on echocardiography
- Associated with low blood pressure, orthostatic hypotension, palpitations
- Benign long-term course

Myxomatous Mitral Valve Disease
- Older age (40-70 yr)
- Predominantly male
- Thickened, redundant valve leaflets
- Mitral regurgitation on physical exam and echocardiography
- High likelihood of progressive disease requiring mitral valve surgery

Secondary Mitral Valve Prolapse
- Marfan syndrome
- Hypertrophic cardiomyopathy
- Ehlers-Danlos syndrome
- Other connective tissue diseases

Modified from Otto CM: *Valvular heart disease,* ed 2, Philadelphia, 2004, Saunders, p. 369.

- Although MVP is more common in women than men, men more often develop severe regurgitation requiring surgical intervention.

PHYSICAL FINDINGS & CLINICAL PRESENTATION

- Mid to late systolic click, heard best at the apex. Midsystolic click is caused by degeneration of the valve resulting in an abnormal ratio between the length of the mitral apparatus and left ventricle (LV) during contraction. When the valve prolapses, it gets caught by the subvalvular structures, causing an abrupt halt that creates the click.
- If regurgitation is present, a crescendo mid to late systolic murmur may be heard that worsens with standing and Valsalva's maneuver.
- Timing of click within the cardiac cycle varies with loading conditions within the left ventricle (i.e., may occur earlier with standing or Valsalva and later with squatting or expiration).
- May be associated with small anteroposterior chest diameter, scoliosis, pectus excavatum, or low BMI.
- Most patients with MVP are asymptomatic; symptoms, if present, consist primarily of chest pain, palpitations, fatigue, dyspnea, and anxiety.
- Neurologic abnormalities (e.g., transient ischemic attack [TIA] or stroke) are rare.
- A spectrum of arrhythmias, mainly paroxysmal supraventricular tachycardia and atrial and ventricular premature beats, etc., is also observed with mitral valve prolapse. There is also an increased association with Wolff-Parkinson-White syndrome and QT prolongation.

ETIOLOGY

- Myxomatous degeneration of connective tissue within mitral valve, usually involving multiple leaflet segments. In contrast, fibroelastic deficiency of single leaflet segment develops in elderly patients.
- Congenital deformity of mitral valve and supportive structures.
- Secondary to other disorders of connective tissue such as Ehlers-Danlos, Marfan, or pseudoxanthoma elasticum; association with other connective tissue disorders suggests MVP result of defective embryogenesis in cells of mesenchymal origin.

Ⓓ DIAGNOSIS

DIFFERENTIAL DIAGNOSIS

- Other valvular abnormalities (especially mitral regurgitation [MR])
- Anxiety/panic disorders
- Pulmonary embolism
- Atypical chest pain

WORKUP

- Medical history and physical examination, with increased suspicion in patients with other findings of connective tissue disorder.
- Two- or three-dimensional echocardiography in patients with a systolic click or murmur on careful auscultation.

- Cardiac MRI is an emerging tool for the evaluation and diagnosis of MVP but has not yet been independently validated.
- ECG is most often normal but may show nonspecific ST-T wave changes, prolonged QT interval, or prominent Q waves.

IMAGING STUDIES

Echocardiography (Fig. 1) shows one or more leaflets prolapsing >2 mm into the left atrium during systole in a long axis view. Mitral leaflets may be thickened (>5 mm) with myxomatous degeneration. MR is typically present, though sometimes only during exertion. If moderate or severe MR is present, findings of dilated left atrium, LV dilation and/or dysfunction, and elevated estimated RV systolic pressures may also be present. There is an increased incidence of secundum-type atrial septal defects (ASDs) in patients with MVP, which may also be identified with echocardiography.

℞ TREATMENT

NONPHARMACOLOGIC THERAPY

Avoidance of stimulants (e.g., caffeine, nicotine) in patients with palpitations. Sometimes, reassurance is sufficient to reduce the severity of symptoms in many patients.

ACUTE GENERAL Rx

β-blockers may be tried in symptomatic patients (e.g., palpitations, chest pain) to decrease the heart

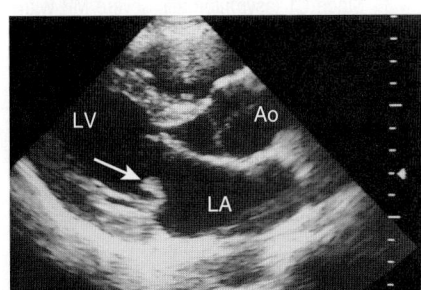
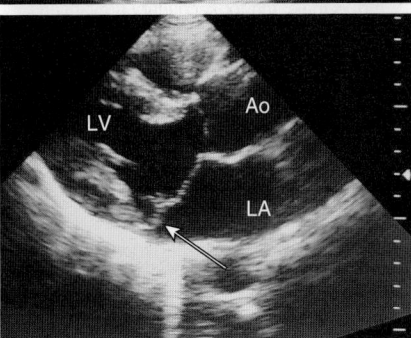

FIG. 1 Mitral valve prolapse. Parasternal long-axis view in diastole *(top)* and systole *(bottom)* in a patient with mitral valve prolapse and myxomatous changes. In the *upper panel,* note the open mitral valve and the diffuse thickening of the posterior mitral valve leaflet *(arrow).* The *lower panel* was recorded in systole. Note that both leaflets prolapse behind the plane of the mitral valve annulus. The prolapse of the posterior leaflet is somewhat more prominent *(arrow). Ao,* Aorta; *LA,* left atrium; *LV,* left ventricle. (From Zipes DP et al [eds]: *Braunwald's heart disease,* ed 7, Philadelphia, 2005, Saunders.)

TABLE 2 Predictors of Clinical Outcome in Mitral Valve Prolapse

Predictor	Survival	Valve Surgery	Arrhythmias or Sudden Death	Endocarditis
Age	+++	+++	–	–
Gender	++	++	–	–
Leaflet thickness or redundancy	+++	+++	++++	++++
Severity of mitral regurgitation	++++	++++	++++	++++
Systolic click	+	–	–	–
Left ventricular dilation	+	++++	++	–
Left atrial dilation	–	++	+	–

Symbols indicate the relative predictive value of each variable for the listed clinical outcomes on a scale of no predictive value (–) to strongly predictive (++++).
From Bonow RO et al: *Braunwald's heart disease: a textbook of cardiovascular medicine*, Philadelphia, 2012, Saunders.

rate and contractility, thus potentially decreasing the stretch on the prolapsing valve leaflets.

CHRONIC Rx

Monitoring for complications:
- Mitral regurgitation (most common complication); on rare occasion may occur acutely due to rupture of chordae tendineae.
- Routine echocardiographic monitoring is indicated at the following intervals with patients with evidence of mitral regurgitation:
  1. Stage B with mild regurgitation—every 3 to 5 years.
  2. Stage B with moderate regurgitation—every 1 to 2 years.
  3. Stage C1 (asymptomatic severe MR without LV dysfunction)—every 6 to 12 months.
- Bacterial endocarditis (risk is three to eight times that of the general population); higher risk in patients with concomitant regurgitation. However, routine antibiotic prophylaxis is not recommended.
- TIA or stroke caused by embolic phenomena (from fibrin and platelet thrombi) in patients with thickened leaflets; risk in young patients is <0.05% per year. If present, aspirin (75-325 mg) is indicated for secondary prevention.

- Cardiac arrhythmias with the vast majority being supraventricular and benign.
- Sudden death (rare); most often associated with acute flail leaflets or caused by ventricular arrhythmias associated with other structural heart disease.
- The incidence of complications of MVP is very low (<1% per year). Mitral leaflet thickness is ≤0.5 mm, young patients <45 yr, and in the absence of mitral systolic murmur or MR on Doppler echocardiography. Table 2 lists variables that are predictors of favorable clinical outcome in mitral valve prolapse.
- Risk factors that predict higher risk of complications are presence of moderate to severe MR, LV ejection fraction <50%, LA dimension >40 mm, age >50 years.

SURGICAL REFERRAL

Surgical referral may be necessary in patients who develop progressive MR with surgical indications as per guidelines for valvular heart disease (see topic on mitral regurgitation).

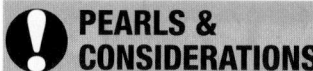

PEARLS & CONSIDERATIONS

COMMENTS
- Recent studies suggest that the prevalence of MVP and its propensity to cause symptoms and serious complications have been overestimated in the past.
- The relationship between MVP syndrome and sudden cardiac death is unclear. The best evidence suggests that there is only a slight risk in subsets of patients with MVP who have severe MR, severe valvular deformity, complex ventricular arrhythmias, QT prolongation, and a history of syncope.
- Asymptomatic patients with MVP and mild or no MR can be evaluated clinically every 3 to 5 yr. High-risk patients (those with symptoms, arrhythmias, or significant regurgitation) should undergo a follow-up examination once a year.
- In 2007, the AHA guidelines for prevention of infectious endocarditis were revised and prophylactic antibiotics are no longer recommended for patients with MVP without previous endocarditis.

PATIENT & FAMILY EDUCATION
www.themitralvalve.org

SUGGESTED READING
Available at www.expertconsult.com

RELATED CONTENT
Mitral Valve Prolapse (Patient Information)

AUTHOR: **UYEN T. LAM, M.D.**

BASIC INFORMATION

DEFINITION

Molar pregnancy (hydatidiform mole) is a premalignant gestational disorder and is included in the spectrum of disorders characterized as gestational trophoblastic disease. Molar pregnancies are classified as complete or partial based on morphologic and pathologic examination. Both complete and partial molar pregnancies have an abnormal placenta with enlargement and swelling of the chorionic villi and hyperplasia of the villous trophoblastic cells. Most molar pregnancies are complete and are characterized by generalized hydropic villous changes with no fetal tissue. Partial moles are characterized by a mixture of large hydropic villi and normal placental tissue and often have fetal tissue present.

The risk of malignant sequelae (gestational trophoblastic neoplasia) for a complete mole is 6% to 32% and for a partial mole is less than 5%.

SYNONYMS

Hydatiform mole

ICD-10CM CODES
O01.0	Classical hydatidiform mole
O01.1	Incomplete and partial hydatidiform mole
O01.9	Hydatidiform mole, unspecified

EPIDEMIOLOGY & DEMOGRAPHICS

INCIDENCE:
- 1/1500 pregnancies in the U.S.

PREDOMINANT SEX AND AGE:
- Females of reproductive age, highest rates at extremes of reproductive ages

RISK FACTORS:
- Extremes of reproductive age (<21 and >40 years)
- Previous molar pregnancy
- History of spontaneous abortion
- Use of combined oral contraceptives

PHYSICAL FINDINGS & CLINICAL PRESENTATION

Complete molar pregnancy:
- 80% to 90% present with vaginal bleeding at 6 to 16 weeks' gestational age
- 28% with uterine enlargement greater than expected for gestational age
- 8% with hyperemesis gravidarum
- 1% with pregnancy-induced hypertension in the first or second trimester
- 15% to 25% with bilateral theca lutein cysts
- 15% will have a beta hCG >100,000 mIU/ml
- <10% with anemia

Partial molar pregnancy:
- 90% present with an incomplete or missed abortion
- 75% present with vaginal bleeding
- <10% will have a beta hCG of >100,000 mIU/ml

ETIOLOGY

Complete molar pregnancy
- Fertilization of an oocyte with absent or inactive maternal chromosomes and duplication of paternal chromosomes (85%-90% are 46, XX) or fertilization of an empty oocyte with 2 sperm (46, XY or XX).
- Diffuse villous enlargement and trophoblastic proliferation with no development of a fetus.

Partial molar pregnancy
- Fertilization of a normal oocyte with 2 sperm (usually 69, XXY or 69, XXX)
- Focal villous edema and trophoblastic proliferation with identifiable fetus

DIAGNOSIS

DIFFERENTIAL DIAGNOSIS

Complete mole, partial mole, ectopic pregnancy, abortion (incomplete or spontaneous), normal intrauterine pregnancy

WORKUP

- Pelvic exam to evaluate for uterine size and bleeding
- Blood pressure to assess for gestational hypertension or preeclampsia (systolic blood pressure >140 or diastolic blood pressure >90)
- Fig. 1 describes an algorithm for the diagnosis and management of molar pregnancy

LABORATORY TESTS

- Quantitative beta human chorionic growth hormone (beta hCG); significantly elevated levels >100,000 will raise suspicion for molar pregnancy
- Complete blood count (CBC) to assess for acute anemia from vaginal bleeding
- Comprehensive metabolic panel to evaluate for renal or liver disease
- TSH to evaluate for hyperthyroidism

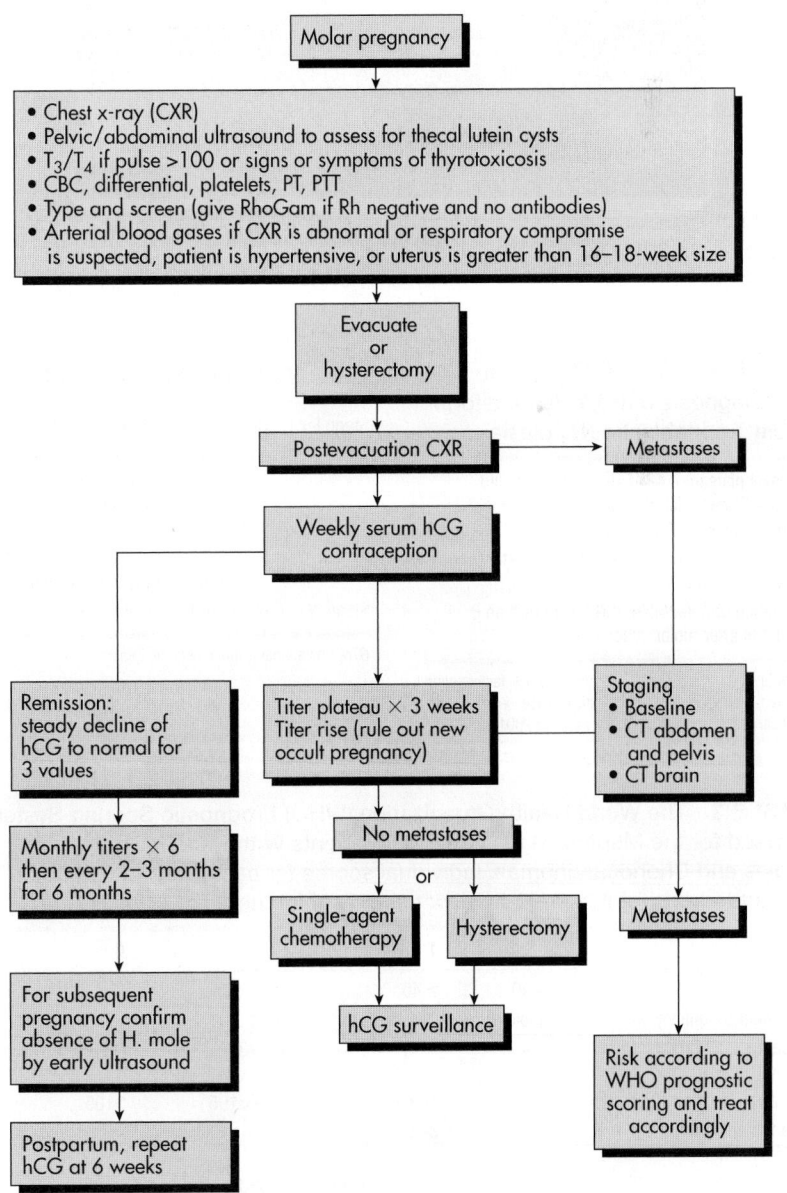

FIG. 1 Algorithm for the management of molar pregnancy. (From Gabbe SG: *Obstetrics*, ed 6, Philadelphia, 2012, WB Saunders.)

- Urinalysis for proteinuria to evaluate for preeclampsia
- Type and screen to evaluate Rh and to prepare for surgery

IMAGING STUDIES

- Pelvic ultrasound (Fig. E2)
  1. Complete moles in the first trimester will demonstrate a complex, echogenic, intrauterine mass containing many small cystic spaces that are secondary to swollen chorionic villi and no identifiable fetus. This is the classic "snowstorm" appearance (Fig. 3).
  2. Partial mole will show a thickened, hydropic placenta with fetal parts.
- Baseline chest x-ray to use for comparison if malignant trophoblastic disease develops

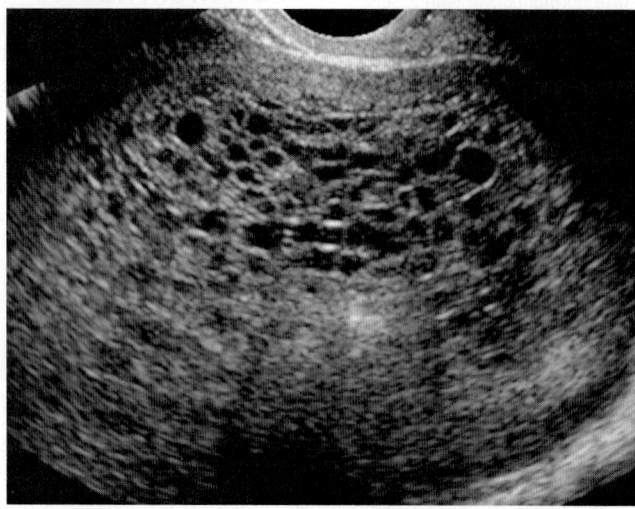

FIG. 3 Complete molar pregnancy: classic appearance. Transabdominal scan shows a vesicular echogenic mass distending the endometrium. The mass is filled with innumerable uniformly distributed cystic spaces that corresponded to hydropic chorionic villi at pathology. (From Rumack CM et al: *Diagnostic ultrasound*, ed 4, Philadelphia, 2011, Mosby.)

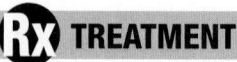 **TREATMENT**

NONPHARMACOLOGIC THERAPY

Surgical uterine evacuation with dilatation and curettage (D&C)

ACUTE GENERAL Rx

D&C, Rh immune globulin if Rh negative

CHRONIC Rx & DISPOSITION

If pathology results are consistent with complete or partial mole, patients must be followed to evaluate for trophoblastic neoplasia. 15% to 20% of complete moles and 1% to 5% of partial moles will develop into trophoblastic neoplasia. Quantitative beta hCG should be followed weekly until three consecutive results show normal levels. After that, check quantitative beta hCG every month for a total of 6 months. Patients should remain on reliable contraception during this time to prevent confusion from a rising beta hCG in the case of a new pregnancy.

Specific criteria by beta hCG have been established by FIGO for diagnosis of postmolar gestational trophoblastic disease (see Tables 1 through 3).

REFERRAL

- If there is concern for a molar pregnancy, the patient should be managed by a gynecologist for uterine evacuation and follow-up.
- If there is a plateau or rise of the beta hCG during follow-up, the patient should be referred to a gynecologic oncologist for treatment with chemotherapy.

SUGGESTED READINGS

Available at www.expertconsult.com

RELATED CONTENT

Spontaneous Miscarriage (Related Key Topic)
Vaginal Bleeding During Pregnancy (Related Key Topic)

AUTHORS: **SHIVANI SHAH, M.D.,** and **PATRICIA W. LO, M.D.**

TABLE 1 The 2002 Criteria for the Diagnosis of Post Hydatidiform Mole Trophoblastic Neoplasia

HCG-level plateau of 4 values ±10% recorded over a 3-week duration (days 1, 7, 14, and 21)

An hCG-level increase of more than 10% of 3 values recorded over a 2-week duration (days 1, 7, and 14)

Persistence of detectable hCG for more than 6 months after molar evacuation

Kohorn EI: The new FIGO 2000 staging and risk factor scoring system for gestational trophoblastic disease: description and critical assessment, *Int J Gynecol Cancer* 2001;11:73–77.

TABLE 2 FIGO Staging of GTN

Stage I	Disease confined to the uterus.
Stage II	GTN extends outside the uterus but is limited to the genital structures (adnexa, vagina, broad ligament).
Stage III	GTN extends to the lungs with or without genital tract involvement.
Stage IV	All other metastatic sites.

GTN, gestational trophoblastic neoplasia.

TABLE 3 The World Health Organization (WHO) Prognostic Scoring System Is Used for the Medical Management of Patients With Partial, Complete Moles and Choriocarcinomas. Individual scores for each prognostic factor are added up. Total score 0-6 = low risk; >7 = high risk.

Figo Scoring	0	1	2	4
Age	<40	≥ 40	-	-
Antecedent pregnancy	Mole	Abortion	Term	-
Interval months from index pregnancy	<4	4-<7	7-<13	≥ 13
Pretreatment serum HCG (IU/L)	<103	103-<104	104-<105	≥105
Large tumor size (including uterus) cm	<3	3-<5	≥5	-
Site of metastases	Lung	Spleen, kidney	Gastrointestinal	Liver, brain
Previous failed chemotherapy	-	-	Single drug	2 or more drugs

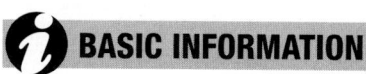

BASIC INFORMATION

DEFINITION

Molluscum contagiosum is a poxvirus infection characterized by discrete skin lesions with central umbilication.

SYNONYMS

MC

ICD-10CM CODES
B08.1 Molluscum contagiosum

EPIDEMIOLOGY & DEMOGRAPHICS

- Molluscum contagiosum spreads by autoinoculation, scratching, or touching a lesion.
- It usually occurs in young children. It is also common in sexually active adults and patients with HIV infection.
- Incubation period varies between 4 and 8 wk.
- Spontaneous resolution in immunocompetent patients can occur after several months.

PHYSICAL FINDINGS & CLINICAL PRESENTATION

- The individual lesion appears initially as a small (2-3 mm), flesh-colored, firm, smooth-surfaced papule with subsequent central umbilication. Lesions are frequently grouped (Fig. 1). The size of each lesion generally varies from 2 to 6 mm in diameter.
- Typical distribution in children involves the face, extremities, and trunk. Mucous membranes are spared.
- Distribution in adults generally involves pubic and genital areas.
- Erythema and scaling at the periphery of the lesions may be present as a result of scratching or hypersensitivity reaction.
- Lesions are not present on the palms and soles.

ETIOLOGY

Viral infection of epithelial cells caused by a poxvirus, molluscum contagiosum

DIAGNOSIS

Diagnosis is usually established by the clinical appearance of the lesions (distribution and central umbilication). A magnifying lens can be used to observe the central umbilication. If necessary, the diagnosis can be confirmed by removing a typical lesion with a curette and examining the content on a slide after adding potassium hydroxide and gentle heating. Staining with toluidine blue will identify viral inclusions.

DIFFERENTIAL DIAGNOSIS

- Verruca plana (flat warts): no central umbilication, not dome shaped, irregular surface, can involve palms and soles
- Herpes simplex: lesions become rapidly umbilicated
- Varicella: blisters and vesicles are present
- Folliculitis: no central umbilication, presence of hair piercing the pustule or papule
- Cutaneous cryptococcosis in AIDS patients: budding yeasts will be present on cytologic examination of the lesions
- Basal cell carcinoma: multiple lesions are absent
- Cellulitis

WORKUP

Careful examination of the papules

LABORATORY TESTS

Generally not indicated in children. Screening for other sexually transmitted diseases is recommended in all cases of genital molluscum contagiosum.

TREATMENT

GENERAL THERAPY

- Therapy is individualized depending on number of lesions, immune status, and patient's age and preference.
- Observation for spontaneous resolution is reasonable in patients with few, small, nonirritated, and nonspreading lesions. Genital lesions should be treated in all sexually active patients.
- Liquid nitrogen cryotherapy.
- Carbon dioxide laser.
- Curettage after pretreatment of the area with combination prilocaine 2.5% with lidocaine 2.5% cream (EMLA) for anesthesia is useful for treatment of a few lesions. Curettage should be avoided in cosmetically sensitive areas because scarring may develop.
- Treatments with liquid nitrogen therapy in combination with curettage are effective in older patients who do not object to some discomfort.
- Application of cantharidin 0.7% to individual lesions covered with clear tape will result in blistering over 24 hr and possible clearing without scarring. This medication should be avoided on facial lesions.
- Other treatment measures include use of imiquimod cream or tretinoin 0.025% gel or 0.1% cream at bedtime, daily use of salicylic acid (Occlusal) at bedtime, and use of laser therapy.
- Trichloroacetic acid peel generally repeated every 2 wk for several weeks is useful in immunocompromised patients with extensive lesions.

DISPOSITION

Most patients respond well to the therapeutic modalities listed previously. Spontaneous resolution can occur after 6 to 9 mo in some immunocompetent patients.

REFERRAL

To dermatology when diagnosis is in doubt or in patients with extensive lesions

PEARLS & CONSIDERATIONS

COMMENTS

Genital molluscum contagiosum in children may be indicative of sexual abuse.

RELATED CONTENT

Molluscum Contagiosum (Patient Information)

AUTHOR: **FRED F. FERRI, M.D.**

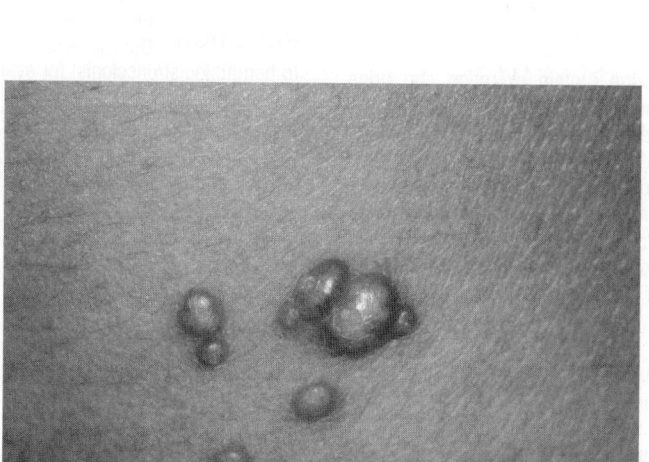

FIG. 1 Grouped molluscum. (From Kliegman RM et al: *Nelson textbook of pediatrics,* ed 19, Philadelphia, 2011, Saunders.)

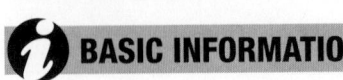 **BASIC INFORMATION**

DEFINITION

MGUS is a premalignant disorder characterized by the clonal expansions of plasma cells that produce monoclonal immunoglobulins or immunoglobulin fragments. The term "monoclonal gammopathy of undetermined significance" (MGUS) is defined by the presence of a serum monoclonal (M) protein less than 3 g/dL and clonal plasma cells less than 10% in the bone marrow. In addition, there must be no evidence of end organ dysfunctions such as renal insufficiency, anemia, hypercalcemia, or bony lesions on skeletal surveys (Table 1).

SYNONYMS

- MGUS
- Non-IgM MGUS
- IgM MGUS
- Light chain MGUS

ICD-10CM CODES
D47.2 Monoclonal gammopathy of
undetermined significance (MGUS)

EPIDEMIOLOGY & DEMOGRAPHICS

INCIDENCE: In the U.S., the estimated age-adjusted incidence of MGUS is higher in men than in women. The annual incidence of MGUS in men is 120 per 100,000 at age 50 yr and increases to 530 per 100,000 at age 80 yr. The incidence for women is lower at 60 per 100,000 at age 50 yr and 370 per 100,000 at age 80 yr.

PREVALENCE: The prevalence of MGUS is associated with increasing age; approximately 1.5% of persons older than 50 yr and 3.0% of persons older than 70 yr have an elevated M protein level without end organ dysfunctions. Studies have shown that when first clinically recognized, MGUS is most likely to have been present undetected for a median duration of more than 10 yr. The prevalence of MGUS is also higher in African Americans. In one study from North Carolina, there was an almost threefold increase in prevalence among the African American population at 8.6% versus 3.6% among the Caucasian population.

PREDOMINANT SEX AND AGE: The median age at diagnosis is about 70 yr. Prevalence is higher in men than in women at any given age.

RISK FACTORS: Race (African American), older age, male sex, or exposure to pesticides. Also, shared environmental and/or genetic defects play an important role, since the relative risk of MGUS in relatives of multiple myeloma or MGUS patients is increased twofold to threefold. The risk of progression into multiple myeloma or related disorders is 1% per year.

PHYSICAL FINDINGS & CLINICAL PRESENTATION

- MGUS typically is detected after a routine blood test reveals an elevated total protein concentration and is a common finding in medical practice.
- Patients are asymptomatic.
- Physical exam is normal.

ETIOLOGY

- The mechanism is unknown, and most cases are sporadic. The cause of malignant transformation of MGUS into multiple myeloma is still not well understood. A variety of factors such as genetic predisposition, cytokine releases, and bone marrow angiogenesis may play a role in the progression of MGUS into multiple myeloma.
- Characterized by a rearrangement of immunoglobulin genes resulting in the production of a monoclonal protein.

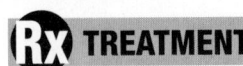 **DIAGNOSIS**

DIFFERENTIAL DIAGNOSIS

- Smoldering myeloma (Table E2)
- Multiple myeloma
- Waldenström's agammaglobulinemia
- Secondary monoclonal gammopathies
  - Chronic liver disease
  - Rheumatologic diseases
  - Chronic myelomonocytic leukemia
  - Chronic neutrophilic leukemia
  - Lichen myxedematosus
- Pyoderma gangrenosum
- AL amyloidosis
- Idiopathic Bence Jones proteinuria

LABORATORY TESTS

- Protein studies with serum free light chain assay
- Serum protein electrophoresis (Fig. E1)
  - IgG most common, followed by IgM and IgA
- 24-hour urine protein excretion and urine electrophoresis
- Serum and urine immunofixation
- Determination of serum free light chain ratio (kappa and lambda free light chains)
- Hemoglobin
- Serum calcium and creatinine
- Examination of the bone marrow aspirate only when clinically indicated

IMAGING STUDIES

- Skeletal survey
- Bone mineral density resting at baseline (MGUS is associated with increased risk of osteoporosis)

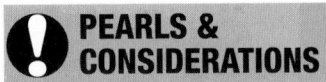 **TREATMENT**

1. Risk stratification
   - Low risk: serum M protein <1.5 g/dL, IgG subtype, normal genetics, free light chain ratio between 0.26 and 1.65. Absolute risk of progression (ARP) at 20 years is 5%.
   - Low-intermediate risk: any 1 factor abnormal. ARP at 20 years is 21%.
   - High-intermediate risk: any 2 factors abnormal. ARP at 20 years is 37%.
   - High risk: more than 3 factors abnormal. ARP at 20 years is 58%.
2. Follow-up by risk category
   - Patients with MGUS should be tested again within 4 to 6 months from the time of first diagnosis to exclude evolving multiple myeloma. Those with low-risk MGUS can be followed up every 1 to 2 yr, whereas those with intermediate- or high-risk MGUS need to be followed up at least annually for life or until they develop a life-expectancy-threatening condition.
3. Reevaluation consists of:
   - Serum protein electrophoresis
   - 24-hour urine protein excretion
   - Hemoglobin
   - Serum creatinine and calcium
   - Careful history and physical examination to look for signs and symptoms known to evolve from MGUS

DISPOSITION

- Risk of myeloma at 25 yr is 30%.
- Annual risk of transformation to myeloma depends on type of M protein:
  - Immunoglobulin MGUS: 1% per year
  - Light-chain MGUS: 0.3% per year
- Risk of infection (bacterial and viral) is twofold compared with healthy controls
- Increased risk of mortality from bacterial infections

REFERRAL

To hematologist/oncologist for evaluation

PEARLS & CONSIDERATIONS

- Approximately 55% of 70-yr-old patients diagnosed as having MGUS have had the condition for more than 10 yr.
- Most patients with MGUS should be monitored every 6 to 12 mo for signs and symptoms of progression.
- There is no indicated treatment.

SUGGESTED READINGS
Available at www.expertconsult.com

AUTHORS: **DONNY V. HUYNH, M.D.,** and **BHARTI RATHORE, M.D.**

TABLE 1 Disease Definitions for the Monoclonal Gammopathies: MGUS and Related Disorders

Type of Monoclonal Gammopathy	Premalignancy with a Low Risk of Progression (1%-2% per year)	Premalignancy with a High Risk of Progression (10% per year)	Malignancy
IgG and IgA (non-IgM) monoclonal gammopathies*	**Non-IgM MGUS** All 3 criteria must be met: Serum monoclonal protein <3 g/dl Clonal bone marrow plasma cells <10%, and Absence of end-organ damage such as hypercalcemia, renal insufficiency, anemia, and bone lesions (CRAB) that can be attributed to the plasma cell proliferative disorder	**Smoldering multiple myeloma** Both criteria must be met: Serum monoclonal protein (IgG or IgA) ≥3 g/dl and/or clonal bone marrow plasma cells ≥10%, and Absence of end-organ damage such as lytic bone lesions, anemia, hypercalcemia, or renal failure that can be attributed to a plasma cell proliferative disorder	**Multiple myeloma** All 3 criteria must be met except as noted: Clonal bone marrow plasma cells ≥10% Presence of serum and/or urinary monoclonal protein (except in patients with true nonsecretory multiple myeloma), and Evidence of end-organ damage that can be attributed to the underlying plasma cell proliferative disorder, specifically Hypercalcemia: serum calcium >11.5 mg/dL or Renal insufficiency: serum creatinine >2 mg/dL or estimated creatinine clearance <40 mL/min Anemia: normochromic, normocytic with a hemoglobin value of >2 g/dL below the lower limit of normal or a hemoglobin value <10 g/dL Bone lesions: lytic lesions or severe osteopenia attributed to a plasma cell proliferative disorder or pathologic fractures
IgM monoclonal gammopathies	**IgM MGUS†** All 3 criteria must be met: Serum monoclonal protein <3 g/dl Clonal bone marrow lymphoplasmacytic cells <10%, and Absence of end-organ damage such as anemia, constitutional symptoms, hyperviscosity, lymphadenopathy, or hepatosplenomegaly that can be attributed to the underlying lymphoproliferative disorder	**Smoldering Waldenström macroglobulinemia** Both criteria must be met: Serum IgM monoclonal protein ≥3 g/dl and/or bone marrow lymphoplasmacytic infiltration ≥10%, and No evidence of anemia, constitutional symptoms, hyperviscosity, lymphadenopathy, or hepatosplenomegaly that can be attributed to the underlying lymphoproliferative disorder	**Waldenström macroglobulinemia** All criteria must be met: IgM monoclonal gammopathy (regardless of the size of the M-protein), and ≥10% bone marrow lymphoplasmacytic infiltration (usually intratrabecular) by small lymphocytes that exhibit plasmacytoid or plasma cell differentiation and a typical immunophenotype (e.g., surface IgM+, CD5+/−, CD10−, CD19+, CD20+, CD23−) that satisfactorily excludes other lymphoproliferative disorders including chronic lymphocytic leukemia and mantle cell lymphoma Evidence of anemia, constitutional symptoms, hyperviscosity, lymphadenopathy, or hepatosplenomegaly that can be attributed to the underlying lymphoproliferative disorder. **IgM myeloma** All criteria must be met: Symptomatic monoclonal plasma cell proliferative disorder characterized by a serum IgM monoclonal protein regardless of size Presence of 10% plasma cells on bone marrow biopsy Presence of lytic bone lesions related to the underlying plasma cell disorder and/or translocation t(11;14) on fluorescence in situ hybridization
Light-chain monoclonal gammopathies	**Light-chain MGUS** All criteria must be met: Abnormal FLC ratio (<0.26 or >1.65) Increased level of the appropriate involved light-chain (increased kappa FLC in patients with ratio >1.65 and increased lambda FLC in patients with ratio <0.26) No immunoglobulin heavy-chain expression on immunofixation Clonal bone marrow plasma cells <10%, and Absence of end-organ damage such as hypercalcemia, renal insufficiency, anemia, and bone lesions (CRAB) that can be attributed to the plasma cell proliferative disorder	**Idiopathic Bence Jones proteinuria†** All criteria must be met: Urinary monoclonal protein on urine protein electrophoresis ≥500 mg/24 h and/or clonal bone marrow plasma cells ≥10% No immunoglobulin heavy-chain expression on immunofixation Absence of end-organ damage such as hypercalcemia, renal insufficiency, anemia, and bone lesions (CRAB) that can be attributed to the plasma cell proliferative disorder	**Light-chain multiple myeloma†** Same as multiple myeloma except no evidence of immunoglobulin heavy-chain expression

FLC, Free light chain; MGUS, monoclonal gammopathy of undetermined significance.
*Occasionally patients with IgD and IgE monoclonal gammopathies have been described and will be considered to be part of this category as well.
†Note that conventionally IgM MGUS is considered a subtype of MGUS, and similarly light-chain multiple myeloma is considered as a subtype of multiple myeloma. Unless specifically distinguished, when the terms MGUS and multiple myeloma are used in general, they include IgM MGUS and light-chain multiple myeloma, respectively.
From Rajkumar SV, et al.: Advances in the diagnosis, classification, risk stratification, and management of monoclonal gammopathy of undetermined significance: implications for recategorizing disease entities in the presence of evolving scientific evidence, *Mayo Clin Proc* 85(10):945-948, 2010.

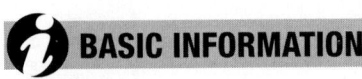

BASIC INFORMATION

DEFINITION

Mononucleosis is a symptomatic infection most commonly caused by Epstein-Barr virus (EBV) and characterized by fever, tonsillar pharyngitis, and lymphadenopathy.

SYNONYMS

IM
Infectious mononucleosis (IM)
EBV
Kissing disease

ICD-10CM CODES

B27 Infections mononucleosis
B27.0 Gamma herpesviral mononucleosis
B27.1 Cytomegaloviral mononucleosis
B27.8 Other infectious mononucleosis
B27.9 Infectious mononucleosis

EPIDEMIOLOGY & DEMOGRAPHICS

INCIDENCE (IN U.S.): 500 cases/100,000 persons/yr. Worldwide, approximately 95% of adults are infected with EBV at some point in life.
PREDOMINANT SEX: Incidence is the same, but occurs earlier in females.
PREDOMINANT AGE: Most common between the ages of 15 and 24 yr.

PHYSICAL FINDINGS & CLINICAL PRESENTATION

- Following an incubation period of 1 to 2 mo, a prodrome may occur, with fever, chills, malaise, and anorexia for several days. This is followed by the classic triad, which includes pharyngitis, fever, and adenopathy. Although fatigue and malaise may be prominent, pharyngitis is usually the most severe symptom. Tonsillitis with marked tonsillar exudates is common.
- Lymphadenopathy is most prominent in the cervical region but may be diffuse.
- Splenomegaly may occur, most commonly during the second wk of illness.
- Rash is uncommon but will occur in nearly all patients who receive ampicillin or amoxicillin.
- At times, IM can present as fever and adenopathy without pharyngitis. Although complications may be severe, they are uncommon and tend to resolve completely. Involvement of the hematologic, pulmonary, cardiac, or nervous system may occur; splenic rupture is rare. IM is usually a self-limited illness, but symptoms of malaise and fatigue may last months before resolving.
- Children are at the highest risk of airway obstruction. This is the most common cause of hospitalization from IM.

ETIOLOGY

The most common cause of IM is primary infection with EBV. Cytomegalovirus (CMV) can cause a similar disease syndrome, but CMV infection often occurs in infancy or early childhood and is minimally symptomatic. Primary EBV infection during childhood also often causes few or no symptoms; persistent fatigue and recurrent/persistent fevers are the most common reasons parents bring symptomatic children to medical care. Infection during childhood is more common in lower socioeconomic groups. The frequency of IM in late adolescence is attributed to the onset of social contact between the sexes. Close personal contact is usually necessary for transmission. Transfer via saliva while kissing may be responsible for many cases. EBV can persist in the oropharynx of patients with IM for up to 18 mo. Transmission may also occur sexually as EBV can be isolated in cervical epithelial cells and male seminal fluid and can also be transmitted by blood transfusion.

DIAGNOSIS

DIFFERENTIAL DIAGNOSIS

- Heterophile-negative IM caused by cytomegalovirus (CMV)
- Bacterial and viral causes of pharyngitis
- Toxoplasmosis
- Acute retroviral syndrome of HIV, lymphoma

WORKUP

Initial testing consists of heterophile antibody (monospot) and CBC with differential. Fig. E1 illustrates a diagnostic algorithm for EBV infection and IM.

LABORATORY TESTS

- A heterophile antibody test is the best initial test for diagnosis of EBV infection (71% to 90% accuracy for diagnosing IM). However, the test has a 25% false negative rate in the first week of illness.
- Increased WBC is common, with a relative lymphocytosis and neutropenia. Atypical lymphocytes (Fig. E2) are the hallmark of IM, but are not pathognomonic. Mild thrombocytopenia is common. A falling hematocrit may signal splenic rupture or severe immune-mediated hemolytic anemia. Elevated hepatocellular enzymes and cryoglobulins occur in many cases. Heterophile antibody, as measured by the monospot test, may be positive at presentation, or may appear later in the course of illness. A negative test should be repeated if clinical suspicion is high; negative results are common in patients symptomatic for <2 wk and children <4 yr. If this test remains negative for 8 wk, other causes of IM are likely. The monospot usually remains positive for 3 to 6 mo but can last >1 yr.
- In addition to the heterophile antibody, virus-specific antibodies may result in response to IM. Determination of these EBV-specific antibodies is rarely necessary to diagnose IM, although early diagnosis in monospot-negative cases may be made by isolating IgM to the viral capsid antigen, which is usually positive during the acute illness.

IMAGING STUDIES

Chest x-ray may rarely show infiltrates. An elevated left hemidiaphragm may occur in cases of splenic rupture.

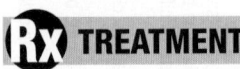

TREATMENT

NONPHARMACOLOGIC THERAPY

- Supportive rest is advocated by some, but effect on outcome is not clear.
- Splenectomy if rupture occurs; transfusions for severe anemia or thrombocytopenia

GENERAL Rx

- Pharmacologic therapy, including corticosteroids, is not indicated in mild illness.
- The use of steroids (Fig. E3) is suggested in patients who have severe thrombocytopenia or hemolytic anemia, or impending airway obstruction as a result of enlarged tonsils. Prednisone, 60 to 80 mg PO qid for 3 days, then tapered over 1 to 2 wk. Dexamethasone may also be used for severe tonsillar enlargement. There is no role for antiviral agents such as acyclovir in the management of IM.

CHRONIC Rx

A rare, chronic form of IM with persistent organ infection and inflammation has been described. This should not be confused with chronic fatigue syndrome, which is unrelated to EBV.

DISPOSITION

Eventual resolution of all symptoms is the rule.

PEARLS & CONSIDERATIONS

COMMENTS

- Contact sports should be avoided during the first month of illness, because splenic rupture can occur, even in the absence of clinically detectable splenomegaly.
- Between 30% and 75% of college freshmen are seronegative for EBV. Each year nearly 20% of susceptible persons become infected and up to 50% of these persons develop IM.

SUGGESTED READINGS

Available at www.expertconsult.com

RELATED CONTENT

Mononucleosis (Patient Information)
Epstein-Barr Virus Infection (Related Key Topic)

AUTHOR: **RUSSELL J. MCCULLOH, M.D.**

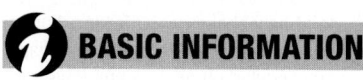 BASIC INFORMATION

DEFINITION

Motion sickness is a clinical syndrome associated with motion or perception of motion. Patients with motion sickness suffer perspiration, nausea, vomiting, increased salivation, and generalized malaise in response to movement.

SYNONYMS

Physiologic vertigo

ICD-10CM CODES
T75.3 Motion sickness

EPIDEMIOLOGY & DEMOGRAPHICS

INCIDENCE (IN U.S.): Common
PEAK INCIDENCE: Any age
PREVALENCE (IN U.S.): Common
PREDOMINANT SEX: Male = female
PREDOMINANT AGE: Any age
GENETICS: Not known to be genetic

PHYSICAL FINDINGS & CLINICAL PRESENTATION

- Vomiting
- Sweating
- Pallor

ETIOLOGY

- Motion (e.g., amusement rides, rides in automobiles or planes)

- Exacerbated by anxiety, fumes (e.g., industrial pollutants), visual stimuli
- Fig. 1 describes a proposed neural pathway resulting in motion sickness

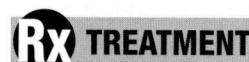 DIAGNOSIS

DIFFERENTIAL DIAGNOSIS

- Acute labyrinthitis
- Gastroenteritis
- Metabolic disorders
- Viral syndrome

WORKUP

None necessary in routine case

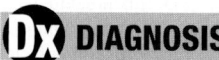 TREATMENT

NONPHARMACOLOGIC THERAPY

- Fixate on far object
- Cease motion
- Avoid reading
- Avoid alcohol

ACUTE GENERAL Rx

- Scopolamine patch is most effective. It should be applied to a hairless area behind the ear every 3 days prn. It should be applied >4 hr before antiemetic effect is required.
- Oral promethazine is effective but highly sedating.
- Over-the-counter oral preparations (e.g., Dramamine) are less effective.

- Meclizine 12.5 to 25 mg q6h may be effective but is very sedating.

CHRONIC Rx

- Rarely chronic
- Symptoms generally resolve completely with cessation of motion exposure.

DISPOSITION

Follow-up is not needed.

REFERRAL

If another diagnosis is suspected (e.g., purulent ear, fever, cranial nerve abnormalities)

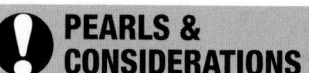 PEARLS & CONSIDERATIONS

COMMENTS

- Many patients with migraine report having had severe motion sickness as a child.
- Improved ventilation, avoidance of large meals before travel, semirecumbent sitting, and avoidance of reading while in motion will minimize the risk of motion sickness.

RELATED CONTENT

Motion Sickness (Patient Information)

AUTHOR: **FRED F. FERRI, M.D.**

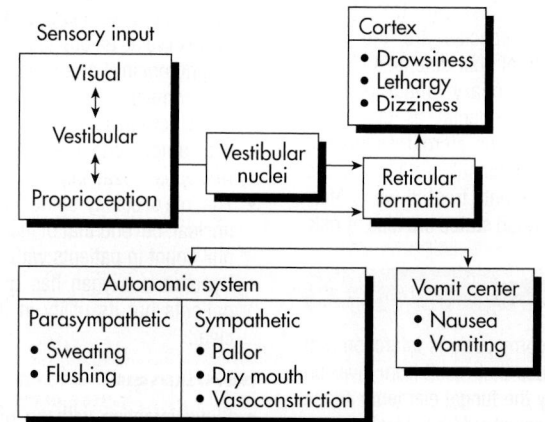

FIG. 1 Proposed neural pathway resulting in motion sickness. (From Kuhn SM: Motion sickness. In Keystone JS, et al.: *Travel medicine*, ed 2, Philadelphia, 2008, Elsevier, pp 435-440.)

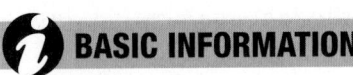

BASIC INFORMATION

DEFINITION

Mucormycosis is a fungal infection by Zygomycetes fungi and includes species in the order Mucorales (*Rhizopus* sp., *Rhizomucor, Cunninghamella, Apophysomyces, Saksenaea, Absidia, Syncephalastrum, Cokeromyces, Mortierella*) and in the order Entomophthorales (*Conidiobolus* and *Basidiobolus*).

SYNONYMS

Zygomycosis

ICD-10CM CODES
B46.5 Mucormycosis, unspecified
B46.1 Rhinocerebral mucormycosis
B46.0 Pulmonary mucormycosis
B46.3 Cutaneous mucormycosis
B46.4 Disseminated mucormycosis

EPIDEMIOLOGY & DEMOGRAPHICS

- These fungi are ubiquitous in nature and can be found in soil and decaying vegetation. Infection is seen in association with underlying conditions, including diabetes mellitus especially with ketoacidosis, hematologic malignancies, stem cell or solid organ transplants, severe burns or trauma, treatment with deferoxamine or iron overload states, steroid treatment, immunodeficiency states (e.g., AIDS), injection drug use, and malnutrition. Immunocompetent hosts may become infected in tropical climates.
- The fungus gains entry to the body most commonly through the respiratory tract. The spores are deposited in the nasal turbinates and may be inhaled into the pulmonary alveoli. In cases of cutaneous mucormycosis, the spores are introduced directly into the skin lesion.
- After a tornado with winds >200 mph struck Joplin, Missouri, in May 2011, there were 13 confirmed cases of mucormycosis (*Apophysomyces trapeziformis),* including five deaths. While two patients had diabetes, none were immunocompromised. It was felt that the fungus entered through wounds sustained during the tornado. Wooden splinters were found in four patients.

PHYSICAL FINDINGS & CLINICAL PRESENTATION

- Rhinocerebral-rhinoorbital-paranasal syndrome is the most common presentation, which presents with fever, facial and orbital pain, headache, diplopia, loss of vision, facial or orbital cellulitis, facial anesthesia, cranial nerve dysfunction, black nasal discharge, epistaxis, and seizure. Physical findings in this situation include proptosis; chemosis; nasal, palatal, or pharyngeal necrotic ulcerations; and retinal infarction. Thrombosis of the cavernous sinus or internal carotid artery may occur. This form of mucormycosis is found most commonly in diabetics, primarily in the presence of acidosis, and in patients with leukemia and neutropenia. Isolated CNS mucormycosis may result from hematogenous spread (can occur with injection drug users).
- Pulmonary mucormycosis can present with pneumonia, lung abscess, pulmonary infarction, pleurisy, pleural effusion, hemoptysis, chills, and fever. This form of mucormycosis is found most commonly in immunocompromised neutropenic hosts after chemotherapy for hematologic malignancies.
- Gastrointestinal zygomycosis presents with abdominal pain, diarrhea, gastrointestinal hemorrhage, ulcers, peritonitis, and bowel infarction. This form of mucormycosis is found most commonly in patients with extreme malnutrition and is believed to arise from ingestion of spores of the fungi.
- Cutaneous zygomycosis presents as nodular lesions (hematogenous seeding) or a wound infection. It primarily involves the epidermis and dermis after use of occlusive dressings that have not been properly sterilized.
- Cardiac mucormycosis is a form of endocarditis.
- Septic arthritis and osteomyelitis
- Brain abscess occurs most often from extension of the fungus from the nose or paranasal sinuses through adjacent bones in severely debilitated patients.
- Disseminated zygomycosis (rare but uniformly fatal)
- Physical findings depend on the location of the infection.

ETIOLOGY & PATHOGENESIS

The cause of mucormycosis is infection by a fungus of the Zygomycetes class (see "Definition"). Rhizopus and mucor species are the most common causes. Normal host defenses include leukocytes and pulmonary macrophages. Quantitative (e.g., neutropenia) or qualitative (e.g., diabetes mellitus or steroid treatment) disruption in the host defenses predisposes the patient to infection. Patients treated with deferoxamine for iron-overload states are also at risk.

DIAGNOSIS

The hallmark of mucormycosis is infarction and necrosis of host tissues that result from invasion of the vasculature by the fungal elements. Black eschars and discharges should be closely evaluated. Diagnosis depends on the demonstration of the organism in the tissue of a biopsy specimen.

DIFFERENTIAL DIAGNOSIS

- Infection of the sites described previously by other organisms (bacterial [including tuberculosis and leprosy], viral, fungal, or protozoan)
- Noninfectious tissue necrosis (e.g., neoplasia, vasculitis, degenerative) of the sites described previously

WORKUP

- Biopsy of infected tissue with direct-light microscopy examination establishes the diagnosis within minutes of the biopsy in the case of nasopharyngeal infection. Fungal hyphae are broad (5- to 15-micron diameter) and irregularly branched and have rare septations, in contrast to molds such as *Aspergillus,* which are narrower, have regular branching, and have many septations.
- Bronchoalveolar lavage or bronchoscopy with biopsy for smear, culture, and histologic examination
- Radiographs and other imaging studies such as CT of symptomatic sites may be required before infection is suspected and tissue specimens are obtained.

TREATMENT

Aggressive correction of underlying disease (e.g., hyperglycemia, high steroid doses, use of immunosuppressive drugs) should be undertaken.

Standard therapy consists of aggressive surgical debridement of involved tissues and antifungal therapy. For invasive mucormycosis recommended treatment is with a lipid formulation of amphotericin B that allows higher doses with less nephrotoxicity. The start dose is 5 mg/kg of liposomal amphotericin B or amphotericin B lipid complex. Doses as high as 10 mg/kg have also been used.

Traditional amphotericin B given IV at a daily dose of 1.0 to 1.5 mg/kg infused over 2 to 4 hr daily for a total of 1 to 4 g can also still be used, but is associated with significant nephrotoxicity and adverse reactions such as fever, chills, myalgias, vomiting, and electrolyte disturbances.

- Other antifungals do not appear to be effective except possibly posaconazole, which may serve as an oral step-down therapy after amphotericin B at a dose of 400 mg bid with a fatty meal.
- Some studies suggest that caspofungin with amphotericin B may be synergistic for *Rhizopus oryzae* infections only.
- The role of colony-stimulating factors remains unclear, beyond that of increasing the neutrophil count in patients with neutropenia.
- Hyperbaric oxygen has been used in some patients but its utility in therapy is still not clear.

PROGNOSIS

- Sinus infection with no underlying disease: 75% survival
- Sinus infection with diabetes: 60% survival
- Sinus infection with renal disease: 25% survival

SUGGESTED READINGS
Available at www.expertconsult.com

AUTHOR: **GLENN G. FORT, M.D., M.P.H.**

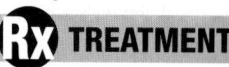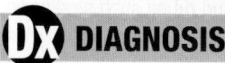

BASIC INFORMATION

DEFINITION

These are gram-negative bacteria that are resistant to at least one antimicrobial in three or more antimicrobial classes (antipseudomonal penicillins, third-generation cephalosporins, fluoroquinolones, carbapenems, and aminoglycosides).

SYNONYMS

CRE: carbapenem-resistant Enterobacteriaceae
ESBL: extended-spectrum beta-lactamases
MDR-GNB: multidrug-resistant gram-negative bacilli
MDRO: multidrug-resistant organisms
NDM-1: New Delhi metallo-beta-lactamase-1

ICD-10CM CODES
Z16.30 Resistance to unspecified antimicrobial drugs
Z16.10 Resistance to unspecified beta lactam antibiotics

EPIDEMIOLOGY & DEMOGRAPHICS

INCIDENCE: There is an increasing incidence of these bacteria in hospitals and long-term care facilities in the U.S. and around the world. ESBL bacteria were first discovered in Europe in 1984 and in the U.S. in 1988. CRE bacteria were first described in the late 1990s in the U.S. The NDM-1 bacteria were first noted in 2009 in Sweden in a patient from India.

PREDOMINANT SEX AND AGE: These bacteria can be seen in any age group. They may be more frequent in women due to increased risk of urinary tract sepsis.

RISK FACTORS: In general, these bacteria are more common in hospitals and long-term care facilities, but they are spread nosocomially through patient care and thus are now entering the community, where the incidence is also increasing. Specific risk factors include:
- Length of stay in the hospital
- Length of ICU stay
- Use of central line catheters
- Abdominal surgery
- Presence of gastrostomy or jejunostomy tube
- Prior administration of any antibiotic
- Prior residence in a long-term care facility
- Presence of indwelling urinary catheter

ETIOLOGY

- Several different classes of MDR-GNRs exist based on their resistance mechanism.
  1. ESBL: These bacteria contain enzymes that break open the beta-lactam ring of penicillins, cephalosporins, and aztreonam and thus inactivate antibiotics from those classes. Enzymes conferring resistance include:
     a. TEM beta-lactamases
     b. SHV beta-lactamases
     c. CTX-M beta lactamases
     d. OXA beta-lactamases
     e. These enzymes are plasmid-mediated and thus can spread from one gram-negative bacteria to another, causing outbreaks in a single institution.

  2. CRE: Enzymes conferring resistance include:
     a. Class A beta-lactamases: encoded on chromosomes or plasmids (e.g., *Klebsiella pneumoniae* carbapenamase [KPC], which has caused outbreaks in hospitals around the world)
     b. Class B: metallo-beta-lactamases (e.g., New Delhi metallo-beta-lactamase-1). Encoded on a mobile plasmid that can spread to other gram-negative bacteria.
     c. Class C and Class D beta-lactamases
  3. *MCR-1* gene: In May 2016, the *MCR-1* gene was reported for the first time in *E. coli* from a patient (urine culture) in the U.S. This gene makes bacteria resistant to the antibiotic colistin, which is used to treat other MDR-GNR organisms. This raises the concern that this plasma-encoded gene could be spread to CRE bacteria.

- *Stenotrophomonas maltophilia*: MDR-GNR that acts as an opportunistic pathogen among mostly hospitalized patients with high morbidity and mortality. It has intrinsic or acquired resistance mechanisms to multiple antibiotic classes and has the ability to adhere to foreign materials and form a biofilm, which escapes host defenses.
- *Acinetobacter* sp. (e.g., *Acinetobacter baumannii*): strains have emerged that are resistant to all commercially available antibiotics. These bacteria have the capability to acquire diverse mechanisms of resistance including:
  1. AmpC beta-lactamases
  2. Beta-lactamases: serine and metallo-beta-lactamases

CLINICAL PRESENTATION

All these resistant bacteria have the capability of causing diverse infections, including
- Pneumonia
- Bacteremia
- Urinary tract sepsis
- Central line–associated infections
- Ventilator-associated pneumonia (VAP)
- Surgical site infections
VAP from *A. baumannii* now accounts for 8.4% of GNR pneumonias in the ICU.

DIAGNOSIS

DIFFERENTIAL DIAGNOSIS

Other gram-negative rods such as:
- *Pseudomonas aeruginosa*
- *Klebsiella pneumoniae* that are not ESBL or CRE by resistance pattern
- *Morganella morganii*
- *Providencia*, *Proteus* sp., *Serratia*

WORKUP

Detection of ESBL and CRE bacteria can pose problems for the clinical microbiology laboratory:
1. To detect ESBL bacteria: automated systems such as Vitek use disk diffusion or broth dilution techniques, or double disk test or E-test strip with clavulanate
2. To detect CRE: modified Hodge test to detect carbapenamase-producing bacteria. Polymerase chain reaction (PCR) testing, pulsed-field

gel electrophoresis (PFGE), and whole genome sequencing (WGS) are useful for detecting CRE.
3. In 2010, testing guidelines with respect to susceptibility involving several beta-lactam antibiotics were changed to better identify these bacteria via automated systems.

LABORATORY TESTS

Clinical testing is the same in infections from these resistant organisms as with nonresistant organisms:
- Cultures of any wounds, blood, sputum, urine, catheter tips
- CBC, liver function tests, urinalysis

IMAGING STUDIES

Studies depend on the clinical presentation but are similar to those for nonresistant bacteria causing infections.

TREATMENT

Because of multidrug resistance, only a few reliable antibiotics are available to treat these infections.
1. ESBL bacteria: carbapenem antibiotics such as imipenem, meropenem, ertapenem, or the cephalosporin cefoxitin or tigecycline.
2. CRE bacteria: selection of antibiotic will depend on testing but tigecycline may be used clinically. Other alternatives include:
   a. IV colistin
   b. *Stenotrophomonas maltophilia*: only available agents are Bactrim (drug of choice), Levaquin, and minocycline
   c. *A. baumannii*: will depend on susceptibility testing, but ampicillin-sulbactam, imipenem or meropenem, or tigecycline can be used for MDR strains. For pan-resistant strains, IV colistin ± rifampin can be used. Inhaled colistin can be used for pneumonia patients.
   d. Newer antibiotics such as ceftolozane/tazobactam and ceftazidime/avibactam offer coverage for some of the resistant enzymes, but not all, and thus they require susceptibility testing to confirm.

DISPOSITION

Morbidity and mortality can be quite high with infections from these MDR bacteria.
1. Nosocomial *Acinetobacter* pneumonia carries a mortality rate of 35% to 70%.
2. *Stenotrophomonas* infections carry a mortality rate of 21% to 69%.
3. ESBL infections carry a mortality rate of 3.7% despite therapy with carbapenem antibiotics.

REFERRAL

- Infectious diseases specialist for selection of best antibiotic choice and follow-up
- Microbiologist for specialized testing and interpretation of results
- Pulmonary specialist for severe forms of pneumonia
- Infection control officer to help prevent spread of these bacteria in an institution

SUGGESTED READINGS
Available at www.expertconsult.com

AUTHOR: **GLENN G. FORT, M.D., M.P.H.**

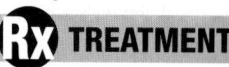
Diseases and Disorders

M

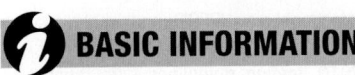

BASIC INFORMATION

DEFINITION

Multifocal atrial tachycardia (MAT) is a supraventricular tachyarrhythmia (rate greater than 100 beats/min) with P waves having at least three or more different morphologies and irregular P-P intervals. An isoelectric baseline further differentiates MAT from atrial fibrillation or atrial flutter.

SYNONYMS

MAT
Chaotic atrial rhythm
Chronic atrial tachycardia
Repetitive multifocal paroxysmal atrial tachycardia
The term *wandering pacemaker* is used for a similar arrhythmia associated with a normal or slow heart rate (<100 beats/min).

ICD-10CM CODES

I47.1 Supraventricular tachycardia

EPIDEMIOLOGY & DEMOGRAPHICS

Estimated prevalence in hospitalized patients of 0.05% to 0.32%. Average age is 70s. Usually associated with underlying pulmonary disease with right atrial electromechanical delay. Chronic obstructive pulmonary disease (COPD) is present in approximately 55% of patients with MAT. It may also be seen in patients with valvular heart disease, pulmonary hypertension, and hypomagnesemia.

PHYSICAL FINDINGS & CLINICAL PRESENTATION

Symptoms:
• Palpitation
• Lightheadedness
• Syncope
• Symptoms of the underlying pulmonary disease
• Physical findings associated with the underlying pulmonary disease

ETIOLOGY

• Exact mechanism unknown
• Exacerbated by underlying pulmonary disease (COPD, hypoxia, pulmonary embolism, pneumonia), cardiac disease, hypercarbia, acidosis, electrolyte disturbances

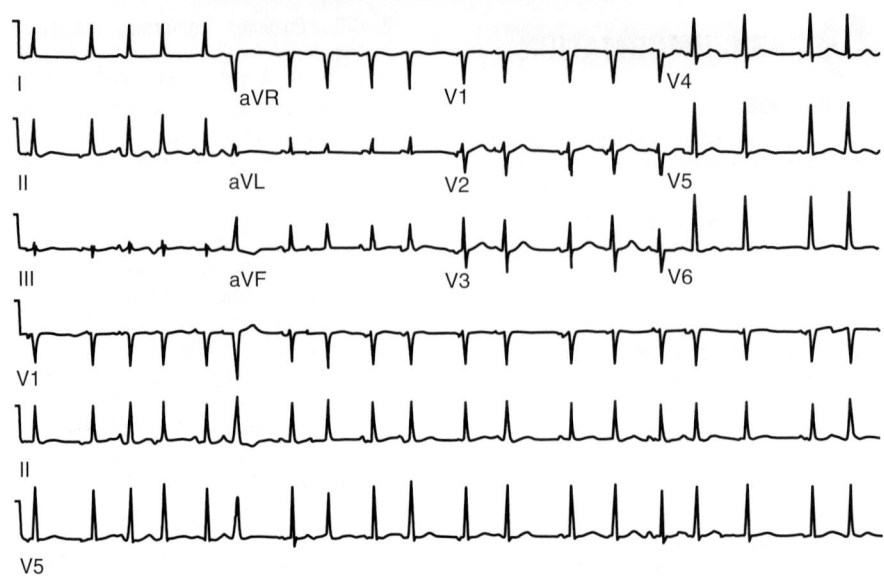

FIG. 1 Surface ECG of multifocal atrial tachycardia. Note the varying morphology of the P waves and the PR intervals. (From Issa Z, et al.: *Clinical arrhythmology and electrophysiology,* ed 2, Philadelphia, 2012, Saunders.)

DIAGNOSIS

DIFFERENTIAL DIAGNOSIS

• Atrial fibrillation
• Atrial flutter with variable AV conduction
• Sinus tachycardia
• Paroxysmal atrial tachycardia
• Extrasystole

WORKUP

• ECG (Fig. 1)
• Chest x-ray
• Pulmonary function tests
• Electrolytes
• Arterial blood gases

TREATMENT

• Correction and/or improvement in the underlying pulmonary or metabolic dysfunction if possible and avoiding drugs such as digoxin, theophylline, etc.
• Electrolyte repletion, especially magnesium and potassium, to normal levels.

• Intravenous magnesium infusion may occasionally be helpful in patients with normal magnesium levels.
• Calcium channel blockers—verapamil may be effective acutely and chronically and is often used as first line in patients with preserved LV function.
• β-blockers are typically contraindicated by obstructive lung disease or acute heart failure.
• If the arrhythmia is asymptomatic, it can be left untreated.
• Direct current cardioversion is ineffective.
• No significant role for antiarrhythmics or catheter ablation.
• In extreme cases of refractory MAT in symptomatic patients who cannot tolerate medical therapy or in MAT resistant to medical therapy, AV nodal ablation with pacemaker implantation has been performed.

SUGGESTED READINGS

Available at www.expertconsult.com

AUTHORS: **BARRY FINE, M.D., Ph.D,** and **JOHN WYLIE, M.D.**

BASIC INFORMATION

DEFINITION

Multiple myeloma (MM) is a plasma cell neoplasm characterized by clonal proliferation of malignant plasma cells in the bone marrow, monoclonal protein in the blood or urine, and associated end-organ dysfunction. Diagnostic criteria for the diagnosis of MM require the following:

1. Presence of ≥20% plasma cells on examination of the bone marrow (or biopsy of a tissue with monoclonal plasma cells).
2. Monoclonal protein in the serum or urine. Occasional patients without detectable monoclonal protein are considered to have nonsecretory myeloma.
3. Evidence of end-organ damage (*c*alcium elevation, *r*enal insufficiency, *a*nemia, or *b*one lesions [CRAB criteria]).

SYNONYMS

MM

ICD-10CM CODES
C90.00 Multiple myeloma not having achieved remission
C90.01 Multiple myeloma in remission
C90.02 Multiple myeloma in relapse

EPIDEMIOLOGY & DEMOGRAPHICS

ANNUAL INCIDENCE:

- Five cases/100,000 persons (blacks affected twice as frequently as whites, males more than females)
- MM accounts for 10% of all hematologic cancers and is the most common primary bone malignancy.
- An estimated 30,330 new cases and 12,650 deaths will occur in 2016 in the U.S.

PREDOMINANT AGE: Peak incidence is in the seventh decade at a median age of 70 yr.

PHYSICAL FINDINGS & CLINICAL PRESENTATION

The patient usually comes to medical attention because of one or more of the following:

- Bone pain (58%) commonly in the back and thorax or pathologic fractures (30%) caused by osteolytic lesions
- Anemia from bone marrow infiltration by plasma cells
- Recurrent infections as a result of impaired neutrophil function and deficiency of normal immunoglobulins (humoral deficiency)
- Nausea and vomiting caused by constipation and uremia
- Delirium resulting from hypercalcemia
- Neurologic complications, such as spinal cord or nerve root compression, blurred vision from hyperviscosity
- Purpura, epistaxis from thrombocytopenia
- Paresthesias, weight loss, generalized weakness

DIAGNOSIS

DIFFERENTIAL DIAGNOSIS

- Metastatic carcinoma to bone marrow
- Lymphoma, non-Hodgkin's
- Bone neoplasms (e.g., sarcoma)
- Monoclonal gammopathy of undetermined significance
- Primary amyloidosis
- Waldenström's macroglobulinemia
- Table 1 compares diagnostic criteria for multiple myeloma variants and monoclonal gammopathy of unknown significance.

LABORATORY TESTS

- Normochromic, normocytic anemia; rouleaux formation on peripheral smear (Fig. 1)

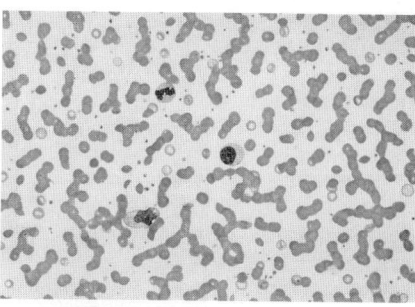

FIG. 1 Increased rouleaux formation is seen in this blood smear from a patient with a large M protein. Marked rouleaux formation is often a clue to the diagnosis of a plasma cell neoplasm, but may be observed in other conditions (Wright-Giemsa stain). (From Jaffe ES et al: *Hematopathology,* Philadelphia, 2011, Saunders.)

TABLE 1 Diagnostic Criteria for Multiple Myeloma, Myeloma Variants, and Monoclonal Gammopathy of Unknown Significance

Monoclonal Gammopathy of Undetermined Significance or Monoclonal Gammopathy, Unattributed/Unassociated

M protein in serum <30 g/L
Bone marrow clonal plasma cells <10%
No evidence of other B cell proliferative disorders
No myeloma-related organ or tissue impairment (no end-organ damage, including bone lesions)

Asymptomatic Myeloma (Smoldering Myeloma)

M protein in serum >30 g/L *or*
Bone marrow clonal plasma cell ≥10%
No related organ or tissue impairment (no end-organ damage, including bone lesions) or symptoms

Symptomatic Multiple Myeloma

M protein in serum or urine*
Bone marrow (clonal) plasma cells* or plasmacytoma
Related organ or tissue impairment (end-organ damage, including bone lesions)

Solitary Plasmacytoma of Bone

No M protein in serum or urine[†]
Single area of bone destruction caused by clonal plasma cells
Bone marrow not consistent with MM
Normal skeletal survey (and MRI of spine and pelvis if done)
No related organ or tissue impairment (no end-organ damage other than solitary bone lesion)[†]

Nonsecretory Myeloma

No M protein in serum or urine with immunofixation
Bone marrow clonal plasmacytosis ≥10% or plasmacytoma
Related organ or tissue impairment (end-organ damage, including bone lesions)

Extramedullary Plasmacytoma

No M protein in serum or urine[†]
Extramedullary tumor of clonal plasma cells
Normal bone marrow
Normal skeletal survey
No related organ or tissue impairment (end-organ damage including bone lesions)

Multiple Solitary Plasmacytomas (± Recurrent)

No M protein in serum or urine[†]
More than one localized area of bone destruction or extramedullary tumor of clonal plasma cells, which may be recurrent
Normal bone marrow
Normal skeletal survey and MRI of spine and pelvis if done
No related organ or tissue impairment (no end-organ damage other than the localized bone lesions)

Myeloma-Related Organ or Tissue Impairment (End-Organ Damage)

Calcium levels increased: serum calcium >0-25 mmol/L above the upper limit of normal or >2-75 mmol/L
Renal insufficiency: creatinine >173 mmol/L
Anemia: hemoglobin 2 g/dl below the lower limit of normal or hemoglobin <10 g/dl
Bone lesions: lytic lesions or osteoporosis with compression fractures (MRI or CT may clarify)
Other: symptomatic hyperviscosity, amyloidosis, recurrent bacterial infections (more than two episodes in 12 months)

CT, Computed tomography; *MM,* multiple myeloma; *MRI,* magnetic resonance imaging.
*If flow cytometry is performed, most plasma cells (>90%) will show a neoplastic phenotype.
[†]A small M component may sometimes be present.
From Hoffman R et al: *Hematology, basic principles and practice,* ed 6, Philadelphia, 2013, WB Saunders.

Diagnosis

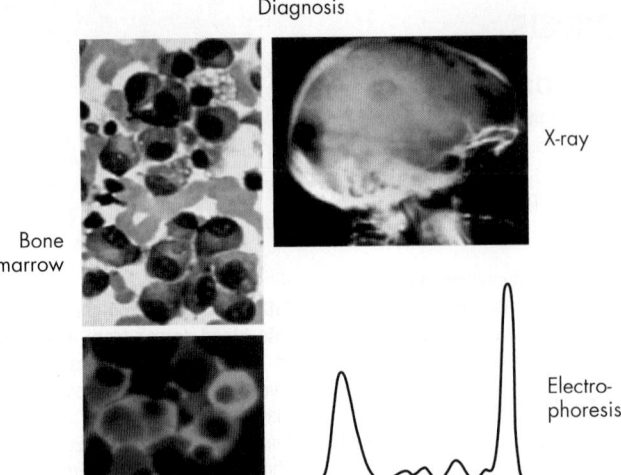

Bone marrow

X-ray

Electro-phoresis

FIG. 2 Common diagnostic features in multiple myeloma. Light chain-restricted plasma cells in a bone marrow aspirate; multiple lytic lesions in a skull radiograph; large monoclonal spike in the g-globulin area in serum electrophoresis. (From Hoffman R et al: *Hematology, basic principles and practice,* ed 5, Philadelphia, 2009, Churchill Livingstone.)

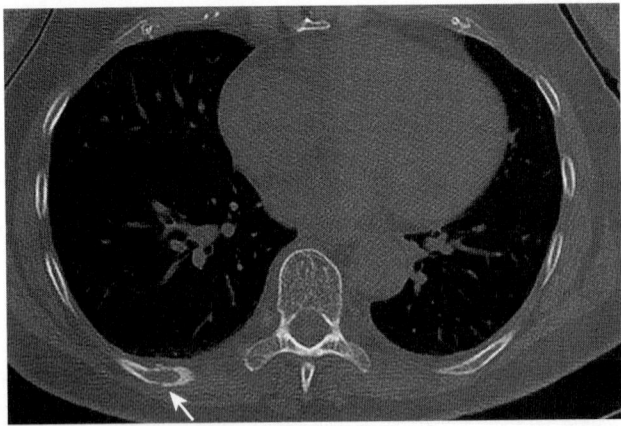

FIG. 3 Rib involvement in multiple myeloma *(arrow).* There is thinning of the cortex and enlargement of a circumscribed area of the rib. Soft tissue Hounsfield units are noted within the lesion. In contrast to osteoporotic or traumatic fractures of the rib, no callus formation is seen. In a whole-body examination, every single rib must be screened by scrolling through it posteriorly to anteriorly. (From Pope TL et al: *Musculoskeletal imaging,* ed 2, Philadelphia, 2015, Saunders.)

- Hypercalcemia is present in 15% of patients at diagnosis.
- Elevated blood urea nitrogen, creatinine, uric acid, and total protein
- Urine protein immunoelectrophoresis: proteinuria from overproduction and secretion of free monoclonal kappa or lambda chains (Bence Jones protein)
- Serum protein immunoelectrophoresis: monoclonal spike (M spike) on protein immunoelectrophoresis in approximately 75% of patients (Fig. 2); decreased levels of normal immunoglobulins (Ig)
  1. The increased immunoglobulins are generally IgG (70%) and IgA (20%).
  2. Approximately 5% to 10% of patients have only increased light chains in the urine by electrophoresis (light chain MM).
  3. A small percentage (<2%) of patients have nonsecreting MM (no increase in immunoglobulins and no light chains in the urine) but have other evidence of the disease (e.g., positive bone marrow examination).
- Elevated serum free light chains (kappa or lambda types) with abnormally elevated or decreased kappa:lambda ratios suggestive of the presence of monoclonal light chain proteins.
- Hyponatremia, serum hyperviscosity (more common with production of IgA)
- Bone marrow examination demonstrates nests or sheets of plasma cells, which comprise >20% of the bone marrow
- Serum beta-2 microglobulin is useful for prognosis because levels >8 mg/L indicate high tumor mass and aggressive disease.
- Elevated serum lactate dehydrogenase at diagnosis define a subgroup of myeloma patients with very poor prognosis.
- Nearly all patients with MM present with abnormal chromosomes identified by fluorescence in situ hybridization (FISH). High-risk patients (<25% of patients at diagnosis) are those with any of the following: deletion 17p, translocation 4:14, translocation 14:16, deletion 13q, or cytogenetic hypodiploidy.

TABLE 2 Durie-Salmon Multiple Myeloma Staging System

Stage	Criteria
I	All of the following: Hemoglobin >10 g/dl Serum calcium <12 mg/dl Normal bone radiograph or solitary lesion Low M-component production IgG level <5 g/dl IgA level <3 g/dl Urine light chain <4 g/24 hr
II	Fitting neither I nor III
III	One or more of the following: Hemoglobin <8.5 g/dl Serum calcium >12 mg/dl Advanced lytic bone lesions High M-component production IgG level >7 g/dl IgA level >5 g/dl Urine light chains >12 g/24 hr

IMAGING STUDIES

Radiograph films of painful areas often demonstrate punched-out lytic lesions or osteoporosis (Fig. 2). CT can identify rib involvement not evident on plain films and differentiate it from osteoporotic and traumatic fractures (Fig. 3). MRI is the preferred technique for suspected spinal compression or soft tissue plasmacytomas. Bone scans may not be useful because MM lesions are not blastic.

STAGING

Table 2 describes a historical multiple myeloma staging system. With use of newer tumor biology factors (see "Disposition") that can affect prognosis, along with tumor burden described in Table 2 and patient-related factors, it is possible to classify patients in three risk groups (high, intermediate, and standard).

🆁🆇 TREATMENT

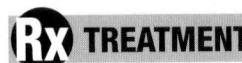

NONPHARMACOLOGIC THERAPY

- Prevention of renal failure with adequate hydration and avoidance of nephrotoxic agents and dye contrast studies

ACUTE GENERAL Rx

- Treatment strategy is initially related to the determination of transplant-eligible patients (Fig. 4).
- All transplant-eligible patients should be considered for approximately 12 weeks of induction chemotherapy with triplet regimens such as the VRD regimen (dexamethasone, lenalidomide, and bortezomib) or the CyBorD regimen (cyclophosphamide, lenalidomide, dexamethasone). Upon demonstration of at least a very good partial response, these patients can undergo stem cell mobilization and collection.
- All patients with high-risk characteristics should be offered autologous stem cell transplant (ASCT) subsequently, provided they have adequate cardiac, pulmonary, and hepatic function. Currently, ASCT can be safely performed in most centers in fit patients up to age 75 years.

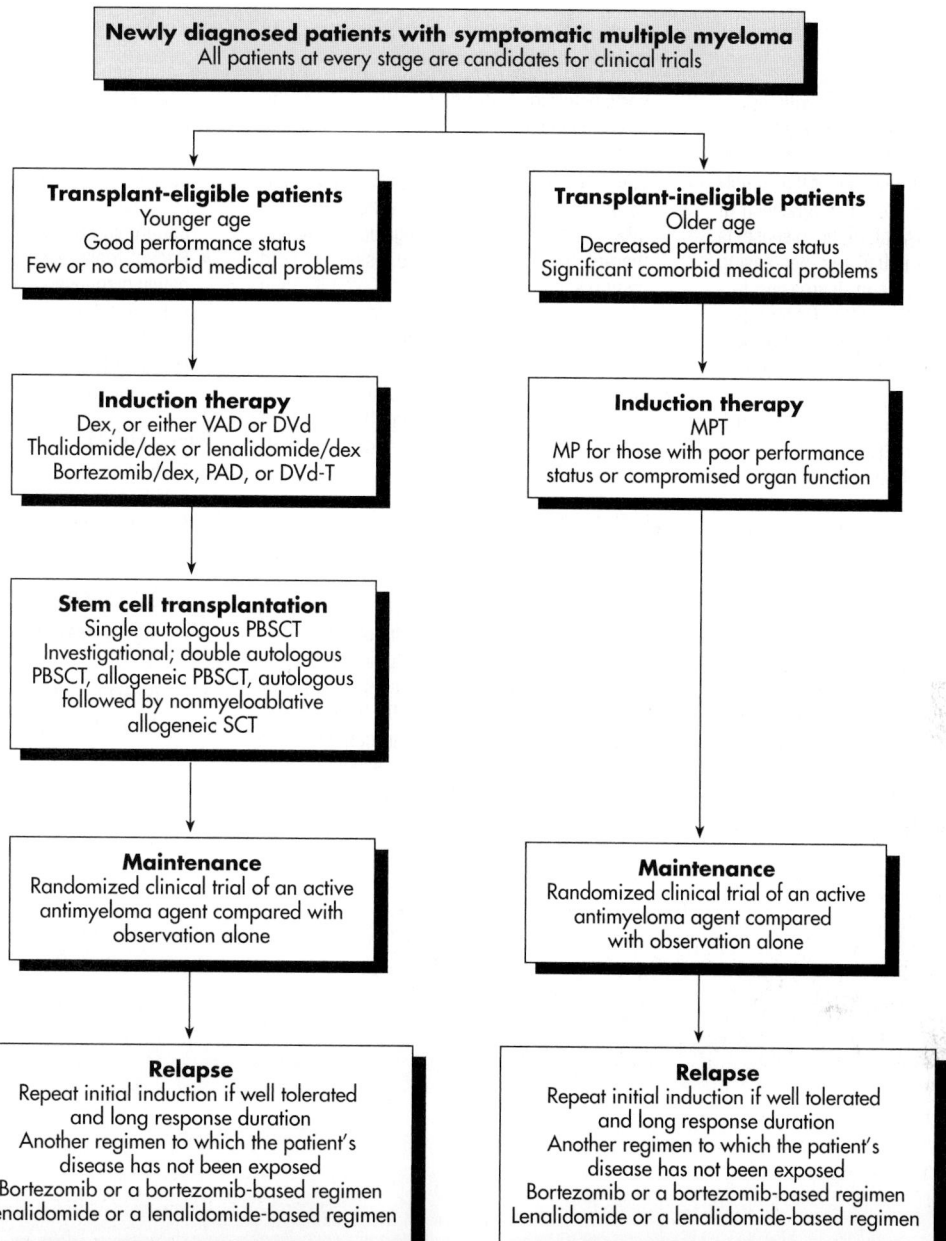

FIG. 4 A treatment algorithm for multiple myeloma. A treatment algorithm for patients who are or are not suitable candidates for stem cell transplantation is presented. Further detail is provided in the text. *Dex,* Dexamethasone; *DVd,* pegylated liposomal doxorubicin with vincristine and oral dexamethasone; *DVd-T,* DVd with thalidomide; *MP,* melphalan and prednisone; *MPT,* melphalan and prednisone with thalidomide; *PAD,* bortezomib with infusional doxorubicin and dexamethasone; *PBSCT,* peripheral blood stem cell transplantation; *SCT,* stem cell transplantation; *VAD,* infusional doxorubicin and vincristine with oral dexamethasone. (Modified from Runge MS, Greganti MA: *Netter's internal medicine,* Philadelphia, 2008, Saunders.)

- It is unclear if all MM patients without high-risk features benefit from upfront ASCT. The duration of median improved survival with single ASCT is estimated to be 12 months. ASCT performed at relapse is also associated with improvement in overall survival.
- Patients should be offered maintenance chemotherapy with either lenalidomide or bortezomib after recovery from ASCT for at least 2 years but potentially indefinitely.
- Induction chemotherapy in patients ineligible for transplantation (age >75 years, high comorbidity index, poor performance status)

can be identical to that offered transplant-eligible patients. Alternatively, less aggressive regimens (doublet regimens or single agents) can be recommended, including the following:
Melphalan, bortezomib, and prednisone (VMP)
Melphalan, lenalidomide, and prednisone (MPR)
Lenalidomide and dexamethasone (RD)
Bortezomib and dexamethasone (VD)
- Therapy for relapsed and refractory myeloma can include second-generation proteasome inhibitors (carfilzomib), immunomodulatory drugs (thalidomide, pomalidomide), and steroids. More recently, elotuzumab, an antibody

targeting signaling lymphocytic activation molecule F7 (SLAMF7), and daratumumab, an antibody targeting CD38 antigen, have both showed responses and survival benefits in relapsed multiple myeloma and are useful options in this setting. The oral proteasome inhibitor ixazomib as well as the histone deacetylase inhibitor panobinostat are also approved in this setting.
- If the relapse occurs more than 6 months after conventional therapy is stopped, the initial chemotherapy regimen can be reinstituted.

- ASCT can be considered as salvage therapy in patients who had stem cells cryopreserved early in the course of the disease.
- Approximately 15% of patients with newly diagnosed MM are recognized incidentally and present without significant symptoms (asymptomatic MM, formerly known as smoldering myeloma). The rate of progression of smoldering MM to symptomatic disease is 10% per year for the initial 5 yr, decreasing to 5% for the next 5 yr, and decreasing further to 1.5% per year thereafter. Observation alone is reasonable in these patients because no survival advantage has been demonstrated by treating them.
- An exception to this may be in high-risk smoldering myeloma patients. A recent trial has shown that early treatment with lenalidomide plus dexamethasone of patients with high-risk smoldering myeloma delays progression to active disease and increases overall survival.

CHRONIC Rx

- Promptly diagnose and treat infections. Common bacterial agents are *Streptococcus pneumoniae* and *Haemophilus influenzae*. Prophylactic therapy against *Pneumocystis jiroveci* with trimethoprim-sulfamethoxazole must be considered in patients receiving chemotherapy and high-dose corticosteroid regimens. Vaccinate against *S. pneumoniae*, influenza, and *H. influenzae*.
- Control hypercalcemia with IV fluids and corticosteroids. Monthly infusions of the bisphosphonate pamidronate or zoledronate provide significant protection against skeletal complications and improve the quality of life of patients with advanced multiple MM. Control pain with analgesics; radiation therapy to treat painful bone lesions or cord compression. Perform surgical stabilization of pathologic fractures. Consider vertebroplasty or kyphoplasty for selected vertebral lesions.
- Treat anemia with erythropoietin.
- Aggressive treatment of reversible causes of renal failure such as dehydration, hypercalcemia, and hyperuricemia.

DISPOSITION

- In patients presenting at an age <60 yr, the 10-year survival is approximately 30%. The median length of survival after diagnosis is now 8 yr. Prognosis is better in asymptomatic patients with indolent or smoldering myeloma. Median survival time is approximately 10 yr in persons with no lytic bone lesions and a serum myeloma protein concentration <3 g/dl. Adverse outcome is associated with increased levels of beta-2 microglobulin, low levels of serum albumin, circulating plasma cells, plasmablastic features in bone marrow, increased plasma cell labeling index, poor cytogenetics (t (4;14) or t (14;16) translocation, deletion 17p).
- Compared with a single ASCT, tandem transplantation (two successive ASCT) improves survival among patients with MM who do not have a very good partial response after undergoing a single transplantation.
- Recent trials reveal that among patients with newly diagnosed myeloma, survival in recipients of a hematopoietic stem cell autograft followed by a stem cell allograft from an HLA-identical sibling is superior to that in recipients of tandem stem cell autografts.

REFERRAL

- To hematologist for management of disease and bone marrow transplant (BMT) specialist for transplantation options and management.

SUGGESTED READINGS
Available at www.expertconsult.com

RELATED CONTENT
Multiple Myeloma (Patient Information)

AUTHOR: **BHARTI RATHORE, M.D.**

BASIC INFORMATION

DEFINITION

Multiple sclerosis (MS) is a chronic predominantly autoimmune demyelinating disease of the central nervous system (CNS) characterized by subacute neurologic deficits correlating with CNS lesions separated in time and space, excluding other possible disease.

Subtypes include:
- **Relapsing-remitting MS (RRMS)** (82%): relapses followed by complete or near-complete recovery, 50% to 85% of which later transition to SPMS
- **Secondary progressive MS (SPMS):** progression of disability with few or no relapses
- **Primary progressive MS (PPMS)** (18%): progression from the onset, rare relapses
- Progressive relapsing or relapsing progressive courses can be incorporated into PPMS or SPMS respectively.
- Relapses are defined as a subacute onset of neurologic dysfunction that lasts for at least 24 hr due to inflammatory demyelination.

Classic rare MS variants include:
- **Marburg variant:** MRI reveals a tumor-like lesion with notable edema in one cerebral hemisphere. Pathology shows severe inflammation with necrosis: typically acute onset with a fulminant, often malignant, course. May also involve peripheral nerves.
- **Balo's concentric sclerosis:** Neuroimaging and pathology show alternating rings of myelination and demyelination resembling an onion bulb macroscopically and microscopically.
- **Schilder's diffuse sclerosis:** childhood onset with one to two large confluent lesions. Some cases were later found to be due to metabolic defects, and many have thus abandoned this disorder.
- **Relapsing optic neuritis**
- **Neuromyelitis optica (Devic's disease):** previously considered a variant, now classified as a distinct demyelinating disease. Lesions primarily involve the optic nerves and spinal cord. Most (75%) are aquaporin-4 receptor Ab positive.

SYNONYMS

MS
Disseminated sclerosis

ICD-10CM CODES
G35 Multiple sclerosis

EPIDEMIOLOGY & DEMOGRAPHICS

PEAK INCIDENCE: 20 to 40 yr in two thirds of patients; it is the most common permanently disabling disorder of the central nervous system in young adults; mean age of onset is 30 yr, range is infancy to 70 yr.
PREVALENCE: More common in people raised in northern latitudes and in certain genetic clusters. Prevalence per 10,000 varies from 20 in southern Europe to 150 to 180 in Canada, northern United States, and northern Europe; and <10 in Asia, Central America, and most of Africa.

PREDOMINANT SEX & AGE: Female/male ratio is 2 to 3:1.
GENETICS: Frequency of MS in dizygotic twins and siblings is 3% to 5% and 20% to 40% in monozygotic twins. Most common associations include human leukocyte antigen classes I and II (*DRB1*1501, DQA1*0102, DQB1*0602*), (*DRB1*0405-DQA1*0301-DQB1*0302* in Mediterranean population). A notable epigenetic interaction between vitamin D and the main MS-linked HLA-DRB1*1501 allele has been elucidated.

PHYSICAL FINDINGS & CLINICAL PRESENTATION

Findings depend on the location of the CNS lesion(s) and may include the following:
- Common: nonspecific complaints such as fatigue, blurred vision, diplopia, vertigo, falls, hemiparesis, paraparesis, monoparesis, numbness, paresthesias, ataxia, cognitive deficits, depression, sexual dysfunction, and urinary dysfunction
- Visual abnormalities: horizontal nystagmus, visual field defects, ***Marcus Gunn pupil*** (i.e., relative afferent papillary defect—normal direct and consensual light reflexes; however, when swinging flashlight from one eye to the other, direct light causes dilatation of pupil of affected eye), ***internuclear ophthalmoplegia*** (paresis of the adducting

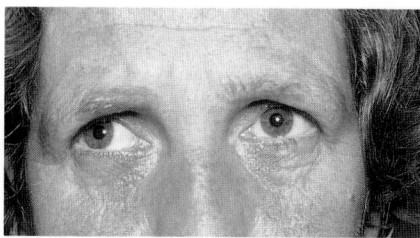

FIG. 1 Internuclear ophthalmoplegia may be an initial feature of brain stem involvement in multiple sclerosis. On lateral gaze to the right, adduction of the left eye is incomplete. On convergence, eye movement was normal. The lesion is in the left medial longitudinal bundle, between the nucleus in the pons and the third nerve nucleus on the opposite side. (From Forbes CD, Jackson WF: *Color atlas and text of clinical medicine,* ed 3, London, 2003, Mosby.)

eye on conjugate lateral gaze with horizontal nystagmus of the abducting eye [Fig. 1])
- Corticospinal tract(s) involvement: leads to upper motor neuron signs such as spasticity, hyperreflexia, clonus, extensor plantar responses, and upper motor neuron pattern of weakness
- Sensory loss: may include partial or full dermatomal loss of pain and temperature, loss of vibration (common) and position sense, or a thoracic band of sensory loss
- Ataxia: intention tremor, dysmetria, dysdiadochokinesis, titubation, inability to tandem gait
- Bladder dysfunction: detrusor hyperreflexia (urge incontinence), flaccidity (neurogenic bladder), and dyssynergia (bladder contracts against a closed sphincter)
- ***Lhermitte's sign:*** flexion of the neck elicits an electrical sensation extending down the spine and occasionally into the extremities
- ***Uhthoff's phenomenon:*** transient worsening of preexisting symptoms with small elevations in body temperature (e.g., during exercise or warm bathing)

ETIOLOGY

Remains unknown but multifactorial with evidence for autoimmunity (autoreactive T and B cells), environmental factors, and genetics (Mendelian and epigenetic). Environmental risk factors during childhood include certain viruses (e.g., Epstein-Barr virus and human herpes virus 6), low UV exposure, and month of birth (higher in spring). Other risk factors include low vitamin D level and smoking.

DIAGNOSIS

- MS: based on revised 2010 McDonald criteria (Table 1)
- RRMS: see Table 1
- PPMS: insidious progression of disability with a positive CSF and either dissemination in both space and time *or* ongoing progression for at least 1 yr

DIFFERENTIAL DIAGNOSIS (TABLE 2)

- Autoimmune: acute disseminated encephalomyelitis (ADEM), postvaccination encephalomyelitis, Devic's disease

TABLE 1 Summary of Revised 2005-2010 McDonald Criteria for Diagnosis of Multiple Sclerosis

RRMS/Clinical Attacks	Clinical Lesions	Paraclinical Testing Needed
2	2	None
2	1	MRI dissemination in space *or* 2 MRI lesions consistent with MS plus positive CSF
1	2	MRI dissemination in time
1	1	MRI dissemination in space *or* 2 MRI lesions consistent with MS plus positive CSF and MRI dissemination in time

Evidence of clinical lesions by physical examination or evoked potentials. *CSF,* Cerebrospinal fluid; *MRI dissemination in space;* ≥1 T2 lesions in 2 of the 4 typical areas for MS lesions—periventricular, juxtacortical, infratentorial or spinal cord; *MRI dissemination in time,* a new lesion at follow-up MRI at any time, or presence of both an enhancing and nonenhancing lesion at any time.

TABLE 2 Conditions That Can Be Mistaken for Multiple Sclerosis and Other Diseases of Myelin

Vascular Disease

Small-vessel cerebrovascular disease
Vasculitides
Arteriovenous malformation
CADASIL
Antiphospholipid antibody syndrome

Structural Lesions

Craniocervical junction, posterior fossa, or spinal tumors
Cervical spondylosis or disc herniation
Chiari malformation or syrinx

Degenerative Diseases

Hereditary myelopathy
Spinocerebellar degeneration

Infections

HTLV-1 infection
HIV myelopathy or HIV-related cerebritis
Neuroborreliosis (e.g., Lyme disease)
JC virus/progressive multifocal leukoencephalopathy
Neurosyphilis

Other Inflammatory Conditions

Systemic lupus erythematosus
Sjögren's syndrome
Sarcoidosis

Monofocal or Monophasic Demyelinating Syndromes

Transverse myelitis
Optic neuritis
Neuromyelitis optica/Devic's disease
Acute disseminated encephalomyelitis

Other Conditions

Hashimoto's thyroiditis with or without encephalopathy
Nonspecific MRI abnormalities related to migraine, aging, or trauma

CADASIL, cerebral autosomal dominant arteriopathy with subcortical infarcts and leukoencephalopathy; *HTLV,* human T-cell lymphotropic virus.
From Goldman L, Schafer AI: *Goldman's Cecil Medicine,* ed 24, Philadelphia, 2012, Saunders.

- Degenerative: subacute combined degeneration of the cord (vitamin B_{12} deficiency), amyotrophic lateral sclerosis, primary lateral sclerosis
- Infections: Lyme disease, neurosyphilis, HIV, tropical spastic paraparesis, progressive multifocal leukoencephalopathy, Whipple's disease
- Inflammatory: systemic lupus erythematosus, vasculitis, sarcoidosis, Sjögren's disease, Behçet's disease, celiac disease
- Inherited metabolic disorders: leukodystrophies
- Mitochondrial: Leber's hereditary optic neuropathy, mitochondrial encephalopathy, lactic acidosis, and strokelike episodes (MELAS)
- Neoplasms: CNS lymphoma, metastases
- Vascular: subcortical infarcts, Binswanger's disease

WORKUP

- Lumbar puncture for cases that are atypical or do not satisfy the diagnostic criteria for MS. Typical CSF abnormalities may include

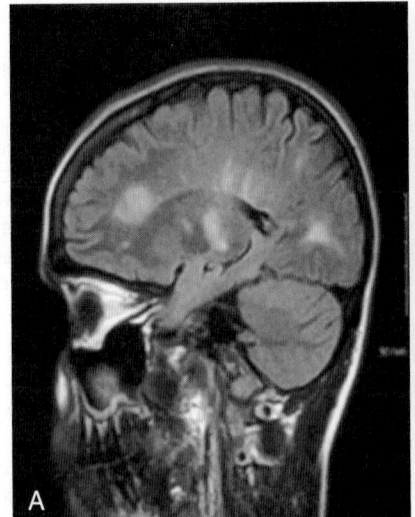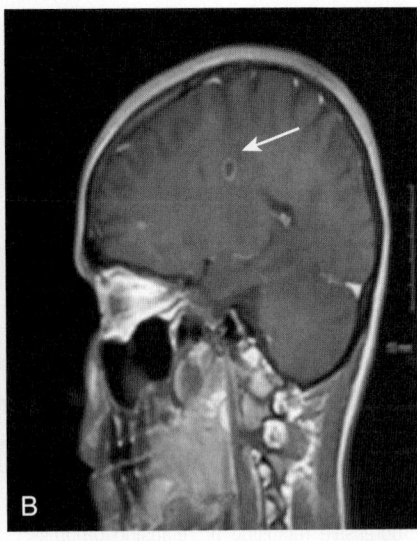

FIG. 2 Multiple sclerosis. A, Sagittal FLAIR image magnetic resonance scan shows multiple lesions in corpus callosum, "Dawson's fingers" (periventricular fingerlike lesions oriented towards the ventricles), along with ovoid and punctuate lesions in the deep white matter. **B,** Gadolinium-enhanced scan shows an enhancing lesion *(arrow).*

increased protein (less than 100 mg/dl), mild elevation of mononuclear white blood cells, and increased IgG synthesis rate. 70% of clinically definite MS (CDMS) have elevated CSF immunoglobulin (Ig) G index and 90% have oligoclonal bands. (Serum needs to be sent to lab simultaneously with CSF for both tests.) False-positive results with IgG index and rarely with positive OCBs can be seen in CNS infections, parainfections, vasculitis, and CNS lymphoma.

- Serum: complete blood count, ESR, chemistry panel, liver function tests, ANA, vitamin B_{12}, vitamin D.
- Consider collagen vascular serum tests, neuromyelitis optica IgG A, Lyme titer, ACE TSH, free T_4, anti–thyroglobulin A, very-long-chain fatty acids, arylsulfatase A.
- Consider optical coherence tomography or evoked potentials (visual, somatosensory and brain stem auditory evoked response).

IMAGING STUDIES

Brain MRI with and without gadolinium is recommended in all cases. Fig. 2 illustrates imaging features of MS. MRI with and without contrast of the cervical and thoracic spine can be helpful. MRI assesses acute and chronic lesions as well as atrophy. A normal MRI of the brain does not conclusively exclude early MS.

(Rx) TREATMENT

NONPHARMACOLOGIC THERAPY

Patient education regarding disease characteristics, treatment options, risks and benefits of treatment, and prognosis. Often patients need intermittent rest periods on a daily basis and when physically active, and avoid exposure to heat, which typically worsens symptoms (not the disease).

Recommend physical therapy for new or worsening weakness, incoordination, or spasticity.

ACUTE GENERAL Rx

Relapses: high-dose IV methylprednisolone (3-5 days of 15 mg/kg/day, with a maximum of 1 g/day), often followed by a 7- to 10-day prednisone or methylprednisolone taper. High-dose corticosteroids do not alter the long-term course of disease. May consider plasmapheresis for refractory cases.

CHRONIC Rx

- FDA-approved therapies are only for relapsing MS; there are none yet approved for progressive MS.
- Disease-modifying injection therapy includes interferon beta-1a (IM Avonex, IM Plegridy, SC Rebif), interferon beta-1b (SC Betaseron, SC Extavia), and glatiramer acetate (SC Copaxone). Common side effects for interferons include flulike symptoms, liver toxicity, and leukopenia; CBC and LFTs (initially q1mo, then q3mo). Common side effects for Copaxone include injection site reactions and benign chest tightness; no serum studies are needed.
- Disease-modifying oral therapy: Consider baseline pregnancy test and infectious tests for all oral therapies, although not required by the FDA, such as VZV Ab, Lyme Ab, TB test, JC virus Ab, hepatitis Ab panel. Also review general risk of infections (hx UTIs, kidney stones, smoking, diabetes, bronchitis, disability, pulmonary function, and age). Typically monthly CBC and liver function tests for 6 mo then q3mo; pregnancy test.
  1. Fingolimod (Gilenya), a sphingosine-1-phosphate receptor modulator and lymphocyte sequester. Possible side effects: liver toxicity, bradycardia with first dose (requiring cardiac monitoring and ECG for at least 8 hr after administration of first dose), arrhythmia, pancytopenia, macular edema (ophtho exam at baseline, 3 months, and thereafter for those with hx DM or uveitis), and reduced pulmonary function. Obtain VZV serology.

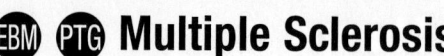
M

2. Teriflunomide (Aubagio), reversible inhibitor of pyrimidine synthesis (enzyme dihydroorotate dehydrogenase). Possible side effects: diarrhea, abnormal liver function tests, nausea, and hair loss; pregnancy category X. Serum levels can be measured, and drug can be eliminated by charcoal or cholestyramine. Obtain TB test.

3. Dimethyl fumarate (Tecfidera), mechanism includes inhibition of transcription of NF-KB. Frequent side effects include nausea, abdominal discomfort, and flushing—especially during the first month—and rarely leukopenia.

- Disease-modifying IV therapy:
  1. Natalizumab (Tysabri) is a monoclonal humanized Ab that binds integrin-$\alpha 4$ interfering with binding to VCAM-1. It has been associated with a *higher* risk of progressive multifocal leukoencephalopathy (JC virus) than other immunomodulatory therapies. Test for JC virus Ab at least annually (every 6 months if history of chemotherapy). If positive, PML is still rare, but risk increases with increased length of therapy, history of chemotherapy, and concomitant immunosuppressants.
  2. For rapidly progressive disability or frequent relapses on other maximum therapy, MS specialist may consider alemtuzumab, cyclophosphamide, or rituximab.

- Symptomatic therapy:
  - Dalfampridine (Ampyra) is a potassium channel blocker recently approved to improve walking speed in patients with MS.
  - Treat spasticity with baclofen or tizanidine. Onabotulinum toxin type A injection

for focal intractable spasticity. Intrathecal baclofen pump for generalized intractable spasticity. Acute worsening may be due to infections such as UTI, injury, recent surgery, or colder temperatures.

- Treat urge incontinence with anticholinergic/muscarinic therapy such as oxybutynin, tolterodine, or solifenacin. Treat urinary retention with tamsulosin. In both cases, rule out a bladder infection.
- Treat dysesthesias with gabapentin or oxcarbazepine.
- Fatigue: consider amantadine 100 mg bid, modafinil, stimulant, or fluoxetine.
- Tremor: clonazepam, carbamazepine, propranolol, or gabapentin.
- Depression and anxiety are common. Consider referring to both a counselor and psychiatrist.

DISPOSITION

Most patients have complete or near-complete recovery weeks to months after a relapse. Typically, 2 relapses occur in RRMS patient per year (75% will have >1 relapse). Although the rate of disease progression is highly variable, there is higher risk of greater long-term disability with higher relapse rate during the first 2-5 yr, poor recovery from initial relapses, older age of onset, involvement of multiple systems, male sex, African-American, and primary progressive disease.

REFERRAL

- Referral to neurologist is highly recommended. Referral to MS specialist should be considered in cases of poor response to therapy and/or if there is concern about complications of therapies.

- Consider referrals for physical, speech, and occupational therapy.
- Consider referral to urology if possible dyssynergia, or not responsive to treatment.

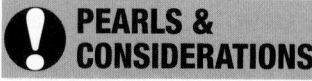 **PEARLS & CONSIDERATIONS**

- Clinically isolated syndrome (CIS): isolated demyelinating event and assessing risk of CDMS 1) in optic neuritis, if brain MRI is completely normal, there is 20% to 25% chance of CDMS over 15 yrs. 2) In CIS, if there are >2 T2 hyperintensities on brain MRI, there is 84% risk, and if there are >2 Gd + lesions there is a 96% risk of CDMS over 18 months.
- Pseudorelapses may occur with heat, fever, or infections (urinary tract infections common in patients with MS).
- Headache, fever, altered mental status, elevated CSF WBCs, or recurrent relapses over days to weeks, raises concern for CNS infection or ADEM.

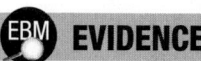 **EVIDENCE**

Available at www.expertconsult.com

SUGGESTED READINGS

Available at www.expertconsult.com

RELATED CONTENT

Multiple Sclerosis (Patient Information)

AUTHORS: **JOSEPH S. KASS, M.D., J.D.,** and **ALEXANDRA DEGENHARDT, M.D., M.M.SC.**

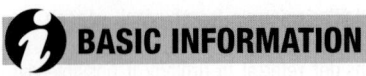

DEFINITION

Mumps is an acute generalized viral infection that is usually characterized by nonsuppurative swelling and tenderness of one or both parotid glands. It is caused by mumps virus, a single-stranded RNA paramyxovirus, of which humans are the only natural host.

SYNONYMS

Viral parotitis
Parotitis

ICD-10CM CODES
B26.0   Mumps orchitis
B26.1   Mumps meningitis
B26.2   Mumps encephalitis
B26.3   Mumps pancreatitis
B26.81   Mumps hepatitis
B26.82   Mumps myocarditis
B26.83   Mumps nephritis
B26.84   Mumps polyneuropathy
B26.85   Mumps arthritis
B26.89   Other mumps complications
B26.9   Mumps without complication

EPIDEMIOLOGY & DEMOGRAPHICS

INCIDENCE (IN U.S.):
- About 300 infections/yr. Sporadic outbreaks still occur in schools, colleges, military posts, or summer camps started by an unvaccinated person.
- Recent mumps outbreaks in the U.S.: at an Ohio university in 2014 (386 cases), at a California university in 2011 (29 cases)
- More than 150,000 cases/yr before licensure of mumps vaccine in 1967

PREDOMINANT SEX: Males = females
PREDOMINANT AGE: 75% of disease in teen-age years
PEAK INCIDENCE: Late winter and early spring months
GENETICS: Congenital infection:

- First-trimester infection is associated with excessive fetal deaths.
- Second- and third-trimester infection is not associated with increased fetal mortality.

Neonatal infection:
- Uncommon
- Uncommon in infants <1 yr because of passive immunity conferred by placental transfer of maternal antibody

PHYSICAL FINDINGS & CLINICAL PRESENTATION

- Prodromal period: includes low-grade fever, malaise, anorexia, and headache
- Parotid swelling (Fig. 1) and tenderness; often the first signs of infection:
  1. Progresses over 2 to 3 days, then opposite side may become involved
  2. Unilateral parotitis in 25% of cases
  3. Considerable pain with parotid swelling, causing trismus and difficulty with mastication and pronunciation
  4. Pain exacerbated by eating or drinking citrus and other acidic foods
  5. Possible fever with parotid swelling, ranging up to 40° C
  6. Parotid swelling, usually resolving within 1 wk
- CNS involvement:
  1. May occur from 1 wk before to 2 wk after the onset of parotitis or even in its absence
  2. Meningitis:
     a. Occurs in 1% to 10% of patients with mumps parotitis
     b. Occurs three times more often in males than females
     c. Symptoms: headache, fever, nuchal rigidity, and vomiting
     d. Full recovery with no sequelae
  3. Encephalitis:
     a. May develop early, as a result of direct viral invasion of neurons, or late, around the second wk after onset of parotitis, and is a postinfectious demyelinating process.

b. Mumps accounted for only 0.5% of viral meningitis.
c. Symptoms: fever, alterations in the level of consciousness, possible seizures, paresis or paralysis, and aphasia. Fever can be quite high (40° to 41° C).
d. Cerebellitis and hydrocephalus are serious complications of mumps encephalitis.
e. May result in permanent sequelae or death.
  4. Other rare neurologic complications include cerebellar ataxia, transverse myelitis, Guillain-Barré syndrome, and facial palsy.
- Epididymoorchitis:
  1. Most common extrasalivary gland complication of mumps in adult men
  2. Occurs in 38% of postpubertal males who have mumps
  3. Most often unilateral but is bilateral in 30% of males who develop this complication
  4. May precede development of parotitis and may be only manifestation of mumps
  5. Two thirds of cases develop during first week of parotitis
  6. Symptoms:
     a. Severe pain, swelling, and tenderness of the testes and scrotal erythema
     b. Fever and chills
  7. Some degree of testicular atrophy in 50% of cases, mo to yr later
  8. Sterility from bilateral orchitis is rare
- Involvement of pancreas and ovaries:
  1. Pancreas: abdominal pain, fever, and vomiting
  2. Ovaries: oophoritis
     a. Occurs in 5% of postpubertal women with mumps
     b. Symptoms include fever, nausea, vomiting, and lower abdominal pain
     c. May rarely result in decreased fertility and premature menopause
- Transient renal impairment: common and manifested by hematuria and polyuria
- Joint involvement:
  1. Migratory polyarthritis is most frequent
  2. Infrequently affects adults with mumps
  3. Occurs rarely in children
  4. Self-limited, with complete resolution
- Deafness:
  1. Most often unilateral, involving high frequencies; may rarely cause bilateral involvement
  2. Most patients recover
  3. Permanent unilateral deafness reported in 1 in 20,000 cases
  4. Labyrinthitis and end lymphatic hydrops also reported
- Myocardial involvement:
  1. Uncommon
  2. Rarely causes progressive and fulminant fatal myocarditis with dilated cardiomyopathy
  3. Refractory arrhythmia and congestive heart failure
  4. Coronary artery involvement

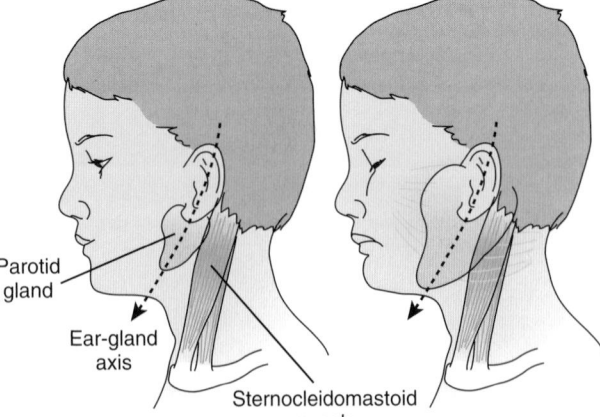

Parotid gland
Ear-gland axis
Sternocleidomastoid muscle

FIG. 1 Schematic drawing of a parotid gland infected with mumps *(right)* compared with a normal gland *(left)*. An imaginary line bisecting the long axis of the ear divides the parotid gland into two equal parts. These anatomic relationships are not altered in the enlarged gland. An enlarged cervical lymph node is usually posterior to the imaginary line. (From Mumps [epidemic parotitis]. In Krugman S et al [eds]: *Infectious diseases in children*, ed 6, St Louis, 1977, Mosby.)

- Eye involvement:
  1. Corneal endotheliitis following mumps parotitis

ETIOLOGY

- Virus is spread via direct contact, droplet nuclei, fomites, or oral or nasal secretions.
- Patients are contagious from 48 hr before to 9 days after parotid swelling.

DX DIAGNOSIS

DIFFERENTIAL DIAGNOSIS

- Other viruses that may cause acute parotitis:
  1. Parainfluenza types 1 and 3
  2. Coxsackie viruses
  3. Influenza A
  4. Cytomegalovirus
- Suppurative parotitis:
  1. Most often caused by *Staphylococcus aureus*
  2. May be differentiated from mumps
     a. Extreme indurations, tenderness and erythema overlying the gland
     b. Ability to express pus from Stensen's duct or massage of parotid
- Other conditions that may occur with parotid enlargement or swelling:
  1. Sjögren's syndrome
  2. Leukemia
  3. Diabetes mellitus
  4. Uremia
  5. Malnutrition
  6. Cirrhosis
- Drugs that cause parotid swelling:
  1. Phenothiazines
  2. Phenylbutazone
  3. Thiouracil
  4. Iodides
- Conditions that cause unilateral swelling:
  1. Tumors
  2. Cysts
  3. Stones causing obstruction
  4. Strictures causing obstruction

WORKUP

- Diagnosis based on history of exposure and physical finding of parotid tenderness with mild to moderate constitutional symptoms.
- Diagnosis is confirmed by a variety of serologic tests or isolation of the virus.

LABORATORY TESTS

- Diagnosis is confirmed by a positive IgM mumps antibody or by fourfold rise between acute and convalescent sera by CF, ELISA, or neutralization tests. However, serologic mumps testing is particularly unhelpful in some vaccinated individuals who can have mumps without having the usual immunoglobulin M (IgM) spike. A polymerase chain reaction (PCR) assay, reverse transcription PCR, also is available.
- Virus can be isolated from the saliva, usually from 2 to 3 days before to 4 to 5 days after the onset of parotitis. Researchers have shown that many cases labeled as "parotitis" are actually caused by other viruses (EB virus, human herpesvirus 6B, human parainfluenza virus).[1]
- Virus can be cultured from CSF in patients with meningitis during the first 3 days of meningeal findings. More rapid confirmation of mumps in the CSF is IgM antibody capture immunoassay and nested PCR assay.
- Virus can be detected in urine during the first 2 wk of infection.
- WBC:
  1. May be normal or possible mild leukopenia with a relative lymphocytosis
  2. Leukocytosis with left shift with extrasalivary gland involvement, such as meningitis, orchitis, or pancreatitis
- Serum amylase:
  1. Elevated in the presence of parotitis
  2. May remain elevated for 2 to 3 wk
  3. May be differentiated from mumps and parotids by isoenzyme analysis or serum pancreatic lipase
- Mumps meningitis:
  1. CSF WBCs from 10 to 2000 WBC/mm^3 with a predominance of lymphocytes
  2. In 20% to 25% of patients, predominance of polymorphonuclear cells
  3. CSF protein normal or mildly elevated
  4. CSF glucose low, <40 mg/dl, in 6% to 30% of patients

RX TREATMENT

NONPHARMACOLOGIC THERAPY

- Supportive treatment
- Adequate hydration and nutrition

ACUTE GENERAL Rx

- Analgesics and antipyretics to relieve pain and fever
- Narcotic analgesics, along with bed rest, ice packs, and a testicular bridge, to relieve pain associated with mumps orchitis
- IV fluids for patients with frequent vomiting associated with mumps pancreatitis or meningitis

DISPOSITION

Most patients recover without incident.

---

[1]Barshey AE et al: Viruses detected among sporadic cases of parotitis, United States 2009-2011, *J Infect Dis* 208:1979, 2013.

REFERRAL

- To a neurologist if significant neurologic complications develop during or following mumps (myelitis, encephalitis, cranial nerve involvement, cerebellar ataxia, etc.)
- To a cardiologist if viral perimyocarditis develops
- To a urologist if orchitis develops

! PEARLS & CONSIDERATIONS

COMMENTS

Prevention:

- Attenuated live mumps virus vaccine has been available since 1967.
  1. Usually given in combination with measles and rubella vaccines (MMR) or as a measles-mumps-rubella-varicella vaccine (MMRV). A monovalent mumps vaccine is no longer available.
  2. Either vaccine should be given at 12 to 15 mo of age and again at 4 to 6 years of age.
  3. Seroconversion in about 100% of infants given the vaccine.
  4. Contraindicated in pregnant women and immunocompromised patients.
  5. Patients with asymptomatic HIV infection and patients with symptomatic HIV infection, in the absence of severe immunosuppression, can safely receive mumps, measles, and rubella (MMR) vaccine.
  6. Adverse events of vaccination include local pain, indurations, thrombocytopenic purpura, Guillain-Barré syndrome, and cerebellar ataxia.
  7. Adults born before 1957 are considered immune. Those born after 1957 who lack documentation of immunization are considered susceptible. Adults can receive two doses 1 month apart.
- The CDC and American Academy of Pediatrics (AAP) recommend that patients with mumps stay home from work or school for 5 days after onset of clinical symptoms.
- Because virus may be shed before the onset of parotid swelling, isolation possibly not of great value in limiting spread of infection. Use droplet precautions as per CDC and AAP.
- Mumps is a notifiable disease in all U.S. states.

SUGGESTED READING

Available at www.expertconsult.com

RELATED CONTENT

Mumps (Patient Information)

AUTHOR: **GLENN G. FORT, M.D., M.P.H.**

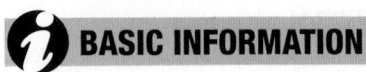

BASIC INFORMATION

DEFINITION

Muscular dystrophy (MD) refers to a heterogeneous group of inherited disorders resulting in characteristic patterns of muscle weakness, some with cardiac involvement. Only disorders with childhood or adult onset are considered here (i.e., excluding congenital myopathies).

SYNONYMS

MD

ICD-10CM CODES
G71.0 Muscular dystrophy

EPIDEMIOLOGY & DEMOGRAPHICS

INCIDENCE:

- Most common childhood MD is Duchenne's muscular dystrophy (DMD) with an incidence of 1/3500 male births.
- Most common adult MD is myotonic dystrophy with an incidence as high as 1/8000.

GENETICS:

- **Dystrophinopathies:** X-linked recessive defect in dystrophin gene resulting in either absence (DMD) or reduced/defective (Becker's MD [BMD]) dystrophin (Fig. 1)
- **Myotonic Dystrophy:** Autosomal dominant (AD) CTG trinucleotide repeat (see "Myotonia")
- **Limb-Girdle Muscular Dystrophy:** The majority are autosomal recessive, also autosomal dominant forms. Associated with deficiencies identified in multiple proteins (sarcoglycan, calpain, dystroglycan, and dysferlin may be most common; also may involve telethonin, lamin A/C, myotilin, and caveolin-3)
- **Emery-Dreifuss Muscular Dystrophy:** X-linked recessive defect in nuclear protein emerin or AR/AD defect in inner nuclear lamina proteins lamin A/C
- **Facioscapulohumeral Muscular Dystrophy:** AD; genetic mutation causes deletion of 3.3 kb repeat
- **Oculopharyngeal Muscular Dystrophy:** AD GCG trinucleotide repeat resulting in deficient mRNA transfer from nucleus

PHYSICAL FINDINGS & CLINICAL PRESENTATION

- **Dystrophinopathies:** Proximal arm and leg weakness with hypertrophic calf muscles (Fig. 2), delayed motor milestones, cognitive impairment, cardiac involvement, progressive course resulting in respiratory complications and respiratory failure
  1. DMD (Fig. 3) onset at 2 to 3 yr old, typically wheelchair-bound by 12 yr
  2. BMD onset at 5 to 15 yr old, ambulatory beyond age 15
- **Myotonic Dystrophy:** Variable age of onset and severity manifesting as predominantly distal weakness with long face, percussion and grip myotonia, temporalis and masseter wasting, ptosis, hypersomnolence, cognitive impairment, and cardiac conduction defects. May be associated with frontal balding, cataracts, impaired glucose tolerance, and male infertility.
- **Limb-Girdle MD:** Phenotypically and genetically heterogenous characterized by proximal hip and shoulder girdle weakness, some genotypes featuring cardiac involvement
- **Emery-Dreifuss MD:** Early adulthood onset with predominantly humeroperoneal weakness, early contractures, and cardiac dysfunction
- **Facioscapulohumeral MD:** Onset typically in late childhood or adolescence with weakness mostly in face and shoulder girdle musculature and possible later, mild involvement of lower extremities
- **Oculopharyngeal MD:** Symptom onset typically in mid-adult life with ptosis, dysphagia, dysarthria, and proximal muscle weakness
- Table 1 shows a classification of muscular dystrophies

DIAGNOSIS

DIFFERENTIAL DIAGNOSIS

Myasthenia gravis, inflammatory myopathy, metabolic myopathy, endocrine myopathy, toxic myopathy, mitochondrial myopathy

WORKUP

- CK
- ECG, Holter monitor, echocardiography
- EMG
- Muscle biopsy with immunohistochemistry useful for diagnosis of dystrophinopathies and limb-girdle MD

- DNA analysis helpful if clinical suspicion is for myotonic, Emery-Dreifuss, facioscapulohumeral, and oculopharyngeal MDs
- Assessment of respiratory parameters, including forced vital capacity (FVC)

TREATMENT

NONPHARMACOLOGIC THERAPY

- Genetic counseling
- Physical, occupational, respiratory, speech therapy as symptoms dictate
- Screening for sleep-disordered breathing with overnight polysomnogram (PSG) if clinically indicated
- Pacemaker placement may be necessary if cardiac conduction defect present

ACUTE GENERAL Rx

Prednisone may modestly prolong ambulation in DMD. A dose of 0.75 mg/kg/day may improve muscle strength and function over 6 months to 2 years. These short-term benefits must be weighed against the side effects of long-term steroid therapy.

CHRONIC Rx

Vigilance to avoid cardiac and respiratory complications, joint contractures

DISPOSITION

Variable course, because severity of phenotype is contingent upon both diagnosis and genotype

REFERRAL

- Surgical referral for correction of scoliosis or contractures may be necessary
- Assessment and follow-up in an MD specialty clinic

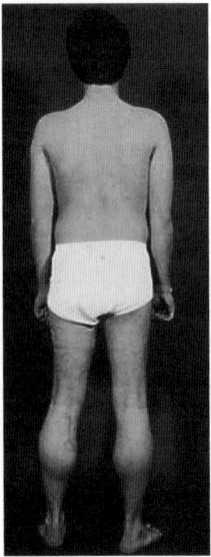

FIG. 2 Becker muscular dystrophy in a 24-year-old male. There is dystrophy of the shoulder girdle and calf pseudohypertrophy. (Courtesy Dr. R. Pascuzzi. From Libby PL et al: *Braunwald's heart disease: a textbook of cardiovascular medicine,* ed 8, Philadelphia, 2007, Saunders.)

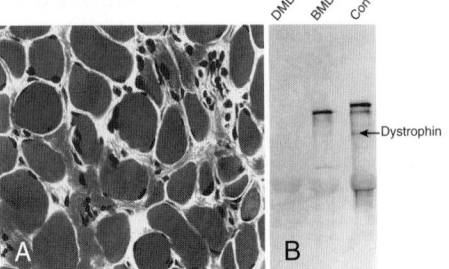

FIG. 1 A, Duchenne muscular dystrophy showing variation in muscle fiber size, increased endomysial connective tissue, and regenerating fibers. **B,** Western blot showing absence of dystrophin in DMD and altered dystrophin size in Becker muscular dystrophy (BMD) compared with control (Con). (Courtesy Dr. L. Kunkel, Children's Hospital, Boston. From Kumar V et al: *Robbins and Cotran pathologic basis of disease,* ed 7, Philadelphia, 2005, Saunders.)

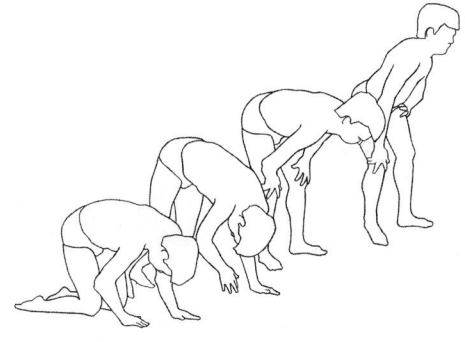

FIG. 3 In Duchenne's muscular dystrophy, the patient will get up from the floor with Gower's maneuver. The boy will "walk up" his body with his hands as he rises. (From Remmel KS et al: *Handbook of symptom-oriented neurology,* ed 3, St Louis, 2002, Mosby.)

❗ PEARLS & CONSIDERATIONS

Formal evaluation by anesthetist is recommended before any operation with general anesthesia in patients with dystrophinopathy.

RELATED CONTENT

Muscular Dystrophy (Patient Information)

AUTHOR: **TAYLOR HARRISON, M.D.**

Diseases and Disorders

TABLE 1 Classification of Muscular Dystrophies

Disease	Genetic Locus	Inheritance	Protein	Outcome
Duchenne/Becker		XR	Dystrophin	Lethal
Emery-Dreifuss		XR	Emerin, lamins A and C	40% lethality
Limb-Girdle Muscular Dystrophies				
LGMD 1A	5q31	AD	Myotilin	With LGMD, less-severe forms can emerge during the first three decades, leading to loss of ambulation after 30 yr of age. The most severe forms start at 3-5 yr of age and progress rapidly.
LGMD 1B	1q11-q21	AD	Laminin A/C	
LGMD 1C	3p35	AD	Caveolin	
LGMD 1D	6q23	AD	—	
LGMD 1E	7q	AD	—	
LGMD 1F	7q32	AD	—	
LGMD 1G	4p21	AD	—	
LGMD 2A	15q15.1-q21.1	AR	Calpain 3	
LGMD 2B	2p13	AR	Dysferlin	
LGMD 2C	13q12	AR	γ-Sarcoglycan	
LGMD 2D	17q12-q21.33	AR	α-Sarcoglycan	
LGMD 2E	4q12	AR	β-Sarcoglycan	
LGMD 2F	5q33-q34	AR	δ-Sarcoglycan	
LGMD 2G	17q11-q12	AR	Telethonin	
LGMD 2H	9q31-q34.1	AR	E3-Ubiquitin ligase (TRIM32)	
LGMD 2I	19q13.3	AR	Fukutin-related protein	
LGMD 2J	2q24.3	AR	Titin	
LGMD 2K	9q34	AR	Protein O-mannosyltransferase	
CMDs with CNS Involvement				
Fukuyama CMD	9q31	AR	Fukutin	LE, 11-16 yr
Walker-Warburg CMD	1p32	AR	O-Mannosyltransferase	LE, <3 yr
Muscle-eye-brain CMD	1p32-34	AR	O-MNAGAT	LE, 10-30 yr
CMDs without CNS Involvement				
Merosin-deficient classic type	6q2	AR	Merosin (laminin A$_2$)	Many patients never walk; others have an LGMD pattern
Merosin-positive classic type	4p16.3	AR	Selenoprotein N1, collagen VI α$_2$	Course stabilizes in late childhood; many continue to walk into adulthood
Integrin-deficient CMD	12q13	AR	Integrin α7	Presents early in infancy with hypotonia and delayed milestones
Other Dystrophies				
Facioscapulohumeral	4q35	AD	—	20% wheelchair bound
Oculopharyngeal	14q11.2-q13	AD/AR	Polyadenylate binding protein nuclear 1	Onset: ≈48 yr, 100% symptomatic by age 70
Myotonic dystrophy	19q13.3	AD	DMPK, CCHC-type zinc finger and CNBP	Onset: 50% show signs by age 20; variable severity

AD, Autosomal dominant; *AR,* autosomal recessive; *CCHC,* cysteine and histidine amino acid sequence in this class of zinc finger; *CMD,* congenital muscular dystrophy; *CNBP,* cellular nucleic acid–binding protein; *CNS,* central nervous system; *DMPK,* dystrophia myotonica-protein kinase; *LE,* life expectancy; *LGMD,* limb-girdle muscular dystrophy; *O-MNAGAT,* O-mannose β-1,2-N-acetylglucosaminyl transferase; *XR,* X chromosome related.
From Firestein G.S.: *Kelley's textbook of rheumatology,* ed 9, Philadelphia, 2013, Saunders.

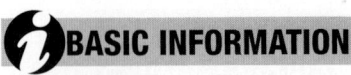

BASIC INFORMATION

DEFINITION

Mushroom poisoning is intoxication resulting from ingestion of poisonous mushrooms.

ICD-10CM CODES
T62.0X1A Toxic effect of ingested mushrooms, accidental (unintentional), initial encounter

EPIDEMIOLOGY & DEMOGRAPHICS

- 5% of all mushrooms are poisonous. Distinction between poisonous and edible mushrooms may be difficult even by experienced persons.
- Common poisonous species include *Amanita, Russula, Gyromitra,* and *Omphalotus* (see Table E1).
- Identification of syndromes is more important than knowing the associated species (Table 2).

PHYSICAL FINDINGS & CLINICAL PRESENTATION

- *Russula* causes confusion, delirium, visual disturbance, tachycardia, and diarrhea within a few hours of ingestion. Prognosis: spontaneous recovery (mortality rate >1%).
- *Amanita* and *Gyromitra* intoxication begins with symptoms of gastroenteritis (nausea, vomiting, diarrhea, and abdominal cramps) approximately 10 hr after ingestion. *Amanita* then causes cardiomyopathy and hepatic and renal failure. *Gyromitra* produces jaundice and seizures. Both mushrooms are associated with a 50% mortality rate.
- *Omphalotus* causes symptoms of gastroenteritis that subside spontaneously within 24 hr.

ETIOLOGY

- *Amanita* contains cytotoxic substances and isoxazoles that are gamma-aminobutyric acid neurotransmitter analogs.
- *Gyromitra* contains a pyridoxine antagonist that disrupts the gastrointestinal mucosa and causes hemolysis.
- *Russula* contains a cholinergic substance.

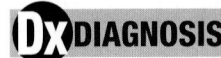 DIAGNOSIS

DIFFERENTIAL DIAGNOSIS

- Food poisoning
- Overdose of prescription or illegal drug
- Other intoxications
- See topic on specific organ failure (e.g., renal or hepatic failure) for differential diagnosis of those conditions

WORKUP

- History
- Inspection and identification of suspected mushrooms
- Mushroom or gastric content analysis (by thin-layer chromatography or radioimmunoassay)

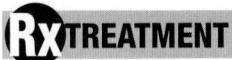 TREATMENT

- Gastric lavage
- Repeated administration of activated charcoal
- Penicillin G or silibinin can be used for *Amanita* mushroom intoxication. Silibinin interferes with hepatic uptake of alpha-amanitine. IV silibinin is not currently available in the U.S. Where available, it is given at a rate of 5 mg/kg IV over 1 hour, followed by 20 mg/kg/day. An oral form of silibinin is available in health food stores as an extract from milk thistle called silymarin. Dose is 1 g PO qid. IV benzyl penicillin reduces hepatocyte uptake of amatoxin.
- Supportive care as needed (may require respiratory assistance, hemodialysis, or emergency liver transplantation)

RELATED CONTENT

Mushroom Poisoning (Patient Information)

AUTHOR: **FRED F. FERRI, M.D.**

Table 2 Mushroom Poisoning Syndromes

Syndrome	Commonly Implicated Mushrooms	Toxins
Short Incubation		
Delirium, restlessness	*Amanita muscaria, Amanita pantherina*	Ibotenic acid, muscimol
Parasympathetic hyperactivity	*Inocybe* spp., *Clitocybe* spp., *Boletus* spp.	Muscarine
Hallucinations, somnolence, dysphoria	*Psilocybe* spp., *Panaeolus* spp., *Conocybe* spp.	Psilocybin
Disulfiram reaction	*Coprinus atramentarius*	Coprine
Gastroenteritis	Many	Various uncharacterized irritants
Long Incubation		
Gastroenteritis, hepatorenal failure	*Amanita phalloides, Amanita virosa,* and other *Amanita; Galerina, Cortinarius,* and *Lepiota* spp.	Cyclopeptides (i.e., amatoxins, phallotoxins)
Gastroenteritis, muscle cramping, hepatic failure, hemolysis, seizures, coma	*Gyromitra* spp.	Gyromitrin
Gastroenteritis, acute renal failure (temporary)	*Amanita smithiana*	Allenic norleucine
Gastroenteritis, acute renal failure (often irreversible)	*Cortinarius* spp.	Orellanine

From Bennett JE et al: *Mandell, Douglas, and Bennett's principles and practice of infectious diseases,* ed 8, Philadelphia, 2015, WB Saunders.

BASIC INFORMATION

DEFINITION

Myasthenia gravis (MG) is an autoimmune disorder that affects postsynaptic neuromuscular transmission classically mediated by antibodies directed against the nicotinic acetylcholine receptor (AChR) of the neuromuscular junction, resulting in a decrease in functional postsynaptic ACh receptors and consequent weakness. More recently, antibodies against muscle-specific tyrosine kinase (MuSK) have been described, which impact both pre- and postsynaptic function of the neuromuscular junction.

ICD-10CM CODES
G70.00	Myasthenia gravis without (acute) exacerbation
G70.01	Myasthenia gravis with (acute) exacerbation
P94.0	Transient neonatal myasthenia gravis

EPIDEMIOLOGY & DEMOGRAPHICS

INCIDENCE (IN U.S.): 8 to 10 cases annually per 1 million persons. It is the most common disorder of neuromuscular junction transmission.
PEAK INCIDENCE: Female, second to third decades; male, sixth to eighth decades
PREVALENCE (IN U.S.): 150 to 250 cases per 1 million.
PREDOMINANT SEX: Females are affected more often than males (3:2) in adults; they are equally affected in the elderly
GENETICS: Increased frequency of HLA-B8, DR3

PHYSICAL FINDINGS & CLINICAL PRESENTATION

- The hallmark of MG is fluctuating weakness worsened with exercise and improved with rest.
- Generalized weakness involving proximal muscles, diaphragm, and neck extensors is common.
- Weakness is confined to eyelids and extraocular muscles in approximately 15% of patients.
- Bulbar symptoms of ptosis, diplopia, dysarthria, and dysphagia are common.
- Reflexes, sensation, and coordination are normal.

ETIOLOGY

Antibody-mediated decrease in nicotinic AChR in the postsynaptic neuromuscular junction resulting in defective neuromuscular transmission and subsequent muscle weakness and fatigue. Early-onset MG is associated with *HLA-DR3*, *HLA-B8*, and non-*HLA* genes. Late-onset MG is associated with *HLA-DR2*, *HLA-B27*, and *HLA-DRB1*. MuSK antibodies have been recognized since 2001 and present with a similar syndrome to AChR MG although they may have more bulbar weakness, proximal muscle atrophy, and either lack of or paradoxical response to pyridostigmine.

DIAGNOSIS

DIFFERENTIAL DIAGNOSIS

Lambert-Eaton myasthenic syndrome, botulism, medication-induced myasthenia, chronic progressive external ophthalmoplegia, congenital myasthenic syndromes, thyroid disease, basilar meningitis, intracranial mass lesion with cranial neuropathy, Miller-Fisher variant of Guillain-Barré syndrome

WORKUP

- Edrophonium (Tensilon) test (Fig. E1): useful in MG patients with ocular symptoms. Cardiac monitoring and atropine ready at the bedside are essential. Patients with MG may also have a positive ice test (Fig. E2).
- Repetitive nerve stimulation: successive stimulation shows decrement of muscle action potential in clinically weak muscle; may be negative in up to 50%.
- Single-fiber electromyography: highly sensitive; abnormal in up to 95% of patients.
- Serum AChR antibodies found in up to 90% of patients.
- A subset of patients with seronegative MG may have MuSK antibodies.

ADDITIONAL TESTS

- Spirometry to document pulmonary function
- CT scan or MRI with contrast of anterior chest to look for thymoma or residual thymic tissue. 10% of patients with MG have a thymoma and the prevalence increases with age.
- Thyroid-stimulating hormone, free T_4 to rule out thyroid disease

TREATMENT

NONPHARMACOLOGIC THERAPY

- Patient education to facilitate recognition of worsening symptoms and impress need for medical evaluation at onset of clinical deterioration
- Avoidance of selected drugs known to provoke exacerbations of MG (beta-blockers, aminoglycoside and quinolone antibiotics, penicillamine, interferons, class I antiarrhythmics [procainamide, quinidine, etc.])
- Prompt treatment of infections, diet modification, and speech evaluation with dysphagia

ACUTE GENERAL Rx

- Symptomatic treatment with acetylcholinesterase inhibitors:
  1. Pyridostigmine 30 to 60 mg PO q4 to 6h initially; onset of effects is 30 min, duration 4 hr. May be titrated up to 120 mg every 4 hr. GI upset is not uncommon with higher doses and may respond to hyoscyamine.
- Immunosuppressive treatment with corticosteroids and azathioprine is first line treatment
  1. Prednisone initiated at 10 to 20 mg qd titrate by 5-mg increments to effect or dose of 1 mg/kg/day with improvement

in 2 to 4 wk and maximal response by 3 to 6 mo
  2. Azathioprine initiated at 50 mg qd titrated to 2 to 3 mg/kg/day with clinical effect in 6 to 12 mo. Azathioprine is not recommended in patients with no thiopurine methyltransferase activity.
- Alternative secondary agents:
  1. Cyclosporine initiated at 5 mg/kg/day with clinical effect within 1 to 2 mo
  2. Mycophenolate mofetil 500 mg twice a day titrated to 2 g/day with clinical effect in 3 to 6 mo, but can be up to 12 mo
  3. Rituximab
- Plasmapheresis and IV immunoglobulin are short-term options for immunotherapy during an exacerbation. There is no significant difference in efficacy between IVIG and plasmapheresis.
- Mechanical ventilation is lifesaving in setting of a myasthenic crisis. Consider elective intubation if forced vital capacity <15 ml/kg, maximal expiratory pressure <40 cm H_2O, or negative inspiratory pressure <25 cm H_2O.

SURGICAL Rx

- In thymomatous MG, thymectomy is indicated in all patients. If the tumor cannot be surgically resected, chemotherapy can be considered for prevention of local invasion and symptom relief.
- For nonthymomatous autoimmune MG, thymectomy may improve clinical outcomes and reduce the need for steroids over a 3-year period. Surgical referral should be considered in patients under 40 without significant medical comorbidities.

DISPOSITION

Course of disease is highly variable. Mortality rate has decreased from 75% to 4.5% over past 4 decades.

REFERRAL

Surgical referral for thymectomy in selected cases (see "Surgical Rx")

PEARLS & CONSIDERATIONS

- Sustained upward or lateral gaze and arm abduction for 120 sec may be necessary to elicit subtle signs on examination.
- Myasthenic patients can worsen rapidly and warrant close, careful observation during an exacerbation.

SUGGESTED READINGS

Available at www.expertconsult.com

RELATED CONTENT

Myasthenia Gravis (Patient Information)

AUTHORS: **RADHIKA SAMPAT, D.O.,** and **TAYLOR HARRISON, M.D.**

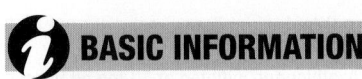

DEFINITION

Myelodysplastic syndromes (MDS) are a group of acquired clonal disorders affecting hematopoietic stem cells and are characterized by altered differentiation and proliferation. Patients present with peripheral blood cytopenias and morphologic abnormalities but have a hypercellular bone marrow upon examination. The increased marrow cellularity reflects ineffective hematopoiesis with inadequate maturation resulting in cytopenias.

CLASSIFICATION

- Several classification systems have been developed as our understanding of MDS has evolved. In 1982, the French-American-British (FAB) classification included refractory anemia (RA), refractory anemia with ringed sideroblasts (RARS), refractory anemia with excess blasts (RAEB), chronic myelomonocytic leukemia (CMML), and refractory anemia with excess blasts in transformation (RAEB-T).
- In 1999, the World Health Organization (WHO) modified the FAB by incorporating newer morphologic insights and cytogenetic findings. It reduced the blast percentage for the diagnosis of acute myeloid leukemia (AML) to 20%, added refractory cytopenia with multilineage dysplasia (RCMD), refined refractory anemia with excessive blasts into types 1 and 2 (RAEB-1, RAEB-2), and added unclassified MDS, and MDS associated with isolated del(5q).
- In 2008, the WHO further modified the classification by subcategorizing MDS into six different categories.

SYNONYMS

MDS
Preleukemia

ICD-10CM CODES
D46.9 Myelodysplastic syndrome, unspecified
D46.C Myelodysplastic syndrome with isolated del(5q) chromosomal abnormality
D46.Z Other myelodysplastic syndromes

EPIDEMIOLOGY & DEMOGRAPHICS

INCIDENCE (IN U.S.): Approximately 80 cases/100,000 persons per yr. An estimated 30,000 new cases are diagnosed annually in the U.S.
PREDOMINANT AGE: More common in elderly patients; median age >65 yr

PHYSICAL FINDINGS & CLINICAL PRESENTATION

- Patients often present with fatigue due to anemia and also with thrombocytopenia and leukopenia.
- Skin pallor, mucosal bleeding, and ecchymosis may be present.
- Fever, infection, and dyspnea are common.

ETIOLOGY

Exposure to radiation, chemotherapeutic agents, benzene, or other organic compounds is associated with myelodysplasia. Table 1 describes predisposing factors and epidemiologic associations of patients with MDS. Up to 40 genes are mutated in MDS with 90% of patients having at least one mutation and a median of two to three mutations detected per patient. These mutations affect specific functional pathways and can be subcategorized into those that affect spliceosome machinery, DNA methylation, chromatin modification, transcription factors, kinase signaling pathways, and DNA repair pathways.

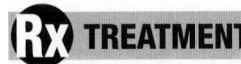 **DIAGNOSIS**

DIFFERENTIAL DIAGNOSIS

- Hereditary dysplasias (e.g., Fanconi's anemia, Diamond-Blackfan syndrome)
- Vitamin B_{12}/folate deficiency
- Exposure to toxins (drugs, alcohol, chemotherapy)
- Renal failure
- Irradiation
- Autoimmune disease
- Paroxysmal nocturnal hemoglobinuria

WORKUP

Diagnostic workup (Fig. 1) includes laboratory evaluation (Table E2) and bone marrow examination (Fig. E2). Cytogenetic analysis (Box E1) by conventional metaphase karyotyping or by MDS FISH assessment should be performed in patients with MDS. Physical examination, medical history, and laboratory tests aiding in diagnosis of MDS are described in Table 3.

TREATMENT

NONPHARMACOLOGIC THERAPY

- Packed red blood cell transfusions in patients with severe symptomatic anemia
- Platelet transfusions in patients with severe thrombocytopenia or those with bleeding episodes

ACUTE GENERAL Rx

- The initial focus of MDS therapy involves stratification of patients into low-, intermediate-, and high-risk states using well-defined and validated risk stratification systems. The original International Prognostic Scoring System (IPSS) incorporated cytopenias, cytogenetics, and blast percentage and is still clinically used. More classification systems have been proposed, and the revised IPSS (IPSS-R) has been created from an evaluation of more than 7000 patients. The IPSS-R utilizes a five-tier risk grouping and accounts for the degree of cytopenias as well as discrimination of bone marrow blast percentage and has 15 cytogenetic subtypes.
- Low-risk patients are treated with supportive care or growth factors.

TABLE 1 Predisposing Factors and Epidemiologic Associations of Patients with Myelodysplastic Syndrome

Heritable

Constitutional Genetic Disorders

Trisomy 8 mosaicism
Familial monosomy 7
Down syndrome (trisomy 21)
Neurofibromatosis 1
Germ cell tumors [embryonal dysgenesis del(12p)]

Congenital Neutropenia

Kostmann syndrome
Shwachman-Diamond syndrome

DNA Repair Deficiencies

Fanconi anemia
Ataxia-telangiectasia
Bloom syndrome
Xeroderma pigmentosum
Pharmacogenomic polymorphisms (GSTq1-null)

Acquired

Senescence

Mutagen Exposure

Alkylator therapy (chlorambucil, cyclophosphamide, melphalan, N-mustards)
Topoisomerase II inhibitors (anthracyclines)
β Emitters (32p)
Autologous stem cell transplantation
Environmental/occupational (benzene)
Tobacco
Aplastic anemia
Paroxysmal nocturnal hemoglobinuria

From Hoffman R et al: *Hematology, basic principles and practice*, ed 5, Philadelphia, 2009, Churchill Livingstone.

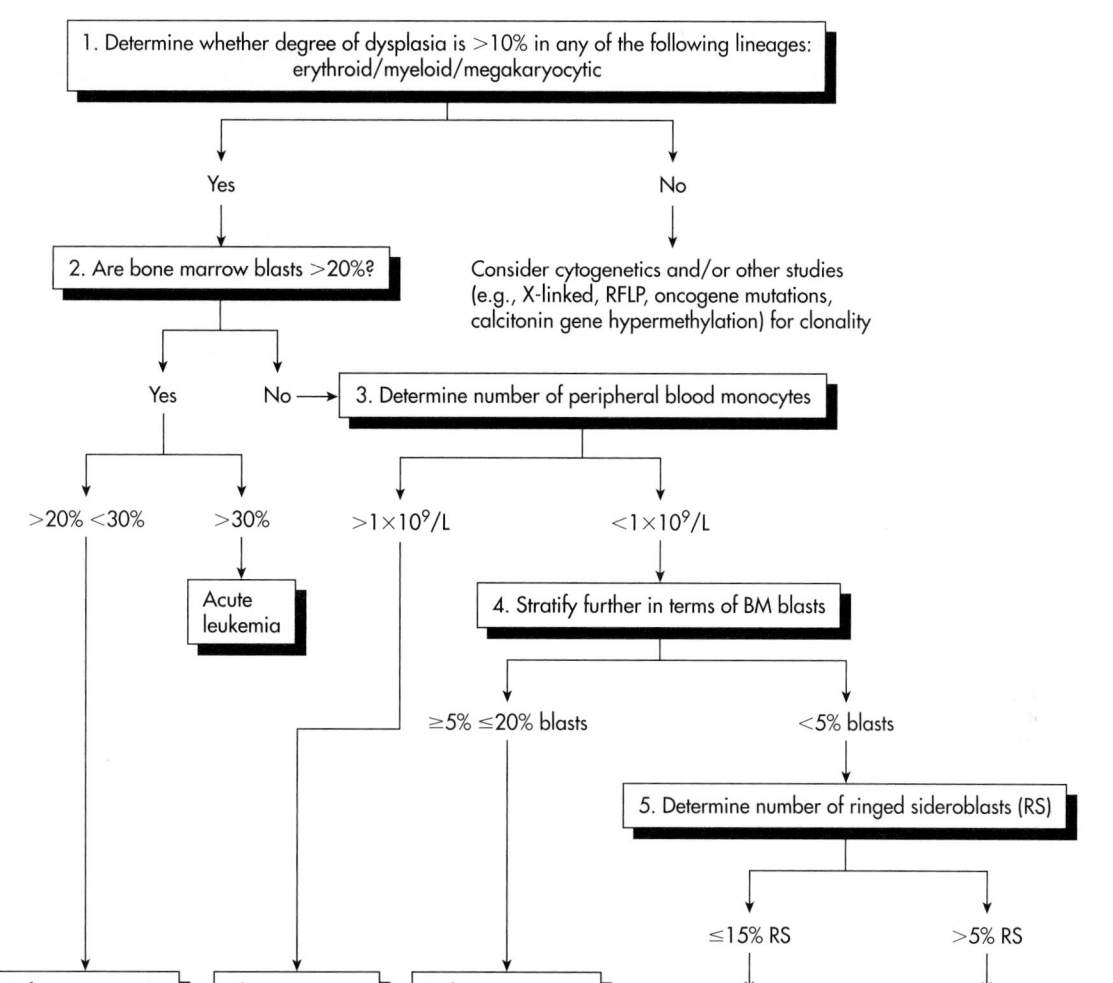

FIG. 1 Myelodysplastic syndrome. *BM blasts,* Bone marrow blastocyst; *RFLP,* restriction fragment length polymorphism. (From Abeloff MD: *Clinical oncology,* ed 3, New York, 2004, Churchill Livingstone.)

- Poor-risk patients are treated with hypomethylating agents along with supportive care.
- Appropriate patients are offered allogeneic stem cell transplantation (Fig. 3) as a potentially curative option with high-volume centers treating patients <80 years old.
- Erythropoietin (10,000 to 40,000 units/week) or pegylated erythropoietin (200-500 mg every 1-3 weeks) is used in patients with symptomatic anemia. Responses with increase in hemoglobin and decreased transfusion requirements are achieved typically in patients who have serum erythropoietin levels <500 U/L and adequate iron stores.
- DNA methyltransferase inhibitors: Azacitidine, a pyrimidine nucleoside analogue of cytidine, has been shown to improve the quality of life for patients and to prolong overall survival. Decitabine, another nucleoside analogue, has also been FDA approved for patients with MDS. These agents may also be useful in preventing the transition of MDS to AML.
- Immunomodulators: Lenalidomide, a novel analogue of thalidomide, has demonstrated

hematologic activity in patients with low-rise MDS who have no response to erythropoietin or who are unlikely to benefit from conventional therapy. Lenalidomide can also reduce transfusion requirements and reverse cytologic and cytogenetic abnormalities in patients who have MDS with the 5q31 deletion.
- Results of chemotherapy are generally disappointing. Combination chemotherapy regimens (e.g., cytarabine plus doxorubicin) that are used to treat AMLs generally induce a complete response in only a minority of patients, and the average duration of response is <1 yr.
- The use of myeloid growth factors (granulocyte colony-stimulating factor [G-CSF], granulocyte-macrophage colony-stimulating factor [GM-CSF]) is reserved for patients with severe neutropenias and high infection risk. Additionally, these CSFs can provide a synergistic effect when used in combination with erythropoietin in terms of improvement in the hemoglobin levels.

CHRONIC Rx

Monitor for infections, bleeding, and complications of anemia. Supportive measures include blood transfusions and erythropoietin for anemia and antibiotics to treat opportunistic infections. Iron overload from frequent transfusions may require iron chelation therapy.

DISPOSITION

- Long-term remission rates in young patients with allogeneic stem cell transplantation approach 40% to 50%.
- The risk of transformation to AML varies with the percentage of blasts in the bone marrow.

REFERRAL

- Hematology referral for all patients with MDS
- Bone marrow transplant physician for evaluation for stem cell transplant eligibility as a potentially curative modality

TABLE 3 Physical Examination, Medical History, and Laboratory Tests Aiding in Diagnosis of Myelodysplastic Syndrome

Medical History

Duration of symptoms
History of blood disease
History of exposure to occupational toxins or cytotoxic agents
Medication history
Alcohol intake
Comorbid conditions

Physical Examination

Pallor
Petechiae
Purpura
Bruising
Tachypnea
Signs of infection
Splenomegaly

Laboratory Testing

Complete blood count with a manual differential
Reticulocyte count
Vitamin B_{12} and folate levels
Consider methylmalonic acid and red blood cell folate levels
Iron, total iron-binding capacity, and ferritin level
Thyroid-stimulating hormone level
Lactate dehydrogenase
Antinuclear antibody
Coombs test and haptoglobin
Serum erythropoietin level
Human leukocyte antigen (histocompatibility antigens) typing in appropriate patients
Paroxysmal nocturnal hemoglobinuria screen

Bone Marrow Testing

Hematopathology
Percentage of blasts on 200 cell aspirate differential
Presence or absence of Auer rods
Percentage of cellularity of bone marrow biopsy
Iron stain on aspirate (ringed sideroblasts)
Iron stain on biopsy (storage)
Dysplastic features (% and number of dysplastic lineages)
Cytogenetics (karyotype of 20 metaphase cells)
Fluorescent in situ hybridization
Flow cytometry (not useful for quantitation)

From Hoffman R et al: *Hematology, basic principles and practice*, ed 5, Philadelphia, 2009, Churchill Livingstone.

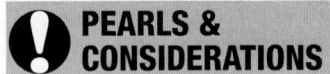

PEARLS & CONSIDERATIONS

COMMENTS

- Somatic point mutations in TP53, EZH2, ETV6, RUNX1, and ASXL1 are predictors of poor overall survival in patients with MDS independent of established risk factors. Patients with cytogenetic abnormalities associated with poor prognosis should be considered for aggressive treatment with allogeneic stem cell transplantation.
- Many younger patients who respond to immunosuppressive therapy with drugs such as antithymocyte globulin and cyclosporine have clonal expansions of cytotoxic CD8+ T cells that suppress normal hematopoiesis, as well as expansion of CD4+ helper T-cell subsets that promote and sustain autoimmunity.
- Nearly 50% of the deaths that result from MDS are the result of cytopenia associated with bone marrow failure.

SUGGESTED READINGS

Available at www.expertconsult.com

RELATED CONTENT

Myelodysplastic Syndrome (Patient Information)

AUTHOR: **RITESH RATHORE, M.D.**

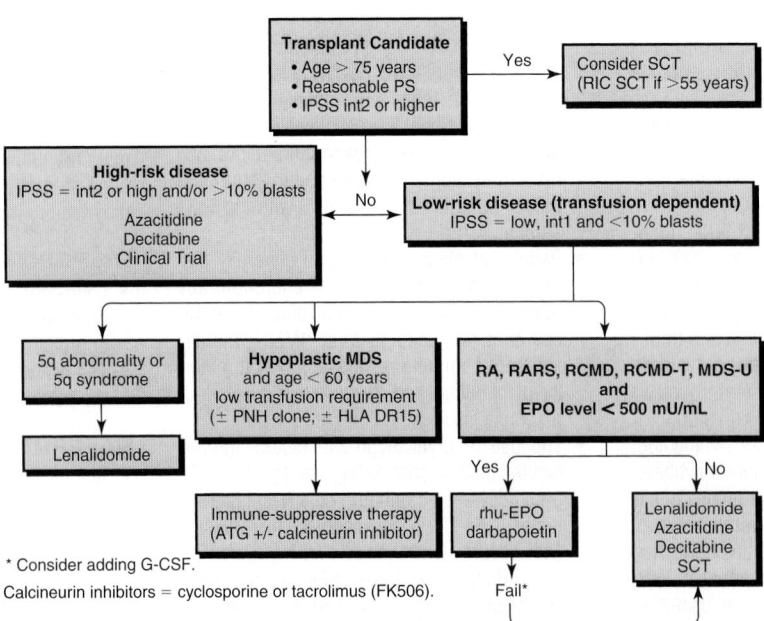

FIG. 3 Algorithm for management of a patient with myelodysplastic syndrome. *PNH,* Paroxysmal nocturnal hemoglobinuria; *PS,* performance status; *RIC,* reduced-intensity conditioning regimen; *SCT,* stem cell transplant. (From Hoffman R et al: *Hematology: basic principles and practice,* ed 5, Philadelphia, 2009, Churchill Livingstone.)

BASIC INFORMATION

DEFINITION

Myocardial infarction (MI) is a clinical syndrome characterized by symptoms of myocardial ischemia, persistent electrocardiographic (ECG) changes, and release of biomarkers of myocardial necrosis resulting from an insufficient supply of oxygenated blood to an area of the heart. According to the European Society of Cardiology/American College of Cardiology, either one of the following criteria for acute evolving or recent MI satisfies the diagnosis:

1. Detection of the rise and/or fall of cardiac biomarker values (preferably cTn) with at least 1 value above the 99th percentile and with at least 1 of the following:
2. Symptoms of ischemia
3. New, or presumed new, significant ST-T changes or new LBBB. New ST elevation at the J point in at least 2 contiguous leads of ≥2 mm (0.2 mV) in men or ≥1.5 mm (0.15 mV) in women in leads V2–V3 and/or of ≥1 mm (0.1 mV) in other contiguous chest leads or the limb leads
4. Development of pathologic Q waves in the ECG
5. Imaging evidence of new loss of viable myocardium or a new regional wall motion abnormality
6. Identification of an intracoronary thrombus by angiography or autopsy
   ○ Pathologic findings of acute MI

MI may be classified as ST-segment elevation MI (STEMI) and non–ST-segment elevation MI [NSTEMI]) depending on the ECG findings on MI presentation. This entry primarily focuses on STEMI. For a discussion of NSTEMI, see "Acute Coronary Syndromes."

The *European Heart Journal* and the *Journal of the American College of Cardiology* published a new definition of acute MI that includes 5 subtypes of acute MI, imaging tests supporting the diagnosis, and biomarker thresholds after percutaneous coronary intervention (PCI) or coronary artery bypass grafting (CABG) in 2012.

- Type 1: Spontaneous MI related to ischemia due to a primary coronary event such as plaque erosion and/or rupture, fissuring, or dissection.
- Type 2: MI secondary to ischemia other than coronary artery disease, due to either increased oxygen demand or decreased supply (e.g., coronary endothelial dysfunction, coronary artery spasm, coronary embolism, anemia, arrhythmias, respiratory failure, hypertension with/without LVH, or hypotension). Also in critically ill patients or in patients undergoing major non-cardiac surgery, elevated values of cardiac biomarkers may appear due to the direct toxic effects of endogenous or exogenous high circulating catecholamine levels.
- Type 3: Sudden unexpected cardiac death, including cardiac arrest, often with symptoms suggestive of myocardial ischemia, accompanied by presumed new ST elevation, new left bundle branch block, or evidence of fresh thrombus in a coronary artery by angiography and/or at autopsy, or death occurring before blood samples could be obtained or

at a time before the appearance of cardiac biomarkers in the blood.

- Type 4a: MI associated with percutaneous coronary intervention. Elevation of cTN >5× percentile of upper reference limit (URL) in patients with normal baseline value, or a rise of cTN >20% if the baseline values are stable and are stable or falling. In addition to either symptoms of ischemia, new ischemic ECG changes or new LBBB, or angiographic loss of a patent coronary artery, persistent slow or no-flow, or embolization, or imaging of new wall motion abnormality.
- Type 4b: MI associated with stent thrombosis as documented by angiography or at autopsy in the setting of myocardial ischemia and with a rise/fall of cardiac biomarker values.
- Type 5: MI associated with coronary artery bypass grafting. Elevation of cardiac biomarker values >10× 99% URL in patients with normal baseline cTn values, in addition to either new pathological Q waves or new LBBB, or new native coronary artery occlusion or imaging of new abnormal wall motion abnormality.

SYNONYMS

MI
Myocardial infarction
ST-elevation MI
Heart attack
Acute myocardial infarction
AMI
Coronary thrombosis
Coronary occlusion

ICD-10CM CODES

I21.01	ST elevation (STEMI) myocardial infarction involving left main coronary artery
I21.02	ST elevation (STEMI) myocardial infarction involving left anterior descending coronary artery
I21.09	ST elevation (STEMI) myocardial infarction involving other coronary artery of anterior wall
I21.11	ST elevation (STEMI) myocardial infarction involving right coronary artery
I21.19	ST elevation (STEMI) myocardial infarction involving other coronary artery of inferior wall
I21.21	ST elevation (STEMI) myocardial infarction involving left circumflex coronary artery
I21.29	ST elevation (STEMI) myocardial infarction involving other sites
I21.3	ST elevation (STEMI) myocardial infarction of unspecified site
I21.4	Non-ST elevation (NSTEMI) myocardial infarction
I22.0	Subsequent ST elevation (STEMI) myocardial infarction of anterior wall
I22.1	Subsequent ST elevation (STEMI) myocardial infarction of inferior wall
I22.2	Subsequent non-ST elevation (NSTEMI) myocardial infarction
I22.8	Subsequent ST elevation (STEMI) myocardial infarction of other sites
I22.9	Subsequent ST elevation (STEMI) myocardial infarction of unspecified site

EPIDEMIOLOGY & DEMOGRAPHICS

INCIDENCE/PREVALENCE (IN U.S.):

- According to data from National Health and Nutrition Examination Survey (NHANES) 2009 to 2012 (National Heart, Lung, and Blood Institute [NHLBI] tabulation), the overall prevalence for MI is 2.8% in U.S. adults ≥20 years of age. MI prevalence is 4.0% for men and 1.8% for women.
- In 2013 in the U.S., coronary heart disease alone caused ≈1 of every 7 deaths. In 2013, 370,213 Americans died of coronary heart disease. Each year, an estimated 660,000 Americans have a new coronary attack (defined as first hospitalized myocardial infarction or coronary heart disease death), and 305,000 have a recurrent attack. It is estimated that an additional 160,000 silent myocardial infarctions occur each year. Approximately every 34 seconds, 1 American has a coronary event, and approximately every 1 minute 24 seconds, an American will die of one.
- Community incidence rates as well as mortality rates from STEMI have declined over the past decade, whereas those for NSTEMI have increased. At present, STEMI comprises approximately 30% to 40% of MI presentations. In-hospital mortality (approximately 5%-6%) and 1-year mortality (approximately 7%-18%). The most common cause of death in adults over the age of 40 is myocardial infarction. A heart attack takes the life of >1,500,000 people each year just in the United States.
- Modifiable risk factors such as hypertension, diabetes, and cigarette smoking have decreased from 2002 to 2009, except for hyperlipidemia, which has shown no significant change. Obesity has increased from 33% to 37.4%.
- Tobacco use remains the second-leading cause of total deaths and disability. The percentage of adults who reported current cigarette use declined from 24.1% in 1998 to 16.9% in 2014; among high school students, the decline was from 36.4% in 1997 to 5.6% in 2013. Still, almost one third of coronary heart disease deaths are attributable to smoking and exposure to secondhand smoke. Patients with first acute MI were found to have an almost threefold increase in cigarette smoking from 2002 to 2009. Cigarette smoking is associated with endothelial dysfunction, prothrombotic defects, and increased oxidative stress.
- It is more prevalent in males between the ages of 45 and 65 yr; no predominant sex after the age of 65
- Women comprised 30% of STEMI patients. They experience more lethal and severe first acute MIs than men regardless of comorbidity, previous angina, or age. Being a woman constituted a strong independent predictor of failure to receive reperfusion therapy, have longer reperfusion times, be less often given the standard of care treatment within 24

hours of presentation, and have higher risk for bleeding with antithrombotic therapy.

- At least one fourth of all MIs are clinically unrecognized. Approximately 23% of patients with STEMI in the U.S. have diabetes mellitus, and three quarters of all deaths among patients with diabetes mellitus are related to coronary artery disease. Diabetes mellitus is associated with higher short- and long-term mortality after STEMI. In the CRUSADE trial, 7% of eligible patients did not receive reperfusion therapy. The most important factor for not providing reperfusion therapy in eligible patients was increasing age.

PHYSICAL FINDINGS & CLINICAL PRESENTATION

Clinical presentation: Myocardial infarction is usually based on a history of substernal pressure type chest pain radiated to the neck, lower jaw, left arm or mid-back lasting 20 min or more that is not completely relieved by sublingual nitroglycerin. The pain may not be severe. Some patients may present with atypical symptoms such as nausea/vomiting, shortness of breath, fatigue, palpitations, and diaphoresis. The elderly in particular may present with dizziness, or syncope. The patients who tend to present with atypical symptoms are more likely to be women, diabetic patients, or elderly patients and less frequently receive reperfusion therapy and other evidence-based therapies than patients with a typical chest pain presentation. Records show that up to 30% of patients with STEMI present with atypical symptoms.

Physical findings:
- Skin may be diaphoretic and exhibit pallor (because of decreased oxygen).

- Rales may be present at the bases of lungs (indicative of heart failure [HF]).
- Cardiac auscultation may reveal an apical systolic murmur caused by mitral regurgitation from papillary muscle dysfunction; S_3 or S_4 may also be present.
- Up to 10% of patients may present with acute pulmonary edema and/or cardiogenic shock.
- Physical examination may be completely normal.

ETIOLOGY

- Coronary atherosclerosis and plaque rupture
- Coronary artery spasm
- Coronary embolism (caused by infective endocarditis, rheumatic heart disease, intracavitary thrombus, atrial fibrillation)
- Periarteritis and other coronary artery inflammatory diseases
- Dissection into coronary arteries (aneurysmal or iatrogenic)
- Calcium supplementation may promote vascular calcification. Studies have shown that calcium supplementation (but not dietary calcium intake) is associated with elevated risk for MI.
- MI with normal coronaries: more frequent in younger patients and cocaine addicts. The risk of acute MI is increased by a factor of 24 during the 60 min after the use of cocaine in persons who are otherwise at relatively low risk. Most patients with cocaine-related MI are young, nonwhite, male cigarette smokers without other risk factors for coronary heart disease and who have a history of repeated cocaine use. Blood and urine toxicology screen for cocaine is recommended in all young patients who present with acute MI.

- Hypercoagulable states, increased blood viscosity (polycythemia vera and autoimmune diseases such as systemic lupus, antiphospholipid syndrome)

DX DIAGNOSIS

DIFFERENTIAL DIAGNOSIS

The various causes of myocardial ischemia are described along with the differential diagnosis of chest pain.

LABORATORY TESTS

- Electrocardiogram (Fig. 1): a 12-lead ECG should be performed and shown to an experienced emergency physician within 10 min of ED arrival for all patients with chest discomfort (or anginal equivalent) or other symptoms suggestive of STEMI. If the initial ECG is not diagnostic for STEMI but the patient remains symptomatic and there is a high clinical suspicion for STEMI, serial ECGs at 5- to 10-minute intervals or continuous 12-lead ST-segment monitoring should be performed to detect the potential development of ST elevation. In patients with inferior STEMI, right-sided ECG leads should be obtained to look for ST elevation suggestive of right ventricular (RV) infarction. The joint ESC/ACCF/AHA committee for the definition of MI established the definition for the diagnosis of ST-elevation MI, which is considered to be present when there is an ST-segment elevation in two contiguous leads, ≥2 mm for men and ≥1.5 mm for women in precordial leads and/or ≥1 mm in limb leads. ST-segment elevation is measured at 0.08 sec after the J point (the junction between

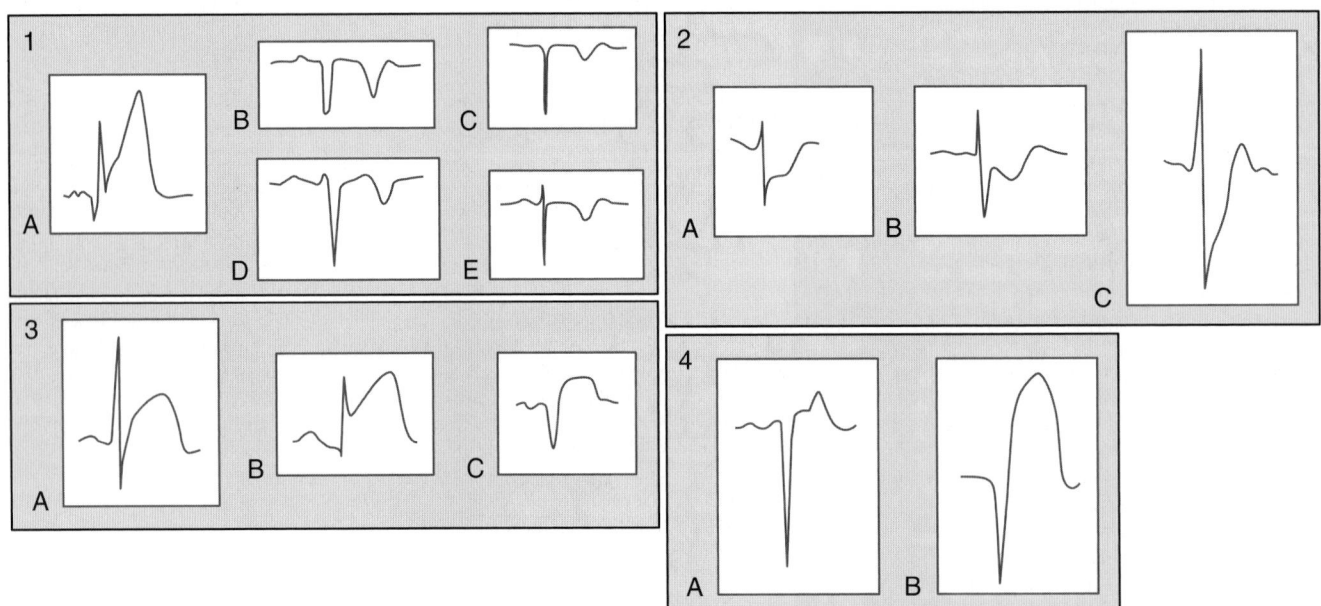

FIG. 1 Electrocardiographic findings of acute myocardial infarction (AMI). 1, T-wave abnormalities of AMI. *A,* Prominent "hyperacute" T wave. *B-E,* T-wave inversions of non–ST-segment elevation MI (NSTEMI). **2,** ST-segment depression. *A,* Flat. *B,* Downsloping. *C,* Upsloping. **3,** ST-segment elevation. *A,* Convex ST-segment elevation. *B,* Obliquely straight ST-segment elevation. *C,* Convex ST-segment elevation. **4,** Pathologic Q waves. *A,* Pathologic Q wave of completed myocardial infarction. *B,* Simultaneous ST-segment elevation with pathologic Q wave 2 hours into the course of ST-segment elevation MI (STEMI). (From Vincent JL et al: *Textbook of critical care,* ed 6, Philadelphia, 2011, Saunders.)

the end of the QRS and the beginning of the ST segment). In addition, ST depression in >2 precordial leads (V1–V4) may indicate transmural posterior injury; multilead ST depression with coexistent ST elevation in lead aVR has been described in patients with left main or proximal left anterior descending artery occlusion.

- New or presumably new LBBB at presentation occurs infrequently, may interfere with ST-elevation analysis, and should not be considered diagnostic of acute myocardial infarction (MI) in isolation.
- ECG findings alone, without laboratory results, are sufficient to diagnose STEMI; therefore, treatment should not be delayed until biomarkers are available.
- Cardiac troponin levels: Cardiac-specific troponin T (cTnT) and cardiac-specific troponin I (cTnI) are generally indicative of myocardial injury with increases in serum levels of >99th percentile of a normal reference population. Detection of a rise and fall pattern of the measurements is essential to the diagnosis of AMI. The rise may occur relatively early after muscle damage (3-6 hr), peak at 12 to 16 hr, and may be present for several days after MI (up to 7 days for cTnI and more than 14 days for cTnT). cTnT or cTnI tests can be falsely positive for myocardial infarction in patients with renal failure, heart failure, myocarditis, aortic dissection, and pulmonary embolism. Recently, highly sensitive troponin assays (hs-cTnI, hs-cTnT) have also been developed to facilitate an early diagnosis of AMI. Most patients can be diagnosed with AMI within the first 2 to 3 hours of presentation. However, an initial negative high-sensitivity troponin at the time of presentation is not sensitive enough to completely rule out AMI. MI can be excluded in most patients by 6 hours of presentation, and guidelines suggest serial samples be obtained every 3 to 6 hours after an initial sample if there is a high degree of suspicion for AMI.
- CK-MB isoenzyme is also a useful marker for MI if troponin levels are not available. It is released in the circulation in amounts that correlate with the size of the infarct. An increased CK-MB value for the diagnosis of MI is defined as a measurement above the 99th percentile of the upper reference limit. CK-MB can be detected within 3 to 8 hr of the onset of chest pain, peak at 12 to 24 hr, and return to baseline levels within 24 to 48 hr. Troponin, however, is the preferred marker for the diagnosis of myocardial necrosis because of its increased sensitivity and specificity as compared to CK-MB. This preference was recommended by the 2007 Joint ESC/ACCF/AHA Task Force for the Definition of Myocardial Infarction. Because troponins need 7 to 14 days to be cleared by the kidneys, they are not sensitive enough to detect a recurrent MI within days from the initial MI. Therefore, CK-MB isoenzyme can be useful in such circumstances.

IMAGING STUDIES
Imaging studies such as a high-quality portable chest x-ray, transthoracic echocardiography, and a contrast chest CT scan should be used to differentiate STEMI from aortic dissection, pulmonary embolism, and other intrathoracic causes of chest pain (i.e., pneumonia and pneumothorax) in patients for whom this distinction is initially unclear, or to assess for complications of AMI such as pulmonary edema. Transthoracic echocardiography may provide evidence of focal wall motion abnormalities and facilitate triage in patients with ECG findings that are difficult to interpret.

RISK ASSESSMENT
Several risk assessment models are available. In the TIMI risk score for STEMI, the mean 30-day mortality was 6.7%. It is composed of eight baseline variables. The risk score showed a >40-fold graded increase in mortality, with scores ranging from 0 to >8 (P <0.0001); 30-day mortality was 0.1% among patients with a score of 0, 2.25 with a score of 5, and >8.8% among patients with a score of 8 or greater. The variables are divided between historical, exam, and presentation:
Historical:
1. Age 65 to 74 (2 points), >75 (3 points),
2. Diabetes/HTN or angina (1 point).
   Exam:
1. SBP <100 mm Hg (3 points),
2. Heart rate >100 bpm (2 points),
3. Killip 2 to 4 (2 points),
4. Weight <67 kg (1 point).
   Presentation:
1. Anterior ST elevation or LBBB (1 point),
2. Time to reperfusion >4 hr (1 point).
   The higher the score, the higher the 30-day mortality rate. Risk assessment is a continuous process that should be repeated throughout hospitalization and at time of discharge.

TREATMENT

NONPHARMACOLOGIC THERAPY
- Limit patient's activity: bed rest with bedside commode for the initial 12 to 24 hr. If the patient remains stable, gradually increase activity.
- Diet: nothing by mouth until stable, then clear liquids as tolerated to advance gradually to a diet tailored to the patient's comorbidities (i.e., diabetes, hypertension, heart failure, hyperlipidemia, renal failure, COPD, etc.).
- Patient education to decrease the risk of subsequent cardiac events, counseling on smoking cessation, dietary restrictions, regular exercise, and medication compliance should be initiated when the patient is medically stable.

ACUTE GENERAL Rx
- Fig. 2 shows a treatment algorithm for STEMI. Assessment and treatment algorithm for non-ST-segment MI is described in Fig. 3. Rationale of the treatment of a patient with STEMI is based on "time is muscle."

Therefore, all communities should create and maintain a regional system of STEMI care that includes assessment and continuous quality improvement of EMS and hospital-based activities. A 12-lead ECG must be done by EMS personnel at the site of first medical contact (FMC).

- Reperfusion therapy should be administered to all eligible patients with STEMI with symptom onset within 12 hours. Indications for primary angioplasty and comparison with fibrinolytic therapy are described in Table 1. Primary PCI (Fig. E4) is the recommended method of reperfusion when it can be performed in a timely fashion by experienced operators with an ideal FMC-to-device time system goal of 90 minutes or less.
- In the absence of contraindications, fibrinolytic therapy (Table 2) should be administered to patients with STEMI at non-PCI-capable hospitals when the anticipated FMC-to-device time at a PCI-capable hospital exceeds 120 minutes because of unavoidable delays. It should be administered within 30 minutes of hospital arrival.
- PCI is superior to thrombolytic therapy and is the standard of care. It is effective and generally results in more favorable outcomes than thrombolytic therapy.
- Primary PCI should be performed in patients with STEMI and persistent ischemic symptoms and who have contraindications to fibrinolytic therapy, irrespective of the time delay from FMC, or in patients with cardiogenic shock or acute severe HF irrespective of time delay from myocardial infarction (MI) onset. Coronary stents (drug-eluting or bare-metal) are useful in patients with STEMI.
- The management of STEMI continues to evolve in a favorable fashion with the advent of bioresorbable stents (BRS). This new technology will in all likelihood overcome the major limitation of current stents, which is delayed thrombosis. BRS will reduce the length of time for long-term dual antiplatelet therapy (DAPT), therefore reducing the risk of bleeding, particularly in the high-risk population. Other BRS advantages are as follows: option to repeat multiple PCIs as surgical revascularization procedures; complete absorption of the stent restoring vascular function, vasomotion; improved feasibility of treating complex lesions; and facilitation of image studies free of metal artifacts.
- The question of culprit vessel vs. complete revascularization during PCI has been brought up since the stent technology was applied to the management of STEMI. The most recent clinical trials and observational studies appear to favor complete revascularization in the setting of STEMI, but the results of larger ongoing trials are necessary to tip the balance one way or the other in terms of mortality and morbidity (contrast use, radiation usage, length of the procedure) in this situation. In the meantime, the approach to each individual patient must be tailored to the patient's characteristics and social circumstances.

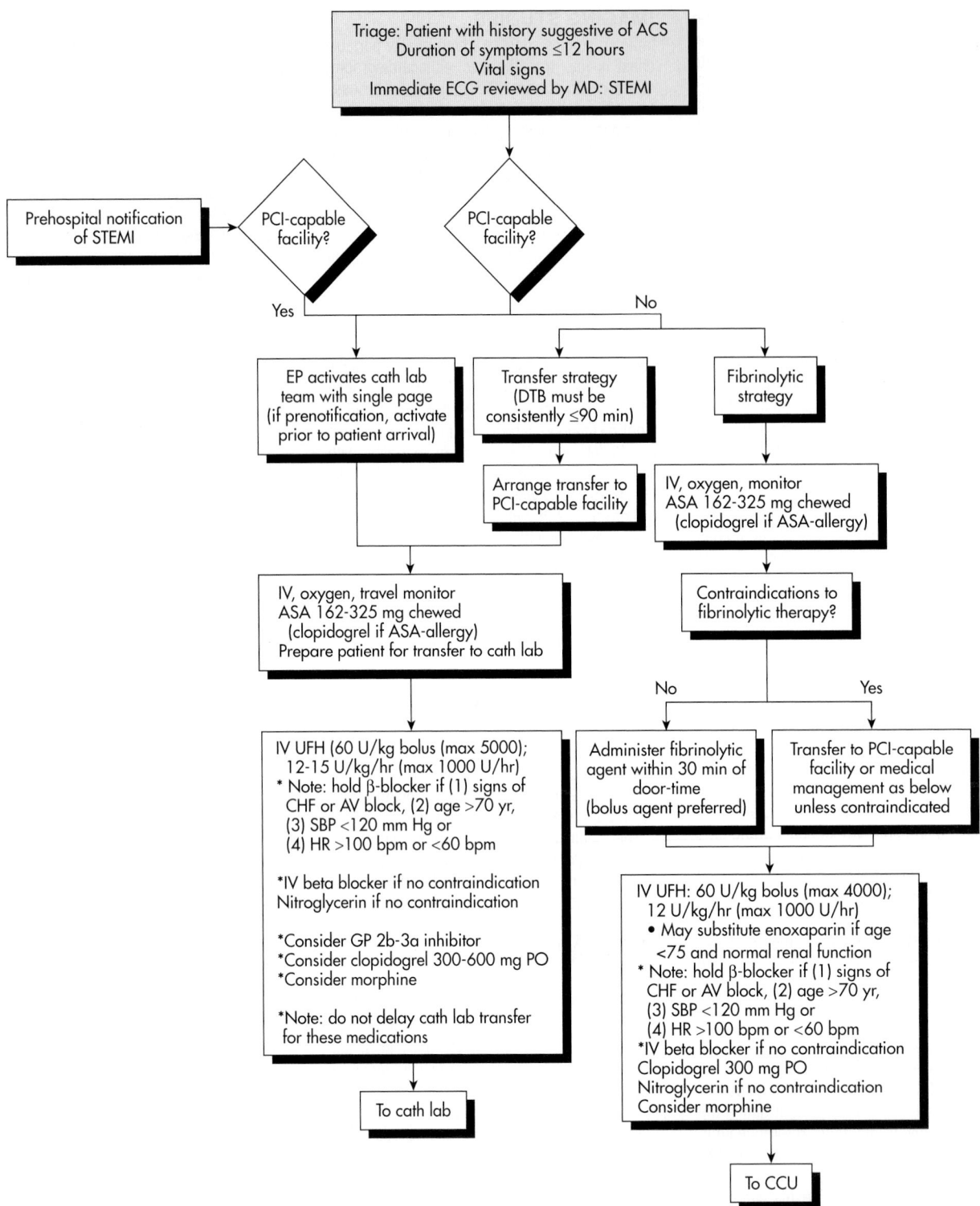

FIG. 2 Assessment and treatment algorithm for ST-segment elevation myocardial infarction (STEMI). *ACS,* Acute coronary syndrome; *ASA,* acetylsalicylic acid; *AV,* atrioventricular; *bpm,* beats per minute; *cath lab,* catheterization laboratory; *CCU,* cardiac care unit; *CHF,* congestive heart failure; *DTB,* door-to-balloon time; *ECG,* electrocardiogram; *EP,* emergency physician; *GP,* glycoprotein; *HR,* heart rate; *IV,* intravenous/intravenous line; *PCI,* percutaneous coronary intervention; *PO,* orally; *SBP,* systolic blood pressure; *UFH,* unfractionated heparin. (From Adams JG et al: *Emergency medicine, clinical essentials,* ed 2, Philadelphia, 2013, Elsevier.)

- For patients presenting to a non–PCI-capable hospital, rapid assessment should be done of (1) the time from onset of symptoms, (2) the risk of complications related to STEMI, (3) the risk of bleeding with fibrinolysis, (4) the presence of shock or severe HF, and (5) the time required for transfer to a PCI-capable hospital and a decision about administration of fibrinolytic therapy reached. Because the effectiveness of thrombolytics is time dependent, these agents should ideally be administered either in the field or within 30 min of the patient's arrival to the emergency department (door-to-needle time).

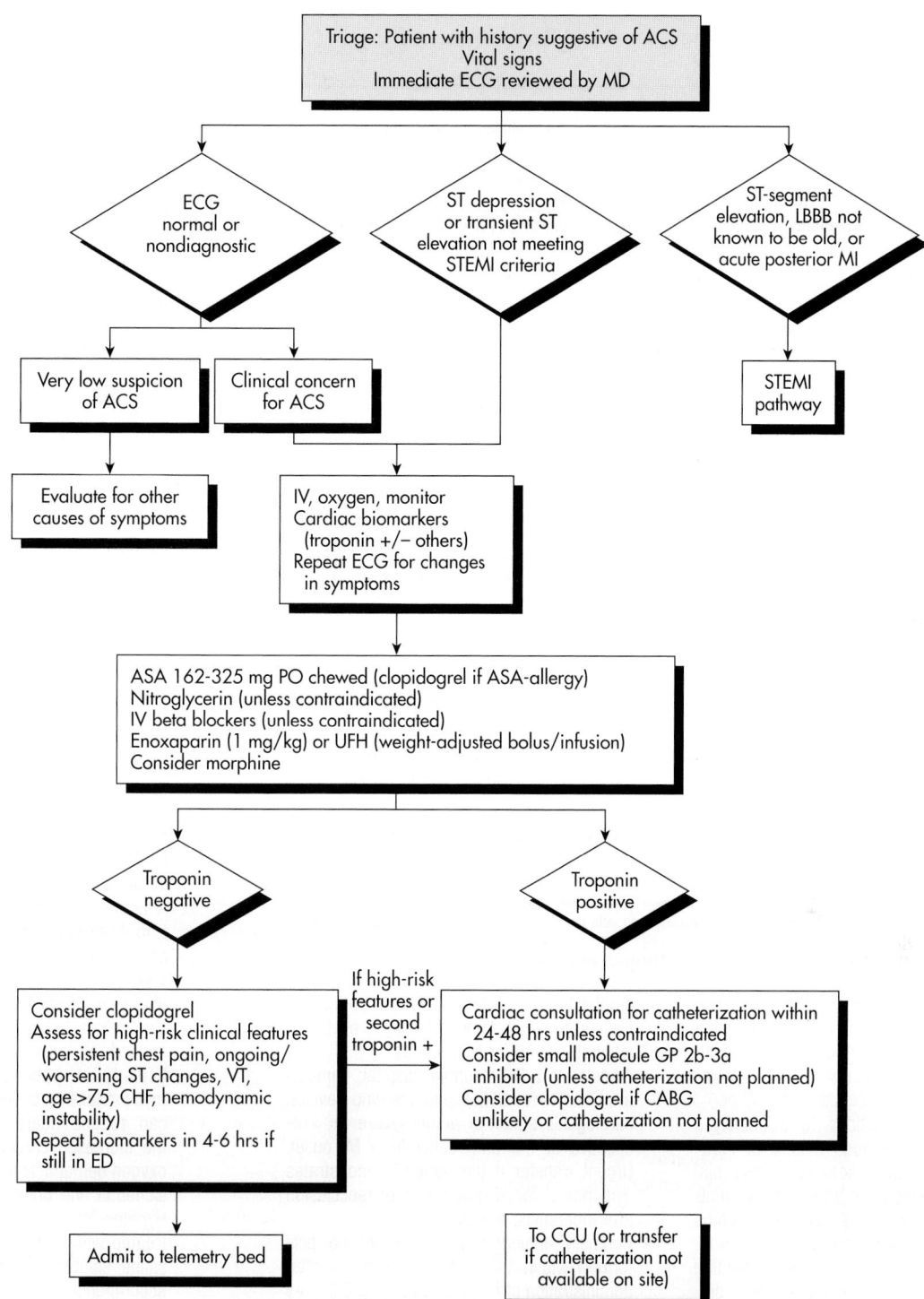

FIG. 3 Assessment and treatment algorithm for non–ST-segment elevation myocardial infarction.
ACS, Acute coronary syndrome; *ASA*, acetylsalicylic acid; *CABG*, coronary artery bypass grafting; *CCU*, cardiac care unit; *CHF*, congestive heart failure; *ED*, emergency department; *ECG*, electrocardiogram; *GP*, glycoprotein; *IV*, intravenous/intravenous line; *LBBB*, left bundle branch block; *MI*, myocardial infarction; *STEMI*, ST-segment elevation myocardial infarction; *UFH*, unfractionated heparin; *VT*, ventricular tachycardia. (From Adams JG et al: *Emergency medicine, clinical essentials,* ed 2, Philadelphia, 2013, Elsevier.)

- Fibrinolytics therapy: if tissue plasminogen activator (t-PA) or reteplase is used, anticoagulants, such as heparin, are given to increase the likelihood of patency in the infarct-related artery for 48 hr and preferably for the duration of the index hospitalization, up to 8 days. In patients receiving fibrinolysis for STEMI, treatment with enoxaparin is superior to treatment with unfractionated heparin for 48 hr but is associated with an increase in major bleeding episodes. In patients receiving streptokinase or APSAC, heparin after thrombolysis is not indicated because it does not offer any additional benefit and can result in increased bleeding complications. Tenecteplase and reteplase are comparable with accelerated infusion recombinant t-PA in terms of efficacy and safety but are more

---

Indications

Alternative recanalization strategy for ST segment elevation or LBBB acute MI within 12 hr of symptom onset (or >12 hr if symptoms persist)

Cardiogenic shock developing within 36 hr of ST segment elevation/Q wave acute MI or LBBB acute MI in patients >75 yr old who can be revascularized within 18 hr of shock onset

Recommended only at centers performing >200 PCI/yr with backup cardiac surgery and for operators performing <75 PCI/yr

Advantages of Primary PCI

Higher initial recanalization rates

Reduced risk of intracerebral hemorrhage

Less residual stenosis; less recurrent ischemia or infarction

Usefulness when fibrinolysis contraindicated

Improvement in outcomes with cardiogenic shock

Disadvantages of Primary PCI (Compared with Fibrinolytic Therapy)

Access, advantages restricted to high-volume centers, operators

Longer average time to treatment

Greater dependence on operators for results

Higher system complexity, costs

LBBB, Left bundle branch block; *MI,* myocardial infarction; *PCI,* percutaneous coronary intervention (includes balloon angioplasty, stenting).
From Goldman L, Schafer AI: *Goldman's Cecil medicine,* ed 24, Philadelphia, 2012, Saunders.

TABLE 2 Dosing Regimens of Commonly Used Thrombolytic Agents

Thrombolytic Agents	Dosing Regimen
t-PA (alteplase)	15 mg bolus IV, followed by 0.75 mg/kg body weight (not to exceed 50 mg) over 30 min, followed by 0.5 mg/kg (not to exceed 35 mg) over 60 min
r-PA (reteplase)	Two 10-U IV boluses, given 30 min apart
TNK–t-PA (tenecteplase)	Single bolus IV 0.5 mg/kg (dose rounded to the nearest 5 mg, ranging from 30 to 50 mg)
Streptokinase	1.5 million U IV over 60 min

IV, Intravenous; *PA,* plasminogen activator; *r-PA,* reteplase plasminogen activator; *TNK–t-PA,* tenecteplase tissue plasminogen activator; *U,* units.
From Andreoli TE et al: *Andreoli and Carpenter's Cecil essentials of medicine,* ed 8, Philadelphia, 2010, Saunders.

convenient because they are administered by bolus injection. Lanoplase and heparin bolus plus infusion are as effective as tPA with regard to mortality rate, but the rate of intracranial hemorrhage is significantly higher.

- Absolute contraindications to thrombolytic therapy (Table 3) include history of intracranial hemorrhage, known intracranial malignant neoplasm or arteriovenous malformation, ischemic stroke within 3 months (except acute ischemic stroke within 4.5 h), suspected aortic dissection, active bleeding or bleeding diathesis (except menses), significant closed head or facial trauma within 3 months, intracranial or intraspinal surgery within 2 months, or severe uncontrolled hypertension (unresponsive to therapy). For streptokinase, this applies to prior treatment within 6 months.
- Relative contraindications: history of chronic severe, poorly controlled hypertension, SBP >180 mm Hg, DBP >110 mm Hg, history of prior ischemic stroke more than 3 months, dementia, known intracranial pathology, traumatic or prolonged CPR (>10 minutes), major surgery <3 weeks, recent internal bleeding within 2 to 4 weeks, noncompressible vascular punctures, pregnancy, active peptic ulcer, oral anticoagulant therapy. After the

administration of thrombolytics, immediate transfer to a PCI-capable facility is advisable without waiting for lytic results.

- Transfer to a PCI-capable hospital: immediate transfer for STEMI patients who develop cardiogenic shock or acute severe HF, irrespective of the time delay from MI onset. Urgent transfer if the patient demonstrates evidence of failed reperfusion or reocclusion after fibrinolytic therapy.
- Coronary angiography should not be performed within the first 2 to 3 hours after administration of fibrinolytic therapy. Coronary artery bypass graft (CABG): urgent CABG is indicated in patients with STEMI and coronary anatomy not amenable to PCI who have ongoing or recurrent ischemia, cardiogenic shock, severe HF, or other high-risk features. CABG is recommended in patients with STEMI at time of operative repair of mechanical defects.
- Therapeutic hypothermia should be started as soon as possible in comatose patients with STEMI and out-of-hospital cardiac arrest caused by ventricular fibrillation (VF) or pulseless ventricular tachycardia, including patients who undergo primary PCI.
- Immediate angiography and PCI when indicated should be performed in resuscitated out-of-hospital patients.

- The use of mechanical circulatory support is reasonable in patients with STEMI who are hemodynamically unstable and require urgent CABG.
- Until the catheterization team is ready or fibrinolytics are administered, medical therapy should be initiated immediately in the emergency department. This includes:
  1. Routine measures
     a. Oxygen: supplemental oxygen should be administered to patients with arterial oxygen desaturation (SaO_2 less than 90%).
     b. Nitroglycerin: increase oxygen supply by reducing coronary vasospasm and decrease oxygen consumption by reducing ventricular preload. Patients with ongoing ischemic discomfort should receive sublingual nitroglycerin every 5 minutes for a total of 3 doses, after which an assessment should be made about the need for intravenous nitroglycerin. Intravenous nitroglycerin is indicated for relief of ongoing ischemic discomfort, control of hypertension, or management of pulmonary congestion. Nitrates should not be administered to patients whose systolic blood pressure is <90 mm Hg or ≥30 mm Hg below baseline or severe bradycardia (<50 beats/min), tachycardia (>100 beats/min), or suspected RV infarction. Nitrates should not be administered to patients who have received a phosphodiesterase inhibitor for erectile dysfunction within the last 24 hr (48 hr for tadalafil).
     c. Adequate analgesia: morphine sulfate 2 to 4 mg IV initially with increments of 2 to 8 mg IV at 5- to 10-min intervals can be given for severe pain unrelieved by nitroglycerin. Morphine can reduce the catecholamine surge caused by anxiety and pain, particularly in patients with anterior myocardial infarctions, which in turn can reduce heart rate and PCWP, the increased cardiac workload and oxygen demand, leading to decreased ischemia and pulmonary congestion. Hypotension from morphine can be treated with careful IV hydration with saline solution. If sinus bradycardia accompanies hypotension, use atropine (0.5 to 1.0 mg IV q5min prn to a total dose of 2.5 mg). Respiratory depression caused by morphine can be reversed with naloxone 0.8 mg. Morphine sulfate and nitroglycerine should be avoided in patients with RV involvement who usually present with bradycardia and hypotension. Pain management in these cases should be provided preferentially with meperidine 25-50 mg intravenously q 4h, in combination with phenergan 12.5 mg to prevent nausea and/or vomiting. Blood pressure support with normal saline solution is of critical importance to maintain adequate

TABLE 3 Contraindications to Thrombolytic Therapy in Acute Myocardial Infarction

Absolute

Suspected aortic dissection
Active bleeding*
Any prior cerebral hemorrhage
Intracranial neoplasm
Cerebral aneurysm or arteriovenous malformation
Ischemic cerebrovascular accident within 3 mo

Relative

Bleeding diathesis, coagulopathy, or anticoagulant use
Major surgery within 3 wk
Puncture of a noncompressible vessel, internal bleeding, or head or major body trauma within previous 2 wk
Nonhemorrhagic stroke or gastrointestinal hemorrhage within 6 mo
Proliferative retinopathy
Active peptic ulcer disease
History of chronic, severe, poorly controlled hypertension
Severe uncontrolled hypertension on presentation (systolic blood pressure >180 mm Hg or diastolic blood pressure >110 mm Hg)
Traumatic or prolonged (>10 min) cardiopulmonary resuscitation
Pregnancy

*Does not include menstrual bleeding.
From Andreoli TE et al: *Andreoli and Carpenter's Cecil essentials of medicine*, ed 8, Philadelphia, 2010, Saunders.

hemodynamics until optimal revascularization is accomplished.

d. Aspirin 162 to 325 mg PO should be crushed and chewed to enhance drug absorption and delivery. It should be given as soon as possible and continued indefinitely, at 81 mg daily. Depending on the clinical and ECG findings, if the patient is suspected to have a coronary anatomy that needs CABG rather than PCI, aspirin should be continued. P2Y12 receptor antagonists should be avoided because they increase the perioperative bleeding risk; on-pump surgery should be deferred for at least 24 hours after clopidogrel and ticagrelor. Off-pump surgery might be considered within 24 hours of clopidogrel or ticagrelor if the benefits of revascularization outweigh the risk of bleeding. However, if the coronary artery disease is likely to benefit from PCI alone, then a loading dose of clopidogrel 600 mg or ticagrelor 180 mg PO should be given as early as possible or prasugrel 60 mg as early as possible and no later than 1 hour after PCI. P2Y12 receptor antagonist should be continued for at least 1 yr after primary PCI with stent for STEMI. Cangrelor is the newest direct-acting P2Y12 platelet receptor inhibitor. It has a similar chemical structure to ATP, with a half-life of 3 to 6 minutes. It is given IV as a bolus plus 120 minutes of infusion at the time of primary PCI in patients who are naïve to P2Y12 receptor antagonists. It was approved by the FDA in 2015 after the CHAMPION PHOENIX trial. Clopidogrel and prasugrel should be started after its infusion is finished. The ticagrelor loading dose can be given during the infusion. New DAPT guidelines call for discontinuation of these drugs at 6 months post PCI since it has been clearly demonstrated

in clinical trial that prolongation of DAPT beyond this period of time does not provide additional benefits in terms of preventing MI and death, and it is actively associated with an increased risk for cardiac mortality secondary to bleeding complications.

2. In patients receiving fibrinolytics only or balloon angioplasty without stent, P2Y12 antagonists can be given for as little as 14 days.

3. Beta-adrenergic blocking agents should generally be given to all patients. Beta-blockers are useful to reduce myocardial oxygen consumption and prevent tachyarrhythmias. Early IV beta blockage (in the initial 24 hr) followed by institution of an oral maintenance regimen is also effective in reducing recurrent infarction and ischemia. Oral beta-blockers should be initiated in the first 24 hr in patients with STEMI who do not have any of the following: signs of HF, evidence of a low-output state, increased risk for cardiogenic shock, or other contraindications for its use (bradycardia, PR interval more than 0.24 seconds, second- or third-degree heart block, active asthma, or reactive airways disease).
They should be continued during and after hospitalization for all patients with STEMI and with no contraindications to their use for at least 2 yr. Patients with initial contraindications to the use of beta-blockers in the first 24 hr after STEMI should be reevaluated to determine their subsequent eligibility. It is reasonable to administer intravenous beta-blockers at the time of presentation to patients with STEMI and no contraindications to their use who are hypertensive or have ongoing ischemia.

4. Anticoagulation therapy: STEMI is due to plaque rupture exposing the underlying collagen platelets that are activated and the coagulation cascade is initiated. IV unfrac-

tionated heparin, bivalirudin, subcutaneous enoxaparin or fondaparinux can be used. In patients at high risk of bleeding, use of bivalirudin is reasonable. Anticoagulation therapy is usually continued for 48 hours after administration of lytic therapy unless streptokinase or APSAC is used.

5. In patients with acute MI, treatment with drug-eluting stents is associated with decreased 2-yr mortality rates and a reduction in the need for repeated revascularization procedures compared with treatment including bare-metal stents.

6. Gp IIb/IIIa inhibitors in the era of DAPT therapy and primary PCI have failed to show benefit with "upstream" treatment. Abciximab might be useful in the presence of large thrombus burden during primary PCI. For patients receiving bivalirudin as the primary anticoagulant, routine adjunctive use of GP IIb/IIIa inhibitors is not recommended but may be considered as adjunctive or "bail-out" therapy in selected cases.

CHRONIC Rx

- Discharge medications in all patients with MI (unless contraindicated) should include antiischemic medications (e.g., nitroglycerin, beta-blocker), lipid-lowering agents, and antiplatelet therapy (aspirin and/or P2Y12 antagonists).

- Aspirin, 81 mg PO daily, but should be continued indefinitely unless not tolerated (e.g., GI bleed). Clopidogrel 75 mg PO daily; ticagrelor, 90 mg bid, or prasugrel, 10 mg PO daily, can be combined with aspirin and should be continued without interruption for a minimum of 30 days after bare-metal stent placement or for 12 months after drug-eluting stent placement; however, aspirin should be continued indefinitely. Combining P2Y12 antagonists with aspirin reduces risk for repeat myocardial infarction and stent thrombosis. If there is an elective surgical intervention pending, it is recommended to defer the surgery until completion of the full course of the P2Y12 antagonist treatment.

- Angiotensin-converting enzyme inhibitors (ACEIs) should be started within the first 24 hours of STEMI to all patients having STEMI with anterior infarction, pulmonary congestion, or LV EF <40%, in the absence of hypotension. They reduce LV dysfunction and dilation and slow the progression to HF during and after acute MI. Angiotensin receptor blockers, ARBs, should be given to patients who have indication but are intolerant of ACEIs. IV formulations of ACEIs should not be given within the first 24 hours of STEMI due to risk of hypotension. ARBs offer no advantage over ACEIs and should be considered only in patients who are intolerant to ACEIs.

1. Commonly used ACEIs are ramipril 2.5 mg PO bid, captopril 12.5 mg PO bid, enalapril 2.5 mg PO bid, and lisinopril 2.5-5 mg PO qd initially, with subsequent titration as needed. Ramipril is associated with a lower mortality rate than most ACEIs.

2. ACEIs may be stopped in patients without complications and no evidence of LV dysfunction after 6 to 8 weeks.

3. ACEIs should be continued indefinitely in patients with impaired LV function (EF <40%) or clinical HF.

- Long-term aldosterone antagonist therapy should be prescribed for post-STEMI patients without significant renal dysfunction (creatinine ≤2.5 mg/dl in men and ≤2.0 mg/dl in women) or hyperkalemia who are already taking an ACEI, a beta-blocker, and have LV EF <40% with symptomatic HF or diabetes.
- Statins should be started as early as possible in all patients with STEMI regardless of lipid panel, not only for their lipid-lowering effects, but also their antiinflammatory properties (JUPITER trial), which can stabilize the ruptured plaque. Atorvastatin 80 mg can be used (PROVE IT-TIMI 22 and MIRACL trials). Fasting lipid panel should be checked during the first 24 hr of hospital course, and the intensive therapy can be stepped down if appropriate. Goal LDL cholesterol is <70 mg/dl. Consider addition of fenofibrate or niacin if triglycerides are significantly elevated. Recent data showed no improvement in outcome with increasing HDL cholesterol therapy using niacin; therefore its use to decrease HDL cholesterol is questionable.

COMPLICATIONS OF STEMI

Cardiogenic shock: emergent revascularization with either PCI or CABG is the recommended treatment.

Sustained ventricular tachycardia: implantable cardioverter-defibrillator therapy (ICD) is indicated before discharge in patients who develop sustained ventricular tachycardia/ventricular fibrillation more than 48 hr after STEMI, provided the arrhythmia is not due to transient or reversible ischemia, reinfarction, or metabolic abnormalities.

Pacing in STEMI: temporary pacing is indicated for symptomatic bradyarrhythmias unresponsive to medical treatment and after revascularization. AV block and bradyarrhythmias in the setting of inferior wall MI are usually transient, will not require long-term pacing, and usually resolve within 2 to 4 weeks of the event. On the contrary, AV block and bradyarrhythmias or new LBBB in the presence of an anterior wall MI is usually a sign of severe disruption of the bundle of His and often requires a permanent pacemaker.

Pericarditis after STEMI: aspirin is recommended for treatment of pericarditis after STEMI. Glucocorticoids and nonsteroidal antiinflammatory drugs are potentially harmful for treatment of pericarditis after STEMI.

EVALUATION OF POST-MI PATIENTS

- Noninvasive testing for ischemia should be performed before discharge to assess the presence and extent of inducible ischemia in patients with STEMI who have not had coronary angiography and do not have high-risk clinical features for which coronary angiography would be warranted. It might be considered before discharge to evaluate the functional significance of a noninfarct artery stenosis previously identified at angiography and/or before discharge to guide the postdischarge exercise prescription.

- Assessment of LV function: LV ejection fraction should be measured in all patients with STEMI.
Echocardiography to rule out presence of mural thrombi in patients suspected of having an extensive infarction (more common with anterior wall MI); contrast echocardiography is added if mural thrombus is suspected.
  1. Assessment of risk for sudden cardiac death: Patients with an initially reduced LV ejection fraction, <40%, who are possible candidates for implantable cardioverter-defibrillator therapy should undergo reevaluation of LV ejection fraction at 90 days (or 42 days if no revascularization was performed). ICD is recommended when LVEF remains <35% in the presence of NYHA class II or III heart failure, or in patients with LVEF <30% regardless of symptoms, if the life expectancy is >1 yr.
- Cardiac rehabilitation/secondary prevention programs are recommended for patients with STEMI
- Lifestyle risk factors modification

DISPOSITION

The prognosis after MI depends on multiple factors:

- New bundle branch block, Mobitz II second-degree block, and third-degree heart block adversely affect outcome.
- Size of infarct: the larger it is, the higher the post-MI mortality rate. Significant myocardial stunning with subsequent improvement of ventricular function occurs in most patients after anterior MI. A lower level of creatine kinase, an estimate of the extent of necrosis, is independently predictive of recovery of function.
- Site of infarct: inferior wall MI carries a better prognosis than anterior wall MI; however, patients with inferior wall MI and right ventricular involvement have a high risk for arrhythmic complications and cardiogenic shock.
- Ejection fraction after MI: the lower the LV ejection fraction, the higher the mortality rate after MI. The risk of death is higher in the first 30 days after MI among patients with LV dysfunction, HF, or both.
- Presence of post-MI angina indicates a high mortality rate.
- Performance on low-level exercise test: the presence of ST-segment changes during the test is a predictor of high mortality rate during the first year.
- Presence of pericarditis during the acute phase of MI increases mortality rate at 1 yr.
- Type A behavior (competitive drive, ambitiousness, hostility) is associated with a lower mortality rate after symptomatic MI.
- The Killip classification is an independent predictor of all-cause 30-day mortality:
  1. Killip class I includes individuals with no clinical signs of HF. Mortality rate is 6%.
  2. Killip class II includes individuals with rales or crackles in the lungs, S₃ gallop, and elevated jugular venous pressure. Mortality rate is 17%.

3. Killip class III describes individuals with frank acute pulmonary edema. Mortality rate is 38%.
4. Killip class IV describes individuals in cardiogenic shock or hypotension (measured as systolic blood pressure <90 mm Hg) and evidence of peripheral vasoconstriction (oliguria, cyanosis, or sweating). Mortality rate is 67%.

- Self-reported moderate alcohol consumption in the year before acute MI is associated with reduced 1-yr mortality rate.
- Discharge medication in patients with MI should include lipid-lowering agents. Statins may also lower vascular inflammation and damage by mechanisms other than reduction of low-density lipoprotein cholesterol. Early initiation of statin treatment in patients with acute MI is associated with reduced 1-yr mortality rate.
- Additional poor prognostic factors include cigarette smoking, history of hypertension or prior MI, presence of ST-segment depression in acute MI, older age, diabetes mellitus, and female sex (especially women >50 yr). Lammintausta and Fonarow reported that single men and women who live alone have a 60% to 70% greater risk of a heart attack. Furthermore, the study showed >160% increase in the risk of sudden death in these groups when compared to people who are married or live with family.
- Renal disease, even mild, as assessed by the estimated glomerular filtration rate, is a major risk factor for cardiovascular complications after MI.
- Although black patients with MI have worse outcomes than their white counterparts, these differences did not persist after adjustment for patient factors and site of care.

⚠ PEARLS & CONSIDERATIONS

COMMENTS

- Approximately 1.5 million patients undergo PCI in the United States each year. Depending on local practices and the diagnostic criteria used, 5% to 30% of these patients have evidence of a periprocedural MI.
- The 12-lead ECG has low sensitivity for the detection of MI if the culprit lesion is in the left circumflex artery (LCX). If the initial 12-lead ECG is not diagnostic and high clinical suspicion for acute coronary syndrome exists it is reasonable to obtain additional posterior chest leads (V₇ to V₉) to detect LCX occlusion.

SUGGESTED READINGS

Available at www.expertconsult.com

RELATED CONTENT

Heart Attack (Patient Information)
Acute Coronary Syndrome (Related Key Topic)
Angina Pectoris (Related Key Topic)
Coronary Artery Disease (Related Key Topic)

AUTHORS: **CLAUDIA SERRANO, M.D.,** and **JUAN A. ESCARFULLER, M.D.**

BASIC INFORMATION

DEFINITION

Myocarditis broadly refers to inflammation of the heart muscle (myocardium). This may result from exposure to discrete external antigens such as viruses, bacteria, parasites, and drugs or from internal triggers such as autoimmune conditions. When cardiac dysfunction ensues, it is then commonly defined as inflammatory cardiomyopathy.

ICD-10CM CODES

I40.0	Infective myocarditis
I40.1	Isolated myocarditis
I40.8	Other acute myocarditis
I40.9	Acute myocarditis, unspecified
A39.52	Meningococcal myocarditis
B26.82	Mumps myocarditis
B33.22	Viral myocarditis
B58.81	Toxoplasma myocarditis
D86.85	Sarcoid myocarditis
I01.2	Acute rheumatic myocarditis
I09.0	Rheumatic myocarditis
I41	Myocarditis in diseases classified elsewhere
I51.4	Myocarditis, unspecified

EPIDEMIOLOGY & DEMOGRAPHICS

- The incidence of focal myocarditis reported at autopsy is 1% to 9% in asymptomatic patients and 50% in patients infected with HIV.
- Myocarditis is a major cause of sudden unexpected death (as high as 8% to 9%) in young adults <40 years of age, especially in cases of idiopathic dilated cardiomyopathy, where myocarditis may account for 10% to 40% of the cases overall.

PHYSICAL FINDINGS & CLINICAL PRESENTATION

- The most common presentations are dyspnea (72% of patients), chest pain (32%), and arrhythmias (18%), which include sinus tachycardia as well as atrial and ventricular premature contractions.
- Chest pain, especially pleuritic and positional, presents when the pericardium is involved.
- Persistent tachycardia out of proportion to fever.
- Faint S_1, S_3, and S_4 gallops on auscultation.
- Murmur of functional mitral regurgitation and functional tricuspid regurgitation caused by severe left ventricular and right ventricular dilatation.
- Pericardial friction rub if associated with pericarditis as in the clinical syndrome of myopericarditis.
- Patients may present with a history of a recent flulike syndrome or nonspecific viral prodrome (fever, arthralgias, malaise, fatigue); children often have a more fulminant presentation than adults. Difficulty breathing is the most common presentation of pediatric myocarditis.
- Congestive heart failure (CHF) symptoms that usually manifest with fatigue and decreased exercise capacity.
- If myocarditis is severe and diffuse and rapid in evolution, it can present with acute CHF symptoms leading to cardiogenic shock and death.
- Signs of biventricular failure (hypotension, hepatomegaly, peripheral edema, distention of neck veins, S_3 sounds, and pulmonary edema).
- Presyncope or syncope secondary to ventricular arrhythmias.
- Sudden cardiac death from ventricular tachycardia/ventricular fibrillation mediated by inflammation and/or a scar, which sets up a reentry-mediated pathway for ventricular arrhythmias.
- Acute coronary syndrome, which can occur due to local coronary spasm and inflammation, and can present on ECG as acute injury pattern or ischemic changes.

ETIOLOGY

- Infection
  1. Viral (adenovirus, parvovirus B19, hepatitis C virus [HCV], Coxsackie B virus, cytomegalovirus, enterovirus, poliovirus, mumps, HIV, and Epstein-Barr virus, etc.). Viruses are the most common cause of myocarditis in developed countries. In the 1980s and 1990s, enteroviruses were frequently associated with myocarditis and dilated cardiomyopathy. In the past 10 years, however, other viruses such as adenovirus, HCV, parvovirus B19, and herpesvirus 6 (HH6) have emerged as the significant pathogens.
  2. Bacterial (*Staphylococcus aureus, Clostridium perfringens,* diphtheria, Mycoplasma and any severe bacterial infection).
  3. Mycotic (*Candida, Mucor, Aspergillus, Blastomyces, Histoplasma*).
  4. Parasitic (*Trypanosoma cruzi*—most common worldwide; *Trichinella, Echinococcus, Amoeba, Toxoplasma*).
  5. Rickettsia rickettsii.
  6. Spirochetal (*Borrelia burgdorferi*–Lyme carditis).
- Rheumatic fever
- Systemic lupus erythematosus
- Granulomatosis with polyangiitis (Wegener's granulomatosis)
- Giant cell arteritis and Takayasu's arteritis
- Drugs (e.g., cocaine, emetine, doxorubicin, sulfonamides, isoniazid, methyldopa, amphotericin B, tetracycline, phenylbutazone, lithium, 5-fluorouracil, phenothiazines, interferon-alfa, nivolumab, ipilimumab, tricyclic antidepressants, cyclophosphamides, smallpox vaccination)
- Toxins (carbon monoxide, ethanol, diphtheria toxin, lead, arsenicals)
- Systemic and collagen-vascular disease (scleroderma, sarcoidosis, celiac disease, Sjögren's syndrome, Kawasaki syndrome, etc.)
- Radiation
- Postpartum status
- Post stem cell transplantation
- Hypersensitivity reactions from insect bites, such as bee and wasp bites; from snake bites; and from tetanus toxoid

DIAGNOSIS (TABLE 1)

DIFFERENTIAL DIAGNOSIS

- Ischemic cardiomyopathy and other, nonischemic cardiomyopathies
- Acute coronary syndromes
- Valvulopathies
- Infiltrative diseases of the myocardium, such as sarcoidosis, amyloidosis, hemochromatosis, and Chagas' disease.

The differential diagnosis of chest pain is described in Section II.

WORKUP

- Medical history: the clinical presentation of myocarditis is nonspecific and can consist of fatigue, palpitations, dyspnea, precordial discomfort, and myalgias.
- Diagnostic workup includes chest x-ray examination, ECG, laboratory evaluation, echocardiogram, cardiac catheterization, cardiac MRI with late gadolinium enhancement, and endomyocardial biopsy (in selected patients on the basis of the likelihood of finding specific treatable disorders such as giant cell myocarditis). Of note, endomyocardial biopsy has a sensitivity of only 10% to 35% using standard histologic criteria. This is due to variability in interpretation and sampling error.

LABORATORY TESTS

- Elevated cardiac troponin is suggestive of myocarditis in patients with clinically suspected myocarditis. Troponin I specificity is 89%; sensitivity is 34% to 53%. A normal level does not rule out the diagnosis.
- Increased creatine kinase (CK) (with elevated MB fraction, lactate dehydrogenase), and aspartate aminotransferase from myocardial necrosis.
- Elevation of cardiac troponin I or T is more common than CK-MB elevation in patients with biopsy-proven myocarditis.
- The elevations of cardiac troponin I were correlated with a short duration (typically less than 1 mo) of CHF symptoms, indicating that the majority of myocardial necrosis occurs early in the disease course.
- Persistent elevations of cardiac biomarkers are indicative of ongoing myocardial necrosis.
- BNP or NT-proBNP is recommended if patient has heart failure symptoms.
- Increased erythrocyte sedimentation rate (nonspecific but may be of value in following the progress of the disease and the response to therapy).
- Increased white blood cell count, again, nonspecific (increased eosinophils if parasitic infection).

TABLE 1 Expanded Criteria for Diagnosis of Myocarditis

Suggestive of myocarditis:	2 positive categories
Compatible with myocarditis:	3 positive categories
High probability of being myocarditis:	all 4 categories positive

(Any matching feature in category = positive for category)

Category I: Clinical Symptoms

Clinical heart failure
Fever
Viral prodrome
Fatigue
Dyspnea on exertion
Chest pain
Palpitations
Presyncope or syncope

Category II: Evidence of Cardiac Structural or Functional Perturbation *in the Absence* of Regional Coronary Ischemia

Echocardiography evidence
Regional wall motion abnormalities
Cardiac dilation
Regional cardiac hypertrophy
Troponin release
High sensitivity (>0.1 ng/mL)
Positive indium In 111 antimyosin scintigraphy
and
Normal coronary angiography *or*
Absence of reversible ischemia by coronary distribution on perfusion scan

Category III: Cardiac Magnetic Resonance Imaging

Increased myocardial T2 signal on inversion recovery sequence
Delayed contrast enhancement after gadolinium-DTPA infusion

Category IV: Myocardial Biopsy—Pathologic or Molecular Analysis

Pathology findings compatible with Dallas criteria
Presence of viral genome by polymerase chain reaction or in situ hybridization

DTPA, Diethylenetriamine penta-acetic acid.
From Bonow R.O., et al.: *Heart disease,* 9th ed, Philadelphia, 2012, Saunders.

- Viral titers (acute and convalescent).
- Cold agglutinin titer, antistreptolysin O titer, blood cultures.
- Lyme disease antibody titer.
- RPR, VDRL.
- Histology on endomyocardial biopsy may reveal histiocytic and mononuclear cellular infiltrates.

IMAGING STUDIES

- Chest x-ray: enlargement of cardiac silhouette with or without pulmonary congestion may be present
- ECG: sinus tachycardia with nonspecific ST-T wave changes unless there is concomitant pericarditis in which the ECG changes are more specific; intraventricular conduction defects and bundle branch blocks are uncommon in typical viral myocarditis but are common manifestations in cardiac sarcoid and idiopathic giant cell myocarditis.
  1. Lyme disease and diphtheria can cause varying degrees of heart block.
  2. Changes mimicking acute myocardial infarction (ST elevations and Q waves) can occur with focal necrosis from myocarditis.
- Echocardiogram:
  1. The most useful test in detecting decreased ventricular function in suspected myocarditis even when subclinical.
  2. Acute severe myocarditis is associated with systolic dysfunction with decreased ejection fraction.
  3. Dilated and hypokinetic chambers
  4. The systolic dysfunction is generally global but may be regional or segmental as in the case of focal myocarditis.
  5. Abnormal tissue Doppler signal can provide additional evidence for the presence of myocarditis.
  6. The echocardiogram can also be helpful with diagnosing coexisting pericardial involvement.
  7. The spheroid dysfunctional ventricle in acute myocarditis tends to remodel to the more normal elliptical shape over several months.
- Cardiac catheterization and angiography:
  1. To rule out coronary artery disease and valvular disease. Coronary angiography is most commonly normal with evidence of minimal or no coronary artery disease.
  2. A right ventricular endomyocardial biopsy can confirm the diagnosis, although a negative biopsy result does not exclude myocarditis owing to the low sensitivity of this test. Recent studies have shown that myocardial biopsy may be unnecessary because immunosuppression therapy based on biopsy results is generally ineffec-

tive. However, if idiopathic giant cell myocarditis is suspected, biopsy can confirm this diagnosis, and immunosuppression therapy is often helpful in this patient cohort.
- Cardiac MRI (Fig. E1):
  1. Can be used to detect myocardial edema and myocyte injury in myocarditis.
  2. Increased focal or global signal intensity can be used to calculate an edema ratio.
  3. Late gadolinium enhancement (LGE) and the presence of increased focal and global myocardial contrast enhancement relative to skeletal muscle.
  4. Any combination of two of the above has a sensitivity and specificity of 76% and 96%, with 85% diagnostic accuracy, and is probably the gold standard for diagnosis of myocarditis, as opposed to routine biopsy.
  5. Cardiac MRI has demonstrated that myocarditis tends to start as a focal process and becomes a more global process over time, with the extent of myocardial enhancement correlating with clinical status and left ventricular function.
  6. Some viral pathogens have focal involvement of the myocardium. Parvovirus B19 involves the subepicardial lateral wall of the left ventricle. HHV6 and especially the combination of HHV6/parvovirus B19 tend to involve the septum and present with more acute and chronic heart failure symptoms.
  7. The pattern of LGE is different from that in ischemic cardiomyopathy. LGE in myocarditis tends to involve the epicardium with variable extension into the midmyocardium and sparing of the endocardium. This is in contrast to ischemic injury, which involves endocardium first with extension outward.
- Indium-111-labeled antimyosin antibody scintigraphy is positive in myocarditis with a sensitivity of up to 65%.

℞ TREATMENT

NONPHARMACOLOGIC THERAPY

- Supportive care is the first line of therapy for patients with myocarditis.
- Restrict physical activity (to decrease cardiac work). Bed rest is advisable during viremia.
- Avoid heavy use of alcohol and use of nonsteroidal antiinflammatory drugs.

ACUTE GENERAL ℞

- Treat underlying cause (e.g., use specific antibiotics for bacterial infection).
- Treat congestive heart failure (CHF) with diuretics, angiotensin-converting enzyme inhibitors (ACE inhibitors), and salt restriction. A beta-blocker may be added once clinical stability has been achieved. Digoxin should be used with caution and only at low doses.
- Patients who are left with an LVEF ≤35% despite optimal medical therapy for 3-9 mo, and who have good functional status with prognosis >1 yr, will benefit from primary

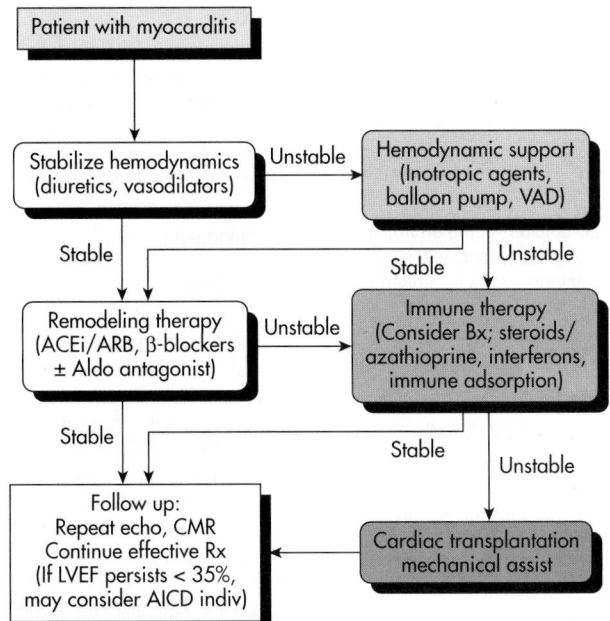

FIG. 2 Treatment algorithms for patients with myocarditis, depending on hemodynamic stability and response to general supportive and remodeling treatment regimen at each step. All patients should have aggressive support and appropriate follow-up. Immune therapy at present is still mainly to support those who have failed to improve spontaneously. *ACEi*, Angiotensin-converting enzyme inhibitors; *AICD*, automatic implantable cardioverter-defibrillator; *Aldo*, aldosterone; *ARB*, angiotensin receptor blockers; *Bx*, biopsy; *CMR*, cardiac magnetic resonance; *indiv*, based on individual assessment of risk versus benefit; *LVEF*, left ventricular ejection fraction; *VAD*, ventricular assist device. (From Bonow RO et al: *Heart disease*, ed 9, Philadelphia, 2012, Saunders.)

prevention therapy with implantable cardioverter-defibrillator (ICD) implantation as in patients with ischemic cardiomyopathy and other nonischemic cardiomyopathies.
- Antiarrhythmics if needed for ventricular arrhythmias. ICD implantation for secondary prevention in patients who have life-threatening ventricular arrhythmias and have good functional status with prognosis >1 yr.
- In patients with chronic CHF from myocarditis, only ACE inhibitors, beta-blockers, and possibly aldosterone receptor antagonists will decrease their mortality in the long term (as with all CHF etiologies).
- Provide anticoagulation to prevent thromboembolism in atrial fibrillation, in severe left ventricular dysfunction with an EF <20%, and in patients with severe segmental wall motion abnormality of the apex.
- Inotropes or mechanical assist devices such as intraaortic balloon pumps, Impella device, and left ventricular assist device (LVAD) if

severe heart failure or if cardiogenic shock persists despite medical therapy.
- Cardiac transplantation in patients with chronic or acute fulminant myocarditis with intractable cardiomyopathy and persistent CHF.
- Corticosteroid use is contraindicated in early infectious myocarditis; it may be justified in only selected patients with intractable CHF, severe systemic toxicity, and severe life-threatening arrhythmias.
- Immunosuppressive drugs (prednisone with cyclosporine/Cytoxan or azathioprine) do not have any significant effect on the prognosis of myocarditis and should not be used in the routine treatment of patients with myocarditis. Immunosuppression may have a role in the treatment of myocarditis from systemic autoimmune disease (e.g., lupus, scleroderma), in idiopathic giant cell myocarditis, sarcoidosis, or myocarditis caused by hypersensitivity reactions, or in severe hemodynamic compromise.

- In patients with ongoing viral genomic expression, preliminary data suggest that treatment with interferons may improve both symptoms and left ventricular function when compared with standard heart failure therapy.
- IV immunoglobulins have been studied, but because of lack of efficacy data, at present there is no indication for their use except in some pediatric cases or those refractory to immunosuppressive therapy.
- A treatment algorithm for patients with myocarditis is described in Fig. 2.

DISPOSITION
- Most patients with acute myocarditis and mild cardiac involvement have a partial or a full clinical recovery. In some cases, however, the process may continue subclinically with eventual progression to a cardiomyopathy. Therefore all patients with myocarditis should be followed up at least initially at intervals of 1 to 3 mo. Of those with advanced cardiac dysfunction, one third will have residual cardiac dysfunction and 25% may progress to cardiac transplantation or death.
- Prognosis is best for patients with fulminant lymphocytic myocarditis (severe hemodynamic compromise, rapid onset of symptoms, or high fever). These patients tend to have complete recovery with total resolution of myocarditis on repeat biopsy.
- In contrast, patients with giant cell myocarditis have an extremely poor prognosis with a median survival of <6 mo, and most require cardiac transplantation.

REFERRAL
Consider heart transplant if intractable CHF develops.

SUGGESTED READINGS
Available at www.expertconsult.com

RELATED CONTENT
Myocarditis (Patient Information)

AUTHORS: **ADAM M. NOYES, M.D.,** and **ARAVIND RAO KOKKIRALA, M.D.**

M

Diseases and Disorders

I

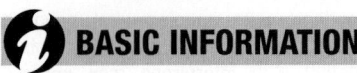 **BASIC INFORMATION**

DEFINITION

Myoclonus is defined as a sudden, brief (<500 ms), and involuntary movement of the extremities, face, and/or trunk. Positive myoclonus is caused by excessive muscle contraction, whereas negative myoclonus is due to a transient loss of postural tone (e.g., asterixis). Myoclonus can be seen in a wide variety of neurologic and systemic disorders.

ICD-10CM CODES
G25.3 Myoclonus

EPIDEMIOLOGY & DEMOGRAPHICS

INCIDENCE: 1.3/100,000 persons
PREVALENCE: 8.6/100,000 persons
PREDOMINANT SEX AND AGE: No gender preference; age at onset varies by the etiology of the myoclonus
GENETICS: Varies by etiology, can be hereditary or sporadic

PHYSICAL FINDINGS & CLINICAL PRESENTATION

- Clinically, myoclonus can be classified by its distribution: focal (only one body part involved), multifocal, segmental (spread to adjacent body parts), axial (muscles innervated by one or several spinal levels), or generalized. It can occur at rest, with maintaining a posture, with action, or with an external stimulus (reflex myoclonus).
- Myoclonus can be due to involvement of the cerebral cortex, brain stem, spinal cord, or peripheral nerve. The causal location may not always influence the characteristics of the myoclonus.
- Negative myoclonus is typically seen in postural muscles of the limbs, causing a bobbing appearance. Asterixis is a form of negative myoclonus.

ETIOLOGY

- The causes of myoclonus are numerous and can be grouped into the categories of physiologic, essential, epileptic, and symptomatic.
- Physiologic myoclonus is a normal phenomenon and includes sleep (hypnic) jerks, hiccups (singultus), and exercise-induced myoclonus.
- Essential myoclonus occurs in the absence of other neurologic symptoms and is usually autosomal dominant. When dystonia is present, it is called myoclonus-dystonia. The myoclonus is often responsive to alcohol in this condition.
- In epileptic myoclonus, seizures dominate the clinical picture. Syndromes include infantile spasms and juvenile myoclonic epilepsy among others.
- Symptomatic or secondary myoclonus comprises myoclonus in the setting of an underlying neurologic disorder or other precipitant. The number of secondary causes

prevents giving a full list, but common etiologies include neurodegenerative diseases (Alzheimer's, atypical forms of parkinsonism), CNS infections (Creutzfeldt-Jakob disease, viral encephalitis), metabolic derangements (uremia, hepatic failure), and drug-induced (selective serotonin reuptake inhibitors [SSRIs], tricyclic antidepressants [TCAs], lithium, stimulants, opioids, gabapentin), autoimmune, paraneoplastic, and post-hypoxic etiologies (myoclonic status epilepticus, Lance-Adams syndrome).

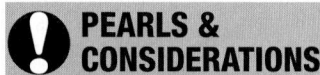 **DIAGNOSIS**

DIFFERENTIAL DIAGNOSIS

- Tremor: a rhythmic oscillation around a point; slower than myoclonus
- Tic: a rapid, patterned movement that, unlike myoclonus, may be briefly suppressed voluntarily or may be accompanied by a premonitory urge
- Dystonia: patterned contractions of agonist/antagonist muscles causing twisting or pulling; slower than myoclonus
- Chorea: typically slower, more complex writhing, patterned movements
- Psychogenic myoclonus: variable in duration and location, distractible, or entrainable

LABORATORY TESTS

- Evaluate for metabolic precipitants (renal and hepatic function, Mg, Ca, thyroid studies, ammonia)
- Toxicology screen (amphetamines, cocaine, opiates/opioids)
- Lumbar puncture if an infectious, inflammatory (including autoimmune), or paraneoplastic CNS process is suspected. Paraneoplastic antibody testing if clinically indicated (i.e., opsoclonus-myoclonus syndrome, limbic encephalitis)
- Electroencephalography (EEG) to evaluate for epileptic/cortical myoclonus
- Electromyography (EMG) may be useful in patients with psychogenic or mixed movement disorders, particularly to characterize subtle myoclonus from a coexistent tremor if there is clinical uncertainty

IMAGING STUDIES

MRI of the brain with and without gadolinium can evaluate for a structural lesion if the myoclonus is cortical. Creutzfeldt-Jakob disease can show diffusion weighted abnormalities in the striatum and cortex.

Rx TREATMENT

NONPHARMACOLOGIC THERAPY

- Treatment should be directed toward correcting the underlying cause if it is reversible (e.g., hepatic or renal failure).
- Carefully remove or decrease potentially causative medications.

ACUTE Rx

Following evaluation for systemic infections and metabolic derangements, myoclonus that is epileptic; interferes with respiration, swallowing, or walking; or causes other severe distress to the patient may be managed acutely with IV formulation antiepileptic drugs such as valproic acid, levetiracetam, or benzodiazepines (lorazepam or midazolam).

CHRONIC Rx

- Clonazepam (preferred over other benzodiazepines for its long half-life), valproic acid, and levetiracetam are typically used for all forms of myoclonus, and often combinations of these medications are more effective.
- If dystonia is present (myoclonus-dystonia), a trial of levodopa is worthwhile although only rarely effective. Anticholinergics may also help dystonia. Botulinum toxin is used for focal dystonia.
- Peripheral focal myoclonus (e.g., hemifacial spasm) can also be helped by botulinum toxin.

DISPOSITION

The ultimate prognosis depends on the etiology of the myoclonus.

REFERRAL

Referral to a general neurologist or movement disorders center is appropriate.

! PEARLS & CONSIDERATIONS

COMMENTS

- When myoclonus is seen with parkinsonism, atypical forms of parkinsonism should be high on the differential, such as dementia with Lewy bodies, corticobasal syndrome, and multiple system atrophy. Myoclonus is only rarely seen in idiopathic Parkinson's disease.
- Symptomatic palatal myoclonus is a specific syndrome that is often associated with a focal brain-stem lesion. In essential palatal myoclonus (no lesion), ear "clicking" is an additional symptom that is not seen in the symptomatic form.

SUGGESTED READING
Available at www.expertconsult.com

AUTHORS: **JENNIFER E. VAUGHAN, M.D.,** and **ANDREW P. DUKER, M.D.**

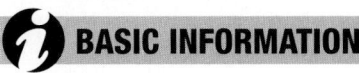

BASIC INFORMATION

DEFINITION

- Myofascial pain syndrome is myalgia characterized by trigger point.
- Trigger point: Trigger points are discrete, focal, hyperirritable spots located in a taut band of skeletal muscle. They produce pain locally and in a referred pattern. Muscle involvement is asymmetric and focal.

SYNONYMS

Chronic myofascial pain
CMP

ICD-10CM CODES
M79.1 Myalgia, myofascial pain syndrome

EPIDEMIOLOGY & DEMOGRAPHICS

- Myofascial pain syndrome is a common painful muscle disorder which can affect any sex at any age. About 85% of the general population at some point suffered from it during their lifetime. It also coexists with other chronic pain conditions.

PHYSICAL FINDINGS & CLINICAL PRESENTATION

- Regional body pain and stiffness; often muscles responsible for body posture are affected. Neck, upper back, and lower back muscles are commonly involved. The most commonly affected muscles are trapezius, scalene, infraspinatus, subscapularis, levator scapulae, piriformis, tensor fasciae latae, iliopsoas, gluteus, and quadratus lumborum. Pain is present at rest and with muscle movement.
- Table 1 lists some distinguishing features of myofascial pain and fibromyalgia.
- Limited range of motion and pain-related weakness of affected muscle.
- Twitch response: Brisk contraction of a taut band of skeletal muscle fibers elicited by snapping palpation of a trigger point in that band producing a taut band.
- One or more trigger points asymmetrical location.
- Referred pain from a trigger point to a zone of reference, but not following dermatomal distribution.
- Resolution of the symptoms with lidocaine injection of the trigger point

ETIOLOGY

- Etiology is unknown. There are several proposed histopathologic mechanisms to account for the development of trigger points, but they are lacking scientific evidence. Most researchers agree that acute trauma or repetitive microtrauma may lead to the development of a trigger point.
- Fig. 1 lists causes of myofascial pain and dysfunction.
- Lack of exercise, prolonged poor posture, vitamin deficiencies, sleep disturbances, and

TABLE 1 Distinguishing Features of Myofascial Pain and Fibromyalgia

	Myofascial Pain	Fibromyalgia
Age distribution	20-40 yr	20-50 yr
Gender distribution	Mainly women	Mainly women
Distribution of pain	Localized; usually unilateral	Generalized; bilaterally symmetric
Tender points	Few	Multiple
Trigger points	Uncommon	Common
Fatigue	Localized muscle fatigue	Generalized fatigue
Sleep disturbance	Common	Common

From Firestein GS, et al: *Kelley's textbook of rheumatology*, ed 9, Philadelphia, 2013, Saunders.

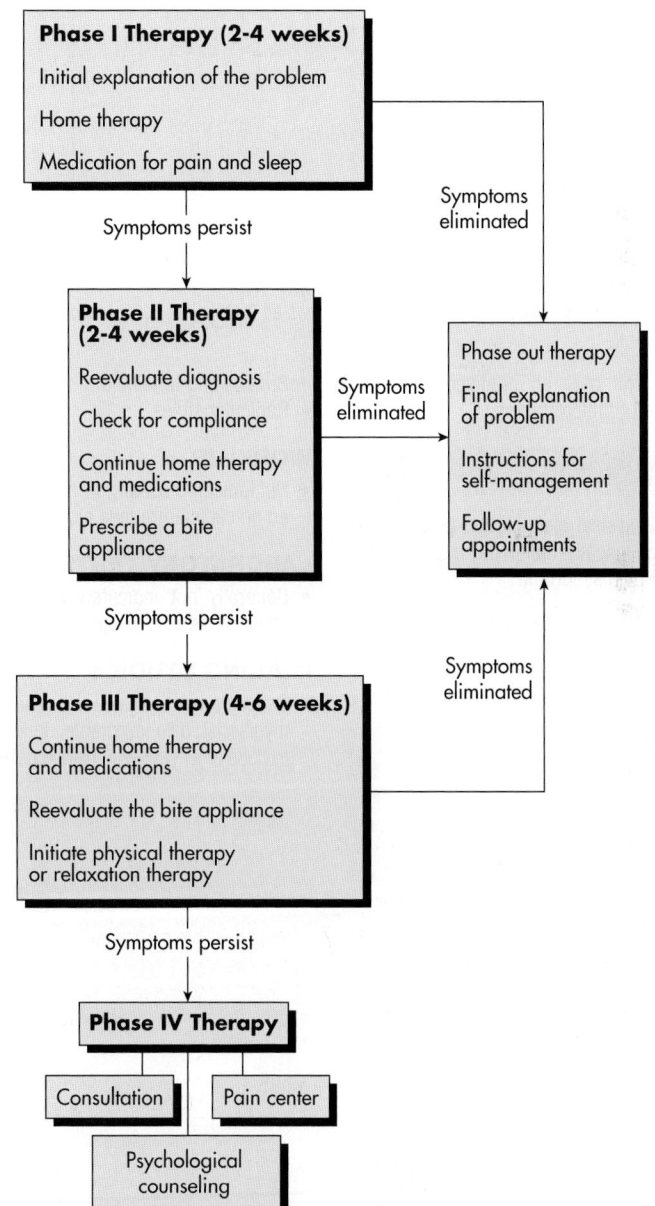

FIG. 1 Management of myofascial pain and dysfunction. Treatments are divided into four phases. If the symptoms are eliminated in any of the first three phases, the ongoing therapy is gradually phased out, and the patient is instructed in continued self-management of the condition. (Modified from Laskin DM, Block S: Diagnosis and treatment of myofascial pain dysfunction [MPD] syndrome, *J Prosthet Dent* 56:75–84, 1986.)

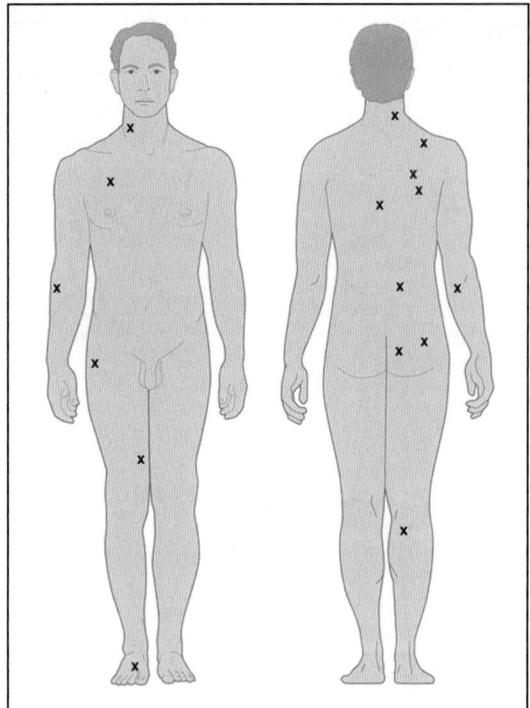

FIG. 2 Most frequent locations of myofascial trigger points. (Adapted from Rachlin E, Rachlin I: *Myofascial pain and fibromyalgia: trigger point management,* ed 2, St Louis, 2002, Mosby.)

joint problems may all predispose to the development of microtrauma.

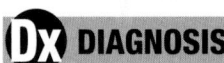 **DIAGNOSIS**

- A detailed physical examination and clinical presentation usually make the diagnosis of myofascial pain syndrome.

DIFFERENTIAL DIAGNOSIS

- Fibromyalgia
- Polymyositis
- Migraine
- Tension headache
- Muscle strain
- Bursitis and tendinitis
- Radiculopathies

WORK-UP

- Not indicated usually, treatment can be started on clinical grounds alone.

LABORATORY TESTS

- Generally not indicated, except to exclude other causes of myalgia.

IMAGING STUDIES

- Generally not indicated in clear-cut cases of myofascial pain syndrome. Indicated only to exclude other causes of pain (e.g., referred pain).

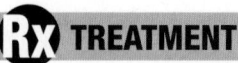 **TREATMENT**

- Spray and stretch therapy: involves passive stretching of the affected muscle. Position patient for maximum decrease in muscle tension, identify trigger points and mark them. Apply vapocoolant spray over entire length of the affected muscle. Passively stretch muscle by applying gentle pressure.
- Physical therapy: TENS unit, ultrasound, massage therapy, myofascial release technique.
- Invasive technique: Trigger point injection with 1% lidocaine is the most commonly used technique.
- NSAIDS and muscle relaxants: short-term use
- Fig. 2 shows the management of myofascial pain and dysfunction.

REFERRAL

An interventional pain management referral is made if trigger point injection is indicated. To physical therapist for increasing ROM and massage therapy.

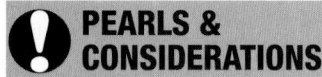 **PEARLS & CONSIDERATIONS**

- Trigger point is commonly misdiagnosed as tender point, which is characteristic finding of fibromyalgia.

Tender point: characterized as non-palpable nodule with symmetric and multiple locations. Tender points are located close to muscle attachment, usually not associated with specific muscle activity. Lacking twitch response and relief of symptoms with localized lidocaine injection.

SUGGESTED READINGS

Available at www.expertconsult.com

AUTHORS: **UZMA NASIR, M.D.,** and **SYEDA M. SAYEED, M.D.**

BASIC INFORMATION

DEFINITION

Myotonia is a type of muscular dystrophy in which relaxation of a muscle after contraction is delayed or prolonged. The most common type of muscular dystrophy with myotonia is myotonic dystrophy. The nondystrophic myotonias (NDMs) are rare disorders (prevalence 1:100,000) caused by mutations in skeletal muscle chloride and sodium channels with the common clinical feature of myotonia without muscle wasting.

SYNONYMS

Myotonic dystrophy

ICD-10CM CODES
G71.1   Myotonic disorders
M62.89 Other specified disorders of muscle
M62.40 Contracture of muscle, unspecified site
G71.12 Myotonia congenita
G71.14 Drug induced myotonia

EPIDEMIOLOGY & DEMOGRAPHICS

- Three to five cases/100,000 persons
- Genetic disorder inherited as an autosomal-dominant illness
- Symptoms usually manifest during adolescence or early adulthood. Cases of infantile myotonic dystrophy have been described.

PHYSICAL FINDINGS & CLINICAL PRESENTATION

- Usual first symptom is distal extremity weakness sometimes associated with muscle stiffness, cramps, or difficulty relaxing grasp.
- Weakness spreads to eventually involve all muscle groups. Flexor neck muscle weakness and masseter and temporal wasting are often prominent features, as is dysarthria.
- Percussion of a muscle produces a slow contraction followed by prolonged relaxation. The myotonic reflex is best tested by percussing the thenar muscles and observing a slow flexion followed by slow relaxation of the thumb.
- As the disease progresses, generalized weakness becomes more pronounced and myotonia becomes less evident.
- Extramuscular involvement:
- Mental retardation of variable severity (may be absent)
- Frontal baldness (Fig. 1)
- Cataracts
- Diabetes mellitus
- Hypogonadism
- Adrenal failure
- Cardiomyopathy
- Infantile myotonic dystrophy presents as neonatal extreme hypotonia with "shark mouth" deformity (upper lip forming an inverted V).

ETIOLOGY & PATHOGENESIS

Genetic disorder encoded on chromosome 19 leading to sustained firing of the muscle membrane, causing prolonged muscle contraction. Myotonic dystrophy 1 (the more common form) is caused by an expanded CTG repeat within the noncoding 3′ untranslated region of the myotonic dystrophy protein kinase (DMPK) gene. The less common form (myotonic dystrophy 2) is caused by an expanded CCTG repeat in the first intron of the zinc finger protein 9 (ZNF9) gene.

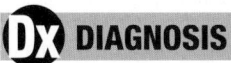

DIAGNOSIS

DIFFERENTIAL DIAGNOSIS

The disease is limited to muscles and causes hypertrophy and stiffness after rest. Muscle function normalizes with exercise. There is no weakness. Symptoms are exacerbated by exposure to cold.

- Myotonia congenita (Thomsen's disease)
- May be autosomal dominant or recessive (two distinct varieties)
- Paramyotonia congenita (autosomal-dominant disease): weakness and stiffness of facial muscles and distal upper extremities, especially or exclusively on cold exposure
- Muscular dystrophies
- Inflammatory myopathies (polymyositis)
- Metabolic muscle diseases
- Myasthenic syndromes
- Motor neuron disease

WORKUP

- History and physical examination usually sufficient
- Muscle enzymes usually abnormal (creatine phosphokinase, aldolase, aspartate aminotransferase)
- Electromyography: typical myotonic "dive bomber" bursts
- Muscle biopsy: type I fiber atrophy, ring fibers, increased central nucleation

TREATMENT

- Phenytoin
- Quinine
- Quinidine
- Procainamide
- Acetazolamide
- Genetic counseling
- Assistive devices, orthotics
- In recent trials,[1] the use of mexiletine resulted in improvement of patient-reported stiffness in patients with nondystrophic myotonias.

DISPOSITION

- In myotonic dystrophy, death is usually caused by the wasting of skeletal muscle and defects in cardiac function.
- Among patients with myotonic dystrophy type 1, an invasive strategy based on systemic electrophysiological studies and prophylactic permanent pacing is associated with longer survival than a non-invasive strategy.[2]

REFERRAL

- To neurologist
- To physical therapy

AUTHOR: **FRED F. FERRI, M.D.**

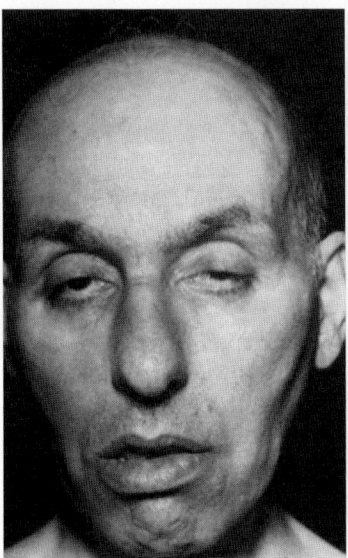
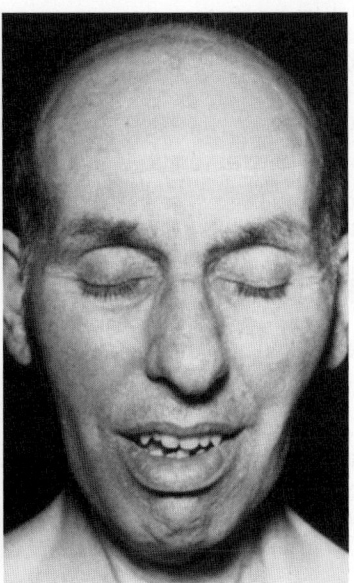

FIG. 1 Myotonic dystrophy with typical myopathic facies, frontal balding, and sunken cheeks. (From Dubowitz V: *Muscle disorders in childhood*, London, 1995, Saunders.)

[1]Statland JM et al: Mexiletine for symptoms and signs of myotonia in nondystrophic myotonia, *JAMA* 308(13): 1357-1365, 2012.
[2]Wahbi K et al: Electrophysiological study with prophylactic pacing and survival in adults with myotonic dystrophy and conduction system disease, *JAMA* 307(12):1292-1301, 2012.

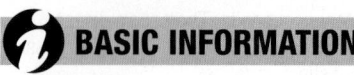

BASIC INFORMATION

DEFINITION

Narcissistic personality disorder (NPD) is characterized by a pattern of grandiosity, need for admiration, and lack of empathy that begins by early adulthood and causes significant distress or impairment in multiple domains of functioning. The individual must meet five or more of the following criteria:

1. Grandiose sense of self-importance. For example, the person may exaggerate achievements and talents or expect recognition as superior without commensurate achievements.
2. Preoccupied with fantasies of unlimited success, power, brilliance, beauty, or ideal love.
3. Views self as "special" and unique and should only associate with other special or highly regarded people and institutions.
4. Requires excessive admiration.
5. Sense of entitlement. For example, unreasonable expectations of especially favorable treatment or automatic compliance with his or her expectations.
6. Interpersonally exploitative.
7. Lacks empathy—unwilling to recognize or identify with the feelings or needs of others.
8. Often envious of others or believes others envious of him or her.
9. Shows arrogant or haughty behaviors.

SYNONYMS

NPD

ICD-10CM CODES
F60.81 Narcissistic personality disorder

EPIDEMIOLOGY & DEMOGRAPHICS

PREVALENCE: Less than 1% of the general population; estimates range from 2% to 16% in the clinical population
PREDOMINANT SEX: More commonly diagnosed in males (up to 3:1)
PREDOMINANT AGE: 20s and 30s

CLINICAL PRESENTATION

- Patients have an underlying sense of inferiority and inadequacy.
- May be related to the failure of parents or parental surrogates to impart a sense of self-worth.
- To avoid these beliefs and their associated painful effects, patients seek to convince self and others that they are special, the best, or unusually talented.
- Astutely aware of status, pecking order.
- Vulnerability in self-esteem makes these patients exquisitely sensitive to criticism, defeat, or perceived weakness, which in turn can lead to feeling humiliated, degraded, and empty.

- These patients react to perceived slights either with more intense grandiosity and admiration-seeking or with disdain and rage. Either approach seeks to bolster their sense of self often by devaluing or criticizing the other person.
- Experiences of self-deflation lead to social withdrawal or depressed mood or to feigned humility that protects grandiosity.
- Interpersonal relationships are typically shallow and limited.
- Although ambition and confidence may lead to high achievement, vocational functioning may be disrupted by intolerance for criticism.

ETIOLOGY

- Limited knowledge about role of genetic loading and neurobiologic vulnerability.
- Prevailing hypotheses focus on impaired development of self as "worthy" because of insufficient affirmation and warmth from parents.

DIAGNOSIS

DIFFERENTIAL DIAGNOSIS

- Mania and hypomania
- Dysthymia and major depressive episode
- Substance-induced euphoria, especially cocaine abuse
- Histrionic, borderline, antisocial, and paranoid personality disorders share common features and are often comorbid
- Personality changes from a general medical condition, including central nervous system processes in the frontal-temporal regions of the brain

WORKUP

- History: collateral information essential to establishing presence of longstanding interpersonal pattern in multiple domains of the patient's life
- Physical examination
- Mental status examination

LABORATORY TESTS

Tests necessary to rule out medical causes of personality changes

IMAGING STUDIES

Those necessary to rule out medical causes of personality changes

TREATMENT

NONPHARMACOLOGIC THERAPY

- Cognitive-behavioral therapy to help patients control rage, manage perceived criticism, and develop social skills
- Psychodynamic psychotherapy to help develop improved self-concept, affect tolerance, and interpersonal functioning

ACUTE GENERAL Rx

Benzodiazepines or low-dose antipsychotics to control rage

CHRONIC Rx

- Selective serotonin reuptake inhibitors for impulsivity or comorbid depression
- Mood stabilizers if comorbid bipolar or to improve impulse control

DISPOSITION

- Severity is variable and course is chronic. The majority of patients obtain greater functioning in fifth decade and beyond when pessimism replaces grandiosity. Often lifelong difficulty maintaining intimate relationships.
- At increased risk for major depressive disorder and substance abuse or dependence (especially cocaine).

REFERRAL

If pharmacotherapy is contemplated

PEARLS & CONSIDERATIONS

COMMENTS

- Illness threatens these patients' image of superiority.
- To defend against this threat, patients may minimize symptoms or deny presence of illness.
- Patients will commonly demand special treatment from senior and well-known physicians.
- Patients may devalue, criticize, or question the behavior or credentials of the treating physician.
- Management guidelines:
  1. Be respectful and nonconfrontational.
  2. Help patient use self-perceived talents in service of treatment.
  3. Do not personalize patient's devaluation, but understand their criticalness as an attempt to manage their own intense insecurity.
  4. Appeal to the patient's narcissism. In other words, agree with the patient that he or she is "entitled" to appropriate care.

SUGGESTED READINGS
Available at www.expertconsult.com

RELATED CONTENT

Narcissistic Personality Disorder (Patient Information)

AUTHOR: **JOHN Q. YOUNG, M.D., M.P.P.**

BASIC INFORMATION

DEFINITION

Narcolepsy is a chronic neurologic sleep disorder characterized by excessive daytime sleepiness and dysregulation of rapid eye movement (REM) sleep. It is the second most common cause of disabling daytime sleepiness after obstructive sleep apnea. Symptoms of REM sleep dysregulation include cataplexy, sleep paralysis, and hallucinations during transition between wake and sleep. Difficulty sleeping with either frequent awakenings or disrupted sleep may also occur.

SYNONYMS

Hypersomnia of central origin
Narcolepsy with cataplexy
Narcolepsy-cataplexy syndrome
Narcolepsy with hypocretin deficiency
Gélineau syndrome

ICD-10CM CODES
G47.419 Narcolepsy without cataplexy
G47.411 Narcolepsy with cataplexy

EPIDEMIOLOGY & DEMOGRAPHICS

INCIDENCE: 0.74/100,000 persons/yr
PREVALENCE: 1 in 2,000 people
PREDOMINANT SEX: Males and females are equally affected.
AGE OF ONSET: Peak 15 to 30 yr (range, 10-55 yr)
GENETICS:
- Associated with human leukocyte antigen (HLA) subtypes, specifically, *DQB1*0602,* which is present in 95% of patients with cataplexy and 96% of patients with hypocretin deficiency.
- Risk of narcolepsy increases 20 to 40 times if a family member is affected.
- Monozygotic twin concordance rate is 17% to 36%, thus indicating an incomplete penetrance and suggesting an environmental factor in the disease process.
RISK FACTORS: Anesthesia, head injury, history of meningitis or encephalitis, family history of narcolepsy, tumor, vascular malformations, stroke, and obesity.

PHYSICAL FINDINGS & CLINICAL PRESENTATION

- Overwhelming urge to sleep with chronic hypersomnia may occur during the day.
- Cataplexy occurs in 60% to 100% of patients with narcolepsy and is reported as a partial or complete loss of voluntary muscle control with preserved consciousness that is precipitated by a strong emotion, more commonly with laughter. This is the most specific symptom and is considered pathognomonic for narcolepsy.
- Hypnagogic (wake to sleep) or hypnopompic (sleep to wake) hallucinations have been reported in 60% to 80% of patients with narcolepsy.

- Sleep paralysis, defined as loss of muscle tone during the transition between sleep and wakefulness, occurs in 60% to 80% of patients with narcolepsy. It may occur with hallucinations and can be interrupted by sensory stimuli.
- Only about one third of patients will have all four symptoms of narcolepsy: chronic daytime sleepiness, cataplexy, hypnagogic hallucinations, and sleep paralysis.
- Fragmented sleep is seen in 60% to 80% of narcolepsy patients and can often be mistaken for insomnia or other intrinsic sleep disorder.
- Other symptoms that have been reported in narcolepsy include automatic behavior or semipurposeful movements in 40% of patients and memory disturbance in 50% of patients.

ETIOLOGY

The loss of hypocretin/orexin signaling, genetic factors, and brain lesions are presently identified factors in the development of narcolepsy.
HYPOCRETIN/OREXIN:
- Loss of hypocretin-1 and hypocretin-2 (also known as orexin-A and orexin-B) producing neurons in the lateral hypothalamus.
- Human cerebrospinal fluid (CSF) levels of hypocretin-1 are low to undetectable in narcoleptics with cataplexy.
- Narcolepsy without cataplexy may have a different cause because CSF hypocretin levels are usually normal in these patients, so there may be a completely separate mechanism in these patients, or it may result from less extensive loss of hypocretin neurons or impaired signaling.
SECONDARY ETIOLOGIES:
- Central nervous system lesions including tumors, vascular malformations, and strokes have all been reported to cause secondary narcolepsy.
- Direct injury to the hypocretin neurons or their projections is the most likely cause of secondary narcolepsy due to central nervous system lesions.
- Narcolepsy has been reported in genetic syndromes, including Prader-Willi syndrome and Niemann-Pick disease type C, as well as paraneoplastic syndromes.

DIAGNOSIS

DIFFERENTIAL DIAGNOSIS

Excessive daytime somnolence:
- Autism
- Autosomal dominant cerebellar ataxia, deafness, and narcolepsy
- Behaviorally induced insufficient sleep syndrome
- Central or obstructive sleep apnea (sleep-disordered breathing)
- Circadian rhythm disorder
- Depression
- Diencephalic lesions
- Drug or alcohol abuse
- Hypothyroidism
- Idiopathic hypersomnia with long or short sleep time
- Inadequate sleep hygiene

- Insufficient sleep
- Increased intracranial pressure Insomnia
- Kleine-Levin syndrome
- Medication effect
- Menstrual-related hypersomnia
- Posttraumatic narcolepsy
- Seizures
- Sleep fragmentation (multiple causes) Cataplexy:
- Seizures
- Periodic paralysis
- Cardiovascular insufficiency
- Psychogenic (multiple causes)
- Lesions of the hypothalamus or brain stem

WORKUP

- Because persistent sleepiness can occur with many conditions, it is important to rule out other sleep disorders.
- Narcolepsy is often diagnosed by clinical history. The Epworth Sleepiness Scale is very useful in determining the degree of excessive daytime sleepiness (Table 1).
- The diagnosis of narcolepsy can be made if there is a clear history of cataplexy in the setting of excessive daytime somnolence, without need for further diagnostic testing. Sleep laboratory testing or possibly laboratory testing is required if these symptoms do not exist, if a diagnosis needs to be confirmed, or if concerns exist for another sleep disorder.
- The medical history should include questions regarding severity of daytime hypersomnia while also evaluating for sleep-disordered breathing, transient muscle weakness triggered by emotion, hallucinations while falling asleep or upon awakening, and inability to move after awakening. The clinical evaluation should also address symptoms of seizures and paraneoplastic disorders while also asking about previous stroke or genetic disorders. A detailed family history is imperative. Hypothalamic dysfunction such as unexplained weight gain, endocrine abnormalities, circadian dysrhythmias, and autonomic nervous system problems may provide useful insight.
- A thorough examination including a detailed neurologic examination should be performed.
- Nocturnal polysomnography followed by a multiple sleep latency test (MSLT) remains the gold standard for the diagnosis of narcolepsy. A drug screen should also be performed to rule out pharmacologic modulations of sleep.

LABORATORY TESTS

HLA subtyping and CSF hypocretin/orexin levels may be attempted in suspected cases of narcolepsy. For a fee, CSF hypocretin/orexin analysis can be performed at the Center for Narcolepsy at Stanford University (med.stanford.edu/psychiatry/narcolepsy). CSF hypocretin levels below 110 pg/mL are indicative of narcolepsy, but normal or high CSF hypocretin levels do not exclude the diagnosis.

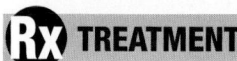 TREATMENT

Narcolepsy can be treated with a combination of behavioral and pharmacologic approaches.

NONPHARMACOLOGIC THERAPY

Avoidance of over-the-counter drugs and illicit drugs, optimal sleep hygiene and scheduled daily naps, and psychosocial support can be used for symptoms of excessive daytime somnolence. However, nonpharmacologic therapy is typically not sufficient for treatment of narcolepsy alone but is often used as adjunct therapy with medications.

PHARMACOLOGIC THERAPY

For excessive daytime somnolence:
- Sodium oxybate: a central nervous system depressant that can be used for the treatment of cataplexy and REM-related symptoms
- Modafinil 200 to 600 mg PO every morning or divided bid
- Armodafinil 150 or 250 mg PO as a single dose in the morning
- Methylphenidate 5 to 15 mg PO bid to tid
- Methylphenidate SR 18 to 54 mg PO every morning or divided bid
- Dextroamphetamine 10 to 60 mg PO qd
- Eldepryl 5 mg PO bid
  For cataplexy:
- Sodium oxybate: a central nervous system depressant that can be used for the treatment of cataplexy and REM-related symptoms

- Fluoxetine 20 mg PO qd initially
- Sertraline 25 mg PO qd initially
- Venlafaxine 25 mg PO qd initially
- Clomipramine 25 mg/day initially
- Protriptyline 5 mg tid initially
- Imipramine 25 to 50 mg/day initially
- Desipramine 10 mg bid initially

DISPOSITION

This is a chronic sleep disorder that may worsen for the first few years and then persist for life.

REFERRAL

Because of the complexity of this disorder and its ever-changing management and treatment, patients should be referred to centers or programs with highly trained sleep specialists with expertise caring for these patients, especially if sodium oxybate (Xyrem) therapy is needed.

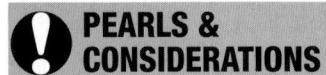

ⓘ PEARLS & CONSIDERATIONS

Many narcoleptics report the onset of symptoms beginning in childhood to early adulthood with a long delay of actual diagnosis on the order of 10 to 15 yr. Typically, excessive daytime sleepiness is the initial symptom followed by REM dysregulation (e.g., cataplexy, sleep paralysis, hypnagogic hallucinations). Patients with narcolepsy also have higher than expected incidence of other sleep disorders, including obstructive sleep apnea, periodic limb movements of sleep, and REM sleep behavior disorder.

COMMENTS

Narcolepsy is a rare disorder that is underdiagnosed. The average time from onset of symptoms to diagnosis is 5 to 15 years. Cataplexy is specific for narcolepsy, but other symptoms of REM dysregulation, including sleep paralysis and hypnagogic or hypnopompic hallucinations, can occur even in normal patients. Sleep-onset REM or REM periods on an MSLT may occur as a result of sleep deprivation or withdrawal from REM-suppressing drugs.

SUGGESTED READINGS
Available at www.expertconsult.com

RELATED CONTENT

Narcolepsy (Patient Information)

AUTHOR: **DON HAYES, JR., M.D., M.S., M.ED.**

TABLE 1 Epworth Sleepiness Scale

How likely are you to doze off or fall asleep in the following situations, in contrast to just feeling tired? This refers to your usual way of life in recent time. Even if you have not done some of these things recently, try to work out how they would have affected you. Use the following scale to choose the most appropriate number for each situation.
0 = would never doze
1 = slight chance of dozing
2 = moderate chance of dozing
3 = high chance of dozing

Situation	Chance of Dozing
Sitting and reading	
Watching TV	
Sitting and inactive in a public place (theater or meeting)	
As a passenger in a car for an hour without a break	
Lying down to rest in the afternoon when circumstances permit	
Sitting and talking to someone	
Sitting quietly after lunch (without alcohol)	
In a car, while stopped for a few minutes in traffic	
Total	

From Johns MW: A new method for measuring daytime sleepiness: the Epworth Sleepiness Scale, *Sleep* 14:540-545, 1991.

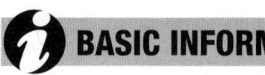

BASIC INFORMATION

DEFINITION

Nasal polyps are a manifestation of chronic rhinosinusitis. Chronic inflammation of the lining of the nasal and sinus cavities results in reactive hyperplasia of the mucosal epithelium in the form of nasal polyps.

SYNONYMS

Nasal polyps
NP
Chronic rhinosinusitis with nasal polyps

ICD-10CM CODES
J33.0 Polyp of nasal cavity

EPIDEMIOLOGY & DEMOGRAPHICS

PEAK INCIDENCE:
- Mean age of onset is 42 yr

PREVALENCE:
- Affects 0.2% to 4.3% of the population.
- Approximately 10% of patients with nasal polyposis have asthma.

PREDOMINANT SEX AND AGE:
- Greater than 2:1 male:female ratio.
- Childhood presentation (age <20) is rare and should prompt evaluation for cystic fibrosis or other pathology.

GENETICS: Some literature suggests there is a genetic component to the disease with an association between HLA-A74 and nasal polyposis.

RISK FACTORS:
- 10% of cases of nasal polyposis are associated with Samter's Triad (asthma, aspirin sensitivity, nasal polyposis).
- Conditions associated with nasal polyps include asthma, bronchiectasis, cystic fibrosis, ciliary dyskinesia syndromes, Churg-Strauss syndrome, allergic fungal sinusitis, and bacterial rhinosinusitis.

CLASSIFICATION: Box 1 describes a classification of nasal polyps.

BOX 1   Classification of Nasal Polyps

1. The antrochoanal polyp, mostly arising from the maxillary sinus and prolapsing into the choana; a commonly large, isolated, unilateral cyst-like noneosinophilic formation
2. Idiopathic unilateral or bilateral; mostly eosinophilic polyps without involvement of the lower airways
3. Bilateral eosinophilic polyposis with concomitant asthma and/or aspirin sensitivity
4. Polyposis with underlying systemic disease such as cystic fibrosis, primary ciliary dyskinesia, Churg-Strauss syndrome, or Kartagener syndrome

From Adkinson NF et al: *Middleton's allergy principles and practice*, ed 8, Philadelphia, 2014, Saunders.

PHYSICAL FINDINGS & CLINICAL PRESENTATION

- Patients usually present with nasal obstruction, anosmia/hyposmia, watery rhinorrhea, and/or post nasal drip.
- Physical Exam
  - Smooth, round, mucosal-lined masses within the nasal cavity, often arising from the middle meatus.
  - Most often bilateral.

ETIOLOGY

- The exact etiology is unclear, but is thought to be multifactorial.
- Cytokine and cellular inflammatory markers found to be largely involved include T-helper 2 (Th-2) cells, eosinophils, IL-5 cytokines, and decreased T-regulatory function.

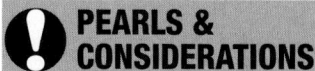

DIAGNOSIS

DIFFERENTIAL DIAGNOSIS

- Possible alternative diagnoses include encephalocele, glioma, inverted papilloma, antrochoanal polyp, and neoplasm.

WORKUP

- Diagnosis can most often be made with history and physical exam.
- Anterior rhinoscopy.
- Nasal endoscopy (Fig. E1).

LABORATORY TESTS

- Allergy testing may be considered based on symptoms and clinical presentation.

IMAGING STUDIES

- CT sinus (Fig. E2): not essential, but recommended for surgical planning if surgery is being considered. Also important to help exclude other diagnoses in the case of unilateral polyps. Findings suggestive of nasal polyps include lobulated cysts or masses in the nasal cavity and partial or complete sinus or nasal cavity opacification.

TREATMENT

ACUTE GENERAL Rx

- Medical management is generally the first consideration in treatment. Goals of treatment are reduction in size of nasal polyps resulting in improvement of symptoms.
  - Nasal corticosteroid sprays are a mainstay of treatment acutely and over the long term.
  - Short courses of oral corticosteroids are reserved for advanced or refractory cases.
  - Antihistamines may be helpful in controlling allergic symptoms but have little effect on nasal polyps.
- Surgical management may be considered for those who have failed medical therapy. Provides symptomatic relief but is rarely curative.
  - High recurrence rate.
  - Nasal polypectomy or more extensive functional endoscopy sinus surgery (FESS) performed by an otolaryngologist.
  - Nasal saline irrigation is important post-operatively and can be continued by the patient as desired.

COMPLEMENTARY & ALTERNATIVE MEDICINE

- There is some evidence that suggests topical intranasal capsaicin may be beneficial in treating nasal polyps.

DISPOSITION

- Patients often require long-term intranasal corticosteroid therapy to reduce nasal inflammation. Recurrence after surgery is common, and the goals of treatment are to reduce symptoms.

REFERRAL

- Referral to an otolaryngologist should be made in cases in which the diagnosis is unclear or the disease is not responsive to standard medical treatments.

PEARLS & CONSIDERATIONS

COMMENTS

- The inferior or middle turbinates are often mistaken for nasal polyps by inexperienced observers.
- When unilateral polyps are identified, histologic evaluation should be undertaken to exclude malignancy or other pathology as described previously.

PREVENTION

- Avoidance of aspirin in sensitive patients.

SUGGESTED READINGS
Available at www.expertconsult.com

AUTHOR: **LOUIS INSALACO, M.D.**

BASIC INFORMATION

DEFINITION

Necrotizing autoimmune myopathy (NAM) is a recently defined subgroup of idiopathic inflammatory myopathies (IIM) that presents with myalgias, weakness, and markedly elevated CPK levels. Most cases of NAM are seen in patients who have a history of statin use, the average duration of which is about three years. The symptoms of NAM may persist long after statins have been discontinued, unlike typical statin-induced myopathy. Unlike with most IIM, there is necrosis but sparse inflammation seen on muscle biopsy. Specific histopathologic findings on muscle biopsy include myophagocytosis with predominant muscle fiber necrosis, prominent regeneration with minimal or no lymphocytic inflammatory infiltrate, and variable deposition of major histocompatibility complex (MHC) class I and membrane attack complex (MAC C5b-9) on small blood vessels (Fig. 1). Macrophages are the only inflammatory cells found, if any. Two specific autoantibodies associated with NAM are anti-signal recognition particle (SRP) and anti-3-hydroxy-3-methylglutaryl-coenzyme-A reductase (HMGCR). Statins have been associated with developing anti-HMGCR in all populations; however, these autoantibodies can be present without statin exposure. Rarely, an individual with NAM can have both the antibodies.

SYNONYM

Immune-mediated necrotizing myopathy
NAM
Necrotizing autoimmune myositis

ICD-10CM CODES
G72.49   Other inflammatory and immune myopathies, not elsewhere classified

EPIDEMIOLOGY & DEMOGRAPHICS

INCIDENCE: Incidence of IIM in a homogenous population is 2.2 to 7.7 per million, and NAM, which is a rare disorder, accounts for 20% of IIM. Anti-SRP–associated NAM accounts for 3% to 6% of IIM, while anti-HMGCR accounts for 5% to 7% of IIM.

PREDOMINANT SEX AND AGE: Primarily affects adults >18 years with mean age at onset around 50 to 60 years, while younger ages of 47 to 49 have been reported in European studies. Also, statin- and cancer-related NAM patients are found to be older (60s). Anti-SRP–positive patients tend to be younger. There is a female predominance.

GENETICS: HLADRB1*11:01 is associated with an increased risk of developing anti-HMGCR NAM in whites and African Americans when exposed to statins. HLADRB1*08:03 may be associated with increased risk of anti-SRP NAM in the Japanese population.

RISK FACTORS:

- Statin exposure: atorvastatin and simvastatin more than others.
- Cancer: GI origin most common as well as lung, thymoma, ovarian, etc.
- CTD: Scleroderma, Sjögren's, and less with systemic lupus erythematosus.
- Infections: Rarely HIV.
- Can occur in association with antisynthetase syndrome.

PHYSICAL FINDINGS & CLINICAL PRESENTATION

Acute (<4 wk) or subacute (<6 mo), but rarely chronic onset of severe symmetrical proximal muscle weakness leading to atrophy. Can involve both shoulder and pelvic girdle. Distal weakness possible, along with myalgias and arthralgias. May be associated with interstitial lung disease and mechanic hands, dysphagia or dyspnea, weight loss, Raynaud's. Case reports of isolated involvement of neck extensors have been reported. Has been associated with antisynthetase syndrome. Diastolic dysfunction and arrhythmias can occur, too.

ETIOLOGY

- The autoimmune nature can be explained by subacute onset, the presence of autoantibodies, and response to immunotherapy. Increased TH1 responses and increased INF-gamma production by macrophages have been proposed. Even after statins are discontinued, immune response is sustained due to high levels of HMGCR expression by regenerating fibers.

DIAGNOSIS

DIFFERENTIAL DIAGNOSIS

- Other conditions that cause muscle weakness and/or elevated muscle enzymes, such as muscular dystrophy, polymyositis, dermatomyositis, inclusion body myopathy, drug-induced myopathy, etc.

WORKUP

- MRI of affected muscle
- Electromyography
- Muscle biopsy

LABORATORY TESTS

- CBC
- Creatine kinase
- Aldolase
- Renal function test
- ALT/AST
- Anti-HMGCR antibody (anti 200/100)
- Anti-SRP antibody

IMAGING STUDIES

- MRI of involved muscles
- CT chest/abdomen/pelvis and other age-appropriate cancer screening
- Echocardiogram, ECG

RX TREATMENT

No guidelines yet exist, and as of now, therapy has to be individualized. Stop statins immediately if they are suspected to be the causative agent. Treatment of underlying malignancy can also ameliorate myopathy. Steroids are the mainstay of therapy; however, steroid monotherapy seldom is effective long-term, so the addition of an immunosuppressant agent should be considered. Aggressive therapy from the beginning is preferred. Options include IVIG, MTX, AZA, MMF, rituximab, cyclosporine, CYC. Relapse can occur.

REFERRAL

- Rheumatology
- Neurology

PEARLS & CONSIDERATIONS

NAM must be considered in patients who have persistent myalgias and weakness after discontinuation of statins. Muscle biopsy is essential for diagnosis.

PREVENTION

Avoid statin rechallenge

PATIENT/FAMILY EDUCATION

Report to your doctor immediately any symptoms of muscle pains and/or weakness at any time after starting statin therapy.

SUGGESTED READINGS
Available at www.expertconsult.com

RELATED CONTENT
Inclusion Body Myositis (Related Key Topic)
Inflammatory Myopathies (Related Key Topic)
Statin-Induced Muscle Syndrome (Related Key Topic)

AUTHOR: **DURKHANI MAHBOOB, M.D.**

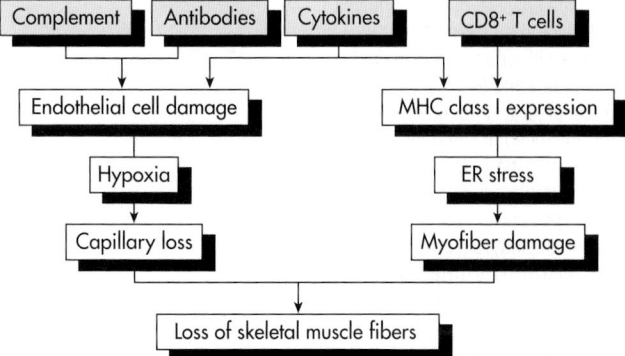

FIG. 1 Mechanisms of muscle fiber damage in myositis. *ER,* endoplasmic reticulum; *MHC,* major histocompatibility complex. Firestein GS et al: *Kelley's textbook of rheumatology,* ed 9, Philadelphia, 2013, Saunders.

BASIC INFORMATION

DEFINITION

Necrotizing fasciitis (NF) is a rapidly spreading bacterial infection of the deep fascia, with associated inflammation, leading to necrosis of subcutaneous tissue planes. This infection can occur in wounds from trauma or surgical wounds or can be spontaneous or idiopathic. There are two clinical types, both of which carry a high rate of morbidity and mortality.

SYNONYMS

NF
Soft tissue gangrene
Flesh-eating bacteria
Fournier's gangrene
Hemolytic streptococcal gangrene

ICD-10CM CODES
M72.6 Necrotizing fasciitis

EPIDEMIOLOGY & DEMOGRAPHICS

PREDOMINANT SEX: Male > female.
PREDOMINANT AGE: 6 to 50 yr; less common in children.

EPIDEMIOLOGY

Invasive group A *Streptococcus* infection occurs at a rate of 3.5 cases per 100,000 persons, with a case fatality rate of around 24%.

PHYSICAL FINDINGS & CLINICAL PRESENTATION

CLINICAL TYPES OF NECROTIZING FASCIITIS:

- Type I: Necrotizing fasciitis: At least one anaerobic species is isolated in conjunction with one or more facultative anaerobic species, such as streptococci (not group A), *and* members of the Enterobacteriaceae
- Anaerobic bacteria, most commonly *Bacteroides* or *Peptostreptococcus* spp.
- Enterobacteriaceae: *Escherichia coli*, *Klebsiella* spp., *Proteus* spp., *Enterobacter* spp.
- Usually associated with diabetes or peripheral vascular disease
- Example of type I: Fournier's gangrene of the perineum
- Type II: Necrotizing fasciitis: Group A *Streptococcus* is isolated alone or in combination with other bacteria, most likely *Staphylococcus aureus*. Also known as hemolytic streptococcal gangrene
  1. Example of type II: Invasive group A *Streptococcus*, associated with virulence factors type 1 and type 3 M protein

EXAMPLES OF NECROTIZING FASCIITIS:

- Fournier's gangrene: Aggressive type I infection of the perineum usually caused by penetration of the gastrointestinal or urethral mucosa by enteric organisms. It can rapidly spread to involve the scrotum, penis, and abdominal wall or gluteal muscles, causing gangrene.

- Clostridial cellulitis: Caused by *Clostridium perfringens* associated by local trauma or surgery and crepitus caused by gas production; generally noted in the skin, with deeper tissues generally spared.

PHYSICAL FINDINGS

Minor skin trauma, toxic-appearing patient:
- Open skin wound.
- Severe pain at injury or surgical site.
- Fever, confusion, weakness, diarrhea.
- Early skin erythema, quickly spreading in hours to days.
- Skin redness changes to purple discoloration.
- Gangrenous skin changes may develop.
- Loosening of skin and subcutaneous skin in association with deep fascial necrosis (Fig. 1). "Woody" induration and crepitus of involved area are characteristics.
- Muscle involvement, thrombosis of blood vessels, and myonecrosis may develop.
- Bullae and gas formation at site.

ETIOLOGY

- NF usually arises from skin damage or trauma. Risk is increased with presence of comorbidities (DM, cancer, liver disease, immunosuppression).
- Polymicrobial: mixture of anaerobes and aerobic enteric gram-negative rods.
- Group A streptococci (*S. pyogenes*).
- *S. aureus*.
- *C. perfringens*.
- *Bacteroides fragilis*.
- *Vibrio vulnificus*.
- Methicillin-resistant *S. aureus* (MRSA), especially community-acquired MRSA.

DIAGNOSIS

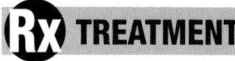

DIFFERENTIAL DIAGNOSIS

- Cellulitis.
- Pyomyositis.
- Gas gangrene.
- A classification of necrotizing skin, soft-tissue, and muscle infections is described in Table 1.

WORKUP

- Diagnosis of necrotizing fasciitis generally requires incision and probing. In patients with necrotizing fasciitis, there is no resistance to probing subcutaneously and there is fascial plane involvement.
- Laboratory tests:
  1. Complete blood cell count (CBC) with differential (leukocytosis, anemia), elevated CRP (≥15 mg/dL), hyponatremia (sodium <135 mEq/L), elevated creatinine (>1.6 mg/dL), hyperglycemia (glucose >180 mg/dL)
  2. Cultures of skin, soft tissue, or debrided tissue, aerobically and anaerobically. Blood cultures are positive in 60% of patients with type II infections and 20% with type I infections.
- Imaging:
  1. Radiographs show subcutaneous gas in fascial planes (Fig. 2).
  2. Computed tomography (CT)/magnetic resonance imaging (MRI) may be helpful because they can detect gas in the tissues.

TREATMENT

- Aggressive surgical debridement of involved necrotic tissues is essential *as soon as possible* to reduce mortality.
- Fasciotomies of extremities may be necessary.
- Immediate start of empiric antibiotics:

  Type I: Piperacillin/tazobactam; carbapenems such as imipenem, meropenem, or doripenem; and third-generation cephalosporin + metronidazole or aminoglycoside + clindamycin are reasonable choices pending cultures. It is important to always have anaerobic coverage.

  Type II: For group A *Streptococcus*, give intravenous (IV) penicillin G, 4 million U q4h in patients who weigh >60 kg with clindamycin, 600 to 900 mg IV q8h.
  1. Clindamycin has the added effect of suppressing toxin production. If MRSA is suspected, add vancomycin, daptomycin, or linezolid.
- Intravenous gammaglobulin (IVIG): 1 g/kg on day 1 and 0.5 g/kg on days 2 and 3 neutralizes circulating streptococcal toxins and has been shown beneficial in severe forms of invasive group A streptococcal infections, although data not definitive.

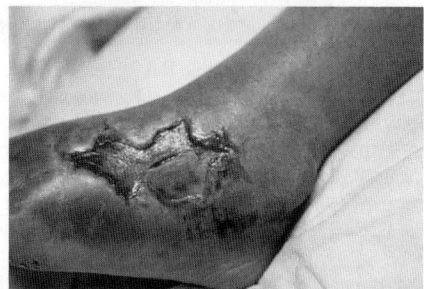

FIG. 1 Necrotizing fasciitis The so-called flesh-eating bacteria, group A β-hemolytic Streptococcus, can cause significant tissue destruction rapidly. This 32-year-old woman had pain, erythema, and swelling of the foot followed by necrotic ulceration over a week. There was no history of trauma. (Courtesy Roger Bitar, MD. From White GM, Cox NH [eds]: *Diseases of the skin, a color atlas and text*, ed 2, St Louis, 2006, Mosby.)

TABLE 1 Classification of Necrotizing Skin, Soft-Tissue, and Muscle Infections

Disease	Bacteriology	Comments
Necrotizing Cellulitis		
Clostridial cellulitis	*Clostridium perfringens*	Local trauma, recent surgery; fascial/deep muscle spared
Nonclostridial cellulitis	Mixed: *Escherichia coli, Enterobacter, Peptostreptococcus* spp., *Bacteroides fragilis*	Diabetes mellitus predisposes; produces foul odor
Meleney's synergistic gangrene	*Staphylococcus aureus*, microaerophilic streptococci	Rare infection; postoperative; slowly expanding, indolent, ulceration in superficial fascia
Synergistic necrotizing cellulitis	Mixed aerobic and anaerobic, including *B. fragilis, Peptostreptococcus* spp.	Diabetes mellitus predisposes; variant of necrotizing fasciitis type I; involves skin, muscle, fat, and fascia
Necrotizing Fasciitis		
Type I	Mixed aerobic and anaerobic; staphylococci, *B. fragilis, E. coli*, group A streptococci, *Peptostreptococcus* spp., *Prevotella, Porphyromonas* spp., *Clostridium* spp.	Usually requires a breach in the mucous membrane layer either through surgery or penetrating injuries or from chronic medical conditions such as diabetes, peripheral vascular disease, malignancy, and anal fissures
Type II	Group A streptococci	Increasing in frequency and severity since 1985; very high mortality; often begins at site of nonpenetrating minor trauma such as a bruise or muscle strain but often no identified precursor
		Predisposing factors: blunt/penetrating trauma, varicella (chickenpox), intravenous drug abuse, surgical procedures, childbirth, nonsteroidal antiinflammatory drug use
Myonecrosis		
Clostridial myonecrosis	*Clostridium* spp.	Predisposing factors: deep/penetrating injury, bowel and biliary tract surgery, improperly performed abortion and retained placenta, prolonged rupture of the membranes, and intrauterine fetal demise or missed abortion in postpartum patients. Recurrent gas gangrene occurs at sites of previous gas gangrene.
Streptococcal myonecrosis	Streptococci	
Special Type of Necrotizing Soft-Tissue Infection		
Fournier's gangrene	Polymicrobial, with *E. coli* the predominant aerobe and *Bacteroides* the predominant anaerobe. Other microflora: *Proteus, Staphylococcus, Enterococcus*, aerobic and anaerobic *Streptococcus, Pseudomonas, Klebsiella*, and *Clostridium*	Necrosis of the scrotum or perineum that starts with scrotal pain and erythema and rapidly spreads onto anterior abdominal wall and gluteal muscle. It is more often seen in diabetics and can be associated with trauma.

From Vincent JL et al: *Textbook of critical care*, ed 6, Philadelphia, 2011, Saunders.

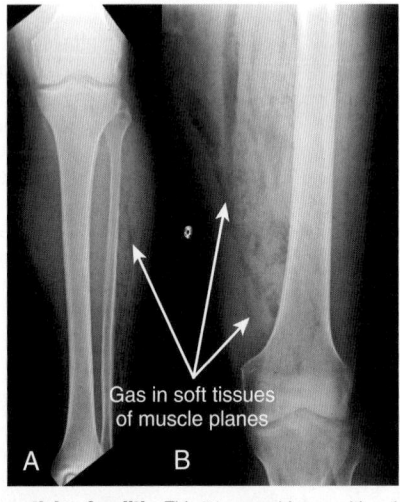
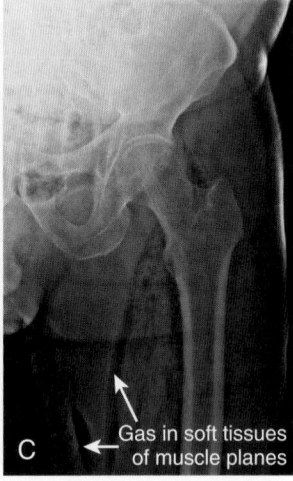

FIG. 2 Necrotizing fasciitis This 71-year-old man with aplastic anemia presented with fevers to 38.9° C, leg weakness, and extreme leg pain. Initially, the patient was thought to have neuropathic pain and weakness, possibly indicating spinal disease such as epidural abscess. He rapidly developed crepitus of his legs. Radiographs of the patient's legs were obtained, followed by noncontrast CT. **A,** Anterior-posterior (AP) tibia and fibula. **B,** AP femur. **C,** AP hip. Air is seen dissecting in muscle planes of the legs. On radiograph, air appears black. Given the wide distribution of air, a focal abscess is unlikely, and necrotizing fasciitis with gas-producing organisms should be suspected. (From Broder JS: *Diagnostic imaging for the emergency physician,* Philadelphia, 2011, Saunders.)

- For Vibrio vulnificus use doxycycline plus ceftazidime; for Aeromonas hydrophila use doxycycline plus ciprofloxacin.
- Hyperbaric oxygen evaluation as an adjunct to surgery and IV antibiotics.

SUGGESTED READINGS

Available at www.expertconsult.com

AUTHOR: **GLENN G. FORT, M.D., M.P.H.**

BASIC INFORMATION

DEFINITION

Nephrotic syndrome is characterized by heavy proteinuria (usually defined as >3.5 g/24 hr), hypoalbuminemia, hyperlipidemia, lipiduria, and edema. Nephrotic-range proteinuria can have many causes that share a common mechanism of glomerular injury leading to proteinuria. Patients with this degree of proteinuria may or may not have the other features of the syndrome.

ICD-10CM CODES
N04.9 Nephrotic syndrome with unspecified morphologic changes
N04.0 Nephrotic syndrome with minor glomerular abnormality
N04.1 Nephrotic syndrome with focal and segmental glomerular lesions
N04.2 Nephrotic syndrome with diffuse membranous glomerulonephritis
N04.3 Nephrotic syndrome with diffuse mesangial proliferative glomerulonephritis
N04.4 Nephrotic syndrome with diffuse endocapillary proliferative glomerulonephritis
N04.5 Nephrotic syndrome with diffuse mesangiocapillary glomerulonephritis
N04.6 Nephrotic syndrome with dense deposit disease
N04.7 Nephrotic syndrome with diffuse crescentic glomerulonephritis
N04.8 Nephrotic syndrome with other morphologic changes

EPIDEMIOLOGY & DEMOGRAPHICS

- Among children (especially those less than 6 years of age), the most common causes of nephrotic syndrome are:
  A) Minimal change disease (MCD) (75% of pediatric cases)
  B) Focal and segmental glomerulosclerosis (FSGS) (7%-20% of cases)
- Among adults, FSGS has now become the most common primary cause of nephrotic-range proteinuria. Membranous nephropathy is now the second most common primary cause of nephrotic syndrome. FSGS is more common in persons of African ancestry, whereas membranous nephropathy is seen more commonly in Caucasians. Overall, diabetic nephropathy remains the most common cause of nephrotic-range proteinuria.

PHYSICAL FINDINGS & CLINICAL PRESENTATION

- Patients usually present with severe lower extremity, periorbital edema, and weight gain.
- Ascites and anasarca can occur.
- Hypercoagulability (i.e., pulmonary embolism [PE]) and risk of infection (i.e., pneumococcal infection) are potential clinical manifestations.

ETIOLOGY

Glomerular diseases have often been grouped into diseases that have a nephrotic vs. nephritic presentation. This artificial delineation has traditionally implied that diseases associated with the "nephritic syndromes" are often associated with subnephrotic proteinuria, a fact that can cause diagnostic confusion, as any glomerular disease can present with nephrotic-range proteinuria. It is better to think of these diseases as having either a noninflammatory sediment (proteinuria alone with no casts or cellular elements) vs. an inflammatory sediment (i.e., those with RBC casts and/or dysmorphic RBCs in conjunction with proteinuria). Fig. E1 details this breakdown. In this chapter, we focus on those primary diseases that present with a noninflammatory sediment (namely, MCD, focal segmental glomerulosclerosis, membranous nephropathy, and amyloidosis) as well as on a primary disease with an inflammatory sediment that often has nephrotic-range proteinuria (membranoproliferative glomerulonephritis [MPGN]). Workup of so-called "nephritic syndrome" as noted by worsening GFR in the setting of proteinuria and hematuria is detailed elsewhere. Important points regarding the most common etiologies of nephrotic syndrome are detailed below and in Table 1.

- MCD: characterized by a bland urine sediment and abrupt onset of disease and equally abrupt remission. Proteinuria can be massive (>20 g daily). NSAID use, lithium, viral infections, and lymphoma have all been associated with secondary forms of MCD.
- FSGS, primary or secondary. Primary FSGS denotes an idiopathic cause that is usually severe and requires immunosuppressive therapy. It is more prevalent in persons of African ancestry. Secondary FSGS refers to FSGS caused by a known etiology (e.g., heroin, sickle cell disease, scarring of any kind from prior injury, obesity, low nephron mass, HIV, etc.). Clinically, primary FSGS is more commonly associated with heavy proteinuria and nephrotic syndrome. By contrast, most cases of secondary FSGS are associated with lower levels of proteinuria (often subnephrotic), higher albumin levels, and less significant edema (e.g., HIV-associated nephropathy is an important exception in that it is associated with heavy proteinuria and rapid progression when untreated). Distinguishing between the two types is important for therapy (see the following).
- Membranous nephropathy: This disorder can be primary or secondary. Primary membranous nephropathy is due to in situ deposition of antibody against a glomerular antigen (in at least 70% of cases the epitope has been found to be phospholipase A2 receptor). Proteinuria may be massive. Secondary membranous nephropathy is often due to infection (e.g., hepatitis B, malaria, schistosomiasis, syphilis), autoimmune disease (e.g., systemic lupus erythematosus [SLE]), medications (e.g., D-penicillamine, gold), and malignancies. Distinguishing between the

two subtypes is important for management (see the following).
- Amyloidosis: Often due to overproduction of a light chain (AL amyloid) or due to a chronic inflammatory state (AA amyloid). Kidney size is often enlarged, and proteinuria may be massive. Congo red staining of amyloid establishes the diagnosis.
- Diabetic nephropathy: Often characterized by slowly progressive proteinuria in the face of retinopathy and preserved kidney size. The correlation between retinopathy, proteinuria, and diabetic nephropathy is very strong in type 1 diabetic patients, and kidney biopsies are usually not undertaken. The relationship is less strong in type 2 diabetes, and the absence of retinopathy does not preclude a diagnosis of diabetic nephropathy.

MPGN: This disorder is usually due to immune complex deposition with complement, or to activation of the alternative complement cascade without immune complexes (e.g., C3 glomerulopathy). Common immune complex causes are from infections (e.g., hepatitis C), autoimmune disorders (e.g., SLE), or dysproteinemias (e.g., monoclonal gammopathies). Distinguishing between these possibilities guides therapy. The urine is associated with heavy proteinuria. Urinary sediment often contains dysmorphic erythrocytes and erythrocyte casts and is also associated with heavy proteinuria.

DIAGNOSIS

DIFFERENTIAL DIAGNOSIS

- Other states that present with edema (CHF, cirrhosis, protein-losing enteropathy, severe malnutrition)
- Glomerulonephritis (those diseases commonly associated with an inflammatory urinary sediment and inflammation of the glomerulus)
- Mimickers of glomerulonephritis (malignant HTN, preeclampsia, antiphospholipid syndrome)

WORKUP

- Evaluation includes determining the rate of change of serum creatinine, quantification of proteinuria by 24-hour collection, and manual examination of the urinary sediment.
- Bland urinary sediment and proteinuria >3.5 g/24 hr should prompt nephrology consultation.
- Serologic tests of use may be a UPEP, SPEP, HIV, hepatitis B surface antigen, hepatitis C virus (HCV) antibody, and antinuclear antibody (ANA). As urinary sediment examination is not 100% sensitive in ruling out an inflammatory process, C3 and C4 can be checked, as complement levels are often low in many inflammatory glomerulonephritides, and are low in MPGN. Low complement levels may change the nature of the differential diagnosis before kidney biopsy.

TABLE 1 Important Clinical, Serological, and Pathological Features of Selected Diseases Causing Nephrotic Syndrome

Disease	Important Clinical Features	Serological Features	Pathological Features
Minimal change disease	Rapid onset with heavy proteinuria and rapid remission with therapy. True steroid resistance is rare and should prompt repeat biopsy to rule out FSGS.	Complements are normal.	Light microscopy shows completely normal kidney architecture. Immunofluorescence microscopy: Normal. Electron microscopy: Diffuse podocyte effacement.
Primary FSGS	Often heavier proteinuria and low serum albumin and edema. Tip lesion subtype and collapsing FSGS often have more explosive onset. Sediment usually bland, but RBCs can be seen. Usually no cellular casts.	Complements are normal.	Light microscopy: Only one glomerulus need show features of FSGS to make diagnosis. Immunofluorescence microscopy: Often devoid of immunoglobulin, although IgM can be seen. Electron microscopy: Often has diffuse podocyte effacement.
Secondary FSGS	Proteinuria is often subnephrotic, or if nephrotic, serum albumin levels are maintained. Minimal edema.	HIV and parvovirus infection can cause phenotype identical to idiopathic collapsing FSGS.	LM: Often shows evidence of glomerulomegaly. Electron microscopy: Foot process effacement is less diffuse.
Primary membranous nephropathy	Often seen in older Caucasian patients. More likely than other forms of nephrotic syndrome to be associated with thrombotic complications. Sediment: bland. RBCs can be found, although RBC casts are usually found.	Serum antiphospholipase A2 receptor antibodies are found in 70% of patients with idiopathic primary membranous nephropathy. Antineutral endopeptidase antibodies are found in a minority of others.	LM: Characterized by thickening of the GBM; "spikes" can be seen on silver stain. Immunofluorescence microscopy: C3 and IgG noted in granular pattern. Newer techniques stain for antiphospholipase A2 receptor antibody *in situ*. Electron microscopy: Associated with subepithelial deposits.
Secondary membranous nephropathy	Associated with **malignancy,** lupus, syphilis, hepatitis B and C, medications (gold, captopril, penicillamine, etc.).	Notable for the absence of antiphospholipase A2 antibodies. ANA, hepatitis B, HCV serologies are helpful. RPR can be sent in context of appropriate history.	Morphology is exactly the same except when examined by EM. On high power, one sees both subendothelial and mesangial deposits in addition to classic subepithelial deposits.
Amyloidosis	Often found with massive proteinuria. Kidney size is enlarged. Bland sediment	UPEP, SPEP, serum free light chains may be positive. The UPEP will show glomerular proteinuria, which can help differentiate from myeloma kidney.	LM: Often notable for nodular pattern. Diagnosis can be made by staining using Congo red or thioflavin T. Immunofluorescence microscopy: Antibody use can differentiate AA from AL amyloid. EM shows characteristic, random 10-nm fibrils.
Diabetes	Often associated with nephrotic-range proteinuria in the setting of retinopathy. Kidney sizes are preserved.	No specific serologic tests are positive.	LM: Nodular pattern often seen, thickened GBM.
MPGN	Often associated with nephrotic-range proteinuria with a "nephritic" sediment. RBC casts often seen along with dysmorphic RBC	C3 and C4 are often low in immune complex MPGN. Immune complex GN warrants checking SPEP, UPEP, as gammopathy is associated with MPGN. Hepatitis B, HCV, ANA, and cryoglobulins are also warranted. C3 alone is low in dense deposit disease and C3 glomerulonephritis, which may prompt specific tests for complement dysregulation.	The key point here is to look at the IF. If immunofluorescence shows both immunoglobulin and complement deposition, the diagnosis is immune complex MGPN. If only complement, the diagnosis is most likely C3 glomerulopathy (either dense deposit disease or C3 glomerulonephritis).

- A newer serological test available to clinicians commercially is an antiphospholipase A2 receptor antibody titer. This test is associated with the development of primary membranous nephropathy but *not* secondary membranous nephropathy. If present, primary membranous nephropathy can suggest a potential diagnosis, determine the need for immunosuppressive therapy (as opposed to merely treating the underlying disease with secondary membranous nephropathy), and potentially allows the practitioner to establish a baseline titer value prior to therapy (to monitor efficacy).
- Ultimately, given that clinical acumen cannot reliably distinguish between various etiologies, a kidney biopsy is usually required, except in very young children where there is a very high likelihood of MCD, or in adults if contraindications are present (coagulopathy).
- Patients should also have a renal ultrasound to document the presence of two kidneys before kidney biopsy is attempted and kidney size is documented.

(Rx) TREATMENT

NONIMMUNOSUPPRESSIVE THERAPY

- Control of proteinuria is key to mitigating risk of progression. Angiotensin-converting enzyme inhibitors or angiotensin II receptor blockers should be titrated upward (except in MCD, where it is not usually given due to complete response). Dual angiotensin-converting enzyme inhibitors and angiotensin II receptor blocker therapy is controversial given a greater risk of hyperkalemia.
- For patients with proteinuria >1 g daily, target blood pressure is <125/75 mm Hg.
- With the exception of MCD, all patients with nephrotic-range proteinuria and hyperlipidemia should be treated with statins if tolerated.
- Although some patients with nephrotic syndrome are hypercoagulable (particularly patients with membranous nephropathy), the

role of prophylactic anticoagulation is not well defined and is controversial. For patients with membranous nephropathy and serum albumin levels <2.0 g/dl, anticoagulation can be considered if bleeding risk is low.
- Patients should be placed on a low sodium diet (<2 g daily) along with diuretics.
- Diuretic resistance is common (from gut wall edema and hypoalbuminemia). More bioavailable diuretics (bumetanide, torsemide) may be beneficial, along with thiazide diuretics.
- To prevent "diuretic braking," diuretics should be dosed at least on a twice-daily basis.

IMMUNOSUPPRESSIVE THERAPY

In general, immunosuppressive therapy is dictated by the identified disorder. Important terms in dealing with the management of nephrotic-range proteinuria due to primary glomerular diseases are listed in Table 2. First-line therapies for each disease are highlighted in the following.
- MCD: First-line therapy in adults is prednisone (1 mg/kg up to 80 mg for minimum of 4

TABLE 2 Important Definitions in Dealing with Treatment of Primary Nephrotic Syndrome

	Adults	Children
Definition		
Complete Remission	Reduction in proteinuria to <0.3 g/24 hours	<4 mg m-2h-1 on at least 3 occasions within 7 days and serum albumin >3.5 g/dl
Partial Remission	Reduction in proteinuria between 0.3 g/24 hour and 3.5 g daily with ≥50% decrease in proteinuria from baseline	Disappearance of edema, increase in serum albumin >3.5 g/dl and persistent proteinuria >4 mg m-2h-1 or >100 mg m-2day-1
Relapse*	Increase in proteinuria to >3.5 g daily after one month of complete or partial remission	Urine dipstick 3+ or proteinuria >40 mg/m²/hour occurring on 3 days within 1 week.
Steroid Dependent*	Two consecutive relapses occurring during therapy or within 14 days of completing therapy	Two relapses of proteinuria within 14 days after stopping or during alternate-day steroid therapy
Steroid Resistant*	Persistence of proteinuria without significant reduction despite prednisone therapy at 1 mg/kg for 16 weeks	Persistence of proteinuria despite prednisone therapy at 60 mg/m² for 4 weeks.

*These definitions only truly apply to diseases such as minimal change disease and FSGS.
Adapted from Cattran DC et al: Cyclosporine in idiopathic glomerular disease associated with the nephrotic syndrome: workshop recommendations, *Kidney Int* 72(12):1429-1447, 2007, and *KDIGO clinical practice guidelines for glomerulonephritis.*

weeks and maximum of 16 weeks with taper over 6 months if response noted). Second-line options include cyclophosphamide and/or cyclosporine.

- FSGS: Primary FSGS is often treated with high-dose prednisone (maximum, 80 mg daily in adults) for 6 months. Alternative regimens include low-dose prednisone with cyclosporine. Mycophenolate mofetil (MMF) has also been used with success in patients with primary FSGS. Newer therapies that have been tried in pilot settings have included exogenous adrenocorticotropic hormone (ACTH) as well as abatacept. While efficacious in some patients, no randomized controlled trials have been done to verify these initial results, so these treatments cannot be recommended as initial therapy at this time. A new randomized controlled trial aims to examine whether a novel agent that blocks both endothelin 1 and angiotensin II receptors (RE-021) has efficacy in treatment of primary FSGS. Treatment of secondary FSGS is based on arresting the underlying cause and nonspecific therapy with blockade of the renin-angiotensin-aldosterone system. Immunosuppression is avoided.
- Membranous nephropathy: Suggested first-line therapy for primary membranous nephropathy involves the Ponticelli protocol for 6 months (intravenous methylprednisolone 1 g/day- for 3 days, then oral prednisone 0.4 mg/kg daily for the remainder of the month for months 1, 3, and 5, and oral cyclophosphamide 1.5-2.5 mg/kg daily on months 2, 4, and 6). Alternative therapy includes low-dose prednisone along with cyclosporine or tacrolimus alone for at least one year. Rituximab may become more commonly used as first-line therapy in the coming years. A novel therapy that can be used is a synthetic depot formulation of ACTH. ACTH may exert effects on the podocyte independent of stimulation of endogenous cortisol production. Given conflicting reports from the U.S. and Europe, exogenous ACTH can be viewed as a last-line resort when all other options have failed, but it is not standard of care. Therapy for secondary membranous nephropathy is directed at treating the underlying cause (malignancy, SLE, etc.).
- Treatment of amyloidosis, diabetes, and MPGN is directed toward the underlying disorder. In rapidly progressive HCV-related MPGN, immunosuppressive therapy with the rituximab or glucocorticosteroids and cyclophosphamide can be administered in addition to treating HCV.

REFERRAL

Nephrology consultation is recommended in all cases of nephrotic syndrome.

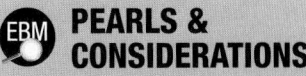

EBM **PEARLS & CONSIDERATIONS**

- Proteinuria >2 g daily generally implies glomerular disease unless multiple myeloma is present. UPEP delineates the character of proteins excreted as tubular, glomerular, or overflow.
- Massive proteinuria (>20 g daily) is rarely seen with inflammatory diseases and generally indicates MCD, FSGS, membranous nephropathy, or amyloidosis.
- Quantification of proteinuria should occur with a 24-hour urine collection with evaluation of urinary creatinine excretion to document validity of the collection. Spot collections have not been validated for heavy proteinuria or in patients with rapidly changing creatinine values. A "spot" urine protein-to-creatinine ratio taken from the 24-hour collection defines the relationship between spot and "true" collections to monitor response to therapy.
- Most noninflammatory processes progress slowly. If a sediment without red blood cell casts is detected with a rapidly increasing serum creatinine and heavy proteinuria, the differential is relatively narrow:
  1. MCD and AIN as seen with NSAID use
  2. Nephrotic syndrome associated with acute tubular necrosis from hypovolemia
  3. Bilateral renal vein thrombosis superimposed on nephrotic syndrome
  4. Myeloma cast nephropathy
  5. Collapsing FSGS/HIV-associated nephropathy

SUGGESTED READINGS

Available at www.expertconsult.com.

RELATED CONTENT

Nephrotic Syndrome (Patient Information)

AUTHOR: **SANJEEV R. SHAH, M.D.**

N

Diseases and Disorders

I

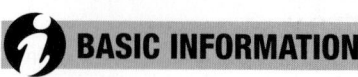

BASIC INFORMATION

DEFINITION

The American Psychological Association's *Diagnostic and Statistical Manual of Mental Disorders,* 5th edition (DSM 5) includes delirium, major neurocognitive disorder, and mild neurocognitive disorder under the grouping *neurocognitive disorders.*

In neurocognitive disorders (NCDs), the primary deficit involves cognitive function. The cognitive dysfunction is acquired rather than developmental and thus represents a decline from a previously attained level of functioning. The NCDs are subtyped according to known or presumed etiologic/pathologic entities underlying the decline. The subtypes may be distinguished by clinical characteristics such as time course, physical examination, and cognitive domains affected. Frequently, more than one NCD exists in a given patient.

In major and mild NCDs, the cognitive deficits are present in one or more cognitive domains. The initial evidence is based on concern brought forth by the patient, a knowledgeable informant, or the clinician and is often supported by performance on objective standardized assessments such as neuropsychological testing. In major NCDs, the deficits interfere with independence in everyday activity, whereas in minor NCDs, the impairment is more modest and does not interfere with capacity for independence in everyday activity.

In the DSM 5, *delirium* is subsumed under the category *neurocognitive disorders.* Although it shares the core feature of acquired deficit in cognitive function, it is discussed as a distinct entity from major and minor neurocognitive disorders and is discussed separately in this text. The DSM IV term *dementia* is subsumed under the entity *major neurocognitive disorder* in the DSM 5, and the DSM IV term *amnestic disorder* and its subtypes are subsumed under the category *major neurocognitive disorder due to another medical condition* in the DSM 5.

Some well-known NCDs include major or mild NCD due to Alzheimer disease, major or mild NCD due to traumatic brain injury, alcohol-induced major NCD, amnestic-confabulatory type disorder (Korsakoff syndrome), and vascular NCD.

ICD-10 CM CODES:
F02.81 Major or mild neurocognitive disorder, with behavior disturbance
F02.80 Major or mild neurocognitive disorder, without behavior disturbance
DSM-5 CODES:
294.11 Major or mild neurocognitive disorder, with behavior disturbance
294.10 Major or mild neurocognitive disorder, without behavior disturbance

EPIDEMIOLOGY & DEMOGRAPHICS

The prevalence varies depending on the etiology of the neurocognitive disorder and age of the patient. Among patients >60 years, the prevalence tends to increase sharply for the most common neurocognitive disorders. Overall prevalence estimates for major NCDs are approximately 1% at 65 years old and as high as 30% at 85 years. Mild NCD prevalence is variable, ranging from 2%-10% at age 65 and 5%-20% at age 85. The strongest risk factor for major and mild NCD is age. Female gender is associated with a higher prevalence in major and mild NCD due to Alzheimer's disease.

PHYSICAL FINDINGS & CLINICAL PRESENTATION

Neurocognitive domains that are affected in NCDs include:
- Complex attention, including sustained attention, divided attention, selective attention, and processing speed.
- Executive functioning, such as planning, decision making, working memory, and mental flexibility
- Learning and memory, including immediate memory, recent memory
- Language skills, such as word finding, naming, grammar, and fluency.
- Perceptual motor skills, including visual construction, praxis, and gnosis.
- Social cognition, including recognition of emotions.

Associated physical findings, time course of illness, and response to treatment depend on etiology of the NCD. Apathy, mood disturbance, and psychosis are recognized as common neuropsychiatric symptoms associated with NCDs. Mood symptoms are common early in the course of NCDs due to Alzheimer's disease and Parkinson's disease, as well as in NCD with Lewy bodies. Psychoses, including delusions and paranoia, occur in mild to moderate stages of NCD with Lewy bodies and in moderate to severe stages of NCD due to Alzheimer's disease. Psychosis, agitation, and other behavioral disturbances lead to increased rate of hospitalization, early admission to assisted living environments or nursing homes, and increased level of caregiver depression and distress. Apathy manifests early in the course of NCDs and is the most common neuropsychiatric symptom of NCD due to Alzheimer's disease across the spectrum of the disease.

ASSOCIATED SIGNS AND SYMPTOMS BY ETIOLOGY

(For each etiology, the criteria are met for major or mild neurocognitive disorder)
- **Alzheimer's disease:** gradual progression with occasional brief plateaus. Impairment in memory and learning are prominent early in the disease. Executive dysfunction is also common. In moderate to severe disease, language and social cognition difficulties are present. Behavior and psychological manifestations such as depression, apathy, irritability, and psychosis are often more distressing to caregivers than the cognitive deficits.
- **Frontotemporal disorder:** Variants are characterized by progressive development of behavioral and personality change and/or language impairment. Patients with behavior variant may present with impaired insight, socially inappropriate behaviors, apathy, hyperorality, or compulsive behaviors. Executive dysfunction includes lack of planning/organization and poor judgment. Learning and memory dysfunction may be spared in the early stages. Language variant, or primary progressive aphasia, is divided into three subtypes: semantic variant, agrammatic/nonfluent variant, and logopenic variant based on characteristics of the language impairment.
- **Lewy body disorder:** Cognitive decline including executive dysfunction occurs prior to or within one year of the onset of parkinsonism motor symptoms. Recurrent, well-formed, and detailed visual hallucinations and fluctuating cognition that can resemble delirium are core features. Mood disturbances, autonomic dysfunction, and REM sleep disorder are suggestive of this diagnosis. Patients with major or mild disorder with Lewy bodies are sensitive to neuroleptics, which can often worsen symptoms and should be used with caution. Individuals with major or mild neurocognitive disorder with Lewy bodies are typically functionally more impaired than would be expected for their cognitive deficits because of the motor and autonomic impairments.
- **Parkinson's disease:** Parkinson's disease onset precedes the onset of major neurocognitive decline by at least one year. Apathy, depression, hallucinations, and REM sleep disorder are suggestive of this diagnosis. The atypical parkinsonian syndrome progressive supranuclear palsy presents with early postural instability and retropulsion, supranuclear gaze palsy, and early cognitive impairment with depression, apathy, and anxiety. Corticobasal degeneration is a progressive asymmetric movement disorder with attentional deficits, slow processing speed, extreme rigidity, aphasia, apraxia, and alien-limb syndrome.
- **Vascular disorder:** The onset of cognitive decline is temporally related to one or more cerebrovascular events. If not the exclusive pathology, cerebrovascular disease is thought to be the dominant pathologic etiology of the NCD. The diagnosis is supported by neuroimaging evidence of parenchymal injury, including large vessel infarcts or hemorrhages, two or more lacunar infarcts outside the brainstem, or confluent white matter lesions attributed to cerebrovascular disease. Patients typically present with decline in processing speed, complex attention, and executive dysfunction. Stepwise and/or fluctuating decline is described. Prominent depression, apathy, and personality changes are common.
- **Traumatic brain injury (TBI):** This NCD presents immediately after the occurrence of or can be attributed to a traumatic brain injury that causes loss of consciousness, posttraumatic amnesia, disorientation, or

neurologic signs such as seizure or hemiparesis. Cognitive presentation may be variable but may include difficulty with complex attention, executive dysfunction or deficits in learning and memory. Associated findings include disturbances in emotional function and personality change. The features of major or mild NCD due to TBI vary by age of patient and specifics of the injury as well as other factors, such as premorbid functioning of the patient.

- **Substance/medication induced:** An NCD that persists beyond the duration of intoxication and acute withdrawal from a substance that is known to be capable of causing the observed impairments. NCD due to alcohol frequently manifests with memory, learning, and executive impairments. Neurocognitive disorders due to alcohol include Wernicke encephalopathy and Korsakoff syndrome. Wernicke syndrome is an acute neurologic disorder caused by thiamine deficiency manifesting with a clinic triad of encephalopathy, oculomotor dysfunction, and gait ataxia. Korsakoff syndrome is a late manifestation of Wernicke syndrome manifesting with dense anterograde and retrograde amnesia. MRI may show mammillary body atrophy. Major or mild NCD may be induced by medication or combinations of medications, including those with sedating and pain-ameliorating properties and those with anticholinergic properties. Particular attention should be paid to review of medications in any patient with major or mild NCD, especially those in the geriatric population.
- **HIV infection:** Neurocognitive deficits may show a subcortical pattern with prominent impairment of executive function with slowed processing speed and difficulty with learning new information.
- **Prion disease:** Neurocognitive deficits occur rapidly, typically over six months. In some variants, prominent psychiatric symptoms such as depression and anxiety may occur prior to neurocognitive deficits. Ataxia, myoclonus, chorea, and a prominent startle reflex are typically present.
- **Huntington's disease:** Early prominent changes in processing speed, organization, and planning rather than learning and memory are common. Behavior changes, changes in mood, anxiety, obsessive-compulsive symptoms, irritability, and apathy often precede motor symptoms.
- **Other medical conditions:** Many medical conditions can cause NCDs. Examples include structural brain lesions such as primary or secondary brain tumors, subdural hematomas or those seen in normal pressure hydrocephalus, hypoxia, infectious causes, endocrine conditions, immune disorders, and metabolic conditions. The temporal association between the onset or exacerbation of the medical condition and the development of the cognitive deficit supports the diagnosis.

DIAGNOSIS

DIFFERENTIAL DIAGNOSIS

Etiology of major or mild NCD is assessed by taking a detailed history from the patient, family members, or other informants, complete physical examination, and ancillary tests, including neuropsychological testing and imaging studies. In some cases, the diagnosis remains unclear, while in other cases, the diagnosis is uncertain early on and becomes clear as the disease progresses. For any patient with a major or mild NCD, the initial differential includes each of the etiologies discussed in this chapter; however, this can often be narrowed by appropriate examination and investigation.

LABORATORY TESTS & IMAGING STUDIES

In all major and mild NCDs, careful history from patient and in most cases, from family and other reliable sources is essential. Detailed physical examination and neuropsychological testing and neuroimaging are indicated. In some cases, serology and lab testing, including B12 and TSH levels, are useful or diagnostic. Biomarkers and genetic screening tests are diagnostic in some cases. Particular attention should be paid to rule out underlying medical causes of the major or mild NCD.

Alzheimer's disease: Detailed history and physical examination including neuropsychological testing often points to the diagnosis. MRI may show hippocampal and temporoparietal cortical atrophy. PET scan may reveal hypometabolism in temporoparietal regions. Cerebrospinal fluid biomarkers include elevated total tau and phosphorylated tau levels with reduced amyloid beta-42. *APOE* testing may support diagnosis in patients with *APOE4* variant. For early onset, autosomal dominant inheritance mutation in *APP, PSEN1*, or *PSEN2* may be detected.

Frontotemporal disorder: In cases with early-onset behavior or language disorders, an MRI or CT scan may show atrophy in frontal lobes and/or corresponding parts of anterior or inferior temporal lobes either bilaterally or asymmetrically. Functional imaging may show hypoperfusion in the corresponding regions. In familial cases, genetic mutations in genes encoding the microtubule-associated protein tau and the granulin gene may confirm the diagnosis.

Lewy body disease: Sleep study may help to confirm a diagnosis of REM sleep behavior disorder. Nuclear medicine testing including SPECT or PET may show low striatal dopamine transporter uptake.

Parkinson's disease: Abnormal dopamine transporter scans are supportive of the diagnosis.

Vascular disorder: Neurologic assessment often reveals a history of stroke or TIA. MRI or CT scan may show significant parenchymal injury attributed to cerebrovascular disease.

TBI: May be associated with abnormal CT or MRI scan showing petechial hemorrhages, subdural or subarachnoid hemorrhage, or evidence of contusion.

Prion disease: May be suspected in patients with appropriate clinical presentation, including rapidly progressive course. MRI may show gray matter hyperintensities in the subcortical region, particularly in the putamen and head of caudate nuclei. EEG reveals periodic synchronous biphasic or triphasic sharp waves complexes. CSF biomarkers including 14-3-3, S100 protein, or neuron-specific enolase is suggestive, though not diagnostic.

Huntington's disease: Genetic testing for CAG repeat is diagnostic.

TREATMENT

- Initial treatment is directed to the underlying etiology.
- Treatment of memory disturbance may be indicated in some causes of major or mild NCDs, such as those caused by Alzheimer's disease.
- Treatment both acutely and chronically is often supportive and aimed at ameliorating behavior and other neuropsychiatric disturbances that may be present.
- Behavioral treatments should be considered first line for most behavior manifestations. Pharmacologic treatments for behavior disturbance have a limited role in improving overall quality of life for most causes of major or minor NCD, although they may have short-term efficacy in acute circumstances.
- Pharmacologic and cognitive behavior treatment may be helpful for associated psychiatric symptoms such as mood disorders, psychosis, and anxiety.
- Patient safety, including risks associated with driving, wandering, and cooking should be addressed early in the course of the illness.
- Family education and support may help reduce the need for a skilled nursing facility and reduce caregiver stress and burnout.
- Cognitive rehabilitation to promote recovery may be helpful.
- Supervised living may ensure appropriate long-term care in late stages of progressive illness.

SUGGESTED READINGS
Available at www.expertconsult.com

RELATED TOPICS
Alzheimer's Disease (Related Key Topic)
Delirium (Related Key Topic)
Human Immunodeficiency Virus (Related Key Topic)
Huntington's Disease (Related Key Topic)
Parkinson's Disease (Related Key Topic)
Progressive Supranuclear Palsy (Related Key Topic)
Traumatic Brain Injury (TBI) (Related Key Topic)
Wernicke Syndrome (Related Key Topic)

AUTHOR: **MICHAEL FRIEDMAN, M.D.**

DEFINITION

Neurofibromatosis (NF) is an autosomal-dominant disorder affecting bone, the nervous system, soft tissue, and skin. There are three major subtypes of NF disorders: NF type 1 (NF1), NF type 2 (NF2), and schwannomatosis (SWN). SWN has only recently been recognized as a distinct disorder; currently very little is known about it.

SYNONYMS

NF1: von Recklinghausen disease, peripheral NF
NF2: bilateral acoustic neurofibromatosis, central NF

ICD-10CM CODES	
Q85.00	Neurofibromatosis, unspecified
Q85.01	Neurofibromatosis, type 1
Q85.02	Neurofibromatosis, type 2

EPIDEMIOLOGY & DEMOGRAPHICS

- Incidence of NF1 (one case/3000 live births), NF2 (one case/25,000 live births).
- Prevalence of NF1 (one case/5000 persons), NF2 (one case/210,000 persons).
- NF1 and NF2 are autosomal dominant; approximately 50% of cases have no family history.
- The two disorders affect approximately 100,000 people in the United States.
- Affects males and females equally.
- NF1 may be associated with optic gliomas, astrocytomas, spinal neurofibromas, pheochromocytomas, and chronic myeloid leukemia.
- NF2 may be associated with meningiomas, spinal schwannomas, and cataracts.
- For SWN, the incidence is one per 30,000 persons, and the disease is mostly sporadic in nature.

PHYSICAL FINDINGS & CLINICAL PRESENTATION

- Common features of NF1 include:
  1. Café-au-lait macules (100% of children by age 2 yr).
     a. Hyperpigmented skin lesions (Fig. 1) occurring anywhere on the body except the face, palms, and soles.
     b. Appear early in life and increase in size and number during puberty.
     c. Are focal or diffuse.
  2. Axillary and inguinal freckling (70%).
  3. Multiple neurofibromas (Figs. 2 and 3) can be soft or firm; three subtypes:
     a. Cutaneous: circumscribed, not specific for NF1.
     b. Subcutaneous: circumscribed, not specific for NF1.
     c. Plexiform: noncircumscribed, thick and irregular; can cause disfigurement of supportive structures and specific for NF1.
  4. Lisch nodule (small hamartoma of the iris) found in >90% of adult cases.

5. Visual defects possibly related to optic gliomas (2% to 5%).
6. Neurodevelopment problems such as learning disability and mental retardation (30% to 40%).
7. Skeletal disorders, including long bone dysplasia, pseudoarthrosis, scoliosis, short stature, and decreased bone mineral density.
- Common features of NF2 include:
  1. Hearing loss and tinnitus related to bilateral acoustic neuromas (>90% of adults).
  2. Cataracts (81%).
  3. Headache (may be due to intracranial meningiomas, which are present in 80% of patients).
  4. Unsteady gait.
  5. Cutaneous and subcutaneous neurofibromas but fewer than in NF1.
  6. Café-au-lait macules (1%).
- Common features of SWN include painful multiple schwannomas of the spinal (74%), peripheral (89%), or cranial nerves *except* the vestibular nerve (9%).

ETIOLOGY

- NF1 is caused by DNA mutations located on the long arm of chromosome 17 responsible for encoding the protein neurofibromin.
- NF2 is caused by DNA mutations located in the middle of the long arm of chromosome 22 responsible for encoding the protein merlin, which is a potent inhibitor of glioma growth.
- Both proteins are speculated to act as tumor suppressors.
- The etiology of SWN remains unclear; however, most cases are attributed to mutations on chromosome 22 that inactivate two distinct tumor suppressor genes.

- NF1 is diagnosed if the person has two or more of the following features:
  1. Six or more café-au-lait macules >5 mm in prepubertal patients and >15 mm in postpubertal patients.
  2. Two or more neurofibromas of any type or one plexiform neurofibroma.
  3. Axillary or inguinal freckling.
  4. Optic glioma.
  5. Two or more Lisch nodules (iris hamartomas).
  6. Sphenoid wing dysplasia or cortical thinning of long bones, with or without pseudoarthrosis.
  7. A first-degree relative (parent, sibling, or child) with NF1 based on the previous criteria.
- NF2 is diagnosed if the person has either of the following two criteria:
  1. Bilateral eighth nerve masses seen by appropriate imaging studies (e.g., CT, MRI).
  2. A first-degree relative with NF2 and either a unilateral eighth nerve mass or two of the following: neurofibroma, meningioma, glioma, schwannoma, or juvenile posterior subcapsular lenticular opacity.
- SWN is diagnosed in an individual >30 yr having either of the following two criteria:
  1. Two nonintradermal schwannomas, no vestibular tumor found on MRI scan, no NF2 mutation.
  2. One nonvestibular schwannoma and a first-degree relative fitting the previous criteria.

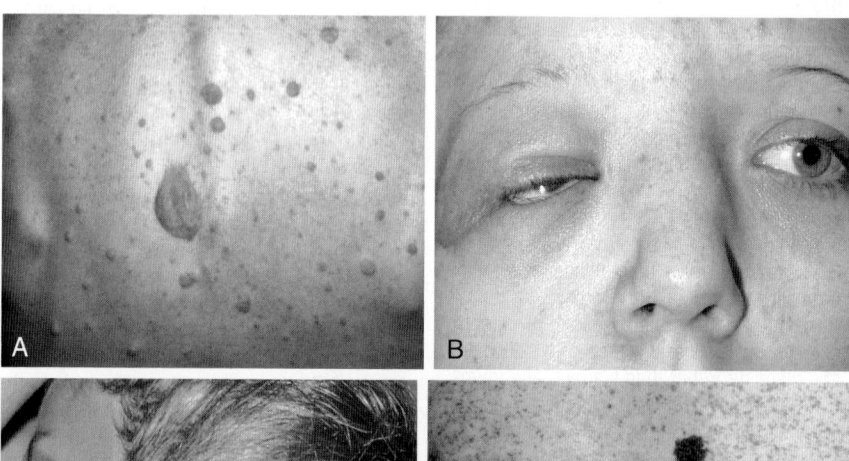

FIG. 1 Systemic features of NF1. A, Discrete neurofibromas. **B,** Nodular plexiform neurofibroma of the eyelid. **C,** Elephantiasis nervosa. **D,** Cafe-au-lait spots. (**C** courtesy S. Kumar Puri. From Kanski JJ, Bowling B: *Clinical ophthalmology, a systematic approach,* ed 7, Philadelphia, 2010, Saunders.)

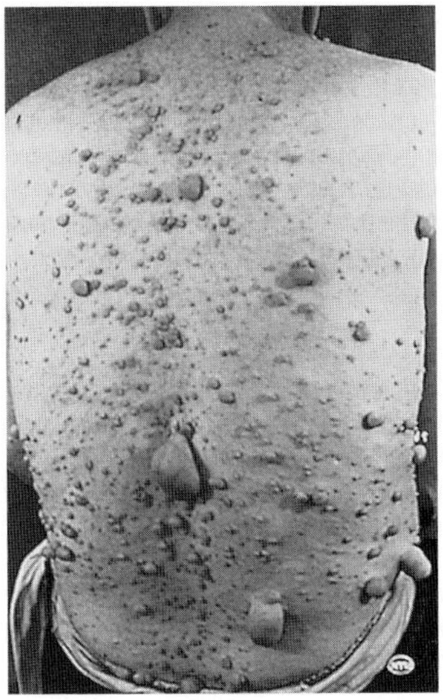

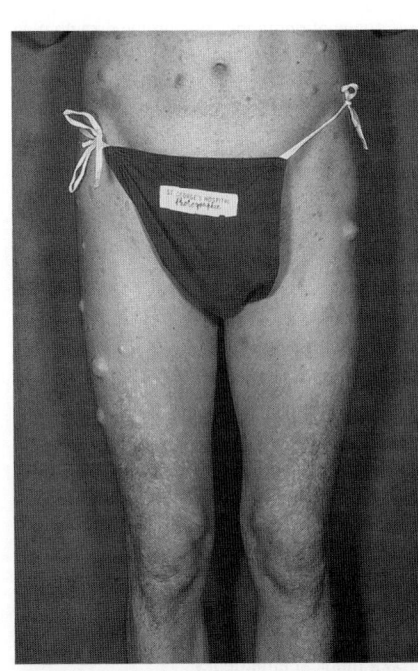

FIG. 2 Nodules. Solid, large (>1 cm), deep-seated mass in dermal or subcutaneous tissues. These nodules are neurofibromas in a patient with neurofibromatosis. (From Goldman L, Ausiello D [eds]: *Cecil textbook of medicine,* ed 22, Philadelphia, 2004, Saunders.)

FIG. 3 Type 1 neurofibromatosis: widespread cutaneous neurofibromata are a prominent feature of the classical variant. (Courtesy of R.A. Marsden, M.D., St George's Hospital, London. From McKee PH, Calonje E, Granter SR [eds]: *Pathology of the skin with clinical correlations,* ed 3, St Louis, 2005, Mosby.)

DIFFERENTIAL DIAGNOSIS
- Abdominal NF.
- Myxoid lipoma.
- Nodular fasciitis.
- Fibrous histiocytoma.
- Segmental NF.

WORKUP
The diagnosis of NF is usually self-evident. Workup is dictated by clinical symptoms in NF1 and usually includes MRI evaluation of the head and spine in NF2 and SWN. In fact, if NF2 is suspected but no vestibular nerve schwannomas are found, the diagnosis points to SWN.

LABORATORY TESTS
- Genetic testing is possible in individuals who desire prenatal diagnosis for NF1. There is no single standard test and multiple tests are required. Results can only tell if an individual is affected but cannot predict the severity of the disease due to variable expression.
- In NF2, linkage analysis testing provides a >99% certainty the individual has NF2.

IMAGING STUDIES
- MRI with gadolinium is the imaging study of choice in both NF1 and NF2 patients. MRI increases detection of optic gliomas, tumors of the spine, acoustic neuromas, and "bright spots" believed to represent hamartomas.
- MRI of the spine is recommended in all patients diagnosed with NF2 to exclude intramedullary tumors.

OTHER TESTS
- Wood lamp examination may be useful in patients with very pale skin for visualizing café-au-lait spots.
- Slit-lamp examination is recommended for children >6 yr to confirm the presence of Lisch nodules and subcapsular opacity.

Rx TREATMENT

Treatment is directed primarily at symptoms and complications of NF1 and NF2. As for SWN, resection should be reserved for tumors that are symptomatic or threaten to cause spinal cord compression.

NONPHARMACOLOGIC THERAPY
- Counseling addressing prognosis and genetic, psychological, and social issues.
- Hearing testing and speech pathology evaluation.

ACUTE GENERAL Rx
- Surgery is usually not done on skin tumors unless cosmetically requested or if suspicion of malignant transformation exists.
- Surgery may be indicated for spinal or cranial neurofibromas, gliomas, or meningiomas.
- Acoustic neuromas can be treated by surgical excision.

CHRONIC Rx
- Radiation may be indicated in optic nerve gliomas and patients whose central nervous system tumors show radiographic progression.
- Stereotactic radiosurgery with a gamma knife may be an alternative approach to surgery for acoustic neuromas.
- Bevacizumab continues to be studied as a treatment option for NF2 meningiomas (which express vascular endothelial growth factor).
- Early trials with selumetinib (AZD6244 or ARRY-142886), an oral selective inhibitor of MAPK (MED) 1 and 2 in children with neurofibromatosis type 1 and inoperable plexiform neurofibromas, reveals benefits from selumetinib without excess toxic effects.

DISPOSITION
- Prognosis varies according to the severity of involvement.
- There is no cure for NF.

REFERRAL
A multidisciplinary team of consultants is needed in patients with NF, including neurosurgeon, otolaryngologist, dermatologist, neurologist, audiologist, speech pathologist, geneticist, and neuropsychologist.

! PEARLS & CONSIDERATIONS

- Friedrich Daniel von Recklinghausen first reported his cases in 1882, although there had been similar accounts dating back to the 1600s.
- A high SPRED1 mutation detection rate has been identified in NF1 mutation-negative families with an autosomal dominant phenotype of CALMs with or without freckling and no other NF1 features.

COMMENTS
For additional information and patient resources, refer to the National Neurofibromatosis Foundation (www.nf.org) or Neurofibromatosis Inc. (www.nfinc.org).

SUGGESTED READINGS
Available at www.expertconsult.com

RELATED CONTENT
Neurofibromatosis Type 1 (Patient Information)
Neurofibromatosis Type 2 (Patient Information)

AUTHORS: **CRAIG BLAKENEY, M.D.,** and **MARK F. BRADY, M.D., M.P.H., M.M.S.**

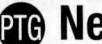

Diseases and Disorders

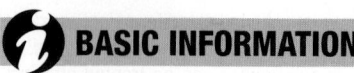
DEFINITION

Neuroleptic malignant syndrome (NMS) is a disorder characterized by hyperthermia, muscular rigidity, autonomic dysfunction, and depressed/fluctuating levels of arousal that evolve over 24 to 72 hr. This occurs as an idiosyncratic adverse reaction to medications that affect the central dopaminergic system, usually D2 receptors blockade.

SYNONYMS

NMS

ICD-10CM CODES
G21.0 Malignant neuroleptic syndrome

EPIDEMIOLOGY & DEMOGRAPHICS

INCIDENCE (IN U.S.): 0.02% to 0.2% annual incidence in psychiatric population.
PREDOMINANT SEX: More than two thirds of patients are male.
PREDOMINANT AGE: Young and middle-aged adults
PREDISPOSING FACTORS:
- History of intake of dopamine antagonists, e.g., antipsychotics

PHYSICAL FINDINGS & CLINICAL PRESENTATION

- Syndrome typically begins abruptly while the patient is taking therapeutic (not toxic) dosages of neuroleptics and reaches maximum severity within 72 hr
- Severe muscle rigidity (hypertonia, cogwheeling, or "lead pipe" rigidity)
- Hyperthermia (38.6° to 42.3° C, usually <40° C)
- Autonomic symptoms: diaphoresis, dysphagia, sialorrhea, skin pallor, urinary incontinence
- Tachycardia, tachypnea
- Labile blood pressure (hypertension or postural hypotension)
- Agitation, catatonia, fluctuating consciousness, obtundation

ETIOLOGY

- Exact etiology is unknown, but it has been suggested that sudden and marked dopamine receptor blockade in nigrostriatal, hypothalamic, mesolimbic, and mesocortical pathways leads to clinical manifestations seen in NMS.
- Neuroleptic drugs have different potencies for inducing NMS:
  1. Typical neuroleptics:
     A. High potency: haloperidol
     B. Medium potency: chlorpromazine, fluphenazine
     C. Low potency: levomepromazine, loxapine
  2. Atypical neuroleptics:
     A. Low potency: risperidone, olanzapine, clozapine, quetiapine

DIAGNOSIS

DIFFERENTIAL DIAGNOSIS

- Infectious: encephalitis, meningitis, brain abscess, rabies, tetanus, sepsis.

- Endocrine: pheochromocytoma, thyrotoxicosis.
- Toxic: substances of abuse (ecstasy, phencyclidine), heavy metals (lead, arsenic), lithium, salicylates.
- Pharmacologic: serotonin syndrome, malignant hyperthermia, drug withdrawal, or overdose.
- Environmental: heatstroke, spider envenomation.
- Neuropsychiatric: catatonia, acute psychosis with agitation, status epilepticus.
- Table E1 summarizes the differential diagnosis of neuroleptic malignant syndrome.

WORKUP

A careful and thorough drug history should be obtained. There is a significant overlap in the features of NMS and serotonin syndrome. The major difference is the presence of hyperreflexia and myoclonus with serotonin syndrome.

LABORATORY TESTS

- Elevated creatine phosphokinase (CPK) (sensitivity 0.71)
- Urinary myoglobin
- Leukocytosis, usually 10,000 to 40,000/mm³
- Electrolytes and renal function
- Blood gases
- Drug levels

TREATMENT

NONPHARMACOLOGIC THERAPY

- Stop all neuroleptic drugs and reinstitute any recently discontinued dopaminergic agonists.
- Respiratory and nutritional support as required.
- Careful fluid balance monitoring with adequate hydration (intravenous in severe cases).
- Active cooling (cooling blanket and antipyretics).
- Skilled nursing care is necessary to prevent decubitus ulcers in bed-confined patients.

ACUTE GENERAL Rx

- Bromocriptine, a dopamine receptor agonist, is the mainstay of therapy for patients with NMS. Initial doses of 2.5 to 10 mg are given IV q8h and are increased by 5 mg/day until clinical improvement is seen. The drug should be continued for at least 10 days after the syndrome has been controlled and then tapered slowly.
- Dantrolene, which blocks calcium efflux from the sarcoplasmic reticulum of skeletal muscles, inhibits the excessive muscle contractions that generate myoglobinemia. Initially, patients can be given 0.25 mg/kg IV q6-12h, followed by a maintenance dose up to 3 mg/kg/day. After 2 to 3 days, patients may be given the drug orally (25 to 600 mg/day in divided doses). Oral dantrolene therapy (50 to 600 mg/day) may be continued for several days afterward.
- Amantadine, an NMDA receptor antagonist with possible dopaminergic properties, can be administered orally at doses of 100 to 200 mg PO bid for moderate to severe cases. As an adjunctive treatment, it has been shown to reduce mortality in comparison to supportive therapy alone.

- IV benzodiazepines (e.g., diazepam 2 to 10 mg, with total daily dose of 10 to 60 mg) to relax muscles and control agitation.
- Electroconvulsive therapy with neuromuscular blockage may be beneficial in pharmacologically refractory cases. Succinylcholine should not be used because it may cause hyperkalemia and cardiac arrhythmias in patients with rhabdomyolysis or dysautonomia.

CHRONIC Rx

- Respiratory care, nutritional support, and physical therapy may be required in more severe cases.
- Appropriate therapy would be required in patients with persistent neuropsychiatric sequelae of NMS (e.g., antidepressants for depression, cognitive behavioral therapy for cognitive deficits, rehabilitation for contractures).

DISPOSITION

- Mortality rate is currently 5% to 10% despite therapeutic measures. Serious sequelae may occur in a further 20%. Complete recovery occurs in >70% of patients.
- Rhabdomyolysis is the most common complication. Other complications include acute kidney injury, respiratory failure, pneumonia, and sepsis.
- Causes of death include cardiac arrhythmias, myocardial infarction, renal failure secondary to rhabdomyolysis, seizures, pulmonary edema, and bronchopneumonia.
- Factors adversely affecting mortality are increased age, acute respiratory failure, renal failure, and core temperature >104° F (40° C).
- Patients should be monitored closely for future complications of pharmacologic therapy.

REFERRAL

If the patient's condition is critical, it is preferable to treat the patient in a medical/neurologic ICU.

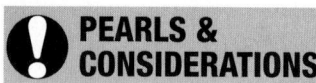 PEARLS & CONSIDERATIONS

COMMENTS

- Early detection and diagnosis lead to a more favorable outcome. Refer to recent consensus diagnostic criteria as a guide. Treatment is a medical emergency.
- Sudden withdrawal from dopaminergic agents (such as those used in Parkinson's disease) may lead to "levodopa withdrawal syndrome" that presents with similar clinical manifestations.

SUGGESTED READINGS
Available at www.expertconsult.com

AUTHORS: **CHLOE MANDER NUNNELEY, M.D.,**
JOSEPH S. KASS, M.D., J.D., and
FARIHA ZAHEER, M.D.

BASIC INFORMATION

DEFINITION

Neuropathic pain is not itself a disease, but rather a symptom that is associated with multiple different diseases. Thus it is not enough to define its presence without searching for a cause. It is defined as the sensation derived from the abnormal discharges of impaired or injured neural structures in either the peripheral or central nervous system. Descriptors include:

- Hyperesthesia: heightened sensitivity to non-painful stimuli (e.g., light touch)
- Hyperalgesia: heightened sensitivity to painful stimuli (e.g., pinprick), or reduced threshold to feel pain
- Allodynia: pain provoked by a stimulus that is not normally painful

SYNONYMS

Neuralgia

ICD-10CM CODES

G58.0	Intercostal neuropathy
G58.7	Mononeuritis multiplex
G58.8	Other specified mononeuropathies
G58.9	Mononeuropathy, unspecified
G60.0	Hereditary sensory and motor neuropathy
G61.9	Inflammatory polyneuropathy, unspecified
G62.0	Drug-induced polyneuropathy
G62.1	Alcoholic polyneuropathy
G62.9	Polyneuropathy, unspecified
G63.2	Diabetic polyneuropathy
G63.5	Polyneuropathy in systemic connective tissue disease
G63.8	Polyneuropathy in other diseases classified elsewhere

EPIDEMIOLOGY & DEMOGRAPHICS

- Estimates of the prevalence of neuropathic pain in the general population range from 1.6% to 8.2%.
- Demographics vary widely depending on etiology, for example:
  1. Postherpetic neuralgia: affects elderly, pain seen in almost 100% of cases
  2. AIDS: 30% of patients affected
  3. Diabetes mellitus: 20% to 24% affected (prevalence rates vary, increasing with longer disease duration)
  4. Fabry disease: affects mostly children, pain in 81% to 90% of patients

PHYSICAL FINDINGS & CLINICAL PRESENTATION

- History: localize the disease with questions
  1. Quality (description) of neuropathic pain: burning, hot or cold, "icy hot," "pins and needles," stinging, lancinating, sharp, shooting
  2. Distribution of symptoms may aid in localization (i.e., "stocking-glove" symptoms in generalized neuropathy, numbness in a peripheral nerve territory in focal neuropathy)

3. Generalized small fiber neuropathy: dysesthesias without numbness common, but many etiologies (e.g., diabetes) cause both small and large fiber dysfunction
4. Large fiber neuropathy (LFPN): coexisting numbness, hyporeflexia, or weakness may be seen, usually worse distally
5. Nerve root: coexisting neck or low back pain that radiates along a specific dermatome; most common cause is structural compression
6. Spinal cord symptoms: coexisting spasticity, bowel or bladder involvement, sensory level
7. Prior history of thalamic stroke in central thalamic pain syndrome (Dejerine-Roussy syndrome)
8. Family history may suggest a genetic cause

- Examination: see Table 1. Table 2 describes joint involvement in neuropathic arthropathy. Fig. 1 illustrates a diagnostic approach to neuropathic pain. Fig. 2 shows a neuropathic ankle.

ETIOLOGY & LABORATORY EVALUATION (TABLE 3)

- Metabolic: diabetes mellitus; malnutrition and alcoholism; vitamin B_{12} deficiency; thiamine deficiency; porphyria; Fabry's disease
- Inflammatory: autoimmune diseases (systemic vasculitides, systemic lupus erythematosus, Sjögren's syndrome, etc.), acute inflammatory demyelinating polyneuropathy (classically presents with ascending weakness and numbness, although pain is also a common feature), chronic inflammatory demyelinating polyneuropathy, sarcoidosis, multiple sclerosis
- Infiltrative: amyloidosis, paraproteinemias (e.g., monoclonal gammopathy of uncertain significance [MGUS] associated neuropathy)
- Infectious: postviral (brachial neuritis), HIV/AIDS, HSV, varicella-zoster virus (VZV; postherpetic neuralgia), Lyme disease, leprosy (thickened nerves and skin lesions), syphilis
- Neoplastic and paraneoplastic-carcinomatous infiltration of nerve/nerve root, anti-Hu
- Drugs/toxins: history of exposure to alcohol, chemotherapeutic agents (paclitaxel, vincristine), isoniazid, metronidazole, or heavy metals (thallium, arsenic)

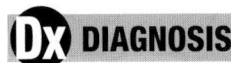 DIAGNOSIS

LABORATORY TESTS

- Fasting blood glucose (FBG)
- 2-hour oral glucose tolerance test (OGTT)

TABLE 1 Examination

Exam Finding	Localization
Pinprick/temperature loss alone	Small fibers only
Pinprick/temperature loss + vibratory/proprioceptive loss	Small and large fibers
Sensory loss and motor dysfunction worse distally than proximal	Large fiber neuropathy
Sensory loss and motor dysfunction along single nerve distribution	Single nerve
Sensory loss and motor dysfunction along multiple single nerves	Multiple mononeuropathies (i.e., mononeuropathy multiplex)
Motor and sensory loss involving multiple nerves belonging to specific region of brachial or lumbar plexus	Plexopathy
Sensory loss along dermatome with multiple myotomal muscles affected	Nerve root lesion
Asymmetric sensory loss without weakness and pseudoathetosis	Dorsal root ganglion
Vibratory/proprioceptive loss without pinprick/temperature loss	Dorsal column dysfunction (from compressive lesion, B_{12} deficiency, or tabes dorsalis from neurosyphilis)
Sensory level with weakness below the level of lesion and long tract signs (spasticity/Babinski's sign)	Spinal cord lesion
Hemisensory hyperalgesia	Contralateral thalamus

TABLE 2 Joint Involvement in Neuropathic Arthropathy

Disease	Site of Involvement
Diabetes mellitus	Midtarsal, metatarsophalangeal, tarsometatarsal
Syringomyelia	Shoulder, elbow, wrist
Amyloidosis	Knee, ankle
Congenital sensory neuropathy	Knee, ankle, intertarsal, metatarsophalangeal
Tabes dorsalis	Knee, hip, ankle
Leprosy	Tarsal, tarsometatarsal

From Hochberg MC et al: *Rheumatology*, ed 5, St Louis, 2011, Mosby.

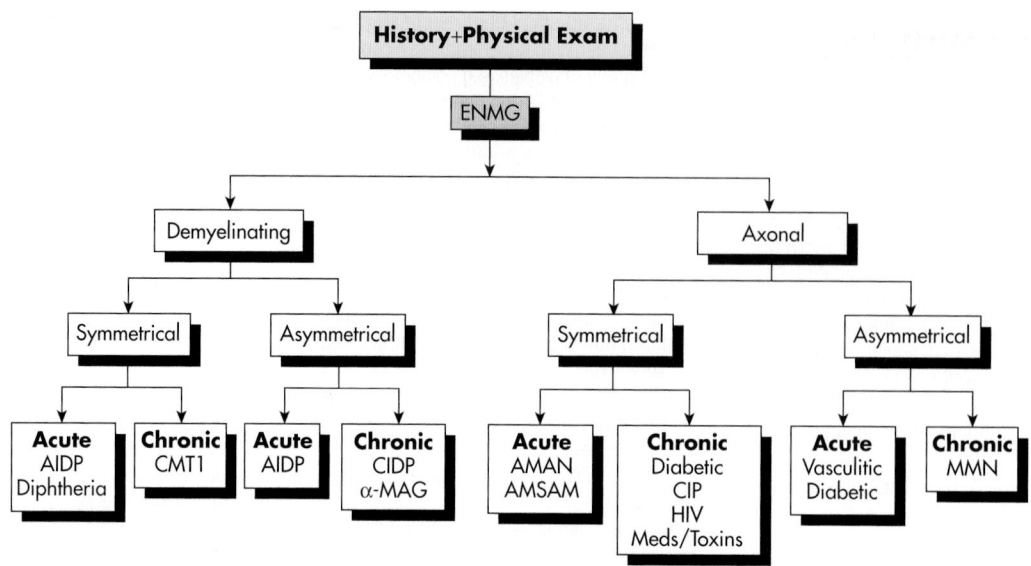

FIG. 1 A systematic approach to evaluate neuropathy. The diseases listed are examples of neuropathies associated with specific neurophysiologic and clinical findings. Diabetic distal, predominantly sensory neuropathies are manifested as chronic axonal neuropathies; acute asymmetric neuropathies can also occur with diabetes. Most neuropathies caused by toxins or by side effects of medication are chronic, symmetric axonal neuropathies. AIDP, AMAN, and AMSAN are subtypes of Guillain-Barré syndrome. These and other examples are discussed in more detail in the text. *AIDP,* Acute inflammatory demyelinating polyradiculoneuropathy; *AMAN,* acute motor axonal neuropathy; *AMSAN,* acute motor and sensory axonal neuropathy; *CIDP,* chronic inflammatory polyradiculoneuropathy; *CIP,* chronic illness polyneuropathy; *CMT1,* Charcot-Marie-Tooth disease type 1, a genetic disorder; *ENMG,* electroneuromyography; *HIV,* human immunodeficiency virus–related neuropathy; α-*MAG,* anti-myelin-associated glycoprotein; *MMN,* multifocal motor neuropathy. (From Goldman L, Schafer AI: *Goldman's Cecil medicine,* ed 24, Philadelphia, 2012, Saunders.)

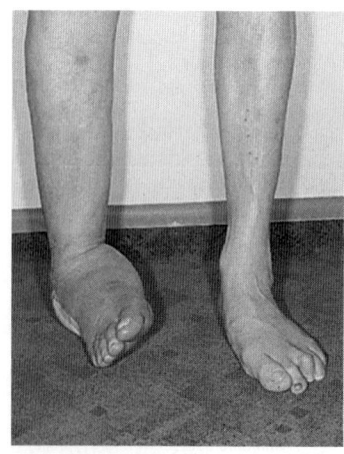

FIG. 2 Neuropathic ankle. Marked instability of the subtalar and midtarsal joints is seen with collapse on weight bearing. (From Hochberg MC et al: *Rheumatology,* ed 5, St Louis, 2011, Mosby.)

- Vitamin B$_{12}$ level
- If B$_{12}$ level normal: serum methylmalonic acid and homocysteine levels
- Serum erythrocyte sedimentation rate (ESR), ANA, SS-A and SS-B, c-ANCA, p-ANCA
- RPR or FTA-ABS
- Serum ACE level (sarcoid)
- HIV antibody
- SPEP, UPEP, immunofixation
- Urine and stool protoporphyrins, if porphyria is suspected clinically
- Hu antibody: can be seen in both small cell and non–small cell lung cancers, may be positive without evidence of lung cancer

- Lumbar puncture: protein elevation, oligoclonal bands, CSF/serum IgG index

ELECTROPHYSIOLOGY STUDIES

- Electrophysiologic testing (electromyography with nerve conduction studies): may be normal in small fiber neuropathies or CNS lesion, but is often abnormal in large fiber neuropathies
- Quantitative sensory testing: abnormal in small and large fiber neuropathy
- Evoked potentials (only if suspicion for spinal cord lesion)

PATHOLOGY STUDIES

- Nerve biopsy is occasionally useful in selected cases, particularly when vasculitis, sarcoidosis, or amyloid neuropathy are in the differential.
- Skin biopsy for intraepidermal nerve fiber (IENF) density may be useful for small fiber neuropathy when other studies are normal.
- Rectal or abdominal fat pad biopsy may show amyloid deposition in systemic amyloidosis.

IMAGING STUDIES

- MRI (with and without contrast):
  1. Of the brain to exclude thalamic pathology if symptoms and signs are consistent with thalamic lesion (hemibody pain)
  2. Of the spinal cord and nerve roots to exclude structural, inflammatory, neoplastic, or infectious causes
  3. Of the lumbar spine to evaluate for arachnoiditis

- If MRI cannot be performed, consider:
  1. CT of the brain for thalamic pathology
  2. CT myelography of the spinal cord to evaluate for structural/neoplastic disease, but only if clinical signs of spinal or nerve root compromise are present

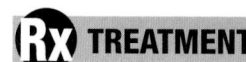 **TREATMENT**

NONPHARMACOLOGIC THERAPY

- Counseling should be initiated at the beginning of therapy to address psychological issues exacerbating physiologic pain
- Physical therapy: especially in cases of chronic neck and low back pain

ACUTE GENERAL Rx

- Antidepressants:
  1. Tricyclic antidepressants (TCAs): nortriptyline preferred over amitriptyline (fewer anticholinergic side effects with nortriptyline). Begin 25 mg PO qd in adults, or 10 mg qd in elderly. Increase dose by 25 mg every week as tolerated until usual maximal effective dose of 150 mg/day.
  2. Duloxetine: begin 30 mg daily, increase to 60 to 120 mg daily. Duloxetine is effective in diabetic neuropathy, post-herpetic neuropathy, and chemotherapy-induced painful peripheral neuropathy.
- Antiepileptics:
  1. Gabapentin: begin 300 mg PO qd, advance to 300 mg PO tid by the end of the first week. Effective dose: higher than 1600 mg/day. Max dose: 1200 mg PO tid.

TABLE 3 Clinical Presentation and Laboratory Findings

Neuropathy Type	Predisposition	Examination Findings	EMG/NCS	Laboratory Analysis
Idiopathic small fiber PN	Age >50	Strength: normal Reflexes: normal Pos/vib: normal Pain/temp: decreased distally	Normal	Serum studies: normal Skin biopsy: abnormal Sudomotor studies: abnormal
Diabetic PN	Longstanding disease Family history	Strength normal to reduced, sensation reduced distally	Abnormal	Abnormal glucose tolerance High fasting glucose
Inherited PN	Family history	Pes cavus, hammer toes, reduced reflexes, sensation reduced distally	Abnormal	Genetic studies may be abnormal, other studies normal
Familial amyloid PN	Family history	Pain/temp loss Reduced reflexes Orthostasis	Abnormal if large fibers affected; also carpal tunnel syndrome	Transthyretin genetic study
Acquired amyloid PN	Monoclonal gammopathy	Pain/temp loss Reduced reflexes Orthostasis	Abnormal if large fibers affected; also carpal tunnel syndrome	SPEP, UPEP, immunofixation abnormal
Fabry's disease	Age Renal failure Strokes	Normal; possible reduced pain/temp sensation	Normal	α-Galactosidase levels in cultured fibroblasts
PN + mixed connective tissue disease	History of lupus, rheumatoid arthritis, Sjögren's syndrome	Reduced reflexes and distal sensation	Abnormal	ANA, RF, SS-A/SS-B may be abnormal
Peripheral nerve vasculitis	Asymmetric disease	Multiple peripheral nerves involved	Abnormal	ANA, RF, SS-A/SS-B, ANCA, cryoglobulins may be abnormal
Paraneoplastic neuropathy	Lung cancer risk factors, chemical exposures	Asymmetric sensory loss, pseudoathetosis, relatively preserved strength	Abnormal	Anti-Hu
Sarcoidosis	Pulmonary sarcoid	Multiple mononeuropathies	Abnormal	Abnormal biopsy, elevated serum ACE, CXR abnormal
Arsenic	Pesticides, copper smelting	Reduced reflexes and distal sensation	Abnormal	Elevated arsenic in plasma, urine, and hair
HIV	Promiscuity, unprotected sex, IV drug abuse, blood transfusion	Variable, but most often reduced reflexes and distal sensation	Abnormal if large fibers involved	HIV antibody

ACE, Angiotensin-converting enzyme; ANA, antibody to nuclear antigens; ANCA, antineutrophil cytoplasmic antibodies; CXR, chest x-ray; EMG, electromyography; HbA1C, glycosylated hemoglobin; HIV, human immunodeficiency virus; IV, intravenous; NCS, nerve conduction studies; PN, polyneuropathy; Pos, position sensation; RF, rheumatoid factor; SPEP, serum protein electrophoresis; SS-A, Sjögren syndrome A; SS-B, Sjögren syndrome B; Temp, temperature sensation; UPEP, urine protein electrophoresis; Vib, vibration sensation.
Adapted from Mendell JR, Sahenk Z: Painful sensory neuropathy, N Engl J Med 348(13):1243, 2003.

2. Carbamazepine: for trigeminal neuralgia. Begin 400 mg PO bid, increase to tid if necessary. Side effects and drug levels help to determine optimal dosing. Risk of aplastic anemia and hyponatremia (monitor CBC and chemistries).
3. Oxcarbazepine: better tolerated than carbamazepine. Start 150 mg PO bid and gradually increase to a dose of 600 mg bid. Maximum dose is 1200 mg bid.
4. Pregabalin: begin 50 mg PO tid, increase slowly to 100 to 200 mg PO tid.
- Analgesics:
  1. Tramadol: 150 mg/day (50 mg tid), increase by 50 mg/wk, max 200 to 400 mg/day.
  2. Morphine (oral): 15 to 30 mg q8h, max 90 to 360 mg/day.
  3. Oxycodone: 20 mg q12h, increase by 10 mg/wk, max 40 to 160 mg/day.
  4. Fentanyl patch: 25 to 100 mcg transdermally q3 days.
- Topical anesthetics:
  1. 5% lidocaine patch, apply to area of pain, max three patches every 12 hr.
  2. Capsaicin is inconsistent in its ability to relieve pain and may exacerbate it. Use not recommended.

- Procedural/surgical: this option is considered mostly when the patient suffers from pain secondary to spinal cord or cauda equina injury. Studies are limited and benefit is not completely established. Procedures should be considered only when all other therapeutic modalities have failed. In addition, the patient should be cautioned that surgical procedures may not result in pain relief and may be associated with significant morbidity and even mortality.
  1. Dorsal root rhizotomy
  2. Nerve blocks
  3. Spinal cord stimulator

DISPOSITION

Prognosis depends on multiple factors, including:
- Etiology of pain
- Treatment of any underlying condition
- Initiation of appropriate (often multiple) therapeutic modalities
- Patient compliance with prescribed regimen
Most care is accomplished in the outpatient setting, except when surgery is required.

REFERRAL

- Pain clinic
- Neurology
- Psychiatry
- Psychology
- Physiatry
- Anesthesiology (nerve blocks)
- Neurosurgery if considering surgical management

⚠ PEARLS & CONSIDERATIONS

- Factitious disorder and malingering frequently manifest with pain complaints. These are diagnoses of exclusion, and require negative evaluation for organic etiologies before diagnosis is made.
- Peripheral neuropathy in diabetics increases the risk of foot ulceration by sevenfold. Abnormal results in monofilament testing and vibratory perception (alone or in combination with the appearance of the feet, ulceration, and ankle reflexes) are the most helpful sign for the detection of LFPN.

SUGGESTED READINGS

Available at www.expertconsult.com

AUTHOR: **JOSEPH S. KASS, M.D., J.D.,** and **GAVIN BROWN, M.D.**

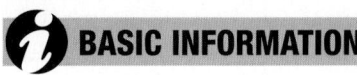

BASIC INFORMATION

DEFINITION

Any disorder affecting the peripheral nervous system, including nerve roots, plexuses, and individual peripheral nerves, that has a genetic basis of inheritance and has been or is capable of being transmitted along generations.

There are many different types of hereditary peripheral neuropathies, including Dejerine-Sottas disease, inherited metabolic neuropathies, hereditary sensory and autonomic neuropathies (HSANs), and hereditary motor neuropathies. Most disorders are diagnosed in infancy or childhood; as such, adult clinicians rarely see these patients. For this reason, this chapter discusses only the hereditary motor and sensory neuropathies that an adult clinician might encounter.

SYNONYMS

Charcot-Marie-Tooth (CMT) disease
Hereditary motor-sensory neuropathy (HMSN)
Hereditary neuropathy with liability to pressure-sensitive palsies (HNPP)

ICD-10CM CODES

G60.0 Hereditary motor and sensory neuropathy
G60.8 Other hereditary and idiopathic neuropathies
G60.9 Hereditary and idiopathic neuropathy, unspecified

EPIDEMIOLOGY & DEMOGRAPHICS

All CMT: approximately 30 per 100,000
- CMT type 1 (demyelinating pathophysiology): 1 in 2500
- CMT type 2 (axonal pathophysiology): 7 in 1000
- CMT type 4 and CMT-X: rare (either axonal or demyelinating pathophysiology)
HNPP: 2 to 5 per 100,000

PHYSICAL FINDINGS & CLINICAL PRESENTATION

CMT: Highly variable
- Age at onset earlier for CMT-1 than CMT-2, but both may present from childhood to old age.
- Severely affected patients have severe distal weakness and muscle atrophy with hand (prominently affecting interossei) and foot deformities (pes cavus, high arched feet, hammer toes).
- Mildly affected patients may have only foot deformity (pes cavus) with little or no weakness/sensory loss.
- Legs can be affected greater than arms, and patients will complain of gait abnormalities (steppage), which cause them to trip and fall.
- Sensory complaints (paresthesias, numbness, dysesthesia) are uncommon despite physical findings of impaired sensation.
- Decreased or absent reflexes.

- Some patients may have postural tremor of the upper limbs.
HNPP (a.k.a. tomaculous neuropathy):
- Age at onset is commonly adolescence.
- Disorder is characterized by recurrent entrapment of peripheral nerves with accompanying signs and symptoms (paresthesias and/or weakness in anatomic distributions). Most common are:
  1. Median nerve at the wrist (carpal tunnel syndrome)
  2. Ulnar nerve at the elbow (cubital tunnel syndrome)
  3. Painless brachial plexopathies
  4. Lateral femoral cutaneous nerve (meralgia paresthetica)
  5. Peroneal nerve at the fibular head
- May be associated with a generalized polyneuropathy.

ETIOLOGY

CMT: more than 30 subgroups have been identified and have various chromosomal abnormalities.
- Most common mutation is PMP-22 duplication, giving rise to CMT 1A demyelinating phenotype.
- Other mutations include P0 (demyelinating) and neurofilament light chain mutations (demyelinating or axonal phenotype)—see the following.
- Updated information may be available at http://www.neuro.wustl.edu/neuromuscular.
HNPP: deletion of chromosome 17p11.2–12.

DIAGNOSIS

DIFFERENTIAL DIAGNOSIS

CMT: other genetic, metabolic, and multisystem disorders including:
- Spinocerebellar ataxias
- Friedreich's ataxia
- Leukodystrophies
- Refsum's disease (elevated serum phytanic acid)
- Distal spinal muscular atrophies and distal myopathies, which can present with pes cavus and other foot deformities
- Chronic inflammatory demyelinating polyneuropathy (CIDP)
HNPP:
- Hereditary neuralgic amyotrophy (HNA), which typically is painful rather than painless. In addition, in HNA, there is no evidence of generalized polyneuropathy.
- Multifocal motor neuropathy with conduction block (MMNCB)—autoimmune-mediated pure motor neuropathy
- Neuropathy associated with renal failure
- Lead neuropathy
- Neuropathy relating to paraproteinemia (demyelinating pathophysiology)

EVALUATION

CMT
- History of gradual onset symptoms is important to distinguish CMT from other forms of neuropathy.

- Detailed family history with *pedigree* is essential. Consider examination of multiple family members.
- History should evaluate for potential heavy metal exposure.
- History of dysesthesias is uncommon and should prompt search for acquired neuropathy or other inherited neuropathies (e.g., Fabry's disease).
HNPP: genetic testing after identification of multiple entrapment neuropathies on EMG and nerve conduction studies

LABORATORY TESTS

- Neurophysiology: electromyography (EMG) and nerve conduction studies (NCSs) must be done first to determine type of pathophysiology: demyelinating or axonal. This will guide genetic testing.
- NCSs in CMT-1 will reveal demyelinating physiology characterized by very slow conduction velocities (around 15 to 30 m/s) with prolonged distal latencies. Inherited demyelinating disorders can be distinguished from acquired demyelinating disorders (e.g., chronic inflammatory demyelinating polyneuropathy or CIDP) by the presence of conduction block in the latter.
- In HNPP, diffusely prolonged distal latencies with superimposed entrapment neuropathies at common sites will be seen on NCSs.
- EMG will reveal reinnervation characterized by long-duration, large-amplitude, polyphasic motor unit potentials (MUPs) with decreased MUP recruitment.
- Genetic tests are available for some CMT subtypes:
  1. CMT-1A: chromosome 17p11-PMP-22 duplication
  2. CMT-1B: chromosome 1q22-P0 mutation
  3. CMT-2E: chromosome 8p21-neurofilament light chain (NF-L) point mutation
  4. CMT-X: connexin 32 mutations
  5. HNPP: chromosome 17p11 deletion, which includes the PMP-22 gene
- Serum and 24-hour urine levels of heavy metals (arsenic, lead, etc.)
- SPEP, UPEP, immunofixation (for paraprotein).
- Anti-GM1 antibody (positive in ~50% of patients with MMNCB).
- Lumbar puncture may reveal elevated CSF protein in CIDP.
- Peripheral nerve biopsy:
  1. Demyelination with "onion bulb formation." Tomaculae, or focal thickening of myelin sheaths, is seen in HNPP
  2. Generally not indicated unless diagnosis is uncertain

IMAGING STUDIES

- Spine plain films: for evaluation of scoliosis.
- MRI: indicated if dissociative sensory loss (dorsal column dysfunction with intact spinothalamic tract function) or if upper motor neuron findings (spasticity, Babinski's sign, clonus, increased tendon reflexes) are present.

- Exclusion of involvement of brain or spinal cord compressive lesions causing arm or leg weakness.
- Some inherited peripheral demyelinating disorders (i.e., CMT-X) are associated with intracerebral white matter abnormalities on MRI.
- Exclusion of structural, infectious, or inflammatory nerve root pathology.

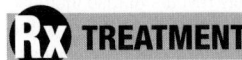 TREATMENT

There is no known cure for any of these disorders. Management is supportive.

NONPHARMACOLOGIC THERAPY

- Physical therapy (PT) and occupational therapy (OT) to provide assistance with gait and coordination.
- PT and OT might provide walking aid such as ankle foot orthosis (AFO), cane, walker, or wheelchair depending on the severity of the neuropathy.
- Wrist splints for superimposed carpal tunnel syndrome.
- Elbow pads (Heelbo Pads) to cushion the ulnar nerve at the elbow.
- Heel-cord strengthening.
- Stretching exercises.
- Analgesics for pain associated with foot deformity.
- Surgical correction of foot deformities by orthopedic surgeons if indicated.

Vincristine may worsen existing neuropathy (important for oncologist to know if patient develops cancer requiring chemotherapy).

SURGICAL TREATMENT

- Patients with HNPP should probably not undergo surgical decompression of the median nerve at the wrist or the ulnar nerve at the elbow; these nerves are sensitive to manipulation. Poor results have been reported with ulnar nerve transposition.
- Anesthesiologists should be aware of HNPP diagnosis in patients undergoing surgery to prevent compression neuropathies from occurring during surgical procedures.

GENETIC COUNSELING

Must be routinely done for patient and family when diagnosis is established. Many aspects of the patient and family's life are affected, including:

- Future progeny of patient and/or patient's parents or children
- Psychosocial aspects including social functioning, marriage, employment
- Financial needs
- Medical and life insurability

PROGNOSIS

- CMT: slowly progressive, and patients often remain ambulatory until late in life. Life expectancy is normal. Patients with

respiratory involvement (i.e., phrenic nerve involvement with diaphragm paresis) may have shorter life expectancy.
- HNPP: benign prognosis.

DISPOSITION

Outpatient care. Routine follow-up appointments should be done initially every 6 mo, and then every 1 to 2 yr.

REFERRAL

- Neurology and/or neuromuscular disease specialist
- Podiatry for recurrent foot problems, including appropriate arches

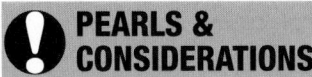 PEARLS & CONSIDERATIONS

PATIENT & FAMILY EDUCATION

Patients can benefit from use of Muscular Dystrophy Association (MDA) resources.

RELATED CONTENT

Charcot-Marie-Tooth Disease (Related Key Topic)
Neuropathic Pain (Related Key Topic)

AUTHORS: **JOSEPH S. KASS, M.D., J.D.,** and **GAVIN BROWN, M.D.**

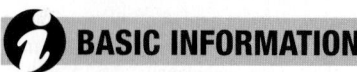

BASIC INFORMATION

DEFINITION

Nonalcoholic fatty liver disease (NAFLD) is a spectrum of diseases based on histopathologic findings and representing a morphologic rather than a clinical diagnosis. It is liver disease occurring in patients who do not abuse alcohol and manifesting histologically by mononuclear cells and/or polymorphonuclear cells, hepatocyte ballooning, and spotty necrosis. Nonalcoholic steatohepatitis (NASH) is a subset of NAFLD. A diagnosis of NAFLD is contingent on the following factors:

1. Alcohol consumption in amounts less than those considered hepatotoxic.
2. Absence of serologic evidence of other hepatic diseases or disorders.
3. Liver biopsy showing predominant macrovesicular steatosis or steatohepatitis.

SYNONYMS

Nonalcoholic steatohepatitis (NASH)
NAFLD
Fatty liver hepatitis
Diabetes hepatitis
Alcohol-like liver disease
Laënnec's disease

ICD-10CM CODES
K76.0 Fatty (change of) liver, not elsewhere classified

EPIDEMIOLOGY & DEMOGRAPHICS

- NAFLD affects 20% to 30% of the general population.
- Increased prevalence in obese persons (57% to 74%), type 2 diabetes mellitus, and hyperlipidemia (primarily hypertriglyceridemia).
- Most common cause of abnormal liver test results in adults in the United States (accounts for up to 90% of cases of asymptomatic ALT elevations).
- 30 million obese adults have steatosis; 8.6 million may have steatohepatitis.
- There is a 3:1 female-to-male predominance.
- Approximately 20% of patients with NAFLD have NASH.

PHYSICAL FINDINGS & CLINICAL PRESENTATION

- Most patients are asymptomatic.
- Patients may report a sensation of fullness or discomfort on the right side of the upper abdomen.
- Nonspecific complaints of fatigue or malaise may be reported.
- Hepatomegaly is generally the only positive finding on physical examination.
- Acanthosis nigricans may be found in children.

ETIOLOGY

- Insulin resistance is the most reproducible factor in the development of NAFLD. High baseline and continuously increasing fasting insulin levels are independent determinants for future development of NFLD.
- Risk factors are obesity (especially truncal obesity), diabetes mellitus, hyperlipidemia.

DIAGNOSIS

DIFFERENTIAL DIAGNOSIS

- Alcohol-induced liver disease (a daily alcohol intake of 20 g in females and 30 g in males [three 12-oz beers or 12 oz of wine] may be enough to cause alcohol-induced liver disease).
- Viral hepatitis.
- Autoimmune hepatitis.
- Toxin- or drug-induced liver disease.

WORKUP

Diagnosis is usually suspected on the basis of hepatomegaly, asymptomatic elevations of transaminases, or "fatty liver" on sonogram of abdomen in obese patients with little or no alcohol use. Liver biopsy will confirm diagnosis and provide prognostic information. It should be considered in patients with suspected advanced liver fibrosis (presence of obesity or type 2 diabetes, AST/ALT ratio 1, age 45 yr).

LABORATORY TESTS

- Elevated ALT, AST: AST/ALT ratio is usually <1, but can increase as fibrosis advances. In advanced fibrosis AST to ALT ratio is >1 and platelet count is low.
- Negative serology for infectious hepatitis; generally normal GGTP and serum alkaline phosphatase.
- Hyperlipidemia (primarily hypertriglyceridemia) may be present.
- Elevated glucose levels may be present.
- Prolonged prothrombin time, hypoalbuminemia, and elevated bilirubin may be present in advanced stages.
- Elevated serum ferritin and increased transferrin saturation may be found in up to 10% of patients; however, hepatic iron index and hepatic iron level are normal.
- Liver biopsy may show a wide spectrum of liver damage, ranging from simple steatosis to advanced fibrosis and cirrhosis.

IMAGING STUDIES

- Ultrasound generally reveals diffuse increase in echogenicity as compared with that of the kidneys; CT scan reveals diffuse low-density hepatic parenchyma.
- Occasionally patients may have focal rather than diffuse steatosis, which may be misinterpreted as a liver mass on ultrasound or CT (Fig. 1); use of MRI in these cases will identify focal fatty infiltration.
- Ultrasound elastography (Fibroscan) can also be used to evaluate hepatic fibrosis.

TREATMENT

NONPHARMACOLOGIC THERAPY

- Weight reduction in all obese patients. The American Gastroenterological Association recommends that the initial target weight loss be 10% of baseline weight at a rate of 1 to 2 lb (0.45 to 0.90 kg) per week.
- Increase physical activity. Vigorous and moderate exercise are equally effective in reducing intrahepatic triglyceride content, the effect being largely mediated by weight loss.
- Alcohol has a deleterious effect on NAFLD and should be avoided.

GENERAL Rx

- Medications to control hyperlipidemia (e.g., fenofibrates for elevated triglycerides) and hyperglycemia (e.g., pioglitazone, insulin, metformin) can lead to improvement in abnormal liver test results.
- A 3-year trial with pioglitazone (30 mg/day), an insulin-sensitizing thiazolidinedione, revealed that pioglitazone treatment was associated with long-term metabolic

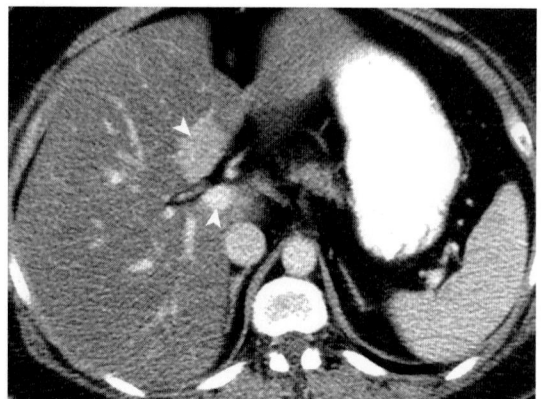

FIG. 1 Focal sparing Two islands of normal parenchyma (*arrowheads*) in segment IVb and the caudate lobe (segment 1) simulate mass lesions in a liver with extensive fatty infiltration. Most of the liver parenchyma shows fatty infiltration, making these islands of normal parenchyma appear of high attenuation by comparison. (Webb WR et al: *Fundamentals of body CT*, ed 4, Philadelphia, 2015, WB Saunders.)

and histologic improvement in patients with prediabetes or type 2 diabetes mellitus and NASH. These results suggest that that NASH progression may be halted and the natural history of the disease may be modified with the use of pioglitazone in patients with prediabetes or type 2 diabetes mellitus.[1]

DISPOSITION

- Patients with pure steatosis on liver biopsy generally have a relatively benign course.
- The presence of steatohepatitis or advanced fibrosis on liver biopsy is associated with a worse prognosis.

---

[1]Cusi K et al: Long-term pioglitazone treatment for patients with nonalcoholic steatohepatitis and prediabetes or type 2 diabetes mellitus: a randomized trial, *Ann Intern Med* 165:305-315, 2016.

REFERRAL

- Liver transplantation should be considered in patients with decompensated, end-stage disease; however, in these patients there may be a recurrence of NAFLD posttransplantation.

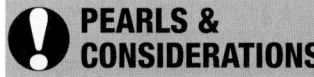 **PEARLS & CONSIDERATIONS**

COMMENTS

- NAFLD is closely associated with metabolic disorders, even in nonobese, nondiabetic subjects. It can be considered an early predictor of metabolic disorders, particularly in the normal-weight population. The presence of metabolic syndrome is a strong predictor of NAFLD.
- NAFLD is associated with an increased risk of incident cardiovascular disease that is independent of the risk conferred by traditional risk factors and components of the metabolic syndrome.

- 10% of patients with NASH have progression to advanced fibrosis. Most common in patients older than 50, ALT > twice normal, BMI >28, triglycerides >150 mg/dL.
- Statins are not contraindicated in patients with NASH.

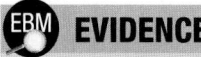 **EVIDENCE**

Available at www.expertconsult.com

SUGGESTED READINGS

Available at www.expertconsult.com

RELATED CONTENT

Fatty Liver (Patient Information)

AUTHOR: **FRED F. FERRI, M.D.**

N

Diseases and Disorders

I

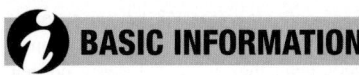

DEFINITION

Nonallergic rhinitis (NAR) is characterized by chronic episodic or perennial symptoms of rhinitis (congestion, rhinorrhea, and postnasal drainage) that are not the result of IgE-mediated events. It is a heterogeneous group of diseases classified into inflammatory (infectious rhinosinusitis, rhinitis with eosinophilia syndrome) and noninflammatory (including but not limited to vasomotor rhinitis, gustatory rhinitis, atrophic rhinitis, rhinitis medicamentosa, hormone-induced rhinitis, rhinitis associated with systemic disease).

SYNONYMS

Chronic nonallergic rhinitis
Idiopathic rhinitis
Intrinsic rhinitis
NAR
Nonallergic-noninfectious chronic rhinitis

ICD-10CM CODES
J30.0 Vasomotor rhinitis
J31.0 Chronic rhinitis (atrophic, granulomatous, hypertrophic, obstructive rhinitis)

EPIDEMIOLOGY & DEMOGRAPHICS

- Nonallergic rhinitis affects approximately 17 to 22 million individuals in the U.S.
- Approximately 50% of patients presenting with rhinitis may have NAR alone or a "mixed form."
  ○ "Mixed nonallergic/allergic rhinitis" may occur in up to an additional 22 million Americans.
- Nonallergic rhinitis typically presents later in life with 70% of patients presenting after 20 years of age. Onset of allergic rhinitis usually occurs in childhood.
- Risk factors for nonallergic rhinitis include female sex and age of >40 years.
- May have genetic component in those individuals whose parents have allergic rhinitis.

PHYSICAL FINDINGS & CLINICAL PRESENTATION

- Physical exam can be completely unremarkable.
- Swollen erythematous turbinates may be present in comparison to pale or violaceous swollen turbinates seen in allergic rhinitis.
- Clear or mucoid nasal secretions.
- Nasal crusting, anosmia (loss of smell), and foul odor from the nares are indicative of atrophic rhinitis.
- Clinical presentation: can be nonspecific but usually consists of nasal congestions and/or rhinorrhea with often associated postnasal drip, sneezing, and throat clearing. Other allergic symptoms including nasal and palatal pruritus and conjunctival symptoms are typically absent.

ETIOLOGY

- NAR is composed of a heterogeneous group of diseases, and each subtype likely has a unique pathogenesis.
  1. Vasomotor rhinitis—frequently triggered by perfumes, strong odors, changes in climate, and smoke but may also occur in absence of defined triggers.
  2. Infectious rhinosinusitis—viral, bacterial, or fungal infections. Typically occurs following an acute viral infection.
  3. Nonallergic rhinitis with eosinophilia syndrome (NARES)—unknown etiology.
  4. Gustatory rhinitis—abnormal vagally mediated rhinitis after ingestion of any food.
  5. Atrophic rhinitis—unknown etiology but bacterial infection is thought to be involved.
  6. Rhinitis medicamentosa—rebound nasal congestion from prolonged use of decongestant/vasoconstrictor agents (phenylephrine, oxymetazoline). Can also occur from cocaine, α-receptor antagonist, or phosphodiesterase-5-selective inhibitors.
  7. Hormone-induced rhinitis—pregnancy-associated, menstrual cycle–associated and oral contraceptive–related hormonal changes.
  8. Rhinitis associated with system disease—severe hypothyroidism, diabetes mellitus.

DIAGNOSIS

DIFFERENTIAL DIAGNOSIS

- Allergic rhinitis (sensitivity to pollens, indoor allergens, occupational allergens)
- Systemic diseases with nasal manifestations (e.g., systemic lupus erythematosus, granulomatous disease, GERD)
- Mechanical obstruction (e.g., deviated septum, nasal polyps, nasal neoplasms, foreign bodies)
- Cerebral spinal fluid (CSF) leak from head trauma, postoperative complication from sinus surgery, or spontaneous leak
- Local allergic rhinitis
- Chronic rhinosinusitis

WORKUP

- A detailed history and physical exam can be helpful to determine if diagnostic testing is necessary. Most cases can be empirically treated without further testing.
- Distinguishing NAR from allergic rhinitis or other forms of rhinitis can be difficult, but a detailed history (lack of allergic symptoms such as sneezing, nasal pruritus) can be helpful. Also, questionnaires, including the Cincinnati Irritant Index Scale, have proven useful in differentiating NAR from allergic rhinitis.
  ○ Because allergic rhinitis cannot be definitively ruled out with history alone, skin testing or assessment for serum-specific IgE should be considered. Adding to the diagnostic complexity, many individuals have a "mixed form" of rhinitis including both allergic and nonallergic types.

- Examination of nasal smears for the presence of neutrophils to rule out an infectious etiology and eosinophils that may suggest an allergic component or NARES.

TREATMENT

NONPHARMACOLOGIC THERAPY

- Identification and avoidance of specific triggers (e.g., smoke/smog, specific foods, perfumes, strong odors, occupational irritants) may provide relief.
- Discontinuing any medication/drugs that could be contributing, including topical decongestants/vasoconstrictors, oral contraceptives (OCPs), cocaine, and alcohol.
- Daily nasal lavage and over-the-counter nasal saline sprays have been shown to improve symptoms.
- Surgical intervention (turbinectomy, vidian nerve resection) can be considered if medical measures fail, but surgery has not proved to be efficacious and involves the risk of complications.

ACUTE AND CHRONIC Rx

- Second-generation antihistamines have not been shown to be beneficial in nonallergic rhinitis. Although first-generation antihistamines may improve rhinorrhea due to their anticholinergic properties, topical therapies including intranasal antihistamines (azelastine, olopatadine), intranasal steroids (fluticasone propionate, triamcinolone, mometasone), and intranasal anticholinergics (ipratropium bromide) have been shown to be most beneficial.
- Treatments should be individualized to the underlying pathophysiology.
  ○ *Vasomotor rhinitis:* Initial therapy typically involves intranasal steroids with the addition of an intranasal antihistamine or intranasal ipratropium bromide if symptoms are not well controlled. A combination intranasal steroid and intranasal antihistamine is now available that may be more convenient.
  ○ *Infectious rhinosinusitis:* Supportive care and intranasal saline spray. May take up to 6 to 8 weeks to improve after resolution of acute infection.
  ○ *Nonallergic rhinitis with eosinophilia syndrome (NARES):* Topical nasal corticosteroids.
  ○ *Gustatory rhinitis:* Preprandial intranasal ipratropium bromide.
  ○ *Atrophic rhinitis:* Frequent irrigation with nasal saline, antibiotics to treat potential underlying bacterial infection; debridement and possible surgical intervention to reduce nasal cavity size can be considered.
  ○ *Rhinitis medicamentosa:* Discontinuation of offending agent (topical decongestant/vasoconstrictor agent, cocaine, α-receptor antagonist or phosphodiesterase-5-selective inhibitors). Patient may require short course of nasal or oral corticosteroids during withdrawal process.

○ *Hormone-induced rhinitis:* Typically resolves with delivery if during pregnancy. Consider discontinuing OCP if offending agent. Nasal saline spray alone can be efficacious.

○ *Rhinitis associated with system disease:* Optimally managing the underlying condition.

- Alternative treatments: topical capsaicin, silver nitrate, and acupuncture.

DISPOSITION

- Most patients experience mild to moderate symptomatic relief with avoidance of triggers and appropriate use of medications. Up to 52% of patients with NAR report worsening symptoms at 3- to 7-year follow-ups. Periodic reevaluations should be performed, as there is evidence supporting increase in comorbidities (asthma, allergic rhinitis, conjunctivitis) with length of NAR diagnosis.

REFERRAL

Referral to allergist and/or ENT may be appropriate when severe symptoms are unresponsive to therapy and/or diagnosis is uncertain.

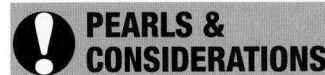

PEARLS & CONSIDERATIONS

COMMENTS

- Nonallergic rhinitis symptoms are nonspecific, and a specific trigger is often never identified. Compared to allergic rhinitis, patients typically lack symptoms of sneezing, nasal pruritus, and conjunctival symptoms.
- Second-generation oral antihistamines are typically not efficacious, and the treatment of nonallergic rhinitis should be individualized based on its underlying pathophysiology.

RELATED CONTENT

Allergic Rhinitis (Patient Information)
Allergic Rhinitis (Related Key Topic)

SUGGESTED READINGS

Available at www.expertconsult.com

AUTHOR: **SHYAM JOSHI, M.D.**

N

Diseases and Disorders

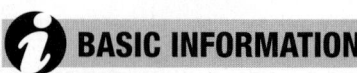

BASIC INFORMATION

DEFINITION

Obesity refers to having an excess amount of body fat in relation to lean body mass, or a body mass index (BMI) of ≥30 kg/m². Overweight is defined as BMI of 25 to 29.9 kg/m² and morbid obesity refers to adults with a BMI ≥40 kg/m². BMI is used as a surrogate measure of obesity. Abdominal obesity is defined as waist circumference >102 cm (40 inches) in men and >88 cm (35 inches) in women.

ICD-10CM CODES
E66.9	Obesity, unspecified
E66.01	Morbid (severe) obesity due to excess calories
E66.09	Other obesity due to excess calories
E66.1	Drug-induced obesity
E66.2	Morbid (severe) obesity with alveolar hypoventilation
E66.8	Other obesity
O99.210	Obesity complicating pregnancy, unspecified trimester
O99.211	Obesity complicating pregnancy, first trimester
O99.212	Obesity complicating pregnancy, second trimester
O99.213	Obesity complicating pregnancy, third trimester
O99.214	Obesity complicating childbirth
O99.215	Obesity complicating the puerperium

EPIDEMIOLOGY & DEMOGRAPHICS

- The World Health Organization first recognized obesity as a worldwide epidemic in 1997. As of 2005, 1.6 billion adults worldwide were classified as overweight, 400 million of whom were obese. It is predicted that the combination of overweight and obesity will soon eclipse public health issues such as malnutrition and infectious diseases as the most significant cause of poor health.
- Worldwide, data from the Global Burden of Disease Study from 1980 to 2013 indicate the prevalence of adult obesity has increased from 28.8% to 36.9% in men and 29.8% to 38% in women. The prevalence of childhood and adolescent obesity has also substantially increased.
- Based on U.S. NHANES data from 2011 to 2012, the prevalence of abdominal obesity was 54%. It is estimated that by 2020, 2 in every 5 adults and 1 in every 4 children in the U.S. will be categorized as obese.
- The present cost of obesity in the U.S. population is estimated at $100 billion annually. Approximately two thirds of people living in the United States are overweight, which is the highest percentage in the world (Marie Ng, 2014).
- For persons with a BMI ≥30 kg/m², all-cause mortality is increased by 50% to 100% above that of persons with BMI in the range of 20 to 25 kg/m².
- Obesity is an independent risk factor for cardiovascular disease (CVD), type 2 diabetes,

hypertension, cancer (particularly colon, prostate, breast, and gynecologic malignancies), sleep apnea, degenerative joint disease, thromboembolic disorders, digestive tract diseases (gallstones), and dermatologic disorders.
- Significant morbidity and risk of death are projected to begin in young adulthood, resulting in >100,000 excess cases of CHD by 2035, even with the most modest projection of future obesity.
- When children enter kindergarten, 12.4% are obese, and another 14.9% are overweight. Data show that incident obesity between the ages of 5 and 14 years is more likely to have occurred at younger ages.[1]
- Obesity in adolescence is significantly associated with increased risk of incident severe obesity in adulthood, with variations by sex and race/ethnicity. Overweight or obese adults who were obese as children have increased risk of type 2 DM, dyslipidemia, hypertension, and carotid artery atherosclerosis.
- Obesity is a major preventable cause of death and disability in the United States (the other is tobacco).
- Extensive data indicate that weight loss can reverse or arrest the harmful effects of obesity.
- In 2013 nearly 180,000 bariatric surgery procedures were performed in the U.S. Of these procedures 42% were laparoscopic sleeve gastrectomy, 34% were Roux-en-Y gastric bypass, and 15% were laparoscopic adjustable gastric banding.

PHYSICAL FINDINGS & CLINICAL PRESENTATION

- Physical examination should assess the degree and distribution of body fat, signs of secondary causes of obesity, and obesity-related comorbidities.
- Increased waist circumference is apparent. Excess abdominal fat is clinically defined as a waist circumference >40 inches (>102 cm) in men and >35 inches (>88 cm) in women (in Asian men and women, >36 inches and >33 inches, respectively). Central obesity is a risk factor for mortality even among individuals with normal BMIs.
- Symptoms associated with hypertension, coronary artery disease (CAD), and diabetes (e.g., polyuria, polydipsia, acanthosis nigricans, retinopathy, and neuropathy) may be present.
- Obesity is associated with cardiac hypertrophy, diastolic dysfunction, and decreased aortic compliance, which are independent predictors of cardiovascular risk.
- Joint pain and swelling are associated with degenerative joint disease secondary to obesity.
- The physical exam and ECG often underestimate the presence and extent of cardiac dysfunction in obese patients. Jugular venous

distention and hepatojugular reflux may not be seen and heart sounds are frequently distant.
- A large quantity of fluid is present in the interstitial space of adipose tissue, as the interstitial space is ~10% of the tissue wet weight. This excess fluid in this compartment if redistributed into the circulation, can have negative repercussions in obese individuals with heart failure. Obese individuals have higher cardiac output and a lower total peripheral resistance than do lean individuals, and obesity is associated with persistence of elevated cardiac filling pressure during exercise.
- Obesity predisposes to heart failure through several different mechanisms: increased total blood volume, increased cardiac output, LVH, left ventricular diastolic dysfunction, and adipositas cordis (excessive epicardial fat and fatty infiltration of the myocardium).

ETIOLOGY

- The pathophysiology of obesity is complex and poorly understood, but includes social, nutritional, physiologic, psychological, and genetic factors.
- Environmental factors such as a sedentary lifestyle and chronic ingestion of excess calories can cause obesity.
- Obesity may be related to genetic factors, which are thought to be polygenic. Genetic studies with adopted children have demonstrated that they have similar BMIs to their biologic parents but not their adoptive parents. Twin studies also demonstrate a genetic influence on BMI.
- Secondary causes of obesity can result from medications (antipsychotics, steroids, and protease inhibitors being common ones) and neuroendocrine disorders (like Cushing's syndrome and hypothyroidism).

DIAGNOSIS

- BMI will establish the diagnosis of obesity. BMI is defined as the adult's weight in kilograms divided by the square of his or her height—and is closely correlated with total body fat content.
- BMI values can categorize patients into three classes of obesity:
  1. Class I (mild): BMI of 30.0 to 34.9 kg/m²
  2. Class II (moderate): BMI of 35.0 to 39.9 kg/m²
  3. Class III (severe): BMI of ≥40 kg/m²
- Although BMI is commonly used to define obesity, it is not a highly accurate indicator of body fat composition in children, who are undergoing rapid changes in height, or in bodybuilders or athletes who have large amounts of muscle tissue.
- Waist circumference or waist-hip ratio is indicative of visceral adipose tissue/intraabdominal fat, which may be more deleterious than overall overweight or obesity.

DIFFERENTIAL DIAGNOSIS

It is important to evaluate obese patients for secondary medical causes of obesity. Hypothalamic disorders, hypothyroidism, Cushing's syndrome,

---
[1]Cunningham SA, et al.: Incidence of childhood obesity in the United States, *N Engl J Med*, 370:403-411, 2014.

insulinoma, depression, and drugs (corticosteroids, antidepressants, second-generation antipsychotics, sulfonylureas, and HIV protease inhibitors) can cause obesity. In children, certain genetic conditions, such as Prader-Willi syndrome, are associated with obesity.

WORKUP

History should be obtained regarding weight change, family history of obesity, and eating and exercise behavior. Assessment for eating disorders and depression should be made. Attention should be directed to the use of nutritional supplements, over-the-counter medications, hormones, diuretics, and laxatives. The workup of an obese patient typically requires laboratory work to assess for risks and complications as well as to rule out underlying causative medical conditions. Fig. E1 describes the evaluation of patients with suspected endocrine cause of obesity.

LABORATORY TESTS

- Obese patients should be assessed for medical consequences of their obesity by screening for metabolic syndrome. This includes measurement of fasting lipid profile, blood pressure, and waist circumference, and screening for diabetes or prediabetes (oral glucose tolerance test, fasting glucose, or hemoglobin A1C).
- Polycythemia might warrant screening for sleep apnea. Liver function tests should be obtained to screen for hepatic steatosis.
- In the proper clinical setting, thyroid function studies and dexamethasone suppression testing will exclude hypothyroidism and Cushing's syndrome as underlying causes of obesity. If insulinoma is suspected, the patient will need to undergo a 72-hour fast to confirm hypoglycemia with inappropriate insulin secretion.
- Obesity is associated with changes in the ECG, including a reduction in voltage and nonspecific ST-T changes that may interfere with diagnosis of left ventricular hypertrophy (LVH) or CAD.

IMAGING STUDIES

- Several methods are available for determining or calculating total body fat but offer no significant advantage over the BMI. These include measurement of total body water, total body potassium, bioelectrical impedance, and dual-energy x-ray absorptiometry.
- Buoyancy testing is an accurate method for determining total body fat composition.

OTHER STUDIES

Obesity increases the risk of obstructive sleep apnea, which, in turn, increases the risks of hypertension, cardiac arrhythmias, CVD, stroke, and heart failure. Therefore one should have a low threshold to screen obese patients for obstructive sleep apnea via sleep study/polysomnography.

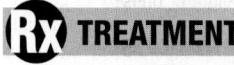 **TREATMENT**

The National Heart, Lung, and Blood Institute (NHLBI) developed guidelines for selecting

TABLE 1 Weight-Loss Treatment Guidelines from the National Heart, Lung, and Blood Institute*

	BMI				
Treatment	25.0-26.9	27.0-29.9	30.0-34.9	35.0-39.9	>40.0
Diet, physical activity, behavioral therapy, or all three	Yes	Yes	Yes	Yes	Yes
Pharmacotherapy†		In patients with obesity-related diseases.	Yes	Yes	Yes
Surgery‡				In patients with obesity-related diseases.	Yes

*Data are from www.nhlbi.nih.gov/guidelines/obesity/ob_home.htm. These guidelines are generally consistent with those from the American Heart Association, the American Medical Association, the American Diabetic Association, the Obesity Society (Practical Guide), the American Diabetes Association, the American Academy of Family Physicians, the American College of Sports Medicine, and the American Cancer Society. BMI denotes body mass index, calculated as the weight in kilograms divided by the square of the height in meters.
†Pharmacotherapy should be considered only in patients who are not able to achieve adequate weight loss with available conventional lifestyle modifications and who have no absolute contraindications for drug therapy.
‡Bariatric surgery should be considered only in patients who are unable to lose weight with available conventional therapy and who have no absolute contraindications for surgery.

treatment strategies for overweight and obese patients based on BMI and comorbidities. They recommend a combination of dietary management, physical activity management, and behavior therapy for anyone with a BMI ≥25 or with a high-risk waist circumference and two or more obesity-associated comorbidities. Pharmacotherapy should be considered for patients with a BMI ≥30 or ≥27 with comorbidities.

Bariatric surgery is indicated for patients with a BMI ≥35 with comorbidities and for any patient with a BMI ≥40 (Table 1).

NONPHARMACOLOGIC THERAPY

- The cornerstones for weight management and reduction are calorie restriction, exercise, and behavioral modification. Assessment of patient's willingness to make changes must be evaluated, as treatment is more likely to succeed in motivated patients.
- The NHLBI guidelines recommend an initial diet to produce a calorie deficit of 500 to 1000 kcal/day. This has been shown to reduce total body weight by an average of 8% over 3 to 12 mo.
- These guidelines recommend the use of a food diary to focus on dietary substitutes.
- Thirty minutes of moderate-intensity activity on 5 or more days of the week results in health benefits for obese individuals. Moreover, several studies indicate that 60 to 80 min of moderate to vigorous physical activity may provide additional benefit.
- Increased physical activity without caloric restriction (minimal or no weight loss) can reduce abdominal (visceral) adipose tissue and improve insulin resistance.
- The key features of the standard behavioral modification program include goal setting, self-monitoring, stimulus

control (modification of one's environment to enhance behaviors that will support weight management), cognitive restructuring (increased awareness of perceptions of oneself and one's weight), and prevention of relapse (weight regain).
- Mammalian sleep is closely integrated with the regulation of energy balance. Trials have shown that the amount of human sleep contributes to the maintenance of fat-free body mass at times of decreased energy intake. Lack of sufficient sleep may compromise the efficacy of typical dietary interventions for weight loss and related metabolic risk reduction.

ACUTE GENERAL Rx

- According to the NHLBI *Guidelines on the Identification, Evaluation, and Treatment of Overweight and Obesity in Adults* and the U.S. Food and Drug Administration (FDA), pharmacotherapy is indicated for:
1. Obese patients with a BMI ≥30.
2. Overweight patients with a BMI of ≥27 and concomitant obesity-related risk factors or diseases, such as hypertension, diabetes, or dyslipidemia.
- Pharmacologic treatment options include:
1. Gastrointestinal lipase inhibitors: Orlistat is the only drug available for long-term treatment of obesity. It blocks the digestion and absorption of ingested dietary fat. It is a reversible inhibitor of pancreatic, gastric, and carboxyl ester lipases and phospholipase A2, which are required for the hydrolysis of dietary fat in the gastrointestinal tract. Side effects include flatulence, fecal incontinence, cramps, and oily spotting. There can also be impairment of absorption of fat-soluble vitamins (A, D, E, K) and beta-carotene. Oxalate-associated acute kidney injury

and rare severe liver injury have also been reported.

2. C serotonin agonists: Lorcaserin is a selective serotonin agonist that acts centrally to reduce appetite, aiding weight loss. Adverse effects include headache, upper respiratory infections, dizziness, and nausea. While there is little evidence of serotonin-associated cardiac valvular disease or pulmonary hypertension (as seen with nonselective serotonergic agonists fenfluramine and dexfenfluramine), long-term data is currently limited.

3. Sympathomimetic medications: Phentermine and diethylpropion are currently approved for short-term treatment of obesity. They reduce food intake by causing early satiety. Side effects include increased blood pressure and increased pulse. They are Schedule IV drugs with a potential for abuse. Other sympathomimetic drugs that have been removed from the market due to concerns about cardiovascular safety are sibutramine, phenylpropanolamine, and ephedrine.

4. Antidepressants: While not FDA-approved for treatment of obesity alone, bupropion and fluoxetine are antidepressants that have been associated with modest weight loss. The FDA has recently approved a fixed-dose combination of bupropion with the opioid receptor antagonist naltrexone. It is called Contrave and approved for use as an adjunct to diet and exercise in patients with BMI ≥30 kg/m^2 or a BMI ≥27 kg/m^2 and one or more weight-related comorbidities (e.g., diabetes, hypertension, dyslipidemia).

5. Antiepileptic drugs: Zonisamide and topiramate (also used in migraine therapy) have been associated with weight loss in clinical trials but are not currently FDA-approved for treatment of obesity alone.

6. Diabetes drugs: While not FDA-approved for treatment of obesity alone, metformin, pramlintide (synthetic human amylin), and glucagon-like polypeptide-1 agonists (GLP-1) (exenatide) have been associated with weight loss in the treatment of individuals with diabetes. The GLP-1 receptor agonist liraglutide (Victoza) is now FDA approved at a higher dose as Saxenda for chronic weight management in adults with BMI ≥30 or a BMI ≥27 with a weight-related comorbidity such as hypertension, dyslipidemia, or diabetes.

CHRONIC Rx

- According to the NHLBI guidelines, surgical intervention is an option for selected patients with clinically severe obesity (a BMI ≥40 or a BMI ≥35 with comorbid conditions), when patients are at high risk for obesity-associated morbidity or death, and when less invasive methods of weight loss have failed.
- Eligible patients should also be at an acceptable risk for surgery, well informed, and motivated.

- Bariatric surgery for weight loss falls into one of three general categories:
- Restrictive surgeries limit the amount of food the stomach can hold and slow the rate of gastric emptying. These include vertical banded gastroplasty and laparoscopic adjustable silicone gastric banding LAGB [Fig. E2]). Band slippage is the most common LAGB complication. Other potential complications include port or tubing malfunction, stomal obstruction, band erosion, pouch dilatation, and port infection. Gastric necrosis of the stomach wall is a rarer late complication that results from ischemia caused by a combination of gastric prolapse—the part of the stomach below the band herniates up through the device (Fig. E3)—and pressure from the band. Gastric bypass has better outcomes than gastric band procedures for long-term weight loss, type 2 diabetes control and remission, hypertension, and hyperlipidemia. These procedures have benefits that include: lower perioperative mortality rate, a quicker recovery period, and no malabsorption issues. However, they are not as effective as gastric bypass for weight reduction and comorbidity improvement.

1. Malabsorptive surgeries reduce nutrient absorption by shortening the length of small intestine. These include jejunoileal bypass and the duodenal switch operation (DS).

2. Restrictive malabsorptive bypass procedures combine the elements of gastric restriction and selective malabsorption. These include Roux-en-Y gastric bypass (considered the gold standard because of its high level of effectiveness and durability) and biliopancreatic diversion. These procedures have higher rates of comorbidity improvement than restrictive surgeries, but can be complicated by malabsorption and nutritional deficiencies

- Compared with usual care, bariatric surgery is associated with reduced number of cardiovascular deaths and lower incidence of cardiovascular events in obese adults. A study on bariatric surgery patients demonstrated a significant reduction in long-term cardiovascular events. Ten-year follow-up estimated relative risk reductions ranging from 18% to 79% according to the Framingham risk score and 8% to 62% with the PROCAM risk score.
- A long-term observational study of obese patients with type 2 diabetes showed that bariatric surgery was associated with higher diabetes remission rates and fewer complications than usual care (Sjostrom et al, 2014). Remission of type 2 DM occurs in 60% to 80% of patients two years after surgery and persists in about 30% of patients 15 years after Roux-en-Y gastric bypass.
- Liposuction is removal of fat by aspiration after injection of physiologic saline. This technique reduces the subcutaneous fat but has failed to improve insulin sensitivity or risk factors for CHD.
- The Maestro Rechargeable System is a subcutaneously implanted device recently FDA approved for weight loss in adults with a BMI of 40 to 45 or with a BMI of ≥35 and at least one obesity-related comorbidity. It utilizes high-frequency electrical pulses to block vagus nerve signals between the brain and stomach. It is less effective than bariatric surgery for weight loss. The list price for the Maestro system is $19,000.

- The AspireAssist device is FDA approved for weight loss in adults ≥22 years old with a BMI of 35 to 55. It requires the insertion of a PEG tube endoscopically and pulled through a percutaneous incision. Thirty minutes after a meal, the patient attaches a connector to it and drains a portion of their stomach content into a toilet. The tube is then flushed with potable water. The connector stops working after 115 cycles (6 weeks) and is replaced at a follow-up appointment. Estimated cost for procedure and follow-ups are $13,000 for first year.

DISPOSITION

- The incidence of venous thromboembolism in the upper tertile of BMI was 2.42 times that of the lowest BMI tertile. Obese patients have a higher incidence of postoperative thromboembolic events when undergoing noncardiac surgery.
- Obesity may be associated with higher rates of postoperative pulmonary complications and poor wound healing.
- Weight-stable obese subjects have an increased risk of arrhythmias and sudden death even in the absence of cardiac dysfunction.
- Obesity and the cardiac autonomic nervous system are intrinsically related. A 10% increase in body weight is associated with a decline in parasympathetic tone accompanied by a rise in mean heart rate. Conversely, a 10% weight loss in severely obese patients is associated with significant improvement in autonomic nervous system cardiac modulation, including decreased heart rate and increased heart rate variability.
- Postmortem Determinants of Atherosclerosis in Youth (PDAY) study data provided convincing evidence that obesity in adolescents and young adults accelerates the progression of atherosclerosis decades before the appearance of clinical manifestations.
- Obesity accelerates the progression of native coronary atherosclerosis and after coronary artery bypass grafting.
- In older adults, obesity is associated with protection against hip fracture, but this protective effect on bone status does not offset the extensive array of potential adverse effects on conditions common in the older population.

REFERRAL

- Obesity is commonly seen in the primary care setting. If pharmacologic therapy is considered, consultation with physicians specializing in obesity and experienced with the use of the drug is recommended. In addition, consultation with nutritionists and behavioral

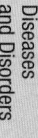

therapists is helpful. A consultation with general surgery is indicated in patients being considered for surgical intervention.

- Recent trials have shown that among adolescents, use of gastric banding compared with lifestyle intervention results in a greater percentage achieving a loss of 50% of excess weight corrected for age. There were associated benefits to health and quality of life.

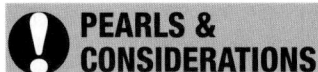
PEARLS & CONSIDERATIONS

COMMENTS

- Enhanced weight-loss counseling helps about one third of obese patients achieve long-term, clinically meaningful weight loss.
- The NHLBI launched the Obesity Education Initiative in January 1991. The overall purpose of the initiative is to help reduce the prevalence of overweight along with the prevalence of physical inactivity to reduce the risk of CHD and overall morbidity and mortality rates from CHD.
- The American Medical Association, in association with the Robert Wood Johnson Foundation and the U.S. Department of Health and Human Services, produced a primer for the assessment and management of adult obesity. The primer consists of 10 booklets that offer practical recommendations for addressing adult obesity in the primary care setting and is available free of charge at: http://www.amaassn.org/ama/pub /physician-resources.
- A recent study on BMI and all-cause mortality in a large prospective study suggests that

optimal BMI range is between 20 and 24.9 (Patel AV, 2014).

- Recent research indicates that brown adipose tissue represents a natural target for the modulation of energy expenditure. The presence of brown adipose tissue in humans may be quantified with the use of ^{18}F-FDG PET-CT. The amount of brown adipose tissue is inversely correlated with BMI, suggesting a potential role of brown adipose tissue in adult human metabolism.
- Obesity, glucose intolerance, and hypertension in childhood are strongly associated with increased rates of premature death from endogenous causes in this population.
- Recent trials have shown that among persons living in a controlled setting, calories alone account for the increase in fat. Protein affected energy expenditure and storage of lean body mass, but not body fat storage.
- There have been no evidence-based studies supporting combination medical therapy for weight loss.
- Data are lacking for the role of pharmacotherapy and bariatric surgery in the elderly population.

PREVENTION

- Prevention of overweight and obesity involves both increasing physical activity and dietary modification to reduce caloric intake.
- There is compelling evidence that prevention of weight regain in formerly obese individuals requires 60 to 90 min of moderate-intensity activity or lesser amounts of vigorous intensity activity.
- Moderate-intensity activity of approximately 45 to 60 min per day, or 1.7 physical activity

level (PAL), is required to prevent the transition to overweight or obesity. For children, even more activity time is recommended.

- Clinicians can help guide patients to develop personalized eating plans and help them recognize the contributions of fat, concentrated carbohydrates, and large portion sizes.
- Clinicians must work with patients to modify other risk factors such as tobacco use, high glycemic intake, and elevated blood pressure to prevent the long-term chronic disease sequelae of obesity.
- Regular screening of body weight and BMI measurements at routine office visits can help identify early weight gain.

PATIENT & FAMILY EDUCATION

Information can be obtained on the American Obesity Association website (http://www.obesity .org) and the American Medical Association website (http://www.ama-assn.org).

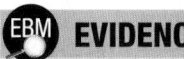
EVIDENCE

Available at www.expertconsult.com

SUGGESTED READINGS
Available at www.expertconsult.com

RELATED CONTENT

Obesity, Female (Patient Information)
Obesity, Male (Patient Information)
Obesity, Child (Patient Information)

AUTHOR: **CRAIG L. BASMAN, M.D.**

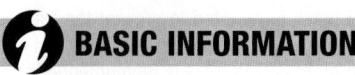

BASIC INFORMATION

DEFINITION

Obsessive-compulsive disorder (OCD) is characterized by obsessions (recurrent and persistent thoughts, urges, or images experienced as intrusive and unwanted) and/or compulsions (repetitive behaviors or mental acts performed in response to obsessions, or according to rules that must be applied rigidly) that are time-consuming (e.g., >1 hr/day) or cause marked impairment or distress. The symptoms are usually perceived as excessive and unreasonable.

SYNONYMS

OCD

ICD-10CM CODES
F42   Obsessive-compulsive disorder
F60.5 Obsessive-compulsive personality disorder

EPIDEMIOLOGY & DEMOGRAPHICS

PEAK INCIDENCE: Mean age at onset is 19.5 yr.
12-MONTH PREVALENCE: 1.2% of adults in the U.S., international prevalence estimates are similar (1.1% to 1.8%).
PREDOMINANT SEX: Slightly more common among females than males in adulthood, although males are more commonly affected in childhood.
PREDOMINANT AGE:
- Modal age of onset for females is between 20 and 29 yr.
- Modal age of onset for males is between 6 and 15 yr.
DISEASE COURSE:
- Condition is chronic with waxing and waning pattern.
- Symptoms typically worsen with stress.
- 15% show progressive deterioration, whereas 5% show an episodic course with little impairment between episodes.
GENETICS:
- OCD is a multifactorial familial condition that involves both polygenic and environmental risk factors.
- Rate of concordance is higher in monozygotic (57%) compared with dizygotic (27%) twins.
- Rate of disorder is also much higher in first-degree relatives of individuals with OCD and Tourette's disorder (8.2%) than in the general population (2%).

PHYSICAL FINDINGS & CLINICAL PRESENTATION

- Persistent and recurrent intrusive and ego-dystonic obsessive ideas, thoughts, urges, or images that are perceived as alien and beyond one's control.
- Frequent experiencing of obsessions related to contamination (e.g., when using the telephone), excessive doubt (e.g., was the door locked?), organization (the need for a particular order), violent impulses (e.g., to yell obscenities in church), or intrusive sexual imagery.
- Compulsive behaviors (e.g., repeated hand washing, checking, rearranging) or mental rituals (e.g., counting, repeating phrases)

meant to temporarily ameliorate anxiety caused by obsessions.
- Obsessions and compulsions almost always accompanied by high anxiety and subjective distress. Both are usually seen as excessive and unreasonable.

ETIOLOGY

- Strong evidence of cortico-striato-thalamo-cortical circuit dysfunction.
- OCD onset may be temporally associated with infectious illness of CNS (e.g., Von Economo's encephalitis, Sydenham's chorea).
- OCD may follow head trauma or other premorbid neurologic condition, including birth hypoxia and Tourette's syndrome.
- Serotonergic, dopaminergic, and glutamatergic systems believed important in some ritualistic instinctual behaviors, with dysfunction of these pathways possibly giving rise to OCD.

DIAGNOSIS

DIFFERENTIAL DIAGNOSIS

- Obsessive-compulsive personality disorder (OCPD) is a maladaptive personality style defined by excessive rigidity, need for order and control, preoccupation with details, and excessive perfectionism. Unlike OCD, OCPD is ego-syntonic.
- Other psychiatric disorders in which obsessive or intrusive thoughts occur (e.g., body dysmorphic disorder, eating disorders, hypochondriasis, phobias, posttraumatic stress disorder).
- Impulse control disorders (e.g., trichotillomania [hair-pulling disorder], excoriation [skin-picking] disorder, pathologic gambling disorder, compulsive shopping, kleptomania, paraphilias/sexual compulsions).
- Neurologic disorders with repetitive behaviors (e.g., Tourette's syndrome, Sydenham's chorea, torticollis, autism).
- Delusions or psychosis, which may be mistaken for obsessive thoughts; unlike OCD, these individuals do not believe their obsessions are unreal and may likely meet criteria for another psychotic spectrum disorder that fully accounts for the obsessions (e.g., schizophrenia).

WORKUP

- Careful history leading to diagnosis.
- In adolescents and children: psychological testing to reveal learning disabilities.
  Screen for presence of past or current tic disorder, and ascertain degree of insight (good or fair, poor, absent/delusional) into OCD beliefs.

TREATMENT

NONPHARMACOLOGIC THERAPY

- Treatment will help ~50% of patients achieve partial remission within the first 6 mo.
- Cognitive-behavioral therapy (CBT), especially exposure/response prevention, is successful in up to 70% of patients, but nearly 25% drop out of treatment because of the initial anxiety the exposures create. Best results

are found for contamination obsessions and washing compulsions.

GENERAL Rx

- Antidepressants with serotonin reuptake blockade, including clomipramine, fluvoxamine, fluoxetine, paroxetine, sertraline, citalopram and escitalopram, venlafaxine, and duloxetine; optimal dosages are typically at the high end of the prescription range. Risk/benefit/alternatives discussion is crucial (e.g., dose-related risk of QT interval prolongation with serotonin reuptake inhibitors in general and clomipramine, citalopram, and escitalopram in particular).
- Clonazepam may be helpful in patients with extreme anxiety.
- Most improve with treatment, but only 20% become symptom-free. No response in 15% of patients.
- Likely indefinite treatment. Relapse is common if medications are discontinued.
- Recent studies suggest that combination CBT and pharmacotherapy yields superior outcomes. More severe symptoms warrant combination therapy.
- Patients who do not respond to first-line treatments and those with comorbid psychosis and/or tic disorders may benefit from augmentation with a first- or second-generation antipsychotic medication (e.g., haloperidol, olanzapine, risperidone).
- Neurosurgical intervention (e.g., cingulotomy, deep brain stimulation) is reserved for the most severely symptomatic and treatment-resistant cases.

DISPOSITION

- Most mild to moderate cases can be managed on a regular outpatient basis. Treatment should typically start with SSRI monotherapy with regular follow-up to assess treatment response and side-effect management. Dose should be increased to maximum tolerated.
- Patient and family education may help improve medical adherence and support.

PEARLS & CONSIDERATIONS

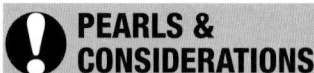

Patients with OCD typically have insight regarding the irrationality of their obsessions and compulsions but lack the ability to control them. This may cause intense shame and avoidance of medical care unless patient education and support are provided. Screen for OCD, especially among patients who present with "depression" or "anxiety."

SUGGESTED READINGS

Available at www.expertconsult.com

RELATED CONTENT

Obsessive-Compulsive Disorder (OCD) (Patient Information)

AUTHOR: **AGUSTIN G. YIP, M.D., PH.D.**

BASIC INFORMATION

DEFINITION

- Opioid addiction/dependence is defined as a cluster of cognitive, behavioral, and physiologic symptoms in which the individual continues use of opiates despite significant opiate-induced problems. Opiate dependence is a chronic, relapsing disorder characterized by repeated self-administration that usually results in opiate tolerance, withdrawal, and compulsive drug use. Tolerance is the need to increase dose to achieve the same effect. Dependence may occur with or without the physiologic symptoms of tolerance and withdrawal.
- There are four stages of addiction:
  1. Stage I, acute drug effects: rewarding effects of drug result from neurobiologic changes in response to the acute drug use. Duration varies from hours to days.
  2. Stage II, transformation to addiction: associated with changes in neuronal function that accumulate with repeated administration and diminish over days or weeks after discontinuation of drug use.
  3. Stage III, relapse after extended periods of abstinence: precipitated by an incubation of cue-induced craving (people, places, and things as triggers) and priming (relapse precipitated by drug exposure).
  4. Stage IV, end-stage addiction: vulnerability to relapse endures for years and results from prolonged changes at the cellular level.
- Pseudoaddiction: undertreatment of pain resulting in "opiate-seeking" behaviors such as "doctor shopping" and multiple emergency department visits. These behaviors disappear with adequate treatment of pain.

SYNONYMS

Opiate addiction
Opiate abuse
Narcotic addiction
Narcotic abuse
Substance use disorder

ICD-10CM CODES
F11.10	Opioid abuse, uncomplicated
F11.120	Opioid abuse with intoxication, uncomplicated
F11.121	Opioid abuse with intoxication delirium
F11.122	Opioid abuse with intoxication with perceptual disturbance
F11.129	Opioid abuse with intoxication, unspecified
F11.14	Opioid abuse with opioid-induced mood disorder
F11.150	Opioid abuse with opioid-induced psychotic disorder with delusions
F11.151	Opioid abuse with opioid-induced psychotic disorder with hallucinations
F11.159	Opioid abuse with opioid-induced psychotic disorder, unspecified
F11.181	Opioid abuse with opioid-induced sexual dysfunction
F11.182	Opioid abuse with opioid-induced sleep disorder
F11.188	Opioid abuse with other opioid-induced disorder
F11.19	Opioid abuse with unspecified opioid-induced disorder

EPIDEMIOLOGY & DEMOGRAPHICS

INCIDENCE: There are more than 980,000 opiate addicts in the U.S.; less than one third are in treatment.

PREVALENCE:
- In 2014, U.S. retail pharmacies dispensed 245 million prescriptions for opioid pain relievers.
- In 2014, 10.3 million persons reported using prescription opioids nonmedically.
- In the U.S., 400,000 persons have used heroin in the past month, and 4 million have reported nonmedical use of prescription pain relievers.
- Emergency department visits involving misuse or abuse of prescription opioids increased 153% between 2004 and 2011.
- Admissions to substance-abuse treatment programs linked to prescription opioids more than quadrupled between 2002 and 2012.
- The percentage of eighth-, tenth-, and twelfth-graders who have used heroin has more than doubled since the late 1990s. This increase has largely been attributed to decreased price and increased purity in the last decade.
- In 2014, nearly 29,000 people died of opiate overdose.
- In March and October 2015, the Drug Enforcement Administration and Centers for Disease Control and Prevention issued nationwide alerts identifying fentanyl, particularly illicitly manufactured fentanyl, as a threat to public health and safety. Illicitly manufactured fentanyl is pharmacologically similar to pharmaceutical fentanyl but is unlawfully produced in clandestine laboratories and obtained via illicit drug markets; it also includes fentanyl analogs. Fentanyl is a synthetic opioid 50 to 100 times more potent than morphine and approved for the management of surgical/postoperative pain, severe chronic pain, and breakthrough cancer pain.
- In the U.S., the opioid analgesic overdose death rate increased from 1.4 to 5.4 per 100,000 adults from 1999 to 2011.

PREDOMINANT SEX: Males abuse opiates more commonly than females, with a male/female ratio of 3:1 for heroin and 1.5:1 for prescription opiates.

PEAK INCIDENCE: The majority of new abusers of opiates are <26 yr.

RISK FACTORS:
- Family history
- Prior history of addiction
- Psychiatric disorders

GENETICS:
- Genetic epidemiologic studies suggest a high degree of heritable vulnerability for opiate dependence.
- Gene polymorphism for dopamine receptor/transporters, opioid receptors, serotonin receptors/transporters, proenkephalin, and catechol-*O*-methyltransferase all appear to be associated with vulnerability to opiate dependence. Future interventions for opiate dependence may include medications identified through genetic research.

PHYSICAL FINDINGS & CLINICAL PRESENTATION

- Physical examination is often noncontributory.
- Small-sized pupils may be the only observable sign of use because only mild tolerance develops for miosis.
- Scars or tracks from chronic IV use may be visible over the veins of the arms, hands, ankles, neck, and breasts.
- Inflamed nasal mucosa or respiratory wheezing may be apparent in patients who are snorting heroin or OxyContin.
- Patients in withdrawal may have more dramatic findings such as tachycardia, hypertension, fever, piloerection (goose flesh), mydriasis, lacrimation, central nervous system (CNS) arousal, irritability, and repeated yawning. In patients with sympathetic overactivity and panic attacks, use of CNS stimulants, such as amphetamines or cocaine, should also be ruled out.
- Although gastrointestinal symptoms of nausea, vomiting, and abdominal pain are common in opiate withdrawal, other causes such as gastroenteritis, pancreatitis, peptic ulcer disease, and intestinal obstruction need to be ruled out.
- The history may provide relevant information in making the diagnosis. Significant findings may include:
  1. A long history of opiate self-administration, typically by the IV or intranasal route but sometimes through smoking as well.
  2. Polysubstance use. Intoxication by drugs other than narcotics (e.g., benzodiazepines, barbiturates) should be ruled out in unconscious patients.
  3. A high incidence of non-opiate-related psychiatric disorders (>80%).
  4. History of problems at work, school, or relationships associated with drug use.
  5. History of legal problems associated with drug use, such as arrest for possession, robbery, or prostitution.
  6. History of interpersonal violence (as perpetrator or victim).
  7. History of physical problems such as skin infections, phlebitis, endocarditis, or liver diseases attributable to acetaminophen toxicity (Vicodin/Percocet) or viral hepatitis. Hepatitis C is the most prevalent bloodborne pathogen. It is present in approximately 90% of opiate-dependent people and is often spread by sharing IV drug paraphernalia or snorting devices. There is also a higher incidence of HIV infection.

ETIOLOGY

Opioid dependence is a biopsychosocial disorder. Pharmacologic, social, genetic, and psychodynamic factors interact to influence abusive behaviors. Pharmacologic factors are especially

TABLE 1   Cage-Aid

1. Have you ever tried to **C**ut down on your alcohol or drug use?
2. Do you get **A**nnoyed when people comment about your drinking or drug use?
3. Do you feel **G**uilty about things you have done while drinking or using drugs?
4. Do you need an **E**ye-opener to get started in the morning?

Two or more questions answered in the affirmative require further assessment. *AID*, adapted to include drugs.
From Bowman S, Eiserman J, Beletsky, L, Stancliff S: Reducing the health consequences of opioid addiction in primary care, *Am J Med* 126, 565-571, 2013.

TABLE 2   Drug Abuse Screening Test (DAST-10)

1. Have you used drugs other than those required for medical reasons?
2. Do you abuse more than one drug at a time?
3. Are you unable to stop using drugs when you want to?
4. Have you ever had blackouts or flashbacks as a result of drug use?
5. Do you ever feel bad or guilty about your drug use?
6. Does your spouse (or parents) ever complain about your involvement with drugs?
7. Have you neglected your family because of your use of drugs?
8. Have you engaged in illegal activities in order to obtain drugs?
9. Have you ever experienced withdrawal symptoms (felt sick) when you stopped taking drugs?
10. Have you had medical problems as a result of your drug use (e.g., memory loss, hepatitis, convulsions, bleeding)?

Two or more questions answered in the affirmative require further assessment.
From Bowman S, Eiserman J, Beletsky, L, Stancliff S: Reducing the health consequences of opioid addiction in primary care, *Am J Med* (2013) 126, 565-571.

prominent in opiate addiction because these drugs are strong reinforcing agents because of their euphoric effects and their ability to reduce anxiety and increase self-esteem and the patient's subjective feelings of improved ability to cope with daily challenges.

(Dx) DIAGNOSIS

DIFFERENTIAL DIAGNOSIS

- Psychiatric disorders (e.g., anxiety, depression, bipolar disorder).
- Acute medical illness (e.g., hypoglycemia, seizure disorder, sepsis, renal or hepatic insufficiency) may mimic opiate withdrawal symptoms.

WORKUP

The history is the most important part of the workup. Useful screening tools are the CAGE-AID (Table 1), the DAST-10 (Table 2), and the CRAFFT (Table 3). The CAGE-AID has a sensitivity of 70% and a specificity of 85% when two questions are answered in the affirmative. The DAST-10 can

TABLE 3   CRAFFT Screening Tool for Adolescents

1. Have you ever ridden in a **C**ar driven by someone (including yourself) who was high or had been using alcohol or drugs?
2. Do you ever use alcohol or drugs to **R**elax, feel better about yourself, or fit in?
3. Do you ever use alcohol or drugs while you are by yourself **A**lone?
4. Do you ever **F**orget things you did while using alcohol or drugs?
5. Do your **F**amily or Friends ever tell you that you should cut down on your drinking or drug use?
6. Have you ever gotten into **T**rouble while you were using alcohol or drugs?

Two or more questions answered in the affirmative require further assessment.
From Bowman S, Eiserman J, Beletsky L, Stancliff S: Reducing the health consequences of opioid addiction in primary care, *Am J Med* 126, 565-571, 2013.

discriminate between current users versus former users. The CRAFFT is a useful screening tool for adolescents. A CRAFFT score of 2 or higher is optimal for identifying any problem (sensitivity 76%, specificity 94%), any disorder (sensitivity 80%, specificity 86%), and drug dependence (sensitivity 92%, specificity 80%).

- Observation of opiate withdrawal is indicative of opiate addiction.
- Observation of purposeful behaviors such as complaints and manipulations directed at getting more drugs and anxiety during withdrawal is suggestive of opiate addiction.
- Screen blood and urine for opiate metabolites.
- Screen for communicable diseases: HIV, hepatitis B and hepatitis C, tuberculosis.
- Screen for endocarditis in patients with newly diagnosed murmurs.

LABORATORY TESTS

- Urine and serum toxicology screen
- Complete blood count
- Chemistries (alanine aminotransferase, aspartate aminotransferase, serum creatinine): elevated liver function test (LFT) results may be from viral hepatitis or acetaminophen toxicity
- Hepatitis screen: if hepatitis C antibody positive, follow up with hepatitis C polymerase chain reaction (viral load) even in patients with normal LFTs
- HIV
- PPD

IMAGING STUDIES

Generally not helpful in routine diagnosis and treatment. Consider echocardiography in patients with heart murmurs and liver sonography or CT scan in patients with elevated LFTs or who are positive for hepatitis C or B (increased risk of hepatocellular carcinoma).

(Rx) TREATMENT

NONPHARMACOLOGIC THERAPY

- Brief counseling interventions during a visit with their primary care physician or OB/

TABLE 4   Basic Components of Opioid Overdose Prevention Education Curriculum

1. Know the signs of an opioid overdose (e.g., unresponsive, limp, slow, shallow breathing, pale or clammy, finger nails or lips turning blue, gurgling)
2. Call 911
3. Administer rescue breathing
4. Administer naloxone if no response and Emergency Medical Services have not yet arrived
5. Stay with the person until help arrives

From Bowman S, Eiserman J, Beletsky, L, Stancliff S: Reducing the health consequences of opioid addiction in primary care, *Am J Med* 126, 565-571, 2013.

GYN have proved efficacious in motivating patients for treatment.
- Therapeutic communities (residential).
- 12-step or other self-help groups (e.g., Alcoholics Anonymous, Narcotics Anonymous).
- Relapse prevention (counseling).
- Opioid prevention education (Table 4)

ACUTE Rx

- Medical withdrawal (not overdosed). Opioid withdrawal alone is not recommended for treatment of opioid use disorder in most patients because of increased risk of overdose death and infectious disease (e.g., HIV through IV drug use) following detoxification.
- Short- (30 days) or long-term (30 to 180 days) protocols.
- Buprenorphine (opioid partial agonist) or methadone (opioid agonist) is initiated in tapering doses.
- Clonidine 0.1 mg bid to tid can be used to minimize autonomic symptoms (sweating) and craving.
- Nonsteroidal antiinflammatory drugs for body and muscle aches.
- The anticholinergic dicyclomine can be used to minimize gastrointestinal hyperactivity.
- Nonbenzodiazepine hypnotics, low-dose atypical antipsychotics (e.g., quetiapine), or low-dose tricyclic antidepressants are effective for promoting adequate sleep.
- Psychosocial supports tailored to patient needs should be offered as an adjunct to medical treatment.

CHRONIC Rx

Opioid antagonist treatment:
- Buprenorphine/naloxone is the preferred first-line treatment. Methadone is an alternative in certain populations.
- Naltrexone: does not stabilize neuronal circuitry like partial or full opioid agonists and generally results in poor outcomes, much like Antabuse for alcohol.
- Opioid partial agonist therapy: buprenorphine (Suboxone, Bunavail).
- Opioid agonist therapy: methadone.
NOTE: Buprenorphine and methadone are both metabolized by the cytochrome P450 3a4 and 2d6 I isoenzyme pathways. Prescribers should be aware of multiple possible drug interactions. Methadone and buprenorphine produce

similar improvements during opioid withdrawal, although buprenorphine is associated with less sedation and respiratory depression. To avoid precipitating more intense withdrawal, buprenorphine should be initiated 12 to 18 hours after the last administration of opioids in patients who misuse shorter-acting opioids (48 hours in patients who are receiving long-acting drugs such as methadone), with initial doses of 4 to 8 mg.[1]

PATIENT SELECTION FOR BUPRENORPHINE OR METHADONE

- Appropriate patients for buprenorphine office-based treatment:
  1. Patients interested (highly motivated) in treatment
  2. Have no major contraindications (see following)
  3. Can be expected to be reasonably compliant with treatment
  4. Understand the benefits and risks of buprenorphine treatment
  5. Willing to follow safety precautions
- Less likely to be appropriate for office-based treatment:
  1. Have comorbid dependence on benzodiazepines or other CNS depressants (including ethylene alcohol)
  2. Have significant untreated psychiatric comorbidities
  3. Have active or chronic suicidal or homicidal ideation or attempts
  4. Have multiple previous treatments with frequent relapses
  5. Have poor response to previous treatment with buprenorphine
  6. Have significant medical complications (e.g., hepatic insufficiency, bacterial endocarditis, active tuberculosis)
- Methadone maintenance: narcotic treatment program (clinic setting) indications
  1. Evidence of opiate addiction >1 yr
  2. Two failed previous treatment attempts
  3. Patients not appropriate for office-based treatment
  4. Eligible without active "use" if prior methadone maintenance patient within previous 2 mo
  5. Pregnancy

DISPOSITION

- Opioid addiction is a chronic, relapsing disease.
- High rate of relapse after "detox."
- Relapse potential after medically supervised withdrawal from methadone:
  1. 90% after 1 yr stable in treatment
  2. 80% after 3 yr stable in treatment
  3. 70% after 5 yr stable in treatment
- Postmarketing surveillance indicates that the diversion and abuse of prescription opioid medications increased between 2002 and

2010 and plateaued or decreased between 2011 and 2013. These findings suggest that the U.S. may be making progress in controlling the abuse of opioid analgesics.[2]

REFERRAL

Refer to addiction medicine specialist or narcotic treatment program when the neurobiologic disease of opioid addiction is identified.

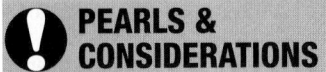

PEARLS & CONSIDERATIONS

COMMENTS

- Methadone maintenance is the gold standard for the pregnant opiate-addicted patient regardless of the duration of the addiction or prior treatment attempts. Detoxification is contraindicated during pregnancy.
- Breastfeeding is encouraged in mothers on methadone maintenance. The American Academy of Pediatrics statement regarding "Transfer of Drugs and Other Chemicals into Human Milk" has placed methadone into the "usually compatible with breastfeeding" group based on the assumption that maternal urine is monitored to detect use of illicit drugs. The U.S. Department of Health and Human Services also recommends that mothers on methadone be encouraged to breastfeed.
- When a physician identifies a patient as a "drug seeker," it is imperative that the physician avoid abruptly stopping the opiate prescription because this will often result in the patient's buying the drugs illegally. These patients should be counseled and referred for treatment.
- Patients on methadone or buprenorphine who have pain resulting from an acute injury will need pain medication in addition to their daily dose of methadone or buprenorphine. They will require higher than usual doses of

pain medications because of opiate receptor blockade attributable to their methadone or buprenorphine use.
- Opiate-dependent patients have a lower pain threshold resulting from hyperalgesia caused by the long-term use of opiates.

PREVENTION

Education is the hallmark of prevention.
- School drug prevention education programs.
- Educate children about their family medical history, including diseases of addiction.
- Address childhood psychiatric disorders to prevent self-medicating.

Opioid overdose
- Naloxone (Narcan) is a competitive mu-opioid receptor antagonist in the brain and is effective for opioid overdose. It is available for IM/IV and intranasal administration. It begins to reverse respiratory depression, sedation, and hypotension 2 to 5 min after IM administration and 1 to 2 min after IV administration.

PATIENT & FAMILY EDUCATION

- Stigma of addictions and treatment often interferes with good treatment.
- Family needs to be educated so they can support the patient's efforts.
- Encourage family meeting with addiction specialist, counselor.
- Recommend support groups for family members. Table 5 identifies organizations providing referral information for patients. Recommendations for integrating risk reduction strategies for addressing opioid misuse in the primary care setting are summarized in Table E6.

SUGGESTED READINGS

Available at www.expertconsult.com

RELATED CONTENT

Drug Abuse (Patient Information)

AUTHOR: **FRED F. FERRI, M.D.**

TABLE 5 Organizations Providing Referral Information for Patients

Organization	Resources/Website
Substance Abuse and Mental Health Services Administration (SAMHSA)	Opioid treatment program directory: http://dpt2.samhsa.gov/treatment/
Physicians who provide buprenorphine	Buprenorphine physician and treatment program locator: http://buprenorphine.samhsa.gov/bwns_locator/
Pain Action	Chronic pain management materials for patients: www.painaction.org
Substance abuse treatment facilities	Substance Abuse treatment facility locator: http://dasis3.samhsa.gov/
Harm Reduction Coalition	Local risk reduction resources and programs, overdose prevention education, and naloxone prescribing information: http://www.harmreduction.org/
Narcotics Anonymous (NA)	General information and meeting information for NA, a 12-step program modeled after Alcoholics Anonymous: www.na.org

From Bowman S, Eiserman J, Beletsky, L, Stancliff S: Reducing the health consequences of opioid addiction in primary care, *Am J Med* 126, 565-571, 2013.

---

[1]Schuckit MA: Treatment of opioid-use disorders, *N Engl J Med* 375:357-368, 2016.

[2]Dart RC et al.: Trends in opioid analgesic abuse and mortality in the United States, *N Engl J Med* 372:241-248, 2015.

ℹ️ BASIC INFORMATION

DEFINITION

Optic neuritis is an inflammation of the optic nerve resulting in impaired visual function.

SYNONYMS

Optic papillitis
Retrobulbar neuritis

ICD-10CM CODES
H46.9 Unspecified optic neuritis
H46.8 Other optic neuritis

EPIDEMIOLOGY & DEMOGRAPHICS

INCIDENCE (IN U.S.): 1 to 5/100,000 person(s) per year; rates vary according to incidence of multiple sclerosis (MS)
PREVALENCE (IN U.S.): Common in patients with MS
PREDOMINANT SEX: Female/male ratio: 1.8:1
PEAK INCIDENCE: 20 to 49 yr, mean 30
GENETICS: Unknown. If due to MS, it is more common in patients with certain HLA blood types and in monozygotic twins of affected siblings.

PHYSICAL FINDINGS & CLINICAL PRESENTATION

- Presentation with acute or subacute (days) visual loss, often accompanied by periocular tenderness that worsens with eye movements.
- **Marcus Gunn pupil** (relative afferent pupillary defect [RAPD]): direct and consensual response is normal; however, when flashlight is swung from eye to eye, the affected eye's pupil dilates to direct light.
- Decreased visual acuity.
- Unilateral visual field abnormalities—often a central scotoma (Fig. E1).
- Color desaturation; red is most often affected.
- Normal fundus examination in 66% cases; disc edema is noted in 33% (Fig. 2). Other abnormalities include uveitis or periphlebitis.
- May have movement or light-induced phosphenes (flashes of light lasting 1 to 2 sec).

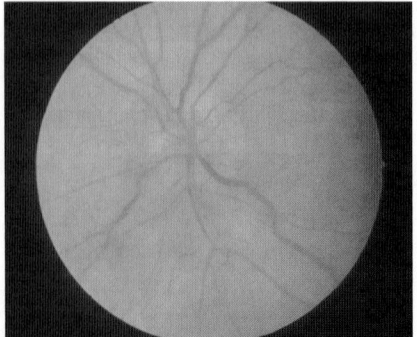

FIG. 2 A case of optic neuritis. The optic disc edema seen here is often not present. Note the otherwise normal fundus. (Courtesy of J. Barton, M.D., Beth Israel Deaconess Medical Center, Boston.)

- Uhthoff's phenomenon (benign exercise- or heat-induced deterioration of vision) is seen in some. Vision may also worsen in bright sunlight.
- Over time the optic disc may atrophy and become pale.

ETIOLOGY

An inflammatory response associated with an infection or autoimmune disease (such as collagen vascular disease, granulomatous disease, MS, or neuromyelitis optica).

🆇 DIAGNOSIS

Diagnosis is clinically established in a young patient with acute onset of monocular vision loss associated with retroorbital pain associated with eye movements and presence of RAPD. Absence of other orbital or ocular pathology is based on clinical examination.

DIFFERENTIAL DIAGNOSIS

For optic neuritis
- Inflammatory: MS, neuromyelitis optica (NMO), sarcoidosis, lupus, Sjögren's, Behçet's, postinfectious, postvaccination, neuroretinitis, acute disseminated encephalomyelitis, paraneoplastic, autoimmune optic neuropathy
- Infectious: syphilis, TB, Lyme disease, *Bartonella,* HIV, CMV, herpes, helminths, chickenpox, Q fever, periorbital infections, *Toxocara* sp.
- Ischemic: anterior and posterior ischemic optic neuropathies, diabetic papillopathy, branch or central retinal artery or vein occlusion
- Drugs and toxins: arsenic, methanol, ethambutol, cyclosporine, etc.
- Mitochondrial: Leber's hereditary optic neuropathy, other mitochondrial

WORKUP

A thorough neurologic examination; dilated ophthalmoscopy.

LABORATORY TESTS

Acute optic neuritis is a clinical diagnosis based on presentation with classical features: acute, painful unilateral loss of vision associated with RAPD in a young person with no other apparent causes such as trauma. In atypical cases additional studies may be considered.
- CBC, ANA, ACE, ESR
- Consider HIV Ab, Lyme titer, RPR, other autoimmune or infectious causes
- Bilateral or recurrent ON: NMO IgG; paraneoplastic CRMP-5-IgG

IMAGING STUDIES

- Contrast-enhanced MRI of the brain is performed to assess the risk of developing MS. Often enhancement of the optic nerve is seen. MRI orbits with thin sections of fat-suppressed sequences may be needed if the patient demonstrates atypical features.
- Consider using optical coherence tomography to follow optic nerve atrophy objectively longitudinally.

℞ TREATMENT

NONPHARMACOLOGIC THERAPY

Assure patient that in most cases there is near complete recovery of vision.

ACUTE Rx

Treat if the visual loss is severe or if there is an abnormal MRI (higher risk of MS). Treatment is with methylprednisolone (MP) 250 mg IV every 6 hr (or 1 g IV daily) for 3 days followed by an oral prednisone taper of 11 days.

CHRONIC Rx

Depends on underlying cause. Disease-modifying treatment when increased risk of developing MS or neuromyelitis optica. See topic "Multiple Sclerosis."

DISPOSITION

Most often vision is worst at the end of week 1, followed by recovery over months. In the Optic Neuritis Treatment Trial (ONTT), 90% had 20/40 or better vision at 1 yr and 3% had 20/200 or worse. Of initial 20/200 or worse cases, only 5% remained in that group at 6 mo.

REFERRAL

- To neurologist for other neurologic signs and to assess risk of developing MS. In ONTT (Optic Neuritis Treatment Trial), risk of MS >15 yr was 72% with ≥1 lesion(s) on MRI, and 25% with a normal MRI
- To ophthalmologist when atypical features or slowly progressive; urgently when other ocular pathology is present or if vision worsens or does not improve after several wk, or pain is severe

❗ PEARLS & CONSIDERATIONS

- Bilateral optic neuritis suggests a systemic inflammatory disorder, infection, NMO, or paraneoplastic, but can also occur in MS.
- Acute bilateral loss of vision with a severe headache or diplopia should raise concern for pituitary apoplexy and/or giant cell arteritis.

🅴🅱🅼 EVIDENCE

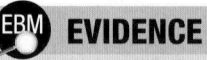
Available at www.expertconsult.com

RELATED CONTENT

Idiopathic Intracranial Hypertension (Related Key Topic)
Multiple Sclerosis (Related Key Topic)

AUTHOR: **SACHIN KEDAR, M.B.B.S., M.D.**

BASIC INFORMATION

DEFINITION

Oral cancers refer to malignant transformation of the oral tissues usually preceded by a process of sequential dysplastic changes leading to the development of squamous carcinoma. Oral squamous cell cancers (OSCC) include oral cavity cancers (lip, floor of mouth, buccal mucosa, anterior tongue, gingivae, hard palate, retromolar trigone), oropharynx cancers (base of tongue, tonsils, soft palate, pharyngeal walls), and hypopharynx cancers (pyriform sinus, postcricoid area, posterior pharyngeal wall)

SYNONYMS

Head and neck cancer
Oral malignant neoplasm
OSCC

ICD-10CM CODES

C01	Malignant neoplasm of base of tongue
C03	Malignant neoplasm of gum
C04	Malignant neoplasm of floor of mouth
C05	Malignant neoplasm of palate
C06	Malignant neoplasm of other and unspecified parts of mouth
C09	Malignant neoplasm of tonsil
C10	Malignant neoplasm of oropharynx
C11	Malignant neoplasm of nasopharynx
C12	Malignant neoplasm of piriform sinus
C13	Malignant neoplasm of hypopharynx
C14	Malignant neoplasm of other and ill-defined sites of lip, oral cavity and larynx
C14.0	Malignant neoplasm of pharynx, unspecified
C14.2	Malignant neoplasm of Waldeyer's ring
C14.8	Malignant neoplasm of overlapping sites of lip, oral cavity and pharynx

EPIDEMIOLOGY & DEMOGRAPHICS

INCIDENCE & PREVALENCE: OSCC comprise the sixth most common cancer in the world. An estimated 530,000 cases are diagnosed annually around the globe, and the rates have been rising, particularly in young people and among minorities. It is estimated that in 2016, approximately 48,330 new cases and 9570 deaths occurred in the U.S. The incidence of oral cancers linked to alcohol and tobacco use has been declining in the U.S., whereas those linked to human papillomavirus (HPV), primarily HPV type 16, are on the rise, especially for cancers located in the tonsils and base of tongue. In developed countries across the world, HPV is increasingly implicated in the growing incidence of oral cancer. In Asian countries where chewing betel nut is customary, oral cancer accounts for up to 40% of cancers in some regions. Squamous cell carcinoma is the most common malignancy that occurs in the oral cavity. Minor salivary gland cancers, lymphomas, and sarcomas are less common.

PREDOMINANT SEX & AGE:

- Male:female ratio is 2.5:1 in the U.S.
- Black males have a higher early incidence in the 50- to 60-yr age group, but with increasing age, white men predominate.

GENETICS: The genes that are critically altered in OSCC include *TP53*, the retinoblastoma family, *p16* and *cyclin D1*. The *TP53*, *CCND1*, and *CDKN2A* genes are established cancer genes in HPV-negative cancers. *TP53* and the genes encoding the Rb family are established cancer genes in HPV-positive cancers. Signaling pathways that are involved in the pathogenesis of oral cancers include that of the human epidermal receptor (HER) family, vascular endothelial growth factor (VEGF) receptor, and signal transducer and activator of transcription 3 (STAT 3). The tumor suppressor gene *TP53* is frequently mutated in HPV-negative tumors.

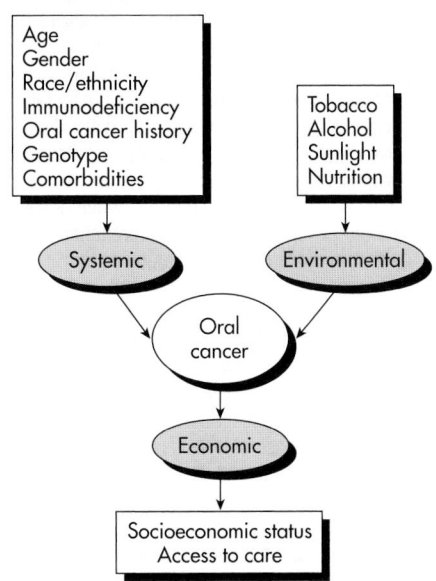

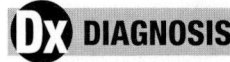

FIG. 1 Risk model for oral cancer. Oral cancer is a multifactorial disease process that includes systemic, environmental, and economic effects. The interplay of these variables ultimately leads to the incidence of this disease. The multifactorial nature of oral cancer should be addressed in the assessment of a patient's risk. (From Jones DL, Rankin KV: Oral cancer and associated risk factors. In Cappelli D Mobley C (eds): *Prevention in clinical oral health care*, St. Louis, 2008, Elsevier, pp 68–77.)

RISK FACTORS (FIG. 1):

- Tobacco use of any kind
- HPV infection (primarily types 16 and 18)
- Alcohol
- Immune deficiency
- Radiation
- Betel nut consumption
- Solar radiation

PHYSICAL FINDINGS & CLINICAL PRESENTATION

- Specific patient complaints may include the following: oral ulcers or mass, choking, difficulty breathing, dysphagia, odynophagia, voice hoarseness, globus sensation, otalgia, ear or nose stuffiness, hemoptysis, trismus, neck mass, and pain in the head/neck region.
- Generalized symptoms and signs may include weight loss, fatigue, anorexia, altered mood, and sleep.
- Clinically, oral cancers can present as:
  1. Erythroplakia (flat red patch); can mimic inflammatory or traumatic lesions
  2. Leukoplakia (white patch; Fig. 2)
  3. Raised lesion
  4. Ulcerated lesion
  5. Warty lesion or growth

DIAGNOSIS

DIFFERENTIAL DIAGNOSIS

- Oral leukoplakia
- Invasive fungal infections
- Chancre of early syphilis and gumma of tertiary syphilis

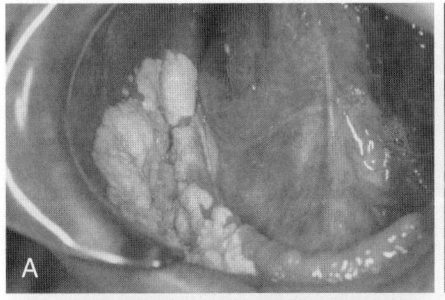
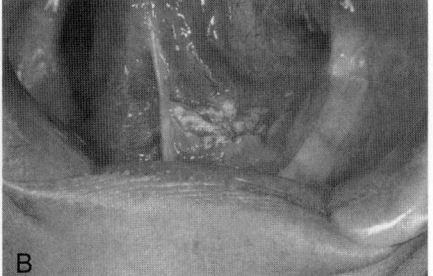
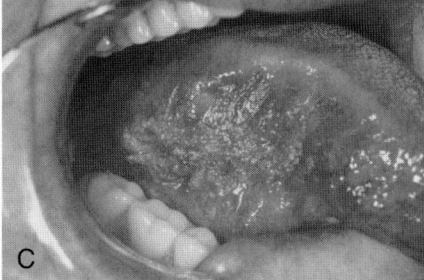

FIG. 2 Squamous cell carcinoma of the oral mucosa. A, Leukoplakia. **B,** Invasive carcinoma of the floor of the mouth. **C,** Invasive carcinoma of the tongue. (Courtesy G. Putnam. In White GM, Cox NH [eds]: *Diseases of the skin: a color atlas and text,* ed 2, St Louis, 2006, Mosby.)

- Chronic ulcer
- Metastatic or locally invading cancers from sinuses or other sites of the body

PATIENT WORKUP

- Primary workup includes either biopsy or fine-needle aspiration (FNA) of the presenting lesion or suspected neck lymph node for histopathologic analysis. HPV assessment with p16 immunohistochemical staining and confirmatory in situ hybridization (ISH) testing is performed when indicated for oropharynx primary tumors.
- Detailed examination of the oral cavity, pharynx, larynx, neck, ears, nose, and cranial nerves should be performed.
- Laryngoscopy and examination under anesthesia are commonly performed.
- Pretreatment evaluation of tumor size, the extent of invasion, and the presence or absence of regional lymph node metastases is critical for planning treatment.
- Laboratory workup can include complete blood count, chemistries including electrolytes, renal panel, liver panel, glucose, and thyroid function.
- Staging workup includes CT or MRI imaging of the head and neck and a chest x-ray. If locoregional or advanced disease is a consideration, the PET scan is typically completed.
- The TNM system is used for staging of OSCC and is subdivided according to primary tumor sites: 1. lip and oral cavity, 2. pharynx.

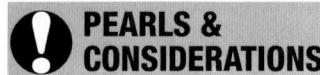 TREATMENT

- Surgery, radiation therapy, and chemotherapy are treatment modalities involved in the treatment plan for OSCC.
- The use of supportive and special therapeutic modalities such as nutritional therapy including feeding gastrostomy, speech and swallowing therapy, reconstructive surgery, and speech prosthesis may be required often.
- For treatment purposes OSCC are classified as early (T1 or T2 lesions), locoregional (T3-4 or any N), or metastatic (M1) stages. Site-specific TNM staging is done as per the primary tumor site (e.g., oral cavity, oropharynx, hypopharynx, etc.)
- After staging completion, the initial treatment considerations include:
  1. Determination of primary tumor resectability (resectable vs. unresectable)
  2. Management of neck nodes

3. Intent of radiation therapy (curative vs. palliative)
4. Need for organ preservation
5. Need for reconstructive surgery
6. Need for chemotherapy
7. HPV status of tumor

- Localized tumors (stage I or II) can be approached by initial surgical resection or definitive radiotherapy. Loco-regionally advanced tumors (stage III and localized IV) that are resectable are typically approached by upfront surgery followed by adjuvant radiation and/or chemotherapy. Unresectable patients are typically treated with definitive chemotherapy and radiotherapy. Patients with distant metastatic disease are treated with systemic chemotherapy, while locally recurrent tumors can be approached with either surgery or chemotherapy or both.
- Surgery is typically associated with less morbidity than radiation therapy. Surgical therapy traditionally involved wide-exposure approaches (mandibulotomy, transpharyngeal access). Newer surgical techniques allow tumor resection through the mouth. Recently, transoral robotic surgery (TORS) has been developed to improve access to oropharyngeal squamous cell carcinomas with excellent oncologic outcomes.
  1. Acute surgical complications can include infection, bleeding, aspiration, wound breakdown, fistula, and flap loss.
  2. Surgical procedures can cause functional deficits in speech and swallowing, but these adverse effects can be minimized by appropriate reconstruction and prostheses.
- Definitive radiation therapy is reserved for patients who cannot tolerate surgery or for whom surgical resection would result in particularly severe functional impairment.
  1. Radiation therapy can include external beam radiation and brachytherapy.
  2. Radiation therapy side effects include mucositis, skin reaction, loss of taste, dysphagia, dental caries and decay, and xerostomia.
  3. Late complications can include skin and soft tissue atrophy and fibrosis, osteoradionecrosis, and trismus.
- Systemic chemotherapy can be administered alone or in combination with radiotherapy, depending on the disease stage. Agents typically used include cisplatin, carboplatin,

5-fluorouracil, taxanes, and the epidermal growth factor receptor (EGFR) antibody cetuximab.
  1. For locally advanced OSCC, the combination of cisplatin and radiotherapy is the regimen of choice.
  2. For metastatic or recurrent OSCC, combination chemotherapy regimens in combination with the EGFR antibody cetuximab have been shown to improve overall survival. More recently, the PD-1 immune checkpoint inhibitors nivolumab and pembrolizumab have been shown to improve survival outcomes in this setting.

DISPOSITION

- Prognosis depends on the staging and resectability of the primary tumor as well as on patient performance status.
- Tumor HPV status is a strong and independent prognostic factor for survival among patients with oropharyngeal cancer.

REFERRAL

Referral to multidisciplinary head and neck cancer team consisting of ENT or head/neck surgeon, radiation oncologist, and medical oncologist.

❗ PEARLS & CONSIDERATIONS

COMMENTS

- Oral and pharyngeal cancer is the sixth most common cancer globally.
- Biopsy is the key for diagnosis.
- Posttreatment surveillance is important.

PREVENTION

- Encourage patients to stop using any type of tobacco and drinking alcohol.
- Examine oral cavities at annual checkups and work up suspicious lesions.

SUGGESTED READINGS
Available at www.expertconsult.com

RELATED CONTENT
Mouth Cancer (Patient Information)

AUTHOR: **RITESH RATHORE, M.D.**

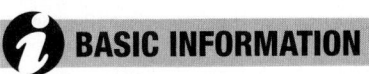

BASIC INFORMATION

DEFINITION

Orchitis is an inflammatory process (usually infectious) involving the testicles. Infection may be viral or bacterial and can be associated with infection of other male sex organs (prostate, epididymis, or bladder) or lower urogenital tract or sexually transmitted diseases often via hematogenous spread. Common causes are:

- Viral: mumps—20% postpubertal; coxsackie B virus
- Bacterial: pyogenic via spread from involving epididymis; bacteria include *Escherichia coli, Klebsiella pneumoniae, P. aeruginosa, Staphylococcus, Streptococcus* or *Rickettsia, Brucella* spp.
- Other:
  1. Viral—HIV-associated, CMV
  2. Fungi
     1. Cryptococcosis
     2. Histoplasmosis
     3. *Candida*
     4. Blastomycosis
     5. Syphilis
  2. *Mycobacterium tuberculosis* and *M. leprae*
  3. Parasitic causes: toxoplasmosis, filariasis, schistosomiasis
- Table 1 describes a classification of epididymitis and orchitis based on etiology.

SYNONYMS

Epididymo-orchitis
Testicular infection
Testicular inflammation

ICD-10CM CODES
N45.9 Orchitis, epididymitis, and epididymo-orchitis without abscess
A54.1 Gonococcal orchitis
A56.1 Chlamydial orchitis
N51.1 Mumps orchitis

EPIDEMIOLOGY & DEMOGRAPHICS

PREDOMINANT SEX: Male
PREDOMINANT ORGANISM: The leading cause of viral orchitis is mumps. The mumps virus rarely causes orchitis in prepubertal males but involves one or both testicles in nearly 30% of postpubertal males.

PHYSICAL FINDINGS & CLINICAL PRESENTATION

- Testicular pain, unilateral or bilateral swelling
- May have associated epididymitis, prostatitis, fever, scrotal edema, erythema, cellulitis
- Inguinal lymphadenopathy
- Acute hydrocele (bacterial)
- Rare development: abscess formation, pyocele of scrotum, testicular infarction
- Spermatic cord tenderness may be present
- Granulomatous

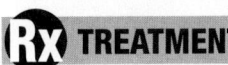 DIAGNOSIS

Clinical presentation as described previously with possible history of acute viral illness or concomitant epididymitis.

DIFFERENTIAL DIAGNOSIS

- Epididymo-orchitis-gonococcal
- Autoimmune disease
- Vasculitis
- Epididymitis
- Mumps, with or without parotitis
- Neoplasm
- Hematoma
- Spermatic cord torsion

LABORATORY TESTS

- CBC with differential
- Urinalysis
- Viral titer—mumps
- Urine culture
- Ultrasound of testicle to rule out abscess

IMAGING STUDIES

Ultrasound if abscess suspected

TREATMENT

- Dependent on cause
- Viral (mumps): observation; bed rest, ice packs, analgesics, and a scrotal sling for support may provide some relief of discomfort that accompanies mumps orchitis
- Bacterial: empiric antibiotic treatment with parenteral antibiotic treatment until pathogen identified: ceftriaxone (250 mg IM once) plus doxycycline (100 mg PO bid for 10 days), in men <35 yr old to cover *Neisseria gonorrhoeae* and *Chlamydia trachomatis*. In homosexual men or men >35 yr old: levofloxacin

500 to 750 mg IV/PO qd for 10 to 14 days *or* ampicillin-sulbactam *or* third-generation cephalosporin or piperacillin/tazobactam.
- Surgery for abscess, pyogenic process

DISPOSITION

Follow-up for evidence of recurrence, hypogonadism, and infertility may be needed with bilateral orchitis.

REFERRAL

- To a urologist if surgical drainage is needed
- To an endocrinologist if hypogonadism develops
- To a fertility specialist if infertility develops

PEARLS & CONSIDERATIONS

Consider tuberculous orchitis if symptoms fail to respond to standard antibacterial therapy, even in the absence of chest radiographic evidence of pulmonary tuberculosis.

SUGGESTED READINGS
Available at www.expertconsult.com

RELATED CONTENT
Orchitis (Patient Information)
Epididymitis (Related Key Topic)
Mumps (Related Key Topic)

AUTHOR: **GLENN G. FORT, M.D., M.P.H.**

TABLE 1 Classification of Epididymitis and Orchitis

Acute Epididymitis or Epididymoorchitis	Granulomatous Epididymitis or Orchitis	Viral Orchitis
Neisseria gonorrhoeae	*Mycobacterium tuberculosis*	Mumps
Chlamydia trachomatis	*Treponema pallidum*	Enteroviruses
Escherichia coli		
Streptococcus pneumoniae	*Brucella* spp.	
Klebsiella spp.	Sarcoid	
Salmonella spp.	Fungal	
Other urinary tract pathogens	Parasitic	
Idiopathic	Idiopathic	

From Cohen J, Powderly WG: *Infectious diseases,* ed 2, St Louis, 2004, Mosby.

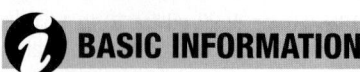

BASIC INFORMATION

DEFINITION

Orthostatic hypotension (OH) is defined as the presence of at least one of the following: a decrease in systolic blood pressure by ≥20 mm Hg or a decrease in diastolic blood pressure by ≥10 mm Hg within 3 min of standing. It is a physical sign that requires further investigation to discern its underlying etiology.

SYNONYMS

Postural hypotension
OH

ICD-10CM CODES
I95.1 Orthostatic hypotension

EPIDEMIOLOGY & DEMOGRAPHICS

- The incidence of OH is increased in older people and in those with diseases associated with autonomic dysfunction (e.g., Parkinson disease, diabetes mellitus) (Table 1).
- OH may cause up to 30% of all syncopal events in the elderly, and OH is associated with an increased risk of heart failure among those aged 45 to 55 yr and an increased risk of cardiovascular disease and all-cause mortality among those aged 55 yr and older.
- There is emerging evidence of an association between orthostatic hypotension and cognitive dysfunction among older adults.

PHYSICAL FINDINGS & CLINICAL PRESENTATION

- Symptoms may include dizziness, lightheadedness, syncope, visual and auditory disturbances, weakness, diaphoresis, pallor, and nausea. OH may also be asymptomatic, especially in older hypertensive patients.
- Associated with increased autonomic activity during meals (from increased splanchnic blood flow), exercise, and hot weather.
- Supine and nocturnal hypertension in patients with OH may indicate an underlying autonomic dysfunction.

ETIOLOGY

- The assumption of an upright posture results in the pooling of approximately 500 mL of blood in the lower extremities due to gravity and decreased venous return, decreased cardiac output, and decreased arterial pressure. The consequent increase in sympathetic tone due to increased carotid baroreceptor activity causes arterial and venous constriction as well as positive inotropic and chronotropic effects, thereby limiting the fall in upright blood pressure. Peripheral vasoconstriction is also mediated by increased activity of the renin-angiotensin system and decreased activity of atrial natriuretic factor.
- Impairment of the baroreceptor reflex, as in central or peripheral autonomic dysfunction and aging, may cause OH because decreased blood pressure cannot be counteracted by the aforementioned regulatory mechanisms.

DIAGNOSIS

DIFFERENTIAL DIAGNOSIS

Common:
- Medications: antihypertensives, antidepressants (tricyclics), antipsychotics (phenothiazines), alcohol, narcotics, barbiturates, insulin, nitrates, PDE-5 inhibitors, alpha-adrenergic antagonists
- Reduced intravascular volume (hemorrhage, dehydration, hyperglycemia, hypoalbuminemia)
- Postprandial effect (especially in the elderly)
- Vasovagal syncope
- Deconditioning

TABLE 1 Causes of Orthostatic Hypotension

Drugs
Diuretics
Alpha-adrenergic blocking drugs
Terazosin (Hytrin), labetalol
Adrenergic neuron blocking drugs
Guanethidine
Angiotensin-converting enzyme inhibitors
Antidepressants
Monoamine oxidase inhibitors
Alcohol
Diuretics
Ganglion-blocking drugs
Hexamethonium, mecamylamine
Tranquilizers
Phenothiazines, barbiturates
Vasodilators
Prazosin, hydralazine, calcium channel blockers
Centrally acting hypotensive drugs
Methyldopa, clonidine

Primary Disorders of Autonomic Failures
Pure autonomic failure (Bradbury-Eggleston syndrome)
Multiple system atrophy (Shy-Drager syndrome)
Parkinson's disease with autonomic failure

Secondary Neurogenic
Aging
Autoimmune disease
Guillain-Barré syndrome, mixed connective tissue disease, rheumatoid arthritis
Eaton-Lambert syndrome, systemic lupus erythematosus
Carcinomatosis autonomic neuropathy
Central brain lesions
Multiple sclerosis, Wernicke encephalopathy
Vascular lesions or tumors involving the hypothalamus and midbrain
Dopamine beta-hydroxylase deficiency
Familial hyperbradykinism
General medical disorders
Diabetes, amyloid, alcoholism, renal failure
Hereditary sensory neuropathies, dominant or recessive
Infections of the nervous system
Human immunodeficiency virus infection, Chagas' disease, botulism, syphilis
Metabolic disease
Vitamin B_{12} deficiency, porphyria, Fabry disease, Tangier disease
Spinal cord lesions

From Bonow RO, et al.: *Braunwald's heart disease: a textbook of cardiovascular medicine*, ed 9, Philadelphia, 2012, Saunders.

- Central autonomic dysfunction (Parkinson's disease)
- Peripheral autonomic dysfunction (diabetes mellitus, Guillain-Barré syndrome)
Uncommon:
- Central autonomic dysfunction (Shy-Drager syndrome)
- Postganglionic autonomic dysfunction: impaired norepinephrine release
- Autoimmune autonomic dysfunction: nicotinic acetylcholine receptor autoantibodies
- Paraneoplastic autonomic dysfunction: anti-Hu antibodies (in small-cell lung cancer)
- Postural tachycardia syndrome (POTS): usually occurs in young women; an abnormally large increase in heart rate is observed in the upright position caused by increased venous pooling from autonomic dysfunction of the lower extremities, but blood pressure is not affected because of an excess of plasma norepinephrine
- Impaired cardiac output (myocardial infarction, aortic stenosis, arrhythmias)
- Cerebrovascular accident
- Adrenal insufficiency
- Deconditioning
- Carotid sinus hypersensitivity
- Anxiety, panic attacks
- Seizures
- Sepsis
- Idiopathic

WORKUP

- Measure supine blood pressure after the patient has been resting comfortably. The duration of time that the patient should spend supine and standing when measuring orthostatic hypotension is controversial. Limited evidence supports having the patient remain supine for 5 to 10 minutes before obtaining the supine blood pressure, followed by blood pressure measurement within 1 minute of standing and again after 3 minutes of standing. The blood pressure cuff must be held at the level of the right atrium; holding the cuff below this level will result in a 5 to 10 mm Hg underestimation of blood pressure.
- Thorough neurologic examination should be performed.
- Rule out treatable causes (e.g., medications, volume depletion).

LABORATORY TESTS

- Hemoglobin and hematocrit
- Consider when treatable causes of OH have been ruled out:
  1. Blood pressure and heart rate monitoring with a tilt table test
  2. Plasma norepinephrine measurements (to distinguish postganglionic from preganglionic autonomic dysfunction)
  3. Other methods, which use the Valsalva maneuver or measure sweating as indirect means of evaluating the autonomic nervous system

IMAGING STUDIES

None

Rx TREATMENT

NONPHARMACOLOGIC THERAPY

- Patient education (leg crossing, prolonged sitting before first standing in the morning, avoid excessive straining and hot baths)
- High-salt diet (e.g., bouillon cubes); caution if history of heart failure
- Liberal fluid intake
- Take needed antihypertensive medications at different times of the day
- Raise the head of the bed at night
- Compression stockings (to include splanchnic circulation)
- Multiple low-carbohydrate meals to avoid postprandial OH
- Avoid large carbohydrate loads and excess alcohol consumption

ACUTE GENERAL Rx

- Correction of volume status
- Review medication list and attempt to eliminate those potentially contributing to OH

CHRONIC Rx

- Fludrocortisone: 0.1 mg/day (may combine with an alpha-1 agonist to lower the dose of each); monitor for electrolyte disturbances and supine hypertension
- Midodrine (alpha-1 agonist): 10 mg three times a day; monitor for supine hypertension
- Erythropoietin (consider if anemic)
- Caffeine (for postprandial hypotension)

OTHER TREATMENTS

- Pyridostigmine (enhances renal sodium reabsorption): 0.2 to 0.6 mg/day (not FDA-approved for this indication)
- Octreotide: 300 to 600 mg/day (not FDA-approved for this indication)
- Indomethacin (prostaglandin inhibitor)
- DDAVP (experimental)
- Droxidopa (used for patients with autonomic dysfunction to increase the availability of norepinephrine) has been FDA approved for treatment of adults with symptomatic neurogenic orthostatic hypotension caused by primary autonomic failure or nondiabetic autonomic neuropathy

⚠ PEARLS & CONSIDERATIONS

COMMENTS

- The presence of OH should always trigger a search for an underlying etiology.
- OH is diagnosed by observing changes in blood pressure, not heart rate.
- Volume depletion should cause an increased heart rate on standing; a lack of heart rate response in this setting suggests autonomic dysfunction.
- Pharmacotherapy with mineralocorticoids may require concomitant potassium replenishment and monitoring for hypertension.
- Evidence to support the efficacy of pharmacologic interventions to treat OH, including midodrine, is limited.

- The etiology of OH is often multifactorial in older patients, but increased susceptibility to volume depletion due to decreased baroreceptor reflexes frequently contributes. Chronic vitamin D deficiency is associated with the development of OH.
- Evidence suggests that nursing home residents with more stringent SBP control (<140 mm Hg) have a lower risk of OH than nursing home residents with less stringent SBP control.
- The physical examination of patients with dizziness, gait disturbance, and/or falls should include an assessment for OH. OH is an independent predictor of unexplained falls in older adults.
- Because OH may be asymptomatic, physical examination of those at risk must include assessment of blood pressure in both the supine and upright positions.

SUGGESTED READINGS

Available at www.expertconsult.com

AUTHOR: **TIMOTHY W. FARRELL, M.D.**

Diseases and Disorders

O

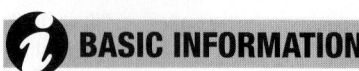

BASIC INFORMATION

DEFINITION
Osgood-Schlatter disease is painful swelling of the growing tibial tuberosity in adolescents.

SYNONYMS
Juvenile osteochondrosis

ICD-10CM CODES
M92.40 Juvenile osteochondrosis of patella, unspecified knee

EPIDEMIOLOGY & DEMOGRAPHICS
PREVALENCE: 4 cases/100 adolescents.
PREDOMINANT SEX: Male/female ratio of 3:1.
PREDOMINANT AGE: Males: ages 13 to 15 years, females: ages 11 to 13 years.

PHYSICAL FINDINGS & CLINICAL PRESENTATION
- Gradual onset of pain and swelling of the tibial tubercle.
- Worsening of pain with athletic activity.
- Tenderness to touch over tibial tubercle, particularly with resisted knee extension.

ETIOLOGY
- Repetitive microtrauma and avulsion of the developing ossification center of the tibial tuberosity.
- Anatomic variants such as patella alta.

DIAGNOSIS

DIFFERENTIAL DIAGNOSIS
- Stress fracture of the proximal tibia.
- Hoffa disease.
- Sinding-Larsen-Johansson syndrome.
- Patellar tendinitis.

WORKUP
- The diagnosis of Osgood-Schlatter disease is made with history and physical examination.
- Imaging may be indicated to exclude fracture or bony tumors.

IMAGING STUDIES
- Lateral x-rays may show separation and fragmentation of the upper tibial epiphysis (Fig. 1).
- Musculoskeletal ultrasound (Fig. 2) can also be used and may be helpful in evaluating soft tissue, tendons, and noncalcified cartilage.

TREATMENT

NONPHARMACOLOGIC THERAPY
- Activity modification with increased periods of rest.
- Physical therapy.

ACUTE GENERAL Rx
- Ice, especially after exercise.

- Nonsteroidal antiinflammatory drugs.
- Quadriceps stretching exercises and cross-training with low-impact sports.

DISPOSITION
- Condition usually heals when the epiphysis closes.
- 90% of patients respond to conservative treatment.
- Recent studies have shown promising results with the use of hyperosmolar dextrose injections in recalcitrant disease.
- Surgery is rarely needed in the treatment of Osgood-Schlatter disease, but can be used for relief of persistent symptoms in which patients have separated ossicles or an abnormally ossified tibial tuberosity.

REFERRAL
Orthopedic consultation is recommended when symptoms persist >6 to 8 weeks with conservative treatment.

PEARLS & CONSIDERATIONS

COMMENTS
Larsen-Johansson disease is a similar disorder. While the diagnosis of Osgood-Schlatter disease is clinical, imaging may be needed to rule out infection, fracture, and malignancy.

SUGGESTED READING
Available at www.expertconsult.com

RELATED CONTENT
Osgood-Schlatter Disease (Patient Information)

AUTHOR: **STEVEN L. BOKSHAN, M.D.**

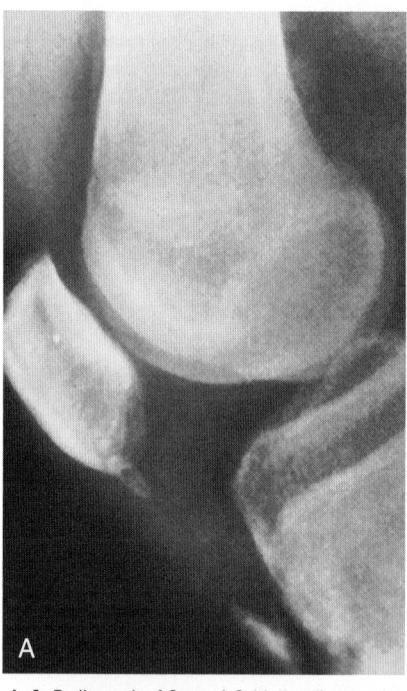
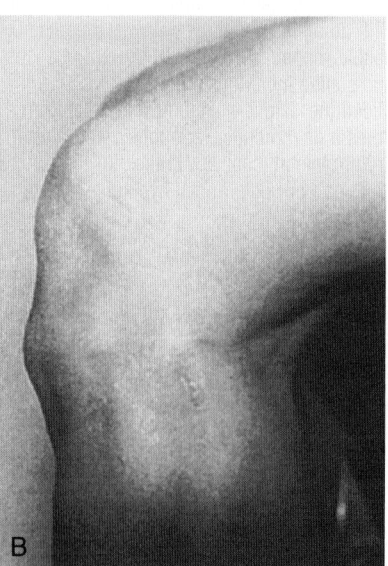

FIG. 1 A, Radiograph of Osgood-Schlatter disease demonstrating thickening of patella tendon, fragmentation of the tibial tubercle, and soft tissue swelling. **B,** Clinical picture of bony prominence anteriorly at the tibial tubercle. (From Scuderi G [ed]: *Sports medicine: principles of primary care,* St Louis, 1997, Mosby.)

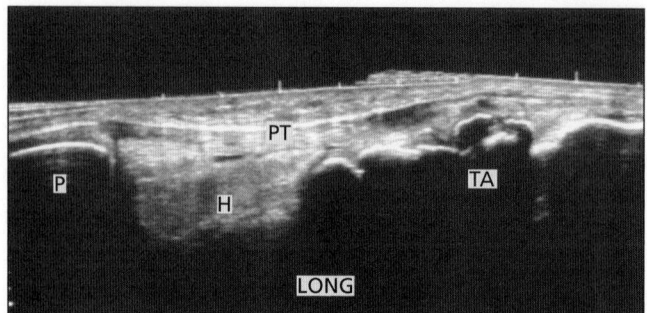

FIG. 2 EFOV of a patient with Osgood-Schlatter disease in the long axis with a knee in extension showing irregularity and fragmentation of the distal tibial apophysis. *P,* Patella; TA, tibial apophysis, PT, patella tendon, H, Hoffa's fat. (From McNally E: *Practical musculoskeletal ultrasound,* ed 1, New York, 2005, Churchill Livingstone, p. 146.)

ℹ BASIC INFORMATION

DEFINITION

Osteoarthritis (OA) is a progressive disease of the joint representing failed repair of joint damage. Intraarticular stresses that lead to joint damage may be initiated by abnormalities in articular cartilage, subchondral bone, ligaments, menisci, periarticular muscles, peripheral nerves, or synovium. The result is the breakdown of cartilage and bone, leading to symptoms of pain, stiffness, and functional disability. The disease is defined as structural abnormalities visualized on plain radiographs and MRI. As an illness, it encompasses a symptom complex of pain, aching, discomfort, stiffness, and sleep disturbance that results in functional limitation, physical disability, and reduced health-related quality of life.

SYNONYMS

Degenerative joint disease (DJD)
DJD
Osteoarthrosis
Arthrosis
OA

ICD-10CM CODES
M15.1	Heberden's nodes (with arthropathy)
M15.2	Bouchard's nodes (with arthropathy)
M15.3	Secondary multiple arthritis
M15.4	Erosive OA
M15.8	Other polyosteoarthritis
M15.9	Polyarthrosis, unspecified
M17	Gonarthrosis (arthrosis of knee)
M18	Arthrosis of first metacarpal joint
M19	Other arthrosis
M19.8	Other specified arthrosis
M19.9	Arthrosis, unspecified

EPIDEMIOLOGY & DEMOGRAPHICS

PREVALENCE: Affects more than 30 million individuals in the U.S.
PREDOMINANT SEX: Prior to age 50, there is almost no gender discrepancy. After age 50, there is increased incidence of OA in females compared to males.
PREDOMINANT AGE: Occurs more frequently after 50 years of age, but it is increasingly being recognized that OA may occur as early as 30 years of age.
GENETICS: 39% to 65% heritability rate in twin studies of women who have generalized OA, concordance rate of 0.64 in monozygotic twins.
RISK FACTORS: Osteoarthritis is considered predominantly a mechanical noninflammatory form of arthritis. Risk factors may be classified as either local or systemic. Local or biomechanical factors include obesity leading to increased load on the articular cartilage, mechanical environment of the joint (includes deformities like pes planus, genu varus and valgus, proprioception at the joint), local joint activity/occupation (textile worker leading to hand OA, high-impact runners leading to knee OA), and muscle weakness (quadriceps weakness leading to knee OA). Systemic risk factors include nutritional factors such as

antioxidant and vitamin D deficiency, hormonal status, high bone mineral density, and genetics (candidate genes being evaluated include IGF-1 gene, cartilage oligomeric protein gene, vitamin D receptor gene). That said, there is no concrete evidence showing that preventing the disease or reducing disease progression can be achieved by supplemental vitamin D, antioxidants, or estrogen.

PHYSICAL FINDINGS & CLINICAL PRESENTATION

- Similar symptoms in most forms: pain generally with activity, stiffness, or gelling (generally short-lived and morning stiffness lasting less than 30 minutes), crepitus
- Joint tenderness, swelling
- Crepitus with motion
- Bouchard's and Heberden's nodes (bony enlargement of the proximal interphalangeal (PIP) and distal interphalangeal (DIP) joints of the hand, respectively) (Fig. E1)
- Pain with range of motion

ETIOLOGY

Primary or idiopathic OA can be monoarticular, oligoarticular, or polyarticular. Secondary OA is due to an identifiable condition such as trauma, mechanical abnormalities, or congenital disorders. Inflammatory arthritis, crystal deposition diseases, metabolic disorders, Paget disease of bone, and osteonecrosis may also contribute to the development of secondary OA.

Ⓓ DIAGNOSIS

DIFFERENTIAL DIAGNOSIS

- Bursitis, tendinitis
- Infectious arthritis
- Crystal arthropathies such as gout and pseudogout
- Inflammatory arthritis such as rheumatoid arthritis (Fig. E2), seronegative arthritis

WORKUP

- No specific laboratory test exists for osteoarthritis.
- Rheumatoid factor, erythrocyte sedimentation rate, complete blood count, and antinuclear antibody tests may be required if inflammatory component is suggested by history.
- Arthrocentesis of swollen joints: synovial fluid examination is generally noninflammatory in character (clear, viscous fluid with normal white cell count)

IMAGING STUDIES

- Plain x-ray of the involved joints is the first step and usually of high diagnostic value.
- Radiographic evaluation (Fig. E3) reveals:
  1. Joint space narrowing
  2. Subchondral sclerosis
  3. New bone formation in the form of osteophytes
- MRI can detect other sources of pain such as synovial thickening, effusions, bone marrow edema, bony attrition, and periarticular lesions.
- Musculoskeletal ultrasound (MSKUS) is emerging as an alternative modality to identify joint damage, presence of osteophytes,

effusions, and noninflammatory synovial proliferation identified using Doppler studies.

℞ TREATMENT

- Optimal use of both pharmacologic and nonpharmacologic measures (Fig. 4) yields best outcome for the management of OA.
- Education and reassurance

NONPHARMACOLOGIC THERAPY
HAND OA:
- Joint protection techniques
- Assistive devices
- Thermal modalities
- Trapeziometacarpal splints

HIP AND KNEE OA:
- Weight loss for overweight patients is probably the most crucial therapy.
- Pedometer step-count of more than 10,000 steps per day has been shown to prevent osteoarthritis.
- Physical therapy includes closed-chain quadriceps strengthening, aerobics, aquatics, and resistance exercises.
- Medial wedge insoles for valgus deformities at the knee.
- Subtalar strapped lateral insoles for varus knees.
- Patellar taping.
- Hinged and unhinged knee braces, offloader knee braces.
- Assistive devices such as canes or walkers.
- Thermal agents.
- Tai chi.

ACUTE GENERAL Rx/ PHARMACOLOGIC Rx

- Hot or cold fomentation.
- Topical applications of capsaicin.
- Topical application of NSAIDs like diclofenac.
- Oral acetaminophen recommended for mild pain.
- Oral NSAIDs definitely more effective than oral acetaminophen. Must consider side effects of NSAIDs, including GI bleeding, cardiovascular toxicity, and renal toxicity. All NSAIDs can increase myocardial infarction risk. Topical NSAIDs are safer than oral NSAIDs.
- Duloxetine if previous initial treatment fails.
- Opioid analgesics including tramadol are recommended only for severe pain that is unresponsive to other treatment modalities.
- Arthrocentesis of the involved joint, followed by intraarticular steroid injection, has been shown to provide short-term relief of symptoms. Clinical studies demonstrate the safety of this approach with regard to the joint.
- Nutritional supplements such as glucosamine and chondroitin are unproven. Most trials indicate that neither glucosamine sulfate nor glucosamine hydrochloride reduces pain compared with placebo in knee or hip osteoarthritis.
- Use of intraarticular hyaluronan injection is controversial. Most trials have shown that hyaluronic acid injections are only minimally better than sham injections in improving pain and function in patients with knee DJD. Positive trials could possibly be influenced by the pharmaceutical industry.

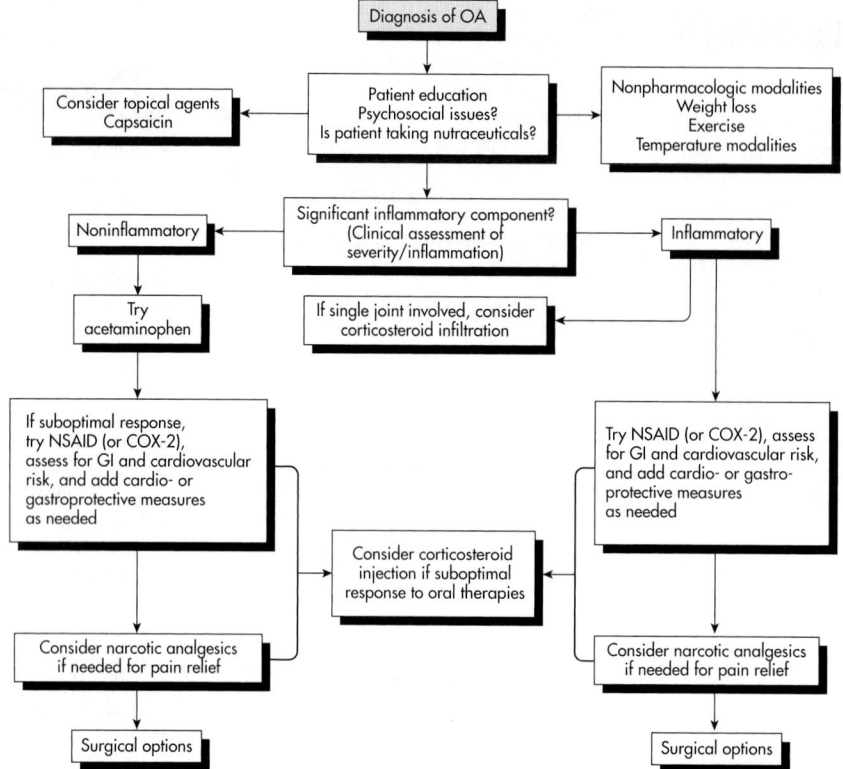

FIG. 4 Algorithm for the management of osteoarthritis (OA). *COX,* Cyclooxygenase; *GI,* gastrointestinal; *NSAID,* nonsteroidal antiinflammatory drug. (Modified from Firestein GS et al: *Kelly's textbook of rheumatology,* ed 9, Philadelphia, 2013, Saunders, Elsevier.)

DISPOSITION

Progression of OA is not always inevitable, and the prognosis is variable depending on the site and extent of the disease.

REFERRAL

Surgical consultation for patients not responding to nonpharmacologic and pharmacologic management. Rheumatology referral could be sought for local injections.

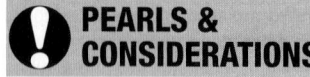

PEARLS & CONSIDERATIONS

COMMENTS

Surgical intervention is generally helpful in degenerative joint disease. Arthroplasty, arthrodesis, and realignment osteotomy are the most common procedures performed. Arthroscopic debridement of the knee appears to be of questionable value. In patients needing hip arthroplasty, resurfacing hip arthroplasty (in which the femoral head is resurfaced with a cap and the neck is preserved) is increasingly popular among younger patients because it results in more hip movement and allows total hip arthroplasty later in the patient's life if necessary.

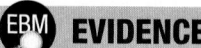 **EVIDENCE**

Available at www.expertconsult.com

SUGGESTED READINGS

Available at www.expertconsult.com

RELATED CONTENT

Osteoarthritis (Patient Information)
Osteoarthritis of the Knee (Patient Information)

AUTHOR: **DEEPAN DALAL, M.D.**

BASIC INFORMATION

DEFINITION

Osteomyelitis is an acute or chronic infection of the bone secondary to the hematogenous or contiguous source of infection or direct traumatic inoculation, which is usually bacterial.

SYNONYMS

Bone infection

ICD-10CM CODES
M86	Osteomyelitis
M86.0	Acute hematogenous osteomyelitis
M86.1	Other acute osteomyelitis
M86.2	Subacute osteomyelitis
M86.3	Chronic multifocal osteomyelitis
M86.6	Other chronic osteomyelitis
M86.9	Osteomyelitis, unspecified

EPIDEMIOLOGY & DEMOGRAPHICS

PREDOMINANT SEX: Male > female
PREDOMINANT AGE: All ages

PHYSICAL FINDINGS & CLINICAL PRESENTATION

HEMATOGENOUS OSTEOMYELITIS:
- Usually occurs in tibia/fibula (children)
- Localized inflammation: often secondary to trauma with accompanying hematoma or cellulitis
- Abrupt fever
- Lethargy
- Irritability
- Pain in involved bone

VERTEBRAL OSTEOMYELITIS:
- Usually hematogenous
- Fever: 50%
- Localized pain/tenderness. Back pain is the most common initial symptom (86% of cases)
- Neurologic defects: motor/sensory (sensory loss, weakness, radiculopathy)

CONTIGUOUS OSTEOMYELITIS:
- Direct inoculation
- Associated with trauma, fractures, surgical fixation
- Chronic infection of skin/soft tissue
- Fever, drainage from surgical site

CHRONIC OSTEOMYELITIS:
- Bone pain
- Sinus tract drainage, nonhealing ulcer
- Chronic low-grade fever
- Chronic localized pain

ETIOLOGY

- *Staphylococcus aureus*
- MRSA: Methicillin-resistant *S. aureus*
- *Pseudomonas aeruginosa*
- Enterobacteriaceae
- *Streptococcus pyogenes*
- Enterococcus
- Mycobacteria
- Fungi
- Coagulase-negative staphylococci
- *Salmonella* (in sickle cell disease)

DIAGNOSIS

DIFFERENTIAL DIAGNOSIS

- Gaucher's disease
- Bone infarction
- Charcot's joint
- Fracture

WORKUP

- ESR, C-reactive protein
- Blood culturing
- Bone culture. A culture of a biopsy specimen has a significantly higher overall diagnostic yield than does a blood culture. Bone samples should be cultured for aerobic and anaerobic bacteria and for fungi
- Pathologic evaluation of bone biopsy for acute/chronic changes consistent with necrosis or acute inflammation
- PCR analysis of specimens obtained by means of biopsy or puncture may be useful for organisms that are difficult to identify (anaerobic bacteria, *Bartonella* sp., *Kingella kingae*); however, broad-range PCR has suboptimal sensitivity and specificity due to contamination and may not provide sufficient information on the susceptibility of the microorganisms to antibiotics

IMAGING STUDIES

- Bone radiograph examination: initial study but not sensitive in early osteomyelitis as may not show changes for as much as 2 wk
- MRI (Fig. 1): most accurate imaging study. CT only if patient has contraindication to MRI
- Triple-phase technetium-99m bone scan (Fig. 2). Typically positive within a few days after onset of symptoms but accuracy is lower than that of MRI
- Gallium scan (Ga-67) scintigraphy with single-photon emission CT (SPECT) has higher accuracy than bone scan but is less sensitive for detection of epidural abscess in vertebral osteomyelitis

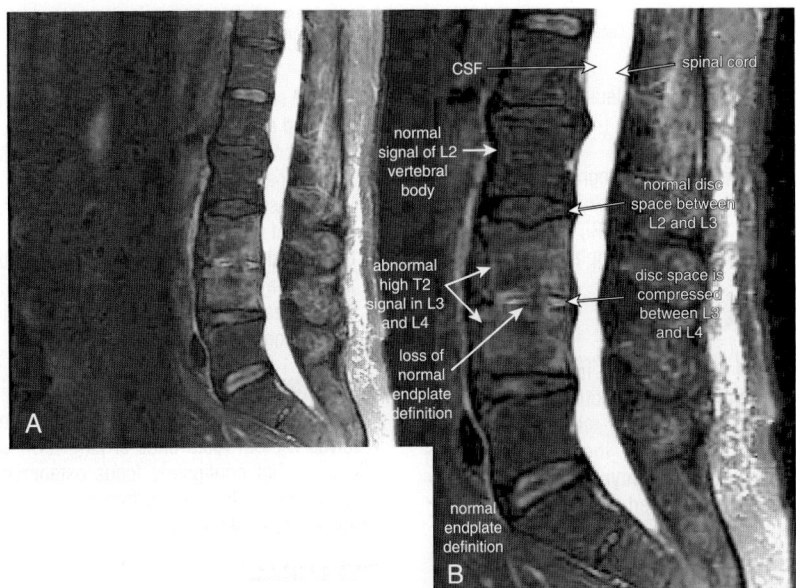

FIG. 1 Osteomyelitis and discitis of L3 and L4. A, T2-weighted fast spin–echo magnetic resonance imaging without contrast demonstrates typical findings of vertebral osteomyelitis and discitis. **B,** Close-up. The inferior endplate of L3 and the superior endplate of L4 are abnormal and ill-defined. The L3 and L4 vertebral bodies show a high T2 signal, indicating an abnormally high fluid content. In comparison, L2 shows a normal marrow signal and appears dark gray due to a normal fat signal. *CSF,* Cerebrospinal fluid. (From Broder JS: *Diagnostic imaging for the emergency physician,* Philadelphia, 2011, Saunders.)

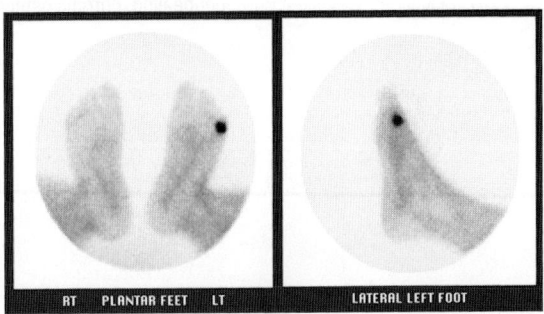

FIG. 2 Osteomyelitis. Intense accumulation of Tc-99m WBCs in proximal phalanx of fifth digit of left foot at 4 hr after injection. (From Specht N [ed]: *Practical guide to diagnostic imaging,* St Louis, 1998, Mosby.)

TABLE 1 Antimicrobial Therapy for Selected Microorganisms in Chronic Osteomyelitis in Adults

Microorganism	First Choice*	Alternative Choice
Methicillin/oxacillin/nafcillin-sensitive staphylococci	Nafcillin sodium or oxacillin sodium 1.5-2 g IV q4- for 4-6 wk *or* cefazolin 1-2 g IV q8h for 4-6 wk	Vancomycin 15 mg/kg IV q12h for 4-6 wk
Methicillin/oxacillin/nafcillin-resistant staphylococci (MRSA)	Vancomycin[†] 15 mg/kg IV q12h for 4-6 wk *or* daptomycin 6 mg/kg IV q24h	Linezolid 600 mg PO/IV q12h *or* levofloxacin[†] 500-750 mg PO/IV daily, plus rifampin 600-900 mg PO for 6 wk if susceptible to both drugs
Penicillin-sensitive streptococci	Aqueous penicillin G 20×10^6 U/24 hr IV either continuously or in six equally divided daily doses *or* ceftriaxone 1-2 g IV q24h *or* cefazolin 1-2 g IV q8h for 4-6 wk	Vancomycin 15 mg/kg IV q12h for 4-6 wk
Enterococci	Aqueous crystalline penicillin G 20×10^6 U/24 hr IV either continuously or in six equally divided daily doses *or* ampicillin sodium 12 g/24 hr IV either continuously or in six equally divided daily doses; the addition of gentamicin sulfate 1 mg/kg IV or IM q8h for 1-2 wk is *optional*	Vancomycin[†] 15 mg/kg IV q12h; the addition of gentamicin sulfate 1 mg/kg IV or IM q8h for 1-2 wk is *optional*
Enterobacteriaceae	Ceftriaxone 1-2 g IV q24h for 4-6 wk or ertapenem 1 g IV q24h	Ciprofloxacin 500-750 mg PO q12h for 4-6 wk or levofloxacin 500-750 mg PO q24h
Pseudomonas aeruginosa	Cefepime 2 g IV q12h, meropenem 1 g IV q8h, or imipenem 500 mg IV q6h for 4-6 wk	Ciprofloxacin 750 mg PO q12h for 4-6 wk or ceftazidime 2 g IV q8h

MRSA, Methicillin-resistant *Staphylococcus aureus*.
*Antimicrobial selection should be based on in vitro sensitivity data, as well as allergies, intolerances, and drug interactions in individual patients.
[†]Doses shown are based on normal renal and hepatic function and may need to be adjusted or serum levels monitored (vancomycin).
Adapted from Berbari EF et al: Osteomyelitis. In Bennett JE et al: *Mandell, Douglas, and Bennett's principles and practice of infectious diseases,* ed 8, Philadelphia, 2015, Saunders.

- Indium-111–labeled leukocyte scintigraphy scan; low sensitivity (<20%) for vertebral osteomyelitis
- Positron-emission tomography (PET) scanning with ^{18}F-fluorodeoxyglucose has high accuracy (similar to MRI) and is useful in patients with metallic implants

(Rx) TREATMENT

- Surgical debridement in biopsy-positive cases will guide direction for antibiotic therapy. This will vary with type of osteomyelitis. Duration of therapy is usually 6 wk for acute osteomyelitis; chronic osteomyelitis may need a longer course of medication
- *S. aureus:* cefazolin IV, nafcillin IV, vancomycin IV (in patient allergic to penicillin)
- *S. aureus* (methicillin resistant): vancomycin IV, linezolid, daptomycin, or
- *Streptococcus* spp.: ceftriaxone, IV penicillin G in sensitive species
- *P. aeruginosa:* cefepime, imipenem/cilastatin, or meropenem
- Enterobacteriaceae: ceftriaxone or ertapenem
- Anaerobes: clindamycin, ticarcillin clavulanate, cefotetan, or metronidazole

- Table 1 summarizes antimicrobial therapy for selected microorganisms in osteomyelitis
- Hyperbaric oxygen therapy: may be useful in chronic osteomyelitis
- Wound-assisted vacuum device may help closure of wound
- Surgical debridement of all devitalized bone and tissue
- Immobilization of affected bone (plaster, traction) if bone is unstable

DISPOSITION

Acute hematogenous osteomyelitis usually resolves without recurrence or long-term complications, but contiguous focus osteomyelitis, bone infections from open fractures, or osteomyelitis frequently recurs.

REFERRAL

- To an orthopedic surgeon if chronic osteomyelitis with need for bone debridement, bone grafting, or stabilization of infected tissue adjacent to a bone fracture
- To an infectious disease specialist for appropriate treatment for difficult-to-treat or recalcitrant infections
- To a hyperbaric oxygen chamber service for nonhealing, chronic osteomyelitis

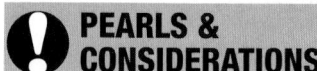 **PEARLS & CONSIDERATIONS**

- Chronic osteomyelitis is one of the most challenging infections to treat; the high failure rate is a consequence of poor vascular supply, nondistensible bone tissue, and limited penetration of bone tissue.
- The optimal duration of therapy for vertebral osteomyelitis is unclear. Trials comparing 6 weeks to 12 weeks of antibiotic treatment in pyogenic vertebral osteomyelitis showed similar cure rates (91%) in both groups.

SUGGESTED READINGS
Available at www.expertconsult.com

RELATED CONTENT
Osteomyelitis (Patient Information)

AUTHOR: **GLENN G. FORT, M.D., M.P.H.**

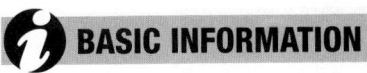

BASIC INFORMATION

DEFINITION

Osteoporosis is a skeletal disorder characterized by a progressive loss of bone mass and a decline in bone quality that results in increased bone fragility and a higher fracture risk. The various types are as follows:

PRIMARY OSTEOPOROSIS: Affects 80% of women and 60% of men with osteoporosis.

- Idiopathic osteoporosis: unknown pathogenesis; may occur in children and young adults.
- Type I osteoporosis (postmenopausal women): characterized by accelerated and disproportionate trabecular bone loss and associated with vertebral body and distal forearm fractures due to estrogen deficiency.
- Type II osteoporosis (involutional): occurs in both men and women aged >70 yr; characterized by both trabecular and cortical bone loss and associated with fractures of the hip, long bone, and vertebrae.

SECONDARY OSTEOPOROSIS: Affects 20% of women and 40% of men with osteoporosis; osteoporosis that exists as a common feature of another disease process, heritable disorder of connective tissue, or drug side effect (see "Differential Diagnosis")

ICD-10CM CODES
M81.0	Age-related osteoporosis without current pathological fracture
M81.4	Drug-induced osteoporosis
M81.5	Idiopathic osteoporosis
M81.6	Localized osteoporosis

EPIDEMIOLOGY & DEMOGRAPHICS

PREVALENCE (IN U.S.):
- Affects more than 10 million people in the U.S.
- Annual incidence of osteoporotic fractures exceeds 1.5 million in the U.S. (70% women)
- Twice as common in women
- Results: institutionalization, death, and costs in excess of $17 billion annually

RISK FACTORS:
- Advanced age
- Previous low-trauma fracture
- Long-term glucocorticoid use
- Low body weight (<58 kg)
- Family history of hip fracture
- Tobacco use
- Excess alcohol use

- Chronic disease states; e.g., diabetes mellitus, androgen deficiency, inflammatory bowel disease, hyperthyroidism, hypercortisolism

PHYSICAL FINDINGS & CLINICAL PRESENTATION

- Most commonly silent with no signs and symptoms
- Insidious and progressive development of dorsal kyphosis *(dowager's hump),* loss of height, and skeletal pain typically associated with fracture; reduced gait speed or grip strength; other physical findings related to other conditions with associated increased risk for osteoporosis such as nodular thyroid, hepatic enlargement, jaundice, cushingoid features (see "Risk Factors")

ETIOLOGY

Normal bone turnover involves balance between process of bone resorption and bone formation. Osteoclasts resorb bone, and osteoblasts secrete bone matrix for building bone. In postmenopausal women, rate of bone turnover increases after loss of ovarian function, leading to progressive bone loss.

Clinical risk factors used in the World Health Organization Fracture Risk Assessment Tool (WHO FRAX) 10-year fracture risk calculator are summarized in Table 1.

DIAGNOSIS

DIFFERENTIAL DIAGNOSIS

- Malignancy (multiple myeloma, lymphoma, leukemia, metastatic carcinoma)
- Primary hyperparathyroidism
- Osteomalacia
- Paget's disease
- Osteogenesis imperfecta: types I, III, and IV

WORKUP

- History and physical examination, with appropriate evaluation for identified risk factors and secondary causes.
- WHO guidelines for the diagnosis of osteoporosis are based on bone mineral density (BMD) measurements of the hip or spine in g/cm^2 and are reported as a T score.
1. Dual-energy x-ray absorptiometry (DEXA) is the gold standard for screening and monitoring changes in BMD due to excellent precision, widespread availability, low cost, and minimal radiation exposure.

2. DEXA (Fig. 1) is indicated in all women 65 years and older and in postmenopausal women younger than 65 years of age who are at risk for fracture (e.g., weight <127 lbs, parental history of hip fracture, use of medications that cause bone loss, smoking, alcoholism, rheumatoid arthritis, or presence of diseases that cause bone loss). Causes of erroneous bone mineral density measures by DEXA in the lumbar spine are summarized in Table 2.
3. Use of FRAX calculator (https://shelf.ac.uk/FRAX/) is proposed by the U.S. Preventive Services Task Force (USPSTF) to determine the need for screening in women between the ages of 50 and 64. If the FRAX 10-year major osteoporotic risk is greater than or equal to 9.3%, the USPSTF recommends screening with DEXA scan.

- Recommendations as to when to repeat bone density testing should be based on initial T scores (Fig. 2). Data from the Study of Osteoporotic Fractures indicates that in women with normal bone density or mild osteopenia, repeat testing might not be necessary for another 10 to 15 yr. For women with moderate osteopenia, a screening interval of 3 to 5 yr may be appropriate. Annual testing may be indicated for women with advanced osteopenia.

LABORATORY TESTS

- Biochemical profile to evaluate renal and hepatic function, primary hyperparathyroidism, and malnutrition.
- CBC: for nutritional status and myeloma.
- TSH to rule out the presence of hyperthyroidism.
- 24-hour urinary calcium levels and 26-hydroxyvitamin D level may be helpful in evaluating for secondary causes of osteoporosis.
- May consider celiac panel and serum protein electrophoresis. Biochemical markers of bone remodeling may be useful to predict rate of bone loss and/or follow therapy response. Specific biochemical markers are followed (e.g., 3-mo interval) to document normalization as a response to therapy.
1. High-turnover osteoporosis: high levels of resorption markers (lysyl pyridinoline, deoxy lysyl pyridinoline, n-telopeptide of collagen cross-links, C-telopeptide of collagen cross-links) and formation markers (osteocalcin and bone-specific alkaline phosphatase); accelerated bone loss responding best to antiresorptive therapy.
2. Low-normal-turnover osteoporosis: normal or low levels of the markers of resorption and formation (see "high turnover osteoporosis" listed previously); no accelerated bone loss; responds best to drugs that enhance bone formation.

IMAGING STUDIES

- BMD determination (see "Workup") should be performed on all women with determined risk factors and/or associated secondary causes; criteria for diagnosis of osteoporosis based on measurement of bone density and T score equivalent cut points are summarized in Table 1.

TABLE 1 1994 WHO Criteria for the Diagnosis of Osteoporosis Based on the Measurement of Bone Density and T Score Equivalent Cut Points

Diagnostic Category	Standard Deviations Below the Young-Adult Mean	T Score
Normal	≤1 SD	Equal to or better than −1
Osteopenia (low bone mass)	Between 1 and 2.5 SD	Between −1 and −2.5
Osteoporosis	≥2.5 SD	Equal to or poorer than −2.5
Severe (established) osteoporosis	≥2.5 SD + a fragility fracture	Equal to or poorer than −2.5 + a fragility fracture

From Hochberg MC et al: *Rheumatology,* ed 5, St Louis, 2011, Mosby.

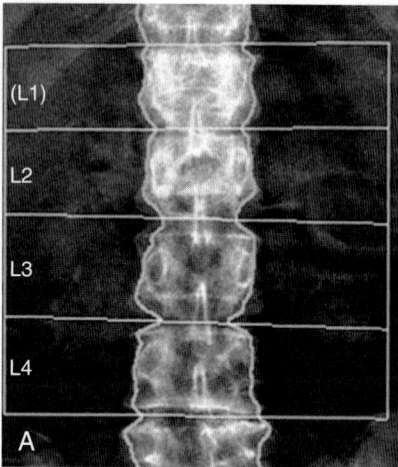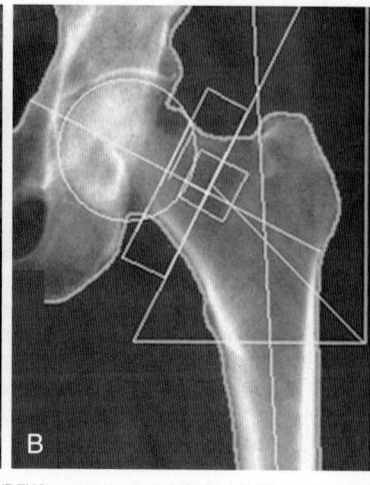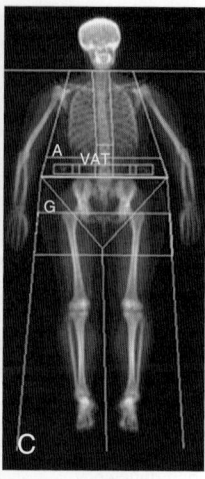

FIG. 1 Dual-energy X-ray absorptiometry (DEXA) provides "areal" bone mineral density (BMD) (g/cm^2) and is currently the gold standard for diagnosis of osteoporosis by bone densitometry (World Health Organization definition T score −2.5 or below) in (**A**) posteroanterior lumbar spine (L1-4) or (**B**) hip (femoral neck or total). **C,** DEXA of the whole body can provide information on total and regional BMD and body composition (fat and muscle mass). Recent additional parameters measured are android A/gynoid G ratio and visceral adipose tissue (VAT). (Pope TL et al: *Musculoskeletal imaging,* ed 2, Philadelphia, 2014, Saunders.)

TABLE 2 Causes of Erroneous Bone Mineral Density Measures by DEXA in the Lumbar Spine

Overestimation of Bone Mineral Density

Extraneous calcification (lymph nodes, aorta)

Degenerative disk and spine disease (osteophytes)

Ankylosing spondylitis

Vertebral fracture

Sclerotic metastases

Vertebral hemangioma

Overlying metal artifacts (navel rings)

Surgical interventions (metallic rods, spinal fusion)

Vertebroplasty

Paget disease

Treatment with strontium ranelate

Underestimation of Bone Mineral Density

Laminectomy

From Pope TL et al: *Musculoskeletal imaging,* ed 2, Philadelphia, 2014, Saunders.

1. Normal: BMD <1 SD of the young adult reference mean
2. Osteopenia: BMD 1 to 2.5 SD below the young adult reference mean
3. Osteoporosis: BMD >2.5 SD below the young adult reference mean
- For patient undergoing treatment: annual BMD to follow response to therapy.
- X-ray exam of appropriate part of skeleton (Figs. E3 and E4) to evaluate clinical osteoporotic fracture only.

Rx TREATMENT

- Osteoporosis based on DEXA measurements of BMD
- History of hip and vertebral fracture

- Osteopenia on DEXA + 10-yr FRAX score of greater than or equal to 3% at hip or reader greater than or equal to 20% of major osteoporotic fracture

NONPHARMACOLOGIC THERAPY

Prevention:
- Identification and minimization of risk factors
- Appropriate diagnosis and treatment of secondary causes
- Behavioral modification: proper nutrition, physical activity, fracture prevention strategies

ACUTE GENERAL Rx

- Vitamin D supplement: 600 IU/day for persons 19 to 70 years of age and 800 IU/day for persons 71 years and older.
- Calcium supplement: The recommended dietary intake of calcium for women 19 to 50 years of age and men 19 to 70 years of age is 1000 mg/day; women older than age 50 and men older than age 70 require 1200 mg/day. Calcium intake above 2500 mg/day (2000 mg/day in persons >50 years of age) should be avoided. Consumption of calcium-rich foods and beverages is the preferred approach to ensuring adequate calcium intake.[1]
- Oral bisphosphonates (alendronate, ibandronate, risedronate): decrease bone resorption by attenuating osteoclast activity. They are first-line therapy for the treatment of most patients with osteoporosis, with proven efficacy to reduce fracture risk. The bisphosphonates differ in binding affinity, dose frequency, and route of administration. To facilitate absorption, most oral bisphosphonates are taken on an empty stomach with a full glass

[1]Bauer DC: Calcium supplements and fracture prevention, *N Engl J Med* 369:1537-1543, 2013.

of water. Patients are instructed to remain in a sitting or standing position for 30 to 60 minutes. Risks include gastroesophageal reflux disease, esophagitis, jaw osteoporosis, and atypical femur fracture.
- Raloxifene (selective estrogen receptor moderator): suppressive effects on osteoclast and bone resorption. Its main use is for prevention of vertebral fractures. It is dosed at 60 mg orally per day. It is ideal for women who cannot tolerate bisphosphonates but are not at high risk for venous thromboembolism or stroke.
- Zoledronic acid: a bisphosphonate given by IV infusion over at least 15 min, 5 mg once/year. It is contraindicated in patients with acute renal failure.
- Teriparatide is a recombinant human parathyroid hormone used for postmenopausal women with osteoporosis who are at high risk for fracture, especially vertebral fractures. It is also used in men with primary or hypogonadal osteoporosis who are at high risk of fracture. It is administered by injection 20 mcg qd SC into the thigh or abdominal wall. Use for >2 yr not recommended. It stimulates bone formation and reduces the risk of fracture but may increase the risk of stroke in older women with osteoporosis. Common side effects include headaches, myalgia, hypercalcemia, and hypercalciuria. Trials involving abaloparatide, a selective activator of the parathyroid hormone type 1 receptor have also shown reduced risk of new vertebral and nonvertebral fractures in postmenopausal women with osteoporosis.
- Biologic agents: Denosumab is a human monoclonal antibody that inhibits osteoclast formation and prevents resorption for treatment of postmenopausal osteoporosis. Dosage is 60 mg subcutaneously every 6 months. Romosozumab is a monoclonal

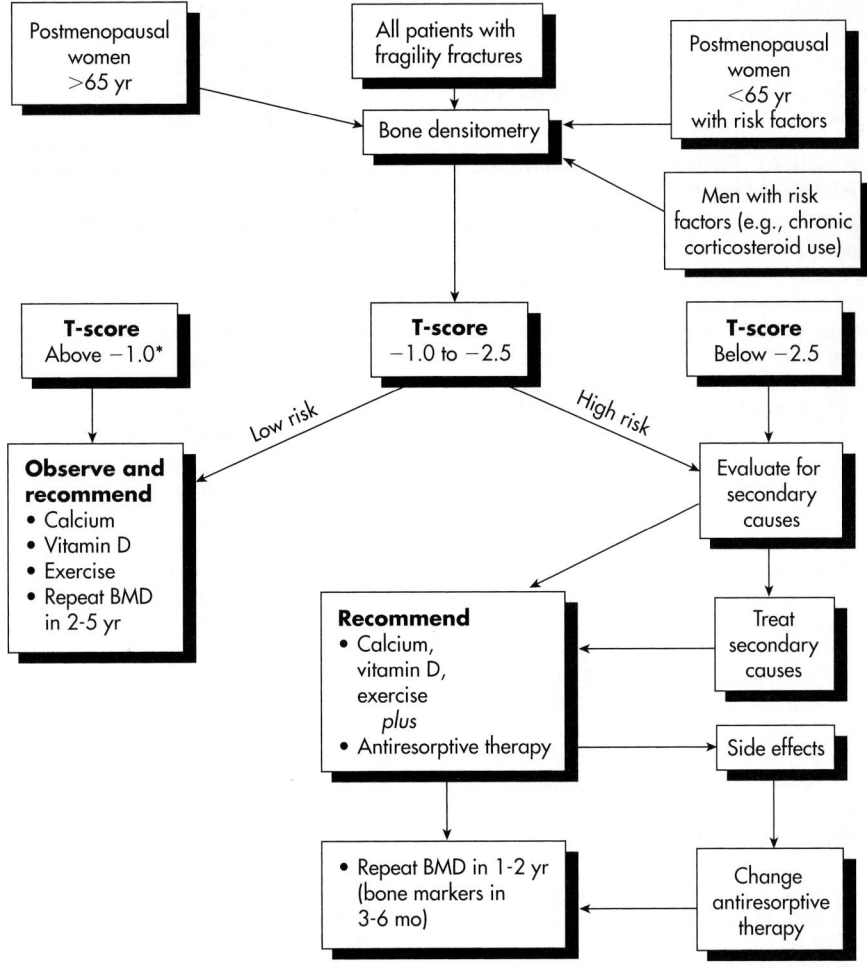

*Patients with fragility fractures and a T-score above −1.0 should be evaluated for other causes
of pathologic fracture.

FIG. 2 Diagnosis and management of osteoporosis. The diagram outlines an approach based largely on evidence from studies of postmenopausal white women, with dual-energy x-ray absorptiometry used to measure bone mineral density *(BMD).* Its application to other populations, including patients with secondary osteoporosis and other methods of assessing BMD, is not established. (Modified from Larsen PR et al: *Williams textbook of endocrinology,* ed 11, Philadelphia, 2008, Saunders.)

antibody that in recent trials increased bone formation and decreased bone resorption by binding to sclerostin.
- Estrogen prescription drugs have been approved for the prevention of postmenopausal osteoporosis.
  - Estrogen (conjugated equine estrogen or equivalent): 0.3 to 0.625 mg/day.
  - Progestin: continuous (e.g., 2.5 mg medroxyprogesterone acetate/day or equivalent) or cyclic (e.g., 10 mg medroxyprogesterone acetate days for 10 days each mo or equivalent) coadministered in women with a uterus in place.
  - Combination estrogen/alendronate or estrogen-progestin/alendronate may be considered in individualized patients on hormone replacement therapy with identified osteoporosis. BMD baseline obtained before onset of therapy and at 1 yr; decrease of 2% or greater results in dosage adjustment or medication change.

CHRONIC Rx
- Lifelong attention to behavior modification issues (nutrition, physical activity, fracture prevention strategies) and compliance with pharmacologic intervention. Recommendations include weight-bearing and muscle-strengthening exercises, smoking cessation, reduced alcohol intake, and adoption of fall prevention strategies.
- There is little evidence to guide physicians about long-term bisphosphonate therapy. Evidence is accumulating that the risk of atypical fracture of the femur increases after 5 years of bisphosphonate use. It is reasonable to consider a drug holiday at 3 to 5 yr in women with moderate risk (T score better than −2.5 and no fractures) and then monitor patients with markers of bone turnover. Continued treatment may be advisable in those at highest risk.
- Continuing need to eliminate high-risk factors when possible and to optimally manage secondary causes of osteoporosis.

DISPOSITION
Goals for diagnosis and treatment include identification of women at risk; initiation of preventive measures for all women lifelong; institution of treatment modalities that will result in a decrease in fracture risk; and reduction of morbidity, mortality, and unnecessary institutionalization, thereby improving quality of independent life and productivity.

REFERRAL
- To reproductive endocrinologist, medical endocrinologist, gynecologist, or rheumatologist if unfamiliar with diagnosis and management of osteoporosis
- If multidisciplinary management is required, to other specialties depending on presence of acute fracture and/or secondary associated disorders

❗ **PEARLS & CONSIDERATIONS**

COMMENTS
- Osteonecrosis of the jaw is a known complication of high-dose IV bisphosphonate therapy for cancer; however, there is considerable debate on whether low-dose bisphosphonates used for osteoporosis can also cause this disorder. Evidence for this is inconclusive.
- Long-term use (>10 yr) of bisphosphonates has been reported to increase risk of atypical subtrochanteric or femoral shaft fractures in several uncontrolled case series. Prodromal symptoms of thigh pain, lack of trauma prior to the procedure, and specific radiologic characteristics (cortical thickening) have been reported. The evidence remains inconclusive. Patients can be reassured that short or intermediate use of bisphosphonates does not increase the risk of atypical femoral fractures. Current strategies should include considering a 12-mo interruption in therapy after 5 yr in patients who are clinically stable and considering teriparatide treatment in individuals who experience an atypical fracture while receiving bisphosphonate therapy.
- Increased risk of esophageal cancer and atrial fibrillation have been reported as possible adverse effects of bisphosphonate therapy.

ⒺⒷⓂ **EVIDENCE**

Available at www.expertconsult.com

SUGGESTED READINGS
Available at www.expertconsult.com

RELATED CONTENT
Osteoporosis (Patient Information)
Bisphosphonate-Related Osteonecrosis of Jaw (Related Key Topic)
Vertebral Compression Fractures (Related Key Topic)

AUTHORS: **DENNIS M. WEPPNER, M.D., RUBEN ALVERO, M.D., AND PATRICIA W. LO, M.D.**

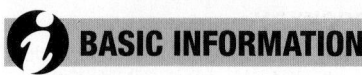

DEFINITION

Otitis externa refers to a variety of conditions causing inflammation and/or infection of the external auditory canal (and/or auricle and tympanic membrane). There are six subgroups of otitis externa:
1. Acute localized otitis externa (furunculosis)
2. Acute diffuse bacterial otitis externa (i.e., "swimmer's ear")
3. Chronic otitis externa
4. Eczematous otitis externa
5. Fungal otitis externa (otomycosis)
6. Invasive or necrotizing (malignant) otitis externa (Fig. 1)

SYNONYMS

See "Definition."

ICD-10CM CODES	
H60.90	Unspecified otitis externa, unspecified ear
H60.2	Malignant otitis externa
H60.3	Other infective otitis externa
H60.5	Acute otitis externa, non-infective
H60.8	Other otitis externa

EPIDEMIOLOGY & DEMOGRAPHICS

INCIDENCE (IN U.S.):
- Among the most common disorders
- Affects 3% to 10% of patients seeking otologic care

PREVALENCE (IN U.S.):
- Diffuse otitis externa is most often seen in swimmers and in hot, humid climates, conditions that lead to water retention in the ear canal. In the United States, 44% of AOE-related healthcare visits occur June to August.
- Necrotizing otitis externa is more common in elderly, diabetics, and immunocompromised patients.

PREDOMINANT SEX: None
PREDOMINANT AGE:
- Occurs at all ages
- Necrotizing otitis externa: typically occurs in elderly: mean age >65 yr

PHYSICAL FINDINGS & CLINICAL PRESENTATION

The two most common symptoms are otalgia, ranging from pruritus to severe pain exacerbated by motion (e.g., chewing), and otorrhea. Patients may also experience aural fullness and hearing loss as a result of swelling with occlusion of the canal. More intense symptoms may occur with bacterial otitis externa, with or without fever, and lymphadenopathy (anterior to tragus). Findings unique to specific forms of the infection include:
- Acute localized otitis externa (furunculosis):
  1. Occurs from infected hair follicles, usually in the outer third of the ear canal, forming pustules and furuncles
  2. Furuncles are superficial and pointing or deep and diffuse
- Impetigo:
  1. In contrast to furunculosis, this is a superficial spreading infection of the ear canal that may also involve the concha and the auricle
  2. Begins as a small blister that ruptures, releasing straw-colored fluid that dries as a golden crust
- Erysipelas:
  1. Caused by group A *Streptococcus*
  2. May involve the concha and canal
  3. May involve the dermis and deeper tissues
  4. Area of cellulitis, often with severe pain
  5. Fever, chills, malaise
  6. Regional adenopathy
- Eczematous or seborrheic otitis externa:
  1. Stems from a variety of dermatologic problems that can involve the external auditory canal
  2. Severe itching, erythema, scaling, crusting, and fissuring possible

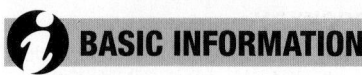

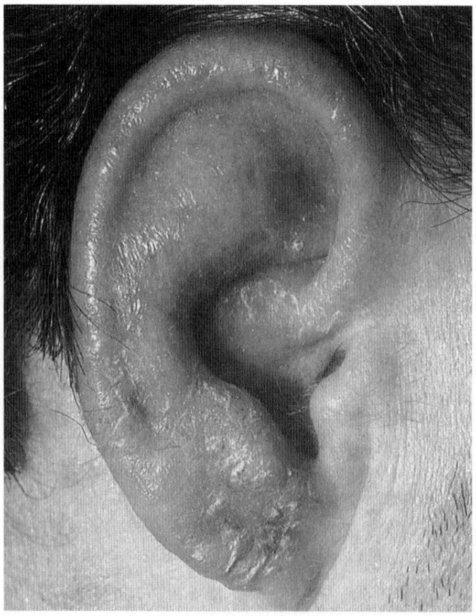

FIG. 1 Malignant external otitis. Severe infection of the ear has occurred after months of chronic inflammation of the pinna. (From Habif TP: *Clinical dermatology: a color guide to diagnosis and therapy,* ed 3, St Louis, 1996, Mosby.)

- Acute diffuse otitis externa (swimmer's ear):
  1. Begins with itching and a feeling of pressure and fullness in the ear that becomes increasingly tender and painful
  2. Mild erythema and edema of the external auditory canal, which may cause narrowing and occlusion of the canal, leading to hearing loss
  3. Minimal serous secretions, which may become profuse and purulent
  4. Tympanic membrane may appear dull and infected
  5. Usually absence of systemic symptoms such as fever, chills
- Otomycosis:
  1. Chronic superficial infection of the ear canal and tympanic membrane
  2. In primary fungal infection, major symptom is intense itching
  3. In secondary infection (fungal infection superimposed on bacterial infection), major symptom is pain
  4. Fungal growth of variety of colors
- Chronic otitis externa:
  1. Dry and atrophic canal
  2. Typically lack of cerumen
  3. Itching, often severe, and mild discomfort rather than pain
  4. Occasionally mucopurulent discharge
  5. With time, thickening of the walls of the canal, causing narrowing of the lumen
- Necrotizing otitis externa (also known as malignant otitis externa). Typically seen in older patients with diabetes or in patients who are immunocompromised.
  1. Redness, swelling, and tenderness of the ear canal
  2. Classic finding of granulation tissue on the floor of the canal and the bone–cartilage junction
  3. Small ulceration of necrotic soft tissue at bone–cartilage junction
  4. Most common symptoms: pain (often severe) and otorrhea
  5. Lessening of purulent drainage as infection advances
  6. Facial nerve palsy often the first and only cranial nerve defect
  7. Possible involvement of other cranial nerves

ETIOLOGY

- Acute localized otitis externa: *Staphylococcus aureus*
- Impetigo:
  1. *S. aureus* including MRSA
  2. *Streptococcus pyogenes*
- Erysipelas: *S. pyogenes*
- Eczematous otitis externa:
  1. Seborrheic dermatitis
  2. Atopic dermatitis
  3. Psoriasis
  4. Neurodermatitis
  5. Lupus erythematosus
- Acute diffuse otitis externa:
  1. Swimming
  2. Hot, humid climates
  3. Tightly fitting hearing aids
  4. Use of ear plugs

5. *Pseudomonas aeruginosa*
6. *S. aureus* including MRSA
- Otomycosis:
  1. Prolonged use of topical antibiotics and steroid preparations
  2. Uncontrolled diabetes mellitus can contribute to risk
  3. *Aspergillus* (80% to 90%)
  4. *Candida*
- Chronic otitis externa: persistent low-grade infection and inflammation
- Necrotizing otitis externa (NOE):
  1. Complication of persistent otitis externa
  2. Extends through Santorini's fissures, small apertures at the bone-cartilage junction of the canal, into the mastoid and along the base of the skull
  3. *P. aeruginosa*

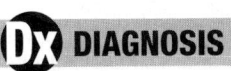 **DIAGNOSIS**

DIFFERENTIAL DIAGNOSIS
- Acute otitis media
- Bullous myringitis
- Mastoiditis
- Foreign bodies
- Neoplasms
- Contact dermatitis
- Eczema
- Ramsey-Hunt syndrome
- Seborrhea
- Otomycosis
- Referred pain

WORKUP
Thorough history and physical examination

LABORATORY TESTS
- Cultures from the canal are usually not necessary unless the condition does not respond to treatment.
- Leukocyte count normal or mildly elevated.
- Erythrocyte sedimentation rate is often quite elevated in malignant otitis externa.

IMAGING STUDIES
- CT scan is the best technique for defining bone involvement and extent of disease in malignant otitis externa.
- MRI is slightly more sensitive in evaluation of soft tissue changes and intracranial extension of infection.
- Gallium scans are more specific than bone scans in diagnosing NOE.
- Follow-up scans are helpful in determining efficacy of treatment.
  NOTE: Expert opinion supports history and physical examination as the best means of diagnosis. Persistent pain that is constant and severe should raise the question of NOE (particularly in the elderly, diabetics, and immunocompromised patients).

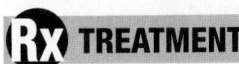 **TREATMENT**

NONPHARMACOLOGIC THERAPY
- Cleansing and debridement of the ear canal with cotton swabs and hydrogen peroxide or other antiseptic solution allows a more thorough examination of the ear.
- If the canal lumen is edematous and too narrow to allow adequate cleansing, a cotton wick or gauze strip inserted into the canal serves as a conduit for topical medications to be drawn into the canal. Usually remove wick after 2 days.
- Local heat is useful in treating deep furunculosis.
- Incision and drainage is indicated in treatment of superficial pointing furunculosis.

ACUTE GENERAL Rx
Topical medications:
- An acidifying agent such as 2% acetic acid (Vosol) inhibits growth of bacteria and fungi
- Topical antibiotics (in the form of otic or ophthalmic solutions) or antifungals, often in combination with an acidifying agent and a steroid preparation
- The following are some of the available preparations:
  1. Neomycin otic solutions and suspensions:
     a. With polymyxin-B-hydrocortisone (Cortisporin)
     b. With hydrocortisone-thonzonium (Coly-Mycin S)
  2. Polymyxin-B-hydrocortisone (Otobiotic)
  3. Quinolone otic solutions:
     a. Ofloxacin 0.3% solution (Floxin Otic)
     b. Ciprofloxacin 0.3% with hydrocortisone (Cipro HC)
  4. Quinolone ophthalmic solutions:
     a. Ofloxacin 0.3% (Ocuflox)
     b. Ciprofloxacin 0.3% (Ciloxan)
  5. Aminoglycoside ophthalmic solutions:
     a. Gentamicin sulfate 0.3% (Garamycin)
     b. Tobramycin sulfate 0.3% (Tobrex)
     c. Tobramycin 0.3% and dexamethasone 0.1% (TobraDex)
  6. Chloramphenicol 0.5% otic solution or 0.25% ophthalmic solution (Chloromycetin)
  7. Gentian violet (methylrosaniline chloride 1%, 2%)
  8. Antifungals:
     a. Amphotericin B 3% (Fungizone lotion)
     b. Clotrimazole 1% solution (Lotrimin)
     c. Tolnaftate 1% (Tinactin)
- Topical preparations should be applied qid (bid for quinolones, antifungals), generally for 3 days after cessation of symptoms (average 10 to 14 days total)
Systemic antibiotics:
- Reserved for when the infection has spread beyond the ear canal
- Treatment usually for 10 days with ciprofloxacin 750 mg q12h or ofloxacin 400 mg q12h, or with antistaphylococcal agent (e.g., dicloxacillin or cephalexin 500 mg q6h). Use Bactrim or clindamycin when MRSA suspected or cultured at one DS twice a day instead of cephalexin or dicloxacillin. For malignant otitis externa (due to *Pseudomonas aeruginosa* in >90% of cases), effective agents are meropenem 1 g IV q8h or ciprofloxacin 400 mg IV q12h or 750 mg PO q12h or cefepime 2 g q12h.

Treatment for NOE:
- Requires prolonged therapy up to 3 mo; whether to use oral parenteral therapy based on clinical judgment
- Oral quinolones, ciprofloxacin 750 mg q12h or ofloxacin 400 mg q12h may be appropriate initial therapy or used to shorten the course of IV therapy
- Intravenous antipseudomonals with or without aminoglycosides are also appropriate
- Local debridement
Pain control:
- May require NSAIDs or opioids
- Topical corticosteroids to reduce swelling and inflammation

CHRONIC Rx
- Patients prone to recurrent infections should try to identify and avoid precipitants to infection.
- Swimmers should try tight-fitting ear plugs or tight-fitting bathing caps and remove all excess water from the ears after swimming.
- Treat underlying systemic diseases and dermatologic conditions that predispose to infection.

DISPOSITION
Inadequate treatment of otitis externa may lead to NOE and mastoiditis.

REFERRAL
To an otolaryngologist:
- NOE
- Treatment failure
- Severe pain

⚠ PEARLS & CONSIDERATIONS

Otitis externa varies in severity from a mild irritation of the external acoustic canal (swimmer's ear) that resolves spontaneously by simply removing the offending agent (stay out of fresh water or wear ear plugs when swimming) to a life-threatening infection with the risk of intracranial extension, gram-negative bacterial meningitis, and severe neurologic impairment with multiple cranial neuropathy. Do not miss severe malignant otitis externa in patients who are diabetic or immunocompromised.

SUGGESTED READINGS
Available at www.expertconsult.com

RELATED CONTENT
Otitis Externa (Patient Information)

AUTHOR: **RUSSELL J. MCCULLOH, M.D.**

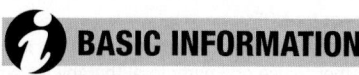

BASIC INFORMATION

DEFINITION

Otitis media is the rapid onset of signs and symptoms of inflammation in the middle ear.

SYNONYMS

Acute suppurative otitis media
Purulent otitis media
Acute otitis media
AOM

ICD-10CM CODES

H65.0 Acute serous otitis media
H65.1 Other acute nonsuppurative otitis media
H65.9 Nonsuppurative otitis media, unspecified
H65.2 Chronic serous otitis media
H65.3 Chronic mucoid otitis media
H65.6 Other chronic nonsuppurative otitis media
H66.0 Acute suppurative otitis media
H66.4 Suppurative otitis media, unspecified
H66.9 Otitis media, unspecified
H66.1 Chronic tubotympanic suppurative otitis media
H66.2 Chronic atticoantral suppurative otitis media

EPIDEMIOLOGY & DEMOGRAPHICS

INCIDENCE (IN U.S.):

- Affects patients of all ages but is largely a disease of infants and young children.
- Affects approximately 80% of all children by age 5 yr.
- Occurs three or more times in one third of all children by age 3 yr.
- Costs associated with otitis media exceed $5 billion, with 40% of the costs occurring from patients ages 1 to 3
- From 1995 to 2006, 80% of children diagnosed with otitis media received an antibiotic at initial visit.
- Nearly 1 in 14 children prescribed an antibiotic for AOM experiences an adverse drug event (e.g., nausea, vomiting, rash, etc.) due to antibiotic use.

PEAK INCIDENCE:

- Between 9 and 15 mo
- Second peak between ages 4 and 6 yr
- Fall, winter, early spring (coincident with peak respiratory virus prevalence in the community)

PREDOMINANT SEX: Males
PREDOMINANT AGE:

- 47% to 60% of all children have their first episode of otitis media during their first year of life and 80% by their fifth birthday.
- Incidence of infection declines with age; seen infrequently in adults.

GENETICS: Familial disposition:

- Native Americans
- Eskimos
- Australian aborigines
- Those with a strong family history

- Immune globulin G (IgG) or subclass deficiencies
  Congenital infection: high incidence in children born with cleft palates and other craniofacial abnormalities
  Other risk factors:
- Day care attendance
- Limited or lack of breastfeeding
- Tobacco smoke exposure

PHYSICAL FINDINGS & CLINICAL PRESENTATION

- Moderate to severe bulging of the tympanic membrane
- Fluid in the middle ear along with signs and symptoms of local inflammation (Figs. 1 and 2).
  1. Erythema with diminished light reflex
- As infection progresses, middle ear exudation occurs (exudative phase); the exudate rapidly changes from serous to purulent (suppurative phase).
  1. Retraction and poor motility of the tympanic membrane, which then becomes bulging and convex
- At any time during the suppurative phase the tympanic membrane may rupture, releasing the middle ear contents (otorrhea).
- Erythema of the tympanic membrane without other abnormalities is not a diagnostic

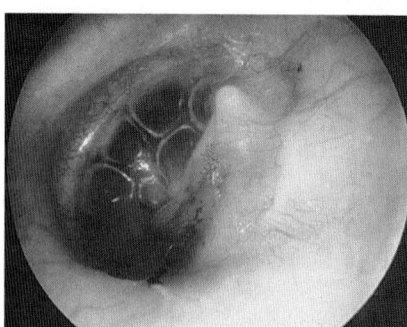

FIG. 1 Otitis media with effusion of left ear. Retracted eardrum, prominent short process of malleus, and air bubbles seen anteriorly through the tympanic membrane. (From Behrman RE: *Nelson textbook of pediatrics,* ed 16, Philadelphia, 1996, Saunders.)

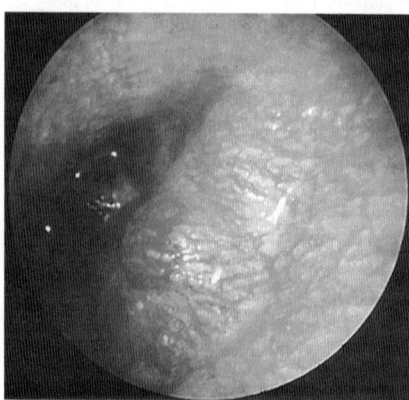

FIG. 2 Acute left otitis media. (From Behrman RE: *Nelson textbook of pediatrics,* ed 16, Philadelphia, 1996, Saunders.)

criterion for acute otitis media (AOM) because it may occur with any inflammation of the upper respiratory tract, crying, or nose blowing.
- Symptoms:
  1. Rapid- or recent-onset otalgia, ranging from slight discomfort to severe, spreading to the temporal region
  2. Ear stuffiness and hearing loss may precede or follow otalgia
  3. Otorrhea if tympanic membrane has ruptured
  4. Vertigo, nystagmus, tinnitus, fever, lethargy, irritability, nausea, vomiting, anorexia
- After an episode of AOM:
  1. Persistence of effusion for weeks or months (called secretory, serous, or nonsuppurative otitis media)
  2. Fever and otalgia usually absent
  3. Hearing loss possible (10 to 50 dB, with predominant involvement of the low frequencies)

ETIOLOGY

- Most common etiologic factor is a viral upper respiratory tract infection, which causes inflammation and dysfunction of the eustachian tube and transient aspiration of nasopharyngeal secretions into the middle ear. Bacterial colonization from the nasopharynx in conjunction with eustachian tube dysfunction leads to infection.
- May occasionally develop as a result of hematogenous spread or by direct invasion from the nasopharynx.
- Conjugated pneumococcal vaccination of children has resulted in decreases in *Streptococcus pneumoniae* causing AOM.
- Most common bacterial pathogens:
  1. *S. pneumoniae* causes approximately 30% of cases and is the least likely of the major pathogens to resolve without treatment.
  2. *Haemophilus influenzae* causes more than 25% of cases.
  3. *Moraxella catarrhalis* causes 10% to 15% of cases.
  4. Of increasing importance, infection caused by penicillin-nonsusceptible *S. pneumoniae* (MIC >0.1 mg/ml), ranging from 8% to 34%. About 50% of PNSSP isolates are penicillin-intermediate (MIC 0.1 to 2.0 mg/ml).
- Viral pathogens:
  1. Respiratory syncytial virus
  2. Rhinovirus
  3. Adenovirus
  4. Influenza
- Others:
  1. *Mycoplasma pneumoniae*
  2. *Chlamydia trachomatis*
  3. *Streptococcus pyogenes* (Latin America)

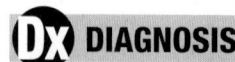 DIAGNOSIS

DIFFERENTIAL DIAGNOSIS

- Otitis externa
- Otitis media with effusion (OME)
- Referred pain

1. Mouth
2. Nasopharynx
3. Tonsils
4. Other parts of the upper respiratory tract
- Section II describes the differential diagnosis of earache

WORKUP

Thorough otoscopic examination. Adequate visualization of the tympanic membrane may require removal of cerumen and debris.
- Tympanometry
  1. Measures compliance of the tympanic membrane and middle ear pressure
  2. Detects the presence of fluid
- Acoustic reflectometry
  1. Measures sound waves reflected from the middle ear
  2. Useful in infants >3 mo
  3. Increased reflected sound correlated with the presence of effusion
  4. Tympanometry and acoustic reflectometry are useful in detection of middle ear effusion but do not provide information regarding infection/inflammation

LABORATORY TESTS

- Tympanocentesis
  1. Not necessary in most cases because the microbiology of middle ear effusions has been shown to be quite consistent
  2. May be indicated in:
     a. Highly toxic patients
     b. Patients who do not respond to treatment in 48 to 72 hr
     c. Immunocompromised patients
- Cultures of the nasopharynx: sensitive but not specific
- Blood counts (generally not necessary): usually show a leukocytosis with polymorphonuclear elevation
- Plain mastoid radiographs: generally not indicated; will reveal haziness in the periantral cells that may extend to entire mastoid
- CT or MRI may be indicated if serious complications suspected (meningitis, brain abscess, severe mastoiditis)

Rx TREATMENT

ACUTE GENERAL Rx

Hydration, avoidance of irritants (e.g., tobacco smoke), nasal systemic decongestants, cool mist humidifier
Antimicrobials:
NOTE: Most uncomplicated cases of AOM resolve spontaneously, without complications. Studies have demonstrated limited therapeutic benefit from antibiotic therapy. Watchful waiting is appropriate for children who look well, can be comforted with supportive care, and are old enough to easily evaluate. Children <24 mo with bilateral AOM should receive antibiotic therapy. Children with severe signs or symptoms (moderate or severe otalgia or otalgia for ≥48 hr or tem-

perature ≥39°C) should also receive antibiotic therapy. When opting to use antibiotic therapy:
- Amoxicillin remains the drug of choice for first-line treatment of uncomplicated AOM despite increasing prevalence of drug-resistant *S. pneumoniae.*
- Treatment failure is defined by lack of clinical improvement of signs or symptoms after 3 days of therapy.
- With treatment failure, in the absence of an identified etiologic pathogen, therapy should be redirected to cover:
  1. Drug-resistant *S. pneumoniae*
  2. β-lactamase–producing strains of *H. influenzae* and *M. catarrhalis*
- Agents fulfilling these criteria include amoxicillin/clavulanate, second-generation (e.g., cefuroxime axetil, cefaclor) or third-generation cephalosporins (e.g., oral cefdinir or cefpodoxime or IM ceftriaxone). Do not use cefaclor, cefixime, loracarbef, and ceftibuten given limited activity against pneumococci.
- TMP/SMX and macrolides have been used as first- and second-line agents, but pneumococcal resistance to these agents is rising (up to 25% resistance to TMP/SMX and up to 10% resistance to erythromycin).
- Cross-resistance between these drugs and the β-lactams exists; therefore patients who do not respond to amoxicillin are more likely to have infections resistant to TMP/SMX and macrolides.
- Fluoroquinolones are not indicated as first- or second-line therapy for AOM and should be avoided in young children due to risks of musculoskeletal effects and limited dosing guidance.
- Treatment should be modified according to cultures and sensitivities when available.
- Generally treatment course is 10 days for children <2 yr and those with severe symptoms, 7 days for children age 2 to 5 yr, and 5 to 7 days for children ≥6 yr.
- Follow up should be tailored to clinical improvement and concern for neurocognitive development delays in at-risk children. Standard follow-up of all cases is no longer required.
- Antibiotic prophylaxis to reduce the frequency of AOM episodes in children with recurrent AOM is not recommended.
  NOTE: Effusions may persist for 8 wk or longer in many cases of adequately treated otitis media.

SURGICAL Rx

- No evidence to support the routine use of myringotomy, but in severe cases it provides prompt pain relief and accelerates resolution of infection.
- Purulent secretions retained in the middle ear can lead to increased pressure that may lead to spread of infection to contiguous areas. Myringotomy to decompress the middle ear is sometimes necessary to avoid complications.

- Complications include mastoiditis, facial nerve paralysis, labyrinthitis, meningitis, and brain abscess.
- Other procedures used for drainage of the middle ear include insertion of a ventilation tube and/or simple mastoidectomy.

CHRONIC Rx

- Myringotomy and tympanostomy tube placement for persistent or recurrent middle ear effusion unresponsive to medical therapy for ≥3 mo if bilateral or ≥6 mo if unilateral.
- Adenoidectomy, with or without tonsillectomy, often advocated for treatment of recurrent otitis media, although indications for this procedure are controversial.
- Long-term complications include tympanic membrane perforations, cholesteatoma, tympanosclerosis, ossicular necrosis, toxic or suppurative labyrinthitis, hearing loss, and intracranial suppuration.

DISPOSITION

Patients can be treated at home as outpatients with the rare exception of patients with evidence of local suppurative complications (e.g., meningitis, acute mastoiditis, brain abscess, cavernous sinus, or lateral vein thrombosis).

REFERRAL

- To otorhinolaryngologist if:
  1. Medical treatment failure
  2. Diagnosis uncertain: adults with one or more episodes of otitis media should be referred for ear-nose-throat evaluation to rule out underlying process (e.g., malignancy)
  3. Any of the above-mentioned acute and chronic complications

! PEARLS & CONSIDERATIONS

COMMENTS

- Otoscopic findings are critical for accurate AOM diagnosis. AOM microbiology has changed with use of pneumococcal conjugate vaccine (PCV13). Antibiotics are modestly more effective than no treatment but cause adverse effects in 4% to 10% of children. Most antibiotics have comparable clinical success.
Prevention:
- Multiple component conjugate vaccines have helped decrease recurrent episodes of AOM
- Breastfeed and bottle-feed infants in an upright position
- Avoidance of irritants (e.g., tobacco smoke)

SUGGESTED READINGS

Available at www.expertconsult.com

AUTHOR: **RUSSELL J. MCCULLOH, M.D.**

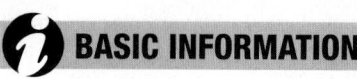

BASIC INFORMATION

DEFINITION

Ovarian cancer is not one disease but a constellation of distinct cancer subtypes, some of which originate outside of the ovary. 90% of tumors are epithelial ovarian cancers, 5% are gram cell tumors, and 5% are sex cord-stromal tumors.

SYNONYMS

Epithelial ovarian cancer
Germ cell tumor
Sex cord stromal tumor
Ovarian tumor of low malignant potential

ICD-10CM CODES
C56.9 Malignant neoplasm of unspecified ovary
C56.1 Malignant neoplasm of right ovary
C56.2 Malignant neoplasm of left ovary

EPIDEMIOLOGY & DEMOGRAPHICS

INCIDENCE: 12.9 to 15.1 cases/100,000 persons; ~25,000 new cases annually. Lifetime risk for developing ovarian cancer is 1.4%. It is the leading cause of gynecologic cancer-related deaths.
PREVALENCE: It is most commonly diagnosed in those 55 to 64 years of age.
RISK FACTORS:
- Low parity, delayed childbearing, smoking, polycystic ovary syndrome, endometriosis, use of talc on the perineum (unlikely), high-fat diet, fertility drugs (unlikely), Lynch II syndrome (nonpolyposis colon cancer, endometrial cancer, breast cancer, and ovarian cancer clusters in first- and second-degree relatives), breast-ovarian familial cancer syndrome, site-specific familial ovarian cancer.
- The strongest risk factors are advancing age and family history of ovarian and breast cancer.
- Factors that decrease the risk of ovarian cancer include previous pregnancy, oral contraceptive pill use, hysterectomy, tubal ligation.

GENETICS: The greatest risk factors of ovarian cancer are a family history and associated genetic syndromes. Familial susceptibility has been shown with the *BRCA1* gene located on 17q12 to 21. This correlates with breast-ovarian cancer syndrome.

PHYSICAL FINDINGS & CLINICAL PRESENTATION

- 60% present with advanced disease
- Abdominal fullness, early satiety, dyspepsia
- Pelvic pain, back pain, constipation
- Pelvic or abdominal mass
- Lymphadenopathy (inguinal)
- Sister Mary Joseph nodule (umbilical mass)

ETIOLOGY

- Can be inherited as site-specific familial ovarian cancer (two or more first-degree relatives have ovarian cancer)
- Breast-ovarian cancer syndrome (clusters of breast and ovarian cancer among first- and second-degree relatives)
- Lynch syndrome
- No family history and unknown etiology in the majority of ovarian cancer cases

DIAGNOSIS

DIFFERENTIAL DIAGNOSIS

- Primary peritoneal cancer mesothelioma
- Benign ovarian tumor
- Functional ovarian cyst
- Endometriosis
- Ovarian torsion
- Pelvic kidney
- Pedunculated uterine fibroid
- Primary cancer from breast, gastrointestinal tract, or other pelvic organ metastasized to the ovary

WORKUP

- Definitive diagnosis made at laparotomy; epithelial ovarian cancer most common type of ovarian cancer (90% of ovarian cancer)
- Careful physical and history, including family history

- Exclusion of nongynecologic etiologies
- Observation of small cystic masses in premenopausal women for regression for 2 mo
- FIGO classification of ovarian carcinoma is described in Table 1.
- Referral to specialists who have extensive training and experience in treating ovarian cancer significantly increases survival after an ovarian cancer diagnosis.

LABORATORY TESTS

- Complete blood count
- Chemistry profile including liver tests and calcium (to evaluate for paraneoplastic syndrome)
- CA-125 or lysophosphatidic acid level. Use of these tests for annual screening is controversial, and most experts warn against universal screening with this marker. Only about 50% of early-stage ovarian cancers will be associated with elevated CA-125. Additionally, false elevations may occur with uterine leiomyoma, endometriosis, pregnancy, and intraabdominal infections. The PLCO cancer screening trial revealed that annual screening based on CA-125 and vaginal ultrasound is ineffective and diagnostic follow-up of false positives resulted in 15% serious complication rate.
- Consider: human chorionic gonadotropin, inhibin, alpha-fetoprotein, neuron-specific enolase, and lactate dehydrogenase in patients at risk for germ cell tumors.
- A panel of 3 serum biomarkers (apolipoprotein A-1 [ApoA-1], transthyretin [TTR], and transferrin [TF]) has been reported useful in distinguishing normal samples from early-stage ovarian cancer with a sensitivity of 84% and normal samples from late-stage ovarian cancer with a sensitivity of 97%.
- *BRCA1/2* testing is recommended for all women with ovarian cancer.

IMAGING STUDIES

- Ultrasound
- Chest x-ray
- CT or MRI of abdomen and pelvis help evaluate extent of disease (Fig. E1)
- Mammogram

TABLE 1	FIGO Classification of Ovarian Carcinoma
Stage I	Growth limited to the ovaries:
	Stage IA: Growth limited to one ovary, no ascites and no tumor present on the external surface; capsule intact
	Stage IB: Growth limited to both ovaries, no ascites and no tumor present on the external surface; capsule intact
	Stage IC: Stage 1A or 1B where there is tumor on the surface of either ovary; or with ruptured capsules or with ascites containing malignant cells or positive peritoneal washings. Surgical spillage of a malignant cyst upgrades the patient to IC, although it is unlikely that this event affects prognosis.
Stage II	Growth involving one or both ovaries with pelvic extension:
	Stage IIA: Extension and/or metastases to the uterus and tubes
	Stage IIB: Extension to other pelvic tissues
	Stage IIC: Stage IIA or IIB with tumor on the surface of either ovary or positive peritoneal washings or malignant ascites
Stage III	Growth involving one or both ovaries with peritoneal implants outside the pelvis or positive retroperitoneal or inguinal lymph nodes:
	Stage IIIA: Microscopic seeding of abdominal peritoneal surfaces
	Stage IIIB: Macroscopic disease outside the pelvis less than 2 cm in diameter
	Stage IIIC: Abdominal implants greater than 2 cm and/or positive nodes
Stage IV	Growth involving one or both ovaries with distant metastases including parenchymal (but not superficial) liver metastases and pleural effusions containing malignant cells

From Symonds EM, Symonds IM: *Essential obstetrics and gynaecology*, ed 4, London, 2004, Churchill Livingstone.

Rx TREATMENT

NONPHARMACOLOGIC THERAPY

Virtually all cases of ovarian cancer involve surgical exploration. This includes:
- Abdominal cytology
- Total abdominal hysterectomy and bilateral salpingo-oophorectomy (except in early stages in which fertility preservation is an issue)
- Omentectomy
- Diaphragm sampling
- Selective lymphadenectomy (pelvic and paraaortic nodes)
- Primary cytoreduction with a goal of residual tumor diameter <<2 cm
- Bowel surgery, splenectomy if needed to obtain optimal (<<2 cm) cytoreduction
- Conventional treatment includes surgical debulking (cytoreduction) followed by chemotherapy. However, patients with low-grade, well-differentiated stage I ovarian cancer do not benefit from adjuvant chemotherapy.

ACUTE GENERAL Rx

- Optimal cytoreduction (debulking) is generally followed by chemotherapy (except in some early-stage disease [stage I without high-risk features is treated with surgery alone]).
- Cisplatin-based combination chemotherapy is used for stage II or greater, 6-mo treatment. Compared with IV paclitaxel plus cisplatin, IV paclitaxel plus intraperitoneal cisplatin and paclitaxel improves survival rates in patients with optimally debulked stage III ovarian cancer.
- Chemotherapy regimens continue to change as research continues. Bevacizumab, a humanized antivascular endothelial growth factor monoclonal antibody, has been shown to be effective in improving progression-free survival in women with ovarian cancer. Trials using bevacizumab during and up to 10 months after carboplatin and paclitaxel chemotherapy have shown prolongation of the median progression-free survival by about 4 months in patients with advanced epithelial ovarian cancer. Olaparib, an oral polymerase inhibitor, has shown

antitumor activity in patients with high-grade serous ovarian cancer with or without BRCA1 and BRCA2 germline mutations. Trials have shown that olaparib or niraparib as maintenance treatment significantly improved progression-free survival among patients with platinum-sensitive, relapsed high-grade serous ovarian cancer.
- Second-look surgery when chemotherapy is complete generally is no longer recommended because this procedure has not been shown to improve survival.
- In most cases, neoadjuvant (presurgical) chemotherapy has no advantage over post-surgical initiation of chemotherapy. However, some trials have shown that neoadjuvant chemotherapy followed by interval debulking surgery is not inferior to debulking surgery followed by chemotherapy as a treatment option for patients with bulky stage IIIC or IV ovarian carcinoma. Complete resection of all macroscopic disease, whether performed as primary treatment or after neoadjuvant chemotherapy, remains the objective whenever cytoreductive surgery is performed.

CHRONIC Rx

- If CA-125 elevated, may have recurrent disease
- Physical and pelvic examinations every 3 mo for 2 yr, every 4 mo during third year, then every 6 mo
- Routine monitoring of CA-125 at every visit does not improve survival and should be reserved for addressing specific clinical concerns
- Yearly Pap smear

DISPOSITION

- Overall 5-yr survival rates remain low because of the preponderance of late-stage disease:
  1. Stage I and II: 80% to 100%
  2. Stage III: 15% to 20%
  3. Stage IV: 5%
- Younger patients (<50 yr) in all stages have a considerably better 5-yr survival than older patients (40% vs. 15%).
- Among women with high-grade serous ovarian cancer, BRCA2 mutation, but not BRCA1

deficiency, is associated with improved survival, improved chemotherapy response, and genome instability compared with BRCA wild-type.
- Among patients with invasive epithelial ovarian cancer (EOC), having a germline mutation in BRCA1 or BRCA2 is associated with improved 5-yr overall survival. BRCA2 carriers have the best prognosis.

COMMENTS

- The U.S. Preventive Services Task Force has concluded that current evidence does not show any mortality benefit to routine screening for ovarian cancer with transvaginal ultrasonography or single-threshold serum CA-125 testing and that the harms of such screening are at least moderate.
- Patients at high risk for developing ovarian cancer (BRCA1/BRCA2 gene mutation, hereditary nonpolyposis colorectal cancer syndrome) should consider prophylactic salpingo-oophorectomy after childbearing is complete. Prophylactic bilateral salpingo-oophorectomy reduces ovarian cancer by 80%. If surgery is declined, the National Comprehensive Cancer Network guidelines recommend intensive surveillance with pelvic and abdominal sonogram and serum CA-125 every 6 mo starting at age 35 or 10 yr earlier than cancer diagnosis in family member.

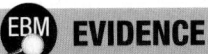 **EVIDENCE**

Available at www.expertconsult.com

SUGGESTED READINGS
Available at www.expertconsult.com

RELATED CONTENT

Ovarian Cancer (Patient Information)
Ovarian Neoplasm, Benign (Related Key Topic)

AUTHOR: **ANTHONY SCISCIONE, D.O.**

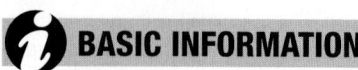

DEFINITION

Benign ovarian neoplasms are often clinically indistinguishable from their malignant counterparts. Therefore, all persistent adnexal masses must be considered malignant until proven otherwise. Nonneoplastic tumors include:
- Germinal inclusion cyst
- Follicle cyst
- Corpus luteum cyst
- Pregnancy luteoma
- Theca lutein cysts
- Sclerocystic ovaries
- Endometrioma
  Neoplastic tumors derived from coelomic epithelium include:
- Cystic tumors: serous cystadenoma, mucinous cystadenoma, mixed forms
- Tumors with stromal overgrowth: fibroma, adenofibroma, Brenner tumor
  Tumors derived from germ cells are dermoids (benign cystic teratomas).

ICD-10CM CODES
D27.9 Benign neoplasm of unspecified ovary
D27.0 Benign neoplasm of right ovary
D27.1 Benign neoplasm of left ovary

EPIDEMIOLOGY & DEMOGRAPHICS

- **Reproductive years:**
  1. Most common benign ovarian neoplasms: serous cystadenoma and benign cystic teratoma
  2. Most common adnexal mass: functional cyst
  3. Risk of malignancy increases after age 40 yr.
- **Infants:** adnexal masses are usually follicular cysts attributable to maternal hormone stimulation that regress during first few months of life.
- **Childhood:**
  1. Adnexal masses are rare
  2. 8% malignant
  3. Almost always dysgerminomas or teratomas (germ cell origin)
  4. Frequency of malignancy inversely correlated with age
- **Adolescence:**
  1. Most common adnexal mass is a functional cyst.
  2. Most common neoplastic ovarian tumor is a benign cystic teratoma.
  3. Solid/cystic adnexal tumors are rare and almost always dysgerminomas or malignant teratomas.

PHYSICAL FINDINGS & CLINICAL PRESENTATION

- Usually asymptomatic
- Pelvic pain or pressure
- Dyspareunia
- Abdominal pain ranging from mild to severe peritoneal irritation
- Increasing abdominal girth or distention
- Adnexal mass of pelvic examination
- Children: abdominal or rectal mass

ETIOLOGY

- Physiologic
- Endometriosis
- Unknown

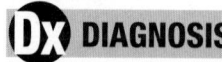

DIFFERENTIAL DIAGNOSIS

- Ovarian torsion
- Malignancy: ovary, fallopian tube, colon
- Uterine fibroid
- Diverticular abscess, diverticulitis
- Appendiceal abscess, appendicitis (especially in children)
- Tubo-ovarian abscess
- Paraovarian cyst
- Distended bladder
- Pelvic kidney
- Ectopic pregnancy
- Retroperitoneal cyst or neoplasm

WORKUP

- Complete history and physical examination
- Pelvic or rectovaginal examination to reveal firm, irregular, mobile mass
- Laparoscopy or laparotomy to establish diagnosis

LABORATORY TESTS

- Pregnancy test
- Serum tumor markers:
  1. Cancer antigen 125 (CA-125)
  2. Alpha-fetoprotein (endodermal sinus tumor, immature teratoma)
  3. Beta-human chorionic gonadotropin
  4. Lactate dehydrogenase (dysgerminoma)

IMAGING STUDIES

Ultrasound (Fig. 1):
- May differentiate adnexal mass from other pelvic masses
- Features that increase risk of malignancy include solid component, papillae, multiple septations or solitary thick septa, ascites, matted bowel, bilaterality, irregular borders
- CT scan with contrast
- Colonoscopy or barium enema, if symptomatic

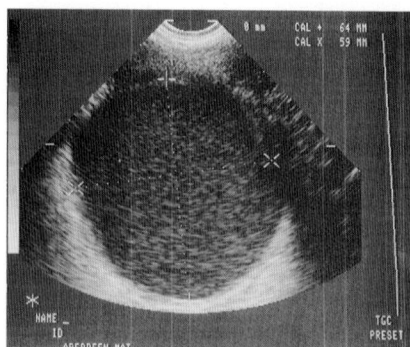

FIG. 1 Ultrasonogram reveals a cyst 6.5 cm across, which was found at laparotomy to be an endometrioma full of altered blood, the so-called chocolate cyst. This may cause cyclical or chronic pelvic pain. (From Greer IA et al: *Mosby's color atlas and text of obstetrics and gynecology,* London, 2000, Harcourt.)

NONPHARMACOLOGIC THERAPY

Repeat pelvic examination, typically with transvaginal pelvic ultrasound, for premenopausal women in 4 to 6 wk to rule out persistent cyst.

ACUTE GENERAL Rx

Indications for surgery:
- Postmenopausal or premenarchal palpable adnexal mass
- Adnexal mass with suspicious ultrasound features
- Premenopausal woman with persistent cyst >5 cm
- Any adnexal mass >8 cm
- Suspected torsion or rupture

CHRONIC Rx

- Depends on diagnosis
- Possible suppression of formation of new cysts by oral contraceptives

DISPOSITION

Depends on diagnosis

REFERRAL

- If malignancy suspected
- If surgery required

SUGGESTED READING
Available at www.expertconsult.com

RELATED CONTENT
Ovarian Cysts (Patient Information)
Ovarian Cancer (Related Key Topic)

AUTHOR: **ANTHONY SCISCIONE, D.O.**

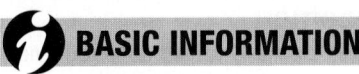

BASIC INFORMATION

DEFINITION

Paget's disease of bone is a focal disorder of chaotic bone remodeling with increased osteoblastic and osteoclastic activity that results in disorganized woven and lamellar bone in one or more skeletal sites. The end result is bone of poor quality that is enlarged, hypervascular, and susceptible to deformation and fracture.

SYNONYMS

Osteitis deformans

ICD-10CM CODES

M88.9	Osteitis deformans of unspecified bone
M88.0	Osteitis deformans of skull
M88.1	Osteitis deformans of vertebrae
M88.869	Osteitis deformans of unspecified lower leg
M88.89	Osteitis deformans of multiple sites
M90.60	Osteitis deformans in neoplastic diseases, unspecified site
M90.679	Osteitis deformans in neoplastic diseases, unspecified ankle and foot
M90.68	Osteitis deformans in neoplastic diseases, other site
M90.69	Osteitis deformans in neoplastic diseases, multiple sites

EPIDEMIOLOGY & DEMOGRAPHICS

Epidemiologic data suggest an origin of Paget's disease in Great Britain spreading to other areas by English colonists beginning in the seventeenth century. Highest prevalence occurs in Eastern and Western Europe and in those who have emigrated to New Zealand, Australia, South Africa, and North America. Paget's is rarely seen in Japanese, Chinese, Asian Indians, sub-Saharan Africans, and Middle Eastern Arabs.

Most commonly diagnosed in those aged >50 years and rare before 40 years.

Prevalence estimates of up to 3% of population aged >50 years and up to 10% in those aged >90 years.

PREDOMINANT SEX: Variable preponderance of males.

PREDOMINANT AGE: Middle or advanced years.

FAMILIAL INCIDENCE: Common, family history positive in up to 40% of cases.

PHYSICAL FINDINGS & CLINICAL PRESENTATION

- Most common sites of involvement: pelvis (70%), lumbar spine (53%), sacrum, femur (55%), skull (42%), tibia (30%) (Fig. E1), humerus, scapula.
- Uncommon: hand, foot, fibula.
- Lesions in one (monostotic) or more bones (polyostotic).
- Gradual progression of disease in affected bone(s) with rare appearance at new site(s).
- Many patients are asymptomatic, but up to 40% of patients who come to medical attention present with bone pain.
- Symptoms and signs include bone and articular pain often related to secondary arthritis, bone deformities and enlargement, increased warmth over pagetic bone, skull enlargement, nerve entrapment or compression syndromes, cranial nerve deficits especially deafness, spinal cord compression and vascular steal syndromes, fissure fractures, fractures, and neoplastic degeneration.

ETIOLOGY

Etiology remains unknown

Extensive epidemiologic and laboratory data are in keeping with potential role of paramyxoviral infection of osteoclasts in a genetically susceptible individual with or without documented genetic mutations.

DIAGNOSIS

Diagnosis is often suspected in asymptomatic patients with isolated elevation of alkaline phosphatase without evidence of liver disease.

DIFFERENTIAL DIAGNOSIS

- Osteosclerosis
- Hyperphosphatasia
- Familial expansile osteolysis
- Fibrous dysplasia
- Skeletal neoplasm (primary or metastatic)
- Osteomalacia with secondary hyperparathyroidism

LABORATORY TESTS

- Increase in serum alkaline phosphatase or bone-specific alkaline phosphatase
- Increase in urine NTx/creatinine ratio or plasma CTx
- Bone biopsy may be necessary to rule out sarcomatous degeneration or metastatic disease

IMAGING STUDIES (FIG. E2)

Bone scintigraphy is the most sensitive test for delineating the extent and site of pagetic lesions but nonspecific in that areas of uptake may be related to arthritis or metastatic lesions. Radiographs (Fig. E3) will further delineate characteristic pagetic changes.

TREATMENT

Indications for therapy include extensive or symptomatic disease; neurologic complications; involvement of weight-bearing bones, skull, vertebrae, and other areas of critical involvement, for example, in proximity to joints; and prevention of excess bleeding from an orthopedic procedure on pagetic bone.

NONPHARMACOLOGIC THERAPY

- Optimization of calcium and vitamin D intake and appropriate guidance regarding ambulatory needs.
- Orthopedic stabilization may be required for patients with pseudofractures.

SPECIFIC THERAPY

Bisphosphonates are the mainstay of therapy and include oral alendronate or risedronate and intravenous pamidronate or zoledronic acid.

- SC salmon calcitonin when bisphosphonates are not tolerated or are contraindicated as in those with GFR of <35 ml/min
- Acetaminophen, aspirin, and nonsteroidal drugs for relief of pain

DISPOSITION

- Without treatment, progression of disease is common
- With treatment, remissions of varying duration in most patients. Bisphosphonates can normalize bone turnover in a high proportion of patients, but evidence that long-term suppression of bone turnover prevents complications or improves the clinical outcome is currently inconclusive.
- Careful and regular clinical and biochemical follow-up at 3- to 6-month intervals with necessity of retreatment in patients with continued pagetic activity or reactivation
- With first ever intravenous dose of pamidronate or zoledronic acid, patients may experience a flu-like syndrome for several days that may be prevented with acetaminophen

SUGGESTED READINGS

Available at www.expertconsult.com

RELATED CONTENT

Paget's Disease of Bone (Patient Information)

AUTHOR: **JOSEPH R. TUCCI, M.D.**

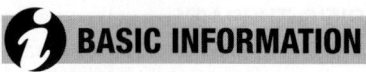

DEFINITION

Paget's disease of the breast is a malignant disease that presents itself as a scaly, sore, eroding, bleeding ulcer of the nipple. It represents an extension of a ductal adenocarcinoma of the breast. Microscopically, typical large clear cells (Paget's cells) with pale and abundant cytoplasm and hyperchromatic nuclei with prominent nucleoli are found in the epidermal layer. Paget's disease is more often associated with primary invasive or in situ carcinoma of the breast.

ICD-10CM CODES
C50.0	Malignant neoplasm of nipple and areola
C50.011	Malignant neoplasm of nipple and areola, right female breast
C50.012	Malignant neoplasm of nipple and areola, left female breast
C50.019	Malignant neoplasm of nipple and areola, unspecified female breast
C50.021	Malignant neoplasm of nipple and areola, right male breast
C50.022	Malignant neoplasm of nipple and areola, left male breast
C50.029	Malignant neoplasm of nipple and areola, unspecified male breast

EPIDEMIOLOGY & DEMOGRAPHICS

- Not common
- Found in one in 100 to 200 breast cancer patients

PHYSICAL FINDINGS & CLINICAL PRESENTATION

- Variable; most often reveals an erythematous, irregularly bordered plaque on the nipple.
- Itching or burning nipple and/or reported lump
- Very minimal scaly lesion that may bleed when scales are lifted
- Typical ulcer located on nipple with serous fluid weeping or small amount of bleeding coming from it (Fig. 1)
- Palpable carcinoma in the breast of some patients

ETIOLOGY

- Exact origin unknown
- Possibly migration of either in situ or invasive carcinoma cells in breast to nipple skin to produce Paget's disease

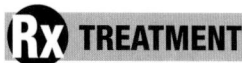

DIAGNOSIS

DIFFERENTIAL DIAGNOSIS

- Chronic dermatitis
- Florid papillomatosis of the nipple or nipple adenoma
- Eczema

WORKUP

- Clinically apparent
- Careful breast examination with diagnosis in mind
- Palpable mass or mammographic lesions in 60% to 70% of patients

A clinical algorithm for the evaluation of nipple discharge is described in Section III, "Breast, Nipple Discharge Evaluation."

LABORATORY TESTS

Biopsy of nipple lesion

IMAGING STUDIES

Mammograms to search for possible primary carcinoma

TREATMENT

NONPHARMACOLOGIC THERAPY

- Fewer patients:
  1. Paget's disease of nipple only finding when mammographically negative breast
  2. Consideration of wide excision of nipple with or without radiation
- Other patients: additional invasive or in situ carcinoma recognized
- Either modified mastectomy or breast conservation treatment
- Presence of underlying in situ or invasive carcinoma in mastectomy specimen of majority of patients

ACUTE GENERAL Rx

Systemic adjuvant therapy depending on extent of invasive carcinoma found

DISPOSITION

- Parallel prognosis to that of breast cancer patient without Paget's disease
- Regular follow-up as in other invasive or in situ carcinoma patients

REFERRAL

At outset, all suspicious nipple lesions should be referred for evaluation and treatment.

SUGGESTED READING
Available at www.expertconsult.com

RELATED CONTENT
Paget's Disease of the Breast (Patient Information)
Breast Cancer (Related Key Topic)

AUTHOR: **RUBEN ALVERO, M.D.**

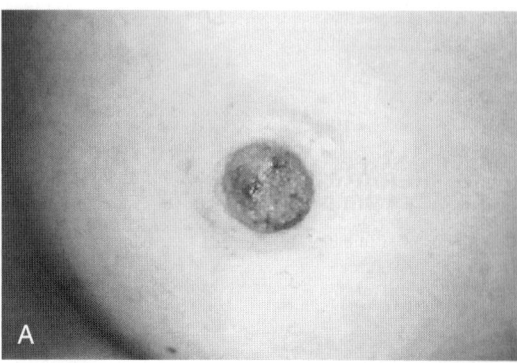 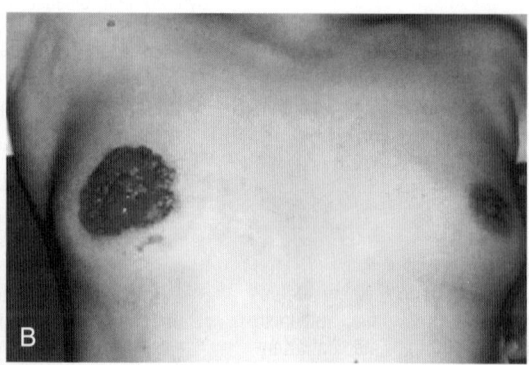

FIG. 1 **A** and **B,** Paget's disease of the nipple. (Courtesy Sehwan Han, M.D.)

BASIC INFORMATION

DEFINITION

Chronic pain is pain that persists for longer than the expected time frame or that is associated with progressive, nonmalignant disease. Pain is an unpleasant sensory and emotional experience associated with actual or potential tissue damage or described in terms of such damage. The perception of pain is influenced by physiologic, psychological, and social factors.

SYNONYMS

Chronic pain management
Nonmalignant chronic pain
Pain management

ICD-10CM CODES
G89.4   Chronic pain syndrome
G89.29 Other chronic pain
G89.21 Chronic pain due to trauma
G89.22 Chronic post-thoracotomy pain
G89.28 Other chronic postprocedural pain
G89.3   Neoplasm related pain (acute)
        (chronic)

EPIDEMIOLOGY & DEMOGRAPHICS

Estimates of the prevalence of chronic pain in the United States vary widely. Data from one national survey (1999-2002 National Health and Nutrition Examination Survey [NHANES]) reported a prevalence of chronic regional and widespread pain of 11% and 3.6%, respectively, while the National Center for Health Statistics estimates that 32.8% of the U.S. population suffers from some form of chronic pain. Chronic pain is the third leading cause of physical impairment in the United States, and related costs are estimated to be tens of billions annually. Patients with chronic pain may also experience changes in mood, depression, sleep disturbances, fatigue, and decreased overall physical functioning.

CLINICAL PRESENTATION

- History: comprehensive patient assessment, including history of present illness (cause of pain, location, timing, characteristics, exacerbating/relieving factors, triggers), past therapies (pharmacologic and nonpharmacologic and outcomes of these therapies), medical history, family and social history, psychiatric history (including history of depression, anxiety, abuse, and/or other psychological disorders), substance use history, allergies, sleep patterns and disturbances, and current medications. Social supports, coping mechanisms, and spirituality can also help guide development of a treatment plan.
- Pain assessment should be performed at each visit; includes pain intensity (1 to 10), response to medication, and attributes of pain. Standardized templates for both initial and follow-up pain assessment have been developed by various organizations. The Brief Pain Inventory is an example of a widely used assessment tool. In addition, a functional

assessment should be performed. Tools such as the Functional Ability Questionnaire (FAQ5) can guide the clinician in determining a patient's functional status. Lastly, consider assessment of a patient's risk for substance abuse.
- Physical examination: directed at systems affected by pain (often musculoskeletal) and neurologic examination.
- Look for contributing factors (e.g., comorbidities, lifestyle factors) and barriers to effective care (e.g., behavioral, social, insurance)

ETIOLOGY

Chronic pain can generally be categorized as originating from one of five etiologies: musculoskeletal, neuropathic, inflammatory, mechanical, or mixed. Chronic pain may include such diagnoses as headache, low back pain, previous trauma, arthritis, neurogenic (e.g., trigeminal neuralgia), psychogenic (related to depression or anxiety), fibromyalgia, reflex sympathetic dystrophy, myofascial pain syndrome, phantom limb pain, idiopathic, or unknown.

DIAGNOSIS

DIFFERENTIAL DIAGNOSIS

- Depends on etiology (musculoskeletal, neuropathic, inflammatory, mechanical, or mixed)
- Depression and anxiety disorders can be both a cause and a result of chronic pain, so temporal association of these disorders is important.

WORKUP

- Workup should be directed at identifying the source of pain
- Laboratory testing, imaging studies, and/or electromyographic studies should be used when etiology of chronic pain is unknown or unclear, when comorbidities are suspected, and as the history and physical examination direct.
- Consider use of random urine drug screens or other tests to screen for presence of illegal drugs, unreported prescribed medications, or alcohol use.

TREATMENT

- Studies increasingly support the application of a multidisciplinary, biopsychosocial approach that addresses the multiple facets of pain and includes the patient's perspective and goals.
- Therapeutic goal is the reduction of pain (elimination of chronic pain is generally unlikely and providers need to discuss these limitations with patients at outset).
- A written care plan that includes methods to address the patient's personal goals, improve sleep, increase physical activity, manage stress, and reduce pain.

NONPHARMACOLOGIC THERAPY

- Exercise (recommended for all patients and tailored to individual abilities and needs)

- Modalities: heat therapy, cold therapy, transcutaneous electrical nerve stimulation (TENS) units, manipulative therapy, cognitive behavioral therapy, psychological counseling, and physical therapy
- Electrostimulation therapy: TENS units
- Behavioral therapies: cognitive behavioral therapy, hypnosis, biofeedback, relaxation therapy
- Music therapy (in conjunction with other types of therapy)
- Surgery

ACUTE GENERAL Rx

- Short-acting antiinflammatory and analgesic medications (e.g., acetaminophen/NSAIDs/ opioids). Avoid use of NSAIDs in patients with hypertension, CHF, or any type of CKD.
- Topical analgesics (lidocaine, NSAIDs, capsaicin)
- Trigger point or joint injections (immediate anesthetic plus long-acting corticosteroids)
- Epidural steroid injections
- Nerve blocks

CHRONIC Rx

- Pain management with long-acting pharmacologic agents is considered a key aspect of therapy but is often underused. Fig. 1 illustrates a strategy for pharmacologic management of pain using the World Health Organization (WHO) analgesic ladder. Fig. E2 describes another algorithm for pain management.
- Long-acting NSAIDs. Table 1 describes adjuvant analgesic drugs for chronic pain.
- Sustained-release opioids (used for moderate to severe pain that has failed other therapeutic interventions): oxycodone, morphine SR, methadone (use with caution), or fentanyl patch; short-acting opioids can be used in conjunction with these agents for management of breakthrough pain. Conversion to a long-acting opioid should be based on an equianalgesic conversion. Table E2 compares morphine milligram equivalent doses for commonly prescribed opioids. Opioids are rarely beneficial in the treatment of inflammatory or mechanical pain and are not indicated for treatment of headaches (http:// www.acpinternist.org/archives/2008/01/extr a/pain_charts.pdf).
- Table 3 provides guidelines for opioid dose selection, conservative initial starting doses for opioid-naïve individuals, and conversion ratios for opioid rotation in patients on chronic opioids. Titration of these medications should not exceed the equivalent of 100 mg morphine/ day to avoid risk of overdose. Box E1 summarizes CDC recommendations for prescribing opioids for chronic pain outside of active cancer and palliative and end-of-life care. Box E2 summarizes the interpretation of recommendation categories and evidence types.
- Antidepressants (tricyclic and selective serotonin reuptake inhibitor)
- Anticonvulsant medications particularly helpful for neuropathic conditions (e.g., carbamazepine, valproic acid, gabapentin, pregabalin)

WHO ANALGESIC LADDER

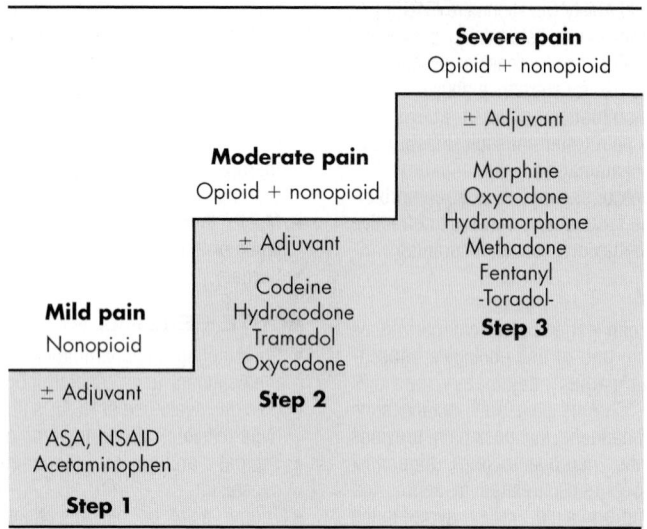

Severe pain
Opioid + nonopioid

± Adjuvant

Morphine
Oxycodone
Hydromorphone
Methadone
Fentanyl
-Toradol-

Step 3

Moderate pain
Opioid + nonopioid

± Adjuvant

Codeine
Hydrocodone
Tramadol
Oxycodone

Step 2

Mild pain
Nonopioid

± Adjuvant

ASA, NSAID
Acetaminophen

Step 1

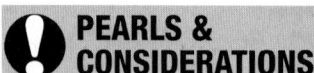

• Advance up the ladder if pain persists

FIG. 1 Strategy for pharmacologic management of pain using the World Health Organization (WHO) analgesic ladder. Multiagent therapy is usually required for optimal pain management. Patients with mild pain should be started on a nonopioid analgesic, and those with moderate pain on a step 2 opioid. Many patients can benefit from the addition of a nonopioid to the opioid (e.g., for bone pain) or an adjuvant agent to the opioid (e.g., for neuropathic pain). If this combination does not produce adequate relief or the patient has severe pain, step 3 opioids should be started initially. Toradol (ketorolac) is a nonsteroidal antiinflammatory drug *(NSAID)* with the pain-relieving potency of a step 3 opioid. Many patients can benefit from the addition of nonopioid analgesics or adjuvants, if indicated. *ASA,* Aspirin. (From Hoffman R et al: *Hematology, basic principles and practice,* ed 5, Philadelphia, 2009, Churchill Livingstone.)

• Implantable methods, epidural and intrathecal drug delivery systems, dorsal column stimulators
• Treatment of insomnia and sleep disorders to reduce pain with standard sleep-inducing agents (trazodone, antihistamines)

COMPLEMENTARY & ALTERNATIVE MEDICINE

Acupuncture and massage (evidence-based for some indications). Acupuncture is most likely to benefit patients with low back pain, neck pain, chronic idiopathic or tension headache, migraine, and knee osteoarthritis.

REFERRAL

• Pain medicine specialist or multidisciplinary pain clinic: useful when primary therapies fail, in patients with complex pain conditions, or for invasive therapies
• Consider referral to an addiction specialist if patient has a history of substance abuse or addiction
• Psychiatry/psychological services for counseling, if needed

! PEARLS & CONSIDERATIONS

• Patient consent should be obtained in the form of a written treatment agreement before initiating treatment. This agreement should outline the goals of therapy, use of a single provider or treatment team and a single pharmacy, limitations on dose and number of prescribed medications, prohibition on use with alcohol or sedating medications, keeping medication safe and secure, prohibition on selling or sharing medication, limitations on refills, compliance with all components of the treatment plan, the role of drug screening, and consequences of nonadherence.
• Follow-up assessment should occur every 1 to 6 mo and include a complete pain assessment (see earlier), review of the type of long-acting analgesic used and dosage, use of breakthrough analgesics, side effects and their management, use of nonpharmacologic therapies, and adjunct medication use.

COMMENTS

• Medication dependence and addiction should not be confused. Most patients receiving chronic opioid therapy can become dependent on these medications for pain relief but opioid addiction does not occur. Patients exhibiting signs of addiction often will seek escalating doses of medication, request refills of prescriptions earlier than planned, and engage in drug-seeking activities (e.g., emergency department visits between prescriptions, seeking multiple prescriptions).
• Side effects need not preclude use of opioid medications and should be anticipated. Antiemetics can aid in controlling nausea. Constipation can be managed with stool softeners and laxatives.
• The emphasis of comprehensive pain management for non–cancer-related chronic pain has led to a fourfold increase in prescribing of opioid medications in the United States. This increase in opiate use has also led to a rise in the misuse and abuse of these medications. Providers should proceed with caution before initiating pain management with opiate medications and should familiarize themselves with processes and tools for pain assessment and medication management. Forty-two states have developed prescription drug monitoring programs (PDMPs) to assist providers in identifying issues of abuse, polypharmacy, and misuse of controlled substances.

PATIENT & FAMILY EDUCATION

National Pain Foundation (http://www.pain-connection.org)
American Pain Foundation (http://www.pain-foundation.org)
National Institutes of Health (http://www.nih.gov)

SUGGESTED READINGS

Available at www.expertconsult.com

RELATED CONTENT

Pain Medications (Patient Information)

AUTHOR: **ANNGENE G. ANTHONY, M.D., M.P.H.**

TABLE 1 Adjuvant Analgesic Drugs for Chronic Pain

Drug	Dosage	Indications	Adverse Effects	Comments
Tricyclic Antidepressants				
Amitriptyline, imipramine, desipramine, nortriptyline	10–150 mg/day	Peripheral neuropathy, postherpetic neuralgia, other types of peripheral neuropathic pain, central pain, facial pain, fibromyalgia, headache prophylaxis, irritable bowel syndrome, and chronic low back pain with or without radiculopathy	Sedation, dry mouth, confusion, weight gain, constipation, urinary retention, ataxia, cardiac conduction delay (QTc prolongation)	First-line agents for neuropathic pain and headache prophylaxis; Secondary amine drugs (e.g., nortriptyline) have fewer side effects than tertiary amines (e.g., amitriptyline); Contraindicated in glaucoma
Serotonin-Norepinephrine Reuptake Inhibitors				
Venlafaxine	75–225 mg/day	Peripheral neuropathy, headache prophylaxis	Sedation, dry mouth, constipation, ataxia, hypertension, hyperhidrosis	Dose adjustment in patients with renal dysfunction
Duloxetine	60–120 mg/day	Peripheral neuropathy, fibromyalgia, chronic back pain	Sedation, dry mouth, constipation, hyperhidrosis	U.S. Food and Drug Administration (FDA)-approved for fibromyalgia and diabetic neuropathy; Contraindicated in glaucoma
Anticonvulsants				
Gabapentin	600–3600 mg/day	Peripheral neuropathy, postherpetic neuralgia, other types of peripheral neuropathic pain, central pain, pelvic pain, headache prophylaxis, radiculopathy, chronic postsurgical pain	Sedation, weight gain, dry mouth, ataxia, edema	First-line agent for neuropathic pain; FDA-approved for postherpetic neuralgia; Effective preemptively for postoperative pain
Pregabalin	150–600 mg/day	Peripheral neuropathy, postherpetic neuralgia, central pain, fibromyalgia	Sedation, weight gain, dry mouth, ataxia, edema	First-line agent for neuropathic pain; FDA-approved for diabetic neuropathy, postherpetic neuralgia, fibromyalgia; Effective preemptively for postoperative pain; Same mechanism of action as gabapentin
Carbamazepine	200–1600 mg/day	Facial neuralgias, diabetic neuropathy	Sedation, ataxia, diplopia, hyponatremia, agranulocytosis, diarrhea, aplastic anemia, hepatotoxicity, Stevens-Johnson syndrome	First-line agent and FDA-approved for trigeminal and glossopharyngeal neuralgia; Contraindicated in patients with porphyria and atrioventricular conduction block
Topiramate	50–400 mg/day	Headache prophylaxis, chronic low back pain with or without radiculopathy	Sedation, ataxia, diplopia, weight loss, diarrhea, metabolic acidosis, kidney stones	First-line agent and FDA-approved for migraine prophylaxis; Often used as appetite suppressant
Corticosteroids (Systemic)				
Prednisone	5–60 mg/day	Inflammatory arthritis, other inflammatory pain conditions (e.g., inflammatory bowel disease), traumatic nerve injury, complex regional pain syndrome	Myriad psychiatric, gastrointestinal, neurologic, and cardiac side effects; immunosuppression, weakness, edema, weight gain, elevated glucose, poor wound healing, others	Stronger evidence supports local (i.e., injection) administration; More effective for acute pain; Strong antiinflammatory effects
Miscellaneous				
Muscle relaxants	Variable depending on drug	Skeletal muscle spasm, acute spinal pain, temporomandibular disorder; Baclofen effective for spasticity, dystonia, and trigeminal neuralgia	Sedation, ataxia, blurred vision, confusion, asthenia, xerostomia and other gastrointestinal effects, palpitations	First-line agents for acute back pain and skeletal muscle spasm
Lidocaine patch	1–3 patches every 12 hr	Postherpetic neuralgia, peripheral neuropathy, other types of neuropathic and possibly myofascial pain associated with allodynia	Minimal systemic side effects when applied appropriately	Second-line agent and FDA-approved for postherpetic neuralgia
Capsaicin cream	0.025% applied three or four times per day	Postherpetic neuralgia, peripheral neuropathy and other types of neuropathic pain, chronic postsurgical pain, arthritis, and other musculoskeletal conditions	Burning on application; Minimal systemic side effects when applied appropriately	FDA-approved for arthritis; Second-line agent for postherpetic neuralgia and third-line agent for peripheral neuropathy; Single application 8% patch providing up to 3 mo of pain relief was recently approved for postherpetic neuralgia
Cannabinoids	Variable depending on drug and delivery route	Strongest evidence is for multiple sclerosis; May be effective for peripheral neuropathy and other types of neuropathic pain spasticity	Myriad psychiatric, neurologic, and cardiac effects; xerostomia, abdominal pain, and other gastrointestinal effects	Fourth-line agent with narrow therapeutic index; Modest analgesic effect comparable to codeine

From Goldman L, Schafer AI: *Goldman's Cecil medicine*, ed 24, Philadelphia, 2012, Saunders.

TABLE 3 Guidelines for Opioid Dose Selection, Conservative Initial Starting Doses for Opioid-Naïve Individuals, and Conversion Ratios for Opioid Rotation in Patients on Chronic Opioids

Opioid Naïve	Morphine SR	Codeine	Oxycodone	Hydrocodone	Hydromorphone	Methadone	Fentanyl	Oxymorphone
Initial dose and range in opioid-naive patient (starting dose range for repeated dosing)*	15 mg (15-30 mg q 8-12h)	30 mg (15-60 mg q 4-6h)	5 mg (5-15 mg q 4-6h)	5 mg (5-10 mg q 4-6h)	2 mg (2-4 mg q 4-6h)	2.5 mg q 6-12h	NA	5 mg q 4-6h
Opioid Tolerant Converting from:	**Morphine PO**	**Codeine**	**Oxycodone**	**Hydrocodone**	**Hydromorphone**	**Methadone**	**Fentanyl**	**Oxymorphone**
Morphine IM 10 mg (the gold standard for opioid comparisons)	20-30 mg	60-90 mg†	5 mg	5-10 mg q 4-6h	2 mg	2.5 mg	25-µg patch/72 hr	5 mg (the gold standard for opioid comparisons)
Morphine SR 30 mg PO q 8-12h, 60-90 mg/24h	30-90 mg q 4h		3-45 mg/24 hr oxycodone, approx 50% of morphine dose	30-45 mg/24 hr	12-18 mg/24 hr	24-hr dose morphine 30-90 mg 4:1 conversion 90-300 mg 8:1 conversion >300 mg 12:1	25-mcg patch/72 hr	5 mg q 12h ER
Codeine 30-60 mg q 4h	15-30 mg q 3-4h		5-7.5 mg q 4h	5-10 mg q 4h	12 mg/24 hr	2.5 mg q 8-12h	12.5-µg patch/72 hr	2.5-5 mg q 4-6h IR
Oxycodone 5 mg q 3-4h	10 mg	30-60 mg q 3-4h		5-10 mg q 4h	12 mg/24 hr	2.5 mg q 8-12h	25-µg patch/72 hr	5 mg q 4-6h IR
Hydrocodone 10 mg q 3-4h	15 mg	30-60 mg q 3-4h	5 mg q 3-4h		12 mg/24 hr		12.5-µg patch/72 hr	2.5-5 mg q 4-6h IR
Hydromorphone 2 mg q 4h	10 mg		5 mg	5-10 mg q 4h		2.5 mg q 8-12h	25-µg patch/72 hr	5 mg q 4-6h IR
Methadone 5 mg q 8h	20 mg SR q 8h		10 mg q 3-4h		4 mg q 4-6h		25-µg patch/72 hr	5 mg q 12h ER
Fentanyl 25 µg/hr patch	90 mg morphine per 24 hr (1 µg to 4 mg morphine)					5 mg q 8-12h		5 mg q12h ER
Oxymorphone ER 5 mg q 12h	15 mg SR q 12h		5 mg q 8-12h	10 mg q 4-6h	12 mg/24 hr	5 mg q 8-12h	25-µg patch/72 hr	

Note: Recommended starting doses are low and should be titrated upward slowly to minimize adverse effects. Limitations of equianalgesic tables exist because they are based on single-dose studies in opioid-naïve individuals. Convert opioid 1 to morphine equivalents and calculate dose of opioid 2 according to conversion ratio then reduce the calculated dose for opioid 2 by 1/3 to 1/2 to ensure safety of the 24-hr total daily dose. Rescue dose is 10% to 20% of daily opioid dose given every 3 to 4 hr as needed. Titration upward for unrelieved pain should be by 25% to 30% of the current 24-hr dose, adjusted by daily amount of rescue medications needed over a several-week period. Equivalent or equianalgesic doses for the different opioid preparations vary in different publications. *ER,* Extended release; *IR,* immediate release.

*Conservative low equianalgesic starting doses for opioid-naïve individuals adapted from published recommendations.

†Doses above 1.5 mg/kg not recommended because of increase in side effects.

From Hochberg MC et al: *Rheumatology,* ed 5, St Louis, 2011, Mosby.

BASIC INFORMATION

DEFINITION

Pancreatic cancer is an adenocarcinoma derived from pancreatic duct epithelium.

ICD-10CM CODES

C25.9	Malignant neoplasm of pancreas, unspecified
C25.0	Malignant neoplasm of head of pancreas
C25.1	Malignant neoplasm of body of pancreas
C25.2	Malignant neoplasm of tail of pancreas
C25.3	Malignant neoplasm of pancreatic duct

EPIDEMIOLOGY & DEMOGRAPHICS

INCIDENCE: In the U.S., it is estimated that there will be 53,000 new cases and 41,780 deaths in 2016. It is the fourth leading cause of cancer-related death in the U.S. The majority of patients present with advanced disease, and less than 20% of patients present with potentially resectable tumors.
PREDOMINANT SEX: Male/female ratio of 2:1
PREDOMINANT AGE: Median age at diagnosis is 71 years

PHYSICAL FINDINGS & CLINICAL PRESENTATION

Presenting symptoms are generally related to location:
Jaundice (60%-70% of pancreatic cancers are located in the head of the pancreas)
Abdominal pain: generally dull upper abdominal pain or vague abdominal discomfort
Weight loss
Anorexia/change in taste, asthenia
Nausea
Uncommonly: depression, gastrointestinal bleeding, acute pancreatitis (from obstruction of the pancreatic duct), back pain
Trousseau syndrome (hypercoagulability in the setting of malignancy) may be initial presentation in some patients.
Physical findings:
Icterus
Cachexia, temporal wasting
Ascites, peripheral lymphadenopathy, hepatomegaly
Excoriations from scratching pruritic skin

ETIOLOGY

Unknown, but several conditions have been associated with pancreatic cancer:
- Smoking
- Alcoholism
- Genetics: 5% to 10% of patients have a family history of the disease
- Genetic syndromes and associated genes: Hereditary pancreatitis (*PRSS1, SPINK1*), Peutz-Jeghers syndrome (*STK11[LKB1]*), familial atypical multiple mole and melanoma syndrome (*p16*), hereditary breast and ovarian cancer syndromes (*BRACA1, BRACA2, PALB2*), ataxia telangiectasia (*ATM*), Li-Fraumeni syndrome (*P53*)
- Gallstones

- Diabetes mellitus (present in at least 50% of patients with pancreatic cancer)
- Chronic pancreatitis
- Diet rich in animal fat
- Occupational exposure: oil refining, paper manufacturing, chemical industry
- Overweight or obesity during early adulthood is associated with a greater risk of pancreatic cancer and a younger age of disease onset. Obesity at an older age is associated with a lower overall survival in patients with pancreatic cancer.
- Possible increased risk for certain type-2 diabetes medications (GLP-1 receptor agonists and DPP-4 inhibitors). However, recent trials have failed to confirm increased risk.

DIAGNOSIS

DIFFERENTIAL DIAGNOSIS

- Common duct cholelithiasis
- Cholangiocarcinoma
- Common duct stricture
- Sclerosing cholangitis
- Primary biliary cirrhosis
- Autoimmune pancreatitis
- Drug-induced cholestasis (e.g., phenothiazines)
- Other pancreatic tumors (islet cell tumor, cystadenocarcinoma, epidermoid carcinoma, sarcomas, lymphomas)

WORKUP

Initial laboratory testing includes complete blood count, serum chemistries. The bile duct antigen CA 19-9 is not used as a screening test but can be utilized as a modality for detecting recurrence and for therapeutic monitoring in patients undergoing therapy.

Routine Laboratory Tests	% Abnormal
Alkaline phosphatase	80
Bilirubin	55
Total protein	15
Amylase	15
Hemoglobin	60

IMAGING STUDIES

Multidetector helical CT with IV administration of contrast is the imaging procedure of choice for initial evaluation. Endoscopic ultrasonography is useful when the diagnosis is strongly suspected and tissue is required for diagnostic purposes. Fine-needle aspiration biopsy combined with endoscopic ultrasonography is the preferred modality for evaluation of cystic or mass lesions to determine malignancy. Endoscopic retrograde cholangiopancreatography (ERCP) is useful in patients with jaundice needing an endoscopic stent to relieve obstruction.

Noninvasive Imaging	% Abnormal
Abdominal ultrasonography	60
Abdominal CT scan (with contrast) (Fig. 1)	90
Abdominal MRI scan	90
Invasive Imaging	
ERCP	90
CT scan or ultrasonography-guided needle aspiration cytology	90-95

STAGING FOR PANCREATIC CANCER

PRIMARY TUMOR (T):

TX	Primary tumor cannot be assessed
T0	No evidence of primary tumor
T1	Tumor <2 cm
T2	Tumor >2 cm, confined to the pancreas
T3	Tumor extends locally beyond the pancreas
T4	Tumor involves celiac or superior mesenteric arteries

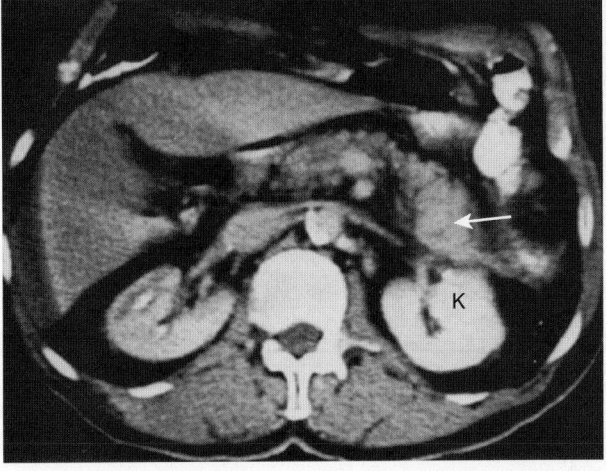

FIG. 1 CT scan of a patient with adenocarcinoma of the body and tail of the pancreas. The tumor *(arrow)* is seen anterior and adjacent to the left kidney *(K)*. At operation, the tumor was invading Gerota's fascia. (From Sabiston D: *Textbook of surgery*, ed 17, Philadelphia, 2005, Saunders.)

LYMPH NODES (N):

NX   Regional lymph nodes cannot be assessed

N0   No regional lymph node metastasis

N1   Regional lymph node metastasis

DISTANT METASTASES (M):

MX   Presence of distant metastasis cannot be assessed

M0   No distant metastasis

M1   Distant metastasis

STAGING GROUPS:

IA   T1, N0, M0

IB   T2, N0, M0

IIAf   T3, N0, M0

IIB   T1-3, N1, M0

III   T4, N0-1, M0

IV   T1-4, N0-1, M1

A clinical/radiographic staging system for adenocarcinoma of the pancreatic head and uncinate process is described in Table 1.

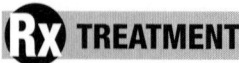

TREATMENT

SURGERY FOR RESECTABLE DISEASE

Curative cephalic pancreatoduodenectomy (Whipple's procedure) for tumors in the head and neck of the pancreas is appropriate for only 10% to 20% of patients whose lesion is <5 cm, solitary, and without locoregional invasion. Surgical mortality rate can be up to 5%. Tumors in the body or tail of the pancreas are removed by means of a distal pancreatectomy, which often includes a splenectomy. Due to the complexity of surgery and risk for significant morbidity and mortality, current guidelines recommend that pancreatic resections be carried out in centers that perform at least 15 to 20 cases annually. In addition, a recent review concluded that high-volume institutions are associated with higher negative-margin status and higher 5-year survival rates, and that patients are more likely to receive multimodality therapy at these centers.

Adjuvant chemotherapy has been demonstrated to improve postoperative survival in multiple randomized trials and is considered the standard approach currently. The use of 5-fluorouracil (5-FU) or gemcitabine for a period of 6 months is currently recommended, with median survival in the 21-month range expected for patients with a complete resection. More recent data have demonstrated that the combination of gemcitabine and capecitabine is superior to gemcitabine alone in this setting. The use of adjuvant radiotherapy in this setting is controversial and is best limited to patients with poor risk features, margin-positive surgery, or with multiple nodal or extranodal tumor involvement. An emerging strategy is the use of neoadjuvant preoperative chemotherapy combined with radiotherapy in patients with resectable pancreatic cancer. Palliative therapeutic ERCP with metal or plastic stents is performed for biliary decompression.

CHEMOTHERAPY

In patients with advanced disease, accepted approaches can include the administration of gemcitabine alone or combined with the oral EGFR inhibitor erlotinib. More recently, a combination therapy regimen consisting of oxaliplatin, irinotecan, fluorouracil, and leucovorin (FOLFIRINOX) offers increased median survival in metastatic pancreatic cancer when compared to gemcitabine (11.1 mo versus 6.8 mo) but at the cost of increased toxicity. A second trial revealed that in patients with metastatic pancreatic cancer, the combination of nab-paclitaxel plus gemcitabine significantly improved overall survival, but rates of peripheral neuropathy and myelosuppression were increased. The liposomal formulation of irinotecan is now also approved in this setting in combination with infusional fluorouracil.

- Poor survival outcomes are seen in patients with poor performance status, significant weight loss, and with liver metastases.
- Combined chemotherapy and radiotherapy can be utilized in the case of patients with locally advanced but unresectable cases and confers a modest improvement in median overall survival.

DISPOSITION

- Adjuvant chemotherapy has a significant survival benefit in patients with resected pancreatic cancer.

- Adjuvant postoperative chemotherapy with gemcitabine or 5-FU significantly delays the development of recurrent disease after complete resection of pancreatic cancer.
- Pancreatic cancer is the most lethal common cancer because it is usually diagnosed at an advanced stage and is resistant to therapy. Median survival for locally unresectable disease is about 14 to 16 months, while the median survival for metastatic disease is 10 to 12 months.

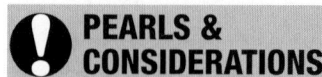

COMMENTS

- The U.S. Preventive Services Task Force (USPSTF) recommends against routine screening for pancreatic cancer in asymptomatic adults by abdominal palpation, ultrasonography, or serologic markers. The USPSTF found no evidence that screening for pancreatic cancer is effective in reducing mortality rates. There is potential for significant harm because of the low prevalence of pancreatic cancer, limited accuracy of available screening tests, invasive nature of diagnostic tests, and poor outcome of treatment. Alcohol consumption, specifically liquor consumption of three or more drinks per day, increases pancreatic cancer mortality independent of smoking.
- Patients should be referred for pancreatic cancer surgery to high-volume medical centers that perform at least 15 to 20 cases a year.
- Adjuvant chemotherapy with either a gemcitabine or 5-fluoruracil (5-FU) regimen for 6 months is proven to improve survival and should be recommended in all patients with a maintained performance status after surgical resection. The role of radiotherapy in the adjuvant setting is best restricted to patients who have a high risk for locoregional recurrence.

RELATED CONTENT

Pancreatic Cancer (Patient Information)

AUTHOR: **RITESH RATHORE, M.D.**

TABLE 1 Clinical/Radiographic Staging System for Adenocarcinoma of the Pancreatic Head and Uncinate Process

Clinical Stage	>AJCC Stage	Tumor-Vessel Relationship On Computed Tomography			
		SMA	Celiac Axis	CHA*	SMV-PV
Resectable (all four are required to be resectable)†	I/II	Normal tissue plane between tumor and vessel	Normal tissue plane between tumor and vessel	Normal tissue plane between tumor and vessel	Patent (may include tumor abutment or encasement)
Borderline resectable (only one of the four required)	III	Abutment	Abutment	Abutment or short segment encasement	May have short segment occlusion if reconstruction possible
Locally advanced (only one of the four required)	III	Encasement	Encasement	Extensive encasement with no technical option for reconstruction	Occluded with no technical option for reconstruction

AJCC, American Joint Commission for Cancer; *CHA*, common hepatic artery; *SMV–PV*, superior mesenteric vein–portal vein confluence. Abutment refers to ≤180 degrees or ≤50% of the vessel circumference; encasement is <180 degrees or <50% of the vessel circumference.

*Assumes normal vascular anatomy; for example, encasement of the CHA is not a limitation in performing PD when there is an uninvolved replaced right hepatic artery arising from the superior mesenteric artery.

†Assumes the technical ability to resect and reconstruct the SMV, PV, or SMV-PV confluence when necessary. Others would consider tumor-vein abutment/encasement, which results in deformity of the vein as borderline resectable.

From Cameron JL, Cameron AM: *Current surgical therapy,* ed 10, Philadelphia, 2011, Saunders.

BASIC INFORMATION

DEFINITION

- Acute pancreatitis is an inflammatory process of the pancreas with intrapancreatic activation of enzymes that may also involve peripancreatic tissue and/or remote organ systems. The diagnosis of acute pancreatitis requires at least 2 of the following criteria: serum amylase or lipase ≥3 times normal, abdominal pain consistent with pancreatitis, and radiographic findings (CT or MRI) of acute pancreatitis.
- Commonly used scoring systems for acute pancreatitis are described in Table 1.

  The **Revised Atlanta Criteria**[1] use early prognostic signs, organ failure, and local complications to define disease severity:
  1. **Mild pancreatitis:** no organ failure, no local or systemic complications, pancreatitis typically resolves in first week
  2. **Moderate pancreatitis:** transient organ failure (≤48 hours) or local complications (e.g., pancreatic necrosis, peripancreatic fluid collections, peripancreatic necrosis) or exacerbation of comorbid disease
  3. **Severe pancreatitis:** persistent organ failure (>48 hours)

  The **BALI Score**[2] evaluates only four variables:
  1. BUN ≥25 mg/dL
  2. Age ≥65 years
  3. LDH ≥300 U/L
  4. Interleukin-6 level ≥300 pg/mL

  These measurements are taken at admission and at 48 hours. Mortality is >25% for a score of 3 and exceeds 50% with a score of 4.

  Severe acute pancreatitis (SAP) is diagnosed by the presence of any of the following four criteria:
  1. Organ failure with one or more of the following: shock (systolic blood pressure <90 mm Hg), pulmonary insufficiency (Pao$_2$ ≤60 mm Hg), renal failure (serum creatinine >2 mg/dl after rehydration), and gastrointestinal bleeding (>500 mL/24 hr)
  2. Local complications such as necrosis, pseudocyst, or abscess
  3. At least three of Ranson's criteria (see below) or
  4. At least eight of the Acute Physiology and Chronic Health Evaluation II (APACHE II) criteria

ICD-10CM Codes
K85.0	Idiopathic acute pancreatitis
K85.1	Biliary acute pancreatitis
K85.2	Alcohol induced acute pancreatitis
K 85.3	Drug induced pancreatitis
K85.6	Other acute pancreatitis
K85.9	Acute pancreatitis, unspecified

[1]Banks PA, et al.: Acute Pancreatitis Classification Working Group: classification of acute pancreatitis-2012: revision of the Atlanta classification and definitions by international consensus, *Gut* 62(1):102-111, 2013.
[2]Spitzer AL, et al.: Applying Ockham's razor to pancreatitis prognostication: a four-variable predictive model, *Ann Surg* 243(3):380-388, 2006.

EPIDEMIOLOGY & DEMOGRAPHICS

- The incidence of pancreatitis is increasing in the U.S. Admissions for acute pancreatitis have increased by 20% over the past 10 years. There are >270,000 cases of acute pancreatitis reported annually in the United States, with nearly 40% due to gallstone disease (most common cause) and 30% due to alcohol.
- Acute pancreatitis is most often secondary to biliary tract disease and alcohol. The rate of pancreatitis continues to rise and ranges from 10 to 45 cases/100,000 in Western countries.
- Incidence in urban areas is twice that of rural areas (20/100,000 persons in urban areas).
- 20% of patients have necrotizing pancreatitis; the remainder have interstitial, or edematous, pancreatitis.
- Drugs are responsible for less than 5% of all cases of acute pancreatitis.

PHYSICAL FINDINGS & CLINICAL PRESENTATION

- Epigastric tenderness and guarding, often radiating to the back; pain usually developing suddenly, reaching peak intensity within 10 to 30 min, severe and lasting several hours without relief
- Hypoactive bowel sounds (from ileus)
- Tachycardia, shock (from decreased intravascular volume)
- Confusion (from metabolic disturbances)
- Fever
- Tachycardia, decreased breath sounds (atelectasis, pleural effusions, acute respiratory distress syndrome [ARDS])
- Jaundice (from obstruction or compression of biliary tract)
- Ascites (from tear in pancreatic duct, leaking pseudocyst)
- Palpable abdominal mass (pseudocyst, phlegmon, abscess, carcinoma)
- Evidence of hypocalcemia (Chvostek's sign, Trousseau's sign)
- Evidence of intraabdominal bleeding (hemorrhagic pancreatitis):
  1. Gray-blue discoloration around the umbilicus (*Cullen*'s sign)
  2. Bluish discoloration involving the flanks (*Grey Turner*'s sign)
- Tender subcutaneous nodules (caused by subcutaneous fat necrosis)

TABLE 1 Commonly Used Scoring Systems: Advantages and Disadvantages

System	Scoring	Advantages	Disadvantages
Ranson's criteria on admission: 1. Age >55 yr 2. WBC >16 × 10⁹/L 3. LDH >350 U/L 4. AST >250 U/L 5. Glucose >200 mg/dl During initial 48 hr: 1. Hgb falls below 10 mg/dl 2. BUN rises by >5 mg/dl 3. Ca <8 mg/dl 4. Pao$_2$ <60 mm Hg 5. Base deficit >4 mEq/L 6. Fluid sequestration >6 L	1 point for each factor listed; score >3 indicates SAP	Well known, relatively easy to calculate	Requires 48 hr to complete evaluation
APACHE II*	Score >8 predicts SAP	Can be calculated within 24 hr of admission	Requires large dataset for processing
BISAP 1. BUN >25 mg/dl 2. Altered mental status 3. Presence of SIRS 4. Age >60 yr 5. Pleural effusions	1 point for each factor listed; score >3 indicates SAP	Ease of use, available within 24 hr of admission	Significantly lower sensitivity than either Ranson's or APACHE II; results in greater likelihood of missing severe AP
CTSI	Based on radiographic data	Excellent predictor of local complications; can show infected pancreatic necrosis	Requires 72 to 96 hr, making it a poor test for guiding decisions at admission

APACHE, Acute Physiology and Chronic Health Evaluation; AST, aspartate aminotransferase; BISAP, Bedside Index for Severity in Acute Pancreatitis; BUN, blood urea nitrogen; Ca, serum calcium; CTSI, Computed Tomography Severity Index; Hgb, hemoglobin; LDH, lactate dehydrogenase; SAP, severe acute pancreatitis; SIRS, systemic inflammatory response syndrome; WBC, white blood cell count.

*Based on diverse variables, including age, physiology, and long-term health; equation available at www.sfar.org/scores2/apache22.html#calcul. Adding body mass index (BMI) to APACHE II (the APACHE 0 score) increases discrimination (1 point added for BMI 26-30; 2 points for BMI >30).

Modified from Cameron JL, Cameron AM: *Current surgical therapy*, ed 10, Philadelphia, 2011, Saunders.
From Cameron JL, Cameron AM: *Current surgical therapy*, ed 10, Philadelphia, 2011, Saunders.

ETIOLOGY

- In >90% of cases: biliary tract disease (calculi or sludge) or alcohol, most common after 5 to 10 yr of heavy drinking
- Drugs (e.g., thiazides, furosemide, corticosteroids, tetracycline, estrogens, valproic acid, metronidazole, azathioprine, methyldopa, pentamidine, ethacrynic acid, procainamide, amiodarone, sulindac, nitrofurantoin, angiotensin-converting enzyme inhibitors, danazol, cimetidine, piroxicam, gold, ranitidine, sulfasalazine, isoniazid, acetaminophen, cisplatin, didanosine, opiates, erythromycin, metformin, GLP-1 receptor agonists, incretin mimetics)
- Abdominal trauma
- Surgery
- Endoscopic retrograde cholangiopancreatography (ERCP)
- Infections (predominantly viral infections)
- Peptic ulcer (penetrating duodenal ulcer)
- Pancreas divisum (congenital failure to fuse of dorsal or ventral pancreas)
- Idiopathic
- Pregnancy
- Vascular (vasculitis, ischemic)
- Hypolipoproteinemia (types I, IV, and V) with triglycerides usually >500 mg/dL
- Hypercalcemia
- Pancreatic carcinoma (primary or metastatic)
- Renal failure
- Hereditary pancreatitis
- Occupational exposure to chemicals: methanol, cobalt, zinc, mercuric chloride, creosol, lead, organophosphates, chlorinated naphthalenes
- Others: scorpion bite, obstruction at ampulla region (neoplasm, duodenal diverticula, Crohn's disease), hypotensive shock, autoimmune pancreatitis

Ⓓⓧ DIAGNOSIS

DIFFERENTIAL DIAGNOSIS

- PUD
- Acute cholangitis, biliary colic
- High intestinal obstruction
- Early acute appendicitis
- Mesenteric vascular obstruction
- DKA
- Pneumonia (basilar)
- Myocardial infarction (inferior wall)
- Renal colic
- Ruptured or dissecting aortic aneurysm
- Mesenteric ischemia

LABORATORY TESTS

Pancreatic enzymes:

Amylase is increased, usually elevated in the initial 3 to 5 days of acute pancreatitis. Isoamylase determinations (separation of pancreatic cell isoenzyme components of amylase) are useful in excluding occasional cases of salivary hyperamylasemia. The use of isoamylase rather than total serum amylase reduces the risk of erroneously diagnosing pancreatitis and is preferred by some as initial biochemical test in patients suspected of having acute pancreatitis.

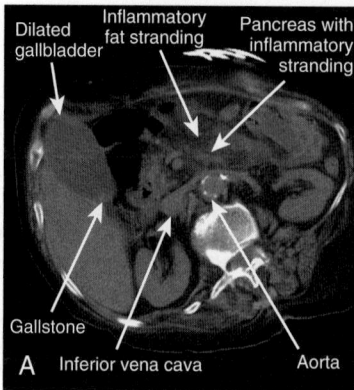
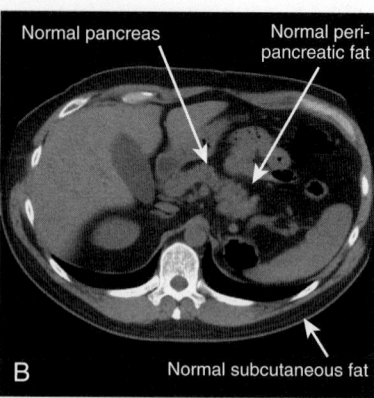

FIG. 1 Gallstone pancreatitis and normal pancreas for comparison, axial CT without contrast. **A,** Gallstone pancreatitis CT. A dilated gallbladder is visible with a hyperdense dependent lesion consistent with a gallstone. The region of the pancreas shows significant inflammatory stranding. In this patient, the pancreas lies just anterior to the left renal vein, which can be seen crossing anterior to the aorta and entering the inferior vena cava. **B,** A normal pancreas is visible. This pancreas is surrounded by uninflamed fat, which is dark (nearly black). Compare this normal fat with normal subcutaneous fat. (From Broder JS: *Diagnostic imaging for the emergency physician,* Philadelphia, 2011, Saunders.)

Urinary amylase determinations are useful to diagnose acute pancreatitis in patients with lipemic serum, to rule out elevated serum amylase caused by macroamylasemia, and to diagnose acute pancreatitis in patients whose serum amylase is normal.

Serum lipase levels are elevated in acute pancreatitis; the elevation is less transient than serum amylase; concomitant evaluation of serum amylase and lipase increases diagnostic accuracy of acute pancreatitis. An elevated lipase/amylase ratio is suggestive of alcoholic pancreatitis.

Elevated serum trypsin levels are diagnostic of pancreatitis (in absence of renal failure).

Serum C-reactive protein at 48 hr is an excellent laboratory marker of severity.

Rapid measurement of urinary trypsinogen-2 (if available) is useful in the emergency department as a screening test for acute pancreatitis in patients with abdominal pain; a negative dipstick test for urinary trypsinogen-2 rules out acute pancreatitis with a high degree of probability, whereas a positive test indicates need for further evaluation.

Interleukin-6 level: worse prognosis with level ≥300 pg/mL.

ADDITIONAL TESTS

- Complete blood count: reveals leukocytosis; hematocrit (Hct) may be initially increased as a result of hemoconcentration; decreased Hct may indicate hemorrhage or hemolysis.
- Blood urea nitrogen (BUN) is increased because of dehydration. Serial BUN measurements are the most valuable lab test for predicting mortality during the initial 48 hr.
- Elevation of serum glucose in a previously normal patient correlates with the degree of pancreatic malfunction and may be related to increased release of glycogen, catecholamines, and glucocorticoid release and decreased insulin release.
- Liver profile: aspartate aminotransferase (AST) and lactate dehydrogenase (LDH) are increased as a result of tissue necrosis; bilirubin and alkaline phosphatase may be increased from common bile duct obstruction. A threefold or greater rise in serum alanine aminotransferase concentrations is an excellent indicator (95% probability) of biliary pancreatitis.
- Serum calcium is decreased as a result of saponification, precipitation, and decreased parathyroid hormone response.
- Arterial blood gases: PaO_2 may be decreased as a result of ARDS, pleural effusion(s); pH may be decreased as a result of lactic acidosis, respiratory acidosis, and renal insufficiency.
- Serum electrolytes: potassium may be increased from acidosis or renal insufficiency; sodium may be increased from dehydration.

IMAGING STUDIES

- Abdominal plain films are useful initially to distinguish other conditions that may mimic pancreatitis (perforated viscus). They may reveal localized ileus (sentinel loop), pancreatic calcifications (chronic pancreatitis), blurring of left psoas shadow, dilation of transverse colon, calcified gallstones.
- Chest x-ray may reveal elevation of one or both diaphragms, pleural effusions, basilar infiltrates, or platelike atelectasis.
- Abdominal ultrasonography is useful in detecting gallstones (sensitivity of 60%-70% for detecting stones associated with pancreatitis). Its availability and noninvasive nature make it the initial imaging study of choice; its major limitation is the presence of distended bowel loops overlying the pancreas.
- CT scan (Fig. 1) is less sensitive than ultrasound in identifying gallstones and exposes the patient to risk of contrast-induced nephropathy. It is, however, superior to ultrasonography in identifying pancreatitis and defining its extent, and it also plays a role in diagnosing pseudocysts (they appear as

TABLE 2 Computed Tomography Severity Index Score for Pancreatitis*

Grade[†]	CT Findings	Score
A	Normal pancreas	0
B	Focal or diffuse enlargement of the pancreas, contour irregularities, heterogeneous attenuation, no peripancreatic inflammation	1
C	Grade B plus peripancreatic inflammation	2
D	Grade C plus a single fluid collection	3
E	Grade C plus multiple fluid collections or gas	4

Percent Necrosis Present on CT	Score
0	0
<33	2
33-50	4
>50	6

*Severity Index Score = Grade score + Percent necrosis score. Maximum score = 10; severe disease = 6 or higher.
[†]Severity of the acute inflammatory process.
From Adams JG, et al.: *Emergency medicine, clinical essentials*, ed 2, Philadelphia, 2013, Elsevier.

a well-defined area surrounded by a high-density capsule); gastrointestinal fistulation or infection of a pseudocyst can also be identified by the presence of gas within the pseudocyst. Sequential contrast-enhanced CT is useful for detection of pancreatic necrosis. The severity of pancreatitis can also be graded by CT scan (Table 2). (A = normal pancreas, B = enlarged pancreas [1 point], C = pancreatic and/or peripancreatic inflammation [2 points], D = single peripancreatic collection [3 points], E = at least two peripancreatic collections and/or retroperitoneal air [4 points]. Percentage of pancreatic necrosis <30% [2 points], 30% to 50% [4 points], >50% [6 points]. The CT severity index is calculated by adding grade points to points assigned for percentage of necrosis.)

- Magnetic resonance cholangiopancreatography (MRCP) has >90% sensitivity for choledocholithiasis and can identify other anatomic abnormalities.
- Endoscopic ultrasonography (EUS) is a minimally invasive test that provides high-resolution imaging of the pancreas. It is useful to identify anatomic abnormalities of the pancreas and has good sensitivity and specificity for small gallstones (≤5 mm).
- ERCP indications: useful to perform biliary sphincterotomy and stone removal in the presence of a retained bile duct stone seen on imaging. The role and timing of ERCP in patients with acute biliary pancreatitis has been controversial. Guidelines from the American College of Gastroenterology suggest that urgent ERCP (within 24 hr of admission) is indicated in patients with biliary pancreatitis who have concurrent acute cholangitis, but it is not needed in most patients who do not have evidence of ongoing biliary obstruction.[3,4]

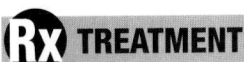 **TREATMENT**

NONPHARMACOLOGIC THERAPY
- Bowel rest with avoidance of liquids or solids during the acute illness
- Avoidance of alcohol and any drugs associated with pancreatitis

ACUTE GENERAL Rx
GENERAL MEASURES:
- Assess severity of pancreatitis (see Table 1).
- Maintain adequate intravascular volume with vigorous IV hydration. Aggressive fluid resuscitation (250-500 mL/hr) with isotonic crystalloids is critical in managing acute pancreatitis.
- Patient should remain NPO until clinically improved, stable, and hungry. Enteral feedings are preferred over total parenteral nutrition. Enteral nutrition reduces mortality, multiple organ failure, systemic infections, and operative interventions more than total parenteral nutrition does in patients with acute pancreatitis. Parenteral nutrition may be necessary in patients who do not tolerate enteral feeding or in whom an adequate infusion rate cannot be reached within 2 to 4 days. Early enteral feeding through a nasogastric (NG) feeding tube is often used instead of an oral diet, but evidence to support this strategy is limited. A recent trial did not show superiority of early NG tube feeding, as compared to oral diet after 72 hours, in reducing the rate of infection or death in patients with acute pancreatitis at high risk for complications.[5]
- Nasogastric suction is useful only in severe pancreatitis to decompress the abdomen in patients with ileus.
- Control pain: IV morphine or fentanyl. Meperidine and hydromorphone are also commonly used narcotics for pain control.
- Correct metabolic abnormalities (e.g., replace calcium and magnesium as necessary).

SPECIFIC MEASURES:
- Pancreatic or peripancreatic infection develops in 40% to 70% of patients with pancreatic necrosis. However, IV antibiotics should not be used prophylactically for all cases of pancreatitis; their use is justified if the patient has evidence of septicemia, pancreatic abscess, or pancreatitis caused by biliary calculi. Their use should generally be limited to 5 to 7 days to prevent development of fungal superinfection. Appropriate empiric antibiotic therapy should cover:
  1. *Bacteroides fragilis* and other anaerobes (cefotetan, cefoxitin, metronidazole, or clindamycin plus aminoglycoside)
  2. *Enterococcus* (ampicillin)
- Surgical therapy has a limited role in acute pancreatitis; it is indicated in the following:
  1. Gallstone-induced pancreatitis: cholecystectomy when acute pancreatitis subsides. However, randomized trials have shown that patients with mild gallstone pancreatitis can undergo cholecystectomy safely during the first 48 hr of hospitalization.
  2. Perforated peptic ulcer.
  3. Necrotizing pancreatitis with infected necrotic tissue is associated with an elevated rate of complications and increased risk of death. Traditional treatment has been open necrosectomy; surgical necrosectomy induces a proinflammatory response and is associated with a high complication rate. Recent trials have shown that a step-up approach consisting of percutaneous drainage followed, if necessary, by minimally invasive retroperitoneal necrosectomy may have a lower rate of complications and death. Endoscopic transgastric necrosectomy, a form of natural orifice transluminal endoscopic surgery, has been shown in recent trials to be effective in reducing the proinflammatory response as well as reducing complications.
- Identification and treatment of complications:
  1. **Pseudocyst:** round or spheroid collection of fluid, tissue, pancreatic enzymes, and blood.
     1. Diagnosed by CT scan or sonography.
     2. Treatment: Pancreatic pseudocysts can be drained surgically or endoscopically. The endoscopic approach is preferable when the patient's anatomy is suitable and an experienced endoscopist is available. CT scan or ultrasound-guided percutaneous drainage (with a pigtail catheter left in place for continuous drainage) can be used, but the recurrence rate is high; the conservative approach is to reevaluate the pseudocyst (with CT scan or sonography) after 6 to 7 wk and surgically drain it if the pseudocyst has not decreased in size.
     3. Generally, pseudocysts <5 cm in diameter are reabsorbed without intervention, whereas those >5 cm require surgical intervention after the wall has matured.

[3]Fogel EL, Sherman S: ERCP for gallstone pancreatitis, *N Engl J Med* 370:150-157, 2014.
[4]Tenner S, et al.: American College of Gastroenterology guidelines: management of acute pancreatitis, *Am J Gastroenterol* 108:1400-1415, 2013.
[5]Bakker OJ, et al.: Early versus on-demand nasogastric tube feeding in acute pancreatitis, *N Engl J Med* 371:1983-1993, 2014.

P

Diseases and Disorders

I

TABLE 3 Prognostic Criteria for Acute Pancreatitis

Ranson's Criteria*	Simplified Glasgow Criteria†	Computed Tomography Criteria‡
On admission: Age >55 yr WBC >16,000/μL AST >250 U/L LDH >350 U/L Glucose >200 mg/dl *48 hr after admission:* Hematocrit decrease by >10 BUN increase by >5 mg/dl Ca^{2+} <8 mg/dl Arterial Po_2 <60 mm Hg Base deficit >4 mEq/L Fluid sequestration >6 L	*Within 48 hr of admission:* Age >55 yr WBC >15,000/μL LDH >600 U/L Glucose >180 mg/dl Albumin <3.2 g/dl Ca^{2+} <8 mg/dl Arterial Po_2 <60 mm Hg BUN >45 mg/dl	Normal Enlargement Pancreatic inflammation Single fluid collection Multiple fluid collection

AST, Aspartate aminotransferase; *BUN,* blood urea nitrogen; *LDH,* lactate dehydrogenase; *WBC,* white blood cells.
*Three or more Ranson's criteria predict a complicated clinical course. Data from Ranson JH, et al.: Prognostic signs and nonoperative peritoneal lavage in acute pancreatitis, *Surg Gynecol Obstet* 143:209-219, 1976.
†Data from Blamey SL, et al.: Prognostic factors in acute pancreatitis, *Gut* 25:1340, 1984.
‡Grades A and B represent mild disease with no risk of infection or death. Grade C represents moderately severe disease with a minimal likelihood of infection and essentially no risk of mortality. Grades D and E represent severe pancreatitis with an infection rate of 30% to 50% and mortality rate of 15%. Data from Balthazar EJ, et al.: Acute pancreatitis value of CT in establishing prognosis, *Radiology* 174:331, 1990.
From Goldman L, Ausiello D (eds): *Cecil textbook of medicine,* ed 24, Philadelphia, 2012, Saunders.

2. **Phlegmon:** represents pancreatic edema. It can be diagnosed by CT scan or sonography. Treatment is supportive because it usually resolves spontaneously.
3. **Pancreatic abscess:** diagnosed by CT scan (presence of bubbles in the retroperitoneum); Gram staining and cultures of fluid obtained from guided percutaneous aspiration usually identify bacterial organism. Therapy is surgical (or catheter) drainage and IV antibiotics (imipenem-cilastatin is the drug of choice).
4. **Pancreatic ascites:** usually caused by leaking of pseudocyst or tear in pancreatic duct. Paracentesis reveals very high amylase and lipase levels in the pancreatic fluid; ERCP may demonstrate the lesion. Treatment is surgical correction if exudative ascites from severe pancreatitis does not resolve spontaneously.
5. Gastrointestinal bleeding: caused by alcoholic gastritis, bleeding varices, stress ulceration, or disseminated intravascular coagulation (DIC).
6. Renal failure: caused by hypovolemia, resulting in oliguria or anuria, cortical or tubular necrosis (shock, DIC), or thrombosis of renal artery or vein.
7. Hypoxia: caused by ARDS, pleural effusion, or atelectasis.

THERAPY OF UNCOMMON FORMS OF PANCREATITIS

1. **Autoimmune pancreatitis (AIP):** Fibro-inflammatory disease characterized by an IgG4 lymphoplasmacytic infiltrate. It is a variant of chronic pancreatitis and it has been associated with other autoimmune disorders (e.g., primary sclerosing cholangitis, Sjögren syndrome). The inflammatory process is generally responsive to corticosteroid therapy. Older men aged 60 to 70 years are primarily affected. Patients present with abdominal pain, weight loss, anorexia, and obstructive jaundice. Immunoglobulin G_4 levels are elevated. Radiographically on CT, the pancreas is diffusely enlarged, with a characteristic smooth, capsule-like rim ("sausage pancreas"). Type II autoimmune hepatitis (idiopathic duct-centric chronic pancreatitis) is associated with inflammatory bowel disease and not related to IgG4 cell deposition.
2. **Hypertriglyceridemic pancreatitis (HTGP):** Beneficial results have been reported with early (within 48 hr) initiation of apheresis with IV heparin and insulin in addition to conventional treatment modalities for acute pancreatitis when there is concomitant hyperglycemia with severe acute pancreatitis.

DISPOSITION

Prognosis varies with the severity of pancreatitis; overall mortality rate in acute pancreatitis is 5% to 10%. Prognostic criteria for acute pancreatitis are described in Table 3.

REFERRAL

- Hospitalization is indicated in moderate to severe cases of pancreatitis.
- Surgical consultation is needed in suspected gallstone pancreatitis, perforated peptic ulcer, or presence of necrotic or infected foci. Acute pancreatitis can generally be attributed to gallstones when patients have both abnormal liver enzymes and gallstones (or sludge) on imaging. Such patients should consider cholecystectomy prior to discharge to prevent recurrent pancreatitis.
- Gastroenterology consultation in severe or recurrent pancreatitis, when ERCP is needed for gallstone pancreatitis, or when the cause of pancreatitis is unclear.

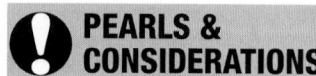

PEARLS & CONSIDERATIONS

- Acute pancreatitis is the most common major complication of ERCP. NSAIDs are potent inhibitors of phospholipase A_2, cyclooxygenase, and neutrophil-endothelial interactions, which play an important role in the pathogenesis of acute pancreatitis. Preliminary trials show that among patients at high risk for post-ERCP pancreatitis, rectal indomethacin (given as two 50-mg indomethacin suppositories administered immediately after ERCP) significantly reduced the incidence of post-ERCP pancreatitis.
- Pancreatic stent placement decreases the risk of post-ERCP pancreatitis.
- Statins reduce risk for pancreatitis in adults. Fibrates do not affect risk for pancreatitis.
- Diabetes mellitus may develop from extensive pancreatic necrosis.

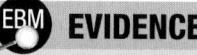 **EVIDENCE**

Available at www.expertconsult.com

SUGGESTED READINGS
Available at www.expertconsult.com

RELATED CONTENT

Acute Pancreatitis (Patient Information)

AUTHOR: **FRED F. FERRI, M.D.**

BASIC INFORMATION

DEFINITION

Chronic pancreatitis is a recurrent or persistent inflammatory process of the pancreas characterized by chronic pain and by pancreatic exocrine and/or endocrine insufficiency. It is classified anatomically as either large-duct disease or small-duct (minimal change) disease.

ICD-10CM CODES
K86.1 Other chronic pancreatitis
K86.0 Alcohol-induced chronic pancreatitis

EPIDEMIOLOGY & DEMOGRAPHICS

- Chronic pancreatitis occurs in approximately five to 10 per 100,000 persons in industrialized countries.
- Average age at diagnosis is 35 to 55 yr; male/female ratio is 5:1.

PHYSICAL FINDINGS & CLINICAL PRESENTATION

- Persistent or recurrent epigastric and left upper quadrant pain that may radiate to the back
- Tenderness over the pancreas, muscle guarding
- Significant weight loss
- Bulky, foul-smelling stools, greasy in appearance
- Epigastric mass (10% of patients)
- Jaundice (5%-10% of patients)

ETIOLOGY

- Chronic alcoholism (most common cause)
- Obstruction (ampullary stenosis, tumor, trauma [with pancreatic duct stricture], pancreas divisum, annular pancreas)
- Tobacco
- Hereditary pancreatitis
- Severe malnutrition
- Idiopathic
- Untreated hyperparathyroidism (hypercalcemia)
- Mutations of the cystic fibrosis transmembrane conductance regulator (CFTR) gene and the TF genotype
- Other genetic mutations (Cationic trypsinogen gene, chymotrypsinogen C gene, calcium-sensing receptor gene, claudin-2 gene, serine protease inhibitor, Kazal type 1 gene)
- **Autoimmune pancreatitis (AIP):** (5% of chronic pancreatitis cases): presents clinically with jaundice (63% of patients) and abdominal pain (35%). CT may reveal diffusely enlarged pancreas, enhanced peripheral rim of hypoattenuation "halo," and low-attenuation mass in head of pancreas. Laboratory values reveal elevated serum immunoglobulin (Ig) G4, elevated serum Ig or gamma-globulin level, presence of antilactoferrin antibody (ALA), anticarbonic anhydrase (ACA) II level, anti-smooth-muscle antibody (ASMA), or antinuclear antibody (ANA).

- **Sclerosing pancreatitis:** a form of chronic pancreatitis characterized by infrequent attacks of abdominal pain, irregular narrowing of the pancreatic duct, and swelling of the pancreatic parenchyma; patients have high levels of serum immunoglobulins (IgG4). Chronic sclerosing pancreatitis is also known as autoimmune pancreatitis.

DIAGNOSIS

DIFFERENTIAL DIAGNOSIS

- Pancreatic cancer
- Peptic ulcer disease
- Cholelithiasis with biliary obstruction
- Malabsorption from other etiologies
- Recurrent acute pancreatitis
- Renal insufficiency
- Intestinal ischemia or infarction
- Other: Crohn's disease, gastroparesis, inflammatory bowel disease

WORKUP

Medical history with focus on alcohol use, laboratory tests, diagnostic imaging

LABORATORY TESTS

- Serum amylase and lipase may be elevated (normal amylase levels, however, do not exclude the diagnosis).
- Hyperglycemia, glycosuria, hyperbilirubinemia, and elevated serum alkaline phosphatase may also be present.
- 72-hr fecal fat determination (rarely performed) reveals excess fecal fat. Fecal elastase test requires only 20 g of stool.
- Secretin stimulation test is the best test for diagnosing pancreatic exocrine insufficiency.
- Lipid panel: significantly elevated triglycerides can cause pancreatitis.
- Serum calcium: hyperparathyroidism is a rare cause of chronic pancreatitis.
- Elevated levels of serum IgG4 are found in sclerosing pancreatitis and AIP.
- Elevated serum Ig or gamma-globulin level, presence of ALA, ACA II level, ASMA, or ANA in AIP.

IMAGING STUDIES

- Plain abdominal radiographs (Fig. E1) may reveal pancreatic calcifications (95% specific for chronic pancreatitis).
- Ultrasound of abdomen may reveal duct dilation, pseudocyst, calcification, and presence of ascites.
- Contrast-enhanced CT scan of abdomen is the initial modality of choice. It is useful to detect calcifications (Fig. E2), evaluate for ductal dilation (Fig. E3), and rule out pancreatic cancer.
- Endoscopic retrograde cholangiopancreatography (ERCP) had been traditionally used to evaluate for the presence of dilated ducts, strictures, pseudocysts, and intraductal stones. However, for the evaluation of pancreatic parenchyma and duct system newer, less invasive modalities such as magnetic

resonance cholangiopancreatography and endoscopic ultrasonography (EUS) are preferred. EUS (Fig. E4) has a sensitivity of 97% and a specificity of 60% for chronic pancreatitis and a very low complication rate. Fine-needle aspiration biopsy combined with EUS is the preferred modality for evaluation of cystic or mass lesions to determine malignancy.

TREATMENT

NONPHARMACOLOGIC THERAPY

- Avoidance of alcohol and tobacco
- Frequent, small-volume, low-fat meals

ACUTE GENERAL Rx

- Avoidance of narcotics if possible (simple analgesics or NSAIDs can be used). Fig. 5 describes an approach to the patient with painful chronic pancreatitis.
- Treatment of steatorrhea with pancreatic supplements (e.g., Pancrease, Creon, pancrelipase titrated prn based on the amount of steatorrhea and patient's weight loss). All non–enteric-coated enzymes should be used with acid-suppressing medications. Proton pump inhibitors and H_2 blockers reduce inactivation of the enzymes from gastric acid.
- Antioxidants (vitamin A, selenium, vitamin E) may be helpful for pain control in chronic pancreatitis.
- Percutaneous or via EUS celiac plexus blockade with corticosteroids or neurolysis with ethanol may provide temporary pain relief.
- Treatment of complications (e.g., type 1 diabetes mellitus).
- Glucocorticoid therapy in patients with AIP and sclerosing pancreatitis can induce clinical remission and significantly decrease serum concentrations of IgG4, immune complexes, and the IgG4 subclass of immune complexes.

CHRONIC Rx

- Surgical intervention may be necessary to eliminate biliary tract disease and improve flow of bile into the duodenum by eliminating obstruction of pancreatic duct.
- ERCP with endoscopic sphincterectomy and stone extraction is useful in selected patients.
- Transduodenal sphincteroplasty or pancreaticojejunostomy in selected patients. Surgery should also be considered in patients with intractable pain.
- Percutaneous or EUS-guided celiac plexus blockade using glucocorticoids is effective in providing short-term pain relief in nearly half of patients.

DISPOSITION

- Long-term survival is poor (50% of patients die within 10 yr from chronic pancreatitis or malignancy).
- Prognosis is best in patients with recurrent acute pancreatitis resulting from cholelithiasis, hyperparathyroidism, or stenosis of the sphincter of Oddi.

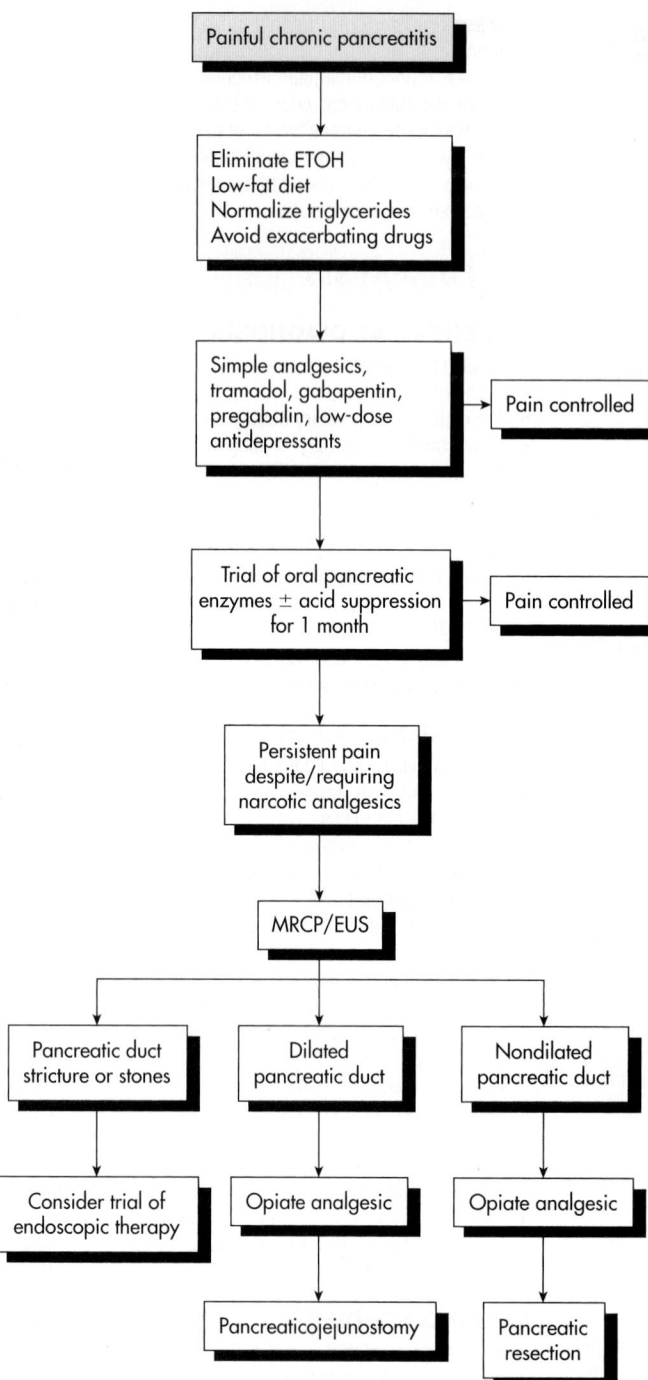

FIG. 5 Approach to the patient with painful chronic pancreatitis. *ETOH,* Alcohol; *EUS,* endoscopic ultrasound; *MRCP,* magnetic resonance cholangiopancreatography. (From Goldman L, Ausiello D [eds]: *Cecil textbook of medicine,* ed 24, Philadelphia, 2012, Saunders.)

REFERRAL

Gastrointestinal referral for ERCP, surgical referral in selected patients (see "Chronic Rx")

RELATED CONTENT

Chronic Pancreatitis (Patient Information)
Malabsorption (Related Key Topic)
Pancreatitis, Acute (Related Key Topic)

AUTHOR: **FRED F. FERRI, M.D**

SUGGESTED READINGS
Available at www.expertconsult.com

BASIC INFORMATION

DEFINITION

- A **panic attack** is a relatively brief, sudden episode of intense fear or apprehension, often associated with a sense of impending doom and various uncomfortable and disquieting physical symptoms. Panic attacks may be uncued ("out of the blue") or cued (i.e., triggered by a particular object or situation). Panic attacks may be present in a variety of different anxiety-related disorders (e.g., phobias, social anxiety, obsessive-compulsive disorder). Table 1 describes criteria for diagnosis of panic attack.
- **Panic disorder** is diagnosed after at least two uncued panic attacks have occurred followed by at least 1 mo (or more) of significant concern about future attacks, worry about their implications, or a major change in behavior related to these attacks. The criteria for diagnosis of panic disorder are summarized in Table 2. **Agoraphobia** is anxiety about, and avoidance of, places or situations in which the ability to escape is perceived to be limited or embarrassing or in which help might not be available in the event of having a panic attack.

SYNONYMS

Anxiety attacks
Fear attacks
Ataque de nervios

ICD-10CM CODES
F41.0 Panic disorder
F40.0 Agoraphobia

EPIDEMIOLOGY & DEMOGRAPHICS

INCIDENCE (IN U.S.): 1% 1-mo incidence of panic attacks
PREVALENCE (IN U.S.):
- 15% to 20% lifetime prevalence of one or more panic attacks.

TABLE 1 Criteria for Diagnosis of a Panic Attack

A discrete period of intense fear or discomfort, in which ≥4 of the following symptoms developed abruptly and reached a peak within 10 min
- Palpitations, pounding heart, or accelerated heart rate
- Sweating
- Trembling or shaking
- Sensations of shortness of breath or being smothered
- Feeling of choking
- Chest pain or discomfort
- Nausea or abdominal distress
- Feeling dizzy, unsteady, light-headed, or faint
- Derealization (feelings of unreality) or depersonalization (being detached from oneself)
- Fear of losing control or going crazy
- Paresthesias (numbness or tingling sensations)
- Chills or hot flashes

From Kliegman RM et al: *Nelson essentials of pediatrics*, ed 5, Philadelphia, 2006, Saunders.

- Panic disorder is much more uncommon, with a lifetime prevalence of 1.5% to 3.5%; chronicity of condition reflected by a similar 1-yr prevalence rate of 1% to 2%.
- Agoraphobia is relatively rare; 0.3% to 1% lifetime prevalence; 30% to 50% of patients diagnosed with panic disorder also have agoraphobia.
- Lower rates of panic disorder are reported among Latinos, African Americans, Caribbean blacks, and Asian Americans (DSM 5)
- Lower estimates for Asian, African, and Latin American countries (0.1%-0.8%) (DSM 5)

PEAK INCIDENCE:
- Chronic condition with a waxing and waning course.
- Bimodal incidence peaks noted, with the first peak between ages 15 and 24 yr and second peak between ages 35 and 44 yr.

PREDOMINANT SEX:
- Women more commonly affected (>85% of clinical population).
- Panic disorder twice as common in women.
- Panic disorder with agoraphobia three times as common in women.

PREDOMINANT AGE:
- Age of onset is typically late adolescence to mid-30s. Onset earlier in males (24 yr) than females (28 yr).
- Onset after age 45 yr is rare and should raise suspicion of different etiology.

GENETICS:
- Risk of developing panic disorder in first-degree relatives of individuals with panic disorder is four to seven times that of general population.
- Findings in twin studies: approximately 60% of contributing factors to panic are genetic.

PHYSICAL FINDINGS & CLINICAL PRESENTATION

Panic disorder
- Present either with a panic attack or with fear and anxiety related to anticipation of a future panic attack or its implications.
- Typical presentation: unexpected, untriggered periods of intense anxiety and fear with associated physiologic changes (e.g., palpitations, sweating, tremulousness, shortness of breath, chest pain, gastrointestinal distress, faintness, derealization, paresthesia). This is accompanied by associated fears of dying, heart attack, stroke, passing out, losing control, or losing one's mind. Panic attacks are often described as "the most terrifying" episode an individual has experienced.
- Emergency or physician visits often occasioned by physical symptoms such as chest pain, dizziness, or difficulty breathing. Thirty percent of patients presenting with chest pain have panic disorder.

TABLE 2 Criteria for Diagnosis of Panic Disorder

1. Recurrent unexpected panic attacks with associated worry or behavior change
2. Not due to effects of a drug, medication, or medical condition

- Patients reporting a fear of dying from a panic attack tend to have more symptomatic panic attacks and agoraphobia.

Agoraphobia:
- Rare complaints to physician. May manifest in missed office visits or tardiness. Patients may request home visits or telephone care.
- Activities usually self-limited by avoiding public situations where the patient believes he or she might experience a panic attack and would be unable to exit readily, such as the following:
  1. Crowded public areas (stores, public transportation, flying, church)
  2. Individual interactions (hairdresser, dentist, neighborhood meetings)
  3. Driving (especially if alone, far from home over bridges, through tunnels, on highways or on isolated roads)
- On exposure to or anticipation of exposure to feared situations, significant anxiety occurs. Anxiety may generate somatic symptoms that trigger a full-blown panic attack. Patients believe that escape from these situations reduces the alarming symptoms, thus reinforcing future avoidance. In actuality, symptom relief stems from adrenaline breaking down in the body after approximately 20 minutes.

ETIOLOGY

Hypotheses (NOTE: There are sufficient data to support each model. Models are not mutually exclusive.)
1. Central dyscontrol of autonomic arousal (typically localized to the locus ceruleus); similar symptoms may be chemically induced with yohimbine, caffeine, or cholecystokinin.
2. Cognitive overreaction (i.e., "catastrophic misinterpretation") to relatively mild or benign physiologic cues that then triggers a genuine autonomic cascade and further misinterpretations.
3. Dysfunction of a central suffocation alarm mechanism; some signs of compensated respiratory alkalosis. Can be experimentally induced with sodium lactate or carbon dioxide.

RISK FACTORS

1. Temperamental. Negative affect and anxiety sensitivity are risk factors for the onset of panic attacks. Severe separation anxiety in childhood may precede the panic disorder.
2. Environmental. Sexual and physical abuse in childhood is common in panic disorder. Most panic sufferers are able to identify a coalescence of stressors preceding their first panic attack.
3. Genetic and physiological. Although the exact genes are unknown, it is believed that multiple genes contribute to the vulnerability to panic attacks.

DIAGNOSIS

DIFFERENTIAL DIAGNOSIS

Medical conditions:
- Endocrinopathies:
  1. Hyperthyroidism
  2. Hyperparathyroidism

3. Pheochromocytoma
4. Carcinoid tumor
- Cardiac and respiratory diseases:
  1. Arrhythmias
  2. Myocardial infarction
  3. Chronic obstructive pulmonary disease
  4. Asthma
  5. Mitral valve prolapse
- Metabolic:
  1. Hypoglycemia
  2. Electrolyte imbalances
  3. Porphyria
- Seizure disorders
- Psychiatric disorders (NOTE: Panic attacks are common in a variety of psychiatric disorders. Panic disorder could be conceptualized as a phobia of the somatic sensations or situations that have become paired with panic attacks.)
  1. Phobias (e.g., specific phobia or social phobia). Note that fear of going on a plane because of crashing would be a specific phobia, whereas fear of going on a plane because one is then trapped and worries about panic is more suggestive of panic disorder with agoraphobia.
  2. Obsessive-compulsive disorder (cued by exposure to the object of the obsession)
  3. Posttraumatic stress disorder (cued by recall of a stressor)
  4. Generalized anxiety disorder (cued by excessive worry)
- Therapeutic (theophylline, steroids) and recreational (cocaine, amphetamine, caffeine, diet pills) drugs and drug withdrawal (alcohol, cannabis, barbiturates, benzodiazepines)

WORKUP
- Emergency presentation: cardiac, respiratory, or neurologic symptoms
- History and physical examination to rule out a concomitant medical or substance-related condition
NOTE: Panic disorder and agoraphobia are not diagnoses of exclusion, but exclusion of other conditions is usually required.

LABORATORY TESTS
- Thyroid profile
- Electrolyte measures, including calcium
- Toxicology screen
- ECG
- Acute cases: possible monitoring and cardiac enzymes to rule out arrhythmia or ischemia

IMAGING STUDIES
- For temporal lobe dysfunction (e.g., temporal lesions or as ictal or interictal manifestation of temporal lobe seizures): brain CT scan or MRI or an electroencephalogram in some patients
- Holter monitor to rule out occult or episodic arrhythmias
- Chest x-ray, arterial blood gases, or pulmonary function tests if respiratory compromise suspected

℞ TREATMENT

NONPHARMACOLOGIC THERAPY
Cognitive-behavioral therapy (CBT), in particular Panic Controlled Treatment, is generally very effective, with strongest results for cognitive restructuring (i.e., challenging catastrophic misinterpretations of somatic symptoms), in vivo or imaginal exposures (i.e., exposure to panic triggers in a controlled graded hierarchical fashion from least to most difficult with the goal of habituation and extinction of the fear response), and interoceptive exposures (i.e., repeated recreation and management of feared somatic sensations via activities such as chair spinning, straw breathing, and hyperventilation). CBT effect sizes are equal to or larger than for pharmacotherapy, attrition rates are lower, and relapse rates are lower. Treatment may take several sessions spread over weeks and may require referral to a behavioral specialist. CBT has been shown to be the most effective intervention for panic disorder with or without agoraphobia across treatment sites.

Traditionally, exposure therapy has relied upon a "desensitization paradigm" (i.e., habituation), in which the goal is to continue exposing an individual to a feared stimulus until the fear is no longer present (e.g., having a person with panic disorder remain in a shopping mall until anxiety has subsided). The assumption has been that habituation is the active ingredient in learning/fear reduction.

New research by Michelle G. Craske, Ph.D., suggests that fear habituation itself is not a predictor or mediator of outcomes when treating anxiety disorders. Craske theorizes that fear reduction during a prolonged exposure does not ensure that a person will not re-experience fear when encountering the feared stimulus in the future (e.g., reducing one's fear in a shopping mall does not ensure that one will not experience fear in other shopping malls). Rather, she suggests that strengthening "inhibitory learning" is the central mechanism of action for fear reduction.

Because of the element of surprise offered by inhibitory learning, cognitive restructuring occurs following an exposure rather than before it. Practicing cognitive restructuring prior to an exposure has been found to actually weaken an exposure. Craske suggests that varying the contexts of an exposure as much as possible is the most effective way to reduce anxiety (e.g., multiple shopping malls, multiple interoceptive exposures). Recent research suggests that an Internet-based mindfulness treatment program might be an effective approach for treating anxiety disorders.

ACUTE GENERAL Rx
- Benzodiazepines, particularly alprazolam: highly effective in the acute setting although long-term use is contraindicated for effective outcome.
- Low-dose alprazolam for patients with rare panic attacks and asymptomatic periods (0.25 to 0.5 mg PO or sublingually prn).
- Start patient on selective serotonin reuptake inhibitor (SSRI) or similar agent and taper patient off benzodiazepine by wk 2 to 3.

CHRONIC Rx
- Preferred pharmacologic agents: antidepressants with a significant serotonin reuptake inhibitory action. Generally start at low dose and titrate upward. Minimum treatment duration is 6 to 8 mo, but many patients need to take medications indefinitely.
  1. SSRIs: paroxetine (10-60 mg/day), sertraline (50-200 mg/day), citalopram (20-60 mg/day), escitalopram (5-30 mg/day), and fluoxetine (5-60 mg/day)
  2. Imipramine (100-300 mg/day)
  3. Venlafaxine (75-225 mg/day)
- Combination CBT plus SSRI has shown good long-term effects and is somewhat better than antidepressants or CBT alone. Combination CBT plus benzodiazepine does not provide any added benefit and may undermine CBT (interoceptive and in-vivo exposures may be less effective if the benzodiazepine is completely controlling the anxiety).

DISPOSITION
- Typical course is chronic but with significant waxing and waning (common to have long periods of remission).
- Presence of agoraphobia associated with a more chronic course.
- Findings with long-term follow-up studies: 6 to 10 yr after treatment some 30% are in remission, 40% to 50% have improved with residual symptoms, and the remainder are either unchanged or worse.

REFERRAL
- If patients do not respond to an SSRI
- Cognitive-behavioral therapy is the preferred treatment.

❗ PEARLS & CONSIDERATIONS
- Patient and family education is an important first step in the management of panic disorder. Education provides more adaptive explanations for the benign somatic sensations paired with panic. Presentation of genetic information and explanation of the benign nature of the physiology of each of the symptoms the patient experiences serve as a good start to allay fears and reduce stigma.
- Resumption of avoided activities or situations is a positive prognostic sign and may promote further therapeutic gains.
- The therapist's adherence to the treatment protocol and the therapeutic alliance established during the first session predict a better outcome for the long-term success of CBT for panic disorder with or without agoraphobia.

SUGGESTED READINGS
Available at www.expertconsult.com

RELATED CONTENT
Panic Disorder (Patient Information)

AUTHOR: **JEFFREY P. WINCZE, PH.D.**

BASIC INFORMATION

DEFINITION

Panniculitis refers to inflammation of subcutaneous fat. Most cases are found in association with a systemic disease. Panniculitis can be separated into groups based on histopathologic characteristics. Panniculitis is classified into lobular or septal panniculitis based on whether the inflammation is seen in the fat lobules or septae, respectively. It can be further classified based on whether the inflammation is found with or without vasculitis (Table 1) and by predominant cell type.

ICD-10CM CODES
M79.3	Unspecified panniculitis
M5400	Panniculitis affecting regions of neck and back, site unspecified
M5401	Panniculitis affecting regions of neck and back, occipito-atlanto-axial region
M5402	Panniculitis affecting regions of neck and back, cervical region
M54.03	Panniculitis affecting regions of neck and back, cervicothoracic region
M54.04	Panniculitis affecting regions of neck and back, thoracic region
M54.05	Panniculitis affecting regions of neck and back, thoracolumbar region
M54.06	Panniculitis affecting regions of neck and back, lumbar region
M54.07	Panniculitis affecting regions of neck and back, lumbosacral region
M54.08	Panniculitis affecting regions of neck and back, sacral and sacrococcygeal region
M54.09	Panniculitis affecting regions, neck and back, multiple sites in spine

EPIDEMIOLOGY & DEMOGRAPHICS

The epidemiology of the various panniculitides varies with each disease process. The most common panniculitis is erythema nodosum (refer to topic "Erythema Nodosum"). Another common panniculitis seen in the clinical setting is lipodermatosclerosis (LDS), which is usually seen in young, overweight females with associated venous insufficiency.

PHYSICAL FINDINGS & CLINICAL PRESENTATION

- Skin lesions can appear as nonspecific areas of erythema or erythematous nodules and/or plaques. The nodules can be palpated beneath the dermis. Ulceration, atrophy, and sclerosis can be associated clinical features of these lesions.
- The lesions are frequently painful and tender to palpation.
- Associated constitutional symptoms such as low-grade fevers, malaise, fatigue, myalgias, and arthralgias may be present.
- These skin findings usually are found on the lower limbs; however, the location of these lesions can vary with each specific panniculitis, that is, erythema nodosum is found on the pretibial areas of the lower extremities (Fig. 1), erythema induratum occurs on the calf, and lupus panniculitis occurs on the upper arms, shoulders, and face.
- Skin findings tend to evolve as the types of inflammatory cells change over the course of a few days.

ETIOLOGY

Panniculitis can be either primary/idiopathic or secondary. Common secondary etiologies can be classified into the following broad categories:

- Infections: bacterial (streptococci), mycobacterial, fungal, parasitic, and viral.
- Inflammatory/connective tissue disease: erythema nodosum, erythema induratum, lipodermatosclerosis, lupus panniculitis, cutaneous polyarteritis nodosa, dermatomyositis-associated panniculitis.
- Malignancy: subcutaneous panniculitis-like type T cell lymphoma.
- Pancreatic disease: pancreatic panniculitis, which is associated with pancreatitis or pancreatic carcinoma.
- Immunodeficiency states: alpha-1 antitrypsin deficiency panniculitis, which is associated with pulmonary and hepatic disease.
- Trauma: cold panniculitis (due to exposure to the cold), traumatic panniculitis, and factitial panniculitis (due to injection of medication or foreign substances into the subcutaneous fat).
- Deposition: calciphylaxis, gout.

Panniculitis can be a sign of an underlying systemic disease. Lupus panniculitis can occur alone or may present before or after the onset of either discoid lupus erythematosus or systemic lupus erythematosus.

DIAGNOSIS

DIFFERENTIAL DIAGNOSIS

- The skin lesions of panniculitis need to be distinguished from other skin lesions that may manifest similarly, such as insect bites, thrombophlebitis, and cellulitis.
- Disorders affecting the deep dermis or fascia (i.e., plaque morphea, eosinophilic fasciitis), benign or malignant tumors manifesting as subcutaneous nodules, and nodules with deep bruising may have similar clinical findings and be difficult to distinguish from panniculitis.

WORKUP

- Diagnosis of panniculitis depends on a thorough history and physical examination, evaluation of patient's risk factors, skin lesion appearance and distribution, as well as any associated clinical findings.
- If the diagnosis is unclear or needs to be confirmed, a deep skin biopsy should be performed. The preferred biopsy is an excisional biopsy, but a large 6- to 8-mm punch biopsy may be sufficient.

Although the above often establishes a diagnosis, there are times when it is difficult to accurately diagnose a specific panniculitis. Different forms of panniculitides have similar clinical findings while others are rare, complicating the presentation. Biopsy specimens may be too superficial to assess for the involvement of the subcutaneous fat or to assess for the presence of vasculitis. Inflammation of the subcutaneous fat is a changing process, with varying histologic findings as well as physical characteristics of skin lesions based on the stage of evolution. Cellular infiltrates may not

---

TABLE 1   Classification of Panniculitis

I. Without prominent vasculitis
  A. Septal inflammation
    1. Lymphocytic and mixed: erythema nodosum and variants.
    2. Granulomatous: palisaded granulomatous diseases, sarcoidosis, subcutaneous infection: tuberculosis, syphilis.
    3. Sclerotic: scleroderma, eosinophilic fasciitis, lipodermatosclerosis, toxins.
  B. Lobular inflammation
    1. Neutrophilic: infection, ruptured folliculitis and cysts, pancreatic fat necrosis.
    2. Lymphocytic: lupus panniculitis, post-steroid panniculitis, lymphoma/leukemia.
    3. Macrophagic: histiocytic cytophagic panniculitis.
    4. Granulomatous: erythema induratum/nodular vasculitis, palisaded granulomatous diseases, sarcoidosis, Crohn's disease.
    5. Mixed inflammation with many foam cells: α1-antitrypsin deficiency, traumatic fat necrosis.
    6. Eosinophilic: eosinophilic panniculitis, arthropod bites, parasites.
    7. Enzymatic fat necrosis: pancreatic enzyme panniculitis.
    8. Crystal deposits: scleredema neonatorum, subcutaneous fat necrosis of the newborn, gout, oxalosis.
    9. Embryonic fat pattern: lipoatrophy, lipodystrophy.
II. With prominent vasculitis (septal or lobular)
  A. Neutrophilic: leukocytoclastic vasculitis, subcutaneous polyarteritis nodosa, thrombophlebitis, ENL.
  B. Lymphocytic: nodular vasculitis, perniosis, angiocentric lymphomas.
  C. Granulomatous: nodular vasculitis/erythema induratum, ENL, granulomatosis with polyangiitis, Churg-Strauss allergic granulomatosis.
III. Mixed patterns

ENL, Erythema nodosum leprosum.
From Lee L, Werth V: The skin and rheumatic diseases: panniculitis. In Firestein G et al (eds): *Kelley's textbook of rheumatology,* ed 9, Philadelphia, 2013, Elsevier Saunders, p. 611.

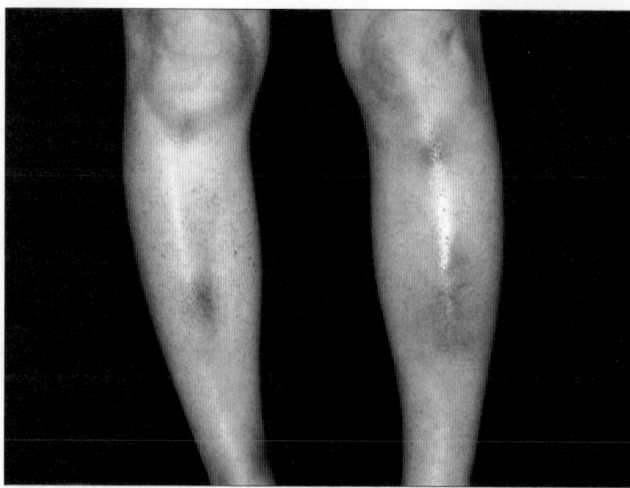

FIG. 1 Erythema nodosum secondary to acute sarcoidosis. (From Hochberg MC et al: *Rheumatology,* ed 5, St Louis, 2011, Mosby.)

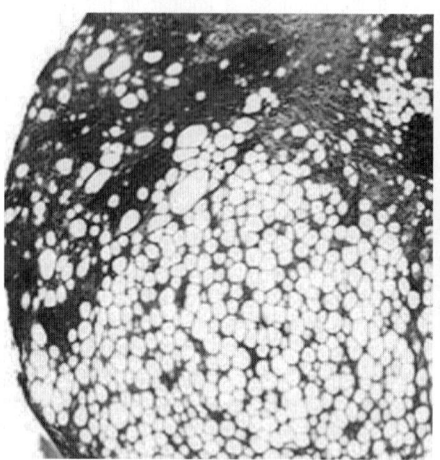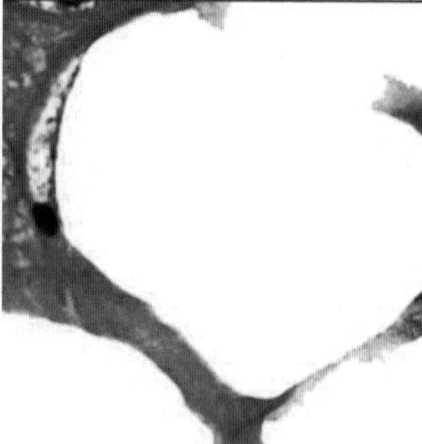

FIG. 2 Mixed lobular and septal panniculitis. (From Hochberg MC et al [eds]: Callen JP and Requena L: Cutaneous vasculitis and panniculitis. In *Rheumatology,* ed 6, Philadelphia, 2015, Elsevier Mosby, pp 1350.)

be confined to one location in the subcutaneous fat, and may overlap between septa and lobules (Fig. 2).

LABORATORY TESTS

Depending on the suspected underlying disorder, the following workup may be considered:
- Throat swab for rapid streptococcal screen, ASO titer, CBC, PPD, chest radiograph, tissue cultures, and histologic stains for organisms
- Amylase, lipase
- Serum alpha-1 antitrypsin level
- ESR, CRP
- Laboratory evaluation for possible connective tissue disease
- Further special studies of biopsy sample if malignancy is suspected

IMAGING STUDIES
- Chest radiography.
- Ankle-brachial index for assessment of peripheral vascular disease.
- Further imaging based on clinical suspicion of disease (i.e., CT scan of abdomen for pancreatitis).

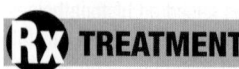 TREATMENT

Treatment of panniculitis is toward treatment of the underlying etiology. Any suspected medications should be discontinued. Appropriate antibiotics to treat underlying infections should be prescribed.

NONPHARMACOLOGIC THERAPY
- Leg elevation, bed rest
- Support stockings

ACUTE GENERAL Rx
- Nonsteroidal antiinflammatory medications (NSAIDs)
- Oral corticosteroids

CHRONIC Rx
- Oral potassium iodide (300-900 mg per day)
- Oral corticosteroids
- Colchicine
- Hydroxychloroquine
- Immunosuppressive medications

REFERRAL
- Dermatology for biopsy of skin lesions
- Specific specialists based on underlying etiology

RELATED CONTENT

Erythema Nodosum (Related Key Topic)

AUTHOR: **JOANNE SZCZYGIEL CUNHA, M.D.**

BASIC INFORMATION

DEFINITION

Paraneoplastic syndromes are a large group of syndromes caused by hormonal, immunologic, or other soluble factors due to the presence of a malignancy. This is in contrast to syndromes that are direct complications of tumors (e.g., superior vena cava syndrome). Findings and symptoms are specific to each syndrome. Paraneoplastic syndromes affect multiple organ systems, but predominantly the central and peripheral nervous systems, endocrine system, kidneys, and skin.

ICD-10CM CODES
G13.0 Paraneoplastic neuromyopathy and neuropathy
G13.1 Other systemic atrophy primarily affecting central nervous system in neoplastic disease
E83.5 Disorders of calcium metabolism
E73.1 Lambert-Eaton syndrome
E73.2 Other myasthenic syndromes in neoplastic disease
E22.2 Syndrome of inappropriate secretion of antidiuretic hormone

EPIDEMIOLOGY & DEMOGRAPHICS
- Paraneoplastic syndromes may affect as many as 8% of cancer patients.
- See Table 1 for epidemiology of each syndrome.

PHYSICAL FINDINGS & CLINICAL PRESENTATION
Hypercalcemia of malignancy
- Nausea/vomiting
- Constipation
- Abdominal pain
- Hypertension
- Anorexia
- Fatigue
- Altered mental status (from confusion to coma)
- Depression/anxiety
- Renal failure

SIADH
- Headache
- Weakness
- Anorexia
- Nausea
- Vomiting
- Memory impairment, irritability, restlessness
- Mental status changes may progress to obtundation or coma if hyponatremia is <125 mEq/L.

Cushing's syndrome
- Rapid weight gain
- Muscle weakness
- Generalized edema
- Centripetal fat distribution, progressing to obesity; limbs are often spared or wasted
- Hypertension
- Characteristic "moon facies" due to accumulation of fat deposition in the cheeks
- Skin atrophy, easy bruising, and purple abdominal striae due to skin fragility
- Hyperpigmentation, notably in sun-exposed areas
- Menstrual irregularity, mild hirsutism in women

Limbic encephalitis (LE)
- Insidious mood or psychiatric changes; hallucinations
- Short-term memory loss
- Hyperthermia or somnolence if hypothalamic involvement
- Two-thirds develop multifocal nervous system involvement

Paraneoplastic Thrombocytosis
- Thrombosis
- Nausea, vomiting
- Paresthesias

Paraneoplastic Erythrocytosis
- Erythroderma
- Post-shower (aquagenic) pruritus
- Plethora

Paraneoplastic cerebellar degeneration (PCD)
- May develop prodrome of dizziness, nausea, vomiting
- Ataxia
- Diplopia
- Dysphagia, dysarthria

Paraneoplastic glomerulonephritis
- Renal failure: oliguric or anuric
- Malaise
- Nausea or vomiting

Lambert-Eaton myasthenic syndrome (LEMS)
- Gradual onset of pelvic girdle and lower-extremity weakness, progressing in caudocranial direction
- Hyporeflexia
- Fatigue
- Mild bulbar dysfunction
- Dysautonomia, especially erectile dysfunction

Myasthenia gravis (MG)
- Ocular symptoms: ptosis and diplopia
- Weakness of facial muscles, notably with fatigable chewing
- Lower-extremity weakness that starts distally and progresses proximally
- May progress to involve muscles of respiration and respiratory crisis

Opsoclonus Myoclonus Syndrome (OMS)
- Truncal ataxia and unsteady gait
- Involuntary and conjugate gaze rapid eye movements (opsoclonus)
- Muscle twitching (myoclonus)
- Other symptoms: irritability, sleep disturbance, dysarthria or mutism

Paraneoplastic dermatologic and rheumatologic syndromes
- Acanthosis nigricans
- Dermatomyositis (DM)
- Erythroderma
- Hypertrophic osteoarthropathy
- Leukocytoclastic vasculitis
- Paraneoplastic pemphigus (PNP)
- Polymyalgia rheumatica (PMR)
- Sweet syndrome (acute febrile neutrophilic dermatosis)

ETIOLOGY
Paraneoplastic endocrine syndromes (PES) are due to tumor production of hormones or peptides that lead to metabolic derangements:
Hypercalcemia of malignancy:
Humoral hypercalcemia of malignancy (HHM): 80% of hypercalcemia of malignancy cases. Most commonly due to production of parathyroid hormone–related peptide (PTHrP) in lung (Table 2) and breast cancer (also

TABLE 1	Epidemiology of Each Paraneoplastic Syndrome	
Condition	**Prevalence**	**Risk Factors**
Hypercalcemia of malignancy	Up to 10%-20% of all cancer patients	Squamous cell cancers (lung, head, and neck), breast, kidney, bladder, and ovarian cancers, lymphoma
Syndrome of inappropriate antidiuretic hormone (SIADH)	Up to 1%-2% of all cancer patients Found in 10%-45% of SCLC patients	SCLC
Cushing's syndrome	Approximately 2% in all cancer patients (50% of these are SCLC)	SCLC Pituitary adenoma, benign and malignant adrenal tumors, carcinoid tumors
Limbic encephalitis (LE)	Less than 1%	SCLC Testicular germ cell tumor Breast cancer Ovarian teratoma
Paraneoplastic cerebellar degeneration	Less than 1%	SCLC Hodgkin's lymphoma Breast cancer
Lambert-Eaton myasthenic syndrome (LEMS)	3% of SCLC patients	SCLC, prostate cancer, lymphoma
Paraneoplastic thrombocytosis	5%-20% of patients with solid tumors	Lung, colorectal, mesothelioma
Paraneoplastic erythrocytosis	4% of patients	Renal cell carcinoma, breast cancer
Paraneoplastic glomerulonephritis	2%-4% of patients	Hodgkin's lymphoma, thymoma, prostate cancer
Myasthenia gravis (MG)	15% of thymoma patients	Thymoma
Opsoclonus myoclonus syndrome (OMS)	Less than 1%	SCLC, breast cancer, ovarian teratoma in adults; neuroblastoma in children

SCLC, Small cell lung cancer.

TABLE 2 Hypercalcemia of Malignancy

Cancer	Frequency (%)	Mechanism
Lung	35	PTHrP
		Local osteolysis
Breast	25	PTHrP
		Local osteolysis
Head and neck	6	PTHrP
Renal	3	PTHrP
		Local osteolysis
Multiple myeloma	15	PTHrP (rare)
		Local osteolysis
		1,25-Dihydroxyvitamin D
Prostate	7	Local osteolysis
Lymphoma	15	1,25-Dihydroxyvitamin D
		PTHrP

PTHrP, Parathyroid hormone related protein.
From Skorecki K et al: *Brenner and Rector's the kidney,* ed 10, Philadelphia, 2016, Elsevier.

seen in renal, bladder, and ovarian cancer). More rarely, can see 1,25-dihydroxyvitamin D production from increased 1α-hydroxylase activity in Hodgkin and non-Hodgkin lymphomas or ectopic production of parathyroid hormone (PTH) by the tumor.

Osteolytic activity: 20% of hypercalcemia of malignancy cases. Tumor cells metastasize, infiltrate bone, and produce local factors that stimulate osteoclast activation.

SIADH: production of antidiuretic hormone (arginine vasopressin, atrial natriuretic peptide) by tumor cells. Due to ectopic ADH production, patients will demonstrate dilute serum in the face of concentrated urine.

Cushing's syndrome: ectopic ACTH promotes excess production of cortisol and other glucocorticoids from the adrenal glands, which do not respond to normal HPA feedback.

Paraneoplastic Erythrocytosis: mediated by inappropriate production of erythropoietin (EPO) and associated with a mutation in the Von Hippel-Lindau gene, commonly seen with renal cell carcinoma. Also reported in hepatocellular carcinoma.

Paraneoplastic Thrombocytosis: mediated by inflammatory cytokines, in particular IL-6, as well as elevated acute-phase reactants ESR and CRP. Elevated thrombopoietin levels may also be seen.

Paraneoplastic Glomerulonephritis: marked by new renal failure in the setting of newly diagnosed malignancy and is not due to direct metastatic involvement of the kidneys or genitourinary system. Diseases include minimal change disease, rapidly progressive glomerulonephritis, focal segmental glomerulonephritis, IgA nephropathy.

Paraneoplastic neurologic syndromes (PNS): are due to immune cross-reactivity between tumor cells and components of the nervous system. Tumor-directed antibodies (onconeural antibodies) are produced by the patient in

response to a developing cancer. These onconeural antibodies and associated onconeural antigen-specific T lymphocytes inadvertently attack components of the nervous system because of antigenic similarity (molecular mimicry).

LE, PCD, LEMS, MG, OMS: cross-reactive autoantibodies against various components of the central and peripheral nervous system

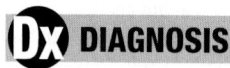 **DIAGNOSIS**

DIFFERENTIAL DIAGNOSIS

Hypercalcemia of malignancy: primary hyperparathyroidism, familial hypocalciuric hypercalcemia, excess calcium intake, vitamin D toxicity, thiazide diuretics. It is important to differentiate between HHM and osteolytic causes of malignancy-associated hypercalcemia because prognosis and response to treatment differ.

SIADH: hypovolemic hyponatremia, volume overload, reset osmostat, psychogenic polydipsia.

Cushing's syndrome: excess glucocorticoid administration, pituitary adenoma, benign or malignant adrenal tumors.

Paraneoplastic Thrombocytosis: reactive thrombocytosis from iron deficiency anemia or inflammation; essential thrombocythemia.

Paraneoplastic Erythrocytosis: polycythemia vera, secondary polycythemia from smoking, high-affinity hemoglobinopathies, or chronic hypoxia (e.g., obstructive sleep apnea).

Paraneoplastic Glomerulonephritis: renal failure from intrinsic injury from nephrotoxic agents (e.g., chemotherapy), postrenal failure from bladder obstruction, or rarely direct metastatic invasion from a primary tumor.

LE, PCD, LEMS, MG, OMS: multiple sclerosis, stroke, meningitis, encephalitis

WORKUP

- History and physical examination. Box 1 summarizes the evaluation and diagnosis of paraneoplastic syndromes.
- Age-appropriate cancer screening
- CT chest, PET in the paraneoplastic neurologic syndromes (PNS)
- EEG, EMG

LABORATORY TESTS

Hypercalcemia of malignancy
- Serum calcium and albumin levels to measure corrected calcium (HHM more common when serum Ca^{2+} >13 mg/dL)
- Ionized serum calcium
- PTH (low to normal)
- PTHrP (elevated)
- $1,25(OH)_2D$ levels (if the above values are inconclusive)

SIADH
- Serum and urine sodium (serum sodium <135 mEq/L or urine sodium >40 mEq/L)
- Serum and urine osmolality (serum osm <280 mOsm/kg of water and/or urine Osm >100 mOsm/kg of water)

Cushing's syndrome
- High-dose dexamethasone suppression: 2 mg dexamethasone by mouth every 6 hr for 72 hr, with measurement of urinary 17-hydroxycorticosteroid at 9 A.M. and midnight days 2 and 3
- Low-dose dexamethasone suppression: 1 mg dexamethasone given with measurement of morning serum cortisol
- Dexamethasone suppression test distinguishes pituitary vs. ectopic source of ACTH: adrenal and ectopic sources are generally non-suppressible
- Potassium and glucose should be monitored closely due to increased risk of hypokalemia and hyperglycemia
- **LE:** Anti-Hu, Anti-Ma2, Anti-CRMP5, Anti-GAD, anti-amphiphysin, CSF analysis, Anti-NMDAR, Anti-SOX2, Anti-SOXB1
- **PCD:** Anti-Yo, Anti-Hu, Anti-Ma, Anti-Ri, Anti-VGCC, Anti-mGluR1, CSF analysis, Anti Tr/Anti-DNER
- **LEMS:** Anti-VGCC (P/Q), CSF analysis
- **MG:** Anti-AchR, Anti-MuSk, CSF analysis
- **OMS:** Anti-Ri
- **Paraneoplastic thrombocytosis:** CBC, liver panel, iron panel, inflammatory markers, ESR, CRP
- **Paraneoplastic erythrocytosis:** CBC, EPO level, peripheral blood smear
- **Paraneoplastic glomerulonephritis:** BMP, urinalysis, urine protein to creatinine ratio, 24-hour urine protein collection, urine sediment analysis

IMAGING STUDIES

Hypercalcemia of malignancy: CT imaging to evaluate for breast lesion, lung mass, or lymphadenopathy

SIADH: CT imaging to evaluate for brain or lung mass

Cushing's syndrome: CT scan, MRI, or octreotide scan

LE, PCD, LEMS, MG: CT chest, FDG-PET scan, MRI

Paraneoplastic erythrocytosis: CT renal mass protocol or renal ultrasound to evaluate for renal cell carcinoma

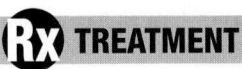 **TREATMENT**

NONPHARMACOLOGIC THERAPY

Hypercalcemia of malignancy
- Treatment of underlying malignancy, either surgical resection or chemotherapy/radiation of identified tumors
- Fluid resuscitation, typically 1 L bolus followed by 200 to 300 mL/hr to achieve euvolemia, followed by maintenance hydration

SIADH
- Surgical resection of identified tumors
- Fluid restriction

Cushing's syndrome
- Surgical resection of identified tumors

LE, PCD, LEMS, MG
- IVIG
- Plasma exchange
- Prednisone and tacrolimus being studied

ACUTE GENERAL Rx

Hypercalcemia of malignancy
- Furosemide intravenously once euvolemia has been reached, although clinical efficacy is debatable
- Bisphosphonates, either pamidronate or zoledronic acid intravenous infusions (treatment side effects are renal dysfunction and osteonecrosis of the jaw). Oral bisphosphonates may be easier to administer in palliative care settings but efficacy is less established.
- Calcitonin weight-based dosing, although tachyphylaxis occurs after 48 hours of administration
- Corticosteroids in cases of myeloma and lymphoma
- Hemodialysis in severe cases

SIADH
- If urine sodium is >308 mOsm/kg and patient develops seizure or obtundation, then sodium replacement with hypertonic saline (3%) is indicated

- Sodium should not be corrected at a rate faster than 9 mEq/L in any 24-hour period or faster than 18 mEq/L in any 48-hour period to decrease chances of osmotic demyelination syndrome. Desmopressin, free water, and/or nephrology consultation may be required for too rapid a correction.

Cushing's syndrome
- Management of volume status and blood pressure with diuretics and antihypertensive agents

CHRONIC Rx

- Chronic treatment is centered on treatment of the underlying malignancy.

Hypercalcemia of malignancy
- Bisphosphonate therapy every 4 weeks in cases of bone metastasis
- Chronic calcitonin use can be considered

SIADH
- Demeclocycline and vasopressin receptor antagonists (vaptans; conivaptan and tolvaptan, although both are approved for initial administration in hospitalized patients only)
- Cessation of any possible causative medications
- Maintain adequate dietary protein and salt intake

    Cushing's syndrome: inhibition of steroid production with ketoconazole, mitotane, metyrapone, aminoglutethimide

    LE/PCD: Glucocorticoids, cyclophosphamide, rituximab

    LEMS: 3,4-diaminopyridine, pyridostigmine, azathioprine

    MG: Pyridostigmine, azathioprine, cyclosporin A, tacrolimus, mycophenolate, rituximab

    Paraneoplastic thrombocytosis: consider prophylactic low-molecular-weight heparin or aspirin if no contraindications exist.

DISPOSITION

Specific to each condition; however, humoral hypercalcemia of malignancy carries a poor overall prognosis with 30-day mortality of 50%.

REFERRAL

Oncology, endocrinology, neurology, nephrology

PEARLS & CONSIDERATIONS

COMMENTS

- Signs or symptoms of a paraneoplastic syndrome may manifest prior to the identification of a malignancy.

- If paraneoplastic syndrome is suspected, a thorough workup for a tumor is indicated.
- With treatment of the primary tumor, the clinical effects of hypercalcemia of malignancy, SIADH, and Cushing's syndrome may improve or resolve.
- Women with anti-NMDAR encephalitis should be evaluated for ovarian malignancy given a strong disease association. Recovery from paraneoplastic anti-NMDAR encephalitis due to ovarian cancer has been reported after salpingo-oophorectomy. For those requiring intensive care, early treatment with cyclophosphamide and/or rituximab has shown to be beneficial.
- The effects of the neurologic paraneoplastic syndromes can be long-term, due to permanent CNS or PNS damage. In neurologic paraneoplastic syndromes, tumor detection can be difficult, since the immune system, which is causing the syndrome, is also keeping the tumor in check.
- Patients with new neurologic deficits after starting a checkpoint inhibitor (e.g., PD-1 inhibitor) may be experiencing drug-induced autoimmunity rather than a paraneoplastic syndrome.

PREVENTION

- Smoking cessation
- Age-appropriate cancer screening

PATIENT & FAMILY EDUCATION

In conditions with autoimmune etiology (LE, PCD, LEMS, MG, OMS), symptoms may not improve even if tumor is identified and treated, as damage to the nervous system may be sustained or permanent.

SUGGESTED READINGS

Available at www.expertconsult.comhttp://www.expertconsult.com/

AUTHORS: **WILLIAM M. RAFELSON, M.D., M.B.A.,** and **JOHN L. REAGAN, M.D.**

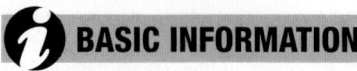

DEFINITION

Idiopathic Parkinson's disease (PD) is a progressive neurodegenerative disorder characterized clinically by rigidity, tremor, postural instability, and slowness of movement (bradykinesia).

SYNONYMS

Paralysis agitans

ICD-10CM CODES

G20	Parkinson's disease
G21.11	Neuroleptic induced parkinsonism
G21.1	Other drug-induced secondary parkinsonism
G21.2	Secondary parkinsonism due to other external agents
G21.3	Postencephalitic parkinsonism
G21.4	Vascular parkinsonism
G21.8	Other secondary parkinsonism
G21.9	Secondary parkinsonism, unspecified

EPIDEMIOLOGY & DEMOGRAPHICS

PREVALENCE:
- Affects more than 1 million people in North America. It is the second most common neurodegenerative disease worldwide.
- In age group <40 yr, <5/100,000 are affected.
- In those aged >70 yr, 700/100,000 are affected.
- Highest incidence in whites, lowest incidence in Asians and African Americans

PHYSICAL FINDINGS & CLINICAL PRESENTATION

- Tremor (Fig. 1)—typically a resting tremor with a frequency of 4 to 6 Hz that is often first noted in the hand as a pill-rolling tremor (thumb and forefinger). Can also involve the leg and lip. Tremor improves with purposeful movement. Usually starts asymmetrically.
- Rigidity—increased muscle tone that persists throughout the range of passive movement of a joint. Rigidity, like resting tremor, is usually asymmetric at onset.
- Akinesia/bradykinesia—slowness in initiating movement
- Postural instability—tested by "pull test." Ask patient to stand in place with back to examiner. Examiner pulls patient back by the shoulders, and proper response would be to take no steps back or very few steps back without falling. Retropulsion is a positive test, as is falling straight back. Postural instability is not usually severe early on. If falls and postural reflexes are greatly impaired early on, then consider other disorders.
- Masked facies (hypomimia)—face seems expressionless, giving the appearance of depression. Decreased blink; often there is excess drooling.
- Gait disturbance
- Stooped posture, decreased arm swing
- Difficulty initiating the first step; small shuffling steps that increase in speed (festinating gait). Steps become progressively faster and shorter while the trunk inclines further forward.
- Other complaints and findings early on include handwriting becoming smaller (micrographia), and voice becoming softer and often "gruffer" (hypophonia).

ETIOLOGY

- Unknown
- Most cases are sporadic. Age is the most common risk factor, although a combination of both environmental and genetic factors likely contributes to disease expression. Rare familial forms with at least seven different genes have been identified; these include the parkin gene, a significant cause of early-onset autosomal recessive PD, and *LRRK2*, the most common cause of familial and sporadic parkinsonism.

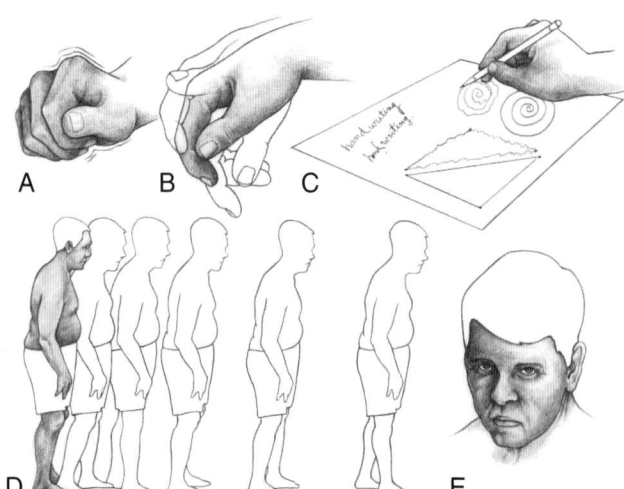

FIG. 1 The parkinsonian syndrome. A, The "pill-rolling" tremor. **B,** Tremor that can worsen with emotional stress. **C,** Handwriting abnormalities, which include micrographia. **D,** Typical posture and gait, which becomes faster (festination). **E,** Lack of facial expression as well as "stare" from decreased blinking. (From Remmel KS et al: *Handbook of symptom oriented neurology,* ed 3, St Louis, 2002, Mosby.)

A clinical diagnosis can be made based on a comprehensive history and physical examination. The four cardinal signs used to diagnose PD are (mnemonic = TRAP):
1. **T**remor (resting, typically 4-6 Hz)
2. **R**igidity, of the cogwheel type
3. **A**kinesia/bradykinesia—slowness of movement
4. **P**ostural instability—failure of postural "righting" reflexes leading to poor balance and falls

One need not demonstrate all four cardinal signs to make a presumptive diagnosis of PD and begin treatment.

DIFFERENTIAL DIAGNOSIS

- Multiple system atrophy—distinguishing features include autonomic dysfunction (including urinary incontinence, orthostatic hypotension, and erectile dysfunction), parkinsonism, cerebellar signs, and normal cognition.
- Dementia with Lewy bodies—parkinsonism with concomitant dementia: patients often have early hallucinations and fluctuations in level of alertness and mental status.
- Corticobasal syndrome—often begins asymmetrically with apraxia, cortical sensory loss in one limb, and sometimes, alien limb phenomenon.
- Progressive supranuclear palsy—tends to have axial rigidity greater than appendicular (limb) rigidity. These patients have early and severe postural instability. Hallmark is supranuclear gaze palsy that usually involves vertical gaze (especially downward) before horizontal.
- Essential tremor—bilateral postural and action tremor.
- Secondary (acquired) parkinsonism:
  1. Iatrogenic—any of the neuroleptics and antipsychotics. The high-potency D_2-blocker neuroleptics are most likely to cause parkinsonism. Quetiapine is an atypical antipsychotic with lower risk of parkinsonism. Metoclopramide can also cause parkinsonism. Abuse of methamphetamine has been recently linked to risk of PD.
  2. Postinfectious parkinsonism—von Economo's encephalitis.
  3. Dementia pugilistica—parkinsonism and dementia after repeated head trauma.
  4. Toxins (e.g., MPTP, manganese, carbon monoxide).
  5. Cerebrovascular disease "vascular parkinsonism" (basal ganglia infarcts); often lower limbs (especially gait) affected more than upper extremities.

WORKUP

1. Identification of clinical signs and symptoms associated with PD (see "Physical Findings") and elimination of conditions that may mimic it with a comprehensive history and physical examination
2. Routine genetic testing is not recommended.

IMAGING STUDIES

Computed tomographic (CT) scan has almost no role in investigations. Magnetic resonance imaging (MRI) of the head may sometimes distinguish between idiopathic PD and other conditions that present with signs of parkinsonism (see "Differential Diagnosis").

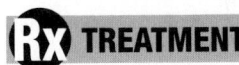 TREATMENT

NONPHARMACOLOGIC THERAPY

- Physical therapy, patient education and reassurance, treatment of associated conditions (e.g., depression) are important. A safe, practical, and reasonable exercise regimen must be encouraged, individualized to the patient's access to resources and motivation. Recent trials reveal that t'ai chi training is effective in reducing balance impairment and falls and improving functional capacity.
- Avoidance of drugs that can induce or worsen parkinsonism: neuroleptics (especially high potency), certain antiemetics (prochlorperazine, trimethobenzamide), metoclopramide, nonselective MAO inhibitors (may induce hypertensive crisis), reserpine, methyldopa

ACUTE GENERAL Rx

- There continues to be controversy whether levodopa or dopamine agonists should be the initial treatment. In younger patients, agonists are usually the drug of choice; in patients >70 yr, levodopa is typically the preferred initial therapy.
- It is appropriate to initiate pharmacotherapy when required by symptoms; prior practice of waiting for limitation of ADLs is now outdated. Fig. E2 describes an approach to patients with parkinsonism.
- Motor complications do develop during the course of the disease and likely reflect the combination of disease progression together with the side effects of dopaminergic medications.

CHRONIC Rx

- Levodopa therapy
  1. Cornerstone of symptomatic therapy—should be used with a peripheral dopa decarboxylase inhibitor (carbidopa) to minimize side effects (nausea, light-headedness, postural hypotension). The combination of the two drugs is marketed under the trade name Sinemet. Levodopa therapy has been found to reduce morbidity and mortality in PD patients.
  2. Usual starting dose is 25/100 mg (carbidopa/levodopa) tid 1 hr before (or after) meals.
  3. Controlled-release preparations (e.g., Sinemet CR) are available, but their use should be deferred to a neurologist.
  4. Stalevo (combination Sinemet and entacapone, a COMT inhibitor). Useful for patients with motor fluctuations (wearing off); has no role in treating early patients with PD.

- Dopamine receptor agonists (ropinirole and pramipexole) are not as potent as levodopa, but they are often used as initial treatment in younger patients to attempt to delay the onset of complications (dyskinesias, motor fluctuations) associated with levodopa therapy. These medications are more expensive than levodopa. In general, they cause more side effects than levodopa, including nausea, vomiting, light-headedness, peripheral edema, confusion, and somnolence. They can also cause impulse control behaviors such as hypersexuality, binge eating, and compulsive shopping and gambling. Presence of these must be assessed at each visit.
  1. Ropinirole: initial dose is 0.25 mg tid
  2. Pramipexole: initial dose is 0.125 mg tid
- MAO-B inhibitors can be used as monotherapy early in the disease or as adjunctive therapy in later stages; they have been shown to have milder symptomatic benefit than dopamine agonists or levodopa. They are well tolerated and easy to titrate. Concurrent use of stimulants and sympathomimetics should be avoided. Certain food restrictions may apply.
  1. Rasagiline: initial dose is 0.5 mg qd, then 1 mg daily. A recent study, ADAGIO, suggests that 1 mg rasagiline may have disease-modifying benefits, but results must be interpreted with caution.
  2. Selegiline: Usual dose, 5 mg bid with breakfast and lunch. Has amphetamine byproduct so has mild stimulant-like effects, which can be beneficial in some patients.
- Amantadine (unclear mechanism of action, but reported to modulate the dopamine and glutamate systems in the CNS) can be used alone early in the disease. It is especially useful in the treatment of dyskinesias. Dosage is 100 mg tid (titrate q week from 100 mg qd). Must adjust for elderly and renal impairment. The most notable side effect, especially in the elderly, is confusion.
- Anticholinergic agents are only helpful in treating tremor and drooling in patients with PD. Potential side effects include constipation, urinary retention, memory impairment, and hallucinations. They should be avoided in the elderly.
  1. Trihexyphenidyl: initial dose, 1 mg PO tid
  2. Benztropine: usual dose, 0.5 to 1 mg qd or bid

SURGICAL OPTIONS

- Pallidal (globus pallidus interna) and subthalamic deep-brain stimulation (subthalamic nucleus) are currently the surgical options of choice for patients with advanced PD; similar improvement in motor function and adverse effects have been reported after either procedure. Compared with ablative procedures, DBS has the advantage of being reversible and adjustable. Thalamic DBS may be useful for refractory tremor. It improves the cardinal motor symptoms, extends medication "on" time, and reduces motor fluctuations during the day. In general, patients are likely to benefit from this therapy if they show a clear response to levodopa. Therefore, when considering DBS, patients should be evaluated for motor response to levodopa by stopping levodopa overnight and evaluating motor response before and after a dose of levodopa.
- Surgery is often limited to patients with disabling, medically refractory problems, and patients must still have a good response to L-dopa to undergo surgery. Yet for many patients, earlier stimulation might provide an improved motor benefit before disability from other symptoms has occurred and should be considered at an earlier stage of PD. DBS results in decreased dyskinesias, fluctuations, rigidity, and tremor.

DISPOSITION

PD usually follows a slowly progressive course leading to disability over the course of several years. However, every patient will progress individually, and patients should be reassured that this diagnosis does not, by definition, result in being either wheelchair- or bed-bound.

REFERRAL

- Neurology consultation is recommended at initial diagnosis of PD.
- Exercise is important for all patients with PD.
- Participation in outpatient physical therapy program is recommended for patients with moderate to advanced disease.

! PEARLS & CONSIDERATIONS

- Asymmetry of symptoms at onset is very useful in distinguishing PD from other causes of parkinsonism.
- Although resting tremor is a common presenting symptom, up to 25% of patients with idiopathic PD do not have classic resting tremor.

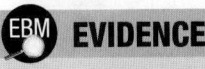 EVIDENCE

Available at www.expertconsult.com

SUGGESTED READINGS

Available at www.expertconsult.com

RELATED CONTENT

Parkinson's Disease (Patient Information)

AUTHORS: **JOSEPH S. KASS, M.D., J.D.,** and **U. SHIVRAJ SOHUR, M.D., PH.D.**

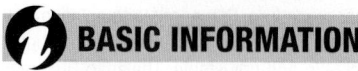

DEFINITION

Paronychia is a localized superficial infection or abscess of the lateral and proximal nail fold. Paronychia may be acute or chronic.

SYNONYMS

Nail bed infection
Nail bed abscess

ICD-10CM CODES
L03.019 Cellulitis of unspecified finger
B37.2   Candidiasis of skin and nail

EPIDEMIOLOGY & DEMOGRAPHICS

- Acute paronychia affects males and females equally.
- Chronic paronychia is more common in females than males (9:1).
- Acute paronychia most often occurs in children.
- Chronic paronychia usually presents in the fifth or sixth decade of life.
- Paronychia is the most common infection of the hand.

PHYSICAL FINDINGS & CLINICAL PRESENTATION

- Acute paronychia usually presents with the sudden onset of redness, swelling, and pain with abscess or cellulitis formation in the nail fold. Fluid with purulence is often present.
- Chronic paronychia is insidious, presenting with mild swelling and erythema of the nail folds.
- Acute paronychia usually involves only one finger.
- Chronic paronychia may involve more than one finger.

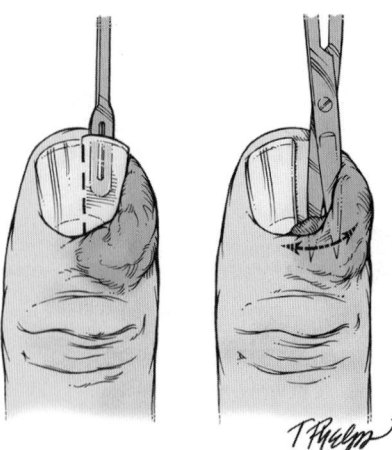

FIG. 1 Surgical drainage of acute paronychia. The lateral nail on the affected side is gently elevated from the nail bed, and a longitudinal strip of nail is removed. If this does not decompress the infection adequately, the margins of the nail fold are opened gently to drain the adjacent soft tissues. (From Cameron JL, Cameron AM: *Current surgical therapy*, ed 10, Philadelphia, 2011, Saunders.)

- Acute paronychia usually involves the thumb.
- Chronic paronychia commonly involves the middle finger.

ETIOLOGY

- Any disruption of the seal between the proximal nail fold and the nail plate can cause paronychial infections.
- Acute paronychia is almost always bacterial in origin (e.g., methicillin-sensitive *Staphylococcus aureus* [most common, but also consider MRSA], *Streptococcus pyogenes*, *Enterococcus faecalis*, *Proteus* and *Pseudomonas* species, and anaerobes).
- Paronychia can also be associated with use of lamivudine and indinavir, which are used in HIV therapy.
- Chronic paronychia is commonly caused by *Candida albicans* (70%), with bacterial organisms accounting for the remaining 30%.
- Trauma, nail biting, hangnails, diabetes, and long-term exposure to water are common predisposing features of paronychia.

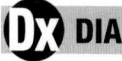 **DIAGNOSIS**

The diagnosis of paronychia is self-evident on physical examination.

DIFFERENTIAL DIAGNOSIS

- Herpetic whitlow caused by herpes simplex
- Pyogenic granuloma
- Viral warts
- Ganglions
- Squamous cell carcinoma

WORKUP

A workup is usually not pursued unless there is treatment failure.

LABORATORY TESTS

- Gram stain and culture any purulent drainage.
- Potassium hydroxide mount may show pseudohyphae.

IMAGING STUDIES

Radiographs of the digit if concerned about osteomyelitis.

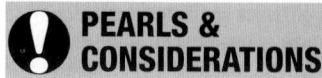 **TREATMENT**

NONPHARMACOLOGIC THERAPY

- For acute paronychia without purulent drainage, warm soaks tid or qid are helpful. If pus is present, surgical drainage is required (Fig. 1).
- For chronic paronychia, avoid frequent immersion in water or exposure to moisture.

ACUTE GENERAL Rx

- Trimethoprim-sulfamethoxazole DS 1 PO bid for 7 days is usually the antibiotic of choice for acute paronychia as it covers methicillin-susceptible *Staphylococcus aureus* strains (MSSA) and methicillin-resistant *S. aureus* (MRSA) strains.

- Alternative antibiotic choices include dicloxacillin 500 mg qid, cephalexin 500 mg qid, clindamycin, and amoxicillin-clavulanate potassium.
- Surgical drainage is indicated if purulent discharge is noted.
- Use local anesthesia such as digital block or ethyl chloride spray.
- A No. 11 blade scalpel is used to lift the lateral perionychium and proximal eponychium off the nail, facilitating drainage.
- If the pus is located beneath the nail, the lateral edge of the nail can be lifted off the nail bed and excised.

CHRONIC Rx

- If no fungal organism is found, tincture of iodine (2 drops bid) helps keep the nail and skin dry.
- Chronic paronychia caused by *Candida albicans* is treated with topical antifungal agents (e.g., miconazole or ketoconazole applied tid).
- Unresponsive cases may be treated with oral itraconazole, fluconazole, or terbinafine, but this should be done in consultation with dermatology and/or infectious disease as it requires prolonged therapy and has significant drug-to-drug interactions.
- One study suggested that topical steroids such as methylprednisone aceponate were more effective than antifungals, implying that the origin is chronic dermatitis, not fungus. Topical tacrolimus ointment 0.1% has also been found effective.
- Surgery may be needed in refractory cases.

DISPOSITION

- Most acute paronychias with appropriate treatment resolve within 7 to 10 days.
- Osteomyelitis is a potential complication of paronychia.
- Untreated chronic paronychia leads to thickening and discoloration with eventual nail loss.

REFERRAL

Chronic paronychia refractory to topical medical therapy is best referred to dermatology and/or infectious disease. A hand surgeon is consulted if abscess drainage or surgery is being considered.

⚠ PEARLS & CONSIDERATIONS

COMMENTS

The gastrointestinal tract, including the mouth and bowel, and the genitourinary tract in women are the usual sources of *C. albicans* in chronic paronychia.

SUGGESTED READING
Available at www.expertconsult.com

RELATED CONTENT
Paronychia (Patient Information)

AUTHOR: **GLENN G. FORT, M.D., M.P.H.**

BASIC INFORMATION

DEFINITION

Patent ductus arteriosus (PDA) is a persistence of the fetal communication between the descending aorta and main pulmonary artery. It is a derivative of the sixth aortic arch. This connection allows for blood to bypass the fetal lungs (which are not participating in gas exchange) and be directed into the descending aorta to supply structures below this region. It usually closes soon after birth under the physiologic effects of elevated oxygen level. Defects can range in size from so small as to be undetectable to large enough to cause volume loading of the left ventricle and pulmonary hypertension.

SYNONYMS

PDA

ICD-10CM CODES
Q25.0 Patent ductus arteriosus

EPIDEMIOLOGY & DEMOGRAPHICS

- Prevalence is 2.9 per 10000 live births. Incidence has increased dramatically due to improved survival of premature infants (especially those born <30 weeks' gestation).
- Female predominance 2:1
- Increased incidence in congenital rubella and with associated cyanotic congenital heart disease

PHYSICAL FINDINGS & CLINICAL PRESENTATION

- Continuous murmur, often referred to as a "machinery-like murmur," which is appreciated over the left scapula and in the left infraclavicular area in patients with left-to-right shunting (Fig. 1).
- The apical impulse may be hyperdynamic if there is significant left-to-right shunting.
- Widened pulse pressure.
- The first heart sound is normal, but the S2 may be split with an accentuated P2 component if there is pulmonary hypertension. An S3 may be appreciated if shunt volume is significant.
- Increased jugular venous pressure (with RV failure):

1. When the defect has resulted in irreversible pulmonary hypertension, there will be no murmur present, but cyanosis and clubbing, particularly of the feet (differential cyanosis), will be present.
- Exertional dyspnea and fatigue.
- Patients with small defects: generally asymptomatic.
- Fig. 2 shows the anatomy of patent ductus arteriosus.

DIAGNOSIS

DIFFERENTIAL DIAGNOSIS

- Rule out other causes of continuous murmurs such as aortopulmonary shunts or window, coronary fistula, ruptured sinus of Valsalva aneurysm, aortic-cameral fistula, and mixed aortic stenosis and regurgitation.
- Coarctation of the aorta will have a murmur over the scapula but arm-leg pressure gradient and hypertension.
  - In patients with Eisenmenger syndrome, consider ASD and VSD in the differential diagnosis.

WORKUP

- ECG:
  1. When the defect is large enough to cause left-sided volume overload there may be LA enlargement, LV hypertrophy
  2. When pulmonary hypertension has occurred, right-axis deviation, RVH and P pulmonale may be present
- Chest x-ray
- Echocardiography (Fig. 3)
- Cardiac magnetic resonance imaging (MRI), or CT
- Cardiac catheterization

IMAGING STUDIES

- Chest x-ray: cardiomegaly, left heart enlargement, increased pulmonary vascular pattern
- Echocardiography with Doppler flow studies is generally diagnostic. The parasternal short-axis and suprasternal views can show the presence of the PDA, the size of the defect, and the direction of shunting. Color flow Doppler may be useful to view even tiny ductus flow. Echocardiography can also show the effect of the PDA on left heart chamber sizes and measure the pulmonary:systemic shunt ratio (Qp:Qs) and determine if pulmonary hypertension has developed

- Transesophageal echocardiography is modestly helpful, especially when patients have poor acoustic windows
- Cardiac MRI and CT: may be useful if echo is not diagnostic; the PDA may be directly visualized and its morphology described with either technique. MRI is gold standard for assessing LV size and function, and it can determine whether the left-sided chambers are enlarged and establish the degree of shunting using phase contrast imaging to determine the Qp:Qs noninvasively. MRI is also useful to assess for associated lesions; cardiac CT can offer similar information at the price of radiation exposure
- Cardiac catheterization: Left- and right-heart catheterization can be used when the diagnosis remains in doubt. It can also help to estimate the degree of left-to-right shunting, establish right-sided pressures, demonstrate the PDA morphology, and attempt closure where technically feasible
- PDAs are classified based on the amount of left-to-right shunting:
  - Small: Qp:Qs <1.5:1
  - Moderate: Qp:Qs 1.5 – 2.2:1
  - Large: Qp:Qs >2.2:1

TREATMENT

PHARMACOLOGIC THERAPY

- NSAIDs (e.g., indomethacin, ibuprofen) may be used to cause PDA closure in the premature infant; the mechanism of action is by inhibition of local prostaglandin synthesis, which is necessary for the duct to remain open in many cases. These are ineffective in term infants and older patients
- Antibiotic prophylaxis is only recommended where there has been previous endocarditis
- Where there is volume overload, patients can be treated with diuretics and digoxin until formal device or surgical closure can be performed
- In older patients with secondary pulmonary hypertension, pulmonary vasodilators can be extremely helpful in improving symptoms and mortality and potentially allowing safe closure of the defect

SURGICAL Rx

- Closure of a PDA is considered if the following are present:
  - Signs of left atrial and/or left ventricular volume overload, or net left-to-right shunting
  - Prior endarteritis
  - PDA should be closed in patients with pulmonary hypertension where the pulmonary arterial pressure is <2/3 of the systemic vascular pressure, or where the pulmonary vascular resistance is <2/3 of the systemic vascular resistance
- Additionally, because >95% of PDAs can successfully be closed percutaneously with a low rate of complications, many advocate closing a PDA when there is the presence of

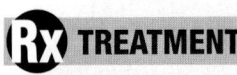

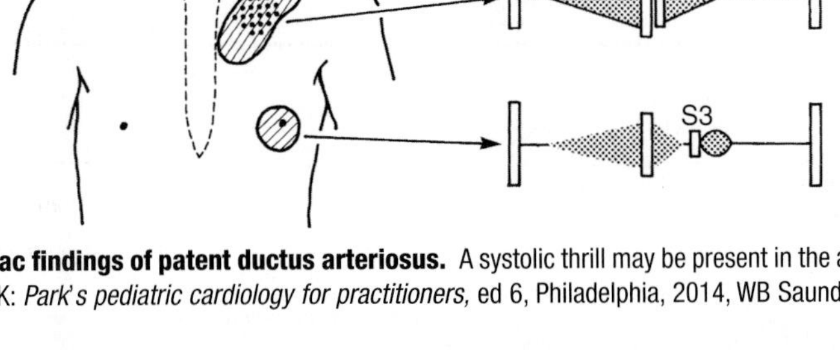

FIG. 1 Cardiac findings of patent ductus arteriosus. A systolic thrill may be present in the area shown by dots. (Park MK: *Park's pediatric cardiology for practitioners,* ed 6, Philadelphia, 2014, WB Saunders.)

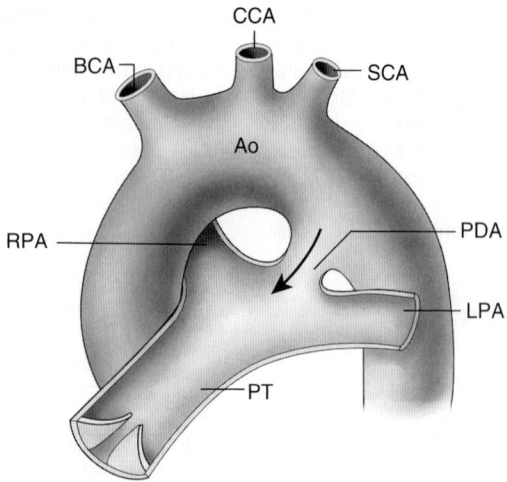

FIG. 2 Anatomy of a patent ductus arteriosus. Note the relationships among the position of the ductus, left subclavian artery, and pulmonary artery bifurcation. *Ao,* Aorta; *BCA,* brachiocephalic; *CCA,* common carotid artery; *LPA,* left pulmonary artery; *PDA,* patent ductus arteriosus; *PT,* pulmonary trunk; *RPA,* right pulmonary artery; *SCA,* subclavian artery. (From Perloff JK, ed: *Clinical recognition of congenital heart disease,* ed 4, Philadelphia, 1994, Saunders.)

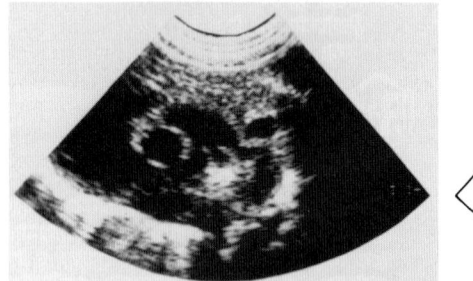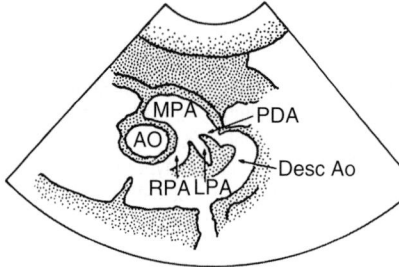

FIG. 3 Parasternal short-axis view demonstrating patent ductus arteriosus (PDA) that connects the main pulmonary artery (MPA) and the descending aorta (Desc Ao). *AO,* Aorta; *LPA,* left pulmonary artery; *RPA,* right pulmonary artery. (Park MK: *Park's pediatric cardiology for practitioners,* ed 6, Philadelphia, 2014, WB Saunders.)

an audible murmur. The chief indication for this "prophylactic closure" is the low but non-zero incidence of infective endocarditis in this condition, although there is no clear evidence to support this procedure and controversy remains
- In patients with pulmonary hypertension, treatment with pulmonary vasodilators should be considered prior to closure
- Device closure is possible in >95% of cases, and various devices are available for these defects. Use of different types depends on morphology of the defect
- Surgical closure may be performed when a patient is undergoing cardiac surgery for other reasons or when the PDA is not suitable for device closure, such as in the case of very large defects or when the child is too small (<6 kg)

- Closure is not indicated in patients with severe pulmonary hypertension, as these patients may require right-to-left shunting to maintain cardiac output.

DISPOSITION

- Long-term outcome depends on the size of the lesion and the associated degree of left-to-right shunting. Defects with a small shunt generally do very well, apart from the possibility of endocarditis. Those with moderate shunts may develop left atrial and left ventricular volume overload and shortness of breath or arrhythmias. Those with a very large shunt may develop heart failure early, then go on to develop Eisenmenger syndrome (fixed pulmonary hypertension with reversal of shunt causing cyanosis) if unrepaired.

- Endocarditis is uncommon and usually occurs at the site where the high-velocity jet lesion enters the PA but generally can be treated medically
- Basic preoperative assessment for patients with adult congenital heart disease (ACHD) should include systemic arterial oximetry, an ECG, chest radiograph, TTE, and blood tests for full blood count and coagulation screen.
- Intracardiac shunts are considered of moderate risk for preoperative evaluation for noncardiac procedure. High-risk features include severe systolic dysfunction (EF <35%), severe pulmonary hypertension (whether primary or secondary), cyanotic heart disease, or severe left-side outlet obstruction.
- Clinical follow-up is recommended for adult patients to exclude residual deficits, pulmonary hypertension and LV dilation and dysfunction, and atrial arrhythmias.
- Patients with small hemodynamically insignificant PDA should be reexamined every 3 to 5 years to assess for cardiopulmonary decompensation.
- Infective endocarditis prophylaxis for dental procedures:
  1. Prophylaxis is not indicated for an unrepaired PDA.
- Prophylaxis is indicated for a repaired PDA in the first 6 months following the repair or where prosthetic material is present and there is a residual defect.
- The estrogen-containing oral contraceptive pill is not recommended in ACHD patients at risk of thromboembolism, such as those with cyanosis related to an intracardiac shunt, atrial fibrillation, severe PAH, or Fontan repair.
- Women with a repaired PDA generally can undergo pregnancy and delivery normally. Those with an unrepaired defect of a size that would ordinarily be repaired are recommended to undergo repair before becoming pregnant.

SUGGESTED READINGS
Available at www.expertconsult.com

RELATED CONTENT
Patent Ductus Arteriosus (PDA) (Patient Information)

AUTHORS: **CRAIG L. BASMAN, M.D.,** and **PAUL LEIS, D.O.**

BASIC INFORMATION

DEFINITION

Pediculosis is lice infestation. Human beings can be infested with three kinds of lice: *Pediculus capitis* (head louse), *Pediculus corporis* (body louse), and *Phthirus pubis* (pubic, or crab, louse). Lice feed on human blood and deposit their eggs (nits) on the hair shafts (head lice and pubic lice) and along the seams of clothing (body lice). Nits generally hatch within 7 to 10 days. Lice are obligate human parasites and cannot survive away from their hosts for longer than 7 to 10 days.

SYNONYMS

Lice

ICD-10CM CODES
B85.2 Pediculosis, unspecified
B85.0 Pediculosis due to Pediculus humanus capitis
B85.1 Pediculosis due to Pediculus humanus corporis
B85.4 Mixed pediculosis and phthiriasis
Z20.7 Contact with and (suspected) exposure to pediculosis, acariasis and other infestations

EPIDEMIOLOGY & DEMOGRAPHICS

- There are 6 to 12 million cases of head lice in the United States yearly. The estimated annual direct and indirect cost of head louse infestation in the United States is $1 billion.
- Lice infestation of the scalp is most common in children (girls affected more often than boys).
- Infestation of the eyelashes is most frequently seen in children and may indicate sexual abuse.
- The chance of acquiring pubic lice from one sexual exposure with an infested partner is >90% (most contagious STD known).
- Body lice is most common in conditions of poor hygiene.

PHYSICAL FINDINGS & CLINICAL PRESENTATION

- Pruritus with excoriation may be caused by hypersensitivity reaction, inflammation from saliva, and fecal material from the lice.

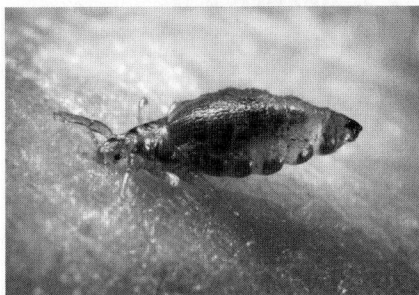

FIG. 1 Body louse, *Pediculus humanus* var. *corporis,* as it was obtaining a blood meal from human host. (Courtesy Public Health Image Library, Centers for Disease Control and Prevention. From Vincent JL et al: *Textbook of critical care,* ed 6, Philadelphia, 2011, Saunders.)

- Nits can be identified by examining hair shafts.
- The presence of nits on clothes is indicative of body lice.
- Lymphadenopathy may be present (cervical adenopathy with head lice, inguinal lymphadenopathy with pubic lice).
- Head lice are most frequently found in the back of the head and neck, behind the ears.
- Scratching can result in pustules and crusting.
- Pubic lice may affect the hair around the anus.

ETIOLOGY

Lice are transmitted by close personal contact or use of contaminated objects (e.g., combs, clothing, bed linen, hats).

DIAGNOSIS

DIFFERENTIAL DIAGNOSIS

- Seborrheic dermatitis
- Scabies
- Eczema
- Other: pilar casts, trichonodosis (knotted hair), monilethrix

WORKUP

Diagnosis is made by seeing the lice (Fig. 1) or their nits. Combing hair with a fine-toothed comb is recommended because visual inspection of the hair and scalp may miss more than 50% of infestations.

LABORATORY TESTS

Wood's light examination is useful to screen a large number of children: live nits fluoresce, empty nits have a gray fluorescence, nits with unborn louse reveal white fluorescence.

TREATMENT

NONPHARMACOLOGIC THERAPY

- Patients with body lice should discard infested clothes and improve their hygiene.
- Combing out nits is a widely recommended but unproven adjunctive therapy.
- Personal items such as combs and brushes should be soaked in hot water for 15 to 30 min.
- Close contacts and household members should also be examined for the presence of lice.

ACUTE GENERAL Rx

The following products are available for treatment of lice:

- Permethrin: available over the counter (1% permethrin [Nix]) or by prescription (5% permethrin [Elimite]); should be applied to the hair and scalp and rinsed out after 10 min. A repeat application 7 days later is generally not necessary in patients with head lice. It can be applied to clean, dry hair and left on overnight (8 to 14 hours) under a shower cap. Resistance to permethrin is now widespread.

- Malathion, an organophosphate, is effective in head lice. It is available by prescription. Use should be avoided in children ≤2 yr. It is not commonly used because of its objectionable odor, fear of flammability, and prolonged application time (8 to 12 hr).
- Spinosad (Natroba) is a newer FDA-approved product for head lice. It is a topical suspension applied to dry hair for 10 min, then rinsed. It may be repeated 7 days later if necessary. It is more effective than permethrin but also much more expensive. It is safe in pregnancy (category B—no evidence of risk in humans).
- Benzyl alcohol lotion, 5% (Ulesfia) can be used for treatment of head lice in patients >6 mo old. The lotion is applied to dry hair and left on for 10 min. Treatment must be repeated after 7 days because the drug is not ovicidal.
- Eyelash infestation can be treated with the application of petroleum jelly rubbed into the eyelashes three times a day for 5 to 7 days. The application of baby shampoo to the eyelashes and brows three or four times a day for 5 days is also effective. The use of fluorescein drops applied to the lids and eyelashes is also toxic to lice.
- In patients who have previously not responded to treatment or in whom resistance with 1% permethrin cream rinse occurs, a 10-day course of trimethoprim-sulfamethoxazole (TMP-SMX) 8 mg/kg/day in divided doses is an effective treatment for head lice infestation, especially for eyelash infestations with *Phthirus pubis*.
- Ivermectin, an antiparasitic drug, given as an oral dose of 400 mcg/kg of body weight on days 1 and 8, is effective for head lice resistant to other treatments (currently not FDA approved for pediculosis). Ivermectin 0.5% lotion is FDA approved as a single-use topical treatment for head lice in patients 6 mo or older. Cost is more than $200 for 4 oz.

PEARLS & CONSIDERATIONS

COMMENTS

- Patients with pubic lice should notify their sexual contacts. Sex partners within the last month should be treated.
- Parents of patients should also be educated that head lice infestation (unlike body lice) does not indicate poor hygiene.

SUGGESTED READINGS

Available at www.expertconsult.com

RELATED CONTENT

Lice (Patient Information)

AUTHOR: **FRED F. FERRI, M.D.**

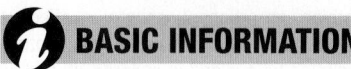

BASIC INFORMATION

DEFINITION

Pelvic abscess is an acute or chronic infection, most commonly involving the pelvic viscera. Treatment requires directed therapy including broad-spectrum antimicrobials and, if medical therapy fails, surgical intervention. There are four categories based on etiologic factors:

- Ascending infection, spreading from cervix through endometrial cavity to adnexa, forming a tuboovarian complex
- Infection occurring in the puerperium, which spreads to the adnexa from the endometrium or myometrium by a hematogenous or lymphatic route
- Abscess complicating pelvic surgery
- Involvement of the pelvic viscera as a result of spread from contiguous organs, such as appendicitis or diverticulitis

SYNONYMS

Tuboovarian abscess (TOA)
Vaginal cuff abscess

ICD-10CM CODES
N70.93 Salpingitis and oophoritis, unspecified
N70.0   Acute salpingitis and oophoritis
N70.1   Chronic salpingitis and oophoritis
K63.0   Abscess of intestine
K65.1   Peritoneal abscess
K68.11 Postprocedural retroperitoneal abscess
K68.12 Psoas muscle abscess
K68.19 Other retroperitoneal abscess

EPIDEMIOLOGY & DEMOGRAPHICS

INCIDENCE:
- 34% of hospitalized patients with pelvic inflammatory disease
- 1% to 2% of patients undergoing hysterectomy, most with vaginal approach
- Peak incidence third to fourth decade

RISK FACTORS: Same risk factors as for pelvic inflammatory disease, although in 30% to 50% of patients there is no prior history of salpingitis before abscess forms.

PHYSICAL FINDINGS & CLINICAL PRESENTATION

- Abdominal or pelvic pain (90%)
- Fever or chills (50%)
- Abnormal bleeding (21%)
- Vaginal discharge (28%)
- Nausea (26%)
- Up to 60% to 80% present in the absence of fever or leukocytosis; absence of these findings should not exclude diagnosis

ETIOLOGY

- Mixed flora of anaerobes, aerobes, and facultative anaerobes, such as *Escherichia coli*, *Bacteroides fragilis*, *Prevotella* spp., aerobic streptococci, and *Peptococcus* and *Peptostreptococcus* spp.

- *Neisseria gonorrhoeae* and *Chlamydia* are the major etiologic bacteria in cervicitis and salpingitis but are rarely found in abscess cavity cultures.
- In elderly patients consider diverticular disease.

DIAGNOSIS

DIFFERENTIAL DIAGNOSIS

- Pelvic neoplasms, such as ovarian tumors and leiomyomas.
- Ovarian torsion.
- Inflammatory masses involving adjacent bowel or omentum, such as ruptured appendicitis or diverticulitis.
- Pelvic hematomas, as may occur after cesarean section or hysterectomy.
- Section III describes the diagnostic approach to patients with a pelvic mass; the differential diagnosis of pelvic mass is described in Section II.
- The differential diagnosis of pelvic pain is described in Section II.
- Pelvic ultrasound or CT scan: commonly used to characterize anatomic abnormalities such as a pelvic mass and to assess for suitability for possible drainage by interventional radiology techniques. Can also be used to follow response to treatment and to assess for resolution of abscess.
- Most common cause of preventable death: physician delay in diagnosis.

LABORATORY TESTS

- CBC with differential
- Aerobic as well as anaerobic cultures of cervix, blood, urine, sputum, peritoneal cavity (if entered), and abscess cavity before starting antibiotics
- Pregnancy test in patients of reproductive age

IMAGING STUDIES

- Sonogram: noninvasive, inexpensive study to confirm diagnosis, estimate size of abscess, and monitor response to therapy; sensitivity >90%
- CT scan: used for both diagnosis and therapy (CT-guided drainage) (Fig. E1)
  1. Useful where sonogram provides insufficient information, as with intraabdominal abscesses
  2. Success rate with CT-guided abscess drainage: unilocular, 90%; multilocular, 40%

TREATMENT

Major concerns:
1. Desire for future fertility
2. Likelihood of rupture of abscess, with resulting peritonitis, septic shock, and morbid sequelae

ACUTE GENERAL Rx

- Clinical quandary is whether patient requires immediate laparoscopic surgery (uncertain diagnosis or suspicion of rupture) or

management with IV antibiotics, reserving surgery for those with inadequate clinical response (e.g., 48 to 72 hr of therapy, with persistent fever or leukocytosis, increasing size of mass, or suspicion of rupture)
- Surgery indicated in poor response to medical therapy. Early surgery may be needed in those with large adnexal masses (>8 cm), or in immunocompromised patients
- Antibiotic combinations:
  1. Clindamycin 900 mg IV q8h or metronidazole 500 mg IV q6-8h plus gentamicin either 5 to 7 mg/kg q24h or 1.5 mg/kg q8h
  2. Alternatives: ampicillin-sulbactam 3 g IV q6h or cefoxitin 2 g IV q6h or cefotetan 2 g IV q12h plus doxycycline 100 mg IV q12h
- During medical management, high index of suspicion for acute rupture, such as acute worsening of abdominal pain or new-onset tachycardia and hypotension, mandating immediate surgical intervention after patient stabilization
- Surgical options:
  1. Laparoscopy with drainage and irrigation
  2. CT-guided drainage (interventional radiology)
  3. Transvaginal colpotomy (abscess must be midline, dissect rectovaginal septum, and be adherent to vaginal fornix)
  4. Laparotomy, including total abdominal hysterectomy with bilateral salpingo-oophorectomy or unilateral salpingo-oophorectomy
  5. Evidence of ruptured tuboovarian abscess is a surgical emergency

DISPOSITION

- Of patients treated with medical therapy, response in 75%, with a 50% pregnancy rate. Pregnancy rate decreases with recurrent episodes.
- No response in 30% to 40%; can be treated with either CT-guided drainage or surgical intervention, keeping in mind that unilateral adnexectomy may give equal chance of cure versus hysterectomy, yet preserve reproductive potential.

REFERRAL

If patient has a tuboovarian abscess, refer to gynecologist.

PEARLS & CONSIDERATIONS

COMMENTS

If *Actinomyces* species is isolated from culture, treatment with penicillin is required for an extended period (6 wk-3 mo).

SUGGESTED READING

Available at www.expertconsult.com

RELATED CONTENT

Pelvic Abscess (Patient Information)
Pelvic Inflammatory Disease (Related Key Topic)

AUTHOR: **MATTHEW J. FAGAN, M.D.**

BASIC INFORMATION

DEFINITION

Pelvic inflammatory disease (PID) is infection and inflammation of the upper female genital tract (including uterus, fallopian tubes, ovaries, and/or pelvic peritoneum) unrelated to pregnancy or surgical intervention. PID can be classified as acute (≤30 days duration), subclinical, or chronic (>30 days duration).

SYNONYMS

PID
Salpingitis
Oophoritis
Adnexitis
Pyosalpinx
Tubo-ovarian abscess
TOA

ICD-10CM CODES

A18.17	Tuberculous female pelvic inflammatory disease
A52.76	Syphilitic pelvic inflammatory disease
A54.2	Gonococcal pelviperitonitis and other gonococcal genitourinary infections
A54.24	Gonococcal female pelvic inflammatory disease
A56.1	Chlamydial infection of pelviperitoneum and other genitourinary organs
A56.11	Chlamydial female pelvic inflammatory disease
N70.0	Acute salpingitis and oophoritis
N70	Salpingitis and oophoritis
N70.0	Acute salpingitis and oophoritis
N70.01	Acute salpingitis
N70.02	Acute oophoritis
N70.03	Acute salpingitis and oophoritis
N70.1	Chronic salpingitis and oophoritis
N70.11	Chronic salpingitis
N70.12	Chronic oophoritis
N70.13	Chronic salpingitis and oophoritis
N70.9	Salpingitis and oophoritis, unspecified
N70.91	Salpingitis, unspecified
N70.92	Oophoritis, unspecified
N70.93	Salpingitis and oophoritis, unspecified
N71.0	Inflammatory disease of uterus, except cervix
N71.0	Acute inflammatory disease of uterus
N71.1	Chronic inflammatory disease of uterus
N71.9	Inflammatory disease of uterus, unspecified
N73.0	Other female pelvic inflammatory diseases
N73.8	Other specified female pelvic inflammatory diseases
N74	Female pelvic inflammatory disorders in diseases classified elsewhere

EPIDEMIOLOGY & DEMOGRAPHICS

INCIDENCE/PREVALENCE: Pelvic inflammatory disease is most often diagnosed in young, sexually active women. The incidence of PID is difficult to ascertain given its broad diagnostic criteria, its propensity to be missed as a diagnosis, and the challenges with follow-up due to patients seeking urgent or emergent care for this condition. The Centers for Disease Control and Prevention estimates 1 million new cases of PID are diagnosed yearly. Severity of illness and hospitalization for PID are decreasing in the U.S. PID has long-term health risks for women including recurrent infection, chronic pelvic pain, pelvic adhesive disease, and tubal disease resulting in ectopic pregnancy and infertility.

RISK FACTORS:
- Sexually active adolescent and young women
- Previous episode of PID
- Prior chlamydial infection
- Multiple or new sexual partners within past 12 months
- Sexual partner diagnosed with sexually transmitted infection (STI)
- Non-use of barrier contraception

CLINICAL PRESENTATION

- Lower abdominal pain
- Abnormal vaginal discharge
- Abnormal uterine bleeding
- Postcoital bleeding
- Dysuria
- Dyspareunia
- Fever
- Nausea and vomiting (suggestive of peritonitis)

PHYSICAL FINDINGS

- Fever
- Abdominal tenderness
- Abnormal vaginal discharge
- Cervical friability
- Cervical motion tenderness
- Adnexal tenderness
- Adnexal mass
- Right upper quadrant tenderness (perihepatitis): 5% of PID cases

Note: Women with PID may be asymptomatic and/or have a benign physical examination.

ETIOLOGY

Pelvic inflammatory disease occurs as a result of ascending infection from the lower genital tract. Infections are often polymicrobial, and although gonorrheal and chlamydial infections are commonly implicated in the development of PID, fewer than 50% of women test positive for these organisms. This is likely due in part to increased STI screening efforts. PID may also arise in the setting of organisms associated with normal vaginal flora such as:
- *Bacteroides fragilis*
- *Escherichia coli* and other enteric gram-negative rods
- *Gardnerella vaginalis*
- *Haemophilus influenzae*

Rarer infectious causes include the following: *Mycoplasma hominis, Ureaplasma urealyticum, Mycobacterium tuberculosis* (an important cause in developing countries), and cytomegalovirus (CMV).

DX DIAGNOSIS

Diagnosis of PID is made when a patient has clinical or pathologic evidence of upper genital tract infection and inflammation. Although no single test or measure reliably diagnoses the spectrum of disorders that comprise PID:
- Providers should maintain a low threshold for diagnosis and treatment of PID given significant long-term health risks associated with the disease, especially if untreated.
- Definitive criteria for diagnosis of PID include:
  1. Laparoscopic abnormalities consistent with PID
  2. Histopathologic evidence of endometritis in women with clinical suspicion for PID
  3. Transvaginal sonography or other imaging techniques showing thickened, fluid-filled tubes, with or without free pelvic fluid or tuboovarian complex
- The CDC suggests that women with risk factors, abdominal or pelvic pain, and any pelvic tenderness (cervical, uterine, and/or adnexal) be treated for PID.

DIFFERENTIAL DIAGNOSIS

- Appendicitis
- Ectopic pregnancy
- Intrauterine/other pregnancy
- Ovarian cyst
- Adnexal torsion
- Endometriosis
- Urinary tract infection (cystitis or pyelonephritis)

WORKUP

History—as in risk factors and clinical presentation, previously

Physical examination—as in physical findings, previously

LABORATORY TESTS

- Wet mount: clue cells, increased white cells
- Gram stain of endocervical exudate: >30 polymorphonuclear cells per high-power field correlates with chlamydial or gonococcal infection
- Endocervical cultures for *N. gonorrhoeae* and *C. trachomatis*
- Fallopian tube aspirate or peritoneal exudate culture if laparoscopy performed
- WBC: leukocytosis
- Elevated acute phase reactants: ESR >15 mm/hr, C-reactive protein
- HCG to rule out intrauterine or ectopic pregnancy
- HIV, with consideration for other STI screening such as RPR, HBsAg, Hep C Ab (HIV increases incidence of TOA)

IMAGING STUDIES

Ultrasonography is commonly used to assess for PID and can be used to determine inpatient vs. outpatient treatment by presence or absence of TOA. Findings include:
- Thick-walled adnexal mass with heterogenous or cystic contents suggestive of abscess
- Dilated fallopian tubes (note that normal fallopian tubes are rarely identified on ultrasonography)
- "Cogwheel sign" indicating thickened fallopian tube walls

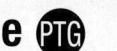

- Heterogenous fluid within the endometrium CT scan (Fig. E1) or MRI may be useful to better characterize adnexal masses and/or rule out other pathology such as appendicitis or renal calculus. Choice of imaging modality will depend on clinical suspicion, logistical access, and associated cost.

PROCEDURES

Endometrial biopsy that reveals endometritis may support a diagnosis of PID. Laparoscopy has been utilized as a gold standard for diagnosing PID, but due to the invasive nature of this procedure and the risks, and costs associated, it is rarely indicated as a diagnostic tool.

℞ TREATMENT

Primary management of PID is medical, with broad-spectrum antibiotics administered in an outpatient setting. Inpatient treatment should be initiated when:

- Surgical emergency is not excluded
- Tuboovarian abscess is present
- Patient is unable or unwilling to complete outpatient treatment (including medication regimen and clinical follow-up)
- Outpatient treatment fails to improve symptoms in 48 to 72 hours
- Pregnancy, immunodeficiency, or other complicating medical condition exists
  Evidence-based guidelines recommended by the CDC for acute PID are as follows:

INPATIENT REGIMENS: Recommended parenteral regimen

- Cefotetan 2 g IV q12h *PLUS*
  Doxycycline 100 mg PO or IV q12h OR
- Cefoxitin 2 g IV q6h PLUS doxycycline 100 mg PO or IV q12h
  OR
- Clindamycin 900 mg IV q8h PLUS gentamicin loading dose IV or IM (2 mg/kg of body weight), followed by a maintenance dose (1.5 mg/kg) q8h. Single daily dosing (3-5 mg/kg) can be substituted.
  Alternative parenteral regimens
- Ampicillin/sulbactam 3 g IV q6h *PLUS*
- Doxycycline 100 mg PO or IV q12h
  When clinical improvement is apparent based on symptoms, physical exam, and laboratory criteria, antibiotics may be transitioned from IV to PO with doxycycline PO or clindamycin PO (depending on the regimen selected) administered to complete 14 days of total antibiotic therapy. If a patient does not improve despite use of a recommended antibiotic regimen, further workup and potential procedural intervention are warranted.

OUTPATIENT REGIMENS: Recommended intramuscular/oral regimens

- Ceftriaxone 250 mg IM in a single dose *PLUS*
- Doxycycline 100 mg PO bid for 14 days
- *WITH or WITHOUT*
- Metronidazole 500 mg PO bid for 14 days

OR

- Cefoxitin 2 g IM in a single dose and probenecid, 1 g PO administered concurrently in a single dose *PLUS*
- Doxycycline 100 mg PO bid for 14 days
- *WITH or WITHOUT*
- Metronidazole 500 mg PO bid for 14 days *OR*
- *OR*
- other third-generation cephalosporin (ceftizoxime or cefotaxime) PLUS
- Doxycycline 100 mg orally bid for 14 days *WITH or WITHOUT*
- Metronidazole 500 mg orally twice a day for 14 days.
  Alternative intramuscular/oral regimen
- Azithromycin 1 g PO once weekly for 2 weeks PLUS ceftriaxone 250 mg IM in a single dose

TREATMENT CONSIDERATIONS

- Antimicrobials should include coverage against *N. gonorrhoeae* and *C. trachomatis* even if these organisms are not identified on culture.
- Due to increasing antibiotic resistance of gonorrhea to fluoroquinolones, these antibiotics should be avoided in the treatment of PID unless the patient has history of severe allergy to components of the recommend regimens and lives in an area where resistant species are not thought to be endemic.
- Women should avoid sexual activity until they and their sexual partners have been adequately treated and symptoms have resolved.
- TOA may require drainage, which may be accomplished by interventional radiology via aspiration or placement of a drain, or by a gynecologist via vaginal or laparoscopic means. Recurrent/persistent TOAs may be managed by total abdominal hysterectomy with bilateral salpingo-oophorectomy after acute treatment of infection.
- Treatment of PID in women with intrauterine devices (IUDs) does not include/require removal of the device unless there is no clinical improvement after 48 to 72 hours of treatment with an approved regimen. IUDs rarely serve as a source for PID, especially greater than 3 weeks after insertion.
- Sexual partners of patients diagnosed with PID or other STIs should be evaluated and treated appropriately. In the setting of PID, treat all sexual partners within 60 days of onset of symptoms. Some states allow for expedited partner therapy (EPT), such that a woman's provider is able to supply her with enough medication to treat herself and her partner(s).
- Treatment of chronic PID may be aimed at a different spectrum of microbes and should be tailored appropriately.

DISPOSITION

- Given the risk of reinfection, all women should be retested for gonorrhea and chlamydia 3 to 6 months after treatment.

- Follow-up includes confirmation of partner treatment, education on use of barrier contraception, and risks of PID and long-term sequelae, including:
  1. Recurrent PID.
  2. Chronic pelvic pain.
  3. Fallopian tubal damage that leads to infertility and/or ectopic pregnancy.
  4. Fitz-Hugh-Curtis syndrome (Fig. E2).
  5. Potential risk for cancer: Limited studies have suggested a small association between PID and ovarian, endometrial, and colon cancer.

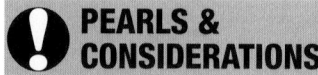

COMMENTS

- Maintain a low threshold for the diagnosis and treatment of PID given the risks for progression to severe infection and to significant and chronic medical and reproductive complications.
- Most patients are candidates for outpatient therapy, but inpatient hospitalization is recommended in select cases.
- Use only CDC-recommended treatment regimens unless contraindicated due to severe patient allergy; in such cases, check local susceptibilities of suspected pathogen.
- Offer HIV and other STI screening to all women with suspected or diagnosed PID.
- IUDs may be retained unless women have failed to improve with 48 to 72 hours of treatment.
- Treat sexual partners of women with PID, with EPT if possible.
- Counsel patients on abstinence until they and their partners have completed treatment.
- Test for reinfection with gonorrhea and chlamydia 3 to 6 months after treatment.

PREVENTION

Women aged <25 years and/or participating in high-risk sexual behavior should be screened annually for chlamydia; studies have shown such screening to reduce cases of PID by > 50%. The importance of minimizing partner exposures and using barrier contraception (either alone or in conjunction with another method) should also be emphasized.

SUGGESTED READINGS
Available at www.expertconsult.com

RELATED CONTENT
Pelvic Inflammatory Disease (Patient Information)
Pelvic Abscess (Related Key Topic)
Chlamydia Genital Infections (Related Key Topic)
Gonorrhea (Related Key Topic)

AUTHORS: **ERIN SMITH, M.D.,** and **GRETCHEN MAKAI, M.D.**

BASIC INFORMATION

DEFINITION

Pelvic organ prolapse (POP) refers to descent of vaginal tissue into the vaginal canal. It results from injury to or weakness in the connective tissue and muscles of the pelvic floor. Modern definitions of POP describe anterior and posterior vaginal wall defects as well as apical defects in pelvic floor connective tissue. Synonyms include terms such as cystocele, rectocele, uterine prolapse, enterocele, and vaginal vault prolapse. Descriptions of this condition as a "dropped bladder," "dropped uterus," or defect in other pelvic organs should be avoided. These types of descriptions do not accurately reflect the pathophysiology of POP and often create confusion and unnecessary stress for patients. Table 1 describes the various types of POP affecting each vaginal compartment with corresponding ICD-10 codes.

SYNONYMS

Vaginal prolapse
Uterine prolapse
Genital prolapse
Uterine descensus
POP
Pelvic floor disorder
PFD

ICD-10CM CODES
N81.4	Uterovaginal prolapse, unspecified
N81.5	Vaginal enterocele
N81.6	Rectocele
N81.I8	Other female genital prolapse
N81.2	Incomplete uterovaginal prolapse
N81.82	Incompetence or weakening of pubocervical tissue

EPIDEMIOLOGY & DEMOGRAPHICS

INCIDENCE AND PREVALENCE: Recent estimates of overall prevalence reveal a rate of 3% to 4% based on objective criteria and physical examination. Prevalence estimates based on nonobjective criteria are often higher. Prevalence increases with age, parity, and BMI. Exact prevalence estimates are difficult to determine due to varying definitions of POP and various diagnostic criteria. POP is common and carries a high burden of disease negatively affecting overall quality of life. The lifetime risk of undergoing surgery due to POP is estimated to be 12%. Annual direct health care costs are high, and repeat operations are common.

GENETICS: Data suggest a heritable component to POP. No specific genes or genetic factors outside of specific connective tissue diseases have been identified. For example, the risk of POP is increased in women with Marfan's syndrome and Ehlers-Danlos syndrome. Because POP is multifactorial and has a long latency, risk estimates based on genetics or family history are difficult to quantify. In general, a genetic susceptibility exists in certain families, which is then affected by external factors to increase an individual woman's risk of POP.

RISK FACTORS: POP has a long latency and is multifactorial. Multiple risk factors have been identified. Some are modifiable, suggesting POP may be preventable. However, many risk factors are not modifiable. Below is a list of the most common risk factors for POP:
- Vaginal childbirth
- Labor
- Pregnancy
- Age
- Chronic obstructive pulmonary disease (COPD) and chronic coughing
- Smoking
- Chronic constipation
- Chronic heavy lifting
- Chronic steroid use
- Connective tissue diseases (Marfan's syndrome, Ehlers-Danlos syndrome)
- Pelvic surgery (including hysterectomy)
- Menopause
- Family history
- Caucasian and Hispanic race

ETIOLOGY

- Muscle injury (levator ani) and connective tissue damage (pubocervical fascia) cause failure of pelvic floor support.
- Increased intraabdominal pressure results in strain on pelvic floor support structures.
- Injury to pelvic floor muscles or connective tissue supports results in uncompensated forces on pelvic floor, resulting in further injury to pelvic floor support structures.
  - Acute (traumatic) injury to pelvic floor support can result from vaginal delivery, labor, or surgery.
  - Chronic injury or strain on pelvic floor connective tissue and muscle can result from conditions such as COPD with chronic coughing or chronic constipation.
  - Neurologic injury from acute or chronic strain on pelvic floor can result in denervation and subsequent muscular atrophy.
  - Diseases or medications that weaken connective tissue (Marfan's syndrome, corticosteroids) can predispose to injury.
  - Hypoestrogenism may weaken pelvic floor tissue and impair ability to heal from injury.
- With injury to pelvic floor support structures, vaginal tissue becomes subjected to the forces from intraabdominal pressure and will stretch and become displaced downward and out through the vaginal opening, resulting in clinical symptoms.

PHYSICAL FINDINGS AND CLINICAL PRESENTATION

- Bulge Symptoms
  - Vaginal pressure.
  - Protrusion from vagina.
- Urinary Symptoms (mainly from obstruction)
  - Urinary hesitancy.
  - Urinary frequency or urgency.
  - Manual reduction of prolapse to complete urination.
  - Incomplete emptying.
  - Weak urinary stream.
- Bowel Symptoms
  - Incomplete defecation.
  - Altered rectal sensation (urgency, lack of sensation).
  - Splinting of vagina/perineum to defecate.
- Sexual Symptoms
  - Dyspareunia.
  - Difficulty with vaginal penetration.
- Other
  - Vaginal bleeding from excoriated vaginal epithelium from chronic exteriorization.
  - Incarcerated prolapse with inability to be manually reduced.

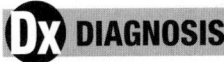

DIAGNOSIS

WORKUP

- Elicit specific symptoms.
- Perform detailed pelvic exam. Examine anterior, posterior, and apical segments of vagina independently.
- POP is dynamic and may not appear the same at various time points or exam conditions.
- Exam is done in standard lithotomy position, and POP is assessed with valsalva during exam.
  - If symptoms are out of proportion to findings, repeat exam in standing position.
- Describe exam findings objectively (Boxes 1, 2, and 3).
  - Quantitatively with POP-Q.
  - Descriptively with Baden-Walker halfway systems.
- Urinary symptoms should be evaluated separately.
  - POP is associated with urinary incontinence but *does not cause* urinary incontinence.
- Evaluate post void residual urine volume in advanced POP (stages 3 and stage 4).
  - Bladder ultrasound or catheterization at time of exam.

TABLE 1 Types of Genital Prolapse

Original Position of Organs	Prolapse	Symptoms (in addition to the general symptoms of discomfort, dragging, the feeling of a "lump," and, rarely, coital problems)
Anterior	Urethrocele Cystocele	Urinary symptoms (stress incontinence, urinary frequency)
Central	Cervix/uterus: 1st, 2nd, and 3rd degree Procidentia	Bleeding and/or discharge from ulceration in association with procidentia
Posterior	Rectocele Enterocele	Bowel symptoms, particularly the feeling of incomplete evacuation and sometimes having to press the posterior wall backward to pass stool

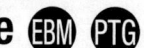

BOX 1 Points of Reference for POP-Q

Point	Description	Range of Values
Aa	3 cm above the hymen on anterior vaginal wall roughly corresponds with the urethrovesical junction.	−3 cm to +3 cm
Ba	The lowest extent of the segment of vagina between point Aa and the apex of the vagina. Unlike point Aa, it is not fixed but will be the same as Aa if point Aa is the most protruding point. In maximal prolapse, it will be the same as point C.	−3 cm to + tvl
C	Most distal edge of cervix (vaginal cuff if uterus/cervix absent).	
D	Posterior fornix (n/a if hysterectomy).	
Ap	3 cm above the hymen on posterior vaginal wall.	−3 cm to +3 cm
Bp	The lowest extent of the segment of vagina between point Ap and the apex of the vagina. Unlike point Ap, it is not fixed but will be the same as Ap if point Ap is the most protruding point. In maximal prolapse it will be the same as point D.	−3 cm to + tvl
GH (Genital Hiatus)	From urethral meatus to inferior hymenal ring.	
PB (Perineal Body)	From inferior hymenal ring to middle of anal orifice.	
TVL	Total Vaginal Length without stretch or Valsalva.	

Key Points: Measure position of six points with respect to the position of the hymen. Points above the hymen (inside) are negative, points below the hymen are positive, and points at the hymen are 0.
Modified from Pemberton J, (ed): *The pelvic floor,* Philadelphia, 2002, WB Saunders, and Bump, et al.: *Am J Obstet Gynecol* 1996:175:13.

BOX 2 POP-Q Examination and Staging

Stage 0	No prolapse.
Stage I	Leading edge ≥1 cm above hymenal ring.
Stage II	Leading edge ≤1 cm above hymenal ring but ≤1 cm below hymenal ring.
Stage III	Most distal point is >1 cm but < (TVL -2) cm below the hymenal ring.
Stage IV	Leading edge ≥ (TVL-2) cm below hymenal ring.

BOX 3 Baden Walker Halfway System

Grade 0	Normal position for each respective site
Grade 1	Descent halfway to the hymen
Grade 2	Descent to the hymen
Grade 3	Descent halfway past the hymen
Grade 4	Maximum possible descent for each site

LABORATORY TESTS

- Not indicated for routine evaluation of POP. Urine testing may be indicated based on presence or absence of urinary tract symptoms.

IMAGING STUDIES

- Not indicated for routine evaluation of POP. Imaging studies for other gynecologic or urologic conditions may be indicated.
- Pelvic ultrasound may be considered in the *absence of POP* in patients with specific symptoms (i.e., pelvic pressure) (Fig. 1).

Rx TREATMENT

NONPHARMACOLOGIC THERAPY
Primary prevention
- Diagnosis and treatment of chronic cough. Correction of constipation.
  - Weight control, nutrition, and smoking cessation counseling.
  - Pelvic muscle exercises.
  - Proper management of vaginal apex at time of hysterectomy in patients without POP.
  - McCall's culdoplasty to prevent vaginal vault prolapse.
- Cesarean delivery NOT indicated for prevention of POP.
  - Untreated urinary retention, even if asymptomatic, can cause bladder infection, reflux, and renal damage.

ACUTE GENERAL TREATMENT
TREATMENT OPTIONS:
- Expectant management is appropriate, except in cases of incomplete bladder emptying associated with POP.
- Pessaries
  - Support device.
  - Silicone, not latex.

- Various shapes and sizes exist.
- Use the simplest and smallest pessary that works.
- 85% of women can be fitted successfully with a pessary.
  - Includes sexually active women.
- Self-care can be learned by the majority of women.
  - Usually remove and clean once per month; otherwise, office visit every 3 months for cleaning and exam.
- Pessary use associated with higher risk of UTI.
- Small vaginal erosions and very mild bleeding or spotting are common side effects.
  - First episode of vaginal bleeding needs evaluation in postmenopausal patients.
- Neglected pessary can cause vaginitis, odor, severe vaginal erosion/bleeding, and fistula.
- Vaginal estrogen may prevent or treat erosions and minimize risk of vaginitis and UTI.

CHRONIC Rx
- Surgery
  - Goals of surgery are to eliminate vaginal bulge and improve associated symptoms.
    - Most reliable symptom resolution is elimination of bulge/protrusion.
    - Resolution of bladder and bowel symptoms is not routinely associated with surgical correction of POP.
  - Evaluate and treat all defects present on exam.
    - Combination defects are the most common presentation.
    - 60% of patients present with multiple defects.
    - Anterior and apical combination is most common.
  - There are multiple ways to classify operations for POP.
  - Obliterative vs. reconstructive procedures:
    - Obliterative procedures remove the vaginal tissue and close off the genital hiatus.
    - High success rates with low morbidity.
    - Option for women who are willing to forgo future vaginal intercourse.
    - Associated with high rates of postoperative incontinence; most surgeons offer anti-incontinence procedure at the same setting.
  - Reconstructive procedures:
    - Restore normal functional anatomy.
    - Subdivided into restorative or compensatory procedures:
      - Restorative procedures use normal anatomic relationships and structures.
      - Compensatory procedures utilize nonanatomic relationships and may or may not use synthetic meshes and graphs.
  - Table 2 categorizes various common procedures for POP.

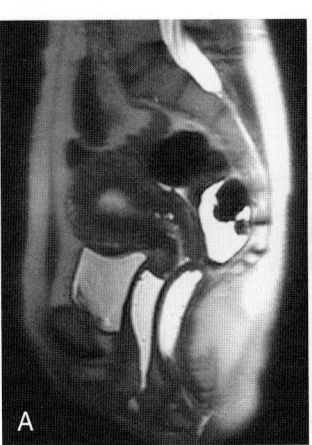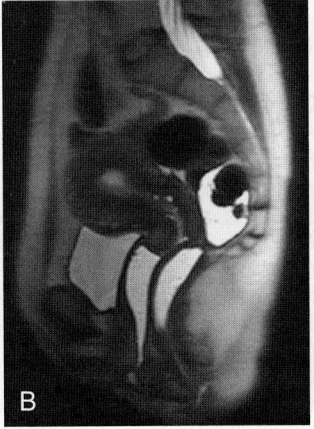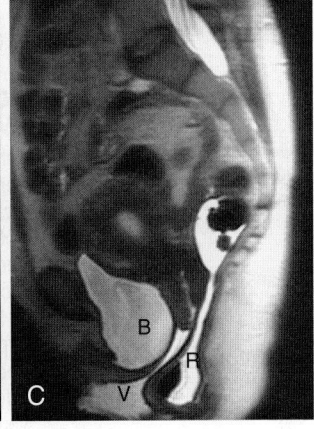

FIG. 1 A, Moderate global pelvic prolapse in a woman with stress urinary incontinence, pelvic heaviness, and constipation after three vaginal deliveries. At rest, all viscera are normally situated in the pelvis. **B,** With Kegel contraction, note that all viscera remain normally situated in the pelvis. **C,** With maximal strain, bladder *(B),* vagina *(V),* and rectum *(R)* are well below the pelvic floor. (From Fielding JR, et al.: *Gynecologic imaging,* Philadelphia, 2011, WB Saunders.)

TABLE 2 Procedures for POP

Classification		Procedure	Compartment(s)
Obliterative		Le Fort colpocleisis	All
		Total colpocleisis	All
Reconstructive	Restorative	Uterosacral ligament suspension	Apex
		Hysteropexy	Apex
		Paravaginal defect repair	Anterior
		Anterior colporrhaphy	Anterior
		Posterior colporrhaphy	Posterior
		Defect-directed posterior repair	Posterior
		Perineorrhaphy	Posterior
	Compensatory		
	Mesh	Sacral colpopexy	All
		Sacral hysteropexy	Apex
		Transvaginal mesh	All
	Nonmesh	Sacrospinous ligament suspension	Apex
			Apex
		Ileococcygeus suspension	Posterior
		Enterocele repair	

○ Hysterectomy alone does not treat POP.
  ■ Often performed concomitantly with POP repair as necessary step to expose critical anatomy.
○ Choice of operation should be tailored to patient's presenting problems, lifestyle, and goals for the surgery.
○ For symptomatic women who desire childbearing: management with pessaries or pelvic muscle exercises is recommended; if surgical correction is required, uterosacral ligament hysteropexy is the preferred method.
  ■ Patients should be counseled that repair will likely break down with subsequent pregnancy.
○ Women without stress incontinence undergoing vaginal surgery for POP are at risk for postoperative urinary incontinence.
○ Use of a prophylactic midurethral sling inserted during vaginal prolapse surgery

has been shown to result in a lower rate of urinary incontinence at 3 and 12 months, but also in a higher rate of adverse events (UTIs, major bleeding complications, incomplete bladder emptying).
○ Abdominal mesh-based repairs and anterior vaginal mesh repairs have superior durability but higher risk and potential for unique complications.
○ Mesh erosion rates have been reported up to 10%, with similar incidence between biologic and synthetic graft. However, synthetic graft erosion often requires surgical revision.

DISPOSITION

• Surgical success rates range between 70% and 95%.
• Up to 30% of patients may require a second operation for POP.
• Untreated POP does not necessarily worsen.

REFERRAL

• To a urogynecologist/gynecologist if surgical intervention is needed or for complex cases involving bladder dysfunction.
• Treating physicians should have special training with synthetic mesh products, if they are used.

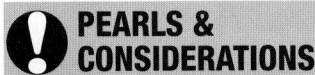 **PEARLS & CONSIDERATIONS**

• POP rarely, if ever, causes pain.
• Stage of POP does not dictate treatment or prognosis.
• Treatment for POP is based on symptoms and patient bother.
• Options for most patients are no treatment, pessary, or surgery.

SUGGESTED READINGS

Available at www.expertconsult.com

RELATED CONTENT

Pelvic Organ Prolapse (Patient Information)
Uterine Prolapse (Patient Information)
Incontinence, Urinary (Related Key Topic)

AUTHORS: **SHIVANI SHAH, M.D.,** and **MATTHEW J. FAGAN, M.D.**

DEFINITION

- *Pemphigus* refers to a group of rare, potentially fatal, chronic, autoimmune blistering diseases of the skin and mucous membranes
- Pemphigus has four main subtypes:
  1. Pemphigus vulgaris (PV) (most common) (Fig. 1)
     1. Pemphigus vegetans, a rare clinical variant of PV
  2. Pemphigus foliaceus (PF)
     1. Pemphigus erythematosus, a variant of PF
  3. Paraneoplastic pemphigus
  4. Immunoglobulin (Ig) A pemphigus

SYNONYMS

Pemphigus
PV
Fogo selvagem: endemic pemphigus foliaceus
Senear-Usher syndrome: pemphigus erythematosus

ICD-10CM CODES
L10.0 Pemphigus vulgaris

EPIDEMIOLOGY & DEMOGRAPHICS

- Pemphigus vulgaris makes up 70% of all pemphigus cases.
- Incidence is approximately one case per 100,000 persons and varies substantially by geographic region.
- More common in Ashkenazi Jews and people of Mediterranean descent.
- Typically occurs in the fourth and fifth decades of life, although range of ages affected is broad and it may occur in the very young or elderly.
- No gender predilection.

PHYSICAL FINDINGS & CLINICAL PRESENTATION

- History:
  1. Multiple oropharyngeal ulcerations and erosions typically occur first (60% of cases), which can then be followed by a more generalized bullous eruption involving the skin within several weeks or months
  2. Blisters are flaccid and rupture easily, leaving painful erosions and ulcerations that may be the predominant clinical finding
  3. Pain associated with oral mucosal blistering often results in dysphagia and hoarseness
  4. Not commonly pruritic
- Physical findings:
  1. Anatomic distribution
     a. Oral mucosa
     b. Can also involve the pharynx, larynx, vagina, penis, anus, and conjunctival mucosa
     c. Generalized cutaneous involvement (Figs. 2 and 3)
  2. Lesion configuration
     a. Mucosal membranes
     b. Any area of the body without any preferential distribution

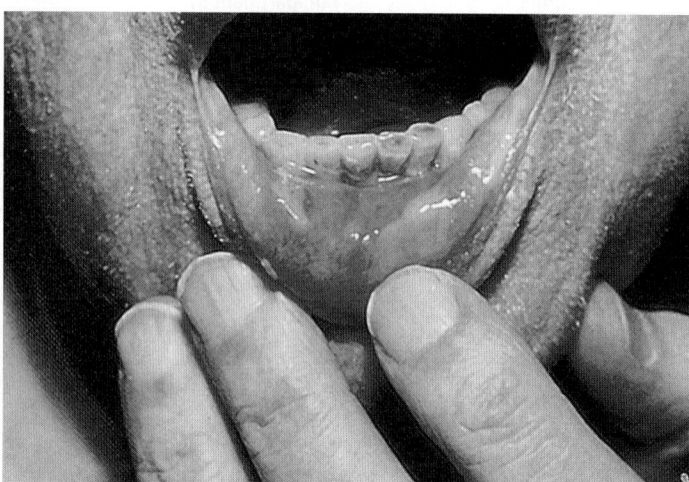

FIG. 1 Pemphigus vulgaris with oral lesions and no intact bullae. (Courtesy Department of Dermatology, University of North Carolina at Chapel Hill. From Goldstein BG, Goldstein AO: *Practical dermatology,* ed 2, St Louis, 1997, Mosby.)

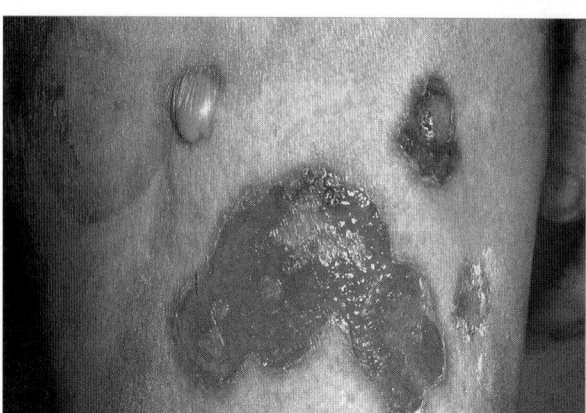

FIG. 2 Pemphigus vulgaris; extensive erosions and blisters are present on the shin. (Courtesy R. A. Marsden, M.D., St. George's Hospital, London. From McKee PH et al [eds]: *Pathology of the skin with clinical correlations,* ed 3, St Louis, 2005, Mosby.)

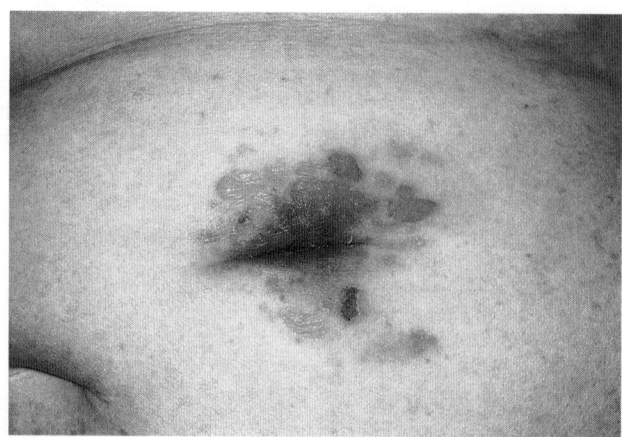

FIG. 3 Pemphigus vulgaris: umbilical lesions showing intact blisters as well as raw erosions. (Courtesy R. A. Marsden, M.D., St. George's Hospital, London. From McKee PH et al [eds]: *Pathology of the skin with clinical correlations,* ed 3, St Louis, 2005, Mosby.)

3. Lesion morphology
   a. Flaccid bullae and vesicles. The **"bulla-spread phenomenon" (Asboe-Hansen sign)** is elicited by pressure on an intact bulla, gently forcing the fluid to spread under the adjacent skin
   b. Erosion with crusting commonly occurs
   c. Large areas of denuded skin with resulting bacterial superinfection
4. Positive **Nikolsky sign:** when the clinician applies lateral pressure to normal-appearing skin at the periphery of active lesions, separation of the superficial epidermis occurs

ETIOLOGY

Autoimmune disease caused by autoantibodies against the cell surface of keratinocytes. The predominant antibody in PV is directed against desmoglein 3; in PF it is directed against desmoglein 1.

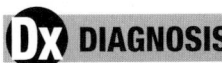 ## DIAGNOSIS

The diagnosis of pemphigus vulgaris should be suspected in patients with painful oral erosions and flaccid bullae or erosions on the skin. The diagnosis is confirmed by histology, immunofluorescence pattern of perilesional skin, indirect immunofluorescence (IIF) testing of serum, or ELISA testing for anti-desmoglein 1 (Dsg1) and anti-Dsg3 autoantibodies.

DIFFERENTIAL DIAGNOSIS

- Bullous pemphigoid (Table 1)
- Cicatricial pemphigoid
- Behçet's syndrome
- Erythema multiforme
- Hailey-Hailey disease
- Aphthous stomatitis
- Bullous lupus erythematosus
- Drug eruptions
- Dermatitis herpetiformis
- Epidermolysis bullosa acquisita
- IgA pemphigus
- Paraneoplastic pemphigus
- Pemphigus foliaceus
- Stevens-Johnson syndrome

WORKUP

Skin biopsy is diagnostic; specimens should be sent for routine histochemical staining and direct immunofluorescence.

LABORATORY TESTS

- Skin biopsy reveals intraepidermal vesicles, also called *acantholysis* (loss of cell adhesion between the epidermal cells).
- Indirect immunofluorescence may detect circulating autoantibodies.
- Direct immunofluorescence studies of perilesional skin demonstrate IgG directed against keratinocyte surfaces in the epidermis.

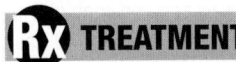 ## TREATMENT

NONPHARMACOLOGIC THERAPY

- Mild soaps and emollients to skin.
- Burow's solution may be useful for weeping erosions.
- Avoid trauma to the skin.
- When there are extensive raw surfaces, daily baths are helpful in removing the thickened crusts and reducing foul odor.
- Soft diet and viscous lidocaine can be used in patients with oral lesions.
- A mixture of equal parts of simethicone (Maalox), elixir of diphenhydramine, and viscous lidocaine is also effective.

ACUTE GENERAL Rx

- For localized disease, topical steroids may be effective.
- For generalized disease, prednisone is the mainstay of therapy and often works rapidly to halt blistering.
  1. Initial dose of prednisone is usually 1 mg/kg/day, then tapered over weeks as blistering decreases.
  2. Steroid-sparing immunosuppressive therapies are often initiated simultaneously with prednisone to minimize the side effects of prolonged corticosteroid therapy.

CHRONIC Rx

- Adjuvant therapy such as immunosuppressants, antiinflammatories, chemotherapeutic agents, and biologics are useful for disease control and to shorten the length of treatment with oral steroids; treatment duration and dosing are determined by clinical response:
  1. Mycophenolate mofetil (MMF) 2 to 3 g daily, or 1 g daily for elderly patients
  2. Azathioprine 50 to 100 mg daily
  3. Dapsone 100 to 200 mg daily

- Refractory disease:
  1. IV Ig
  2. Rituximab (anti-CD20 monoclonal antibody)
  3. Plasmapheresis

DISPOSITION

- Medication is continued until clinical disease is suppressed and pemphigus antibody disappears from serum. A negative DIF test once the antibody is no longer present is predictive of sustained remission.
- Before the use of oral corticosteroids, pemphigus was usually a fatal disease with most patients dying within 5 yr of diagnosis.
- Combined corticosteroids and adjuvant therapy have decreased mortality rates to <10%.
- Death generally occurs from sepsis or complications related to medical therapy.

REFERRAL

Dentist
Dermatology
Ophthalmology
Otolaryngology

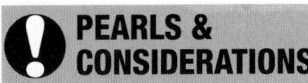 ## PEARLS & CONSIDERATIONS

COMMENTS

- PV, unlike bullous pemphigoid, is a disease of middle-aged persons.
- Prednisone is the mainstay for treatment.

RELATED CONTENT

Pemphigus Vulgaris (Patient Information)

AUTHOR: **KACHIU C. LEE, M.D., M.P.H.**

TABLE 1 Differentiation of Pemphigus Vulgaris and Bullous Pemphigoid

Characteristics	Pemphigus Vulgaris	Bullous Pemphigoid
Age	Usually occurs in middle-aged persons	>60 yr
Site	Oral mucosa, face, chest, groin	Flexural areas, groin, axilla; less often involving mucosal surfaces
Findings	Flaccid bullae and erosions, intraepidermal blisters, IgG autoantibodies against keratinocyte surfaces	Intact bullae, subepidermal blisters, IgG autoantibodies against hemidesmosomal antigens
Treatment	Prednisone 1 mg/kg/day with adjuvant immunosuppressant agents; refractory disease may require intravenous immunoglobulin, plasmapheresis, or rituximab	Prednisone 1 mg/kg/day with adjuvant immunosuppressant therapy; localized disease may be controlled with topical steroids
Prognosis	>90% respond; steroid side effects significant	>90% respond; remissions and recurrences common

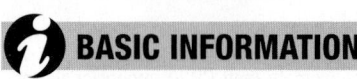

BASIC INFORMATION

DEFINITION

Peptic ulcer disease (PUD) is an ulceration in the stomach or duodenum resulting from an imbalance between mucosal protective factors and various mucosal damaging mechanisms (see "Etiology").

SYNONYMS

PUD
Duodenal ulcer (DU)
Gastric ulcer (GU)

ICD-10CM CODES

K25.3 Acute gastric ulcer without hemorrhage or perforation
K25.7 Chronic gastric ulcer without hemorrhage or perforation
K26.3 Acute duodenal ulcer without hemorrhage or perforation
K26.7 Chronic duodenal ulcer without hemorrhage or perforation
K27.0 Acute peptic ulcer, site unspecified, with hemorrhage
K27.1 Acute peptic ulcer, site unspecified, with perforation
K27.2 Acute peptic ulcer, site unspecified, with both hemorrhage and perforation
K27.3 Acute peptic ulcer, site unspecified, without hemorrhage or perforation
K27.4 Chronic or unspecified peptic ulcer, site unspecified, with hemorrhage
K27.5 Chronic or unspecified peptic ulcer, site unspecified, with perforation
K27.6 Chronic or unspecified peptic ulcer, site unspecified, with both hemorrhage and perforation
K27.7 Chronic peptic ulcer, site unspecified, without hemorrhage or perforation
K27.9 Peptic ulcer, site unspecified, unspecified as acute or chronic, without hemorrhage or perforation
P78.82 Peptic ulcer of newborn
Z87.11 Personal history of peptic ulcer disease

EPIDEMIOLOGY & DEMOGRAPHICS

- Incidence: 250,000 to 500,000 (200,000 to 400,000 duodenal; 50,000 to 100,000 gastric) annually; duodenal ulcer/gastric ulcer ratio is 4:1.
- Anatomic location: <90% of duodenal ulcers occur in the first portion of the duodenum; gastric ulcers occur most frequently in the lesser curvature near the incisura angularis.

PHYSICAL FINDINGS & CLINICAL PRESENTATION

- Physical examination is often unremarkable.
- Patient may have epigastric tenderness, tachycardia, pallor, hypotension (from acute or chronic blood loss), nausea and vomiting (if pyloric channel is obstructed), board-like abdomen and rebound tenderness (if perforated), and hematemesis or melena (with a bleeding ulcer). Box 1 describes key symptoms and signs of peptic ulcer.

ETIOLOGY

Often multifactorial. The following are common mucosal damaging factors:

- *Helicobacter pylori* infection. *H. pylori* is the major cause of PUD. It is found in more than 70% of patients with duodenal ulcers and gastric ulcers in the United States. Rates are much higher (>90%) in other parts of the world. Eradication of *H. pylori* markedly reduces peptic ulcer recurrence.
- Medications (NSAIDs, glucocorticoids). Risk factors for development of NSAID-related ulcers are described in Table 1.
- Incompetent pylorus or lower esophageal sphincter
- Bile acids
- Impaired proximal duodenal bicarbonate secretion
- Decreased blood flow to gastric mucosa
- Acid secreted by parietal cells and pepsin secreted as pepsinogen by chief cells
- Cigarette smoking
- Alcohol

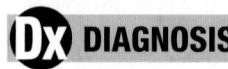 DIAGNOSIS

DIFFERENTIAL DIAGNOSIS

- Gastroesophageal reflux disease
- Cholelithiasis syndrome
- Pancreatitis
- Gastritis
- Nonulcer dyspepsia
- Neoplasm (gastric carcinoma, lymphoma, pancreatic carcinoma)
- Angina pectoris, myocardial infarction, pericarditis
- Dissecting aneurysm
- Other: high small-bowel obstruction, pneumonia, subphrenic abscess, early appendicitis

WORKUP

Comprehensive history and physical exam to exclude other diagnoses. Diagnostic modalities include endoscopy or upper GI series. Endoscopy is preferred and remains the gold standard for diagnosis of PUD. The presence of a mucosal break ≥5 mm in the stomach or duodenum confirms the diagnosis.

LABORATORY TESTS

- Routine laboratory evaluation is usually unremarkable.
- Anemia may be present in patients with significant GI bleeding.
- *H. pylori* testing by endoscopic biopsy, urea breath test, stool antigen test (*H. pylori* stool antigen), or specific antibody test is recommended:

BOX 1 Key Symptoms and Signs of Peptic Ulcer

Uncomplicated Ulcer
No symptoms ("silent ulcer" in up to 40% of cases)
Epigastric pain
Pain may radiate to the back, thorax, other parts of abdomen (cephalad most likely, caudad least likely)
Pain may be nocturnal (most specific), "painful hunger" relieved by food, or continuous (least specific)
Nausea
Vomiting
Heartburn (mimics or associated with gastroesophageal reflux)

Complicated Ulcer
Acute perforation
Severe abdominal pain
Shock
Abdominal boardlike rigidity (and rebound and other signs of peritoneal irritation)
Free intraperitoneal air
Hemorrhage
Hematemesis and/or melena
Hemodynamic changes, anemia
Previous history of ulcer symptoms (80%)
Gastric outlet obstruction
Satiation, inability to ingest food, eructation
Nausea, vomiting (and related disturbances)
Weight loss

TABLE 1 Risk Factors for Development of NSAID-Related Ulcers

Definite

Advanced age
History of ulcer
Concomitant corticosteroid therapy
Concomitant anticoagulation therapy
High doses of NSAIDs
Serious systemic disorders

Possible

Concomitant infection with *Helicobacter pylori*
Cigarette smoking
Consumption of alcohol

NSAIDs, Nonsteroidal antiinflammatory drugs.

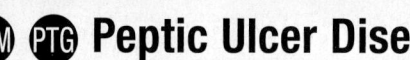

1. Serologic testing for antibodies to *H. pylori* is easy and inexpensive; however, the presence of antibodies demonstrates previous but not necessarily current infection. Antibodies to *H. pylori* can remain elevated for months to years after infection has cleared; therefore antibody levels must be interpreted in light of the patient's symptoms and other test results (e.g., PUD seen on upper GI series).

2. The urea breath test documents active infection (sensitivity and specificity >90%). The patient ingests a small amount of urea labeled with carbon 13 or carbon 14. If urease is present (produced by the organism), the urea is hydrolyzed and the patient exhales labeled carbon dioxide that is then collected and measured. This test is more expensive and not as readily available. Use of proton pump inhibitors (PPI) within 2 wk of the urea breath test may interfere with test results. A new card test for ^{14}C urea is available and provides a testing option in primary care settings. It uses a flat breath card that is read by a small analyzer.

3. Histologic evaluation of endoscopic biopsy samples is considered by many the gold standard for accurate diagnosis of *H. pylori* infection. However, detection of *H. pylori* depends on the site and number of biopsy samples, the method of staining, and experience of the pathologist.

4. Stool antigen test is an ELISA that identifies *H. pylori* antigen in a stool specimen through a polyclonal anti–*H. pylori* antibody. It is as accurate as the urea breath test for diagnosis of active infection and follow-up evaluation of patients treated for *H. pylori*. A negative result on the stool antigen test 6 wk after completion of therapy identifies patients in whom eradication of *H. pylori* was successful.

- Additional laboratory evaluation is indicated only in specific cases (e.g., amylase level in suspected pancreatitis, serum gastrin level in suspected Zollinger-Ellison [ZE] syndrome).

IMAGING STUDIES

Conventional upper GI barium studies identify approximately 70% to 80% of PUD; accuracy can be increased to approximately 90% by using double contrast.

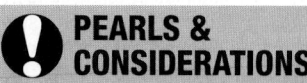 **TREATMENT**

NONPHARMACOLOGIC THERAPY

- Stop smoking; smoking increases the risk of PUD, decreases the healing rate, and increases the frequency of recurrence.
- Avoid NSAIDs and alcohol.
- Special diets have been proved unrelated to ulcer development and healing; however, avoid foods that cause symptoms.

ACUTE GENERAL Rx

Eradication of *H. pylori,* when present, can be accomplished with various regimens (see "*Helicobacter pylori* Infection")

PUD patients testing negative for *H. pylori* should be treated with antisecretory agents:
- H_2 receptor antagonists (H_2RAs): ranitidine, famotidine, and nizatidine are all effective; they are usually given in split dose or at nighttime.
- PPIs: can also induce rapid healing; they are usually given 30 min before meals.

Antacids and sucralfate are also effective agents for the treatment and prevention of PUD.

CHRONIC Rx

Maintenance therapy in peptic ulcer patients is indicated in the following situations:
- Persistent smokers
- Recurrent ulcerations
- Long-term treatment with NSAIDs, glucocorticoids
- Elderly or debilitated patients
- Aggressive or complicated ulcer disease (e.g., perforation, hemorrhage)
- Asymptomatic bleeders

Misoprostol therapy (100 μg qid with food, increased to 200 μg qid if well tolerated) can also be used for the prevention of NSAID-induced gastric ulcers in all patients on long-term NSAID therapy; it is contraindicated in women of childbearing age because of its abortifacient properties. PPIs are at least as effective as misoprostol and more effective than H_2 receptor antagonists at healing ulcers and maintaining remission in patients on long-term NSAIDs.

DISPOSITION

- The recurrence rate for untreated PUD is ~60% (>70% in smokers). Treatment decreases the recurrence rate by nearly 30%.
- Patients with recurrent ulcers should be re-treated for an additional 8 wk and then placed on maintenance therapy with H_2RAs, PPIs, sucralfate, or antacids.
- An ulcer is considered refractory to treatment if healing is not evident after 8 wk for duodenal ulcers and 12 wk for gastric ulcers. In these patients maximum acid inhibition (e.g., esomeprazole 40 mg bid) is preferred over continued therapy with standard antiulcer therapy.
- Eradication of *H. pylori* (when present) is indicated in all patients. A negative stool antigen test for *H. pylori* 6 wk after treatment accurately confirms cure of *H. pylori* infection with reasonable sensitivity in initially seropositive healthy subjects.
- Screening for ZE syndrome should also be considered in patients with multiple recurrent ulcers; in patients with ZE, the serum gastrin level is >1000 pg/ml and the basal acid output is usually >15 mEq/hr.
- Surgery for refractory ulcers is now only rarely performed; it consists of highly selective vagotomy for duodenal ulcers or ulcer removal with antrectomy or hemigastrectomy without vagotomy for gastric ulcers.

REFERRAL

- GI referral for patients requiring endoscopy
- Surgical referral for patients with nonhealing ulcers despite appropriate medical therapy

⓵ **PEARLS & CONSIDERATIONS**

COMMENTS

- Patients with gastric ulcers should generally have repeat endoscopy after 8 to 12 wk of antisecretory therapy to document healing and test exfoliative cytology for gastric carcinoma. Patients with duodenal ulcers and those with low risk gastric ulcers such as young patients on NSAIDs generally do not require endoscopic surveillance.
- After endoscopic treatment of bleeding peptic ulcers, bleeding recurs in up to 20% of patients. PPI administration intravenously by continuous infusion substantially reduces the risk of recurrent bleeding. High-dose IV esomeprazole (80 mg IV bolus followed by 8 mg/hr infusion over 72 hr) given after successful endoscopic therapy to patients with high-risk peptic ulcer bleeding has been reported to reduce recurrent bleeding at 72 hr and to maintain sustained clinical benefits for up to 30 days.
- Among low-dose aspirin recipients who had peptic ulcer bleeding, continuous aspirin therapy may increase the risk for recurrent bleeding; however, mortality was reported higher among those who stopped aspirin therapy and were at risk for cardiovascular events.
- Patients with bleeding ulcers due to low-dose aspirin taken for secondary cardiovascular prevention should resume the use of aspirin within 1 to 7 days after the bleeding stops. Patients with bleeding ulcers due to *H. pylori* infection should receive treatment for this infection and, after eradication is confirmed, discontinue antisecretory medications. Patients with bleeding ulcers due to NSAIDs other than low-dose aspirin should discontinue NSAIDs; if NSAIDs must be resumed, a COX-2 selective NSAID plus a PPI should be used.[1]

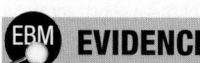 **EVIDENCE**

Available at www.expertconsult.com

SUGGESTED READING

Available at www.expertconsult.com

RELATED CONTENT

Peptic Ulcer (Patient Information)
Helicobacter pylori Infection (Related Key Topic)

AUTHOR: **FRED F. FERRI, M.D.**

[1]Laine L: Clinical practice. Upper gastrointestinal bleeding due to a peptic ulcer, *N Engl J Med* 374:2367-2376, 2016

Diseases and Disorders

P

I

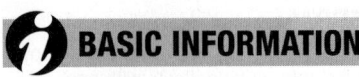

DEFINITION

Pericarditis is the inflammation (or infiltration) of the pericardium. Acute pericarditis is a syndrome characterized by chest pain, and it may have pathognomonic pericardial friction rub on auscultation and specific electrocardiogram (ECG) changes. Chronic pericarditis can lead to infiltration of the pericardium and cause restrictive filling of the ventricles and heart failure.

ICD-10CM CODES
I30.0 Acute nonspecific idiopathic pericarditis
I30.1 Infectious pericarditis
I30.8 Other forms of acute pericarditis
I30.9 Acute pericarditis, unspecified
I301.0 Chronic adhesive pericarditis
I31.1 Chronic constrictive pericarditis
I31.3 Pericardial effusion (non-inflammatory)
I31.9 Diseases of pericardium, unspecified (tamponade)
I31.2 Hemopericardium

EPIDEMIOLOGY & DEMOGRAPHICS

- Most common form of pericardial disease worldwide.
- Pericarditis is responsible for 5% of patients admitted from the emergency room for chest pain and for approximately 0.1% of hospitalized patients.
- Increased incidence found in males and in adults compared with children.

PHYSICAL FINDINGS & CLINICAL PRESENTATION

- Chest pain: characteristically sharp, pleuritic, positional (due to rubbing of inflamed pericardial layers). It is improved by sitting up and leaning forward.
- A pericardial friction rub is pathognomonic for acute pericarditis. It is best heard with the patient sitting up and leaning forward and by pressing the diaphragm of the stethoscope at the lower left sternal border during inspiration. It consists of three short, scratchy sounds, corresponding to a systolic, diastolic, and late diastolic component. In many patients, the rub is not clearly triphasic.
- Classic tamponade physical findings include hypotension, jugular venous distention, and muffled heart sounds (Beck's triad). In addition, tachycardia and pulsus paradoxus are usually present.

ETIOLOGY

- Etiology is dichotomized into infectious and noninfectious causes. The epidemiological background of the patient is important.
- While *M. tuberculosis* is the most common cause in the developing world, 80% to 90% of cases of pericarditis in the developed world are either idiopathic or viral.
- Other infectious agents (bacterial [1%-%2], HIV, fungal, parasitic [amebic, toxoplasmosis]).

- Systemic autoimmune (systemic lupus erythematosus, rheumatoid arthritis, scleroderma, vasculitis, dermatomyositis): 3% to 4%.
- Neoplasm (primary or metastatic [breast, lung, leukemia, lymphoma]): 7% to 13%.
- Drug-induced: procainamide, hydralazine, phenytoin, isoniazid, rifampin, doxorubicin, mesalamine, adalimumab.
- Metabolic: uremia, myxedema.
- Posttraumatic: postpericardiotomy, post pacemaker lead placement, post catheter ablation, post CPR, coronary percutaneous intervention.
- Perimyocardial infarction (Dressler's syndrome, usually 2 weeks post MI).

DIAGNOSIS

DIFFERENTIAL DIAGNOSIS

- Angina pectoris and acute coronary syndrome.
- Myopericarditis/perimyocarditis.
- Dissecting aortic aneurysm.
- Pulmonary causes: embolism, infarction, pneumothorax, pneumonia with pleurisy.
- Gastrointestinal causes: hepatitis, cholecystitis, GERD, esophageal spasm or rupture.
- Musculoskeletal strain.

WORKUP

Diagnosis of pericarditis requires at least two of the four following clinical criteria:
- Typical pleuritic chest pain
- Pericardial friction rub
- Suggestive ECG changes (ST segment elevation, PR depression)
- New or worsening pericardial effusion

LABORATORY TESTS

Laboratory tests may help elucidate the underlying cause and are adjunctive to the clinical criteria previously.
- Inflammatory markers: Erythrocyte sedimentation rate, C-reactive protein (CRP), and complete blood count with differential are elevated in pericarditis.
- Basic metabolic profile.
- Cardiac biomarkers (troponin I and T) when elevated indicate involvement of the myocardium, i.e., myopericarditis).
The following tests may be useful when specific etiologies of pericarditis are suspected:
- HIV.
- PPD.
- Antinuclear antibody, rheumatoid factor.
- Routine viral studies are not indicated since they are low yield.

PERICARDIAL SAMPLING

Indications for echocardiogram- or fluoroscopy-guided pericardiocentesis are:
- Tamponade physiology.
- Moderate to large pericardial effusion with symptoms, or refractory to medical therapy.
- Suspicion of a neoplastic, bacterial, or tuberculous process.
- Evidence of constrictive or effusive-constrictive pericarditis.

- Pericardiocentesis is for diagnostic and therapeutic purposes. The pericardial fluid should be analyzed for RBC, WBC, gram stain, culture, cytology, glucose, pH, LDH, and protein. In select cases, consider checking triglyceride or PCR for tuberculosis.
- Pericardial biopsy may be helpful in recurrent pericardial effusion with an elusive diagnosis and when malignancy or tuberculosis is suspected.

IMAGING STUDIES

- ECG: Changes in the ECG reflect inflammation of the epicardium, since the parietal pericardium is electrically inert. The ECG changes are staged as follows:
  1. Stage I (Acute phase): hours to few days. PR-segment depression (PR elevation in aVR) and diffuse concave ST-segment elevations, which can be distinguished from acute MI by the lack of reciprocal changes and the absence of Q waves.
  2. Stage II (Intermediate phase): seen in first week with return of PR and ST segments to baseline.
  3. Stage III (Intermediate): T-wave inversion in leads previously showing ST-segment elevation (Fig. 1).
  4. Stage IV (Late phase): normalization of the ECG or indefinite persistence of T-wave inversions.
- ECG is required to evaluate for pericardial effusion (present in 50% to 60% of patients) (Fig. 2). It is also important for the diagnosis of tamponade and constrictive pericarditis.Chest x-ray: done primarily to rule out abnormalities of the mediastinum or lung fields that may cause chest pain. Cardiac silhouette may appear enlarged in patients with pericardial effusion if ≥200 mL of fluid has accumulated (Fig. 3). Calcifications around the heart may be seen with chronic constrictive pericarditis.
- Computerized tomography: evaluation of associated pleuropulmonary and extrathoracic diseases and pericardial calcifications.
- MRI (Fig. 4) may be useful in patients with chronic constrictive pericarditis and when malignancy is suspected.

TREATMENT

NONPHARMACOLOGIC THERAPY

- Physical activity restriction until pain abates and normalization of CRP, ECG, and echo.
- Athletes should avoid competitive activity for 3 months (experts' consensus).
- Patient education regarding potential complications: e.g., cardiac tamponade, recurrent pericarditis (which can occur in up to one third of patients), and chronic constrictive pericarditis.

ACUTE GENERAL Rx

- High-dose aspirin (650 to 1000 mg tid) or NSAIDs (e.g., ibuprofen 600-800 mg tid, indomethacin 50 mg tid) for a month are the first line of treatment. NSAIDs should be avoided in patients with recent MI, CHF, acute renal failure, and upper GI bleed.

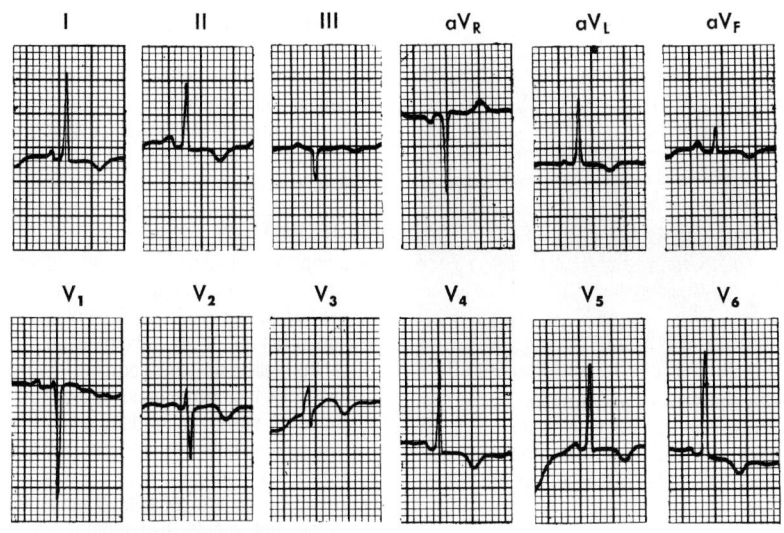

FIG. 1 **Pericarditis, evolving pattern.** Note the diffuse T-wave inversions in leads I, II, III, aVL, aVF, and V2 to V6. (From Goldberg AL [ed]: *Clinical electrocardiography*, ed 5, St Louis, 1994, Mosby.)

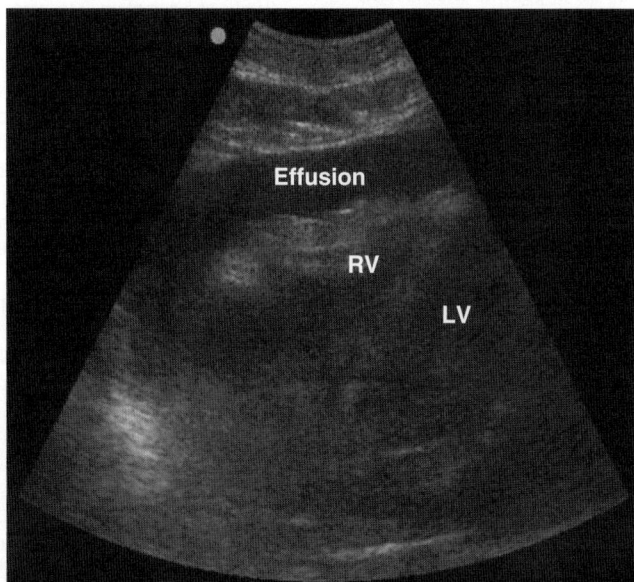

FIG. 2 **Bedside ultrasound showing large pericardial effusion.** *LV,* Left ventricle; *RV,* right ventricle. (From Adams JG et al: *Emergency medicine, clinical essentials,* ed 2, Philadelphia, 2013, Elsevier.)

- Colchicine 0.5 to 0.6 mg bid for 3 months should be used as adjunctive therapy. Current evidence (COPE, CORE, CORP, ICAP, CORP-2 trials) supports the effectiveness of colchicine in symptomatic relief and prevention of recurrent pericarditis.
- Corticosteroids should be used only as second-line treatment. They are associated with severe adverse effects, more hospitalizations, and higher rates of recurrences.
- Low- to moderate-dose (0.25-0.5 mg/kg/day) systemic steroid therapy for a month, followed by taper, is restricted to patients with rheumatologic disease, failure, or contraindication to NSAID/colchicine.
- Immunosuppressors such as azathioprine, intravenous immunoglobulins, and a biological agent such as Anakinra are treatment options for patients with refractory recurrent pericarditis.

- Pericardiectomy and pericardiotomy at specialized centers are reserved for recurrent cardiac tamponade or refractory pericarditis.
- Avoidance of anticoagulants (increased risk of hemopericardium).

TREATMENT OF UNDERLYING CAUSE:
- Bacterial pericarditis: systemic antibiotics and drainage of pericardium
- Collagen vascular disease: prednisone
- Uremic: dialysis

POTENTIAL COMPLICATIONS FROM PERICARDITIS:
1. **Chronic constrictive pericarditis**:
   a. Physical examination: Signs of right heart failure—hepatomegaly, splenomegaly, ascites, pedal edema, scrotal edema, possible anasarca, jugular venous distention, Kussmaul's sign (paradoxical increase in jugular venous distention during inspiration), pericardial knock (early diastolic filling sound heard 0.06 to 0.1 sec after S2), and clear lungs.

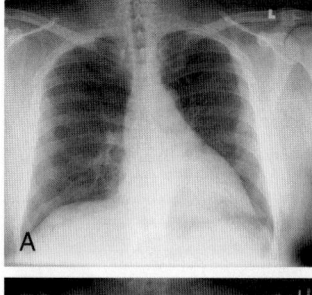

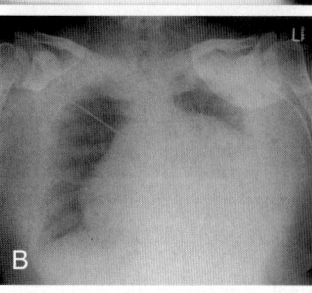

FIG. 3 **Chest x-ray. A,** Patient's chest radiograph 1 year before presentation with cardiac tamponade. **B,** Same patient's chest radiograph on presentation to the emergency department with cardiac tamponade. (From Adams JG et al: *Emergency medicine, clinical essentials,* ed 2, Philadelphia, 2013, Elsevier.)

   b. ECG: Low QRS voltage, nonspecific ST-segment changes, biatrial enlargement.
   c. Chest radiograph: Mild alveolar edema, pleural effusions, biatrial enlargement, pericardial calcification (seen in tuberculous pericarditis).
   d. Echocardiography: May show thickened pericardium (>4 mm). Respiratory variation over the mitral, tricuspid, pulmonary vein, and hepatic vein flow is suggestive of constrictive pericarditis. Respiration-related shifting of ventricular septum attributed to the variable venous return and the ventricular interdependence is seen. Medial mitral annular e' velocity is increased relative to the lateral e'.[1]
   e. Hemodynamics: Elevation of right-sided filling pressures, equalization of diastolic pressures as well as prominent "x" and rapid "y" descent in the atrial tracing are seen in constrictive pericarditis. Right ventricular pressure tracing typically shows a "dip and plateau" (square root sign) that is due to the unimpeded early filling of the RV with an abrupt halt to the late diastolic filling by the stiff pericardium. Discordance of right ventricular and left ventricular systolic pressures during respiration is also suggestive of constrictive pericarditis.
   f. Therapy: Complex surgical stripping or removal of both layers of the constricting pericardium improves the functional class in the majority of late survivors, but has high operative mortality.[2]

[1] Welch TD, Ling LH, Espinosa RE, et al: Echocardiographic diagnosis of constrictive pericarditis. *Circ Cardiovasc Imaging* 7(3):526-534, 2014.
[2] Vustarini N, Chen C, Mazine A, et al: Pericardiectomy for constrictive pericarditis: 20 years of experience at the Montreal Heart Institute, *Ann Thorac Surg* 100(1):107-113, 2015.

P

Diseases and Disorders

I

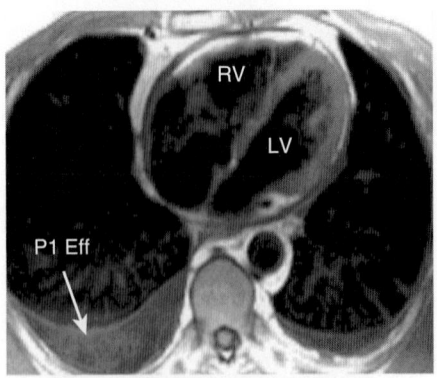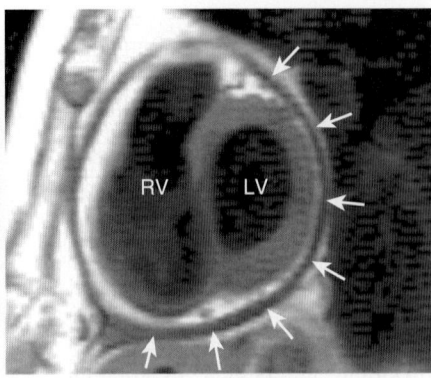

FIG. 4 Cardiovascular magnetic resonance in a patient with constrictive pericarditis. On the *right* is a basal short-axis view of the ventricles showing a thickened pericardium encasing the heart *(arrows)*. On the *left* is a transaxial view, again showing the thickened pericardium, particularly over the right heart, but also a pleural effusion *(P1 Eff)*. *LV,* Left ventricle; *RV,* right ventricle. (From Zipes DP et al [eds]: *Braunwald's heart disease,* ed 7, Philadelphia, 2005, Saunders.)

2. **Cardiac tamponade:** Occurs in 5% to 15% of patients with idiopathic pericarditis, but in up to 60% of those with neoplastic, tuberculous, or purulent pericarditis.
   a. Signs and symptoms: Dyspnea, orthopnea, chest pain, fatigue.
   b. Physical examination: Beck's triad (distended neck veins, distant heart sounds, hypotension), decreased apical impulse, diaphoresis, tachypnea, tachycardia, narrowed pulse pressure, or pulsus paradoxus (decrease in systolic blood pressure ≥10 mm Hg during inspiration; most specific sign).
   c. ECG: Decreased amplitude of the QRS complex, electrical alternans (occurs more frequently with large neoplastic effusions).
   d. Chest x-ray: Cardiomegaly ("water-bottle" configuration of the cardiac silhouette may be seen) with clear lungs; may be normal when acute tamponade occurs rapidly in the absence of prior pericardial effusion.
   e. Echocardiography: May show diastolic collapse of the right ventricle and/or the right atrium, respiratory inflow variation over the mitral valve and tricuspid valve (due to transmission of respiratory changes in intrathoracic pressure to the ventricles), or paradoxical wall motion of interventricular septum may also be seen.
   f. Hemodynamics: Equalization of diastolic pressures within chambers of the heart, elevation of right atrial pressure with a prominent "x" but no significant "y" descent.

   g. Therapy: Immediate pericardiocentesis with the use of echocardiography, fluoroscopy, or CT. In patients with recurrent effusions (e.g., neoplasms), placement of a percutaneous drainage catheter or pericardial window may be necessary. Volume repletion might be necessary, and the avoidance of high PEEP is important.

3. **Effusive-constrictive pericarditis:** Uncommon syndrome characterized by concomitant tamponade caused by tense pericardial effusion and constriction caused by the visceral pericardium.
   a. Signs and symptoms: Similar to features of tamponade and/or constriction. Pulsus paradoxus is often present. This is not seen in constrictive pericarditis because inspiration (fall in thoracic pressure) cannot be transmitted to the right atrium. Kussmaul's sign and the pericardial knock are typically absent.
   b. Echocardiography: Typically not sensitive enough to distinguish effusive-constrictive pericarditis from other types.
   c. Cardiac catheterization: Mixed picture with features of constriction and tamponade. Before drainage, "y" descent is usually less prominent than expected and right atrial "v" wave persists. After drainage, may continue to have elevated right atrial and pulmonary wedge pressures.
   d. Therapy: Extensive epicardiectomy (with disruption of the visceral layer of pericardium) is the procedure of choice in symptomatic patients.

4. **Myopericarditis:** Myocarditis and pericarditis may coexist in 20% to 30% of patients presenting with pericarditis. The laboratory hallmark is the elevation of cardiac enzymes. Overall, myopericarditis has a good prognosis with very low rates of morbidity, mortality, and heart failure.

DISPOSITION

- Complete resolution of pain and other signs and symptoms during the initial 3 wk of therapy occurs in 70% to 90% of cases.
- Admission is highly recommended if any of the following poor prognostic features (high risk factors) is present: fever >38° C, subacute onset, large pericardial effusion/tamponade, failure to respond to 1 wk of outpatient treatment.
- The following are considered moderate risk factors but should also prompt admission: myopericarditis, trauma, immunosuppression, oral anticoagulant therapy.
- Recurrent pericarditis occurs after 4 to 6 weeks of a symptom-free interval after a first episode of pericarditis. Incidence is reported as 10% to 15% and increases to 50% in patients who are not on colchicine.
- Incessant pericarditis is defined as pericarditis lasting for >4-6 weeks but <3 months without remission, while chronic pericarditis is pericarditis lasting for >3 months.
- In patients with pericardial effusion after cardiac surgery, use of NSAIDs is not recommended because they have not been shown to reduce the size of the effusions or prevent late cardiac tamponade. The COPPS trial suggested that prophylactic colchicine may reduce the risk of developing a postpericardiotomy pericarditis.

 EVIDENCE

Available at www.expertconsult.com

SUGGESTED READINGS

Available at www.expertconsult.com

RELATED CONTENT

Pericarditis (Patient Information)
Cardiac Tamponade (Related Key Topic)

AUTHOR: **MAXWELL EYRAM AFARI, M.D.**

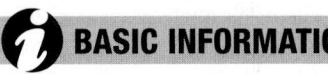
BASIC INFORMATION

DEFINITION

Peripheral arterial disease (PAD) refers to atherosclerotic, inflammatory, occlusive, and aneurysmal diseases involving the abdominal aorta and its branch arteries. (This topic focuses on lower-extremity PAD.)

SYNONYMS

PAD
Peripheral vascular disease (PVD)
Arteriosclerosis obliterans
Atherosclerotic occlusive disease
Atherosclerosis of the extremities
Peripheral arterial stenosis
Vasoocclusive disease of the legs
Chronic critical limb ischemia

ICD-10CM CODES
I70	Atherosclerosis
I70.2	Atherosclerosis of native arteries of the extremities
I70.21	Atherosclerosis of native arteries of extremities with intermittent claudication
I70.22	Atherosclerosis of native arteries of extremities with rest pain
I70.3	Atherosclerosis of unspecified type of bypass graft(s) of the extremities
I73	Other specified peripheral vascular diseases
I73.8	Other specified peripheral vascular diseases
I73.9	Peripheral vascular disease, unspecified
I79	Disorders of arteries, arterioles, and capillaries in diseases classified elsewhere

EPIDEMIOLOGY & DEMOGRAPHICS

- There are >202 million patients afflicted with PAD globally; and 8-12 million patients are affected in the U.S.
- Approximately 4.3% to 5.28% of the adult population over the age of 40 has PAD, and the prevalence is nearly equal in men and women. It increases with age, from 5.28% in those aged 40 to 49 yr to 18.83% in those aged 70 to 79 yr. However, symptoms of claudication are more likely to be present in males with PAD (50%) vs. women with PAD (25%).
- As per the PARTNERS study, the prevalence of PAD in patients >70 yr or 50 to 69 yr with history of smoking or diabetes was 29%.
- Risk factors that increase risk of PAD according to a 2013 meta-analysis of 112,027 studied patients include:
  - Smoking (odds ratio 2.72)
  - Diabetes (odds ratio 1.88)
  - Hypertension (odds ratio 1.55)
  - Hypercholesterolemia (odds ratio 1.19)
- Smoking is three times more likely to lead to PAD than CAD. Conversely, the association of HTN and hyperlipidemia with PAD is lower

than that with CAD and cerebrovascular disease.
- Black race/ethnicity has greater prevalence according to NHANES data (odds ratio 2.83)
- Patients with newly diagnosed PAD are six times more likely to die within the next 10 yr when compared with patients without PAD.
- The total annual costs associated with the hospitalization of patients with PAD in the U.S. exceed $21 billion; and account for ~13% of all Medicare Part A and B expenditures.

PHYSICAL FINDINGS & CLINICAL PRESENTATION

- Peripheral arterial disease may present in a variety of ways:
  - 20% to 50%: Asymptomatic.
  - 10% to 35%: Intermittent claudication (IC), defined as aching pain, cramping, weakness, numbness, or heaviness of the leg induced by exercise, relieved by rest.
  - 1% to 2%: Critical limb ischemia (CLI), defined as rest pain, aching or burning, or tissue loss with nonhealing ulceration, necrosis, or gangrene (Fig. 1).
  - 40% to 50%: Atypical symptoms of involving the calf, thigh, or buttock.
- Physical findings include:
  - Diminished pulses and/or cool skin temperature of lower extremities.
  - Bruits heard over the distal aorta, iliac, or femoral arteries.
  - Change in skin color (dependent rubor in critical limb ischemia; livedo reticularis in ischemia of embolic etiology).
  - Trophic changes of hair loss, brittle nails, and muscle atrophy.

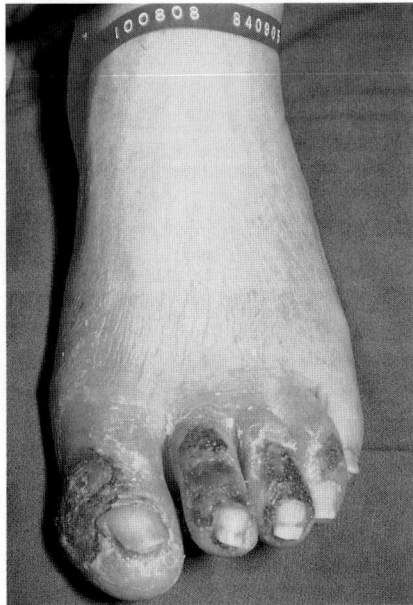

FIG. 1 Ischemic skin ulcer induced by trauma from shoes. This patient with peripheral arterial occlusive disease suffered severe superficial skin necrosis of several toes because of shoes that were too tight. (From Crawford MH et al [eds]: *Cardiology*, ed 2, St Louis, 2004, Mosby.)

ETIOLOGY

PAD is primarily the result of atherosclerotic narrowing of the arterial lumen that results in impaired blood flow to the lower-extremity tissues. Symptoms initially manifest with exercise as metabolic demands increase. Critical limb ischemia (CLI), defined by rest pain or ischemic gangrene, may develop gradually from progressive atherosclerosis or in a subacute fashion from multisegmental atherothrombosis or atheroembolization. In contrast, acute limb ischemia (ALI) is marked by a sudden onset of symptoms in a previously asymptomatic patient with an underlying embolic predisposition.

DIAGNOSIS

DIFFERENTIAL DIAGNOSIS

- Spinal stenosis
- Musculoskeletal disorder
- Lumbar spinal stenosis or nerve root compression (neurogenic or pseudoclaudication)
- Peripheral neuropathy
- Reflex sympathetic dystrophy
- Raynaud's disease
- Compartment syndrome
- Deep venous thrombosis
- Popliteal entrapment syndrome
- Direct vascular injury

WORKUP

- Thorough history, including symptoms regarding walking impairment, claudication, ischemic rest pain, or nonhealing wounds in patients ≥70 yr or those ≥50 yr with a history of smoking and/or diabetes:
- Careful physical examinations include:
  - Measurement of blood pressure in both arms and notation of asymmetry.
  - Palpation and recording of carotid pulses, upstroke, amplitude, and presence of bruits.
  - Auscultation and palpation of abdomen for bruits, aortic pulsation, and diameter.
  - Palpation of brachial, radial, ulnar, femoral, popliteal, dorsalis pedis, and posterior tibial pulses. Pulse intensity should be recorded as follows: 0, absent; 1+, diminished; 2+, normal; 3+, bounding.
  - Auscultation of femoral arteries for the presence of bruits.
  - Extremities should be inspected for color, temperature, integrity of the skin, hair loss, and hypertrophic nails.
- Classification/staging system for PAD:
  - Fontaine's staging system (Table 1):
    I: Asymptomatic
    IIa: Mild claudication
    IIb: Moderate-severe claudication
    III: Ischemic rest pain
    IV: Ulceration or gangrene
  - Rutherford's categories:
    1. Grade 0, Category 0: Asymptomatic
    2. Grade I, Category 1: Mild claudication
    3. Grade I, Category 2: Moderate claudication
    4. Grade I, Category 3: Severe claudication

5. Grade II, Category 4: Ischemic rest pain
6. Grade III, Category 5: Minor tissue loss
7. Grade IV, Category 6: Major tissue loss

- Resting ankle-brachial index (ABI) is the first-line noninvasive test to establish a diagnosis of PAD in individuals with symptoms or signs suggestive of disease (individuals with one or more of the following exertional leg symptoms: nonhealing wounds, age >65 yr, or age >50 yr with smoking or diabetes history). ABI should be measured in both legs in all new patients (Fig. 2).
- Exercise ABI is recommended if resting ABI is borderline or normal (>0.9) and symptoms of claudication are suggestive.
- The severity of PAD is based on the ABI at rest and during treadmill exercise (1 to 2 mph, 5 min, or symptom limited).
  - Noncompressible: >1.40
  - Normal: 1.00 to 1.40 at rest

TABLE 1 Fontaine Classification of Peripheral Artery Disease

Stage	Symptoms
I	Asymptomatic
II	Intermittent claudication
IIa	Pain free, claudication walking >200 m
IIb	Pain free, claudication walking <200 m
III	Rest and nocturnal pain
IV	Necrosis, gangrene

From Bonow RO et al: *Braunwald's heart disease: a textbook of cardiovascular medicine,* ed 9, Philadelphia, 2012, Saunders.

- Borderline: 0.91 to 0.99 at rest
- Mild: ABI at rest 0.71 to 0.90 or ABI during exercise 0.50 to 0.90
- Moderate: ABI at rest 0.41 to 0.70 or ABI during exercise 0.20 to 0.50
- Severe: ABI at rest <0.40 or ABI during exercise <0.20
- Toe-brachial index should be used in patients suspected of PAD with unreliable ABI due to stiff noncompressible vessels. A TBI of <0.70 is the most frequently recommended threshold for an abnormal result; however, this has not been as rigorously studied or validated against angiographic and clinical outcomes as the ABI cutoff of ≤0.90.
- Routine screening for lower-extremity PAD in the absence of risk factors, history, signs, or symptoms is not recommended.

LABORATORY TESTS

- Laboratory tests can help identify risk factors and allow for their modification. These include lipid profile, hemoglobin A_{1C}, homocysteine levels, fibrinogen, D-dimer, and CRP.

PHYSIOLOGIC TESTING AND IMAGING STUDIES

- The diagnosis of PAD can be confirmed by measuring the ABI or Toe-Brachial Index.
- Rest or exercise pulse volume recordings (PVRs) and segmental limb pressures are also useful. PVRs measure volume of limb flow per pulse in different segments of the limb (e.g., thigh, calf, ankle, metatarsal, and toes). They help to assess the location and severity of the lesion with alterations in the pulse volume contour and amplitude indicating proximal arterial obstruction.

- Duplex ultrasound (DUS) incorporates anatomic and physiologic evaluation by combining 2D ultrasound to visualize arterial segments and pulse wave Doppler to sample blood flow velocities at specific locations in the arterial lumen.
- Conventional contrast angiography remains the gold standard modality, but duplex ultrasonography, computed tomography angiography (CTA), and magnetic resonance angiography (MRA) have largely replaced catheter-based angiography in anatomic assessment for revascularization. Contrast angiography (Fig. E3) is now reserved for patients with PAD who are being considered for endovascular revascularization. It allows assessment of translesional pressure gradients prior to percutaneous intervention.
- Carotid intima-media thickness and brachial artery flow-mediated dilation have shown promise but have not been widely applied.

(RX) TREATMENT

The treatment goal in patients with PAD is to focus on cardiovascular risk-factor reduction to decrease morbidity and mortality as well as to improve limb-related symptoms. There are also medical and surgical approaches to management of limb-related symptoms.

MEDICAL THERAPY

LOWERING CARDIOVASCULAR RISK FACTORS, MORBIDITY, AND MORTALITY:

- Smoking cessation should be emphasized in patients with PAD at each visit with assistance of behavioral and pharmacologic treatment (Class I).
- Proper foot care, including use of appropriate footwear, chiropody/podiatric medicine, daily foot inspection, skin cleansing, and use of topical moisturizing creams, should be encouraged, and skin lesions and ulcerations should be addressed urgently in all patients with diabetes and lower-extremity PAD (Class I).
- Antiplatelet therapy is indicated to reduce risk of myocardial infarction, stroke, and vascular death in individuals with symptomatic PAD with either aspirin (75 to 325 mg) or clopidogrel (75 mg) (Class I) and in asymptomatic patients (Class IIa). No clear benefit has been observed with combination aspirin and clopidogrel therapy.
- Warfarin is not indicated except in select postsurgical bypass conditions.
- Lipid-lowering therapy in patients with lower limb PAD has been shown to help slow disease progression, alleviate symptoms, and improve walking distance. The 2013 ACC/AHA Guideline on the Treatment of Blood Cholesterol recommends that patients with atherosclerotic PAD receive moderate- to high-dose statin therapy in order to lower risk of cardiovascular events regardless of baseline cholesterol values. Prior guidelines

---

How to Perform and Calculate the ABI

Partners Program ABI Interpretation
Above 0.90— Normal
0.71–0.90— Mild Obstruction
0.41–0.70— Moderate Obstruction
0.00–0.40— Severe Obstruction

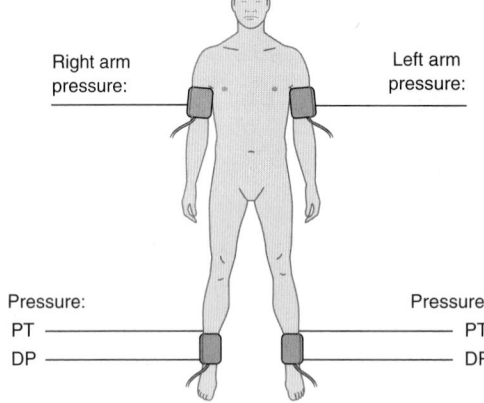

Right arm pressure: Left arm pressure:

Pressure: Pressure:
PT   PT
DP   DP

RIGHT ABI   **LEFT ABI**

$$\frac{\text{Higher right ankle pressure}}{\text{Higher arm pressure}} = \frac{\text{mm Hg}}{\text{mm Hg}} \quad = \quad \frac{\text{Higher left ankle pressure}}{\text{Higher arm pressure}} = \frac{\text{mm Hg}}{\text{mm Hg}} =$$

EXAMPLE

$$\frac{\text{Higher ankle pressure}}{\text{Higher arm pressure}} = \frac{92 \text{ mm Hg}}{164 \text{ mm Hg}} = 0.56 \quad \text{See ABI Chart}$$

FIG. 2 Performing pressure measurements and calculating the ankle-brachial index (ABI). To calculate the ABI, systolic pressures are determined in both arms and both ankles with the use of a handheld Doppler instrument. The highest readings for the dorsalis pedis (DP) and posterior tibial (PT) arteries are used to calculate the index. (From Goldman L, Schafer AI: *Goldman's Cecil medicine,* ed 24, Philadelphia, 2012, Saunders.)

have recommended goal LDL cholesterol of <100 mg/dL and possibly <70 mg/dL in high-risk patients.

- Management of hypertension with a goal of <140/90 mm Hg or <130/80 mm Hg if the patient has diabetes or chronic renal disease. Ramipril use has been reported to improve walking ability and quality of life in PAD patients with intermittent claudication.
- Aggressive control of blood sugar in diabetic patients with PAD is recommended, although studies have failed to demonstrate a beneficial effect on intensive insulin therapy in lowering risk of PAD.

TREATMENT OF CLAUDICATION:

- Exercise therapy: Supervised exercise-training may be as beneficial as stent revascularization in symptomatic improvement. Patients should be prescribed exercise for a minimum of 30 to 45 min, in sessions performed at least three times per week for a minimum of 12 wk.
  - Pharmacologic therapy:
    1 Cilostazol (100 mg bid) is indicated as effective therapy for enabling pain-free and maximal walking distance (Class 1). It is a phosphodiesterase (PDE-3) inhibitor that reduces platelet aggregation and causes vasodilatation. It may have an added benefit of reducing restenosis and repeat revascularization following endovascular therapy. Cilostazol is contraindicated in patients with systolic heart failure.
    2 Pentoxifylline is approved as second-line alternative therapy for symptomatic relief of PAD symptoms. Its clinical effectiveness is marginal and not well established.
    3 Naftidrofuryl, a serotonin 5HT2 receptor antagonist, has favorable vasoactive and rheological properties with few adverse effects. It is approved for use in Europe for the treatment of claudication.
    4 Ticagrelor, an inhibitor of platelet P2Y12 receptor has not been shown to be superior to clopidogrel for the reduction of cardiovascular events in symptomatic PAD.

REVASCULARIZATION

There is no difference in clinical outcomes in percutaneous vs. surgical revascularization in iliac and femoropopliteal disease except for the higher morbidity with surgery and greater re-interventions in the percutaneous approach.
- The 2011 ACC/AHA guidelines on PAD have suggested that the following factors be considered prior to revascularization with either percutaneous/endovascular or surgical methods:
  1 Considerations in percutaneous/endovascular treatment:
    1 In patients with a vocational- or lifestyle-limiting disability due to intermittent claudication despite optimal medical therapy when clinical features suggest a reason-

able likelihood of symptomatic improvement with endovascular intervention.
    2 Although the 2011 ACC/AHA guidelines recommend endovascular intervention as the preferred therapy for TASC (TransAtlantic Inter-Society Consensus) type A iliac and femoropopliteal arterial lesions, technological and procedural advancements in endovascular therapy in the last decade have led to greater success rates in more complex lesions, thus making it a low-risk alternative to vascular surgery in patients with multiple comorbidities.
    3 Endovascular therapy is preferred in patients aged <50 yr due to a higher risk of graft failure after surgical therapy than older patients.
    4 Endovascular intervention is not indicated as prophylactic therapy in an asymptomatic patient with lower-extremity PAD.
    5 Stenting is effective as primary therapy for common iliac artery stenosis and occlusions, and in external iliac artery stenoses and occlusions, but not for infra-inguinal disease in the femoral, popliteal, and tibial arteries where it should be reserved for those who fail balloon dilatation.
  2 Considerations in surgical revascularization:
    1 Individuals with claudication symptoms who have a significant functional disability that is vocational or lifestyle limiting. These patients need to also be unresponsive to exercise or pharmacotherapy and should have a reasonable likelihood of symptomatic improvement with an acceptable surgical risk.
    2 Iliac or femoropopliteal disease with long segments; multifocal segments; long segment occlusions; and eccentric, calcified stenosis, which are less amenable to percutaneous interventions.
    3 Surgical intervention is not indicated to prevent progression to limb-threatening ischemia in patients with intermittent claudication as generally claudication does not progress to severe ischemia.
    4 Prior to any surgical therapy, patients should have a preoperative cardiovascular risk evaluation as it is a high-risk surgery and is associated with a higher morbidity compared to percutaneous revascularization.

DISPOSITION

Risk factors for atherosclerosis should be assessed, and appropriate modification instituted. Focus should be placed on smoking cessation, dietary adjustment, and pharmacotherapy for dyslipidemia, hyperglycemia, and hypertension. All patients with PAD should receive aspirin therapy unless contraindicated. Revascularization should be considered for refractory lifestyle-limiting symptoms.

REFERRAL

Consultation with vascular medicine, vascular surgery, or other physicians with expertise in PAD

is recommended in patients with rest pain, functional disability from pain, ABI <0.50 at rest, or any physical signs of limb ischemia or gangrene.

❶ PEARLS & CONSIDERATIONS

COMMENTS

- PAD remains underdiagnosed and undertreated.
- Patients with PAD are at markedly higher risk of future coronary, cerebrovascular, and other vascular events.
- Medical treatment is aimed mainly at cardiovascular risk factor modification, except for cilostazol.
- Studies of the natural history of claudication show the relative safety of initial conservative treatment of PAD in the absence of critical limb ischemia.
- When PAD limits a patient's ability to walk and exercise, percutaneous revascularization can be considered.
- Exercise training is an important and often neglected treatment strategy that has proven beneficial in improving functional status, reducing symptoms, and improving quality of life. Exercise capacity alone is the strongest predictor of mortality in patients with PAD.
- Surgical intervention should be considered in patients who meet the criteria for intervention but have lesions that are not amenable to PTA/stenting or in older patients with a low surgical risk. Advances in endovascular therapy have broadened the range of revascularization options for refractory claudication and critical and acute limb ischemia in patients with multiple comorbidities.

PREVENTION

Cardiovascular disease is the major cause of death in patients with intermittent claudication. Therefore, the treatment of claudication is directed not only at improving walking distance but also at reducing cardiovascular risk.

PATIENT & FAMILY EDUCATION

The following organizations offer more information about PAD:
- American College of Cardiology (http://www.acc.org)
- Vascular Disease Foundation (http://www.vdf.org)

SUGGESTED READINGS
Available at www.expertconsult.com

RELATED CONTENT
Peripheral Arterial Disease (Patient Information)

AUTHORS: **CHRIS W. PAN, M.D., M.B.A., M.S.,** and **PRANAV M. PATEL, M.D.**

P

Diseases and Disorders

I

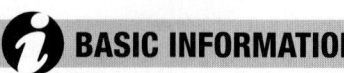

DEFINITION

A perirectal abscess is a localized inflammatory process that can be associated with infections of soft tissue and anal glands based on anatomic location. Perianal and perirectal abscesses may be simple or complex, causing suppuration. Infections in these spaces may be classified as superficial perianal or perirectal with involvement in the following anatomic spaces: ischiorectal, intersphincteric, perianal, and supralevator. The Parks classification of anorectal abscess is subdivided into intersphincteric, transsphincteric, suprasphincteric, and extrasphincteric abscess (Fig. 1).

SYNONYMS

Rectal abscess
Perianal abscess
Anorectal abscess

ICD-10CM CODES
K61.0 Anal abscess
K61.1 Rectal abscess

EPIDEMIOLOGY & DEMOGRAPHICS

INCIDENCE (IN U.S.): Commonly encountered
PREDOMINANT SEX: Male > female
PREDOMINANT AGE: All ages
PEAK INCIDENCE: Not seasonal; common
GENETICS: None known

PHYSICAL FINDINGS & CLINICAL PRESENTATION

- Localized perirectal or anal pain—often worsened with movement or straining
- Perirectal erythema or cellulitis
- Perirectal mass by inspection or palpation
- Fever and signs of sepsis with deep abscess
- Urinary retention

ETIOLOGY

- Polymicrobial aerobic and anaerobic bacteria involving one of the anatomic spaces (see "Definition"), often associated with localized trauma
- Microbiology: most bacteria are polymicrobial, mixed enteric, and skin flora

- Predominant anaerobic bacteria:
  1. *Bacteroides fragilis*
  2. *Peptostreptococcus* spp.
  3. *Prevotella* spp.
  4. *Porphyromonas* spp.
  5. *Clostridium* spp.
  6. *Fusobacterium* spp.
- Predominant aerobic bacteria:
  1. *Staphylococcus aureus*
  2. *Streptococcus* spp.
  3. *Escherichia coli*
  4. *Enterococcus* spp.

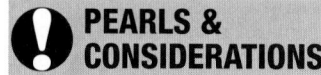 DIAGNOSIS

Many patients will have predisposing underlying conditions including:
- Malignancy or leukemia
- Immune deficiency
- Diabetes mellitus
- Recent surgery
- Steroid therapy

DIFFERENTIAL DIAGNOSIS

- Neutropenic enterocolitis
- Crohn's disease (inflammatory bowel disease)
- Pilonidal disease
- Hidradenitis suppurativa
- Tuberculosis or actinomycosis; Chagas' disease
- Cancerous lesions
- Chronic anal fistula
- Rectovaginal fistula
- Proctitis—often STD-associated, including syphilis, gonococcal, chlamydia, chancroid, condylomata acuminata
- AIDS-associated: Kaposi's sarcoma, lymphoma, CMV

WORKUP

- Examination of rectal, perirectal/perineal areas
- Rule out necrotic process and crepitance suggesting deep tissue involvement
- Local aerobic and anaerobic culture
- Blood cultures if toxic, febrile, or compromised
- Possible sigmoidoscopy

IMAGING STUDIES

Usually not indicated unless extensive disease is suspected. CT has a sensitivity of 77% and is relatively poor in detecting a perirectal abscess in immunocompromised patients.

TREATMENT

ACUTE GENERAL Rx

- Incision and drainage of abscess
- Debridement of necrotic tissue
- Rule out need for fistulectomy
- Local wound care—packing
- Sitz baths
- Antibiotic treatment: directed toward coverage for mixed skin and enteric flora

OUTPATIENT—ORAL:
- Trimethoprim/sulfamethoxazole DS bid or ciprofloxacin 500 mg bid or levofloxacin 500 mg q24h plus metronidazole 500 mg q8h x 7 to 10 days
- Amoxicillin/clavulanic acid 875 to 1000 mg 1 tabs bid
- Clindamycin 150 to 300 mg PO q6 to 8h ± ciprofloxacin

INPATIENT—INTRAVENOUS:
- Piperacillin/tazobactam 3.375 g IV q6 to 8h
- Ampicillin/sulbactam 1.5 to 3 g IV q6h
- Cefotetan 1 to 2 g IV q8h
- Imipenem or meropenem 500 to 1000 mg IV q8h

DISPOSITION

Follow-up with a general surgeon or infectious disease physician is often warranted.

REFERRAL

- General surgeon or colorectal surgeon for drainage.
- AIDS specialist may be needed for perirectal complications of HIV infection.
- Gastroenterologist follow-up may be warranted in Crohn's disease with perirectal fistula and other complications.

PEARLS & CONSIDERATIONS

Perirectal abscess may be a presenting manifestation of type 2 diabetes mellitus in older adults. Check the blood sugar in patients to exclude the possibility of undiagnosed diabetes mellitus.

SUGGESTED READINGS
Available at www.expertconsult.com

RELATED CONTENT
Perirectal Abscess (Patient Information)

AUTHOR: **GLENN G. FORT, M.D., M.P.H.**

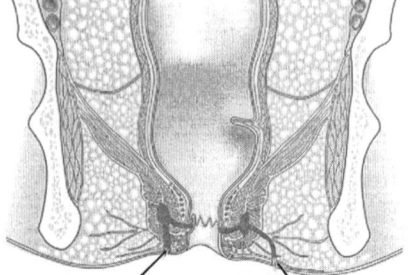

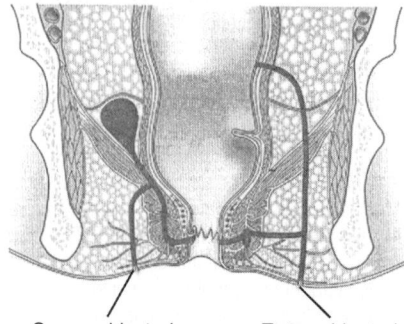

Intersphincteric   Trans-sphincteric   Suprasphincteric   Extrasphincteric

FIG. 1 Parks classification of anorectal abscess. (From Cameron JL, Cameron AM: *Current surgical therapy*, ed 10, Philadelphia, 2011, Saunders.)

BASIC INFORMATION

DEFINITION

Peritonitis refers to the acute onset of severe abdominal pain caused by peritoneal inflammation.

Secondary peritonitis is a localized (abscess) or diffuse peritonitis originating from a defect in abdominal viscus.

SYNONYMS

Acute abdomen
Surgical abdomen

ICD-10CM CODES
K65.0	Generalized (acute) peritonitis
K65.8	Other peritonitis
K65.9	Peritonitis, unspecified
A18.31	Tuberculous peritonitis
A54.85	Gonococcal peritonitis
A74.81	Chlamydial peritonitis
K35.2	Acute appendicitis with generalized peritonitis
K35.3	Acute appendicitis with localized peritonitis
K65.2	Spontaneous bacterial peritonitis
N73.3	Female acute pelvic peritonitis
N73.4	Female chronic pelvic peritonitis
N73.5	Female pelvic peritonitis, unspecified
P78.1	Other neonatal peritonitis

EPIDEMIOLOGY & DEMOGRAPHICS

Common presentation as a result of diverse etiologies; for example, 5% to 10% of the population has acute appendicitis at some point in their lives.

PHYSICAL FINDINGS & CLINICAL PRESENTATION

- Acute abdominal pain
- Abdominal distention and ascites
- Abdominal rigidity, rebound, and guarding
- Fever, chills
- Exacerbation with movement
- Anorexia, nausea, and vomiting
- Constipation
- Decreased bowel sounds
- Hypotension and tachycardia
- Tachypnea, dyspnea

ETIOLOGY

- Microbiology: most common is gram-negative bacteria (*Escherichia coli, Enterobacter, Klebsiella, Proteus*), gram-positive bacteria (enterococci, streptococci, staphylococci), anaerobic bacteria (*Bacteroides, Clostridium*), and fungi

- Acute perforation peritonitis: gastrointestinal perforation, intestinal ischemia, pelvic peritonitis, and other forms
- Postoperative peritonitis: anastomotic leak, accidental perforation, and devascularization
- Posttraumatic peritonitis: after blunt or penetrating abdominal trauma

DIAGNOSIS

DIFFERENTIAL DIAGNOSIS

- Postoperative: abscess, sepsis, bowel obstruction, injury to internal organs
- Gastrointestinal: perforated viscus, appendicitis, inflammatory bowel disease, infectious colitis, diverticulitis, acute cholecystitis, peptic ulcer perforation, pancreatitis, bowel obstruction
- Gynecologic: ruptured ectopic pregnancy, pelvic inflammatory disease, ruptured hemorrhagic ovarian cyst, ovarian torsion, degenerating leiomyoma
- Urologic: nephrolithiasis, interstitial cystitis
- Miscellaneous: abdominal trauma, penetrating wounds, infections caused by intraperitoneal dialysis

WORKUP

- Acute peritonitis is mainly a clinical diagnosis based on patient history and physical examination.
- Laboratory and imaging studies (see "Laboratory Tests") assist in determining the need for and type of intervention.
- If patient is hemodynamically unstable, immediate diagnostic laparotomy should be performed in lieu of adjuvant diagnostic studies.

LABORATORY TESTS

- Complete blood count: leukocytosis, left shift, anemia
- SMA7: electrolyte imbalances, kidney dysfunction
- Liver function tests: ascites from liver disease, cholelithiasis
- Amylase: pancreatitis
- Blood cultures: bacteremia, sepsis
- Peritoneal cultures: infectious etiology
- Blood gas: respiratory versus metabolic acidosis
- Ascitic fluid analysis: exudate versus transudate
- Urinalysis and culture: urinary tract infection
- Cervical cultures for gonorrhea and *Chlamydia*
- Urine/serum human chorionic gonadotropin

IMAGING STUDIES

- Abdominal series: free air from perforation, small or large bowel dilation from obstruction, identification of fecalith

- Chest x-ray examination: elevated diaphragm, pneumonia
- Pelvic/abdominal ultrasound: abscess formation, abdominal mass, intrauterine versus ectopic pregnancy, identify free fluid suggestive of hemorrhage or ascites
- CT: mass, ascites

TREATMENT

NONPHARMACOLOGIC THERAPY

- IV hydration to correct dehydration, hypovolemia
- Blood transfusion to correct anemia from hemorrhage
- Nasogastric decompression, especially if obstruction is present
- Oxygen: intubation if necessary
- Bed rest

ACUTE GENERAL Rx

- Surgery to correct underlying pathology, such as controlling hemorrhage, correcting perforation, draining abscess
- Broad-spectrum antibiotics to cover both gram-negative aerobic and gram-negative anaerobic bacteria:
  1. Mild-moderate disease: piperacillin-tazobactam 3.375 g IV q6h or 4.5 g IV q8h *or* ticarcillin-clavulanate 3.1 g IV q6h. Alternative agents are ciprofloxacin 400 mg IV q12h or levofloxacin 750 mg IV q24h *plus* metronidazole 1 g IV q12h.
  2. Severe life-threatening disease: imipenem 500 mg IV q6h or meropenem 1 g IV q8h. Alternative agents are ampicillin *plus* metronidazole *plus* ciprofloxacin.
- Pain control: morphine or meperidine as needed (hold until diagnosis confirmed)

DISPOSITION

Depends on etiology of peritonitis, age of patient, coexisting medical disease, and duration of process before presentation

REFERRAL

Surgical consultation is required in all cases of acute peritonitis.

AUTHOR: **RUBEN ALVERO, M.D.**

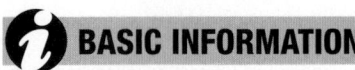

BASIC INFORMATION

DEFINITION

Spontaneous bacterial peritonitis (SBP) is an inflammatory reaction of the peritoneum secondary to the presence of bacteria or other microorganisms. More specifically, SBP is defined as an ascitic fluid infection without an evident intraabdominal surgically treatable source occurring primarily in patients with advanced cirrhosis of the liver.

SYNONYMS

Primary peritonitis
SBP

ICD-10CM CODES
K65.2 Spontaneous bacterial peritonitis

EPIDEMIOLOGY & DEMOGRAPHICS

PREVALENCE: The prevalence of SBP in cirrhotic patients admitted to the hospital has been estimated at 10% to 30%.
PREDOMINANT SEX: Males affected more often than females.

PHYSICAL FINDINGS & CLINICAL PRESENTATION

- Acute fever with accompanying abdominal pain/ascites, nausea, vomiting, diarrhea.
- In cirrhotic patients, presentation may be subtle with a low-grade temperature (100° F) with or without abdominal abnormalities.
- In patients with ascites, a heightened degree of awareness is necessary for detection
- Jaundice and encephalopathy.
- Deterioration of mental status and/or renal function.

ETIOLOGY

- *Escherichia coli.*
- *Klebsiella pneumoniae.*
- *Streptococcus pneumoniae.*
- *Streptococcus* and *Enterococcus* spp.
- *Staphylococcus aureus.*
- Anaerobic pathogens: *Bacteroides, Clostridium* organisms.
- Other: fungal, mycobacterial, viral.

DIAGNOSIS

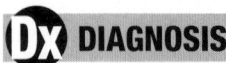

The diagnosis of SBP is established by a positive ascitic fluid bacterial culture and an elevated ascitic fluid absolute polymorphonuclear leukocyte count (≥250 cells/mm³).

DIFFERENTIAL DIAGNOSIS

- Appendicitis (in children).
- Perforated peptic ulcer.

- Secondary bacterial peritonitis.
- Peritoneal abscess.
- Splenic, hepatic, or pancreatic abscess.
- Cholecystitis.
- Cholangitis.

WORKUP

Paracentesis and ascitic fluid analysis will confirm diagnosis (see "Laboratory Tests").

LABORATORY TESTS

Ascitic fluid analysis reveals the following:
- Cell count with an absolute polymorphonuclear cell count >250/mm³.
- Presence of bacteria on Gram stain.
- pH <7.31.
- Lactic acid >32 mg/dl.
- Protein <1 g/dl.
- Glucose >50 mg/dl.
- Lactate dehydrogenase <225 mU/mL.
- Positive culture of peritoneal fluid.
- Measurement of the serum/ascites/albumin gradient: The serum/ascites/albumin gradient indirectly measures portal pressure. The albumin concentration of ascitic fluid and serum must be obtained on the same day. The ascitic fluid value is subtracted from the serum value to obtain the gradient. If the difference (not a ratio) is >1.1 g/dl, the patient has portal hypertension, with 97% accuracy. If the difference is <1.1 g/dl, portal hypertension is not present. The majority of patients with SBP have portal hypertension as a result of cirrhosis.

IMAGING STUDIES

- Abdominal ultrasound: if there is clinical difficulty in performing paracentesis.
- CT scan: to rule out secondary peritonitis (if indicated) and to exclude abscess, mass.

TREATMENT

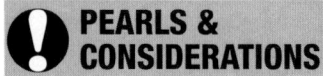

ACUTE GENERAL Rx

- Cefotaxime (2 g IV q8h) or ceftriaxone (2 g IV q24h). Alternative agents include ticarcillin-clavulanate, piperacillin-tazobactam, cefoxitin, and meropenem. Continue therapy for 5 to 7 days. Repeat diagnostic paracentesis can be done at day 2. Repeat paracentesis at 48 hr will demonstrate a significant decrease in polymorphonuclear count in patients with SBP. If ascites PMN count decreases by at least 25% at day 2, IV therapy can be switched to PO (levofloxacin 500-750 mg qd) to complete 7 days of therapy if organisms are susceptible.
- IV albumin (1.5 g/kg of body weight upon initial diagnosis and 1 g/kg of albumin on day 3) if BUN >30 mg/dL, serum creatinine >1 mg/dl, bilirubin >4 mg/dL.

PROPHYLAXIS

- Ciprofloxacin 500 mg PO qd or levofloxacin 250 mg PO qd.
- Alternative therapy: TMP-SMX one double-strength tablet PO qd.
- Rifaximin 1200 mg a day was shown in a recent study to be superior to norfloxacin.
- Prophylaxis should be continued until disappearance of ascites or until liver transplantation.

DISPOSITION

- The overall mortality rate from an episode of SBP is 20%, and following an episode, the 1-year mortality rate approaches 70%.

REFERRAL

- To a gastroenterologist for management of ascites and prevention of recurrent SBP.
- To an infectious disease specialist for management of difficult-to-treat infections, antibiotic-resistant bacterial infections, or antibiotic drug intolerance.

PEARLS & CONSIDERATIONS

COMMENTS

- Renal failure is a major cause of morbidity in cirrhotic patients with SBP. The use of IV albumin (1.5 g/kg at the time of diagnosis and 1 g/kg on day 3) may lower the rate of renal failure and mortality in patients with SBP.
- The criteria for the diagnosis of SBP require that abdominal paracentesis be performed and ascitic fluid be analyzed before a diagnosis of SBP can be made.
- Culturing ascitic fluid as if it were blood (with bedside inoculation of at least 10 mL of ascitic fluid directly into blood culture bottles at the bedside) has been shown to significantly increase the culture positivity of the ascitic fluid in the 80% to 100% range.
- Avoid therapeutic paracenteses during active infection.
- Positive blood cultures in an individual with ascites require exclusion of a peritoneal source by paracentesis.
- Follow-up paracentesis is indicated only in selected cases (worsening clinical status, nosocomial SBP, infection with atypical organism, recent β-lactam exposure).

SUGGESTED READINGS

Available at www.expertconsult.com

AUTHOR: **GLENN G. FORT, M.D., M.P.H.**

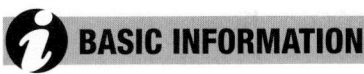

BASIC INFORMATION

DEFINITION

Peritonsillar abscess is an acute infection located between the capsule of the palatine tonsil and the superior constrictor muscle of the pharynx.

SYNONYMS

Quinsy
PTA

ICD-10CM CODES
J36 Peritonsillar abscess

EPIDEMIOLOGY & DEMOGRAPHICS

INCIDENCE (IN U.S.): 30:100,000/yr for ages 5 to 59. For adolescents, the incidence is 40:100,000/yr. It is the most common deep infection of the head and neck in children and adolescents, accounting for at least 50% of cases.

PEAK INCIDENCE: Bimodal frequency during the year, with highest occurrence from November to December and April to May.

PREVALENCE: 45,000 cases/yr in the United States

PREDOMINANT SEX: Male > female

PREDOMINANT AGE: Highest incidence is adults aged 20 to 40 yr.

RISK FACTORS: Smoking, periodontal disease, oropharyngeal or dental infection, male gender

PHYSICAL FINDINGS & CLINICAL PRESENTATION

- There is often a delay of 2 to 5 days between abscess formation and local and systemic symptoms
- Sore throat, which may be severe and unilateral (Table 1)
- Dysphagia and odynophagia
- Otalgia on the side of abscess
- Foul-smelling breath
- Facial swelling
- Drooling
- Headache
- Fever
- Trismus: the examination of the pharynx can be limited by trismus
- Hoarseness, muffled voice (also called "hot potato voice")
- Tender submandibular and anterior cervical lymph nodes
- Tonsillar hypertrophy with likely peritonsillar edema
- Contralateral deflection of the uvula: the distinguishing feature of peritonsillar abscess is inferior medial displacement of the infected tonsil with contralateral deviation of the uvula (Fig. 1)
- Stridor

ETIOLOGY

- Peritonsillar abscess is usually a complication of tonsillitis or acute bacterial pharyngitis caused by blockage of salivary ducts. Tonsillitis → peritonsillar cellulitis → peritonsillar abscess
- Group A β-hemolytic *Streptococcus* is the most common bacterial cause, accounting for 15% to 30% of cases in children and 5% to 10% of cases in adults.
- Less common aerobic causes are *Staphylococcus aureus, Haemophilus influenzae, Neisseria* species.
- The most common anaerobic organism is *Fusobacterium.*

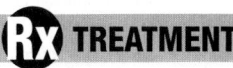

DIAGNOSIS

DIFFERENTIAL DIAGNOSIS

- Hypertrophic tonsillitis
- Infectious mononucleosis
- Peritonsillar cellulitis
- Retropharyngeal abscess
- Epiglottitis
- Dental abscess (retromolar)
- Lymphoma
- Ludwig's angina
- Tubercular granuloma
- Cervical adenitis
- Diphtheria
- Foreign body
- Neoplasm

WORKUP

- Based on history and physical exam. Aspiration of pus established diagnosis of peritonsillar abscess
- Consider additional testing if presentation is less clear.

LABORATORY TESTS

- Consider rapid strep antigen testing and/or pharyngeal culture and sensitivity.
- Aspiration of the abscess for culture and sensitivity (see "Treatment" for role of aspiration in tx)
- Consider lab testing for mononucleosis (patients with peritonsillar abscess have a 20% incidence of mononucleosis)

IMAGING STUDIES

- Consider ultrasound, CT scan (Fig. 2), or MRI to help differentiate abscess from cellulitis or mass when diagnosis is unclear.
- Intraoral ultrasound may improve diagnosis and aspiration of PTA compared with visual inspection in adult patients.
- MRI provides better soft-tissue differentiation than CT.

TREATMENT

NONPHARMACOLOGIC THERAPY

- Drainage of the abscess by needle aspiration or by surgical incision and drainage. Intraoral ultrasound-guided needle aspiration is a useful adjunct in the presence of trismus

ACUTE GENERAL Rx

- Aspiration or surgical drainage AND antibiotics for 10 to 14 days

TABLE 1 Clinical Differentiation of Common Conditions Arising as Sore Throat

Feature	Viral Pharyngitis	Bacterial Tonsillitis	Peritonsillar Abscess	Epiglottitis
Tonsillar Enlargement	Usual	Rare	None	None
Tonsillar Exudates	Occasional (mononucleosis)	Usual	Often	None
Tonsillar Asymmetry	None	None	Usual	None
Trismus (Inability to Open Jaw)	None	None	Usual	None
Cervical Adenopathy	Occasional	Usual (tender)	Usual (tender)	None
Tender Larynx	Rare	None	None	Usual

From Goldman L, Schafer AI: *Goldman's Cecil Medicine*, ed 24, Philadelphia, 2012, Saunders.

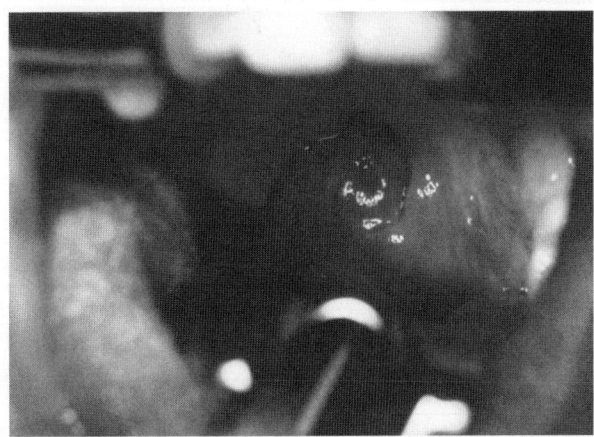

FIG. 1 Peritonsillar abscess with uvular displacement to the right. (Marx JA, et al.: *Rosen's emergency medicine*, ed 8, Philadelphia, 2014, WB Saunders.)

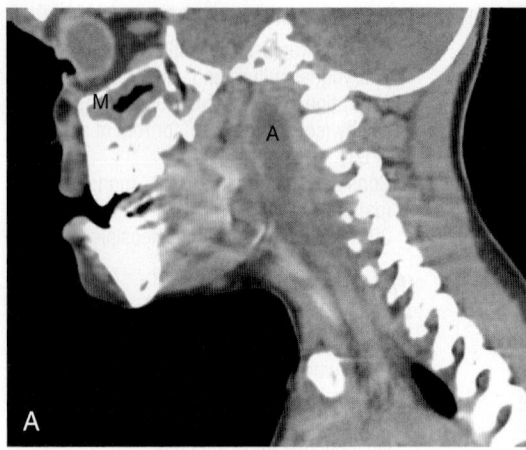
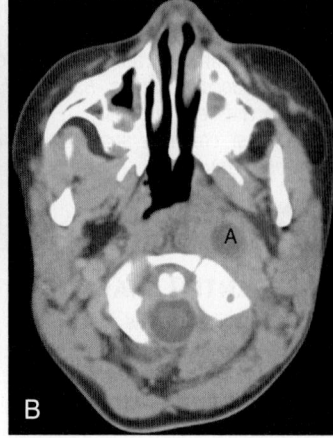

FIG. 2 CT of parapharyngeal abscess in a 3-yr-old child. A, Sagittal section demonstrating parapharyngeal abscess *(A)* and mucosal swelling *(M)* in the maxillary sinus. **B,** Coronal section of parapharyngeal abscess *(A).* (From Kliegman RM, et al.: *Nelson textbook of pediatrics*, ed 19, Philadelphia, 2011, Saunders.)

- Initial antibiotics should cover group A *Streptococcus* and anaerobes
- Intravenous
  1. Piperacillin/tazobactam or ticarcillin/clavulanate. If penicillin allergic, use IV clindamycin (600-900 mg IV q8h).
  2. Ampicillin-sulbactam 3 g q6h
  3. Penicillin G 10 million units q6h AND metronidazole 500 mg q6h (may use clindamycin 900 mg q8h if penicillin allergic)
- OR oral
  1. Amoxicillin-clavulanic acid 875 mg twice daily
  2. Penicillin VK 500 mg 4 times daily AND metronidazole 500 mg 4 times daily
  3. Clindamycin 600 mg twice daily or 300 mg 4 times daily
- Selection of antibiotics should be guided by culture and sensitivity of the organism. Consulting local antimicrobial guidelines for resistance profiles is also advisable for empiric coverage before culture results are available.

CHRONIC Rx

- Tonsillectomy can be considered 3 to 6 mo after diagnosis of peritonsillar abscess with or without the diagnosis of recurrent tonsillitis.
- Though rare, in adults and children with an acute case of peritonsillar abscess and a history of recurrent pharyngitis or previous peritonsillar abscess, a specialist may recommend a *quinsy or hot tonsillectomy,* an immediate removal of the tonsils after starting IV antibiotics.

DISPOSITION

- Successful treatment is defined by symptomatic improvement in sore throat, fever, and/or tonsillar swelling within 24 hr of intervention.
- Treatment failure is defined by lack of symptomatic improvement or worsening despite 24 hr of antimicrobial therapy (with or without surgical drainage).

REFERRAL

- Consider ENT or diagnostic radiology for drainage of abscess.
- Consider ENT for tonsillectomy if criteria are met.

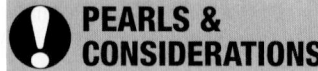

PEARLS & CONSIDERATIONS

COMMENTS

- Risk for a recurrence is immediate (within 4 days) and long term (2 to 3 yr).
- Most recurrences occur shortly after the initial presentation, suggesting continued infection rather than recurrence.
- Overall recurrence rate is 10% to 15%.
- Supportive treatment for pain control and hydration. Newer reports suggest a single dose of dexamethasone (10 mg) administered following needle aspiration will reduce pain at 24 hours as compared with placebo (see "Suggested Readings").

PREVENTION

- Adequate treatment of peritonsillar abscess.
- Up to 30% of patients with peritonsillar abscess meet criteria for tonsillectomy.

PATIENT/FAMILY EDUCATION

Advise family members to call with any trouble breathing, swallowing, or talking.

SUGGESTED READINGS

Available at www.expertconsult.com

AUTHORS: **PETER J. SELL, D.O.,** and **AMITY RUBEOR, D.O.**

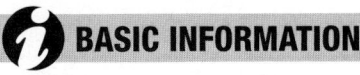

BASIC INFORMATION

DEFINITION

Pertussis is a prolonged bacterial infection of the upper respiratory tract characterized by paroxysms of an intense cough.

SYNONYMS

Whooping cough

ICD-10CM CODES

A37.90 Whooping cough, unspecified species without pneumonia
A37.00 Whooping cough due to Bordetella pertussis without pneumonia
A37.01 Whooping cough due to Bordetella pertussis with pneumonia
A37.10 Whooping cough due to Bordetella parapertussis without pneumonia
A37.11 Whooping cough due to Bordetella parapertussis with pneumonia
A37.80 Whooping cough due to other Bordetella species without pneumonia
A37.81 Whooping cough due to other Bordetella species with pneumonia
A37.90 Whooping cough, unspecified species without pneumonia
A37.91 Whooping cough, unspecified species with pneumonia

EPIDEMIOLOGY

INCIDENCE (IN U.S.): Case reports from 2015 were 18,166, including five deaths. This represents a decrease in the number of case reports compared with each of the 3 previous years. The reported rates were 32,971 and 28,639 in 2014 and 2013, respectively. In 2012, there were 48,277 cases reported, which is the highest rate reported since 1955. The highest incidence, in 2015, was among infants <6 months (150.9/100,000), but rates in adolescents 13 to 15 years of age have been increasing in recent years.

PEAK INCIDENCE
- Childhood
- Usually affects children aged <1 yr
- Increasing infections seen in adolescence

PREDOMINANT AGE:
- 50% in children aged <1 yr
- 20% in children aged >15 yr
- Classically an infection of infants and young children, pertussis is often overlooked as a cause of chronic cough in adults. However, a resurgence of pertussis has been observed in recent years, with nearly 50% of all cases identified in adolescents and adults, likely due to waning immunity and decreased effectiveness of acellular vaccines in early childhood compared to older, whole-cell-derived vaccines.

PHYSICAL FINDINGS & CLINICAL PRESENTATION

- Infection is characterized by 3 phases: catarrhal, paroxysmal, and convalescent
- Catarrhal phase: Usually begins with a 1- to 2-wk prodrome that resembles a common cold. This phase may be mild or absent in adolescents and adults given partial immunity from prior immunization
- After this initial phase, increased production of mucus occurs. Excessive lacrimation and conjunctival infection should heighten the suspicion for pertussis
- Paroxysmal phase: Increased mucus production is followed by an intense, paroxysmal cough, ending with gasps and an inspiratory whoop
- In some children, apnea, cyanosis, and anoxia are noted; posttussive gagging and vomiting are characteristic of pertussis
- Cases can be severe and life-threatening in young infants, particularly children <6 months old
- When prolonged, frank exhaustion and even apnea occur. The paroxysmal phase lasts from 2 wk to 2 mo
- Convalescent phase: Lasts over 2 months and is characterized by cough of decreasing severity
- See Box 1 for complications of pertussis

ETIOLOGY

Bordetella pertussis, a gram-negative rod that adheres to human cilia and respiratory epithelia

DIAGNOSIS

DIFFERENTIAL DIAGNOSIS

- Croup
- Epiglottitis
- Foreign body aspiration
- Bacterial pneumonia
- Viral pneumonia

WORKUP

Pertussis is often overlooked as a cause of chronic cough, especially in adolescents and adults. The presence of posttussive emesis and/or inspiratory whoop increases the likelihood of pertussis but only modestly. Therefore, clinicians must use their overall impression in pursuing the diagnosis.

- Enzyme-linked immunosorbent assay for detection of antibody to pertussis. Polymerase chain reaction (PCR) is the most sensitive method for rapid detection of pertussis. PCR

BOX 1   Pertussis Complications

Periorbital edema
Subconjunctival hemorrhage
Petechiae
Epistaxis
Hemoptysis
Subcutaneous emphysema
Pneumothorax
Pneumomediastinum
Diaphragmatic rupture
Umbilical and inguinal hernias
Rectal prolapse

From Marx J, et al.: Rosen's emergency medicine: concepts and clinical practice, ed 7, Philadelphia, 2010, Mosby.

---

testing should be used only to confirm a diagnosis in persons with signs and symptoms consistent with pertussis. PCR testing sensitivity declines and is unlikely to be positive after 1 month of infection. PCR testing after 5 days of treatment with antibiotics can cause false-negative results and is generally not recommended
- Blood cultures in hospitalized patients
- Chest x-ray
- Culture of bacteria, usually from nasopharynx by aspiration or by swabbing the posterior nasopharynx with a polyester-tipped, rayon-tipped, or nylon-flocked swab
- Immunofluorescent staining of nasopharyngeal secretions
- Serologic tests for immunoglobulin G (IgG) or A (IgA) are available. A twofold increase between acute and convalescent sera is considered proof of seroconversion. A single elevated IgG or IgA titer is considered diagnostic when no acute serum is available. Can be useful for diagnosis later in illness.

LABORATORY TESTS

Complete blood count, which usually demonstrates marked lymphocytosis:
- Up to 18,000 white blood cells
- 70% to 80% lymphocytes

IMAGING STUDIES

Chest x-ray examination is of value if secondary bacterial pneumonia is suspected.

TREATMENT

ACUTE GENERAL Rx

- Intensive supportive care:
  1. Adequate hydration
  2. Control of secretions
  3. Maintenance of airway
- Antibiotics (Table 1) are indicated even though their ability to alter the course of the disease is controversial.
  1. Azithromycin 500 mg on day 1, followed by 250 mg for days 2 to 5. Erythromycin 50 mg/kg/day for 14 days. Recent literature reports indicate that a 7-day treatment regimen may be as effective as a 14-day course of erythromycin. TMP/SMX 320/1600 mg per day in divided doses can be used in patients with allergy or intolerance to macrolides.
  2. Although unproved, dexamethasone 1 mg/kg/day in four doses for severe, life-threatening paroxysms.
  3. Ceftriaxone 75 mg/kg/day in two doses for broad coverage of secondary bacterial pneumonias.
  4. Close observation of infants <6 months old as risk for apnea is high in this age group.
- Vaccination is successful in preventing the disease: universal vaccination is advised for all children and adults. The Advisory Committee on Immunization Practices (ACIP) updated Tdap recommendations to include a single dose of Tdap vaccine in place of routine Td for adults age 19-64 yr and a single-dose Tdap for adults 65 yr and older

TABLE 1 Recommended Antimicrobial Treatment and Postexposure Prophylaxis for Pertussis, by Age Group

| Age Group | Primary Agents | | Alternate Agent* | |
	Azithromycin	Erythromycin	Clarithromycin	TMP-SMZ
<1 mo	Recommended agent. 10 mg/kg/day in a single dose for 5 days (only limited safety data available)	Not preferred. Erythromycin is substantially associated with infantile hypertrophic pyloric stenosis. Use if azithromycin is unavailable; 40-50 mg/kg/day in 4 divided doses for 14 days	Not recommended (safety data unavailable)	Contraindicated for infants aged <2 mo (risk for kernicterus)
1-5 mo	10 mg/kg/day in a single dose for 5 days	40-50 mg/kg/day in four divided doses for 14 days	15 mg/kg/day in two divided doses for 7 days	Contraindicated at age <2 mo. For infants aged ≥2 mo: TMP 8 mg/kg/day plus SMZ 40 mg/kg/day in two divided doses for 14 days
Infants aged ≥6 mo and children	10 mg/kg in a single dose on day 1 (maximum 500 mg), then 5 mg/kg/day (maximum 250 mg) on days 2-5	40 mg/kg/day (maximum 1-2 g/day) in four divided doses for 14 days	15 mg/kg/day in 2 divided doses (maximum 1 g/day) for 7 days	TMP 8 mg/kg/day plus SMZ 40 mg/kg/day in two divided doses for 14 days
Adolescents and adults	500 mg in a single dose on day 1 then 250 mg/day on days 2-5	2 g/day in four divided doses for 14 days	1 g/day in two divided doses for 7 days	TMP 320 mg/day, SMZ 1600 mg/day in two divided doses for 14 days

*Trimethoprim-sulfamethoxazole (TMP-SMZ) can be used as an alternative agent to macrolides in patients aged ≥2 mo who are allergic to macrolides, who cannot tolerate macrolides, or who are infected with a rare macrolide-resistant strain of *Bordetella pertussis*.
From Centers for Disease Control and Prevention: Recommended antimicrobial agents for treatment and postexposure prophylaxis of pertussis: 2005 CDC guidelines, *MMWR Morbid Mortal Wkly Rep* 54:1-16, 2005.

who have or will have close contact with an infant (<12 mo). The ACIP also recommends that all pregnant women receive a dose of Tdap with every pregnancy, preferably during weeks 27 to 36 of gestation.
• Azithromycin, clarithromycin, or erythromycin is recommended for all household contacts and should be given to all persons at high risk of severe disease from pertussis and who were in contact with a pertussis case within 21 days of cough onset: TMP/SMX in two oral doses per day for those intolerant to macrolides.

DISPOSITION
Close attention to accepted vaccination schedules is the best prevention.

REFERRAL
To intensive care setting for life-threatening infections:

• Pulmonologist
• Infectious disease specialist

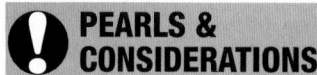 **PEARLS & CONSIDERATIONS**

• The diagnosis of pertussis in a young child is easily recognized, but in adults pertussis can be a subtle diagnosis and is often missed. The tip-off is often a persistent, hacking, and productive cough with minor or no fever in a previously healthy person that lasts <2 wk.
• Approximately 11% of pertussis cases in the pediatric population are attributable to vaccine refusal, dispelling the myth that herd immunity protects children whose parents refuse pertussis vaccine.

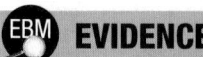 **EVIDENCE**

Available at www.expertconsult.com

SUGGESTED READINGS
Available at www.expertconsult.com

RELATED CONTENT
Pertussis (Patient Information)

AUTHORS: **JOEL P. WADDELL, D.O.,** and **RUSSELL J. MCCULLOH, M.D.**

BASIC INFORMATION

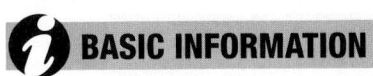

DEFINITION

- A hamartomatous polyp is a benign intestinal growth that may contain all components of the intestinal mucosa. In gastrointestinal polyposis, multiple such polyps coexist within the intestinal tract, and associated manifestations are usually also present.
- Juvenile polyps are benign polyps composed of cystic dilations of glandular structures within the fibroblastic stroma of the lamina propria. They may cause bleeding or intussusception.
- Commonly recognized syndromes are Peutz-Jeghers syndrome, juvenile polyposis syndrome, Cowden's disease, Bannayan-Ruvalcaba-Riley syndrome, and Cronkhite-Canada syndrome. Other, lesser known inherited hamartomatous polyposis syndromes are hereditary mixed polyposis syndrome, intestinal ganglioneuromatosis and neurofibromatosis (variant of von Recklinghausen's syndrome), Devon family syndrome, basal cell nevus syndrome, and tuberous sclerosis (may involve gastrointestinal tract). Table 1 describes general features of some inherited colorectal cancer syndromes.

ICD-10CM CODES
D12.6 Colon, unspecified (adenomatosis of colon, hereditary polyposis)

EPIDEMIOLOGY

- Colonic adenomas, the precursors of nearly all colorectal cancers, are found in nearly 40% of patients by age 60 yr.
- 25% of men and 15% of women who undergo colonoscopy are found to have one or more adenomas.
- Detection of any adenoma in patients <60 yr confers an increased risk of colorectal cancer (by a factor of 2.6) in their first-degree relatives.

PHYSICAL FINDINGS & CLINICAL PRESENTATION

PEUTZ-JEGHERS SYNDROME (PJS):

- Transmission: autosomal dominant with incomplete penetrance. The syndrome is caused in the majority of patients by a germline mutation of the *STK11/LKB1* tumor suppression gene on chromosome 19P13.
- Disease expression:
  1. Stomach, small and large intestinal hamartomas with bands of smooth muscle in the lamina propria
  2. Pigmented lesions around mouth (lips and buccal mucosa [Fig. 2]), nose, hands, feet, genitals, and perineal areas
  3. Ovarian tumors
  4. Sertoli cell testicular tumors
  5. Airway polyps
  6. Pancreatic cancer
  7. Breast cancer
  8. Urinary tract polyps
- Cumulative lifetime cancer risk
  1. Colon cancer: 39%
  2. Stomach cancer: 29%
  3. Small intestine cancer: 13%
  4. Pancreatic cancer: 36%
  5. Breast cancer: 54%
  6. Ovarian cancer: 10%
  7. Sertoli cell tumor: 9%
  8. Overall cancer risk: 93%
- Clinical manifestation:
  1. Gastrointestinal, small-bowel obstruction, intussusception, gastrointestinal bleeding
  2. See chapters on relevant malignancies for their signs and symptoms

DIAGNOSIS: The diagnosis of PJS is made with any of four major criteria:
1. Two or more histologically confirmed PJS polyps
2. Any number of PJS polyps and a family history of PJS
3. Characteristic mucocutaneous pigmentation and a family history of PJS, or
4. Any number of PJS polyps and characteristic mucocutaneous pigmentation

JUVENILE POLYPOSIS SYNDROME:
- Transmission: autosomal dominant
- Disease expression
  1. Solitary juvenile polyps numbering 10 or more in the rectum or throughout the gastrointestinal tract; the polyps are smooth and covered with normal epithelium
  2. Various congenital abnormalities coexist in 20%
- Cumulative cancer risk is increased (may be as high as 50%)
- Clinical manifestation
  1. Intestinal obstruction
  2. Intussusception
  3. Gastrointestinal bleeding

COWDEN'S DISEASE:
- Transmission: autosomal dominant, rare
- Disease expression
  1. Juvenile intestinal polyposis
  2. Orocutaneous hamartomas
  3. Fibrocystic breast disease and breast cancer
  4. Goiter and thyroid cancer
  5. Facial tricholemmomas (papules) in 83%
- Cumulative cancer risk
  1. Gastrointestinal: same as general population
  2. Thyroid: 3% to 10%
  3. Breast: 25% to 50%

BANNAYAN-RUVALCABA-RILEY SYNDROME:
- Transmission: autosomal dominant, rare
- Disease expression
  1. Juvenile intestinal polyposis
  2. Macrocephaly
  3. Developmental delay
  4. Penile pigmented spots
  5. Cumulative cancer risk unknown

CRONKHITE-CANADA SYNDROME:
- Transmission: acquired
- Age of onset: midlife

TABLE 1 General Features of Some Inherited Colorectal Cancer Syndromes

Syndrome	Polyp Histology	Polyp Distribution	Age of Onset	Risk of Colon Cancer	Genetic Lesion	Clinical Manifestations	Associated Lesions
Familial adenomatous polyposis (Fig. 1)	Adenoma	Large intestine, duodenum	16 yr (range, 8-34 yr)	100%	5q (*APC* gene)	Rectal bleeding, abdominal pain, bowel obstruction	Desmoids, CHRPE
Peutz-Jeghers syndrome	Hamartoma	Large and small intestine	First decade	Slightly above average	19p (*STK11* gene)	Possible rectal bleeding, abdominal pain, intussusception	Orocutaneous melanin pigment spots, other tumors
MUTYH-associated polyposis	Adenoma	Large intestine, duodenum	45-50 yr (range, 13-60 yr)	75% (range, 50%-100%)	1p (*MYH* gene)	Rectal bleeding, abdominal pain, bowel obstruction	CHRPE, osteomas
Juvenile polyposis	Hamartoma (rarely adenoma)	Large and small intestine	First decade	≈9%	*PTEN, SMAD4, BMPR1*	Possible rectal bleeding, abdominal pain, intussusception	Pulmonary AVMs
Hereditary nonpolyposis colon cancer	Adenoma	Large intestine	40 yr (range, 18-65 yr)	30%	Mismatch repair genes+*	Rectal bleeding, abdominal pain, bowel obstruction	Other tumors (e.g., ovary, uterus, pancreas, stomach)

AVM, Arteriovenous malformation; *CHRPE*, congenital hypertrophy of the retinal pigment epithelium; *MUTYH*, mutY homolog (*Escherichia coli*).
*Including *hMSH2, hMSH3, hMSH6, hMLH1, hPMS1,* and *hPMS2.*
From Goldman L, Schafer AI: *Goldman's Cecil medicine,* ed 24, Philadelphia, 2012, Saunders.

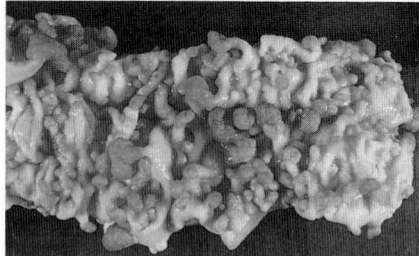

FIG. 1 Familial adenomatous polyposis. This disorder is marked by the development of hundreds of large bowel adenomas, as seen in this segment of large bowel, which is covered with adenomas of various sizes. It usually arises in the second and third decades. (From Skarin AT: *Atlas of diagnostic oncology*, 4th ed, St Louis, 2010, Mosby, 2010.)

- Disease expression
  1. Diffuse gastrointestinal juvenile polyposis (50%-95% of cases)
  2. Chronic diarrhea and protein-losing enteropathy (the entire intestinal mucosa may be inflamed), which leads to abdominal pain, weight loss, and various complications of malnutrition
  3. Dystrophic nails
  4. Alopecia
  5. Hyperpigmentation
- Cumulative cancer risk: same as the average population

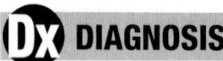 DIAGNOSIS

Diagnosis is suggested in many cases by family history and confirmed by colonoscopy and physical findings described previously.

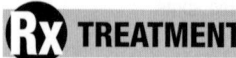 TREATMENT

GENERAL Rx/SURVEILLANCE

Peutz-Jeghers syndrome:
- Colonoscopies with polypectomies and upper endoscopy every 2 to 3 years beginning in teen years
- MRI or endoscopic ultrasound of the pancreas every 1 to 2 years beginning at age 30
- Screening for breast cancer, testicular cancer, possibly ovarian cancer
- Surveillance of small bowel with capsule endoscopy or CT or magnetic resonance enterography every 2 to 3 years starting at age 8 to 10 years.

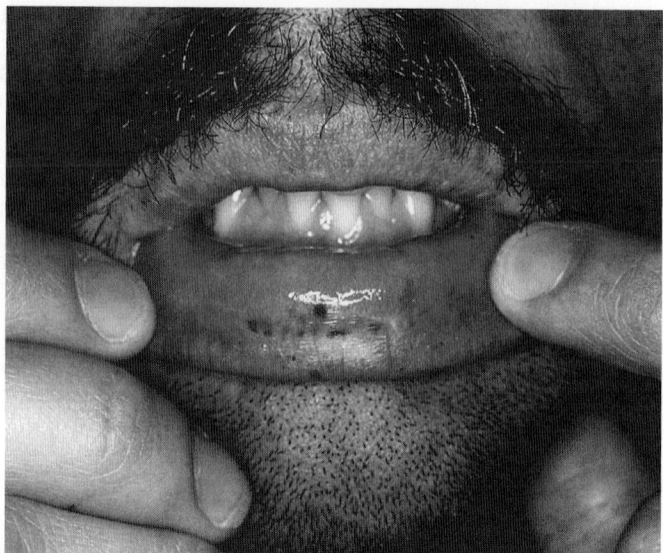

FIG. 2 Peutz-Jeghers syndrome, macular pigmentation of lower lip. (James WD et al: *Andrews' diseases of the skin*, ed 12, Philadelphia, 2016, WB Saunders.)

Juvenile polyposis syndrome:
- Colonoscopies with polypectomies and upper endoscopy every 2 to 3 years beginning at age 15
- Total colectomy if numerous polyps
- Esophagogastroscopies and polypectomies

Cowden's disease:
- Rigorous breast cancer screening or prophylactic simple bilateral mastectomy with reconstruction.

Cronkhite-Canada syndrome:
- Progressive malabsorption syndrome is the hallmark of this syndrome, and no specific treatment exists. Enteral or parenteral feeding is the cornerstone of management and can result in remission.
- Other syndromes
  - Serrated polyposis syndrome: colonoscopy yearly
  - PTEN hamartoma tumor syndrome: Colonoscopy every 5 years beginning at age 35

DISPOSITION

- The screening of first-degree relatives of patients with colonic adenomas detected before 60 yr of age is controversial. Some recommend beginning colonoscopic screening at age 40 yr or 10 yr younger than the age at diagnosis of the youngest person in the family with an adenoma.
- Recommended interval between colonoscopies from the U.S. Consensus Guidelines for Colonoscopic Surveillance after Polypectomy are as follows:
  1. 10 yr for small, rectal hyperplastic polyps
  2. 5 to 10 yr for one to two low-risk adenomas (tubular adenomas <1 cm)
  3. 3 yr for low-risk adenomas or any high-risk adenoma (large [≥1 cm] or histologically advanced adenomas [tubulovillous or villous adenomas or villous adenomas and those with high-grade dysplasia])
  4. <3 yr for presence of >10 adenomas
  5. 2 to 6 mo for inadequately removed adenomas

RELATED CONTENT

Peutz-Jeghers Syndrome (Patient Information)
Colorectal Cancer (Related Key Topic)
Familial Adenomatous Polyposis and Gardner Syndrome (Related Key Topic)
Lynch Syndrome (Related Key Topic)

AUTHOR: **FRED F. FERRI, M.D.**

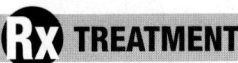 BASIC INFORMATION

DEFINITION

Peyronie's disease is an abnormal curvature and shortening of the penis during an erection. This is caused by scarring of the tunica albuginea of the corpora cavernosa.

SYNONYMS

Plastic induration of the penis
Penile fibromatosis

ICD-10CM CODES
N48.6 Induratio penis plastica

EPIDEMIOLOGY & DEMOGRAPHICS

- Peyronie's disease occurs in approximately 1% of men.
- It is commonly seen between the ages of 45 and 60 yr.
- A genetic predisposition has been suggested.
- There are no incidence and prevalence data available in the literature.

PHYSICAL FINDINGS & CLINICAL PRESENTATION

- Painful erections
- Tenderness over the scar tissue area
- Erectile dysfunction
- Curvature of the erected penis interfering with penetration
- Dupuytren's contracture is a commonly associated finding in patients with Peyronie's disease

ETIOLOGY

- Specific cause is unknown. It is believed that scar tissue forms on either the dorsal or ventral midline surface of the penile shaft. The scar restricts expansion at the involved site, causing the penis to bend or curve in one direction.
- The precipitating factor appears to be trauma from repetitive microvascular injury caused by vigorous sexual intercourse, accidents, or prior surgeries (e.g., transurethral or radical prostatectomy, cystoscopy).

DX DIAGNOSIS

Diagnosis is based on the clinical findings.

DIFFERENTIAL DIAGNOSIS

- The history differentiates congenital from acquired curvatures of the penis.
- Other causes of erectile dysfunction must be excluded, including metabolic, diabetic, thyroid, and renal causes, in addition to hypogonadism and hyperprolactinemia.

WORKUP

History and physical examination alone will usually establish the diagnosis of Peyronie's disease.

LABORATORY TESTS

There are no specific blood tests to diagnose Peyronie's disease. Electrolytes, blood urea nitrogen, creatinine, glucose, thyroid function tests (thyroid-stimulating hormone, T_3U, T_4), testosterone, and prolactin levels are blood tests to exclude other medical causes of erectile dysfunction.

IMAGING STUDIES

Imaging studies are not specific.

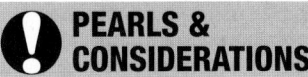 TREATMENT

NONPHARMACOLOGIC THERAPY

A conservative approach of reassurance and observation is taken at first because the disease process may be self-limiting.

ACUTE GENERAL Rx

Although not substantiated by direct randomized, controlled clinical trials, the following treatment modalities have been tried:

- Vitamin E 400 mg bid.
- Paraaminobenzoic acid 12 g/day.
- Colchicine 0.6 mg bid for 2 to 3 wk.
- Fexofenadine 60 mg bid for 3 mo.
- Steroid injection into the scar tissue.
- Collagenase injection into the scar tissue.
- Radiation to the scar tissue area.
- Extracorporeal shockwave therapy (ESWT): Current evidence on the safety, but not the efficacy, of ESWT appears adequate. From comparative studies, the main benefits of ESWT were the alleviation of pain and reduction of angulation of the penis. In one comparative study, 10 of 20 patients receiving ESWT had a decrease in the curvature of at least 30%. Case series evidence also suggested some improvement of sexual performance.
- Other medications that can be helpful include verapamil, tamoxifen, and interferon.

CHRONIC Rx

In patients who have progressed to intractable pain with erection or erectile dysfunction, surgical treatment with excision of the plaque and skin grafting may be indicated. Boxes 1 and 2 summarize indications for surgery and preoperative consent. An algorithm for the surgical management of Peyronie's disease is described in Fig. 1.

DISPOSITION

Peyronie's disease evolves slowly and in some cases can resolve on its own. Waiting for 1 yr before proceeding with surgical attempts is recommended.

REFERRAL

A urologic consultation is recommended in patients with progressive symptoms and erectile dysfunction.

! PEARLS & CONSIDERATIONS

COMMENTS

- Peyronie's disease is not commonly seen in younger patients because they are able to sustain intracorporeal pressures high enough to stretch the scar tissue, preventing it from deforming the penis during erection.
- Trauma from buckling of the erected penis is thought to be the precipitant cause of scar formation and Peyronie's disease. It is found more often in men who are sexually very active and vigorous, having sexual intercourse daily or almost daily.
- Sexual positions with the woman being on top or thrusting the penis into the anterior vaginal wall are thought to increase the chances of developing Peyronie's disease.

RELATED CONTENT

Peyronie's Disease (Patient Information)

AUTHOR: **TANYA ALI, M.D.**

BOX 1 Indications for Surgery

- Stable deformity for at least 6 months from onset of symptoms
- Inability to engage in satisfactory penetrative sexual intercourse because of deformity and/or inadequate rigidity
- Failed conservative treatment
- Desire for most rapid and reliable result

From Wein AJ et al: *Campbell-Walsh urology*, ed 11, Philadelphia, 2016, Elsevier.

BOX 2 Preoperative Consent

Set expectations regarding outcome:
- Persistent or recurrent curvature: The goal is "functionally straight" (curvature <20 degrees).
- Change in length: The result is more likely shorter with plication than with grafting.
- Diminished rigidity
  - ≥5% in all studies—grafting more than plication
  - ≥30% if suboptimal preoperative rigidity—dependent on preoperative erectile quality
- Decreased sexual sensation
  - Typically resolves in 1 to 6 months
  - Rarely compromises orgasm or ejaculation

From Wein AJ et al: *Campbell-Walsh urology*, ed 11, Philadelphia, 2016, Elsevier.

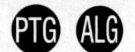

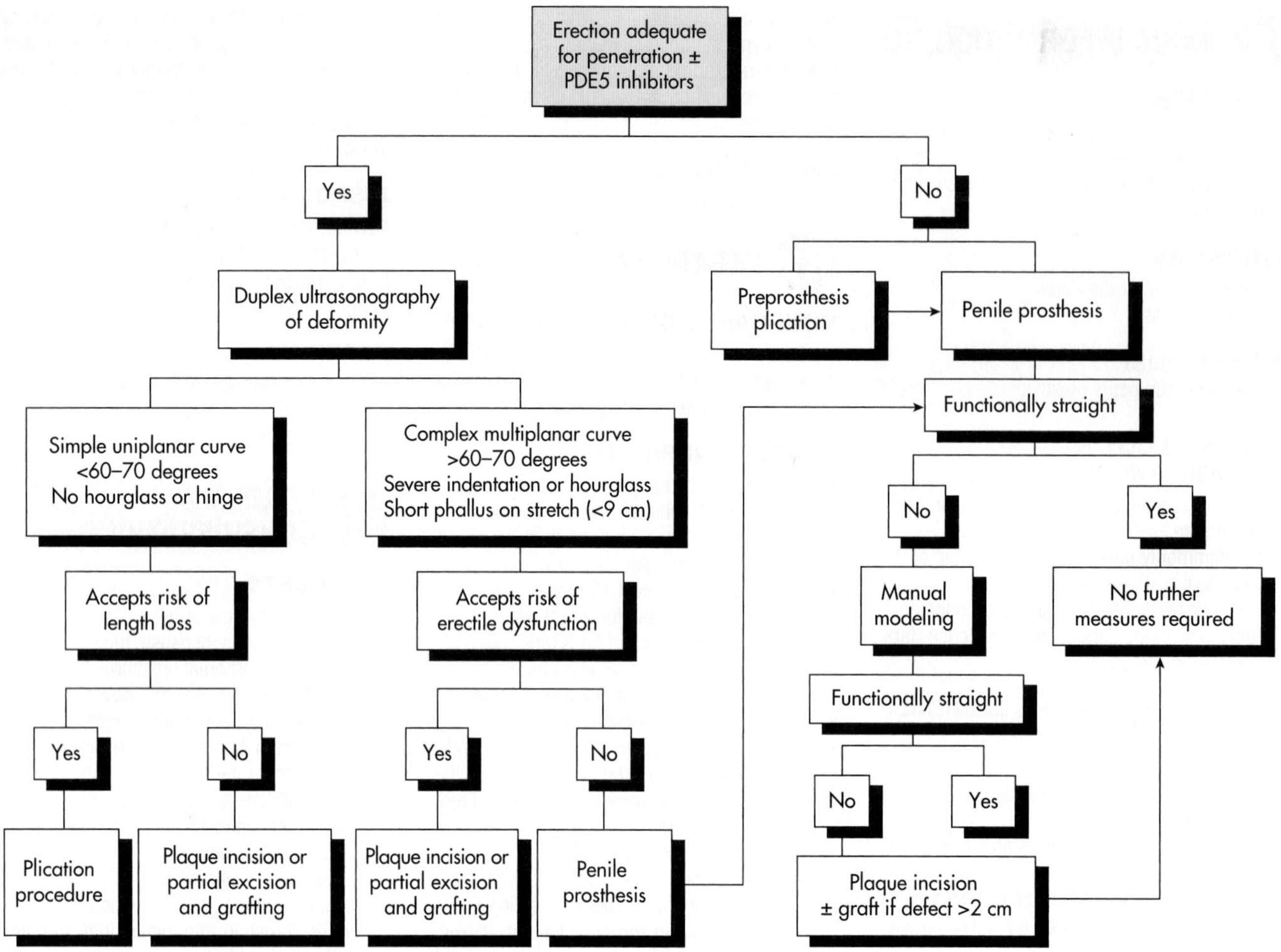

FIG 1 Algorithm for the surgical management of Peyronie's disease. *PDE5,* phosphodiesterase type 5. (From Wein AJ et al: *Campbell-Walsh urology,* ed 11, Philadelphia, 2016, Elsevier.)

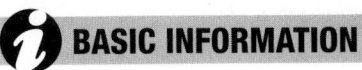

BASIC INFORMATION

DEFINITION

Inflammation of the pharynx or tonsils

SYNONYMS

Sore throat
Group A streptococci (GAS)
Pharyngitis
Tonsillitis
GABHS

ICD-10CM CODES

J02.9 Acute pharyngitis, unspecified
J03.0 Acute tonsillitis
J03.9 Acute tonsillitis, unspecified
J04.0 Acute laryngitis

EPIDEMIOLOGY & DEMOGRAPHICS

- Acute pharyngitis accounts for 1.3% of outpatient visits to health care providers in the United States and is diagnosed in two million persons in the outpatient setting each year in the United States.

PEAK INCIDENCE: Late winter/early spring (GAS infections)

PREDOMINANT SEX: Females = males

PREDOMINANT AGE:

- All ages affected
- Streptococcal pharyngitis most common among school-age children (5-15 yr of age). GAS are responsible for 5% to 15% of cases of pharyngitis in adults and 20% to 30% of cases in children (5-15 yr of age).

PHYSICAL FINDINGS & CLINICAL PRESENTATION

- Pharynx:
  1. May appear normal to severely erythematous
  2. Tonsillar hypertrophy and exudates commonly seen but do not indicate etiology
- Viral infection:
  1. Rhinorrhea
  2. Conjunctivitis
  3. Cough
- Bacterial infection, especially GAS:
  1. High fever
  2. Systemic signs of infection
- Herpes simplex or enterovirus infection: vesicles
- Streptococcal infection:
  1. Rare complications:
     a. Scarlet fever
     b. Rheumatic fever
     c. Acute glomerulonephritis
  2. Extension of infection: tonsillar, parapharyngeal, or retropharyngeal abscess presenting with severe pain, high fever, trismus
- Streptococcal tonsillitis is manifested as acute onset of fever, headache, neck pain, odynophagia, sore throat, otalgia, red tongue with enlargement of papillae, sore throat, red swollen uvula, and tender anterior cervical adenitis.

- Peritonsillar abscess (accumulation of pus between the tonsil and its capsule) is the most common complication of acute tonsillitis. Clinical signs include deformed posterior pharynx, medial displacement of the uvula, trismus, and muffled voice (hot-potato voice).
- Table 1 describes seven danger signs in patients with sore throat.

ETIOLOGY

- Viruses:
  1. Respiratory syncytial virus
  2. Influenza A and B
  3. Epstein-Barr virus
  4. Adenovirus
  5. Herpes simplex
- Bacteria:
  1. GAS: *Streptococcus pyogenes.* β-Hemolytic GAS are the most common cause of acute tonsillitis.
  2. *Neisseria gonorrhoeae*
  3. Fusobacterium necrophorum (10% of pharyngitis): highest incidence in patients aged 15 to 30 years
- Other organisms:
  1. *Mycoplasma pneumoniae*
  2. *Chlamydophila pneumoniae*
  3. *Arcanobacterium haemolyticum*

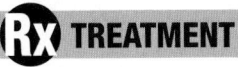

DIAGNOSIS

DIFFERENTIAL DIAGNOSIS

- Sore throat associated with granulocytopenia, thyroiditis
- Tonsillar hypertrophy associated with lymphoma
- Section II describes the differential diagnosis of sore throat.

WORKUP

The Centor criteria to identify patients at risk for GAS consists of (1) fever subjective or measured >38.1° C (100.5° F), (2) absence of cough, (3) tonsillar exudates, (4) tender anterior cervical lymphadenopathy. Patients with ≤1 criteria are at low risk and do not need additional testing. The McIsaac criteria adds 1 point for ages 3 to 14 and subtracts a point for ages ≥45 yr.

- Rapid streptococcal antigen test (culture should be performed if rapid test negative)

TABLE 1 Seven Danger Signs in Patients with Sore Throat

1. Persistence of symptoms longer than 1 wk without improvement
2. Respiratory difficulty, particularly stridor
3. Difficulty in handling secretions
4. Difficulty in swallowing
5. Severe pain in the absence of erythema
6. A palpable mass
7. Blood, even in small amounts, in the pharynx or ear

From Andreoli TE et al: *Andreoli and Carpenter's Cecil essentials of medicine,* ed 8, Philadelphia, 2010, Saunders.

- Throat swab for culture to exclude *S. pyogenes, N. gonorrhoeae* (requires specific transport medium) in selected cases

LABORATORY TESTS

- Bloodwork is only rarely necessary
- Complete blood count with differential
  1. May help support diagnosis of bacterial infection when diagnosis is unclear
  2. Streptococcal infection suggested by leukocytosis >15,000/mm^3
- Viral cultures, serologic studies rarely needed
- Monospot if diagnosis is unclear

IMAGING STUDIES

Seldom indicated. If necessary to distinguish between tonsillitis and peritonsillar abscess, CT or MRI of the neck can be done.

TREATMENT

NONPHARMACOLOGIC THERAPY

- Fluids
- Salt water gargles

ACUTE GENERAL Rx

- Analgesics: aspirin (adults) or acetaminophen or ibuprofen (adults and children).
- If streptococcal infection proven or suspected:
  1. Amoxicillin 500 mg BID or penicillin V 500 mg PO bid for 10 days or benzathine penicillin 1.2 million U IM once (adults). Children: penicillin V 250 mg bid or tid
  2. Azithromycin 500 mg on day 1 then 250 mg on days 2 through 5 or erythromycin 500 mg PO bid or 250 mg qid for 10 days if penicillin allergic
- If gonococcal infection proven or suspected: ceftriaxone 250 mg IM once.
- Amoxicillin 500 mg tid for 10 days is the primary antibiotic treatment of streptococcal tonsillitis. Macrolides or clindamycin can be used in penicillin-allergic patients.
- Treatment of peritonsillar abscess is drainage through needle or incision.
- Avoid quinolones, sulfonamides, and tetracyclines due to treatment failures.

CHRONIC Rx

- Recurrent streptococcal infections are common and may represent reinfection from other household members, including pets.
- There is no conclusive evidence from randomized clinical trials that tonsillectomy is superior to antibiotic therapy for recurrent tonsillitis in adults.
- Tonsillopharyngitis is generally managed in an outpatient setting with follow-up arranged in 1 to 2 wk. Admission to the hospital is indicated for local suppurative complications (peritonsillar abscess; lateral pharyngeal or posterior pharyngeal abscess; impending airway closure; or inability to swallow food, medications, or water).

REFERRAL
- To otolaryngologist:
  1. If peritonsillar or other abscess is suspected
  2. If tonsillar hypertrophy persists

SUGGESTED READINGS
Available at www.expertconsult.com

RELATED CONTENT
Sore Throat (Patient Information)

Strep Throat (Patient Information)
Tonsillitis (Patient Information)

AUTHOR: **GLENN G. FORT, M.D., M.P.H.**

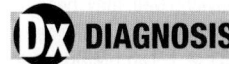

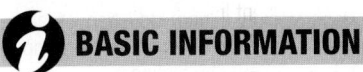

DEFINITION

Pheochromocytomas are catecholamine-producing tumors that originate from the chromaffin cells of the adrenergic system. While they generally secrete both norepinephrine and epinephrine, norepinephrine is usually the predominant amine.

SYNONYMS

Paraganglioma

ICD-10CM CODES
C74.9 Malignant neoplasm of adrenal gland, unspecified
C75.9 Malignant neoplasm of endocrine gland, unspecified
E27.5 Adrenomedullary hyperfunction

EPIDEMIOLOGY & DEMOGRAPHICS

- Incidence: 0.05% of population; peak incidence in 30s and 40s.
- Approximately 25% of patients with apparently sporadic pheochromocytoma may be carriers of mutations.
- Approximately 25% of pheochromocytomas are familial and associated with genetic disorders (Table 1). Pheochromocytoma is a feature of two disorders with an autosomal-dominant pattern of inheritance:
  1. Multiple endocrine neoplasia (MEN) type 2
  2. Von Hippel-Lindau disease: angioma of the retina, hemangioblastoma of the central nervous system, renal cell carcinoma, pancreatic cysts, and epididymal cystoadenoma

- Pheochromocytomas occur in 5% of patients with neurofibromatosis type 1.

PHYSICAL FINDINGS & CLINICAL PRESENTATION

- Hypertension: can be sustained (55%) or paroxysmal (45%).
- Headache (80%): usually paroxysmal in nature and described as "pounding" and severe.
- Palpitations (70%): can be present with or without tachycardia.
- Hyperhidrosis (60%): most evident during paroxysmal attacks of hypertension.
- Physical examination may be entirely normal if done in a symptom-free interval; during a paroxysm the patient may demonstrate marked increase in both systolic and diastolic pressure, profuse sweating, visual disturbances (caused by hypertensive retinopathy), dilated pupils (from catecholamine excess), paresthesias in the lower extremities (caused by severe vasoconstriction), tremor, and tachycardia.
- Orthostatic hypotension is common among patients with pheochromocytoma due to reduction of blood volume and desensitization of adrenergic receptors by the chronic excess of catecholamines.

ETIOLOGY

- Catecholamine-producing tumors that are usually located in the adrenal medulla.
- Specific mutations of the RET protooncogene cause familial predisposition to pheochromocytoma in MEN 2.
- Mutations in the von Hippel-Lindau tumor suppressor gene (VHL gene) cause familial

disposition to pheochromocytoma in von Hippel-Lindau disease.
- Recently identified genes for succinate dehydrogenase subunit D (SDHD) and succinate dehydrogenase subunit B (SDHB) predispose carriers to pheochromocytoma and globus tumors.

DIAGNOSIS

DIFFERENTIAL DIAGNOSIS

- Anxiety disorder
- Thyrotoxicosis
- Amphetamine or cocaine abuse
- Carcinoid
- Essential hypertension

WORKUP

Laboratory evaluation and imaging studies to locate the neoplasm (Fig. 1). Misdiagnosis of pheochromocytoma is common. Correct interpretation of biochemical tests and imaging is crucial to a correct diagnosis.

LABORATORY TESTS

- Although there is no consensus on the best test, plasma-free metanephrines have been suggested as the test of first choice for excluding the tumor. Elevated plasma concentrations of normetanephrines or metanephrine have a sensitivity of up to 100%, but the specificity is markedly lower (85%).
- 24-hr urine collection will also show increased metanephrines (90% sensitivity, 95% specificity); the accuracy of the 24-hr urinary levels for metanephrines can be improved by indexing urinary metanephrine levels by urine creatinine levels.

TABLE 1 Autosomal Dominant Syndromes Associated with Pheochromocytoma and Paraganglioma

Syndrome	Gene	Gene Locus	Protein Product	Protein Function	Gene Mechanism	Typical Tumor Location
SDHD (familial paraganglioma type 1)*	SDHD	11q23	SDH D subunit	ATP production	Tumor suppressor	Skull base and neck; occasionally adrenal medulla, mediastinum, abdomen, pelvis
Familial paraganglioma type 2*	SDHAF2	11q13.1	Flavination cofactor	ATP production	Tumor suppressor	Skull base and neck; occasionally abdomen and pelvis
SDHC (familial paraganglioma type 3)	SDHC	1q21	SDH C subunit	ATP production	Tumor suppressor	Skull base and neck
SDHB (familial paraganglioma type 4)	SDHB	1p36.1-35	SDH B subunit	ATP production	Tumor suppressor	Abdomen, pelvis and mediastinum; rarely adrenal medulla, skull base, and neck
MEN1	MEN1	11q13	Menin	Transcription regulation	Tumor suppressor	Adrenal medulla
MEN2A and MEN2B	RET	10q11.2	RET	Tyrosine kinase receptor	Protooncogene	Adrenal medulla, bilaterally
Neurofibromatosis type 1	NF1	17q11.2	Neurofibromin	GTP hydrolysis	Tumor suppressor	Adrenal-periadrenal
von Hippel-Lindau disease	VHL	3p25-26	VHL	Transcription elongation suppression	Tumor suppressor	Adrenal medulla, bilaterally; occasionally paraganglioma
Familial pheochromocytoma	FP/TMEM127	2q11	Transmembrane protein	Regulation of the mTORC1 signaling complex	Tumor suppressor	Adrenal medulla

ATP, Adenosine triphosphate; GTP, guanosine triphosphate; MEN, multiple endocrine neoplasia; SDH, succinate dehydrogenase.
*Associated with maternal imprinting.
From Melmed S: Williams textbook of endocrinology, ed 12, Philadelphia, 2011, Saunders, Elsevier.

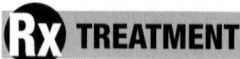

IMAGING STUDIES

- Abdominal CT scan (Fig. E2) with and without contrast (88% sensitivity) is useful in locating pheochromocytomas >0.5 inch in diameter (90% to 95% accurate).
- MRI with contrast: pheochromocytomas demonstrate a distinctive MRI appearance (up to 100% sensitivity); MRI may become the diagnostic imaging modality of choice.
- Scintigraphy with 131 or 1-123 I-MIBG (up to 100% sensitivity) (Fig. E2): this norepinephrine analog localizes in adrenergic tissue; it is particularly useful in locating extraadrenal pheochromocytomas.
- 6-[18F]Fluorodopamine positron emission tomography is reserved for cases in which clinical symptoms and signs suggest pheochromocytoma and results of biochemical tests are positive but conventional imaging studies cannot locate the tumor. It is also used for identification of metastatic disease.

Rx TREATMENT

GENERAL Rx

Laparoscopic adrenalectomy (surgical resection for both benign and malignant disease):

1. Preoperative stabilization with combination of alpha-adrenergic blocking agents (phenoxybenzamine, prazosin, doxazosin, or terazosin), beta-blocker, and liberal fluid and salt intake starting 10 to 14 days before surgery. Beta-blockers should be avoided until patients receive adequate alpha-adrenergic blockade for several days to avoid hypertensive crisis due to unopposed alpha stimulation. Amlodipine or verapamil can be added to beta-blockers if blood pressure control is still inadequate. Table E2 describes orally administered drugs to treat pheochromocytoma.

2. Hypertensive crisis preoperatively and intraoperatively can be controlled with nitroprusside. Table E3 summarizes intravenously administered drugs used to treat pheochromocytoma.

⊘ PEARLS & CONSIDERATIONS

COMMENTS

- Obtaining a detailed family history is important because 25% of pheochromocytomas are familial.
- Screening for pheochromocytoma should be considered in patients with any of the following:
  1. Malignant hypertension
  2. Poor response to antihypertensive therapy
  3. Paradoxical hypertensive response
  4. Hypertension during induction of anesthesia, parturition, surgery, or thyrotropin-releasing hormone testing
  5. Hypertension associated with imipramine or desipramine
  6. Neurofibromatosis (increased incidence of pheochromocytoma)
- All patients with pheochromocytoma should be screened for MEN-2 and von Hippel-Lindau disease with the pentagastrin test, serum parathyroid hormone, ophthalmoscopy, MRI of the brain, CT scan of the kidneys and pancreas, and ultrasonography of the testes.
- In patients with pheochromocytoma, routine analysis for mutations of *RET, VHL, SDHD,* and *SDHB* is indicated to identify pheochromocytoma-associated syndromes.

SUGGESTED READINGS

Available at www.expertconsult.com

RELATED CONTENT

Pheochromocytoma (Patient Information)
Hypertension (Related Key Topic)

AUTHORS: **BRETT PATRICK, M.D., MARK F. BRADY, M.D., M.P.H., M.M.S,** and **FRED F. FERRI, M.D.**

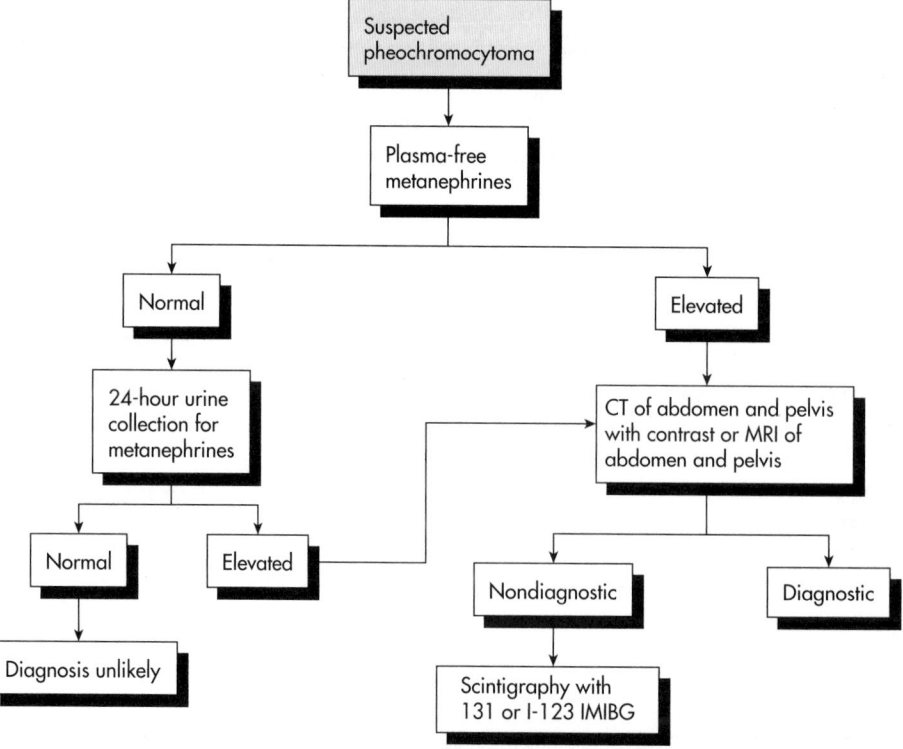

FIG. 1 Pheochromocytoma. *CT,* Computed tomography; *IMIBG,* iodine metaiodobenzyl guanidine; *MRI,* magnetic resonance imaging.

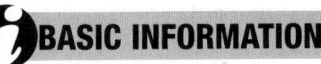

BASIC INFORMATION

DEFINITION

Specific phobias are anxiety disorders characterized by an excessive, persistent fear elicited by a specific object or situation that is then avoided or tolerated with intense distress. The provoking stimulus may be a specific object, such as an animal or insect; natural environments, such as heights or water; or a specific situation, such as the sight of blood, the receipt of an injection, or being in a tunnel or on a bridge. Social anxiety disorder (formerly named social phobia) is a specific, separately diagnosed disorder characterized by a fear of being embarrassed, humiliated, or rejected in social or performance situations. Agoraphobia also is a separately diagnosed disorder, characterized by an intense anxiety about being in a place or situation from which they would not be able to escape in the event of a panic attack or panic-like symptoms. Such situations include being in enclosed/crowded spaces or being more than a certain distance from home alone. If agoraphobia is present in individuals with panic disorder, both diagnoses are given.

SYNONYMS

Simple phobia (obsolete name for specific phobia)
Phobias named for the provoking stimulus, such as arachnophobia (fear of spiders) and acrophobia (fear of heights)

Specific phobias are codes:
ICD-10CM CODES
F40.1 Social phobias
F40.2 Specific phobias
F40.8 Other phobic anxiety disorders
F40.9 Phobic anxiety disorder, unspecified
Agoraphobia:
ICD-10CM CODES
F40.00

EPIDEMIOLOGY & DEMOGRAPHICS

PEAK INCIDENCE: The majority of cases of specific phobia tend to onset prior to age 10; median onset is from ages 7-10.
PREVALENCE (IN U.S.):
- Specific phobias are prevalent in 7% to 9% of the general population (12-month prevalence rate).
- Agoraphobia is prevalent in approximately 1.7% of the general population per year.
PREDOMINANT SEX AND AGE:
- Females with specific phobias outnumber males 2:1, though rates vary by phobia.
- Agoraphobia is more prevalent in women than men (2:1).
- Most specific phobias have childhood onset, although it is possible for them to develop at any age.
- Situational phobias tend to have a later age of onset compared to natural environment, animal, or blood-injection phobias.

- Onset of agoraphobia typically occurs in late adolescence or early adulthood; two thirds of cases onset prior to age 35.
GENETICS: Specific phobia is more common in first-degree relatives.

PHYSICAL FINDINGS & CLINICAL PRESENTATION

- When approaching the phobic stimulus, the experience of extreme anxiety is often accompanied by autonomic symptoms such as tachycardia, tremor, and diaphoresis; depersonalization may occur. In blood or injection phobias, symptoms are often followed by a parasympathetic response that can cause vasovagal syncope.
- Specific phobias frequently occur with other anxiety disorders.

ETIOLOGY

There is no clear etiology and likely is a combination of factors including temperamental (e.g., behavioral inhibition, neuroticism), environmental (e.g., negative encounters with the feared stimulus, parental overprotection), and genetic.

DIAGNOSIS

DIFFERENTIAL DIAGNOSIS

- Social anxiety disorder is distinguished from specific phobias in that what is feared is humiliation or embarrassment in social interaction or performance situations, rather than fear of a specific object or environment.
- Panic attacks (with or without agoraphobia): anxiety symptoms seen in specific phobia may resemble symptoms of panic attacks, but the stimulus in the specific or social situation is clear, whereas panic attacks do not have a clearly associated provoking stimulus (i.e., they occur unexpectedly in the absence of a trigger).
- Posttraumatic stress disorder (PTSD): anxiety and physiologic arousal associated with specific cues from the traumatic event defining the PTSD may resemble the symptoms induced by a phobia.
- Psychotic disorders can present with a fear of being in public that arises from delusions.

WORKUP

- History: usually diagnostic. This should include information about other medical disorders, medications, any history of past trauma, and substance abuse. Fig. 1 describes a diagnostic decision tree for specific phobias.
- Physical examination: to confirm absence of cardiovascular abnormalities such as arrhythmias or evidence of endocrinologic reasons for hyperarousal such as an enlarged or tender thyroid gland.

LABORATORY TESTS

No specific laboratory tests are indicated.

IMAGING STUDIES

No specific imaging studies are recommended.

TREATMENT

NONPHARMACOLOGIC THERAPY

- Cognitive-behavioral therapy (CBT) and exposure-based treatments have been effective for treating specific phobia in controlled trials and are considered an appropriate first-line treatment.
- Behavioral treatments sometimes involve relaxation training, often paired with visualization and progressive desensitization.
- Success rates in treating specific phobias are higher when the phobia is not complicated by other anxiety disorders.

ACUTE GENERAL Rx

- Although benzodiazepines provide rapid relief of anxiety associated with exposure to provoking stimuli, they are associated with adverse effects including somnolence, accidents, abuse, and dependence, and thus are not recommended as a first-line treatment.

CHRONIC Rx

- If the phobic stimulus is rarely encountered, benzodiazepines used on an as-needed basis can be an appropriate long-term treatment; however, there is a risk of abuse and dependence that makes them a less desirable choice for long-term treatment.

COMPLEMENTARY & ALTERNATIVE MEDICINE

No definitive evidence supports complementary or alternative medicines in the treatment of phobic disorders.

DISPOSITION

Phobic disorders are generally present for life, although outpatient-based treatment may effectively reduce symptoms.

REFERRAL

Recommended for confirmation of diagnosis and for evaluation for psychotherapy and other treatment modalities.

SUGGESTED READINGS
Available at www.expertconsult.com

RELATED CONTENT

Phobias (Patient Information)
Panic Disorder, With or Without Agoraphobia (Related Key Topic)
Posttraumatic Stress Disorder (Related Key Topic)
Social Anxiety Disorder (Related Key Topic)

AUTHOR: **KRISTY L. DALRYMPLE, PH.D.**

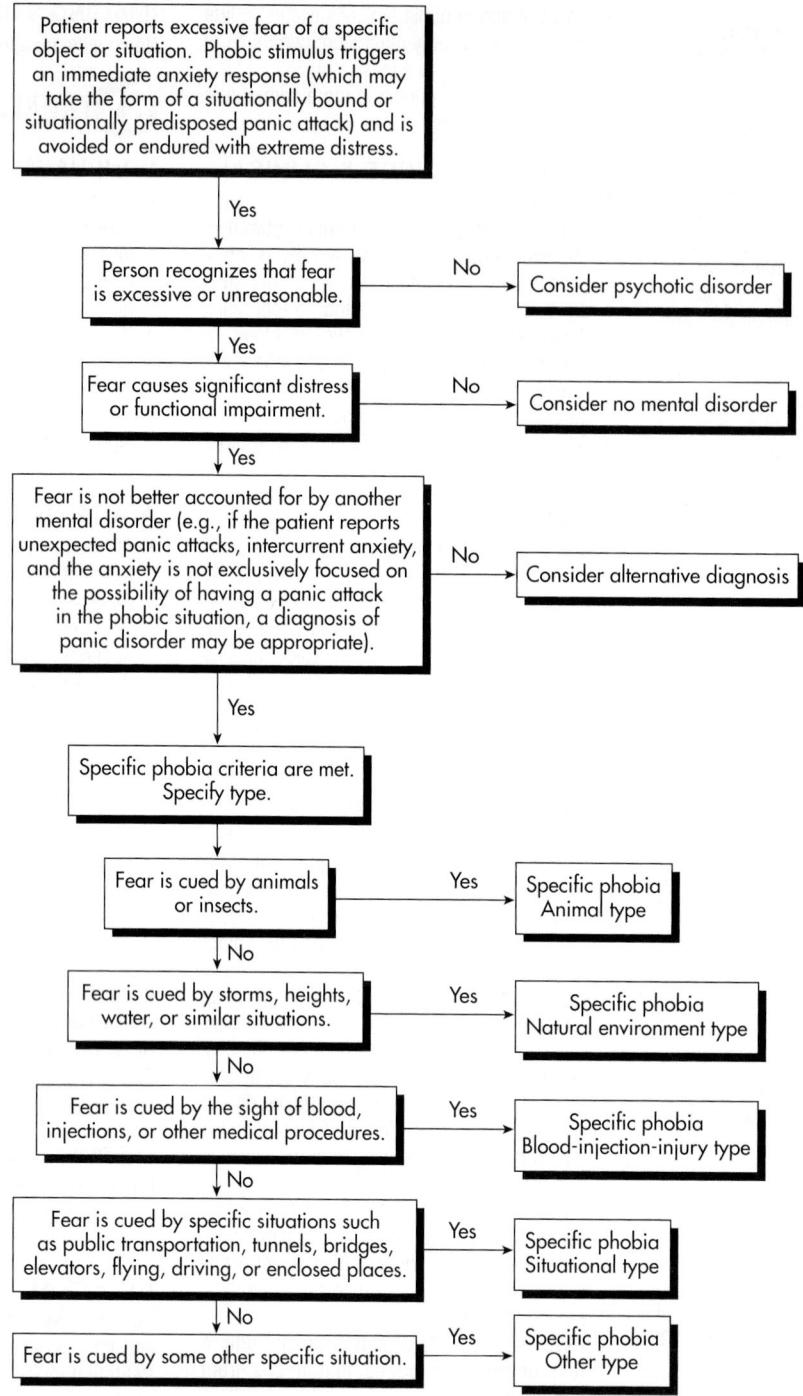

FIG. 1 Specific phobia: diagnostic decision tree. (From Lieberman, K: Social and specific phobias. In Lieberman K. (ed.): *Psychiatry behavioral science and clinical essentials: a companion to Tasman*, Philadelphia, 2000, Saunders, p. 368-378.)

ⓘ BASIC INFORMATION

DEFINITION

From the Latin words *pilus,* meaning "hair," and *nidus,* meaning "nest."

A *pilonidal sinus* is a short tract extending from the skin surface that contains hair and skin debris. It is most commonly found in the intergluteal fold sacrococcygeal region, but it can also occur in the interdigital area, umbilicus, chest wall, and scalp. An *acute pilonidal abscess* consists of pus and a wall of edematous fat. A chronic *pilonidal cyst* develops from a chronic abscess of long duration as a thin and flat lining of epithelium grows into the cavity from the skin surface.

SYNONYMS

Jeep disease: During World War II, many soldiers developed pilonidal cysts thought to be caused by hours of riding on Jeeps.
Pilonidal sinus
Pilonidal cyst

ICD-10CM CODES
L05	Pilonidal cyst
L05.0	Pilonidal cyst with abscess
L05.9	Pilonidal cysts without abscess

EPIDEMIOLOGY & DEMOGRAPHICS

INCIDENCE: 26 cases per 100,000 persons
PREDOMINANT SEX: Males are more commonly affected than females (2.2:1).
AVERAGE AGE OF PRESENTATION: 21 yr
RISK FACTORS:
- Male sex
- Local trauma or irritation
- Family predisposition
- Obesity
- Sedentary lifestyle
- Occupation requiring prolonged sitting or excessive exposure to hair (barbers)
- Local hirsutism
- Poor hygiene
- Increased sweat activity

PHYSICAL FINDINGS & CLINICAL PRESENTATION

- Asymptomatic pits or pores in the natal cleft (Fig. E1).
- Tenderness after physical activity or prolonged sitting.
- Acute pilonidal abscess presents as a hot, tender, fluctuant swelling just lateral to the midline over the sacrum that may exude pus through the midline pit.
- Acute pilonidal abscess in 20% of patients with pilonidal disease.
- Chronic pilonidal may have recurrent pain and drainage.
- Chronic pilonidal abscess in 80% of patients with pilonidal disease.
- Infrequently, systemic reaction: occasionally fever, leukocytosis, and malaise.

ETIOLOGY

- Currently believed to be acquired rather than congenital.
- Drilling of hair shed from the perineum or the head into sebaceous or hair follicles in the natal cleft.
- Drilling is facilitated by the friction of the natal cleft.
- Subsequent infection by skin organisms leads to pilonidal abscess.

ⒹⓍ DIAGNOSIS

DIFFERENTIAL DIAGNOSIS

- Perianal abscess arising from the posterior midline crypt
- Hidradenitis suppurativa
- Skin abscess: furuncle or carbuncle
- Folliculitis
- Anorectal fistula
- Anal complication of Crohn's disease
- Case report of squamous cell carcinoma arising from neglected chronic pilonidal sinuses

WORKUP

- Diagnosis is based on history and physical examination.
- Midline pits present behind the anus overlying the sacrum and coccyx.
- Broken hairs are often seen extruding from the midline pits.
- Insert probe in pilonidal sinus in path away from the anus.
- Complicated anal fistula may be angulating posteriorly before passing into a retrorectal abscess, but thorough examination of the anal cavity usually discloses point of origin.

ⓇⓍ TREATMENT

NONPHARMACOLOGIC THERAPY

Prevention of exacerbations:
1. Local hygiene.
2. Avoidance of prolonged sitting position.
3. Weight reduction.
4. Early in the infection, sitz baths may decrease pain and decrease the chance that a cyst may develop into an abscess.
5. Treatment of an symptomatic sinus is not indicated.

Treatment of Acute Abscess
- Procedure of choice for first-episode acute abscess: simple incision and drainage in an outpatient setting. Box E1 describes surgical options for the treatment of pilonidal sinus.
- Cure rate of about 50% within 5 weeks; recurrence rate 20% to 55%
- Antibiotics: generally not indicated, except for the treatment of cellulitis or in patients with immunosuppression, high risk of endocarditis, MRSA, or underlying systemic disease
- First-generation cephalosporin plus metronidazole is the antibiotic regimen of choice

TREATMENT OF CHRONIC OR RECURRENT DISEASE

Elective treatment of pilonidal disease:
1. Minimal surgery:
   a. Remove hair from midline pits and shave buttocks.
   b. May use a fine wire brush with local anesthesia to clear the pits and any lateral openings of granulation tissue and hair (Fig. E2).
   c. Keep area clean.
2. Fistulotomy and curettage:
   a. Used when minimal surgery does not control episodes of suppuration
   b. Pass probe to outline the pilonidal sinus and open tract surgically
   c. Curette granulation tissue at the base of the sinus and excise edges of the skin
   d. Keep open granulating wound meticulously clean and allow to heal
   e. If complete healing does not take place, use a skin graft or advancement flap to close the defect
3. Marsupialization:
   a. This is the treatment of choice for chronic pilonidal disease.
   b. Wide excision of the pilonidal area is performed, including all affected skin and subcutaneous tissues down to the presacral fascia.
   c. Wound is left open, allowed to marsupialize, or closed as a primary procedure.
   d. Give antibiotics for 24 hr (particularly those directed against *Staphylococcus* and *Bacteroides* species).
4. Other procedures:
   a. Excision and primary closure or closure with skin grafts or flaps: Z-plasty, V-Y advancement flap, rhomboid flap, gluteus maximus myocutaneous flap
   b. Bascom procedure (follicle removal and lateral drainage)
   c. Recurrence rate for excision (most definitive procedure): 1% to 6%
   d. Incidence of squamous cell carcinoma in a chronic, recurrent pilonidal sinus is rare (<1%)

REFERRAL

- Emergency department for incision and drainage for an acute abscess
- General surgeon for elective treatment or management of chronic or recurrent disease

⚠ PEARLS & CONSIDERATIONS

COMMENTS

Because of significant associated morbidity, the elective surgical procedures outlined are performed only after the potential risks versus benefits are carefully weighed by a general or colorectal surgeon.

RELATED CONTENT

Pilonidal Cyst (Patient Information)

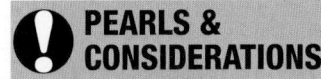

AUTHOR: **MARIA E. SOLER, M.D., M.P.H., M.B.A.**

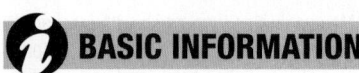

BASIC INFORMATION

DEFINITION

Pinworms are a noninvasive infestation of the intestinal tract by *Enterobius vermicularis*, a helminth of the nematode family. It is a small (1 cm in length), white, thread-like roundworm that typically inhabits the cecum, appendix, and adjacent areas of the ileum and ascending colon.

SYNONYMS

Enterobiasis
Oxyuriasis

ICD-10CM CODES
B80 Enterobiasis

EPIDEMIOLOGY & DEMOGRAPHICS

- Most common intestinal nematode; approximately 30,000 cases annually in the United States.
- Worldwide distribution, but most common in temperate climates.
- The prevalence of pinworm infection is lowest in infants and reaches highest infection rate in school-age children (ages 5-14 yr).
- Eggs are infective within 6 hr of oviposition and may remain so for 20 days.
- Clusters are found in families, institutionalized persons, and homosexual men.

PHYSICAL FINDINGS & CLINICAL PRESENTATION

- Most infested persons are asymptomatic.
- Perianal itching is the most common reported symptom, with scratching leading to excoriation and sometimes secondary infection.
- The vagina may become infested with pinworms.
- Rarely insomnia, irritability, anorexia, and weight loss are described.
- Granulomas have been described in various organs resulting from worms wandering outside the intestines and dying there.

ETIOLOGY & PATHOGENESIS

- *E. vermicularis* is highly prevalent throughout the world, particularly in countries of the temperate zone. Human beings are the only host for this worm. Infestation is by fecal-oral route; ingested eggs hatch in the stomach and the larvae migrate to the colon, where they mature. Gravid female worms containing an average of 10,000 ova migrate to the perianal skin at night, lay their eggs there, and die. The eggs embryonate within 6 hr and cause itching; scratching causes egg deposition under fingernails, from which they can contaminate food or lead to autoreinfection. Ova may also be airborne and collect in dust that may be on the floor or on furniture.
- *E. vermicularis* may be transmitted between sexual partners, especially those engaging in oral-anal sex.

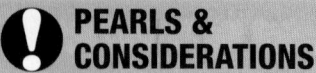

DIAGNOSIS

DIFFERENTIAL DIAGNOSIS

- Perianal itching related to poor hygiene
- Hemorrhoidal disease and anal fissures
- Perineal yeast/fungal infections
  Section II describes the causes of pruritus ani.

WORKUP

Identification of adult worms or eggs. *E. vermicularis* ova are ovoid but flattened on one side and measure approximately 56 × 27 micrometers (Fig. 1). The eggs can be identified on transparent tape placed on the perianal skin on awakening. (NOTE: Five consecutive negative tests rule out the diagnosis.) A single examination detects 50% of infections, three examinations detect 90%, and five examinations detect 99%.

TREATMENT

- Single dose of mebendazole (100 mg) with a repeat dose given after 2 wk results in cure rates of 90% to 100%.
- Single dose of albendazole (400 mg) with a second dose given 2 wk later is also highly effective.
- Pyrantel pamoate (11 mg/kg up to 1 g) can prevent against *E. vermicularis*. It is available as a suspension and has minimal toxicity (mild transient gastrointestinal symptoms, headache, drowsiness). A repeat dose after 2 wk is recommended because of the frequency of reinfection and autoinfection.
- Other infected family members, classmates, or residents of long-term care facilities should be treated at the same time as the index case.

PEARLS & CONSIDERATIONS

- Eosinophilia is not observed in most cases because tissue invasion does not occur.
- Good hand hygiene is the most effective method of prevention.
- Frequent changing of underclothes, bed clothes, and bed sheets is helpful to decrease risk of autoinfection.
- Personal hygiene and cleanliness are crucial. Fingernails should be cut short and scrubbed frequently.

RELATED CONTENT

Pinworms (Patient Information)

AUTHOR: **FRED F. FERRI, M.D.**

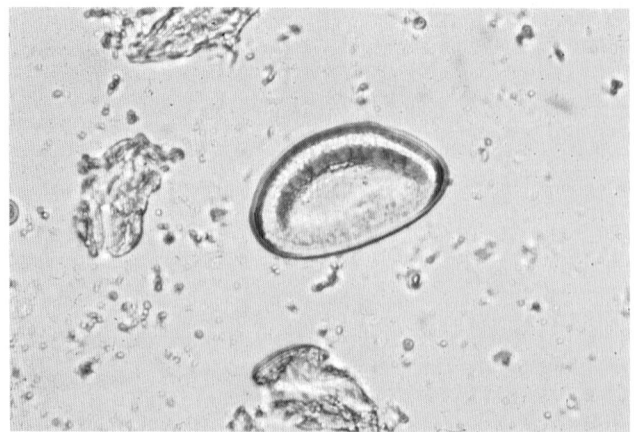

FIG. 1 Enterobius vermicularis embryonated egg. Note larva inside (40 × 10 μm). (From Gorbach SL et al [eds]: *Infectious diseases*, ed 2, Philadelphia, 1998, Saunders.)

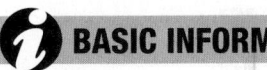

BASIC INFORMATION

DEFINITION

Pituitary adenoma is a benign neoplasm of the anterior lobe of the pituitary that causes symptoms, either by excess secretion of hormones or by a local mass effect as the tumor impinges on other, nearby structures (e.g., optic chiasm, hypothalamus, pituitary stalk). Pituitary adenomas are classified by their size, function, and features that characterize their appearance. Microadenomas are <10 mm in size, macroadenomas are ≥10 mm in size, and giant adenomas are ≥40 mm in size.

- *Acromegaly* is the disease state characterized by a pituitary adenoma that secretes growth hormone (GH).
- A *prolactinoma* secretes prolactin (PRL).
- *Cushing's disease* is a disease state of hypersecretion of adrenocorticotropic hormone (ACTH).
- *Thyrotropin-secreting pituitary adenomas* secrete primarily thyroid-stimulating hormone (TSH).
- *Nonsecretory pituitary adenomas* are those in which the neoplasm is a space-occupying lesion whose secretory products do not cause a specific disease state.

ICD-10CM CODES
D35.2 Benign neoplasm of pituitary gland

EPIDEMIOLOGY & DEMOGRAPHICS

CLASSIFICATION (BY HORMONE SECRETED):
- PRL only: 35%.
- No hormone: 30%.
- GH only: 20%.
- PRL and GH: 7%.
- ACTH: 7%.
- Luteinizing hormone (LH), follicle-stimulating hormone (FSH), TSH: 1%.

PREVALENCE/INCIDENCE:
- Pituitary adenomas: up to 10% to 15% of all intracranial neoplasms; 3% to 27% at autopsy series.
- Prolactinomas: up to 20% in women with unexplained primary or secondary amenorrhea. Prolactinomas account for 32% to 62% of pituitary adenomas.
- GH-secreting pituitary adenoma: 50 to 60 cases per 1 million persons. They account for 8% to 16% of pituitary tumors.
- Thyrotropin-secreting pituitary adenoma: 1% of pituitary adenomas with a slight female/male predominance of 1.7:1
- Corticotropin-secreting pituitary adenomas: female/male predominance of 8:1 but overall uncommon diagnosis, accounting for 2% to 6% of adenomas.

PHYSICAL FINDINGS & CLINICAL PRESENTATION

PROLACTINOMAS:
- Females:
  1. Galactorrhea.
  2. Amenorrhea.
  3. Oligomenorrhea with anovulation.
  4. Infertility.
  5. Estrogen deficiency and associated osteopenia.
  6. Decreased vaginal lubrication.
- Males:
  1. Large tumors more common as a result of delayed diagnosis.
  2. Possible impotence, decreased libido, or hypogonadism.
  3. Galactorrhea rare because males lack the estrogen-dependent breast growth and differentiation.

GH-SECRETING PITUITARY ADENOMA: ACROMEGALY:
- Coarse facial features.
- Oily skin.
- Prognathism.
- Carpal tunnel syndrome.
- Osteoarthritis.
- History of increased hat, glove, or shoe size.
- Decreased exercise capacity.
- Visual field deficits.
- Diabetes mellitus.

CORTICOTROPIN-SECRETING PITUITARY ADENOMA: CUSHING'S DISEASE:
- Usually present when the tumor is small (1 to 2 mm).
- 50% of the tumors <<5 mm.
- Other symptoms:
  1. Truncal obesity.
  2. Round facies (moon face).
  3. Dorsocervical fat accumulation (buffalo hump).
  4. Hirsutism.
  5. Acne.
  6. Menstrual disorders.
  7. Hypertension.
  8. Striae.
  9. Bruising.
  10. Thin skin.
  11. Hyperglycemia.

THYROTROPIN-SECRETING PITUITARY ADENOMA:
- In males, larger, more invasive, and more rapidly growing tumors that present later in life.
- Other symptoms: thyrotoxicosis, goiter, visual impairment.

NONSECRETORY PITUITARY ADENOMAS (ENDOCRINE INACTIVE PITUITARY ADENOMA):
- Usually large at the time of diagnosis.
- Symptoms:
  1. Bitemporal hemianopsia as a result of compression of the optic chiasm.
  2. Hypopituitarism from compression of the pituitary gland.
  3. Hypogonadism in men and in premenopausal women.
  4. Cranial nerve deficits caused by extension into the cavernous sinus.
  5. Hydrocephalus from extension into the third ventricle, compressing the foramen of Monro.
  6. Diabetes insipidus resulting from compression of the hypothalamus or pituitary stalk (a rare complication).

ETIOLOGY

Benign neoplasms of epithelial origin

DIAGNOSIS

DIFFERENTIAL DIAGNOSIS

PROLACTINOMA:
- Pregnancy.
- Postpartum puerperium.
- Primary hypothyroidism.
- Breast disease.
- Breast stimulation.
- Drug ingestion (especially phenothiazines, antidepressants, haloperidol, methyldopa, reserpine, opiates, amphetamines, and cimetidine).
- Chronic renal failure.
- Liver disease.
- Polycystic ovarian disease.
- Chest wall disorders.
- Spinal cord lesions.
- Previous cranial irradiation.

ACROMEGALY: Ectopic production of GH-releasing hormone from a carcinoid or other neuroendocrine tumor

CUSHING'S DISEASE:
- Diseases that cause ectopic sources of ACTH overproduction (including small-cell carcinoma of the lung, bronchial carcinoid, intestinal carcinoid, pancreatic islet cell tumor, medullary thyroid carcinoma, or pheochromocytoma).
- Adrenal adenomas, adrenal carcinoma.
- Nelson's syndrome.

THYROTROPIN-SECRETING PITUITARY ADENOMAS: Primary hypothyroidism.

NONSECRETORY PITUITARY ADENOMA: Nonneoplastic mass lesions of various etiologies (e.g., infectious, granulomatous).

WORKUP

Pituitary adenomas should be identified at an early stage so that effective treatment can be implemented.

Screening tests for functional pituitary adenomas are described in Table 1.

PROLACTINOMA: First step: measurement of basal PRL levels (practitioners should be aware of discriminatory values in their own institutions).
- Elevated PRL levels are correlated with tumor size.
- Level >200 ng/ml indicates likely prolactinoma, with levels of 100 to 200 ng/ml being equivocal and possibly associated with medications or other sources.
- Basal PRL levels between 20 and 100 suggest a microadenoma as well as other conditions such as psychotropic drug ingestion, recent breast examination, and even a recent meal.
- Basal level <<20 ng/ml is usually considered normal. Each laboratory should develop its own normative values, however, and practitioner should refer to these values.
- Threshold level for obtaining imaging such as MRI should be developed by individual providers depending on the level of specificity and sensitivity desired.

ACROMEGALY:
- First screening tests are the measurement of the serum insulin-like growth factor I level, postprandial serum GH, and TRH stimulation test.

TABLE 1 Screening Tests for Functional Pituitary Adenomas

Disorder	Test	Comments
Acromegaly	IGF1 OGTT with GH obtained at 0, 30, and 60 min.	Interpret IGF1 relative to age- and gender-matched controls. Normal subjects should suppress GH to <1 µg/L.
Prolactinoma	Serum PRL level.	A level >500 µg/L is pathognomonic for macroprolactinoma. If >200 µg/L, prolactinoma is likely.*
Cushing's disease	24-hr UFC Nighttime salivary cortisol dexamethasone (1 mg) at 11 PM and fasting plasma cortisol measured at 8 AM ACTH assay	Ensure that urine collection is total and accurate by measuring urinary creatinine. Free salivary cortisol reflects circadian rhythm, and elevated levels may indicate Cushing's disease. Normal subjects suppress to <1.8 µg/dL. Distinguishes adrenal adenoma from ectopic ACTH or Cushing's disease.
TSH-secreting tumor	TSH measurement Free T_4 by dialysis Total T_3.	If T_4 or T_3 is elevated and TSH is measurable or elevated, a TSH-secreting tumor may be present.

ACTH, adrenocorticotropic hormone; *GH*, growth hormone; *IGF1*, insulin-like growth factor type 1; *OGTT*, oral glucose tolerance test; *PRL*, prolactin; *T3*, triiodothyronine; *T4*, thyroxine; *TSH*, thyroid-stimulating hormone; *UFC*, urinary free cortisol.
*Risperidone may result in prolactin levels >200 µg/L.
From Melmed S et al: *Williams textbook of endocrinology*, ed 12, Philadelphia, 2011, WB Saunders.

- Follow with an oral glucose tolerance test.
- Failure to suppress serum GH to <2 ng/ml with an oral load of 100 g glucose is considered conclusive.
- A GH-releasing hormone level >300 ng/ml is indicative of an ectopic source of GH.

CUSHING'S DISEASE:
- Measurement of late-night salivary cortisol level is the best screening test.
- Normal or slightly elevated corticotropin levels ranging from 20 to 200 pg/ml; normal is 10 to 50 pg/ml (normative data should be developed by each institution for its population).
- Level <<10 pg/ml usually indicates an autonomously secreting adrenal tumor.
- Level >>200 pg/ml suggests an ectopic corticotropin-secreting neoplasm.
- Cushing's disease can be assessed by absence of cortisol suppression with the low-dose dexamethasone test but with the presence of cortisol suppression after the high-dose test. As a method to distinguish Cushing's disease from an ectopic source of ACTH, this test is robust.
- 24-hr urine collection should demonstrate an increased level of cortisol excretion.

THYROTROPIN-SECRETING PITUITARY ADENOMA:
- Highly sensitive thyrotropin assays, which evaluate the presence of thyrotoxicosis, are one way to detect a thyrotropin-secreting tumor.
- Free alpha subunit is secreted by >80% of tumors, with the ratio of the alpha subunit to thyrotropin <1.
- With central resistance to thyroid hormone, ratio is <1, and the sella is normal.

- Laboratory tests show elevated serum levels of both T_3 and T_4.

NONSECRETORY PITUITARY ADENOMA:
- Visual field testing.
- Assessment of the pituitary and organ function to determine if there is hypopituitarism or hypersecretion of hormones (even if the effects of hypersecretion are subclinical).
- TRH to provoke secretion of FSH, LH, and LH-beta-subunit; will not elicit response in normal persons.
- Exclusion of Klinefelter's syndrome in patient with longstanding primary hypogonadism, elevated gonadotropin levels, and enlargement of the sella.

IMAGING STUDIES

Study of choice: MRI of the pituitary (Fig. E1) and hypothalamus. If an MRI shows the tumor impinging on the optic chiasm then formal visual field testing is indicated.
- When evaluating Cushing's disease, small size at the onset of symptoms noted.
- MRI, in this case, only 60% sensitive at best and may yield false-positive results.
- CT scan only when MRI is unavailable or is otherwise contraindicated.

Rx TREATMENT

NONPHARMACOLOGIC THERAPY
SURGERY:
- Selective transsphenoidal resection of the adenoma (Table 2) is the treatment of choice for acromegaly, Cushing's disease, and thyrotropin-secreting pituitary adenomas, all of which tend to be microadenomas at the time of onset of symptoms.

TABLE 2 Transsphenoidal Pituitary Surgery

Primary Indications

General

Visual tract or central nervous system compression arising from within sella
Relief of compressive hypopituitarism by presenting, residual, or recurrent tumor tissue
Tumor recurrence after surgery or irradiation
Pituitary hemorrhage
Cerebrospinal fluid leak
Resistance to medical therapy
Intolerance of medical therapy
Personal choice
Desire for immediate pregnancy with macroadenoma
Requirement for diagnostic tissue histology

Specific

Acromegaly
Cushing's disease
Clinically nonfunctioning macroadenoma
Prolactinoma
Nelson's syndrome
TSH-secreting adenoma

Side Effects

Transient

Diabetes insipidus
Cerebrospinal fluid leak and rhinorrhea
Inappropriate ADH secretion
Arachnoiditis
Meningitis
Postoperative psychosis
Local hematoma
Arterial wall damage
Epistaxis
Local abscess
Pulmonary embolism
Narcolepsy

Permanent (up to 10%)

Diabetes insipidus
Total or partial hypopituitarism
Visual loss
Inappropriate ADH secretion
Vascular occlusion
CNS damage: oculomotor palsy, hemiparesis, encephalopathy
Nasal septum perforation

Surgery-Related Mortality (up to 1%)

Brain, hypothalamic
Vascular damage
Postoperative meningitis
Cerebrospinal fluid leak
Pneumocephalus
Acute cardiopulmonary disease
Anesthesia-related
Seizure

ADH, Antidiuretic hormone; *CNS*, central nervous system; *TSH*, thyroid-stimulating hormone.
From Melmed S et al: *Williams textbook of endocrinology*, ed 12, Philadelphia, 2011, WB Saunders.

- Macroadenomas, such as the nonsecretory pituitary adenoma, may also be surgically removed, but risk of recurrence is greater with these tumors and adjunctive therapy such as irradiation may also be necessary.
- Bilateral adrenalectomy has been performed in patients with Cushing's disease after failure of other therapies; complications requiring

lifelong hormone replacement or Nelson's syndrome (rapid enlargement of pituitary tumor due to adrenal resection) may occur.

RADIOTHERAPY:
- Radiotherapy is used primarily as adjuvant treatment. It is reserved for patients who have not responded to surgical treatment and who still have symptoms of the adenoma.
- Used with varying degrees of success in all the different pituitary adenomas.
- Radiotherapy complications include long-term hypopituitarism (40% of patients) and secondary neoplasms (1.5% of patients).

ACUTE GENERAL Rx

PROLACTINOMA:
- For prolactinomas, initial therapy is generally dopamine agonists. Bromocriptine, a dopamine analogue, is generally given orally in divided doses of 1.5 to 10 mg. Cabergoline is given once or twice weekly. It is better tolerated and more effective than bromocriptine for tumor shrinkage but more expensive.
- Side effects include orthostatic hypotension, nausea, and dizziness; avoided by beginning with low-dose therapy.
- Other compounds include pergolide mesylate, a long-acting ergot derivative with dopaminergic properties, as well as other nonergot derivatives.

ACROMEGALY:
- Somatostatin analogues: octreotide, lanreotide administered as monthly injections.
- Cabergoline or bromocriptine can also be used. They have modest activity but can be administered orally and are less expensive than somatostatin analogues.
- Pegvisomant can also be used to normalize IGF-1 levels.

CUSHING'S DISEASE:
- Ketoconazole, which inhibits the cytochrome P-450 enzymes involved in steroid biosynthesis, is effective in managing mild to moderate disease in daily oral doses of 600 to 1200 mg.
- Metyrapone and aminoglutethimide can be used to control hypersecretion of cortisol but are generally used when preparing a patient for surgery or while waiting for a response to radiotherapy.

THYROTROPIN-SECRETING PITUITARY ADENOMA:
- Ablative therapy with either radioactive iodide or surgery is indicated.
- Treatment directed to the thyroid alone may accelerate growth of the pituitary adenoma.
- Octreotide has been shown to be effective in doses similar to those used for acromegaly.

NONSECRETORY PITUITARY ADENOMA:
- There is no role for medical therapy at this time.

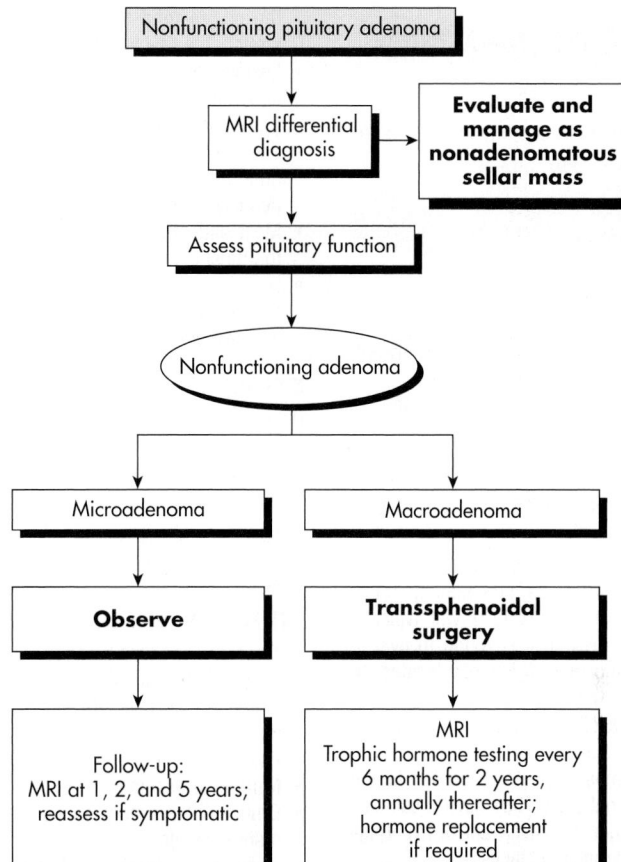

FIG. 2 **Management of nonfunctioning pituitary adenomas.** Skilled interpretation of magnetic resonance images is crucial to diagnosing a nonadenomatous mass such as a meningioma, aneurysm, or other sellar lesion. (From Melmed S et al: *Williams textbook of endocrinology*, ed 12, Philadelphia, 2011, WB Saunders.)

- Surgery and radiotherapy may be indicated. An algorithm for the management of nonfunctioning pituitary adenomas is described in Fig. 2.

CHRONIC Rx
For all pituitary adenomas:
- Careful follow-up is important. Patients undergoing transsphenoidal microsurgical resection should be seen in 4 to 6 wk to ensure that the adenoma has been completely removed and that the endocrine hypersecretion is resolved.
- If there is good clinical response, patient should be monitored yearly for recurrence and to follow the level of the hypersecreted hormone.
- Patients who have undergone irradiation should have close follow-up with backup medical therapy because response to radiotherapy may be delayed; incidence of hypopituitarism also increases with time.

- Surgical resection is not indicated in pituitary incidentalomas that are microadenomas since only 10% will experience tumor growth.

SUGGESTED READINGS
Available at www.expertconsult.com

RELATED CONTENT
Evaluation of Suspected Pituitary Tumor (Algorithm, Section III)
Pituitary Adenoma (Patient Information)
Acromegaly (Related Key Topic)
Amenorrhea (Related Key Topic)
Cushing's Disease and Syndrome (Related Key Topic)
Galactorrhea (Related Key Topic)
Prolactinoma (Related Key Topic)

AUTHOR: **RUBEN ALVERO, M.D.**

P

Diseases
and Disorders

I

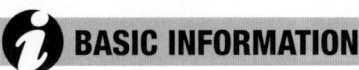

BASIC INFORMATION

DEFINITION
Pityriasis is a common self-limiting skin eruption of unknown etiology.

ICD-10CM CODES
L42 Pityriasis rosea

EPIDEMIOLOGY & DEMOGRAPHICS
- Most cases of pityriasis rosea occur between ages 10 and 35 yr; mean age is 23 yr.
- The incidence of disease is highest in the fall and spring.
- Female/male ratio is 1.5:1.

PHYSICAL FINDINGS & CLINICAL PRESENTATION
- Initial lesion (herald patch), an annular pink patch with trailing scale, precedes the eruption by approximately 1 to 2 wk; typically measures 3 to 6 cm; it is round to oval in appearance and most frequently located on the trunk (Fig. 1).
- Eruptive phase follows within 2 wk and peaks after 7 to 14 days.
- Lesions are most frequently located in the lower abdominal area. They have a salmon-pink appearance in whites and a hyperpigmented appearance in blacks.
- Most lesions are 4 to 5 mm in diameter; center has a "cigarette paper" appearance; border has a characteristic ring of scale (collarette). When stretched across the long axis, the scales tend to fold across the lines of stretch, the so-called "hanging curtain sign."
- Lesions occur in a symmetric distribution and follow the cleavage lines of the trunk (Christmas tree pattern).
- The number of lesions varies from a few to hundreds. They generally disappear spontaneously after 3 to 8 weeks.
- Most patients are asymptomatic; pruritus is the most common symptom.
- History of recent fatigue, headache, sore throat, and low-grade fever is present in approximately 25% of cases.

ETIOLOGY
Unknown, possibly viral exanthem. Active replication of human herpesvirus (HHV)-6 and HHV-7 has been demonstrated in mononuclear cells of lesional skin.

DIAGNOSIS

DIFFERENTIAL DIAGNOSIS
- Tinea corporis (can be ruled out by potassium hydroxide examination).
- Secondary syphilis (absence of herald patch, positive serologic test for syphilis).
- Psoriasis.
- Nummular eczema.
- Drug eruption: medications that may cause rashes similar to pityriasis rosea include clonidine, captopril, interferon, bismuth, barbiturates, gold, hepatitis B vaccine, and imatinib mesylate.
- Other viral exanthem.
- Seborrheic dermatitis.
- Eczema.
- Lichen planus.
- Tinea versicolor (the lesions are more brown and the borders are not as ovoid).
- Erythema migrans.

WORKUP
Presence of herald lesion and characteristic rash are diagnostic. Skin biopsy is generally reserved for atypical cases.

LABORATORY TESTS
Generally not necessary; serologic test for syphilis if clinically indicated.

TREATMENT

NONPHARMACOLOGIC THERAPY
The disease is self-limited and generally does not require any therapeutic intervention.

ACUTE GENERAL Rx
- Use calamine lotion or oral antihistamines in patients with significant pruritus. Corticosteroid lotions or creams also provide some relief from itching.
- Use prednisone tapered over 2 wk in patients with severe pruritus.
- Direct sun exposure or use of ultraviolet light within the first week of eruption is beneficial in decreasing the severity of disease.
- One small trial showed improvement of rash and pruritus with erythromycin 250 mg qid for 2 weeks.

DISPOSITION
- Spontaneous complete resolution of the rash within 4 to 8 wk.
- Recurrence rare (<2% of cases).

PEARLS & CONSIDERATIONS

COMMENTS
Reassure patient that the disease is not contagious and its course is benign.

SUGGESTED READING
Available at www.expertconsult.com

RELATED CONTENT
Pityriasis Rosea (Patient Information)

AUTHOR: **FRED F. FERRI, M.D.**

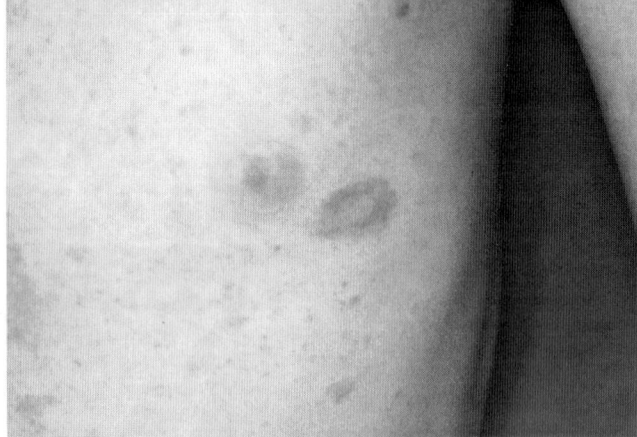

FIG. 1 Herald patch and surrounding pityriasis rosea. (From Kliegman RM et al: *Nelson textbook of pediatrics,* ed 19, Philadelphia, 2011, Saunders.)

BASIC INFORMATION

DEFINITION

Placenta previa is the presence of placental tissue over the internal cervical os. Four degrees of this abnormality (Fig. 1) have been traditionally defined; however, the accurate localization of the placental edge in relation to the discrete point of the internal os with transvaginal sonography makes the following terms outmoded:
1. Total placenta previa: the internal os is covered completely.
2. Partial placenta previa: the internal os is partially covered.
3. Marginal placenta previa: the edge of the placenta is at the margin of the internal os.
4. Low-lying placenta: the placental edge is <2 cm from, but not covering, the internal os.

Placenta previa should be described by the distance that the placental edge covers the internal os.

ICD-10CM CODES
O44   Placenta previa
O44.0 Placenta previa specified as without hemorrhage
O44.1 Placenta previa specified as with hemorrhage

EPIDEMIOLOGY & DEMOGRAPHICS

INCIDENCE: 0.26% to 0.7% of pregnancies in the surgically naïve uterus

1.2% to 4.2% in uteri with history of at least one prior cesarean delivery or greater than two prior cesarean deliveries, respectively

RISK FACTORS:
- Previous placenta previa
- Previous cesarean delivery (after one cesarean delivery, the risk is 1% to 4%; after four or more, the risk approaches 10%)
- Multiparity
- Multiple gestation
- Smoking and cocaine use
- Previous intrauterine surgical procedure or Asherman syndrome
- Abnormal or large placenta

PHYSICAL FINDINGS & CLINICAL PRESENTATION

The classic presentation of placenta previa is painless vaginal bleeding, usually in the second

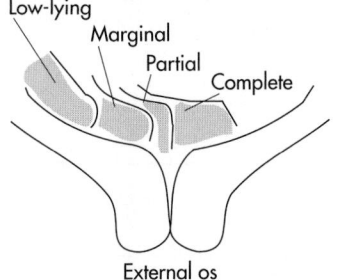

FIG. 1 Depiction of degrees of placenta previa. (From Weissleder R et al: *Primer of diagnostic imaging,* St Louis, 2007, Mosby.)

or third trimester. Uterine contractions may or may not be present. On physical examination, the uterus is soft and pain free. The fetus is often in breech, transverse lie, or high. Fetal distress is usually not present.

DIAGNOSIS

DIFFERENTIAL DIAGNOSIS
- Morbidly adherent placenta (accreta, increta, percreta)
- Vasa previa
- Abruptio placentae
- Vaginal or cervical trauma
- Labor
- Local malignancy

WORKUP
- Do *not* perform a digital vaginal examination.
- The diagnosis of placenta previa can seldom be firmly established by physical examination alone. A speculum examination in a hospital setting to exclude any local bleeding may be performed.
- This diagnosis should not be dismissed until thorough evaluation, including sonography (preferably transvaginal unless the previa is clearly central), has completely excluded its presence.

LABORATORY TESTS
- A complete blood count can be used to monitor hemoglobin and hematocrit.
- A Kleihauer-Betke preparation of maternal blood in all Rh-negative women and Rh-immune globulin when indicated

IMAGING STUDIES
- The simplest and safest method of placental localization is transabdominal sonography with confirmatory imaging by transvaginal ultrasonography (TVS). Transabdominal ultrasound alone is inaccurate in the diagnosis of placenta previa and should be used only as a screening tool. TVS (Fig. 2) has become the gold standard for the diagnosis of placenta previa. It is safe even in the presence of active bleeding. Translabial (transperineal) imaging is an alternative technique by experienced providers. A distance of <20 mm from placental edge to interior cervical os is becoming a new criterion for performing term cesarean delivery in women with placenta previa.
- MRI has also been effective in detecting placenta previa, although sonography remains the preferred method due to lower cost, widespread availability, and well-established accuracy.

TREATMENT

NONPHARMACOLOGIC THERAPY
- In preterm pregnancies with no active bleeding, close observation and expectant management are indicated. In those with active bleeding, conservative management, including blood transfusions for severe bleeds, is

appropriate. The woman should stay in the hospital for at least 48 hr after the bleeding has stopped.
- Once diagnosed, and if prior to 32 weeks' gestation, a follow-up ultrasound should be performed at 32 weeks to determine whether a previa is still present, as many will have resolved by this gestational age. If resolution of previa is noted, transvaginal ultrasonography with color and pulsed Doppler is recommended to exclude the possibility of vasa previa.
- Pelvic rest should be prescribed as long as placenta previa remains the diagnosis. Bed rest is recommended by some providers..

ACUTE GENERAL Rx
- Initial assessment for signs of maternal hemodynamic compromise or hemorrhagic shock; large-bore IV access with crystalloid fluid resuscitation.
- Assess fetal status and gestational age by sonogram and continuous fetal heart rate monitoring.
- Cross-matched blood should be made available during bleeding episodes; if the hemorrhage is severe, cesarean delivery is indicated despite fetal immaturity.
- Tocolytic therapy may be considered in those women in preterm labor, as well as the administration of corticosteroids to enhance fetal lung maturity.
- Magnesium sulfate therapy for fetal neuroprotection should be considered in those with symptomatic preterm (less than 32 weeks) placenta previa if the decision has been made to likely deliver the patient within 24 hours. Emergent delivery should not be delayed to administer magnesium.

CHRONIC Rx
- Cesarean delivery is necessary in nearly all cases of placenta previa.
- Uncontrollable hemorrhage after placental removal should be anticipated as a result of the poorly contractile nature of the lower uterine segment. The need for hysterectomy to control bleeding should be discussed with the patient before delivery.

DISPOSITION
Because of the unpredictable nature of placenta previa, not all women with placenta previa can be treated expectantly.

REFERRAL
Affected women and their families should be aware of all signs and symptoms that would necessitate immediate transport to the hospital. The possibility of hysterectomy should also be discussed early during pregnancy.

PEARLS & CONSIDERATIONS

COMMENTS
Third-trimester measurement of the distance from the placental edge to the internal cervical os by TVS commonly is used to gauge

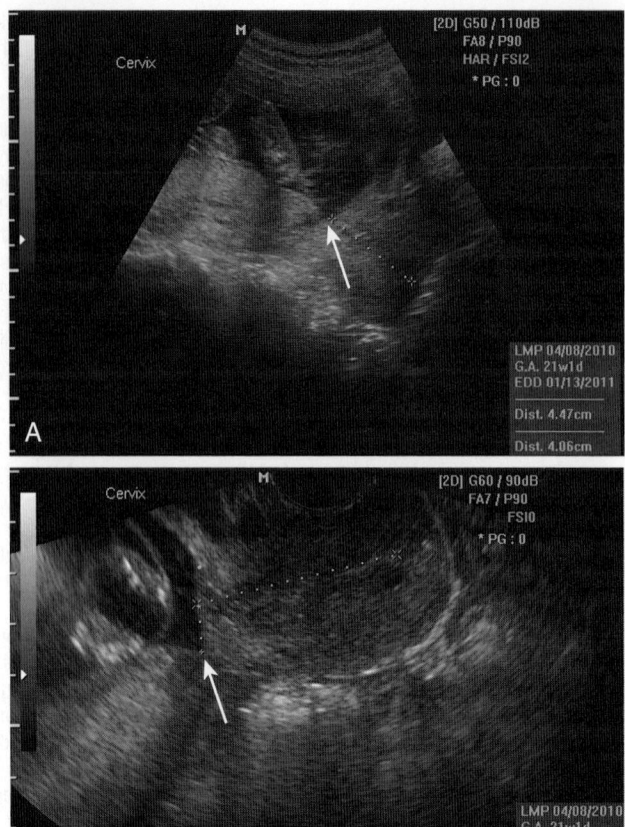

FIG. 2 Transabdominal and transvaginal ultrasounds of marginal placenta previa. *Arrows* identify placental edge. (Courtesy K. Francois. From Gabbe SG: *Obstetrics*, ed 6, Philadelphia, 2012, WB Saunders.)

the likelihood of need for cesarean section. The decision to offer women with a placenta that is situated 11 to 20 mm away a trial of labor remains controversial. Recent reports by Vergani et al indicate that more than two thirds of women with a placental edge to cervical os distance of >10 mm fewer than 28 days before delivery can deliver vaginally without increased risk of hemorrhage.

SUGGESTED READING

Available at www.expertconsult.com

RELATED CONTENT

Placenta Previa (Patient Information)
Vaginal Bleeding During Pregnancy (Related Key Topic)

AUTHOR: **SONYA S. ABDEL-RAZEQ, M.D.**

BASIC INFORMATION

DEFINITION

Plantar fasciitis is chronic degeneration of the plantar fascia rather than a true inflammatory condition. This disorder may be better classified as a fasciosis rather than a fasciitis due to histologic findings. Three bands—medial, central, and lateral—make up the plantar fascia; each band is separated by an intermuscular septum. The plantar fascia is composed of longitudinal collagen fibers that arise from the calcaneal tuberosity and extend distally into five digital bands at the metatarsophalangeal joints. Normal plantar fascia thickness is ~3 mm. The function of the plantar fascia is to provide dynamic shock absorption, medial longitudinal arch support, and protection to underlying anatomic structures. The plantar fat pad protects and cushions the origin and insertion of the plantar fascia.

Patients with plantar fasciitis have pain that is typically elicited along the medial calcaneal tuberosity on which the medial band of the plantar fascia inserts or along the coursing of the plantar fascia (Fig. 1).

SYNONYMS

Heel spur syndrome

ICD-10CMCODES	
M72.2	Plantar fascial fibromatosis
M77.30	Calcaneal spur, unspecified foot
M77.31	Calcaneal spur, right foot
M77.32	Calcaneal spur, left foot

EPIDEMIOLOGY & DEMOGRAPHICS

INCIDENCE: In the U.S., it is estimated that greater than two million people suffer from and are treated for plantar fasciitis on an annual basis. Most patients seek their primary care physicians for initial consultation. Studies have shown that plantar fasciitis resolves in 80% of patients who do not seek any medical treatment during a 12-month period.

PREDOMINANT SEX: Predominance of plantar fasciitis varies according to studies.
PREDOMINANT AGE: Most prevalent from ages 40 to 60 but can occur at any age.
RISK FACTORS: Rapid increase in activity, weight gain, obesity, pes cavus or pes planus foot type, prolonged standing, excessive running, abrupt change in activity, trauma, and ambulating on hard surfaces barefoot.

PHYSICAL FINDINGS & CLINICAL PRESENTATION

- Pain can be localized to the heel or radiate along the course of the plantar fascia.
- Pain is often described as sharp, deep, and achy.
- Post-static dyskinesia: experience heel pain with the first few steps in the morning and with standing after sitting for a prolonged period of time.
- Symptoms typically improve with ambulation secondary to the plantar fascia being in a nontaut position.
- Passive ankle dorsiflexion can cause discomfort in the proximal plantar fascia.
- Pain at the plantar medial tubercle upon palpation.
- Plantar fascial thickness may be present.

ETIOLOGY

- Factors that contribute to increased tension along the plantar fascia band create not only inflammation but also fasciosis. Calcaneal heel spurs may or may not be present and are more of an incidental finding than a factor related to the etiology of plantar fasciitis.
- Decrease in ankle dorsiflexion (equinus, pseudoequinus).
- Intrinsic biomechanical factors: Forefoot varus, compensated rearfoot varus, rearfoot varus, flexible forefoot valgus, compensated forefoot valgus, tibial varum, excessive femoral anteversion.
- Poor footwear.
- Prolonged standing/walking occupations.
- Heel pad atrophy.
- Ambulating barefoot on hard surfaces.
- Exercising on uneven terrain.
- Overtraining.
- Obesity.

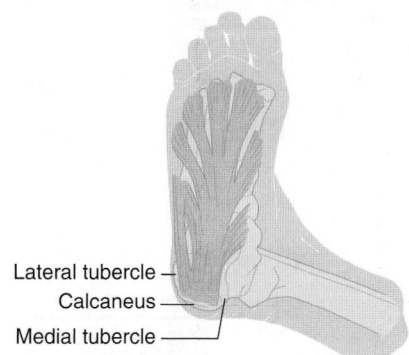

FIG. 1 Plantar view of origin and insertion of plantar fascia. (From Frontera WR: *Essentials of physical medicine and rehabilitation,* ed 2, Philadelphia, 2008, Saunders.)

Lateral tubercle
Calcaneus
Medial tubercle

DIAGNOSIS

DIFFERENTIAL DIAGNOSIS

- Calcaneal fracture
- Tarsal tunnel syndrome
- Foreign body
- Bone cyst or bone tumor
- Bone contusion
- Posterior tibial tendon dysfunction
- Flexor hallucis longus tendonitis
- Plantar fascial fibromatosis
- Rheumatoid arthritis
- Seronegative arthropathies including reactive arthritis, psoriatic arthritis, and ankylosing spondylitis
- Plantar fascial rupture
- Bursitis of the plantar heel
- Baxter's neuritis

STUDIES

- Weight-bearing x-rays: to evaluate for osseous abnormalities including tumors, fractures (lateral, oblique, anterior-posterior, calcaneal axial views)
- MRI to evaluate soft tissue and osseous structures in greater anatomic detail without any exposure to radiation
- CT to evaluate osseous structure abnormalities such as tarsal coalitions and osteocartilaginous lesions in greater anatomic detail
- Bone scan to evaluate for stress fractures
- Ultrasound to evaluate for soft-tissue structure anomalies or abnormalities
- Nerve conduction tests to evaluate for nerve disorders such as tarsal tunnel syndrome

TREATMENT

- Supportive shoe gear with appropriate modifications (e.g., gel heel cup for comfort).
- Custom-molded orthotics (rearfoot posting to correct for rearfoot varus or valgus).
- Physical therapy: ultrasound, iontophoresis, electrical stimulation (TENS unit); stretching, strengthening, and proprioception exercises.
- Ice, NSAIDs, Medrol Dosepak, activity reduction.
- Low-dye strapping/taping.
- Weight reduction in those who are overweight.
- Stretching before activities.
- Corticosteroid injection.
- Botulin toxin injection: inhibits the release of acetylcholine in overactive muscles.
- Platelet-rich plasma injection (Fig. 2).
- Dorsiflexion night splint to maintain ankle joint at 90 degrees (stretches plantar fascia).
- Manual deep foot massage.
- Heel lifts or heel cup if the etiology is Achilles equinus.
- Severe cases may require a CAM boot or short leg cast for 4 to 6 weeks of immobilization.
- Recalcitrant cases may require surgical intervention (endoscopic plantar fasciotomy or open plantar fasciectomy).
- Pulsed radiofrequency electromagnetic field therapy.

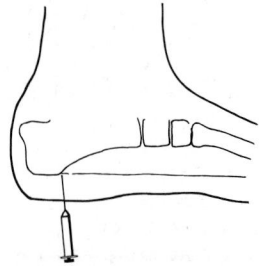

FIG. 2 Injection site for plantar fasciitis. Injection should be through the sole into the area of maximum tenderness. A 25- or 27-gauge needle should be used and the medication injected slowly because some pain may occur. (From Mercier L: *Practical orthopedics,* ed 5, St Louis, 2002, Mosby.)

- Extracorporeal shock-wave therapy (ESWT): last option before surgical intervention in those who have failed all other conservative treatment modalities. MOA: increases proliferation of growth factors; inhibits demyelinated plantar sensory nerves; reduces calcification within the plantar fascia; increases peripheral blood circulation, angiogenesis, neovascularization in the degenerative tissue of the heel.

DISPOSITION

Higher success rates for treating plantar fasciitis are associated with early recognition from astute physicians. It is absolutely imperative to recognize the biomechanical components when assessing plantar fasciitis. Pathology that is not recognized early typically involves a longer treatment course, and those cases that are recalcitrant to conservative treatment modalities tend to need surgical intervention.

REFERRAL

- For biomechanical exam, orthotics, or surgical consult (podiatric surgeon and/or foot and ankle orthopedic surgeon).
- Physical therapy can be used as an adjunct to conservative treatment measures.

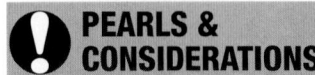 **PEARLS & CONSIDERATIONS**

COMMENTS

Caution: Plantar fasciitis is commonly misdiagnosed. The cases that are recalcitrant to treatment need to be reevaluated to exclude other etiologies.

PREVENTION

- Avoid sitting for prolonged periods of time without stretching.
- Avoid wearing nonsupportive shoe gear.

- Avoid abrupt change and intensity in physical activity.
- Perform stretches before any exercises or strenuous activity.
- Seek early medical attention with onset of heel pain.

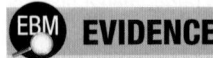 **EVIDENCE**

Available at www.expertconsult.com

SUGGESTED READINGS

Available at www.expertconsult.com

RELATED CONTENT

Plantar Fasciitis (Patient Information)

AUTHOR: **BRANDI KIMBLE, D.P.M.**

BASIC INFORMATION

DEFINITION

Pleurisy refers to the inflammation of the parietal pleura. This inflammation results in pleuritic chest pain that is characteristically worsened with respiration or movement.

SYNONYMS

Pleuritis

ICD-10CM CODES
R09.1 Pleurisy

EPIDEMIOLOGY & DEMOGRAPHICS

INCIDENCE: One of the most common causes of pleuritic chest pain is viral pleurisy. However, there are a variety of disorders that may result in pleurisy. Infectious diseases, rheumatologic disorders, thromboembolic events, and trauma may all lead to pleural inflammation. Therefore, the incidence of pleurisy varies in accordance with the underlying etiology.

PHYSICAL FINDINGS & CLINICAL PRESENTATION

- The defining characteristic of pleurisy is chest pain that worsens with respiration, coughing, or sneezing.
- Pleuritic chest pain is typically described as sharp or stabbing. However, pleuritic chest pain may also be described as dull pain, burning pain, or a "catch" while breathing.
- Movements of the trunk or chest wall may exacerbate pain. Patients with pleurisy may locate the position of minimal discomfort and remain still in that position.
- Dyspnea may be associated with pleurisy.
- Physical exam may be remarkable for a pleural friction rub.
- Decreased breath sounds, rales, or egophony may be appreciated if pneumonia is the underlying etiology of the patient's pleurisy.

ETIOLOGY

- Pleurisy is caused by inflammation of the parietal pleura. The visceral pleura is not innervated by nociceptors. However, injury or inflammation at the periphery of the lung parenchyma often results in inflammation of the overlying parietal pleura. The parietal pleura, which lines the rib cage and the lateral portion of each hemidiaphragm, is innervated by intercostal nerves; therefore pain is localized to the cutaneous distribution of those nerves (over the chest wall). The parietal pleura of the central diaphragm is innervated by fibers that travel with the phrenic nerve; therefore pain associated with inflammation in this area is referred to the ipsilateral shoulder or neck.
- Various underlying etiologies may result in pleurisy, including:
  1. Thromboembolism (pulmonary embolism).
  2. Viral infection (coxsackieviruses, respiratory syncytial virus [RSV], cytomegalovirus [CMV], adenovirus, Epstein-Barr virus [EBV], parainfluenza, influenza).
  3. Bacterial infection (pneumonia or tuberculous pleuritis).
  4. Fungal infection (coccidioidomycosis, histoplasmosis).
  5. Rheumatologic disease (rheumatoid arthritis, systemic lupus erythematosus [SLE]).
  6. Medications.
  7. Malignancy of the lung or pleura.
  8. Trauma (rib fracture).
  9. Hereditary (familial Mediterranean fever, sickle cell disease).

DIAGNOSIS

DIFFERENTIAL DIAGNOSIS

- Cardiac: myocardial infarction, ischemia, pericarditis.
- Intraabdominal process: pancreatitis, cholecystitis.
- Thromboembolic: pulmonary embolism, infarction of lung parenchyma.
- Traumatic/mechanical: rib fracture or pneumothorax.
- Viral infection: viral infections may lead to epidemic pleurodynia (also known as Bornholm's disease). Implicated viruses include coxsackieviruses, RSV, CMV, adenovirus, EBV, parainfluenza, influenza. Of note, viral pleurisy is a diagnosis of exclusion.
- Bacterial infection: pneumonia or tuberculous pleurisy.
- Fungal infection: coccidioidomycosis, histoplasmosis.
- Rheumatologic disease: rheumatoid arthritis, SLE.
- Medications: drug-induced lupus.
- Hereditary causes: familial Mediterranean fever, sickle cell disease.
- Malignancy: malignancy affecting the lung or pleura.
- Uremia.

WORKUP

- A thorough history and physical exam of all patients presenting with pleuritic chest pain should be taken. The time course of the patient's symptoms can provide valuable diagnostic clues. Acute onset of symptoms is suggestive of traumatic injuries, spontaneous pneumothorax, pulmonary embolism, or myocardial infarction. Subacute onset of symptoms suggests a potential infectious, rheumatologic, or medication-induced cause. Viral pleurisy is often associated with prodromal symptoms of upper respiratory infection. Chronic or recurrent symptoms suggest a potential malignant, tuberculous, or hereditary cause.
- Chest x-ray to evaluate for pneumonia, pneumothorax, or pleural effusion.
- ECG to evaluate for infarction, ischemia, or pericarditis.
- Evaluation for pulmonary embolism should be undertaken if clinical suspicion exists.

LABORATORY TESTS

- Laboratory testing varies based on suspected underlying etiology. Consider CBC, Chem 7, and D-Dimer testing depending on clinical presentation.
- If a pleural effusion is present, diagnostic thoracentesis may provide valuable diagnostic clues to the underlying etiology.

IMAGING STUDIES

- Chest x-ray.
- ECG.
- CT chest in selected patients.

TREATMENT

- Treatment of pleurisy consists of pain control as well as treating the underlying condition.
- NSAIDs are the preferred first-line agent to control pain associated with pleurisy. Human studies have been limited to trials using indomethacin for pain control, although an NSAID class effect is presumed.
- Indomethacin 50 mg orally up to three times a day has been found to be effective in relieving pain and is associated with an improvement in mechanical lung function.

AUTHOR: **CHAKRAVARTHY REDDY, M.D.**

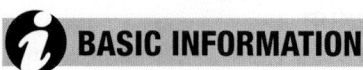

BASIC INFORMATION

DEFINITION

Aspiration pneumonia is a vague term that refers to pulmonary abnormalities following abnormal entry of endogenous or exogenous substances in the lower airways. It is generally classified as:

- Aspiration (chemical pneumonitis)
- Primary bacterial aspiration pneumonia
- Secondary bacterial infection of chemical pneumonitis

SYNONYMS

Aspiration pneumonia

ICD-10CM CODES
J69.0 Pneumonitis due to inhalation of food and vomit

EPIDEMIOLOGY & DEMOGRAPHICS

INCIDENCE (IN U.S.):
- 20% to 35% of all pneumonias.
- 5% to 15% of all community-acquired pneumonias.

PEAK INCIDENCE: Elderly patients in hospitals or nursing homes.

PREVALENCE (IN U.S.): Unknown (unreliable data).

PREDOMINANT SEX: Males and females affected equally.

PREDOMINANT AGE: Elderly.

PHYSICAL FINDINGS & CLINICAL PRESENTATION

- Shortness of breath, tachypnea, cough, sputum, fever after vomiting, or difficulty swallowing.
- Rales, rhonchi, often diffusely throughout lung.

ETIOLOGY

Complex interaction of etiologies, ranging from chemical (often acid) pneumonitis after aspiration of sterile gastric contents (generally not requiring antibiotic treatment) to bacterial aspiration.

COMMUNITY-ACQUIRED ASPIRATION PNEUMONIA:

- Generally results from predominantly anaerobic mouth bacteria (anaerobic and microaerophilic streptococci, fusobacteria, gram-positive anaerobic nonspore-forming rods), *Bacteroides* species (*melaninogenicus, intermedius, oralis, ureolyticus*), *Haemophilus influenzae,* and *Streptococcus pneumoniae*
- Rarely caused by *Bacteroides fragilis* (of uncertain validity in published studies) or *Eikenella corrodens*
- High-risk groups: the elderly; alcoholics; IV drug users; patients who are obtunded; stroke victims; and those with esophageal disorders, seizures, poor dentition, or recent dental manipulations.

HOSPITAL-ACQUIRED ASPIRATION PNEUMONIA:

- Often occurs among elderly patients and others with diminished gag reflex; those with nasogastric tubes, intestinal obstruction, or ventilator support; and especially those exposed to contaminated nebulizers or unsterile suctioning.
- High-risk groups: seriously ill hospitalized patients (especially patients with coma, acidosis, alcoholism, uremia, diabetes mellitus, nasogastric intubation, or recent antimicrobial therapy, who are frequently colonized with aerobic gram-negative rods); patients undergoing anesthesia; those with strokes, dementia, or swallowing disorders; the elderly; and those receiving antacids or H_2 blockers (but not sucralfate).
- Hypoxic patients receiving concentrated O_2 have diminished ciliary activity, encouraging aspiration.
- Causative organisms:
  1. Anaerobes listed above, although in many studies gram-negative aerobes (60%) and gram-positive aerobes (20%) predominate.
  2. *E. coli, P. aeruginosa, S. aureus* including MRSA, *Klebsiella, Enterobacter, Serratia, Proteus* spp., *H. influenzae, S. pneumoniae, Legionella,* and *Acinetobacter* spp. (sporadic pneumonias) in two thirds of cases.
  3. Fungi, including *Candida albicans,* in <1%.

DIAGNOSIS

DIFFERENTIAL DIAGNOSIS

- Other necrotizing or cavitary pneumonias (especially tuberculosis, gram-negative pneumonias).
- See "Pulmonary Tuberculosis."

WORKUP

- Chest x-ray.
- Complete blood count (CBC), blood cultures.
- Sputum Gram stain and culture.
- Consideration of tracheal aspirate.

LABORATORY TESTS

- CBC: leukocytosis often present.
- Sputum Gram stain.
  1. Often useful when carefully prepared immediately after obtaining suctioned or expectorated specimen, examined by experienced observer.
  2. Only specimens with multiple white blood cells and rare or absent epithelial cells should be examined.
  3. Unlike nonaspiration pneumonias (e.g., pneumococcal), multiple organisms may be present.
  4. Long, slender rods suggest anaerobes.
  5. Sputum from pneumonia caused by acid aspiration may be devoid of organisms.
  6. Cultures should be interpreted in light of morphology of visualized organisms.

IMAGING STUDIES

- Chest x-ray often reveals bilateral, diffuse, patchy infiltrates and posterior segment upper lobes. Chemical pneumonitis typically affects the most dependent regions of the lungs.
- Aspiration pneumonia of several days' or longer duration may reveal necrosis (especially community-acquired anaerobic pneumonias) and even cavitation with air-fluid levels, indicating lung abscess.

TREATMENT

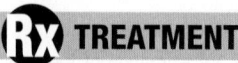

NONPHARMACOLOGIC THERAPY

- Airway management to prevent repeated aspiration.
- Ventilatory support if necessary.

ACUTE GENERAL Rx

Acute aspiration of acidic gastric contents without bacteria may not require antibiotic therapy; consult infectious disease or pulmonary expert.

- Community-acquired anaerobic aspiration pneumonia: clindamycin (600 mg IV twice daily followed by 300 mg q6h orally). Intravenous penicillin G (1 to 2 million U q4 to 6h) can also still be used. Alternative oral agents include: amoxicillin-clavulanate (875 mg orally twice daily), amoxicillin plus metronidazole or oral moxifloxacin (400 mg orally once daily). Do not use metronidazole alone, as this is associated with high failure rates.
- Nursing home aspirations: levofloxacin 500 to 750 mg qd or piperacillin-tazobactam 3.375 g q6h or cefepime 2 g q8h ± vancomycin if MRSA suspected or known.
- Hospital-acquired aspiration pneumonia:
  1. Piperacillin-tazobactam 3.375 g IV q6h, or meropenem 1 g IV q 8h ± vancomycin IV to cover MRSA. Alternative agents are ceftriaxone 2 g IV q24h plus metronidazole 500 mg IV q8h.
  2. Knowledge of resident flora in the microenvironment of the aspiration within the hospital is crucial to intelligent antibiotic selection; consult infection control nurses or hospital epidemiologist.
  3. Confirmed *Pseudomonas* pneumonia should be treated with antipseudomonal beta-lactam agent (piperacillin/tazobactam, cefepime) plus an aminoglycoside until antimicrobial sensitivities confirm that less toxic agents may replace the aminoglycoside.
  4. Do not use metronidazole alone for anaerobes.

DISPOSITION

Repeat chest x-ray in 6 to 8 wk in most patients.

REFERRAL

For consultation with infectious disease and/or pulmonary experts for patients with respiratory distress, hypoxia, ventilatory support, pneumonia in more than one lobe, or necrosis or cavitation on x-ray examination or for those not responding to antibiotic therapy within 2 to 3 days.

SUGGESTED READINGS
Available at www.expertconsult.com

RELATED CONTENT
Aspiration Pneumonia (Patient Information)

AUTHOR: **GLENN G. FORT, M.D., M.P.H.**

BASIC INFORMATION

DEFINITION

Bacterial pneumonia is an infection involving the lung parenchyma. It can be community acquired or nosocomial (see Box 1).

SYNONYMS

Community-acquired pneumonia
CAP
Legionella pneumonia

ICD-10CM CODES

J15.9	Unspecified bacterial pneumonia
J69.0	Pneumonitis due to inhalation of food and vomit
J15.9	Unspecified bacterial pneumonia
J13	Pneumonia due to *Streptococcus pneumoniae*
J15.1	Pneumonia due to *Pseudomonas*
J15.20	Pneumonia due to staphylococcus, unspecified
J15.0	Pneumonia due to *Klebsiella pneumoniae*
J14	Pneumonia due to *Haemophilus influenzae*
J15.211	Pneumonia due to methicillin-susceptible *Staphylococcus aureus*
J15.212	Pneumonia due to methicillin-resistant *Staphylococcus aureus*
J15.6	Pneumonia due to other aerobic Gram-negative bacteria
J15.7	Pneumonia due to *Mycoplasma pneumoniae*

EPIDEMIOLOGY & DEMOGRAPHICS

- The incidence of community-acquired pneumonia (CAP) is 1 in 100 persons. CAP is the most common infectious cause of death in the U.S.
- The incidence of health care facility–acquired pneumonia (HCAP) is 8 cases per 1000 persons annually.
- Primary care physicians see an average of 10 cases of pneumonia annually.
- Hospitalization rate for pneumonia is 15% to 20%. Incidence is highest among the oldest adults.
- Most cases of pneumonia occur in the winter and in elderly patients.

PHYSICAL FINDINGS & CLINICAL PRESENTATION

- Fever, tachypnea, chills, tachycardia, cough; pleurisy in the case of pleural effusion.
- Presentation varies with the cause of pneumonia, the patient's age, and the clinical situation:
  1. Patients with streptococcal pneumonia usually present with high fever, shaking chills, pleuritic chest pain, cough, and copious production of rusty-appearing purulent sputum. Pleurisy and parapneumonic effusions are also common. Potential complications include bacteremia, empyema, and distant infections (e.g., meningitis).
  2. *Mycoplasma pneumoniae:* insidious onset; headache; dry, paroxysmal cough that is worse at night; myalgias; malaise; sore throat; extrapulmonary manifestations (e.g., erythema multiforme, aseptic meningitis, urticaria, erythema nodosum) may be present.
  3. *Chlamydia pneumoniae:* persistent, nonproductive cough, low-grade fever, headache, sore throat.
  4. *Legionella pneumophila:* high fever, mild cough, mental status change, myalgias, diarrhea, respiratory failure.
  5. MRSA pneumonia: often preceded by influenza, may present with shock and respiratory failure.
  6. Elderly or immunocompromised hosts with pneumonia may initially present with only minimal symptoms (e.g., low-grade fever, confusion); respiratory and nonrespiratory symptoms are less commonly reported by older patients with pneumonia.
  7. In general, auscultation of patients with pneumonia reveals crackles and diminished breath sounds.
  8. Percussion dullness is present if the patient has pleural effusion.
  9. The clinical impression of pneumonia has an overall sensitivity of 70% to 90%; specificity ranges from 40% to 70%.

ETIOLOGY

- *Streptococcus pneumoniae* (10%-15% of CAP cases): incidence has been declining due to widespread use of pneumococcal vaccination and reduced rate of cigarette smoking.
- *Haemophilus influenzae* (3%-10% of CAP cases)
- *L. pneumophila* (1%-5% of adult pneumonias) (2%-8% of CAP cases)
- *Klebsiella, Pseudomonas, Escherichia coli*
- *Staphylococcus aureus* (3%-5% of CAP cases)
- Atypical organisms such as *M. pneumoniae, C. pneumoniae,* and *L. pneumophila* implicated in up to 40% of cases of CAP
- Influenza infection is one of the important predisposing factors to *S. pneumoniae* and *S. aureus* pneumonia; gram-negative organisms cause >80% of nosocomial pneumonias
- Predisposing factors:
  1. Chronic obstructive pulmonary disease: *H. influenzae, S. pneumoniae, Legionella, Moraxella catarrhalis*
  2. Seizures: aspiration pneumonia
  3. Compromised hosts: *Legionella*, gram-negative organisms
  4. Alcoholism: *Klebsiella, S. pneumoniae, H. influenzae*
  5. HIV: *S. pneumoniae*
  6. IV drug addicts with right-sided bacterial endocarditis: *S. aureus*
  7. Older patient with comorbid diseases: *C. pneumoniae*

DIAGNOSIS

DIFFERENTIAL DIAGNOSIS

- Viral pneumonias: Viral pneumonias/pneumonitis are on the rise. Several viruses alone or in combination can cause pneumonias in adults. Influenza is the predominant virus, but respiratory syncytial virus (RSV), parainfluenza viruses, adenoviruses, rhinoviruses, coronaviruses, and human metapneumovirus are all possible etiologies. The diagnosis is based on clinical suspicion, negative bacterial workup, and/or respiratory cultures, serologies, or rapid PCR testing.
- Exacerbation of chronic bronchitis
- Pulmonary embolism or infarction
- Lung neoplasm
- Bronchiolitis
- Sarcoidosis
- Hypersensitivity pneumonitis
- Pulmonary edema
- Drug-induced lung injury
- Fungal pneumonias
- Parasitic pneumonias
- Atypical pneumonia
- Tuberculosis

WORKUP

Laboratory evaluation and chest x-ray. Table 1 summarizes diagnostic testing for CAP. Useful tools for assessing severity of illness are the *CURB-65* (see "Disposition") and *Pneumonia Severity Index* (Fig. 1 and Box 2). Poor prognostic indicators are hypotension (SBP <90 or DBP <60), respiratory rate >30/min, hyperpyrexia (>40° C), or hypothermia (<35° C). None of these indices is as valuable as clinical judgment of the physician.

- Laboratory Tests: Complete blood count with differential; white blood cell count is elevated, usually with left shift.
- Blood cultures (hospitalized patients only): positive in approximately 20% of cases of pneumococcal pneumonia.
- Pneumococcal urinary antigen test can be used to detect the C-polysaccharide antigen of *S. pneumoniae*. It is a useful tool in the treatment of hospitalized adult patients with CAP.
- When suspecting *Legionella,* a respiratory specimen culture on special media and/or a urinary antigen should be requested.
- Serologic testing for HIV in selected patients.
- Serum electrolytes (hyponatremia in suspected *Legionella* pneumonia), BUN, creatinine.
- Serum procalcitonin level: May be helpful to distinguish pneumonia from heart failure in patients presenting to the emergency department with acute dyspnea. The procalcitonin level is significantly higher in patients with pneumonia than in those without.[1]
- Pulse oximetry or arterial blood gases: hypoxemia with partial pressure of oxygen <60 mm Hg while the patient is breathing room air, a standard criterion for hospital admission.

IMAGING STUDIES

Chest x-ray (Fig. 2): findings vary with the stage and type of pneumonia and the hydration of the patient:

- Classically, pneumococcal pneumonia presents with a segmental lobe infiltrate.
- Diffuse infiltrates on chest x-ray can be seen with *L. pneumophila* (Fig. E3), *M. pneumoniae,*

---

[1]Alba GA, et al: Diagnostic and prognostic utility of procalcitonin in patients presenting to the emergency department with dyspnea, *Am J Med* 129:96, 2016.

viral pneumonias, *P. jirovecii (carinii),* miliary tuberculosis, aspiration, aspergillosis.
- An initial chest x-ray is also useful to rule out the presence of any complications (pneumothorax, empyema, abscesses).

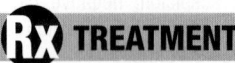 TREATMENT

NONPHARMACOLOGIC THERAPY
- Avoidance of tobacco use
- Oxygen to maintain partial oxygen pressure in arterial blood >60 mm Hg
- IV hydration, correction of dehydration
- Assisted ventilation in patients with significant respiratory failure

ACUTE GENERAL Rx
- Initial antibiotic therapy should be based on clinical, radiographic, and laboratory evaluation.

- Macrolides (azithromycin or clarithromycin) or doxycycline is recommended for empiric outpatient treatment of CAP as long as the patient has not received antibiotics within the past 3 months and does not reside in a community in which the prevalence of macrolide resistance is high. Box 3 summarizes empirical therapy regimens for severe CAP. The treatment of choice in suspected *Legionella* pneumonia is either a quinolone (e.g., moxifloxacin) or a macrolide (e.g., azithromycin) antibiotic.
- In the hospital setting, patients admitted to the general ward can be treated empirically with a second- or third-generation cephalosporin (ceftriaxone, cefotaxime, or cefuroxime) plus a macrolide (azithromycin or clarithromycin) or doxycycline. An antipseudomonal quinolone (levofloxacin or

moxifloxacin) can be substituted in place of the macrolide or doxycycline.
- Empiric therapy in ICU patients: IV beta-lactam (ceftriaxone, cefotaxime, ampicillin-sulbactam) plus an IV quinolone (levofloxacin, moxifloxacin) or IV azithromycin.
- In hospitalized patients at risk for *P. aeruginosa* infection, empiric treatment should consist of an antipseudomonal beta-lactam (meropenem, doripenem, imipenem, or piperacillin-tazobactam) with or without a second antipseudomonal agent such as an aminoglycoside or an antipseudomonal quinolone.
- In patients with suspected methicillin-resistant *S. aureus,* vancomycin or linezolid is effective.
- Steroids: A meta-analysis published in 2015 by Siemieniuk et al showed that in hospitalized adults with CAP, systemic steroid therapy may reduce mortality, the need for mechanical ventilation, and length of hospital stay. Based on those results and several other supportive studies, corticosteroids (i.e., methylprednisolone 0.5 mg/kg IV q12h for 5 days) are recommended by several experts in hospitalized adult patients presenting with severe CAP, as long as no major contraindications for steroid usage are present.
- Duration of treatment ranges from 5 to 14 days. Trials have shown that in adults hospitalized with community-acquired pneumonia, stopping antibiotic treatment after 5 days in clinically stable patients is reasonable and noninferior to usual care. Hematogenous *Staphylococcus* infection, abscesses, and cavitary lesions might require prolonged antibiotic therapy, sometimes until radiological resolution is documented.

BOX 1   Classification of Pneumonia

Community-Acquired Pneumonia (CAP)
An alveolar infection that develops in the outpatient setting or within 48 hours of admission to a hospital.

Nosocomial Pneumonia
Hospital-Acquired Pneumonia (HAP)
Pneumonia occurring ≥48 hours after hospital admission and not incubating at the time of admission.

Ventilator-Associated Pneumonia (VAP)
Pneumonia occurring ≥48 hours after endotracheal intubation and mechanical ventilation.

Health Care–Associated Pneumonia (HCAP)
Pneumonia in patients with one or more of the following risk factors for multidrug-resistant (MDR) bacteria: (1) hospitalization for ≥2 days in an acute care facility within 90 days before infection; (2) residence in a nursing home or long-term care facility; (3) antibiotic therapy, chemotherapy, or wound care within 30 days before current infection; (4) hemodialysis treatment at a hospital or clinic; (5) home infusion therapy or home wound care; or (6) family member with infection due to MDR pathogen.

From Parrillo JE, Dellinger RP: *Critical care medicine: principles of diagnosis and management in the adult,* ed 4, Philadelphia, 2014, Saunders.

TABLE 1   Diagnostic Testing for Community-Acquired Pneumonia (CAP)

Test	Sensitivity	Specificity	Comment
Chest radiograph	65%-85%	85%-95%	CT is more sensitive to infiltrates. Recommended for all patients.
Computed tomography	Gold standard	Not infection specific	Should not be done routinely but helpful to identify cavitation and loculated pleural fluid. Recommended in the evaluation of nonresponding patients.
Blood cultures	10%-20%	High when positive	Usually shows pneumococcus (in 50%-80% of positive samples) and defines antibiotic susceptibility. Recommended in patients with severe CAP, particularly if not on antibiotic therapy at the time of testing.
Sputum Gram stain	40%-100% depending on criteria	0%-100% depending on criteria	Can correlate with sputum culture to define predominant organism and can be used to identify unsuspected pathogens. Recommended if sputum culture is obtained. May not be able to narrow empirical therapy choices.
Sputum culture			Use if suspect drug-resistant or unusual pathogen, but positive result cannot separate colonization from infection. Obtain via tracheal aspirate in all intubated patients.
Oximetry or arterial blood gas			Both define severity of infection, need for oxygen; if hypercarbia is suspected, a blood gas sample is needed. Recommended in severe CAP.
Serologic testing for *Legionella,* *Chlamydia pneumoniae,* *Mycobacterium pneumoniae,* viruses			Accurate, but usually requires acute and convalescent titers collected 4-6 wk apart. Not routinely recommended.
Legionella urinary antigen	50%-80%		Specific to serogroup 1, but the best acute diagnostic test for *Legionella.*
Pneumococcal urinary antigen	70%-100%	80%	False positives if recent pneumococcal infection. Can increase sensitivity with concentrated urine.
Serum procalcitonin			Not a routine test, but if done, should be measured with the highly sensitive Kryptor assay. May help guide duration of therapy and need for ICU admission.

From Vincent JL et al: *Textbook of critical care,* ed 6, Philadelphia, 2011, Saunders

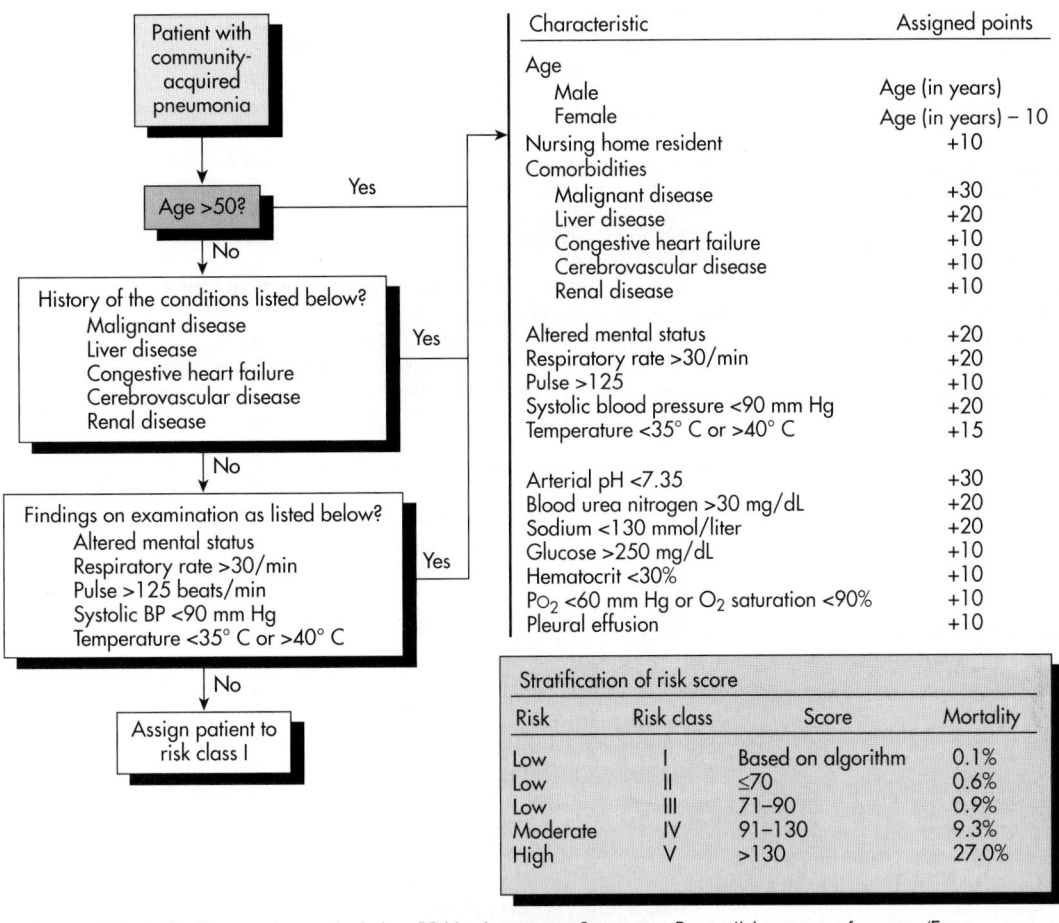

Characteristic	Assigned points
Age	
Male	Age (in years)
Female	Age (in years) − 10
Nursing home resident	+10
Comorbidities	
Malignant disease	+30
Liver disease	+20
Congestive heart failure	+10
Cerebrovascular disease	+10
Renal disease	+10
Altered mental status	+20
Respiratory rate >30/min	+20
Pulse >125	+10
Systolic blood pressure <90 mm Hg	+20
Temperature <35° C or >40° C	+15
Arterial pH <7.35	+30
Blood urea nitrogen >30 mg/dL	+20
Sodium <130 mmol/liter	+20
Glucose >250 mg/dL	+10
Hematocrit <30%	+10
Po_2 <60 mm Hg or O_2 saturation <90%	+10
Pleural effusion	+10

Algorithm flowchart:
- Patient with community-acquired pneumonia
- Age >50? → Yes (to Characteristic table)
- No ↓
- History of the conditions listed below?
  - Malignant disease
  - Liver disease
  - Congestive heart failure
  - Cerebrovascular disease
  - Renal disease → Yes
- No ↓
- Findings on examination as listed below?
  - Altered mental status
  - Respiratory rate >30/min
  - Pulse >125 beats/min
  - Systolic BP <90 mm Hg
  - Temperature <35° C or >40° C → Yes
- No ↓
- Assign patient to risk class I

Stratification of risk score			
Risk	Risk class	Score	Mortality
Low	I	Based on algorithm	0.1%
Low	II	≤70	0.6%
Low	III	71–90	0.9%
Moderate	IV	91–130	9.3%
High	V	>130	27.0%

FIG. 1 The Pneumonia severity index. *BP*, blood pressure; *O₂*, oxygen; *Po₂*, partial pressure of oxygen. (From Sellke FW et al: *Sabiston & Spencer surgery of the chest*, ed 9, 2016, Elsevier.)

BOX 2 Severe pneumonia: diagnostic criteria[1]

Major Criteria
Invasive mechanical ventilation
Use of vasopressors to maintain blood pressure

Minor Criteria
Respiratory rate ≥30 breaths/min
    Multilobar infiltrates
    New-onset confusion/disorientation
    Uremia (BUN >20 mg/dl)
    Leukopenia (WBC count <4000 cells/μL)
    Pao_2/Fio_2 ratio ≥250
    Thrombocytopenia (platelet count <100,000 cells/μL)
    Hypothermia (core temperature <36° C)
    Hypotension requiring aggressive fluid resuscitation
ATS/IDSA, American Thoracic Society/Infectious Diseases Society of America; *BUN*, blood urea nitrogen; *WBC*, white blood cell.

[1]According to ATS/IDSA 2007 guidelines.
From Parrillo JE, Dellinger RP: *Critical care medicine: principles of diagnosis and management in the adult*, ed 4, Philadelphia, 2014, Saunders.

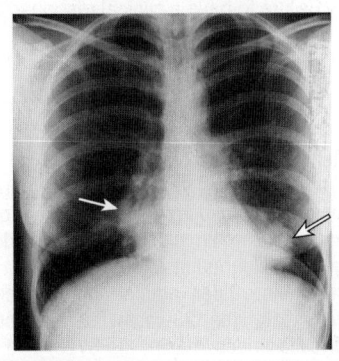

FIG. 2 *Streptococcus pneumoniae* pneumonia, bilateral lower zone consolidation (*arrows*). Although pneumococcal pneumonia is typically unifocal, multifocal involvement is not uncommon. (From Grainger RG et al: *Grainger and Allison's diagnostic radiology*, ed 4, London, 2001, Harcourt.)

CHRONIC Rx

Parapneumonic effusion and empyema can be managed with chest tube placement for drainage. Instillation of fibrinolytic agents (streptokinase, urokinase, or, more commonly, tissue plasminogen activator [TP]) along with DNase (i.e., dornase alfa) twice a day by chest tube may facilitate the drainage of effusions not responding to chest tube drainage alone. A thoracoscopic debridement or a surgical decortication may be necessary in resistant cases.

DISPOSITION

- Most patients respond well to antibiotic therapy. Risk factors for a poor outcome from CAP are summarized in Box 4.
- Indications for hospital admission are:
  1. Hypoxemia (oxygen saturation <90% while patient is breathing room air)
  2. Hemodynamic instability
  3. Inability to tolerate medications
  4. Active coexisting condition requiring hospitalization. A criterion often used to determine hospital admission is known as the "CURB-65": **C**onfusion, B**U**N >19.6 mg/dl, **R**espiratory rate >30 breaths/min, systolic **B**P <90 mg Hg, and diastolic BP ≤60 mm Hg, age ≥**65**. Patients are generally admitted to the hospital if they fulfill 2 or more criteria and to the ICU if they have 3 or more criteria

❗ PEARLS & CONSIDERATIONS

COMMENTS

- Use of gastric acid suppressive therapy (H₂ receptor antagonists, proton pump inhibitors [PPIs]) has been reported to increase the risk of CAP. It has been reported that PPI therapy started within the previous 30 days is associated with an risk for CAP, whereas longer-term current use is not. Recent studies have

P

Diseases and Disorders

I

BOX 3 Empirical Therapy Regimens for Severe Community-Acquired Pneumonia

No Pseudomonal Risk Factors

Selected β-lactam (cefotaxime, ceftriaxone)

plus

Intravenously administered macrolide *or* quinolone (moxifloxacin or levofloxacin[1])

Pseudomonal Risk Factors Present

Selected antipseudomonal β-lactam (cefepime, piperacillin/tazobactam, imipenem, meropenem)

plus

Ciprofloxacin or levofloxacin

or

Selected antipseudomonal β-lactam

plus

Aminoglycoside

plus

Intravenously administered macrolide or antipneumococcal quinolone (moxifloxacin or levofloxacin)

[1]For patients with normal renal function, the recommended dose of levofloxacin is 750 mg daily. Note: Although routine MRSA coverage is not recommended for all severe community-acquired pneumonia, consider CA-MRSA, especially after influenza and with bilateral necrotizing pneumonia, and if suspected, treat by adding either linezolid or the combination of vancomycin and clindamycin.

From Vincent JL et al: *Textbook of critical care,* ed 6, Philadelphia, 2011, Saunders.

failed to confirm increased risk of CAP with PPI use and have shown that risk of CAP is higher during 30 days before PPI prescription than during the 30 days after PPI prescription.[2]

- Causes of slowly resolving or nonresolving pneumonia:
  1. Difficult to treat infections: viral pneumonia, *Legionella,* pneumococci or staphylococci with impaired host response, tuberculosis, fungi
  2. Neoplasm: lung, lymphoma, metastasis
  3. Congestive heart failure
  4. Pulmonary embolism
  5. Immunologic or idiopathic: Wegener granulomatosis, pulmonary eosinophilic syndromes, systemic lupus erythematosus
  6. Drug toxicity (e.g., amiodarone)
- If patients with pneumonia don't improve within a reasonable time frame, repeat films should be taken promptly. In those with complete clinical recovery, it is reasonable to wait 6 to 8 wk before repeating

[2]Othman F, et al.: Community acquired pneumonia incidence before and after proton pump inhibitor prescription, *BMJ* 355:i5813, 2016.

BOX 4 Risk Factors for a Poor Outcome from Community-Acquired Pneumonia

Patient-Related Factors
- Male sex
- Absence of pleuritic chest pain
- Nonclassic clinical presentation
- Neoplastic illness
- Neurologic illness
- Age >65 years
- Family history of severe pneumonia or death from sepsis

Abnormal Physical Findings
- Respiratory rate >30 breaths/min on admission
- Systolic (<90 mm Hg) or diastolic (<60 mm Hg) hypotension
- Tachycardia (>125 beats/min)
- High fever (>40° C) or afebrile
- Confusion

Laboratory Abnormalities
- Blood urea nitrogen >19.6 mg/dl
- Leukocytosis or leukopenia (<4000/mm³)
- Multilobar radiographic abnormalities
- Rapidly progressive radiographic abnormalities during therapy
- Bacteremia
- Hyponatremia (<130 mmol/L)
- Multiple organ failure
- Respiratory failure
- Hypoalbuminemia
- Thrombocytopenia (<100,000/mm³)
- Arterial pH <7.35
- Pleural effusion

Pathogen-Related Factors
- High-risk organisms:
  ○ Type III pneumococcus, *Staphylococcus aureus,* gram-negative bacilli (including *Pseudomonas aeruginosa*), aspiration organisms, severe acute respiratory syndrome
- Possibly high levels of penicillin resistance (minimal inhibitory concentration of at least 4 mg/L) in pneumococcus

Therapy-Related Factors
- Delay in initial antibiotic therapy (more than 4-6 hours)
- Initial therapy with inappropriate antibiotic therapy
- Failure to have a clinical response to empirical therapy within 72 hours

From Vincent JL et al: *Textbook of critical care,* ed 6, Philadelphia, 2011, Saunders.

the radiograph to document clearing of the infiltrate. The benefit of routine radiography after pneumonia has been questioned due to the low 1-yr incidence of lung cancer. Opponents propose a selective approach limiting follow-up chest x-ray to middle-aged and older adults.

- Prevention: Older adults should receive sequentially the 23-valent pneumococcal polysaccharides vaccine (PPSV23) and the pneumococcal conjugated vaccine (PCV13). The ACIP recommends giving the PCV13 first to be followed after a year by the PPSV23. This recommendation includes patients younger than 65 years with some defined risk factors (end-stage renal disease, sickle cell disease, congenital or acquired asplenia, HIV infection, congenital or acquired immunodeficiency, nephrotic syndrome, leukemia, lymphoma, Hodgkin's disease, generalized malignancy, iatrogenic immunosuppression, solid organ transplant, multiple myeloma, CSF leak, cochlear implant).
- Prevention: In season, patients should also receive influenza vaccination.

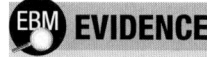 **EVIDENCE**

Available at www.expertconsult.com

SUGGESTED READINGS

Available at www.expertconsult.com

RELATED CONTENT

Bacterial Pneumonia (Patient Information)
Pneumonia, Aspiration (Related Key Topic)
Pneumonia, Mycoplasma (Related Key Topic)

AUTHOR: **NAIM AOUN, M.D.**

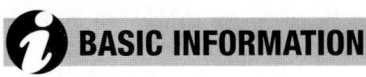 BASIC INFORMATION

DEFINITION

Mycoplasma pneumonia is an infection of the lung parenchyma caused by a small bacterium, *Mycoplasma pneumoniae.*

SYNONYMS

Primary atypical pneumonia
Eaton's pneumonia
Walking pneumonia

ICD-10CM CODES
J15.7 Pneumonia due to *Mycoplasma pneumoniae*

EPIDEMIOLOGY & DEMOGRAPHICS

INCIDENCE (IN U.S.):

- It is a frequent cause of community-acquired pneumonia (CAP), accounting for up to 37% of CAP in patients treated as outpatients and 10% of pneumonia in persons requiring hospitalization. CDC estimates 2 million cases a year with 100,000 pneumonia-related hospitalizations.
- Many cases probably resolve without coming to medical attention.
- Incidence is estimated at one case per 1000 persons annually.
- Incidence is estimated to at least triple every (approximately) 5 yr during epidemics.

PEAK INCIDENCE:

- Some increased incidence in fall to early winter.
- Seems more prevalent in temperate climates.

PREVALENCE (IN U.S.):

- Estimated to be present in one in every five patients hospitalized for pneumonia (generally a self-limited disease, so its true prevalence is unknown).
- Estimated to cause 7% of all cases of pneumonia and approximately half the cases in those aged 5 to 20 yr.

PREDOMINANT SEX: Equal distribution

PREDOMINANT AGE:

- Most commonly affected: school-age children and young adults (ages 5-20 yr).
- Occurs in older adults as well, especially with household exposure to a young child.
- More severe infections in affected elderly patients.

GENETICS: Familial disposition:

- None known.
- May be more severe in patients with sickle cell anemia.
- Neonatal infection: severe respiratory distress, sometimes requiring intubation, attributed to this disease in infants.

PHYSICAL FINDINGS & CLINICAL PRESENTATION

- Nonexudative pharyngitis (common).
- Headache, otalgia common.
- Fever may be mild or not present.
- Rhonchi or rales without evidence of consolidation (common) in lower lung zones.
- Associated with bullous myringitis (nonspecific finding; perhaps no more frequently than in other pneumonias).
- Skin rashes in up to one fourth of patients
  1. Morbilliform.
  2. Urticaria.
  3. Erythema nodosum (unusual).
  4. Erythema multiforme (unusual).
  5. Stevens-Johnson syndrome (rare).
- Muscle tenderness (<50% of the patients).
- On examination (and confirmed with testing):
  1. Mononeuritis or polyneuritis.
  2. Transverse myelitis.
  3. Cranial nerve palsies.
  4. Meningoencephalitis.
- Lymphadenopathy and splenomegaly.
- Conjunctivitis.
- Table 1 summarizes the clinical manifestations of *Mycoplasma pneumoniae.*

ETIOLOGY

Infection is spread person-to-person via respiratory droplets or secretions with an incubation period of 1 to 4 wk.

(DX) DIAGNOSIS

DIFFERENTIAL DIAGNOSIS

- *Chlamydia* (now known as *Chlamydophila) pneumoniae.*
- *Chlamydophila psittaci.*
- *Legionella* spp.
- *Coxiella burnetii.*
- Several viral agents.
- Q fever.
- *Streptococcus pneumoniae.*
- Pulmonary embolism or infarction.

WORKUP

- Chest x-ray (Fig. 1).
- Thorough history and physical examination.
- Laboratory tests.
- Evaluation guided by symptoms and findings.

LABORATORY TESTS

- White blood cells (WBCs):
  1. WBC count >10,000/mm^3 in approximately one fourth of patients.
  2. Differential count nonspecific.
  3. Leukopenia rare.
- Cold agglutinins:
  1. Detected in approximately 50% to 70% of all patients within 1 to 2 weeks after infection; highest in children with yield decreasing with age. Since neither sensitive nor specific, the use of cold agglutinins has come into question.
  2. Also may be found in:
     a. Lymphoproliferative diseases.
     b. Influenza.
     c. Mononucleosis.
     d. Adenovirus infections.
     e. Occasionally, Legionnaires' disease.
  3. Titers typically >1:64.
     a. May be detectable with bedside testing.
     b. Appear between days 5 and 10 of the illness (so may be demonstrable when patient is first examined) and disappear within 1 mo.
- Complement fixation testing assay specific for mycoplasma antigens of paired sera (fourfold rise) or a single titer ≥1:32 in patients with pneumonia and a compatible history:
  1. Considered diagnostic in the appropriate clinical setting.
  2. Other assays include ELISA, antigen capture-enzyme immunoassay, and PCR; if available, is considered diagnostic test of choice.
- Culture of the organism from specimens.
  1. Only truly specific test for infection.
  2. Technically difficult and done reliably by few laboratories.
  3. May require weeks to get results.
- Sputum
  1. Often no sputum produced for laboratory testing.
  2. When present, Gram-stained specimens show polymorphonuclear cells without organisms.
- Infection occasionally complicated by pancreatitis or glomerulitis.
- Disseminated intravascular coagulation is a rare complication.
- Electrocardiographic evidence of pericarditis or myocarditis may be present.

IMAGING STUDIES

- Predilection for lower lobe involvement (upper lobes involved in less than a fourth), with radiographic abnormalities frequently out of proportion to those on physical examination (Fig. 2).
- Small pleural effusions in approximately 30% of patients.

TABLE 1	Clinical Manifestations of *Mycoplasma Pneumoniae* Infection
Respiratory tract	Pharyngitis, laryngitis, acute bronchitis, bronchopneumonia
Skin and mucosa	Maculopapular and vesicular exanthema, urticaria, purpura, erythema nodosum, erythema multiforme, Stevens-Johnson syndrome
Central nervous system	Meningitis, meningoencephalitis, acute psychosis, cerebellitis, Guillain-Barré syndrome?
Parenchymatous organs	Pancreatitis, diabetes mellitus, nonspecific reactive hepatitis, subacute thyroiditis?
Miscellaneous	Hemorrhagic bullous myringitis, hemolytic anemia, pericarditis, thromboembolism?

Some association remains uncertain.
From Cohen J, Powderly WG: *Infectious diseases,* ed 2, St Louis, 2004, Mosby.

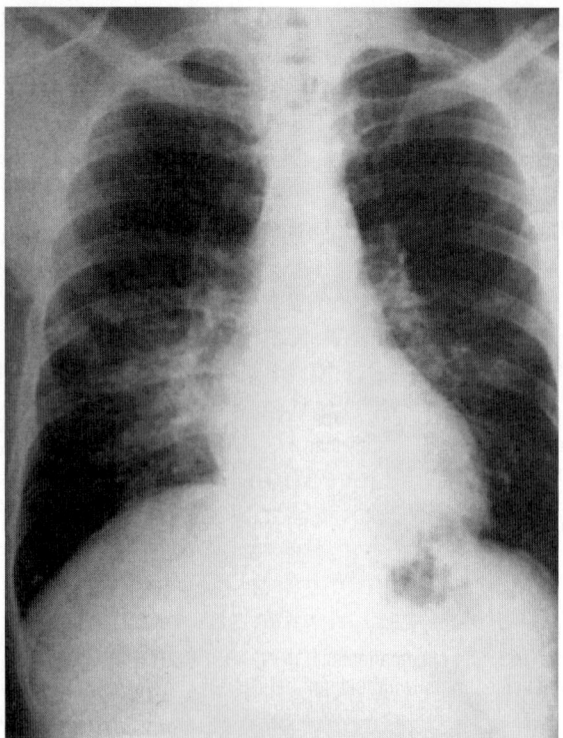

FIG. 1 Radiographic findings in *Mycoplasma pneumoniae* pneumonia are nonspecific. Bilateral bronchopneumonia occurred in this patient. (From Mason RJ et al: *Murray and Nadel's textbook of respiratory medicine*, ed 5, Philadelphia, 2010, Saunders.)

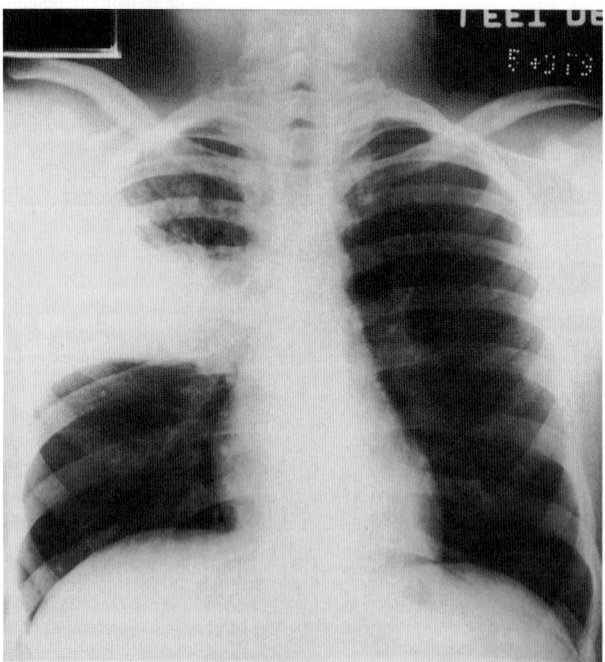
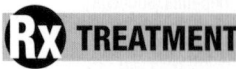

FIG. 2 Localized airspace opacification resulting from *Mycoplasma pneumoniae*. (From Specht N [ed]: *Practical guide to diagnostic imaging,* St Louis, 1998, Mosby.)

- Large effusions: rare.
- Infiltrates: patchy, unilateral, and with a segmental distribution, although multilobar involvement may be seen.
- Evidence of hilar adenopathy on chest radiographs in 20% to 25%.
- Rare cases reported:
  1. Associated lung abscess.
  2. Residual pneumatoceles.
  3. Lobar collapse.
  4. Hyperlucent lung syndrome.

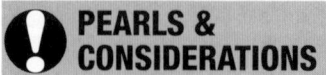 **TREATMENT**

ACUTE GENERAL Rx

- Therapy: azithromycin 500 mg qd × 3 or 500 mg initially, then 250 mg daily for 4 days for adults. For children: 10 mg/kg in one dose on first day, then 5 mg/kg in one dose for 4 days or clarithromycin: 500 mg bid for 10 days in adults, 15 mg/kg per day in two divided doses for 10 days in children. Alternatives include erythromycin (500 mg qid) for adults or 30 to 40 mg/kg per day in four divided doses in children or doxycycline: 2 to 4 mg/kg per day in one or two divided doses for 10 days, maximum daily dose: 100 to 200 mg, but this agent cannot be used in young children or women of childbearing age. Respiratory fluoroquinolones such as Levaquin or moxifloxacin are alternative agents for treatment in adults but should not be used in young children.
- Therapy shortens the duration and severity of symptoms and may hasten radiographic clearing, but the disease is self-limiting.
- Macrolide resistance is becoming a concern, especially in Asia.

CHRONIC Rx

- Effective antimicrobial therapy does not eliminate the organism from the respiratory secretions, which may be positive for weeks.
- Serum antibody response does not necessarily provide lifelong immunity.
- Chronic symptoms do not occur, although clinical relapses may occur 7 to 10 days after the initial response and may be associated with new areas of infiltration.

DISPOSITION

- Clinical improvement is almost universal within 10 days.
- Infiltrates generally clear within 5 to 8 wk.
- Rare deaths are likely attributable to underlying medical diseases.
- Person-to-person spread can be minimized by avoiding open coughing, especially in enclosed areas. Azithromycin prophylaxis can prevent infection in close contacts of patients.

REFERRAL

- Not responding to treatment.
- Severe infection.
- Severe extrapulmonary manifestations.
- Multilobe involvement accompanied by respiratory embarrassment (very rare).

❗ PEARLS & CONSIDERATIONS

COMMENTS

X-ray resolution complete by 8 wk in approximately 90% of patients.

SUGGESTED READINGS

Available at www.expertconsult.com

RELATED CONTENT

Mycoplasma Pneumonia (Patient Information)
Pneumonia, Bacterial (Related Key Topic)

AUTHOR: **GLENN G. FORT, M.D., M.P.H.**

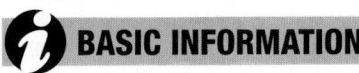

DEFINITION

Pneumocystis jiroveci pneumonia (PJP) is a respiratory infection caused by the fungal pathogen *P. jiroveci* (formerly known as *P. carinii*).

SYNONYMS

Pneumocystis jiroveci pneumonia
PCP
PJP

ICD-10CM CODES
B59 Pneumocystosis

EPIDEMIOLOGY & DEMOGRAPHICS

INCIDENCE (IN U.S.):
- Seen primarily in the setting of acquired immunodeficiency syndrome (AIDS).
- Approximately 95% of cases occur in HIV infected individuals with CD4 counts <200/mm^3.
- Also seen in other immunocompromised patients with severe cell-mediated immune deficiency (congenital T-cell deficiency, acute leukemia, lymphoma, bone marrow or organ transplant deficiency).
- May be associated with prednisone use (usually higher than 20 mg/day).
- Rituximab use has been associated with PJP in HIV-negative patients, most of whom have hematologic cancers.

PEAK INCIDENCE: Age 20 to 40 years (parallel to AIDS epidemic).
PREDOMINANT SEX: Equal incidence when adjusted for HIV status.
PREDOMINANT AGE:
- 20 to 40 years
GENETICS: Neonatal infection:
- Most frequent opportunistic infection among HIV-infected children.
- Neonatal occurrence unusual.

PHYSICAL FINDINGS & CLINICAL PRESENTATION

- Fever, cough, shortness of breath present in almost all cases. May be subacute or insidious.
- Lungs frequently clear to auscultation, although rales occasionally present.
- Cyanosis and pronounced tachypnea in severe cases.
- Hemoptysis unusual.
- Spontaneous pneumothorax is possible.

ETIOLOGY

- *P. jiroveci* (formerly *P. carinii*) recently reclassified as a fungal organism (previously classified as a protozoan) (Fig. E1).
- Reactivation of dormant infection.
- Extrapulmonary involvement rare but possible.

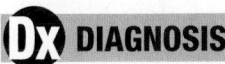

DIFFERENTIAL DIAGNOSIS

- Other opportunistic respiratory infections:
  1. Tuberculosis
  2. Histoplasmosis
  3. Cryptococcosis
  4. Mycobacterium avium complex (MAC)
- Nonopportunistic infections:
  1. Bacterial pneumonia
  2. Viral pneumonia
  3. Mycoplasma pneumonia
  4. Legionella
- Occurs almost exclusively in the setting of profound depression of cellular immunity.

WORKUP

- Chest x-ray (Fig. 2) or chest CT (Fig. E3).
- Arterial blood gases.
- Because *Pneumocystis* cannot be cultured, diagnosis relies on detection of the organism by colorimetric or immunofluorescent stains or PCR.
- Cannot be cultured. Sputum examination for cysts of PJP and to exclude other pathogens.
- Bronchoscopy with bronchoalveolar lavage or lung biopsy for diagnosis if sputum examination is negative or equivocal. Stains such as the methenamine silver stain or toluidine blue O are used to identify the organism.
- Fig. 4 describes an algorithm for the diagnostic evaluation and management of patients with suspected *Pneumocystis* pneumonia.

LABORATORY TESTS

- Arterial blood gas monitoring.
- Elevated lactate dehydrogenase in majority of cases.
- HIV antibody test and CD4 cell count if cause of underlying immune deficiency state is unclear.
- Beta-D-glucan testing may be positive (92% sensitivity, 86% specificity).

IMAGING STUDIES

- PJP may appear as diffuse, unilateral, bilateral, or interstitial infiltrates on chest x-ray or CT. Imaging may be normal in up to one quarter of individuals. Pneumothoraces may also occur.

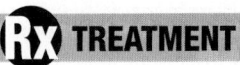

NONPHARMACOLOGIC THERAPY

- Supplemental oxygen.
- Ventilation support if needed.
- Prompt thoracotomy if pneumothorax develops.

ACUTE GENERAL Rx

For confirmed or suspected PJP:
- Trimethoprim-sulfamethoxazole (15-20 mg/kg trimethoprim and 75-100 mg/kg sulfamethoxazole qd) PO or IV per day divided and given q6 to 8h.
- Pentamidine (4 mg/kg IV qd) (severe cases with a contraindication to trimethoprim/sulfamethoxazole). Careful monitoring is required, can cause nephrotoxicity, numerous electrolyte disturbances, and cardiac arrhythmias.
- Either regimen with prednisone (40 mg PO bid):
  1. If arterial oxygen pressure <70 mm Hg.
  2. If arterial-alveolar oxygen pressure difference >35 mm Hg.
  3. Dose tapered to 20 mg bid after 5 days and 20 mg qd after 10 days.
- Therapy continued for three weeks.
- Alternative therapies available for patients unable to tolerate conventional therapy:
  1. Dapsone/trimethoprim
  2. Clindamycin/primaquine
  3. Atovaquone
- Table 1 summarizes causes of deterioration in an HIV-infected patient receiving treatment for PJP.

CHRONIC Rx

- After completion of therapy, prophylaxis should be maintained with trimethoprim-sulfamethoxazole (one single-strength tablet PO qd or double-strength three times weekly) until the CD4 cell count is >200 for three months.

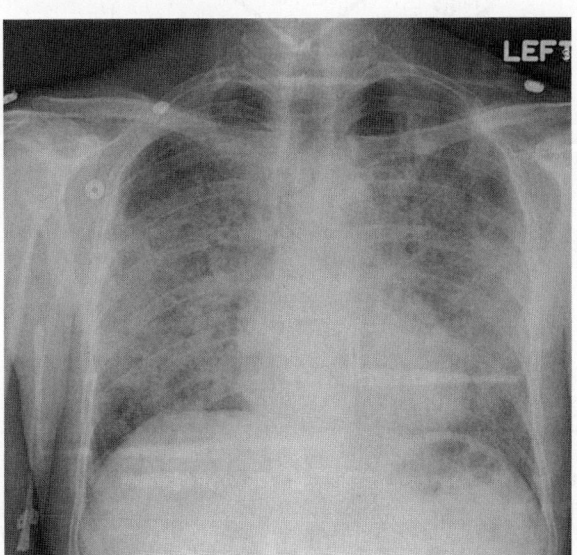

FIG. 2 Chest radiograph showing diffuse interstitial infiltrate in a patient with *Pneumocystis jiroveci* pneumonia. (From Firestein GS et al [eds]: *Kelly's textbook of rheumatology*, ed 9, Philadelphia, 2013, Saunders.)

TABLE 1 Causes of Deterioration in an HIV-Infected Person Receiving Treatment for PJP

Etiology	Explanation
Severe Progressive PCP	
Iatrogenic	Pulmonary edema due to IV fluid overload when giving TMP-SMX IRIS following early initiation of ART
Side effects of therapy	Anemia (e.g., caused by TMP-SMX), methemoglobinemia (e.g., caused by dapsone, primaquine)
Inadequate therapy	Incorrect dosage or route of administration Adjuvant glucocorticoids not given for treatment of moderate or severe PCP
Postbronchoscopy	Sedation Pneumothorax
Pneumothorax	Spontaneous Associated with intubation and positive pressure ventilation
Copathology in lung	Bacterial infection Pulmonary Kaposi sarcoma Intercurrent pulmonary embolism
Wrong diagnosis	Empiric diagnosis of PCP, and correct diagnosis is another pathology (e.g., bacterial pneumonia)

ART, Antiretroviral therapy; _HIV_, human immunodeficiency virus; _IRIS_, immune reconstitution inflammatory syndrome; _IV_, intravenous; _PJP_, _Pneumocystis jiroveci_ pneumonia; _TMP-SMX_, trimethoprim-sulfamethoxazole.
Bennett JE et al: _Mandell, Douglas, and Bennett's principles and practice of infectious diseases_, ed 8, Philadelphia, 2015, WB Saunders.

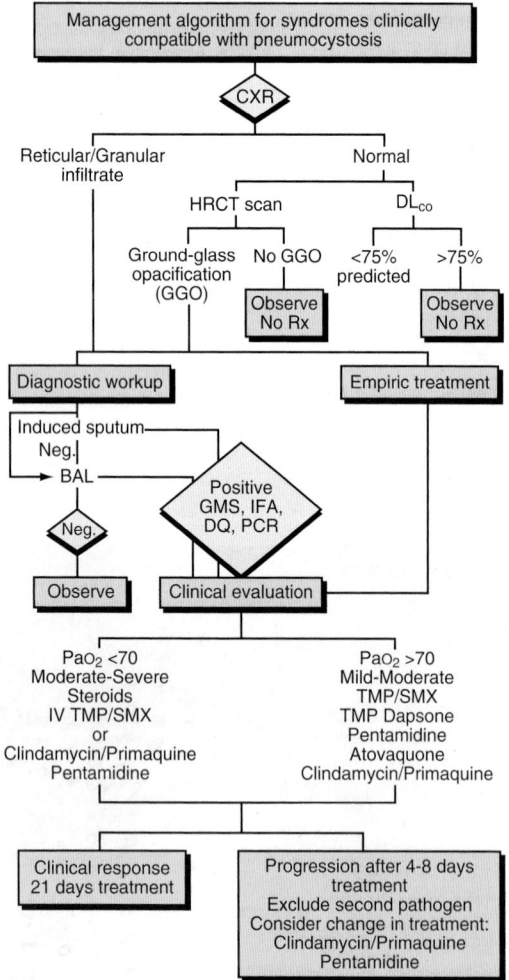

FIG. 4 Algorithm for the diagnostic evaluation and management of patients with suspected _Pneumocystis_ pneumonia. _BAL_, Bronchoalveolar lavage; _CXR_, chest x-ray; _DL_$_{CO}$, single-breath diffusing capacity for carbon monoxide; _DQ_, Diff-Quik (stain); _GGO_, ground-glass opacities; _GMS_, Gomori methenamine silver (stain); _HRCT_, high-resolution computed tomography; _IFA_, immunofluorescent antibody (stain); _IV_, intravenous; _PCR_, polymerase chain reaction; _Rx_, treatment; _TMP/SMX_, trimethoprim-sulfamethoxazole. (Bennett et al: _Mandell, Douglas, and Bennett's principles and practice of infectious diseases_, ed 8, Philadelphia, 2015, WB Saunders.)

- Patients intolerant of this therapy should be treated with dapsone (100 mg PO qd) or atovaquone (1500 mg PO qd).
- Inhaled pentamidine (300 mg monthly by standardized nebulizer) is less effective and is reserved for patients intolerant to other forms of prophylaxis.

DISPOSITION

After completion of therapy, long-term ambulatory follow-up is mandatory to provide secondary prevention of PJP (see "Chronic Rx" previously) and management of the underlying immunodeficiency syndrome.

REFERRAL

- To pulmonologist for bronchoscopy if diagnosis cannot be confirmed by sputum examination.
- To an infectious disease specialist if case is severe or difficult to manage.

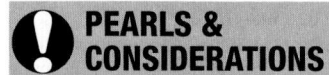 **PEARLS & CONSIDERATIONS**

COMMENTS

- All patients, especially those with severe infection or intolerant of conventional therapy, should be followed by a physician experienced in the management of PJP and, if appropriate, in the long-term management of HIV infection or other underlying disease.
- Severe and life-threatening hypoglycemia may occur 1 or 2 weeks after start of IV pentamidine. Monitor closely and advise the patient of symptoms of hypoglycemia.

RELATED CONTENT

Pneumocystis Pneumonia (Patient Information)
Acquired Immunodeficiency Syndrome (Related Key Topic)

AUTHOR: **PHILIP A. CHAN, M.D., M.S.**

BASIC INFORMATION

DEFINITION

Viral pneumonia is a lung infection caused by any of a large number of viral pathogens. The most important viruses are discussed in this chapter.

SYNONYMS

Viral pneumonia
Nonbacterial pneumonia
Atypical pneumonia

ICD-10CM CODES
J12.9 Viral pneumonia, unspecified
J12.89 Other viral pneumonia

EPIDEMIOLOGY & DEMOGRAPHICS

INCIDENCE (IN U.S.):
- Influenza virus:
  1. 10% to 20% of population in temperate zones infected during 1 to 2 month epidemics occurring yearly during winter months.
  2. Up to 50% infected during pandemics.
  3. Secondary bacterial pneumonia develops in a small percentage of infected persons.
- Incidence of other important viral pathogens that cause pneumonia can vary widely depending on setting and geography.

PEAK INCIDENCE:
- Influenza:
  1. Winter months for influenza A
  2. Year round for influenza B
  3. Peak of pneumonia seen weeks into the outbreak of infection
- Respiratory syncytial virus (RSV) and parainfluenza virus:
  1. Winter and spring
- Adenovirus:
  1. Endemic (military)
- Varicella:
  1. Spring in temperate zones
- Measles:
  1. Year round
- Cytomegalovirus (CMV):
  1. Year round

PREVALENCE (IN U.S.):
- Often related to immune status of the population or presence of an epidemic
- Normal hosts (estimates):
  1. 86% of cases of pneumonia resulting in hospitalization in American adults
  2. 16% of pediatric pneumonias managed as outpatients
  3. 49% of hospitalized infants with pneumonia
- Important problem in hosts with impaired immunity

PREDOMINANT SEX:
- Equal predominance.
- Male sex may predispose to more severe respiratory disease in RSV infection.

PREDOMINANT AGE:
- Influenza:
  1. Overall incidence greatest at age 5 years
  2. Lower incidence with increasing age

  3. The most serious sequelae in those with chronic medical illnesses, especially cardiopulmonary disease
  4. Hospitalizations greatest in infants and adults aged >64 years
- RSV and parainfluenza virus:
  1. Young children (as the major cause of pneumonia)
  2. Occurs throughout life
- Adenoviruses:
  1. Young children
  2. Adults, primarily military recruits
- Varicella:
  1. Approximately 16% of adults (not infected in childhood) who contract chickenpox
  2. Acute varicella during pregnancy more likely to be complicated by severe pneumonia
  3. 90% of reported varicella pneumonia cases are in adults (highest incidence ages 20 to 60 years)
- Measles:
  1. Young adults and older children who received a single vaccination (5% failure rate)
  2. Measles during pregnancy more likely to be complicated by pneumonia
  3. Underlying cardiopulmonary diseases and immunosuppression predispose to serious pneumonia complicating measles
  4. Before availability of measles vaccine, 90% of pneumonias in those <10 years
  5. Currently more than one third of patients >14 years in the U.S.
  6. 3% to 50% of measles cases are complicated by pneumonia
- CMV:
  1. Neonatal through adult
  2. Immunosuppression is key predisposing factor

GENETICS: Familial disposition:
- Close contact, not genetics, is important in acquisition
- Congenital anomalies and immunosuppression worsen course of RSV pneumonia

Congenital infection:
- CMV is the most common intrauterine infection in the U.S.
- Pneumonia occurs occasionally in infants with symptomatic congenital infection.

Neonatal infection:
- Severe RSV pneumonia
- Adenovirus pneumonia
  1. 5% to 20% mortality rate
  2. Can lead to residual restrictive or obstructive functional abnormalities
- "Varicella neonatorum"
  1. Disseminated visceral disease including pneumonia
  2. May develop in neonates whose mothers develop peripartum chickenpox
- CMV pneumonia
  1. Generally fatal
  2. Associated with severe cerebral damage in this population

PHYSICAL FINDINGS & CLINICAL PRESENTATION

1. Influenza:
   - Fever, cough, or sore throat (referred to as influenza-like illness [ILI])
   - Uncomfortable or lethargic appearance

   - Prominent dry cough (rarely hemoptysis)
   - Flushed integument and erythematous mucous membranes
   - Rales or rhonchi
2. RSV and parainfluenza:
   - Fever
   - Tachypnea
   - Prolonged expiration
   - Wheezes and rales
3. Adenoviruses:
   - Hoarseness
   - Pharyngitis
   - Tachypnea
   - Cervical adenitis
4. Measles:
   - Conjunctivitis
   - Rhinorrhea
   - Koplik's spots (white lesions on the buccal mucosa)
   - Exanthem (maculopapular rash that starts on the head, then moves down to rest of body)
   - Pneumonitis
     a. May occur as a complication in 3% to 4% of adolescents and young adults
     b. Coincident with rash
     c. May also develop after apparent recovery from measles
   - Fever
   - Dry cough
5. Varicella:
   - Fever
   - Maculopapular or vesicular rash (all lesions at the same stage)
     a. Becomes encrusted
     b. Pneumonia typical 1 to 6 days after rash appears
     c. Pneumonia (Fig. E1) accompanied by cough and occasionally hemoptysis
   - Few auscultatory abnormalities noted on examination of the lungs
6. CMV:
   - Fever
   - Paroxysmal cough
   - Occasional hemoptysis
   - Diffuse adenopathy when pneumonia occurs after transfusion

ETIOLOGY

Viral infection can lead to pneumonia in both immunocompetent and immunocompromised hosts.

DIAGNOSIS

DIFFERENTIAL DIAGNOSIS

- Bacterial pneumonia, which frequently complicates (i.e., can follow or be simultaneous with) viral pneumonia
- Other causes of atypical pneumonia:
  1. *Mycoplasma* spp.
  2. *Chlamydia* spp.
  3. *Coxiella* spp.
  4. Legionnaires' disease
In certain patient populations (e.g., immunocompromised), consider fungal infections, tuberculosis, or atypical mycobacterium.
- Acute respiratory distress syndrome (ARDS)
- Physical findings and associated hypoxemia confused with pulmonary emboli

WORKUP

- Information about the current prevalent strain of influenza virus can be obtained from local health departments or from the Centers for Disease Control and Prevention.
- Influenza and other viruses may be cultured from respiratory secretions during the initial few days of the illness (special media and techniques necessary).
- Respiratory viral panels that use PCR-based assays to test for a variety of viruses are extremely sensitive and are becoming the test of choice.
- Rapid flu tests have a 50% sensitivity in diagnosing influenza (a negative test does not mean the patient does not have influenza).
- Measles and adenovirus pneumonia are usually diagnosed clinically and can be confirmed with serology.
- CMV may be grown in culture or PCR amplified from bronchoalveolar lavage samples. An algorithm for the workup and management of suspected severe influenza pneumonia in the critical care unit is described in Fig. E2. Open lung biopsy is required for a definite diagnosis of CMV pneumonia.

LABORATORY TESTS

- Sputum Gram stain (usually produced in scanty amounts) typically shows few polymorphonuclear leukocytes and few bacteria.
- White blood cell count may vary from leukopenic to modest elevation, usually without a leftward shift.
- Disseminated intravascular coagulation occasionally complicates adenovirus type 7 pneumonia.
- Multinucleated giant cells on Tzanck preparation of an unroofed vesicular lesion are useful in diagnosing varicella in a patient with an infiltrate (also found in herpes simplex).
- Severe immunosuppression is associated with symptomatic CMV pneumonia (usually reactivation of latent infection or in previously seronegative recipients from the donor).
- Hypoxemia may be profound.
- Cultures may be helpful in identifying superinfecting bacterial pathogens.
- When they occur, parapneumonic pleural effusions are exudative.

IMAGING STUDIES

- Chest radiographs may demonstrate a spectrum of findings from ill-defined, patchy, or generalized interstitial infiltrates, which can be associated with ARDS.
- A localized dense alveolar infiltrate suggests a superimposed bacterial pneumonia.
- Small calcified nodules may develop as a radiographic residual of varicella pneumonia.

Rx TREATMENT

NONPHARMACOLOGIC THERAPY

General:
- Measures to diminish person-to-person transmission
- Modified bed rest

- Maintenance of adequate hydration
- Possible ventilation support for severe pneumonia or ARDS

Influenza:
- Yearly prophylactic strain-specific influenza vaccination can be given to prevent infection.
- Live, attenuated influenza vaccines administered by nose drops as effective as injected inactivated viral vaccines.

RSV:
- Isolation techniques are important in limiting spread of RSV infections.
- Immunoglobulins with a high RSV-neutralizing antibody titer are beneficial in treatment.

Adenoviruses:
- Intestinal inoculation of respiratory adenoviruses has been used to successfully immunize military recruits.
- Although they produce no disease in recipients, the viruses may be shed chronically and may infect others at a later date.
- These vaccines are not available for civilian populations.

Varicella:
- Live, attenuated varicella vaccine has been successfully used in clinical trials.
- Varicella-zoster immune globulin should be administered within 4 days of exposure to prevent or modify the disease in susceptible persons.
- Non-immunized persons exposed to varicella are potentially infectious between 10 and 21 days after exposure.

Measles:
- Effective measles vaccine is available.
  1. The vaccine should be administered at age 15 months.
  2. A second dose should be administered at the time of school entry.
- Live, attenuated vaccine or gamma-globulin can prevent measles in unvaccinated persons if administered early after exposure.
- Vitamin A given PO for two days reduces morbidity and mortality rates from measles in exposed children.

Severe acute respiratory syndrome (SARS)-associated coronaviruses:
- No vaccine currently available.
- Supportive care: ribavirin ineffective, use of steroids or interferon-alpha of unclear value.

ACUTE GENERAL Rx

- **General:** Administer appropriate antibiotics for bacterial superinfections.
- **Influenza:**
  1. Amantadine and rimantadine for influenza A (not active against influenza B). Early use can speed recovery from small airway dysfunction, but whether it influences the development or course of pneumonia is uncertain.
  2. The neuraminidase inhibitors oseltamivir and zanamivir are effective if given in the first 48 hours of symptoms of influenza; their efficacy in established influenza pneumonia is unclear.
  3. Aerosolized ribavirin or amantadine may have a role in treating severe influenza pneumonia, but they have not been approved for this indication.

- **RSV and parainfluenza:**
  1. Ribavirin aerosol may be effective for severe RSV pneumonia.
  2. There is no approved antiviral therapy for parainfluenza virus pneumonia.
- **Adenoviruses:** no effective agent; some case reports of cidofovir use but unproved.
- **Varicella:**
  1. Varicella pneumonia can be treated with IV acyclovir.
  2. Adults who develop chickenpox should be considered for acyclovir treatment, which may prevent the development of pneumonia.
- **Measles:** no effective antimeasles agent.
- **CMV:**
  1. Acyclovir can prevent CMV infection in renal transplant recipients.
  2. Ganciclovir and foscarnet, with or without CMV hyperimmune globulin, show promise in the treatment of serious CMV infection, including pneumonia, in compromised hosts.

DISPOSITION

- Supportive therapy is useful.
- Death is possible during acute illness.
- Residual functional abnormalities may be persistent or develop into or predispose to chronic respiratory diseases in later life.
- Morbidity and mortality rates after most viral pneumonias are increased by bacterial superinfection.

REFERRAL

- Uncertainty about the diagnosis in a compromised host.
- Symptoms or findings are progressive.
- Severe respiratory compromise, diffuse infiltrates, or the development of ARDS.

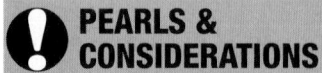

PEARLS & CONSIDERATIONS

COMMENTS

- Influenza spreads by close contact and by small droplets transmitted by cough.
- RSV is effectively transmitted by fomites and by direct contact (little by aerosol).
- Varicella is transmitted by direct contact or by aerosol.
- Of the three major forms of parainfluenza viruses (types 1 to 3), type 3 is the most common cause of viral pneumonia; types 1 and 2 primarily cause laryngotracheitis.
- Recent evidence indicates that a newly discovered virus known as metapneumovirus is a common cause of upper respiratory infections worldwide; this virus can cause pneumonia.

RELATED CONTENT

Viral Pneumonia (Patient Information)
Cytomegalovirus Infection (Related Key Topic)
Influenza (Related Key Topic)
Varicella (Related Key Topic)

AUTHOR: **PHILIP A. CHAN, M.D., M.S.**

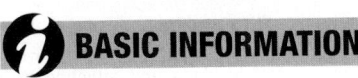

BASIC INFORMATION

DEFINITION

A spontaneous pneumothorax (SP) is defined as air in the pleural space, collapsing the lung without a precipitating event. This can be primary SP (otherwise healthy people without any obvious underlying lung disease) or secondary SP (with underlying lung disease).

SYNONYMS

Primary spontaneous pneumothorax
Secondary spontaneous pneumothorax

ICD-10CM CODES

J93.0	Spontaneous tension pneumothorax
J93.11	Primary spontaneous pneumothorax
J93.12	Secondary spontaneous pneumothorax
J93.81	Chronic pneumothorax
J93.83	Other pneumothorax
J93.9	Pneumothorax, unspecified
J95.811	Postprocedural pneumothorax
P25.1	Pneumothorax originating in the perinatal period
S27.0XXA	Traumatic pneumothorax, initial encounter
S27.0XXD	Traumatic pneumothorax, subsequent encounter
S27.0XXS	Traumatic pneumothorax, sequela

EPIDEMIOLOGY & DEMOGRAPHICS

- Approximately 20,000 new cases of SP occur each year in the United States.
- SP is more common in men than women (6:1).
- Incidence of primary SP is 7.4 per 100,000 in men and 1.2 per 100,000 in women.
- Incidence of secondary SP is 6.3 per 100,000 in men and 2.0 per 100,000 in women.
- SP is commonly seen in tall, thin young men aged 20 to 40 yr.
- Risk factors include smoking, family history, Marfan's syndrome, homocystinuria, and thoracic endometriosis.
- Anorexia nervosa is thought to be a risk factor due to pulmonary parenchymal consequences of malnutrition.

PHYSICAL FINDINGS & CLINICAL PRESENTATION

- Sudden onset of pleuritic chest pain (90%), usually at rest and no relationship between the onset of pneumothorax and physical activity, which often becomes dull after a few hours.
- Pain is usually unilateral and can be sharp and agonizing and associated with considerable apprehension.
- Dyspnea (80%), which often resolves within 24 hr, despite persistence of pneumothorax.
- Cough (10%).
- Asymptomatic (5%); may take up to 7 days to come to medical attention.
- Tachycardia.
- Hypoxemia.
- Hypercapnia is rare because the alveolar ventilation is maintained by the contralateral lung.
- Decreased chest excursion on the affected side.
- Diminished breath sounds.
- Subcutaneous emphysema may be present.
- Hyperresonance on percussion.

ETIOLOGY

- In primary SP, rupture of small blebs and bullae, usually located near the apex of the upper lobes, is a common cause.
- In secondary SP, chronic obstructive pulmonary disease is the most common cause, but it can also be associated with pneumonia, bronchogenic carcinoma, mesothelioma, sarcoidosis, tuberculosis, cystic fibrosis, and many other lung diseases (Fig. 1).

Dx DIAGNOSIS

Established by the chest x-ray (Fig. 2).

DIFFERENTIAL DIAGNOSIS

- Pleurisy.
- Pulmonary embolism.
- Myocardial infarction.
- Pericarditis.
- Asthma.
- Pneumonia.

WORKUP

CXR

LABORATORY TESTS

Arterial blood gases may show hypoxemia and hypocapnia as a result of hyperventilation.

IMAGING STUDIES

- SP is usually confirmed by upright CXR:
  1. A white visceral pleural line. The absence of vessel markings peripheral to this line helps differentiate from mimicking conditions such as an overlying skin fold. A lateral width of 1 cm corresponds to 27% pneumothorax, and 2 cm occupies 49% of the hemithorax.
  2. The left lateral decubitus position is the most sensitive and the supine position the least sensitive. Inspiratory and expiratory films have equal sensitivities.
  3. As little as 50 mL of air can be detected on upright film.

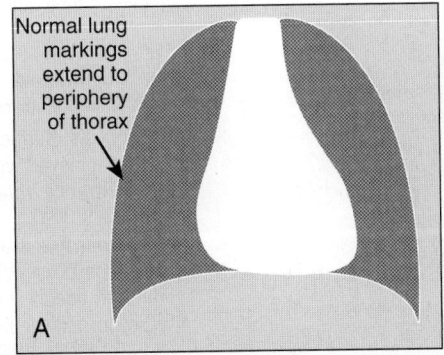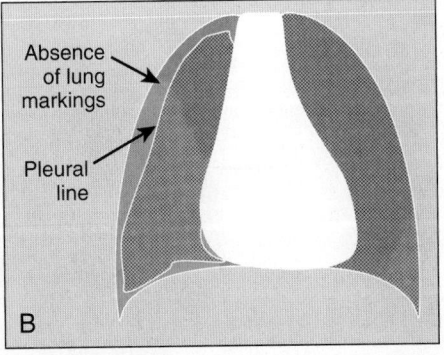

FIG. 1 Pneumothorax. A, Schematic of normal lung. **B,** Schematic of pneumothorax. Pneumothoraces can range in size from tiny to massive. Because of the variability in their size and location, pneumothoraces can be difficult to detect on chest x-ray. For example, a pneumothorax that is anterior or posterior rather than lateral may be hidden on frontal chest x-ray, particularly one taken in the supine position. An upright chest x-ray should be obtained if possible. An expiratory film is thought to be more sensitive, because the lung and thorax decrease in size during expiration, but air trapped in the pleural space remains the same size and thus appears relatively larger. Subtle pneumothoraces may not be visible on chest x-ray. In some cases, subcutaneous air may be the only visible clue to underlying lung injury. CT is extremely sensitive for pneumothorax, although controversy remains over the proper management of pneumothoraces seen only on CT. Ultrasound is also thought to be more sensitive than chest x-ray for detection of pneumothorax, although, again, the management of pneumothorax seen only on ultrasound is uncertain because this is a relatively newly described method of detection. The chest x-ray findings of pneumothorax include a lack of the normal lung markings, which should be visible to the periphery of the chest wall. Sometimes a line marking the boundary of the lung and visceral pleura is visible, although this can be confused with ribs and with the medial margin of the scapula. Depending on the degree of pneumothorax and lung collapse, the lung parenchyma may appear denser than the opposite side. In extreme cases of tension pneumothorax, the pressure exerted by the air in the pleural space may begin to displace other structures, including the diaphragm and mediastinum. In tension pneumothorax, the hyperinflated hemithorax may also have abnormally positioned ribs, with a position more horizontal than usual. (From Broder JS: *Diagnostic imaging for the emergency physician,* Philadelphia, 2011, Saunders.)

- Tension pneumothorax (Fig. 3) is a medical emergency and should be suspected when the patient is hemodynamically unstable or with contralateral tracheal and mediastinal deviation and ipsilateral flattening or inversion of the diaphragm on the CXR (Fig. E4).
- CT scan is considered acceptable for a patient with recurrent pneumothorax or persistent air leak, and for planning surgery.

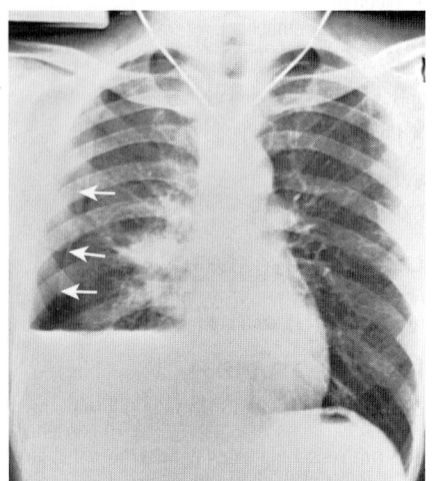

FIG. 2 Chest radiograph shows right hydropneumothorax. Horizontal line in lower right hemithorax is interface between air and liquid in pleural space. *Arrows* point to visceral pleura above level of effusion. There is air in pleural space between visceral pleura and chest wall. (From Weinberg SE et al: *Principles of pulmonary medicine,* ed 5, Philadelphia, 2008, Saunders.)

- Lung ultrasound has emerged as a rapid and accurate screening tool for pneumothorax. The lung point sign, a sonographic representation of the point of the chest wall where the pleural layers readhere, is 100% specific to confirm the diagnosis.[1]

RX TREATMENT

INITIAL MANAGEMENT

- 100% oxygen administration reduces the partial pressure of nitrogen in pleural capillaries, consequently quadrupling the rate of pneumothorax absorption, and should be administered to all patients with pneumothorax.
- Further treatment is based on the size of the pneumothorax.
  1. If the pneumothorax is small (<2 cm between lung and chest wall on CXR) and the patient is asymptomatic, the patient can be treated with observation alone. Repeat imaging should be performed to ensure stability/resorption of the pneumothorax.
  2. If the pneumothorax is large (>2 cm), or if the patient is symptomatic with chest pain and dyspnea, initial management should focus on removing air from the pleural space. Needle aspiration is the treatment of choice in the clinically stable patient.
- Needle aspiration can be done at the bedside using a large-bore angiocatheter needle or commercially available catheter aspiration

---

[1]Aspler A, et al.: Double-lung point sign in traumatic pneumothorax, *Am J Emerg Med* 32:819, 2014.

kit. The needle is introduced in the second intercostal space midclavicular line. The catheter is left in place and attached to a three-way stopcock and a large syringe. Air is aspirated until resistance is met or the patient experiences significant coughing. Repeat CXR is done immediately after aspiration and again in 4 to 24 hr to document reexpansion of the lung. If the pneumothorax fails to resolve with aspiration, repeated aspiration is reasonable for primary spontaneous pneumothorax.
- If there is improvement but not complete resolution of pneumothorax after the aspiration, the catheter can be attached to a Heimlich (one-way) valve to allow further lung expansion. Some stable patients can be discharged home with this device in place if close follow-up monitoring can be obtained. Chest tube insertion has been recommended for patients with primary SP who are unsuccessful in controlling symptoms by simple aspiration or catheter aspiration. Most patients can be managed with small chest tubes (<12 Fr). The chest tube can be connected to a water seal device, with or without suction, and left in position until the pneumothorax has resolved.
- An algorithmic approach to the treatment of primary spontaneous pneumothorax is outlined in Fig. 5.

PREVENTION

- Approximately 25% to 50% of patients with primary SP with have a recurrence within 1 yr.
- Prevention of spontaneous pneumothorax is surgical intervention or instillation of sclerosing agents through a chest tube.
- Indication for the surgical intervention is second ipsilateral SP, first contralateral SP, simultaneous bilateral SP, persistent air leak (>5-7 days), failure of lung reexpansion by the chest tube, and professions at risk (e.g., pilots, divers).
- The current recommended surgical approach is the use of video-assisted thoracoscopy (VATS) with bullectomy and pleurodesis. Surgical chemical pleurodesis is best achieved with sterile talc. The overall recurrence rate is estimated at <5% after VATS.
- Instillation of a sclerosing agent through a chest tube: doxycycline and talc slurry are the preferred agents; minocycline is considered to be an acceptable agent. The recurrence rates for the instillation of sclerosing agents (minocycline 5 mg/kg in 50 ml of normal saline or doxycycline 500 mg in 50 ml of normal saline) are higher than for VATS-guided therapy (<25%). Therefore this mode of therapy should be reserved for patients who are poor surgical candidates.

DISPOSITION

- Smoking cessation should be advised.
- Death from primary SP is uncommon. In patients with secondary SP and chronic obstructive pulmonary disease, mortality rates range from 1% to 16%.

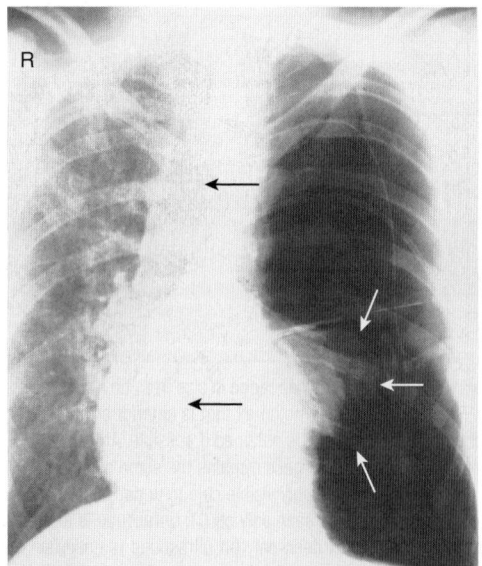

FIG. 3 Tension pneumothorax. On this PA chest radiograph, the left hemithorax is very dark or lucent because the left lung has collapsed completely *(white arrows).* The tension pneumothorax can be identified by the fact that the mediastinal contents, including the heart, are shifted toward the right *(black arrows),* and the left hemidiaphragm is flattened and depressed. (From Mettler FA et al: *Primary care radiology,* Philadelphia, 2000, Elsevier.)

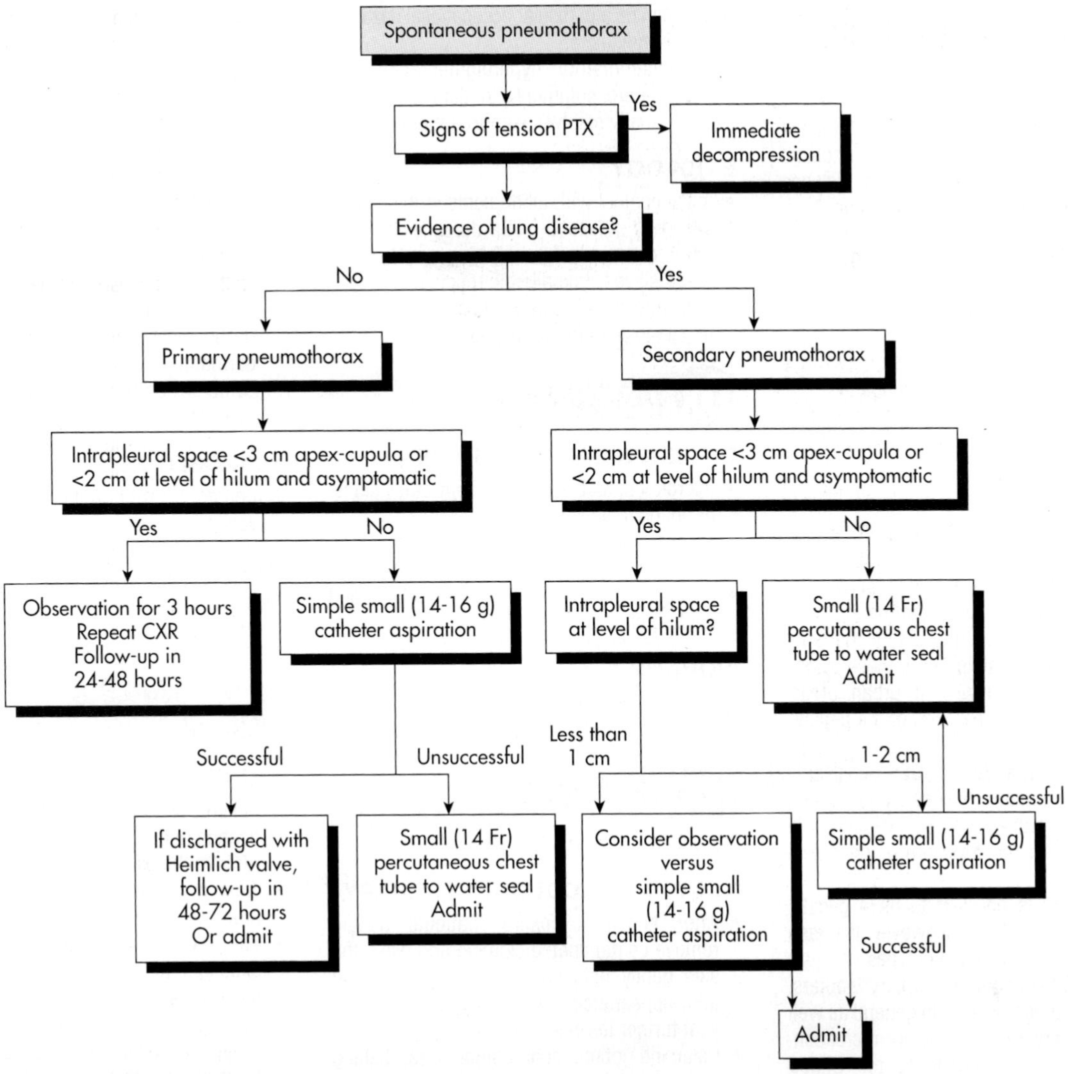

Spontaneous pneumothorax

Signs of tension PTX → Yes → Immediate decompression

Evidence of lung disease?

No → Primary pneumothorax

Yes → Secondary pneumothorax

Primary pneumothorax:
Intrapleural space <3 cm apex-cupula or <2 cm at level of hilum and asymptomatic

Yes → Observation for 3 hours
Repeat CXR
Follow-up in 24-48 hours

No → Simple small (14-16 g) catheter aspiration

Successful → If discharged with Heimlich valve, follow-up in 48-72 hours Or admit

Unsuccessful → Small (14 Fr) percutaneous chest tube to water seal Admit

Secondary pneumothorax:
Intrapleural space <3 cm apex-cupula or <2 cm at level of hilum and asymptomatic

Yes → Intrapleural space at level of hilum?

No → Small (14 Fr) percutaneous chest tube to water seal Admit

Less than 1 cm → Consider observation versus simple small (14-16 g) catheter aspiration

1-2 cm → Simple small (14-16 g) catheter aspiration

Unsuccessful → (to Small percutaneous chest tube)

Successful → Admit

FIG. 5 Algorithmic approach to the treatment of primary spontaneous pneumothorax. *CXR,* Chest radiograph. (From Adams JG et al: *Emergency medicine: clinical essentials,* ed 2, Philadelphia, 2013, Elsevier.)

REFERRAL

A pulmonary specialist and surgical consultation are recommended.

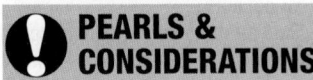 **PEARLS & CONSIDERATIONS**

- The rate of pleural air absorption is approximately 1.25% of the volume of the hemithorax per day. Therefore the interval for complete resolution of pneumothorax with observation can be estimated.
- Catamenial pneumothorax is a rare condition characterized by recurrent SP coinciding with the onset of menses. It usually affects the right lung and is believed to be caused by endometriosis with involvement of the diaphragm and/or pleura. It is believed to be hormonally related, and treatment is aimed at endometrial suppression.

COMMENTS

- Patients with AIDS and *Pneumocystis jiroveci* infection have a high incidence of SP. Treatment typically requires chest tube placement and either thoracoscopy or open thoracotomy.

 EVIDENCE

Available at www.expertconsult.com
SUGGESTED READINGS
Available at www.expertconsult.com

RELATED CONTENT

Pneumothorax (Patient Information)

AUTHOR: **HISASHI TSUKADA, M.D., PH.D.**

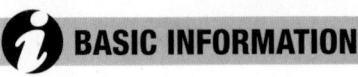

BASIC INFORMATION

DEFINITION

Poison ivy dermatitis is a contact dermatitis caused by exposure to urushiol, the oil of plants of the genus *Toxicodendron,* which includes poison ivy, poison oak, and poison sumac.

SYNONYMS

Rhus dermatitis
Toxicodendron dermatitis

ICD-10CM CODES
L23.7 Allergic contact dermatitis due to plants, except food

EPIDEMIOLOGY & DEMOGRAPHICS

INCIDENCE: Affects 10 million to 40 million Americans annually.
PEAK INCIDENCE: More frequent in months when outdoor activity is more common.
PREVALENCE: From 50% to 75% of the adult population is clinically sensitive to these plants. Sensitivity rates are lower in urban areas. (Tolerance is found in 10%-15% of the population.)
PREDOMINANT SEX AND AGE: Sensitization occurs most commonly between ages 8 and 14 yr. Sensitivity wanes with age, especially in individuals with limited exposure or prior mild reactions.
GENETICS: There is believed to be a genetic susceptibility to sensitivity; however, the rash occurs in all ethnicities and skin types.
RISK FACTORS: Firefighters, forestry workers, farmers, and outdoor workers in general as well as those who participate in outdoor recreation. These plants are indigenous to the United States, Canada, and Mexico, and cases are most common in these areas.

PHYSICAL FINDINGS & CLINICAL PRESENTATION

- Patients typically present with intense pruritus and rash. The patient may not be aware of exposure to the plant.
- Symptoms typically peak from 1 to 14 days after exposure depending on the degree of exposure and thickness of affected skin.
- Dermatitis may initially present as erythema and may develop into papules, vesicles, and bullae.
- Lesions may be found in the classic linear configuration, typically in exposed areas likely to have been in contact with plants (Fig. E1). Atypical appearance or location of dermatitis is more common with secondary exposure, such as through pets or infected tools or clothing.
- Face and genital involvement may present with significant edema.
- Inhalation of urushiol aerosolized by fire can cause significant respiratory tract inflammation.

This can be a particular occupational hazard of forest firefighters.
- Postinflammatory hyperpigmentation may occur, more commonly in dark skin types. This usually resolves with treatment.

ETIOLOGY

- Initial contact with oil of plants in this genus, which is released with damage to plant parts, causes a classic T-lymphocyte–mediated delayed-type allergic reaction.
- Subsequent exposures cause a cell-mediated cytotoxic immune response.

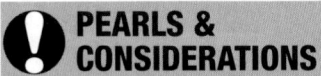

DIAGNOSIS

DIFFERENTIAL DIAGNOSIS

- Allergic contact dermatitis from other plants or nonplant substances.
- Irritant contact dermatitis.
- Nummular dermatitis.
- Arthropod reactions, including scabies and bedbug bites.

WORKUP

Typically not needed. Diagnosis is based on characteristic rash and possibly history of exposure.

TREATMENT

Prevention is the most effective treatment.

NONPHARMACOLOGIC THERAPY

- After known exposure, patients should remove contaminated clothing and wash the skin gently with soap and water. Washing after appearance of dermatitis does not prevent further lesions.
- Calamine lotion, cool compresses, baking soda, or colloidal oatmeal baths may provide symptomatic relief.
- Keep nails short and clean to help prevent secondary bacterial infection.
- Exposed clothing, as well as tools, pets, and equipment, should be washed with soap and water to prevent secondary exposure.

ACUTE GENERAL Rx

- Topical steroids are generally not helpful. They may be effective for symptom management in mild, early cases with erythema and pruritus but no vesiculation.
- Topical antibiotics should be avoided.
- Use of antihistamines for associated pruritus may be effective, but this has not been extensively studied.
- Systemic corticosteroids offer significant relief in moderate to severe *Rhus* dermatitis, including generalized rash or severe facial or genital involvement.
- Effective dosing of oral prednisone is 1 mg/kg/day over 7 to 10 days (maximum 60 mg initial dose), with tapering over an additional 7 to 10 days.

- Inadequate doses or too-rapid tapering of systemic steroids may cause symptom rebound.
- IM treatment with long-acting triamcinolone suspension may be considered for patients intolerant of oral therapy.

CHRONIC Rx

- Recurrence may be caused by repeated exposure to fomites, including contaminated clothing, equipment, or pets.
- Secondary bacterial infection of the skin is the most common complication of *Rhus* dermatitis. Staph and strep are the most common pathogens, but MRSA must be considered.

DISPOSITION

Untreated *Rhus* dermatitis will resolve in 1 to 3 weeks.

REFERRAL

Refer to dermatology if there is diagnostic confusion.

PEARLS & CONSIDERATIONS

PREVENTION

- Patients should be educated regarding identification and avoidance as well as washing to remove the oil after known exposure.
- Total avoidance of the plants may not be practical.
- The use of barrier creams applied before exposure to prevent dermatitis may be of some benefit, particularly in potential occupational (therefore predictable) exposure.
- Products available for postexposure prophylaxis are effective; however, equal efficacy may be obtained from less expensive liquid dishwashing soap.
- Desensitization has not been found to be effective.

PATIENT & FAMILY EDUCATION

- "Leaves of three, let it be," is a helpful reminder for patients.
- Patient education material, including access to photographs of the leaves of these plants in a variety of seasons and conditions, may be useful.

SUGGESTED READING
Available at www.expertconsult.com

RELATED CONTENT
Poison Ivy (Patient Information)
Contact Dermatitis (Related Key Topic)

AUTHOR: **MARGARET TRYFOROS, M.D.**

BASIC INFORMATION

DEFINITION

Polyarteritis nodosa (PAN) is a systemic vasculitic syndrome involving medium-sized to small arteries, characterized histologically by necrotizing inflammation of the arterial media and inflammatory cell infiltration. It is not associated with antineutrophil cytoplasmic antibodies (ANCA).

SYNONYMS

Periarteritis nodosa
PAN
Necrotizing arteritis

ICD-10CM CODES
M30.0 Polyarteritis nodosa

EPIDEMIOLOGY & DEMOGRAPHICS

- Incidence is 1/100,000 persons annually.
- Increased incidence in patients with hepatitis B surface antigen or hepatitis C virus.
- Male:female ratio of 1.5:1.
- Commonly occurs between ages 40 and 60 yr.
- Can also occur in children.
- No racial predilection is observed.
- Prevalence is 2 to 33/1,000,000.
- Is also associated with hairy cell leukemia.

PHYSICAL FINDINGS & CLINICAL PRESENTATION

- Typical presentation is subacute in >90% of cases.
- Weight loss.
- Nausea, vomiting, headache.
- Testicular pain or tenderness.
- Myalgias, weakness, or leg tenderness in 24% to 80% of cases.
- Neuropathy (mononeuritis multiplex), foot drop.
- Cutaneous manifestations like tender nodules, livedo reticularis, palpable purpura, ulceration of digits.
- Abdominal pain after meals, hematemesis, hematochezia, occasionally with diarrhea and gastrointestinal bleeding in severe cases.
- Asymmetric polyarthritis (tending to involve large joints of lower extremities); true synovitis occurs only in a minority of patients.
- Presence of lung vasculitis suggests other causes.
- Fever (PAN is often a cause of fever of unknown origin) can range from intermittent, low-grade fevers to high fevers with chills.
- Chest pain secondary to ischemic infarcts in the coronary arteries, pericarditis, cardiomyopathy, and arrhythmias are seen with cardiac involvement.
- Tachycardia is common and often striking.
- Hypertension secondary to renal ischemia, perirenal hematomas.

ETIOLOGY

- Unknown.
- Hepatitis B virus–associated PAN appears to be an immune complex–mediated disease.
- Hepatitis C, hairy cell leukemia, and human immunodeficiency virus are also associated in some cases.

DIAGNOSIS

DIFFERENTIAL DIAGNOSIS

- Cryoglobulinemia.
- Systemic lupus erythematosus.
- Infections (e.g., subacute bacterial endocarditis, trichinosis, *Rickettsia*).
- Lymphoma.
- Henoch-Schönlein purpura (IgA vasculitis).
- Granulomatosis with polyangiitis (Wegener granulomatosis).
- Microscopic polyangiitis.
- Kawasaki disease.
- Eosinophilic granulomatosis with polyangiitis (EGPA).
- Giant cell arteritis.
- Human immunodeficiency virus.
- Drug-induced vasculitis.

WORKUP

- Laboratory evaluation, arteriography, and biopsy of small or medium-sized arteries can confirm diagnosis. Clinical manifestations are variable and depend on the arteries involved and the organs affected (e.g., kidney involvement occurs in >80% of cases). Table 1 summarizes investigations for patients with suspected PAN.
- The presence of any three of the following 10 items allows the diagnosis of PAN with a sensitivity of 82% and a specificity of 86%:
    1. Weight loss >4 kg.
    2. Livedo reticularis.
    3. Testicular pain or tenderness.
    4. Myalgias, weakness, or leg tenderness.
    5. Neuropathy.
    6. Diastolic blood pressure <90 mm Hg.
    7. Elevated blood urea nitrogen (BUN) or creatinine.
    8. Positive test for hepatitis B virus.
    9. Arteriography revealing small or large aneurysms and focal constrictions between dilated segments.
    10. Biopsy of small or medium-sized artery containing necrotizing inflammatory infiltrate.

TABLE 1 Investigations for Patients With Suspected Polyarteritis Nodosa (PAN)

Test	Supports Diagnosis of PAN	Supports an Alternative Diagnosis	Comment
Elevated C-reactive protein	+		Supports the presence of systemic inflammation
Elevated sedimentation rate	+		Supports the presence of systemic inflammation
Elevated serum creatinine	+/−	+/−	Raised serum creatinine, typically without hematuria or proteinuria on urinalysis, may indicate renal ischemia or infarction. Significant proteinuria or hematuria (especially red cell casts) would suggest glomerular disease, which is *not* a feature of PAN
Abnormal liver function tests	+		May suggest hepatitis, either from HBV or as a result of ischemic hepatitis from PAN affecting the hepatic arteries
Positive HBV serology	+		Seen in HBV PAN
Anemia	+		Due to chronic inflammation or from gastrointestinal blood loss
Positive ANCA		+	A positive ANCA would suggest an alternative type of vasculitis such as granulomatosis with polyangiitis or MPA
Elevated creatine kinase	+/−	+/−	Normal or mildly elevated, despite any muscle involvement
Blood cultures		+	To exclude endocarditis or other infective mimic of vasculitis
Positive HCV serology and cryoglobulins		+	HCV associated with a skin limited manifestation of PAN, but typically it is associated with a small vessel vasculitis related to cryoglobulinemia
Positive rheumatoid factor and ACPA		+	To rule out rheumatoid arthritis, especially in the context of a patient presenting predominantly with arthritis
Positive ANA and anti-dsDNA		+	In patients with clinical features consistent with SLE or other connective tissue disease
HIV positive		+	

ACPA, Anticitrullinated protein antibody; *ANA,* antinuclear antibody; *ANCA,* antineutrophil cytoplasm antibody; *dsDNA,* double-stranded deoxyribonucleic acid; *ESR,* erythrocyte sedimentation rate; *HBV,* hepatitis B virus; *HCV,* hepatitis C virus; *HIV,* human immunodeficiency virus; *MPA,* microscopic polyangiitis; *SLE,* systemic lupus erythematosus.
From Firestein GS et al: *Kelly's textbook of rheumatology,* ed 9, Philadelphia, 2013, Saunders.

LABORATORY TESTS

- Elevated BUN or creatinine, positive test for hepatitis B virus or hepatitis C.
- Elevated erythrocyte sedimentation rate and C-reactive protein, anemia, elevated platelets, eosinophilia, proteinuria, hematuria.
- Biopsy of small or medium-sized artery of symptomatic sites (muscle, nerve) is >90% specific. Biopsy of the gastrocnemius muscle and sural nerve is commonly performed.
- Circumferential or segmental vessel wall involvement with necrotizing mixed cell inflammation with fibrinoid necrosis is characteristic lesion of active PAN.
- Assays for antinuclear antibody and rheumatoid factor are negative; however, low, nonspecific titers may be detected.
- Serum and urine immunofixation electrophoresis for monoclonal gammopathy and human immunodeficiency virus should also be tested for alternative diagnoses.

IMAGING STUDIES

Arteriography can be done in patients with negative biopsies or if there are no symptomatic sites. Mesenteric angiography will reveal aneurysmal dilation of the renal, mesenteric (Fig. 1), or hepatic arteries. Less invasive techniques, such as computed tomography (CT) and MRI angiography, also help evaluate the extent and resolution of the disease.

Nerve conduction studies are useful in patients with neuropathy suggesting PAN, helping to evaluate nerves or muscles to biopsy.

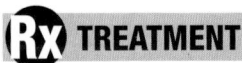

TREATMENT

NONPHARMACOLOGIC THERAPY

Low-sodium diet in hypertensive patients.

ACUTE GENERAL Rx

- Prednisone 1 to 2 mg/kg/day with higher doses initially, then tapering the doses slowly with overall course of average 9 months or longer.
- Patients with isolated cutaneous involvement may be treated with steroids alone or in combination with methotrexate.

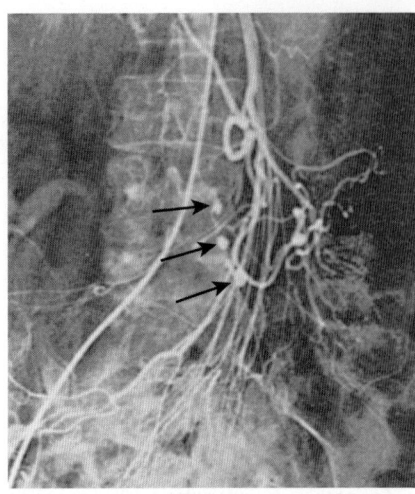

FIG. 1 Superior mesenteric arteriogram in patients with polyarteritis. Several small aneurysms *(arrows)* are present in branches of superior mesenteric artery. (Courtesy Dr. A.W. Stanson. From Harris ED et al: *Kelley's textbook of rheumatology,* ed 7, 2005, Saunders.)

- Severe PAN with multiorgan involvement treated with a combination of cyclophosphamide 1.5 to 2 mg/kg per day and glucocorticoids has shown good disease outcomes. Once patient achieves stable remission, transition to a less toxic immunomodulatory therapy such as methotrexate or azathioprine, along with tapering doses of oral prednisone, is indicated for chronic therapy.
- In conditions where the disease is resistant to cyclophosphamide glucocorticoids, pulse steroids for few months then switching to alternate agents such as mycophenolate, azathioprine or methotrexate is tried.
- If hepatitis B is identified, then appropriate antiviral treatment (interferon alpha-2b or lamivudine with or without plasma exchange) is initiated.
- Plasma exchange has been shown to have a limited role in treatment of severe forms of acute hepatitis B–associated PAN.

CHRONIC Rx

Monitoring for infections and potential complications such as thrombosis, infarction, or organ necrosis. Hypertension in patients with renal involvement in PAN is treated with angiotensin-converting enzyme inhibitor.

DISPOSITION

The 5-yr survival is <20% in untreated patients. Treatment with corticosteroids increases survival to approximately 50%. Use of both corticosteroids and immunosuppressive drugs may increase 5-yr survival to >80%. Poor prognostic signs are severe renal or gastrointestinal involvement. Prognosis is better in patients with cutaneous PAN without systemic involvement. Patients on cyclophosphamide should have regular white cell count monitoring for leukopenia. Cyclophosphamide can cause increased risk of infertility, myelodysplasia, lymphoma, bladder malignancy, and when given in combination of high-dose corticosteroids can predispose patients to infection with *Pneumocystis jiroveci (carinii)* pneumonia. Therefore, close follow-up and PCP prophylaxis are recommended.

REFERRAL

Patients with suspected diagnosis of PAN should be immediately referred to a rheumatologist.

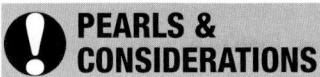

PEARLS & CONSIDERATIONS

- After treatment, patients should be followed up closely for relapse throughout their lifetime.
- Smoking cessation, exercise, and lifestyle modifications should be discussed to decrease vascular complications.

SUGGESTED READINGS

Available at www.expertconsult.com

AUTHORS: **SYEDA M. SAYEED, M.D.**

BASIC INFORMATION

DEFINITION

Autosomal dominant polycystic kidney disease (ADPKD) is a systemic inherited disorder due to mutations in either the *PKD1* or *PKD2* gene. These mutations lead to cyst formation and growth in multiple organs including kidneys, liver, and pancreas. ADPKD is also associated with multiple gastrointestinal and cardiovascular abnormalities. It is the most common inherited kidney disease, and its prevalence is more common than that of Huntington's disease, hemophilia, sickle cell disease, cystic fibrosis, myotonic dystrophy, and Down syndrome combined.

SYNONYMS

Adult polycystic kidney disease
Autosomal dominant polycystic kidney disease
ADPKD

ICD-10CM CODES
Q61.3 Polycystic kidney, unspecified
Q61.2 Polycystic kidney, adult type
Q61.19 Other polycystic kidney, infantile type
Z82.71 Family history of polycystic kidney

EPIDEMIOLOGY & DEMOGRAPHICS

- Most common single genetic cause of chronic kidney disease (CKD)
- Mendelian dominant disorder
- Affects all ethnic groups equally worldwide
- Approximately 85 percent of ADPKD individuals have a mutation on chromosome 16 (*PKD1* locus), and 15% have a mutation located on chromosome 4 in the *PKD2* gene. 3% of the ADPKD population has mutations in the glucosidase, alpha, neutral AB form (*GANAB*) gene located on chromosome 11q12.3.
- Each child of an affected parent has a 50% chance of inheriting the mutated gene.
- The disease has 100% penetrance and does not skip generations.

INCIDENCE:
- Between 1 in 400 and 1000 live births in the U.S.

GENETICS: ADPKD is caused by a mutation in the *PKD1* gene located on the short arm of chromosome 16, which lies next to the *TSC2* gene. The gene encoding polycystin-1 (PC1) plays a vital role in cell-cell and cell-matrix interactions and primary ciliary function. Mutations in *PKD1* lead to an alteration in the differentiation of epithelial cells and the abnormal phenotypic expressions characteristic of ADPKD. ADPKD is less commonly caused by a mutation in the *PKD2* gene located on chromosome 4. *PKD2* encodes the protein polycystin-2 (PC2), which is involved in intracellular calcium signaling. *PKD2* patients typically have milder disease with later onset of end-stage renal disease (ESRD), death, and hypertension. Polycystin 1 and 2 form a single functional complex through interactions of their intracellular carboxy termini. Consequently, a mutation of either *PKD1* or *PKD2* results in a similar phenotype.

- ADPKD is also caused by mutations in the *GANAB* gene in 3% of ADPKD patients. This gene is located on chromosome 11q12.3 and is expressed in the kidney and liver. The *GANAB* gene encodes the catalytic subunit of glucosidase II (GIIα). GII is thought to play an important role in PC1 maturation. Cystogenesis is likely caused by disruption in PC1 maturation. Usually these patients have very mild PKD and mild to severe polycystic liver disease.

CLINICAL PRESENTATION

ADPKD is a systemic disorder, and symptoms relate primarily to the kidney cyst burden and extrarenal involvement, including polycystic liver disease and vascular complications. Total kidney volume (TKV) and cyst volume in ADPKD increase exponentially over time in patients with ADPKD.

RENAL MANIFESTATIONS

Many patients with ADPKD are asymptomatic. The diagnosis is established by either the identification of an afflicted family member, asymptomatic screening (approximately 40%), or renal imaging performed for another reason. Patients may present with gross hematuria, flank mass/pain, polyuria/nocturia, fever due to a kidney or lower urinary tract infection, nephrolithiasis, or blood pressure elevation. All of these complications are manifested through increased cyst burden or TKV.

Gross hematuria occurs in 35% to 50% of patients with ADPKD and is associated with increased TKV. Hematuria is also caused by rupture of a cyst into the collecting system or is secondary to nephrolithiasis. Nephrolithiasis occurs in approximately 27% of ADPKD patients, and is due in part to low levels of urinary citrate. Kidney stones may present as flank pain or hematuria, which is commonly microscopic.

Polyuria, nocturia, and increased thirst in ADPKD occur from impaired urinary concentrating ability and increases in circulating vasopressin levels.

Proteinuria is not a common feature of ADPKD and is usually less than 1 g/day. However, the presence of detectable proteinuria and microalbuminuria is correlated with increased TKV and more severe kidney disease.

Urinary tract infections are common in patients with PKD but do not appear to be more common than in the general population. Renal cyst infections are specific to ADPKD, and patients typically present with localized flank pain, fevers, and nausea and vomiting, similar to pyelonephritis.

Acute flank pain can be caused by a kidney stone, kidney, or liver cyst rupture or hemorrhage. Chronic pain is typically due to enlarged kidneys, either unilaterally or bilaterally.

CARDIAC MANIFESTATIONS

Hypertension occurs in 60% of patients with ADPKD prior to any substantial decline in kidney function and appears earlier in males than in females. Hypertension in ADPKD is due to upregulation of renin-angiotensin-aldosterone system (RAAS). Hypertension is a predictor of worse renal outcome and is associated with cardiovascular morbidity and mortality. Cardiac valvular abnormalities occur in 25% to 30% of patients and include mitral valve prolapse and aortic regurgitation.

EXTRARENAL MANIFESTATIONS

1. The prevalence of intracranial aneurysms (ICA) in ADPKD is approximately 5% and increases to as high as 20% in patients with a first-degree relative with a known intracranial aneurysm rupture.
2. Rupture of an ICA is a serious complication of PKD and may produce significant permanent morbidity or death. Routine screening for ICA is recommended for patients with a family history of ICA or intracerebral bleed, or for patients with warning symptoms such as a sentinel headache.
3. In addition to kidney cysts, cysts can develop in the liver, pancreas, and seminal vesicles. Hepatic cysts are common and occur in up to ~85% of ADPKD patients by the age of 30 years. Hepatic cysts represent the most common extrarenal manifestation of ADPKD. Liver cystic disease is typically asymptomatic and develops slightly later than kidney cysts in ADPKD. However, hepatic cysts can cause serious complications including pain, infection, bleeding, and biliary obstruction. Liver cysts continue to grow and expand after patients reach ESRD.
4. Colonic diverticula and abdominal or inguinal hernias occur more frequently in ADPKD patients.
5. Seminal vesical cysts have been reported to occur in up to 40% of men with ADPKD, but are not associated with changes in fertility.
6. Patients with ADPKD may be at an increased risk of developing liver, colon, and kidney cancer. However, there is not much evidence to change cancer screening guidelines for patients with PKD.

NATURAL HISTORY

- Patients with *PKD1* mutations have faster disease progression than patients with PKD2 mutations, and the median age of onset of ESRD is 54 years in *PKD1* patients and 74 years in PKD2 patients.
- Other clinical risk factors associated with progressive kidney disease in ADPKD include male sex, onset of hypertension before 35 years of age, early onset of gross hematuria, presence of proteinuria or microalbuminuria, increased urinary sodium excretion, and increased low-density lipoprotein cholesterol (LDL) levels. However, all of these risk factors are mediated through cyst burden or TKV.
- Data from the Consortium of Radiologic Imaging studies of Polycystic Kidney Disease (CRISP) indicate that the decline in renal blood flow and the increases in TKV and cyst volume are strong predictors of future renal functional decline and progression to CKD stage 3. Baseline height-adjusted TKV of 600 ml/m predicts the risk of developing stage 3 CKD within 8 years. Patients with ADPKD can be classified into categories 1A-1E based on height-adjusted TKV limits for

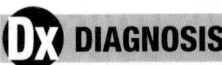

their ages. Patients in class 1A are at a low risk for renal function decline, and patients in class 1C-1E are at a high risk for progressive disease. This classification helps physicians identify patients with severe disease.

DIAGNOSIS

Ultrasound of the kidneys is the most commonly used imaging modality for screening and diagnosis and is inexpensive, readily available, noninvasive, and free of radiation. CT and MRI are also used, but typically in the setting of acute complications. CT scan and MRI are more sensitive than ultrasound, with cyst detection at <1 cm in size.

The following diagnostic criteria are used for diagnosis of ADPKD in asymptomatic individuals at risk for development of ADPKD (i.e., those with positive family history of ADPKD):

1. Individuals 15 to 39 years of age: At least three unilateral or bilateral kidney cysts.
2. Individuals 40 to 59 years of age: At least two cysts in each kidney.
3. Individuals older than 60 years of age: At least four cysts in each kidney.

With no family history of ADPKD, there is no definitive number of cysts and/or cyst location that provides an unequivocal diagnosis. The diagnosis is strongly suspected when multiple and bilateral kidney cysts are present along with hepatic cysts.

Genetic testing can be done to diagnose ADPKD when imaging results are equivocal and when a definitive diagnosis is required in a young individual such as a potential living donor.

DIFFERENTIAL DIAGNOSIS

- Multiple benign simple cysts
- Autosomal-recessive PKD
- Familial juvenile nephronophthisis
- Medullary cystic or UMOD (uromodulin) disease
- Medullary sponge kidney
- Tuberous sclerosis
- von Hippel-Lindau syndrome
- Acquired cystic kidney disease

LABORATORY TESTS

- Hemoglobin and hematocrit may be elevated because of increased erythropoietin production but are typically similar to levels in other patients with CKD.
- Urinalysis can show microscopic hematuria and proteinuria (seldom >1 g per day).
- With decreased kidney function, blood urea nitrogen and creatinine are elevated.
- Platelet counts can be mildly reduced in patients with extensive polycystic liver disease.
- Metabolic acidosis, hyperparathyroidism, and hyperphosphatemia are all associated with CKD in ADPKD.

TREATMENT

NONPHARMACOLOGIC THERAPY

- Restriction of dietary salt (<2 g sodium/24 h) and calories is recommended.

- Cyclic adenosine monophosphate (cAMP) contributes to cyst formation and growth in ADPKD. Vasopressin stimulates the production of cAMP. Increasing water intake to greater than 3 L/day can suppress vasopressin. Increasing water intake is recommended in all ADPKD patients with preserved renal function. However, in patients with CKD, serum sodium should be monitored.

ACUTE GENERAL Rx

- The treatment of gross hematuria is typically supportive with bed rest, hydration, and analgesics. Antihypertensive medications should be stopped during this time.
- Extracorporeal shock wave lithotripsy (ESWL) has been used in patients with small obstructing kidney stones (<2 cm in diameter) in the renal pelvis or calyces. Percutaneous nephrolithotomy is another potential option.
- Infections are treated with antibiotics that penetrate cysts such as fluoroquinolones, Bactrim, vancomycin, and chloramphenicol.

CHRONIC GENERAL Rx

- Data from the HALT-PKD trial showed that in young individuals with preserved kidney function, strict BP control of <110/75 mm Hg was associated with slower increase in TKV, reduced urinary albumin excretion, and a greater reduction of left ventricular mass index.
- For all ADPKD patients, the goal BP is <130/80 mm Hg. For young, healthy patients with ADPKD and with intact kidney function, the goal BP target can be <110/75 mm Hg.
- ACE inhibitors or angiotensin receptor blockers are the first drug of choice for treatment of hypertension.
- Hyperlipidemia should be aggressively treated with LDL-cholesterol targets <80 mg/dl.
- Pretransplant unilateral or bilateral nephrectomy is recommended only in select patients with recurrent infections, significant kidney enlargement causing limitation of daily activities, and malnutrition.
- For patients with ESRD, peritoneal or hemodialysis can be used as a bridge to kidney transplantation.

New therapies impacting cyst growth:

- A number of compounds that impact the cyst growth are being tested in ADPKD.
- Vasopressin receptor 2 antagonist tolvaptan was shown to significantly decrease the kidney volume in a phase 3 double-blind, placebo-controlled randomized trial involving patients with PKD and preserved renal function. Further trials are being planned to test the safety and efficacy of tolvaptan.
- A small trial involving the somatostatin analogue octreotide long-acting repeatable depot (octreotide-LAR) showed that there was significantly less increase in TKV in the octreotide group compared to placebo.

REFERRAL

- Patients with ADPKD should be referred at time of diagnosis to a nephrologist for

ongoing care. Urology can also be consulted in patients with nephrolithiasis for recurrent episodes of gross hematuria, or the consideration for nephrectomy before transplantation. Genetic counseling should be offered if patients plan to start a family or are considering having their children screened. Individuals at risk for ADPKD should undergo pretest and posttest counseling if they are found to have ADPKD.

PEARLS & CONSIDERATIONS

- ADPKD is the most common single genetic cause of chronic kidney disease.
- TKV increases exponentially over time, and the increase in TKV is a strong predictor of future renal function decline.
- Increasing water intake to >3 L per day is recommended in patients with ADPKD and preserved renal function.
- Strict blood pressure control is recommended in all patients with ADPKD.

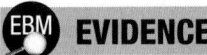 EVIDENCE

Available at www.expertconsult.com

SUGGESTED READINGS
Available at www.expertconsult.com

RELATED CONTENT
Polycystic Kidney Disease (Patient Information)

AUTHORS: **BHARATHI V. REDDY, M.D.,** and **ARLENE CHAPMAN, M.D.**

BASIC INFORMATION

DEFINITION

Polycystic ovary syndrome (PCOS) is characterized by an accumulation of incompletely developed follicles in the ovaries due to anovulation and associated with ovarian androgen production. In its complete form, it is associated with polycystic ovaries, amenorrhea, hirsutism, and obesity. Criteria for PCOS according to published definitions are described in Table 1.

SYNONYMS

Polycystic ovarian syndrome
Stein-Leventhal syndrome
PCOS

ICD-10CM CODES
E28.2 Polycystic ovarian syndrome

EPIDEMIOLOGY & DEMOGRAPHICS

- 6% to 25% of reproductive-age women (most common endocrine disorder in this population).
- Symptoms usually begin around the time of menarche, and the diagnosis is often made during adolescence or young adulthood.
- Increased risk of endometrial and ovarian cancers.
- PCOS is the most common cause of anovulatory infertility

PHYSICAL FINDINGS & CLINICAL PRESENTATION

- Oligomenorrhea or amenorrhea.
- Dysfunctional uterine bleeding.
- Infertility.
- Hirsutism (Fig. E1).
- Acne, alopecia, acanthosis nigricans (Fig. E2).
- Obesity (40% only), predominantly abdominal obesity.
- Insulin resistance (type 2 diabetes mellitus).
- Hypertension.

ETIOLOGY & PATHOGENESIS

Elevated serum luteinizing hormone (LH) concentrations and an increased serum LH/follicle-stimulating hormone (FSH) ratio result either from an increased gonadotropin-releasing hormone hypothalamic secretion or less likely from a primary pituitary abnormality. This results in dysregulation of androgen secretion and increased intraovarian androgen, the effect of which in the ovary is follicular atresia, maturation arrest, polycystic ovaries, and anovulation. Hyperinsulinemia is a contributing factor to ovarian hyperandrogenism, independent of LH excess. A role for insulin growth factor (IGF) receptors has been postulated for the association of PCOS and diabetes. Fig. 3 illustrates the pathologic mechanisms in PCOS.

DIAGNOSIS

The diagnosis of PCOS excludes secondary causes (androgen-producing neoplasm, hyperprolactinemia, adult-onset congenital adrenal hyperplasia).
Clinical:
- The symptoms, signs, and biochemical features of PCOS vary greatly among women and may change over time.
- PCOS is the most common cause of chronic anovulation with estrogen present. A positive progesterone withdrawal test establishes the presence of estrogen. Medroxyprogesterone (Provera) 10 mg qd is administered for 5 days and bleeding occurs if estrogen is present.
- The presence of oligomenorrhea, hirsutism, obesity, and documented polycystic ovaries establishes the diagnosis.

DIFFERENTIAL DIAGNOSIS

Causes of amenorrhea:
- Primary (unusual in PCOS).
  1. Genetic disorder (Turner's syndrome).
  2. Anatomic abnormality (e.g., imperforate hymen).
- Secondary
  1. Pregnancy.
  2. Functional (cause unknown, anorexia nervosa, stress, excessive exercise, hyperthyroidism, less commonly hypothyroidism, adrenal dysfunction, pituitary dysfunction, severe systemic illness, drugs such as oral contraceptives, estrogens, or dopamine agonists).
  3. Abnormalities of the genital tract (uterine tumor, endometrial scarring, ovarian tumor).

LABORATORY TESTS

- Glucose tolerance test at the initial presentation and every 2 yr thereafter (rule out diabetes mellitus). Impaired glucose tolerance is very common, occurring in approximately 30% of women with PCOS.
- Fasting lipid panel (rule out dyslipidemia), alanine aminotransferase, aspartate aminotransferase (rule out hepatic steatosis).
- Elevated LH/FSH ratio >2.5.
- Prolactin level elevation in 25%.
- Elevated androgens (testosterone [free and total levels], DHEA-S) (rule out androgen-secreting tumor).
- Other: thyroid-stimulating hormone (rule out hypothyroidism), 17-hydroxyprogesterone (rule out congenital adrenal hyperplasia), 24-hr urine for cortisol and creatinine (rule out Cushing's syndrome).
- TSH
- Table 2 summarizes laboratory testing to exclude other causes of ovulatory dysfunction and hyperandrogenism.

IMAGING STUDIES

Pelvic ultrasound (Fig. E4) (or CT scan) reveals the presence of twofold to fivefold ovarian enlargement with a thickened tunica albuginea, thecal hyperplasia, and 20 or more subcapsular follicles from 1 to 15 mm in diameter (Fig. E5). It is important to note that having polycystic ovaries alone does not make the diagnosis of PCOS because 20% of women with polycystic ovaries have no symptoms.

TABLE 1 Criteria for Polycystic Ovary Syndrome According to Published Definitions

	NICHD/NIH/1990	Rotterdam 2003	AE-PCOS/2009
Diagnostic criteria	Requires simultaneous presence of:	Requires the presence of at least two criteria:	Requires the presence of:
	Clinical and/or biochemical hyperandrogenism Menstrual dysfunction	Clinical and/or biochemical hyperandrogenism Ovulatory dysfunction PCOM	Hyperandrogenism and/or hyperandrogenemia Ovarian dysfunction: oligoovulation or anovulation and/or polycystic ovaries
Exclusion criteria	Congenital adrenal hyperplasia, androgen-secreting tumors, Cushing's syndrome, and hyperprolactinemia	Congenital adrenal hyperplasia, androgen-secreting tumors, and Cushing's syndrome	21-hydroxylase-deficient nonclassic adrenal hyperplasia, androgen-secreting neoplasms, androgenic–anabolic drug use or abuse, the hyperandrogenic-insulin resistance-acanthosis nigricans syndrome, thyroid dysfunction, and hyperprolactinemia
Clinical traits	Hirsutism, acne, and alopecia	Hirsutism, acne, and androgenic alopecia	Hirsutism
PCOM	Not included	At least one ovary showing either:	At least one ovary showing either:
		Twelve or more follicles of 2-9 mm in diameter Ovarian volume, 10 mL	Twelve or more follicles of 2-9 mm in diameter Ovarian volume, 10 mL

AE-PCOS, Androgen Excess and PCOS Society; *NICHD/NIH,* National Institute for Child Health and Human Development/National Institutes of Health; *PCOM,* polycystic ovarian morphology.
From Fielding JR et al: *Gynecologic imaging,* Philadelphia, 2011, Saunders.

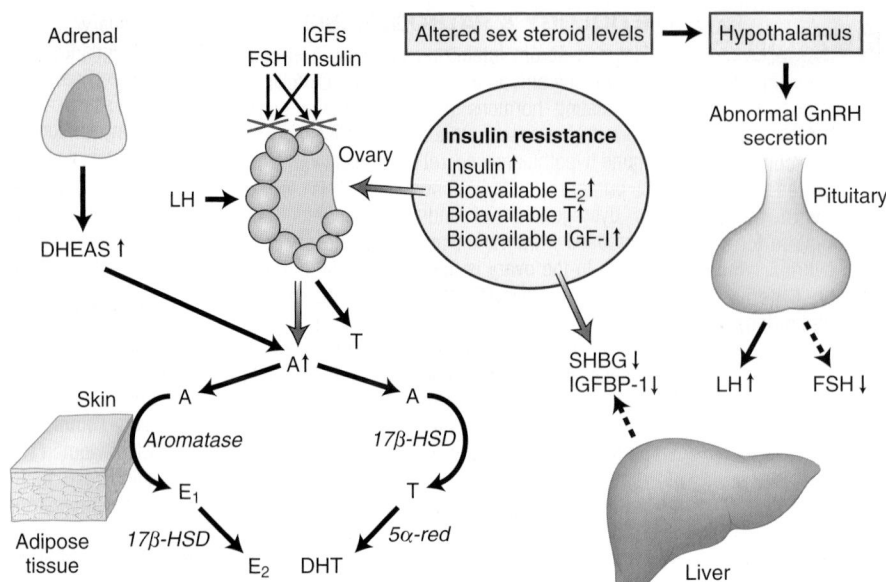

Peripheral and target tissues

FIG. 3 Pathologic mechanisms in polycystic ovary syndrome (PCOS). A deficient in vivo response of the ovarian follicle to physiologic quantities of follicle-stimulating hormone (*FSH*), possibly because of an impaired interaction between signaling pathways associated with FSH and insulin-like growth factors (*IGFs*) or insulin, may be an important defect responsible for anovulation in PCOS. Insulin resistance associated with increased circulating and tissue levels of insulin and bioavailable estradiol (E_2), testosterone (*T*), and IGF1 gives rise to abnormal hormone production in a number of tissues. Oversecretion of luteinizing hormone (*LH*) and decreased output of FSH by the pituitary, decreased production of sex hormone–binding globulin (*SHBG*) and IGF-binding protein 1 (*IGFBP-1*) in the liver, increased adrenal secretion of dehydroepiandrosterone sulfate (*DHEAS*), and increased ovarian secretion of androstenedione (*A*) all contribute to the feed-forward cycle that maintains anovulation and androgen excess in PCOS. Excessive amounts of E_2 and T arise primarily from the conversion of A in peripheral and target tissues. T is converted to the potent steroids estradiol or DHT (dihydrotestosterone). Reductive 17β-hydroxysteroid dehydrogenase (17β-HSD) enzyme activity may be conferred by protein products of several genes with overlapping functions; 5α-reductase (5α-red) is encoded by at least two genes, and aromatase is encoded by a single gene. *GnRH*, Gonadotropin-releasing hormone. (From Melmed S et al: *Williams textbook of endocrinology*, ed 12, Philadelphia, 2011, Saunders.)

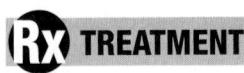 **TREATMENT**

The goal is to interrupt the self-perpetuating abnormal hormone cycle:
- Reduction of ovarian androgen secretion by laparoscopic ovarian wedge resection. Laparoscopic ovarian surgery (laparoscopic ovarian drilling [LOD]) is a useful alternative that does not trigger ovarian hyperstimulation.
- Reduction of ovarian androgen secretion by using oral contraceptives or LH-releasing hormone (LHRH) analogs.
- Weight reduction for all obese women with PCOS. Loss of abdominal fat seems to be crucial to restore ovulation.
- FSH stimulation with clomiphene HMG or pulsatile LHRH.
- Urofollitropin (pure FSH) administration.
- Metformin improves ovulation, insulin sensitivity, and possibly hyperandrogenemia. Choice of treatment:
- The management of hirsutism without risking pregnancy includes oral contraceptives, glucocorticoids, LHRH analogs, or spironolactone (an antiandrogen). Finasteride and

flutamide may be similarly effective in reducing hirsutism as spironolactone.
- Pregnancy can be achieved with clomiphene (alone or with glucocorticoids, human chorionic gonadotropin, or bromocriptine), HMG, urofollitropin, pulsatile LHRH, or ovarian wedge resection. Metformin may also induce ovulation. Recent trials comparing the aromatase inhibitor letrozole to clomiphene for infertility have shown higher live-birth and ovulation among infertile women with PCOS treated with letrozole. When considering in vitro fertilization (IVF), the transfer of fresh embryos is generally preferred over the transfer of frozen embryos; however, a recent trial among infertile women with PCOS undergoing IVF revealed that frozen-embryo transfer is associated with a higher rate of live birth, a lower risk of the ovarian hyperstimulation syndrome, and a higher risk of preeclampsia after the first transfer than with fresh-embryo transfer.[1]

[1]Chen ZJ et al: Fresh versus frozen embryos for infertility in the polycystic ovary syndrome, *N Engl J Med* 375:523-533, 2016.

- Psychological screening for depression is recommended. Women with PCOS are fourfold more likely to have abnormal depression scores.
- Table 3 describes a mnemonic for assessment and management of PCOS.

DISPOSITION
- Table 4 summarizes metabolic complications in PCOS.

SUGGESTED READINGS
Available at www.expertconsult.com

RELATED CONTENT
Polycystic Ovarian Syndrome (Patient Information)

AUTHOR: **FRED F. FERRI, M.D.**

TABLE 2 Laboratory Testing to Exclude Other Causes of Ovulatory Dysfunction and Hyperandrogenism

Lab	Evaluation for:	Comment
Total and/or bioavailable testosterone	Androgen-secreting tumor	Measure if there are symptoms concerning for an androgen-secreting tumor or if biochemical evidence of hyperandrogenism is needed to make the diagnosis of polycystic ovary syndrome. Rapid progression or a total testosterone >200 ng/dl should prompt a workup for an androgen-secreting tumor.
Dehydroepiandrosterone sulfate	Androgen-secreting tumor	Measure if there are symptoms concerning for an androgen-secreting tumor. Although modest elevations in dehydroepiandrosterone sulfate can be seen in polycystic ovary syndrome, rapid progression or greater elevations should prompt a workup for an adrenal androgen-secreting tumor.
Morning 17-hydroxyproges-terone	Late-onset congenital adrenal hyperplasia	This disorder is caused by a partial adrenal enzyme defect that leads to impaired cortisol production, compensatory elevation in adrenocorticotropic hormone, and subsequent excess androgen production. Symptoms may mimic polycystic ovary syndrome. Normal values <200 ng/dl. If higher than this, adrenocorticotropic hormone stimulation test recommended.
24-hour urine for cortisol and creatinine; dexamethasone suppression test; salivary cortisol	Cushing's syndrome	Consider ruling out Cushing's syndrome in women with an abrupt change in menstrual pattern, later-onset hirsutism, or other evidence of cortisol excess such as hypertension, facial plethora, supraclavicular fullness, hyperpigmented striae, and fragile skin.
Prolactin	Hyperprolactinemia	May be accompanied by galactorrhea. Consider ruling this out in all women with irregular menstrual cycles.
Thyroid function studies	Hyperthyroidism or hypothyroidism	Consider ruling out thyroid dysfunction in all women with irregular menstrual cycles.

From Setji TL, Brown AJ: Polycystic ovary syndrome: update on diagnosis and treatment, *Am J Med* 127:912-919, 2014.

TABLE 3 MY PCOS: Mnemonic for Assessment and Management of Polycystic Ovary Syndrome (PCOS)

	Assessment	Management
Metabolic	2-hour glucose tolerance test with 75 grams oral glucose, measuring serum glucose at time 0 and 120 min. Lipid profile Liver function tests (if other risk factors for nonalcoholic fatty liver disease)	Lifestyle intervention: diet, exercise, and weight loss (if overweight or obese) Metformin for abnormal glucose tolerance not controlled with lifestyle Statin therapy if patient meets criteria (Adult Treatment Panel-III or American College of Cardiology/American Heart Association guidelines)
Cycle control	Ask about menstrual pattern; normal cycle length is 28 days (range 21-35)	If amenorrhea for 3 months or more, induce withdrawal bleed with progesterone (after negative pregnancy test) Hormonal therapy Examples: • Estrogen-containing oral contraceptives (monthly cycling, seasonal cycling, continuous use) • Vaginal ring • Patch • Progestin-only pill (smokers, hypertension) • Progestin-eluting intrauterine device (Mirena) • Progesterone prn to induce withdrawal bleeding (medroxyprogesterone acetate 10 mg daily for 10-14 days, micronized progesterone 400 mg daily for 10-14 days) • Metformin (second-line therapy)
Psychosocial	Screen for depression, disordered eating Affirm that polycystic ovary syndrome is an important medical issue; provide nonjudgmental support Discuss stress management Reinforce self-care behaviors	Mental health referral and/or antidepressant therapy may be warranted if depression or disordered eating is identified
Cosmetic	Ferriman-Gallwey score as guide to assess hirsutism Evaluate for acne and male pattern hair loss Serum androgen levels if uncertain about degree of hirsutism or atypical symptoms	Estrogen-containing hormonal contraception Antiandrogens such as spironolactone or finasteride. Teratogenic; only use with contraception) Cyproterone acetate (not available in the U.S.) Eflornithine hydrochloride 13.9% cream Laser or electrolysis Topical treatment for acne Minoxidil 2.5% or 5% for male pattern hair loss
Ovulation and fertility	Counsel that fertility is reduced in polycystic ovary syndrome, but patients typically not infertile Assess fertility goals	If subfertility is an issue, consider referral to Reproductive Endocrine for possible clomiphene citrate therapy Metformin has limited role
Sleep apnea	Screen for sleep apnea: daytime somnolence, morning headache, reflux symptoms, snoring, observed interrupted breathing	Refer for sleep study Continuous positive airway pressure therapy recommended if sleep apnea diagnosed

PCOS, Polycystic ovary syndrome.
From Setji TL, Brown AJ: Polycystic ovary syndrome: Update on diagnosis and treatment, *Am J Med* 127:912-919, 2014.

TABLE 4   Metabolic Complications in Polycystic Ovary Syndrome

Abnormal glucose tolerance (impaired glucose tolerance or type 2 diabetes)	30% of obese polycystic ovary syndrome women have impaired glucose tolerance, and 10% have type 2 diabetes by age 40. In thin women with polycystic ovary syndrome, 10% have impaired glucose tolerance, and 1.5% have type 2 diabetes.
Obesity	Prevalence of obesity varies considerably in women with polycystic ovary syndrome. Previously, prevalence rates of obesity were estimated based on populations of women with polycystic ovary syndrome seeking care. A recent study comparing patients presenting for care in a polycystic ovary syndrome clinic with an unselected population evaluated during a preemployment physical suggests that obesity and overweight may not be more common in polycystic ovary syndrome. In that study, 63.7% of polycystic ovary syndrome clinic patients were obese, compared with 28% of unselected women with polycystic ovary syndrome identified during screening, and 28% of nonpolycystic ovary syndrome controls. Polycystic ovary syndrome symptoms, including hyperandrogenism and oligo-ovulation, are exacerbated by obesity.
Metabolic syndrome	33%-50% of U.S. women with polycystic ovary syndrome have metabolic syndrome compared to only 12% in a similarly aged National Health and Nutrition Examination Survey population. In contrast, only 8.2% of women with polycystic ovary syndrome in Italy met criteria for metabolic syndrome. Thus, metabolic syndrome varies by geographic location, a finding likely related to different body mass index, though other causes including genetics and diet could also be playing a part.
High blood pressure	Data have been conflicting, but a large Kaiser Permanente study demonstrated that hypertension or elevated blood pressure was more than twice as common in women with polycystic ovary syndrome (27% vs. 12%).
Dyslipidemia	Dyslipidemia is more prevalent in women with polycystic ovary syndrome compared to controls (15% vs. 6%). In a metaanalysis, triglyceride values were 26 mg/dl higher (95% CI 17-35), low-density lipoprotein cholesterol was 12 mg/dl higher (95% CI 10-16), and high-density lipoprotein-cholesterol was 6 mg/dl lower (95% CI 4-9) in women with polycystic ovary syndrome compared with controls. Women with polycystic ovary syndrome also have higher concentrations and proportions of small, dense low-density lipoprotein cholesterol.
Nonalcoholic fatty liver disease and nonalcoholic steatohepatitis	Nonalcoholic fatty liver disease and nonalcoholic steatohepatitis have recently been recognized as a potential complication in women with polycystic ovary syndrome. Prevalence of fatty liver disease in polycystic ovary syndrome women has been estimated to be 15%-55%, depending on the diagnostic parameter used (level of serum alanine aminotransferase or ultrasound). Individuals that may be at higher risk of nonalcoholic fatty liver disease including nonalcoholic steatohepatitis include those with metabolic syndrome, insulin resistance, and possibly hyperandrogenemia.
Cardiovascular disease	Many studies demonstrate abnormal surrogate markers of cardiovascular disease in women with polycystic ovary syndrome. However, data regarding cardiovascular disease risk are conflicting with some studies suggesting an increased risk in women with polycystic ovary syndrome, whereas other studies have not found this difference in cardiovascular risk. While it is important to recognize and treat cardiovascular risk factors in this population, further research of cardiovascular risk and complications is still needed to clarify the long-term risk.

CI, Confidence interval.

From Setji TL, Brown AJ: Polycystic ovary syndrome: update on diagnosis and treatment, *Am J Med* 127:912-919, 2014.

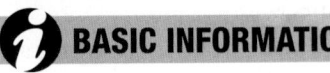 BASIC INFORMATION

DEFINITION

Polycythemia vera is a disorder of the myeloid/erythroid stem cell resulting in erythropoietin-independent proliferation of erythrocytes.

SYNONYMS

PV
Primary polycythemia
Vaquez disease

ICD-10CM CODES
D45 Polycythemia vera

EPIDEMIOLOGY & DEMOGRAPHICS

INCIDENCE: 1 case per 100,000 persons. Occurs most commonly in patients aged 50 to 75 years. Mean age at onset is 60 yr; men are affected more often than are women.

PHYSICAL FINDINGS & CLINICAL PRESENTATION

Polycythemia vera has a latent, proliferative, and spent phase. The patient generally comes to medical attention because of symptoms associated with increased blood volume and viscosity or impaired platelet function:

- Impaired cerebral circulation resulting in headache, vertigo, blurred vision, dizziness, transient ischemic attack, cerebrovascular accident
- Fatigue, poor exercise tolerance
- Pruritus, particularly after bathing (caused by overproduction of histamine)
- Bleeding: epistaxis, upper gastrointestinal bleeding (increased incidence of peptic ulcer disease)
- Abdominal discomfort from splenomegaly; hepatomegaly may be present
- Hyperuricemia may result in nephrolithiasis and gouty arthritis
- Nearly 20% of patients experience arterial or venous thrombosis as their initial symptom. Hepatic brain thrombosis or portal vein thrombosis should raise suspicion for PV. The physical examination may reveal:
- Facial plethora, congestion of oral mucosa, ruddy complexion
- Enlargement and tortuosity of retinal veins
- Splenomegaly (found in >75% of patients)

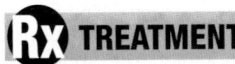 DIAGNOSIS

DIFFERENTIAL DIAGNOSIS

Smoking:
- Polycythemia is caused by increased carboxyhemoglobin, resulting in left shift in the hemoglobin (Hgb) dissociation curve.
- Laboratory evaluation shows increased hematocrit (Hct), RBC mass, erythropoietin level, and carboxyhemoglobin.
- Splenomegaly is not present on physical examination.

Hypoxemia (secondary polycythemia):
- Living for prolonged periods at high altitudes, pulmonary fibrosis, congenital cardiac lesions with right-to-left shunts.
- Laboratory evaluation shows decreased arterial oxygen saturation and elevated erythropoietin level.
- Splenomegaly is not present on physical examination.

Erythropoietin-producing states:
- Renal cell carcinoma, hepatoma, cerebral hemangioma, uterine fibroids, polycystic kidneys.
- The erythropoietin level is elevated in these patients, and the arterial oxygen saturation is normal.
- Splenomegaly may be present with metastatic neoplasms.

Stress polycythemia (Gaisböck's syndrome, relative polycythemia):
- Laboratory evaluation demonstrates normal RBC mass, arterial oxygen saturation, and erythropoietin level; plasma volume is decreased.
- Splenomegaly is not present on physical examination.

Hemoglobinopathies associated with high oxygen affinity:
- An abnormal oxyhemoglobin-dissociation curve (P50) is present.

WORKUP

PV is suspected when the hemoglobin level exceeds 18.5 g/dl in men or 16.5 g/dl in women after secondary causes have been excluded. Recent developments in molecular biology have identified a single, acquired point mutation in the Janus kinase 2 (*JAK2*) gene in the majority of patients with polycythemia vera and other pH-negative myeloproliferative disorders. The *JAK2* mutation is found in >95% of patients with polycythemia vera and can be used for diagnostic purposes. Testing for the *JAK2 V617F* mutation with polymerase chain reaction assay is now available. In patients with high hematocrit (>52% in men or >48% in women) and in the absence of coexisting secondary erythrocytosis, the presence of the *JAK2* mutation is sufficient for the diagnosis of polycythemia vera.

The World Health Organization diagnostic criteria for polycythemia vera are described in Table 1.

LABORATORY TESTS

- Elevated RBC count (>6 million/mm^3), elevated Hgb (>18 g/dl in men, >16 g/dl in women), elevated Hct (<54% in men, <49% in women)
- Increased white blood cell count (often with basophilia; basophilia is a strong predictor of PV instead of a reactive state); thrombocytosis is found in the majority of patients
- Elevated leukocyte alkaline phosphatase, serum vitamin B$_{12}$ (due to increased levels of transcobalamin III produced in proliferating leukocytes), and uric acid levels (due to DNA turnover in the marrow)
- Low serum erythropoietin level
- Peripheral blood smear: may reveal basophils or immature myeloid forms
- Bone marrow aspiration revealing RBC hyperplasia (Fig. E1) and absent iron stores

Rx TREATMENT

NONPHARMACOLOGIC THERAPY

Phlebotomy to keep Hct >45% in men and >42% in women is the mainstay of therapy. Phlebotomy, however, has no effect on the development of myelofibrosis.

ACUTE GENERAL Rx

- Add aspirin in patients younger than 60 years without prior thromboembolic event.
- Hydroxyurea can be used in conjunction with phlebotomy in patients older than 60 years to decrease the incidence of thrombotic events.
- Interferon-alpha-2b is also effective in controlling RBC values without significant side effects.
- Box 1 describes an algorithm for management of patients with polycythemia vera.
- Recent trials have shown that ruxolitinib, a Janus kinase (JAK) 1 and 2 inhibitor was superior to standard therapy in controlling the hematocrit, reducing the spleen volume and improving symptoms associated with polycythemia vera.

TABLE 1 World Health Organization 2008 Diagnostic Criteria for Polycythemia Vera

Major Criteria

1. Hemoglobin (Hgb) >18.5 g/dl (men), >16.5 (women); *or* Hgb or hematocrit (Hct) >99% reference range for age, sex, or altitude of residence; *or* Hgb >17 g/dl (men), >15 g/dl (women) if associated with a sustained increase of ≥2 g/dl from baseline that cannot be attributed to correction of iron deficiency; *or* elevated red cell mass (>25% above mean normal predicted value)
2. Presence of *JAK2 V617F* or similar mutation

Minor Criteria

1. Bone marrow trilineage myeloproliferation
2. Subnormal serum erythropoietin level
3. Endogenous erythroid colony formation in vitro

Either both major criteria and one minor criterion *or* the first major criterion and two minor criteria must be met for diagnosis of polycythemia vera.

From Andreoli TE et al: *Andreoli and Carpenter's Cecil essentials of medicine,* ed 8, Philadelphia, 2010, Saunders.

BOX 1   Algorithm for Management of Patients with Polycythemia Vera

Low-risk young patients (age <60 years) and no history of thrombosis, platelet count <1.5 × 10⁶ mm³

Phlebotomy + low-dose aspirin (81 mg/day) to maintain hematocrit lower than 45% in males and lower than 42% in females. Aspirin should not be used in patients with histories of a hemorrhagic episode or with extreme thrombocytosis (>1.5 × 10⁶ mm³) or acquired von Willebrand syndrome.

↓

Thrombosis or hemorrhage
Systemic symptoms
Severe pruritus refractory to histamine antagonists
Painful splenomegaly

↓

Hydroxyurea 15-20 mg/kg (unless younger than 40 years, pregnant, intolerant to hydroxyurea; consider pegylated INF)

↓

Pegylated INF 45 to 180 μg/wk or INF (3 × 10⁶ units three times a week; alter dose depending on response and toxicity). Consider the use of pegylated INF, which can be administered once weekly.

↓

If platelet control is inadequate or patient cannot tolerate interferon, one option is the use of anagrelide. However, the use of this drug is controversial. In this case, supplemental phlebotomy is required to maintain hematocrit lower than 45% in males and lower than 42% in females, and the use of hydroxyurea should be considered, especially if patient continues to have thrombotic episodes.

↓

If the patient has increasing splenomegaly, systemic symptoms, or repeated thromboses despite adequate dose of hydroxyurea (2-3 g/day), start busulfan, 4 to 6 mg/day orally for 4 to 8 weeks. It should be mentioned that the sequential use of hydroxyurea and busulfan may be associated with an increased risk of leukemia. Supplemental phlebotomy may be required.

Painful splenomegaly

↓

Splenectomy + continued systemic therapy

↓

High-risk patients (age >60 years), previous thrombosis, platelet count >1.5 × 10⁶ mm³

Phlebotomy to hematocrit of 42% in females and 45% in males

Aspirin (81 mg/day) to be given only in patients with platelet counts <1.5 × 10⁶ mm²

Myelosuppressive therapy with hydroxyurea 30 mg/kg orally for 1 week

Then 15 to 20 mg/kg

↓

If patient continues to have thrombotic episodes and has extreme thrombocytosis or cannot tolerate hydroxyurea

Consider pegylated INF 45 to 180 μg/wk or add busulfan 4 to 6 mg/d orally for 4 to 8 weeks.

If on busulfan, stop when blood counts are normalized or platelet count is lower than 300,000 mm³.

Occasional supplemental phlebotomy if hematocrit is >42% in females and greater than 45% in males; when patient relapses (patient is symptomatic), initiate busulfan therapy again at same dose.

Patient age >70 years

Phlebotomy + low-dose aspirin + hydroxyurea

↓

No response or poor compliance

Busulfan 4 to 6 mg/day orally for 4 to 8 weeks. Stop when blood counts are normalized or platelet count is lower than 300,000 mm³.

From Hoffman R.: *Hematology, basic principles and practice*, 6th ed, Philadelphia, 2013, Saunders.

CHRONIC Rx

- Patient education regarding need for lifelong monitoring and treatment.
- Adjunctive therapy: treatment of pruritus with antihistamines, control of significant hyperuricemia with allopurinol, reduction of gastric hyperacidity with antacids of H_2 blockers, low-dose aspirin to treat vasomotor symptoms in patients without bleeding diathesis. Low-dose aspirin can safely prevent thrombotic complications in patients with polycythemia vera and should be given to all patients in absence of contraindications.

DISPOSITION

- The median survival time without treatment is 6 to 18 mo after diagnosis; phlebotomy extends the average survival time to 12 yr.
- Patients with polycythemia vera with a hematocrit <45% have a significantly lower rate of cardiovascular death and major thrombosis than those with hematocrit of 45% to 50%.
- Prognosis is worse in patients >60 yr and those with a history of thrombosis.

SUGGESTED READINGS

Available at www.expertconsult.com

RELATED CONTENT

Polycythemia Vera (Patient Information)

AUTHOR: **BHARTI RATHORE, M.D.**

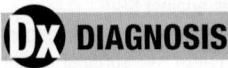 **BASIC INFORMATION**

DEFINITION

Polymyalgia rheumatica (PMR) is an inflammatory condition characterized by neck, shoulder girdle, and pelvic girdle muscle pain and stiffness of at least four weeks' duration. PMR can occur alone or in conjunction with giant cell arteritis (GCA).

SYNONYMS

Anarthritic rheumatoid syndrome
PMR

ICD-10CM CODES
M35.3 Polymyalgia rheumatica

EPIDEMIOLOGY & DEMOGRAPHICS

PREVALENCE: 60 to 80/100,000; Scandinavian and Northern European populations are high risk.
PREDOMINANT SEX: Female/male ratio of 2:1.
PREDOMINANT AGE: Age greater than 50 years with peak between seventh and eight decade. Unlikely in those less than 50 years old.

PHYSICAL FINDINGS & CLINICAL PRESENTATION

- Typically, abrupt onset of muscle pain, symmetric myalgias, and stiffness.
- Neck, shoulders, lower back, hips, thighs, and occasionally trunk and arms are involved. Shoulders are usually affected first.
- Patients often note severe pain and stiffness during the night, with difficulty rising and dressing.
- Constitutional symptoms of fatigue, malaise, weight loss, loss of appetite, and depression may accompany pain and stiffness.
- Physical exam shows passive range of motion is preserved, strength testing is normal; subdeltoid and subacromial bursitis most prominent finding, minimal joint synovitis.
- Fever, chills, night sweats, visual disturbances, headaches, or jaw claudication should raise suspicion of giant cell arteritis and be further evaluated.

ETIOLOGY

Appears related to the presence of HLA-D4 haplotype, which is associated with global activation of the innate immune system and circulating monocytes that produce IL-1 and IL-6, leading to inflammation.

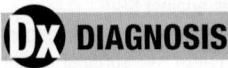 **DIAGNOSIS**

DIFFERENTIAL DIAGNOSIS
See Box 1.

WORKUP

- Initial laboratory evaluation: ESR, CRP, CBC, CPK.
- ESR >40 in majority of patients.
- CBC may show a normocytic, normochromic anemia and thrombocytosis.
- Clinical diagnosis: Symptoms of stiffness, aching, pain, increased ESR and CRP
- An algorithm for diagnosing polymyalgia rheumatica without giant cell arteritis is described in Fig. E1.
- Table 1 describes diagnostic criteria for PMR.

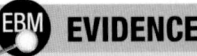 **TREATMENT**

ACUTE GENERAL Rx

- Prednisone 15 to 20 mg/day with dramatic improvement in symptoms in 24 to 48 hrs.
- Dose adjustment may be necessary for weight, symptom severity, coexisting conditions such as diabetes mellitus, hypertension, or heart failure.
- If symptoms persist after 1 week, increase dose by 5 mg.
- If nighttime symptoms are bothersome, consider divided dose (A.M. and P.M.). Ongoing symptoms require consideration of alternative diagnosis.
- Initial prednisone dose should be maintained for 4 to 8 weeks.
- Steroid dose may be reduced by 20% every month if patient remains symptom free.
- ESR and CRP should be monitored for disease activity and steroid dose adjustment after 2 months of treatment.
- When dose reaches 10 mg/day, taper slowly by 1 mg/month. Flares, typical during tapering, can be managed by increasing prednisone by 10% to 20%.
- A proton pump inhibitor or H2R blocker should be initiated with glucocorticoids.
- Attention should be paid to bone health. Calcium and vitamin D supplementation should be started early and bisphosphonates used if indicated by bone density measurement.

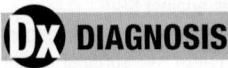 **PEARLS & CONSIDERATIONS**

Patients with PMR should be monitored carefully for the development of giant cell arteritis. Patients who have incomplete response to treatment with prednisone or have an evolving pattern of pain and swelling should be reevaluated for the possibility of a different diagnosis.

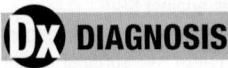 **EVIDENCE**

Available at www.expertconsult.com

SUGGESTED READINGS
Available at www.expertconsult.com

RELATED CONTENT
Polymyalgia Rheumatica (PMR) (Patient Information)
Giant Cell Arteritis (Related Key Topic)
Vasculitis, Systemic (Related Key Topic)

AUTHOR: **ALISHA LAKHANI, M.D., M.P.H.**

BOX 1 Differential Diagnosis of Polymyalgia Rheumatica

Rheumatoid arthritis
Rotator cuff syndrome
Osteoarthritis of shoulder and hip joints
Fibromyalgia
Polymyositis/dermatomyositis
Spondyloarthritis
Systemic lupus erythematosus
Vasculitides
Paraneoplastic myalgias
Infection-associated myalgias
RS3PE (remitting seronegative symmetric synovitis and pitting edema)
Parkinson's disease
Hypothyroidism

From Hochberg M: *Rheumatology,* ed 4, Philadelphia, 2007, Mosby.

TABLE 1 Polymyalgia Rheumatica: Diagnostic Criteria

Chuang et al 1982	Healey 1984
- Age of onset = 50 yr or older - Erythrocyte sedimentation rate >40 mm/h - Bilateral aching and stiffness for =1 mo and involving two of the following areas: neck or torso, shoulders or proximal regions of the arms, and hips or proximal aspects of the thighs - Exclusion of all other diagnoses causing PMR-like symptoms	- Age of onset = 50 yr or older - Erythrocyte sedimentation rate >40 mm/h - Pain persisting for =1 mo and involving two of the following areas: neck, shoulders, and pelvic girdle - Absence of other diseases capable of causing the musculoskeletal symptoms - Morning stiffness lasting >1 hr - Rapid response to prednisone (=20 mg/day)??

From Hochberg M: *Rheumatology,* ed 4, Philadelphia, 2007, Mosby.

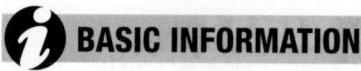

DEFINITION

Clinically significant portal hypertension is defined as a portal vein pressure >10 mm Hg, most commonly attributable to liver disease.

SYNONYMS

None

ICD-10CM CODES
K76.6   Portal hypertension

EPIDEMIOLOGY & DEMOGRAPHICS

- Incidence of portal hypertension is not known.
- Cirrhosis is the most common cause of portal hypertension in the United States.
- Portal hypertension is developed by >90% of patients with cirrhosis.
- Alcoholic and viral liver diseases are the most common causes of cirrhosis and portal hypertension in the United States.
- Schistosomiasis is the main cause of portal hypertension outside the United States.
- Esophageal varices may appear when portal vein pressure rises to >10 mm Hg.
- Variceal hemorrhage is the most serious complication of portal hypertension and may occur when portal pressures rise >12 mm Hg.

PHYSICAL FINDINGS & CLINICAL PRESENTATION

- Jaundice.
- Ascites (Fig. 1).
- Spider angiomata.
- Testicular atrophy.
- Gynecomastia.
- Palmar erythema.
- Dupuytren's contracture.
- Asterixis (with advanced liver failure).

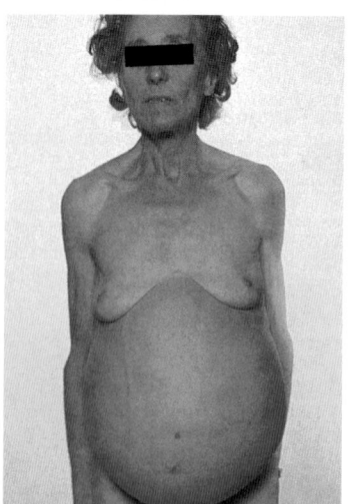

FIG. 1 Ascites secondary to portal hypertension. Note the dilated collateral vein running up the right side of the abdomen. (From Forbes A et al [eds]: *Atlas of clinical gastroenterology,* ed 3, Oxford, 2005, Mosby.)

- Irritability, encephalopathy.
- Splenomegaly.
- Dilated veins in the anterior abdominal wall.
- Venous pattern on the flanks.
- Caput medusae (tortuous collateral veins around the umbilicus).
- Hemorrhoids.
- Hematemesis.
- Melena.
- Pruritus.

ETIOLOGY

Pathophysiologically caused by:
1. Conditions resulting in an increased resistance to flow.
   ○ **Prehepatic** (e.g., portal vein thrombosis, splenic vein thrombosis, congenital stenosis).
   ○ **Hepatic** (e.g., cirrhosis, alcoholic liver disease, primary biliary cirrhosis, schistosomiasis).
   ○ **Posthepatic** (e.g., Budd-Chiari syndrome, constrictive pericarditis, inferior vena cava obstruction, cor pulmonale, tricuspid regurgitation).
2. Conditions leading to increase in portal blood flow.
   ○ Splanchnic arterial vasodilation accompanying portal hypertension, mediated by local release of nitric oxide.
   ○ Arterial-portal venous fistulae.

Table 1 summarizes the etiology of portal hypertension.

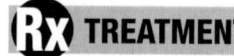 **DIAGNOSIS**

- The diagnosis of portal hypertension is made on clinical grounds after a comprehensive history and physical examination.
- Noninvasive and invasive procedures confirm diagnosis and determine the severity of portal hypertension.

DIFFERENTIAL DIAGNOSIS

- Ascites from infection, neoplasm, or other inflammatory processes.
- Obesity.
- Abdominal organomegaly.

WORKUP

The workup of portal hypertension includes blood tests and noninvasive imaging studies to determine if the cause of portal hypertension is prehepatic, hepatic, or posthepatic. Ascitic fluid analysis is a key part of the diagnosis.

LABORATORY TESTS

- Complete blood count with platelets.
- Liver function tests with serum albumin.
- Prothrombin and partial thromboplastin times.
- Hepatitis B surface antigen and antibody.
- Hepatitis C antibody.
- In selected cases: iron, total iron-binding capacity, and ferritin; antinuclear antibody, anti–smooth muscle antibodies, antimitochondrial antibody, ceruloplasmin, alpha-1 antitrypsin.

- Ascitic fluid analysis: a serum-ascites albumin gradient ≥1.1 mg/dl suggests portal hypertension. Polymorphonuclear cells ≥250 cells/mL or positive Gram stain or culture suggest complicating spontaneous bacterial peritonitis (SBP).

IMAGING STUDIES

- Duplex-Doppler ultrasound is effective in screening for portal hypertension.
- Less commonly, CT/MRI/MRA scanning (Figs. 2 and E3) or liver-spleen nuclear medicine scanning can be used if the results from ultrasound are equivocal.
- Upper endoscopy is the most reliable test documenting the presence of esophageal varices.

Rx TREATMENT

The treatment of portal hypertension is complex and involves measures to reduce the hypertension directly, minimize volume overload, correct underlying disorders, and prevent complications (most notably SBP and variceal bleeding).

NONPHARMACOLOGIC THERAPY

Dietary sodium restriction to generally 2000 mg/day forms the basis of therapy to limit fluid overload.

ACUTE GENERAL Rx

- For tense ascites, serial large-volume paracentesis (LVP) is generally recommended. The use of albumin infusion (8 to 10 g/L of ascites fluid removed) during LVP >5 L has been shown to reduce the incidence of postparacentesis circulatory dysfunction, although its use remains somewhat controversial.
- IV diuretics, typically furosemide and spironolactone, are used to achieve natriuresis and net negative salt and water balance. Renal function and serum electrolytes are monitored frequently, with transition to an oral regimen for long-term therapy.
- SBP is treated with IV antibiotics directed against enteric bacteria.
- Acute variceal hemorrhage is treated with crystalloid and blood product resuscitation, IV octreotide, terlipressin/vasopressin or somatostatin, and urgent upper endoscopy, often with sclerotherapy or band ligation. Patients with acute variceal hemorrhage should receive antibiotic prophylaxis against SBP.
- Traditionally, a transjugular intrahepatic portosystemic shunt (TIPS) or surgical shunt placement may be considered in patients not responding to above measures. However, recent data show early TIPS placement improved outcomes in acute variceal hemorrhage.

CHRONIC Rx

- Dietary sodium restriction in combination with diuretics: the typical ratio of furosemide 40 mg to spironolactone 100 mg retains normal serum potassium levels in most patients.

TABLE 1 Etiology of Portal Hypertension

Condition	Site of Increased Resistance	FHVP	WHVP	HVPG	SPP	Liver Disease
Cirrhosis	Intrahepatic sinusoidal	Normal	Increased	Increased	Increased	Yes
Alcoholic hepatitis	Intrahepatic sinusoidal	Normal	Increased	Increased	Increased	Yes
Extrahepatic portal, splenic, or mesenteric vein thrombosis	Extrahepatic presinusoidal	Normal	Normal	Normal	Increased	No
Early primary biliary cirrhosis, PSC, sarcoid, schistosomiasis, congestive heart failure, non-cirrhotic portal fibrosis, NRH	Intrahepatic presinusoidal	Normal	Normal/?raised	Normal/?raised	Increased	No
Hemochromatosis, peliosis, infiltrative disease, acute fatty liver of pregnancy	Intrahepatic sinusoidal hypertension	Normal	Increased	Increased	Increased	Yes
Venoocclusive disease, posttransplant rejection	Intrahepatic postsinusoidal hypertension	Normal	?Increased	?Decreased	Increased	Yes
Budd-Chiari syndrome (noncirrhotic)	Extrahepatic postsinusoidal hypertension	Increased	Increased	Normal	Increased	Depends on severity
Constrictive pericarditis, inferior vena cava obstruction, congenital inferior vena cava web, right heart failure	Extrahepatic postsinusoidal hypertension	Increased	Increased	Normal	Increased	Depends on severity

FHVP, Free hepatic venous pressure; *HVPG,* hepatic venous pressure gradient; *SPP,* systolic pulse pressure; *WHVP,* wedged hepatic venous pressure.
From Vincent JL et al: *Textbook of critical care,* ed 6, Philadelphia, 2011, Saunders.

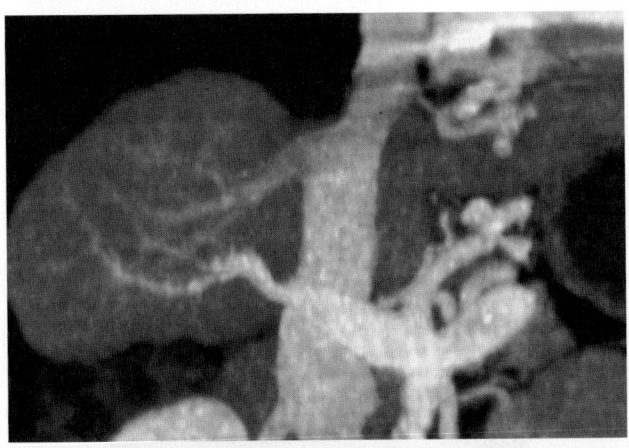

FIG. 2 MR angiography showing portal hypertension with collaterals. The shrunken liver and collateral are obvious. (From Forbes A et al [eds]: *Atlas of clinical gastroenterology,* ed 3, St Louis, 2005, Mosby.)

- Nonselective beta-blockers (propranolol and nadolol) in dosages sufficient to reduce the resting heart rate by 25% have been shown to be effective in primary prophylaxis for first-time variceal bleeding and for preventing recurrent variceal bleeding. Dosages are usually given bid and decreased if heart rate falls to <55 beats/min or systolic blood pressure drops to <90 mm Hg. The addition of a long-acting nitrate (e.g., isosorbide-5-mononitrate) has been shown to improve portal hemodynamics. Findings of a prospective trial of beta-blockers to prevent the formation of varices were negative. The combination of beta-blockade plus endoscopic esophageal variceal banding is superior to either intervention alone.
- Intermittent LVP may be needed in "diuretic resistant" patients.

- Patients with prior SBP merit lifelong antibiotics for secondary prevention.
- Abstinence from alcohol or treatment for hepatitis B or hepatitis C. Vaccination for hepatitis A and B as appropriate.
- Hepatic transplantation is an option in selected patients.

DISPOSITION

- The most common complication associated with portal hypertension is variceal bleeding. The risk of bleeding from varices is approximately 15% at 1 yr.
- Development of the hepatorenal syndrome (HRS) is associated with high near-term mortality. In particular, HRS may complicate SBP, which emphasizes the importance of making the diagnosis of SBP and instituting appropriate prophylaxis.

REFERRAL

Consultation with a gastroenterologist is recommended in all patients with portal hypertension to screen for esophageal varices.

⊘ PEARLS & CONSIDERATIONS

Splanchnic arterial vasodilation is increasingly recognized as an important component of the pathophysiology of portal hypertension and ascites. There may be vasodilation in other capillary beds as well; of note, pulmonary arteriolar vasodilation can create a significant shunt fraction and resultant hypoxemia in the absence of chest radiograph or CT chest evidence of parenchymal disease. The diagnosis is suspected when otherwise unexplained hypoxia arises in a patient with cirrhosis, along with platypnea (dyspnea worse when sitting upright) and orthodeoxia (desaturation with upright posture). The diagnosis is confirmed by echocardiography with agitated saline, in which there is delayed appearance of bubbles in the left heart after injection into a peripheral vein.

COMMENTS

Portal hypertension and its complications carry significant morbidity and mortality rates. Emphasize ethanol abstinence, provide vaccinations and prophylactic therapy where indicated, and consider early referral to a specialist for assistance with management and consideration for hepatic transplantation.

SUGGESTED READING

Available at www.expertconsult.com

AUTHOR: **MEL L. ANDERSON, M.D.**

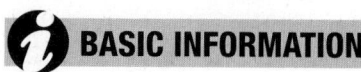

BASIC INFORMATION

DEFINITION

Portal vein thrombosis (PVT) is thrombotic occlusion of the portal vein. The thrombus can also involve segments of the mesenteric veins and/or the splenic vein.

SYNONYMS

Pylethrombosis
PVT

ICD-10CM CODES

I81 Portal vein thrombosis

EPIDEMIOLOGY & DEMOGRAPHICS

- Occurs with equal frequency in children (peak age: 6 yr) and adults (peak age: 40 yr)
- Occurs in 8% to 25% of patients with decompensated cirrhosis

PHYSICAL FINDINGS & CLINICAL PRESENTATION

- Acute PVT may present with sudden onset of fever and abdominal pain (when there is mesenteric extension).
- Upper gastrointestinal hemorrhage (hematemesis and/or melena) caused by esophageal varices.

ETIOLOGY & PATHOPHYSIOLOGY

In children: umbilical sepsis (pathophysiology unknown). In adults:
1. Hypercoagulable states:
   - Antiphospholipid syndrome.
   - Neoplasm (common cause).
   - Paroxysmal nocturnal hemoglobinuria.
   - Myeloproliferative diseases.
   - Oral contraceptives.
   - Polycythemia vera.
   - Pregnancy.
   - Protein S or C deficiency.
   - Sickle cell disease.
   - Thrombocytosis.
2. Inflammatory diseases:
   - Crohn's disease.
   - Pancreatitis.
   - Ulcerative colitis.
3. Complications of medical intervention:
   - Ambulatory dialysis.
   - Chemoembolization.
   - Liver transplantation.
   - Partial hepatectomy.
   - Sclerotherapy.
   - Splenectomy.
   - Transjugular intrahepatic portosystemic shunt.
4. Infections:
   - Appendicitis.
   - Diverticulitis.
   - Cholecystitis.

5. Miscellaneous:
   - Cirrhosis (common cause).
   - Bladder cancer.

Pathophysiology: PVT results in portal hypertension, leading to esophageal and gastrointestinal varices. The liver sustained by the hepatic artery maintains normal function.

DIAGNOSIS

DIFFERENTIAL DIAGNOSIS

Causes of upper gastrointestinal hemorrhage and abdominal pain are described in Section II.

WORKUP

- Abdominal ultrasound with Doppler (Fig. 1) or MRI may show the PVT. Abdominal ultrasound color Doppler imaging has a 98% negative predictive value and is considered the imaging modality of choice in diagnosing PVT.
- Determination of underlying cirrhosis of the liver should be the foremost step. It is crucial to differentiate acute from chronic PVT because chronic PVT does not require treatment.
- Esophagogastroscopy typically shows esophageal varices.
- Laboratory evaluation for hypercoagulable state is not cost-effective in patients with cirrhosis.

TREATMENT

- Anticoagulation data on thrombolytic therapy are inconclusive and there is no formal recommendation for or against anticoagulation in acute PVT. However, anticoagulation is generally recommended for patients with extension of PVT into the superior mesenteric vein to prevent intestinal infarction. In patients with chronic PVT and concomitant cirrhosis, long-term anticoagulation is generally not recommended.
- Variceal sclerotherapy or banding.
- Surgical mesocaval or splenorenal shunt.
- The roles of thrombolysis and transjugular intrahepatic portosystemic shunt continue to evolve.

REFERRAL

- To surgeon to rule out intestinal infarction.
- To gastroenterologist.

SUGGESTED READINGS

Available at www.expertconsult.com

AUTHOR: **FRED F. FERRI, M.D.**

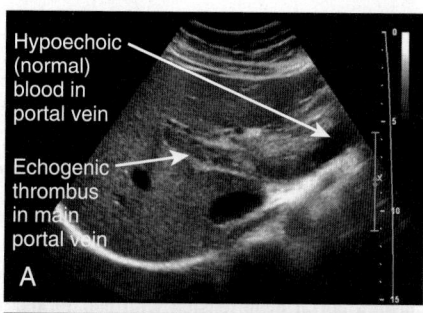

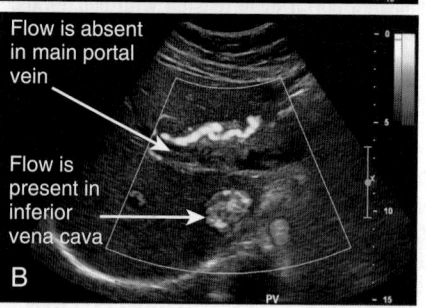

FIG. 1 Portal vein thrombosis: ultrasound. This 22-year-old female, 2 months postpartum, presented with 1 week of right upper quadrant pain. Ultrasound was performed to evaluate for suspected cholecystitis or symptomatic cholelithiasis. Instead, portal vein thrombosis was discovered. The postpartum state is a risk factor for this condition. Hypercoagulable states and inflammatory or neoplastic abdominal conditions, including pancreatitis and abdominal malignancies, also can result in portal vein thrombosis. **A,** Ultrasound gray scale image showing thrombus in the main portal vein. **B,** Doppler ultrasound showing no flow within the portal vein. (From Broder JS: *Diagnostic imaging for the emergency physician*, Philadelphia, 2011, Saunders.)

BASIC INFORMATION

DEFINITION

Postconcussive syndrome (PCS) refers to non-specific neurologic, cognitive, and psychological symptoms that result from traumatic brain injury (TBI) and persist beyond the expected recovery period. There is no consensus regarding the duration of symptoms to make the diagnosis, but symptoms usually manifest or significantly worsen within a few days following head trauma and persist for weeks to months. PCS can also follow moderate and severe brain injury, although it is more commonly associated with mild brain injury or concussion. Concussion is an acute trauma-induced alteration of mental function lasting <24 hours, with or without preceding loss of consciousness.

SYNONYMS

PCS
Postconcussion syndrome
Posttraumatic nervous instability or brain injury
Postcontusion syndrome or encephalopathy
Status post commotio cerebri

ICD-10CM CODES
F07.81 Postconcussional syndrome

EPIDEMIOLOGY & DEMOGRAPHICS

- Incidence is approximately 27 cases per 100,000 persons/year.
- From 30% to 80% of patients with mild to moderate brain injury will experience some symptoms of PCS.
- Usually reported in the young, ages 20 to 30 years old.
- Risk factors include female sex, low socioeconomic status, anxiety sensitivity, previous TBI, severe bodily injury from TBI, headaches, and unsettled court cases.

PHYSICAL FINDINGS & CLINICAL PRESENTATION

- Symptoms start within a few days to weeks after the head injury and usually persist after 3 months. 15% of patients will have persistent symptoms 1 year later.
- At least three of the following symptoms after TBI are required to meet ICD-10 criteria:
  1. Headache (usually of fronto-occipital location and showing characteristics of tension or migraine headache). The International Headache Society suggests that coding and attribution of headaches with characteristics of primary headaches but in the setting of an inciting event should be attributed to the event, unless there was a known history of the headache and the inciting event was seen as aggravating/initiating the preexisting migraine/tension headache.
  2. Fatigue
  3. Dizziness and/or vertigo
  4. Impaired memory
  5. Difficulty in concentrating
  6. Insomnia
  7. Irritability
  8. Lowered tolerance of stress, emotion, or alcohol
- Other associated symptoms: noise sensitivity, neck pain, nondermatomal paresthesias, interference with social role functioning.
- Focal neurologic deficits are typically absent on examination.

ETIOLOGY

- The inciting TBI may occur as a result of events such as falls, motor vehicle accidents, military injuries, and contact sports.
- The primary injury triggers a slew of pathophysiological changes at the cellular level secondary to the axonal stretching and injury, leading to alterations in membrane and intracellular physiology, thereby affecting neurotransmission. These changes are believed to be a factor in determining whether the outcome will be an apparent normal recovery or persistent postconcussion symptoms.
- Postmortem findings reveal diffuse axonal injury as the primary pathologic finding, along with small petechial hemorrhages and local edema.
- A psychogenic origin has been suggested by a number of empiric and clinical observations; however, limitations in methodology and differing definitions preclude firm conclusions. Prior history of anxiety is a strong risk factor for occurrence of PCS.

DIAGNOSIS

A careful history, a nonfocal neurologic examination, and normal neurologic testing will usually establish the diagnosis.

DIFFERENTIAL DIAGNOSIS

- Headache (dissection of the vertebral artery, occipital neuralgia)
- Epidural hematoma
- Subdural hematoma
- Skull fracture
- Cervical spine disk disease
- Whiplash
- Cerebrovascular accident
- Depression
- Anxiety

WORKUP

To exclude other causes of neurologic symptoms after TBI:
- Normal results of electroencephalography
- Normal evoked potentials
- Neuropsychological testing, which often reveals difficulties in concentration, memory, language, and executive function

LABORATORY TESTS

Various biomarkers in blood and cerebrospinal fluid and genetic testing have been proposed and studied in patients with TBI, but these tests are not specific and are not routinely used.

IMAGING STUDIES

- There is no imaging modality to diagnose PCS. PCS is primarily a clinical diagnosis. The American College of Emergency Physicians' clinical policy regarding neuroimaging in adults with mild traumatic brain injury is summarized in Box 1.
- 10% of CT scans of the head following mild TBI are abnormal, showing mild subarachnoid hemorrhage, subdural hemorrhage, or contusions.

BOX 1 American College of Emergency Physicians' Clinical Policy Regarding Neuroimaging in Adults With Mild Traumatic Brain Injury

A noncontrast head CT is indicated (level one recommendation) in adults with LOC or posttraumatic amnesia only if at least one of the following is present:
- Headache
- Vomiting
- Age older than 60 years
- Drug or alcohol intoxication
- Deficits in short-term memory
- Physical evidence of trauma above the clavicle
- Posttraumatic seizure
- GCS score below 15
- Focal neurologic deficit
- Coagulopathy

A noncontrast head CT should be considered (level two recommendation) in head trauma patients with no LOC or posttraumatic amnesia if any of the following is present:
- Focal neurologic deficit
- Vomiting
- Severe headache
- Age 65 years or older
- Physical signs of a basilar skull fracture
- GCS score below 15
- Coagulopathy
- A dangerous mechanism (e.g., ejection from motor vehicle, pedestrian struck, fall of more than 3 feet or 5 stairs)

CT, computed tomography; *GCS*, Glasgow Coma Scale; *LOC*, loss of consciousness.
From Marx J et al: *Rosen's emergency medicine: concepts and clinical practice*, ed 7, Philadelphia, 2010, Mosby.

- MRI of the head after an mTBI is abnormal in 30% of patients with normal CT scans and may show irregular brain contours or old cerebral contusions.
- Recent improvements in imaging modalities, including diffuse tensor imaging (DTI) and susceptibility weighted imaging (SWI) in MRI, functional MRI (fMRI), and metabolic imaging such as magnetic resonance spectroscopy (MRS), positron emission tomography (PET), and single-photon emission computed tomography (SPECT) imaging, appear to be promising in elucidating the underlying pathophysiology of TBI and PCS, although they have not found a major role in clinical practice yet.
- None of the imaging modalities have been able to predict the occurrence of PCS in patients with mild TBI.

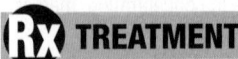 **TREATMENT**

PCS must be recognized as a physiologic and psychological problem and treated accordingly. Treatment should be individualized to target the patient's particular symptoms and is typically completed on an outpatient basis. Some symptoms may be refractory to treatment.

NONPHARMACOLOGIC Rx

- Early reassurance and patient education are major components of treatment. Explanation of symptoms and expectations, combined with early follow-up with reassurance, may hasten resolution of symptoms.
- Graduated physical activity is preferred over prolonged cognitive and physical rest. Light aerobic activity that avoids risk for reinjury has been shown beneficial in mitigating refractory concussion symptoms. Physical and occupational therapy may be beneficial.
- Cognitive behavioral therapy may be effective in treating symptoms.

- Avoidance of alcohol, narcotics, and sleep deprivation.

PHARMACOLOGIC THERAPY

- Supportive symptomatic care may include the use of nonnarcotic analgesics and antiemetics.
- Amitriptyline has been widely used for posttraumatic tension-type headaches as well as for nonspecific symptoms such as irritability, dizziness, insomnia, and depression.
- Posttraumatic migraine-type headaches can be treated with a trial of propranolol or amitriptyline alone or in combination.
- Depression can be treated with selective serotonin reuptake inhibitors but may not respond as well when compared with patients without PCS who have depression.

DISPOSITION

- Most patients improve after mild TBI without any residual deficits within 3 months.
- Although good improvement is typically seen within the first 6 months, patients can continue to show improvement for up to 12 to 18 months.
- Patients with very severe brain injuries (low Glasgow Coma Scale [GCS] score) and prolonged anterograde amnesia are at increased risk of development of some degree of permanent cognitive and personality disturbance.
- Predictors for the development of persistent PCS include:
  1. Female sex
  2. Ongoing litigation (conflicting studies)
  3. Low socioeconomic status
  4. Prior headaches
  5. Prior TBI
  6. Prior psychiatric illnesses, particularly anxiety

REFERRAL

Early consultations with psychologists, psychiatrists, neurologists, and rehabilitation specialists in an outpatient setting may be beneficial.

⚠ PEARLS & CONSIDERATIONS

- PCS starts within a few days after the injury.
- Recognizing depression and treating pain symptoms early in the course may help prevent the development of persistent PCS (>1 year).
- The severity of the trauma does not clearly predict the risk of PCS.
- The severity of brain injury is usually documented by initial GCS score, duration of loss of consciousness, and duration of amnesia; however, there is a move toward tests of function, such as neuropsychological testing or fMRI.

COMMENTS

- Attempts to determine how much of a role psychological and/or neurologic factors play in the PCS are important but very difficult.
- No medication at hospital discharge has been proved to change the natural course of the disease.
- Engaging in physical activity within 7 days after concussion is associated with a lower rate of persistent postconcussive symptoms.

SUGGESTED READINGS

Available at www.expertconsult.com

RELATED CONTENT

Post-concussion Syndrome (Patient Information)
Concussion (Related Key Topic)
Traumatic Brain Injury (Related Key Topic)

AUTHORS: **CHLOE MANDER NUNNELEY, M.D., JOSEPH S. KASS, M.D., J.D.,** and **PRASHANTH KRISHNAMOHAN, M.B.B.S, M.D.**

BASIC INFORMATION

DEFINITION

- Postherpetic neuralgia (PHN) is a pain syndrome that results as a complication of herpes zoster (HZ). HZ, also known as shingles, is a painful vesicular eruption in a dermatomal distribution. HZ is caused by the reactivation of varicella zoster virus (VZV) in someone with a known history of varicella. PHN is pain and/or dysesthesia that persist for 3 or more months at the site of resolved HZ.

ICD 10-CM CODES
B02.29 Other postherpetic nervous system involvement

EPIDEMIOLOGY & DEMOGRAPHICS

INCIDENCE: PHN occurs in approximately 9% to 34% of HZ patients. It is the most frequent chronic complication of herpes zoster and the most common neuropathic pain disorder resulting from infection. In one study, approximately 60% of patients with HZ developed PHN at age 60 years, and 75% developed PHN at age 70 years. In another study, the incidence of PHN at 9 years post-HZ eruption was 21%.

PEAK INCIDENCE: Unknown

PREDOMINANT SEX AND AGE:
- PHN occurs equally in males and females.
- The likelihood of developing PHN significantly increases with advancing age.

GENETICS:
- Family history of HZ is considered a risk factor for HZ, with higher risk if multiple family members have had HZ.

RISK FACTORS:
- Advanced age
- Greater severity of HZ prodromal pain
- Greater severity of pain during acute HZ eruption
- Location—specifically ophthalmic (V1) location and brachial plexus
- Severe immunosuppression

PHYSICAL FINDINGS & CLINICAL PRESENTATION

- HZ typically presents as a painful vesicular eruption in a dermatomal distribution. Rarely, HZ can occur subclinically with dermatomal pain in the absence of a rash.
- PHN is pain that continues for 3 months at the dermatomal site of the resolved HZ. The pain may be described as burning, stabbing, shooting, or shock-like.
- Patients may note an amplified response to stimuli at the site of PHN, with increased pain response (hyperalgesia), pain to typically non-noxious stimuli (allodynia), or focal changes in autonomic function (e.g., increased sweating).
- Physical examination should include a comparison of sensory function in the affected dermatome with that on the contralateral side.

ETIOLOGY

- PHN is associated with damage and scarring to the dorsal root ganglion secondary to inflammation related to active herpes zoster infection.

DIAGNOSIS

DIFFERENTIAL DIAGNOSIS

Zoster sine herpete (subclinical HZ without skin eruption)

TREATMENT

ACUTE GENERAL Rx

- Administration of acyclovir or valacyclovir within 72 hours of HZ onset is thought to help reduce the likelihood of developing PNH. However, one Cochrane review paper found no difference with acyclovir administration.
- A single published study supports the use of amitriptyline (25 mg daily) as an adjunct to an antiviral agent in acute HZ to decrease the incidence of PHN and the pain associated with subsequent PHN.
- A suggestive non-controlled study with co-administration of valacyclovir and gabapentin during acute HZ reduced the incidence of PHN as well.
- Corticosteroids do NOT prevent PHN.

CHRONIC Rx

TOPICAL TREATMENTS:
- Lidocaine 5% patches may be used for mild pain.
- Capsaicin 0.075% cream (although little reported efficacy) 5 times per day.
- Capsaicin 8% patch has greater efficacy, but overall analgesia may be minimal at best, with 1/3 of patients unable to tolerate the agent due to burning, stinging, and erythema. However, a single 60-minute treatment with high concentration capsaicin patch was found in one study to reduce PHN for up to 12 weeks regardless of concomitant systemic neuropathic pain medication use.

ORAL TREATMENTS: First line:
- Gabapentinoids (gabapentin, pregabalin) are the only FDA-approved oral therapy for PHN and are some of the most commonly used first-line therapies for chronic PHN pain. Gabapentin may be administered in the immediate-release or extended-release formulation. Dosing includes gabapentin 300 mg 3 times a day (titrating up to max 3600 mg/day) and pregabalin 75 mg nightly (titrating up to 300 mg twice daily).
- Tricyclic antidepressants such as amitriptyline (25 mg/day, increased 25 mg every night to a maximum of 75 mg/night), desipramine (10-25 mg/day, increased every 3 days as needed to a maximum of 150 mg/day) and nortriptyline (10-25 mg/day increased by 25 mg/day weekly as needed to maximum of 75 mg day) are another first line treatment. These medications have a delayed onset of action and may not work as well in patients with certain types of pain, such as burning pain or allodynia. They have a considerable side effect profile. Their use in elderly patients should be carefully considered. A recent study showed the combination of gabapentin and nortriptyline was more efficacious than either drug as monotherapy for neuropathic pain.

Second Line:
- Opiates (e.g., controlled-release oxycodone): side effects, the possibility of misuse, and the potential for abuse must be weighed.

Other Modalities:
- Dorsal root entry zone (DREZ) lesions have been used with an improvement rate of 20% in long-term studies.
- For recalcitrant cases, epidural corticosteroids and nerve blocks, botulinum toxin, and cryotherapy
- Fig. 1 describes a treatment algorithm for HZ and PHN.

COMPLEMENTARY AND ALTERNATIVE MEDICINE:
- Acupuncture
  - Studies on acupuncture and PHN pain have had varying results; however, the only randomized, controlled study showed no significant difference in pain reduction between control and treatment groups.

REFERRAL

- For complicated cases, dermatology, neurology, and/or pain management input can be helpful.

PEARLS & CONSIDERATIONS

COMMENTS

- Careful consideration of treatment side effects and drug interactions is needed.
- The natural history of PHN is slow resolution, and most individuals respond to medical therapy. However, a subtype of patients may develop severe, long-lasting pain that is recalcitrant to medical therapy.
- In a questionnaire study of 385 adults age >65 years old with persistent acute pain, the mean duration of PHN was 3.3 years.

PREVENTION

- Vaccination
  - A live-attenuated VZV vaccine (Zostavax®) is effective in reducing the risk for both HZ and PHN (11 and 43 needed to vaccinate to prevent a case of HZ or PHN, respectively), with the main benefit being the reduction of morbidity caused by PHN. Vaccination reduces the risk of PHN by 67% in patients >60 years old.
  - FDA-approved 50 and older; currently, the CDC recommends at age 60 regardless of history of chicken pox.
  - Data still insufficient regarding long-term prevention of HZ and PHN given efficacy likely wanes over time.

PATIENT/FAMILY EDUCATION

- The only well-documented means of preventing PHN is the prevention of herpes zoster through vaccination.
- Patients should understand both the benefits and the potential adverse effects of treatment.
  - They should be informed that pain relief will likely not be immediate.
  - Frequent reassessment may be needed, and drug doses should be increased as necessary.

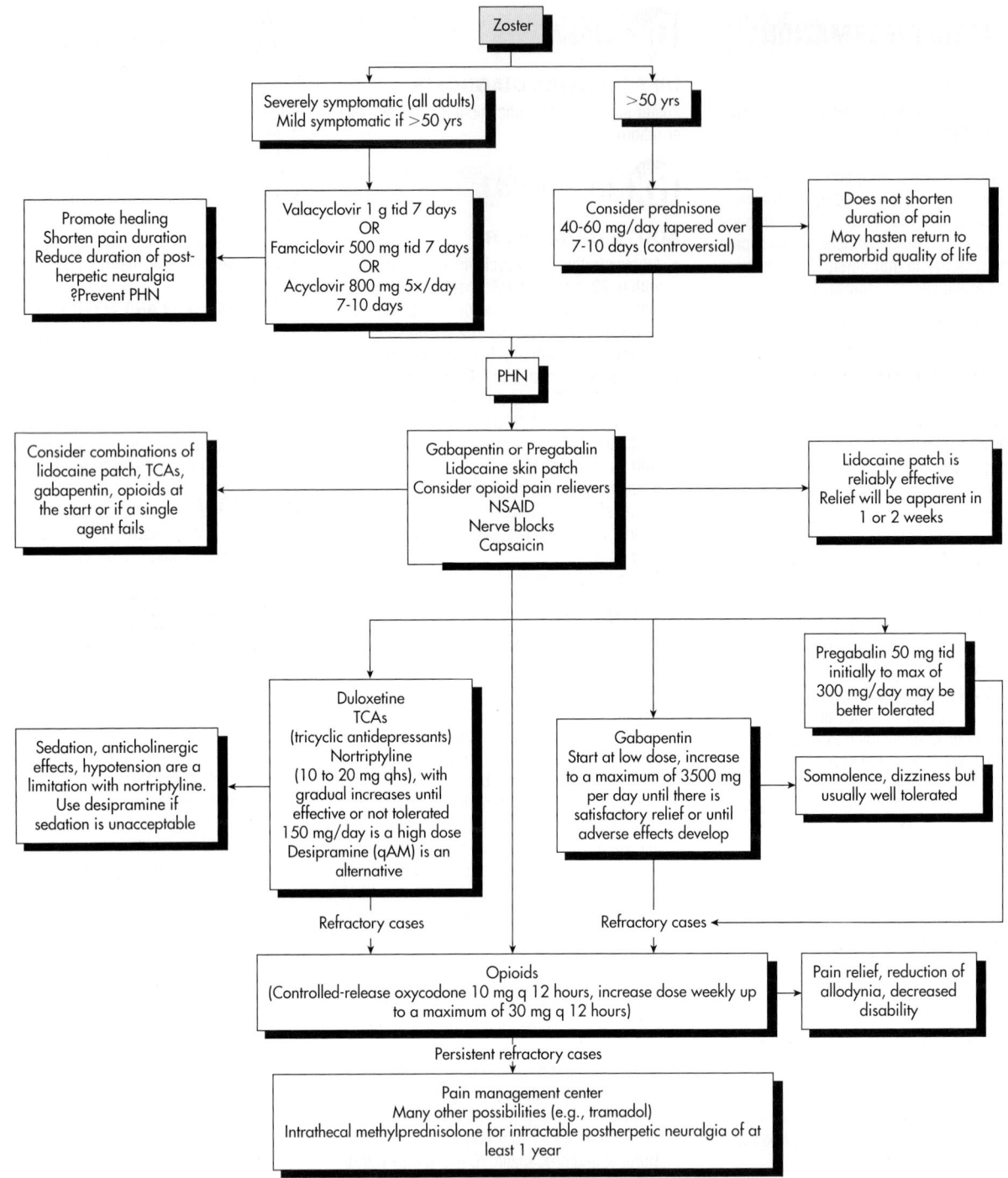

FIG. 1 Treatment of herpes zoster and postherpetic neuralgia. *NSAID,* Nonsteroidal antiinflammatory drug; *PHN,* postherpetic neuralgia. (Modified from Habif TA: *Clinical dermatology,* ed 4, St Louis, 2004, Mosby.)

RELATED CONTENT

Herpes Zoster (Related Key Topic)
Peripheral Neuropathy (Related Key Topic)

SUGGESTED READINGS

Available at www.expertconsult.com

AUTHORS: **EMILY Z. HEJAZI, M.D., M.S.,** and **LISA K. PAPPAS-TAFFER, M.D.**

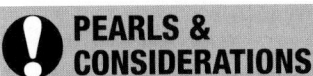

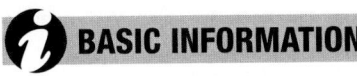

DEFINITION
Major or minor depressive episodes occurring within 3 to 12 months of delivery

SYNONYMS
Postpartum blues
Postpartum depression
Postpartum psychosis

ICD-10CM CODES
F53: includes postpartum depression and postpartum psychosis
090.6: includes postpartum blues, postpartum dysphoria and sadness

EPIDEMIOLOGY & DEMOGRAPHICS
INCIDENCE: Approximately half a million women in the U.S. are affected annually by postpartum depression.
PREVALENCE: Perinatal depression affects 1 in 7 women
GENETICS: A family history of mood disorders is a risk factor for postpartum depression
RISK FACTORS: Risk factors include depression or anxiety during pregnancy, traumatic birth experiences, stressful life events during pregnancy or the postpartum period, infant NICU admission or preterm delivery, poor social support, history of depression, and problems with breastfeeding.

PHYSICAL FINDINGS & CLINICAL PRESENTATION
Patients present with depressed or irritable mood, decreased interest in activities, appetite and sleep changes, weight changes, decreased energy, excessive guilt or feelings of worthlessness, psychomotor agitation or retardation, and possibly suicidal/homicidal ideation. The diagnosis of major depressive episode requires that symptoms be present nearly every day for two weeks and that the woman experiences a decline from a previous level of functioning.

ETIOLOGY
The decline in reproductive hormones following delivery is believed to contribute to the development of postpartum depression in some women. In addition, women with a history of depression, stressful life events, and a family history of mood disorders have an increased risk of both depression and postpartum depression.

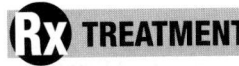

DIFFERENTIAL DIAGNOSIS
- Hyperthyroid
- Hypothyroid
- Postpartum blues: syndrome with weepiness and sadness usually occurring shortly after delivery and resolving by 10 days postpartum.
- Postpartum psychosis: usually occurs between 1 to 2 weeks post-delivery and is characterized by extreme disorganization of thought, hallucinations, and bizarre behavior. It requires rapid intervention as there is a real risk of suicide or infanticide
- Bipolar disorder

WORK-UP
- History and physical examination
- Screening all postpartum women with a screening instrument such as the Edinburgh Postnatal Depression Scale (specific to the postpartum period and takes less than 5 minutes to complete) or the Patient Health Questionnaire 9
- In any patient with postpartum depression, screening for bipolar disorder

LABORATORY TESTS
There are no diagnostic laboratory tests.

IMAGING STUDIES
None

TREATMENT

NONPHARMACOLOGIC THERAPY
- Psychotherapy: studies have shown psychotherapy to be equally effective to fluoxetine.

ACUTE GENERAL Rx
- Therapy with a selective serotonin reuptake inhibitor should be considered as first-line treatment because of low risk of toxic effects with overdose and ease of dosing. However, if patient has had good success with another medication in the past, then it is appropriate to restart that medication. Start at half the recommended dose and increase after 4 days, with gradual up-titration until therapeutic effects are seen.
- A single medication is favored over multiple medications in order to decrease exposure to the fetus/neonate.
- Sertraline is the first-line selective serotonin reuptake inhibitor recommended for breastfeeding mothers secondary to existing evidence suggesting little risk for infants. There is, however, no evidence of adverse infant effects from mothers taking sertraline, paroxetine or fluvoxamine. Fluoxetine may be present in higher levels in breast milk and breastfed infants.
- Tricyclic antidepressants do not appear to pass in significant amounts into breastfeeding infants and their use appears to be safe. Data regarding atypical antidepressants and breastfeeding is limited.

CHRONIC Rx
- Medical therapy should be continued until at least 6 months after remission.
- Long-term therapy should be considered for women with a history of 3 or more episodes of depression.

DISPOSITION
- Without treatment, the duration of postpartum depression averages seven months.
- Fifteen percent to 85% of women will experience at least one relapse after completing medical therapy.

REFERRAL
- Consider referral to psychiatrist if a patient demonstrates no improvement after six weeks of drug therapy or experiences a relapse.
- Prompt or urgent referral to psychiatrist is indicated if a patient has signs/symptoms of postpartum psychosis, bipolar disorder, or expresses suicidal/homicidal ideation.

PEARLS & CONSIDERATIONS

COMMENTS
- Depression and anxiety both during and after pregnancy can have negative effects not only on the mother but also on her fetus, new baby, and family. Low birth weight, decreased fetal growth, increased NICU admission rates, increased nenonate crying, and decreased developmental scores have been seen with these disorders when untreated. In addition, depression is associated with increased smoking, alcohol, and drug use, which can have negative effects on the infant and family. These factors should be taken into account when counseling women about medical therapy.
- Selective serotonin reuptake inhibitors do pass through breast milk but are present in very small quantities compared with the transplacental exposure infants receive in utero. Adverse infant effects are extremely rare; however, long-term data is lacking.

PREVENTION
In a patient with a history of postpartum depression, recurrence risk is approximately 25%. These patients should be screened for depression both during and after pregnancy. It is reasonable to initiate prophylactic therapy in patients with a history of depression, and they should have close postpartum follow-up for early identification of depressive episodes.

PATIENT/FAMILY EDUCATION
National Women's Health Information Center: www.womenshealth.gov
Postpartum Support International: www.postpartum.net
Center for Disease Control and Prevention: http://www.cdc.gov/reproductivehealth/depression/

RELATED CONTENT
Depression, Major (Related Key Topic)

SUGGESTED READINGS
Available at www.expertconsult.com

AUTHOR: **CLAIRE SCHULTZ, M.D.**

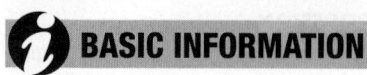

BASIC INFORMATION

DEFINITION

Postpartum hemorrhage (PPH) is classically defined as estimated blood loss >500 ml after a vaginal birth or >1000 ml after a cesarean section. Primary PPH is hemorrhage within the first 24 hr after delivery. Secondary PPH is hemorrhage after 24 hr and within 6 to 12 wk.

SYNONYMS

Obstetric hemorrhage
PPH

ICD-10CM CODES
O72.1 Other immediate postpartum hemorrhage
O72.2 Delayed and secondary postpartum hemorrhage

EPIDEMIOLOGY & DEMOGRAPHICS

INCIDENCE: 4% to 6%
PREDOMINANT SEX AND AGE: Female of reproductive age
RISK FACTORS: Prolonged labor, augmented labor, rapid labor, history of PPH, episiotomy, preeclampsia, multiple gestation, macrosomic infant, operative delivery, chorioamniotis, bleeding dyscrasia, Asian or Hispanic ethnicity

PHYSICAL FINDINGS & CLINICAL PRESENTATION (TABLE 1)

- Bleeding is generally brisk at time of delivery.
- Examination findings include boggy uterus with continued passage of clot or blood with fundal pressure.
- Objective findings can also include hypotension, tachycardia, and oliguria with substantial blood loss.

ETIOLOGY

- Primary: uterine atony (>80%), retained placenta, coagulopathies, lacerations
- Secondary: subinvolution of placental site, retained products, infection, coagulopathies

DIAGNOSIS

WORKUP

- Bladder should be emptied
- Bimanual examination to evaluate for atony; massage if it is present
- Examination to verify that no lacerations are present, including cervical examination with necessary lighting and retractors
- Ultrasonography at bedside to evaluate for retained tissue or clot
- Examination to verify that placenta is intact

LABORATORY TESTS

Significant hemorrhage can lead to disseminated intravascular coagulation (DIC). If DIC is suspected, complete blood count and coagulation panels should be ordered. Similarly, if coagulopathy is suspected, evaluation of clotting factors should be ordered.

IMAGING STUDIES

Ultrasonography can be used to scan for retained products, including clot or placenta. It can be performed to assess the need for more invasive measures, such as instrumentation or a manual sweep.

TREATMENT

Medical management with uterotonics is generally the first line of treatment:
- Oxytocin (IV, 10-40 units diluted into IV solution, or 10 units IM); often given prophylactically immediately after delivery (preferred)
- Methergine (IM, 0.2 mg)
- Hemabate (IM, 0.25 mg)
- Misoprostol (400-800 mcg sublingually or rectally)

NONPHARMACOLOGIC THERAPY

Secondary management includes the following:
- Packing with gauze, Foley catheter, or tamponade balloon
- Uterine curettage for suspected retained products
- Uterine artery embolization
- Ensure adequate IV access
- Surgical management with laparotomy
  1. Hypogastric artery ligation
  2. Bilateral uterine artery ligation (O'Leary sutures)
  3. B-lynch sutures
  4. Hysterectomy

ACUTE GENERAL Rx

- Uterotonics, surgical management, embolization, blood transfusion. Fig. 1 outlines the management of postpartum hemorrhage.
- Table 2 describes therapeutic response to initial fluid resuscitation. Dosing regimen for oxytocic drugs is summarized in Table 3. Blood product replacement is described in Box 1.

CHRONIC Rx

For anemia: ferrous sulfate supplementation to support new red blood cell production

TABLE 1 Presentation of Symptoms in Postpartum Hemorrhage

% Blood loss (ml)	Systolic blood pressure (mm Hg)	Signs and symptoms
10-15 (500-1000)	Normal	Tachycardia, palpitations, dizziness
15-25 (1000-1500)	Low-normal	Tachycardia, weakness, diaphoresis
25-35 (1500-2000)	70-80	Restlessness, pallor, oliguria
35-45 (2000-3000)	50-70	Collapse, air hunger, anuria

From Vincent JL et al: *Textbook of critical care*, ed 6, Philadelphia, 2011, WB Saunders.

TABLE 2 Therapeutic Response to Initial Fluid Resuscitation

Response	Description	Follow-up treatment
Rapid response	<20% of blood volume lost	No additional fluids or blood are needed.
Transient response	20%-40% of blood volume lost; responds to initial fluid bolus but later has worsening vital signs	Continue fluids and consider blood transfusions.
Minimal or no response	Ongoing severe hemorrhage with >40% blood volume lost	Continue aggressive fluid and blood product replacements.

From Vincent JL et al: *Textbook of critical care*, ed 6, Philadelphia, 2011, WB Saunders.

TABLE 3 Dosing Regimens for Oxytocic Drugs

Drug	Regimens
Oxytocin (Pitocin)	5-unit IV bolus
	Add 20-40 units oxytocin to 1 L of fluids
	10 units intramyometrially
Methylergonovine (Methergine)	0.2 mg IM every 2-4 hr
Ergonovine (Ergotrate Maleate)	100-125 mcg IM or intramyometrially every 2-4 hr
	200-250 mcg IM
	Total dose 1.25 mg
Carboprost (Hemabate)	250 mcg IM or intramyometrially every 15-90 min
	Total dose 2 mg
Misoprostol	800 mcg PR or 800 mcg of sublingual misoprostol

IM, Intramuscular; *IV*, intravenous; *PR*, per rectum.
From Vincent JL et al: *Textbook of critical care*, ed 6, Philadelphia, 2011, WB Saunders.

DISPOSITION

- The patient should be closely watched for at least 24 hr after a postpartum hemorrhage. Vital signs should be monitored for evidence of hemodynamic stability and appropriate response to anemia. Serial laboratory tests can be performed in the setting of concern for ongoing bleeding.
- Morbidity can include shock, acute respiratory distress syndrome, Sheehan's syndrome, and loss of fertility.

REFERRAL

During the course of a postpartum hemorrhage, the anesthesiology department should be notified and adequate nursing should be available. Early considerations should be made to notify obstetricians. If bleeding is brisk or estimated blood loss is considerable, preparation should be made for transfusion of blood products, including drawing blood for typing and notifying the blood bank.

SUGGESTED READING

Available at www.expertconsult.com

AUTHOR: **LEO HAN, M.D., M.P.H.**

P

Diseases and Disorders

I

BOX 1 Blood Product Replacement

Cross-matched blood
Type-specific or "saline cross-matched" blood
Compatible ABO and Rh blood types
Rh-negative blood is preferable.
Warm the blood, if possible, especially if the rate of infusion is >100 ml/min or if the total volume transfused is high; cold blood is associated with an increased incidence of arrhythmias and paradoxical hypotension.
Administer calcium if blood is transfused rapidly at >100 ml/min because of binding of calcium by anticoagulants in banked blood.
Give 6-10 units fresh frozen plasma (FFP) for every 10 units of packed red blood cell transfusions.
Give 10-12 units of platelets if the platelet count decreases to <50 × 109/L.
Cryoprecipitate can be given to replace fibrinogen in addition to the FFP.
Consider 60-120 mcg/kg intravenous bolus injection of recombinant activated factor VII (rFVIIa).

From Vincent JL et al: *Textbook of critical care,* ed 6, Philadelphia, 2011, WB Saunders.

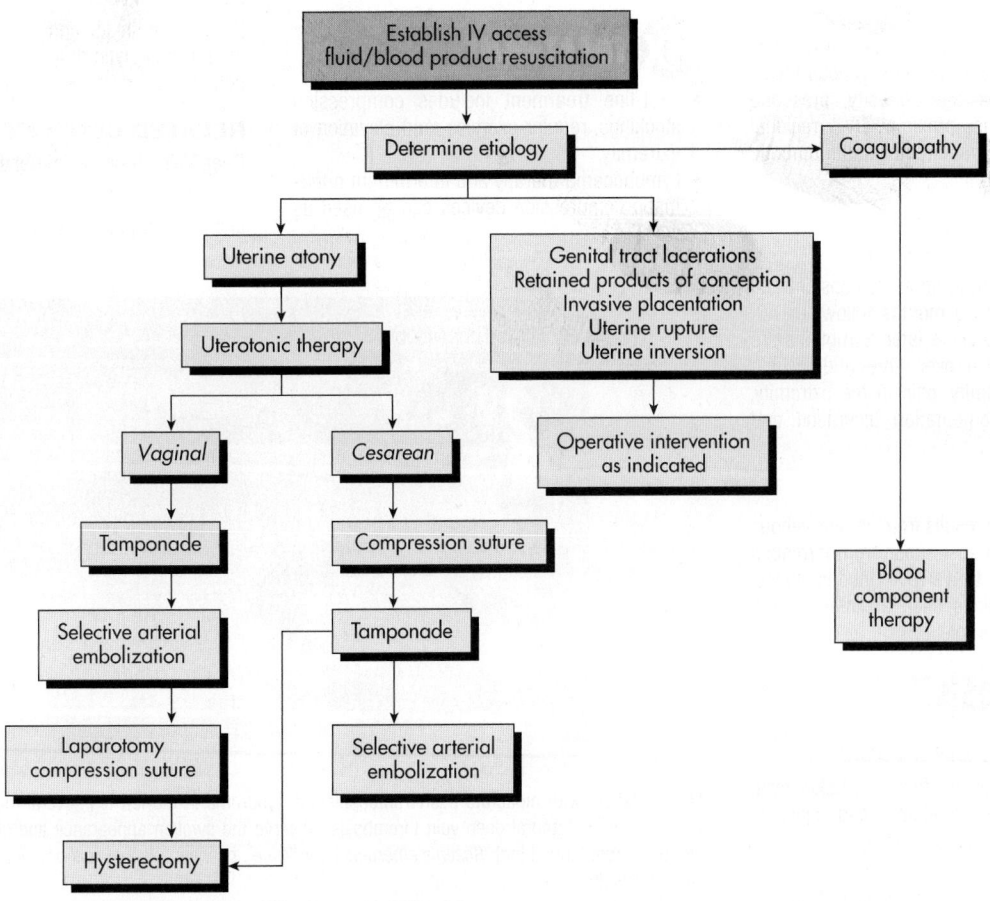

FIG. 1 Management of postpartum hemorrhage. (From Gabbe SG: *Obstetrics,* ed 6, Philadelphia, 2012, WB Saunders.)

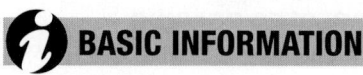

BASIC INFORMATION

DEFINITION

A delayed complication of deep vein thrombosis (DVT) that leads to signs and symptoms of venous insufficiency.

SYNONYMS

Post-phlebitic syndrome
Chronic venous insufficiency

ICD-10CM CODES
I87.001	Postthrombotic syndrome without complications of right lower extremity
I87.002	Postthrombotic syndrome without complications of left lower extremity
I87.003	Postthrombotic syndrome without complications of bilateral lower extremities

EPIDEMIOLOGY AND DEMOGRAPHICS

INCIDENCE:
- 23%-60% of people with DVT will experience post-thrombotic syndrome, often within 2 yr of DVT.

PREVALENCE:
- Unknown

PREDOMINANT SEX:
- Slightly female predominance

RISK FACTORS:
- Symptomatic DVT, postoperative DVT, recurrent DVT, underlying primary venous insufficiency, younger age, obesity, presence of varicose veins, proximal DVT, residual thrombus, and inadequate antithrombotic treatment.

PHYSICAL FINDINGS AND CLINICAL PRESENTATION

Symptoms can be intermittent or constant and often appear weeks to months following DVT, but can occur up to years later. Symptoms are generally progressive over time and include edema in the extremity, pain in the extremity, changes in skin pigmentation, ulceration, and venous dilatation.

ETIOLOGY

Venous insufficiency results from chronic venous hypertension due to obstruction from thrombus and reflux related to valvular incompetence. Inflammatory cytokines such as interleukin 6 are thought to play a role.

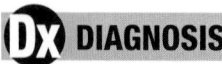 **DIAGNOSIS**

DIFFERENTIAL DIAGNOSIS

DVT, primary venous insufficiency, Baker cyst, tumor, lymphedema, lipedema, and injury to extremity.

WORKUP

Clinical diagnosis based on history of DVT and signs and symptoms of chronic venous insufficiency. The Villalta scale can be used in cases when the diagnosis is uncertain. It is the mostly widely used scoring system for both diagnosing postthrombotic syndrome (PTS) and assessing its severity.
- Entails five patient symptoms (pain, leg cramps, heaviness in extremity, paresthesia, and pruritus) and six physical signs (pretibial edema, skin induration, hyperpigmentation, pain with calf compression, venous ectasia, and redness) (Fig. 1).
- Scored on a scale of 0 to 3 (0 = none, 1 = mild, 2 = moderate, 3 = severe).
- Total score ranges from 0 to 33; a ≥5 is consistent with a diagnosis of PTS.
  ○ PTS can also be diagnosed if a venous ulcer is present independent of total score.
- Severity is assessed based on score in which 5 to 9 is mild, 10 to 14 is moderate, and 15 to 33 is severe.

LABORATORY TESTS

None presently used.

IMAGING TESTS

Venous duplex ultrasonography or compression ultrasonography can be done to look for prior evidence of DVT but is not necessary to make the diagnosis.

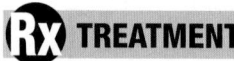 **TREATMENT**

- First-line treatment includes compression stockings, regular exercise, and elevation of extremity.
- Lymphedema therapy and intermittent pneumatic compression devices can be used as well.

- Skin care is important, particularly in cases with eczematous changes. Moisturizing lotions can be used in conjunction with mild potency corticosteroids.
- Diuretics have a limited role but can decrease edema in some patients.
- Surgical repair is generally reserved for severe cases and for those with nonhealing ulcers. Surgical options include angioplasty, venous bypass, or endophlebectomy.

DISPOSITION

- Chronic venous insufficiency can impair quality of life and is often a chronic condition.
- Early treatment with anticoagulation may decrease the risk of postthrombotic syndrome.
- Early use of compression stockings can reduce symptoms of venous insufficiency and halt progression.

REFERRAL

Lymphedema clinic, interventional radiology, and vascular surgery.

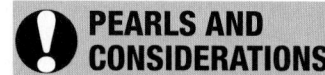 **PEARLS AND CONSIDERATIONS**

COMMENTS

Compression stockings have the most evidence both for preventing post-thrombotic syndrome and for treatment once the syndrome has developed.

PREVENTION

Evidence both for and against early treatment with thrombolytic drugs to prevent post-thrombotic syndrome.

RELATED CONTENT

Deep Vein Thrombosis (Related Key Topic)
Venous Insufficiency, Chronic (Related Key Topic)

AUTHOR: **LYNN PESTA, M.D.**

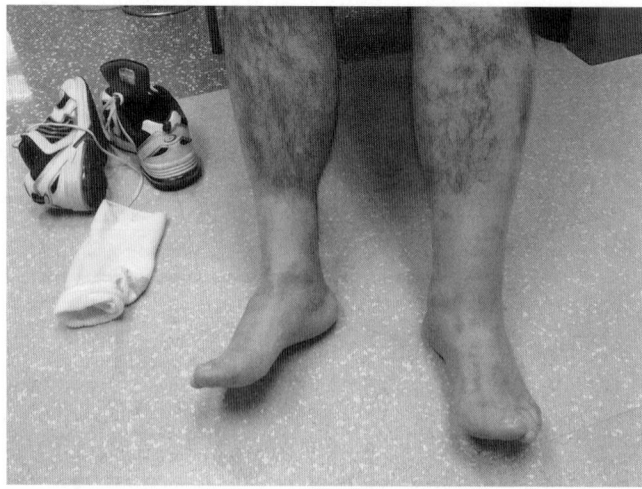

FIG. 1 Patient with moderate postthrombophlebitic syndrome in the left leg several months after diagnosis with a common femoral deep vein thrombosis. Observe the swollen appearance and slight color change in the foot. (From Marx J [ed]: *Rosen's emergency medicine : concepts and clinical practice,* ed 7, London, 2009, Elsevier Health Sciences.)

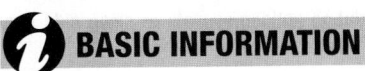 BASIC INFORMATION

DEFINITION

Posttraumatic stress disorder (PTSD) develops in some people after witnessing or experiencing a traumatic event that involves actual or threatened injury to self or others. Symptoms continue longer than a month after the event or may have delayed onset and include intrusive thoughts, nightmares, flashbacks, avoidance of things associated with the trauma, hypervigilance, sleep disturbance, and negative changes in mood and cognition. These symptoms cause distress and a decline in interpersonal, social, and occupational functioning. People with PTSD may feel numb or irritable, may be easily startled or frightened, and sometimes isolate themselves from others. They are at risk for comorbid psychiatric illness, substance abuse, and suicide.

SYNONYMS (HISTORICAL)

Soldier's heart
Effort syndrome
Shell shock
Concentration camp syndrome

ICD-10CM CODES
F43.10 Post-traumatic stress disorder, unspecified
F43.11 Post-traumatic stress disorder, acute
F43.12 Post-traumatic stress disorder, chronic

EPIDEMIOLOGY & DEMOGRAPHICS

INCIDENCE: Fewer than 10% of individuals who have experienced a traumatic event will develop PTSD.
PREVALENCE (IN U.S.):

- 12-month prevalence in the U.S. 3% to 6%. Estimated lifetime prevalence 7.8% to 12.3%.
- Prevalence among high-risk populations (e.g., combat veterans or victims of violent crimes) up to 58%.
- Comorbidity is common: depression, anxiety, substance use, and somatic symptom disorder.
- Factors most associated with development are previous traumatic experience and subsequent life stress and perceived lack of social support.

PREDOMINANT AGE AND SEX:
- No predisposing age factors.
- Twice as many women as men are affected (prevalence 10%-14% for women and 5%-6% for men). More than 50% of cases in women are related to sexual assault.

GENETICS: Twin studies have demonstrated genetic vulnerability related to combat.

PHYSICAL FINDINGS & CLINICAL PRESENTATION

Core symptom clusters include intrusion, avoidance, negative mood and cognition, hyperarousal, and sometimes dissociative symptoms. Individuals present with different variations of these symptoms. Symptoms must occur for >1 month and result in significant distress and functional impairment.
Key PTSD symptoms:
1. Distressing memories or dreams of the event. Note: Children older than 6 years may express this symptom in repetitive play.
2. Flashbacks.
3. Intense distress after reminders of the event.
4. Avoidance due to trauma-related thoughts or feelings.
5. Persistent negative trauma-related emotions.
6. Feeling detached.
7. Aggressive or reckless behavior.
8. Hypervigilance.
9. Problems with concentration or sleep.
10. Depersonalization.

ETIOLOGY

- Common types of trauma: violent personal assault, natural disaster, military combat, rape, motor vehicle accident, childhood abuse and neglect, critical illness or hospitalization in ICU, severe physical injury, diagnosis of life-threatening illness.
- Risk factors: previous trauma, initial severity of reaction to event, psychiatric history, childhood abuse or neglect, poor social support, gender, age.
- Interpersonal violence is more likely to cause PTSD than events such as motor vehicle accidents or natural disasters.
- Severity of physical injury is a weaker predictor of PTSD than the psychological distress; stress duration is the most important factor.
- Proposed mechanisms include activation of the amygdala, disruption of prefrontal cortex modulation of the amygdala, and excessive stress-induced HPA and alpha-1 receptor activation.

Fig. 1 illustrates a hypothesized relationship between "stressors" and the development of syndromes

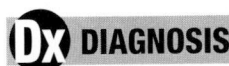 DIAGNOSIS

Diagnosis is made when the stressor is consistent with DSM-5 definition (follows), and the individual experiences symptoms of re-experiencing, avoidance, negative mood and cognition, and arousal and reactivity as defined under "Clinical Presentation." The symptoms must be present for >1 month, must cause impairment

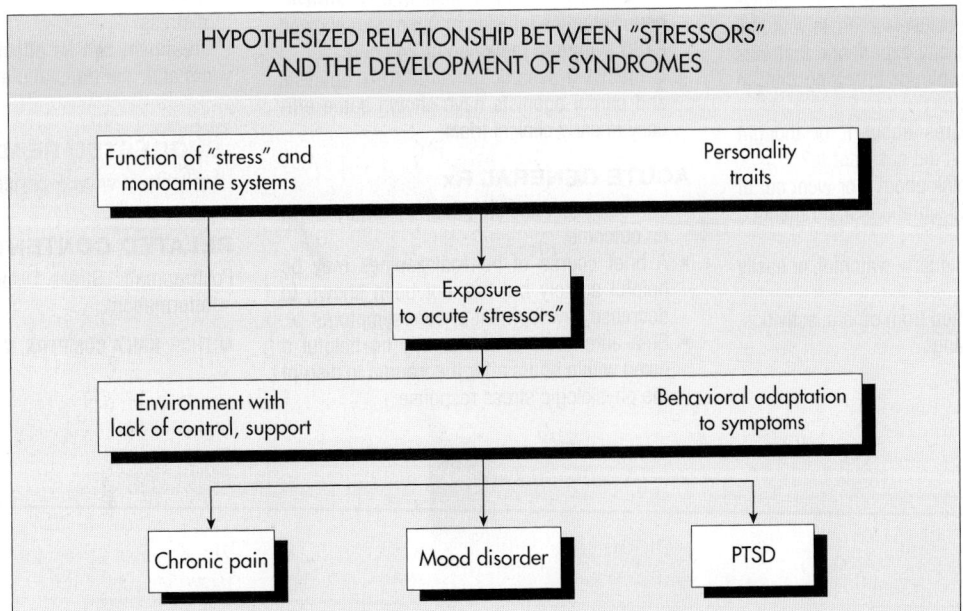

FIG. 1 The hypothesized relationship between "stressors" and the development of syndromes such as fibromyalgia, posttraumatic stress disorder, and depression. (From Hochberg MC et al: *Rheumatology*, ed 5, St Louis, 2011, Mosby.)

in functioning, and must not be attributable to substance use or other medical conditions. Subtypes include dissociative (PTSD criteria and depersonalization or derealization) and delayed onset (PTSD criteria starting at least six months after the event.)

Definition of Stressor

Exposure to death, threatened death, actual or threatened serious injury, or actual or threatened sexual violence, as follows (one required):
1. Directly experiencing the event.
2. Witnessing the event occur to others.
3. Indirectly, by learning that a close relative or close friend was exposed to trauma. If the event involved actual or threatened death, it must have been violent or accidental.

Repeated or extreme indirect exposure to aversive details of the event(s), usually in the course of professional duties (e.g., first responders collecting body parts; professionals repeatedly exposed to details of child abuse).

DIFFERENTIAL DIAGNOSIS

- Adjustment disorders: precipitating stress is less catastrophic and psychological reaction is less specific
- Mood disorder: depression or bipolar Anxiety disorder
- Somatic symptom or conversion disorder (functional neurological symptom disorder)
- Psychotic disorder
- Traumatic brain injury

WORKUP

- Among self-report questionnaires and structured diagnostic instruments, the best validated is the Posttraumatic Diagnostic Scale.
- Laboratory and imaging are not clinically useful.
- Primary care PTSD (PC-PTSD) screen recommended by the Veterans Administration.
  "Yes" answers to three of four of the following questions is a positive screen. In your life, have you ever had any experience that was so frightening, horrible, or upsetting that, in the past month, you:
  have had nightmares about it or thought about it when you did not want to?
  tried hard not to think about it or went out of your way to avoid situations that reminded you of it?
  were constantly on guard, watchful, or easily startled?
  felt numb or detached from others, activities, or your surroundings?

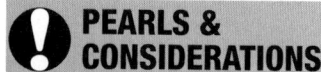
TREATMENT

- Trauma-focused CBT with sensitivity to pacing, readiness, containment, dissociation, and coping skills can decrease symptom intensity and frequency.
- Prolonged exposure (PE), a type of CBT that includes education on stress response and the recounting of the event, including sensory details.
- Group therapy.
- Eye movement desensitization reprocessing (EMDR).
- Couples therapy when appropriate.
- Transcranial magnetic stimulation (TMS) is being evaluated as a possible effective treatment modality.

MEDICATIONS

There is no definitive cure for PTSD, and individuals have varying responses to different medications. Sertraline and paroxetine, both SSRIs, are the only FDA-approved medications for PTSD. Other medication use is off-label with differing levels of evidence to support use. Medications are used to target symptoms and the physiologic changes associated with PTSD.
- SSRIs: sertraline, paroxetine, fluoxetine.
- SNRIs: venlafaxine, duloxetine.
- Other antidepressants: mirtazapine.
- Alpha-adrenergic receptor blockers: Prazosin may decrease nightmares; guanfacine may be helpful in treating arousal symptoms.
- Atypical antipsychotics have had mixed results in clinical trials. Risperidone been shown to be effective in some studies. Other antipsychotics, particularly quetiapine and olanzapine, are sometimes used off-label as monotherapy or augmentation to target individual patient symptoms such as paranoia, extreme anxiety, or angry outbursts.
- Ketamine: A recent clinical trial of intravenous ketamine infusion at 0.5 mg/kg showed PTSD symptom reduction at 24 hours
- N-methyl-D-aspartic acid (NMDA) agonists and partial agonists have shown some efficacy in early clinical trials.

ACUTE GENERAL Rx

- Immediate postincident debriefing may worsen outcome.
- A brief course of benzodiazepines may be helpful acutely but has not been shown to decrease development of core symptoms.
- Beta-adrenergic blockers may be helpful if given within hours after the trauma to disrupt the physiologic stress response.

- Sedating antidepressants or sleep aids may be helpful for initial insomnia.

COMPLEMENTARY & ALTERNATIVE APPROACHES

Acupuncture has been shown to be effective in decreasing symptoms of PTSD.

DISPOSITION

- Recovery rates are highest in the first 12 mo after onset.
- Average duration of symptoms is 36 mo for those who undergo treatment and 64 mo for those never treated.
- 50% chance of remission at 2 yr; 50% have chronic symptoms.
- Predictors of chronic course include previous trauma, premorbid psychiatric function, panic reaction at time of event, prolonged terror, or dissociation at time of event.

REFERRAL

Because early intervention improves outcome, refer to psychiatry as soon as diagnosis made.

⚠ PEARLS & CONSIDERATIONS

- PTSD can be associated with suicidal ideation and attempts.
- PTSD can be associated with aggressive and violent behavior.
- Traumatic medical experiences such as being in the ICU, myocardial infarction, or an emergent cesarean section can cause PTSD.
- Individuals with PTSD are at risk for comorbid psychiatric disorder, including substance abuse.
- Among combat veterans of recent wars, there is a 41% co-occurrence with mild TBI.
- PTSD may vary culturally and present as culturally specific syndromes and idioms of distress.

Treatment can be effective even if it begins years after the traumatic event occurred.

SUGGESTED READINGS

Available at www.expertconsult.com

RELATED CONTENT

Posttraumatic Stress Disorder (PTSD) (Patient Information)

AUTHOR: **KAILA COMPTON, M.D., PH.D.**

ⓘ BASIC INFORMATION

DEFINITION

Precocious puberty is defined as sexual development occurring before age 8 yr in females and 9 yr in males.

SYNONYMS

Pubertas praecox

ICD-10CM CODES
E30.1 Precocious puberty

EPIDEMIOLOGY & DEMOGRAPHICS

INCIDENCE: Estimated to be between 1 in 5000 to 1 in 10,000.

PREDOMINANT SEX: Females are affected 5 times more often than males for the idiopathic variant; for other causes, dependent on the underlying etiology.

GENETICS: The genetics for some of the etiologies of precocious puberty is known. Deficiency of *MKRN3* causes central precocious puberty in humans.

PHYSICAL FINDINGS & CLINICAL PRESENTATION

- In females: breast development, pubic hair development, accelerated growth, menarche.
- In males: increase in testicular volume and penile length, pubic hair development, accelerated growth, muscular development, acne, change in voice, penile erections.

ETIOLOGY

- Central (GnRH-dependent, "true precocious puberty")
  ○ Idiopathic (74%)—diagnosis of exclusion
  ○ CNS problem (7%)
    ■ Tumor, encephalitis, head trauma, hydrocephalus
- Peripheral (GnRH-independent, incomplete, pseudopuberty)
  ○ Ovarian cyst or tumor (11%)
  ○ McCune-Albright syndrome (5%)
  ○ Adrenal feminizing or masculinizing (2%)
  ○ Ectopic gonadotropin production (0.5%)
  ○ Severe hypothyroidism (very rare)

Ⓓ DIAGNOSIS

DIFFERENTIAL DIAGNOSIS

- Most common diagnoses to consider: premature thelarche and premature adrenarche (incomplete puberty).
- Constitutional precocity—onset near 8 years of age, familial.
- Gonadotropin hormone-releasing hormone (GnRH)-dependent precocious puberty: idiopathic, CNS tumors, hypothalamic hamartomas, neurofibromatosis, tuberous sclerosis, hydrocephalus, status after acute head injury, ventricular cysts, status after CNS infection.

- GnRH-independent precocious puberty: congenital adrenal hyperplasia, adrenocortical tumors (males), McCune-Albright syndrome (females), gonadal tumors, ectopic human chorionic gonadotropin (hCG)-secreting tumors (chorioblastoma, hepatoblastoma), exposure to exogenous sex steroids, severe hypothyroidism.
- Table 1 summarizes the differential diagnosis of sexual precocity.

WORKUP

Priorities:
- Rule out life-threatening disease (neoplasm of central nervous system [CNS], gonad, adrenal).
- Establish velocity of process.
- Thorough history and physical examination are essential to determine if the patient has true precocious puberty. Particular attention should be paid to growth, development, order of appearance of the secondary sexual characteristics, pubertal development in family members, medications, neurologic symptoms, Tanner staging, abdominal and neurologic examination. Flowcharts for diagnosing sexual precocity in females and males are shown in Figs. 1 and 2.

LABORATORY TESTS

- GnRH stimulation testing will help determine if dependent or independent cause.
- Sex hormone studies: luteinizing hormone, follicle-stimulating hormone, hCG, testosterone (males), estrogen (females). Levels of sex steroids should be determined in the morning, with use of assays that have detection limits adapted to pediatric values. In girls, serum estradiol levels are highly variable and have a rather low sensitivity for the diagnosis of precocious puberty.
- Free T_4, thyroid-stimulating hormone (TSH)

IMAGING STUDIES

- Bone age: left hand/wrist x-ray establishes severity of process.
- CT scan or MRI of the brain to evaluate for CNS pathology.
- Consideration of pelvic ultrasound in female patients to evaluate for ovarian cysts or tumors.
- Abdominal imaging with CT scan if intraabdominal pathology suspected.

℞ TREATMENT

NONPHARMACOLOGIC THERAPY

- Good communication with the parents is essential to care.
- Psychological support for the child may be needed with regard to self-image and problems with peer acceptance. Because appearance is ahead of age, social and emotional difficulties may occur. Sexual abuse is a particular point of concern.

ACUTE GENERAL Rx

There is no acute therapy for precocious puberty.

CHRONIC Rx

Therapy depends on the etiology of precocious puberty. For the treatment of central or gonadotropin-dependent precocious puberty depot GnRH agonists (leuprorelin, leuprolide, triptorelin, goserelin, histrelin, buserelin) are effective.

- Leuprolide is given 0.25 to 0.3 mg/kg with a 7.5 mg minimum IM every 4 wk. Local side effects include pain, erythema, and inflammatory reactions. Other side effects include headaches and menopausal-like symptoms (asthenia, hot flashes).
- For other CNS lesions and extragonadal tumors, therapy is dependent on the type of lesion, location of the lesion, and the overall prognosis of the underlying problem.
- For severe hypothyroidism, treatment with thyroid hormone will result in regression of the sexual development. The child will subsequently undergo appropriate pubertal development later in life.
- For familial male gonadotropin-independent precocious puberty, the androgen-synthesis inhibitor ketoconazole can be used at doses of 600 mg/day divided tid, or a combination of the aromatase inhibitors testolactone or anastrozole and spironolactone can be used.

DISPOSITION

- For true precocious puberty and some CNS lesions, long-term outcome is usually very good. When drug therapy is instituted, it is continued until a time when further pubertal development is appropriate. It is then discontinued, allowing the child to progress through puberty.
- For other cases, long-term outcomes depend on the prognosis of the underlying cause.

REFERRAL

- Initial workup can be instituted by the primary care provider.
- Referral to an endocrinologist is indicated for most children because they will need long-term management, monitoring, and treatment.
- Attention to the emotional needs of the child is important.

SUGGESTED READINGS
Available at www.expertconsult.com

RELATED CONTENT
Precocious Puberty (Patient Information)

AUTHOR: **RUBEN ALVERO, M.D.,** and **GEORGE KOVALEVSKY, M.D.**

TABLE 1 Differential Diagnosis of Sexual Precocity

	Plasma Gonadotropins	LH Response to GnRH	Serum Sex Steroid Concentration	Gonadal Size	Miscellaneous
Gonadotropin-Dependent					
True precocious puberty	Prominent LH pulses (premature reactivation of GnRH pulse generator)	Pubertal LH response initially during sleep	Pubertal values of testosterone or estradiol	Normal pubertal testicular enlargement or ovarian and uterine enlargement	MRI of brain to rule out CNS tumor or other abnormality; skeletal survey for McCune-Albright syndrome (by US)
Incomplete Sexual Precocity (Pituitary Gonadotropin-Independent)					
Males					
Chorionic gonadotropin-secreting tumor in males	High hCG, low LH	Prepubertal LH response	Pubertal value of testosterone	Slight to moderate uniform enlargement of testes	Hepatomegaly suggests hepatoblastoma; CT scan of brain if chorionic gonadotropin-secreting CNS tumor suspected
Leydig cell tumor in males	Suppressed	No LH response	Very high testosterone	Irregular, asymmetric enlargement of testes	
Familial testotoxicosis	Suppressed	No LH response	Pubertal values of testosterone	Testes symmetric and >2.5 cm but smaller than expected for pubertal development; spermatogenesis occurs	Familial; probably sex-limited, autosomal dominant trait
Virilizing congenital adrenal hyperplasia	Prepubertal	Prepubertal LH response	Elevated 17-OHP in CYP21 deficiency or elevated 11-deoxycortisol in CYP11B1 deficiency	Testes prepubertal	Autosomal recessive, may be congenital or late-onset form, may have salt loss in CYP21 deficiency or hypertension in CYP11B1 deficiency
Virilizing adrenal tumor	Prepubertal	Prepubertal LH response	High DHEAS and androstenedione values	Testes prepubertal	CT, MRI, or US of abdomen
Premature adrenarche	Prepubertal	Prepubertal LH response	Prepubertal testosterone, DHEAS, or urinary 17-ketosteroid values appropriate for pubic hair stage 2	Testes prepubertal	Onset usually after 6 yr of age; more frequent in CNS-injured children
Females					
Granulosa cell tumor (follicular cysts may present similarly)	Suppressed	Prepubertal LH response	Very high estradiol	Ovarian enlargement on physical examination, CT, or US	Tumors often palpable on physical examination
Follicular cyst	Suppressed	Prepubertal LH response	Prepubertal to very high estradiol	Ovarian enlargement on physical examination, CT, or US	Single or recurrent episodes of menses and/or breast development; exclude McCune-Albright syndrome
Feminizing adrenal tumor	Suppressed	Prepubertal LH response	High estradiol and DHEAS values	Ovaries prepubertal	Unilateral adrenal mass
Premature thelarche	Prepubertal	Prepubertal LH, pubertal	Prepubertal or early estradiol response	Ovaries prepubertal	Onset usually before 3 yr of age
Premature adrenarche	Prepubertal	Prepubertal LH response	Prepubertal estradiol; DHEAS or urinary 17-ketosteroid values appropriate for pubic hair stage 2	Ovaries prepubertal	Onset usually after 6 yr of age; more frequent in brain-injured children
Late-onset virilizing congenital adrenal hyperplasia	Prepubertal	Prepubertal LH response	Elevated 17-OHP in basal or corticotropin-stimulated state	Ovaries prepubertal	Autosomal recessive
In Both Sexes					
McCune-Albright syndrome	Suppressed	Suppressed	Sex steroid pubertal or higher	Ovarian (on US); slight testicular enlargement	Skeletal survey for polyostotic fibrous dysplasia and skin, examination for café au lait spots
Primary hypothyroidism	LH prepubertal; FSH may be slightly elevated	Prepubertal FSH may be increased	Estradiol may be pubertal	Testicular enlargement; ovaries cystic	TSH and prolactin elevated; T₄ low

CNS, Central nervous system; *CT*, computed tomography; *CYP*, P450 cytochrome isoenzyme; *DHEAS*, dehydroepiandrosterone sulfate; *GnRH*, gonadotropin-releasing hormone; *hCG*, human chorionic gonadotropin; *LH*, luteinizing hormone; *17-OHP*, 17-hydroxyprogesterone; *T₄*, thyroxine; *TSH*, thyrotropin; *US*, ultrasonography.
From Melmed S et al: *Williams textbook of endocrinology,* ed 12, Philadelphia, 2011, WB Saunders.

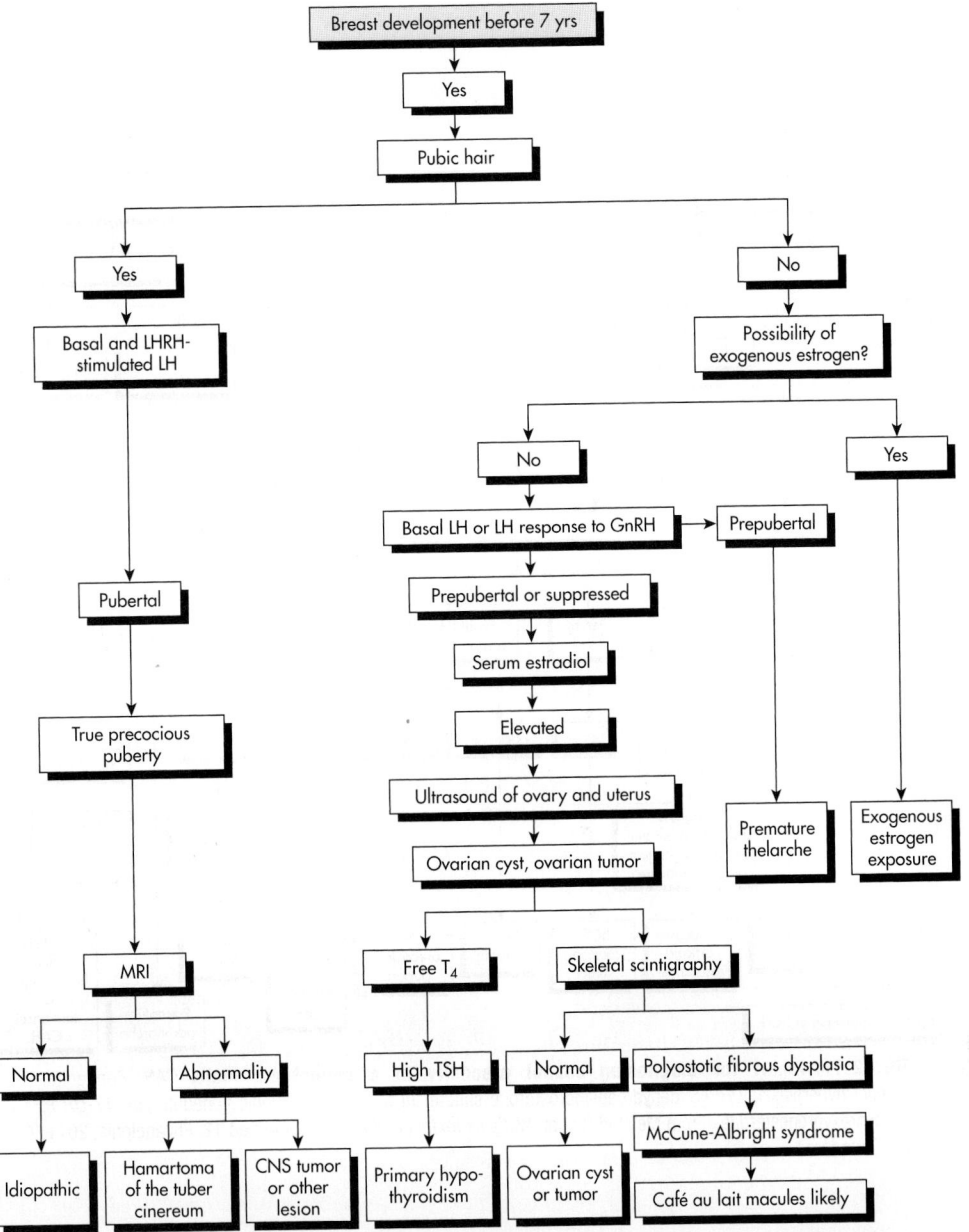

FIG. 1 Flowchart for diagnosing sexual precocity in girls. *CNS*, Central nervous system; *FSH*, follicle-stimulating hormone; *LH*, luteinizing hormone; T₄, thyroxine; *TSH*, thyroid-stimulating hormone. (From Melmed S et al: *Williams textbook of endocrinology*, ed 3, Philadelphia, 2011, WB Saunders.)

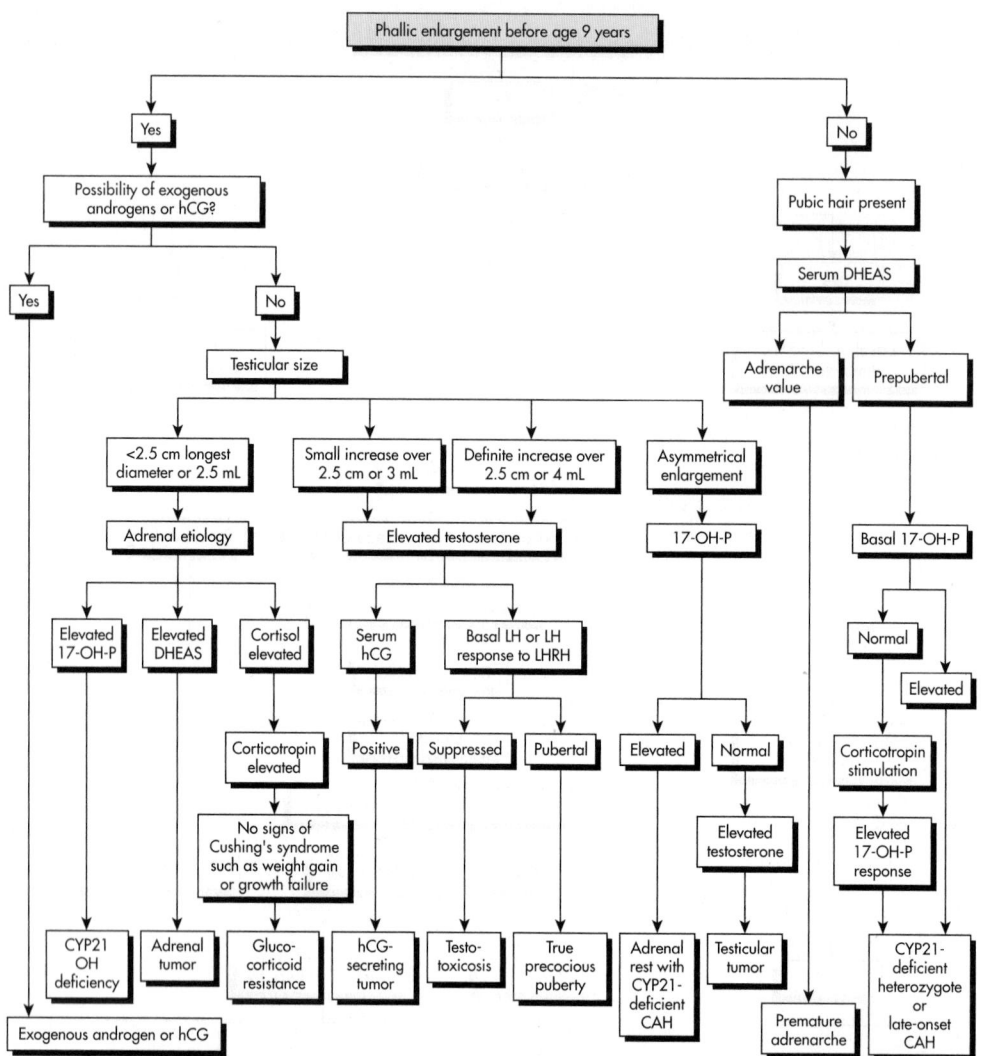

FIG. 2 Flowchart for diagnosing sexual precocity in a phenotypic male. *CAH*, Congenital adrenal hyperplasia; *DHEAS*, dehydroepiandrosterone sulfate; *hCG*, human chorionic gonadotropin; *17-OH-P*, 17-hydroxyprogesterone. (From Melmed S et al: *Williams textbook of endocrinology*, ed 12, Philadelphia, 2011, WB Saunders.)

BASIC INFORMATION

DEFINITION

Preeclampsia involves the presence of hypertension with other associated comorbidities in a pregnant woman. In 2013, the American College of Obstetrics and Gynecology (ACOG) Task Force on Hypertension in Pregnancy revised the criteria, making preeclampsia a hypertensive disorder and one where the presence of proteinuria was no longer needed to make the diagnosis. The task force reinforced the importance of hypertension as a necessary condition and deemphasized proteinuria. In the absence of proteinuria, thrombocytopenia, renal insufficiency, impaired liver function, pulmonary edema, and cerebral or visual symptoms could substitute as criteria.

Additionally, the task force emphasized the categories employed in prior ACOG bulletins:

1. Preeclampsia: Hypertension with or without proteinuria, but with the presence of one of the previously mentioned comorbidities
2. Preeclampsia with severe features (see Table 1)
3. Chronic hypertension: hypertension predating pregnancy
4. Gestational hypertension: hypertension in pregnancy after 20 wk without proteinuria or any of the previously mentioned comorbidities
5. Chronic hypertension with superimposed preeclampsia: The presence of chronic hypertension with new onset of signs and symptoms meeting criteria for preeclampsia Table 1 summarizes the criteria for the diagnosis of severe preeclampsia.
6. Atypical preeclampsia: onset prior to 20 wk; onset after 48 hours postpartum; gestational proteinuria with symptoms of preeclampsia, hemolysis, thrombocytopenia, or elevated liver enzymes

SYNONYMS

Pregnancy-induced hypertension
Toxemia of pregnancy

ICD-10CM CODES

O11.1 Pre-existing hypertension with pre-eclampsia, first trimester
O11.2 Pre-existing hypertension with pre-eclampsia, second trimester
O11.3 Pre-existing hypertension with pre-eclampsia, third trimester
O11.9 Pre-existing hypertension with pre-eclampsia, unspecified trimester
O14.00 Mild to moderate pre-eclampsia, unspecified trimester
O14.02 Mild to moderate pre-eclampsia, second trimester
O14.03 Mild to moderate pre-eclampsia, third trimester
O14.10 Severe pre-eclampsia, unspecified trimester
O14.12 Severe pre-eclampsia, second trimester
O14.13 Severe pre-eclampsia, third trimester
O14.90 Unspecified pre-eclampsia, unspecified trimester
O14.92 Unspecified pre-eclampsia, second trimester
O14.93 Unspecified pre-eclampsia, third trimester

EPIDEMIOLOGY & DEMOGRAPHICS

INCIDENCE: 2% to 7% in primigravidas, up to more than 50% in multigravidas with risk factors
RISK FACTORS: See Table 2.
GENETICS: Positive correlation with maternal and paternal family history

PHYSICAL FINDINGS & CLINICAL PRESENTATION

- Preeclampsia typically presents with hypertension and proteinuria, most commonly in the third semester of pregnancy.
- May be asymptomatic.
- Generalized swelling or nondependent edema, possibly manifested by rapid weight gain (>4 lb/wk), even in the absence of edema, is common but is nonspecific and is seen in many normal pregnancies.
- Auscultation of pulmonary rales.
- Right upper quadrant pain (HELLP syndrome [hemolysis, elevated liver enzymes, and low platelet count] or subcapsular liver hematoma).
- Hyperreflexia or clonus.
- Vaginal bleeding (placental abruption).
- Chronic fetal compromise manifested by intrauterine growth restriction or acute fetal compromise manifested by nonreassuring fetal testing.
- Wide range of symptoms attributable to multiorgan system dysfunction, involving hepatic, hematologic, renal, pulmonary, and central nervous systems.

- Possibility of severe disease despite "normal" blood pressure readings, so a high index of suspicion must be maintained in high-risk situations.

ETIOLOGY

- Exact etiology or toxic substance is unknown.
- Theories:
  1. Imbalance between thromboxane A_2 (vasoconstrictor and platelet aggregator) and prostacyclin (vasodilator)
  2. Abnormal trophoblastic invasion of spiral arteries
  3. Increased sensitivity to angiotensin II by the muscular walls of the arteries
  4. Excess circulating soluble fms-like tyrosine kinase 1 (*sFlt1*), which binds placental growth factor (PIGF) and vascular endothelial growth factor (VEGF), may have a pathogenic role
- Potential secondary effects of the metabolic, inflammatory endothelial alternatives in preeclampsia are described in Table 3.

DIAGNOSIS

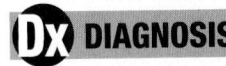

DIFFERENTIAL DIAGNOSIS

- Acute fatty liver of pregnancy
- Appendicitis
- Diabetic ketoacidosis
- Gallbladder disease
- Gastroenteritis
- Glomerulonephritis
- Hemolytic-uremic syndrome
- Hepatic encephalopathy
- Hyperemesis gravidarum
- Idiopathic thrombocytopenia
- Thrombotic thrombocytopenic purpura
- Nephrolithiasis
- Pyelonephritis
- Peptic ulcer disease
- Systemic lupus erythematosus

TABLE 1 Criteria for the Diagnosis of Severe Preeclampsia

In patients with preeclampsia, **severe preeclampsia** can be diagnosed if any one of the following criteria is present:

Blood pressure ≥160 mm Hg systolic or ≥110 mm Hg diastolic on two separate occasions at least 4 hr apart
Serum creatinine >1.1 mg/dl or a doubling of the serum creatinine
New onset of cerebral or visual disturbances
Pulmonary edema
Hepatocellular injury (serum transaminases at least twice normal) or severe persistent right upper quadrant or epigastric pain
Thrombocytopenia <100,000

TABLE 2 Risk Factors for Preeclampsia

- Nulliparity
- Age >40 years
- Pregnancy with assisted reproduction
- Interpregnancy interval >7 years
- Family history of preeclampsia
- Woman born small for gestational age
- Obesity/gestational diabetes
- Multifetal gestation
- Preeclampsia in a previous pregnancy
- Poor outcome in a previous pregnancy
- Fetal growth restriction, placental abruption, fetal death
- Preexisting medical-genetic conditions
- Chronic hypertension
- Renal disease
- Type 1 (insulin-dependent) diabetes mellitus
- Antiphospholipid antibody syndrome
- Factor V Leiden mutation

From Gabbe SG, et al: *Obstetrics*, ed 7, 2016, Philadelphia, Elsevier.

- Viral hepatitis
- Medications or medication withdrawal

WORKUP

Hypertension
- Two blood pressure measurements with the patient in lateral recumbent position at least 4 hr apart, with an absolute pressure ≥140 mm Hg systolic or ≥90 mm Hg diastolic.
- A single blood pressure ≥160 mm Hg systolic or ≥110 mm Hg diastolic.

Hypertension can thus be confirmed in a brief period to allow for immediate treatment of the blood pressure.

Proteinuria
- ≥300 mg per 24-hr urine collection
- Protein/creatinine ratio ≥0.3
- 1+ on dipstick ONLY IF OTHER METHODS NOT AVAILABLE
- In the absence of proteinuria, preeclampsia may be diagnosed with new onset of hypertension and one of the following:
  ○ Platelet count less than 100,000/mL
  ○ Serum creatinine concentrations greater than 1.1 mg/dL, or doubling of serum Cr levels in the absence of other renal disease
  ○ Elevated serum liver transaminases to twice the normal concentration
  ○ Pulmonary edema
  ○ Cerebral or visual symptoms
- Because of the insidious nature of the disease with potential for multiple organ involvement, as well as its prevalence, complete evaluation for preeclampsia in any pregnant patient presenting with central nervous system derangement or gastrointestinal symptoms after 20 wk of gestation
- Evaluation for associated conditions such as disseminated intravascular coagulation, hepatic dysfunction, or subcapsular hematoma
- Fig. 1 outlines a management plan for patients with severe preeclampsia

TABLE 3 Potential Secondary Effects of the Metabolic, Inflammatory Endothelial Alternatives in Preeclampsia

CVS	Increased peripheral resistance leading to hypertension; increased vascular permeability and reduced maternal plasma volume.
Lungs	Laryngeal and pulmonary edema.
Renal	Glomerular damage leading to proteinuria, hypoproteinemia, and reduced oncotic pressure, which further exacerbates the hypovolemia. May develop acute renal failure ± cortical necrosis.
Clotting	Hypercoagulability, with increased fibrin formation and increased fibrinolysis (i.e., disseminated intravascular coagulation).
Liver	HELLP syndrome hepatic rupture.
CNS	Thrombosis and fibrinoid necrosis of the cerebral arterioles. Eclampsia (convulsions), cerebral hemorrhage, and cerebral edema.
Fetus	Impaired uteroplacental circulation, potentially leading to FGR, hypoxemia, and intrauterine death.

CVS, Cardiovascular system; *CNS,* central nervous system; *FGR,* fetal growth restriction; *HELLP,* hemolysis, elevated liver enzymes, low platelets.
(From Drife J, Magowan B: *Clinical obstetrics and gynecology,* Philadelphia, 2004, WB Saunders.)

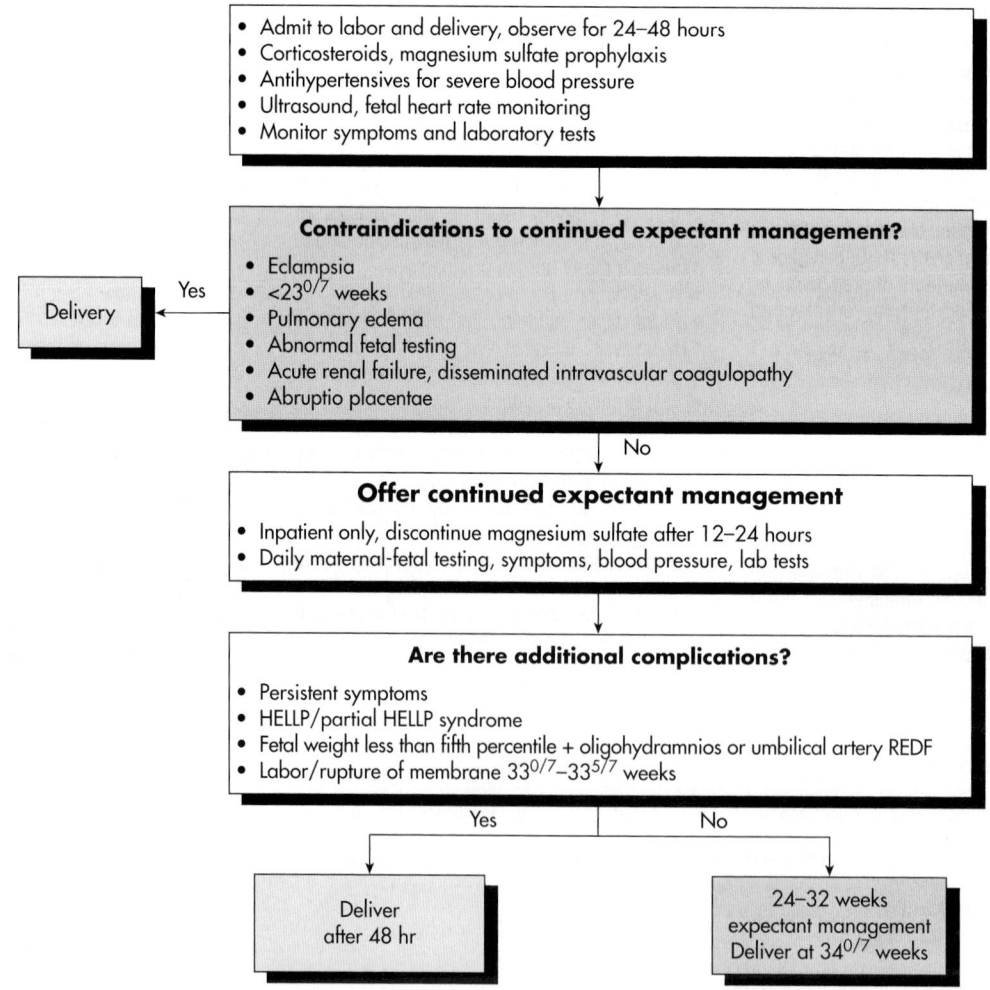

FIG. 1 Management plan for patients with preeclampsia with severe features before 34 weeks' gestation. *HELLP,* hemolysis, elevated liver enzymes, and low platelets; *REDF,* reversed end-diastolic flow. (From Gabbe, SG et al: *Obstetrics: Normal and problem pregnancies,* ed 7, Philadelphia, 2017, Elsevier.)

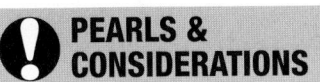

LABORATORY TESTS

- High-risk patients: Baseline assessment of renal function (24-hr urine collection for protein and creatinine clearance), platelets, blood urea nitrogen, creatinine, liver function tests (LFTs), and uric acid should be obtained at the first prenatal visit.
- Complete blood count (hemoglobin, hematocrit, platelets) may show signs of volume contraction or HELLP syndrome.
- LFTs (aspartate aminotransferase, alanine aminotransferase, lactate dehydrogenase) are useful in evaluation for HELLP syndrome or to exclude important differentials.
- Hyperuricemia or increased creatinine may indicate decreasing renal function.
- Prothrombin time, partial thromboplastin time, and fibrinogen should be checked to rule out disseminated intravascular coagulation.
- Peripheral smear may demonstrate microangiopathic hemolytic anemia.
- Complement levels can be used to differentiate from an acute exacerbation of a collagen-vascular disease.
- The ratio of soluble FMS-like tyrosine kinase 1 (sFlt-1) to placental growth factor (PIGF) is elevated in pregnant women before the clinical onset of preeclampsia. Increased levels of sFlt1 and reduced levels of PIGF predict subsequent development of preeclampsia. An sFlt-1:PIGR ratio of 38 or lower can be used to predict the short-term absence of preeclampsia in women in whom the syndrome is suspected clinically.[1]

IMAGING STUDIES

- CT scan of head if atypical presentation of eclampsia or preeclampsia with atypical cerebral symptoms, possibility of intracerebral bleed, or prolonged postictal state
- Sonogram of fetus to evaluate for intrauterine growth restriction (Fig. 2), amniotic fluid, placenta
- Sonogram of maternal liver if subcapsular hematoma suspected

Rx TREATMENT

ACUTE GENERAL Rx

Delivery is the treatment of choice and the only cure for the disease. This must be taken in the context of the gestational age of the fetus, severity of the preeclampsia, and the likelihood of a successful induction and reliability of patient.

- Administer magnesium sulfate 4 to 6 g IV loading dose, with 1 to 2 g/hr maintenance (or phenytoin at 10-15 mg/kg loading dose, then 200 mg IV q8h starting 12 hr after loading dose if a contraindication to magnesium sulfate).
- Hydralazine 10 mg IV, labetalol hydrochloride 20 to 40 mg IV, nifedipine 20 mg SL can be used for acute blood pressure control.

- Continuous fetal monitoring.
- Epidural is anesthesia of choice for pain management in labor or cesarean section.
- All patients undergoing induction of labor or cesarean section should receive antiseizure medications if disease is severe.

CHRONIC Rx

- Preeclampsia without severe features <37 wk: close observation for worsening maternal or fetal condition, with delivery at 37 wk. If 24 to 36 wk, consider antenatal corticosteroids.
- Severe preeclampsia: delivery in the presence of maternal or fetal compromise, labor, or 34 wk; at 24 to 34 wk consider steroids with very close monitoring, and at <24 wk consider termination of pregnancy. Risks of expectant management include severe worsening of disease, eclampsia, abruption placenta, stillbirth, HELLP syndrome, ICU admission, and pulmonary edema.
- Contraindications to expectant management include eclampsia, HELLP syndrome, pulmonary edema, DIC, abrutpio placenta, uncontrollable severe hypertension, fetal demise, and nonreassuring fetal status.
- Labetalol, hydralazine, and Procardia are the drugs of choice for long-term blood-pressure control during pregnancy.

DISPOSITION

Preeclampsia is a progressive and unpredictable disease process; a course of expectancy should be managed with caution. Up to 20% of patients who have seizures are normotensive.

REFERRAL

Obstetric management is indicated because of the insidious nature of the disease, with transfer of all cases <34 wk to a facility with a level three nursery.

⚠ PEARLS & CONSIDERATIONS

COMMENTS

- Low-dose aspirin, beginning as early as the second trimester, decreases the risk of preeclampsia, preterm birth, and intrauterine growth retardation in women who are at high risk of preeclampsia. The American College of Obstetricians and Gynecologists (ACOG) and the U.S. Preventive Services Task Force (USPSTF) recommend the use of low-dose aspirin (81 mg/day) as preventive medication after 12 wk of gestation in women who are at high risk for preeclampsia.
- Although the absolute risk of end-stage renal disease (ESRD) in women who have had preeclampsia is low, preeclampsia is a marker for an increased risk of subsequent ESRD.
- The development of preeclampsia may be one of the earliest identifiable risk markers for potential future cardiovascular disease in women. It has been shown that women who develop preeclampsia have a higher incidence of cardiovascular risk factors including components of the metabolic syndrome within 1 yr of delivery.

SUGGESTED READINGS

Available at www.expertconsult.com

RELATED CONTENT

Preeclampsia (Patient Information)
Eclampsia (Related Key Topic)
Hypertension (Related Key Topic)

AUTHOR: **PHILLIP A. SHLOSSMAN, M.D.**

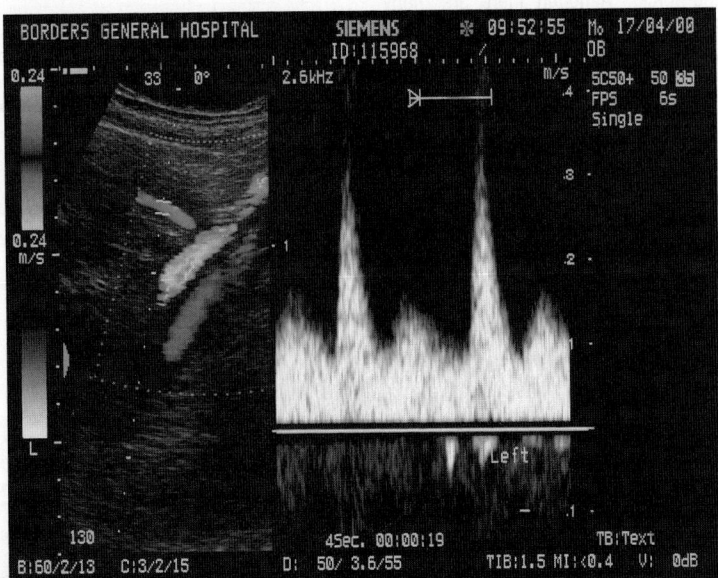

FIG. 2 Task Force on Hypertension in Pregnancy. American College of Obstetricians and Gynecologists. Hypertension in Pregnancy. http://www.acog.org/Resources-And-Publications/Task-Force-and-Work-Group-Reports/Hypertension-in-Pregnancy, November 2013.

[1]Zeisler H et al: Predictive value of the sFlt-1:PIGF ratio in women with suspected preeclampsia, *N Engl J Med* 374:13-22, 2016.

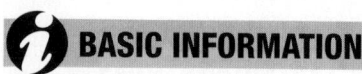

DEFINITION

Premature rupture of membranes (PROM) is defined as rupture of membranes at term before the onset of labor.

SYNONYMS

Preterm premature rupture of membranes (prior to 37 weeks)
PROM

ICD-10CM CODES
042 Premature rupture of membranes

EPIDEMIOLOGY & DEMOGRAPHICS

INCIDENCE: Affects approximately 8% of all pregnancies.
RISK FACTORS: Intraamniotic infection, low socioeconomic status, second and third trimester bleeding, low body mass index, nutritional deficiencies, connective tissue disorders, maternal cigarette use, cervical conization or cerclage, short cervix, pulmonary disease in pregnancy, uterine overdistention, amniocentesis, prior history of PROM, prior history of preterm delivery.

PHYSICAL FINDINGS & CLINICAL PRESENTATION

- Patients will classically present complaining of leakage or gush of fluid from the vagina. Patients may also present with contractions and vaginal bleeding. Additional symptoms can include fever, chills or abdominal pain if there is concurrent infection. Ultrasound will often demonstrate oligohydramnios.

ETIOLOGY

- Premature rupture of membranes at term may occur due to physiologic changes in addition to uterine contractions causing shearing forces. Although there are many risk factors for PROM, it often occurs in the absence of any known risk factor.

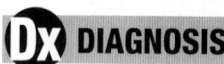 **DIAGNOSIS**

DIFFERENTIAL DIAGNOSIS

Differential diagnosis includes leakage of urine or vaginal discharge.

WORKUP

- Sterile speculum examination demonstrating pooling of fluid in posterior fornix, visualization of fluid coming out of the cervix during Valsalva maneuver, basic vaginal pH, and characteristic ferning pattern of vaginal fluid that is dried on a microscope. Table 1 summarizes bedside testing for premature rupture of membranes.
- Care should be taken to avoid any procedure that may introduce infection, so digital examination should be avoided unless patient is in active labor or delivery is imminently planned. This is of particular importance in preterm PROM.

- Fig. 1 shows initial assessment and management of women with premature rupture of the membranes.

LABORATORY TESTS

- pH test: sample vaginal fluid from posterior fornix. Normal vaginal pH is 4.5 to 6.0. pH of amniotic fluid is 7.1 to 7.3. False positive test can occur in presence of blood or semen, antiseptic of bacterial vaginosis.
- Microscopy: visualization of ferning of vaginal fluid allowed to dry on the microscope slide. False positive test can occur if cervical mucus is sampled.

- Commercially available tests: AmniSure and other tests are available and demonstrate good sensitivity and specificity; however, per the American College of Obstetrics and Gynecology, these should be considered ancillary to standard evaluation.

IMAGING STUDIES

- Abdominal ultrasound: evaluation of amniotic fluid volume either by maximum vertical pocket or amniotic fluid index. Oligohydramnios or low fluid volume in itself should not be considered diagnostic of PROM.

TABLE 1 Bedside Testing for Premature Rupture of Membranes

Method	Result
Nitrazine	Amniotic fluid (pH >6.5) will turn nitrazine paper blue; normal vaginal secretions (pH <5.5) will leave nitrazine paper yellow.
Ferning	Amniotic fluid crystallizes.
Smear combustion	Amniotic fluid, when flamed, turns white and crystallizes.
	Vaginal secretions caramelize and turn brown.

From Marx J et al: Rosen's emergency medicine: concepts and clinical practice, ed 7, Philadelphia, 2010, Mosby.

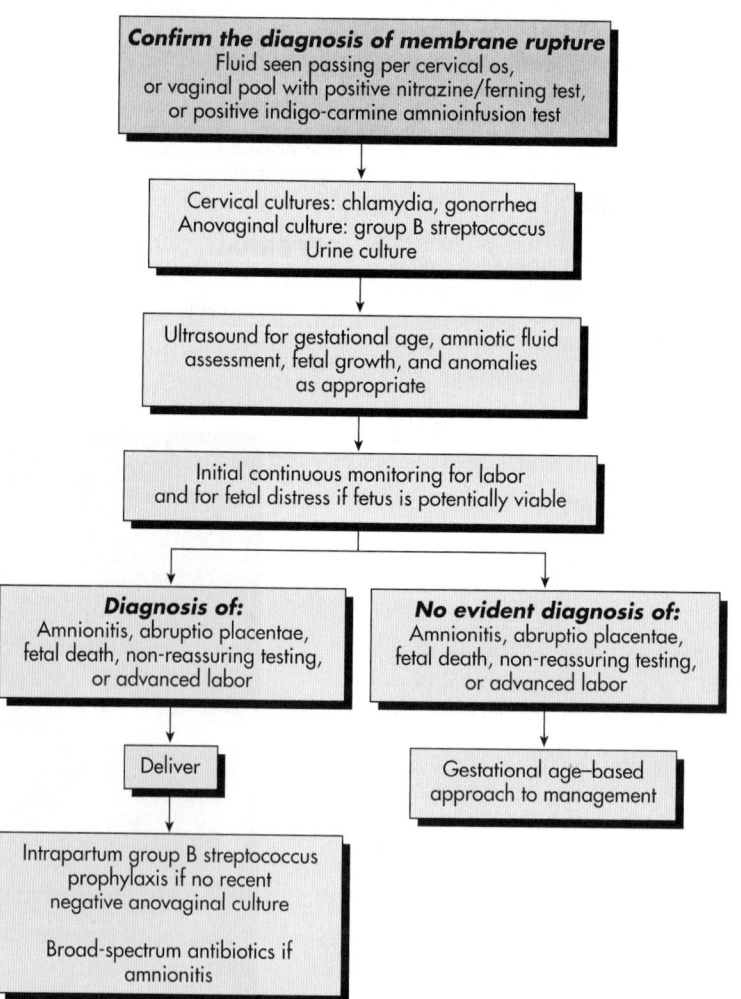

FIG. 1 Initial assessment and management of women with preterm premature rupture of the membranes. (From Mercer BM: Preterm premature rupture of the membranes: diagnosis and management. *Clin Perinatol* 31:765, 2004.)

- Amniotic fluid dye test: This is considered the gold standard in diagnosis of PROM, used in clinical scenario of suspected preterm PROM with equivocal testing. Indigo carmine dye is injected via ultrasound guidance into the amniotic sac, and diagnosis made if blue dye passes into vagina.

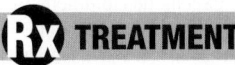 **TREATMENT**

NONPHARMACOLOGIC THERAPY

- All patients with PROM should have prompt evaluation of gestational age, fetal well-being via NST monitoring, and fetal presentation. In a patient with evidence of intraamniotic infection or fetal distress, prompt delivery is recommended. Close monitoring and consideration of delivery is recommended if there is concern for placental abruption.
- Collect swab for evaluation of GBS status.

ACUTE GENERAL Rx

Term PROM:
- Any patient diagnosed with PROM at term should proceed toward delivery. Induction of labor has been shown to decrease time to delivery, risk of chorioamnionitis, endometritis, and NICU admissions, with no increase in rate of operative delivery.
- A period of expectant management can be offered in select patients who decline induction and have been appropriately counseled.
- Routine induction agents may be used. The most researched agents for induction in setting of PROM include oxytocin and prostaglandins. Oxytocin has been shown to be associated with lower rates of chorioamnionitis.

- GBS prophylaxis should be provided in GBS-positive individuals or individuals with GBS-unknown status and concurrent risk factors

Preterm PROM:
- 34 weeks or above: Clinician should proceed toward delivery as in term patients
- 24 to 34 weeks:
  1. Administration of betamethasone for fetal lung maturity
  2. Administration of prophylactic antibiotics to prolong latency period, consisting of 7-day course of parenteral and oral therapy. Current guidelines recommend ampicillin or amoxicillin and erythromycin.
  3. Expectant management until 34 weeks, unless fetal lung maturity is demonstrated between 32 to 34 weeks.
  4. Magnesium sulfate administration if delivery is imminent and <32 weeks
  5. GBS prophylaxis in setting of GBS unknown/GBS positive if delivery is expected.

CHRONIC Rx

- Hospitalization with expectant management is recommended for all patients with preterm PROM. Ongoing maternal and fetal surveillance in a hospital setting allows for quick recognition of infection, labor, or fetal compromise secondary to cord compression.

DISPOSITION

- Most women with preterm PROM will proceed to deliver within one week despite medical interventions. Latency period is generally longer when PROM occurs at an earlier gestational age.

- Clinical chorioamnionitis develops in 13% to 16% of preterm PROM. This risk is increased with earlier PROM as well as with an increase in the number of digital vaginal examinations.
- Complications of preterm PROM are related mostly to complications of prematurity, and decrease with increasing gestational age at time of delivery. The most common complications include respiratory distress, neonatal infection, intraventricular hemorrhage, and necrotizing enterocolitis.
- There is a 1% to 2% risk of antenatal demise in the setting of preterm PROM.

REFERRAL

- Consultation with an Ob-Gyn is recommended in the setting of preterm PROM.

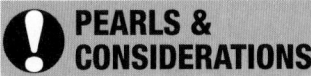 **PEARLS & CONSIDERATIONS**

PREVENTION

- Patients with a history of preterm delivery (with or without PROM) may benefit from administration of progesterone supplementation in future singleton pregnancy starting at 16 to 24 weeks to prevent preterm delivery.

SUGGESTED READINGS

Available at www.expertconsult.com

RELATED CONTENT

Abruptio Placentae (Related Key Topic)
Premature Labor (Related Key Topic)

AUTHOR: **CLAIRE SCHULTZ, M.D.**

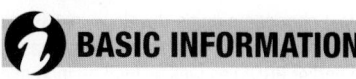

BASIC INFORMATION

DEFINITION

Premenstrual syndrome (PMS) consists of various somatic and physical complaints that develop during the luteal phase of the menstrual cycle and that are of sufficient severity to interfere with daily functioning and/or interpersonal relationships. The symptoms resolve shortly after the onset of menses.

SYNONYM

PMS

ICD-10CM CODES
N94.3 Premenstrual tension syndrome

EPIDEMIOLOGY & DEMOGRAPHICS

- Premenstrual disorders affect about 12% of reproductive-age women, although as many as 80% of women will report at least one somatic or affective symptom during their luteal phase (see Table 1).
- Severe cases of premenstrual dysphoric disorder (PMDD), which is more of a psychiatric diagnosis, occur in approximately 1.3% to 5.3% of women.
- The prevalence of PMS is not associated with age, race, or socioeconomic status.
- Those seeking treatment for PMS are usually in their 30s or 40s.
- Based on some identical twinning studies, a genetic component is thought to exist, but no genes have been identified.
- The natural history of PMS has not been clearly elucidated.

PHYSICAL FINDINGS & CLINICAL PRESENTATION

- Diverse and potentially disabling symptoms. Table 1 summarizes common symptoms of PMS.
- Associated with multiple psychological, physical, and behavioral symptoms
- Most frequent reason for seeking treatment: emotional symptoms

- Most common emotional symptoms: depression, irritability, anxiety, labile moods, anger, crying easily, sadness, extreme sensitivity, nervous tension
- Most common physical symptoms: headache, bloating, cramps, breast tenderness, migraines, fatigue, weight gain, aches and pains, palpitations
- Most common behavior symptom: food cravings
- Other behavioral symptoms: increased appetite, increased alcohol intake, decreased motivation, decreased efficiency, avoidance of activities, staying home, sleep changes, libido changes, forgetfulness, decreased concentration

ETIOLOGY

- Etiology is poorly understood. The syndrome is thought to result from steroid hormone effects on serotonin, Υ-aminobutyric acid, dopamine systems, and the renin-aldosterone system, thus causing some of the bloating symptoms.
- Because of the multifactorial, multiorgan nature of PMS, a single etiologic cause is unlikely.

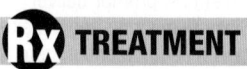 DIAGNOSIS

DIFFERENTIAL DIAGNOSIS

- A diagnosis of exclusion, so other medical or psychological disorders should be ruled out.
- Common disorders to rule out: depression or anxiety, anemia, migraines, endometriosis, thyroid disease.

WORKUP

- History.
- Physical examination.
- Laboratory studies to rule out alternative diagnosis.
- If no alternative diagnosis, confirm by either history of regular menses, basal body temperature charting, or elevated luteal progesterone that patient is ovulatory.
  1. If she is not ovulating, it is not PMS.

2. A prospective questionnaire given over two menstrual cycles has been found to be the most accurate way to assess the presence of PMS or PMDD. If symptoms are not occurring only in the luteal phase, it is not PMS and further investigation is needed.
   a. If symptoms occur in the follicular phase, patient has premenstrual exacerbation of another condition.
   b. If symptoms do not occur in the follicular phase, diagnosis of PMS is confirmed.

LABORATORY TESTS

- None available to specifically confirm the diagnosis of PMS
- Thyroid function tests to rule out thyroid disease

TREATMENT

NONPHARMACOLOGIC THERAPY

- Individualization of the treatment plan to maximize therapeutic response. Fig. 1 describes a summary of treatment approaches to PMS.
- Psychosocial intervention:
  1. Education
  2. Stress management
  3. Environmental changes
  4. Adequate rest and sleep
  5. Regular exercise
- Nutritional recommendations:
  1. Regularly eaten, well-balanced meals.
  2. Adequate amounts of protein, fiber, and complex carbohydrates; low fat.
  3. Avoidance of foods that are high in salt and simple sugars; may promote water retention, weight gain, and physical discomfort.
  4. Avoidance of alcohol and illicit drugs; may worsen emotional lability.
  5. Calcium supplementation (1000 mg/day for women 19 to 50 yr, 1300 mg/day for girls 14 to 18 yr) to reduce the physical and emotional symptoms.
  6. The data are mixed regarding the benefits of vitamin D supplementation in reducing PMS symptoms, so more studies are needed.
  7. Pyridoxine (vitamin B_6) 80 mg qd to improve depression, fatigue, and irritability has been suggested in small studies.

ACUTE GENERAL Rx

Suppression of ovulation:
- Oral contraceptives: one pill per day; continuous use associated with better treatment effect
- Progestin-only oral contraceptive: one pill per day
- Oral micronized progesterone: 100 mg every morning and 200 mg every evening on days 17 through 28 of menstrual cycle
- Progestin suppository: 200 to 400 mg bid on days 17 through 28 of menstrual cycle
- Medroxyprogesterone: 150 mg IM q3mo
- Levonorgestrel implants: surgical insertion every 5 yr
- Transdermal estradiol: one or two 100-µg patches every 3 days
- Danazol: 100 to 200 mg/day (ovulation not suppressed at this dose); has significant side-effect profile

---

TABLE 1 Common Symptoms of Cyclic Premenstrual Syndrome

Somatic Symptoms

Abdominal bloating	Constipation or diarrhea
Acne	Headache
Alcohol intolerance	Peripheral edema
Breast engorgement and tenderness	Weight gain
Clumsiness	

Emotional and Mental Symptoms

Anxiety	Insomnia
Change in libido	Irritability
Depression	Lethargy
Fatigue	Mood swings
Food cravings (especially salt and sugar)	Panic attacks
Hostility	Paranoia
Inability to concentrate	Violence toward self and others
Increased appetite	Withdrawal from others

From Goldman L, Schafer AI: *Goldman's Cecil medicine,* ed 24, Philadelphia, 2012, WB Saunders.

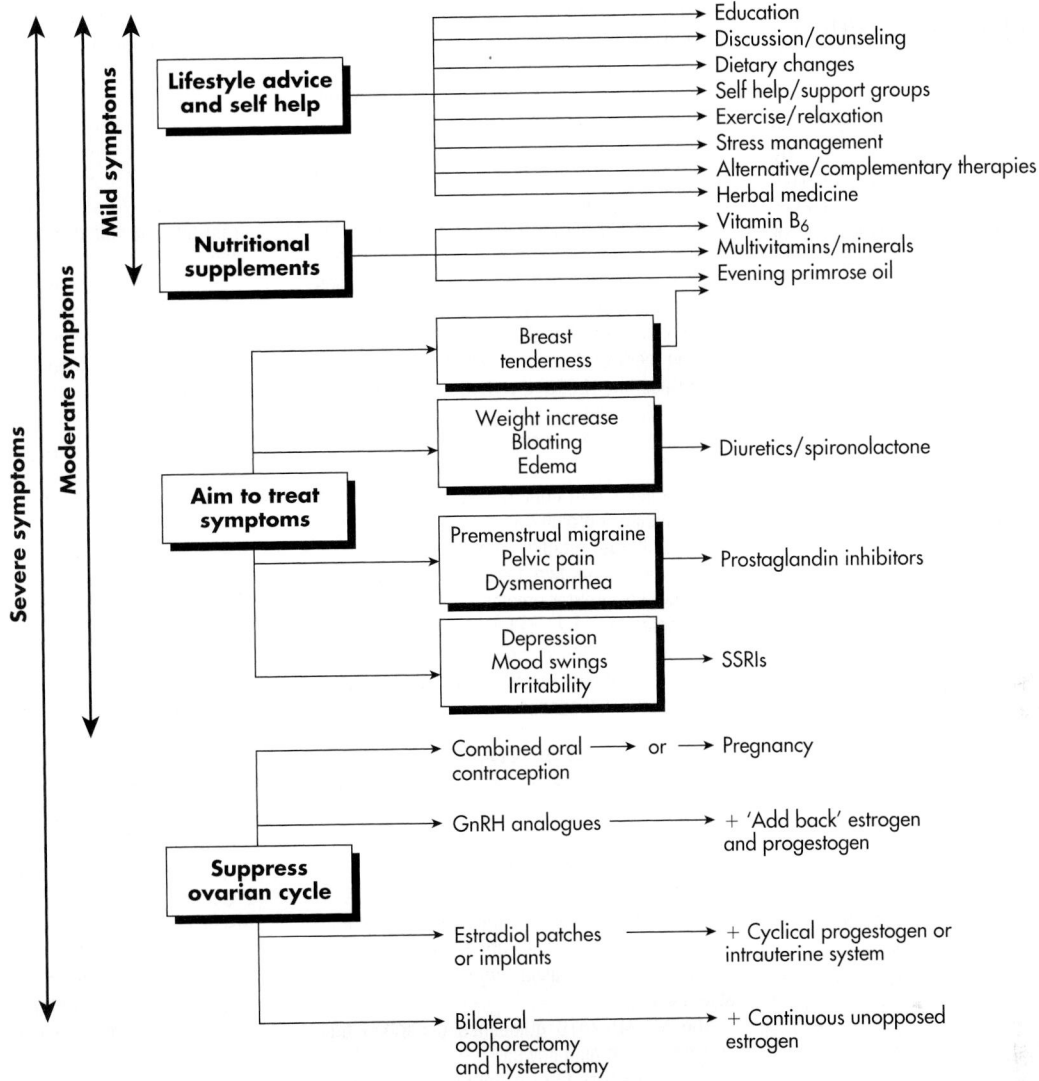

FIG. 1 Summary of treatment approaches to PMS. (Modified from Andrews G: Premenstrual syndrome. In Andrews G. (ed): *Women's sexual health*, Oxford, 2005, Elsevier.)

- Gonadotropin-releasing hormone (GnRH) agonists: daily by intranasal spray or monthly by depot injection; profound hypoestrogenism, concerns for osteoporosis and vasomotor symptoms Suppression of physical symptoms:
- Spironolactone: 25 to 50 mg bid on days 14 through 28 of menstrual cycle—need a reliable form of birth control
- Mefenamic acid
  1. For fluid retention: 250 mg tid on days 24 through 28 of cycle
  2. For pain: 500 mg tid on days 19 through 28 of cycle
- Bromocriptine: 5 mg/day on days 10 through 26 of cycle
- Naproxen: 550 mg bid on days 17 through 28 of cycle, Naprosyn-500 mg bid on days 17 through 28 of cycle Suppression of psychological symptoms:
- SSRI, or serotonergic antidepressants, are first-line treatment for PMS/PMDD, treating mostly the psychological aspects but also some physical aspects.
- Sertraline, paroxetine, fluoxetine, citalopram, escitalopram.

- In 2013 the *Cochrane Reviews* reported a statistically significant benefit over placebo when taken either continuously or in the luteal phase.
- Serotonin-norepinephrine reuptake inhibitors (SNRI) such as venlafaxine; use is off-label, but onset of action is quick and has been found to be helpful.
- Seroquel: smaller studies
- Wellbutrin: not as effective as the other options

CHRONIC Rx

- Therapy is largely trial and error, with the goal of providing effective treatment with the safest therapy. Provider should initially attempt to ameliorate the most pronounced symptom(s).
- For severe intractable PMS: bilateral oophorectomy; give trial of GnRH therapy or danazol before surgery (bilateral oophorectomy should be exceedingly rare).
- Estrogen replacement therapy recommended postoperatively to reduce the risk of osteoporosis, heart disease, and genitourinary atrophy.

DISPOSITION

Improved symptoms in 90% of women over time

REFERRAL

- For counseling with a psychologist or psychiatrist if underlying psychiatric disorder is discovered (cognitive-behavioral therapy)
- To a gynecologist if surgical therapy is contemplated

SUGGESTED READINGS

Available at www.expertconsult.com

RELATED CONTENT

Premenstrual Syndrome (Patient Information)
Dysmenorrhea (Related Key Topic)
Premenstrual Dysphoric Disorder (Related Key Topic)

AUTHOR: **ADRIENNE B. NEITHARDT, M.D.**

DEFINITION

A pressure injury is localized damage to the skin and underlying soft tissue over a bony prominence and can be related to a medical or other device. It can present as intact skin or an open ulcer. The injury occurs as a result of intense and/or prolonged pressure, or pressure in combination with shear.

SYNONYMS

Decubitus ulcers
Pressure sores
Bedsores
Pressure ulcers

ICD-10CM CODES

L89   Pressure ulcers
Subcategories of codes determined by stage and location of ulcer
L89.153   Example: Stage 3 ulcer of sacral area
L98.491   Non-pressure chronic ulcer of skin of other sites limited to breakdown of skin
L98.492   Non-pressure chronic ulcer of skin of other sites with fat layer exposed
L98.493   Non-pressure chronic ulcer of skin of other sites with necrosis of muscle
L98.494   Non-pressure chronic ulcer of skin of other sites with necrosis of bone
L98.499   Non-pressure chronic ulcer of skin of other sites with unspecified severity

EPIDEMIOLOGY & DEMOGRAPHICS

- The incidence of pressure injury varies by clinical setting.
- An estimated 2.5 million cases of pressure ulcers are treated each year in acute care facilities across the U.S.
- Development of pressure injury results in increased hospital length of stays by 7 to 10 days, and these patients are three times more likely to be discharged to long-term care facilities.
- Patients who develop pressure injury tend to be older patients (mean age of 71) and have multiple medical problems to include dementia, diabetes, urinary or fecal incontinence, and nutritional deficiencies.
- Occurs in all health care settings including hospitals, nursing homes, and residential homes. The reported rates upon admission to a nursing home range from 10% to 35%. The incidence rate is highest in institutions with lower staffing levels of registered nurses and certified nursing assistants, reflecting emphasis on health care resources more than medical decision-making.
- In December 2008, the Centers for Medicare and Medicaid Services discontinued reimbursement for hospital-acquired pressure ulcers.
- Associated with impaired quality of life with significant morbidity and mortality. One-year mortality rate roughly approaches 40%.
- Pain occurs in two thirds of patients with Stage 2 or greater pressure injury.
- Complicated by cellulitis, osteomyelitis, abscesses, sepsis, sinus tracts, heterotrophic calcification, systemic amyloidosis, and squamous cell cancer.

CLINICAL PRESENTATION

There are a number of staging systems that have been developed and utilized to describe the stages of pressure injury. The most commonly used system is the National Pressure Ulcer Advisory Panel (NPUAP). The European Pressure Ulcer Advisory Panel (EPUAP) recommends similar stages except for the presence of suspected deep tissue injury and unstageable ulcers.

The NPUAP 2016 guidelines described the staging system as follows:

Stage 1 Pressure Injury: Nonblanchable erythema of intact skin

Skin is intact with a localized area of nonblanchable erythema, which may appear different in darkly pigmented skin. The presence of blanchable erythema or changes in sensation, temperature, or firmness may precede visual changes. Color changes do not include purple or maroon discoloration; these may indicate deep tissue pressure injury.

Stage 2 Pressure Injury: Partial-thickness skin loss with exposed dermis

The wound bed is viable, pink or red, moist, and may also present as an intact or ruptured serum-filled blister. Adipose (fat) is not visible, and deeper tissues are not visible. Granulation tissue, slough, and eschar are not present. These injuries commonly result from adverse microclimate and shear in the skin over the pelvis and shear in the heel. This stage should not be used to describe moisture-associated skin damage, including incontinence-associated dermatitis, intertriginous dermatitis, medical adhesive–related skin injury, or traumatic wounds (skin tears, burns, abrasions).

Stage 3 Pressure Injury: Full-thickness skin loss

At this stage there is full-thickness loss of skin with adipose visible in the ulcer; granulation tissue and epibole (rolled wound edges) are often present. Slough and/or eschar may be visible. The depth of tissue damage varies by anatomical location; areas of significant adiposity can develop deep wounds. Undermining and tunneling may occur. Fascia, muscle, tendon, ligament, cartilage, and/or bone are not exposed. If slough or eschar obscures the extent of tissue loss, this is an unstageable pressure injury.

Stage 4 Pressure Injury: Full-thickness skin and tissue loss

At this stage there is full-thickness skin and tissue loss with exposed or directly palpable fascia, muscle, tendon, ligament, cartilage, or bone in the ulcer. Slough and/or eschar may be visible. Epibole (rolled edges), undermining, and/or tunneling often occur. Depth varies by anatomical location. If slough or eschar obscures the extent of tissue loss, this is an unstageable pressure injury (Fig. 1).

Unstageable Pressure Injury: Obscured full-thickness skin and tissue loss

Unstageable pressure injury is full-thickness skin and tissue loss in which the extent of tissue damage within the ulcer cannot be confirmed because it is obscured by slough or eschar. If slough or eschar is removed, a Stage 3 or Stage 4 pressure injury will be revealed. Stable eschar (i.e., dry, adherent, intact without erythema or fluctuance) on the heel or ischemic limb should not be softened or removed.

Deep Tissue Pressure Injury: Persistent nonblanchable deep red, maroon, or purple discoloration

Deep tissue pressure injury consists of intact or nonintact skin with a localized area of persistent nonblanchable deep red, maroon, or purple discoloration, or with epidermal separation revealing a dark wound bed or blood-filled blister. Pain and temperature change often precede skin color changes. Discoloration may appear different in darkly pigmented skin. This injury results from intense and/or prolonged pressure and shear forces at the bone-muscle interface. The wound may evolve rapidly to reveal the actual extent of tissue injury, or it may resolve with-

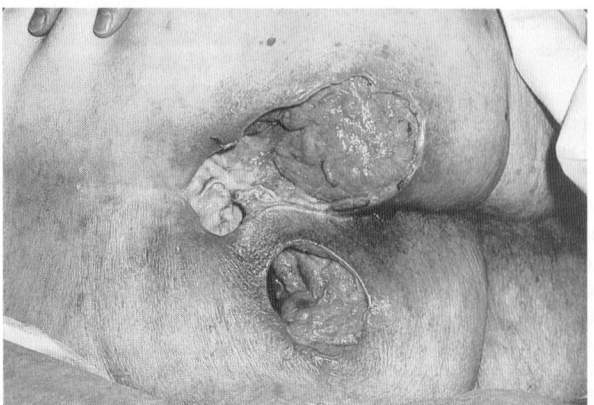

FIG. 1 Natural Debridement of Pressure Injury at 2 Weeks. (From Tallis R, Fillit H: *Brockelhurst's textbook of geriatric medicine and gerontology*, ed 6, London, 2003, Churchill Livingstone.)

out tissue loss. If necrotic tissue, subcutaneous tissue, granulation tissue, fascia, muscle, or other underlying structures are visible, a full-thickness pressure injury is indicated (unstageable, Stage 3 or Stage 4). Do not use deep tissue pressure injury to describe vascular, traumatic, neuropathic, or dermatologic conditions.

Medical Device–Related Pressure Injury

Medical device–related pressure injuries result from the use of devices designed and applied for diagnostic or therapeutic purposes. The resultant pressure injury generally conforms to the pattern or shape of the device. The injury should be staged using the staging system.

Mucosal Membrane Pressure Injury

Mucosal membrane pressure injury is found on mucous membranes with a history of a medical device in use at the location of the injury. Due to the anatomy of the tissue, these ulcers cannot be staged.

PATHOGENESIS

The development of a pressure injury is a complex process that involves external forces to intact skin resulting in ischemia. The most common sites include the sacrum, heels, and buttocks. The tolerance of soft tissue for pressure and shear may also be affected by immobility, microclimate, nutrition, perfusion, incontinence, comorbidities including sensory deficits, and the condition of the soft tissue. Body mass index (BMI) has an important role in the risk for pressure injury. Underweight (BMI <19 kg/m^2) and morbidly obese (BMI >40 kg/m^2) patients are at high risk for pressure injury formation. Diseases that affect tissue perfusion such as peripheral vascular disease, diabetes mellitus, and heart failure pose a heightened risk for pressure injury development. However, it is important to note that patients with poor arterial flow in addition to liver failure, sepsis, and acute respiratory distress syndrome may be presenting with acute skin failure (ASF) rather than pressure injury. Unlike pressure injury, ASF is not considered preventable. Kennedy Terminal Ulcer (KTU) has also been described in the literature as an unavoidable skin breakdown or skin failure that occurs as part of the dying process. There have been no studies differentiating KTUs from ASF at this time.

Complications of untreated pressure injury include sinus tract formation, heterotrophic calcification, systemic amyloidosis from chronic inflammation, and squamous cell cancer, particularly in a nonhealing pressure injury.

Dx DIAGNOSIS

DIFFERENTIAL DIAGNOSIS

- Venous insufficiency ulcers
- Arteriooclusive ulcers
- Diabetic ulcers
- Neuropathic ulcers
- Skin cancer
- Cellulitis and erysipelas
- Kennedy terminal ulcers (KTU)
- Acute skin failure (ASF)
- Incontinence-associated dermatitis (IAD)
- Perineal dermatitis

DIAGNOSTIC WORKUP

A thorough physical examination of the identified areas of skin damage should be performed. These areas should be evaluated for their length, width, and depth and for the presence of sinus tracts, undermining, tunneling, fistulas, exudate, and necrotic tissue as well as any evidence for healing such as the formation of granulation tissue. Adequate documentation is a must. Additionally, it is equally important to rule out infection, as this would impair wound healing. Cellulitis, abscess, and osteomyelitis should be ruled out.

LABORATORY TESTS

- Directed at identifying causes, risk factors, and/or any complications arising from the pressure injury (e.g., abscess or osteomyelitis).
- Cultures of wound bed are not believed to be helpful and should be avoided. Deep tissue biopsy is the gold standard to rule out osteomyelitis.
- Markers for malnutrition include prealbumin, albumin, transferrin, lymphocyte count, and total cholesterol level.
- Complete blood count may be obtained if systemic infection is suspected.

IMAGING STUDIES

- Ultrasound is not proven to be effective.
- Plain radiographs, MRI, and triple-phase bone scan may help identify osteomyelitis when clinically suspected.
- A comparison study of 44 patients scheduled for open biopsy did not show MRI to have superior diagnostic benefit over plain radiography.

Rx PREVENTION & TREATMENT

Conduct a structured risk assessment:

- Identify high-risk patients using standardized risk assessment scales and risk prediction tools (e.g., Braden and Norton in the U.S., Waterlow scale in the U.K., Cubbin and Jackson scale for ICU patients).
- Practice meticulous skin inspection and good skin care for at-risk patients.
- Focus on controlling the microclimate (moisture and temperature).
  1. Minimize prolonged skin exposure to moisture, urine, or stool.
  2. Treat dry, cracked skin.
- Use repositioning and pressure-reducing devices (e.g., foam mattresses, air-fluidized beds, low–air loss beds, pillows, or foam wedges when in bed or in a chair).
  1. Patient repositioning (based on individual tissue tolerance): A recent multicenter trial demonstrated no difference in pressure ulcer formation in high-risk nursing home patients turned at 2-, 4-, and 6-hour intervals when on a high-density foam mattress.
  2. Bed surface
     a. Two randomized controlled trials (RCTs) found that use of air-fluidized beds contributed to the healing of a greater number of pressure injuries after 15 days compared with standard care.
     b. Systematic review revealed no differences in rate of pressure injury healing with the use of either alternating-pressure mattresses or low–air loss beds compared with standard care.
  3. Pressure-relieving overlays: One RCT demonstrated that a viscoelastic pad on the operating table significantly reduced incidence of postoperative pressure injuries compared with a standard operating table.
  4. Foam alternatives
     a. Forty-one RCTs demonstrated that patients lying on standard hospital mattresses are more likely to develop pressure injuries than those patients lying on higher-specification foam mattresses.
        ○ Use adequate support surfaces while in bed or in a chair to prevent "bottoming out" (defined as less than 1 inch between patient and support surface; measured by putting hand under support surface and feeling thickness to patient).
        ○ Recent systematic review of pressure ulcer prevention strategies showed poor methodology in most studies. Use of support surfaces, repositioning, optimized nutrition, and sacral skin moisturizing was most appropriate.

The 2010 consensus statement from the National Pressure Ulcer Advisory Panel established that some pressure injuries are unavoidable in situations where pressure cannot be relieved and perfusion cannot be improved. The 2014 consensus identified risk factors in specific situations that may lead to the development of unavoidable pressure injuries. These include the following: impaired tissue oxygenation, cardiovascular instability, hypovolemia, sepsis, anasarca, peripheral vascular disease (venous vs. arterial), sensory impairment, immobility, end-of-life skin failure, multiorgan failure.

NONPHARMACOLOGIC THERAPY

- Pressure injuries should be cleaned at each dressing change.
- Avoid agents that are cytotoxic to epithelial cells (e.g., iodine, iodophor, sodium hypochlorite, hydrogen peroxide, acetic acid, alcohol).
- Wound irrigation should not exceed 15 psi and is best done with an 18-gauge angiocatheter. Necrotic tissue should be debrided quickly because it delays wound healing and increases risk of infection.
  ○ Do not debride hard, dry, stable eschar on heels or ischemic limbs.

- No single dressing or product is superior; should be used to keep ulcer bed moist and protect it from urine/stool. Silver dressings (which are felt to be antimicrobial), topical phenytoin, and growth factors should be limited to difficult-to-heal wounds, chronic ulcers, and extensive burns given their extra cost and limited scientific validation. Reduce pressure by using foam mattress, dynamic support surface (e.g., low–air loss bed), and frequent repositioning (e.g., every 2 hours or, in cases of poor perfusion, more frequently).
- Hyperbaric oxygen, ultrasound, ultraviolet, electromagnetic therapy, and low-energy radiation either are ineffective or have not been extensively evaluated for efficacy.
- Negative pressure devices (VAC devices) may help in wounds that have significant drainage. They also may improve healing by promoting angiogenesis, improving tissue perfusion, and decreasing bacterial count. Calcium alginate and foam dressings may also be beneficial for such wounds.
- Although correcting poor nutrition has been shown to be beneficial, a recent large investigation demonstrated that feeding tube insertion did not prevent or heal pressure ulcers, but increased the risk for developing a pressure ulcer.
- Minimize or promptly remove urinary and/or fecal contamination.
- Use a standardized assessment tool to monitor wound healing on a weekly basis. Examples of monitoring scales include the Pressure Sore Status Tool (PSST) and Pressure Ulcer Scale for Healing (PUSH) in addition to the NPUAP staging system.
- No RCTs have compared debridement versus NO debridement in the treatment of pressure ulcers.
  - Thirty-two RCTs have compared different debridement agents, but there is insufficient evidence to promote the use of one particular agent.
  - One RCT demonstrated ulcers treated with collagenase healed significantly more quickly than those treated with hydrocolloid.
  - One RCT comparing honey-treated dressings with dressings soaked with saline showed faster healing times with the honey-treated group.
  - A meta-analysis and one RCT found significant benefit in rates of healing with use of hydrocolloid dressings versus traditional saline gauze dressings but not over other forms such as hydrogels, foam dressings, or collagenase.

- No benefit was found with nutritional and vitamin supplements, artificial nutrition, or ultrasound therapy.

ACUTE GENERAL Rx

- Management of pressure injury is directed by its staging.
- The cornerstone of therapy involves the use of appropriate wound dressings, pressure-reducing devices, treatment of infection, debridement, and surgical consultation when appropriate.
- All pressure ulcers are colonized with bacteria. Clinically evident infections should be assessed with culture and treated appropriately with topical and systemic antibiotics.
- Adjunctive therapies such as electrical stimulation, negative pressure wound therapy, therapeutic ultrasound, hyperbaric oxygen, topical oxygen, and application of growth factors to the wound are continually being investigated.
- Pain medications are necessary because pressure injuries are often painful. One study found that excruciating pain was more prevalent in nursing home residents with pressure injuries. Local factors that may be contributing to pain such as ischemia, infection, or breakdown of surrounding skin should be properly addressed.

CHRONIC Rx

- Continue vigilance with pressure reduction because pressure ulcers can recur with minimal trauma.
- There are no randomized trials available to identify whether repositioning makes a difference in the healing rates of pressure ulcers or what the optimal repositioning regimen should be.
- Consider radiologic evaluation for infected ulcer bed, occult osteomyelitis, or abscess.

COMPLEMENTARY & ALTERNATIVE MEDICINE

Vitamin C, zinc, and multivitamin supplements may be beneficial for patients with nutritional deficiencies. However, their efficacy has not been conclusively demonstrated. Anabolic steroids are sometimes recommended in patients with weight loss and protein depletion. However, the evidence is not conclusive as of yet.

DISPOSITION

- When systematic risk assessments are done and preventive measures are followed, most pressure injuries can be prevented. Most

ulcers heal when appropriate management strategies are followed.
- Stage 4 pressure injuries in high-risk patients (e.g., paraplegics) can take months or years to heal.

REFERRAL

- Physical and occupational therapists to improve bed and chair mobility
- Wounds with necrotic tissue need referral to providers trained in sharp debridement
- Role of plastic surgeons for operative repair for large Stage 3 or 4 ulcers that do not respond to optimal care
- To a specialty wound care center for nonhealing complex pressure injuries

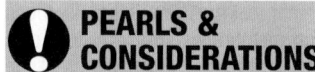

⚠ PEARLS & CONSIDERATIONS

COMMENTS

- Up to 10% of older persons will have a pressure injury.
- Because 70% of pressure injuries occur in older persons, the approach should be similar to other multifactorial geriatric syndromes with an interprofessional team approach. Identify and reduce all modifiable risk factors for pressure injuries.
- Treat the pain associated with pressure injuries.
- Proper skin care, use of support surfaces, mobilization, and nutritional support are key for prevention and treatment.
- Clinical studies have not revealed if any one dressing product is superior.
- Nonhealing ulcers require assessment for debridement, infection, abscess, and/or referral to a wound center.

PATIENT & FAMILY EDUCATION

- Educate patient and family members on the risk factors for pressure injury formation.
- Encourage mobility and adequate nutritional intake as well as avoidance of bed rest.

SUGGESTED READINGS
Available at www.expertconsult.com

RELATED CONTENT
Bed Sores (Patient Information)

AUTHORS: **MARY-BETH WELESKO, M.S., A.P.R.N.-B.C.**, and **NOELLE MARIE JAVIER, M.D.**

BASIC INFORMATION

DEFINITION

Preterm labor is defined as regular contractions that result in cervical dilation or effacement prior to 37 wk gestation.

SYNONYMS

Premature labor

ICD-10CM CODES
O60.0 Preterm labor without delivery
O60.1 Preterm spontaneous labor with preterm delivery
O60.2 Preterm spontaneous labor with term delivery

EPIDEMIOLOGY & DEMOGRAPHICS

INCIDENCE: The incidence of preterm births in the U.S. has increased over the past two decades from 9.5% in 1981 to 12.7% in 2006. Between 40% and 45% of these births follow spontaneous preterm labor; either the remaining preterm births result from preterm premature rupture of membranes (PPROM), or they occur secondary to maternal or fetal indications.

PREDOMINANT SEX AND AGE: Pregnant women at the extremes of reproductive age (<17 yr and >35 yr) are at greatest risk.

GENETICS: A genetic component has been suggested. Women with sisters who have had preterm births and women with grandparents who were born preterm may be at increased risk for having preterm deliveries themselves. Single-nucleotide polymorphisms have also been associated with preterm labor.

RISK FACTORS: Risk factors for premature labor include a prior preterm delivery, intrauterine infection, systemic or genital tract infections, interpregnancy interval (<6 mo), short cervical length (<25 to 30 mm), low pre-pregnancy BMI (<19.8 kg/m²), age <17 yr or >35 yr), a history of elective pregnancy termination, history of prior stillbirth, African-American ethnicity, vaginal bleeding, polyhydramnios or oligohydramnios, multiple gestation, structural abnormalities of the uterus, history of cervical cone biopsy or loop electrocautery excision, in vitro fertilization or ovulation induction, tobacco use, heavy alcohol consumption, cocaine use, heroin use, and psychological or social stress.

PHYSICAL FINDINGS & CLINICAL PRESENTATION

Presenting symptoms include increased pelvic pressure, abdominal cramping or contractions, increased vaginal discharge, vaginal spotting, or leakage of fluid.

ETIOLOGY

Causes of premature labor are varied and often difficult to determine. Premature labor may be secondary to infection, systemic illness, trauma, anatomic abnormalities (i.e., uterine anomaly such as lateral fusion defects like unicornuate or bicornuate uterus), or a combination of factors. It is thought that cervical ripening is the most common first step to premature labor or delivery. Subsequently, decidual-membrane activation occurs, as do contractions (Box 1).

DIAGNOSIS

DIFFERENTIAL DIAGNOSIS

The differential should include premature labor, preterm rupture of membranes, preterm contractions (contractions prior to 37 wk gestation that do not result in cervical change), and abdominal pain or cramping secondary to other medical conditions. There are many conditions that may cause preterm contractions or premature labor. These include:
- Infection
  1. Chorioamnionitis
  2. Genital tract infections, including bacterial vaginosis, gonorrhea, chlamydia
  3. Urinary tract infections, including pyelonephritis, cystitis, or asymptomatic bacteriuria
  4. Gastroenteritis
- Trauma
- Placental abruption
- Illicit drug use
- Preterm premature rupture of membranes
- Appendicitis
- Nephrolithiasis
- Pancreatitis
- Cholelithiasis

WORKUP
- History and physical exam to rule out trauma, abuse, other causes of abdominal pain, and infection

- Fetal heart rate monitoring and tocometry to determine fetal status and contraction frequency
- Speculum exam to visually assess the cervix and assess for rupture of membranes, bleeding, infection, or advanced cervical dilation
  1. If the patient is <35 wk gestation, a Fetal Fibronectin (FFN) test should be collected prior to performing a digital exam or transvaginal ultrasound. A FFN test can help predict preterm delivery if the patient has a cervical length on transvaginal ultrasound of <30 mm.
- Digital exam to determine cervical dilation and effacement, and fetal station

LABORATORY TESTS
- CBC
- Urine analysis and culture
- Urine toxicology screen
- Collect tests for GBS, gonorrhea, and *Chlamydia*
- Perform a wet prep for yeast, bacterial vaginosis, and *Trichomonas*
- Fetal fibronectin
- Consider PT, PTT, INR, CMP, amylase, and lipase
- Amniocentesis may be performed if an intraamniotic infection is suspected

IMAGING STUDIES

A formal ultrasound is indicated to determine estimated fetal weight, fetal presentation, amniotic fluid volume, placental location and appearance, and cervical length.

TREATMENT

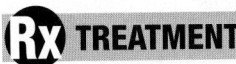

Patients with premature labor should be delivered promptly when an intraamniotic infection is

---

BOX 1   Factors Linked to Preterm Labor

Demographic and Psychosocial
Extremes of age (>40 yr, teenagers)
Lower socioeconomic status
Tobacco use
Cocaine abuse
Prolonged standing (occupation)
Psychosocial stressors

Reproductive and Gynecologic
Prior preterm delivery
Diethylstilbestrol exposure
Multiple gestations
Anatomic endometrial cavity anomalies
Cervical incompetence
Low pregnancy weight gain
First-trimester vaginal bleeding
Placental abruption or previa

Surgical
Prior reproductive organ surgery
Prior paraendometrial surgery other than genitourinary (appendectomy)

Infectious
Urinary tract infections
Nonuterine infections
Genital tract infections (bacterial vaginosis)

From Marx JA et al: *Rosen's emergency medicine: concepts and clinical practice*, ed 7, Philadelphia, 2010, Elsevier.

suspected or when they have cervical dilation >5 cm, a persistently nonreassuring fetal heart rate tracing, intrauterine growth restriction, or vaginal bleeding concerning for placental abruption.

NONPHARMACOLOGIC THERAPY
- Smoking cessation
- Bedrest, activity restriction, and pelvic rest are often recommended, but there are insufficient data to support this practice.

ACUTE GENERAL Rx
- Antenatal administration of corticosteroids between 24 wk and 33 6/7 wk gestation is recommended for women at risk of preterm delivery to prevent neonatal respiratory distress syndrome and decrease the incidence of intraventricular hemorrhage and necrotizing enterocolitis.
- Numerous tocolytic agents have been used in an attempt to inhibit contractions (Box 2). Although efficacy is unclear, they can be utilized during an observation period in an effort to prolong gestation for administration of steroids or to transfer the mother to a facility capable of caring for preterm infants. This, of course, assumes there are no maternal or fetal medical contraindications to use of tocolytic drugs and no indications for rapid delivery. The most commonly used tocolytics are beta-mimetics (terbutaline), magnesium sulfate, calcium channel blockers (nifedipine), or prostaglandin synthetase inhibitors (indomethacin, ketorolac, sulindac). Table 1 summarizes side effect profiles of tocolytic agents.

- Routine antibiotic use has failed to show benefit in the absence of a known infection. But all mothers in preterm labor (without a documented negative group B strep culture) should be given antibiotics to prevent neonatal infection.
- Intravenous magnesium sulfate has been shown to decrease cerebral palsy in children exposed antenatally with premature labor or premature rupture of the membranes.

CHRONIC Rx
- Patients with a history of prior spontaneous preterm birth may be candidates for

---

BOX 2 Commonly Used Tocolytic Agents

Magnesium sulfate
4-6 g IV bolus over 30 min
2-4 g/hr IV infusion
 Terbutaline
5-10 mg PO q4-6h
0.25-0.5 mg SC q30 min-6 h
10-80 µg/min IV
 Ritodrine[1]
10 mg PO q2-4 h
5-10 mg IM q2-4 h
50-350 µg/min IV
 Isoxsuprine
20 mg PO q4-6 h
0.05-0.5 mg/min IV

[1] Ritodrine is currently discontinued in the U.S. *IV*, Intravenously; *PO*, orally; *SC*, subcutaneously. From Marx JA et al: *Rosen's emergency medicine: concepts and clinical practice*, ed 7, Philadelphia, 2010, Elsevier.

---

prophylactic use of 17 alpha-hydroxyprogesterone caproate between 16 wk and 36 wk gestation.
- Patients with a history of preterm birth and short cervix may also be candidates for prophylactic or rescue cerclage.
- There is no evidence supporting the use of maintenance tocolytic therapy.

REFERRAL
- Women who present in preterm labor should be referred to an obstetrician and transferred to a facility with a neonatal intensive care unit.
- For women who present for prenatal care with a history of preterm delivery, early referral to an obstetrician is also recommended.

 **EVIDENCE**

Available at www.expertconsult.com

SUGGESTED READINGS
Available at www.expertconsult.com

RELATED CONTENT
Abruptio Placentae (Related Key Topic)
Breech Birth (Related Key Topic)

AUTHOR: **ANTHONY SCISCIONE, D.O.**

TABLE 1 Side Effect Profiles of Tocolytic Agents

	Side Effects		
Agent or Class	**Maternal**	**Fetal or Neonatal**	**Contraindications**
β-adrenergic receptor agonists	Tachycardia and hypotension, tremor (39% vs. 4% with placebo), shortness of breath (15% vs. 1% with placebo), chest discomfort (10% vs. 1% with placebo), pulmonary edema (0.3%), hypokalemia (39% vs. 6% with placebo), hyperglycemia (30% vs. 10% with placebo)	Tachycardia	Tachycardia-sensitive maternal cardiac disease, poorly controlled diabetes mellitus
Magnesium sulfate	Flushing, diaphoresis, nausea, loss of deep-tendon reflexes (at doses of 9.6 to 12 mg/dL), respiratory paralysis (at doses of 12 to 18 mg/dL), cardiac arrest (at doses of 24 to 30 mg/dL); when used with calcium channel blockers, suppression of heart rate, contractility and left ventricular systolic pressure, and neuromuscular blockade	Conflicting data with regard to effect on perinatal mortality	Myasthenia gravis
Calcium channel blockers	Dizziness, flushing, hypotension when used with magnesium sulfate, suppression of heart rate, contractility, and left ventricular systolic pressure and neuromuscular blockade; elevation of hepatic aminotransferase levels		Hypotension, preload-dependent cardiac lesions (e.g., aortic insufficiency)
Cyclo-oxygenase inhibitors	Nausea, esophageal reflux, gastritis, and emesis; platelet dysfunction (rarely of clinical significance in patients without underlying bleeding disorder)	In utero closure of ductus arteriosus (risk associated with use for >48 hr), patent ductus arteriosus in neonate (conflicting data)	Platelet dysfunction or bleeding disorder, hepatic or renal dysfunction, gastrointestinal or ulcerative disease, asthma (in women with hypersensitivity to aspirin)
Oxytocin receptor antagonists	Hypersensitivity injection-site reactions	For atosiban, an increased rate of fetal or infant death (may be attributable to the lower gestational age of infants in the atosiban group)	None
Nitric oxide donors	Dizziness, flushing, hypotension		Hypotension, preload-dependent cardiac lesions (e.g., aortic insufficiency)

From Gabbe SG et al: *Obstetrics: normal and problem pregnancies*, ed 6, Philadelphia, 2012, Saunders.

BASIC INFORMATION

DEFINITION

- Primary angiitis of the CNS (PACNS) is the preferred name for vasculitis that is confined to the CNS.
- CNS vasculitis is considered secondary when it occurs in the context of a systemic inflammatory disease, such as a systemic vasculitis or systemic lupus erythematosus (SLE), or an infectious process such as varicella zoster virus.
- PACNS predominantly affects small- and medium-sized arteries of the brain parenchyma, spinal cord, and leptomeninges, resulting in symptoms and signs of CNS dysfunction.
- It is defined by inflammation of the cerebral vasculature without angiitis in other organs.

SYNONYMS

PACNS
CNS vasculitis

ICD-10CM CODES
I67.7 Cerebral endarteritis

EPIDEMIOLOGY & DEMOGRAPHICS

INCIDENCE: PACNS is a rare disease.
A retrospective analysis of 101 patients with PACNS reported an annual incidence rate of 2.4 cases per 1,000,000 person-years.
PREDOMINANT SEX: There is a 2:1 male predominance among reported cases.
PREDOMINANT AGE: The median age at diagnosis is 50 years, although PACNS can occur at almost every age.

PHYSICAL FINDINGS & CLINICAL PRESENTATION

- PACNS is characterized by a long prodromal period, with few patients presenting acutely.
- The vasculitis can affect any part of the CNS, causing the clinical manifestations to be highly variable and nonspecific.
- Headache is the most commonly reported symptom, usually subacute and insidious, in contrast to the sudden-onset thunderclap headache that is observed with reversible cerebral vasoconstriction syndromes (RCVS).
- Other symptoms include cognitive impairment, stroke, and transient ischemic attack.
- Patients with PACNS who develop strokes usually present with more than a single stroke in different anatomic territories.
- Other, less common symptoms may appear, including cranial neuropathies, ataxia, and seizure.
- Signs and symptoms suggestive of systemic vasculitis, such as peripheral neuropathy, fever, weight loss, or rash, are usually lacking.
- Spinal cord involvement occurs alone or coincides with parenchymal brain involvement.
- Angiitis affecting the spinal cord usually presents as a myelopathy, with pain, motor weakness, and sensory findings.
- Symptoms and signs of untreated PACNS progress over the course of months.

ETIOLOGY

- The cause of PACNS is unknown.
- Several potential etiologic agents or mechanisms have been proposed, but understanding of the cause of PACNS remains highly speculative.
- Various infectious agents have been proposed as etiologic factors, such as varicella zoster virus, West Nile virus, *Mycoplasma gallisepticum*, and HIV.
- Cerebral amyloid angiopathy and PACNS have been described together in some patients, and associations between amyloid deposition have also been proposed as a trigger.
- Although the cause of PACNS is unknown, inflammation of the CNS causes the vessels to become narrowed, occluded, and thrombosed, resulting in tissue ischemia and necrosis of the territories of the involved vessels.
- PACNS is more likely to affect blood vessels in the cerebral cortex and leptomeninges than subcortical regions.
- Blood vessels supplying cranial nerves may also be involved.

DIAGNOSIS

- The diagnosis of PACNS is based upon a constellation of symptoms and signs in the setting of supportive studies and the exclusion of alternative diagnoses.
- The diagnosis can usually be made when all of the following are present:
  - An acquired otherwise unexplained neurologic deficit
  - Evidence of either classic angiographic or histopathologic features of angiitis within the CNS (Fig. E1)
  - No evidence of systemic vasculitis or any other condition that could elicit the angiographic or pathologic findings

DIFFERENTIAL DIAGNOSIS

- PACNS can be mimicked closely in both its clinical presentation and radiologic manifestations by a number of other disorders (Tables 1 and 2). The most frequent mimic of PACNS is a group of disorders known collectively as the reversible cerebral vasoconstriction syndromes (RCVS).
- Systemic vasculitis affecting the brain such as Behçet's disease and polyarteritis nodosa.
- Other rheumatic diseases affecting the brain such as Sjögren's syndrome and systemic lupus erythematosus.
- Infections such as tuberculosis, HIV and *Borrelia burgdorferi*, hepatitis, cysticercosis, actinomyces, *Treponema pallidum*
- Atherosclerosis
- Cerebral emboli
- Moyamoya disease
- Susac syndrome

WORK-UP

LABORATORY TESTS

- Laboratory testing and serological assays (Table 3) are used primarily to exclude other etiologies of CNS dysfunction.

- Analysis of the cerebrospinal fluid (CSF) is a crucial part of the evaluation of patients with potential PACNS and should be performed in all patents unless there are contraindications.
- The CSF is abnormal in 80% to 90% of patients with pathologically documented disease.
- CSF findings are nonspecific but most commonly include an elevated CSF protein and a modest lymphocytic pleocytosis.
- Table 4 describes an algorithmic approach to the diagnosis of PACNS.

IMAGING STUDIES

- Various neuroimaging modalities can be used to assess for both parenchymal and vascular abnormalities in the evaluation of suspected PACNS.
- Magnetic resonance imaging (MRI) should be performed in all patients.
- The selection of additional neuroimaging modalities depends on the initial MRI findings and individual patient characteristics.
- Conventional angiography (Fig. E2) remains an important part of the diagnostic testing for suspected PACNS.
- Angiography can detect segmental narrowing in multiple vessels that are typical of, though not pathognomonic for, PACNS, and help

---

TABLE 1 Clinical Syndromes of Cerebral Vasculitis

Primary CNS vasculitis/primary angiitis of the nervous system
Granulomatous angiitis of the CNS
Secondary CNS vasculitis
Systemic vasculitis
Behçet's disease
Necrotizing arteritis of the polyarteritis type
Systemic granulomatous vasculitis/antineutrophil cytoplasmic antibody: associated vasculitis
Giant cell arteritis
Hypersensitivity vasculitis and cryoglobulinemic vasculitis
Connective tissue diseases
Systemic lupus erythematosus
Sjögren's syndrome
Rheumatoid arthritis
Mixed connective tissue disease/overlap syndrome
Scleroderma
Sarcoidosis
Infection-associated cerebral vasculitis
Virus (varicella-zoster virus, West Nile virus, cytomegalovirus, hepatitis B and C viruses)
Retroviral infection/HIV-1
Spirochete (*Treponema pallidum*, *Borrelia burgdorferi*)
Fungi (*Aspergillus*, *Coccidioides*, *Histoplasma*)
Bartonella
Rickettsia
Bacterial meningitis
Mycoplasma
Mycobacterium tuberculosis
Protozoal (amebiasis, cysticercosis)
Cerebral vasculitis associated with amyloidosis
Amyloid angiitis
Cerebral vasculitis associated with paraneoplastic disorders
Paraneoplastic angiitis

From Hochberg MC et al: *Rheumatology* ed 5, St Louis, 2011, Mosby.

TABLE 2 Disorders That Mimic PACNS

Reversible cerebral vasoconstriction syndromes
Intracranial atherosclerosis
Cerebral embolism
Intracranial vertebral artery dissection
Susac syndrome
Cerebral autosomal dominant arteriopathy with subcortical infarcts and leukoencephalopathy (CADASIL)
Moyamoya disease
Acute multifocal placoid pigment epitheliopathy (AMPPE)
Mitochondrial encephalopathy, lactic acidosis, and stroke-like illness (MELAS)
Progressive multifocal leukoencephalopathy (PML) and reversible posterior leukoencephalopathy syndrome (RPLS)

From Hochberg MC et al: *Rheumatology* ed 5, St Louis, 2011, Mosby.

TABLE 3 Laboratory Evaluation of Suspected PACNS

General studies
Complete blood cell count
Complete metabolic panel and hepatic function test
Erythrocyte sedimentation rate
C-reactive protein
Lipid panel
Urinalysis and urine microalbumin level
Urine toxicology screen
Prothrombin and thromboplastin time
Proteins S and C
Serum and urine protein electrophoresis and serum immunoglobulin electrophoresis
Quantitative immunoglobulin
Acute hepatitis panel for hepatitis B and C virus
HIV
Serology panel
Rheumatoid factor
Antinuclear antibody
Antibodies to Ro/SSA, La/SSB, Sm, and RNP antigens
Anticardiolipin antibody and lupus anticoagulant
Serum complement level: C2, C3, C4, and CH_{50}
Antibody to double-stranded (ds)-DNA
Antineutrophil cytoplasmic antibody
Angiotensin-converting enzyme
Lyme titer (enzyme-linked immunosorbent assay and Western blot)
Serum cryoglobulins
Treponema pallidum, rapid plasma reagent (RPR), and fluorescent treponemal antibody (FTA)
CSF studies
Protein
Glucose
Cell count
IgG level and index
Oligoclonal bands
Venereal Disease Research Laboratory (VDRL)
Viral antibodies and antigens and polymerase chain reaction (PCR) for West Nile virus, cytomegalovirus, herpes simplex and herpes zoster, and HIV
Lyme titer
Antineutrophil cytoplasmic antibody titer
Angiotensin-converting enzyme level
India ink, Gram stain, and routine cultures including acid-fast *Bacillus* stain

From Hochberg MC et al: *Rheumatology* ed 5, St Louis, 2011, Mosby.

TABLE 4 An Algorithmic Approach to the Diagnosis of PACNS

1. *Is there a known systemic disease?*
   a. Systemic vasculitis, connective tissue diseases
   b. Infection: HIV, viral, bacterial, Lyme, syphilis, mycobacterial, fungal, protozoal
   c. Malignant hypertension, eclampsia, infective endocarditis, atrial myxoma/thrombus, patent foramen ovale, disrupted carotid plaques
   d. Neoplasm: intravascular lymphoma, lymphoid granulomatosus
   e. Drug exposure and illicit drug use
   f. Recent trauma, neurosurgery, intracranial dissection
2. *Is there abnormal MRI (brain, leptomeninges)?*
   a. Vasculitis, vascular disorders including stroke syndrome or arterial venous malformation, demyelinating syndrome, sarcoidosis, infection, neoplasm
3. *Is there abnormal cerebrospinal fluid (pleocytosis)?*
   a. Acute, recurrent, and chronic meningitis; partially treated bacterial (pyogenic), HIV, viral, syphilis, Lyme, mycobacterial, fungal, protozoal
   b. Non-infectious: PML, sarcoidosis, Behçet disease, neoplasm
4. *Is there abnormal conventional cerebral angiography?*
   a. True vasculitis: PACNS, systemic vasculitis
   b. Infection
   c. RCVS
   d. Neoplasm
   e. Subarachnoid hemorrhage
   f. Trauma
5. *Is there abnormal biopsy with inflammation?*
   a. True vasculitis: PACNS, secondary vasculitis
   b. Perivascular inflammation: demyelinating syndrome, undersampled vasculitis, infection (PML, SSPE, VZV), lymphoma
   c. Neoplasm: lymphoma, metastatic malignancy

HIV, human immunodeficiency virus; *MRI,* brain magnetic resonance imaging; *PML,* progressive multifocal leukoencephalopathy; *RCVS,* reversible cerebral vasoconstriction syndrome; *SSPE,* subacute sclerosing panencephalitis; *VZV,* varicella-zoster virus. Small vessel PACNS may have normal cerebral angiography. However, PACNS is unlikely in the context of normal brain MRI and normal cerebrospinal fluid studies.
From Hochberg MC et al: *Rheumatology* ed 5, St Louis, 2011, Mosby.

further rule out alternative diagnoses such as atherosclerosis, moyamoya, and dissection. These tests may also be helpful in selecting a location for brain biopsy if needed.
- A brain biopsy should be performed in most patients with suspected PACNS. A biopsy will help histologically identify PACNS (Fig. E1) as well as exclude other lesions or vasculitis mimics, particularly infection or malignancy.

Rx TREATMENT

ACUTE GENERAL Rx
- PACNS should be treated with a combination of glucocorticoids and cyclophosphamide (Grade 2C).
- Treatment of atypical PACNS should be individualized according to the severity and the extent of the neurologic deficit.
- The response to treatment is monitored by periodic reassessment of symptoms, neurologic findings, and neuroimaging abnormalities.
- It is important to differentiate between disease damage and disease progression. Neurologic deficits due to cerebral or cerebellar infarction may resolve slowly or not at all.
- For some patients, a response to treatment may only be indicated by symptomatic improvement (e.g., resolution of headache) but not the resolution of magnetic resonance (MR) lesions.
- A lack of new lesions on MRI is a more reliable way to assess for progression of the disease.
- A follow-up MR should be obtained 4 to 6 wk after beginning treatment, then every 3 to 6 mo throughout therapy, and subsequently according to the evolution of the disease.

CHRONIC Rx
We recommend the use of measures to prevent osteoporosis and *Pneumocystis* infections during the treatment of PACNS (Grade 1A).

DISPOSITION
Usually inpatient due to severe disease presentation

REFERRAL
Rheumatology, neurology, infectious diseases

! PEARLS & CONSIDERATIONS

- PACNS predominantly affects small- and medium-sized arteries of the brain parenchyma, spinal cord, and leptomeninges, resulting in symptoms and signs of CNS dysfunction.
- The most frequent mimic of PACNS is a group of disorders known collectively as the reversible cerebral vasoconstriction syndromes (RCVS).
- The diagnosis of PACNS is based upon a constellation of symptoms and signs in the setting of supportive studies and the exclusion of alternative diagnoses.
- CSF findings are nonspecific but most commonly include an elevated CSF protein and a modest lymphocytic pleocytosis.
- PACNS should be treated with a combination of glucocorticoids and cyclophosphamide (Grade 2C).

SUGGESTED READINGS
Available at www.expertconsult.com

AUTHOR: **CATHERINE E. NAJEM, M.D.**

BASIC INFORMATION

DEFINITION

Primary biliary cholangitis (PBC), previously known as primary biliary cirrhosis is a chronic, variably progressive cholestatic liver disease most often affecting middle-aged women and characterized by autoimmune destruction of intrahepatic bile ducts leading to portal inflammation, hepatic cell necrosis, fibrosis, cirrhosis, and ultimately, liver failure.

SYNONYMS

PBC
Primary biliary cirrhosis
Biliary cirrhosis
Nonsuppurative destructive cholangitis
Autoimmune cholangiopathy PBC

ICD-10CM CODES
K74.3 Primary biliary cirrhosis

EPIDEMIOLOGY & DEMOGRAPHICS

INCIDENCE:
- PBC affects all races and accounts for up to 2% of deaths from cirrhosis worldwide.
- Annual incidence rates range from 2.3 to 58 cases per million.

PREVALENCE: Prevalence is greatest in the U.K., Scandinavia, Canada, and the U.S. and varies tremendously by geographic areas, ranging from 19 to 492 cases per million. Disease burden seems to be increasing, which may be a result of better detection rather than true rise in disease incidence.

PREDOMINANT SEX: Female to male ratio of up to 10:1.

PREDOMINANT AGE: Onset typically occurs between the ages of 30 and 60 yr, and it is uncommon before age 25 yr.

PREDOMINANT RACE: Predominantly Caucasian but can be seen in other races.

GENETICS:
- Although there are no clearly identified genetic factors associated with PBC, there is a clear familial occurrence. Prevalence among familial clustering of PBC is 3.8% to 9%. The concordance rate among monozygotic twins is 63%.
- Up to 84% of patients with PBC have at least one other autoimmune disorder, such as thyroiditis, Sjögren's syndrome, rheumatoid arthritis, Raynaud's phenomenon, scleroderma, systemic lupus erythematosus, pernicious anemia, celiac disease, autoimmune thrombocytopenia purpura and other autoimmune diseases. A variant form of PBC exists as an overlap syndrome with autoimmune hepatitis (AIH).
- PBC is closely associated with a greater risk of hepatocellular carcinoma as well as an overall greater risk of cancer.

ETIOLOGY

- Although the cause of PBC remains unknown, it is believed to require both a genetic susceptibility as well as an environmental trigger, ultimately leading to the modification of mitochondrial proteins triggering a persistent T lymphocyte–mediated attack on intralobular bile duct epithelial cells.
- PBC is associated most strongly with HLA alleles DRA, DRB1, DPB1, DQB1, BTNL2, and c6orf10, but there is a great deal of variation among ethnicities.
- Possible environmental triggers include cigarette smoking, environmental pollutants, radiation, urinary tract infections, reproductive hormone replacement, and toxic waste sites (particularly exposure to halogenated hydrocarbons), as well as xenobiotics found in food additives and cosmetics.
- A group of autoantigens collectively known as the "M2 subtype," are peptides that play a major role in the early pathogenesis of PBC. The enzyme complex subunit PDC-E2 is one of the key autoantigens in this group. Patients with PBC have a tenfold increased concentration of PDC-E2 specific cytotoxic $CD8^+$ lymphocytes in their livers compared to their blood, and antimitochondrial antibodies (AMAs), which are the serologic hallmark of this disease, react to the PDC-E2 subunit. In addition, biliary epithelial cells handle PDC-E2 in a unique way that exposes them to immune-mediated attack by PDC-E2-oriented cytotoxic T cells. Future therapies may be specific immunomodulation directed at these peptides.
- In addition to the T lymphocyte–mediated direct destruction of small bile ducts, secondary damage to hepatocytes results from the chronic accumulation of bile acids.

PHYSICAL FINDINGS & CLINICAL PRESENTATION

Clinical stages:
- Asymptomatic
- Symptomatic
- Cirrhotic
- Hepatic failure

Symptoms:
- 50% to 65% of patients may be asymptomatic; about one third to half of these patients will develop symptoms in five yr, 80% in ten yr and 95% in 20 yr. Nearly 25% of symptomatic patients at diagnosis will progress to liver failure within 10 yr without treatment.
- Fatigue (20%-85% of patients) and pruritus (20%-75% of patients) are the usual presenting symptoms.
- Fatigue can be chronic and correlated with daytime somnolence and autonomic dysfunction.
- Pruritus is worse at night with constricting, coarse garments, and in association with dry skin and hot, humid weather. The cause is unknown, but histamine, elevated bile salt concentration, endogenous opioids, lysophosphatidic acid and female steroid hormones and their metabolites have been controversially discussed as potential causes. Pruritus may first occur during pregnancy but is distinguished from pruritus of pregnancy because it persists into the postpartum period and beyond.
- Other common symptoms include dyslipidemia (75-95%), sicca symptoms (26%-73%), jaundice (10%-60%), xanthomas (15%-50%), osteoporosis (35%), scleroderma (6%), unexplained right upper quadrant pain (10%), Hashimoto's thyroiditis (13%), and manifestations of portal hypertension.
- Musculoskeletal complaints caused by inflammatory arthropathy in 40% to 70% of patients: 5% to 10% experience development of chronic rheumatoid arthritis, and 10% experience development of "arthritis of PBC."
- Steatorrhea may be seen in advanced disease.

Physical Examination:
- Variable: Findings depend on stage of disease at time of presentation; patients at the early stage may be completely unaffected.
- Excoriations may be present.
- Hepatomegaly (verifiable in up to 80%) and splenomegaly (up to 35%) can worsen with disease progression.
- Xanthomas and jaundice generally appear in advanced disease. Kayser-Fleischer rings are rare and result from copper retention. Hyperpigmentation of the skin due to melanin deposition may be present.
- Late physical findings mirror those of cirrhosis: spider nevi, caput medusae, temporal and proximal limb wasting, ascites, palmar erythema, digital clubbing, gynecomastia, and edema.

DIAGNOSIS

The diagnosis of PBC can be established when two of the following three criteria are met.
- Positive serum AMA, titer >1:40
- Biochemical evidence of cholestasis (mainly alkaline phosphatase elevation ≥1.5 times the upper limit of normal)
- Characteristic liver histology

DIFFERENTIAL DIAGNOSIS

- Drug-induced cholestasis
- PBC-AIH overlap syndrome: reported in 1%-19% of patients initially diagnosed with PBC; transition from stable PBC to AIH and vice versa also seen
- Other etiologies of chronic liver disease and cirrhosis, such as alcoholic cirrhosis, chronic viral hepatitis, primary sclerosing cholangitis, AIH, sarcoidosis, hepatic amyloidosis, chemical/toxin-induced cirrhosis, other hereditary or familial disorders (e.g., cystic fibrosis, α-1-antitrypsin deficiency)
- Biliary obstruction
- Secondary biliary cirrhosis or secondary sclerosing cholangitis

WORKUP

History, physical examination, laboratory evaluation, liver biopsy

LABORATORY TESTS

- AMAs found in 95% of patients with PBC and are 98% specific.

- Antinuclear antibodies (ANAs) and AMAs found in approximately 50% of patients. In approximately 10% of patients, AMAs are absent (AMA-negative PBC). Nearly all of these patients have ANA or AMAs, or both.
- Cholestatic pattern of liver biochemical markers; markedly increased alkaline phosphatase (of hepatic origin). Alkaline phosphatase levels along with bilirubin levels correlate with the risk of liver transplantation or death.
- γ-Glutamyl transpeptidase is increased.
- Serum IgM levels are increased (lower in AMA-negative PBC).
- Bilirubin level is normal early on and increases with disease progression (direct and indirect) in 60% of patients. Increased serum bilirubin level is a poor prognostic indicator.
- Aminotransferase level may be normal and, if increased, is rarely more than five times the upper limit of normal.
- Markedly increased serum lipids in more than 50% of patients. Total cholesterol may surpass 1000 mg/dl. No increased risk for death from atherosclerosis seen, possibly because of high levels of LP-X, an antiatherogenic low-density lipoprotein, very-high-density lipoprotein levels, and low serum levels of lipoprotein(a).
- Percutaneous liver biopsy confirms or rules out the diagnosis, allows staging, but is not essential to make diagnosis or to initiate medical therapy in patients with typical liver chemistry and positive AMA test.
- Histology is not uniform, so histologic stage is based on the most advanced lesion present.
  1. Stage I: Lymphocytic infiltration of the epithelial cells of the small bile ducts with granuloma-like lesions, limited to portal triads (bridging fibrosis)
  2. Stage II: Extension of inflammatory cells to periportal parenchyma, ductular prolif-

eration, invasion by foamy macrophages, and development of biliary piecemeal necrosis
  3. Stage III: Fibrous septa link portal triads
  4. Stage IV: Frank cirrhosis with regenerative nodules; hyaline deposits and accumulation of stainable copper are also seen

IMAGING STUDIES

If history, physical examination, blood tests, and liver biopsy are all consistent with PBC, neither imaging nor cholangiography is necessary (Fig. 1).

PROGNOSIS

- Median survival was ~10 yr but may be getting longer with earlier diagnosis and initiation of treatment.
- The median time of progression from stage I or II disease to cirrhosis with no medical treatment is ~2 yr.
- Neither presence nor total titer level of AMAs predicts survival, disease progression, or response to therapy.
- Prognostic laboratory measures: Serum bilirubin is the best predictor of survival and the most heavily weighted factor in prognostic models.
- Response to ursodiol therapy can be prognostic: Patients with a decrease in alkaline phosphatase level of at least 40% or to the reference range after 1 yr of treatment with ursodeoxycholic acid (UDCA) may have a prognosis similar to an age-matched healthy population. Similarly, the Mayo Risk score, a predictor of short-term survival probability (http://www.mayoclinic.org/gi-rst/mayomodel1.html), can also reliably predict life expectancy when calculated after 6 mo of ursodiol therapy.

Poorer prognosis exists with jaundice, advanced histologic stage, advanced age, edema, esophageal varices, coagulopathy, and ascites.

🆁🆇 TREATMENT

- Treatment is according to the clinical stage of the disease.
- Asymptomatic stage: Follow liver function tests every 3 mo. Once alkaline phosphatase is elevated up to 1.5 x ULN, begin UDCA at 13 to 15 mg/kg/day in 2-3 divided doses regardless of histologic stage. Side effects may include headaches, dizziness, diarrhea or constipation, dyspepsia, nausea, weight gain of approximately 5 lbs during the first 1 to 2 yr, back pain, and upper respiratory infections. Watch for interactions with fibric acid derivatives, bile-acid sequestrants, estrogen derivatives, as well as aluminum hydroxide, which may interfere with the therapeutic effect or serum concentration of UDCA. Efficacy is best if started during stage I or II disease but should be started at any stage of disease. Lifelong therapy is currently recommended, but benefits are still observed if therapy is interrupted and restarted.
- Treatment also includes treatment of associated conditions such as pruritus, osteoporosis, increased low-density lipoprotein level, malabsorption, vitamin deficiencies, anemia, hypothyroidism, and any eventual complications of cirrhosis.
- 33% of patients will not respond to medical therapy and will proceed to liver transplantation, which is the only definitive treatment for this disease.

ACUTE GENERAL Rx

- Symptomatic stage: Goals of treatment are resolution of symptoms such as pruritus, treatment of chronic cholestatic complications, and delay of progression to liver failure.
- Ursodiol can significantly improve bilirubin and alkaline phosphatase levels, prolong survival without liver transplantation, and delay progression of liver fibrosis and development of portal hypertension.
- The addition of colchicine, methotrexate, or fibrates has not been found to be of benefit to mortality or time to liver transplantation in controlled trials.
- Recent trials have shown that obeticholic acid administered with ursodiol or as monotherapy for 12 months decreases alkaline phosphatase and bilirubin levels.
- Prednisone, azathioprine, penicillamine, cyclosporine, silymarin and mycophenolate mofetil are no longer used because of limited efficacy and/or significant toxicity.
- For the pruritus of PBC, cholestyramine resin (4 g/dose; maximum, 16 g/day) reduces pruritus in most patients but must be given at least 4 hrs before ursodiol to avoid reducing the efficacy of that drug. Antihistamines at bedtime help nighttime symptoms. Rifampin

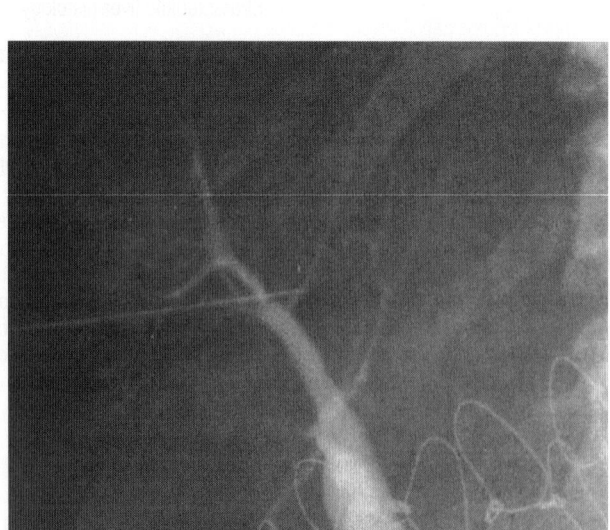

FIG. 1 Primary biliary cholangitis demonstrated by endoscopic retrograde cholangiopancreatography. (From Berk RN, Ferrucci Jr JT, Leopold GR: Radiology of the gallbladder and bile ducts: diagnosis and intervention, Philadelphia, 1983, Saunders.)

(150-300 mg bid), oral opiate antagonists such as naltrexone (12.5-50 mg daily) and sertraline (75-100 mg daily) can be used for pruritus refractory to bile acid sequestrants. Intractable pruritus can be an indication for liver transplantation.

CHRONIC Rx

- Liver function tests should be checked every 3 to 6 mo.
- Management of sicca syndrome: Artificial tears can be used initially for dry eyes. Saliva substitutes can be used for xerostomia and dysphagia; pilocarpine or cevimeline can be used for refractory cases. Moisturizers can be given for vaginal dryness.
- Treatment/Prevention of osteopenia/osteoporosis: Patients with PBC should be provided 1000 to 1500 mg calcium daily in divided doses and 1000 IU of vitamin D daily in the diet and as supplements if needed. Weight-bearing exercises are also recommended. Bone densitometry should be done every 2 to 4 yr. Alendronate (70 mg weekly) should be considered if patients are osteopenic in the absence of acid reflux or known varices.
- Hyperlipidemia is common in patients with PBC. However, there is no elevated risk of cardiovascular disease. Statins are safe in patients who may need treatment even if liver chemistry is abnormal.
- Vitamin A, K, and E deficiencies can be clinically important in advanced cases and respond to oral replacement.
- Upper endoscopy to assess for varices is indicated every 2 to 3 yr in patients with cirrhosis or Mayo risk score >4.1. Nonselective beta-blockers or endoscopic banding can be considered for prevention of variceal hemorrhage.
- Regular screening for hepatocellular carcinoma with ultrasound and α-fetoprotein every 6 to 12 mo is recommended for patients with cirrhosis.
- Liver transplantation is the only effective treatment for patients with liver failure. Indications for transplantation include hepatic decompensation (ascites, encephalopathy, jaundice), hepatocellular carcinoma fulfilling Milan criteria (see "Hepatocellular Carcinoma"), and intractable pruritus. Liver transplant should also be considered when the Mayo risk score ≥7.8, MELD score >12, and bilirubin approaches 6.
- The outcome of liver transplantation for patients with PBC is more favorable than that of nearly all other liver disease categories. The survival rates are 93%, 90%, and 79% at 1, 5, and 10 yr, respectively. Although recurrent disease may develop in up to 30% of patients after liver transplantation over 10 yr, patient and graft survival is usually not affected.

DISPOSITION

Definitive treatment requires liver transplantation; survival is 7 to 16 yr depending on symptoms at time of diagnosis.

REFERRAL

Gastroenterology and/or hepatology for treatment, evaluation for liver transplantation, and management of portal hypertension

SUGGESTED READINGS

Available at www.expertconsult.com

RELATED CONTENT

Primary Biliary Cirrhosis (PBC) (Patient Information)

AUTHORS: **JEANETTE G. SMITH, M.D.,** and **NICOLETTE J. RODRIGUEZ, M.D., M.P.H**

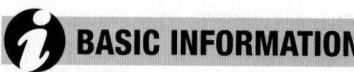

DEFINITION

- Women younger than 40 yr of age with amenorrhea, oligomenorrhea, or dysfunctional uterine bleeding for 4 mo or more along with follicle stimulating hormone (FSH) levels in the menopausal range meet diagnostic criteria for primary ovarian insufficiency.
- Menopause younger than the age of 40 yr.

SYNONYMS

Hypergonadotropic hypogonadism
Premature ovarian failure
Premature menopause
Gonadal dysgenesis

ICD-10CM CODES

E28.3	Primary ovarian failure
E28.9	Ovarian dysfunction, unspecified
E28.310	Symptomatic premature menopause
E28.39	Other primary ovarian failure

EPIDEMIOLOGY & DEMOGRAPHICS

INCIDENCE: Affects 1% to 4% of the female population in the U.S.
PREDOMINANT AGE: 1:250 incident cases by age 35 and 1:100 by age 40

PHYSICAL FINDINGS & CLINICAL PRESENTATION

- The most common presentation is disturbance in menstrual pattern due to intermittent ovarian function.
- Between 5% and 30% of affected women have another affected female relative.
- Between 10% and 30% of affected women already have a concurrent autoimmune condition, the most common of which is hypothyroidism.
- Symptoms of estrogen deficiency include hot flashes, night sweats, poor concentration, drying of the vagina, and infertility.
- Physical exam may reveal stigmata of an autoimmune condition such as vitiligo, thyroid enlargement, or Turner's syndrome (webbed neck, short stature, and high-arched palate).

ETIOLOGY (SEE TABLE 1)

Idiopathic in 95% of cases

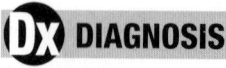

DIAGNOSIS

DIFFERENTIAL DIAGNOSIS

- Pregnancy
- Causes of secondary amenorrhea include eating disorder, exercise, drugs, sarcoidosis, polycystic ovarian disease, hypothalamic amenorrhea, hyperprolactinemia/prolactinoma, and Cushing's disease.

WORKUP

- After pregnancy is ruled out, the initial evaluation should include the measurement of serum prolactin, FSH, and thyrotropin (TSH) levels.

- If the FSH level is in the menopausal range (>40 uIU/ml by radioimmunoassay), the test should be repeated in 1 month along with a serum estradiol measurement to confirm the diagnosis of primary ovarian insufficiency.

LABORATORY TESTS

Once a diagnosis of premature ovarian failure is made, other evaluations include:

- Autoimmune disorders, adrenal insufficiency (seen in 3% of cases): serum anti-adrenal and anti-21 hydroxylase antibodies should be measured.
- Hypothyroidism: serum TSH, T_4, and anti-TPO antibodies
- All cases should be screened for osteoporosis by DXA for bone mineral density.
- A karyotype analysis should be performed for all patients to look for chromosomal defects including Turner's variant or deletions of the X chromosome.
- Permutations for the fragile X syndrome (FMR1 gene) should be checked for as well.

IMAGING STUDIES

Pelvic ultrasound has no proven benefit in the management of these patients.

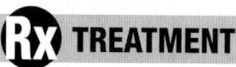

TREATMENT

NONPHARMACOLOGIC THERAPY

Counseling or patient support group should be offered to all women with low self-esteem and depression due to the psychological scar left by the diagnosis.

ACUTE GENERAL Rx

- Physiologic estrogen and progestin replacement is reasonable in the cases of young women until they reach the age of natural menopause.
- A dose of 100 mcg of estradiol per day, administered by transdermal patch, achieves average estradiol level observed in normal menstruating women and effectively treats symptoms.
- Cyclic medroxyprogesterone at a dose of 10 mg per day for 12 days each month is the preferred progestin to provide protection against endometrial cancer.

TABLE 1 Mechanisms and Causes of Primary Ovarian Insufficiency

Accelerated Follicular Depletion

Genetic: Turner's syndrome, fragile X premutations, galactosemia Toxic: Chemotherapy, radiation, infections such as mumps or cytomegalovirus Autoimmune: Polyglandular failure, hypothyroidism, Addison's disease, vitiligo, myasthenia gravis

Abnormal Follicular Stimulation

Gonadotropin receptor function: follicle stimulating hormone/luteinizing hormone receptor mutation Enzyme defects: Aromatase deficiency Luteinized follicles

---

- Pregnancy may occur while a woman is taking estrogen and progesterone therapy and the therapy should be stopped immediately if the pregnancy test is found to be positive.

CHRONIC Rx

- Intake of 1200 mg of elemental calcium and 800 units of vitamin D_3 per day should be encouraged to prevent bone loss. A serum 25-hydroxyvitamin D level of 30 ng per ml or higher should be maintained.
- Patients with positive tests for adrenal antibodies should be evaluated annually for adrenal insufficiency by corticotropin stimulation test.
- Patients who wish to avoid pregnancy should use a barrier method or an IUD.
- Options for parenthood include adoption, foster parenthood, egg donation, and embryo donation.

DISPOSITION

Women with the known diagnosis should be encouraged to maintain a lifestyle that optimizes bone and cardiovascular health, including regular weight-bearing exercises, adequate intake of calcium (1200 mg daily) and vitamin D (800 IU daily), healthy diet to prevent obesity, and screening for cardiovascular risk factors.

REFERRAL

Referral to gynecologist and reproductive endocrinologist may be helpful in patients who decide to pursue parenthood.

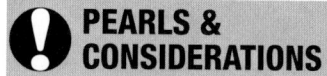

PEARLS & CONSIDERATIONS

COMMENTS

- Common etiologies should be ruled out, including chromosomal abnormalities, fragile X premutations, and autoimmune causes.
- Management directed at symptom resolution and bone protection primarily, but should include psychosocial support for women facing this devastating diagnosis.

PREVENTION

Early diagnosis of primary ovarian insufficiency important for osteoporosis prevention and possibly prevention of coronary artery disease.

PATIENT & FAMILY EDUCATION

www.pofsupport.org
poi.nichd.nih.gov

SUGGESTED READING

Available at www.expertconsult.com

AUTHOR: **PRIYA BANSAL, M.D., M.P.H.**

BASIC INFORMATION

DEFINITION

Primary sclerosing cholangitis (PSC) is a chronic idiopathic progressive cholestatic liver disease characterized by segmental fibrosing and inflammation of intrahepatic and extrahepatic bile ducts complicated by recurrent cholangitis, cholangiocarcinoma (CCA), cirrhosis, and portal hypertension.

SYNONYMS

Chronic obliterative cholangitis
Fibrosing cholangitis
Stenosing cholangitis
PSC

ICD-10CM CODES
K83.0 Cholangitis
K83.0 Disease of biliary tract, unspecified

EPIDEMIOLOGY & DEMOGRAPHICS

- The incidence and prevalence of PSC are 0.9 to 1.3 cases and 8.5 to 16.2 cases per 100,000 population, respectively.
- About 65% of patients with PSC are men.
- Mean age of presentation is 30 to 40 yr.
- 60% to 80% of patients with PSC also have inflammatory bowel disease (IBD). 4% to 5% of patients with ulcerative colitis (UC) will develop PSC. PSC is an independent risk factor for developing colon cancer in patients with IBD.
- PSC can coexist with other autoimmune liver diseases. Autoimmune hepatitis (AIH) and PSC overlap syndrome can be seen in young adults and children.
- Cholangiocarcinoma is present in 1% to 2% of PSC patients at diagnosis. The lifetime risk is 5% to 10%.
- The median survival from time of diagnosis is 10 to 15 yr without liver transplantation.

PHYSICAL FINDINGS & CLINICAL PRESENTATION

- Most patients are asymptomatic (15%-40%) at the time of diagnosis with normal physical findings. However, many patients will have abnormal liver tests and a known diagnosis of IBD.
- More than 75% of asymptomatic patients develop symptoms, the most common of which are nonspecific pruritus (70%) and fatigue (70%). Physical findings of symptomatic patients may reveal jaundice, skin excoriation and hyperpigmentation from scratching, hepatosplenomegaly, and xanthelasma. Other symptoms include abdominal discomfort, steatorrhea, jaundice, and weight loss, which are concerning for advanced PSC, sepsis, or mechanical obstruction (i.e., cholangitis), and malignancy (i.e., cholangiocarcinoma).
- Patients can also present with advanced liver disease and decompensated cirrhosis (i.e., ascites, spontaneous bacterial peritonitis, hepatic encephalopathy, and variceal hemorrhage) or hepatic failure. In patients with cirrhosis, physical findings may reveal a shrunken nodular liver and evidence of portal hypertension.

ETIOLOGY

- The cause of PSC is unknown, but the most likely mechanism is immunologic priming in a genetically susceptible patient causing phenotypic expression of PSC.
- Genetic and immunologic factors are supported by reports of familial occurrence of this disorder and increased frequency of HLA B8 and DR3. Genome-wide association studies have discovered novel loci associated with PSC, but the functional aspects of these genes are still unknown.
- Portosystemic inflammation caused by translocation of the gut microbiota is an increasing area of research. The close association with UC and PSC may be secondary to gut-activated T lymphocytes in IBD causing portal inflammation because of overlapping adhesion molecules in the gut and liver. Furthermore, intestinal dysbiosis in PSC has also been seen and remains an area of ongoing research.

DIAGNOSIS

Diagnosis is based on characteristic cholangiographic findings in combination with clinical, biochemical, and in some cases histologic features. It is increasingly common to diagnose PSC based on imaging with magnetic resonance cholangiopancreatography (MRCP). Liver biopsy is now rarely used to diagnose disease. Table 1 describes staging of PSC. Work is being done that enables a diagnosis to be made based on biomarkers such as microRNA and fecal microbiota profiles.

DIFFERENTIAL DIAGNOSIS

- Surgical biliary trauma
- Ischemic cholangitis
- Intraarterial chemotherapy (5-FU/floxuridine)
- AIDS-related cholangiopathy
- Choledocholithiasis
- Recurrent pyogenic cholangitis
- Cholangiocarcinoma
- IgG4-associated cholangitis (IAC)
- Diffuse intrahepatic metastasis
- Histiocytosis X

TABLE 1 Staging of Primary Sclerosing Cholangitis

Stage	Description
I—Portal	Portal edema, inflammation, ductal proliferation; abnormalities do not extend beyond the limiting plate
II—Periportal	Periportal fibrosis with or without inflammation extending beyond the limiting plate
III—Septal	Septal fibrosis, bridging necrosis, or both
IV—Cirrhotic	Biliary cirrhosis

From Cameron JL, Cameron AM: *Current surgical therapy*, ed 10, Philadelphia, 2011, Saunders.

WORKUP

History, physical examination, laboratory evaluation, imaging studies, and possible liver biopsy

LABORATORY TESTS

- Serum biochemical tests usually indicate cholestasis with predominant elevation in the serum alkaline phosphatase (three to ten times the upper limit of normal). However, this value can vary and be normal during the disease course. Serum aminotransferase levels are elevated in the majority of patients (two to three times the upper limits of normal). Serum bilirubin is usually normal at the time of diagnosis unless the patient has advanced stricturing disease; an initial elevation of bilirubin at diagnosis may be related to worse prognosis.
- A wide range of autoantibodies can be detected in patients with PSC; however, they are nonspecific for PSC, including the perinuclear antineutrophil cytoplasmic antibody (pANCA), autoantibodies such as antinuclear antibody (ANA), and anti-smooth muscle antibody (ASMA). Anti-mitochondrial antibody (AMA), which is characteristic of primary biliary cirrhosis, is *NOT* found in PSC and can be helpful in excluding PSC. Serum IgG levels are useful in the diagnosis of PSC-AIH overlap syndrome and IAC with autoimmune pancreatitis. In particular, elevated levels of IgG4 are found in 10% to 20% of PSC patients, with a subset of these patients displaying features of autoimmune pancreatitis. PSC patients with elevated IgG4 seem to respond to corticosteroid therapy, and hence all patients with PSC should be tested once for IgG4.

IMAGING STUDIES

- Cholangiography, with MRCP or ERCP, is considered to be the gold standard for the diagnosis of PSC. Characteristic findings

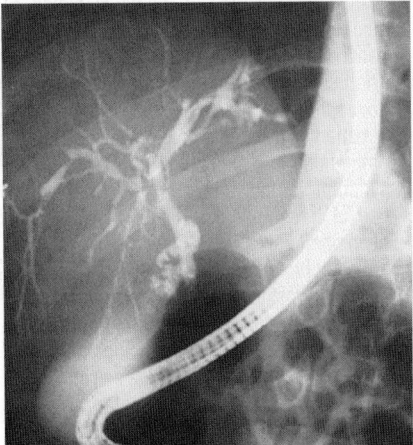

FIG. 1 A 29-year-old male patient who was diagnosed with PSC 5 years previously. Both the intra- and extrahepatic bile ducts are involved at cholangiography. (From Parlak E et al: An endoscopic finding in patients with primary sclerosing cholangitis: retraction of the main duodenal papilla into the duodenum wall, *Gastrointest Endosc* 65[3]:535, 2007.)

reveal segmental fibrosis of bile ducts with saccular dilatation of normal intervening areas resulting in a "beads-on-a-string" appearance (Fig. 1).

- Magnetic resonance cholangiopancreatography (MRCP) has an overall diagnostic accuracy rate of 90%. It is the first imaging modality of choice when PSC is suspected because endoscopic retrograde cholangiopancreatography (ERCP) can be associated with serious complications (i.e., pancreatitis and cholangitis).
- Liver biopsy is not necessary for the diagnosis of PSC in patients with typical cholangiographic findings, except for small duct PSC, which makes up 5% of patients with PSC. Biopsies are subject to sample variation, and the typical "onion skin"–type periductal fibrosis finding is rare. Liver biopsy may help in the diagnosis of PSC-AIH overlap syndrome, small-duct PSC (normal cholangiogram), or IAC.

Rx TREATMENT

- No medical therapy has been established to be effective in halting the disease progression of PSC.
- Ursodeoxycholic acid (UDCA) has shown variable benefit in randomized controlled trials. Although biochemical improvement has been seen with UDCA, there has been no proven benefit on survival. In two trials, high-dose UDCA (28-30 mg/kg/day) was associated with colorectal dysplasia, liver transplantation, and varices. Therefore, high-dose UDCA is *NOT* universally recommended as medical therapy in patients with PSC. A trial of medium- or low-dose UDCA ~20 mg/kg/day is used by some clinicians, since some trials have shown biochemical response.
- Oral vancomycin may show clinical and biochemical response in pediatric patients, but no randomized clinical trial has been performed.
- Management of PSC patients is aimed at symptom relief and management of complications from PSC (i.e., obstruction/strictures).
- The use of corticosteroids and other immunosuppressive agents is not recommended in patients with PSC alone; however, it is recommended in patients with PSC-AIH overlap syndrome or elevated IgG4.
- Use of tumor necrosis factor inhibitors has been ineffective in PSC. Other monoclonal antibody therapies targeting lymphocyte trafficking, tyrosine kinase signaling, and liver fibrosis are being studied. Furthermore, other targets for treatment are ongoing and aimed at bile acid synthesis and mast cell inhibition.
- Bile acid–based therapeutic approaches are currently in clinical trials, including peroxisome proliferator-activated receptor agonists and farnesoid X receptor agonists.

ACUTE GENERAL Rx

- With mild pruritus, skin emollients and antihistamines are recommended as the first-line treatment. With moderate or severe pruritus, bile acid sequestrants (i.e., cholestyramine 16

g/day) are the preferred choice for the initial management of pruritus. Alternative agents for pruritus refractory to bile acid sequestrants include rifampicin 150 to 300 mg twice daily, naltrexone 50 mg daily, sertraline 75 to 100 mg daily, or phenobarbital 90 mg at bedtime.
- Patients who present with increasing serum bilirubin and/or worsening pruritus, progressive bile duct dilatation on imaging studies, or cholangitis need to be evaluated for dominant strictures with imaging. A dominant stricture is a stenosis >1.5 mm in the common bile duct or ≥1 mm in the hepatic duct.
- ERCP with brushings, cytology, and fluorescent in situ hybridization (FISH) is recommended to evaluate dominant strictures for cholangiocarcinoma. Once malignancy is excluded, balloon dilatation with or without stenting is recommended to treat symptoms. Routine stenting is not required, but short-term stenting may be helpful in patients with severe stricture. If ERCP is unsuccessful, percutaneous cholangiopancreatography with stenting should be considered.
- In noncirrhotic patients with dominant strictures refractory to endoscopic or percutaneous management, surgery should be considered, although this may complicate future liver transplantation surgery.
- Antibiotic usage is recommended in patients with dominant strictures/obstructions both acutely and for long-term prophylaxis in patients with recurrent cholangitis.

CHRONIC Rx

- Avoidance of alcohol and vaccination against hepatitis A and B are advised.
- Patients with PSC are at risk for osteoporosis and osteopenia. At time of diagnosis, a DEXA scan is recommended and should be repeated in 2 to 4 yr. Calcium (1000 to 1500 mg) and vitamin D 600 to 800 IU daily are recommended for patients with osteopenia, and the addition of bisphosphonate is recommended in patients with osteoporosis.
- Patients with newly diagnosed PSC should have a full colonoscopy with biopsies to exclude concurrent IBD and for surveillance of colorectal cancer. In patients with IBD, continued surveillance colonoscopy with biopsies, or chromoendoscopy, at 1- to 2-yr intervals is recommended. In patients without IBD, a suggested 3- to 5-yr surveillance interval has been recommended due to an increased risk of colorectal cancer.
- Cholangiocarcinoma (CCA) development is common in PSC. PSC patients with biochemical or symptomatic deterioration should be evaluated for CCA. Surveillance for CCA with annual MRCP and CA19-9 has been recommended by some authorities. Abnormal values should prompt further investigation of dominant strictures with ERCP. Although CA19-9 may detect CCA, even high levels (>129 U/mL) may lack specificity since one-third of patients did not have CCA after 30 months of follow up. These differences may in part be due to genotypic differences in *FUT2/3* alleles that affect expression of CA19-9.

- Annual transabdominal ultrasound is recommended due to the increased risk of gallbladder malignancy. If masses or polyps >8 mm are detected, cholecystectomy should be performed.
- Patients with cirrhosis are recommended to have gastroesophageal variceal and hepatocellular carcinoma (HCC) surveillance at regular intervals.
- With advanced disease, fat-soluble vitamin deficiencies such as A, E, and D should be assessed.
- In cases of HCC and CCA, depending on underlying liver disease, resection versus liver transplantation would be required.

DISPOSITION

Liver transplantation is the only effective treatment for patients with end-stage liver disease, portal hypertension, liver failure, and recurrent or intractable bacterial cholangitis. Survival is excellent, with 90% and 80% survival rates at 1 and 5 yr, respectively. The recurrence of PSC after transplant is reportedly 5% to 20%. Transplant referral is warranted when MELD exceeds 14 or greater, or with worsening cholangitis or intractable pruritus.

REFERRAL

Gastroenterology and/or hepatology for treatment of PSC, management of its complications, surveillance of associated malignancy, and evaluation for liver transplantation.

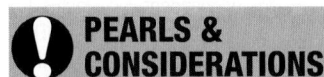

PEARLS & CONSIDERATIONS

- Management of PSC targets symptom relief, complications of PSC, cirrhosis, early carcinoma detection, and timely referral for liver transplantation.
- High-dose UDCA is not universally recommended for treatment of PSC.
- Patients are at increased risk for the development of colorectal cancer, gallbladder cancer, and cholangiocarcinoma and need surveillance.
- Patients with PSC and ulcerative colitis have more common right-sided colon involvement and greater risk of pouchitis after colectomy with an ileal pouch-anal anastomosis.
- In patients with cirrhosis, surveillance for gastroesophageal varices and HCC is recommended.
- Liver transplant remains the only definitive therapy for complications of PSC.

SUGGESTED READINGS
Available at www.expertconsult.com

RELATED CONTENT
Ulcerative Colitis (Related Key Topic)

AUTHORS: **MICHAL GANZ, M.D.**, and **AMANDA PRESSMAN, M.D.**

ⓘ BASIC INFORMATION

DEFINITION

Prolactinomas are monoclonal tumors that secrete prolactin.

ICD-10CM CODES
D35.2 Benign neoplasm of pituitary gland
E22.8 Other hyperfunction of pituitary gland

EPIDEMIOLOGY & DEMOGRAPHICS

INCIDENCE: Most common pituitary tumor; nearly 30% of all pituitary adenomas secrete enough prolactin to cause hyperprolactinemia.
PREDOMINANT SEX: Microadenomas are more common in women; macroadenomas are found more frequently in men.

PHYSICAL FINDINGS & CLINICAL PRESENTATION

- Men: decreased facial and body hair, infertility, small testicles; may also have decreased libido, erectile dysfunction, and delayed puberty (caused by decreased testosterone as a result of inhibition of gonadotropin secretion).
- Women: physical examination may be normal; history may reveal amenorrhea, galactorrhea (Fig. E1), oligomenorrhea, and anovulation.
- Both sexes: visual field defects and headache may occur depending on size of tumor and its expansion.

ETIOLOGY

Prolactin-secreting pituitary adenomas: microadenomas (<10 mm diameter) or macroadenomas (>10 mm diameter). No risk factors have been identified for sporadic prolactinomas. Rarely prolactinomas can be part of multiple endocrine neoplasia (MEN) type 1 syndrome.

Ⓓ DIAGNOSIS

DIFFERENTIAL DIAGNOSIS

Secretion of prolactin is under tonic inhibitory control by hypothalamic dopamine. Hyperprolactinemia may be caused by the following:

- Drugs: risperidone, phenothiazines, methyldopa, reserpine, monoamine oxidase inhibitors, androgens, progesterone, cimetidine, tricyclic antidepressants, haloperidol, meprobamate, chlordiazepoxide, estrogens, narcotics, metoclopramide, verapamil, amoxapine, cocaine, oral contraceptives
- Hepatic cirrhosis, renal failure, primary hypothyroidism
- Ectopic prolactin-secreting tumors (hypernephroma, bronchogenic carcinoma)
- Infiltrating diseases of the pituitary (sarcoidosis, histiocytosis)
- Head trauma, chest wall injury, spinal cord injury
- Polycystic ovary disease, pregnancy, nipple stimulation
- Idiopathic hyperprolactinemia, stress, exercise

WORKUP

- The diagnosis of prolactinoma is established by demonstration of an elevated serum prolactin level (after exclusion of other causes of hyperprolactinemia) and radiographic evidence of a pituitary adenoma.
  1. Normal mean prolactin levels are 8 ng/ml in women and 5 ng/ml in men.
  2. Prolactin levels >100 ng/ml are suspicious for prolactinoma. Most macroprolactinomas raise prolactin levels >250 ng/ml and levels >300 ng/ml are virtually diagnostic of prolactinomas.
  3. Prolactin levels can vary with time of day, stress, sleep cycle, and meals. More accurate measurements can be obtained 2 to 3 hr after awakening, preprandially, and when patient is not distressed.
  4. Serial measurements are recommended in patients with mild prolactin elevations.
- TSH, free T_4, BUN, Creat, ALT, AST are useful tests. Pregnancy test in all women of childbearing age.
- All patients with prolactinomas should undergo visual field testing. Serial evaluation is recommended, particularly during pregnancy in patients with macroadenomas.

IMAGING STUDIES

- MRI with gadolinium enhancement is the procedure of choice in the radiographic evaluation of pituitary disease.
- In absence of MRI, a radiographic diagnosis is best accomplished with a high-resolution CT scanner and special coronal cuts through the pituitary region.

ⓡ TREATMENT

NONPHARMACOLOGIC THERAPY

Pregnancy and breastfeeding should be avoided because they can encourage tumor growth.

ACUTE GENERAL Rx

- Management of prolactinomas depends on their size and encroachment on the optic chiasm and other vital structures, the presence or absence of gonadal dysfunction, and the patient's desires regarding fertility. Patients with microprolactinomas without symptoms of hypogonadism do not require treatment. Fig. 2 describes a management algorithm for prolactinomas.
- Medical therapy is preferred when fertility is an important consideration. Prolactinomas are treated with the dopamine agonists (DA) bromocriptine and cabergoline.
  1. Bromocriptine: initial dose is 0.625 mg at bedtime for the first week. After 1 wk, add morning dose of 1.25 mg. Gradually increase dose by 1.25 mg/wk until dose of 5 to 10 mg/day is achieved. Bromocriptine decreases size of the tumor and generally lowers the prolactin level into the normal range when the initial serum prolactin is <500 ng/ml. Side effects of bromocriptine are nausea, constipation, dizziness, and nasal stuffiness. Bromocriptine appears to be safe during pregnancy.
  2. Cabergoline is a longer-acting dopamine agonist that is more expensive but may be more effective and better tolerated than bromocriptine; initial dose is 0.25 mg twice weekly.
  3. After therapy is initiated, MRI should be repeated in 1 year for microprolactinomas if the prolactin level normalizes. For macroprolactinomas, MRI is repeated after 2 months and every 6 to 12 months until stable on serial studies.
- Transsphenoidal resection: option in an infertile patient who cannot tolerate bromocriptine or cabergoline or when medical therapy is ineffective. The success rate depends on the location of the tumor (entirely intrasellar), experience of the neurosurgeon, and size of the tumor (<10 mm in diameter); the recurrence rate may reach 80% within 5 yr. Possible complications of transsphenoidal surgery vary with experience and skill of the neurosurgeon and tumor anatomy and include transient diabetes insipidus, hypopituitarism, cerebrospinal fluid rhinorrhea, and infections (meningitis, wound infection).
- Pituitary irradiation is useful as adjunctive therapy of macroadenomas (>10 mm in diameter) and in patients with persistent hypersecretion after surgery. Potential complications include cranial nerve damage, radionecrosis, and cognitive abnormalities.
- Stereotactic radiosurgery (gamma knife) has become popular as a modality in the treatment of prolactinomas. A high dose of ionizing radiation is delivered to the tumor through multiple ports. Its advantage is minimal irradiation to surrounding tissues. Proximity of the tumor to the optic chiasm limits this therapeutic modality.

CHRONIC Rx

- Patients on medical therapy require periodic measurement of prolactin levels. An attempt to reduce the dose of bromocriptine or cabergoline can be made after the prolactin level has been normal for 2 yr. An MRI scan of the pituitary should be obtained to rule out tumor enlargement within 6 mo of initiation of tapering regimen.
- Evaluation and monitoring of pituitary function are recommended after transsphenoidal surgery.

DISPOSITION

- Transsphenoidal surgery will result in a cure in nearly 50% to 75% of patients with microadenomas and 10% to 20% of patients with macroadenomas.
- Nearly 20% of microprolactinomas resolve during long-term dopamine agonist treatment.

❗ PEARLS & CONSIDERATIONS

COMMENTS

- Patients must be monitored for several years after surgery because up to 50% of

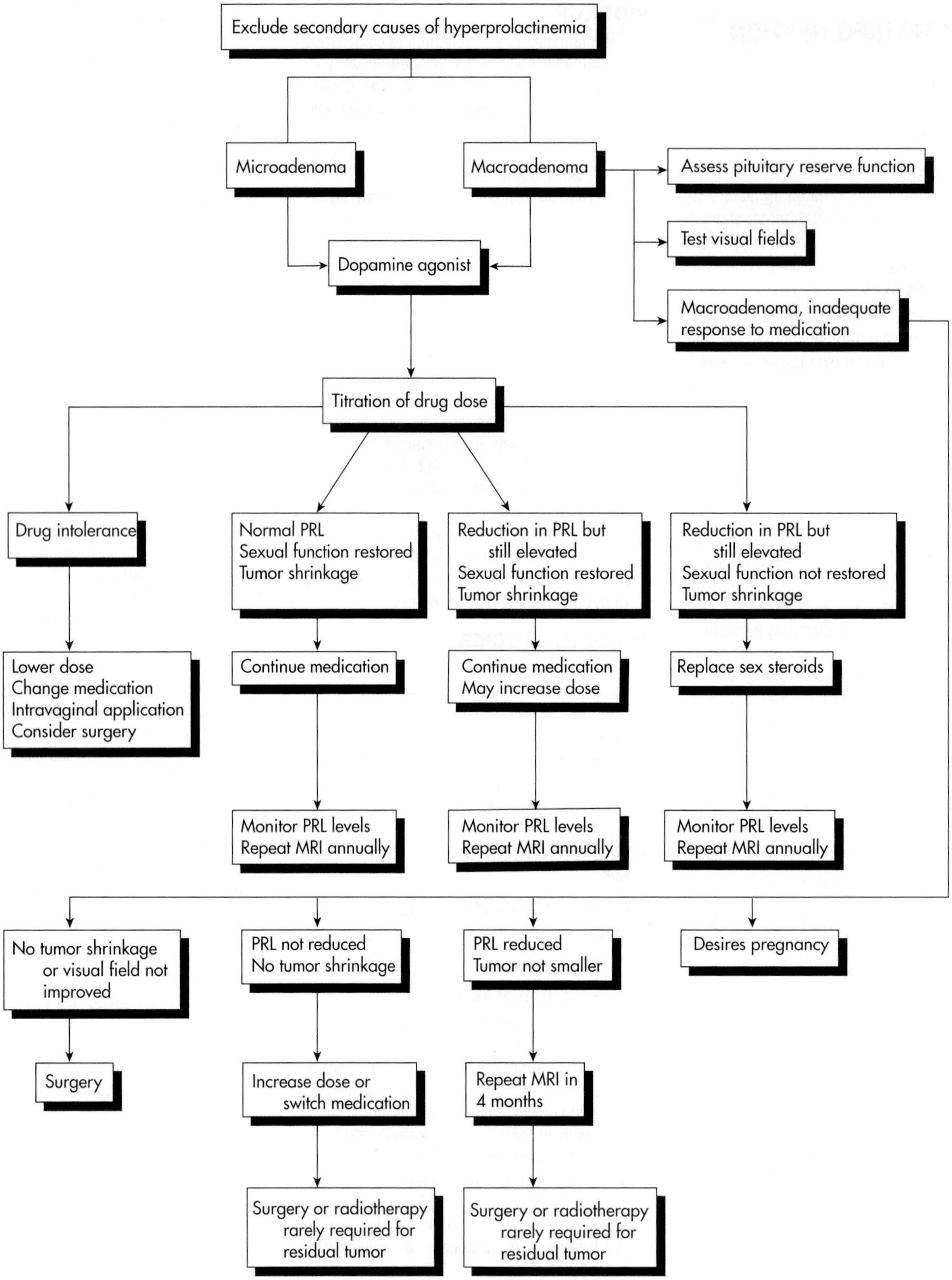

Exclude secondary causes of hyperprolactinemia

Microadenoma

Macroadenoma

Assess pituitary reserve function

Test visual fields

Macroadenoma, inadequate response to medication

Dopamine agonist

Titration of drug dose

Drug intolerance

Normal PRL
Sexual function restored
Tumor shrinkage

Reduction in PRL but
still elevated
Sexual function restored
Tumor shrinkage

Reduction in PRL but
still elevated
Sexual function not restored
Tumor shrinkage

Lower dose
Change medication
Intravaginal application
Consider surgery

Continue medication

Continue medication
May increase dose

Replace sex steroids

Monitor PRL levels
Repeat MRI annually

Monitor PRL levels
Repeat MRI annually

Monitor PRL levels
Repeat MRI annually

No tumor shrinkage
or visual field not
improved

PRL not reduced
No tumor shrinkage

PRL reduced
Tumor not smaller

Desires pregnancy

Surgery

Increase dose or
switch medication

Repeat MRI in
4 months

Surgery or radiotherapy
rarely required for
residual tumor

Surgery or radiotherapy
rarely required for
residual tumor

FIG. 2 Prolactinoma management. After secondary causes of hyperprolactinemia have been excluded, subsequent management decisions are based on clinical imaging and biochemical criteria. *MRI,* Magnetic resonance imaging; *PRL,* prolactin. (Modified from Larsen PR et al: *Williams textbook of endocrinology,* ed 11, Philadelphia, 2008, Saunders.)

microadenomas and nearly 90% of macroadenomas can recur.
- Pituitary microadenomas are found in 10.9% of autopsies, and 44% of these microadenomas are prolactinomas.

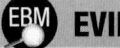 **EVIDENCE**

Available at www.expertconsult.com

SUGGESTED READING

Available at www.expertconsult.com

RELATED CONTENT

Prolactinoma (Patient Information)
Pituitary Adenoma (Related Key Topic)

AUTHOR: **FRED F. FERRI, M.D.**

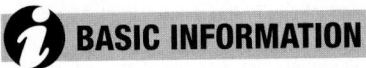

BASIC INFORMATION

DEFINITION & CLASSIFICATION

Prostate cancer is a neoplasm involving the prostate. Various classifications have been developed to evaluate malignancy potential and prognosis.

- The degree of malignancy varies with the stage:
  1. Stage A: Confined to the prostate, no nodule palpable.
  2. Stage B: Palpable nodule confined to the gland.
  3. Stage C: Local extension.
  4. Stage D: Regional lymph nodes or distant metastases.
- In the Gleason classification, two histologic patterns are independently assigned numbers 1 to 5 (best to least differentiated). These numbers are added to give a total tumor score between 2 and 10. Prognosis is best for highly differentiated tumors (e.g., Gleason score 2 to 4) compared with most poorly differentiated tumors (Gleason score 7 to 10).
- Another commonly used classification is the Tumor-Node-Metastasis (TNM) classification of prostate cancer.
- Table 1 summarizes the definition of risk groups and biopsy criteria.

ICD-10CM CODES
C61   Malignant neoplasm of prostate
D07.5 Carcinoma in situ of prostate

EPIDEMIOLOGY & DEMOGRAPHICS

- Prostate cancer has surpassed lung cancer as the most common nonskin cancer in men.
- In the United States, more than 220,000 new cases are diagnosed yearly, and nearly 30,000 males die from prostate cancer each year (second leading cause of death from cancer in U.S. men).
- Incidence of prostate cancer increases with age: uncommon <50 yr; 80% of new cases are diagnosed in patients aged ≥65 yr. Widespread PSA testing has doubled the incidence of prostate cancer and the lifetime risk for prostate cancer to approximately 16%. Prostate cancer is also diagnosed earlier, and the incidence of clinically "silent" T1 tumors has increased from 17% in 1989 to 48% in 2001 since the advent of PSA screening.

Currently, approximately 80% of prostate cancer cases are diagnosed as localized disease and only 4% as metastatic disease.

- Prostate cancer is found at autopsy in more than half of U.S. men older than 50 years but is the cause of death in only 3%.
- Average age at time of diagnosis is 72 yr.
- Blacks in the United States have the highest incidence of prostate cancer in the world (one in every nine males).
- Incidence is low in Asians.
- Approximately 9% of all prostate cancers may be familial. Obesity is a risk factor for prostate cancer. High-fat, low-fiber diet increases risk. High insulin levels may also increase the risk of prostate cancer. Dietary supplementation with vitamin E has been reported to significantly increase the risk of prostate cancer among healthy men. Linkage studies have implicated chromosome 17p21-22 as a possible location of a prostate-cancer susceptibility gene. Germline mutations in *HOXB13* are associated with a significantly increased risk of hereditary prostate cancer.
- Mortality rates of prostate cancer have declined substantially in the past 15 yr from 34% in 1990 to <20% currently.

PHYSICAL FINDINGS & CLINICAL PRESENTATION

- Generally silent disease until it reaches advanced stages.
- Bone pain and pathologic fractures may be initial symptoms of prostate cancer.
- Local growth can cause symptoms of outflow obstruction.
- Digital rectal examination (DRE) may reveal an area of increased firmness; 10% of patients will have a negative DRE.
- Prostate may be hard, fixed, with extension of tumor to the seminal vesicles in advanced stages.

DX DIAGNOSIS

DIFFERENTIAL DIAGNOSIS

- Benign prostatic hypertrophy
- Prostatitis
- Prostate stones

LABORATORY TESTS

- Measurement of prostate-specific antigen (PSA) is controversial in early diagnosis of prostate cancer. PSA screening is associated with psychological harm, and

its potential benefits remain uncertain. In asymptomatic men with no history of prostate cancer, screening using PSA does not reduce all-cause mortality or death from prostate cancer. Normal PSA is found in >20% of patients with prostate cancer, whereas only 20% of men with PSA levels between 4 ng/ml and 10 ng/mL have prostate cancer. Most guidelines encourage a shared decision-making approach between patient and physician regarding PSA testing. Available evidence favors clinician discussion of the pros and cons of PSA screening with average-risk men aged 65 to 69 yr. Only men who express a definite preference for screening should have PSA testing. Rather than widespread annual PSA screening, a reasonable approach may be to focus on high-risk men (those with PSA levels ≥2 ng/ml at age 60). The American Cancer Society recommends offering the PSA test and DRE yearly to men aged ≥50 yr who have a life expectancy of at least 10 yr. Earlier testing, starting at age 40 to 45 yr, is recommended for men at high risk (e.g., blacks, men with family history of prostate cancer). An isolated elevation in PSA level should be confirmed several weeks later before proceeding with further testing, including prostate biopsy. Screening for prostate cancer in men aged ≥75 yr is controversial and generally not recommended. The American College of Physicians (ACP) recommends that clinicians should not screen for prostate cancer using the PSA in average-risk men under age 50, men over age 69, or men with a life expectancy of <10 to 15 yr. The U.S. Preventive Services Task Force (USPSTF) recommends against PSA-based screening for prostate cancer in all age groups. According to the USPSTF:

1. The magnitude of harms from screening (e.g., falsely high PSA levels, psychological effects, unnecessary biopsies, overdiagnosis of indolent tumors) is "at least small."
2. The magnitude of treatment-associated harms (i.e., adverse effects of surgery, radiation, and hormonal therapy) is "at least moderate."
3. The 10-yr mortality benefit of PSA-based prostate cancer screening is "small to none."
4. The overall balance of benefits and harms results in "moderate certainty that PSA-based screening has no net benefit."

- Free PSA: the use of serum free PSA for prostate screening has been proposed by some urologists as a means to decrease unwarranted biopsies without missing a significant number of prostate cancers. This approach is based on the higher free PSA in men with benign prostatic hyperplasia and the higher protein-bound PSA levels in men with prostate cancer. For example, in men with total PSA levels of 4 to 10 ng/ml, the cancer probability is 0.25, but if the percentage of free PSA is ≤17%, the probability of cancer increases to 0.45.

TABLE 1 Definition of Risk Groups

Risk Group	Clinical Stage	PSA (ng/mL)	Gleason Score	Biopsy Criteria
Low	T1a or T1c	<10	2-6	Unilateral or <50% of core involved
Intermediate	T1b, T1c, or T2a	<10	3 + 4 = 7	Bilateral
High	T1b, T1c, T2b, or T3	10-20	4 + 3 = 7	>50% of core involved or perineural invasion or ductal differentiation
Very high	T4	>20	8-10	Lymphovascular invasion or neuro-endocrine differentiation

From Wein AJ et al: *Campbell-Walsh urology*, ed 11, Philadelphia, 2016, Elsevier.

- PSA velocity: the rate of increase of serum PSA over time (PSA velocity) can aid in the diagnosis of prostate cancer. A yearly PSA velocity >0.75 ng/ml increases the likelihood of later malignancy when total PSA is still within normal range. Proper interpretation of PSA velocity requires at least three PSA measurements over an 18-month period because most PSA variations are physiologic. Recent trials have cast a doubt on the value of PSA velocity by showing that adding PSA velocity as a trigger for biopsy did not improve predictive accuracy beyond that of using PSA threshold values alone.
- Age-adjusted PSA: there is evidence that the current threshold of 4.0 ng/ml is inadequate for younger men, because in a recent study 22% of men with PSA levels between 2.6 and 4.0 were found to have prostate cancer. The concept of age-related cutoffs remains controversial. Lowering the upper limit of normal for PSA would improve sensitivity but decrease specificity.
- Prostatic acid phosphatase can be used for evaluation of nonlocalized disease.
- Prostate cancer gene 3 (PCA3) is overexpressed in prostate cancer cell, and high levels are suggestive of prostate cancer. Measurement of PCA3 in urine specimens collected after digital exams is helpful to make decisions about prostate biopsy in men with elevated PSA.
- Transrectal biopsy and fine-needle aspiration of prostate can confirm the diagnosis. Indications for biopsy include an abnormal PSA level, an abnormal DRE, or a previous biopsy specimen that showed prostatic intraepithelial neoplasia or prostatic atypia. The number of cores taken is patient specific, typically including a minimum of 10 cores. Prostate volume negatively affects cancer detection rate (23% in glands >50 cm^3, 38% in glands <50 cm^3).

IMAGING STUDIES

- Bone scan is useful to evaluate bone metastasis (present or eventually develops in almost 80% of patients). However, according to the American Urological Association (AUA), the routine use of bone scanning is not required for staging of prostate cancer in asymptomatic men with clinically localized cancer if the PSA level is ≤20 ng/ml.
- CT scan, MRI, and transrectal ultrasonography may be useful in selected patients to assess extent of prostate cancer. High-resolution MRI with magnetic nanoparticles has been used for the detection of small and otherwise undetectable lymph node metastases in patients with prostate cancer. However, according to the AUA, transrectal ultrasonography adds little to the combination of PSA and DRE. Similarly, CT and MRI imaging are generally not indicated for cancer staging in men with clinically localized cancer and PSA <25 ng/ml. With regard to pelvic lymph node dissection in staging, the AUA states that it

may not be required in patients with PSA levels <10 ng/ml and when PSA level is <20 ng/ml and the Gleason score is <6.

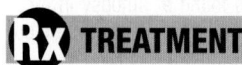 **TREATMENT**

NONPHARMACOLOGIC THERAPY

Watchful waiting is reasonable in selected patients with early-stage (T-IA) and projected life expectancy <10 yr or in patients with focal and moderately differentiated carcinoma.

ACUTE GENERAL Rx

- Therapeutic approach varies with the following:
  1. Stage of the tumor.
  2. Patient's life expectancy.
  3. General medical condition.
  4. Patient's treatment preference (e.g., patient may be opposed to orchiectomy).
- The optimal treatment of clinically localized prostate cancer is unclear. It is important to remember that all forms of treatment have potential adverse effects. Management requires careful consideration of the potential benefits and harms of intervention, the patient's age, health status, and individual preferences. Table 2 summarizes recommended treatment based on risk group and life expectancy.
  1. Radical prostatectomy is generally performed in patients with localized prostate cancer and life expectancy >10 yr. Radical prostatectomy reduces disease-specific mortality, overall mortality, and the risks of metastasis and local progression. The absolute reduction in the risk of death after 10 yr is small, but the

TABLE 2 Recommended Treatment

Risk Group	Life Expectancy (Years)	Recommended Treatment
Low	0-5	AS, HT
	5-10	AS, RT, HT, O
	>10	RP, RT, AS, O
Intermediate*	0-5	AS, HT, RT, O
	5-10	RT, HT, RP, O
	>10	RP, RT, O, HT
High*	0-5	AS, RT + HT, O
	5-10	RT + HT, HT, RP, O
	>10	RT + HT, RP + RT + HT, HT
Very high*	0-5	AS, RT + HT, O
	5-10	H, RT + HT, ST
	>10	RT + HT, RP + RT + HT, HT, ST, IT

*If there is more than a 20% probability of positive lymph nodes, AS, HT, ST + HT.

AS, active surveillance; HT, hormone therapy; IT, investigational multimodal therapy; O, others; RP, radical prostatectomy; RT, radiation therapy; ST, systemic therapy.
From Wein AJ et al: Campbell-Walsh urology, ed 11, Philadelphia, 2016, Elsevier.

reductions in the risks of metastasis and local tumor progression are substantial. Postoperative complications of radical prostatectomy include urinary incontinence (10%-20% depending on degree of neurovascular bundle and urethral preservation, patient age, and correct mucosal apposition) and erectile dysfunction (percentage >50% and varies with patient age, preoperative erectile dysfunction, stage of tumor at time of surgery, and preservation of neurovascular bundle). Lower complication rates occur in hospitals that perform a large number of prostatectomies. Fewer men will have postsurgical erectile dysfunction after unilateral or bilateral nerve-sparing surgery. In men undergoing prostatectomy, robotic-assisted laparoscopic surgery represents an alternative to open retropubic radical prostatectomy. Despite advertisements that suggest that there are fewer complications after robotic surgery, recent data show that sexual dysfunction occurs postoperatively in about 88% of patients who have undergone robotic-assisted or conventional prostatectomy and that incontinence problems are more prevalent (33%) with robotic surgery than with open retropubic radical prostatectomy (RPP) (27%). Trials have shown that prostatectomy is preferred over "watchful waiting" in patients with localized prostate cancer detected by PSA if the PSA level is >10 ng/ml. In this subgroup, the 10-year mortality is 48.4% with prostatectomy versus 61.6% with watchful waiting. In men who have low-risk disease (PSA level <10 mcg/L, stage <T2a, Gleason score ≤3 + 3), and <6% risk for prostate cancer–specific death at 15 yr, watchful waiting (WW) and active surveillance (AS) are reasonable and underutilized options.

  2. Radiation therapy (external-beam irradiation or brachytherapy with implantation of radioactive pellets [iodine-125 or palladium-103 seeds] into the prostate gland) represents an alternative in patients with localized prostate cancer, especially poor surgical candidates or patients with a high-grade malignancy. The efficacy of brachytherapy is comparable to external radiation. In patients receiving external-beam radiation, a total dose of 79.2 Gy (high dose) compared with a total dose of 70.2 Gy (conventional dose) has been reported to lower the risk of recurrence without increased risk of morbidity and mortality. Newer radiation treatments such as intensity-modulated radiation therapy (IMRT) and proton therapy are becoming increasingly popular and replacing the older technique of conformal radiation therapy over the past 10 years. Trials have shown that among patients with nonmetastatic prostate cancer, the use of IMRT compared with conformal therapy is associated

with less gastrointestinal morbidity and fewer hip fractures but more erectile dysfunction; IMRT compared with proton therapy is associated with less GI morbidity. Patients with localized prostate cancer and high risk for extraprostatic disease and disease recurrence (e.g., Gleason score ≤7 with multiple positive biopsy cores and clinical stage T1b-T2b) may benefit (increased overall survival) with the addition of 6 mo of androgen suppression therapy to radiation therapy.

3. Watchful waiting is reasonable in patients who are too old or too ill to survive longer than 10 yr. If the cancer progresses to the point where it becomes symptomatic, palliation can be attempted with several methods. Conservative management is also reasonable for patients with Gleason score of 2 to 4 because these patients do not have a shortened life expectancy and treatment is associated with long-term side effects. Watchful waiting also appears to be safe in older men with less-aggressive disease. Individual preferences play a central role in the decision whether to treat or to pursue active surveillance.

- Patients with advanced disease and projected life expectancy <10 yr are candidates for radiation therapy and hormonal therapy (diethylstilbestrol, luteinizing hormone–releasing hormone analogs, antiandrogens, bilateral orchiectomy).
- Recommended treatment of patients with regional metastatic prostate cancer with projected life expectancy ≥10 yr includes radiation therapy and hormonal therapy.
- Prostate cancer is an androgen-receptor-dependent disease, and the blocking of androgen-receptor signaling is an effective treatment modality. Table 3 summarizes major circulating androgens. Androgen deprivation therapy (ADT) is the mainstay of treatment for metastatic prostate cancer. Adverse effects of ADT include decreased libido, impotence, hot flashes, osteopenia with increased fracture risk, metabolic alterations, and changes in mood and cognition. Adjuvant treatment with luteinizing hormone-releasing hormone (LHRH) agonists (goserelin, leuprolide, or triptorelin) plus antiandrogens (flutamide, bicalutamide, or nilutamide), when started simultaneously with external-beam radiation, improves local control and survival in patients with locally advanced prostate cancer. Pamidronate inhibits osteoclast-mediated bone resorption and prevents bone loss in the hip and lumbar spine in

men receiving treatment for prostate cancer. Gonadotropin-releasing hormone (GnRH) receptor antagonists can be used for rapid medical castration of men with advanced prostate cancer. Degarelix is an injectable GnRH agonist useful to suppress testosterone in patients with prostate cancer who are not good candidates for LHRH agonists and refuse surgical castration. Assessment of bone density and treatment with once-weekly oral alendronate can prevent and improve the bone loss that occurs in men receiving ADT for prostate cancer.

- Docetaxel plus prednisone or docetaxel plus estramustine can be used in metastatic hormone–refractory prostate cancer. Newer treatments for hormone-refractory prostate cancer (castration-resistant cancer) include immunotherapy with sipuleucel and cabazitaxel, a microtubule inhibitor that interferes with cell mitosis and replication. Both agents can prolong survival but adverse effects can be severe and both agents are very expensive. Abiraterone is an oral agent that blocks biosynthesis of androgens by inhibiting CYP17, an enzyme required for androgen biosynthesis. It has been FDA approved for oral treatment, in combination with prednisone, of metastatic castration-resistant prostate cancer in patients previously treated with docetaxel.
- Enzalutamide is a newer nonsteroidal antiandrogen. Trials have shown it to be highly effective in extending survival in patients with metastatic castration-resistant prostate cancer. It can be used sequentially with other agents such as docetaxel, abiraterone, cabazitaxel, and immunotherapy. Radium-223, an alpha emitter, selectively targets bone metastases and has been found effective in improving survival in men with castration-resistant prostate cancer and bone metastases.
- The poly(adenosine diphosphate [ADP]-ribose) polymerase (PARP) inhibitor has shown a high response rate in patients whose prostate cancers were no longer responding to standard treatments and who had defects in DNA-repair genes.

CHRONIC Rx

- Patients should be monitored at 3- to 6-mo intervals with clinical examination and PSA for the first year, then every 6 mo for the second year, then yearly if stable. For patients who have undergone radical prostatectomy, a rising PSA level suggests evidence of residual or recurrent prostate cancer. Salvage radiotherapy may potentially cure patients

with disease recurrence after radical prostatectomy. Recent trials have shown that addition of 24 months of antiandrogen therapy with daily bicalutamide to salvage radiation therapy results in significantly higher rates of long-term overall survival and lower incidences of metastatic prostate cancer and death from prostate cancer than radiation therapy plus placebo.[1]

- Chest radiography and bone scan should be performed yearly or sooner if patient develops symptoms.

DISPOSITION

- Prognosis varies with the stage of the disease and the Gleason classification (see "Definition"). For patients between ages 65 and 69 yr at diagnosis and a Gleason score of 2 to 4, the probability of dying from prostate cancer 15 yr after diagnosis is 0.06 and that of dying from other causes is 0.56. If the Gleason score is 7 to 10, the probability of dying from prostate cancer increases to 0.72 and from other causes varies from 0.25 to 0.36.
- The ploidy of the tumor also has prognostic value; prognosis is better with diploid tumor cells and worse with aneuploid tumor cells.
- For grade 1 tumors, the extended 10-yr, disease-specific survival is similar for patients with prostatectomy (94%), radiotherapy (90%), and conservative management (93%); survival rate is better with surgery than with radiotherapy or conservative management in patients with grade 2 or 3 localized prostate cancer.
- Expression of the gene EZH2 has been identified as an important factor in the determination of the aggressiveness of prostate cancer. A recent study revealed that expression of the EZH2 gene may be a better predictor of clinical failure than Gleason score, tumor stage, or surgical margin status. Testing for EZH2 protein in prostate cancer tissue may be useful to determine prognosis and direct treatment.
- Preoperative PSA level and PSA velocity have prognostic significance. Men whose PSA level increases by >2.0 mcg/mL during the year before the diagnosis of cancer may have a relatively high risk of death from prostate cancer despite undergoing radical prostatectomy.
- Extraprostatic disease is detected at radical prostatectomy in 38% to 52% of patients and is associated with a risk of disease

[1]Shirley WV, et al.: Radiation with or without antiandrogen therapy in recurrent prostate cancer, *N Engl J Med* 376:417-428, 2017.

Source	Androgen	Amount Produced/Day (mg)	Relative Potency	Relative Potency/Amount Produced
Testes	Testosterone	6.6	100	15.2
Testes and peripheral tissues	Dihydrotestosterone	0.3	160-190	533-633
Adrenal glands	Androstenedione	1.4	39	27.9
Adrenal glands	Dehydroepiandrosterone	29	15	0.5

TABLE 3 Major Circulating Androgens

From Wein AJ et al: *Campbell-Walsh urology*, ed 11, Philadelphia, 2016, Elsevier.

TABLE 4 Common Pain Syndromes in Metastatic Castration-Resistant Prostate Cancer

Pain Syndrome	Initial Management	Other Therapeutic Alternatives
Localized bone pain	Pharmacologic pain management	Surgical stabilization of pathologic fractures or extensive bone erosions
	Localized radiotherapy (special attention to weight-bearing areas, lytic metastasis, and extremities)	Epidural metastasis and cord compression should be evaluated in all patients with focal back pain
		Radiopharmaceuticals should be considered if local radiation therapy fails
Diffuse bone pain	Pharmacologic pain management	Corticosteroids
	"Multispot" or wide-field radiotherapy	Bisphosphonates or RANK ligand inhibitors
	Radiopharmaceuticals	Calcitonin
		Chemotherapy
Epidural metastasis and cord compression	High-dose corticosteroids	Pharmacologic pain management
	Radiation therapy	Physical therapy for recovery of neurologic function
	Surgical decompression and stabilization are indicated in high-grade epidural compressions, extensive bone involvement, or recurrence after irradiation.	
Nerve plexopathies caused by direct tumor extension or previous therapy (rare)	Pharmacologic pain management	Tricyclic antidepressants (amitriptyline)
	Radiation therapy (if not previously used)	Anticonvulsants (gabapentin, pregabalin)
	Neurolytic procedures (nerve blocks)	
Miscellaneous neurogenic causes: postherpetic neuralgia, peripheral neuropathies	Complete neurologic evaluation	Tricyclic antidepressants (amitriptyline)
	Pharmacologic pain management	Anticonvulsants (gabapentin, pregabalin)
	Discontinuation of neurotoxic drugs: docetaxel, platinum compounds	
Other uncommon pain syndromes: extensive skull metastasis with cranial nerve/skull base involvement, extensive painful liver metastasis, or pelvic masses	Radiation therapy	Chemotherapy
	Pharmacologic pain management	Intrathecal chemotherapy may ameliorate symptoms of meningeal involvement
	Corticosteroids (cranial nerve involvement)	

RANK, receptor activator of nuclear factor-κB.
From Wein AJ et al: *Campbell-Walsh urology,* ed 11, Philadelphia, 2016, Elsevier.

recurrence, progression, and death. In these patients, adjuvant radiotherapy results in significantly reduced risk of PSA relapse and disease recurrence; however, the improvements in metastases-free survival and overall survival are not statistically significant. Table 4 summarizes common pain syndromes in metastatic castration-resistant prostate cancer.

- The Prostate Cancer Prevention trial revealed that the use of 5-alpha-reductase inhibitors lowers the incidence of prostate cancer but also increases the incidence of high-grade tumors (Gleason score >7). It is possible that these agents delay diagnosis of prostate cancer by lowering PSA levels and decreasing prostate size. The trade-off inherent

in using 5-alpha-reductase inhibitors for prostate cancer prevention is risk of one additional high-grade cancer in order to avert three or four lower-grade cancers. Based on these results, the FDA's Oncologic Drugs Advisory Committee concluded that finasteride and dutasteride do not have a favorable risk-benefit profile for chemoprevention of prostate cancer in healthy men.

- Patients undergoing prostatectomy are more likely to have urinary incontinence than those undergoing radiotherapy at 2 years and 5 years. However, at 15 years there are no significant relative differences in disease-specific functional outcomes among men undergoing prostatectomy or radiotherapy.

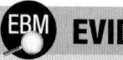 **EVIDENCE**

Available at www.expertconsult.com

SUGGESTED READINGS

Available at www.expertconsult.com

RELATED CONTENT

Prostate Cancer (Patient Information)

AUTHOR: **FRED F. FERRI, M.D.**

BASIC INFORMATION

DEFINITION

Benign prostatic hyperplasia (BPH) is the benign growth of the prostate, generally originating in the periureteral and transition zones, with subsequent obstructive and irritative voiding symptoms. Histologically, BPH refers to the proliferation of smooth muscle, epithelium, and stromal cells within the transition zone of the prostate that surrounds the proximal urethra.

SYNONYMS

Benign prostate hyperplasia
BPH
Prostatic hypertrophy

ICD-10CM CODES
N40.0 Enlarged prostate without lower urinary tract symptoms
N40.1 Enlarged prostate with lower urinary tract symptoms
N40.2 Nodular prostate without lower urinary tract symptoms
N40.3 Nodular prostate with lower urinary tract symptoms

EPIDEMIOLOGY & DEMOGRAPHICS

- 80% of men have evidence of BPH by age 80 yr.
- Medical and surgical intervention for problems caused by BPH is required in <20% of males by age 75 yr.
- Transurethral resection of the prostate (TURP) is the tenth most common operative procedure (<400,000/yr in U.S.).

- 10% to 30% of men with BPH have occult prostate cancer.

PHYSICAL FINDINGS & CLINICAL PRESENTATION

- Digital rectal examination (DRE) reveals enlargement of the prostate.
- Focal enlargement may be indicative of malignancy.
- There is poor correlation between size of prostate and symptoms (BPH may be asymptomatic if it does not encroach on the urethral lumen).
- Most patients with BPH report difficulty in initiating urination (hesitancy), decrease in caliber and force of stream, incomplete emptying of bladder often resulting in double voiding (need to urinate again a few minutes after voiding), postvoid "dribbling," and nocturia.

ETIOLOGY

Multifactorial; a functioning testicle is necessary for development of BPH (as evidenced by the absence in males who were castrated before puberty).

DIAGNOSIS

DIFFERENTIAL DIAGNOSIS

- Prostatitis
- Prostate cancer
- Strictures (urethral)
- Medications interfering with the muscle fibers in the prostate and also with bladder function
  - Opiates: impaired autonomic function
  - Decongestants: increased sphincter tone
  - Antihistamines: decreased parasympathetic tone
  - Tricyclic antidepressants: anticholinergic effects
- Neurogenic bladder
- Bladder cancer

WORKUP

Symptom assessment (use of American Urological Association [AUA] Symptom Index for BPH [Table 1]), laboratory tests, and imaging studies. Fig. E1 describes a diagnostic approach to patients with BPH.

LABORATORY TESTS

- Prostate-specific antigen (PSA): protease secreted by epithelial cells of the prostate; elevated in 30% to 50% of patients with BPH. Testing for PSA increases detection rate for prostate cancer and tends to detect cancer at an earlier stage. However, the PSA test does not discriminate well between patients with symptomatic BPH and those with prostate cancer, particularly if the cancer is pathologically localized and curable. The test may also trigger additional evaluation, including ultrasound biopsy of the prostate. Asymptomatic men with PSA levels >2 ng/ml do not need annual testing. According to the AUA, PSA testing and DRE should be offered to any asymptomatic man <50 yr with a life expectancy of 10 yr. PSA testing can also be offered at an earlier age in men at higher risk of prostatic cancer (e.g., first-degree relatives with prostate cancer; African American race).
- Measurement of "free" PSA is useful to assess the probability of prostate cancer in patients with normal DRE and total PSA

TABLE 1 International Prostate Symptom Score (I-PSS)

Symptom	Not at All	Less Than 1 Time in 5	Less Than Half the Time	About Half the Time	More Than Half the Time	Almost Always	Total Score
Incomplete emptying: Over the past month, how often have you had a sensation of not emptying your bladder completely after you finished urinating?	0	1	2	3	4	5	
Frequency: Over the past month, how often have you had to urinate again <2 hr after you finished urinating?	0	1	2	3	4	5	
Intermittency: Over the past month, how often have you found you stopped and started again several times when you urinated?	0	1	2	3	4	5	
Urgency: Over the past month, how often have you found it difficult to postpone urination?	0	1	2	3	4	5	
Weak stream: Over the past month, how often have you had a weak urinary stream?	0	1	2	3	4	5	
Straining: Over the past month, how often have you had to push or strain to begin urination?	0	1	2	3	4	5	
	None	1 Time	2 Times	3 Times	4 Times	5 or More Times	
Nocturia: Over the past month, how many times did you most typically get up to urinate from the time you went to bed at night until the time you got up in the morning?	0	1	2	3	4	5	

Total I-PSS score =

between 4 and 10 ng/ml. In these patients the global risk of prostate cancer is 25%. However, if the free PSA is >25%, the risk of prostate cancer decreases to 8%, whereas if the free PSA is <10%, the risk of cancer increases to 56%. Free PSA is also useful to evaluate the aggressiveness of prostate cancer. A low free PSA percentage generally indicates a high-grade cancer, whereas a high free PSA percentage is generally associated with a slower-growing tumor.

- Elevated measurement of prostate cancer gene 3 (*PCA3*) in urine specimens collected after digital exam is helpful in deciding about prostate biopsy in men with elevated PSA (increased *PCA3* = increased likelihood of prostate cancer).
- Urinalysis, urine culture, and sensitivity to rule out infection (if suspected).
- Blood urea nitrogen and creatinine to rule out postrenal insufficiency.

IMAGING STUDIES

- Transrectal ultrasound may be indicated in patients with palpable nodules or significant elevation of PSA. It is also useful to estimate prostate size. BPH may also be evident in suprapubic ultrasound and MRI.
- Uroflowmetry may be used to determine relative impact of obstruction on urine flow. Urethral pressure profile is useful to predict prostatic hypertrophy within the urethral lumen.
- Pressure flow studies, although invasive, are particularly helpful in patients whose history and/or examination suggest primary bladder dysfunction as a cause of symptoms of prostatism. They are also useful in patients for whom a distinction between prostatic obstruction and impaired detrusor contractility may affect the choice of therapy. However, pressure flow studies may not be useful in the workup of the usual patient with symptoms of prostatism.
- Postvoid residual urine measurement has not been proved useful in predicting the need for or response to treatment; it may be useful in monitoring the course of the disease in patients who elect nonsurgical treatment.
- Urethral cystoscopy is an option during later evaluation if invasive treatment is being planned.

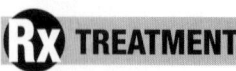
TREATMENT

NONPHARMACOLOGIC THERAPY

- Avoidance of caffeine or any other foods that may exacerbate symptoms
- Avoidance of medications that may exacerbate symptoms (e.g., most cold and allergy remedies)

GENERAL Rx

- Asymptomatic patients with prostate enlargement caused by BPH generally do not require treatment. Patients with mild to moderate symptoms are candidates for pharmacologic treatment (see the following). For patients who have specific complications from BPH,

prostate surgery is usually the most appropriate form of treatment. However, surgery may result in significant complications (e.g., incontinence, infection).

- Alpha-blockers (e.g., tamsulosin, alfuzosin, doxazosin, prazosin, terazosin) relax smooth muscle of the bladder neck and prostate and can increase peak urinary flow rate. They have no effect on the size of the prostate. Alpha-1 blockers are useful in symptomatic patients to relieve symptoms of obstruction by causing relaxation of smooth muscle tone in the prostatic capsule, urethra, and bladder neck.
- Hormonal manipulation with finasteride, a 5-alpha-reductase inhibitor that blocks conversion of testosterone to dihydrotestosterone, can reduce the size of the prostate. Usual dose is 5 mg qd. Treatment requires ≥6 mo for maximal effect.
- Dutasteride is also a 5-alpha-reductase inhibitor useful to decrease prostate size and improve urinary flow. In addition to inhibiting the isoform of 5-alpha-reductase located in the prostate, the medication inhibits a second isoform and reduces dihydrotestosterone formation in the skin and liver. Usual dose is 0.5 mg qd.
- Tadalafil 2.5 to 5 mg qd has been FDA-approved to treat patients with signs and symptoms of BPH and patients with both ED and signs and symptoms of BPH. Tadalafil can potentiate the hypotensive effect of alpha-blockers and should not be used in combination with alpha-blockers.
- The dietary supplement saw palmetto is commonly used for relief of symptoms of BPH. Recent trials using 160 mg of saw palmetto bid did not improve symptoms of BPH. This contrasts with the positive findings of many previous studies. Trials with higher dose-ranging protocols are currently in progress.
- TURP is the most commonly used surgical procedure for BPH. It is recommended for patients unresponsive to medical therapy who have renal insufficiency, recurrent UTIs, bladder stones, or gross hematuria. Transurethral incision of the prostate (TUIP), a procedure almost equivalent in efficacy, is limited to patients whose estimated resection tissue weight would be 30 g or less. TUIP can be performed in an ambulatory setting or during a 1-day hospitalization. Open prostatectomy is typically performed on patients with very large prostates. A prostatic urethral lift implant (UroLift) is now available for BPH. It is placed transurethrally at the site of obstruction to open the urethra by compressing the obstructing prostatic lobes and holding them permanently retracted with suture-based implants.
- Laser therapy for BPH is a less invasive alternative to TURP; YAG laser enucleation has minimal effect on potency, libido, or patient satisfaction with his sex life and is associated with retrograde ejaculation. However, recent studies indicate that at least in the initial 7 mo after surgery, TURP is moderately more effective than laser therapy in relieving symptoms of BPH.

- Transurethral needle ablation with radiofrequency to remove periurethral prostate tissue is being increasingly used in patients with prostate volume >60 mL and moderate symptoms. It has a low morbidity rate, but treatment failure is approximately 25% at 5 yr and <80% at 10 yr.
- Balloon dilation of the prostatic urethra is less effective than surgery for relieving symptoms but is associated with fewer complications. It is a reasonable treatment option for patients with smaller prostates and no middle lobe enlargement.
- Surgery need not be the treatment of last resort for most patients; that is, patients need not undergo other treatments for BPH before they can have surgery. However, recommending surgery on the grounds that a patient's surgical risk will "only increase with age" is generally inappropriate.

DISPOSITION

With appropriate therapy, symptoms improve or stabilize in <70% of patients with BPH.

REFERRAL

Urology referral for patients with severe or intolerable symptoms and for any patient suspected of having prostate cancer (10%-30% of men with BPH)

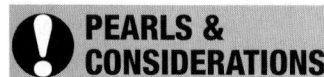
PEARLS & CONSIDERATIONS

COMMENTS

- Emerging technologies for treating BPH, including transurethral holmium laser enucleation, transurethral electrovaporization, and transurethral microwave thermotherapy of the prostate, appear promising; however, long-term effectiveness has not yet been demonstrated.
- The increase in the use of pharmacologic management has resulted in <30% reduction in the total number of TURP procedures.
- Combined drug therapy for BPH with an alpha-blocker and a 5-alpha-reductase inhibitor is superior to monotherapy with either agent.
- Saw palmetto extract is ineffective for BPH symptoms. Trials have shown that even at three times the standard dosing, saw palmetto extract had no greater effect than placebo on improving lower urinary symptoms associated with BPH.

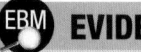
EVIDENCE

Available at www.expertconsult.com

SUGGESTED READINGS

Available at www.expertconsult.com

RELATED CONTENT

Enlarged Prostate (Patient Information)

AUTHOR: **FRED F. FERRI, M.D.**

BASIC INFORMATION

DEFINITION

Prostatitis refers to inflammation of the prostate gland. There are four major categories:
1. Acute bacterial prostatitis (type I).
2. Chronic bacterial prostatitis (type II).
3. Chronic prostatitis/pelvic pain syndrome (CP/CPPS) (type III): subdivided into type IIIA (inflammatory) and IIIB (noninflammatory).
4. Asymptomatic inflammatory prostatitis (type IV).

ICD-10CM CODES
N41.0 Acute prostatitis
N41.1 Chronic prostatitis

EPIDEMIOLOGY & DEMOGRAPHICS

- 50% of men will have symptoms of prostatitis in their lifetime.
- Prostatitis accounts for >8% of visits to urologists and 1% of visits to primary care physicians.
- The prevalence of chronic bacterial prostatitis is 5% to 10%.
- CP/CPPS is the most common of the clinically defined prostatitis syndromes, with prevalence ranging from 9% to 12% of men.
- Acute bacterial prostatitis accounts for 10% of all cases of prostatitis.

PHYSICAL FINDINGS & CLINICAL PRESENTATION

1. Acute bacterial prostatitis:
   ○ Sudden or rapidly progressive onset of:
      1. Dysuria.
      2. Frequency.
      3. Urgency.
      4. Nocturia.
      5. Perineal pain that may radiate to the back, rectum, or penis.
   ○ Hematuria or a purulent urethral discharge may occur.
   ○ Occasionally urinary retention complicates the course.
   ○ Fever, chills, and signs of sepsis can also be part of the clinical picture.
   ○ On rectal examination the prostate is typically tender.
2. Chronic bacterial prostatitis:
   ○ Characterized by positive culture of expressed prostatic secretions. May cause symptoms such as suprapubic, low back, or perineal pain; mild urgency, frequency, and dysuria with urination; and possibly recurrent urinary tract infections.
   ○ May be asymptomatic when the infection is confined to the prostate.
   ○ May present as an increase in severity of baseline symptoms of benign prostatic hypertrophy (BPH).
   ○ When cystitis is also present, urinary frequency, urgency, and burning may be reported.
   ○ Hematuria may be a presenting complaint.
   ○ In elderly men, new onset of urinary incontinence may be noted.

3. CP/CPPS:
   ○ Presents similarly with pain in the pelvic region lasting >3 mo. Symptoms also can include pain in the suprapubic region, low back, penis, testes, or scrotum.
   ○ The symptoms can be of variable severity and may include lower urinary tract symptoms, sexual dysfunction, and reduced quality of life.

ETIOLOGY

1. Acute bacterial prostatitis:
   ○ Acute, usually gram-negative infection of the prostate gland. *E. coli* is the most commonly isolated organism.
      1. Generally associated with cystitis.
      2. Results from the ascent of bacteria into the urethra.
   ○ Occasionally the route of infection is hematogenous or a lymphatogenous spread of rectal bacteria.
   ○ Consider *Neisseria gonorrhoeae* or *Chlamydia trachomatis* in young patients (age <35 yr) with risk of sexually transmitted disease (STD).
2. Chronic bacterial prostatitis:
   ○ Often asymptomatic. *E. coli* is the most commonly isolated organism.
   ○ Exacerbation of symptoms of BPH caused by the same mechanism as in acute bacterial prostatitis.
3. CP/CPPS:
   ○ Type IIIA: refers to symptoms of prostatic inflammation associated with the presence of white blood cells in prostatic secretions with no identifiable bacterial organism.
   ○ *Chlamydia* infection may be etiologically implicated in some cases.
   ○ Type IIIB: refers to symptoms of prostatic inflammation with no or few white blood cells in the prostatic secretion.
   ○ Its cause is unknown. Spasm in the bladder neck or urethra may be responsible for the symptoms.

DIAGNOSIS

DIFFERENTIAL DIAGNOSIS

- BPH with lower urinary tract symptoms
- Prostate cancer
- Interstitial cystitis/bladder pain syndrome
- Pelvic floor dysfunction
- Bladder cancer
- Urolithiasis
- UTI
- Proctitis

WORKUP

- Rectal examination:
  1. Tender prostate most suggestive of acute bacterial prostatitis.
  2. Enlarged prostate common in chronic bacterial prostatitis.
  3. Normal prostate is consistent with chronic bacterial prostatitis and CP/CPPS.
- Expression of prostatic secretions by prostate massage is contraindicated in acute

bacterial prostatitis but is appropriate in the other three situations.

LABORATORY TESTS

- Urinalysis.
- Urine culture and sensitivity.
- Bacterial localization studies can be performed but are cumbersome and impractical in most clinical settings.
- Cell count and culture of expressed prostatic secretions.
- Prostate-specific antigen (PSA) is not used to diagnose prostatitis and is not recommended unless a nodule is present on digital examination. A rapid rise over baseline should raise the possibility of prostatitis even in the absence of symptoms. In such cases, a follow-up PSA after treatment of prostatitis is appropriate.
- Complete blood count and blood cultures if fever, chills, or signs of sepsis exist.

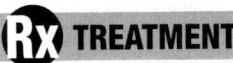 TREATMENT

1. Acute bacterial prostatitis:
   ○ Uncomplicated (with risk of STD, age <35 yr): ceftriaxone 250 mg IM × 1 dose *or* cefixime 400 mg PO × 1 *then* doxycycline 100 mg bid × 10 days.
   ○ Uncomplicated with low risk of STD: levofloxacin 500 mg qd or ciprofloxacin 500 mg bid × 10 to 14 days.
2. Chronic bacterial prostatitis:
   ○ First-line choice is a quinolone (ciprofloxacin or levofloxacin) for 4 wk.
   ○ Trimethoprim-sulfamethoxazole (TMP-SMX) is second-line choice for 1 to 3 mo if the organism is sensitive. Tissue penetration for TMP-SMX is not as good as quinolones, and there is evidence of increasing uropathogenic resistance.
3. CP/CPPS:
   ○ No specific treatment. A brief course of NSAIDs may be tried until urine localization cultures are completed. Alfuzosin may reduce symptoms in men who have not received prior therapy with an alpha-blocker.
   ○ Recent trials have shown modest improvement with quinolones (possibly secondary to their antiinflammatory and analgesic effects), but antibiotics are not generally effective and should be avoided in patients who are afebrile and have normal urinalysis results.

SUGGESTED READINGS
Available at www.expertconsult.com

RELATED CONTENT
Prostatitis (Patient Information)

AUTHOR: **FRED F. FERRI, M.D.**

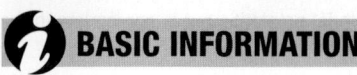

DEFINITION

Calcium pyrophosphate dihydrate crystal deposition (CPPD) disease refers to the precipitation of calcium pyrophosphate dihydrate (CPP) in connective tissues that may be asymptomatic or may be associated with several clinical syndromes, including acute and chronic arthritis. CPP was formerly abbreviated and commonly referred to as "CPPD" because the dihydrate is necessary for crystallization, but the abbreviation is now reserved for "CPP deposition." Alternative names representing specific clinical or radiographic features of CPPD disease include pseudogout, chondrocalcinosis, and pyrophosphate arthropathy.

Pseudogout/acute CPP crystal arthritis is used to describe acute attacks of CPP crystal-induced arthritis that clinically resembles the arthritis that is commonly encountered in urate gout. The term "acute CPP crystal arthritis" is now preferred in place of "pseudogout."

Chondrocalcinosis (CC) refers to radiographic calcification in hyaline cartilage and/or fibrocartilage and does not confirm the diagnosis of CPP-related arthritis as it can be present in other types of crystal deposition diseases or be asymptomatic.

Pyrophosphate arthropathy is the term used for a chronic structural arthropathy related to CPPD deposition.

SYNONYMS

Calcium pyrophosphate dihydrate crystal deposition disease
CPP crystal deposition disease
CPPD
CC
Chondrocalcinosis
Pyrophosphate arthropathy

ICD-10CM CODES
M11.2 Other chondrocalcinosis
M11.9 Crystal arthropathy, unspecified
M11.8 Other specified crystal arthropathies
M11.1 Familial chondrocalcinosis

EPIDEMIOLOGY & DEMOGRAPHICS

PREVALENCE:
- The epidemiology of CPPD crystal deposition is described in Table 1.
- Most linked with advancing age (average age of 72)

GENETICS: Associated with *ANKH* (ankylosis human) gene, which functions to transport inorganic pyrophosphate (PPi) out of cells. Familial mutations can increase extracellular PPi and lead to onset of CPPD disease in third or fourth decade of life.

PHYSICAL FINDINGS & CLINICAL PRESENTATION

- *Acute CPP crystal arthritis/pseudogout:* monoarticular attacks most commonly involve the knee but can be polyarticular. Patients, especially the elderly, can have systemic manifestations such as fever and altered mental status. Situations that may trigger acute CPPD crystal arthritis are described in Box E1.
- Asymptomatic disease ("asymptomatic CPPD")
- Pseudogout ("acute CPP crystal arthritis")
- Pseudo-RA ("chronic CPP crystal inflammatory arthritis"): symmetric polyarthritis
- Pseudo-OA, with or without superimposed acute attacks ("OA with CPPD")
- Pseudo-neuropathic joint disease
- Crowned-dens syndrome caused by crystal deposition in the ligamentum flavum of the cervical spine either asymptomatic or causing acute neck pain
- "Pseudo-polymyalgia rheumatica (pseudo-PMR)": pain and stiffness in the neck and shoulder girdle mimicking PMR

ETIOLOGY

- Idiopathic
- Familial
- Trauma
- Hemochromatosis
- Metabolic and endocrine disorders: hyperparathyroidism, hypophosphatasia, hypomagnesemia, Gitelman syndrome, gout, ochronosis, acromegaly, Wilson's disease, familial hypocalciuric hypercalcemia, X-linked hypophosphatemic rickets

TABLE 1 Epidemiology of Calcium Pyrophosphate Dihydrate Crystal Deposition

Age association	Rises with age
Sex distribution	(F:M) 1:1
Chondrocalcinosis prevalence	8.1% (age range 63 to 93)
Pyrophosphate arthropathy prevalence	3.4% (age range 40 to 89)
Geography	Appears ubiquitous
Genetic associations	Mutations of *ANKH* gene on chromosome 5p (CCAL2) and unknown genes on chromosome 8q (CCAL1)

From Hochberg MC et al: *Rheumatology*, ed 5, St Louis, 2011, Mosby.

DIFFERENTIAL DIAGNOSIS

- Gouty arthritis
- Septic arthritis
- RA
- PMR

Table 2 describes metabolic diseases predisposing to CPPD disposition. Section II describes the differential diagnosis of acute monoarticular and oligoarticular arthritis and crystal-induced arthritides. An algorithm for evaluation and treatment of CPPD is shown in Fig. 1.

LABORATORY TESTS

- Arthrocentesis with presence of weakly positive birefringent rhomboid-shaped crystals by compensated polarized light microscopy (Fig. E2)
- Synovial fluid should always be analyzed for cell count with differential, crystals, Gram stain, and culture because acute CPP crystal arthritis/pseudogout and septic arthritis can coexist.
- Evaluate for possible metabolic cause, especially in younger patients aged <55 yr or patients with florid polyarticular disease. Box 2 describes screening blood tests for metabolic diseases associated with CPPD crystal deposition.

IMAGING STUDIES

- Plain radiographs often reveal CC located parallel to subchondral bone.
  - Classic locations for CC (Fig. E3) include knee menisci (Fig. E4), wrist triangular fibrocartilage, symphysis pubis, and glenoid and acetabular labra.
- Musculoskeletal ultrasound can detect deposition of CPP crystals within the hyaline cartilage and/or fibrocartilage. In contrast to urate crystal deposits in gout, CPP crystals often deposit within the substance of the hyaline cartilage and fibrocartilage, providing a means to distinguish CPP from urate deposition that occurs on the surface of the hyaline cartilage as seen in gout (Fig. E5).

TABLE 2 Metabolic Diseases Predisposing to Calcium Pyrophosphate Dihydrate Deposition

	CC	Pseudogout	Chronic PA
Hemochromatosis	Yes	Yes	Yes
Hyperparathyroidism	Yes	Yes	No
Hypophosphatasia	Yes	Yes	No
Hypomagnesemia	Yes	Yes	No
Gout	Possibly	Possibly	No
Acromegaly	Possibly	No	No
Ochronosis	Yes	Yes	No
Familial hypocalciuric hypercalcemia	Possibly	No	No
X-linked hypophosphatemic rickets	Possibly	Possibly	Possibly

CC, Chondrocalcinosis; *PA*, pyrophosphate arthropathy.

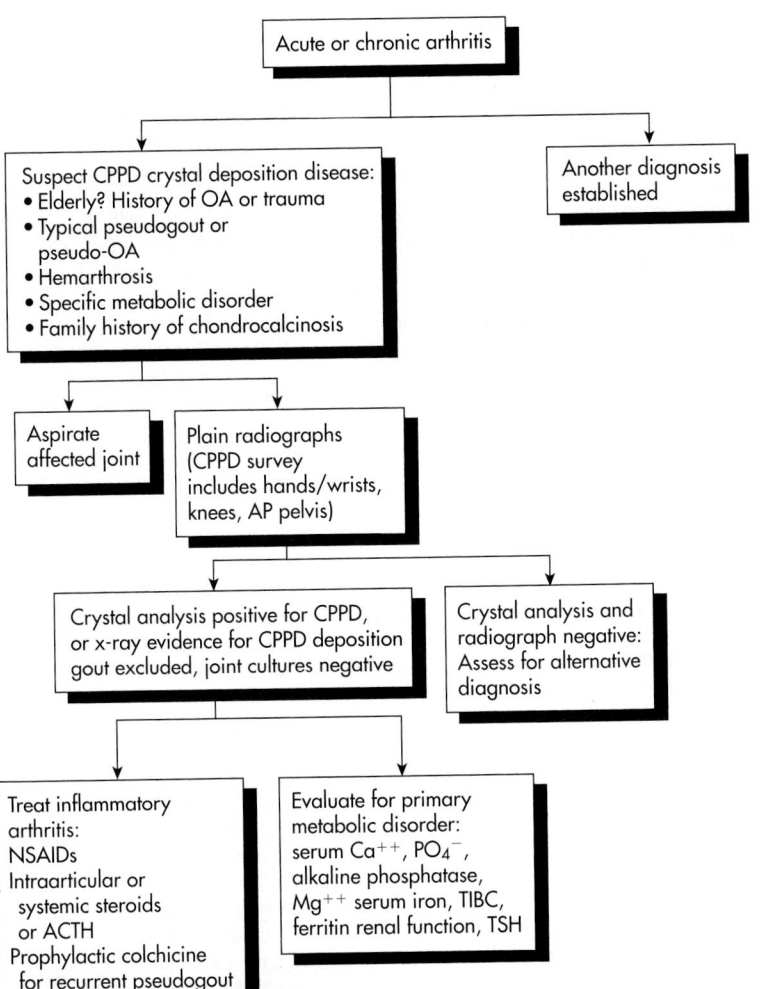

FIG. 1 Algorithm for evaluation and treatment of calcium pyrophosphate dihydrate disease. *ACTH,* Adrenocorticotropic hormone; *AP,* anteroposterior; *CPPD,* calcium pyrophosphate deposition; *NSAIDs,* nonsteroidal antiinflammatory drugs; *OA,* osteoarthritis; *TIBC,* total iron-binding capacity; *TSH,* thyroid-stimulating hormone. (From Harris ED et al: *Kelley's textbook of rheumatology,* ed 7, Philadelphia, 2005, Saunders.)

BOX 2 Screening Blood Tests for Metabolic Diseases Associated with Calcium Pyrophosphate Dihydrate Crystal Deposition

Calcium
Alkaline phosphatase
Magnesium
Ferritin, iron, transferrin
Liver function
Thyroid-stimulating hormone

From Hochberg MC et al: *Rheumatology,* ed 5, St Louis, 2011, Mosby.

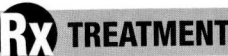 **TREATMENT**

P

Diseases and Disorders

NONPHARMACOLOGIC THERAPY
General measures such as immobilization of inflamed joint

ACUTE GENERAL Rx
- Monoarticular pseudogout:
  1. Aspiration followed by corticosteroid injection (often superior to systemic treatment in the elderly)
- Polyarticular pseudogout:
  1. Oral corticosteroids, colchicine, or NSAIDs, if not contraindicated.

CHRONIC GENERAL Rx
Prophylaxis: daily low-dose colchicine 0.6 mg twice daily or once daily as tolerated
- Pseudo-RA or refractory disease: hydroxychloroquine or methotrexate
- Anakinra (Interleukin-1 receptor antagonist): treatment and prophylaxis of polyarticular acute CPP crystal arthritis unresponsive to oral corticosteroids
- Treat underlying metabolic disease

DISPOSITION
Structural joint damage may occasionally occur, requiring arthroplasty in rare cases.

REFERRAL
Rheumatology

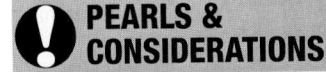 **PEARLS & CONSIDERATIONS**

COMMENTS
Acute CPP crystal arthritis/pseudogout attacks have been reported to occur in the setting of surgical procedures, diuresis, bisphosphonate administration, and hyaluronate joint injections.

SUGGESTED READINGS
Available at www.expertconsult.com

RELATED CONTENT
Pseudogout (Patient Information)
Gout (Related Key Topic)

AUTHORS: **NICOLE B. YANG, M.D.,** and **ANTHONY M. REGINATO, PH.D., M.D.**

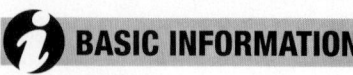

BASIC INFORMATION

DEFINITION

Psoriasis is a chronic skin disorder characterized by excessive proliferation of keratinocytes, resulting in the formation of thickened scaly plaques, itching, and inflammatory changes of the epidermis and dermis. The various forms of psoriasis include guttate, pustular, and arthritis variants.

ICD-10CM CODES
L40 Psoriasis
L40.4 Guttate psoriasis
L40.1 Generalized pustular psoriasis
L40.8 Other psoriasis
L40.9 Psoriasis unspecified
L40.54 Psoriatic juvenile arthropathy
L40.0 Psoriasis vulgaris

EPIDEMIOLOGY & DEMOGRAPHICS

- Psoriasis affects 1% to 3% of the world's population. Most patients have limited psoriasis involving <5% of their body surface.
- There is a strong association between psoriasis and human leukocyte antigens (HLAs) B13, B17, and B27 (pustular psoriasis).
- Peak age of onset is bimodal (adolescents and at age 60 yr).
- Men and women are affected equally.

PHYSICAL FINDINGS & CLINICAL PRESENTATION

- Approximately 85% of patients with psoriasis have mild-to-moderate disease.
- The primary psoriatic lesion is an erythematous papule topped by a loosely adherent scale. Scraping the scale results in several bleeding points (Auspitz sign).
- Chronic plaque psoriasis generally manifests with symmetric, sharply demarcated, erythematous, silver-scaled patches affecting primarily the intergluteal folds, elbows, scalp, fingernails, toenails, and knees (Fig. 1). This form accounts for 80% of psoriasis cases.
- Psoriasis can also develop at the site of any physical trauma (sunburn, scratching). This is known as Koebner's phenomenon.
- Nail involvement is common (pitting of the nail plate), resulting in hyperkeratosis, onychodystrophy with onycholysis.
- Pruritus is variable; soreness and bleeding may occur.
- Joint involvement can result in sacroiliitis and spondylitis.
- Guttate psoriasis is generally preceded by streptococcal pharyngitis and manifests with multiple droplike lesions on the extremities and the trunk.
- Adverse effect on psychological and social functioning, with affected persons often feeling stigmatized.

ETIOLOGY

- Unknown, but there is a strong genetic component and high heritability. There are at least nine chromosomal loci with linkage to psoriasis. These loci are called psoriasis

susceptibility 1 through 9 (PSORS1-PSORS9). PSORS1 locus in the major histocompatibility complex (MHC) region on chromosome 6 is considered the most important susceptibility locus and is believed to account for 35% to 50% of the heritability of the disease.
- Familial clustering (genetic transmission with a dominant mode with variable penetrants).
- One third of persons affected have a positive family history.
- A high prevalence of celiac disease has been noted in patients with psoriasis.

DIAGNOSIS

DIFFERENTIAL DIAGNOSIS

- Contact dermatitis.
- Atopic dermatitis.
- Stasis dermatitis.
- Tinea.
- Nummular dermatitis.
- Candidiasis.
- Mycosis fungoides.
- Cutaneous systemic lupus erythematosus.
- Secondary and tertiary syphilis.
- Drug eruption.
- Dermatomyositis (DM).
- Lupus erythematosus (LE).
- Seborrheic dermatitis.
- Pityriasis rosea.
- Lichen planus.

WORKUP

- Diagnosis is clinical. Blood work is rarely needed.
- Skin biopsy is rarely necessary.

LABORATORY TESTS

Generally not necessary for diagnosis.

TREATMENT

NONPHARMACOLOGIC THERAPY

- Sunbathing generally leads to improvement.
- Eliminate triggering factors (e.g., stress, certain medications [e.g., lithium, beta-blockers, antimalarials]). Severe emotional stress tends to aggravate psoriasis.
- Patients with psoriasis benefit from a daily bath in warm water followed by application of a cream or ointment moisturizer. Regular use of an emollient moisturizer limits evaporation of water from the skin and allows the stratum corneum to rehydrate itself.
- PUVA therapy (see "General Treatment").
- Local hyperthermia has been used successfully to clear psoriatic plaques, but relapse is common.
- Occlusive treatment with surgical tape or dressings is effective as monotherapy or in combination with topical medications.

GENERAL Rx

Therapeutic options vary according to the extent of disease. Approximately 70% to 80% of all patients can be treated adequately with topical therapy.

- Patients with limited disease (<20% of the body) can be treated with the following:
  1. Topical steroids: disadvantages are brief remissions, expense, and decreased effect with continued use. Salicylic acid can be compounded by pharmacist in concentrations of 2% to 10% and used in combination with a corticosteroid to decrease the amount of scale.
  2. Calcipotriene: a vitamin D analogue effective for moderate plaque psoriasis. Adults should comb the hair, apply solution to the lesions, and rub it in, avoiding uninvolved skin. Disadvantages include its cost and potential burning and skin irritation. It should not be used concurrently with salicylic acid because calcipotriene is inactivated by the acidic nature of salicylic acid. Taclonex ointment and enstilar aerosol foam formulation are a combination of calcipotriene and the high-potency corticosteroid betamethasone dipropionate. They are well tolerated and more effective than either agent used alone but also much more expensive.
  3. Tar products (Estar, LCD, Psorigel) can be used overnight and are most effective when combined with ultraviolet B (UVB) light (Goeckerman regimen).
  4. Anthralin: useful for chronic plaques; can result in purple-brown staining; best used with UVB light.
  5. Retinoids such as tazarotene 0.05%, 0.1% cream or gel, are effective in thinning plaques but are expensive and can cause irritation.
  6. Other useful measures include tape or occlusive dressing, UVB and lubricating agents, and interlesional steroids.
- Therapeutic options for persons with generalized disease (affecting >20% of the body) and for those with inadequate response to topical agents:
  1. UVB light exposure three times a week: this therapy does not require administration of a systemic drug (unlike psoralen plus ultraviolet A [PUVA]), but to be effective, it requires removal of scale with keratolytic agents and emollients.
  2. Oral PUVA administered two to three times weekly is effective for generalized disease. It is often considered in patients for whom narrow-band UVB therapy is ineffective. However, many PUVA treatments are required, necessitating frequent office visits, and it may be associated with phototoxicity, such as erythema and blistering, and increased risk of skin cancer.
- Systemic treatments include methotrexate 25 mg/wk for severe psoriasis. Etretinate (a synthetic retinoid) is most effective for palmar-plantar pustular psoriasis. Dose is 0.5 to 1 mg/kg/day. It can cause liver enzyme and lipid abnormalities and is teratogenic.
- Apremilast is a phosphodiesterase type-4 inhibitor used in moderate to severe plaque psoriasis. Side effects include diarrhea, nausea, headache, and worsening depression.
- Cyclosporine is also effective in severe psoriasis; however, relapses are common.

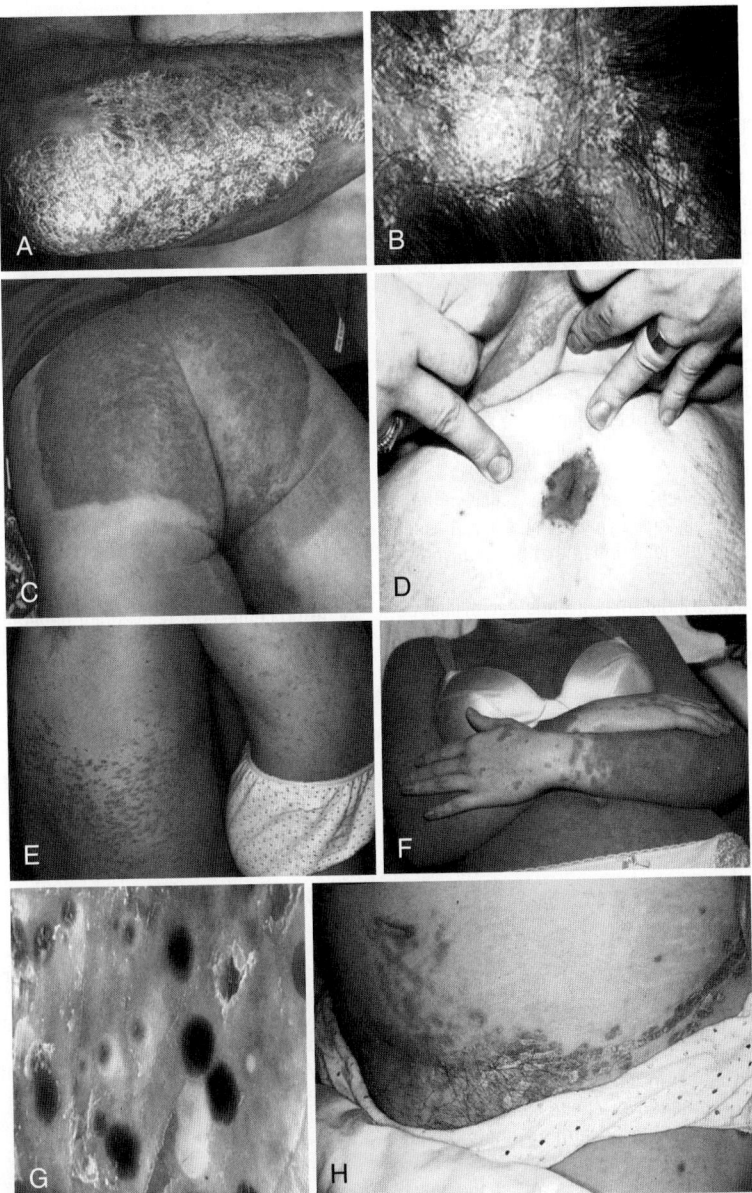

FIG. 1 Clinical phenotypes in psoriasis: plaque psoriasis (psoriasis vulgaris). A, At extensor surface of elbow and on scalp (**B**). **C,** Genital psoriasis. **D,** Inframammary and umbilical flexural psoriasis. **E,** Guttate psoriasis in a father and child. **F,** Erythrodermic psoriasis on the trunk and upper limbs. **G,** Pustular psoriasis on the foot. **H,** The Koebner phenomenon on a surgical abdominal wound. (From Firestein GS et al: *Kelly's textbook of rheumatology,* ed 9, Philadelphia, 2013, Saunders.)

24 wk can also lead to a reduction in severity of plaque psoriasis. Efalizumab, a humanized monoclonal antibody that inhibits the activation of T cells, has also been reported to produce significant improvement in plaque psoriasis treatment period. Adalimumab—a fully human, anti-TNF-alpha monoclonal antibody—has been reported to be effective for joint and skin manifestations of psoriasis.
- Newer biologic agents in patients with moderate to severe plaque psoriasis are ustekinumab (an interleukin-12 and interleukin-23 blocker), brodalumab, ixerizumab, and secukinumab anti–interleukin-17 receptor antagonists, and briakinumab, a monoclonal antibody against the p40 molecule shared by interleukin-12 and interleukin-23, which is overexpressed in psoriatic skin lesions.

DISPOSITION

The course of psoriasis is chronic, and the disease may be refractory to treatment.

REFERRAL

- Dermatology referral is recommended in all patients with generalized disease.
- Hospital admission may be necessary for severe diffuse or poorly responsive psoriasis. The Goeckerman regimen combines daily application of tar with UVB exposure and can result in prolonged remissions.

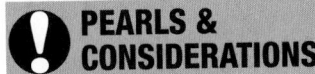 **PEARLS & CONSIDERATIONS**

COMMENTS

Psoriasis is more emotionally than physically disabling for most patients. Counseling may be indicated, particularly when it affects younger patients.

EBM **EVIDENCE**

Available at www.expertconsult.com

SUGGESTED READINGS
Available at www.expertconsult.com

RELATED CONTENT

Psoriasis (Patient Information)
Psoriatic Arthritis (Related Key Topic)

AUTHOR: **FRED F. FERRI, M.D.**

- Chronic plaque psoriasis may be treated with alefacept, a recombinant protein that selectively targets T lymphocytes. Treatment with alefacept for 12 wk (0.025, 0.075, or 0.150 mg/kg of body weight IV weekly) may result in significant improvement. Some

patients also demonstrate a sustained clinical response after the cessation of treatment. This medication is very expensive (a 12-wk course can cost >$8000).
- TNF inhibitors: Treatment with etanercept, a tumor necrosis factor (TNF) antagonist, for

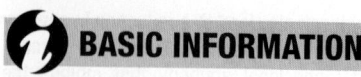

BASIC INFORMATION

DEFINITION

Psoriatic arthritis (PsA) is an inflammatory arthropathy occurring in association with cutaneous psoriasis. It is often included in a class of disorders called the *seronegative spondyloarthropathies,* a family of diseases characterized by inflammation of the spine, peripheral joints, and entheses (sites of insertion of tendon into bone). Classifications of psoriatic arthritis are described in Table 1.

ICD-10CM CODES
L40.5+	Arthropathic psoriasis
L40.54	Psoriatic juvenile arthropathy
L40.52	Psoriatic arthritis mutilans

EPIDEMIOLOGY & DEMOGRAPHICS

INCIDENCE: 6 per 100,000 per year in the general population
PREVALENCE: 0.1% to 0.2% overall, variable estimates of 7% to 30% of patients with psoriasis (psoriasis incidence varies by population but overall estimated prevalence of 1% to 2% of general population)
PREDOMINANT SEX: Equal male/female distribution
PREDOMINANT AGE: Symptom onset generally age 30 to 55 yr.

PHYSICAL FINDINGS & CLINICAL PRESENTATION

- Arthritis, dactylitis, spondylitis, and enthesitis occur in the setting of known psoriasis.
- Joint symptoms predate skin psoriasis in about 15% of patients.
- Arthritis is inflammatory in nature, commonly characterized by prolonged morning stiffness, joint erythema, warmth, or swelling including joint effusions.
- Distribution of joint involvement follows five classically described patterns (Box 1).

- Often more than one pattern will occur simultaneously, and patterns can evolve over time in an individual patient. Subtypes of psoriatic arthritis are described in Box 1. The distal interphalangeal (DIP) joints and spine are each affected in 40% to 50% of cases.
- Dactylitis refers to diffuse swelling of a digit, either finger or toe, which is typically the result of inflammation in both small joints of the digit as well as associated digital tendons. Dactylitis is common in psoriatic arthritis and occurs in approximately 30% to 40% of patients during the course of disease.
- Enthesitis commonly occurs at the Achilles tendon insertion into the calcaneus as well as the insertion of the plantar fascia. Findings on physical exam may include swelling and tenderness.
- Dystrophic changes of the nails (pitting, onycholysis, leukonychia may occur in association with joint inflammation in involved digits.
- Spondyloarthritis may include sacroiliitis, as well as inflammation of the axial spine, but is generally less likely to cause contiguous fusion to the extent seen in ankylosing spondylitis.
- Ocular inflammation including conjunctivitis and uveitis can also occur in some patients with PsA.

ETIOLOGY

Unknown

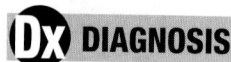 DIAGNOSIS

DIFFERENTIAL DIAGNOSIS

- Rheumatoid arthritis.
- Erosive osteoarthritis.
- Crystal arthritis including gout and pseudogout.
- Other seronegative spondyloarthropathies including reactive arthritis, enteropathic arthritis, and ankylosing spondylitis.
- The differential diagnosis of spondyloarthropathies is described in Section III.

WORKUP

- Diagnosis generally made on clinical grounds based on history, exam, and radiographic findings given lack of specific lab findings. An algorithm for the diagnosis of psoriatic arthritis is described in Fig. 1.
- Early diagnosis may be difficult to establish when the arthritis develops before skin lesions appear.

LABORATORY TESTS

- No specific/diagnostic lab tests
- Acute phase reactants such as ESR and CRP may be elevated, although less commonly than in patients with rheumatoid arthritis.
- Anemia of chronic disease may be seen.
- Rheumatoid factor (RF), while generally negative, can be present in >10% of patients.
- *HLA B27* is significantly more common in patients with axial inflammation (note that *HLA B27* positivity is present in up to 8% of general population).
- Arthrocentesis of active joint generally demonstrates inflammatory synovial fluid and absence of crystals.

IMAGING STUDIES

- Radiographic findings (Fig. E2) of involved joints may include soft tissue swelling, joint space narrowing, subluxation, erosive changes, and new bone formation such as periostitis and fusion.

BOX 1   Subtypes of Psoriatic Arthritis

Distal interphalangeal joint–predominant arthritis (10%) (Fig. 3).
Symmetric polyarthritis–predominant arthritis (5%-20%).
Asymmetric oligoarthritis or monoarthritis (70%-80%).
Axial disease–predominant (spondylitis and/or sacroiliitis) (5%-20%).
Arthritis mutilans (rare).

From Hochberg MC et al: *Rheumatology,* ed 5, St Louis, 2011, Mosby.

TABLE 1   Classifications of Psoriatic Arthritis

Moll and Wright	Classification Criteria for Psoriatic Arthritis (Caspar)*		
	Points	Category	Description
Presence of psoriasis and: An inflammatory arthritis (peripheral arthritis and/or sacroiliitis or spondylitis) The (usual) absence of serologic tests for rheumatoid factor	2	Current psoriasis or personal or family history of psoriasis	Psoriatic skin or scalp disease confirmed by dermatologist or rheumatologist; history of psoriasis from patient, family physician, dermatologist, rheumatologist, or other qualified practitioner; patient-reported history of psoriasis in first- or second-degree relative
	1	Psoriatic nail dystrophy on current physical examination	Includes onycholysis, pitting, and hyperkeratosis
	1	Negative for rheumatoid factor	Enzyme-linked immunosorbent assay or nephelometry preferred (no latex) using local laboratory reference range
	1	Current dactylitis or history of dactylitis documented by a rheumatologist	Swelling of entire digit
	1	Radiographic evidence of juxta-articular new bone formation	Ill-defined ossification near joint margins excluding osteophyte formation on plain radiographs of hand or foot

*Psoriatic arthritis is diagnosed when ≥3 points are assigned in the presence of inflammatory articular disease (joint, spine, or entheseal).
From Hochberg MC et al: *Rheumatology,* ed 5, St Louis, 2011, Mosby.

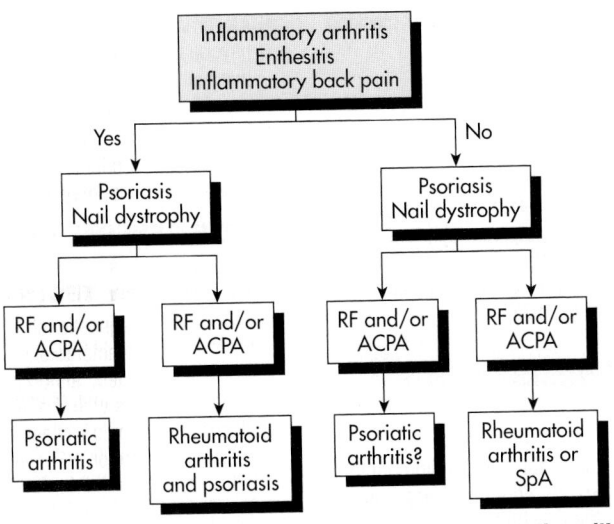

FIG. 1 Algorithm to be used in the diagnosis of individual patients presenting with possible psoriatic arthritis. Some patients may present with typical articular manifestations of psoriatic arthritis but in the absence of skin or nail disease. They can be diagnosed as having definite psoriatic arthritis only when psoriasis subsequently develops. *ACPA,* Anticitrullinated protein antibody; *RF,* rheumatoid factor; *SpA,* spondyloarthropathy. (From Firestein GS et al: *Kelly's textbook of rheumatology,* ed 9, Philadelphia, 2013, Saunders.)

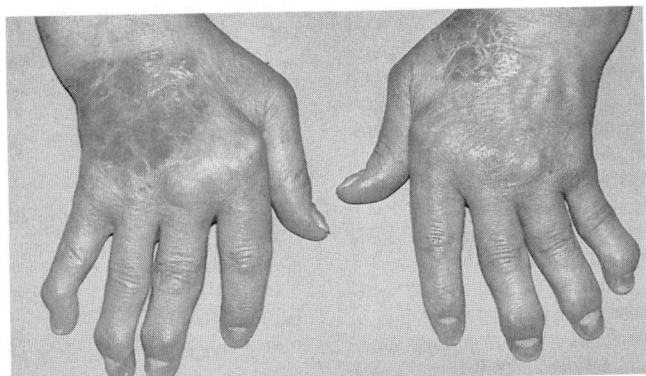

FIG. 3 The hands of a woman with symmetric polyarthritis. Initially this was indistinguishable from rheumatoid disease, but note the distal interphalangeal joint involvement, which is uncommon in rheumatoid arthritis, as well as the skin psoriasis. (From Klippel J et al [eds]: *Primary care rheumatology,* London, 1999, Mosby.)

- Severe digital erosive change with adjacent heterotopic bone formation may give rise to "pencil in cup" deformity seen in arthritis mutilans.
- Findings in patients with spondylitis may include sacroiliitis and development of vertebral syndesmophytes that often bridge adjacent vertebral bodies.
- Musculoskeletal ultrasound may be helpful in the evaluation of an inflamed enthesis or joint.
- MRI may be helpful in the evaluation of sacroiliitis or spinal involvement.

Rx TREATMENT

ACUTE GENERAL Rx
- NSAIDs may be used for mild symptoms or limited involvement.

- Intraarticular corticosteroid injections can be used as adjunctive therapy in involved joints.

CHRONIC Rx
The choice of therapeutic agents in psoriatic arthritis depends on the types of clinical manifestations by an individual patient as not all agents are effective for all types of clinical manifestations. For example, inflammation at the enthesis and spine are not responsive to traditional oral disease-modifying agents such as methotrexate or leflunomide but are responsive to tumor necrosis factor (TNF) blocking agents such as infliximab, adalimumab, and etanercept.
- NSAIDs may be used for mild or limited disease.

- In patients with several sites of active peripheral joint disease, elevated acute phase reactants, or with evidence of erosive changes on imaging, traditional DMARDs such as methotrexate, sulfasalazine, and leflunomide should be considered early in disease.
- In patients with peripheral arthritis who fail to respond to traditional DMARD therapy, additional therapy with a tumor necrosis factor (TNF) inhibitor should be considered. Current FDA-approved TNF inhibitors for psoriatic arthritis include etanercept, infliximab, adalimumab, golimumab, and certolizumab pegol.
- In patients with predominant axial disease not responsive to NSAIDs, anti-TNF therapy should be considered for initial disease-modifying therapy.
- Enthesitis and dactylitis are poorly responsive to oral DMARD therapy but, like spondylitis, will often respond to anti-TNF therapy.

Advanced therapies are now available for patients who fail to respond to oral DMARDs and anti-TNF treatment. Ustekinumab, a human IgG monoclonal antibody that binds to the p40 subunit of interleukin-12 and -23 and is responsible for T-helper-17 inflammatory cell suppression, and secukinumab, an IL-17 inhibitor, effectively treat psoriasis and psoriatic arthritis and are FDA approved as alternative biologic treatments for psoriatic arthritis in patients resistant to TNF-inhibitor therapy. Recent trials involving brodalumab, an anti-IL17RA monoclonal antibody and ixekizumab, an anti-IL-17 monoclonal antibody, have shown significantly positive response rates. Another agent recently approved is apremilast, an oral phosphodiesterase 4 (PDE 4) inhibitor that has been demonstrated to be effective in psoriatic arthritis.

REFERRAL
Rheumatology for confirmation of diagnosis and management

ⓘ PEARLS & CONSIDERATIONS
- Patients frequently have a positive family history of psoriasis or psoriatic arthritis.
- Severity of skin psoriasis and activity of inflammatory arthritis are frequently discordant.

SUGGESTED READINGS
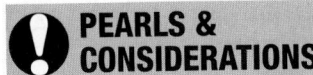
Available at www.expertconsult.com

RELATED CONTENT
Psoriatic Arthritis (Patient Information)

AUTHOR: **SYEDA M. SAYEED, M.D.**

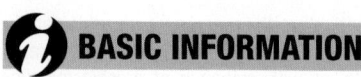

BASIC INFORMATION

DEFINITION

Psychosis is a state in which external reality is distorted by delusions and/or hallucinations (a delusion is a fixed false idiosyncratic belief; a hallucination is a false auditory, visual, olfactory, tactile, or taste perception).

SYNONYMS

Psychosis is a key finding in many mental illnesses, such as brief psychotic disorder, delusional disorder, schizoaffective disorder, schizophrenia, schizophreniform disorder, or shared psychotic disorder. Psychosis can also present as part of the evolution of a mood disorder (depression and bipolar disorder), a sign of an underlying medical condition, or a manifestation of a toxic state, i.e., abuse of substances or withdrawal state.

ICD-10CM CODES

F09	Unspecified organic or symptomatic mental disorder.
F10.5	Psychotic disorder due to psychoactive substance use
F05	Delirium not induced by alcohol and other psychoactive substances.
F06.0	Organic hallucinosis.
F32.3	Major depressive disorder, single episode, severe with psychotic features.
F30.2 and F31.2	Manic episode with psychosis and bipolar affective disorder with psychosis.

EPIDEMIOLOGY & DEMOGRAPHICS

One-year prevalence: 4.5 per 1000. The (demographics of) psychosis depends on the underlying disorder.

PHYSICAL FINDINGS & CLINICAL PRESENTATION

History:
- Past and current medical history important to identify potential medical etiologies.
- Medication use.
- Use of illicit substances or alcohol.
- Identification of functional and social impairment.
- Behavior that is odd or unpredictable; patient may be acting based on misinterpretation of their reality or false perceptions (delusions or hallucinations).

Examination:
- Examine for symptoms of:
  1. Mood disorder: delusions or hallucinations are usually congruent with the mood (e.g., auditory hallucinations in a depressed patient may tell the patient what a terrible person he is).
  2. Altered or disorganized thought pattern: usually reflected in disorganized speech (including word salad, thought blocking, rhyming, clang associations).
  3. Lack of insight into problems.
  4. Signs of Parkinson's disease, dementia.

ETIOLOGY

- Involves an interaction among:
  1. Dopaminergic overactivity (particularly in the mesolimbic, nigrostriatal, and mesocortical systems).
  2. Environmental, social, or childhood factors.
  3. Genetic predisposition.

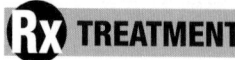

DIAGNOSIS

WORKUP

- Evaluate for potential confounding factors. Fig. 1 describes an algorithmic approach to evaluation of the psychotic patient.
- Underlying mental disorder: schizophrenia, major depression, brief psychotic disorder, delusional disorder, schizoaffective disorder, schizophreniform disorder.
- Underlying personality disorder: borderline, paranoid, schizoid, schizotypal.
- Underlying medical conditions: infections ranging from UTIs to HIV/AIDS, Parkinson's disease, Huntington's disease, leprosy, malaria, sarcoidosis, systemic lupus erythematosus, prion disease, hypoglycemia, postpartum state, cerebrovascular event, temporal lobe epilepsy, brain neoplasm.
- Medications: systemic steroids, anticonvulsants, antiparkinsonian medications, some chemotherapy, scopolamine.
- Underlying dementia: Alzheimer's disease, Lewy body dementia, vascular dementia.
- Illicit drugs (usually with chronic use; can be caused by intoxication or withdrawal): LSD, PCP, cocaine, gamma-hydroxybutyrate (GHB; withdrawal), alcohol, amphetamines, and marijuana. New substances of abuse (e.g., "bath salts," synthetic cannabinoids) may not be detected by current toxicology panels.
- Traumatic brain injury.
- Intensive care unit stay: hypoxia, decreased cardiac output, infection, medications, sleep deprivation, alteration of diurnal cycle, sensory deprivation or overload, pain.
- Emotional stress.

LABORATORY TESTS

Consider checking chemistry panel (calcium), complete blood count, UA, liver function tests, cortisol, HIV, rapid plasma reagin, thyroid-stimulating hormone, toxicology screen, lumbar puncture (LP).

IMAGING STUDIES

Consider chest x-ray (rule out sarcoid), electroencephalography, head CT or MRI.

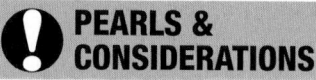

TREATMENT

Nonpharmacologic Therapy
- Cognitive-behavioral therapy.
- Social and behavioral skills training.
- Training for self-management of disease.
- Aforementioned strategies favored over psychoanalytic techniques given the relative inability for abstract thought and lack of insight in psychotic patients.
- Family intervention, including education and strategies to reduce emotional expression.
- Counseling for substance abuse.

ACUTE GENERAL Rx

- Antipsychotics, such as haloperidol and consider combining with anticholinergics like benztropine to reduce side effects if such arise; low doses should control first episode. Use with caution in elderly patients because adverse effects limit effectiveness. Second-generation antipsychotics are also useful starting with low doses. Alternative formulations are available; e.g., rapid injectable form or oral disintegrating tablets.
- Benzodiazepines if agitation is severe.
- Discontinue offending medication if present.

CHRONIC Rx

Second-generation antipsychotics may reduce the incidence of tardive dyskinesia but may increase incidence of metabolic disorders compared with first-generation antipsychotics. Multicenter trials showed similar efficacy between first and second generation. Consider economic factors, including insurance formulary, when selecting a maintenance regimen.

DISPOSITION

Prognosis varies according to etiology of psychosis. In general, the more severe and longer the psychotic episode, the worse the prognosis.

REFERRAL

Patient should be admitted for acute stabilization if actively psychotic to prevent harm to self and others as well as ensure administration of medications.

PEARLS & CONSIDERATIONS

- Delusions and/or hallucinations are hallmarks of psychosis.
- Rule out medical or drug causes of psychosis.
- Antipsychotics are the mainstay of acute and chronic treatment.
- Consider alternatives to antipsychotics in elderly or intellectually disabled patients (see "Nonpharmacologic Therapy").

SUGGESTED READINGS

Available at www.expertconsult.com

RELATED CONTENT

Psychosis (Patient Information)
Delirium (Related Key Topic)

AUTHORS: **ARNALDO A. BERGES, M.D.,** and **RICHARD J. GOLDBERG, M.D., M.S.**

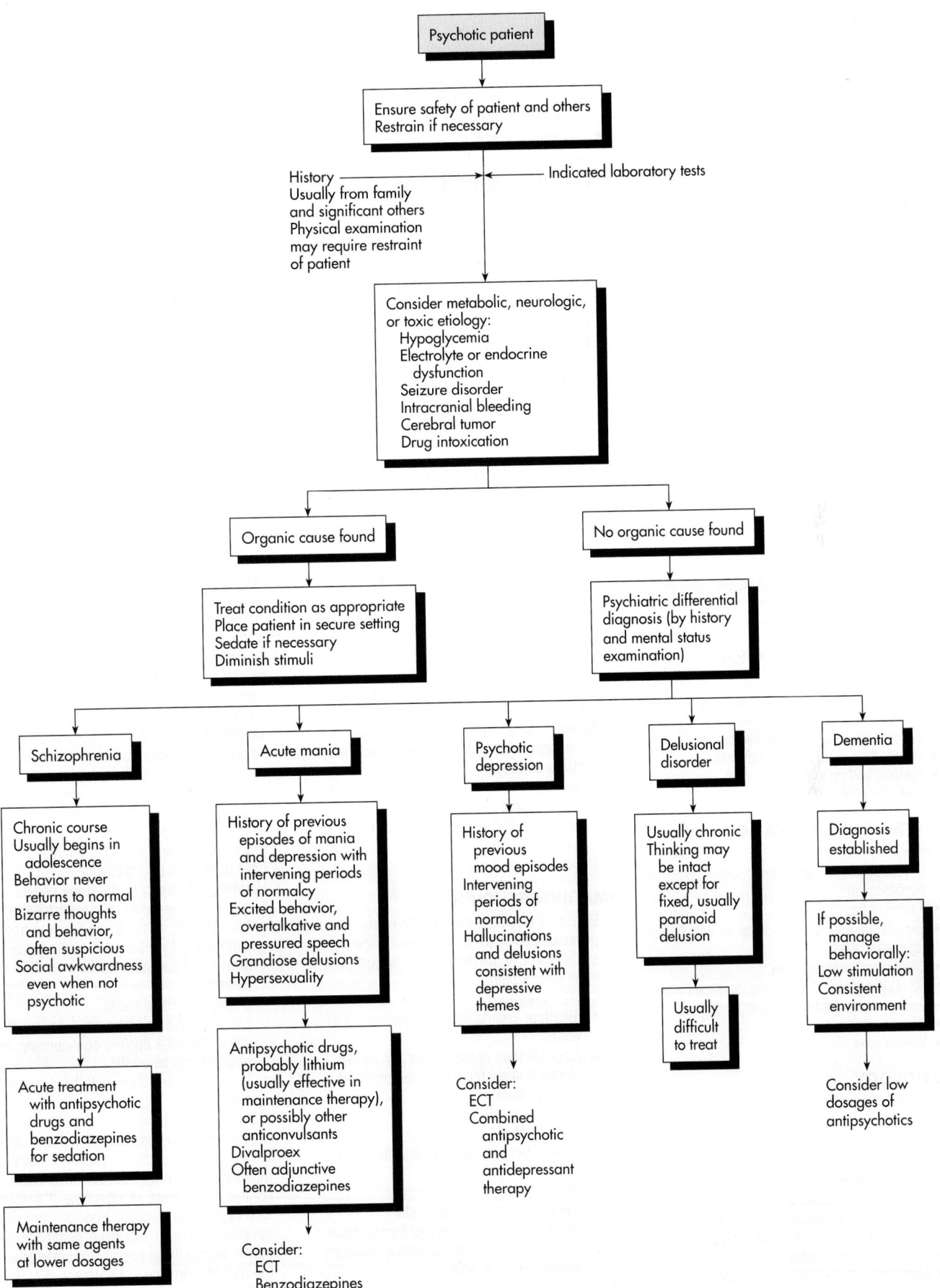

FIG. 1 Evaluation of psychotic patient. *ECT,* Electroconvulsive therapy. (Modified from Greene HL et al [eds]: *Decision making in medicine,* ed 2, St Louis, 1998, Mosby.)

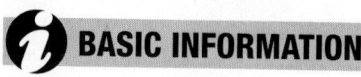

DEFINITION

Acute cardiogenic pulmonary edema (ACPE) is a life-threatening condition that may occur when there is elevated left ventricular (LV) filling pressure related to systolic or diastolic LV dysfunction.

SYNONYMS

CPE
Cardiogenic pulmonary edema
Acute cardiogenic pulmonary edema
ACPE
Acute heart failure (AHF) with pulmonary edema
Acute diastolic heart failure with pulmonary edema
Acute systolic heart failure with pulmonary edema

ICD-10CM CODES
I50.1 Left ventricular failure
J68.1 Pulmonary edema due to chemicals, gases, fumes and vapors
J81.0 Acute pulmonary edema
J81.1 Chronic pulmonary edema

EPIDEMIOLOGY & DEMOGRAPHICS

- Leading cause of hospitalization (6.5 million hospital days in the United States each year).
- In-hospital mortality rate is 10% to 20%, particularly when associated with acute MI.

CLINICAL PRESENTATION

- Altered mental status.
- Dyspnea (exertional or at rest, paroxysmal nocturnal dyspnea, orthopnea).
- Cough and wheezing (cardiac asthma).
- Diaphoresis, cold and clammy skin.
- Perioral and peripheral cyanosis.
- Pink, frothy sputum.

PHYSICAL EXAMINATION FINDINGS

- Hypertension (in cardiogenic shock could be hypotensive).
- Tachycardia.
- Elevated jugular venous pressure with hepatojugular reflex.
- Bilateral pulmonary rales.
- S3 gallop and/or S4/laterally displaced apex.
- Abdominal distention/ascites.
- Peripheral edema.
- Weight gain.

ETIOLOGY

Common causes of acute pulmonary edema include the following:
- Acute myocardial infarction.
- Poor dietary compliance or medication nonadherence.
- Atrial and ventricular arrhythmias.
- Valvular heart disease (mitral stenosis or regurgitation, aortic stenosis or regurgitation).
- Renal and liver disease.
- Endocrine (thyrotoxicosis, obesity, metabolic syndrome, diabetes).
- Toxic (cocaine, alcohol, chemotherapy agents, ephedra).
- Peripartum cardiomyopathy.
- Infections (myopericarditis, endocarditis, HIV, Chagas').
- Uncontrolled hypertension.
- Structural heart disease (ventricular septal defect, infiltrative heart disease).
- Pulmonary embolism.

DIAGNOSIS

DIFFERENTIAL DIAGNOSIS

- Noncardiogenic pulmonary edema (see Fig. E1).
- Viral pneumonitis and other pulmonary infections.
- Pulmonary embolism.
- Exacerbation of asthma.
- Exacerbation of chronic obstructive pulmonary disease.
- Sarcoidosis.
- Pulmonary fibrosis.
- Lymphangitic carcinomatosis.

LABORATORY TESTS

- Arterial blood gases (ABGs): respiratory and metabolic acidosis, decreased Pa_{O_2}, increased Pa_{CO_2}, low pH. (NOTE: The patient may initially show respiratory alkalosis as a result of hyperventilation in attempts to maintain Pa_{O_2}.)
- BNP and NT-pro BNP add diagnostic value to the history and physical examination as evidenced in the Breathing Not Properly [BNP] study.
- Cardiac biomarkers: troponin T or I if suspicion for acute coronary syndrome.
- Basic metabolic profile: hyponatremia indicates severe heart failure; renal impairment dictates therapy.
- Complete blood count: anemia can trigger acute pulmonary edema.
- Glucose, Hb A1C, fasting lipid profile, TSH for risk stratification.
- Urinalysis.

IMAGING STUDIES

- ECG: May elucidate the specific cause of the pulmonary edema. Causes may include ischemia/infarct, arrhythmias, LV hypertrophy, atrial enlargement.
- Chest x-ray (Fig. 2):
  1. Bilateral interstitial and alveolar infiltrates.
  2. Cephalization of the pulmonary vessels.
  3. Kerley B lines; fluffy perihilar infiltrates.
  4. Pleural effusions.
  5. Enlarged cardiac silhouette.
- Echocardiogram:
  1. Assess left and right ventricular systolic function.
  2. Determine diastolic dysfunction.
  3. Evaluate valvular abnormalities.
  4. Noninvasive assessment of hemodynamic status. E/e' >15 suggests capillary wedge pressure >15.
- Right heart catheterization (RHC): May be useful for tailored therapy in cardiogenic shock or for diagnosis in patients with unclear hemodynamics. PCWP and PA diastolic pressures are elevated, while the mixed venous oxyhemoglobin saturation is typically low. Pulmonary artery catheter failed to demonstrate benefit in overall mortality and hospitalization in the ESCAPE trial.

TREATMENT

ACUTE GENERAL Rx

Nonpharmacologic Treatment
- Heart failure teaching.
- Sodium restriction. Restriction in patients with American College of Cardiology/American Heart Association class C and D heart failure is controversial with conflicting data.
- Fluid restriction (1.5-2 L), especially in patients with hyponatremia.
- Risk factor modification (blood pressure control).
- Oxygen supplementation if signs of hypoxia.
- Noninvasive ventilation (continuous positive airway pressure [CPAP]) or bilevel noninvasive positive-pressure ventilation [NPPV]) reduces dyspnea and may reduce the need for endotracheal intubation. They improve oxygenation and lower carbon dioxide. Positive pressure ventilation (invasive or noninvasive) decreases preload and afterload and reduces the work of breathing, while positive end expiratory pressure improves oxygenation.

Pharmacologic-preload reducers:
1. Diuretics: initiate at a low dose and increase to achieve increased urine output or weight loss (0.5 to 1.0 kg daily). Furosemide is the most common diuretic. In the DOSE trial (*NEJM* March 3, 2011), there are no significant differences in global assessment of symptoms or in the change in renal function when diuretic therapy was administered by bolus as compared with continuous infusion or at a high dose as compared with a low dose. Torsemide and bumetanide tend to have better oral bioavailability.
2. Nitrates: particularly useful if the patient has concomitant chest pain or is hypertensive.
   a. Nitroglycerin: 0.4-0.8 mg SL or nitroglycerin spray may be given immediately on arrival and repeated multiple times if the patient remains symptomatic and blood pressure remains stable.
   b. 2% nitroglycerin ointment: 1 to 3 inches out of the tube applied continuously; absorption may be erratic.
   c. IV nitroglycerin: Start at 0.2-0.4 mcg/kg/min.
3. Morphine: 2 to 4 mg IV, SC, or IM; may repeat q15min prn. It decreases venous return, anxiety, and systemic vascular resistance (naloxone should be available at bedside to reverse the effects of morphine if respiratory depression occurs). However, potential adverse effects of morphine administration may outweigh these physiologic benefits, and the role of morphine in treatment of ACPE is controversial.

Pharmacologic-vasodilator therapy:
1. Nitroprusside: useful for afterload reduction in hypertensive patients.

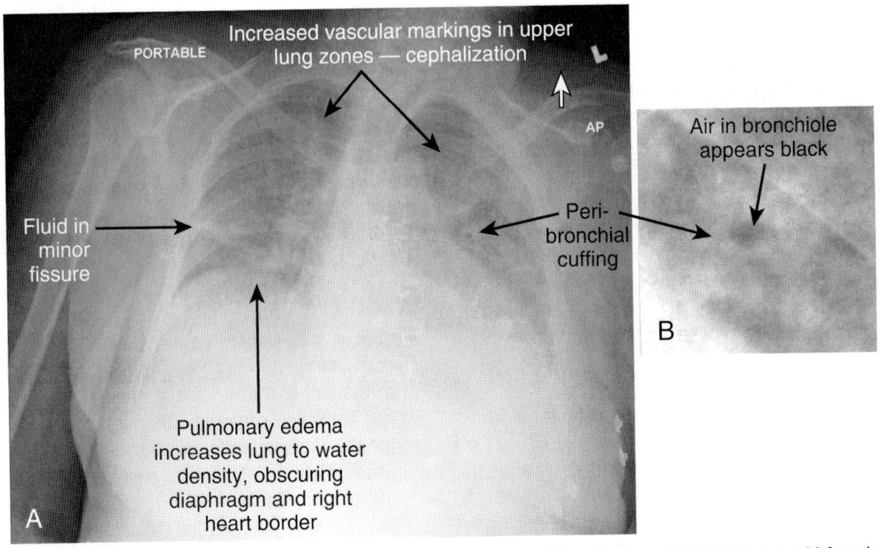

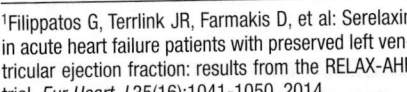

FIG. 2 Pulmonary edema. A, Anterior-posterior chest x-ray. **B,** Close-up from **A.** This 53-year-old female with end-stage renal disease missed dialysis and presented to the emergency department. Her examination demonstrated bilateral rales. Her x-ray shows mild cardiomegaly, bilateral interstitial opacities, and cephalization of the pulmonary vascular markings. The minor fissure appears thickened. These findings are consistent with pulmonary edema. In addition, peribronchial cuffing is present. As discussed elsewhere, this is a nonspecific thickening of the bronchial wall that can occur from edema in the setting of heart failure, asthma, viral illness, or even infections such as pertussis. The thickened wall appears white, whereas the air-filled bronchiole appears black and has a circular short-axis cross section. (From Broder JS: *Diagnostic imaging for the emergency physician,* Philadelphia, 2011, Saunders.)

a. Reduces left and right ventricular afterloads and thus improves left- and right-sided volumes.
b. Start at low dose 0.5 µg/kg/min with an arterial line in place.
c. Monitor for cyanide toxicity.
2. Nesiritide (recombinant human BNP), a potent vasodilator in the venous and arterial vessels, including coronary vasculature, produces significant reduction in venous and ventricular filling pressures and mildly increases cardiac output. However, its high cost and potential safety concerns, including increased mortality, have limited its use.
3. Serelaxin, an experimental drug, which is a recombinant form of relaxin-2, increases production of NO and binds to endothelial B receptor on endothelial cells causing vasodilation. It can be used effectively for pulmonary edema from both systolic and diastolic heart failure.[1]
Pharmacologic-vasopressors
Patients with profound hypotension benefit from vasopressors.
1. Norepinephrine: It is a powerful vasoconstrictor with small inotropic effect.

2. Dopamine: Low doses (0.5-3 µg/kg/min) increase blood flow to coronary, renal, and cerebral beds. Intermediate doses (3-10 µg/kg/min) increase cardiac contractility. High doses (10-20 µg/kg/min) have a pressor effect. Neither low-dose dopamine nor nesiritide improved diuresis or renal function when added to standard diuretics in ROSE-AHF trial.[2] In the treatment of shock, dopamine is associated with more arrhythmias (SOAP II trial).
Pharmacologic-Inotropes
1. Dobutamine: potent inotrope, mild chronotropic effects. Dose ranges from 2.5 to 20 mcg/kg/min.
2. Phosphodiesterase inhibitors (amrinone, milrinone, and enoximone [not available in U.S.]) may be useful in refractory cases. Milrinone may be associated with increased hypotension and new atrial arrhythmias with increased mortality in patients with ischemia.
3. Levosimendan is a novel agent that increases myocardial contractility and produces peripheral vasodilation through calcium sensitization. In REVIVE-II and SURVIVE trials, levosimendan has been shown to sig-

nificantly increase cardiac output, reduce PCWP and afterload, and improve dyspnea compared with standard care.
4. Potential future therapies: istaroxime, natriuretic peptides, adenosine antagonists, vasopressin antagonists, endothelin antagonists.
Mechanical support:
1. Intraaortic balloon pump (IABP): decreases afterload, increases coronary blood flow. The IABP-SHOCK II trial failed to demonstrate reduction in all-cause mortality in patients with cardiogenic shock.
2. Impella: Axial-flow pump on a pigtail catheter that crosses the aortic valve and unloads the left ventricle. It has been shown to improve hemodynamics.
3. Tandem heart device: Oxygenated blood is pumped into the femoral artery. It can provide 3.5-4.5 L/min of cardiac output.
4. Extracorporeal membrane oxygenation: destination therapy or bridge to transplant.
5. Ultrafiltration/aquapheresis if diuretic resistant.

DISPOSITION
Admit to ICU/CCU if:
1. Need for intubation.
2. Signs and symptoms of hypoperfusion.
3. SpO$_2$ <90% despite supplemental oxygen.
4. Use of accessory muscles/RR >25/min
5. Heart rate <40 or >130, SBP <90

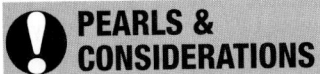
PEARLS & CONSIDERATIONS

COMMENTS
Accumulated evidence still favors the use of noninvasive ventilation, especially CPAP, in patients with ACPE, especially as this therapy reduces dyspnea and helps correct metabolic abnormalities more rapidly than standard oxygen therapy. The role of morphine in the treatment of ACPE has come into question.

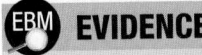
EVIDENCE

Available at www.expertconsult.com

SUGGESTED READINGS
Available at www.expertconsult.com

RELATED CONTENT
Heart Failure (Related Key Topic)

AUTHOR: **MAXWELL EYRAM AFARI, M.D.**

[1]Filippatos G, Terrlink JR, Farmakis D, et al: Serelaxin in acute heart failure patients with preserved left ventricular ejection fraction: results from the RELAX-AHF trial. *Eur Heart J* 35(16):1041-1050, 2014.

[2]Chen HH et al: Low-dose dopamine or low-dose nesiritide in acute heart failure with renal dysfunction: the ROSE acute heart failure randomized trial, *JAMA* 310(23):2533-2543, 2013.

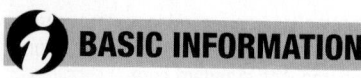

BASIC INFORMATION

DEFINITION

Pulmonary embolism (PE) refers to the lodging of a thrombus or other embolic material from a distant site in the pulmonary circulation. A classification of acute pulmonary embolism is described in Table 1.

SYNONYMS

Pulmonary thromboembolism
PE

ICD-10CM CODES

I26	Pulmonary embolism
I26.01	Septic pulmonary embolism with acute cor pulmonale
I26.09	Other pulmonary embolism with acute cor pulmonale
I26.90	Septic pulmonary embolism without acute cor pulmonale
I26.99	Other pulmonary embolism without acute cor pulmonale
I27.82	Chronic pulmonary embolism
Z86.711	Personal history of pulmonary embolism

EPIDEMIOLOGY & DEMOGRAPHICS

- 650,000 cases of PE occur in the U.S. each year (increased incidence in women and with advanced age); annually, as many as 100,000 people in the U.S. die from acute PE, and the diagnosis is often not made until after autopsy. The incidence of PE is increasing with the increasing use of spiral CT scans, with a lower severity of illness and lower mortality, suggesting the increase is caused by earlier diagnosis.
- More than 90% of pulmonary emboli originate in the deep venous system of the lower extremities.
- Pulmonary thromboembolism is associated with >200,000 hospitalizations. 8% to 10% of victims of PE die within the first hr.

PHYSICAL FINDINGS & CLINICAL PRESENTATION

- Most common symptom: dyspnea (82%-85%).
- Tachypnea (30%-60%).
- Cough (30%-40%)
- Wheezing (20%)
- Chest pain: may be nonpleuritic or pleuritic (infarction) (40%-49%).
- Syncope (massive PE) (10%-14%).
- Fever, diaphoresis, apprehension.
- Hemoptysis (2%).
- Evidence of DVT may be present (e.g., swelling and tenderness of extremities).
- Cardiac examination may reveal: tachycardia (23%), increased pulmonic component of S2, murmur of tricuspid insufficiency, right ventricular heave, right-sided S3.
- Pulmonary examination: may demonstrate rales, localized wheezing, friction rub.

ETIOLOGY

- Thrombus, fat, or other foreign material
- Risk factors for PE:
  1. Prolonged immobilization, reduced mobility.
  2. Postoperative state, major surgery.
  3. Trauma to lower extremities, immobilizer, or cast.
  4. Estrogen-containing birth control pills, hormone replacement therapy.
  5. Prior history of DVT or PE.
  6. CHF.
  7. Pregnancy and early puerperium.
  8. Visceral cancer (lung, pancreas, alimentary and genitourinary tracts).
  9. Spinal cord injury.
  10. Advanced age.
  11. Obesity.
  12. Hematologic disease (e.g., factor V Leiden mutation, antithrombin III deficiency, protein C deficiency, protein S deficiency, lupus anticoagulant, polycythemia vera, dysfibrinogenemia, paroxysmal nocturnal hemoglobinuria, acquired protein C resistance without factor V Leiden, G20210A prothrombin mutation).
  13. COPD, diabetes mellitus, acute medical illness.
  14. Prolonged air travel.
  15. Central venous catheterization.
  16. Autoimmune diseases (SLE, IBD, RA).

DIAGNOSIS

DIFFERENTIAL DIAGNOSIS

- Myocardial infarction.
- Pericarditis.
- Pneumonia.
- Pneumothorax.
- Chest wall pain.
- GI abnormalities (e.g., peptic ulcer, esophageal rupture, gastritis).
- CHF
- Pleuritis.
- Anxiety disorder with hyperventilation.
- Pericardial tamponade.
- Dissection of aorta.
- Asthma.

WORKUP

- Clinical assessment alone is insufficient to diagnose or rule out PE. It is also important to remember that no single noninvasive test has both high sensitivity and high specificity for PE. Consequently, in addition to clinical assessment, most patients require an imaging test to diagnose PE. Figs. 1 and 2 are diagnostic algorithms for suspected PE. The Wells prediction rules can be used to estimate the probability of PE. Each of the following findings is assigned a score:
  1. Clinical signs/symptoms of deep vein thrombosis (score = 3.0).
  2. No alternate diagnosis as likely or more likely than PE (score = 3.0).
  3. Heart rate >100/min (score = 1.5).
  4. Immobilization or surgery in last 4 weeks (score = 1.5).
  5. Previous history of DVT or PE (score = 1.5).
  6. Hemoptysis (score = 1.0).
  7. Cancer actively treated within last 6 months (score = 1.0).
- The probability of PE is high if total score is >6, moderate if 2-6; and low if <2.
- The modified Wells score divides PE as likely (>4 points) or unlikely (<4 points).
- A low clinical probability of PE in association with a normal plasma D-dimer measurement essentially rules out PE, and further imaging is not needed. If clinical probability is intermediate or high, and/or the D-dimer measurement is abnormal, further workup with imaging is needed.
- CT pulmonary angiography (CTPA) (see Fig. 3) is an excellent diagnostic modality (83% sensitivity and 96% specificity).
- V/Q scan is reserved for patients with clinically significant contrast allergies or renal insufficiency, or when CTPA is not available.
- Pulmonary angiogram (gold standard) can confirm the diagnosis, but is rarely used.
- Serial compressive duplex ultrasonography of lower extremities can be used in patients with "low-probability" lung scan and high clinical suspicion (see "Imaging Studies"). It is useful if positive; negative results do not exclude PE.

LABORATORY TESTS

- ABGs may reveal hypoxemia and respiratory alkalosis (decreased Pao_2 and $Paco_2$ and increased pH); normal results do not rule out PE.
- Alveolar-arteriolar (A-a) oxygen gradient, a measure of the difference in oxygen concentration between alveoli and arterial blood, may be elevated. However, a normal A-a gradient does not rule out PE.

TABLE 1 Classification of Acute Pulmonary Embolism

Classification	Presentation	Therapy
Massive PE	Systolic blood pressure <90 mm Hg or poor tissue perfusion or multisystem organ failure plus right or left main pulmonary artery thrombus or "high clot burden"	Thrombolysis or embolectomy or inferior vena caval filter plus anticoagulation
Submassive PE	Hemodynamically stable but moderate or severe right ventricular dysfunction or enlargement	Addition of thrombolysis, embolectomy, or filter remains controversial
Small to moderate PE	Normal hemodynamics and normal right ventricular size and function	Anticoagulation

From Bonow RO et al: *Heart disease*, ed 9, Philadelphia, 2012, Saunders.

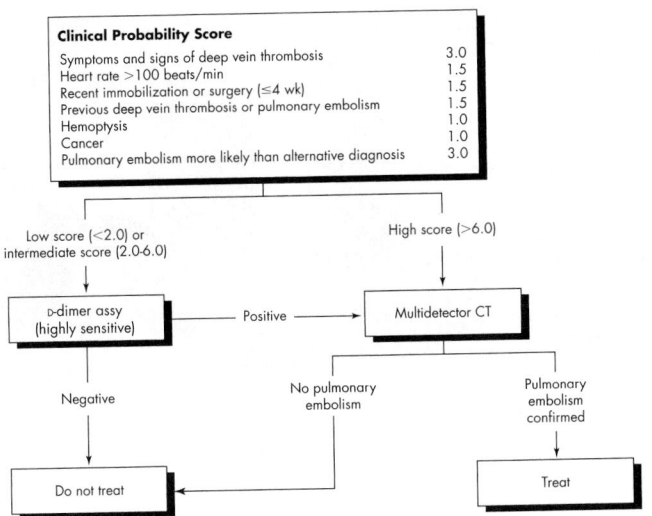

FIG. 1 Diagnostic algorithm for suspected pulmonary embolism in a patient without hypotension or shock. This assessment of clinical probability is based on the Wells score (which has a range of 0 to 12.5, with higher scores indicating higher clinical probability). The revised Geneva score may be used as an alternative. If a moderately sensitive latex-derived D-dimer assay is used instead of the highly sensitive enzyme-linked immunosorbent D-dimer assay, pulmonary embolism can be ruled out only in patients with a low clinical probability. Alternatively, the Wells score can be dichotomized, classifying pulmonary embolism as unlikely (≤4.0) or likely (>4.0). For patients in whom pulmonary embolism is considered unlikely, either a highly sensitive or a moderately sensitive D-dimer assay can be used to rule out the diagnosis without need for further testing. If multidetector CT pulmonary angiography, with or without venography, is negative in a patient with a high clinical probability, the possibility of a false-negative result should be considered and further testing performed to rule out pulmonary embolism. Options include serial venous ultrasonography, ventilation-perfusion lung scanning, and pulmonary angiography. If a multidetector CT scan shows only subsegmental defects in a patient with a low clinical probability, the possibility of a false-positive result should be considered, and further testing (e.g., venous ultrasonography) should be performed to confirm the diagnosis. This may also apply to patients with an intermediate clinical probability, although the need for further tests is less well established for these patients. (From Konstantinides S: Acute pulmonary embolism, *N Engl J Med* 359:2804-2813, 2008.)

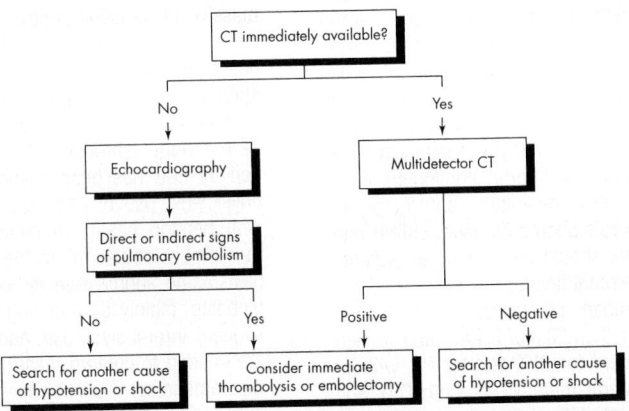

FIG. 2 Emergency diagnostic workup for suspected pulmonary embolism in a patient with hypotension or shock. A direct sign of pulmonary embolism on a transthoracic or transesophageal echocardiogram is the presence of thrombi in the right atrium, right ventricle, or pulmonary artery. Thrombi may protrude into the left atrium through a patent foramen ovale. Indirect signs include right ventricular dysfunction (identified by the finding of dilation, free-wall hypokinesia, or paradoxical septal wall motion); a systolic pressure gradient between the right ventricle and the right atrium of more than 30 mm Hg; and a pulmonary arterial flow acceleration time of less than 80 msec. When direct or indirect signs of pulmonary embolism are present, immediate treatment (without further diagnostic tests) is justified, particularly if CT angiography is still not available and arterial hypotension or shock persists. Adapted from the 2008 Guidelines on the Diagnosis and Management of Acute Pulmonary Embolism of the European Society of Cardiology. Since validation of diagnostic algorithms in prospective trials excluded hemodynamically unstable patients, these recommendations reflect expert opinion. (From Konstantinides S: Acute pulmonary embolism, *N Engl J Med* 359:2804-2813, 2008.)

- High-sensitivity plasma D-dimer measurement: D-dimer assays by ELISA detect the presence of plasmin-mediated degradation products of fibrin that contain cross-linked D fragments in the whole blood or plasma. A normal plasma D-dimer level is useful to exclude PE in patients with a low pretest probability of PE. However, it cannot be used to "rule in" the diagnosis because it increases with many other disorders (e.g., metastatic cancer, trauma, sepsis, postoperative state). Plasma D-dimer can also be used in conjunction with lower-extremity compression ultrasonography in patients with indeterminate V/Q and spiral CT scans. Absence of DVT and presence of a normal D-dimer level in these settings generally rules out clinically significant PE.
- Elevated cardiac troponin levels also occur in patients with PE because of right ventricular dilation and myocardial injury; therefore, PE should be considered in the differential diagnosis of all patients presenting with chest pain or dyspnea and elevated cardiac troponin levels.
- Elevated serum BNP levels in patients with acute PE may reflect RV overload.
- ECG is abnormal in 85% of patients with acute PE. Frequent abnormalities are sinus tachycardia; nonspecific ST-segment or T-wave changes; S-1, Q-3, T-3 pattern (10% of patients); S-1, S-2, S-3 pattern; T-wave inversion in V_1 to V_6; acute RBBB; new-onset atrial fibrillation; ST segment depression in lead II; right ventricular strain. A right ventricular strain pattern on ECG in patients with PE and normal blood pressure is associated with adverse short-term outcome and adds incremental prognostic value to echocardiographic evidence of right ventricular function.

IMAGING STUDIES

- Chest x-ray may be normal; suggestive findings include elevated diaphragm, pleural effusion, dilation of pulmonary artery, infiltrate or consolidation, abrupt vessel cut-off, oligemia distal to the PE (*Westermark sign*), or atelectasis. A wedge-shaped consolidation in the middle and lower lobes is suggestive of a pulmonary infarction and is known as *Hampton's hump.*
- CT angiography is an accurate, noninvasive tool in the diagnosis of PE at the main, lobar, and segmental pulmonary artery levels. A major advantage of CT angiography over standard pulmonary angiography is its ability to diagnose intrathoracic disease other than PE that may account for the patient's clinical picture. It is also less invasive, less costly, and more widely available. Its major shortcoming is its poor sensitivity for subsegmental emboli.
- V/Q Lung scan (in patient with normal chest x-ray examination): This test must be interpreted within the pretest probability of having a PE.

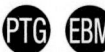

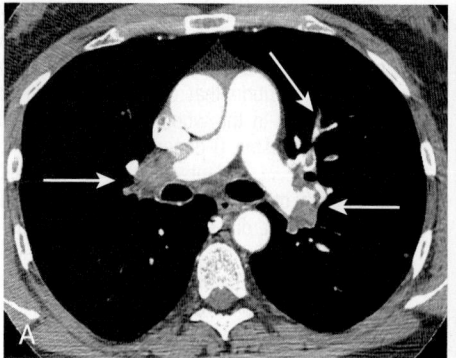 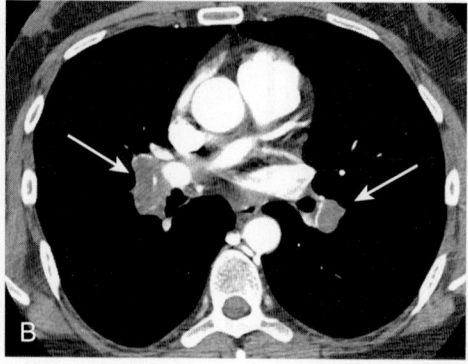 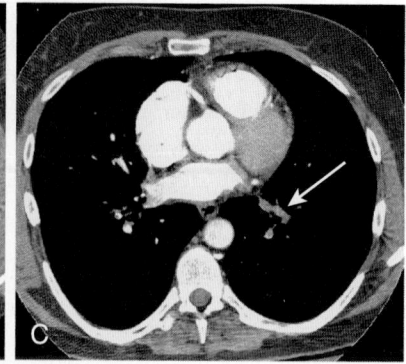

FIG. 3 A 46-year-old woman presented with acute shortness of breath and hypoxia. Chest radiograph was normal. A, Chest computed tomography shows a low-attenuation filling defect in left and right main pulmonary arteries *(arrows)* and left upper lobe segmental artery *(arrow)*, representing massive pulmonary embolism. Emboli extend to left and right interlobar arteries *(arrows)*, as well as a left lower lobe segmental artery *(arrow)*, seen in **B** and **C**, respectively. (From Vincent JL et al: *Textbook of critical care,* ed 6, Philadelphia, 2011, Saunders.)

1. A normal lung scan rules out PE.
2. A ventilation-perfusion mismatch is suggestive of PE, and a lung scan interpretation of high probability is confirmatory (Fig. E4).
3. If the clinical suspicion of PE is high and the lung scan is interpreted as low probability, moderate probability, or indeterminate, a pulmonary arteriogram is diagnostic; a positive arteriogram confirms diagnosis; a positive compressive duplex ultrasonography for DVT obviates the need for an arteriogram, because treatment with IV anticoagulants is indicated in these patients; the overall sensitivity of compressive ultrasonography for DVT in patients with PE is 29%, specificity 97%; adding ultrasonography in patients with a nondiagnostic lung scan prevents 9% of angiographies; however, this improvement in efficacy is achieved at the cost of unnecessary anticoagulant therapy in 26% of patients who have false-positive ultrasonography results.

- Angiography: pulmonary angiography is the historic gold standard; however, it is invasive, expensive, and not readily available in some clinical settings. False-positive pulmonary angiograms may result from mediastinal disorders such as radiation fibrosis and tumors.
- Gadolinium-enhanced magnetic resonance angiography (MRA/MRV) of the pulmonary arteries has a moderate sensitivity and high specificity for the diagnosis of PE at experienced centers, but obtaining acceptable images is technically challenging and should only be performed if other imaging tests are contraindicated.
- Echocardiography: useful for identifying patients with PE who may have poor prognosis. Moderate or severe hypokinesis, persistent pulmonary hypertension, patent foramen ovale, and free-floating right heart thrombus are markers for increased risk of death or recurrent thrombosis. Such patients should be considered for thrombolysis or embolectomy.

Rx TREATMENT

NONPHARMACOLOGIC THERAPY
Correction of risk factors (see "Etiology") to prevent future PE.

ACUTE GENERAL Rx
Patients with acute PE should be initially stratified according to risk (Table 1) so that higher-risk therapies (e.g., thrombolysis, embolectomy) are offered to patients with the greatest chance of benefit.

- Anticoagulants are recommended as initial therapy in patients with small to moderate PE.
- Anticoagulant drugs for initial treatment of PE are described in Table E2. Unfractionated heparin (UFH) (IV or subcutaneous), subcutaneous low-molecular-weight heparin (LMWH), or subcutaneous fondaparinux is recommended for the initial treatment for at least 5 days. If IV unfractionated heparin is used, a bolus dose (80 U/kg) followed by a weight-based (18 U/kg/hr) continuous infusion to achieve therapeutic anti-factor Xa (or aPTT) levels should be used. LMWH and fondaparinux should be avoided in patients with severe renal failure.
- Oral rivaroxaban, a factor Xa inhibitor (15 mg bid for 3 wk, then 20 mg/d), has been studied as a treatment for DVT and for PE, without prior parenteral therapy. For both DVT and PE, treatment with rivaroxaban alone was noninferior to treatment with LMWH followed by a vitamin K antagonist with regard to the endpoint of recurrent venous thromboembolism. Use of rivaroxaban should be avoided in patients with severe renal failure.
- Dabigatran, a direct thrombin inhibitor (150 mg twice a day), has been recently approved for the treatment of PE from data assembled from the RECOVER, REMEDYSM, and RESONATE trials. Dabigatran met its noninferiority efficacy endpoints with improved safety margins (bleeding) compared to warfarin. All trial recipients received heparin bridge to start their anticoagulation.

- Apixaban, a Factor Xa inhibitor (10 mg twice a day for a week, followed by 5 mg twice a day), was recently approved for the treatment of acute PE based on the data in the AMPLIFY and AMPLIFY-EXT trials, in which apixaban met its noninferiority mark in terms of efficacy and improved safety compared to warfarin.
- Thrombolytic agents (urokinase, tPA, streptokinase): provide rapid resolution of clots with increased risk of major bleeding (up to 3% incidence of intracranial hemorrhage); thrombolytic agents are the treatment of choice in patients with massive PE who are hemodynamically unstable and with no contraindication to their use. The use of thrombolytic agent in the treatment of hemodynamically stable patients with acute submassive PE remains controversial, although there is some evidence that half-dose tPA has some efficacy. Use of the thrombolytic agents alteplase (100 mg IV over 2-hr period) in normotensive patients with moderate or severe right ventricular dysfunction identified by ECG has been advocated by some physicians. Use of alteplase in conjunction with heparin has been shown to improve the clinical course of stable patients who have acute submassive PE without internal bleeding, mainly by reducing need for subsequent thrombolytic use. Additional studies are needed to confirm these findings before recommending routine use of this therapeutic approach. The Pulmonary Embolism Thrombolysis (PEITHO) trial revealed that in patients with intermediate risk of pulmonary embolism, fibrinolytic therapy prevented hemodynamic compensation but increased the risk of major hemorrhage and stroke.
- Long-term treatment for PE not associated with malignancy can be carried out with warfarin therapy or rivaroxaban.
- For PE associated with malignancy, LMWH is recommended for long-term therapy.
- For PE occurring in the setting of a reversible risk factor, anticoagulation should be continued for 3 mo. For patients with an unprovoked PE, longer-term anticoagulation should be considered, and indefinite long-term

anticoagulation should be used in patients with recurrent unprovoked PE. Important factors to consider in the decision to extend anticoagulation include the patient's risk of bleeding and patient preferences after an informed discussion of risks and benefits.

- If thrombolytics and anticoagulants are contraindicated (e.g., GI bleeding, recent CNS surgery, recent trauma) or if the patient continues to have recurrent PE despite anticoagulation therapy, vena caval interruption is indicated by transvenous placement of an inferior vena caval filter.
- IVC filters are also strongly associated with reduced in-hospital fatality rate in stable patients who received thrombolytic therapy. It seems prudent to consider a vena cava filter in patients with PE who are receiving thrombolytic therapy.
- Acute pulmonary artery surgical embolectomy or catheter-based thrombectomy may be indicated in a patient with massive PE who cannot receive thrombolytic therapy. Pulmonary embolectomy is also recommended for those whose critical status does not allow sufficient time for thrombolytic therapy to be effective and for those who remain unstable after receiving fibrinolysis.
- Recent guidelines from the Clinical Guidelines Committee of the American College of Physicians for the Evaluation of Patients with Suspected Acute Pulmonary Embolism recommend the following:[1]
  1. Use of validated clinical prediction rules to estimate pretest probability in patients in whom acute PG is being considered.
  2. Not obtaining a D-dimer measurement or imaging studies in patients with low pretest probability of PE and who meet all pulmonary embolism rule-out criteria.
  3. Obtaining a high-sensitivity D-dimer measurement as the initial diagnostic test in patients who have an intermediate pretest probability of PE or in patients

---

[1]Raja AS, et al: Evaluation of patients with suspected acute pulmonary embolism: best practice advice from the Clinical Guidelines Committee of the American College of Physicians, *Ann Intern Med* 163:701-711, 2015.

with low pretest probability of PE who do not meet all pulmonary embolism rule-out criteria. Clinicians should not use imaging studies as the initial test in patients who have a low or intermediate pretest probability of PE.
  4. Use age-adjusted D-dimer thresholds (age × 10 ng/mL rather than a generic 500 ng/mL) in patients older than 50 years to determine whether imaging is warranted.
  5. Clinicians should not obtain any imaging studies in patients with a D-dimer level below the age-adjusted cutoff.
  6. CTPA should be obtained in patients with high pretest probability of PE. Ventilation-perfusion scans should be reserved for patients who have a contraindication to CTPA or if CTPA is not available.
  7. A D-dimer measurement should not be obtained in patients with a high pretest probability of PE.

CHRONIC Rx

- Elimination of risk factors (see "Etiology").
- Patients with unprovoked DVT/PE have a high rate of recurrent VTE. Longer durations of chronic anticoagulation after unprovoked DVT/PE result in lower rates of recurrent DVT/PE while on anticoagulation, but benefits are lost once anticoagulation is halted. The use of indefinite anticoagulation in selected individuals with apparently unprovoked DVT/PE must be weighed against ongoing bleeding risk and other factors.
- A recent study demonstrated that aspirin (100 mg daily) is superior to placebo in preventing recurrence of venous thromboembolism in patients with a first-ever unprovoked venous thromboembolism (VTE) who had already completed 6 to 18 months of oral anticoagulation. This suggests that aspirin could be offered as an alternative to oral anticoagulants for prevention of recurrent VTE in patients who refuse to or cannot continue oral anticoagulant therapy but who have a high risk of recurrent VTE.
- Trials involving extending the treatment time of the novel oral anticoagulants (rivaroxaban,

dabigatran, and apixaban) all showed superior efficacy and reduced morbidity compared to placebo as well as similar rate of major bleeding (though increased all bleeding).

DISPOSITION

- Mortality can be reduced to <10% by rapid and effective treatment. Stratification of risk of death associated with PE and severity-adjusted treatment is described in Table E3.
- Mortality from recurrent pulmonary emboli is 8% with effective treatment and >30% in patients with untreated pulmonary emboli.

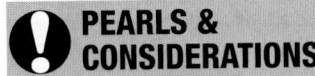

COMMENTS

- Use of clinical prediction rules in association with D-dimer testing may reduce the use of unnecessary imaging in patients in whom PE is unlikely.
- Massive PE (PE associated with hypotension, shock, or circulatory arrest) remains the clearest situation in which thrombolytics should be employed. Submassive PE (PE associated with right ventricular dysfunction or injury but without hypotension) remains an area of controversy with regards to thrombolytic use.

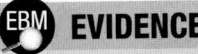

Available at www.expertconsult.com

SUGGESTED READINGS
Available at www.expertconsult.com

RELATED CONTENT
Pulmonary Embolism (PE) (Patient Information)
Deep Vein Thrombosis (Related Key Topic)
Hypercoagulable State (Related Key Topic)

AUTHOR: **CHAKRAVARTHY REDDY, M.D.**

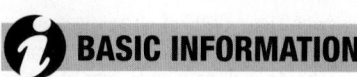

BASIC INFORMATION

DEFINITION

Pulmonary hypertension (PH) is defined as the presence of an elevated mean pulmonary arterial pressure (PAP) >25 mm Hg at rest. Pulmonary hypertension is classified into five major groups: idiopathic pulmonary arterial hypertension (Group 1), pulmonary hypertension due to left heart disease (Group 2), pulmonary hypertension due to lung disease (Group 3), pulmonary hypertension due to chronic thromboembolic disease (Group 4), and miscellaneous (Group 5).

Pulmonary arterial hypertension (PAH) is a syndrome defined as mean pulmonary pressure >25 mm Hg with pulmonary capillary wedge pressure <155 mm Hg and a pulmonary vascular resistance >3 Wood units on right heart catheterization. Idiopathic pulmonary arterial hypertension (IPAH) is diagnosed when PAH is present without any apparent cause. It is a highly morbid disease characterized by progressive obliteration of precapillary arterioles. Pulmonary hypertension from lung disease is covered under the separate topic Cor Pulmonale.

SYNONYMS

PH
Pulmonary arterial hypertension
Idiopathic pulmonary arterial hypertension
IPAH
Associated pulmonary arterial hypertension
PAHA, also known as secondary pulmonary hypertension
Heritable pulmonary arterial hypertension
HPAH
Group I Pulmonary Hypertension

ICD-10CM CODES
I27.0 Primary pulmonary hypertension
I27.2 Other secondary pulmonary hypertension

EPIDEMIOLOGY & DEMOGRAPHICS

- IPAH is rare, occurring in one to two cases per 1 million people per year, with an overall prevalence estimated at 15 to 50 per 1 million.
- IPAH is more common in women than men (3:1), usually presenting in the third to fourth decades of life.
- In adults the most common cause of pulmonary hypertension is due to left-sided heart disease (Group 2).
- Prevalence of secondary PAH could range from 8% to 12% in cases of scleroderma, 0.5% of HIV, 23% to 53% of mixed connective tissue disorders, and 1% to 4% cases of systemic lupus erythematosus.

PHYSICAL FINDINGS & CLINICAL PRESENTATION

- Insidious, may go undetected for years.
- Exertional dyspnea most common presenting symptom (60%).
- Fatigue and weakness.
- Syncope, classically exertion-related or after a warm shower with peripheral vasodilation.
- Chest pain.
- Hoarse voice from compression of recurrent laryngeal nerve by an enlarged pulmonary artery (Ortner's syndrome).
- Loud P2 component of the second heart sound and paradoxical splitting of second heart sound.
- Right-sided S4.
- Jugular venous distention.
- Abdominal distention and ascites.
- Prominent parasternal (right ventricular [RV]) impulse.
- Holosystolic tricuspid regurgitation murmur heard best along the left fourth parasternal line that increases in intensity with inspiration.
- Peripheral edema.

ETIOLOGY

- The etiology of IPAH is unknown. APAH (associated PAH) has several known risk factors: connective tissue disorders, portal hypertension and liver cirrhosis, appetite-suppressant drugs (fenfluramine), hemoglobinopathies, and infections including schistosomiasis and HIV disease. Schistosomiasis, sickle cell disease, and HIV disease may be the most common causes of PH worldwide, although pulmonary venous hypertension from left ventricular failure and PH related to COPD are more common causes of PH in developed nations.
- Several genetic abnormalities have been associated with HPAH (heritable PAH), many of which are mutations in the genes that code for members of the tumor growth factor-beta family of receptors (BMPR-II, ALK-1, endoglin) on chromosome 2q33. A recent study[1] has identified the association of a novel gene, KCNK3, with familial and idiopathic pulmonary arterial hypertension.
- Heritable PAH is an autosomal-dominant disease with variable penetrance, affecting only about 10% to 20% of carriers.
- Several factors play a role in the pathogenesis of PAH, including a genetic predisposition, endothelial cell dysfunction, abnormalities in vasomotor control, thrombotic obliteration of the vascular lumen, and vascular remodeling through cell proliferation and matrix production.
- SSRI use in late pregnancy is associated with increased persistent PHA in newborns.
- The updated clinical classification of pulmonary hypertension is described in Table 1.

DIAGNOSIS

- PAH is a hemodynamic diagnosis involving the detection of elevated pressure in the pulmonary arteries and elevated pulmonary vascular resistance in the pulmonary vascular bed, occurring in the absence of significant pulmonary venous hypertension; characterization of this abnormality determines its etiology.

TABLE 1 Updated Clinical Classification of Pulmonary Hypertension

Group 1

Pulmonary arterial hypertension

Idiopathic pulmonary arterial hypertension

Heritable

BMPR2

ALK1, endoglin (with or without hereditary hemorrhagic telangiectasia)

Unknown

Drug- and toxin-induced

Associated with:

Connective tissue diseases

HIV infection

Portal hypertension

Congenital heart diseases

Schistosomiasis

Chronic hemolytic anemia

Persistent pulmonary hypertension of the newborn

Pulmonary veno-occlusive disease with left to right shunts and/or pulmonary capillary hemangiomatosis

Group 2

Pulmonary hypertension owing to left heart disease

Systolic dysfunction

Diastolic dysfunction

Valvular disease

Group 3

Pulmonary hypertension owing to lung diseases and/or hypoxia

Chronic obstructive pulmonary disease

Interstitial lung disease

Other pulmonary diseases with mixed restrictive and obstructive pattern

Sleep-disordered breathing

Alveolar hypoventilation disorders

Chronic exposure to high altitude

Developmental abnormalities

Group 4

Chronic thromboembolic pulmonary hypertension

Group 5

Pulmonary hypertension with unclear multifactorial mechanisms

Hematologic disorders: myeloproliferative disorders, splenectomy

Systemic disorders: sarcoidosis, pulmonary Langerhans cell histiocytosis: lymphangioleiomyomatosis, neurofibromatosis, vasculitis

Metabolic disorders: glycogen storage disease, Gaucher's disease, thyroid disorders

Others: tumoral obstruction, fibrosing mediastinitis, chronic renal failure on dialysis

ALK1, Activin receptor-like kinase type 1; *BMPR2,* bone morphogenetic protein receptor type 2; *HIV,* human immunodeficiency virus.

From Simonneau G et al: Updated clinical classification of pulmonary hypertension, *J Am Coll Cardiol* 54:S43-S54, 2009.

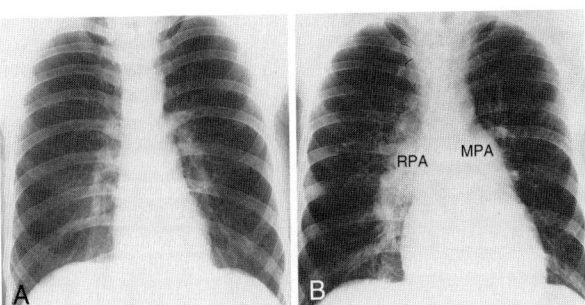

FIG. 1 Progressive pulmonary arterial hypertension. This patient initially presented with a relatively normal chest radiograph **(A).** However, several years later **(B)** there is increasing heart size and marked dilation of the main pulmonary artery *(MPA)* and right pulmonary artery *(RPA).* Rapid tapering of the arteries as they proceed peripherally is suggestive of pulmonary hypertension and is sometimes referred to as pruning. (From Mettler FA [ed]: *Primary care radiology,* Philadelphia, 2000, WB Saunders.)

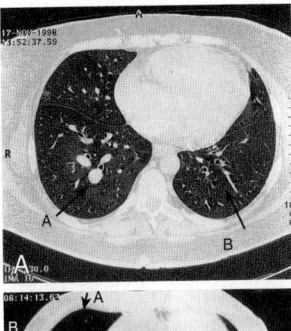

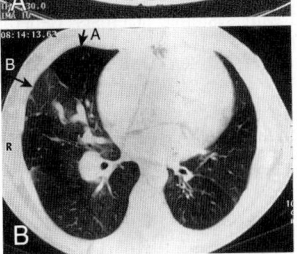

FIG. 2 Chest computed tomographic scans in a patient with chronic thromboembolic pulmonary hypertension. A, Helical scan with contrast medium enhancement of the pulmonary vasculature shows a marked disparity in vessel size between the involved vessels *(A),* which are enlarged from thrombus, and the uninvolved vessels *(B).* **B,** Non-contrast-enhanced high-resolution scan illustrates a marked mosaic pattern manifest by differences in density of regions of the lung parenchyma reflecting the perfused areas *(B)* and the nonperfused areas *(A),* also consistent with underlying thromboembolic disease. (From Zipes DP et al [eds]: *Braunwald's heart disease,* ed 7, Philadelphia, 2005, WB Saunders.)

- Right-sided heart catheterization must be performed in all patients suspected of having PAH to establish the diagnosis and to assess pulmonary hemodynamics including reactivity response to vasodilators.
- IPAH is a diagnosis of exclusion; causes that lead to Groups 2-5 pulmonary hypertension must be ruled out.

DIFFERENTIAL DIAGNOSIS
The differential diagnosis is as listed under "Etiology."

EVALUATION
- Consists of establishing the diagnosis and etiology.
- Echocardiography with Doppler technique can provide a noninvasive but limited estimation of systolic PAP. Common findings include tricuspid regurgitation, right heart enlargement, abnormal movement of septum and, rarely, pericardial effusion. However, the diagnosis of PH cannot be established by echocardiography alone, as echocardiography can overestimate or underestimate PAP.
- ECG shows RV enlargement, strain pattern, and right axis deviation.
- Chest radiograph (Fig. 1) shows enlarged central pulmonary arteries and right heart enlargement. Chest radiography is abnormal in 90% of patients at diagnosis.
- A normal chest radiograph does not rule out the diagnosis. High-resolution computed tomography (CT) (Fig. 2) can assist in the evaluation for emphysema or interstitial lung disease. Ventilation-perfusion lung scan has high sensitivity for chronic thromboembolic disease. The diagnosis should be confirmed by pulmonary angiography, which has high specificity.
- Pulmonary function tests may show obstructive (airway disease) and/or restrictive disease (parenchymal disease) depending on etiology. Diffusion capacity of carbon monoxide in the lung is reduced due to pulmonary vascular destruction in PAH.
- In asymptomatic patients the severity of pulmonary arterial hypertension (PAH) disease should be evaluated in a systematic and consistent manner, using a combination of World Health Organization (WHO) functional class (FC), exercise capacity, and echocardiographic, laboratory, and hemodynamic variables to inform therapeutic decisions.
- Right heart catheterization is required to assess pulmonary hemodynamics, exclude shunts and left heart disease, and perform acute vasoreactivity response testing.
- Symptomatic patients with PAH, in the absence of contraindications, should undergo acute vasoreactivity testing using a short-acting agent at a center with experience in the performance and interpretation of vasoreactivity testing. Screening for the presence of PAH with Doppler echocardiography is warranted in individuals with a known predisposing genetic mutation or first-degree relative with IPAH, connective tissue diseases (especially scleroderma), congenital heart disease with left-to-right shunt, or portal hypertension undergoing evaluation for orthotopic liver transplantation.
- Determining the degree of functional impairment, as assessed by the WHO functional classification system (Classes I-IV) and the 6-min walk test (6MWT), is a useful way to monitor disease progression and assess response to treatment.

LABORATORY TESTS
- Complete blood count is usually normal in PAH but may show secondary polycythemia.
- Arterial blood gases show low PO_2 and oxygen saturation.
- Overnight oximetry and/or sleep study to rule out sleep apnea or hypopnea.
- Other blood tests: antinuclear antibody (ANA), antineutrophil cytoplasmic antibodies (ANCA), anti-Scl-70, anticentromere, ribonucleoprotein antibody levels, and rheumatoid factor (RF) to screen for underlying connective tissue disease, HIV serology, liver function tests, and antiphospholipid antibodies.
- Brain natriuretic peptide (BNP) level can provide prognostic information, with elevation in BNP level being associated with increased mortality.
- Ventilation-perfusion lung scan has high sensitivity for chronic thromboembolic PAH. The diagnosis should be confirmed by pulmonary angiography, which has high specificity.

TREATMENT
- Most of the evidence in management of PAH is limited to IPAH/HPAH. There is some evidence in treatment of PAHA associated with connective tissue disease, especially scleroderma, and congenital heart disease. The recommendations for treating PAH associated with other causes are limited to case studies and expert opinions.
- There is some evidence for the use of advanced therapies for sarcoidosis-associated PH. The heterogeneity of sarcoid-associated PH complicates the interpretation.

NONPHARMACOLOGIC THERAPY
- Oxygen therapy to improve alveolar oxygen flow in both idiopathic and secondary PH. Goal oxygen saturation >90%.
- Avoidance of vigorous exercise and pregnancy.

GENERAL TREATMENT:
1. Diuretics (e.g., furosemide 40-80 mg qd) improve dyspnea by reducing preload and peripheral edema. Avoid excessive diuresis in patients who are preload dependent.
2. Digoxin 0.25 mg qd has been used in patients with IPAH with inconclusive benefits. There is no conclusive data regarding the use of beta blockers, ACE inhibitors, or ARB in IPAH unless required by comorbidities such as concurrent hypertension.

3. Evidence for the use of oral anticoagulation with warfarin for IPAH is derived mostly from retrospective single-center experience. Data from RCT and registries remain heterogenous and inconclusive. Recently, a large multicenter observational longitudinal registry of patients with IPAH (REVEAL Registry) assessed the effect of warfarin treatment on survival and found no benefit; it also found poorer survival in patients with PAH associated with systemic sclerosis. Generally, patients with IPAH who are undergoing IV prostaglandin therapy are anticoagulated if there are no contraindications to anticoagulation, as they are at high risk for catheter-related thrombosis. There are no data regarding the role of novel oral anticoagulants in IPAH.

4. Iron deficiency is common and is associated with reduced exercise capacity; it should be closely monitored and replenished as needed.

CHRONIC Rx

• Acute vasoreactivity response testing should be done in all patients at the time of right heart catheterization. Epoprostenol, adenosine, or nitric oxide is generally used to assess the response. A positive response is a fall in mean PAP of >10 mm Hg to a value of <40 mm Hg, with increased or unchanged cardiac output. Fewer than 10% of patients are responders in IPAH.

• The positive responders may benefit from treatment with calcium channel blockers (diltiazem, amlodipine, or nifedipine). Verapamil is not recommended because of its negative inotropic effects. All patients should be reassessed in 6 to 8 wk to demonstrate sustained benefit from the calcium channel blocker.

• Calcium channel blockers (CCBs) should not be used empirically to treat PAH in the absence of demonstrated acute vasoreactivity because of potential severe side effects.

• If patients do not show an adequate response, additional PAH therapy should be started.

PROSTANOIDS

• These synthetic prostacyclin analogues act as potent vasodilators of pulmonary arteries and inhibitors of platelet aggregation. They all have shown improvement in symptoms, exercise capacity including 6MWD, and hemodynamics. They are ideal for class III and IV patients.

1. Epoprostenol: IV formulation with very short half-life. It is the only drug that improves mortality. It requires long-term IV access with associated risks of infection and thrombosis. Rapid tachyphylaxis with dose escalation is seen. Common side effects include jaw pain, abdominal cramping, and diarrhea. Limited evidence exists for use in secondary PAH patients.

2. Treprostinil: IV and SQ formulation with longer half-life. Main disadvantage is pain at SQ pump site (no long-term evidence for IV formulation). Treprostinil is also available as a nebulized inhaled solution.

3. Iloprost: aerosolized formulation with short half-life requiring 6 to 8 treatments/day. Well tolerated, with flushing and jaw pain being the most frequent side effects.

4. Beraprost: PO formulation. Not approved in the U.S.

5. Selexipag: PO formulation, selective prostacyclin IP receptor agonist. Although the mode of action is similar, the chemical structure is different. In a recent RCT, selexipag showed reduction in death from any cause and from complications related to pulmonary hypertension.

RIOCIGUAT: GUANYLATE CYCLASE STIMULATORS

Guanylate cyclase stimulators enhance cGMP production and in preclinical studies show antiproliferative and antiremodeling properties in animal models. These oral agents are useful for class II and III patients and have shown favorable results on exercise capacity, hemodynamics, WHO functional class, and time to clinical worsening without any mortality benefit. The most serious side effect is syncope.

• **Endothelin receptor antagonists (ERAs):**
1. Activation of the endothelin system results in vasoconstriction by acting on the pulmonary vascular smooth muscles. These oral pulmonary vasodilators require monthly liver function tests, and often the response is delayed by weeks. Thus, it is not an ideal starting therapy for WHO class IV patients. It is effective in class II and III patients and improves symptoms, exercise capacity, and hemodynamics without any improvement in mortality.
2. Bosentan (nonselective endothelin A and B receptor blocker): Sitaxsentan and ambrisentan (selective endothelin A receptor blockers).
3. Macitentan: Nonselective endothelin receptor antagonist. Showed significant reduction in composite end point of death in patients with IPAH. It has no liver toxicity but can cause reduction in hemoglobin.

• **Phosphodiesterase (PDE-5) inhibitors:**
1. These are oral agents that act by inhibiting phosphodiesterase type 5 enzyme (PDE-5), resulting in increased concentration of nitric oxide. Highly effective in WHO class II patients, both in IPAH and scleroderma-associated PAH. Improve symptoms, exercise capacity including 6MWD, hemodynamics, and time to clinical worsening. Most side effects are related to vasodilation including headache, flushing, and epistaxis.
2. Sildenafil is administered as 20 mg PO tid. Tadalafil dose is 40 mg once daily.

• **Prostacyclin agonists:**
1. Selexipag and treprostinil are oral prostacycline IP receptor agonists approved for PAH. Epoprostenol is available IV and iloprost and tyvaso are available via inhalation.

Caveats to treatment depending on WHO class of symptoms are as follows:

According to consensus definition, patients with PAH who demonstrate acute vasoreactivity should be considered candidates for a trial of therapy with an oral calcium channel blocker (CCB), except in the case of right heart failure or other contraindications.

CCBs should not be used empirically to treat PAH in the absence of demonstrated acute vasoreactivity, as described previously.

• For treatment-naive PAH patients with WHO functional class FC II or III symptoms who are not candidates for, or who have failed CCB therapy, monotherapy should be initiated with an approved ERA, phosphodiesterase-5 (PDE5) inhibitor, or the soluble guanylate cyclase stimulator riociguat.

• For treatment-naive PAH patients with WHO functional Class FC III symptoms who have evidence of rapid progression of their disease or other markers of a poor clinical prognosis, consideration of initial treatment with a parenteral prostanoid is recommended.

• For treatment-naive PAH patients in WHO class FC IV who are unable, or do not desire, to manage parenteral prostanoid therapy, treatment with an inhaled prostanoid in combination with an ERA is recommended.

• For WHO class FC III or IV PAH patients with unacceptable clinical status despite established PAH-specific monotherapy, addition of a second class of PAH therapy to improve exercise capacity is recommended. Such patients should be evaluated at centers with expertise in the evaluation and treatment of complex patients with PAH.

• Combination therapies: considered when there is no improvement or deterioration on monotherapy. The FDA has approved the use of ambrisentan and tadalafil together as the first two-drug regimen for PAH. Starting dose is 5 mg for ambrisentan and 20 mg for tadalafil once daily.

• Bosentan + inhaled iloprost (STEP trial) showed some benefit over monotherapy.

• IV epoprostenol + oral bosentan (BREATH-2 trial) did not show much difference.

• IV epoprostenol + oral sildenafil (PACES trial) showed benefit over monotherapy.

INVASIVE RX

Lung transplantation and heart-lung transplantation are other options in patients with end-stage class IV disease.

• Atrial septostomy may be performed as a bridge to transplant. The defect can be closed at the time of transplantation. Atrial septostomy is recommended for individuals with a room air SaO_2 >90% who have severe right-sided heart failure (with refractory ascites) despite maximal diuretic therapy, or who have signs of impaired systemic blood flow (such as syncope) from reduced left heart filling.

• Extracorporeal membrane oxygenation (ECMO) is also commonly used as a bridge to transplant.

• Lung transplant recipients with IPAH had survival rates of 73% at 1 yr, 55% at 3 yr, and 45% at 5 yr.

TREATMENT OF SECONDARY PAH, APAH:

• Directed toward cause. Some situations merit mention.

• PAH with uncorrected congenital heart disease: Eisenmenger's syndrome. Medical

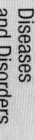

treatment generally ineffective. Heart-lung transplantation required in most patients. PH may persist after surgical correction of congenital heart disease, and pulmonary vasodilators can be effective therapies in this patient population.

- PAH with scleroderma: selective pulmonary vasodilators are effective.
- PAH with lung disease or hypoxia: oxygen therapy, for hypoxemia, CPAP (for OSA), control of primary disease process.
- PAH with chronic thromboembolic disease: may consider pulmonary vasodilators after anticoagulation and pulmonary thromboendarterectomy (or if thromboendarterectomy is not an option) if continued symptoms and elevation in PVR and transpulmonary gradient.
- PAH with HIV: control of viral load by antiretroviral therapy.

FOLLOW-UP

Regular follow-up at 3-mo intervals with clinical assessment: WHO class and 6MWT, 6 to 12 mo objective assessment of RV function by ECG and cardiac catheterization studies.

DISPOSITION

- The 6MWT is predictive of survival in patients with idiopathic PAH. A baseline 6MWT <250 m is associated with a 50% risk of death at 2 yr. Drop in O_2 saturation >10% during the test increases mortality risk 2.9 times over a median follow-up of 26 mo.
- A BNP level ≥350 pg/mL at baseline evaluation is associated with a 25% risk of death at 2 yr.
- WHO class II and III patients with PAH have a mean survival of 3.5 yr.
- WHO class IV patients have a mean survival of 6 mo.
- As per the REVEAL (Registry to Evaluate Early and Long-term Pulmonary Arterial Hypertension Disease Management) risk score, poor prognostic signs include:
  1. Signs of RV failure.
  2. WHO functional class III or IV.
  3. Walk a distance of <165 meters in 6-min walk test.

4. Peak VO2 <15 ml/min/kg in cardiopulmonary testing.
5. Elevated BNP levels >180 pg/ml.
6. Presence of pericardial effusion.
7. TAPSE [tricuspid annular plane systolic excursion] <2 cm on echo of right ventricle.
8. Right atrial pressure >20 mm Hg or pulmonary vascular resistance of >32 Wood units on right heart catheterization.
9. Increased heart rate >92 or BP <109 mm Hg.
10. Male gender >60 years of age.
11. Concomitant renal dysfunction with estimated glomerular filtration rate ≤30/mL/min/m.
12. Diffusion capacity of lung for carbon monoxide (DLCO) <33%.

REFERRAL

If the diagnosis of IPAH/HPAH is suspected, a consultation with a pulmonary specialist is recommended. PHA may require disease-specific consultations. Advanced cases need to be transferred to transplant centers.

PEARLS & CONSIDERATIONS

- The exertional dyspnea of PAH is typically described by patients as being relentlessly progressive over several months to a year, often out of proportion to, or in the absence of, underlying heart or lung disease.
- Over 20% of patients in the Registry to Evaluate Early and Long-term PAH Disease Management had symptoms for more than 2 years before PAH was recognized. Consideration of the diagnosis of PAH in the differential diagnosis of unexplained dyspnea, especially in younger individuals, is essential.
- Chest x-ray may reveal evidence of interstitial fluid or fibrosis within the lungs in cases of secondary PH. IPAH is not associated with infiltrates on chest radiograph.

COMMENTS

- RV systolic pressure (RVSP) as estimated by echocardiography is not a good indicator of the presence of PAH because RVSP increases with age and body mass index. Athletically conditioned men also have a higher resting RVSP. Thus, these measurements can be misleading.
- Abrupt development of pulmonary edema during acute vasodilator testing suggests pulmonary venoocclusive disease or pulmonary capillary hemangiomatosis and is a contraindication to long-term vasodilator treatment.
- In advanced PAH, heart rate increase is the main compensatory mechanism and reflects increased sympathetic tone. A higher heart rate at rest is an important marker of prognosis and should be assessed at frequent intervals after initiation of treatment for PAH.

FUTURE DIRECTIONS

- Serotonin receptor modulators, platelet-derived growth factor, and Rho kinase inhibitors.
- Gene analysis to identify genes that determine individual disease susceptibility and help identify targeted therapy.

EBM EVIDENCE

Available at www.expertconsult.com

SUGGESTED READINGS

Available at www.expertconsult.com

RELATED CONTENT

Pulmonary Hypertension (Patient Information)

AUTHOR: **WAJIH A. SYED, M.D.**

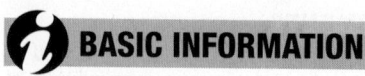 BASIC INFORMATION

DEFINITION

Pulseless electrical activity (PEA) is defined as the presence of organized cardiac electrical activity without sufficient mechanical contraction to produce a palpable pulse.

SYNONYMS

Electromechanical dissociation (EMD)

ICD-10CM CODES

I46.9 Cardiac arrest, cause unspecified
I49.9 Cardiac arrhythmia, unspecified

EPIDEMIOLOGY & DEMOGRAPHICS

- Accounts for about 35% of cardiac arrest cases.
- Increasingly recognized as the cause of sudden cardiac death in patients with implantable cardioverter-defibrillators.

PHYSICAL FINDINGS & CLINICAL PRESENTATION

PRIMARY PEA:
- Organized electrical activity (not VT/VF).
- No detectable pulse.

SECONDARY PEA: As in primary PEA and may also have:
- Bradycardia: drug overdose.
- Tachycardia: hypovolemia, massive PE.
- Decreased jugular venous pressure (JVP): hypovolemia.
- Elevated JVP and no pulse with CPR: cardiac tamponade, massive PE, tension pneumothorax.
- Absent unilateral breath sounds and tracheal deviation: tension pneumothorax.
- Cyanosis: hypoxia.

ETIOLOGY

PRIMARY PEA: Myocardial electromechanical uncoupling secondary to advanced heart muscle disease.

SECONDARY PEA: Because of changes in the loading conditions of the heart, ischemia, myocardial depressants
- Massive MI.
- Massive PE.
- Hypovolemia.
- Cardiac tamponade.
- Tension pneumothorax.
- Hypoxia.
- Hypothermia.
- Acidosis.
- Hyperkalemia/hypokalemia.

- Drug overdose: β-blockers, calcium channel blockers, digoxin, tricyclic antidepressants, benzodiazepines, opioids.

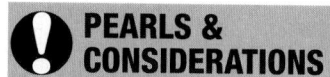 DIAGNOSIS

WORKUP

- Stabilizing patient and workup to establish etiology should proceed simultaneously.
- History, physical examination, laboratory tests, imaging studies.

LABORATORY TESTS

- CBC, potassium, magnesium, CK-MB, troponin, toxicology screen.
- Arterial blood gas.
- ECG (Fig. 1):
  Low voltage: tamponade.
  Right heart strain: PE, pneumothorax.
  Arrhythmias: MI, metabolic abnormalities, drug effects.
  ST changes, Q waves: MI.

IMAGING STUDIES

- Chest radiograph: rule out pneumothorax, aortic dissection.
- Echocardiogram: rule out tamponade, ischemia (LV contractility, wall motion), valve dysfunction, tumors, and clots. May help diagnose aortic dissection and PE and assess intravascular volume status.
- Abdominal radiograph or ultrasound: rule out ruptured abdominal aortic aneurysm.

TREATMENT

Identifying and treating a reversible cause is critical.

Physiologic parameters can help monitor quality of CPR and detect the return of spontaneous circulation (ROSC). Suggested methods include quantitative waveform capnography, arterial relaxation diastolic pressure, arterial pressure monitoring, or central venous oxygen saturation.

NONPHARMACOLOGIC THERAPY

- Activate emergency response service.
- Begin CPR; ensure high quality, minimize interruptions. Perform CPR for 2 min between pauses to assess rhythm and circulation.
- Attach cardiac monitor/defibrillator.
- Obtain IV/intraosseous (IO) access.
- Consider advanced airway placement.
- Confirm absence of blood flow with Doppler ultrasound, arterial line, or bedside echocardiogram.

ACUTE GENERAL Rx

- Treat specific cause if known.
- Give 100% oxygen.
- Epinephrine 1 mg IV push/IO, q3 to 5min.
- Give normal saline (20 mL) bolus after peripheral IV administration of medication to improve its distribution.
- Medication can be given via endotracheal tube if IV/IO access cannot be obtained; IV/IO routes preferred because they provide more predictable drug delivery and pharmacologic effects. Give 2 to 2.5× the IV dose in 10 ml of sterile water.
- If rhythm changes to VF or pulseless VT.
  1. Defibrillate.
  2. For refractory VF or pulseless VT consider amiodarone.
- If achieve ROSC, initiate postcardiac arrest care.

DISPOSITION

Of hospitalized patients who develop PEA, <15% survive to discharge. Survival rates much lower in patients with prehospital PEA. Survivors often have poor neurologic outcomes.

REFERRAL

As needed for underlying condition.

! PEARLS & CONSIDERATIONS

- The benefit of epinephrine in PEA resuscitation is uncertain; it may be associated with worse neurologic outcomes and increased long-term mortality. However, the 2015 American Heart Association guidelines support its continued use.
- Use of steroids in resuscitation and postresuscitation shock may improve neurologic outcomes and survival to hospital discharge for patients with in-hospital cardiac arrest.
- Targeted temperature management (32° to 36° C for 24 hr) may improve neurologic outcomes and reduce mortality in comatose cardiac arrest survivors.
- Termination of resuscitation guidelines exist for out-of-hospital cardiac arrest. Similar guidelines for in-hospital cardiac arrest are not available; termination of resuscitation is based on multiple patient factors.
- Prognosis may be guided by testing, but no single exam finding or test is definitive; a multimodal approach is needed. Delay testing for at least 72 hr after ROSC. In addition to neurologic examination (corneal and pupillary reflexes, motor response), testing may include median nerve somatosensory-evoked potentials, EEG, biomarkers, and neuroimaging. Prognostication is more difficult in patients treated with hypothermia; wait >72 hr after return to normothermia before attempting to predict outcome.

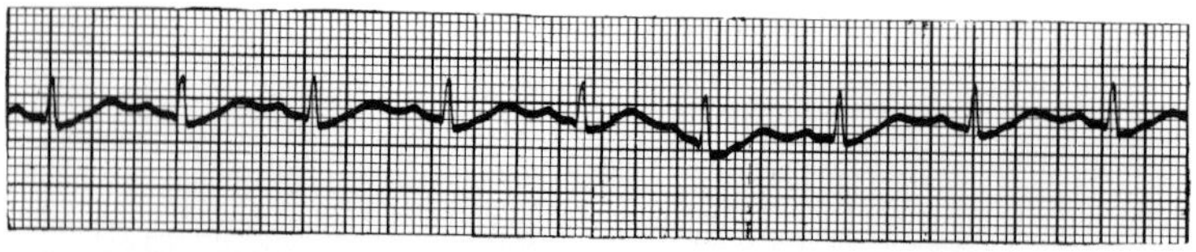

SUGGESTED READINGS

Available at www.expertconsult.com

FIG. 1 Sinus rhythm with pulseless electrical activity (PEA). Although the ECG showed sinus rhythm, the patient had no pulse or blood pressure. In this case the PEA was a result of depressed myocardial function after a cardiac arrest. (From Goldberg AL: *Clinical electrocardiography,* ed 5, St Louis, 1994, Mosby.)

AUTHOR: **SUDEEP K. AULAKH, M.D.**

BASIC INFORMATION

DEFINITION

Ascending infection of a bacterial pathogen infecting the renal pelvis and kidney. Primarily presenting clinically as a urinary tract infection (UTI) characterized by painful urination (dysuria) concomitantly with flank pain/tenderness, nausea, vomiting, and/or fever. The elderly may also present with failure to thrive, unexplained anorexia, other organ system decompensation, and generalized deterioration.

CONSISTS OF TWO GROUPS

Uncomplicated. Can be treated as an outpatient with oral antibiotics.

COMPLICATED: Requires inpatient treatment with IV antibiotics. Hospitalization indicated for persistent vomiting, progression of uncomplicated UTI, suspected sepsis, immunosuppression, or urinary tract obstruction. This is a potentially life-threatening infection that can lead to renal parenchymal damage; timely diagnosis and management can significantly impact patient outcome.

Acute pyelonephritis
Pyonephrosis
Renal carbuncle
Lobar nephronia
Acute bacterial nephritis

ICD-10CM CODES
N10	Acute tubulo-interstitial nephritis
N11	Chronic tubulo-interstitial nephritis
N11.0	Nonobstructive reflux-associated chronic pyelonephritis
N11.1	Chronic obstructive pyelonephritis
N11.8	Other chronic tubulo-interstitial nephritis
N11.9	Chronic tubulo-interstitial nephritis, unspecified
N12	Tubulo-interstitial nephritis, not specified as acute or chronic
N20.9	Calculus pyelonephritis

Use additional code (B95-B97) to identify infectious agent.

EPIDEMIOLOGY & DEMOGRAPHICS

INCIDENCE (IN U.S.): Pyelonephritis is extremely common in U.S. (10,000 cases per year). The highest incidence occurs in the summer months. Pyelonephritis is responsible for 9.1% to 31% of severe sepsis cases annually depending on geographic area. Mortality averages 16.1% annually, ranging from 5% for ages <25 years to 43% for ages >64 years.
PREDOMINANT SEX: Women are five times more likely to be hospitalized than men until age 65 years. Afterward, in males, the difference in prevalence narrows. Risk factors associated with pyelonephritis in healthy women are sexual intercourse (three or more times weekly over the previous 30 days), a new sex partner in the past year, use of spermicide, urinary tract infection (UTI) in the past 12 mo, a mother with a history of UTI, diabetes mellitus, and urinary incontinence. Urinary tract obstruction is the most important risk factor for a complicated UTI.
PREDOMINANT AGE: Trimodal distribution described in women
- Females, ages 0 to 4 years
- Women, ages 15 to 35 years, especially if sexually active.
- Gradual increase in frequency again after age 50 years, with a peak at 80 years of age Bimodal distribution in men
- Boys, ages 0 to 4 years
- Gradual increase after age 35 years to peak at 85 years

GENETICS: Congenital urologic structural disorders associated with vesicoureteral reflux predispose to infections at an early age (<5 years), and may produce renal scarring in most males and some females. Pyelonephritis may produce an Ask-Upmark kidney, segmental renal hypoplasia, which is found more often in young females with severe hypertension.

PHYSICAL FINDINGS & CLINICAL PRESENTATION

Diagnosis established by clinical presentation, history, and physical examination.

Diagnosis is suspected in cases of lower urinary tract symptoms (e.g., urinary frequency, urgency, and dysuria) accompanied by any of the following:
- Fever, rigors, chills (fever may not be present in the elderly or immunosuppressed)
- Flank pain
- Hematuria: Gross hematuria is rare with acute pyelonephritis and should raise suspicion for acute cystitis, papillary necrosis, or a lower genitourinary malignancy
- Toxic appearance
- Nausea and vomiting
- Headache
- Diarrhea

Physical examination notable for costovertebral angle tenderness with exquisite flank pain. Flank pain is a nearly universal finding; its absence should raise suspicion for an alternative diagnosis. Patients presenting with nephrolithiasis/ureterolithiasis usually do not present with costovertebral angle tenderness; instead, abdominal or suprapubic tenderness may be present.

ETIOLOGY

Ascending infections from intestinal bacteria that colonize the perineum and vulva in women account for most of the infections. Much less commonly, bacteria and viruses may produce a hematogenously induced pyelonephritis, as with bacterial septic emboli.
- Gram-negative bacilli cause 95% of cases (e.g., *E. coli* and *Klebsiella* spp).
- Other, more unusual gram-negative organisms may be causative, particularly after urinary-tract instrumentation (e.g., *Enterobacter, Serratia,* and *Proteus mirabilis, Pseudomonas,* among others).
- Resistant gram-negative organisms or even fungi such as *Candida* species appear in hospitalized patients with indwelling catheters.
- Gram-positive organisms such as enterococci and, rarely, *Staphylococcus saprophyticus.*
- *Staphylococcus aureus* indicates hematogenous spread to the kidneys.
- Viruses generally are limited to the lower tract.
- Urea-splitting organisms results in the production of ammonia, bicarbonate, and carbonate; generate an alkaline urine; facilitates crystal formation from supersaturation of carbonate apatite (staghorn calculus). As the staghorn calculus grows, it leads to infection, obstruction, or both.

In the elderly, *E. coli* is less common (60%), whereas diabetics develop infections from *Klebsiella* spp, *Enterobacteriaceae, Clostridia,* or *Candida* species.

During the past decade, community-acquired bacteria (particularly *E. coli*) that produce extended-spectrum beta-lactamases have emerged as a cause of acute pyelonephritis worldwide. The most common risk factors for these uropathogens include frequent visits to health care centers, recent use of antimicrobials (e.g., cephalosporins and fluoroquinolones), older age, immunosuppression, recurrent pyelonephritis, nephrolithiasis, and comorbid conditions such as diabetes mellitus and recurrent UTIs.

DIAGNOSIS

DIFFERENTIAL DIAGNOSIS

Differential diagnosis includes any of the following:
- Abdominal abscess
- Acute abdomen
- Appendicitis
- Basilar pleural process
- Diverticulitis
- Endometriosis
- Lower rib fracture
- Metastatic disease
- Musculoskeletal disorders
- Nephrolithiasis
- Pancreatitis
- Papillary necrosis
- Pelvic inflammatory disease
- Pulmonary infarctions
- Renal corticomedullary necrosis
- Renal vein thrombosis
- Retroperitoneal hemorrhage or abscess
- Herpes zoster
- Splenic abscess or infarct
- Urinary tract obstruction
- Vascular pathology

WORKUP

Evaluation includes prostate health assessment in older males.

URINALYSIS

Performed on a clean-catch voided or catheterized specimen if unable to void or cooperate. Dipstick and microscopic examination must be performed on a fresh specimen for preservation of formed elements (e.g., cells, casts, and microorganisms). Most cases demonstrate pyuria and positive leukocyte esterase in association with positive blood reaction and microhematuria. Leukocyte casts are generally of renal origin but are not always present.

URINE CULTURE

Clean midstream cultures are obtained from all patients suspected of having acute pyelonephritis to guide antibiotic therapy. However, a "clean catch" specimen may not be necessary, as recent evidence demonstrates no significant difference in the number of contaminated or unreliable culture results when collected with or without preparatory cleansing. Obtain a catheterized urine sample if the patient is unable to void, is uncooperative, or has a change in mental status. There is no difference in colony counts or organisms between catheterized and midstream voiding samples.

More than 95% of acute pyelonephritis cases exhibit more than 10^5 colony-forming units of a single bacterium per ml of urine. However, it is important to obtain an accurate history regarding the timing of culture acquisition and prior antibiotic administration. A negative culture with classic clinical and radiological findings does not rule out acute pyelonephritis as shown by a prospective study with only 23.5% positive urine cultures in 196 patients with clinical and radiological evidence of acute pyelonephritis. A urine gram stain may aid in the choice of empiric antimicrobial therapy pending urine culture. If gram-positive cocci are seen, one should consider *Enterococcus* species or *Staphylococcus saprophyticus* as causative.

Posttreatment urinalysis and culture are unnecessary if symptomatic improvement occurs, but these should be obtained when symptoms do not improve substantially within 2 to 3 days after initiation of antibiotic treatment, or if symptoms recur within 2 wk of therapy. Urinary tract imaging is recommended in these cases.

BLOOD CULTURES

Cultures are obtained in patients admitted to the hospital but may not be routinely required in uncomplicated cases. Approximately 15% to 30% of patients with acute pyelonephritis are bacteremic. The elderly and those with complicated acute pyelonephritis are more likely to develop bacteremia and sepsis.

Urine cultures yield a causative organism in almost all cases of acute pyelonephritis; thus, a positive blood culture may be diagnostically redundant. However, if an alternate diagnosis to acute pyelonephritis is suspected, such as endometriosis, intraabdominal or psoas abscesses, or cholangitis, blood cultures should be considered.

RADIOLOGY

Most uncomplicated cases of acute pyelonephritis do not require imaging studies, unless symptoms do not improve or there is recurrence. Abdominal radiographs (i.e., kidney, ureter, and bladder x-ray [KUB]) are of limited use in acute pyelonephritis, unless staghorn calculi are present. Retrograde or antegrade

pyelography is helpful in severe obstruction that is not demonstrated noninvasively. Voiding cystourethrography demonstrates vesicoureteral reflux and is generally performed routinely only in children.

Recommendations for radiologic tests
- Healthy patients with uncomplicated pyelonephritis do not typically require radiologic workup if therapeutic response occurs with 72 hr of antibiotic therapy.
- If no response to therapy occurs within 72 hr, abdominal CT is the study of choice.
- Diabetics and immunocompromised patients should undergo precontrast and postcontrast abdominal and pelvic CT scans (Fig. 1) within 24 hr of diagnosis when there is not a prompt response to therapy.
- Ultrasound is reserved for patients in whom exposure to contrast or radiation is considered hazardous. There is a high false negative rate for renal abscess with ultrasound. In a prospective study of acute pyelonephritis of 213 patients submitted for CT/NMR study, 50 patients (23.5%) had a renal abscess, yet only two were detected by ultrasound.
- All other adults with complicated cases (i.e., history of stones or other urologic conditions, prior urologic surgery, repeated episodes of pyelonephritis) should be evaluated early by CT scan.
- Helical CT scans detect calculi with high sensitivity.
- Urologic imaging studies should be conducted in all young men and boys.

Because of the risk of contrast nephropathy, caution should be considered when administering contrast to patients taking metformin or with chronic kidney disease. When evaluating kidney function, consider basing diagnostic decisions on eGFR rather than serum creatinine, especially in the elderly. Patients with acute pyelonephritis and an acutely elevated baseline serum creatinine may warrant CT imaging as part of an evaluation to rule out obstruction. If concern remains when administering iodinated radiocontrast or gadolinium-based medium (increased risk of nephrogenic sys-

temic fibrosis), particularly when GFR is <30 ml/min/1.73 m^2, consider retrograde or antegrade pyelography.

The primary purpose of imaging is to identify underlying structural abnormalities, such as occult obstruction from a stone or abscess, and serious complications, such as emphysematous pyelonephritis. In a prospective study of 213 patients with acute pyelonephritis, there were no differences in frequency of fever, leukocytosis, C-reactive protein, pyuria, urine cultures, and duration of symptoms prior to hospitalization for positive or negative CT scans. Thus, systematic CT or NMR is necessary to exclude an anatomical abnormality such as noted previously, and such an abnormality cannot be predicted on the basis of clinical, biochemical, or culture parameters. Emphysematous pyelonephritis is a necrotizing infection that produces intraparenchymal kidney gas identifiable by renal imaging that is associated with high mortality. Risk factors include diabetes mellitus and/or urinary tract obstruction. Gas-forming bacteria, most commonly *E. coli*, produce gas that is usually restricted within Gerota's fascia. If gas is localized to the kidney, mortality is 60%. If gas spreads to the perinephric space, mortality is 80%. In emphysematous pyelitis, the mortality is 20%. This must be differentiated from a renal abscess that can also be associated with gas collection. With drainage and antibiotic treatment, a renal abscess has a favorable prognosis.

LABORATORY TESTS

Basic metabolic profile on all patients with suspected acute pyelonephritis to assess renal function. CBC with differential count. If the diagnosis is in doubt, other laboratory tests may be appropriate to clarify the differential diagnosis (e.g., lipase, transaminase, and β-HCG levels).

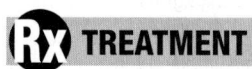

ACUTE GENERAL Rx
Uncomplicated acute pyelonephritis

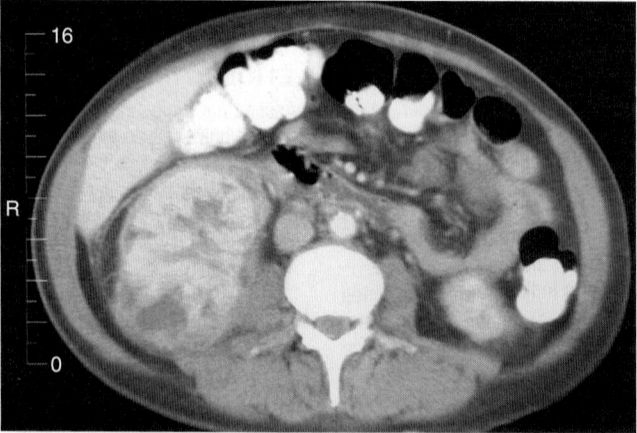

FIG. 1 Acute pyelonephritis: contrast material–enhanced computed tomographic (CT) scan. The heterogeneous CT nephrogram shows the diffuse involvement of the right kidney. Stranding and some fluid are visible in the perinephritic space with thickening of Gerota's fascia. (From Skorecki K et al: *Brenner & Rector's the Kidney*, ed 10, Philadelphia, 2016, Elsevier.)

Close outpatient follow-up is possible with minimal gastrointestinal symptoms and the ability to maintain fluid intake and oral medications. Prompt antibiotic therapy prevents progression of infection and must be initiated following acquisition of appropriate cultures.

Begin empiric therapy based on risk of adverse effects, local community bacterial profiles, and resistance rates. Antibiotics are revised after urine culture results are available.

The concept of requiring long-term treatment of acute pyelonephritis has been questioned. Women with acute pyelonephritis were randomized to oral treatment with ciprofloxacin 500 mg twice daily for 7 days or 14 days, and 27% of these patients experienced bacteremia from *E. coli*. No differences in the cure rates were found (87% and 96%, respectively).

Outpatient regimens

- Fluoroquinolones preferred in communities where local prevalence of resistant *E. coli* is ≤10%.
- Ciprofloxacin 500 mg PO twice daily or 1000 mg extended-release form PO daily for 7 days.
- Levofloxacin 750 mg PO daily for 5 days.
- The initial dose may be administered IV (ciprofloxacin 400 mg or levofloxacin 500 mg). Alternative treatment with trimethoprim/ sulfamethoxazole 160/800 mg PO twice daily for 14 days.

Because of the high prevalence of resistance to oral beta-lactam antibiotics and trimethoprim/ sulfamethoxazole, these agents usually are reserved for cases where susceptibility results are known, but additional factors (e.g., allergy history, potential drug-drug interactions, drug availability) may require empiric treatment with these agents before susceptibility results are known. For such cases, a long-acting, broad-spectrum parenteral drug ([e.g., ceftriaxone 1 gram or gentamicin 5 mg/kg) may be administered as a one-time dose or longer until sensitivities of the organism are known. If the local fluoroquinolone resistance prevalence to *E. coli* exceeds 10%, an initial IV dose of ceftriaxone or gentamicin is recommended, followed by an oral fluoroquinolone regimen.

Significant clinical improvement during appropriate empiric antibiotic therapy should occur within 48 to 72 hr. If improvement does not occur, a complication of acute pyelonephritis or an alternative diagnosis such as an abscess, emphysematous pyelonephritis, or an obstructing calculus should be considered. Any unexpected change in the clinical picture warrants immediate investigation with a CT or MRI scan, with potential for surgical intervention.

Complicated Acute Pyelonephritis

- Hospitalization is indicated for the following reasons:
  1. Toxic patients
  2. Complicated infections
  3. Diabetes or otherwise immunosuppressed
  4. Suspected bacteremia

Inpatient care includes supportive care, monitoring of culture results, adjustment of antibiotic regimen, and IV volume repletion as required. IV antibiotics are continued until defervescence

and clinical improvement occurs, with subsequent conversion to an oral antibiotic regimen for a total duration of antibiotic administration of 10 to 14 days.

1. IV antibiotic options for more toxic patients pending cultures include ceftriaxone (1-2 g once daily), IV ciprofloxacin (400 mg every 12 hr) or IV levofloxacin (500-750 mg IV once daily), piperacillin/tazobactam (3.375 g IV every 6 hr) or carbapenems such as meropenem or imipenem (500 mg IV every 6-8 hr).
2. Ceftazidime 1-2 g IV every 8 hr, piperacillin/ tazobactam, and carbapenems are optimal choices for *Pseudomonas* due to increasing *Pseudomonas* resistance to ciprofloxacin.
3. Aminoglycosides (2 mg/kg IV loading dose followed by 1 mg/kg IV every 8-12 hr adjusted for kidney function) are potentially nephrotoxic and are used only if there is no better alternative. Vancomycin 1 g IV every 12 hr, linezolid 600 mg IV or PO every 12 hr, or daptomycin 4-6 mg/kg IV daily for gram-positive cocci (e.g., enterococci, staphylococci).
4. Ampicillin 1 to 2 g IV every 4 to 6 hr for ampicillin-sensitive enterococci with an aminoglycoside for synergy. Urinary obstruction is promptly drained by nephrostomy tube. Surgical drainage of abscess formation(s). Pregnant females with acute pyelonephritis are hospitalized and treated initially with a second- or third-generation cephalosporin.

RENAL ABSCESSES (RENAL CARBUNCLES)

Cortical abscesses historically required surgical drainage; however, using current antibiotics is commonly sufficient for cure.

- Semisynthetic penicillin, cephalosporin, fluoroquinolone, or vancomycin, with guidance from culture and sensitivity results.
  1. Parenteral therapy for 10 to 14 days followed by oral therapy for 2 to 4 wk.
  2. Fever should resolve in 5 to 6 days and pain within 24 hr.
  3. If there is no clinical response within 48 hr, percutaneous or open drainage should be considered. More extreme measures are sometimes needed including enucleation or nephrectomy.

CORTICOMEDULLARY ABSCESSES

- Parenteral therapy for at least 48 hr is typically successful.
- May require incision and drainage and, possibly, nephrectomy.
- If clinical defervescence occurs, IV antibiotic treatment may be switched to complete a 2-wk course of oral antibiotic therapy.

PERINEPHRIC ABSCESS

- Serious complication with mortality in the 25% to 50% range
- Requires early recognition, surgical drainage, and parenteral antibiotics (not adequate alone) to reduce mortality.

- Initial antibiotic therapy should include an aminoglycoside and an antistaphylococcal agent.
  1. If *Pseudomonas* species grow in culture or is suspected, add an antipseudemonal beta-lactam antibiotic to the aminoglycoside.
  2. For enterococcus, an aminoglycoside and ampicillin are recommended.
- Reported with tuberculosis or fungi as rare causes.
- Nephrectomy may be considered with clinical deterioration despite aggressive therapy.

CALCULI-RELATED INFECTIONS

Organisms may survive within calculi making these cases especially problematic.

- With acute infection, calculi must be removed immediately using cystoscopy or open surgical procedure.
  1. Surgical observation is not recommended as mortality is 28% with observation versus 7.2 % in surgical treated group.
- In staghorn calculi, it is optimal to remove the entire stone (as remaining fragments are still infected and may recur).
  1. Urease inhibitors are effective at reducing stone formation.
     a. Limited by long-term toxicity with neurosensory, hematologic, and dermatologic adverse side effects.

RENAL PAPILLARY NECROSIS

- Admission for parenteral antibiotics
  1. Initial therapy should cover *E. coli*, *Enterobacter*, *Proteus*, and *Klebsiella* species pending culture results.
  2. For more serious infections, also cover *Pseudomonas* and *Enterococcus*.
  3. Empiric therapy agent options include:
     a. Aminoglycosides
     b. Cefotaxime
     c. Ceftriaxone
     d. Ceftazidime
     e. Cefepime
     f. Piperacillin-tazobactam
     g. Imipenum-cilastin
     h. Meropenem
     i. Ciprofloxacin
  4. Continue parenteral therapy until fever and clinical symptoms defervesce (typically 14 days).

CHRONIC Rx

- Repair underlying structural problems, especially when kidney function is compromised.
  1. Reflux
  2. Obstruction
  3. Suspect nephrolithiasis
- Avoid urinary catheters.

DISPOSITION

- If pyelonephritis is uncomplicated with no significant GI symptoms, it can readily be treated on an outpatient basis with close monitoring of therapeutic response(s) in 48 to 72 hr.
- If pyelonephritis is complicated, if symptoms persist for >48 to 72 hr, or any of

the following exist, admission is warranted: significant GI symptoms that preclude oral therapy, patient is pregnant, urinary tract obstruction, suspected renal or perinephric abscess, bacterial sepsis, diabetes or other immunocompromised states, recurrent or refractory pyelonephritis, or infection with an unusual or antibiotic-resistant microorganism.

- If signs or symptoms are consistent with sepsis, consider intensive care unit admission.
- Acute pyelonephritis may be fatal when complications develop, such as emphysematous pyelonephritis (20%-80% mortality rate), perinephric abscess (20%-50% mortality rate), or sepsis syndrome (>25% overall mortality rate).
- Acute deterioration or nonresponse to conventional therapy may be due to a complication, resistant organism, or unrecognized comorbidity.
- Diabetic patients with acute pyelonephritis are prone to bacteremia, longer hospital stays, and higher mortality, and diabetics should be considered complicated patients.

- Patients >65 years are associated with higher mortality, septic shock, bedridden status, and immunosuppression. In males, mortality is also increased with the use of antibiotics in the previous month.

REFERRAL

- To a surgeon for suspected abscess
- Infectious disease for resistant organisms and poor response to routine antibiotic therapy as outlined
- Urology to correct underlying urologic problems (e.g., reflux and hydronephrosis)
- Nephrology consult if renal dysfunction is present or for nephrolithiasis workup
- Critical care medicine if patient requires ICU admission

PEARLS & CONSIDERATIONS

- Consider acute pyelonephritis in anyone presenting with urinary symptoms, flank pain, and fever.

- Obtain a urinalysis and culture before starting empiric antibiotic therapy, and adjust treatment pending antibiotic sensitivity testing.
  Evaluate clinical response in 48 to 72 hr during outpatient therapy. If no or tardy improvement, continue evaluation to rule out urinary tract obstruction.
- Urology consultation in all cases of urinary tract obstruction or detection of urinary tract gas (e.g., emphysematous pyelonephritis).
- Treat all diabetics as complicated acute pyelonephritis.

RELATED CONTENT

Pyelonephritis (Patient Information)

AUTHOR: **NELSON KOPYT, D.O.**

BASIC INFORMATION

DEFINITION

Ramsay Hunt syndrome is a localized herpes zoster infection involving the seventh nerve and geniculate ganglia, resulting in hearing loss, vertigo, and facial nerve palsy.

SYNONYMS

Herpes zoster oticus
Geniculate herpes
Herpetic geniculate ganglionitis

ICD-10CM CODES
B02.21 Postherpetic geniculate ganglionitis

EPIDEMIOLOGY & DEMOGRAPHICS

PREDOMINANT SEX: Equal sex distribution
PREDOMINANT AGE:
- Increasingly common with advancing age
- Rare in childhood

PHYSICAL FINDINGS & CLINICAL PRESENTATION

- Characteristic vesicles:
  1. On pinna
  2. In external auditory canal (Fig. 1)
  3. In distribution of the facial nerve and, occasionally, adjacent cranial nerves
- Facial paralysis on the involved side
- Auditory symptoms include mild to severe tinnitus, deafness, vertigo, and nystagmus.

ETIOLOGY

- Reactivation of dormant infection with varicella-zoster virus after primary varicella
- Herpetic inflammation of the geniculate ganglion is thought to be the cause of this syndrome.

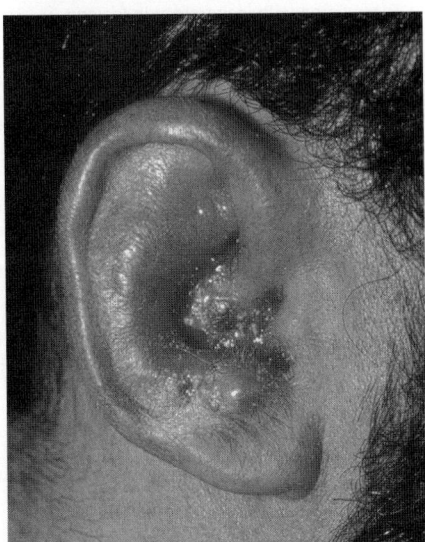

FIG. 1 Herpes zoster of the geniculate ganglion resulting in vesicles on the ear (as shown here) and tympanic membrane occurs in Ramsay Hunt syndrome. Both seventh and eighth cranial nerve functions may be affected. (From White GM, Cox NH [eds]: *Diseases of the skin: color atlas and text*, ed 2, St Louis, 2006, Mosby.)

DIAGNOSIS

- Usually made by recognition of the clinical features detailed previously
- Viral culture and/or microscopic examination of specimens taken from active vesicles

DIFFERENTIAL DIAGNOSIS

- Herpes simplex
- External otitis
- Impetigo
- Enteroviral infection
- Guillain-Barre syndrome
- Bell's palsy of other etiologies, such as Lyme disease
- Acoustic neuroma (before appearance of skin lesions)
  The differential diagnosis of headache and facial pain is described in Section II.

WORKUP

If the diagnosis is in doubt, confirm varicella-zoster virus infection.

LABORATORY TESTS

- Generally not necessary
- Viral culture of specimens of vesicular fluid and scrapings of the vesicle base
- Tzanck preparation, which may reveal multinucleated giant cells
- Direct immunofluorescent staining of scrapings

IMAGING STUDIES

MRI may demonstrate enhancement of the facial and vestibulocochlear nerves before appearance of vesicles.

TREATMENT

ACUTE GENERAL Rx

- Use of corticosteroids is controversial.
- Acyclovir (800 mg PO five times qd for 10 days), famciclovir (500 mg tid for 7 days), or valacyclovir (1 g q8h for 7 days) may hasten healing.
- Use of prednisone (60 mg PO qd for 7 days or on a tapering regimen, 40 mg PO for 2 days, 30 mg for 7 days, followed by tapering course) is recommended by some authors but its use remains controversial.
- Analgesics should be used as indicated.

CHRONIC Rx

- Duloxetine and amitriptyline are effective in postherpetic pain.
- Other agents for postherpetic pain include gabapentin and pregabalin.
- Narcotic analgesics may occasionally be necessary.

DISPOSITION

Recurrences are unusual.

REFERRAL

To otolaryngologist: patients with persistent facial paralysis for potential surgical decompression of the facial nerve

PEARLS & CONSIDERATIONS

COMMENTS

Immunodeficiency states, particularly HIV infection, should be considered in:
- Younger patients
- Severe cases
- Patients with a history of specific risk behavior

SUGGESTED READING

Available at www.expertconsult.com

RELATED CONTENT

Ramsay Hunt Syndrome (Patient Information)
Herpes Zoster (Related Key Topic)

AUTHOR: **GLENN G. FORT, M.D., M.P.H.**

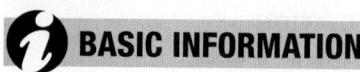

DEFINITION

Raynaud's phenomenon (RP) is a vasospastic disorder that causes an exaggerated response to cold temperatures and/or emotional stress, resulting in episodic digital ischemia. It presents as a cold-induced, symmetric, sharply demarcated white or blue discoloration of the distal fingers or toes, followed by erythema at a variable time after rewarming.

SYNONYMS

Primary Raynaud's phenomenon or Raynaud's disease
Secondary Raynaud's phenomenon

ICD-10CM CODES
I73.0 Raynaud's syndrome
I73.00 Raynaud's syndrome without gangrene
I73.01 Raynaud's syndrome with gangrene

EPIDEMIOLOGY & DEMOGRAPHICS

- RP is classified clinically into primary or secondary forms and affects approximately 3% to 5% of the general population, 15% of children younger than 12 yr, and less than 1% of adults older than 60 yr.
- Occurs more commonly in colder climates.
- Primary RP usually occurs between the ages of 12 and 25 yr.
- It is more likely to affect women than men (4:1).
- 5% to 15% of patients with primary Raynaud's phenomenon develop a secondary cause later in the course of the disease (mostly a connective tissue disorder).
- Secondary RP tends to begin after age 35 to 40 yr.
- Secondary RP occurs in more than 90% of patients with scleroderma and in approximately 30% of patients with systemic lupus erythematosus or Sjögren's syndrome.

PHYSICAL FINDINGS & CLINICAL PRESENTATION

- The typical manifestation of RP is the biphasic color response of the digits to cold exposure and rewarming, which may or may not be accompanied by pain. RP most often affects the hand (Fig. 1).
  1. White (pallor) or blue (cyanotic) discoloration of the digit(s) resulting from vasospasm on cold or vibration exposure.
  2. Red (rubor) with or without pain and paresthesia when vasospasm resolves and blood returns to the digit.
- Color changes can sometimes be induced by placing the hand in an ice bath, although this is not recommended as a diagnostic maneuver because responses may be inconsistent even in patients with definite RP.
- Color changes are well delineated, symmetric, and usually bilateral, involving fingers and toes. The index, middle, and ring fingers are commonly involved and the thumb infrequently; however, if the thumb is involved, that suggests secondary causes of RP.
- Fingertips are most often involved, but feet, ears, nose, tongue, and nipples can also be affected.
- Patients with RP may exhibit a violaceous or reticular pattern of skin of arms and legs, sometimes with regular, unbroken circles (livedo reticularis).
- Duration of attacks can range from seconds to hours and averages 15 to 20 min.
- Chronic skin changes resulting from repeated attacks may include skin thickening and brittle nails. Ulcerations and, rarely, gangrene may occur.
- Physical examination should also include examination for symptoms associated with autoimmune disease, such as fever, rash, arthritis, dry eyes, dry mouth, myalgias, or cardiopulmonary abnormalities.

ETIOLOGY

- Primary RP can also be called idiopathic Raynaud's phenomenon, primary Raynaud's syndrome, or Raynaud's disease. It occurs in the absence of any associated disease.
- With primary RP, the possibility that another first-degree family member is affected is reported as approximately 25%.
- Secondary RP is associated with an underlying pathologic condition or disorder, use of certain drugs, or related occupation. Secondary RP is associated with:
  1. CREST syndrome (calcinosis, RP, esophageal involvement, sclerodactyly, and telangiectasia)
  2. Scleroderma, Sjögren's syndrome, mixed connective tissue disease, polymyositis, and dermatomyositis
  3. Primary pulmonary hypertension
  4. Systemic lupus erythematosus, arteritis
  5. Rheumatoid arthritis
  6. Thromboangiitis obliterans (Buerger's disease)
  7. Drugs (beta-blockers, ergotamine, methysergide, vinblastine, bleomycin, oral contraceptives, nicotine, clonidine, cocaine, caffeine, vinyl chloride, tegafur, interferon alfa, interferon beta)
  8. Hematologic disorders (polycythemia, cryoglobulinemia, cold agglutinins, paraproteinemia, cryofibrinogenemia)
  9. Carpal tunnel syndrome
  10. Use of tools that vibrate
  11. Endocrine disorders (hypothyroidism, carcinoid syndrome, pheochromocytoma, metabolic syndrome)
  12. Estrogen replacement therapy without progesterone
  13. Hypercoagulable states, protein C, protein S, antithrombin III deficiency, factor V Leiden deficiency, and antiphospholipid syndrome
  14. Poliomyelitis is a rare cause
  15. Primary biliary cirrhosis
  16. Vasospastic disorders (migraines, Prinzmetal angina)
  17. Malignancies (angiocentric lymphoma, ovarian cancer)

Clinical criteria:
- Definite RP: repeated episodes of biphasic color change on cold exposure
- Possible RP: Uniphasic color changes plus numbness or paresthesia on cold exposure
- No RP: No color change on cold exposure

The suggested criteria for primary RP are:
- Symmetric attacks
- Absence of tissue necrosis, ulceration, gangrene, or peripheral vascular disease
- Absence of a secondary cause on the basis of a patient's history and general physical examination
- Negative nail-fold capillary examination
- Negative test for antinuclear antibody (ANA)
- Normal erythrocyte sedimentation rate (ESR)

Secondary RP is suggested by the following findings:
- Onset of symptoms after age 30 yr
- Male gender
- Episodes that are painful, asymmetric, or associated with ischemic skin lesions
- Clinical features suggestive of a connective-tissue disease
- Elevated specific autoantibody tests and ESR
- Evidence of microvascular disease on microscopy of nail-fold capillaries

DIFFERENTIAL DIAGNOSIS

- Neurogenic thoracic outlet syndrome or carpal tunnel syndrome
- Frostbite or cold weather injury
- Medication reaction (ergotamine, chemotherapeutic agents)
- Atherosclerosis, thromboembolic disease
- Buerger's disease, embolic disease
- Acrocyanosis
- Livedo reticularis
- Injury from repetitive motion

WORKUP

- Fig. 2 describes an approach to diagnosis of Raynaud's phenomenon. Once the diagnosis of RP is established, differentiating primary from secondary is helpful in treatment and prognosis.
- Patients who are younger when their symptoms occur, have a normal history and physical examination and normal nail-fold

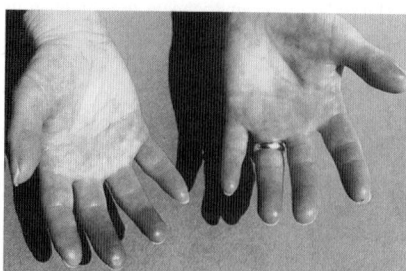

FIG. 1 Raynaud's phenomenon. Sharply demarcated cyanosis of the fingers with proximal venular congestion (livedo reticularis) is seen. (From Klippel J et al [eds]: *Primary care rheumatology,* London, 1999, Mosby.)

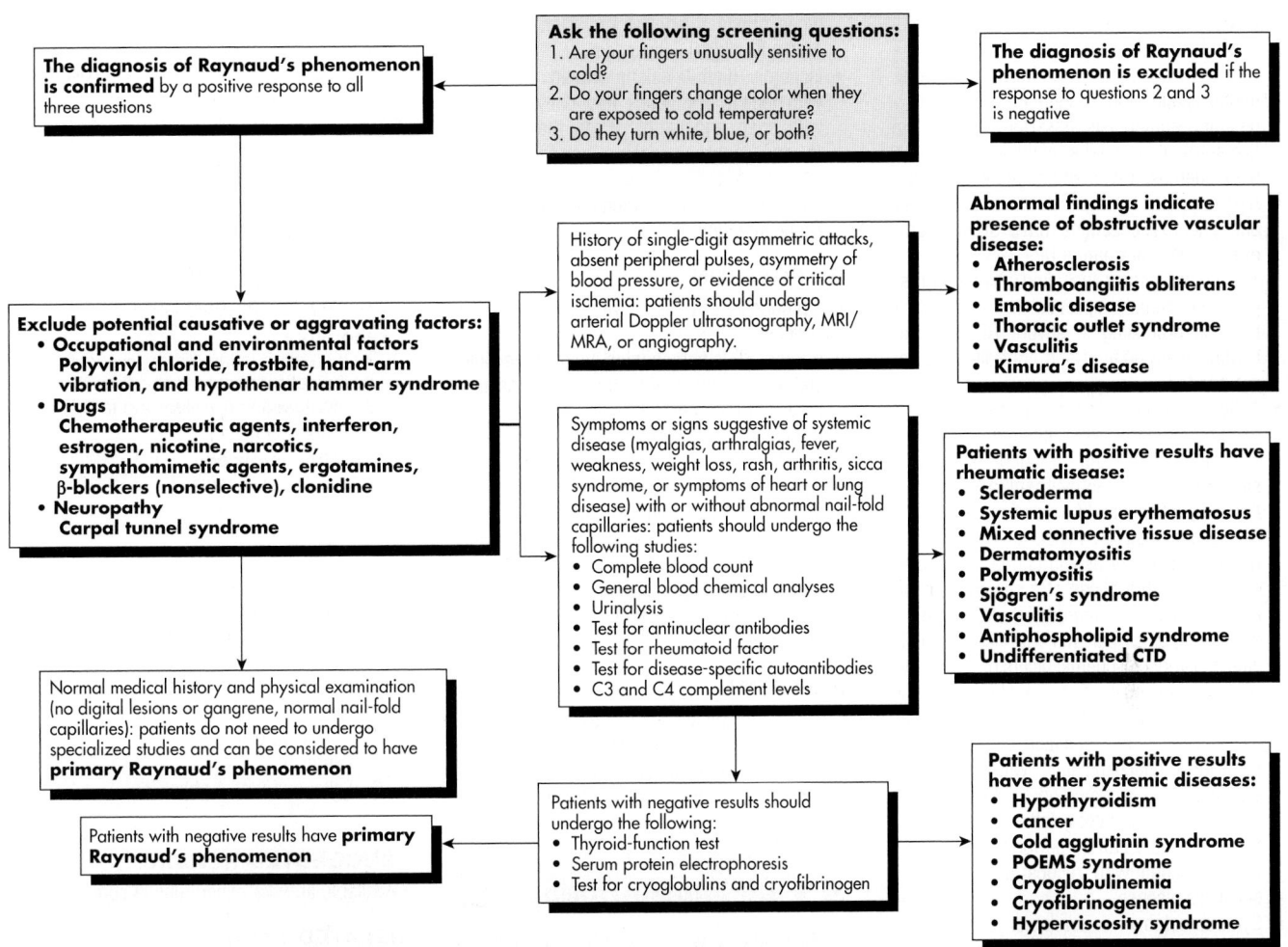

FIG. 2 Approach to diagnosis of Raynaud's phenomenon. *CTD,* Connective tissue disease; *MRA,* magnetic resonance angiography; *MRI,* magnetic resonance imaging; *POEMS,* polyneuropathy, organomegaly, endocrinopathy, monoclonal gammopathy, and skin changes. (From Firestein GS et al [eds]: *Kelly's textbook of rheumatology,* ed 9, Philadelphia, 2013, Saunders.)

capillaries, and have no history of digital ischemic lesions can be considered as having primary RP. These patients can be monitored clinically without any further testing.

- If a secondary cause of RP is suspected, appropriate laboratory testing is recommended (see "Laboratory Tests"). Secondary RP has associated abnormal nail-fold microscopy.

LABORATORY TESTS

- CBC, serum electrolytes, blood urea nitrogen, creatinine, ESR, ANAs, VDRL antibody test, rheumatoid factor, and urinalysis should be included in the initial evaluation.
- If the history, physical examination, and initial laboratory tests suggest a possible secondary cause, specific serologic testing (e.g., anticentromere antibodies, anti-Scl 70, cryoglobulins, complement testing, and serum protein electrophoresis) may be indicated.
- Noninvasive vascular testing includes finger systolic blood pressures, segmental blood pressure measurements, cold recovery time (measure vasoconstrictor and vasodilator responses of finger to cold), fingertip thermography, and laser Doppler with thermal challenge (measures relative change in skin blood flow with ambient warming).

IMAGING STUDIES

- The diagnosis of RP should not be made on the basis of laboratory tests, and imaging studies should not replace a good history and physical examination.
- Duplex ultrasound can image the palmar arch and digital arteries for patency.
- Magnetic resonance angiography is useful for imaging larger arteries.
- Contrast angiography is the gold standard for arterial imaging.
- Nail-fold capillary microscopy can differentiate primary from secondary RP.
- Videomicroscopy and thermography are also useful for diagnosis of RP.

Rx TREATMENT

NONPHARMACOLOGIC THERAPY

- Avoid drugs that may precipitate RP (see "Etiology").
- Avoid cold exposure and sudden temperature shifts. Use warm gloves, hats, and garments during the winter months or before going into cold environments (e.g., air-conditioned rooms).
- Avoid stressful situations, and use relaxation techniques in preventing RP attacks.

ACUTE GENERAL Rx

- Acute measures to terminate an attack include rotating the arms in a windmill pattern, placing the hands under warm water or in a warm body fold such as the axilla, and the swing-arm maneuver.
- Medications are indicated in the treatment of RP if there are signs of critical ischemia or if the quality of life of the patient is affected to the degree that activities of normal living are no longer possible and preventive techniques do not work.

CHRONIC Rx

- Dihydropyridine calcium channel blockers (e.g., nifedipine, amlodipine, felodipine, nisoldipine, isradipine) are the most effective pharmacologic treatment for RP and are the drugs of choice.
- Nifedipine is most often prescribed at a dose of 10 to 20 mg 30 min before cold exposure. If symptoms occur with long duration, nifedipine XL 30 to 180 mg PO qd is often effective.
- Some potential therapeutic options include direct vasodilators such as nitroprusside, hydralazine, papaverine, minoxidil, niacin, and griseofulvin. Topical 1% nitroglycerin or topical l-arginine, ethyl nicotinate, hexyl nicotinate,

R

I

thurfyl salicylate may also be useful, particularly if low blood pressure is a concern.

- Phosphodiesterase inhibitors (cilostazol, pentoxifylline, and sildenafil), angiotensin 2 receptor antagonists (losartan), and selective serotonin reuptake inhibitors (fluoxetine) have been used with some limited success.
- Alpha receptor antagonists such as prazosin and phenoxybenzamine have shown some effectiveness in treating RP.
- The prostaglandins, including inhaled iloprost, IV epoprostenol, alprostadil, and tadalafil, may be promising in severe RP. However, additional experience and controlled studies are needed.
- Antioxidants like zinc gluconate have been used to decrease tissue damage.
- N-Acetylcysteine and probucol have been shown to lead to improvement in RP.
- Anticoagulation with IV unfractionated heparin or subcutaneous low-molecular-weight heparin and addition of aspirin can be considered during the acute phase of a severe ischemic event. Aspirin (81 mg/day) therapy can be considered in all patients with secondary RP with a history of ischemic ulcers or thrombotic events; however, caution should be exercised because aspirin can theoretically worsen vasospasm by the inhibition of prostacyclin. Long-term anticoagulation with heparin or warfarin is not recommended unless there is evidence of a hypercoagulable state.
- Bypass surgery can be performed for severe RP associated with reconstructible arterial occlusive disease.
- Sympathectomy is available for unreconstructible occlusive disease or pure vasospastic disease refractory to medical treatment.
- Microsurgical revascularization of the hand and digital reconstruction may improve digital vascular perfusion and heal digital ulcers

when proximal arterial occlusion is associated with digital vasospasm.

- Ischemic digital lesions should be treated with topical antibiotics and daily cleansing with soap and water. Digits that progress to dry gangrene should be permitted to undergo autoamputation. Surgical amputation is limited for intractable pain or deep tissue infection.

DISPOSITION

The prognosis of patients with RP depends on the etiology.

- Primary RP is fairly benign, usually remaining stable and controlled with nonpharmacologic medical treatment.
- Remission of primary RP can occur spontaneously.
- Patients with secondary RP, specifically those with scleroderma, CREST syndrome, or thromboangiitis obliterans, may develop severe ischemic digits with ulceration, gangrene, and autoamputation.
- Box 1 summarizes features suggestive of progression of Raynaud's phenomenon.

REFERRAL

- Rheumatology consult is indicated if secondary collagen vascular disease is diagnosed.
- Vascular surgery consult is indicated if ulcers, gangrene, or threatened digit loss is noted.

❗ PEARLS & CONSIDERATIONS

- Most patients with RP can be managed by a primary care provider.
- It is important to differentiate primary from secondary forms. Secondary forms may become manifest as far out as 10 yr from the diagnosis of RP. It is important to take

BOX 1   Features Suggestive of Progression of Raynaud's Phenomenon

Clinical
- Older age at onset (>35 yr)
- Recurrence of chilblains as adult
- Vasospasm all year round
- Asymmetric attacks
- Sclerodactyly
- Digital ulceration
- Finger pulp pitting scars

Laboratory
- Increased inflammatory markers
- Detection of autoantibodies
- Increased von Willebrand factor antigen

Nail fold microscopy
- Abnormal vessels

From Hochberg MC et al: *Rheumatology*, ed 5, St Louis, 2011, Mosby.

immediate action during an attack, and patients are encouraged to:
1. Keep warm
2. Not use tobacco products
3. Avoid aggravating medications
4. Control stress
5. Exercise
6. Follow up with a physician

SUGGESTED READING
Available at www.expertconsult.com

RELATED CONTENT
Raynaud's Phenomenon (Patient Information)

AUTHORS: **SYEDA M. SAYEED, M.D.,** and **FRED F. FERRI, M.D.**

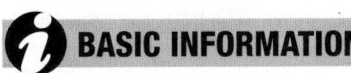

BASIC INFORMATION

DEFINITION

Reiter's syndrome is one of the seronegative spondyloarthropathies, so called because serum rheumatoid factor is not present in these forms of inflammatory arthritis. Its characteristic clinical trial consists of urethritis, conjunctivitis, and arthritis. Hans Reiter was a Nazi war criminal and many believe that he should no longer be given name recognition to designate this syndrome. There is an international consensus that the term *reactive arthritis* (ReA) should replace the name "Reiter's syndrome" to describe this constellation of signs and symptoms. Unfortunately, the original name is still associated with the syndrome. Reiter's syndrome is an asymmetric polyarthritis that affects mainly the lower extremities and is associated with one or more of the following:

- Urethritis
- Cervicitis
- Dysentery
- Inflammatory eye disease
- Mucocutaneous lesions

SYNONYMS

Reiter's disease
Reactive arthritis
Seronegative spondyloarthropathy

ICD-10CM CODES

M02.30 Reiter's disease, unspecified site

EPIDEMIOLOGY & DEMOGRAPHICS

INCIDENCE (IN U.S.): 0.0035% annually of men ≤50 yr
PEAK INCIDENCE: Most common in the third decade
PREDOMINANT SEX: Male
PREDOMINANT AGE: 20 to 40 yr
GENETICS: Familial disposition: strongly associated with HLA-B27 (63% to 96%)

PHYSICAL FINDINGS & CLINICAL PRESENTATION

- Polyarthritis
  1. Affecting the knee and ankle
  2. Commonly asymmetric
- Heel pain and Achilles tendinitis, especially at the insertion of the Achilles tendon
- Plantar fasciitis
- Large effusions
- Dactylitis, or "sausage toe"
- Urethritis
- Uveitis or conjunctivitis; uveitis can progress to blindness without treatment
- Keratoderma blennorrhagicum, circinate balanitis
  1. Hyperkeratotic lesions on soles of the feet (Fig. E1), toes, penis (Fig. E2), hands
  2. Closely resembles psoriasis
- Aortic regurgitation similar to that seen in ankylosing spondylitis

ETIOLOGY

- Epidemic Reiter's syndrome after outbreaks of dysentery has been well described.
- Genetically susceptible HLA-B27 individuals are at risk for developing Reiter's syndrome after infection with certain pathogens:
  1. *Salmonella*
  2. *Shigella*
  3. *Yersinia enterocolitica*
  4. *Chlamydia trachomatis*
- Symptom complex indistinguishable from Reiter's syndrome has been described in association with HIV infection.

DIAGNOSIS

DIFFERENTIAL DIAGNOSIS

- Ankylosing spondylitis
- Psoriatic arthritis
- Rheumatoid arthritis
- Gonococcal arthritis-tenosynovitis
- Rheumatic fever
- Serum sickness
- Gout
- Chronic mucocutaneous candidiasis

WORKUP

- X-ray examination of affected joints
- Synovial fluid examination and culture
- Careful examination of eyes and skin
- Cultures for gonococcus (urethral, cervical, stool)

LABORATORY TESTS

- Elevated but nonspecific erythrocyte sedimentation rate
- No specific laboratory tests to diagnose Reiter's syndrome
- Do not use HLA-B27 testing as a diagnostic tool

IMAGING STUDIES

Plain radiographs:
- Juxtaarticular osteopenia of affected joints
- Erosions and joint space narrowing in more advanced disease
- Periostitis and reactive new bone formation at the insertions of the Achilles tendon and the plantar fascia
- Sacroiliitis:
  1. Unilateral or bilateral
  2. Indistinguishable from ankylosing spondylitis
- Vertebral bridging osteophytes

TREATMENT

NONPHARMACOLOGIC THERAPY

Physical therapy to maintain range of motion of the spine and other joints

ACUTE GENERAL Rx

- Flares treated with nonsteroidal antiinflammatory drugs such as indomethacin (25-50 mg PO tid). Refractory cases can be treated with methotrexate or infliximab.
- Mucocutaneous lesions are visually self-limited and clear with topical corticosteroids.

Acitretin or cyclosporine can be used for refractory 84-inch lesions.
- Enteric or urethral infection should be treated with appropriate antibiotic coverage.
- Uveitis should be treated with steroid eye drops in consultation with an ophthalmologist.
- Achilles tendinitis and plantar fasciitis should be treated with injections of methylprednisolone (40-80 mg).
- Sulfasalazine (500-1000 mg PO bid, then titrate up to maximum 3 g/day) may be effective.
- Careful monitoring for the following is essential:
  1. Gastrointestinal toxicity
  2. Hypersensitivity
  3. Bone marrow suppression
- Persistent and uncontrolled disease should be managed with cytotoxic drugs (methotrexate, azathioprine) in consultation with a rheumatologist.

CHRONIC Rx

Chronic disease is best managed by a team approach with the collaboration of a rheumatologist or other experienced physician and physical therapist.

DISPOSITION

- Recurrences are frequent, even with treatment.
- Long-term sequelae:
  1. Persistent polyarthritis
  2. Chronic back pain
  3. Heel pain
  4. Progressive iridocyclitis
  5. Aortic regurgitation

REFERRAL

- To ophthalmologist if uveitis is suspected
- To rheumatologist if arthritis and tendinitis fail to improve rapidly after a course of nonsteroidal antiinflammatory drugs

PEARLS & CONSIDERATIONS

COMMENTS

- Infection with HIV is associated with particularly severe cases of Reiter's syndrome.
- HIV testing is recommended, especially if risk factors such as unprotected sexual activity or IV drug use are identified.

SUGGESTED READINGS

Available at www.expertconsult.com

RELATED CONTENT

Reiter's Syndrome (Patient Information)

AUTHOR: **GLENN G. FORT, M.D., M.P.H.**

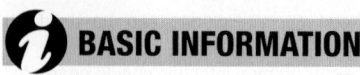

BASIC INFORMATION

DEFINITION

Renal abscess and perinephric abscess are a purulent complication of an underlying urinary infection of the ascending tract with an obstructed pyelonephritis. Predisposing factors include diabetes and renal stones. There is lobar necrosis with renal abscess and perirenal fat necrosis in perinephric abscess.

SYNONYMS

Intrarenal abscess
Perinephric abscess
Kidney abscess

ICD-10CM CODES
N15.1 Renal and perinephric abscess

EPIDEMIOLOGY & DEMOGRAPHICS

INCIDENCE: Ranges from 1 to 10 per 10,000 hospital admissions
PREDOMINANT SEX AND AGE: In one study median age was 59.8 years
RISK FACTORS: Diabetes and renal stones

PHYSICAL FINDINGS & CLINICAL PRESENTATION

- Symptoms include fever, flank pain, abdominal pain, and urinary frequency or dysuria.
- At times renal abscess can present insidiously in the elderly or persons with diabetes.

ETIOLOGY

These infections may be a complication of a urinary tract infection that ascends to the upper tract, usually due to gram-negative bacteria, or a complication of a bacteremia with hematogenous seeding to the kidney, usually secondary to a *Staphylococcus aureus* infection.

DIAGNOSIS

DIFFERENTIAL DIAGNOSIS

- Acute pyelonephritis with papillary necrosis
- Acute lobar nephronia: acute nonsuppurative renal infection
- Renal cell carcinoma
- Malakoplakia: rare granulomatous inflammatory disease seen with *Escherichia coli* infection
- Emphysematous pyelonephritis: gas formation within the renal parenchyma caused by infection by facultative anaerobes or *Candida* spp.

WORKUP

Combination of laboratory tests and imaging

LABORATORY TESTS

- Blood cultures, urine cultures, urinalysis, and CBC are basic tests.
- Elevated ESR or C-reactive protein may be marker for a deep-seated infection.

IMAGING STUDIES

- Ultrasound may show thick-walled fluid-filled cavity in renal parenchyma. A perinephric abscess is confined to the perinephric space by Gerota's fascia.
- CT with contrast is preferred over ultrasound for the diagnosis (Fig. 1).
- MRI and nuclear scans are of limited value.

TREATMENT

Antibiotic therapy and, when necessary, interventional radiology or surgical drainage procedure

NONPHARMACOLOGIC THERAPY

- Therapy for a renal abscess greater than 5 cm in diameter should be percutaneous drainage by CT- or US-guided therapy along with intravenous antibiotics.
- A perinephric abscess should be drained percutaneously with CT or US guidance.
- At times a nephrectomy may be required for severe cases, usually in diabetic patients.

ACUTE GENERAL Rx

A renal abscess less than 5 cm in diameter can be treated successfully with targeted intravenous therapy (92% success rate for abscess 3-5 cm in diameter). Antibiotic choices are

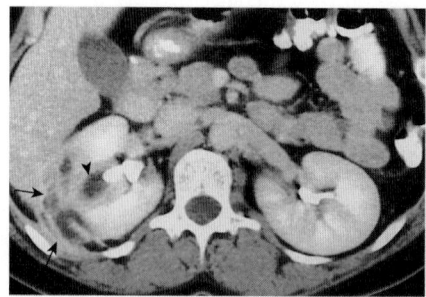

FIG. 1 Renal abscess. Contrast-enhanced CT scan shows an abscess in the medulla of the kidney *(arrowhead)* with penetration and extension into the perinephric space *(arrows)*. (Courtesy L. Towner.)

based on culture results but initially should target gram-negative bacteria unless infection is secondary to staphylococcal bacteremia. Empiric antibiotic therapy in geographic areas where fluoroquinolone resistance rates are <10% consists of ciprofloxacin 400 mg IV loading dose. In areas with high fluoroquinolone resistance rates, ceftriaxone 1 g IV is appropriate. If perinephric abscess is associated with staphylococcal bacteremia, give IV nafcillin if methicillin-susceptible *Staphylococcus aureus* (MSSA) or vancomycin 1 g IV q12h if methicillin-resistant *S. aureus*.

CHRONIC Rx

Antibiotic therapy generally continues for 2 to 3 weeks, some of which can be completed with oral therapy.

DISPOSITION

Antibiotics such as trimethoprim-sulfamethoxazole and quinolone antibiotics penetrate well in the kidney and are ideal oral agents for therapy.

REFERRAL

Interventional radiology, urologic surgeon, and infectious diseases consult

PEARLS & CONSIDERATIONS

COMMENTS

This diagnosis should be considered in patients who are being treated for pyelonephritis with appropriate antibiotics and fail to respond clinically after 5 days.

PREVENTION

Early and targeted therapy for urinary tract infections, especially in diabetic patients

RELATED CONTENT

Pyelonephritis (Related Key Topic)
Urinary Tract Infection (Related Key Topic)

AUTHOR: **GLENN G. FORT, M.D., M.P.H.**

BASIC INFORMATION

DEFINITION

Renal artery stenosis (RAS) is the progressive narrowing of the renal artery, which is most commonly due to atherosclerosis or fibromuscular dysplasia (FMD). RAS is an important, potentially reversible cause of hypertension, ischemic nephropathy, and destabilizing cardiac syndromes. RAS increases the risk of renal artery occlusion via progression of the severity of the stenosis.

SYNONYMS

Fibromuscular disease
FMD
RAS
Renovascular disease

ICD-10CM CODES
I70.1   Atherosclerosis of renal artery
I15.0   Renovascular hypertension
I77.9   Disorder of arteries and arterioles, unspecified
Q27.1   Congenital renal artery stenosis

EPIDEMIOLOGY & DEMOGRAPHICS

- RAS:
  1. Atherosclerotic RAS (ARAS) accounts for about 90% of cases. True prevalence is unknown.
     a. General population autopsy studies: 10%, 27% over 50 years; hypertensive patients: 0.2% to 5%.
     b. In the general population >65 years of age, the prevalence is 6.8% by Doppler ultrasound (5.5% of women, 9.1% of men, 6.7% of African Americans, and 6.9% of Caucasians). Of those with ARAS, 12% had bilateral disease.
     c. In patients with malignant hypertension, the prevalence is 43% in Caucasians and 7% in African Americans. In patients with mild hypertension, the prevalence is <1%.
     d. In patients with peripheral artery disease, the prevalence is 22% to 59%.
  2. FMD accounts for approximately 10% of chronic RAS. It is typically seen in women (90%). FMD was previously thought to be a disease of the young and healthy with few risk factors, but recent data suggest an average age of diagnosis of 54 years, and 26% have bilateral disease.

ETIOLOGY

RAS:
- Atherosclerosis: Atherosclerotic renal artery stenosis is a process similar to atherosclerosis in other vascular beds with similar risk factors: family history, smoking, diabetes, hypertension, and hyperlipidemia. ARAS most often involves the ostium and proximal third of the main renal artery.
- Fibromuscular dysplasia (FMD) (Fig. 1): etiology unknown. Classified into three categories based on the layer of arterial wall affected: medial (>90%), intimal (<10%), adventitial (<1%). FMD typically involves the distal main renal artery and intrarenal branches.

PATHOGENESIS

- Pathogenesis of fibromuscular dysplasia is unknown. Fibromuscular dysplasia involves abnormal constrictions and dilations of the renal artery, leading to a typical "string of beads" finding on angiography.
- The pathogenesis of atherosclerotic RAS is similar to that of atherosclerosis in other vascular beds.
- The pathogenesis of renovascular hypertension is related to the neurohormonal cascade resulting from renal ischemia. The macula densa of the kidney senses a decreased systemic blood pressure caused by the reduced blood flow through the stenotic artery. Renal hypoperfusion or ischemia produces an increase in plasma renin that converts angiotensin I to angiotensin II, producing vasoconstriction and aldosterone secretion, sodium retention, and potassium wasting. Hypertension results and can be self-sustaining, even in the case of unilateral RAS, because of hypertensive damage to the contralateral kidney.
- The pathogenesis of ischemic nephropathy is a topic of current debate. Whether renal dysfunction develops purely from persistent ischemia related to progressively narrowed vessels or from repetitive small ischemic insults and upregulation of inflammatory mediators is yet to be fully elucidated.
- "Flash" or sudden-onset pulmonary edema, a manifestation usually seen in bilateral ARAS, results from sodium and water retention as well as upregulation of the sympathetic nervous system.

NATURAL HISTORY

- RAS caused by fibromuscular dysplasia rarely causes renal artery occlusion or ischemic nephropathy.
- ARAS rarely progresses to total occlusion. One study of serial ultrasounds of patients with RAS demonstrated that those with >60% stenosis progressed to total occlusion in 1 year in only 5% of cases; an additional 11% progressed after 2 years.

PHYSICAL FINDINGS & CLINICAL PRESENTATION

Progressive RAS
- Renal artery stenosis should be considered in any white female aged <30 years with hypertension not attributed to any other cause, or in any patient aged >50 years with new-onset refractory hypertension, or with stable hypertension that has abruptly and significantly worsened.
- Renal artery stenosis most often presents as a clinically asymptomatic finding. Manifestations can include renovascular hypertension, ischemic nephropathy, or flash pulmonary edema.
- Flash pulmonary edema in the absence of cardiac disease most often indicates severe bilateral renal artery stenosis.
- Renovascular hypertension should be considered if blood pressure control remains suboptimal on a medication regimen that includes 3 maximally dosed medications, including a diuretic.

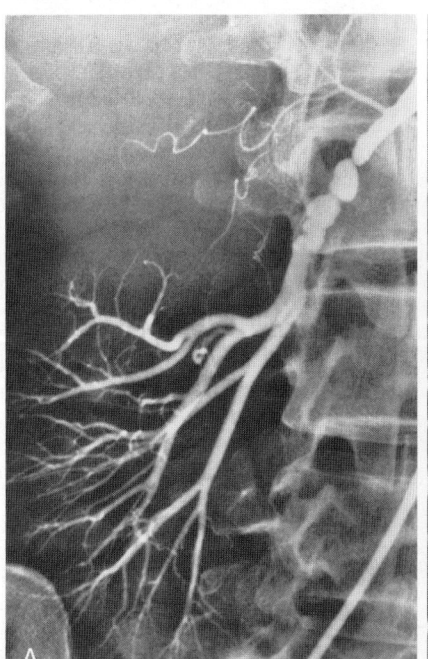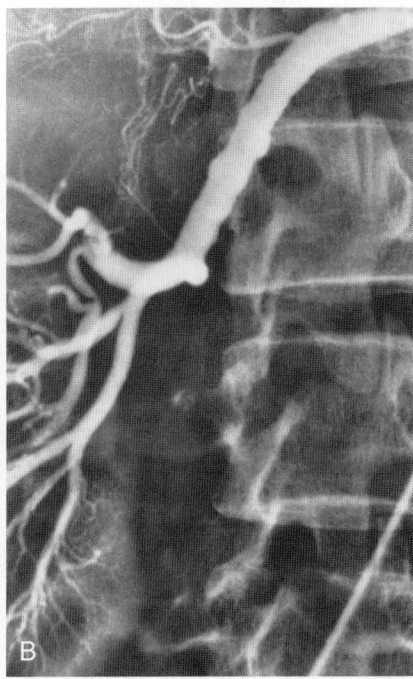

FIG. 1 Fibromuscular dysplasia. A, Selective renal arteriogram illustrating the beaded appearance of fibromuscular dysplasia with multiple webs characteristic of medial fibroplasia in a 39-yr-old woman. **B,** Selective injection of the same renal artery after technically successful percutaneous transluminal renal angioplasty. (Courtesy Michael McKusick, M.D., Mayo Clinic, Rochester, Minnesota. From Floege J et al: *Comprehensive clinical nephrology,* ed 4, Philadelphia, 2010, Saunders.)

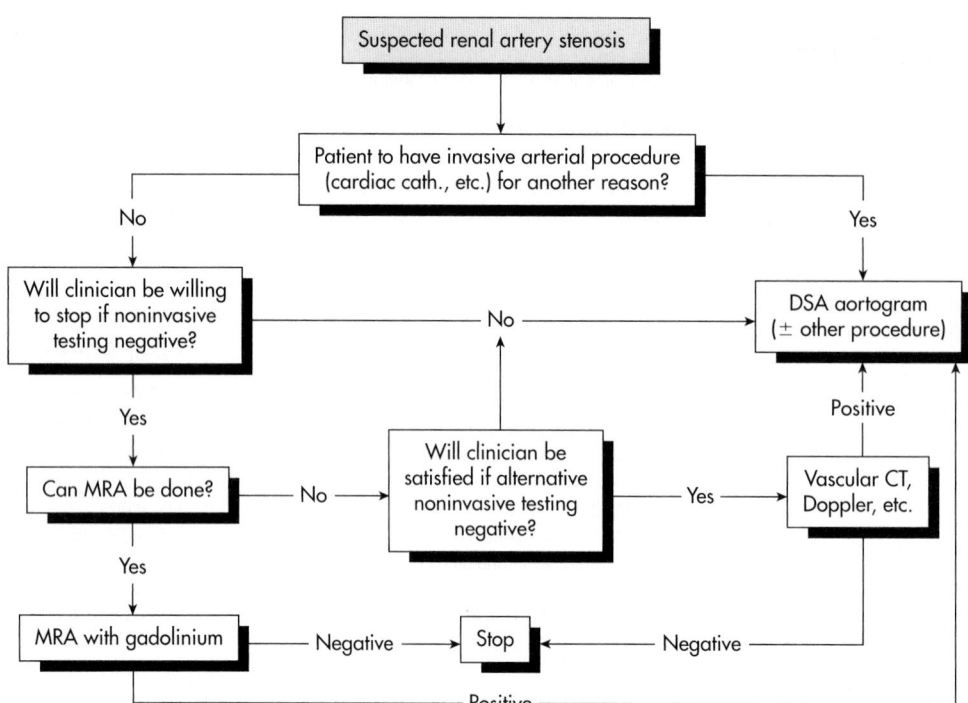

FIG. 2 Approach to the anatomic evaluation of renal artery stenosis. Once stenosis is suspected, if the patient is to have another invasive arterial procedure, noninvasive imaging is deferred and a low-volume digital subtraction aortogram *(DSA)* is done at the time of that procedure. In other cases, the clinician should assess whether a negative noninvasive test would be sufficient evidence to acquit the renal arteries. If so, noninvasive testing should be performed. If not, consideration should be given to DSA and selective angiography. *Cath,* Catheterization; *CT,* computed tomography; *MRA,* magnetic resonance angiography. (From Zipes DP et al [eds]: *Braunwald's heart disease,* ed 7, Philadelphia, 2005, Saunders.)

- Ischemic nephropathy should be considered if kidney function is rapidly deteriorating or parenchymal sizes are decreasing on serial imaging, particularly with bilateral disease.
- Acute elevation of serum creatinine (>30%) after starting angiotensin–converting-enzyme inhibitors (ACEIs) or angiotensin type 1 receptor blockers (ARBs) may be seen in bilateral disease.
- A bruit heard in either upper quadrant on abdominal auscultation may suggest RAS. Patients with atherosclerotic RAS will often have bruits heard in other vascular beds.

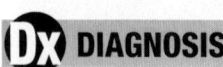 **DIAGNOSIS**

SCREENING

American College of Cardiology and American Heart Association (ACC/AHA) guidelines for identification of patients who should be screened for RAS:

- Onset of hypertension at age <30 years or severe hypertension at age >55 years
- Clinical findings that suggest secondary hypertension as opposed to essential hypertension in the absence of a more likely cause of secondary hypertension such as pheochromocytoma
- Malignant hypertension: hypertension with coexistent evidence of acute end-organ damage (acute renal failure, acute decompensated heart failure, new visual or neurologic disturbance, and/or advanced retinopathy)

- Accelerated hypertension: sudden and persistent worsening of previously controlled hypertension
- Resistant hypertension: full doses of a 3-drug regimen that includes a diuretic
- Sudden unexplained pulmonary edema
- New azotemia or acute kidney injury following initiation of an ACEI or ARB
- Unexplained atrophic kidney or variation in size of both kidneys by >1.5 cm, smaller kidney likely affected by RAS

Consider screening when renal asymmetry is noted with kidney lengths differing by ≥1.5 cm

LABORATORY TESTS

- Basic chemistry panel including sodium, potassium, blood urea nitrogen, and serum creatinine
- Urinalysis
- Renal vein renin sampling helps determine whether one or both kidneys are overproducing renin in cases of suspected renovascular hypertension (RVH). A positive result has strong predictive value. However, 50% of patients with no evidence for lateralization can still respond to unilateral intervention. This procedure is rarely performed except in specialized hypertension centers.

IMAGING STUDIES

- Duplex Doppler ultrasonography, CT angiography, and magnetic resonance angiography (MRA) are effective diagnostic screening methods. The choice of imaging modality will

depend on the availability of the diagnostic tool, the experience and local accuracy of each modality, patient characteristics including body size, renal function, and contrast allergy, and the presence of prior stents. Fig. 2 describes an approach to the anatomic evaluation of RAS. An approach to the angiographic evaluation and treatment of RAS is described in Fig. 3.

RENAL DOPPLER ULTRASOUND:

- Renal Doppler is a noninvasive, inexpensive screening study, and it can determine whether a stenosis of >60% is present.
- Abnormal results in RAS
  - Peak systolic velocity (PSV) >250 cm/sec
  - Peak diastolic velocity >150 cm/sec
  - Renal-to-aortic ratio (RAR) >3.5
  - Acceleration time >100 msec
  - Exact definitions of a positive renal Doppler for RAS will vary by institution.
- Compared to renal angiography, Doppler studies have shown varied performance, with a sensitivity of 84% to 98% and a specificity of 62% to 99%.
- Limitations include high user variability. Valid test performance requires technicians who perform a high volume of these tests to reduce user error. If significant user variability exists at certain institutions, renal Doppler may be excluded from diagnostic algorithm. Patients with a large body habitus may have limited imaging results. It is not as sensitive or specific as MR or CT methods. Detection of RAS is limited to identifying whether stenosis of 60% to 99% is present.

Renal Artery Stenosis Evaluation

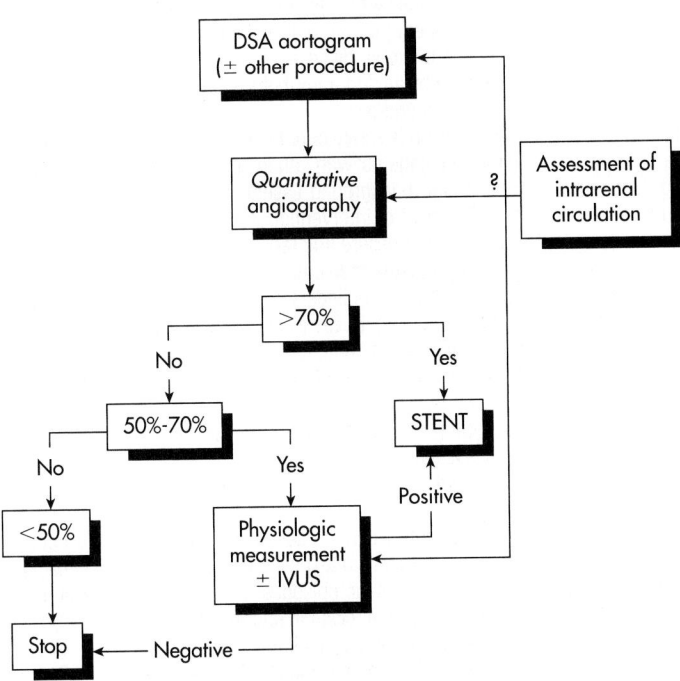

FIG. 3 Approach to the angiographic evaluation and treatment of renal artery stenosis. Once a digital subtraction aortogram *(DSA)* is performed, confirming the presence of renovascular disease, quantitative angiography, and objective evaluation of the severity of stenosis should be performed. Very severe (>70% diameter stenosis) lesions are subjected to revascularization, and mild lesions (<50% diameter stenosis) are not. It is believed that the intermediate lesion should be assessed with physiologic evaluation and/or an additional anatomic documentation of severity, such as intravascular ultrasound *(IVUS)*. The absence of translesional flow acceleration or a pressure gradient should mitigate the desire to intervene. (From Zipes DP et al [eds]: *Braunwald's heart disease,* ed 7, Philadelphia, 2005, Saunders.)

- Duplex Doppler is a good modality for monitoring patency after a stent has been placed.

MAGNETIC RESONANCE ANGIOGRAPHY:

– MRA (Fig. 4) provides good visualization of both main and accessory renal arteries. The test has high sensitivity (90%-100%) and a specificity of 76% to 94%. It is superior to renal Doppler ultrasonography and equivalent to CT angiography.

– Benefits include the lack of exposure to iodine contrast or radiation.

– Limitations include claustrophobia, high cost, and inability to image within a previously placed metallic stent. In addition, gadolinium exposure is relatively contraindicated in CKD patients with an estimated glomerular filtration rate (GFR) <30 ml/min per 1.73 m^2 due to the risk of inducing nephrogenic systemic fibrosis.

COMPUTED TOMOGRAPHY ANGIOGRAPHY:

- CT angiography is rapid and effective. When compared with angiography, CT has a sensitivity of 59% to 96% and a specificity of 82% to 99%. It is superior to renal Doppler and equivalent to MRA. Contrast uptake in kidneys can also be used to estimate viability of affected kidneys.

- CT has good spatial resolution and can detect restenosis through metal stents.

- CTA can be used more easily than MRA in obese or claustrophobic patients.

- Limitations include radiation exposure and potentially nephrotoxic, iodinated radiocontrast medium exposure to CKD patients. Heavily calcified arteries may appear narrower than in actuality.

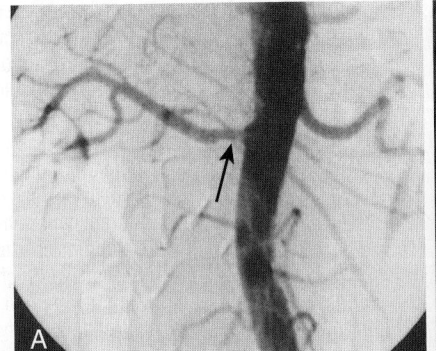
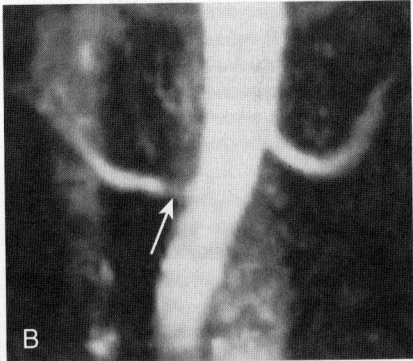

FIG. 4 Renal arteriograms. A, Conventional renal digital subtraction (DSA) showing mild renal stenosis *(arrows)* on the right. **B,** Magnetic resonance angiogram (MRA) of the same patient. The stenosed segment *(arrows)* is clearly seen in this coronal projection. (Courtesy Dr. W. Gedroyc. From Souhami RL, Moxham J: *Textbook of medicine,* ed 4, London, 2002, Churchill Livingstone.)

DIRECT ANGIOGRAPHY:

- IV digital subtraction angiography (DSA) has an 88% sensitivity and 90% specificity. It is the gold standard for anatomic diagnosis of RAS. It is not a first-line screening tool, but it is recommended after a positive noninvasive test. DSA is also used for patients with a high clinical suspicion for RAS and inconclusive noninvasive tests and in whom the decision has already been made that correction of stenosis will produce clinical benefit. DSA allows for angioplasty with stenting during the same procedure. Renal fractional flow reserve at the time of DSA can evaluate the severity of RAS during maximal vasodilatation.

- This modality is reserved for patients with a high likelihood of intervention.

- Limitations include its invasive nature, requiring intraaortic catheterization that may lead to aortic and renal artery trauma with possible dissection, rupture, thrombosis, or embolization.

- Procedure requires a skilled interventionalist (radiologist, cardiologist, or vascular surgeon) knowledgeable in RAS.

- Procedure requires iodinated contrast and must be used cautiously with CKD. Carbon dioxide contrast imaging and limiting image acquisition number reduce kidney injury risk.

NUCLEAR RENOGRAPHY (WITHOUT CAPTOPRIL):
- A noninvasive test conducted when renal atrophy is present to document differential kidney function. This can be useful when determining whether to revascularize an atrophic kidney or to remove it in renovascular hypertension. Atrophic kidneys with <20% differential renal function are unlikely contributors to ongoing worsening kidney function but may still contribute to renovascular hypertension.

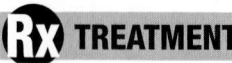 **TREATMENT**

ACUTE GENERAL Rx

RAS:

The treatment of renal artery stenosis must be targeted to the clinical presentation.
- Asymptomatic RAS requires no treatment.
- Patients with chronic hypertension in the setting of incidentally discovered RAS require only antihypertensive medical therapy.
- Patients in whom RVH is suspected should be initially treated with antihypertensive therapy, specifically medications that block the renin-angiotensin-aldosterone system. As discussed below, failure to control blood pressure on an aggressive regimen represents a reason to consider renal revascularization.
- Patients with ischemic nephropathy should be considered for intervention only if the renal function is rapidly declining or flash pulmonary edema develops in the setting of bilateral renal artery stenosis.

PHARMACOLOGIC THERAPY

- Because of the activation of the renin-angiotensin-aldosterone system in RAS, ACEIs or ARBs are recommended and well tolerated (92%) for the treatment of RVH. Kidney function should be monitored carefully when initiating or titrating these medications, particularly when bilateral RAS (78% tolerability) or unilateral stenosis with solitary kidney is present to avoid precipitating AKI.
- Diuretics should be considered in patients with congestive heart failure or flash pulmonary edema.
- Antiplatelet therapy and statin therapy in patients with atherosclerotic RAS

NONPHARMACOLOGIC THERAPY

- If either blood pressure cannot be controlled by medications alone, flash pulmonary edema occurs, or there is rapid decline in renal function, referral for renal angiography, angioplasty, and stenting may be indicated.
- Angioplasty without stenting is insufficient for atherosclerotic lesions due to a high failure rate of adequate dilation of the artery or a high rate of restenosis.
- Occasionally a kidney that has lost its function due to RAS may cause refractory hypertension. This situation would be discovered only by renal vein renin sampling in a patient with unilateral renal atrophy. In such cases, nephrectomy of the atrophied kidney may be the best method to control blood pressure.

- Rarely is renal artery bypass required.
- If RAS is suspected as the cause of flash pulmonary edema or rapidly declining kidney function, bilateral disease is likely, and, if confirmed by angiography, both renal arteries should be stented.
- Hypertension is rarely cured with revascularization in patients with atherosclerotic RAS due to high background essential hypertension. The goal of intervention is to gain control of blood pressure and reduce the number of blood pressure medications.
- The ACC/AHA guidelines for clinical indications of renal artery revascularization in the presence of significant stenosis include:
  1. Accelerated, resistant, or malignant hypertension (class IIa)
  2. Hypertension with unilateral small kidney (class IIa)
  3. Hypertension with intolerance to medication (class IIa)
  4. Treatment of cardiac destabilization syndromes such as unexplained heart failure exacerbations or episodes of flash pulmonary edema (class I), and refractory or unstable angina (class IIa)
  5. Progressive chronic kidney disease with bilateral RAS or RAS associated with a solitary functioning kidney (class IIa)
- Many patients who meet these criteria will not demonstrate a beneficial response to renal revascularization. Careful selection of patients for angiography and intervention must be made.
- Randomized, controlled trials (e.g., ASTRAL, CORAL, DRASTIC, and STAR) have not shown benefit to percutaneous therapy compared to medical therapy, with end points of blood pressure control, renal function, and cardiovascular events. However, these trials did have several inherent limitations.
  1. DRASTIC trial was a small angioplasty-only trial that demonstrated no difference in blood pressure, but it did show decrease in daily doses of antihypertensive drugs and number of drugs in the intervention group. Cross-over was high from the medication arm to the intervention arm.
  2. The ASTRAL trial was a moderate-sized trial of stenting versus medication in RAS that showed no difference in blood pressure control or in the number of antihypertensive medications required to achieve blood pressure control. RAS severity was only moderate in the study population, decreasing the likelihood of finding a positive result.
  3. CORAL is a large, prospective, multicenter trial comparing stenting versus medication in severe RAS (>60% stenosis). This study confirms that with atherosclerotic renal artery stenosis and hypertension, clinical outcomes are not improved by stenting and that renal artery stenting is futile in general. RAS severity was moderate in many patients and may have diluted the beneficial effects of intervention on those with severe RAS.

  4. Follow-up of the CORAL population at 3 years failed to show any difference in blood pressure control, change in GFR, end-stage renal disease, or death with stenting vs. medical therapy.
- With these limitations in mind, there is no prospective, randomized, controlled trial that has shown a benefit in any subgroup of patients with renal artery stenosis of revascularization over medical management. Therefore, it is recommended that the decision to refer a patient for revascularization be made by specialists who are practiced and skilled in handling hypertension and renal artery stenosis.

FIBROMUSCULAR DYSPLASIA

- Medical therapy should include an ACEI or ARB to control blood pressure unless severe bilateral disease is present (rare).
- RVH from fibromuscular dysplasia (FMD) is often cured by renal artery revascularization because many younger patients do not have background essential hypertension.
- In most cases, patients should be referred for renal artery angioplasty regardless of whether blood pressure can be controlled medically.
- Stenting is not appropriate in patients with FMD because angioplasty alone usually yields a durable result. In addition, recurrence of FMD is common, and the presence of stents may hinder additional interventions.
- Renal artery bypass may be necessary in patients whose FMD recurs multiple times or in whom angioplasty failed to yield an improvement in blood pressure.

DISPOSITION & REFERRAL

- Patients with uncontrolled hypertension on multiple agents should be referred for management by a hypertension specialist.
- Percutaneous intervention for atherosclerotic RAS must be reserved for selected patients until further data are available.

! PEARLS & CONSIDERATIONS

- Renal artery stenosis is most commonly an incidental finding and clinically silent.
- Renal artery stenosis may present as hypertension, renal dysfunction, or both, or flash pulmonary edema.
- Stenting is inappropriate for most patients with RAS. Consideration should be made only in high-risk patients and after consultation with a specialist in the field.
- The modality for the type of imaging should depend on the expertise of the institution.

SUGGESTED READINGS

Available at www.expertconsult.com

RELATED CONTENT

Renal Artery Stenosis (Patient Information)
Hypertension (Related Key Topic)

AUTHOR: **JAMES F. SIMON, M.D.**

BASIC INFORMATION

DEFINITION

Renal cell carcinoma (RCC) is a primary carcinoma originating in the renal parenchyma from the malignant transformation of proximal renal tubular epithelial cells. Most renal cell cancers are of clear cell type; papillary tumors comprise 15% of renal cancers, and chromophobe cancers make up 10%.

SYNONYMS

Hypernephroma
RCC
Renal cell adenocarcinoma

ICD-10CM CODES
C64.9 Malignant neoplasm of kidney, except renal pelvis
C64.1 Malignant neoplasm of right kidney, except renal pelvis
C64.2 Malignant neoplasm of left kidney, except renal pelvis
C64.9 Malignant neoplasm of unspecified kidney, except renal pelvis
C65.9 Malignant neoplasm of renal pelvis

EPIDEMIOLOGY & DEMOGRAPHICS

INCIDENCE: In 2016, an estimated 62,700 new cases and 14,240 deaths were expected in the U.S. Two percent of cases of renal cancer are associated with inherited syndromes.
PREDOMINANT SEX: Male:female ratio is approximately 2:1.
PREDOMINANT AGE: Peak incidence is at age 50 to 70 years.

PHYSICAL FINDINGS & CLINICAL PRESENTATION

Patients are often asymptomatic until they have advanced disease. The classic presentation of RCC includes the triad of flank pain, hematuria, and a palpable abdominal mass, but currently this now represents an unusual presentation. Current presenting findings in RCC include:

Hematuria	50%-60%
Elevated erythrocyte sedimentation rate	50%-60%
Abdominal mass	25%-45%
Anemia	20%-40%
Flank pain	35%-40%
Hypertension	20%-40%
Weight loss	30%-35%
Fever	5%-15%
Hepatic dysfunction	10%-15%
Classic triad (hematuria, abdominal mass, flank pain)	5%-10%
Hypercalcemia	3%-6%
Erythrocytosis	3%-4%
Varicocele	2%-3%

ETIOLOGY

Hereditary forms:
- Familial renal carcinoma.
- Renal carcinoma associated with Von Hippel-Lindau disease.
- Hereditary papillary renal cell carcinoma.

Risk factors:
- Cigarette smoking.
- Obesity.
- Phenacetin-containing analgesics.
- Asbestos, lead, Thorotrast, and chromium exposure.
- Gasoline and other petroleum products.
- Role of the *VHL* gene on chromosome 3.

DIAGNOSIS

DIFFERENTIAL DIAGNOSIS

- Transitional cell carcinomas of the renal pelvis (8% of all renal cancers).
- Wilms' tumor.
- Other primary renal carcinomas and sarcomas.
- Renal cysts.
- Retroperitoneal tumors.

WORKUP

LABORATORY TESTS:
- Urinalysis: hematuria.
- Complete blood count: anemia or erythrocytosis.
- Nonmetastatic hepatic dysfunction with elevated alkaline phosphatase, prolonged prothrombin time, and hypoalbuminemia.
- Hypercalcemia (caused by parathyroid-related protein).

IMAGING STUDIES

Nearly 50% of renal cancers are now detected because a renal mass is incidentally detected on radiographic evaluation.
- Renal ultrasound.
- Abdominal CT scan with contrast (Fig. 1 and Fig. 2); CT-guided biopsy is generally not necessary for diagnosis of solid masses >4 cm (high likelihood of cancer).
- MRI.
- Renal arteriogram.
- Intravenous pyelography.

STAGING
See Table 1.

COMMON SITES OF METASTASES

Lung	50%-60%
Bone	30%-40%
Regional nodes	15%-30%
Main renal vein	15%-30%
Perirenal fat	10%-20%
Adrenal (ipsilateral)	10%-15%
Vena cava	10%-15%
Brain	10%-15%
Adjacent organs (colon, pancreas)	10%
Kidney (contralateral)	2%

TREATMENT

- Surgery
  1. Surgical nephrectomy (open procedure or laparoscopic approach) is the only effective management for stages I, II, and some stage III tumors. Although radical nephrectomy had long been the standard treatment, retrospective studies have shown that partial rather than radical nephrectomy is associated with improved survival and is appropriate for patients with renal cell neoplasms <4 cm that are not adjacent to the renal pelvis or invading the vena cava.
  2. Laparoscopic robotic-assisted nephrectomy has been adopted in multiple centers, primarily for nephron-sparing surgery in the case of tumors <4 cm. Advantages include less blood loss, minimal effects on renal function, and similar oncologic outcomes. Disadvantages include increased costs and limitations in tumor size and locations eligible for robotic surgery.
  3. Various forms of partial nephrectomy may be available for patients with bilateral cancers or with a solitary kidney.

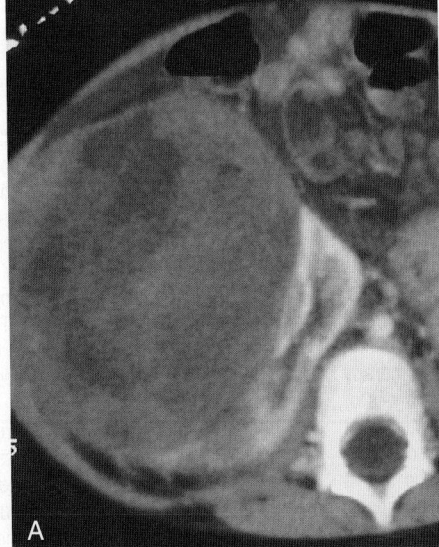
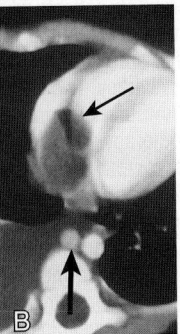

FIG. 1 Renal cell carcinoma. Ultrasound demonstrates a 17-mm hyperreflective mass in the left kidney with posterior shadowing. (From Grainger RG et al [eds]: *Grainger & Allison's diagnostic radiology*, ed 4, London, 2001, Harcourt.)

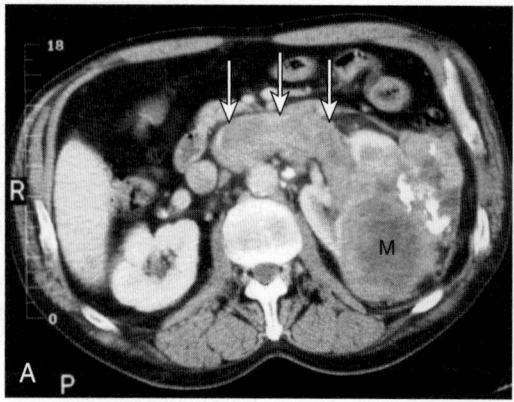
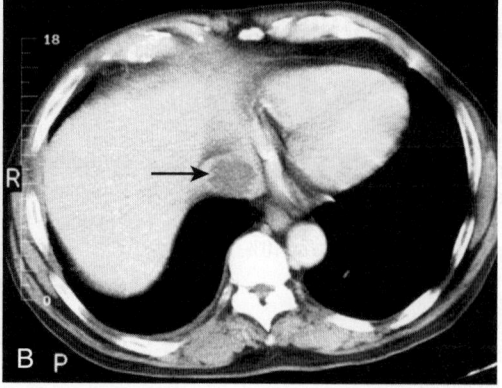

FIG. 2 Renal cell carcinoma. In this patient, the computed tomography scan at the midportion of the kidneys (**A**) demonstrates a large left renal mass (*M*) that extends into the renal vein and into the inferior vena cava (*arrows*). **B**, An image at the level of the base of the heart shows that the tumor thrombus (*arrow*) extends into the right atrium. (From Mettler FA Jr: *Essentials of radiology,* 3 ed, 2014, Saunders.)

TABLE 1   TNM Staging of Renal Cell Carcinomas

T Stage	Description
Tx	Tumor cannot be assessed
T1: tumor ≤7 cm, limited to kidney	1a: tumor <4 cm
	1b: tumor ≥4 cm but ≤7 cm
T2: tumor >7 cm, limited to kidney	2a: tumor >7 cm but ≤10 cm
	2b: tumor >10 cm
T3: tumor extending into major veins or perinephric tissue but not into adrenal gland or beyond Gerota's fascia	3a: tumor extends to renal vein/branches or invades perirenal and/or renal sinus fat
	3b: tumor extends into IVC below diaphragm
	3c: tumor extends into IVC above diaphragm or wall of IVC
T4	Tumor invades beyond Gerota's fascia (including contiguous extension into ipsilateral adrenal gland)
N stage	
Nx	Regional nodes cannot be assessed
N1	No regional nodes involved
N2	Metastasis in regional node(s)
M stage	
M0	No distant metastases
M1	Distant metastasis present
Stage	**TNM grouping**
I	T1N0M0
II	T2N0M0
III	T1-2N1M0 or T3N0-1M0
IV	T4N0-3M0-1 or Tx-4N0-2M1

4. The role of nephrectomy in patients with metastatic RCC is somewhat controversial, and the procedure should probably be reserved for patients who have a good performance status and low risk score, and who are candidates for systemic targeted therapy. Two randomized trials' data showed that nephrectomy before immunotherapy improved survival in patients compared with immunotherapy alone. A recent retrospective analysis of national U.S. data has suggested that 30% of patients undergo nephrectomy in the era of targeted therapies and that it may be associated with a survival benefit.
- Angioinfarction, cryoablation, or radiotherapy (for palliation).
- Chemotherapy: In patients with unresectable disease, monoclonal antibody inhibitors of vascular endothelial growth factor (VEGF) such as bevacizumab, mTOR kinase inhibitors such as everolimus and temsirolimus, and the tyrosine kinase inhibitors axitinib, sunitinib, pazopanib, and sorafenib can be used as first-line therapy or sequential therapy. Typically, patients are offered sequential therapy with either of these agents until maximum response duration or onset of major toxicity from each agent. The majority of responses with these agents are typically either partial or stable disease, and relapse is the norm.
- Immunotherapy: High-dose interleukin-2 therapy may achieve a 15% response rate, which is often durable and associated with long-term survival in highly selected patients with excellent performance status. The severe toxicities associated with this therapy and the requirement for specialized treatment centers have put limits on the use of this approach.
- Checkpoint inhibitors: The PD-1 inhibitor nivolumab has demonstrated an overall survival benefit in patients previously treated with targeted therapies.
- Cabozantinib, an inhibitor of the c-met oncogene, has also shown improved survival in patients with relapsed metastatic renal carcinoma.

PROGNOSIS

The 5-year survival rate among patients with kidney cancer has increased from 57% in 1987-1989 to 74% in 2006-2012. The prognosis of surgically treated patients is shown in the following:

TNM Stage	5-yr Survival (%)
I	95
II	88
III (renal vein or vena cava)	50-60
III (nodal involvement)	15-25
IV	5-20

REFERRAL

- To urologist for staging and surgery
- To medical oncologist if metastatic disease is present.

CLINICAL PEARLS

- Patients should be considered for nephron-sparing surgery in case of smaller tumors (<4 cm).
- Laparoscopic robotic-assisted surgery is utilized for standard nephron-sparing surgery routinely; it is utilized for central tumors and tumors >4 cm in some experienced centers.
- Adjuvant therapy utilizing tyrosine kinase inhibitors has showed mixed results when used in the postresection setting and is not approved for use in this setting. An intergroup study showed no survival benefit, whereas a smaller study limited to high-risk patients showed a progression-free survival benefit.
- High-dose interleukin-2 can lead to long-term remissions in 10% to 15% of carefully selected patients.

RELATED CONTENT

Kidney Cancer (Patient Information)

AUTHOR: **BHARTI RATHORE, M.D.**

BASIC INFORMATION

DEFINITION

Renal tubular acidosis (RTA) is a group of chronic diseases characterized by hyperchloremic metabolic acidosis (HCMA) produced by an inability of the renal tubules either to excrete hydrogen ion (H^+) or to retain bicarbonate ion (HCO_3-). Factors differentiating types of RTA are described in Table 1. Four main types of RTA are described:

- Type I (classic, distal RTA): abnormality in distal tubule hydrogen secretion, resulting in hypokalemic HCMA.
- Type II (proximal RTA): decreased proximal tubule bicarbonate reabsorption, resulting in hypokalemic HCMA.
- Type III (mixed RTA): rare autosomal recessive disorder with features of distal and proximal RTA.
- Type IV (hyporeninemic, hypoaldosteronism RTA): aldosterone deficiency or a disease of the cortical collecting duct characterized by decreased distal sodium reabsorption and decreased distal tubule acidification hyperkalemic HCMA.

SYNONYMS

RTA

ICD-10CM CODES
N25.89 Other disorders resulting from impaired renal tubular function

EPIDEMIOLOGY & DEMOGRAPHICS

RTA type IV affects primarily adults, whereas RTA types I and II are more frequent in children.

PHYSICAL FINDINGS & CLINICAL PRESENTATION

- Examination may be normal.
- Reduced skin turgor may be present from polyuria and dehydration.
- Muscle weakness and aches, paralysis, and arrhythmias from hypokalemia may occur.
- Low back pain and bone pain may be present in patients with abnormalities of calcium and phosphorus metabolism (RTA II).
- Failure to thrive or delayed growth in children.
- Some patients may present with sensorineural deafness in RTA type I (mutations of H^+-ATPase).

ETIOLOGY

- Type I RTA: inherited as a primary disorder with mutation of the basolateral chloride-bicarbonate exchanger (*SLC4A1* gene) or apical proton-ATPase (H^+-ATPase). Acquired causes: autoimmune disorders (SLE, Sjögren's syndrome); primary biliary cirrhosis and other liver diseases; medications (amphotericin, NSAIDs, lithium carbonate, ifosfamide); genetic disorders (Ehlers-Danlos syndrome, Marfan syndrome, hereditary elliptocytosis); toxins (toluene); disorders with nephrocalcinosis (primary hyperparathyroidism, vitamin D intoxication, idiopathic hypercalciuria); and tubulointerstitial disease (renal transplantation, renal medullary cystic disease, obstructive uropathy, chronic urinary tract infections, and analgesic nephropathy).
- Type II RTA: inherited disorders such as proximal tubule cell sodium bicarbonate co-transporter (NBCe1) defect, carbonic anhydrase type 2 deficiency, and Fanconi's syndrome (caused by cystinosis, Wilson disease, hereditary fructose intolerance, Lowe's and Fanconi-Bickel syndrome, Dent diseases, tyrosinemia, galactosemia). Acquired causes: hyperparathyroidism, multiple myeloma, amyloidosis, light chain deposit diseases, heavy metals (copper, lead, mercury, and cadmium), chronic rejection of a transplanted kidney, and medications (acetazolamide, topiramate, outdated tetracycline, ifosfamide, Retrovir, didanosine, aminoglycosides).
- Type III RTA: rare inherited recessive disorder with carbonic anhydrase (CA) 2 deficiency, drugs (topiramate).
- Type IV RTA: inherited disorders such as pseudohypoaldosteronism type I or type II (Gordon syndrome). Acquired causes: diabetes mellitus, HIV/AIDS, sickle cell disease, obstructive uropathy, lupus, amyloidosis, adrenal insufficiency, kidney transplant rejection, drugs (spironolactone, eplerenone, amiloride, angiotensin–converting-enzyme [ACE] inhibitors, angiotensin receptor blockers [ARBs], trimethoprim, pentamidine, heparin, NSAIDs, calcineurin inhibitors [cyclosporine, tacrolimus]).

DIAGNOSIS

DIFFERENTIAL DIAGNOSIS: EXTRARENAL ORIGIN

- Diarrhea with significant bicarbonate loss.
- External loss of biliary and pancreatic secretions.

- Gastrointestinal-urinary diversion procedures (e.g., ureterosigmoidostomy, ileal conduit).
- Respiratory acidosis.
- Drugs: calcium chloride, magnesium sulfate, cholestyramine.

WORKUP

Detection of HCMA by serum electrolyte and arterial blood gas (ABG) analysis followed by evaluation of potential causes (see "Etiology"). Fig. 1 describes an approach to the patient with RTA.

LABORATORY TESTS

- ABG reveals metabolic acidosis.
- Anion gap is normal.
- Serum potassium is low in RTA types I and II, normal in type III, and high in type IV.
- First-morning urine pH is >5.5 in RTA type I, <5.5 in types II and III, and <5.5 (low mineralocorticoid secretion) or >5.5 (collecting duct abnormality) in RTA type IV.
- Urinary anion gap (UAG) is an indirect evaluation of urinary ammonium excretion, which differentiates renal from extrarenal causes of normal anion gap metabolic acidosis (e.g., diarrhea). UAG is 0 or positive in all types of RTA.

$$UAG = U_{(Na + K)} - U_{Cl}$$

UAG is valid only if U_{Na} >20 mEq/L and urine pH <6.5.
- Urine osmolar gap (UOG) is an independent surrogate of urinary ammonium concentration and is not affected by the presence of other nonreabsorbable anions (e.g., keto acids, 5-oxoproline/pyroglutamic acid, bicarbonate, or hippurate).

Calculated U_{NH4}^+ = 0.5 (measured Uosm – calculated Uosm [2 (Na + K) + urea in mg/dl/2.8 + glucose in mg/dl/18]).
- Calculated urine ammonium ≥75 mEq/L denotes intact renal tubular function and supports an extrarenal origin of HCMA.

TABLE 1   Contrasting Features and Diagnostic Studies in Renal Tubular Acidosis

Finding	Types of Renal Tubular Acidosis		
	Proximal (Type II)	Classical Distal (Type I)	Generalized Distal Dysfunction (Type IV)
Plasma potassium	Low	Low	High
Urine pH during metabolic acidosis (ABG pH <7.3)	<5.5	>5.5	<5.5 or >5.5
Urine net charge	Positive	Positive	Positive
Fanconi's lesion	Present	Absent	Absent
Fractional bicarbonate excretion	10%-15%	2%-5%	5%-10%
(U – B) PCO₂	Normal	Low	Low
H⁺-ATPase defect		Low	
HCO₃–/Cl– transporter defect		High	
Amphotericin B		Normal	
Response to therapy	Least responsive	Responsive	Less responsive
Associated features	Fanconi's syndrome	Nephrocalcinosis/ hypergammaglobulinemia	Chronic kidney disease

ATPase, Adenosine triphosphatase; (U – B) PCO₂, urine minus blood CO₂ tension.
Modified from DuBose TD: Disorders of acid-base balance. In *Brenner and Rector's the kidney*, ed 9, Philadelphia, 2011, WB Saunders.

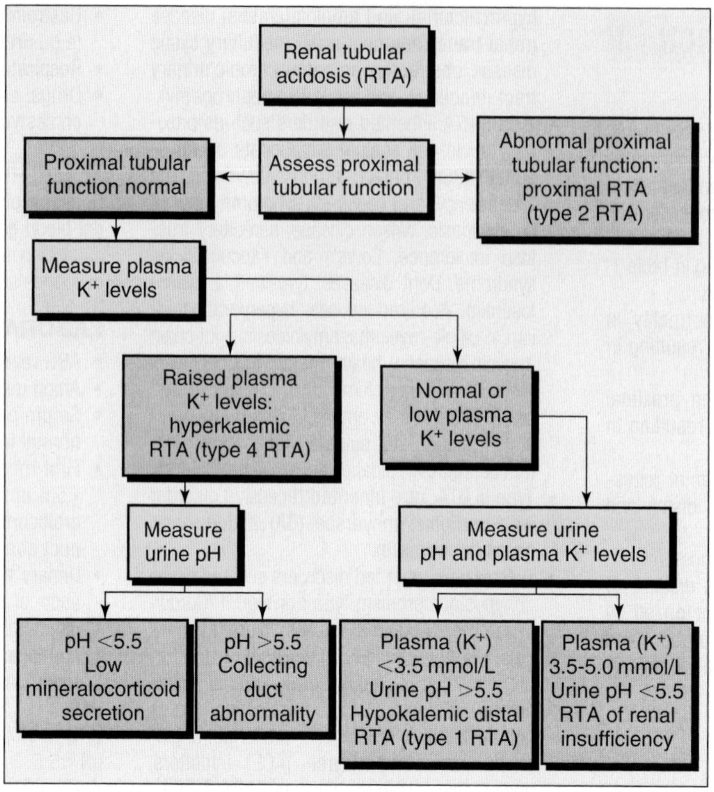

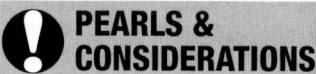

FIG. 1 Approach to the patient with renal tubular acidosis. (From Floege J et al: *Comprehensive clinical nephrology,* ed 4, Philadelphia, 2010, WB Saunders.)

- Calculated urine ammonium ≤25 mEq/L denotes inappropriately low concentration. (UOG cannot be used if there are other neutral substances in the urine (e.g., mannitol, alcohols) or if there is a urinary tract infection caused by bacteria that produce urease.
- Additional studies include urine and serum calcium.
- Parathyroid hormone measurement when primary hyperparathyroidism is suspected (type II RTA).

IMAGING STUDIES
- Plain abdominal radiographs for evaluation of nephrocalcinosis
- Kidney ultrasound to determine kidney sizes or presence of stones
- Noncontrast-enhanced CT scan in patients with nephrocalcinosis or nephrolithiasis

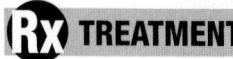 **TREATMENT**

ACUTE GENERAL Rx
- Types I and II are treated with oral sodium bicarbonate (1-2 mEq/kg/day in RTA type I,

2-4 mEq/kg/day in RTA type II) titrated to correct metabolic acidosis (serum bicarbonate >22 mEq/L).
- Potassium supplementation is required for hypokalemic patients.
- Type IV RTA can be treated with diuretics to lower elevated potassium levels and with sodium bicarbonate to correct significant acidosis. Fludrocortisone 0.1 to 0.3 mg/day can be used to correct mineralocorticoid deficiency.

CHRONIC Rx
- Monitor potassium levels in RTA type IV.
- Monitor for bone disease (osteomalacia) in RTA type II.
- Monitor for nephrolithiasis and nephrocalcinosis in RTA type I.

DISPOSITION
- Prognosis varies with the associated conditions (see "Etiology").
- Untreated distal RTA may result in hypocalcemia, hypophosphatemia, nephrolithiasis, and nephrocalcinosis.

PEARLS & CONSIDERATIONS

1. NAGMA: Check for urine ammonium (urine anion and osmolar gaps) to differentiate nonrenal vs. renal causes of HCMA.
2. Examine serum potassium to differentiate between RTA Types 1 or 2 vs. Type IV.
3. In Type IV hyperkalemic RTA, carefully review medication list and rule out urinary obstruction, especially in elderly males.

COMMENTS
Patient education material can be obtained from the National Kidney and Urologic Diseases Information Clearinghouse, Box NKUDIC, Bethesda, MD 20893.

SUGGESTED READING
Available at www.expertconsult.com

AUTHORS: **JIAN LI, M.D., PH.D.,** and **BAHA AL-ABID, M.D.**

BASIC INFORMATION

DEFINITION

Renal vein thrombosis is the thrombotic occlusion of one or both renal veins.

ICD-10CM CODES
I82.3 Embolism and thrombosis of renal vein

EPIDEMIOLOGY & DEMOGRAPHICS

- Incidence unknown; probably an underdiagnosed condition.
- May occur at any age with no gender preference.
- Epidemiology tied to the underlying cause.

PHYSICAL FINDINGS & CLINICAL PRESENTATION

Acute bilateral renal vein thrombosis:
- Back and bilateral flank pain.
- Acute renal failure.

Acute unilateral renal vein thrombosis:
- Flank pain.
- Decline in renal function.
- Hematuria.
- Increase in the amount of proteinuria if associated with nephrotic syndrome.

Chronic unilateral renal vein thrombosis:
- May be silent.
- Pulmonary emboli and hemolysis.
- Back pain.
- Deep vein thrombosis in lower extremities.
- Edema.
- Glycosuria.
- Hyperchloremic acidosis.
- Left varicocele (if the left renal vein is thrombosed).
- Dilated abdominal veins.

ETIOLOGY & PATHOGENESIS

- Extrinsic compression by a tumor or retroperitoneal mass.
- Invasion of the renal vein or inferior vena cava by tumor (almost always renal cell cancer).
- Trauma.
- Hypercoagulable states.
- Dehydration.
- Glomerulopathies (membranous glomerulonephritis, crescentic glomerulonephritis, systemic lupus erythematosus, amyloidosis) especially in the presence of nephrotic syndrome when the serum albumin is <2 g/dl.

NOTE: For unknown reasons, diabetic nephropathy is not commonly associated with renal vein thrombosis even if the nephrotic syndrome is present.

A controversy has existed regarding whether the renal vein thrombosis association with nephrotic syndrome is a complication of nephrotic syndrome or whether renal vein thrombosis occurring in the setting of increased renal vein pressure (e.g., with congestive heart failure, constrictive pericarditis, or extrinsic compression) can independently cause proteinuria. Current evidence is that renal vein thrombosis does not cause nephrotic syndrome.

DIAGNOSIS

DIFFERENTIAL DIAGNOSIS

The diagnosis of renal vein thrombosis does not include any differential consideration. The differential diagnosis is that of proteinuria. Renal vein thrombosis should be considered if proteinuria worsens or if renal function worsens in a patient with glomerulonephritis. Renal vein thrombosis should also be considered in patients with pulmonary emboli and no lower-extremity deep vein thrombosis.

WORKUP

Clinical suspicion (see "Differential Diagnosis") and imaging studies.

IMAGING STUDIES

- Abdominal ultrasound.
- Abdominal MRI or CT with contrast (Fig. 1).
- Renal arteriography (delayed films during venous phase).
- Selective renal vein venography (inferior venacavogram images should be obtained before advancing the catheter in the vena cava because clots, if present, could be dislodged).
- Renal biopsy may be indicated if evidence of nephritis is present (e.g., active urinary sediment).

TREATMENT

- Anticoagulation in acute renal vein thrombosis to prevent pulmonary emboli and in attempt to improve renal function and decrease proteinuria.
- Thrombolytic therapy or surgical thrombectomy has also been reported to be effective
- The value of anticoagulation in chronic renal vein thrombosis is dubious except in nephrotic patients with membranous glomerulonephritis with profound hypoalbuminemia where prolonged prophylactic anticoagulation may be of benefit even if renal vein thrombosis has not been documented.

PROGNOSIS

Probable worsening of the underlying glomerulonephritis by acute renal vein thrombosis; the effect of chronic renal vein thrombosis is unclear.

AUTHOR: **FRED F. FERRI, M.D.**

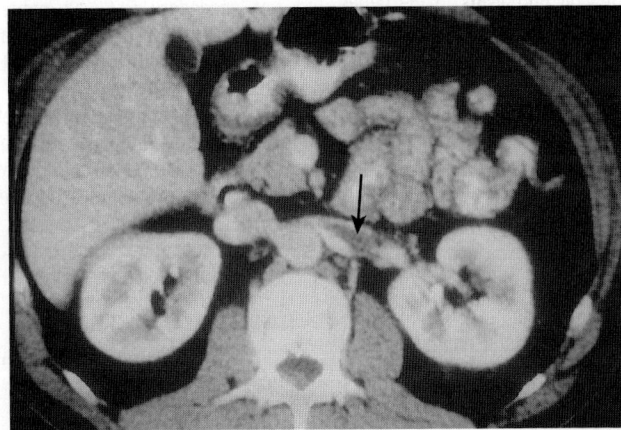

FIG. 1 Renal vein thrombus in a patient with nephritic syndrome. Contrast medium–enhanced CT at the level of the renal vein shows thrombus in the left renal vein (arrow). (From Grainger RG, et al, [eds]: *Grainger & Allison's diagnostic radiology,* ed 4, Philadelphia, 2001, Churchill Livingstone.)

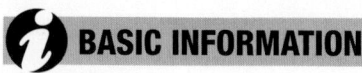

BASIC INFORMATION

DEFINITION

Restless legs syndrome (RLS) is an awake phenomenon consisting of an urge to move legs, usually associated with feeling of discomfort in legs. Symptoms typically are present only at rest and at least partially improve with movement. Additionally, symptoms are usually worse at night. RLS can result in sleep disturbance with associated executive dysfunction and depression.

SYNONYMS

RLS
Wittmaack-Ekbom syndrome

ICD-10CM CODES
G25.81 Restless legs syndrome

EPIDEMIOLOGY & DEMOGRAPHICS

PREVALENCE: Average prevalence rate is 1% to 29%. Prevalence estimates in Europe are around 10%, and 0.1% to 12% in East Asian population.
PEAK PREVALENCE: 10% in persons aged 30 to 79 and 19% in persons aged 80 or above.
PREDOMINANT SEX: Early-onset RLS is more common in females, with 2:1 female/male ratio.
PREDOMINANT AGE: Prevalence of RLS increases with age, and it is more commonly seen in the elderly population.
GENETICS: Genetic basis of RLS has been reported, particularly in early-onset RLS.
- Autosomal dominant disorder
- Common among first-degree relatives
- RLS associated with certain sequences in chromosome 6p, 12q, 14q, 9p, 20p, 2p, 16p
- These include polymorphisms in the genes *BTBD9, MEIS1, PTPRD, MAP2K5, SKOR1,* and *TOX3*

RISK FACTORS: Diabetes mellitus (most consistent risk factor for RLS), iron deficiency anemia (IDA), end-stage renal disease (ESRD) requiring hemodialysis, pregnancy, rheumatoid arthritis, Parkinson's disease, neuropathy, and myelopathy

CLASSIFICATION

- Primary RLS is without any obvious cause, with no associated disorder.
- Secondary RLS results from other medical conditions; the most frequently found associations are pregnancy, IDA, ESRD, and Parkinson disease.

PHYSICAL FINDINGS & CLINICAL PRESENTATION

- Wide spectrum of severity of clinical manifestations has been reported in RLS.
- Most common symptom is unpleasant sensations in legs ("dysesthesias"), reported as discomfort or "creepy-crawling" sensations, mostly bilateral. Arms are occasionally involved.
- There is an extreme urge to move legs and relief is sustained as long as the movement continues.
- Symptoms are worse at night or evening. Best sleep is usually early in the morning.

ETIOLOGY

The exact etiology remains unknown. Pharmacologic, pathologic, physiologic, and imaging studies have implicated dopaminergic pathways, brain iron metabolism, and endogenous opioid pathways.

DX DIAGNOSIS

DIFFERENTIAL DIAGNOSIS

- Periodic limb movement disorder (PLMD)
- Nocturnal leg cramps
- Painful peripheral neuropathy
- Akathisia
- Positional discomfort
- Volitional movements, foot tapping, leg rocking

WORKUP

- Diagnosis of RLS is based on established clinical criteria (Table 1) and normal neurologic examination.
- Testing is done to determine possible cause of secondary RLS. All patients with RLS should be screened for iron deficiency.
- Polysomnography to document periodic limb movements during sleep
- Leg activity monitors to determine limb movements during sleep but they are unable to distinguish periodic limb movements from periodic movements associated with sleep apnea.
- Nerve conduction studies and electromyography for associated peripheral neuropathy

LABORATORY TESTS

- Iron status: serum ferritin, total iron binding capacity, percent saturation
- CBC for anemia in case of iron deficiency
- Metabolic panel: blood urea nitrogen and serum creatinine for renal insufficiency

IMAGING STUDIES

No imaging studies are required for diagnosis for RLS.

Rx TREATMENT

Treatment options for RLS include:
- Dopaminergic agents, levodopa, and dopamine agonists help to ameliorate RLS symptoms, decrease periodic limb movements, and improve sleep. Dopamine agonists, pramipexole and ropinirole, are first-line agents in the treatment of RLS.
- Rotigotine patch (Neupro) is also effective and FDA-approved for moderate to severe RLS.
- Anticonvulsants, such as gabapentin, have been shown to be effective in multiple studies. A recent trial has shown that pregabalin is also effective and well tolerated for RLS.[1] Limited case reports reveal use of lamotrigine and topiramate in patients who are intolerant to other agents.
- Opiates, mostly methadone, are generally reserved as last line of treatment.
- Iron replacement should be started in case of iron deficiency. Iron supplements are indicated even with low-normal ferritin levels (<45 ng/mL).

NONPHARMACOLOGIC THERAPY

- Avoidance of caffeine, alcohol, nicotine, and medications that exacerbate RLS (selective serotonin reuptake inhibitors, dopamine blocking agents, stimulants)
- Physical and mental activity
- Good sleep hygiene

ACUTE GENERAL Rx

Once the diagnosis of RLS is considered based on clinical criteria as mentioned in Table 1 and causes impairment of quality of life, a dopamine agonist (bromocriptine, pramipexole, or ropinirole) should be started at low dose and then gradually tapered depending on tolerance. Dopaminergic medications have the potential to cause iatrogenic worsening (augmentation) of RLS with long-term treatment.

REFERRAL

Refer to neurologist if diagnosis is uncertain or an underlying disorder is suspected.

SUGGESTED READINGS
Available at www.expertconsult.com

RELATED CONTENT

Restless Legs Syndrome (Patient Information)

AUTHOR: **FARIHA ZAHEER, M.D.**

TABLE 1 Diagnostic Criteria for Restless Legs Syndrome

Minimal Criteria
1. Desire to move the legs usually associated with paresthesias.
2. Motor restlessness, as characterized by floor pacing, leg rubbing, stretching, and flexing.
3. Worse at rest, with relief by activity.
4. Worse at night.

Additional Criteria
1. Sleep disturbances, as difficulty in sleep onset and maintaining sleep, daytime fatigue, or somnolence.
2. Involuntary movements, as periodic limb or leg movements in sleep and periodic or aperiodic limb movements while awake.
3. Neurologic examination is normal in idiopathic restless legs syndrome.
4. Clinical course may begin at any age but most severe in middle and older age.
5. Family history suggests autosomal dominant mode of inheritance in 1/3 of the cases.

From Stiansy K et al: Clinical symptomatology and treatment of restless leg syndrome and periodic limb movement disorder, *Sleep Med Rev* 6(4):253-265, 2002.

[1]Allen RP et al: Comparison of pregabalin with pramipexole for restless legs syndrome, *N Engl J Med* 370:621-631, 2014.

BASIC INFORMATION

DEFINITION

Retropharyngeal abscess is a soft tissue infection of the throat that involves retropharyngeal space and that primarily affects children. The anatomic boundaries of the retropharyngeal space are the buccopharyngeal fascia (middle layer of the deep cervical fascia) anteriorly and the alar fascia (deep layer of the deep cervical fascia) posteriorly (Fig. 1). The space begins at the skull base superiorly and ends inferiorly where the two fasciae fuse at the level between the first and second thoracic vertebrae.

ICD-10CM CODES
J39.0   Retropharyngeal and parapharyngeal abscess

EPIDEMIOLOGY & DEMOGRAPHICS

Retropharyngeal abscess occurs most commonly in children between the ages of 2 and 4 yr, analogous to suppurative cervical adenitis. 70% of cases are in patients under the age of 6, and 50% are in patients under the age of 3 years. This represents the peak age group for numerous viral upper respiratory tract infections and their attendant complications, acute otitis media and sinusitis. Retropharyngeal space infection is less common in older children and adults because the lymph nodes generally atrophy by puberty.

PHYSICAL FINDINGS & CLINICAL PRESENTATION

- The onset of a retropharyngeal infection may be insidious, with little more than fever, irritability, drooling, a muffled voice (dysphonia), or possibly nuchal rigidity.
- The acute symptoms relate to pressure and inflammation produced by the abscess on either the airway or the upper digestive tract and pharynx. The patient may have intense dysphagia, drooling, and odynophagia, or there may be some element of respiratory distress from edema and inflammation of the airway (stridor, tachypnea, or both).
- Unwillingness to move the neck because of discomfort is often a prominent presenting feature and should lead to consideration of retropharyngeal abscess if the child is febrile and irritable.
- Extension of the neck is usually affected more than flexion. This causes the patient to hold his or her neck stiffly or to present with torticollis.
- Trismus is unusual.
- On physical examination it may be possible to appreciate midline or unilateral swelling of the posterior pharyngeal wall. The mass may be fluctuant to the examining finger, and care must be taken to avoid rupture of the abscess into the upper airway.

Complications are numerous and could be fatal; these include airway obstruction, septicemia, thrombosis of the internal jugular vein, carotid artery rupture, and acute necrotizing mediastinitis. Aspiration with resultant pneumonia may complicate retropharyngeal abscess if rupture of the abscess occurs and empties into the airway. Infection can spread from one space in the neck to another.

The most dreaded complication is jugular vein suppurative thrombophlebitis (Lemierre's syndrome), in which the vessels of the carotid sheath become infected, leading to bacteremia and spread of infection to the lungs, brain, and mediastinum.

ETIOLOGY

- The retropharyngeal space comprises two chains of lymph nodes that drain the nasopharynx, adenoids, posterior paranasal sinuses, middle ear, and eustachian tube. Accordingly, suppurative infections in these areas may provide the seeds for infection for retropharyngeal abscess.
- The predominant bacterial species are *Streptococcus pyogenes* (group A *Streptococcus*), *Staphylococcus aureus,* and respiratory anaerobes (including *Fusobacteria, Prevotella,* and *Veillonella* species). *Haemophilus* species are also occasionally found.
- In young children, infection usually reaches this space by lymphatic spread from a septic focus in the pharynx or sinuses.
- In adults, infection may reach the retropharyngeal space from either local or distant sites. Penetrating trauma (e.g., from chicken bones or iatrogenic) is the usual source of local spread. More distant sources of infection include odontogenic sepsis and peritonsillar abscess (now a rare cause).

DIAGNOSIS

DIFFERENTIAL DIAGNOSIS

- Cervical osteomyelitis
- Pott's disease
- Meningitis
- Calcific tendonitis of the long muscle of the neck

LABORATORY STUDIES

- CBC with differential.
- Blood cultures may be considered in refractory cases or for severe symptoms.

IMAGING STUDIES

- A lateral neck film should be obtained and can be helpful in delineating the presence of a retropharyngeal abscess and may demonstrate cervical lordosis; the retropharyngeal space is considered widened and pathologic

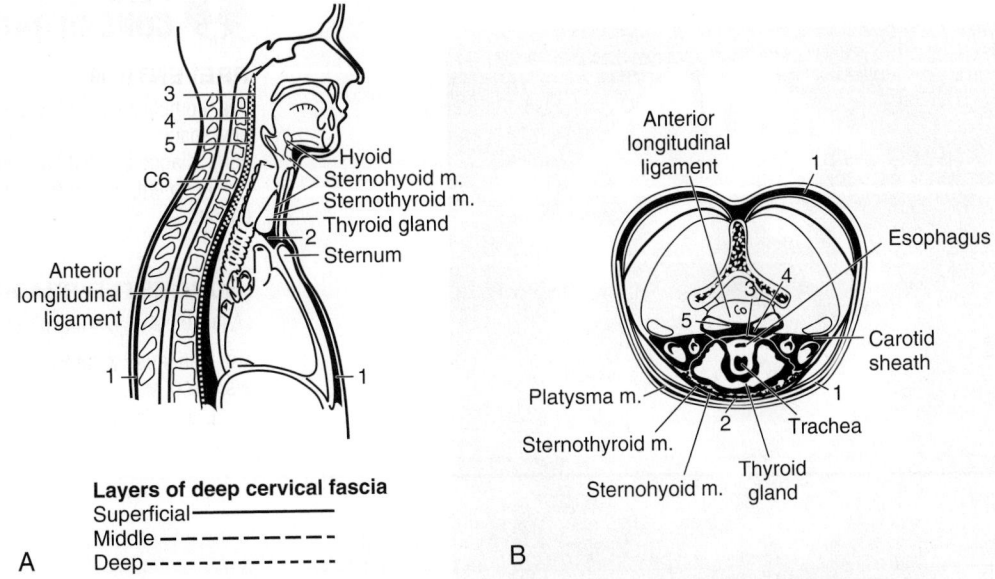

FIG. 1 Relation of various cervical fascial spaces to the superficial and deep layers of the cervical fascia.
A, Cross section of the neck at the level of the thyroid isthmus. **B,** Coronal section in the suprahyoid region of the neck. *1,* Superficial space; *2,* pretracheal space; *3,* retropharyngeal space; *4,* "danger" space; *5,* prevertebral space.

if it is greater than 7 mm at C2 or 14 mm at C6 (Fig. 2).

- There must be attention to technical issues when performing the study, especially in children. The film should be a perfect lateral, and the child must keep the neck in extension during inspiration to avoid a false thickening of the retropharyngeal space. Crying, particularly in infants, may also cause false thickening of the retropharyngeal space.
- CXR should be considered to evaluate for mediastinitis or aspiration pneumonia.
- A CT scan of the neck is useful for patients with moderate or high suspicion of having a deep neck space abscess. It is the most useful imaging modality to identify abscesses in the retropharyngeal space, but it is not perfect. Both the sensitivity and specificity of the CT scan in predicting the presence of drainable purulent material are quite variable from study to study, ranging between 68% and 100%.

- The CT scan provides more information than the plain radiograph because it can generally differentiate between retropharyngeal cellulitis and retropharyngeal abscess and can demonstrate extension of the retropharyngeal abscess to contiguous spaces in the neck. Findings on CT common to both cellulitis and abscess are a low-density core, soft tissue swelling, obliterated fat planes, and mass effect. Findings on CT scan that are indicative of abscess are "complete rim enhancement" and scalloping of the abscess borders (Fig. 3). The abscess may be seen as a mass impinging on the posterior pharyngeal wall.
- MRI of the neck is rarely used for diagnosis, especially in the pediatric population because of the longer time to acquire the study and the need for sedation in the younger population. T2-weighted images may identify and localize areas of pus for drainage or aspiration. Gadolinium enhancement is important to

accurately define the soft tissue component. It also can be useful for distinguishing inflammatory from congenital or neoplastic lesions. Magnetic resonance angiography can be helpful for imaging vascular lesions, such as jugular thrombophlebitis.

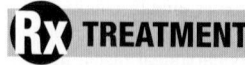

TREATMENT

ACUTE GENERAL & CHRONIC Rx

- When the CT findings suggest cellulitis or phlegmon, a trial of IV antibiotic therapy without drainage is initiated, and the child is monitored as an inpatient for 48 hours. If the child is clinically improved, consider discharge home with a course of oral antibiotics. If the clinical course is not improved or is worse, a repeat CT scan should be obtained, and surgical drainage or prolonged IV antibiotic therapy may be warranted. Some investigators also support a trial of IV antibiotic therapy alone when small abscesses are identified by CT scans, as long as the airway is not compromised.
  - Ampicillin-sulbactam (300 mg/kg/day IV divided q6h) or clindamycin (25-40 mg/kg/day IV divided q8h) are effective antimicrobial selections. In adults, ampicillin-sulbactam 3 g IV q6h or clindamycin 600 mg IV q8h. Antibiotics should be adjusted as culture data become available, and oral therapy is continued to complete at least a 14-day course.
- Surgical intervention has historically played a prominent role in the management of retropharyngeal abscess in conjunction with antibiotic therapy. Prompt surgical drainage is indicated when there is a large hypodense area suggestive of an abscess or when a patient has not responded to parenteral therapy alone.

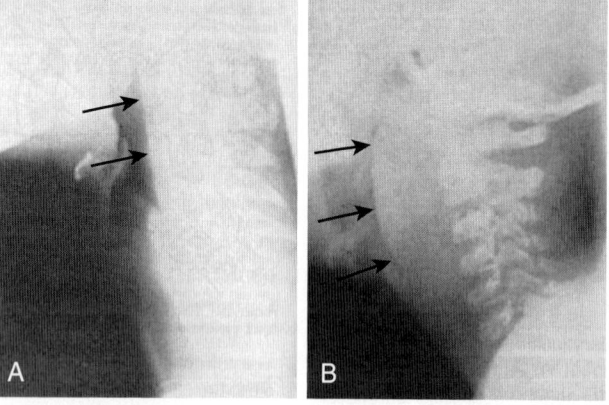

FIG. 2 Lateral radiographs of the neck show normal lateral cervical view **(A)** and expansion of the prevertebral soft tissues by a retropharyngeal abscess **(B).**

PEARLS & CONSIDERATIONS

PREVENTION

The complications of deep neck infection in any space are numerous and potentially fatal. Early diagnosis, with prompt and appropriate management, is key to avoiding these complications.

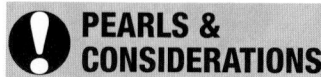

SUGGESTED READINGS

Available at www.expertconsult.com

AUTHORS: **RUBY K. SATPATHY, M.D.**, and **LOUIS INSALACO, M.D.**

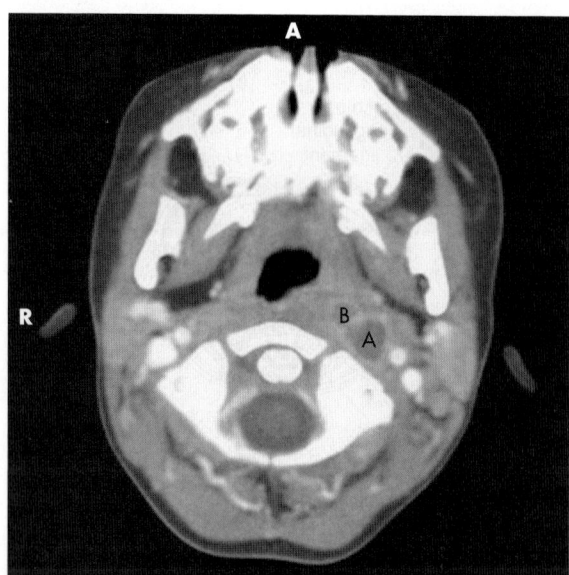

FIG. 3 CT scan of a retropharyngeal abscess (*A* and *B*) demonstrates a low-density core, soft tissue swelling, obliterated fat planes, mass effect, and rim enhancement.

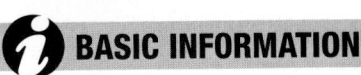 BASIC INFORMATION

DEFINITION

Rh incompatibility occurs when a pregnant woman has Rh-negative blood and her baby has Rh-positive blood. This situation causes risk of isoimmunization.

ICD-10CM CODES
036.0910 Maternal care for other rhesus isoimmunization, first trimester, not applicable or unspecified
T80.4 Rh incompatibility reaction
T80.4 Unspecified complication following infusion, transfusion, and therapeutic injection

EPIDEMIOLOGY & DEMOGRAPHICS

INCIDENCE:
- The absence of the D antigen (Rh negative blood type) occurs in 15% of whites, 7% of blacks, and less than 1% of the Native American and Asian populations. If the father's blood type is not known, the chance that an Rh − pregnant woman is bearing an Rh + fetus is approximately 60%.
- Of those pregnancies complicated by Rh incompatibility, the risk of maternal isoimmunization to the D antigen is approximately 8% for each ABO-compatible pregnancy if no prophylaxis is given.
- Maternal-fetal ABO incompatibility is somewhat protective against Rh isoimmunization.

GENETICS: Five major loci determine Rh status: C, D, E, c, e. The presence of the D antigen results in an Rh + individual, while its absence results in an Rh − individual. Of Rh + fathers, 45% are homozygotes, and 55% are heterozygotes. For homozygous Rh + fathers, the probability of an Rh + offspring is 100%. The probability for heterozygotes is approximately 50%.

RISK FACTORS:
- RhD-negative woman.
- Antepartum: fetal-to-maternal transfusion.
- Intrapartum: fetal-to-maternal transfusion, spontaneous abortion, ectopic pregnancy, abruptio placentae, abdominal trauma, chorionic villus sampling, amniocentesis, percutaneous umbilical blood sampling (PUBS), external cephalic version, manual removal of the placenta, therapeutic abortion, autologous blood product administration.
- Maternal history of hydrops or sensitization to RhD.

ETIOLOGY

The initial response to D antigen exposure is production of immunoglobulin (Ig) M (molecular weight 900,000) that does not cross the placenta. With a repeated exposure, IgG (MW 160,000) is produced. Hemolysis in the fetus results once maternal IgG is present in the fetal circulation by crossing the placenta. This may produce erythroblastosis fetalis or hemolytic disease in the newborn, resulting in antepartum or neonatal death or neurologic damage to the fetus because of hyperbilirubinemia and kernicterus.

DX DIAGNOSIS

LABORATORY TESTS

ABO and Rh blood type and an antibody screen as part of the initial prenatal profile.
- If antibody screen negative:
  1. Repeat antibody screen at 28 weeks of gestation.
  2. Obtain neonatal blood type after delivery.
  3. If Rh incompatibility is confirmed by the neonatal blood type, a Kleihauer-Betke/flow cytometry or rosette test should be performed to determine the amount of fetomaternal transfusion in the following high-risk circumstances: abruptio placentae, placenta previa, cesarean delivery, intrauterine manipulation, manual removal of the placenta.
- If anti-D antibody screen is positive:
  1. Maternal indirect Coombs test is needed to determine antibody titer.
  2. Determine paternal Rh status and zygosity.
  3. If father is heterozygous, PUBS or amniotic fluid is needed to determine fetal Rh status.

IMAGING STUDIES

Ultrasound evaluation may show subcutaneous edema, ascites, pleural effusion, pericardial effusion, or hepatomegaly. It can diagnose hydrops fetalis, but it cannot predict it.

Doppler ultrasound of middle cerebral artery can predict moderate to severe anemia.

RX TREATMENT

PREVENTION OF D ISOIMMUNIZATION

- 50 mcg of D immunoglobulin: after spontaneous or induced abortion or ectopic pregnancy <13 weeks' gestation.
- 300 mcg of D immunoglobulin (protects against 30 ml of fetal blood).
  1. After spontaneous or induced abortion >13 weeks' gestation, amniocentesis, chorionic villous sampling, PUBS, external cephalic version, or other intrauterine manipulation.
  2. As antepartum prophylaxis at 28 weeks' gestation. Maternal anti-D prophylaxis does not cause hemolysis in the fetus or newborn.
  3. At 40 weeks' gestation or at delivery if the neonate is D- or Du-positive.
  4. If Kleihauer-Betke or rosette test confirms >30 ml of fetal red blood in maternal circulation, additional D immunoglobulin is indicated. Confirm adequacy of therapy by a maternal indirect Coombs test 48 to 72 hr after Rh immune globulin is given.

MANAGEMENT OF D ISOIMMUNIZED PREGNANCIES

- Serial amniocentesis for assessment of amount of fetal bilirubin in fluid (OD_{450}) after 25 weeks' gestation with interpretation of the Delta OD_{450} according to criteria established by Liley.
- PUBS if ultrasonographic evidence of hydrops, rising zone II Delta OD_{450} values on amniocentesis, or maternal history of a severely affected child.
- Intrauterine exchange transfusion if severe anemia is documented remote from term.
- Initiation of steroids for lung maturation at 28 weeks in severely affected pregnancies with delivery at lung maturity.
- Delivery as soon as lung maturation is achieved in mild to moderately affected pregnancies.

Fig. 1 shows an algorithm for clinical management of a patient with red cell sensitization in the first affected pregnancy and Fig. 2 shows an algorithm for clinical management of a patient with red cell sensitization and a previously affected fetus or infant.

DISPOSITION

Survival of nonhydropic infants is 90%. Of infants with hydrops, 82% survive.

REFERRAL

Refer all Rh isoimmunized pregnancies to a tertiary care center before 18 to 20 weeks of gestation.

SUGGESTED READING

Available at www.expertconsult.com

AUTHORS: **HUSSAIN MOHAMMAD H. NASERI, M.D.**, and **BHARTI RATHORE, M.D.**

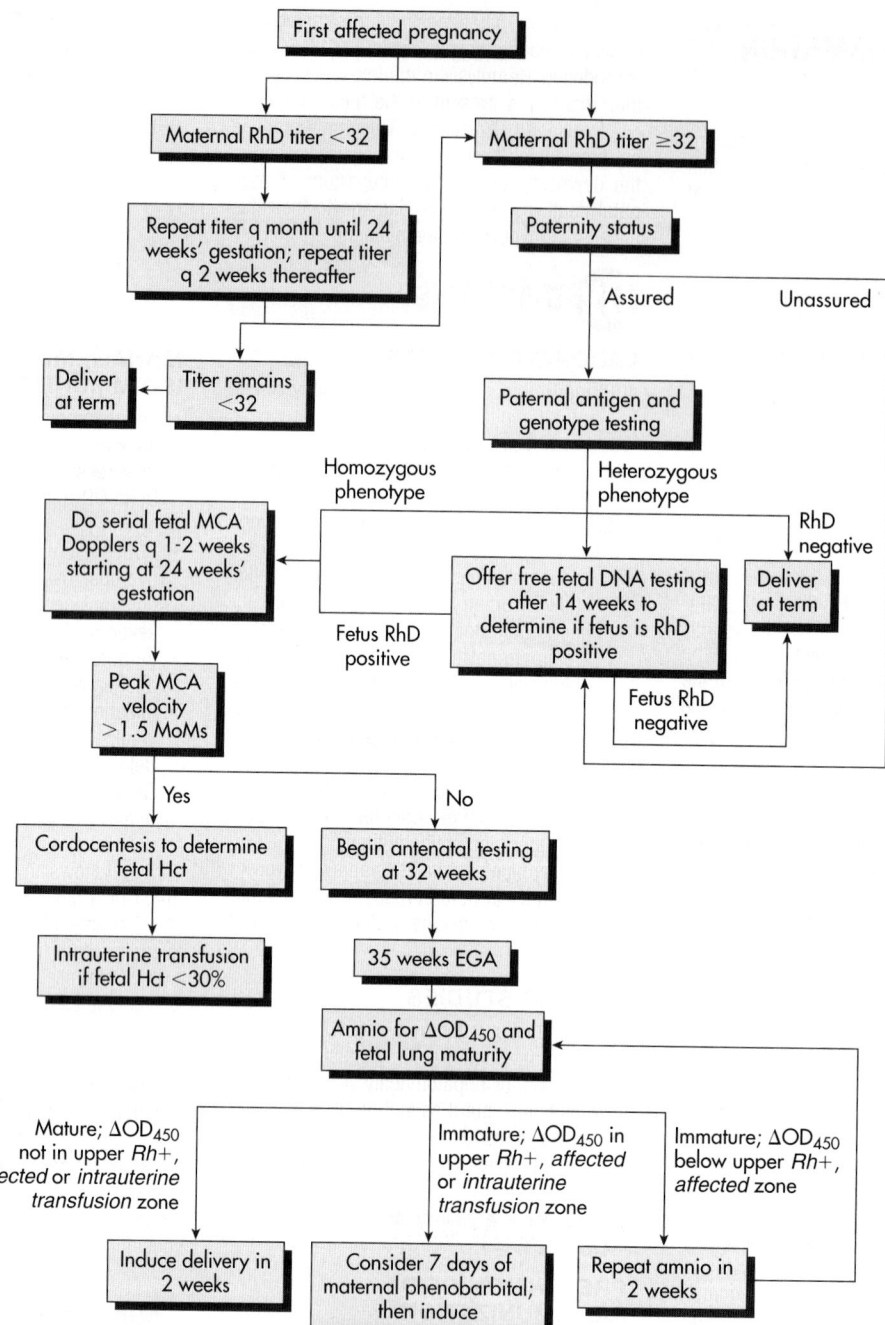

FIG. 1 Algorithm for clinical management of a patient with red cell sensitization in the first affected pregnancy. (From Gabbe SG: *Obstetrics*, ed 6, Philadelphia, 2012, Saunders.)

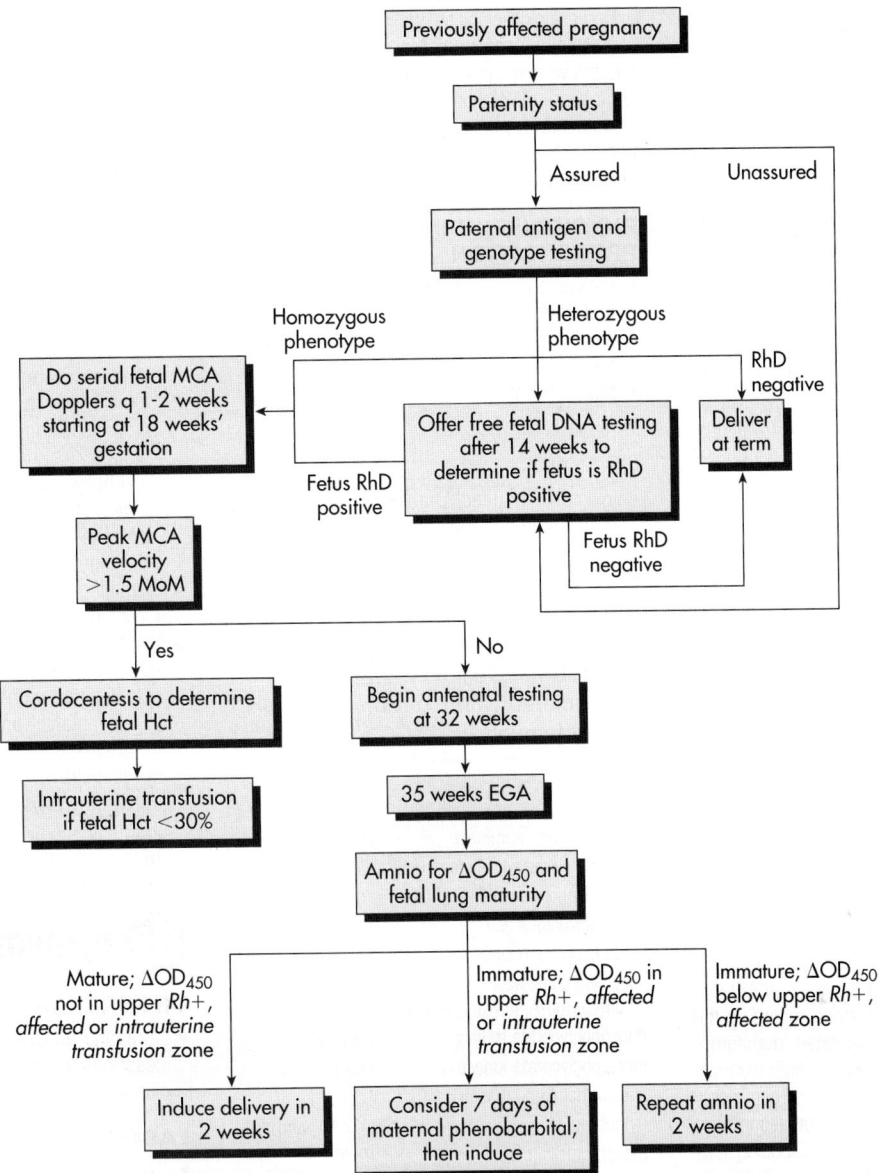

FIG. 2 Algorithm for clinical management of a patient with red cell sensitization and a previously affected fetus or infant. (From Gabbe SG; *Obstetrics*, 6 ed, Philadelphia, 2012, Saunders.)

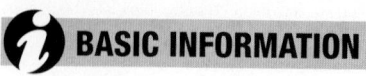

BASIC INFORMATION

DEFINITION

Rhabdomyolysis is a syndrome characterized by striated muscle lysis with resulting muscle damage and leakage of intracellular contents into the circulation. The presentation may range from asymptomatic elevation of creatine kinase (CK) to severe muscle injury with irreversible renal failure with long-term dialysis dependency. In general, 5- to 10-fold elevations of CK levels, muscle pain, and myoglobinuria in an appropriate clinical setting (see the following) are sufficient criteria for the diagnosis of rhabdomyolysis. Acute renal injury occurs from a combination of factors, including volume depletion, tubular obstruction, direct heme-induced proximal tubular cell injury, or associated renal vasoconstriction.

ICD-10CM CODES
M62.82 Rhabdomyolysis (idiopathic)
T79.6 Traumatic ischemia of muscle
M62.89 Other specified disorders of muscle

EPIDEMIOLOGY & DEMOGRAPHICS

PREDOMINANT AGE: Incidence of 1 in 10,000 in the U.S.

Rare in children. Increased risk with advanced age, i.e., >80 years.

Reported incidence of AKI with rhabdomyolysis is 10% to 15%.

7% to 10% of cases of AKI are due to rhabdomyolysis.

MORTALITY RATE: 5% to 8%.

Prognosis is better in the absence of AKI.

ONSET: There is limited evidence regarding the onset of physical exertion-induced rhabdomyolysis. Exercise levels exceeding usual exercise tolerance levels for individuals are commonly causative. Extracellular volume depletion and vasoconstriction are common predisposing features. Patients with risk factors (e.g., metabolic myopathies, advanced age) develop symptoms associated with rhabdomyolysis within 2 to 6 hours after activity; patients without such risk factors become symptomatic around 12 to 36 hours after muscle injury. The presence of concurrent electrolyte abnormalities such as hypokalemia, hyponatremia, hypernatremia, hypomagnesemia, hypophosphatemia, and hypocalcemia from whichever cause are predisposing.

CK levels rise within 2 to 12 hours of the onset of muscle injury, peak generally by 24 to 72 hours, and decline, on average, 3 to 5 days after cessation of muscle injury. Peak CK concentrations may predict development of renal injury. In patients with rhabdomyolysis secondary to malignant hyperthermia, CK concentrations peak approximately 14 hours after an acute episode.

Cholesterol-lowering therapy with a "statin" agent is common, and clinical rhabdomyolysis is reported in less than 0.1% of cases, although myalgia is a frequent complaint. Among the statins, pravastatin has been reported to have a lower risk of rhabdomyolysis, presumably due to its lower lipid solubility. The average duration of statin therapy before the onset of myopathy is 6 months with symptom resolution, with normalization of serum CK concentrations occurring in days to weeks following drug discontinuation. The average time for onset of rhabdomyolysis after addition of fibrate to statin therapy is 32 days.

PHYSICAL FINDINGS & CLINICAL PRESENTATION

- Classic triad: 1) muscle pain, 2) weakness, and 3) dark urine from myoglobinuria
- Muscle tenderness is present only 50% of the time
- Muscle swelling
- Muscular rigidity
- Fever
- Altered consciousness
- In statin-induced rhabdomyolysis, fatigue (74%) is nearly as common as muscle pain (88%)
- Oliguria or anuria in the presence of renal injury

TABLE 1 Genetic Mutations Associated with Exertional Rhabdomyolysis

Gene	
Ryanodine receptor 1	RyR1
Myoadenylate deaminase	AMPDA1
Carnitine palmitoyltransferase II	CPT2
Myophosphorylase	PYGM
Phosphofructokinase	PFKM
Phosphorylase b kinase	PHKA1
Very long chain acyl coenzyme-A dehydrogenase	ACAD9
Phosphoglycerate mutase	PGAMM
Phosphoglycerate kinase	PGK1
Lactate dehydrogenase	LDHA
Cytochrome c oxidase	COX I, II, and III
Cytochrome b (complex III)	CYTB
Mitochondrial tRNA	Mt-tRNA
β-Sarcoglycan	SGCB

From Goldman L, Schafer AI: *Goldman's Cecil medicine*, ed 24, Philadelphia, 2012, Saunders.

ETIOLOGY

Causes can be divided into three categories:
1) Traumatic or muscle compression
   a. High-current electrical injury
   b. Crush injury and compartment syndrome
   c. Tourniquet and limb ischemia
   d. Reperfusion after revascularization procedures for ischemia
   e. Extensive surgical (spinal) dissection, bariatric surgery
2) Nontraumatic exertional
   a. Exercise: Genetically predisposing mutations associated with exertional rhabdomyolysis are described in Table 1.
   b. Sickle cell trait, rarely; usually additional predisposing factors are involved (e.g., BMI >30 kg/m², tobacco use, statin use, antipsychotic use, high altitude).
   c. Heat stroke.
   d. Metabolic myopathies.
   e. Malignant hyperthermia and neuroleptic malignant syndrome.
   f. Seizure activity.
3) Nontraumatic, nonexertional
   a. Drug-induced (statins alone, combination of statins with fibrates, or erythromycin, simvastatin and amiodarone, amphetamines, haloperidol)
   b. Alcoholism
   c. Hypothyroidism
   d. Infectious and inflammatory myositis
   Table 2 summarizes the various causes of rhabdomyolysis.

DIAGNOSIS

DIFFERENTIAL DIAGNOSIS

- "Creatine Kinase Elevation" in Section IV describes a clinical algorithm for the evaluation of CK elevation.

LABORATORY TESTS

- Creatine kinase: Usually CK is 5 to 10 times the upper limit of normal and typically peaks 24 to 72 hours after the initial insult (Fig. 1). Levels >15,000 IU/L are more likely to be associated with renal injury. However, in patients with concomitant risk

TABLE 2 Causes of Rhabdomyolysis

Muscle Injury/Ischemia	Trauma, Pressure Necrosis, Electric Shock, Burns, Acute Vascular Disease
Myofiber exhaustion	Seizures, excessive exercise, heat exhaustion
Toxins	Alcohol, cocaine, heroin, amphetamines, Ecstasy, phencyclidine, snakebite
Drugs	Statins, fibrates, zidovudine, neuroleptic malignant syndrome, azathioprine, theophylline, lithium, diuretics
Electrolyte disorders	Hypophosphatemia, hypokalemia, excess water shifts (hyperosmolality)
Infections	Viral (influenza, HIV, Coxsackievirus, Epstein-Barr virus), bacterial (*Legionella, Francisella, Streptococcus pneumoniae, Salmonella, Staphylococcus aureus*)
Familial	McArdle's disease, carnitine palmitoyl transferase deficiency, malignant hyperthermia
Other	Hypothyroidism, polymyositis, dermatomyositis

From Floege J et al: *Comprehensive clinical nephrology*, ed 4, Philadelphia, 2010, Saunders.

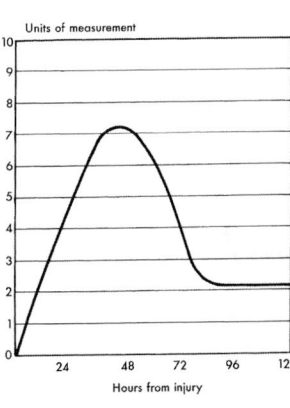

FIG. 1 Typical creatine kinase elimination curve. (From Rosen P [ed]: *Emergency medicine,* ed 4, St Louis, 1998, Mosby.)

factors such as hypokalemia or volume depletion, CK levels as low as 5000 U/L have been associated with AKI.

- Myoglobin: Excreted in urine with visible changes in urine ("port wine") at levels >100 to 300 mg/dl. Myoglobinuria can be suspected by a positive urine dipstick test for blood and minimal or no microhematuria. Due to its more rapid hepatic metabolism, myoglobin lacks sensitivity in detecting rhabdomyolysis; therefore, serum or urine myoglobin is not measured to establish diagnosis. Blood urea nitrogen and creatinine help monitor the severity of AKI.
- Potassium, calcium, phosphorus, and uric levels are released from damaged muscle, and levels should be monitored.
- Calcium: hypocalcemia from influx and deposition of calcium in damaged muscle tissue. Hypercalcemia may follow resolution of rhabdomyolysis from subsequent release of muscle-sequestered calcium back into the circulation and increased gastrointestinal calcium absorption from enhanced vitamin D production.
- Anion gap metabolic acidosis may occur from release of organic acids and phosphates from damaged muscle.
- Urinalysis: Myoglobin is detected as blood on dipstick, but RBCs are absent on microscopy. Presence of pigmented tubular casts establishes acute tubular necrosis.
- Unlike most other causes of acute tubular necrosis, rhabdomyolysis may result in a fractional excretion of sodium (FENa) of <1% due to renal vasoconstriction.
- Box 1 summarizes laboratory abnormalities observed with rhabdomyolysis.

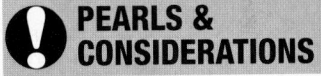 **TREATMENT**

ACUTE GENERAL Rx

- Identify precipitating factor(s) and discontinuation of drugs or toxins that might be a contributing factor.
- Early, aggressive, high-volume IV fluid replacement with normal saline. Extracellular fluid volume loading and diuresis reduce the risk for renal damage by elimination of urate and phosphate that can precipitate in the

BOX 1   Laboratory Abnormalities Observed With Rhabdomyolysis

Potassium
Elevated
Risk for acute kidney injury

Bicarbonate
Decreased (20 mEq/L)
Metabolic acidosis

Uric Acid
Elevated (>7 mg/dl)
Marker of acute renal failure

Sodium
Usually normal
Can decrease with mannitol therapy
Use serum osmolality values as a guide

Phosphate
Elevated
Risk for precipitation of calcium phosphate
May need phosphate binders if phosphate >7 mg/dl

Creatine Kinase
Elevated
Associated with creatine kinase level of 15 to 75,000

Blood Urea Nitrogen
Elevated (>20 mg/dl)

Creatinine
Elevated

Calcium
Initially low
Rebound phase may demonstrate hypercalcemia

Liver Function Tests
Occasionally elevated
Serum aspartate transaminase, lactate dehydrogenase, aldolase, muscle enzyme levels elevated

Troponin
Normal
Suspect myocardial damage as a cause (or effect) if elevated
7% false-positive rate for troponin I

Anion Gap
Sometimes elevated
May predict acute kidney injury

Prothrombin Time, Partial Thromboplastin Time, D-Dimer
Disseminated intravascular coagulation in up to 30% of severe cases
Associated with greater mortality

From Adams JG et al. *Emergency medicine, clinical essentials,* ed 2, Philadelphia, 2013, Elsevier.

kidneys. Fig. 2 describes a treatment algorithm for rhabdomyolysis.
- Fasciotomy is indicated in compartment syndrome for preservation of muscle and nerve function; the procedure rapidly decompresses compartment syndrome.
- Initiate volume repletion with normal saline at a rate of 200 to 1000 ml/hour depending on the clinical circumstances and severity of muscle damage. Titrate to maintain a urine output of at least 200 ml/hr. Consider treatment with mannitol (up to 200 g/day with cumulative dose up to 800 g) to GFR, diuresis, and scavenge free radicals. Typically, a 20% mannitol infusion at a dose of 0.5 g/kg is given over a 15-min period followed by an infusion at 0.1 g/kg/hour. Discontinue mannitol and volume resuscitation if diuresis (>20 ml/hour) is not established. Maintain volume repletion until myoglobinuria stops (negative urine dipstick blood test) or plasma CK levels decrease to <5000 U/L.
- Correct hypocalcemia if symptomatic or hyperkalemia is severe enough to produce electrocardiographic changes.
- Treatment of all electrolyte imbalances.
- Urine alkalinization (urine pH 6-7 by dipstick while maintaining serum pH at ~7.50) is controversial, but it appears helpful in research models when administered early in the course of rhabdomyolysis. Urine alkalinization may prevent renal tubular myoglobin precipitation and reduce lipid peroxidation, reactive oxygen species formation, and myoglobin-induced vasoconstriction.
- Initiation of renal replacement therapy is guided by the severity of renal injury and electrolyte imbalances. The use of continuous renal replacement therapy or high-flux membranes to enhance myoglobin clearance has not been validated.

DISPOSITION

Early diagnosis and management are required to avoid AKI, which occurs in 30% of cases. Rhabdomyolysis accounts for 7% to 10% of all cases of AKI in the U.S.

REFERRAL

Renal consultation and surgical consultation if compartment syndrome develops

PEARLS & CONSIDERATIONS

COMMENTS

- Statin-induced rhabdomyolysis occurs 12 times more frequently when statins are combined with fibrates than when used alone.
- Short-term, high-dose glucocorticoid steroid administration (500-1000 mg methylprednisolone) has been used for treatment of alcohol-induced rhabdomyolysis, refractory to volume repletion. This treatment may be efficacious in cases of severe rhabdomyolysis by retarding secondary leukocyte inflammatory muscle injury.

SUGGESTED READINGS
Available at www.expertconsult.com

RELATED CONTENT
Rhabdomyolysis (Patient Information)
Statin-Induced Muscle Syndrome (Related Key Topic)

AUTHORS: **JUNIOR UDUMAN, M.D.,** and **REDDY SINGASANI, M.D.**

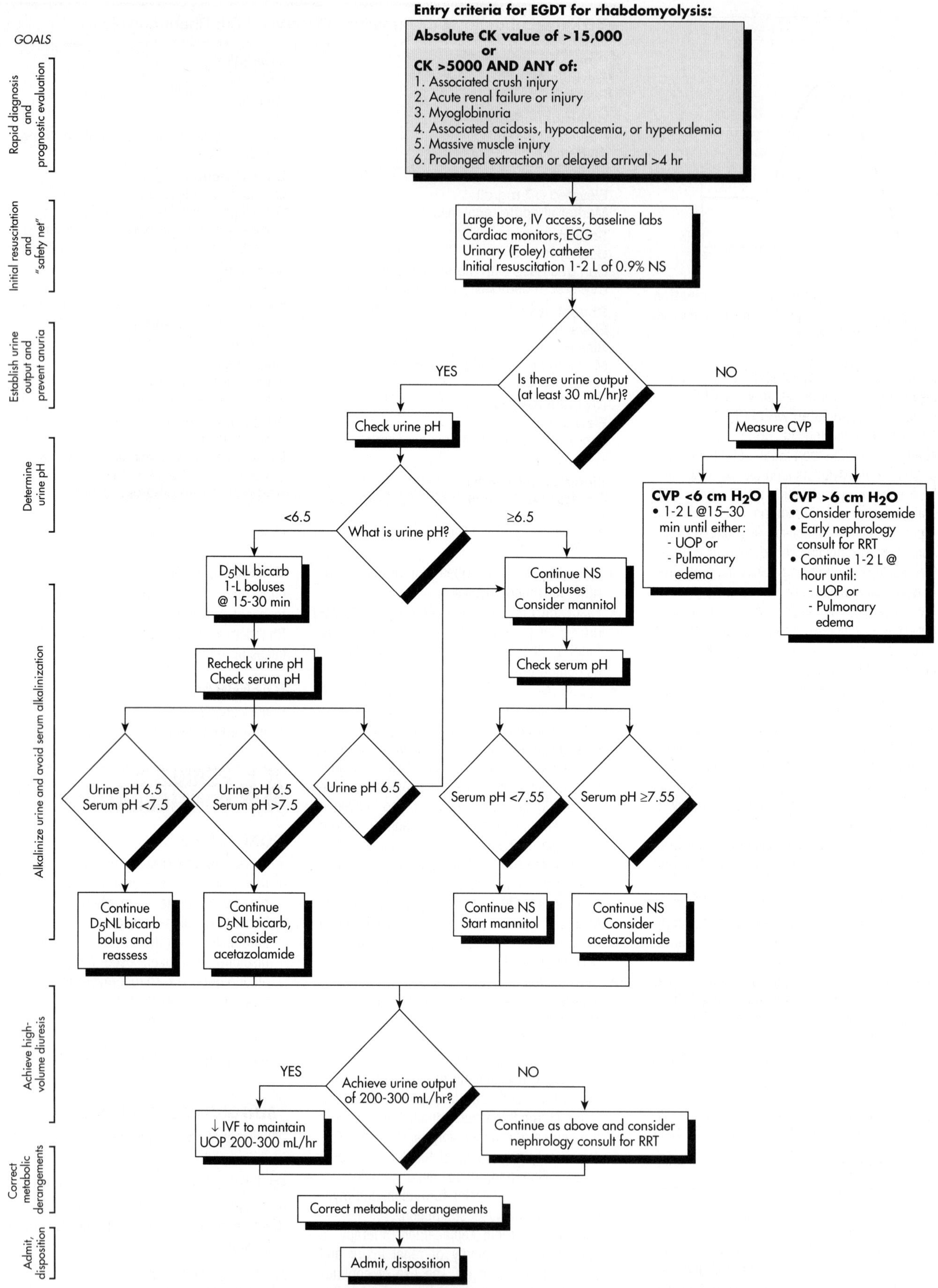

GOALS

Rapid diagnosis and prognostic evaluation

Entry criteria for EGDT for rhabdomyolysis:

Absolute CK value of >15,000
or
CK >5000 AND ANY of:
1. Associated crush injury
2. Acute renal failure or injury
3. Myoglobinuria
4. Associated acidosis, hypocalcemia, or hyperkalemia
5. Massive muscle injury
6. Prolonged extraction or delayed arrival >4 hr

Initial resuscitation and "safety net"

Large bore, IV access, baseline labs
Cardiac monitors, ECG
Urinary (Foley) catheter
Initial resuscitation 1-2 L of 0.9% NS

Establish urine output and prevent anuria

Is there urine output (at least 30 mL/hr)?

YES → Check urine pH

NO → Measure CVP

CVP <6 cm H₂O
- 1-2 L @15–30 min until either:
  - UOP or
  - Pulmonary edema

CVP >6 cm H₂O
- Consider furosemide
- Early nephrology consult for RRT
- Continue 1-2 L @ hour until:
  - UOP or
  - Pulmonary edema

Determine urine pH

What is urine pH?

<6.5 → D₅NL bicarb 1-L boluses @ 15-30 min

≥6.5 → Continue NS boluses Consider mannitol

Recheck urine pH Check serum pH

Check serum pH

Alkalinize urine and avoid serum alkalinization

Urine pH 6.5 Serum pH <7.5

Urine pH 6.5 Serum pH >7.5

Urine pH 6.5

Serum pH <7.55

Serum pH ≥7.55

Continue D₅NL bicarb bolus and reassess

Continue D₅NL bicarb, consider acetazolamide

Continue NS Start mannitol

Continue NS Consider acetazolamide

Achieve high-volume diuresis

Achieve urine output of 200-300 mL/hr?

YES → ↓ IVF to maintain UOP 200-300 mL/hr

NO → Continue as above and consider nephrology consult for RRT

Correct metabolic derangements

Correct metabolic derangements

Admit, disposition

Admit, disposition

FIG. 2 Early goal-directed therapy for rhabdomyolysis. *CK,* Creatine kinase; *CVP,* central venous pressure; *D5NL bicarb,* 5% dextrose in normal sodium bicarbonate solution; *EGDT,* early goal-directed therapy; *IV,* intravenous; *IVF,* intravenous fluid; *NS,* normal saline; *RRT,* renal replacement therapy; *UOP,* urinary output. (From Adams JG et al: *Emergency medicine, clinical essentials,* 2nd ed, Philadelphia, Elsevier 2013.)

BASIC INFORMATION

DEFINITION

Rheumatoid arthritis (RA) is a systemic auto-immune disease characterized by inflammatory polyarthritis which affects peripheral joints, especially the small joints of the hands and feet. It is a chronic, progressive disease in which untreated inflammation may lead to cartilage and bone erosions and joint destruction resulting in functional impairment.

SYNONYMS

RA

ICD-10CM CODES
M06.9	Rheumatoid arthritis, unspecified
M05.10	Rheumatoid lung disease with rheumatoid arthritis of unspecified site
M05.20	Rheumatoid vasculitis with rheumatoid arthritis of unspecified site
M05.30	Rheumatoid heart disease with rheumatoid arthritis of unspecified site
M05.39	Rheumatoid heart disease with rheumatoid arthritis of multiple sites
M05.40	Rheumatoid myopathy with rheumatoid arthritis of unspecified site
M05.49	Rheumatoid myopathy with rheumatoid arthritis of multiple sites
M05.50	Rheumatoid polyneuropathy with rheumatoid arthritis of unspecified site
M05.59	Rheumatoid polyneuropathy with rheumatoid arthritis of multiple sites
M05.60	Rheumatoid arthritis of unspecified site with involvement of other organs and systems
M05.69	Rheumatoid arthritis of multiple sites with involvement of other organs and systems
M05.70	Rheumatoid arthritis with rheumatoid factor of unspecified site without organ or systems involvement
M05.79	Rheumatoid arthritis with rheumatoid factor of multiple sites without organ or systems involvement
M05.80	Other rheumatoid arthritis with rheumatoid factor of unspecified site

EPIDEMIOLOGY & DEMOGRAPHICS

INCIDENCE: Annual incidence in northern Europe and the United States 0.15 to 0.60 per 1000.

TYPICAL AGE AT DIAGNOSIS: Usually fourth or fifth decade. Steadily increases with age until the mid-70s.

PREVALENCE: 0.5% to 1.0% of the worldwide population, with different rates in different ethnic groups.

PREDOMINANT SEX: *Females > males (2-3:1).*

RISK FACTORS: Female gender, age, tobacco use, silica exposure, and obesity.

PHYSICAL FINDINGS & CLINICAL PRESENTATION

Initial presentation:

- Pain, swelling, warmth in one or more peripheral joints, frequently with symmetric small joint involvement, often associated with >1 hour of morning stiffness and constitutional symptoms such as fatigue, malaise, low-grade fevers, and weight loss occurring over a period of weeks to months. A subset of patients can also present with acute-onset polyarthritis instead of insidious symptoms.
- Most common joints involved include metacarpophalangeal (MCP) joints, proximal interphalangeal (PIP) joints, and metatarsophalangeal (MTP) joints as well as wrists.
- Other affected joints involved include elbows, shoulders, hips, knees, and ankles.
- Distal interphalangeal (DIP) joints are spared.
- Sacroiliac and vertebral joints are spared, except for the C1 and C2 articulations.

Chronic longstanding disease:

- "Swan-neck" (DIP flexion and PIP hyperextension), "boutonniere" (DIP hyperextension and PIP flexion), and "Z-thumb" (MCP flexion and IP hyperextension) deformities (Fig. 1), ulnar deviation and subluxation of the MCP joints (Fig. 2) as well as radial deviation of the wrists.
- C1-C2 (atlantoaxial) inflammation can lead to odontoid erosion and transverse ligament laxity/rupture, resulting in atlantoaxial subluxation and cord compression.

- Joint damage of wrists, elbows, shoulders, hips, and knees can lead to severe osteoarthritis, necessitating joint surgery and/or replacement.

Extraarticular manifestations:

- Secondary Sjögren's syndrome (~35%): immune-mediated inflammation of lacrimal and salivary glands, resulting in dry mouth (xerostomia) and eyes (keratoconjunctivitis sicca).
- Rheumatoid nodules (25%): nontender, firm nodules on extensor surfaces and pressure points, usually in rheumatoid factor positive (RF+) disease. Histopathology demonstrates palisading histiocytes surrounding a central area of fibrinoid necrosis.
- Felty's syndrome: RA with splenomegaly and leukopenia. Most patients are positive for HLA-DR4 and RF.

Pulmonary disease:

- Pleural disease (exudative effusions, pleuritis).
- Interstitial lung disease (up to 10% clinically significant).
- Bronchiolitis obliterans.
- Cryptogenic organizing pneumonia.
- Pulmonary nodules. A combination of RA and pneumoconiosis is called Caplan syndrome.

Neuromuscular:

- Entrapment neuropathy (carpal tunnel, tarsal tunnel, cubital tunnel most commonly involved).
- Mononeuritis multiplex.
- Peripheral neuropathy. Cervical myelopathy and cord compression in atlantoaxial subluxation.
- Pachymeningitis (rare).
  ○ Vasculitis.

Cardiac disease:

- Pericarditis (most common).
- Myocarditis.
- Valvular nodules.
- There is an increased risk of cardiovascular disease compared to the general population, probably due to accelerated atherosclerosis from systemic inflammation.

Ocular disease:

- Keratoconjunctivitis sicca (dry eye, without dry mouth) (10%).
- Episcleritis, scleritis, scleral thinning, scleromalacia perforans, ulcerative keratitis.

  Amyloidosis: occurs in longstanding, poorly controlled RA. Usually presents as nephrotic syndrome. Can affect heart, kidney, liver, spleen, intestines, and skin.

  Osteoporosis.

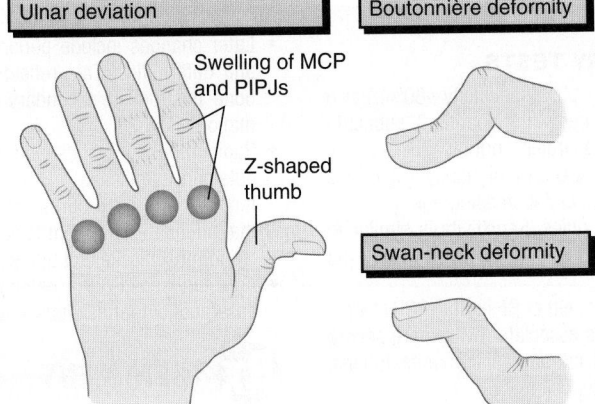

FIG. 1 Characteristic hand deformities in rheumatoid arthritis. *MCP*, Metacarpophalanges; *PIPJs*, proximal interphalangeal joints. (From Ballinger A: *Kumar & Clark's essentials of clinical medicine,* ed 6, Edinburgh, 2012, Saunders.)

Labels in figure: Ulnar deviation; Swelling of MCP and PIPJs; Z-shaped thumb; Boutonnière deformity; Swan-neck deformity

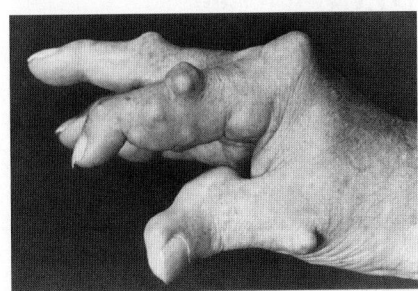

FIG. 2 Rheumatoid arthritis. Hand of a 60-year-old man with seropositive rheumatoid arthritis. There are fixed deformities and gross rheumatoid nodules. (From Canoso JJ: *Rheumatology in primary care,* Philadelphia, 1997, Saunders.)

ETIOLOGY

The exact cause of RA remains unknown despite extensive research. It is likely that a combination of genetic, hormonal, and environmental factors lead to aberrant immune activation and inflammatory response in the joint. A common genetic background plays a role in susceptibility to disease, as twins and first-degree relatives of RA patients are at increased risk of developing the disease compared to the general population. Patients with HLA-DR4, DR1, and DR14 alleles have increased susceptibility to RA; in particular, one amino acid sequence in the DR β chain, known as the shared epitope, is overrepresented in these patients. Other identified genetic associations include polymorphisms in *PTPN22, PADI4, CTLA4, TRAF1-C5, STAT4, TNFAIP3*. Epigenetic factors are also likely to be involved. Multiple environmental factors have also been implicated as possible etiologic factors, including cigarette smoking, silica exposure, and low socioeconomic class. Infectious agents such as *P. gingivalis*, Epstein-Barr virus, and parvovirus B19 have also been reported as possible triggers.

Stages of disease development presumably include:

- Initiation of the innate immune response through toll-like receptor (TLR) activation by a stimulating signal.
- Perpetuation of inflammatory response through activation of the adaptive immune system. There is migration of inflammatory cells (autoreactive B and T cells, monocytes) into the joint space, activation of macrophage-like and fibroblast-like synoviocytes, and development of a "synovial pannus," a thickened synovial membrane.
- The pannus releases proinflammatory cytokines (TNF-α, IL-1, IL-6, IL-15, IL-17, IL-18) as well as proteases, which erode cartilage and bone. Bone erosions are caused mainly by osteoclasts, which express the receptor activator of NF-κB (RANK). TNF-α, IL-1, and IL-17 promote the expression of RANK ligand (RANKL) on T cells and fibroblast-like synoviocytes.
- Many of the new "biologic" disease-modifying antirheumatic drugs (DMARDs) are engineered to target these cytokines (see treatment section).

DIAGNOSIS

The American College of Rheumatology and the European League against Rheumatism developed new classification criteria for RA in 2010. These are based on a point system where patients with score ≥6/10 are considered to have "definite RA." Four variables constitute the new criteria:

1. The number and size of involved joints (0 to 5 points, with higher scores for a larger number of small joints affected).
2. Levels of rheumatoid factor (RF) and anti-cyclic citrullinated peptide (CCP) antibody (0 to 3 points, with a higher score for a high-titer positive RF or anti-CCP).

TABLE 1 Factors Useful for Differentiating Early Rheumatoid Arthritis from Osteoarthritis

	Rheumatoid Arthritis	Osteoarthritis
Age at onset	Childhood and adults, peak incidence in 50s	Increases with age
Predisposing factors	Susceptibility epitopes (HLA-DR4, HLA-DR1, HLA-DR14)	Trauma
	Polymorphisms, epigenetic factors, infectious agents	Congenital abnormalities (e.g., shallow acetabulum)
	Smoking, silica exposure	
Early symptoms	Morning stiffness, pain, swelling	Pain increases through the day and with use
Joints involved	Wrists, MCP, PIP, and MTP joints; DIP joints are almost never involved.	DIP joints (Heberden's nodes), PIP joints (Bouchard's nodes), carpometacarpal joints, weight-bearing joints (hips, knees)
Physical findings	Soft tissue swelling, warmth	Bony osteophytes, minimal soft tissue swelling early on, crepitus
Radiologic findings	Periarticular osteopenia, marginal erosions	Subchondral sclerosis, osteophytes
Laboratory findings	Increased CRP, RF, and anti-CCP antibody, anemia, thrombocytosis	Normal

anti-CCP, anticitrullinated protein; *CRP-RF*, C-reactive protein-rheumatoid factor; *DIP*, distal interphalangeal joint; *MCP*, metacarpophalangeal joint; *MTP*, metatarsophalangeal joint; *PIP*, proximal interphalangeal joint.

3. Elevated erythrocyte sedimentation rate (ESR) or C-reactive protein (CRP) (1 point).
4. Symptom duration ≥6 weeks (1 point).

DIFFERENTIAL DIAGNOSIS

- Infectious causes: parvovirus B19, hepatitis B, hepatitis C, poststreptococcal reactive arthritis, acute rheumatic fever.
- Connective tissue diseases: systemic lupus erythematosus, scleroderma, mixed connective tissue disease, Sjögren's syndrome.
- Seronegative spondyloarthropathies.
- Calcium pyrophosphate deposition (CPPD or "pseudo-RA").
- Polyarticular gout.
- Polymyalgia rheumatica.
- Remitting seronegative symmetric synovitis with pitting edema (RS3PE) can resemble seronegative RA in elderly patients.
- Hemochromatosis.
- Paraneoplastic syndrome.
- Osteoarthritis, a degenerative arthritis that lacks prolonged morning stiffness and that usually lacks synovitis, should not be confused with RA (see Table 1).

LABORATORY TESTS

- RF (sensitivity ~60%; specificity ~80%). False positives are seen with hepatitis C, subacute bacterial endocarditis, primary biliary cirrhosis, sarcoidosis, malignancy, Sjögren's syndrome, SLE, and increasing age.
- Anti-CCP antibodies. Sensitivity is similar to RF, but it is more specific for RA than RF (up to 95%-98%).
- The presence of either RF or anti-CCP ("seropositive RA") is associated with more severe disease, more extraarticular manifestations, and worse prognosis.
- Elevated ESR and/or CRP. Will decline with treatment; thus can be used to monitor

disease activity along with physical examination and clinical presentation.
- CBC with differential. Possible anemia of chronic disease and thrombocytosis.
- Hypoalbuminemia and hypergammaglobulinemia.
- ANA is present is 20% to 30% of patients. However, complement will usually be normal or increased, in contrast to patients with systemic lupus erythematosus. Many patients will have secondary Sjögren's syndrome (positive ANA with negative SSA and SSB).
- Inflammatory synovial fluid with >2000 PMNs. Of note, patients with RA have an increased risk of developing septic arthritis. Hence, synovial fluid with white blood cells >50,000 cells/mm^3 is concerning for an infectious process and must always be ruled out.

IMAGING STUDIES

Plain radiography:
- Early changes include soft tissue swelling, symmetrical joint space narrowing, and periarticular osteopenia.
- Later changes include periarticular erosions and deformities. This reflects cartilage and bone destruction secondary to pannus formation (Fig. 3).
- Radiographs of hands and feet should be obtained at disease onset and repeated to monitor disease progression and to ensure that adequate treatment is achieved.

MRI and musculoskeletal ultrasound:
- Are more sensitive for detecting erosive disease and joint effusions/synovitis.

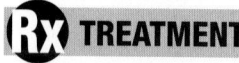 TREATMENT

- Early identification and treatment of RA with DMARDs is crucial. More than half of patients

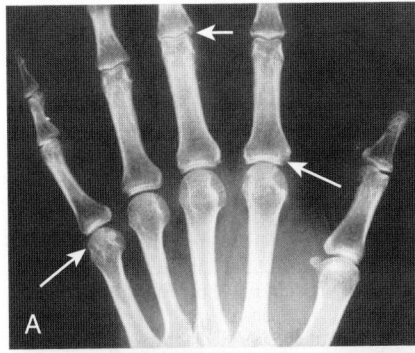

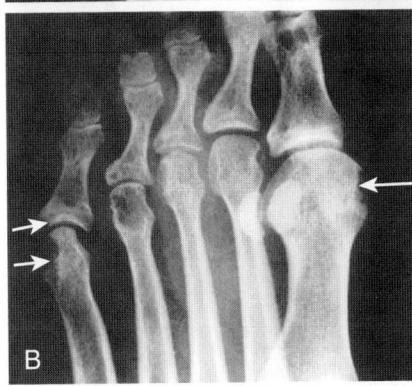

FIG. 3 Rheumatoid arthritis. A, Periarticular osteopenia and marginal erosions in metacarpophalangeal joints and a proximal interphalangeal joint *(arrows)*. **B,** In the same patient, marginal erosions at metatarsal heads. (From Canoso JJ: *Rheumatology in primary care,* Philadelphia, 1997, Saunders.)

have radiographic joint damage within 2 years of disease onset, but early aggressive treatment with DMARDs and/or biologic agents is associated with decreased progression of synovitis and bone erosions, and with decreased disability. Fig. 4 describes the American College of Rheumatology recommendations for treatment of rheumatoid arthritis. Goal of therapy is to "treat to a target" of low disease activity or remission.

- There are several tools to measure disease activity and define remission in rheumatoid arthritis, including (but not limited to) the following: Clinical Disease Activity Index (CDAI), Simplified Disease Activity Index (SDAI), Disease Activity Score (DAS) 28, Routine Assessment of Patient Index Data 3 (RAPID3), Stanford Health Assessment Questionnaire (HAQ), and Patient Activity Scale (PAS).

ACUTE GENERAL Rx

- NSAIDs: can be used initially to relieve pain and mild inflammation, or used later in the disease course for additional control of mild pain. NSAIDs are not disease modifying.
- Corticosteroids: oral or intraarticular, frequently used initially to reduce inflammation rapidly until oral DMARD treatments take effect. They may also be used during acute flares or in low doses for additional control of inflammation. The use of corticosteroids at

the lowest dose possible and shortest duration is recommended. Corticosteroids have many side effects, including but not limited to weight gain, increased risk of diabetes, osteoporosis, cataract formation, peptic ulcer disease (especially when used in combination with NSAIDs), and avascular necrosis.

CHRONIC Rx

- DMARDs: Can be classified into "nonbiologic" and "biologic" treatments.
  ○ Nonbiologic DMARDs: most commonly used agents are methotrexate (MTX), hydroxychloroquine (HCQ), sulfasalazine (SSZ), and leflunomide (LEF). Most of these are associated with potential toxicity and require close monitoring. They are also slow-acting drugs that require >8 weeks to become fully effective.
  ○ MTX is the most commonly used DMARD worldwide for the treatment of RA. It is effective as monotherapy in only 30% of patients with RA.
  ○ "Triple therapy"—MTX, HCQ, and SSZ—has been shown to be superior to MTX alone.
- Biologic DMARDs: newer biologically engineered therapies, which target cytokines and cells involved in the RA inflammatory response. Major side effects include an increased risk of severe infection, most notably reactivation of tuberculosis with anti-TNF agents. A negative PPD or interferon γ-release assay is a prerequisite to initiate therapy. Biologic DMARDs are most effective when used in combination with a nonbiologic DMARD, usually MTX.
- The five approved tumor necrosis factor α inhibitors (TNFI) include infliximab, etanercept, adalimumab, certolizumab pegol, and golimumab.
- Abatacept (CTLA-4Ig) is a recombinant protein that prevents costimulatory binding of antigen presenting cell to T cell, preventing T cell activation.
- Tocilizumab (anti–IL-6) is a monoclonal antibody against the IL-6 receptor.
- Tofacitinib (JAK3 inhibitor) inhibits the JAK-STAT intracellular signaling pathway, thus preventing the production of inflammatory mediators. The first oral biologic DMARD, it can be used as monotherapy or in combination with MTX. Recent trials with baricitinib, an oral reversible inhibitor of janus kinase JAK1 and JAK2 have shown significant improvement in patients with RA who have had an inadequate response to methotrexate.
- Rituximab (anti-CD20) is a monoclonal antibody against the CD20 antigen on B lymphocytes.
- Treatment recommendations in RA patient with high-risk comorbidities:
  ○ TNFI should be avoided in patients with congestive heart failure, as it can worsen the condition.
  ○ In patients with hepatitis B, immunosuppressive therapy can be safely prescribed along with concomitant antiviral therapy.
  ○ Treatment of hepatitis C patients with RA should be done following standard

guidelines in collaboration with gastroenterology/hepatology. Immunosuppressive therapy can be used safely in conjunction with antiviral therapy; avoidance of DMARDs such as MTX and LEF should be taken into consideration.
  ○ In patients with a history of skin cancer, DMARDs are recommended over the use of biologics. For patients with previously treated lymphoproliferative disorders, use of rituximab should be considered first, as well as combination DMARDs and non-TNF biologics. One should avoid TNFI, as there is an increased risk of lymphoma with these agents. Recommendations for treatment of patients with previously treated solid organ malignancy are the same as for patients without the condition.

Immunization, cardiovascular disease prevention (smoking cessation, blood pressure control, cholesterol control), and osteoporosis prevention (with calcium and vitamin D supplementation and bisphosphonate therapy) should be addressed in all RA patients.

DISPOSITION

- Remissions and exacerbations are common, but condition is chronically progressive in the majority of cases.
- Joint degeneration and deformity often lead to disability. Joint replacement is indicated for patients with severe joint damage whose symptoms are poorly controlled by medical management.
- Early and aggressive diagnosis and treatment are crucial in preventing or slowing joint destruction.

REFERRAL

- Early referral to rheumatologist.
- Orthopedic consultation for corrective surgery.

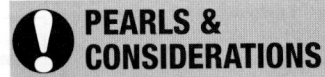 **PEARLS & CONSIDERATIONS**

RA sometimes develops acutely in the postpartum patient; conversely, as high as 75% of pregnant RA patients will experience remission during pregnancy.

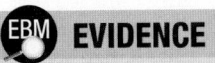 **EVIDENCE**

Available at www.expertconsult.com

SUGGESTED READINGS
Available at www.expertconsult.com

RELATED CONTENT
Rheumatoid Arthritis (Patient Information)

AUTHOR: **EDITH GARNEAU, M.D., M.SC.**

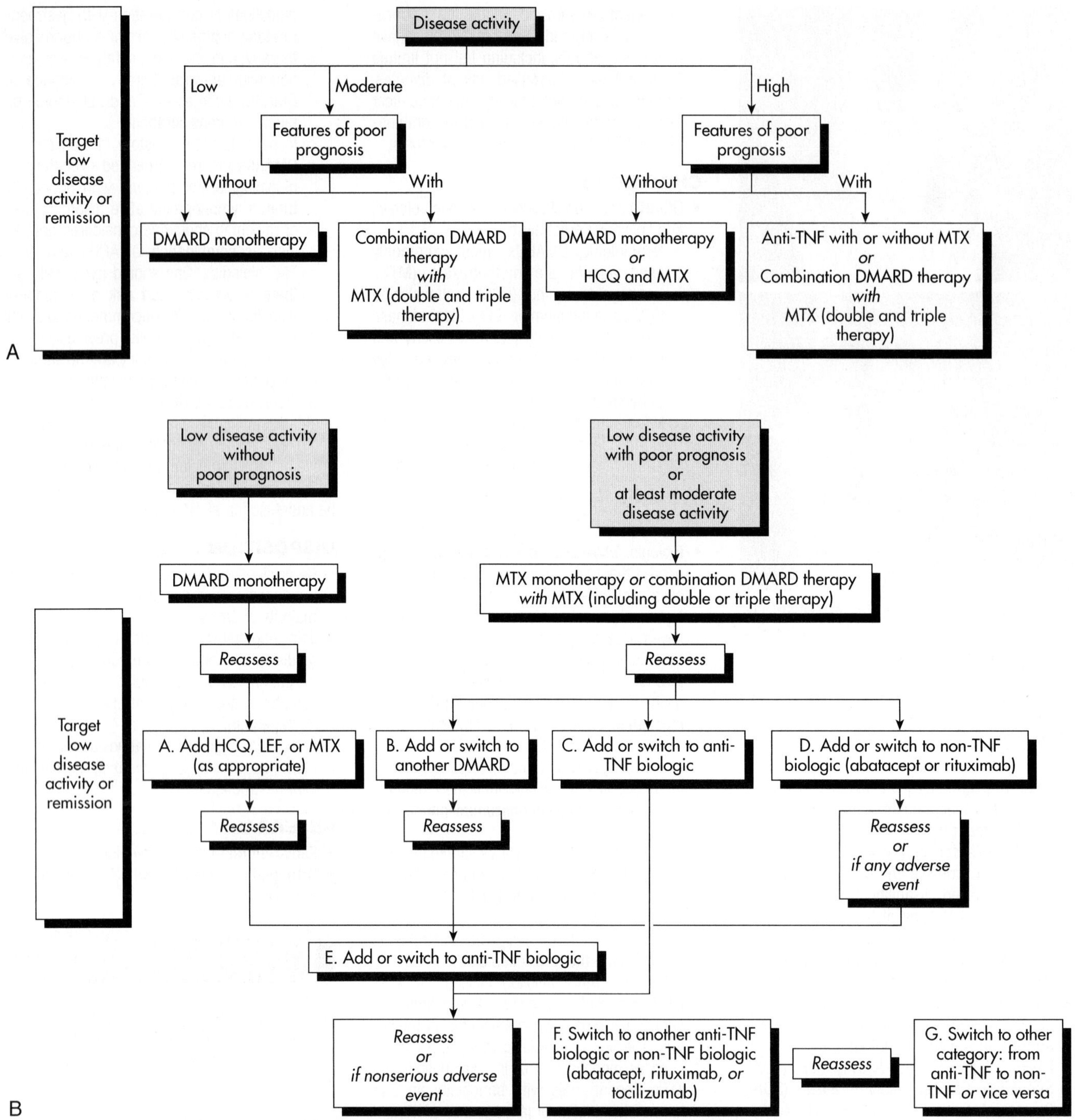

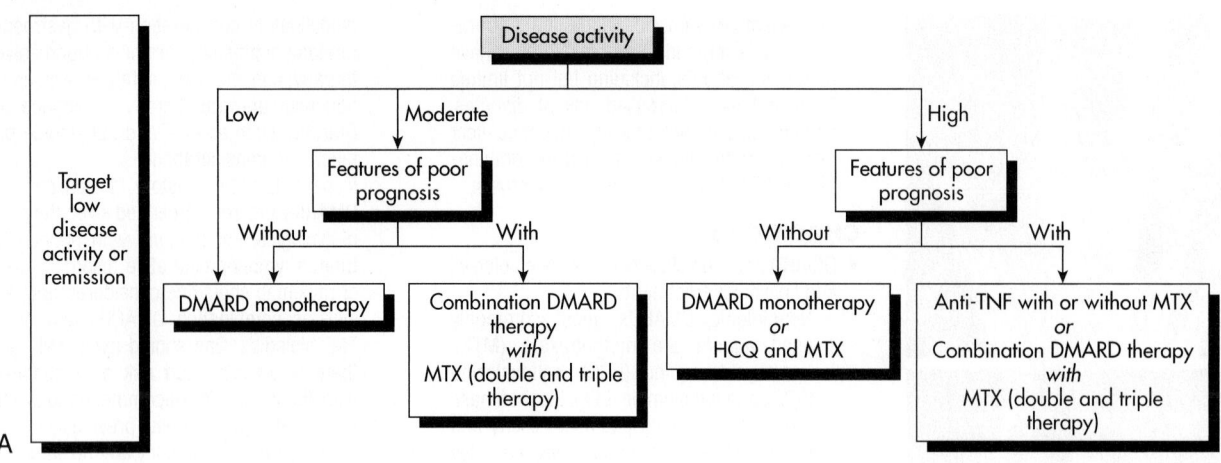

FIG. 4 American College of Rheumatology recommendations for treatment of rheumatoid arthritis. A, Early disease. **B,** Established disease. *DMARD,* Disease-modifying antirheumatic drug; *HCQ,* hydroxychloroquine; *LEF,* leflunomide; *MTX,* methotrexate; *TNF,* tumor necrosis factor. (From Firestein GS: et al. [eds]: *Kelly's textbook of rheumatology,* ed 9, Philadelphia, 2013, Saunders.)

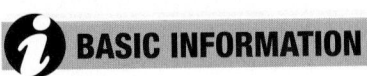

BASIC INFORMATION

DEFINITION

Rocky Mountain spotted fever (RMSF) is a life-threatening, tick-borne febrile illness caused by infection with *Rickettsia rickettsii*. The infection occurs when *R. rickettsii* in the salivary glands of a vector tick is transmitted into the dermis, spreading and replicating in the cytoplasm of endothelial cells and eliciting widespread vasculitis and end-organ damage.

SYNONYMS

RMSF

ICD-10CM CODES
A77.0 Spotted fever due to Rickettsia rickettsii

EPIDEMIOLOGY & DEMOGRAPHICS

INCIDENCE: 0.18 to 0.32 cases per 100,000 person-years. Infections have been reported throughout the United States.

PREVALENCE: Most prevalent in the Southeast, followed by the South Central states, but seen anywhere (Fig. 1). It has recently been reported in eastern Arizona, with common brown dog ticks *(Rhipicephalus sanguineus)* implicated as a vector of *R. rickettsii.*

PREDOMINANT SEX: Affects both genders equally.

PREDOMINANT AGE: Occurs at any age, but more likely in children ages 5 to 14 yr.

PHYSICAL FINDINGS & CLINICAL PRESENTATION

- Incubation: 2 to 14 days
- First symptoms: fever, headache, malaise, myalgias

Common History, Signs, or Symptoms	%
Tick bite	65
Fever	100
Rash	90
Rash on palms and soles (Fig. 2)	80
Headache	90
Myalgia	75
Nausea or vomiting	60
Abdominal pain	40
Conjunctivitis	30
Edema	20
Pneumonitis	15
Any severe neurologic complication (including stupor, delirium, seizures, ataxia, papilledema, focal neurologic deficits, and coma)	30

- Rash: a petechial rash is the hallmark of RMSF
  1. Appears during first 3 days in 50%; by day 5, 80% have it. No rash in 10%.
  2. Initial appearance: blanching erythematous macules on wrists and ankles that then spread to trunk, palms, and soles (Fig. 3). The rash involves palms and soles in more than 30% of cases and usually spares the face.
  3. Lesions may evolve into papules and eventually become nonblanching (petechiae or palpable purpura).
- Gastrointestinal symptoms:
  1. Nausea, vomiting, and abdominal pain are common.
  2. Occasionally may mimic an "acute abdomen" (e.g., appendicitis, cholecystitis).
  3. Mild hepatitis.
- Cardiopulmonary involvement:
  1. Interstitial pneumonitis.
  2. Myocarditis.

- Renal problems:
  1. Prerenal azotemia.
  2. Interstitial nephritis.
  3. Glomerulonephritis.
- Neurologic involvement:
  1. Encephalitis (confusion, lethargy, delirium).
  2. Ataxia.
  3. Convulsion.
  4. Cranial nerve palsy.
  5. Speech impediment.
  6. Hemiparesis or paraparesis.
  7. Spasticity.
- Fulminant RMSF:
  1. Early, widespread vascular necrosis leading to multisystem illness and death.

ETIOLOGY & PATHOGENESIS

- Infectious agent: *R. rickettsii* (an intracellular bacterium).
- Vector: dog tick and wood tick (vertical transmission exists in ticks, but horizontal transmission involving rodents represents an important reservoir for the agent). In the United States *R. rickettsii* is transmitted mainly by the American dog tick *(Dermacentor variabilis)* and the Rocky Mountain wood tick *(D. andersoni).*
- Pathogenesis: the spread of *R. rickettsii* is hematogenous with attachment to the vascular endothelium, causing a vasculitis. The manifestations of this illness are caused by increased vascular permeability.

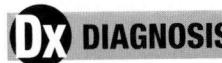

DIAGNOSIS

DIFFERENTIAL DIAGNOSIS

Influenza A, enteroviral infection, typhoid fever, leptospirosis, infectious mononucleosis, viral hepatitis, sepsis, ehrlichiosis, gastroenteritis, acute abdomen, bronchitis, pneumonia, meningococcemia, disseminated gonococcal infection, secondary syphilis, bacterial endocarditis, toxic shock syndrome, scarlet fever, rheumatic fever, measles, rubella, typhus, rickettsialpox, Lyme disease, drug hypersensitivity reactions, idiopathic thrombocytopenic purpura, thrombotic thrombocytopenic purpura, Kawasaki dis-

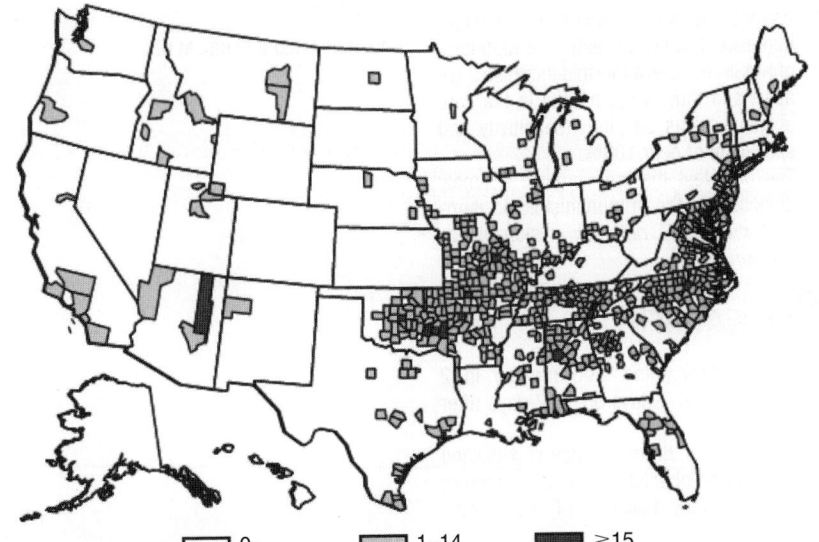

FIG. 1 Spotted fever rickettsiosis. Number of reported cases, by county, United States, 2010. (From Centers for Disease Control and Prevention: Summary of notifiable diseases—United States, 2010, *MMWR Morb Mortal Wkly Rep* 59[53]:1-111, 2012.)

Legend: 0 | 1–14 | ≥15

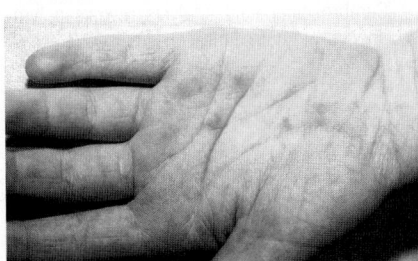

FIG. 2 Palmar rash associated with Rocky Mountain spotted fever. (From Walker DH, Raoult D: *Rickettsia rickettsii* and other spotted fever group rickettsiae [Rocky Mountain spotted fever and other spotted fevers]. In Mandell GL et al [eds]: *Principles and practice of infectious diseases,* ed 5, New York, 2000, Churchill Livingstone.)

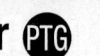
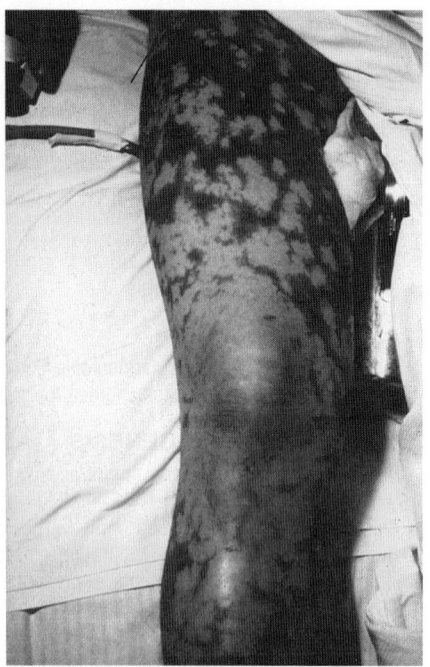

FIG. 3 Late appearance of rash: Rocky Mountain spotted fever manifesting on lower extremity. (Courtesy of Theodore Woodward, MD. From Marx JA et al: *Rosen's emergency medicine: concepts and clinical practice,* 7 ed, Philadelphia, 2010, Elsevier.)

ease, immune complex vasculitis, connective tissue disorders.

WORKUP

- Consider RMSF in any patient with an acute febrile illness with headache and myalgia, especially with an associated history of tick exposure. Absence of rash does not rule out the diagnosis.
- Rickettsial antibodies take several weeks to develop; therefore, serologic testing is of limited utility in acute illness.
- Box 1 shows the diagnostic criteria for Rocky Mountain spotted fever.

LABORATORY TESTS

- Thrombocytopenia and elevated aminotransferase are common (see the following).
- Cerebrospinal fluid analysis reveals a lymphocyte-predominant pleocytosis.

Routine Tests	%
White cell count	
<10,000/mm³	72
>10% bands	69
Platelet count	
<150,000/mm³	52
<99,000/mm³	32
Serum sodium value <132 mEq/L	56

BOX 1   Diagnostic Criteria for Rocky Mountain Spotted Fever

Laboratory Criteria
- Serologic evidence of a significant change in serum antibody titer reactive with *Rickettsia rickettsii* antigens between paired serum specimens, as measured by a standardized assay conducted in a commercial, state, or reference laboratory.
- Demonstration of *R. rickettsii* antigen in a clinical specimen by immunohistochemical methods.
- Detection of *R. rickettsii* DNA in a clinical specimen by the polymerase chain reaction (PCR) assay.
- Isolation of *R. rickettsii* from a clinical specimen in cell culture.
   For confirmed cases, a significant change in titer must be determined by the testing laboratory; examples of commonly used measures of significant change include, but are not limited to, a fourfold or greater change in antibody titer as determined by indirect immunofluorescent antibody (IFA) assay or an equivalent change in optical density measured by enzyme-linked immunosorbent assay (EIA or ELISA).

Case Classification (CDC Case Definition, 2004)
Confirmed: The patient has a clinically compatible illness that is laboratory confirmed.
Probable: The patient has a clinically compatible illness and serologic evidence of antibody reactive with *R. rickettsii* in a single serum sample at a titer considered indicative of current or past infection (cutoff titers are determined by individual laboratories).

CDC, Centers for Disease Control and Prevention.
From Diagnosis and management of tickborne rickettsial diseases: Rocky Mountain spotted fever, ehrlichioses, and anaplasmosis—United States. *MMWR Recomm Rep* 55(RR-4):18, 2006, and from Marx JA et al: *Rosen's emergency medicine: concepts and clinical practice,* 7 ed, Philadelphia, 2010, Elsevier.

Routine Tests	%
Aspartate aminotransferase ≥2× normal	62
Alanine aminotransferase ≥2× normal	39
Bilirubin value >1.4 mg/dl	30
Cerebrospinal fluid	
Opening pressure ≥250 mm H₂O	14
Glucose value ≤50 mg/dl	8
Protein value ≥50 mg/dl	35
White cell count ≥5/mm³	38
Mononuclear cell predominance	46
Polymorphonuclear cell predominance	50

- Etiologic tests:
   1. Antibody titers to *R. rickettsii* (by indirect fluorescent antibody test). The diagnosis of RMSF requires a fourfold increase 2 wk apart and thus is not helpful in the care of the patients despite a sensitivity and specificity of near 100%.
   2. The only test that can provide a timely diagnosis is the immunohistologic demonstration of *R. rickettsii* in skin biopsy specimens.

Rx TREATMENT

- Oral or IV doxycycline, 200 mg/day in 2 divided doses for 7 days or for 2 days after defervescence.
- Chloramphenicol, 50 mg/kg/day in 4 divided doses; chloramphenicol may be preferred during pregnancy because of the effects of doxycycline on fetal bones and teeth; therapy continued for at least 2 days after defervescence.

PROGNOSIS

Fatality rate: 1% to 4% (five times greater if treatment is initiated after day 5 of illness, which is more likely in the absence of rash and during seasonal nonpeak tick activity). Long-term sequelae seen in patients who recover from severe RMSF: paraparesis, hearing loss; peripheral neuropathy; bladder and bowel incontinence; cerebellar, vestibular, and motor dysfunction; language disorders; limb amputation; and scrotal pain after cutaneous necrosis.

RELATED CONTENT

Rocky Mountain Spotted Fever (Patient Information)

AUTHOR: **FRED F. FERRI, M.D.**

BASIC INFORMATION

DEFINITION

Rosacea is a chronic skin disorder characterized by papules and pustules affecting the face and often associated with flushing and erythema.

SYNONYMS

Acne rosacea

ICD-10CM CODES
L71   Rosacea
L71.9   Rosacea unspecified
L71.1   Rhinophyma
L71.8   Other rosacea
L71.0   Perioral dermatitis

EPIDEMIOLOGY & DEMOGRAPHICS

- Rosacea occurs in 1 in 20 Americans.
- Onset often between ages 30 and 50 yr
- More common in people of Celtic origin; however, this disease may be overlooked in nonwhites because skin pigmentation results in atypical presentation.
- Female/male ratio of 3:1.

PHYSICAL FINDINGS & CLINICAL PRESENTATION

- Facial erythema, presence of papules, pustules, and telangiectasia.
- Excessive facial warmth and redness are the predominant presenting symptoms.
- Itching is generally absent.
- Comedones are absent (unlike acne).
- Women are more likely to show symptoms on the chin and cheeks, whereas in men the nose is commonly involved.
- Ocular findings (mild dryness and irritation with blepharitis, conjunctival injection, burning, stinging, tearing, eyelid inflammation, swelling, and redness) are present in 50% of patients.

Rosacea can be classified into four major subtypes:
1. Erythematotelangiectatic (vascular): erythema in central part of face, telangiectasia, flushing.
2. Papulopustular (inflammatory): presence of dome-shaped erythematous papules and small pustules, in addition to facial erythema, flushing, and telangiectasia.
3. Phymatosis (Fig. 1): presence of thickened skin with prominent pores that may affect the nose (rhinophyma), chin (gnathophyma), forehead (metophyma), eyelids (blepharophyma), and ears (otophyma).
4. Ocular: conjunctival injection, sensation of foreign body in the eye, telangiectasia and erythema of lid margins, scaling.

ETIOLOGY

- Unknown but believed to involve the vasculature.
- Hot drinks, alcohol, and sun exposure may accentuate the erythema by causing vasodilation of the skin.
- Flare-ups may also result from reactions to medications (e.g., simvastatin, angiotensin-converting enzyme inhibitors, vasodilators, fluorinated corticosteroids), stress, extreme heat or cold, wind, humidity, strenuous exercise, spicy drinks, menstruation.

DIAGNOSIS

DIFFERENTIAL DIAGNOSIS

- Drug eruption.
- Acne vulgaris.
- Contact dermatitis.
- Systemic lupus erythematosus.
- Carcinoid flush.
- Idiopathic facial flushing.
- Seborrheic dermatitis.
- Facial sarcoidosis.
- Photodermatitis.
- Mastocytosis.
- Perioral dermatitis.
- Granulomas of the skin.

WORKUP

Diagnosis is based on clinical findings. Distinguishing features between acne and rosacea are the presence of telangiectasia and deep diffuse erythema and absence of comedones in rosacea.

TREATMENT

NONPHARMACOLOGIC THERAPY

- Avoid alcohol, excessive sun exposure, and hot drinks of any type.
- Use of mild, nondrying soap is recommended; local skin irritants should be avoided.
- Sunscreens are an important component of therapy and should be applied each morning.
- Daily circular massage for several minutes of the central portion of the face is helpful in decreasing lymphedema and inflammation in this area.
- Reassure patient that rosacea is completely unrelated to poor hygiene.
- Vascular laser surgery is effective for telangiectasia.
- Surgical options are available for telangiectasia and rhinophyma and include dermabrasion, laser ablation, heated scalpel, electrocautery, and radiofrequency electrosurgery.

GENERAL Rx

- Several classes of drugs are used in treatment of rosacea, including the metronidazole family, the tetracycline family, ivermectin cream, and azelaic acid.
- Vascular rosacea: topical therapy with metronidazole aqueous gel (MetroGel) applied bid is effective as initial therapy for mild cases. A new 1% formulation of metronidazole (Noritate) applied daily may improve patient compliance. Clindamycin lotion (Cleocin), sulfacetamide, or erythromycin 2% solution may also be effective. Brimonidine (Mirvaso) is a selective alpha$_2$-adrenergic receptor agonist FDA-approved as a gel preparation for topical treatment of adults with persistent facial erythema of rosacea.
- Pustular and ocular rosacea: systemic antibiotics (doxycycline 100 mg qd or tetracycline 250 mg qid until symptoms diminish, then taper off). Minocycline 50 to 100 mg qd should be used only in resistant cases because this medication is expensive. Oral metronidazole (200 mg qd to bid) for 4 to 6 wk is also effective. A 1% cream formulation of the antiparasitic drug ivermectin (Soolantra) is effective for papulopustular rosacea with minimal adverse effects. After 3 months of therapy, it will produce clearing of rosacea lesions in up to 80% of patients with moderate to severe symptoms. Its mechanism of action is unknown, but it may be due to the combination of its antiinflammatory effects and its antiparasitic effects on the Demodex mite, which may contribute to the symptoms of rosacea. Cost may be a limiting factor ($320 for one 30-g tube).
- Isotretinoin (Accutane) 0.5 to 1 mg/kg/day in two divided doses for 15 to 20 wk can be used for refractory papular and pustular rosacea; use of retinoids may, however, worsen erythema and telangiectasis.

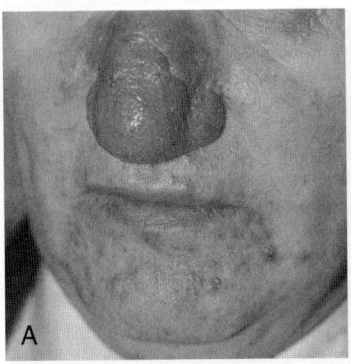
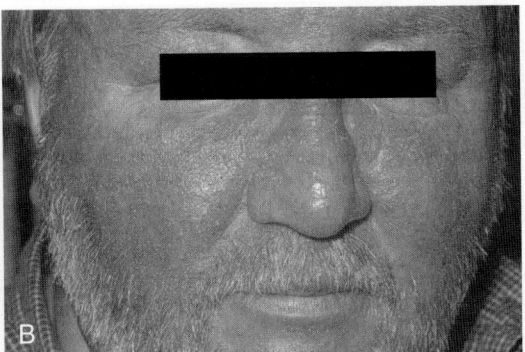

FIG. 1 Severe rosacea. A, Note the scattered papules on the face and the confluent involvement of the nose. Alcohol ingestion is not related to this appearance. **B,** Note the severe inflammation with confluent redness and significant edema. (From White GM, Cox NH [eds]: *Diseases of the skin, a color atlas and text,* ed 2, St Louis, 2006, Mosby.)

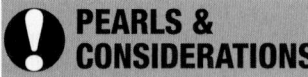

- Erythema and flushing may respond to low-dose clonidine (0.05 mg bid).
- Treatment of phymatous rosacea: oral tetracyclines, oral isotretinoin, ablative/pulsed dye laser therapy, electrosurgery.
- Treatment of ocular rosacea: topical or oral tetracyclines, artificial tears, and/or lid cleansing for eyelid hygiene.

DISPOSITION

- Rosacea is often resistant to initial treatment and recurrent. Periods of remission and relapse are common.
- The progression of rosacea is variable. Typical stages include:
  1. Facial flushing.
  2. Erythema and/or edema and ocular symptoms.
  3. Papules and pustules.
  4. Rhinophyma.

 PEARLS & CONSIDERATIONS

COMMENTS

- The course of the disease is typically chronic, with remissions and relapses.
- Patients with resistant cases may have *Demodex folliculorum* mite infestation or tinea infection (diagnosis can be confirmed with potassium hydroxide examination); the role of *D. folliculorum* in rosacea is unclear. These mites can sometimes be found in large numbers in the lesions; however, their numbers do not generally decline with treatment.

- Rosacea can result in emotional and social stigmas, especially because many people associate rosacea and rhinophyma with alcohol abuse.
- Early consultation with an ophthalmologist is recommended in patients with suspected ocular involvement.

EVIDENCE

Available at www.expertconsult.com

SUGGESTED READINGS

Available at www.expertconsult.com

RELATED CONTENT

Rosacea (Patient Information)

AUTHOR: **FRED F. FERRI, M.D.**

BASIC INFORMATION

DEFINITION

Roseola is a benign viral illness found in infants and characterized by high fevers that last 3 or 4 days, followed by defervescence, and development of a macular or maculopapular rash.

SYNONYMS

Exanthem subitum.
Sixth disease.
Roseola infantum.
Pseudorubella.
Human herpesvirus 6 (HHV-6), human herpesvirus 7 (HHV-7).

ICD-10CM CODES
B08.2 Exanthema subitum (sixth disease)

EPIDEMIOLOGY & DEMOGRAPHICS

- Nearly one third of all infants develop roseola before the age of 2 yr.
- Peak prevalence is between 7 and 13 mo.
- More than 90% of children older than 2 yr of age are seropositive for the virus causing roseola.
- Roseola is spread from person to person. It is not known how it is spread, but it must be very efficiently spread and presumably via the respiratory tract.
- There is no predilection for gender or time of year.
- Like other herpesviruses, HHV-6 induces a lifelong latent infection in humans.

PHYSICAL FINDINGS & CLINICAL PRESENTATION

- Typically the child develops a high fever, usually up to 104° F (40° C), that lasts for 3 to 5 days.
- Fever may be associated with a runny nose, irritability, and fatigue.
- A rash appears within 48 hr of defervescence; it begins on the neck or trunk and then spreads to the extremities, and persists for a few hours to 2 days.
- Faint pink maculopapular rash that blanches when palpated (Fig. E1) and generally nonpruritic. The mucous membranes are spared.
- Other common findings: cervical and/or occipital adenopathy, erythematous tympanic membranes, anorexia.
- Nagayama spots: red papules on the soft palate or base of the uvula.
- Seizures.
- Less common: febrile seizures (≤6% of cases), cough, diarrhea, aseptic meningitis.

ETIOLOGY

- Roseola is usually caused by human herpesvirus-6 (HHV-6) in the great majority of cases but other causes include human herpesvirus-7, enteroviruses, adenoviruses, and parainfluenza virus type 1. A small percentage of children may have primary infection with HHV-7.
- The incubation period is between 5 and 15 days.

DIAGNOSIS

The diagnosis of roseola is usually made by the clinical presentation as stated previously. It can be confirmed serologically by indirect immunofluorescence assays, ELISA, neutralization assays, and immunoblot. Viral culture is the gold standard to document active viral replication but is expensive, time consuming, and available only in research laboratories.

DIFFERENTIAL DIAGNOSIS

- Rubeola (measles).
- Rubella.
- Fifth disease (erythema infectiosum) caused by parvovirus B19.
- Enteroviral infections.
- Drug eruption.
- Mononucleosis.
- All causes of fever (e.g., otitis media, pneumonia, and urinary tract infection).
- Meningitis.

WORKUP

- If unsure of the diagnosis of roseola in a febrile infant, a fever workup is done to rule out other infectious causes.
- The decision to proceed with a fever workup is a clinical judgment call.

LABORATORY TESTS

- CBC with differential usually shows relative neutropenia and mild atypical lymphocytosis.
- Erythrocyte sedimentation rate (ESR), blood cultures as indicated.
- Urinalysis and urine cultures.
- Stool cultures if diarrhea is present.
- Lumbar puncture if needed to rule out meningitis in patients with mental status changes.
- Commercial assays can be used to detect HHV-6-specific IgG antibody responses but IgM assays are not always reliable for acute infection.
- A PCR real-time assay is available to quantify viral DNA in blood and body fluids, but it is generally reserved to detect reactivation of virus in immunocompromised patients, such as hematopoietic stem cell transplant patients.

IMAGING STUDIES

Chest x-ray to rule out pneumonia.

TREATMENT

NONPHARMACOLOGIC THERAPY

- Supportive care.
- Maintain hydration by drinking clear fluids: water, fruit juice, lemonade, and so forth.
- Sponge bath with lukewarm water if febrile.

ACUTE GENERAL Rx

- Acetaminophen 10 to 15 mg/kg per dose at 4-hr intervals for fever.
- Ibuprofen 5 to 10 mg/kg per dose at 6-hr intervals (maximal dose 600 mg).

CHRONIC Rx

Roseola is a viral disease that is short lasting; chronic treatment is usually not an issue.

DISPOSITION

- Roseola is generally a benign, self-limited disease that usually lasts approximately 1 wk.
- Complications, although rare, can occur and include:
  1. Febrile seizures.
  2. Meningitis.
  3. Encephalitis.
  4. Pneumonitis.
  5. Hepatitis.

REFERRAL

Subspecialty consultation is made with the appropriate discipline if any of the previously mentioned complications occur (e.g., neurology for seizures).

PEARLS & CONSIDERATIONS

COMMENTS

- A child with fever and rash should be excluded from day care.
- HHV-6 is named accordingly because it is the sixth herpesvirus discovered after herpes simplex 1 (HSV-1), HSV-2, cytomegalovirus (CMV), Epstein-Barr virus (EBV), and varicella-zoster virus (VZV).
- Roseola is called sixth disease because it represents the sixth childhood "exanthem"; the other five are measles, scarlet fever, rubella, Dukes disease, and erythema infectiosum.

SUGGESTED READING
Available at www.expertconsult.com

RELATED CONTENT
Roseola (Patient Information)

AUTHOR: **GLENN G. FORT, M.D., M.P.H.**

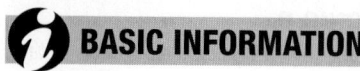

BASIC INFORMATION

DEFINITION

Salivary gland neoplasms are benign or malignant tumors of a salivary gland (parotid, submandibular, or sublingual).

SYNONYMS

These tumors are often named according to their histologic type (see "Diagnosis").

ICD-10CM CODES

C08.9 Malignant neoplasm of major salivary gland, unspecified
C07 Malignant neoplasm of parotid gland
C08.0 Malignant neoplasm of submandibular gland
C08.1 Malignant neoplasm of sublingual gland

EPIDEMIOLOGY & DEMOGRAPHICS

INCIDENCE: One to two cases per 100,000 person-years (1% of all head and neck tumors).
DISTRIBUTION:

- Parotid gland, 85% (80% are benign).
- Submandibular gland, 10% (55% are benign).
- Sublingual and minor glands, 5% (35% are benign).

PHYSICAL FINDINGS & CLINICAL PRESENTATION

- Parotid gland:
  1. Painless swelling overlying the masseter muscle (under the temporomandibular joint).
  2. Pain.
  3. Facial nerve palsy.
  4. Cervical lymph nodes.
  5. Mass in oral cavity.
- Submandibular gland: swelling under anterior portion of the mandible.
- Sublingual gland: intraoral swelling under the tongue, medial to the mandible.

DIAGNOSIS

PATHOLOGY

HISTORY

Benign Tumors.

- Mixed tumor (usually parotid).
- Adenolymphoma (Warthin's tumor).
- Pleomorphic adenoma.
- Capillary hemangioma, lymphangioma (in children).
- Intraductal papilloma.
- Other (e.g., myoepithelioma, canalicular adenoma, basal cell adenoma).

MALIGNANT TUMORS

- Mucoepidermoid carcinoma (most common malignant tumor of the parotid gland).
- Adenoid cystic carcinoma.
- Adenocarcinoma.
- Malignant mixed tumor.
- Squamous cell carcinoma.
- Other.

STAGE (TNM):

T_0	No evidence of primary tumor
T_1	Tumor <2 cm
T_2	Tumor 2 to 4 cm
T_3	Tumor 4 to 6 cm
T_4	Tumor >6 cm

All subdivided into

- Without local extension.
- With local extension.

N_0	No lymph node metastasis
N_1	Single ipsilateral node <3 cm
N_2	Ipsilateral, contralateral, or bilateral node <6 cm
N_3	Any node >6 cm
M_0	No distant metastasis
M_1	Distant metastasis
Stage I	T_{1a} or $_{2a}N_0M_0$
Stage II	$T_{1b,2b,3a}$ N_0M_0
Stage III	$T_{3b,4a}$ N_0M_0 or any T except $_{4b}N_1M_0$
Stage IV	T_{4b} any N any M or any T $N_{2,3}M_0$ or any T, any N_1M_1

WORKUP

- Fine-needle aspiration. The sensitivity, specificity, and accuracy of parotid gland aspirates are approximately 92%, 100%, and 98%, respectively.
- Imaging by CT scan or MRI (Fig. 1).
- Open biopsy (rarely indicated).

TREATMENT

Malignant tumors:

- Surgery is the mainstay of treatment; gland resection and neck dissection if lymph nodes are involved.
- A lateral lobectomy with preservation of facial nerve should be considered for tumors confined to the superficial lobe of the parotid gland. Gross tumor should not be left in situ, but if the facial nerve is able to be preserved by "peeling" tumor off the nerve, it should be attempted, followed by radiation therapy for microscopic disease.
- Postoperative radiation is indicated for high-grade malignancies demonstrating extraglandular disease, perineural invasion, direct invasion of surrounding tissues, or regional metastases.
- Chemotherapy.
  Benign tumors: surgery for tumor resection.

PROGNOSIS OF MALIGNANT TUMORS

Five-year survival rates:

- Mucoepidermoid carcinoma: 75% to 95%.
- Adenoid cystic carcinoma: 40% to 80%.
- Adenocarcinoma: 20% to 75%.
- Malignant mixed tumor: 35% to 75%.
- Squamous cell carcinoma: 25% to 60%.

PEARLS & CONSIDERATIONS

COMMENTS

Salivary gland neoplasms most often present as slow-growing, well-circumscribed masses. Pain, rapid growth, nerve weakness, fixation to skin or underlying muscle, and paresthesias usually are indicative of malignancy.

RELATED CONTENT

Salivary Gland Tumors (Patient Information)

AUTHOR: **BHARTI RATHORE, M.D.**

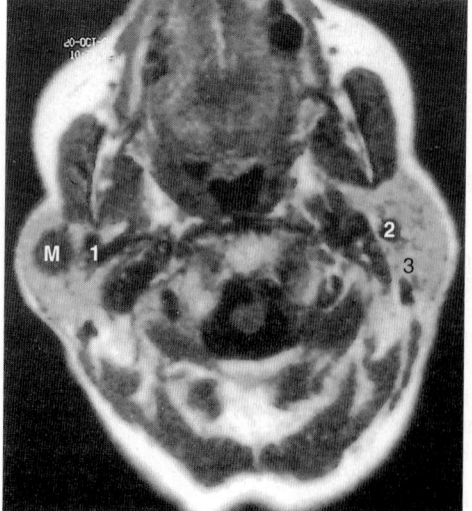

FIG. 1 Pleomorphic Adenoma of Parotid Gland. Pleomorphic adenoma in the right parotid (M) is a well-defined, low-signal intensity mass on the axial T_1-weighted MRI. Note displacement of the retromandibular vein **(1)** medially by the mass compared with the normal left retromandibular vein **(2)**. The left facial nerve **(3)** branching through the normal left parotid is seen. (From Skarin AT: *Atlas of diagnostic oncology*, ed 4, St Louis, 2010, Mosby.)

BASIC INFORMATION

DEFINITION
Salmonellosis is an infection caused by one of several serotypes of a gram-negative bacillus of the genus *Salmonella*. Current *Salmonella* nomenclature is described in Table 1.

SYNONYMS
Typhoid fever
Paratyphoid fever
Enteric fever

ICD-10CM CODES
A02.0 *Salmonella* enteritis
A02.1 *Salmonella* sepsis
A02.2 Localized *Salmonella* infections
A02.8 Other specified *Salmonella* infections
A0.9 *Salmonella* infection, unspecified

EPIDEMIOLOGY & DEMOGRAPHICS
INCIDENCE (IN U.S.):
- Epidemiologically, the clinical syndromes are divided into those that cause a typhoidal type of infection (systemic illness with fever and abdominal pain) such as *Salmonella typhi* and those that do not: nontyphoidal *Salmonella* infections (gastroenteritis) such as *S. enteritidis*, *S. newport*, and *S. typhimurium*.
- Estimated 1 million cases/yr of nontyphoidal salmonellosis in the United States (leading cause of foodborne illness in the U.S.). In 2009, contaminated peanut butter and peanut products caused a nationwide *Salmonella typhimurium* outbreak in 46 states, affecting more than 700 people.
- Largest outbreak of gastroenteritis syndrome (nontyphoidal): 200,000 who ingested contaminated milk.
- Approximately 500 cases of *Salmonella typhi* infection are reported each year, of which nearly 80% is associated with foreign travel.

PEAK INCIDENCE: Summer and fall.
PREDOMINANT AGE:
- <20 yr old.
- >70 yr old.
- Highest rates of infection in infants, especially neonates.

GENETICS
Neonatal infection.
- Highly susceptible to infection with nontyphoidal *Salmonella*.

PHYSICAL FINDINGS & CLINICAL PRESENTATION

- Infections
  1. Localized to GI tract (gastroenteritis).
  2. Systemic (typhoid fever).
  3. Localized outside of GI tract.
- **Gastroenteritis**
  1. Incubation period: 12 to 48 hr.
  2. Nausea, vomiting.
  3. Diarrhea, abdominal cramps.
  4. Fever.
  5. Bacteremia: occurs mostly in the immunocompromised host or those with underlying conditions, including HIV infection.
  6. Self-limited illness lasting 3 or 4 days.
  7. Colonization of GI tract persistent for months, especially in those treated with antibiotics.
- **Typhoid fever**
  1. Incubation period of few days to several wk.
  2. Prolonged fever, often with a stepwise-increasing temperature pattern.
  3. Myalgias.
  4. Headache, cough, sore throat.
  5. Malaise, anorexia.
  6. Abdominal pain.
  7. Hepatosplenomegaly.
  8. Diarrhea or constipation early in the course of illness.
  9. Rose spots (faint, maculopapular, blanching lesions) sometimes seen on chest or abdomen.
- Untreated disease
  1. Fever lasting 1 to 2 mo.
  2. Main complication: GI bleeding caused by perforation from ulceration of Peyer's patches in the ileum.
  3. Rare complications:
     a. Mental status changes.
     b. Shock.
  4. Relapse rate of approximately 10%.
- Infections outside GI tract
  1. Can occur in virtually any location.
  2. Usually occur in patients with underlying diseases.
  3. Endocarditis, endovascular infections are caused by seeding of atherosclerotic plaques or aneurysms.
  4. Hepatic or splenic abscesses in patients with underlying disease in these organs.
  5. Urinary tract infections in patients with renal TB or schistosomiasis.
  6. *Salmonellae* are a frequent cause of gram-negative meningitis in neonates.
  7. Osteomyelitis in children with hemoglobinopathies (particularly sickle cell disease).

ETIOLOGY

- More than 2000 serotypes of *Salmonella* exist, but only a few cause disease in humans. Host factors and conditions predisposing to the development of systemic disease with nontyphoidal *Salmonella* strains are described in Table 2.
- Raw produce is an increasingly recognized vehicle for salmonellosis. In 2008 there was a large outbreak of *Salmonella* Saintpaul involving 1500 persons, of whom 21% were hospitalized and 2 died. It was due to contaminated jalapeno and serrano peppers. More recently outbreaks of human *Salmonella* infections have been increasingly associated with contact with live poultry.
- Some found only in humans are the cause of enteric fever.
  1. *S. typhi.*
  2. *S. paratyphi.*
- Some responsible for gastroenteritis and frequently isolated from raw meat and poultry and uncooked or undercooked eggs.
  1. *S. typhimurium.*
  2. S. enteritidis.
- *S. choleraesuis* is a prototype organism that causes extraintestinal nontyphoidal disease.
- Transmission generally via ingestion of contaminated food or drink.
- Outbreaks of gastroenteritis related to contaminated poultry, meat, and dairy products are common.
- Typhoid fever is a systemic illness caused by serotypes exclusive to humans.
  1. Acquisition by ingestion of food or water contaminated by other humans
  2. Most cases in the United States are:
     a. Acquired during foreign travel: 80% of cases.
     b. Acquired by ingestion of food prepared by chronic carriers, many of whom have acquired the organism outside of the United States.

TABLE 2 Host Factors and Conditions Predisposing to the Development of Systemic Disease with Nontyphoidal *Salmonella* Strains

Neonates and young infants (≤3 mo of age)
HIV/AIDS
Other immunodeficiencies and chronic granulomatous disease
Immunosuppressive and corticosteroid therapies
Malignancies, especially leukemia and lymphoma
Hemolytic anemia, including sickle cell disease, malaria, and bartonellosis
Collagen vascular disease
Inflammatory bowel disease
Achlorhydria or use of antacid medications
Impaired intestinal motility
Schistosomiasis, malaria
Malnutrition

From Kliegman RM et al: *Nelson textbook of pediatrics*, ed 19, Philadelphia, 2011, Saunders.

TABLE 1 *Salmonella* Nomenclature

Traditional Usage	Formal Name	CDC Designation
S. typhi	*S. enterica** subsp. enterica ser. Typhi	*S.* ser. Typhi
S. dublin	*S. enterica* subsp. enterica ser. Dublin	*S.* ser. Dublin
S. typhimurium	*S. enterica* subsp. enterica ser. Typhimurium	*S.* ser. Typhimurium
S. choleraesuis	*S. enterica* subsp. enterica ser. Choleraesuis	*S.* ser. Choleraesuis
S. marina	*S. enterica* subsp. houtenae ser. Marina	*S.* ser. Marina

CDC, Centers for Disease Control and Prevention; *ser.*, serovar; *subsp.*, subspecies.
*Some authorities prefer *S. choleraesuis* or *S. enteritidis* rather than *S. enterica* to describe the species.
From Kliegman RM et al: *Nelson textbook of pediatrics*, ed 19, Philadelphia, 2011, Saunders.

Dx DIAGNOSIS

DIFFERENTIAL DIAGNOSIS

- Other causes of prolonged fever:
  1. Malaria.
  2. TB.
  3. Brucellosis.
  4. Amebic liver abscess.
- Other causes of gastroenteritis:
  1. Bacterial: *Shigella, Yersinia, Campylobacter* spp.
  2. Viral: Norwalk virus, rotavirus.
  3. Parasitic: *Entamoeba histolytica, Giardia lamblia.*
  4. Toxic: *enterotoxigenic E. coli, Clostridium difficile.*

WORKUP

- Typhoid fever
  1. Cultures of blood, stool, urine; repeat if initially negative.
  2. Blood cultures are more likely to be positive early in the course of illness.
  3. Stool and urine cultures are more commonly positive in the second and third wk of illness.
  4. Highest yield with bone marrow biopsy cultures: 90% positive.
  5. Serology using Widal's test is helpful in retrospect, showing a fourfold increase in convalescent titers.
- Gastroenteritis: stool cultures.
- Extraintestinal localized infection:
  1. Blood cultures.
  2. Cultures from the site of infection.

LABORATORY TESTS

- Neutropenia is common.
- Transaminitis is possible.
- Culture to grow organism: blood, body fluids, biopsy specimens.

IMAGING STUDIES

- Not routinely indicated.
- Radiographs of bone may be suggestive of osteomyelitis (particularly in patients with sickle cell disease and bone infarctions).
- CT scan or sonogram of abdomen:
  1. May reveal hepatic or splenic abscesses or pleural involvement.
  2. May reveal aortic aneurysm.

Rx TREATMENT

NONPHARMACOLOGIC THERAPY

Adequate hydration and electrolyte replacement in people with diarrhea.

ACUTE GENERAL Rx

Treatment decisions must consider the severity of infection and the risk for extraintestinal disease.

- Typhoid fever:
  1. Levofloxacin 750 mg PO/IV q24h or ciprofloxacin 500 mg PO bid or 400 mg IV bid for 7 to 10 days. Should not be used as first line in patients from South Asia due to resistance unless known to be susceptible.
  2. Ceftriaxone 2 g IV qd for 7 to 14 days or cefixime (20-30 mg/kg/day orally divided into q12h dosing for 7-14 days).
  3. Another alternative agent: azithromycin (1 g orally then 500 mg daily for 5-7 days)
  4. Children: see Table 3. In general, quinolones are avoided in children unless a multidrug-resistant strain is involved due to concerns of possible cartilage damage. Another alternative for children: azithromycin (10-20 mg/kg to 1 g maximum once daily for 5-7 days)
  5. If tests show susceptibility, can also use amoxicillin or Bactrim in adults and children.
  6. Dexamethasone 3 mg IV initially, followed by 1 mg IV q6h for eight doses for patients with shock or mental status changes.
- Gastroenteritis:
  1. Usually not indicated for gastroenteritis alone because this illness usually self-limited.
  2. Treatment may prolong the carrier state and is discouraged for healthy patients <50 yr of age who have relatively mild disease.
  3. Prophylactic treatment for patients who are at high risk of developing complications from bacteremia (see Table 3).
     a. Neonates.
     b. Patients with hemoglobinopathies.
     c. Patients with atherosclerosis.
     d. Patients with aneurysms.
     e. Patients with prosthetic devices.
     f. Immunocompromised patients.

CHRONIC Rx

- Carrier states are possible in those with typhoid fever.
- More common in people >60 yr of age and in people with gallstones.
- Usual site of colonization is the gallbladder.
- Treatment should be considered for those with persistently positive stool cultures and for food handlers.
- Suggested regimens for eradication of carrier state:
  1. Ciprofloxacin 500 mg PO bid for 4 wk.
  2. SMX/TMP 1 to 2 DS tabs PO bid for 6 wk (if susceptible).
  3. Amoxicillin 2 g PO q8h for 6 wk (if susceptible).
- Cholecystectomy may be required in carriers with gallstones who fail medical therapy, but this is rarely indicated for nontyphoidal salmonellosis currently.
- Prolonged course of oral therapy or lifetime suppression for patients with AIDS who have chronic infection.

DISPOSITION

- Typhoid fever
  1. Treated patients usually respond to therapy; small percentage of chronic carriers.
  2. Untreated patients may have serious complications.
- Gastroenteritis
  1. Usually self-limited.
  2. May be recurrent or persistent in AIDS patients.

REFERRAL

- If gastroenteritis is persistent or recurrent.
- If there is evidence of extraintestinal infection, typhoid fever, or chronic carriers.

! PEARLS & CONSIDERATIONS

COMMENTS

- Fluoroquinolones remain the most reliably effective class of antibiotics for empiric therapy despite increasing resistance. Fluoroquinolones should not be used in children or pregnant women.
- Infections should be reported to local health departments.
- Recent outbreaks in the United States have been traced back to raw tomatoes, peanut butter, pet turtles, and frozen pot pies.

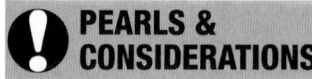 **EVIDENCE**

Available at www.expertconsult.com

SUGGESTED READINGS

Available at www.expertconsult.com

RELATED CONTENT

Salmonellosis (Patient Information)
Typhoid Fever (Related Key Topic)

AUTHOR: **GLENN G. FORT, M.D., M.P.H.**

TABLE 3 Treatment of *Salmonella* Gastroenteritis

Organism and Indication	Dose and Duration of Treatment
Salmonella infections in infants <3 mo of age or immunocompromised persons (in addition to appropriate treatment for underlying disorder)	Cefotaxime 100-200 mg/kg/day every 6 hr for 5-14 days or Ceftriaxone 75 mg/kg/day once daily for 7 days or Ampicillin 100 mg/kg/day every 6 hr for 7 days or Cefixime 15 mg/kg/day for 7-10 days

From Kliegman RM et al: *Nelson textbook of pediatrics*, ed 19, Philadelphia, 2011, Saunders.

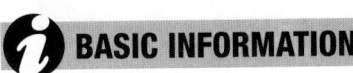 BASIC INFORMATION

DEFINITION

Sarcoidosis is a chronic multisystem granulomatous disease characterized histologically by the presence of nonspecific, noncaseating granulomas.

SYNONYMS

Boeck's sarcoid

ICD-10CM CODES
D86   Sarcoidosis
D86.0 Sarcoidosis of lung
D86.1 Sarcoidosis of lymph nodes
D86.2 Sarcoidosis of lung with sarcoidosis of lymph nodes
D86.3 Sarcoidosis of skin
D86.8 Sarcoidosis of other and combined sites
D86.9 Sarcoidosis, unspecified

EPIDEMIOLOGY & DEMOGRAPHICS

INCIDENCE (IN U.S.): Incidence is 11 in 100,000 in whites and 35 in 100,000 in blacks; presents most commonly in the winter and early spring. (The adjusted annual incidence among black Americans is roughly three times higher than among white Americans [35.5 cases/100,000, as compared with 10.9/100,000] and is likely more chronic and fatal in black Americans.)
PREDOMINANT SEX: Increased incidence in females.
PREDOMINANT AGE: 20 to 40 yr.
GENETICS: Familial clustering has been described. Having a first-degree relative with sarcoidosis increases the risk for disease fivefold (ACCESS study). There have been reports of association between sarcoidosis and gene products, specifically HLA class II antigens, encoded by HLA-DRB1 and DQB1 alleles.

PHYSICAL FINDINGS & CLINICAL PRESENTATION

- Clinical manifestations often vary with the stage of the disease and degree of organ involvement. Patients may be asymptomatic, but a chest radiograph may demonstrate findings consistent with sarcoidosis (see "Imaging Studies"). Nearly 50% of patients with sarcoidosis are diagnosed by incidental findings on chest radiograph. Thoracic involvement occurs in >90% of patients with sarcoidosis.
- Frequent manifestations:
  1. Pulmonary manifestations: dry, nonproductive cough; dyspnea; chest discomfort.
  2. Constitutional symptoms: fatigue, weight loss, anorexia, malaise, night sweats.
  3. Visual disturbances: blurred vision, ocular discomfort, conjunctivitis, iritis, uveitis (65% of patients).
  4. Dermatologic manifestations (30% of patients): erythema nodosum (10% of patients), macules, papules, subcutaneous nodules, hyperpigmentation, lupus pernio (indurated violaceous lesions on the nose, lips, ears, and cheeks that can erode into underlying cartilage and bone) (Fig. E1).
  5. Myocardial disturbances, arrhythmias, cardiomyopathy, various conduction abnormalities, and pericardial effusion. Cardiac sarcoidosis is much more common than clinically appreciated and is found in up to 25% of patients in the United States.
  6. Splenomegaly, hepatomegaly.
  7. Rheumatologic manifestations: arthralgias have been reported in up to 40% of patients.
  8. **Löfgren's syndrome**, consisting of arthritis, erythema nodosum, and bilateral hilar adenopathy, occurs in 9% to 34% of patients.
  9. Neurologic and other manifestations: cranial nerve palsies, diabetes insipidus, meningeal involvement, parotid enlargement, hypothalamic and pituitary lesions, peripheral adenopathy. Neurosarcoidosis is detected in up to 25% of patients and can occur in the absence of apparent disease elsewhere. The presence of anterior uveitis, parotiditis, fevers, and facial nerve palsy is known as **Heerfordt syndrome.**

ETIOLOGY

Unknown. A cardinal feature of sarcoidosis is the presence of CD4+ T cells that interact with antigen-presenting cells to initiate the formation and maintenance of granulomas. Multiple lines of evidence suggest that sarcoidosis may result from the interaction of multiple genes with environmental exposures or infection.

DX DIAGNOSIS

DIFFERENTIAL DIAGNOSIS

- Tuberculosis.
- Lymphoma.
- Hodgkin's disease.
- Metastases.
- Pneumoconioses.
- Enlarged pulmonary arteries.
- Infectious mononucleosis.
- Lymphangitic carcinomatosis.
- Idiopathic hemosiderosis.
- Alveolar cell carcinoma.
- Pulmonary eosinophilia.
- Hypersensitivity pneumonitis.
- Fibrosing alveolitis.
- Collagen disorders.
- Parasitic infection.
  Section II describes the differential diagnosis of granulomatous lung disease and a classification of granulomatous disorders.

WORKUP

- No pathognomonic diagnostic test exists for sarcoidosis, so the diagnosis remains one of exclusion. Workup is aimed at excluding critical organ involvement, determining extent and severity of disease, and excluding other disease. The presence of noncaseating granulomas does not establish the diagnosis, because conditions such as tuberculosis and malignancies, among others, can cause granulomas. A complete neurologic and ophthalmologic examination is mandatory. A complete occupational and environmental exposure history is recommended.
- Initial laboratory evaluation should include complete blood count, serum chemistries (alanine aminotransferase, aspartate aminotransferase, alkaline phosphatase, electrolytes, blood urea nitrogen, creatinine, serum calcium), urinalysis, 24-hour urinary excretion of calcium, CRP, ESR, and tuberculin skin test.
- Chest radiograph and ECG should also be obtained in all patients with sarcoidosis.
- Pulmonary function testing: spirometry, diffusion capacity of carbon monoxide–single breath.
- Biopsy should be done on accessible tissues suspected of sarcoid involvement (conjunctiva, skin, lymph nodes); bronchoscopy with transbronchial biopsy (85% diagnostic yield) is often performed in patients without any readily accessible site. Endobronchial ultrasound-guided fine-needle aspiration of intrathoracic lymph nodes also has high diagnostic yield and makes use of mediastinoscopy usually unnecessary. Among patients with suspected Stage I/II pulmonary sarcoidosis undergoing tissue confirmation, the use of endosonographic nodal aspiration compared with bronchoscopic biopsy resulted in greater diagnostic yield.

LABORATORY TESTS

Laboratory abnormalities:
- Hypergammaglobulinemia, anemia, leukopenia may be present.
- Liver function test abnormalities are common, e.g., elevated alkaline phosphatase.
- Hypercalcemia (11% of patients), hypercalciuria (40% of patients; attributable to increased gastrointestinal absorption, abnormal vitamin D metabolism, and increased calcitriol production by sarcoid granuloma).
- Angiotensin-converting enzyme: elevated in approximately 75% of patients with untreated sarcoidosis; nonspecific and poor sensitivity; generally not useful as a diagnostic tool or in following the course of the disease.
- Serum adenosine deaminase (ADA); serum amyloid A (SAA) elevated but nonspecific.

IMAGING STUDIES

- Chest radiograph (Fig. E2): pulmonary sarcoidosis is classified based on radiographic pattern. Adenopathy of the hilar and paratracheal nodes is a frequent finding. Parenchymal changes may also be present, depending on the stage of the disease (stage 0, normal radiograph; stage I, bilateral hilar adenopathy; stage II, stage I plus pulmonary infiltrate; stage III, pulmonary infiltrate without

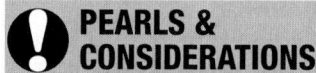

adenopathy; stage IV, advanced fibrosis with evidence of "honeycombing," hilar retraction, bullae, cysts, and emphysema).

- Pulmonary function tests (spirometry and diffusing capacity of the lung for carbon dioxide): may be normal or may reveal a restrictive ventilatory defect with reduced forced vital capacity, reduced DLCO, or both. Endobronchial sarcoidosis may exhibit obstructive physiology, depending on severity.
- For patients without apparent lung involvement, ^{18}F-fluorodeoxyglucose positron emission tomography (FDG-PET) is useful in identifying sites for diagnostic biopsy.
- CT imaging, more specifically high-resolution CT, may help detect early parenchymal abnormalities. It is indicated when the chest radiograph is atypical for sarcoidosis.
- FDG-PET and MRI with gadolinium are useful in patients with suspected cardiac and neurologic involvement.
- Gallium-67 scan: represents an older testing modality. It will localize in areas of granulomatous infiltrates; however, it is not specific and not necessary. The "panda" sign (localization in the lacrimal and salivary glands, giving a "panda" appearance to the face) is suggestive of sarcoidosis.
- Bronchoscopy: Flexible bronchoscopy and bronchoalveolar lavage (BAL) with transbronchial biopsy (showing noncaseating granulomas) are traditional methods for the minimally invasive diagnosis of sarcoidosis. With hilar adenopathy, endobronchial ultrasound is the preferred method for lymph node sampling. BAL may show predominantly lymphocytosis, elevated ADA levels, and elevated CD4:CD8 ratio (4:1).
- Mediastinoscopy: Rarely used nowadays for lymph node sampling and diagnosis.

Rx TREATMENT

GENERAL Rx

- Many patients with sarcoidosis will not require any treatment. In general, treatment should be instituted when organ function is threatened. Corticosteroids (Table 1) are the mainstay of therapy when treatment is required (e.g., prednisone 40 mg qd for 8 to 12 wk with gradual tapering of the dose to 10 mg qod over 8 to 12 mo); corticosteroids should be considered in patients with severe symptoms (e.g., dyspnea, chest pain); hypercalcemia; ocular, central nervous system, or cardiac involvement; or progressive pulmonary disease. Patients with interstitial lung disease benefit from oral steroid therapy for 6 to 24 mo.
- A lack of benefit from steroid therapy may be due to the presence of irreversible fibrotic disease. Patients with progressive disease refractory to corticosteroids may be treated with methotrexate 7.5 to 15 mg

TABLE 1 Indications for Use of Corticosteroids in Sarcoidosis

Disorder	Treatment
Iridocyclitis	Corticosteroid eye drops; local subconjunctival deposit of cortisone
Posterior uveitis	Oral prednisone
Pulmonary involvement	Steroids rarely recommended for stage I; typically used if infiltrate remains static or worsens over 3-mo period or the patient is symptomatic
Upper airway obstruction	Rare indication for intravenous steroids
Lupus pernio	Oral prednisone shrinks the disfiguring lesions
Hypercalcemia	Responds well to corticosteroids
Cardiac involvement	Corticosteroids usually recommended if patient has arrhythmias or conduction disturbances
Central nervous system involvement	Response is best in patients with acute symptoms
Lacrimal/salivary gland involvement	Corticosteroids recommended for disordered function, not gland swelling
Bone cysts	Corticosteroids recommended if symptomatic

From Andreoli TE (ed): *Cecil essentials of medicine*, ed 8, Philadelphia, 2010, Saunders.

once per week or another immunosuppressant such as azathioprine or mycophenolate mofetil.

- Hydroxychloroquine is effective for chronic disfiguring skin lesions, hypercalcemia, and neurologic involvement.
- Nonsteroidal antiinflammatory drugs are useful for musculoskeletal symptoms and erythema nodosum.
- Pulmonary rehabilitation in patients with significant respiratory insufficiency. Consider liver and lung transplantation in patients unresponsive to conventional treatment.
- Pulmonary hypertension is a dreaded complication of advanced pulmonary sarcoidosis. The prognosis for patients with sarcoidosis-associated pulmonary hypertension is not known.

DISPOSITION

- The majority of patients with sarcoidosis have spontaneous remission within 2 yr and do not require treatment. Their course can be followed by periodic clinical evaluation, chest radiographs, and pulmonary function tests.
- Blacks have increased rates of pulmonary involvement, a worse long-term prognosis, and more frequent relapses.
- Up to one third of patients have unrelenting disease, leading to clinically significant organ impairment. Adverse prognostic factors in sarcoidosis include age of onset >40 yr, cardiac involvement, neurosarcoidosis, progressive pulmonary fibrosis, chronic hypercalcemia, chronic uveitis, involvement of nasal mucosa, nephrocalcinosis, and presence of cystic bone lesions and lupus pernio.

REFERRAL

Ophthalmologic examination is indicated in all patients with suspected sarcoidosis because ocular findings (iridocyclitis, uveitis, conjunctivitis, and keratopathy) are found in ≥25% of documented cases.

⊘ PEARLS & CONSIDERATIONS

COMMENTS

- Serial spirometry and measurement of DLCO can be useful in following response to therapy and disease progression.
- Approximately 15% to 20% of patients with lung involvement advance to irreversible lung impairment (bronchiectasis, cavitation, progressive fibrosis, pneumothorax, and respiratory failure). Death from pulmonary failure occurs in 5% to 7% of patients with sarcoidosis.
- Newer treatment approaches are aimed at targeting mechanisms involving CD4 type 1 helper T cells.
- The diagnosis of sarcoidosis should be reconsidered in the presence of atypical manifestations or persistent/progressive disease despite appropriate therapy.
- Diagnostic biopsy may not be necessary in most patients presenting with asymptomatic bilateral lymphadenopathy (with no other evidence of malignancy), in those with Lofgren syndrome, or in those with Heerfordt syndrome.

SUGGESTED READINGS
Available at www.expertconsult.com

RELATED CONTENT
Sarcoidosis (Patient Information)

AUTHOR: **IMRANA QAWI, M.D.**

BASIC INFORMATION

DEFINITION

Sarcomas are heterogenous groups of malignant tumors of connective tissue, with more than 100 distinct entities. They show a wide range of differentiation—blood vessels (angiosarcoma), fat tissue (liposarcoma), and bone (osteosarcoma), among others. Sarcomas can be classified into two basic types: soft tissue sarcoma (STS) and primary bone sarcoma. Affecting virtually all tissues, they are more common in soft tissues, but 75% occur in the limbs. Sarcomas of bone are extremely rare. There are three histiogenic types: osteosarcoma, Ewing's sarcoma, and chondrosarcoma.

ICD-10CM CODES
C40   Malignant neoplasm of bone and articular cartilage of limbs
C41   Malignant neoplasm of bone and articular cartilage of other unspecified sites
C22.3 Angiosarcoma of liver
C49.9 Malignant neoplasm of connective and soft tissue, unspecified
C49.0 Malignant neoplasm of connective and soft tissue of head, face, and neck

EPIDEMIOLOGY & DEMOGRAPHICS

INCIDENCE: Soft tissue sarcoma: 30 cases per million per annum.
Sarcoma of bone: 8 cases per million per annum.
  Soft tissue sarcoma can occur at any age.
- In the U.S. there are 7800 new cases per year.
- Incidence increases with age.
- Average age of diagnosis is 57 yr.
- Men and women are affected equally.
- Soft tissue sarcomas represent <1% of all newly diagnosed malignancies.
Sarcomas of bone represent 0.2% of all new cancers.
- About 2600 new cases in the U.S. each year.
  Osteosarcoma and Ewing's sarcoma (the two most common bone tumors) occur predominantly during childhood and adolescence.
GENETICS: See "Etiology."

PHYSICAL FINDINGS & CLINICAL PRESENTATION

- Bone sarcomas. Clinical presentation usually includes:
  1. Pain—at rest or at night.
  2. Swelling or mass at the site.
  3. Pathologic fractures.
- Soft tissue sarcomas:
  Present with painless mass (usually >5 cm).
  Mass grows slowly for months or years.

ETIOLOGY

- Most sarcomas arise sporadically.
- Genetic predispositions:

1. Familial retinoblastoma (mutation of the *RBI* gene at 13q14) predisposes to osteosarcoma.
2. Neurofibromatosis type 1 (mutation of *NF1* gene at 17q11) predisposes to malignant peripheral nerve sheath tumor (malignant schwannomas and neurofibrosarcomas).
3. Diaphyseal aclasis (an autosomal inherited condition) is associated with increased risk of peripheral chondrosarcoma.
- Environmental causes:
  1. Previous radiotherapy (e.g., for cervical or breast cancer): predisposes to sarcoma 4 to 10 yr after exposure.
  2. Chronic lymphedema: associated with the development of angiosarcoma.
  3. Exposure to chemicals (e.g., dioxins, phenoxyacetic herbicides, vinyl chloride increase the risk of hepatic angiosarcoma).
  4. Viruses (e.g., human herpesvirus 8 plays a role in the development of Kaposi's sarcoma).
  5. Foreign body (shrapnel, medical implants).

DIAGNOSIS

WORKUP

- Soft tissue sarcoma: any unexplained superficial soft tissue mass >5 cm, or any deep-seated soft tissue mass should be regarded as malignant until proven otherwise.
- Bone sarcoma: patients with unexplained bone pain, persistent bone tenderness, or nonmechanical bone pain (especially when it disturbs sleep or rest) have bone cancer until proven otherwise.
- Patients with suspected spontaneous fracture or recurrence of the fracture with minor trauma should be considered as having bone cancer.
- Referral to a sarcoma treatment center of all patients with a suspected sarcoma is recommended.

IMAGING STUDIES

- A chest spiral CT scan is compulsory for staging purposes. Chest spiral CT helps detect lung metastasis, since metastasis through blood to the lungs is the principal form of spread.
- Staging aids in estimating prognosis, survival, and plan management.
- The American Joint Committee on Cancer (AJCC) and International Union Against Cancer (IUCC) are widely used for staging classification.
- Soft tissue sarcoma.
- Magnetic resonance imaging (MRI) is the initial imaging modality of choice, especially for soft tissue sarcoma of the extremities, trunk, and head and neck. CT with IV contrast is also useful for diagnosis.
- Ultrasound is used to help differentiate between benign and suspicious lesions.
- Bone sarcoma.
- Radiograph (Fig. 1) is the initial imaging of choice. It helps to rule out bone tumor, shows calcification, and reveals bone erosions. Fig. 2 summarizes radiographic features that may help differentiate benign from malignant lesions.
- A multidisciplinary approach is essential. The team should include radiologist, surgeons, pathologist, medical oncologist, and radiation therapists.

BIOPSY

- In nearly all cases a biopsy is needed to establish a tissue diagnosis.
- Multiple core needle biopsies are usually done.
- An excisional biopsy may be used for superficial lesions <5 cm.
- In carefully selected cases an open biopsy may be done (rarely used because of its high complication rate).
- For difficult to palpate or necrotic soft sarcomas, ultrasound or computed tomography (CT)–guided biopsies are performed.
- Biopsy results are interpreted collaboratively by the specialist sarcoma pathologist, surgeon, and radiologist together.

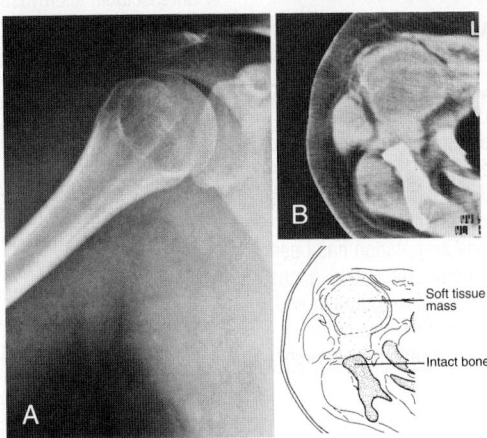

FIG. 1 Fibrosarcoma. A, Anteroposterior plain film of the shoulder of a 40-year-old woman with a history of an enlarging mass in the right axilla shows an ill-defined mass adjacent to the lateral border of the scapula. **B,** CT section with contrast enhancement shows the extent of the mass and the lack of bone involvement. The tumor proved to be a fibrosarcoma. (From Skarin AT: *Atlas of diagnostic oncology*, ed 3, St Louis, 2003, Mosby.)

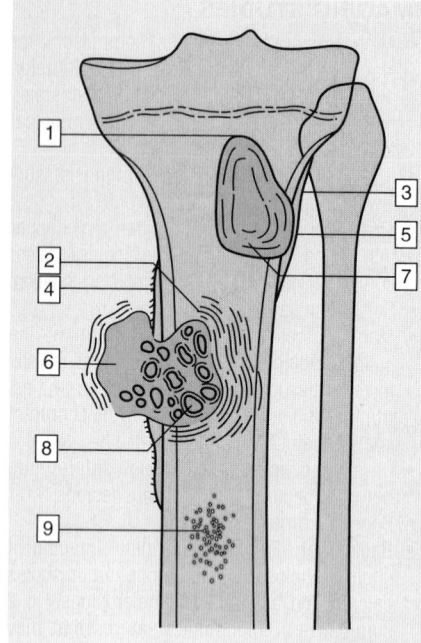

Feature	Benign (slow-growing process)	Malignant (aggressive process)
Border	1. Sharply outlined, sclerotic (narrow zone of transition)	2. Poorly defined (wide zone of transition)
Periosteal reaction	3. Solid, uninterrupted	4. Interrupted (sunburst, Codman triangle)
Soft tissue extension/mass	5. Absent or contained by shell of periosteal new bone	6. Frank extension through destroyed periosteum
Type of bone destruction	7. Geographic: uniformly destroyed area with sharply defined border	8. "Moth-eaten" (likely malignant): destroyed areas with ragged borders
		9. Permeative (aggressive/malignant): ill-defined destruction spreading through marrow space

FIG. 2 Benign versus malignant bone lesions. The radiographic features illustrated may help differentiate benign from malignant lesions. (From Bullough PG, Vigorita VJ: *Atlas of orthopedic pathology.* Baltimore/New York, 1984, University Park Press/Gower Medical Publishing, in Skarin AT: *Atlas of diagnostic oncology,* 4 ed, St Louis, 2010, Mosby, 2010.)

HISTOLOGIC DIAGNOSIS

- Treatment planning is guided by a histologic diagnosis.
- Histologic diagnosis is made according to the World Health Organization (WHO) classification.
- WHO has defined >50 histologic subtypes of soft tissue sarcoma.
- Newer methods such as immunocytochemistry and cytogenetics can aid diagnosis. They identify tumor lineage.

(Rx) TREATMENT

Treatment depends on the extent of the disease and falls into several groups.

ACUTE GENERAL Rx

- Tumors treated by surgery: for example, in most adults soft tissue sarcoma and sarcoma of bone are not sensitive to chemotherapy.
  1. Surgery must be done by surgeon trained to treat this disease.
  2. Wide excision with negative margins is the standard surgical procedure.
  3. For bone sarcomas amputation has been the standard procedure. Recent advances permit the avoidance of amputation with limb-sparing surgery followed by reconstruction by endoprosthetic replacement.

- Chemotherapy followed by local therapy: for example, osteosarcoma.
  1. Early chemotherapy to reduce disseminated micrometastasis and tumor size.
  Systemic chemotherapy regimens for advanced soft tissue sarcoma typically comprise multiple drugs such as the MAID regimen (mesna, doxorubicin, ifosfamide, dacarbazine) and the AIM regimen (doxorubicin, ifosfamide, mesna). Single-agent therapy with either doxorubicin or ifosfamide is also appropriate in the palliative setting. More recently, pazopanib, a tyrosine kinase inhibitor, has been approved in patients with metastatic or recurrent sarcoma. Trabectedin, an agent derived from a marine organism, has now been approved in metastatic or unresectable leiomyosarcoma or liposarcoma.
- Follow-up of bone sarcoma after treatment includes:
  1. Periodic monitoring with radiographs and other imaging modalities.
  2. CT scan of the chest.
  3. Bone scan.
- Follow-up of soft tissue sarcoma (extremities):
  1. Physical exam detects 97% of recurrence.
  2. Physical exam is done every 3 to 6 mo for 3 yr, then every 6 mo for the next 2 yr for stage II and III cancers, then annually.
  3. Imaging.
- Stage I: CXR every 6 to 12 mo.

- Stages II and III: image the primary site with MRI or CT.
- Chest x-ray or chest CT every 3 to 6 mo for 5 yr, then annually.

REFERRAL

- Sarcomas are relatively uncommon yet comprise a wide variety of different entities; as such, evaluation by multidisciplinary oncology teams with expertise in this field is recommended.
- Treatment and follow-up guidelines have been published by the National Comprehensive Cancer Network (www.nccn.org).

SUGGESTED READINGS
Available at www.expertconsult.com

AUTHOR: **BHARTI RATHORE, M.D.**

BASIC INFORMATION

DEFINITION

Scabies is a contagious disease caused by the mite *Sarcoptes scabiei*.

ICD-10CM CODES
B86 Scabies

EPIDEMIOLOGY & DEMOGRAPHICS

- Scabies is generally acquired by sleeping with or in the bedding of infested individuals.
- It is generally associated with poor living conditions and is also common in hospitals and nursing homes.

PHYSICAL FINDINGS & CLINICAL PRESENTATION

- Primary lesions are caused when the female mite burrows within the stratum corneum, laying eggs within the tract she leaves behind; burrows (linear or serpiginous tracts, see Fig. E1) end with a minute papule or vesicle.
- Primary lesions are most commonly found in the web spaces of the hands, wrists, buttocks, scrotum, penis, breasts, axillae, and knees. They are often confused with eczema (Fig. E2).
- Secondary lesions result from scratching or infection.
- Intense pruritus, especially nocturnal, is common; it is caused by an acquired sensitivity to the mite or fecal pellets and is usually noted 1 to 4 wk after the primary infestation.
- Examination of the skin may reveal burrows, tiny vesicles, excoriations, inflammatory papules.
- Widespread and crusted lesions (Norwegian or crusted scabies) may be seen in elderly and immunocompromised patients (Fig. E3). Pruritus may be mild or absent due to impaired host immune response.
- Table 1 summarizes the different presenting forms of scabies.

ETIOLOGY

- Human scabies is caused by the mite *S. scabiei*, var. *hominis* (Fig. E4). After impregnation on the skin surface, the gravid female burrows in the stratum corneum within 30 min and gradually extends the tract along the boundary with the stratum granulosum depositing 10 to 25 oval eggs in a 4- to 5-wk period. The eggs hatch in 3 to 5 days, and larvae move to the skin surface and mature in 2 to 3 wk, resuming the cycle.
- Clinical manifestations result from a delayed type IV hypersensitivity reaction to the mete, eggs, saliva, or scybala.

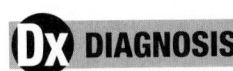 DIAGNOSIS

DIFFERENTIAL DIAGNOSIS

- Pediculosis.
- Atopic dermatitis.
- Flea bites.
- Seborrheic dermatitis.
- Dermatitis herpetiformis.
- Contact dermatitis.
- Nummular eczema.
- Syphilis.
- Other insect infestation.

WORKUP

Diagnosis is made on the clinical presentation and on the demonstration of mites, eggs, or mite feces.

LABORATORY TESTS

- Microscopic demonstration of the organism, feces, or eggs: a drop of mineral oil may be placed over the suspected lesion before removal; the scrapings are transferred directly to a glass slide; a drop of potassium hydroxide is added and a cover slip is applied.
- Skin biopsy is rarely necessary to make the diagnosis.

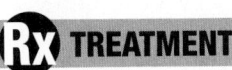 TREATMENT

NONPHARMACOLOGIC THERAPY

Clothing, underwear, and towels used in the 48 hr before treatment must be laundered.

ACUTE GENERAL Rx

- Permethrin 5% cream is usually effective with one treatment; it should be massaged into the skin from head to soles of feet and applied under fingernails and toenails (it's best if applied in the evening and left overnight to maximize exposure); remove 8 to 14 hr later by washing. Repeat in 1 to 2 wk. Permethrin is safe for children >2 mo old.
- A single dose (150-200 μg/kg in 6-mg tablets) of ivermectin, an antihelmintic agent, is also effective for the treatment of scabies. It is the best treatment for generalized crusted scabies. Three to seven doses of ivermectin given on days 1, 2, 8, 9, 15, 22, and 28 may be needed for crusted scabies.

TABLE 1 Different Presenting Forms of Scabies

Presenting Forms of Scabies	Specific High-Risk Populations	Clinical Manifestations	Limited Differential Diagnoses
Classic scabies (scabies vulgaris)	Infants and children; sexually active adults; men who have sex with men	Intense generalized pruritus, worse at night; inflammatory pruritic papules localized to finger webs, flexor aspects of wrists, elbows, axillae, buttocks, genitalia, female breasts; lesions and pruritus spare the face, head, and neck; secondary lesions include eczematization, excoriation, impetigo	Dermatitis herpetiformis, drug reactions, eczema, pediculosis corporis, lichen planus, pityriasis rosea
Scalp scabies	Infants and children; institutionalized older adults; AIDS patients; patients with preexisting crusted scabies	Atypical crusted papular lesions of the scalp, face, palms, and soles	Dermatomyositis, ringworm, seborrheic dermatitis
Crusted scabies (Norwegian scabies, scabies norvegica, scabies crustosa)	Institutionalized older adults; institutionalized developmentally disabled (Down syndrome); homeless, especially HIV-positive; all immunocompromised patients, particularly those with AIDS or positive for HIV or HTLV-1; transplant recipients; patients on prolonged systemic corticosteroids and chemotherapy	Psoriasiform hyperkeratotic papular lesions of the scalp, face, neck, hands, feet, with extensive nail involvement; eczematization and impetigo common	Contact dermatitis, drug reactions, eczema, erythroderma, ichthyosis, psoriasis
Nodular scabies	Sexually active adults; men who have sex with men; HIV-positive men > HIV-positive women	Violaceous pruritic nodules localized to male genitalia, groin, axillae, representing hypersensitivity reaction to mite antigens	Acropustulosis, atopic dermatitis, Darier's disease, lupus erythematosus, lymphomatoid papulosis, papular urticaria, necrotizing vasculitis, secondary syphilis

AIDS, Acquired immunodeficiency syndrome; *HIV*, human immunodeficiency virus; *HTLV-1*, human T cell lymphotropic virus type 1.
From Bennett JE et al: *Mandell, Douglas, and Bennett's principles and practice of infectious diseases*, ed 8, Philadelphia, 2015, WB Saunders.

TABLE 2 Currently Recommended Treatment for Scabies

Scabicides	FDA Approved?	Pregnancy Category*	Dosing Schedule	Safety Profile	Contraindications
5% Permethrin cream (Actin, Nix, Elimite)	Yes	B	Apply from neck down; wash off after 8-14 hr; good residual activity, but second application recommended after 1 wk	Excellent; itching and stinging on application	Prior allergic reactions; infants <2 mo of age; breastfeeding
1% Lindane lotion or cream	Yes	B	Apply 30-60 mL from neck down; wash off after 8-12 hr; no residual activity; increasing drug resistance	Potential for central nervous system toxicity from organochloride poisoning, usually manifesting as seizures, with overapplication and ingestions	Preexisting seizure disorder; infants and children <6 mo of age; pregnancy; breastfeeding
10% Crotamiton cream or lotion (Eurax)	Yes	C	Apply from neck down on 2 consecutive nights; wash off 24 hr after second application	Excellent; not very effective; exacerbates pruritus	None
2%-10% Sulfur in petrolatum ointments	No	C	Apply for 2-3 days, then wash	Excellent; not very effective	Preexisting sulfur allergy
10%-25% Benzoyl benzoate lotion	No	None	Two applications for 24 hr with 1-day to 1-wk interval	Irritant; exacerbates pruritus; can induce contact irritant dermatitis and pruritic cutaneous xerosis	Preexisting eczema
0.5% Malathion lotion (Ovide), 1% malathion shampoo (unavailable in the U.S.)	No	B	95% ovicidal; rapid (5 min) killing; good residual activity; increasing drug resistance	Flammable 78% isopropyl alcohol vehicle stings eyes, skin, mucosa; increasing drug resistance; organophosphate poisoning risk with overapplication and ingestions	Infants and children <6 mo of age; pregnancy; breastfeeding
Ivermectin (Stromectol)	Yes	C	200 μg/kg single PO dose, may be repeated in 14-15 days; not ovicidal, second dose on day 14 or 15 highly recommended; recommended for endemic or epidemic scabies in institutions and refugee camps	Excellent; may cause nausea and vomiting; take on empty stomach with water	Safety in pregnancy uncertain; probably safe during breastfeeding; not recommended for children younger than 5 yr of age or weighing <15 kg

*U.S. Food and Drug Administration (FDA) safety in pregnancy categories: A, safety established; B, presumed safe; C, uncertain safety; D, unsafe; X, highly unsafe.
From Bennett JE et al: *Mandell, Douglas, and Bennett's principles and practice of infectious diseases*, ed 8, Philadelphia, 2015, WB Saunders.

- Pruritus generally abates 24 to 48 hr after treatment but can last up to 2 wk; oral antihistamines are effective in decreasing postscabietic pruritus.
- Topical corticosteroid creams may hasten the resolution of secondary eczematous dermatitis.
- If the patient is a resident of an extended care facility, it is important to educate the patients, staff, family, and frequent visitors about scabies and the need to have full cooperation in treatment. Scabicide should be applied to all patients, staff, and frequent visitors, whether symptomatic or not; symptomatic family members of staff and visitors should also receive treatment.
- Table 2 summarizes currently recommended treatment for scabies.

DISPOSITION

Refractory cases usually are seen with immunocompromised hosts or patients with underlying skin diseases. **Norwegian scabies** refers to a highly contagious variant often found in institutions caring for physically and mentally disabled individuals.

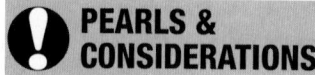 **PEARLS & CONSIDERATIONS**

COMMENTS

- Lindane is potentially neurotoxic and should not be used on infants or pregnant women (permethrin is safe in pregnancy and infants over two months old).
- Sexual partners should be notified and treated.

SUGGESTED READINGS

Available at www.expertconsult.com

RELATED CONTENT

Scabies (Patient Information)

AUTHOR: **FRED F. FERRI, M.D.**

BASIC INFORMATION

DEFINITION

Scarlet fever is a rash involving the skin and tongue and complicating streptococcal group A pharyngitis.

SYNONYMS

Scarlatina
SF

ICD-10CM CODES
A38   Scarlet fever
A38.9 Scarlet fever, uncomplicated
A38.0 Scarlet fever with otitis media
A38.1 Scarlet fever with myocarditis
A38.8 Scarlet fever with other complications

EPIDEMIOLOGY & DEMOGRAPHICS

- Same as streptococcal pharyngitis; namely, children ages 5 to 15 yr. May also complicate impetigo.
- Most common in cooler climates during the late fall, winter, and early spring.
- Most cases follow tonsillitis or pharyngitis; however, it has also been reported after wounds ("surgical scarlet fever"), burns, and pelvic or puerperal infections.

PHYSICAL FINDINGS & CLINICAL PRESENTATION

- Diffuse erythema, beginning on face and spreading to neck, back, chest, rest of trunk, and extremities (Fig. 1, *A*). Most intense on inner aspects of arms and thighs.
- Erythema blanches, but nonblanching petechiae may be present or produced by a tourniquet.
- Strawberry or raspberry tongue (Fig. 1, *B, C*).
- Rash lasts approximately 1 wk and then desquamates.
- Febrile illness with headache, malaise, anorexia, and pharyngitis begins after a 2- to 4-day incubation period.
- Scarlatinal rash begins 1 or 2 days after the onset of pharyngitis.

ETIOLOGY

Caused by group A beta-hemolytic *Streptococcus* infection, which produces one of three erythrogenic toxins (NOTE: Some streptococcal species have the ability to cause both scarlet fever and rheumatic fever).

DIAGNOSIS

DIFFERENTIAL DIAGNOSIS

- Viral exanthems (covered in Section II)
- Kawasaki disease
- Toxic shock syndrome
- Drug rashes
  See differential diagnosis of "Pharyngitis" in Section I.

WORKUP

- Identification of group A *Streptococcus* by throat culture
- Streptolysin O antibody titers

TREATMENT

- Penicillin 250 mg PO qid for 10 days or erythromycin 250 mg PO qid for 10 days in penicillin-allergic patients. A clinical response can be expected in 24 to 48 hr.
- Benzathine penicillin 1 to 2 million U IM once; may be used for a patient who cannot swallow pills.

COMPLICATIONS (RARE)

- Peritonsillar abscess.
- Mastoiditis.
- Otitis media.
- Pneumonia.
- Sepsis and distant foci of infection.
- Acute rheumatic fever.
- Inability to swallow liquids or upper airway obstruction requiring hospitalization.
  NOTE: Failure to respond to penicillin should raise doubt about the diagnosis because *Streptococcus* may be carried in the pharynx without causing infection.

PEARLS & CONSIDERATIONS

COMMENTS

Patients with antibodies against the toxin are spared the rash but still develop other symptoms of the infection (e.g., sore throat).

RELATED CONTENT

Scarlet Fever (Patient Information)

AUTHOR: **FRED F. FERRI, M.D.**

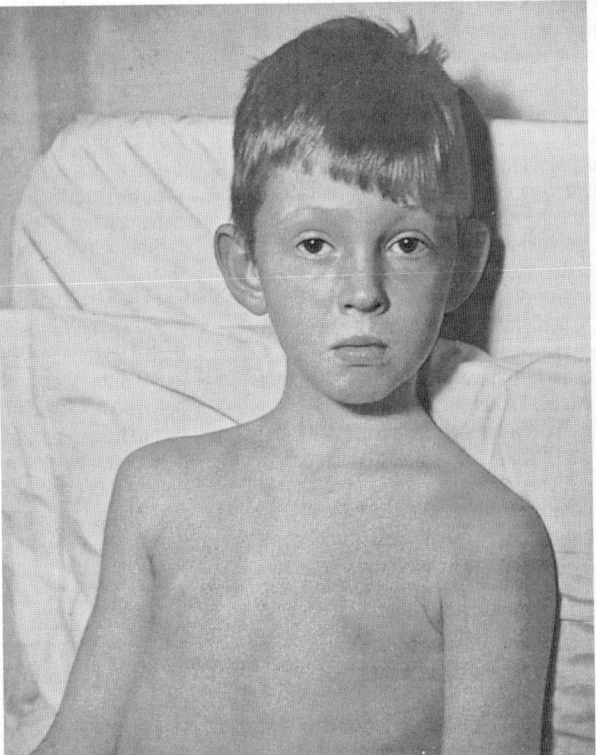
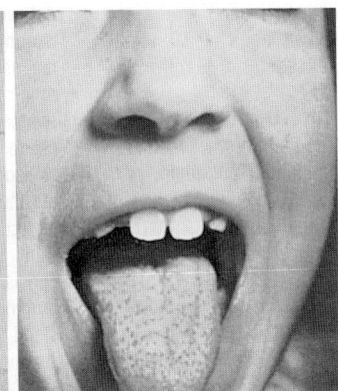
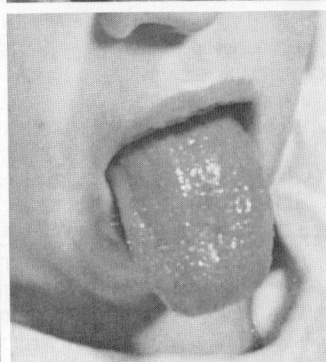

FIG. 1 Scarlet fever. *A,* Punctate, erythematous rash (second day). ***B,*** White strawberry tongue (first day). ***C,*** Red, strawberry tongue (third day). (Courtesy Dr. Franklin H. Top, Professor and Head of the Department of Hygiene and Preventive Medicine, State University of Iowa, College of Medicine, Iowa City, IA; and Parke, Davis & Company's Therapeutic Notes. From Gershon AA et al: *Krugman's infectious diseases of children,* ed 11, Philadelphia, 2004, Mosby.)

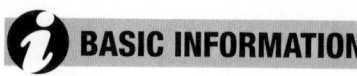

BASIC INFORMATION

DEFINITION

Schizophrenia is a disorder that causes significant distortions in thinking, perception, speech, and behavior. Characteristics include psychosis, apathy, social withdrawal, and cognitive impairment, which result in significant social impairment.

SYNONYMS

Dementia praecox

ICD-10CM CODES
F20   Schizophrenia
F20.0 Paranoid schizophrenia
F20.1 Hebephrenic schizophrenia
F20.2 Catatonic schizophrenia
F20.3 Undifferentiated schizophrenia
F20.5 Residual schizophrenia
F20.6 Simple schizophrenia
F20.8 Other schizophrenia
F20.9 Schizophrenia, unspecified

EPIDEMIOLOGY & DEMOGRAPHICS

INCIDENCE: 0.2 per 1000.
PREVALENCE: 0.5%; lifetime prevalence risk, 0.4%.
PREDOMINANT SEX: Males have a more severe illness with earlier onset. Prevalence in males approximately 1.4 times higher.
PREDOMINANT AGE:
- Age of onset of psychotic symptoms is the early 20s for males and the late 20s for females.
- Age of onset of negative symptoms is usually earlier (i.e., the mid-teenage years).
PEAK INCIDENCE: Between ages of 16 and 30 yr.
GENETICS:
- Genetics accounts for 70% of risk; the remaining 30% associated with other factors such as urban environments, migration, or cannabis use.
- First-degree relatives have a 10 times greater chance of becoming schizophrenic.
- Discordant rates among identical twins are higher than expected with the simple inheritance pattern.
- Associations with several chromosomes have been described, but none has been replicated.
- Evidence exists that triple nucleotide repeat expansion (e.g., such as that seen with Huntington's disease) may play a role in the inheritance of the disease.

PHYSICAL FINDINGS & CLINICAL PRESENTATION

- Schizophrenia is best defined as a dementing illness that begins early in life and that progresses slowly throughout the lifetime.
- Frequent structural brain imaging findings include the enlargement of the ventricular system, a loss of brain volume and cortical gray matter, and an alteration of the white matter tracts.
- The initial "negative" symptoms of adolescence (prodromal phase)—cognitive decline, social withdrawal and awkwardness, loss of motivation and pleasure, and loss of emotional expressiveness—begin after a period of normal development.
- During early adulthood, positive symptoms of psychosis and thought disturbance occur; psychotic symptoms then wax and wane throughout life. Treatment ameliorates positive symptoms, but generally does little for negative ones.
- The condition is also accompanied by cognitive impairment, including problems with attention and concentration, psychomotor speed, learning, memory, and executive functions (e.g., abstract thinking, problem solving, planning).
- Social and occupational dysfunction can be profound.

ETIOLOGY

- The basic determination of whether this is a degenerative or developmental condition has not been made.
- The major hypothesis is that abnormality of the mesocortical pathways produces the hypofrontality and the negative symptoms. This occurs along with a compensatory hyperactivation of the mesolimbic pathways, which produces the positive symptoms of psychosis.

DIAGNOSIS

DIFFERENTIAL DIAGNOSIS

- Schizophrenia is diagnosed when an individual has experienced at least 6 mo (1 mo if using ICD-10 criteria) of hallucinations, delusions, thought disorders, catatonia, or negative symptoms (e.g., avolition, anhedonia, social isolation, affective flattening).
- Any medical condition, medicine, or substance that can affect brain homeostasis can cause psychosis; this is distinguished from schizophrenia by a relatively brief course and an alteration in mental status that suggests an underlying delirium.
- Other neurologic conditions that have psychosis as the initial presentation (e.g., Huntington's disease) need to be ruled out.
- Mood disorders with psychosis: these are indistinguishable from schizophrenia cross-sectionally but have a longitudinal course that includes full recovery.
- Delusional disorder involves nonbizarre delusions and lacks the thought disturbance, hallucinations, and negative symptoms of schizophrenia.
- Autism in the adult has an early age of onset and lacks significant hallucinations or delusions.

WORKUP

- History and physical examination to help determine whether the psychosis is primary or secondary.
- Neurologic examination to uncover the soft neurologic signs (e.g., clumsiness, cortical thumb, loss of fine motor movements) that are common with schizophrenia.

LABORATORY TESTS

- No laboratory tests are specific.
- Laboratory examinations (e.g., chemistry profile, blood count, sedimentation rate, toxicology screen, and urinalysis) are geared toward excluding a primary medical condition or toxic state. Note that new common drugs of abuse may not be detectable with regular screening tests.

IMAGING STUDIES

- CT or MRI of the brain during the initial workup; repeated if the course of the illness varies from what is expected.
- EEG may reveal slowing when psychosis is the result of an encephalopathy. Findings can be similar as a result of common medication use for treatment of psychosis.

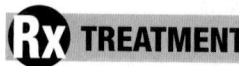 TREATMENT

NONPHARMACOLOGIC THERAPY

- Significant social support is required by most schizophrenic patients, but available support services are grossly inadequate. Schizophrenic patients constitute nearly one third of all homeless individuals and approximately 5% of the incarcerated population. They usually require help with basic social, occupational, and interaction skills.
- Family stress can precipitate relapse and re-hospitalization. Family interventions can reduce morbidity.
- Cognitive behavioral therapy can reduce the severity of both psychotic and negative symptoms.
- Illness management training for patients can increase medication adherence and reduce symptom distress.
- Integrated treatment that includes assertive community treatment, family involvement programs, and social skills training reduces the severity of both psychotic and negative symptoms, reduces comorbid substance misuse, reduces hospital days, increases adherence to treatment, and increases satisfaction with treatment.

ACUTE GENERAL Rx

- Acute psychosis is usually adequately controlled with antipsychotic agents.
- Few differences in effectiveness exist between first-generation antipsychotics (e.g., haloperidol, perphenazine, fluphenazine, chlorpromazine) and second-generation antipsychotics (e.g., risperidone, olanzapine, quetiapine, ziprasidone, aripiprazole, clozapine, lurasidone) for nonrefractory patients. First-generation antipsychotics are slightly more likely than second-generation antipsychotics to cause a parkinsonian state and eventual tardive dyskinesia (rate of tardive dyskinesia, 15%-30%). Antiparkinsonian drugs (e.g., benztropine, amantadine) are used to ameliorate the parkinsonism. Risperidone has been shown to be superior to haloperidol for the prevention of acute psychotic relapse.

- Sedatives (i.e., benzodiazepines and, to a lesser degree, barbiturates) can be used transiently if a patient is in an agitated state.

CHRONIC Rx

- Relapse prevention is a major goal of treatment. Noncompliance is common and leads to high relapse rates. Antipsychotic agents usually must be continued at the same doses that controlled psychosis. For noncompliant patients, long-acting injectable preparations given biweekly, monthly, or every three months can be used.
- Most patients frequently switch among antipsychotics; there is considerable individual variability with regard to antipsychotic response and vulnerability to specific adverse effects.
- Clozapine is more effective than other agents for treatment-refractory patients. However, it requires monitoring to prevent life-threatening adverse effects. Olanzapine may also be more effective than less expensive first-generation drugs but has substantial adverse metabolic effects. Lurasidone is a newer second-generation antipsychotic that appears to be better tolerated, but longer-term studies are needed.
- Neurocognitive improvement associated with antipsychotic treatment among patients with schizophrenia is small and does not differ between first-generation and second-generation antipsychotics.
- Antiparkinsonian agents may also need to be continued for the long term.
- Tardive dyskinesia (i.e., choreoathetoid movements of the muscles of tongue and face and occasionally of other muscle groups) can occur in as many as 30% of patients with the long-term use of neuroleptics.
- The negative symptoms of schizophrenia can resemble depression. In addition, depressive disorders may occur in schizophrenic patients. Antidepressant treatment of the negative symptoms is usually not effective. However, antidepressants can improve the symptoms of a comorbid depressive episode.

- Mood stabilizers (e.g., lithium, valproate, carbamazepine) are of little use unless the patient has a comorbid impulse control disorder.
- Substance abuse is a major problem for more than a third of schizophrenic patients. More than half of these patients smoke cigarettes. Unfortunately, these individuals do poorly in traditional substance abuse treatment programs. Specialized "dual-diagnosis" programs with highly structured aftercare are required.
- Specific antipsychotic medications have been associated with weight gain (i.e., olanzapine and clozapine) and QT prolongation. Hyperlipidemia and diabetes mellitus are associated with second-generation antipsychotics, and hyperprolactinemia is associated with first-generation antipsychotics. (Risperidone, a second-generation antipsychotic, can also produce hyperprolactinemia.) Clozapine is associated with agranulocytosis and a decrease in intestinal motility. Metabolic status and weight should be screened before the start of treatment and at regular intervals.
- Patients with schizophrenia have a higher lifetime incidence of suicide, with 20% attempting on one or more occasions and 5% to 6% completing suicide. Comorbid use of substances and hopelessness are associated risk factors. Clozapine has shown the ability to decrease the incidence of suicidal attempts in schizophrenia patients.
- Several 1st and 2nd generation antipsychotics are available in long-acting injectable preparations that may be helpful in addressing issues of poor compliance or difficulty when treatment needs to be supervised.

DISPOSITION

- The positive symptoms of as many as 20% to 30% of schizophrenic patients do not respond to available treatments. A much higher fraction of patients experience relapse as a result of poor compliance.

- Negative symptoms are responsible for the 50% to 70% of patients in whom deterioration in occupational and social function continues.
- Approximately 10% of schizophrenic patients will complete suicide.
- The course of the illness is most strongly predicted by the level of social development attained at the onset of psychosis.
- Schizophrenic patients die 12 to 15 years sooner than the average population, mostly as a result of physical causes related to a lack of access to health care or as a result of health risk factors (e.g., smoking, obesity).

REFERRAL

- If hospitalization is required.
- If patient is noncompliant.
- If patient is resistant to treatment.

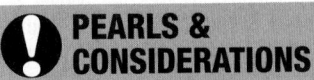 **PEARLS & CONSIDERATIONS**

- Rule out delirium caused by medical conditions, medications, or substance abuse before diagnosing an individual's psychotic behavior as schizophrenia.
- All antipsychotic medications have high discontinuation rates in chronic schizophrenia treatment. Olanzapine and clozapine may be more effective than other antipsychotics for chronic treatment, but they have significant side effects.
- Significant social support is required for most patients with schizophrenia. Nonpharmacologic therapy should be used in conjunction with pharmacotherapy.

SUGGESTED READINGS
Available at www.expertconsult.com

RELATED CONTENT
Schizophrenia (Patient Information)

AUTHOR: **ARNALDO A. BERGES, M.D.**

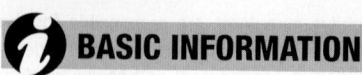

BASIC INFORMATION

DEFINITION

Scleritis is inflammation of the sclera (the fibrous layer of the eye underlying the conjunctiva and episclera). It is characterized by edema and cellular infiltration of the entire thickness of the sclera.

Classification of immune:
1. Anterior nonnecrotizing scleritis: can be subdivided into diffuse or nodular.
2. Anterior necrotizing scleritis with inflammation: can be subdivided into vasoocclusive, granulomatous, or surgically induced. Aggressive form of scleritis. Average age of onset is 60 yr. Bilateral in 60% of patients.
3. Scleromalacia perforans: typically affects elderly women with longstanding rheumatoid arthritis.
4. Posterior scleritis: involves the deeper tissues of the eye and is potentially blinding. Age of onset is often under 40 yr. Bilateral in 35% of cases.

SYNONYMS

Anterior scleritis
Diffuse nodular, necrotizing scleritis
Scleromalacia perforans
Scleral melt syndrome

ICD-10CM CODES
H15.0 Scleritis
H15.1 Episcleritis

EPIDEMIOLOGY & DEMOGRAPHICS

PEAK INCIDENCE: Increases with increasing age.
INCIDENCE (IN U.S.): Busy ophthalmologists may see one or two cases a year
PREVALENCE (IN U.S.): Relatively rare.
PREDOMINANT SEX: 61% women.
PREDOMINANT AGE: 52 yr.

PHYSICAL FINDINGS & CLINICAL PRESENTATION

- Deep, boring (dull) eye pain that may awaken patient from sleep.
- Photophobia.
- Tearing.
- Painful eye movements.
- Globe is tender to touch.
- Conjunctival injection (Fig. 1).
- Thinning of the sclera.
- An underlying systemic autoimmune disease is found in >50% of patients. Most common rheumatic problem is rheumatoid arthritis. Most patients with systemic disease are diagnosed before development of scleritis.

ETIOLOGY

- Inflammatory (seen with rheumatoid arthritis, granulomatosis with polyangiitis [Wegener granulomatosis], relapsing polychondritis, polyarteritis nodosa), lupus, sarcoidosis.
- Allergic.
- Infectious scleritis (herpes zoster, tuberculosis, Lyme disease, syphilis, *Pseudomonas aeruginosa, Nocardia,* leprosy) is uncommon, accounting for 4% to 18% of cases
- Approximately 50% of patients with scleritis have an underlying systemic disease (vasculitis, infectious disease).

DIAGNOSIS

DIFFERENTIAL DIAGNOSIS

Most common causes are rheumatoid arthritis and other collagen-vascular diseases.
- Occasionally there are allergic, infectious, or traumatic causes.
- Conjunctivitis, iritis, and episcleritis should be considered in the differential diagnosis. Patients with episcleritis generally have less pain and vision is unaffected.

WORKUP

- Eye examination.
- Visual field examination.
- Workup for autoimmune disease (e.g., vasculitis, collagen vascular diseases)

LABORATORY TESTS

Rheumatoid factor, antinuclear antibody, erythrocyte sedimentation rate, ANCA (c-ANCA, p-ANCA), antiphospholipid antibodies, may be useful for underlying etiology.

IMAGING STUDIES

Usually not necessary; CT scan of orbit may be useful in selected patients for collagen vascular disease or vasculitis.

TREATMENT

NONPHARMACOLOGIC THERAPY

- Bandage lenses.
- Surgery if thinning of the sclera is severe to prevent eye rupture.

ACUTE GENERAL Rx

Immunotherapy:
- Steroids (topical, periocular, and systemic).
- Cycloplegic drops.
- Nonsteroidal antiinflammatory drugs (topical and systemic); systemic more effective than topical.
- Cytotoxic agents (cyclophosphamide, azathioprine, mycophenolate mofetil, methotrexate).
- Immune modulators (cyclosporin, tacrolimus).
- Specific antibodies (infliximab, rituximab).

CHRONIC Rx

- Systemic corticosteroids can be given for the underlying disease.
- Local steroids may be helpful. Topical steroids should be used judiciously since these can potentiate the collagenase activity and worsen the scleral loss.
- Control underlying disease.

DISPOSITION

Urgent referral to ophthalmologist because this disorder can be a sight-threatening condition.

REFERRAL

Should be managed by ophthalmologist; complications of scleritis can be severe, including scleral melt, inflammation, corneal involvement.

PEARLS & CONSIDERATIONS

COMMENTS

Necrotizing scleritis can be an ominous diagnosis because these patients often have other severe underlying debilitating vasculitic disease processes.

SUGGESTED READINGS
Available at www.expertconsult.com

AUTHOR: R. SCOTT HOFFMAN, M.D.

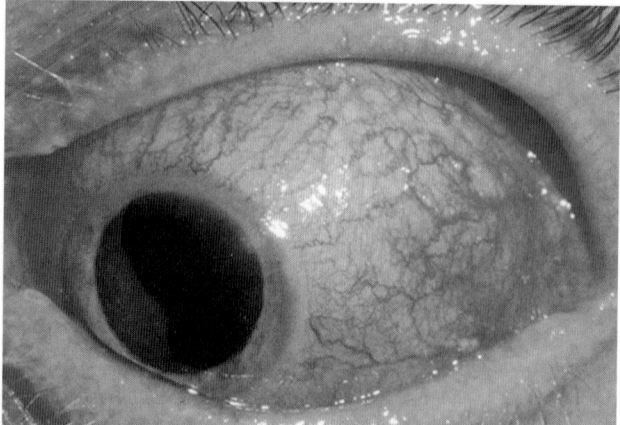

FIG. 1 In diffuse anterior scleritis, widespread injection of the conjunctival and deep episcleral vessels occurs. (From Palay D [ed]: *Ophthalmology for the primary care physician,* St Louis, 1997, Mosby.)

BASIC INFORMATION

DEFINITION

Scleroderma or systemic sclerosis (SSc) is a term used to describe a connective tissue disorder that is characterized by thickening and fibrosis of the skin. It is divided into two forms: localized scleroderma and systemic sclerosis. Skin thickening without any organ involvement is known as localized scleroderma and includes three subset conditions (see Box 1). Systemic sclerosis includes skin fibrosis along with variable severe involvement of diverse internal organs. It is further divided into two major subgroups: (1) limited cutaneous SSc (lcSSc), which involves skin thickening of the face, neck, and distal to the elbows and knees; and (2) diffuse cutaneous SSc (dcSSc), which affects the skin in a more generalized distribution including the proximal and distal extremities, face, neck, and trunk. Table 1 compares localized scleroderma and SSc.

SYNONYMS

SSc

Systemic sclerosis

Morphea applies to localized scleroderma that affects only the skin

Scleredema is a disease of the skin that is distinct from scleroderma

ICD-10CM CODES
M34.0   Progressive systemic sclerosis
M34.1   CREST syndrome

BOX 1   Classification of Scleroderma

I. Localized scleroderma
   A. Morphea
   B. Linear scleroderma
   C. Scleroderma en coup de sabre
II. Systemic sclerosis
   A. Limited cutaneous systemic sclerosis
   B. Diffuse cutaneous systemic sclerosis

From Hochberg MC et al: *Rheumatology*, ed 5, St Louis, 2011, Mosby.

M34.2   Systemic sclerosis induced by drug and chemical
M34.81   Systemic sclerosis with lung involvement
M34.82   Systemic sclerosis with myopathy
M34.83   Systemic sclerosis with polyneuropathy
M34.89   Other systemic sclerosis
M34.9   Systemic sclerosis, unspecified
L94.0   Localized scleroderma (morphea)
L94.1   Linear scleroderma

EPIDEMIOLOGY & DEMOGRAPHICS

Incidence and prevalence of SSc varies between studies due to variations between geographic regions and time periods.

INCIDENCE: There are an estimated 2.3 to 22.8 cases per 1 million persons per year, but many mild cases go unrecognized.

PREVALENCE: 50 to 300 cases per 1 million persons.

PREDOMINANT SEX: Female/male ratio of 4:1.

PREDOMINANT AGE: 30 to 50 years old

DISTRIBUTION: Worldwide

PHYSICAL FINDINGS & CLINICAL PRESENTATION

PHYSICAL FINDINGS:

1. Skin
   ○ Initial presentation of puffy hands and fingers may occur in some patients.
   ○ Tightening of the skin begins on the hands and then progresses to the forearms, face, and neck. The skin is shiny, taut, and sometimes red, with loss of creases and hair. Skin thickening involving the fingers or toes is known as sclerodactyly (Fig. E1). Skin involvement in scleroderma is classified as lcSSc or dcSSc, depending on the distribution of the skin thickening (see previously) (Fig. E2). Fig. E3 illustrates the method used to quantify skin thickness in scleroderma.
   ○ Skin tightening may limit movement by causing flexion contractures of the fingers, wrists, and elbows. Perioral skin tightening (Fig. E4) results in decreased oral aperture,

furrowing around the lips, and dry membranes.
   ○ Pigmentary skin changes (hypo- or hyper-pigmentation) may occur.
   ○ Telangiectasias (dilated capillaries) may be seen on face, hands, mucous membranes (Fig. E4) and trunk.
   ○ Subcutaneous calcinosis.
   ○ In dsSSc patients, the skin fibrosis can soften to normal skin (occurring two years after onset of skin manifestation), and joint mobility can improve.
   ○ Skin atrophy and thinning can also occur in the late stages of SSc.

2. Musculoskeletal
   ○ Arthralgias and swelling
   ○ Symmetric inflammatory arthritis
   ○ Myalgias
   ○ Myopathy
   ○ Tendon friction rubs (physical exam finding of a palpable rub felt over tendon sheaths–fingers, wrists, elbows, knees, and/or ankles)

3. Gastrointestinal involvement
   ○ Esophageal dysmotility with heartburn
   ○ Esophageal stricture with dysphagia and odynophagia
   ○ Delayed gastric emptying
   ○ Gastrointestinal bleeding from mucosal telangiectasias, gastric antral vascular ectasias, or gastritis
   ○ Small bowel dysmotility with abdominal cramps, bloating, and diarrhea
   ○ Colon dysmotility with constipation
   ○ Intestinal bacterial overgrowth resulting in irregular bowel movements (diarrhea alternating with constipation)
   ○ Pseudoobstruction (functional ileus)
   ○ Primary biliary cirrhosis (see "Primary Biliary Cirrhosis" in Section I)

4. Pulmonary
   ○ Interstitial lung disease (ILD): pulmonary fibrosis with symptoms of dyspnea and nonproductive cough as well as fine inspiratory crackles on examination. Seen in both lcSSc and dcSSC, but it is more common and severe in dcSSC.

   Pulmonary arterial hypertension (PAH): presenting with dyspnea and/or fatigue. Can be identified in both lcSSc and dcSSc, but it is more commonly seen in lcSSc.

5. Cardiac
   ○ Pericarditis or pericardial effusion
   ○ Myositis or myocardial fibrosis that can lead to congestive heart failure or arrhythmias
   ○ Left or right systolic or diastolic dysfunction

6. Renal
   ○ Rapidly progressive renal failure also known as scleroderma renal crisis (SRC): new-onset hypertension, anemia with schistocytes on peripheral blood smear, thrombocytopenia and renal insufficiency with active urinary sediment and proteinuria

7. Vascular
   ○ Raynaud phenomenon (RP): vasospasm of the fingers with exposure to cold, resulting in color changes of the digits along with numbness/tingling and pain or discomfort.

TABLE 1   Comparison of Localized Scleroderma and Systemic Sclerosis

Feature	Localized Scleroderma/ Morphea	Systemic Sclerosis
Skin findings	Patches or linear distribution of thickened skin	Sclerodactyly ± proximal skin thickening
Raynaud's phenomenon	Absent	Present
Digital ischemic changes	Absent	Usually present (digital pitting scars or ulcers, loss of fingerpad substance)
Internal organ disease	Absent	Present
Antinuclear antibody	Positive in ≥50% of cases	Positive in ≥85% of cases
Scleroderma-specific autoantibodies*	Negative	Positive in 60% of cases
Biopsy—histologic findings	Dermal fibrosis	Dermal fibrosis

*Scleroderma-specific antibodies include antibodies to centromere, topoisomerase-1 (Scl 70), and RNA polymerase III.
From Hochberg MC et al: *Rheumatology*, ed 5, St Louis, 2011, Mosby.

○ Complications of this vascular involvement include: digital pitted scars or ulcers (Fig. E5), nonreversible ischemic changes with impending tissue loss, dry gangrene, and auto-amputation.

○ Nailfold capillary abnormalities: seen with nailfold capillaroscopy, including capillary dilatation, avascularity, or "drop out" of capillaries.

8. Other organ involvement
○ Hypothyroidism
○ Erectile dysfunction
○ Sjögren's syndrome
○ Entrapment neuropathies
○ Depression

CLINICAL PRESENTATION:
- Raynaud's phenomenon: initial complaint in 70% of patients (NOTE: The prevalence of Raynaud's phenomenon is 5% to 10% in the general population; most cases do not progress to scleroderma)
- Finger or hand swelling that is sometimes associated with carpal tunnel syndrome
- Arthralgias/arthritis
- Internal organ involvement

LcSSc (previously known as CREST syndrome):
○ Calcinosis, Raynaud's syndrome, Esophageal dysmotility, Sclerodactyly Telangiectasias— skin fibrosis is limited to the distal extremities. This acronym is now considered obsolete by many because it does not accurately reflect the burden of internal organ involvement.

ETIOLOGY

The etiology of this condition is unknown, but genetic and environmental factors (infectious agents, occupational exposures, drugs) contribute to the manifestation of the disease. Genetic profiles show clustering of different alleles according to the subtype of SSc.

Pathologically, small- and medium-sized arteries become injured, leading to fibrin deposition and ultimately luminal occlusion, causing chronic tissue hypoxia. There is also an abnormal selection of fibroblasts and aberrant control of connective tissue synthesis by fibroblasts and other cells. This fibrosis occurs in different organs, causing dysfunction and eventual failure. Although there are characteristic autoantibodies detected, it is not clear that they directly participate in the pathogenesis of the disease.

Dx DIAGNOSIS

The American College of Rheumatology (ACR) and European League Against Rheumatism (EULAR) have created criteria as a guide in diagnosing and classifying SSc. These include a scoring system for both clinical and laboratory findings (sclerodactyly, fingertip lesions, telangiectasias, abnormal nailfold capillaries, Raynaud's phenomenon, PAH/ILD, and SSc-related autoantibodies).

DIFFERENTIAL DIAGNOSIS
DERMATOLOGIC:
- Scleredema
- Amyloidosis
- Porphyria cutanea tarda
- Eosinophilic fasciitis
- Reflex sympathetic dystrophy
- Nephrogenic systemic fibrosis
SYSTEMIC:
- Idiopathic pulmonary fibrosis
- Primary pulmonary hypertension
- Primary biliary cirrhosis
- Cardiomyopathies
- Gastrointestinal dysmotility problems
- Systemic lupus erythematosus and overlap syndromes

WORKUP
Laboratory tests and imaging studies

LABORATORY TESTS
- Antinuclear antibodies (ANA): nucleolar (more common), homogeneous, or speckled patterns.
- Rheumatoid factor positive in 20% of patients.
- Routine biochemistry tests may indicate specific organ involvement (e.g., liver, kidney, muscle).

The following extractable nuclear antigens are either present or absent in SSc:
- Anticentromere antibodies: generally positive in one third of patients with lcSSc.
- Anti-Scl-70 antibody: positive in 40% of patients with dcSSc and has an increased risk of developing ILD.
- Anti-RNA polymerase III antibody: portends a worse prognosis and extensive skin fibrosis and increases risk of developing SRC.
- Autoantibodies against ribonucleoprotein (anti-RNP): positive in 20% of patients.
- Negative antibody to native DNA
- Negative anti-smooth muscle antibody

IMAGING AND OTHER STUDIES
1. Arthritis: joint radiographs
2. Gastrointestinal
   ○ Endoscopy (diagnostic procedure of choice; may be therapeutic)
   ○ Cine-esophagography (in rare circumstances)
   ○ Barium swallow (occasionally indicated)
   ○ Esophageal manometry (almost never necessary)
3. Pulmonary
   ○ Chest x-ray
   ○ Pulmonary function tests (especially single-breath diffusion capacity for carbon monoxide)
   ○ Thoracic high-resolution computed tomography (HRCT) scan
   ○ Bronchoscopy with biopsy
   ○ Bronchoalveolar lavage
4. Cardiac
   ○ ECG
   ○ Ambulatory (Holter) ECG monitoring

○ Echocardiography
○ Cardiac catheterization
5. Kidney: renal biopsy
6. Skin: skin biopsy
7. Vascular: nailfold capillaroscopy

Rx TREATMENT

Currently, there is no disease-modifying therapy available for SSc. Generally, the internal organ involvement of the disease is treatable. Fig. 6 illustrates management strategies in SSc. Immunosuppressive agents are used in individual patients. Prednisone should be used with extreme caution, especially in doses >20 mg/day. Table 2 summarizes current recommendations for treatment of scleroderma.

1. Raynaud's syndrome:
   ○ Keep hands and body warm
   ○ Avoid smoking
   ○ Calcium channel blockers (i.e., long-acting dihydropyridines)
   ○ Peripheral $\alpha 1$-adrenergic blockers
   ○ Angiotensin II receptor blockers
   ○ Pentoxifylline
   ○ Phosphodiesterase inhibitors
   ○ Stellate ganglion blockades
   ○ Digital sympathectomy
2. Arthralgias: nonsteroidal antiinflammatory drugs or low-dose corticosteroids (5-10 mg of prednisone per day)
3. Myositis: methotrexate or azathioprine with low-dose corticosteroids
4. Skin: for extensive skin fibrosis, immunomodulatory drugs have been used such as methotrexate, mycophenolate mofetil, and cyclophosphamide, but have not been proved to be beneficial
5. Esophageal reflux
   ○ H_2-receptor blockers
   ○ Proton pump inhibitors
6. Interstitial lung disease
   ○ Cyclophosphamide for symptomatic scleroderma-related ILD
   ○ Mycophenolate mofetil and rituximab have been reported to be beneficial but are still being studied in clinical trials
   ○ Lung transplantation for patients with advanced pulmonary involvement
7. Pulmonary hypertension
   ○ Oxygen
   ○ Diuretics (with caution)
   ○ Prostacyclins (epoprostenol, iloprost, treprostinil)
   ○ Endothelin-1 receptor inhibitors (bosentan, ambrisentan)
   Phosphodiesterase 5 inhibitors (sildenafil, tadalafil)
8. Renal involvement
   ○ Angiotensin-converting enzyme inhibitors
   ○ Dialysis
   ○ Renal transplantation

REFERRAL

Rheumatology consultation is indicated. Consider pulmonary, cardiology, or gastrointestinal consultations depending on organ involvement.

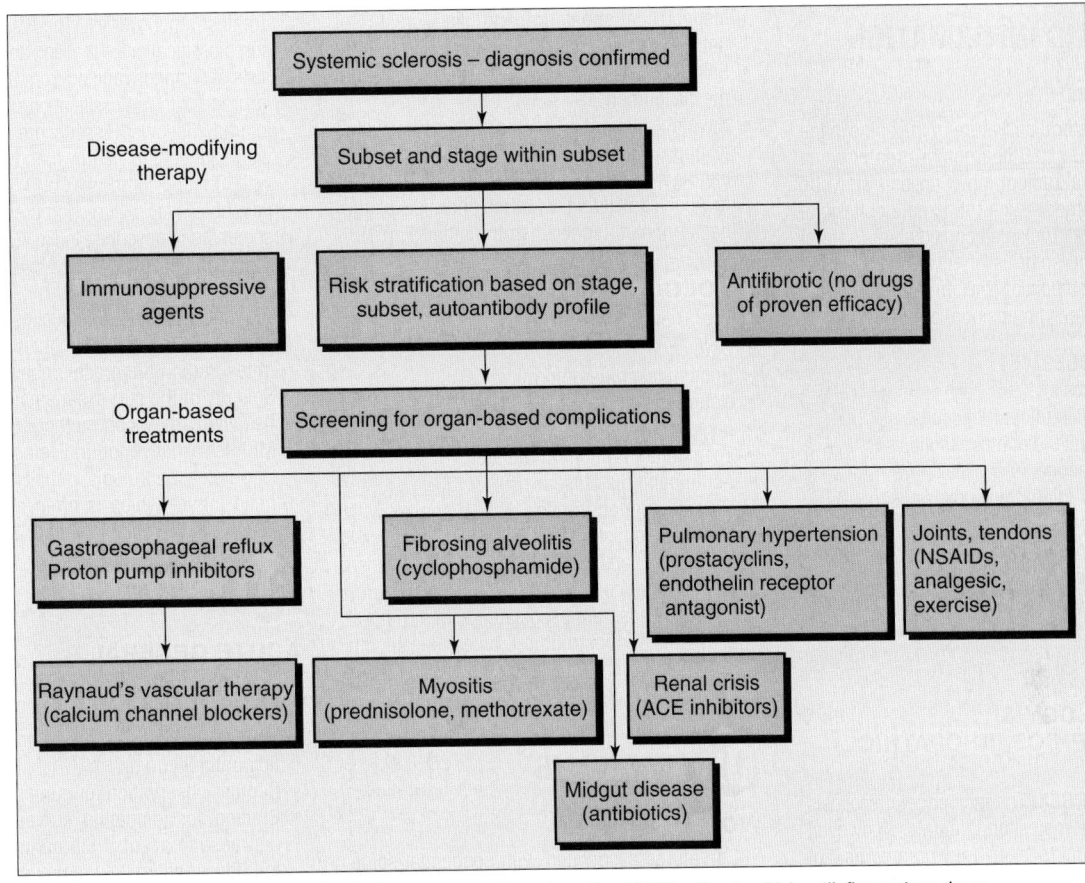

FIG. 6 Management strategies in systemic sclerosis. *NSAIDs,* Nonsteroidal antiinflammatory drugs.
(From Hochberg MC et al: *Rheumatology,* ed 5, St Louis, 2011, Mosby.)

TABLE 2 Current Recommendations for Treatment of Scleroderma

Manifestation	Primary Therapy	Alternative/Second-Line Therapy
Raynaud's phenomenon	Vasodilators (CCB) Antiplatelet	PDE5 inhibitors, prostacyclin, endothelin antagonists
Hypertensive renal disease	ACE inhibitors	ARBs, CCB, prostacyclin, renal transplant (wait at least 24 mo)
GI involvement	**Upper GI** Dental/periodontal care, lifestyle modifications, proton pump inhibitors, prokinetics	EGD to treat stenosis and/or GAVE
	Lower GI Probiotics, rotational antibiotics	Total parenteral nutrition
Skin	Mycophenolate mofetil, cyclophosphamide	IVIG, ATG, research trial (severe cases)
Interstitial lung disease	Cyclophosphamide, mycophenolate mofetil, azathioprine	Research trial
Pulmonary arterial hypertension	PDE5 inhibitors, endothelin antagonists, prostacyclin	Combination therapy, atrioseptostomy, lung transplant, research trial
Cardiac involvement	Heart failure therapy, diuretics, CCB	Immunosuppression (myocardial inflammation)
Joints	Prednisone, methotrexate, TNF inhibitors	IVIG (if contractures and rubs are present), PT/OT
Muscles	Prednisone, methotrexate, azathioprine	IVIG
Psychosocial	Antidepressants, pain control, sleep control	Support group

ACE, Angiotensin-converting enzyme; *ARBs,* angiotensin receptor blockers; *ATG,* antithymocyte globulin; *CCB,* calcium channel blockers; *EGD,* esophagogastroduodenoscopy; *GAVE,* gastric antral vascular ectasia; *GI,* gastrointestinal; *HSCT,* hematopoietic stem cell transplantation; *IVIG,* intravenous immunoglobulin; *PDE5,* phosphodiesterase-5 inhibitor; *PT/OT,* physical therapy/occupational therapy; *TNF,* tumor necrosis factor.
From Firestein GS et al: *Kelly's textbook of rheumatology,* ed 9, Philadelphia, 2013, Saunders.

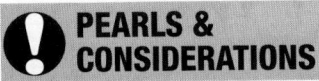 **PEARLS & CONSIDERATIONS**

COMMENTS

• A recent trial of autologous hematopoietic stem cell therapy (HSCT) versus monthly cyclophosphamide in patients with early diffuse cutaneous systemic sclerosis showed better long-term event-free survival and overall survival at a median follow-up of approximately 6 years and clinically meaningful improvements in objective and patient-reported outcome measures at 2 years with HSCT. However, there was greater treatment-related mortality.

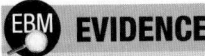 **EVIDENCE**

Available at www.expertconsult.com

RELATED CONTENT

Scleroderma (Patient Information)

AUTHOR: **JOANNE SZCZYGIEL CUNHA, M.D.**

DEFINITION

Scoliosis is a lateral curvature of the spine in the upright position of 10 degrees or greater when measured on a radiograph. Scoliosis may be classified as either structural (fixed, nonflexible) or nonstructural (flexible, correctable). Lateral curvature of the spine is often associated with lordosis and rotation of the affected vertebrae, leading to a three-dimensional deformity.

ICD-10CM CODES	
M41	Scoliosis
M41.0	Infantile idiopathic scoliosis
M41.1	Juvenile idiopathic scoliosis
M41.3	Thoracogenic scoliosis
M41.20	Other idiopathic scoliosis, site unspecified
M41.80	Other forms of scoliosis, site unspecified
Q67.5	Congenital deformity of spine
M41.40	Neuromuscular scoliosis, site unspecified

EPIDEMIOLOGY & DEMOGRAPHICS (IDIOPATHIC FORM)

PREDOMINANT SEX: The incidence of scoliosis is the same in males and females; however, females have up to a 10-fold greater risk of curve progression. Females are roughly seven times as likely to require orthopedic surgical intervention for idiopathic scoliosis.
PREVALENCE: 1.5% to 3% of adolescents.
PREDOMINANT AGE:
- Onset variable.
- Most curves found in adolescents (age ≥11 years).

PHYSICAL FINDINGS & CLINICAL PRESENTATION

- Record patient age (in years plus months) and height.
- Perform neurologic examination to rule out neuromuscular disease.
- Inspect the shoulders and iliac crests to determine if they are level.
- Palpate the spinous processes to determine their alignment.
- Have the patient bend forward at the waist to approximately 45 degrees with the arms hanging free (Adams' position); observe from the back to detect whether one side of the back appears higher than the other (Fig. 1).

ETIOLOGY

- 90% unknown, usually referred to as *idiopathic* (genetic).
- Congenital spine deformity.
- Neuromuscular disease.
- Leg-length inequality.
- Local inflammation or infection.
- Acute pain (disk disease).
- Chronic degenerative disk disease with asymmetric disk narrowing.

Curves of an idiopathic nature or those accompanying congenital deformity or neuromuscular disease are associated with structural changes. The nonstructural types (leg-length discrepancy, inflammation, or acute pain) disappear when the offending disorder is corrected.

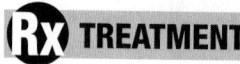 **DIAGNOSIS**

WORKUP

- Curvatures associated with congenital spine abnormalities, neuromuscular disease, and other less common forms of scoliosis can usually be identified by history or associated radiographic or physical findings.
- The diagnosis of scoliosis is suspected on the basis of physical examination and confirmed by radiography performed while the patient is in a standing position. Physical examination with the Adams' forward bend test and scoliometer measurement can identify scoliosis, and the radiologic testing for Cobb angle measurement can confirm the diagnosis. The Cobb angle is measured on a thoraco-lumbar radiograph and is defined as the intersecting angle between lines drawn from the two vertebrae with the greatest amount of tilt. The Risser grade measures ossification of the iliac apophysis. It consists of 5 grades ranging from 25% ossification in grade 1 to full ossification of the apophysis in grade 5. Lower Risser scores are associated with higher spinal growth potential. Patients with Risser scores of 0 or 1 are at greatest risk of scoliosis curve progression. Scoliosis screening is described in Fig. 2.

IMAGING STUDIES

- Diagnosis of idiopathic scoliosis is confirmed by a Cobb angle greater than 10 degrees as measured on a thoracolumbar radiograph.
- Severity of the curve is measured in degrees, usually by the Cobb method (Fig. 3).
- MRI is usually not indicated unless there is pain, a neurologic deficit, or a left thoracic curve (which is often associated with an underlying spinal disorder).

Rx **TREATMENT**

ACUTE GENERAL Rx

- Treatment or correction of cause if curve is nonstructural.
- Early detection is key in treating genetic (idiopathic) curve.
- Regular observation for curves <20 degrees.
- Bracing for idiopathic curves of 25 to 45 degrees in patients with an immature skeleton (Risser score 0-2) to prevent progression.
- Surgery for idiopathic curves >45 degrees in patients with an immature skeleton.

DISPOSITION

- The larger the curve at detection, the greater the chance of progression.
- Progression is more common in young children who are beginning their growth spurt.
- Curves in females are more likely to progress.
- Curves <20 degrees will improve spontaneously >50% of the time.
- Failure to diagnose and treat these curves may allow progressive deformity, pain, and cardiopulmonary compromise to develop.
- Spinal deformities >50 degrees in adults may progress and eventually become painful or compromise pulmonary function.
- There is no difference in the rate of back pain in the general population and patients with adolescent idiopathic scoliosis.

REFERRAL

Refer for orthopedic consultation if structural curve >20 degrees is present or if structural curve <20 degrees progresses 5 degrees or more upon follow-up evaluation.

! **PEARLS & CONSIDERATIONS**

COMMENTS

- Congenital scoliosis has a high incidence of cardiac and urinary tract abnormalities.
- Bracing is not intended to completely straighten the idiopathic curve. It may

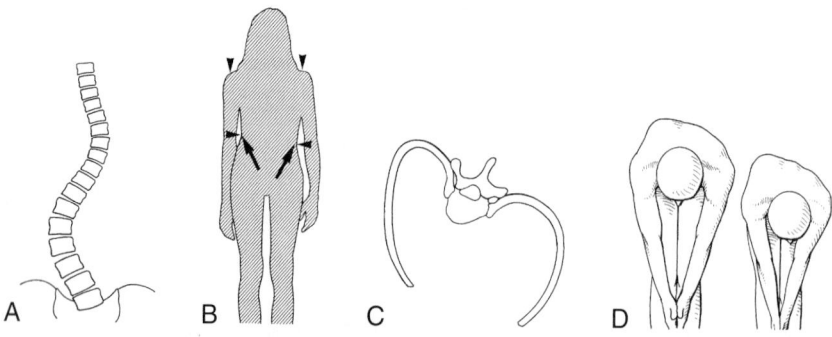

FIG. 1 Structural changes in idiopathic scoliosis. A, As curvature increases, alterations in body configuration develop in both the primary and compensatory curve regions. **B,** Asymmetries of shoulder height, waistline, and the elbow-to-flank distance are common findings. **C,** Vertebral rotation and associated posterior displacement of the ribs on the convex side of the curve are responsible for the characteristic deformity of the chest wall in scoliosis patients. **D,** In the school screening examination for scoliosis, the patient bends forward at the waist. Rib asymmetry of even a small degree is obvious. (From Scoles PV: Spinal deformity in childhood and adolescence. In Behrman RE, Vaughn VC III [eds]: *Nelson textbook of pediatrics,* ed 5, Philadelphia, 1989, Saunders.)

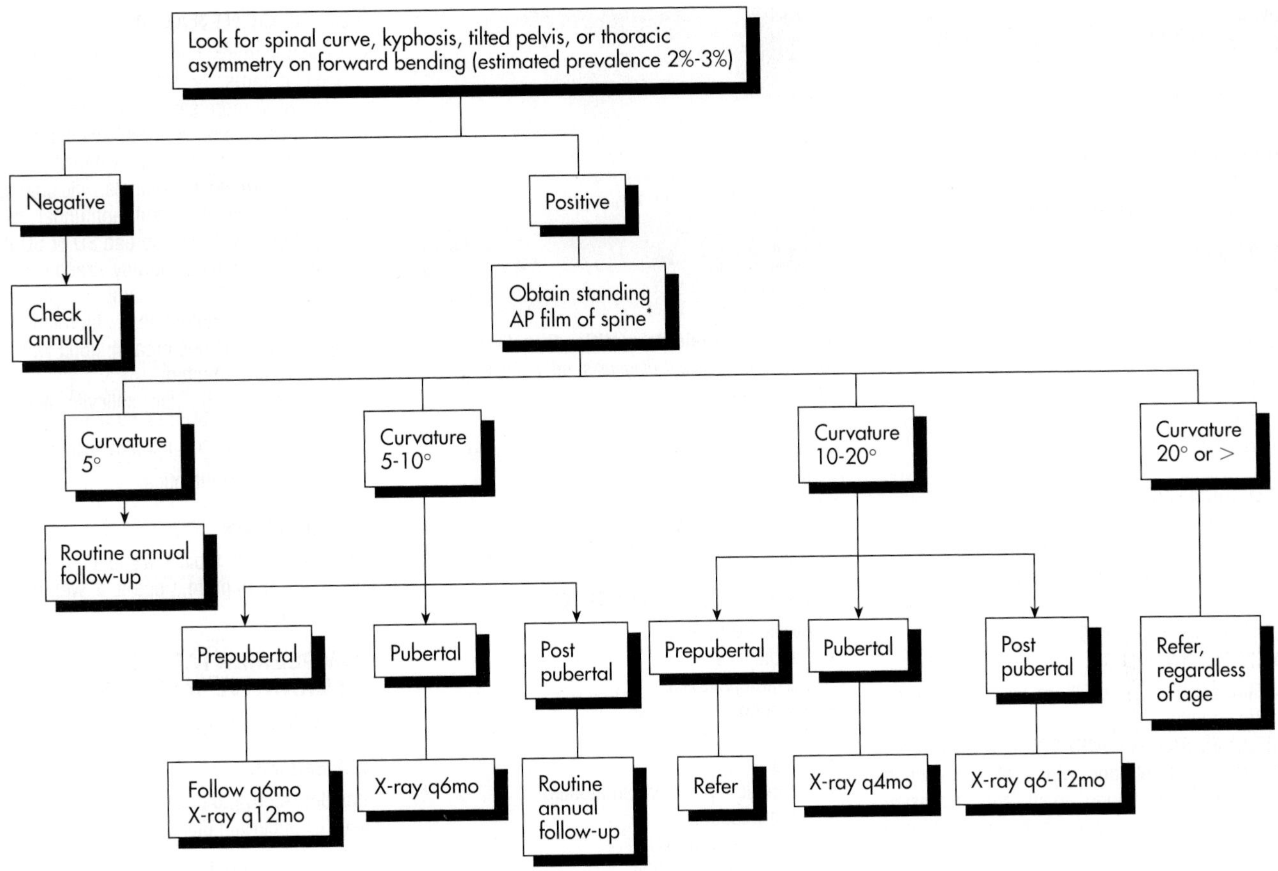

Look for spinal curve, kyphosis, tilted pelvis, or thoracic asymmetry on forward bending (estimated prevalence 2%-3%)

Negative

Positive

Check annually

Obtain standing AP film of spine*

Curvature 5°

Curvature 5-10°

Curvature 10-20°

Curvature 20° or >

Routine annual follow-up

Prepubertal

Pubertal

Post pubertal

Prepubertal

Pubertal

Post pubertal

Refer, regardless of age

Follow q6mo X-ray q12mo

X-ray q6mo

Routine annual follow-up

Refer

X-ray q4mo

X-ray q6-12mo

*Cobb method of angle measurement.

1. Find the lowest vertebra whose bottom tilts toward concavity of curve.
2. Erect a perpendicular line from extension of bottom surface.
3. Find highest vertebra as in #1 and erect perpendicular from extension of top surface.
4. Measure intersecting angle = angle of scoliosis.

FIG. 2 Scoliosis screening and follow-up. *AP,* Anteroposterior. (From Driscoll C [ed]: *The family practice desk reference,* ed 3, St Louis, 1996, Mosby.)

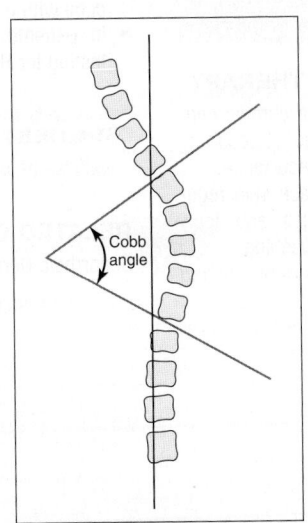

FIG. 3 Cobb angle. This is measured using the superior and inferior end plates of the most tilted vertebrae at the end of each curve. (From Tschudy MM, Arcara KM: *The Harriet Lane handbook,* ed 19, Philadelphia, 2012, Mosby.)

improve the curvature, but is mainly used to stabilize and prevent progression.
• The initial Cobb angle magnitude (≥25 degrees) is the most important predictor of long-term curve progression.

SUGGESTED READINGS
Available at www.expertconsult.com

RELATED CONTENT
Scoliosis (Patient Information)

AUTHOR: **GREGORY ELIA, M.D.**

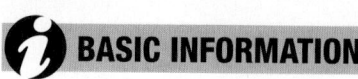

BASIC INFORMATION

DEFINITION

Seborrheic dermatitis (SD) is a common, inflammatory skin condition characterized by a mild to severe rash with scaling and erythema that occurs in areas of the skin rich in sebaceous glands.

SYNONYMS

SD
Dandruff
Cradle cap (Fig. E1)
Sebopsoriasis
Seborrheic eczema
Pityriasis capitis
Seborrhea

ICD-10CM CODES
L21.9 Seborrheic dermatitis, unspecified
L21.1 Seborrheic infantile dermatitis
L21.8 Other seborrheic dermatitis

EPIDEMIOLOGY & DEMOGRAPHICS

PREVALENCE: Affects 3% to 5% of otherwise healthy adults
PREDOMINANT SEX AND AGE: Can occur from infancy through old age, with peak incidence in adolescents and young adults and increasing again after age 50 yr. More common in men than women.
RISK FACTORS: More common in patients with HIV/AIDS, Parkinson's disease, other neurologic disorders, mood disorders, chronic alcoholic pancreatitis, hepatitis, cancer, and genetic disorders (e.g., Down syndrome). Occurs more often during winter season.

PHYSICAL FINDINGS & CLINICAL PRESENTATION

- Mild, greasy scaling of the scalp and nasolabial folds (Fig. 2); postauricular skin, beard area, eyebrows, trunk, and sometimes the central face. Blepharitis, otitis externa, and coexisting acne vulgaris or pityriasis may also be present. Itching and stinging of lesions can occur. Increased occurrence during times of stress or sleep deprivation.
- The scale often has a yellow, greasy appearance.

ETIOLOGY

- Fungal infections of the *Malassezia* species have been associated with SD, and the skin changes are thought to result from an inflammatory response to Malassezia yeast.
- Altered immune function may play a role. Patients with SD may show upregulation of

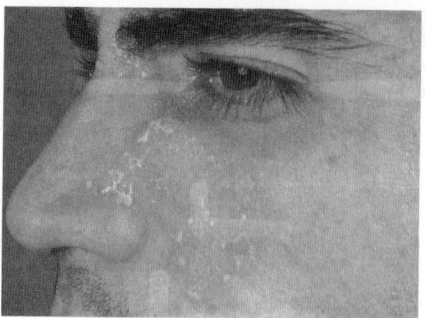

FIG. 2 **Seborrheic dermatitis.** (From Swartz MH: *Textbook of physical diagnosis,* ed 7, Philadelphia, 2014, Saunders, 2014.)

interferon (IFN)-α, expressed interleukin-6 (IL-6), expressed IL-1β, and IL-4.

DIAGNOSIS

DIFFERENTIAL DIAGNOSIS

- Atopic dermatitis.
- Candidiasis.
- Dermatophytosis.
- Impetigo.
- Psoriasis.
- Rosacea.
- Systemic lupus erythematosus.
- Tinea infection.
- Contact dermatitis.
- Nummular dermatitis.

WORKUP

- Diagnosis usually based on clinical identification of lesions.
- Skin biopsies can be performed, if warranted, to distinguish SD from similar disorders.

LABORATORY TESTS

- Microscopic examination with special stains can be used to determine whether yeast cells are present in keratinocytes.
- HIV testing.

TREATMENT

NONPHARMACOLOGIC THERAPY

- Patient education that SD is a chronic condition and treatment is aimed at resolving lesions but does not prevent recurrence.
- General recommendations: wash skin regularly, soften and remove scales, and apply moisturizing emollients after washing.
- Scale removal can be accomplished through the application of mineral or olive oil and removed with a comb or brush after 1 hr.

ACUTE GENERAL Rx

- Topical steroids: can be in the form of shampoos, creams, or ointments. Can be used alone or in more severe SD with antifungals.
- Antifungals (e.g., Nizoral, selenium sulfide, ketoconazole [the most evidence for effectiveness among antifungals], ciclopirox, fluconazole). Reserve oral antifungal therapy for patients with widespread SD or SD that is refractory to topical therapy. Itraconazole 200 mg/day for 7 days is a sample oral regimen.
- Calcineurin inhibitors (e.g., tacrolimus ointment, pimecrolimus cream): good when face and ears are affected.
- Keratolytics (e.g., tar, salicylic acid, zinc pyrithione).
- Treatment of any secondary bacterial infection with oral antibiotics.

CHRONIC Rx

Recalcitrant SD: topical azole combined with desonide regimen (limit use to 2 wk), pimecrolimus cream.

COMPLEMENTARY & ALTERNATIVE MEDICINE

Tea tree oil (melaleuca oil).

REFERRAL

Consider referral to dermatology for recalcitrant cases or uncertain diagnosis

PEARLS & CONSIDERATIONS

- Use a combination of topical steroids and antifungal cream for severe SD.
- Limit use of steroids to 2-wk course of treatment due to risk of cutaneous atrophy and telangiectasias.
- SD of the scalp can be treated with an antifungal (e.g., 2% ketoconazole) or keratolytic shampoo. Limit use of antifungal shampoos to twice a week to prevent drying of the scalp. Alternate the use of antifungal shampoos with a moisturizing shampoo.
- In patients with widespread SD, consider testing for HIV infection.

SUGGESTED READINGS
Available at www.expertconsult.com

RELATED CONTENT
Seborrheic Dermatitis (Patient Information)

AUTHOR: **ANNGENE ANTHONY, M.D., M.P.H.**

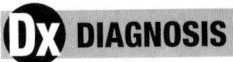

BASIC INFORMATION

DEFINITION

Absence seizures are a type of generalized seizures, characterized by brief episodes of staring with impairment of consciousness (absence). They usually last a few seconds, up to 20 to 30 sec. The onset and the end of the seizures are sudden. Usually the patients are not aware of them and resume the activity they were doing before the seizure. The electroencephalogram signature of absence seizures consists of a generalized 3-Hz spike and slow wave discharges.

SYNONYMS

Childhood absence epilepsy
Petit mal epilepsy
Absence seizures

ICD-10CM CODES
G40.309 Generalized idiopathic epilepsy and epileptic syndromes, not intractable, without status epilepticus
G40.009 Localization-related (focal) (partial) idiopathic epilepsy and epileptic syndromes with seizures of localized onset, not intractable, without status epilepticus
G40.019 Localization-related (focal) (partial) idiopathic epilepsy and epileptic syndromes with seizures of localized onset, intractable, without status epilepticus
G40.109 Localization-related (focal) (partial) symptomatic epilepsy and epileptic syndromes with simple partial seizures, not intractable, without status epilepticus
G40.119 Localization-related (focal) (partial) symptomatic epilepsy and epileptic syndromes with simple partial seizures, intractable, without status epilepticus
G40.209 Localization-related (focal) (partial) symptomatic epilepsy and epileptic syndromes with complex partial seizures, not intractable, without status epilepticus
G40.219 Localization-related (focal) (partial) symptomatic epilepsy and epileptic syndromes with complex partial seizures, intractable, without status epilepticus

EPIDEMIOLOGY & DEMOGRAPHICS

INCIDENCE: 1 to 10 cases per 100,000 population.
PEAK INCIDENCE: 6 to 7 yr.
PREVALENCE: Represents up to 18% of all pediatric epilepsy syndromes.
PREDOMINANT SEX AND AGE: More common in girls than in boys, absences typically begin between 4 and 8 yr.

PHYSICAL FINDINGS & CLINICAL PRESENTATION

- Patients with absence seizures usually have normal physical and neurologic examinations.
- During the seizures, the patients are unresponsive and can have motor phenomena (automatisms, eye blinks, mouth and hand movements).
- Absence seizures are not associated with postictal confusion.
- They may be triggered by hyperventilation associated with activity.
- Tonic clonic seizures are not usually a feature of this syndrome. If this is the case, other etiologies should be investigated, such as juvenile absence epilepsy, juvenile myoclonic epilepsy, complex partial seizures, etc.

ETIOLOGY

Genetic.

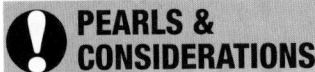 DIAGNOSIS

DIFFERENTIAL DIAGNOSIS

- Juvenile absence epilepsy.
- Juvenile myoclonic epilepsy.
- Complex partial seizures.
- Nonepileptic spells comprised of staring.

WORKUP

- EEG with hyperventilation and photic stimulation is crucial in the diagnosis.
- Ambulatory EEG and video EEG are recommended for patients with diagnostic uncertainty.

LABORATORY TESTS

No specific studies needed.

IMAGING STUDIES

- MRI of the brain should be performed in all epilepsy patients, especially if the EEG does not show the typical characteristic of absence seizures (3-Hz spike and slow wave discharges).
- CT scans of the head should be avoided in children due to unnecessary exposure to radiation and low yield of the test except when MRI cannot be obtained.

TREATMENT

The medication of choice based on the best current evidence available is ethosuximide, followed by valproic acid and lamotrigine.

NONPHARMACOLOGIC THERAPY

Not applicable.

GENERAL Rx

- Ethosuximide: initial dose: 10 mg/kg/day; then after 7 days, 20 mg/kg.
- Valproic acid (Depakote): initial dose: 5 to 10 mg/kg/day (divided bid), maximum dose 60 mg/kg/day
- Lamotrigine: dose for patients on no other antiepileptic drugs. Wk 1 and 2: 0.3 mg/kg/day. Wk 3 and 4: 0.6 mg/kg/day. Wk 5 onward: increase every 1 to 2 wk by 0.6 mg/kg/day. Maintenance: 4.5 to 7.5 mg/kg/day. Warning: should be used with caution due to the potential

for toxicity and Stevens-Johnson syndrome. Patients on other antiepileptic drugs can also have severe adverse reactions (e.g., valproic acid can cause increased levels of lamotrigine).

CHRONIC Rx

- Children with recurrent seizures require chronic treatment.
- If children are seizure free for a period of 1 to 2 yr, a trial on no medications should be considered; children, unlike adults, can "outgrow" seizures.

COMPLEMENTARY & ALTERNATIVE MEDICINE

Not applicable.

DISPOSITION

- Response to treatment is excellent.
- Absence seizures tend to remit in teenage years.
- Epilepsy can be considered as resolved once 10 years have elapsed since the last event, including 5 years free from medications.

REFERRAL

Patients with epilepsy and seizures should be referred for a consultation by a neurologist, preferably one specializing in epilepsy.

PEARLS & CONSIDERATIONS

COMMENTS

- Absence seizures can be present in other epilepsy syndromes.
- Valproic acid should be avoided in girls and women with childbearing potential due to the risk of teratogenicity.
- Carbamazepine and phenytoin should be avoided in the treatment of absence seizures, since these medications may worsen seizures and could provoke absence status epilepticus.
- All women of childbearing age taking antiepileptic drugs should take folic acid supplementation (1-4 mg/day) for the prevention of neural tube defects.

PREVENTION

Sleep deprivation and alcohol consumption should be avoided.

PATIENT & FAMILY EDUCATION

- Patients with ongoing seizures are forbidden to drive; check state regulations and laws regarding driving and epilepsy.

SUGGESTED READING

Available at www.expertconsult.com

RELATED CONTENT

Absence Seizures (Patient Information)

AUTHOR: **PATRICIO SEBASTIAN ESPINOSA, M.D., M.P.H.**

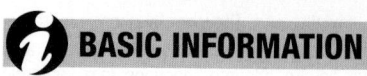

DEFINITION

Febrile seizures are seizures that occur in febrile children (fever of at least 100.4° F [38° C]) between the ages of 6 and 60 months in the absence of infection of the central nervous system (CNS), metabolic disturbance, or history of neonatal seizures or a previous unprovoked seizures. Febrile seizures are subdivided into 2 categories: simple and complex. Simple febrile seizures last <15 min, are generalized (without a focal component), and occur once in a 24-hr period, whereas complex febrile seizures are prolonged (>15 min), show focal neurologic signs, or occur more than once in 24 hr.

SYNONYMS

Febrile convulsions
Febrile seizures

ICD-10CM CODES
R56.0 Febrile convulsions

EPIDEMIOLOGY & DEMOGRAPHICS

INCIDENCE: Febrile seizures are the most common seizures of childhood. 2% to 5% of children will have a febrile seizure by age 60 mo. Simple febrile seizures represent 65% to 90% of febrile seizures.
PREDOMINANT SEX AND AGE: Slightly more common in boys than girls.
PEAK INCIDENCE: 6 to 60 mo
PREVALENCE: Represents up to 18% of all pediatric epilepsy syndromes

PHYSICAL FINDINGS & CLINICAL PRESENTATION

- Children with febrile seizures have normal physical and neurologic examinations.
- Viral illnesses are the predominant cause of febrile seizures.

ETIOLOGY

- Viral infections are a common cause of fever that triggers febrile seizures.
- Febrile seizures tend to occur in families. Although clear evidence exists for a genetic basis of febrile seizures, the mode of inheritance is unknown.
- Febrile seizures are likely multifactorial with genetic and environmental factors.

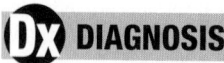 DIAGNOSIS

DIFFERENTIAL DIAGNOSIS

- CNS infection (i.e., meningitis).
- Epilepsy.

WORKUP

- It is important to first investigate whether an underlying infection exists. Fig. 1 describes guidelines for febrile seizure evaluation.
- In patients with simple self-limited febrile seizures with rapid return to consciousness and a normal neurologic examination, further workup is not routinely recommended.
- In patients with complex febrile seizures, laboratory workup and brain imaging are recommended.
- EEG is not routinely recommended in the evaluation of a neurologically healthy child with simple partial seizures.

LABORATORY TESTS

- Routine blood workup (CBC with differential, CMP, electrolytes), blood and urine cultures are often performed, but there is no evidence that these tests are necessary for identifying the cause of a simple febrile seizure.
- CSF analysis: lumbar puncture guidelines (American Academy of Pediatrics).
- Lumbar puncture should be performed in children with febrile seizures and signs and symptoms of meningitis (e.g., neck stiffness, Kernig sign, Brudzinski sign), or if the patient history or examination suggests the presence of meningitis or intracranial infection.
- In infants 6 to 12 months of age with febrile seizures, lumbar puncture is an option if they have not received the recommended *Haemophilus influenza* type b (Hib) or pneumococcal vaccinations, or if their immunization status is unknown.
- Lumbar puncture is also considered an option in children with febrile seizures pretreated with antibiotics.

IMAGING STUDIES

- MRI of the brain is not required in the routine evaluation of patients with simple febrile seizures.
- Imaging of the brain should be considered in children with complex febrile seizures and in children with focal neurologic deficits.
- CT scans of the head should be avoided in children, if possible, due to exposure to radiation and the relative low yield of the test compared with MRI. CT scans of the head are reserved for neurologic emergencies and are adjusted for weight in children.

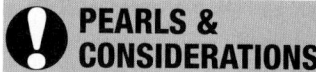 TREATMENT

Febrile seizures do not usually require antiepileptic drug treatment.

NONPHARMACOLOGIC THERAPY

Not applicable

GENERAL Rx

Symptomatic treatment of fever.

CHRONIC Rx

No chronic treatment for febrile seizures is recommended.

COMPLEMENTARY & ALTERNATIVE MEDICINE

Not applicable.

DISPOSITION

- Treatment is not recommended.
- Febrile seizures should stop by age 60 months.
- Risk of recurrence in the first 2 years after an initial febrile seizure is 15% to 70%.

REFERRAL

Patients with recurrent febrile seizures need to be referred for a consultation by a pediatric neurologist.

PEARLS & CONSIDERATIONS

COMMENTS

- It is crucial to find out the etiology of the fever and to treat it appropriately.
- Patient with seizures and fever after age 60 mo are not classified as febrile seizures.

PREVENTION

Antipyretics do not reduce the recurrence risk of febrile seizures. However, fever should be treated and worked up independently of the diagnosis of febrile seizures.

PATIENT & FAMILY EDUCATION

- Children with febrile seizures do not need antiepileptic drug treatment.
- Patient education and information can be obtained at the Epilepsy Foundation: www.epilepsyfoundation.org. Parents should be reassured that children without underlying developmental problems will usually not have lasting neurologic effects from febrile seizures.

SUGGESTED READINGS
Available at www.expertconsult.com

RELATED CONTENT
Fever Seizures (Patient Information)

AUTHOR: **PATRICIO SEBASTIAN ESPINOSA, M.D., M.P.H.**

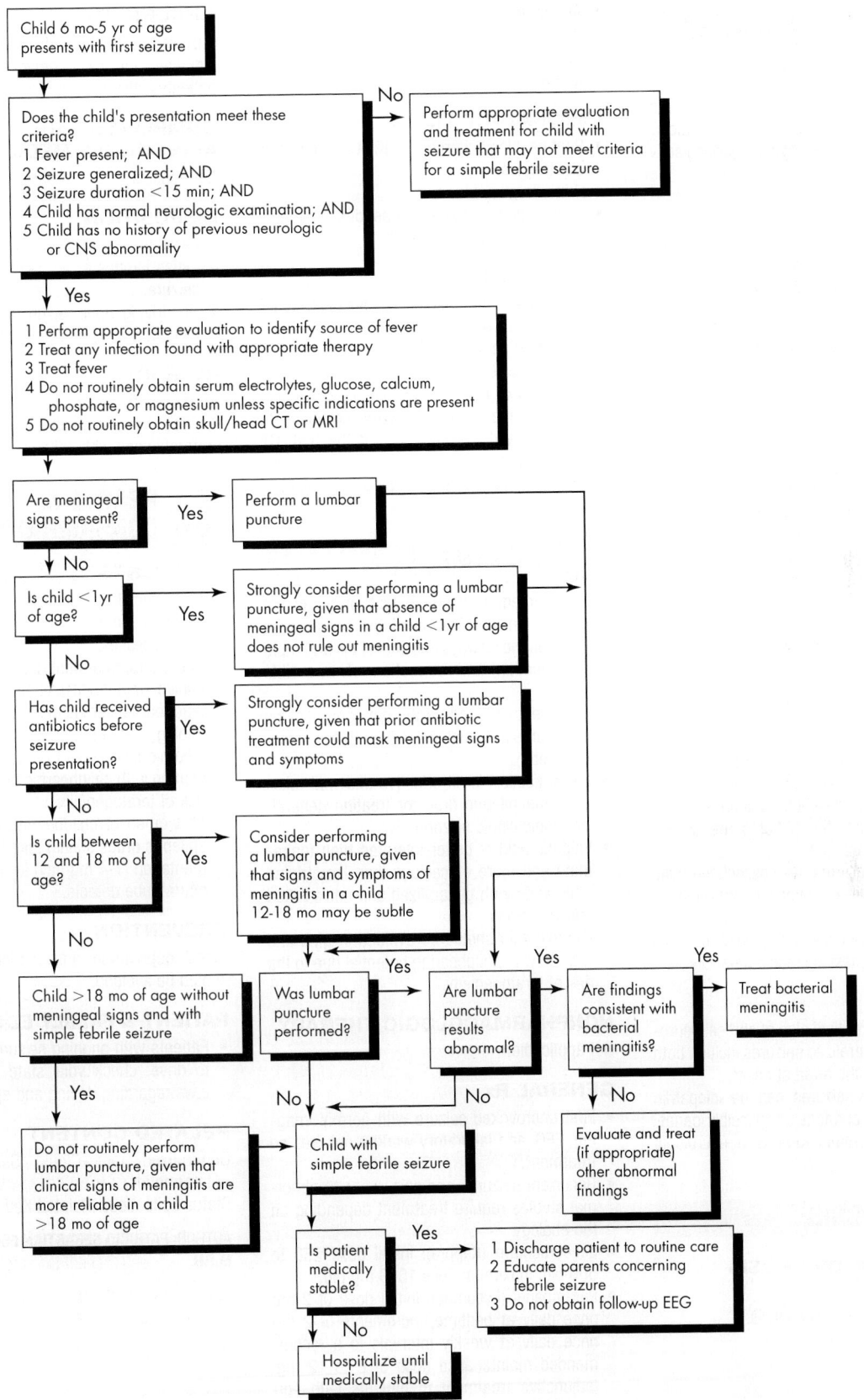

FIG. 1 Guidelines for febrile seizure evaluation. (From Custer JW, Rau RE: *The Harriet Lane handbook,*
ed 18, St Louis, 2009, Mosby.)

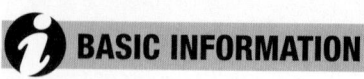

DEFINITION

Tonic clonic seizures are characterized by sudden loss of consciousness, muscle contraction (tonic phase) followed by rhythmic jerking activity (clonic phase).

SYNONYMS

Convulsive seizures
Grand mal seizures
Generalized tonic clonic seizures

ICD-10CM CODES

G40.6 Grand mal seizures, unspecified
G41.0 Grand mal status epilepticus

EPIDEMIOLOGY & DEMOGRAPHICS

INCIDENCE: 30 to 50 cases per 100,000 person-yr (epilepsy incidence).
PEAK INCIDENCE: Not applicable.
PREVALENCE: 5 to 8 cases per 1000 persons (epilepsy incidence).
PREDOMINANT SEX AND AGE: No gender preference.

PHYSICAL FINDINGS & CLINICAL PRESENTATION

- Patients with tonic clonic seizures usually have normal physical and neurologic examinations.
- During the seizures, the patients are unresponsive and can have violent postures with severe repetitive muscle contractions.
- After the seizure, the patients are usually lethargic and confused.
- Tonic clonic seizures are associated with injuries, bladder incontinence, and tongue biting.
- Focal postictal weakness may point toward a focal neurologic lesion (Todd's paralysis).

ETIOLOGY

- Seizures are a cardinal sign of cortical neurologic injury. Generalized seizures include both hemispheres of the brain at onset.
- The etiology of seizures can be idiopathic (likely genetic), cryptogenic (possibly genetic), and symptomatic (due to a neurologic injury/infection).

DIAGNOSIS

DIFFERENTIAL DIAGNOSIS

- Convulsive syncope.
- Psychogenic nonepileptic spells.
- EPI
- TIA
- Vertigo

WORKUP

- EEG. An EEG can help confirm the presence of epilepsy but cannot be used to exclude the diagnosis.

- Ambulatory EEG and/or video EEG recommended for patients with diagnostic uncertainty.
- MRI of the brain.

LABORATORY TESTS

- Routine blood workup (CBC, CMP, glucose, electrolytes).
- Urine drug screen.
- Lumbar puncture is recommended in patients with suspicion of meningitis.

IMAGING STUDIES

- Neurodiagnostic imaging studies such as CT of the head or, preferably, MRI of the brain should be performed in all patients with first unprovoked seizure.
- CT scans of the head should be avoided in children due to unnecessary exposure to radiation and the low yield of the test. CT scans of the head are reserved for neurologic emergencies and are adjusted for weight in children.

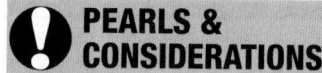

- The immediate management of a seizure focuses on stabilization of the patient with focus on the airways and vital signs and rapid identification and correction of reversible causes.
- Treatment is based on the type and etiology of seizures (i.e., metabolic disturbance, infectious, etc.).
- Levetiracetam is an effective and well-tolerated antiepileptic drug for treating generalized tonic clonic seizures.
- Valproic acid is better tolerated than topiramate and more efficacious than lamotrigine in patients with generalized and unclassified epilepsy types.
- Valproic acid should be avoided in girls and women with childbearing potential due to the risk of teratogenicity.

NONPHARMACOLOGIC THERAPY

Not applicable.

GENERAL Rx

- First unprovoked seizure with normal imaging, EEG, and laboratory workup requires no treatment.
- Recurrent seizures and seizures with abnormal studies require treatment depending on the etiology.
- Levetiracetam (Keppra): Initial dose 250 to 500 bid, maximum dose 1500 mg bid.
- Perampanel (Fycompa): Initial dose of 2 mg once daily at bedtime, increments of 2 mg once daily at weekly intervals to a recommended maintenance dose of 8 to 12 mg. (adjunctive treatment in patients with epilepsy 12 years of age and older).
- Valproic acid (Depakote): Initial dose: 10 to 15 mg/kg/day (divided bid), maximum dose 60 mg/kg/day.

CHRONIC Rx

Chronic treatment with antiepileptic drugs is indicated for ≥2 unprovoked seizures or in patients with one seizure with abnormal workup.

COMPLEMENTARY & ALTERNATIVE MEDICINE

Not applicable.

DISPOSITION

- Patients should avoid situations that may cause injuries or accidents in the event of a seizure.
- No driving until seizure-free in accordance with local laws and regulations.

REFERRAL

Patients with epilepsy and seizures should be referred for a consultation by a neurologist, preferably one with epilepsy training.

PEARLS & CONSIDERATIONS

COMMENTS

- It is crucial to understand that tonic clonic seizures can occur in variety of acute neurologic diseases.
- Successful treatment depends on the correct choice of antiepileptic drugs based on the type (partial versus generalized in onset) and etiology of the seizures.
- Valproic acid should be avoided in girls and women with childbearing potential due to the risk of teratogenicity.
- All women of childbearing age taking antiepileptic drugs should take folic acid supplementation (1-4 mg/day) for the prevention of neural tube defects.

PREVENTION

Sleep deprivation and alcohol consumption should be avoided.

PATIENT & FAMILY EDUCATION

- Patients with ongoing seizures are forbidden to drive; check your state regulations and laws regarding driving and epilepsy.

RELATED CONTENT

Generalized Tonic-Clonic Seizures (Patient Information)
Status Epilepticus (Related Key Topic)

AUTHOR: **PATRICIO SEBASTIAN ESPINOSA, M.D., M.P.H.**

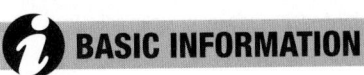

BASIC INFORMATION

DEFINITION

Partial seizures are characterized by focal cortical discharges that provoke seizure symptoms related to the area of the brain involved. Simple partial seizures do not cause impairment of consciousness. However, partial seizures can evolve into complex partial and/or tonic clonic seizures.

SYNONYMS

Simple partial seizures
Focal seizures
Partial seizures

ICD-10CM CODES
G40.0 Localization-related (focal) (partial) idiopathic epilepsy and epileptic syndromes with seizures of localized onset
G40.109 Localization-related (focal) (partial) symptomatic epilepsy and epileptic syndromes with simple partial seizures, not intractable, without status epilepticus

EPIDEMIOLOGY & DEMOGRAPHICS

INCIDENCE: 30 to 50 cases per 100,000 person-yr
PREVALENCE: 5 to 8 cases per 1000 persons
PREDOMINANT SEX AND AGE: No gender preference

PHYSICAL FINDINGS & CLINICAL PRESENTATION

- Patients with partial seizures usually have normal physical and neurologic examinations unless the focal seizures are due to a structural abnormality such as a stroke, where the patient will have a neurologic exam consistent with the area of CNS structural damage.
- During partial seizures the patients are conscious, unless there is spread of the epileptic focus causing secondary generalization and unresponsiveness. A focal seizure can evolve to a generalized tonic clonic seizure. Clues to this progression include a subjective aura before the onset of convulsion, unilateral shaking, and head turning to one side (versive head turning).
- Patients with partial seizures can experience postictal weakness/paralysis that usually resolves within 24 hr (Todd's paralysis). However, focal neurologic deficits may also be indicative of a structural brain lesion.
- Manifestations of complex partial seizures may include automatisms (semipurposeful behaviors) such as fumbling of fingers or lip smacking.

ETIOLOGY

- Seizures in general are a cardinal sign of cortical neurologic injury.
- The etiology of partial seizures can be idiopathic (likely genetic), cryptogenic (unknown, possibly genetic), and symptomatic (due to a neurologic injury).
- Frequent causes of partial seizures are tumor, stroke, CNS infections (cysticercosis, abscesses), arteriovenous malformations (AVMs), traumatic brain injury, cortical malformations, and others.

DIAGNOSIS

DIFFERENTIAL DIAGNOSIS

- Transient ischemic attack.
- Movement disorders.
- Psychogenic nonepileptic spells.
- Migraines.

WORKUP

- EEG. Ambulatory EEG and/or video EEG recommended for patients with diagnostic uncertainty.

LABORATORY TESTS

Routine blood workup (CBC, CMP, glucose, electrolytes) may be considered in appropriate clinical situations.

IMAGING STUDIES

- In the acute setting, a CT scan of the head is high yield to rule out space-occupying lesions.
- MRI of the brain with a defined epilepsy protocol should be performed in all patients with recurrent seizures.

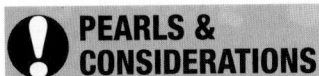

TREATMENT

- Carbamazepine traditionally has been the standard initial drug treatment for partial seizures. However, newer antiepileptic drugs have better side effect profiles.
- Eslicarbazepine is indicated for the treatment of partial-onset seizures as monotherapy or adjunctive therapy. The recommended initial dose of eslicarbazepine is 400 mg once daily. For some patients, treatment may be initiated at 800 mg once daily if the need for seizure reduction outweighs an increased risk of adverse reactions. Increase the dose in weekly increments of 200 mg, based on clinical response and tolerability, to a recommended maintenance dose of 800 to 1600 mg once daily.
- Lacosamide is indicated as monotherapy or adjunctive therapy in patients with partial-onset seizures. The initial recommended dose is 50 mg twice daily; increase at weekly intervals by 50 mg twice daily, up to a recommended maintenance dose of 100 to 200 mg twice daily. An alternate loading dose schedule: 200 mg PO/IV as a single dose, followed 12 hr later by starting 100 mg PO/IV bid × 1 week; then increase dose at weekly intervals by 50 mg bid, up to a recommended dose of 150 to 200 mg bid.
- Lamotrigine and levetiracetam are effective and well-tolerated antiepileptic drugs for treating partial seizures.
- Other antiepileptic drugs (e.g., perampanel, oxcarbazepine, ezogabine) may be used by an epilepsy specialist in specific cases.
- Surgical treatments (e.g., temporal lobectomy in mesial temporal sclerosis) may be indicated in refractory cases of partial seizures.

GENERAL Rx

- After a first unprovoked seizure with normal examination, imaging, and EEG, no treatment may be necessary.
- Recurrent seizures and seizures with abnormal studies require treatment in the form of medicines, consideration of surgery, or with approved medical devices.

DISPOSITION

- Response to treatment often depends on the etiology of the partial seizures.
- 47% of patients become seizure free with monotherapy and 67% with polytherapy.
- Patients who do not respond to three drugs should be referred to an Epilepsy Center for consideration of surgical treatment.
- No driving until seizure free in accordance with local laws and regulations.

REFERRAL

Patients with epilepsy and seizures should be referred for a consultation by a neurologist, preferably one with a special interest in epilepsy.

PEARLS & CONSIDERATIONS

COMMENTS

- Successful treatment depends on the correct choice of antiepileptic drugs based on patient's gender and comorbidities.
- Valproic acid should be avoided in girls and women with childbearing potential due to the risk of teratogenicity.
- All women in childbearing age taking antiepileptic drugs should take folic acid supplementation (1-4 mg/day) for the prevention of neural tube defects.

PREVENTION

- Sleep deprivation and alcohol consumption should be avoided.
- Drug compliance is compulsory to prevent seizure recurrence.

PATIENT & FAMILY EDUCATION

- Patient education and information can be obtained at the Epilepsy Foundation: www.epilepsyfoundation.org.
- Patients should be counseled on general seizure precautions such as swimming, bathing, and heights.

RELATED CONTENT

Partial Motor Seizures (Patient Information)

AUTHOR: **PATRICIO SEBASTIAN ESPINOSA, M.D., M.P.H.**

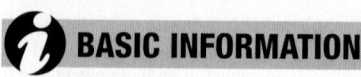

BASIC INFORMATION

DEFINITION

Sepsis is an exaggerated inflammatory response to an infectious stimulus. It is generally caused by generalized bacterial or fungal infection and characterized by evidence of infection, fever or hypothermia, hypotension, and evidence of end-organ compromise. The Sepsis Definitions Task Force has recently updated definitions for sepsis and septic shock. A major change in the new definitions is the elimination of mention of SIRS*. According to the new definitions, sepsis is now defined as evidence of infection plus life-threatening organ dysfunction, clinically characterized by an acute change in 2 points or greater in the SOFA score**. The new clinical criteria for septic shock include sepsis with fluid, unresponsive hypotension, serum lactate level greater than 2 mmol/L, and the need for vasopressors to maintain mean arterial pressure of 65 mm Hg or greater.[1,2]

SYNONYMS

Septicemia
Sepsis syndrome
Severe sepsis
Systemic inflammatory response syndrome
Septic shock

ICD-10CM CODES
A41.9   Sepsis, unspecified organism
A41.50 Gram-negative sepsis, unspecified

---

*SIRS (Systemic Inflammatory Response Syndrome): Variables in SIRS criteria include respiratory rate (breaths/min), white blood cell count (10^9/L), hands (%), heart rate (beats/min), temperature (°C), and arterial carbon dioxide tension (mm Hg). Score range is 0-4.

**SOFA (Sequential [Sepsis-Related] Organ Failure Assessment): Variables in SOFA criteria include PaO_2/FIO_2 ratio, Glasgow Coma Scale score, mean arterial pressure (mm Hg), administration of vasopressors with type/dose/rate of infusion, serum creatinine (mg/dL) or urine output (mL/d), bilirubin (mg/dL), and platelet count (10^9/L). Score range is 0-24.

[1]Abraham E: New definitions for sepsis and septic shock: continuing evolution but with much still to be done, *JAMA* 315(8):757-759, 2016.
[2]Shankar-Hari M, et al.: Developing a new definition and assessing new clinical criteria for septic shock: for the Third International Consensus Definitions for Sepsis and Septic Shock (Sepsis-3), *JAMA* 315(8):775-787, 2016.

A41.2	Sepsis due to unspecified *Staphylococcus*
A41.4	Sepsis due to anaerobes
A41.51	Sepsis due to *Escherichia coli* [E. coli]
A41.52	Sepsis due to Pseudomonas
A54.86	Gonococcal sepsis
B37.7	Candidal sepsis
A32.7	Listerial sepsis
A40.0	Sepsis due to streptococcus, group A
A40.1	Sepsis due to streptococcus, group B
A40.3	Sepsis due to Streptococcus pneumoniae
A40.8	Other streptococcal sepsis
A40.9	Streptococcal sepsis, unspecified
A41.01	Sepsis due to Methicillin susceptible *Staphylococcus aureus*
A41.02	Sepsis due to Methicillin resistant *Staphylococcus aureus*

EPIDEMIOLOGY & DEMOGRAPHICS

INCIDENCE (IN U.S.):
- Exact incidence is unknown.
- More than 1 million cases sepsis occur each year in the U.S.

PREDOMINANT SEX: Males slightly more commonly affected than females.

PREDOMINANT AGE:
- Neonatal period.
- Patients >65 yr of age account for 60% of all cases of sepsis.

GENETICS:
- Familial disposition: a great variety of congenital immunodeficiency states and other inherited disorders may predispose to septicemia.
- Neonatal infection: incidence is high in neonatal period.

PHYSICAL FINDINGS & CLINICAL PRESENTATION

- Fever or hypothermia.
- Hypotension.
- Tachycardia.
- Tachypnea.
- Altered mental status.
- Bleeding diathesis.
- Skin rashes.
- Symptoms that reflect primary site of infection: urinary tract, GI tract, CNS, respiratory tract.

- Table 1 describes some clinical signs and symptoms of sepsis.

ETIOLOGY

- Disseminated infection with a great variety of bacteria:
  - A. Gram-negative bacteria.
    1. *Escherichia coli.*
    2. *Klebsiella spp.*
    3. *Pseudomonas aeruginosa.*
    4. *Proteus spp.*
    5. *Neisseria meningitides.*
  - B. Gram-positive bacteria.
    1. *Staphylococcus aureus (including MRSA).*
    2. *Streptococcus spp.*
    3. *Enterococcus* spp.
- Less common infections:
  1. Fungal.
  2. Viral.
  3. Rickettsial.
  4. Parasitic.
- Sepsis is a complex dysregulation of both inflammation and coagulation. There is activation of coagulation, inflammatory cytokines, complement, and kinin cascades with release of a variety of vasoactive endogenous mediators.
- Predisposing host factors:
  1. General medical condition.
  2. Extremes of age.
  3. Immunosuppressive therapy.
  4. Recent surgery.
  5. Granulocytopenia.
  6. Hyposplenism.
  7. Diabetes.
  8. Instrumentation.

Dx DIAGNOSIS

DIFFERENTIAL DIAGNOSIS

- Cardiogenic shock.
- Acute pancreatitis.
- Pulmonary embolism.
- Systemic vasculitis.
- Toxic ingestion.
- Exposure-induced hypothermia.
- Fulminant hepatic failure.
- Collagen-vascular diseases.

TABLE 1   Clinical Signs and Symptoms of Sepsis

Infection	General	Inflammatory	Hemodynamic	Tissue Perfusion
Documented or suspected	Temperature >38°C or <36°C Heart rate >90 beats/min Respiratory rate ≥20 breaths/min Altered mental status Hyperglycemia Third spacing of fluid	WBC count <4000 or >12,000 cells/mcL or ≥10% bands	Hypotension: systolic blood pressure <90 mm Hg MAP <70 mm Hg SVo_2 >70 CI >3.5 L/min/m²	Hypoxemia: (Pao_2/Fio_2 <300) Acute oliguria (urine output <0.5 mL/kg/hr) Coagulopathy Abnormal liver function tests Platelet count <100,000 cells/μL Lactic acidosis Skin mottling

CI, Cardiac index; *MAP,* mean arterial pressure; *SVo₂,* mixed venous oxygen saturation; *WBC,* white blood cell.
From Cameron JL, Cameron AM: *Current surgical therapy,* ed 10, Philadelphia, 2011, Saunders.

WORKUP

- Evaluation should focus on identifying a specific pathogen and localizing the site of primary infection.
- Hemodynamic, metabolic, coagulation disorders should be carefully characterized.
- Intensive monitoring.

LABORATORY TESTS

- Cultures of blood and examination and culture of sputum, urine, wound drainage, stool, and CSF, depending on the presenting signs and symptoms for each patient.
- CBC with differential, coagulation profile.
- Routine chemistries, LFTs.
- ABGs, lactic acid level; procalcitonin can be useful as a marker of bacterial infection as a cause of the sepsis.
- Urinalysis.

IMAGING STUDIES

- Chest x-ray.
- Other radiographic and radioisotope procedures according to suspected site of primary infection.

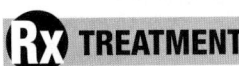 TREATMENT

NONPHARMACOLOGIC THERAPY

- Tissue oxygenation: mixed venous oxygen saturation maintained >70% if possible; early mechanical ventilation with low tidal volume (6 ml/kg predicted body weight) to protect lung parenchyma from overstretching and "volutrauma." Recommended plateau pressure for sepsis-related ARDS is ≤30 cm H_2O.
- Focal infection should be drained if possible, and potentially infected catheters should be removed.

ACUTE GENERAL Rx

- Blood pressure support, rapid IV fluid resuscitation and vasopressors, if needed, with the goal of reestablishing a mean arterial blood pressure >65 mm Hg; reduction in blood lactate and improved mixed venous oxygen saturation >70% within 6 hr of recognition of septic shock is associated with improved survival. If possible, measure vena cava oxygen saturation (ScvO₂) to assess adequacy of resuscitation. If the ScvO₂ is <70%, consider packed red blood cell transfusion to achieve Hct >30%. Start inotropic agents if ScvO₂ is <70% despite transfusion and adequate fluid resuscitation.
  1. IV hydration; crystalloids are as effective as colloids as resuscitation fluids. Use the fluid challenge technique to evaluate the effect (and safety) of fluid administration. For sepsis-induced hypoperfusion, give 30 ml/kg of IV crystalloids within 3 hours, with additional fluid based on frequent reassessment using dynamic variables (e.g., passive leg raise test or pulse or stroke volume variations induced by mechanical ventilation) rather than previous guidelines using target-specific

values of central venous pressure. Fluid administration should be discontinued when the response to fluids is no longer beneficial. Most patients need 4 to 6 L of fluid in the first 6 hours. Trials have shown that resuscitation with balanced crystalloids or albumin compared with other fluids seems to be associated with reduced mortality and that albumin replacement in addition to crystalloids alone does not improve the rate of survival at 28 and 90 days.
  2. Therapy with vasopressors if mean arterial blood pressure of >65 mm Hg cannot be maintained by hydration alone. Use norepinephrine as a first-choice vasopressor and target a mean arterial pressure (MAP) of 65 mm Hg.
- Correction of acidosis by improving the tissue perfusion, not by giving bicarbonate
  1. Mechanical ventilation as needed.
- Antibiotics:
  1. Directed at the most likely sources of infection. Table 2 describes initial antibiotic recommendations for septic patients.
  2. Should generally provide broad coverage of gram-positive and gram-negative bacteria (or fungi if clinically indicated).
  3. Antibiotics should be administered within 1 hr of the diagnosis of septic shock—this is a medical emergency.
- The role of corticosteroids in the acute management of septicemia has long been debated. Previous trials had shown that corticosteroid therapy improved hemodynamic outcomes in patients with severe septic shock. Patients with relative adrenal insufficiency may benefit from low-dose therapy with hydrocortisone (200 mg IV by continuous infusion for 7 days). Recent trials, however, revealed that hydrocortisone did not improve survival or reversal of shock, either overall or in patients who did not have a response to corticotropin, although hydrocortisone hastened reversal of shock in patients in whom shock was reversed. Until definitive data are available, the decision to administer corticosteroids for septic shock should be based on the individual patient's severity of illness versus risk of corticosteroid administration. Current evidence and guidelines support limiting the use of IV hydrocortisone for patients with septic shock to these instances with fluid resuscitation and vasopressor therapy are inadequate to restore hemodynamic stability.[1] The corticotropin (ACTH) stimulation test is not helpful and should not be used to determine the need for corticosteroid in these patients.
- Blood transfusion: A lower hemoglobin threshold is preferred. Trials have shown that among patients with septic shock, mortality at 90 days and rates of ischemic events and use of life support is similar among those assigned to blood transfusion at a higher

hemoglobin threshold (hemoglobin level of 9 g/dl or less) and those assigned to blood transfusion at a lower threshold (hemoglobin level of 7 g/dl or less).

CHRONIC Rx

- Adjust antibiotic therapy on the basis of culture results.
- In general, continue antibiotic therapy for a minimum of 7 to 10 days.
- Infection source control (e.g., removal of catheter/device suspected to be infected).
- If hyperglycemia develops during treatment start continuous insulin IV infusion, maintain blood glucose in the 110 to 180 mg/dl level, and avoid insulin-induced hypoglycemia.

DISPOSITION

- All patients with sepsis should be hospitalized and given access to intensive monitoring and nursing care.
- Among adults with suspected infection admitted to an ICU, an increase in SOFA score of 2 or more has greater prognostic accuracy for in-hospital mortality than SIRS criteria or the qSOFA score.[2]

REFERRAL

- To infectious diseases expert.
- To physician experienced in critical care.

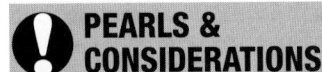 PEARLS & CONSIDERATIONS

COMMENTS

- Mortality rises quickly if antibiotic therapy is not instituted promptly (preferably within 1 hr of onset of shock) and metabolic derangements are not treated aggressively.
- Human recombinant activated protein C (drotrecogin alfa activated) was taken off the market as a treatment for sepsis after follow-up studies showed no added benefit to standard sepsis care.
- On October 1, 2015, the Centers for Medicare and Medicaid Services (CMS) and the Joint Commission (TJC) launched a Sepsis Core Measure for all 4000 TJC-accredited U.S. hospitals. Core measure performance is an integral part of ongoing TJC accreditation for hospitals, and core measure compliance on sepsis is publicly reported by CMS.

SUGGESTED READINGS

Available at www.expertconsult.com

AUTHORS: **GLENN G. FORT, M.D., M.P.H.,** and **FRED F. FERRI, M.D.**

[1]Yende S, Thompson T: Evaluating glucocorticoids for sepsis. Time to change course, *JAMA* 316(17):1769–1770, 2016.

[2]Raith EP, et al.: Prognostic accuracy of the SOFA score, SIRS criteria, and qSOFA score for in-hospital mortality among adults with suspected infection admitted to the intensive care unit, *JAMA* 310(3):290–300, 2016.

Diseases and Disorders

I

TABLE 2 Empirical Antibiotic Options for Patients With Severe Sepsis or Septic Shock

	Suspected Source				
	Lung	**Abdomen**	**Skin/Soft Tissue**	**Urinary Tract**	**Source Uncertain**
Major Community-Acquired Pathogens	*Streptococcus pneumoniae* *Haemophilus influenzae* *Legionella* *Chlamydia pneumoniae*	*Escherichia coli* *Bacteroides fragilis*	*Streptococcus pyogenes* *Staphylococcus aureus* Polymicrobial	*E. coli* *Klebsiella* species *Enterobacter* species *Proteus* spp. Enterococci	
Empirical Antibiotic Therapy	Moxifloxacin *or* levofloxacin *or* azithromycin *plus* cefotaxime *or* ceftazidime *or* cefepime *or* piperacillin-tazobactam	Imipenem *or* meropenem *or* doripenem *or* piperacillin-tazobactam ± aminoglycoside If biliary source: piperacillin-tazobactam, ampicillin-sulbactam, *or* ceftriaxone with metronidazole	Vancomycin *or* daptomycin *plus either* imipenem *or* meropenem *or* piperacillin-tazobactam; ± clindamycin (see text)	Ciprofloxacin *or* levofloxacin (if gram-positive cocci, use ampicillin *or* vancomycin ± gentamicin)	Vancomycin *plus either* doripenem *or* ertapenem *or* imipenem *or* meropenem
Major Commensal or Nosocomial Microorganisms	Aerobic gram-negative bacilli	Aerobic gram-negative rods Anaerobes *Candida* spp.	*Staphylococcus aureus* (? MRSA) Aerobic gram-negative rods	Aerobic gram-negative rods Enterococci	Consider MDRO if in area of high prevalence. Consider echinocandin if neutropenic or indwelling intravascular catheter
Empirical Antibiotic Therapy	Imipenem *or* meropenem *or* doripenem *or* cefepime (if *Acinetobacter baumannii* or carbapenem-resistant *Klebsiella* in ICU, add colistin)	Imipenem *or* meropenem ± aminoglycoside (consider echinocandin)	Vancomycin *or* daptomycin *plus* imipenem-cilastatin *or* meropenem *or* cefepime, ± clindamycin	Vancomycin *plus* imipenem *or* meropenem *or* cefepime	Cefepime *plus* vancomycin ± caspofungin

Dosages for intravenous administration (normal renal function):

*Imipenem-cilastatin, 0.5-1.0g q6-8h

*Meropenem, 1-2g q8h

*Doripenem, 0.5g q8h

Piperacillin-tazobactam, 3.375g q4h or 4.5g q6h

Vancomycin, load 25-30mg/kg, then 15-20 q8-12h

Cefepime, 1-2g q8h

Levofloxacin, 750mg q24h

Ciprofloxacin, 400mg q8-12h

Moxifloxacin, 400mg qd

Ceftriaxone, 2g q24h

Caspofungin, 70mg, followed by 50mg q24h

Colistin: loading dose = 5mg/kg body weight. For maintenance dosing, see University of California, Los Angeles Dosing Protocol: www.infectiousdiseases-ucla-affiliated.org/Intranet/FILES/ColistinDosing.pdf

ICU, Intensive care unit; *MDRO*, multidrug-resistant organisms; *MRSA*, methicillin-resistant *Staphylococcus aureus*.

For MDRO, resistance usually includes carbapenems.

* Carbapenems are less susceptible to extended-spectrum β-lactamases; base choice on local resistance pattern.

From Bennett JE et al: Mandell, Douglas, and Bennett*'s principles and practice of infectious diseases,* ed 8, Philadelphia, 2015, WB Saunders.

BASIC INFORMATION

DEFINITION

Septic arthritis is a highly destructive form of joint disease most often caused by hematogenous spread of organisms from a distant site of infection. Direct penetration of the joint as a result of trauma or surgery and spread from adjacent osteomyelitis may also cause bacterial arthritis. Any joint in the body may be affected.

SYNONYMS

Infectious arthritis
Bacterial arthritis
Pyogenic arthritis

ICD-10CM CODES
M00.9 Pyogenic arthritis, unspecified

EPIDEMIOLOGY & DEMOGRAPHICS

INCIDENCE (IN U.S.): Unknown.
PREVALENCE (IN U.S.): Unknown.
PREDOMINANT SEX: Gonococcal arthritis in females.
PREDOMINANT AGE: Gonococcal arthritis in sexually active adults.
PEAK INCIDENCE:
- Gonococcal arthritis: young adults.
- Other bacterial causes: all ages.

PHYSICAL FINDINGS & CLINICAL PRESENTATION

- Hallmark: acute onset of monoarticular joint pain, erythema, heat, and immobility.
- Limited range of motion of the joint.
- Effusion, with varying degrees of erythema and increased warmth around the joint.
- Single joint affected in 80% to 90% of cases of nongonococcal arthritis.
- Gonococcal dermatitis-arthritis syndrome.
  1. Typical pattern is a migratory polyarthritis or tenosynovitis.
  2. Small pustules on the trunk or extremities.
- Febrile patient at presentation.
- Most commonly affected joints in adult: knee and hip, but any joint may be involved; in children: hip.

ETIOLOGY

- Bacteria spread from another locus of infection.
  1. Highly vascular synovium is invaded by hematogenously spread bacteria.
  2. WBC enzymes cause necrosis of synovium, cartilage, and bone.
  3. Extensive joint destruction is rapid if infection is not treated with appropriate IV antibiotics and drainage of necrotic material.
- Predisposing factors: rheumatoid arthritis, prosthetic joints, advanced age, immunodeficiency (HIV, DM, immunosuppressive drugs), gout, sexual activity (gonococcal arthritis), skin infections, cutaneous ulcers (contiguous spread), recent joint surgery, recent

intraarticular infection. Fig. E1 illustrates routes by which bacteria can reach the joint.
- The most common nongonococcal organisms are staphylococci (40%), streptococci (28%), and gram-negative bacilli (19%). Less common are mycobacteria (8%), gram-negative cocci (3%), anaerobes (1%), and gram-positive bacilli (1%).
- Staphylococci (*S. aureus* and coagulase-negative staphylococcal species) account for >50% of prosthetic-hip and prosthetic-knee infections. *S. aureus* is very common in patients with rheumatoid arthritis.

DIAGNOSIS

DIFFERENTIAL DIAGNOSIS

- Gout.
- Pseudogout.
- Trauma.
- Hemarthrosis.
- Rheumatic fever.
- Adult or juvenile rheumatoid arthritis.
- Spondyloarthropathies such as reactive arthritis (Reiter's syndrome).
- Osteomyelitis.
- Viral arthritides.
- Septic bursitis.
- Lyme disease caused by *Borrelia burgdorferi.*

WORKUP

- Joint aspiration, Gram stain, and culture of the synovial fluid. Fig. 2 describes an algorithm for synovial fluid analysis in septic arthritis.
- Immediate arthrocentesis before other studies are undertaken or antibiotics instituted. Synovial fluid should be evaluated at bedside and then sent for lab evaluation.

LABORATORY TESTS

- Joint fluid analysis.
  1. Synovial fluid leukocyte count is usually elevated >50,000 cells/mm³ with > 80% polymorphonuclear cells.
  2. Counts are highly variable, with similar findings in gout, pseudogout, or rheumatoid arthritis. Lower WBC counts can occur in joint replacement, disseminated gonococcal disease, and peripheral leukopenia.
  3. Synovial fluid glucose or protein is not helpful because results are not specific for septic arthritis. The differential diagnosis of synovial fluid abnormalities is described in Section IV.
  4. PCR testing: useful for detection of uncommon organisms (e.g., Lyme disease).
  5. Crystal analysis: septic arthritis can coexist with crystal arthropathy; therefore, the presence of crystals does not preclude a diagnosis of septic arthritis.
- Blood cultures: positive in 25% to 50% of patients with septic arthritis.
- Culture of possible extraarticular sources of infection.
- Elevated peripheral WBC count, ESR (nonspecific), C-reactive protein (CRP) (nonspecific).

When elevated, ESR and CRP may be useful to monitor therapeutic response.
- If gonococcus is suspected, perform nucleic acid amplification tests (NAATs) on synovial fluid.

IMAGING STUDIES

- Radiograph of the affected joint (Fig. E3): useful to rule out osteomyelitis, fractures, chondrocalcinosis, or inflammatory arthritis.
- MRI: findings that suggest an acute intraarticular infection include the combination of bony erosions with marrow edema.
- CT scan: useful for early diagnosis of infections of the spine, hips, and sternoclavicular and sacroiliac joints.
- Ultrasound: can be useful for detecting effusions in joints that are more difficult to examine (e.g., hip).

TREATMENT

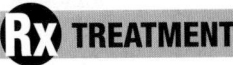

NONPHARMACOLOGIC THERAPY

- Affected joints aspirated daily to remove necrotic material and to follow serial WBC counts and cultures.
- If no resolution with IV antibiotics and closed drainage: open debridement and lavage, particularly in nongonococcal infections.
- Prevention of contractures:
  1. After acute stage of inflammation, range-of-motion exercises of the affected joint.
  2. Physical therapy helpful.

ACUTE GENERAL Rx

- IV antibiotics immediately after joint aspiration and Gram stain of the synovial fluid. Empiric antibiotic therapy (Table E1) is based on organism found on Gram stain of synovial fluid:
  1. Gram-positive cocci: vancomycin: 15 to 20 mg/kg IV q8 to 12h. Keep trough levels at 15 to 20 mcg/ml.
  2. Gram-negative cocci: ceftriaxone: 1 to 2 g IV q day in adults (children: 50 to 100 mg/kg IV q day).
  3. Gram-negative rods: ceftriaxone, cefepime: 1 to 2 g IV q8 to 12 h in adults (children: 100-150 mg/kg/day divided in q8h dosing), piperacillin-tazobactam: 4-5 g q6h. Aztreonam or fluoroquinolones can be used in patients with allergy to penicillin or cephalosporins.
  4. Negative Gram stain: vancomycin plus either cefepime or a carbapenem such as meropenem: 1 g IV q8h in adults (children: 60 mg/kg/day divided in q8h dosing) or ertapenem.

SUGGESTED READINGS
Available at www.expertconsult.com

RELATED CONTENT
Septic Arthritis (Patient Information)

AUTHOR: **GLENN G. FORT, M.D., M.P.H.**

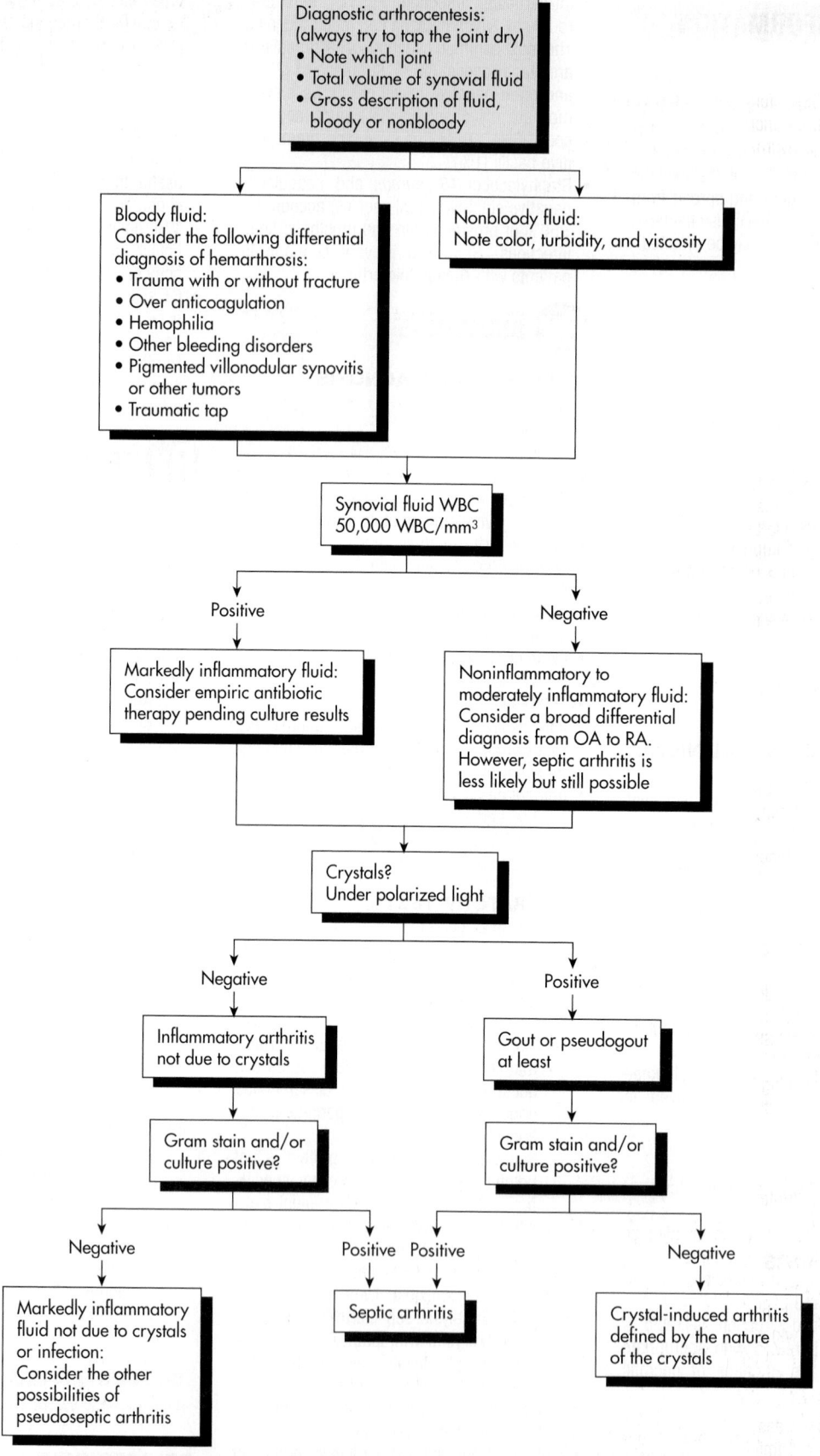

FIG. 2 Algorithm for synovial fluid analysis in septic arthritis. *OA*, osteoarthritis; *RA*, rheumatoid arthritis; *WBC*, white blood cell count. (From Harris ED et al: *Kelley's textbook of rheumatology*, ed 7, Philadelphia, 2005, Saunders.)

BASIC INFORMATION

DEFINITION

Serotonin syndrome (SS) refers to a group of symptoms resulting from increased concentrations of serotonin (5-hydroxytryptamine) in the CNS. SS is a drug-induced disorder that is classically characterized by a change in mental status and alteration in neuromuscular activity and autonomic function.

SYNONYMS

SS
Hyperserotonemia
Serotonergic syndrome
Serotonin toxicity

ICD-10CM CODES
Y49	Adverse effects due to psychotropic drugs
Y49.0	Adverse effects due to tricyclic and tetracyclic antidepressants
Y49.1	Adverse effects due to monoamine-oxidase-inhibitor antidepressants
Y49.2	Adverse effects due to other and unspecified antidepressants
Y49.3	Adverse effects due to phenothiazine antipsychotics and neuroleptics
G25.89	Other specified extrapyramidal and movement disorders

EPIDEMIOLOGY & DEMOGRAPHICS

- The incidence of SS is not known.
- SS is seen in all age groups.
- SS classically occurs in patients receiving two or more serotonergic drugs, but it can also occur with monotherapy—selective serotonin reuptake inhibitor (SSRI) monotherapy has an incidence of 0.5 to 0.9 cases of SS per 1000 patient-mo. Although there is an FDA alert, it has been argued that there is a lack of sufficient evidence showing that SSRIs and triptans cause serious SS.
- Concomitant use of an SSRI with a monoamine oxidase inhibitor (MAOI) poses the greatest risk of developing SS.
- Combination of SSRIs with other serotonergic drugs (e.g., tryptophan, illicit drugs like cocaine and MDMA, "Ecstasy") or drugs with serotonergic properties (e.g., methylene blue, lithium, meperidine, triptans, linezolid) may also lead to SS.

PHYSICAL FINDINGS & CLINICAL PRESENTATION

- Findings of clonus with hyperreflexia in the setting of recent (<5 wk) use of serotonergic agents strongly suggest the diagnosis of SS.
- Symptoms can manifest within minutes to hours after starting a new psychopharmacologic treatment, increasing the dose of a serotonergic drug, or administering a second serotonergic drug.
- Clonus (inducible, spontaneous, and ocular) is the key finding in establishing a diagnosis of SS.

- Classic triad of clinical features:
  1. Neuromuscular excitation: hyperreflexia, clonus, muscle rigidity, respiratory failure.
  2. Autonomic nervous system excitation: nausea/vomiting, diarrhea, hypertension, tachycardia, diaphoresis, fever >38° C (100° F), severe hyperthermia.
  3. Altered mental status: anxiety, agitation, confusion, coma.

ETIOLOGY

- Hyperstimulation of the brain stem and spinal cord serotonin receptors leading to the neuromuscular and autonomic symptoms.
- Psychopharmacologic drugs—in particular, fluoxetine and sertraline co-administered with MAOI (e.g., tranylcypromine and phenelzine)—have been cited as a common cause of SS. Triptans (serotonin-receptor agonists used in the treatment of migraines) may also precipitate the SS when used in combination with SSRIs and serotonin-norepinephrine reuptake inhibitors (SNRIs). Box 1 describes classes of medications that produce SS.

BOX 1 Classes of Medications That Produce Serotonin Syndrome in Psychiatric Patients

Selective serotonin reuptake inhibitors
Monoamine oxidase inhibitors
Atypical antipsychotics
Heterocyclic antidepressants
Trazodone
Dual-uptake inhibitors
Psychostimulants
Buspirone
Mood stabilizers
Analgesics
Antiemetics
Cough suppressants
Dietary supplements

From Goldman L, Schafer AI: *Goldman's Cecil medicine*, ed 24, Philadelphia, 2012, Saunders.

DIAGNOSIS

- SS is a clinical diagnosis. There are no specific laboratory tests for SS. A high index of suspicion along with a detailed medication history is the mainstay of diagnosis.
- Diagnostic criteria: most accurate is Hunter Serotonin Toxicity Criteria (sensitivity 84%, specificity 97%, confirmation by toxicologist). Sternbach's diagnostic criteria (Table 1) are also commonly used.
- To fulfill Hunter criteria a patient must have consumed a serotonergic drug and have one of the following:
  1. Spontaneous clonus.
  2. Inducible clonus plus agitation or diaphoresis.
  3. Ocular clonus plus agitation or diaphoresis.
  4. Tremor and hyperreflexia.
  5. Temperature >38° C (100° F) plus hypertonia plus ocular clonus or inducible clonus.

DIFFERENTIAL DIAGNOSIS

- Neuroleptic malignant syndrome (NMS), substance abuse (e.g., cocaine, amphetamines), anticholinergic toxicity, thyroid storm, infection (e.g., meningitis, encephalitis), alcohol and opioid withdrawal.
- Classic features in differentiation of NMS from SS are that SS develops over 24 hr, involves neuromuscular hyperactivity, and begins to resolve within 24 hr with appropriate therapy, whereas NMS develops gradually over days to weeks, involves sluggish neuromuscular response, and resolves over an average period of 1 wk to 10 days.

WORKUP

- Because SS is a clinical diagnosis, there is no laboratory test that confirms the diagnosis, and serum serotonin concentration does not correlate with the clinical picture. Other causes are described in "Differential Diagnosis." Thus,

---

TABLE 1 Criteria to Determine Serotonin Syndrome and Toxicity

Sternbach's diagnostic criteria for serotonin syndrome	1. Recent addition or increase of proserotonergic medication 2. At least three of the following: ○ Agitation ○ Ataxia ○ Diaphoresis ○ Diarrhea ○ Hyperreflexia ○ Hyperthermia ○ Mental status changes ○ Myoclonus ○ Shivering ○ Tremor 3. Neuroleptic agent not added or dose increased before the onset of symptoms 4. Diagnosis of infections, withdrawal, and other poisoning or metabolic disruptions excluded
Hunter's criteria for serotonin toxicity (context of serotonergic medications)	1. If patient has spontaneous clonus, serotonin toxicity present 2. If no spontaneous clonus, one of the following needed for a diagnosis of serotonin toxicity: ○ Inducible clonus *and* agitation *or* diaphoresis ○ Ocular clonus *and* agitation *or* diaphoresis ○ Tremor *and* hyperreflexia ○ Temperature >38° C *and* ocular clonus *or* inducible clonus

From Adams JG et al: *Emergency medicine, clinical essentials*, ed 2, Philadelphia, 2013, Elsevier.

all patients should have blood tests and diagnostic imaging studies to rule out infectious, toxic, and metabolic causes.

- Additional laboratory tests are performed to exclude complicating features of SS (e.g., renal failure secondary to rhabdomyolysis).

LABORATORY TESTS

- CBC with differential to rule out sepsis.
- Electrolytes, BUN, and creatinine to rule out acidosis and renal failure.
- Blood and urine toxicology screen, including acetaminophen and salicylate levels if overdose was intentional.
- Thyroid function tests.
- Creatine-phosphokinase (CPK) with isoenzymes.
- Urine and blood cultures.
- ECG because ventricular rhythm disturbance is a potentially fatal complication.
- Cerebrospinal fluid studies to rule out meningitis.

IMAGING STUDIES

Imaging studies are not specific in the diagnosis of SS and are only ordered to exclude other causes with similar clinical presentations as SS.

Rx TREATMENT

- Once a diagnosis of SS is established, consultation with a medical toxicologist, clinical pharmacologist, and/or poison control center should be sought.
- Management includes:
  1. Discontinue use of all potential precipitating drugs.
  2. Provide supportive management.
  3. Control agitation.
  4. Administer serotonin antagonists.
  5. Control autonomic instability.
  6. Control hyperthermia.
  7. Reassess the need to resume the use of the serotonergic agent once the symptoms have resolved.

NONPHARMACOLOGIC THERAPY

- Discontinuation of the drug is the mainstay of therapy.
- Treatment is supportive: maintaining oxygenation and blood pressure and monitoring respiratory status. Hypotensive patients may require both IV fluids and vasopressor therapy.
- Patients who are severely hyperthermic with temperatures >41° C (106° F) should be given IV sedation, paralyzed, and intubated. Cooling blankets can be used for patients with mild to moderate hyperthermia. There is no role for acetaminophen here.
- Intubation is recommended for patients unable to protect their airways as a result of mental status changes or seizures.

ACUTE GENERAL Rx

- Benzodiazepines for control of agitation are preferred to physical restraints.
  1. Lorazepam 1 to 2 mg IV every 30 min has been used effectively in treating agitation, muscle rigidity, myoclonus, and seizure complications.
  2. Diazepam is an alternative choice.
- Blood pressure management with short-acting agents such as esmolol and nitroprusside.
- Serotonin antagonists should be titrated to clinical effectiveness in patients for whom nonpharmacologic therapy and benzodiazepines are not achieving adequate response, although substantial and rigorous data are lacking.
  1. Cyproheptadine 4 mg tablet or 2 mg/5 ml syrup is given 12 mg initially followed by 2 mg every 2 hr until therapeutic response is achieved in adults (up to 32 mg/day); children ages 7 to 14 should receive 4 mg every 6 hr (up to 16 mg/day), children ages 2 to 6 should receive 2 mg every 6 hr (up to 12 mg/day), and children younger than 2 yr should receive a maximum of 0.25 mg/kg/day as 0.06 mg/kg every 6 hr.
  2. Atypical antipsychotic agents with serotonin antagonist properties (e.g., olanzapine 10 mg SL) have been tried with some success.
  3. Chlorpromazine 50 to 100 mg IM may be considered in severe cases, but intravenous fluid loading is essential to prevent hypotension.

CHRONIC Rx

For patients not requiring hospital admission, cyproheptadine and lorazepam can be given in an oral dose on a prn basis with close follow-up.

DISPOSITION

- SS is a potentially life-threatening condition if not recognized early, although it does exist on a spectrum.
- Prompt diagnosis and withdrawal of the medication result in improvement of symptoms within 24 hr.
- Seizures, rhabdomyolysis, hyperthermia, ventricular arrhythmia, respiratory arrest, and coma are all complicating features of SS.

REFERRAL

All cases of SS secondary to psychotropic medications should be referred to a psychiatrist.

PREVENTION

Modify prescription practices by avoiding multidrug regimens.

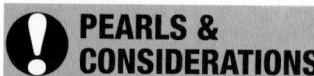 **PEARLS & CONSIDERATIONS**

The combined use of SSRIs and MAOIs is contraindicated.

COMMENTS

- The use of SSRIs and other serotonergic agents is not an absolute contraindication; however, prompt withdrawal of the medication is recommended if any symptoms suggesting SS occur.
- SS is usually found in patients being treated for depression, bipolar disorders, obsessive-compulsive disorder, attention-deficit disorder, and Parkinson's disease.
- It is important to note the existence of several drugs that may not be recognized as serotonergic (e.g., linezolid, dextromethorphan, sumatriptan, tramadol, methadone, St. John's wort) but that can increase the risk of serotonin syndrome when taken concurrently with an SSRI or SNRI.

SUGGESTED READINGS
Available at www.expertconsult.com

AUTHORS: **FRAZER GRANT, M.D.,** and
MARK F. BRADY, M.D., M.P.H., M.M.S.

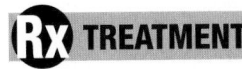 BASIC INFORMATION

DEFINITION

Sexual assault is any sexual act performed by one person on another without consent, resulting from the use of force, the threat of force or from the victim's inability to give consent.

SYNONYMS

Rape

ICD-10CM CODES
Y05 Sexual assault by bodily force
Z04.41 Encounter for examination and observation following alleged adult rape
Z04.42 Encounter for examination and observation following alleged child rape

EPIDEMIOLOGY & DEMOGRAPHICS

INCIDENCE: 17.6% of women, 3% of men
PEAK INCIDENCE: As high as 25%
PREVALENCE (IN U.S.): 17.7 million women, 2.8 million men
PREDOMINANT SEX AND AGE: Female, ages 16 to 24
RISK FACTORS: Alcohol/drug consumption, prior history of being sexually/physically abused, multiple sexual partners, involvement in sex work, poverty, incarceration/institutionalization, mental retardation

PHYSICAL FINDINGS & CLINICAL PRESENTATION

- Extragenital trauma: 70%: bruises, abrasions, erythema on thigh, arms, face, neck
- Anogenital trauma: 27%: injury to breasts, external genitalia, vagina, anus, rectum
- Physical findings more likely if examined within 72 hr of event, if event occurred outdoors, and if perpetrator was unknown

Dx DIAGNOSIS

WORKUP

Preliminary issues and strategies in preparing for taking the history from a sexual assault victim (SAV) are described in Box 1. Consent issues are summarized in Box 2.

- History
  1. Circumstances of assault: date, time, location
  2. Physical description of perpetrator
  3. Areas of trauma, specifically details of oral, vaginal, anorectal contact, or penetration
  4. Condom use
  5. Ejaculation: presence or absence
  6. Presence of bleeding in victim or perpetrator
  7. Recent consensual sexual activity
  8. Showering, bathing, changing of clothes since event
- Physical examination
  1. Ideally performed by individual trained to perform sexual assault examinations, i.e.,

SANE (Sexual Assault Nurse Evaluation) providers: www.sane-sart.com
2. Physical exam can take 3 to 6 hr to complete
3. Components
   - Physical examination of entire body
   - Forensic evidence collection
   - STD evaluation and treatment
   - Pregnancy risk evaluation
   - Care of injuries
4. General physical exam components
   - Documentation of any physical trauma, including photographs
   - Colposcopy: may reveal areas of minor genital trauma
   - Wood's light: to reveal foreign debris or semen
5. Forensic evaluation: not required, but should be offered; written informed consent needed
   - Commercially made specimen collection kits available: once completed, kits need to be sealed and handled according to kit instructions
   - U.S.: States required to provide free specimen collection
   - Samples of blood, saliva, mucosal swabs: buccal/vaginal/rectal, fingernail scrapings/clippings, hair specimens
   - Clothing: if unchanged since event
- Box 3 summarizes potential specimens to be gathered for forensic evidence collection.

- Fig. 1 describes an algorithm for emergency department management of patients after sexual assault.

LABORATORY TESTS

- Pregnancy test (if applicable)
- STD testing
  1. GC/CT: recommended for all, may be excluded if individual elects prophylactic treatment
  2. Wet mount or vaginal swab for *Trichomonas*
  3. Baseline HIV/hepatitis/syphilis testing: individual basis
  4. Retest for HIV/syphilis at 6 wk, 3 mo, and 6 mo from incident

IMAGING STUDIES

Use of imaging studies as dictated by other injuries sustained for diagnosis/treatment of fractures, soft tissue, and other traumatic injuries

Rx TREATMENT

NONPHARMACOLOGIC THERAPY

Acute crisis counseling: to support mental health needs of victim in immediate post-assault period

ACUTE GENERAL Rx

- Sexually transmitted infections
  1. Empiric treatment recommended secondary to poor follow-up rates

---

BOX 1 Preliminary Issues and Strategies in Preparing for Taking the History from a Sexual Assault Victim (SAV)

Provide quiet, confidential, safe environment.
   Briefly review the interview and examination process in private with the SAV.
   Explain the sensitive, personal, embarrassing nature of questions and the right to be interviewed without family or friends.
   Show concern for the SAV's immediate comfort (e.g., if thirsty, take oral swabs first so SAV may drink).
   Provide advocacy.
   Try to conduct the interview the same way.
   Leave difficult questions until the end; some may need to be repeated during appropriate parts of the physical examination.
   Explain why you are asking the question and the possible responses.
   Explain that all questions will be asked.

From Marx JA et al: *Rosen's emergency medicine*, ed 8, Philadelphia, 2014, WB Saunders.

BOX 2 Consent Issues in Sexual Assault Cases

Consents should specify that the sexual assault victim's signature acknowledges the following:
- That hospitals and health care professionals are mandated reporters and that an anonymous Jane Doe report can be made
- Receipt of information about victim compensation funds
- Specific understanding of the examination and evidence collection procedures
- Specific understanding of the use of photography in documenting physical and genital injuries
- That information collected will be sent to law enforcement and is obtainable by defense counsel
- That data without patient identity can be collected for valid educational and scientific interest
- That consent may be withdrawn at any time
- That there is no charge for the examination, whether reported to law enforcement or not

From Marx JA et al: *Rosen's emergency medicine*, ed 8, Philadelphia, 2014, WB Saunders.

2. Gonorrhea: ceftriaxone 250 mg IM *or* cefixime 400 mg PO
3. *Chlamydia:* azithromycin 1 g (single dose) *or* doxycycline 100 mg bid × 7 days
4. Trichomoniasis: metronidazole 2 g PO (single dose)

- Hepatitis B
  1. If perpetrator known to be infected: HBIG + Hep B vaccination
  2. If perpetrator disease status unknown: Hep B vaccination alone
  3. If victim has already been vaccinated with documented immunity: no treatment necessary
- HIV
  1. Use of antiretrovirals after sexual assault is controversial.
  2. Overall risk of acquiring HIV is unknown but higher in certain situations.
     1. Male-on-male rapists
     2. Assault occurring in area with high local prevalence
     3. Multiple assailants
     4. Anal sexual assault
     5. Presence of trauma, bleeding, or genital lesions in either victim/assailant
  3. Antiretroviral drugs should be offered in all situations.
  4. Ideally, antiretrovirals are initiated within 4 hr; should not start if >72 hr.
- Pregnancy
  1. Pregnancy risk is estimated to be 5% per rape in women age 12 to 45.
  2. Emergency contraception should be offered in all cases.
     - Levonorgestrel: 0.75 mg q12h for two doses or 1.5 mg single dose
     - Yuzpe regimen: 100 mcg ethinyl estradiol + 0.5 mg levonorgestrel, repeated in 12 hr
     - Ulipristal (selective progesterone receptor modulator): preferred method when >72 hr from assault
  3. Antiemetics: EC + antibiotics for STD prophylaxis commonly causes nausea.

CHRONIC Rx

- No chronic prescriptions
- Long-term psychiatric counseling may be needed.

REFERRAL

Mental health professional

EBM EVIDENCE

Available at www.expertconsult.com

SUGGESTED READINGS

Available at www.expertconsult.com

RELATED CONTENT

Chlamydia Genital Infections (Related Key Topic)
Contraception (Related Key Topic)
Gonorrhea (Related Key Topic)
Syphilis (Related Key Topic)
Human Immunodeficiency Virus (Related Key Topic)

AUTHOR: **SARAH L. CHISHOLM, M.D.**

BOX 3 Potential Specimens to Be Gathered for Forensic Evidence Collection

Clothing
- Each article of clothing should be packaged in a separate paper bag to avoid cross-contamination.
- If the patient has changed her clothing, only underwear should be collected.

Known blood sample
- Crime laboratory assesses for the secretor status and blood type of the patient.

Toxicology testing (urine and blood)
- For use in cases in which drug-facilitated sexual assault is suspected.
- Collect for evaluation less than 72 to 96 hr after the assault (the time varies by crime laboratory).

Oral swabs and smears
- Collect for evaluation up to 24 hr after the assault.

Head hair combings

Fingernail scrapings

Foreign material collection

Swabs of bite marks or areas where the assailant's mouth touched the patient

Pubic hair combings

External genital swabs

Vaginal swabs and smears
- Cervical sampling should be considered for evaluation between 96 and 120 hr after the assault.

Perianal swabs

Anorectal swabs and smears
- Collect for evaluation up to 24 hr after the assault.

Forensic photography
- Three views per injury, one with a ruler for scale

From Adams JG et al: *Emergency medicine: clinical essentials*, ed 2, Philadelphia, 2013, Elsevier.

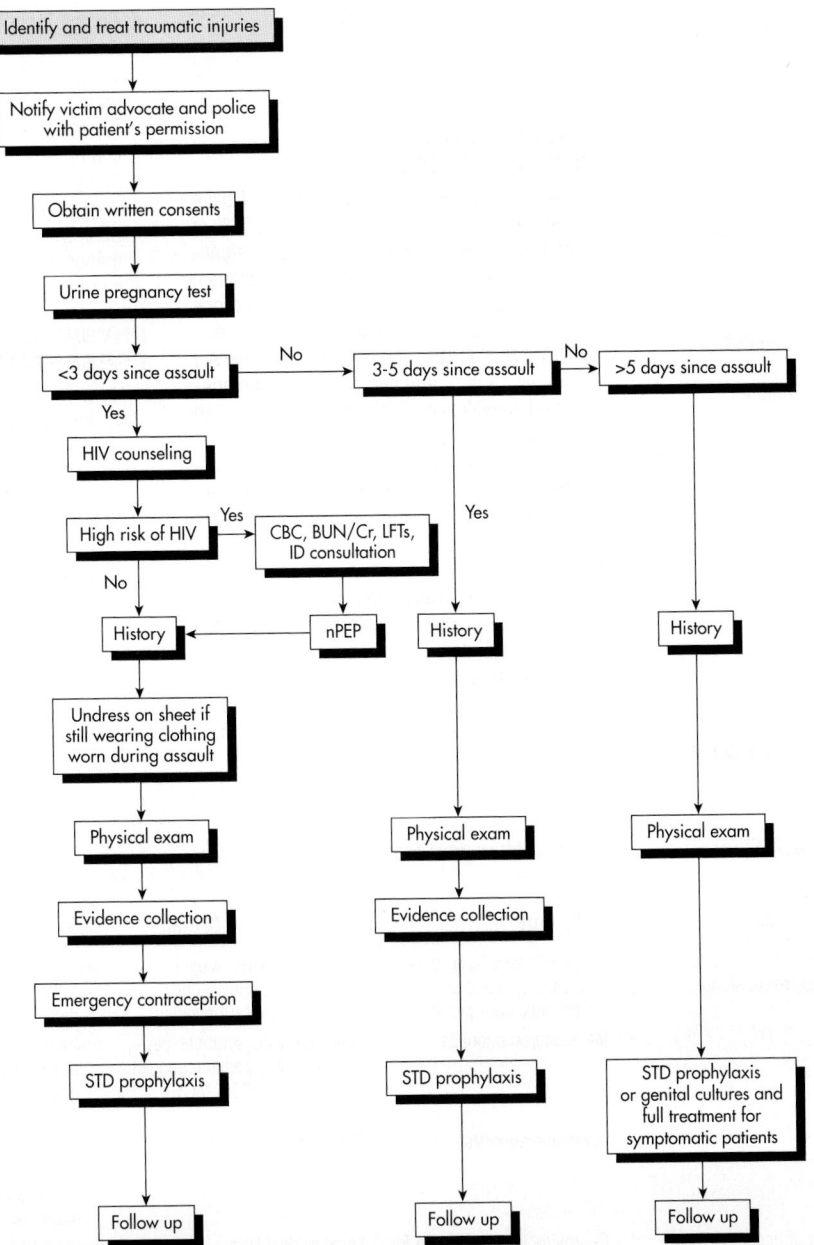

FIG. 1 Emergency department management of patients after sexual assault. *BUN*, Blood urea nitrogen; *CBC*, complete blood count; *Cr*, creatinine; *HIV*, human immunodeficiency virus; *LFTs*, liver function tests; *nPEP*, nonoccupational postexposure prophylaxis; *STD*, sexually transmitted disease. (From Adams JG et al: *Emergency medicine, clinical essentials,* ed 2, Philadelphia, 2013, Elsevier.)

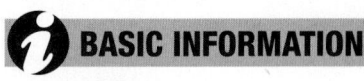

BASIC INFORMATION

DEFINITION

A sexual dysfunction in a woman is any disorder that interferes with female sexuality and that causes marked distress to that person. These disorders are generally categorized into five types:

1. Hypoactive sexual desire disorder (most common)
2. Sexual arousal disorder
3. Orgasmic disorders
4. Sexual pain disorders (including dyspareunia, vaginismus, and vulvodynia)
5. Anxiety about sexual performance

Female sexual dysfunction is also further categorized as lifelong (primary) or acquired (secondary), situational (e.g., current partner) or generalized (all partners and settings).

SYNONYMS

Female sexual dysfunction
Hypoactive sexual desire disorder
HSDD

ICD-10CM CODES
R37   Sexual dysfunction, unspecified
F52.0 Hypoactive Sexual Desire Disorder

F52.31 Female orgasmic disorder
N94.1   Dyspareunia
N94.81 Vulvodynia

EPIDEMIOLOGY & DEMOGRAPHICS

INCIDENCE: According to the National Health and Social Life Survey, in 1999, ~20% to 50% of women reported some form of sexual dysfunction during their lifetimes. One third of women reported a decrease in sexual interest, and one fourth reported an inability to achieve orgasm.

PREVALENCE (TABLE 1): A more recent survey of women 18 yr of age and older found an age-adjusted prevalence of any sexual problem to be ~43%.

PREDOMINANT AGE: Sexually related personal distress was more common in middle-aged women (aged 45-64) than in younger or older women.

RISK FACTORS:
- Correlates of distressing sexual problems include poor self-assessed health, low education level, depression, anxiety, thyroid conditions, and urinary incontinence.
- Obesity and overweight body status have been associated with lower sexual satisfaction and desire.

- Comorbid conditions such as arthritis, diabetes mellitus, hypertension, malignancy, neuromuscular disorders, renal failure, and gynecologic (e.g., chronic pelvic pain) and dermatologic conditions (e.g., lichen sclerosis, psoriasis) can contribute to sexual dysfunction.
- Aging is associated with decreased sexual responsiveness, sexual activity, and libido.
- Decreased hormonal levels associated with menopause can cause decreased vaginal lubrication and dyspareunia.

PHYSICAL FINDINGS & CLINICAL PRESENTATION

- History:
  1. Important to obtain the patient's definition of the dysfunction, including its onset and duration; to determine whether the dysfunction is situational or global; and to determine whether more than one dysfunction exists and the interrelationship among the dysfunctions. Dysfunction is diagnosed if the symptoms are causing distress to the patient.
- Related medical and gynecologic conditions (including prior gynecologic surgery)
- Psychosocial factors, including sexual abuse, sexual orientation, depression and anxiety, status of current relationships and sexual

---

TABLE 1   Investigational Pharmacotherapy for Women's Sexual Dysfunctions

Sexual Dysfunction	Mechanisms of Dysfunction	Drug Type	Off-Label and Investigational Drugs	Comments
Sexual interest/desire disorder	Loss of brain's arousability to sexual stimuli	Drugs with specific serotonin receptor subtype or agonist/antagonist profile	Flibanserin: 5-HT1A agonist and 5-HT2A antagonist, weak partial D4 agonist	Flibanserin is now FDA approved for treatment of hypoactive sexual desire disorder
Subjective arousal disorder		Melanocortin agonists	Bremelanotide: synthetic peptide, α-MSH analog agonist at MC1R, MC3R, MC4R	Small RCT showed benefit for women's arousal disorder with in-home use of nasal drug 45 min before sex. Sponsor has discontinued trials.
Combined arousal disorder		Dopamine agonists	Bupropion	One small 4-mo study in nondepressed premenopausal women showed increased arousability and sexual response, no increase in initial desire.
Genital arousal disorder: Estrogen deplete	Loss of genital vasocongestion in response to sexual stimulation	To provide local substrate for estrogen and testosterone intracrine synthesis	Local vaginal DHEA	Phase 3 RCT showed increased maturation of vaginal epithelium, lower pH, and sexual benefit in all domains of response from local vaginal DHEA for 12 wk.
		Selective tissue estrogenic activity regulator with androgenic and progestogenic properties	Tibolone	RCT of dysfunctional women showed tibolone marginally superior to 50 µg/140 µg combined transdermal estradiol/norethisterone.
				Major problem is distinguishing the subgroup of women with genital arousal disorder who have reduced genital vasocongestion. Small RCTs in diabetes and MS showed only modest benefit from sildenafil.
Genital arousal disorder despite estrogen replete	Loss of genital vasocongestion in response to sexual stimulation	To enhance the action of NO–PDEIs	Sildenafil, tadalafil, vardenafil	
Serotoninergic antidepressant–associated orgasmic disorder	Former orgasmic response absent or extremely delayed	PDEIs	Sildenafil	8-wk RCT with very strict entry criteria showed benefit from 50-100 mg sildenafil.

D4, Dopamine 4 receptor; *DHEA,* dehydroepiandrosterone; *5-HT,* serotonin; *ISSWSH,* International Society for the Study of Women's Sexual Health; *MC1R,* melanocortin-1 receptor; *MS,* multiple sclerosis; *MSH,* melanocyte-stimulating hormone; *NO,* nitric oxide; *PDEIs,* phosphodiesterase inhibitors; *RCTs,* randomized controlled trials.
From Melmed S: *Williams textbook of endocrinology,* ed 12, Philadelphia, 2011, Saunders.

activity, personal and family beliefs about sexuality

- Current medications including OTC and herbal preparations, alcohol, tobacco and drug use, and birth control method.
- Physical examination:
  1. The gynecologic examination can aid in identifying signs of decreased estrogen and androgen levels, infection, endometriosis, pelvic floor dysfunction, and systemic disease
  2. Other body systems as indicated (e.g., cardiovascular, thyroid)

ETIOLOGY

- Chronic medical conditions (e.g., diabetes, coronary vascular disease, arthritis, urinary incontinence)
- Medication induced (e.g., antihypertensives, selective serotonin reuptake inhibitors [SSRIs]). SSRIs are the most common medications linked to sexual dysfunction.
- Gynecologic conditions (e.g., cystitis, posthysterectomy, gynecologic cancers, breast cancer [femininity/self-image issues; chemotherapy effects], postpregnancy, postmenopausal)
- Psychosocial (e.g., religion, taboos, identity conflicts, guilt, relationship problems, abuse, rape, life stressors)
- Fig. 1 illustrates the four phases of the human sexual response as postulated by Masters and Johnson.

Dx DIAGNOSIS

DIFFERENTIAL DIAGNOSIS

- Depression
- Psychosocial stressors
- Medical disease (e.g., thyroid dysfunction)

LABORATORY TESTS

- Cervical cultures and vaginal swabs for infectious disease
- Pap smear
- Appropriate laboratory tests if comorbid or chronic disease is suspected
- No utility to monitoring androgen levels before or after treatment

IMAGING STUDIES

Appropriate imaging studies if comorbid or chronic disease is suspected

Rx TREATMENT

NONPHARMACOLOGIC THERAPY

- Education including a discussion of normal sexual behavior
- Stress management
- Activities to enhance stimulation and eliminate routine
- Distraction techniques
- Noncoital behavior
- Position changes (e.g., female astride)
- Lubricants (e.g., nonpetroleum based). There are several over-the-counter lubricants and

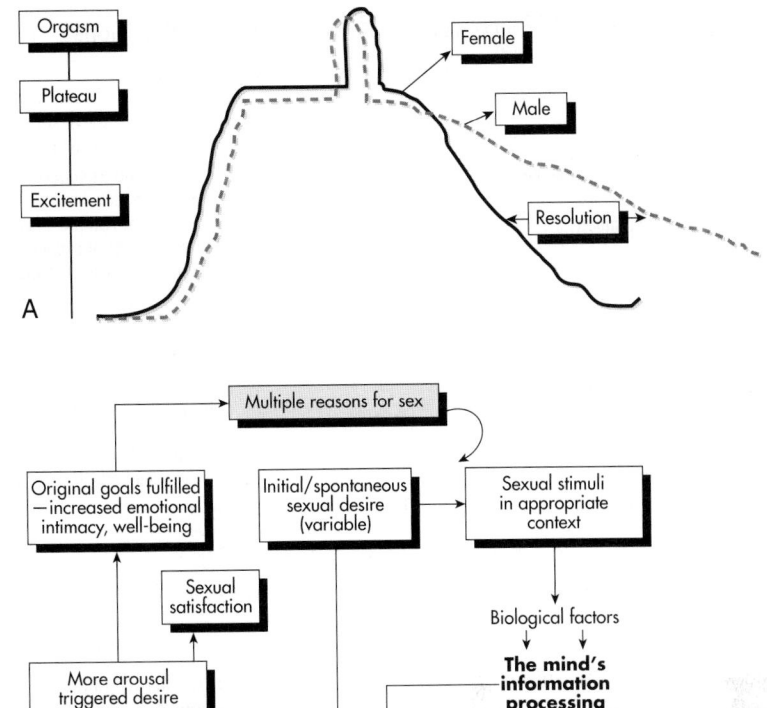

FIG. 1 A, The four phases of the human sexual response cycle as postulated by Masters and Johnson. Because the resolution phase is prolonged considerably in men, men can experience refractoriness to further stimulation for varying lengths of time before they can achieve another orgasm. As discussed in the text, understanding of the human sex response cycle has evolved substantially since the publication of this work. **B,** The circular human response cycle of overlapping phases. It is increasingly recognized that the human sexual response involves much more complexity, circularity, and flexibility than is reflected in Masters and Johnson's original model. "Desire" may or may not be present initially; it can be triggered during the experience. Arousal and desire overlap. Multiple psychologic and biologic factors influence the information processing of sexual stimuli. Underlying this processing may be the individual's unique tendency for excitation versus inhibition. *ANS,* autonomic nervous system. (From Melmed S: *Williams textbook of endocrinology,* ed 12, Philadelphia, 2011, Saunders.)

massage oils, some of which are hypoallergenic, that can be safely applied to female genitalia

ACUTE GENERAL Rx

NSAIDs before intercourse for sexual pain disorders

CHRONIC Rx

- Treat underlying medical, gynecologic, or psychological conditions.
- Reduce comorbidities, including weight loss.
- Increase physical activity (associated with increased satisfaction and sexual engagement).
- For medication-induced conditions, decrease dose or change medication.
- For postmenopausal women or those with hypoestrogenism, try estrogen replacement therapy with or without progesterone. Local vaginal estrogen therapy is preferred over systemic therapy. Estrogen replacement is associated with improvements in dyspareunia and vaginal dryness.
- For postmenopausal vaginal and/or vulvar atrophy, ospemifene has been associated with improved sexual function.

- Transdermal testosterone therapy: results show increase in satisfying sexual activity and sexual desire. Must weigh risks (hirsutism, acne, virilization, and cardiovascular complications) vs. benefits of use.
- Sildenafil (evidence from RCTs for use in patients with neurodegenerative disease and antidepressant-induced FSD after traditional therapy has failed). Data are conflicting. Phosphodiesterase inhibitors may increase blood flow to the genitalia but generally appear to have little benefit in treating arousal disorders. Sildenafil has been helpful in patients with SSRI-induced sexual dysfunction.
- Bupropion 300 to 400 mg/day was shown to increase sexual arousal and orgasm completion in a recent trial. In addition, adjunctive treatment with bupropion significantly improved key aspects of sexual function in women with SSRI-induced sexual dysfunction.
- Behavioral therapy (e.g., cognitive-behavioral therapy to reduce anxiety) and mindfulness-based interventions can treat low sexual desire and arousal disorders.

TABLE 2 Prevalence and Definition of Female Sexual Dysfunctions

	Prevalence*	Definition†
Hypoactive sexual desire/low libido	9%-60%	Diminished feelings of sexual interest or desire, absence of sexual thoughts, and/or lack of receptivity to sexual activity‡
Sexual arousal disorder/sex not pleasurable	5%-51%	**Genital Female Sexual Arousal Disorder (GFSAD):** Disruption of clitoral erection, vaginal vasocongestion, vaginal lubrication
Difficulty with genital lubrication	8%-60%	**Psychological Female Sexual Arousal Disorder (PFSAD):** Absent or markedly diminished feelings of excitement or pleasure in response to sexual stimuli
		Mixed Female Sexual Arousal Disorder: GFSAD and PFSAD
Persistent genital arousal disorder	~1%	Persistent, recurrent, intrusive, and/or distressing sensations of genital arousal not related to sexual stimulation and that do not resolve after orgasm
Female orgasmic disorder	7%-65%	Lack of experience of orgasm or diminished orgasm intensity despite high sexual arousal after a period of sufficient sexual stimulation and arousal
Sexual pain disorders	4%-42%	**Dyspareunia:** Persistent/recurrent pain with attempted/complete vaginal entry with a penis, finger, or other object
		Vaginismus: Vaginal spasm or pain in response to penetration with a penis, finger, or other object despite a desire for penetration to occur‡
Anxiety about sexual performance	6%-16%	N/A

*Laumann et al, 1999; Nicolosi et al, 2005, 2006a, 2006b; Shifren et al, 2008; West et al, 2008; Witting et al, 2008; Garvey et al, 2009.
†Waldinger et al, 2009; Basson et al, 2010b.
‡The term *vaginismus* is no longer preferred, as it includes significant semantic baggage as a psychological disorder.
From Wein AJ et al: *Campbell-Walsh urology*, ed 11, Philadelphia, 2016, Elsevier.

- Flibanserin (Addyi) has recently been approved to treat hypoactive sexual desire disorder. It is an agonist at serotonin 5-HT receptors and an antagonist at 5-HT$_{2A}$ receptors. Its mechanism of action in treating HSDD is unknown. The recommended dose is 100 mg once daily at bed time. Side effects include hypotension, syncope, and CNS depression. Consumption of alcohol increases risk of side effects and is contraindicated. It is mostly effective with approximately 10% of women reporting "much" or "very much" improvement in HSDD symptoms.

- Table 1 summarizes investigational pharmacotherapy for women's sexual dysfunctions.

REFERRAL

- Gynecologic referral for conditions that may be amenable to surgical therapy
- Psychological referral for conditions (e.g., depression, abuse) that may benefit from counseling or psychotherapy
- Social services referrals for active abuse issues

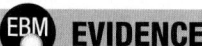 **EVIDENCE**

Available at www.expertconsult.com

SUGGESTED READINGS

Available at www.expertconsult.com

RELATED CONTENT

Female Sexual Dysfunction (Patient Information)
Hypoactive Sexual Desire Disorder (Related Key Topic)

AUTHOR: **ANNGENE ANTHONY, M.D., M.P.H.**

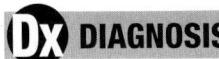 BASIC INFORMATION

DEFINITION

Shaken baby syndrome is a potentially life-threatening and severe form of abuse in which an infant or child is violently shaken. Intracranial injury is caused by rapid acceleration and rotation of the cranium (sometimes associated with impact on a solid object which leads to rapid angular deceleration). The classic injury pattern associated with shaking includes diffuse subdural hemorrhage, retinal hemorrhages, and diffuse brain injury (Fig. E1). The diagnosis is often difficult to make because the clinical manifestations are nonspecific, perpetrators are unlikely to report a history of trauma, and there may be little to no external signs of injury.

SYNONYMS

Shaken infant syndrome
Abusive head trauma
Nonaccidental head injury

ICD-10CM CODES

T74.1	Physical abuse
T74.4	Shaken infant syndrome, initial encounter
T74.4XXD	Shaken infant syndrome, subsequent encounter
T74.4XXS	Shaken infant syndrome, sequela

EPIDEMIOLOGY & DEMOGRAPHICS

INCIDENCE: Most common cause of death or serious neurologic injury resulting from child abuse. It is specific to infancy, when children have unique anatomic features. A population-based study conducted in the United States showed an incidence of abusive head trauma in children <2 yr of 17 per 100,000 persons with a higher incidence in the first year of life compared to the second. Population-based studies in Europe show similar incidence in the first yr.
PEAK INCIDENCE: Shaken babies are typically younger than 1 yr; with median age of 4 mo.
PREVALENCE: ~25% of clinically diagnosed babies with shaken baby syndrome die, and ~80% of the remaining suffer lifelong neurologic damage.
PREDOMINANT SEX: About 60% of identified victims of shaking injury are male. Children of families who live at or below the poverty level are at an increased risk for these injuries as well as any type of child abuse.
RISK FACTORS: History of abuse, history of domestic violence, low socioeconomic status, perinatal illness, incessant crying, and family dysfunction. The perpetrators in 65% to 90% of cases are males and are most commonly the father.

PHYSICAL FINDINGS & CLINICAL PRESENTATION

In several retrospective series, no history of a traumatic event was offered in 64% to 97% of cases. One study of 364 children with shaken baby syndrome found that 40% had no signs of external injury on initial evaluation. Majority will have an abnormal neurologic examination. Generally present with nonspecific symptoms (i.e., seizures, failure to thrive, vomiting associated with lethargy or drowsiness, decreased feeding, hypothermia, bradycardia, hypertension or hypotension, respiratory irregularities, apnea, coma or death). Retinal and cranial hemorrhages and brain injury are hallmarks of the syndrome. Other signs of abuse such as skull fractures, occult fractures (particularly of ribs and long bone diaphysis), abdominal injury and hearing loss, may be present.

ETIOLOGY

Angular deceleration forces cause primary parenchymal injury including traumatic axonal injury. Neuropathology and imaging techniques have established the cause of brain injury as hypoxic ischemic encephalopathy.

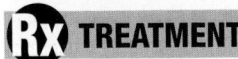 DIAGNOSIS

DIFFERENTIAL DIAGNOSIS

Head trauma from other etiology vs. infection vs. bleeding disorder vs. other etiology

WORKUP

Imaging of the brain, skeletal survey

LABORATORY TESTS

CBC, chemistry, coagulation study, lumbar puncture if meningitis is considered

IMAGING STUDIES

Initial study of unenhanced CT scan and skeletal survey. MRI should be done as follow up in patients with abnormal CT findings and is indicated for infants who are asymptomatic but require neuroimaging after finding noncranial injuries.

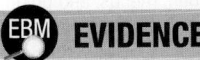 TREATMENT

Treatment focused on targeting specific injuries and also on prevention of future injuries.

NONPHARMACOLOGIC THERAPY

Admission to a hospital for observation.

ACUTE GENERAL Rx

Supportive care and interventions as dictated by the clinical, laboratory, and imaging findings

CHRONIC Rx

Counseling, working with the child's school to optimize academic development

REFERRAL

Neurologist and neurosurgery (if needed)

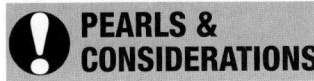 PEARLS & CONSIDERATIONS

PREVENTION

The National Center on Shaken Baby Syndrome offers a prevention program. Additionally, researchers like Harvey Karp have suggested ideas.

PATIENT & FAMILY EDUCATION

Shaken baby syndrome can result in lifelong, irreversible injuries. Prevention is a key component. Infants crying most commonly leads to shaking. Therefore the National Center on Shaken Baby Syndrome offers a prevention program, the **Period of Purple Crying,** which seeks to help parents and other caregivers understand crying in normal infants. By defining and describing the sometimes inconsolable infant crying that can sometimes cause stress, anger, and frustration in parents and caregivers, the program hopes to educate and empower people to prevent abusive head trauma.

Another method that may help is one suggested by author Dr. Harvey Karp's "five S's":
1. Shushing: use "white noise" or rhythmic sounds that mimic the constant whir of noise in the womb.
2. Side/stomach positioning: place the baby on the left side to help digestion.
3. Sucking: let the baby breast-feed or bottle-feed, or give the baby a pacifier or finger to suck on.
4. Swaddling: wrap the baby up snugly in a blanket to help him or her feel more secure.
5. Swinging gently: rock in a chair, use an infant swing, or take a car ride to help duplicate the constant motion the baby felt in the womb.

EBM EVIDENCE

Available at www.expertconsult.com

SUGGESTED READINGS

Available at www.expertconsult.com

AUTHORS: **PRIYA SARIN GUPTA, M.D., M.P.H.,** **LEANNA R. GARBUS, O.M.S. III,** and **POOJA VERMA, M.D.**

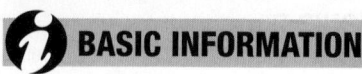

BASIC INFORMATION

DEFINITION

Shigellosis is an inflammatory disease of the bowel caused by one of four species of *Shigella*. It is the third most common cause of diarrhea in the United States after *Salmonella* and *Campylobacter* and the most common cause of bacillary dysentery in the United States.

SYNONYMS

Bacillary dysentery

ICD-10CM CODES
A03.9 Shigellosis, unspecified
A03.0 Shigellosis due to Shigella dysenteriae
A03.1 Shigellosis due to Shigella flexneri
A03.2 Shigellosis due to Shigella boydii
A03.3 Shigellosis due to Shigella sonnei
A03.8 Other shigellosis

EPIDEMIOLOGY & DEMOGRAPHICS

INCIDENCE (IN U.S.): 6.59 cases per 100,000 population with approximately 450,000 cases/yr
PREDOMINANT SEX: Male homosexuals at increased risk.
PREDOMINANT AGE: Shigellosis predominantly affects children with 28 cases per 100,000 population in children <4 yr old and 25.67 cases per 100,000 population in children aged 4 to 11.
PEAK INCIDENCE: Summer.
GENETICS: Neonatal infection: rare but severe.

PHYSICAL FINDINGS & CLINICAL PRESENTATION

- Possibly asymptomatic, but incubation period can range from 1 to 7 days with an average of 3 days.
- Mild illness that is usually self-limited, resolving in a few days.
- High fever.
- Watery diarrhea. Dysentery (abdominal cramps, tenesmus, and numerous, small-volume stools with blood, mucus, and pus).
- Descending intestinal tract illness, reflecting infection of small bowel first and then the colon.
- Severe disease is more common in children and elderly and outside of the United States.
- Complications of severe illness:
  1. Seizures.
  2. Megacolon.
  3. Intestinal perforation.
  4. Death.
- Extraintestinal manifestations are uncommon (reactive arthritis in up to 3% of patients).

- Bacteremia is more common in children; in adults it has been described in patients with AIDS, the elderly, and diabetics.
- Hemolytic-uremic syndrome (HUS): can be caused by *S. dysenteriae* 1.
- Reactive arthritis, sometimes as part of Reiter's syndrome following *S. flexneri* infection.

ETIOLOGY

- *Shigella:* gram-negative rod bacteria that are less susceptible to stomach acid and thus as few as 10 to 100 bacteria can cause disease. The bacteria invade colonic tissue and cause inflammation.
  1. *S. flexneri.*
  2. *S. dysenteriae.*
  3. *S. sonnei.*
  4. *S. boydii.*
- *S. sonnei* is the most commonly isolated species in the United States (over 75% of cases), and it usually causes a mild watery diarrhea.
- Direct person-to-person transmission is thought to be the most common route. Outbreaks among men who have sex with men have occurred because of direct or indirect oral-anal contact.
- Contaminated food or water may transmit disease.
- Outbreaks have occurred in day care centers, a community wading pool frequented by toddlers, and residential institutions.

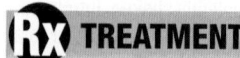

DIAGNOSIS

DIFFERENTIAL DIAGNOSIS

- May mimic other bacterial gastroenteritis, such as *Clostridium difficile*, *Salmonella*, *Campylobacter*, and *Yersinia*.
- Dysentery can also be caused by *Entamoeba histolytica*.
- Bloody diarrhea may resemble disease caused by invasive *E. coli* (IEC).
- Hemolytic-uremic syndrome caused by enterohemorrhagic *E. coli* (O157:H7).

LABORATORY TESTS

- The diagnosis is established by bacterial stool culture.
- Stool should be cultured from fresh samples, because the yield is increased by processing the specimen soon after passage. The best yield is from the mucoid part of the stool.
- Serology is available but rarely useful.
- Polymerase chain reaction (PCR) is available but due to cost used mainly for outbreak investigations.
- Fecal leukocyte preparation may show WBCs.
- Total WBCs may be low, normal, or high. Leukemoid reactions can occur in children.

- Blood cultures should be obtained in patients with severe disease or sepsis syndromes.

IMAGING STUDIES

Abdominal radiographs may suggest megacolon or perforation in rare, severe cases.

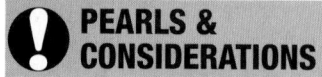

TREATMENT

NONPHARMACOLOGIC THERAPY

- Adequate hydration.
- Electrolyte replacement.

ACUTE GENERAL Rx

Antibiotics recommended in all patients with positive stool cultures:
- To shorten course of illness.
- To limit transmission of illness.
- For adults: Pending susceptibilities, ciprofloxacin 750 mg PO bid for 3 days or levofloxacin 500 to 750 mg q day for 3 days should be used. An alternative is azithromycin 500 mg q day for 3 days.
- For children: IV ceftriaxone (50 mg/kg/day) for 5 days in cases of severe disease. For oral therapy, can use cefixime: 8 mg/kg/day as single daily dose or divided q12h for 5 days *or* azithromycin: 10 mg/kg/day in a single daily dose for 3 days. A short course of an oral quinolone can also be used safely although they are not approved for children.

DISPOSITION

- Most disease is self-limited and resolves without treatment.
- Severe illness may be fatal.

REFERRAL

For severe illness or complications.

PEARLS & CONSIDERATIONS

COMMENTS

- Shigella is one cause of "gay bowel syndrome."
- Illness is worsened by agents that decrease intestinal motility.
- Food handlers, child care providers, and health care workers should have a negative stool culture documented following treatment.

SUGGESTED READING
Available at www.expertconsult.com

RELATED CONTENT
Shigellosis (Patient Information)

AUTHOR: **GLENN G. FORT, M.D., M.P.H.**

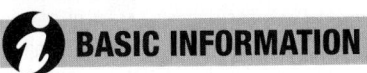

BASIC INFORMATION

DEFINITION

Short bowel syndrome (SBS) is a malabsorption syndrome that results from extensive small intestinal resection or congenital causes (Table 1).

SYNONYMS

Short bowel
SBS

ICD-10CM CODES
K91.2 Postsurgical malabsorption, not elsewhere classified

EPIDEMIOLOGY & DEMOGRAPHICS

- Parallels Crohn's disease (see "Crohn's Disease" in Section I), which is the most common cause of the syndrome in adults.
- In children, two thirds of short bowels are related to congenital abnormalities (intestinal atresia, gastroschisis, volvulus, aganglionosis) and one third are related to necrotizing enterocolitis.
- Prevalence: 10,000 to 20,000 cases are estimated to exist in the United States.

PHYSICAL FINDINGS & CLINICAL PRESENTATION

- Diarrhea and steatorrhea
- Weight loss
- Anemia related to iron or vitamin B_{12} absorption
- Bleeding diathesis related to vitamin K malabsorption
- Osteoporosis/osteomalacia related to vitamin D and calcium malabsorption
- Hyponatremia, hypokalemia
- Hypovolemia
- Other macronutrient or micronutrient deficiency states

ETIOLOGY

- Extensive bowel resection for treatment of the conditions mentioned previously (see "Epidemiology"). SBS typically does not occur until less than 200 cm of healthy small intestine remains. Risk for SBS is decreased if colon is intact.
- Congenital (Table 1).

The human intestine is 3 to 8 m in length. Removal of up to half of the small intestine produces no disruption in nutrient absorption, and most patients can maintain nutritional balance on oral feeding if they have more than 100 cm (3 ft) of jejunum. Similarly, 100 cm of intact jejunum can maintain a normal water, sodium, and potassium balance under normal circumstances. The presence of an intact colon can compensate for some small intestine loss.

Site-specific functions:
- Calcium, magnesium, phosphorus, iron, and vitamins are absorbed in the duodenum and proximal jejunum.
- Vitamin B_{12} and bile acids are absorbed in the ileum. The resection of more than 60 cm of ileum results in vitamin B_{12} malabsorption. The loss of more than 100 cm results in fat malabsorption (from the loss of bile acids).
- The loss of gastrointestinal endocrine hormones can affect intestinal motility.
- Intestinal bacterial overgrowth may also occur, especially if the ileocecal valve is lost.

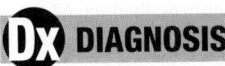

DIAGNOSIS

Presence of macronutrient and/or micronutrient loss in a patient with a known history of bowel resection

DIFFERENTIAL DIAGNOSIS

Because the history of significant bowel resection is typically known, there is no differential diagnosis. If that history is not known, all causes of weight loss, malabsorption, and diarrhea must be considered.

TABLE 1 Causes of Short Bowel Syndrome

Congenital
Congenital short bowel syndrome
Multiple atresias
Gastroschisis
Bowel resection
Necrotizing enterocolitis
Volvulus with or without malrotation
Long-segment Hirschsprung disease
Meconium peritonitis
Crohn's disease
Trauma

From Kliegman RM et al: *Nelson textbook of pediatrics*, ed 19, Philadelphia, 2011, Saunders.

TABLE 2 Management Strategies for Short Bowel Syndrome

1. Acute phase
   a. Treat postoperative complications
   b. Maintain full support via the parenteral route
   c. Initiate low-rate trophic enteral feeds
   d. Document amount and site of remaining bowel and underlying disease
2. Early adaptation (up to 1 yr postsurgery)
   a. Increase enteral nutrition to tolerance; supplement with glutamine
   b. Achieve permanent parenteral access, if indicated
   c. Maximize antiperistaltic agents
   d. Octreotide for high-output ostomy or fistula
   e. Dietary counseling
   f. Clinical trials of trophic growth factors
3. Long-term adaptation (>1 yr postsurgery)
   a. Recruit bypassed bowel
   b. Bowel-lengthening procedure (Bianchi or STEP)
   c. Monitor for development of TPN-associated complications, and refer for transplant before recurrent sepsis, thrombosis, or end-stage liver disease

From Cameron JL, Cameron AM: *Current surgical therapy*, ed 10, Philadelphia, 2011, Saunders.

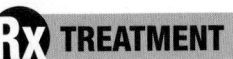

TREATMENT

Extensive small bowel resection with colectomy (<100 cm of jejunum)
- Rx: long-term total parenteral nutrition (TPN). Some patients can switch to oral intake after 1 to 2 yr of TPN. In jejunostomy patients, excessive fluid loss can be reduced with H_2 blockers, proton pump inhibitors, or octreotide. Micronutrients are supplemented.

Extensive small bowel resection with partial colectomy (usually patients with Crohn's disease)
- Rx: oral intake alone is possible in all patients with >100 cm of jejunum. In addition to vitamin B_{12} deficiency, these patients often have diarrhea. Consider lactose malabsorption and bacterial overgrowth treated, respectively, with lactose restriction and antibiotics (tetracycline 250 mg tid or metronidazole 500 mg tid for 2 wk). Nonspecific antidiarrheal agents may also be indicated (e.g., Imodium or codeine). The patient must be monitored for micronutrient losses.
- Table 2 summarizes management strategies for SBS. Intestinal transplantation is performed mostly in children at selective centers.
- FDA-approved medications for SBS in patients receiving nutritional support are:
  1. Recombinant growth hormone somatropin (Zorbtive): effective in increasing weight and reducing parenteral nutrition volume. These effects do not persist when the drug is stopped.
  2. Teduglutide (Gattex), a recombinant DNA analog of glucagon-like peptide-2. It promotes mucosal growth in the small bowel through stimulation of crypt cell proliferation and inhibition of enterocyte apoptosis. This drug may have to be continued indefinitely for effects to persist.

COMPLICATIONS
- Oxalate kidney stones
- Cholesterol gallstones
- D-Lactic acidosis

PROGNOSIS
- Directly dependent on the extent of the bowel resection and in the case of Crohn's disease by the underlying illness
- Whether the colon remains in continuity with the small bowel is an important factor in the patient's ability to adapt after significant small bowel resection.

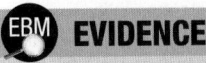

EVIDENCE

Available at www.expertconsult.com

RELATED CONTENT

Short Bowel Syndrome (Patient Information)
Malabsorption (Related Key Topic)

AUTHOR: **FRED F. FERRI, M.D.**

DEFINITION

Short QT syndrome (SQTS) is a genetically inherited disorder of cardiac repolarization characterized by a severely shortened QT interval on the ECG, leading to atrial and ventricular arrhythmias and sudden cardiac death in affected individuals. This is a primary electrical disorder and patients have structurally normal hearts.

SYNONYMS

SQTS

ICD 10CM CODES

I45.89 Other specified conduction disorders

EPIDEMIOLOGY AND DEMOGRAPHICS

- Unknown; disease described for the first time only in 2000 (Gussak et al., 2000)
- This is primarily because, while there is near-unanimity on what constitutes the upper limit of a normal QT interval, no such consensus exists about the lower limit. In most (but not all) cases of the SQTS, the QT or QTc (corrected QT interval) has been <360 msec; however, there are many individuals with that QT interval who are clinically unaffected. Consequently, the incidence and prevalence is unknown, especially given the extremely small number of individuals diagnosed with the syndrome.
- Genetics: the disease is genetically heterogeneous and transmitted in an autosomal dominant fashion. So far, six variants have been identified. Three represent gain of function mutations, and three represent loss of function mutations. SQT1 is the most common variant described, due to a mutation in the cardiac ion channel KCNH2(HERG).

PHYSICAL FINDINGS AND CLINICAL PRESENTATION

- Seen across all age groups, though most patients are children or young adults.
- Syncope and cardiac arrest are the most common presenting features. Syncope is likely due to ventricular arrhythmias. Sudden death can happen with exercise as well as at rest. Cardiac arrest is often the first manifestation of the disease with a peak incidence in the first year of life.
- Atrial fibrillation and flutter are well described as being part of the syndrome.
- A significant percentage of patients are asymptomatic

ETIOLOGY

- Cardiac repolarization abnormality
- Genetic channelopathy transmitted via autosomal dominant mode, caused by missense mutations on genes (six identified so far)
- Mutations cause an increase in net outward current from either a reduction in inward depolarizing currents INa or ICa or augmentation of outward repolarizing currents I to I K1, I K-ATP, I ACh, I Kr or I Ks. The resultant shortening of the action potential causes a shortening of the effective refractory period,

with subsequent increased susceptibility of both atrial and ventricular muscle to premature depolarizations that lead to AF and VF.
- Acquired causes—see "Differential Diagnosis"

DX DIAGNOSIS

- Per the most recent 2013 HRS guidelines:
  - 1. SQTS is diagnosed in the presence of a QTc ≤330 ms.
  - 2. SQTS can be diagnosed in the presence of a QTc ≤360 ms and one or more of the following: a pathogenic mutation, family history of SQTS, family history of sudden death at age ≤40, survival of a ventricular tachycardia/ventricular fibrillation episode in the absence of heart disease.
- A proposed scoring system (Table 1) for the diagnosis of SQTS incorporates the above criteria but has not yet been fully endorsed by the current guidelines.
- The differential diagnosis of a short QT includes various conditions such as hyperkalemia, hypercalcemia, acidosis, digitalis toxicity, effect of acetylcholine or epinephrine, sinus tachycardia, or hyperthermia. All these are possible causes of an acquired short QT interval that must be ruled out before a diagnosis of SQTS can be entertained.

WORKUP

- Evaluation of any survivor of sudden death starts with a detailed history and physical examination, with particular emphasis on family history. Many patients with SQTS have unexplained syncope or palpitations prior to

resuscitated sudden death. Atrial fibrillation is common in SQTS patients and a family history of lone AF should also be sought, in addition to resuscitated VF arrest.
- Physical examination is mostly normal in patients with SQTS.
- ECG findings in SQTS include not only an abnormally short QT interval (usually <360 msec), but usually also a short or even absent ST interval, with the T-wave appearing to emanate directly from the S-wave. T-waves are usually any combination of tall, narrow, and symmetric, with a prolonged Tpeak-Tend ratio (Fig. 1). Another feature to look for is the lack of adaptation of the QT interval to the heart rate (diminished rate dependence) as a result of which the corrected QT interval can be misleading; therefore, QT measurement on resting ECG in SQTS is more accurate with heart rate as close to 60 as possible.
- Echocardiogram and cardiac MRI should be performed to confirm a lack of structural heart disease.
- Holter recordings and stress tests can document a lack of variation of the QT interval in relation to the RR cycle; this is an important aspect of establishing the diagnosis. The QT interval shortens only slightly with increasing heart rates, so the QT and QTc values approach normal levels during faster heart rates. The QT fails to lengthen at slower heart rates.
- At electrophysiology study, the atrial and ventricular refractory periods are usually very short (140-200 msec at a CL of 400-600 msec). Sustained atrial fibrillation

---

TABLE 1 SQTS Diagnostic Criteria

	Points
QT$_c$, msec	
<370	1
<350	2
<330	3
Jpoint-Tpeak interval <120 msec	1
Clinical history	
History of sudden cardiac arrest	2
Documented polymorphic VT or VF	2
Unexplained syncope	1
Atrial fibrillation	1
Family history	
First- or second-degree relative with high-probability SQTS	2
First- or second-degree relative with autopsy-negative sudden cardiac death	1
Sudden infant death syndrome	1
Genotype	
Genotype positive	2
Mutation of undetermined significance in a culprit gene	1

VF, ventricular fibrillation; *VT*, ventricular tachycardia.
A minimum of 1 point must be obtained in the electrocardiographic section in order to obtain additional points.
High-probability SQTS: ≥4 points; intermediate-probability SQTS: 3 points, low-probability SQTS: ≤2 points. Electrocardiogram: must be recorded in the absence of modifiers known to shorten the QT. Jpoint-Tpeak interval must be measured in the precordial lead with the greatest amplitude T-wave. Clinical history: events must occur in the absence of an identifiable etiology, including structural heart disease. Points can only be received for 1 of cardiac arrest, documented polymorphic VT, or unexplained syncope. Family history: points can only be received once in this section.
Adapted from Gollob MH, Redpath CJ, Roberts JD: The short QT syndrome: proposed diagnostic criteria, *J Am Coll Cardiol* 57(7):802-812, 2011.

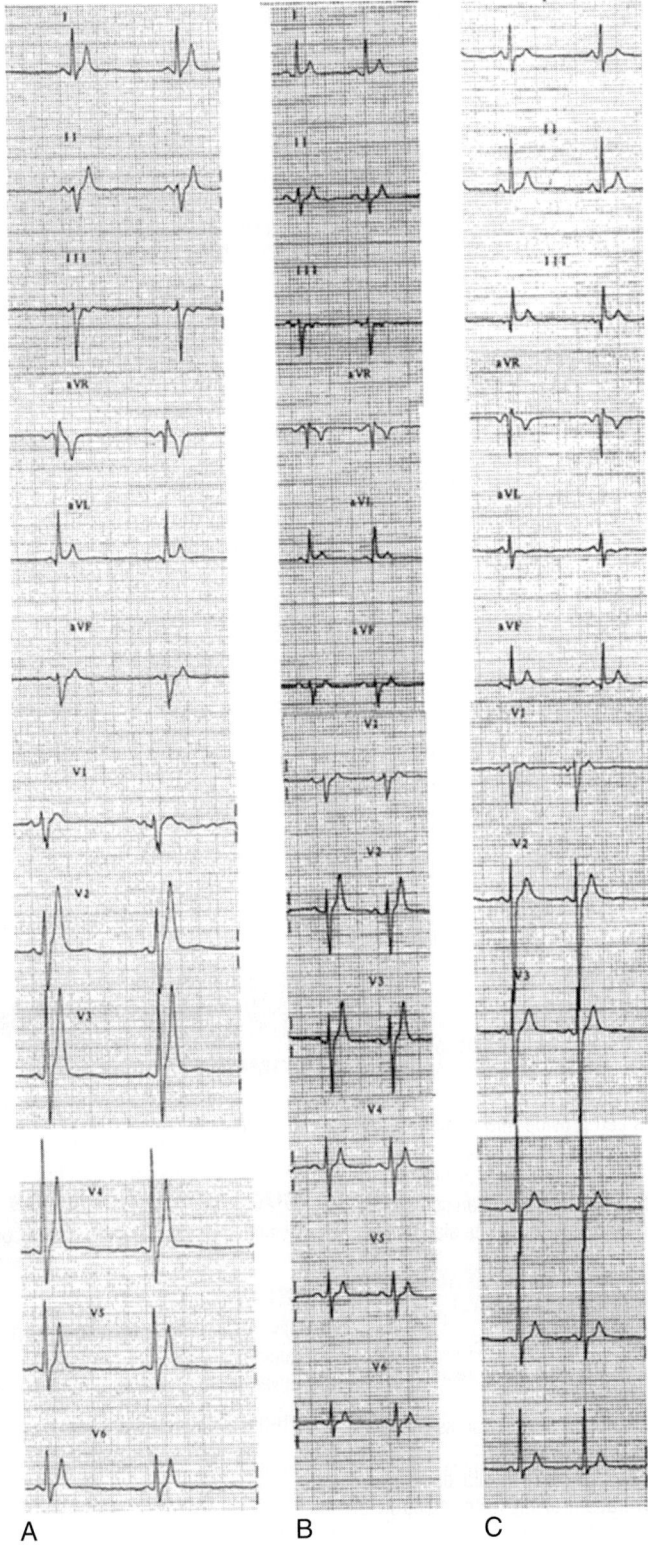

FIG. 1 Twelve-lead ECG (25 mm/s paper speed) of family 1 patients. A, Patient 1 (IV, 3): sinus rhythm, heart rate 52 beats per minute (bpm); left-axis deviation, QT 280 msec. **B,** Patient 2 (IV, 2): sinus rhythm, heart rate 96 bpm; left-axis deviation, QT 220 msec. **C,** Patient 3 (V, 1): sinus rhythm with mean heart rate 92 bpm, QT 260 msec. (Adapted with permission from Gaita F et al: Short QT syndrome: a familial cause of death, *Circulation* 108:965-970, 2003.)

or flutter with rapid ventricular rates is often induced with programmed stimulation in the atrium. The inducibility of VF in SQTS patients at EPS is about 60%. EPS has a role in adding to the diagnosis by demonstrating short A and V refractory periods (also seen in other channelopathies such as Brugada syndrome), but given its low sensitivity it cannot be used for risk stratification.

LABORATORY TESTS

Genetic testing is recommended for all patients in whom a diagnosis of SQTS is suspected. This is especially true if they have a clinical or family history of syncope or sudden death.

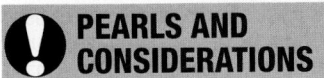 TREATMENT

- There is no significant clinical data on how to approach patients with an isolated short QT interval but no family or clinical history or genotype criterion (low and intermediate probability of SQTS). Risk stratification of these patients is not possible at this time; however, they should be referred to an electrophysiologist with expertise on this topic for comprehensive testing, including genetic testing.
- Patients with QT <330 msec and one criterion from clinical/family history or genetic testing fall in the high probability category of SQTS and hence a higher-risk subgroup for sudden cardiac death. An ICD implant is recommended in this group for secondary and possibly also primary prevention against sudden cardiac death.
- SQTS is a highly lethal disease and survivors of cardiac arrest are at high risk for subsequent events. ICD implantation is strongly recommended in this group.
- A peculiar issue in patients with SQTS implanted with an ICD is double counting of peaked T-waves that are closely coupled to the QRS complex. This often leads to inappropriate ICD shocks. Most ICDs have programming modifications that can be turned on to get around this problem.
- Pharmacologic therapy is usually only advised in patients with multiple and frequent appropriate ICD shocks.
- However, they may be the mainstay of therapy in patients in whom an ICD cannot be implanted for various reasons, including in children in whom technical challenges are significant.
- While many drugs, such as flecainide, sotalol, ibutilide, hydroquinone, and amiodarone, have been used in an attempt to increase the QT interval, most of the available data favor hydroquinidine as the drug of choice across all forms of the SQTS.

REFERRAL

Consultation with an electrophysiologist is strongly recommended if SQTS is suspected.

⊘ PEARLS AND CONSIDERATIONS

- SQTS is a rare genetic syndrome causing arrhythmias and sudden death.
- Should be suspected in patients with QT interval <360 msec presenting with syncope, sudden cardiac death, or atrial fibrillation and a family history of the same.

AUTHORS: **SIMON GRINGUT, M.D.,** and **JOYDEEP GHOSH, M.D.**

Diseases and Disorders

I

BASIC INFORMATION
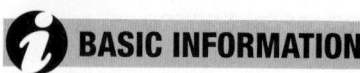

DEFINITION

Sialadenitis is an inflammation of one or multiple salivary glands. It may present as acute or chronic disease with multiple potential etiologies. This section focuses mainly on the workup and management of acute sialadenitis.

ICD-10CM CODES
K11.20 Sialadenitis, unspecified

EPIDEPIDEMIOLOGY & DEMOGRAPHICS
INCIDENCE:
- Accounts for approximately 0.01% to 0.02% of hospital admissions.
- 30% to 40% of affected patients are postoperative patients.
- Parotid gland is most frequently affected, followed by the submandibular glands (Fig. E1).

PREDOMINANT SEX AND AGE
- Affects men and women equally.
- Patients are usually in the sixth and seventh decades of life.

PHYSICAL FINDINGS & CLINICAL PRESENTATION
- Pain and swelling of the affected salivary gland.
- Increased pain with meals.
- Erythema and localized tenderness at the duct opening.
- Massage may express purulent discharge from duct orifice.
- Induration and pitting of the skin, with involvement of the masseteric and submandibular spatial planes in severe cases.

ETIOLOGY
- Ductal obstruction is generally from salivary stasis and increased salivary viscosity as a result of dehydration, medication-induced xerostomia, or poor dental hygiene. This predisposes patients to retrograde migration of bacteria, which can then lead to suppurative sialadenitis.
- Acute suppurative sialadenitis is a bacterial infection of the salivary gland. Most frequent infecting organisms are *Staphylococcus aureus* (50%-90% of cases), streptococcal species, *Haemophilus influenzae, and E. coli*; more recently, anaerobic infections have been increasing in prevalence.
- Recent surgery, Sjögren's syndrome, diabetes mellitus, hypothyroidism, renal failure, trauma, radiation therapy, chemotherapy, dehydration, and chronic illness are predisposing factors.

- Mumps is the most common cause of non-suppurative acute sialadenitis. Majority of cases (>80%) occur in children younger than 15 years.

DIAGNOSIS

DIFFERENTIAL DIAGNOSIS
- Salivary gland neoplasm.
- Ductal stricture.
- Sialolithiasis.
- Decreased salivary secretion as a result of medications (e.g., amitriptyline, diphenhydramine, anticholinergics).
- Dental infections.
- Lymphoma.
- Cervical adenitis.
- Infected branchial cleft or sebaceous cysts.

WORKUP
- Generally not necessary. Fig. E2 describes a diagnostic algorithm.
- Ultrasound or CT scan in patients not responding to medical treatment.

LABORATORY TESTS
- Generally not indicated.
- Complete blood count with differential to possibly reveal leukocytosis with left shift.
- Mumps antibodies if there is clinical suspicion.
- Culture of purulent drainage from salivary duct opening or percutaneously should be obtained to provide useful information in tailoring antibiotic therapy if the patient is not responding to empiric therapy.

IMAGING STUDIES
- Ultrasound or CT scan may be needed in patients with no improvement or clinical worsening after 48 to 72 hours of medical therapy. This can provide information on the presence of a drainable collection.
- Sialography should not be performed during the acute phase, as it can worsen symptoms.
- MRI is also of little utility in acute sialadenitis.

TREATMENT

Nonpharmacologic therapy—these interventions are crucial in expediting resolution of symptoms.
- Massage of the gland: may express pus and relieve some of the pressure.
- Hydration with intravenous fluid or aggressive oral hydration along with electrolyte repletion.

- Warm compresses.
- Oral cavity irrigations.
- Administration of sialagogues such as lemon drops or vitamin C lozenges.

ACUTE GENERAL Rx
- Amoxicillin-clavulanate 500 to 875 mg bid or cefuroxime 250 to 500 mg bid should be given for 10 days. Clindamycin is an alternative choice in patients allergic to penicillin.
- In patients coming from nursing homes or in cases of nosocomial infections, consider empiric treatment with vancomycin given the prevalence of methicillin-resistant *S. aureus.*
- IV antibiotics (e.g., cefoxitin, nafcillin) can be given in severe cases.
- Patients generally improve with 48 to 72 hours of medical treatment. If there is no improvement, consider imaging with CT or ultrasound.
- Surgical drainage is indicated for the rare cases that are refractory to medical management and that are found to have an abscess on CT or ultrasound.

DISPOSITION
Complete recovery unless the patient has underlying obstruction (e.g., ductal stricture, tumor, or stone)

REFERRAL
- To ear-nose-throat specialist for cases refractory to appropriate medical therapy.
- For salivary gland incision and drainage, which may be necessary in resistant cases.

PEARLS & CONSIDERATIONS

COMMENTS
Prevention of dehydration will decrease the risk of sialadenitis.

SUGGESTED READINGS
Available at www.expertconsult.com

RELATED CONTENT
Salivary Gland Inflammation (Patient Information)
Sialolithiasis (Related Key Topic)
Salivary Gland Neoplasm (Related Key Topic)

AUTHOR: **LOUIS INSALACO, M.D.**

BASIC INFORMATION

DEFINITION

Sialolithiasis is the existence of hardened intra-luminal deposits in the ductal system of a salivary gland.

SYNONYMS

Salivary gland stone
Salivary calculus

ICD-10CM CODES
K11.5 Sialolithiasis

EPIDEMIOLOGY & DEMOGRAPHICS

Affects patients mostly in the fifth to eighth decades and occurs most commonly in the submandibular gland (80%); less than 20% of occurrences are located in a parotid gland.

PHYSICAL FINDINGS & CLINICAL PRESENTATION

- Symptoms: colicky postprandial pain and swelling of a salivary gland. Tends to have a remitting/relapsing course.
- Signs: swelling and tenderness of a salivary gland. The stone may be felt with bimanual palpation of the floor of the mouth or inner cheek (Fig. E1).

ETIOLOGY

- The cause is unknown. Contributing factors include saliva stagnation, sialadenitis (inflammation of a salivary gland), ductal inflammation, or injury (Fig. 2).
- Gout is a known cause of salivary gland calculi.
- Salivary calculus composition is mainly calcium phosphate and carbonate, often combined with small proportions of magnesium, zinc, ammonium salts, and organic materials or debris.

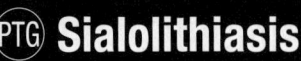 DIAGNOSIS

DIFFERENTIAL DIAGNOSIS

- Lymphadenitis.
- Salivary gland tumor.
- Salivary gland bacterial (*Staphylococcus* or *Streptococcus*), viral (mumps), or fungal infection (sialadenitis).
- Noninfectious salivary gland inflammation (e.g., Sjögren's syndrome, sarcoidosis, lymphoma).
- Salivary duct stricture.
- Dental abscess.

IMAGING STUDIES

- X-ray: 90% of submandibular stones are radiopaque and will show up on x-ray. 90% of parotid stones are radiolucent and will not show up on x-ray.

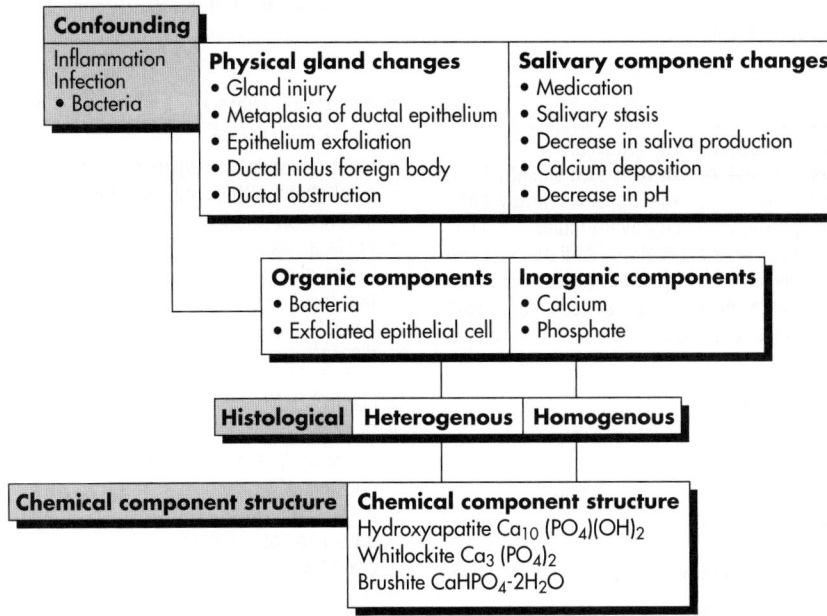

FIG. 2 Algorithm of clinical findings and pathogenesis of sialolithiasis. (From Lee LT, Wong YK: Sialolithiasis in minor salivary glands, *J Oral Maxillofac Surg*, 2010.)

- Non–contrast-enhanced computed tomography is very useful in detecting nearly all salivary stones.
- Ultrasound can detect 90% of salivary stones >2 mm.
- Sialography has a 95% to 100% sensitivity in detecting stones, although it is more invasive than the above options and requires contrast injection into the affected duct.

(Rx) TREATMENT

- Nonsurgical management is usually the first-line treatment.
  - Warm compresses, gland massages, sialogogues (lemon wedges, sour candies), IV or oral hydration.
  - Antibiotics if associated bacterial sialadenitis is present.
- Surgical treatment
  - The surgical approach depends on the location of the stone. Submandibular stones in the distal aspect of the duct that are palpable may be excised transorally under local anesthesia. More proximal stones may require removal of the submandibular gland. Sialendoscopy is a newer technique where a semirigid endoscope and specialized instruments and/or lasers are used to visualize and remove the stones. Stones in the parotid duct also may be accessible via the transoral approach or may require parotidectomy.

Sialoendoscopy is also an option for parotid stones.
- Extracorporeal shock wave lithotripsy is an alternative technique that breaks up the stones into smaller fragments that can be secreted naturally through the duct.

REFERRAL

To otorhinolaryngologist.

RELATED CONTENT

Salivary Gland Stones (Patient Information)
Sialoadenitis (Related Key Topic)
Primary Gland Neoplasm (Related Key Topic)

SUGGESTED READINGS
Available at www.expertconsult.com

AUTHOR: **LOUIS INSALACO, M.D.**

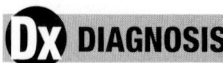
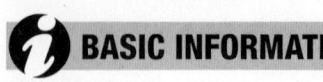 **BASIC INFORMATION**

DEFINITION

Sinus node dysfunction is a group of cardiac rhythm disturbances characterized by abnormalities of the sinus node, including (1) chronic, inappropriate bradycardia; (2) sinus pauses, arrest, or exit block; (3) sinoatrial exit block; and (4) alternating sinus bradycardia with paroxysmal supraventricular tachyarrhythmias (frequently atrial fibrillation) known as tachycardia-bradycardia syndrome. When sinus node dysfunction is associated with symptoms, it is called sick sinus syndrome (SSS).

SYNONYMS

Sinus pause
Sinus arrest
Tachycardia-bradycardia syndrome
Sinoatrial exit block
SSS
Bradycardia-tachycardia syndrome

ICD-10CM CODES
I49.5 Sick sinus syndrome

EPIDEMIOLOGY & DEMOGRAPHICS

- In children: associated with congenital and acquired heart disease, particularly after cardiac surgery.
- In adults: it is primarily a disease of the elderly secondary to idiopathic degenerative disease. A recent population study has suggested that white race, increased BMI, prolonged baseline QRS or right bundle branch block, HTN, or other cardiovascular diseases are associated with increased incidence of sick sinus syndrome.

PHYSICAL FINDINGS & CLINICAL PRESENTATION

- Light-headedness, syncope, presyncope, palpitations. Other manifestations include dyspnea on exertion and worsening angina.
- Physical examination may be normal or reveal abnormalities (e.g., signs of congestive heart failure, heart murmurs, or gallop sounds) associated with the underlying heart disease.

ETIOLOGY

- Sinus node fibrosis is the primary etiology, which may also affect the atrioventricular node, the His bundle, or its branches.
- Polypharmacy should be considered, and obtaining an accurate medicine list is essential.
- In addition, acute coronary syndromes, diseases of the SA nodal artery, inflammatory and infiltrative diseases such as hemochromatosis, amyloidosis, collagen vascular diseases (SLE and scleroderma), epicardial and pericardial diseases, medications (beta-blockers, calcium channel blockers, methyldopa, cimetidine, clonidine, lithium, and antiarrhythmics), trauma following cardiac surgery, hypothyroidism, hypothermia, hypoxia, sepsis, muscular dystrophies (myotonic dystrophy, Friedreich ataxia), infectious etiologies such as Lyme disease, increased intracranial pressure.

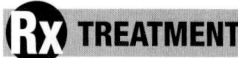 **DIAGNOSIS**

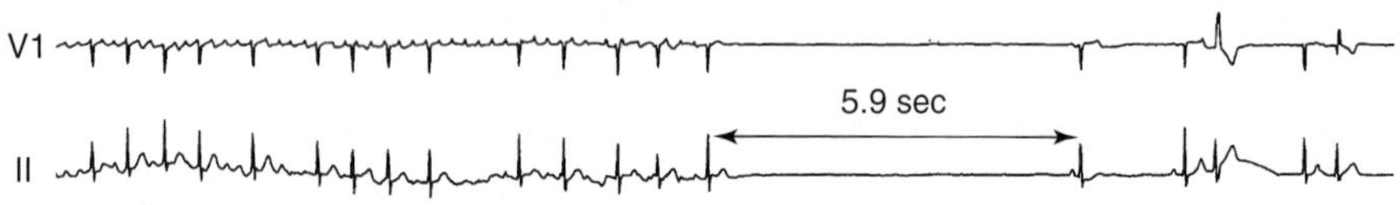

DIFFERENTIAL DIAGNOSIS

- Bradycardia: atrioventricular block
- Tachycardia: atrial fibrillation or atrial flutter
- Sinus tachycardia
- Medication toxicity

WORKUP

- ECG (Fig. 1)
- Ambulatory cardiac rhythm monitoring
- 24-hour ambulatory ECG (Holter) with diary to correlate symptoms to findings
- Event recorder or a loop recorder if symptoms are less frequent
- Exercise stress testing to evaluate the severity of chronotropic incompetence
- Electrophysiologic testing, including sinus nodal recovery time and sinoatrial conduction time

Rx **TREATMENT**

- Permanent pacemaker placement is primarily indicated if bradycardia is symptomatic. Indications for permanent pacemaker in sinus node dysfunction are described in Table 1.
- In tachycardia-bradycardia syndrome, drug treatment is indicated for tachycardia, primarily with AV node blocking agents after placement of the permanent pacemaker.

REFERRAL

To cardiologist

SUGGESTED READINGS
Available at www.expertconsult.com

AUTHORS: **AMANDA C. DORAN, M.D., PH.D.,** and **DANIEL R. FRISCH, M.D.**

V1

5.9 sec

II

FIG. 1 Tachycardia-bradycardia syndrome. Two surface ECG leads show atrial fibrillation that spontaneously terminates followed by a 5.9-second pause before sinus rhythm resumes. The patient became light-headed during this period. (From Issa Z et al: *Clinical arrhythmology and electrophysiology,* ed 2, Philadelphia, 2012, Saunders.)

TABLE 1	Indications for Permanent Pacing in Sinus Node Dysfunction
Class	**Indications**
I	• Sinus node dysfunction with documented symptomatic bradycardia or sinus pauses • Symptomatic sinus bradycardia that is iatrogenic and will occur as a consequence of essential long-term therapy of a type and dose of drugs for which there are no acceptable alternatives. • Symptomatic chronotropic incompetence.
IIa	• Sinus node dysfunction, occurring spontaneously or as a result of necessary drug therapy, with a heart rate of less than 40 beats/min when a clear association between significant symptoms consistent with bradycardia has not been documented. • Unexplained syncope when sinus abnormalities are observed or provoked with electrophysiologic study.
IIb	• A chronic heart rate of less than 40 beats/min, while awake, in the minimally symptomatic patient.
III	• Sinus node dysfunction in asymptomatic patients, including those in whom substantial sinus bradycardia (heart rate of less than 40 beats/min) is a consequence of long-term drug treatment. • Sinus node dysfunction in which symptoms suggestive of bradycardia are clearly documented as not associated with a slow heart rate. • Symptomatic bradycardia associated with nonessential drug therapy.

ACC, American College of Cardiology; *AHA,* American Heart Association; *HRA,* Heart Rhythm Society.
Adapted from ACC/AHA/HRS 2008 revised guidelines.

BASIC INFORMATION

DEFINITION

- Sickle cell disease (SCD) is a hemoglobin-opathy characterized by the production of hemoglobin S caused by substitution of the amino acid valine for glutamic acid in the sixth position of the gamma-globin chain. When exposed to lower oxygen tension, red blood cells (RBCs) assume a sickle shape, resulting in stasis of RBCs in capillaries. Painful crises are caused by ischemic tissue injury resulting from obstruction of blood flow produced by sickled erythrocytes. Vasoocclusive crises are the main reason for hospital admission of children with sickle cell disease.
- Patients with SCD include those who are homozygous for sickle cell hemoglobin (HbSS), also called sickle cell anemia (SCA) and those with one sickle hemoglobin gene plus a gene from another abnormal hemoglobin type (e.g., HbSβ±thalassemia, HbSC).

SYNONYMS

Sickle cell anemia
SCA
SCD
Hemoglobin S disease

ICD-10CM CODES
D57.1	Sickle-cell disease without crisis
D57.20	Sickle-cell/Hb-C disease without crisis
D57.211	Sickle-cell/Hb-C disease with acute chest syndrome
D57.212	Sickle-cell/Hb-C disease with splenic sequestration
D57.219	Sickle-cell/Hb-C disease with crisis, unspecified
D57.3	Sickle-cell trait
D57.40	Sickle-cell thalassemia without crisis
D57.411	Sickle-cell thalassemia with acute chest syndrome
D57.412	Sickle-cell thalassemia with splenic sequestration
D57.419	Sickle-cell thalassemia with crisis, unspecified
D57.80	Other sickle-cell disorders without crisis
D57.811	Other sickle-cell disorders with acute chest syndrome
D57.812	Other sickle-cell disorders with splenic sequestration
D57.819	Other sickle-cell disorders with crisis, unspecified

EPIDEMIOLOGY & DEMOGRAPHICS

- Sickle cell hemoglobin S is transmitted by an autosomal-recessive gene. In African Americans, the incidence of sickle cell anemia at birth is 1 in 600 and the incidence of all genotypes of sickle cell disease is 1 in 300. Approximately 90,000 people in the United States have sickle cell disease.
- Sickle cell trait occurs in approximately 300 million people worldwide, with the highest prevalence of approximately 30%

to 40% in sub-Saharan Africa. In the United States, it is found in nearly 10% of black Americans.
- It is estimated that 2000 babies are born with sickle cell disease in the United States each year, and worldwide 275,000 infants are born with the disease annually.
- There is no predominant sex.

PHYSICAL FINDINGS & CLINICAL PRESENTATION

- Physical examination is variable depending on the degree of anemia and presence of acute vasoocclusive syndromes or neurologic, cardiovascular, genitourinary, and musculoskeletal complications. Table 1 summarizes organ damage seen in sickle cell disease.
- Pain in adults with sickle cell disease is the rule rather than the exception and is far more prevalent and severe than reported in older large-scale surveys.
- There is no clinical laboratory finding that is pathognomonic of painful crisis of sickle cell disease. The diagnosis of a painful episode is made solely on the basis of the medical therapy and physical examination.
- Bones are the most common site of pain. Dactylitis, or hand-foot syndrome (acute, painful swelling of the hands and feet), is the first manifestation of sickle cell disease in many infants. Irritability and refusal to walk are other common symptoms. After infancy, musculoskeletal pain can be symmetric, asymmetric, or migratory, and it may or may not be associated with swelling, low-grade fever, redness, or warmth.

TABLE 1 Organ Damage Seen in Sickle Cell Disease

Organ Or System	Injury
Skin	Stasis ulcer
Central nervous system	Cerebrovascular accident
Eye	Retinal hemorrhage, retinopathy
Cardiac	Congestive heart failure
Pulmonary	Intrapulmonary shunting, embolism, infarct, infection
Vascular	Occlusive phenomenon at any site
Liver	Hepatic infarct, hepatitis resulting from transfusion, hepatic sequestration, intrahepatic cholestasis
Gallbladder	Increased incidence of bilirubin gallstones caused by hemolysis
Spleen	Acute sequestration
Urinary	Hyposthenuria, hematuria
Genital	Decreased fertility, impotence, priapism
Skeletal	Bone infarcts, osteomyelitis, aseptic necrosis
Placenta	Insufficiency with fetal wastage
Leukocytes	Relative immunodeficiency
Erythrocytes	Chronic hemolysis

From Marx J et al: *Rosen's emergency medicine: concepts and clinical practice,* ed 7, Philadelphia, 2010, Mosby.

- In both children and adults, sickle vaso-occlusive episodes are difficult to distinguish from osteomyelitis, septic arthritis, synovitis, rheumatic fever, or gout.
- When abdominal or visceral pain is present, care should be taken to exclude sequestration syndromes (spleen, liver) or the possibility of an acute condition such as appendicitis, pancreatitis, cholecystitis, urinary tract infection, pelvic inflammatory disease, or malignancy.
- Pneumonia develops during the course of 20% of painful events and can present as chest and abdominal pain. In adults chest pain may be a result of vasoocclusion in the ribs and often precedes a pulmonary event. The lower back is also a frequent site of painful crisis in adults.
- The acute chest syndrome manifests with chest pain, fever, wheezing, tachypnea, and cough. Chest radiograph may reveal pulmonary infiltrates. Common causes include infection (*Mycoplasma, Chlamydia,* viruses), infarction, and fat embolism.
- Musculoskeletal and skin abnormalities seen in sickle cell anemia include leg ulcers (particularly on the malleoli) and limb-girdle deformities caused by avascular necrosis of the femoral and humeral heads. Osteonecrosis of the heads of the femur and humerus is found in nearly 50% of adults with sickle cell disease.
- Endocrine abnormalities include delayed sexual maturation and late physical maturation, especially evident in boys.
- Neurologic abnormalities on examination may include seizures and altered mental status. Strokes occur in about 10% of children and adults with sickle cell anemia and approximately 35% of children with sickle cell anemia have cerebrovascular disease.
- Infections, particularly involving *Salmonella, Mycoplasma,* and *Streptococcus,* are relatively common.
- Severe splenomegaly as a result of sequestration often occurs in children before splenic atrophy.

DIAGNOSIS

DIFFERENTIAL DIAGNOSIS

- Thalassemia
- Iron-deficiency anemia, leukemia
- The differential diagnosis of patients presenting with a painful crisis is discussed in "Physical Findings"

WORKUP

- Screening of all newborns regardless of racial background is performed in the United States. Screening can be performed with sodium metabisulfite reduction test (Sickledex test).
- Hemoglobin electrophoresis will also confirm the diagnosis and is useful to identify hemoglobin variants such as fetal hemoglobin and hemoglobin A_2.
- Sickle cell disease encompasses genotypes associated with hemolysis and vasoocclusive

crisis. Hemoglobin electrophoresis results, mean corpuscular volume, erythrocyte morphology, and degree of anemia can be used to differentiate among the sickle cell syndromes.

- For prenatal diagnosis, initial step is identification of parenteral globin gene mutation by DNA-based testing. If positive, then DNA-based testing of chorionic villus sampling or amniotic fluid cells is performed.

LABORATORY TESTS

- Anemia (resulting from chronic hemolysis), reticulocytosis, leukocytosis, and thrombocytosis are common.
- Elevations of bilirubin and lactate dehydrogenase are also common.
- Peripheral blood smear may reveal sickle cells, target cells, poikilocytosis, and hypochromia (Fig. 1).
- Elevated blood urea nitrogen and creatinine may be present in patients with progressive renal insufficiency.
- Urinalysis may reveal hematuria and proteinuria. Patients with SCD should be screened for microalbuminuria and proteinuria with spot urine testing by 10 yr of age.

IMAGING STUDIES

- Chest x-ray is useful in patients presenting with chest syndrome. Cardiomegaly may be present on chest x-ray.
- MRI or bone scan is useful to rule out suspected osteomyelitis (usually the result of *Salmonella*).
- CT scan or MRI of brain is not indicated in asymptomatic adults and children with SCD but is often needed in patients with neurologic complications such as transient ischemic attack, cerebrovascular accident, seizures, or altered mental status.
- Transcranial Doppler ultrasonography (TCD) is a useful commodity to identify children with sickle cell anemia who are at risk for stroke. There should be an annual screening starting at age 2 until age 16. Patients determined to be at risk (transcranial Doppler velocity ≥200 cm/s) should be enrolled in long-term transfusion programs. These are effective in reducing risk of stroke by >90%. In adults magnetic

resonance angiography (MRA) can be used instead of TCD to identify those at risk for stroke.
- Doppler echocardiography may be helpful in diagnosing pulmonary hypertension but has a low positive predictive value. Screening for vasculopathy is done by estimating the tricuspid regurgitant jet velocity (TRV). Elevated values are predictive of early mortality. The prevalence of pulmonary hypertension when right heart catheterization is performed is approximately 6% in adults with sickle cell disease.

℞ TREATMENT

NONPHARMACOLOGIC THERAPY

- Patients should be instructed to avoid conditions that may precipitate sickling crisis, such as hypoxia, infections, acidosis, and dehydration.
- Maintain adequate hydration (PO or IV).
- Correct hypoxia.

ACUTE GENERAL Rx

- Aggressively diagnose and treat suspected infections (*Salmonella* osteomyelitis and pneumococcal infections occur more often in patients with sickle cell anemia because of splenic infarcts and atrophy). Combination therapy with a cephalosporin and erythromycin plus incentive spirometry and bronchodilators is useful in patients with acute chest syndrome.
- Provide pain relief during the vasoocclusive crisis. The fear of creating or perpetuating addiction or being deceived by patients often causes physicians to prescribe subtherapeutic dosages of opioids. However, available evidence suggests that the prevalence of drug addiction among patients with sickle cell anemia is no higher than in the overall U.S. population. Medications should be administered on a fixed time schedule with a dosing interval that does not extend beyond the duration of the desired pharmacologic effect.

1. Meperidine is contraindicated in patients with renal dysfunction or central nervous system disease because its metabolite, normeperidine (which is excreted by the kidneys), can cause seizures.
2. Narcotics (e.g., morphine 0.1 mg/kg IV q3-4h or 0.3 mg/kg PO q4h) should be given on a fixed schedule (not prn for pain), with rescue dosing for breakthrough pain as needed.
3. Except when contraindications exist, concomitant use of nonsteroidal antiinflammatory drugs should be standard treatment.
4. Nurses should be instructed not to give narcotics if the patient is heavily sedated or respirations are depressed.
5. When the patient shows signs of improvement, narcotic drugs should be tapered gradually to prevent withdrawal syndrome. It is advisable to observe the patient on oral pain relief medications for 12 to 24 hr before discharge from the hospital.
6. Analgesic medications should be used in combination with psychological, behavioral, and physical modalities in the management of sickle cell disease.
   - Incentive spirometry is recommended in patients hospitalized for a vasoocclusive crisis.
- Aggressively diagnose and treat any potential complications (e.g., septic necrosis of the femoral head, priapism, bony infarcts, and acute chest syndrome).
- Overall strategies for the management of acute chest syndrome are described in Table 2.
- Hydroxyurea (15 mg/kg body weight per day in patients with normal creatinine clearance) increases hemoglobin F levels and reduces the incidence of vasoocclusive complications. It is generally well tolerated. Side effects consist primarily of mild, reversible neutropenia. There is strong evidence to support use of hydroxyurea therapy in patients 9 mo and older to decrease the frequency of

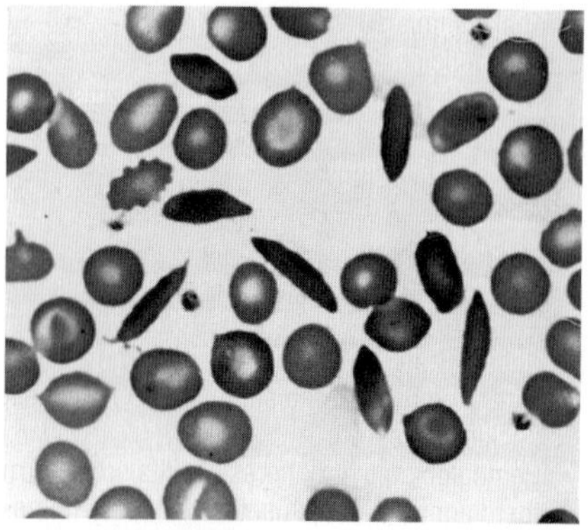

FIG. 1 Photomicrograph of peripheral blood smear with sickle cells, typical of sickle cell anemia. (From Andreoli TE [ed]: *Cecil essentials of medicine,* ed 4, Philadelphia, 1997, Saunders.)

TABLE 2   Overall Strategies for the Management of Acute Chest Syndrome

Prevention

Incentive spirometry and periodic ambulation in patients admitted for vasoocclusive crises, surgery, or febrile episodes
Watchful waiting in any hospitalized child or adult with sickle cell disease (pulse oximetry monitoring and frequent respiratory assessments)
Avoidance of overhydration
Intense education and optimum care of patients who have sickle cell anemia and asthma

Diagnostic Testing and Laboratory Monitoring

Blood cultures
Nasopharyngeal samples for viral culture (respiratory syncytial virus, influenza)
Blood counts every day and appropriate chemistries
Continuous pulse oximetry
Chest radiographs

Treatment

Blood transfusion (simple or exchange)
Supplemental O_2 for drop in pulse oximetry by 4% over baseline, or values <90%
Empirical antibiotics (cephalosporin and macrolide)
Continued respiratory therapy (incentive spirometry and chest physiotherapy as necessary)
Bronchodilators and steroids for patients with asthma
Optimum pain control and fluid management

From Kliegman RM et al: *Nelson textbook of pediatrics,* ed 19, Philadelphia, 2011, Saunders.

vasoocclusive crises and acute chest syndrome. Hydroxyurea therapy is also strongly recommended for adults with three or more vasoocclusive crises during any 12-month period, with SCD pain or chronic anemia interfering with daily activities, or with severe or recurrent episodes of acute chest syndrome. It should be avoided in patients with existing leukopenia, thrombocytopenia, or severe hypoplastic anemia. It is indicated for adults with sickle cell anemia who have moderate to severe disease, typically those with three or more acute painful crises or episodes of the acute chest syndrome in the previous year.

- Replace folic acid (1 mg PO qd) due to loss from increased utilization of folic acid stores due to chronic hemolysis. Sickle cell patients also often have mineral and vitamin deficiencies (calcium, zinc, and vitamins A, C, D, and E) and may need vitamin and nutritional supplementation.

CHRONIC Rx

- Guidelines for prompt management of fever, infections, pain, and specific complications should be reviewed.
- Genetic counseling is recommended in all cases.
- Silent cerebral infarcts are the most common neurologic injury in children with sickle cell anemia and are associated with the recurrence of an infarct (stroke or silent cerebral infarct) and impaired cognition. A recent trial revealed that regular blood-transfusion therapy significantly reduced the incidence of cerebral infarct in children with sickle cell anemia. Additional research is required before these results can be translated into medical practice to develop a balance between stroke prevention and avoidance of unnecessary transfusions. Exchange transfusions may be necessary for patients with acute neurologic signs, in aplastic crisis, or undergoing surgery. The target hemoglobin level is 10 to 11 g/dl (hematocrit 30%). Transfusing to a higher Hb/Hct should be avoided due to associated hyperviscosity if there is a substantial portion of HbS in the blood. Indications for transfusion in sickle cell disease are described in Table 3. Serum ferritin level should be monitored quarterly. Iron overload due to blood transfusions (transfusional hemosiderosis) can be treated with chelating agents (deferoxamine [SC infusion], deferasirox [PO], and deferiprone [PO]).
- Gene therapy for patients with sickle cell disease represents a novel approach. Recently a patient was successfully treated with lentiviral vector-mediated addition of an antisickling β-globin gene into autologous hematopoetic stem cells. Fifteen months after treatment, the level of therapeutic antisickling β-globin remained high (approximately 50% of the beta-like globin chains) without recurrence of sickle cell crises and with correction of the biologic hallmarks of the disease.[1]

- Angiotensin-converting enzyme inhibitor therapy is recommended for microalbuminuria in adults with SCD.
- Children and adults with proliferative sickle cell retinopathy should be referred to specialists for consideration of laser photocoagulation.
- Allogeneic stem cell transplantation can be curative in young patients with symptomatic sickle cell disease; however, the death rate from the procedure is nearly 10%, the marrow recipients are likely to be infertile, and there is an undefined risk of chemotherapy-induced malignancy. Myeloablative stem cell transplantation is generally limited to children under age 16 with severe disease.
- Penicillin V 125 mg PO bid should be administered by age 2 mo and increased to 250 mg bid by age 3 yr. Penicillin prophylaxis can be discontinued after age 5 yr except in children who have had splenectomy.
- Table 4 summarizes disease-modifying treatments to consider.

REFERRAL

- Hospitalization is generally recommended for most crises and complications.

TABLE 3 Indications for Transfusion in Sickle Cell Disease

	Duration	Consensus	Method	Goal*
Stroke, acute	Single	+	Ex	HbS <30%
Stroke, ongoing care	Chronic	+	Either	HbS <30%
High-velocity transcranial Doppler	Chronic	+	Either	HbS <30%
ACS, initial episode	Single	+	Dir > Ex	Hgb 10
ACS, recurrent	6-12 mo	+	Either	
Pulmonary hypertension	Chronic	+	Either	
Multiorgan failure	Single	+	Ex	
Major surgery	Single	+	Dir	Hgb 10
Acute anemia	Single	+	Dir	
Recurrent spleen sequestration	Chronic	+		
Sepsis/meningitis	Single	+	Dir	
Severe chronic pain	6-12 mo	+		
Congestive heart failure	Chronic	+		
Silent infarct with abnormal neuropsychology	Chronic	−		
Pregnancy		−		
Anemia/renal failure	Chronic	−		
Leg ulcers	6-12 mo	−		
Severe growth delay		−		
Severe eye disease		−		
Priapism		−		

ACS, Acute chest syndrome; *Dir*, direct; *Ex*, exchange; *Hb*, hemoglobin type; *Hgb*, hemoglobin concentration; +, consensus reached; −, consensus not reached.
*Goal of transfusion if a consensus has been reached.
From Fuhrman BP et al: *Pediatric critical care*, ed 4, Philadelphia, 2011, Saunders.

TABLE 4 Disease-Modifying Treatments to Consider*

Robust Clinical Data	**Penicillin Prophylaxis**
	Streptococcus pneumoniae vaccination
	Hydroxyurea
	Chronic exchange transfusion
	Iron chelation for chronic iron overload[†]
Limited clinical data	Folate supplementation[‡]
	Haemophilus influenzae vaccination
	Influenza vaccination
	Erythropoietin
	Phlebotomy
Experimental	Hb F reactivation with decitabine, histone deacetylase inhibitors, or Imids
	Erythropoietin for chronic relative reticulocytopenia
	Nutritional supplements and antioxidants (e.g., glutamine, zinc, multivitamins)
	N-acetylcysteine

Hb F, Fetal hemoglobin.
*See text for specific indications and limitations.
[†]Best data from thalassemia patient experience.
[‡]Risks minimal (however, can mask vitamin B_{12} deficiency). Therefore, it is generally done.
From Hoffman R: *Hematology, basic principles and practice*, ed 6, Philadelphia, 2013, Saunders.

[1]Ribeil JA, et al.: Gene therapy in a patient with sickle cell disease, *N Engl J Med* 376:848–865, 2017.

- Psychosocial counseling and support structures should be developed.
- At least yearly evaluation by a hematologist competent in sickle cell anemia is recommended in all patients with sickle cell anemia. Children with transcranial Doppler ultrasonography >170 cm per second should be referred to a subspecialist with expertise in long-term transfusion therapy for stroke prevention.
- Referral to a nephrologist if proteinuria is detected (>300 mg/24 h).
- Patients with pulmonary hypertension should follow up with a cardiologist and a pulmonologist.
- Referral to an ophthalmologist for an annual dilated retinal examination beginning at 10 yr of age. Persons with normal dilated retinal exam should be rescreened at 1- to 2-yr intervals.

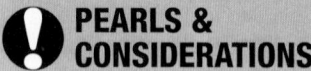

PEARLS & CONSIDERATIONS

COMMENTS

- Pain in adults with sickle cell disease is the rule rather than the exception and needs to be treated appropriately.
- A recent phase 2 trial for the prevention of pain crises in sickle cell disease involving crizanlizumab, an antibody against the adhesion molecule p-selectin revealed a significantly lower rate of sickle cell-related pain crises than placebo and was associated with a low incidence of adverse events.[2]
- Patients and their families should receive genetic counseling and should be made

[2]Ataga KI, et al.: Crizanlizumab or the prevention of pain crises in sickle cell disease, *N Engl J Med* 376:429–439, 2017

aware of the difference between sickle cell trait and sickle cell disease.
- Regular immunizations and pneumococcal vaccination are recommended. The prophylactic administration of penicillin soon after birth and the timely administration of pneumococcal and *Haemophilus influenzae* type b vaccines have resulted in a significant decline in the incidence of these infections. The heptavalent conjugated pneumococcal vaccine (Prevan) should be administered from 2 mo of age. The 23-valent unconjugated pneumococcal vaccine is given from age 2 yr and can be boosted once 3 yr later. Influenza vaccination can be given after 6 mo of age.
- Patients should be instructed on a well-balanced diet and appropriate folic acid supplementation.
- The presence of dactylitis, Hb 7, or leukocytosis in the absence of infection during the first 2 yr of life indicates a higher risk of severe sickle cell disease later in life.
- Among patients with sickle cell disease, acute chest syndrome is commonly precipitated by fat embolism and infection, especially community-acquired pneumonia. Among older patients and those with neurologic symptoms, the syndrome often progresses to respiratory failure.
- Poloxamer 188, a nonionic surfactant with hemorheologic and antithrombotic properties, has been reported to produce a significant but relatively small decrease in the duration of painful episodes and an increase in the proportion of patients who achieved resolution of the symptoms. A more significant effect was observed in patients who received concomitant hydroxyurea.

- Pulmonary hypertension is a complication of chronic hemolysis and is associated with a high risk of death. It can be detected by Doppler echocardiography in more than 30% of adult patients with sickle cell disease. Cardiac catheterization will confirm the diagnosis. It is resistant to hydroxyurea therapy.
- Neurocognitive brain dysfunction is common in sickle cell disease. Trials have shown that compared with healthy controls, adults with sickle cell disease have a poorer cognitive performance, which is associated with anemia and age.
- Among patients with sickle cell disease hospitalized with vasoocclusive pain crisis, the use of inhaled nitric oxide compared with placebo did not improve time to crisis resolution.
- The average life span of individuals with sickle cell trait is similar to that of the general population. However, it is associated with a higher incidence of renal medullary cancer.

SUGGESTED READINGS
Available at www.expertconsult.com

RELATED CONTENT
Sickle Cell Anemia (Patient Information)

AUTHOR: **BHARTI RATHORE, M.D.**

BASIC INFORMATION

DEFINITION

Silicosis is a lung disease attributable to the inhalation of silica (silicon dioxide) in crystalline form (quartz) or in cristobalite or tridymite forms.

SYNONYMS

Pneumoconiosis caused by silica

ICD-10CM CODES
J62.8 Pneumoconiosis due to other dust containing silica

EPIDEMIOLOGY & DEMOGRAPHICS

- Occupational disease affecting men and women involved in gathering, milling, processing, or using silica-containing rock or sand. Jobs that can lead to silicosis are described in Box 1.
- According to the Occupational Safety and Health Administration (OSHA), an estimated 200,000 miners and 1.7 million others have experienced an occupational exposure to silica.
- African Americans have a seven times greater rate of developing silicosis compared with whites at the same exposure. The annual number of silicosis deaths declined 40% from 185 in 1999 to 111 in 2013, but the decline appears to have leveled off during 2010 to 2013, according to the Centers for Disease Control.

PHYSICAL FINDINGS & CLINICAL PRESENTATION

- There are three patterns of silicosis: acute, chronic, and accelerated.
- Simple silicosis may be asymptomatic with the only manifestation being an abnormal chest radiograph.
- Acute silicosis is also known as silicoproteinosis. Develops several weeks to <5 years after silica exposure. Presents with rapid onset of cough, weight loss, fatigue, and pleuritic chest pain.
- Chronic silicosis will present with cough, dyspnea, and sputum production in 35% of the cases. It is the most common clinical presentation, and onset is after decades of repeated exposure.

BOX 1   Jobs That Can Lead to Silicosis

Mining: surface or underground mining (tunneling)
Milling: ground silica for abrasives and filler
Quarrying
Sandblasting (e.g., of buildings, preparing steel for painting)
Pottery; ceramic or clay work
Grinding, polishing using silica wheels
Stone work
Foundry work: grinding, molding, chipping
Refractory brick work
Glass making: to polish and as an abrasive
Boiler work: cleaning boilers
Manufacture of abrasives

From Goldman L, Schafer AI: *Goldman's Cecil medicine,* ed 24, Philadelphia, 2012, Saunders.

- Accelerated silicosis may have an initial asymptomatic phase followed by increasing frequency of symptoms parallel with worsening radiographic abnormalities. Develops <10 years after initial high-level exposure.

ETIOLOGY

- Silica particles are ingested by alveolar macrophages, which in turn release oxidants causing cell injury and cell death, attract fibroblasts, and activate lymphocytes, increasing immunoglobulins in the alveolar space.
- Hyperplasia of alveolar epithelial cells occurs.
- Collagen accumulates in the interstitium.
- Neutrophils also accumulate and secrete proteolytic enzymes, which leads to tissue destruction and emphysema.
- Silica dust may be carcinogenic (not proven).
- Exposure to silicosis predisposes to tuberculosis.
- Some patients develop rheumatoid silicotic pulmonary nodules and may have arthritic symptoms of rheumatoid arthritis (Caplan's syndrome). Scleroderma has also been associated with silicosis.

DIAGNOSIS

DIFFERENTIAL DIAGNOSIS

- Other pneumoconiosis, berylliosis, hard metal disease, asbestosis
- Sarcoidosis
- Tuberculosis
- Interstitial lung disease
- Hypersensitivity pneumonitis
- Lung cancer
- Langerhans' cell granulomatosis (histiocytosis X)
- Granulomatous pulmonary vasculitis

WORKUP

- History of occupational exposure
- Chest radiograph (Fig. 1)

Acute silicosis:
- Chest radiograph demonstrates bilateral, diffuse ground-glass opacities.
- Chest CT demonstrates diffuse nodular and patchy consolidative opacities with enlargement of hilar lymph nodes.
- Milky and lipoproteinaceous effluent is seen on bronchoalveolar lavage (BAL).

- Lung biopsy is not necessary in the setting of a definite exposure history.
- Exclusion of other causes like pulmonary edema, alveolar hemorrhage, and pulmonary alveolar proteinosis is necessary.

Chronic silicosis:
- Chest radiograph demonstrates multiple small, rounded opacities (<10 cm in diameter) distributed in the upper lung zones.
- Progressive massive fibrosis (PMF) refers to coalescence of the nodules of chronic silicosis with calcified hilar adenopathy.
- Pulmonary function tests (PFT) shows mixed obstructive and restrictive defect.
- High resolution CT scan (HRCT), bronchoscopy, and lung biopsies have limited diagnostic role unless atypical radiographic features are noted.

Accelerated silicosis
- Radiographic pattern is that of simple silicosis, although development of radiographic abnormalities is more rapid. This has greater risk for PMF.

TREATMENT

- Treatment is symptomatic (supplemental O_2 for hypoxemia, bronchodilators, antibiotics for infections).
- Prevention (industrial hygiene).
- Smoking cessation.
- Supportive measures (oxygen, bronchodilators).
- Vaccination against influenza and pneumococcus.
- Whole-lung lavage may have a role in acute silicoproteinosis.
- Treatment of associated tuberculosis if present.
- Consider lung transplant for patients who develop chronic respiratory failure.

Associated Complications
- Silicosis is associated with increased risk of mycobacterial tuberculosis, chronic necrotizing aspergillosis, lung cancer, rheumatic disorders, and chronic airflow obstruction.

RELATED CONTENT

Silicosis (Patient Information)

AUTHORS: **FAHAD FAROOQ, M.D.,** and **SAMAAN RAFEQ, M.D.**

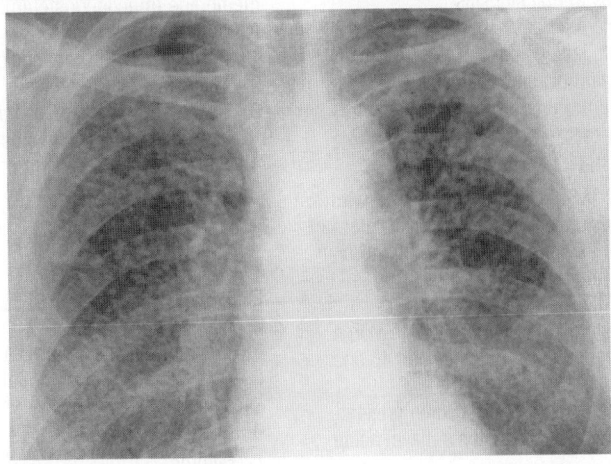

FIG. 1 Simple silicosis. There are multiple small (2- to 4-mm) nodules distributed throughout the lungs, with an upper lobe predominance. (From McLoud TC: *Thoracic radiology: the requisites,* St Louis, 1998, Mosby.)

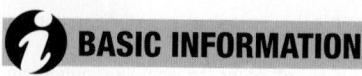

BASIC INFORMATION

DEFINITION

Sinusitis is inflammation of the mucous membranes lining one or more of the paranasal sinuses. The various presentations are:
- Acute sinusitis: infection lasting <4 wk, with complete resolution of symptoms.
- Subacute infection: lasts from 4 to 12 wk, with complete resolution of symptoms.
- Recurrent acute infection: episodes of acute infection lasting <30 days, with resolution of symptoms, which recur at intervals at least 10 days apart.
- Chronic sinusitis: inflammation of the paranasal sinuses and nasal cavities lasting >12 wk, with persistent upper respiratory symptoms. It accounts for 1% to 2% of total physician encounters.
- Acute bacterial sinusitis superimposed on chronic sinusitis: new symptoms that occur in patients with residual symptoms from prior infection(s). With treatment, the new symptoms resolve but the residual ones do not.

SYNONYMS

Rhinosinusitis: sinusitis is almost always accompanied by inflammation of the nasal mucosa; thus it is now the preferred term.

ICD-10CM CODES
J32.9	Chronic sinusitis, unspecified
J01.90	Acute sinusitis, unspecified
J01.00	Acute maxillary sinusitis, unspecified
J01.01	Acute recurrent maxillary sinusitis
J01.10	Acute frontal sinusitis, unspecified
J01.11	Acute recurrent frontal sinusitis
J01.20	Acute ethmoidal sinusitis, unspecified
J01.21	Acute recurrent ethmoidal sinusitis
J01.30	Acute sphenoidal sinusitis, unspecified
J01.31	Acute recurrent sphenoidal sinusitis
J01.80	Other acute sinusitis
J01.81	Other acute recurrent sinusitis
J01.91	Acute recurrent sinusitis, unspecified
J32.0	Chronic maxillary sinusitis
J32.1	Chronic frontal sinusitis
J32.2	Chronic ethmoidal sinusitis
J32.3	Chronic sphenoidal sinusitis
J32.8	Other chronic sinusitis

EPIDEMIOLOGY & DEMOGRAPHICS

INCIDENCE (IN U.S.): Seems to correlate with the incidence of upper respiratory tract infections and higher in women than men; 30 million cases a year in the United States.

PEAK INCIDENCE:
- Fall, winter, spring: September through March
- In adults: greatest incidence between 45 and 74 years of age
- Approximately 6% to 7% of children presenting with respiratory symptoms have acute sinusitis.

PHYSICAL FINDINGS & CLINICAL PRESENTATION

- Patients often give a history of a recent upper respiratory illness with some improvement, then a relapse.
- Mucopurulent secretions in the nasal passage:
  1. Purulent nasal and postnasal discharge lasting 7 to 10 days
  2. Facial tightness, pressure, or pain
  3. Nasal obstruction
  4. Headache
  5. Decreased sense of smell
  6. Purulent pharyngeal secretions, brought up with cough, often worse at night
- Erythema, swelling, and tenderness over the infected sinus in a small proportion of patients:
  1. Diagnosis cannot be excluded by the absence of such findings.
  2. These findings are not common, and do not correlate with number of positive sinus aspirates.
- Intermittent low-grade fever in about half of adults with acute bacterial sinusitis.
- Toothache is a common complaint when the maxillary sinus is involved.
- Periorbital cellulitis and excessive tearing with ethmoid sinusitis:
  1. Orbital extension of infection: chemosis, proptosis, impaired extraocular movements
- Characteristics of acute sinusitis in children with upper respiratory tract infections:
  1. Persistence of symptoms
  2. Cough
  3. Bad breath
- Symptoms of chronic sinusitis (may or may not be present):
  1. Nasal or postnasal discharge
  2. Fever
  3. Facial pain or pressure
  4. Headache
- Nosocomial sinusitis is typically seen in patients with nasogastric tubes or nasotracheal intubation.

ETIOLOGY

- Each of the four paranasal sinuses is connected to the nasal cavity by narrow tubes (ostia), 1 to 3 mm in diameter; these drain directly into the nose through the turbinates. The sinuses are lined with a ciliated mucous membrane (mucoperiosteum).
- Acute viral infection:
  1. Infection with the common cold or influenza
  2. Mucosal edema and sinus inflammation
  3. Decreased drainage of thick secretions/obstruction of the sinus ostia
  4. Subsequent entrapment of bacteria
     a. Multiplication of bacteria
     b. Secondary bacterial infection
- Other predisposing factors:
  1. Tumors
  2. Polyps
  3. Foreign bodies
  4. Congenital choanal atresia
  5. Other entities that cause obstruction of sinus drainage
  6. Allergies
  7. Asthma

- Dental infections lead to maxillary sinusitis.
- Viruses recovered alone or in combination with bacteria (in 16% of cases):
  1. Rhinovirus
  2. Coronavirus
  3. Adenovirus
  4. Parainfluenza virus
  5. Respiratory syncytial virus
- The principal bacterial pathogens in sinusitis are *Streptococcus pneumoniae*, nontypable *Haemophilus influenzae*, and *Moraxella catarrhalis*.
- In the remainder of cases *Streptococcus pyogenes*, *Staphylococcus aureus*, beta-hemolytic streptococci, and mixed anaerobic infections (*Peptostreptococcus*, *Fusobacterium*, *Bacteroides*, *Prevotella* spp.) are found.
- Infection is polymicrobial in about one third of cases.
- Anaerobic infections are seen more often in cases of chronic sinusitis and in cases associated with dental infection; anaerobes are unlikely pathogens in sinusitis in children.
- Fungal pathogens are isolated with increasing frequency in immunocompromised patients but remain uncommon pathogens in the paranasal sinuses. Fungal pathogens include: *Phaeohyphomycosis*, *Aspergillus*, *Pseudallescheria*, *Sporothrix*, and *Zygomycetes* spp.
- Nosocomial infections: occur in patients with nasogastric tubes, nasotracheal intubation, cystic fibrosis, and immunocompromised state.
  1. *S. aureus* (including MRSA)
  2. *Pseudomonas aeruginosa*
  3. *Klebsiella pneumoniae*
  4. *Enterobacter* spp.
  5. *Proteus mirabilis*
- Organisms typically isolated in chronic sinusitis:
  1. *S. aureus*
  2. *S. pneumoniae*
  3. *H. influenzae*
  4. *P. aeruginosa*
  5. Anaerobes

DIAGNOSIS

DIFFERENTIAL DIAGNOSIS
- Temporomandibular joint disease
- Migraine headache
- Cluster headache
- Dental infection
- Trigeminal neuralgia
- Allergic rhinitis
- Drugs (cocaine, decongestant overuse)
- Gastroesophageal reflux disease
- Wegener granulomatosis
- Cystic fibrosis

WORKUP
- The diagnosis is generally based on clinical signs and symptoms (purulent rhinorrhea and facial pain). Radiologic tests and cultures are not recommended initially and should be considered only when treatment is ineffective and sinusitis persists.

- In the normal healthy host, the paranasal sinuses should be sterile. Although the contiguous structures are colonized with bacteria and likely contaminate the sinuses, the mucociliary lining functions to remove these bacteria.
- Gold standard for diagnosis: recovery of bacteria in high-density $\geq 10^4$ colony-forming units/ml from a paranasal sinus, in the setting of a patient with history of upper respiratory infection and symptoms persisting for 7 to 10 days. Sinus aspiration is the best method for obtaining cultures; however, it must be performed by an otorhinolaryngologist and is not practical for the primary care practitioner. Therefore, most diagnoses are based on the clinical history and presentation, possibly supported by radiologic evaluations.
  1. Overall, standard radiographs are of limited use in diagnosis, although negative films are strong evidence against the diagnosis
  2. CT scans:
     a. Much more sensitive than plain radiographs in detecting acute changes and disease in the sinuses
     b. Recommended for patients requiring surgical intervention, including sinus aspiration; it is a useful adjunct to guide therapy
  3. Transillumination:
     a. Used for diagnosis of frontal and maxillary sinusitis
     b. Absence of light transmission indicates that sinus is filled with fluid
     c. Dullness (decreased light transmission) is less helpful in diagnosing infection
  4. Endoscopy:
     a. Used to visualize secretions coming from the ostia of infected sinuses
     b. Culture collection via endoscopy often contaminated by nasal flora; not nearly as good as sinus puncture
  5. Sinus puncture:
     a. Gold standard for collecting sinus cultures
     b. Generally reserved for treatment failures, suspected intracranial extension, and nosocomial sinusitis

Rx TREATMENT

NONPHARMACOLOGIC THERAPY

To help promote sinus drainage:
- Air humidification with vaporizers (for steam) or humidifiers (for a cool mist)
- Application of hot, wet towel over the face
- Sipping hot beverages
- Hydration

ACUTE GENERAL Rx

- Sinus drainage:
  1. Nasal vasoconstrictors, such as phenylephrine nose drops, 0.25% or 0.5%
  2. Topical decongestants should not be used for more than a few days because of the risk of rebound congestion
  3. Systemic decongestants
  4. Corticosteroids: Nasal or systemic corticosteroids, such as nasal beclomethasone. Oral corticosteroids combined with

antibiotics may be associated with modest benefit for short-term relief of symptoms in adults with severe symptoms of acute sinusitis compared with antibiotics alone. Oral corticosteroids as monotherapy are not associated with improved clinical outcomes in adults with clinically diagnosed acute sinusitis.[1]
  5. Nasal irrigation, with hypertonic or normal saline (saline may act as a mild vasoconstrictor of nasal blood flow)
  6. Use of antihistamines has no proven benefit, and the drying effect on the mucous membranes may cause crusting, which blocks the ostia, thus interfering with sinus drainage
- Analgesics, antipyretics

Antimicrobial therapy:
- Most cases of acute sinusitis have a viral cause and will resolve within 2 wk without antibiotics.
- Current treatment recommendations favor symptomatic treatment for those with mild symptoms. 85% of persons have a reduction or resolution of symptoms within 7 to 15 days without antibiotic therapy. Physicians grossly overprescribe antibiotics for presumed bacterial sinusitis despite a much higher prevalence of viral infections.
- Antibiotics should not be prescribed for mild to moderate sinusitis within the first week of illness. They should be reserved for those with severe symptoms who meet the criteria for diagnosis of sinusitis.
- Antibiotic therapy is usually empiric, targeting the common pathogens:
  1. First-line antibiotics in children include amoxicillin or amoxicillin/clavulanate. For adults amoxicillin/clavulanate or doxycycline is first-line agent, with quinolones (levofloxacin or moxifloxacin) reserved as second-line agents unless patient is penicillin allergic.
  2. Second-line antibiotics include the newer macrolides: clarithromycin, and oral cephalosporins: cefuroxime axetil, cefprozil, cefaclor, loracarbef, but high rate of resistance of *S. pneumoniae* is a concern with these agents as is *H. influenzae* resistance with TMP-SMX and azithromycin such that they should no longer be used as first-line agents.
  3. For patients with uncomplicated acute sinusitis, the less expensive first-line agents appear to be as effective as the costlier second-line agents.
- Hospitalization and IV antibiotics may be required for more severe infection and those with suspected intracranial complications. Broader-spectrum antibiotic coverage may be indicated in severe cases, to cover for MRSA, *Pseudomonas*, and fungal pathogens.
- Duration of therapy generally 5 to 7 days in adults rather than 10 to 14 days as recommended in the past.

Optimal duration of treatment in children varies from 10 to 28 days.

Surgery:
- Surgical drainage indicated
  1. If intracranial or orbital complications suspected
  2. Many cases of frontal and sphenoid sinusitis
  3. Chronic sinusitis recalcitrant to medical therapy
- Surgical debridement imperative in the treatment of fungal sinusitis

Complications:
- Untreated, sinusitis may lead to a number of serious, life-threatening complications.
- Intracranial complications include meningitis, brain abscess, and epidural and subdural empyema.
- Intracranial sequelae are more common with frontal and ethmoid infections.
- Extracranial complications include orbital cellulitis, blindness, orbital abscess, osteomyelitis.
- Extracranial sequelae are more commonly seen with ethmoid sinusitis.

CHRONIC Rx

- Chronic sinusitis: Evidence supports daily high-volume saline irrigation with topical corticosteroid therapy at a first-line therapy for chronic sinusitis. A short course of systemic corticosteroids (1-3 wk), short course of doxycycline (3 wk), or a leukotriene antagonist may be considered in patients with nasal polyps. A prolonged course (3 mo) of macrolide antibiotic may be considered for patients without polyps.[2]
- Surgical intervention may be necessary in nonresponders

REFERRAL

- To infectious disease specialist if failure to respond to initial therapy
- To otorhinolaryngologist for:
  1. Failure to respond to therapy
  2. Suspected fungal infection
  3. Suspected intracranial or orbital complications

! PEARLS & CONSIDERATIONS

- Recurrent sinusitis is usually related to anatomic defects, poor drainage, or immunocompromised states; such patients deserve a thorough workup by an ENT specialist and/or an infectious disease specialist.
- Nosocomial sinusitis from obstruction by nasotracheal or nasogastric tubes is not uncommon and can be difficult to recognize in patients in critical care units.

SUGGESTED READINGS

Available at www.expertconsult.com

RELATED CONTENT

Sinusitis (Patient Information)

AUTHOR: **GLENN G. FORT, M.D., M.P.H.**

[1]Venekamp RP, et al.: Systemic corticosteroid therapy for acute sinusitis, *JAMA* 313(12):1258-1259, 2015.

[2]Rudmik L, Soler ZM: Medical therapies for adult chronic sinusitis: a systematic review, *JAMA* 314(9):926-939, 2015.

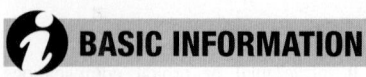

BASIC INFORMATION

DEFINITION

Sjögren's syndrome (SS) is a chronic autoimmune disorder that targets exocrine glands. It is characterized by lymphocytic and plasma cell infiltration and destruction of salivary and lacrimal gland, resulting predominantly in dry eyes and dry mouth, but it can affect other organ systems as well.

Primary and secondary forms have been described:
- Primary: dry mouth (xerostomia) and dry eyes (xerophthalmia) develop as isolated entities.
- Secondary: associated with other autoimmune connective tissue diseases.

SYNONYMS

SS
Sicca syndrome
Keratoconjunctivitis sicca
Sicca complex
Dry eye syndrome/dysfunctional tear syndrome

ICD-10CM CODES
M35.00 Sicca syndrome, unspecified
M35.01 Sicca syndrome with keratoconjunctivitis
M35.02 Sicca syndrome with lung involvement
M35.03 Sicca syndrome with myopathy
M35.04 Sicca syndrome with tubulo-interstitial nephropathy
M35.09 Sicca syndrome with other organ involvement

EPIDEMIOLOGY & DEMOGRAPHICS

INCIDENCE: 4 per 100,000; of these cases, 70% had primary SS.
PREVALENCE: Prevalence is 0.2% to 2.7% of population; secondary SS is also common and can affect up to 19% of patients with systemic lupus erythematosus (SLE) and 26% to 31% of rheumatoid arthritis (RA) and scleroderma patients.
PREDOMINANT SEX: Female/male ratio is approximately 10:1
PREDOMINANT AGE: Peak incidence is in the fourth and fifth decade, but SS can occur in all ages.

RISK FACTOR: Seen in all races/ethnicities, but more common in Caucasians.

PHYSICAL FINDINGS & CLINICAL PRESENTATION

- Diagnosis of SS is based on the presence of at least two of three objective diagnostic tests below:
  1. Positive serum levels of anti-SS-A/Ro and/or anti-SS-B/La or a positive rheumatoid factor and antinuclear antibody (ANA) titer of at least 1:320.
  2. Salivary gland biopsy exhibiting focal sites of inflammation. One or more sites of inflammation per 4 mm^2 is considered to be positive.
  3. Keratoconjunctivitis sicca with ocular staining score of three or more (the dissipation rate of a specialized dye that is applied to the tear film that bathes the surface of the eye; a score of three or more is considered to be positive).
- Dry mouth with dry lips (cheilosis), erythema of tongue (Fig. 1) and other mucosal surfaces, carious teeth
- Dry eyes (conjunctival injection, corneal ulceration, blurred vision, decreased luster, enlargement of lacrimal glands, and irregularity of the corneal light reflex)
- Salivary gland enlargement and dysfunction, with subsequent difficulty in chewing and swallowing food and in speaking without frequent water intake, thickened saliva, and burning sensation in mouth
- Leukocytoclastic vasculitis may be present.
- Skin ulceration, photosensitivity, and allergic drug eruptions
- Extraglandular involvement occurs in 50% of patients. There are multiple systemic manifestations associated with SS, which include the following:
  1. Dyspareunia and pruritus can occur secondary to vaginal dryness.
  2. Pulmonary involvement includes interstitial lung disease (e.g., NSIP), chronic obstructive pulmonary disease, lymphocytic interstitial pneumonitis, fibrosis, and xerotrachea.

  3. Gastrointestinal conditions such as celiac disease, esophageal dysmotility, type I autoimmune hepatitis, primary biliary cirrhosis, and pancreatitis can occur.
  4. Renal manifestations include renal tubular acidosis, Fanconi syndrome, glomerulonephritis, and interstitial nephritis.
  5. Neurologic involvement including peripheral neuropathy and trigeminal neuropathy.
  6. Musculoskeletal symptoms including arthralgias and polymyopathy.
  7. Hematologic conditions such as lymphoma and pancytopenia. Nearly 5% of patients develop B-cell lymphoma.
  8. RA and other connective tissue diseases are present in secondary SS.
  9. Autoimmune thyroiditis may be observed in patients with SS.

ETIOLOGY

Sjögren's syndrome is an autoimmune disorder of unclear etiology. It is associated with certain HLA-DQ and HLA-DR alleles. It has been postulated that viral agents (e.g., hepatitis C and Epstein-Barr virus) may trigger the clinical manifestations. The pathogenesis involves a complex interplay of several factors, including genetic and epigenetic controls of immune homeostasis and gene expression, age, gender, and environmental insults.

DIAGNOSIS

DIFFERENTIAL DIAGNOSIS

- Medication-related dryness (e.g., anticholinergics, antihistamines).
- Age-related exocrine gland dysfunction.
- Mouth breathing.
- Anxiety.
- HIV infection.
- Hepatitis C infection.
- Diabetes mellitus.
- Chronic sialadenitis.
- Acromegaly.
- Type V hyperlipidemia.
- Graft-versus-host disease.
- Other: sarcoidosis, primary salivary hypofunction, radiation injury, amyloidosis.
- IgG4-related disease.
- Ocular herpetic lesions, blepharitis, corneal abrasions.
- An algorithm for the diagnosis of SS is provided in Fig. 2.

WORKUP

Workup involves ocular and oral examination and laboratory and radiographic testing to demonstrate the following criteria for diagnosis of primary and secondary SS.
PRIMARY:
- Symptoms and objective signs of ocular dryness:
  1. Schirmer's test (Fig. 3): <5 mm wetting per 5 min
  2. Positive rose-bengal or fluorescein staining of cornea and conjunctiva to demonstrate keratoconjunctivitis sicca
  3. Tear breakup time and tear osmolality measured after instillation of fluorescein

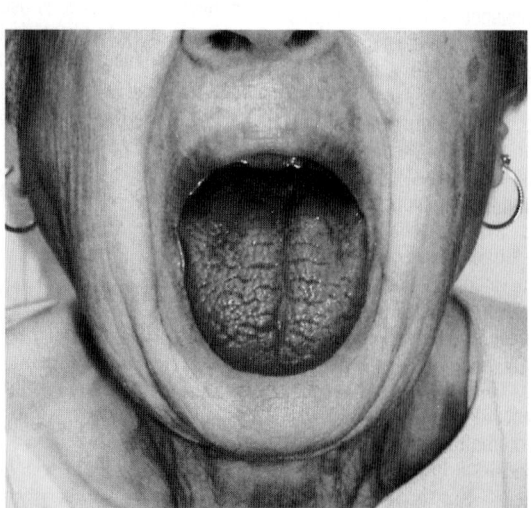

FIG. 1 "Crocodile tongue" in a patient with Sjögren's syndrome. (From Noble J: *Primary care medicine*, ed 3, St Louis, 2001, Mosby.)

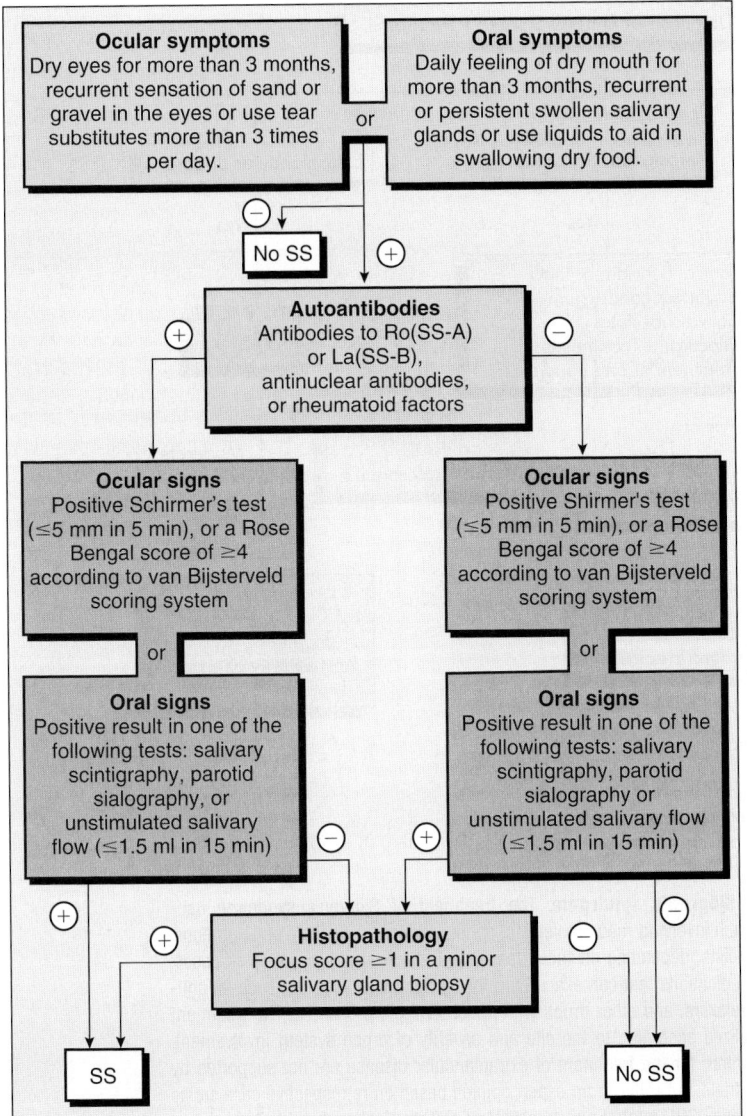

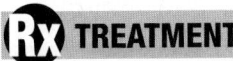

FIG. 2 Suggested algorithm for the diagnosis of Sjögren's syndrome. Exclusion criteria include hepatitis C or human immunodeficiency virus infection, sarcoidosis, graft-versus-host disease, preexisting lymphoma, previous head or neck irradiation, and use of anticholinergic drugs. (From Hochberg MC et al: *Rheumatology*, ed 5, St Louis, 2011, Mosby.)

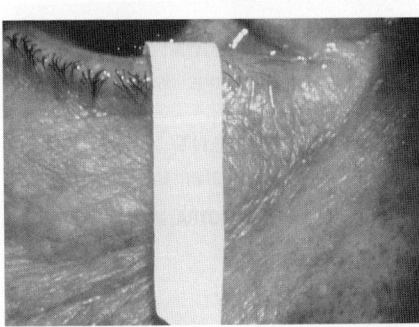

FIG. 3 Schirmer test in a patient with Sjögren's syndrome. Wetting of less than 5 mm/5 min of the filter paper strip is shown. (From Hochberg MC et al: *Rheumatology*, ed 5, St Louis, 2011, Mosby.)

- Symptoms and objective signs of dry mouth:
  1. Decreased parotid flow using Lashley cups or other methods
  2. Abnormal biopsy result of minor salivary gland (focus score >1 based on average of four assessable lobules)
  3. Assessment of rate of saliva production in which collection of ≤1.5 mL after two expectorations 15 min apart is considered positive
- Evidence of systemic autoimmune disorder:
  1. Elevated rheumatoid factor (70%-90% of patients)
  2. Elevated titer of ANA >1:320 (80% of patients)
  3. Presence of anti-SS-A (Ro) (>60% of patients) or anti-SS-B (La) antibodies (40% of patients)

SECONDARY:
- Characteristic signs and symptoms of SS
- Clinical features sufficient to allow a diagnosis of RA, SLE, polymyositis, or scleroderma

LABORATORY TESTS

- Positive ANA (80% of patients) with autoantibodies anti-SS-A and anti-SS-B may be present.
- Additional laboratory abnormalities may include elevated erythrocyte sedimentation rate, anemia, abnormal liver function studies, elevated serum beta$_2$ microglobulin levels, rheumatoid factor, hypergammaglobulinemia, antibodies to double-stranded DNA (in cases with proteinuria), depressed C3 and C4, and the presence of cryoglobulins (30% of patients).
- A definite diagnosis of SS can be made with a salivary gland biopsy showing focal lymphocytic sialadenitis with focus score of 1 per 4 mm^2 of glandular tissue.
- Salivary gland ultrasound can be done to characterize changes in salivary gland parenchyma. Diseased gland shows hypoechoic areas with convex borders.
- MRI of the gland shows inhomogeneous parenchyma. Finding correlates with biopsy of the gland.

Rx TREATMENT

NONPHARMACOLOGIC THERAPY

- Adequate fluid replacement. Ameliorate skin dryness by gently blotting dry after bathing, leaving a small amount of moisture, and then applying a moisturizer.
- Increased environmental moisture by using humidifiers
- Proper oral hygiene (daily topical fluoride use, antimicrobial mouth rinses, and stabilization of oral cavity pH) to reduce the incidence of caries.
- Sugar-free chewing gum and sour lemon lozenges to stimulate salivary secretion.
- Periodic dental and ophthalmologic evaluations to screen for complications

GENERAL Rx

- Use artificial tears frequently.
- The muscarinic agonist pilocarpine (5 mg PO qid) is useful to improve dryness.
- Cyclosporine 0.05% ophthalmic emulsion may also be useful for dry eyes.
- Cevimeline, a cholinergic agent with muscarinic agonist activity, 30 mg PO tid is effective for the treatment of dry mouth in patients with SS.
- Hydroxychloroquine alone or in conjunction with methotrexate may be useful for arthralgias and cutaneous manifestations.
- Oral cyclosporine only improves the symptoms of subjective dryness.
- Tumor necrosis factor (TNF) antagonists have not shown benefit in short-duration placebo-controlled trials.
- Rituximab (RTX) has shown some improvement in oral dry mouth symptoms, relieving marked salivary and lacrimal gland swelling in a retrospective review and showing possible reduced fatigue in a randomized clinical trial.
- Propionic acid gel can be used for vaginal dryness.
- Systemic manifestations are treated according to symptoms and complications.

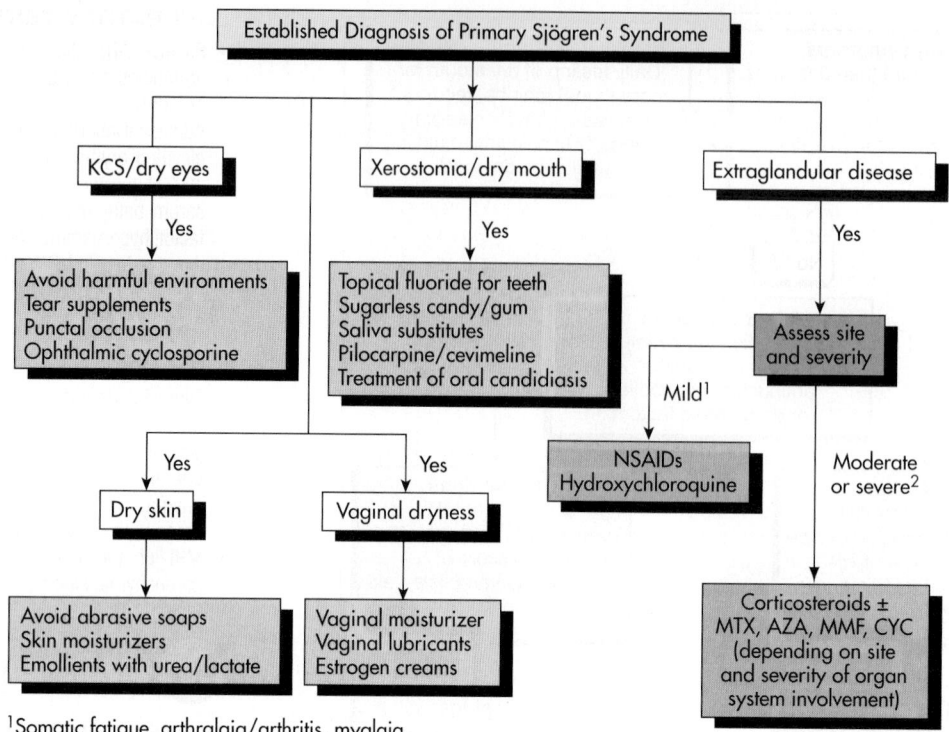

Established Diagnosis of Primary Sjögren's Syndrome

KCS/dry eyes — Yes →
- Avoid harmful environments
- Tear supplements
- Punctal occlusion
- Ophthalmic cyclosporine

Xerostomia/dry mouth — Yes →
- Topical fluoride for teeth
- Sugarless candy/gum
- Saliva substitutes
- Pilocarpine/cevimeline
- Treatment of oral candidiasis

Extraglandular disease — Yes →
Assess site and severity

Mild[1] → NSAIDs / Hydroxychloroquine

Moderate or severe[2] → Corticosteroids ± MTX, AZA, MMF, CYC (depending on site and severity of organ system involvement)

Dry skin — Yes →
- Avoid abrasive soaps
- Skin moisturizers
- Emollients with urea/lactate

Vaginal dryness — Yes →
- Vaginal moisturizer
- Vaginal lubricants
- Estrogen creams

[1] Somatic fatigue, arthralgia/arthritis, myalgia, palpable purpura without skin ulceration

[2] NSIP or LIP, interstitial nephritis, PNS involvement with motor weakness, systemic necrotizing vasculitis, CNS involvement with focal deficits or severe cognitive dysfunction

FIG. 4 Treatment algorithm for Sjögren's syndrome. The treatment of Sjögren's syndrome usually requires a multidisciplinary approach involving rheumatologists, ophthalmologists, dentists/oral surgeons, otolaryngologists, and other subspecialists, depending on the extent of extraglandular disease. In all cases, it is prudent to minimize the use of medications that can exacerbate the symptoms of dryness, such as antihistamines, antidepressants, muscle relaxers, and other drugs with anticholinergic properties. The treatment of extraglandular disease is individualized according to the site and severity of organ system involvement. The approaches indicated in the algorithm for the treatment of extraglandular disease are not supported by evidence from randomized, controlled trials, but rather from expert opinion based on retrospective case series and clinical experience. *AZA*, Azathioprine; *CNS*, central nervous system; *CYC*, cyclophosphamide; *KCS*, keratoconjunctivitis sicca; *LIP*, lymphocytic interstitial pneumonitis; *MMF*, mycophenolate mofetil; *MTX*, methotrexate; *NSAIDs*, nonsteroidal antiinflammatory drugs; *NSIP*, nonspecific interstitial pneumonitis; *PNS*, peripheral nervous system. (From Firestein GS et al: *Kelly's textbook of rheumatology*, ed 9, Philadelphia, 2013, Saunders.)

- Cyclophosphamide, azathioprine, and mycophenolate mofetil are generally reserved for life-threatening extraglandular manifestations.
- Fig. 4 describes a treatment algorithm for Sjögren's syndrome.

REFERRAL
- Rheumatology referral is generally indicated.
- Referral should be made to an oncologist when lymphoma is suspected.

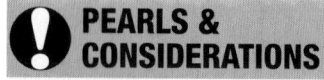

PEARLS & CONSIDERATIONS

COMMENTS
- Unusual presentations of SS may occur in association with polymyalgia rheumatica, chronic fatigue syndrome, fever of unknown origin, and inflammatory myositis.
- The most serious complication of primary SS is the development of non-Hodgkin's lymphoma and other lymphoproliferative disorders, which occur at a 10- to 44-fold increased rate as compared to age-matched controls.
- The presence of parotid gland enlargement, rheumatoid factor, low C4, cryoglobulinemia, lymphopenia, and higher levels of disease activity as measured by EULAR Sjogren's syndrome disease activity index (ESSDAI) predicts a higher lymphoma risk.

EBM EVIDENCE

Available at www.expertconsult.com

SUGGESTED READINGS

Available at www.expertconsult.com

RELATED CONTENT

Sjögren's Syndrome (Patient Information)

AUTHOR: **PIEUSHA MALHOTRA, M.D.**

BASIC INFORMATION

DEFINITION

The *International Classification of Sleep Disorders, Second Edition,* classifies sleep-disordered breathing disorders into three categories: central sleep apnea syndrome, obstructive sleep apnea (OSA), and sleep-related hypoventilation/hypoxic syndromes. The American Academy of Sleep Disorders defines OSA as repetitive episodes of upper airway obstruction that occur during sleep and that are typically associated with oxyhemoglobin desaturations.

SYNONYMS

Sleep apnea syndrome
Sleep-disordered breathing
Obstructive sleep apnea syndrome
Obstructive sleep apnea–hypopnea syndrome
OSA

ICD-10CM CODES
G47.30 Sleep apnea, unspecified
G47.31 Primary central sleep apnea
G47.33 Obstructive sleep apnea (adult) (pediatric)
G47.37 Central sleep apnea in conditions classified elsewhere
G47.39 Other sleep apnea
P28.3 Primary sleep apnea of newborn

EPIDEMIOLOGY & DEMOGRAPHICS

OSA is a common disease in the U.S. Data from the Wisconsin Cohort Study indicated that the current prevalence of moderate to severe sleep-disordered breathing (apnea-hypopnea index, measured as events/hour, ≥15) is 10% among 30- to 49-year-old men; 17% among 50- to 70-year-old men; 3% among 30- to 49-year-old women; and 9% among 50- to 70-year-old women.[1] The prevalence of OSA with associated excessive daytime somnolence is approximately 3% to 7% in adult men and 2% to 5% in adult women.[2] The prevalence is higher in obese and hypertensive patients. The prevalence of OSA in the general pediatric population is estimated to be 1% to 6%. However, in obese children and adolescents, OSA is reported to occur in 19% to 61%. Risk factors include obesity and craniofacial and upper airway soft tissue abnormalities, retrognathia, and potential risk factors include heredity, current tobacco smoking, nasal congestion, and diabetes.

PHYSICAL FINDINGS & CLINICAL PRESENTATION

- Nocturnal symptoms, including nocturia and angina pectoris
- Snoring that can be loud, habitual, and bothersome to others
- Witnessed apneas that often interrupt snoring and end with a snort
- Gasping, choking, or smothering sensations that arouse the patient from sleep
- Restless sleep associated with frequent arousals
- Daytime symptoms:
  1. Nonrestorative sleep
  2. Not feeling refreshed upon awakening
  3. Morning headache
  4. Dry mouth or throat upon awakening
  5. Excessive daytime sleepiness, typically during quiet activities
  6. Daytime fatigue or tiredness
  7. Problems with memory, concentration, and cognitive function, especially with executive functioning
  8. Easily angered, short tempered, and inattentive
  9. Hyperactivity in children
  10. Symptoms of fibromyalgia
- Systemic hypertension (HTN)
- Obesity (body mass index >30 kg/m^2)
- History of insulin resistance or type 2 diabetes mellitus
- Mood swings, irritability, anxiety, depression
- Decreased libido and impotence
- Neck circumference (which is a surrogate for central obesity) of >43 cm (17 in) in men and >37 cm (15 in) in women
- Erythematous oropharynx because of snoring.
- Adenotonsillar hypertrophy, excessive soft tissue, high-arched hard palate, pendulous uvula, prominent tongue, large degree of overjet, and retrognathia or micrognathia can be present.
- Narrowing of lateral airway walls is independent predictor of OSA in men but not women.
- Craniofacial skeletal abnormalities can lead to OSA, particularly among children and non-obese adults.
- A positive family history increases an individual's risk with each additional close family member with OSA.

ETIOLOGY

- Narrowing of upper airway as a result of obesity or increased peripharyngeal fat deposition, retrognathia and/or micrognathia, adenotonsillar hypertrophy, macroglossia, or neuromuscular weakness
- Upper airway muscular weakness as a result of neuromuscular disorders, primary CNS disorders (e.g., stroke), or metabolic disorders
- Other diseases associated with the development of OSA (e.g., hypothyroidism, acromegaly)

DIAGNOSIS

DIFFERENTIAL DIAGNOSIS

- Anemia
- Anxiety or panic disorder
- Behaviorally induced insufficient sleep syndrome
- Cardiac or heart disease
- Central sleep apnea
- Circadian rhythm disorder
- Depression
- Drug or alcohol abuse
- Gastroesophageal reflux
- Hypothyroidism
- Idiopathic hypersomnia with long or short sleep time
- Inadequate sleep hygiene
- Insomnia
- Medication effect
- Narcolepsy
- Nocturnal asthma
- Nocturnal gastroesophageal reflux
- Nocturnal seizures
- Obesity-hypoventilation syndrome (i.e., Pickwickian syndrome)
- Parasomnias
- Parkinson's disease
- Periodic limb movement disorder
- Primary snoring
- Pulmonary or lung disease
- Restless legs syndrome
- Shift work sleep disorder
- Sleep fragmentation (multiple causes)

WORKUP

- Evaluation should include questions about snoring, witnessed apneas, gasping or choking episodes, restless sleep, and excessive daytime sleepiness. Fig. 1 describes the Epworth Sleepiness Scale, an instrument that evaluates the likelihood of dozing in eight different situations in the preceding 30 days.
- Mood swings and personality changes should be addressed.
- Job performance and difficulty driving or previous motor vehicle accidents related to excessive daytime sleepiness should be discussed.
- Additional concerns include morning dry mouth/throat, morning headaches, alcohol intake, weight gain, mood or personality changes.
- A thorough drug history should include muscle relaxants and sedatives.
- A family history should target any family members with OSA.
- Physical exam is frequently normal in patients with OSA except for the presence of obesity, enlarged neck circumference, and HTN.
- OSA is confirmed by nocturnal polysomnography (PSG), which is the gold standard for diagnosis. The PSG (Fig. 1) should be performed during the patient's typical sleeping hours; it should include all stages of sleep as well as sleep in the supine position.
- The severity of the OSA is determined by the apnea-hypopnea index (AHI) (Table 1), which is derived from the total number of apneas and hypopneas divided by the total sleep time.
- Recommended severity cutoff levels for the AHI in adult patients are as follows:
  1. Mild: 5 to 15 respiratory events per hour (with symptoms)
  2. Moderate: 15 to 30 respiratory events per hour
  3. Severe: >30 respiratory events per hour
- In children, the cutoff values for severity are lower than adult values
- Criteria for the treatment of mild OSA often require symptoms, including excessive daytime sleepiness, cardiovascular disease, HTN, and mood swings.
- In certain patients, portable sleep studies or pulse oximetry may be an effective alternative to PSG for evaluation of OSA.

Epworth Sleepiness Scale	
Situation	**Score**
Sitting and reading	
Watching TV	
Sitting inactive in public place	
Passenger in car	
Lying down to rest in afternoon	
Sitting talking to someone	
Sitting after lunch without alcohol	
In a car, stopped for minutes in traffic	
Total (normal #10)	

Dozing
0 = Never
1 = Slight chance
2 = Moderate chance
3 = High chance

FIG. 1 Polysomnographic tracing of a patient with obstructive sleep apnea during two minutes of non–rapid eye movement sleep. Displayed are airflow in the upper airway ("nasal flow"), recorded with a nasal pressure transducer; respiratory effort ("abdomen"), recorded by inductance plethysmography; and oxygen saturation of hemoglobin (SpO$_2$), recorded with pulse oximetry. (From Goldman L, Schafer AI: *Goldman's Cecil medicine,* ed 24, Philadelphia, 2012, WB Saunders.)

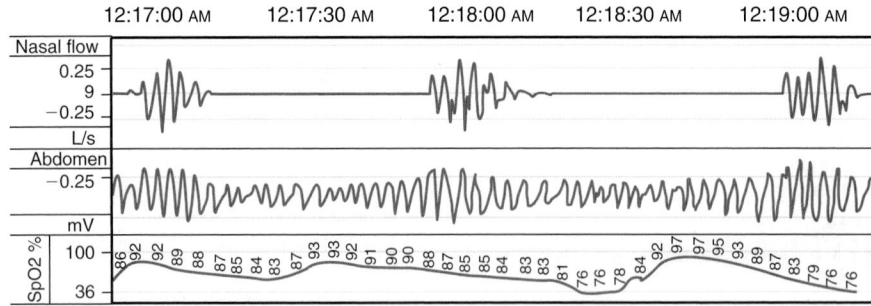

FIG. 2 The Epworth Sleepiness Scale. This instrument asks patients about their likelihood of dozing in eight different situations over the past month. (From Mason RJ et al: *Murray and Nadel's textbook of respiratory medicine,* ed 5, Philadelphia, 2010, WB Saunders.)

LABORATORY TESTS

- Arterial blood gas testing should be performed if a patient has suspected pulmonary HTN or cor pulmonale to rule out daytime hypoxemia or hypercapnia.
- Thyroid-stimulating hormone level should be obtained if hypothyroidism is suspected.
- Fasting glucose level is recommended because OSA increases the risk of developing diabetes independent of other risk factors.
- CBC is helpful to look for anemia; iron studies if anemia is detected and ferritin level if concomitant RLS is present.
- Pulmonary function testing if pulmonary disorder is suspected or to assess severity of neuromuscular disease, if present.
- ECG or echocardiogram is indicated if a cardiac disorder (e.g., arrhythmia, pulmonary HTN) is suspected.

IMAGING STUDIES

- Plain radiography of the neck can be helpful to assess the soft tissues of patients with suspected anatomic abnormalities.
- Chest x-ray if pulmonary disease is suspected.

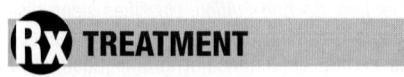 **TREATMENT**

NONPHARMACOLOGIC THERAPY

- Behavioral modifications:
  1. Weight loss in overweight and obese patients. Weight loss is effective for reducing the severity of OSA, and if significant, it may potentially allow some patients to discontinue continuous positive airway pressure (CPAP) therapy.
  2. A 10% weight gain predicted an approximate 32% increase in the AHI and sixfold increase in the odds of developing moderate to severe sleep disordered breathing.
  3. A 10% weight loss predicted a 26% decrease in the AHI.
  4. Weight loss with bariatric surgery may improve OSA in some patients, but its definitive role remains unclear. In a recent trial in obese patients with OSA, the use of bariatric surgery compared with conventional weight loss therapy did not result in a statistically greater reduction in AHI despite major differences in weight loss.
  5. Exercise without weight loss may improve OSA.
  6. Avoid alcohol for 4 to 6 hr before bedtime.
  7. Avoid muscle relaxants and sedating medications.
  8. Sleep hygiene training, especially avoiding sleep deprivation
  9. Avoid or eliminate supine sleeping positions.
  10. Avoid medications that may worsen OSA.
- Medical treatment:
  1. CPAP is the primary therapy for OSA. It delivers a constant airway pressure that acts as a pneumatic splint that relieves the upper airway obstruction.
  2. Other methods of delivering positive pressure include:
  3. Bilevel positive airway pressure (BiPAP), which delivers a preset inspiratory and expiratory airway pressure.
  4. Auto titrating positive airway pressure (APAP), which increases or decreases the level of pressure in response to change in airflow, a vibratory snore, or change in circuit pressure.
  5. Adaptive servo ventilation provides a varying amount of inspiratory pressure superimposed on a low level of CPAP.
  6. Oral appliance constructed by a reputable and qualified dentist may be effective for the treatment of mild OSA in certain patients, especially those with retrognathia. Mandibular advancement devices (MADs) are a good alternative to CPAP in patients who are unable to tolerate CPAP. Trials have shown that although CPAP is more effective than MADs in reducing AHI (4.5 vs 11 events/h, respectively), self-reported

TABLE 1 Definitions*

Events

Apnea: Cessation of breathing lasting 10 seconds or longer. Obstructive: continued respiratory effort with paradoxical motion of rib cage and abdomen; central: absent respiratory effort.

Hypopnea: Different definitions used. Two alternative definitions are part of the scoring criteria advanced by the American Academy of Sleep Medicine:

1. Score a hypopnea if all of the following are present:
   a. Nasal pressure signal excursions; drop ≥30% of baseline for at least 10 seconds.
   b. There is a ≥4% desaturation from pre-event baseline.
   c. At least 90% of the event's duration must meet the amplitude reduction of criteria for hypopnea.
2. Score a hypopnea if all of the following are present:
   a. Nasal pressure signal excursions; drop ≥50% of baseline for at least 10 seconds.
   b. There is a ≥3% desaturation from pre-event baseline *or* the event is associated with an arousal. (The latter does not require a desaturation.)
   c. At least 90% of the event's duration must meet the amplitude reduction of criteria for hypopnea.

Respiratory Effort–Related Arousal (RERA): Pattern of progressively more negative esophageal pressure terminated by a sudden change in pressure to a less negative level and an arousal; events last 10 seconds or longer.

Metrics of Severity

Apnea-Hypopnea Index: Average number of apneas plus hypopneas per hour of sleep.
Respiratory Disturbance Index: Average number of apneas plus hypopneas plus RERAs per hour of sleep.

Consensus Definitions of Severity

Normal: <5 episodes/hr
Mild sleep apnea: ≥5 and <15 episodes/hr
Moderate sleep apnea: ≥15 and <30 episodes/hr
Severe sleep apnea: ≥30 episodes/hr

Concept of Sleep Apnea Syndrome

Sleep-disordered breathing with complaint of excessive sleepiness.

*See also American Academy of Sleep Medicine.
From Mason RJ et al: *Murray and Nadel's textbook of respiratory medicine*, ed 5, Philadelphia, 2010, WB Saunders.

adherence with use of MADs is higher (6.5 vs 5.2 h/night for CPAP use). Important health outcomes were similar after 1 month of optimal MAD and CPAP treatment in patients with moderate-severe OSA, which may be explained by the greater efficacy of CPAP being offset by inferior compliance relative to MAD, resulting in similar effectiveness. There was no overall difference between MADs and CPAP with respect to improvement in blood pressure, daytime sleepiness, or quality of life.

7. Optimal treatment of allergic rhinitis is needed; nasal irrigation with saline followed by nasal corticosteroids is often helpful.
8. Symptoms of excessive daytime sleepiness may linger and require further investigation or medical therapy.
9. Patients should be considered for surgery if multiple attempts at CPAP therapy have failed and if an oral appliance is not an option. If the patient opts for surgery, ensure that it is performed by a reputable and qualified otolaryngologist and is based on the location of airway collapse.

- Surgical treatment
  ○ Surgery is done to correct specific anatomic areas of narrowing: nasal, pharyngeal, and tongue base/hypopharynx
  ○ Adenotonsillectomy is often curative for children with OSA.

  ○ Nasal septoplasty/turbinectomy should be considered for patients with nasoseptal deformities.
  ○ Uvulopalatopharyngoplasty, which involves resection of the uvula and the soft palate, is effective for a small number of patients. However, predicting which patients will benefit is difficult.
  ○ The latest available treatment is hypoglossal nerve stimulation (by surgical placement of an implant in the upper chest), which recruits lingual muscles, reduces pharyngeal collapsibility, and decreases upper airway resistance[4]
  ○ Tracheostomy is typically reserved for patients with very severe OSA who failed medical therapy or who have cor pulmonale.

DISPOSITION

- The short-term prognosis for excessive daytime sleepiness and snoring is good to excellent with the regular use of nasal CPAP, but no studies have been performed to address the long-term effects in a large population of patients.
- Residual symptoms of excessive daytime sleepiness can occur in some patients with OSA despite regular CPAP use. This has led the FDA to approve modafinil for the management of residual sleepiness.

REFERRAL

- Highly trained sleep specialists with expertise in caring for patients with OSA are recommended, especially for complex cases.
- Surgical referral to otolaryngology should be considered for children with adenotonsillar hypertrophy and for adults who are unresponsive to weight loss and CPAP therapy.
- Referral to a qualified dentist for treatment with an oral appliance may be useful for certain patients with mild OSA.

⚠ **PEARLS & CONSIDERATIONS**

- OSA is a common disorder that is underrecognized and underdiagnosed, so the identification of risk factors is crucial for making the correct diagnosis.
- The prevalence of OSA increases among women after menopause.
- The single most effective therapy for OSA is nasal CPAP.
- Patients with OSA are more vulnerable than healthy persons to the effects of alcohol consumption and sleep restriction with regard to various driving performance variables.
- OSA is a risk factor for systemic and pulmonary hypertension, stroke, atrial fibrillation, and coronary artery disease. In patients with untreated HTN and OSA, the use of CPAP results in small but statistically significant reductions in blood pressure. Therapy with CPAP has not been shown to prevent cardiovascular events in patients with moderate-to-severe obstructive sleep apnea and established cardiovascular disease.
- OSA may also be an independent risk factor for peptic ulcer bleeding.
- Ethnic differences may exist for some populations, with South Asians having a higher prevalence and risk for cardiovascular side effects.

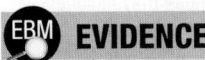 **EVIDENCE**

Available at www.expertconsult.com

SUGGESTED READINGS
Available at www.expertconsult.com

RELATED CONTENT

Sleep Apnea (Patient Information)

AUTHORS: **GRACE REBECCA PAUL, M.B.B.S., M.D.,** and **DON HAYES JR., M.D., M.S., M.ED.**

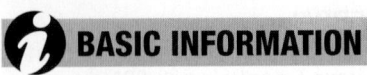

BASIC INFORMATION

DEFINITION

- Mechanical obstruction means the blockage of the intestinal lumen, preventing the passage of luminal contents through the gut tube.
- This may be either:
  a) Simple obstruction: in which the lumen may be *partially* or *completely blocked* but with intact intestinal blood flow
  b) Strangulated obstruction
     1. This is a surgical emergency.
     2. Usually the obstruction is complete, blood flow to the obstructed segment is cut off, and tissue necrosis and gangrene may occur.

ICD-10CM CODES

K56.6	Other and unspecified intestinal obstruction
K56.9	Ileus, unspecified
K56.5	Intestinal adhesions (bands) with obstruction
K56.4	Other impaction of intestine
K56.3	Gallstone ileus
K56.2	Volvulus
K5.1	Intussusception
K56	Paralytic ileus and intestinal obstruction

EPIDEMIOLOGY & DEMOGRAPHICS

- The most frequently encountered surgical disorder of the small intestines is mechanical small bowel obstruction (SBO).
- 75% of all cases of small bowel obstruction are due to intraabdominal adhesion related to prior abdominal surgery, such as appendectomy, colorectal surgery, and gynecologic procedures.

PREDOMINANT SEX AND AGE: None

PHYSICAL FINDINGS & CLINICAL PRESENTATION

PHYSICAL FINDINGS: These may include:
- Abdominal distention, especially in distal bowel obstruction
- Hyperactive bowel sounds (an early occurrence)
- Hypoactive bowel sounds (late finding)
- Hernia
- Rectal examination may reveal
  1. Blood (suggestive of neoplasm or strangulation)
  2. Masses (may suggest obturator hernia)

CLINICAL PRESENTATION: There are four key symptoms: abdominal pain, vomiting, distention, and constipation
- Abdominal pain
  1. Often crampy; intermittent
  2. Constant pain (that is, change in pain's character) signifies serious complication
- Nausea
- Vomiting (bilious vomiting seen in proximal obstructions)
- Diarrhea (early finding)
- Constipation (a late finding)
- Fever, tachycardia, and peritoneal signs (these late findings may be seen with strangulation or intestinal ischemia)

- It is important to perform serial abdominal examinations to detect changes early.

ETIOLOGY

- Postoperative adhesions (may cause acute obstruction usually within one month of surgery; or chronic obstructions can occur years later)
- Incarcerated inguinal hernia
- Malignant tumor
- IBD
- Gallstone ileus
- Stricture
- Cystic fibrosis
- Volvulus
- In children consider pyloric stenosis, intussusception, congenital atresia

DIAGNOSIS

DIFFERENTIAL DIAGNOSIS

- Acute cholangitis
- Cholecystitis
- Gastroenteritis
- Inflammatory bowel disease
- Diverticulitis
- Endometriosis
- Mesenteric ischemia
- Pancreatitis
- Dysmenorrhea
- Ovarian torsion

WORKUP

- During the initial evaluation of patients with suspected SBO, the primary objectives are to gauge the degree of metabolic derangement and volume depletion and to assess the need for and expediency of surgery. As with many surgical conditions, determining the correct diagnosis and management strategy hinges on a focused yet thorough history and physical examination.

LABORATORY TESTS

- Laboratory abnormalities are not diagnostic of bowel obstruction but instead may indicate complications of obstruction. Essential laboratory tests include:
  1. Basic metabolic panel
  2. CBC: hemoconcentration, leukocytosis
  3. Urinalysis
  4. Serum amylase: may be elevated
  5. LDH
  6. Hepatic panel
  7. Type and cross-match (in anticipation of possible surgical intervention)

IMAGING STUDIES

- Initial radiographic evaluation begins with plain x-ray films of the abdomen (supine and upright) and an upright chest radiograph. An upright chest radiograph is of paramount importance to inspect for pneumoperitoneum and also for evidence of aspiration in a patient with a history of vomiting. A supine and upright plain abdominal x-ray in patients with suspected small bowel obstruction may show:
  1. Ladder-like pattern of dilated small bowel loops with air-fluid levels (Fig. 1) indicating small bowel obstruction
  2. Accumulation of air and fluid proximal and clearance of fluid and air distal to the post of obstruction
- Enteroclysis (a fluoroscopic x-ray of the small intestine) is useful in detecting obstruction and can distinguish partial from complete blockage and adhesions from metastases.
- CT scan is the study of choice if the patient has fever, tachycardia, abdominal pain, and leukocytosis. It can reveal the etiology of the obstruction: abscess, inflammatory process, extra-luminal pathology, and/or metastases.
- CT can elucidate the cause, such as the presence of a mass (Fig. 2) or a hernia with subsequent obstruction (Fig. 3). In addition, CT has high sensitivity for detecting

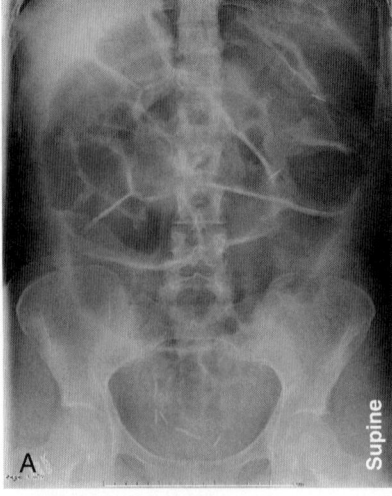
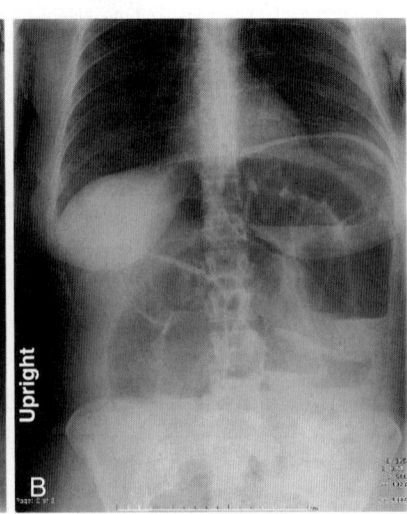

FIG. 1 A, Supine film showing dilated loops of small bowel in a patient with small bowel obstruction. **B,** Upright abdominal film revealing multiple air-fluid levels and small bowel dilation, consistent with a diagnosis of small bowel obstruction. (From Marx J: *Rosen's emergency medicine: concepts and clinical practice*, ed 6, Philadelphia, 2006, Saunders.)

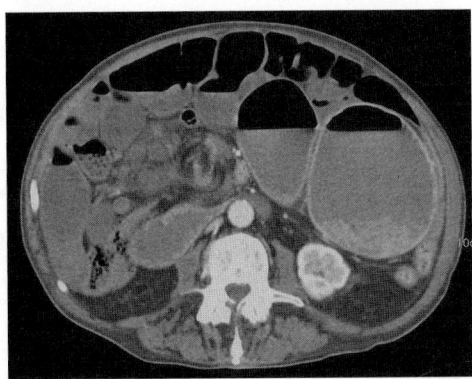

FIG. 2 CT scan of small bowel volvulus with notable mesenteric torsion. (From Cameron JL, Cameron AM: *Current surgical therapy*, ed 10, Philadelphia, 2011, Saunders.)

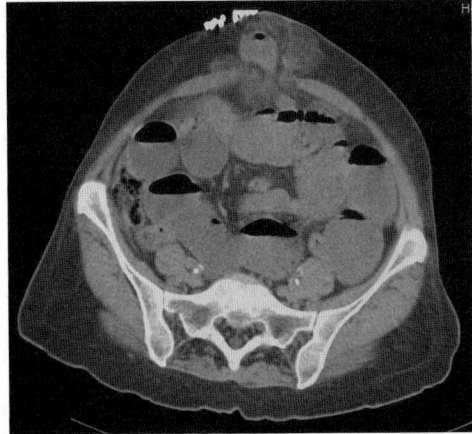

FIG. 3 CT scan of complete small bowel obstruction due to incisional hernia. (From Cameron IL, Cameron AM: *Current surgical therapy*, ed 10, Philadelphia, 2011, Saunders.)

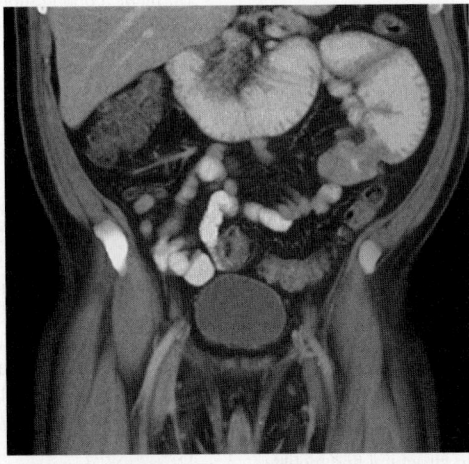

FIG. 4 Coronal image of CT scan showing mass in proximal small bowel with decompressed loops of small bowel distal to obstruction. (From Cameron JL, Cameron AM: *Current surgical therapy*, ed 10, Philadelphia, 2011, Saunders.)

impractical in the patient with gastrointestinal (GI) distress who is nauseated and vomiting.

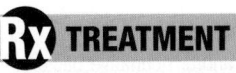 **TREATMENT**

EMERGENCY ROOM CARE

- Vigorous fluid resuscitation and correction of electrolyte disorders underpin the initial therapeutic goals of both nonoperative and preoperative management strategies. Placing a Foley catheter to measure urinary output, establishing adequate intravenous access, and reassessing hemodynamic and electrolyte status are all essential in the initial management.
- Initial treatment consists of:
  1. Designate the patients nothing by mouth ("NPO")
  2. Fluid resuscitation (with isotonic Ringer's or normal saline solution)
  3. Bowel decompression (via nasogastric [NG] tube placement): a standard NG tube provides symptomatic relief, prevents added gas and fluid accumulation proximally, and enables the serial assessment of antegrade fluid movement.
  4. Pain management
  5. Antiemetic administration
  6. Surgical consultation: must be done early
  7. Antibiotic administration

NONSURGICAL INPATIENT CARE

- Continue NG suction.
- Provide adequate fluid.

  Patients with low-grade partial SBOs are prone to spontaneous resolution with conservative interventions such as bowel rest, NG decompression, and appropriate fluid resuscitation. For partial or simple obstructions resolution usually occurs within 72 hr.

SURGICAL CARE

More than 25% of inpatients admitted because of SBO will require an operation. Patients with complete or high-grade partial SBO are most likely to need surgery, with less than 20% successfully managed nonoperatively. Surgery is indicated in:

- Strangulated obstruction (which is a surgical emergency)
- Simple complete obstruction: after failed nonoperative care

AUTHOR: **DANIEL K. ASIEDU, M.D., PH.D.**

strangulation and pneumoperitoneum indicative of a perforation and is particularly useful in the early postoperative setting to rule out ischemia, intraabdominal abscess, or morbidity as the underlying cause. It is also useful in patients with a history of malignancy to differentiate potentially recurrent disease from adhesions (Fig. 4).

- CT enterography, in which intraluminal distention is achieved with administration of large volumes of oral contrast such as water-methylcellulose solution, can be useful. This modality is most often used to diagnose patients with Crohn's disease–related strictures, and its benefit is high-resolution imaging of the bowel wall; however, it is

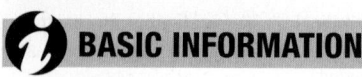

BASIC INFORMATION

DEFINITION

Small bacterial overgrowth (SIBO) is the presence of excessive native and/or nonnative bacteria in the small intestine (bacterial count >10^5/mL) causing chronic diarrhea and malabsorption.

SYNONYM

Bacterial overgrowth syndrome
SIBO

ICD-10CM CODES
K90.4   Malabsorption due to intolerance, NEC
K90.89 Other intestinal malabsorption

EPIDEMIOLOGY & DEMOGRAPHICS

PREVALENCE: The prevalence of SIBO is varied based on the population studied and the diagnostic tests used. It has shown to be prevalent in up to 12.5% to 20% of the healthy population using glucose and lactulose breath test.
PREDOMINANT SEX AND AGE: SIBO affects predominantly the elderly population. The elderly population has decreased gastric secretion and hypomotility due to age-associated decline as well as increased use of motility-altering medications.
RISK FACTORS:
- Advanced age is a known risk factor as there is thought to be an age-associated decline in GI motility.
- Patients with irritable bowel syndrome have a higher prevalence of SIBO compared to the general population. Initial studies have shown up to 65% to 80% of IBS patients with confirmed SIBO with an abnormal lactulose breath test.
- Other risk factors include UGI tract surgery, inflammatory bowel disease, chronic pancreatitis, immunodeficiency, liver disease, and obesity.

PHYSICAL FINDINGS & CLINICAL PRESENTATION

- Patients will present with nonspecific findings, which include abdominal distention, bloating, and/or pain. Other common symptoms include diarrhea and subsequent weight loss and weakness.
- The severity of symptoms reflects the extent of bacterial overgrowth.
- Severe malabsorption can present as symptoms secondary to vitamin deficiencies. Fat-soluble vitamin deficiencies can present as night blindness (vitamin A), osteomalacia and hypocalcemia (vitamin D), or prolonged bleeding (vitamin K). Bacterial overgrowth can affect vitamin B12 absorption in the ileum leading to neuropathies with sensory ataxia.

ETIOLOGY

Disorders that disrupt protective mechanisms against bacterial burden predispose patients to SIBO.
- Patients with structural or anatomical abnormalities are at greater risk. These include patients with small bowel diverticula, small intestinal strictures, surgical blind loops, ileocecal resections, or gastric resections (increasing common cause of SIBO).
- Motility disorders predispose to SIBO because of the ineffective clearance of bacteria from the proximal bowel into the colon. Examples of this include gastroparesis and small bowel dysmotility, both suggestive of poorly controlled diabetes. Long-standing celiac disease can also interfere with small bowel motility.
- It is thought that recent antibiotic use as well as antacid medication can alter the normal bacterial flora in the small intestine, contributing to SIBO.

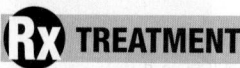

DIAGNOSIS

DIFFERENTIAL DIAGNOSIS

- Celiac disease
- Chronic pancreatitis
- Inflammatory bowel disease
- Irritable bowel syndrome
- Tropical sprue
- Whipple's disease
- Lactose intolerance

WORK-UP

- Diagnostic testing should include workup for diarrhea, anemia, and malabsorption. While endoscopy with jejunal aspirate and culture was a diagnostic tool of choice, its role is limited because of low specificity. While breath tests have their limitations as well, they are noninvasive and easy to perform.

LABORATORY TESTS

- Breath tests have become more commonplace in diagnosing SIBO. Typically fermenting bacteria reside in the colon. In SIBO, fermenting bacteria is present in the small intestine as well. A carbohydrate test dose (typically lactulose or glucose) is given and its byproduct (hydrogen) is measured as it is excreted in the breath. In SIBO, exhaled hydrogen concentrations rise early.
- Standard anemia workup is essential. CBC may suggest macrocytic anemia secondary to B12 deficiency.
- Nutritional status should be evaluated with albumin levels.
- Stool evaluation can aid in the diagnosis as well. An increase in fecal fat may be suggestive of SIBO. Stool WBC, culture, ova, and parasites should be ordered as well to rule out other infectious etiology.

IMAGING STUDIES

- Endoscopic evaluation of the small intestine can be useful in finding structural and motility causes of bacterial overgrowth such as diverticula and strictures. Small bowel biopsy may aid in the diagnosis of celiac disease as well.
- Jejunal aspirate cultures via endoscopy are considered a standard of diagnosis. Aspirate cultures that exceed 10^5 organisms/ml suggest the presence of SIBO.
- There are several limitations to jejunal aspirate cultures. Bacterial overgrowth is not uniform and may be in inaccessible areas to endoscopist and can easily be missed. Contamination from oropharyngeal flora can lead to false-positive tests. Also endoscopy is an invasive test and other methods of testing such as a breath test may be a more practical initial approach.

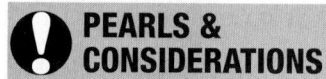

TREATMENT

The goal is to treat the underlying cause and treat the bacterial overgrowth with antibiotic therapy.

NONPHARMACOLOGIC THERAPY

- Structural disorders such as strictures, fistula, and diverticula may require surgical intervention.

ACUTE GENERAL Rx

- 7- to 10-day course of antibiotic therapy with rifaximin, amoxicillin-clavulanate, or metronidazole and ciprofloxacin has been shown to be beneficial.
- Nutritional support with vitamin replacement and dietary modification (lactose-free diet).

CHRONIC Rx

- Recurrence is common after antibiotic therapy. These patients may require subsequent courses of antibiotic therapy.
- Avoid using antacid medication.
- Avoid drugs that reduce GI motility (opioids).
- Consider lactose-free diet if the response to antimicrobial agents is incomplete.

DISPOSITION

- Prognosis is dependent on underlying cause of SIBO. Although recurrence rate is high, antibiotic therapy remains the mainstay of therapy.

REFERRAL

- Gastroenterology consultation for small bowel evaluation.
- Surgical consultation with an underlying structural disorder.

PEARLS & CONSIDERATIONS

COMMENTS

- SIBO is due to a disruption of protective mechanisms against bacterial burden
- Look for risk factors including UGI tract surgery, structural disorders, IBD, IBS, and disorders decreasing GI motility.
- Diagnosis can be made with hydrogen breath test or endoscopic jejunal aspirate culture.
- Treatment is with antibiotics.
- The combination of vitamin B12 deficiency (due to bacterial consumption) and an elevated serum folate level (due to bacterial production) is suggestive of SIBO.

RELATED CONTENT

Small Intestinal Bacterial Overgrowth (Patient Information)
Irritable Bowel Syndrome (Related Key Topic)
Malabsorption (Related Key Topic)

SUGGESTED READINGS
Available at www.expertconsult.com

AUTHOR: **GEORGE CHOLANKERIL, M.D.**

BASIC INFORMATION

DEFINITION

Somatic symptom disorder is a new diagnostic entity subsumed within DSM-5 under somatic symptom and related disorders and replaces somatization disorder. Patients with these disorders are usually encountered in primary medical settings, and thus the diagnoses have been reconceptualized to make them more useful for nonpsychiatric providers. Previous criteria overemphasized the concept of the medically unexplained symptom, which has now been dropped in favor of incorporating affective, cognitive, and behavioral components to more accurately reflect the clinical picture. In this particular condition, patients often present with one or more somatic symptoms that are perceived as distressing and significantly disrupt daily life, and they interpret or understand bodily symptoms as harmful and threatening. It is crucial to understand that somatic symptoms without a medical explanation are not sufficient to make the diagnosis.

SYNONYMS

Functional syndrome
Nonorganic symptoms
Medically unexplained symptoms
Somatization syndrome
Somatoform disorder

DSM 5 and ICD-10CM CODES
DSM V: 300.82 Somatic symptom disorder
ICD10CM: F45.9 Somatoform disorder

EPIDEMIOLOGY & DEMOGRAPHICS

INCIDENCE: Not known.
PEAK INCIDENCE: Not known.
PREVALENCE: Estimated to be around 5% to 7%
PREDOMINANT SEX AND AGE: Females tend to report more somatic symptoms.
GENETICS: Not known but thought to contribute along with other factors.
RISK FACTORS: Tendency to experience negative affect (neuroticism), limited education, lower socioeconomic status, recent stressful life events, childhood adversity, or abuse.

PHYSICAL FINDINGS & CLINICAL PRESENTATION

- These patients usually present with multiple somatic symptoms that are distressing and disrupt life and function. Symptoms can be specific, such as localized pain, but often are not. These somatic symptoms can coexist with another medically diagnosable condition. They present with high levels of anxiety about their symptoms, which they focus on excessively and perceive as unduly threatening. They have a high level of utilization of medical services.

ETIOLOGY

- Thought to be the result of multiple contributing factors such as genetic predisposition, early traumatic experiences, learning, and cultural and social issues.

Dx DIAGNOSIS

DIFFERENTIAL DIAGNOSIS

- Other medical conditions: Symptoms of unknown etiology are insufficient to make the diagnosis of somatic symptom disorder.
- Illness anxiety disorder: Distress about the meaning of the complaint, not the symptom itself.
- Conversion disorder: Voluntary motor or sensory symptom not compatible with known neurological condition.
- Factitious disorder: Falsification of physical or psychological symptoms or induction of injury/disease.
- Mood and anxiety disorders.
- Obsessive-compulsive disorder: Intrusive thoughts, images about the symptoms.
- Delusional disorder: If beliefs about somatic symptoms are rigid and firmly held.
- Malingering.

WORKUP

Rule out general medical conditions. With patients suspected or known to experience recurrent somatic symptoms, a conservative approach that limits the use of tests is best, as testing may only serve to reinforce the underlying beliefs about the nature of the symptoms.

LABORATORY TESTS

- No specific laboratory test is required, except as indicated by history and physical examination.

IMAGING STUDIES

- No specific imaging test is required, except as indicated by history and physical examination.

Rx TREATMENT

NONPHARMACOLOGIC THERAPY

- Establish a therapeutic alliance with the patient.
- Validate concerns and suffering.
- Elicit expectations and help set goals that are realistic.

ACUTE GENERAL Rx

- Brief examination that focuses on complaint area.
- Explore current psychosocial issues.
- Provide empathy and support.

- Benefit from antidepressant medication for somatic symptoms is unclear, but this benefit may be independent of depression.
- Serotonergic and noradrenergic transmission mediates endogenous analgesic mechanisms via descending inhibitory pathways in the central nervous system and may play a role in the heightened pain sensitivity seen in many of these patients.

CHRONIC Rx

- Single provider to manage overall care.
- Provide empathy and support while reinforcing previously set goals, particularly restoration of function.
- Regular follow-up to support therapeutic relationship.
- Avoid invasive or extensive testing unless clinically warranted.
- Treat coexisting mood and anxiety disorders.

DISPOSITION

- This is a chronic condition with frequent exacerbations requiring close follow-up.

REFERRAL

- To a psychiatrist and/or a psychotherapist if patient is psychologically minded and open to referral.

PEARLS & CONSIDERATIONS

- Some mental disorders may initially manifest with somatic symptoms; with multiple somatic symptoms, there is a higher likelihood of psychopathology.
- It is important to elicit the patient's own explanatory models for his or her symptoms.
- When more psychological explanations are reported, the patient is more likely to be disabled.
- Some patients have a negative self-perception that can persist and is a strong predictor of poor outcome.
- Patients may have catastrophic thinking and may be hostile to previous doctors, whom they may blame.
- Help patients reframe thoughts and keep focus on restoring function rather than on diagnosis and elimination of symptoms.

SUGGESTED READINGS
Available at www.expertconsult.com

AUTHOR: **DWAYNE R. HEITMILLER, M.D.**

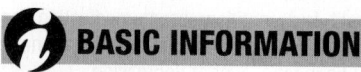

BASIC INFORMATION

DEFINITION

Spasticity is an exaggerated tone that displays a velocity-dependent increase in resistance of muscles to a passive stretch stimulus.

SYNONYMS

Hypertonicity

ICD-10CM CODES
M62.838	Other muscle spasm
G81.10	Spastic hemiplegia affecting unspecified side
R25.0	Abnormal head movements
R26.0	Ataxic gait
G81.10	Spastic hemiplegia affecting unspecified side
G83.9	Paralytic syndrome, unspecified
G80.9	Cerebral palsy, unspecified

EPIDEMIOLOGY & DEMOGRAPHICS

INCIDENCE: Spasticity affects between 47% and 70% of people with multiple sclerosis, 32% to 36% of those with spinal cord injury, approximately 20% of those with stroke, more than 90% with cerebral palsy, and approximately 50% of patients with traumatic brain injury.

PREDOMINANT SEX AND AGE: Spasticity is not affected by sex, race, or age group, nor is it more prevalent in any of those groups.

RISK FACTORS: Multiple sclerosis, stroke, spinal cord injury, cerebral palsy, traumatic brain injury

PHYSICAL FINDINGS & CLINICAL PRESENTATION

- Patient may present with impaired gait, impaired limb function, decreased mobility, or discomfort due to increased muscle tone.
- While increased tone may preserve strength in the affected muscles, function may be impaired, especially fine motor. Examine active and passive motion, reflexes, and functions:
  1. Strength may be normal or decreased. Isometric strength is typically greater than concentric strength.
  2. Tone may be variably increased to passive range of motion (modified Ashworth scale; see Table 1).
  3. Reflexes are typically brisk.
  4. Patient may have accompanying extensor plantar signs, clonus, or spontaneous flexor spasms.
  5. Function may be impaired or enhanced due to increased tone.

TABLE 1 Modified Ashworth Scale

0	No increase in muscle tone
1	Slight increase in muscle tone, manifested by a catch and release or by minimal resistance at the end range of motion when the part is moved in flexion or extension/abduction or adduction
1+	Slight increase in muscle tone, manifested by a catch, followed by minimal resistance throughout the remainder (less than half) of the range of motion
2	More marked increase in muscle tone through most of the range of motion, but the affected part is easily moved
3	Considerable increase in muscle tone, passive movement is difficult
4	Affected part is rigid in flexion or extension (abduction or adduction)

From Stein J: Spasticity. In Frontera WR et al (eds): *Essentials of physical medicine and rehabilitation*, ed 2, Philadelphia, 2008, Saunders.

ETIOLOGY

Upper motor neuron injury, most commonly due to multiple sclerosis, stroke, spinal cord injury, cerebral palsy, traumatic brain injury

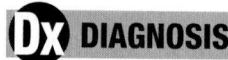 DIAGNOSIS

DIFFERENTIAL DIAGNOSIS

Rigidity, clonus, dystonia, dyskinesia, myotonia, tetanus, muscle contracture, cramps

WORKUP

- A diagnosis is established clinically.
- Investigate reversible exacerbating causes of spasticity: underlying infection, bladder distention, bowel impaction, fracture, pain.

LABORATORY TESTS

Urinalysis, complete blood count, metabolic panel

IMAGING STUDIES

Chest x-ray, abdominal x-ray series, bladder ultrasound

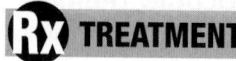 TREATMENT

First treat reversible causes of spasticity (see "Workup"), then proceed to physical and pharmacologic therapeutics. Lastly, consider surgical intervention in severe, refractory cases.

NONPHARMACOLOGIC THERAPY

- Physical therapeutics include range of motion and muscle stretching, serial casting or orthotics, muscle cooling, electrical stimulation.
- Surgical procedures include tenotomy, tendon lengthening, and tendon transfers. More invasive surgical interventions include peripheral neurectomy, myelotomy, and rhizotomy.

ACUTE GENERAL Rx

- Oral medications: baclofen, tizanidine, diazepam, dantrolene (Table E2)
- Other interventions: intrathecal baclofen, botulinum toxin intramuscular injections, chemical nerve blocks (with bupivacaine, phenol, or ethyl alcohol)

COMPLEMENTARY & ALTERNATIVE MEDICINE

EMG biofeedback

DISPOSITION

Typically nonprogressive, but medications may lose efficacy after long duration of use. Drug holidays (with use of alternate spasmolytic) may be beneficial.

REFERRAL

- Physicians: neurologist or physiatrist with expertise in botulinum toxin injection and/or intrathecal spasmolytic therapy is recommended when oral medications are ineffective or not tolerated.
- Physical and occupational therapy

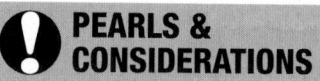 PEARLS & CONSIDERATIONS

- Assess whether the spasms recently increased in severity or intensity (as would occur with reversible exacerbating causes).
- Consider whether patient's tone is beneficial or detrimental to patient's functionality or overall health status.
- Spasticity may assist posture and mobility, as well as maintain muscle mass and bone mineralization, reduce dependent edema, and prevent deep venous thromboses.
- Spasticity may impair patient's functionality, interfere with activities of daily living, interfere with sleep, and cause discomfort.
- Monitor liver function with dantrolene and tizanidine, as these drugs may cause hepatotoxicity.

AUTHOR: **SACHIN KEDAR, M.B.B.S., M.D.**

BASIC INFORMATION

DEFINITION

Spinal cord compression is characterized by direct compression of the spinal cord within the spinal canal. This may result in the neurologic loss of function from compression of the spinal cord in the cervical, thoracic, and upper lumbar spinal canal or from compression of the cauda equina in the lower lumbar spinal canal. Fig. 1 illustrates a schematic demarcation of levels of principal dermatomes shown as distinct segments. Depending on the underlying etiology, symptoms may develop gradually or acutely and may result in complete or incomplete deficits. Neurologic deficits related to compression of the cord itself are referred to as myelopathy, while deficits cause by compression on nerve roots are described as radiculopathy.

- Signs and symptoms of myelopathy
  - Upper motor neuron signs (Hoffman's sign, inverted radial reflex, Babinski sign, spasticity, hyperreflexia) in chronic cases
  - Weakness
  - Sensory deficits
  - Clumsiness, difficult ambulation, broad-based gait
- Signs and symptoms of radiculopathy
  - Lower motor neuron signs (hyporeflexia, hypotonicity, fasciculations, muscle atrophy)
  - Weakness
  - Sensory deficits

Incomplete spinal cord lesions may classically present in distinct syndromic patterns (Table 1), for example, as follows:

- Anterior cord syndrome
- Brown-Séquard syndrome
- Cauda equina syndrome (not a true example of spinal cord compression but rather of cauda equina compression, affecting lumbosacral nerve roots (lower motor neurons)
- Central cord syndrome
- Conus medullaris syndrome

SYNONYMS

Central cord syndrome
Anterior cord syndrome
Brown-Sequard syndrome
Acute spinal cord compression
Cauda equina syndrome
Conus medullary syndrome

ICD-10CM CODES
S14.13XX Anterior cord syndrome
G83.81 Brown-Séquard syndrome
G83.4 Cauda equina syndrome
S14.12XX Central cord syndrome
G95.81 Conus medullaris syndrome

EPIDEMIOLOGY AND DEMOGRAPHICS

Dependent on etiology of cord compression

Degenerative spine disorders (i.e., degenerative disk disease, spinal stenosis, spondylolisthesis) are more common with increasing age, although they can affect any age group. Epidemiology and demographics are dependent on the type of degenerative changes.

TUMOR

Epidemiology dependent entirely on tumor type. Malignant tumors in the spinal cord are most commonly metastatic disease, although primary musculoskeletal tumors are possible. The spine is the third-most common site for tumor metastases, after the lung and liver. Common metastatic lesions to the spine include lung cancer, breast cancer, prostate cancer, cancer of the GI tract, multiple myeloma, and lymphoma.

INFECTION

Diskitis/osteomyelitis may progress to epidural abscess, causing spinal cord compression and neural compromise. Epidural abscess incidence is approximately 0.2 to 3.0 per 10,000 hospital admissions. *Staphylococcus aureus* is the most common offending organism. Risk factors include increasing age, diabetes mellitus, end-stage renal disease, chronic hepatitis/cirrhosis, known endocarditis, immunocompromise, and IV drug abuse.

SPINAL CORD INJURY (SCI):

Occurred most commonly in males with a mean age of 37 years in 2010. Alcohol plays a major role in at least 25% of SCI.

INCIDENCE: 12,400 new cases/year in 2010 in the U.S.

PREVALENCE: 250,000 persons in 2005 in the U.S.

COST (IN U.S.): >$5 billion/year

RISK FACTORS: Underlying spinal disease can predispose to SCI:

- Spondyloarthropathy, especially ankylosing spondylitis
- Diffuse idiopathic skeletal hyperostosis (DISH)
- Congenital spinal disorders
- Preexisting spinal canal stenosis or compromise
- Atlantoaxial instability
- Osteoporosis
- Rheumatoid arthritis (cervical spine)

PHYSICAL FINDINGS & CLINICAL PRESENTATION

Clinical features reflect the amount of spinal cord involvement:

- Weakness, sensory changes (dependent on level of compression/lesion/injury).
- Myelopathy if cord involvement, radiculopathy if nerve root involvement (may involve both).
- *Central cord syndrome (most common incomplete spinal cord injury):* Motor impairment greater in upper than in lower extremities, variable degree of sensory loss below the injury level. Weakness and poor hand dexterity especially common. Classically occurs after mild trauma including cervical hyperextension in the setting of preexisting cervical spondylosis.
- *Anterior cord syndrome (worst prognosis of incomplete spinal cord injury):* Affects the anterior or ventral 2/3 of the spinal cord, sparing the dorsal columns. May be caused by a vascular injury to the anterior spinal artery or by a flexion/compression injury.

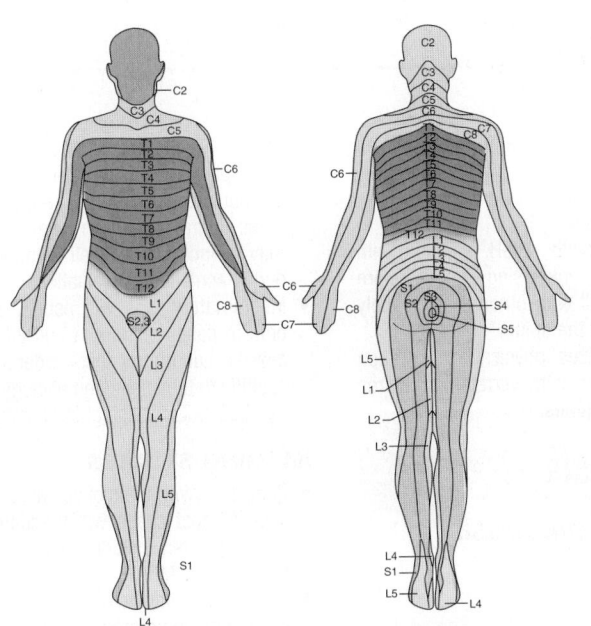

Levels of principal dermatomes

C5	Clavicles	T10	Level of umbilicus
C5,6,7	Lateral parts of upper limbs	T12	Inguinal or groin regions
C8, T1	Medial sides of upper limbs	L1,2,3,4	Anterior and inner surfaces of lower limbs
C6	Thumb	L4,5 S1	Foot
C6,7,8	Hand	L4	Medial side of great toe
C8	Ring and little fingers	S1,2, L5	Posterior and outer surfaces of lower limbs
T4	Level of nipples	S1	Lateral margin of foot and little toe
		S2,3,4	Perineum

FIG. 1 Schematic demarcation of levels of principal dermatomes shown as distinct segments. There is actually considerable overlap between any two adjacent dermatomes. (From Goldman L, Schafer AI: *Goldman's Cecil medicine,* ed 24, Philadelphia, 2011, Saunders.)

TABLE 1 Spinal Cord Syndromes

Syndrome	Sensory	Motor	Sphincter Involvement
Central cord syndrome	Variable	Upper extremity weakness, distal > proximal	Variable
Brown-Séquard syndrome	Ipsilateral position and vibration sense loss, Contralateral pain and temperature sensation loss	Motor loss ipsilateral to cord lesion	Variable
Anterior cord syndrome	Loss of pin and touch sensation Vibration, position sense preserved	Motor loss or weakness below cord level	Variable
Transverse cord syndrome—complete	Loss of sensation below level of cord injury	Loss of voluntary motor function below cord level	Sphincter control lost
Cauda equina syndrome	Saddle anesthesia may be present, or sensory loss may range from patchy to complete transverse pattern	Weakness may be of lower motor neuron type	Sphincter control impaired

From Marx JA et al: *Rosen's emergency medicine*, ed 8, Philadelphia, 2014, WB Saunders.

Impairment usually is worse in the lower extremities than upper extremities. Physical manifestations include motor, pain, and temperature loss below the lesion. Proprioception and vibratory sense may be preserved as dorsal columns are preserved.

• *Brown-Séquard syndrome:* Rare in isolation. Caused by injury to either half of the spinal cord and resulting in the loss of motor function, position, vibration, and light touch on the side of injury as well as loss of pain and temperature sense on the contralateral side.

• *Conus medullaris syndrome:* Results in variable motor loss in the lower extremities with loss of bowel and bladder function.

• *Cauda equina syndrome:* Low back pain, weakness in bilateral lower extremities, saddle anesthesia, and loss of voluntary bladder and/or bowel control, often presenting as bladder retention and/or bowel incontinence.

ETIOLOGY

• Trauma (most SCIs result from high-speed motor vehicle accidents, falls, sports injuries, or violence)
• Tumor
• Infection (e.g., epidural abscess)
• Inflammatory processes
• Degenerative disk disease with associated spinal stenosis
• Acute disk herniation
• Cystic abnormalities
• Ankylosing spondylitis, DISH. Patients with underlying DISH or ankylosing spondylitis are at high risk of SCI with otherwise relatively minor fractures of the spine.
• Table 2 summarizes physical examination findings associated with vertebral fractures and spinal cord injuries.

Dx DIAGNOSIS

DIFFERENTIAL DIAGNOSIS
• See "Etiology."

WORKUP
• Signs and symptoms of spinal cord or cauda equina compression often indicate urgent surgical conditions and thus require urgent imaging and early referral for assessment by a spine specialist.
• In cases of acute trauma in which spinal cord injury is suspected, patient should undergo full trauma evaluation following advanced trauma life support protocol in emergency room setting. With suspected injury to the cervical spine, the patient should be immobilized in a hard cervical collar or in-line traction at all times during evaluation. Log-roll precautions may be indicated as well to immobilize spine during acute injury evaluation.
• Inflammatory labs will usually be elevated both in cases of trauma and infectious processes. Laboratory tests ordered should be specific to the suspected etiology or differential diagnosis for spinal cord compression.

IMAGING STUDIES
• Signs and symptoms of spinal cord compression in most cases will mandate advanced imaging, often including CT and CT myelogram and/or MRI. Plain x-rays may be helpful; however, normal plain films do not negate the need for further advanced imaging in the setting of signs and symptoms of spinal cord compression or spinal cord injury.
• In the trauma setting, after primary and secondary surveys, fine-cut helical CT scans with axial, coronal, and sagittal reconstructions have replaced plain cervical radiographs in most trauma centers as the initial evaluation of choice in detecting fractures of the cervical spine.

TABLE 2 Physical Examination Findings Associated with Vertebral Fractures and Spinal Cord Injuries

Injury	Physical Examination Area	Associated Findings
Vertebral fracture	Spine	Tenderness of the neck and/or back. Examine the entire spine because vertebral fractures may occur in multiples.
	Neurologic	See spinal cord injury below.
	Chest	*Thoracic spine fractures:* check for chest tenderness, unequal breath sounds, and arrhythmia, which are suggestive of an associated intrathoracic injury or myocardial contusion.
	Abdomen/pelvis	*Thoracolumbar and lumbar spine fractures:* check for abdominal or pelvic tenderness. For instance, up to 50% of patients with a transverse process fracture and 33% of patients with a Chance fracture have concurrent intraabdominal pathology. A transverse area of ecchymosis on the lower abdominal wall (seat belt sign) increases the chance of an abdominopelvic injury.
	Extremity	*Thoracolumbar and lumbar spine fractures:* check for calcaneal tenderness because 10% of calcaneal fractures are associated with a low thoracic or lumbar fracture. Mechanistically, these areas are fractured as a result of axial loading.
Spinal cord injury	Neurologic, motor (anterior column)	Assess motor function on a scale of 0 to 5. The *motor level* is defined as the most caudal segment with at least 3/5 strength. Injuries to the first eight cervical segments result in tetraplegia (previously known as quadriplegia); lesions below the T1 level result in paraplegia.
	Neurologic, sensory (spinothalamic tract)	Assess sensory function via pinprick and light touch on the following scale: 0 = absent; 1 = impaired; 2 = normal. The *sensory level* is defined as the most caudal segment of the spinal cord with normal sensory function. The highest intact sensory level should be marked on the patient's spine to monitor for progression.
	Neurologic, sensory (dorsal column)	Assess vibratory sensory function on a scale of 0 to 2 by using a tuning fork over bony prominences. Assess position sense (proprioception) by flexing and extending the great toe.
	Neurology, deep tendon reflex	On a scale of 0 to 4, assess the deep tendon reflexes in the upper (biceps, triceps) and lower (patellar, Achilles) extremities.
	Anogenital	Assess rectal tone, sacral sensation, signs of urinary or fecal retention or incontinence, and priapism. Also check the anogenital reflexes: an *anal wink* (S2-S4) is present if the anal sphincter contracts in response to stroking the perianal skin area. The *bulbocavernosus reflex* (S3-S4) is elicited by squeezing the glans penis or clitoris (or pulling on an inserted Foley catheter), which results in reflexive contraction of the anal sphincter.
	Head-to-toe examination	A spinal cord injury may mask a patient's ability to perceive and localize pain. Imaging of high-risk areas, such as the abdomen, and areas of bruising or swelling may be required to exclude occult injuries.

From Adams JG et al: *Emergency medicine, clinical essentials,* ed 2, Philadelphia, 2013, Elsevier.

- Detection of injury to any part of the spine during trauma evaluation mandates full imaging evaluation of the entire spine, as noncontiguous injuries are common.
- While CT scan is excellent at imaging bony structures and detecting fractures, MRI provides more detailed imaging of the soft-tissue structures, including neural structures, discoligamentous structures, the posterior ligamentous complex, and paraspinal soft tissues. MRI is very sensitive for detecting ligamentous injury, spinal cord edema, spinal cord compression from soft-tissue structures, epidural hematoma, diskitis, osteomyelitis, and epidural abscess (Fig. E2). Of note, gadolinium contrast may increase the sensitivity of the MRI study for the detection of tumors or infections.

Rx TREATMENT

- Depending on the etiology of spinal cord compression as well as the specific signs and symptoms during physical examination and history-taking, urgent surgical decompression and/or stabilization may be indicated. Referral to a spine specialist is indicated in most cases of spinal cord compression.
- Corticosteroids: Controversial in cases of acute spinal cord injury. Methylprednisolone was thought to reduce the amount of secondary injury that occurs after SCI and was

previously used in many trauma centers. However, current evidence is insufficient to support corticosteroids for this use, and most spine trauma centers no longer utilize steroids in cases of acute spinal cord injury.
- Vasopressors: Current evidence supports the use of vasopressors in cases of spinal cord injury to maintain spinal cord perfusion and to prevent ischemic damage to the cord. The ideal mean arterial pressure and duration of treatment are yet to be defined. Both the treatment modality and the injury itself mandate admission to ICU level of care in most cases for close monitoring.

DISPOSITION

Indicators regarding prognosis:
- Patients with acute traumatic SCI need monitoring in the ICU and evaluation for potential life-threatening complications, including cardiovascular instability and respiratory failure.
- In general, the greater the distal motor and sensory sparing, the greater the expected recovery.
- In most cases of spinal cord compression and/or spinal cord injury, the primary goal of surgical decompression and/or stabilization should be to spare the remaining functional levels and to prevent worsening of the injury. Return of function should not be guaranteed.

- Prophylaxis against deep vein thrombosis and pulmonary embolism should always be provided. In acute injuries to the spine or postoperatively, this may consist of mechanical prophylaxis including TEDs and SCDs. Pharmacologic deep vein thrombosis/pulmonary embolism prophylaxis is often held initially to prevent development of epidural hematoma.

REFERRAL

- Signs and symptoms of spinal cord or cauda equina compression often indicate urgent surgical conditions and thus require urgent imaging and early referral for assessment by a spine specialist.

SUGGESTED READINGS

Available at www.expertconsult.com

RELATED CONTENT

Spinal Stenosis (Patient Information)
Spinal Stenosis, Lumbar (Related Key Topic)
Spinal Epidural Abscess (Related Key Topic)
Lumbar Disk Syndrome (Related Key Topic)

AUTHOR: **DANIEL BRIAN CARLIN REID, M.D., M.P.H.**

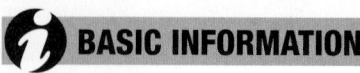

BASIC INFORMATION

DEFINITION

A spinal epidural abscess (SEA) is a focal suppurative infection occurring in the spinal epidural space.

SYNONYM

SEA

ICD-10CM CODES
G06.1 Intraspinal abscess and granuloma

EPIDEMIOLOGY & DEMOGRAPHICS

INCIDENCE (IN U.S.):
- 2 to 25 cases/100,000 hospitalized patients/yr
- May be increasing over the past 3 decades

PREDOMINANT AGE
- Median age of onset approximately 50 yr (35 yr in intravenous drug users)
- Peak incidence in seventh and eighth decades of life

PHYSICAL FINDINGS & CLINICAL PRESENTATION
- The presentation of SEA can be nonspecific.
- Fever, malaise, and back pain are the most consistent early symptoms.
- Pain is often focal. It may initially be mild but can progress to become severe.
- As the disease progresses, root pain can occur, followed by motor weakness, sensory changes, bladder and bowel dysfunction, and paralysis.
- Physical findings may be limited to fever or spinal tenderness.
- The evolution to neurologic deficits can occur as quickly as a few hours, or over weeks to months.
- Once paralysis occurs, it may quickly become irreversible without the appropriate intervention.

ETIOLOGY
- Pyogenic bacteria account for the majority of cases in the United States. Immigrants from TB-endemic areas may present with tuberculous SEAs. Fungi and parasites can also cause this condition. The most common causative organism is *Staphylococcus aureus*. Gram-negative bacilli and anaerobes may be seen if the infection has a urinary or GI source.
- Most posterior SEAs are thought to originate from distant focus (e.g., skin and soft tissue infections), while anterior SEAs are commonly associated with diskitis or vertebral osteomyelitis. No source was found in approximately one third of cases.
- Associated predisposing conditions include diabetes mellitus, alcoholism, cancer, AIDS, and chronic renal failure, or following epidural anesthesia, spinal surgery or trauma, prolonged epidural catheter placement, paraspinal glucocorticoid or analgesic injections, acupuncture, or IV drug use. No predisposing condition is found in approximately 20% of patients.

- Damage to the spinal cord can be caused by direct compression of the spinal cord, vascular compromise, bacterial toxins, and inflammation.

DIAGNOSIS

DIFFERENTIAL DIAGNOSIS
- Herniated disk
- Vertebral osteomyelitis and diskitis
- Metastatic tumors
- Meningitis

LABORATORY TESTS
- WBC may be normal or elevated.
- ESR is usually elevated over 30 mm/hr.

- Blood cultures are positive in approximately 60% of patients with SEA.
- CSF cultures are positive in 19%, but lumbar puncture is unnecessary, and may be contraindicated.
- Once imaging is done, CT-guided aspiration or open biopsy should be done to determine causative organism. Abscess content culture is positive in 90% of patients.

IMAGING STUDIES
- MRI with gadolinium is the imaging modality of choice (Fig. 1); CT scan with contrast may show the abscess (Fig. 2) but is less sensitive than MRI.

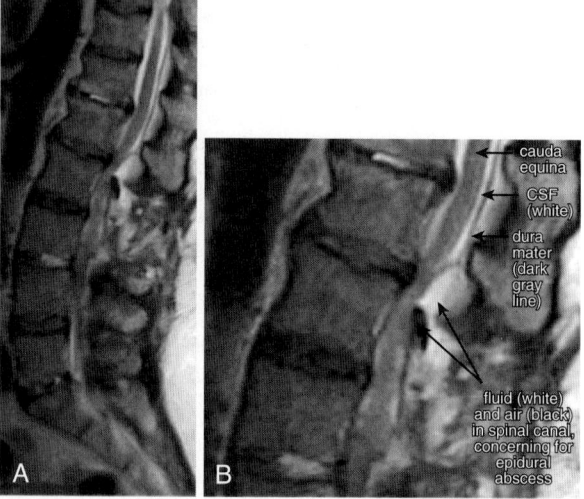

FIG. 1 Same patient as in Fig. 2, in whom noncontrast computed tomography showed air in the spinal canal, concerning for epidural abscess. Magnetic resonance imaging (MRI) of the lumbar spine without contrast was performed, as the patient was in acute renal failure. **A,** This T_2-weighted sagittal MR image provides useful information even without gadolinium contrast. **B,** Close-up. On T_2-weighted MRI sequences, fluid including cerebrospinal fluid *(CSF)* appears white. Fat-containing tissues such as bone marrow and the spinal cord or cauda equina appear dark gray. Calcified bone appears nearly black due to an absence of resonating protons. Air appears completely black for the same reason. The midline sagittal image shows the cauda equina to be impinged upon by an epidural fluid collection containing air—an epidural abscess. The dura mater is visible as a thin, dark gray line parallel to the spinal cord. It is indented in the region of the epidural abscess. (From Broder JS: *Diagnostic imaging for the emergency physician,* Philadelphia, 2011, Saunders.)

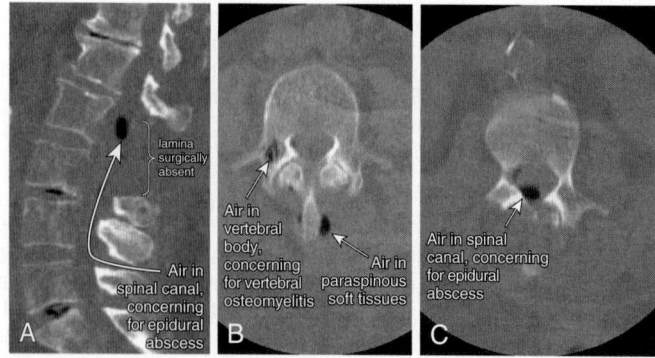

FIG. 2 This 67-year-old female presented with delirium and fever. Three months prior, she had undergone lumbar laminectomy, and her wound had been treated with a wound VAC dressing. Magnetic resonance imaging was not initially available, so noncontrast computed tomography (CT) was performed. Noncontrast CT is excellent at delineating air, which appears black on bone windows. **A,** The midsagittal view demonstrates air *(black)* in the spinal canal at the L2 and L3 levels. On the axial views **(B, C),** air is visible in the spinal canal, in paraspinal soft tissues, and within the vertebral body. These findings are concerning for a paraspinal infection that has developed into an epidural abscess with vertebral osteomyelitis. (From Broder JS: *Diagnostic imaging for the emergency physician,* Philadelphia, 2011, Saunders.)

- CT with myelography is more sensitive for cord compression.

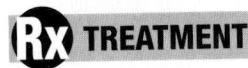 **TREATMENT**

NONPHARMACOLOGIC THERAPY

- Surgical decompression is the mainstay of treatment. Decompression within the first 24 hr has been related to an improved prognosis.
- Nonsurgical treatment is effective in some patients, but failure rate may be excessive. This approach should not be considered and should only be attempted in the absence of signs of compressive myelopathy and with very careful follow-up.

ACUTE GENERAL Rx

- In addition to surgery, antibiotics directed at the most likely organism should be initiated. Fig. 3 describes an algorithm for the management of patients with SEA.
- If the organism is unknown, broad coverage against staphylococci, streptococci, and gram-negative bacilli should be initiated. Empiric antimicrobial therapy typically includes vancomycin plus an antipseudomonal cephalosporin or carbapenem. The regimen can be adjusted according to culture results. Therapy should continue for at least 4 to 6 wk.

CHRONIC Rx

Neurologic deficits may remain despite aggressive treatment.

DISPOSITION

Irreversible paralysis and death can occur in up to 25% of patients.

REFERRAL

All cases should be referred to a neurosurgeon and an infectious disease specialist.

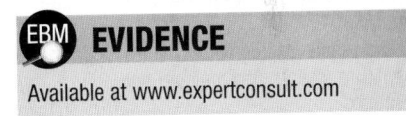 **PEARLS & CONSIDERATIONS**

- It is critically important to recognize this process early; the prognosis is generally excellent if treatment is initiated while symptoms are localized and before evidence of myelopathy develops.
- The likelihood of success postsurgery is low in patients who have developed complete paralysis for longer than 36 hours.

EBM EVIDENCE

Available at www.expertconsult.com

AUTHOR: **GLENN G. FORT, M.D., M.P.H.**

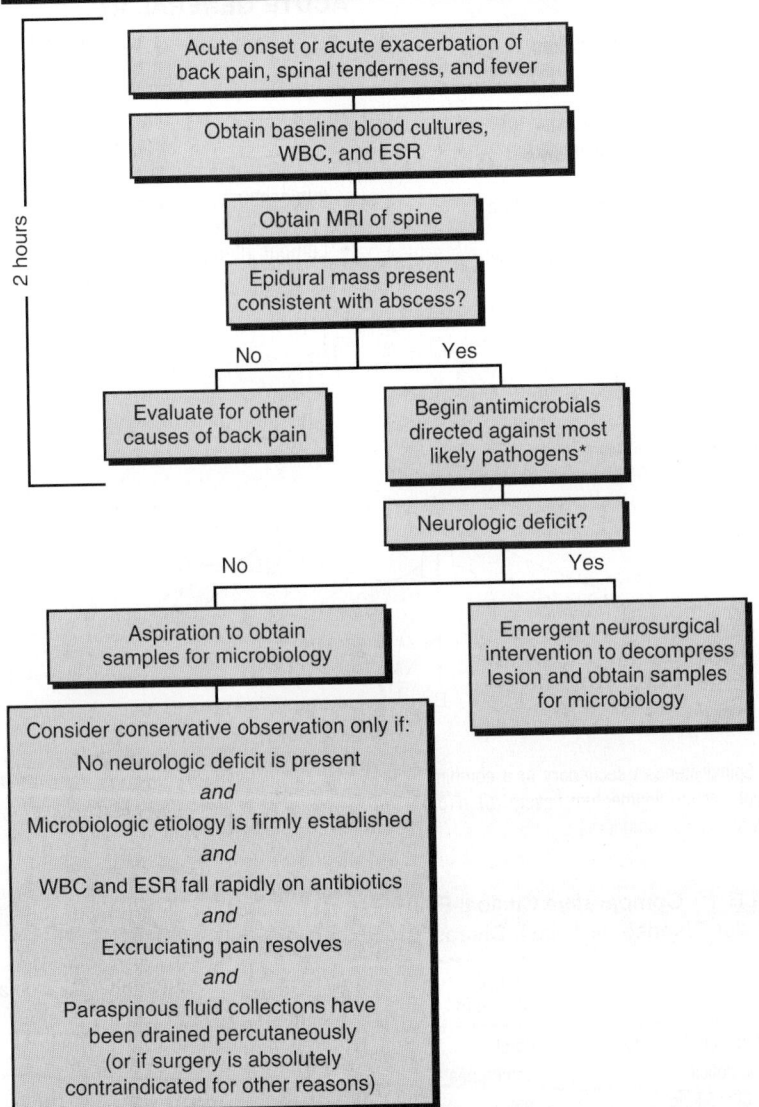

FIG. 3 Algorithm for the management of patients with spinal epidural abscess syndrome. If magnetic resonance imaging *(MRI)* cannot be performed, myelography, high-contrast computed tomography (CT), or CT-myelography may be an acceptable alternative to localize an epidural abscess. *If abscess drainage can be performed promptly, antimicrobial drugs may be withheld until specimens for microbial analysis are obtained. *ESR,* Erythrocyte sedimentation rate; *WBC,* white blood cell. (From Vincent JL et al: *Textbook of critical care,* ed 6, Philadelphia, 2011, Saunders.)

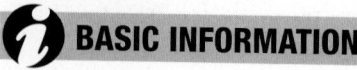

DEFINITION

Lumbar spinal stenosis (LSS) is an anatomical impairment characterized by narrowing of the spinal canal or nerve root foramen.

SYNONYMS

Central spinal stenosis
Lateral spinal stenosis
Spondylosis
Lumbar spinal stenosis
LSS

ICD-10CM CODES
M48.06 Spinal stenosis, lumbar region

EPIDEMIOLOGY & DEMOGRAPHICS

More common between 50 and 60 yr of age

PHYSICAL FINDINGS & CLINICAL PRESENTATION

- Symptoms caused by direct mechanical compression or indirect vascular compression of the nerve roots or the cauda equina.
- Neurogenic claudication: leg, buttock, or back pain precipitated by walking and relieved by sitting.
- Pain may radiate down to ankles and is associated with numbness, tingling, and weakness.
- Taking a flexed posture reduces symptoms because it increases the available space in the lumbar spinal canal.
- Decreased lumbar extension.
- Normal peripheral pulses.
- Positive Romberg's sign (decreased proprioception).
- Wide-based gait.
- Reduced knee and ankle reflex.
- Urine incontinence.

ETIOLOGY

Spinal stenosis may be primary or secondary (Fig. 1)
- Primary stenosis (congenital or developmental narrowing)
  1. Idiopathic
  2. Achondroplasia
  3. Morquio-Ullrich syndrome
- Secondary stenosis (acquired)
  1. Degenerative (hypertrophy of the articular processes, disk degeneration, ligamentum flavum hypertrophy, spondylolisthesis)
  2. Fracture/trauma
  3. Postoperative (postlaminectomy)
  4. Paget's disease
  5. Ankylosing spondylitis
  6. Tumors
  7. Acromegaly

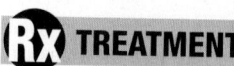

DIFFERENTIAL DIAGNOSIS

- Osteoarthritis of the knee or hip
- Acute cauda equina syndrome, resulting from compression by epidural abscess or tumors
- Pain and weakness caused by multiple myeloma or osteomyelitis
- Intermittent claudication—peripheral vascular disease
- Peripheral neuropathy such as that caused by a herniated nucleus pulposus
- Scoliosis or spondylolisthesis
- Rheumatoid diseases: ankylosing spondylitis, Reiter's syndrome, fibromyalgia
- Table 1 compares clinical features of spinal stenosis, peripheral vascular disease, and disk disease.

WORKUP

History, physical examination, and specific imaging studies

IMAGING STUDIES

- Lumbar spine film sensitivity 66%, specificity 93%.
- Ultrasound of the spinal canal has also been used.
- CT scan of the lumbosacral spine: sensitivity (75%-85%), specificity (80%).
- MRI of the lumbosacral spine (Fig. 2): sensitivity (80%-90%), specificity (95%).
- Myelogram: sensitivity (77%), specificity (72%). Absolute stenosis is defined as the anterior-posterior (AP) diameter of the spinal canal <10 mm. Relative stenosis: 10 to 12 mm AP diameter.
- Electromyography (EMG) and nerve conduction velocity (NCV) are additional studies particularly useful in differentiating peripheral neuropathy from lumbar spinal stenosis.

TREATMENT

NONPHARMACOLOGIC THERAPY

- Physiotherapy
- Lumbar corsets
- Back exercises
- Abdominal muscle strengthening
- Aquatic exercises

ACUTE GENERAL Rx

- Surgery should be considered in patients with significant compression of nerve roots as determined by MRI or CT and incapacitating symptoms limiting activities of daily living or bladder and bowel incontinence.
- Surgical procedures include decompressive laminectomy, arthrodesis, hemilaminectomy, and medial facetectomy.
- Lumbar interspinous process decompression using X-STOP device: a titanium oval spacer

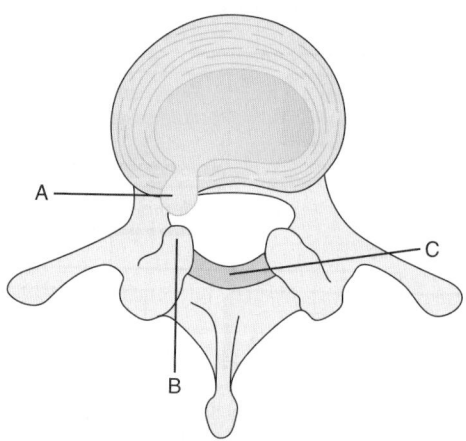

FIG. 1 Spinal stenosis secondary to a combination of disk herniation *(A),* facet joint hypertrophy *(B),* and hypertrophy of the ligamentum flavum *(C).* (From Firestein GS et al: *Kelly's textbook of rheumatology,* ed 9, Philadelphia, 2013, Saunders.)

TABLE 1 Comparative Clinical Features of Spinal Stenosis, Peripheral Vascular Disease, and Disk Disease

Feature	Spinal Stenosis	Disk Prolapse	Peripheral Vascular Disease
Reduced straight leg raise	Rarely	Usually	No
Neurologic deficit	Sometimes	Often	No
Leg pain on walking	Yes	Usually	Yes
Leg pain on sitting	No	Yes	No
Pain relief on standing still	No	No	Yes
Pain relief on sitting	Yes	No	Yes
Numbness/paresthesia	Yes	Yes	Sometimes

From Carr A, Hamilton W: *Orthopedics in primary care,* ed 2, Philadelphia, 2005, Butterworth-Heinemann.

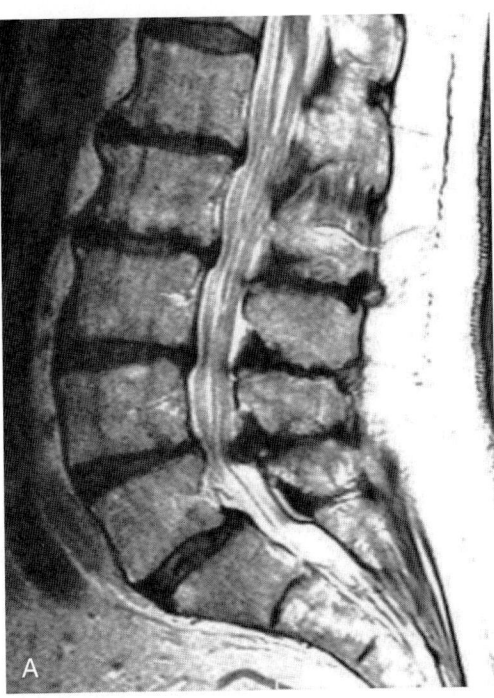
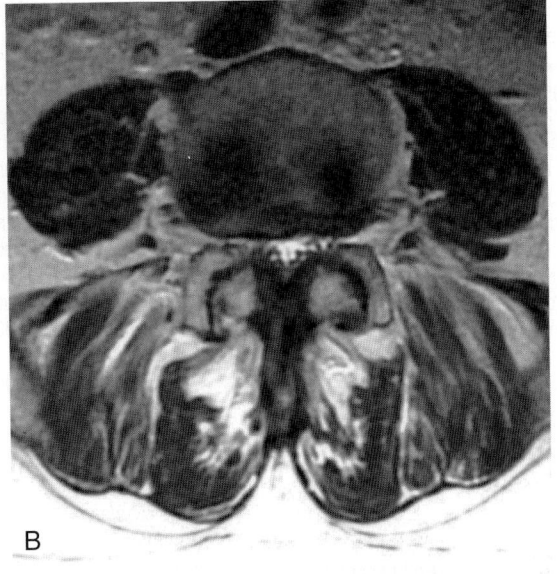

FIG. 2 Degenerative spinal stenosis. A, The sagittal T2-weighted magnetic resonance image shows decreased anteroposterior diameter of the neural canal at the L4-5 level due to redundancy of the ligamentum flavum. **B,** The axial image through the L4-5 disk shows decreased cross-sectional area of the thecal sac from hypertrophic changes of the facet joints posterolateral to the thecal sac. (Courtesy Dr. John Crues, University of California, San Diego.)

placed between the two adjacent spinous processes of the affected level; provides an unloading distractive force to the stenotic middle column part of the motion segment.

- There is little value in adding fusion to decompression surgery. For most patients, spinal stenosis surgery should be limited to decompression when no overt instability is present. Trials have shown that fusion for the treatment of spinal stenosis should be restricted to patients who have proven spinal instability, as confirmed on flexion-extension radiographs; vertebral destruction caused by trauma, tumors, infections, or spinal deformities, such as congenital spondylolisthesis or adult scoliosis.[1]

CHRONIC Rx

- Conservative therapy with NSAIDs (ibuprofen 800 mg PO tid, naproxen 500 mg PO bid) may be tried for symptomatic relief in addition to acetaminophen.
- Epidural glucocorticoid injections are widely used to treat symptoms of lumbar spinal stenosis; however, rigorous data are lacking regarding the effectiveness and safety of these injections. A recent trial revealed that in the treatment of lumbar spinal stenosis, epidural injection of glucocorticoids plus lidocaine offered minimal or no short-term benefit as compared with epidural injection of lidocaine alone.

DISPOSITION

- Approximately 20% of patients having surgery require repeat surgery within 10 yr. Nearly one third of these patients continue to experience pain.
- The natural history of spinal stenosis is one of slow progression. Although not very common, cord compression with resultant bowel and bladder incontinence and paresis can occur.
- Operative treatment in patients with LSS has been reported as being more effective in reducing pain and disability than nonoperative treatment. However, in a recent randomized trial comparing surgery vs. nonsurgical treatment of lumbar spinal stenosis, surgical decompression and a physical therapy regimen yielded similar effects among patients with LSS who were surgical candidates. Patients and health care providers should engage in shared decision-making conversations that include full disclosure of evidence involving surgical and nonsurgical treatments for LSS.[2]

REFERRAL

- Patients who have spinal stenosis should be referred to an orthopedic surgeon specializing in back surgery or to a neurosurgeon.
- Pain clinic referrals should be made if surgery is contraindicated or if the patient does not want surgery.

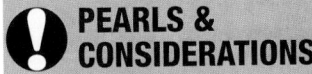

PEARLS & CONSIDERATIONS

COMMENTS

- Approximately one third of patients have coexisting peripheral vascular disease.
- The severity of cauda equina constriction is directly related to the walking ability and the pain intensity in the legs and back.
- Spinal stenosis is also a cause of chronic low back pain in the young.

SUGGESTED READINGS

Available at www.expertconsult.com

RELATED CONTENT

Spinal Stenosis (Patient Information)

AUTHOR: **JORGE A. VILLAFUERTE, M.D.**

[1]Peul WC, et al.; Moojen WA: Fusion for spinal stenosis, safeguard or superfluous surgical implant? *N Engl J Med* 374(15):1478-1479, 2016.

[2]Delitto A et al: Surgery versus nonsurgical treatment of lumbar spinal stenosis: a randomized trial, *Ann Intern Med* 162:465-473, 2015.

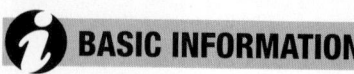

BASIC INFORMATION

DEFINITION

Spontaneous miscarriage is fetal loss before week 20 of pregnancy, calculated from the patient's last menstrual period or the delivery of a fetus weighing <500 g. Early loss is before menstrual week 12, whereas late loss refers to losses from weeks 12 to 20.

Miscarriage can also be classified as incomplete (partial passage of fetal tissue through partially dilated cervix), complete (spontaneous passage of all fetal tissue), threatened (uterine bleeding without cervical dilation or passage of tissue), inevitable (bleeding with cervical dilation without passage of fetal tissue), or missed abortion (intrauterine fetal demise without passage of tissue).

Recurrent miscarriage involves three or more spontaneous pregnancy losses before week 20. It affects approximately 1% of couples attempting to conceive. However, in actual practice, most reproductive experts consider two spontaneous pregnancy losses sufficient to initiate an evaluation for habitual or recurrent spontaneous abortion, since the risk of another loss is similar at this point and the emotional stress is high. As many as 5% of couples and probably even a higher proportion of couples in which the woman is over the age of 35 are affected by two or more consecutive miscarriages.

SYNONYMS

Spontaneous abortion
Miscarriage
Spontaneous pregnancy loss

ICD-10CM CODES
003.9   Complete or unspecified spontaneous abortion without complication
003.89 Complete or unspecified spontaneous abortion with other complications

EPIDEMIOLOGY & DEMOGRAPHICS

INCIDENCE: 10% to 20% of clinically recognized pregnancies; 80% of miscarriages occur in the first trimester. Recurrent miscarriage occurs in <1% of couples attempting to have children.

ETIOLOGY

- In a general overview, the etiology can be classified in terms of maternal (environmental) and fetal (genetic) factors, with the majority of miscarriages being related to genetic or chromosomal causes.

GENETICS

- Fetal chromosomal aneuploidy and polyploidy account for the overwhelming majority of first-trimester losses.
- Autosomal trisomy accounts for the majority of abnormalities, followed by monosomy X, tetraploidy, and, lastly, structural chromosomal abnormalities.

- The incidence of trisomy increases as maternal age increases.

MATERNAL CAUSES

- Uterine anomalies: Mullerian abnormalities such as unicornuate, bicornuate, or septated uterus are associated with increased miscarriage risk, although rates vary in different studies. A septated uterus is most highly associated with recurrent loss and can be surgically corrected and thus is important to diagnose. Other intrauterine pathologies such as synechiae, leiomyomas, or prior DES exposure is important to rule out also.
- Incompetent cervix (iatrogenic or congenital, associated with 20% of mid-trimester losses).
- Antiphospholipid antibody syndrome.
- Uncontrolled diabetes mellitus.
- Rare or controversial causes include HLA associations between mother and father; infections such as tuberculosis, *Chlamydia*, and *Ureaplasma*; smoking and alcohol use; irradiation; progesterone deficiency; and environmental toxins. Most of the literature is observational in nature, which may skew risk factor data.
- With two or more spontaneous miscarriages, a karyotype can be performed on the products of conception to evaluate for aneuploidy, which may be associated with a balanced translocation in one of the parents, and which has a substantially increased risk for abortion (depending on the actual type of translocation); if the pregnancy is carried to term, it has a 3% to 5% risk for an unbalanced karyotype. In patients with habitual abortion, evaluation for anatomic defects such as uterine septum and for antiphospholipid syndrome (lupus anticoagulant, beta 2 glycoprotein IgG/IgM, and anticardiolipin antibody) IgG/IgM should also be obtained.

RISK FACTORS

- Vaginal bleeding, especially >3 d, carries with it a 15% to 20% chance of miscarriage.
- Advancing maternal age.
- 2 or more prior miscarriages.
- Significant underlying maternal health issues such as uncontrolled diabetes, thyroid disease, or other endocrine disturbances.
- Illicit substance use.
- Obesity.
- Alcohol, smoking, and excessive caffeine intake.
- Use of fluconazole in pregnancy is associated with a statistically significant increased risk of spontaneous miscarriage.

PHYSICAL FINDINGS & CLINICAL PRESENTATION

- Profuse bleeding and cramping have a higher association with miscarriage than bleeding without cramping, which is more consistent with a threatened miscarriage.
- Cervical dilation with history or finding of fetal tissue at cervical os may be present.

- In cases of missed abortion, uterine size may be smaller than menstrual dating, in contrast to molar gestation, where size may be greater than dates.
- The presence of nausea and vomiting in early pregnancy is associated with a reduced risk for pregnancy loss.

DIAGNOSIS

DIFFERENTIAL DIAGNOSIS

- Normal pregnancy
- Hydatidiform molar gestation
- Ectopic pregnancy
- Dysfunctional uterine bleeding
- Pathologic endometrial or cervical lesions

WORKUP

- All patients with bleeding in the first trimester should have an evaluation for possible ectopic pregnancy.
- If there are three early, prior pregnancy losses, a workup and treatment for recurrent miscarriage should begin before next conception. If there is a strong history for second-trimester loss, consideration for cerclage should be given if the history is consistent with incompetent cervix (e.g., painless cervical dilation).
- Most providers will initiate an evaluation for couples who have had 2 previous losses.
- One unexplained fetal loss beyond 10 weeks or 1 birth before 34 weeks because of preeclampsia should prompt an evaluation for antiphospholipid antibody syndrome.

LABORATORY TESTS

- Type and antibody screen are used to evaluate the need for Rh immune globulin.
- Recurrent pregnancy loss: During the preconception period in patients with recurrent pregnancy loss, hemoglobin A_{1c}, TSH, prolactin, anticardiolipin antibody, lupus anticoagulant, 20210A beta 2 glycoprotein antibodies, karyotyping, and anatomic evaluation with hysterosalpingography, or saline ultrasonography to assess for uterine septum. With increasing age, oocyte quality is a factor, and some practitioners will perform day 3 of the menstrual cycle FSH and anti-müllerian hormone to assess for diminished ovarian reserve. Progesterone level <5 mg/dl suggests nonviable gestation vs. >25 mg/dl, which suggests a good prognosis.

IMAGING STUDIES

Transvaginal sonogram (preferred) can be used with menstrual dating and serum quantitative human chorionic gonadotropin to document pregnancy location, fetal heart presence, gestational sac size, and adnexal pathology.

TREATMENT

NONPHARMACOLOGIC THERAPY

Depending on the patient's clinical status, desire to continue the pregnancy, and certainty of

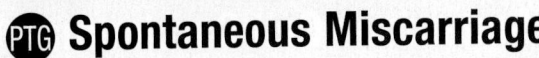

the diagnosis, expectant management can be considered. In pregnancies <6 wk or >14 wk, complete expulsion of fetal tissue usually occurs, and surgical intervention such as D&C can be avoided.

ACUTE GENERAL Rx

- Incomplete miscarriage between 6 and 14 wk can be associated with great blood loss; these patients should undergo D&C.
- In cases of missed abortion, if fetal demise has occurred >6 wk before or gestational age is >14 wk, there is an increased risk of hypofibrinogenemia with disseminated intravascular coagulation. Thus D&C or manual vacuum aspiration should be performed early in the disease course. Consider use of misoprostol (Cytotec) 200 mg PO q6h as an alternative approach if patient desires a less invasive approach.
- Rh-negative patients should be given RhoGAM 50 mcg IM to prevent Rh isoimmunization.

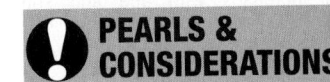

PEARLS & CONSIDERATIONS

Spontaneous pregnancy loss is recommended as a replacement for the term *abortion* and to acknowledge the emotional aspects of losing a pregnancy.

SUGGESTED READINGS
Available at www.expertconsult.com

RELATED CONTENT

Miscarriage (Patient Information)

AUTHOR: **ADRIENNE B. NEITHARDT, M.D.**

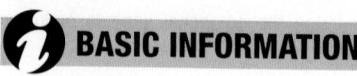
DEFINITION

Squamous cell carcinoma (SCC) is a malignant tumor of the skin arising in the epithelium.

SYNONYMS

SCC
Skin cancer

ICD-10CM CODES

C44.5	Malignant neoplasm of skin of trunk
C44.4	Malignant neoplasm of skin of scalp and neck
D04	Carcinoma in situ of skin
C44.9	Malignant neoplasm of skin, unspecified
C44.0	Malignant neoplasm of skin of lip
C44.2	Malignant neoplasm of skin of ear and external auricular canal
C44.3	Malignant neoplasm of skin of other and unspecified parts of skin
C44.02	Squamous cell carcinoma of skin of lip
C44.121	Squamous cell carcinoma of skin of unspecified eyelid, including canthus
C44.122	Squamous cell carcinoma of skin of right eyelid, including canthus
C44.129	Squamous cell carcinoma of skin of left eyelid, including canthus
C44.221	Squamous cell carcinoma of skin of unspecified ear and external auricular canal
C44.222	Squamous cell carcinoma of skin of right ear and external auricular canal
C44.229	Squamous cell carcinoma of skin of left ear and external auricular canal
C44.320	Squamous cell carcinoma of skin of unspecified parts of face
C44.321	Squamous cell carcinoma of skin of nose
C44.329	Squamous cell carcinoma of skin of other parts of face
C44.42	Squamous cell carcinoma of skin of scalp and neck
C44.520	Squamous cell carcinoma of anal skin
C44.521	Squamous cell carcinoma of skin of breast
C44.529	Squamous cell carcinoma of skin of other part of trunk
C44.621	Squamous cell carcinoma of skin of unspecified upper limb, including shoulder
C44.622	Squamous cell carcinoma of skin of right upper limb, including shoulder
C44.629	Squamous cell carcinoma of skin of left upper limb, including shoulder
C44.721	Squamous cell carcinoma of skin of unspecified lower limb, including hip
C44.722	Squamous cell carcinoma of skin of right lower limb, including hip
C44.729	Squamous cell carcinoma of skin of left lower limb, including hip
C44.82	Squamous cell carcinoma of overlapping sites of skin

EPIDEMIOLOGY & DEMOGRAPHICS

- SCC is the second most common cutaneous malignancy, comprising 20% of all cases of nonmelanoma skin cancer.
- Incidence is highest in lower latitudes (e.g., southern U.S., Australia).
- Male/female ratio is 2:1.
- Incidence increases with age and sun exposure.
- In black patients, SCC are 20% more common than basal cell carcinomas (BCC).
- Average age at diagnosis is 66 yr.

PHYSICAL FINDINGS & CLINICAL PRESENTATION

- SCC frequently begins at the site of actinic keratosis and commonly affects the scalp, neck region, back of hands (Fig. 1), superior surface of the pinna, and the lip (Fig. 2). On the lower lip, SCC often develops on actinic cheilitis. A history of smoking is a significant predisposing factor.
- The lesion may have a scaly, erythematous macule or plaque. (Fig. 3)
- Telangiectasia, central ulceration may also be present (Fig. 4). The ulcer may be superficial and hidden by a crust. Removal of the crust may reveal a well-defined papillary base.
- Most SCCs present as exophytic lesions that grow over a period of months.
- Although most SCCs are relatively slow growing and nonaggressive, some (2%-5%) can exhibit rapid growth and metastases. Aggressive tumors are more common in immunocompromised patients and when arising from scars, burns, or prior injury (Marjolin's ulcer). Presence of SCC on ears, lips, or size >2 cm are high-risk features of SCC.

ETIOLOGY

Risk factors include ultraviolet B radiation, immunosuppression (kidney transplant recipients have a significantly increased risk), arsenic exposure, HPV infection, medications (azathioprine, sorafenib, tumor necrosis factor [TNF] inhibitors), discoid LE, erosive lichen planus, chronic ulcers, prior radiation exposure, and tobacco abuse.

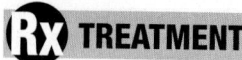 **DIAGNOSIS**

DIFFERENTIAL DIAGNOSIS

- Keratoacanthomas
- Actinic keratosis
- Amelanotic melanoma
- Basal cell carcinoma
- Benign tumors
- Healing traumatic wounds
- Spindle cell tumors
- Warts

WORKUP

Diagnosis is made by full-thickness skin biopsy (incisional or excisional).

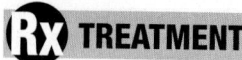 **TREATMENT**

ACUTE GENERAL Rx

- Electrodesiccation and curettage for small SCCs (<2 cm in diameter), superficial tumors, and lesions located in extremity and trunk.
- Tumors thinner than 4 mm can be managed by simple local removal.
- Lesions 4 to 8 mm thick or those with deep dermal invasion should be excised.
- Tumors penetrating the dermis can be treated with several modalities, including excision and Mohs' surgery, radiation therapy, and chemotherapy. Mohs' surgery is commonly used for lesions on the face.
- Metastatic SCC can be treated with cryotherapy and combination of chemotherapy using 13-*cis*-retinoic acid and interferon-alpha 2A.

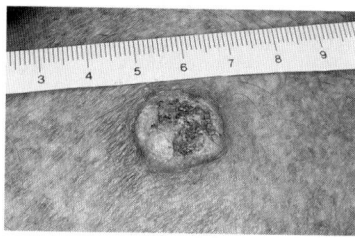

FIG. 1 Squamous cell carcinoma. (From James WD et al: *Andrews' diseases of the skin*, ed 12, Philadelphia, 2016, Elsevier.)

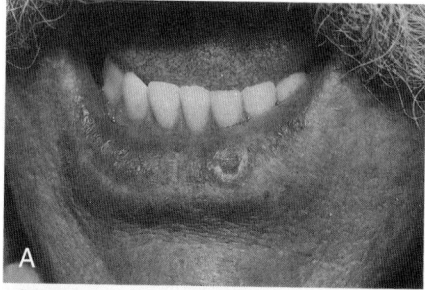
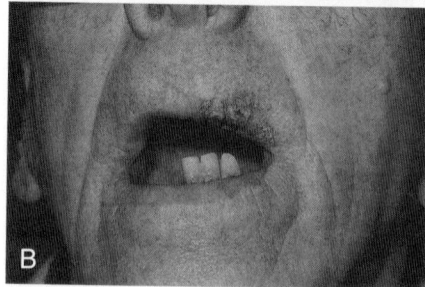

FIG. 2 Squamous cell carcinoma of the lip. The lower lip (**A**) is a relatively commonly affected site. Smoking is a risk factor for this site, and the prognosis is poorer compared to similar-sized lesions at other sun-exposed sites. Treatment is usually by wedge excision or with radiotherapy. By contrast, the upper lip margin (**B**) is a relatively uncommon site. The chronic trauma from the patient's only three teeth may have been relevant. (From White GM, Cox NH [eds]: *Diseases of the skin, a color atlas and text*, ed 2, St Louis, 2006, Mosby.)

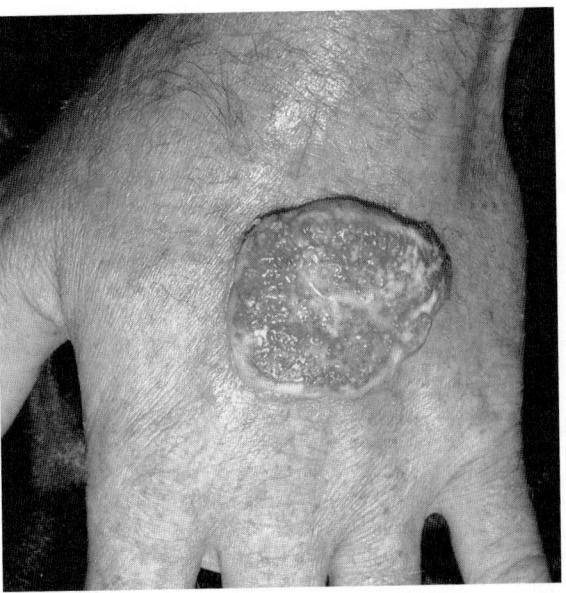

FIG. 3 A cutaneous squamous cell carcinoma (invasive, well differentiated with keratoacanthomatous features) on the leg of a 61-year-old woman, presenting after 3 wk of treatment with vemurafenib for metastatic lung cancer. (From Callen JP et al: *Dermatologic signs of systemic disease*, ed 5, Philadelphia, 2017, Elsevier.)

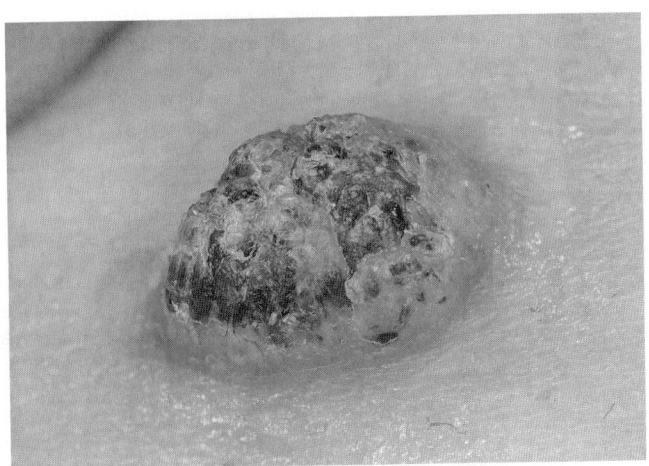

FIG. 4 Squamous cell carcinoma. Nodular hyperkeratotic lesion with central erosion. (From Noble J et al: *Textbook of primary care medicine*, ed 3, St Louis, 2001, Mosby.)

DISPOSITION

- Survival is related to size, location, degree of differentiation, immunologic status of the patient, depth of invasion, and presence of metastases. Risk factors for metastasis include lesions on the lip or ear, increasing lesion depth, and poor cell differentiation.
- Patients whose tumors penetrate through the dermis or exceed 8 mm in thickness are at risk of tumor recurrence.
- The most common metastatic locations are regional lymph nodes, liver, and lung.
- Tumors on the scalp, forehead, ears, nose, and lips also carry a higher risk.
- The rate of SCC metastasis from all skin sites ranges from 0.5% to 5.2%.
- SCCs originating in the lip and pinna metastasize in 10% to 20% of cases.
- 5-year survival for metastatic SCC is 34%.

REFERRAL

Oncology referral for metastatic SCC

⚠ PEARLS & CONSIDERATIONS

COMMENTS

- SCC arising in areas of prior radiation, thermal injury, and areas of chronic ulcers or chronic draining sinuses are more aggressive and have a higher frequency of metastasis than those originating in actinic damaged skin.
- Oral retinoids may be useful as a preventive strategy in patients with immunosuppression.
- Nicotinamide (500 mg bid, available over the counter) mitigates some of the deleterious effects of UV radiation and has been reported to lower the incidence of nonmelanoma skin cancer (NMSCO) by 23%.[1]

EBM EVIDENCE

Available at www.expertconsult.com

RELATED CONTENT

Squamous Cell Carcinoma (Patient Information)

AUTHOR: **FRED F. FERRI, M.D.**

[1]Chen AC, et al: A phase 3 randomized trial of nicotinamide for skin cancer chemoprevention, *N Engl J Med* 373:1618, 2015.

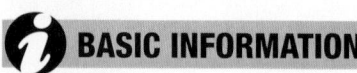

BASIC INFORMATION

DEFINITION

Statin-induced muscle syndromes (SIMS) include myopathy, myalgia, myositis, and rhabdomyolysis. Definitions for these syndromes are inconsistent in the medical literature.

- Myopathy: a general term defined as any disease of muscles.
- Myalgia: muscle weakness or pain without serum creatinine kinase elevation.
- Myositis: muscle weakness or pain with an increased serum creatinine kinase level.
- Rhabdomyolysis: muscle weakness or pain and a marked serum creatinine kinase level usually greater than 10 times the upper limit of normal and serum creatinine elevation as well as signs of brown urine and elevated urine myoglobin. A rare **immune-mediated necrotizing myopathy (IMNM)**, also known as **statin-associated autoimmune myopathy**, has also been associated with the use of statins with symptoms persisting after discontinuation of the drug. This condition presents with symmetric proximal arm and leg weakness and severe elevations of muscle enzymes.

SYNONYMS

Statin-induced myopathies
Statin-induced myositis
Statin-induced myalgias
Statin-induced rhabdomyolysis
Statin-associated autoimmune myopathy

ICD-10CM CODES	
M60.9	Myositis, unspecified
M62.82	Rhabdomyolysis
G72.2	Myopathy due to other toxic agents
G72.9	Myopathy, unspecified
G72.81	Critical illness myopathy
G72.89	Other specified myopathies
M60.89	Other myositis, multiple sites

EPIDEMIOLOGY & DEMOGRAPHICS

INCIDENCE: Risk of statin-induced rhabdomyolysis is 1.2 per 10,000 persons/yr. Rhabdomyolysis risk of death is 0.15 deaths per 1 million prescriptions. SIMS most commonly occur in people aged 51 to 75, which may reflect the pattern of statin use. Statin-associated autoimmune myopathy occurs in an estimated 2 or 3 of every 100,000 patients treated with statins.

PEAK INCIDENCE: Patients on high-dose statins have a 0.9% incidence of statin-induced rhabdomyolysis.

PREVALENCE: The prevalence of statin-induced myalgias is about 1% to 5%, similar to placebo in clinical trials, although observational studies have suggested a prevalence of 10% or higher. Statins may cause elevated transaminases (ALT, AST) at a prevalence of 0.5% to 2.0% and rhabdomyolysis ~0.08%.

PREDOMINANT SEX AND AGE: The mean age of hospitalized patients with statin-induced myopathy or rhabdomyolysis was 64 yr and was slightly more common in women (56%).

GENETICS: Interpatient variability exists in the activity of the *CYP3A4* gene for the metabolism of simvastatin, atorvastatin, and lovastatin. Homozygous carriers of CYP2D6 (poor metabolizers) had a higher rate of discontinuation of simvastatin due to muscle syndromes compared with the CYP2D6 wild-type genotype; patients taking atorvastatin and having a muscle event were more likely to have the CYP2D6*4 allele. SLCO1B1 polymorphisms encode for the organic anion transport of statins into the liver cells. The variant C allele may increase the risk of the SLCO1B1 statin–induced myopathy. A statin-associated autoimmune myopathy has shown a link to class II HLA allele DRB1*11:01 in the development of anti-HMG coA reductase antibodies, leading to an increase in expression of the antibodies in the muscles of patients exposed to statins. Some data exist on deficiencies in ubiquinone (coenzyme Q10) in patients with a mutation in the *COQ2* gene.

RISK FACTORS: Small body frame; age over 80 yr; women, particularly frail elderly women; patients taking multiple drugs, especially gemfibrozil, niacin, cyclosporine, itraconazole, ketoconazole, erythromycin, clarithromycin, verapamil, amiodarone; renal or liver impairment; pharmacogenetic variability; hypothyroidism; excessive alcohol intake; vigorous exercise; severe infections; excessive grapefruit juice ingestion; inherited defects of muscle metabolism such as carnitine palmityl transferase II deficiency, McArdle's disease, and myoadenylate deaminase deficiency; acquired myopathies such as postpoliomyelitis syndrome; lipophilic statins (simvastatin, atorvastatin, lovastatin); multiple conditions such as diabetes; and drugs of abuse (amphetamines, heroin, cocaine, phencyclidine).

PHYSICAL FINDINGS & CLINICAL PRESENTATION

- Myopathy can occur at any time, although it is more common within the first 4 weeks of therapy.
- Proximal generalized muscle aches, body aches, and pains, and may be mild or severe.
- Dark-colored urine
- Muscle cramps, spasms, tenderness, or stiffness
- Unusually tired or weak
- Nocturnal cramping
- Tendon pain

ETIOLOGY

- History of current statin use
- May be explained by one of three deficiencies of end products of the 3-hydroxy-3-methyl-glutaryl-coA reductase pathway: cell signaling and apoptosis, mitochondrial function and ubiquinone concentrations, and cholesterol concentrations and cell membrane integrity.
- The risk may be enhanced by drug interactions that interfere with hepatic metabolism and gut wall transport of interacting medications and by pharmacodynamic effects.
- Underlying metabolic muscle disorder may predispose a patient to develop myopathy.

- Patients with statin-associated autoimmune myopathy have been found to have anti-HMG-CoA reductase antibodies even prior to exposure to statin therapy.

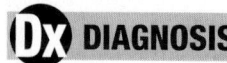

DIAGNOSIS

DIFFERENTIAL DIAGNOSIS

Bursitis, tendinitis, radiculopathy, osteoarthritis, muscle strain, myofascial pain, hypothyroidism, proton-pump inhibitor-induced polymyositis, viral illness, polymyositis, and polymyalgia rheumatica

WORKUP

Workup consists of a thorough history, including exercise history, urine color, medication history, and physical exam to palpate tenderness and obtain blood tests to evaluate muscle and kidney damage.

LABORATORY TESTS

If severe myopathy or rhabdomyolysis is suspected:

- Elevated CPK, positive serum myoglobin, elevated BUN, serum creatinine, AST, ALT, LDH, and potassium
- Urine creatinine, positive casts, and hemoglobin in urine with absence of red blood cells
- Consider electrocardiogram and assessment of calcium, phosphate, and uric acid.

If mild to moderate myopathy is suspected:

- Monitor TSH and CPK levels; CPK may only be elevated when sudden severe myopathy occurs.
- If the patient has brown or dark urine or elevated CPK, monitor BUN and serum creatinine.
- In statin-associated autoimmune myopathy, the creatine kinase level is usually ≥10 times the upper limit of normal. In these patients, muscle biopsy specimens will be positive for autoantibodies against HMG-CoA reductase.

IMAGING STUDIES

- Not recommended
- In statin-associated autoimmune myopathy, electromyography shows small-amplitude motor-unit potentials with increased spontaneous activity characteristic of an active myopathic process. Muscle edema is evident on MRI.[1]

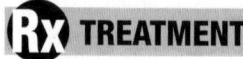

TREATMENT

NONPHARMACOLOGIC THERAPY

- Treatment of rhabdomyolysis is generally supportive in nature (see "Rhabdomyolysis" topic).

ACUTE GENERAL Rx

- Stop statin therapy immediately if muscle symptoms occur. Check history, potential drug-drug interactions, CPK, TSH, renal function, hepatic function, and urinalysis.

[1]Mammen AL: Statin-associated autoimmune myopathy, *N Engl J Med* 374:664-669, 2016.

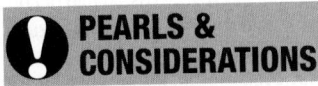

- If patients have suspected rhabdomyolysis, they should be hospitalized and treated with supportive therapy and monitoring of complications.
- If CPK <10× the upper limit of normal without symptoms, continue statin therapy at the same or lower dosage
- If CPK <10× the upper limit of normal with intolerable symptoms, discontinue statin.
- If CPK >10× the upper limit of normal, discontinue statin.

Box 1 describes recommendations of the National Lipid Association Statin Safety Assessment Task Force regarding statin and muscle safety.

CHRONIC Rx

- After stopping the statin and symptom or CPK resolution, which may take up to 4 months, consider the same statin at a lower dosage or a different statin at an equivalent or lower dosage.
- When restarting therapy, consider statins such as low-dose rosuvastatin; pravastatin; and alternate-day dosing of rosuvastatin or atorvastatin.
- If patient had rhabdomyolysis secondary to statin therapy, consider nonstatin treatments.
- If the patient develops myopathy after a second trial of therapy, statin treatment should be permanently discontinued and nonstatin cholesterol-lowering therapy initiated.
- For IMNM (statin-associated autoimmune myopathy), immunosuppressive therapy with prednisone (1 mg per kilogram of body weight per day) and at least one agent (methotrexate, azathioprine, or mycophenolate mofetil) have been used. In resistant cases, IV immune globulin or another agent such as rituximab may be added.

COMPLEMENTARY & ALTERNATIVE MEDICINE

- The effect of coenzyme Q10 on reducing or preventing SIMS remains controversial. Given its safety, coenzyme Q10 can be recommended if the actions listed under "Chronic Rx" are insufficient to continue the use of the statin and if the muscle symptoms have been limited to myalgias. Use coenzyme Q10 with caution in patients taking warfarin, as its anticoagulant effect may be decreased.
- A 2015 meta-analysis of observational studies reported that vitamin D levels were lower in patients with statin-induced myalgias than in individuals who did not have these symptoms.
- In a study of 282 patients with vitamin D levels less than 32 ng/ml and with myalgia-myositis from statins, vitamin D supplementation (median 50,000 IU D_3/week) for 6 months improved symptoms and statin tolerance in 74% to 85% of patients.

DISPOSITION

- Usually resolves within 1 wk up to 4 mo after discontinuing statin therapy.
- Once the patient has a full recovery, an alternative statin can be tried.

- Statins should not be restarted in IMNM.

REFERRAL

- If rhabdomyolysis is suspected, immediate referral for hospitalization is suggested.

⊙ PEARLS & CONSIDERATIONS

COMMENTS

SIMS are usually mild and will resolve within a few wk after discontinuing statin therapy. However, such syndromes may progress to rhabdomyolysis.

PREVENTION

- Follow the 2013 AHA/ACC treatment guidelines to achieve the appropriate percent reduction in LDL cholesterol and limit the concomitant use of fibrates with statins.
- Discontinue statin therapy prior to and during surgical procedures.
- If patient requires a short-term therapy with an interacting medication such as an azole antifungal, temporarily discontinue statin therapy until interacting therapy is completed.
- If statin–fibric acid therapy is warranted, fenofibrate is preferred over gemfibrozil to decrease risk of myopathy.
- Baseline liver function testing before initiation of statin therapy and only if clinically indicated thereafter

PATIENT & FAMILY EDUCATION

- Inform patients to promptly report muscle weakness, unexpected muscle pain, or brownish urine.
- Ensure that the pharmacist and/or primary care physician checks for drug-drug interactions with every new prescription, including those from dentists and physicians from other specialties.
- Coenzyme Q10 may lessen milder muscle symptoms from statins, but patients should inform their physician and pharmacist if they decide to use this supplement.
- A recent clinical trial comparing lipid-lowering efficacy for two nonstatin therapies, ezetimibe and evolocumab, among patients with statin intolerance revealed that evolocumab resulted in a significantly greater reduction in LDL-C levels after 24 weeks. Further studies are needed to assess long-term efficacy and safety.[1]

SUGGESTED READINGS

Available at www.expertconsult.com

RELATED CONTENT

Rhabdomyolysis (Related Key Topic)

AUTHORS: **LISA COHEN, M.D.,** and **ANNE L. HUME, PHARM.D.**

[1]Nissen SE et al: Efficacy and tolerability of evolocumab vs ezetimibe in patients with muscle-related statin intolerance: the GAUSS-3 randomized clinical trial, *JAMA* 315(15):1580-1590, 2016.

BOX 1 Recommendations to Health Care Professionals Regarding Statin and Muscle Safety

- Whenever muscle symptoms or an increased CK level is encountered in patients receiving statin therapy, health professionals should attempt to rule out other causes, because these are most likely to explain the findings. Other common causes include increased physical activity, trauma, falls, accidents, seizure, shaking chills, hypothyroidism, infections, carbon monoxide poisoning, polymyositis, dermatomyositis, alcohol abuse, and drug abuse (cocaine, amphetamines, heroin, or PCP).
- Obtaining a pretreatment, baseline CK level can be considered in patients who are at high risk of experiencing muscle toxicity (e.g., older patients or those combining a statin with an agent known to increase myotoxicity), but this is not routinely necessary in other patients.
- It is unnecessary to measure CK levels in asymptomatic patients during the course of statin therapy, because marked, clinically important CK elevations are rare and are usually related to physical exertion or other causes.
- Patients receiving statin therapy should be counseled about the increased risk of muscle symptoms, particularly if initiation of vigorous, sustained endurance exercise or a surgical operation is being contemplated; they should be advised to report such muscle symptoms to a health professional.
- Creatine kinase measurements should be obtained in symptomatic patients to help gauge the severity of muscle damage and facilitate decision of whether to continue therapy or alter doses.
- In patients who develop intolerable muscle symptoms with or without CK elevation and for whom other etiologies have been ruled out, the statin should be discontinued. Once symptoms disappear, the same or different statin at the same or a lower dose can be restarted to test the reproducibility of symptoms. Recurrence of symptoms with multiple statins and doses requires initiation of other lipid-altering therapy.
- In patients who develop tolerable muscle symptoms or have no symptoms but have a CK level <10 × ULN, statin therapy may be continued at the same or reduced doses and symptoms may be used as the clinical guide to stop or continue therapy.
- In patients who develop rhabdomyolysis (CK >10,000 IU/L or >10 × ULN with an elevation in serum creatinine or need for intravenous hydration therapy), statin therapy should be stopped. Intravenous hydration therapy in a hospital should be instituted if indicated for patients experiencing rhabdomyolysis. Once patients recover, risk vs. benefit of statin therapy should be carefully reconsidered.

CK, Creatine kinase; *PCP,* phencyclidine; *ULN,* upper limit of normal.
From McKenney JM et al: Final conclusions and recommendations of the National Lipid Association Statin Safety Assessment Task Force, *Am J Cardiol* 97(suppl 8A):89C-94C, 2006.

Diseases and Disorders

I

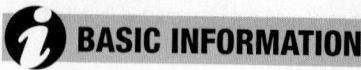

BASIC INFORMATION

DEFINITION

Status epilepticus is a medical neurologic emergency. It is historically defined as 30 min of continuous seizure activity or two or more seizures without full recovery of consciousness between seizures. However, in practice a continuous seizure that lasts >5 min is treated as status epilepticus.

SYNONYMS

Convulsive status epilepticus
Nonconvulsive status epilepticus

ICD-10CM CODES
G41   Status epilepticus
G40.301 Generalized idiopathic epilepsy
         and epileptic syndromes, not
         intractable, with status epilepticus

EPIDEMIOLOGY & DEMOGRAPHICS

INCIDENCE: 40 to 100 cases per 100,000 persons
PEAK INCIDENCE: It is most common among children younger than 1 yr and adults older than 60 yr.
PREDOMINANT SEX AND AGE: No gender preference

PHYSICAL FINDINGS & CLINICAL PRESENTATION

- Patients can present with repetitive tonic clonic movements of the body (convulsive status epilepticus); other patients are comatose and nonresponsive (nonconvulsive status epilepticus).
- Patients may also present with lethargy, intermittent confusion, and involuntary movements.

ETIOLOGY

- Status epilepticus can be the result of an acute neurologic injury, such as stroke, meningitis, brain tumor, etc.
- In patients with epilepsy, abrupt discontinuation of antiepileptic drugs can result in status epilepticus.
- See Table 1 for causes of status epilepticus.

TABLE 1   Causes of Status Epilepticus

- Stroke (ischemic/hemorrhagic)
- CNS infections
- Traumatic head injury
- CNS toxicity: certain medications, drugs, ethanol
- Brain tumors or other mass lesions
- Metabolic disturbances: hypoglycemia, hyponatremia
- Abrupt discontinuation of antiepileptic drugs in patient with epilepsy
- Cryptogenic

CNS, Central nervous system.

DIAGNOSIS

DIFFERENTIAL DIAGNOSIS

- Convulsive syncope
- Encephalopathies: metabolic, infectious, toxic, etc.
- Nonepileptic spells

WORKUP

- ABCs
- ICU admission
- Emergent electroencephalogram (EEG)
- Continuous video EEG in refractory cases
- Investigation of the patient with status epilepticus is summarized in Box 1.

LABORATORY TESTS

- Routine blood workup (CBC, CMP, glucose, electrolytes)
- Urine drug screen
- Lumbar puncture and CSF analysis in patients with suspected meningitis

IMAGING STUDIES

- Immediate CT scan of the head
- MRI of the brain should be performed once the patient is in a stable condition.

TREATMENT

- Patients with continuous seizure activity over 3 min need intravenous lorazepam 0.1 mg/kg at 2 mg/min (or diazepam 0.2 mg/kg at 5 mg/min only when lorazepam is not available).
- In the absence of intravenous access, intramuscular administration of midazolam 10 mg in an adult is a superior alternative.
- Failure of response to lorazepam or midazolam is referred to as established status epilepticus and should be followed by intravenous fosphenytoin 20 mg/kg (PE) at a rate not greater than 150 mg/min. An alternate to fosphenytoin is phenytoin 20 mg/kg IV at up to 50 mg/min as tolerated. Vital signs should be monitored during the infusion.
- If seizures continue, intravenous valproate, levetiracetam, lacosamide, brivaracetam, phenobarbital, midazolam, and propofol are alternatives. Many of these drugs remain under investigation, and superiority of any one agent is not established.

BOX 1   Investigation of the Patient with Status Epilepticus

To Be Performed in All Patients with Status Epilepticus
- Serum glucose, electrolytes, calcium, magnesium
- Blood gas, serum osmolality
- Toxicology screen (serum and urine)
- Antiepileptic drug levels
- Complete blood count (RBC, differential WBC, platelet count)
- Liver enzymes, serum ammonium
- Blood culture
- Lumbar puncture, including:
  1. Opening pressure
  2. Cell count, Gram stain, smear for acid-fast bacilli
  3. Viral and bacterial cultures
  4. PCR for herpesvirus
- EEG, preferably continuous monitoring with video
  1. To monitor for subtle or subclinical seizures
  2. To guide antiepileptic drug therapy
  3. To localize the epileptogenic brain region (focal slowing or epileptiform activity)

To Be Considered in Patients with Status Epilepticus
- Structural neuroimaging (CT, MRI)
  1. To diagnose acute infarction, hemorrhage, vascular malformation, encephalitis, abscess, neurocysticercosis, neoplasm
  2. In nonlesional cases, may localize the epileptogenic zone by evidence of focal edema in the affected cortical region
  3. To assess the degree of cerebral edema and diagnose impending uncal or transtentorial herniation
  4. MR angiography may identify CNS vasculitis, especially in medium or large vessel disease
- Functional neuroimaging (PET, SPECT)
  1. In nonlesional cases, may identify the epileptogenic zone
- Cerebral angiography
  1. To identify small vessel CNS vasculitis, which may not be visible on MR angiography
- Rheumatologic workup for vasculitides
- ESR, C-reactive protein, rheumatoid factor, serum complement levels, antineutrophil cytoplasmic antibodies
- Brain biopsy
  1. To diagnose cerebral vasculitis (granulomatous compared with nongranulomatous)
  2. To identify malformations of cortical development

CNS, Central nervous system; CT, computed tomography; EEG, electroencephalography; ESR, erythrocyte sedimentation rate; MRI, magnetic resonance imaging; PCR, polymerase chain reaction; PET, positron emission tomography; RBC, red blood cell; SPECT, single-photon emission computed tomography; WBC, white blood cell.
From Fuhrman BP et al: *Pediatric critical care*, ed 4, Philadelphia, 2011, Saunders.

**A. Prolonged Seizures and Status Epilepticus
in Infants (Age > 1 Month), Children, and Adolescents**

Seizure onset

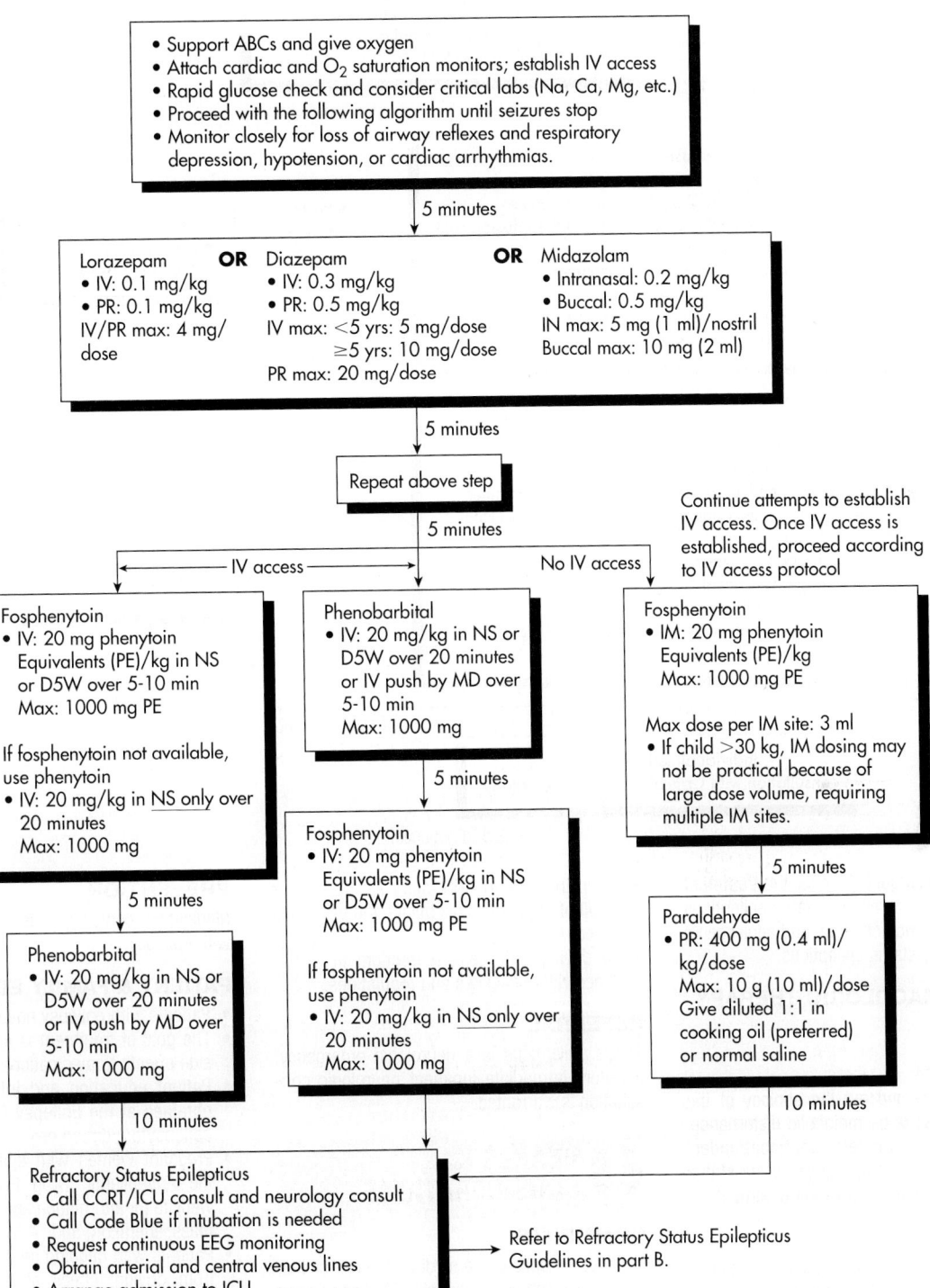

- Support ABCs and give oxygen
- Attach cardiac and O$_2$ saturation monitors; establish IV access
- Rapid glucose check and consider critical labs (Na, Ca, Mg, etc.)
- Proceed with the following algorithm until seizures stop
- Monitor closely for loss of airway reflexes and respiratory depression, hypotension, or cardiac arrhythmias.

5 minutes

Lorazepam **OR** Diazepam **OR** Midazolam
- IV: 0.1 mg/kg
- PR: 0.1 mg/kg
IV/PR max: 4 mg/ dose

- IV: 0.3 mg/kg
- PR: 0.5 mg/kg
IV max: <5 yrs: 5 mg/dose
≥5 yrs: 10 mg/dose
PR max: 20 mg/dose

- Intranasal: 0.2 mg/kg
- Buccal: 0.5 mg/kg
IN max: 5 mg (1 ml)/nostril
Buccal max: 10 mg (2 ml)

5 minutes

Repeat above step

5 minutes

IV access — No IV access

Continue attempts to establish IV access. Once IV access is established, proceed according to IV access protocol

Fosphenytoin
- IV: 20 mg phenytoin Equivalents (PE)/kg in NS or D5W over 5-10 min
Max: 1000 mg PE

If fosphenytoin not available, use phenytoin
- IV: 20 mg/kg in NS only over 20 minutes
Max: 1000 mg

Phenobarbital
- IV: 20 mg/kg in NS or D5W over 20 minutes or IV push by MD over 5-10 min
Max: 1000 mg

Fosphenytoin
- IM: 20 mg phenytoin Equivalents (PE)/kg
Max: 1000 mg PE

Max dose per IM site: 3 ml
- If child >30 kg, IM dosing may not be practical because of large dose volume, requiring multiple IM sites.

5 minutes

5 minutes

Fosphenytoin
- IV: 20 mg phenytoin Equivalents (PE)/kg in NS or D5W over 5-10 min
Max: 1000 mg PE

If fosphenytoin not available, use phenytoin
- IV: 20 mg/kg in NS only over 20 minutes
Max: 1000 mg

Phenobarbital
- IV: 20 mg/kg in NS or D5W over 20 minutes or IV push by MD over 5-10 min
Max: 1000 mg

Paraldehyde
- PR: 400 mg (0.4 ml)/ kg/dose
Max: 10 g (10 ml)/dose
Give diluted 1:1 in cooking oil (preferred) or normal saline

5 minutes

10 minutes

10 minutes

Refractory Status Epilepticus
- Call CCRT/ICU consult and neurology consult
- Call Code Blue if intubation is needed
- Request continuous EEG monitoring
- Obtain arterial and central venous lines
- Arrange admission to ICU

Refer to Refractory Status Epilepticus Guidelines in part B.

FIG. 1 Guidelines for the treatment of prolonged seizures and status epilepticus in infants (age >1 month), children, and adolescents. (From The Hospital for Sick Children, Toronto, Canada. In Fuhrman BP et al: *Pediatric critical care*, ed 4, Philadelphia, 2011, Saunders.)

B. Refractory Status Epilepticus in Infants (Age > 1 Month), Children, and Adolescents

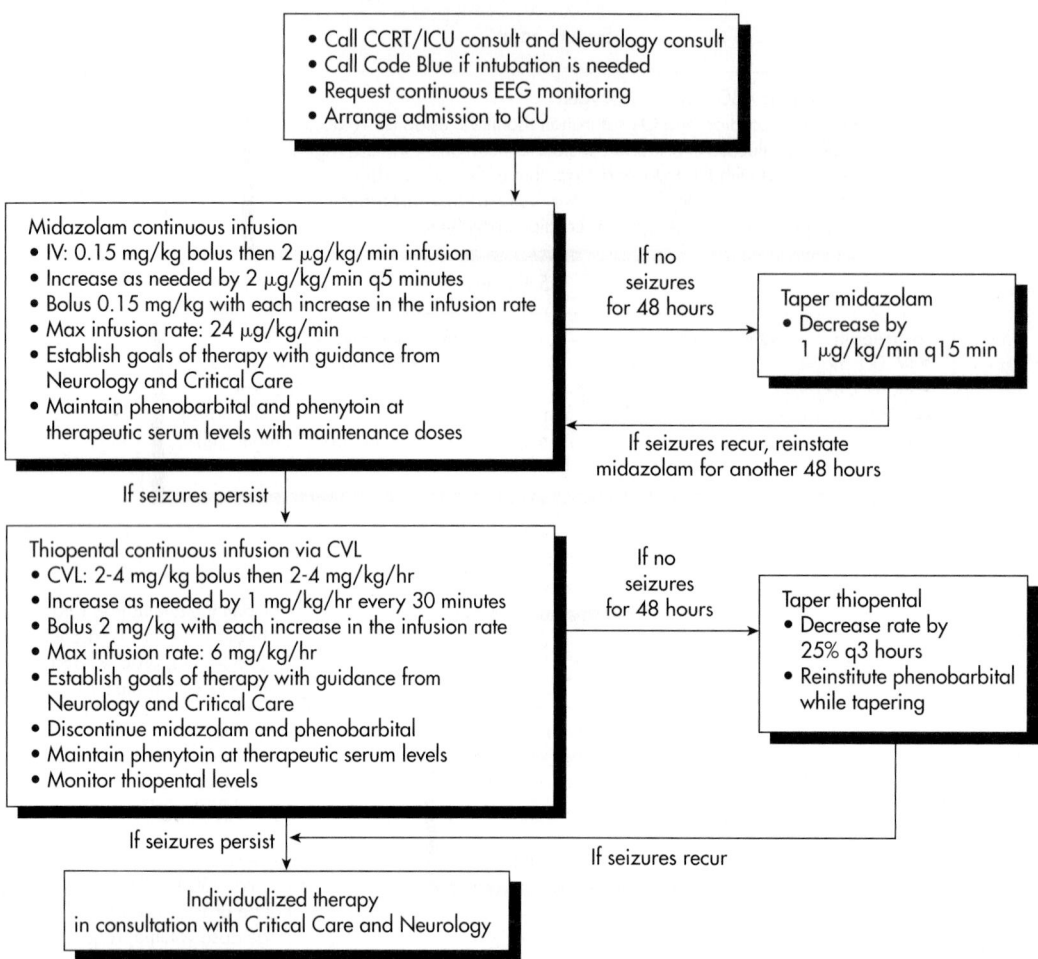

FIG. 1 (Continued)

- Fig. 1 describes guidelines for the treatment of prolonged seizures and status epilepticus in infants (>1 mo), children, and adolescents and refractory status epilepticus.

NONPHARMACOLOGIC THERAPY
None

GENERAL Rx
It is important to find out the etiology of the status epilepticus (e.g., metabolic disturbance, infection). The appropriate treatment/understanding of the underlying cause of the status epilepticus will impact successful treatment.

CHRONIC Rx
- Chronic treatment of status epilepticus depends on underlying etiology.
- Patient with status epilepticus due to epilepsy will need chronic treatment.

COMPLEMENTARY & ALTERNATIVE MEDICINE
Not applicable

DISPOSITION
- Response to treatment depends on the etiology of the status epilepticus.

- When there is no CNS injury as a cause or result of the status epilepticus, the prognosis is good.
- No driving until seizure freedom in accordance with local laws and regulations.

REFERRAL
Status epilepticus is a neurologic emergency; therefore immediate inpatient neurologic consultation is warranted.

⊘ PEARLS & CONSIDERATIONS

COMMENTS
- Status epilepticus is a medical emergency that carries a high risk of mortality. Mortality among patients who present in status epilepticus is 15% to 22%. Among those who survive, functional ability will decline in 25% of cases.
- Continuous video EEG is crucial in the treatment of these patients because some of them may not be clinically seizing (convulsing) but electrographically they may still have subclinical repetitive seizures or subclinical status epilepticus.

PREVENTION
Medication compliance is crucial in patients with epilepsy.

PATIENT & FAMILY EDUCATION
- Patients with epilepsy have normal lives.
- The goal of treatment is no seizures and no side effects to medications.
- Patient education and information can be obtained at the Epilepsy Foundation: www.epilepsyfoundation.org
- Pregnant women with epilepsy should visit the Antiepileptic Drug Pregnancy Registry website for information and assistance: www.massgeneral.org/aed
- Patients with ongoing seizures are forbidden from driving; check state regulations and laws regarding driving and epilepsy.

AUTHOR: **PATRICIO SEBASTIAN ESPINOSA, M.D., M.P.H.**

BASIC INFORMATION

DEFINITION

Stevens-Johnson syndrome (SJS) is a rare, severe vesiculobullous form of erythema multiforme (EM) affecting the skin, mouth, eyes, and genitalia. SJS is defined as affecting <10% of body surface area (BSA). When it affects 10% to 30% of BSA, it is known as SJS-toxic epidermal necrolysis (TEN) overlap syndrome. TEN affects >30% of BSA.

SYNONYMS

SJS
Herpes iris
Febrile mucocutaneous syndrome

ICD-10CM CODES
L51.1 Stevens-Johnson syndrome

EPIDEMIOLOGY & DEMOGRAPHICS

- SJS affects predominantly children and young adults.
- Male/female ratio is 2:1.
- Prevalence: 1:100,000 for SJS and 1:1,000,000 for TEN

PHYSICAL FINDINGS & CLINICAL PRESENTATION

- The cutaneous eruption generally occurs within 8 wk of drug initiation and is generally preceded by vague, nonspecific symptoms of low-grade fever and fatigue (influenza-like symptoms) occurring 1 to 14 days before the skin lesions. Cough is often present. Fever may be high during the active stages.
- Enlarging red-purple macules or papules and bullae generally occur on the conjunctiva, mucous membranes of the mouth (Fig. 1), nares, and genital regions. Lesions rapidly spread to their maximum extent usually within 2 days.
- Corneal ulcerations may result in blindness.
- Ulcerative stomatitis results in hemorrhagic crusting.
- Nikolsky sign (shearing off of epidermis with pressure on skin) can be present.
- Flat, atypical target lesions or purpuric maculae may be distributed on the trunk or be widespread (Fig. 2).

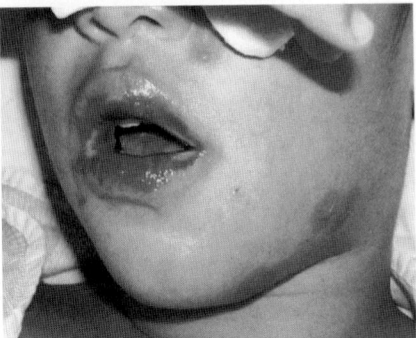

FIG. 1 Lip changes found in Stevens-Johnson syndrome associated with *Mycoplasma pneumoniae* infection. (From Kliegman RM et al: *Nelson textbook of pediatrics*, ed 19, Philadelphia, 2011, Saunders.)

- The pain from oral lesions may compromise fluid intake and result in dehydration.
- Thick, mucopurulent sputum and oral lesions may interfere with breathing.

ETIOLOGY

- Drugs (e.g., phenytoin, sulfonamides, lamotrigine, sertraline, NSAIDs, tramadol, allopurinol, β-lactam antibiotics, phenobarbital) are the most common cause.
- Upper respiratory tract infections (e.g., *Mycoplasma pneumoniae*) and HSV infections have also been implicated.

DIAGNOSIS

DIFFERENTIAL DIAGNOSIS

- Toxic erythema (drugs or infection)
- Pemphigus
- Pemphigoid
- Urticaria
- Hemorrhagic fevers
- Serum sickness
- *Staphylococcus* scalded-skin syndrome
- Behçet's syndrome

WORKUP

- Diagnosis is generally based on clinical presentation and characteristic appearance of the lesions.
- Skin biopsy is generally reserved for when classic lesions are absent and diagnosis is uncertain. Biopsy reveals epidermal necrolysis but cannot distinguish between SJS, TEN, and EM.

LABORATORY TESTS

CBC with differential, cultures in cases of suspected infection

IMAGING STUDIES

Chest x-rays may show patchy changes in patients with pulmonary involvement.

TREATMENT

NONPHARMACOLOGIC THERAPY

- Withdrawal of any potential drug precipitants
- Careful skin nursing to prevent secondary infection

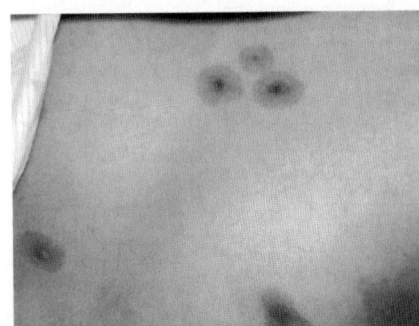

FIG. 2 Classic erythema multiforme skin lesions found in Stevens-Johnson's syndrome associated with *Mycoplasma pneumoniae* infection. (From Kliegman RM et al: *Nelson textbook of pediatrics*, ed 19, Philadelphia, 2011, Saunders.)

ACUTE GENERAL Rx

- Treatment of associated conditions (e.g., acyclovir for HSV infection, azithromycin for *Mycoplasma* infection)
- Antihistamines for pruritus
- Treatment of the cutaneous blisters with cool, wet Burow's compresses
- Relief of oral symptoms by frequent rinsing with lidocaine (Xylocaine Viscous)
- Liquid or soft diet with plenty of fluids to ensure proper hydration
- Treatment of secondary infections with antibiotics
- Corticosteroids: use remains controversial and there is a clear risk of sepsis; they should be used only in severe cases early in the disease; when used, prednisone 20 to 30 mg bid until new lesions no longer appear, then rapidly tapered
- Topical steroids: may use to treat papules and plaques; however, should not be applied to eroded areas
- Vitamin A: may be used for lacrimal hyposecretion
- Consider IVIG in severe cases.

DISPOSITION

- Prognosis varies with severity of disease. It is generally good in patients with limited disease; however, mortality rate may approach 10% in patients with extensive involvement. A severity of illness score known as SCORETEN that incorporates increased glucose level (>252 mg/dl), increased BUN (>28 mg/dl), electrolytes (serum bicarbonate <20 mEq/L), age (>40 yr), immunosuppression (presence of cancer), involvement >10% of BSA, and increased heart rate (>120 beats/min) can be used to calculate mortality risk.
- Oral lesions may continue for several months.
- Scarring and corneal abnormalities may occur in 20% of patients.

REFERRAL

- Management of SIS is similar to those with extensive burns. Hospital admission in a unit used for burn care is recommended in severe cases.
- Urethral involvement may necessitate catheterization.
- Ocular involvement should be monitored by an ophthalmologist.

SUGGESTED READINGS
Available at www.expertconsult.com

RELATED CONTENT

Stevens-Johnson's Syndrome (Patient Information)
Toxic Epidermal Necrolysis (Related Key Topic)

AUTHOR: **FRED F. FERRI, M.D.**

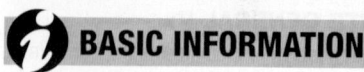

BASIC INFORMATION

DEFINITION

Stomatitis is inflammation involving the oral mucous membranes. Mucositis is inflammation and ulceration of the mucous membranes. It is most commonly seen in the mouth but can occur anywhere in the GI, genitourinary (GU), or respiratory tract. It is most often due to side effects of chemotherapy or radiation therapy (Fig. E1) in cancer patients.

SYNONYMS

Heterogeneous grouping of unrelated illnesses, each with its own designation(s)

ICD-10CM CODES
K12	Stomatitis and related lesions
K12.1	Other forms of stomatitis
K13.0	Other and unspecified lesions of oral mucosa
K12.0	Recurrent oral aphthae
B37.0	Candidal stomatitis
A69.0	Necrotizing ulcerative stomatitis
B08.4	Enteroviral vesicular stomatitis with exanthem
B08.61	Bovine stomatitis
B37.0	Candidal stomatitis
K12.30	Oral mucositis (ulcerative), unspecified
K12.31	Oral mucositis (ulcerative) due to antineoplastic therapy
K12.32	Oral mucositis (ulcerative) due to other drugs
K12.33	Oral mucositis (ulcerative) due to radiation
K12.39	Other oral mucositis (ulcerative)

PHYSICAL FINDINGS & CLINICAL PRESENTATION

WHITE LESIONS:
- Candidiasis (thrush).
- Caused by yeast infection (Candida albicans).
- Examination: white, curdlike material (Fig. E2) that when wiped off leaves a raw bleeding surface.
- Epidemiology: seen in the very young and the very old, those with immunodeficiency (AIDS, cancer), persons with diabetes, and patients treated with antibacterial agents.
- Other.
  1. Leukoedema: filmy opalescent-appearing mucosa, which can be reverted to normal appearance by stretching. This condition is benign.
  2. White sponge nevus: thick, white corrugated folds involving the buccal mucosa. Appears in childhood as an autosomal dominant trait. Benign condition.
  3. Darier's disease (keratosis follicularis): white papules on the gingivae, alveolar mucosa, and dorsal tongue. Skin lesions also present (erythematous papules). Inherited as an autosomal dominant trait.
  4. Chemical injury: white sloughing mucosa.
  5. Nicotine stomatitis: whitened palate with red papules.
  6. Lichen planus: linear, reticular, slightly raised striae on buccal mucosa. Skin is involved by pruritic violaceous papules on forearms and inner thighs.
  7. Discoid lupus erythematosus: lesion resembles lichen planus.
  8. Leukoplakia: white lesions that cannot be scraped off; 20% are premalignant epithelial dysplasia or squamous cell carcinoma.
  9. Hairy leukoplakia: shaggy white surface that cannot be wiped off; seen in HIV infection, caused by Epstein-Barr virus.

RED LESIONS:
- Candidiasis may present with red lesions instead of the more frequent white. Median rhomboid glossitis is a chronic variant.
- Benign migratory glossitis (geographic tongue): area of atrophic depapillated mucosa surrounded by a keratotic border. Benign lesion, no treatment required.
- Hemangiomas.
- Histoplasmosis: ill-defined, irregular patch with a granulomatous surface, sometimes ulcerated.
- Allergy.
- Anemia: atrophic reddened glossal mucosa seen with pernicious anemia.
- Erythroplakia: red patch usually caused by epithelial dysplasia or squamous cell carcinoma.
- Burning tongue (glossopyrosis): normal examination; sometimes associated with denture trauma, anemia, diabetes, vitamin B_{12} deficiency, psychogenic problems.

DARK LESIONS (BROWN, BLUE, BLACK):
- Coated tongue: accumulation of keratin; harmless condition that can be treated by scraping.
- Melanotic lesions: freckles, lentigines, lentigo, melanoma, Peutz-Jeghers syndrome, Addison's disease.
- Varices.
- Kaposi's sarcoma: red or purple macules that enlarge to form tumors; seen in patients with AIDS.

RAISED LESIONS:
- Papilloma.
- Verruca vulgaris.
- Condyloma acuminatum.
- Fibroma.
- Epulis.
- Pyogenic granuloma.
- Mucocele.
- Retention cyst.

BLISTERS:
- Primary herpetic gingivostomatitis (Fig. E3).
- Caused by herpes simplex virus type 1 or, less frequently, type 2.
- Course: day 1: malaise, fever, headache, sore throat, cervical lymphadenopathy; days 2 and 3: appearance of vesicles that develop into painful ulcers of 2 to 4 mm in diameter; duration of up to 2 wk.
- Recurrent intraoral herpes: rare; recurrences typically involve only the keratinized epithelium (lips).
- Pemphigus and pemphigoid.
- Hand-foot-mouth disease: caused by coxsackievirus group A.
- Erythema multiforme.
- Herpangina: caused by echovirus.
- Traumatic ulcer.
- Primary syphilis.
- Perlèche (or angular cheilitis).
- Recurrent aphthous stomatitis (canker sores): most common oral mucosa lesion; may be associated with many systemic diseases.
- Behçet's syndrome (aphthous ulcers, uveitis, genital ulcerations, arthritis, and aseptic meningitis).
- Reiter's syndrome (conjunctivitis, urethritis, and arthritis with occasional oral ulcerations).
- Unknown cause.

Course: solitary or multiple painful ulcers may develop simultaneously and heal over 10 to 14 days. The size of the lesions and the frequency of recurrences are variable.

DIAGNOSIS

WORKUP
- White lesions: candidiasis (thrush) diagnosis: ovoid yeast and hyphae seen in scrapings treated with KOH culture.
- Blisters:
  1. Exfoliative cytology.
  2. Viral culture.
  3. Immunofluorescence for herpes antigen.

TREATMENT

White lesions: candidiasis (thrush) treatment:
- Topical with nystatin or clotrimazole.
- Systemic with ketoconazole or fluconazole.
Blisters:
- Supportive.
- Consider acyclovir.

Recurrent intraoral herpes/aphthous ulcerations: topical corticosteroids (dexamethasone ointment applied to the identified ulcer tid) or systemic steroids for severe cases.

RELATED CONTENT

Stomatitis (Patient Information)

AUTHOR: **FRED F. FERRI, M.D.**

BASIC INFORMATION

DEFINITION

Ischemic stroke is the sudden onset of a focal neurologic deficit as a result of cerebral ischemia resulting in cell death. The purpose of this chapter is to help the provider make decisions about the management of the acute stroke patient within the first several hours of symptoms; this is the crucial time for definitive treatment interventions.

SYNONYMS

Stroke
Brain attack
Cerebrovascular accident (this is a nonspecific term and should not be used.)

ICD-10CM CODES
I63	Cerebral infarction
I63.3	Cerebral infarction due to thrombosis of cerebral arteries
I63.4	Cerebral infarction due to embolism of cerebral arteries
I63.5	Cerebral infarction due to unspecified occlusion or stenosis of cerebral arteries
I63.6	Cerebral infarction due to cerebral venous thrombosis, nonpyogenic
I63.8	Other cerebral infarction
I63.9	Cerebral infarction, unspecified
I67.89	Other cerebrovascular disease

EPIDEMIOLOGY & DEMOGRAPHICS

INCIDENCE:
- ~800,000 new or recurrent strokes occur each year in the U.S.
- Stroke is the number five cause of death (130,000 deaths every year) and the leading cause of long-term disability in the U.S.

PREVALENCE: There are ~4.5 million stroke survivors in the U.S.

RISK FACTORS: Hypertension, dyslipidemia, diabetes mellitus, and smoking are the four major risk factors. Other risk factors include atrial fibrillation (most common cause of cardioembolic stroke), mechanical heart valve, patent foramen ovale, recent myocardial infarction, metabolic syndrome, carotid artery stenosis, vertebral artery stenosis, intracranial artery stenosis, hypercoagulable states, subclinical atrial tachyarrhythmias without clinical atrial fibrillation, sickle cell disease, and obesity.

GENETICS: Multifactorial

PHYSICAL FINDINGS & CLINICAL PRESENTATION

Clinical presentation varies with the artery and region of CNS affected. Below is a noncomprehensive list of common stroke syndrome presentations based on the cerebral vascular territory affected. Please note that this list is not comprehensive and that all findings for a particular syndrome may not be listed here.

- Large- to medium-sized arteries:
  1. Left middle cerebral artery: right face, arm, and leg weakness and sensory loss with aphasia (expressive, receptive, or both); possible hemianopia
  2. Right middle cerebral artery: left face, arm, and leg weakness and sensory loss with hemineglect; possible hemianopia
  3. Basilar artery: typically an acute loss of consciousness preceded by vertigo, nausea, vomiting, and diplopia; quadriparesis or quadriplegia may be seen, including "locked-in" syndrome
  4. Posterior cerebral artery: unilateral hemianopia; blindness with anosognosia (Anton syndrome) if bilateral
  5. Anterior cerebral artery: unilateral leg weakness and sensory loss
  6. Posterior inferior cerebellar artery: lateral medullary (Wallenberg's) syndrome—ipsilesional loss of pinprick and temperature on the face and contralateral loss of pinprick and temperature on the body; ipsilesional Horner's syndrome and ipsilesional palatal weakness with resulting dysphagia, dysarthria. Also with vertigo, nystagmus, ataxia.
  7. **Lacunar syndrome:** no cortical signs are present in lacunar syndromes.
     - Pure motor hemiparesis: typically due to an ischemic lesion in either the internal capsule or pons.
     - Pure sensory stroke: typically due to an ischemic lesion of the thalamus.
     - Ataxic hemiparesis: ataxia out of proportion to the hemiparesis; typically due to an ischemic lesion of either the internal capsule or pons.
     - Sensorimotor stroke: typically due to ischemic lesion involving both the thalamus and internal capsule.
     - Dysarthria–clumsy hand syndrome: multiple localizations possible but typically the pons; facial weakness, dysarthria, and mild clumsiness and weakness of the hand.

ETIOLOGY

Etiologies include atherosclerosis, cardioembolism, artery-to-artery embolism, small-vessel lipohyalinosis, arteritis, arterial dissection, and vasospasm.

DIAGNOSIS

DIFFERENTIAL DIAGNOSIS

The differential diagnosis of acute ischemic stroke includes hemorrhagic stroke (intracerebral hemorrhage), seizure with postictal paralysis, migraine with hemiparesis, syncope, hypoglycemia, hypertensive encephalopathy, and conversion disorder.

LABORATORY TESTS

- Immediate (Box 1): CBC, metabolic panel that includes blood glucose and renal function, PT/INR, aPTT, troponin I, and urinalysis. Blood glucose is the only test required before initiation of IV tPA.
- National Institutes of Health Stroke Scale: a brief, focused neurologic examination aimed at providing a numeric estimate of the severity of stroke; can be performed by any health care provider trained in its use; may increase the likelihood of the correct assessment of stroke
- ECG and telemetry monitoring
- Echocardiogram to look for potential cardiogenic source of embolism, infective endocarditis and intracardiac shunts

---

BOX 1   Immediate Diagnostic Studies: Evaluation of a Patient With Suspected Acute Ischemic Stroke

All Patients
Noncontrast brain computed tomographic scan (magnetic resonance imaging, if available)
Blood glucose level[1]
Serum electrolyte and renal function tests
Electrocardiography
Markers of cardiac ischemia
Complete blood count, including platelet count[2]
Prothrombin time/international normalized ratio
Activated partial thromboplastin time
Oxygen saturation

Selected Patients
Hepatic function tests
Toxicology screen
Blood alcohol level
Pregnancy test
Arterial blood gas tests (if hypoxia is suspected)
Chest radiography (if lung disease is suspected)
Lumbar puncture (if subarachnoid hemorrhage is suspected and computed tomography scan is negative for blood)
Electroencephalogram (if seizures are suspected)

[1] Only test recommended before initiation of IV rtPA.
[2] Although it is desirable to know the results of these tests before giving a patient tissue plasminogen activator, thrombolytic therapy should not be delayed while awaiting the results unless (1) there is clinical suspicion of a bleeding abnormality or thrombocytopenia; (2) the patient has received heparin or warfarin; or (3) the patient's use of anticoagulants is not known.

From Christensen H et al: Abnormalities on ECG and telemetry predict stroke outcome at 3 months, *J Neurol Sci* 234:99–103, 2005.

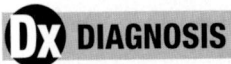

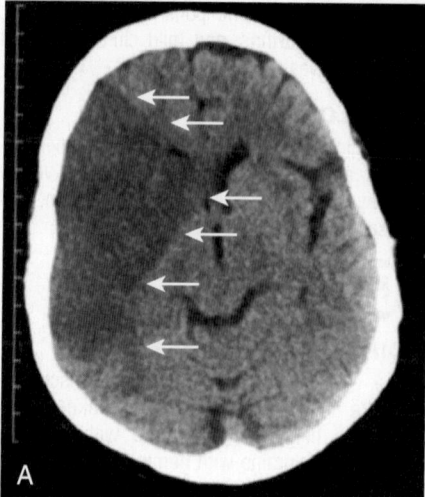 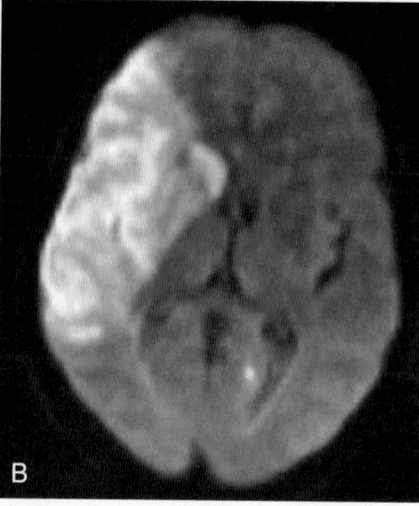

FIG. 1 Large right middle cerebral artery infarct on an unenhanced computed tomographic scan **(A)** and a diffusion-weighted magnetic resonance image **(B)**. There is a mass effect, and this patient is at risk for cerebral herniation syndromes.

TABLE 1 Imaging Modalities for Stroke

Imaging Modality	Advantage	Disadvantage
Cerebral catheter angiography	• Allows for the definitive assessment of cerebral circulation (gold standard) • Allows for the deployment of intra-arterial thrombolysis and thrombectomy devices if a thrombus is found • Allows for the assessment of collateral circulation	• Invasive (significant risks) • High cost • Not available at all facilities
Doppler studies	• Noninvasive • May be performed at the patient's bedside	• Can be limited by the patient's body habitus • Operator dependent
Magnetic resonance angiography	• Excellent view of the large arteries of the neck and brain • No contrast material needed	• Cannot be performed in patients who are critically ill, who are unable to tolerate supine positioning, who have a pacemaker or other ferromagnetic hardware, or who are claustrophobic
Magnetic resonance perfusion	• Assesses cerebral hemodynamics • May show ischemic penumbra (i.e., the area of the brain that may be saved by timely intervention)	• Not commonly available • Not well standardized
CT angiography	• Excellent view of the large arteries of the neck and brain • Similar to magnetic resonance angiography with regard to resolution	• Requires intravenous contrast
CT perfusion	• Assesses cerebral hemodynamics • May show ischemic penumbra (i.e., the area of the brain that may be saved by timely intervention)	• Challenging to interpret in some cases • Not routinely available at many facilities • Requires intravenous contrast

IMAGING STUDIES

- Immediate (Fig. 1): computed tomography (CT) of the head without contrast to rule out hemorrhage.
- MRI of the brain with stroke protocol to assess the extent of stroke (because CT typically will not show an ischemic stroke for several hours), but it is rarely needed in the hyperacute setting to determine reperfusion strategy, although some newer techniques like diffusion and perfusion MR are being utilized for this purpose at some centers.
- Several other neuroimaging studies are useful during the early stages of acute stroke to assess whether there is a thrombus that is amenable to intervention (Table 1).

Cross reference: see "Transient Ischemic Attack" for general workup, which is identical to that for ischemic stroke.

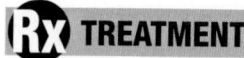

NONPHARMACOLOGIC THERAPY
GENERAL CONSIDERATIONS:
- Airway and breathing should be maintained.
- Supplemental oxygen should be provided to keep the oxygen saturation at ≥92%.
- Pneumatic compression devices or pharmacologic means should be applied to help prevent deep venous thrombosis.
- Avoid any and all oral intake until swallowing is clearly unimpaired; this helps to avoid aspiration pneumonia.
- Early mobilization for rehabilitation is desirable.
- Consider neurosurgical intervention for craniectomy in select cases. Typical cases in which craniectomy may be performed include cerebellar ischemia with compression of the brain stem and/or the fourth ventricle as well as large middle cerebral artery ischemia. Available evidence suggests that it may be better to perform early hemicraniectomy (<48 hr) to achieve better outcomes. Decompressive hemicraniectomy has shown good benefit in terms of mortality but not much benefit in terms of disability and functional outcomes.

ACUTE GENERAL Rx
INTRAVENOUS THROMBOLYSIS:
- IV t-PA, or alteplase, is the only medical therapy approved by the U.S. FDA for the treatment of acute ischemic stroke.
- The time window for administration is generally accepted to be within 4.5 hours of symptom onset, although the FDA indication is still within 3 hours. The American Heart Association/American Stroke Association recommends a t-PA administration window of up to 4.5 hours with certain additional exclusion criteria when compared to the 3-hour administration.
- There are strict criteria for the administration of IV t-PA (see Box 2).
- The protocol is weight based, with 90 mg being the maximum allowable dose.
- The risk of brain hemorrhage with IV t-PA is about 6% in stroke patients.

IMMEDIATE CATHETER CEREBRAL ANGIOGRAPHY FOR ENDOVASCULAR INTERVENTION
(Figs. 2 and 3): Methods available:
- The Merci clot retrieval system, cleared by the FDA in 2004, was the first device for clot retrieval in acute stroke. However, recanalization rates were only modest, and poorly designed clinical trials failed to demonstrate improved outcomes over standard thrombolytic therapy. Subsequently, several new devices have been developed for mechanical clot retrieval with excellent recanalization rates. Multiple randomized clinical trials published in the last two to three years using these newer devices on a carefully selected patient population with large vessel

BOX 2 Three-Hour Criteria for Tissue Plasminogen Activator (Alteplase [Activase]) Use in Patients with Thromboembolic Stroke

Criteria for considering TPA as a treatment option:
- Clinical presentation consistent with an ischemic stroke with clearly demonstrable neurologic deficits
- Noncontrast CT head without evidence of hemorrhage
- Time since onset of symptoms (or last known normal if time of onset not known) clearly <3 hr (3-4.5 hr with additional exclusion criteria) before TPA administration would begin
- Age ≥18 years

Criteria for excluding TPA as a treatment option:
- Absolute exclusion criteria:
- Historic and clinical findings suggestive of subarachnoid hemorrhage, even if CT scan is normal
  1. Sudden, severe headache, often with a loss of consciousness at onset
  2. Vomiting
- Active internal bleeding, increased risk of bleeding, or known bleeding diathesis, including those resulting from:
  1. Recent use of warfarin with an INR of ≥1.7
  2. Use of heparin within 48 hr with a prolonged aPTT
  3. Current use of direct thrombin inhibitors or factor Xa inhibitors
  4. Platelet count of <100,000/mm³
  5. History of intracranial hemorrhage
  6. Known intracranial neoplasm, arteriovenous malformation or aneurysm
  7. Arterial puncture at a noncompressible site within the past 7 days
- Stroke, intracranial surgery, or head trauma within the previous 3 mo
- Systolic blood pressure >185 mm Hg or diastolic blood pressure >110 mm Hg that does not decrease below that range with treatment
- Blood glucose <50 mg/dl or >400 mg/dl
- CT findings:
  1. Evidence of intracranial hemorrhage
  2. Hypodensity or effacement of the sulci in one third of the territory of the middle cerebral artery
- Relative exclusion criteria:
  - Major surgery or serious trauma within the preceding 14 days
  - Acute myocardial infarction (recent within the previous 3 months) or postmyocardial infarction pericarditis
  - GI or GU bleeding within the past 21 days
  - Seizure at stroke onset
  - Rapidly improving neurologic signs or Isolated mild neurologic deficits
  - Patient who is pregnant or lactating
- Additional exclusion criteria for administering IV tPA in the 3-4.5 hour window
  - Age >80 years
  - High stroke scale on presentation (NIHSS >25)
  - Current use of oral anticoagulants regardless of INR
- Prior history of stroke and diabetes mellitus

aPTT, Activated partial thromboplastin time; *CT*, computed tomography; *GI*, gastrointestinal; *GU*, genitourinary; *INR*, international normalized ratio; *TPA*, tissue plasminogen activator.
Modified from Rakel RE [ed]: *Principles of family practice*, ed 6, Philadelphia, 2002, Saunders.

occlusions in the anterior circulation have demonstrated improved neurologic outcomes with endovascular treatment.
- The American Heart Association/American Stroke Association recently published an update of its original guidelines on acute ischemic stroke, recommending endovascular treatment (Class I: Level A evidence) for highly selected patients.
- Intraarterial tissue plasminogen activator (t-PA) is used routinely for up to 6 hours after the onset of symptoms, although it is not approved by the U.S. FDA for this purpose.

Pearls and caveats:
- Multimodal therapy (i.e., thrombectomy and intraarterial t-PA) is sometimes performed.
- Endovascular treatment may be performed for select cases in which intravenous (IV) TPA has failed to recanalize an occluded artery.

- Endovascular intervention may be an option for cases in which there are systemic contraindications to IV t-PA.
- Endovascular intervention is useful only for large, accessible thrombi. Therefore, if a stroke patient is a candidate for IV t-PA, then he or she should probably receive IV t-PA.
- One can reasonably expect an endovascular recanalization rate of 60% in appropriate patients when used alone. Combining the Solitaire device with other endovascular approaches has shown recanalization rates close to 88% in recent studies (Solitaire).
- Complications can ensue from the endovascular procedure itself, including an intracerebral hemorrhage rate that is similar to that associated with IV t-PA. A recent meta-analysis revealed that among patients with acute ischemic stroke, endovascular therapy with mechanical thrombectomy versus standard medical care with t-PA

was associated with improved functional outcomes and higher rates of angiographic revascularization, but no significant difference in symptomatic intracranial hemorrhage or all-cause mortality at 90 days.[1]
- Endovascular intervention is typically available only at comprehensive stroke centers.
- Some practitioners use perfusion imaging (i.e., CT perfusion and magnetic resonance perfusion) to assess whether there is salvageable brain tissue before performing a mechanical thrombectomy. In some cases, use of perfusion imaging may lead to a dramatic expansion of traditional time windows; this practice is currently being studied in clinical trials.
- Fever: Fever is harmful during acute stroke. Ascertaining and addressing the cause while lowering an elevated temperature is strongly advised.

HYPERTENSION: Elevated blood pressure is common during acute stroke, and it often subsides without specific therapy. In general, hypertension is not treated acutely unless it is extremely high (e.g., >220 mm Hg systolic blood pressure); there is evidence of hypertension-induced organ damage; or thrombolysis is being considered, in which case the blood pressure needs to come down (if it can be safely accomplished) to <185/110 mm Hg. It is risky to decrease blood pressure dramatically and quickly in the presence of acute ischemic stroke as it can cause an extension of the infarcted tissue into the ischemic penumbra. A 15% to 25% decrease over the first 24 hours is recommended.

HYPOTENSION: The presence of systemic hypotension in acute ischemic stroke portends a poor outcome. The cause should be sought, and volume depletion should be corrected with normal saline. Cardiac arrhythmias should be treated. Induced hypertension with vasopressor agents may be useful for select cases with an ischemic penumbra that is at risk, but caution is strongly advised.

HYPOGLYCEMIA: Hypoglycemia can mimic stroke. Prompt assessment of serum glucose level and replacement as necessary are important.

HYPERGLYCEMIA: The presence of hyperglycemia worsens ischemic stroke outcome. Hyperglycemia should be managed aggressively.

ANTIPLATELET THERAPY: Oral, rectal, or feeding tube administration of aspirin (325 mg/day) within 48 hours of stroke onset is advised to decrease the likelihood of a repeat ischemic stroke. Other oral antiplatelet regimens approved for secondary stroke prophylaxis (e.g., clopidogrel, aspirin plus extended-release dipyridamole) will also suffice and may be superior in the long term. In patients with acute ischemic stroke and atrial fibrillation, full dose anticoagulation with heparin infusion or low molecular weight heparin should be avoided in

[1]Badhiwala JH, et al.: Endovascular thrombectomy for acute ischemic stroke: a meta-analysis, *JAMA* 314(17):1832–1843, 2015.

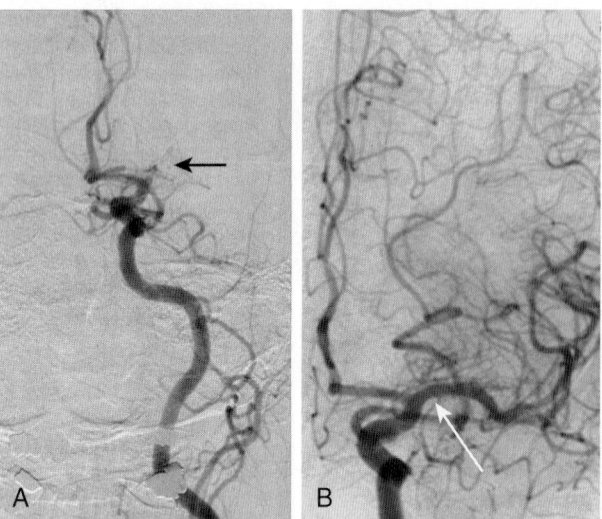

FIG. 2 A, A catheter angiogram showing left middle cerebral artery occlusion, which caused severe stroke symptoms for several hours. **B,** The artery was opened with the Merci clot retrieval system, and this resulted in normal flow.

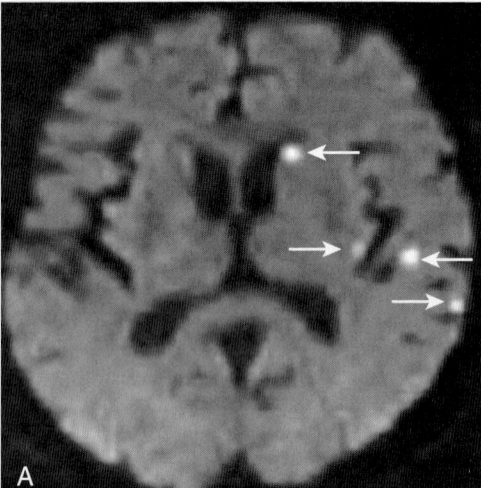 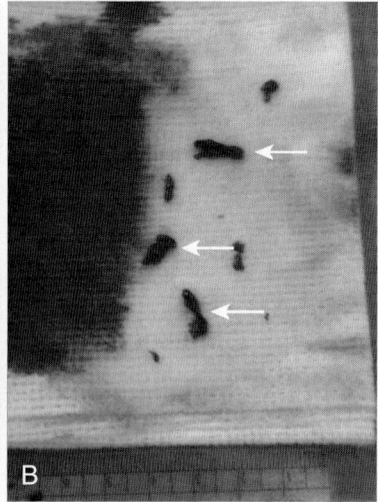

FIG. 3 A, A diffusion-weighted magnetic resonance image of the same patient as shown in previous figure, this time showing only mild left cerebral ischemia after intervention. The patient was clinically normal. **B,** Thrombi removed from the middle cerebral artery with the use of the Merci clot retrieval system.

the acute setting, as this could potentially harm the patient by causing symptomatic intracranial hemorrhage, and there is very little evidence to suggest any benefit. However, chronic anti-coagulation is indicated after the acute period has passed.

DISPOSITION

Patients with acute ischemic stroke should be cared for in a stroke unit or an intensive care unit. Nurses with skills in stroke care and telemetry monitoring should be routine. Once the patient is stable and the workup is complete, rehabilitation should be arranged.

REFERRAL

Patients with acute ischemic stroke should be transported to a hospital in which providers are skilled in stroke care. Depending on the severity and duration of symptoms, the patient may qualify for immediate endovascular intervention at a comprehensive stroke center, even if he or she is not a candidate for IV TPA. If complications from brain edema develop, further evaluation by a neurosurgeon may be helpful during the acute phase.

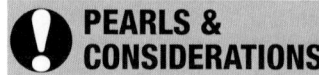

PEARLS & CONSIDERATIONS

PREVENTION

- The prevention of acute ischemic stroke depends on the aggressive management of risk factors in individual patients.
- Cross reference: stroke, secondary prevention
- Paroxysmal atrial fibrillation is common in patients with cryptogenic stroke. A recent study found that noninvasive ambulatory ECG monitoring for 30 days significantly improved the detection of atrial fibrillation by a factor of >5 and nearly doubled the rate of anticoagulant treatment compared to the standard practice of short-duration ECG monitoring

PATIENT & FAMILY EDUCATION

Patients and families need to be taught about ways to reduce the risk for recurrent stroke, including lifestyle modifications. Education about rehabilitation goals, when appropriate, should also be accomplished.

SUGGESTED READINGS

Available at www.expertconsult.com

RELATED CONTENT

Algorithm for the emergency evaluation of a patient with suspected stroke (Algorithm, Section III)
Stroke (Patient Information)

AUTHORS: **JOSEPH S. KASS, M.D., J.D.,** and **PRASHANTH KRISHNAMOHAN, M.B.B.S., M.D.**

BASIC INFORMATION

DEFINITION

Hemorrhagic stroke is the sudden onset of a focal neurologic deficit caused by hemorrhage into or around the brain.

SYNONYMS

Intracerebral hemorrhage (ICH)
Intracranial hemorrhage
Cerebrovascular attack (This is a nonspecific term and should not be used.)
The term *subarachnoid hemorrhage* refers to a specific location for hemorrhage, which commonly occurs as a result of a ruptured aneurysm. Please see "Subarachnoid Hemorrhage" for additional information.

ICD-10 CM CODES
I61	Intracerebral hemorrhage
I61.0	Intracerebral hemorrhage in hemisphere, subcortical
I61.1	Intracerebral hemorrhage in hemisphere, cortical
I61.2	Intracerebral hemorrhage in hemisphere, unspecified
I61.3	Intracerebral hemorrhage in brainstem
I61.4	Intracerebral hemorrhage in cerebellum
I61.5	Intracerebral hemorrhage, intraventricular
I61.6	Intracerebral hemorrhage, multiple localized
I61.9	Nontraumatic intracerebral hemorrhage, unspecified

EPIDEMIOLOGY & DEMOGRAPHICS

INCIDENCE: There are approximately 795,000 new or recurrent strokes per year in the U.S., of which approximately 10% are hemorrhagic.[1]
RISK FACTORS:
- Hypertension
- Anticoagulant use
- Thrombolysis
- Alcoholism
- Illicit drug use (e.g., cocaine)
- Cerebral amyloid angiopathy
- Increased age
- African American race
- Low cholesterol, LDL, and triglycerides
- Minuscule increase in absolute risk from antiplatelet therapy
- Questionable effect of chronic kidney disease and selective use of serotonin reuptake inhibitors

GENETICS: Multifactorial

PHYSICAL FINDINGS & CLINICAL PRESENTATION

The presentation varies with the region of the brain that is affected. The following are common locations for hemorrhage:
- Basal ganglia
- Cerebellum
- Pons
- Lobar (i.e., amyloid angiopathy)

- The ICH score is a widely used grading scale to estimate mortality based on CT scan results. Parameters used to calculate the ICH score include Glasgow Coma Scale (GCS) (0 to 2 points) at presentation, patient age ≥80 (1 point), ICH volume ≥30 mL (1 point), presence of intraventricular blood (1 point), and infratentorial origin of blood (1 point). Scores range from 0 to 6 with a score of 0 conferring 0% mortality and a score of 6 with estimated 100% mortality.

ETIOLOGY

- Rupture of vessels
- Aneurysm
- Arteriovenous malformation
- Brain tumor
- Amyloid angiopathy

DIAGNOSIS

DIFFERENTIAL DIAGNOSIS

- Ischemic stroke
- Seizure with postictal paralysis
- Syncope
- Migraine with hemiparesis
- Conversion disorder

LABORATORY TESTS

- CBC, metabolic panel including blood glucose and renal function, PT/INR, aPTT, urinalysis, and toxicology screens
- ECG and telemetry monitoring

IMAGING STUDIES

- Immediate: CT scanning of the head without contrast is highly sensitive for hemorrhage (Fig. 1).
- CT or MR angiogram to rule out an underlying vascular malformation. CT spot sign on the CTA has been shown to be a reliable early predictor of hematoma expansion.
- MRI of the brain with a gradient echo sequence is also highly sensitive for hemorrhage, including intracerebral microhemorrhages that may not be visible with computed

tomography scanning. MRI may also help to identify underlying brain tumors or vascular malformations, especially if the bleeding occurs at atypical sites.

TREATMENT

NONPHARMACOLOGIC THERAPY

- Urgent neurosurgical evaluation is needed in many cases either for evacuation of the hematoma or for relieving raised intracranial pressure by procedures such as EVD placement or decompressive surgeries.
- Surgery should be performed promptly for cases of cerebellar hemorrhage of >3 cm when the patient is deteriorating clinically, showing brain stem edema or hydrocephalus.
- Surgery for lobar or deep brain clots may be considered for select cases, although the level of evidence for efficacy is not high. Currently, guidelines recommend standard craniotomy for patients with lobar clots >30 ml within 1 cm.
- Recent innovative surgical techniques, such as instillation of thrombolytic agents for intraventricular hemorrhage and minimally invasive surgery for hematoma evacuation, appear to be promising. Clinical trials are currently in progress to assess whether these approaches improve mortality and neurologic outcomes.

ACUTE GENERAL Rx

The cornerstones of medical management of acute intracerebral hemorrhage include:
Control of hypertension
Correction of coagulopathy
Management of elevated intracranial pressure
Treatment of seizures

Hypertension (Box 1): Blood pressure should be quickly lowered by 15% and then gradually and safely brought to the individual patient's target range. In theory, this may diminish the expansion of the hematoma. More aggressive control of systolic blood pressure (SBP) to 140 or less in the acute setting has been shown to be safe in clinical trials (INTERACT2 trial) with slightly

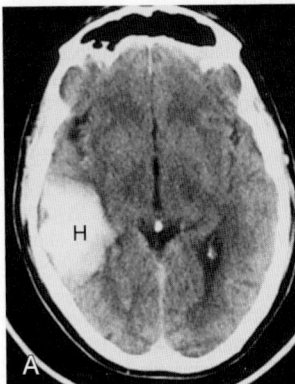
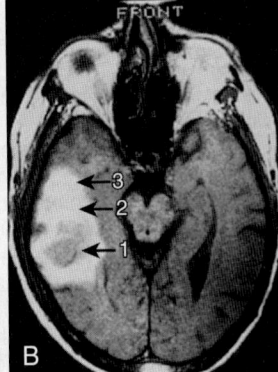
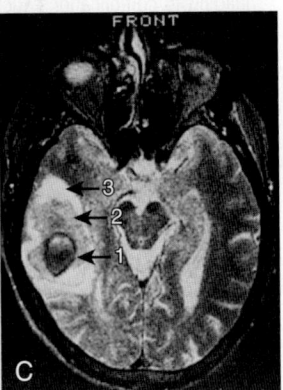

FIG. 1 Hemorrhage. Axial CT image **(A)** demonstrates a large area of acute hemorrhage *(H)* in right temporal lobe. T_1-weighted **(B)** and T_2-weighted **(C)** MRI scans demonstrate the hemorrhage in various stages of breakdown. Center of lesion is dark on T_1- and T_2-weighted images, indicating oxyhemoglobin *(1)*. Intermediate zone is bright on T_1-weighted image and gray on T_2-weighted image, indicating intracellular methemoglobin *(2)*. Outer rim is bright on both T_1- and T_2-weighted images, indicating extracellular methemoglobin *(3)*. (From Vincent JL et al: *Textbook of critical care*, ed 6, Philadelphia, 2011, Saunders.)

BOX 1 Suggested Recommended Guidelines for the Treatment of Elevated Blood Pressure in Patients with Spontaneous Intracerebral Hemorrhage

1. SBP of >200 mm Hg or MAP of >150 mm Hg: Consider the aggressive reduction of BP with continuous intravenous infusion, with BP monitoring every 5 min.
2. SBP of >180 mm Hg or MAP of >130 mm Hg with evidence or suspicion of elevated ICP: Consider ICP monitor and reducing BP with intermittent or continuous intravenous medications to keep cerebral perfusion pressure >60 to 80 mm Hg.
3. SBP of >180 mm Hg or MAP of >130 mm Hg without evidence or suspicion of elevated ICP: Consider a modest reduction of BP (e.g., MAP of 110 mm Hg or target blood pressure of 160/90 mm Hg) with intermittent or continuous intravenous medications, and clinically reexamine the patient every 15 min.

BP, Blood pressure; *ICP,* intracranial pressure; *MAP,* mean arterial pressure; *SBP,* systolic blood pressure.
Modified from Broderick J et al: Guidelines for the management of spontaneous intracerebral hemorrhage in adults: 2007 update, *Stroke* 38:2001-2023, 2007.

improved outcomes compared to less aggressive BP control (target SBP <180) and is currently recommended by the American Heart Association/American Stroke Association guidelines. Evidence suggests that a more sustained BP control with continuous IV medications might be more beneficial than using intermittent medications resulting in significant BP variability. The most recent guidelines, published in 2015, state that for ICH patients presenting with SBP between 150 and 220 mm Hg and without contraindication to acute BP treatment, acute lowering of SBP to 140 mm Hg is safe and can be effective for improving functional outcome. For ICH patients presenting with SBP >220 mm Hg, it may be reasonable to consider aggressive reduction of BP with a continuous intravenous infusion and frequent BP monitoring.

Correction of Coagulopathy
- Early hematoma expansion has been associated with poor outcome.
- Protamine sulfate is used to treat cases of heparin-induced intracerebral hemorrhage. Protamine dosage is 1 mg IV for every 100 units of heparin administered in the previous 2 to 3 hours (maximum dose is 50 mg).
- Prothrombin concentrate complex (PCC) is now recommended for reversal of warfarin-associated ICH. FFP may also be used for this purpose, although it carries the disadvantage of administering more volume, potentially leading to complications such as pulmonary edema and slightly longer times to reversal of coagulopathy compared to PCC. Vitamin K should be administered IV along with flash-frozen plasma (FFP)/PCC for sustained effects. Routine use of recombinant factor VII concentrates is not recommended due to insufficient evidence and concern for increased risk of thromboembolic events.
- Idarucizumab (Praxbind) is a humanized monoclonal antibody fragment that can be used for urgent reversal of the anticoagulant effect of the direct thrombin inhibitor dabigatran (Pradaxa).
- Andexanet alfa, a recombinant modified human factor X2 decoy protein has been effective for reversion of the anticoagulant effect of apixaban (Eliquis), rivaroxaban (Xarelto), and edoxaban (Savaysa).

- Recommendations for thrombolytic-associated intracerebral hemorrhage treatment include the consideration of the infusion of platelets and cryoprecipitate.
- Hemostatic therapy has not been shown convincingly to improve outcomes, despite reducing hematoma expansion. Efforts are under way to identify patients at high risk of early hematoma expansion by using clinical and radiographic information to determine who may benefit from more aggressive hemostatic intervention.

Elevated intracranial pressure: This condition should be treated with a graded approach, which may include the elevation of the head of the bed, analgesia/sedation, hyperventilation, and osmotic therapy. In patients clinically suspected to have elevated ICP or with GCS <8, invasive monitoring of the ICP may be required. If conservative treatment fails to control ICP, EVD placement or other decompressive procedures like craniotomy should be pursued.

Seizures: If seizures occur, they should be treated aggressively, including with intravenous medications, if needed. Although widely practiced, routine use of prophylactic antiepileptic medications is not recommended. Continuous EEG monitoring should be employed in patients with suspected seizures or unexplained low levels of consciousness.

Supportive Treatment:
- Hyperglycemia: a high blood glucose level predicts a worse outcome. Markedly elevated glucose levels should be lowered to <200 mg/dl.
- Antipyretics should be administered for fever in addition to searching for a cause of the fever.
- Care should be taken to avoid hypoxia. Airway and ventilatory management should happen early and concurrently with the primary management of ICH.
- Pneumatic compression devices should be applied to help prevent deep venous thrombosis. Chemical DVT prophylaxis can be started after 48 to 72 hours in most situations once the bleed has been determined to be stable.
- Early mobilization for rehabilitation is desirable.

DISPOSITION
For large hemorrhages or unstable patients, immediate referral to a stroke center

REFERRAL
Patients with hemorrhagic stroke should be transported to a hospital where providers are skilled in the treatment of stroke and cerebrovascular diseases including the availability of neurosurgery services and neurocritical care. Depending on the severity and duration of symptoms, the patient may require neurosurgical intervention.

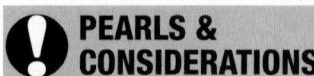

❗ PEARLS & CONSIDERATIONS

- Outcomes are inversely correlated with hemorrhage size.
- Specific reversal agents may be useful for warfarin-, heparin-, NOAC-, or thrombolysis-associated hemorrhage.
- No procoagulant medications have yet been shown to be safe and effective for the mitigation of spontaneous intracerebral hemorrhage in placebo-controlled trials.

PREVENTION
- Prevention depends on the aggressive management of risk factors in individual patients, including hypertension, smoking, alcohol use, and cocaine use.
- Non–vitamin K oral anticoagulants (NOACs) dabigatran, apixaban, rivaroxaban, and edoxaban are uniformly associated with an overall reduced risk of iatrogenic ICH when used for stroke prevention in atrial fibrillation when compared to warfarin. Any of the currently available NOACs can be considered first line for patients at high risk for ICH.[1]

PATIENT & FAMILY EDUCATION
Patients and families need to understand that most patients will not soon achieve functional independence and that rehabilitation will be a long process. Education about avoiding antithrombotic agents should be stressed as appropriate for individual circumstances.

SUGGESTED READINGS
Available at www.expertconsult.com

RELATED CONTENT
Stroke (Patient Information)

AUTHORS: **A. BASIT KHAN, B.A., JOSEPH S. KASS, M.D., J.D.,** and **PRASHANTH KRISHNAMOHAN, M.B.B.S., M.D.**

[1]Chatterjee S et al.: New oral anticoagulants and the risk of intracranial hemorrhage: traditional and Bayesian meta-analysis and mixed treatment comparison of randomized trials of new oral anticoagulants in atrial fibrillation, *JAMA Neurol* 70(12):1486-1490, 2013.

BASIC INFORMATION

DEFINITION

Secondary prevention of stroke involves preventing the recurrence of a cerebral vascular ischemic or hemorrhagic stroke after a primary event and early rehabilitation. It now includes preventive treatments after a transient ischemic event (reversible symptoms with no MRI findings after 24 hours).

SYNONYMS

Brain attack
Stroke
Cerebral thrombosis
Cerebral hemorrhage
Brain infarct

ICD-10CM CODES

I65.2 Occlusion and stenosis of carotid artery
I65.0 Occlusion and stenosis of vertebral artery
I65.9 Occlusion and stenosis of unspecified precerebral artery
I66   Occlusion and stenosis of cerebral artery, not resulting in cerebral infarction
I65.1 Occlusion and stenosis of basilar artery

EPIDEMIOLOGY

Stroke is the third leading cause of death in the U.S. Each year, there are a total of 800,000 strokes, of which approximately 200,000 are recurrent strokes. Thus, secondary prevention of ischemic stroke remains good treatment strategy. Secondary prevention is specifically targeted toward modifiable risk factors.
RISK FACTORS: Age is the most important non-modifiable risk factor. Modifiable risk factors include hypertension, hyperlipidemia, cigarette smoking, excessive alcohol consumption, physical inactivity, obesity (i.e., a body mass index of >25 kg/m^2), illegal drug use (amphetamines, cocaine), and diabetes mellitus.
GENETICS: Multifactorial and strong family correlation if idiopathic strokes occur in parents <65 years old.

PHYSICAL FINDINGS & CLINICAL PRESENTATION

- Stroke can have a varied presentation. Typically, the individual has a sudden definable loss of motor, sensory, visual, or cognitive functions that have a clear time of onset and that are noticed by others or by the individuals themselves.
- Physical findings such as weakness and/or numbness in one limb or on one side of the body, facial droop, visual field loss, or the inability to understand or communicate with others raises one's suspicion of a stroke event.

ETIOLOGY

- Strokes are broadly divided into ischemic or hemorrhagic (i.e., intraparenchymal or subarachnoid hemorrhage).

- Ischemic strokes can be caused by large-vessel atherosclerosis, cardioembolic, such as in atrial fibrillation or cardiomyopathy, or small vessel disease such as lacunar stroke. Rare causes such as recreational drug use (e.g., cocaine abuse); arterial dissection; and hypercoagulable states need to be considered when ischemic stroke occurs in younger individuals.
- The most common cause of intracerebral hemorrhage is uncontrolled hypertension. Spontaneous rupture of a brain aneurysm causes subarachnoid hemorrhage.

DIAGNOSIS

DIFFERENTIAL DIAGNOSIS

- Seizure and postictal states
- Complicated migraine
- Hypoglycemia
- Brain tumor
- Psychogenic disorder

WORKUP

- Blood glucose level HBA1c
- APTT, PT/INR, CBC, and CMP
- Fasting lipid panel
- Hypercoagulability tests for young stroke patients with no obvious risk factors

IMAGING STUDIES

- Computed tomography scanning of the head without contrast can differentiate between ischemic and hemorrhagic stroke. MRI of the brain is a more specific and prognostic study.
- Carotid ultrasound and transcranial Doppler are used to detect large-vessel atherosclerosis. Magnetic resonance and computed tomography angiography are good alternatives.
- Echocardiogram and ECG can be used to detect a cardioembolic source.

TREATMENT

The secondary prevention of stroke is targeted toward modifiable risk factors. These include lifestyle modifications such as appropriate diet, exercise, weight loss, and smoking cessation, avoidance of heavy alcohol use, and risk factor modification as listed in the following. All patients with noncardioembolic ischemic stroke or transient ischemic attack (TIA) should be on aspirin (50 to 325 mg/day), a combination of aspirin and extended-release dipyridamole, or clopidogrel. A consultation with a neurologist should be considered for young stroke patients and for patients with no obvious cause or with stroke from unusual causes (e.g., hypercoagulable states, dissections). Treatment with a combination of Plavix and aspirin in secondary stroke prevention when no other pressing medical conditions require their use is no longer recommended; this was published in the MATCH trial.

PREVENTING STROKE IN SPECIFIC CONDITIONS

Cardioembolic strokes as a result of atrial fibrillation (AF) have two first-line drug therapies:

warfarin and dabigatran. Warfarin remains a first-line therapy with an international normalized ratio (INR) between 2.0 and 3.0. Dabigatran at a dosing regimen of 150 mg twice a day has efficacy equal to that of warfarin without the need for routine monitoring of INR. The U.S. Food and Drug Administration approved dabigatran for nonvalvular AF. Recently the newer antithrombotic agents such as rivaroxaban and apixaban have been introduced for nonvalvular AF. Expert consult by a neurologist is recommended before starting these newer agents. It is important to note that these agents do not have an effect on the PT/INR or APTT in cases where there is a bleed, and no standard effective reversal therapy is available.

1. For patients with contraindications to anticoagulants, aspirin (325 mg/day) is recommended. The Active-A trial suggested that a combination of aspirin and clopidogrel is slightly better than aspirin alone for those unable to tolerate warfarin.
2. Cardioembolic strokes as a result of a prosthetic metallic valve: anticoagulant therapy with warfarin is recommended with a goal INR between 2.5 and 3.5.
3. Strokes as a result of large-vessel atherosclerosis (i.e., symptomatic carotid stenosis): for patients with recent TIA or ischemic stroke within the last 6 months and ipsilateral severe (70%-99%) carotid artery stenosis, carotid endarterectomy (CEA) performed by a surgeon is recommended and results in a perioperative morbidity and mortality rate of <6%. For patients with recent TIA or ischemic stroke and ipsilateral moderate (50%-69%) carotid stenosis, CEA is recommended within 14 days of the event. When the degree of stenosis is <50%, there is no indication for CEA. Carotid stenting is not indicated except for cases in which surgery is high risk. Current trials are comparing carotid enterectomy versus carotid stenting. As of 2013, the Carotid Revascularization Endarterectomy Versus Stenting Trial (CREST) has shown no inferiority of stenting versus endarterectomy, and stenting may favor younger patients (<75 yr) or those at higher surgical risk for complications.
4. Symptomatic intracranial atherosclerosis: treatment with aspirin has proven effective and just as efficacious as warfarin in both the WASID and WARSS studies. The utility of angioplasty and stenting in patients with symptomatic intracranial atherosclerosis is available at several stroke centers but remains investigational (Fig. 1). In April 2011 the NINDS stopped enrollment into the symptomatic intracranial artery stenosis stenting trial (SAMMPRIS).
5. Patent foramen ovale (PFO): the American Academy of Neurology's new 2016 guidelines recommend medical therapy for stroke patients with PFO. Antiplatelet therapy is recommended in cases of cryptogenic strokes.
6. Intracerebral hemorrhage: for immediate management, please refer to the chapter on intracerebral hemorrhage. Antiplatelet agents should be held for 3 to 4 weeks and

can be restarted if there is a compelling indication such as nonvalvular atrial fibrillation. The American Stroke Association/American Heart Association 2010 guideline recommends avoiding long-term anticoagulation (e.g., warfarin, heparin) after spontaneous lobar intracerebral hemorrhage, but antiplatelet therapy (e.g., aspirin, clopidogrel, Aggrenox) may be considered in all cases of intracerebral hemorrhage where there is a definite indication. Consider a neurology consultation in these cases.

PREVENTING LONG-TERM COMPLICATIONS AFTER A STROKE

Evaluation by a physical, occupational, and speech therapist will reduce the long-term disability that can follow a stroke event. The American Stroke Association 2010 guideline recommends a multidisciplinary approach to rehabilitation. Studies have shown an improved survival and recovery. Home-based rehabilitation can be considered after discussion with the rehabilitation specialist.

RISK FACTOR MODIFICATION

1. Hypertension: antihypertensive treatment is recommended for both the prevention of recurrent stroke and the prevention of other vascular events in persons who have had an ischemic stroke or a TIA. Absolute target blood pressure level and reduction are uncertain and should be individualized. Blood pressure should be lowered gradually over a period of months to prevent cerebral hypoperfusion and extension of stroke. Lifestyle modifications as listed previously should be included as part of a comprehensive antihypertension treatment plan.

2. Diabetes: the goal for the hemoglobin A_{1c} level should be <7%. For type 2 diabetics, diet and exercise can prove very beneficial. Type 1 diabetics can also benefit from diet and compliance with their insulin regimen. Uncontrolled hyperglycemia can lead to acceleration of both intracranial and extracranial arteriosclerosis. Always consider consulting a diabetic educator.

3. Hyperlipidemia: for patients with ischemic stroke or TIA with elevated cholesterol levels, statin agents are recommended. The target goals for cholesterol lowering are an LDL-C level of <100 mg/dl and an LDL-C level of <70 mg/dl for very high-risk persons with multiple risk factors (e.g., both coronary artery disease and diabetes).

4. Cigarette smoking: absolute cessation is required. Try to offer pharmacologic therapy or counseling services to the patient. Secondhand tobacco exposure is just as dangerous, so inquire about secondhand exposure.

5. Obesity: weight reduction may be considered for all overweight ischemic stroke and TIA patients to maintain the goal of a body mass index of between 18.5 and 24.9 kg/m^2 and a waist circumference of <35 in for women and <40 in for men.

6. Excessive alcohol consumption: patients with ischemic stroke or TIA who are heavy drinkers should eliminate or reduce their consumption of alcohol. Light to moderate levels of no more than two drinks per day for men and one drink per day for nonpregnant women may be considered.

DISPOSITION

Secondary stroke prevention is a multifaceted approach of lifestyle modification and pharmacologic intervention that is aimed at preventing or limiting disability.

REFERRAL

For complicated recurrent strokes, a referral to a neurologist who specializes in stroke is recommended.

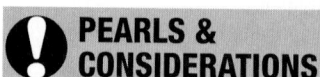

The modification of risk factors is the best preventive measure for stroke. Lifestyle modification is a very important aspect of secondary stroke prevention. Always consider the patient's ability to afford the therapy and prescribed follow-up tests. Experience teaches us that patients sometimes will not let us know about their ability to afford therapies unless we inquire.

PREVENTION

Prevention is the goal of treatment, and compliance is the most important factor. Review risk factor reduction and pharmacologic therapy as previously discussed.

PATIENT/FAMILY EDUCATION

More information can be obtained from the following sources:
- American Heart Association, National Center, 7272 Greenville Avenue, Dallas, TX 75231
- American Stroke Association, 1-888-4-STROKE or 1-888-478-7653
- H.O.P.E. for Stroke, 250 Duck Pond Drive, Wantagh, NY 11793, 516-804-8495

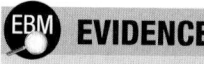 **EVIDENCE**

Available at www.expertconsult.com

SUGGESTED READINGS

Available at www.expertconsult.com

RELATED CONTENT

Stroke (Patient Information)
Transient Ischemic Attack (Related Key Topic)

AUTHOR: **NAWAZ K.A. HACK, M.D.**

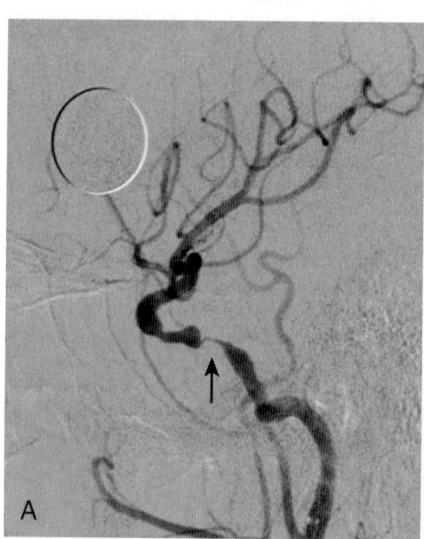
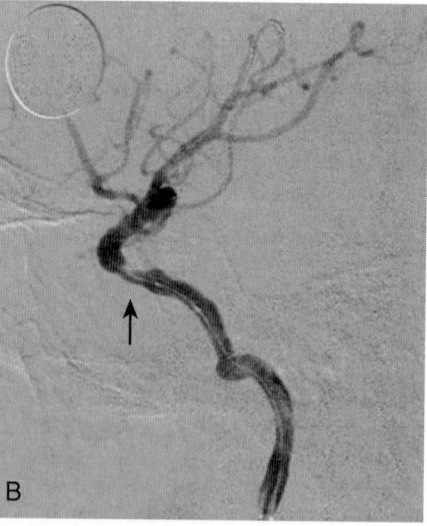

FIG. 1 A, Intracranial high-grade symptomatic stenosis. **B,** This patient failed aggressive medical therapy and responded only to angioplasty and stenting.

BASIC INFORMATION

DEFINITION

A hordeolum is an acute inflammatory process affecting the eyelid and arising from the meibomian (posterior) or Zeis (anterior) glands. It is most often infectious and usually caused by *Staphylococcus aureus*. When infection involves the meibomian glands, it is called meibomianitis.

SYNONYMS

Hordeolum
Meibomianitis

ICD-10CM CODES

H00.011	Hordeolum externum right upper eyelid
H00.012	Hordeolum externum right lower eyelid
H00.013	Hordeolum externum right eye, unspecified eyelid
H00.014	Hordeolum externum left upper eyelid
H00.015	Hordeolum externum left lower eyelid
H00.016	Hordeolum externum left eye, unspecified eyelid
H00.019	Hordeolum externum unspecified eye, unspecified eyelid
H00.021	Hordeolum internum right upper eyelid
H00.022	Hordeolum internum right lower eyelid
H00.023	Hordeolum internum right eye, unspecified eyelid
H00.024	Hordeolum internum left upper eyelid
H00.025	Hordeolum internum left lower eyelid
H00.026	Hordeolum internum left eye, unspecified eyelid
H00.029	Hordeolum internum unspecified eye, unspecified eyelid

EPIDEMIOLOGY & DEMOGRAPHICS

INCIDENCE (IN U.S.): Unknown.
PREVALENCE (IN U.S.): Unknown.
PREDOMINANT SEX: No gender predilection.
PREDOMINANT AGE: May occur at any age.
NEONATAL INFECTION: Rare in the neonatal period.
PEAK INCIDENCE: May occur at any age.

PHYSICAL FINDINGS & CLINICAL PRESENTATION

- Abrupt onset with pain and erythema of the eyelid.
- Localized, tender mass in the eyelid (Fig. 1).
- May be associated with blepharitis.
- External hordeolum: points toward the skin surface of the lid and may spontaneously drain.
- Internal hordeolum: can point toward the conjunctival side of the lid and may cause conjunctival inflammation.

ETIOLOGY

- 75% to 95% of cases are caused by *S. aureus*, which includes MRSA strains.
- Occasional cases are caused by *Streptococcus pneumoniae*, other streptococci, gram-negative enteric organisms, or mixed bacterial flora.

DIAGNOSIS

DIFFERENTIAL DIAGNOSIS

- Eyelid abscess.
- Chalazion.
- Allergy or contact dermatitis with conjunctival edema.
- Acute dacryocystitis.
- Herpes simplex infection.
- Cellulitis of the eyelid.

LABORATORY TESTS

- Generally, none are necessary.
- If incision and drainage are performed, specimens should be sent for bacterial culture.

TREATMENT

NONPHARMACOLOGIC THERAPY

External stye (eyelash follicle): Usually responds to warm compresses and will drain spontaneously.

ACUTE GENERAL Rx

- Systemic antibiotics generally not necessary.
- For internal stye, use hot packs *plus* oral dicloxacillin 500 mg qid × 7 days. If suspecting MRSA, use trimethoprim-sulfamethoxazole DS bid in place of dicloxacillin. In patients with hospital-acquired infection, consider linezolid 600 mg PO bid.
- For external stye, topical erythromycin ophthalmic ointment applied to the lid margins two to four times daily until resolution may be helpful in some cases.
- Incision and drainage: rarely needed but should be considered for progressive infections.

DISPOSITION

- Usually sporadic occurrence.
- Possible relapse if resolution is not complete.

REFERRAL

- For evaluation by an ophthalmologist if visual acuity or ocular movement is affected or if the diagnosis is in doubt.
- For surgical drainage if necessary.

PEARLS & CONSIDERATIONS

COMMENTS

Seborrheic dermatitis may coexist with hordeolum.

SUGGESTED READINGS

Available at www.expertconsult.com

RELATED CONTENT

Chalazion (Patient Information)
Stye (Hordeolum) (Patient Information)

AUTHOR: **GLENN G. FORT, M.D., M.P.H.**

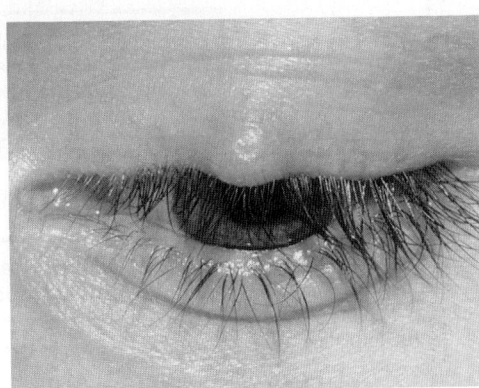

FIG. 1 External stye. (From Palay D [ed]: *Ophthalmology for the primary care physician*, St Louis, 1997, Mosby.)

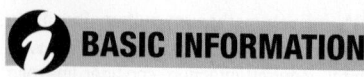

BASIC INFORMATION

DEFINITION

Subarachnoid hemorrhage (SAH) is defined as hemorrhage into the subarachnoid space surrounding the brain. This can be either nontraumatic or traumatic in nature. Here we will focus upon nontraumatic subarachnoid hemorrhage. Box 1 describes the Hunt and Hess clinical classification of patients presenting with aneurysmal SAH.

SYNONYMS

Subarachnoid bleed
SAH

ICD-10CM CODES
I60	Subarachnoid hemorrhage
I60.1	Subarachnoid hemorrhage from middle cerebral artery
I60.2	Subarachnoid hemorrhage from anterior communicating artery
I60.3	Subarachnoid hemorrhage from posterior communicating artery
I60.4	Subarachnoid hemorrhage from basilar artery
I60.5	Subarachnoid hemorrhage from vertebral artery
I60.7	Subarachnoid hemorrhage from intracranial artery, unspecified

EPIDEMIOLOGY & DEMOGRAPHICS

INCIDENCE: Nontraumatic: 6 to 8 cases/100,000 persons per yr
PREDOMINANT SEX: Women aged >55 yr were found to have a 25% greater risk of developing SAH compared with men of the same age.
PREDOMINANT AGE: The mean age at onset is 55 yr.
PEAK INCIDENCE: Most aneurysmal SAH occurs in people who are between the ages of 55 and 60 yr.
GENETICS:
- First-degree relatives have a 5 to 12 times greater risk of developing SAH compared with the general population.
- Autosomal dominant polycystic kidney disease is known to be associated with cerebral aneurysms in 8% of cases; screening is recommended in families with this condition in which one family member has experienced a ruptured aneurysm.
- Collagen vascular diseases such as Marfan syndrome, Ehler Danlos syndrome have also been implicated in the formation of aneurysms.

RISK FACTORS: Although genetics seem to play a factor in SAH, lifestyle factors are more important for determining overall risk. These risk factors include smoking, hypertension, oral contraception, pregnancy, and amphetamine/cocaine use.

PHYSICAL FINDINGS & CLINICAL PRESENTATION

- The primary symptom is a sudden, severe headache in 97% of cases. This is classically described as the "worst headache of my life" and also called a thunderclap headache. This headache may be associated with nausea/vomiting, neck pain, seizure, or complete loss of consciousness.
- 30% to 60% of patients report a history of headaches during the weeks preceding the actual hemorrhage event. These are most likely sentinel bleeds that represent microhemorrhages.
- Altered mental status and coma may result from the direct effect (hemorrhagic mass effect), but more likely is the result of acutely increased intracranial pressure.
- A posterior communication aneurysm may present as oculomotor (cranial nerve III) palsy, even in a nonruptured setting.
- Table E1 describes the World Federation of Neurologic Surgeons clinical classification of SAH.

ETIOLOGY

- Trauma is the most common cause of SAH; a ruptured aneurysm is the most common cause of spontaneous SAH (75%-80% of spontaneous SAH).
- Idiopathic SAH, also known as angiogram-negative SAH, accounts for 5% to 20% of spontaneous SAH. In these cases, no angiographic cause of the hemorrhage is found. This entity is also known as benign perimesencephalic SAH and is thought to occur due to rupture of venous plexus in the cisterns surrounding the brain stem.
- Other causes of spontaneous SAH include arteriovenous malformations, bleeding into preexisting tumors, vasculitis, and cerebral artery dissection.
- Cocaine abuse, sickle cell anemia, coagulopathies, and pituitary apoplexy can also result in SAH.

DIAGNOSIS

DIFFERENTIAL DIAGNOSIS

- Intracerebral hemorrhage as a result of trauma, intratumoral bleed, ischemic stroke with hemorrhagic conversion, venous hemorrhage associated with venous sinus thrombosis, mycotic aneurysm rupture.
- Other causes: thunderclap headaches such as idiopathic thunderclap headache, migraine headache, sexual headache, cough headache, exertional headache, secondary causes including, but not limited to, pituitary apoplexy or acute hydrocephalus.

WORKUP

IMAGING STUDIES:

- Computed tomography (CT) of the head (Fig. 1) shows hemorrhage in more than 95% of cases, especially during the acute phase (i.e., 24-48 hr) after the onset of bleeding. Box 2 describes the Fisher grade of SAH on initial CT (Fisher III being associated with highest risk of vasospasm). About 3% to 5% of SAH may be missed on initial CT of the head. MRI head, specifically FLAIR sequence, is helpful in detecting subarachnoid blood if clinically suspected.
- Lumbar puncture should be performed in all cases of suspected SAH with "normal CT of the head" between 6 and 12 hours after the onset of the headache for highest yield. The following suggest SAH:
  1. An RBC count of more than 100,000/m³ in tubes 1 AND 4. This is to differentiate from a traumatic tap in which there will be a drop in RBC count from tube 1 to 4.
  2. Presence of xanthochromia or bilirubin in the cerebrospinal fluid.
  3. SAH can also be excluded by the following two criteria: CSF RBC count < 2000 × 10^6/L and no xanthochromia.

BOX 1   Hunt and Hess Clinical Classification of Subarachnoid Hemorrhage

I	Asymptomatic or mild headache and neck stiffness
II	Moderate to severe headache and neck stiffness ± cranial nerve palsy
III	Mild focal deficit, lethargy, or confusion
IV	Stupor, moderate to severe hemiparesis
V	Deep coma, extensor posturing

From Vincent JL et al: *Textbook of critical care*, ed 6, Philadelphia, 2011, Saunders.

BOX 2   Fisher Grade of Subarachnoid Hemorrhage on Initial Computed Tomography

1	No blood detected
2	Diffuse or vertical layers <1 mm thick
3	Localized subarachnoid clot and/or vertical layers ≥1 mm thick
4	Intraparenchymal or intraventricular clot with diffuse or no SAH

Modified Fisher CT Rating Scale

1	Minimal or diffuse thin SAH without IVH
2	Minimal or thin SAH with IVH
3	Thick cisternal clot without IVH
4	Thick cisternal clot with IVH

CT, Computed tomography; IVH, intraventricular hemorrhage; SAH, subarachnoid hemorrhage.
From Vincent JL et al: *Textbook of critical care*, ed 6, Philadelphia, 2011, Saunders.

- CT angiogram
- Digital subtraction angiography with 3D processing when indicated is the gold standard for diagnosis of etiology in subarachnoid hemorrhage.

LABORATORY TESTS

- Basic laboratory values, including CBC, chemistry panel, prothrombin time, partial thromboplastin time, and platelet count
- Serum troponin to evaluate for severe cardiac stress; elevated troponins indicate cardiac ischemia secondary to catecholamine surge and is associated with poor outcome.
- Patients with SAH are prone to developing cerebral salt wasting, resulting in hyponatremia. Sodium levels should be monitored frequently.

Rx TREATMENT

NONPHARMACOLOGIC THERAPY

- Airway, breathing, and circulation
- Once stabilized, good neurologic exam
- Cerebrospinal fluid drainage may be required for patients who develop hydrocephalus and increased intracranial pressure. It is also recommended for patients with Hunt and Hess grade 3 or higher.

ACUTE GENERAL Rx

- Critical care management: initial management strategies are geared toward stabilizing the patient and preventing re-hemorrhage and hydrocephalus. Re-hemorrhage is associated with very high mortality rates.
- Blood pressure control: Tight blood pressure control is paramount before securing the aneurysm to protect against re-rupture. Blood pressure control can be achieved with the use of antihypertensive infusions such as intravenous nicardipine. A systolic blood pressure of less than 140 mm Hg is recommended. Placement of arterial line is recommended. After securing of the aneurysm, liberalization of blood pressure parameters is the standard.

- Pain control: using short-acting and less-sedating medications (e.g., codeine, low-dose morphine).
- Seizures occur in about 3% of patients during the acute phase; use of prophylactic antiepileptics is controversial and not recommended, but patients presenting with seizures should be treated appropriately with anticonvulsants.
- Vasospasm: cerebral vasospasm is a morbid complication leading to cerebral ischemia, disability, and death after SAH. It typically develops between day 4 and 14 (but may occur up to day 21) after the hemorrhage, and it reaches a peak on day 6 to 8. Treatment strategies include:
  1. Current medical therapy for vasospasm focuses upon hypertension, with typical mean arterial pressure goals of 90 to 100 (after aneurysm is secured) and with euvolemia instead of hypervolemia, as the latter was found to lead to significant cardiopulmonary and hemodynamic complications. "Triple H" therapy—*H*ypertension, *H*ypervolemia, and *H*emodilution—was originally employed to maintain cerebral perfusion, but it has fallen out of favor due to its many complications. Rather, nimodipine (60 mg q4h or 30 mg q2h if blood pressure is low) has been shown to improve outcomes if it is administered between days 4 and 21 after the hemorrhage, even if it does not significantly reduce the amount of vasospasm detected on angiography.
  2. Statins are no longer recommended for vasospasm prevention.
  3. Intraarterial therapies such as intraarterial calcium channel blockers and balloon angioplasty may be employed as needed.
- In cases of aneurysmal SAH, treatment focuses on occlusion/exclusion of the aneurysm to prevent rebleeding. The most common treatment methods are:
  1. Microsurgical clipping: performed through a craniotomy by placing a clip around the neck of the aneurysm.
  2. Endovascular coiling: performed via digital subtraction angiography; it consists of deploying platinum coils inside the aneurysm or stents in the parent artery to cause

thrombosis of the aneurysmal sac. Most aneurysms are currently treated endovascularly. New stentlike devices called flow diverters (Pipeline) are now also being used.

CHRONIC Rx

- Management of reversible risk factors mentioned above (smoking, hypertension, drug use).
- Management of neurologic disability through physical therapy and rehabilitation.

DISPOSITION

- SAH is often associated with a poor outcome with a death rate between 30% and 40%; 10% to 15% of patients die before they reach the hospital.
- Almost half of those who survive hospitalization have cognitive impairments or disability that affect their lifestyles.

REFERRAL

Patients should be managed in a cerebrovascular center that maintains capacity to perform open surgical and endovascular procedures, with a critical care unit experienced in caring for neurosurgical patients.

(!) PEARLS & CONSIDERATIONS

COMMENTS

- "Thunderclap" headaches should be considered SAH till proven otherwise and evaluated by CT of the head with/without LP. MRI FLAIR sequence is also a helpful modality.
- All SAH should be managed in a critical care setting (preferably neurocritical care unit) with neurosurgical care available.
- Measures to prevent rebleeding include adequate control of blood pressure and aneurysm treatment with the use of coiling or clipping.

PREVENTION

Controlling some of the modifiable risk factors, including smoking and blood pressure, may help to decrease the risk of aneurysmal rupture.

PATIENT & FAMILY EDUCATION

- SAH is a devastating condition, with most survivors developing significant neurologic or cognitive deficits. A good support system and an adequate physical and cognitive rehabilitation program may prove useful to survivors.
- Screening may be useful for patients with two or three first-degree relatives with SAH.

(EBM) EVIDENCE

Available at www.expertconsult.com

SUGGESTED READING

Available at www.expertconsult.com

RELATED CONTENT

Subarachnoid Hemorrhage (Patient Information)

AUTHORS: **FARHAN A. MIRZA, M.B.B.S.,** and **JUSTIN F. FRASER, M.D.**

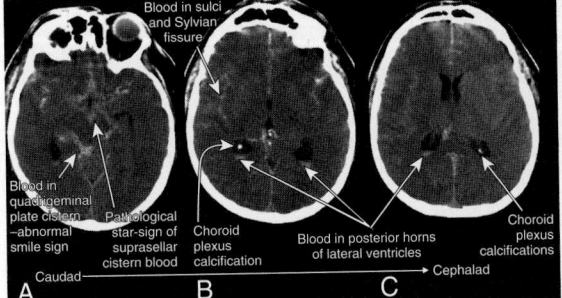

FIG. 1 Subarachnoid hemorrhage (SAH), noncontrast CT, brain windows. Acute SAH appears white on noncontrast computed tomography (CT) brain windows. **A** through **C,** nonconsecutive axial slices, progressing from caudad to cephalad. In this case of diffuse SAH, note the presence of subarachnoid blood filling the sulci, as well as extending into the cisterns, Sylvian fissures, and even lateral ventricles. In **A,** blood *(white)* fills the suprasellar cistern. This star-shaped structure is normally filled with CSF *(black).* The quadrigeminal plate cistern is normally a smile-shaped black crescent, filled with CSF, but in this case is filled with blood. Extremely bright calcifications in the choroid plexus of the posterior horns of the lateral ventricles are common, normal findings—do not mistake these for hemorrhage. Note their similarity in density to bone of the calvarium. (From Broder JS: *Diagnostic imaging for the emergency physician,* Philadelphia, 2011, Saunders.)

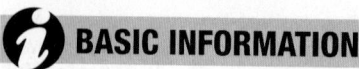

BASIC INFORMATION

DEFINITION

Subclavian steal syndrome is an occlusion or severe stenosis of the proximal subclavian artery leading to decreased antegrade flow or retrograde flow in the ipsilateral vertebral artery and neurologic symptoms referable to the posterior circulation.

SYNONYMS

Proximal subclavian (or innominate) artery stenosis or occlusion

ICD-10CM CODES
G45.8 Other transient cerebral ischemic attacks and related syndromes

EPIDEMIOLOGY & DEMOGRAPHICS

- Similar to that of other manifestations of atherosclerosis (coronary artery disease, cerebrovascular disease, or peripheral vascular disease)
- Affects middle-aged persons (men somewhat younger than women on average) with arteriosclerotic risk factors, including family history, smoking, diabetes mellitus, hyperlipidemia, hypertension, and sedentary lifestyle

PHYSICAL FINDINGS & CLINICAL PRESENTATION

Symptoms:
- Many patients are asymptomatic.
- Upper-extremity ischemic symptoms: fatigue, exercise-related aching, coolness, numbness of the involved upper extremity.

- Neurologic symptoms are reported by 25% of patients with known unilateral subclavian steal. These include brief spells of:
  1. Vertigo
  2. Diplopia
  3. Decreased vision
  4. Oscillopsia
  5. Gait unsteadiness
  These spells are only occasionally provoked by exercising the ischemic upper extremity (classic subclavian steal). Left subclavian steal is more common than right, but the latter is more serious.
- Posterior circulation stroke related to subclavian steal is rare.
- Innominate artery stenosis can cause decreased right carotid artery flow and cerebrovascular symptoms of the anterior cerebral circulation, but this is uncommon.
Physical findings:
- Delayed and smaller volume pulse (wrist or antecubital) in the affected upper extremity
- Lower blood pressure in the affected upper extremity
- Supraclavicular bruit
  NOTE: Inflating a blood pressure cuff will increase the bruit if it originates from a vertebral artery stenosis and decrease the bruit if it originates from a subclavian artery stenosis.

ETIOLOGY & PATHOGENESIS

Etiology:
- Atherosclerosis
- Arteritis (Takayasu's disease and temporal arteritis)
- Embolism to the subclavian or innominate artery
- Cervical rib
- Long-term use of a crutch

- Occupational (baseball pitchers and cricket bowlers)
  Pathogenesis: the vertebral artery originates from the subclavian artery. For subclavian steal to occur, the occlusion must be proximal to the takeoff of the vertebral artery. On the right side, only a small distance separates the bifurcation of the innominate artery and the takeoff of the vertebral artery, explaining why the condition occurs less commonly on the right side. Occlusion of the innominate artery must affect right carotid artery flow.

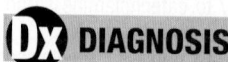

The carotid arteries should be evaluated at least noninvasively in all cases.

DIFFERENTIAL DIAGNOSIS

- Posterior circulation transient ischemic attack or stroke
- Upper-extremity ischemia
  1. Distal subclavian artery stenosis or occlusion
  2. Raynaud's syndrome
  3. Thoracic outlet syndrome

WORKUP

- Noninvasive upper-extremity arterial flow studies
- Doppler sonography of the vertebral, subclavian, and innominate arteries
- Arteriography, magnetic resonance arteriogram (Fig. 1)

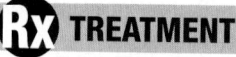

- In most patients the disease is benign and requires no treatment other than atherosclerosis risk factor modification and aspirin. Symptoms tend to improve over time as collateral circulation develops.
- Vascular surgical reconstruction requires a thoracotomy; it may be indicated in innominate artery stenosis or when upper-extremity ischemia is incapacitating.

AUTHOR: **FRED F. FERRI, M.D.**

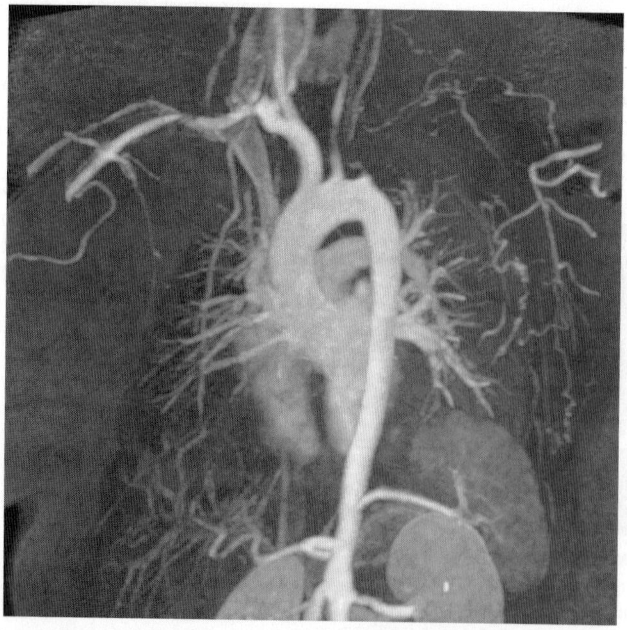

FIG. 1 Magnetic resonance arteriogram demonstrating diffuse moderate stenosis of the proximal left common carotid and proximal occlusion of the left subclavian artery coming off the aortic arch with development of an extensive collateral network. (From Hochberg MC et al: *Rheumatology*, ed 5, St Louis, 2011, Mosby.)

ℹ️ BASIC INFORMATION

DEFINITION

A subdural hematoma (SDH) is a collection of blood or blood products between the arachnoidal layer and the dura or meningeal layer surrounding the brain. Subdural hematomas can be acute (ASDH) or chronic (CSDH) and vary significantly in presentation and treatment.

SYNONYMS

Subdural hemorrhage

ICD-10CM CODES
S06.5   Traumatic subdural hemorrhage
I62.03 Chronic subdural hematoma
I62.01 Acute subdural hematoma

EPIDEMIOLOGY & DEMOGRAPHICS

INCIDENCE:
- The exact incidence of ASDH is unknown, but it is commonly seen in patients with head injury.
- CSDH is most common in the elderly with an estimated incidence of 1.72 to 13.1 per 100,000.

PREVALENCE: Unknown

PREDOMINANT AGE AND SEX:
- Peak incidence of CSDH is in the eighth decade and is notably higher in males.
- ASDHs usually present in the trauma setting and can happen in all age groups. In particular, shaken baby syndrome can be associated with SDH in the infant population.

RISK FACTORS:
- Trauma and antithrombotic therapy are the most common risk factors for ASDH and CSDH.
- Brain atrophy secondary to advanced age and alcoholism are common risk factors, especially with the coagulopathy/thrombocytopenia seen in chronic alcoholics.
- Intracranial hypotension associated with CSF shunts or leaks is uncommon but can result in acute or chronic SDH.

PHYSICAL FINDINGS & CLINICAL PRESENTATION

Symptoms vary on the basis of acuity, size, and location. Acute traumatic SDHs are often seen in traumatic brain injury patients, and their Glasgow Coma Scale may vary according to the extent of brain injury, size of hematoma, and associated compression. When associated with a midline shift (i.e., >5 mm), they can cause signs of cerebral herniation (e.g., ipsilateral pupil dilation, contralateral weakness) requiring prompt surgical evacuation.
- Patients with CSDH may present with diverse nonspecific symptoms such as headaches, confusion, aphasia, hemiparesis, TIA-like symptoms, and seizures.

ETIOLOGY

SDH is usually the result of shearing and tearing of a bridging vein between the brain parenchyma and the dura mater. Other causes of bleeding into the subdural space include contusion, extension of parenchymal hemorrhage. In the setting of spontaneous SDH, other vascular abnormalities, such as AV malformation, aneurysm, and dural AV fistula, should be kept in mind.

Dx DIAGNOSIS

DIFFERENTIAL DIAGNOSIS

CSF hygromas, abscesses, and tumor infiltrations

WORKUP
- Clinical assessment: patient history, including medications, specifically anticoagulants/antiplatelets; alcohol abuse; recent trauma; cancer; and recent bacterial infections
- Neurologic examination: Glasgow Coma Scale, cranial nerves, motor/sensory exam CT head

LABORATORY TESTS

Assessment of the patient's coagulation status including CBC with platelet count, prothrombin time, partial thromboplastin time and liver function test (especially with a history of alcoholism or liver failure)

IMAGING STUDIES

CT head (Fig. 1): demonstrates the classic crescentic collection between the brain and inner table. For comatose and trauma patients, include a cervical spine CT scan. ASDH is usually hyperdense, whereas a CSDH is usually hypodense on noncontrast CT. Contrast is only needed if there are concerns about tumor or infection.

Rx TREATMENT

- Correction of underlying coagulopathy, if present (e.g., Coumadin/ASA/clopidogrel reversal)
- Admission for overnight monitoring in the setting of acute SDH
- The majority of SDH can be managed without surgery in awake patients with normal neurologic examinations.

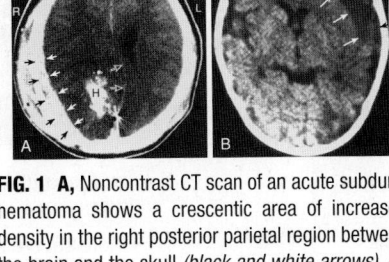

FIG. 1 A, Noncontrast CT scan of an acute subdural hematoma shows a crescentic area of increased density in the right posterior parietal region between the brain and the skull *(black and white arrows)*. An area of intraparenchymal hemorrhage *(H)* is also seen. **B,** A chronic subdural hematoma for a different patient is shown. There is an area of decreased density in the left frontoparietal region *(arrows)* that effaces the sulci, compresses the anterior horn of the left lateral ventricle, and shifts the midline somewhat to the right. (From Mettler FA [ed]: *Primary care radiology*, Philadelphia, 2000, Saunders.)

- Medical management of CSDH using antifibrinolytic therapy with tranexamic acid 650 mg per day is showing promising results. Studies will continue to evaluate its efficacy as a medical therapy for SDH.
- Seizure prophylaxis with phenytoin or levetiracetam for seven days should be considered in almost all cases, as there is underlying injury to the brain tissue associated with acute subdural hematoma. The irritative effects of blood products on the brain can also contribute to seizures, in both acute and chronic subdural hematomas. If seizures do occur, video EEG monitoring should be instituted and aggressive treatment undertaken.

NONPHARMACOLOGIC THERAPY

Surgical treatment is indicated in:
- ASDHs measuring >10 mm in thickness with a midline shift >5 mm on CT scan and a compromised neurologic status should be evacuated.
- In CSDH with a mass effect, a clear change in the neurologic examination from baseline, and/or enlargement of the hematoma size, evacuation via craniotomy or burr hole should be considered.

DISPOSITION

Depending on the size and location of the SDH and the examination of the patient, observation can range from the ICU to outpatient management. When observation of the patient is considered, clinical examinations should be serially performed. Patient baseline and follow-up clinical examinations are more important than CT scan findings.

REFERRAL

Neurosurgical and operative consultation should be made available.

❗ PEARLS & CONSIDERATIONS

COMMENTS
- Many elderly patients have small CSDHs or hygromas. Unless these are associated with seizures or clinical or radiographic progression, they are usually not emergent and usually do not require neurosurgical intervention. Recurrence after surgical management for CSDH is common.
- SDHs in elderly patients can have a mixed hyperdense and hypodense appearance on noncontrast CT scan; this finding is suggestive of subdural membranes and chronic components.

PATIENT & FAMILY EDUCATION

Individuals with SDHs are at higher risk seizure, so surveillance is important.

RELATED CONTENT

Subdural Hematoma (Patient Inform
AUTHORS: **FARHAN A. MIRZA, M.B.P**
JUSTIN F. FRASER, M.D.

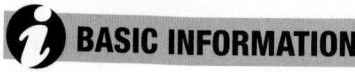
DEFINITION

Superior vena cava (SVC) syndrome is a set of symptoms that results when a mediastinal mass compresses the SVC or the veins that drain into it, resulting in obstruction of blood flow from the head, neck, upper torso, or extremities to the right atrium.

SYNONYM

SVC

ICD-10CM CODES	
I87.1	Compression of vein
S25.20XA	Unspecified injury of superior vena cava, initial encounter
S25.29XA	Other specified injury of superior vena cava, initial encounter

EPIDEMIOLOGY & DEMOGRAPHICS

- SVC syndrome occurs in 15,000 persons in the United States every year.
- More than 50% of patients present with SVC on presentation of malignancy.
- Mirrors lung cancer (especially small cell carcinoma) and lymphoma (see "Lung Neoplasm" and "Lymphoma" in Section I).

PHYSICAL FINDINGS & CLINICAL PRESENTATION

The pathophysiology of the syndrome involves increased pressure in the venous system draining into the SVC producing edema of the head, neck, and upper extremities. Symptoms develop over a period of 2 weeks in one third of patients and include:

- Shortness of breath
- Chest pain
- Cough

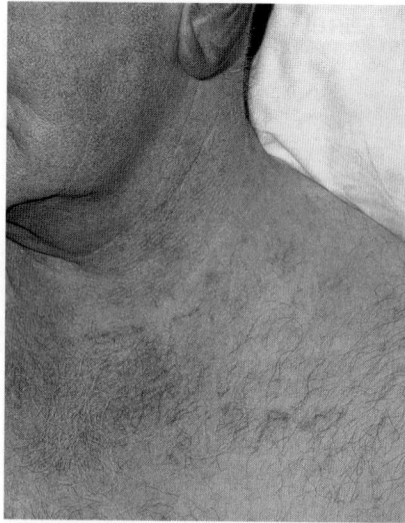

FIG. 1 Superior vena cava obstruction causing dilated veins and plethora of the upper trunk and neck in a patient with bronchial carcinoma. Patients with superior vena cava obstruction are occasionally referred to dermatologists with suspected contact allergy (eyelid swelling) or angioedema (facial or hand swelling). (From White GM, Cox NH [eds]: *Diseases of the skin, a color atlas and text*, ed 2, St Louis, 2006, Mosby.)

- Dysphagia, hoarseness, stridor
- Headache
- Syncope
- Visual trouble
  Signs:
- Chest wall vein distention (Fig. 1)
- Neck vein distention
- Facial edema, facial plethora
- Upper-extremity swelling
- Cyanosis

ETIOLOGY

- Lung cancer (65% of all cases, of which half are small cell lung cancer)
- Lymphoma (15%)
- Thymoma
- Tuberculosis
- Goiter
- Aortic aneurysm (arteriosclerotic or syphilitic)
- SVC thrombosis
  1. Primary: associated with a central venous catheter
  2. Secondary: complication of SVC syndrome associated with one of the above-mentioned causes
- Inflammatory process, fibrosing mediastinitis
- Fig. 2 illustrates the anatomy of superior vena cava syndrome. Table 1 summarizes common malignancies associated with SVC syndrome in adults.

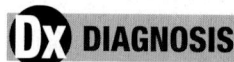 **DIAGNOSIS**

CT scan of the chest with contrast (Fig. 3) is the most useful diagnostic study. MRI is usually adequate to establish the diagnosis of

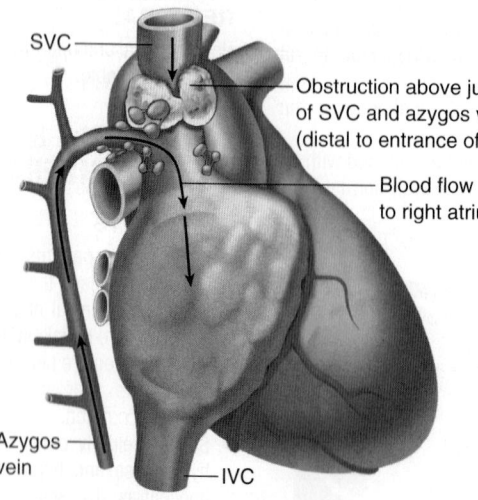

SVC — Obstruction above junction of SVC and azygos vein (distal to entrance of SVC)

Blood flow to right atrium

Azygos vein — IVC

Obstruction in SVC (proximal to entrance of SVC)

Manifestations of supra-azygos SVC obstruction

- Distended arm and neck veins
- Edema of neck, face, and arms
- Congested mucous membranes (mouth)
- Dilated, tortuous vessels on upper chest and back

Manifestations of infra-azygos SVC obstruction

- More severe symptoms but all of the features for obstruction distal to entrance of SVC
- Dilation of collateral vessels on anterior and posterior abdominal wall with downward blood flow into IVC, then back to heart

A   B

FIG. 2 A... the face, ne... **Superior vena cava (SVC) syndrome.** Lymph nodes may obstruct blood return above the entrance of the azygos vein **(A)**, resulting in edema of flow through th... and distended veins in the neck and arms and over the upper chest. Obstruction below the return of the azygos vein **(B)** results in retrograde (Modified from Sk... through collateral veins to the inferior vena cava (IVC), with all the symptoms and signs in **A** plus dilation of the veins over the abdomen as well. ...d): *Atlas of diagnostic oncology*, ed 3, Philadelphia, 2003, Elsevier.)

TABLE 1 Malignancies Associated with Superior Vena Cava (SVC) Syndrome in Adults*

Neoplastic Diagnosis	Percentage of SVC	Percentage of Disease-Associated SVC
Lung cancer, stage 3B or 4:	48-81	
Small cell lung cancer		15-45
Squamous cell cancer		20-25
Adenocarcinoma		5-25
Large cell carcinoma		4-30
Lymphoma:	2-21	
Diffuse large cell lymphoma		64
Lymphoblastic lymphoma		33
Breast cancer	11	

*Includes lung cancer, lymphomas, and metastases from other solid tumors. 75% to 85% of patients with SVC have neoplastic disease.
From Zipes DP et al (eds): *Braunwald's heart disease,* ed 7, Philadelphia, 2005, Saunders.

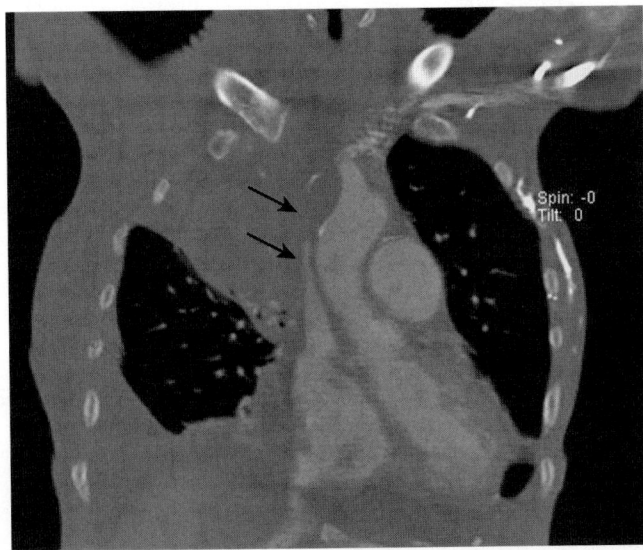

FIG. 3 Computed tomography scan showing blockage of the superior vena cava *(arrows).* (From Adams JG et al: *Emergency medicine, clinical essentials,* ed 2, Philadelphia, 2013, Elsevier.)

SVC obstruction and to assist in the differential diagnosis of probable cause.

DIFFERENTIAL DIAGNOSIS

The syndrome is characteristic enough to exclude other diagnoses. The differential diagnosis concerns the underlying etiologies listed previously.

WORKUP

- Chest radiograph (mediastinal widening, pleural effusion)
- Chest CT with contrast or MRI (in patient who cannot tolerate contrast medium)
- Venography: warranted only when an intervention (e.g., stent or surgery) is planned

- Percutaneous needle biopsy, endobronchial ultrasound-guided needle biopsy, or mediastinoscopy are usually the initial diagnostic modalities used to establish a histologic diagnosis

Rx TREATMENT

- Tissue diagnosis is usually needed before commencing therapy. EBUS is now considered the first step in evaluation. Mediastinoscopy would be considered if EBUS is non-diagnostic or there is high clinical suspicion for lymphoma.
- Management is guided by the severity of the symptoms and the underlying etiology.
- Emergency empiric radiation is indicated in critical situations such as respiratory failure or central nervous system signs associated with increased intracranial pressure.
- Treatment of the underlying malignancy:
  1. Radiotherapy: the majority of tumors causing SVC syndrome are sensitive to radiotherapy
  2. Systemic chemotherapy
- Anticoagulant or fibrinolytic therapy in patients who do not respond to cancer treatment within a week or if an obstructing thrombus has been documented.
- Loop diuretics are often used, but their effect is limited.
- Upright positioning and fluid restriction until collateral channels develop and allow for clinical regression are useful modalities for SVC syndrome secondary to benign disease.
- Steroids (dexamethasone 4 mg q6h) may be useful in reducing the tumor burden in lymphoma and thymoma after definitive diagnosis is made.
- Percutaneous self-expandable stents that can be placed under local anesthesia with radiologic manipulation are useful in the treatment of SVC syndrome to bypass the obstruction, especially in cases associated with malignant tumors.
- Surgical bypass grafting is infrequently used to treat SVC syndrome.

REFERRAL

To a thoracic surgeon, pulmonary specialist, or oncologist

AUTHOR: **GAETANE MICHAUD, M.D.**

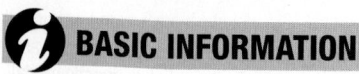

DEFINITION

Supraventricular tachycardia (SVT) is a group of rapid regular tachyarrhythmia. There are three major categories of SVT:

1. Atrial Tachycardia (AT): an arrhythmia that originates from the atrium and does not involve the AV node. This is usually a focal arrhythmia. In some, the underlying mechanism may be reentry, either with a small circuit (microreentry) or a large circuit (macroreentry).
2. AV nodal reentrant tachycardia (AVNRT).
3. AV reentrant tachycardia (AVRT) (Fig. 1). The latter two are reentrant arrhythmia that always involve the AV node as part of the circuit (Fig. 1).

Other forms of arrhythmia that involve the atria, such as atrial fibrillation and atrial flutter, have distinct electrocardiographic features and will not be discussed here. Rare forms of SVT such as inappropriate sinus tachycardia, sinus mode reentry tachycardia, and junctional tachycardia are beyond the scope of this chapter.

SYNONYMS

SVT
Paroxysmal supraventricular tachycardia
PSVT

ICD-10CM CODES
I47.1 Supraventricular tachycardia

EPIDEMIOLOGY & DEMOGRAPHICS

SVT is most commonly diagnosed between the ages of 12 and 30. SVT occurs most commonly in patients with no prior cardiac conditions. AVNRT is the most common type of SVT in both genders and at all ages. It occurs most commonly in young women. AVRT is the second most common SVT, and it is typically diagnosed in younger patients as compared to the age of patients with AVNRT. AT is more commonly associated with structural heart disease.

PHYSICAL FINDINGS & CLINICAL PRESENTATION

- Patients may be either symptomatic or asymptomatic.

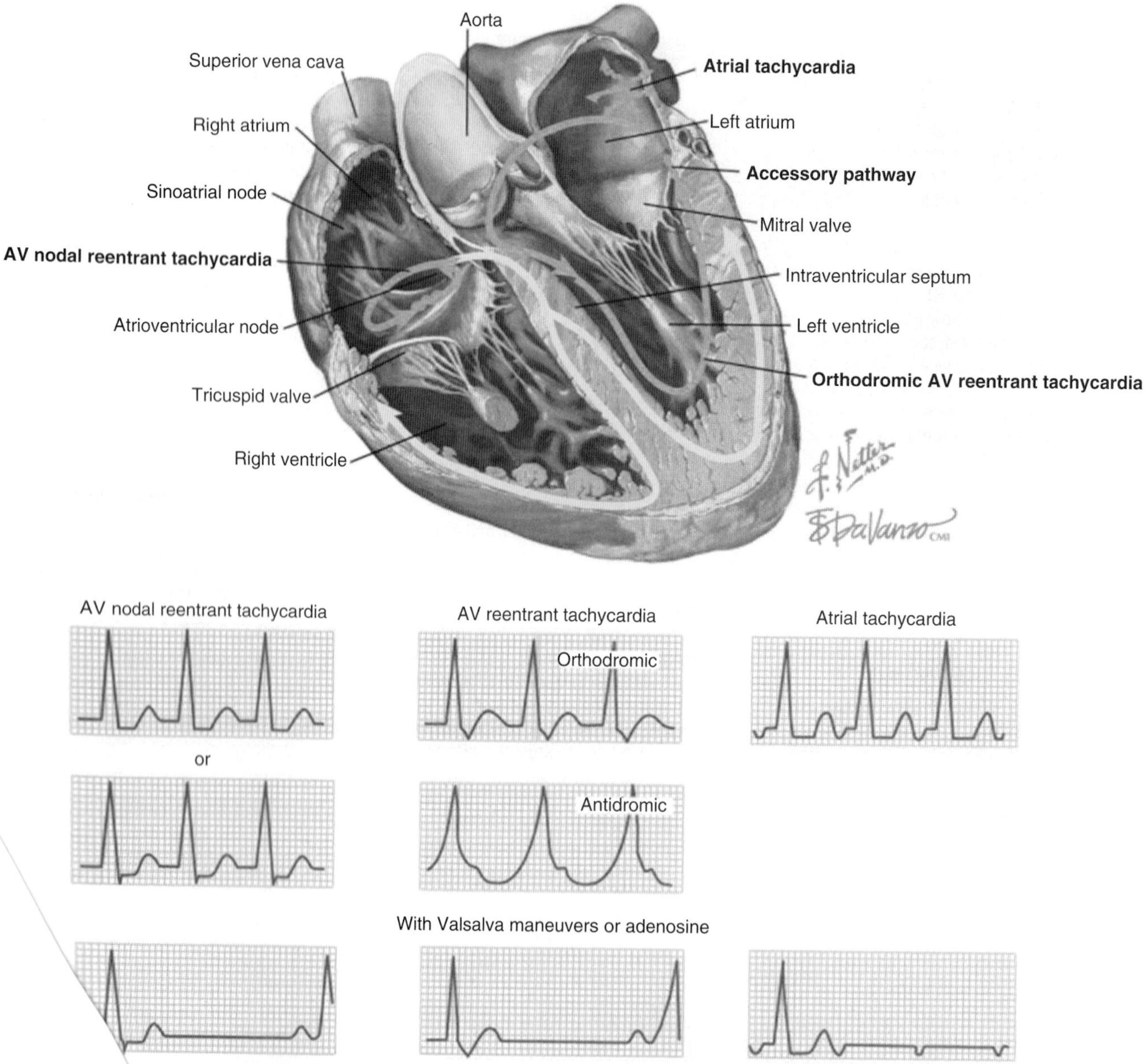

FIG. 1 Typical electrocardiographic recordings and anatomic representation of the common supraventricular tachycardias. *AV,* Atrioventricular. (From *Netter's cardiology*, ed 2, Philadelphia, 2010, Saunders. Adapted from Delacretaz E: Clinical practice: supraventricular tachycardia, *N Engl J Med* 354:1039–1051, 2006.)

- Patient may be aware of "fast" regular heartbeat (but sometimes complain of irregular heartbeat: palpitations); may complain of weakness, dyspnea, dizziness, chest pain, presyncope or, rarely, syncope.
- Patients with AVNRT may complain of neck pounding during the episode due to simultaneous contraction of the atrial and ventricles with closed AV valves and hence sharp increase in atrial and neck venous pressure.
- In some cases the episodes can be triggered by physical activity or psychological stress, but in others there may not be an obvious trigger. In patients with AVNRT, sometimes the arrhythmia is reproducibly initiated when bending forward to pick up an item from the floor.
- Hemodynamic status during the arrhythmia may vary and depend on the patient's comorbidities and presence of underlying structural heart disease. Usually, patients are hemodynamically stable.
- Physical examination is most commonly normal and unrevealing, except rapid regular heart rate and occasionally hypotension. In patients with AVNRT sharp tall jugular vein A waves may be seen when the right atrium contracts against a closed tricuspid valve.

ETIOLOGY (SEE FIG. 1)

- AVNRT: Dual electrical pathways within the AV node. In typical AVNRT the anterograde limb conducts slowly (slow pathway) and the retrograde limb has fast conduction properties (fast pathway), and vice versa in atypical AVNRT.
- AVRT is accessory pathway mediated, either orthodromic (antegrade through the AV node and retrograde through the accessory pathway) or, much less commonly, antidromic (antegrade through the accessory pathway and retrograde through the AV node). In the case of antidromic tachycardia, the QRS will be wide and fully preexcited. In some patients, the presence of accessory pathway is not evident on the baseline ECG (concealed accessory pathway), while in others it is manifest in the baseline ECG, presenting the typical features of the Wolff-Parkinson-White (WPW) syndrome.
- Atrial fibrillation and atrial flutter are covered in separate chapters.
- Paroxysmal atrial tachycardia and multifocal atrial tachycardia: abnormal automaticity of atrial tissue or triggered activity. In some cases (especially in patients who underwent previous cardiac surgery such as valve replacement or ASD closure), the underlying mechanism is macroreentrant AT.

Dx DIAGNOSIS AND DIFFERENTIAL DIAGNOSIS

The diagnosis of SVT relies principally on the 12-lead ECG. Every patient should have a 12-lead ECG done. Typically patients with SVT will present with a narrow complex QRS

tachycardia with a ventricular rate faster than 100 beats per minute (bpm) and typically faster than 130-150 bpm.

- P wave morphology can be useful in discriminating rhythms. P waves with a similar axis to the sinus node can be atrial tachycardias and sinus tachycardias. P waves with retrograde depolarization of the atria (seen as inverted in the inferior leads) can be seen in AVNRT, AVRT, and atrial tachycardia. Sawtooth P waves are indicative of classical counterclockwise typical type I flutter, and an absence of P waves with irregular R-R intervals points to atrial fibrillation. Variable (>3) morphologies of P wave are suggestive of multifocal atrial tachycardia. Wide QRS complex (>0.12 sec) with initial slurring (delta wave) during sinus rhythm and short PR (<0.12 sec) is characteristic of Wolff-Parkinson-White syndrome.

In typical AVNRT, due to the small size of the circuit within the AV node and the fast retrograde conduction, there is simultaneous depolarization of the ventricles and atria, thus making the P wave "buried" in the QRS and therefore not visible or inscribed very close to the QRS at the final part of the QRS complex, and sometimes creating a "pseudo terminal S wave" usually seen in leads II, III, and aVF and "pseudo terminal R waves" at the end of the QRS in V1 and avR (Fig. 1).

In orthodromic AVRT, the P wave is usually visible close after the QRS due to the rapid conduction properties of the accessory pathway (short RP tachycardia). In AT, the P wave is usually noticed farther away after the QRS (long RP tachycardia) (Fig. 1).

Other diagnostic maneuvers that may assist in the differential diagnosis are vagal maneuvers (such as carotid sinus massage or giving IV AV nodal blocking agents such as adenosine or verapamil) to produce AV nodal conduction block. This will terminate reentrant arrhythmia dependent on the AV node—AVNRT and AVRT—but not AT, which will continue, albeit with nonconducted P waves.

Other arrhythmias that present with narrow complex tachycardia like PSVT are:

1. Fascicular VT.

2. Junctional tachycardias.
3. Artifact such as with Parkinson's.

SVT can conduct with bundle branch block (BBB) and wide QRS due to preexisting BBB on the baseline ECG or due to aberrant conduction (rapid rate–dependent BBB). When a patient presents with wide QRS tachycardia, VT must be excluded first. Features to distinguish SVT from ventricular tachycardia are outlined in Table 1.

WORKUP

- Electrocardiography.
- Echocardiography to exclude structural heart disease.
- Thyroid function tests.
- Complete blood count to exclude anemia or infection as a causative trigger for the event.
- In most cases the workup will be negative, with no underlying cardiac or systemic pathology and no clear triggers for an acute episode.
- Holter or event monitor to document the arrhythmias if they are paroxysmal and not documented yet.

Rx TREATMENT

NONPHARMACOLOGIC THERAPY

If the patient is hemodynamically unstable, prompt synchronized cardioversion with an external defibrillator using 50 to 100 J should be performed.

If the patient is stable, Valsalva maneuver in the supine position is the most effective way to terminate most types of SVT; carotid sinus massage (after excluding occlusive carotid disease and murmurs over the carotid arteries) is also commonly used to elicit vagal efferent impulses. These are effective in terminating AVRT, AVNRT, and some types of atrial tachycardia, but in the case of sinus tachycardia, atrial flutter, and atrial fibrillation, they only transiently slow down AV conduction without terminating the actual tachycardia.

PHARMACOLOGIC THERAPY

- Adenosine is useful for treatment of orthodromic AVRT and AVNRT and can uncover

TABLE 1 Features That May Differentiate Ventricular Tachycardia from Supraventricular Tachycardia with Aberrancy

Helpful Features	Implications
Positive QRS concordance	Diagnostic of VT
Presence of AV dissociation, capture beats, or fusion beats	Diagnostic of VT
Atypical RBBB (monophasic R, QR, RS, or triphasic QRS in V_1; R:S ratio <1, QS or QR, monophasic R in V_6)	Suggests VT
Atypical LBBB (R >30 min or R to S [nadir or notch] >60 min in V_1 or V_2; R:S ratio <1, QS or QR in V_6)	Suggests VT
Shift of axis from baseline	Suggests VT
History of CAD	Suggests VT
QRS during tachycardia identical to QRS during sinus rhythm	Suggests SVT
Termination with adenosine	Suggests SVT

AV, Atrioventricular; *CAD,* coronary artery disease; *LBBB,* left bundle branch block; *RBBB,* right bundle branch block; *VT,* ventricular tachycardia.

From Andreoli TG et al (eds): *Andreoli and Carpenter's Cecil essentials of medicine,* ed 8, Philadelphia,

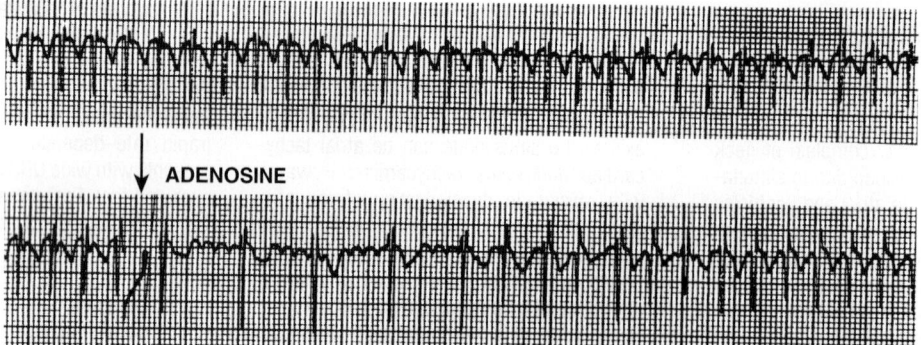

FIG. 2 Adenosine can uncover the mechanism of supraventricular tachycardia. A 3-month-old infant developed an extremely fast, narrow QRS complex tachycardia and a heart rate of 220 beats/min after insertion of a central line through a jugular vein. Adenosine produced a transient atrioventricular block and unmasked very rapid atrial fibrillation waves (570 beats/min). (From Park MK: *Park's Pediatric cardiology for practitioners*, ed 6, Philadelphia, Elsevier, 2014.)

the underlying rhythm in paroxysmal atrial tachycardia (Fig. 2); it is the first choice of therapy for treatment of almost all episodes of SVT unresponsive to vagal maneuvers. The dose is 6 mg given as a rapid IV bolus; tachycardia is usually terminated within a few seconds. If this fails, may repeat with 12 mg IV bolus. Contraindications are second- or third-degree atrioventricular block; WPW with atrial fibrillation; sick sinus syndrome; and chronic use of drugs such as dipyridamole, theophylline, or aminophylline; and heart transplant. Adenosine may cause broncho-spasm in asthmatics.
- Verapamil 5 to 10 mg IV is given over 5 min; if no effect, may repeat in 30 min.
  1. Verapamil should be used cautiously in patients with SVT associated with hypo-tension.
  2. Slow injection of calcium chloride (10 ml of a 10% solution given over 5 to 8 min before verapamil administration) decreases the hypotensive effect without compromising its antiarrhythmic effect.
- Metoprolol (IV 5 mg/2 min up to 15 mg) or esmolol (500 µg/kg IV bolus, then 50 µg/kg/min) may be effective in the treatment of SVT.
- IV digoxin (0.75 to 1 mg slow IV loading in increments of 0.25 mg over several hours) if other agents are not effective.
  1. Digoxin, beta-blockers, and calcium-channel blockers should be avoided in patients with pre-excitation syndrome and antidromic AVRT or atrial fibrillation to avoid increased conduction through the accessory pathway.

- A recent trial comparing "standard Valsalva" (patient placed in a semirecumbent [45-degree] position and directed to strain to 40 mm Hg pressure for 15 seconds by forced expiration and to stay in the semirecumbent position for 60 sec) to "modified Valsalva" (patients asked to strain in the same way in the semirecumbent position but immediately afterward asked to lay flat and raise their legs to 45 degrees for 15 sec) found that the modified Valsalva was more effective than the standard Valsalva maneuver for restoring sinus rhythm in patients with supraventricu-lar tachycardia.[1]

CHRONIC TREATMENT

The goal is prevention of recurrent episodes. In patients with infrequent and minimally symp-tomatic episodes without preexcitation, providing treatment is optional only during acute episodes. In patients with recurrent symptomatic episodes, regular treatment with beta-blockers, nondihy-dropyridines, or calcium channel blockers can be tried; if these fail, class Ic antiarrhythmics are an option. It is also possible to treat patients who have infrequent symptomatic episodes with a "pill-in-the-pocket" strategy with either beta-blockers or other antiarrhythmics. Patients who fail antiarrhythmic therapy, or develop side effects due to medications, or refuse medical therapy should be referred for catheter ablation.

---

[1]Appelbaum A, et al.: Revert trial collaborators: postur-al modification to the standard Valsalva maneuver for emergency treatment of supraventricular tachycar-dias (REVERT): a randomized controlled trial, *Lancet* 386:1747-1753, 2015.

This is a highly effective mode of treatment with low risk of complications.

DISPOSITION

Most patients respond well with resolution of the SVT upon treatment (see "Acute General Rx"). Some patients may need chronic AV block-ing agents for recurrence.

REFERRAL

Radiofrequency ablation (RFA) is the procedure of choice in symptomatic patients who are refractory to medical therapy especially in AVRT, AVNRT, and atrial flutter. RFA has high efficacy rates (single procedure success is 93.2%), low all-cause mortality (0.1%), and low adverse events (2.9%). Despite high reported success rates, RFA appears to be underused in clinical practice.

❶ PEARLS & CONSIDERATIONS

SUGGESTED READINGS
Available at www.expertconsult.com

RELATED CONTENT
Supraventricular Tachycardia (Patient Information)

AUTHORS: **MOTI HAIM, M.D., BARRY FINE, M.D., PH.D.,** and **YUVAL KONSTANTINO, M.D.**

BASIC INFORMATION

DEFINITION

Syncope is the transient loss of consciousness with spontaneous recovery that results from an acute global reduction in cerebral blood flow. There are 3 major types: neurally mediated, orthostatic, and cardiac. Syncope is a symptom, and the goal is to distinguish lethal causes from benign causes of transient loss of consciousness.

ICD-10CM CODES
R55 Syncope and collapse

EPIDEMIOLOGY & DEMOGRAPHICS

- Syncope accounts for 3% to 5% of emergency department visits.
- 30% of the adult population will experience at least one syncopal episode during their lifetimes.
- Incidence of syncope is highest in elderly men and young women.
- 15% of children and adolescents experience syncope; less than 5% have cardiac causes.

PHYSICAL FINDINGS & CLINICAL PRESENTATION

- Blood pressure: if low, consider orthostatic hypotension; if unequal in both arms (difference >20 mm Hg), consider subclavian steal or dissecting aneurysm. (NOTE: Blood pressure [BP] and heart rate should be recorded in the supine and standing positions, waiting at least 5 minutes between each position.) If there is a drop in BP but no change in heart rate (HR), the patient may be taking a beta-blocker or may have an autonomic neuropathy.
- Pulse: if patient has tachycardia, bradycardia, or irregular rhythm, consider arrhythmia.
- Heart: if there are murmurs present, consider syncope attributable to left ventricular outflow obstruction (aortic stenosis or idiopathic hypertrophic subaortic stenosis); if there are jugular venous distention and distal heart sounds, consider cardiac tamponade.
- Carotid sinus pressure: can be diagnostic if it reproduces symptoms and other causes are excluded; a pause >3 sec or a systolic BP drop >50 mm Hg without symptoms or <30 mm Hg with symptoms when sinus pressure is applied separately on each side for <5 sec is considered abnormal. This test should be avoided in patients with carotid bruits or cerebrovascular disease. ECG monitoring, IV access, and bedside atropine should be available when carotid sinus pressure is applied.

ETIOLOGY

- Neurally mediated syncope: most common type, accounting for two-thirds of cases. It includes vasovagal, situational, carotid hypersensitivity, and postexertional syncope.
  1. Psychophysiologic (emotional upset, panic disorders, hysteria, hyperventilation)
  2. Visceral reflex (micturition, defecation, food ingestion, coughing, ventricular contraction, glossopharyngeal neuralgia)
  3. Carotid sinus pressure
  4. Reduction of venous return caused by Valsalva maneuver
- Orthostatic hypotension (10% of cases)
  1. Hypovolemia
  2. Vasodilator medications
  3. Autonomic neuropathy (diabetes, amyloid, Parkinson's disease, multisystem atrophy)
  4. Pheochromocytoma
  5. Carcinoid syndrome
- Cardiac (10%-20%)
  1. Reduced cardiac output
     a. Left ventricular outflow obstruction (aortic stenosis, hypertrophic cardiomyopathy)
     b. Obstruction to pulmonary flow (pulmonary embolism, pulmonic stenosis, primary pulmonary hypertension)
     c. Myocardial infarct with pump failure
     d. Cardiac tamponade
     e. Mitral stenosis
     f. Reduction of venous return (atrial myxoma, valve thrombus)
     g. Beta-blocker therapy
  2. Arrhythmias or asystole
     a. Extreme tachycardia (>160-180 beats/min)
     b. Severe bradycardia (<30-40 beats/min)
     c. Sick sinus syndrome
     d. Atrioventricular block (second or third degree)
     e. Ventricular tachycardia or fibrillation
     f. Long QT syndrome
     g. Pacemaker malfunction
     h. Psychotropic medications and beta-blockers

DIAGNOSIS

DIFFERENTIAL DIAGNOSIS

1. Seizure (see "Workup")
2. Vertebrobasilar transient ischemic attack (TIA) usually manifests as diplopia, vertigo, or ataxia but not loss of consciousness. Isolated episodes of transient loss of consciousness (TLOC) without accompanying neurologic symptoms are unlikely to be TIAs.
3. Recreational drugs or alcohol.
4. Functional causes, such as stress and somatoform disorders.
5. Sleep disorders, such as sleep attacks and narcolepsy, are also in the differential for TLOC.
6. Head trauma.

WORKUP

The history is crucial to diagnosing the cause of syncope and may suggest a diagnosis that can be evaluated with directed testing. History is also important to determine other etiologies for TLOC, such as seizure. Fig. E1 describes an algorithm for syncope evaluation.
- Sudden LOC: consider cardiac arrhythmias.
- Gradual LOC: consider orthostatic hypotension, vasodepressor syncope, hypoglycemia.
- History of aura before LOC or prolonged confusion (>1 min), amnesia, or lethargy after LOC suggests seizure rather than syncope.

- Patient's activity at the time of syncope:
  1. Micturition, coughing, defecation: consider syncope caused by decreased venous return.
  2. Turning head or while shaving: consider carotid sinus syndrome.
  3. Physical exertion in a patient with murmur: consider aortic stenosis.
  4. Arm exercise: consider subclavian steal syndrome.
  5. Assuming an upright position: consider orthostatic hypotension.
- Associated events:
  1. Chest pain: consider myocardial infarction, pulmonary embolism.
  2. Palpitations: consider arrhythmias.
  3. Incontinence (urine or fecal) and tongue biting are associated with seizure or syncope.
  4. Brief, transient shaking after LOC may represent myoclonus from global cerebral hypoperfusion and not seizures. However, sustained tonic/clonic muscle action is more suggestive of seizure.
  5. Focal neurologic symptoms or signs point to a neurologic event such as a seizure with residual deficits (e.g., Todd's paralysis) or cerebral ischemic injury.
  6. Psychologic stress: syncope may be vasovagal.
- Review current medications, particularly antihypertensive and psychotropic drugs.
- All patients presenting with syncope require electrocardiography, orthostatic vital signs, and QT interval monitoring.

LABORATORY TESTS

Routine blood tests rarely yield diagnostically useful information and should be done only if they are specifically suggested by the results of the history and physical examination. Box E1 describes possibly useful tests. The following are commonly ordered tests:
- Pregnancy test in women of childbearing age
- Complete blood count to look for anemia and signs of infection
- Electrolytes, blood urea nitrogen, creatinine, magnesium, and calcium to look for electrolyte abnormalities and evaluate fluid status
- Serum glucose level
- Cardiac troponins, especially if the patient gives a history of chest pain before the syncopal episode
- Drug and alcohol levels with suspected toxicity

IMAGING STUDIES

- ECG to rule out arrhythmias; may be diagnostic in 5% to 10% of patients.
- Echocardiography.
- If seizure is suspected, CT scan and/or M the head and electroencephalogram useful.
- If head trauma or neurologic signs nation, CT or MRI may be helpful is
- If arrhythmias are suspected, ring is monitor or admission to a syncope appropriate. In general, H rarely useful, revealing

in <3% of cases. Loop recorders that can be activated after syncopal episode to retrieve information about the cardiac rhythm during the preceding 4 min add considerable diagnostic yield in patients with unexplained syncope.

- Implantable cardiac monitors that function as permanent loop recorders or implantable cardioverter-defibrillators, which are placed subcutaneously in the pectoral region with the patient under local anesthesia, are useful in patients with cardiac syncope.
- Electrophysiologic studies may be indicated in patients with structural heart disease and/or recurrent syncope.

TILT-TABLE TESTING

- Useful to support a diagnosis of neurally mediated syncope. Patients age >50 yr should have stress testing before tilt-table testing. Positive results would preclude tilt-table testing.
- Indicated in patients with recurrent episodes of unexplained syncope as well as patients in high-risk occupations (e.g., pilots, bus drivers) (Fig. 2). The test is also useful for identifying patients with prominent bradycardic response who may benefit from implantation of a permanent pacemaker. The test is contraindicated in patients with recent stroke, MI, and severe coronary or carotid disease.
- It is performed by keeping the patient strapped in an upright posture on a tilt table with footboard support. The angle of the tilt table varies from 60 to 80 degrees. The duration of upright posture during tilt-table testing varies from 25 to 45 min.
- The hallmark of neurally mediated syncope is severe hypotension associated with a paradoxic bradycardia triggered by a specific stimulus. The diagnosis of neurally mediated syncope is likely if upright tilt testing reproduces these hemodynamic changes in <15 min and causes presyncope or syncope.

PSYCHIATRIC EVALUATION

- May be indicated in young patients without heart disease who have frequently recurring transient loss of consciousness and other somatic symptoms.
- Generalized anxiety disorder, pain disorder, and major depression predispose patients to neurally mediated reactions and may result in syncope.

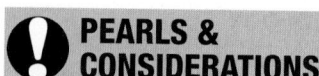 **TREATMENT**

NONPHARMACOLOGIC THERAPY

- Ensure proper hydration; consider compression stockings and salt tablets in appropriate patients.
- Eliminate medications that may induce hypotension.

ACUTE GENERAL Rx

- Varies with the underlying etiology of syncope (e.g., pacemaker in patients with syncope resulting from complete heart block).
- Syncope caused by orthostatic hypotension is treated with volume replacement in patients with intravascular volume depletion. Also consider midodrine to promote venous return by adrenergic-mediated vasoconstriction and Florinef for its mineralocorticoid effects to increase intravascular volume.

DISPOSITION

Prognosis varies with the age of the patient and the etiology of the syncope. In general:
- Benign prognosis (very low 1-yr morbidity rate) in patients:
  1. Age <30 yr and having noncardiac syncope
  2. Age <70 yr and having vasovagal or psychogenic syncope or syncope of unknown cause

- Poor prognosis (high mortality and morbidity rates) in patients with cardiac syncope, with presenting systolic BP <90 mm Hg.
- Patients with the following risk factors have a higher 1-yr mortality rate: abnormal ECG, history of ventricular arrhythmia, history of congestive heart failure.

REFERRAL

Hospital admission in elderly patients without prior history of syncope or unknown etiology of their syncope and in any patients suspected of having cardiac syncope, with presenting systolic BP <90 mm Hg.

⊘ PEARLS & CONSIDERATIONS

COMMENTS

- Section III, "Palpitations, Dizziness, and/or Syncope," describes an algorithmic approach to the patient.
- The etiology of syncope is identified in <50% of cases during the initial evaluation.
- A thorough history and physical examination are the most productive means of establishing a diagnosis in patients with syncope.

ⓔⓑⓜ EVIDENCE

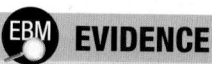
Available at www.expertconsult.com

SUGGESTED READINGS
Available at www.expertconsult.com

RELATED CONTENT
Syncope (Patient Information)
Orthostatic Hypotension (Related Key Topic)

AUTHORS: **JOSEPH S. KASS, M.D., J.D.,** and **TZU-CHING (TEDDY) WU, M.D., M.P.H.**

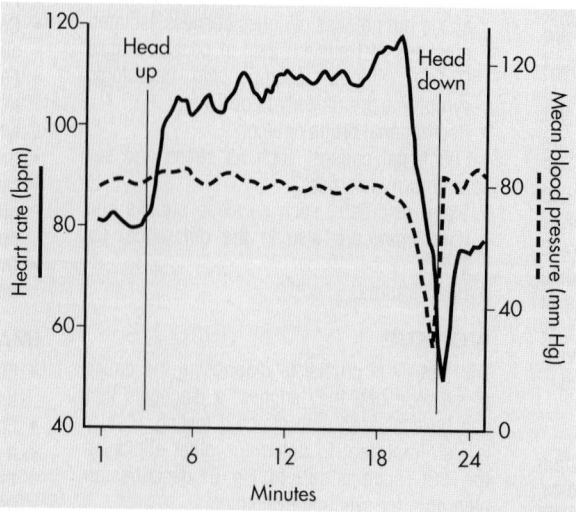

FIG. 2 Head-up tilt test performed on an 18-year-old woman with a history of syncope associated with pain, preceded by a prodrome of dizziness, graying vision, and diaphoresis. A similar prodrome preceded syncope during the test. Note the precipitous and nearly simultaneous decline of heart rate and blood pressure after an initial rise in heart rate. Vital signs returned to normal rapidly after the head was lowered. (Courtesy Robert F. Sprung, University of Utah. In Goldman L, Ausiello D [eds]: *Cecil textbook of medicine,* ed 22, Philadelphia, 2004, Saunders.)

BASIC INFORMATION

DEFINITION

The appropriate (osmotically driven) physiologic response to serum hypotonicity is the inhibition of hypothalamic osmoreceptors, resulting in suppression of antidiuretic hormone (ADH) synthesis and release, and excretion of increased volumes of dilute urine. The consequent decrease in total body water (TBW) with minimal decreases in total body stores of sodium and potassium (i.e., total body cation) increases the serum sodium (S_{Na}) (mEq/L) towards normal. The syndrome of inappropriate antidiuresis (SIAD) is defined by the occurrence of "inappropriately" concentrated urine in patients with hypotonic hyponatremia and normal extracellular fluid volume (ECFV). The S_{Na} is primarily determined by the ratio of total exchangeable cations, sodium ($TBNa_e$) plus potassium (TBK_e) to TBW as depicted by the following equation.

$$S_{Na} = \frac{TBNa_e + TBK_e}{TBW}$$

Hyponatremia results from either loss of total body cations (numerator), increased TBW (denominator), or both. In the syndrome of inappropriate antidiuresis (SIAD), expanded TBW in the presence of normal total body cations produces hyponatremia. The severity of hyponatremia associated with SIAD reflects the severity of the defect in urinary dilution and the magnitude of electrolyte-free fluid intake. Hemodynamic stimuli known to stimulate ADH release preclude a diagnosis of SIAD, and this group of disorders includes those with decreased ECFV (decreased TB_{Na}), hypotension, and decreased effective arterial blood volume (EABV). This latter group is characterized by an increased ECFV (equivalent to an increased TBNa) and includes congestive heart failure, nephrotic syndrome, and cirrhosis.

The term *syndrome of inappropriate antidiuretic hormone* has been supplanted by SIAD because 10% to 15% of SIADH patients have suppressed or undetectable serum ADH concentrations; the remainder demonstrate nonosmotic stimulation of ADH. The group with suppressed ADH is postulated to have increased sensitivity of renal collecting duct principal cells to ADH (gain of function mutations of the AVP V2 receptor), secretion of other ADH-like peptides and/or changes in renal hemodynamics that decrease delivery of sodium and water to distal diluting sites. Establishing a diagnosis of SIAD does not require the measurement of ADH levels or the demonstration of high serum ADH concentrations. Patients with hypothyroidism and adrenal insufficiency are conventionally excluded from the definition of SIAD. Drugs that impair free water excretion constitute another cause of SIAD that some categorize as a separate diagnostic entity. SIAD cannot be diagnosed in patients with acute or chronic kidney disease or recent use of loop diuretics. However, thiazide-induced hyponatremia is considered a drug-induced form of SIAD or SIAD-type physiology.

SYNONYMS

SIADH
Syndrome of inappropriate antidiuretic hormone secretion
Syndrome of inappropriate ADH release
Inappropriate secretion of antidiuretic hormone

ICD 10-CM CODES
E22.2 Syndrome of inappropriate secretion of antidiuretic hormone

EPIDEMIOLOGY & DEMOGRAPHICS

INCIDENCE: Hyponatremia occurs in 15% to 20% of hospitalized patients and is caused by SIAD in approximately half of cases. The adjusted odds ratio for in-hospital mortality in patients with hyponatremia at hospital admission is 1.47 (95% confidence interval 1.33-1.62). The effect is significant regardless of severity of hyponatremia and persists at 1 and 5 years of follow-up.

PHYSICAL FINDINGS & CLINICAL PRESENTATION

- Clinical ECF volume is normal. Patients are hemodynamically stable and there is no evidence of edema, ascites, pleural or pericardial effusions, or other evidence of third-spacing.
- Manifestations of the precipitating cause or underlying disease may be evident (e.g., history of marathon running or other extreme endurance exercise with excessive fluid intake, fever and delirium following the use of 3,4-methylenedioxy-methamphetamine [MDMA, ecstasy]), stigmata of alcoholism or malnutrition, fever and/or localizing symptoms related to pneumonia or other pulmonary disease, or headaches and visual field defects from an intracranial mass).
- Delirium, lethargy, or seizures may be present if hyponatremia occurs rapidly (within <24 hr). Diminished reflexes and extensor plantar responses may occur with severe hyponatremia.
- Neurologic abnormalities including ataxia, mood changes, and proximal muscle weakness are frequent in chronic hyponatremia, but abnormalities may be subtle, even when hyponatremia is relatively severe (defined as S_{Na} <120 mEq/L).

ETIOLOGY

- Drugs: thiazide diuretics and selective serotonin reuptake inhibitor (SSRI) antidepressants are the two most common causes of drug-related hyponatremia. Narcotic analgesics, carbamazepine, phenothiazines, tricyclic antidepressants, MDMA (ecstasy), nicotine, clofibrate, haloperidol, NSAIDs, nicotine, MAO inhibitors, chlorpropamide, vasopressin, desmopressin, oxytocin, chemotherapeutic agents (vincristine, vinblastine, cyclophosphamide) are additional causes.
- Neoplasms: lung, oropharynx, stomach, duodenum, pancreas, brain, thymus, bladder, prostate, endometrium, mesothelioma, lymphoma, Ewing's sarcoma.

- Pulmonary disorders: pneumonia, aspergillosis, pulmonary abscess, TB, bronchiectasis, emphysema, cystic fibrosis, status asthmaticus, respiratory failure associated with positive-pressure breathing.
- Intracranial pathology: trauma, neoplasms, infections (meningitis, encephalitis, brain abscess), hemorrhage, hydrocephalus, multiple sclerosis, Guillain-Barré syndrome.
- Postoperative period: surgical stress, positive pressure ventilation, anesthetic agents.
- Other: acute intermittent porphyria, psychosis, delirium tremens, general anesthesia, endurance exercise.
- Table 1 summarizes common etiologies of the syndrome of inappropriate antidiuresis.

DIFFERENTIAL DIAGNOSIS

- Solute-limited water excretion ("tea-and-toast" diet, beer-drinker's potomania)
- Hyponatremia associated with subclinical hypovolemia
- Primary polydipsia
- Endocrine disorders (hypothyroidism, adrenal insufficiency)
- Hypokalemia (due to decreased TBK_e)
- Hypertonic hyponatremia (hyperglycemia, iatrogenic administration of mannitol, sorbitol, glycine)
- Hyponatremia associated with subclinical heart or liver disease
- Factitious ("pseudohyponatremia" caused by extreme hyperproteinemia or hyperlipidemia)
- Reset osmostat (osmoreceptors secrete ADH at a lower sodium concentration; diagnosis of exclusion)

WORKUP

- Normal ECFV by history and physical examination. No history of large-volume electrolyte and/or fluid losses. No generalized edema, ascites, or large pleural effusions.
- Laboratory evaluation (see "Laboratory Tests") is consistent with excessive ADH secretion or sensitivity in the absence of osmotic or hemodynamic stimuli for ADH secretion.
- Normal thyroid, adrenal, and cardiac function.
- No recent or concurrent use of loop diuretics.
- Failure to correct hyponatremia after 0.9% saline infusion.
- Correction of hyponatremia through fluid restriction alone is possible but unlikely because low urine volumes severely limit urinary free water loss.
- Diagnostic criteria for SIADH are described in Table 2.

LABORATORY TESTS

- Normal or low BUN, creatinine
- Normal TSH
- S_{Na} < lower limit of normal
- Decreased serum osmolality (<275 mOsm/kg)
- Decreased uric acid
- Urine osmolality >100 mOsm/kg with plasma hypotonicity
- Urine sodium usually >40 mEq/L with normal dietary salt intake

TABLE 1 Common Etiologies of the Syndrome of Inappropriate Antidiuretic Hormone Secretion (SIADH)

Tumors

Pulmonary/mediastinal (bronchogenic carcinoma, mesothelioma, thymoma)

Extrapulmonary (duodenal carcinoma, pancreatic carcinoma, ureteral/prostate carcinoma, uterine carcinoma, nasopharyngeal carcinoma, leukemia)

Central Nervous System Disorders

Mass lesions (tumors, brain abscesses, subdural hematoma)

Inflammatory diseases (encephalitis, meningitis, systemic lupus erythematosus, acute intermittent porphyria, multiple sclerosis)

Degenerative/demyelinating diseases (Guillain-Barré syndrome, spinal cord lesions)

Miscellaneous (subarachnoid hemorrhage, head trauma, acute psychosis, delirium tremens, pituitary stalk section, transsphenoidal adenomectomy, hydrocephalus)

Drug-Related

Stimulated release of AVP (nicotine, phenothiazines, tricyclics)

Direct renal effects and/or potentiation of AVP antidiuretic effects (desmopressin, oxytocin, prostaglandin synthesis inhibitors)

Mixed or uncertain actions (ACE inhibitors, carbamazepine and oxcarbazepine, chlorpropamide, clofibrate, clozapine, cyclophosphamide, 3,4-methylenedioxymethamphetamine ["ecstasy"], omeprazole; serotonin reuptake inhibitors, vincristine)

Pulmonary

Infections (tuberculosis, acute bacterial and viral pneumonia, aspergillosis, empyema)

Mechanical/ventilatory causes (acute respiratory failure, COPD, positive-pressure ventilation)

Other Causes

Acquired immunodeficiency syndrome (AIDS) and AIDS-related complex

Prolonged strenuous exercise (marathon, triathlon, ultramarathon, hot-weather hiking)

Senile atrophy

Idiopathic

ACE, Angiotensin-converting enzyme; *AVP,* arginine vasopressin; *COPD,* chronic obstructive pulmonary disease.
From Melmed S: *Williams textbook of endocrinology,* ed 12, Philadelphia, 2011, Saunders.

TABLE 2 Diagnostic Criteria for the Syndrome of Inappropriate Antidiuretic Hormone Release.

Essential Diagnostic Criteria

Decreased extracellular fluid effective osmolality (<270 mOsm/kg)

Inappropriate urinary concentration (>100 mOsm/kg)

Clinical normovolemia

Elevated urinary sodium concentration under conditions of normal salt and water intake

Absence of adrenal, thyroid, or pituitary insufficiency

Absence of chronic kidney disease

Absence of diuretic use

Supplemental Criteria

Abnormal water loading test (inability to excrete at least 90% of a 20-ml/kg water load in 4 hr and/or failure to dilute urine osmolality to <100 mOsm/kg)

Plasma vasopressin level inappropriately elevated relative to the plasma osmolality

No significant correction of SNa with volume expansion, but improvement after fluid restriction

From Floege J et al: *Comprehensive clinical nephrology,* ed 4, Philadelphia, 2010, Saunders.

IMAGING STUDIES

Not routinely required for diagnosis of SIAD. In relevant clinical circumstances, imaging may be required to facilitate diagnosis of underlying pulmonary or central nervous system (CNS) disease associated with SIAD, or to rule out other intracranial pathology in cases of severe encephalopathy.

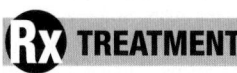 **TREATMENT**

NONPHARMACOLOGIC THERAPY

With mild SIAD, reasonable degrees of fluid restriction (10-15 ml/kg/day) combined with increased solute loads (diets that are high in protein, sodium chloride, and potassium chloride) may increase free water clearance sufficiently until an underlying cause is determined or until definitive therapy is initiated. Nonpharmacologic therapy is seldom sufficiently rapid or effective to constitute the sole therapy of severe or symptomatic acute hyponatremia.

ACUTE GENERAL Rx
PHARMACOLOGIC THERAPY

Rate of Correction. All patients with moderate to severe hyponatremia warrant intense serial monitoring of S_{Na}, and urine volume and chemistry (osmolality, K, and Na) during the initial 48 hr of admission and during active therapy to make sure that recommended rates of correction are achieved but not exceeded.

The level of nursing intensity may require the resources of an ICU or step-down unit, even if patients are minimally symptomatic. The vast majority of patients with SIAD have chronic hyponatremia (developing over a period of greater than 24 hr) that is associated with mild symptoms because adequate time for brain compensation has elapsed. In this case, the most important therapeutic principle is to avoid rapid rates of correction that can cause severe neurologic injury due to osmotic demyelination syndrome. Sodium correction rates should not exceed 6 to 8 mEq/L/day in chronic hyponatremia, and the S_{Na} should be actively lowered in patients who experience increases of >10 mEq/L over a 24-hour period. If SIAD is present, free water loss and the rate of change of S_{Na} should be slow and predictable during administration of normal or hypertonic saline because urine volume will remain relatively low. If the patient has unrecognized volume contraction that is repaired by NaCl infusion, or if the underlying cause of SIAD resolves rapidly, a simultaneous aquaresis (isolated free water loss) may transpire with very rapid rates of S_{Na} elevation.

In the minority of patients with acute hyponatremia (duration <24 hr), excessive rates of correction are of minimal concern, and the goal is to repair the hyponatremia rapidly enough to prevent or reduce the severity of acute cerebral edema. In this circumstance the S_{Na} should be increased by 4-6 mEq/L within the first 3 hr if symptoms are mild-moderate and within the first 1 hr if symptoms are severe (seizures, coma, obtundation).

Acute Hyponatremia. The rapid correction of serum sodium mandated in acute hyponatremia requires 3% saline, despite the patient's normal volume status, as total body sodium can be increased more rapidly than TBW can be decreased. Infusion of each 1 ml/kg body weight of 3% saline infusion (513 mEq/L) increases the serum sodium level by approximately 0.8 to 1 mEq/L (with greater S_{Na} increases in patients with smaller TBW). The infusion volume and rate should reflect the therapeutic goals outlined previously. Furosemide, 20 to 40 mg IV, may be adjunctive by increasing urinary loss of free water as infused sodium is excreted and by helping prevent symptomatic increases in ECFV.

Chronic Hyponatremia. The goal of therapy in chronic hyponatremia due to SIAD is to restore TBW to normal while maintaining already normal quantities of TBK_e and $TBNa_e$. This is accomplished by following these steps:

1. Select a target S_{Na} based on the current S_{Na} and a safe rate of correction (see "Rates of Correction").
2. Estimate the patient's current TBW (L) (see next paragraph and following example).
3. Calculate the TBW (L) that equates with the target S_{Na} selected in Step 1.
4. Calculate net 24-hr electrolyte-free water excretion required to attain the TBW (L) determined in Step 3.
5. Estimate other sources of water intake and loss including insensible losses. Then, add to/subtract from the estimated net electrolyte-free water (Step 4) to determine the net target electrolyte-free water excretion.
6. Select an appropriate strategy (direct ADH V2 receptor antagonist or combined use of a

loop diuretic with electrolyte replacement) to achieve the target electrolyte-free water.

Calculation of S_{Na} demonstrates that in euvolemic patients (including in SIAD) the ratio of TBW (L)/ weight (kg) increases 1.85% for every 10 mEq/L decrease in S_{Na}. The following example demonstrates the calculations required to determine the target TBW and free water loss required to achieve the appropriate S_{Na} target after 24 hr of therapy in a patient with chronic hyponatremia.

Example: A minimally symptomatic 70-year-old woman chronically taking chlorthalidone and an SSRI develops S_{Na} 115 mEq/L.

Step 1 (Target serum sodium)
Target S_{Na} after 24 hours = Current S_{Na} + 6 = 121 mEq/L

Step 2 (Estimate current TBW)
Current weight = 75 kg
Baseline (normal) TBW fraction = 0.5 L/kg body weight (50%)
Current TBW fraction = 0.5 L/kg body weight + (140-115) x .00185 = 0.546 L/kg (54.6 %)
Current TBW = 75 x 0.546 = 41 L

Step 3 (Target TBW)
Using and rearranging Eq. 751-1,

S_{Na} (mEq/L) = Cat_{TB} (mEq) /TBW (L) Target
115 mEq/L = Cat_{TB} (mEq) /41 L
Cat_{TB} = 115 mEq/L × 41 L = 4715 mEq

The targeted S_{Na} of 121 mEq/L
would correspond with
TBW (L) = 4715 (mEq/L) /121mEq/L = 38.9 L

Step 4 (Target net free water loss)
Target *net free water loss* at 24 hours = Current TBW (L) – Target TBW (L) = 41 L– 38.9 L = 2.1 L

Step 5 (Target total free water loss)
Target *total urine free water excretion* (includes allowance for 1 L oral fluid intake and 0.5 L insensible loss) = 2.1 L + 1 L – 0.5 L = 2.6 L

Step 6 (Therapeutic Strategy)
Furosemide and Saline Strategy. The classical treatment strategy for SIAD is to increase urine volume and electrolyte-free water loss via furosemide-induced diuresis, which also restricts urine tonicity (i.e., total of urinary [Na] + [K] concentrations) to approximately 75 mEq/L. Urinary losses of Na and K are then replaced in higher concentrations than that excreted to effect net electrolyte-free water loss. The fol-

lowing table illustrates the urine output and replacement solution (0.9% or 3% NaCl) volumes required in this patient to achieve the target S_{Na}.
Target Total Furosemide-Induced Urinary Free
Water Excretion = 2.5 L
(Urine Na + K = 75 mEq/L)

Replacement Solutions	Cation (NaCl) mEq/L	Net Free Water Loss/L Urine	Target Urine Output (L/24 hr)	Volume (L/ 24 hr) to Replace Electrolyte Loss
0.9% Saline	154	1 – (75/154) = 0.5	2.5/0.5 = 5.0	0.5 L/L UOP × (5 L) = 2.5 L
3% Saline	513	1 – (75/513) = 0.85	2.5/0.85 = 2.94	0.15 L/L UOP × 2.94 = 0.44 L

Periodic monitoring of S_{Na}, urine volume, and urine chemistries (osmolality, sodium, and potassium) is critical to ensure that urine volumes do not exceed targets and that S_{Na} is increasing at the predicted rate.

Use of Direct Vasopressin Receptor Antagonists. Conivaptan (20 mg IV × 1 followed by continuous IV infusion of 20-40 mg/day for 2–4 days) and tolvaptan (15-60 mg/day PO, titrated daily from 15 mg as required) are selective type 2 vasopressin receptor (V_2) antagonists. Compared to furosemide and NaCl infusions, their use is relatively straightforward and convenient for patients and medical personnel. Urinary electrolyte losses are minimal, meaning that their *dosing can be titrated to produce urine output equal to the actual targeted total urine free water loss* (Step 5). Therapeutic effects occur relatively quickly, enabling relatively rapid evaluation and titration of dosing for inpatients provided that S_{Na} and urine output are closely monitored. The medications expense may be offset by a reduction in hospital length-of-stay.

CHRONIC Rx

- When SIAD is chronic, fluid restriction (ideally <15 ml/kg) may be needed indefinitely, in conjunction with high dietary electrolyte and protein content, which increases obligatory free water losses through osmotic diuresis.
- NaCl tablets and protein powders achieve the same goal. Monthly monitoring of electrolytes

is recommended in patients with chronic SIAD.
- Demeclocycline 300 to 600 mg PO twice daily effectively increases electrolyte-free water excretion in some patients. Contraindicated in hepatic disease.

DISPOSITION

- Mortality exceeding 40% has been reported in patients with S_{Na} <110 mEq/L.
- Hospital readmission rates are common in chronic SIAD when an underlying cause cannot be eliminated, especially if patients are unwilling or unable to restrict their fluid intake and follow dietary recommendations.
- Growing evidence suggests that even mild to moderate chronic hyponatremia has been associated with bone loss, falls, and increased fracture risk, especially in elderly patients.

REFERRAL

Urgent emergency department evaluation and hospital admission are appropriate for moderate to severe hyponatremia due to SIAD, especially if it is acute or symptomatic, or if therapy is being initiated. Because of the high risk of complications from overly aggressive or ineffective treatment, referral to a nephrologist, endocrinologist, or critical care physician is recommended.

SUGGESTED READING
Available at www.expertconsult.com

RELATED CONTENT
Syndrome of Inappropriate Secretion of Antidiuretic Hormone (Patient Information)

AUTHORS: **MARK D. FABER, M.D.,** and **MUHAMMAD FAROOQ, M.D**

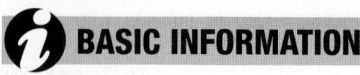
DEFINITION

Syphilis is a systemic sexually transmitted treponemal disease, with acute and chronic manifestations, characterized by primary skin lesions; secondary eruption involving skin and mucous membranes; long periods of latency; and late lesions of the skin, bone, viscera, central nervous system, and cardiovascular system.

SYNONYMS

Lues

ICD-10CM CODES
A51.0 Primary genital syphilis
A51.1 Primary anal syphilis
A51.2 Primary syphilis of other sites
A51.3 Secondary syphilis of skin and mucous membranes
A51.4 Other secondary syphilis
A51.5 Early syphilis, unspecified
A52   Late syphilis
A52.0 Cardiovascular syphilis
A52.1 Symptomatic neurosyphilis
A52.3 Asymptomatic neurosyphilis
A52.3 Neurosyphilis, unspecified
A53.9 Syphilis, unspecified

EPIDEMIOLOGY & DEMOGRAPHICS

- Most commonly diagnosed in people 20 to 30 years old.
- More prevalent in men than women.
- Rates reached historic lows in the U.S. in 2000 but began increasing among males in 2001, and increase has continued. Rates are disproportionately higher among black and Hispanic men who have sex with men (MSM) compared with white MSM and among young MSM.
- Usually more prevalent in urban areas and among people of lower socioeconomic status.
- Nearly 20,000 new cases were reported in the U.S. in 2014.
- Communicability is indefinite and variable. Communicable during primary, secondary, and latent mucocutaneous lesions in up to first 4 yr of latency. Most probable congenital transmission occurs in early maternal syphilis. Adequate penicillin treatment ends infectivity within 24 to 48 hr.

PHYSICAL FINDINGS & CLINICAL PRESENTATION

PRIMARY SYPHILIS:
- Characteristic lesion is a painless chancre on genitalia, mouth, or anus (Fig. 1); atypical primary lesions may occur.
- May appear 10 days to 12 weeks (usually 3 weeks) after exposure and may resolve without treatment within 6 weeks.

SECONDARY SYPHILIS:
- Bacteremia associated with generalized lymphadenopathy and a characteristic maculopapular rash including palms, soles, and mucous membranes. Constitutional, flulike symptoms may also occur.
- 60% to 80% have maculopapular lesions on palms and soles.
- 21% to 58% have mucocutaneous or mucosal lesions (pharyngitis, tonsillitis, "mucous patch" lesion on oral and genital mucosa).
- Condylomata lata intertriginous papules form at areas of friction and moisture, such as the vulva.
- Occurs 4 to 6 weeks after appearance of chancre. Resolves within 1 week to 12 months.

LATENT SYPHILIS: EARLY VS. LATE LATENT:
- Generally asymptomatic.
- Seroreactivity without other evidence of primary, secondary, or tertiary disease.
- Not sexually transmitted but may be transmitted from a pregnant woman to her fetus.
- In the first year, symptoms or signs of secondary syphilis may occur without a patient's being contagious.
- Early latent: <12 months from acquisition.
- Late latent: >12 months from acquisition.

TERTIARY SYPHILIS:
- Characterized by gummas (nodular, ulcerative lesions) that can involve the skin, mucous membranes, skeletal system, and viscera.
- Manifestations of cardiovascular syphilis include aortitis, aneurysm, or aortic regurgitation.
- Neurosyphilis may be asymptomatic or symptomatic. Tabes dorsalis, meningovascular syphilis, general paralysis, or insanity may occur. Iritis, choroidoretinitis, and leukoplakia may also occur.

ETIOLOGY

- *Treponema pallidum*, a spirochete
- Spread by sexual intercourse or by intrauterine transfer

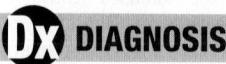
DIFFERENTIAL DIAGNOSIS

- Other genitoulcerative diseases such as herpes, chancroid (see Section II)
- See Section III for a clinical algorithm for the evaluation of genital ulcer disease

WORKUP

Confirmation is primarily through laboratory diagnosis.
- Culture of lesions
- Serologic testing (see the following lab tests)
- Cerebrospinal fluid (CSF) testing

LABORATORY TESTS

- Dark-field microscopy of fluid from lesion to look for treponeme is the definitive method for diagnosis of early syphilis.
- Serologic testing:
  - Nontreponemal tests: venereal disease research laboratory (VDRL) or rapid plasma reagin (RPR).
  - Treponemal tests: fluorescent treponemal antibody absorbed (FTA-ABS) tests, the *T. pallidum* passive particle agglutination (TP-PA) assay, various enzyme immunoassays (EIAs), chemiluminescence immunoassays, immunoblots, or rapid treponemal assays.

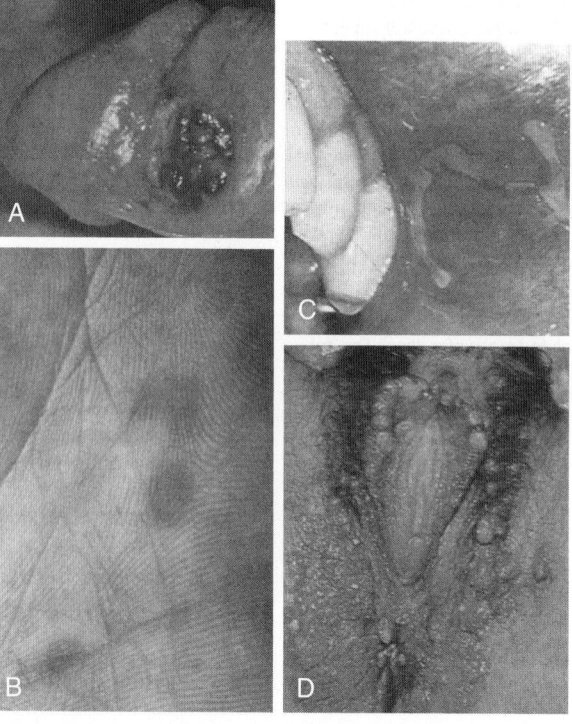

FIG. 1 Syphilis lesions. A, Chancre in primary syphilis. **B,** Palmar lesions of a coppery color in secondary syphilis. **C,** Mucous patch in secondary syphilis. **D,** Condylomata lata in secondary syphilis. (**A, C,** and **D** from Forbes CD, Jackson WF: *Color atlas and text of clinical medicine,* ed 3, London, 2003, Mosby. **B** from Habif TP et al: *Skin disease: diagnosis and treatment,* St Louis, 2001, Mosby.)

- Antibody titers can assess for response to treatment and for reinfection in previously treated patients.
- Screening with nontreponemal tests; confirmation with treponemal testing.
- When the nontreponemal test is negative despite a positive screen, an additional treponemal screen may be helpful. Trials have shown that two positive treponemal screens help identify a population with likely prior or current syphilis, and treatment of these patients may be justifiable.
- In patients with neurosyphilis, serologic criteria for response to therapy is a fourfold or greater decrease in VDRL titer over 6 to 12 months.
- Lumbar puncture (LP) for cerebrospinal fluid VDRL (CSF-VDRL) in patients with evidence of latent syphilis. When reactive in the absence of substantial contamination of CSF with blood, it is considered diagnostic of neurosyphilis. The Centers for Disease Control and Prevention indications for LP are neurologic symptoms, treatment failure, any eye or ear involvement, or evidence of active syphilis (aortitis, gumma, iritis).
- HIV testing in all patients.

Rx TREATMENT

ACUTE GENERAL Rx

- Primary, secondary, early latent:
  - Penicillin G benzathine 2.4 million U IM.
  - Infants and children: benzathine penicillin G 50,000 units/kg IM, up to the adult dose of 2.4 million units in a single dose.
  - Nonpregnant penicillin-allergic patients: doxycycline 100 mg bid × 14 days.
  - Azithromycin 2 g PO × 1 dose: only if penicillin and doxycycline are not options. Contraindicated in MSM, persons with HIV, or pregnant women.
  - Careful clinical and serologic follow-up of persons receiving any alternative therapy is essential.
  - Persons with a penicillin allergy whose compliance with therapy or follow-up cannot be ensured should be desensitized and treated with benzathine penicillin.

- With HIV infection: benzathine penicillin G 2.4 million units IM × 1 dose.
- Late latent syphilis, latent syphilis of unknown duration, tertiary syphilis (not neurosyphilis) in adults:
  - Penicillin G benzathine 2.4 million U IM q wk × 3 wk.
  - Nonpregnant penicillin-allergic patients: doxycycline 100 mg PO bid × 4 wk.
  - With HIV infection: benzathine penicillin G 2.4 million units IM weekly for 3 wk.
- Neurosyphilis:
  - Aqueous crystalline penicillin G 18 to 24 million U/day, administered as 3 to 4 million U IV q4h or continuous infusion for 10 to 14 days.
  - Alternative regimen: procaine penicillin 2.4 million U IM/day plus probenecid 500 mg PO qid, both for 10 to 14 days.
- Congenital syphilis:
  - Aqueous crystalline penicillin G 50,000 U/kg/dose IV q12h × first 7 days of life and q8h after that for a total of 10 days OR procaine penicillin G 50,000 U/kg/dose IM/day × 10 days.

DISPOSITION

- Repeat quantitative nontreponemal tests at 3, 6, and 12 mo to ensure adequate treatment. Pregnancy requires monthly tests until delivery.
- If a fourfold increase in titer occurs, if initial high titer fails to drop by fourfold within a year, or signs persist, retreatment may be indicated. Because treatment failure may be the result of unrecognized CNS infection, CSF examination can be considered in such situations. For retreatment, weekly infusions of benzathine penicillin G 2.4 million units IM for 3 wk is recommended, unless CSF examination indicates that neurosyphilis is present.
- Pregnant women without a fourfold drop in titer in a 3-mo period need to be retreated.
- Cases should be reported to local or state health department for referral, follow-up, and partner notification.

REFERRAL

- Pregnant and possible congenital syphilis

- Pregnant and allergic to penicillin, with need to be desensitized
- Late latent syphilis with serious central nervous system, cardiovascular, or other organ system compromise

! PEARLS & CONSIDERATIONS

- Jarisch-Herxheimer reaction (fever, myalgia, tachycardia, hypotension) may occur within 24 hr of treatment.
- One third of untreated patients develop central nervous system and/or cardiovascular sequelae.
- Up to 80% of those treated during late stages remain seropositive indefinitely.
- Treponemal tests remain positive even after adequate therapy.
- Male circumcision does not decrease the incidence of syphilis (unlike HIV, HSV-2, and HPV infection).
- Partner notification and treatment:
  1. Persons who are exposed within 90 days preceding the diagnosis of primary, secondary, or early latent syphilis in a sex partner might be infected even if seronegative; therefore, such persons should be treated presumptively.
  2. Persons who were exposed ≥90 days before the diagnosis of syphilis in a sex partner should be treated presumptively if serologic test results are not available immediately and the opportunity for follow-up is uncertain.

SUGGESTED READINGS
Available at www.expertconsult.com

RELATED CONTENT
Syphilis (Patient Information)
Tabes Dorsalis (Related Key Topic)

AUTHOR: **NICOLE A. ROBERTS, M.D.**

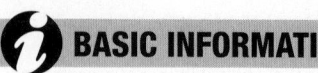

DEFINITION

- Systemic lupus erythematosus (SLE) is a chronic inflammatory disorder characterized by autoantibody production responsible for antibody-mediated and immune complex deposition tissue damage. SLE involves multiple organs and systems and has heterogeneous disease patterns. Relapses and remissions are a common feature.

SYNONYMS

SLE
Lupus

ICD-10CM CODES

M32	Systemic lupus erythematosus
M32.0	Drug-induced systemic lupus erythematosus
M32.8	Other forms of systemic lupus erythematosus
M32.9	Systemic lupus erythematosus, unspecified
M32.10	Systemic lupus erythematosus, organ or system involvement unspecified
M32.11	Endocarditis in systemic lupus erythematosus
M32.12	Pericarditis in systemic lupus erythematosus
M32.13	Lung involvement in systemic lupus erythematosus
M32.14	Glomerular disease in systemic lupus erythematosus
M32.15	Tubulo-interstitial nephropathy in systemic lupus erythematosus
M32.19	Other organ or system involvement in systemic lupus erythematosus

EPIDEMIOLOGY & DEMOGRAPHICS

INCIDENCE: Varies across gender, race/ethnic groups, and geography from 20 to 70 cases per 100,000 persons. Prevalence higher among African Americans, Asian Americans, and Hispanics. There are an estimated 350,000 people with SLE in the U.S.
PREDOMINANT SEX: Female/male ratio is 9:1. The ratio is highest in reproductive age group, and about half of that in patients younger than 16 and older than 55.
PREDOMINANT AGE: Mean age at diagnosis is 31.

PHYSICAL FINDINGS & CLINICAL PRESENTATION

- Constitutional: unexplained fever (rare in active SLE), fatigue (80% to 100% patients), malaise (see Table 1).
- Mucocutaneous lesions (more than 80% of patients): Acute (associated with + Ro antibody): malar rash sparing nasolabial folds (acute cutaneous lupus) (Fig. 1); annular or papulosquamous rash (subacute cutaneous lupus) (Fig. 2); Chronic: raised erythematous patches with subsequent edematous plaques and adherent scales (discoid

TABLE 1 Potential Clinical Manifestations of Systemic Lupus Erythematosus

Target Organ	Potential Clinical Manifestations
Constitutional	Fatigue, anorexia, weight loss, fever, lymphadenopathy
Musculoskeletal	Arthritis, myositis, arthralgias, myalgias, avascular necrosis, osteoporosis
Skin	Malar rash, discoid rash, photosensitive rash, cutaneous vasculitis, livedo reticularis, periungual capillary abnormalities, Raynaud's phenomenon, alopecia, oral and nasal ulcers
Renal	Hypertension, proteinuria, hematuria, edema, nephrotic syndrome, renal failure
Cardiovascular	Pericarditis, myocarditis, conduction system abnormalities, Libman-Sacks endocarditis
Neurologic	Seizures, psychosis, cerebritis, stroke, transverse myelitis, depression, cognitive impairment, headaches, pseudotumor, peripheral neuropathy, chorea, optic neuritis, cranial nerve palsies
Pulmonary	Pleuritis, interstitial lung disease, pulmonary hemorrhage, pulmonary hypertension, pulmonary embolism
Hematologic	Immune-mediated cytopenias (hemolytic anemia, thrombocytopenia or leukopenia), anemia of chronic inflammation, hypercoagulability, thrombocytopenic thrombotic microangiopathy
Gastroenterology	Hepatosplenomegaly, pancreatitis, vasculitis affecting bowel, protein-losing enteropathy
Ocular	Retinal vasculitis, scleritis, episcleritis, papilledema

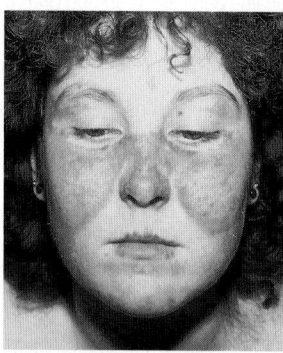

FIG. 1 Acute cutaneous lupus erythematosus (LE) (systemic LE). The classic butterfly rash occurs in 10% to 50% of patients with acute LE. (From Habif TP: *Clinical dermatology: a color guide to diagnosis and therapy,* ed 3, St Louis, 1996, Mosby.)

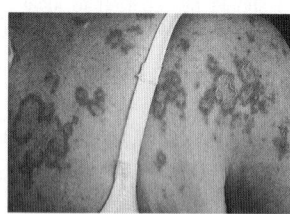

FIG. 2 Subacute cutaneous lupus. (From Hochberg MC et al: *Rheumatology,* ed 4, St Louis, 2008, Mosby.)

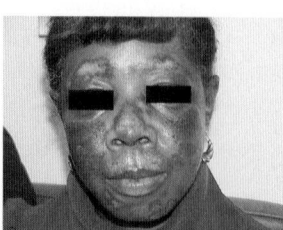

FIG. 3 Discoid lupus erythematosus. (From Firestein GS et al: *Kelley's textbook of rheumatology,* ed 8, Philadelphia, 2008, Saunders.)

cutaneous lupus), lupus profundus, lupus tumidus (Fig. 3); alopecia, photosensitivity, nasal, or oropharyngeal ulcerations (classically painless, but discoid lesions may be painful); Raynaud's phenomenon; leukocytoclastic vasculitis, chilblains; livedo reticularis or livedo racemosa (secondary to antiphospholipid antibody syndrome); skin biopsy hallmark: interface dermatitis.
- Musculoskeletal (about 90% of lupus patients): arthralgias are more common than true arthritis, but nonerosive deforming arthritis is not rare; myositis.
- Cardiac: pericardial rub (pericarditis) is most common; valvular heart disease: valve nodules and thickening (Libman-Sacks endocarditis); congestive heart failure, myocarditis, premature atherosclerotic heart disease.
- Pulmonary: pleuritis (most common), acute or chronic pneumonitis, diffuse alveolar hemorrhage, pulmonary hypertension.
- Gastrointestinal: dysphagia, mesenteric vasculitis, peritonitis, pancreatitis, hepatitis.
- Neuropsychiatric: headache, psychosis, seizure, acute confusional states, peripheral or cranial neuropathy, transverse myelitis, stroke (may be associated with antiphospholipid syndrome), cognitive dysfunction.
- Hematologic (about 50% of lupus patients): anemia (hemolytic, anemia of chronic disease, aplastic anemia), thrombocytopenia, leukopenia, lymphadenopathy, secondary antiphospholipid antibody syndrome.
- Renal: acute renal failure, proteinuria, nephritic syndrome, nephrotic syndrome.

ETIOLOGY

Lupus may develop in genetically susceptible individuals, triggered by endogenous and exogenous factors. SLE susceptibility involves MHC class II polymorphism with commonly observed association with HLA-DR-2, DR3, DR4, and DR8. SLE is also associated with inherited deficiencies of C1q, C2, C4a, others. There is predilection for familial clustering of SLE with risk in monozygotic twins—about 25% to 50%—and 5% in dizygotic twins. Environmental factors such as UV light, Epstein-Barr virus infection, and tobacco smoking may have a triggering role. Autoantibody production is the hallmark of disease development and diagnosis of SLE. Evidence supports the improper processing of nuclear proteins and nucleic acid from cell death. Impairments in neutrophil cell death via a process termed NET-osis (nuclear extracellular trap) contribute to the accumulation of nuclear debris. This, in turn, can lead to the presentation of self-nuclear material to plasmacytoid dendritic cells. Plasmacytoid dendritic cells propagate antibody and immune complex production via a type I interferon-dependent mechanism.

Dx DIAGNOSIS

DIFFERENTIAL DIAGNOSIS

- Rheumatoid arthritis, mixed connective tissue disease, systemic vasculitis
- Neoplastic disorder
- Hematologic malignancy, paraneoplastic syndrome
- Systemic infection
- Other: thrombotic thrombocytopenic purpura/hemolytic uremic syndrome, primary antiphospholipid antibody syndrome

EVALUATION

The diagnosis of SLE is suspected when any four or more of the following 1997 American College of Rheumatology (ACR) criteria (sensitivity 86%, specificity 93%) are present. These criteria were developed for research purposes, and diagnosis should be made on clinical grounds. The 2012 Systemic Lupus International Collaborating Clinics (SLICC) Classification Criteria (sensitivity 94%, specificity 92%) is also a validated tool for the diagnosis of SLE.

1997 ACR Criteria
- Malar rash
- Discoid rash
- Photosensitivity (recurrence of unusual skin rash in sun-exposed areas)
- Oral or nasopharyngeal painless ulceration, observed by physician
- Arthritis (nonerosive)
- Serositis (pleuritis, pericarditis)
- Renal disorder (persistent proteinuria >0.5 g/day, or ≥3+ on dipstick if quantification not performed; cellular casts)
- Neurologic disorder (seizures, psychosis [in absence of offending drugs or metabolic derangement])
- Hematologic disorder:
  1. Hemolytic anemia with reticulocytosis
  2. Leukopenia (<4000/mm^3 total on two or more occasions)
  3. Lymphopenia (<1500/mm^3 on two or more occasions)
  4. Thrombocytopenia (<100,000/mm^3 in the absence of offending drugs)
- Immunologic disorder:
  1. Anti–double-stranded DNA antibody (anti-dsDNA)
  2. Anti-Smith antibody (anti-Sm)

3. Antiphospholipid antibodies (anticardiolipin IgM or IgG, lupus anticoagulant, anti-beta-2 glycoprotein IgM or IgG, or false-positive fluorescent treponemal antibody absorption test or *Treponema pallidum* immobilization for 6 months)
- Antinuclear antibody (ANA): an abnormal titer of ANA by immunofluorescence or equivalent assay at any time in the absence of drugs known to be associated with drug-induced lupus syndrome

2012 SLICC Criteria
SLE can be diagnosed if:
I. Biopsy-proven nephritis with either ANA or anti-dsDNA antibodies
II. *or*
III. Patient satisfies four clinical criteria, requiring at least one clinical and at least one immunologic criterion
IV. Clinical Criteria
  1. Acute cutaneous lupus (malar rash, bullous lupus, toxic epidermal necrolysis, photosensitive lupus rash, maculopapular lupus, subacute cutaneous lupus)
  2. Chronic cutaneous lupus (discoid, hypertrophic verrucous, panniculitis, mucosal lupus, lupus tumidus, chilblains lupus, lichen planus)
  3. Oral ulcers or nasal ulcers
  4. Nonscarring alopecia
  5. Synovitis (more than two joints or inflammatory arthralgias of more than two joints)
  6. Serositis (pleurisy for more than 1 day, pericardial pain for more than 1 day)
  7. Renal (>500 mg proteinuria/24 hours) or RBC casts)
  8. Neurologic (seizures, psychosis, mononeuritis multiplex, myelitis, peripheral or cranial neuropathy, acute confusional state)
  9. Hemolytic anemia
  10. Lymphopenia (<1000/mm^3 at least once)

11. Thrombocytopenia (<100,000/mm^3 at least once)
V. Immunologic Criteria
  1. ANA
  2. Anti-dsDNA (>2× laboratory reference range)
  3. Anti-Smith
  4. Antiphospholipid antibodies (lupus anticoagulant, RPR, anti-cardiolipin IgA, IgG, IgM, anti-β2 glycoprotein IgA, IgG, IgM)
  5. Low complement
  6. Direct Coombs test in the absence of hemolytic anemia

LABORATORY TESTS

Suggested initial laboratory evaluation of suspected SLE:
  ANA
- Complete blood count with differential, blood urea nitrogen and serum creatinine, urinalysis, ESR, PTT, complements (C3, C4)

Consider additional laboratory testing in a patient with strong suspicion for systemic lupus:
- Anti-dsDNA, anti-Smith, anti-SSA, anti-SSB, anti-RNP antibodies. Table 2 summarizes autoantibodies and clinical significance in SLE.
- Lupus anticoagulant, RPR, anticardiolipin antibodies, anti-beta-2 glycoprotein antibodies especially in patients with thrombotic events or recurrent miscarriages
- Urinalysis for RBC, cellular casts
- Random spot urine protein: urine creatinine ratio, 24-hour urine protein collection if proteinuria; >0.5 or >500 mg/24 hours is abnormal, respectively.
  Direct Coombs test

IMAGING STUDIES

- Chest x-ray for evaluation of pulmonary involvement (pleural effusion, pulmonary infiltrates)
- Electrocardiogram for chest pain
- Echocardiogram if murmur, evidence of new or unexplained congestive heart failure, or suspected pericarditis

TABLE 2 Autoantibodies and Clinical Significance in Systemic Lupus Erythematosus (SLE)

Autoantibody	Prevalence in SLE	Clinical Significance
Antinuclear Antibody		
Anti-dsDNA	60%	95% specificity for SLE; fluctuates with disease activity; associated with glomerulonephritis
Anti-Smith	20%-30%	99% specificity for SLE; associated with anti-U1RNP antibodies
Anti-U1RNP	30%	Antibody associated with mixed connective tissue disease and lower frequency of glomerulonephritis
Anti-Ro/SSA	30%	Associated with Sjögren's syndrome, photosensitivity, SCLE, neonatal lupus, congenital heart block
Anti-La/SSB	20%	Associated with Sjögren's syndrome, SCLE, neonatal lupus, congenital heart block, anti-Ro/SSA
Antihistone	70%	Also associated with drug-induced lupus
Antiphospholipid	30%	Associated with arterial and venous thrombosis, pregnancy morbidity

SCLE, Subacute cutaneous lupus erythematosus.
From Firestein GS et al: *Kelley's textbook of rheumatology,* ed 9, Philadelphia, 2013, Saunders.

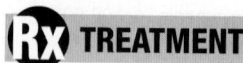 **TREATMENT**

NONPHARMACOLOGIC THERAPY

- Avoidance of sunlight and use of high-SPF sunscreen (>35).
- Screening and counseling for modifiable cardiovascular risk factors such as cigarette smoking and uncontrolled HTN.
- Counseling for pregnancy planning for patients of childbearing age.
- Calcium and vitamin D supplementation for prevention of early osteoporosis.

GENERAL Rx

- Treatment should be targeted toward the involved organ(s).
- Limited and defined courses of corticosteroids are useful for a variety of SLE symptoms. Steroid therapy should be restricted to acute or subacute control of symptoms, due to the increased cardiovascular risk and increased organ damage associated with chronic steroid use.
- Consider checking G6PD in certain ethnic groups more predisposed to antimalarial-induced hemolytic anemia.
- Hydroxychloroquine has best evidence for reducing flares, organ damage, lipids, thrombosis; improving survival, augmenting action of mycophenolate mofetil (MMF) in lupus nephritis, and preventing seizures. Additional useful medications are listed in the following:
- Methotrexate or azathioprine is used as steroid-sparing drug. Indications for immunosuppressive therapy in SLE are described in Tables 3 and 4.
- Joint pain and mild serositis are generally well controlled with nonsteroidal antiinflammatory drugs or low-dose corticosteroids. Hydroxychloroquine and methotrexate are

also effective for arthritis. Leflunomide and rituximab may be considered for difficult arthritis.
- Cutaneous manifestations
  1. Topical or intradermal corticosteroids are helpful for individual discoid lesions, especially in the scalp.
  2. Hydroxychloroquine alone or in combination with quinacrine and/or chloroquine could be considered for refractory skin disease.
- Hematologic manifestations
  1. Corticosteroids are first-line therapy.
  2. Azathioprine can be used for thrombocytopenia or hemolytic anemia. Check for TPMT genetic mutation before the first use.
  3. Intravenous immunoglobulin (IVIG) or rituximab may be considered for severe leukopenia, autoimmune hemolytic anemia, or autoimmune thrombocytopenia.
- Central nervous system manifestations.
  1. Headaches are treated symptomatically. Most headaches will not be SLE-related and should be treated accordingly.
  2. Anticonvulsants and antipsychotics may be indicated.
  3. Standard therapy for other neuropsychiatric SLE symptoms is not established.
- Renal disease (Class III, IV, or IV/V with cellular crescents lupus nephritis; see Table 5). INDUCTION: 6-month treatment
- The typical treatment induction period is 6 months. The use of intravenous cyclophosphamide (CYC) with corticosteroids given at monthly intervals is more effective in preserving renal function than is treatment with glucocorticoids alone. Low-dose "Euro-Lupus" protocol may be equally efficacious and less toxic for certain populations (e.g., Caucasians) than high-dose regimen. MMF

is considered equivalent to CYC based on high-quality studies, with better tolerability and fertility profile. MMF may be preferred in African Americans and Hispanics. MMF or azathioprine is a good option for treatment maintenance.
- Severe nonrenal organ disease:
  1. Evidence from systematic randomized controlled trials for nonrenal lupus treatment is comparatively limited.
  2. High-dose intravenous CYC is used as induction treatment. Azathioprine or MMF may be used as maintenance.
  3. IVIG may be considered in severe disease especially when concomitant infection is present.
  4. Plasmapheresis or plasma exchange may be considered in critical situations: first-line therapy in Guillain-Barre syndrome, TTP, second line for SLE-related hemolytic anemia, cerebritis, and DAH. Infectious complications are common.
- Therapy targeting B cells
  1. Rituximab anti-CD 20 monoclonal antibody: randomized controlled trials for rituximab as an adjunct induction agent were negative in terms of both renal and nonrenal outcomes.
  2. Epratuzumab: an anti-CD 22 agent, it is in the late stages of clinical trials with satisfactory data for improvement in areas of mucocutaneous, renal, and neuropsychiatric SLE.
  3. Belimumab: decreases activation of B cells; when used in addition to standard therapy, patients on belimumab showed improvement in cutaneous and musculoskeletal disease. Belimumab-treated patients had decreased SLE activity, a reduced time to disease flare, and lower glucocorticoid exposure. Safety data were good. Patients with central nervous system or serious kidney disease were excluded.
  4. Abatacept: downregulates T cell activation; data is limited about improvement in arthritis, fatigue, sleep if added to routine therapy.
  5. Interferon therapy: interferon α (INFα) has been linked to increased disease activity in SLE. INFα blocking therapies are in phase II clinical trials. Sifalimumab, a monoclonal antibody against INFα, reduced moderate to severe mucocutaneous involvement in SLE and decreased active joint count and fatigue scores in preliminary data analysis.

DISPOSITION

- Most patients with SLE experience remissions and exacerbations.
- Five-year survival rate has improved to more than 90% in patients with newly diagnosed SLE since the advent of potent immunosuppressive therapy. The 15-year survival rate is now 85%.
- Early death related to SLE activity and infections; late death due to CVD.
- Lupus nephritis progression rate to ESRD in 10% to 30% within 15 years.

TABLE 3 Indications for Immunosuppressive Therapy in Systemic Lupus Erythematosus

General Indications

Involvement of major organs or extensive involvement of nonmajor organs (skin) refractory to other agents, or both

Failure to respond to or inability to taper corticosteroids to acceptable doses for long-term use

Specific Organ Involvement

Renal

Proliferative or membranous nephritis (nephritic or nephritic syndrome), or both

Hematologic

Severe thrombocytopenia (platelets <20,000/mm³)

Thrombotic thrombocytopenic purpura–like syndrome

Severe hemolytic or aplastic anemia, or immune neutropenia not responding to glucocorticoids

Pulmonary

Lupus pneumonitis or alveolar hemorrhage, or both

Cardiac

Myocarditis with depressed left ventricular function, pericarditis with impending tamponade

Gastrointestinal

Abdominal vasculitis

Nervous system

Transverse myelitis, cerebritis, optic neuritis, psychosis refractory to corticosteroids, mononeuritis multiplex, severe peripheral neuropathy

From Firestein GS et al: *Kelly's textbook of rheumatology*, ed 9, Philadelphia, 2013, Saunders.

TABLE 4 Recommended Immunosuppressive Therapy for Major Organ Involvement in Systemic Lupus Erythematosus

Disease Severity	Induction Therapy	Maintenance Therapy
Mild	High-dose GC (0.5-1 mg/kg/day prednisone ×4-6 wk, tapered to 0.125 mg/kg every other day within 3 mo) alone or in combination with AZA (1-2 mg/kg/day)	Low-dose GC (prednisone ≤0.125 mg/kg on alternative days) alone or with AZA (1-2 mg/kg/day)
	If no remission within 3 mo, treat as moderately severe	Consider further gradual tapering at the end of each year of remission
Moderate	MMF (2 g/day) (or AZA) with GC as above; if no remission after the first 6-12 mo, treat as severe	MMF tapered to 1.5 g/day for 6-12 mo and then to 1 g/day; consider further tapering at the end of each year in remission Alternative: AZA (1-2 mg/kg/day)
Severe	Pulse IV-CYC alone or in combination with pulse IV-MP for the first 6 mo (background GC 0.5 mg/kg/day for 4 wk, then taper)	Quarterly pulses of IV-CYC for at least 1 year beyond remission
	If no response, consider adding RTX or switch to MMF	Alternative: AZA (1-2 mg/kg/day), MMF (1-2 g/day)

AZA, Azathioprine; *CYC,* cyclophosphamide; *GC,* glucocorticoid; *IV,* intravenous; *MMF,* mycophenolate mofetil; *MP,* methylprednisolone; *RTX,* rituximab.
From Firestein GS et al: *Kelley's textbook of rheumatology,* ed 9, Philadelphia, 2013, Saunders.

TABLE 5 Severity of Lupus Nephritis*

Proliferative Disease

Mild	Type III without severe histologic features (e.g., crescents, fibrinoid necrosis); low chronicity index (i.e., ≤3); normal renal function; nonnephrotic-range proteinuria
Moderately severe	Mild disease as defined above with partial or no response after the initial induction therapy or delayed remission (>12 months), or Focal proliferative nephritis with adverse histologic features or reproducible increase of at least 30% in serum creatinine levels, or Diffuse proliferative nephritis (class IV) without adverse histologic features
Severe	Moderately severe as defined above but not remitting after 6 to 12 months of therapy, or Proliferative disease with impaired renal function and fibrinoid necrosis or crescents in >25% of glomeruli, or Mixed membranous and proliferative nephritis, or Proliferative nephritis with high chronicity alone or in combination with high activity (chronicity index >4 or chronicity index >3 and activity index >10), or Rapidly progressive glomerulonephritis (doubling of serum creatinine within 2 to 3 months)

Membranous Nephropathy

Mild	Nonnephrotic-range proteinuria with normal renal function
Moderate	Nephrotic-range proteinuria with normal renal function at presentation
Severe	Nephrotic-range proteinuria with impaired renal function at presentation (at least 30% increase in serum creatinine)

*Concomitant therapy with corticosteroids or other immunosuppressive drugs may modify urinary sediment and/or histologic findings and should be taken into consideration.
From Hochberg MC et al: *Rheumatology,* ed 5, St Louis, 2011, Mosby.

- African Americans, Asian Americans, and Hispanic Americans in general have a worse prognosis. The leading cause of death in SLE patients in developed countries is premature atherosclerosis. The quality of life for many SLE patients is poor due to fatigue, chronic pain, and cognitive impairment.

REFERRAL

- Rheumatology consultation for all patients with SLE
- Hematology consultation for patients with significant hematologic abnormalities (e.g., severe hemolytic anemia or thrombocytopenia)
- Nephrology consultation in patients with proteinuria and/or suspected renal involvement
- Dermatology consultation for patients with unexplained or unusual skin rash
- Cardiology consultation for patients with lupus carditis, arrhythmias

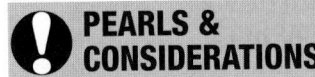 **PEARLS & CONSIDERATIONS**

- Arthritis in SLE often has no prolonged morning stiffness and is not erosive on x-rays; reversible joint deformities in lupus are termed Jaccoud's arthropathy.
- Myocardial infarction is 50 times more common in young female patients than in age-matched control group.
- Prevent adverse effects of medications: consider prophylaxis for infections and appropriate vaccinations, ensure yearly Pap and other cancer screening as clinically indicated; for patients taking CYC, intervention to preserve bladder and fertility should be considered; manage bone health.

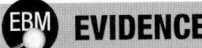 **EVIDENCE**

Available at www.expertconsult.com

SUGGESTED READINGS

Available at www.expertconsult.com

RELATED CONTENT

Systemic Lupus Erythematosus (Patient Information)

AUTHOR: **KATARZYNA GILEK-SEIBERT, M.D., RH.M.S.U.S.**

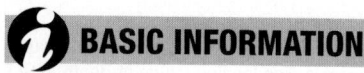

BASIC INFORMATION

DEFINITION

Takayasu's arteritis is a rare type of chronic idiopathic systemic granulomatous large-vessel vasculitis that primarily affects the aorta and its main branches. Systemic inflammation of involved vessels leads commonly to stenosis, occlusion, dilation, and aneurysms in the arterial wall.

SYNONYMS

Pulseless disease
Aortitis syndrome
Aortic arch arteritis
Nonspecific aortoarteritis

ICD-10CM CODES
M31.4 Aortic arch syndrome [Takayasu]

EPIDEMIOLOGY & DEMOGRAPHICS

A worldwide survey revealed that Takayasu's arteritis is prevalent in Asia and Middle Eastern countries. The incidence of Takayasu's arteritis is greatest in East Asia. In the U.S., the incidence is 2.6 per 1 million persons. The highest prevalence of Takayasu's arteritis has been described in Japan, where all cases of Takayasu's arteritis are registered by the government, and it has been estimated that 100 to 200 new cases occur each year.

The female/male ratio is 8:1. The age of onset is usually between 10 and 40 yr of age, with three quarters of patients presenting between the age of 10 and 20 years old.

PHYSICAL FINDINGS & CLINICAL PRESENTATION

Clinical signs and symptoms originate from both the systemic inflammation and from local vascular complications. Takayasu's arteritis is manifested with clinically nonspecific signs and symptoms of systemic inflammation. Systemic inflammations are common in the early phase of the disease and include general fatigue, weight loss, generalized arthralgias and myalgias, and low-/high-grade fever. Vascular symptoms are rare at presentation, and localized symptoms and signs vary depending on the location of the affected arteries.

- Table 1 summarizes common symptoms and signs in Takayasu's arteritis.
- The systemic stage of Takayasu's arteritis manifests as nonspecific inflammatory symptoms, including the following:
  1. Low-grade fever
  2. Malaise
  3. Weight loss
  4. Fatigue
  5. Arthralgia and myalgia
- The occlusive stage of Takayasu's arteritis may progress to stenosis or aneurysm of the aorta and its primary branches, and may manifest as a variety of clinical signs and symptoms, such as:
  1. Arm or leg claudication, weakness, and numbness
  2. Amaurosis fugax, diplopia, headache, orthostasis, vertigo, memory loss, trouble thinking, or syncope
  3. Angina or myocardial infarction
  4. Vascular bruits of the carotid artery, subclavian artery, and aorta
  5. Discrepancy of blood pressures between the upper extremities, typically of ≥10 mm Hg
  6. Diminished or absent pulses, ischemic ulcerations, or gangrene in advanced disease
  7. Hypertension
  8. Retinopathy
  9. Aortic insufficiency as a result of aortic root dilatation and aneurysm formation
  10. Weakness of the arterial walls may give rise to localized aneurysms/dissection.

ETIOLOGY

- The cause of Takayasu's arteritis is poorly understood. Cell-mediated mechanisms (cytotoxic T cell, macrophage, natural killer cells, and others) are thought to be important to the pathogenesis. Some HLA alleles have been reported to be associated with Takayasu's arteritis in a Japanese patient. Positive associations with HLA-B52, HLA-B39, and HLA-B67 have been identified, suggesting an immunogenetic component.
- Cytokines (such as tumor necrosis factor-alpha [TNF-α], interleukin-6 [IL-6], and interferon-gamma [IFN-γ]), a variety of chemokines, and other proteins (including perforin and matrix metalloproteinases) are involved in induction and amplification of the inflammatory response and tissue injury. Infiltration by inflammatory cells (lymphocytes, macrophages, and multinucleated giant cells) into the vasa vasorum and media of the large elastic arteries (Fig. E1) leads to production of matrix metalloproteinases (MMP), which cause destruction of elastic fibers in the arterial wall, neovascularization, and other inflammatory changes. An intermediate stage, driven in part by TNF-alpha, leads to mucopolysaccharide deposition and proliferation of fibroblasts and smooth muscle cells causing intimal hypertrophy. With chronic disease, inflammatory lesions progress to either thick fibrotic calcified narrowings (≥90% of cases) or aneurysms if fibrosis is insufficient and the arterial wall is instead thinned and dilated (≥25% of cases).
- Infection, in particular, tuberculosis, has been implicated in the pathogenesis of Takayasu's disease with several studies reporting an increased incidence of caseating granulomas in Takayasu patients. Additional immunologic studies lend support to a pathogenic role of CD4 and CD8 T-cells in this patient population.

TABLE 1 Common Symptoms and Signs (%) in Takayasu's Arteritis

Symptom/Sign	Japan (n = 52)	India (n = 106)	China (n = 530)	Korea (n = 129)	USA (n = 60)	Mexico (n = 107)
Fatigue/constitutional	27%	—	—	34%	43%	78%
Weight loss	—	9%	—	11%	20%	22%
Musculoskeletal	6%	5%	—	—	53%	53%
Claudication	13%	—	25%	21%	90%	29%
Headache	31%	44%	—	60%	42%	57%
Visual changes	6%	12%	10%	20%	30%	8%
Syncope/dizziness	40%	26%	14%	36%	35%	13%
Palpitations	23%	19%	—	23%	10%	43%
Dyspnea	21%	26%	11%	42%	—	72%
Carotidynia	21%	—	—	2%	32%	—
Hypertension	33%	77%	60%	40%	35%	72%
Bruit	—	35%	58%	37%	80%	94%
Decreased pulses	62%	—	37%	55%	60%	96%
Asymmetric blood pressure	—	—	—	—	47%	—

From Hochberg MC et al: *Rheumatology,* ed 5, St Louis, 2011, Mosby.

TABLE 2 Pathologic Characteristics of Selected Forms of Vasculitis

	Takayasu's Arteritis	Polyarteritis Nodosa	Wegener's Granulomatosis	Churg-Strauss Syndrome	Henoch-Schönlein Purpura	Cutaneous Leukocytoclastic Angiitis
Vessels involved	Elastic (large) or muscle (medium-sized) arteries	Medium-sized and small muscle arteries	Small arteries and veins; sometimes medium-sized vessels	Small arteries and veins; sometimes medium-sized vessels	Capillaries, venules, arterioles	Capillaries, venules, arterioles
Organ involvement	Aorta, aortic arch and major branches, pulmonary arteries	Skin, peripheral nerve, gastrointestinal tract, other viscera	Upper respiratory tract, lungs, kidneys, skin, eyes	Upper respiratory tract, lungs, heart, peripheral nerves	Skin, joints, gastrointestinal tract, kidneys	Skin, joints
Type of vasculitis and inflammatory cells	Granulomatous with some giant cells; fibrosis in chronic stages	Necrotizing, with mixed cellular infiltrate	Necrotizing or granulomatous (or both); mixed cellular infiltrate plus occasional eosinophils	Necrotizing or granulomatous (or both); prominent eosinophils and other mixed infiltrate	Leukocytoclastic, with some lymphocytes and variable eosinophils; IgA deposits in affected tissues	Leukocytoclastic, with occasional eosinophils

From Goldman L, Schafer AI: *Goldman's Cecil medicine*, ed 24, Philadelphia, 2012, Saunders.

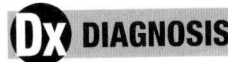 **DIAGNOSIS**

Diagnostic criteria for Takayasu's arteritis were established by the American College of Rheumatology in 1990. A diagnosis is made if at least three of the six criteria are present; this results in a sensitivity of 91% and specificity of 98%. The criteria are:

- Age of disease onset <40 yr
- Claudication of the extremities
- Decreased brachial artery pulse
- Systolic blood pressure difference ≥10 mm Hg between left and right arms
- Bruit over one or both of the subclavian arteries or the abdominal aorta
- Abnormal arteriogram, not related to arteriosclerosis or fibromuscular dysplasia

Recent advances in diagnostic clinical tests, especially imaging modalities, and new biomarkers have improved the accuracy of diagnosis, and new immunosuppressive agents are increasingly applied to this disease.

DIFFERENTIAL DIAGNOSIS

Table 2 describes pathologic characteristics of selected forms of vasculitis. Other causes of inflammatory arteritis must be excluded:

- Temporal arteritis (giant cell arteritis)
- Syphilis
- Tuberculosis
- Systemic lupus erythematosus
- Rheumatoid arthritis
- Buerger's disease
- Behçet's disease
- Marfan syndrome
- Ehlers-Danlos syndrome
- Cogan's syndrome
- Kawasaki disease
- Spondyloarthropathies

WORKUP

Any young patient with findings of absent pulses and loud bruits merits a workup for Takayasu's arteritis. Although there are no blood tests specific for Takayasu's arteritis, the most useful markers for diagnosis of Takayasu's arteritis are nonspecific inflammatory biomarkers including C-reactive protein (CRP) and erythrocyte sedimentation rate (ESR). In most patients, the diagnosis is made by clinical findings and imaging of the arterial branches. Recent advances in imaging modalities allow not only early diagnosis but also detailed assessment of vascular lesions. Contrast-enhanced magnetic resonance angiography (MRA) or CT angiography (CTA) allows noninvasive imaging of the aorta and its major branches and is useful for detecting stenosis and dilatation of the aorta and its major branches. CTA or MRA can also reveal thickening of aortic walls, and this characteristic finding can be a clue for the diagnosis. Three-dimensional reconstructions of the whole aorta and neck arteries using CTA are especially useful for surveying lesions. Ultrasound and FDG-PET are commonly used for diagnosis as well as in serial monitoring of disease activity.

LABORATORY TESTS

- ESR and serum CRP levels are usually elevated, but can be normal even in the setting of active vasculitis.
- A CBC may reveal a normal or elevated white blood cell count as well as anemia.
- Immunologic studies may include elevated immunoglobulins (IgG and IgA) and complement components (C3 and C4).
- Hypercoagulation and increase in platelet aggregation
- Recent studies have attempted to establish a link between elevated levels of various interleukins and other inflammatory markers and active disease.

IMAGING STUDIES

- Imaging of the entire aorta and major branch vessels using angiography, CTA or MRA
- CTA can detect changes in the vessel wall and provide an accurate representation of luminal diameters.

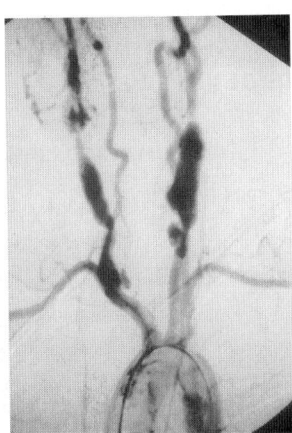

FIG. 2 Angiogram of a child with Takayasu's arteritis that shows massive bilateral carotid dilation, stenosis, and poststenotic dilation. (From Behrman RE: *Nelson textbook of pediatrics*, ed 16, Philadelphia, 2000, Saunders.)

- MRA provides information on vessel lumen and wall thickening, cardiac morphology and function, and myocardial tissue characterization.
- Angiography (Fig. 2) can show the narrowing of the aorta and its branches, aneurysm formation, poststenotic dilation, and the development of any collateral circulation. Angiographic findings are classified into five types:
  1. Type I: lesions that involve only branches of the aortic arch
  2. Type IIa: lesions that involve the ascending aorta, the aortic arch, and its branches
  3. Type IIb: lesions from IIa plus the thoracic descending aorta
  4. Type III: lesions that involve the thoracic descending aorta, abdominal aorta, and/or renal arteries
  5. Type IV: lesions that involve the abdominal aorta and/or renal arteries
  6. Type V: lesions that involve the entire aorta and its branches

- Chest radiography: pathologic changes of the aorta are often visible, with areas of alternating stenosis and dilation seen. Segmental calcification outlining areas of aortic narrowing is characteristic of Takayasu's disease.
- Ultrasound: carotid, thoracic, and abdominal ultrasound are useful adjunctive imaging studies to diagnose the occlusive disease that results from Takayasu's arteritis. The addition of Doppler is helpful to assess blood flow and absent pulses.
- Positron emission tomography using radioisotope fluorodeoxyglucose (FDG-PET) as a marker for tissue with high glucose uptake has shown promising results in terms of specificity and sensitivity.

℞ TREATMENT

- To date there have been no controlled clinical trials evaluating the efficacy or safety of different agents in the acute or chronic treatment of Takayasu's arteritis.
- Treatment of Takayasu's arteritis consists of two parts: induction and maintenance of remission and management of arterial complications.

ACUTE GENERAL Rx

- High-dose glucocorticoids are first-line therapy for suppressing systemic symptoms and stopping disease progression. Prednisone (40-60 mg PO daily or 1 mg/kg/day) can be used for 3 months or intravenous steroids can be administered initially.
- Patients are monitored for symptoms and the ESR is followed. Attempts to taper prednisone can be made with resolution of constitutional symptoms, significant decline in the ESR and C-reactive protein levels, and in accordance with imaging studies.
- The majority of patients require a second agent to achieve and sustain remission with steroid dose reduction. Commonly used second-line agents include methotrexate, azathioprine, and cyclophosphamide.
- Strong observational evidence supports use of TNF-α inhibitors in treating patients refractory to initial therapies and in those patients unable to taper steroids.
- As for TNF-α inhibitors, etanercept, adalimumab and infliximab are available and a majority of patients appear to respond to TNF-α inhibitors.
- Limited experience with other biologic agents, including the IL-6 inhibitor tocilizumab and the B-cell inhibitor rituximab, has shown promising results in certain patient groups.

CHRONIC Rx

Patients with Takayasu's arteritis are monitored closely for signs of relapse and disease complications with clinical assessment, inflammatory biomarkers (e.g., ESR and CRP), and imaging.

Multiple indexes exist for the assessment of disease activity, including the NIH criteria for active disease, the Disease Extent Index-Takayasu (DEI-Tak), and the Indian Takayasu's Arteritis Score (ITAS).

- Treatment of hypertension in these patients can be difficult, especially since typically there is concurrent glucocorticoid therapy and there is the potential for renovascular hypertension. Special monitoring should be employed when using ACE inhibitors due to the high frequency of renal artery stenosis in this population.
- Percutaneous angioplasty or bypass grafts should be considered for irreversible arterial stenoses with severe ischemia (cardiac or cerebral), severe hypertension in renal artery stenosis, or aneurysmal enlargement with risk of rupture. Five-year arterial complication rate after surgical or endovascular revascularization is 44%; the likelihood of complications increases sevenfold when inflammation is present at the time of revascularization.
- There have been positive data regarding drug-eluting stents, and in particular sirolimus-covered stents, likely related to the synergistic effect of its antiproliferative and immunosuppressive properties.
- Studies of coronary artery angioplasty and stenting in this population are limited, due to a high frequency of coronary lesions that are near the ostia; a large number of these patients have surgical interventions as opposed to percutaneous interventions.
- Aortic regurgitation may require valve replacement or repair by surgery, although the need to manipulate friable tissue can lead to complications such as valvular detachment after replacement.

DISPOSITION

- Immunosuppressant therapy may achieve clinical remission.
- No studies have proved that treatment results in regression of stenosis, although there are limited case reports describing the return of pulses with treatment.
- With the addition of a second agent for patients with treatment resistance or relapse, 50% remission has been seen.
- Quality of life is comparable to that of patients with rheumatoid arthritis or ankylosing spondylitis.
- The prognosis and vascular complications of Takayasu's arteritis are improving. Fatal or serious complications have diminished during the past decade.
- Mortality results are mixed, with high rates in reports from Asia and lower rates in studies performed in the United States (2%). In the absence of major complications (MI, stroke, severe HTN, heart failure, aneurysm), 5-year

survival rates reach 95%. In the presence of major complications, 5-year survival is 50% to 70%.

- Death can occur suddenly from a ruptured aneurysm, a myocardial infarction, or a cerebrovascular accident.

Pregnancy may exacerbate cardiovascular complications and can increase the risk for maternal and fetal morbidity and mortality. Heart failure, embolism, and thrombosis are common complications during pregnancy. If a pregnant woman is diagnosed with the disease, oxytocin should be injected to the corpus uteri directly (when needed), and the intravenous route should be avoided. It is important to maintain the mother's blood pressure in a stable range and to avoid fluctuations in hemodynamics.

REFERRAL

Whenever the diagnosis of vasculitis is suspected, a rheumatology consultation is appropriate. Vascular surgery and cardiology consultations are recommended for any evidence of carotid, peripheral, or coronary artery disease or if a large abdominal aneurysm is found.

❗ PEARLS & CONSIDERATIONS

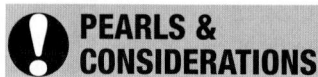

With long-term glucocorticoid use, consider measures to protect against bone loss. Bisphosphonates have been studied prospectively with corticosteroid use in this fashion; remember to ensure adequate dietary calcium and vitamin D intake as well.

COMMENTS

The long-term prognosis of patients with treated Takayasu's disease varies by geography, and 10-yr survival ranges from 80% to 96%.

SUGGESTED READINGS
Available at www.expertconsult.com

RELATED CONTENT
Vasculitis, Systemic (Related Key Topic)

AUTHORS: **HIRO KAWATA, M.D.,** and **PRANAV M. PATEL, M.D.**

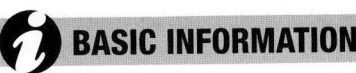 BASIC INFORMATION

DEFINITION

Takotsubo cardiomyopathy, also known as stress cardiomyopathy (SC), is a syndrome characterized by transient systolic and diastolic dysfunction with a characteristic ballooning of the apical and/or mid segments of the left ventricle (LV). It mimics acute myocardial infarction (MI); however, the difference lies in the absence of epicardial coronary occlusion. Typically, but not always, it is preceded by severe illness or intense emotional, physical, or psychological stress. Initially described in the 1990s in Japan, the systolic LV on left angiogram has a distinctive shape similar to a *tako-tsubo* pot with a narrow neck and round bottom, used by fishermen to trap octopi. The variants of SC include apical (81.7%), midventricular (14.6%), basal/reverse takotsubo (2.2%), and focal (1.5%).

SYNONYMS

Stress cardiomyopathy (SC)
Left ventricular apical ballooning syndrome (LVABS)
Ampulla cardiomyopathy
Broken heart syndrome

ICD-10CM CODES
I51.81 Takotsubo syndrome

EPIDEMIOLOGY & DEMOGRAPHICS

INCIDENCE: Uncertain, although increasingly reported. The recurrence rate is 11.4% over 4 years after initial presentation. Occurs mostly in summer; few cases in winter.
PREVALENCE: Studies suggest that it comprises 0.7% to 2.5% of cases presenting with acute coronary syndrome (ACS).
PREDOMINANT SEX AND AGE: Postmenopausal women (90%) are predominantly affected. Mean age 66.8 years
RISK FACTORS: Frequently, but not always, triggered by severe medical illness or intense emotional or physical stress (death of loved ones, domestic abuse, fierce arguments, financial hardships, severe pain, natural disasters, etc.). Chronic stress or distress could also trigger Takotsubo cardiomyopathy. Familial case series have raised the possibility of a genetic predisposition.

PHYSICAL FINDINGS & CLINICAL PRESENTATION

- Acute substernal chest pain, dyspnea, and syncope are the most common presenting complaints (International Takotsubo Registry study).
- Electrocardiographic (ECG) changes or elevated cardiac biomarkers may be noted; can mimic acute coronary syndrome.
- Heart failure (30%), arrhythmias (tachy and brady), cardiogenic shock, and sudden cardiac death are possible complications.

ETIOLOGY

Not well established. The proposed mechanisms for an acute and reversible ventricular dysfunction include the following:
- Coronary spasm: abnormality in endothelial-dependent vasodilation, resulting in excessive vasoconstriction leading to coronary vasculature spasm.
- Microvascular dysfunction/aborted MI: transient coronary occlusion by a fast-dissolving clot with spontaneous reperfusion.
- Abnormal myocardial architecture: increased beta-adrenoreceptors in the apex and increased surface area of the apex due to trabeculations. Fig. 1 depicts the interplay among triggers, pathogenic factors, and predisposing factors in SC.

DIAGNOSIS

Mayo Clinic proposed criteria (2008) for diagnosis of SC: All 4 criteria required to make diagnosis.
- Transient hypokinesis, akinesis, or dyskinesis of the left ventricular midsegments with or without apical involvement (Fig. 2). The regional wall motion abnormalities extend beyond a single epicardial vascular distribution; a stressful trigger is often, but not always, present.
- Absence of obstructive coronary disease or angiographic evidence of acute plaque rupture. If present, the wall motion abnormalities should not be in the distribution of the coronary disease.
- New ECG abnormalities (ST-segment elevation and/or T-wave inversion) or modest elevation in cardiac troponins. Absence of pheochromocytoma or myocarditis.

DIFFERENTIAL DIAGNOSIS

- Acute MI
- Cardiac syndrome X/microvascular angina
- Prinzmetal's angina
- Myocarditis
- Cocaine abuse
- Cerebrovascular disease with Takotsubo-like myocardial dysfunction
- Pheochromocytoma

WORKUP

- A high index of suspicion is required when a postmenopausal woman presents with ACS after intense stress.
- Cardiology consult should be immediately obtained.
- Obstructive coronary artery disease needs to be ruled out.

LABORATORY TESTS

- Cardiac biomarkers (troponin, CK-MB) are often modestly elevated, but typically less than MI.
- Beta natriuretic peptide (BNP) levels are also commonly elevated.

IMAGING STUDIES

- Electrocardiogram findings could include ST elevation, depression, T-wave inversion, QT prolongation, and abnormal Q waves.
- Echocardiography (ECHO) typically shows the characteristic apical ballooning. Contrast ECHO is quite useful to exclude apical thrombus.
- SC is a diagnosis of exclusion. Left heart catheterization should be done to exclude obstructive coronary artery disease.
- Cardiac magnetic resonance imaging can show the absence of late gadolinium enhancement in contrast to MI (subendocardial delayed hyperenhancement).
- Positron emission tomography: some recent studies have demonstrated inverse flow metabolism mismatch in regions with dysfunction.
- Histopathologic findings: interstitial infiltrates of mononuclear lymphocytes and macrophages with fibrosis and contraction band necrosis. Typically, atherosclerotic epicardial artery occlusion and MI is a coagulation necrosis.

COMPLICATIONS

- Approximately 20% have in-hospital complications including heart failure, cardiogenic shock (requiring mechanical support),

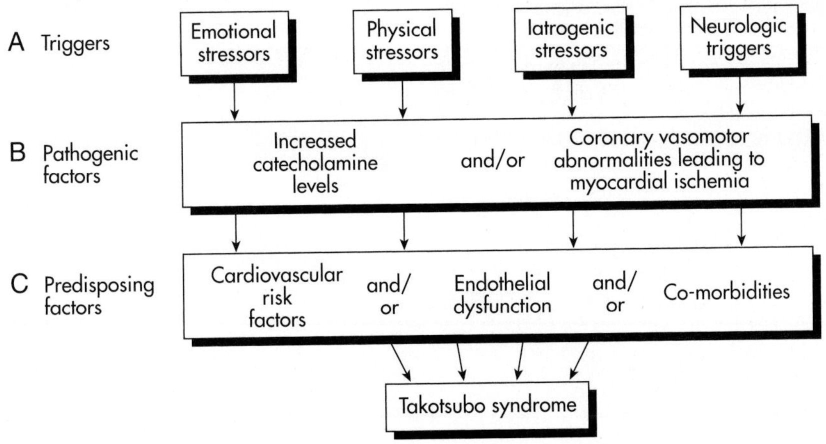

FIG. 1 The interplay among triggers, pathogenic factors, and predisposing factors in Takotsubo disease. (From Pelliccia F et al: Takotsubo syndrome (stress cardiomyopathy): an intriguing clinical condition in search of its identity, *Am J Med* 127:699-704, 2014.)

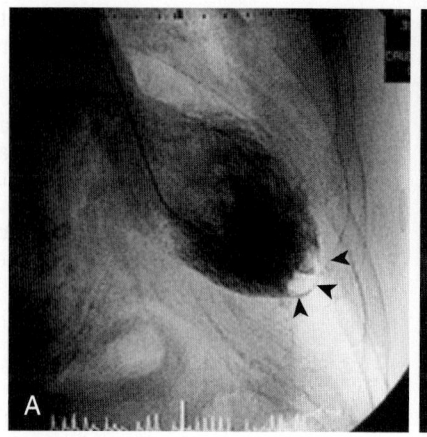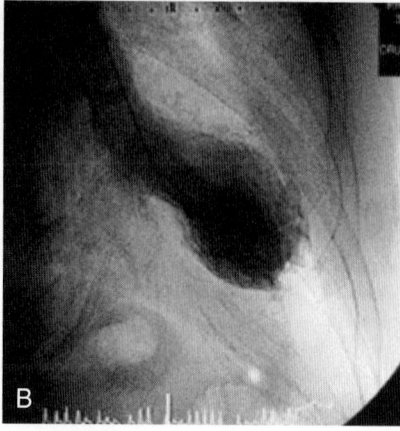

FIG. 2 A and **B,** Left ventriculogram showing apical ballooning characteristic of stress-induced cardiomyopathy. (From Mitsuma W et al: *JACC* 51(1): cover, 2008.)

life-threatening arrhythmias, acute mitral regurgitation, LV outflow tract (LVOT) obstruction, free wall rupture, and death.
- The presence of physical triggers, left ventricular ejection fraction <45%, acute neurologic or psychiatric disease, and first troponin >10× upper limit of normal predict high in-hospital complications.
- A reduced left ventricular ejection fraction is a common finding (86.5%) with recovery seen in days to weeks.
- The prognosis is worse for males.
- Even short-term LV dysfunction can lead to intraventricular thrombus formation (2.5%). This carries a great risk of cerebrovascular accident and distant embolization during the recovery phase.

Rx TREATMENT

There is lack of consensus on the treatment of Takotsubo cardiomyopathy. Initially, patients should be treated for presumptive acute coronary syndrome until this is excluded. Patients should be treated with goal-directed medical therapy for systolic dysfunction (beta-blockers, ACE inhibitors or angiotensin II receptor blockers, aldosterone antagonists).

NONPHARMACOLOGIC THERAPY

Supportive care such as the elimination of the physical or emotional trigger is important.

ACUTE GENERAL Rx

- Patients who are hemodynamically stable should be started on a beta-blocker, ACE inhibitor/angiotensin II receptor blockers, and diuretics if signs of volume overload.
- Patients in shock should get urgent ECHO to determine presence of LVOT obstruction.
- Patients in cardiogenic shock without significant LVOT obstruction may benefit from an intraaortic balloon pump (IABP).
- Patients who are in cardiogenic shock with significant LVOT obstruction may benefit from cautious fluid resuscitation (if no significant pulmonary congestion) and the use of beta-blockers (reduce contractility of basal segments).
- IABP and inotropes will likely worsen the LVOT obstruction.

CHRONIC Rx

- Continued medical therapy and repeat ECHO (in 4-6 wk) to ensure normalization of systolic function (most patients normalize by this time).

- Duration of medical therapy is debatable. A period of 3 to 6 months has been suggested.
- Three months of anticoagulation is suggested if an intraventricular thrombus is detected.
- Recently published data could not find the protective effect of β-blockers in preventing the occurrence or recurrence of SC.
- Ace inhibition is associated with increased survival.

DISPOSITION

Carries a favorable prognosis compared to STEMI or NSTEMI; in-hospital mortality is approximately 2%. The recurrence rate is around 11%.

In a Medicare cohort, patients ≥85 years of age had higher in-hospital, 30-day, 1-year mortality, and 30-day readmission rates; hence, the need for good discharge planning is key.

REFERRAL

Follow-up with a cardiologist is suggested.

❗ PEARLS & CONSIDERATIONS

COMMENTS

- The term *takotsubo* is the Japanese name for an octopus trap (*tako-tsubo*), which has a similar shape of the LV in systole during a left ventriculogram (see Fig. 2).
- Patients with takotsubo cardiomyopathy have a higher prevalence of neurologic or psychiatric disorders than those with an acute coronary syndrome.

PREVENTION

Minimizing stress may reduce incidence but no data to support this.

SUGGESTED READINGS
Available at www.expertconsult.com

AUTHOR: **MAXWELL EYRAM AFARI, M.D.**

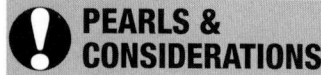

BASIC INFORMATION

DEFINITION

Four species of adult tapeworm (cestodes) may infect humans as the definitive host: *Taenia saginata* (beef tapeworm), *Taenia solium* (pork tapeworm), *Diphyllobothrium latum* (fish tapeworm), and *Hymenolepis nana*. In addition, several tapeworms (*T. solium, T. crassiceps, T. multiceps*) can infect human tissue in their larval form, resulting in cysticercosis, and others infect in their intermediate forms, resulting in hydatid disease (see "Echinococcosis" in Section I). Table 1 describes common cestode parasites of humans, their typical vectors, and their usual symptoms.

SYNONYMS

Cysticercosis (larval infection by *T. solium*)

ICD-10CM CODES
B68.0 *Taenia solium* taeniasis
B68.1 *Taenia saginata* taeniasis
B68.9 Taeniasis unspecified
B70.0 Diphyllobothriasis
B71.9 Cestode infection, unspecified

EPIDEMIOLOGY & DEMOGRAPHICS

INCIDENCE (IN U.S.):
- Diagnosed primarily in immigrants, particularly those from Latin America and Southeast Asia
- Varies widely by country of origin and dietary practices

PREVALENCE (IN U.S.):
- *T. saginata:* <0.1%
- *D. latum:* <0.05%
- *T. solium:* <0.1%
- *H. nana:* sporadic, often in setting of outbreak

PREDOMINANT SEX: Equal sex distribution

PREDOMINANT AGE:
- *T. saginata, T. solium, D. latum:* 20 to 39 yr of age
- *H. nana* in setting of institution outbreaks: children

PHYSICAL FINDINGS & CLINICAL PRESENTATION

Adult worms
1. Attach to bowel mucosa via suckers, hooks, or grooves depending on species
2. Feed and grow, producing digestive/body/reproductive segments called proglottids
3. Cause minimal or no symptoms or sequelae but occasionally can cause nausea, anorexia, or epigastric pain.
Cysticercosis: larval infection by *T. solium*
1. Mass lesions of brain (neurocysticercosis), soft tissue, viscera
2. Neurocysticercosis may cause seizures, hydrocephalus (due to ventricle obstruction)
Prolonged infection with *D. latum*
1. Vitamin B$_{12}$ deficiency
2. Megaloblastic anemia

ETIOLOGY

TAPEWORM:
- Adult worms consist of a head (scolex), neck, and hundreds or thousands of proglottids. Each proglottid contains male and female reproductive organs, including eggs.
- Adult worm resides in small or large bowel; proglottids and eggs are passed in stool.
- *T. saginata* may produce up to 100,000 eggs/proglottid and *T. solium* up to 50,000 eggs/proglottid.
- Eggs are ingested by the animal intermediate host (Fig. 1).
- Eggs hatch into larvae.
- Larvae perforate the host intestinal wall and disseminate into skeletal muscle, brain, viscera.
- Develop into cysticerci (scolex inside a cyst) over several weeks
- Humans eat infected beef *(T. saginata)*, pork *(T. solium)*, or fish *(D. latum)*.
- Larval scolex attaches to intestinal wall and mature into adults within the GI lumen.
- *H. nana* infection is acquired by ingesting eggs in human or rodent feces.

CYSTICERCOSIS:
- Humans ingest eggs of *T. solium* in food contaminated with human feces that contain the eggs.
- Eggs hatch into larvae in gut and cross intestinal wall.
- Larvae disseminate widely through tissues (particularly soft tissue and CNS) forming cystic lesions containing either viable or nonviable larvae.

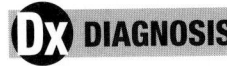 DIAGNOSIS

WORKUP

- Stool examination for eggs or proglottids (tapeworm)
  1. Eggs of *Taenia* spp. cannot be differentiated by microscopy, but the species can be identified through examination of the proglottids in stool.
  2. Eggs of *Taenia* spp. are round and measure 30 to 40 micrometers.
- Cerebral CT scan (neurocysticercosis)
- Serum antibody (neurocysticercosis) with high sensitivity with multiple cysts (94%) but

---

TABLE 1 Common Cestode Parasites of Humans, Their Typical Vectors, and Their Usual Symptoms

Parasite Species	Developmental Stage Found in Humans	Common Name	Transmission Source	Symptoms Associated with Infection
Diphyllobothrium latum	Tapeworm	Fish tapeworm	Plerocercoid cysts in freshwater fish	Usually minimal; with prolonged or heavy infection, vitamin B$_{12}$ deficiency
Hymenolepis nana	Tapeworm, cysticercoids	Dwarf tapeworm	Infected humans	Mild abdominal discomfort
Taenia saginata	Tapeworm	Beef tapeworm	Cysts in beef	Abdominal discomfort, proglottid migration
Taenia solium	Tapeworm	Pork tapeworm	Cysticerci in pork	Minimal
Taenia solium (Cysticercus cellulosae)	Cysticerci	Cysticercosis	Eggs from infected humans	Local inflammation, mass effect; if in central nervous system, seizures, hydrocephalus, arachnoiditis
Echinococcus granulosus	Larval cysts	Hydatid cyst disease	Eggs from infected dogs	Mass effect leading to pain, obstruction of adjacent organs; less commonly, secondary bacterial infection, distal spread of daughter cysts
Echinococcus multilocularis	Larval cysts	Alveolar cyst disease	Eggs from infected canines	Local invasion and mass effect leading to organ dysfunction; distal metastasis possible
Taenia multiceps	Larval cysts	Coenurosis, bladder worm	Eggs from infected dogs	Local inflammation and mass effect
Spirometra mansonoides	Larval cysts	Sparganosis	Cysts from infected copepods, frogs, snakes	Local inflammation and mass effect

Bennett JE et al: *Mandell, Douglas, and Bennett's principles and practice of infectious diseases*, ed 8, Philadelphia, 2015, WB Saunders.

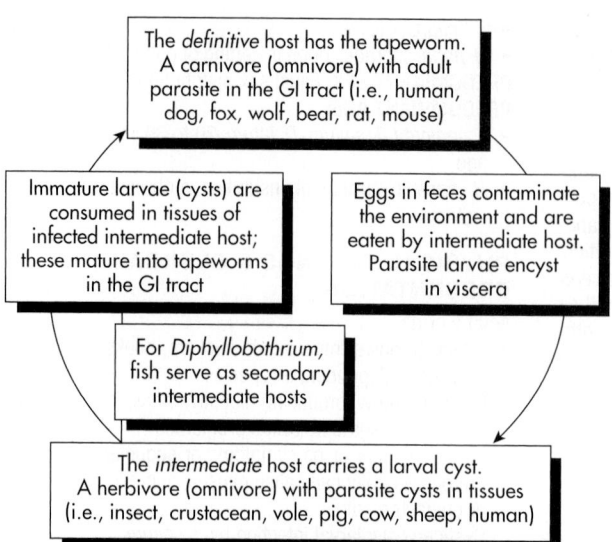

FIG. 1 Cestode parasites alternate larval and adult stages in two different hosts. *GI*, Gastrointestinal. (Bennett JE et al: *Mandell, Douglas, and Bennett's principles and practice of infectious diseases*, ed 8, Philadelphia, 2015, WB Saunders.)

low with a single cyst or calcified cysts (as low as 28%)
- CBC may show eosinophilia

IMAGING STUDIES
- Tapeworm: incidental finding on upper GI series
- Neurocysticercosis:
  1. Cerebral cysts are readily demonstrated by CT scan or MRI.
  2. Calcified lesions are an incidental finding.

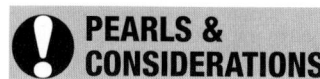 **TREATMENT**

ACUTE GENERAL Rx
- All adults and children with intestinal tapeworm infections should be treated with a single oral dose of praziquantel.
  1. *T. solium:* 5 to 10 mg/kg
  2. *T. saginata:* 5 to 10 mg/kg
  3. *D. latum:* 5 to 10 mg/kg
  4. *H. nana:* 25 mg/kg and a repeat dose 7 to 10 days later if heavy infection
- Praziquantel acts by causing changes in the teguments of the worms, allowing increased permeability to calcium ions, which then accumulate inside worm and cause paralysis.
- Repeat stool screening at 1 and 3 mo to confirm cure.
- Can use purgatives adjunctively to hasten clearance of deceased worms from intestine

- An alternative therapy to praziquantel for tapeworm infections is niclosamide, 2 g PO once for adults and 1 g for children 11 to 34 kg and 1.5 g for children over 34 kg.
- Therapy that may be considered for symptomatic cysticercosis:
  1. May regress spontaneously (i.e., no treatment)
  2. Surgery, especially in cases of ventricular obstruction (neurocysticercosis)
  3. Albendazole 10 to 15 mg/kg/day PO divided in two doses for 8 days
  4. Praziquantel 50 to 100 mg/kg/day PO for 15 to 30 days divided in three doses
  5. Use of steroids in neurocysticercosis may reduce CNS inflammation and increase levels of albendazole in CNS.
- Therapy contraindicated with:
  1. Ocular infections
  2. Cerebral infections in which local inflammation caused by destruction of the parasite may cause significant damage/inflammation
- Adjunctive antiepileptics may be necessary for neurocysticercosis

CHRONIC Rx
- Retreatment if required
- Avoidance of undercooked pork, meat, or fish
- Cysticercosis: proper hand washing, proper disposal of human waste

DISPOSITION
- Neurologic follow-up for patients with neurocysticercosis
- Ophthalmologic follow-up for patients with ocular involvement

REFERRAL
Patients treated for neurocysticercosis should be evaluated by a physician experienced in managing this infection, if possible.

❗ PEARLS & CONSIDERATIONS

COMMENTS
T. solium is the most dangerous of the tapeworms because of the potential for cysticercosis by means of autoinfection.

SUGGESTED READINGS
Available at www.expertconsult.com

RELATED CONTENT
Tapeworm Infection (Patient Information)
Cysticercosis (Related Key Topic)

AUTHOR: **RUSSELL J. MCCULLOH, M.D.**

BASIC INFORMATION

DEFINITION

Tardive dyskinesia (TD) is a syndrome of involuntary movements associated with the long-term use of antipsychotic medication, particularly first-generation antipsychotics. Patients exhibit rapid, repetitive, stereotypic movements that mostly involve the oral, lingual, trunk, and limb areas.

SYNONYMS

Orofacial dyskinesia
Tardive syndrome
TD

ICD-10CM CODES
G24.01 Drug induced subacute dyskinesia

EPIDEMIOLOGY & DEMOGRAPHICS

- The disorder is caused by dopamine-blocking antipsychotics (e.g., haloperidol) and antiemetics (e.g., metoclopramide, prochlorperazine, and promethazine).
- With first-generation antipsychotics, at least 20% of patients are affected with TD, and ~5% are expected to develop TD with each year of antipsychotic treatment.
- The incidence of TD with second-generation antipsychotics is reduced only by about one third. With the increasing use of these medications, TD remains a serious problem.
- Risk increases with the duration of antipsychotic treatment, in female and in elderly patients, in patients with brain damage or dementia, with concurrent anticholinergic use, and in patients with nonschizophrenia diagnoses.

PHYSICAL FINDINGS & CLINICAL PRESENTATION

- TD is classically described as a chronic condition of insidious onset, but symptoms are variable over time and may even improve despite continued antipsychotic therapy.
- The condition typically appears with the reduction or withdrawal of the antipsychotic medications.
- TD classically involves stereotypic movements of the mouth and tongue, including lip smacking and puckering, tongue twisting and protrusion, and facial grimacing.
- TD may also involve slow, writhing movements of the trunk or choreoathetotic movements of the fingers and toes.
- The involuntary mouth movements associated with TD may be suppressed by voluntary actions (e.g., putting food in the mouth, talking).
- Variants of TD with similar treatment include tardive dystonia (e.g., torticollis, blepharospasm), tardive myoclonus, tardive akathisia, and tardive tics.

ETIOLOGY

TD is caused by chronic exposure to dopamine receptor antagonists that is thought to result in the upregulation of dopamine receptors in the basal ganglia as well as damage to striatal cholinergic neurons. Dysfunction of striatal GABAergic interneurons has also been implicated. It has been proposed that dopamine receptor hypersensitivity and neurodegenerative changes might cause altered synaptic plasticity of excitatory synapses onto striatal interneurons, resulting in an imbalance between the direct and indirect basal ganglia pathways.

DIAGNOSIS

DIFFERENTIAL DIAGNOSIS

- Acute extrapyramidal symptoms (e.g., short-term withdrawal dyskinesias, parkinsonism, akathisia)
- Basal ganglia movement disorders (e.g., Huntington's chorea, Tourette's syndrome, levodopa-induced dyskinesia in Parkinson's disease, Wilson's disease)
- Autoimmune diseases (Sydenham's chorea, multiple sclerosis)
- Other causes of neurologic damage (e.g., lead or mercury toxicity, HIV, neurosyphilis, head injury, neurodegeneration from illicit substances)
- Mannerisms associated with disorganized type or catatonic type schizophrenia
- Hyperthyroidism-induced choreoathetosis
- Edentulous dyskinesias and improperly fitted dentures
- Rabbit syndrome (a rare variant of extrapyramidal symptoms with rapid vertical orofacial movements without tongue involvement); may respond to anticholinergic agents

WORKUP

TD is a diagnosis of exclusion, with emphasis on a complete neuropsychiatric and medication history and a thorough physical examination.

IMAGING STUDIES

Standard brain imaging is normal in patients with TD.

TREATMENT

ACUTE GENERAL Rx

- Treatment is predicated on prevention: limit the indications for antipsychotics; use the lowest effective dose; discontinue the drugs, when feasible; and monitor patients frequently. Anticholinergic medications may worsen symptoms.
- Switch to second-generation antipsychotics, if possible.

CHRONIC Rx

- If continued antipsychotic treatment is needed, switching to clozapine or quetiapine is the preferred initial treatment.
- For mild to moderate TD, clonazepam, amantadine, acetazolamide, pyridoxal 5-phosphate, vitamin B_6, and gingko biloba may be helpful, although controlled trial evidence remains weak.
- For severe or persistent TD, tetrabenazine, a centrally acting synaptic dopamine depleter, is becoming a first-line treatment option. The prodrug of an isomer of tetrabenazine, valbenazine, was recently granted breakthrough drug status by the FDA.
- For disabling TD, deep brain stimulation of the subthalamic nucleus or internal globus pallidus seems to provide significant symptom reduction without exacerbation of psychiatric symptoms.
- TD is potentially irreversible in nearly two thirds of patients; thus, patients undergoing long-term treatment with dopamine receptor–blocking medications require frequent monitoring and aggressive management at the onset of TD symptoms.

REFERRAL

Movement disorder specialist consultation if symptoms are severe

PEARLS & CONSIDERATIONS

- After removal of the causative medication, symptoms of tardive dyskinesia can take months to resolve or may become permanent (higher risk in elderly, female sex, prolonged use, and higher dose of causative medication).
- First-generation antipsychotics should be resumed to treat TD in the absence of active psychosis only as a last resort for persistent, disabling, and treatment-resistant TD.
- Avoid anticholinergic medications (e.g., benztropine), which may exacerbate TD symptoms.
- Recent evidence suggests increased overall mortality among patients with TD, which highlights the need for referral for more aggressive specialized interventions.

SUGGESTED READINGS

Available at www.expertconsult.com

RELATED CONTENT

Tardive Dyskinesia (Patient Information)

AUTHOR: **JOHN A. GRAY, M.D., PH.D.**

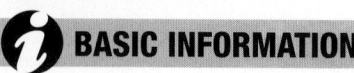

BASIC INFORMATION

DEFINITION

Temporomandibular joint (TMJ) syndrome refers to a group of disorders leading to symptoms of the TMJ. Temporomandibular joint disorders (TMD) can be classified as intraarticular (within the joint) or extraarticular (involving the surrounding musculature). The TMJ is a diarthrotic joint, meaning neither joint can move independently of the other because each is hinged at both ends. The joint is a true synovial joint capable of two actions of movement: translational and rotational. The articulating surfaces are the glenoid fossa of the temporal bone and the condylar process of the mandible, with the articular disk interposed between the two.

SYNONYMS

Temporomandibular dysfunction
Painful temporomandibular joint
TMJ
Temporomandibular disorders (TMD)

ICD-10CM CODES
N26.60 Temporomandibular joint disorder, unspecified

EPIDEMIOLOGY & DEMOGRAPHICS

- 15% to 25% of the population have symptoms of TMJ disorders at some point in their lives.
- Females are affected more often than males (up to 4:1 ratio).
- Occurs between the second and fourth decades of life.
- Usually unilateral, affecting either side with equal frequency.

PHYSICAL FINDINGS & CLINICAL PRESENTATION:

- Symptoms may appear or be worse during stressful life events.
  - Often unilateral pain in the muscles of mastication, usually described as a "dull" ache
  - Otalgia
  - Odontalgia
  - Headaches (frontal, temporal, retroorbital)
  - Tinnitus
  - Dizziness
  - Clicking or popping sounds with movement of the TMJ
  - Joint locking
- Physical exam findings
  - Tender to palpation over TMJ in external auditory meatus or preauricular region anterior to tragus
  - Limited jaw opening or trismus
  - Clicking or popping of TMJs with joint mobility
  - Lateral deviation of mandible
  - TMJ crepitus

ETIOLOGY

- Myofascial pain-dysfunction syndrome: the most common cause of TMJ syndrome and results from teeth grinding and clenching the jaw (bruxism)
- Internal TMJ derangement: abnormal connection of the articular disk to the mandibular condyle as a result of disk displacement or chronic dislocations

- Degenerative joint disease
- Rheumatoid arthritis
- Gouty arthritis
- Pseudogout
- Ankylosing spondylitis
- Trauma (i.e., fractures)
- Congenital defects (i.e., aplasia, hypoplasia)
- Prior surgery (orthodontic, intraarticular steroid injection)
- Tumors

DIAGNOSIS

Can be made based on history and physical examination in most cases.

DIFFERENTIAL DIAGNOSIS

Includes the list provided above. Myofascial pain-dysfunction syndrome, internal TMJ derangement, and degenerative joint disease represent >90% of all causes of TMJ syndrome. Others not mentioned include dental problems such as dental caries, loss of posterior teeth support, and Eagle's syndrome (stylohyoid syndrome, carotidynia, and trigeminal neuralgia). Alternative diagnoses such as otitis, mastoiditis, salivary gland disorders, migraine headache, sinusitis, postherpetic neuralgia, trigeminal neuralgia, glossopharyngeal neuralgia, and giant cell arteritis should always be excluded.

WORKUP

The diagnosis is based largely on history and physical examination findings. Radiographic imaging evaluation is used to exclude anatomic or systemic causes of disease when conservative management has failed.

LABORATORY TESTS

Laboratory examination is often not needed but may be helpful in ruling out certain conditions. CBC if infection is suspected. Rheumatoid factor if rheumatoid arthritis is suspected.

IMAGING STUDIES

- Plain radiographs: the most common views are the panoramic, transorbital, and transpharyngeal in both opened and closed positions.
- CT scan is highly accurate in diagnosing osseous derangements of the TMJ.
- MRI is the procedure of choice and has replaced arthrography in cases of disabling pain or if locking occurs. It is used to determine disk position and morphology along with degenerative bony changes.
- Arthrography is helpful in looking for meniscus involvement but is seldom performed anymore, as it is more invasive and less accurate than MRI for TMJ imaging.

TREATMENT

NONPHARMACOLOGIC THERAPY

- Soft diet to rest the muscles of mastication
- Heat 15 to 20 min 4 to 6 times per day
- Massage of the masseter and temporalis muscles
- Formed splints or bite appliances to reduce compression of retrodiscal tissue (Fig. E1)
- Range-of-motion exercises

- Cognitive-behavioral therapy and biofeedback have been shown to reduce pain.
- Acupuncture

ACUTE GENERAL Rx

- Nonsteroidal antiinflammatory drugs: ibuprofen 800 PO mg tid PRN or naproxen 500 mg PO bid prn, titrated to relieve symptoms
- Muscle relaxants or benzodiazepines at bedtime: diazepam 2.5 to 5 mg PO tid PRN or amitriptyline 5 to 100 mg PO qd PRN
- In degenerative joint disease of the TMJ, intraarticular steroid injection can be tried
- Botulism toxin injections into the masticatory muscles
- Arthrocentesis with joint lavage and lysis of adhesions (Fig. E2)
- In patients with pain and clicking in the TMJ that is unresponsive to nonsurgical treatment, the disc should be repositioned arthroscopically or by open surgery (discoplasty) (see "Chronic Rx")

CHRONIC Rx

- Most of the above treatments are used for myofascial pain-dysfunction syndrome; however, they can be applied to other causes of TMJ syndrome. Surgery is usually a measure of last resort in patients who do not respond to nonpharmacologic and acute general treatment. Absolute indications for surgical therapy include neoplasms, growth abnormalities, and joint ankylosis.
- Surgical procedures include:
  1. Meniscoplasty
  2. Meniscectomy
  3. Subcondylar osteotomy
  4. TMJ reconstruction

DISPOSITION

The course depends on the underlying etiology; however, less than 5% of adults with temporomandibular symptoms develop chronic symptoms.

REFERRAL

All patients with TMJ syndrome refractory to conservative nonpharmacologic and acute therapy should be referred to a periodontist, oral maxillofacial surgeon, or ear-nose-throat surgeon.

PEARLS & CONSIDERATIONS

Patients with rheumatoid arthritis involving the TMJ usually have bilateral involvement.

COMMENTS

Frequently, emotional stress initiates the myofascial pain-dysfunction, which accounts for 85% of all cases of TMJ syndrome.

SUGGESTED READING
Available at www.expertconsult.com

RELATED CONTENT

Temporomandibular Joint (TMJ) Syndrome (Patient Information)

AUTHORS: **RYAN W. ZUZEK, M.D., DOUGLAS BURTT, M.D.,** and **LOUIS INSALACO, M.D.**

BASIC INFORMATION

DEFINITION

Testicular neoplasms are primary cancers originating in a testis.

SYNONYMS

Testis tumor
Testicular neoplasms

ICD-10CM CODES

C62.00 Malignant neoplasm of unspecified undescended testis
C62.01 Malignant neoplasm of undescended right testis
C62.02 Malignant neoplasm of undescended left testis
C62.10 Malignant neoplasm of unspecified descended testis
C62.11 Malignant neoplasm of descended right testis
C62.12 Malignant neoplasm of descended left testis
D40.10 Neoplasm of uncertain behavior of unspecified testis
D40.11 Neoplasm of uncertain behavior of right testis
D40.12 Neoplasm of uncertain behavior of left testis

EPIDEMIOLOGY & DEMOGRAPHICS

INCIDENCE: 5.4 cases per 100,000 men annually. White men have the highest incidence at 6.3 cases/100,000 men. Testicular cancer is the most common cancer diagnosis in men between 15 and 35 yr. The incidence has been gradually increasing since 1975.

PREVALENCE: 1% to 2% of all cancers in males.

PREDOMINANT AGE: Can occur in any age but most common in young adults; average age for embryonal cell carcinoma: 30 yr; average age for seminoma: 36 yr.

PHYSICAL FINDINGS & CLINICAL PRESENTATION

- Testicular cancer typically presents as a painless mass in the testis. Any mass within the testicle should be considered cancer until proven otherwise. It may be found by the patient, who brings it to the attention of a physician, or it may be found by a physician on a routine examination.
- Symptoms other than scrotal or testicular swelling are typically absent unless the cancer has metastasized (10% of patients at diagnosis). Occasionally a patient may report scrotal fullness or heaviness. About 10% of patients present with acute pain. Back pain secondary to enlarged retroperitoneal lymph nodes can occur. Gynecomastia from tumors that secrete beta-human chorionic gonadotropin (hCG) is found in 5% of men with testicular cancer.
- Testicular palpation should be performed with two hands. Transillumination may distinguish a solid mass (e.g., cancer) and a fluid-filled lesion (e.g., hydrocele or spermatocele). The mass is nontender; indeed, it is less sensitive than a normal testicle.

ETIOLOGY, CLASSIFICATION, & PATHOLOGY

- Cryptorchidism (undescended testes) is a major risk factor even if corrected by orchiopexy; however, treatment of undescended testis before puberty decreases the risk of testicular cancer from fivefold to twofold. Other risk factors are family history (risk is 8 to 10 times as high in a brother of a person with testicular cancer), genetic disorders (Down's syndrome, testicular dysgenesis syndrome), Klinefelter's syndrome, infertility, tobacco use, and white race (risk is highest among whites and lowest among blacks).
- Classification: testicular cancers can be classified as pure seminomas or nonseminomatous germ cell tumors (embryonic carcinoma, choriocarcinoma, yolk sac carcinoma, teratoma).
- Pathology: germ cell tumors account for >95% of testicular cancers.

Cell Type	Frequency (%)
Seminoma	42
Embryonal cell carcinoma	26
Teratocarcinoma	26
Teratoma	5
Choriocarcinoma	1

- Other rare types:
  1. Yolk sac carcinoma.
  2. Mixed germ cell tumors.
  3. Carcinoid tumor.
  4. Sertoli cell tumors.
  5. Leydig cell tumors.
  6. Lymphoma.
  7. Metastatic cancer to the testes.
- TNM staging system for testicular cancer
  1. T_0: No apparent primary.
  2. T_1: Testis only (excludes rete testis).
  3. T_2: Beyond the tunica albuginea.
  4. T_3: Rete testis or epididymal involvement.
  5. T_4: Spermatic cord.
     1. Spermatic cord.
     2. Scrotum.
- N_0: No nodal involvement.
- N_1: Ipsilateral regional nodal involvement.
- N_2: Contralateral or bilateral abdominal or groin nodes.
- N_3: Palpable abdominal nodes or fixed groin nodes.
- N_4: Juxtaregional nodes.
- M_0: No distant metastases.
- M_1: Distant metastases present.

The clinical stages consist of stage I, with tumor confined to the testis; stage II, with positive regional lymph nodes; and stage III, with metastases. Fig. 1 shows the clinical staging of testicular cancer.

DIAGNOSIS

DIFFERENTIAL DIAGNOSIS

- Spermatocele.
- Varicocele.
- Hydrocele.
- Epididymitis/orchitis.
- Epidermoid cyst of the testicle.
- Epididymis tumors.
- Inguinal hernia.
- Hematocele or testicular rupture.
- Torsion of testicular appendage.
- Skin cancer.

WORKUP

Physical examination, laboratory tests, and imaging studies (see Section III, "Testicular Mass"). A radical inguinal orchiectomy is diagnostic and therapeutic. Immunohistochemical analysis is used to determine the histologic composition of the tumor. Staging involves CT of chest, abdomen, and pelvis and measurement of beta subunit of human chorionic gonadotropins (β-hCG), alpha-fetoprotein, and lactate dehydrogenase.

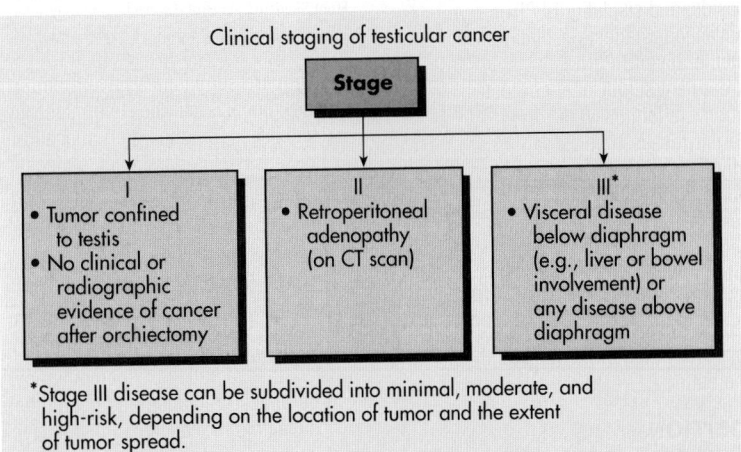

FIG. 1 Clinical Staging of Testicular Cancer. The AJCC TNM staging system is less commonly used, because it is based upon histologic evaluation of the orchidectomy specimen and retroperitoneal periaortic lymph node dissection. Because the latter may not be performed in every patient, the clinical staging system is generally more practical. (From Skarin AT. *Atlas of diagnostic oncology,* ed 4, St Louis, 2010, Mosby.)

LABORATORY TESTS

- Serum hCG: elevated in approximately 20% of patients with pure seminomas.
- Serum alpha-fetoprotein (AFP): elevated in nonseminoma tumors, never elevated in patients with pure seminomas.
  One or both of these tumor markers will be elevated in 70% of cases of testicular cancer.
- Serum lactate dehydrogenase (LDH) level: elevated with rapid turnover of malignant cells.
- Testicular biopsy contraindicated.

IMAGING STUDIES

- Testicular ultrasound.
- CT scan of chest, pelvis, and abdomen.
- MRI of the brain in patients with neurologic symptoms.
- PET scan is not recommended (frequent false positives).

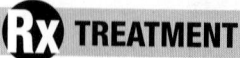 **TREATMENT**

- Seminoma
  1. Stage I: Most patients with clinical stage 1 are cured with orchiectomy. Radical orchiectomy plus one cycle of single-agent carboplatin chemotherapy or radiation therapy (RT) to the paraaortic lymph nodes was the standard of treatment for many years but has been eliminated in many instances and most patients are treated with active surveillance post-orchiectomy. More relapses are associated with surveillance (20% vs. 4% with radiotherapy or chemotherapy), but long-term survival approaches 100% irrespective of initial option chosen.[1]
  2. Stage IIA or IIB: RT or cisplatin-based chemotherapy (e.g., cisplatin, bleomycin, etoposide).
- Nonseminoma
  1. Stage IA: radical orchiectomy plus nerve-sparing retroperitoneal lymph node dissection (RPLND).
  2. Stage IB: Same as stage IA plus two cycles of chemotherapy (bleomycin, etoposide, and cisplatin [BEP]).
  3. Advanced stages: cisplatin-based chemotherapy or RPLND.
- Posttreatment surveillance for testicular cancer survivors (annually).
  1. Fertility assessment.
  2. Physical examination and skin examination (increased risk of dysplastic nevi).
  3. Testicular examination (3%-4% risk of second testicular cancer).
  4. Serum tumor markers (hCG, AFP).
  5. Abdominal and pelvic CT every 3 to 4 months for 2 years, every 6 to 12 months in third and fourth year, and annually thereafter.

DISPOSITION

- The overall cure for testicular cancer is >95% (80% for metastatic disease). Patients

[1]Hanna NH, Einhorn LH: Testicular cancer, discoveries and updates, *N Engl J Med* 371:2005-2016, 2014.

TABLE 1 International Germ Cell Consensus Criteria for Testicular Cancer

Nonseminoma	Seminoma
Good Prognosis	
Testis/retroperitoneal primary	Any primary site
And	*And*
No nonpulmonary visceral metastases	No nonpulmonary visceral metastases
And	*And*
Good markers—all of	Normal AFP, any hCG, any LDH
• AFP < 1000 ng/ml and	
• hCG < 5000 IU/L (1000 ng/mL) and	
• LDH < 1.5 × upper limit of normal	
58% of nonseminomas	90% of seminomas
5-year PFS 89%	5-year PFS 82%
5-year survival 92%	5-year survival 86%
Intermediate Prognosis	
Testis/retroperitoneal primary	Any primary site
And	*And*
No nonpulmonary visceral metastases	Nonpulmonary visceral metastases
And	*And*
Intermediate markers—any of	Normal AFP, any hCG, any LDH
• AFP ≥ 1000 and ≤ 10,000 ng/ml or	
• hCG ≥ 5000 IU/L and ≤ 50,000 IU/L or	
• LDH ≥ 1.5 × normal and ≤ 10 × normal	
28% of nonseminomas	10% of seminomas
5-year PFS 75%	5-year PFS 67%
5-year survival 80%	5-year survival 72%
Poor Prognosis	
Mediastinal primary	No patients classified as poor prognosis
Or	
Nonpulmonary visceral metastases	
Or	
Poor markers—any of	
• AFP > 10,000 ng/ml or	
• hCG > 50,000 IU/L (10,000 ng/mL) or	
• LDH > 10 × upper limit of normal	
16% of nonseminomas	
5-year PFS 41%	
5-year survival 48%	

AFP, α-fetoprotein; *hCG*, human chorionic gonadotrophin; *LDH*, lactate dehydrogenase; *PFS*, progression-free survival.
From Skarin AT: *Atlas of diagnostic oncology*, ed 4, St Louis, 2010, Mosby.

with pure seminomas have a better prognosis. Prognosis can be determined by criteria established by the International Germ Cell Consensus Criteria (Table 1). Because treatment produces favorable outcomes even in advanced stages, the U.S. Preventive Services Task Force recommends against screening asymptomatic men for testicular cancer. There is also an increased risk for metabolic syndrome (insulin resistance, hypertension, dyslipidemia, abdominal obesity) after radiation or chemotherapy.

- Therapeutic radiation and chemotherapy are risk factors for cancers of thyroid, lymphoma, kidney, pancreas, stomach, and leukemia. There is also an increased risk for metabolic syndrome (insulin resistance, hypertension, dyslipidemia, abdominal obesity) after radiation or chemotherapy.

 EVIDENCE

Available at www.expertconsult.com

SUGGESTED READING

Available at www.expertconsult.com

RELATED CONTENT

Testicular Cancer (Patient Information)

AUTHOR: **BHARTI RATHORE, M.D.**

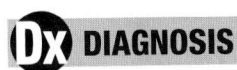 BASIC INFORMATION

DEFINITION

Testicular torsion is a twisting of the spermatic cord leading to cessation of testicular blood flow, ischemia, and infarction if left untreated.

SYNONYMS

Spermatic cord torsion

ICD-10CM CODES
N44.03 Torsion of testis, unspecified

EPIDEMIOLOGY & DEMOGRAPHICS

INCIDENCE: Affects 1 in 4000 males <25 yr
PREDOMINANT AGE: Two thirds of all cases occur between the ages of 12 and 18 yr but may occur at any age, including antenatally.

PHYSICAL FINDINGS & CLINICAL PRESENTATION

- Typical sequence is sudden onset of hemiscrotal pain, then swelling, nausea, and vomiting without fever or urinary symptoms.
- Physical examination may reveal a tender firm testis, high-riding testis, horizontal lie of testis, absent cremasteric reflex, and no pain with elevation of testis. Absence of the cremasteric reflex (stroking or pinching the medial thigh causing contraction of cremaster muscle and elevation of testis) is the most sensitive physical finding.
- Painless testicular swelling occurs in 10%.
- One out of three patients reports previous episodes of spontaneously remitting scrotal pain.
- In the neonate, testicular torsion should be presumed in patients with a painless, discolored hemiscrotal swelling.
- In rare cases, torsion may involve an undescended testicle. In such situations an empty hemiscrotum is palpated with a tender lump in the inguinal area.

ETIOLOGY

- There are three types of testicular torsion (Fig. E1): extravaginal, caused by nonadherence of the tunica vaginalis to the dartos layer; intravaginal torsion, caused by malrotation of the spermatic cord with the tunica vaginalis; and torsion of the testis below the epididymis. Intravaginal torsion accounts for 90% of cases.
- Torsion usually occurs in the absence of any precipitating events. Trauma accounts for <10% of cases.

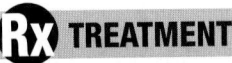 DIAGNOSIS

Diagnosis made mainly by clinical suspicion (Table 1). Color Doppler ultrasound evaluation or a nuclear testicular scan (Fig. E2) may help with diagnosis. Ultrasonography shows absent or decreased blood flow; scintigraphy reveals decreased perfusion on symptomatic side.

DIFFERENTIAL DIAGNOSIS

See Fig. E3.

- Torsion of the testicular appendages (appendix testis)
- Testicular tumor
- Epididymitis
- Incarcerated inguinoscrotal hernia
- Orchitis
- Spermatocele
- Hydrocele, varicocele

WORKUP

The diagnosis is usually based on history and physical examination.

IMAGING STUDIES

- Radionuclide scrotal scanning (technetium-99m): cold testicle (Fig. E2)
- Doppler ultrasonic stethoscope (Doppler flowmetry) (Fig. E4)

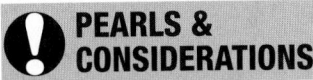 TREATMENT

Surgical derotation of the spermatic cord followed by bilateral testicular fixation with nonabsorbable sutures. If affected testis is nonviable, orchiectomy of affected testis and orchiopexy of contralateral side are performed. Attempts at manual detorsion should not delay surgical consultation.

PROGNOSIS

- The degree of ischemia depends on the duration of torsion and the degree of rotation of the spermatic cord.
- There is an 80% testicular salvage rate if detorsion occurs within 12 hr of onset.
- After 24 hr, irreversible testicular infarction is expected.
- Because contralateral testes can be affected (immunologic process), if treatment delayed and blood flow does not return after detorsion, some recommend orchiectomy of the infarcted testicle.

! PEARLS & CONSIDERATIONS

- Manual detorsion by external rotation of the testis toward the thigh can be attempted for adolescent intravaginal torsion if an operating facility is not readily available.
- Extravaginal torsion is diagnosed in the newborn. Intravaginal torsion can occur at any age but is usually diagnosed in males ages 12 to 18 yr.

RELATED CONTENT

Testicular Torsion (Patient Information)

AUTHOR: **FRED F. FERRI, M.D.**

TABLE 1 Differentiation of Testicular Torsion, Epididymitis, and Appendage Torsion

	Testicular Torsion	Epididymitis*	Appendage Torsion
Historical Features			
Age	Peak incidence in neonatal and adolescent groups but may occur at any age	Primarily adolescents and adults but may occur at any age	Typically prepubertal boys
Risk factors	Undescended testicle (neonate), rapid increase in testicular size (adolescent), failure of previous orchiopexy	Sexual activity or promiscuity, GU anomalies, GU instrumentation	Presence of appendages
Pain onset	Sudden	Gradual	Gradual or sudden
Previous episodes of similar pain	Possible (spontaneous detorsion)	Unlikely	Occasional
History of trauma	Possible	Possible	Possible
Nausea, vomiting	More likely	Less likely	Less likely
Dysuria	Less likely	More likely	Less likely
Physical Findings			
Fever	Less likely	More likely, particularly with advanced disease (epididymoorchitis)	Less likely
Location of swelling and tenderness	Testicle, progressing to diffuse hemiscrotal involvement	Epididymis, progressing to diffuse hemiscrotal involvement	Localized to head of affected testicle or epididymis
Cremasteric reflex	Testicular torsion less likely if present	May be present or absent	May be present or absent
Testicle position	High-riding testicle, transverse alignment	Normal position, vertical alignment	Normal position, vertical alignment
Pyuria	Less likely	More likely	Less likely

GU, Genitourinary.
*Including epididymoorchitis.
From Adams JG et al: *Emergency medicine, clinical essentials*, ed 2, Philadelphia, 2013, Elsevier.

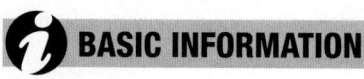

BASIC INFORMATION

DEFINITION

Thalassemias are a heterogeneous group of disorders of hemoglobin synthesis that have in common a deficient synthesis of one or more of the polypeptide chains of the normal human hemoglobin, resulting in a quantitative abnormality of the hemoglobin thus produced. Table 1 describes the various thalassemias. There are no qualitative changes such as those encountered in the hemoglobinopathies (e.g., sickle cell disease).

SYNONYMS

Mediterranean anemia
Cooley's anemia

ICD-10CM CODES
D56   Thalassemia
D56.0 Alpha thalassemia
D56.1 Beta thalassemia
D56.2 Delta-beta thalassemia
D56.3 Thalassemia trait
D56.4 Hereditary persistence of fetal
       hemoglobin (HPFH)
D56.8 Other thalassemias
D56.9 Thalassemia, unspecified

EPIDEMIOLOGY & DEMOGRAPHICS

- Thalassemia is among the most common genetic disorder worldwide. Approximately 4.83% of the world's population carry globin variants, including 1.67% of the population that are heterozygous for alpha-thalassemia and beta-thalassemia.
- The highest concentration of alpha-thalassemia is found in Southeast Asia and the African west coast. For example, the prevalence is 5% to 10% in Thailand. It is also common among blacks, with a prevalence of approximately 5%.
- The worldwide prevalence of beta-thalassemia is approximately 3%; in certain regions of Italy and Greece the prevalence reaches 15% to 30%. This high prevalence can be found in Americans of Italian or Greek descent.
- The distribution of thalassemia in Europe and Africa parallels that of malaria, suggesting that thalassemic persons are more resistant to the parasite, thus permitting evolutionary survival advantage.

CLASSIFICATION

Beta-thalassemia:
- Beta (+) thalassemia (suboptimal beta-globin synthesis)
- Beta (o) thalassemia (total absence of beta-globin synthesis)
- Delta-beta-thalassemia (total absence of both delta-globin and beta-globin synthesis)
- Lepore hemoglobin (synthesis of small amounts of fused delta-beta-globin and total absence of delta- and beta-globin)
- Hereditary persistence of fetal hemoglobin (HPHF) (increased hemoglobin F synthesis and reduced or absence of delta- and beta-globin)
Alpha-thalassemia:
- Silent carrier (three alpha-globin genes present)
- Alpha-thalassemia trait (two alpha-globin genes present)
- Hemoglobin H disease (one alpha-globin gene present)
- Hydrops fetalis (no alpha-globin gene)
- Hemoglobin constant sprint (elongated alpha-globin chain)
Thalassemic hemoglobinopathies:
- Hb Terre Haute, Hb Quong Sze, HbE, Hb Knossos

PHYSICAL FINDINGS & CLINICAL PRESENTATION

Beta-thalassemia:
- Heterozygous beta-thalassemia (thalassemia minor): no or mild anemia, microcytosis and hypochromia, mild hemolysis manifested by slight reticulocytosis and splenomegaly

---

TABLE 1   The thalassemias

Thalassemia	Globin Genotype	Features	Expression	Hemoglobin Analysis
α-Thalassemia				
1 gene deletion	-,α/α,α	Normal	Normal	Newborn: Bart's 1%-2%
2 gene deletion trait	-,α/-,α -, -/α,α	Microcytosis, mild hypochromasia	Normal, mild anemia	Newborn: Bart's 5%-10%
3 gene deletion hemoglobin H	-,-/-,α	Microcytosis, hypochromic	Mild anemia, transfusions not required	Newborn: Bart's 20%-30%
2 gene deletion 1 Constant Spring	-,-/α,α^Constant Spring	Microcytosis, hypochromic	Moderate to severe anemia, transfusion, splenectomy	2%-3% Constant Spring, 10%-15% hemoglobin H
4 gene deletion	-,-/-,-	Anisocytosis, poikilocytosis	Hydrops fetalis	Newborn: 89%-90% Bart's with Gower 1 and 2 and Portland
Nondeletional	α,α/α,α^variant	Microcytosis, mild anemia	Normal	1%-2% variant hemoglobin
β-Thalassemia				
β⁰ or β⁺ heterozygote: trait	β⁰/A, β⁺/A	Variable microcytosis	Normal	Elevated A_2, variable elevation of F
β⁰-Thalassemia	β⁰/β⁰, β⁺/β⁰, E/β⁰	Microcytosis, nucleated RBC	Transfusion dependent	F 98% and A_2 2% E 30%-40%
β⁺-Thalassemia severe	β⁺/β⁺	Microcytosis, nucleated RBC	Transfusion dependent/thalassemia intermedia	F 70%-95%, A_2 2%, trace A
Silent	β⁺/A	Microcytosis	Normal with only microcytosis	A_2 3.3%-3.5%
β⁺/β⁺	Hypochromic, microcytic	Mild to moderate anemia	A_2 2%-5%, F 10%-30%	
Dominant (rare)	B⁰/A	Microcytosis, abnormal RBCs	Moderately severe anemia, splenomegaly	Elevated F and A_2
d-Thalassemia	A/A	Normal	Normal	A_2 absent
(dβ)⁰-Thalassemia	(dβ)⁰/A	Hypochromic	Mild anemia	F 5%-20%
(dβ)⁺-Thalassemia Lepore	β^Lepore/A	Microcytosis	Mild anemia	Lepore 8%-20%
Lepore	β^Lepore/β^Lepore	Microcytic, hypochromic	Thalassemia intermedia	F 80%, Lepore 20%
γdβ-Thalassemia	(γ^Adβ)⁰/A	Microcytosis, microcytic, hypochromic	Moderate anemia, splenomegaly, homozygote: thalassemia intermedia	Decreased F and A_2 compared with db-thalassemia
γ-Thalassemia	(γ^Aγ^G)⁰/A	Microcytosis	Insignificant unless homozygote	Decreased F
Hereditary Persistence of Fetal Hemoglobin				
Deletional	A/A	Microcytic	Mild anemia	F 100% homozygotes
Nondeletional	A/A	Normal	Normal	F 20%-40%

From Kliegman RM et al: *Nelson textbook of pediatrics*, ed 19, Philadelphia, 2011, Saunders.

- Homozygous beta-thalassemia (thalassemia major): intense hemolytic anemia; transfusion dependency; bone deformities (skull and long bones); hepatomegaly; splenomegaly; iron overload leading to cardiomyopathy, diabetes mellitus, and hypogonadism; growth retardation; pigment gallstones; susceptibility to infection
- Thalassemia intermedia caused by combination of beta- and alpha-thalassemia or beta-thalassemia and Hb Lepore: resembles thalassemia major but is milder
  Alpha-thalassemia:
- Silent carrier: no symptoms.
- Alpha-thalassemia trait: microcytosis only.
- Hemoglobin H disease: moderately severe hemolysis with microcytosis and splenomegaly.
- The loss of all four alpha-globin genes is incompatible with life (stillbirth of hydropic fetus). Note: Pregnancies with hydrops fetalis are associated with a high incidence of toxemia.

ETIOLOGY

- Beta-thalassemia: it is caused by more than 200 point mutations and, rarely, by deletions. The reduction of beta-globin synthesis results in redundant alpha-globin chains (Heinz bodies), which are cytotoxic and cause intramedullary hemolysis and ineffective erythropoiesis. The pathophysiology of beta-thalassemia is illustrated in Fig. E1. Fetal hemoglobin may be increased.
- Alpha-thalassemia: duplication of the α-globin chain on chromosome 16 results in 4α-globin genes ($\alpha\alpha/\alpha\alpha$); α-thalassemia results from deletion of one or more of these. There are several mutations that can result in insufficient amounts of alpha-globin available for combination with non–alpha-globins.

Dx DIAGNOSIS

LABORATORY TESTS
Beta-thalassemia:
- Microcytosis (mean cell volume: 55-80 fL)
- Normal red blood cell (RBC) distribution width index (RDW)

- Smear: nucleated RBCs, anisocytosis, poikilocytosis, polychromatophilia, Pappenheimer and Howell-Jolly bodies
- Hemoglobin electrophoresis: absent or reduced hemoglobin A, increased fetal hemoglobin, variable increase in the amount of hemoglobin A_2
- Markers of hemolysis: elevated indirect bilirubin and lactate dehydrogenase, decreased haptoglobin
  Alpha-thalassemia:
- Microcytosis in the absence of iron deficiency
- Hemoglobin electrophoresis normal except for the presence of hemoglobin H in hemoglobin H disease (Table 2)

Rx TREATMENT

- Thalassemia minor: no treatment, but avoid iron administration for incorrect diagnosis of iron deficiency.
- Beta-thalassemia major (and hemoglobin H disease):
1 Transfusion therapy: monthly erythrocyte transfusions should be initiated for hemoglobin levels less than 7 g/dL (70 g/L). Guidelines for transfusion therapy recommend administration of 10 to 15 ml/kg of RBC every 2 to 4 weeks to maintain the pretransfusion hemoglobin level above 9 to 10.5 g/dl. Use of leukoreduced RBCs that have been stored for less than 7 to 10 days is preferred. Use of first-degree relatives as blood donors should be avoided.
2 Chelation therapy: Transfusion hemosiderosis is the major cause of late morbidity and mortality in patients with thalassemia major. Each unit of packed RBCs contains approximately 250 mg of iron. Chelation of iron can be accomplished with desferrioxamine (by IV or subcutaneous administration, 8-12 hr nightly, 5-6 days a week at a dose of 2-6 g/day with a portable infusion pump). Deferiprone, an oral chelating agent, can be used as a second-line treatment of iron overload caused by blood transfusions (transfusional hemosiderosis).

3 Splenectomy for hypersplenism if present.
4 Bone marrow transplantation. Allogenic hematopoietic stem cell transplantation (HSCT) should be considered in patients with severe forms before the onset of end-organ damage. Although hematopoietic stem cell transplantation is the only curative approach for thalassemia, it has been limited by the high cost and scarcity of human leukocyte antigen–matched donors. Before transplantation, it is necessary to administer myeloablative regimens to eradicate the endogenous thalassemic bone marrow. Commonly used agents are hydroxyurea, azathioprine, fludarabine, busulfan, and cyclophosphamide.
5 Hydroxyurea may increase the level of hemoglobin F.

! PEARLS & CONSIDERATIONS

- Polymerase chain reaction can be used to detect point mutations or deletions in chorionic villous samples, enabling first-trimester, DNA-based testing for thalassemia.
- Preimplantation genetic diagnosis can be extended to human leukocyte antigen typing on embryonic biopsies, allowing the selection of an embryo that is not affected by thalassemia and that may also serve as a stem cell donor for a previously affected child within the same family.

SUGGESTED READING
Available at www.expertconsult.com

AUTHOR: **BHARTI RATHORE, M.D.**

Diseases and Disorders

I

TABLE 2 Distinguishing Laboratory Features of α- and β-Thalassemias

Diagnosis*	BCB Prep†	HbA₂‡	HbF	HbH	Hb Barts in Newborn§
Normal	–	nl	nl	nl	–
α-Thalassemia	+	nl	nl	nl or ↑	+
β-Thalassemia	–	nl or ↑	nl or ↑	nl	–

Hb, Hemoglobin type; *nl*, normal; ↑, increased; –, negative; +, positive. Can be negative for a one α-globin deletion (silent carrier), for compound heterozygotes with combined α- and β-thalassemia, and other hemoglobinopathies (e.g., HbE or HbS). Table shows typical results; exceptions occur.
*All forms of α-or β-thalassemia are pooled; specific results will vary.
†Brilliant cresyl blue (*BCB*) or inclusion body prep. Results vary by lab, but this can be done semiquantitatively. This can be negative when a one α-globin deletion (silent carrier) is present. This assay is unreliable in the presence of other hemoglobins (e.g., HbS or HbE). This can be negative when α- and β-thalassemia are simultaneously present.
‡HbA₂ results vary depending on laboratory method.
§Hb Barts increases with the degree of α-thalassemia.
From Fuhrman: *Pediatric critical care*, ed 4. Philadelphia, 2010, Elsevier.

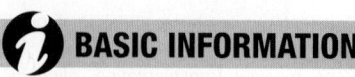

BASIC INFORMATION

DEFINITION

Thoracic outlet syndrome (TOS) describes a condition producing upper extremity symptoms believed to result from neurovascular compression at the thoracic outlet (Fig. 1). Three types are described on the basis of point of compression: (1) cervical rib and scalenus syndrome, in which abnormal scalene muscles or the presence of a cervical rib may cause compression; (2) costo-clavicular syndrome, in which compression may occur under the clavicle; and (3) hyperabduction syndrome, in which compression may occur in the subcoracoid area. The compression occurs in three anatomical structures: arteries, veins, and nerves. TOS usually is caused by a combination of two factors: (1) having abnormal anatomy that creates compression in the thoracic outlet, (2) having some injury at the thoracic outlet.

- Neurogenic TOS: Caused by compression of brachial nerve plexus
- Arterial TOS: Caused by subclavian artery compression
- Venous TOS: Caused by compression of sub-clavian vein

SYNONYMS

TOS

ICD-10CM CODES
G54.0 Brachial plexus disorders

EPIDEMIOLOGY & DEMOGRAPHICS

PREVALENCE: TOS is an uncommon disorder. Varies from source to source; presence of cervical ribs in 0.5% to 1% of population (50% bilateral), but most are asymptomatic. Approximately 90% of all TOS disorders are neurogenic, and the remaining 10% are arterial or venous.

PREDOMINANT SEX: Females affected more often than males (ratio of 3.5:1)

PREDOMINANT AGE: Rare in those aged <20 yr

PHYSICAL FINDINGS & CLINICAL PRESENTATION

- Symptoms and signs are related to the degree of involvement of each of the various structures at the level of the first rib.
- True venous or arterial involvement is not common.
- Diagnosis is most often used in the consideration of neural pain affecting the arm, which suggests involvement of the brachial plexus.
  1. Arterial compression: pallor, paresthesias, diminished pulses, coolness, Raynaud's phenomenon, digital gangrene, supracla-vicular bruit or mass, and stroke
  2. Venous compression: edema and pain, thrombosis causing superficial venous dilation in the shoulder area
  3. Neurologic compression: Pain and/or par-esthesia of neck, shoulder region, arm or hand, depending on the root involved with difficulty; intrinsic weakness and diminished sensation on examination

4. Possible supraclavicular tenderness
5. Provocative tests (Adson's, Wright's): may reproduce pain but are of disputed use-fulness

ETIOLOGY

- Congenital cervical rib or fibrous extension of cervical rib (Fig. 2)
- Abnormal scalene muscle insertion
- Drooping of shoulder girdle from generalized hypotonia or trauma
- Narrowed costoclavicular interval as a result of downward and backward pressure on shoulder (sometimes seen in individuals who carry heavy backpacks), poor posturing, pregnancy
- Acute venous thrombosis with exercise (effort thrombosis)
- Bony abnormalities of first rib
- Abnormal fibromuscular bands
- Malunion of clavicle fracture

DIAGNOSIS

DIFFERENTIAL DIAGNOSIS

- Carpal tunnel syndrome
- Cervical radiculopathy

- Brachial neuritis
- Ulnar nerve compression (cubital tunnel syndrome)
- Complex regional pain syndrome
- Superior sulcus tumor

WORKUP

Fig. 3 describes a diagnostic algorithm for thoracic outlet syndrome. Except for venous or arterial pathology, no ancillary diagnostic tests are reliable for diagnostic confirmation.

IMAGING STUDIES

- Electromyography, nerve conduction velocity studies to rule out carpal tunnel syndrome, cervical radiculopathy
- Ultrasound for initial evaluation for arterial or venous thoracic outlet syndrome
- Cervical spine radiographs to rule out cervical disk disease
- Chest radiograph to rule out lung tumor
- Computed tomography (CT) for detailed anatomical relationship of vascular structure to surrounding muscles and bones
- Contrast-enhanced magnetic angiography can be very useful in assessing vessel imaging while using provocative arm positions

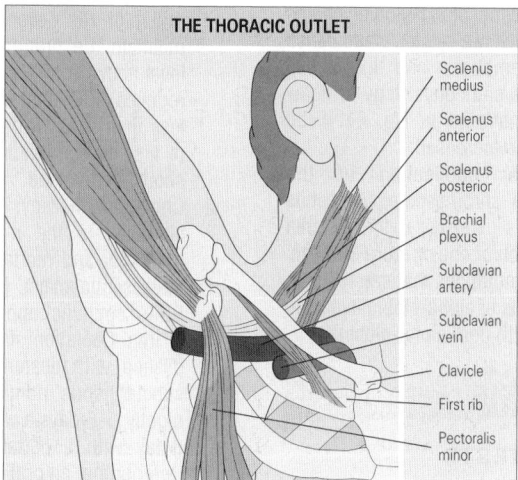

FIG. 1 The thoracic outlet. Three narrow channels of the outlet include the scalene triangle, the costo-clavicular passage, and the pectoralis minor attachment at the coracoid process. (From Hochberg MC et al: *Rheumatology,* ed 5, St Louis, 2011, Mosby.)

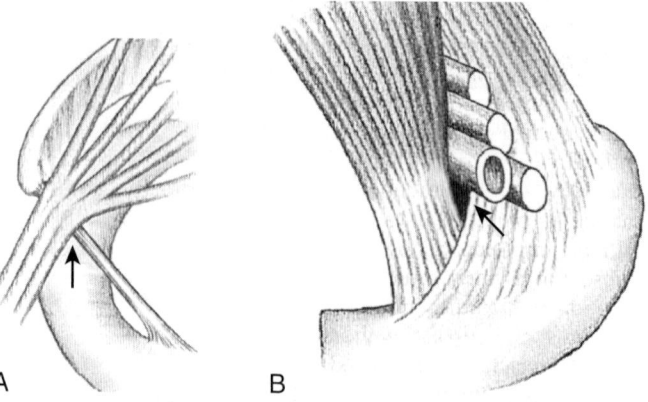

FIG. 2 A, Compression caused by a cervical rib *(arrow).* **B,** Abnormal scalene muscle insertions that may cause compression at the cervicobrachial region *(arrow).* (From Mercier LR: *Practical orthopedics,* ed 5, St Louis, 2000, Mosby.)

Diseases
and Disorders

I

- Arteriography or venography (Fig. 4) can be used for dynamic studies while performing upper extremity maneuvers and also performing thrombolysis, if needed

℞ TREATMENT

ACUTE GENERAL Rx

- Sling for pain relief
- Physical therapy modalities plus shoulder girdle–strengthening exercises
- Postural reeducation
- Nonsteroidal antiinflammatory drugs
- Muscle relaxants

CHRONIC Rx

Surgical treatment is indicated:
- After failure of physical therapy
- With complications such as thrombosis, aneurysms
- With neurologic compressions
- With sympathetic cervical rib

Surgical options
- Thoracic outlet decompression
- Cervical rib resection
- Thoracic sympathetectomy
- Vascular repair
- Catheter-directed thrombolysis

DISPOSITION

- Nonsurgical treatment: often successful for patients with pain as the primary symptom
- Complications of surgical treatment include transient dysesthesia, venous injury, arterial injuries, or brachial plexus injuries.

REFERRAL

For vascular surgery consultation when venous or arterial impairment is present

❗ PEARLS & CONSIDERATIONS

COMMENTS

- True thoracic outlet syndrome is probably an uncommon condition.
- Diagnosis is often used to describe a wide variety of clinical symptoms.
- Considerable disagreement exists regarding the frequency of this disorder.

RELATED CONTENT

Thoracic Outlet Syndrome (Patient Information)

AUTHOR: **HISASHI TSUKADA, M.D., PH.D.**

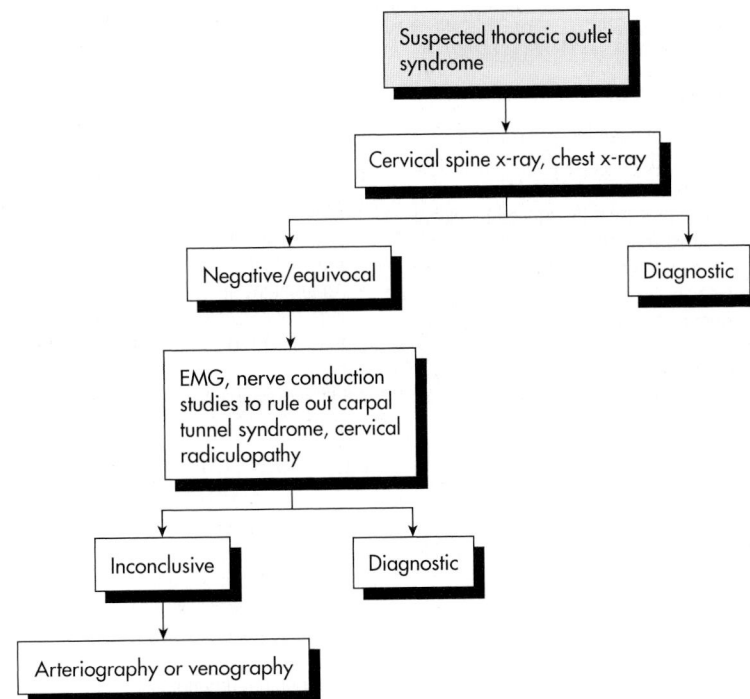

FIG. 3 **Thoracic outlet syndrome.** *EMG*, Electromyogram.

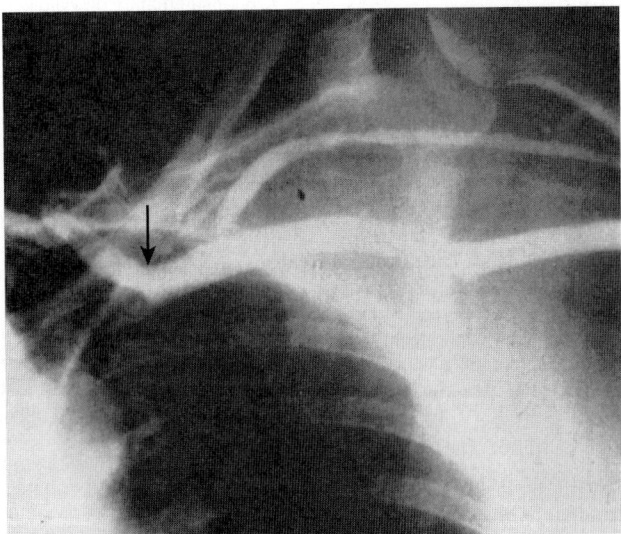

FIG. 4 Phlebogram showing total occlusion (*arrow*) with minimal collateral circulation of the left subclavian vein resulting from thoracic outlet compression. At operation, no thrombus was present in the vein, and obstruction was relieved by removing the first rib. (From Sellke FW et al.: *Sabiston & Spencer surgery of the chest*, ed 9, Philadelphia, 2016, Elsevier.)

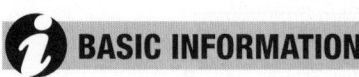

BASIC INFORMATION

DEFINITION

Thrombocytosis is defined by an elevated platelet count (>450,000/ml) in peripheral blood. It is caused by overproduction of platelets (reactive thrombocytosis), or it may be caused by clonal expansion of megakaryocytes (clonal thrombocytosis). Reactive thrombocytosis is driven by excessive cytokines induced by various stimuli, such as trauma or inflammation. The latter is defined as chronic myeloproliferative disorders (CMPD), of which four subgroups are well characterized: chronic myelogenous leukemia (CML), polycythemia vera (PV), primary myelofibrosis (PMF), and essential thrombocythemia (ET). In addition, platelet count can be spuriously elevated in some conditions (see differential diagnosis). Extreme thrombocytosis is defined as platelet count >1 million/ml.

SYNONYMS

Thrombocythemia
Essential thrombocythemia
ET

ICD-10CM CODES

D47.3 Essential (hemorrhagic)
        thrombocythemia
D75.89 Other specified diseases of blood
        and blood-forming organs
D75.9 Disease of blood and blood-forming
        organs, unspecified
D77   Other disorders of blood and blood-
        forming organs in diseases classified
        elsewhere

EPIDEMIOLOGY & DEMOGRAPHICS

Reactive thrombocytosis is much more frequent than clonal thrombocytosis (70% vs. 22% in one series).
Epidemiology for essential thrombocythemia:
INCIDENCE: 2.5 cases/100,000 population/yr
PREVALENCE: Estimated as 24 cases/100,000 population
PREDOMINANT SEX AND AGE: The median age at diagnosis is 60 yr. Female/male ratio is 2:1.

PHYSICAL FINDINGS & CLINICAL PRESENTATION

- Regardless of the cause, a high platelet count may be associated with vasomotor symptoms such as headache, visual disturbances, dizziness, atypical chest pain, acral dysesthesia, and erythromelalgia.
- Thrombotic and bleeding complications can occur.
- Symptoms and complications are much more likely to occur in association with autonomous thrombocytosis than reactive thrombocytosis.
- The degree of thrombocytosis does not predict the likelihood of autonomous thrombocytosis, and does not generally correlate to the risk of thrombosis.
- Splenomegaly is common with CMPD.

- Coexistent leukocytosis and erythrocytosis are common with CML and PV.
- Disease transformation from ET to PV, PMF, and acute myeloid leukemia (AML) is uncommon.

ETIOLOGY

- Essential thrombocythemia, a myeloproliferative neoplasm, is a clonal disorder of a multipotent hematopoietic progenitor cell.
- Abnormality in JAK2-STAT pathway (including *JAK2, CALR,* and *MPL* gene mutations) may play a role in pathogenesis of CMPD.

DIAGNOSIS

DIFFERENTIAL DIAGNOSIS

- Spurious thrombocytosis
  1. Mixed cryoglobulinemia
  2. Circulating cytoplasmic fragments in patients with leukemia, lymphoma, or severe hemolysis or burns can be counted as platelets
- Reactive thrombocytosis
  1. Benign hematologic disorders
  2. Acute hemorrhage, iron deficiency anemia, hemolytic anemia
  3. Chronic infection, such as tuberculosis
  4. Acute and chronic inflammatory disorders
  5. Rheumatologic disorders
  6. Inflammatory bowel disease
  7. Celiac disease
  8. Functional and surgical asplenia
  9. Tissue damage
  10. Trauma, thermal burn
  11. Myocardial infarction
  12. Acute pancreatitis
  13. Recent surgery
  14. Renal failure, nephrotic syndrome
  15. Exercise
  16. Medications, such as vincristine, epinephrine

- Clonal thrombocytosis
  1. CML
  2. PV
  3. PMF
  4. Myelodysplastic syndrome (5q-syndrome)
  5. AML with inv(3), t(3;3)
  6. Essential thrombocytosis (Box 1)

WORKUP

- Comprehensive history and physical examination to exclude many of the common causes of reactive thrombocytosis: history and physical examination suggestive of acute blood loss, iron deficiency, acute or chronic infection/inflammation, medication use, asplenia, malignancy, and trauma should be evaluated. Fig. E1 describes a diagnostic algorithm for thrombocytosis. The diagnosis of ET is evolving, but it classically requires platelet counts >450 × 10³/ml on two separate occasions >4 weeks apart, absence of Philadelphia chromosome, and exclusion of secondary causes of thrombocytosis.
- Repeat CBC with peripheral blood smear and bone marrow biopsy (Figs. 2 and E3) to exclude spurious thrombocytosis.

LABORATORY TESTS

- CBC with peripheral blood smear: Howell-Jolly bodies and target cells are present in patients with asplenia; nucleated RBC, teardrop RBC and WBC precursors in patients with PMF
- Serum ferritin level: low ferritin level suggests iron deficiency
- Serum C-reactive protein (CRP), ESR, and plasma fibrinogen: nonspecific markers of infection or inflammation
- Philadelphia chromosome or BCR-ABL rearrangement: positive in CML
- Serum erythropoietin assay: low to normal in PV and ET

BOX 1 World Health Organization Diagnostic Criteria for Essential Thrombocythemia

Diagnosis requires that all of the following criteria be met:
- Sustained platelet count ≥450 × 10⁹/L[1]
- Bone marrow biopsy specimen showing proliferation mainly of the megakaryocytic lineage, with increased numbers of enlarged, mature megakaryocytes; no significant increase or left shift of neutrophil granulopoiesis or erythropoiesis
- Failure to meet the WHO criteria for polycythemia vera,[2] primary myelofibrosis,[3] BCR-ABL1–positive chronic myelogenous leukemia,[4] myelodysplastic syndrome,[5] or other myeloid neoplasms
- Demonstration of JAK2 V617F or other clonal marker; or, in the absence of JAK2 V617F, no evidence of reactive thrombocytosis[6]

[1] Sustained during the workup process.
[2] Requires the failure of iron replacement therapy to increase the hemoglobin level to the polycythemia vera range in the presence of decreased serum ferritin. Exclusion of polycythemia vera is based on hemoglobin and hematocrit levels; red cell mass measurement is not required.
[3] Requires the absence of relevant reticulin fibrosis, collagen fibrosis, peripheral blood leukoerythroblastosis, or markedly hypercellular marrow accompanied by megakaryocyte morphology typical for primary myelofibrosis—small to large megakaryocytes with an aberrant nuclear-to-cytoplasmic ratio and hyperchromatic, bulbous, or irregularly folded nuclei and dense clustering.
[4] Requires the absence of BCR-ABL1.
[5] Requires the absence of dyserythropoiesis and dysgranulopoiesis.
[6] Causes of reactive thrombocytosis include iron deficiency, splenectomy, surgery, infection, inflammation, connective tissue disease, metastatic cancer, and lymphoproliferative disorders.
From Swerdlow SH et al (eds): *WHO classification of tumours of haematopoietic and lymphoid tissues,* Lyon, France, 2008, IARC Press.

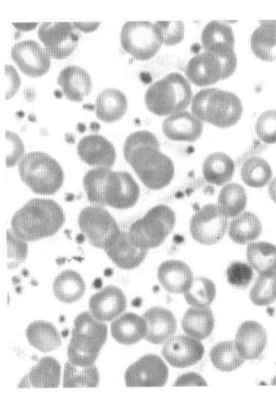

FIG. 2 Essential thrombocythemia: peripheral blood smear. The peripheral blood smear in ET shows a marked thrombocytosis with anisocytosis (varying sizes) of the platelets. (From Hoffman R et al: *Hematology: basic principles and practice,* ed 5, Philadelphia, 2009, Churchill Livingstone.)

- JAK2 mutation analysis: PV and ET; JAK2 mutation is found in 95% to 99% of patient with PV, in 40% to 60% of patients with PMF, and in about 50% of patients with ET
- MPL and CALR mutation analysis: Frequency is reported as 4% and 15% to 32%, respectively, in ET
  - These mutations are associated with differences in prognosis and risk of thrombosis and are mutually exclusive.
- Bone marrow chromosome analysis: 5q-syndrome and other myelodysplastic syndrome, CML.
- Bone marrow exam in ET may show clusters of abnormal megakaryocytes and increased reticulin fibrosis (see Fig. E3).

℞ TREATMENT

No therapies are known to alter survival or leukemic transformation in ET. Reactive thrombocytosis has been rarely associated with thrombosis or bleeding and generally does not require specific therapy.

ACUTE GENERAL Rx

- Vasomotor symptoms easily manageable with low-dose aspirin (<100 mg/day)
- Bleeding
  1. Discontinue any platelet antiaggregating agent, such as aspirin or nonsteroidal anti-inflammatory agents.
  2. Evaluate for disseminated intravascular coagulopathy and coagulation factor

deficiency. Acquired factor V deficiency is occasionally present in association with autonomous thrombocytosis. In that case, treat with fresh frozen plasma infusion.
  3. In case of extreme thrombocytosis (platelet count generally >1,000,000/uL [1000×10⁹/L]), acquired von Willebrand disease may occur. Immediate definitive therapy with a platelet-lowering agent is essential in this instance. Platelet pheresis should be reserved for cases of acute thrombosis or bleeding.
- Thrombosis
  1. Arterial or venous thrombosis occurs in 20% to 30% of patients.
  2. If the platelet count is >800,000/m³, platelet apheresis coupled with a platelet-lowering agent should be considered with the goal of platelet count <400,000/mm³.
  3. Anticoagulant therapy for 3 months to indefinite based on the presence or absence of additional thrombophilic defects.

CHRONIC Rx

Treatment strategies for ET are based on the presence or absence of risk factors for thrombosis. Smoking cessation and obesity management should be discussed with all patients with ET. In low-risk patients (age <60 yr, no history of thrombosis or hemorrhage, platelet count <1 million/mL), observation may be adequate. Treatment with low-dose aspirin is indicated in low-risk patients with vasomotor symptoms or with other indications for aspirin use. The cytoreductive therapy along with low-dose aspirin therapy is indicated in high-risk patients (age >60 yr and/or with previous history of thrombosis).

- Low-dose aspirin (81 mg/day) may be safe and effective in preventing vascular events. It is also effective in preventing recurrent vascular events in high-risk patients and in treating the vasomotor symptoms.
- Cytoreductive therapy
  1. Hydroxyurea (HU) versus anagrelide: HU plus aspirin is suggested to be safer and more effective than anagrelide plus aspirin in regard to thrombosis, bleeding, and transformation to PMF at 5 yr in a randomized trial. Monitor liver function tests and the degree of neutropenia or anemia with HU therapy.

  2. The incidence of leukemic conversion in patients with ET treated with HU alone is reported as <1%. Interferon alpha may be effective for controlling platelet count in patients failing treatment with HU.

DISPOSITION

Although long survival is expected in patients with ET, it is inferior to the sex- and age-matched U.S. population.

An International Prognostic Score for Essential thrombocythemia (IPSET) was proposed by International Working Group on Myelofibrosis Research and Treatment based on age, WBC count, and history of thromboembolism at diagnosis.

REFERRAL

Refer to hematologist/oncologist when platelet count is consistently elevated >450,000/mm³ without causes for reactive thrombocytosis.

❗ PEARLS & CONSIDERATION

COMMENTS

- Some patients with clinically apparent ET have Philadelphia chromosome or BCR-ABL rearrangement, even in the absence of other features of CML. It is suggested that it should be tested in all ET patients due to its potential therapeutic implications.
- The risk of bleeding with aspirin use in patients with ET is increased when the platelet count is >1 million/ml.
- A recent trial has shown complete hematologic response in patients with ET treated with the telomerase inhibitor imetelstat, although long-term responses and side effects are still unclear.

PATIENT & FAMILY EDUCATION

Smoking cessation is encouraged in both patients with ET and reactive thrombocytosis.

SUGGESTED READINGS
Available at www.expertconsult.com

AUTHORS: **VICTORIA BROWN, M.D.,** and **JOHN L. REAGAN, M.D.**

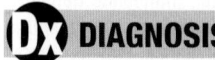

BASIC INFORMATION

DEFINITION

Superficial venous thrombophlebitis (SVT) is an inflammation of a vein with subsequent secondary thrombus formation. SVT most frequently involves superficial veins of the leg, but any superficial vein can be affected. SVT has been reported to occur in 125,000 people in the United States per year; however, the actual incidence is likely far greater. SVT is not always a benign condition. SVT should be regarded as the superficial venous manifestation of a systemic process known as venous thromboembolism (DVT, PE).

SYNONYMS

SVT
Superficial phlebitis
Superficial suppurative thrombophlebitis
Suppurative thrombophlebitis

ICD-10CM CODES
I80.00 Phlebitis and thrombophlebitis of superficial vessels of unspecified lower extremity
I80.8   Phlebitis and thrombophlebitis of other sites
I80.9   Phlebitis and thrombophlebitis of unspecified site

EPIDEMIOLOGY & DEMOGRAPHICS

- Approximately 30% to 45% of patients diagnosed with SVT are men with an average age of 54 yr.
- Approximately 55% to 70% of patients diagnosed with SVT are women with an average age of 58 yr.
- The overall recurrence of SVT is 18% over an average observation period of 15 mo, equally involving varicose and nonvaricose veins.
- The lifetime incidence of SVT in those with untreated varicose veins has been estimated at 25% to 50%.

PHYSICAL FINDINGS & CLINICAL PRESENTATION

- Subcutaneous vein is palpable as a tender cord or "wormlike" mass with increased warmth and erythema.
- Induration, redness, and tenderness are localized along the course of the vein. This linear appearance rather than circular appearance is useful to distinguish thrombophlebitis from other conditions (cellulitis, erythema nodosum).
- There is some swelling of the overlying skin and subcutaneous tissue but without generalized edema of the limb.
- Low-grade fever may be present.

ETIOLOGY

- In the lower extremity, 70% of SVT occurs in patients with varicose veins, with the great saphenous vein being most commonly involved (60%-80%).
- Intravenous catheters and infusion of caustic drugs are the most common cause of upper-extremity SVT.

- Malignancy
- Pregnancy/puerperium
- Hypercoagulable states
- Previous
- DVT/SVT
- OCP (oral contraceptive pill)/HRT (hormone replacement therapy)

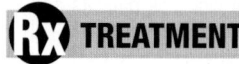

DIAGNOSIS

DIFFERENTIAL DIAGNOSIS

- Lymphangitis
- Cellulitis
- Erythema nodosum
- Panniculitis
- Acute lipodermatosclerosis

WORKUP

The clinical investigation includes not only the local findings but also the presence of varicose veins with or without the stigmata of chronic venous insufficiency. Today, duplex ultrasound is the most important additional diagnostic tool.

IMAGING STUDIES

- Duplex ultrasound offers the advantage of being inexpensive, noninvasive, and repeatable for follow-up examination.
- Ultrasonography confirms the diagnosis, shows the location of the thrombus and its location regarding the saphenofemoral and/or saphenopopliteal junctions.
- Ultrasound examination of patients with SVT has revealed that a concomitant DVT can exist in 15% to 20%.
- In up to 25% of these patients, the DVT may not be contiguous with the SVT and may be found in the contralateral leg.
- Therefore bilateral duplex exam is recommended in all cases of SVT that involve the main trunk of the great saphenous vein (GSV) or small saphenous vein (SSV).

TREATMENT

NONPHARMACOLOGIC THERAPY

- Warm, moist compresses
- Do not restrict activity. Immediate mobilization with walking exercises.

ACUTE GENERAL Rx

- Treatment guidelines for SVT are not well established because of the lack of controlled clinical trials. In general, the primary goal of management should be to prevent thrombus extension and the risk of venous thromboembolism. All other therapy is directed at patient comfort.
- In patients with migratory SVT, recurrent SVT, or SVT without varicose veins, the underlying condition should be investigated and treatment directed accordingly.
- The most common cause of upper-extremity SVT is an intravenous catheter. Treatment starts with removal of the cannula and application of warm compresses. The resultant lump may persist for months. No anticoagulant therapy is required.

- In patients with lower-extremity SVT in a varicose vein branch, control of pain with analgesics and the use of gradient compression stockings are usually sufficient. Patients are encouraged to continue their usual daily activities.
- Many investigators favor systemic anticoagulation when there is superficial thrombosis of 5 cm or more in length, the thrombus is within 1 cm of the saphenous junctions, or more than 5 cm of the saphenous trunk is involved, as shown by duplex ultrasonography.
- The 2012 American College of Chest Physicians guidelines recommend the use of fondaparinux (1 mg/kg/day) for 45 days over no anticoagulation in patients with lower-extremity SVT within 1 cm of the saphenofemoral or saphenopopliteal junction.
- In the case of patients with varicose veins secondary to saphenous vein reflux, a catheter vein ablation procedure should be performed only after the acute SVT episode is over in order to avoid the thromboembolic complications induced by such procedures.

DISPOSITION

Clinical improvement within 10 to 14 days

REFERRAL

Referral to vascular surgeon or phlebologist with vascular lab

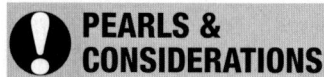

PEARLS & CONSIDERATIONS

SUPERFICIAL SUPPURATIVE THROMBOPHLEBITIS

- Superficial suppurative thrombophlebitis is associated with an intravenous catheter or multiple puncture sites secondary to IV drug abuse and is located primarily in the upper extremity.
- Clinical presentation is similar to that of non-suppurative SVT but with associated fever, leukocytosis, and/or septicemia.
- Most cases of intravenous catheter sepsis are not complicated by suppurative thrombophlebitis; local IV catheter site infections occur in about 7% of cases and septicemia is found in only 1 of every 400 IV catheterizations.
- The incidence of peripheral vein suppurative thrombophlebitis is highest in patients with specific risk factors such as burns, steroids, and IV drug abuse.
- Treatment consists of antibiotics with adequate coverage of gram-negative rods and *Staphylococcus aureus*, including MRSA. Initial empirical treatment is with IV vancomycin 1 g q12h *plus* ceftriaxone 1 g IV q24h. Alternative regimen consists of daptomycin 6 mg/kg IV q 12h *plus* ceftriaxone 1 g IV q24h.

SUGGESTED READINGS

Available at www.expertconsult.com

RELATED CONTENT

Thrombophlebitis (Patient Information)

AUTHOR: **FRANK G. FORT, M.D.**

BASIC INFORMATION

DEFINITION

Thrombotic thrombocytopenic purpura (TTP) is a rare disorder characterized by thrombocytopenia (often accompanied by purpura) and microangiopathic hemolytic anemia; neurologic impairment, renal dysfunction, and fever may also be present.

SYNONYMS

TTP

ICD-10CM CODES
M31.1 Thrombotic microangiopathy

EPIDEMIOLOGY & DEMOGRAPHICS

- TTP primarily affects females aged between 18 and 50 yr.
- The incidence of acquired TTP in adults is 2.9 cases per million per year. Incidence in children is 0.1 cases per million per year. There is increased incidence in HIV/AIDS and during pregnancy.

PHYSICAL FINDINGS & CLINICAL PRESENTATION

- The disease often begins as a flulike illness ultimately followed by clinical and laboratory abnormalities.
- Most patients present with nonspecific constitutional symptoms (weakness, nausea, abdominal pain, vomiting).
- Purpura (secondary to thrombocytopenia).
- Jaundice, pallor (from hemolysis).
- Mucosal bleeding.
- Fever.
- Fluctuating levels of consciousness (caused by thrombotic occlusion of the cerebral vessels). However, one third of patients have no neurologic abnormalities.
- Renal failure and neurologic events are usually end-stage features.

ETIOLOGY

- Acquired TTP is an autoimmune disorder caused by autoantibody inhibition of ADAMTS13 activity. Hereditary TTP (also called Upshaw-Schulman syndrome) is caused by homozygous or compound heterozygous ADAMTS13 mutations.
- Many drugs, including clopidogrel, penicillin, antineoplastic agents (gemcitabine, mitomycin C, cyclosporine) oral contraceptives, quinine, and ticlopidine, have been associated with TTP. Other precipitating causes include infectious agents, pregnancy, malignancies, allogeneic bone marrow transplantation, and neurologic disorders.

DIAGNOSIS

DIFFERENTIAL DIAGNOSIS

- Disseminated intravascular coagulation (DIC)
- Malignant hypertension
- Vasculitis
- Eclampsia or preeclampsia
- Hemolytic-uremic syndrome (typically encountered in children, often after a viral infection)
- Gastroenteritis as a result of a serotoxin-producing serotype of *Escherichia coli*
- Medications: clopidogrel, ticlopidine, penicillin, antineoplastic chemotherapeutic agents, oral contraceptives

WORKUP

- A comprehensive history, physical examination, and laboratory evaluation usually confirm the diagnosis.

LABORATORY TESTS

- Severe anemia and thrombocytopenia (platelet count <50,000 or >50% reduction from previous counts). Peripheral blood smear (Fig. E1) reveals numerous red cell fragments (schistocytes).
- Elevated blood urea nitrogen and creatinine.
- Evidence of hemolysis: elevated reticulocyte count, indirect bilirubin, lactate dehydrogenase, decreased haptoglobin.
- Urinalysis: hematuria (red blood cells [RBCs] and RBC casts in urine sediment) and proteinuria.
- Peripheral smear: severely fragmented RBCs (schistocytes). More than 4% RBC fragments in the peripheral blood.
- No laboratory evidence of DIC (normal fibrin degradation product, fibrinogen).
- The diagnosis of hereditary TTP requires documentation of ADAMTS13 deficiency and an absence of ADAMTS13 autoantibody inhibitor, and confirmation requires documentation of ADAMTS13 mutations. Diagnostic criteria for acquired TTP are the presence of microangiopathic hemolytic anemia and thrombocytopenia without another apparent cause. An ADAMTS13 level indicating less than 10% of normal activity supports the clinical diagnosis of acquired TTP.

TREATMENT

ACUTE GENERAL Rx

- Discontinue potential offending agents. Initiate ADAMTS13 replacement by plasma infusion in patients with hereditary TTP.
- The American Association of Blood Banks, the American Society for Apheresis, and the British Committee for Standards in Haematology recommend daily plasma exchange with replacement of 1.0 to 1.5 times the predicted plasma volume of the patient as standard therapy for TTP. The British guidelines recommend that plasma exchange therapy be continued for a minimum of 2 days after the platelet count returns to normal (>150,000 cells/m^3).
- High-dose plasma infusion (25 mL/kg/day) may be useful only if plasma exchange cannot be promptly started and for patients with very severe or refractory disease between plasma exchange sessions. High-dose plasma infusions can cause volume overload in patients with renal insufficiency.
- Patients with hereditary TTP who experience severe plasma allergic reactions have been effectively treated with plasma-derived factor VIII concentrate that contains ADAMTS13.
- Corticosteroids (prednisone 1 to 2 mg/kg/day) may be effective alone in patients with mild disease or may be administered concomitantly with plasmapheresis plus plasma exchange with fresh frozen plasma.
- The monoclonal antibody rituximab has also been used for treatment of TTP.
- Platelet transfusions are contraindicated except in severely thrombocytopenic patients with documented bleeding or those who are facing surgery or other invasive procedures in the setting of severe thrombocytopenia.
- Use of antiplatelet agents (acetylsalicylic acid, dipyridamole) is controversial.
- Splenectomy is performed in refractory cases.
- Dialysis is rarely required.

CHRONIC Rx

- Relapsing TTP may be treated with plasma exchange.
- Remission of chronic TTP that is unresponsive to conventional therapy has been reported after treatment with cyclophosphamide and the monoclonal antibody rituximab.
- Splenectomy done while the patients are in remission has been used in some centers to decrease the frequency of relapse in TTP.

DISPOSITION

- Survival of patients with TTP currently exceeds 80% with plasma exchange therapy.
- Relapse occurs in 20% to 40% of patients who have TTP in remission.

PEARLS & CONSIDERATIONS

COMMENTS

- The diagnosis of TTP/hemolytic-uremic syndrome should be considered in pregnant women with vague neurologic, gastrointestinal, or renal symptoms in either the obstetric triage or emergency department areas.
- TTP is fatal in 90% of patients without therapy.
- Trials with caplacizumab, an anti-von Willebrand factor humanized single-variable-domain immunoglobulin, have shown that for acquired TTP, caplacizumab induces a faster resolution of the acute TTP episode than placebo and the platelet-protective effect of caplacizumab was maintained during the treatment period.[1]

SUGGESTED READINGS

Available at www.expertconsult.com

RELATED CONTENT

Hemolytic Uremic Syndrome (Related Key Topic)

AUTHOR: **BHARTI RATHORE, M.D.**

[1]Pyvandi F, et al.: Caplacizumab for acquired thrombotic thrombocytopenic purpura, *N Engl J Med* 374:511–522, 2016.

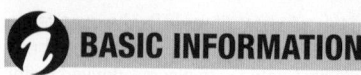

BASIC INFORMATION

DEFINITION

Thyroid carcinoma is a primary neoplasm of the thyroid. There are four major types of thyroid carcinoma: papillary, follicular, anaplastic, and medullary.

SYNONYMS

Papillary carcinoma of thyroid
Follicular carcinoma of thyroid
Anaplastic carcinoma of thyroid
Medullary carcinoma of thyroid

ICD-10CM CODES
C73   Malignant neoplasm of thyroid gland
D09.3 Carcinoma in situ of thyroid and other endocrine glands
D34   Benign neoplasm of thyroid gland
D44.0 Neoplasm of uncertain behavior of thyroid gland

EPIDEMIOLOGY & DEMOGRAPHICS

- Thyroid cancer is the most common endocrine cancer, with over 48,000 new cases in the United States and approximately 1100 deaths. The incidence of thyroid cancer is rising at a faster rate than any other type of malignancy.
- Female/male ratio is 3:1.
- Median age at diagnosis: 45 to 50 yr.
- Occult thyroid cancer is identified in 20% of autopsy specimens.

PHYSICAL FINDINGS & CLINICAL PRESENTATION

- Presence of thyroid nodule
- Hoarseness and cervical lymphadenopathy
- Painless swelling in the region of the thyroid

ETIOLOGY

- Risk factors: prior neck irradiation
- Multiple endocrine neoplasia II (medullary carcinoma)
- Inherited syndromes associated with thyroid cancer are described in Table 1
- GLP-1 receptor agonists for the treatment of type 2 DM (e.g., exenatide, albiglutide) can increase the risk of medullary thyroid carcinoma (MTC)

TABLE 1   Inherited Syndromes Associated With Thyroid Cancer

Multiple endocrine neoplasia (MEN) 2A and 2B
Isolated familial medullary thyroid cancer
Gardner syndrome
Familial adenomatous polyposis
Carney complex
Cowden syndrome
Familial nonmedullary thyroid cancer

From Cameron JL, Cameron AM: *Current surgical therapy*, ed 10, Philadelphia, 2011, Saunders.

- Although formerly thought to be a single entity, papillary thyroid carcinoma encompasses several tumor types that have mutually exclusive mutations. BRAF V600E accounts for 60% of these mutations.

DIAGNOSIS

DIFFERENTIAL DIAGNOSIS

- Multinodular goiter
- Lymphocytic thyroiditis
- Ectopic thyroid

WORKUP

The workup of thyroid carcinoma includes laboratory evaluation and diagnostic imaging. However, diagnosis is confirmed with fine-needle aspiration or surgical biopsy. At diagnosis the vast majority of thyroid cancers are well differentiated, with excellent prognosis. The characteristics of thyroid carcinoma vary with the type:

- Papillary carcinoma (85%):
  1. Most frequently occurs in women during second or third decades
  2. Histologically, psammoma bodies (calcific bodies present in papillary projections) are pathognomonic; found in 35% to 45% of papillary thyroid carcinomas
  3. Majority are not papillary lesions but mixed papillary follicular carcinomas
  4. Spread is by lymphatics and by local invasion
- Follicular carcinoma (10%):
  1. More aggressive than papillary carcinoma
  2. Incidence increases with age
  3. Tends to metastasize hematogenously to bone, producing pathologic fractures
  4. Tends to concentrate iodine (useful for radiation therapy)
- Anaplastic carcinoma (1%):
  1. Very aggressive neoplasm
  2. Two major histologic types: small cell (less aggressive, 5-yr survival approximately 20%) and giant cell (death usually within 6 mo of diagnosis)
- MTC (4%):
  1. Unifocal lesion: found sporadically in elderly patients
  2. Bilateral lesions: associated with pheochromocytoma and hyperparathyroidism; this combination is known as MEN-II and is inherited as an autosomal-dominant disorder

LABORATORY TESTS

- Thyroid function studies are generally normal. Thyroid-stimulating hormone (TSH), T4, and serum thyroglobulin levels should be obtained before thyroidectomy in patients with confirmed thyroid carcinoma. Serum thyroglobulin levels can be useful postoperatively to monitor recurrence of thyroid carcinoma (Fig. E1).
- Increased plasma calcitonin assay in patients with medullary carcinoma (tumors produce thyrocalcitonin). RET proto-oncogene sequencing and measurement of plasma free metanephrine

and normetanephrine levels to rule out coexistent pheochromocytoma are recommended in all patients with medullary thyroid cancer.

- Fine-needle aspiration biopsy is the best method to assess a thyroid nodule (see "Thyroid Nodule" in Section I).

IMAGING STUDIES (FIG. E2)

- Thyroid ultrasound can detect solitary solid nodules that have a high risk of malignancy. However, a negative ultrasound does not exclude diagnosis of thyroid carcinoma.
- Thyroid scanning with iodine-123 or technetium-99m can identify hypofunctioning (cold) nodules, which are more likely to be malignant. However, warm nodules can also be malignant.

STAGING

- Stage I: thyroid cancer of any size without distal spread in patient under age 45. In patients 45 years or older, tumor size ≤2 cm without local invasion or positive cervical lymph nodes
- Stage II: distal spread in patient younger than 45 years. In patients 45 years or older, tumors >2 cm but <4 cm without local invasion or positive cervical lymph nodes
- Stage III: tumors >4 cm in patient over 45 years of age
- Stage IV: distal spread in patient over 45 years of age

TREATMENT

ACUTE GENERAL Rx

- Papillary carcinoma:
  1. Total thyroidectomy is indicated if the patient has:
     a. Extrapyramidal extension of carcinoma
     b. Papillary carcinoma limited to thyroid but a positive history of irradiation to the neck
     c. Lesion >2 cm
  2. Lobectomy with isthmectomy may be considered in patients with intrathyroid papillary carcinoma <2 cm and no history of neck or head irradiation; surgery should be followed with suppressive therapy with thyroid hormone because these tumors are TSH responsive. The accepted practice is to suppress serum TSH concentrations to <0.1 microunit/ml in patients with persistent disease, suppression to 0.1 to 0.5 microunit/ml in patients who are disease free but are at high risk of recurrence, and a goal TSH level of 0.3 to 2.0 microunits/ml in patients who are disease free and have a low risk of recurrence.
  3. Radioiodine ablation reduces rates of death and recurrence (Table 2). Radioiodine is administered for stages III and IV disease.
- Follicular carcinoma:
  1. Total thyroidectomy followed by TSH suppression, as previously noted

2. Radiotherapy with iodine-131 followed by thyroid suppression therapy with triiodothyronine is useful in patients with metastasis (Table 2)

- Anaplastic carcinoma:
  1. At diagnosis, this neoplasm is rarely operable; palliative surgery is indicated for extremely large tumor compressing the trachea.
  2. Management is usually restricted to radiation therapy or chemotherapy (combination of doxorubicin, cisplatin, and other antineoplastic agents) (Table 2); these measures rarely provide significant palliation.

- Medullary carcinoma:
  1. Thyroidectomy should be performed, followed by TSH suppression.
  2. Vandetanib, an oral tyrosine kinase inhibitor, was recently FDA-approved for treatment of symptomatic or progressive, unresectable, locally advanced or metastatic medullary thyroid cancer. It is not recommended for treatment of asymptomatic or less aggressive disease due to its many serious side effects.
  3. Patients and their families should be screened for pheochromocytoma and hyperparathyroidism.

DISPOSITION

Prognosis varies with the type of thyroid carcinoma: 5-yr survival approaches 80% for follicular carcinoma and is approximately 5% with anaplastic carcinoma (see Table 3).

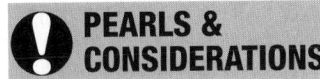

PEARLS & CONSIDERATIONS

COMMENTS

- Family members of patients with medullary carcinoma should be screened; DNA analysis for the detection of mutations in the *RET* gene structure permits the identification of *MEN IIA* gene carriers.
- Motesanib, an oral inhibitor of vascular endothelial growth factor (VEGF) receptors, has been reported effective in inducing partial responses in patients with advanced or metastatic differentiated thyroid cancer that is progressive.
- While there is little controversy regarding the benefit of radioactive iodine in iodine-avid advanced-stage well-differentiated thyroid cancer, the indications for radioactive iodine following total thyroidectomy in patients with very low risk disease is controversial. Proponents argue that its use may destroy

microscopic metastases while opponents counter that the risk of secondary cancer due to radioactive iodine is not warranted in patients whose prognosis is typically excellent.

- Metastatic thyroid cancers that are refractory to radioiodine (iodine-131) are associated with a poor prognosis. Recent trials have shown that the selective mitogen-activated protein kinase (MAPK) pathway antagonist selumetinib produces clinically meaningful increases in iodine uptake and retention in some patients with thyroid cancer that is refractory to radioiodine. In recent phase 2 trials, lenvatinib has also shown significant improvements in progression-free survival and response rate among patients with iodine-131 refractory thyroid cancer.

SUGGESTED READINGS

Available at www.expertconsult.com

RELATED CONTENT

Thyroid Cancer (Patient Information)
Thyroid Nodule (Related Key Topic)

AUTHOR: **BHARTI RATHORE, M.D.**

Diseases
and Disorders

I

TABLE 2 Indications for Iodine-131 Treatment in Patients With Papillary, Follicular, or Hürthle Cell Thyroid Carcinoma after Initial Definitive Near-Total Thyroidectomy

No Indication

Adult patients at very low risk for cause-specific mortality or relapse: complete surgical resection, favorable histology, and limited extent of disease (e.g., PTC patients with MACIS scores <6; patients with tumor size <1 cm, N0, and M0).

Definite Indications

Distant metastasis at diagnosis
Incomplete tumor resection
Complete tumor resection but high risk for mortality or recurrence (e.g., PTC patients with MACIS scores ≥6 and pTNM stage II/III FTC or HCC)

Probable Indications

Incomplete surgery (less than near-total thyroidectomy, no lymph node dissection)
PTC or FTC in a child younger than 16 yr
If PTC, tall cell or columnar cell variant and diffuse sclerosing variant
If FTC, widely invasive or poorly differentiated tumor
Bulky nodal metastases

FTC, Follicular thyroid carcinoma; *HCC,* Hürthle cell carcinoma; *MACIS,* scoring system based on metastasis, age, completeness of resection, invasion, and size; *PTC,* papillary thyroid carcinoma; *pTNM,* pathologic tumor-node-metastasis classification.
From Melmed S et al (eds): *Williams textbook of endocrinology,* ed 12, Philadelphia, 2011, Saunders.

TABLE 3 Characteristics of Thyroid Cancers

Type of Cancer	Percentage of Thyroid Cancers	Age of Onset (Yr)	Treatment	Prognosis
Papillary	88	40-80	Thyroidectomy, followed by radioactive iodine ablation and TSH suppression	Good
Follicular	10	45-80	Thyroidectomy, followed by radioactive iodine ablation and TSH suppression	Fair to good
Medullary	3-4	20-50	Thyroidectomy and central compartment lymph node dissection and TSH suppression	Fair
Anaplastic	1	50-80	Isthmusectomy followed by palliative x-ray treatment	Poor
Lymphoma	<1	25-70	X-ray therapy and/or chemotherapy	Fair

From Andreoli TE et al: *Andreoli and Carpenter's Cecil essentials of medicine,* ed 8, Philadelphia, 2010, Saunders.

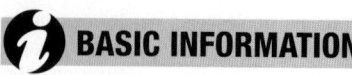

DEFINITION

A thyroid nodule is an abnormality found on physical examination of the thyroid gland; nodules can be benign (70%) or malignant.

ICD-10CM CODES
E04.1   Nontoxic single thyroid nodule.
E05.2   Thyrotoxicosis with toxic single thyroid nodule.
E05.11 Thyrotoxicosis with toxic single thyroid nodule with thyrotoxic crisis or storm

EPIDEMIOLOGY & DEMOGRAPHICS

- Palpable thyroid nodules occur in 4% to 7% of the population.
- Thyroid nodules can be found in 50% of autopsies; however, only one in 10 is palpable.
- Malignancy is present in 5% to 15% of all thyroid nodules and in 7% to 9% of palpable nodules.
- Incidence of thyroid nodules increases after 45 yr. They are found more frequently in women (5% of women; 1% of men).
- History of prior head and neck irradiation increases the risk of thyroid cancer.
- Increased likelihood that nodule is malignant: nodule increasing in size or >3 cm, regional lymphadenopathy, fixation to adjacent tissues, age <40 yr, symptoms of local invasion (dysphagia, hoarseness, neck pain, male sex, family history of thyroid cancer or polyposis [Gardner syndrome]), rapid growth during levothyroxine therapy, microcalcification within the nodule, and high intranodular vascular flow.

PHYSICAL FINDINGS & CLINICAL PRESENTATION

- Palpable, firm, and nontender nodule in the thyroid area should prompt suspicion of carcinoma. Signs of metastasis are regional lymphadenopathy and inspiratory stridor.
- Signs and symptoms of thyrotoxicosis can be found in functioning nodules.

ETIOLOGY

- History of prior head and neck irradiation.
- Family history of pheochromocytoma, carcinoma of the thyroid, and hyperparathyroidism (medullary carcinoma of the thyroid is a component of MEN-II).

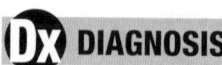

DIAGNOSIS

DIFFERENTIAL DIAGNOSIS

- Thyroid carcinoma.
- Multinodular goiter.
- Thyroglossal duct cyst.
- Epidermoid cyst.
- Laryngocele.
- Nonthyroid neck neoplasm.
- Branchial cleft cyst.

WORKUP

- Ultrasonography is an inexpensive and effective modality to stratify malignancy risk.
- Fine-needle aspiration (FNA) biopsy is the best diagnostic study; the accuracy can be >90%, but it is directly related to the level of experience of the physician and the cytopathologist interpreting the aspirate. FNA is not routinely recommended for thyroid nodules <1 cm in diameter unless there are significant risk factors (see above).
- FNA biopsy is less reliable with thyroid cystic lesions; surgical excision should be considered for most thyroid cysts not abolished by aspiration.
- A diagnostic approach to thyroid nodule is described in Fig. 1. Preoperative, ultrasonically guided FNA accurately classifies 62% to 85% of thyroid nodules as benign; however, 15% to 30% of aspirations yield indeterminate cytologic findings. Table 1 describes the probability of malignancy at histology based on FNA biopsy cytology.

LABORATORY TESTS

- Serum TSH should be obtained in all patients with thyroid nodules. If suppressed, obtain free T4 and free T3 and thyroid scan to rule out "hot nodule," indicative of hyperthyroid adenoma. Less than 1% of hyperfunctioning nodules are malignant. Typically FNA biopsy is not necessary in hot nodules.
- Thyroid-stimulating hormone (TSH), T4, and serum thyroglobulin levels should be obtained before thyroidectomy in patients with confirmed thyroid carcinoma on FNA biopsy.
- Serum calcitonin at random or after pentagastrin stimulation is useful when suspecting medullary carcinoma of the thyroid and in anyone with a family history of medullary thyroid carcinoma.
- Serum thyroid autoantibodies (see "Thyroiditis" in Section I) are useful in patients with multinodular goiter and when suspecting thyroiditis.
- Molecular analysis of thyroid tissue for the presence of BRAF and RAS mutations and for RET/PTC and PAX8-PPAR gamma 1 gene rearrangements can be used as a diagnostic tool, since 60% to 70% of thyroid cancers harbor at least one genetic mutation. The gene expression classifier profile can be used to identify a subpopulation of patients with a low likelihood of cancer, thereby avoiding unnecessary surgery in patients with indeterminate FNA. The gene expression classifier test has a high negative predictive value for cytologically indeterminate nodules (95% for an atypical or follicular lesion of undetermined significance, 94% for a follicular neoplasm, and 85% for a lesion suggestive of cancer).

IMAGING STUDIES

- Thyroid ultrasound (Fig. E2) is useful to evaluate the size of the thyroid and the number, composition (solid versus cystic), and dimensions of the thyroid nodule; solid thyroid nodules have a higher incidence of malignancy, but cystic nodules can also be malignant. The three characteristics on thyroid ultrasound most predictive of cancer are nodules >2 cm, microcalcifications, and entirely solid nodules.
- Thyroid scan can be performed with technetium-99m pertechnetate, iodine-123, or iodine-131. Iodine isotopes are preferred because up to 35% of nodules that appear functioning on pertechnetate scanning may appear nonfunctioning on radioiodine scanning. A thyroid scan:
  1. Classifies nodules as hyperfunctioning (hot), normally functioning (warm), or nonfunctioning (cold); cold nodules have a higher incidence of malignancy.
  2. Scan has difficulty evaluating nodules near the thyroid isthmus or at the periphery of the gland.
  3. Normal tissue over a nonfunctioning nodule might mask the nodule as "warm" or normally functioning.
- Both thyroid scan and ultrasound provide information about the risk of malignant neoplasia based on the characteristics of the thyroid nodule, but their value in the initial evaluation of a thyroid nodule is limited because neither provides a definite tissue diagnosis.

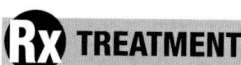

TREATMENT

GENERAL Rx

- Evaluation of results of FNA:
  1. Normal cells: may repeat biopsy during present evaluation or reevaluate patient after 3 to 6 mo of suppressive therapy (L-thyroxine, prescribed in doses to suppress the TSH level to 0.1-0.5).
     a. Failure to regress indicates increased likelihood of malignancy.
     b. Reliance on repeat FNA biopsy is preferable to routine surgery for nodules not responding to thyroxine.
- Indeterminate: use of gene expression classifier profile. If suspicious, perform surgery; if benign, monitor with subsequent repeat FNA and gene expression classifier profile.
- Malignant cells: surgery.

DISPOSITION

Variable with results of FNA biopsy.

REFERRAL

Surgical referral for FNA biopsy.

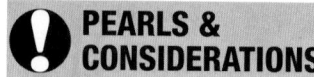

PEARLS & CONSIDERATIONS

COMMENTS

- Most solid, benign nodules grow; therefore, an increase in nodule volume alone is not a reliable predictor of malignancy.
- Thyroid nodules incidentally identified on fluorodeoxyglucose-PET (FDG-PET) scan done for other disorders has a much higher malignancy rate (30%-50%).

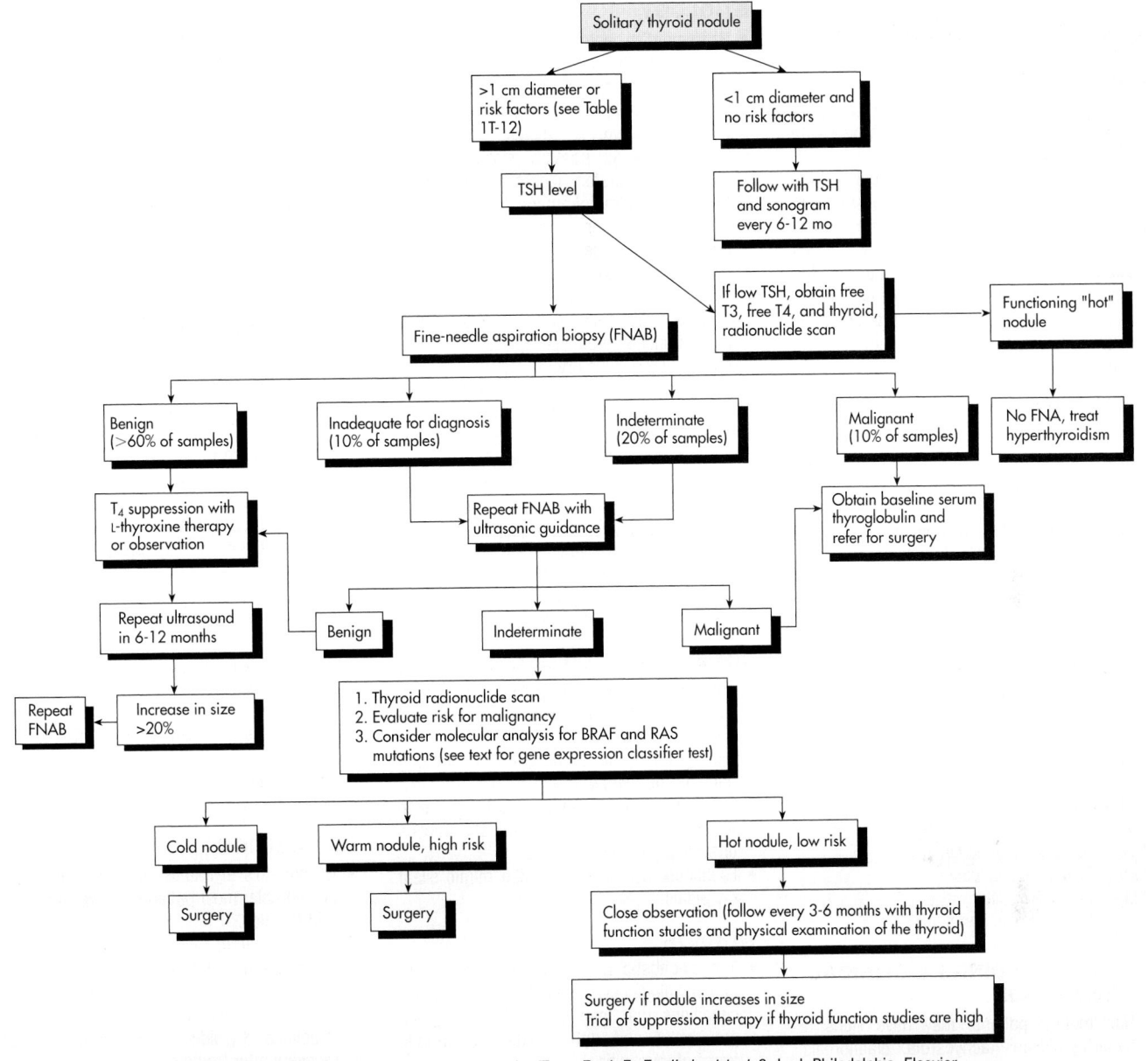

FIG. 1 Diagnostic algorithm for thyroid nodule. (From Ferri, F: *Ferri's best test*, 3rd ed, Philadelphia, Elsevier, 2014.)

TABLE 1   Clinical and Ultrasound Findings in Favor of Malignant Thyroid Nodules

Clinical Features	Ultrasound Findings
History	Higher Suspicion
Young age (<20 yr) or older age (>60 yr)	Hypoechoic lesions
Male gender	Irregular margins
Neck irradiation during childhood or adolescence	Presence of microcalcifications
Rapid growth	Absence of halo
Recent changes in speaking, breathing, or swallowing	Internal or central blood flow
Family history of thyroid malignancy or MEN2	
Physical Examination	Low Suspicion
Firm and irregular consistency of nodule	Echo-free (cystic) lesion
Fixation to underlying or overlying tissues	Spongiform lesion
Vocal cord paralysis	
Regional lymphadenopathy	

From Melmed S, Polonsky KS, Larsen PR, et al: *Williams textbook of endocrinology*, ed 12, Philadelphia, 2011, Elsevier.

- Surgery is indicated in hard or fixed nodule, presence of dysphagia or hoarseness, and rapidly growing solid masses regardless of "benign" results on FNA.
- Suppressive therapy of malignant thyroid nodules postoperatively with thyroxine is indicated. The use of suppressive therapy for benign solitary nodules is controversial.

SUGGESTED READINGS

Available at www.expertconsult.com

RELATED CONTENT

Thyroid Nodule (Patient Information)
Thyroiditis (Related Key Topic)
Thyroid Cancer (Related Key Topic)

AUTHOR: **FRED F. FERRI, M.D.**

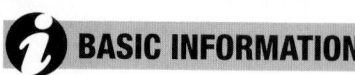

BASIC INFORMATION

DEFINITION

Thyroiditis is an inflammatory disease of the thyroid. It is a multifaceted disease with various etiologies, different clinical characteristics (depending on the stage), and distinct histopathology. Thyroiditis can be subdivided into three common types (Hashimoto's, painful, and painless) and two rare forms (suppurative and Riedel's). To add to the confusion, there are various synonyms for each form, and there is no internationally accepted classification of autoimmune thyroid disease.

SYNONYMS

Hashimoto's thyroiditis: chronic lymphocytic thyroiditis, chronic autoimmune thyroiditis, lymphadenoid goiter

Painful subacute thyroiditis: subacute thyroiditis, giant cell thyroiditis, de Quervain's thyroiditis, subacute granulomatous thyroiditis, pseudogranulomatous thyroiditis

Painless postpartum thyroiditis: subacute lymphocytic thyroiditis, postpartum thyroiditis

Painless sporadic thyroiditis: silent sporadic thyroiditis, subacute lymphocytic thyroiditis

Infectious thyroiditis: acute suppurative thyroiditis, bacterial thyroiditis, microbial inflammatory thyroiditis, pyogenic thyroiditis

Riedel's thyroiditis: fibrous thyroiditis

ICD-10CM CODES

E06.3 Autoimmune thyroiditis
E06.1 Subacute thyroiditis
E06.9 Thyroiditis, unspecified
E06.0 Acute thyroiditis
E06.5 Other chronic thyroiditis

PHYSICAL FINDINGS & CLINICAL PRESENTATION

- Hashimoto's: patients may have signs of hyperthyroidism (tachycardia, diaphoresis, palpitations, weight loss) or hypothyroidism (fatigue, weight gain, delayed reflexes) depending on the stage of the disease. Usually there is diffuse, firm enlargement of the thyroid gland; the gland may also be of normal size (atrophic form with clinically manifested hypothyroidism).
- Painful subacute: exquisitely tender, enlarged thyroid, fever; signs of hyperthyroidism are initially present; signs of hypothyroidism can subsequently develop.
- Painless thyroiditis: clinical features are similar to subacute thyroiditis except for the absence of tenderness of the thyroid gland.
- Suppurative: patient is febrile with severe neck pain, focal tenderness of the involved portion of the thyroid, erythema of the overlying skin.
- Riedel's: slowly enlarging hard mass in the anterior neck; often mistaken for thyroid cancer; signs of hypothyroidism occur in advanced stages.

ETIOLOGY

- Hashimoto's: autoimmune disorder that begins with the activation of CD4 (helper) T-lymphocytes specific for thyroid antigens. The etiologic factor for the activation of these cells is unknown.
- Painful subacute: possibly postviral; usually follows a respiratory illness not considered to be a form of autoimmune thyroiditis
- Painless thyroiditis: frequently occurs postpartum
- Infectious (suppurative): infectious etiology, generally bacterial, although fungi and parasites have also been implicated; often occurs in immunocompromised hosts or after a penetrating neck injury
- Riedel's: fibrous infiltration of the thyroid; etiology unknown
- Drug induced: typically painless due to lithium, interferon-alfa, amiodarone, interleukin-2
- Radiation thyroiditis: occurs 5 to 10 days after treatment with radioactive iodine; it is painful and may result in transient exacerbation of hyperthyroidism

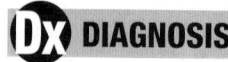

DIAGNOSIS

DIFFERENTIAL DIAGNOSIS

- The hyperthyroid phase of Hashimoto's, subacute, and silent thyroiditis can be mistaken for Graves' disease.
- Riedel's thyroiditis can be mistaken for carcinoma of the thyroid.
- Painful subacute thyroiditis can be mistaken for infections of the oropharynx and trachea or for suppurative thyroiditis.
- Factitious hyperthyroidism can mimic silent thyroiditis.

WORKUP

- The diagnostic workup includes laboratory and radiologic evaluation to rule out other conditions that may mimic thyroiditis (see previously) and differentiate the various forms of thyroiditis.
- The patient's medical history may be helpful in differentiating the various types of thyroiditis (e.g., presentation after childbirth is suggestive of silent [postpartum, painless] thyroiditis; occurrence after a viral respiratory infection suggests subacute thyroiditis; history of penetrating injury to the neck indicates suppurative thyroiditis).

LABORATORY TESTS

- Thyroid-stimulating hormone, free T_4: may be normal or indicative of hypothyroidism or hyperthyroidism depending on the stage of the thyroiditis.
- White blood cell (WBC) with differential: increased WBC with left shift occurs with subacute and suppurative thyroiditis.
- Antimicrosomal antibodies: detected in >90% of patients with Hashimoto's thyroiditis and 50% to 80% of patients with silent thyroiditis.
- Serum thyroglobulin levels are elevated in patients with subacute and silent thyroiditis;

this test is nonspecific but may be useful in monitoring the course of subacute thyroiditis and distinguishing silent thyroiditis from factitious hyperthyroidism (low or absent serum thyroglobulin level).

IMAGING STUDIES

Twenty-four–hour radioactive iodine uptake (RAIU) is useful to distinguish Graves' disease (increased RAIU) from thyroiditis (normal or low RAIU). Table E1 summarizes factors that influence 24-hr thyroid iodide uptake.

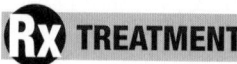

TREATMENT

ACUTE GENERAL Rx

- The duration of the thyrotoxic phase of thyroiditis is usually 3 to 6 wk. This phase is followed by a hypothyroid phase typically lasting up to 12 wk.
- Treat hypothyroid phase with levothyroxine 25 to 50 mcg/day initially and monitor serum thyroid-stimulating hormone initially every 6 to 8 wk.
- Control symptoms of hyperthyroidism with beta-blockers (e.g., propranolol 20-40 mg PO q6h).
- Control pain in patients with subacute thyroiditis with nonsteroidal antiinflammatory drugs. Prednisone 20 to 40 mg qd may be used if nonsteroidals are insufficient, but it should be gradually tapered off over several weeks.
- Use IV antibiotics and drain abscess (if present) in patients with suppurative thyroiditis.

DISPOSITION

- Hashimoto's thyroiditis: long-term prognosis is favorable; most patients recover their thyroid function.
- Painful subacute thyroiditis: permanent hypothyroidism occurs in 10% of patients.
- Painless thyroiditis: 6% of patients have permanent hypothyroidism.
- Infectious thyroiditis: there is usually full recovery after treatment.
- Riedel's thyroiditis: hypothyroidism occurs when fibrous infiltration involves the entire thyroid.

REFERRAL

Surgical referral in patients with compression of adjacent neck structures and in some patients with infectious (suppurative) thyroiditis

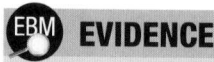

Available at www.expertconsult.com

RELATED CONTENT

Thyroiditis (Patient Information)

AUTHOR: **FRED F. FERRI, M.D.**

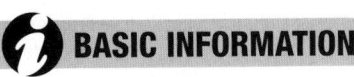

BASIC INFORMATION

DEFINITION

Tinea capitis is a dermatophyte infection of hair shaft and follicles of the scalp, eyebrows, and eyelashes. It is a form of superficial mycosis. Etiologic agents are fungal species of the genera *Microsporum* and *Trichophyton*.

SYNONYMS

Ringworm of the scalp, ringworm of the head, gray patch tinea capitis, black dot tinea capitis, tinea tonsurans, herpes tonsurans, kerion, favus

ICD-10CM CODES
B35.0 Tinea barbae and tinea capitis

EPIDEMIOLOGY & DEMOGRAPHICS

Tinea capitis primarily affects prepubertal children with peak age between 3 and 7 yr old. Adult cases are rare, possibly because of the fungistatic effect of the sebum found in older persons. Urban living, large family size, low socioeconomic status, and crowded living conditions may contribute to an increased incidence of tinea capitis. The elderly and immunocompromised individuals have an increased risk of infection. The incidence of the disease varies worldwide; however, it has is relatively low in the United States. It is reportedly widespread in parts of central and South America, India, and Africa.

In the United States, peak incidence occurs in school-aged children of low socioeconomic status, with African-American male children accounting for the greatest proportion of cases. About 3% to 8% of American children are affected, and 34% of household contacts are asymptomatic carriers.

PHYSICAL FINDINGS & CLINICAL PRESENTATION

- Classic triad of scalp scaling, alopecia, and cervical adenopathy
- Most forms of tinea capitis begin with one or few round patches of scale or alopecia.
- Primary lesions include plaques, papules, pustules, or nodules on the scalp (usually occipital region).
- Secondary lesions include scales, alopecia (usually reversible), erythema, exudates, and edema.

- Scalp pruritus may be present.
- Fever, pain, and lymphadenopathy (commonly postcervical) may occur with inflammatory lesions.
- Different clinical patterns of tinea capitis have been described:
  1. Gray patch: Lesions are scaly and well demarcated. The hairs within the patch break off a few millimeters above the scalp. One or several lesions may be present; sometimes the lesions join to form larger ones.
  2. Black dot: Early lesions with erythema and scaling patch are easily overlooked until areas of alopecia develop. Hairs within the patches break at the surface of the scalp, leaving behind a pattern of swollen black dots.
  3. Kerion (Fig. 1): inflamed, exudative, pustular, boggy, tender nodules exhibiting marked edema, and hair loss seen in severe tinea capitis. Caused by immune response to the fungus. May lead to some scarring.
  4. Favus: production of scutula (hair matted together with dermatophyte hyphae and keratin debris), characterized by yellow cup-shaped crusts around hair shafts. A fetid odor may be present.

ETIOLOGY

Although fungi of the *Microsporum* or *Trichophyton* genera cause most cases of tinea capitis, causative species vary between geographical areas and across time. *T. tonsurans* is the predominant cause of tinea capitis, present in more than 90% of cases in North and Central America. *Microsporum canis*, *M. audouinii*, and *Trichophyton mentagrophytes* are less common. The most common causative species for black dot tinea capitis is *T. tonsurans*, while gray patch tinea capitis tends to be caused by *M. audouinii* and *M. canis*. Infection of the hair shaft is preceded by invasion of the stratum corneum of the scalp. Transmission of *T. tonsurans* occurs from person-to-person via infected persons or asymptomatic carriers, fallen infected hairs, animal vectors, and fomites. *M. audouinii* is commonly spread by dogs and cats. Infectious fungal particles may remain viable for many months. Even though the organism remains viable on combs, hairbrushes, and other fomites for long periods of time, the role

of fomites in spreading the infection may vary in different geographic areas.

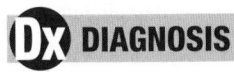

DIAGNOSIS

DIFFERENTIAL DIAGNOSIS

Seborrheic dermatitis and psoriasis may be confused with tinea capitis. Other conditions that resemble tinea capitis include alopecia areata, impetigo, pediculosis, trichotillomania, traction alopecia, folliculitis, pseudopelade, seborrhea/atopic dermatitis, psoriasis, carbuncles, pyoderma, lichen ruber planus, and lupus erythematosus; these should also be considered in the differential. Table 1 highlights distinctive features of conditions that may be confused for tinea capitis.

WORKUP

- KOH testing of hair shaft extracted from the lesion, not the scale, because the *T. tonsurans* spores attach to or reside inside hair shafts and will rarely be found in the scales.
- Wood's ultraviolet light fluoresces blue-green on hair shafts for Microsporum infections but will fail to identify *T. tonsurans*.
- Fungal culture of hairs and scales on fungal medium such as Sabouraud's agar may be used to confirm the diagnosis, especially if uncertain.
- Histology of biopsies with fungal staining in cases where mycology tests are negative because of treatment initiation.

TREATMENT

- Griseofulvin is the gold standard FDA-approved treatment. Published studies show mean efficacy for griseofulvin treatment of about 68% for *Trichophyton* species and 88% for *Microsporum*. It is less costly than other drug options and has an excellent long-term safety profile. Micronized and ultramicronized preparations are absorbed better, and side effects are infrequent, especially when administered with fatty meals. Periodic monitoring of hematologic, liver, and renal function may be indicated, especially in prolonged treatment over 8 wk.
  Children: Griseofulvin is approved for children older than 2 yr of age: microsize griseofulvin 10 to 25 mg/kg PO per day in one single dose or two divided doses (maximum, 1 g/day; for tinea capitis, higher doses [20-25 mg/kg/day] have been recommended) or ultramicrosize griseofulvin, 5 to 15 mg/kg PO per day (maximum, 750 mg/day), in one single dose or two divided doses. Optimally, griseofulvin is given after a meal containing fat (e.g., peanut butter or ice cream). Recommended treatment length is 6 to 8 wk and should be continued 2 wk beyond clinical resolution (until hair regrowth occurs). Some children may require higher doses to achieve clinical cure.
  Adults and elderly persons: microsize griseofulvin 500 mg PO per day in one single dose or divided doses. The other option is ultramicrosize griseofulvin 375 mg PO per

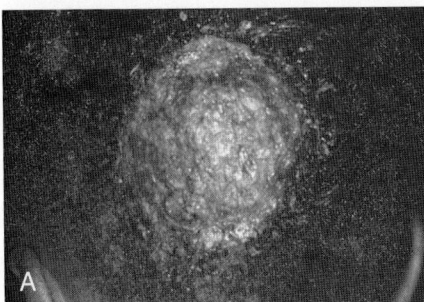
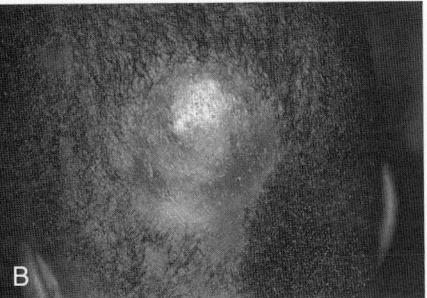

FIG. 1 A, Kerion. Boggy granulomatous mass of the scalp. **B,** Scarring after kerion. (From Kliegman RM et al: *Nelson textbook of pediatrics,* ed 19, Philadelphia, 2011, Saunders.)

TABLE 1 Differential Diagnosis of Tinea Capitis

Disorder	Differentiating Features
Psoriasis	Red skin with thick, uniform, silvery scale, sharply demarcated; often psoriasis at other body sites also
Dermatitis	Main possibility is seborrheic dermatitis: usually more diffuse and has uniform fine scaling, rather than localized areas; doesn't typically cause alopecia or significant inflammation. May also be present on the face, especially the nasolabial fold, or as otitis externa. Atopic dermatitis is generally diffuse on scalp and almost inevitably present at other sites, but may coexist with tinea capitis, especially in children.
Pityriasis amiantacea	Thick sheets of asbestos-like scale, very adherent, generally a solitary patch. This may occur in various dermatoses.
Lichen simplex	Usually nape of neck; cobblestoned or lichenified skin thickening, with broken hairs that are not coated with scale
Alopecia areata	Usually not inflamed (may be mildly so), not scaly, usually sharply defined. "Exclamation mark" hairs occur but are not coated with fungus; "cadaverized" hairs especially cause difficulty, as they mimic black dot alopecia.
Scarring alopecias	Examples: discoid lupus erythematosus, lichen planus of scalp; cause perifollicular inflammation around intact hairs; usually associated with lesions at other sites also. Dissecting cellulitis of scalp is also in this differential.
Bacterial infections	Impetigo causes crusting but little inflammation, and hairs are intact; carbuncle is deeper and very tender but may be in the differential of kerion
Trichotillomania	Broken hairs of unequal length, but hair shafts themselves and the scalp are normal
Damage from hairdressing processes	Usually clear from the timescale
Neoplasm	May be in the differential of kerion; usually slower-growing and mainly on elderly, balding scalp, whereas kerion is in children or young adults with previously intact hair

From White GM, Cox NH (eds): *Diseases of the skin, a color atlas and text,* ed 2, St Louis, 2006, Mosby.

day in one single dose or divided doses. Recommended treatment length is 4 to 6 weeks.

- Newer alternative treatments: oral terbinafine, itraconazole, or fluconazole are comparable in efficacy and safety to griseofulvin, with possibly shorter treatment and better patient compliance. Preferred when resistant or when an allergy to griseofulvin is of concern. Monitoring of CBC, liver function tests, and renal function may be indicated.
  1. Terbinafine—4-wk course of therapy as effective as with griseofulvin. Dosages are 67.5 mg/day for patients weighing <20 kg; 125 mg/day for patients weighing 20 to 40 kg; and 250 mg for patients weighing >40 kg.
  2. Itraconazole—3.5 mg/kg daily for 4 to 6 wk or pulse therapy of 5 mg/kg daily for 1 wk each month for 2 to 3 mo (not approved for children)
  3. Fluconazole—the only oral antifungal agent approved for children <2 yr, 6 mg/kg/day for 6 wk in children (3-6 wk in adults) or 8 mg/kg weekly for 8 to 12 wk (cap at 150 mg weekly for adults)
- The adjuvant use of antifungal shampoos may be recommended for all patients and household contacts. Shampoo like selenium sulfide 2.5% used for 5 min or ketoconazole shampoo used 2 to 3 times/wk can help prevent infection or eradicate asymptomatic carrier state by inhibiting fungal growth.
- Severe inflammatory kerion can be managed with additional prednisone 40 mg daily (1 mg/kg/day in children) and tapering over 2 wk.

- Prompt treatment is indicated, as is examination of siblings and other household contacts for evidence of tinea capitis.
- Recommend follow-up visit every 2 to 4 wk with Wood's light, microscopic study, and fungal culture. A mycologic documented cure is the goal of treatment.
- Pets that are infected or asymptomatic carriers should be treated.
- Children receiving treatment for tinea capitis may attend school once they start therapy with griseofulvin or other effective systemic agent.

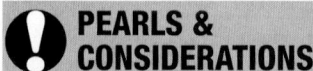 **PEARLS & CONSIDERATIONS**

- Systemic antifungal therapy is required for tinea capitis because topical antifungal medications are not effective.
- Shaving of the head, haircuts, or wearing a cap or scarf during treatment is unnecessary.
- Sharing of combs, hair ribbons, and hairbrushes should be discouraged.

COMMENTS

- Confirming the diagnosis of tinea capitis with a laboratory specimen is important because misdiagnosis will result in delay or improper treatment.
- Patients and their families should look for sources of infections and disinfect contaminated objects such as combs, brushes, towels, and headgear. Avoid sharing personal hygiene utensils.
- Culture of hairs and scalp dander facilitates carrier identification and prevention.

SUGGESTED READING

Available at www.expertconsult.com

RELATED CONTENT

Tinea Capitis (Patient Information)

AUTHORS: **PRIYA SARIN GUPTA, M.D., M.P.H., NADINE MBUYI, M.D.,** and **ALVARO M. RIVERA, M.D.**

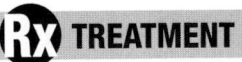

BASIC INFORMATION

DEFINITION

Tinea corporis is a dermatophyte fungal infection caused by the genera *Trichophyton* or *Microsporum*. Tinea corporis includes all superficial dermatophyte infections of the skin other than those involving the scalp, beard, face, hands, feet, and groin.

SYNONYMS

Ringworm
Body ringworm
Tinea circinata

ICD-10CM CODES
B35.4 Tinea corporis

EPIDEMIOLOGY & DEMOGRAPHICS

- The disease is more common in warm climates.
- There is no predominant age or sex.

PHYSICAL FINDINGS & CLINICAL PRESENTATION

- Typically appears as single or multiple annular lesions with an advancing scaly border (Fig. 1); the margin is slightly raised, reddened, and may be pustular.
- The central area becomes hypopigmented and less scaly as the active border progresses outward (Fig. 2), thus the name "ringworm."
- The trunk and legs are primarily involved.
- Pruritus is variable.
- It is important to remember that recent topical corticosteroid use can significantly alter the appearance of the lesions.

- Tinea gladiatorum is a common problem for wrestlers.

ETIOLOGY

Trichophyton rubrum is the most common pathogen. Other common causes in the U.S. are *M. canis* and *T. mentagrophytes.*

DIAGNOSIS

DIFFERENTIAL DIAGNOSIS

- Pityriasis rosea
- Erythema multiforme
- Psoriasis
- Cutaneous systemic lupus erythematosus
- Secondary syphilis
- Nummular eczema
- Eczema
- Granuloma annulare
- Lyme disease
- Tinea versicolor
- Contact dermatitis

WORKUP

Diagnosis is usually made on clinical grounds. It can be confirmed by direct visualization under the microscope of a small fragment of the scale using wet mount preparation and potassium hydroxide solution; dermatophytes appear as translucent branching filaments (hyphae) with lines of separation appearing at irregular intervals.

LABORATORY TESTS

- Microscopic examination of hyphae
- Mycotic culture is usually not necessary.
- Biopsy is indicated only when the diagnosis is uncertain and the patient has not responded to treatment.
- HIV (widespread tinea corporis may be a presenting sign of AIDS)

TREATMENT

NONPHARMACOLOGIC THERAPY

Affected areas should be kept clean and dry.

ACUTE GENERAL Rx

- Various creams are effective; the application area should include normal skin approximately 2 cm beyond the affected area:
  1. Butenafine cream applied qd for 14 days
  2. Terbinafine cream applied bid for 7-14 days
  3. Other effective topical agents are sulconazole, miconazole, clotrimazole, ketoconazole, naftifine, ciclopirox olamine, and efinaconazole.
- Systemic therapy is reserved for severe cases and is usually given up to 4 wk; commonly used agents:
  1. Fluconazole, 150 mg once a week for 4 wk
  2. Terbinafine, 250 mg qd for 7-14 days
  3. Itraconazole 200 mg/day for 1 wk

DISPOSITION

Majority of cases resolve without sequelae within 3 to 4 wk of therapy.

REFERRAL

Dermatology referral in patients with persistent or recurrent infections

RELATED CONTENT

Ringworm (Patient Information)
Tinea Capitis (Related Key Topic)
Tinea Cruris (Related Key Topic)

AUTHOR: **FRED F. FERRI, M.D.**

Diseases and Disorders

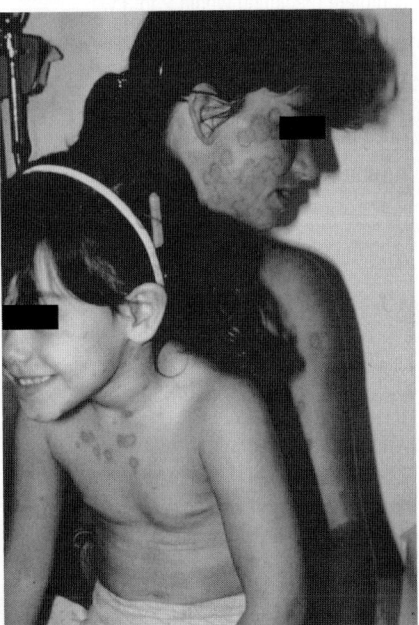

FIG. 1 Tinea corporis. (Courtesy of David Effron, MD.)

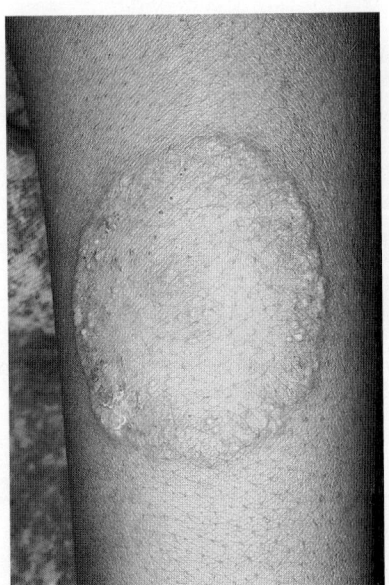

FIG. 2 Annular lesion (tinea corporis). Note raised erythematous, scaling border and central clearing. (From Noble J et al: *Textbook of primary care medicine,* ed 3, St Louis, 2001, Mosby.)

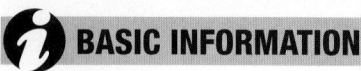
BASIC INFORMATION

DEFINITION
Tinea cruris is a dermatophyte infection of the groin.

SYNONYMS
Jock itch
Groin ringworm
Crotch itch

ICD-10CM CODES
B35.6 Tinea cruris

EPIDEMIOLOGY & DEMOGRAPHICS
- Most common during the summer in adolescent and young adult males.
- Males are affected more frequently than females; however, it has become more common in postpubertal females who are overweight or who often wear tight jeans or pantyhose.
- The infection often coexists with tinea pedis.

PHYSICAL FINDINGS & CLINICAL PRESENTATION
- It begins as a small erythematous, and scaling or crusted patch that spreads peripherally.
- Erythematous plaques have a half-moon shape and a scaling border.
- The acute inflammation tends to move down the inner thigh and usually spares the scrotum; in severe cases the fungus may spread onto the buttocks.
- Itching may be severe.
- Red papules, vesicles, and pustules may be present.
- An important diagnostic sign is the advancing well-defined border with a tendency toward central clearing (Fig. 1).

ETIOLOGY
- Dermatophytes of the genera *Trichophyton, Epidermophyton,* and *Microsporum. T. rubrum* and *E. floccosum* are the most common infecting agents.
- Transmission from direct contact (e.g., infected persons, animals). The patient's feet should be evaluated as a source of infection because tinea cruris is often associated with tinea pedis.

DIAGNOSIS

DIFFERENTIAL DIAGNOSIS
- Candidal intertrigo
- Psoriasis
- Seborrheic dermatitis
- Erythrasma
- Contact dermatitis
- Tinea versicolor

WORKUP
Diagnosis is based on clinical presentation and demonstration of hyphae microscopically using potassium hydroxide.

LABORATORY TESTS
- Microscopic examination
- Cultures are generally not necessary.

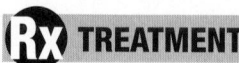
TREATMENT

NONPHARMACOLOGIC THERAPY
- Keep infected area clean and dry.
- Boxer shorts are preferred to briefs. The reduction of perspiration and enhancement of evaporation from the crural area are necessary prophylactic measures.

ACUTE GENERAL Rx
- Various topical antifungal agents are available:
  1. Butenafine cream, applied qd × 14 days
  2. Terbinafine cream, applied bid × 14 days
- Drying powders (e.g., miconazole nitrate) may be useful in patients with excessive perspiration.
- Oral antifungal therapy is generally reserved for cases unresponsive to topical agents or can be used along with topical agents in severe cases. Effective medications are fluconazole 200 mg qd × 7 days or 150 mg once a week for 4 wks, terbinafine 250 mg qd × 14 days, or itraconazole 200 mg/day for 7 days.

DISPOSITION
Most cases respond promptly to therapy with complete resolution within 2 to 3 wk.

RELATED CONTENT
Tinea Cruris (Patient Information)
Tinea Capitis (Related Key Topic)
Tinea Corporis (Related Key Topic)

AUTHOR: **FRED F. FERRI, M.D.**

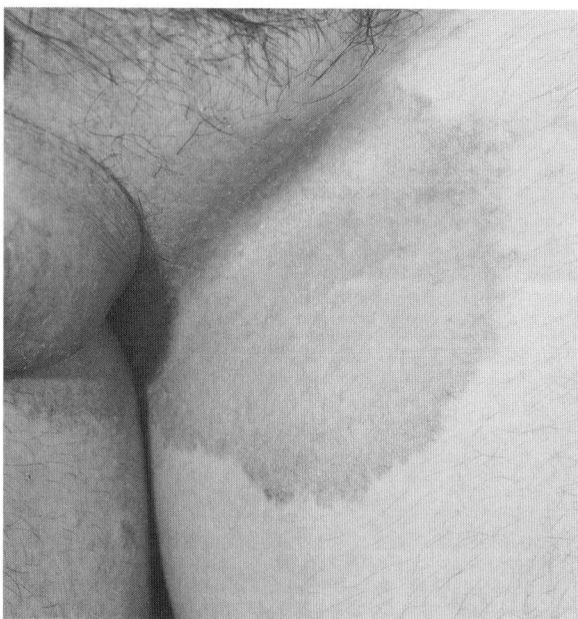

FIG. 1 Tinea cruris. A half-moon–shaped plaque has a well-defined, scaling border. (From Habif TB: *Clinical dermatology: a color guide to diagnosis and therapy*, ed 3, St Louis, 1996, Mosby.)

ℹ️ BASIC INFORMATION

DEFINITION

Tinea pedis is a dermatophyte infection of the feet.

SYNONYMS

Athlete's foot

ICD-10CM CODES
B35.3 Tinea pedis

EPIDEMIOLOGY & DEMOGRAPHICS

- Most common dermatophyte infection
- Increased incidence in hot humid weather; occlusive footwear is a contributing factor
- Occurrence is rare before adolescence
- More common in adult males

PHYSICAL FINDINGS & CLINICAL PRESENTATION

- Typical presentation is variable and ranges from erythematous scaling plaques (Fig. 1) and isolated blisters to interdigital maceration.
- The infection usually starts in the interdigital spaces of the foot. Most infections are found in the toe webs or on the soles.
- Fourth or fifth toes are most commonly involved.
- Pruritus is common and is most intense after removal of shoes and socks.
- Infection with *Trichophyton rubrum* often manifests with a "moccasin" distribution affecting the soles and lateral feet.

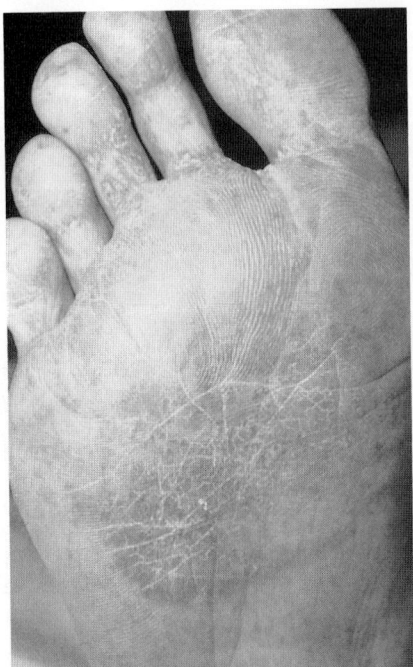

FIG. 1 Tinea pedis. (From Goldstein BG, Goldstein AO: *Practical dermatology,* ed 2, St Louis, 1997, Mosby.)

Tinea pedis caused by trichophyton mentagrophytes (interdigitale) can present with:
1. Erythema and desquamation between the toes.
2. Multilocular bullae involving the thin skin of the plantar arch and along the sides of the feet and heel.
3. White superficial onychomycosis.

ETIOLOGY

- Dermatophyte infection caused by *T. rubrum, Trichophyton mentagrophytes,* or less commonly *Epidermophyton floccosum*
- There may be an autosomal dominant predisposition to this form of infection.

Ⓓ DIAGNOSIS

DIFFERENTIAL DIAGNOSIS

- Contact dermatitis
- Toe web infection (bacterial or candidal infection)
- Eczema
- Psoriasis
- Keratolysis exfoliativa
- Juvenile plantar dermatosis

WORKUP

- Diagnosis is usually made by clinical observation.
- Laboratory testing, when performed, generally consists of a simple potassium hydroxide preparation with mycologic examination under a light microscope to confirm the presence of dermatophytes.

LABORATORY TESTS

- Microscopic examination of a scale or the roof of a blister with 10% KOH under low or medium power will reveal hyphae.
- Mycologic culture is rarely indicated in the diagnosis of tinea pedis.
- Biopsy is reserved for when the diagnosis remains in question after testing or failure to respond to treatment.

℞ TREATMENT

NONPHARMACOLOGIC THERAPY

- Hyperhidrosis is a predisposing factor for tinea pedis. Keep infected area clean and dry. Aerate feet by using sandals when possible.
- Use 100% cotton socks rather than nylon socks to reduce moisture.

- Areas likely to become infected should be dried completely before being covered with clothes.

ACUTE GENERAL Rx

- Benzylamines: butenafine HCl 1% cream applied bid for 1 wk or qd for 4 wk is effective in interdigital tinea pedis.
- Allylamines: terbinafine cream applied bid × 14 days, or naftifine 1% cream applied qd or naftifine gel applied bid for 4 wk produces a significantly high cure rate.
- Imidazoles: econazole, ketoconazole, miconazole, luliconazole, and clotrimazole cream are also effective agents. Clotrimazole 1% cream is an over-the-counter treatment. It should be applied to affected and surrounding area bid for up to 4 wk.
- Ciclopirox and tolnaftate are other antifungal agents available in cream, suspension, or gel. Tolnaftate is also available as a lotion, spray, or powder.
- When using topical preparations, the application area should include normal skin approximately 2 cm beyond the affected area.
- Areas of maceration can be treated with Burow's solution soaks for 10 to 20 min bid followed by foot elevation.
- Oral agents (fluconazole 150 mg once per week for 4 wk, terbinafine 250 mg/day for 14 days, itraconazole 200 mg bid × 7 days, or griseofulvin 500-1000 mg/day for 14 days) can be used in combination with topical agents in resistant cases.

❗ PEARLS & CONSIDERATIONS

- Use of tolnaftate powder (Tinactin) or Zeasorb medicated powder on the feet after bathing may be helpful in preventing recurrent tinea pedis in susceptible persons.
- Combination therapy of antifungal and corticosteroid (clotrimazole/betamethasone [Lotrisone]) should only be used when the diagnosis of fungal infection is confirmed and inflammation is a significant issue.
- Nystatin is not effective and should not be used.

RELATED CONTENT

Athlete's Foot (Patient Information)

AUTHOR: **FRED F. FERRI, M.D.**

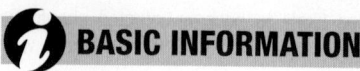

BASIC INFORMATION

DEFINITION

Tinea unguium is defined as a persistent fungal infection affecting the toenails and fingernails.

SYNONYMS

Onychomycosis
Ringworm of the nails

ICD-10CM CODES
B35.1 Tinea unguium

EPIDEMIOLOGY & DEMOGRAPHICS

- Tinea unguium is most commonly found in people between the ages of 40 and 60 yr.
- Tinea unguium rarely occurs before puberty.
- Incidence: 20 to 100 cases/1000 population.
- Toenail infection is 4 to 6 times more common than fingernail infection.
- Tinea unguium affects men more often than women.
- Occurs more frequently in patients with diabetes, peripheral vascular disease, and any

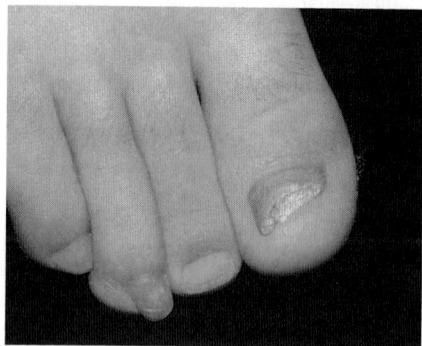

FIG. 1 Distal subungual onychomycosis in a 5-year-old. Note how heavily infected nails occur adjacent to totally normal nails. Cutting back the big toe's nail plate has revealed the friable subungual debris. This material is the most desirable for culture. (From White GM, Cox NH [eds]: *Diseases of the skin, a color atlas and text,* ed 2, St Louis, 2006, Mosby.)

conditions resulting in the suppression of the immune system.
- Occlusive footwear, physical exercise followed by communal showering, and incompletely drying the feet predispose the individual to developing tinea unguium.

PHYSICAL FINDINGS & CLINICAL PRESENTATION

- Tinea unguium causes nails to become thick, brittle, hard, distorted, and discolored (yellow to brown color) (Fig. 1). Eventually, the nail may loosen, separate from the nail bed, and fall off (Fig. 2).
- Tinea unguium is frequently associated with tinea pedis (athlete's foot).

ETIOLOGY

- The most common causes of tinea unguium are dermatophyte, yeast, and nondermatophyte molds.
- The dermatophyte *Trichophyton rubrum* accounts for 80% of all nail infections caused by fungus.
- *Trichophyton interdigitale* and *Trichophyton mentagrophytes* are other fungi causing tinea unguium.
- The yeast *Candida albicans* is responsible for 5% of the cases of tinea unguium and tends to involve fingernails more than toenails.
- Nondermatophyte molds *Scopulariopsis brevicaulis* and *Aspergillus niger,* although rare, can also cause tinea unguium.
- Tinea unguium is classified according to the clinical pattern of nail bed involvement. The main types are:
  1. Distal and lateral subungual tinea unguium (DLSO)
  2. Superficial tinea unguium
  3. Proximal subungual tinea unguium
  4. Endonyx tinea unguium
  5. Total dystrophic tinea unguium

DIAGNOSIS

The diagnosis of tinea unguium is based on the clinical nail findings and confirmed by direct microscopy and culture.

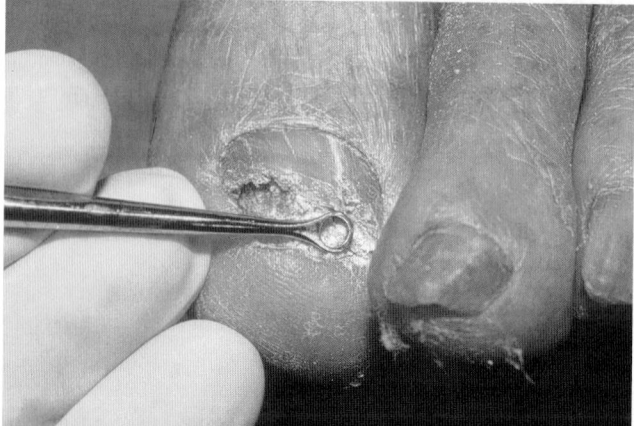

FIG. 2 Collection of nail for culture. The subungual debris is the most valuable material for culture. After the nail is cut back, a curette may be used. Clippings of the nail may be added to the culture. (From White GM, Cox NH [eds]: *Diseases of the skin, a color atlas and text,* ed 2, St Louis, 2006, Mosby.)

DIFFERENTIAL DIAGNOSIS

- Psoriasis
- Contact dermatitis
- Lichen planus
- Subungual keratosis
- Paronychia
- Infection (e.g., *Pseudomonas*)
- Trauma
- Peripheral vascular disease
- Yellow nail syndrome

WORKUP

The workup of suspected tinea unguium is directed at confirming the diagnosis of tinea unguium by visualizing hyphae under the microscope by KOH prep or by culturing the organism. Although the standard for the diagnosis of fungal nail disease is a positive result on microscopic examination and culture of nail clippings with subungual debris or from surface debris in superficial white tinea unguium, treatment is often prescribed in the absence of confirmatory findings.

LABORATORY TESTS

- KOH prep: specificity is high but sensitivity is variable
- Fungal cultures on Sabouraud medium: culture may take 4 to 6 wk
- Dermatophyte test medium (DTM): an alternative to Sabouraud's that takes only 3 to 7 days and can be done in office setting. A color change indicates dermatophyte growth.
- Nail plate biopsy with periodic acid–Schiff (PAS) stain
- Blood tests are not specific in the diagnosis of tinea unguium and therefore not useful

IMAGING STUDIES

- Imaging studies are not very specific in making the diagnosis of tinea unguium and not useful.
- If an infection is present and osteomyelitis is a consideration, an x-ray of the specific area and a bone scan may help establish the diagnosis.

CLASSIFICATION

- The Onychomyosis Severity Index (OSI) is a new classification system for grading the severity of tinea unguium.
- The OSI score is obtained by multiplying the score for the area of involvement (range, 0-5) by the score for the proximity of the disease to the matrix (range, 1-5). Ten points are added for the presence of a longitudinal streak or a patch (dermatophytoma) or for >2 mm of subungual hyperkeratosis.
- Mild tinea unguium corresponds to a score of 1 to 5; moderate to a score of 6 to 15; severe to a score of 16 to 35.

TREATMENT

NONPHARMACOLOGIC THERAPY

- Surgical removal of the nail plate is a treatment option; however, the relapse rate is high.

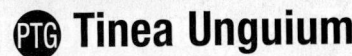

- Prevent reinfection by wearing properly fitted shoes, avoiding public showers, and keeping feet and nails clean and dry.
- Short-pulse laser therapy is fungicidal and is a newer treatment modality for tinea unguium. Most patients will require two to four treatments, each lasting 15 to 30 min. Laser therapy is useful in patients with contraindications to oral agents. It is, however, expensive ($250-$1000 per treatment) and not covered by most insurance plans.

ACUTE GENERAL Rx

- Topical antifungal creams are used for early superficial nail infections.
  1. Miconazole 2% cream applied over the nail plate bid
  2. Clotrimazole 1% cream bid
  3. Ciclopirox: topical antifungal nail lacquer can be used for moderate tinea unguium that spares the lunula. Success rate <10%.
  4. Efinaconazole 10% topical solution (Jublia) is modestly effective in treating toenail tinea unguium due to *Trichophyton rubrum* and/or *Trichophyton mentagrophytes*. Dosage is 1 drop (2 drops for big toenail) once daily for 48 wk. Cost and formulary are limiting factors with this agent.
  5. Tavaborole 5% solution (Kerydin) is an oxaborole antifungal drug approved by the U.S. Food and Drug Administration (FDA) for topical treatment of toenail tinea unguium due to *T. rubrum* or *T. mentagrophytes*. It is applied to affected toenails once daily for 48 wk. It is modestly effective but much more expensive than topical ciclopirox 8% nail lacquer.

- Oral agents
  1. Terbinafine
     a. For toenails: 250 mg/day for 3 mo
     b. For fingernails: 250 mg/day for 6 wk
  2. Itraconazole
     a. For toenails: 200 mg PO daily for 3 mo
     b. For fingernails: 200 mg PO daily for 6 wk
  3. Fluconazole: not as effective as terbinafine or itraconazole
     a. For toenails: 150 to 300 mg once weekly for 18 to 26 wk
     b. For fingernails: 150 to 300 mg once weekly for 12 to 16 wk
- All oral agents used for tinea unguium require periodic monitoring of liver function blood tests. Patients should be advised to watch for symptoms of drug-induced hepatitis (anorexia, fatigue, nausea, right upper quadrant pain) while taking these oral antifungal agents. They should stop their medication and contact their physician immediately if symptoms occur.
- Itraconazole is contraindicated in patients taking cisapride, astemizole, triazolam, midazolam, and terfenadine. Statins should be discontinued during itraconazole therapy. Itraconazole requires gastric acidity for absorption; patients should be advised not to take oral antacids, H_2 blockers, or proton pump inhibitors while taking itraconazole.
- Fluconazole is contraindicated in patients taking cisapride and terfenadine.
- Oral antifungal agents should not be initiated during pregnancy.

DISPOSITION

- Spontaneous remission of tinea unguium is rare.
- A disease-free toenail is reported to occur in approximately 25% to 50% of patients treated with the oral antifungal agents mentioned previously.

REFERRAL

- Podiatry consultation is indicated in diabetic patients for proper instruction in foot care, footwear, and nail debridement or surgical removal of the toenail.
- Dermatology consultation is indicated in patients refractory to treatment or if another diagnosis is considered (e.g., psoriasis).

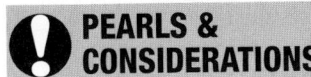

PEARLS & CONSIDERATIONS

COMMENTS

- The growth of fungus on an infected nail typically begins at the end of the nail and spreads under the nail plate to infect the nail bed as well.
- Carefully consider the informational insert regarding drug-drug interactions and contraindications before initiating oral antifungal agents.
- Meta-analysis showed cure rates with the oral agents as follows: terbinafine (about 75%), itraconazole (60%-65%), and fluconazole (about 50%).

SUGGESTED READINGS

Available at www.expertconsult.com

RELATED CONTENT

Nail Fungus (Patient Information)
Ringworm (Patient Information)

AUTHOR: **GLENN G. FORT, M.D., M.P.H.**

Diseases and Disorders

T

I

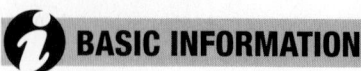

BASIC INFORMATION

DEFINITION

Tinea versicolor is a fungal infection of the skin caused by the yeast *Pityrosporum orbiculare (Malassezia furfur)*.

SYNONYMS

Pityriasis versicolor

ICD-10CM CODES
B36.0 Pityriasis versicolor

EPIDEMIOLOGY & DEMOGRAPHICS

- Increased incidence in adolescence and young adulthood
- More common during the summer (hypopigmented lesions are more evident when the skin is tanned)

PHYSICAL FINDINGS & CLINICAL PRESENTATION

- Most lesions begin as multiple small, circular macules of various colors (Fig. 1) on the trunk and upper arms.
- The macules may be darker or lighter than the surrounding normal skin and will scale with scraping.
- Most frequent site of distribution is trunk.
- Facial lesions are more common in children (forehead is most common facial site).
- Eruption is generally of insidious onset and asymptomatic.
- Lesions may be hyperpigmented in blacks.
- Lesions may be inconspicuous in fair-complexioned individuals, especially during the winter.
- Most patients become aware of the eruption when the involved areas do not tan (Fig. 2).
- Mild itching and inflammation around the patches may be present.
- Facial lesions may occur in infants and immunocompromised patients.

ETIOLOGY

The infection is caused by *Malassezia* species (*M. globosa, M. restricta, M. sympodialis, M. furfur, M. obtusa,* and *M. slooffiae*) Factors that favor proliferation are pregnancy, malnutrition, immunosuppression, oral contraceptives, and excess heat and humidity.

DIAGNOSIS

DIFFERENTIAL DIAGNOSIS

- Vitiligo
- Pityriasis alba
- Secondary syphilis
- Pityriasis rosea
- Seborrheic dermatitis
- Postinflammatory hyperpigmentation or hypopigmentation
- Pityriasis rubra pilaris
- Syphilis
- Hansen's disease

WORKUP

Diagnosis is based on clinical appearance. The *Malassezia* fungus is easily demonstrated in

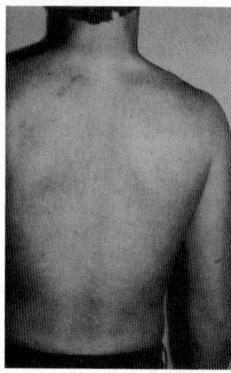

FIG. 1 Tinea versicolor. (Courtesy David Effron, M.D.)

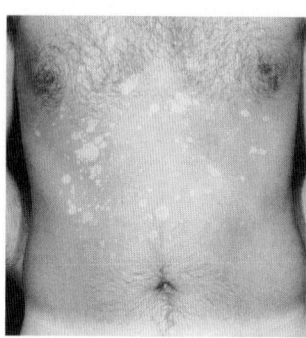

FIG. 2 The classic presentation of tinea versicolor with white, oval, or circular patches on tan skin. (From Habif TB: *Clinical dermatology: a color guide to diagnosis and therapy*, ed 3, St Louis, 1996, Mosby.)

scraping of the profuse scales that cover the lesions. Identification of hyphae and budding spores ("spaghetti and meatballs" appearance) with microscopy confirms diagnosis.

LABORATORY TESTS

Microscopic examination with potassium hydroxide confirms diagnosis.

TREATMENT

NONPHARMACOLOGIC THERAPY

Sunlight accelerates repigmentation of hypopigmented areas.

ACUTE GENERAL Rx

- Topical treatment: selenium sulfide 2.5% suspension (Selsun or Exsel) applied daily for 30 min for 7 consecutive days results in a cure rate of 80% to 90%. The scalp can be shampooed monthly with selenium sulfide to reduce scalp colonization.
- Antifungal topical agents (e.g., miconazole, ciclopirox, clotrimazole) are also effective.
- Oral treatment can be given along with topical agents but is generally reserved for resistant cases. Effective agents are ketoconazole 200 mg qd for 5 days, or single 400-mg dose (cure rate >80%), fluconazole 400 mg given as a single dose (cure rate >70% at 3 wk after treatment), or itraconazole 200 mg/day for 7 days.

DISPOSITION

The prognosis is good, with eradication of the fungus usually occurring within 3 to 4 wk of treatment; however, recurrence is common. After initial therapy, use of monthly application of selenium sulfide may lower risk of recurrence.

PEARLS & CONSIDERATIONS

COMMENTS

Patients should be informed that the hypopigmented areas will not disappear immediately after treatment and that several months may be necessary for the hypopigmented areas to regain their pigmentation.

RELATED CONTENT

Tinea Versicolor (Patient Information)

AUTHOR: **FRED F. FERRI, M.D.**

BASIC INFORMATION

DEFINITION

Tinnitus is a perceived sound in the absence of acoustic stimulus external to the head. It may be unilateral, bilateral, or lateral dominant. It is commonly described as a ringing, buzzing, roaring, hissing, whistling, humming, cricket-like, or pulsing sound. It is frequently a symptom associated with hearing loss, Ménière's disease, acoustic neuroma, drug toxicity, depression, or an autoimmune inner ear disease. The sound may be internal and perceived only by the patient, called subjective or tonal tinnitus, or it may be heard by both the patient and the examiner, called objective or nontonal tinnitus.

ICD-10CM CODES
H93.1   Tinnitus
H93.2   Other abnormal auditory perceptions
H93.11 Tinnitus, right ear
H93.12 Tinnitus, left ear
H93.13 Tinnitus, bilateral
H93.19 Tinnitus, unspecified ear

EPIDEMIOLOGY & DEMOGRAPHICS

PREVALENCE:
- The American Tinnitus Association reports 50 to 60 million Americans have tinnitus for >6 mo.
- Prevalence increases steadily with age, peaking for persons aged 60 to 69 years.
- Prevalence in the U.S. based on National Health Interview Survey (NHIS) in 1996
  1. 2.98% all ages
  2. 0.26% for persons <18 yr old
  3. 1.6% for persons aged 18 to 44 yr
  4. 5.96% for persons aged 45 to 64 yr: 7.7% males, 4.3% females
  5. 9.6% for persons aged 65 to 74 yr: 12% males, 7.7% females
  6. 7.6% for persons >75 yr: 11.4% males, 5.3% females
  7. 2:1 South/Northeast regions
- Up to 18% of people in industrialized societies are mildly affected by chronic tinnitus, and 0.5% report tinnitus having a severe effect on their daily life.
- Only 20% of patients with persistent tinnitus ever seek medical evaluation.

PREDOMINANT SEX AND AGE: Persons most affected are male, Caucasian, elderly, persons with hearing impairment, persons living in southern U.S. For military veterans, tinnitus is the third most common service-related disability.

RISK FACTORS: Any condition causing hearing loss or damage to the auditory system can produce tinnitus. Cochlear damage from exposure to noise is the most common cause. Exposure to ototoxic drugs is also important.

PHYSICAL FINDINGS & CLINICAL PRESENTATION

- History should focus on exposure to loud noises, evidence of hearing loss, and ototoxic drugs.
- Patient should be screened for depression.
- Patient who complains of sound in ear may also complain of ear pain or fullness.
- Objective tinnitus is pulsatile and coincides with patient's pulse.
- Physical examination should focus on HEENT, neck, and neurologic exam.
- There may be no significant physical findings.

ETIOLOGY

- The mechanism behind tinnitus is poorly understood. It may originate at any point along the auditory pathway. Causes of tinnitus include injured cochlear hair cells, spontaneous activity in auditory nerve fibers, hyperactivity in the auditory nuclei in the brain stem, or a reduction in the suppressive activity of the central auditory cortex.
- Medications implicated in causing tinnitus include salicylates, NSAIDs, aminoglycosides, loop diuretics, valproate, quinine, chemotherapeutic agents, cisplatin, vincristine, and heavy metals such as lead.

DIAGNOSIS

DIFFERENTIAL DIAGNOSIS

- Subjective/tonal tinnitus:
  1. Otologic: tympanic membrane disorder, inner ear disorder (hair cells, organ of Corti), Ménière's disease
  2. Ototoxic medications
  3. Neurologic: multiple sclerosis, head trauma, cochlear nerve lesion, acoustic schwannoma, neurofibroma, meningioma
  4. Metabolic: thyroid disorder, hyperlipidemia (leading to plaque formation), vitamin B_{12} deficiency
  5. Psychogenic: depression, anxiety, fibromyalgia
  6. Infectious: otitis media, Lyme disease, meningitis, syphilis
- Objective/nontonal tinnitus:
  1. Vascular: arterial bruit, venous hum, arteriovenous malformation, vascular tumors
  2. Neurologic: contraction of muscles of the eustachian tube, contraction of the stapedius muscle, contraction of the tensor tympani muscles, or a palatal myoclonus, glomus jugulare tumor
  3. Conductive: patulous (wide-open) eustachian tube

WORKUP*

- Audiometry
- Tympanometry
- Electronystagmography is used to evaluate for Ménière's disease.
- An algorithm for tinnitus evaluation is described in Figs. E1 and E2.

LABORATORY TESTS

Evaluate for metabolic abnormalities: TSH, CBC, B_{12}, and lipid panel.

IMAGING STUDIES

- CT/MRI: to evaluate for subjective tinnitus
- MRI/MRA: to evaluate objective tinnitus
- Imaging should not be part of routine management. Clinicians must distinguish patients with bothersome tinnitus from patients with nonbothersome tinnitus. For patients without persistent and bothersome tinnitus, audiometric testing is optional.

TREATMENT

NONPHARMACOLOGIC THERAPY

- It is best to avoid exposure to excessive noise, ototoxic agents, and to wear protective equipment in noisy environments, or mask the tinnitus through amplification of normal sounds with a hearing aid. Habituation techniques such as tinnitus retraining therapy may help. Cognitive behavioral therapy helps patients cope with tinnitus distress through biofeedback.
- Recent trials involving brain stimulation in the form of repetitive transcranial magnetic stimulation (rTMS have shown reduction in the perception or severity of tinnitus).[1]

ACUTE GENERAL Rx

- If the tinnitus is severe enough to cause suicidal symptoms, immediate referral to a psychiatrist and an otolaryngologist is recommended to minimize the time to diagnosis and optimize treatment.
- Patients with persistent symptoms or tinnitus accompanied by visual changes or headache should be evaluated for tumors such as acoustic neuroma.
- Clinicians should not routinely recommend anxiolytics, anticonvulsants, or intratympanic medications.

CHRONIC Rx

There is insufficient evidence to support the use of any medication, vitamin, or nutritional supplement to treat tinnitus. Empirical use of over-the-counter supplements or prescription medications should be discouraged.

DISPOSITION

Clinical course is variable. About 20% to 25% of patients with chronic tinnitus consider it a significant problem. Individualized tinnitus management programs can be beneficial in most patients.

PEARLS & CONSIDERATIONS

PREVENTION

- Avoid loud, chronic noise and ototoxic drugs.
- Higher caffeine intake is associated with a lower risk of incidence of tinnitus in women.

EVIDENCE

Available at www.expertconsult.com

RELATED CONTENT

Tinnitus (Patient Information)

AUTHORS: **VICKY H. BHAGAT, M.D., M.P.H.** and **DAWN HOGAN, M.D.**

[1]Folmer RL, et al: Repetitive transcranial magnetic stimulation treatment for chronic tinnitus: a randomized clinical trial, *JAMA Otolaryngol Head Neck Surg* 141(8):716-722, 2015.

BASIC INFORMATION

DEFINITION

The term *Torsade de Pointes* (TdP) refers to a polymorphic ventricular tachycardia (VT) associated with a prolonged QT interval and electrocardiographically characterized by QRS complexes of changing amplitude that appear to twist around the isoelectric line, hence the name *Torsade de Pointes*, or "twisting of the points" (Fig. 1).

Torsade is typically initiated by a short-long-short sequence of ventricular beats but can also be initiated by a short-coupled variant. Typically, TdP occurs in the setting of a markedly prolonged QT interval (>500 msec); the QTc prolongs even further during the long diastolic interval of a compensatory pause, leading to a polymorphic VT with a ventricular rate of 160 to 250 beats per minute, irregular RR intervals, and a cycling of the QRS axis through 180 degrees every 5 to 20 beats. It may be repetitive, nonsustained, or sustained and may degenerate into ventricular fibrillation. In some cases, the result is sudden cardiac death.

SYNONYMS

Torsades
TdP

ICD-10CM CODES
I47.2 Ventricular tachycardia

EPIDEMIOLOGY & DEMOGRAPHICS

INCIDENCE: The precise incidence of TdP is unclear but accounts for fewer than 5% of all sudden cardiac arrests. In congenital long QT syndromes (LQTS), TdP may occur in up to 6% cases at rest and 9% of cases during an exercise test. Among drug-induced causes of TdP, the incidence may vary between <1% in cases of antibiotics and antipsychotics to 2% to 4% when caused by class III anti-arrhythmics such as sotalol, ibutilide, and dofetilide.

PREDOMINANT SEX AND AGE: Because testosterone shortens the QT interval, women have a longer baseline QT interval, which is believed to be the reason for a two- to threefold increased incidence of TdP in women.

GENETICS: Of the congenital LQTS channelopathies, long QT syndromes 1, 2, and 3 account for >70% of all cases. In general, the risk of TdP increases as the QT lengthens; however, there are also genotype-phenotype relationships that help define risk; for example, LQTS3 carries a higher risk of TdP than LQTS1. Similarly, the Jervell and Lange-Nielsen syndrome and Romano-Ward syndrome may lead to TdP.

It is also likely that genetic factors are at play in acquired LQT and in the development of TdP. For example, in large populations, the QT interval prolongs very little with the administration of QT-prolonging drugs such as fluoroquinolones; however, certain individuals will have markedly exaggerated QT prolongation that leads to TdP; this is likely due to some underlying genetic factor.

RISK FACTORS: TdP in patients with congenital LQTS is often initiated by an external trigger (Table 1). Triggers can include exercise, noise, emotion, sudden waking from sleep by an alarm clock, telephone ringing, thunder, swimming, or diving. TdP in LQT1 patients is classically triggered by vigorous exercise or swimming; in LQT2 by emotion, pregnancy, or noise; and in LQT3 when at rest or asleep. Risk factors for drug-induced TdP are outlined in Table 2.

The risk factors for developing TdP in patients with acquired long QT are extensive and are outlined in Table 3.

PATHOPHYSIOLOGY:

- Changes in the balance of transmembrane ionic currents lead to lengthening of the QT interval and to abnormal action potentials called early afterdepolarizations (EADs). An EAD, in the setting of electrical instability induced by the prolonged QT, initiates the torsades. Perpetuation may be caused by transmural entry, triggered activity, or abnormal automaticity. A distinct group of cells called the M cells, located in the mid-myocardium, has a less rapid delayed rectifier potassium current (IKr), and the cells are central to the genesis of TdP.
- Drugs with the potential to cause TdP most frequently inhibit the rapid potassium channels and result in prolongation of the action potential duration, producing a prolonged QT on ECG.

PHYSICAL FINDINGS & CLINICAL PRESENTATION

- Clinical features depend on whether the TdP is caused by acquired or congenital long QT syndrome. Congenital LQTS patients may have certain specific triggers, such as noise, exercise, and emotions (see "Risk Factors").
- Symptoms of the tachycardia itself include palpitations, pre-syncope, syncope (sometimes with jerking movements from myoclonus, often misinterpreted as seizures), and sudden cardiac death (SCD).
- Patients resuscitated from SCD have an especially ominous prognosis, with a relative risk of 12.9% of experiencing another cardiac arrest.

ETIOLOGY

The etiology or triggers of TdP may be congenital or acquired causes of QT prolongation (see Table 1). For a comprehensive list of drugs that can cause or have the potential to cause TdP, see "Patient/Family Education."

DIAGNOSIS

DIFFERENTIAL DIAGNOSIS

Other causes of syncope.

Other causes of broad complex tachycardia such as:
- Polymorphic VT.
- Wolff-Parkinson-White (WPW) syndrome with rapid atrial fibrillation.
- ECG artifact.

WORKUP

- ECG and telemetry are the mainstays of diagnosing TdP as they detect the arrhythmia, the preceding prolonged QT interval, and the long-short cycles that trigger it.
- Determination and treatment of the etiology of TdP (see Table 1) is key.

LABORATORY TESTS

- Electrolytes: assess for hypokalemia, hypocalcemia, and hypomagnesemia.
- Thyroid function tests.
- Genetic studies if suspicion of congenital LQT syndrome.

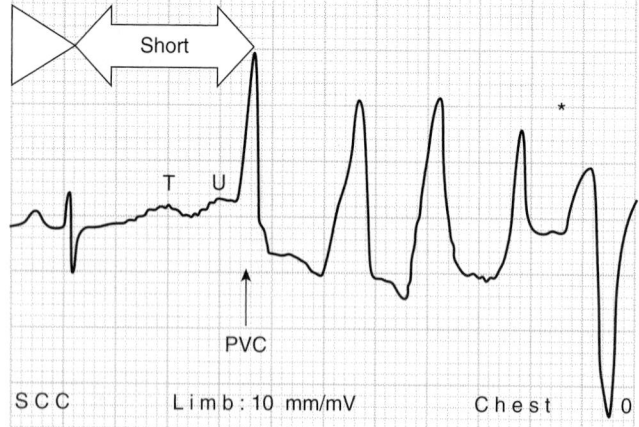

FIG. 1 Onset of Torsade de Pointes during the recording of a standard 12-lead ECG in a young male with a history of drug addiction treated with chronic methadone therapy who presented to a hospital emergency department after ingesting an overdose of prescription and over-the-counter drugs from his parent's drug cabinet. Classic ECG features evident in this rhythm strip include a prolonged QT interval with distorted T-U complex, initiation of the arrhythmia after a short-long-short cycle sequence by a PVC that falls near the peak of the distorted T-U complex, "warm-up" phenomenon with initial R-R cycles longer than subsequent cycles, and abrupt switching of QRS morphology from predominantly positive to predominantly negative complexes (asterisk). (From Drew BJ et al: Prevention of Torsade de Pointes in hospital settings: a scientific statement from the American Heart Association and the American College of Cardiology Foundation, *J Am Coll Cardiol* 55;934-947, 2010.)

TABLE 1 Causes and Triggers of Torsade de Pointes

Congenital	• Romano-Ward syndrome [autosomal dominant] • Jervell and Lange-Nielsen syndrome [autosomal recessive] • LQTS channelopathies
Acquired	
Metabolic syndromes	• Hypokalemia • Hypocalcemia • Hypomagnesemia • Starvation • Anorexia nervosa • Liquid protein diets • Hypothyroidism
Bradyarrhythmias	• Sinus node dysfunction • Second- or third-degree AV block
Antiarrhythmic drugs	• Quinidine • Procainamide • Disopyramide • Amiodarone and dronedarone • Sotalol • Dofetilide, ibutilide, azimilide
Antimicrobial drugs	• Erythromycin, clarithromycin, azithromycin • Pentamidine • Azole antifungals like voriconazole • Fluoroquinolones such as levofloxacin & moxifloxacin • Chloroquine
Antihistaminics	• Terfenadine • Astemizole
Psychiatric drugs	• Phenothiazines • Thioridazine • Tricyclic antidepressants • Haloperidol • Risperidone • Selective serotonin reuptake inhibitors
Antineoplastic agents	• Tyrosine kinase inhibitors such as sunitinib, dasatinib • Vorinostat • Arsenic
Gastric motility agents	• Cisapride, domperidone
Opioid dependence drugs	• Methadone
Other factors	• Myocardial ischemia • Hypothermia • Intracranial disease • HIV infection • Connective tissue disease with anti-Ro/SSA antibodies • Periodic paralysis (Andersen syndrome) • Cocaine

TABLE 2 Risk Factors for Drug-Induced Torsade de Pointes

- Congenital long QT
- Female gender
- Electrolyte abnormalities (hypokalemia, hypomagnesemia, hypocalcemia)
- Diuretic use
- Bradycardia
- Cardiac hypertrophy
- Myocardial fibrosis
- Congestive heart failure
- Renal and liver insufficiency
- Coadministration of drugs blocking P450 isoenzyme CYP3A4
- High doses or rapid intravenous infusion of the drug
- Baseline electrocardiographic abnormalities (prolonged QT, T-wave lability)

From Gowda RM et al: Torsades de Pointes: the clinical considerations, *Int J Cardiol* 96(1):1-6, 2004.

TABLE 3 Risk Factors for Torsade de Pointes in Hospitalized Patients

- Clinically recognizable risk factors
- QTc >500 msec
- LQT2-type repolarization: notched or "bifid" T-wave
- Use of QT-prolonging drugs
- Concurrent use of more than one QT-prolonging drug
- Rapid infusion by intravenous route
- Structural heart disease
- Congestive heart failure
- Myocardial infarction
- Advanced age
- Female sex
- Hypokalemia
- Hypomagnesemia
- Hypocalcemia
- Treatment with diuretics
- Impaired hepatic drug metabolism
- Bradycardia
- Sinus bradycardia, heart block, incomplete heart block with pauses
- Premature QRS complexes leading to short-long-short cycles
- Multiple clinically recognizable risk factors
- Occult (latent) congenital LQTS
- Genetic polymorphisms

From Drew BJ et al. Prevention of Torsade de Pointes in hospital settings: a scientific statement from the American Heart Association and the American College of Cardiology Foundation, *Circulation* 121(8):1047, 2010.

IMAGING STUDIES
- Echocardiography to rule out structural heart disease as a cause of VT.
- Stress test to rule out myocardial ischemia. Stress ECG with dynamic assessment of the QT interval during varying heart rates may be diagnostic of long QT syndromes and related TdP.
- CT scan of the head if intracranial disease is suspected.
- Fig. 2 shows TdP in a teenage patient with long QT syndrome.

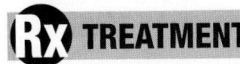 **TREATMENT**

The cornerstone of treatment comprises intravenous magnesium and acceleration of the heart rate, either by mechanical overdrive pacing or by infusion of isoproterenol. Withdrawal of causative drugs and correction of underlying causes such as electrolyte imbalances, hypothermia, and ischemia are also important.

NONPHARMACOLOGIC THERAPY
- Withdrawal of any offending drugs and correction of electrolyte abnormalities are recommended in patients presenting with TdP (Class I recommendation).
- Temporary atrial or ventricular overdrive pacing is a Class I recommendation for all causes of TdP if intravenous magnesium fails.
- Acute and long-term pacing is recommended for patients presenting with TdP due to heart block and symptomatic bradycardia (Class 1) or those with recurrent pause-dependent torsades (Class IIa).
- Active internal and external rewarming if hypothermia is the etiology.
- If TdP degenerates into ventricular fibrillation, defibrillation and advanced cardiac life support protocol should be followed.

ACUTE Rx
- Intravenous magnesium sulfate 1 to 2 g given over 1 to 2 min is first-line therapy for patients who present with LQTS and few episodes of TdP (Class IIa). Magnesium is not likely to be effective in patients with a normal QT interval
- Isoproterenol is reasonable as temporary treatment in patients with acute disease who present with recurrent pause-dependent TdP and who do not have congenital LQTS (Class IIa).
- Beta-blockade combined with pacing is reasonable acute therapy for patients who

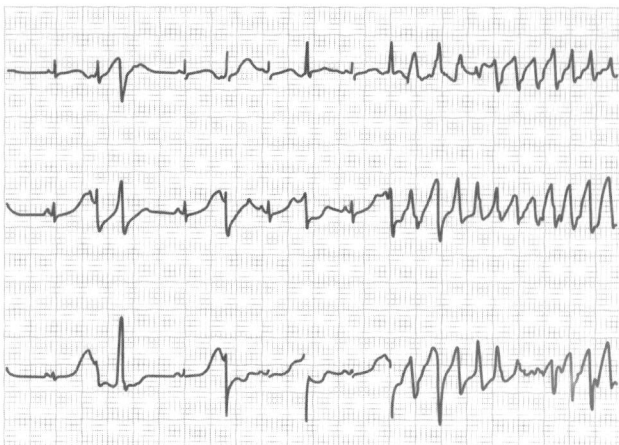

FIG. 2 Torsade de Pointes in a teenage patient with long QT syndrome. This arrhythmia is associated with no pulse and results in syncope. It often terminates spontaneously, but otherwise rapidly degenerates to ventricular fibrillation. (From Fuhrman: *Pediatric critical care,* ed 4, 2010, Elsevier.)

present with TdP and sinus bradycardia (Class IIa).
- Potassium repletion to 4.5 to 5 mmol/L may be considered for patients who present with TdP and hypokalemia (Class IIb).
- Intravenous lidocaine, oral mexiletine, or phenytoin may be considered in patients who present with LQT3 and TdP (Class IIb).
- TdP is usually self-limited, and cardioversion should be performed only as a last resort in the setting of pulseless VF because of the high likelihood of immediate recurrence of the TdP after cardioversion.

CHRONIC Rx
- TdP resulting from congenital LQTS is treated with beta-blockade, pacing, and implantable cardioverter-defibrillator (ICD) in high-risk cases. For patients who continue to have syncope despite maximal drug therapy, cervical-thoracic sympathectomy may be considered.
- Long-term pacing is recommended for patients presenting with TdP due to heart block and symptomatic bradycardia.
- Avoid use of QT-prolonging drugs.
- Lifestyle modification in case of congenital LQTS.

- In patients with eating disorders, nutritional rehabilitation will correct the QT prolongation over the long term (3-18 mo).
- Psychiatric evaluation of patients with drug overdose and eating disorders.

DISPOSITION
Patients with TdP should be monitored in an intensive care setting.

REFERRAL
Patients should have an urgent cardiology consultation.

⊘ PEARLS & CONSIDERATIONS

COMMENTS
- Identification of the etiology for TdP is key in diagnosis, management, and prognosis of this condition.
- Drugs associated with TdP vary greatly in their risk for arrhythmia; an updated list can be found at https://crediblemeds.org. The risk-benefit ratio should be assessed for each individual to determine whether the potential therapeutic benefit of a drug outweighs the risk for TdP.

- Risk factors for drug-induced TdP include older age, female sex, heart disease, electrolyte disorders (especially hypokalemia and hypomagnesemia), renal or hepatic dysfunction, bradycardia or rhythms with long pauses, treatment with more than one QT-prolonging drug, and genetic predisposition.
- After initiation of a drug associated with TdP, ECG signs indicative of risk for arrhythmia include an increase in QTc from predrug baseline of >60 msec, marked QTc interval prolongation >500 msec, T-U wave distortion that becomes more exaggerated in the beat after a pause, visible T-wave alternans, new-onset ventricular ectopy, and couplets and nonsustained polymorphic ventricular tachycardia initiated in the beat after a pause.

PREVENTION
The 2011 AHA/ACC scientific statement on prevention of TdP suggests a strategy of documenting the QTc interval before and at least every 8 to 12 hr after the initiation, increased dose, or overdose of QT-prolonging drugs. If QTc prolongation is observed, documentation of more frequent measurements is recommended. The duration of QTc monitoring depends upon the duration of treatment with the QT-prolonging drug and the drug half-life.

PATIENT/FAMILY EDUCATION
- Patients should be educated about avoiding use of QT-prolonging drugs. A complete list of these drugs can be found at https://crediblemeds.org
- First-degree relatives of all patients with congenital LQTS should undergo genetic testing.
- Congenital LQTS patients should avoid certain specific triggers (e.g., swimming and exercise in LQTS 1 and LQTS 2 and acoustic stimuli in LQTS 2).
- It is recommended that all patients affected by LQTS avoid competitive sports activity.

RELATED TOPICS
Long QT Syndrome (Related Key Topic)

AUTHOR: **CHRISTOPHER PICKETT, M.D.**

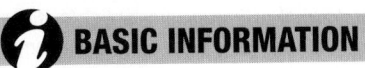 **BASIC INFORMATION**

DEFINITION

Tourette's syndrome (TS) is an inherited neuropsychiatric disorder characterized by motor, vocal, and phonic tics that change during the course of illness. Onset of symptoms is typically before the age of 18.

Tics are sudden, brief, intermittent, involuntary or semi-voluntary movements (motor tics), or sounds (phonic or vocal tics) that mimic fragments of normal behavior.

SYNONYMS

Gilles de la Tourette syndrome
TS
Tourette's disorder

> **ICD-10CM CODES**
> F95.2 Combined vocal and multiple motor tic disorder [de la Tourette]

EPIDEMIOLOGY & DEMOGRAPHICS

PREVALENCE (IN U.S.): Unknown; estimates range from 0.3% to 0.9% in children.
PREDOMINANT SEX: Approximate male:female ratio of 4:1.
PREDOMINANT AGE: Typical age of onset is between 2 and 15 years (mean 5-7 years).

PHYSICAL FINDINGS & CLINICAL PRESENTATION

- Neurologic examination is normal.
- Vocal and phonic tics are characterized as simple (e.g., clearing of throat, sniffing, grunting, sucking) or complex (e.g., repetition of short phrases, swearing [coprolalia]).
- Motor tics can be simple (e.g., blinking, grimacing, head jerking) or complex (e.g., gesturing). Tics wax, wane, change over time, and are often suppressed for short periods. Commonly, they are preceded by an urge to perform the tic.
- TS is often associated with a variety of behavioral symptoms, most commonly attention deficit hyperactivity disorder (ADHD) and obsessive-compulsive disorder (OCD).

TS can be diagnosed using the DSM 5 criteria as follows:
1. Both multiple motor and one or more vocal tics must be present at some time during the illness, although not necessarily concurrently.
2. The tics may wax and wane in frequency but have persisted for more than one year since first tic onset.
3. Age at onset is less than 18 years.
4. Disturbance is not attributable to the direct physiologic effects of a substance (e.g., stimulants) or another medical condition (e.g., Huntington's disease or postviral encephalitis).

ETIOLOGY

The exact pathogenesis is unknown. Genetic predisposition is likely as there is a strong family history of OCD or TS in patients with tics, and twin studies provide evidence for the importance of genetic factors. Recent analysis of linkage in a two-generation pedigree has led to the identification of a mutation in the HDC gene encoding I-histidine decarboxylase, the rate-limiting enzyme in histamine biosynthesis, pointing to a role for histaminergic neurotransmission in the mechanism and modulation of TS and tics (Fig. 1. Immunologic dysfunction is also being explored in the pathogenesis of this complex disorder.

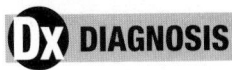 **DIAGNOSIS**

DIFFERENTIAL DIAGNOSIS

- Sydenham's chorea: occurs after infection with group A *Streptococcus.*
- Pediatric autoimmune neuropsychiatric disorder associated with group A streptococci (PANDAS).
- Sporadic tic disorders: tics tend to be motor or vocal but not both.
- Head trauma.
- Drug intoxication: many drugs are known to induce or exacerbate tic disorders, including

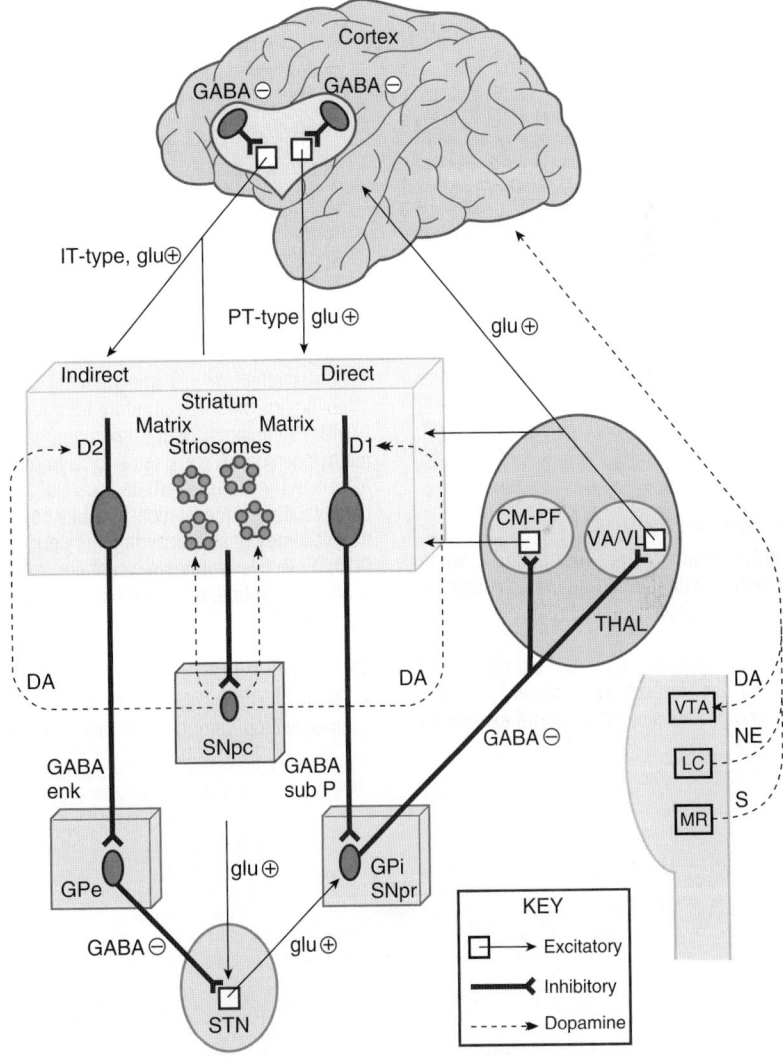

FIG. 1 The cortico-striatal-thalamo-cortical pathway and ascending cortical inputs. Hypothesized abnormalities have included disorders of excess excitation or diminished inhibition, disruptions in frontal cortex, striatum, or striosomes, and abnormalities of various synaptic neurotransmitters. *CM-PF,* Centromedian-parafascicular complex; *DA,* dopamine; *enk,* enkephalins; *GABA,* gamma-aminobutyric acid; *glu,* glutamate; *GPe,* globus pallidus externa; *GPi,* globus pallidus interna; *IT,* intra telencephalic; *LC,* locus ceruleus; *MR,* median raphe; *NE,* norepinephrine; *PT,* pyramidal tract; *S,* serotonin; *SNpc,* substantia nigra pars compacta; *SNpr,* substantia nigra pars reticulata; *STN,* subthalamic nucleus; *sub P,* substance P; *THAL,* thalamus; *VA/VL,* ventral anterior/ventral lateral nuclei; *VTA,* ventral tegmental area. (From Harris K and Singer HS. Tic disorders: neural circuits, neurochemistry, and neuroimmunology. *J Child Neurology* 2006;21:678–689.)

methylphenidate, amphetamines, pemoline, anticholinergics, and antihistamines.
- Postinfectious encephalitis.
- Inherited disorders: Huntington's disease, Hallervorden-Spatz disease, and neuroacanthocytosis. These conditions should have other observed abnormalities on neurologic examination.

WORKUP

Clinical observation and history to confirm diagnosis.

LABORATORY TESTS

No definitive laboratory tests.

IMAGING STUDIES

CT scan and MRI of brain are unremarkable in TS and unnecessary if the neurologic examination is within normal limits.

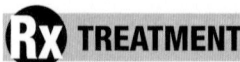 **TREATMENT**

NONPHARMACOLOGIC THERAPY

Multidisciplinary: education of parents, teachers, psychologists, and school nurses is essential. Cognitive behavioral therapy, termed habit-reversal treatment, is efficacious in suppressing tics.

ACUTE GENERAL Rx

Dopamine-blocking agents may be used to acutely reduce the severity of tics. However, these agents carry a risk of side effects, such as acute dystonic reactions.

CHRONIC Rx

Tics only require long-term treatment when they interfere with an individual's psychosocial, educational, and occupational function.
TICS:
- Alpha-2 agonists, such as clonidine and guanfacine, are used for treatment of motor tics and are considered by some experts as

first-line medications because of their favorable adverse effect profile. However, they are more beneficial for treatment of behavioral symptoms and are preferred for patients with predominant psychiatric disorders.
- Haloperidol and pimozide are the only U.S. Food and Drug Administration-approved neuroleptics for the treatment of tics in TS. Pimozide is started at a dose of 0.5 to 1.0 mg at night and increased every 5 to 7 days to a therapeutic dose of 2 to 8 mg. Haloperidol is started at a dose of 0.25 to 0.5 mg and can be increased to 1 to 4 mg depending on response and side effects. Use of neuroleptics carries a small but significant risk of tardive dyskinesia.
- Tetrabenazine is a dopamine-depleting agent that can be used effectively in TS patients to control tics. Tetrabenazine does not cause many of the typical side effects of neuroleptic medication. However, severe depression may occur with use of tetrabenazine.
- Dopamine agonists include ropinirole and pramipexole. A few small, open-label studies have found that, in low doses, these medications may be effective in reducing tic severity.
- Botulinum toxin (local injection) is effective for focal tics like eye blinking and neck and shoulder tics. The benefits are temporary, lasting 3 to 6 months.
- Surgical treatment with deep brain stimulation is effective in some patients with disabling tics that are refractory to medications.

ADHD: Stimulants (e.g., dextroamphetamine, methylphenidate) are useful for symptoms of ADHD but may exacerbate tics in 25% of patients. These medications should be used if troublesome behavioral symptoms persist.
OCD: Selective serotonin reuptake inhibitors, such as fluoxetine, are the most effective treatment for OCD.

DISPOSITION

- The intensity and frequency of tics typically diminishes during the later teenage years.

- One third of patients will achieve significant remission, although complete, lifelong remission is rare.
- One third will have mild, persistent, but "non-impairing" tics.

REFERRAL

Neurologist to confirm the initial diagnosis and for treatment in difficult cases.

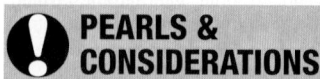 **PEARLS & CONSIDERATIONS**

- Tics do not need treatment unless they interfere with an individual's ability to function.
- Greater improvement in symptom severity among children with TS and chronic tic disorder has been reported with a comprehensive behavioral intervention compared with supportive therapy and education.
- An important part of treatment is appropriate evaluation and therapy of coexisting conditions (e.g., ADHD, OCD).
- Deep brain stimulation has shown promising results as an alternative therapy in patients with medically refractory disease.

COMMENTS

Patient education may be obtained from the Tourette's Syndrome Association, 4240 Bell Blvd., Bayside, NY 11361-2864; 800-237-0717 or 718-224-2999; http://www.tsa-usa.org.

SUGGESTED READINGS

Available at www.expertconsult.com

RELATED CONTENT

Tourette's Syndrome (Patient Information)

AUTHORS: **ALEXANDRA BUFFIE, M.D., JOSEPH S. KASS, M.D., J.D.,** and **FARIHA ZAHEER, M.D.**

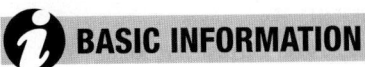

BASIC INFORMATION

DEFINITION

Toxic megacolon is a rare but severe complication of colonic inflammation, usually inflammatory bowel disease (IBD). It is characterized by total or segmental nonobstructive colonic distention (>6 cm) associated with systemic toxicity of inflammatory or infectious etiology.

SYNONYMS

Toxic dilation of the colon

ICD 10-CM CODES
K59.3 Megacolon, not elsewhere classified
A04.7 Megacolon due to *Clostridium difficile*

EPIDEMIOLOGY & DEMOGRAPHICS

INCIDENCE: Varies depending on etiology. Incidence in patients with ulcerative colitis (UC) is between 7% and 10% and approximately 1% and 5% in patients with Crohn's. *Clostridium difficile* infections may be complicated by toxic megacolon in up to 3% of cases.
PEAK INCIDENCE: N/A
PREVALENCE: N/A
PREDOMINANT SEX AND AGE: With increasing rates of *Clostridium difficile* (*C. diff*) infections due to overuse of antibiotics and hypervirulent strains, patients ages 65 and older are at higher risk for developing toxic megacolon as a result of *C. diff* infection.
GENETICS: There are no known genetic factors that predispose patients to developing toxic megacolon associated with an inflammatory or infectious etiology.
RISK FACTORS: Major risk factors include inflammatory, infectious, and ischemic conditions of the colon, especially in individuals who are immunocompromised. Other risk factors include hypokalemia, use of narcotics or antidiarrheal agents, pregnancy, and recent instrumentation (such as colonoscopy).

PHYSICAL FINDINGS & CLINICAL PRESENTATION

- Patients with toxic megacolon usually appear severely ill. Clinical symptoms are similar to those of IBD and acute colitis and may include abdominal pain, diarrhea (usually bloody), and vomiting.
- Physical exam findings may include a distended, tender, and tympanic abdomen with reduced or absent bowel sounds. The patient may also present with signs of shock such as fever, tachycardia, mental status changes, and hypovolemia.
- Laboratory findings may include leukocytosis, anemia, and electrolyte abnormalities such as hypokalemia and hypoalbuminemia.

ETIOLOGY

- Most common etiologies are inflammatory conditions such as UC, Crohn's, and Behcet's disease.
- Infections such as *C. diff, Salmonella, Shigella, E. coli,* cytomegalovirus, and *Entamoeba* can also be complicated by toxic megacolon.
- Other less common etiologies include ischemic colitis, malignancy such as lymphoma, and Kaposi's sarcoma. In general, toxic megacolon is more likely to be associated with pancolitis than segmental colitis (Box 1).

DIAGNOSIS

DIFFERENTIAL DIAGNOSIS

- Ischemic colitis, Crohn's disease, ulcerative colitis

WORKUP

- General principles of workup include physical examination to evaluate for an acute abdomen, laboratory testing to detect electrolyte abnormalities, and plain radiography to evaluate for colonic dilatation.
- Clinical criteria for toxic megacolon, proposed by Jalan et al. in 1969, are still used. A diagnosis can be made if radiographic evidence of colonic distention >6 cm is present with at least three of the following: fever >38°C, heart rate >120, leukocytosis >10.5, or anemia. In addition, at least one of the following must also be present: dehydration, altered level of consciousness, electrolyte abnormalities, or hypotension.

LABORATORY TESTS

- Initial testing should include a CBC, full chemistry panel, lactic acid, coagulation panel, liver function panel, and a type and screen.

IMAGING STUDIES

- All patients should initially receive a plain abdominal radiograph (Fig. 1) to assess for colonic dilatation. Common findings include mucosal irregularity, loss of haustrations, "thumb printing" due to bowel wall edema, and thickening of the colonic wall with a continuous segment of air-filled colon >6 cm in diameter. The transverse or right colon is usually the most dilated segment seen.
- Computed tomography (CT) has been increasingly used to assess disease extent

BOX 1   Disorders Associated With Toxic Megacolon.

- Inflammatory bowel disease
  1. Ulcerative colitis
  2. Crohn's disease
- Infectious colitis
  1. *Salmonella, Shigella*, amoebic colitis
  2. *Clostridium difficile*
  3. Cytomegalovirus colitis
  4. HIV infection
- Cancer chemotherapy
- Ischemia

HIV, Human immunodeficiency virus.

From Vincent JL et al: *Textbook of critical care,* ed 6, Philadelphia, 2011, Saunders.

and for surgical planning (Fig. 2). It can also be helpful when differentiating between the various etiologies of toxic megacolon and to assess for complications such as intraabdominal hemorrhage or abscess.

TREATMENT

Treatment includes both medical and surgical options. Principles of initial management include treating the underlying cause and managing symptoms of shock with early surgical and gastroenterology consultation.

NONPHARMACOLOGIC THERAPY

- Surgery may be required in up to 50% of patients with toxic megacolon who do not show clinical improvement within 24-48 hr. The preferred first-line surgical treatment is subtotal colectomy with an end ileostomy. Other options include total proctocolectomy or colon decompression via the Turnbull method.
- Timing of surgical treatment is still controversial, with many advocating for aggressive medical treatment and observation before surgical intervention. Definitive indications for early surgical treatment include perforation, persistent colonic hemorrhage, or rapid clinical deterioration.

ACUTE GENERAL Rx

- Medications that impact colonic motility such as anticholinergics, opioids, and antidiarrheal agents should be discontinued and avoided.
- Electrolyte abnormalities, dehydration, and anemia are common clinical findings and should be addressed early. Fluid resuscitation with an isotonic solution (normal saline or lactated Ringer's) and correction of electrolyte disturbances (especially hypokalemia) can help prevent worsening atony of the colonic wall. Patients with anemia from colonic hemorrhage should receive blood transfusion.
- Patients with systemic signs of infection or a suspected infectious etiology should receive broad-spectrum antibiotics. Infections due to *C. diff* should be treated with vancomycin (oral or rectal) or metronidazole (oral or IV). Toxic megacolon due to cytomegalovirus should be treated with ganciclovir IV.
- Patients with inflammatory etiologies such as UC or Crohn's should receive high-dose IV steroids, either hydrocortisone 100 mg IV or methylprednisolone 60 mg IV. Steroids should not be used in patients with a confirmed infectious etiology.
- There are currently no data to support empiric treatment of toxic megacolon due to IBD with cyclosporine or infliximab. These treatment options should be reserved for patients who are not steroid responsive and should be limited to one attempt at clinical improvement so as not to delay surgical intervention.

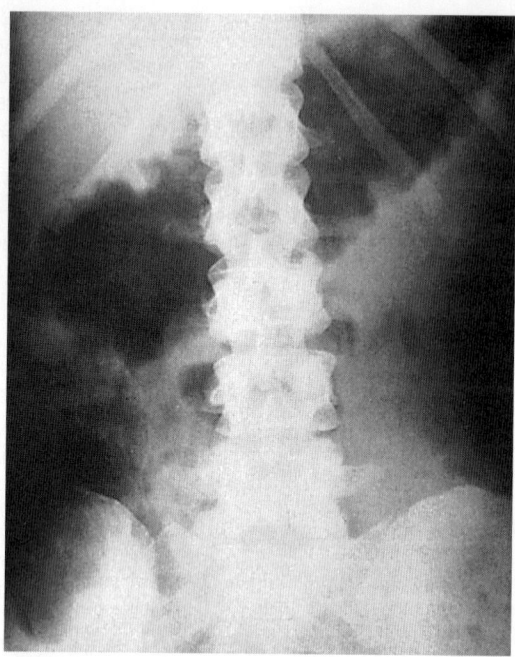

FIG. 1 Toxic megacolon secondary to ulcerative colitis. The smooth indentations seen along the margin of the colon represent pseudopolyps. (From Marx, JA, et al. (eds): *Rosen's emergency medicine: concepts and clinical practice*, ed 7, Philadelphia, 2010, Elsevier.)

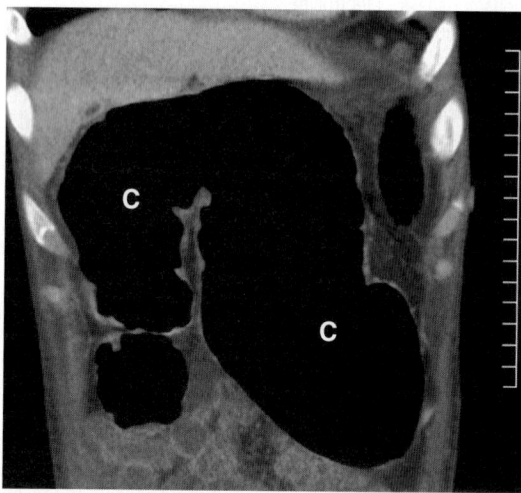

FIG. 2 Toxic megacolon. In a young patient with severe ulcerative colitis, coronal computed tomography demonstrates marked dilatation of the colon (*C*) with thinning of its walls. The diameter of the lumen of the colon exceeds 7 cm. This finding places the patient at high risk of colon perforation. (From Webb WR et al: *Fundamentals of body CT*, ed 4, Philadelphia, 2015, WB Saunders.)

CHRONIC Rx

- Patients with IBD will need continued treatment for the underlying disease process once the acute processes associated with toxic megacolon have resolved.

COMPLEMENTARY AND ALTERNATIVE MEDICINE

- N/A

DISPOSITION

- All patients with toxic megacolon will require admission, possibly to the intensive care unit, depending on their clinical presentation.

REFERRAL

- Surgical consultation in all cases.
- All patients with toxic megacolon due to newly diagnosed IBD who are discharged from the hospital should be referred to a gastroenterologist for continued treatment.

PEARLS & CONSIDERATIONS

COMMENTS

- Early recognition and treatment of toxic megacolon is critical given the associated high morbidity and mortality.
- Anticholinergic medications, antidiarrheal agents, and opioids can precipitate or worsen toxic megacolon.
- Management includes medical and surgical treatment with inpatient hospitalization and treatment of the underlying cause.

PREVENTION

- Prevention focuses on treatment of underlying causes of colitis to prevent complications such as toxic megacolon.

SUGGESTED READINGS

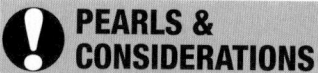

Available at www.expertconsult.com

RELATED CONTENT

Crohn's Disease (Related Key Topic)
Clostridium difficile Infection (Related Key Topic)
Small Bowel Obstruction (Related Key Topic)
Ulcerative Colitis (Related Key Term)

AUTHOR: **STEVEN ROUGAS, M.D., M.S.**

BASIC INFORMATION

DEFINITION

Toxic shock syndrome (TSS) is an acute febrile illness resulting in multiple organ system dysfunction caused most commonly by a bacterial exotoxin. Disease characteristics also include hypotension, vomiting, myalgia, watery diarrhea, vascular collapse, and an erythematous sunburnlike cutaneous rash that desquamates during recovery.

SYNONYMS

TSS

ICD-10CM CODES
A48.3 Toxic shock syndrome

EPIDEMIOLOGY & DEMOGRAPHICS

- Case reported incidence peak: 14 cases per 100,000 menstruating women annually in 1980; has since fallen to 1 case per 100,000 persons
- Occurs most commonly between ages 10 and 30 yr in healthy, young, menstruating white females
- Case fatality ratio of 3%

PHYSICAL FINDINGS & CLINICAL PRESENTATION

- Fever (>38.0° C)
- Diffuse macular erythrodermatous rash that involves both skin and mucous membranes, resembles sunburn, and also involves the palms and soles. The rash then desquamates 1 to 2 wk after disease onset in survivors
- Orthostatic hypotension
- Gastrointestinal symptoms: vomiting, diarrhea, abdominal tenderness
- Constitutional symptoms: myalgia, headache, photophobia, rigors, altered sensorium, conjunctivitis, arthralgia
- Respiratory symptoms: dysphagia, pharyngeal hyperemia, strawberry tongue
- Genitourinary symptoms: vaginal discharge, vaginal hyperemia, adnexal tenderness
- End-organ failure
- Severe hypotension and acute renal failure
- Hepatic failure
- Cardiovascular symptoms: disseminated intravascular coagulation, pulmonary edema, acute respiratory distress syndrome (ARDS), endomyocarditis, heart block

ETIOLOGY

- Menstruation-associated TSS: 45% of cases associated with tampons, diaphragm, or vaginal sponge use.
- Non–menstruation-associated TSS: 55% of cases associated with puerperal sepsis, post–cesarean section endometritis, mastitis, sinusitis, wound or skin infection, septorhinoplasty (nasal packings), pelvic inflammatory disease, respiratory infections following influenza, enterocolitis, and burns.

- Causative agent: *Staphylococcus aureus* infection of a susceptible individual (10% of population lacking sufficient levels of antitoxin antibodies), which liberates the disease mediator TSST-1 (exotoxin). While most cases are caused by methicillin-susceptible *S. aureus* (MSSA), cases of TSS from methicillin-resistant *S. aureus* (MRSA) have occurred, particularly those due to the more virulent community-associated MRSA strains.
- *S. aureus* exotoxins are superantigens that can activate large numbers of T cells (up to 20% at one time) resulting in a massive cytokine production: interleukin (Il-1), Il-2, TNF, and interferon gamma that then mediate the signs and symptoms of the disease.
- Other causative agents: coagulase-negative staphylococci producing enterotoxins B or C, and exotoxin A–producing group A beta-hemolytic streptococci.

DIAGNOSIS

DIFFERENTIAL DIAGNOSIS

- Staphylococcal food poisoning
- Septic shock
- Mucocutaneous lymph node syndrome
- Scarlet fever
- Rocky Mountain spotted fever
- Meningococcemia
- Toxic epidermal necrolysis
- Kawasaki syndrome
- Leptospirosis
- Legionnaires' disease
- Hemolytic-uremic syndrome
- Stevens-Johnson syndrome
- Scalded skin syndrome
- Erythema multiforme
- Acute rheumatic fever

WORKUP

Broad-spectrum syndrome with multiorgan system involvement and variable but acute clinical presentation, including the following diagnostic criteria for staphylococcal toxic shock syndrome:

- Fever (>38° C)
- Classic desquamating rash (1-2 wk)

- Hypotension/orthostatic systolic blood pressure ≤90 mm Hg
- Syncope
- Negative throat and cerebrospinal fluid cultures
- Negative serologic test for Rocky Mountain spotted fever, rubeola, and leptospirosis
- Clinical involvement of three or more of the following:
  1. Cardiopulmonary: ARDS, pulmonary edema, endomyocarditis, second- or third-degree atrioventricular block
  2. Central nervous system: altered sensorium without focal neurologic findings
  3. Hematologic: thrombocytopenia (platelets <100,000)
  4. Liver: elevated liver function test results
  5. Renal: >5 cells/high-power field, negative urine cultures, azotemia, and increased creatinine (double normal)
  6. Mucous membrane involvement: vagina, oropharynx, conjunctiva
  7. Musculoskeletal: myalgia, creatine phosphokinase twice normal
  8. Gastrointestinal: vomiting, diarrhea

For streptococcal toxic shock syndrome the diagnostic criteria is as follows:

- Definite case: Isolation of group A β-hemolytic streptococci (GABHS) from a sterile site
- Probable case: Isolation of GABHS from a nonsterile site.
- Hypotension: Presence of two of the following findings:
  - Acute kidney injury or failure
  - Elevated aminotransferase
  - Erythematous macular rash, soft tissue necrosis
  - Coagulopathy, including thrombocytopenia and disseminated intravascular coagulation
  - Acute respiratory distress syndrome

LABORATORY TESTS

- Pan culture (cervix and vagina, throat, nasal passages, urine, blood, cerebrospinal fluid, wound) for *Staphylococcus, Streptococcus* (Table 1), and other pathogenic organisms
- Electrolytes to detect hypokalemia, hyponatremia
- Complete blood count with differential and clotting profile for anemia (normocytic or

TABLE 1 Staphylococcal versus Streptococcal Toxic Shock Syndrome

Feature	Staphylococcal	Streptococcal
Age	Primarily 15-35 yr	Primarily 20-50 yr
Gender	Higher frequency in women	Men and women equally affected
Severe pain	Rare	Common
Hypotension	100%	100%
Erythroderma rash	Very common	Less common
Renal failure	Common	Common
Bacteremia	Low frequency	60%
Tissue necrosis	Rare	Common
Predisposing factors	Tampons, surgery	Cuts, burns, varicella
Thrombocytopenia	Common	Common
Mortality rate	<3%	30%-70%

From Mandell GL et al: *Principles and practice in infectious diseases*, ed 7, Philadelphia, 2008, Churchill Livingstone.

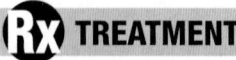

normochromic), thrombocytopenia, leukocytosis, coagulopathy, and bacteremia

- Chemistry profile to detect decreased protein, increased aspartate aminotransferase, increased alanine aminotransferase, hypocalcemia, elevated blood urea nitrogen and creatinine, hypophosphatemia, increased lactate dehydrogenase, increased creatine phosphokinase
- Urinalysis to detect white blood cells (>5 cells/high-power field), proteinemia, microhematuria
- Arterial blood gases to assess respiratory function and acid-base status
- Serologic tests considered for Rocky Mountain spotted fever, rubeola, and leptospirosis

IMAGING STUDIES

- Chest x-ray to evaluate pulmonary edema
- ECG to evaluate arrhythmia
- Sonography, CT scan, or MRI considered if pelvic abscess or tuboovarian abscess suspected

℞ TREATMENT

NONPHARMACOLOGIC THERAPY

- For optimal outcome: high index of suspicion and early and aggressive supportive management in an ICU setting
- Aggressive fluid resuscitation (maintenance of circulating volume, cardiac output, systolic blood pressure)
- Thorough search for a localized infection or nidus: incision and drainage, debridement, removal of tampon or vaginal sponge
- Central hemodynamic monitoring, Swan-Ganz catheter, and arterial line for surveillance of hemodynamic status and response to therapy
- Foley catheter to monitor hourly urine output
- Possible military antishock trousers as temporary measure
- Acute ventilator management if severe respiratory compromise
- Renal dialysis for severe renal impairment
- Surgical intervention for indicated conditions (i.e., ruptured tubo-ovarian abscess, wound abscess, mastitis)
- Hyperbaric oxygen treatment can be used adjunctively.

ACUTE GENERAL Rx

- Isotonic crystalloid (normal saline solution) for volume replacement following "7-3" rule (refers to the response in millimeters of mercury [mm Hg] of the pulmonary artery wedge pressure to volume replacement).

- Electrolyte replacement (K+, C+)
- Packed red blood cells, coagulation factor replacement, fresh frozen plasma to treat anemia or dilation and curettage.
- Vasopressor therapy for hypotension refractory to fluid volume replacement (e.g., dopamine beginning at 2 to 5 µg/kg/min)
- Steroids have been used but are not generally recommended due to lack of evidence of benefit.
- It is not clear whether antibiotics alter the course of acute TSS. Most authors recommend that patients receive 10 to 14 days of combination antibiotic therapy. In staphylococcal TSS, effective agents are clindamycin (900 mg IV every 8 hr in adults or 25 to 40 mg/kg per day in children) plus vancomycin (adults: 30 mg/kg per day IV in two divided doses; children: 40 mg/kg per day IV in four divided doses). Oxacillin or nafcillin sodium (2 g IV every 4 hr in adults; children: 100 to 150 mg/kg per 24 hr divided in four doses) can be used instead of vancomycin if TSS due to MSSA. An alternative to vancomycin is linezolid.
- In streptococcal TSS, effective agents are penicillin G 24 million units/day in divided doses *plus* clindamycin 900 mg IV q8h. Alternative agents are ceftriaxone 2 g IV q24h *plus* clindamycin 900 mg IV q8h.
- Broad-spectrum antibiotic including gram-negative coverage added if concurrent sepsis suspected with TSS.
- Intravenous immune globulin (IVIG): while no controlled trials exist, most authors recommend IVIG (400 mg/kg in a single dose administered over several hours) in severe cases of TSS that are not responding to fluids or vasopressors. It may neutralize superantigen and decrease tissue damage.
- Tetracycline added if considering Rocky Mountain spotted fever.

CHRONIC Rx

- Severely ill patient: may require prolonged hospitalization and supportive management with gradual recovery and/or sequelae from severe end-organ involvement (ARDS or renal failure requiring dialysis)
- Majority of patients: complete recovery
- Early-onset complications (within 2 wk):
  1. Skin desquamation
  2. Impaired digit sensation
  3. Denuded tongue
  4. Vocal cord paralysis
  5. Acute tubular necrosis
  6. ARDS
- Late-onset complications (after 8 wk):
  1. Nail splitting and loss
  2. Alopecia

  3. Central nervous system sequelae
  4. Renal impairment
  5. Cardiac dysfunction
- Recurrent TSS:
  1. More common in menstruation-related cases.
  2. Less common in patients treated with beta-lactamase–resistant antistaphylococcal antibiotics.
  3. Patients with history of TSS: if suspect signs and symptoms occur, have high index of suspicion and low threshold for evaluation and treatment.
  4. Screen for nasal carriage of *S. aureus* in patients with *S. aureus* TSS and treat with mupirocin in those with positive cultures.

PREVENTION

- Avoidance of tampons or use of low-absorbency tampons only (<4 hr in situ) and alternate with napkins
- Education for patients concerning signs and symptoms of TSS
- Avoidance of tampons for patients with history of TSS

DISPOSITION

- Complete recovery for most patients
- Long-term management of early- and late-onset complications for minority of patients

REFERRAL

- For multidisciplinary management, involving primary physician, gynecologist, internist, infectious disease specialist, and other supportive care specialists
- To tertiary-level hospital

❗ PEARLS & CONSIDERATIONS

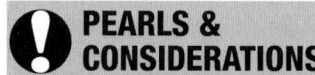

COMMENTS

Antibiotic prophylaxis against invasive group A streptococcal infection with benzathine penicillin G plus rifampin, clindamycin, or azithromycin is recommended for immunocompromised household contacts of patients with streptococcal TSS-like syndrome.

SUGGESTED READINGS

Available at www.expertconsult.com

RELATED CONTENT

Toxic Shock Syndrome (Patient Information)

AUTHOR: **GLENN G. FORT, M.D., M.P.H.**

BASIC INFORMATION

DEFINITION

Toxoplasmosis is an infection caused by the protozoal parasite *Toxoplasma gondii*.

ICD-10CM CODES
B58.9 Toxoplasmosis, unspecified
B58.3 Pulmonary toxoplasmosis
B58.89 Toxoplasmosis with other organ involvement
P37.1 Congenital toxoplasmosis

EPIDEMIOLOGY & DEMOGRAPHICS

INCIDENCE (IN U.S.):
- 3% to >50% of healthy adults (seroprevalence)
- Increases with age
- Increases with certain activities
  1. Slaughterhouse workers
  2. Cat owners
- Increases with certain geographic locations: high prevalence of cats

PREDOMINANT SEX: Equal gender distribution

PREDOMINANT AGE:
- Infancy (congenital infection)
- Prevalence increases with age

PEAK INCIDENCE: Temperate climates

GENETICS: Congenital infection: 400 to 4000 cases/year in the United States
- Incidence and severity vary with the trimester of gestation during which the mother acquired infection.
  1. 10% to 25% (first trimester)
  2. 30% to 54% (second trimester)
  3. 60% to 65% (third trimester)
- Congenital infection occurring in the first trimester is the most severe.
- 89% to 100% of infections in the third trimester are asymptomatic.
- Risk to the fetus is not correlated with symptoms in the mother.

PHYSICAL FINDINGS & CLINICAL PRESENTATION
- Acquired (immunocompetent host)
  1. 80% to 90% asymptomatic
  2. Adenopathy (usually cervical)
  3. Fever
  4. Myalgias
  5. Malaise
  6. Sore throat
  7. Maculopapular rash
  8. Hepatosplenomegaly
  9. Chorioretinitis rare
- Acquired (in patients with AIDS, CD4 count <100)
  1. 89% of symptomatic cases
     a. Encephalitis
     b. Intracerebral mass lesions
  2. Pneumonitis
  3. Chorioretinitis
  4. Other end organ
- Acquired (immunocompromised patients)
  1. Encephalitis
  2. Myocarditis (especially in heart transplant patients)

3. Pneumonitis
- Ocular infection in the immunocompetent host
  1. Congenital infection
  2. Blurred vision
  3. Photophobia
  4. Pain
  5. Loss of central vision if macula involved
  6. Focal necrotizing retinitis
  7. Typically presents in second or third decade
- Congenital
  1. Results from acute infection acquired by the mother within 6 to 8 weeks before conception or during gestation
  2. Usually, asymptomatic mother
  3. No sign of disease
  4. Chorioretinitis
  5. Blindness
  6. Epilepsy
  7. Psychomotor or mental retardation
  8. Intracranial calcifications
  9. Hydrocephalus
  10. Microcephaly
  11. Encephalitis
  12. Anemia
  13. Thrombocytopenia
  14. Hepatosplenomegaly
  15. Lymphadenopathy
  16. Jaundice
  17. Rash
  18. Pneumonitis
  19. Most infected infants are asymptomatic at birth

ETIOLOGY
- *Toxoplasma gondii*
  1. Ubiquitous intracellular protozoan
  2. Present worldwide
  3. Cat is the definitive host (Fig. E1)
- Human infection
  1. Ingestion of oocysts shed by cats in soil, litter boxes, vegetables
  2. Ingestion of inadequately cooked meat containing tissue cysts
  3. Vertical transmission

DIAGNOSIS

DIFFERENTIAL DIAGNOSIS
- Lymphadenopathy
  1. Infectious mononucleosis
  2. Cytomegalovirus (CMV) mononucleosis
  3. Cat-scratch disease
  4. Sarcoidosis
  5. Tuberculosis
  6. Lymphoma
  7. Metastatic cancer
- Cerebral mass lesions in immunocompromised host
  1. Lymphoma
  2. Tuberculosis
  3. Bacterial abscess
- Pneumonitis in immunocompromised host
  1. *Pneumocystis jiroveci (carinii)* pneumonia
  2. Tuberculosis
  3. Fungal infection

- Chorioretinitis
  1. Syphilis
  2. Tuberculosis
  3. Histoplasmosis (competent host)
  4. CMV
  5. Syphilis
  6. Herpes simplex
  7. Fungal infection
  8. Tuberculosis (AIDS patient)
- Myocarditis
  1. Organ rejection in heart transplant recipients
- Congenital infection
  1. Rubella
  2. CMV
  3. Herpes simplex
  4. Syphilis
  5. Listeriosis
  6. Erythroblastosis fetalis
  7. Sepsis

WORKUP
- Acute infection, immunocompetent host
  1. CBC
  2. *Toxoplasma* serology (IgG, IgM) in serial blood specimens 3 weeks apart
  3. Lymph node biopsy if diagnosis uncertain
- Immunocompromised host
  1. CNS symptoms
     a. Cerebral CT scan or MRI if CNS symptoms present
     b. Spinal tap, if safe
     c. Brain biopsy if no response to empiric therapy
  2. Ocular symptoms
     a. Funduscopic examination
     b. Serologic studies
     c. Rarely, vitreous tap
  3. Pulmonary symptoms
     a. Chest x-ray examination
     b. Bronchoalveolar lavage
     c. Transbronchial or open-lung biopsy
  4. Myocarditis
     a. Cardiac enzymes
     b. Electrocardiogram
     c. Endomyocardial biopsy for definitive diagnosis
- Toxoplasmosis in pregnancy (Fig. 2)
  1. Initial maternal screening with IgM and IgG
     a. If negative, mother at risk of acute infection and should be retested monthly
     b. If both IgG and IgM positive, obtain IgA and IgE ELISA, AC/HS test
     c. IgA and IgE ELISA, AC/HS test elevated in acute infection
     d. Ig high for 1 year or more
     e. IgG repeated 3 to 4 weeks later to determine if titer is stable
  2. Acute maternal infection not excluded or documented
     a. Fetal blood sampling (for culture, Ig, IgA, IgE)
     b. Amniotic fluid polymerase chain reaction (PCR)
  3. Fetal ultrasound every other weeks if maternal infection documented
- Congenital toxoplasmosis (Fig. 3)
  1. Placental histology
  2. Specific IgM or IgA in infant's blood

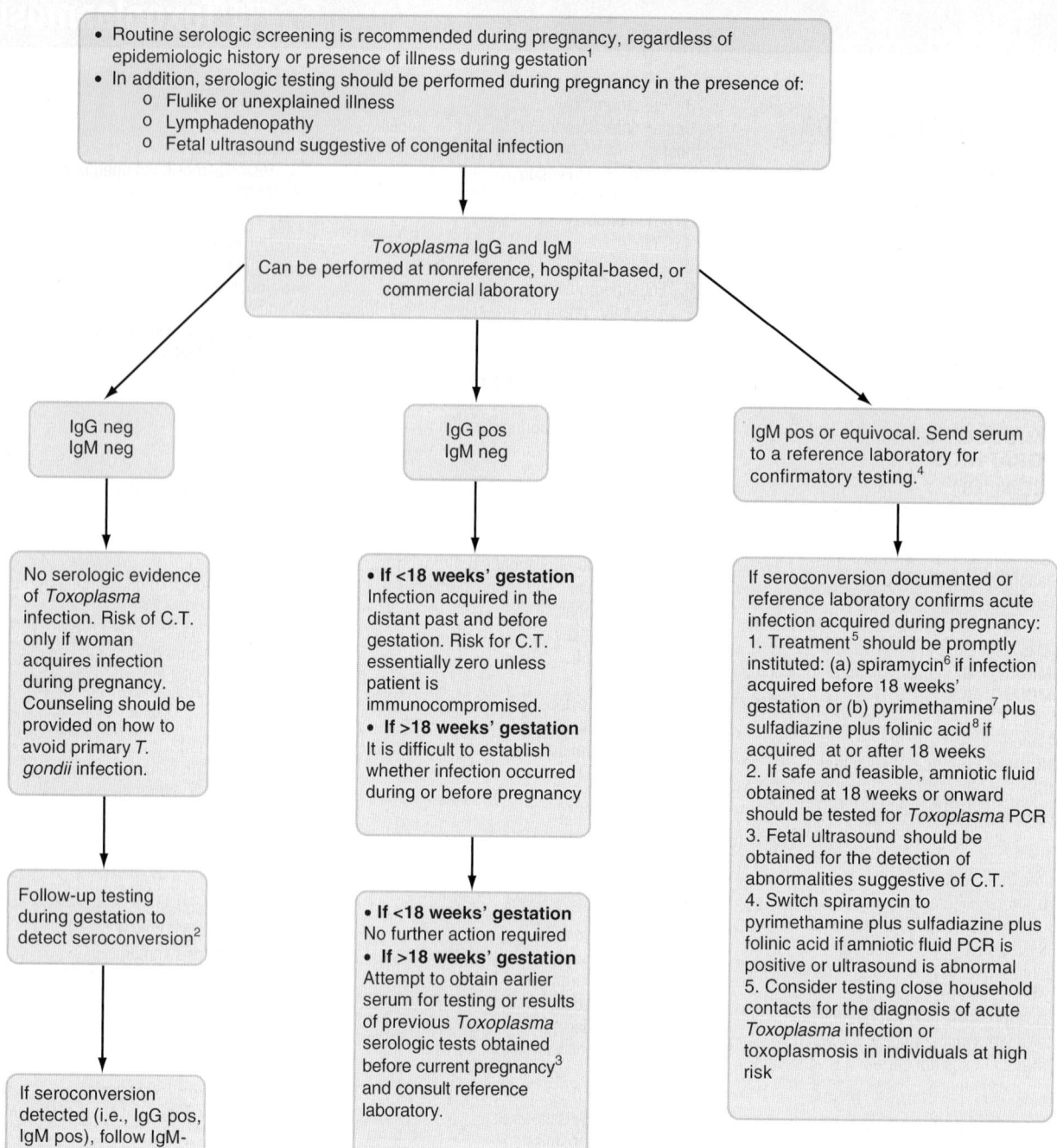

FIG. 2 Diagnostic approach and management algorithm of toxoplasmosis during pregnancy. Most of the initial serologic screening can be accomplished by nonreference or commercial laboratories. Only positive immunoglobulin M results should be considered for additional testing and consultation with medical experts at a reference laboratory. *CT*, Congenital toxoplasmosis; *IgG*, immunoglobulin G; *IgM*, immunoglobulin M; *neg*, negative test result; *pos*, positive test result.[1] Up to 50% of women who acquire *Toxoplasma* infection during gestation do not have a known risk factor for acute infection or an illness suggestive of toxoplasmosis. Thus, to identify all women at risk, serologic screening should be performed in all pregnant women, along with other routine screening tests.[2] In a recent study from Lyon, France, monthly screening of seronegative pregnant women was reported to significantly decrease the risk of vertical transmission and of clinical signs at 3 years of age. Consider consultation with a physician expert in management of toxoplasmosis during pregnancy (e.g., in the U.S., Palo Alto Medical Foundation–*Toxoplasma* Serology Laboratory [PAMF-TSL], www.pamf.org/serology/; 650-853-4828; e-mail, toxolab@pamf.org; or U.S. [Chicago] National Collaborative Treatment Trial Study [NCCTS]; 773-834-4152).[4] Consider sending serum sample to a reference laboratory (e.g., PAMF-TSL).[5] Treatment regimens vary by country. The pyrimethamine-sulfadiazine–folinic acid regimen should not be offered to any pregnant woman before 12 weeks of gestation because of potential teratogenicity. In some centers in Europe, this regimen is offered at 14 weeks of gestation or later; in the U.S., it is recommended at 18 weeks or later.[6] Spiramycin is not commercially available in the U.S. It can be obtained at no cost and after consultation (with PAMF-TSL or the NCCTS through the U.S. Food and Drug Administration).[7] When using pyrimethamine, folic acid should be discontinued from the prenatal multivitamins. Folic acid can potentially counteract the antiparasitic effect of the drug.[8] Folic acid should not be erroneously used instead of folinic acid. (Bennett JE et al: *Mandell, Douglas, and Bennett's principles and practice of infectious diseases,* ed 8, Philadelphia, 2015, WB Saunders.)

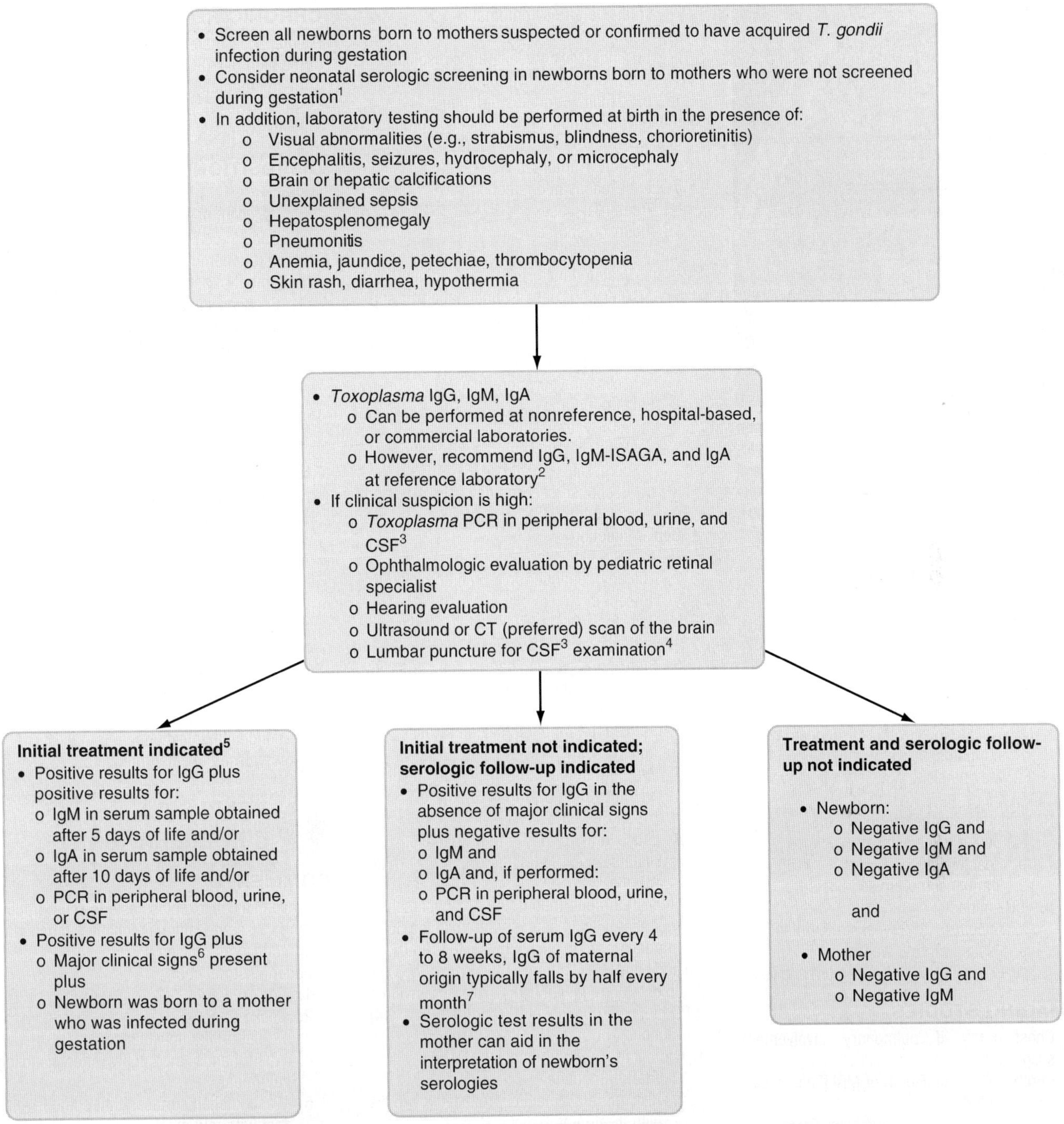

- Screen all newborns born to mothers suspected or confirmed to have acquired *T. gondii* infection during gestation
- Consider neonatal serologic screening in newborns born to mothers who were not screened during gestation[1]
- In addition, laboratory testing should be performed at birth in the presence of:
  - Visual abnormalities (e.g., strabismus, blindness, chorioretinitis)
  - Encephalitis, seizures, hydrocephaly, or microcephaly
  - Brain or hepatic calcifications
  - Unexplained sepsis
  - Hepatosplenomegaly
  - Pneumonitis
  - Anemia, jaundice, petechiae, thrombocytopenia
  - Skin rash, diarrhea, hypothermia

- *Toxoplasma* IgG, IgM, IgA
  - Can be performed at nonreference, hospital-based, or commercial laboratories.
  - However, recommend IgG, IgM-ISAGA, and IgA at reference laboratory[2]
- If clinical suspicion is high:
  - *Toxoplasma* PCR in peripheral blood, urine, and CSF[3]
  - Ophthalmologic evaluation by pediatric retinal specialist
  - Hearing evaluation
  - Ultrasound or CT (preferred) scan of the brain
  - Lumbar puncture for CSF[3] examination[4]

Initial treatment indicated[5]
- Positive results for IgG plus positive results for:
  - IgM in serum sample obtained after 5 days of life and/or
  - IgA in serum sample obtained after 10 days of life and/or
  - PCR in peripheral blood, urine, or CSF
- Positive results for IgG plus
  - Major clinical signs[6] present plus
  - Newborn was born to a mother who was infected during gestation

Initial treatment not indicated; serologic follow-up indicated
- Positive results for IgG in the absence of major clinical signs plus negative results for:
  - IgM and
  - IgA and, if performed:
  - PCR in peripheral blood, urine, and CSF
- Follow-up of serum IgG every 4 to 8 weeks, IgG of maternal origin typically falls by half every month[7]
- Serologic test results in the mother can aid in the interpretation of newborn's serologies

Treatment and serologic follow-up not indicated

- Newborn:
  - Negative IgG and
  - Negative IgM and
  - Negative IgA

  and

- Mother
  - Negative IgG and
  - Negative IgM

FIG. 3 Diagnostic approach and management algorithm of the newborn whose mother has been suspected or confirmed to have acquired toxoplasmosis during gestation. *CSF,* Cerebrospinal fluid; *CT,* computed tomography; *IgG, IgM,* and *IgA,* immunoglobulins G, M, and A, respectively; *ISAGA,* immunosorbent agglutination assay; *PCR,* polymerase chain reaction. [1] Consider consultation with a physician expert in management of toxoplasmosis during pregnancy (e.g., in the U.S., Palo Alto Medical Foundation–*Toxoplasma* Serology Laboratory [PAMF-TSL], www.pamf.org/serology/; 650-853-4828; e-mail, toxolab@pamf.org; or U.S. [Chicago] National Collaborative Treatment Trial Study, 773-834-4152). [2] Consider sending serum sample to a reference laboratory (e.g., PAMF-TSL). [3] If lumbar puncture is clinically indicated, deemed safe, and feasible. [4] In an attempt to confirm the diagnosis of congenital toxoplasmosis, CSF should be sent for cell count and differential (congenital toxoplasmosis is one of the few causes of eosinophilic meningitis), protein (congenital toxoplasmosis is one of the few causes of extreme elevation of CSF protein), glucose, and *T. gondii* PCR. [5] The recommended regimen is pyrimethamine plus sulfadiazine plus folinic acid (see text). [6] Major clinical signs are referred here: chorioretinitis, brain calcifications, and hydrocephalus. [7] Maternally transferred IgG antibodies usually decline and disappear within 6 to 12 months of life. (Bennett JE et al: *Mandell, Douglas, and Bennett's principles and practice of infectious diseases,* ed 8, Philadelphia, 2015, WB Saunders.)

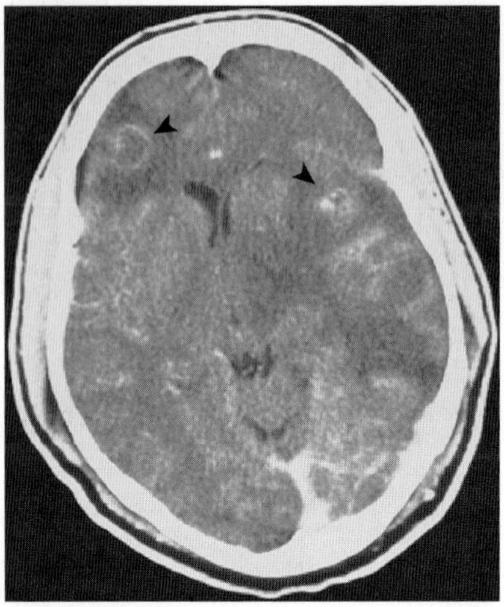

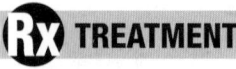

FIG. 4 Toxoplasmic encephalitis in person who has AIDS. A cranial CT scan shows bilateral contrast-enhanced ring lesions with peripheral edema and mass effect. (From Cohen J, Powderly WG: *Infectious diseases,* ed 2, St Louis, 2004, Mosby.)

LABORATORY TESTS

- Antibody studies
  1. More than one test necessary to establish diagnosis of acute toxoplasmosis
  2. IgM antibody
     a. Appears 5 days into infection
     b. Peaks at 2 weeks
     c. Falls to low level or disappears within 2 months
     d. May persist at low levels for 1 year or more
  3. Antibody not measurable
     a. Ocular toxoplasmosis
     b. Reactivation
     c. Immunocompromised hosts
  4. IgG antibody
     a. Appears 1 to 2 weeks after infection
     b. Peaks at 6 to 8 weeks
     c. Gradually declines over months to years

IMAGING STUDIES

- Chest x-ray if pulmonary involvement suspected
- Cerebral CT scan (Fig. 4) or MRI if encephalitis suspected

Rx TREATMENT

NONPHARMACOLOGIC THERAPY

- Selected cases of ocular infection
  1. Photocoagulation
  2. Vitrectomy
  3. Lentectomy
- Selected cases of congenital cerebral infection
  1. Ventricular shunting

ACUTE GENERAL Rx

- Acute infection, immunocompetent host
  1. No treatment, unless severe and persistent symptoms or vital organ damage
- Acute infection, immunocompromised host, non-AIDS

1. Treat even if asymptomatic
2. Duration
   a. Until 4 to 6 weeks after resolution of all signs and symptoms
   b. Usually 6 months or longer
- Reactivated infection, immunocompromised host, non-AIDS
  1. Treat if symptomatic
- Acute or reactivated infection, AIDS
  1. Treat in all cases
  2. Induction course
     a. 3 to 6 weeks.
     b. Maintenance therapy continued for life; consider discontinuation of suppressive therapy if the patient has a good response to antiretroviral therapy and if the CD4 count remains >200 cells/mm^3 for more than 3 months.
  3. Empiric therapy
     a. AIDS with positive IgG
     b. Multiple ring-enhancing lesions on cerebral CT scan or MRI
     c. Response seen by day 7 in 71% and day 14 in 91%
- Ocular infection
  1. Treat in all cases
  2. Therapy continued for 1 month or longer if needed
  3. Response seen in 70% within 10 days
  4. Retreat as needed
  5. Steroids may be indicated in patients with signs or symptoms of increased intracranial pressure
  6. Surgical treatment in selected cases
- Treatment regimens
  1. Pyrimethamine 200 mg loading dose once PO, then 50 mg (<60 kg) to 75 mg (>60 kg) q day; plus
  2. Leucovorin 10 to 20 mg PO qid, plus
  3. Sulfadiazine 1 (<60 kg) to 1.5 g (>60 kg) PO q6h

Other treatment options (if sulfa hypersensitivity or allergy is present): pyrimethamine 50 to 75 mg/day PO with leucovorin 10 to 20 mg/day PO and either (1) clindamycin 600 mg q6h PO or IV (up to 1200 mg IV) q6h, or (2) clarithromycin 1 g PO bid, or (3) dapsone 100 mg/day PO, or (4) atovaquone 750 mg PO q6h.

- Acute infection in pregnancy
  1. Treat immediately
  2. Risk of fetal infection reduced by 60% with treatment
     a. First trimester
        i. Spiramycin 3 g PO qid in two to four divided doses
        ii. Sulfadiazine 4 g PO qid in four divided doses
     b. Second and third trimester
        i. Sulfadiazine as previously described, *plus*
        ii. Pyrimethamine 25 mg PO qid, *plus*
        iii. Leucovorin 5 to 15 mg PO qid
        iv. Spiramycin as previously described
- Congenital infection
  1. Sulfadiazine 50 mg/kg PO bid, *plus*
  2. Pyrimethamine 2 mg/kg PO for 2 days, then 1 mg/kg PO, three times weekly, *plus*
  3. Leucovorin 5 to 20 mg PO three times weekly
  4. Minimum duration of treatment: 12 month

CHRONIC Rx

Maintenance therapy in AIDS patients because of the high risk (80%) of relapse
1. Pyrimethamine 25 mg PO qid
2. Sulfadiazine 500 mg PO qid
3. Leucovorin 10 to 20 mg PO qid

DISPOSITION

- Prognosis
  1. Excellent in the immunocompetent host
  2. Good in ocular infection (although relapses are common)
- Treatment of acute infection in pregnancy
  1. Reduces incidence and severity of congenital toxoplasmosis
- Treatment of congenital infection
  1. Improvement in intellectual function
  2. Regression of retinal lesions
- AIDS
  1. 70% to 95% response to therapy

REFERRAL

- To infectious disease expert:
  1. Immunocompromised hosts
  2. Pregnant women
  3. Difficulty in making a diagnosis or deciding on treatment
- To pediatric infectious disease expert:
  1. Congenital infection
- To obstetrician:
  1. Pregnant seronegative mother
  2. Acute seroconversion
- To ophthalmologist:
  1. Congenital infection
  2. Any case of ocular infection

① PEARLS & CONSIDERATIONS

COMMENTS

- Prevention of toxoplasmosis is most important in seronegative pregnant women and immunocompromised hosts.
- Patient instructions:
  1. Cook meat to 66° C.
  2. Cook eggs.
  3. Do not drink unpasteurized milk.
  4. Wash hands thoroughly after handling raw meat.
  5. Wash kitchen surfaces that come in contact with raw meat.
  6. Wash fruits and vegetables.
  7. Avoid contact with materials potentially contaminated with cat feces.

SUGGESTED READING

Available at www.expertconsult.com

RELATED CONTENT

Toxoplasmosis (Patient Information)

AUTHOR: **PHILIP A. CHAN, M.D., M.S.**

BASIC INFORMATION

DEFINITION

Acute hemolytic transfusion reaction (AHTR) is acute intravascular hemolysis most commonly caused by an alloantibody in a recipient's plasma to a cognate antigen in the donor red cells. The most common alloantibodies are to ABO antigens, but alloantibodies to minor blood group antigens have also been implicated. Typically the alloantibodies are of the IgM class but complement fixing IgGs may also cause such a reaction. The clinical features vary but commonly there is high fever, chills, nausea, and backache. Red urine may be passed. The plasma shows hemoglobinemia, and the direct Coombs test can be positive or negative. Delayed hemolytic reactions are usually caused by an anamnestic alloantibody response upon re-exposure to cognate erythrocyte antigen. They are typically IgG and commonly non-complement fixing. They usually occur 1 to 10 days after transfusion. In delayed transfusion reactions, hemoglobinemia is unusual and the only manifestations may be fever and the finding of a newly positive indirect antiglobulin (indirect Coombs test) and or the presence of a positive direct Coombs test. Delayed reactions can be clinically silent (called delayed serological hemolytic reactions) or manifest with fever, chills, nausea, or vomiting. There is no specific treatment other than supportive care.

SYNONYMS

AHTR
DSTR
DHTR
Acute hemolytic transfusion reaction

ICD-10CM CODES
T80.9 Unspecified complication following infusion, transfusion and therapeutic injection
T80.3 ABO incompatibility reaction
T80.4 Rh incompatibility reaction
T80.8 Other complications following infusion, transfusion, and therapeutic injection

EPIDEMIOLOGY & DEMOGRAPHICS

- Acute intravascular hemolysis occurs in one to five per 50,000 transfusions.
- Delayed reactions occur about 1: 1500 red cell transfusions.

PHYSICAL FINDINGS & CLINICAL PRESENTATION

- Hypotension
- Pain at the infusion site
- Fever, tachycardia, chest pain, dyspnea, dizziness, bronchospasm
- Lower back pain due to ischemic muscle pain or vasospasm rather than kidney pain from developing renal failure
- Severe reactions may occur in surgical patients under anesthesia who are unable to give any warning signs.
- Table 1 summarizes signs and symptoms of acute adverse reactions to blood transfusion
- Patients with delayed hemolytic transfusion reactions typically do not present as a clinical emergency. In most cases presentation is with a low-grade fever from the generation of IL-1 or other proinflammatory cytokines. Hemoglobinuria and hemoglobinemia are rarely present unless the amount of incompatible blood infused is excessive.

ETIOLOGY

Most fatal hemolytic reactions are caused by clerical errors and mislabeled specimens.

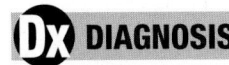 DIAGNOSIS

DIFFERENTIAL DIAGNOSIS

- Septic reaction
- Transfusion-related acute lung injury

MANAGEMENT

The transfusion must be stopped immediately. The blood bank must be notified, and the donor transfusion bag must be returned to the blood bank along with a freshly drawn posttransfusion specimen.

LABORATORY TESTS

- The direct antiglobulin test (DAT) is usually positive in a delayed reaction but preparation of an eluate will help identify the offending antibody.
- In some delayed reactions, the only finding is a positive indirect Coombs test, and the implicated alloantibody can be identified in an antibody panel.
- In acute reactions, the urine may show hemoglobinuria (wine-colored urine), and the plasma hemoglobinemia (pink plasma).
- Labs: Decreased hematocrit and serum haptoglobin (haptoglobin low to 0 mg/dl). Elevated LDH, indirect bilirubin and creatinine, if acute.
- In acute cases, monitor coagulation status (PT, aPTT, fibrinogen) for disseminated intravascular coagulation.

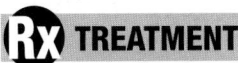 TREATMENT

NONPHARMACOLOGIC THERAPY

- Stop transfusion immediately. Test anticoagulated blood from the recipient for the presence of free hemoglobin in the plasma (Table 2).
- Monitor vital signs closely, and maintain IV access with a suitable crystalloid or colloid solution.
- Maintain an adequate airway.

ACUTE GENERAL Rx

- Treatment is supportive and consists of fluid resuscitation, vasopressor support, and mannitol.
- Vigorous IV hydration (0.9% NaCl or some other suitable crystalloid solution) to maintain urine flow at >100 ml/hr until hypotension is corrected and hemoglobinuria clears. IV furosemide may be necessary to maintain adequate renal flow.
- The addition of mannitol may prevent renal damage (controversial). Mannitol, if chosen, must be used with caution; if acute tubular necrosis occurs before mannitol infusion, pulmonary edema may occur as a result of the acute increase in intravascular volume secondary to fluid expansion.

TABLE 1 Signs and Symptoms of Acute Adverse Reactions to Blood Transfusion

Reaction	Fever	Chills/ Rigors	Nausea/ Vomiting	Chest Discomfort/ Pain	Facial Flushing	Wheezing/ Dyspnea	Back/ Lumbar Pain	Discomfort at Infusion Site	Hypotension
Acute hemolytic	X	X	X	X	X	X	X	X	X
Febrile nonhemolytic	X	X		X	X				
Nonimmune hemolysis									
Acute lung injury	X			X		X			X
Allergic									
Massive transfusion complications									
Anaphylaxis	X	X	X	X	X	X	X	X	X
Passive cytokine infusion	X	X	X			X			
Hypervolemia						X			
Bacterial sepsis	X	X	X				X	X	X
Air embolus				X		X			

From Goldman L, Bennett JC [eds]: *Cecil's textbook of medicine*, ed 22, Philadelphia, 2004, Saunders.

TABLE 2 Components of the Protein C Anticoagulant Pathway

Protein (Amino Acids)	Molecular Mass (kd)	Subunits (Amino Acids)	Domains	Special Functions
Protein C (417)	62	Light chain (155)		
Heavy chain (262)	Gla, 2 EGFs			
AP and SP	Zymogen to APC; anticoagulant, antiinflammatory, and anti-apoptotic protease, which cleaves factor V/activated factor V and activated factor VIII and PAR1			
Protein S (635)	75	Single chain	Gla, TSR, 4 EGFs, SHBG (2 LamG domains)	Cofactor to APC; cofactor to tissue factor pathway inhibitor; binds C4b-binding protein; binds to apoptotic cells; stimulates phagocytosis
Thrombomodulin (554)	75	Single chain	Lectin, hydrophobic, 6 EGFs, S/T-rich, transmembrane, cytoplasmic tail	In membrane of all endothelium; cofactor to thrombin in activation of protein C and thrombin activatable fibrinolysis inhibitor; antiinflammatory
Endothelial protein C receptor (221)	50	Single chain	MHC/CD1	In membrane of endothelium; binds Gla domain of protein C; stimulates protein C activation by thrombin–thrombomodulin and PAR1 cleavage by APC
Factor V (2196)	330	Single chain	A1, A2, B, A3, C1, C3	Precursor to procoagulant activated factor V and to anticoagulant APC; cofactor in activated factor VIII degradation
Factor VIII (2332)	330	Heavy chain (1313)		
Light chain (684)	A1, A2, B, A3, C1, C3	Precursor to procoagulant-activated factor VIII; cofactor in the tenase complex		
C4b-binding protein (4078)	570	7 α chains (549)		
1 β chain (235)	8 CCPs			
3 CCPs	α-Chains are cofactors to factor I, an enzyme regulating the complement system; β-chain binds to protein S			
Protein C inhibitor (387)	60	Single chain	Serpin	Inhibitor of APC and other proteases; stimulated by heparin
α₁ Antitrypsin (394)	60	Single chain	Serpin	Inhibitor of APC and other proteases

The total numbers of amino acids in the mature proteins are given in parenthesis. The molecular masses are approximate and include posttranslational modifications such as carbohydrate side chains. Factor VIII is synthesized as single chain but processed to two chains with heterogeneity of heavy chains; the number of amino acids refers to the longest heavy chain of factor VIII. References to different proteins and their properties are given in the text; some of the information is derived from protein databases available on the Internet. http://www.ncbi.nlm.nih.gov/; http://www.expasy.org/
APC, Activated protein C; *EGF,* epidermal growth factor; *Gla,* γ-carboxyglutamic acid; *PAR,* protease-activated receptor 1; *S/T-rich,* serine/threonine-rich; *TSR,* thrombin-sensitive region.
From Hoffman R, et al.: *Hematology: basic principles and practice,* ed 5, Philadelphia, 2009, Saunders.

- Monitor for the presence of disseminated intravascular coagulation. PT, aPTT, and fibrinogen levels should be closely monitored.
- If sepsis is suspected, culture as appropriate.

DISPOSITION

Mortality rate is 3% to 10% in severe transfusion reactions.

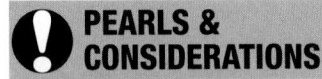 **PEARLS & CONSIDERATIONS**

COMMENTS

Hemolysis caused by minor antigen systems is generally less severe and may be delayed 1 to 10 days after transfusion.

AUTHOR: **JOSEPH SWEENEY, M.D.**

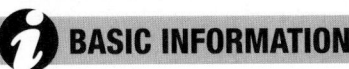 BASIC INFORMATION

DEFINITION

A clinical syndrome lasting up to 24 hours, of sudden onset, severe anterograde and variable retrograde amnesia without loss of other neurologic function.

SYNONYMS

TGA

ICD-10CM CODES
G45.4 Transient global amnesia

EPIDEMIOLOGY & DEMOGRAPHICS

INCIDENCE (IN U.S.): 3.4 to 10.4 per 100,000 people.
PEAK INCIDENCE: Most between ages 50 to 70 and equally common in men and women. In population older than 50 the incidence increases to 23.5 per 100,000 per year. TGA is also more common in individuals with migraine.[1]
RECURRENCE RATE: 2.9% to 23.8%

PHYSICAL FINDINGS & CLINICAL PRESENTATION[2]

- Cannot recall novel episodic information, repeatedly asking the same questions
- No impairment in consciousness or cognition, no focal neurologic deficit
- Complex procedural memory is often preserved (i.e., driving)
- Triggers include Valsalva maneuver, immersion in cold or hot, sexual intercourse, emotional stress
- Typically a single attack that is self-limited, with amnestic gap of the duration of episode
- Those with recent head injury or epilepsy diagnosis are excluded

ETIOLOGY

- Several proposed mechanisms of pathophysiology:
- Hypoperfusion or arterial ischemia of the hippocampi

- Internal jugular venous flow reversal causing venous hypertension to the medial temporal lobe[1]
- Migraine phenomena with cortical spreading depression

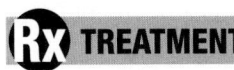 DIAGNOSIS

DIFFERENTIAL DIAGNOSIS

- Posterior cerebral artery transient ischemic attack: can be associated with confusion or memory loss. Commonly with vascular risk factors and other focal neurologic signs (homonymous hemianopsia, aphasia, hemiparesis, hemisensory loss, hemi-body pain, oculomotor nerve palsy or vertical gaze palsy).
- Transient epileptic amnesia: epilepsy syndrome, consisting of atypical TGA or recurrent attacks of amnesia, often less than one hour and upon waking, responsive to antiepileptic medications. Associated with olfactory hallucinations or oral automatisms. Interictal EEG may be abnormal. Hippocampal atrophy on MRI may be seen.
- Dissociative fugue, or transient dissociative amnesia: extensive retrograde amnesia, loss of personal identity may occur, unlike in TGA where such is preserved.
- Hypoglycemia: metabolic dysfunction can cause impairment in consciousness, focal signs or prolonged cognitive impairment unlike TGA.

WORKUP

- Largely a clinical diagnosis, workup should focus on exclusion of vascular or epileptic source of symptoms.
- Collateral history of witnessed event and exclusion of prior event.
- Cognitive examination with evaluation of registration, delayed recall and orientation.
- Careful cranial nerve examination to exclude posterior circulation stroke.

---

[1]Arena JE, et al.: Transient global amnesia, *Mayo Clin Proc* 90(2):264–272, 2015.

LABORATORY TESTS

- Complete blood count with erythrocyte sedimentation rate and C-reactive protein.
- Serum chemistries, including lipid profile.

DIAGNOSTIC STUDIES

- MRI of the brain may show reversible T2 hyperintensity or diffusion restriction exclusive to the hippocampi.
- EEG to exclude epileptiform activity.

Rx TREATMENT

NONPHARMACOLOGIC THERAPY

Self-limited, not requiring specific pharmacologic or nonpharmacologic treatment

ACUTE GENERAL Rx

- Investigate as an emergency.

CHRONIC Rx

- Does not lead to long-term sequela of memory loss. Complete recovery of cognitive function has been reported 5 days to 6 months after the episode.[2]
- Low risk of subsequent ischemic cerebral stroke or seizures.

DISPOSITION

Due to the benign nature of transient global amnesia rarely is continued follow up necessary.

REFERRAL

Referral to a neurologist is necessary when the diagnosis is uncertain or with atypical features of the clinical presentation

AUTHOR: **RITUPARNA DAS, M.D.**

---

[2]Arena JE, et al.: Long-term outcome in patients with transient global amnesia: a population-based study, *Mayo Clin Proc* 92(3):399–405, 2017.

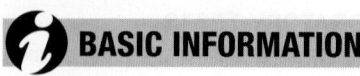
DEFINITION

Transient ischemic attack (TIA) is a transient episode of neurologic dysfunction caused by focal brain, spinal cord, or retinal ischemia without acute infarction on MRI. TIA symptoms typically resolve within 60 min and almost always within 24 hours.

SYNONYMS

TIA
Amaurosis fugax
Ophthalmologic TIA
"Mini-stroke"
Pre-stroke

ICD-10CM CODES

G45.9   Transient cerebral ischemic attack, unspecified
G45.8   Other transient cerebral ischemic attacks and related syndromes
Z86.73 Personal history of transient ischemic attack (TIA), and cerebral infarction without residual deficits

EPIDEMIOLOGY & DEMOGRAPHICS

INCIDENCE: 49 to 83 cases per 100,000 persons annually
PEAK INCIDENCE: After age 60 year
PREVALENCE: 200,000 to 500,000 persons in the United States. The annual risk of stroke after either a TIA or minor stroke is approximately 3% to 4%.
PREDOMINANT SEX AND RACE: Males > females; African American > Caucasian
RISK FACTORS: Same as for ischemic stroke

PHYSICAL FINDINGS & CLINICAL PRESENTATION

TIAs often present with ipsilateral transient monocular blindness (amaurosis fugax), contralateral numbness or weakness, contralateral homonymous hemianopsia, and/or aphasia.

ETIOLOGY

Embolic (cardioembolism in 10%-15%) large vessel atherothrombotic disease (20%-25%) lacunar disease, hypoperfusion, hypercoagulable state, arteritis

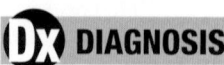 **DIAGNOSIS**

DIFFERENTIAL DIAGNOSIS

Seizures, hypoglycemia, complicated migraine, intracranial hemorrhage, mass lesion, vestibular disease, Bell's palsy, meningitis, multiple sclerosis, subdural hematoma, brain abscess, cervical or lumbar spine disease, conversion disorder

WORKUP

Given the high risk of stroke within the first 48 hours following TIA (up to 10%), hospital admission for workup is advised. Fig. 1 describes a TIA algorithm. The American Heart Association recommends that the ABCD2 score be used in the evaluation of TIA. It consists of 1 point for age ≥60 years, 1 point for BP ≥140 mm Hg systolic or ≥90 mm Hg diastolic, clinical features (2 points for unilateral weakness, 1 point for speech impairment), duration of TIA (2 points for duration ≥60 min, 1 point for duration 10-59 min), presence of diabetes mellitus (1 point). According to the guidelines, it is reasonable to hospitalize patients with TIA if they present within 72 hours and have an ABCD2 score ≥3. There is some debate about the usefulness of this scale since it fails to account for changes seen on echocardiogram, carotid Dopplers, or ECG that may place the patient at more imminent risk of stroke (carotid stenosis, Afib, cardiac thrombus, etc.). Alternatives to this scoring system are being investigated.

LABORATORY TESTS

Complete blood count, basic metabolic panel, prothrombin time, activated partial thromboplastin time, sedimentation rate, fasting lipid panel, serum glucose and hemoglobin A_{1c} (to detect latent diabetes mellitus), and TSH.

IMAGING STUDIES

- CT scan should be obtained to exclude hemorrhage; MRI with diffusion weighting if immediately available.
- Imaging of the vessels should be obtained via magnetic resonance angiography (MRA) head and neck, computed tomography angiography (CTA) head and neck, or carotid Doppler/transcranial Doppler (CD/TCD).
  1. If symptoms are referable to the posterior circulation, MRA or CTA should be obtained in lieu of CD/TCD.
  2. Transthoracic echocardiogram should be obtained.
  3. An echocardiogram with bubble should be obtained in all patients younger than 50 years with TIA symptoms.
- Electrocardiogram should be obtained to exclude the presence of arrhythmias, namely atrial fibrillation.
  At least 24 hours of heart rhythm monitoring should be accomplished to screen for arrhythmia. Many stroke centers now utilize prolonged ambulatory cardiac rhythm monitoring over several weeks to months to identify paroxysmal atrial fibrillation in select patients when there is a high index of clinical suspicion.
- Paroxysmal atrial fibrillation is common in patients with TIA. A recent study found that noninvasive ambulatory ECG monitoring for 30 days significantly improved the detection of atrial fibrillation by a factor of more than five and nearly doubled the rate of anticoagulant treatment as compared with the standard practice of short-duration ECG monitoring.

R **TREATMENT**

NONPHARMACOLOGIC THERAPY

- Carotid endarterectomy or carotid stenting should be considered for patients found to have carotid stenosis of ≥50% as the cause for TIA. Please refer to the "Carotid Stenosis" chapter for more information.

- The practice of intracranial angioplasty and stenting has largely declined following the publication of negative results from clinical trials and is only used in select patients who fail maximal medical management with aggressive platelet inhibition, strict risk factor control such as hyperlipidemia, hypertension, diabetes mellitus, weight loss, treatment of sleep apnea, and smoking cessation among others.

ACUTE GENERAL Rx

- In the absence of contraindications, patients with atrial fibrillation should be considered for anticoagulation with intravenous heparin (or therapeutic lovenox) along with warfarin until target INR between 2.0 and 3.0 is achieved.
- Although no compelling evidence exists for the use of heparin in the acute treatment of TIAs without cardioembolic source, patients who develop recurrent symptoms within the same vascular territory that increase in duration, severity, and/or frequency (crescendo TIA/stuttering TIA) may benefit from its use pending cardiac and vascular imaging and identification of a possible source.

CHRONIC Rx

- Chronic therapy should be aimed at modifying the four major risk factors: hypertension, dyslipidemia, diabetes mellitus, and smoking cessation.
- Antiplatelet therapy should be used to reduce the risk of recurrent TIAs or subsequent stroke. Three antiplatelet agents are commonly used in stroke prevention: aspirin, aspirin/dipyridamole, and clopidogrel. All are reasonable choices but practitioners should consider their individual patient's comorbidities when selecting an antiplatelet agent.
- Dose-adjusted warfarin (INR 2.0-3.0) is indicated for prevention of future strokes in atrial fibrillation patients. The direct thrombin inhibitor dabigatran and the direct factor Xa inhibitors apixaban and rivaroxaban have been approved as alternative treatments to warfarin for stroke prevention in atrial fibrillation.

! **PEARLS & CONSIDERATIONS**

- Despite complete symptom resolution, 20% to 50% of patients clinically suspected to have suffered a TIA have evidence of acute tissue infarction on MRI.
- Dual antiplatelet therapy in acute TIA and minor stroke is being evaluated. A recent trial revealed that among patients with TIA or minor stroke who can be treated within 24 hours after the onset of symptoms, the combination of clopidogrel and aspirin is superior to aspirin alone for reducing the risk of stroke in the first 90 days and does not increase the risk of hemorrhage.
- Previous studies conducted between 1987 and 2003 estimated the risk of stroke or an acute coronary syndrome was 12% to 20%

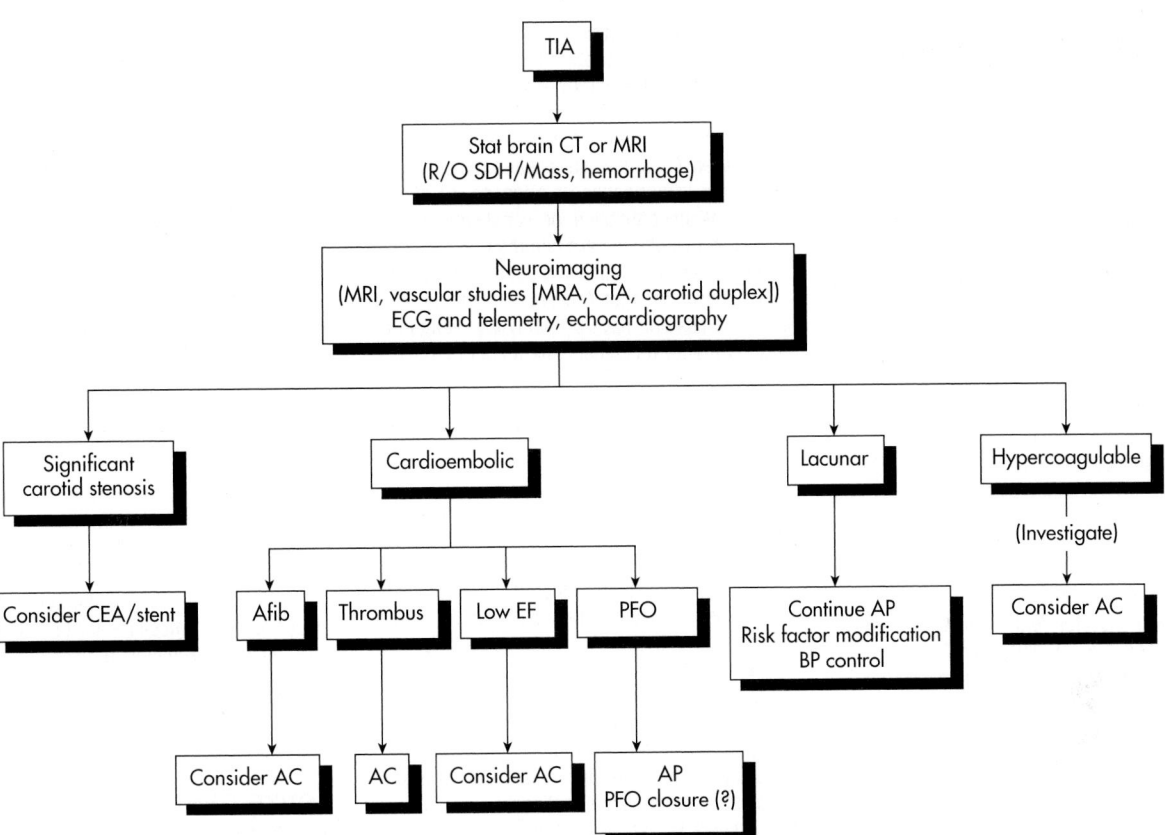

FIG. 1 Transient ischemic attack (TIA). *AC,* Anticoagulation; *AP,* antiplatelet; *ASA,* aspirin; *BP,* blood pressure; *CEA,* carotid endarterectomy; *CTA,* CT angiography; *EF,* ejection fraction; *MRA,* magnetic resonance angiography; *PFO,* patent foramen ovale; *SDH,* subdural hematoma.

during the first 3 months after a TIA. New data estimate the 1-year risk to be 6.2%. Multiple infarctions on brain imaging, large-artery atherosclerosis, and an ABCD[2] score of 6 or 7 were each associated with more than a doubling of the risk of stroke.[1]

PREVENTION
- A healthy lifestyle and management of cardiovascular risk factors should be encouraged.
- The identification of insulin resistance as a risk factor for stroke and myocardial infarction raises the possibility that pioglitazone, which improves insulin sensitivity,

might benefit patients with cerebrovascular disease. In a recent trial involving patients without a history of ischemic stroke or TIA, the risk of stroke or MI was lower among patients who received pioglitazone than among those who received placebo. Pioglitazone was also associated with a lower risk of diabetes but with a higher risk of weight gain, edema, and fracture.[2]

PATIENT/FAMILY EDUCATION

Patients should be counseled on the early signs of stroke symptoms and instructed to promptly seek medical attention if they develop symptoms concerning for stroke. Patients should

be encouraged to pursue a healthy lifestyle to include exercise and smoking cessation. In addition, patients should take an active role in controlling blood pressure and blood glucose. Further educational materials can be found online at http://www.strokecenter.org/.

SUGGESTED READINGS
Available at www.expertconsult.com

RELATED CONTENT
Transient Ischemic Attack (TIA) (Patient Information)

AUTHORS: **ANGAD JOLLY,**
JOSEPH S. KASS, M.D., J.D., and
PRASHANTH KRISHNAMOHAN, M.B.B.S., M.D.

[1]Amarenco P, et al.: One-year risk of stroke after transient ischemic attack or minor stroke, *N Engl J Med* 374:1533–1542, 2016.

[2]Kernan WN, et al: Pioglitazone after ischemic stroke or transient ischemic attack, *N Engl J Med* 374:1321-1331, 2016.

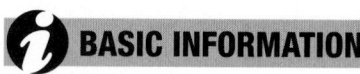

DEFINITION

Demyelination in a transverse region of the spinal cord due to an inflammatory process that leads to sensory and motor changes below the lesion and autonomic dysfunction. The term "transverse myelitis" of late refers to any cause of inflammatory myelopathy, irrespective of severity or degree of structural or functional interruption of pathways through a transverse spinal cord section. Patients usually experience bandlike symptoms, which is classically an area of altered sensation or pain in a horizontal (i.e., transverse) band usually at the dermatomal level corresponding to the lesion within the cord. Transverse myelitis that extends across three or more segments of the cord is referred to as longitudinally extensive transverse myelitis. The pathologic hallmark of transverse myelitis is the presence of focal collections of lymphocytes and monocytes with varying degrees of demyelination, axonal injury, and astroglial and microglial activation within the spinal cord.

SYNONYMS

Idiopathic transverse myelitis
TM

ICD-10CM CODES
G37.3   Acute transverse myelitis in demyelinating disease of central nervous system
G04.89 Other myelitis

EPIDEMIOLOGY & DEMOGRAPHICS

INCIDENCE: Annual incidence ranges from 1.3 to 8 cases per million. The incidence increases to 24.6 cases per million annually if causes of acquired demyelination such as multiple sclerosis (MS) are included.
PREVALENCE: Unknown
PREDOMINANT SEX: None, but female preponderance seen in cases associated with multiple sclerosis.
GENETICS: No genetic predisposition has been shown.
PEAK INCIDENCE: Can occur at any age. Bimodal peak in the incidence between 10 to 19 yr and 30 to 39 yr. 20% of cases occur in children with a bimodal peak of incidence between 0 to 2 yr and 5 to 17 yr.
RISK FACTORS: Infection, vaccination

PHYSICAL FINDINGS & CLINICAL PRESENTATION

- The clinical signs are caused by an interruption in ascending and descending neuroanatomic pathways in the transverse plane of the spinal cord, and a resulting sensory level is characteristic of transverse myelitis.
- Rapid onset of symmetric or asymmetric paraparesis or paraplegia of the lower extremities over a few days, ascending paresthesia, sensory level at the trunk, back pain, sphincter dysfunction, and positive Babinski, which can be bilateral. The arms may also be involved but less than the legs in most cases. In the acute phase the weakness is

flaccid, with diminished deep tendon reflexes mimicking a peripheral neuropathy.
- One third to one half of patients present with localizing back pain.
- There is progression to nadir of clinical deficits between 4 hr and 21 days after symptom onset.
- Urinary incontinence or retention, GI disturbances (incontinence or constipation), and sexual dysfunction are common.
- Acute flaccid myelitis is a subtype of myelitis in which patients present with acute limb weakness and have primarily involvement of gray matter on spinal cord imaging.

ETIOLOGY

- Can be idiopathic demyelination (15%-30%) or demyelination secondary to neurologic and systemic conditions.
- Secondary causes include postinfection, postvaccination, acute demyelinating encephalomyelitis (where transverse myelitis tends to be monophasic), and others such as multiple sclerosis, neuromyelitis optica (NMO), mixed connective tissue disorders, sarcoidosis, and paraneoplastic conditions, which can be progressive or relapsing.
- About 50% of patients have had a recent upper respiratory infection.
- Epstein-Barr virus and cytomegalovirus are most common viral infections.
- Hepatitis B, varicella, enterovirus, rhinovirus, mycoplasma, syphilis, measles, Lyme disease are less common.

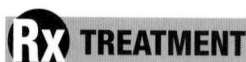

DIFFERENTIAL DIAGNOSIS

- MS
- Neuromyelitis optica (NMO)
- Spinal cord tumors
- Herniated or slipped discs
- Spinal stenosis
- Abscess
- Vascular malformation

WORKUP

Transverse myelitis (TM) should be suspected in patients with a history of rapid (hours to days) onset of motor weakness and sensory abnormalities with bladder or bowel dysfunction that is referable to the spinal cord. The dysfunction is bilateral (not necessarily symmetric) and there is a clearly defined sensory (dermatomal) level. It is important to distinguish idiopathic TM from TM due to MS or neuromyelitis optica because idiopathic TM does not relapse and does not require long-term immunomodulatory therapy.

IMAGING STUDIES

- Gadolinium-enhanced magnetic resonance imaging (MRI) of brain and MRI of the entire spine (Fig. E1). This will show demyelinating lesion on T_2 with contrast enhancement. In MS there is a short segment lesion (less than three vertebral segments) that is dorsally located. Longitudinally extensive transverse myelitis that spans more than three or more segments of the cord is typical of NMO.
- Computed tomography (CT) of the spine should be obtained if MRI is unavailable.

- CT myelogram may also be obtained.
- Chest CT scan if sarcoidosis is suspected.

LABORATORY TESTS

- Lumbar puncture looking for CSF pleocytosis, oligoclonal bands for MS, aquaporin 4 antibodies, or infection such as varicella zoster virus PCR and enterovirus PCR.
- ANA, hepatitis B serology, Lyme disease titer, VDRL, SSA, SSB, anticardiolipin antibody, copper, vitamin B_{12}, treponemal antibody.
- Serum NMO-IgG and myelin oligodendrocyte glycoprotein (MOG) antibodies to evaluate for neuromyelitis optica.

Rx TREATMENT

Corticosteroids (IV methylprednisone 1 g/day for 3-7 days) are the first-line treatment for transverse myelitis; IVIG, plasma exchange, cyclophosphamide, and rituximab are other acute therapies used, although there is no evidence-based medicine for use of corticosteroids, plasma exchange, or IVIG.

NONPHARMACOLOGIC THERAPY

- Physical therapy
- Respiratory and oropharyngeal support

ACUTE GENERAL Rx

- High-dose IV corticosteroid (e.g., methylprednisolone 1000 mg/day for 3-5 days).
- Rescue therapy with plasma exchange may be helpful in patients who do not respond to corticosteroids.
- Combination therapy with plasmapheresis and corticosteroids or other immunosuppressive agents (e.g., cyclophosphamide) may also be effective.
- Naproxen, ibuprofen for pain.

CHRONIC Rx

- Baclofen, tizanidine, or some other muscle relaxant for muscle spasms
- Gabapentin for pain
- Low-molecular-weight heparin for DVT prophylaxis in patients with immobility

DISPOSITION

- One third of patients with transverse myelitis will have complete recovery, one third will have fair recovery, and one third have permanent disability and do not recover. Recurrence or relapse is possible.
- Patients who need further care, including those with urinary retention, may need home nursing assistance. Some patients may benefit from rehabilitation, either inpatient or outpatient.

REFERRAL

- Consider physical therapy.
- Consider occupational therapy.
- Consider rehabilitation services.
- Consider psychiatric consultation (high incidence of long-term mood and anxiety disorders).

SUGGESTED READING
Available at www.expertconsult.com

AUTHOR: **PADMAJA SUDHAKAR, M.B.B.S.**

BASIC INFORMATION

DEFINITION

Impact to the head resulting in varying levels of cellular and macroscopic changes, detected with clinical examination supplemented by imaging studies. Maas et al have proposed this definition: "brain damage resulting from external forces, as a consequence of direct impact, rapid acceleration or deceleration, a penetrating object (e.g., gunshot) or blast waves from an explosion. The nature, intensity, direction, and duration of these forces determine the pattern and extent of damage."

SYNONYMS

TBI
Head injury
Concussion
Intracranial contusion

ICD-10CM CODES

S06.9 X0A	Intracranial injury
S06.1X7A	Traumatic cerebral edema with loss of consciousness of any duration with death due to brain injury prior to regaining consciousness, initial encounter
S06.2X9A	Diffuse traumatic brain injury with loss of consciousness of unspecified duration, initial encounter
S06.300A	Unspecified focal traumatic brain injury without loss of consciousness, initial encounter
S06.305A	Unspecified focal traumatic brain injury with loss of consciousness greater than 24 hours with return to pre-existing conscious level, initial encounter
S06.309A	Unspecified focal traumatic brain injury with loss of consciousness of unspecified duration, initial encounter

EPIDEMIOLOGY & DEMOGRAPHICS

Traumatic brain injury (TBI) is a worldwide leading cause of mortality in young individuals. Urbanization and increasing use of motor vehicles has led to an overall increase in TBI, especially in high-income and developing countries.
INCIDENCE: Globally, more than 10 million people suffer TBI resulting in mortality or requiring hospitalization each year. By the year 2020, it is projected that TBI will surpass many diseases as the major cause of death and disability worldwide. TBI likely accounts for 9% of global mortality and is a threat to health in every country in the world. The financial burden of TBI has been estimated to be greater than $60 billion per year in the United States alone. According to estimates from the CDC, about 2.5 million emergency department visits, including deaths and hospitalizations, were associated with TBI in 2010.
PREVALENCE: The prevalence of TBI in the United States has been estimated at approximately 5.3 million. In the European Union with 330 million inhabitants, approximately 7,775,000 new TBI cases occur each year.

According to the CDC, combined rates of TBI-related hospitalizations, emergency department visits, and deaths have risen from 521/100,000 in 2000 to 823.7/100,000 in 2010.
PEAK INCIDENCE: Approximate incidence in the US per CDC data is 103/100,000 population. In the European Union, this is estimated to be at 235/100,000.
PREDOMINANT SEX AND AGE: TBI occurs more frequently in young adults, particularly males 15 to 25 years of age, and has a high cost to society because of life years lost as a result of death and disability.
GENETICS: Work on the genetic basis and the susceptibility it affords in traumatic brain injury is being currently studied. The most recognized association between a genetic polymorphism and outcome involves the apolipoprotein E (apo E) gene. The ε4 allele has been associated with poorer outcome after TBI. The same isoform is associated with Alzheimer's and increased deposition of amyloid beta lipoprotein after TBI. TBI and apo E ε4 synergistically are also associated with a 10-fold increased risk for Alzheimer's as well as larger intracerebral hematomas and greater ischemia after TBI.
RISK FACTORS: N/A.

PHYSICAL FINDINGS & CLINICAL PRESENTATION

TBI patients can present with a spectrum of clinical symptoms including nausea, vomiting, headache, seizures, altered mental status, and/or coma. Stigmata of trauma, including bruises, scalp lacerations, and periorbital or mastoid ecchymosis suggesting skull base fractures, are telltale signs of possible underlying traumatic brain injury. Box 1 describes risk stratification in patients with minor head trauma. The spectrum of TBI is most commonly assessed using the Glasgow Coma Scale (GCS), which ranges from 3 to 15 and utilizes eye, motor, and verbal exams (Table 1).

ETIOLOGY

Etiology in most cases is impact related. Mechanical falls, motor vehicle accidents, and assaults resulting in direct or indirect trauma to the head from acceleration and rotational forces result in brain injury.

DIAGNOSIS

DIFFERENTIAL DIAGNOSIS

Differential diagnosis of TBI is quite limited; however, there are several considerations and diagnoses considered as a possibility within the realm of TBI. These are enumerated in the imaging section.

WORKUP

TBI workup is always a part of the advanced trauma life support (ATLS) protocol. Primary and secondary survey followed by imaging studies constitutes the standardized approach to TBI. Focused TBI workup includes:
- History: including timing of injury, duration of loss of consciousness if applicable, seizures (if any), comorbidities, use of anticoagulants and antiplatelet agents (requires reversal in the event of intracranial blood on imaging).

- Neurological examination: Glasgow Coma Scale, cranial nerves, motor/sensory exam. Assess for scalp lacerations, specifically overlying a skull fracture as well as CSF otorrhea or rhinorrhea.
- CT imaging of the head if there is a significant history of impact to the head, polytrauma, positive loss of consciousness, or stigmata of trauma to the head.

LABORATORY TESTS

Basic labs including CBC, basic metabolic panel, prothrombin time, activated partial thromboplastin time, urine drug screen, and ethanol blood level. Upcoming tests for platelet function analysis for unknown antiplatelet use are also being performed for early reversal with platelet replacement. These tests focus on an individual's responsiveness to antiplatelet agents and are available at most academic institutions. There are no current laboratory biomarkers for

---

BOX 1   Risk Stratification in Patients With Minor Head Trauma

High Risk
Focal neurologic findings
Asymmetrical pupils
Skull fracture on clinical examination
Multiple trauma
Serious, painful, distracting injuries
External signs of trauma above the clavicles
Initial Glasgow Coma Scale score of 14 or 15
Loss of consciousness
Posttraumatic confusion or amnesia
Progressively worsening headache
Vomiting
Posttraumatic seizure
History of bleeding disorder or anticoagulation
Recent ingestion of intoxicants
Unreliable or unknown history of injury
Previous neurologic diagnosis
Previous epilepsy
Suspected child abuse
Age above 60 years or below 2 years

Medium Risk
Initial Glasgow Coma Scale score of 15
Brief loss of consciousness
Posttraumatic amnesia
Vomiting
Headache
Intoxication

Low Risk
Currently asymptomatic
No other injuries
No focality on examination
Normal pupils
No change in consciousness
Intact orientation and memory
Initial Glasgow Coma Scale score of 15
Accurate history
Trivial mechanism
Injury less than 24 hours ago
No or mild headache
No vomiting
No preexisting high-risk factors

From Marx JA et al: *Rosen's emergency medicine*, ed 8, Philadelphia, 2014, WB Saunders.

TBI severity, but a search for such a biomarker is an area of intense research.

IMAGING STUDIES (TABLE 2)

CT imaging forms the current cornerstone of imaging modalities for head trauma. Usually, in addition to a plain CT of the head (Fig. 1), CTA head/neck and CT of the spine is helpful if arterial or C-spine injury is suspected, respectively. Other imaging modalities such as MRI can be helpful in certain situations but are typically adjuncts in the acute setting to CT-guided management. Canadian CT head rules are a useful guide in determining utility of obtaining a CT scan. These are based on risk factors:

HIGH-RISK:
1. Failure to reach GCS of 15 within 2 hours
2. Suspected open or any signs of basal skull fracture
3. More than two episodes of vomiting
4. Age older than 65

LOW RISK:
1. Dangerous mechanism of injury or poly-trauma
2. Loss of consciousness lasting >30 minutes
Pathologies that can be identified with imaging are noted in the following:
- Primary extraaxial: epidural, subdural, subarachnoid hemorrhage
- Primary intraaxial: axonal injury, cortical contusion, intracerebral or intraventricular hemorrhage, encephalomalacia (from prior TBI or vascular insult)
- Skull fracture: Linear, depressed, open, involving frontal sinus or skull base
- Penetrating brain injury: Gunshot wounds, sharp objects resulting in parenchymal and vascular injury
- Vascular injury: dissection, traumatic carotid-cavernous fistula (CCF), dural arteriovenous fistula (dAVF), pseudoaneurysm formation
- Secondary acute injury: diffuse cerebral swelling/dysautoregulation (seen more commonly in children from posttraumatic hyperemia), infarction, infection from penetrating trauma, brain herniation from mass lesion or cerebral edema
- Secondary chronic injury: hydrocephalus (posttraumatic due to disruption of normal CSF absorption pathways), encephalomalacia, CSF leak (from skull base fractures, manifests as otorrhea or rhinorrhea, leptomeningeal cyst (seen most commonly in infants, skull fracture resulting in underlying dural injury)

Rx TREATMENT

Prevention of secondary injury is the primary goal of prehospital and early in-hospital management. Most common mechanisms of secondary injury are either intracranial (ICP, hematoma) or systemic (hypoxia, hypovolemia, hypotension). Early categorization of head trauma patients according to the severity (based on GCS) and transport to facilities equipped with personnel and technology to deal with issues pertaining to head trauma has improved the overall management of head injury patients and prevention of secondary injury. Airway, breathing, and circulation, however, still remain the most important parameters to be stabilized and both directly and indirectly affect GCS and overall outcome. Trauma guidelines suggest intubation should be performed in any patient with a GCS of 8 or less to prevent hypoxemia and hypercapnia. Intravenous fluid resuscitation should also be started early to prevent hypovolemia resulting in hypotension, shown to double mortality. Transfer to and care in a Level I trauma center are associated with better outcomes.

Details of in-hospital management including critical care and surgical intervention is beyond the scope of this text. Some important points are summarized below.

TABLE 1 Glasgow Coma Scale (GCS)

Adult		Infant	
Eye Opening	**E**	**Eye Opening**	
Spontaneous	4	Spontaneous	
To speech	3	To speech	
To pain	2	To pain	
No response	1	No response	
Best Motor Response	**M**	**Best Motor Response**	
Obeys verbal command	6	Normal movements	
Localizes to pain	5	Localizes to pain	
Withdraws to pain	4	Withdraws to pain	
Flexion (decorticate)	3	Flexion (decorticate)	
Extension (decerebrate)	2	Extension (decerebrate)	
No response	1	No response	
Best Verbal Response	**E**	**Best Verbal Response**	
Oriented speech	5	Coos, babbles	
Disoriented speech	4	Cries but consolable	
Inappropriate words	3	Persistently irritable	
Incomprehensible sounds	2	Grunts to pain/restless	
No response	1	No response	

Mild TBI: GCS 13-15, Moderate TBI: GCS 9-12, Severe TBI GCS 8 or less.
GCS can range from 3 to 15. If intubated, then verbal component is replaced by 'T'. Best possible score if intubated is 10T, and worst is 3T.
In obtunded patients, pain stimulus can be central or peripheral. In patients with suspected spinal cord injury and paralysis, central stimulus to elicit facial grimace can be used to assess motor and eye component.

TABLE 2 Comparison of Head Imaging Modalities

	Computed Tomography Scans	Magnetic Resonance Imaging	Angiography	Skull Radiography
Advantages	Fast Patient accessible for monitoring Defines acute hemorrhages, mass effects, bone injuries, hydrocephalus, intraventricular blood, edema	Defines contusions and pericontusion edema, post-traumatic ischemic infarction, brainstem injuries	Helps localize acute traumatic lesions Defines vascular injuries, injuries to venous sinuses Detects mass effects	Readily available May help screen some patients for further imaging studies
Disadvantages	Artifacts arise from patient's movement, foreign bodies Streak artifacts may obscure brainstem or posterior fossa	Slow Patients not easily accessible for monitoring Does not define most acute hemorrhagic lesions Not useful for bone injuries	Does not define nature of acute lesion Does not detect infratentorial masses	Does not indicate presence or absence of intracranial injury
Indications	Acute severe head trauma Acute moderate head trauma Suspected depressed skull fracture High-risk minor head trauma Suspected child abuse in minor head trauma Deteriorating neurologic status	Persistent symptoms with postconcussive syndrome Suspected post-traumatic ischemic infarction Suspected contusions not seen on CT scan	Suspected vascular injury CT scan not available	CT scan may not be done Penetrating head trauma

CT, Computed tomography.
From Marx: *Rosen's emergency medicine: concepts and clinical practice,* J.A. Marx, R.S. Hockberger, R.M. Walls, et al. (eds.) 7 ed, 2010, Elsevier.

1. ATLS protocol (airway, breathing, circulation, disability, exposure)
2. Ventilatory support
3. Optimization of oxygenation, ventilation, and fluid status
4. CT head (Fig. E2) to evaluate for mass lesion (hematoma) or cerebral edema. These findings may necessitate either surgical intervention or ICP monitor placement. ATLS guidelines recommend maximum 30 minutes between initial assessment and CT head.
5. In case of either a severe TBI (GCS 8 or less) or a moderate TBI (GCS 8 to 13) with an unreliable neurological exam, patients should be admitted to the intensive care unit for frequent neurological checks. TBI guidelines suggest ICP monitor placement for GCS 8 or less to monitor intracranial pressure closely. ICP monitors are of various kinds, and the most commonly used include external ventricular drain, intraparenchymal pressure monitor, and a bolt device with brain tissue oxygen pressure monitoring with fiberoptic pressure monitor. Recent research has also supported the use of brain tissue oxygen monitoring for severe TBI patients. Surgical decompression may involve evacuation of hematoma (epidural, subdural intraparenchymal contusion) through craniotomy alone (replacement of bone after completion of operation) versus decompressive craniectomy (complete removal of bone without replacement) in certain cases where cerebral edema is out of proportion to the presence of mass lesion. Skull fractures are treated depending on the morphology of the fracture. Open, depressed fractures require surgical debridement and elevation in most cases, in addition to broad-spectrum antibiotics.
6. Avoid electrolyte imbalance, especially hyponatremia and hyperglycemia, which may contribute to cerebral edema and increase intracranial pressure.
7. Elevation of head of bed to allow better venous drainage to reduce intracranial pressure.
8. ICP management, which may include the following: drainage of cerebrospinal fluid via external ventricular drain, surgical hematoma evacuation, administration of hyperosmotic fluids to reduce edema, pharmacologic sedation and paralysis, pentobarbital-induced coma, and surgical decompression of the brain. In patients with traumatic brain injury, hypothermia can reduce intracranial hypertension, but recent trials in patients with an intracranial pressure of more than 20 mm Hg after TBI, therapeutic hypothermia, plus standard care to reduce intracranial pressure did not result in outcomes better than those with standard care alone. The new TBI guidelines do not recommend hypothermia.[1]
9. Prevention of seizures in the acute setting. The most commonly used and studied drug is phenytoin. Indications for acute seizure prophylaxis in severe head trauma are described in Box 2. Levetiracetam (Keppra) is also a beneficial antiepileptic now commonly used in the TBI setting. Seizure prophylaxis, however, has not shown to prevent long-term development of traumatic epilepsy.
10. DVT prophylaxis is recommended in almost all patients on hospital day 1 in addition to sequential compression devices (SCDs) for immobile or bedbound patients to prevent DVTs.
11. Early initiation of parenteral nutrition.
12. Early tracheostomy for ventilator-dependent patients is recommend to reduce mechanical ventilation days.

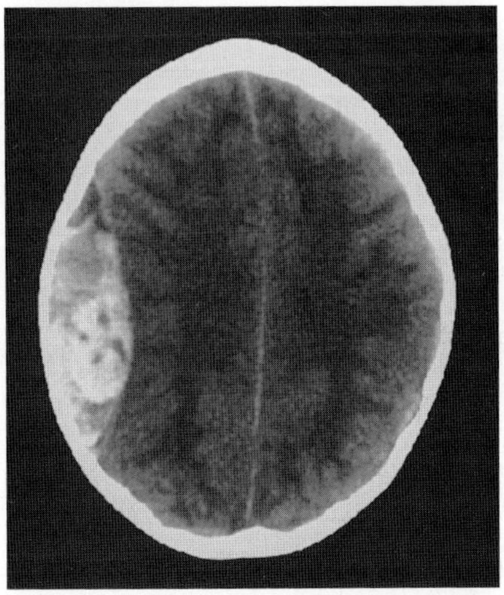

CHRONIC Rx

- Patients suffering from TBI are shown to benefit from neurocognitive, occupational, and physical therapy. The Glasgow Outcome Scale is a comprehensive measure of severity and eventual outcome of brain injury. Posttraumatic amnesia, age, length of coma, GCS score within the first 24 hours, and imaging study scales are some of the factors affecting outcome and dictating long-term prognosis.
- Chronic treatment addresses several sequelae of TBI, including, but not limited to, the following: dysautonomia, agitation, sleep disturbance, posttraumatic epilepsy, spasticity, dysphagia, syndrome of the trephined, posttraumatic hydrocephalus, apathy, fecal/urinary incontinence, headache, and neuropathic pain syndromes.

COMPLEMENTARY AND ALTERNATIVE MEDICINE

Currently, there are no proven drugs that improve outcomes after TBI. Several pro-drugs are under study, with the hopes to have a single TBI cocktail that would enhance repair at the cellular and molecular pathway level. Neurostimulants such as amantadine, bromocriptine, amphetamine, and methylphenidate are used in the rehabilitation phase with anecdotal data, but good RCTs are lacking in this area.

DISPOSITION

Depending on severity of head injury, patients may require admission to a rehabilitation facility or discharge to home with outpatient neurocognitive therapy.

REFERRAL

Early transfer to a Level 1 Trauma Center with neurosurgical personnel if high-risk findings are noted on clinical exam or CT head, and is associated with better outcomes.

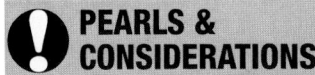

PEARLS & CONSIDERATIONS

TBI is major healthcare issue. Guidelines have been developed to address TBI in a timely and effective fashion. Clinical acumen and judgment, however, is irreplaceable and should be exercised for better patient care and outcomes. Early recognition of high-risk patients and early imaging and early evaluation at a Level 1 Trauma Center by a specialist are associated with improved outcomes. The goal of healthcare providers in the field or in the community is to identify patients who need this attention.

PATIENT/FAMILY EDUCATION

- Brain Injury Association of America http://www.biausa.org/
- Brain Injury Resource Center http://www.headinjury.com/linktbisup.htm

RELATED CONTENT

Concussion (Related Key Topic)
Postconcussive Syndrome (Related Key Topic)

AUTHORS: **FARHAN A. MIRZA, M.B.B.S.,** and **JUSTIN F. FRASER, M.D.**

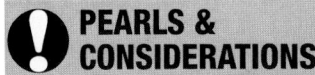

FIG. 1 Non–contrast-enhanced computed tomography scan of acute epidural hematoma at the level of right midconvexity. There is an associated mass effect and moderate midline shift. (From Marx: *Rosen's emergency medicine: concepts and clinical practice,* J.A. Marx, R.S. Hockberger, R.M. Walls, et al. (eds.) 7 ed, 2010, Elsevier.)

BOX 2 Indications for Acute Seizure Prophylaxis in Severe Head Trauma

Depressed skull fracture
Paralyzed and intubated patient
Seizure at the time of injury
Seizure at emergency department presentation
Penetrating brain injury
Severe head injury (Glasgow Coma Scale score ≤8)
Acute subdural hematoma
Acute epidural hematoma
Acute intracranial hemorrhage
Prior history of seizures

---

[1]Andrews PJD et al.: Hypothermia for intracranial hypertension after traumatic brain injury, *N Engl J Med* 373:2103-2112, 2015.

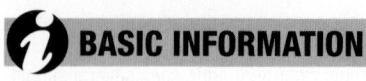

BASIC INFORMATION

DEFINITION

Traveler's diarrhea (TD) is defined as 3 or more loose-to-watery stools, with or without associated fever, abdominal cramps, and vomiting, within a 24-hr period. It develops during or within 10 days of traveling to developing areas of the world.

SYNONYMS

TD
Enterotoxigenic *E. coli*
Enteroaggregative *E. coli*
Infectious diarrhea
Postinfectious irritable bowel syndrome

ICD-10CM CODES
A09 Infectious diarrhea

EPIDEMIOLOGY & DEMOGRAPHICS

Traveler's diarrhea is mostly caused by bacteria and other pathogens in food and water

At least 1 episode of diarrhea occurs in 40% to 50% of travelers during their stay abroad. Table 1 describes pathogens and epidemiologic features associated with traveler's diarrhea

INCIDENCE: High risk (>20%): South and Southeast Asia, Africa (except South Africa), South and Central America, and Mexico

Moderate risk (10%-20 %): Caribbean Islands, South Africa, Central and East Asia (including Russia and China), Eastern Europe, and the Middle East, including Israel.

Low risk (<10%): Northern and Western Europe, Australia, New Zealand, United States, Canada, Singapore, Japan.

PEAK INCIDENCE:
- Peak incidence occurs during the first week of travel and progressively declines after that
- Seasonal variation does exist for TD, with lower rates in the winter months

PREVALENCE: Acute and chronic diarrhea account for a third of medical visits by returned travelers as per the GeoSentinel database.

PREDOMINANT SEX AND AGE:
- Travelers in their 30s are at highest risk, possibly secondary to more adventurous travel
- Gender does not seem to influence the risk for TD
- Infants and toddlers are more likely to have a more severe form of TD and are more likely to need hospitalization

GENETICS: Travelers with the O blood group are at higher risk for diarrhea caused by Norovirus and *Shigella*

RISK FACTORS:
- Gastric acid protects against enteropathogens, so medications that reduce gastric acid secretion (i.e., PPI or H2-receptor blockers) are known to increase risk for TD by a factor of 12
- Immunocompromised travelers such as those with HIV/AIDS are at higher risk for parasitic infections
- Backpackers are at higher risk than those staying at a resort
- Food bought from street vendors or prepared by persons not wearing gloves carries a higher risk

PHYSICAL FINDINGS & CLINICAL PRESENTATION

- The clinical presentation does not allow determination of infectious cause
- 90% of cases occur within 2 weeks of stay
- Acute watery diarrhea predominates in 90% of patients
- Signs of invasive infection, including fever and bloody/mucoid diarrhea, occur in 3% to 30%
- Most patients report 3 to 5 bowel movements a day, but in 20% a higher frequency of up to 20 daily bowel movements occurs
- Nausea (10%-70%), vomiting (4%-36%), abdominal cramps/tenesmus (80%), urgency (90%)
- Other: myalgia, arthralgia, headache
- Average episode resolves in 3 to 5 days

- Prolonged symptoms lasting more than a week: 8% to 15%; chronic diarrhea >30 days: 1% to 3%
- Severe episodes may result in electrolyte imbalance (K+ loss)
- 50% of all travelers are incapacitated for at least 24 hours, but up to 20% are ill in bed for 1 to 2 days.

ETIOLOGY

- *E. coli* (Table E2): Accounts for up to 60% of all cases of TD and is most prevalent in Central and South America, South Asia, and Africa. Table E3 summarizes etiology of traveler's diarrhea in Latin America, Africa, and Asia.
  - Enterotoxigenic *E. coli* (ETEC): produce heat labile and heat stable toxin and are the most common cause, accounting for 10% to 45% of cases. Frequently seen in Latin America, Africa, and South Asia.
  - Enteroaggregative *E. coli* (EAEC): more commonly seen in Latin America.
  - Other *E. coli* (enteropathogenic [EPEC], enteroinvasive [EIEC], enterohemorrhagic [EHEC]: Shiga toxin-producing or diffuse adhering *E. coli* are much less common.
- *Campylobacter*: 2% to 32% of cases. More common in Southeast Asia, where it is more frequent than ETEC.
- Shigella: 2% to 9%. More common in Africa.
- Salmonella: <5% of cases except in Asia, where it is seen in up to 10% of cases.
- Other bacteria: *Aeromonas, Arcobacter, Plesiomonas*, enterotoxigenic *Bacteroides fragilis, Vibrio cholera*, noncholera vibrios.
- Viral pathogens:
  - Norovirus: up to 17% of cases from Caribbean and Africa.
  - Rotavirus: 4% to 7% of cases.
- Protozoans:
  - *Entamoeba histolytica*: more common in South and Southeast Asia.
  - *Giardia lamblia*: more common in South and Southeast Asia, especially Nepal.
  - *Cryptosporidium, Cyclospora, Isospora*.

TABLE 1 Pathogens and Epidemiologic Features Associated With Traveler's Diarrhea

Organism	Approximate Percentage of Cases (%)	Epidemiologic Features
Enterotoxigenic *Escherichia coli*	15-50	Most important causative agent of traveler's diarrhea overall; not diagnosed by routine microbiologic methods
Enteroaggregative *E. coli*	20-35	Not diagnosed by routine microbiologic methods
Shigella spp. and enteroinvasive *E. coli*	10-25	Most important causes of dysentery. Enteroinvasive *E. coli* not diagnosed by routine microbiologic methods
Nontyphoidal *Salmonella* spp.	5-10	
Campylobacter jejuni	3-15	More common in Asia; antimicrobial resistance a concern
Aeromonas	5	
Plesiomonas	5	
Giardia lamblia	<2	Affects hikers and campers who drink from contaminated freshwater streams
Cryptosporidium hominis/parvum	<2	Occasional large-scale waterborne outbreaks
Cyclospora cayetanensis	<2	
Vibrio cholerae		Ongoing outbreaks in Haiti and Zimbabwe, and endemic in many countries in Asia; rare cause of disease in travelers
Norovirus		Outbreaks on cruise ships
Entamoeba histolytica		May cause liver abscess

From Bennett JE et al: *Mandell, Douglas, and Bennett's principles and practice of infectious diseases*, ed 8, Philadelphia, 2015, WB Saunders.

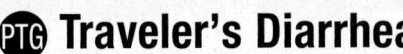

Dx DIAGNOSIS

DIFFERENTIAL DIAGNOSIS

- Malaria
- Dengue fever
- Influenza
- Rocky Mountain spotted fever
- Irritable bowel syndrome
- Inflammatory bowel disease
- Shellfish poisoning
- Mushroom poisoning

WORKUP

- Most cases of TD are self-limiting, do not require workup, and are treated symptomatically without regard to etiologic agent.
- In patients with diarrhea, fever, and colitic symptoms (bloody stools, cramping), a stool culture should be obtained to look for specific bacterial pathogens.

LABORATORY TESTS

- Stool culture ×3 for bacterial pathogens.
- Stool for ova and parasites to help identify protozoans. Special stains such as modified acid fast or trichrome stain may be necessary for *Cryptosporidium, Cyclospora,* and *Isospora.*
- Blood cultures in patients with systemic illness to rule out *Salmonella* species.

Rx TREATMENT

NONPHARMACOLOGIC THERAPY

- Fluid replacement to treat volume depletion of diarrhea is important.
- Mild cases: alternate fluids that contain salts and fluids that contain sugars, such as broths or fruit juices. Pedialyte is effective as an over-the-counter product.
- Severe cases: Oral rehydration solution (ORS) packets are available in most pharmacies. They should be mixed with clean water to replace lost electrolytes and are used until patient is urinating regularly. An alternative home-based solution can be made with: ½ teaspoon of salt, ½ teaspoon of baking soda, and 4 tablespoons of sugar in one liter of clean water.

ACUTE GENERAL Rx

- Antisecretory agents may reduce symptoms but do not treat underlying cause
  - Bismuth subsalicylate: 1 dose of 525 mg (2 tablets of Pepto-Bismol) PO every 30 min up to 8 doses a day. Can reduce number of bowel movements by 50%.

- Loperamide: 4 mg PO, then 2 mg after each loose bowel movement, not to exceed 16 mg per day. Use for up to 48 hrs. Has antisecretory and antimotility effect. Antimotility drugs should not be used in cases of bloody diarrhea or dysentery (increased risk of colitis and colonic perforation). When used, they should be given only in conjunction with antimicrobial therapy.
- Antibiotics are warranted only for moderate to severe diarrhea (i.e., >4 bowel movements a day, fever, or blood, pus, or mucus in stool. Antibiotics can reduce duration of diarrhea by 1 to 2 days.
  - Fluoroquinolones are considered first-line agents for bacterial causes of TD. Cannot be used in children under 15 and in pregnant women:
    1. Ciprofloxacin: 500 mg twice a day for 1 to 3 days
    2. Levaquin: 500 mg a day for 1 to 3 days
  - Azithromycin: preferred agent for children and pregnant women. Dose of 1 gram PO single dose. Particularly effective against quinolone-resistant *Campylobacter* infections in Southeast Asia.
  - Rifaximin: 200 mg PO TID for 3 days for children age>12 and adults is effective for afebrile, noncolitic diarrhea such as ETEC. Does not treat *Salmonella, Shigella,* or *Campylobacter.*
- Concerns of use of antibiotics
  - Widespread use of antibiotics has led to resistance. Tetracycline and sulfa agents such as Bactrim are no longer used due to widespread resistance
  - Antibiotic treatment may lead to prolonged colonization in infections with *Salmonella* and nontyphoid *Salmonella*
  - In cases of EHEC (Shiga toxin production) treatment with quinolones, but not rifaximin, may increase risk of complications such as hemolytic uremic syndrome
  - *Clostridia difficile* infection can occur with use of antibiotics

PREVENTION BY ANTIBIOTICS AND NONANTIBIOTIC AGENTS

- Antibiotic prophylaxis can be considered for certain groups, such as persons with underlying illness, athletes, and politicians for up to 2 to 3 weeks. Ciprofloxacin 250 to 500 mg a day is effective in preventing 90% of TD. Rifaximin dosed daily has been shown to help prevent TD for U.S. travelers to Mexico, but not as effectively as Ciprofloxacin

- Bismuth subsalicylate can be used. It must be given 4× daily and can cause black tongue and stools. As it contains salicylates, it can interact with anticoagulants and lead to toxicity in patients on long-term salicylate therapy
- Probiotics are being studied for their potential use but evidence of their effectiveness is limited

REFERRAL

- Infectious diseases physician for more difficult cases lasting more than 72 hours.

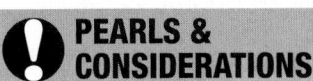 PEARLS & CONSIDERATIONS

- Travelers on cruises have lower incidence of TD than land-based trips, but cruise ship passengers and staff are at higher risk of large outbreaks of Norovirus that are difficult to contain. Norovirus infection needs only a low inoculum of virus to cause illness, and the virus is relatively resistant to cleaning
- In up to 40% of cases of TD, no pathogen is identified
- *Giardia* is the most frequent cause of long-lasting TD

PREVENTION

- There are oral and injectable vaccines against *Salmonella typhi* available in the U.S.
- Dukoral oral vaccine is available in some countries such as Canada and Australia and in Europe to help prevent cholera and ETEC.

PATIENT/FAMILY EDUCATION

- Food hygiene education: Wash hands often, especially after going to bathroom and before eating. Avoid raw fruits and vegetables (unless peeled and washed in clean water). Avoid undercooked meats, fish, and seafood. Avoid tap water and ice. Choose beverages in factory-sealed containers (such as bottled water and carbonated soft drinks). Try to avoid buffet-style foods.

SUGGESTED READINGS

Available at www.expertconsult.com

RELATED CONTENT

Traveler's Diarrhea (Patient Information)

AUTHOR: **GLENN G. FORT, M.D., M.P.H.**

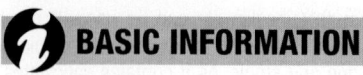

BASIC INFORMATION

DEFINITION

Trigeminal neuralgia is an intense, usually unilateral, paroxysmal, stabbing pain in the sensory distribution of the trigeminal (cranial nerve V) nerve.

SYNONYMS

Tic douloureux ("painful tics/spasms")

ICD-10CM CODES
G50.0 Trigeminal neuralgia

EPIDEMIOLOGY & DEMOGRAPHICS

INCIDENCE: 4 per 100,000
PEAK INCIDENCE: Incidence increases with age and peaks at 67 years of age; onset in 90% of patients is after age 40.
PREVALENCE: 155 in 1 million
PREDOMINANT SEX AND AGE: Male/female ratio is 1:1.5.
RISK FACTORS: Most cases are idiopathic; age and multiple sclerosis are risk factors.

PHYSICAL FINDINGS & CLINICAL PRESENTATION

- Patients present with paroxysmal, unilateral facial pain that is usually described as shock-like, stabbing, or electric (Fig. 1).
- Pain can be spontaneous or triggered by touch, an air current, or activities such as shaving, eating, or brushing teeth.
- In severe cases, facial spasms can accompany the pain.
- Pain is usually described in distribution of the second (V2-maxillary) and third (V3-mandibular) divisions of the trigeminal nerve.
- The pain seldom lasts more than a few seconds to a minute.
- There is usually no sensory or motor loss.

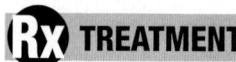

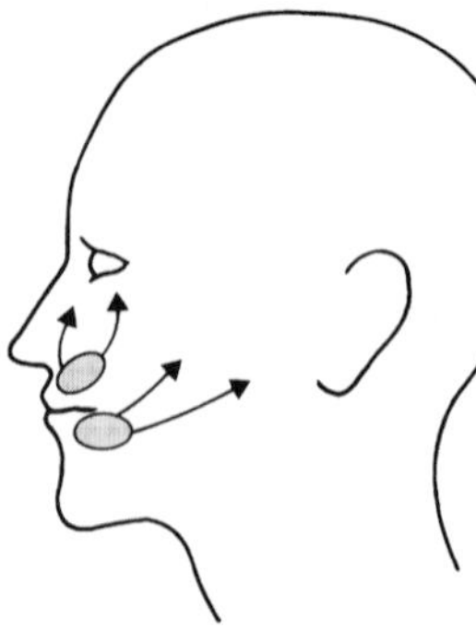

FIG. 1 Trigeminal neuralgia. The two most common sites of origin and radiation of pain are shown: mouth-ear and nose-orbit. Pain usually starts in the region of the encircled area and radiates in the directions shown. (From Souhami RL, Moxham J: *Textbook of medicine,* ed 4, London, 2002, Churchill Livingstone.)

ETIOLOGY

- Idiopathic or "classical": cause usually unknown, likely an aberrant artery or vein compressing cranial nerve V at or near the pons. Neurovascular contact is also commonly found incidentally on imaging in asymptomatic individuals.
- Secondary: accounts for up to 15% of cases; caused by nonvascular lesions such as a demyelinating plaque from multiple sclerosis or compression from a tumor near the pons.
- Box 1 summarizes causes of trigeminal neuralgia

DIAGNOSIS

DIFFERENTIAL DIAGNOSIS

- Trigeminal neuropathy
- Primary stabbing headache
- Short-lasting unilateral neuralgiform headache with conjunctival injection and tearing (SUNCT)
- Postherpetic neuralgia
- Glossopharyngeal neuralgia
- Dental pain

WORKUP

Trigeminal neuralgia is a clinical diagnosis (see previously).

IMAGING STUDIES

Neuroimaging (MRI) should be considered in young patients (<40 years) with atypical symptoms (sensory loss, bilateral symptoms). MRI is useful to identify potential compressors or demyelinating causes.

TREATMENT

PHARMACOLOGIC Rx

- Carbamazepine 400 to 800 mg, 2 to 3 times daily divided dosing is the recommended

---

BOX 1 Causes of Trigeminal Neuralgia

Classical
Neurovascular compression by an artery or vein

Symptomatic
Saccular aneurysm
  Arteriovenous malformation
  Tumors/mass-lesions at cerebellopontine angle
- Vestibular schwannoma
- Meningioma
- Epidermoid
Primary demyelinating disorders
- Multiple sclerosis
- Charcot-Marie-Tooth disease (rare)
Infiltrative disorders
- Trigeminal amyloidoma
Nondemyelinating lesions
- Small infarct or angioma in the brainstem
Familial

Modified from Adams JG et al: *Emergency medicine, clinical essentials,* ed 2, Philadelphia, 2013, Elsevier.

---

initial treatment. This can be titrated to pain relief by 100 to 200 mg every 3 days to a maximum of 1200 mg divided bid or tid.
- Oxcarbazepine can be used if carbamazepine is not tolerated due to side effects. Other medications include baclofen, phenytoin, gabapentin, clonazepam, lamotrigine, and levetiracetam.
- Drug combinations can be tried when one medication is partially effective before proceeding with secondary intervention.
- Spontaneous remissions may be seen in trigeminal neuralgia, and therefore periodic medication tapers should be considered if the patient is pain free.
- In the elderly population, caution should be used when initiating and titrating the above medications. Caution and extensive counseling should also be used in women of childbearing age when initiating treatment with anti-seizure medications.

NONPHARMACOLOGIC THERAPY

Patients with refractory pain eventually need secondary intervention such as microvascular decompression, selective nerve fiber destruction (rhizotomy), glycerol injection, thermal lesioning, chemical ablation, or gamma knife radiosurgery. Microvascular decompression is the only available nondestructive procedure and is effective in 75% of patients, and possesses observed long-term benefits.

DISPOSITION

- Most patients are responsive to initial pharmacologic treatment. Spontaneous remission is possible.
- Medical management is eventually ineffective in 30% to 50% of patients.

REFERRAL

Referral to a neurologist is appropriate if there is uncertainty about diagnosis or if symptoms are refractory to conservative management.

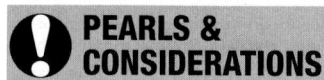

PEARLS & CONSIDERATIONS

In a young patient with trigeminal neuralgia, secondary causes such as multiple sclerosis should be considered, and an MRI of the head obtained. In secondary disease, initial therapy should address underlying secondary causes.

SUGGESTED READING
Available at www.expertconsult.com

RELATED CONTENT
Trigeminal Neuralgia (Patient Information)

AUTHOR: **JONATHAN H. SMITH, M.D.**

BASIC INFORMATION

DEFINITION

Greater trochanteric pain syndrome (GTPS) is a term used to describe chronic pain overlying lateral aspect of the hip. There are overlaps of trochanteric bursitis (TB) and GTPS. Unlike TB, GTPS is rarely accompanied by the principal symptoms of inflammation including erythema, edema, and rubor. GTPS often mimics pain generated from other sources, including myofascial pain, degenerative joint disease, and spinal pathology. Components of GTPS include tendinopathies, tendinous tears, bursal inflammation, and effusion.

SYNONYMS

Greater trochanteric pain syndrome
GTPS
Trochanteric bursitis
Trochanteric tendinitis

ICD-10CM CODES
M70.60 Trochanteric bursitis, unspecified hip
M70.61 Trochanteric bursitis, right hip
M70.62 Trochanteric bursitis, left hip

EPIDEMIOLOGY & DEMOGRAPHICS

- This commonly diagnosed regional pain syndrome is estimated to affect between 10% and 25% of the general population.
- In the primary care setting, the incidence of greater trochanteric pain is reported to be around 1.8 patients per 1000 per year.
- Incidence peaks between the fourth and sixth decades of life but can occur at any age.
- Occurs in females more often than males (ratio of 4:1).
- One study found the prevalence of GTPS to be 17.6%, being higher in women and in patients with coexisting LBP, OA, ITB tenderness and obesity.

PHYSICAL FINDINGS & CLINICAL PRESENTATION

- GTPS typically presents as chronic, persistent pain in the lateral hip and/or buttock that is exacerbated by lying on affected side, prolonged standing, driving, climbing stairs, running, or other high-impact activities.
- Pain may radiate along lateral aspect to the knee.
- Tenderness along the lateral or posterior aspect of the greater trochanter (Fig. 1).

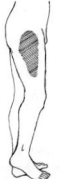

FIG. 1 Typical location of pain in trochanteric bursitis syndrome. This is also a frequent pain radiation site for lumbar spine lesion, various nerve compression syndromes, and hip disease, particularly in osteonecrosis of the femoral head. (From Canoso JJ: *Rheumatology in primary care,* Philadelphia, 1997, Saunders.)

- Pain is reproduced with resisted hip abduction.
- Pain is produced by palpation, flexion, abduction, and external rotation (positive Patrick's/FABER test).

ETIOLOGY

- GTPS can be caused by repetitive high-intensity use of the tensor fasciae and gluteus medius over the outer femur. Trauma, falls, infection (tuberculosis and bacterial), and crystal deposition can precipitate the disease.
- It can occur when other conditions such as osteoarthritis of the knee and hip, RA, sacroiliac joint disorders, leg length discrepancy, ankle sprain, and bunions of the feet cause changes in the patient's gait placing varus stress on the hip joint.
- It can also occur as a complication resulting from arthroscopic surgery of the hip (estimated 1.4% of cases).

DIFFERENTIAL DIAGNOSIS

- Piriformis tendinopathy
- L2-L3 lumbar radiculopathy, and lumbar facet syndrome
- Iliotibial band syndrome
- Osteoarthritis of the hip
- Osteonecrosis of the hip
- Stress fracture of the femoral neck
- Meralgia paresthetica
- Acetabular labral tear
- Iliopsoas bursitis
- Osteomyelitis
- Metastatic bone disease
- Septic or pyogenic arthritis
- Gluteal medius tendon tears

WORKUP

Since there is a wide differential for lateral hip pain, GTPS can be a challenging diagnosis to reach. Complete neurologic and musculoskeletal examination should be performed, including back, bilateral hip, knee, and observation of gait. Usually tenderness to palpation over the greater trochanter and pain with abduction resistance and positive Patrick's/FABER test are found.

LABORATORY TESTS

Are not indicated in straightforward cases.

IMAGING STUDIES

- Plain radiography: Plain x-rays are usually normal, but other potential causes can be excluded, including OA, femoroacetabular impingement, fractures. Calcifications over the greater trochanter may be seen in 40% of patients presenting with GTPS.
- Ultrasound: Simple, dynamic, inexpensive test that can be very useful in establishing cause of lateral hip pain.
- CT and MRI will depict both osseous and soft tissue pathology but are usually not warranted unless suspect associated conditions that would affect treatment decisions. MRI shows increased signal in bursitis.

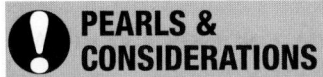

TREATMENT

Most cases of GTPS are self-limiting and tend to resolve with conservative measures.

NONPHARMACOLOGIC THERAPY

- Physical therapy and iliotibial band stretching exercises can reduce irritation of the trochanteric bursa area.
- Warm compressors.
- Ultrasound therapy.
- Cryotherapy.
- Treat gait disturbance by knee brace, shoe lift, ankle supports, and foot orthotics for the specific underlying conditions.

ACUTE GENERAL Rx

- NSAIDs for pain relief: ibuprofen 800 mg PO tid or naproxen 500 mg PO bid.
- Topical corticosteroids delivered by percutaneous phonophoresis.
- Corticosteroid injection.
- Regional anesthetic block can be used as a treatment and may also help differentiate from referred pain.

CHRONIC Rx

- Most patients respond to NSAIDs and/or nonpharmacologic therapy.
- Steroid injection: ~70% of patients respond after first injection and >90% respond to two injections.
- 25% of patients receiving steroid injection may develop a relapse.
- While the majority of patients with GTPS will improve with nonoperative management, endoscopic iliotibial band release, trochanteric bursectomy, and gluteal tendon repair may be effective treatment for severe recalcitrant cases.

REFERRAL

- Physical therapy.
- Rheumatology or orthopedics referral if steroid injection therapy is indicated.
- Orthopedics for possible bursectomy in chronic refractory cases.

PEARLS & CONSIDERATIONS

Patients with GTPS will commonly report "hip" pain. The physical examination readily distinguishes GTPS from other hip pathologies. Relief of pain with local corticosteroid injection is helpful in differentiating trochanteric bursitis from referred pain.

COMMENTS

- The absence of limitation in range of motion differentiates trochanteric bursitis from degenerative joint disease of the hip.
- Localization of pain over the lateral hip and thigh differentiates trochanteric bursitis from meralgia paresthetica located over the anterolateral thigh and osteoarthritis located over the inner thigh groin area.

SUGGESTED READINGS
Available at www.expertconsult.com

RELATED CONTENT

Trochanteric Bursitis (Patient Information)

AUTHOR: **RASHA B. ALQADI, M.D.**

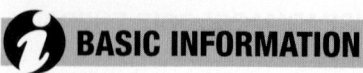
DEFINITION

Miliary tuberculosis (TB) is an infection of disseminated hematogenous disease, caused by the bacterium *Mycobacterium tuberculosis* (MTB), and is often characterized as resembling millet seeds on pathologic or radiologic examination. Extrapulmonary disease may occur in virtually every organ site.

SYNONYM

Disseminated TB

ICD-10CM CODES
A19.9 Miliary tuberculosis, unspecified

EPIDEMIOLOGY & DEMOGRAPHICS

INCIDENCE (IN U.S.): >38% of AIDS patients with TB have disseminated disease, often with concurrent pulmonary and extrapulmonary active sites. (See "Tuberculosis, Pulmonary" in Section I.)

PREVALENCE (IN U.S.):
- Undetermined
- Highest prevalence
  1. AIDS patients
  2. Minorities
  3. Children
  4. Foreign-born persons
  5. Elderly

PREDOMINANT SEX:
- No specific predilection
- Male predominance in AIDS, shelters, and prisons reflected in disproportionate male TB incidence

PREDOMINANT AGE: Predominantly among 24 to 45 yr

PEAK INCIDENCE: HIV-positive patients, regardless of age

PHYSICAL FINDINGS & CLINICAL PRESENTATION

- See also "Etiology"
- Common symptoms
  1. High intermittent fever (93%)
  2. Night sweats (79%)
  3. Weight loss (85%)
  4. Dyspnea (64%)
  5. Cough (82%)
- Symptoms referable to individual organ systems may predominate
  1. Meninges
  2. Pericardium
  3. Liver
  4. Kidney
  5. Bone
  6. GI tract
  7. Lymph nodes
  8. Serous spaces
     a. Pleural
     b. Pericardial
     c. Peritoneal
     d. Joint
  9. Skin
  10. Lung: cough, shortness of breath

- Adrenal insufficiency possible, caused by infection of adrenal gland
- Pancytopenia
  1. With fever and weight loss *or*
  2. Without other localizing symptoms or signs *or*
  3. With only splenomegaly
- TB hepatitis
  1. Tender liver
  2. Obstructive enzymes (alkaline phosphatase) elevated out of proportion to minimal hepatocellular enzymes (SGOT, SGPT) and bilirubin
- TB meningitis
  1. Gradual-onset headache
  2. Minimal meningeal signs
  3. Malaise
  4. Low-grade fever (may be absent)
  5. Sudden stupor or coma
  6. Cranial nerve VI palsy
- TB pericarditis
  1. Effusions resembling TB pleurisy
  2. Cardiac tamponade
- Skeletal TB
  1. Large joint arthritis (with effusions resembling TB pericarditis)
  2. Bone lesions (especially ribs)
  3. Pott's disease
     a. TB spondylitis, especially of lower thoracic spine
     b. Paraspinous TB abscess
     c. Possible psoas abscess
     d. Frequent cord compression (often relieved by steroids)
- Genitourinary TB
  1. Renal TB
     a. Papillary necrosis
     b. Destruction of renal pelvis
     c. Strictures of upper third of ureters
     d. Hematuria
     e. Pyuria with misleading bacterial cultures
     f. Preserved renal function
  2. TB orchitis or epididymitis
     a. Scrotal mass
     b. Draining abscess
  3. Chronic prostatic TB
- GI TB
  1. Diarrhea
  2. Pain
  3. Obstruction
  4. Bleeding
  5. Especially common with AIDS
  6. Bowel lesions
     a. Circumferential ulcers
     b. Short strictures
     c. Calcified granulomas
     d. TB mesenteric caseous adenitis
     e. Abscess, but rare fistula formation
     f. Often difficult to distinguish from granulomatous bowel disease (Crohn's disease)
- TB peritonitis
  1. Fluid resembles TB pleurisy
  2. PPD often negative
  3. Tender abdomen
  4. Doughy peritoneal consistency, often with ascites
  5. Peritoneal biopsy indicated for diagnosis

- TB lymphadenitis (scrofula)
  1. May involve all node groups
  2. Common adenopathies
     a. Cervical
     b. Supraclavicular
     c. Axillary
     d. Retroperitoneal
  3. Biopsy generally needed for diagnosis
  4. Surgical resection of nodes may be necessary
  5. Especially common with AIDS
- Cutaneous TB
  1. Skin infection from autoinoculation or dissemination
  2. Nodules or abscesses
  3. Tuberculids (possibly allergic reactions)
  4. Erythema nodosum
- Miscellaneous presentations
  1. TB laryngitis
  2. TB otitis
  3. Ocular TB
     a. Choroidal tubercles
     b. Iritis
     c. Uveitis
     d. Episcleritis
  4. Adrenal TB
  5. Breast TB

ETIOLOGY

- See also "Pulmonary Tuberculosis" in Section I.
- MTB, a slow-growing, aerobic, non–spore forming, nonmotile acid-fast bacillus
- Humans are the only reservoir for MTB.
- Pathogenesis:
  1. Acid-fast bacilli (AFB) (MTB) are ingested by macrophages in alveoli, then transported to regional lymph nodes where spread is contained.
  2. Some AFB reach the bloodstream and disseminate widely.
  3. Immediate active disseminated disease may ensue or a latent period may develop.
  4. During latent period, T-cell immune mechanisms contain infection in granulomas until later reactivation occurs as a result of immunosuppression or other undefined factors in conjunction with reactivated pulmonary TB or alone.
- Miliary TB may occur as a consequence of the following:
  1. Primary infection: inability to contain primary infection leads to a hematogenous spread and progressive disseminated disease.
  2. In late chronic TB and in those with advanced age or poor immunity, a continuous seeding of the blood may develop and lead to disseminated disease.

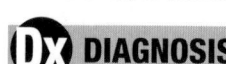 **DIAGNOSIS**

DIFFERENTIAL DIAGNOSIS

Widespread sites of possible dissemination associated with myriad differential diagnostic possibilities:
- Lymphoma

- Typhoid fever
- Brucellosis
- Other tumors
- Collagen-vascular disease

WORKUP

- Prompt evaluation is essential
- Sputum for AFB stain and culture and chest x-ray
- High-resolution CT is more sensitive for miliary TB than CXR
- PPD, which may be negative in immunocompromised patients
- Fluid analysis and mycobacterial culture wherever available
  1. Sputum
  2. Blood: particularly helpful in patients with AIDS
  3. Urine
  4. CSF
  5. Pleural
  6. Pericardial
  7. Peritoneal
  8. Gastric aspirates
- Biopsy of any involved tissue is advisable to make immediate diagnosis
  1. Transbronchial biopsy preferred and easily accessible
  2. Bone marrow
  3. Lymph node
  4. Scrotal mass if present
  5. Any other involved site
  6. Positive granuloma or AFB on biopsy specimen is diagnostic
- Imaging studies as needed

LABORATORY TESTS

- Culture and fluid analysis as described previously
- Smear-negative sputum often is positive weeks later on culture
- CBC is usually normal

- ESR is usually elevated

IMAGING STUDIES

- Chest x-ray examination (may or may not be positive) (see "Tuberculosis, Pulmonary" in Section I)
- CT scan or MRI of brain and spinal cord (Fig. 1)
  1. Tuberculoma
  2. Basilar arachnoiditis
- Barium studies of bowel

Rx TREATMENT

NONPHARMACOLOGIC THERAPY

- Bed rest during acute phase of treatment
- High-calorie, high-protein diet to reverse malnutrition and enhance immune response to TB
- Isolation in negative-pressure rooms with high-volume air replacement and circulation (with health care provider wearing proper protective 0.5- to 1-micron filter respirators)
  1. Until three consecutive sputum AFB smears are negative, if pulmonary disease coexists
  2. Isolation not required for closed-space TB infections such as peritonitis and scrofula.

ACUTE GENERAL Rx

- See "Tuberculosis, Pulmonary" in Section I.
- Therapy should be initiated immediately. Do not wait for definitive diagnosis.
- More rapid response to chemotherapy by disseminated TB foci than cavitary pulmonary TB.
- Treatment for 6 months with INH plus rifampin plus PZA.
  1. Treatment for 12 months often required for bone and renal TB.

  2. Prolonged treatment often required for CNS and pericardial.
  3. Prolonged treatment often required for all disseminated TB in infants.
- Compliance (rigid adherence to treatment regimen) is the chief determinant of success.
  1. Supervised directly observed therapy (DOT) is recommended for all patients.
  2. Supervised DOT is mandatory for unreliable patients.
- Steroids are often helpful additions in fulminant miliary disease with the hypoxemia and DIC.

CHRONIC Rx

- Generally not indicated beyond treatment described previously
- Prolonged treatment supervised by infectious disease expert required in a few complicated infections caused by resistant organisms

DISPOSITION

- Monthly follow-up by physician experienced in TB treatment
- Confirm sensitivity testing, and alter treatment appropriately (see "Tuberculosis, Pulmonary" in Section I)

REFERRAL

- To infectious disease expert for:
  1. HIV-positive patient
  2. Patient with suspected drug-resistant TB
  3. Patient previously treated for TB
  4. Patient whose fever has not decreased and sputum (if positive) has not converted to negative in 2 to 4 wk
  5. Patients with overwhelming pulmonary or extrapulmonary TB
- To pulmonary, orthopedic, or GI physicians for examinations or biopsy

! PEARLS & CONSIDERATIONS

COMMENTS

- Consider acute TB in critically ill patients with enigmatic acute respiratory distress syndrome, shock, or DIC.
- All contacts (especially close household contacts and infants) should be properly tested for PPD conversions >3 months following exposure.
- Those with positive PPD should be evaluated for active TB and properly treated or given prophylaxis.

EBM EVIDENCE

Available at www.expertconsult.com

SUGGESTED READINGS

Available at www.expertconsult.com

RELATED CONTENT

Pulmonary Tuberculosis (Related Key Topic)

AUTHOR: **GLENN G. FORT, M.D., M.P.H.**

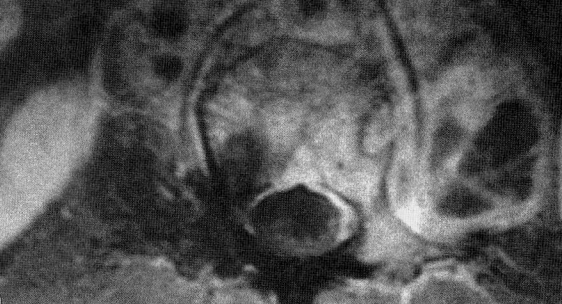
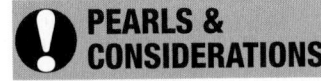
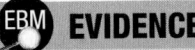

FIG 1 A and **B,** Magnetic resonance images of tuberculous spinal osteomyelitis with scalloping of the vertebrae (tuberculous caries) and paraspinal "cold" abscesses. (From Grainger RG, Allison D: *Grainger & Allison's diagnostic radiology, a textbook of medical imaging,* ed 4, London, 2001, Churchill Livingstone.)

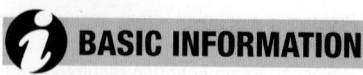

BASIC INFORMATION

DEFINITION

Pulmonary tuberculosis (TB) is an infection of the lung and, occasionally, surrounding structures, caused by the bacterium *Mycobacterium tuberculosis* (MTB). Multidrug-resistant (MDR) TB is defined as disease caused by strains of MTB that are at least resistant to treatment with isoniazid and rifampin; extensively drug-resistant (XDR) TB refers to disease caused by MDR strains that are also resistant to treatment with any fluoroquinolone and any of the injectable drugs used in the treatment of second-line anti-TB drugs.

SYNONYMS

TB

ICD-10CM CODES
A15.0 Tuberculosis of lung

EPIDEMIOLOGY & DEMOGRAPHICS

INCIDENCE (WORLDWIDE):
- One third of the world's population is infected with TB, and it is still one of the deadliest diseases known to humans.
- In 2014, 9.6 million people worldwide developed TB, which led to 1.5 million deaths. Overall 13% of cases of TB involved coinfection with HIV.
- In 2014 HIV and TB coinfection led to 430,000 deaths, and there are more than 300,000 cases of multidrug-resistant TB worldwide.
- Sub-Saharan Africa has the highest rates of active TB per capita.
- Absolute number of cases is highest in Asia, with India and China having the greatest burden of disease globally.

INCIDENCE (IN U.S.):
- In 2014, there were 9421 cases of TB in the U.S. for a rate of 2.9 cases/100,000 persons; both the number of TB cases reported and the case rate decreased compared to 2013. This represents a 1.5% decline in cases and a 2.2% decline in incidence.
- >90% of new cases each yr from reactivated prior infections
- 9% newly infected
- Only 10% of patients with purified protein derivative (PPD) conversions (higher [8%/yr] in HIV-positive patients) will develop TB, most within 1 to 2 yr
- Two thirds of all new cases in racial and ethnic minorities
- 80% of new cases in children in racial and ethnic minorities
- Occurs most frequently in geographic areas and among populations with highest AIDS prevalence
  1. Urban blacks and Hispanics between 25 and 45 yr old
  2. Poor, crowded urban communities
- Nearly 36% of new cases from new immigrants
- In 2014 in the U.S., 1.3% of cases were MDR TB (91 cases), which is a decline from 8.2% in 2008. Overall, 88% of the cases of MDR TB in 2014 were in foreign-born persons.

PREVALENCE (IN U.S.):
- Estimated 10 million people infected
- Varies widely among population groups

PREDOMINANT SEX:
- No specific predilection
- Male predominance in AIDS, shelters, and prisons reflected in disproportionate male incidence

PREDOMINANT AGE:
- Ages 24 to 45
- Childhood cases common among minorities
- Nursing home outbreaks among elderly

PEAK INCIDENCE:
- Infancy
- Teenage years
- Pregnancy
- Elderly
- HIV-positive patients at highest risk regardless of age

GENETICS:
- Populations with widespread low native resistance have been intensely infected when initially exposed to TB.
- Following elimination of those with least native resistance, incidence and prevalence of TB tends to decline.

PHYSICAL FINDINGS & CLINICAL PRESENTATION

- See "Etiology"
- Primary pulmonary TB infection generally asymptomatic
- Reactivation pulmonary TB
  1. Fever
  2. Night sweats
  3. Cough
  4. Hemoptysis
  5. Scanty nonpurulent sputum
  6. Weight loss
- Progressive primary pulmonary TB disease: same as reactivation pulmonary TB
- TB pleurisy
  1. Pleuritic chest pain
  2. Fever
  3. Shortness of breath
- Rare massive, suffocating, fatal hemoptysis secondary to erosion of pulmonary artery within a cavity (Rasmussen's aneurysm)
- Chest examination
  1. Not specific
  2. Usually underestimates extent of disease
  3. Rales accentuated following a cough (posttussive rales)

ETIOLOGY

- MTB, a slow-growing, aerobic, non-spore-forming, nonmotile bacillus, with a lipid-rich cell wall
  1. Lacks pigment
  2. Produces niacin
  3. Reduces nitrate
  4. Produces heat-labile catalase
  5. MTB staining, acid-fast and acid-alcohol fast by Ziehl-Neelsen method, appearing as red, slightly bent, beaded rods 2 to 4 microns long (acid-fast bacilli [AFB]), against a blue background
  6. Polymerase chain reaction (PCR) to detect <10 organisms/ml in sputum (compared with the requisite 10,000 organisms/ml for AFB smear detection)
  7. Culture
     a. Growth on solid media (Löwenstein-Jensen; Middlebrook 7H11) in 2 to 6 wk
     b. Growth in liquid media (BACTEC, using a radioactive carbon source for early growth detection) often in 9 to 16 days
     c. Enhanced in a 5% to 10% carbon dioxide atmosphere
  8. DNA fingerprinting (based on restriction fragment length polymorphism [RFLP])
     a. Facilitates immediate identification of MTB strains in early growing cultures
     b. False negatives possible if growth suboptimal
  9. Humans are the only reservoir for MTB
  10. Transmission
      a. Facilitated by close exposure to high-velocity cough (unprotected by proper mask or respirators) from patient with AFB-positive sputum and cavitary lesions, producing aerosolized droplets containing AFB, which are inhaled directly into alveoli
      b. Occurs within prisons, nursing homes, and hospitals
- Pathogenesis
  1. AFB (MTB) ingested by macrophages in alveoli, then transported to regional lymph nodes, where spread is contained
  2. Some AFB may reach bloodstream and disseminate widely
  3. Primary TB (asymptomatic, minimal pneumonitis in lower or midlung fields, with hilar lymphadenopathy) essentially an intracellular infection, with multiplication of organisms continuing 2 to 12 wk after primary exposure, until cell-mediated hypersensitivity (detected by positive skin test reaction to tuberculin PPD) matures, with subsequent containment of infection
  4. Local and disseminated AFB thus contained by T-cell–mediated immune responses
     a. Recruitment of monocytes
     b. Transformation of lymphocytes with secretion of lymphokines
     c. Activation of macrophages and histiocytes
     d. Organization into granulomas, where organisms may survive within macrophages (Langhans' giant cells), but within which multiplication essentially ceases (95%) and from which spread is prohibited
  5. Progressive primary pulmonary disease
     a. May immediately follow the asymptomatic phase
     b. Necrotizing pulmonary infiltrates
     c. Tuberculous bronchopneumonia
     d. Endobronchial TB
     e. Interstitial TB
     f. Widespread miliary lung lesions
  6. Postprimary TB pleurisy with pleural effusion
     a. Develops after early primary infection, although often before conversion to positive PPD

b. Results from pleural seeding from a peripheral lung lesion or rupture of lymph node into pleural space

c. May produce a large (sometimes hemorrhagic) exudative effusion (with polymorphonuclear cells early, rapidly replaced by lymphocytes), frequently without pulmonary infiltrates

d. Generally resolves without treatment

e. Portends a high risk of subsequent clinical disease, and therefore must be diagnosed and treated early (pleural biopsy and culture) to prevent future catastrophic TB illness

f. May result in disseminated extrapulmonary infection

7. Reactivation pulmonary TB
   a. Occurs months to years following primary TB
   b. Preferentially involves the apical posterior segments of the upper lobes and superior segments of the lower lobes
   c. Associated with necrosis and cavitation of involved lung, hemoptysis, chronic fever, night sweats, weight loss
   d. Spread within lung occurs via cough and inhalation

8. Reinfection TB
   a. May mimic reactivation TB
   b. Ruptured caseous foci and cavities, which may produce endobronchial spread

9. MTB in both progressive primary and reactivation pulmonary TB
   a. Intracellular (macrophage) lesions (undergoing slow multiplication)
   b. Closed caseous lesions (undergoing slow multiplication)
   c. Extracellular, open cavities (undergoing rapid multiplication)
   d. INH and rifampin are bactericidal in all three sites
   e. Pyrazinamide (PZA) especially active within acidic macrophage environment
   f. Extrapulmonary reactivation disease also possible

10. Rapid local progression and dissemination in infants with devastating illness before PPD conversion occurs

11. Most symptoms (fever, weight loss, anorexia) and tissue destruction (caseous necrosis) from cytokines and cell-mediated immune responses

12. MTB has no important endotoxins or exotoxins

13. Granuloma formation related to tumor necrosis factor (TNF) secreted by activated macrophages

DX DIAGNOSIS

DIFFERENTIAL DIAGNOSIS
- Necrotizing pneumonia (anaerobic, gram-negative)
- Histoplasmosis
- Coccidioidomycosis
- Melioidosis
- Interstitial lung diseases (rarely)
- Cancer
- Sarcoidosis
- Silicosis
- Rare pneumonias
  1. *Rhodococcus equi* (cavitation)
  2. *Bacillus cereus* (50% hemoptysis)
  3. *Eikenella corrodens* (cavitation)

WORKUP
- Sputum for AFB stains
- Chest x-ray (Fig. E1)
- PPD (tuberculin skin test [TST])
  1. Recent conversion from negative to positive within 3 mo of exposure is highly suggestive of recent infection.
  2. Single positive PPD is not helpful diagnostically.
  3. Negative PPD never rules out acute TB.
  4. Be certain that positive PPD does not reflect "booster phenomenon" (prior positive PPD may become negative after several yr and return to positive only after second repeated PPD; repeat second PPD within 1 wk), which thus may mimic skin test conversion.
  5. Positive PPD reaction is determined as follows:
     a. Induration after 72 hr of intradermal injection of 0.1 ml of 5 TU-PPD
     b. 5-mm induration if HIV-positive (or other severe immunosuppressed state affecting cellular immune function), close contact of active TB, fibrotic chest lesions
     c. 10-mm induration if in high–medical risk groups (immunosuppressive disease or therapy, renal failure, gastrectomy, silicosis, diabetes), foreign-born high-risk group (Southeast Asia, Latin America, Africa, India), low socioeconomic groups, IV drug addict, prisoner, health care worker
     d. 15-mm induration if low risk
  6. Anergy antigen testing (using mumps, *Candida,* tetanus toxoid) may identify patients who are truly anergic to PPD and these antigens, but results are often confusing. Not recommended.
  7. Patients with TB may be selectively anergic only to PPD.
  8. Positive PPD indicates prior infection but does not itself confirm active disease.
- Interferon gamma release assays (IGRAs): diagnostic test for latent TB infection, known as the Quantiferon test (QFT-G). This is a blood test that measures interferon response to specific MTB antigens. The test is approved by the U. S. Food and Drug Administration (FDA) and may assist in distinguishing true positive reactions from individuals with latent TB, from PPD reactions related to nontuberculous mycobacteria; prior BCG vaccination; or difficult-to-interpret skin-test results from people with dermatologic conditions or immediate allergic reactions to PPD. The diagnostic utility of the test as a replacement or supplement to the standard PPD is not yet fully determined. When IGRA is used for routine screening, positive results should be repeated routinely due to a high rate of false-positive results. The enzyme-linked immunospot assay (Elispot plus) incorporating a novel antigen, RV3879c, when used in combination with tuberculin testing, has been reported to enable rapid exclusion of active infection in patients with moderate to high pretest probability of TB. Other IGRAs now available for detection of TB using blood include QFT-GIT and the T-spot TB test.

- The Xpert MTB/RIF is an automated molecular test for *Mycobacterium tuberculosis* (MTB) and resistance to rifampin (RIF) that provides sensitive detection of TB and rifampin resistance directly from untreated sputum in less than 2 hr with minimal hands-on time.

LABORATORY TESTS
- Sputum for AFB stains and culture
  1. Induced sputum if patient not coughing productively
- Sputum from bronchoscopy if high suspicion of TB with negative expectorated induced sputum for AFB
  1. Positive AFB smear is essential before or shortly after treatment to ensure subsequent growth for definitive diagnosis and sensitivity testing
  2. Consider lung biopsy if sputum negative, especially if infiltrates are predominantly interstitial
- AFB stain-negative sputum may grow MTB subsequently
- Gastric aspirates reliable, especially in HIV-negative patients
- CBC
  1. Variable values
     a. WBCs: low, normal, or elevated (including leukemoid reaction: >50,000)
     b. Normocytic, normochromic anemia often
  2. Rarely helpful diagnostically
- ESR usually elevated
- Thoracentesis
  1. Exudative effusion
     a. Elevated protein
     b. Decreased glucose
     c. Elevated WBCs (polymorphonuclear leukocytes early, replaced later by lymphocytes)
     d. May be hemorrhagic
  2. Pleural fluid usually AFB-negative
  3. Pleural biopsy often diagnostic—may need to be repeated for diagnosis
  4. Culture pleural biopsy tissue for AFB
- Bone marrow biopsy is often diagnostic in difficult-to-diagnose cases, especially miliary TB

IMAGING STUDIES
- Chest x-ray
  1. Primary infection reflected by calcified peripheral lung nodule with calcified hilar lymph node
  2. Reactivation pulmonary TB
     a. Necrosis
     b. Cavitation (especially on apical lordotic views)
     c. Fibrosis and hilar retraction
     d. Bronchopneumonia

e. Interstitial infiltrates
f. Miliary pattern
g. Many of the previous findings may also accompany progressive primary TB.
3. TB pleurisy
a. Pleural effusion, often rapidly accumulating and massive
4. TB activity not established by single chest x-ray examination
5. Serial chest x-ray examinations are excellent indicators of progression or regression

Rx TREATMENT

NONPHARMACOLOGIC THERAPY

- Increased rest during acute phase of treatment
- High-calorie, high-protein diet to reverse malnutrition and enhance immune response to TB
- Isolation in negative-pressure rooms with high-volume air replacement and circulation, with health care provider wearing proper protective 0.5- to 1-micron filter respirators, until three consecutive sputum AFB smears are negative

ACUTE GENERAL Rx

- Compliance (rigid adherence to treatment regimen) chief determinant of success
  1. Supervised directly observed therapy (DOT) recommended for all patients and mandatory for unreliable patients
- Preferred adult regimen: DOT
  1. Isoniazid (INH) 15 mg/kg (max 900 mg), rifampin 600 mg, ethambutol (EMB) 30 mg/kg (max 2500 mg), and pyrazinamide (PZA) (2 g [<50 kg]; 2.5 g [51 to 74 kg]; 3 g [>75 kg]) thrice weekly for 6 mo
  2. Alternative, more complicated DOT regimens
- Rifapentine, a rifampin derivative with a much longer serum half-life, was shown to be as effective when administered weekly (with weekly isoniazid) as conventional regimens for drug-sensitive pulmonary TB in non–HIV-infected patients.
- Short-course daily therapy: adult
  1. HIV-negative patient: 6 mo total therapy (2 mo INH 300 mg, rifampin 600 mg, and EMB 15 mg/kg [max 2500 mg]) and PZA (1.5 g [<50 kg]; 2 g [51-74 kg]; 2.5 g [>75 kg]) daily and until smear negative and sensitivity confirmed; then INH and rifampin daily for 4 mo
  2. HIV-positive patient: 9 mo total therapy (2 mo INH, rifampin, EMB, and PZA daily until smear negative and sensitivity confirmed; then INH and rifampin qid for 7 mo)
  3. Continue treatment at least 3 mo following conversion to negative cultures.
- Drug resistance (often multiple drug resistance TB [MDRTB]) increased by:
  1. Prior treatment
  2. Acquisition of TB in developing countries

3. Homelessness, incarceration
4. AIDS, IVDA
5. Known contact with MDRTB
- Never add single drug to failing regimen.
- Never treat TB with fewer than two to three drugs or two to three new additional drugs.
- Other medications used in MDR or XDRTB include moxifloxacin, cycloserine, aminoglycosides such as amikacin or kanamycin, clarithromycin, PAS, and ethionamide.
- Bedaquiline, a diarylquinoline antimycobacterial, is used for treatment of MDR-TB. Recommended dose is 400 mg once daily for 2 wk, followed by 200 mg 3×/wk for weeks 3 to 24. Bedaquiline is administered in combination with ≥3 drugs to which it is susceptible.
- Monitor for clinical toxicity (especially hepatitis).
  1. Patient and physician awareness that anorexia, nausea, right upper quadrant pain, and unexplained malaise require immediate cessation of treatment
  2. Evaluation of liver function testing
     a. Minimal SGOT/SGPT elevations without symptoms generally transient and not clinically significant
- Preventive treatment for PPD conversion only (infection without disease)
  1. Must be certain that chest x-ray examination is negative and patient has no symptoms of TB
  2. Most important groups
     a. HIV-positive and other severely immunocompromised patients
     b. Close contact with active TB
     c. Recent converter
     d. Old TB on chest x-ray examination
     e. IV drug addict
     f. Medical risk factor
     g. High-risk foreign country
     h. Homeless
  3. The traditional preventive therapy for persons with latent *M. tuberculosis* consists of INH 300 mg daily for 9 mo (at least 12 mo if HIV-positive patient). The CDC has issued recommendations for a new regimen consisting of isoniazid and rifapentine administered once a week for 12 wk as directly observed therapy. Studies have demonstrated that this regimen is as effective as 9 mo of isoniazid therapy for preventing tuberculosis. Patients who should not receive this regimen include children younger than 2 years, persons with HIV infection taking antiretroviral therapy, pregnant women or those who may become pregnant during the course of treatment, and patients who have latent *M. tuberculosis* infection that is presumed to be resistant to isoniazid or rifampin.
- Infants generally given prophylaxis immediately if recent contact with active TB (even if infant PPD negative), then retested with PPD in 3 mo (continuing INH if PPD becomes positive and stopping INH if PPD remains negative)

- Chronic, stable PPD (several yr) given INH prophylaxis generally only if patient is <35 yr
  1. INH toxicity may outweigh benefit
  2. Individualize decision
- Preventive therapy for suspected INH-resistant organisms is unclear.
- Pyridoxine (Vitamin B6) supplementation (25-50 mg daily) should be added to INH regimens in patients predisposed to neuropathy such as alcohol use, diabetes, uremia, malnutrition, and HIV.

CHRONIC Rx

- Generally not indicated beyond treatment described previously
- Prolonged treatment, supervised by infectious disease expert, in a few very complicated infections caused by resistant organisms

DISPOSITION

- Monthly follow-up by physician experienced in TB treatment
- Confirm sensitivity testing and alter treatment appropriately
- Frequent sputum samples until culture is negative
- Confirm chest x-ray regression at 2 to 3 mo

REFERRAL

- To infectious disease expert for:
  1. HIV-positive patient
  2. Patient with suspected drug-resistant TB
  3. Patients previously treated for TB
  4. Patients whose fever has not decreased and sputum has not converted to negative in 2 to 4 wk
  5. Patients with overwhelming pulmonary or extrapulmonary TB
- To pulmonologist for bronchoscopy or pleural biopsy

! PEARLS & CONSIDERATIONS

COMMENTS

- All contacts (especially close household contacts and infants) should be properly tested for PPD conversions during 3 mo following exposure.
- Those with positive PPD should be evaluated for active TB and properly treated or given prophylaxis.
- Previous treatment is a common risk factor for XDR and MDR TB.

SUGGESTED READINGS

Available at www.expertconsult.com

RELATED CONTENT

Tuberculosis (TB) (Patient Information)
Tuberculosis, Miliary (Related Key Topic)

AUTHOR: **GLENN G. FORT, M.D., M.P.H.**

BASIC INFORMATION

DEFINITION

Acute tubular necrosis (ATN) is a form of acute kidney injury (AKI) characterized by acute tubular cell injury and dysfunction. It is the most common form of AKI. ATN may be secondary to ischemic injury, nephrotoxic injury, or septic injury or may be multifactorial.

SYNONYMS

Acute tubular necrosis
ATN
Acute tubular injury
Ischemic or nephrotoxic acute renal failure (ARF)

ICD-10CM CODES
N17.0 Acute kidney failure with tubular necrosis
N17.2 Acute kidney failure with medullary necrosis
N19 Unspecified kidney failure

EPIDEMIOLOGY & DEMOGRAPHICS

- Most common cause of AKI among hospitalized patients.
- In the ICU setting, more than 50% of cases will require renal replacement therapy.
- The in-hospital mortality rate is approximately 50%.
- Risk factors: advanced age, diabetes mellitus, chronic kidney disease, preexisting hypovolemia or poor renal perfusion.
- Early recognition of ATN is important to prevent further tubular injury by repeated exposure to nephrotoxins.

PHYSICAL FINDINGS & CLINICAL PRESENTATION

- Physical examination is nonspecific
- Suspect ischemic ATN in the setting of hemorrhage, hypotension, recent surgery, and/or sepsis
- Suspect nephrotoxic ATN in the setting of iodinated radiocontrast imaging, nephrotoxic medications, rhabdomyolysis, hemolysis, or multiple myeloma
- Classic progression of ischemic ATN includes three phases, but can be highly variable:
  1. Initiation phase (hours to days): Renal hypoperfusion, evolving ischemia. Acute decrease in glomerular filtration rate (GFR), sudden rise in BUN and serum creatinine, and/or decrease in urine output.
  2. Maintenance phase (1-2 weeks): Renal cell injury established, GFR stabilizes, and at its nadir, urine output is at its lowest rate (usually 40-400 ml/day). ATN is complicated by hyperkalemia, metabolic acidosis, uremia, and sodium and/or fluid overload. Patients are at an increased risk of infection, and approximately 25% of deaths from ATN occur during its maintenance phase.
  3. Recovery phase (>2 weeks): Tubular cell repair and regeneration, with gradual, partial or complete return of kidney function to baseline levels; often associated with marked osmotic diuresis.

PATHOLOGIC FINDINGS

- Vacuolization and loss of brush border in proximal tubular cells, basement membrane disruption, sloughing of tubular cells, and occlusion of the tubular lumen by casts. Interstitial edema and mild leukocyte accumulation are variably present.

ETIOLOGY

- Diagnosis of exclusion. Prerenal, postrenal, and other intrinsic parenchymal causes of AKI must be ruled out.
- Ischemic processes that contribute to ATN include hypotension, shock, prolonged prerenal azotemia, and surgery.
- Renal hypoperfusion may occur without systemic hypotension (normotensive AKI)
- Medications: NSAIDs, COX-2 inhibitors, antimicrobial drugs (acyclovir, foscarnet, tenofovir, cidofovir, adefovir, aminoglycosides, amphotericin B, pentamidine), calcineurin inhibitors, cisplatin, ifosfamide, angiotensin–converting-enzyme inhibitors, angiotensin II receptor blockers, and intravenous immunoglobulin.
- Iodinated radiocontrast medium (contrast nephropathy).
- Hemoglobin and myoglobin (rhabdomyolysis, transfusion reactions).
- Heavy metals.
- Synthetic cannabinoids.
- Cast nephropathy secondary to multiple myeloma.

DIAGNOSIS

DIFFERENTIAL DIAGNOSIS

Prerenal disease (e.g., hypovolemia, cirrhosis, nephrosis, heart failure), postrenal disease (e.g., obstructive nephropathy), intrinsic renal vascular diseases (e.g., thrombotic thrombocytopenic purpura [TTP], hemolytic uremic syndrome [HUS], scleroderma, and malignant hypertension, renal infarction from aortic dissection or systemic thromboembolism), acute glomerulonephritis, acute interstitial nephritis, and atheroembolic renal disease.

LABORATORY TESTS & FINDINGS

- Urinalysis with specific gravity <1.015, and low-grade albuminuria with more severe ATN.
- Urine osmolality <450 mOsm/kg (usually <350 mOsm/kg). Urine sediment examination with muddy brown casts and tubular epithelial cells.
- Fractional excretion of sodium (FE_{Na}) typically is >1% to 2% (= $[(U_{Na} \times P_{Cr})/(P_{Na} \times U_{Cr})] \times 100\%$).

- Multiple biomarkers for early diagnosis of ATN are currently under investigation, but none as yet are suitable for routine clinical use.

IMAGING STUDIES

No specific studies are indicated, but appropriate studies may be ordered to diagnose the etiology of ATN (e.g., CT scan to search for an infectious process that may be the cause of AKI in a septic patient) or rule out other causes of AKI (e.g., kidney ultrasound to rule out obstruction).

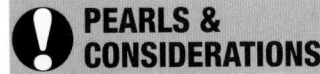 TREATMENT

ACUTE GENERAL Rx

Treatment is etiology specific. Hemodynamic abnormalities should be corrected and potentially nephrotoxic agents discontinued. Renal replacement therapy may be required until renal function is restored. There is no significant evidence that diuretic administration reduces the requirement for dialysis or improves renal recovery. However, diuretic use may facilitate fluid balance.

DISPOSITION

Kidney function typically recovers within 2 to 3 weeks from onset. Outcomes are variable and depend on premorbid kidney function, mechanism of injury, and superimposed renal insults. Patients with nonoliguric ATN have a better prognosis than patients with oliguric ATN. Patients may remain dialysis dependent for up to 3 months before the tubules regenerate. Of patients surviving an ATN episode (~50%), approximately 5%-10% never recover kidney function and remain dialysis dependent.

REFERRAL

Nephrology consultation

PEARLS & CONSIDERATIONS

COMMENTS

Some patients with ATN may have FE_{Na} <1%: patients taking ACEIs, ARBs, or NSAIDs; cirrhosis; heart failure; radiocontrast injury; heme pigment–induced injury (e.g., myoglobinuria or hemoglobinuria); and early sepsis.

PREVENTION

- Aggressive restoration of intravascular volume in hypovolemic surgical/trauma patients
- Discontinuation of potentially nephrotoxic agents
- Low volumes of nonionic radiocontrast agents with isotonic intravenous fluid administration (e.g., sodium chloride or sodium bicarbonate) before and after contrast delivery

RELATED CONTENT

Acute Kidney Injury (Related Key Topic)

AUTHOR: **LENAR YESSAYAN, M.D., M.S.**

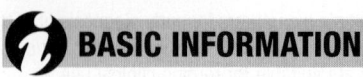

BASIC INFORMATION

DEFINITION

- Tumor lysis syndrome (TLS) is an oncologic emergency referring to the acute release of potentially dangerous intracellular contents, from breakdown of tumor cells, into the systemic circulation.
- It is recognized as a constellation of metabolic disturbances that occur most commonly in the setting of rapid tumor cell lysis induced by cancer-targeted treatment (chemotherapy and/or other interventions such as embolization or radiation). Additionally, spontaneous rapid tumor cell turnover has caused TLS without precipitation by chemotherapy.
- Syndrome characterized by hyperuricemia, hyperphosphatemia, hypocalcemia, hyperkalemia, and acute kidney injury (AKI), often with progressive oliguria.
- In the current 2004 classification system of Cairo and Bishop, TLS can be defined as laboratory or clinical:
  1. **Laboratory TLS** is defined by the presence of at least two of the following biochemical variables within 3 days before or 7 days after initiation of chemotherapy despite adequate hydration and the use of uric acid–lowering agents. Laboratory TLS is clinically silent.
     - Hyperuricemia
       - Results from the rapid release and catabolism of intracellular nucleic acids.
       - Purine nucleic acids are metabolized to hypoxanthine, xanthine, and finally, uric acid.
       - In an acidic environment, uric acid can precipitate in the renal tubular lumen causing obstruction.
     - Hyperkalemia
     - Hyperphosphatemia
       - Phosphate may precipitate with calcium to form calcium phosphate stones in renal tubules.
     - Hypocalcemia
       - Occurs secondary to precipitation with phosphorus.
  2. **Clinical TLS** occurs when laboratory TLS is complicated by at least one of the following clinical complications (severe renal impairment, cardiac arrhythmias, central nervous system toxicity, and/or death) that are not attributed to chemotherapy regimen.

ICD-10CM CODES
E88.3 Tumor lysis syndrome

EPIDEMIOLOGY & DEMOGRAPHICS

INCIDENCE: Unknown, but it is the most common disease-related emergency encountered by physicians who treat children or adults with hematologic cancers. The incidence depends on cancer mass (greater mass correlates with greater cellular content release at cell death), patient characteristics (e.g., preexisting chronic kidney disease, volume depletion, hypotension), and supportive care.

PREVALENCE:
- Varies
- Increased frequency is associated with bulky, aggressive, and treatment-sensitive tumors

PREDOMINANT SEX AND AGE:
- No sex predilection exists.
- Occurs in all age groups. Older adults are more susceptible because of impaired renal function with age.

GENETICS: No known racial predilection

RISK FACTORS:
- High tumor burden
  1. Large-size tumor
  2. LDH >1500 IU/L
  3. WBC >25,000/mm^3
  4. Risk of TLS is further stratified by tumor type:
     - High risk
       - Burkitt's lymphoma
       - High-grade non-Hodgkin's lymphoma
       - Lymphoblastic lymphoma
       - T-cell acute leukemia
       - Other acute leukemias
     - Moderate risk
       - Low-grade lymphoma treated with chemotherapy/radiation/corticosteroids
       - Multiple myeloma
       - Breast carcinoma treated with chemotherapy/hormonal therapy
       - Small-cell lung carcinoma
       - Germ-cell tumors (e.g., seminoma, ovarian)
     - Low risk
       - Low-grade lymphoma treated with interferon
       - Merkel cell carcinoma
       - Adenocarcinoma of the gastrointestinal tract
- Administration of certain agents, including:
  1. Paclitaxel
  2. Hydroxyurea
  3. Etoposide
  4. Fludarabine
- Extensive bone marrow involvement
- Elevated pretreatment uric acid, potassium, or phosphorus levels
- Tumor highly sensitive to treatment
- Volume depletion
- Chronic kidney disease
- Decreased urine output
- Acidic urine
- Tumor involvement of the kidney/renal vasculature)
- Advanced age

ETIOLOGY

Most commonly occurs in patients with acute leukemias, bulky solid tumors, or high-grade lymphomas.
- Can occur spontaneously or after antitumor intervention (chemotherapy, radiation, etc.)
- Associated with administration of certain chemotherapeutic agents (whether intravenous, intrathecal, etc.):
  1. Paclitaxel
  2. Hydroxyurea
  3. Etoposide
  4. Fludarabine
- Spontaneous TLS:
  1. Rare
  2. Lysis of tumor cells without chemotherapy or in setting of minimal chemotherapy (e.g., steroid monotherapy in case of lymphomas)
  3. Related to rapid cell turnover rate
  4. Can be associated with pregnancy; fever; and rarely, generalized anesthesia in predisposed individuals
  5. Hyperphosphatemia may not recur because of the reutilization of released phosphorus for resynthesis of newer tumor cells

PHYSICAL FINDINGS & CLINICAL PRESENTATION

CLINICAL PRESENTATION:
Patients may present with a number of symptoms either before starting chemotherapy or commonly within 3 days after initiating cytotoxic treatment. Common symptoms include:
- Nausea
- Vomiting
- Edema
- Shortness of breath (from fluid overload or CHF)
- Lethargy or weakness
- Seizure
- Syncope
- Muscle cramp
- Tetany

PHYSICAL FINDINGS

- Associated with specific metabolic abnormalities, including hyperkalemia, hyperphosphatemia, hyperuricemia, and hypocalcemia
- Findings often overlap for these metabolic derangements
  1. Hyperkalemia:
     - Generalized weakness
     - Paresthesias
     - Paralysis
     - ECG abnormalities, including:
       - Peaked T waves
       - Flattened P waves
       - Widened QRS complexes
       - Bradycardia
     - Cardiac arrhythmias, including:
       - Ventricular tachycardia
       - Ventricular fibrillation
       - Asystole
       - Pulseless electrical activity
     - Cardiac arrest
  2. Hyperphosphatemia
     - Oliguric or anuric AKI
     - Cardiac arrhythmias
  3. Hypocalcemia
     - Paresthesias
     - Tetany
     - Muscle twitching
     - Chvostek's sign (nonspecific)
     - Trousseau's sign (more specific)
       - Occluding the arterial blood flow in the arm with the blood pressure cuff for 1 to 5 minutes
       - Positive test if thumb adducts and the phalangeal joints extend

- Bronchospasm
- ECG abnormalities, including:
  - Inverted T waves
  - Prolonged QT interval
  - Ventricular arrhythmias
  - Heart block
- Cardiac arrest

ETIOLOGY

- Can occur spontaneously or after initiation of therapy in patients with:
  1. Acute leukemias
  2. Bulky solid tumors
  3. High-grade lymphomas
- Administration of certain agents:
  1. Paclitaxel
  2. Hydroxyurea
  3. Etoposide
  4. Fludarabine
- It has been reported in some cancer patients who received:
  1. Intrathecal administration of chemotherapy
  2. Rare causes: pregnancy, fever, and rarely general anesthesia in predisposed individuals

DX DIAGNOSIS

DIFFERENTIAL DIAGNOSIS

See "Acute Kidney Injury" topic in Section I.

LABORATORY TESTS

- Early identification of abnormal laboratory values is required as this may prevent or reduce complications of TLS.
- Laboratory TLS is defined by the presence of at least two of the following biochemical criteria within 3 days before or 7 days after initiation of chemotherapy despite adequate volume repletion or use of uric acid-lowering agents:
  1. Uric acid
     - >8.0 mg/dl in adults or above the upper limit of the normal range for age in children
  2. Phosphorus
     - >4.5 mg/dl in adults or >6.5 mg/dl in children
  3. Potassium
     - >6.0 mEq/L
  4. Calcium
     - Corrected calcium <7.0 mg/dl or ionized calcium <1.12 mg/dl
- Patients should have careful and frequent laboratory and clinic monitoring
  1. Perform frequent ECGs or continuous cardiac monitoring for arrhythmia detection
  2. Monitor renal status closely and follow daily weights and fluid intakes and outputs
  3. Monitor BUN, creatinine, phosphorus, potassium, calcium, uric acid, and LDH in high-risk patients before and up to 72 hours after initiating therapy
     - If evidence of TLS develops, laboratory parameters should be checked twice daily

IMAGING STUDIES

- Consider abdominal/renal ultrasound if kidney failure present
- Consider CT chest/abdominal/pelvis to evaluate for underlying malignancies

RX TREATMENT

GENERAL PRINCIPLES

- "Prevention is always better than cure" is highly relevant regarding TLS treatment.
- Identify high-risk patients (by assessing the extent of tumor burden, kidney function, and pathologic findings) to initiate prophylactic measures in timely fashion. Delayed treatment may lead to life-threatening conditions.
- Optimal treatment involves preservation of renal function. It also includes the prevention of cardiac dysrhythmias and neuromuscular irritability.
- If possible, all metabolic derangements should be corrected before starting cancer treatment.
- Prevention for high-risk patients without TLS
  1. Prompt, vigorous volume repletion and uricosuric agents are mainstays of therapy
     - Volume repletion
       - Prevents volume depletion and corrects electrolyte derangement
       - Fluid intake (whether oral or intravenous) should be maintained at 2–3 L/m^2 per day
       - Begin 24 to 48 hours before initiating cancer treatment and continue for up to 72 hours after treatment
       - If IV fluids are required, isotonic solutions are appropriate (e.g., 0.9% saline or 1 L D$_5$W plus 3 amps of NaHCO$_3$)
       - Maintain urine output at 80–100 ml/m^2/hr
       - Patients with underlying cardiac or kidney dysfunction should be monitored for volume overload and necessity for loop diuretics
     - Hypouricemic agents (e.g., allopurinol and rasburicase)
       - Allopurinol
         - Xanthine oxidase inhibitor which prevents the conversion of xanthine and hypoxanthine to uric acid
         - Prophylactic dose is 600 mg/day PO or IV while treatment dose is 600 to 900 mg/day
         - In patients with high-grade liquid tumors, Allopurinol prophylaxis may cause xanthine nephropathy/nephrolithiasis
           - Low serum uric acid levels and high urinary xanthine levels aid in diagnosis
           - Consideration for reduction/cessation of allopurinol therapy should then be considered
       - Rasburicase
         - Recombinant urate oxidase, which is used when uric acid levels cannot be lowered by standard measures

- Given IV or IM dosages from 50 to 100 U/kg/day for 1–5 days
- Should not be administered at same time as allopurinol, because allopurinol reduces uric acid levels and may reduce rasburicase efficacy
- Contraindicated in pregnancy and glucose-6-phosphate dehydrogenase deficiency because it can cause severe hemolysis
  - Urinary alkalinization
    - Uric acid more soluble at urinary alkaline pH
    - Remains controversial and has fallen out of favor
    - Contraindicated with hyperphosphatemia because of risk of calcium phosphate deposition leading to stones/nephrocalcinosis

TREATMENT OF PATIENTS WITH TUMOR LYSIS SYNDROME

- Principles:
  1. Early consultations for nephrology and critical care teams
  2. Preventive measures as indicated previously
  3. Aggressive treatment of electrolyte disturbances to prevent cardiac arrhythmias and neuromuscular irritability
     - Arrhythmias tend to be resistant to conventional therapy
     - Arrhythmias are a leading cause of death in patients with severe TLS
  4. Treatment of kidney failure
- Management of electrolyte disturbances:
  1. Multiple, coexisting electrolyte abnormalities may make conservative management strategies difficult
     - Systemic alkalinization may be required for concurrent hyperphosphatemia, hyperuricemia, and acidemia; however, alkalinization may worsen coexisting hypocalcemia
  2. Hyperuricemia:
     - Hypouricemic agents including allopurinol or rasburicase
  3. Hyperkalemia
     - Low potassium diet
     - IV calcium chloride/gluconate for ECG changes of hyperkalemia
     - IV infusions of glucose and insulin to shift potassium into intracellular compartments
     - Oral potassium-exchange resins
     - Hemodialysis
  4. Hyperphosphatemia
     - Low phosphorus diet
     - IV infusion of glucose and insulin to shift phosphorus to intracellular compartment
     - Oral phosphorus binders
  5. Hypocalcemia
     - Treat only if neuromuscular irritability is present
     - IV calcium chloride/gluconate

- ■ Calcitriol can be used if the serum phosphorus level is normal, but is a relatively slow form of therapy
- Management of kidney failure:
  1. Perform standard workup for kidney failure, including urinalysis, urine microscopy, urinary electrolytes, kidney ultrasound, etc.
  2. Supportive care with IV fluids and diuretics (if required).
  3. Consider early dialysis if above methods fail (especially if cardiac abnormalities are present).

REFERRAL

- Nephrology
- Critical care

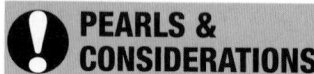
PEARLS & CONSIDERATIONS

COMMENTS

- TLS is an oncologic emergency, which can occur spontaneously, or, more commonly, in the setting of chemotherapy-related tumor cell lysis.

- TLS is associated with the release of several intracellular contents, including potassium, phosphorus, and uric acid.
- Because of simultaneous renal failure, these products are retained to pathological levels, leading to cardiac and neurological abnormalities.
- Common risk factors associated with TLS include patients with highly proliferative tumors and large tumor burdens (e.g., high-grade lymphomas and acute leukemias), and preexisting metabolic derangements and renal failure.
- High-risk patients should have prophylactic measures initiated 24 to 48 hours prior to starting cytotoxic drugs.
- These prophylactic measures include aggressive intravenous volume repletion and administration of uricosuric drugs.
- All patients should undergo frequent laboratory testing and frequent monitoring of vital signs, intakes and outputs, and cardiac/neurological abnormalities.

- Complications of TLS could include continued electrolyte disturbances, renal failure and associated uremia, cardiac arrhythmias, and pulmonary edema secondary to aggressive hydration.

SUGGESTED READING

Available at www.expertconsult.com

AUTHORS: **JESSE GOLDMAN, M.D.,**
SANDEEP AGARWAL, M.D., and
CHRISTOPHER R. KERN, D.O.

BASIC INFORMATION

DEFINITION

Ulcerative colitis (UC) is an idiopathic, remitting and relapsing, chronic inflammatory bowel disease that starts in the rectum and extends proximally.

SYNONYMS

UC
Inflammatory bowel disease (IBD)
Idiopathic proctocolitis
Pancolitis

ICD-10CM CODES
K51.0   Ulcerative pancolitis
K51.2   Ulcerative proctitis
K51.3   Ulcerative rectosigmoiditis
K51.5   Left-sided colitis
K51.90 Ulcerative colitis, unspecified, without complications
K51.80 Other ulcerative colitis without complications
K51.811 Other ulcerative colitis with rectal bleeding
K51.812 Other ulcerative colitis with intestinal obstruction
K51.813 Other ulcerative colitis with fistula
K51.814 Other ulcerative colitis with abscess
K51.818 Other ulcerative colitis with other complication
K51.819 Other ulcerative colitis with unspecified complications
K51.911 Ulcerative colitis, unspecified with rectal bleeding
K51.912 Ulcerative colitis, unspecified with intestinal obstruction
K51.913 Ulcerative colitis, unspecified with fistula
K51.914 Ulcerative colitis, unspecified with abscess
K51.918 Ulcerative colitis, unspecified with other complication
K51.919 Ulcerative colitis, unspecified with unspecified complications

EPIDEMIOLOGY & DEMOGRAPHICS

INCIDENCE: The incidence of UC is 9 to 12 cases per 100,000 persons per year in the U.S.; worldwide, the estimated incidence ranges from 1.2 to 20.3 cases per 100,000 person-years and its prevalence ranges from 7.6 to 246.0 per 100,000 persons. It is most common between ages 15 and 40 yr, with a second peak between 50 and 80 yr. The disease affects men and women at similar rates. Infection with nontyphoid salmonella or campylobacter is associated with an 8-10 time higher risk of developing ulcerative colitis in the following year. Worldwide UC is more common than Crohn's disease.

PREVALENCE: The prevalence of UC is 7.6 to 246.0 cases per 100,000 per year. Higher prevalence in Ashkenazi Jewish descendants.

GEOGRAPHIC DISTRIBUTION: The highest incidence and prevalence of IBD are seen in northern Europe and North America, and the lowest in continental Asia.

GENETICS:
- Both specific and nonspecific gene variants are associated with UC.
- There are 47 loci associated with UC, of which 19 are specific for UC and 28 are shared with Crohn's disease.
- Abnormalities in humoral and cellular adaptive immunity are also found in UC.

ETIOLOGY AND PATHOGENESIS

Accumulating evidence suggests that it may result from an inappropriate inflammatory response to environmental triggers and immune dysregulation involving CD4+ T-cell Th2 response in a genetically susceptible host.

PHYSICAL FINDINGS & CLINICAL PRESENTATION

- Patients with UC often present with acute onset of bloody diarrhea accompanied by tenesmus, fever, and dehydration. At presentation 40% of adults have proctitis, 40% have left-sided colitis, and 20% have pancolitis.
- Abdominal distention and tenderness may indicate the presence of complications such as toxic megacolon.
- The onset of symptoms is typically acute and is generally followed by periods of spontaneous remission and frequent relapses.
- Fever, evidence of dehydration may be present during the acute flare-up.
- Evidence of extraintestinal manifestations may be present in nearly 25% of patients: liver disease, sclerosing cholangitis, iritis, uveitis, episcleritis, arthritis, erythema nodosum, pyoderma gangrenosum, aphthous stomatitis.

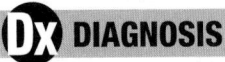

DIAGNOSIS

DIFFERENTIAL DIAGNOSIS

- Crohn's disease (Table 1)
- Bacterial infections (Table 2)
    1. Acute: Campylobacter, Yersinia, Salmonella, Shigella, Chlamydia, Escherichia coli, Clostridium difficile, gonococcal proctitis
    2. Chronic: Whipple's disease, tuberculosis, enterocolitis
- Irritable bowel syndrome
- Protozoal and parasitic infections (amebiasis, giardiasis, cryptosporidiosis)
- Neoplasm (intestinal lymphoma, carcinoma of colon)
- Ischemic bowel disease
- Diverticulitis
- Celiac sprue, lymphocytic or collagenous colitis, radiation enteritis, endometriosis
- Solitary rectal ulcer
- Acute self-limited colitis
- Medication (NSAIDs, chemotherapy)

WORKUP

An accurate diagnosis of UC should define the extent and severity of inflammation. Diagnostic workup includes:
- Comprehensive history, physical examination
- Laboratory tests (see "Laboratory Tests")

TABLE 1 Comparison of Crohn's Disease and Ulcerative Colitis

Feature	Crohn's Disease	Ulcerative Colitis
Rectal bleeding	Sometimes	Common
Diarrhea, mucus, pus	Variable	Common
Abdominal pain	Common	Variable
Abdominal mass	Common	Not present
Growth failure	Common	Variable
Perianal disease	Common	Rare
Rectal involvement	Occasional	Universal
Pyoderma gangrenosum	Rare	Present
Erythema nodosum	Common	Less common
Mouth ulceration	Common	Rare
Thrombosis	Less common	Present
Colonic disease	50%-75%	100%
Ileal disease	Common	None except backwash ileitis
Stomach-esophageal disease	More common	Chronic gastritis can be seen
Strictures	Common	Rare
Fissures	Common	Rare
Fistulas	Common	Rare
Toxic megacolon	None	Present
Sclerosing cholangitis	Less common	Present
Risk for cancer	Increased	Greatly increased
Discontinuous (skip) lesions	Common	Not present
Transmural involvement	Common	Unusual
Crypt abscesses	Less common	Common
Granulomas	Common	None
Linear ulcerations	Uncommon	Common

From Kliegman RM et al: *Nelson textbook of pediatrics*, ed 19, Philadelphia, 2011, Saunders.

TABLE 2 Infectious Agents Mimicking Inflammatory Bowel Disease

Agent	Manifestations	Diagnosis	Comments
Bacterial			
Campylobacter jejuni	Acute diarrhea, fever, fecal blood, and leukocytes	Culture	Common in adolescents, may relapse
Yersinia enterocolitica	Acute → chronic diarrhea, right lower quadrant pain, mesenteric adenitis-pseudoappendicitis, fecal blood, and leukocytes Extraintestinal manifestations, mimics Crohn's disease	Culture	Common in adolescents as fever of unknown origin, weight loss, abdominal pain
Clostridium difficile	Postantibiotic onset, watery → bloody diarrhea, pseudomembrane on sigmoidoscopy	Cytotoxin assay	May be nosocomial Toxic megacolon possible
Escherichia coli 0157:H7	Colitis, fecal blood, abdominal pain	Culture and typing	Hemolytic-uremic syndrome
Salmonella	Watery → bloody diarrhea, food borne, fecal leukocytes, fever, pain, cramps	Culture	Usually acute
Shigella	Watery → bloody diarrhea, fecal leukocytes, fever, pain, cramps	Culture	Dysentery symptoms
Edwardsiella tarda	Bloody diarrhea, cramps	Culture	Ulceration on endoscopy
Aeromonas hydrophila	Cramps, diarrhea, fecal blood	Culture	May be chronic Contaminated drinking water
Plesiomonas	Diarrhea, cramps	Culture	Shellfish source
Tuberculosis	Rarely bovine, now *Mycobacterium tuberculosis* Ileocecal area, fistula formation	Culture, purified protein derivative, biopsy	Can mimic Crohn's disease
Parasites			
Entamoeba histolytica	Acute bloody diarrhea and liver abscess, colic	Trophozoite in stool, colonic mucosal flask ulceration, serologic tests	Travel to endemic area
Giardia lamblia	Foul-smelling, watery diarrhea, cramps, flatulence, weight loss; no colonic involvement	"Owl"-like trophozoite and cysts in stool; rarely duodenal intubation	May be chronic
AIDS-Associated Enteropathy			
Cryptosporidium	Chronic diarrhea, weight loss	Stool microscopy	Mucosal findings not like inflammatory bowel disease
Isospora belli	As in *Cryptosporidium*		Tropical location
Cytomegalovirus	Colonic ulceration, pain, bloody diarrhea	Culture, biopsy	More common when on immunosuppressive medications

From Kliegman RM et al: *Nelson textbook of pediatrics*, ed 19, Philadelphia, 2011, Saunders.

- Colonoscopy to establish the presence of mucosal inflammation; typical endoscopic findings in UC are areas of continuous friable mucosa; diffuse, uniform erythema replacing the usual mucosal vascular pattern; and pseudopolyps. The transition from abnormal to normal tissue tends to be abrupt. Rectal involvement is invariably present if the disease is active. Pathologic findings suggestive of UC include crypt abscesses and atrophy, mucin depletion, basal plasmacytosis, basal lymphoid aggregates, increased lamina propria cellularity, and Paneth cell metaplasia.

LABORATORY TESTS

- Anemia and high erythrocyte sedimentation rate (in severe colitis) are common but normal levels do not rule out the disorder.
- Potassium, magnesium, calcium, and albumin may be decreased.
- Antineutrophil cytoplasmic antibodies (ANCA) with a perinuclear staining pattern (pANCA) can be found in >45% of patients; there is an increased frequency in treatment-resistant left-sided colitis, suggesting a possible association between these antibodies and a relative resistance to medical therapy in patients with UC.
- Calprotectin is a protein that is measured in feces as a marker of intestinal mucosa leukocyte activity that may be useful for screening

of patients with suspected IBD. Trials have shown that based on a pretest probability of IBD of 32% in adults, an abnormal fecal calprotectin test would increase the posttest probability to 91% and a normal result would reduce the probability to 3%.
- Fecal lactoferrin is also a sensitive marker of intestinal inflammation.
- Stool examinations for ova and parasites, stool culture, and testing for *Clostridium difficile* toxin and *E. coli* 0157:H7 may be useful to eliminate other causes of diarrhea in selected patients with risk factors.

IMAGING STUDIES

Image studies (plain radiography, CT scan [Fig. 1]) are generally reserved for suspected complications such as perforation of bowel or toxic megacolon.

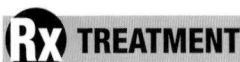 **TREATMENT**

NONPHARMACOLOGIC THERAPY

- Correct nutritional deficiencies; total parenteral nutrition with bowel rest may be necessary in severe cases. Folate supplementation may reduce the incidence of dysplasia and cancer in chronic UC.
- Avoid oral feedings during acute exacerbation to decrease colonic activity; a low-roughage diet may be helpful in early relapse.

- Psychotherapy is useful in most patients. Referral to self-help groups is also important because of the chronicity of the disease and the young age of the patients.

ACUTE GENERAL Rx

The therapeutic options vary with the degree of disease (mild, severe, fulminant) and areas of involvement (distal, extensive).

- Mild disease can be treated with 5-aminosalicylate agents (mesalamine, olsalazine, balsalazide, sulfasalazine). It can be administered as an enema (40 mg once daily at bedtime for 3-6 wk) or suppository (500 mg bid) for patients with distal colonic disease. Oral forms in which the 5-acetyl salicylic acid is in a slow-release or pH-dependent matrix (Pentasa 1 g qid, Asacol 800 mg PO tid) can deliver therapeutic concentrations to the more proximal small bowel or distal ileum. Olsalazine can be useful for maintenance of remission of UC in patients intolerant to sulfasalazine. Usual dose is 500 mg bid taken with food. Balsalazide is indicated for mild to moderately active UC. Usual dose is three 750-mg capsules tid. Probiotics may also be helpful in inducing remission in mild-to-moderate UC.
- Mild-to-moderate UC is often treated with a combination of rectal and oral 5-aminosalicylate. Refractory patients are candidates for

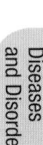

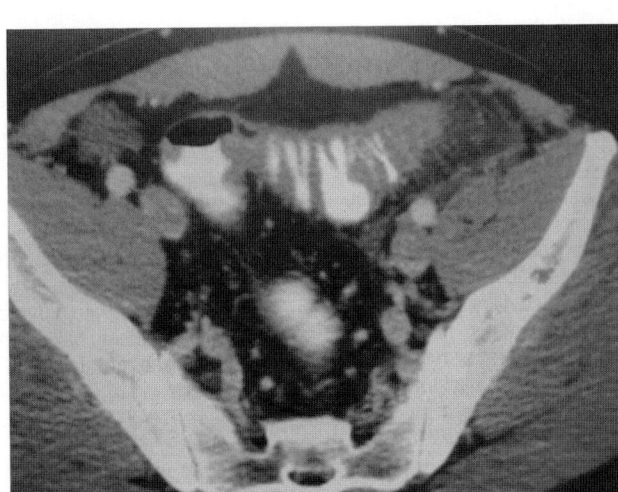

FIG. 1 Computed tomography scan showing colonic wall thickening in a patient with ulcerative colitis. (From Adams JG, et al: *Emergency medicine, clinical essentials*, ed 2, Philadelphia, 2013, Elsevier.)

oral glucocorticoids or immunosuppressive agents (e.g., cyclosporine).

- Severe disease usually responds to oral corticosteroids (e.g., prednisone 40-60 mg/day); the FDA has recently approved an extended-release formulation of the corticosteroid budesonide for induction of remission in mild to moderate ulcerative colitis. Corticosteroid suppositories or enemas are also useful for distal colitis. The immunosuppressant azathioprine also provides effective long-term treatment for Crohn's disease.

- Biological agents are emerging treatment options for the management of ulcerative colitis. Infliximab, a chimeric monoclonal antibody, has been shown to be effective in patients who have not responded to corticosteroid therapy. Newer TNF inhibitors include adalimumab (ADA), golimumab, and vedolizumab for treatment of moderate-to-severe ulcerative colitis. Head-to-head trials of these biologic agents are necessary to establish the best therapeutic option.

- Fulminant disease generally requires hospital admission and parenteral corticosteroids (e.g., IV hydrocortisone 100 mg q6h). When bowel movements have returned to normal and the patient is able to eat normally, oral prednisone is resumed. IV cyclosporine can also be used in severe refractory cases; renal toxicity is a potential complication.

- Surgery is indicated in patients who do not respond to intensive medical therapy. Proctocolectomy is usually curative in these patients and also eliminates the high risk of developing adenocarcinoma of the colon (10%-20% of patients develop it after 10 yr with the disease). Total proctocolectomy with ileal pouch-anal anastomosis (IPAA) is the procedure of choice for most patients who require elective surgery, since it preserves anal sphincter function. Continent ileostomy is an alternative procedure.

CHRONIC Rx

- Colonoscopic surveillance and multiple biopsies should be instituted approximately 10 yr after diagnosis because of the increased risk of colon carcinoma.

- Erythropoietin is useful in patients with anemia refractory to treatment with iron and vitamins.

- In patients on long-term steroid therapy, periodic bone density scans are recommended to screen for glucocorticoid-induced osteoporosis.

DISPOSITION

- The natural history of the disease is one of remission and episodic flares.

- The clinical course is variable. ~66% of patients will achieve clinical remission with medical therapy, and nearly 80% of treatment-compliant patients maintain remission. 15% to 20% of patients eventually require colectomy. Pouchitis is the most common long-term complication of IPAA (up to 40% of patients). >75% of patients treated medically will experience relapse.

REFERRAL

- Gastrointestinal consultation for initial diagnostic sigmoidoscopy/colonoscopy in suspected cases

- Surgical referral for patients with severe disease unresponsive to medical therapy

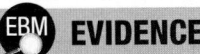 **EVIDENCE**

Available at www.expertconsult.com

SUGGESTED READINGS

Available at www.expertconsult.com

RELATED CONTENT

Ulcerative Colitis (Patient Information)

AUTHOR: **FRED F. FERRI, M.D.**

Diseases and Disorders

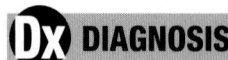

DEFINITION

Deep vein thrombosis of the upper extremity (UEDVT) refers to the thrombosis of the subclavian, axillary, and brachial veins (Fig. 1). UEDVT has become more common due to the increased use of central venous catheters (CVCs), cardiac pacemakers, and defibrillators.

SYNONYMS

UEDVT
Upper extremity deep venous thrombosis

ICD-10CM CODES
I82.621	Acute embolism and thrombosis of deep veins of right upper extremity
I82.622	Acute embolism and thrombosis of deep veins of left upper extremity
I82.623	Acute embolism and thrombosis of deep veins of upper extremity, bilateral

EPIDEMIOLOGY & DEMOGRAPHICS

- UEDVT accounts for approximately 10% of all cases of deep vein thrombosis, resulting in an annual incidence of 0.4 to 1 case per 10,000 people.
- Complications of upper extremity deep vein thrombosis include pulmonary embolism (6%), recurrent venous thromboembolism (between 4% and 8%), and postthrombotic syndrome (15%).
- The overall 3-mo mortality rate of patients with UEDVT is 11%, which is significantly high compared to patients with lower extremity DVT.

RISK FACTORS:
- Prior line infection
- Obstructed central venous catheter
- Upper extremity surgery
- Casting of the arm with immobility
- Malignancy

PHYSICAL FINDINGS & CLINICAL PRESENTATION

Patients with upper extremity deep vein thrombosis most commonly present with swelling, discoloration, or both, and pain and tenderness to palpation of the affected upper limb. Most thrombotic episodes secondary to indwelling central venous catheters (CVCs) remain subclinical and are only discovered during workup of catheter sepsis, catheter malfunction, or pulmonary embolism.

ETIOLOGY

- Primary UEDVT is a rare disorder (2 per 100,000 persons per year) and includes idiopathic thrombosis and thrombosis associated with the thoracic outlet syndrome (TOS) or effort (Paget-Schroetter syndrome). TOS refers to compression of the neurovascular bundle as it exits the thoracic inlet. Effort thrombosis is frequently associated with TOS and occurs in young and physically active individuals.
- In contrast, individuals with idiopathic UEDVT have no known cause or underlying disease; however, it may be associated with an occult cancer.
- Secondary UEDVT represents the majority of cases and occurs in patients with CVCs, pacemakers, or cancer.

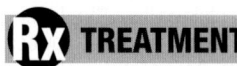 **DIAGNOSIS**

DIFFERENTIAL DIAGNOSIS

The differential diagnosis includes superficial thrombophlebitis, cellulitis, venous congestion due to external vein compression, and lymphedema.

WORKUP

Clinical signs and symptoms are often nonspecific or unreliable. A venogram, once the gold standard, is no longer used; compression ultrasonography is now the preferred imaging exam for these patients.

LABORATORY TESTS

The D-dimer test cannot be recommended for use in screening patients with suspected upper extremity deep vein thrombosis because many of these patients have coexisting conditions that are associated with an elevated D-dimer level.

IMAGING STUDIES

Compression ultrasonography (Fig. 2), which relies on the noncompressibility of a thrombosed vein, is the preferred imaging modality for patients suspected of upper extremity deep vein thrombosis. A complete examination of the internal jugular vein, the brachial and axillary vein, as well as the subclavian vein distal to the clavicle is needed. The superficial veins, the cephalic and basilic, should also be insonated at their confluence with the deep system. A recent systemic review reported a sensitivity of 97% and a specificity of 96% for the diagnosis of UEDVT with ultrasonography.

Rx **TREATMENT**

No randomized controlled trials have been performed to determine the optimal treatment and duration for patients with UEDVT.

NONPHARMACOLOGIC THERAPY

In patients with catheter-associated thrombosis of the upper extremity, routine catheter removal is not recommended. Removal is indicated when there is a nonworking catheter, infection, or a contraindication to anticoagulation therapy.

ACUTE GENERAL Rx

For acute upper extremity DVT, anticoagulation therapy should be started promptly on either UFH or LMWH, while simultaneously beginning vitamin K antagonists (warfarin). Warfarin treatment should be continued for at least 3 mo, with a goal INR of 2.0 to 3.0. The ultimate treatment duration with warfarin follows the same guidelines as treatment with an LEDVT. Alternatives to warfarin may include the oral factor Xa inhibitors rivaroxaban, apixaban, or edoxapan; or dabigatran, a direct oral thrombin inhibitor.

Although prophylaxis is not routinely recommended, dosing 1 mg of warfarin beginning 3 days before subsequent CVC placement should be considered if patient requires a future CV.

For patients with extensive swelling, recent onset of functional impairment, and low risk for bleeding complications, catheter-directed thrombolysis should be considered. Mechanical catheter interventions (aspiration, thrombectomy, balloon angioplasty, or stenting) or surgical procedures (thrombectomy, venoplasty,

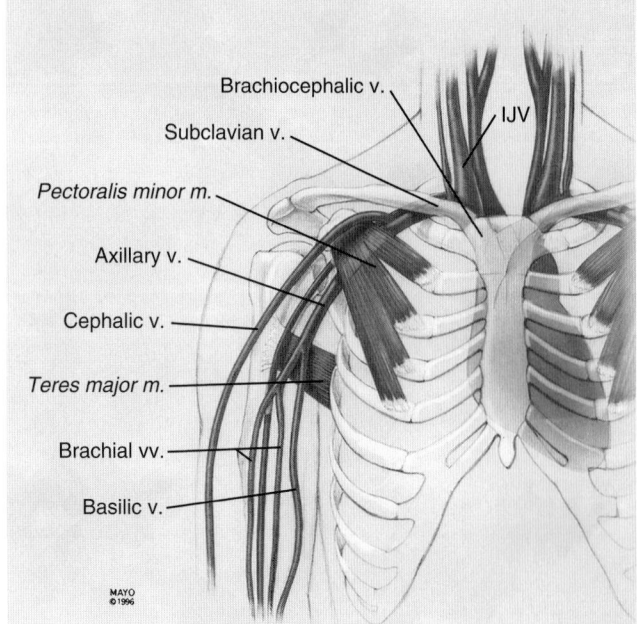

FIG. 1 Anatomy of the upper extremity veins. *IJV,* Internal jugular vein. (From Rumack CM et al: *Diagnostic ultrasound,* ed 4, Philadelphia, 2011, Elsevier.)

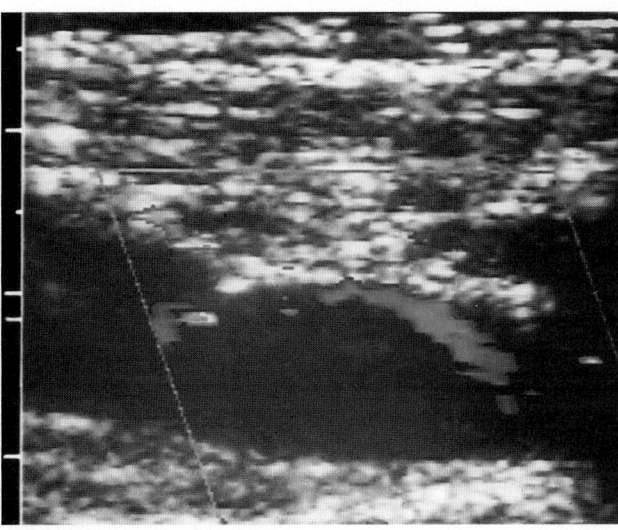

FIG. 2 Acute subclavian vein thrombosis. Color flow Doppler sonography of the subclavian vein shows extensive hypoechoic thrombus with minimal peripheral flow remaining. (From Rumack CM et al: *Diagnostic ultrasound*, ed 4, Philadelphia, 2011, Elsevier.)

venous bypass, or decompression at the venous thoracic outlet) should be considered only for patients with persistent evidence of severe DVT after anticoagulation therapy or thrombolysis, and only in settings with sufficient expertise and resources.

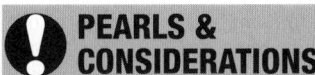

PEARLS & CONSIDERATIONS

- Diagnosing UEDVT rapidly and accurately is essential to preventing thrombotic related morbidity and mortality.

- Catheter factors that increase the incidence of UEDVT include large luminal diameter, multiple ports, incorrect positioning, bacteremia, and prior line infection.
- The use of compression arm sleeves is recommended only in patients with persistent symptoms or in the postthrombotic syndrome.

PREVENTION

At this time, there is no convincing evidence to support routine thromboprophylaxis in patients with central venous catheters; therefore, routine pharmacological prophylaxis is not recommended.

SUGGESTED READING

Available at www.expertconsult.com

RELATED CONTENT

Deep Vein Thrombosis (Related Key Topic)
Pulmonary Embolism (Related Key Topic)
Thoracic Outlet Syndrome (Related Key Topic)

AUTHOR: **FRANK G. FORT, M.D.**

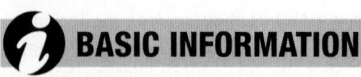

BASIC INFORMATION

DEFINITION

Urethritis is a well-defined clinical syndrome manifested by dysuria, a urethral discharge, or both.

SYNONYMS

Gonococcal urethritis
GCU

ICD-10CM CODES
A54.00 Gonococcal infection of lower genitourinary tract, unspecified

EPIDEMIOLOGY & DEMOGRAPHICS

- The major single specific etiology of acute urethritis is *Neisseria gonorrhoeae,* producing gonococcal urethritis (GCU). Urethritis of all other etiologies is called *nongonococcal urethritis* (NGU).
- NGU is twice as common as GCU in the U.S. NGU is the most common sexually transmitted disease (STD) syndrome occurring in men, accounting for 6 million office visits annually. NGU is more frequently encountered in higher socioeconomic groups. GCU is more common in homosexual males than heterosexual males with acute urethritis.
- *N. gonorrhoeae* is a gram-negative, kidney-shaped diplococcus with flattened opposed margins. The urethra is the most common site of infection in all men. In the United States, the rates of gonorrhea are 40 times higher in black adolescent males than in white adolescent males. In heterosexual men, the pharynx is infected in 7%, and in homosexual men the pharynx is infected in 40% and the rectum in 25%. A single episode of intercourse with an infected partner carries a transmission risk of 20% for males; female partners of an infected male will contract the disease 80% of the time.

PHYSICAL FINDINGS & CLINICAL PRESENTATION

- Symptoms of GCU: urethral discharge and dysuria are the most common symptoms. There is complaint of urethral itching. Prostatic involvement can cause frequency, urgency, and nocturia. It can involve the epididymis through spreading down the vas deferens, causing acute epididymitis.
- Incubation period: 3 to 10 days. Without treatment, urethritis persists for 3 to 7 wk, with 95% of men becoming asymptomatic after 3 mo. GCU is asymptomatic in up to 60% of contacts.
- Signs of GCU: yellow-brown discharge, meatal edema, urethral tenderness to palpation. Rectal bleeding with pus is seen with gonococcal proctitis. Periurethritis leading to urethral stenosis can occur. Disseminated infection can occur. Tenosynovitis and arthritis can occur. Rarely, hepatitis, myocarditis, endocarditis, and meningitis can occur.

DIAGNOSIS

DIFFERENTIAL DIAGNOSIS

- NGU
- Herpes simplex virus

LABORATORY TESTS

- Nucleic acid amplification tests (NAATs): these tests have largely replaced culture in many settings where persons are screened for asymptomatic genital infection. They are not more sensitive than culture for detecting *N. gonorrhoeae* in cervical or urethral specimen; however, they have specificities of >99% and retain sensitivity when used to test voided urine or self-collected vaginal swabs. The performance of NAATs with respect to overall sensitivity, specificity, and ease of specimen transport is better than that of any of the other tests available for the diagnosis of chlamydial and gonococcal infections. NAATs should be used to detect chlamydia and gonorrhea except in cases of child sexual assault involving boys and rectal and oropharyngeal infections in prepubescent girls and when evaluating a potential gonorrhea treatment failure, in which case culture and susceptibility testing might be required.
- Calcium alginate or rayon swab on a metal shaft (not cotton-tipped swabs, which are bactericidal) of the urethra should be performed anywhere from 2 to 4 hr after voiding to prevent bacterial washout with voiding. Gram staining with modified Thayer-Martin media is indicated. Cultures of the pharynx and rectum when indicated.
- Concomitant serologic testing for syphilis on all patients.
- Concomitant *Chlamydia* testing on all patients.
- Offer of HIV counseling and testing to all patients.

TREATMENT

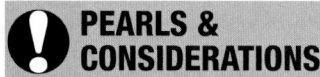

NONPHARMACOLOGIC THERAPY

Behavioral management: avoid intercourse until cure has been attained and sexual partners have been evaluated and treated.

ACUTE GENERAL Rx

- Ceftriaxone 250 mg IM × 1 dose *plus* azithromycin 1 g orally single dose. Doxycycline 100 mg orally twice/day for 7 days can be substituted for azithromycin in cases of allergy to azithromycin.

Alternative regimens:

- Cefixime 400 mg PO × 1 dose *plus* azithromycin 1 g orally single dose. Cure rate with this regimen is lower than ceftriaxone plus azithromycin because cefixime does not provide as high, nor as sustained, bactericidal blood levels as a 250 mg dose or ceftriaxone. Doxycycline 100 mg orally twice/day for 7 days can be substituted for azithromycin in cases of allergy to azithromycin.

- Resistance to penicillins, fluoroquinolones, sulfonamides, cephalosporins, and tetracyclines is now widespread.
- The use of azithromycin as the second antimicrobial is preferred over doxycycline due to the high prevalence of tetracycline resistance.
- The proportion of gonorrhea cases in heterosexual men that are fluoroquinolone resistant (QRNG) has reached 6.7%, an 11-fold increase from 0.6% in 2001. Fluoroquinolone antibiotics are no longer recommended to treat gonorrhea in the U.S.
- Dual treatment for gonococcal and chlamydial infections is based on theory and expert opinion rather than evidence from clinical trials.

CHRONIC Rx

Postgonococcal urethritis (PGU): reinfection is the most common cause of recurrence. Repeat swab and culture of the urethra, pharynx, and rectum (where applicable) are mandatory. Persistence of polymorphonuclear cells (PMNs) with the absence of gram-negative intracellular diplococci suggests a diagnosis of PGU. This occurs when GCU is treated with a regimen that is ineffective against coincident chlamydial infection; it represents NGU after GCU. The syndrome should be treated as NGU. Persistence of *N. gonorrhoeae* by smear or culture requires treatment for *N. gonorrhoeae.*

PEARLS & CONSIDERATIONS

COMMENTS

- Partner notification: the names and contact information of sexual partners should be gathered at the time of the visit and referred to the health department or the patient notifies the contact directly. Expedited partner treatment is recommended by the Centers for Disease Control and Prevention (CDC) and approved in several states. This consists of giving prescriptions to the infected patient for their partner(s) who has not been evaluated by a physician and is unlikely to seek medical care.
- On examination of the urethral smear, the presence of small numbers of PMNs provides objective evidence of urethritis. The complete absence of PMNs on a urethral smear argues against urethritis. If in addition to the PMNs there are gram-negative, intracellular diplococci, the diagnosis of gonorrhea is established.

SUGGESTED READINGS
Available at www.expertconsult.com

RELATED CONTENT
Evaluation of patients with dysuria and/or urethral/vaginal discharge (Algorithm, Section III)
Gonococcal Urethritis (Patient Information)
Gonorrhea (Related Key Topic)

AUTHOR: **ANTHONY SCISCIONE, D.O.**

BASIC INFORMATION

DEFINITION

Nongonococcal urethritis (NGU) is urethral inflammation caused by any of several organisms.

SYNONYMS

NGU
Nongonococcal urethritis

ICD-10CM CODES
A56.0 Chlamydial infection of lower genitourinary tract
N34.1 Nonspecific urethritis

EPIDEMIOLOGY & DEMOGRAPHICS

- Occurrence is 50% in sexually transmitted disease clinics. *Chlamydia trachomatis* is the most common notifiable disease in the U.S., with >1.3 million infections reported to the Centers for Disease Control and Prevention (CDC) in 2010.
- NGU most commonly affects men in a higher socioeconomic class, affecting heterosexual men more frequently than homosexual men.
- NGU carries a greater morbidity rate than gonococcal urethritis (GCU).

PHYSICAL FINDINGS & CLINICAL PRESENTATION

- Incubation period: 2 to 35 days
- Symptoms: dysuria, whitish-clear urethral discharge (Fig. E1), and urethral itching. The onset of symptoms in NGU is less acute than GCU. The majority of persons with *C. trachomatis* infection are not aware of their infection because they do not have symptoms that would prompt them to seek medical care.
- Signs: whitish-clear urethral discharge, meatal edema, and erythema. Infected women manifest pyuria, and the disease can present as acute urethral syndrome.

COMPLICATIONS

Epididymitis in heterosexual men may be linked to nonbacterial prostatitis, proctitis in homosexual men, or Reiter's syndrome.

ETIOLOGY

- Most common agent is *Chlamydia* spp., an obligate intracellular parasite possessing both DNA and RNA, which replicates by binary fission. It causes 20% to 50% of NGU cases. Two species exist:
  1. *Chlamydia psittaci*
  2. *Chlamydia trachomatis* with its 15 serotypes:
     Serotypes A through C cause hyperendemic-blinding trachoma.
     Serotypes D through K cause genital tract infection.
     Serotypes L1 through L3 cause lymphogranuloma venereum.
- Other causes of NGU: *Mycoplasma genitalium* (found in 44% of treatment failures); *Ureaplasma urealyticum*, causing 15% to 30% of the cases of NGU; *Trichomonas vaginalis*; and herpes simplex virus. The cause of 20% of the cases of NGU has not been identified.
- Asymptomatic infection occurs in 28% of the contacts of women with chlamydial cervical infection.

DIAGNOSIS

DIFFERENTIAL DIAGNOSIS

- GCU
- Herpes simplex virus
- Trichomoniasis

LABORATORY TESTS

- Requires demonstration of urethritis and exclusion of infection with *N. gonorrhoeae*.
- Nucleic acid amplification tests (NAATs): these tests have replaced culture in many settings where persons are screened for asymptomatic genital infection. The performance of NAATs with respect to overall sensitivity, specificity, and ease of specimen transport is better than that of any of the other tests available for the diagnosis of chlamydial and gonococcal infections. NAATs should be used to detect chlamydia and gonorrhea except in cases of child sexual assault involving boys, rectal and oropharyngeal infections in prepubescent girls, and when evaluating a potential gonorrhea treatment failure, in which case culture and susceptibility testing might be required.
- Chlamydia culture: The appearance of PMNs on urethral smear confirms the diagnosis of urethritis. Because *Chlamydia* is an intracellular parasite of the columnar epithelium, the best specimen for culture is an endourethral swab taken from an area 2 to 4 cm inside the urethra. For culture, a Dacron-tipped swab is used; avoid calcium alginate or cotton swabs. The organism can only be grown in tissue culture, which is expensive.

TREATMENT

Because it is impossible to differentiate among the common etiologies of NGU, the condition is treated syndromically, including in the initial treatment regimen those drugs effective against the common causative agents. In patients with isolated uncomplicated NGU, recommended regimens are azithromycin 1 g orally single dose or doxycycline 100 mg bid × 7 days. In patients with confirmed urethritis and unclear etiology, concurrent treatment for gonorrhea and *Chlamydia* is recommended. In these patients, uncomplicated infections of the urethra can be treated with combination of a single 1-g dose of oral azithromycin or 100 mg doxycycline bid × 7 days *plus*

- Cefixime 400 mg PO × 1 dose (ceftriaxone is preferred over cefixime) or
- Ceftriaxone 250 mg IM × 1 dose
  Recommended regimen in pregnancy is azithromycin, 1 g orally as a single dose. Repeat test 3 wk after completion of treatment to confirm cure.
- In areas where *T. vaginitis* is prevalent, men who have sex with women and have persistent or recurrent urethritis should be presumably treated with metronidazole 2 g orally in a single dose of tinidazole 2 g orally in a single dose.

PEARLS & CONSIDERATIONS

COMMENTS

Partner notification: The names and contact information of all sexual partners within preceding 60 days should be gathered at the time of the visit and referred to the health department, or the patient notifies the contacts directly. Expedited partner treatment is recommended by the CDC and approved in several states. This consists of giving prescriptions to the infected patient for their partner(s) who have not been evaluated by a physician and are unlikely to seek medical care.

SUGGESTED READINGS

Available at www.expertconsult.com

RELATED CONTENT

Evaluation of Patients with Dysuria and/or Urethral or Vaginal Discharge (Algorithm in Section III)
Nongonococcal Urethritis (Patient Information)
Cervicitis (Related Key Topic)
Chlamydia Genital Infections (Related Key Topic)

AUTHORS: **RUBEN ALVERO, M.D.,** and **PHILIP J. ALIOTTA, M.D.**

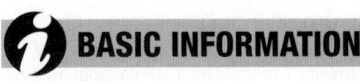

BASIC INFORMATION

DEFINITION

Urinary tract infection (UTI) is a term that encompasses a broad range of clinical entities that have in common a positive urine culture. A conventional threshold is growth of >100,000 colony-forming units per milliliter from a midstream-catch urine sample. In symptomatic patients, a smaller number of bacteria (between 100 and 10,000 colony-forming units per milliliter of midstream urine) are recognized as an infection.

SYNONYM

UTI

ICD-10CM CODES
N39.0	Urinary tract infection, site not specified
N99.521	Infection of other external stoma of urinary tract
N99.531	Infection of other stoma of urinary tract
N30.00	Acute cystitis without hematuria
N30.30	Trigonitis without hematuria
N30.20	Other chronic cystitis without hematuria

CLASSIFICATION

- Uncomplicated UTI: occurs in a normal urinary tract and resolves rapidly with conventional antimicrobials. Patients have a low risk of upper UTI.
- Complicated UTI: occurs in patients with coexisting pathology (strictures, stones, comorbidities [diabetes mellitus, multiple sclerosis, spinal cord injuries]). Patients are considered at high risk for upper UTI.
- First infection: the first documented UTI; tends to be uncomplicated and is easily treated.
- Unresolved bacteriuria: UTI in which the urinary tract is not sterilized during therapy. Main causes are bacterial resistance, patient noncompliance with medication, mixed bacterial infection, rapid reinfection, azotemia, infected stones, Münchausen syndrome, and papillary necrosis.
- Bacterial persistence: UTI in which the urine cultures become sterile during therapy, but a persistent source of infection gives rise to reinfection by the same organism. Causes include infected stone, chronic bacterial prostatitis, atrophic infected kidney, vesicovaginal or enterovesical fistulas, obstructive uropathy, infected pyelocaliceal diverticula, infected ureteral stump after nephrectomy, infected necrotic papillae from papillary necrosis, infected urachal cysts, infected medullary sponge kidney, urethral diverticula, and foreign bodies.
- Reinfection: UTI in which a new infection occurs with new pathogens at variable intervals after a previous infection has been eradicated.
- Relapse: the less common form of recurrent infection; occurs within 2 wk of treatment when the same organism reappears in the same site as the previous infection. Relapsing infections of the urinary tract most commonly occur in pyelonephritis, kidney obstruction from a stone, foreign body, and prostatitis.

EPIDEMIOLOGY & DEMOGRAPHICS

INCIDENCE:

- UTI is the most common bacterial infection encountered in the ambulatory care setting in the U.S. The self-reported annual incidence of UTI in women is 12%, and by age 32 half of all women report having had at least one UTI.
- In neonates: more common in boys as a result of anatomic abnormalities such as the posterior urethral valves.
- In preschool children: more common in girls (4.5% vs. 0.5% for boys).
- In adulthood: more common in women, with a 1% to 3% prevalence in nonpregnant women. Table 1 describes factors modulating risk for acute uncomplicated UTIs in women. In pregnancy at 12 wk, the incidence of asymptomatic bacteriuria is similar to nonpregnant women, at 2% to 10%. However, 25% to 30% of pregnant women with untreated asymptomatic bacteriuria develop acute pyelonephritis, especially in the second and third trimesters, and have a pyelonephritic recurrence rate of 10%. In adults aged ≥65 yr, at least 10% of men and 20% of women have bacteriuria.

PHYSICAL FINDINGS & CLINICAL PRESENTATION

Typical symptoms of UTI include:
1. Urinary frequency, urgency
2. Dysuria
3. Suprapubic pain
4. Gross or microscopic hematuria

- The probability of cystitis is greater than 50% in women with any symptom of UTI and greater than 90% in women who have dysuria and frequency without vaginal symptoms.
- Clinical symptoms alone can be used to make the diagnosis of uncomplicated UTI in women without a urine culture.
- When negative cultures are associated with significant pyuria, vaginal discharge, or hematuria, infections with *Chlamydia trachomatis, Neisseria gonorrhoeae,* and *Trichomonas vaginalis* should be considered.
- Acute pyelonephritis presents with fever, flank or abdominal pain, chills, malaise, and vomiting. It is these systemic symptoms that distinguish pyelonephritis from cystitis. Complications of acute pyelonephritis are renal abscess, perinephric abscess, emphysematous pyelonephritis, and pyonephrosis.

ETIOLOGY & PATHOGENESIS

- Ascending infection via the urethra with bacterial flora from the genital and gastrointestinal tracts is the major pathway for UTI in women.
- Other risk factors: incomplete bladder emptying due to neurologic disease, bladder outlet obstruction or urethral stricture, renal failure, diabetes, vesicoureteral reflux, fistula, urinary diversion, infected stones, age, pregnancy, instrumentation, and poor patient compliance.
- Catheters: all patients who require a long-term Foley catheter eventually develop significant levels of bacteriuria. Treatment is reserved for individuals who become symptomatic (leukocytosis, fever, chills, malaise, loss of appetite, etc.) Using prophylactic antibiotics to treat patients who have chronic catheters is not indicated because of the risk of acquiring bacteria resistant to antibiotic therapy.
- Once bacteria reach the urinary tract, three factors determine whether symptomatic infection occurs (Box E1). These factors also determine the anatomic level of the UTI:
1. Virulence of the microorganism
2. Inoculum size
3. Adequacy of the host defense mechanisms

- Urinary pathogens: in 95% of UTIs the infecting organism is a member of the Enterobacteriaceae, enterococci, or, in young women, *Staphylococcus saprophyticus. Escherichia coli* is the most common pathogen (85% of UTI cases). In contrast, the organisms that commonly colonize the distal urethra and skin of both men

TABLE 1 Factors Modulating Risk for Acute Uncomplicated Urinary Tract Infections in Women

Host Determinants	Uropathogen Determinants
Behavioral: sexual intercourse, use of spermicidal products, recent antimicrobial use, suboptimal voiding habits	*Escherichia coli* virulence determinants: P, S, Dr, and type I fimbriae; hemolysin; aerobactin; serum resistance
Genetic: innate and adaptive immune response, enhanced epithelial cell adherence, antibacterial factors in urine and bladder mucosa, nonsecretor of ABO blood group antigens, P_1 blood group phenotype, reduced CXCR1 expression, previous history of recurrent cystitis	
Biologic: estrogen deficiency in postmenopausal women, micturition	

From Floege J, et al.: *Comprehensive clinical nephrology,* ed 4, Philadelphia, 2010, Saunders.

and women and the vagina of women are *Staphylococcus epidermidis,* diphtheroids, lactobacilli, *Gardnerella vaginalis,* and a variety of anaerobes that rarely cause UTIs. In general, the isolation of two or more bacterial species from a urine culture signifies a contaminated specimen unless the patient is being managed with an indwelling catheter or urinary diversion or has a chronic complicated infection.

- Defense mechanisms against cystitis: low urine pH and high urine osmolarity, mucopolysaccharide glycosaminoglycan protective layer, normal bladder that empties completely, and low vaginal pH due to the presence of estrogen and resulting colonization of the genital tract by lactobacillus.
- In uncomplicated, nonpregnant patients, cystitis rarely progresses to pyelonephritis or other serious infections such as bacteremia.

Dx DIAGNOSIS (FIG. 1)

DIFFERENTIAL DIAGNOSIS

- Vaginitis
- Urethritis (gonococcal, nongonococcal, *Trichomonas*)
- Interstitial cystitis (painful bladder syndrome)
- Pelvic inflammatory disease
  Nephrolithiasis Structural urethral abnormalities such as diverticulum or stricture

LABORATORY TESTS

- Urinalysis with microscopic evaluation of clean-catch urine for bacteria and pyuria. The presence of ≥10 leukocytes/μl of unspun urine from a midstream catch indicates UTI.
- Dipstick urinalysis with the presence of nitrites or leukocyte esterase is indicative

of UTI. However, dipstick urinalysis may not be useful in symptomatic patients with typical symptoms and a negative dipstick urinalysis does not exclude the diagnosis of UTI such cases.

- Urine culture and sensitivity are useful in complicated UTIs and to help guide therapy in women who fail initial therapy. They are generally not needed in uncomplicated UTIs.

IMAGING STUDIES

- Warranted only if renal infection or genitourinary abnormality is suspected
- CT urogram, voiding cystourethrogram, renal sonogram, and intravenous pyelogram
- Specialty examination: cystoscopy and retrograde pyelography to rule out obstructive uropathy

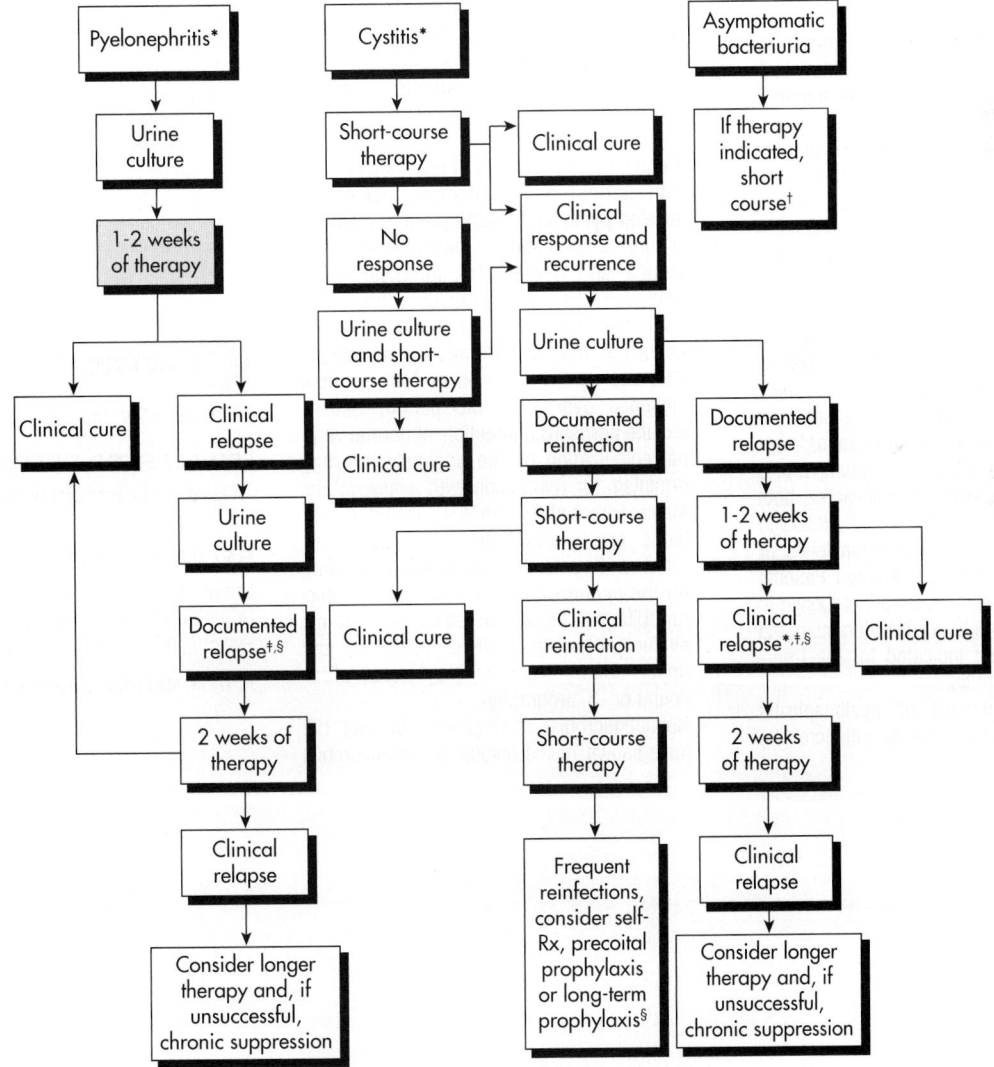

*Consider imaging studies in all men and in women with complicated urinary tract infection.
†No therapy except for renal transplant patients or prior to urologic procedures. Follow-up culture only in transplant patients.
‡Evaluate men for chronic bacterial prostatitis.
§Consider imaging studies in women.

FIG. 1 Approach to the management of urinary tract infection in nonpregnant adults. (From Bennett JE, et al.: *Mandell, Douglas, and Bennett's principles and practice of infectious diseases,* ed 8, Philadelphia, 2015, Saunders.)

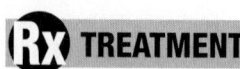 **TREATMENT**

NONPHARMACOLOGIC THERAPY

- Urinary analgesics such as phenazopyridine and aggressive hydration.

ACUTE GENERAL Rx

- First-line antimicrobials for uncomplicated UTI as recommended by the Infectious Disease Society of North America, the American Urologic Society, and ACOG include: nitrofurantoin, trimethoprim plus sulfamethoxazole (TMP-SMX), or fosfomycin.
- Antimicrobial stewardship and drug resistance needs to be considered when choosing antibiotic therapy. Empiric treatment with TMP-SMX is considered appropriate when resistance rates are below 20%. Nitrofurantoin continues to have the lowest rates of antimicrobial resistance. Beta lactam antibiotics may be appropriate in cases of known patient hypersensitivity to conventional first-line agents.
- Conventional therapy of 3 days, with 5 to 7 days for nitrofurantoin is generally appropriate (Fig. E2).
- High rates of resistance and the potential for serious side effects should limit the use of fluoroquinolone antimicrobials. The US FDA has warned against the use of fluoroquinolone antibiotics for routine infections when suitable alternatives are available.
- Pyelonephritis may be treated as an outpatient in stable, well-hydrated patients with close follow-up. Antimicrobial selection is ideally based on urine culture results. Empiric treatment with fluoroquinolone antimicrobials or TMP-SMX is acceptable. Initiation of treatment in the emergency room setting with a single parenteral dose of a long-acting beta lactam or aminoglycoside antibiotic followed by oral treatment with fluoroquinolones or TMP-SMX is an acceptable regimen. Patients should be assessed for a proper response to treatment within 48 hours. Nitrofurantoin and fosfomycin are not indicated for the treatment of pyelonephritis.
- Inpatient management of pyelonephritis should begin with parenteral antimicrobials followed by transition to oral agents based on clinical response and culture results.
- Pyelonephritis requires a total duration of 10 to 14 days of therapy, although evidence exists that 7 to 10 days may be equally effective in low-risk patients.

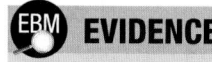 **PEARLS & CONSIDERATIONS**

COMMENTS

- Asymptomatic bacteriuria occurs commonly in postmenopausal women. Treatment of asymptomatic bacteriuria with antimicrobials is discouraged because it seldom resolves and can result in the development of drug-resistant organisms. Patients with cloudy or foul-smelling urine should be encouraged to aggressively hydrate to eliminate these symptoms. Postmenopausal women with vaginal atrophy can be treated with vaginal estrogen to reduce the incidence of bacteriuria. Exceptions include immunocompromised patients, patients with structural urinary tract abnormalities, and pregnant patients.
- Pregnancy: 25% to 30% of pregnant women with untreated asymptomatic bacteriuria develop pyelonephritis. All pregnant women should be screened for asymptomatic bacteriuria and treated. Nitrofurantoin, TMP-SMX, and beta lactam antibiotics are appropriate first-line choices in pregnancy.
- Recurrent UTI: two or more symptomatic UTIs over a 6-mo period or four or more episodes over a 12-mo period. Causes include unresolved infection, abnormal vaginal colonization by the originally infecting organism, or reinfection with a new strain. Management of recurrent UTI includes antibiotic prophylaxis, intermittent self-treatment, and postcoital prophylaxis depending on the circumstances. Patients with recurrent UTIs can be considered for an anatomic evaluation including office cystoscopy and upper urinary tract imaging (renal ultrasound or CT urography).
- Nonantimicrobial strategies to prevent UTI have shown mixed results. Nonantimicrobial agents with antiseptic effects on the lower urinary tract include cranberry supplements with vitamin C, D-mannose, and methenamine. Studies demonstrating clinical effectiveness of these agents show at best modest effects with few side effects.

ANTIMICROBIAL RESISTANCE:

- Because of the overuse of antibiotics, organisms once sensitive to a number of antimicrobial agents are now increasingly resistant, making effective management of UTI and pyelonephritis more difficult and potentially more dangerous. Most important has been the increasing resistance to trimethoprim plus sulfamethoxazole (TMP-SMX), the current primary care provider drug of choice for acute uncomplicated UTI in women.
- Fluoroquinolone use for the treatment of acute cystitis in women should be avoided when suitable alternatives exist. The US FDA has changed the labeling of quinolone antibiotics to reflect this recommendation.
- When choosing a treatment regimen, physicians should consider such factors as:
  1. In vitro susceptibility
  2. Adverse effects on individual patients
  3. Adverse effects on the population (stewardship)
  4. Cost-effectiveness
  5. Resistance rates in their respective communities

(EBM) **EVIDENCE**

Available at www.expertconsult.com

SUGGESTED READINGS

Available at www.expertconsult.com

RELATED CONTENT

Urinary Tract Infection (Patient Information)
Urinary Tract Infection (Child) (Patient Information)
Pyelonephritis (Related Key Topic)

AUTHOR: **MATTHEW J. FAGAN, M.D.**

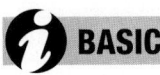

BASIC INFORMATION

DEFINITION

Urolithiasis is the presence of calculi within the urinary tract from the kidney to the urethra. The five major types of urinary stones are calcium oxalate (70%-80%), calcium phosphate (10%-20%), uric acid (10%), struvite (7%), and cystine (1%) (Table 1).

SYNONYMS

Kidney stones
Kidney calculi
Ureteral stones
Ureteral calculi
Nephrolithiasis
Ureterolithiasis

ICD-10CM CODES
N20.9 Urinary calculus, unspecified
N20.0 Calculus of kidney
N20.1 Calculus of ureter
N20.2 Calculus of kidney with calculus of ureter
N21.0 Calculus in bladder
N21.1 Calculus in urethra
N21.8 Other lower urinary tract calculus
N21.9 Calculus of lower urinary tract, unspecified

EPIDEMIOLOGY & DEMOGRAPHICS

- In the U.S., the lifetime prevalence of nephrolithiasis is approximately 10% in males and females.
- Peak incidence occurs in the fourth to sixth decade of life.
- Stone prevalence is increasing and females now have stones almost as often as males.
- Between 1 and 2 million emergency department visits annually are due to kidney stones and renal colic.
- The incidence of symptomatic nephrolithiasis is greatest during the summer as a result of

increased temperature, with an increased risk of dehydration and urinary concentration.
- Calcium oxalate or mixed calcium oxalate/calcium phosphate stones account for nearly 70% to 80% of stones.

PHYSICAL FINDINGS & CLINICAL PRESENTATION

Stones may be asymptomatic, or they may cause the following signs and symptoms as a result of obstruction:
- Acute, often severe, flank pain (renal colic).
- Nausea and vomiting.
- Hematuria, gross or microscopic.
- Patients are unable to find a position of comfort.
- Pain radiating from the flank downward and anteriorly with referred pain to the groin and genitalia with stone progression down the ureter.
- Urinary urgency and frequency with distal ureteral stones can mimic a urinary tract infection.
- Fever and chills may accompany acute colic with superimposed infection.

ETIOLOGY

- Urine supersaturation of various solutes and stone constituents is the driving force in kidney stone formation. All urine contains dissolved stone solutes, which can precipitate under conditions that supersaturate the urine, such as low urine volume, low or high urine pH, and elevated urine solute levels.
- Low urine volume is a common issue in many stone formers.
- Idiopathic hypercalciuria.
- Hyperparathyroidism with resulting hypercalcemia and hypercalciuria.
- Malabsorption (e.g., inflammatory bowel disease) with increased oxalate absorption.
- Chronic diarrheal states.
- Gastric bypass surgery.
- Primary hyperoxaluria: genetic, rare, and usually presenting as a childhood disorder.
- Low urine pH due to metabolic syndrome (e.g., overweight, diabetes), often causes uric acid stones.
- Medullary sponge kidney.
- Hyperuricosuria (e.g., metabolic defects, dietary excess) (Box E1).
- Type I (distal tubule) renal tubular acidosis (>1% of calcium phosphate stones).
- Chronic infections with urease-producing organisms (e.g., *Proteus, Providencia, Pseudomonas, Klebsiella*). Struvite, or magnesium ammonium phosphate crystals, is produced when the urinary tract is colonized by bacteria, producing elevated concentrations of ammonia (Box E2).
- Cystinuria, autosomal recessive, and 1% of stones.
- Medications including protease inhibitors (e.g., indinavir, ritonavir), topiramate, and chronic laxative overuse.
- Anatomic changes predisposing to urinary stasis, including malrotated and horseshoe kidney.

DIAGNOSIS

DIFFERENTIAL DIAGNOSIS

- Urinary tract infection
- Pyelonephritis
- Diverticulitis
- Pelvic inflammatory disease
- Ovarian pathology
- Dysmenorrhea
- Factitious (illicit substance-seeking behavior), often with recurrent stone formers
- Appendicitis
- Small-bowel obstruction
- Ectopic pregnancy
- Constipation
- Malignancy (primary urinary tract or retroperitoneal lymphadenopathy causing ureteral/kidney obstruction)
- Musculoskeletal back pain

The differential diagnosis of obstructive uropathy is described in Section II.

WORKUP

- Fig. E1 describes an algorithm for evaluation of suspected renal colic.
- Stone composition of recovered stones should be determined by infrared spectroscopy or X-ray crystallography.
- A clinical algorithm for the evaluation of nephrolithiasis is described in Fig. E2.
- Box E3 describes events in the medical history that may be significant with regard to urolithiasis.

LABORATORY TESTS

- Urinalysis: Hematuria may be present, but its absence does not exclude stones. Urine pH may help identify stone type: pH >7.5 is associated with struvite stones; pH <5.5 is generally associated with uric acid stones, and low serum bicarbonate concentration with urine pH ≥6 is consistent with a renal tubular acidosis.
- Urine culture and sensitivity results should be obtained in all patients.
- Serum chemistries include electrolytes, BUN, creatinine, calcium, phosphate, uric acid, and may consider parathyroid hormone.
- Additional tests: 24-hr urine collection for volume, creatinine, calcium, uric acid, phosphate, oxalate, and citrate excretion is generally reserved for patients with recurrent stones, young patients, or bilateral stones. A 24-hr urine collection may be appropriate for motivated, first-time stone patients interested in preventing recurrent stones.

IMAGING STUDIES

- Common diagnostic modalities for renal colic are summarized in Table 2. Noncontrast CT scanning has the greatest sensitivity and specificity. Ultrasonography may be an adequate initial study in many instances, especially in patients known to have a history of stones and in patients where radiation should be avoided (e.g., pregnancy and children).

TABLE 1 Stone Composition and Relative Occurrence

Stone Composition	Occurrence (%)
Calcium-containing stones	
Ca oxalate	60
Mixed Ca oxalate/hydroxyapatite	20
Brushite	2
Non–calcium containing stones	
Uric acid	7
Magnesium ammonium phosphate (struvite)	7
Cystine	1-3 (10% of stones in children)
Xanthine	<1
Medication-related stones	<1

From Lipshultz LI et al: *Urology and the primary care practitioner*, ed 3, Philadelphia, 2008, Elsevier.

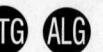

TABLE 2 Common Diagnostic Imaging Modalities for Renal Colic

Modality	Information Provided	Radiation Dose	Contrast	Approximate Cost	Time
CT	Renal stones, including size and position of stones and evidence of obstruction. Alternative diagnoses, such as AAA, appendicitis, and free air	4-10 mSv	No	$750-$1000	Less than 5 min to perform, 30 min for interpretation
CT with IV contrast	Same as noncontrast CT. Delineation of renal mass lesions. Additional information about vascular dissections and mesenteric ischemia	4-10 mSv	Yes	$750-$1000	Less than 5 min, after delay to measure creatinine
CT with IV and oral contrast	Same as CT with IV contrast. Potentially improved diagnosis of bowel abnormalities	4-10 mSv	Yes	$750-$1000	Less than 5 min, after delay of approximately 2 hr to ingest oral contrast
Intravenous urogram	Structural and functional information about obstruction. Rarely, identification of other pathology, such as AAA	1.5 mSv	Yes	$350	Approximately 75 min
X-ray	Possible identification of stone, but not useful for hydronephrosis or most other pathology	0.5-1 mSv	No	$250	Less than 5 min
Ultrasound	Identification of hydronephrosis or hydroureter. Possible identification of stone. Used to assess for AAA or biliary disease	No	No	$150	Approximately 15-30 min—bedside ultrasound is quicker

CT, Computed tomography; *IV,* intravenous.
From Lipshultz LI et al: *Urology and the primary care practitioner,* ed 3, Philadelphia, 2008, Elsevier.

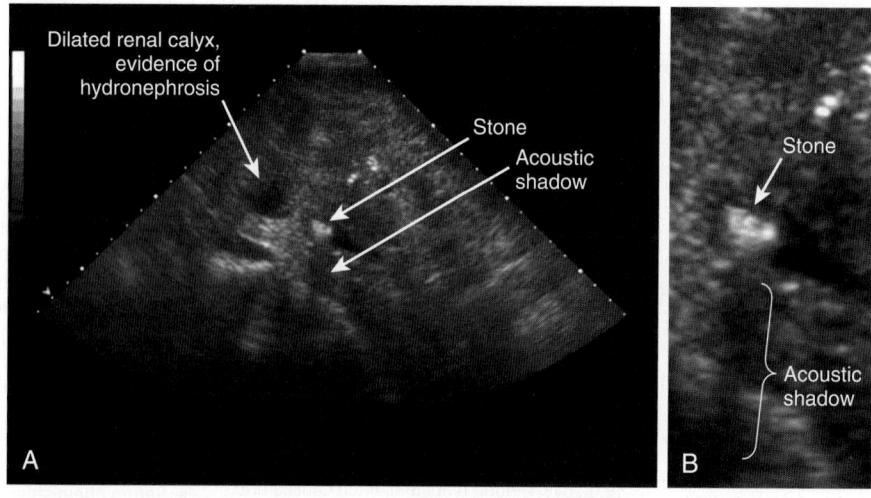

FIG. 3 Ultrasound of renal stone. Ultrasound can be used to assess for renal stones and complications such as hydronephrosis. Stones can be difficult to detect, whereas hydronephrosis is usually readily observed. Because stones are dense, they reflect sound and prevent its through transmission. As a result, stones are echogenic (bright) on ultrasound, and cast an acoustic shadow (black). **A,** Short-axis view of kidney. **B,** Close-up. (From Broder JS: *Diagnostic imaging for the emergency physician,* Philadelphia, 2011, Saunders.)

- Kidney ultrasound (Fig. 3): Initial ultrasonography is associated with lower cumulative radiation exposure than initial CT, without significant differences in serious adverse events, pain scores, return emergency department visits, or hospitalizations. It is reasonable to use ultrasonography as the initial imaging modality in suspected nephrolithiasis; however, a CT scan is the optimal test for planning surgical management of stones. Accuracy of sonography in detecting distal ureteral stones is variable due to variable stone size, body habitus, and expertise of the technician and radiologist. The absence of an ipsilateral ureteral jet supports for a condition of renal blockage, but is not pathognomonic.

- Unenhanced (noncontrast) helical CT scanning (Fig. E4), is rapid and accurate (sensitivity, nearly 100%; specificity, 94%-96%) and can identify all stone types in all locations except for indinavir stones, which are now quite rare, since indinavir is no longer commonly used. These stones are not radiopaque and contrast-enhanced CT may be required to diagnose them.
- Abdominal radiography can identify radiopaque stones (e.g., calcium-containing but not radiolucent uric acid stones), and 20 to 30% of stones will not be visible.
- CT scans may be ordered by urologists planning surgical intervention because a CT yields information on adjacent organs and

stone density that ultrasound and plain film radiography cannot reveal.

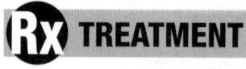 **TREATMENT**

ACUTE GENERAL Rx

- Diagnosis with labs and imaging
- Pain control: NSAIDs are excellent drugs for managing renal colic (e.g., ketorolac). Opiates may be required for severe pain.
- IV fluids and antiemetics may be required.
- Patients that cannot be pain controlled may require urgent kidney drainage (ureteral stent by a urologist or nephrostomy tube placement). For patients that have a stone with a

high probability of passage, medical expulsive therapy with α-blockers or calcium channel blockers (used less often due to side effects) may be helpful. New Level 1 evidence suggests that medical expulsive treatment may not be superior to placebo; however, numerous older studies have shown benefit to passage of distal stones >5 mm in size with the use of medical expulsive therapy.

PREVENTION

- Increase low-calorie fluid intake. Generally, patients at increased risk for the development of stones should increase fluid intake to maintain a urine volume of 2.5 to 3 L/day.
- RDA of dietary calcium 800-1200 mg/day is recommended. Lower calcium consumption results in less gut oxalate binding and more colonic oxalate absorption, which in turn increases urinary oxalate and risk for calcium-based stones. Limiting animal protein to one serving daily is often recommended.
- Greater fruit and vegetable intake increases urinary excretion of citrate (stone inhibitor).
- Dietary sodium restriction is recommended to <2 g daily because this decreases calcium excretion.
- Dietary oxalate restriction in patients with hyperoxaluria.
- Increased dietary citrate (e.g., lemons, oranges).
- Stone specific therapy:
  1. Uric acid calculi can be prevented or even dissolved with urine pH over 6 to 6.5. This is often accomplished with potassium citrate, taken two or three times daily with food.
  2. Calcium stones:
     - In general, cannot be dissolved and either remain, pass, or are removed.
     - With hypercalciuria, thiazide diuretics and low-sodium diet are appropriate. Potassium citrate supplementation for patients with calcium stones and low 24-hr urine citrate excretion. Potassium citrate may also be effective with calcium stones even when urine citrate excretion is not low.
     - Urate-lowering treatment for patients with hyperuricosuria but not hypercalciuria.

  3. Struvite stones:
     - Surgical interventions are usually required. Shock wave lithotripsy (SWL), percutaneous nephrolithotomy (PCNL), and/or ureteroscopy will usually be needed, depending on stone size and configuration.
     - Urease inhibitor treatment by acetohydroxamic acid in patients who are not rendered stone free or are poor surgical candidates. This agent is poorly tolerated and infrequently used in contemporary practice.
  4. Cystine stones
- High fluid intake of 3 to 4 L daily is the principal therapy. Urine alkalinization to pH >6.5–7 with potassium citrate. Thiol drugs such as penicillamine and tiopronin reduce the poorly soluble cystine to a soluble cysteine–drug complex. Tiopronin is better tolerated than penicillamine.
- Surgical Therapy:
  ○ Surgical treatment is needed for patients with: severe pain unresponsive to medication, possible infection from an obstructing stone, acute kidney injury from ureteral obstruction, refractory nausea/vomiting, and prolonged kidney obstruction (i.e., risk of irreversible renal damage).
  ○ Ureteral stones can often be managed with ureteroscopy or SWL.
  ○ Stones in the kidney can be managed with ureteroscopy or SWL if <1 to 2 cm in size and in a favorable location. As a stone become larger and more complex, PCNL becomes the preferred means of management.
  ○ Indications for PCNL are described in Table E3.
- Fig. E5 describes the management of ureteral stones.
- Guidelines for ureteral stone treatment:
  1. Proximal ureteral stones <1 cm diameter: SWL or ureteroscopy preferred.
  2. Proximal ureteral stones >1 cm diameter: SWL, ureteroscopy, or PCNL for complex and/or large stones.
  3. Distal ureteral stones <1 cm diameter: SWL or ureteroscopy, although ureteroscopy is generally preferred.
  4. Distal ureteral stones >1 cm diameter: SWL or ureteroscopy. Ureteroscopy is generally preferred.

Fig. E5 describes an approach to the management of ureteral calculi.

CHRONIC Rx

Maintenance of proper hydration and dietary restrictions (see "Acute General Rx")

DISPOSITION

- >50% to 80% of patients will pass a ureteral stone within 4 to 6 weeks of presentation
- Stone recurrence is variable and based on size, location, and number of stones, along with patient comorbidities and stone-forming tendencies. The Recurrence of Kidney Stone (ROKS) nomogram was developed to predict recurrence in first-time stone formers.

REFERRAL

Urology referral is appropriate when spontaneous passage is unlikely, when a patient cannot be discharged from the emergency department, or when patients have complicated or recurrent stones.

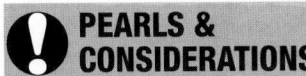 **PEARLS & CONSIDERATIONS**

COMMENTS

- Use the ROKS nomogram to calculate recurrence risk in first-time stone-formers.
- Approximately 75% to 80% of patients will not need admission or surgery for a ureteral stone.
- Patients should be referred to a urologist if they have multiple stones at presentation, complex stones, or have had multiple prior episodes.

SUGGESTED READINGS
Available at www.expertconsult.com

RELATED CONTENT
Kidney Stones (Patient Information)
Urinary Tract Infection (Patient Information)

AUTHOR: **LAMA NAZZAL, M.D., M.SC.,** and **PETER L. STEINBERG, M.D.**

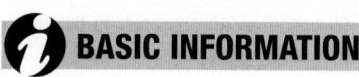

DEFINITION

Urticaria is a pruritic rash involving the epidermis and the upper portions of the dermis caused by localized capillary vasodilation and caused by the release of histamine and other vasoactive mediators. It is followed by transudation of protein-rich fluid in the surrounding tissue and manifesting clinically with the presence of raised erythematous, circumscribed lesions with central pallor. Urticaria is classified according to its chronicity into acute (<6-wk duration) and chronic (>6-wk duration).

SYNONYMS

- Hives
- Wheals

ICD-10CM CODES
L50.0 Allergic urticaria
L50.1 Idiopathic urticaria
L50.2 Urticaria due to cold and heat
L50.8 Other urticaria
L50.9 Urticaria, unspecified
L50.6 Contact urticaria

EPIDEMIOLOGY & DEMOGRAPHICS

- 15% to 20% of the population will have at least one episode of urticaria during their lifetime.
- The etiology of chronic urticaria (hives lasting >6 wk) is determined in only 5% to 20% of cases.
- Incidence is increased in atopic patients.

PHYSICAL FINDINGS & CLINICAL PRESENTATION

- Presence of elevated, erythematous, or white circumscribed lesions that change in size and shape over time in no specific distribution; they are characterized by extreme pruritus and evanescent in nature, with individual lesions generally lasting <24 hr in duration and disappear without scarring. If the patient has persistent symptoms, new lesions typically have a novel distribution.
- Annular configuration with central pallor (Fig. 1).
- Angioedema occurs in approximately 40% of cases of urticaria and is caused by mast cell mediator release in the subcutaneous tissue and deep dermis.

ETIOLOGY

- Food allergies (e.g., shellfish, eggs, strawberries, nuts, legumes, milk).
- Medication allergies (e.g., penicillin, aspirin, sulfonamides, hormone therapy).
- Insect sting allergies.
- Systemic diseases (e.g., systemic lupus erythematosus, serum sickness, autoimmune thyroid disease, urticaria pigmentosa).
- Infections (viral infections such as hepatitis B and C, fungal infections, chronic bacterial infections, helminthic); viral upper respiratory infections are the predominant cause.
- Physical stimuli (e.g., pressure urticaria, exercise-induced, solar urticaria, cold urticaria, cholinergic).
- Contact (nonimmunologic) urticaria (e.g., caterpillars, plants).
- Other: pregnancy, cryoglobulinemia, hair bleaches, chemicals, saliva, cosmetics, perfumes, pemphigoid, emotional stress, malignancy (lymphomas, endocrine tumors).
- Idiopathic urticaria is diagnosed in 50% of patients with chronic urticaria.

DX DIAGNOSIS

DIFFERENTIAL DIAGNOSIS

- Erythema multiforme
- Erythema marginatum
- Erythema infectiosum
- Urticarial vasculitis
- Herpes gestationis
- Drug eruption
- Multiple insect bites
- Bullous pemphigoid
- Mastocytosis
- Mast cell activation syndrome

WORKUP

- It is useful to determine whether hives are acute or chronic; a medical history focused on various etiologic factors is necessary before embarking on extensive laboratory testing.
- Most cases of acute urticaria resolve spontaneously and diagnostic testing is not required. However, in patients with acute urticaria, it is crucial to consider anaphylaxis before further workup of urticaria because this may require urgent management.
- Fig. 2 The etiology of chronic urticaria (CU) is often never determined, and no diagnostic testing may be necessary based on a detailed history and physical examination. Targeted laboratory testing based on clinical findings is appropriate.

LABORATORY TESTS

- If history consistent with allergen-induced urticaria, skin testing with allergic extracts and screening for dermatographism by attempting to elicit a wheal after application of linear skin pressure should be performed only after withholding antihistamines for 36 to 72 hr to prevent false-negative results.
- CBC with differential, ESR, TSH, and liver function tests should be considered only in patients with chronic urticaria and a remarkable history or physical exam for an underlying condition. Even with extensive testing, the cause of chronic urticaria is rarely established.
- Measurement of C4, C1 inhibitor antigenic level, and function and C1q may be helpful in patients who present with angioedema alone. In these patients, C1 inhibitor deficiency should be considered.
- Skin biopsy is helpful in patients with fever, arthralgias, and elevated erythrocyte sedimentation rate. Histologic evidence of leukocytoclasia (neutrophilic infiltration with fragmentation of nuclei) is indicative of urticarial vasculitis.
- When food or contact allergy is suspected in acute urticaria, testing can be performed using skin prick, immunoCAP, and radioallergosorbent testing.

Rx TREATMENT

NONPHARMACOLOGIC THERAPY

- Remove suspected etiologic agents (e.g., stop aspirin and all nonessential drugs) and avoid any foods that may have been observed to precipitate an attack.

ACUTE URTICARIA Rx

- Oral antihistamines: Use of second-generation nonsedating antihistamines (e.g., loratadine 10 mg/day, fexofenadine 180 mg/day) or second-generation sedating antihistamines (e.g., cetirizine 10 mg qd, levocetirizine 5 mg qd) is preferred over first-generation antihistamines (e.g., hydroxyzine, diphenhydramine). Higher doses of second-generation antihistamines may be required to achieve adequate control of symptoms.
- H_2 receptor antagonists (cimetidine, ranitidine, famotidine) or leukotriene receptor antagonists (montelukast) can be added to H_1 antagonists in refractory cases.
- Doxepin (a tricyclic antidepressant that blocks both H1 and H2 receptors) 25 to 75 mg qhs may be effective in patients with chronic urticaria.
- Oral corticosteroids should be reserved for refractory cases (e.g., prednisone 20 mg qd or 20 mg bid).

CHRONIC URTICARIA Rx

Step-care approach for management of nonsedating chronic urticaria is described in Figs. E3 and E4 and in topic "Urticaria, Chronic".

- Step 1: Monotherapy with second-generation antihistamines (see "Acute General Rx"). Avoidance of triggers (e.g., NSAIDs, physical factors).
- Step 2: One of more of the following:
  Dose advancement of second-generation antihistamine.
  Add another second-generation antihistamine.
  Add H2 antagonist.
  Add leukotriene receptor antagonist.
  Add first-generation antihistamine to be taken at bedtime
- Step 3: Dose advancement of potent antihistamine (e.g., hydroxyzine, diphenhydramine, doxepin) as tolerated
- Step 4: Add an alternate agent such as omalizumab (a monoclonal antibody that inactivates free IgE and downregulates surface IgE receptors), cyclosporine, or other antiinflammatory agents or immunosuppressants.
- Patient should be evaluated at each visit and if symptoms are well managed, should be considered for step down in treatment.

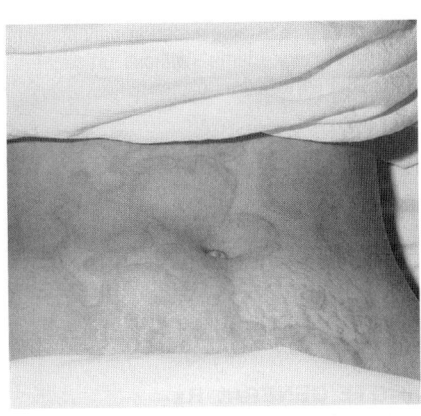

FIG. 1 Wheal (urticaria). Note central clearing, giving annular configuration. (From Noble J et al: *Textbook of primary care medicine*, ed 3, St Louis, 2001, Mosby.)

DISPOSITION

- Most cases of urticaria resolve within 6 wk.
- More than 50% of patients may not achieve satisfactory control of CU with antihistamines alone and may require additional therapies Median duration of CU is between 3 to 5 yr, but it can often be present for much longer durations.

! PEARLS & CONSIDERATIONS

COMMENTS

Topical treatment (e.g., starch baths or oatmeal baths) may be temporarily soothing in selected patients; however, they are not recommended for long-term control of chronic urticaria.

If individual urticarial lesions leave residual ecchymoses or pigmentation, consider skin biopsy to evaluate for urticarial vasculitis.

Avoid NSAIDs in all CU patients because up to 30% of these patients will experience exacerbation of CU symptoms and angioedema.

SUGGESTED READINGS

Available at www.expertconsult.com

RELATED CONTENT

Hives (Patient Information)
Urticaria, Chronic (Related Key Topic)

AUTHORS: **SHYAM JOSHI, M.D.**, and **FRED F. FERRI, M.D.**

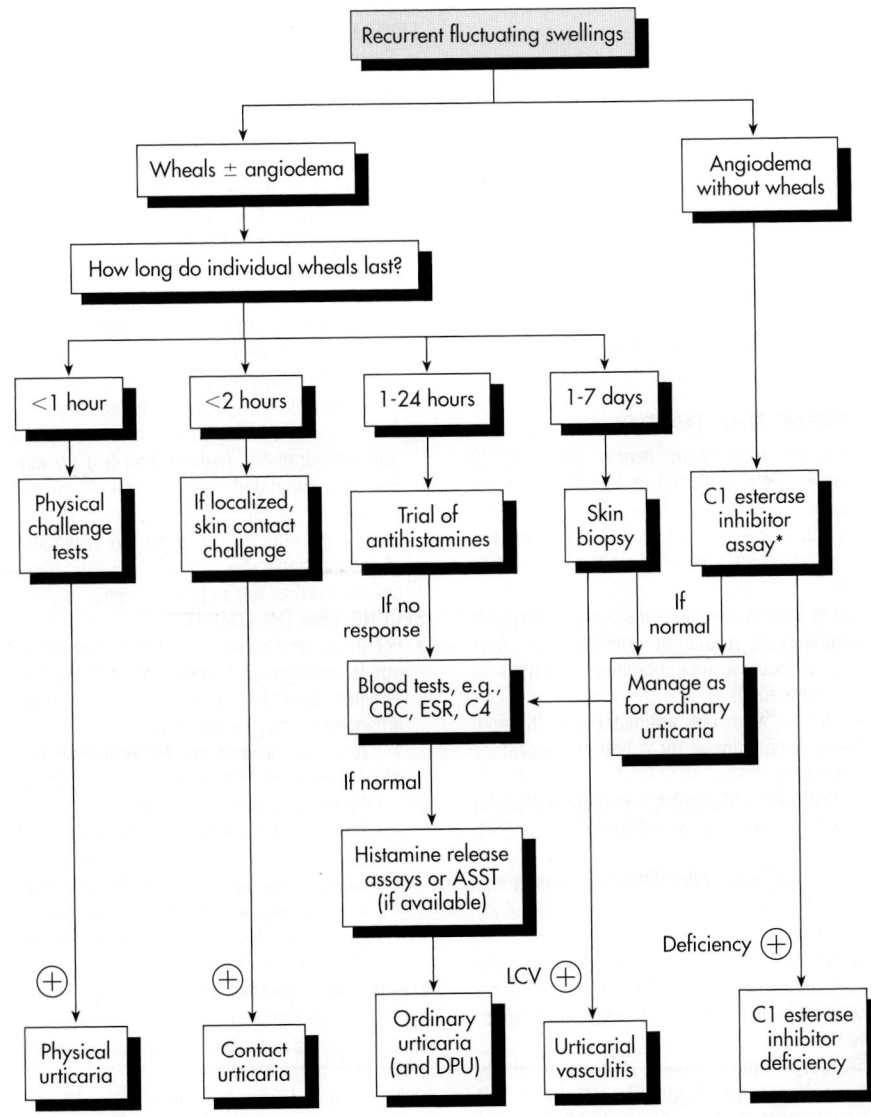

*Amount and function.

FIG. 2 Approach to the diagnosis of chronic urticaria. *ASST,* Autologous serum skin test; *CBC,* complete blood count; *DPU,* delayed pressure urticaria; *ESR,* erythrocyte sedimentation rate. (From Bolognia JL et al: *Dermatology,* St Louis, 2003, Mosby.)

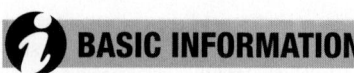

BASIC INFORMATION

DEFINITION

Chronic urticaria (CU) is the occurrence of hives (edematous, pruritic pink wheals of variable size and shape) that have been present continuously or intermittently for at least 6 weeks. Some patients may also experience angioedema (deep swelling, often painful). CU can be associated with autoimmune conditions but is often idiopathic. When no underlying cause is found, CU has been referred to as chronic idiopathic urticaria (CIU).

SYNONYMS

Chronic hives
CU
CIU
Chronic idiopathic urticaria

ICD 10-CM CODES
ICD 10 L50.8   Other Urticaria: Chronic Urticaria

EPIDEMIOLOGY & DEMOGRAPHICS

INCIDENCE: 1.4 % per year.
PREVALENCE: Lifetime prevalence is 1.8%. The period prevalence in the last 12 months is 0.6% to 0.8%. CU occurs in 0.1% to 0.3% of children.
PREDOMINANT SEX AND AGE: There is a 2:1 female to male predominance. The mean age is 40 yr.
GENETICS: Patients with demonstrable histamine-releasing autoantibodies have a very strong association with HLA-DR4 and the associated allele HLA-DQ8.
RISK FACTORS: None

PHYSICAL FINDINGS & CLINICAL PRESENTATION

- CU lesions are edematous, pink or red wheals of variable size and shape with surrounding erythema and are usually pruritic. Individual urticarial lesions usually resolve within 24 hr, but new lesions may be developing simultaneously.
- Angioedema typically appears as brawny nonpitting edema, often without well-defined margins and erythema commonly affecting the lips, tongue, eyelids, and genitalia. This is often described as painful rather than pruritic.

ETIOLOGY

- CU results from cutaneous mast cells releasing histamine. It is often triggered by immunoglobulin E (IgE), components of the complement cascade, endogenous peptides, endorphins, and enkephalins.
- More than 30% of patients have autoimmune manifestations, including specific IgG antibodies against the $Fc\epsilon RI\alpha$ subunit of the high-affinity IgE receptor or IgG antibodies against IgE itself, thyroid autoimmunity, or positive autologous serum skin test (ASST).
- Activation of the coagulation cascade, including increased levels of prothrombin fragment F112 and D-dimer, has been noted in patients with CU and may be a marker for CU severity.
- Chronic infections such as hepatitis B and C, Epstein-Barr virus (EBV), herpes simplex virus, and helminthic parasitic infections have been implicated.

DIAGNOSIS

DIFFERENTIAL DIAGNOSIS

- Urticarial vasculitis
- Erythema multiforme
- Drug eruptions
- Still's disease
- Insect bites

WORKUP

- Complete history and physical exam: Questioning about new drugs, travel, infection, health status, and a complete review of systems (including fever, arthralgias, abdominal pain, bone pain, weight loss, and cold/heat sensitivity) is important. Determining if an individual lesion resolves within 24 hours, whether lesions are tender or itchy, and whether lesions leave a purpuric mark is important (to screen for urticarial vasculitis).
- Fig. 1 describes an algorithm for the diagnosis and management of chronic urticaria.

LABORATORY TEST(S)

- In a recent systemic review analyzing 29 studies (6462 patients), a causative internal disease was detected in 1.6% of patients with CU, with no association between the number of tests ordered and the detection rate.
- Aside from a complete history and physical examination, a trial of antihistamine therapy without further diagnostic testing is recommended.
- In those who fail antihistamine therapy, there is consensus for a limited laboratory workup:
  ○ CBC with differential, complete metabolic panel (creatinine, liver function tests), ESR, TSH.
  ○ Typically also check G6PD, hepatitis B and C, HIV, and age-appropriate malignancy screening.
- A skin biopsy may be performed in cases of suspected urticarial vasculitis or urticaria with atypical historical or physical findings.
- NOTE:
Testing for autoantibodies to the high-affinity IgE receptor, autoantibodies to IgE, ASST, and the autologous plasma skin test (APST) is not routinely recommended because it has not been clearly demonstrated that these tests identify a distinct subgroup of patients with CU nor that there is a different response to therapy based on these results.

- C4 testing is recommended in patients with isolated angioedema (without urticaria) to rule out C1 inhibitor deficiency.

IMAGING STUDIES

None

TREATMENT

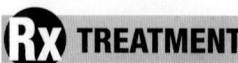

NONPHARMACOLOGIC THERAPY

Elimination of any suspected medications, herbal products, etc.

ACUTE GENERAL Rx

- Oral corticosteroids are not recommended as long-term treatment because of their detrimental effects over prolonged periods. However, they may be necessary for 3 to 7 days to abort severe, acute flares.

CHRONIC Rx
FIRST-LINE TREATMENT:
- Second-generation nonsedating H1-antagonist antihistamines
  1. Loratadine 10 mg, fexofenadine 180 mg, cetirizine 10 mg, levocetirizine 2.5 mg, desloratadine 5 mg twice daily.
  2. These are the mainstay of treatment (50%-95% of patients achieve satisfactory disease control with one or a combination of antihistamines only). The typical starting dose is twice daily. If no improvement after 2 weeks, there is current data supporting dose-escalation to fourfold on-label dosing. Studies have shown routine (rather than episodic) use is important for efficacy.
- Sedating H1-antagonist antihistamines (diphenhydramine, hydroxyzine) are no longer recommended as first-line treatment given their potential for sedation and anticholinergic effects, as well as the availability of second-generation agents. However, these can be used as adjuncts at bedtime.

SECOND-LINE TREATMENT:
- For those who do not respond to monotherapy H1-antagonist, a combination of antihistamines, both second-generation H1 and H2 antagonists, may be necessary:
  1. A second nonsedating H1 antihistamine.
  2. Addition of H2 blockade (ranitidine, famotidine, and cimetidine).
  3. Addition of doxepin 25-50 mg at night or twice daily (which is a potent H1/H2 blocker) may be necessary. Of note, doxepin can prolong PR interval and worsen conduction defects; an EKG before initiation may be warranted.

THIRD-LINE TREATMENT: Choice of agent depending on histologic infiltrate (e.g., neutrophilic), patient's comorbidities, and preferences. If failed the above treatments, patients are typically considered refractory CIU.

IMMUNOMODULATING AGENTS

- Addition of leukotriene-receptor antagonist (e.g., montelukast 10 mg/day).
- Dapsone 25 to 500 mg/day (typically 100 mg/day starting dose). Must check for G6PD and

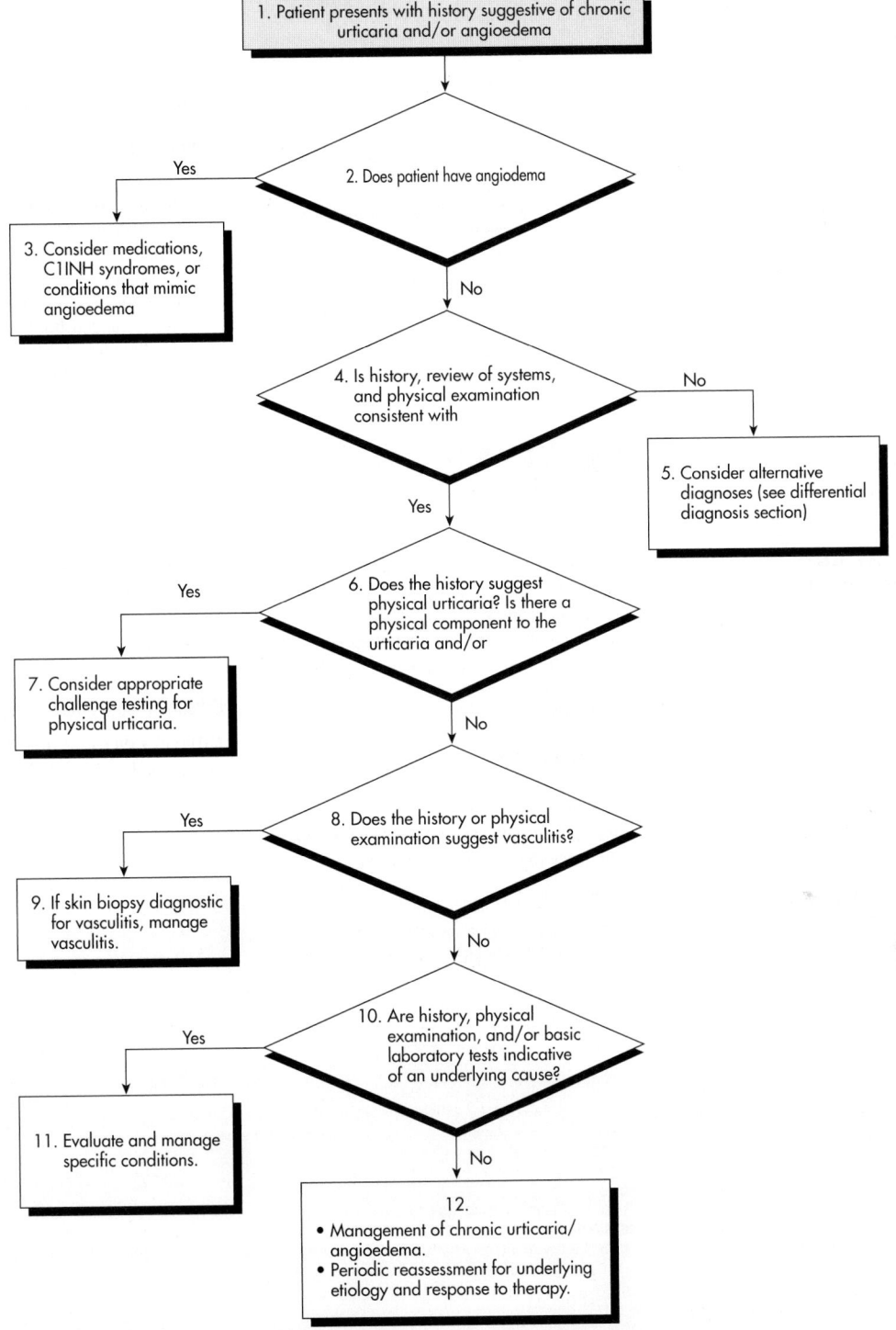

FIG. 1 Algorithm for the diagnosis and management of chronic urticaria. (From Bernstein JA, Lang DM, Khan DA, et al. The diagnosis and management of acute and chronic urticaria: 2014 update, *J Allergy Clin Immunol* 133[5]:1270-1277, 2014.)

monitor labs. Limited use in patients with anemia. Side effects include peripheral neuropathy, methemoglobinemia, agranulocytosis, and systemic drug hypersensitivity. Improvement is generally noted within days to weeks.

- Hydroxychloroquine 200 mg twice daily (can start with dapsone or sulfasalazine because of slow onset on the order of 3 months). Must monitor for retinal toxicity.

- Sulfasalazine 500 mg twice daily (then uptitrate to 1 g twice daily). Good option if patient is anemic and cannot tolerate dapsone.

BIOLOGIC AGENTS

- Omalizumab 300 mg subcutaneous injection every 4 weeks
  1. A monoclonal IgG antibody that binds free IgE. Approved in both the U.S. and EU for the treatment of antihistamine-resistant CIU in March 2014 (Table 1).

IMMUNOSUPPRESSIVE AGENTS

- Mycophenolate mofetil 500 to 1500 mg twice daily
- Cyclosporine (3-5 mg/kg per day for 3-6 months). Limited by nephrotoxic potential. Should not be used longer than a year.

TABLE 1 Features of Basophil Responder and Nonresponder Phenotypes in Chronic Idiopathic Urticaria

Histamine Release–Associated Feature	Observed Reaction	
	CIU Responder	CIU Nonresponder
Release to optimal dose of cross-linking anti-IgE	>10% of cellular histamine content	≤10% of cellular histamine content
Dose response to anti-IgE in active disease	Similar to normal	Tenfold higher dose for maximal release
Phosphatase levels relative to normal	Reduced SHIP-1 levels	Increased SHIP-2 levels
Kinase levels	Syk similar to normal	Syk same as or below normal
Sensitivity to anti-IgE in remission	Increased sensitivity at low end of dose response	Increased sensitivity and maximal release

CIU, Chronic idiopathic urticaria; *IgE,* Immunoglobulin E; *SHIP-1, SHIP-2,* SH1, SH2 domain–containing inositol 5-phosphatases.
Adkinson NF, et al.: *Middleton's allergy: principles and practice,* ed 8, Philadelphia, 2014, Elsevier/Saunders.

Phototherapy
- In a recent study, narrow band UVB (NB-UVB) was effective and safe in steroid-dependent patients with chronic refractory urticaria.

COMPLEMENTARY AND ALTERNATIVE MEDICINE
- A combination of ear acupuncture and conventional filiform needle acupuncture has been reported.

DISPOSITION
N/A

REFERRAL
Dermatology and/or allergy and immunology referral for patients who fail antihistamine therapy or in whom there is a concern for urticarial vasculitis.

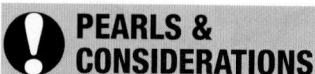

PEARLS & CONSIDERATIONS

COMMENTS
- In atypical cases, given a patient's history or appearance, a skin biopsy for histologic evaluation can be helpful.
- Antihistamine blockade response can often be determined by the presence of dermatographism on exam (wheal produced by scratching).

PREVENTION
- Measures that increase vasodilation such as alcoholic drinks, excessive ambient temperature, heavy clothing, hot baths or showers, and spicy food should be avoided.

- Up to 15% of CU patients experience an exacerbation of their disease after taking aspirin or other cyclooxygenase-1 (COX-1) inhibitors. Patients should be cognizant of such reactions to these medications.

PATIENT/FAMILY EDUCATION
1. A cause is typically not identified.
2. Patients should be aware that the course of disease is unpredictable and may last months to years. However, reassurance should be given that 50% of patients experience remission within 1 yr. In one study, the duration of disease ranged from 1 to 5 yr in 8.7% and more than 5 yr in 11.3% of patients.
3. CIU is different from acute urticaria in etiology, and it is typically not a dietary cause. That said, some providers feel that pseudoallergens in foods can play a role in exacerbations but do not recommend a pseudoallergen-free diet.

SUGGESTED READINGS
Available at www.expertconsult.com

RELATED TOPICS
Hives (Patient Information)
Urticaria (Related Key Topic)

AUTHORS: **EMILY Z. HEJAZI, M.D., M.S.,** and **LISA K. PAPPAS-TAFFER, M.D.**

BASIC INFORMATION

DEFINITION

Uterine fibroids, or leiomyomas, are benign tumors of muscle cells of the myometrium and connective tissue. The incidence of malignancy is less than 1 in 1000. They are typically discrete nodular tumors that vary in size and number.

Fibroids are classified by location in the uterus relative to the myometrium.

- Subserosal: located directly underneath the uterine serosa
- Intramural: located in the myometrium proper
- Submucosal: also known as intracavitary as they are located adjacent to the endometrium and protrude into the uterine cavity
- Pedunculated: located on a pedicle or stalk, either from the serosa or in the cavity

Fibroids can also be located within the cervix, broad ligament, or diffusely in the body such as within the abdomen on peritoneum or within skin. Parasitic fibroids acquire a blood supply from a nonuterine source (Fig. 1).

SYNONYMS

Uterine leiomyomas
Uterine myomas

ICD-10CM CODES
D25.0 Submucous leiomyoma of uterus
D25.1 Intramural leiomyoma of uterus
D25.2 Subserosal leiomyoma of uterus
D25.9 Leiomyoma of uterus, unspecified

EPIDEMIOLOGY & DEMOGRAPHICS

- Estimated prevalence of 20% to 50% of reproductive age women by time of menopause.
- The most common benign solid pelvic tumor diagnosed in women and the most common reason for benign hysterectomy.
- More common in African American women than in Caucasian women.
- May occur singly but are often multiple.
- Less than 50% of all fibroids are estimated to produce symptoms.
- Frequently diagnosed incidentally on pelvic examination.
- There is increased familial incidence.
- Potential to enlarge during pregnancy as well as regress after menopause.
- Approximately 200,000 hysterectomies, 30,000 myomectomies, and thousands of selective uterine-artery embolizations and high-intensity focused ultrasound procedures are performed annually in the U.S. to remove or destroy uterine fibroids.[1]

PHYSICAL FINDINGS & CLINICAL PRESENTATION

- Enlarged, irregular uterus on pelvic examination
- Presenting symptoms

1. Abnormal uterine bleeding (most common)
2. Chronic pelvic pain (dysmenorrhea, dyspareunia, pelvic pressure)
3. Bulk symptoms (bloating, increase in abdominal girth)
4. Anemia
5. Acute pain (torsion of pedunculated fibroid, infarction, and degeneration)
6. Urinary symptoms (frequency from bladder pressure, partial ureteral obstruction, complete ureteral obstruction, incontinence in setting of prolapse)
7. GI symptoms (rectosigmoid compression with constipation or intestinal obstruction, pain with defecation)
8. Prolapse through cervix of pedunculated submucosal fibroid
9. Infertility

ETIOLOGY

Not well understood. It is suggested that fibroids arise from an original single smooth muscle cell in the myometrium. Each individual fibroid is monoclonal (all the cells are derived from one progenitor myocyte). Malignant degeneration of preexisting leiomyoma is extremely uncommon (<0.5%). There is a racial disparity in the prevalence, suggesting a genetic component, with most fibroids having a normal chromosomal makeup. A small group of women have an autosomal dominant disorder, hereditary leiomyomatosis and renal cell carcinoma syndrome, in which there is a genetic mutation in the fumarate hydratase gene, causing diminished suppressor function in fibroid formation.

DIAGNOSIS

DIFFERENTIAL DIAGNOSIS

- Ovarian mass (neoplastic, nonneoplastic, endometrioma)
- Adenomyosis
- Endometrial polyp
- Leiomyosarcoma
- Inflammatory mass (reproductive organ or GI origin)
- Pregnancy

WORKUP

- Complete pelvic examination, including speculum exam as well as bimanual exam
- Estimation of size of uterus/mass and location of fibroids via imaging
- Endometrial sampling may be indicated (biopsy or dilation and curettage) when abnormal bleeding and pelvic mass are present
- If significant urinary symptoms are prominent, intravenous pyelogram to rule out impingement on urinary system

LABORATORY TESTS

- Pregnancy test
- Complete blood count
- BUN/creatinine
- TSH

IMAGING STUDIES

- Pelvic ultrasound (Fig. 2) is useful as a primary diagnostic modality. Transvaginal ultrasound commonly has higher diagnostic accuracy.
- MRI scan is helpful in planning treatment if malignancy is strongly suspected. Also important to localize fibroids, especially if myomectomy is contemplated. Size, number, and location of fibroids are also important if a minimally invasive myomectomy is considered.
- Diagnostic hysteroscopy can be performed in the office and may provide direct evidence of intrauterine pathology or submucosal leiomyoma that distorts uterine cavity.

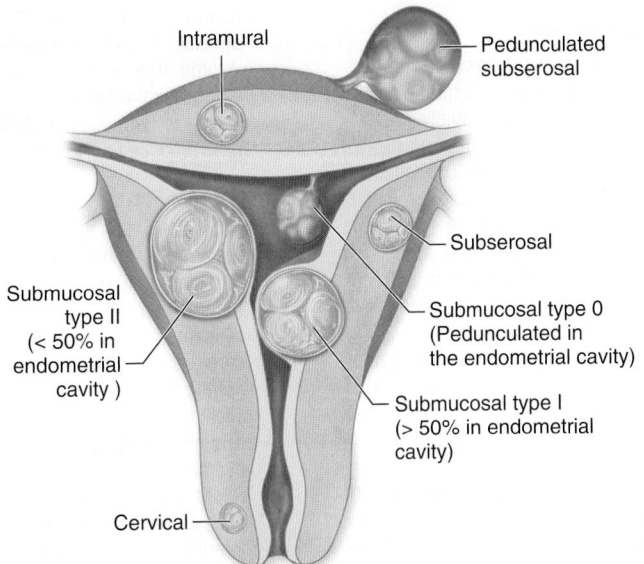

FIG. 1 Drawing of uterus in the coronal plane, illustrating possible location of uterine leiomyomas.
(From Fielding JR et al: *Gynecologic imaging,* Philadelphia, 2011, Saunders.)

[1]Bulun SE: Uterine fibroids, *N Engl J Med* 369:1344-1355, 2013.

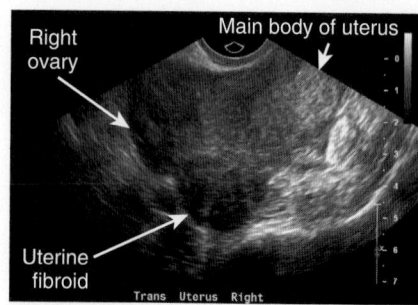

FIG. 2 Fibroid uterus: endovaginal ultrasound. Ultrasound is the primary modality used for evaluation of uterine fibroids (leiomyomas). Typical features include a well-circumscribed appearance. Fibroids may be hypoechoic or hyperechoic relative to the uterus. They may be exophytic or intramural, or they may project into the uterine cavity. Whereas malignant uterine tumors may invade adjacent structures, a fibroid is contained within the uterine serosa. Uterine tumors, both benign and malignant, can show central necrosis, which usually appears hypoechoic with ultrasound. In this 38-year-old woman, the fibroid is exophytic. The right ovary lies adjacent and is difficult to distinguish in this case. (From Broder JS: *Diagnostic imaging for the emergency physician,* Philadelphia, 2011, Saunders.)

- Saline infusion sonography can be helpful in determining location and degree of intrusion into uterine cavity.

℞ TREATMENT

Management should be based on primary symptoms and may include observation with close follow-up, temporizing surgical therapies, embolization, medical management, or definitive surgical procedures. Treatment is generally indicated if bleeding is requiring blood transfusions, renal function is affected by size of the enlarged fibroid uterus, or when symptoms are present and are severe enough to be unacceptable to the patient.

NONSURGICAL Rx

- Patient observation and follow-up with periodic repeat pelvic examinations to ensure that tumors are not growing rapidly.
- Gonadotropin-releasing hormone (GnRH) agonist use results in 40% to 60% reduction in uterine volume within 3 mo of initiating treatment. Hyperestrogenism, reversible bone loss, and hot flushes are associated with use. Limit to short-term use and consider low-dose progesterone replacement to minimize hypoestrogenic effects.
  1. Regrowth and return of bleeding symptoms occurs in approximately 50% of women treated within a few months after cessation.
  2. Indications for GnRH:
     a. Fertility preservation in women with large myomas before attempting conception or preoperative myectomy treatment
     b. Anemia treatment to normalize hemoglobin before surgery
     c. Women approaching menopause to avoid surgery
     d. Preoperative for large myomas to make vaginal hysterectomy, hysteroscopic resection/ablation, or laparoscopic destruction more feasible
     e. Women with medical contraindications for surgery
  3. Personal or medical indications for delaying surgery: Use of GnRH agonists may alter the consistency of the fibroid, making myomectomy more challenging.
- Progestational agents may also result in decrease in uterine size and amenorrhea, allowing iron therapy to treat anemia with limited success.
  1. Progesterone IUD can be used to treat menorrhagia, but intracavitary fibroids may be a relative contraindication.
  2. Ulipristal acetate, not yet available in the U.S. for treatment of fibroids, is a selective progesterone-receptor modulator that acts on progesterone receptors in myometrial and endometrial tissue and inhibits ovulation without causing large effects on estradiol levels or antiglucocorticoid activity. Recent trials have shown that treatment with ulipristal acetate for 13 wk effectively controlled excessive bleeding due to uterine fibroids and reduced the size of the fibroids.
- Tranexamic acid is an oral antifibrinolytic agent that prevents fibrinolysis of menstrual fluid and is a nonhormonal option to decrease menorrhagia by 40% to 65%. Side effects include abdominal cramps, headaches, fatigue, and increase risk of venous thromboembolism.
- Other drugs used and under investigation
  1. Danazol: androgen and multienzyme inhibitor of steroidogenesis
  2. Mifepristone: antiprogesterone shown to reduce the fibroid volume by 40% to 50% with amenorrhea
  3. Raloxifene: selective estrogen receptor modulator, either alone or with a GnRH agonist, shown to reduce the fibroid volume 70% up to 1 yr but only in postmenopausal women
  4. Fadrozole: aromatase inhibitor reported to have produced a 71% reduction in volume

SURGICAL Rx

- Indications
  1. Abnormal uterine bleeding with anemia refractory to hormonal therapy
  2. Chronic pain with severe dysmenorrhea, dyspareunia, or lower abdominal pressure/pain
  3. Acute pain, torsion, or prolapsing submucosal fibroid
  4. Urinary symptoms or signs such as hydronephrosis
  5. Rapid uterine enlargement premenopausal or any growth after menopause
  6. Infertility or recurrent pregnancy loss with submucous leiomyoma as only finding
  7. Enlarged uterus with compression symptoms or discomfort
- Procedures
  1. Hysterectomy (definitive procedure): vaginal, laparoscopic, robotic, or abdominal approach, dependent on surgical preference/expertise and uterine size.
  2. Myomectomy (to preserve fertility or due to patient preference): may be performed via abdominal, laparoscopic, or robotic approach.
  3. Vaginal myomectomy for prolapsed pedunculated submucous fibroid.
  4. Hysteroscopic resection: Typically at least 50% of the fibroid must be intracavitary for a hysteroscopic approach to be successful.
  5. Myolysis: Radio-frequency energy is used to ablate an individual fibroid and destroy the blood supply to that fibroid. Currently approved in the U.S. as a laparoscopic procedure performed under ultrasound guidance.
  6. Uterine artery embolization (UAE): safe and effective short-term alternative to surgery, but its less invasive nature should be balanced against a higher rate for treatment failure or complications at 5 yr (32%) versus the surgery group (4%). Age 40 yr and under at embolization and history of previous myomectomy are significant predictors of embolization failure. If the patient wishes to preserve future fertility, UAE should not be performed.
  7. Endometrial ablation: performed specifically to decrease menorrhagia
  8. MRI-guided focus ultrasound surgery for fibroids is a noninvasive thermoablative procedure that allows high-energy ultrasound waves to converge on a fibroid localized by MRI. Note, there is limited availability of this procedure.

COMPLICATIONS

- Red degeneration occurs when the fibroid outgrows its blood supply leading to hemorrhage in the center of the fibroid. This is typically seen in the second trimester of pregnancy but is a rare occurrence.
- Leiomyosarcoma (<0.1%). Recent concern has been voiced by the U.S. Food and Drug Administration (FDA) regarding the use of morcellation in minimally invasive surgery because of the possibility of spreading occult malignancy in the peritoneal cavity.

REFERRAL

Consultation with gynecologic oncologist if suspicious of malignancy

SUGGESTED READINGS

Available at www.expertconsult.com

RELATED CONTENT

Uterine Fibroids (Patient Information)
Dysfunctional Uterine Bleeding (Related Key Topic)

AUTHORS: **NIMA R. PATEL, M.D., M.S.,** and **TERRI Q. HUYNH, M.D.**

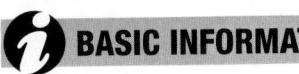

BASIC INFORMATION

DEFINITION

Cancers of the uterine corpus include tumors from the endometrium (endometrial cancers) and tumors as a result of abnormal proliferation of cells originating from the mesenchymal, or connective tissue, elements of the uterine wall (myometrium).

SYNONYMS

Leiomyosarcomas
Endometrial stromal sarcoma
Malignant mixed Müllerian tumors
Adenosarcomas

ICD-10CM CODES

C54.1 Malignant neoplasm of endometrium
C54.0 Malignant neoplasm of isthmus uteri
C54.8 Malignant neoplasm of overlapping sites of corpus uteri

EPIDEMIOLOGY & DEMOGRAPHICS

INCIDENCE: 17.1 cases per 1 million females. Endometrial cancer remains the most common gynecologic malignancy in the U.S.
PREVALENCE: Uterine sarcoma accounts for <5%of all cancers of the uterine corpus and is associated with poor prognosis.
MEAN AGE AT DIAGNOSIS: 52 yr
RISK FACTORS: Box 1 describes risk factors for uterine sarcoma

PHYSICAL FINDINGS & CLINICAL PRESENTATION

- Abnormal vaginal bleeding is the most common symptom.
- May also present as pelvic pain or pressure and pelvic mass on examination.

BOX 1   Risk Factors for Uterine Sarcoma

Nulliparity
Obesity
History of pelvic radiation
Exposure to tamoxifen

From Fielding JR et al: *Gynecologic imaging,* Philadelphia, 2011, Saunders.

- May appear as tumor protruding through the cervix as a fungating mass.
- Vaginal discharge may also be a presenting symptom.
- Rapidly enlarging uterus or pelvic mass.

ETIOLOGY

- The exact etiology is unknown.

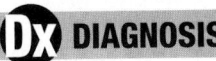

DIAGNOSIS

DIFFERENTIAL DIAGNOSIS

Leiomyoma

WORKUP

Diagnosis is made histologically by biopsy for abnormal bleeding.

LABORATORY TESTS

Chest radiography, CT scans, and MRI are used to evaluate metastatic lesions.

BOX 2   Uterine Sarcoma Prognostic Factors

Tumor stage
Tumor grade
Tumor size
Patient age
Vascular space involvement
Mitotic count
Residual disease at surgery
Adjuvant chemotherapy

From Fielding JR et al: *Gynecologic imaging,* Philadelphia, 2011, Saunders.

BOX 3   Uterine Sarcoma: Key Points

The disease mainly affects postmenopausal women.
Most patients present early with postmenopausal bleeding.
The primary treatment is hysterectomy.
Adjuvant radiotherapy to the pelvis is used if poor prognosis features in stage 1 or if spread has occurred beyond the corpus.

From Greer IA et al: *Mosby's color atlas and text of obstetrics and gynecology,* London, 2001, Harcourt.

IMAGING STUDIES

- Chest x-ray is usually done as routine preoperative testing.
- CT scans (Fig. E1) and MRI are useful for assessing tumor spread once diagnosis is made.

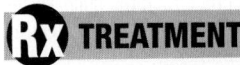

TREATMENT

NONPHARMACOLOGIC THERAPY

- Surgical excision is the mainstay of treatment.
- Grade and stage of tumor affect prognosis.
- The benefit of adjuvant radiotherapy in stage I endometrial adenocarcinoma to improve pelvic disease control and improve survival remains controversial despite several phase 3 trials.
- Chemotherapeutic agents have produced only partial and short-term responses.

DISPOSITION

- Survival varies with each type of sarcoma but is generally very poor. Box 2 describes uterine prognostic factors.
- Five-year survival for leiomyosarcoma ranges from 48% for stage I to 0% for stage IV.
- Five-year survival for malignant mixed mesodermal tumor ranges from 36% for stage I to 6% for stage IV.

REFERRAL

Uterine sarcoma should be managed by a gynecologic oncologist and radiation oncologist. Key points in the management of uterine sarcoma are described in Box 3.

SUGGESTED READING

Available at www.expertconsult.com

RELATED CONTENT

Uterine Cancer (Patient Information)
Endometrial Cancer (Related Key Topic)

AUTHORS: **TONI PICERNO, D.O.,** and **ANTHONY SCISCIONE, D.O.**

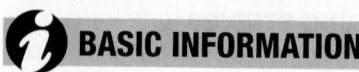

DEFINITION

Uveitis is inflammation of the uveal tract, including the iris, ciliary body, and choroid. It may also involve other contiguous structures such as the sclera, cornea, retina, and vitreous humor (Fig. 1).

SYNONYMS

Anterior uveitis (iritis, iridocyclitis)
Intermediate uveitis (pars planitis)
Posterior uveitis (choroiditis)
Acute or chronic uveitis
Granulomatous or nongranulomatous uveitis

ICD-10CM CODES
H20.0	Acute and subacute iridocyclitis
H20.1	Chronic iridocyclitis
20.8	Other iridocyclitis
H20.9	Unspecified iridocyclitis
H44.131	Sympathetic uveitis, right eye
H44.132	Sympathetic uveitis, left eye
H44.133	Sympathetic uveitis, bilateral
H44.139	Sympathetic uveitis, unspecified eye

EPIDEMIOLOGY & DEMOGRAPHICS

INCIDENCE (IN U.S.): Common; busy ophthalmologist will see two or more cases per week.
PEAK INCIDENCE: Middle age or older.
PREVALENCE (IN U.S.): 17 cases per 100,000 persons
PREDOMINANT SEX: None
PREDOMINANT AGE: 38 yr. Although uveitis is less common in children than adults, it is believed to be more severe with an increased risk for vision-threatening complications.

PHYSICAL FINDINGS & CLINICAL PRESENTATION

- Symptoms of uveitis depend on the site of involvement and whether process is acute or insidious:
  1. Acute anterior uveitis: pain and photophobia. Vision may not be affected initially.

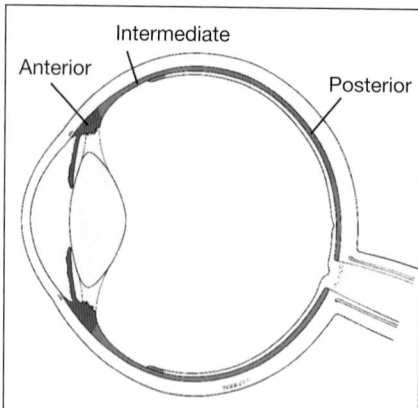

FIG. 1 Anatomic classification of uveitis. (From Kanski JJ, Bowling B: *Clinical ophthalmology, a systematic approach,* ed 7, Philadelphia, 2010, Saunders.)

  2. Posterior uveitis: floaters, hazy vision. Involvement of the retina may produce blind spots or flashing lights.
  3. Insidious anterior uveitis: symptoms may not be present until scarring cataracts and loss of vision occur.
- Photophobia
- Blurred visual acuity
- Irregular pupil
- Hazy cornea
- Abnormal cells and flare in anterior chamber or vitreous humor noted with slit lamp examination
- Retinal hemorrhage, vascular sheathing
- Conjunctival injection, particularly around the iris (ciliary flush)
- Keratitic precipitates (white precipitates on the posterior surface of the cornea)
- Hazy vitreous
- Retinal inflammation
- Iris nodules

ETIOLOGY

- Infections: herpes simplex and zoster virus, cytomegalovirus, toxoplasmosis, tuberculosis, syphilis, HIV
- Systemic disorders (autoimmunity): sarcoidosis, Behçet syndrome, HLA-B27–associated diseases (e.g., ankylosing spondylitis, psoriatic arthritis), inflammatory bowel disease, juvenile idiopathic arthritis (Fig. E2)
- Idiopathic (>50% of patients)

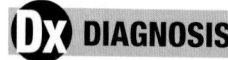 DIAGNOSIS

DIFFERENTIAL DIAGNOSIS

- Glaucoma
- Conjunctivitis
- Retinopathy or neovascular glaucoma
- Keratitis
- Scleritis
- Episcleritis
- Masquerading syndromes: lymphoma, uveal melanoma, metastases (breast, lung, renal), leukemia, retinitis pigmentosa, retinoblastoma

WORKUP

- Comprehensive eye examination including slit lamp exam, dilated ophthalmoscopy

LABORATORY TESTS

- Complete blood count
- Laboratory tests for specific inflammatory causes cited previously in "Workup" (e.g., antinuclear antibody, erythrocyte sedimentation rate, syphilis (VDRL), HLA-B27, purified protein derivative, Lyme titer, angiotensin converting enzyme [ACE])
- Urinalysis

IMAGING STUDIES

- Chest radiograph in suspected sarcoidosis, tuberculosis, histoplasmosis
- Sacroiliac radiograph in suspected ankylosing spondylitis

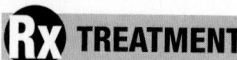 TREATMENT

ACUTE GENERAL Rx

- Corticosteroids are the mainstay of therapy for noninfectious causes. The route and dosage of medication depends on the location of inflammation, the severity, and the presence of systemic disease. Cycloplegic drops (cyclopentolate, homatropine BID to QID) and topical steroids (prednisone acetate 1% 1 gtt qh during day, prn at night until favorable response, then q4 to 6h); avoid topical corticosteroids in infectious uveitis. Periocular corticosteroid injections can be used for posterior disease; they have the advantage of achieving high intraocular levels of steroids without the systemic side effects of oral corticosteroids.
- Antibiotics for bacterial infections and antiviral agents, when infection is suspected, should be started to prevent retinal damage.
- Systemic steroids if appropriate for the underlying disease. Systemic corticosteroid therapy is generally reserved for patients with systemic disorders and those with bilateral disease that is refractory to local medication or those with major ocular disability or retinitis.
- Antimetabolites when indicated. Immunosuppressive medications used in steroid-dependent or refractory uveitis include methotrexate, sulfasalazine, azathioprine, cyclosporine, and tacrolimus. These medications can have significant toxicity and should be prescribed only by physicians experienced with their use.
- High-dose IV daclizumab has been reported as effective in reducing active inflammation in active juvenile idiopathic arthritis (JIA)-associated anterior uveitis. Additional trials are needed to better assess efficacy and safety. Phase 3 trials with adalimumab as a glucocorticoid-sparing agent for the treatment of noninfectious uveitis revealed a lower risk of uveitic flare or visual impairment and more adverse events and serious adverse events than placebo.[1]

REFERRAL

Urgent referral to ophthalmologist for diagnosis and treatment

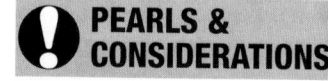 PEARLS & CONSIDERATIONS

COMMENTS

Chronic anterior uveitis is the most common form of intraocular inflammation in children. JIA is the most common cause.

SUGGESTED READING
Available at www.expertconsult.com

AUTHOR: **R. SCOTT HOFFMAN, M.D.**

[1]Jaffe GJ, et al.: Adalimumab in patients with active noninfectious uveitis, *N Engl J Med* 375:932–943, 2016.

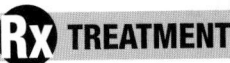 BASIC INFORMATION

DEFINITION

Bleeding per vagina at any time during pregnancy must be regarded as abnormal and is associated with an increased likelihood of pregnancy complications.

ICD-10CM CODES

O20.8	Other hemorrhage in early pregnancy
O20.9	Hemorrhage in early pregnancy, unspecified
O03.9	Complete or unspecified spontaneous abortion
O44.10	Placenta previa with hemorrhage, unspecified trimester
O45.8X9	Other premature separation of placenta, unspecified trimester

EPIDEMIOLOGY & DEMOGRAPHICS

- Common in U.S. and occurs in women of childbearing age.
- 20% to 25% of patients have vaginal spotting/bleeding in the first trimester.
- Early vaginal bleeding increases the risk of miscarriage (50%) and preterm birth.
- Ectopic pregnancy is the leading cause of maternal mortality in the first trimester.
- 1% to 2% of all pregnancies in the U.S. are ectopic with a recent increased risk of cesarean scar pregnancies.
- After one ectopic pregnancy, the chance of recurrence is 7% to 15%.
- Average reported frequency for placental abruption is about 1 in 150 deliveries.
- Recurrence rate for abruption in subsequent pregnancies is 6% to 17% after one episode, increasing to 25% after two episodes.
- Incidence of placenta previa is 1 in 200 deliveries (0.5%) at term.
- Vasa previa is uncommon (1 in 2500-5000 pregnancies) though associated with significant fetal compromise.

PHYSICAL FINDINGS & CLINICAL PRESENTATION

- Bleeding: ranges from scant to life-threatening with hemodynamic instability
- Color: brown to bright red
- Can be painless or painful (cramps, back pain, severe abdominal pain)
- Fetal compromise: ranges from none to fetal demise

DX DIAGNOSIS

DIFFERENTIAL DIAGNOSIS

- Any gestational age:
  1. Cervical lesions: polyps, decidual reaction, neoplasia
  2. Vaginal trauma
  3. Cervicitis/vulvovaginitis
  4. Postcoital trauma
  5. Bleeding dyscrasias
  6. Gestation <20 wks:
  7. Implantation bleeding
  8. Spontaneous abortion
  9. Presence of intrauterine device
  10. Ectopic pregnancy (including cesarean scar pregnancy)
  11. Molar pregnancy
  12. Low-lying placenta/placenta previa
- Gestation >20 wks:
  1. Molar pregnancy
  2. Placental disorders (low-lying placenta, placenta previa, placenta accreta)
  3. Placental abruption
  4. Vasa previa
  5. Marginal separation of the placenta
  6. Preterm labor
  7. Preterm labor
  8. Bloody show at term
  9. Uterine rupture
- Section II describes the differential diagnosis of vaginal bleeding in pregnancy.

WORKUP

- Gestation<20 wks (Section III, "Bleeding, Early Pregnancy"):
  1. Pelvic examination with vaginal/cervical cultures if appropriate
  2. Laparoscopy (if indicated)
  3. Laparotomy (rarely required)
  4. Ultrasound to verify viable intrauterine pregnancy when β-hCG levels achieve threshold values (≥1500 mIU/ml for transvaginal sonography)
  5. If viable intrauterine pregnancy, evaluate pregnancy and uterine cavity including placenta and placental location
- Gestation >20 wks:
  1. Before pelvic examination, ultrasound for placental location, placental cord insertion, and placental evaluation
  2. If placenta previa or low-lying placenta, no bimanual examination
  3. If viable fetus, evaluation of fetal well-being as appropriate based on gestational age
  4. If suspected preterm labor, evaluate as clinically appropriate

LABORATORY TESTS

- Urine pregnancy test: If positive, get quantitative beta human chorionic gonadotropin (β-hCG). The following are typical although not entirely exclusive patterns:
  1. Early pregnancy: follow serially every 48 hr
  2. Normal pregnancy: β-hCG doubles approximately every 48 hr
  3. Spontaneous abortion: β-hCG level will fall
  4. Ectopic pregnancy: β-hCG level will rise inappropriately (less than expected; threshold increase over 48 hr should be ≥66%)
  5. Molar pregnancy: β-hCG level is higher than expected for gestational age
- CBC
- Blood type and screen (Rh-negative patients need RhoGAM)
- Coagulation profile (particularly if moderate to heavy bleeding)
- Cervical/vaginal cultures, wet mount
- Pap smear for cervical malignancy; caution with biopsy, because cervix can bleed extensively

IMAGING STUDIES

Ultrasound:
- 5 to 6 wk: gestational sac (transvaginally); β-hCG >>1500 mIU/ml is discriminatory level for seeing a singleton gestation
- 6 to 7 wk: fetal cardiac activity
- Molar pregnancy: characteristic cluster of cysts
- Evidence of subchorionic hemorrhage
- Location of placenta and placental cord insertion (if >20wks)
- Degree of placental separation: difficult to assess

Rx TREATMENT

NONPHARMACOLOGIC THERAPY

- Pelvic rest: no coitus, douching, or tampons
- Counseling: genetic, bereavement (if indicated)
- For viable fetuses, ultrasound assessment of fetal growth and assessment of fetal well-being
- Bedrest, if >20 wk (recent studies show limited to no benefit of bedrest and possible increased medical and psychological risk to patients on activity restriction)

ACUTE GENERAL Rx

- Hemodynamic stabilization
- Emergency D&C, laparoscopy, laparotomy, or cesarean delivery as necessary

REFERRAL

- If patient is unstable and needs emergency OB/GYN management and/or surgery
- If patient has suspected ectopic or molar pregnancy, because immediate surgical treatment or medical intervention is indicated
- Perinatal consultation for high-risk pregnancies (placental disorders, placental abruption)

SUGGESTED READINGS

Available at www.expertconsult.com

RELATED CONTENT

Abruptio Placentae (Related Key Topic)
Cervical Insufficiency (Related Key Topic)
Ectopic Pregnancy (Related Key Topic)
Molar Pregnancy (Related Key Topic)
Placenta Previa (Related Key Topic)
Sheehan's Syndrome (Related Key Topic)
Spontaneous Miscarriage (Related Key Topic)

AUTHOR: **JENNIFER B. MERRIMAN, M.D.,** and **NAOMI HAUSER, M.P.H., M.D.**

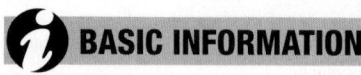

BASIC INFORMATION

DEFINITION

An abnormal passageway between the vagina and another epithelialized surface (Fig. 1)

SYNONYM

Vaginal sinus

ICD-10CM CODES
N82.0 Vesicovaginal fistula
N82.2 Fistula of vagina to small intestine
N82.3 Fistula of vagina to large intestine
N82.9 Female genital tract fistula, unspecified

EPIDEMIOLOGY & DEMOGRAPHICS

INCIDENCE: After benign hysterectomy: <1% (0.08%-0.26%); after radical hysterectomy: 1% to 4%. Incidence is difficult to estimate in developing countries because of lack of medical care and medical follow-up after obstetric care.

PREVALENCE: Rare in the developed world from obstetric complications, but in developing countries, the best estimate of prevalence is as high as 124 in 100,000.

RISK FACTORS: *In developing countries*
- Obstetric trauma
- Prolonged, protracted labor
- Cephalopelvic disproportion causing ischemia and necrosis of the tissue between the fetal head and maternal pubic bone

In developed countries
- Hysterectomy, especially with the following:
  1. Extensive bladder dissection
  2. Iatrogenic injury of the bowel or bladder
  3. Prolonged operating times
  4. Laparoscopic approach has the greatest risk, vaginal approach the lowest
  5. Large blood loss
  6. Large volume uterus
  7. Coexisting pelvic adhesions distorting the normal pelvic anatomy

- Obstetric trauma
  1. Rectovaginal fistulas are primarily related to severe vaginal lacerations. Risk factors for such include:
     ○ Primiparity
     ○ Midline episiotomies
     ○ Increasing birth weights
     ○ Use of vaginal forceps
  2. Bladder injury related to uterine rupture
- Invasive cancer
- Pelvic radiation, directly proportional to dosimetry
  ○ Also as a result of tumor necrosis after therapy
- Chronic inflammatory disease
  1. Crohn disease
  2. Diverticulitis
- Pelvic infection
  1. Tuberculosis
  2. Syphilis
  3. Lymphogranuloma venereum
- Trauma
- Previous pelvic surgery
- Diabetes mellitus
- Age >50, likely as a result of poor tissue quality from menopausal estrogen deficiency, although some studies have refuted this.
- Tobacco usage
- Foreign bodies
  ○ Suburethral slings for stress urinary incontinence have increased the incidence of urethrovaginal fistula

PHYSICAL FINDINGS & CLINICAL PRESENTATION

- Flatus, stool, or urine per vagina
- Frequent urinary tract infections
- Mucopurulent malodorous discharge per vagina
- Dyspareunia
- Perineal pain
- Recurrent vaginal infections

ETIOLOGY

- Obstetric
  1. Incompletely repaired or unidentified vaginal lacerations

  2. Prolonged pressure between the fetal head and the maternal pubic bone, causing tissue necrosis
- Gynecologic
  1. Extensive dissection about the urinary tract, including unidentified injury
  2. Poor-quality tissue with prolonged healing as a result of estrogen deficiency, infection, malignancy, or prior radiation therapy

DIAGNOSIS

DIFFERENTIAL DIAGNOSIS

- Rectal or urinary incontinence
- Pelvic inflammatory disease
- Vaginal infection
- Vaginal fistula
  1. Vesicovaginal
  2. Urethrovaginal
  3. Ureterovaginal
  4. Rectovaginal
- Urinary tract infection

WORKUP

- Thorough history and physical exam, specifically, questioning about Crohn disease symptomology; constitutional symptoms such as weight loss and fatigue, with malignancy in mind
- Obtaining of past medical records specific to obstetric and surgical procedures
- Evaluation of patient's rectal and urinary continence
- Physical exam, looking for extraintestinal signs consistent with Crohn disease; lymphadenopathy; inspection of perineum and perianal area for evidence of abscess, obvious fistula, or scarring; pelvic exam including lighted speculum exam for any vulvar, vaginal, or cervical anomaly, excluding PID
  ○ For rectovaginal fistulas: Can use gel mixed with methylene blue massaged into the rectal tissues; if visualized vaginally can aid in localizing fistulous tract
- Administration of IV indigo carmine or fluorescein (if seen vaginally, diagnostic of vesicovaginal fistula)
- Biopsy of fistula tract

LABORATORY TESTS

- Urinalysis
- Urine culture
- Complete blood count
- Wet prep
- Gonococcal and chlamydial testing

IMAGING STUDIES

- Proctoscopy for suspected rectovaginal fistula
- Vaginogram (Fig. 2)
- Cystoscopy
- CT of the abdomen and pelvis to exclude malignancy (especially in women with no history of obstetric trauma, previous fistula, IBD, or known pelvic malignancy) (Fig. 2)
- Endoanal ultrasound, with or without hydrogen peroxide contrast injected into the suspected fistula tract
- Magnetic resonance imaging
- Intravenous urogram
- Retrograde ureteropyelography

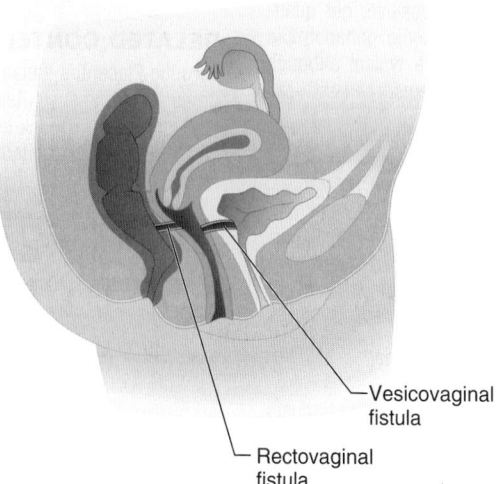

Vesicovaginal fistula

Rectovaginal fistula

FIG. 1 The two most common types of vaginal fistulas are vesicovaginal and rectovaginal. (From Fielding JR et al: *Gynecologic imaging,* Philadelphia, 2011, Saunders.)

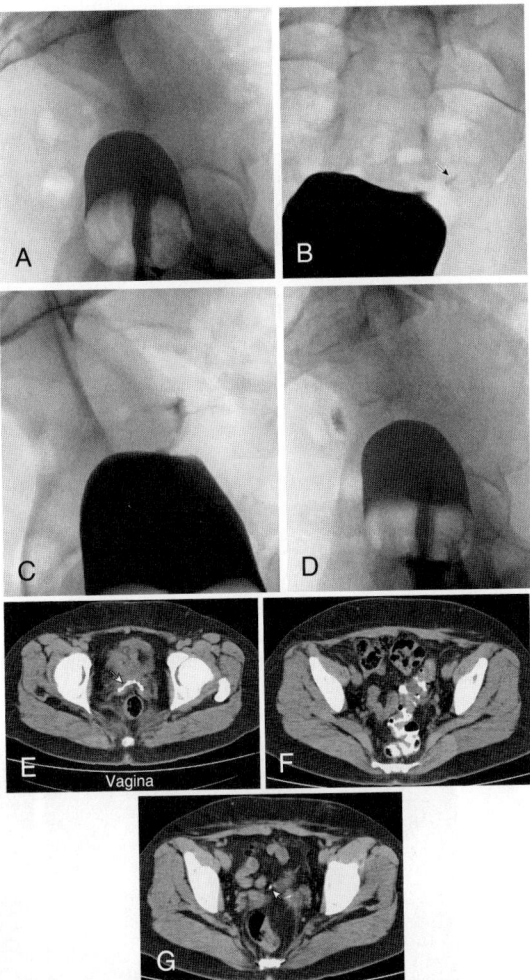

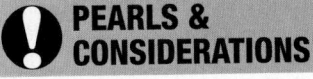

FIG. 2 A 44-year-old woman with gas and stool per vaginum 1 year after hysterectomy. Vaginal fistula was treated medically. **A,** Vaginogram, patient in left lateral position. **B,** Vaginogram, patient supine. The left apical vaginal fistula has just started to fill with contrast agent (*arrow*). **C,** Contrast agent is extending horizontally, likely in a loop of bowel. **D,** Vaginogram, patient in left lateral position, demonstrates small fistula to a loop of bowel, likely the rectosigmoid colon based on its relationship to the sacrum. **E,** Unenhanced computed tomographic (CT) scan of the pelvis immediately after the vaginogram demonstrates residual contrast agent in the vagina (*arrow*). **F,** CT scan confirms contrast agent from the vagina in the rectosigmoid colon. **G,** CT scan demonstrates 3 mm diameter short fistula to the rectosigmoid (*arrow*). (From Fielding JR et al: *Gynecologic imaging,* Philadelphia, 2011, Saunders.)

(Rx) TREATMENT

NONPHARMACOLOGIC THERAPY
- Tension-free surgical repair, with multiple documented approaches
  1. Transvaginal
  2. Perineal
  3. Abdominal
  4. Laparoscopic
  5. Robot assisted
  6. Transrectal
  7. Transanal endoscopy
- If vesicovaginal identified early:
  1. Prolonged urinary catheter placement, greater than 3 weeks

ACUTE GENERAL Rx
- Treatment of urinary or vaginal infection
- Estrogen replacement therapy, local vs. systemic if no contraindications

- Surgical repair of fistula with subsequent pelvic rest for 4 to 6 wk
- Minimizing Valsalva maneuvers

CHRONIC Rx
- If initial surgical management fails, repeat operations tailored to the cause of the fistula would be indicated, such as advancement flaps, sphincteroplasty, coloanal anastomosis (for rectovaginal fistula), gracilis flap.

DISPOSITION
- Cure rates after surgical repair vary in the literature, especially with the type of fistula repaired. With early intervention, estimated cure rates are between 84% and 100% in developed countries.

REFERRAL
- If there is concern for vaginal fistula, the patient should be managed by a surgeon familiar with fistula surgery for repair and follow-up. Consider consulting with a urologist, colorectal surgeon, gynecologic oncologist, or urogynecologist.

(!) PEARLS & CONSIDERATIONS

PREVENTION
- Prompt repair of obstetric lacerations
- Screen patients most at risk before surgery
- Avoid urologic complications in surgery (e.g., injury to bladder or ureters)
- Perform cystoscopy with complicated hysterectomy dissections to identify defects immediately

SUGGESTED READINGS
Available online at www.expertconsult.com

AUTHOR: **AMBER N. FONTENOT FERRISS, M.D.**

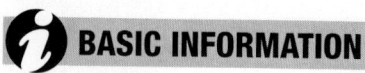

BASIC INFORMATION

DEFINITION

Vaginal malignancy is an abnormal proliferation of vaginal epithelium demonstrating malignant cells below the basement membrane.

SYNONYMS

Squamous cell carcinoma of the vagina
Adenocarcinoma of the vagina
Melanoma of the vagina
Sarcoma of the vagina
Endodermal sinus tumor

ICD-10CM CODE
C52 Malignant neoplasm of vagina

EPIDEMIOLOGY & DEMOGRAPHICS

INCIDENCE: 0.42 cases per 100,000 persons
PREVALENCE: Vaginal cancer is the second rarest gynecologic cancer. It comprises 2% of malignancies of the female genital tract.
MEAN AGE AT DIAGNOSIS: Predominantly a disease of menopause. Mean age at diagnosis is 60 yr.

PHYSICAL FINDINGS & CLINICAL PRESENTATION

- Majority of cases are asymptomatic
- Postmenopausal vaginal bleeding and/or vaginal discharge are the most common symptoms
- May also present as pelvic pain or pressure, dyspareunia, dysuria, malodor, or postcoital bleeding
- May present as a vaginal lesion or abnormal Pap smear

ETIOLOGY

- The exact etiology is unknown.
- Most vaginal cancers are related to infection with HPV. HPV is implicated in 9 of 10 vaginal cancers and vaginal intraepithelial neoplasias. Cervical cancers have a similar risk factor. Vaginal intraepithelial neoplasia is believed to be a precursor for squamous cell carcinoma of the vagina.
- Long-term pessary use has been associated with vaginal malignancy.
- Prior pelvic radiation may be a risk factor.
- Clear-cell adenocarcinoma may be related to in utero diethylstilbestrol exposure (DES). Treatment of pregnant women with DES ended in the early 1970s, and it is anticipated that this spike in clear cell tumors will abate in the future.

DIAGNOSIS

DIFFERENTIAL DIAGNOSIS

- Extension from other primary carcinoma more common than primary vaginal cancer
- Vaginitis

WORKUP

- Diagnosis is made histologically by biopsy.
- Colposcopy and biopsy should follow suspicious Pap smear.
- Cystoscopy, proctosigmoidoscopy, chest radiography, IV urography, and barium enema may be used for clinical staging.
- CT scan (Fig. 1), FDG, PET scan, and MRI are used to evaluate spread.
- Staging I to IV (Fig. 2).

IMAGING STUDIES

- Chest radiography, IV urography, and barium enema are used for staging.
- CT scan and MRI are good for assessing tumor spread.

TREATMENT

NONPHARMACOLOGIC THERAPY

- Radiation therapy is the mainstay of treatment.
- Stage I tumors that are small and confined to the posterior, upper third of the vagina may be treated with radical surgery.
- Other stages require a whole-pelvis, interstitial, and/or intracavitary radiation therapy.
- Chemotherapy is used in conjunction with radiotherapy in rare select cases.

DISPOSITION

Five-year survival ranges from 80% for stage I to 17% for stage IV.

REFERRAL

Vaginal cancer should be managed by a gynecologic oncologist and radiation oncologist.

SUGGESTED READINGS
Available at www.expertconsult.com

RELATED CONTENT

Vaginal Cancer (Patient Information)

AUTHOR: **ANTHONY SCISCIONE, D.O.**

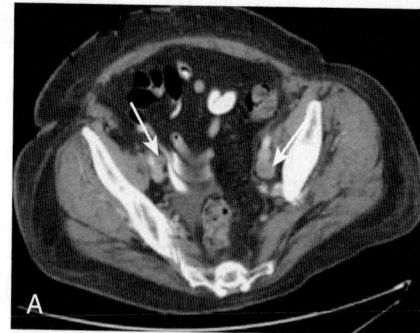
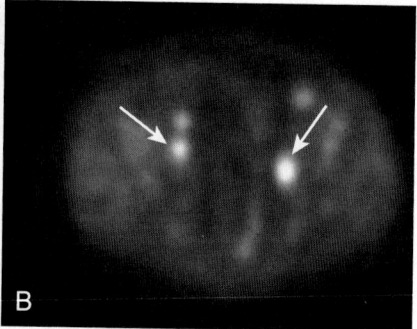

FIG. 1 **Vaginal cancer with lymphadenopathy. A,** CT of pelvis showing mildly enlarged external iliac nodes suggestive of metastases *(arrows).* **B,** Axial FDG PET scan showing hypermetabolic nodes as hyperintense spots confirming metastases. (From Abeloff MD: *Clinical oncology,* ed 3, Philadelphia, 2004, Churchill Livingstone.)

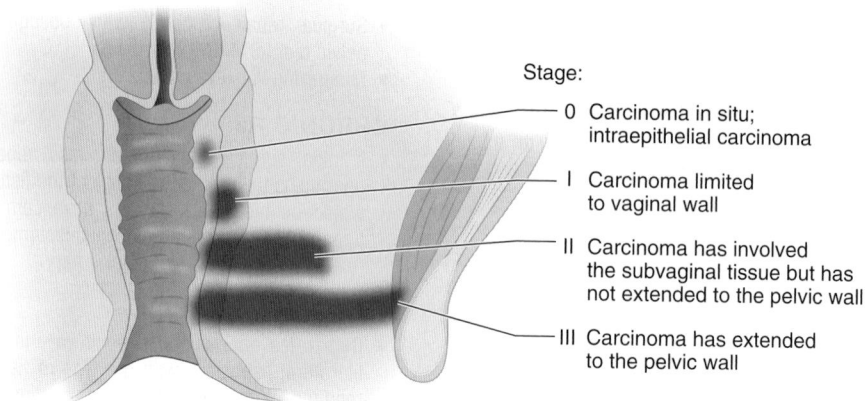

Stage:
0 Carcinoma in situ; intraepithelial carcinoma
I Carcinoma limited to vaginal wall
II Carcinoma has involved the subvaginal tissue but has not extended to the pelvic wall
III Carcinoma has extended to the pelvic wall

FIG. 2 **Staging system for vaginal cancer.** Metastatic disease that involves the bladder or rectum is stage IV-a. Metastatic disease beyond the pelvis is stage IV-b. (From Copeland LJ: *Textbook of gynecology,* ed 2, Philadelphia, 2000, Saunders.)

BASIC INFORMATION

DEFINITION

Vaginismus refers to the involuntary spasm of the vaginal, introital, and/or levator ani muscles, preventing penetration or causing painful intercourse. The vaginal spasm or pain may be in response to penetration with a penis, finger, or other object despite a desire for penetration to occur. The term "vaginismus" is no longer preferred, as it includes significant baggage as a psychological disorder and in DSM-5 the terms "vaginismus" and "dyspareunia" have been combined into the term "genito-pelvic pain/penetration disorder".

SYNONYM

Genitopelvic pain/penetration disorder

ICD-10CM CODES
N94.1   Vaginismus
F52.5   Non-organic vaginismus
F52.5   Vaginismus not due to a substance or known physiological condition

EPIDEMIOLOGY & DEMOGRAPHICS

INCIDENCE: Estimated at 11.7% to 42% of women presenting to sexual dysfunction clinics.
PREVALENCE: Affects approximately 1 in 200 women.
PREDOMINANT SEX: Affects only females.
RISK FACTORS: Any previous sexual trauma, including incest or rape.

PHYSICAL FINDINGS & CLINICAL PRESENTATION

- Fear of pain with coitus.
- Dyspareunia.
- Orgasmic dysfunction.

ETIOLOGY

- Learned conditioned response (Fig. 1) to real or imagined painful vaginal experience (e.g., traumatic speculum examination, incest, rape)
- Vaginitis
- Pelvic inflammatory disease
- Endometriosis
- Anatomic anomalies
- Atrophic vaginitis
- Mucosal tears
- Inadequate lubrication
- Focal vulvitis
- Painful hymenal tags
- Scarring secondary to episiotomy
- Skin disorders
- Topical allergies
- Postherpetic neuralgia

DIAGNOSIS

WORKUP

- Thorough history (including sexual history)
- Careful pelvic examination
- Behavioral therapy

TREATMENT

NONPHARMACOLOGIC THERAPY

- Deconditioning the response by systematic self-administered progressive dilation techniques using fingers or dilators
- Behavioral and/or psychosexual therapy

ACUTE GENERAL Rx

- Botulinum toxin therapy given locally has been shown to relieve the perineal muscle spasms associated with vaginismus, allowing resumption of intercourse.
  1. Acts by preventing neuromuscular transmission, causing muscle weakness.

2. Considered experimental treatment for vaginismus at this time.
- Cause should be determined by history and explained to the patient so that she understands the mechanics of the muscle spasms.
- Patient must be motivated to desire painless vaginal insertion for such reasons as pleasurable coitus, tampon insertion, or gynecologic examination.
- Patient (and her partner) must be willing to patiently undergo the process of systematic desensitization and counseling.

DISPOSITION

A high percentage of successfully treated patients

REFERRAL

To a gynecologist or sex therapist

PEARLS & CONSIDERATIONS

COMMENTS

- May uncover early sexual abuse or an aversion to sexuality in general
- American Association of Sex Educators, Counselors and Therapists, 11 Dupont Circle, NW, Washington, DC, 20036
- Sex Information and Education Council of the United States (SIECUS), 90 John St., New York, NY 10038

RELATED CONTENT

Dyspareunia (Related Key Topic)

AUTHOR: **RUBEN ALVERO, M.D.**

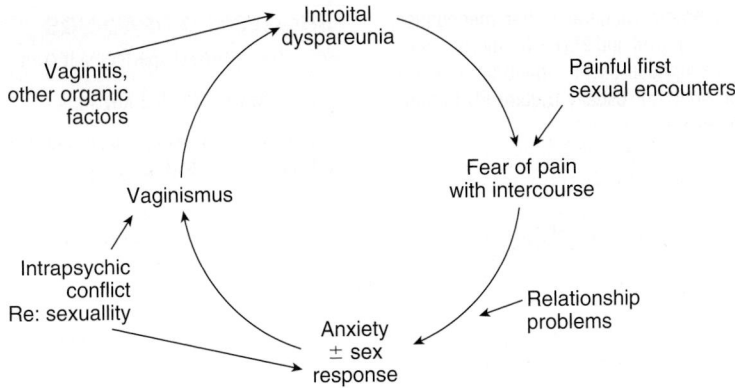

FIG. 1 Dyspareunia and vaginismus cycle. (From Lentz GM: *Emotional aspects of gynecology sexual dysfunction, eating disorders, substance abuse, depression, grief, loss; comprehensive gynecology*, St Louis, 2007, Mosby.)

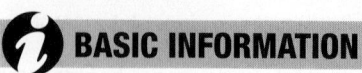

DEFINITION

Estrogen-deficient vulvovaginitis is the irritation and/or inflammation of the vulva and vagina because of progressive thinning and atrophic changes secondary to estrogen deficiency (Fig. 1).

SYNONYMS

Atrophic vaginitis
Vulvovaginal atrophy

ICD-10CM CODE
N95.2 Post-menopausal atrophic vaginitis

EPIDEMIOLOGY & DEMOGRAPHICS

- Seen most often in postmenopausal women
- Average age of menopause is 52 yr
- Up to half of postmenopausal women are symptomatic, but a quarter of these will not seek treatment

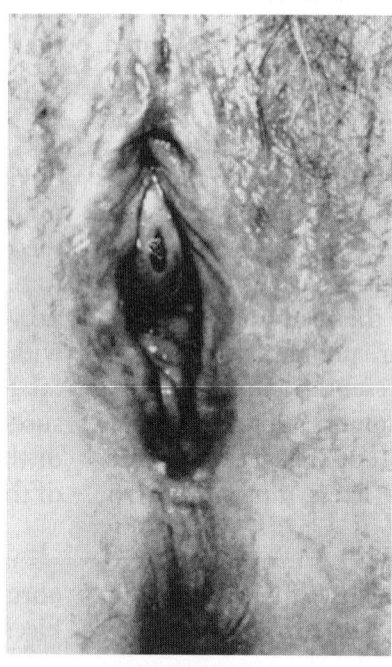

FIG. 1 Advanced postmenopausal atrophy of the vulva in a 72-year-old woman. (From Symonds EM, Macpherson MBA: *Color atlas of obstetrics and gynecology,* St Louis, 1994, Mosby.)

PHYSICAL FINDINGS & CLINICAL PRESENTATION

- Thinning of pubic hair, labia minora and majora
- Decreased secretions from the vestibular glands, with vaginal dryness
- Regression of subcutaneous fat
- Vulvar and vaginal itching
- Dyspareunia
- Dysuria and urinary frequency
- Vaginal spotting

ETIOLOGY

- Estrogen deficiency. Estrogen is essential to maintaining the urogenital environment. Postmenopausal thinning of the vaginal epithelium and increase in subepithelial connective tissue result in loss of rugal folds and elasticity. Reduced blood flow also contributes to a decline in vaginal secretions.
- Smoking and use of antiestrogen medications (e.g., aromatase inhibitors) increase the risk of vulvovaginal atrophy.

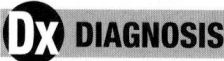

DIFFERENTIAL DIAGNOSIS

- Infectious vulvovaginitis
- Squamous cell hyperplasia
- Lichen sclerosus
- Vulvar malignancy
- Vaginal malignancy
- Cervical and endometrial malignancy
- Irritant contact dermatitis

WORKUP

- Pelvic examination
- Speculum examination
- Pap smear
- Possible endometrial biopsy if bleeding
- Possible vulvar or vaginal biopsy in the event of suspicious lesion

LABORATORY TESTS

FSH and estradiol: generally after menopause, estradiol <15 pg/ml and FSH >40 mIU/ml (diagnosis of menopause usually made on a clinical basis and does not usually require FSH and/or estradiol testing)

Rx TREATMENT

NONPHARMACOLOGIC THERAPY

- Avoidance of contact irritants such as scented soaps and feminine hygiene products
- Avoidance of synthetic undergarments, tight-fitting clothing

GENERAL Rx

- Regular use of vaginal moisturizers (e.g., Replens) can decrease vaginal itching and irritation.
- Use of water or silicone-based personal lubricants (e.g., Astroglide) during intercourse is useful to reduce dyspareunia.
- Conjugated estrogen vaginal cream intravaginally. Estradiol vaginal cream (Estrace).
  2 to 4 g/day × 2 wk then
  1 to 2 g/day × 2 wk then
  1 to 2 g × 2-3 days/wk
- Vagifem (estradiol vaginal tablets) 25 mg inserted intravaginally daily for 2 wk then twice weekly. May take up to 12 wk to feel the full benefits of the medication.
- Conjugated estrogen vaginal cream: 2 to 4 g qd (3 wk on, 1 wk off) for 3 to 5 mo.
- Hormone replacement therapy (HT): use ultra-low doses. Estrogen use should be reviewed every 3 to 6 mo, with an attempt to taper or discontinue its use.
- Estraderm patch 0.05 mg ×2 per week.
- If uterus present:
  1. Estrogen +2.5 mg PO Provera qd *or*
  2. Estrogen +5 to 10 mg PO Provera 14 days each mo

DISPOSITION

The symptoms should be improved with the therapy. Caution for vaginal bleeding if uterus present.

REFERRAL

To obstetrician/gynecologist if vaginal bleeding

SUGGESTED READINGS
Available at www.expertconsult.com

Pruritus Vulvae (Related Key Topic)

AUTHOR: **RUBEN ALVERO, M.D.,** and **ELIZABETH M. ZADZIELSKI, M.D., M.B.A.**

BASIC INFORMATION

DEFINITION
Inflammation of the vagina or vulva caused by a fungal infection.

SYNONYMS
Candidiasis, vulvovaginal
Monilial vulvovaginitis
Vulvovaginal candidiasis
VVC
Vulvovaginitis

ICD-10CM CODE
B37.3 Candidiasis of vulva and vagina

EPIDEMIOLOGY
- The lifetime incidence of fungal vaginitis is 75%.
- This is the second most common cause of vaginitis.

PHYSICAL FINDINGS & CLINICAL PRESENTATION
- Intense vulvar and vaginal pruritus or burning
- External dysuria
- Dyspareunia edema and erythema
- Thick, white discharge ("cottage cheese" discharge)
- May be asymptomatic

ETIOLOGY
- *Candida albicans* is responsible for 80% to 95% of vaginal fungal infections.
- In recurrent fungal vaginitis, *Candida tropicalis* and *Candida glabrata* are the most common non-*albicans Candida* species that can induce vaginitis.

PREDISPOSING RISK FACTORS
- Pregnancy
- Diabetes mellitus
- Antibiotics
- Immunosuppression

DIAGNOSIS

DIFFERENTIAL DIAGNOSIS
- Bacterial vaginosis
- *Trichomonas* vaginitis
- Atrophic vaginitis

Section II describes the differential diagnosis of vaginal discharges and infections.

WORKUP
- History and physical examination
- Pelvic and speculum examination: pseudohyphae or blastospores on 10% KOH preparation (positive in 50%-70% of individuals with yeast infection)
- Vaginal pH <4.5
Perform vaginal cultures if the infection is recurrent.
Section III, "Vaginal Discharge," describes the evaluation of discharge.
Classification of vulvovaginal candidiasis
- Uncomplicated: infrequent episodes, mild to moderate symptoms, caused by *C. albicans*, nonpregnant patient and without medical complications.
- Complicated: recurrent episodes (>4 per year), severe symptoms, non-albicans Candida, women with diabetes, immunosuppression, severe medical illness, other vulvovaginal conditions and/or pregnancy.

TREATMENT

ACUTE GENERAL Rx
- Cure rate of the various azole derivatives 85% to 90%; little evidence of superiority of one azole agent over another.
- Oral therapy may cause gastrointestinal intolerance, headache, and liver function test elevations. Topical treatments may cause local side effects, such as burning and irritation. Fluconazole 150 mg PO × 1 is preferred treatment.
- Miconazole 200-mg suppository, one suppository ×3 days, 100 mg suppository x7 days, 1200 mg suppository x 1 day, or 2% vaginal cream, one applicatorful (5 g) intravaginally qhs × 7.
- Clotrimazole 200-mg vaginal tablet, one tablet intravaginally qhs ×3 or 100-mg vaginal tablet one tablet intravaginally qhs ×7, or 500 mg suppository x 1 day, or 1% vaginal cream (5g) intravaginally qhs ×7 or 2% vaginal cream intravaginally (5 g) x 3 days.
- Tioconazole 6.5% ointment (Vagistat), one applicator intravaginally × 1 or 2% vaginal cream, one applicator (5 g) intravaginally x 3 days.

- In pregnant patient, treat with 7-day course of topical imidazole.

CHRONIC Rx (FOUR OR MORE SYMPTOMATIC EPISODES ANNUALLY)
- Resistance or recurrence:
If recurrence is due to *C. albicans* treat with 7 to 14 days of fluconazole and then continue with fluconazole 150 mg PO weekly for 6 months.
- Ketoconazole 200 mg PO bid × 5 to 14 days
- Boric acid 600-mg capsule intravaginally bid × 14 days
- Clotrimazole 500 mg vaginal tablet weekly or 200 mg vaginal tablet twice per week.
- Prophylactic regimens
  1. Clotrimazole one 500-mg vaginal tablet each month
  2. Ketoconazole 200 mg PO bid × 5 days each month
  3. Fluconazole 150 mg PO × 1 each month
  4. Miconazole 100-mg vaginal tablet × 2 weekly

PEARLS & CONSIDERATIONS

COMMENTS
- No evidence that treating a woman's male sexual partner significantly improves woman's infection or reduces her rate of relapse.

SUGGESTED READINGS
Available at www.expertconsult.com

RELATED CONTENT
Candidiasis (Patient Information)
Vaginal Yeast Infection (Patient Information)
Candidiasis, Cutaneous (Related Key Topic)
Pruritus Vulvae (Related Key Topic)
Vaginitis, Prepubescent (Related Key Topic)

AUTHORS: **REBECCA RINKO, D.O.,** and **EMILY K. SAKS, M.D., M.S.C.E.**

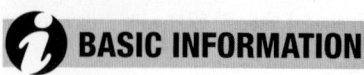

BASIC INFORMATION

DEFINITION

Prepubescent vulvovaginitis is an inflammatory condition of the vulva and vagina.

SYNONYMS

Vulvovaginitis

ICD-10CM CODES
N76.0 Acute vaginitis
N76.1 Subacute and chronic vaginitis

EPIDEMIOLOGY & DEMOGRAPHICS

- Most common gynecologic problem of pre-menarchal girls.
- Prepubertal girls are susceptible to irritation and trauma because of the absence of protective hair and labial fat pads, as well as a lack of estrogenization leading to atrophic vaginal mucosa.
- Symptoms of vulvovaginitis and introital irritation and discharge account for 80% to 90% of gynecologic visits.
- Nonspecific etiology in approximately 75% of children with vulvovaginitis.
- Majority of vulvovaginitis in girls involves a primary irritation of the vulva with secondary involvement of the lower third of the vagina.

PHYSICAL FINDINGS & CLINICAL PRESENTATION

Vulvar pain, dysuria, pruritus
1. Discharge is not a primary symptom.
2. If present, vaginal discharge may be foul smelling or bloody.

ETIOLOGY

- Most commonly attributed to poor hygiene or nonspecific irritants
- Infections
  1. Bacterial
  2. Protozoal/parasitic
  3. Mycotic
  4. Viral
- Endocrine disorders
- Labial adhesions
- Skin disorders
- Sexual abuse
- Allergic substance
- Trauma

- Foreign body
- Masturbation
- Constipation
  Section II describes the differential diagnosis of vaginal discharge in prepubertal girls.

DIAGNOSIS

DIFFERENTIAL DIAGNOSIS

- Physiologic leukorrhea
- Foreign body
- Bacterial vaginosis
- Fungal vulvovaginitis
- Sexual abuse and possibly an associated sexually transmitted infection such as gonorrhea, chlamydia, or trichomonas
- Pinworms

WORKUP

- Pelvic, genital examination
- Speculum examination
- Rectal examination
- Vaginoscopy if considering a foreign body
- KOH and normal saline preparation of discharge
- Knee-chest position for examination may be easier for the child to tolerate during an examination
  Section III, "Vaginal Discharge," describes the evaluation of discharge.

LABORATORY TESTS

- Urinalysis to rule out urinary tract infection and diabetes
- Cultures including sexually transmitted diseases

TREATMENT

NONPHARMACOLOGIC THERAPY

- Avoid tight clothing
- Perineal hygiene
- Avoid irritant chemicals
- Reassurance

ACUTE GENERAL Rx

- Canddiasis: fluconazole 150 mg PO, one dose
- Group A beta *Streptococcus* and *Streptococcus pneumoniae*: penicillin V potassium 125 to 250 mg PO qid × 10 days.
- *Chlamydia trachomatis*: for children <45 kg, treat with erythromycin base or

ethylsuccinate 50 mg/kg/day PO qid × 14 days. For children ≥45 kg, treat with azithromycin 1 g PO single dose or doxycycline 100 mg PO bid × 7 days.
- *Neisseria gonorrhoeae*: for children ≤45 kg, treat with ceftriaxone 25 to 50 mg/kg IV or IM in a single dose. Children >45 kg should be treated with ceftriaxone 250 mg IM plus azithromycin 1 g PO once.
- *Staphylococcus aureus*: amoxicillin-clavulanate 20 to 40 mg/kg/day PO × 7 to 10 days.
- *Haemophilus influenzae*: amoxicillin 20 to 40 mg/kg/day PO × 7 days.
- *Trichomonas*: metronidazole 125 mg (15 mg/kg/day) tid PO × 7 to 10 days.
- Pinworms: mebendazole 100-mg tablet chewable, repeat in 2 wk.
- Labial agglutination: spontaneous resolution or topical estrogen cream for 7 to 10 days. High degree of efficacy with topical estrogen hormone.

CHRONIC Rx

See "Referral."

DISPOSITION

Further education:
- Discuss appropriate hygiene
- If sexually active, discuss pregnancy prevention and safe sexual practices. If there is suspicion of sexual abuse, report to child protective services.

REFERRAL

- To obstetrician/gynecologist, preferably a physician with specialized training in pediatric and adolescent gynecology if available
- To pediatrician

SUGGESTED READINGS
Available at www.expertconsult.com

RELATED CONTENT
Chlamydia Genital Infection (Related Key Topic)
Pruritus Vulvae (Related Key Topic)
Vaginitis, Fungal (Related Key Topic)
Vaginitis, *Trichomonas* (Related Key Topic)
Vaginosis, Bacterial (Related Key Topic)

AUTHOR: **MARGARET R. HINES, M.D.**

BASIC INFORMATION

DEFINITION

Trichomonas vulvovaginitis is the inflammation of vulva and vagina caused by *Trichomonas* spp.

SYNONYMS

Trichomonas vaginalis
Trichomoniasis
TV

ICD-10CM CODE
A59.01 Trichomonal vulvovaginitis

EPIDEMIOLOGY & DEMOGRAPHICS

- Acquired through sexual contact
- Diagnosed in
  1. 50% to 75% of prostitutes
  2. 5% to 15% of women visiting gynecology clinics
  3. 7% to 32% of women in sexually transmitted disease (STD) clinics
  4. 5% of women in family planning clinics
  5. 13% of black women, 1.8% of non-Hispanic white women
  6. >11% of women ≥40 years old
- Most prevalent nonviral sexually transmitted infection in the U.S.

PHYSICAL FINDINGS & CLINICAL PRESENTATION

These symptoms and physical findings may or may not be present depending on the case:
- Yellow-green, malodorous vaginal discharge
- Vaginal and/or vulvar pruritus
- Dysuria
- Dyspareunia
- Intense erythema of the vaginal mucosa
- Cervical petechiae ("strawberry cervix")
- Some infected men may have symptoms of urethritis, epididymitis, or prostatitis
- Asymptomatic in ~50% of women and 90% of men

ETIOLOGY

Single-cell protozoan *Trichomonas vaginalis*

RISK FACTORS

- Multiple sexual partners
- History of previous STDs
- HIV infection

DIAGNOSIS

DIFFERENTIAL DIAGNOSIS (TABLE 1)

- Bacterial vaginosis
- Fungal vulvovaginitis
- Atrophic vulvovaginitis
- Vaginal or cervical infection with other sexually transmitted infections such as gonorrhea or chlamydia

WORKUP

- Pelvic examination
- Speculum examination

- Mobile trichomonads seen on normal saline preparation (Fig. 1): 30% to 70% sensitivity
- Elevated pH (>5) of vaginal discharge
- Culture is considered the traditional gold standard laboratory test for diagnosis of TV.
- Nucleic acid amplification tests (NAATs) have been developed that combine excellent performance characteristics with a more rapid turnaround time compared with culture.
- APTIMA assays utilize target capture and transcription-mediated amplification (TMA) to selectively purify, amplify, and detect species-specific 16 S ribosomal RNA. APTIMA *Trichomonas vaginalis* transcription-mediated amplification may be a better laboratory test than culture based on sensitivity and time frame for results.

LABORATORY TESTS

- NAAT is highly sensitive. The APTIMA *T. vaginalis* assay is FDA cleared for detection of *T. vaginalis* from vaginal, endocervical, and urine specimens from women (95%-100% clinical sensitivity and specificity). The OSOM Trichomonas Rapid Test on vaginal secretions provides results in 10 min with sensitivity of 82% to 95% and specificity of 97% to 100%.
- Microscopic evaluation of wet preparations of genital secretions: convenient and low cost but low sensitivity (51%-65%) in vaginal specimen with even lower sensitivity if there is a delay in evaluating slides.

TREATMENT

NONPHARMACOLOGIC THERAPY

Condom use: best way to prevent trichomoniasis is through consistent and correct use of condoms during all penile-vaginal sexual encounters

ACUTE GENERAL Rx

- Preferred initial treatment: metronidazole 2 g PO × 1 *or* tinidazole single 2-g oral dose in both sexes. Treatment of the sexual partner is essential to prevent reinfection.
- Alternative regimen: Metronidazole 500 mg PO bid × 7 days.
- Alcohol consumption should be avoided during treatment with metronidazole (at least 24 hr after completion of therapy) and tinidazole (at least 72 hr after completion of therapy) to reduce possibility of disulfiram-like reaction.

CHRONIC Rx

- For persistent infections, the CDC recommends first trying metronidazole 500 mg PO bid × 7 days.
- If treatment is still unsuccessful, proceed with metronidazole or tinidazole 2 g PO daily × 7 days.
- Allergy, intolerance, or adverse reactions: alternatives to metronidazole or tinidazole are not recommended. Patients who are allergic to nitroimidazoles can be managed by desensitization.

TABLE 1 Differential Diagnosis of Vaginitis in Women

	VAGINAL DISCHARGE	pH	WHITE BLOOD CELLS	MICROSCOPY	SYMPTOMS
Normal	White, thick, smooth	≤4.5	Absent	Lactobacilli	None
Candidiasis	White, thick, curdlike	≤4.5	Absent	Mycelia	Vulvar pruritus, external or superficial dysuria
Trichomoniasis	Frothy or purulent	≥4.5	Present	Mobile trichomonads present Amine odor	Vulvar erythema and edema, punctate strawberry lesions on cervix
Bacterial vaginosis	Thin, white homogeneous	≥4.5	Absent	Paucity of lactobacilli (75% of patients) Amine odor Clue cells	Fishy odor and increased vaginal discharge

Wein AJ et al: *Campbell-Walsh urology*, ed 11, Philadelphia, 2016, Elsevier.

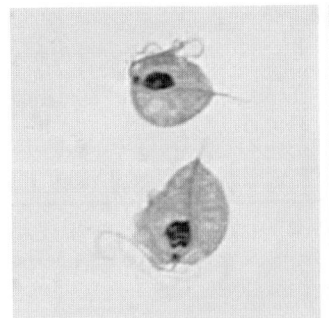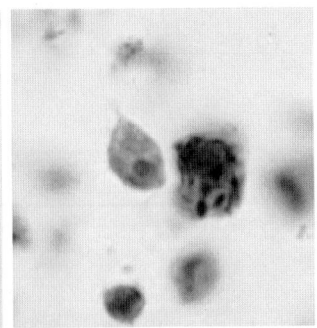

FIG. 1 *Trichomonas vaginalis* trophozoites stained with Giemsa *(left)* and iron hematoxylin *(right)*. (From the Centers for Disease Control and Prevention: *Laboratory identification of parasites of public health concern, Trichomoniasis.* www.dpd.cdc.gov/dpdx/HTML/ImageLibrary/Trichomoniasis_il.htm. Accessed August 30, 2010.)

- Pregnancy:
  1. Associated with adverse outcomes (i.e., premature rupture of membranes, preterm delivery), although it is unclear whether treatment decreases the incidence of these outcomes.
  2. Treat with metronidazole 2 g PO × 1 day; avoid tinidazole as there is little known about tinidazole in pregnancy.

DISPOSITION

- *Trichomonas* infection is considered an STD; therefore, treatment of the sexual partner is necessary.

- *T. vaginalis* infection is associated with two- to threefold increased risk for HIV acquisition
- *T. vaginalis* infection in pregnancy is associated with premature rupture of membranes, preterm birth, and delivery of low birthweight infants.

REFERRAL

To obstetrician/gynecologist for recurrence and pregnancy.

SUGGESTED READINGS

Available at www.expertconsult.com

RELATED CONTENT

Trichomoniasis (Patient Information)
Pruritus Vulvae (Related Key Topic)

AUTHOR: **MARGARET R. HINES, M.D.**

ⓘ BASIC INFORMATION

DEFINITION

Bacterial vaginosis (BV) is a polymicrobial infection in which anaerobic bacteria overgrow and replace the normal hydrogen peroxide–producing lactobacilli, resulting in thin, gray, and malodorous vaginal discharge.

SYNONYMS

Bacterial vaginosis
BV
Nonspecific vaginitis
Gardnerella vaginalis vaginitis

ICD-10 CODES
N76.0 Acute vaginitis
N77.1 Vaginitis, vulvitis and vulvovaginitis in diseases classified elsewhere

EPIDEMIOLOGY & DEMOGRAPHICS

- 50% to 75% of patients are asymptomatic
- Most common organisms include *Gardnerella vaginalis, Mycoplasma hominis, Bacteroides* species, *Peptostreptococcus* species, *Fusobacterium* species, *Prevotella* species, and *Atopobium vaginae* and other anaerobes.
- May be associated with low birthweight, premature rupture of membranes (PROM), and prematurity.
- Associated with pelvic inflammatory disease (PID), postprocedural gynecologic infections, and acquisition of HIV and herpes simplex virus infections in nonpregnant women.
- BV may recur in 30% within the first 3 months after treatment, which may be due to:
  1. Persistence of pathogenic bacteria
  2. Reinfection from exogenous sources including sexual partners
  3. Failure of the normal lactobacillus-dominant flora to reestablish
- Risk factors: sexual activity including females who partner with females, douching, tobacco use, lack of condom use, and lack of vaginal lactobacilli.

PHYSICAL FINDINGS & CLINICAL PRESENTATION

- A thin, dull, and gray homogeneous discharge (Fig. E1)
- Characterized by a "fishy" odor from the vagina

ETIOLOGY

- It is unclear how the vaginal floral imbalance occurs and the role sexual activity plays in the pathogenesis of BV
- *G. vaginalis* may be important in epithelial biofilm formation
- Ethnicity and age may contribute to the vaginal microbial environment

ⒹⓍ DIAGNOSIS

WORKUP

Amsel's criteria:
- Sensitivity of 92% and specificity of 77%:
  1. Thin, gray, and homogeneous, malodorous discharge that adheres to the vaginal walls.
  2. Vaginal pH >4.5.
  3. Positive amines test.
     a. Conducted by placing wet mount specimen and adding 10% potassium hydroxide, which creates a fishy odor, otherwise known as the 'whiff test."
  4. More than 20% of the epithelial cells are clue cells.
- Cultures are unnecessary.
- Gram stain of vaginal secretions is the gold standard for diagnosis (Fig. 2).
- Other tests include Affirm VPIII and the OSOM BVBlue test.
- Rule out other causes such as vulvar diseases and atrophic vaginitis.

ⓇⓍ TREATMENT

ACUTE GENERAL Rx

- Recommended regimens:
  1. Metronidazole 500 mg PO bid for 7 days *or*
  2. 0.75% metronidazole gel one full applicator (5 gm) intravaginally once a day for 5 days *or*

  3. 2% clindamycin cream one full applicator (5 gm) intravaginally at bedtime for 7 days
- Alternate regimens:
  1. Clindamycin 300 mg PO bid for 7 days or clindamycin ovules intravaginally once at bedtime for 3 days. May be associated with antimicrobial resistance.
- Disulfiram-type reactions may occur while taking oral or topical metronidazole and patients should be advised to avoid alcohol while undergoing treatment.
- Sexual partners: it is not necessary to treat male partners of affected females; however, females who partner with females need to be aware of the signs and symptoms of BV, and treatment is indicated in this population if symptoms occur.
- Treatment in pregnancy:
  1. Symptomatic pregnant patients with BV should be treated to relieve bothersome symptoms.
  2. Some experts believe oral therapy is superior to topical therapy in pregnancy secondary to the potential subclinical upper genital tract infection protection.
  3. There is no evidence that metronidazole or clindamycin have any teratogenic effect during pregnancy.
- Recurrent BV:
  1. Condom use may help reduce the risk of recurrence.
  2. Chronic suppressive therapy has been proven to reduce the development or recurrence of BV.

❗ PEARLS & CONSIDERATIONS

- BV is the most common cause of vaginitis in reproductive women.
- BV has been associated with pelvic inflammatory disease, post-hysterectomy vaginal cuff cellulitis, and postabortal infection; therefore, it is reasonable to treat asymptomatic women who are to undergo hysterectomy and pregnancy termination.
- ACOG, USPSTF, and CDC all agree to not routinely screen and treat all pregnant women with asymptomatic BV to prevent preterm birth.

SUGGESTED READINGS
Available at www.expertconsult.com

RELATED CONTENT
Bacterial Vaginal Infections (Patient Information)

AUTHORS: **MELISSA L. DAWSON, D.O., M.S.,** and **EMILY K. SAKS, M.D., M.S.C.E.**

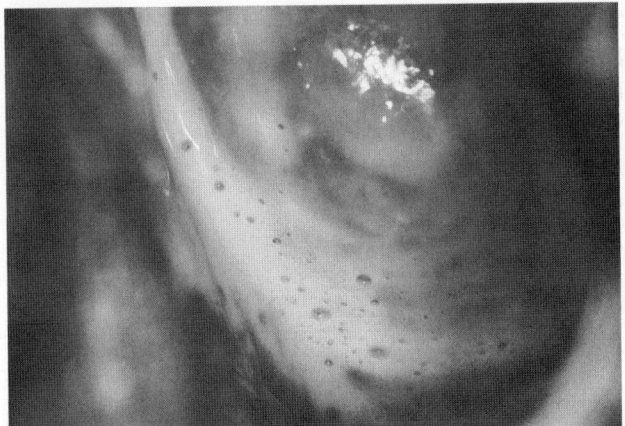

FIG. 2 Clue cells characteristic of bacterial vaginosis, squamous epithelial cells whose borders are obscured by bacteria. (From Carlson K [ed]: *Primary care of women,* St Louis, 1995, Mosby.)

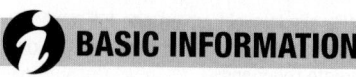

BASIC INFORMATION

DEFINITION

Enterococci are gram-positive, facultative anaerobic organisms usually oval in shape and can be seen as single cells, pairs, or chains. Vancomycin-resistant *Enterococcus* (VRE) are enterococci that have become resistant to vancomycin and several antibiotics normally used to treat enterococcal infections.

SYNONYM

VRE

ICD-10CM CODES
Z16.39 Resistance to other specified antimicrobial drug

EPIDEMIOLOGY & DEMOGRAPHICS

INCIDENCE: VRE may be associated with the use of specific classes of antibiotics.
PEAK INCIDENCE: VRE was first reported in Europe in 1986, and there has been a steady rise in the incidence of enterococcal strains resistant to vancomycin. In 2007, 80% of *E. faecium* isolates and 7% of *E. faecalis* isolates were resistant to vancomycin.
PREVALENCE: 80% of *E. faecium* are VRE; 69% of *E. faecalis* are VRE.
RISK FACTORS:
- Prior antimicrobial therapy, especially vancomycin
- Prolonged hospitalization
- Chronic medical conditions, renal failure
- Invasive devices
- ICU stay
- Colonization: VRE colonize the gastrointestinal tract; can be found on skin or perirectal swab culture or stool culture

PHYSICAL FINDINGS & CLINICAL PRESENTATION

Patients may be asymptomatic and have gastrointestinal colonization; it can be associated with diarrhea. In hospitalized patients, infection is associated with colonization and can cause wound infections, bacteremia, abscesses (intraabdominal), and, rarely, pneumonia and urinary tract infections.

ETIOLOGY

- The Clinical and Laboratory Standards Institute uses the following MIC definitions for vancomycin susceptibility and resistance in enterococci:
  1. Vancomycin susceptible: ≤4 mcg/ml
  2. Vancomycin resistant: ≥32 mcg/ml
  3. Vancomycin intermediate: 8 to 16 mcg/ml (vancomycin not recommended)

- Enterococci are primarily found in the human digestive tract and female genital tract, where they make up a significant portion of the normal bacterial population in healthy people. Enterococci can cause urinary tract, wound, bloodstream, heart valve, and brain infections. In the great majority of cases, VRE infections occur in hospitalized patients who have compromised immune systems. Most cases of VRE are caused by the *E. faecium* strains that have acquired resistance when they came in contact with other bacteria and shared genetic information.
- VRE is most commonly transmitted from one patient to another by health care workers whose hands have become contaminated inadvertently with feces or fluids of a person carrying the organism. VRE are not airborne but can survive on surfaces for several weeks.

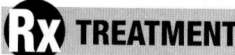 DIAGNOSIS

DIFFERENTIAL DIAGNOSIS

- Other bacterial pathogens in blood, wounds, or urine
- Once colonized, increased incidence to become infected

LABORATORY TESTS

- VRE rectal culture
- VRE stool culture
- Blood, urine, and wound cultures

TREATMENT

- For rectal or stool colonization, therapy is not recommended
- Therapy is complicated by the fact that strains exhibit inherent resistance to many commonly used antibiotics.
- More than 80% of vancomycin-resistant *E. faecium* strains are also resistant to ampicillin.
- In symptomatic patients, if VRE strains are known to be susceptible, potential therapeutic agents include
  - Linezolid: 600 mg IV or PO q12h
  - Daptomycin: 4 mg/kg/day IV
  - Quinupristin-dalfopristin (Synercid) only effective for *E. faecium* strains with no activity for *E. faecalis* strains: 7.5 mg/kg q8 to 12h. Can cause severe myalgias and arthralgias and venous irritation that often requires use of a central line, which has limited the use of this antibiotic.
- The Healthcare Infection Control Practices Advisory Committee recommends that three negative stool/rectal cultures be obtained at weekly intervals to remove a patient from contact precautions.

REFERRAL

To infectious disease specialist

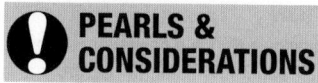

PEARLS & CONSIDERATIONS

COMMENTS

- Patients who are colonized with VRE have about an 8% rate of developing a true VRE infection in hospital or after discharge. The rate is higher in immunocompromised and severely ill patients.
- Incidence increases with comorbidity and hospitalization.
- The number of patients already colonized with VRE in a defined geographic area (colonization pressure) is the most significant factor for predicting new acquisition of VRE.
- An association between VRE colonization and *Clostridium difficile* infection has been reported in patients with hematologic malignancies.

PREVENTION

- Hand hygiene: most important and practical method of preventing spread in hospital environment. Soap and water (used as a 30-sec wash) and alcohol-based hand rubs are effective, as is chlorhexidine.
- Cohorting and isolation techniques: use of private rooms and use of gowns and gloves has been shown to decrease the risk of spread of multidrug-resistant bacteria.
- Cleaning contaminated objects or surfaces with standard hospital disinfectants, antibiotic management (prudent vancomycin use), and surveillance also help prevent spread.

RELATED CONTENT

Health Care-Related Infections (Related Key Topic)

AUTHOR: **GLENN G. FORT, M.D., M.P.H.**

BASIC INFORMATION

DEFINITION

Varicella is a viral illness that is characterized by the acute onset of a generalized vesicular rash and fever.

SYNONYM

Chickenpox

ICD-10CM CODES

B01.9	Varicella without complication
B01.8	Varicella with other complications
B01.0	Varicella meningitis
B01.11	Varicella encephalitis and encephalomyelitis
B01.12	Varicella myelitis
B01.2	Varicella pneumonia
B01.81	Varicella keratitis
B01.89	Other varicella complications
Z20.820	Contact with and (suspected) exposure to varicella

EPIDEMIOLOGY & DEMOGRAPHICS

- Varicella is extremely contagious. More than 90% of unvaccinated contacts become infected.
- The incubation period of chickenpox ranges from 9 to 21 days.
- The peak incidence is during the springtime.
- The predominant age is 5 to 10 yr.
- The infectious period begins 2 days before the onset of clinical symptoms and lasts until all of the lesions have crusted.
- Most patients will have lifelong immunity after an attack of chickenpox; protection from the virus after a varicella vaccine is approximately 6 yr.

PHYSICAL FINDINGS & CLINICAL PRESENTATION

- Findings vary with the clinical course. Initial symptoms consist of fever, chills, backache, generalized malaise, and headache.
- Symptoms are generally more severe in adults.
- Initial lesions generally occur on the trunk (centripetal distribution) and occasionally on the face; these lesions consist primarily of 3- to 4-mm red papules with an irregular outline and a clear vesicle (Fig. 1) on the surface (i.e., the appearance of dewdrops on a rose petal).

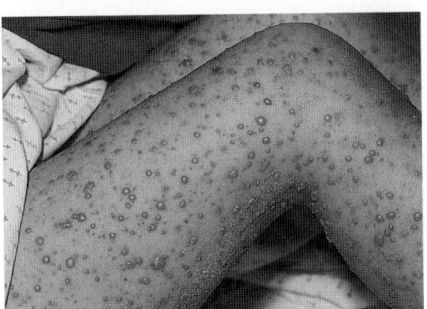

FIG. 1 Chickenpox. (From Swartz, MH: *Textbook of physical diagnosis*, 7 ed, Philadelphia, 2014, Saunders.)

- Intense pruritus generally accompanies the initial stage.
- New lesion development generally ceases by the fourth day, with subsequent crusting by the sixth day.
- Lesions generally spread to the face and the extremities (i.e., centrifugal spread).
- Patients generally present with lesions that are in different stages at the same time.
- Crusts generally fall off within 5 to 14 days.
- The fever is usually highest during the eruption of the vesicles; the patient's temperature generally returns to normal after the disappearance of vesicles.
- Signs of potential complications (e.g., bacterial skin infections, neurologic complications, pneumonia, hepatitis) may be present on physical examination.
- Mild constitutional symptoms (e.g., anorexia, myalgias, headaches, restlessness) may be present; these are most common among adults.
- Excoriations may be present if scratching is prominent.

ETIOLOGY

Varicella-zoster virus is a human herpes virus III that can manifest with either varicella or herpes zoster (i.e., shingles, which is a reactivation of varicella).

DIAGNOSIS

DIFFERENTIAL DIAGNOSIS

- Other viral infection.
- Impetigo.
- Scabies.
- Drug rash.
- Urticaria.
- Dermatitis herpetiformis.
- Smallpox.

WORKUP

The diagnosis is usually made on the basis of the patient's history and clinical presentation.

LABORATORY TESTS

- Laboratory evaluation is generally not necessary.
- The CBC may reveal leukopenia and thrombocytopenia.
- Serum varicella titers (i.e., a significant rise in the serum varicella immunoglobulin G antibody level), skin biopsies, or Tzanck smears are used only when diagnosis is in question.

TREATMENT

NONPHARMACOLOGIC THERAPY

- Use antipruritic lotions for symptomatic relief.
- Avoid scratching to prevent excoriations and superficial skin infections.
- Use a mild soap for bathing.
- Hands should be washed often.

ACUTE GENERAL Rx

- Use acetaminophen for fever and myalgias; aspirin should be avoided because of the associated increased risk of Reye's syndrome.

- Oral acyclovir (20 mg/kg qid for 5 days) initiated at the earliest sign (i.e., within 24 hr of illness) is useful for healthy, nonpregnant individuals 13 yr old or older to decrease the duration and severity of signs and symptoms. Immunocompromised hosts should be treated with intravenous acyclovir 500 mg/m^2 or 10 mg/kg q8h for 7 to 10 days.
- Varicella is most contagious from 2 days before to a few days after the onset of the rash. Varicella vaccine is available for children and adults; protection lasts at least 6 yr. Healthy, nonimmune adults and children exposed to varicella-zoster virus should receive prophylaxis with live attenuated varicella vaccine (Varivax). Patients with HIV or other immunocompromised patients should not receive the live attenuated vaccine.
- Exposed patients with contraindications to varicella vaccine can be treated with varicella-zoster immunoglobulin (VariZIG), which effectively prevents varicella in susceptible individuals. The dose is 12.5 U/kg IM up to a maximum of 625 U. VariZIG must be administered as early as possible after presumed exposure (i.e., within 10 days) for postexposure prophylaxis of varicella.
- Pruritus from chickenpox can be controlled with antihistamines (e.g., hydroxyzine 25 mg q6h) and antipruritic lotions (e.g., calamine).
- Oral antibiotics are not routinely indicated and should be used only in patients with secondary infection and infected lesions; the most common infective organisms are *Streptococcus* sp. and *Staphylococcus* sp.

DISPOSITION

- The course is generally benign in immunocompetent adults and children.
- Infants who develop chickenpox are incapable of controlling the infection and should be given varicella-zoster immunoglobulin or gamma globulin if VariZIG is not available.

PEARLS & CONSIDERATIONS

COMMENTS

- VariZIG can be obtained from the nearest regional Red Cross Blood Center or the Centers for Disease Control and Prevention in Atlanta.
- Varicella immunization is recommended for all who have not had chickenpox; the dosage for adults and adolescents (>13 yr old) is two 0.5 ml doses 4 to 8 wk apart.

RELATED CONTENT

EVIDENCE

Available at www.expertconsult.com

Chickenpox (Patient Information)

AUTHOR: **FRED F. FERRI, M.D.**

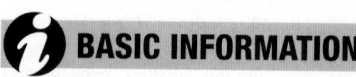

BASIC INFORMATION

DEFINITION

Veins in the leg are soft, thin-walled tubes that return blood back to the heart. This is accomplished by the presence of one-way valves and the action of the calf pump. Superficial venous insufficiency develops when venous return is impaired by valvular incompetence, obstruction, or calf muscle pump failure.

Varicose veins, the most common clinical manifestation of chronic venous disease, are bulging (>3 mm in diameter), tortuous conduits (Fig. 1). Reticular veins, often called "feeder veins," are bluish subdermal veins about 1 to 3 mm in diameter that give rise to telangiectasia. Spider veins or telangiectasias are very small (≤1 mm in diameter) thread veins found commonly in clusters on the surface of the skin.

SYNONYMS

Chronic venous disorder

ICD-10CM CODES

I83.90 Asymptomatic varicose veins of unspecified lower extremity
I83.899 Varicose veins of unspecified lower extremities with other complications

EPIDEMIOLOGY

PREVALENCE: One large U.S. cohort study found the biannual incidence of varicose veins was 3% in women and 2% in men.

The prevalence of varicose veins in Western populations was estimated in one study to be about 25% to 30% in women and 10% to 20% in men.
RISK FACTORS:
Gender: female
Genetics: family history of varicose veins
Increasing age
Multiple pregnancies

SYMPTOMS AND PHYSICAL FINDINGS

Leg complaints consistent with chronic venous disease include aching, heaviness, subjective swelling, cramps, itching, tingling, and pain. These symptoms can be exacerbated by menses, heat, and prolonged standing.

CLINICAL PRESENTATION

- Chronic vein disease is the result of the introduction of high pressures into a normal low-pressure superficial venous system.
- This increased pressure or venous hypertension causes superficial veins to distend to such a degree that vein valves fail to close, causing reflux and pooling of blood in surface veins.
- Manifested clinically by two syndromes:
  1. Junctional: failure of the terminal valve at the intersection between the saphenous vein trunks and the deep system. If the great saphenous vein is involved, large varicose veins are found mainly above medial knee or calf. When the small saphenous vein is involved, large varicose veins are found in posterior knee or calf area. If the anterior accessory of great saphenous vein is involved, large varicose veins are found mainly in anterior or lateral thigh.
  2. Perforator: failure of valves located in perforating vein. Large varicose veins are found most commonly in medial calf and proximal thigh region.

CLASSIFICATION

Chronic venous disease can now be classified using the Clinical-Etiology-Anatomy-Pathophysiology (CEAP) criteria to allow a precise description of the type of venous disease being discussed and provide an orderly framework for decision making (Table 1).

ETIOLOGY

- The underlying etiology of varicose veins remains uncertain.
- Important structural changes that occur: failure of vein valve function and vein wall dilation from fragmentation of the muscle layer.

COMPLICATIONS

- Superficial venous thrombophlebitis (SVT): a very common disorder with an incidence of 125,000 new cases per year in the U.S. The most frequent predisposing risk factors are varicose veins. The clinical findings include the presence of erythema, tenderness, and a palpable cord. Pain, increased warmth, and swelling are also present. Diagnosis is made by ultrasonography, which is useful to identify associated deep vein thrombosis that can occur in approximately 15% of patients. The location of the SVT determines the course of treatment; if the proximal great saphenous vein (GSV) is involved, a 1-mo course of low-molecular-weight heparin plus compression stockings has been found to be more effective than vein ligation. If SVT involves branch varicosities, treatment is usually symptomatic (control of pain).
- Bleeding is a more common complication than traditionally suspected. It is associated with thin-walled ectatic veins known as "blue blebs" that are found predominantly in the medial lower calf and ankle region. The best emergency treatment consists of pressure wrapping and not suture ligation, which results in delayed healing of the bleeding site. Sclerotherapy of these veins is the definitive treatment to prevent further bleeding.
- Dermal pathology of prolonged chronic venous disease (CEAP classes 4, 5, and 6).
  1. Varicose eczema: see "Venous Ulcers" section.
  2. Atrophie blanche: see "Venous Ulcers" section.
  3. Lipodermosclerosis: see "Venous Ulcers" section.
  4. Venous stasis ulcer: see "Venous Ulcers" section.

DIAGNOSIS

DIFFERENTIAL DIAGNOSIS

Other conditions that cause leg pain:
- Stress fracture
- Arthritis hip/knee joint
- Gout
- Degenerative disk disease of lower back
- Intermittent claudication secondary to peripheral arterial disease (PAD)
- Medications such as allopurinol and statins
Other conditions that cause leg swelling:
- Cellulitis
- Soft tissue injury to leg/ankle/foot

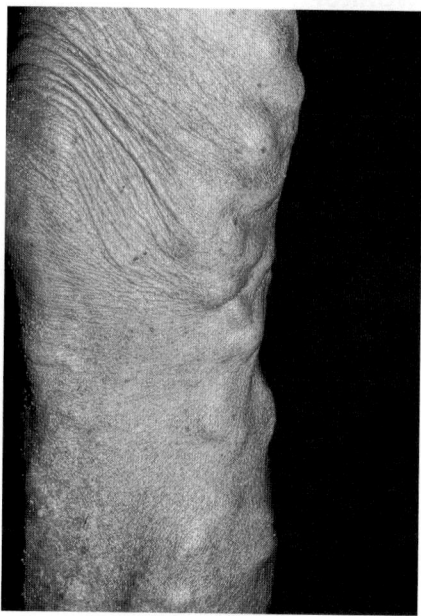

FIG. 1 Varicose veins. (From White GM, Cox NH [eds]: *Diseases of the skin, a color atlas and text,* ed 2, St Louis, 2006, Mosby.)

TABLE 1 CEAP Classification of Chronic Venous Disease

C: Clinical

C_0: no visible or palpable signs of venous disease
C_1: telangiectasias or reticular veins
C_2: varicose veins
C_3: edema
C_4: pigmentation or eczema
C_5: healed venous ulcer
C_6: active venous ulcer

E: Etiology

c: congenital
p: primary
s: secondary or post thrombotic
n: no venous cause identified

A: Anatomy

s: superficial veins
p: perforator veins
d: deep veins
n: no venous location identified

P: Pathophysiology

r: reflux
o: obstruction
r,o: reflux and obstruction
n: no venous pathophysiology identified

- Obesity
- Diabetes
- Advancing age
- Medications such as calcium channel blockers, steroids, MAO inhibitors, and tricyclics

WORKUP

The diagnosis of chronic venous disorders is predominantly clinical. Initial evaluation consists of a thorough history and physical exam with classification of disease according to the CEAP criteria.

LABORATORY TESTS

Laboratory tests are not useful in patients with varicose veins.

IMAGING STUDIES

Duplex ultrasonography:
- Gold-standard imaging modality for the diagnosis, prognostic evaluation, pretreatment mapping, and posttreatment assessment of therapeutic intervention.
- Duplex ultrasound is used to identify and quantify points of valvular reflux within the superficial venous system.
- Assessment of valvular reflux is done with patient in the upright position, which physiologically approximates the condition in which valvular reflux occurs.
- Reverse flow of greater than 0.5 sec after distal compression is considered abnormal.

Other tests:
- Air plethysmography: may be useful in patients who have reflux in both superficial and deep venous systems or in patients with an unusual presentation of leg pain.
- Venography: has been largely replaced by duplex ultrasonography but still retains a critical role in the evaluation of chronic venous insufficiency prior to venous reconstruction.

Rx TREATMENT

CONSERVATIVE THERAPY:
- Aerobic exercise regularly for 30 min a day.
- Elevate legs above heart level to reduce swelling.

- Flex ankles frequently at work and during air travel or long car travel.
- Maintain proper weight.
- Graduated compression stockings (below knee) to alleviate symptoms in patients who are not candidates or do not desire to undergo treatment of their varicose veins.

SCLEROTHERAPY:
- Small- to medium-sized varicose veins such as spider veins and reticular varices in the absence of reflux in saphenous trunks are best treated with liquid sclerotherapy.
- The three principal sclerosants used in the U.S. are hypertonic saline, sodium tetradecyl sulfate, and the newly FDA-approved solution, polidocanol.
- These agents are injected into vessels using 27-gauge or 30-gauge needles at concentrations of 23.4%, 0.1%, or 0.5%, respectively, causing injury to the endothelium with the resultant disappearance of the vein over period of time (usually 8-12 wk).

AMBULATORY PHLEBECTOMY:
- A procedure in which large varicose vein branches are removed with special hook instruments through a small puncture—incisions are made with an 18-gauge needle or No. 11 blade
- Performed safely under local anesthesia in an office setting and offers excellent cosmetic results and relief of symptoms
- Most commonly performed in conjunction with endovenous ablation procedures

ENDOVENOUS ABLATION:
- Ablation of diseased saphenous vein trunks, large incompetent tributaries, or perforating veins can be achieved by using:
  1. Radiofrequency energy.
  2. Laser energy.
  3. Ultrasound-guided foam sclerotherapy.
- The first two accomplish thermal injury to the vein in situ via an intraluminal catheter or bare-tipped laser wire. Chemical ablation uses a solution (polidocanol or sodium tetradecyl sulfate) that is injected directly into the vein in the form of foam.
- Endovenous ablation can be performed in an office setting using local anesthesia. Patients

can return to their normal daily activities immediately.
- The efficacy of these endovenous ablation procedures has been borne out by numerous published reports with occlusion rates over 95% and reflux free rates over 5-yr follow-up of 86%. A recent trial comparing ultrasound-guided foam sclerotherapy and endovenous laser ablation revealed that quality of life measures were generally similar among the study groups, with the exception of a slightly worse disease-specific quality of life in the foam group than in the surgery group. Both treatments had similar efficacy, but complications were less frequent after laser treatment and ablation rates were lower after foam treatment.

DISPOSITION

- It is important that the physician educate the patient to understand that varicose veins are a chronic and progressive disease.
- Any treatment is at best palliative, as patients in time will develop varicose veins in other areas.

REFERRAL

To either a phlebologist, preferably board certified by the newly created American Board of Phlebology, or a residency-trained vascular surgeon.

SUGGESTED READINGS
Available at www.expertconsult.com

RELATED CONTENT
Varicose Veins (Patient Information)
Thrombophlebitis, Superficial Venous (Related Key Topic)

AUTHOR: **FRANK G. FORT, M.D.**

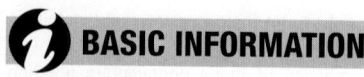

BASIC INFORMATION

DEFINITION

Vasculitis refers generically to inflammation occurring within the walls of blood vessels. Blood vessel inflammation can result in either perforation of affected vessels with hemorrhage into adjacent structures or thrombosis with subsequent ischemia and infarction of supplied tissues. Vasculitis can occur as a primary process or secondary to another connective tissue disease, infection, or drug exposure. The systemic vasculitides are a heterogeneous group of disorders (Table E1) characterized by blood vessel inflammation affecting vessels of varying size and location resulting in a wide range of clinical manifestations dictated largely by which vessels are affected (Fig. E1). Vasculitis

---

TABLE 2 Classification Scheme of Vasculitides According to Size of Predominant Blood Vessels Involved

- Primary vasculitides
- Predominantly large vessel vasculitides
- Takayasu's arteritis
- Giant cell arteritis (temporal arteritis)
- Cogan's syndrome
- Behçet's disease*
- Predominantly medium-sized vessel vasculitides
- Polyarteritis nodosa
- Cutaneous polyarteritis nodosa
- Buerger's disease
- Kawasaki disease
- Primary angiitis of the central nervous system
- Predominantly small vessel vasculitides
- Immune complex mediated
- Goodpasture's disease (anti-glomerular basement membrane disease)†
  - Cutaneous leukocytoclastic angiitis ("hypersensitivity vasculitis")
  - Henoch-Schönlein purpura
  - Hypocomplementemic urticarial vasculitis
  - Essential cryoglobulinemia‡
  - Erythema elevatum diutinum
- ANCA-associated disorders§
  - Granulomatosis with polyangiitis (Wegener granulomatosis)‡
  - Microscopic polyangiitis‡
  - Eosinophilic granulomatosis with polyangiitis (Churg-Strauss syndrome)‡
  - Renal-limited vasculitis
Secondary forms of vasculitis
Miscellaneous small vessel vasculitides
Connective tissue disorders‡ (rheumatoid vasculitis, lupus erythematosus, Sjögren's syndrome, inflammatory myopathy)
Inflammatory bowel disease
Paraneoplastic
Infection
Drug-induced vasculitis: ANCA-associated, other

ANCA, Antineutrophil cytoplasmic antibody.
*May involve small, medium-sized, and large blood vessels.
†Immune complexes formed in situ, in contrast to other forms of immune complex–mediated vasculitis.
‡Frequent overlap of small and medium-sized blood vessel involvement
§Not all forms of these disorders are always associated with ANCA.
From Firestein G et al: *Kelley's textbook of rheumatology,* ed 8, Philadelphia, 2008, Saunders.

---

is traditionally classified according to the size of the blood vessels predominantly affected (Table 2). Several of these are covered in individual chapters including chapters on granulomatosis with polyangiitis (GPA), polyarteritis nodosa (PAN), giant cell arteritis (GCA), Takayasu's arteritis, and Henoch-Schönlein purpura (HSP). Severity varies between and within specific vasculitides from a relatively benign, self-limited process to severe, life-threatening multisystem organ involvement with significant morbidity and mortality.

SYNONYMS

None

ICD-10CM CODES
M30.0   Polyarteritis nodosa
M30.3   Mucocutaneous lymph node syndrome [Kawasaki]
M31.30   Wegener's granulomatosis without renal involvement
M31.6   Other giant cell arteritis
M31.4   Aortic arch syndrome [Takayasu]

EPIDEMIOLOGY & DEMOGRAPHICS

- The epidemiology and demographics of the various vasculitides vary by the individual disease and, where applicable, are covered under the relevant disease chapters.
- The most common form of systemic vasculitis in the U.S. is giant cell arteritis, with an approximate incidence of 170 cases per 1 million per year in individuals older than 50 years.
- Antineutrophil cytoplasmic antibodies (ANCA)-associated vasculitis is significantly less common with aggregate incidence estimated at approximately 20 per million in the U.S.
- Age distribution can demonstrate significant variability between the vasculitides as shown by the fact that GCA generally does not occur before age 50, while 90% of cases of HSP occur in the pediatric population, and 80% of patients with Kawasaki disease are under age 5.
- Although genetic factors clearly play a role in disease susceptibility, familial cases of vasculitis are rare.

PHYSICAL FINDINGS & CLINICAL PRESENTATION

- Clinical presentation often includes nonspecific constitutional symptoms including fever, malaise, headache, and weight loss.
- Signs and symptoms are generally dictated by the tropism of involved vessels.
- Skin manifestations of vasculitis include petechiae, palpable purpura (Fig. 2), subcutaneous nodules, livedo reticularis, ulcerations, and digital ischemia.
- Kidney involvement of medium-sized and large vessel vasculitis is often in the form of renovascular hypertension. Glomerulonephritis may be seen in small vessel vasculitis.
- Pulmonary small vessel involvement can cause alveolar hemorrhage, which can present with cough, dyspnea, and alveolar hemorrhage.

- Mononeuritis multiplex is the characteristic finding of vasculitis affecting the vasa nervorum of the peripheral nervous system.
- Gastrointestinal involvement of the mesenteric vasculature can cause postprandial pain, bleeding, and perforation.
- Arthritis, while nonspecific, can be present.
- Significant clinical variability exists between the various vasculitides, although overlapping symptoms may be seen.

ETIOLOGY

Most forms of systemic vasculitis are of unknown etiology. Cryoglobulinemia vasculitis is often secondary to hepatitis C infection, and cutaneous leukocytoclastic vasculitis is often related to a drug exposure.

DIAGNOSIS

DIFFERENTIAL DIAGNOSIS

- Infective endocarditis
- Atrial myxoma
- Cholesterol emboli
- Malignancy
- Hypercoagulopathy
- Congenital collagen vascular disorder

WORKUP

- The diagnosis of most forms of systemic vasculitis relies on the history and physical examination as well as supportive laboratory testing. Table 3 describes differential diagnostic features of selected forms of small vessel vasculitis.
- Tissue biopsy is important in establishing an accurate diagnosis; biopsy sites should target affected tissues.

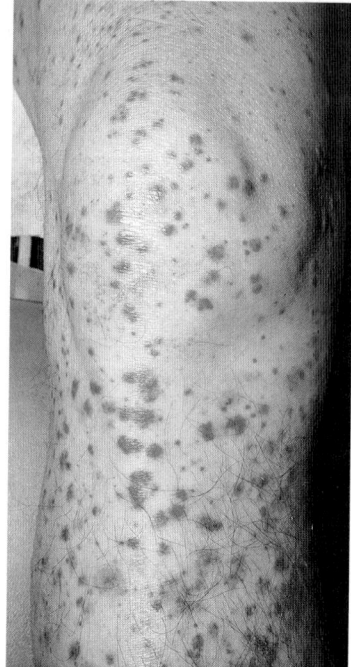

FIG. 2 Leukocytoclastic vasculitis, palpable purpura. (From James W et al: *Andrews' diseases of the skin, clinical dermatology,* ed 10, Philadelphia, 2005, Saunders.)

TABLE 3 Differential Diagnostic Features of Selected Forms of Small Vessel Vasculitis

Features	Microscopic Polyangiitis (MPA)	Granulomatosis with Polyangiitis (GPA)	Eosinophilic Granulomatosis with Polyangiitis	Henoch-Schönlein Purpura (HSP)	Cryoglobulinemic Vasculitis
Vasculitic signs and symptoms	+	+	+	+	+
IgA-dominant immune deposits	–	–	–	+	–
Cryoglobulins in blood and vessels	–	–	–	–	–
Antineutrophil cytoplasmic antibodies in blood	+	+	+	–	–
Necrotizing granulomas	–	+	+	–	–
Asthma and eosinophils	–	–	+	–	–

From Floege J et al: *Comprehensive clinical nephrology*, ed 4, Philadelphia, 2010, Saunders.

- Imaging such as mesenteric angiography can be supportive and may obviate the need for tissue biopsy.

LABORATORY TESTS

- Laboratory markers of systemic inflammation include an elevated erythrocyte sedimentation rate (ESR), C-reactive protein (CRP), and an anemia of chronic disease.
- ANCA targeting myeloperoxidase (MPO) and proteinase 3 (PR3) are frequently found in several small vessel vasculitides, including GPA (Wegener), microscopic polyangiitis (MPA), and Churg-Strauss syndrome (CSS).
- Hepatitis C antibodies and rheumatoid factor are often present in cryoglobulinemic vasculitis.
- Urinalysis in patients with glomerulonephritis due to small vessel ANCA-associated vasculitis will generally demonstrate hematuria with active urinary sediment with red blood cell casts and proteinuria.

IMAGING STUDIES

- Angiography can demonstrate vascular narrowing and aneurysm formation in suspected medium-size and large-vessel vasculitis.
- Pulmonary and sinus CT scans can demonstrate active pulmonary and upper airway disease in ANCA-associated vasculitis.

Rx TREATMENT

Treatment of vasculitis depends on the specific type of vasculitis and is tailored to the severity of disease activity.

ACUTE GENERAL Rx

- Systemic corticosteroids are generally required to gain initial control of active disease although mild cases of drug-induced cutaneous leukocytoclastic vasculitis can often be treated with NSAIDs and cessation of the offending medication.
- GCA, HSP, and vasculitis limited to the skin, including cutaneous PAN, can often be managed without further immunosuppression.
- Major organ-threatening disease in systemic vasculitis has traditionally been treated with oral or intravenous cyclophosphamide.
- Studies have demonstrated noninferiority of rituximab compared to cyclophosphamide in ANCA-associated vasculitis with major organ involvement, and it is approved for this use.
- Rituximab with prednisone has also recently been shown to be effective in the treatment of relapsing flares of disease activity in ANCA-associated vasculitis.
- Less severe disease such as granulomatosis with polyangiitis limited to the upper airways can be managed with methotrexate rather than cyclophosphamide.
- Trimethoprim/sulfamethoxazole should be used to prevent *Pneumocystis carinii* infection with concurrent immunosuppressive therapy.
- The goal of acute therapy is to induce remission of disease activity and is generally continued for 1 to 2 mo once this is achieved, at which point chronic therapy is used to prevent disease relapse.

CHRONIC Rx

- The goal of chronic therapy is to prevent disease relapse and minimize medication side effects.
- Steroids are gradually tapered as allowed by disease activity.
- Immunomodulatory agents such as methotrexate or azathioprine are commonly used for maintenance therapy in place of cyclophosphamide to reduce side effects.

- Cryoglobulinemic vasculitis due to chronic hepatitis C will often improve with treatment of the underlying viral infection.
- Rituximab may also be an appropriate remission maintenance agent in ANCA-associated vasculitis, although frequency of dosing and duration of therapy are not yet well characterized.

DISPOSITION

Varies widely among the various vasculitides

REFERRAL

Systemic vasculitis care is generally coordinated by a rheumatologist. Renal, pulmonary, neurologic, and gastrointestinal consultation is often needed when vasculitis involves these organ systems. Isolated cutaneous leukocytoclastic vasculitis is often managed by dermatology.

SUGGESTED READINGS

Available at www.expertconsult.com

RELATED CONTENT

Cogan's Syndrome (Related Key Topic)
Cryoglobulinemia (Related Key Topic)
Eosinophilic Granulomatosis with Polyangiitis (Related Key Topic)
Giant Cell Arteritis (Related Key Topic)
Granulomatosis with Polyangiitis (Related Key Topic)
Henoch-Schönlein Purpura (Related Key Topic)
Kawasaki Disease (Related Key Topic)
Microscopic Polyangiitis (Related Key Topic)
Polyarteritis Nodosa (Related Key Topic)
Takayasu's Arteritis (Related Key Topic)

AUTHORS: **NICOLE B. YANG, M.D.**, and **ANTHONY M. REGINATO, PH.D., M.D.**

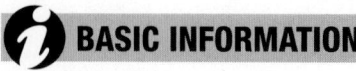

DEFINITION

The spectrum of chronic venous disease (CVD) ranges from varicose veins to leg edema and skin manifestations consisting of hyperpigmentation, eczema, lipodermatosclerosis, and venous ulcer. These latter venous-specific skin changes constitute an advanced form of CVD known as chronic venous insufficiency (CVI).

SYNONYMS

Stasis dermatitis
Postthrombotic syndrome (PTS)

ICD-10CM CODES
I87.2   Venous insufficiency (chronic) (peripheral)
I87.8   Other specified disorders of veins
I87.9   Disorder of vein, unspecified
I83.10 Varicose veins of unspecified lower extremity with inflammation

EPIDEMIOLOGY & DEMOGRAPHICS

- From 10% to 35% of adults in the United States have some form of CVI.
- Venous ulcers are the complication of CVI that results in the greatest morbidity and affects 4% of people over the age of 65.
- The population-based costs to the U.S. government for CVI treatment and venous ulcer care have been estimated at >$1 billion a year.
- In addition, 4.6 million workdays per year are lost to chronic venous-related diseases.

PHYSICAL FINDINGS & CLINICAL PRESENTATION

The spectrum of cutaneous changes of CVI in the affected leg include:
- Varicose eczema: the most common and earliest sign, this involves the skin above the medial ankle and consists of pruritic, red, and scaly eczematous patches and plaques (Fig. 1).
- Hyperpigmentation: caused by the breakdown of red blood cells and leads to hemosiderin deposition and dark staining of the skin (Fig. 2).
- Atrophie blanche: usually presents as hypopigmented white patches with focal red punctate dots or telangiectasia surrounded by hyperpigmentation. Skin in this condition is avascular and prone to ulceration (Fig. 3).
- Lipodermatosclerosis: a chronic, brawny induration of the skin and underlying fat that usually involves the skin from medial malleolus up to the lower border of the calf. Progression of the disease leads to an "inverted champagne bottle" appearance. The induration and lack of perfusion of the skin in this area make it susceptible to ulcer formation (Fig. 4).

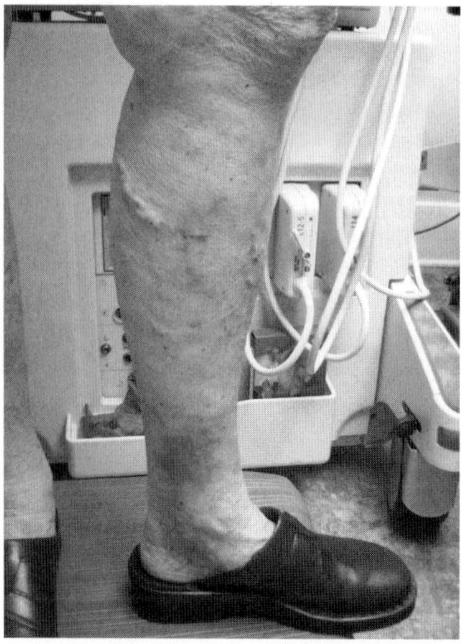

ETIOLOGY

- CVI occurs as a result of sustained venous hypertension in the leg, which can be caused by the following:
1. Primary: vein valve failure with reflux in the superficial venous system or perforating veins (most common cause of CVI).
2. Secondary: post-thrombotic syndrome in which a deep vein thrombosis causes outflow obstruction or
3. Combination of the two previous processes.
- This sustained elevation in venous pressure or venous hypertension results in pathologic effects in the skin and subcutaneous tissues such as edema, eczema, hyperpigmentation, fibrosis, and ultimately venous ulceration.

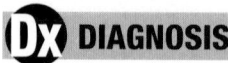
DIAGNOSIS

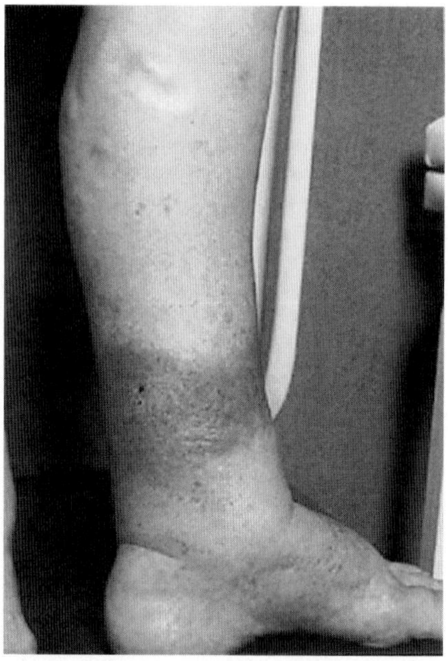

The diagnosis and evaluation of CVI are directed primarily by a detailed history and physical examination.

DIFFERENTIAL DIAGNOSIS

- Contact dermatitis.
- Atopic dermatitis.
- Cellulitis.
- Dermatophyte infection.
- Pretibial myxedema.
- Nummular eczema.
- Xerosis.
- Asteatotic eczema.

WORKUP

The primary goal is to identify the cause of sustained venous hypertension. Fig. 5 describes the evaluation and management of chronic venous insufficiency.

LABORATORY TESTS

Generally not indicated

IMAGING STUDIES

- Evaluation of the patient is performed in the standing position with duplex ultrasonography to identify reflux in the superficial, deep, and perforating veins as well as obstruction of the deep veins.

FIG. 1 Varicose eczema.

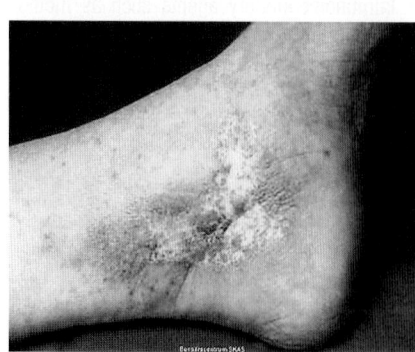
FIG. 2 Hyperpigmentation.

FIG. 3 Atrophie blanche.

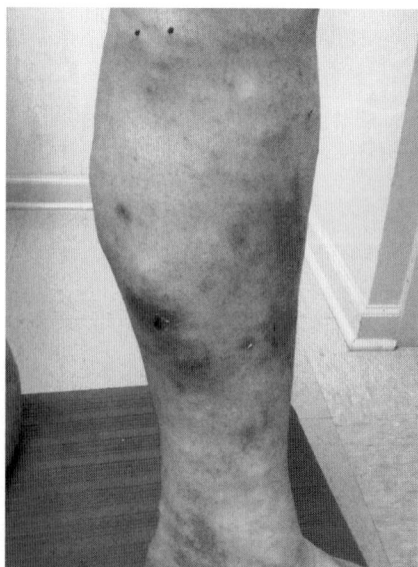
FIG. 4 Lipodermosclerosis.

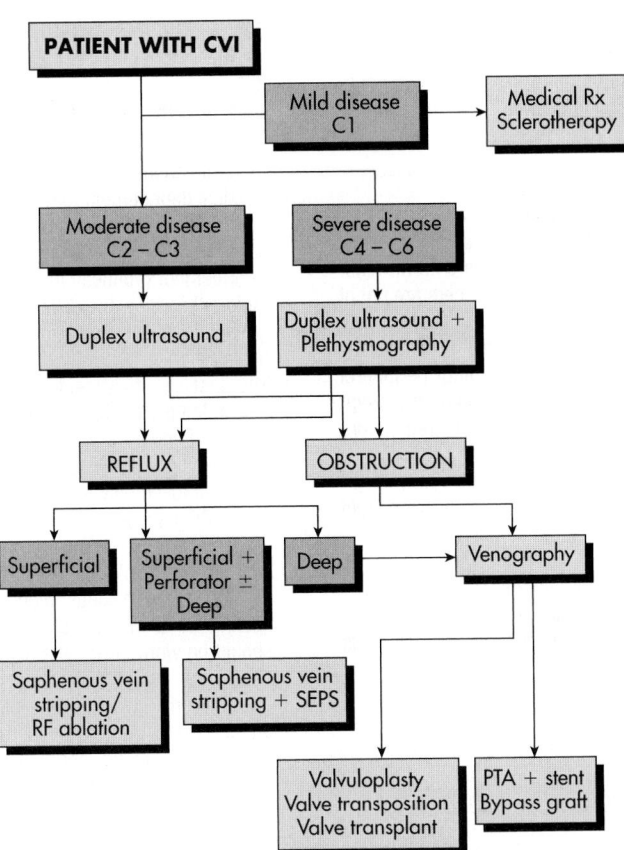

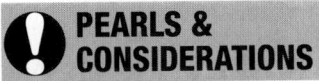

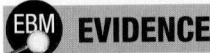

FIG. 5 Evaluation and management of chronic venous insufficiency. (From Cameron JA: *Current surgical therapy "varicose veins"*, Philadelphia, 2004, Saunders.)

- No exam of a leg with CVI is complete without palpation of pulses and/or determination of ankle-brachial index (ABI).

Rx TREATMENT

NONPHARMACOLOGIC THERAPY

- Leg elevation above heart level for 30 min 3 to 4 times a day.
- Weight reduction because obesity is a risk factor for DVT and CVI.
- Walking exercises to improve calf function.
- Physical therapy to improve ankle joint mobility.
- For weeping skin lesions, wet-to-dry dressing changes.

ACUTE GENERAL Rx

- The fundamental role of compression in the treatment of CVI is well recognized and has been validated by randomized controlled trials (RCTs).
- The beneficial effects of gradient compression stockings (decrease in edema and control of discomfort) are due to their effect on microvascular hemodynamics and Starling forces.

- Below-knee compression stocking with a gradient of at least 20 to 30 mm Hg will control edema, alleviate pain, and improve the quality of life in CVI patients.
- Compression stockings are contraindicated in patients with an ABI of <0.6.
- Some patients (acute lipodermatosclerosis) may benefit from nonelastic compression with the Unna gel paste gauze boot to alleviate their symptoms and acute increase in their swelling. The Unna boot is changed once a week.
- Topical corticosteroid creams or ointments (e.g., triamcinolone 0.12% bid) may be used to help reduce inflammation and itching. Steroids should never be applied to ulcer.
- Antibiotics should only be used when treating a clinically apparent, culture-proved infection. Most secondary infections are the result of *Staphylococcus* or *Streptococcus* organisms.
- Diuretics have no role in the treatment of CVI-related edema.

CHRONIC Rx

- While conservative care is fundamental, patients with CVI should be considered for correction of their underlying venous hypertension.

- The majority of patients with CVI have superficial vein or perforator vein reflux as their underlying pathology and would benefit from the newer vein ablation procedures listed below.
  1. Endovenous ablation of superficial (saphenous) or perforator vein reflux.
  2. RF ablation with VNUS closure.
  3. Endovenous laser therapy (EVLT).
  4. Ultrasound-guided foam sclerotherapy.

COMPLEMENTARY & ALTERNATIVE MEDICINE

Several groups of drugs have been evaluated in the treatment of CVI, including coumarins, flavonoids, and saponosides (horse chestnut extracts). These drugs have venoactive properties and are widely used in Europe but are not approved for use in the United States. The precise mechanism of action is not known. Horse chestnut seed extract has been found, in the short term, to be as effective as compression stockings in reducing pain and edema, but long-term efficacy has not been established.

REFERRAL

- Phlebology.
- Vascular surgery.
- Indications for referral.
  1. Skin and subcutaneous changes consistent with CVI.
  2. Associated peripheral arterial insufficiency (PAD).
  3. Longstanding varicose vein disease.
  4. Consideration for vein ablation procedure.

! PEARLS & CONSIDERATIONS

COMMENTS

1. Inflammatory skin changes from CVI are irreversible. The goal of therapy is to eliminate venous hypertension and prevent progression.
2. Venous ulcers are often an end-stage manifestation of CVI. Refer to "Venous Ulcers" for more information.

EBM EVIDENCE

Available at www.expertconsult.com

SUGGESTED READING

Available at www.expertconsult.com

RELATED CONTENT

Stasis Dermatitis (Patient Information)
Varicose Veins (Related Key Topic)
Venous Ulcers (Related Key Topic)

AUTHOR: **FRANK G. FORT, M.D.**

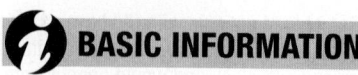

BASIC INFORMATION

DEFINITION

Venous ulcers are defined as chronic defects of the skin that fail to heal spontaneously and persist for longer than 4 weeks. Venous ulcers account for about 70% of all lower-extremity ulcerations. They are usually located in the "gaiter" region and can be accompanied by varicose veins, edema, hyperpigmentation, and lipodermatosclerosis. Venous ulceration develops in patients as a result of sustained venous hypertension.

SYNONYM

Stasis ulcers

ICD-10CM CODES
I87.2	Venous insufficiency (chronic) (peripheral)
L97.909	Non-pressure chronic ulcer of unspecified part of unspecified lower leg with unspecified severity

EPIDEMIOLOGY & DEMOGRAPHICS

In industrialized nations, up to 1.5% of the population will suffer from venous ulcers. In patients ≥65 yr, the incidence increases to 4%. In the United States, >500,000 people suffer from stasis ulcers.

RISK FACTORS

- Obesity.
- Increasing age.
- Family history of chronic venous insufficiency.
- History of deep venous thromboembolism.

PHYSICAL FINDINGS & CLINICAL PRESENTATION

Venous ulcers are most commonly located in the lower leg just above the ankle (gaiter region). They are a partial-thickness, irregularly shaped wound with well-defined borders with granulation tissue and fibrin present in the ulcer base (Fig. 1). Venous ulcers are relatively painless and are surrounded by brown-stained skin and/or dry, itchy, and reddened skin. In about 50% of patients, there are visible varicose veins in an aching, swollen leg.

ETIOLOGY

The exact mechanism of the role of venous hypertension in the etiology of venous ulcers is not certain. Hemodynamic forces such as venous hypertension, circulatory stasis, and modified conditions of shear stress appear to play an important role in an inflammatory reaction accompanied by leukocyte activation that clinically leads to fibrosclerotic remodeling of the skin and then to ulceration.

DIAGNOSIS

DIFFERENTIAL DIAGNOSIS

- Arterial ulcer.
- Neurotrophic ulcers (located predominantly in the foot).
- Vasculitis.
- Pyoderma gangrenosum.
- Ulcerated skin tumors like basal cell or squamous cell carcinoma (Marjolin ulcer).
- Rheumatoid arthritis.

WORKUP

- The history and clinical signs and symptoms of leg ulcers are often misleading and may not differentiate venous ulcers from other leg ulcers; about 30% of leg ulcers are not of venous origin.
- Measurement of the ankle-brachial index (ABI) is essential in excluding peripheral arterial disease (PAD), which can be present in 20% of patients and is required before starting compression therapy. Arterial insufficiency is suggested by an ABI <0.9.
- Patients with lower-extremity ulcers should also be evaluated for diabetes.
- Coagulation defects have been found in 40% of patients with leg ulcers. This finding suggests that many patients with leg ulcers have a known or suspected history of deep venous thrombosis and a thrombophilia workup is indicated.
- If vasculitis is suspected, a biopsy of the edge of the ulcer can confirm the diagnosis.
- Any wound that has failed to improve after therapy of 4 wk should have a biopsy to rule out malignancy.

IMAGING STUDIES

- Evaluation of patients with venous leg ulcer should include duplex sonography to identify reflux in the superficial, deep, and perforating veins as well as possible obstruction of the deep veins.
- If the ulcer appears to be infected, consider tissue for culture, plain x-ray films, and bone scan to evaluate for osteomyelitis.

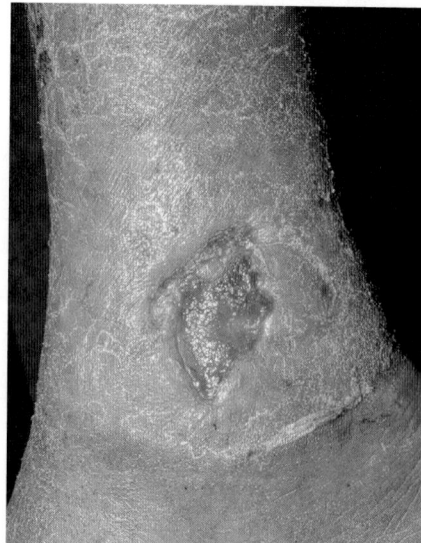

FIG. 1 Stasis ulcer. Any ulcer in this location with surrounding edema, redness, and scale is typical of a stasis ulcer. (From White GM, Cox NH [eds]: *Diseases of the skin, a color atlas and text,* ed 2, St Louis, 2006, Mosby.)

TREATMENT

NONPHARMACOLOGIC THERAPY

- Fig. 2 describes an algorithm for the treatment of venous ulcers.
- Surgical debridement to remove all nonviable material can be accomplished in the office setting with the use of a topical Xylocaine gel. Debridement produces the release of growth factors that allow the development of healthy granulation tissue and the initiation of the healing process.
- The first-line treatment of ulcers includes below-knee compression stockings to improve venous return to the heart, thereby decreasing edema, inflammation, and tissue ischemia (used only if the ABI is between 0.6 and 0.85 because compression can cause limb ischemia).
- There is Level A evidence that graduated compression stockings alone can lead to healing of a venous ulcer. The stockings should be worn during the day and removed at night.
- Regular, brisk walking 30 min a day, five times a week is recommended.
- Elevate leg above heart level and raise the foot of bed with 3-in blocks to reduce edema.
- Role of surgery: in a randomized controlled trial, endovenous catheter ablation of superficial reflux showed no improvement in the healing rate of ulcers but did demonstrate a reduction of ulcer recurrence from 28% to 12% at 12 mo.

ACUTE GENERAL Rx

- Dressings are used under compression stockings to provide a clean, moist environment to promote healing.
- Modern, more complex dressings have been developed and include occlusive and semiocclusive dressings, classified according to their physical composition and ability to control wound drainage.
- Semiocclusive dressings have varying ability to absorb wound drainage. Some examples of this type are hydrocolloids (DuoDerm), hydrogels (DuoDerm hydrogel), foam dressings (Allevyn), and alginates.
- Biologic wound dressings (Apligraf) and tissue-engineered products (Oasis) have been developed, and these products can either directly provide growth factors or indirectly stimulate growth factors in the ulcer bed.
- Pentoxifylline (800 mg tid) has been shown to be an effective adjuvant to compression therapy as reported in a meta-analysis of nine clinical trials.
- Skin grafting should be considered for large or refractory ulcers as long as the wound is clean and there is healthy granulation tissue.
- Published randomized clinical trials on the value of the different types of dressings in the management of leg ulcers have not

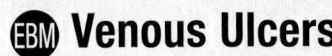

shown effects on ulcer healing. Despite the lack of evidence to support their use, modern dressings remain a part of the standard of care. Decisions regarding their use should be based on local cost of the dressings and the physician's clinical experience.

- Trials involving the use of weekly, low-dose, high-frequency ultrasound for hard-to-heal venous leg ulcers do not support adding therapeutic ultrasound to standard care for venous leg ulcers.

DISPOSITION

The overall prognosis for this condition is poor; the healing rate depends on the initial size of the ulcer. Although 65% to 70% of venous ulcers are healed within 6 mo, the 5-yr recurrence rate of healed venous ulcers can be as high as 40%. Maintenance of lifelong compression therapy is recommended.

REFERRAL

All patients should be evaluated weekly during the first month of therapy. Nonhealing ulcers with little to no improvement should also be referred to a wound care clinic.

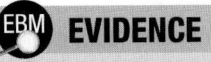 **EVIDENCE**

Available at www.expertconsult.com

SUGGESTED READINGS

Available at www.expertconsult.com

AUTHOR: **FRANK G. FORT, M.D.**

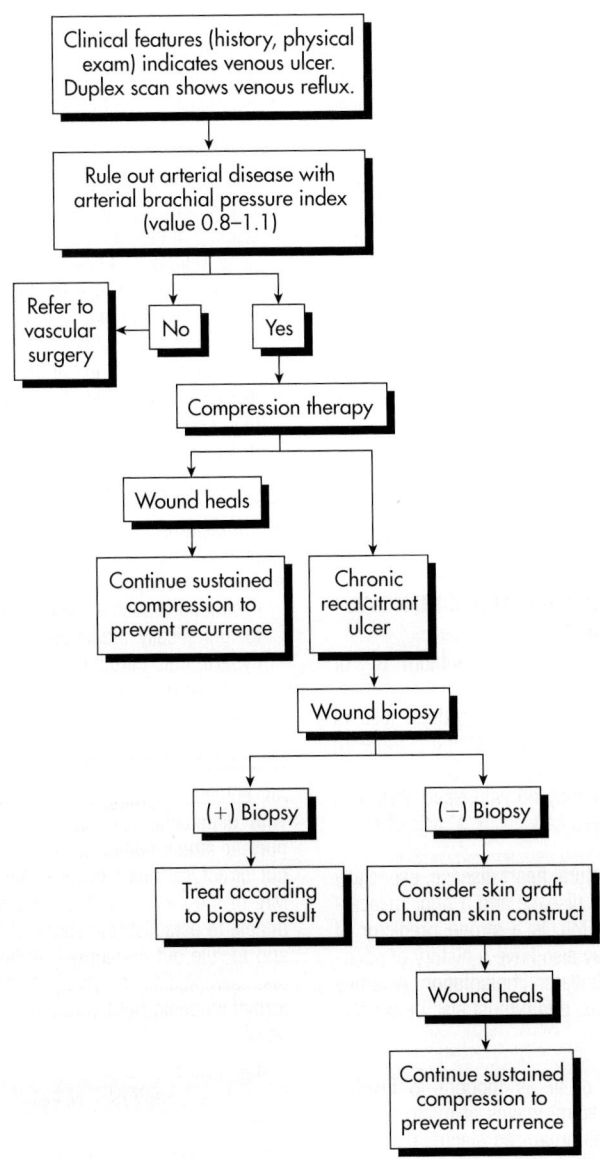

FIG. 2 Scheme for treatment of venous ulcer. (From *Venous stasis ulcers; Conn's current therapy*, St Louis 2008; Elsevier.)

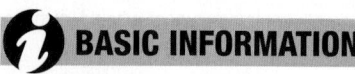
DEFINITION

Ventricular fibrillation (VF) is a rapid, disorganized ventricular arrhythmia that results in no meaningful cardiac output or blood pressure and, if not rapidly interrupted, death. The ECG appearance of VF can evolve rapidly over the course of minutes as the heart becomes more ischemic. Upon initiation, QRST complexes in VF often appear coarse with grossly irregular oscillating complexes of variable rate, axis, and morphology. As VF continues, the QRST complexes become finer, lower amplitude, and slower, eventually resulting in asystole. VF is the leading mechanism of sudden cardiac death.

ICD-10CM CODES
I49.01 Ventricular fibrillation

EPIDEMIOLOGY & DEMOGRAPHICS

INCIDENCE: The true incidence of VF is impossible to know because the majority of these episodes result in sudden cardiac death in unmonitored patients. Sudden cardiac death, as determined by death certificate analysis, is estimated to account for 400,000 to 450,000 deaths per year in the U.S. In small studies in which patients were wearing monitoring at the time of death, the majority of sudden cardiac deaths were caused by VF (60%-70%). The true proportion of sudden cardiac deaths caused by VF is highly dependent on the population studied.

RISK FACTORS:
- The majority (~85%) of sudden cardiac death and VF occurs in patients with coronary artery disease or systolic dysfunction, with 15% of VF occurring in a "normal" heart at autopsy.
- After the age of 35 yr, coronary artery disease predominates as cause of VF; before the age of 35, inherited channelopathies and mild trauma-induced (commotio cordis) etiologies are more common.
- 60% to 70% of patients with VF have CAD.
- 50% of patients with sudden cardiac arrest presenting for cardiac catheterization have an acute artery occlusion.

RISK FACTORS FOR VF IN PATIENTS PRESENTING WITH ACUTE MI

- STEMI
- Baseline repolarization abnormalities
- Larger infarcts
- Hypokalemia
- Male sex
- Inferior infarcts
- Absence of pre-infarct angina

ETIOLOGIES OF VF IN ABSENCE OF STRUCTURAL OR CORONARY HEART DISEASE

- **Long QT syndrome:** estimated prevalence of 1:2000 to 1:5000; the diagnosis is made based on combination of ECG findings and clinical and family history collectively

compiled as Schwartz criteria. Typically inherited as autosomal dominant mutation with variable penetrance, making genetic testing helpful for confirming diagnosis or screening family members.
- **Short QT syndrome:** inherited syndrome characterized by both a short QTc (<350 ms in males and 360 ms in females) and symptomatic atrial fibrillation and VF.
- **Brugada syndrome:** prevalence is 5 to 50:10,000 of autosomal dominant inherited mutation characterized by a classic Brugada pattern on ECG in leads V1-2 combined with syncope or clinical sudden death. The ECG pattern is mutable and not always present within the patient and genetic testing is limited.
- Wolff-Parkinson-White syndrome: 2% to 3% of sudden cardiac arrest due to WPW caused by AF conducting down bypass tract degenerating into VF.
- Idiopathic VF: diagnosis of exclusion typified by VF induced by early coupled PVCs typically emanating from conduction system. Notably suppressed by isoproterenol and quinidine.
- Early repolarization syndrome: typified by 1-mm ST elevation in two sequential inferior or lateral leads. This ECG pattern is quite nonspecific, occurring in 5% to 10% of general population and increasing risk of sudden death by threefold, or roughly 0.3%.
- Commotio cordis: VF as a result of low-velocity projectile impact on the chest wall inducing VF in the absence of sudden death. This is uncommon and occurs in young, typically male individuals.

PHYSICAL FINDINGS & CLINICAL PRESENTATION

- Patients are unconscious, without BP or pulse.
- Witnesses may describe a sudden loss of consciousness, without breathing along with a cyanotic appearance.
- Seizure activity may be witnessed after loss of consciousness caused by a lack of cerebral perfusion.
- History of structural heart disease, especially coronary artery disease and a prior myocardial infarction (MI), is a strong predictor of VF. Patients may also have a history of pacemaker or defibrillator implantation. A family history of sudden death must also be sought.

ETIOLOGY

The mechanism of VF is thought to involve multiple rotating spiral waves of micro reentry without any overall organized electrical activity. This is distinctly different from the predominant mechanism of monomorphic ventricular tachycardia, which is reentry around a fixed zone of slow conduction, typically ventricular scar. VF results from a substrate of heterogeneous repolarization and a triggering event such as critically timed PVC. Repolarization of the heart is an active process requiring ATP to obtain and maintain a negative resting membrane potential via NA/K ATPase ion channels. By depriving a significant amount of myocardium

to oxygen and thus the ability to generate ATP, ischemia can provide both the substrate of VF by impairing the ischemic areas to fully repolarize and allow for a triggering event by allowing spontaneous depolarization. Genetic conditions such as Long QT syndrome can also predispose to VF in absence of ischemia by providing more heterogeneous repolarization within the myocardium.

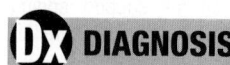
DIFFERENTIAL DIAGNOSIS

Differential diagnosis of an ECG suspicious of VF includes:
- ECG artifact
- Atrial fibrillation with aberration
- Polymorphic ventricular tachycardia

WORKUP

- Lab testing should especially focus on checking K and Mg levels as well as ischemia workup of cardiac biomarkers and ECG when sinus rhythm has been restored.
- A full 12-lead ECG of the tachycardia should always be obtained, whenever possible, and compared to the ECG in sinus rhythm if there is any uncertainty about the diagnosis.
- Ischemia evaluation is paramount, and cardiac catheterization should be performed in most cases.

LABORATORY TESTS

- Potassium, magnesium, and cardiac biomarkers.
- Genetic testing should be reserved for specific situations such as when there is a concern for genetically mediated conditions such as hypertrophic cardiomyopathy, catecholaminergic polymorphic ventricular tachycardia, or Brugada syndrome.

IMAGING STUDIES

An echocardiogram and ischemia evaluation with diagnostic coronary angiography and/or nuclear stress testing is recommended to rule out structural heart disease and ischemia. An MRI of the heart is indicated if these tests are unable to establish the cause of the arrhythmia and to rule out cardiomyopathies such as cardiac sarcoidosis, amyloid, LV noncompaction, arrhythmogenic right ventricular dysplasia, and so on.

TREATMENT

ACUTE GENERAL Rx

Patients with VF are hemodynamically unstable and require emergent unsynchronized defibrillation along with appropriate high-quality CPR as per ACLS protocols.

Antiarrhythmic therapy with IV amiodarone and/or IV lidocaine is appropriate, particularly if patients have more than one event. IV lidocaine is particularly effective if VF is mediated by cardiac ischemia. Cardiac catheterization is recommended provided no contraindications exist.

IV beta blockers are also recommended provided the patient is not in shock and blood pressure is permissive. If the patient had a prolonged down time and was unresponsive after appropriate CPR a hypothermia protocol should be considered to aid in neurologic recovery. If the patient is having multiple episodes of VF despite these measures and is still awake between episodes, sedation and intubation are appropriate to reduce adrenergic drive. Cardiac electrophysiology consultation is appropriate for management of VF.

Electrolyte supplementation is essential if hypokalemia or hypomagnesemia is detected.

CHRONIC Rx

After acute stabilization has occurred, chronic treatment is dependent on circumstances surrounding VF. If VF occurred within 48 hr of a large MI, then relief of ischemia via PCI, CABG, or lytic therapy is the primary treatment. A patient who has a well-defined ischemic trigger that has been satisfactorily treated likely will not require an implantable cardiac defibrillator, but a wearable external defibrillator could be considered under certain circumstances. Patients with VF in the periinfarction period who survive to hospital discharge have a prognosis similar to patients without arrhythmias in the periinfarction period. ICD implantation is recommended in patients when there is not a clearly reversible trigger, such as acute MI, commotio cordis, or drug overdose. If an inherited ion channelopathy is suspected, such as long QT, Brugada syndrome, or CPVT, genetic testing should be performed, but an ICD is appropriate even before definitive diagnosis is made for secondary prevention of sudden death from VF. If cardiac sarcoid, hypertrophic cardiomyopathy, arrhythmogenic right ventricular cardiomyopathy is suspected, consideration of cardiac MRI before ICD implantation is reasonable. If a patient is subsequently diagnosed with inherited arrhythmia syndrome, familial screening should be discussed with the patient.

Cardiac echocardiography plays an important role in long-term risk stratification as well. If a patient's EF remains <35% 3 mo after appropriate revascularization and institution of appropriate heart failure therapy (ACE, beta-blocker therapy), then consideration of ICD is appropriate at that time.

Chronic therapy with antiarrhythmic medications such as amiodarone, mexiletine, or sotalol may be needed even after ICD implantation if the patient presents with multiple appropriate shocks. Continued focus on the trigger of VF such as ischemia or electrolyte disturbance is also critical. Cardiac ablation has been described in rare cases if a distinct triggering PVC is isolated, but this is not as commonly employed as ablation for VT.

DISPOSITION

Patients with sustained VF should be managed in an ICU because of the risk of degeneration to a hemodynamically unstable rhythm. A cardiologist or cardiac electrophysiologist should be consulted.

REFERRAL

All patients with VF should be referred to a cardiologist or a cardiac electrophysiologist.

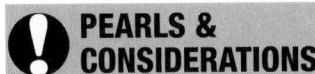

PEARLS & CONSIDERATIONS

COMMENTS

- Effective VF treatment is strongly dependent on identifying and treating the inciting trigger (i.e., ischemia, cardiogenic shock) while using antiarrhythmic therapy IV amiodarone +/- IV lidocaine for stabilization.
- Hypothermia protocol should be considered in patients who have return of spontaneous circulation after VF arrest who remain comatose upon presentation.

- ICDs are indicated for secondary prevention of VF independent of the substrate in the absence of a clearly reversible trigger.
- In the peri-infarction period, VT, particularly VT occurring 48 hr after MI, is far more predictive of subsequent out-of-hospital sudden death than VF and as such often warrants earlier ICD therapy consideration.
- In managing patients with multiple VF events (VF storm), therapies to reduce adrenergic drive are important, such as IV beta blockers as BP tolerates, aggressive IV sedation with propofol or Versed, or fentanyl along with intubation and electrolyte repletion.
- In patients with suspected long QT or Brugada syndrome, VF storm may be managed differently than VF in an ischemic setting or with structural cardiomyopathy. Long QT syndrome VF storm may prompt use of isoproterenol, magnesium repletion, and consideration of atrial pacing to prevent bradycardia. In treating Brugada syndrome VF storm, use of isoproterenol, quinidine, and treatment of fever if it exists can be helpful.

PATIENT/FAMILY EDUCATION

Patients with familial or genetic causes of ventricular arrhythmias should have family screening of first-degree relatives.

SUGGESTED READING

Available at www.expertconsult.com

RELATED CONTENT

Arrhythmogenic Right Ventricular Dysplasia (Related Key Topic)
Brugada Syndrome (Related Key Topic)
Hypertrophic Cardiomyopathy (Related Key Topic)
Long QT Syndrome (Related Key Topic)
Torsade de Pointes (Related Key Topic)

AUTHOR: **SHAW NATAN, M.D.**

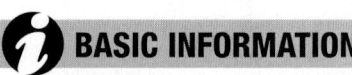

DEFINITION

- *Ventricular septal defect* (VSD) refers to an abnormal communication through the septum that separates the right and left ventricles of the heart.
- VSDs may be large or small, single or multiple.
- VSDs are located at various anatomic regions of the septum and classified as follows:
  1. Membranous (75%-80%): This is the most common type of defect, and it extends into the membranous portion of the interventricular septum. The septal leaflet of the tricuspid valve may become adherent and form a "pouch" of the septum that can limit the left-to-right shunting and lead to self-closure.
  2. Muscular or trabecular (5%-20%): This defect is entirely surrounded by muscular tissue. Often has less hemodynamic impact, and spontaneous closure is common.
  3. Canal or inlet (8%): This defect commonly lies beneath the septal leaflet of the tricuspid valve; associated with Down syndrome.
  4. Subarterial, outlet, infundibular, or supracristal (5%-7%): This is the least common type of defect. It is usually found beneath the aortic valve, and it may lead to aortic regurgitation. High prevalence in Asian population.

SYNONYM

VSD

ICD-10 CODES
Q21.0 Ventricular septal defect
I23.2 Ventricular septal defect as current complication following acute myocardial infarction

EPIDEMIOLOGY & DEMOGRAPHICS

- VSDs are one of the most common congenital heart abnormalities.
- VSD accounts for ~25% of all congenital heart defects in children and for approximately 10% of defects in adults (the decrease is a result of spontaneous closure that occurs by adulthood, with the majority occurring prior to 3 UTIs of age).
- The prevalence of VSD is 3 to 3.5 infants per 1000 live births and 0.5/1000 adults.
- VSD is found with equal frequency among both males and females.
- VSD may be associated with the following conditions:
  1. Atrial septal defect (35%)
  2. Patent ductus arteriosus (22%)
  3. Coarctation of the aorta (17%)
  4. Subvalvular aortic stenosis (4%)
  5. Subpulmonic stenosis, usually associated with progressive aortic regurgitation caused by prolapse of the aortic cusp through the defect

- Multiple VSDs are more prevalent among patients with tetralogy of Fallot and double-outlet right ventricular defects.

PHYSICAL FINDINGS & CLINICAL PRESENTATION

- Clinical presentation depends on the direction and volume of the VSD shunt, which is dictated by the size of the defect and the ratio of the pulmonary vascular resistance. Fig. 1 illustrates the physiology of VSD.
  1. Defects of ≤25% of the aortic annulus diameter are small defects. These typically involve small left-to-right shunts, no left ventricular volume overload, and no pulmonary artery hypertension (PAH).
  2. Defects that are 25% to 75% of aortic annulus diameter are considered to be moderate in size. Small to moderate left-to-right shunting, mild to moderate left ventricular volume overload, and mild or no pulmonary artery hypertension are seen. Patients may have symptoms of congestive heart failure that may improve with medical therapy or with age as the defect decreases in size relative to increasing body size.

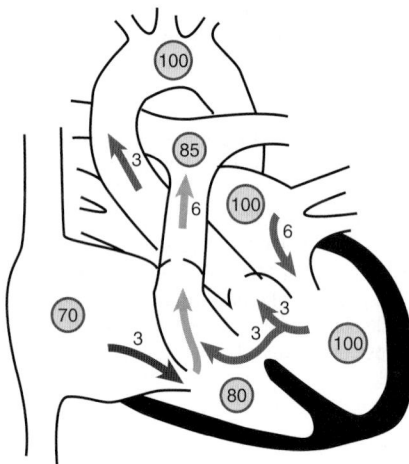

FIG. 1 Physiology of a large ventricular septal defect (VSD). Circled numbers represent oxygen saturation values. The numbers next to the arrows represent volumes of blood flow (in L/min/m²). This illustration shows a hypothetical patient with a pulmonary-to-systemic blood flow ratio (Qp:Qs) of 2:1. Desaturated blood enters the right atrium from the vena cava at a volume of 3 L/min/m² and flows across the tricuspid valve. An additional 3 L of blood shunts left to right across the VSD, the result being an increase in oxygen saturation in the right ventricle. Six liters of blood is ejected into the lungs. Pulmonary arterial saturation may be further increased because of incomplete mixing at right ventricular level. Six liters returns to the left atrium, crosses the mitral valve, and causes a mid-diastolic flow rumble. Three liters of this volume shunts left to right across the VSD, and 3 L is ejected into the ascending aorta (normal cardiac output). (From Kliegman RM et al: *Nelson textbook of pediatrics*, ed 19, Philadelphia, 2011, Saunders.)

3. Defects of ≥75% of the aortic annulus diameter usually have moderate to large left-to-right shunting, left ventricular volume overload, and pulmonary artery hypertension. These patients usually have a history of congestive heart failure, or they may possibly develop right-to-left shunting in the setting of Eisenmenger's syndrome during late childhood, adolescence, or young adulthood.
- Infants may be asymptomatic at birth because of elevated pulmonary artery resistance. During the first few weeks of life, pulmonary arterial resistance decreases, thereby allowing for more left-to-right shunting through the VSD. This results in a subsequent increase in flow into the lungs, the left atrium, and the left ventricle, which can potentially cause left ventricular volume overload. Tachypnea, failure to thrive, and congestive heart failure may then ensue.
- In adults with VSD, the shunt is left to right in the absence of pulmonary stenosis and pulmonary hypertension. Patients typically manifest symptoms of left-sided heart failure from left ventricular volume overload (e.g., shortness of breath, orthopnea, dyspnea on exertion).
- A spectrum of physical findings may be seen, including the following:
  1. Machine-like holosystolic murmur that is heard best along the left sternal border
  2. Murmur becomes shorter as right heart pressures increase
  3. Systolic thrill
  4. Mid-diastolic rumble heard at the apex
  5. S_3 heart sound
  6. Rales
- With the development of pulmonary hypertension, the following occur:
  1. An augmented pulmonic component of the S_2 heart sound
  2. Cyanosis, clubbing, right ventricular heave, and signs of right heart failure (i.e., as seen with Eisenmenger's complex, with a reversal of the shunt in a right-to-left direction)

ETIOLOGY

- VSD is usually congenital but can be acquired.
- Acquired VSD may result from postsurgical residual leak, trauma, or myocardial infarction.
- Postinfarct ventricular septal defect (PIVSD) typically occurs 1 to 5 days after the event in 0.2% of patients in the current fibrinolytic or primary angioplasty era.

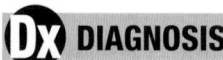 **DIAGNOSIS**

The diagnosis of VSD can be suspected during a physical examination. Imaging studies—particularly transthoracic echocardiography with color Doppler—establish the diagnosis.

DIFFERENTIAL DIAGNOSIS

On the basis of the physical examination alone, the diagnosis of VSD may be confused with other causes of systolic murmurs, such as mitral regurgitation, tricuspid regurgitation, aortic stenosis, pulmonary stenosis, and hypertrophic cardiomyopathy.

WORKUP

Any person who is suspected of having a VSD should undergo an ECG, a chest radiograph, and an echocardiogram.

LABORATORY TESTS

- Laboratory tests are not specific but may offer insight into the severity of the disease.
- The CBC may show polycythemia, especially in patients with Eisenmenger's complex.
- Arterial blood gas results may demonstrate hypoxemia, which does not correct with supplemental oxygen.

IMAGING STUDIES

- ECG findings vary in accordance with the size of the VSD and depending on whether pulmonary hypertension is present. With large VSDs with pulmonary hypertension, right-axis deviation is seen, along with evidence of right ventricular hypertrophy and left atrial enlargement.
- Chest x-ray findings in patients with VSD include the following:
  1. Cardiomegaly that results from left ventricular volume overload that directly relates to the magnitude of the shunt
  2. The enlargement of the proximal pulmonary arteries along with the redistribution and pruning of the distal pulmonary vessels as a result of sustained pulmonary hypertension (Fig. 2, A)
- Echocardiography is the imaging modality of choice for the diagnosis of VSD:
  1. Two-dimensional echocardiography and color Doppler display the size and location of the VSD (Fig. 2, B), the chamber sizes, ventricular function, the presence of aortic valve prolapse or regurgitation, outflow tract obstruction, and the presence of tricuspid regurgitation.
  2. Continuous-wave Doppler approximates the gradient between the left and right ventricles and estimates the pulmonary artery pressure.

3. The magnitude of the shunt can be determined by the calculation of the pulmonary-to-systemic flow ratio with the use of echocardiography.
- Heart catheterization is primarily indicated to assess operability of VSD patients with PAH based on their pulmonary vascular resistance (PVR) and in patients in whom the noninvasive testing was inconclusive, and further information, such as quantification of shunting and assessment of pulmonary pressures, is required.
- MRI, computed tomography or (3D) transesophageal echocardiography can be useful to assess the pulmonary artery, the pulmonary vein, and the aortic anatomy and to confirm the anatomy of unusual VSDs (e.g., inlet or apical defects) that are not seen well with conventional echocardiography.

Rx TREATMENT

The decision to close a VSD depends on the type, size, and shunt severity as well as the patient's pulmonary vascular resistance, functional capacity, and associated valvular abnormalities.

NONPHARMACOLOGIC THERAPY

- Young children and adults with a small, asymptomatic VSD with a large left-to-right ventricular pressure gradient, a pulmonary-to-systemic blood flow ratio (Qp/Qs) of less than 1.4:1, and no evidence of pulmonary hypertension can be observed (i.e., restrictive defect).
- Oxygen for hypoxemia and a low-salt diet are recommended for patients with congestive heart failure.

ACUTE GENERAL & CHRONIC Rx

Closure of the VSD is indicated for the following patients:
- Infants with congestive heart failure. Unrestrictive VSDs require surgical intervention within the first 2 yr of life to prevent pulmonary hypertension.
- Children between the ages of 1 and 6 yr with persistent VSD and a Qp/Qs of >2:1. Adults with a Qp/Qs of ≥2 and clinical evidence of

left ventricular volume overload (class I, level of evidence: B), positive history of infective endocarditis (IE) (class I, level of evidence: C), adults with a Qp/Qs of >1.5 with pulmonary artery pressure that is less than two thirds of the systemic pressure and pulmonary vascular resistance that is less than two thirds of the systemic vascular resistance (class IIa, level of evidence: B), and adults with a Qp/Qs of >1.5 in the presence of left ventricular systolic or diastolic failure (class IIa, level of evidence: B). Surgical closure is not indicated for VSD with severe irreversible PAH with high PVR (class III, level of evidence: B). Although the exact PVR at which a child with VSD and pulmonary arterial hypertension is considered inoperable has not been determined, the consensus is that a PVR of <4 Wood units/m² is considered optimal. PVR of between 4 and 8 wood units/m² is considered on a case-by-case basis. There are no definitive guidelines on the use of vasoreactivity as a preoperative predictor, but a >20% decrease in PVR during vasodilator testing is considered a positive response. Some progress has been made in attempts to use pharmacotherapy to decrease PVR to allow for surgical correction.

Surgical closure with Dacron or Gore-Tex patches or primary surgical closure has long been the gold standard of therapy. It has low operative mortality (<2%) at experienced centers. However, surgery still carries a small risk of complete heart block (CHB), postpericardiotomy syndrome, wound infection, and neurologic sequelae related to cardiopulmonary bypass. The transcatheter approach to VSD closure is becoming an increasingly accepted modality of treatment for appropriately selected patients. Some studies have shown similar success rates for both surgical and percutaneous closures, and there are significantly fewer complications, days in the hospital, and blood transfusions after percutaneous closures. For patients with difficult vascular access, a periventricular approach using a partial median sternotomy allows for a less invasive repair, often without cardiopulmonary bypass.

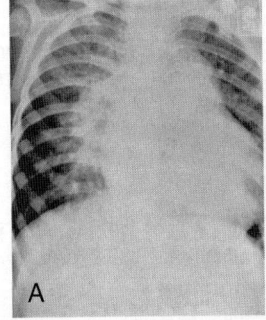
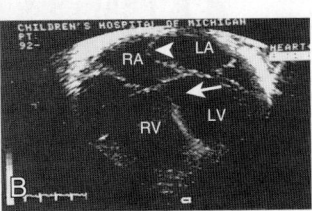

FIG. 2 A, Chest roentgenogram of a child with a large ventricular septal defect, large pulmonary blood flow, and pulmonary hypertension but only mild elevation of peripheral vascular resistance. This is reflected in the evidence of left and right ventricular enlargement, the enlargement of the main pulmonary artery, and a marked increase in pulmonary blood flow. **B,** Apical four-chamber echocardiographic view of ventricular septal defect *(large arrow).* The small arrow points to the interatrial septum. *LA,* Left atrium; *LV,* left ventricle; *RA,* right atrium; *RV,* right ventricle. (**A** from Pacifico AD et al: Surgical treatment of ventricular septal defect. In Sabiston DC Jr, Spencer FC [eds]: *Surgery of the chest,* ed 5, Philadelphia, 1990, Saunders. **B** courtesy of Richard Humes, M.D., Children's Hospital of Michigan, Detroit.)

Catheter-based closure in muscular VSD may be considered, especially if the VSD is remote from the tricuspid valve and the aorta, if the VSD is associated with severe left-sided heart chamber enlargement, or if there is PAH (class IIb, level of evidence: C). Device closure is indicated in residual defects after prior attempts at surgical closure, restrictive VSDs with either a significant left-to-right shunt (Qp/Qs >1.5:1) or history of IE, trauma, or iatrogenic artifacts after surgical replacement of the aortic valve.

Surgery still remains the treatment of choice in patients with large defects, coexistent congenital anomalies requiring surgical correction, and defects with close proximity to the aortic valve. Subpulmonic VSDs may require surgery due to the increased risk of aortic valve prolapse. Perimembranous VSD with more than trivial aortic regurgitation should be referred to surgery. Availability of early reperfusion therapy has led to a decline in incidence of periinfarct VSDs. Surgical closure remains the gold standard in the acute setting or for large (>15 mm) septal ruptures. In the subacute or chronic setting, small or medium PIVSD (<15 mm) can be treated with percutaneous closure with comparable mortality to surgery. Percutaneous closure may also be considered as a temporizing measure to clinically stabilize patients prior to surgical correction. VSDs post myocardial infarctions generally arise within 3 to 5 days of the acute event, and even earlier following reperfusion therapy. PIVSDs usually carry a high mortality rate of ~95% of those treated medically and ~50% with surgical repair. Surgical management within 10 days has better outcomes than waiting for cardiac stabilization.

DISPOSITION

- The natural history of an isolated VSD depends on the type of defect, its size, and any associated abnormalities.
- ~75% to 80% of small VSDs close spontaneously by the time the patient reaches the age of 10 yr.
- Only 10% to 15% of large VSDs will close spontaneously.
- Large VSDs that are left untreated may lead to arrhythmias, congestive heart failure, pulmonary hypertension, and Eisenmenger's complex.
- Eisenmenger's complex carries a poor prognosis, with most patients dying before the age of 40 yr.
- Issues to monitor in adults with unrepaired or repaired and catheter-closed VSDs include the following:
  1. Development of aortic regurgitation
  2. Assessment of associated coronary artery disease
  3. Development of tricuspid regurgitation
  4. Assessment of the degree of left-to-right shunting (in unrepaired or residual VSD after repair)

5. Ventricular dysfunction
6. Assessment of pulmonary pressure
7. Development of subpulmonary stenosis (usually as a result of a double-chambered right ventricle)
8. Development of discrete subaortic stenosis
9. Development of arrhythmia or heart block
10. Thromboembolic complications
11. Infective endocarditis
- After closure, late survival is excellent when ventricular function is normal. Pulmonary artery hypertension may improve, progress, or remain the same. Late operations may be required for tricuspid or aortic regurgitation.

REFERRAL

All infants and children diagnosed with VSD should be referred to a pediatric cardiologist. Adults with VSD should be referred to an adult cardiologist. Cardiothoracic surgeons who have experience with congenital heart disease surgery should be consulted if surgery is indicated.

FOLLOW-UP

- Adults with no residual VSD, no associated lesions, and normal pulmonary artery pressure do not require continued follow-up at a regional adult congenital heart disease (ACHD) center except on referral from the patient's cardiologist or physician.
- Adults with VSD with residual heart failure, shunts, PAH, AR, or RV outflow tract (RVOT) or LV outflow tract (LVOT) obstruction should be seen at least annually at an ACHD regional center (class I, level of evidence: C).
- Adults with a small residual VSD and no other lesions should be seen every 3 to 5 yr at an ACHD regional center (class I, level of evidence: C).
- Adults with device closure of a VSD should be followed up every 1 to 2 yr at an ACHD center depending on the location of the VSD and other factors (class I, level of evidence: C).
- Patients who develop bifascicular block or transient trifascicular block after VSD closure are at risk in later years for the development of complete heart block and should be followed up yearly by history and ECG and have periodic ambulatory monitoring and/or exercise testing.

❗ PEARLS & CONSIDERATIONS

COMMENTS

- A loud murmur does not imply a large VSD. Small, hemodynamically insignificant VSDs can cause loud murmurs.
- In patients with Eisenmenger's complex, the right-to-left shunting across the VSD

is usually not associated with an audible murmur.
- The risk of patients with unrepaired VSD developing infective endocarditis is 4%. The risk is higher if aortic insufficiency is present.
- For patients with endocarditis, routine antibiotic prophylaxis for dental or surgical procedures is no longer indicated for isolated VSDs, except in the following circumstances:
  1. In the presence of complex congenital heart disease with cyanosis
  2. In the presence of a residual VSD after surgical closure
  3. During the first 6 mo after surgical patch or percutaneous transcatheter closure
- Any patient with a newly diagnosed murmur or hemodynamic compromise after a myocardial infarction should undergo evaluation for possible VSD.
- Pregnancy with a VSD is generally well tolerated in women with small VSDs, no pulmonary artery hypertension, and no associated lesions. Women with large shunts may experience arrhythmias, ventricular dysfunction, and the progression of pulmonary hypertension.
- Women with VSDs and severe pulmonary artery hypertension or Eisenmenger's physiology should be counseled against pregnancy because of associated excessive maternal and fetal mortality. Small perimembranous VSDs (without left heart dilatation) and corrected VSDs have a good prognosis during pregnancy, when LV function is preserved. Prepregnancy evaluation of the presence of a (residual) defect, cardiac dimensions, and an estimation of pulmonary pressures is recommended. Preeclampsia may occur more often than in the normal population. Usually follow-up twice during pregnancy is sufficient, and spontaneous vaginal delivery is appropriate.

SUGGESTED READINGS
Available at www.expertconsult.com

RELATED CONTENT
Ventricular Septal Defect (VSD) (Patient Information)

AUTHORS: **JOHANNES STEINER, M.D.,** and **TRACE BARRETT, M.D.**

BASIC INFORMATION

DEFINITION

Ventricular tachycardia (VT) can be classified based on time (duration) or morphology.

Nonsustained ventricular tachycardia (NSVT) is defined as beats originating from the ventricle, lasting from 3 to 30 seconds or for <30 seconds, at a rate >100/min.

Sustained ventricular tachycardia is defined as above but lasts >30 seconds or produces symptoms in the patient and/or requires early intervention due to hemodynamic embarrassment.

Ventricular tachycardia can be monomorphic or polymorphic (see Fig. 1), and the etiology, significance, and treatment of these two types of VT are different.

SYNONYMS

VT
Nonsustained paroxysmal ventricular tachycardia (NSVT)
Sustained ventricular tachycardia
Ventricular tachycardia, monomorphic
Ventricular tachycardia, nonsustained
Ventricular tachycardia, paroxysmal
Ventricular tachycardia, polymorphic
Ventricular tachycardia, sustained

ICD-10CM CODES
I47.2 Ventricular tachycardia

EPIDEMIOLOGY & DEMOGRAPHICS

INCIDENCE: The actual incidence and prevalence of VT in the general population is unknown. VT, especially NSVT, can be seen in both structurally normal and abnormal hearts, although it is far more common in the latter. In apparently healthy, asymptomatic individuals, the incidence is estimated at 0% to 3% (1).

For details on incidence of NSVT in various cardiac conditions, please refer to Table 1.

RISK FACTORS: The presence of structural heart disease is a strong risk factor for VT, but there are multiple, specific types of VT seen in patients without any structural heart disease.

PHYSICAL FINDINGS & CLINICAL PRESENTATION

• Patients may be asymptomatic, or they may present with any combination of palpitations, dizziness, syncope, chest pain, shortness of breath, seizures, or even cardiac arrest.
• History of structural heart disease, especially coronary artery disease and a prior

TABLE 1 Reported Prevalence of Nonsustained Ventricular Tachycardia in Different Cardiac Conditions

Condition	Prevalence
Apparently healthy individuals	0-3%
Non-ST ACS (2 to 9 days after admission)	18-25%
Acute MI (early phase)	45-75%
Reperfused acute MI (later than 1 week)	7-13%
Heart failure (LVEF <30-40%)	30-80%
DCM	40-50%
HCM	25-80%
Significant valve disease	≤25%
Hypertension	8%
Hypertension and left ventricular hypertrophy	12%-28%

DCM, Dilated cardiomyopathy; *HCM,* hypertrophic cardiomyopathy; *LVEF,* left ventricular ejection fraction; *MI,* myocardial infarction; *Non-ST ACS,* non–ST-segment elevation acute coronary syndrome.
From Saksena S et al.: *Electrophysiological disorders of the heart,* ed 2, Philadelphia, Elsevier (Table 43.1).

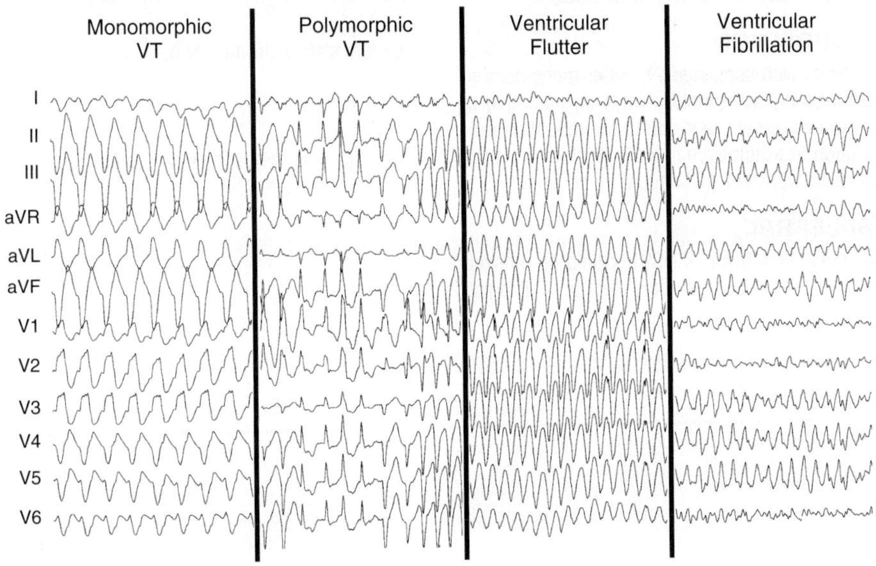

myocardial infarction, is a strong predictor of VT. Patients may also have a history of pacemaker or defibrillator implantation. A family history of sudden death must also be sought.
• Physical findings of AV dissociation may be seen by the astute observer. These include cannon A waves in the neck and variability in intensity of heart sounds. The patient may also present physical findings of congestive heart failure including an S3 gallop, pedal edema, or crackles at the lung bases.
Fig. E2 shows initiation and termination of VT by means of programmed ventricular stimulation.

ETIOLOGY

Sustained monomorphic VT is mostly caused by reentry around a scar in the ventricular wall. The scar is most commonly the result of an old myocardial infarction, but arrhythmogenic RV cardiomyopathy (ARVC), nonischemic dilated cardiomyopathy, sarcoidosis, Chagas disease, tuberculosis, surgical incisions for repair of congenital heart disease and ventricular volume reduction surgery can all cause scars in the myocardium. Fibrosis in the scar creates areas of anatomical conduction block, and fibrosis between surviving myocytes reduces cell-to-cell coupling, thereby distorting the path of propagation and causing areas of slow conduction, which promotes reentry.

Monomorphic VT can also be seen in patients without any evidence of structural heart disease (idiopathic VT). This subgroup represents 10% of all patients with VT and includes RVOT VT and fascicular VT. Common sites of origin of idiopathic VT include the right ventricular outflow tract (most common), the left ventricular outflow tract, the regions near the anterior and posterior left fascicles, and the papillary muscles.

Polymorphic VT is usually the result of active myocardial ischemia, electrolyte abnormalities (hypokalemia, hypomagnesemia) or genetic conditions such as LQTS, BRS, and CPVT. It may also be seen in HCM, various types of nonischemic cardiomyopathy, and idiopathic VF. The mechanisms are poorly understood but likely involve an initiating trigger that interacts with multiple rotors in the substrate to maintain the arrhythmia.

DIAGNOSIS

DIFFERENTIAL DIAGNOSIS

Differential diagnosis of an ECG suspicious of VT includes:
• SVT with aberrancy, either with a preexisting bundle branch block or a rate-related bundle branch block
• SVT in a patient taking anti-arrhythmic drugs, e.g., IA or IC agents
• Antidromic tachycardia from ventricular preexcitation
• Ventricular paced rhythms
• ECG artifact
The following ECG characteristics strongly favor VT as opposed to SVT: Northwest axis, QRS

FIG. 1 Surface ECG of different types of VT. (From Issa, Miller, Zipes [eds]: *Clinical arrhythmology and electrophysiology,* ed 1, p. 405, Fig. 18.1, Philadelphia, Saunders, Elsevier.)

width >160 ms, AV dissociation, fusion beats, and capture beats. The last three are highly specific for VT.

WORKUP

- Lab testing should especially focus on checking K and Mg levels.
- A full 12-lead ECG of the tachycardia should always be obtained, whenever possible, and compared to the ECG in sinus rhythm if there is any uncertainty about the diagnosis.
- This should be followed by an echocardiogram and ischemia evaluation with diagnostic coronary angiography and/or nuclear stress testing. Exercise testing should be performed because it may aid in provoking as well as establishing patient response to exercise-induced arrhythmias, including catecholaminergic VT.
- An MRI of the heart is indicated if these tests are unable to establish the cause of the arrhythmia.
- Ambulatory ECG, event monitors, and implantable recorders are appropriate to evaluate for QT interval changes and T-wave alternans, judge therapy, evaluate risk, and to allow for symptom-rhythm correlation.
- Electrophysiologic testing is useful for the inducibility of VT, to guide ablation, the evaluation of drug effects, the assessment of the risk of recurrent VT, the loss of consciousness with arrhythmia as a suspected cause, and the assessment of indications for ICD therapy.

LABORATORY TESTS

- Potassium, magnesium
- Genetic testing should be reserved for specific situations, i.e., when there is a concern for genetically mediated conditions such as HCM, CPVT, or BRS

IMAGING STUDIES

An echocardiogram and ischemia evaluation with diagnostic coronary angiography and/or nuclear stress testing is recommended to rule out structural heart disease and ischemia. An MRI of the heart is indicated if these tests are unable to establish the cause of the arrhythmia, to rule out cardiomyopathies such as cardiac sarcoidosis, amyloid, LV noncompaction, arrhythmogenic right ventricular dysplasia, etc.

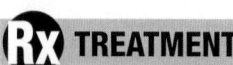 **TREATMENT**

ACUTE GENERAL Rx

Patients with VT may become hemodynamically unstable very quickly. In such situations emergency synchronized cardioversion (or defibrillation for polymorphic rhythms) is needed. Those who subsequently become pulseless or unresponsive should be managed as per standard ACLS resuscitation protocols.

If the patient is hemodynamically stable, either IV amiodarone, lidocaine (especially if there is a suspicion of ongoing ischemia) or procainamide may be used. In the case of a patient with sustained monomorphic VT and a known structurally normal heart, IV beta blockers or calcium blockers may be used. It must be remembered that use of all these agents may be associated with hemodynamic deterioration and an external defibrillator must be made available at all times.

Electrolyte supplementation is essential if hypokalemia or hypomagnesemia is detected.

CHRONIC Rx

An implantable cardioverter-defibrillator (ICD) is indicated for all cases of hemodynamically untolerated monomorphic VT in patients with structural heart disease or prior MI (in the absence of a successful catheter ablation that eliminates all VT, which is usually possible only in patients with normal LVEF and stable VT), since it indicates the presence of a scar and risk of subsequent arrhythmias. Patients with idiopathic VT and structurally normal hearts generally do not require an ICD, but in cases of syncope associated with VT that cannot be successfully treated with ablation, it may be considered. For polymorphic VT, a reversible cause such as ischemia or electrolyte disturbances can sometimes be found, and an ICD may not be appropriate under these circumstances.

Chronic therapy with antiarrhythmic medications such as amiodarone, mexiletine, or sotalol may be needed even after ICD implantation if the patient presents with multiple appropriate shocks. Cather ablation of VT, particularly if performed early after first appropriate ICD discharge, is also very effective in preventing further ICD discharges and is associated with improved acute and long-term outcomes.

DISPOSITION

Patients with sustained VT, either monomorphic or polymorphic, should always be managed in an intensive care unit due to the risk of degeneration to a hemodynamically unstable rhythm. An electrophysiologist should be consulted.

REFERRAL

All patients with VT or NSVT should be referred to a cardiologist or a cardiac electrophysiologist.

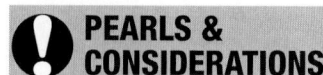 **PEARLS & CONSIDERATIONS**

COMMENTS

- Use of antiarrhythmic drugs, especially IC agents, to treat NSVT is associated with increased mortality (CAST trial), while beta blockers have been shown to be helpful.
- In patients with coronary disease, NSVT has not been shown to have an adverse significance if LVEF is >40%. If the EF is below 40%, the MUSTT trial showed a benefit of EP-guided ICD therapy over antiarrhythmic agents such as mexiletine, propafenone, sotalol, or amiodarone. Patients with LVEF <35% are candidates for prophylactic ICD implantation based on the MADIT II and SCDHeFt trials.
- In hypertrophic cardiomyopathy, NSVT does seem to confer an increased risk of sudden death, especially if symptomatic, prolonged, or repetitive.
- There are certain conditions in which NSVT does not seem to have an adverse significance and does not predict sudden cardiac death. These include nonischemic dilated cardiomyopathy, mitral valve prolapse, mitral regurgitation, and absence of structural heart disease.

PATIENT/FAMILY EDUCATION

Patients with familial or genetic causes of ventricular tachycardia should have family screening of first-degree relatives.

RELATED TOPICS

Arrhythmogenic Right Ventricular Dysplasia (Related Key Topic)
Brugada Syndrome (Related Key Topic)
Long QT Syndrome (Related Key Topic)
Torsade des Pointes (Related Key Topic)

SUGGESTED READINGS

Available at www.expertconsult.com

AUTHOR: **SIMON GRINGUT, M.D.**

BASIC INFORMATION

DEFINITION

Vertebral compression fractures (VCFs) are defined as fractures of spinal vertebrae in which a bony surface is driven toward another bony surface. These fractures are classified as radiographic reductions in vertebral body height of more than 15%.

SYNONYMS

Thoracolumbar vertebral compression fractures
Osteoporotic fractures

ICD-10 CODES

M80.0	Post-menopausal osteoporosis with pathologic fracture
M80.4	Drug-induced osteoporosis with pathological fracture
M80.5	Idiopathic osteoporosis with pathological fracture
M80.8	Other osteoporosis with pathological fracture
M80.9	Unspecified osteoporosis with pathological fracture
S32.009A	Unspecified fracture of unspecified lumbar vertebra, initial encounter for closed fracture
S22.009A	Unspecified fracture of unspecified thoracic vertebra, initial encounter for closed fracture

EPIDEMIOLOGY & DEMOGRAPHICS

~700,000 VCFs occur in the United States each year, and they affect up to 25% of postmenopausal women. They are the most common complication of osteoporosis. The prevalence increases with age, reaching a peak of 40% to 50% among women aged >80 yr. Compression fractures are also a major concern among men, although their rates of VCF are lower.

RISK FACTORS:

- Modifiable: tobacco or alcohol use, osteoporosis, estrogen deficiency (i.e., early menopause, bilateral oophorectomy, premenopausal amenorrhea for >1 yr), frailty, impaired vision, abusive situations, inadequate physical activity, low body mass index, and deficiency of vitamin D or calcium.
- Nonmodifiable: advanced age, female gender, dementia, Caucasian descent, history of fractures in adulthood and among first-degree relatives, and falls.

PHYSICAL FINDINGS & CLINICAL PRESENTATION

- Asymptomatic: Most VCFs are asymptomatic, except for height loss or kyphosis (i.e., dowager's hump [Fig. 1]), which is often a sign of multiple VCFs and height loss of >6 cm has a sensitivity/specificity of 94% and 30%, respectively, for VCF.
- Symptomatic: When symptomatic, VCFs usually present as acute back pain after activity (e.g., bending, lifting) or coughing; neck strain and radicular rib pain may also be present.

ETIOLOGY

- VCFs take place when the combination of bending and the axial load on the spine exceed the strength of the vertebral body.
- The primary etiology of VCF is osteoporosis, though a pathologic fracture from an underlying malignancy, typically metastatic disease, must be ruled out.

DIAGNOSIS

DIFFERENTIAL DIAGNOSIS

- Osteoporosis
- Malignancy, most often metastases
- Hyperparathyroidism
- Osteomalacia
- Granulomatous diseases (e.g., tuberculosis)
- Hematologic/oncologic diseases (e.g., multiple myeloma, primary bone malignancy)

WORKUP

- Only one third of VCFs are diagnosed. Guidelines for patient selection for vertebral fractural assessment are described in Box 1.
- VCFs can be clinically suspected from the history and physical alone, though they are often diagnosed incidentally by imaging performed for another indication.
- There may or may not be a specific injury or a remembered event that led to the VCF.

LABORATORY TESTS

Tests to rule out infection or cancer may be helpful, such as a CBC, an erythrocyte sedimentation rate, an alkaline phosphatase level, and a C-reactive protein level; these tests can be reserved for individuals for whom there is clinical suspicion.

IMAGING STUDIES

- Plain frontal and lateral radiographs (x-rays) are the initial imaging method (Fig. 1) and may be sufficient, particularly when no neurologic abnormalities are present. MRI and computed tomography (CT) scans may be uncomfortable or painful for the patient, especially during the acute phase.
- Although CT scans are not routinely necessary for the diagnosis, they can be helpful for visualizing fractures that are not seen on plain films, for evaluating the integrity of the posterior vertebral wall, for ruling out other causes of back pain, for detecting spinal canal narrowing, and for assessing instability.
- MRI may be useful when spinal cord compression is suspected, if neurologic symptoms are present, or to distinguish malignancy from osteoporosis (e.g., in patients <55 yr with VCF after minimal or no trauma).
- Bone density studies may be helpful to determine the severity of osteoporosis, which is a key risk factor for future fractures.

TREATMENT

NONPHARMACOLOGIC THERAPY

- Physical therapy.

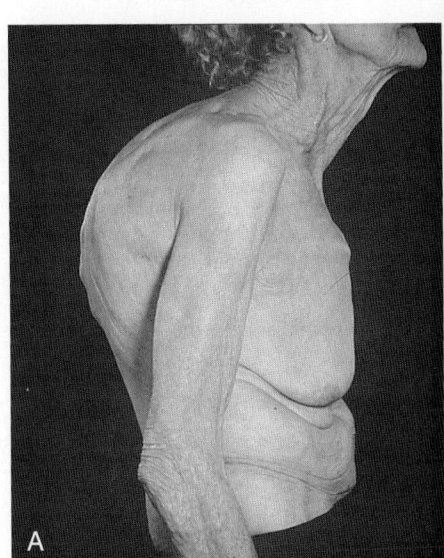
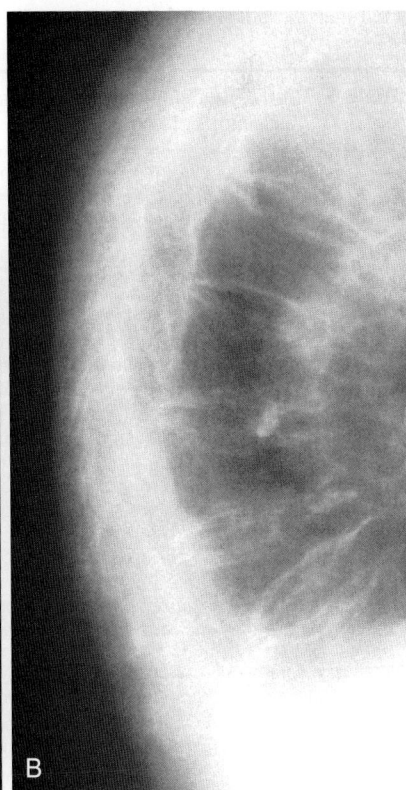

FIG. 1 Dowager's hump. A, Marked thoracic kyphosis due to multiple osteoporotic fractures in an elderly woman with corresponding radiograph (**B**). (From Hochberg MC et al [eds]: *Rheumatology*, ed 3, St Louis, 2003, Mosby.)

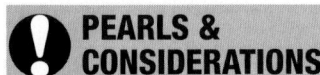
- External back braces: Frequently recommended to relieve pain and improve mobility, however, controlled trials have not shown any effect in patients with vertebral compression fractures.
- Exercise programs: Getting active as soon as possible is extremely important for both short- and long-term recovery.

ACUTE GENERAL Rx

- Analgesics are first line for pain control, including acetaminophen and opioids (oral or parenteral), and pain can be expected to diminish over 4 to 6 wk.
- Nonsteroidal antiinflammatory drugs are helpful but must be used with caution among elderly patients or when contraindicated.
- Muscle relaxants should be used judiciously because they have significant side effects, particularly in the elderly.
- Intranasal calcitonin (200 units once daily, alternating nostrils) has been shown in some small trials to hasten relief from pain when used as an adjunct to oral analgesics, and a 2- to 4-wk course may be useful for patients who do not achieve adequate control with oral analgesics alone.
- Early mobilization with physical therapy is important for recovery and prevention of subsequent fractures.
- The efficacy of vertebroplasty versus kyphoplasty versus conservative treatment remains controversial.
- Percutaneous vertebroplasty involves the injection of acrylic bone cement into the affected vertebral body in an effort to stabilize the fracture and reduce pain, whereas

in kyphoplasty, a high-pressure inflatable bone tamp or balloon is expanded within the body of the affected vertebra to restore prefracture vertebral height before the injection of bone cement. These two procedures were thought to be helpful in patients who did not respond to conservative therapy; however, further studies showed them to be no more effective than sham procedures (Buchbinder et al., 2009; Kallmes et al., 2009). Nonetheless, Klazen et al. (2010) demonstrated in an open-label prospective randomized trial that for the subgroup of patients with acute osteoporotic VCFs and persistent pain, percutaneous vertebroplasty may provide immediate pain relief, sustained for at least a year, which may be significantly greater than that achieved with conservative treatment. Zampini (2010) showed in a nonrandomized cohort study that elderly patients who underwent kyphoplasty were more likely to be discharged home. McCullough et al. (2013) analyzed Medicare claims of patients with VCF treated with kyphoplasty or vertebroplasty compared with medical management and found no difference in mortality or major medical outcomes but decreased health care utilization in the conservatively managed group. These procedures are still in their infancy, and more answers should be forthcoming as to their efficacy, as well as questions regarding the amount of time that conservative therapy alone should be pursued and which procedure, if any, should be advised. Most current guidelines recommend 4 to 6 wk of medical therapy before

pursuing surgical intervention in neurologically intact VCF.

CHRONIC Rx

Osteoporosis should be treated with the reduction of risk factors (e.g., smoking, alcohol), diet, exercise, calcium and vitamin D supplements, and with medications used to treat osteoporosis (e.g., bisphosphonates).

REFERRAL

Referral is indicated for neurologic abnormalities, unremitting pain, instability, continued disability, or when the investigation of the cause of the fracture reveals serious underlying pathology.

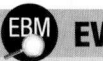 **PEARLS & CONSIDERATIONS**

Prevention of osteoporosis and conservative therapy remain the mainstay of treatment.

COMMENTS

- VCFs should be suspected in anyone aged >50 yr with the acute onset of low back pain. There are many opportunities for diagnosis and treatment that are easy to miss, especially for males.
- Solitary vertebral fractures higher than T7 are unusual and should raise suspicion for other pathologic causes.
- Diagnosing and treating osteoporosis reduce the incidence of VCFs.
- Getting people with VCF physically active as soon as possible will be efficacious both acutely and in the long term.
- In general, VCF will be best managed through a partnership of the patient, the primary care physician, an orthopedist, a physical therapist, a dietitian, and a social worker.

PREVENTION

Reducing the effects of modifiable risk factors is key.

EBM EVIDENCE

Available at www.expertconsult.com

SUGGESTED READINGS

Available at www.expertconsult.com

AUTHOR: **THOMAS J.T. ANDERSON, M.D.**

BOX 1	2007 ISCD Guidelines for Patient Selection for Vertebral Fractural Assessment

- Postmenopausal women with low bone mass (osteopenia) by BMD criteria, *plus* any one of the following: age >70 yr, historical height loss >4 cm (1.6 in), or prospective height loss >2 cm (0.8 in), self-reported vertebral fracture (not previously documented)
- Two or more of the following: age 60 to 69 yr, self-reported prior non-vertebral fracture, historical height loss of 2 to 4 cm, or chronic systemic diseases associated with increased risk of vertebral fractures (e.g., moderate to severe COPD or COAD, seropositive rheumatoid arthritis, Crohn's disease)
- Men with low bone mass (osteopenia) by BMD criteria, *plus* any one of the following: age >80 yr, historical height loss >6 cm (2.4 in), prospective height loss >3 cm (1.2 in), self-reported vertebral fracture (not previously documented)
- Two or more of the following: age 70 to 79 yr, self-reported prior non-vertebral fracture, historical height loss of 3 to 6 cm, on pharmacologic androgen deprivation therapy or following orchiectomy, chronic systemic diseases associated with increased risk of vertebral fractures (e.g., moderate to severe COPD or COAD, seropositive rheumatoid arthritis, Crohn's disease)
- Women or men on chronic glucocorticoid therapy (equivalent to 5 mg or more of prednisone daily for 3 mo or longer)
- Postmenopausal women or men with osteoporosis by BMD criteria, if documentation of one or more vertebral fractures will alter clinical management

BMD, Bone mineral density; *COAD*, chronic obstructive airways disease; *COPD*, chronic obstructive pulmonary disease; *ISCD*, International Society for Clinical Densitometry.

Reproduced with permission from the International Society for Clinical Densitometry.
From Hochberg MC et al: *Rheumatology*, ed 5, St Louis, 2011, Mosby.

BASIC INFORMATION

DEFINITION

Vestibular neuronitis is a syndrome of sudden-onset dysfunction of the peripheral vestibular system, often severe, with prolonged vertigo, nausea, and vomiting.

SYNONYMS

Vestibular neuritis
Acute neuritis
Neurolabyrinthitis
Vestibular neuropathy

ICD-10CM CODES
H81.2   Vestibular neuronitis
H81.23 Vestibular neuronitis, bilateral
H81.20 Vestibular neuronitis, unspecified ear
H81.21 Vestibular neuronitis, right ear
H81.22 Vestibular neuronitis, left ear

EPIDEMIOLOGY & DEMOGRAPHICS

Vestibular neuritis is the second most common cause of peripheral vestibular vertigo with an incidence of about 3.5:100,000 population. Although etiology remains uncertain, it is thought to result from viral infection causing selective inflammation of the vestibular nerve. Infectious origin is supported by the fact that it occurs in epidemics, may affect several family members, and occurs more commonly in spring and early summer. The male-to-female ratio is nearly 1:1. There is selective damage to the superior part of the vestibular labyrinth, supplied by the superior vestibular portion of the eighth cranial nerve.

PHYSICAL FINDINGS & CLINICAL PRESENTATION

Course: develops acutely over a period of hours and resolves over periods of days or weeks, although long-term sequelae may occur, such as residual imbalance and nonspecific dizziness persisting for months. Symptoms include vertigo, spontaneous peripheral nystagmus, positive head-thrust test, and imbalance. Patients report intense sensation of rotation and difficulty standing and walking and tend to veer toward the affected side; autonomic symptoms occur with pallor, sweating, nausea, and vomiting.

ETIOLOGY

Etiology remains uncertain but viral and postviral inflammatory disorders are suspected. Herpes zoster, reactivation of herpes simplex type I, and other viruses have been implicated, but evidence is circumstantial.

DIAGNOSIS

DIFFERENTIAL DIAGNOSIS

- Labyrinthitis: similar symptoms of vertigo, with the addition of unilateral hearing loss
- Labyrinthine infarction
- Acoustic neuroma
- Perilymph fistula
- Brain stem and cerebellar infarction
- Migraine-associated vertigo
- Meniere disease
- Multiple sclerosis

WORKUP

- Patient may fall toward affected side when attempting ambulation or during Romberg tests.
- Hallpike maneuver: checking for nystagmus and asking about recreation of vertigo symptoms
- Head-thrust test: grasp patient's head, apply brief small-amplitude rapid head turn, first to one side and then the other; patient fixates on examiner's nose: positive test is lack of corrective eye movements ("saccades") on affected side. A positive test supports the diagnosis of vestibular neuronitis.
- Laboratory testing and imaging are generally not indicated but may help rule out other etiologies

LABORATORY TESTS

- Electronystagmography (ENG): a battery of eye movement tests that may provide an objective assessment of the vestibular and oculomotor systems and may help localize the lesion's site
- Audiogram: normal

IMAGING STUDIES

Brain imaging: CT or MRI—normal

TREATMENT

NONPHARMACOLOGIC THERAPY

Vestibular exercises, when tolerated, will accelerate recovery.

ACUTE GENERAL Rx

Most treatments are empirical and related to symptoms. Further studies are needed.

- Corticosteroids: corticosteroids are often prescribed, although a recent Cochrane Review finds that there is insufficient evidence for administration. Some studies have shown that glucocorticoids administered within 3 days after onset of vestibular neuronitis may improve long-time recovery of vestibular function and reduce the length of hospital stay and may improve the caloric extent and recovery of canal paresis.

- Antihistamines: e.g., meclizine, dimenhydrinate, promethazine
- Anticholinergics: scopolamine
- Antiemetics: droperidol, prochlorperazine
- Benzodiazepines: e.g., diazepam, valium, lorazepam
- Valacyclovir, either alone or in combination, is likely ineffective in treating vestibular neuronitis.

CHRONIC Rx

- Vestibular rehabilitation exercises
- Anti-GABA agents
- Antihistamines

DISPOSITION

Most patients can be treated as outpatients, but inpatient care may be required in cases where vomiting is uncontrollable. If dehydrated because of severe vomiting, sufferers may require brief parenteral therapy.

REFERRAL

- ENT: if diagnosis uncertain, and if these patients are at risk for benign paroxysmal positional vertigo (BPPV) subsequently; also if symptoms linger
- Neurology: if question of central origin or migraine

PEARLS & CONSIDERATIONS

COMMENTS

- Diagnosis unlikely to be vestibular neuronitis if hearing is impaired or other neurologic signs and symptoms are present.
- Although patients may recover from dramatic acute symptoms, subtle vestibular deficits may linger for prolonged period, if not indefinitely (i.e., residual imbalance and nonspecific dizziness).
- Program of vestibular habituation head movement exercises can reduce imbalance symptoms.

PATIENT & FAMILY EDUCATION

Vestibular Disorders Association: http://www.vestibular.org

SUGGESTED READINGS

Available at www.expertconsult.com

RELATED CONTENT

Benign Paroxysmal Positional Vertigo (Related Key Topic)
Meniere's Disease (Related Key Topic)
Labyrinthitis (Related Key Topic)

AUTHOR: **ROCCO J. RICHARDS, M.D.**

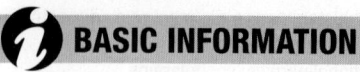

- Vitamin D is a hormone and a steroid and, by definition, not a vitamin. There are two forms of vitamin D: vitamin D_2 and vitamin D_3.
- Vitamin D_2 (ergocalciferol) is mainly found in some plant foods.
- Vitamin D_3 (cholecalciferol) is produced in skin exposed to ultraviolet (UV) B radiation from sunlight (Fig. 1). Gloson, Whistler, and DeBoot independently described rickets in the mid-seventeenth century. Sniadecki first reported the association of rickets with inadequate exposure to sunlight in 1822.
- The major functions of vitamin D include:
  1. Increasing calcium and phosphorus absorption from the small intestines.
  2. Promoting the maturation of osteoclast to resorb calcium from bones.

DEFINITION

Vitamin D deficiency is characterized by impaired bone mineralization. It is classified as a serum 25-hydroxyvitamin D (25[OH]D) level of <20 ng/ml (50 nmol/L).

The consequences of vitamin D deficiency include:
- Bone disease (rickets, osteoporosis, low bone mass)
- May impair reproductive success
- Decrease the ability to combat infection (especially TB, influenza, viral infection)
- May induce or worsen autoimmune disorders
- May increase the incidence of death due to heart disease, IBD, fracture, and cancer of the breast, colon, and prostate

SYNONYMS

The sunshine vitamin
The antirachitic factor
Cholecalciferol

ICD-10CM CODES
E55.9 Vitamin D deficiency, unspecified

EPIDEMIOLOGY & DEMOGRAPHICS

INCIDENCE:
- Vitamin D insufficiency is very high among older adults and hospitalized and institutionalized people.
- Worldwide deficiency and insufficiency affect about 1 billion people.
- Children and young adults: 40% to 50% of preadolescent Caucasian girls, and Hispanic and African American adolescents, are vitamin D deficient.

PEAK INCIDENCE: In the United States, 40% to 100% of the elderly are vitamin D deficient.

60% of nursing home residents may be vitamin D deficient.

PREVALENCE: 42% of African American girls and women 15 to 49 yr old have 25(OH)D levels <20 ng/dl.

PREDOMINANT SEX AND AGE:
- Decreased skin production of vitamin D with age
- Increased prevalence among darker-skinned individuals

RISK FACTORS:
1. Age (due to decreased ability to produce D_3)
2. Sunshine-deficient areas (geographic location, living in higher latitudes)
3. Dark-skinned individuals (melanin competes with vitamin D_3 precursors for UV photons and thus decreases pre-D_3 formation)
4. Obese individuals
5. Institutionalized individuals
6. Pregnant and lactating women
7. Use of sunscreen (sun radiation that causes skin cancer also produces pre-vitamin D_3 in skin)
8. Patients on certain medications that antagonize vitamin D action (phenobarbital, phenytoin)
9. Intestinal resection
10. Severe chronic liver diseases (such as cirrhosis)
11. Kidney disease (e.g., nephritic syndrome)
12. Sarcoidosis and lymphomas (increased catabolism of 25[OH]D to 1,25[OH]2D)
13. Intestinal malabsorption disease (caused by celiac sprue, cystic fibrosis, Whipple's disease)

PHYSICAL FINDINGS & CLINICAL PRESENTATION

- Rickets—seen in children; caused by defective mineralization in the skeleton (Fig. E2).
  1. Bowing of the legs
  2. Leg bone pain
  3. Delayed growth
  4. Seizure due to hypocalcemia
- Osteomalacia—seen in adults
  1. Periosteal bone pain (best detected by putting firm pressure on tibia or sternal bones)
  2. Proximal muscle weakness
  3. Chronic muscle aches/pain
- Fracture with very minimal trauma (brittle and easily broken bones)
- Severe hypocalcemia—especially in late vitamin D deficiency leading to seizure tetany
- Hypophosphatemia
- Neuromuscular
- Paresthesia
- Tetany
- Muscle cramps

ETIOLOGY

- Inadequate exposure to sunlight, such as:
  1. During winter
  2. In nursing home and health care institution residents
  3. With excessive use of sunscreen
- Medications:
  1. Individuals on certain medications, such as phenobarbital, phenytoin, and rifampin (antagonize vitamin D action/increase vitamin D catabolism)
- Diseases and disease states:
  1. Diseases causing vitamin D malabsorption:
     Cystic fibrosis
     Whipple's disease
     Celiac sprue
  2. Diseases increasing vitamin D catabolism:
     Lymphoma
     Sarcoidosis
  3. Intestinal resection
  4. Decreased 25(OH)D production:
     Kidney disease
     Liver cirrhosis

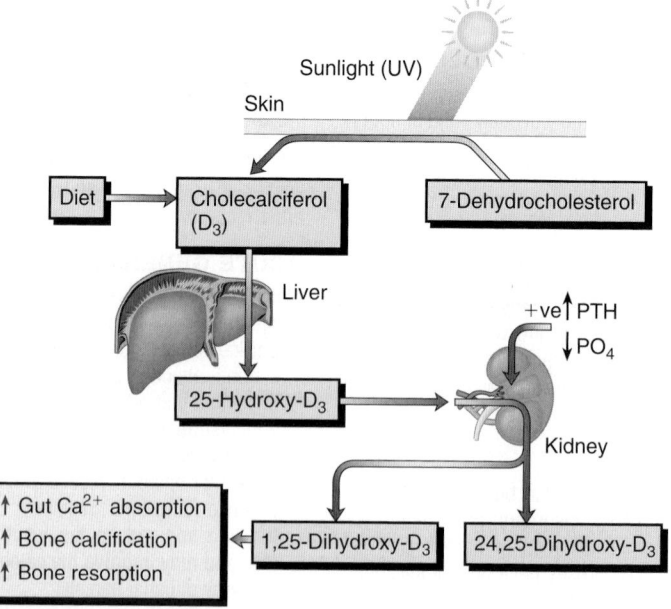

FIG. 1 The metabolism and actions of vitamin D. The primary source of vitamin D in humans is photoactivation in the skin of 7-dehydrocholesterol to cholecalciferol, which is then converted first in the liver to 25-hydroxyvitamin D and subsequently in the kidney to the much more active form, 1,25-dihydroxycholecalciferol (1,25[OH]$_2$,D$_3$). Regulation of the latter step is by PTH, phosphate, and feedback inhibition by 1,25(OH)$_2$,D$_3$. This step can also occur in lymphomatous and sarcoid tissue, resulting in the hypercalcemia that may complicate these diseases. (From Ballinger A: *Kumar & Clark's essentials of clinical medicine,* ed 6, Edinburgh, 2012, Saunders.)

Dx DIAGNOSIS

DIFFERENTIAL DIAGNOSIS

- Arthritis
- Fibromyalgia

WORKUP

- Population-wide screening for vitamin D deficiency is not recommended because evidence to support this practice is lacking.
- Screening is needed for individuals at risk (osteoporosis, history of falls, obese persons, pregnant and lactating women, diseases causing vitamin D malabsorption, African Americans). Workup involves blood and urine tests as well as radiography, as outlined in the next section.

LABORATORY TESTS

- Serum 25(OH)D: this is the best test to determine vitamin D status.
- Parathyroid hormone (PTH): increased levels in vitamin D insufficiency. It is a marker of vitamin D insufficiency.
- Increased (serum or bone) alkaline phosphatase.
- Decreased 24-hour urine calcium (patient should not be on a thiazide).

IMAGING STUDIES

- Radiographs may show:
  1. Pseudofractures of the pelvis, femur, metatarsals
  2. Nontraumatic fractures
- Bone density:
  1. Decreased bone mineral density (osteopenia or osteoporosis).

Rx TREATMENT

NONPHARMACOLOGIC THERAPY

- Natural sources of vitamin D. These include:
  1. Exposure to sunlight. A mild sunburn is equivalent to consuming 10,000 to 25,000 IU of dietary vitamin D.
  2. Dietary sources are not enough to meet daily requirements. Oily fish such as salmon, cod, and mackerel are rich sources of vitamin D_3.
- Foods fortified with vitamin D.
  1. Mainly fortified dairy products.
  2. Fortified orange juice.

ACUTE GENERAL Rx

- Treating deficiency (general population):
  1. 50,000 IU of vitamin D every week for 8 weeks, or
  2. 6000 IU daily to achieve a serum level of 25(OH)D of at least 30 ng/ml.

- Maintenance measures after treatment (general population): 1500 to 2000 IU daily.
- Treating deficiency (obese patients, patients with malabsorption syndromes, or those taking certain medications, as indicated earlier).
  1. 6000 to 10,000 IU daily.
- Maintenance measures after treatment (obese patients, patients with malabsorption syndromes, or those taking certain medications, as indicated earlier):
  1. 3000 to 6000 IU daily.
- After treating deficiency, recheck 25(OH)D in 12 to 14 weeks.

If deficiency persists after several attempts at treatment, try UV B light therapy

REFERRAL

Referral to an endocrinologist is recommended if there is no response to treatment.

PREVENTION

- Food fortification with vitamin D_2 or vitamin D_3.
- Adequate sun exposure, for example, exposure in the middle of the day (between 10:00 AM and 3:00 p.m.).
- Vitamin D supplementation (per the Endocrine Society):
  1. Infants (age range 1-12 mo) require at least 400 IU/day of vitamin D
  2. Children (age range 1-18 yr) require 600 IU/day of vitamin D
  3. Adult supplementation (adults 19-70 yr): 600 IU of vitamin D daily
  4. Adult supplementation (persons ≥70 yr): 800 IU of vitamin D daily
  5. Exceptions: pregnant or lactating women, obese persons, and patients on antiseizure medications, steroids, antifungals, and AIDS medications should be given 2× to 3× more vitamin D
- Screening: recommended only for individuals at high risk for vitamin D deficiency such as blacks and Hispanics, obese individuals (BMI >30 kg/m²), patients with osteoporosis, the elderly, and patients with certain chronic diseases (see "Risk Factors"). According to the U.S. Preventive Services Task Force (USPSTF), current evidence is insufficient to assess the balance of benefits and harms of screening for vitamin D deficiency in asymptomatic adults.

! PEARLS & CONSIDERATIONS

- In the U.S., vitamin D supplements are available by prescription as vitamin D_2 (ergocalciferol) or over the counter as vitamin D_3 (cholecalciferol, usually in 400-1000-IU doses). Both vitamin D_2 and vitamin D_3 are

acceptable as supplements. On average, oral vitamin D_3 raises blood levels more than does vitamin D_2.
- Upper limit of maintenance tolerability in healthy adults is 4000 IU a day. More than 4000 IU of vitamin D daily in nondeficient individuals increases the risk of harm. High-level supplements (>10,000 IU daily) are associated with kidney and tissue damage.
- Vitamin D supplementation is recommended for fall prevention. High-dose vitamin D supplementation (≥800 IU daily) has been shown to be favorable in the prevention of hip fracture and any nonverbetral fracture in persons 65 years of age or older.
- Prescribing more than the recommended daily amount to improve quality of life or prevent cardiovascular disease or death is not advised.
- Trials have shown that low vitamin D levels are associated with depressive symptoms, especially in persons with a history of depression. These findings suggest that measuring vitamin D levels may be useful in patients with a history of depression.
- Vitamin D supplementation, administered with calcium, has been shown to lower the risk for falling and improve muscle strength in the elderly, especially in older vitamin D–deficient women who are at high baseline risk for falling.
- The treatment of vitamin D insufficiency in asymptomatic persons might reduce mortality risk in institutionalized elderly persons and risks for falls but not fractures.
- Recent data suggest that vitamin D deficiency is associated with the risk of developing certain cancers (including breast, colon, and prostate).
- Vitamin D deficiency is associated with some autoimmune diseases (types 1 and 2 diabetes, metabolic syndrome, multiple sclerosis).

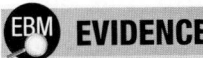

EBM EVIDENCE

Available at www.expertconsult.com

SUGGESTED READINGS

Available at www.expertconsult.com

RELATED CONTENT

Vitamin D Deficiency (Patient Information)
Rickets (Related Key Topic)
Vitamin Deficiency (Related Key Topic)

AUTHOR: **DANIEL K. ASIEDU, M.D., PH.D.**

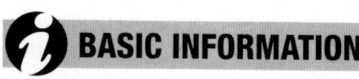

DEFINITION

Vitamins are organic compounds that cannot be synthesized by humans but are required as nutrients in minute amounts. Vitamins have several different functions: They may regulate cell growth and differentiation, as catalysts, as antioxidants, and as co-enzymes. Vitamins are classified as either fat soluble (vitamins A, D, E, K) or water soluble (B group of vitamins and C). Deficiency of most vitamins is rare in Western countries. Certain groups may be prone to vitamin deficiency, and these are discussed here. Vitamin D deficiency is discussed in a separate topic.

SYNONYMS

Vitamin A: retinol
Vitamin E: alpha tocopherol
Vitamin K: phytonadione or menadiol
Vitamin B_1: thiamine
Vitamin B_2: riboflavin
Niacin: vitamin B_3; nicotinic acid
Vitamin B_5: pantothenic acid
Vitamin B_6: pyridoxine; pyridoxal phosphate
Folic acid: vitamin B_9; folate
Vitamin B_{12}: cyanocobalamin
Vitamin C: ascorbic acid

ICD-10CM CODES	
E50	Vitamin A deficiency
E51	Thiamine deficiency
E53	Deficiency of other B group vitamins
E55	Vitamin D deficiency
E56	Other vitamin deficiencies
E56.0	Deficiency of vitamin E
E56.1	Deficiency of vitamin K
E53.0	Riboflavin deficiency
E52	Niacin deficiency [pellagra]
E53.1	Pyridoxine deficiency
E53.8	Deficiency of other specified B group vitamins
E54	Ascorbic acid deficiency

EPIDEMIOLOGY & DEMOGRAPHICS

Deficiency can occur in all age groups but is most common in the elderly.
- Vitamin A deficiency: Affects 250 million preschool children worldwide.
- Vitamin K deficiency: Varies by geographic regions; no race predilection; affects both sexes equally. Encountered often in infants.
- Vitamin B_1 (thiamine) deficiency: Incidence is unknown; no sex, race, or age predilection.
- Vitamin B_5 (pantothenic acid) deficiency: Rare, as it is present in all foods.
- Vitamin B_{12} (cobalamin) deficiency: Relatively common. Occurs in all age groups but more common in the elderly.
- Vitamin B_9 (folic acid) deficiency: Mandatory fortification started in 1998. Prevalence before fortification 16% and after 0.5%. Neural tube defect associated with low maternal folate status during pregnancy. Pregnant women and the elderly are at greatest risk of folic acid deficiency.

- Vitamin C (ascorbic acid) deficiency: Smokers and low-income persons are at increased risk. Fig. 1 shows environmental and nutritional factors in disease.

PHYSICAL FINDINGS & CLINICAL PRESENTATION

- Vitamin A: xerophthalmia, xerosis of the cornea, keratomalacia, Bitot spots (abnormal squamous cell proliferation and keratinization of the conjunctiva), nyctalopia (poor adaptation to darkness)/night blindness, poor bone growth, dry skin and hair, follicular hyperkeratosis (caused by blockage of hair follicles by keratin), pruritus, broken fingernails.
- Vitamin K: clinical manifestation usually occurs if hypoprothrombinemia is present. Major symptom is bleeding to minor trauma. Also can show easy bruisability, epistaxis, hematoma, or gum bleeding.
- Vitamin E: nerve dysfunction (ataxia; hyporeflexia, peripheral neuropathy); bone weakness.
- Vitamin B_1 (thiamine):
  1. Nervous system (dry beriberi): peripheral neuropathy, Wernicke encephalopathy, Korsakoff syndrome.
  2. Cardiovascular (wet beriberi): edema, chest pain, increased heart rate (HR), lowered blood pressure (BP).
  3. Gastrointestinal (GI): anorexia; constipation.
- Vitamin B_2 (riboflavin):
  1. Cheilosis (chapping and fissure of the lip)
  2. Glossitis (sore red tongue)
  3. Oily, scaly rashes on nasolabial folds, eyelids, scrotum, labia majora
  4. Red itchy eyes
  5. Anemia
  6. Peripheral neuropathy
- Vitamin B_3 (niacin):
  1. Pellagra (4 *D*s—diarrhea, dermatitis, dementia, and ultimately death).
  2. Hyperpigmentation of sun-exposed skin.
  3. "Raw beef" swollen and painful tongue.
- Vitamin B_6: seborrheic dermatitis; glossitis, cheilosis, impaired proprioception; sensory ataxia, seizure.
- Vitamin B_{12}: Neurologic symptoms including peripheral neuropathy, ataxia, paresthesia; subacute degeneration of the spinal cord (demyelination of the dorsal column). Patients may also have dementia, depression, and weakness. Glossitis and GI symptoms such as nausea, vomiting, and anorexia are also common.
- Vitamin B_9 (folic acid):
  1. Patchy hyperpigmentation of skin (especially between fingers and toes) and mucous membranes
  2. Moderate fever (temp <102° F) despite the absence of infection
  3. Neural tube defect
  4. Angular stomatitis
  5. Red, beefy, smooth, and shiny tongue.
- Vitamin C: scurvy (poor wound healing, petechiae, follicular hyperkeratosis, fatigue, bleeding gums, weight loss, bone abnormalities [Fig. E2]).

ETIOLOGY

- Fat-soluble vitamins (vitamins A, D, E, K):
  1. Decreased ingestion, malnutrition, eating disorders.
  2. Diseases that affect fat absorption decrease the absorption of fat-soluble vitamins—for example, cystic fibrosis, celiac sprue, inflammatory bowel disease, cholestasis, hepatobiliary disease, small bowel surgery.
  3. Change in vitamin metabolism:
    1. Alcoholism
    2. Drugs such as cholestyramine, warfarin, anticonvulsants, antibiotics (e.g., cephalosporins)
    3. Chronic kidney disease
  2. Increased risk in:
    1. Vegans
    2. Recent immigrants
    3. Refugees
    4. Toddlers/preschoolers living below the poverty line
- Water-soluble vitamins (the B group of vitamins and vitamin C)—there are several etiologic factors, including:
  1. Inadequate intake
  2. Decreased absorption
  3. Alcoholism
  4. Pregnancy/lactation
  5. Peritoneal dialysis
  6. Medications (e.g., isoniazid, phenothiazines, tricyclic antidepressants)
  7. Malabsorption
  8. Low income
  9. Advanced age
- Vitamin B_{12} deficiency—caused by:
  1. Insufficient dietary intake, as in strict vegans
  2. Decreased absorption secondary to intrinsic factor deficiency, decreased intrinsic factor secretion, gastric atrophy, gastrectomy
  3. Terminal ileum disease such as celiac disease, enteritis, tropical sprue
- Folic acid deficiency—increased needs can lead to deficiency (e.g., pregnancy, lactation, malignancy).
- Derangement of folate metabolism by:
  1. Medication (e.g., methotrexate)
  2. Disease (e.g., hypothyroidism)
  3. Increased excretion: as seen in alcoholics

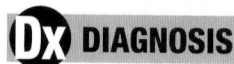 DIAGNOSIS

WORKUP/LABORATORY TESTS

- General initial laboratory tests include:
  1. Complete blood cell count (CBC).
     Liver function tests (LFTs).
     Basic metabolic panel (BMP).
     Albumin.
  2. Measurement of serum levels of the specific vitamin in question.
- Specific tests may be considered in the following cases:
  1. Vitamin A:
  2. Serum retinol level (best test, a direct measure, expensive)

Vitamin	Function	Consequences of deficiency
A	Retinal function, epithelial growth control	Night blindness, keratomalacia, xerophthalmia
B$_1$ (thiamine)	Co-enzyme	Beri beri, Wernicke's encephalopathy
B$_2$ (riboflavin)	Co-enzyme	Dermatitis, glossitis, keratitis, neuropathy, confusion
B$_6$ (pyridoxine)	Co-enzyme	Neuropathy
B$_{12}$ (cobalamin)	Nucleic acid synthesis	Megaloblastic anemia Subacute combined degeneration of spinal cord
Niacin	Co-enzyme NAD, NADP	Pellagra (diarrhea, dermatitis, and dementia)
Folate	Co-enzyme in nucleic acid synthesis	Megaloblastic anemia, villous atrophy of gut
Vitamin C	Co-factor in hydroxylation	Scurvy
Vitamin D	Calcium and phosphate absorption	Rickets (childhood) Osteomalacia (adults)
Vitamin E	Antioxidant	Spinocerebellar degeneration
Vitamin K	Co-factor for coagulation factor synthesis	Bleeding due to coagulation defects

FIG. 1 Environmental and nutritional factors in disease. (From Stevens A: *Core pathology,* St Louis, 2009, Elsevier.)

Retinol binding protein (easier to perform, less expensive)
Dark-adaptation threshold test.
Vitamin K:
○ Prothrombin time/partial thromboplastin time (PT/PTT).
○ Prothrombin.
○ Des-gamma-carboxyprothrombin (most sensitive test).
Niacin: urine-*N*-methylnicotinamide (level <0.8 mg/day indicates niacin deficiency).
Vitamin B$_{12}$:
○ Serum vitamin B$_{12}$ <100 pg/mL is diagnostic of vitamin B$_{12}$ deficiency.
○ Serum methylmalonic acid, which is elevated in B$_{12}$ deficiency.
○ Antiparietal antibody.
○ Intrinsic factor antibody is decreased.
○ Blood smear shows macrocytosis and hypersegmentation of megaloblasts.
○ CBC shows increased mean corpuscle volume (MCV).
○ Megaloblastic anemia.
Folic acid:
○ Check serum folate level

○ Additional testing includes checking for serum homocysteine level, which will be elevated.
○ Red cell folate level shows chronic folate status.

℞ TREATMENT

Most of the vitamins are available over the counter individually or in different multivitamin formulations.
• Specific vitamins:
• Vitamin A deficiency: treat with oral supplementation 10,000 IU daily.
  1. Consume vitamin A–rich foods such as liver, beef, carrots, oranges, mangoes.
  2. 5 servings of fruit and vegetables give enough carotenoids for a day.
• Vitamin K deficiency: treatment depends on the severity of bleeding, administered subcutaneously (SQ) or intramuscularly (IM).
• Vitamin B$_1$ (thiamine) deficiency: give intramuscular thiamine 50 mg for several days.
  1. If B$_1$ deficiency is suspected and patient needs intravenous glucose, give thiamine

first before intravenous glucose. This prevents the development of Korsakoff psychosis.
• Vitamin B$_{12}$ deficiency: give 1000 mcg IM daily for 7 days, then once a week for 1 month, then once a month indefinitely.
  1. A potential option is oral supplementation.
• Folic acid deficiency: daily requirement is 400 to 1000 mcg (1 mg) daily.
  1. Centers for Disease Control and Prevention (CDC) recommend that women of childbearing age take 400 mcg of folic acid daily.

SUGGESTED READING

Available at www.expertconsult.com

RELATED CONTENT

Anemia, Pernicious (Related Key Topic)
Rickets (Related Key Topic)
Vitamin D Deficiency (Related Key Topic)
Wernicke Syndrome (Related Key Topic)

AUTHOR: **DANIEL K. ASIEDU, M.D., PH.D.**

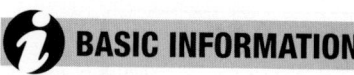

DEFINITION

Vitiligo is the acquired loss of epidermal pigmentation that is characterized histologically by the absence of epidermal melanocytes. There are 6 types based on the extent and distribution of the involved areas: localized (single or few macules in one anatomic area), segmental, generalized, universal (entire body surface is depigmented), acrofacial (fingers, lips), and mucosal.

ICD-10CM CODES
L80 Vitiligo

EPIDEMIOLOGY & DEMOGRAPHICS

PREVALENCE: Vitiligo affects 0.5% to 2% of the population; it is the most common depigmenting disorder.

PREDOMINANT AGE: Vitiligo can begin at any age, but the age at onset is <20 yr for half of patients. Peak onset is between ages 10 and 30. Onset is usually earlier in females.

GENETICS: A positive family history is present in 25% to 30% of patients, and both sexes are equally affected. There are no differences in the rates of occurrence with regard to skin type or race; however, it occurs in more than 8% in some regions of India.

PHYSICAL FINDINGS & CLINICAL PRESENTATION

- Hypopigmented and depigmented lesions (Fig. 1) favor sun-exposed regions, intertriginous areas, genitalia, and sites over bony prominences.
- Areas around the body orifices are also frequently involved.
- The lesions tend to be symmetric.
- Segmental vitiligo (20% of childhood cases and 5% of adult cases) often has a dermatomal or quasidermatomal distribution.
- Vitiligo lesions may occur at trauma sites (i.e., Koebner's phenomenon).
- The hair in affected areas may be white.
- The margins of the lesions are usually well demarcated; when a ring of hyperpigmentation is seen, the term *trichrome vitiligo* is used.
- The term *marginal inflammatory vitiligo* is used to describe lesions with raised borders.

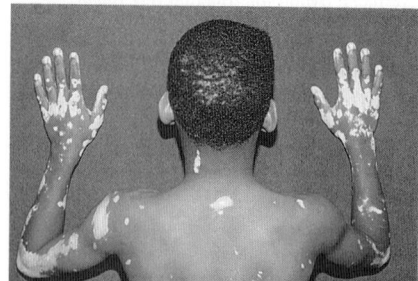

FIG. 1 Multiple, sharply demarcated, symmetric, depigmented areas of vitiligo. (From Behrman RE: *Nelson textbook of pediatrics,* Philadelphia, 2006, Saunders.)

- Initially the disease is limited, but the lesions tend to become more extensive over time.
- Focal vitiligo may affect nondermatomal areas (e.g., glans penis).
- Vitiligo may begin around pigmented nevi and produce a halo (i.e., Sutton's nevus); in such cases, the central nevus often regresses and disappears over time.

ETIOLOGY & PATHOGENESIS

- Three pathophysiologic theories:
  1. Autoimmune theory (i.e., autoantibodies against melanocytes)
  2. Neural theory (i.e., neurochemical mediators selectively destroy melanocytes)
  3. Self-destructive process in which melanocytes fail to protect themselves against cytotoxic melanin precursors
- Although vitiligo is considered to be an acquired disease, 25% to 30% of cases are familial. The mode of transmission is unknown; the condition seems to be polygenic or autosomal dominant with incomplete penetrance and variable expression.
- Associated disorders:
  1. Alopecia areata
  2. Type 1 diabetes mellitus
  3. Adrenal insufficiency
  4. Hyperthyroidism and hypothyroidism
  5. Mucocutaneous candidiasis
  6. Pernicious anemia
  7. Polyglandular autoimmune syndromes
  8. Melanoma
  9. Iritis and retinal pigmentary abnormalities

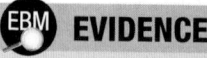

DIFFERENTIAL DIAGNOSIS

- Acquired hypopigmentation disorders:
  1. Chemical-induced (e.g., chloroquine, imatinib, phenolic-catecholic derivatives [e.g., adhesives, deodorants, latex gloves, lacquer resins, varnish, soap antioxidants, insecticides, printing ink, paints, motor oil additives, disinfectants])
  2. Halo nevus
  3. Idiopathic guttate hypomelanosis
  4. Leprosy
  5. Leukoderma associated with melanoma
  6. Pityriasis alba
  7. Postinflammatory hypopigmentation
  8. Tinea versicolor
  9. Vogt-Koyanagi syndrome (i.e., vitiligo, uveitis, and deafness)
  10. Melasma
  11. Mycosis fungoides
- Congenital hypopigmentation disorders:
  1. Albinism, partial (piebaldism)
  2. Albinism, total
  3. Nevus anemicus
  4. Nevus depigmentosus
  5. Tuberous sclerosis
  6. Ito's hypomelanosis

WORKUP

- Inquire about a personal and family history of autoimmune disease.

- A Wood's light examination may enhance the lesions of light-skinned individuals.

TREATMENT

Treatment is indicated primarily for cosmetic purposes when depigmentation causes emotional or social distress. Depigmentation is more noticeable among patients with darker complexions. Combination therapies are associated with more improved repigmentation than monotherapies.

- Cosmetic masking agents (e.g., Dermablend, Covermark) or stains (e.g., Dy-O-Derm, Vitadye)
- Sunless tanning lotions (e.g., dihydroxyacetone)
- Repigmentation (This is achieved by the activation and migration of melanocytes from hair follicles; therefore, skin with little or no hair responds poorly to treatment.)
- Narrow-band ultraviolet B radiation (This is the preferred treatment for nonsegmental vitiligo. It is given twice weekly [not on successive days] during sessions that last from 5 to 10 min. The best results are achieved on the face, trunk, and limbs.)
- Psoralens and sunlight (e.g., PUVAsol)
- Topical mid-potency steroids (e.g., triamcinolone 0.1% or desonide 0.05% cream qd for 3 to 4 mo)
- Topical calcineurin inhibitors for face and neck lesions
- Intralesional steroid injection
- Systemic steroids (e.g., betamethasone 5 mg qd on two consecutive days per wk for 2-4 mo)
- Total depigmentation in cases of extensive vitiligo with 20% monobenzyl ether or hydroquinone (This is a permanent procedure, and patients will require lifelong protection from sun exposure.)
- Topical immunomodulators (e.g., tacrolimus, pimecrolimus) (These substances can also induce the repigmentation of vitiliginous skin lesions. However, their potential for systemic immunosuppression or for increasing the risk of skin cancer or other malignancies remains to be defined.)
- Calcipotriol, which is a synthetic analog of vitamin D_3 (This has also been used in combination with ultraviolet light or clobetasol, with limited results.)
- Surgical techniques can be applied to limited lesions

EVIDENCE

Available at www.expertconsult.com

SUGGESTED READING
Available at www.expertconsult.com

RELATED CONTENT
Vitiligo (Patient Information)

AUTHOR: **FRED F. FERRI, M.D.**

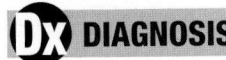

BASIC INFORMATION

DEFINITION

Von Willebrand's disease is an inherited disorder of hemostasis characterized by a quantitative or qualitative deficiency in Von Willebrand factor (vWF), a protein product of a gene located on the short arm of chromosome 12. The vWF factor is mostly synthesized in endothelial cells. Von Willebrand's disease results from a failure to synthesize or secrete vWF or an accelerated clearance of vWF. vWF is the carrier protein for clotting factor VIII (FVIII:C). vWF binds to subendothelial collagen and also causes platelets to aggregate by acting as a ligand for glycoprotein IB on the platelet surface. This latter activity is measured in the laboratory by a test called the ristocetin cofactor (RCF). vWF circulates in plasma as a multimeric protein consisting of protomers attached by disulfide bonds. By definition, vWD is present if the level of vWF is <30% of normal. A clinical entity known as low vWF exists when the level is between 30% and 60%. Previously, this was considered mild vWD. There are several subtypes of Von Willebrand's disease. The most common type (80% of cases) is Type I, where levels of vWF, FVIII:C, and RCF are reduced but concordant. There are four Type 2 subtypes: Type 2A, Type 2B, Type 2N, and Type 2M. All the Type 2 variants are due to a qualitative defect in vWF and show a discordancy between levels of RCF and FVIII:C. Type 3 is rare, and either an autosomal recessive disorder or double heterozygote and characterized by a near-complete quantitative deficiency of vWF and very low FVIII:C. Acquired vWD disease is a rare disorder that presents with mucocutaneous bleeding abnormalities and no clinical family history. It is often accompanied by a hematoproliferative or autoimmune disorder. Successful treatment of the associated illness can reverse the clinical and laboratory manifestations.

SYNONYMS

Pseudohemophilia
vWD

ICD-10CM CODES
D68.0 Von Willebrand's disease

EPIDEMIOLOGY & DEMOGRAPHICS

- Autosomal-dominant disorder.
- Most common inherited bleeding disorder.
- Prevalence is 0.6% to 1.3% in general population, according to screening studies; estimates based on referral for symptoms of bleeding suggest a prevalence of 1 case per 10,000 persons.

PHYSICAL FINDINGS & CLINICAL PRESENTATION

- Generally normal physical examination.
- Mucosal bleeding (gingival bleeding, epistaxis) and gastrointestinal bleeding may occur.
- Easy bruising.

- Postpartum bleeding, bleeding after surgery or dental extraction, menorrhagia.
- Increased incidence of endometriosis (likely related to backflow of menses), miscarriages.

ETIOLOGY

Quantitative or qualitative deficiency of vWF (see "Definition").

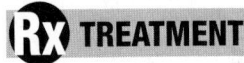

DIAGNOSIS

The diagnosis of Von Willebrand's disease generally requires two criteria: (1) a personal history, family history, or physical evidence of mucocutaneous bleeding and (2) a qualitative or quantitative decrease in functional activity of Von Willebrand's disease. The American Society of Hematology states that a definitive diagnosis of vWD may be made if vWF antigen levels are <30 IU/dl.

DIFFERENTIAL DIAGNOSIS

Platelet function disorders, clotting factor deficiencies.

WORKUP

- Laboratory evaluation (see "Laboratory Tests").
- Initial testing includes prothrombin time (normal), partial thromboplastin time (normal or slightly increased), platelet count (normal), and PFA-100.

- Subsequent tests include vWF level (decreased), factor VIII:C (decreased), and ristocetin cofactor (increased in Type 2B) (Table 1).

LABORATORY TESTS

- Decreased factor VIII coagulant activity.
- Decreased vWF antigen or ristocetin cofactor.
- Normal platelet number and morphology.
- Prolonged bleeding time, or more commonly PFA-100.
- Type 2A Von Willebrand's disease can be distinguished from Type I by absence of medium- and high-molecular-weight multimers.
- Type 2B Von Willebrand's disease is distinguished from Type I by the absence of high-molecular-weight multimers.
- Type 2N is a defect in the factor VIII:C binding and has normal vWF levels but very low factor VIII:C with normal multimer pattern
- Type 2M is a defect in binding to platelets (low RCF) but normal multimers.

TREATMENT

NONPHARMACOLOGIC THERAPY

- Avoidance of aspirin and other nonsteroidal antiinflammatory drugs.
- Use of antifibrinolytics such as tranexamic acid, especially for menorrhagia or oral bleeding.

TABLE 1 Genetic and Laboratory Findings in Von Willebrand's Disease

Parameter Type	BT	VIII-C	vW-Ag	R-Cof	RIPA	Multimer Structure	Mode of Inheritance
I (classic)	P	R	R	R	R	Normal	AD
II							
A	P	N/R	N/R	R	R	Abnormal	AD
B	P	N/R	N/R	N/R	I	Abnormal	AD
III	P	R	R	R	R	Variable	AR

AD, Autosomal dominant; AR, autosomal recessive; BT, bleeding time; I, increased; N/R, normal or reduced; P, prolonged; R, reduced; R-Cof, ristocetin cofactor; RIPA, ristocetin-induced platelet aggregation (agglutination); vW-Ag, Von Willebrand antigen (protein); VIII-C, factor VIII coagulant activity.
From Behrman RE: Nelson textbook of pediatrics, ed 17, Philadelphia, 2004, Saunders.

TABLE 2 Causes of Acquired Von Willebrand Syndrome

Pathophysiologic Category*	Disease or Association
Antibodies to vWF	Monoclonal gammopathies, lymphoproliferative disorders, or autoimmune diseases such as systemic lupus erythematosus
Shear-induced vWF conformational changes leading to increased proteolysis of vWF	Aortic valvular stenosis, ventricular septal defect, hypertrophic obstructive cardiomyopathy, left ventricular assist device, or primary pulmonary hypertension
Markedly elevated blood platelet count	Essential thrombocythemia, polycythemia vera, myeloid metaplasia with myelofibrosis, or other myeloproliferative disorders
Removal of vWF from circulation by aberrant binding to tumor cells	Wilms' tumor and certain lymphoproliferative or plasma cell proliferative disorders
Decreased vWF synthesis	Hypothyroidism
Drugs associated with AVWS	Ciprofloxacin, valproic acid, hydroxyethyl starch, or griseofulvin

AVWS, Acquired Von Willebrand syndrome; vWF, Von Willebrand factor.
*Pathophysiologic categories are listed in descending order of approximate prevalence.
Goldman L, Schafer AI: Goldman's Cecil medicine, ed 24, Philadelphia, 2012, Saunders

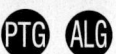

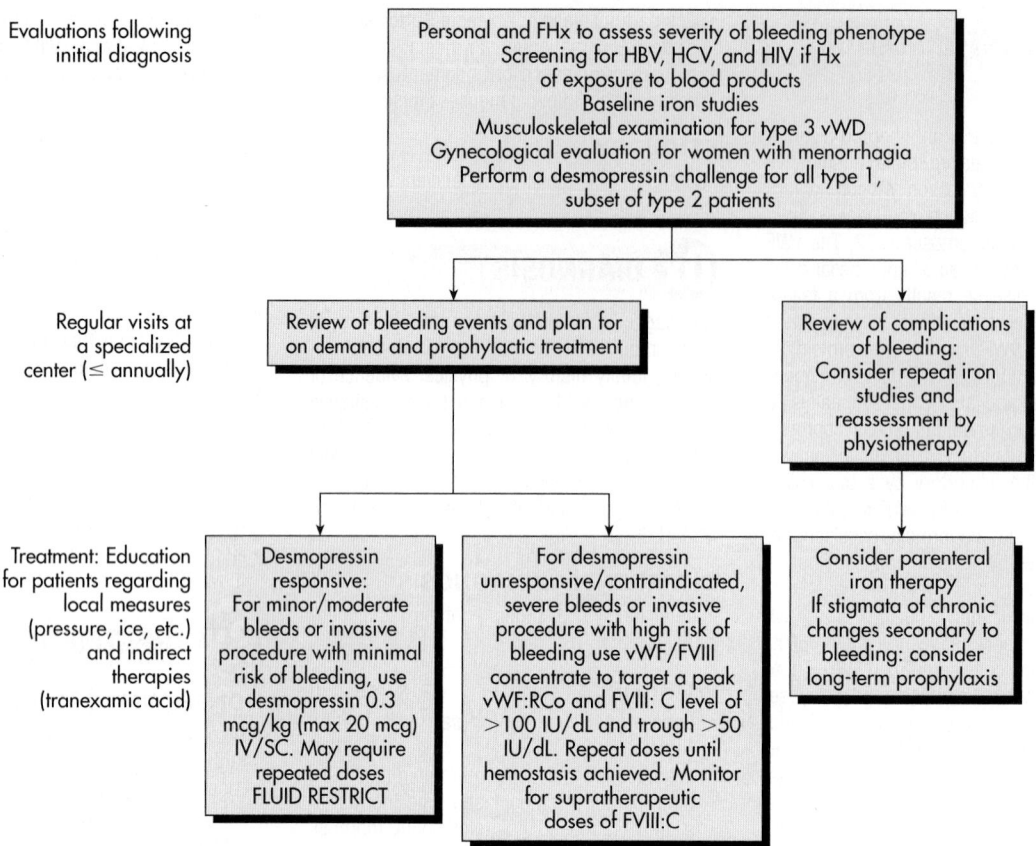

Evaluations following initial diagnosis

Personal and FHx to assess severity of bleeding phenotype
Screening for HBV, HCV, and HIV if Hx of exposure to blood products
Baseline iron studies
Musculoskeletal examination for type 3 vWD
Gynecological evaluation for women with menorrhagia
Perform a desmopressin challenge for all type 1, subset of type 2 patients

Regular visits at a specialized center (≤ annually)

Review of bleeding events and plan for on demand and prophylactic treatment

Review of complications of bleeding: Consider repeat iron studies and reassessment by physiotherapy

Treatment: Education for patients regarding local measures (pressure, ice, etc.) and indirect therapies (tranexamic acid)

Desmopressin responsive: For minor/moderate bleeds or invasive procedure with minimal risk of bleeding, use desmopressin 0.3 mcg/kg (max 20 mcg) IV/SC. May require repeated doses FLUID RESTRICT

For desmopressin unresponsive/contraindicated, severe bleeds or invasive procedure with high risk of bleeding use vWF/FVIII concentrate to target a peak vWF:RCo and FVIII: C level of >100 IU/dL and trough >50 IU/dL. Repeat doses until hemostasis achieved. Monitor for supratherapeutic doses of FVIII:C

Consider parenteral iron therapy If stigmata of chronic changes secondary to bleeding: consider long-term prophylaxis

FIG. 1 Approach to the management of Von Willebrand's disease. (From Hoffman R: *Hematology, basic principles and practice,* ed 6, Philadelphia, 2013, Saunders.)

GENERAL Rx

- Treatment of Von Willebrand's disease is based on normalizing factor VIII levels and Von Willebrand factor at the time of spontaneous bleeding or before an intervention.
- Use of DDAVP: DDAVP binds to V2 receptors in certain endothelial cells and causes the release of vWF. This is suitable for the management of the milder forms of vWD. Dose is 0.3 mcg/kg in 100 mL of normal saline solution IV infused >20 min. DDAVP is also available as a nasal spray

(dose of 150 mcg spray administered to each nostril) as a preparation for minor surgery and management of minor bleeding episodes.
- When a patient undergoes surgery or receives repeated therapeutic doses of concentrates, use of a vWF concentrate such as Humate-P or a new recombinant vWF (Vonvendi) may need to be administered.
- Fig. 1 summarizes the approach to the management of Von Willebrand's disease

SUGGESTED READINGS

Available at www.expertconsult.com

RELATED CONTENT

Von Willebrand's Disease (Patient Information)

AUTHOR: **JOSEPH SWEENEY, M.D.**

BASIC INFORMATION

DEFINITION

Waldenström macroglobulinemia (WM) is an indolent B-cell lymphoplasmacytic lymphoma (LPL) characterized by lymphoplasmacytic infiltration in the bone marrow (BM) and other organs, and a monoclonal immunoglobulin M (IgM) paraprotein in the serum. Less than 5% of LPL secrete IgG, IgA, or light chains. Rare nonsecretory cases may exist.

SYNONYMS

WM
Monoclonal macroglobulinemia
Lymphoplasmacytic lymphoma

ICD-10CM CODES
C88.0 Waldenström macroglobulinemia

EPIDEMIOLOGY & DEMOGRAPHICS

- Accounts for 2% of all hematologic cancers
- 1500 new cases diagnosed every year in the U.S.
- Overall incidence: 3.4 per million person-year in men, 1.7 per million person-year in women
- Median age at diagnosis: 72 years
- More common among men than women and among whites than blacks

PHYSICAL FINDINGS & CLINICAL PRESENTATION

- 30% to 50% of patients can be asymptomatic at presentation.
- Weakness, fatigue, and pallor, usually associated with anemia (50%).
- Fever, night sweats, and weight loss (30%).
- Peripheral neuropathy associated with IgM demyelinating antibodies, usually affecting the feet symmetrically (20%).
- Lymphadenopathy (15%).
- Hepatosplenomegaly (15%).
- Hyperviscosity syndrome, characterized by headaches, recurrent nosebleeds, blurry

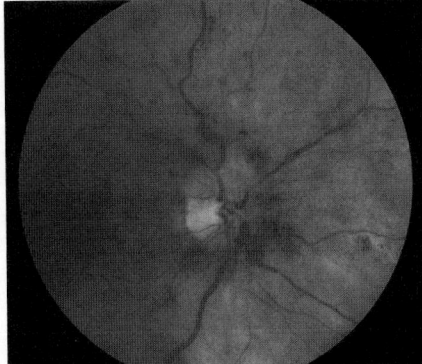

FIG. 1 Hyperviscosity syndrome. Right eye retinal image in a patient with Waldenström's macroglobulinemia and hyperviscosity syndrome showing sausaging (focal venular dilations), intraretinal hemorrhages, microaneurysms, and peripapillary cotton wool spots and disc swelling (papilledema). (From Goldman L, Schafer AI: *Goldman's Cecil medicine,* ed 24, Philadelphia, 2011, Saunders.)

vision due to retinal hemorrhages (10%); retinal vein link: sausage shaped (Fig. 1).
- Acrocyanosis, livedo reticularis, and purpura (Fig. 2), usually associated with symptomatic cryoglobulinemia (5%-10%).
- Peripheral ulcerations associated with severe cryoglobulinemia.
- Hemolytic anemia caused by cold agglutinin disease (5%).
- Amyloidosis causing renal dysfunction, neuropathy, and/or cardiac dysfunction (<5%).
- Meningeal signs caused by CNS involvement by WM (Bing Neel syndrome; 1%).

ETIOLOGY

- The main risk factor for development of WM is having IgM monoclonal gammopathy of unknown significance (MGUS).
- Multiple reports suggest familial clustering in about 20% of the patients, which indicates a genetic predisposition to WM and other blood cancers.
- Approximately 20% of the patients have an Ashkenazi Jewish ancestry.
- Radiation exposure, occupational chemicals, viral infection (hepatitis C), and chronic inflammatory stimulation have been suggested, but there is insufficient evidence to substantiate these hypotheses.
- There is a twofold to threefold increased risk of WM in people with a personal history of autoimmune diseases.

Dx DIAGNOSIS

The diagnosis of WM is usually established by laboratory blood tests and by bone marrow (BM) biopsy. Diagnosis requires demonstration of lymphoplasmacytic lymphoma involving the BM space and the presence of an IgM M protein. MYD88 L265P is a commonly recurring mutation in WM seen in >90% of the patients with WM and 50% to 80% of patients with IgM MGUS and can be useful in differentiating WM from other IgM-secreting B-cell disorders such as marginal zone lymphoma, IgM multiple myeloma, and atypical forms of chronic lymphocytic leukemia and follicular lymphoma. Non-L265P MYD88 mutations have also been described and should be excluded in patients who test negative for MYD88 L265P by PCR-based assays. Mutations in the *CXCR4* gene

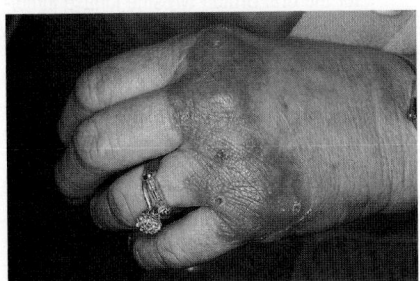

FIG. 2 Nonpalpable purpura of hyperglobulinemic purpura of Waldenström's hypergammaglobulinemia. (From Hochberg MC et al: *Rheumatology,* ed 5, St Louis, 2011, Mosby.)

have been described in 40% of patients, and may impact clinical presentation and response to ibrutinib treatment.

DIFFERENTIAL DIAGNOSIS

- IgM MGUS
- Marginal zone lymphoma
- IgM multiple myeloma
- Atypical chronic lymphocytic leukemia
- Atypical follicular lymphoma

WORKUP

In any patient suspected of having WM, specific blood tests (CBC, erythrocyte sedimentation rate [ESR], serum or urine protein electrophoresis [SPEP or UPEP, respectively], IgM level, beta 2-microglobulin, serum viscosity) should be ordered. BM biopsy confirms the diagnosis. *MYD88* mutation testing can be helpful to support the diagnosis of WM.

LABORATORY TESTS:

- CBC with differential:
  1. Anemia is a common finding, with a median hemoglobin value of approximately 10 g/dl. WBC count is usually normal; thrombocytopenia can occur.
  2. Peripheral smear may reveal "stacked coin" rouleaux formations and malignant lymphoid cells in some patients.
- Elevated ESR.
- SPEP: homogeneous M spike (monoclonal gammopathy).
- Immunoelectrophoresis: confirms IgM responsible for the M spike. Table 1 describes physicochemical and immunologic properties of the monoclonal IgM protein in WM.
- Serum IgM levels are high, generally >3000 mg/dl.
- High serum beta 2-microglobulin levels are associated with poor prognosis.
- Serum viscosity. Hyperviscosity usually occurs when the serum viscosity is four times the viscosity of normal serum; classic feature although presents in only 10% of cases.
- Cryoglobulins or cold agglutinins may be present.
- BM biopsy: BM reveals infiltration by a lymphoplasmacytic cell population constituted by small lymphocytes with evidence of plasmacytoid and plasma cell differentiation. The BM infiltration should be confirmed by immunophenotypic studies (flow cytometry and immunohistochemistry) showing the following profile: sIgM+CD19+CD20+CD22+CD79+.

IMAGING STUDIES

- CT of the chest, abdomen, and pelvis may show lymphadenopathy, hepatosplenomegaly, and rarely, extralymphatic/extramedullary areas of disease.

Rx TREATMENT

- Because of the incurable nature of WM, the aim of treatment is to relieve symptoms and reduce the risk of organ damage. Initiation of therapy should not be based on the IgM levels alone because this may not correlate with either disease burden or symptomatic status.

TABLE 1 Physicochemical and Immunologic Properties of Monoclonal Immunoglobulin Protein in Waldenström's Macroglobulinemia

Properties of Monoclonal Immunoglobulin Protein	Diagnostic Condition	Clinical Manifestations
Pentameric structure	Hyperviscosity	Headaches, blurred vision, epistaxis, retinal hemorrhages, impaired mentation, and intracranial hemorrhage
Prescription on cooling	Cryoglobulinemia (type I)	Raynaud's phenomenon, acrocyanosis, ulcers, purpura, and cold urticaria
Autoantibody activity to myelin-associated glycoprotein, ganglioside M1, and sulfatide moieties on peripheral nerve sheaths	Peripheral neuropathies	Sensorimotor neuropathies, painful neuropathies, ataxic gait, and bilateral foot drop
Autoantibody activity to immunoglobulin G	Cryoglobulinemia (type II)	Purpura, arthralgias, renal failure, and sensorimotor neuropathies
Autoantibody activity to red blood cell antigens	Cold agglutinins	Hemolytic anemia, Raynaud's phenomenon, acrocyanosis, and livedo reticularis
Tissue deposition as amorphous aggregates	Organ dysfunction	Skin: bullous skin disease, papules, and Schnitzler syndrome Gastrointestinal: diarrhea, malabsorption, and bleeding Kidney: proteinuria and renal failure (light-chain component)
Tissue deposition as amyloid fibrils (light-chain fibrils commonly the largest component)	Organ dysfunction	Fatigue, weight loss, edema, periorbital purpura, hepatomegaly, macroglossia, and organ dysfunction of the involved organs: heart, kidney, liver, and peripheral sensory and autonomic nerves

From Hoffman R et al: *Hematology, basic principles and practice,* ed 5, Philadelphia, 2009, Churchill Livingstone.

Patients with smoldering or asymptomatic WM and preserved hematologic function should be observed without therapy.
- Initiation of therapy is appropriate for patients with constitutional symptoms. Considerations for the initiation of treatment include the following: significant adenopathy or organomegaly, symptomatic hyperviscosity, moderate to severe neuropathy, amyloidosis, cryoglobulinemia, cold-agglutinin disease, hemoglobin concentration <10 g/dl, or evidence of disease transformation.
- Treatment is directed at both hyperviscosity and the lymphoproliferative disorder itself.

NONPHARMACOLOGIC THERAPY

Asymptomatic patients do not require treatment, and these patients should be monitored periodically for the onset of symptoms or changes in blood tests (e.g., worsening anemia, thrombocytopenia, rising IgM levels, and serum viscosity). Plasmapheresis should be the initial treatment in patients with symptoms of hyperviscosity or cryoglobulinemia followed immediately by more definitive therapy.

INITIAL Rx
- Treatment of the lymphoproliferative disorder includes single or combination therapy. There is no universally agreed upon standard of care:

1. Combination regimens include BDR (bortezomib, dexamethasone, rituximab), CaRD (carfilzomib, dexamethasone, rituximab), CDR (cyclophosphamide, dexamethasone, rituximab, cyclophosphamide), and bendamustine/rituximab. These should be used in patients with severe constitutional symptoms, symptomatic bulky disease, hyperviscosity, or profound hematologic compromise. Response rates are >80% with any of these regimens.
2. Rituximab, a monoclonal anti-CD20 antibody, can be used in symptomatic patients with modest hematologic compromise, IgM-related neuropathy, or hemolytic anemia unresponsive to corticosteroids. Response rates are 40% to 50%.
3. In April 2015, the FDA granted approval for the oral Bruton tyrosine kinase inhibitor ibrutinib to be used in patients with symptomatic WM. The response rate to ibrutinib is 90%, with a median time to response of 4 weeks. Major responses are absent in patients who do not carry the MYD88 mutation. The response is delayed in patients who carry any *CXCR4* mutation.

RX ON RELAPSED/REFRACTORY DISEASE
- Rituximab can be used as maintenance therapy.
- Refractory patients can be retried on original therapy if length of response from initial therapy is >3 years. If the response from the initial therapy was <3 years, alternative first-line agents can be used.
- Other treatment options: fludarabine, ofatumumab, thalidomide, everolimus, and clinical trials. Autologous stem cell transplantation should be considered in patients with highly refractory disease.

DISPOSITION
- The progression of WM is slow and insidious, with median survival from time of diagnosis of about 10 years.
- Younger patients tend to have more prolonged survival.
- About 10% to 20% of patients die from progression of the disease.
- Some patients develop acute myelogenous leukemia, usually secondary to exposure to chemotherapy, and some patients can develop more aggressive lymphomas.
- The risk of thyroid cancer, kidney cancer, and melanoma is increased in patients with WM.
- A staging system using age, serum beta 2-microglobulin concentration, hemoglobin levels, platelet counts, and serum IgM concentration before treatment provides insight into prognosis and survival.

REFERRAL

A hematology consultation is helpful in guiding future workup, treatment, and monitoring. Participation in clinical trials is highly encouraged in patients with WM.

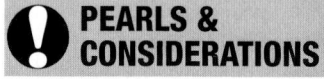 **PEARLS & CONSIDERATIONS**

COMMENTS
- WM was first described in 1944 by the Swedish physician Jan Gösta Waldenström, who also described the X-linked Bruton agammaglobulinemia.

SUGGESTED READINGS
Available at www.expertconsult.com

AUTHORS: **JORGE J. CASTILLO, M.D.,** and **STEVEN P. TREON, M.D., PH.D.**

BASIC INFORMATION

DEFINITION

Warts are benign epidermal lesions caused by human papillomavirus (HPV).

SYNONYMS

Verruca vulgaris (common warts)
Verruca plana (flat warts)
Condyloma acuminatum (venereal warts)
Verruca plantaris (plantar warts)
Mosaic warts (cluster of many warts)
HPV infection

ICD10CM CODES

B07.9 Viral wart, unspecified
B07.8 Other viral warts
A63.0 Anogenital (venereal) warts
B07.0 Plantar wart

EPIDEMIOLOGY & DEMOGRAPHICS

- Risk factors include use of communal showers, occupational handling of meat, and immunosuppression. Common warts occur most frequently in children and young adults.
- Anogenital warts are most common in young, sexually active patients. Genital warts are the most common viral sexually transmitted disease in the United States, with up to 79 million Americans carrying the causative virus, and 14 million persons are newly infected each year in the U.S.
- Persistent infection with oncogenic HPV types can cause cervical cancer in women as well as other anogenital and oropharyngeal cancers in women and men. 66% of cervical cancers, 55% of vaginal cancers, 79% of anal cancers, and 62% of oropharyngeal cancers are attributable to HPV types 16 or 18.
- Common warts are longer lasting and more frequent in immunocompromised patients (e.g., lymphoma, AIDS, immunosuppressive drugs).
- Plantar warts occur most frequently at points of maximal pressure (over the heads of the metatarsal bones or on the heels).

PHYSICAL FINDINGS & CLINICAL PRESENTATION

- Common warts (Fig. E1) have an initial appearance of a flesh-colored papule with a rough surface; they subsequently develop a hyperkeratotic appearance with black dots on the surface (thrombosed capillaries). They may be single or multiple and are most common on the hands.
- Warts obscure normal skin lines (important diagnostic feature). Cylindrical projections from the wart may become fused, forming a mosaic pattern.
- Flat warts generally are pink or light yellow, slightly elevated, and often found on the forehead, back of hands, mouth, and beard area. They often occur in lines corresponding to trauma (e.g., a scratch), are often misdiagnosed (particularly when present on the face), and are inappropriately treated with topical corticosteroids.
- Filiform warts have a fingerlike appearance with various projections; they are generally found near the mouth, beard, or periorbital and paranasal regions.
- Plantar warts are slightly raised and have a roughened surface; they may cause pain when walking; as they involute, small hemorrhages (caused by thrombosed capillaries) may be noted.
- Genital warts (Fig. E2) are generally pale pink with several projections and a broad base. They may coalesce in the perineal area to form masses with a cauliflower-like appearance. Intraanal warts occur predominantly in patients who have had receptive anal intercourse, in contrast with perianal warts (Fig. 3), which may occur in men and women without a history of anal sex.
- Genital warts on the cervical epithelium can produce subclinical changes that may be noted on Pap smear or colposcopy.

ETIOLOGY

- HPV infection; >150 types of viral DNA have been identified. Transmission of warts is by direct contact. Approximately 40 different types of HPV are transmitted through sexual contact.
- Genital warts: 90% are caused by HPV types 6 or 11. HPV types 16, 18, 31, 33, and 35 are found occasionally in visible genital warts (usually as coinfections with HPV 6 or 11) and can be associated with foci of high-grade, intraepithelial neoplasia, particularly in persons who are infected with HIV infection. In addition to warts on genital areas, HPV types 6 and 11 have been associated with conjunctival, nasal, oral, and laryngeal warts.

DIAGNOSIS

DIFFERENTIAL DIAGNOSIS

- Molluscum contagiosum
- Condyloma latum
- Acrochordon (skin tags) or seborrheic keratosis
- Epidermal nevi
- Hypertrophic actinic keratosis
- Squamous cell carcinomas
- Acquired digital fibrokeratoma
- Varicella-zoster virus in patients with AIDS
- Recurrent infantile digital fibroma
- Plantar corns (may be mistaken for plantar warts)

WORKUP

- Diagnosis is generally based on clinical findings.
- Suspect lesions should be biopsied.
- The application of 3% to 5% acetic acid, which causes skin color to turn white, has been used by some providers to detect HPV-infected genital mucosa. However, acetic acid application is not a specific test for HPV infection. Therefore, the routine use of this procedure for screening to detect mucosal changes attributed to HPV infection is not recommended.

LABORATORY TESTS

- Screening for cervical cancer with cytology, which is performed by either Pap smear or liquid-based cytology. Screening guidelines recommend starting screening at age 21. Annual cytology is recommended until at least three normal cytology results are obtained.
- Colposcopy with biopsy is recommended in patients with cervical squamous cell changes.

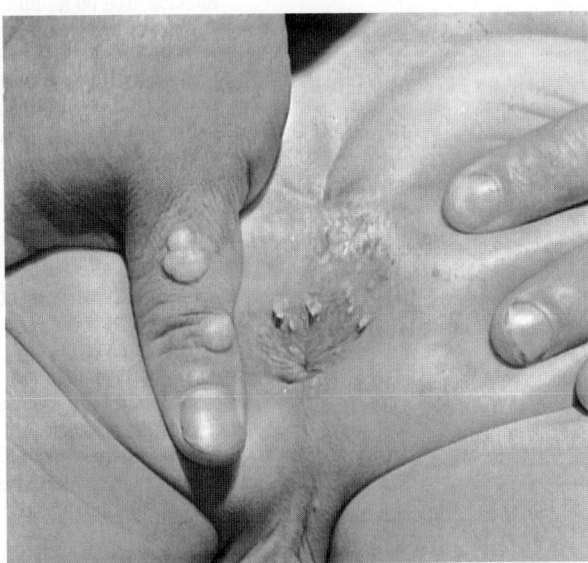

FIG. 3 Common warts of the hand in a mother and perianal condylomata acuminata in her son. (From Meneghini CL, Bonifaz E: *An atlas of pediatric dermatology,* Chicago, 1986, Year Book Medical Publishers.)

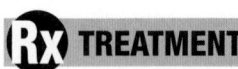

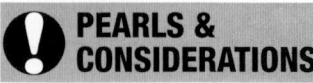 **TREATMENT**

NONPHARMACOLOGIC THERAPY

- Importance of use of condoms to reduce transmission of genital warts should be emphasized.
- Watchful waiting is an acceptable option in the treatment of nongenital cutaneous warts because many warts will disappear without intervention over time. However, many patients often request treatment because of social stigma or discomfort.
- Plantar warts that are not painful do not need treatment.
- Factors that influence selection of treatment include wart size, wart number, anatomic site of the wart, wart morphology, patient preference, cost of treatment, convenience, adverse effects, and provider experience. Factors that might affect response to therapy include the presence of immunosuppression and compliance with therapy.

GENERAL Rx

- Common warts:
  1. Application of topical salicylic acid 17%. Soak area for 5 min in warm water and dry. Apply thin layer once or twice daily for up to 12 wk, avoiding normal skin. Bandage.
  2. Liquid nitrogen and electrocautery are also common methods of removal. Cure rates for cryotherapy are 50% to 70% after three to four treatments.
  3. Blunt dissection can be used in large lesions or resistant lesions.
  4. Duct tape occlusion is also effective for treating common warts. It is cut to cover warts and left in place for 6 days. It is removed after 6 days and the warts are soaked in water and then filed with pumice stones. New tape is applied 12 hr later. This treatment can be repeated until warts resolve.
  5. Recalcitrant warts can be treated with injection of *Candida* or mumps skin antigen into the wart every 3 to 4 wk for up to three treatments, photodynamic therapy with aminolevulinic acid, pulsed dye laser, and intralesional bleomycin.
- Filiform warts: surgical removal is necessary.
- Flat warts: generally more difficult to treat.
  1. Tretinoin cream applied at bedtime over the involved area for several weeks may be effective.
  2. Application of liquid nitrogen.
  3. Electrocautery.
  4. 5-Fluorouracil cream applied once or twice a day for 3 to 5 wk is also effective. Persistent hyperpigmentation may occur after Efudex use.
- Plantar warts:
  1. Salicylic acid therapy (e.g., Occlusal-HP). Soak wart in warm water for 5 min, remove loose tissue, dry. Apply to area, allow to dry, reapply. Use once or twice daily; maximum 12 wk. Use of 40%

salicylic acid plasters (Mediplast) is also a safe, nonscarring treatment; it is particularly useful in treating mosaic warts covering a large area.
  2. Blunt dissection is also a fast and effective treatment modality.
  3. Laser therapy can be used for plantar warts and recurrent warts; however, it leaves open wounds that require 4 to 6 wk to fill with granulation tissue.
  4. Interlesional bleomycin is also effective but generally used when all other treatments fail.
- Genital warts:
  1. Can be effectively treated with 20% podophyllin resin in compound tincture of benzoin applied with a cotton tip applicator by the treating physician and allowed to air dry. The treatment can be repeated weekly if necessary.
  2. Podofilox (Condylox 0.5% gel) is available for application by the patient. Local adverse effects include pain, burning, and inflammation at the site.
  3. Cryosurgery with liquid nitrogen delivered with a probe or as a spray is effective for treating smaller genital warts.
  4. Carbon dioxide laser can also be used for treating primary or recurrent genital warts (cure rate >90%).
  5. Imiquimod cream, 5%, is a patient-applied immune response modifier effective in the treatment of external genital and perianal warts (complete clearing of genital warts in >70% of females and >30% of males in 4-16 wk). Sexual contact should be avoided while the cream is on the skin. It is applied 3 times per wk before normal sleeping hours and is left on the skin for 6 to 10 hr.
  6. Sinecatechins (Veregen), a botanical drug product, is also effective for treatment of external genital and perianal warts. Formulation is a 15% ointment applied to affected area tid for up to 16 wk.
- Application of trichloroacetic acid or bichloracetic acid 80% to 90% is also effective for external genital warts. A small amount should be applied only to warts and allowed to dry, at which time a white "frosting" develops. This treatment can be repeated weekly if necessary.

DISPOSITION

- Warts can be effectively treated with the previous modalities with complete resolution in the majority of patients; however, the recurrence rate is high.
- Cervical carcinomas and precancerous lesions in women are associated with genital papillomavirus infection.
- Squamous cell anal cancer is also associated with a history of genital warts.

REFERRAL

- Dermatology referral for warts resistant to conservative therapy
- Surgical referral in selected cases

- Sexually transmitted disease counseling for patients with anogenital warts

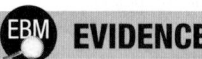 **PEARLS & CONSIDERATIONS**

COMMENTS

- Subungual and periungual warts are generally more resistant to treatment. Dermatology referral for cryosurgery is recommended in resistant cases.
- Examination of sex partners is not necessary for the management of genital warts because no data indicate that reinfection plays a role.

PREVENTION

- Two HPV vaccines (Gardasil, Gardasil-9, Cervarix) have been licensed in the United States. ACIP recommends routine vaccination with HPV4 or HPV2 for females aged 11 to 12 years and HPV4 for males aged 11 to 12 years. Vaccination is also recommended for females aged 13 to 26 years and for males aged 13 through 21 years who were not vaccinated previously. Males aged 22 through 26 may be vaccinated. ACIP recommends vaccination of men who have sex with men and immunocompromised persons (including those with infection) through age 26 years if not previously vaccinated. The 9-valent HPV vaccine (Gardasil-9) is approved for use in girls and women 9-26 years old and boys 9-15 years old. It is indicated to prevent diseases associated with HPV infection with types 6, 11, 16, 18, 31, 33, 45, 52, and 58. It appears to be more effective than the other 2 currently available vaccines. It consists of two doses. The first dose is administered at 11 to 12 years of age, and the second dose 6 to 12 months later. However, if the second dose is given less than 5 mo apart, a third dose will be needed at age 9 to 14. Patients with a weak immune system and in those starting vaccination at age 15 to 26 years will need three doses.
- Male circumcision decreases heterosexual transmission of HPV.

EBM EVIDENCE

Available at www.expertconsult.com

SUGGESTED READINGS
Available at www.expertconsult.com

RELATED CONTENT

Human Papillomavirus Infection (Patient Information)
Warts (Patient Information)
Condyloma Acuminatum (Related Key Topic)

AUTHOR: **FRED F. FERRI, M.D.**

BASIC INFORMATION

DEFINITION

Wolff-Parkinson-White (WPW) syndrome is a congenital heart condition in which, in addition to the normal electrical conduction through the atrioventricular (AV) node, there is an accessory pathway (AP) that connects the atria to the ventricles resulting in ventricular preexcitation. Patients with WPW syndrome have ECG findings of preexcitation, including short PR interval <120 ms, the presence of a delta wave and arrhythmias, which may be atrioventricular (AV) reentrant tachycardia, atrial fibrillation (AF), or both. Patients with the WPW pattern have characteristic ECG findings of preexcitation without evidence of arrhythmia.

SYNONYMS

Preexcitation syndrome
WPW

ICD-10CM CODES
I45.6 Pre-excitation syndrome

EPIDEMIOLOGY & DEMOGRAPHICS

- The prevalence of a WPW pattern on the surface ECG is 0.1% to 0.3% in the general population. The prevalence is increased to 0.55% in first-degree relatives of affected patients. It is estimated that approximately 65% of adolescents and 40% of individuals older than 30 yr with WPW pattern on a resting ECG are asymptomatic.
- The prevalence of WPW is higher among males and decreases with age.
- Most patients with WPW have structurally normal hearts, but it may also occur in patients with congenital heart disease, most notably in patients with Ebstein's anomaly, which is associated with right-side AP and often multiple and slowly conducting APs.

PHYSICAL FINDINGS & CLINICAL PRESENTATION

- The physical examination is usually unremarkable.
- Symptoms are typically related to tachyarrhythmias, including the following:
  1. Palpitations, anxiety, dyspnea, chest pain or tightness
  2. Syncope or near syncope
  3. Sudden cardiac death
- The common arrhythmias in WPW syndrome are:
  1. Supraventricular tachycardia: AV reciprocating tachycardia (AVRT). This is the most common arrhythmia, further classified as orthodromic AVRT (narrow complex tachycardia, with antegrade conduction through the AVN, that occurs in 70% of symptomatic patients), or antidromic AVRT (wide complex tachycardia with antegrade conduction via the AP, which occurs in 4%-5% of patients).

  2. AF (~10%-38%), the second most common tachycardia, can be complicated by a very rapid ventricular response due to conduction over the AP, which can lead to ventricular fibrillation (VF) and sudden death. This risk is dependent on the antegrade refractory period of AP during AF.
- The risk of sudden death in symptomatic patients with WPW syndrome is estimated to be approximately 0.25% per year or 3% to 4% over a lifetime.
- In a meta-analysis including approximately 2000 subjects with asymptomatic WPW, children had a sudden death rate of 1.9 compared with 0.9 in adults per 1000 patient years of follow-up. This incidence is comparable with the estimated 0.1% per year risk of death in the general population in Europe, Japan, and the United States.

ETIOLOGY & PATHOGENESIS

- APs are thought to be an embryologic remnant, as substantiated by reports of SVT in uterus and by a greater prevalence of WPW in newborns and infants.
- Left free wall APs are most common followed by posteroseptal, right free wall, and anteroseptal locations.
- Some patients with WPW syndrome (~5%-10%) have multiple APs.
- If the accessory pathway is capable of anterograde conduction, two parallel routes of AV conduction are possible: one is subject to delay through the AV node, and the other occurs without delay through the AP and results in preexcitation of the ventricle. The resulting QRS complex is a fusion beat, as a portion of the ventricle is preexcited and activated via the AP giving rise to the delta wave, and the remainder of the ventricle is activated by the normal activation pathway (Fig. 1).
- Reciprocating tachycardias occur when conduction is anterograde in one pathway (usually the normal AV pathway, i.e., orthodromic

AVRT) and retrograde in the other (usually the AP) as a result of different refractory periods. This is usually initiated by a premature atrial or ventricular depolarization.

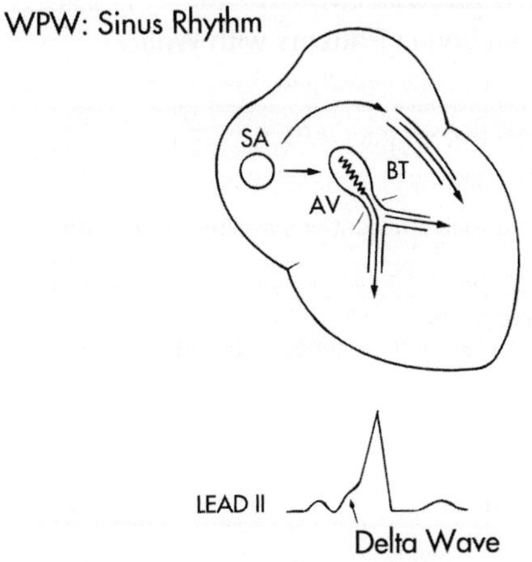

DIAGNOSIS

- Three basic features characterize the ECG abnormalities associated with WPW pattern (Fig. 2):
  1. PR interval <120 ms
  2. QRS complex can be >120 ms with a slurred, slowly rising onset of QRS in some leads (delta wave) and a normal terminal QRS portion. The width of the QRS complex depends on the amount of preexcitation ventricular tissue.
  3. Secondary ST-T wave changes directed in an opposite direction to the major delta and QRS vectors may be present.
- ECG patterns with abnormal QRS complexes and ST and T changes can mask or mimic myocardial infarction (in particular posteroseptal AP with negative delta waves in the inferior wall, which mimics old inferior wall myocardial infarction), bundle branch block, or ventricular hypertrophy.
- Most commonly seen tachycardia (orthodromic AVRT) is characterized by a normal QRS with a regular rate of 150 to 250 bpm. Onset and termination are abrupt.
- Variants of preexcitation:
  1. Lown-Ganong-Levine syndrome is characterized by a short PR interval, a narrow QRS complex without a delta wave, and a clinical syndrome of paroxysmal SVTs, which can be regular SVTs, atrial flutter, or fibrillation. Postulated mechanisms to the short PR interval include a variant of the normal, enhanced sympathetic tone or specialized intranodal fibers with enhanced AV nodal conduction.

WPW: Sinus Rhythm

FIG. 1 With Wolff-Parkinson-White *(WPW)* syndrome, an abnormal accessory conduction pathway called a *bypass tract (BT)* connects the atria and the ventricles. (From Goldberger AL [ed]: *Clinical electrocardiography: a simplified approach,* ed 6, St Louis, 1999, Mosby.)

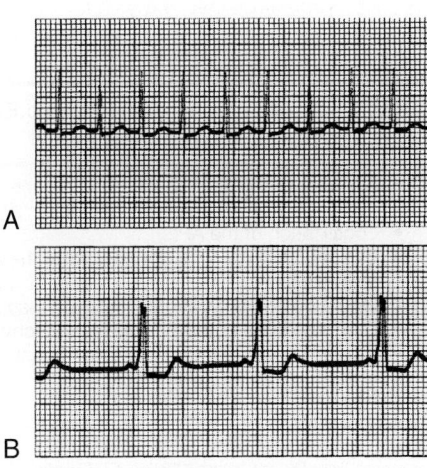

FIG. 2 A, Supraventricular tachycardia in a child with Wolff-Parkinson-White syndrome. Note the normal QRS complexes during the tachycardia. **B,** Later, the typical features of Wolff-Parkinson-White syndrome are apparent: a short P-R interval, a delta wave, and a wide QRS. (From Behrman RE: *Nelson textbook of pediatrics,* ed 18, Philadelphia, 2007, Saunders.)

2. Atriofascicular accessory pathway (Mahaim fiber): a slowly conducting AP with AV-nodal like properties, which connects the right atrium with the right bundle branch or the apical myocardium. In the baseline state, minimal or no preexcitation may be present. During preexcitation the QRS appears like a typical LBBB pattern.
3. Nodoventricular or nodofascicular APs: rare variants that connect the AV node and the ventricle or the bundle branch appropriately.

- An electrophysiology study is the gold standard to confirm the diagnosis, determine the location, and assess the conduction properties of the AP.

RISK STRATIFICATION

- Intermittent and abrupt loss of preexcitation on a beat-to-beat basis is indicative of lower risk, assessed with Holter monitoring or with an exercise stress test. The loss of preexcitation after administration of the antiarrhythmic drug procainamide has also been used to indicate a low-risk subgroup.
- In patients with a persistent preexcitation pattern, EP study is the procedure of choice for risk stratification.

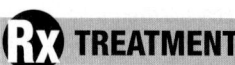 **TREATMENT**

- Goals of electrophysiologic evaluation in patients with WPW syndrome are described in Box 1.

ACUTE MANAGEMENT

- Urgent cardioversion, for an acute tachycardia episode with hemodynamic instability.
- Narrow QRS tachycardia (c/w orthodromic AVRT):

1. Vagal maneuvers and/or IV adenosine.
2. IV beta blockers, diltiazem, or verapamil can be administered for regular and narrow QRS tachycardia, implying antegrade conduction via the AV node, when the patient is hemodynamically stable and IV adenosine is ineffective.

- Wide QRS complex tachycardias (WCTs):

1. Most commonly caused by atrial fibrillation with antegrade conduction via the AP and the AV node. AV nodal blocking therapies (i.e., beta blockers, calcium channel blockers, digoxin, and adenosine) are potentially dangerous and should be avoided in these cases because of the risk of causing VF by enhancement of the ventricular response through the accessory pathway when the AV node is blocked and the blood pressure is lowered.
2. Stable patients with preexcited AF can be managed with IV procainamide. Electrical cardioversion should be performed if the patient is hemodynamically unstable.
3. In a patient with WCT due to antidromic tachycardia, drug treatment may be directed at the AP or at the AV node because both are critical components of the tachycardia circuit.

- Long-term management:
- Asymptomatic:

1. In low-risk patients with intermittent loss of preexcitation, AP effective refractory period (APERP) ≥250, or shortest preexcited RR interval (SPERRI) ≥250 ms, no therapy is required.
2. In high-risk patients with APERP ≤250 ms or SPERRI ≤250 ms, competitive athletes, or high-risk occupation (i.e., pilots), ablation should be considered.

- Symptomatic:
1. Patients who presented with aborted sudden cardiac death, preexcited tachycardia (i.e., atrial fibrillation, flutter, atrial tachycardia), or syncope suggestive of cardiac origin should undergo an electrophysiology study for further characterization and ablation of the AP accordingly.
2. Patients with symptomatic palpitations or documented AVRT should be offered an electrophysiology study and ablation of the AP to prevent recurrence and to allow the patient to avoid long-term medical therapy.
   - Ongoing management for stable patients with history of orthodromic AVRT who are not candidates for, or prefer not to undergo, catheter ablation:
   - Class IC antiarrhythmics (flecainide, propafenone), in the absence of structural heart disease.
   - Class III antiarrhythmics (amiodarone, sotalol).
   - Oral beta blockers, diltiazem, or verapamil.

SUGGESTED READINGS
Available at www.expertconsult.com

RELATED CONTENT
Wolff-Parkinson-White Syndrome (Patient Information)

AUTHORS: **YUVAL KONSTANTINO, M.D.,** and **MOTI HAIM, M.D.**

BOX 1 Goals of Electrophysiologic Evaluation in Patients with Wolff-Parkinson-White Syndrome

- Confirmation of the presence of an accessory bypass tract (AP)
- Evaluation for the presence of multiple APs
- Localization of the AP(s)
- Evaluation of the refractory period of the AP and its implications for life-threatening arrhythmias
- Induction and evaluation of tachycardias
- Demonstration of the AP role in the tachycardia
- Evaluation of other tachycardias not dependent on the presence of the AP
- Ablation of the AP, when indicated.

From Issa Z et al: *Clinical arrhythmology and electrophysiology,* ed 2, Philadelphia, 2012, Saunders.

BASIC INFORMATION

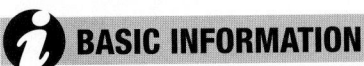

DEFINITION

Zika virus infection is a mosquito-borne flavivirus that has recently emerged as a global public health threat. The infection usually causes subclinical or mild flulike illness, but severe manifestations such microcephaly in babies born to infected mothers and Guillain-Barre syndrome in adults can occur. There is no treatment or vaccine at this time.

SYNONYMS

Zika fever
Zika virus disease

ICD-10CM CODES
A92.8 Other specified mosquito-borne viral fevers
A92.5 Zika virus disease

EPIDEMIOLOGY & DEMOGRAPHICS

INCIDENCE:
- Zika virus has been declared a public health emergency, with more than 20 countries and territories reporting local transmission of the virus in 2016.
- Brazil alone had reported more than 1.3 million people infected with the virus by June 2016.
- In the U.S., local mosquito-borne transmission has occurred in Puerto Rico, U.S. Virgin Islands, and American Samoa; more than 15,000 cases were reported by September 2016, including 31 cases of Guillain-Barré.
- By September 2016, there were 59 locally acquired cases in Florida. There have also been more than 2900 travel-associated cases in the U.S., of which seven had Guillain-Barré and 24 were sexually transmitted. There were 17 cases of live birth defects in babies and five in fetuses of women in the U.S. who were infected abroad as of September 2016. Events are evolving.

PEAK INCIDENCE:
- As a mosquito-borne disease, it is more common in warmer months of the year.

PREVALENCE:
- In an outbreak in Yap islands, 70% of the population was infected in a 13-wk period of time.

RISK FACTORS: The virus can be transmitted in different ways:
- Most common is through the bite of an infected mosquito.
- Maternal-fetal transmission.
- Sexual contact: vaginal, anal, and oral sex. Virus may persist in semen >2 mo.
- Blood transfusion.
- Organ or tissue transplant.

PHYSICAL FINDINGS & CLINICAL PRESENTATION

- Incubation period varies from 3 to 14 days.
- Some 80% of patients will be asymptomatic but can still subsequently develop complications.

- Symptomatic patients will present with:
  1. Mild fever, myalgia, headache
  2. Arthralgias (small joints of hands and feet)
  3. Abdominal pain
  4. Edema
  5. Lymphadenopathy
  6. Retroorbital pain, conjunctivitis
  7. Cutaneous macular-papular rash
- Complications of Zika virus infection
  1. Neurologic complications: meningoencephalitis and Guillain-Barre syndrome in adults.
  2. Neonatal microcephaly: Patients may have mild developmental delays to cerebral palsy.
     a. In Brazil, the incidence of microcephaly increased to 2% to 8% but is still being studied.
     b. Degree of abnormalities may depend on trimester of pregnancy when the infection starts.
     c. 30% of infected pregnant woman may have adverse fetal findings, including fetal death, in utero growth delay with or without microcephaly, optic nerve damage, and ventricular calcifications.
  3. The Zika virus is neurotropic and can cross the blood-brain barrier.

ETIOLOGY

- Zika virus: a flavivirus in the same family as yellow fever virus, dengue virus, West Nile virus.
- First discovered in a febrile rhesus macaque monkey in the Zika forest in Uganda in 1947.
- First human cases discovered in 1954 in Nigeria but cases rare outside of Africa and Southeast Asia until 2007 when first large outbreak occurred in Yap (Micronesia) and then in French Polynesia (2013).
- Zika virus arrived in the Americas in May 2015 in Bahia, Brazil.
- An association with Guillain Barre was noted in French Polynesia, but the association with microcephaly was first noted in September 2015 in Brazil.
- Vector for transmission is the *Aedes aegypti* mosquito, which lives in tropical and subtropical regions including southern U.S., and possibly the *Aedes albopictus* mosquito, which lives in temperate regions, including mid-Atlantic states in the U.S., as well as tropical areas.

DIAGNOSIS

DIFFERENTIAL DIAGNOSIS

- Viral causes of arthritis:
  1. Dengue fever: similar clinical presentation and transmitted by same mosquito
  2. Chikungunya virus: similar presentation, albeit with high fever and intense pain in hands, feet, knees, and back; also transmitted by same mosquito
  3. Parvovirus
  4. Rubella

- Measles
- Leptospirosis
- Malaria
- Rickettsial infections: African tick bite fever and relapsing fever

WORKUP

- Zika virus infection should be suspected in patients with typical clinical manifestations and a history of exposure to the virus via travel/residence in endemic area or sexual contact with a person from endemic area.
- Fig. 1 illustrates a testing algorithm for a pregnant woman with a history of travel to an area with ongoing Zika virus transmission.
- A testing algorithm for a pregnant woman with possible Zika exposure not residing in an area with active Zika virus transmission is described in Fig. 2.
- A testing algorithm for a pregnant woman residing in an area with active Zika virus transmission with or without clinical illness consistent with Zika virus disease is illustrated in Fig. 3.
- Box 1 summarizes recommended Zika virus laboratory testing for infants and children when indicated.
- Recommended clinical evaluation and laboratory testing for infants with possible congenital Zika virus infection is summarized in Box 2.

LABORATORY TESTS

- Zika virus reverse transcriptase polymerase chain reaction (Zika RT-PCR) in serum or urine in acute infection
  1. Serum: only positive if viremic (3 to 7 days after start of symptoms)
  2. Urine: positive for up to 14 days after start of symptoms
- Zika serology: Zika virus IgM ELISA for patients presenting longer than 14 days of symptoms; Zika virus IgG ELISA
- It should be noted that there is cross-reactivity with other flaviviruses; dengue and yellow fever can lead to false positives.

IMAGING STUDIES

- Fetal ultrasound is used to screen for fetal Zika virus infection complications.
- Fetal abnormalities may be seen as early as 18 to 20 wk of gestation but more likely detected in late second and early third trimester.
- Fetal microcephaly is described as a head circumference ≥3 standard deviations below the mean for gestational age by the Society for Maternal-Fetal Medicine and <3rd percentile for gestational age by the Centers for Disease Control and Prevention (CDC).

TREATMENT

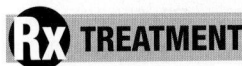

NONPHARMACOLOGIC THERAPY

- Rest and hydration

ACUTE GENERAL Rx

1. Acetaminophen can be used for fever but not aspirin or NSAIDS until dengue virus has been ruled out. Aspirin increases risk of hem-

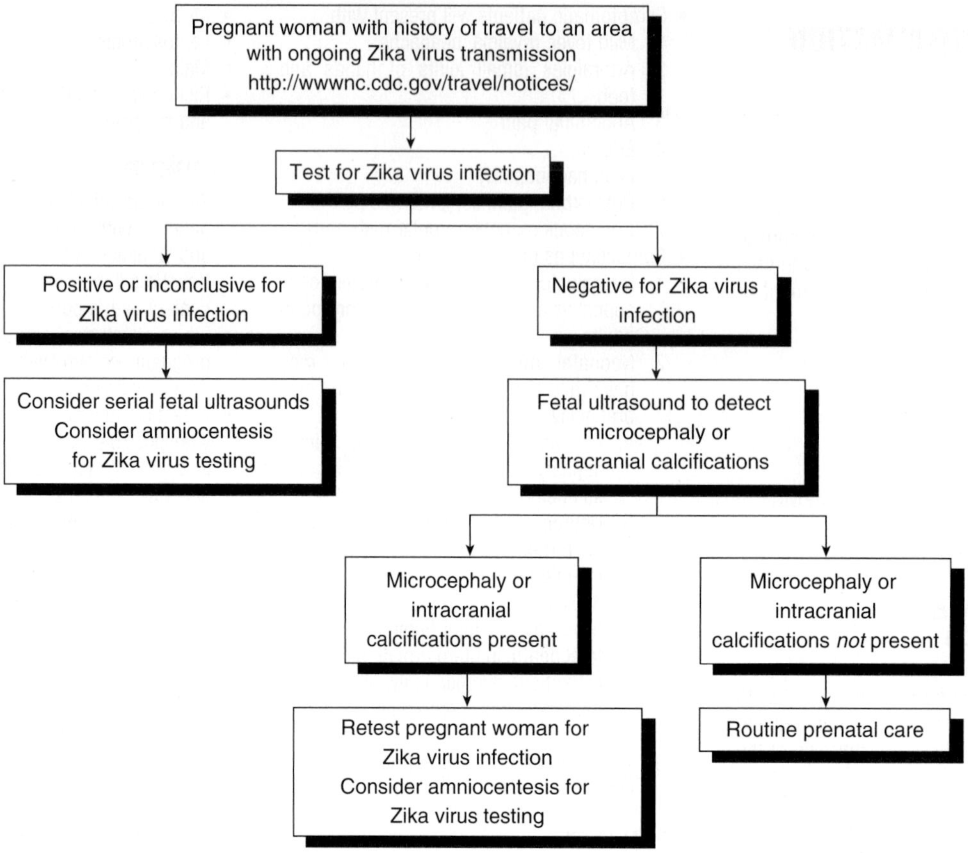

Pregnant woman with history of travel to an area
with ongoing Zika virus transmission
http://wwwnc.cdc.gov/travel/notices/

Test for Zika virus infection

Positive or inconclusive for
Zika virus infection

Negative for Zika virus
infection

Consider serial fetal ultrasounds
Consider amniocentesis
for Zika virus testing

Fetal ultrasound to detect
microcephaly or
intracranial calcifications

Microcephaly or
intracranial
calcifications present

Microcephaly or
intracranial
calcifications *not* present

Retest pregnant woman for
Zika virus infection
Consider amniocentesis for
Zika virus testing

Routine prenatal care

* Testing is recommended for pregnant women with clinical illness consistent with Zika virus disease, which includes two or more of the following signs or symptoms: acute onset of fever, maculopapular rash, arthralgia, or conjunctivitis during or within 2 weeks of travel. Testing includes Zika virus reverse transcription-polymerase chain reaction (RT-PCR), and Zika virus immunoglobulin M (IgM) and neutralizing antibodies on serum specimens (http://www.aphl.org/Materials/CDCMemo_Zika_Chik_Deng_Testing_011916.pdf). Because of the overlap of symptoms and areas where other viral illnesses are endemic, evaluation for dengue or chikungunya virus infection is also recommended.

† Testing can be offered to pregnant women without clinical illness consistent with Zika virus disease. If performed, testing should include Zika virus IgM, and if IgM test result is positive or indeterminate, neutralizing antibodies on serum specimens. Testing should be performed 2–12 weeks after travel.

§ Laboratory evidence of maternal Zika virus infection: 1) Zika virus RNA detected by RT-PCR in any clinical specimen; or 2) positive Zika virus IgM with confirmatory neutralizing antibody titers that are ≥4-fold higher than dengue virus neutralizing antibody titers in serum. Testing is considered inconclusive if Zika virus neutralizing antibody titers are <4-fold higher than dengue virus neutralizing antibody titers.

¶ Fetal ultrasounds might not detect microcephaly or intracranial calcifications until the late second or early third trimester of pregnancy.

** Amniocentesis is not recommended until after 15 weeks of gestation. Amniotic fluid should be tested for Zika virus RNA by RT-PCR. The sensitivity and specificity of RT-PCR testing on amniotic fluid are not known.

FIG. 1 Updated interim guidance: testing algorithm*,†,§,¶,** for a pregnant woman with history of travel to an area with ongoing Zika virus transmission. (From MMWR, Feb 12, 2016, vol 65, no.5. Figure 1 page 124.)

orrhage, and NSAIDS should not be used in pregnancy. Aspirin should be avoided in children due to risk of Reye's syndrome.
2. Antihistamines can be used to control rash in patients with a rash.
3. At this time, there is no specific antiviral agent.

REFERRAL

To an expert in obstetrics and gynecology to evaluate a pregnant woman who may have been exposed to the Zika virus. Recommended long-term follow-up for infants with possible congenital Zika virus infection are summarized in Box 3.

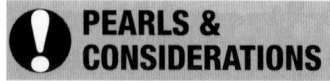

PEARLS & CONSIDERATIONS

• The *Aedes* mosquitos can also transmit dengue and chikungunya viruses.

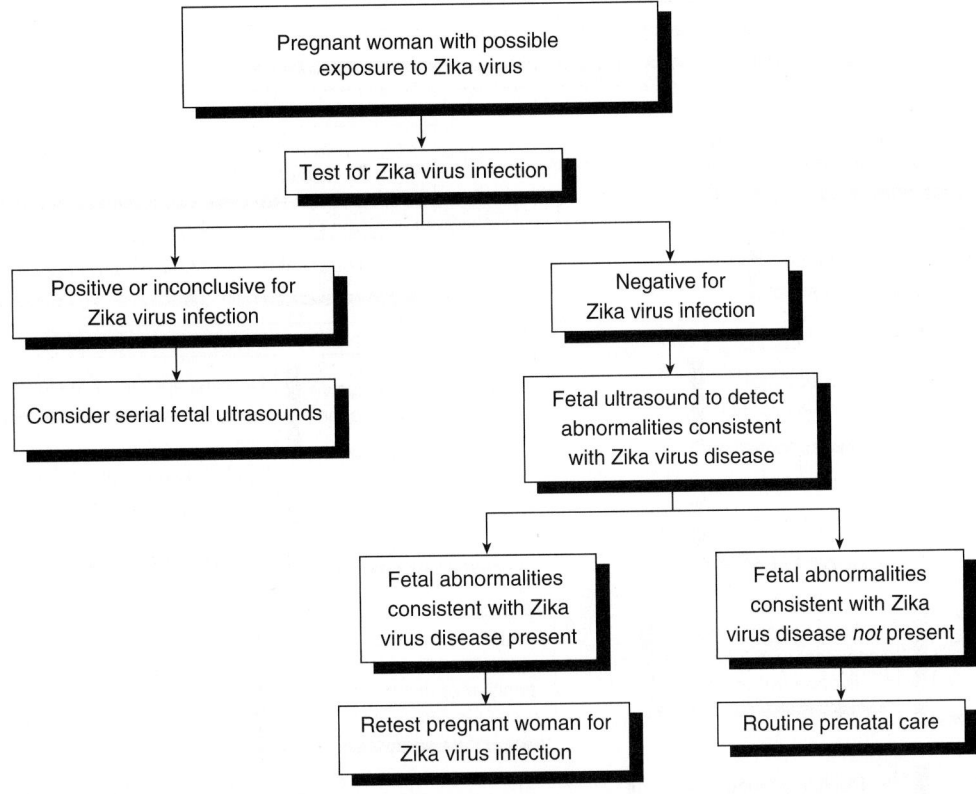

* Testing is recommended for pregnant women with clinical illness consistent with Zika virus disease, including one or more of the following signs or symptoms: acute onset of fever, rash, arthralgia, or conjunctivitis during or within 2 weeks of travel or possible sexual exposure. Testing includes Zika virus reverse transcription-polymerase chain reaction (RTPCR), and Zika virus immunoglobulin M (IgM) and neutralizing antibodies on serum specimens. More information is available at http://www.aphl.org/Materials/CDCMemo_Zika_Chik_Deng_Testing_011916.pdf. Because of the overlap of symptoms and areas where other viral illnesses are endemic, evaluate for possible dengue or chikungunya virus infection.

† Testing can be offered to pregnant women without clinical illness consistent with Zika virus disease. If performed, testing should include Zika virus IgM, and if IgM test result is positive or indeterminate, neutralizing antibodies on serum specimens. Testing should be performed 2–12 weeks after travel.

§ Laboratory evidence of maternal Zika virus infection: 1) Zika virus RNA detected by RT-PCR in any clinical specimen; or 2) positive Zika virus IgM with confirmatory neutralizing antibody titers that are ≥4-fold higher than dengue virus neutralizing antibody titers in serum. Testing is considered inconclusive if Zika virus neutralizing antibody titers are <4-fold higher than dengue virus neutralizing antibody titers.

¶ Fetal abnormalities consistent with Zika virus disease include microcephaly, intracranial calcifications, and brain and eye abnormalities. Fetal ultrasounds might not detect abnormalities until late second or early third trimester of pregnancy

** Possible exposure to Zika virus includes travel to an area with active Zika virus transmission (http://wwwnc.cdc.gov/travel/notices), or sex (vaginal intercourse, anal intercourse, or fellatio) without a condom with a man who traveled to, or resided in, an area with active Zika virus transmission. Testing is not currently recommended for pregnant women with possible sexual exposure to Zika virus if both partners are asymptomatic.

FIG. 2 Updated interim guidance: testing algorithm*,†,§,¶ for a pregnant woman with possible Zika virus exposure** not residing in an area with active Zika virus transmission. (From MMWR, April 1, 2016, vol 65, no.12. Figure 1 page 319.)

- CDC maintains a service to help physicians deal with a pregnant woman and infants exposed to the Zika virus: 1-800-CDC-INFO.
- Vaccine development is ongoing but no currently available vaccine.
- Aerial spraying with EPA-registered insecticides has been a strategy implemented in the Florida outbreak, along with other mosquito-control strategies.

COMMENTS

- Zika virus is already impacting blood donations for people who have traveled to affected area or live in affected areas. Travelers may need to postpone donations for at least 28 days. New guidelines by the U.S. Food and Drug Administration (FDA) call for testing blood donors in areas where active Zika virus transmission has occurred.

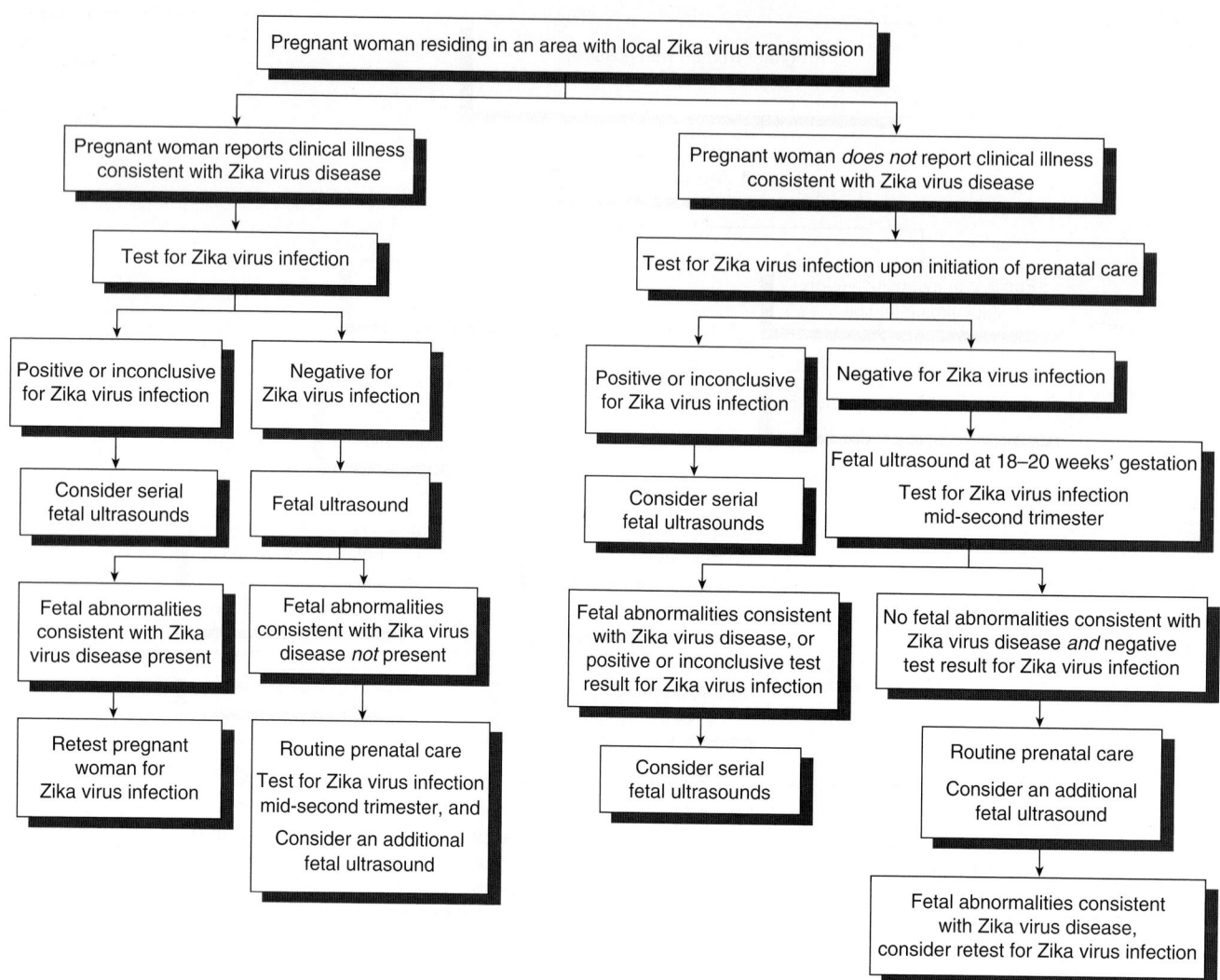

* Tests for pregnant women with clinical illness consistent with Zika virus disease include Zika virus reverse transcription-polymerase chain reaction (RT-PCR), and Zika virus immunoglobulin M (IgM) and neutralizing antibodies on serum specimens. More information is available at http://www.aphl.org/Materials/CDCMemo_Zika_Chik_Deng_Testing_011916.pdf. Because of the overlap of symptoms and areas where other viral illnesses are endemic, evaluate for possible dengue or chikungunya virus infection. If chikungunya or dengue virus RNA is detected, treat in accordance with existing guidelines. Timely recognition and supportive treatment for dengue virus infections can substantially lower the risk of medical complications and death. Repeat Zika virus testing during pregnancy is warranted if clinical illness consistent with Zika virus disease develops later in pregnancy.

† Testing can be offered to pregnant women without clinical illness consistent with Zika virus disease. If performed, testing should include Zika virus IgM, and if IgM test result is positive or indeterminate, neutralizing antibodies on serum specimens. Results from serologic testing are challenging to interpret in areas where residents have had previous exposure to other flaviviruses (e.g., dengue, yellow fever) because of cross-reactivity with other flaviviruses.

§ Laboratory evidence of maternal Zika virus infection: 1) Zika virus RNA detected by RT-PCR in any clinical specimen; or 2) positive Zika virus IgM with confirmatory neutralizing antibody titers that are ≥4-fold higher than dengue virus neutralizing antibody titers in serum. Testing would be considered inconclusive if Zika virus neutralizing antibody titers are <4-fold higher than dengue virus neutralizing antibody titer.

¶ Fetal abnormalities consistent with Zika virus disease include microcephaly, intracranial calcifications, and brain and eye abnormalities. Fetal ultrasounds might not detect abnormalities until late second or early third trimester of pregnancy.

** http://wwwnc.cdc.gov/travel/notices/. Local health officials should determine when to implement testing of asymptomatic pregnant women based on information about levels of Zika virus transmission and laboratory capacity.

†† Clinical illness is consistent with Zika virus disease if one or more signs or symptoms (acute onset of fever, rash, arthralgia, or conjunctivitis) are present.

FIG. 3 Updated interim guidance: testing algorithm*,†,§,¶ for a pregnant woman residing in an area with active Zika virus transmission,** with or without clinical illness†† consistent with Zika virus disease. (From MMWR, April 1, 2016, vol 65, no.12. Figure 2 page 320.)

BOX 1 Recommended Zika Virus Laboratory Testing for Infants and Children When Indicated*,†,§

For possible congenital Zika virus infection
- Test infant serum for Zika virus RNA, Zika virus immunoglobulin M (IgM) and neutralizing antibodies, and dengue virus IgM and neutralizing antibodies. The initial sample should be collected either from the umbilical cord or directly from the infant within 2 days of birth, if possible.
- If cerebrospinal fluid is obtained for other studies, test for Zika virus RNA, Zika virus IgM and neutralizing antibodies, and dengue virus IgM and neutralizing antibodies.
- Consider histopathologic evaluation of the placenta and umbilical cord with Zika virus immunohistochemical staining on fixed tissue and Zika virus reverse transcription-polymerase chain reaction (RT-PCR) on fixed and frozen tissue.
- If not already performed during pregnancy, test mother's serum for Zika virus IgM and neutralizing antibodies, and dengue virus IgM and neutralizing antibodies.

For possible acute Zika virus disease
- If symptoms have been present for <7 days, test serum (and, if obtained for other reasons, cerebrospinal fluid) for Zika virus RNA by RT-PCR.
- If Zika virus RNA is not detected and symptoms have been present for ≥4 days, test serum (and, if obtained for other reasons, cerebrospinal fluid) for Zika virus IgM and neutralizing antibodies, and dengue virus IgM and neutralizing antibodies.

* Indications for testing for congenital infection include (1) an infant with microcephaly or intracranial calcifications born to a woman who traveled to or resided in an area with Zika virus transmission while she was pregnant or (2) an infant born to a mother with a positive or inconclusive test result for Zika virus infection.
† Indications for testing during acute disease include
Infants and children <18 years who (1) traveled to or resided in an affected area within the past 2 wk and (2) have ≥2 of the following manifestations: fever, rash, conjunctivitis, or arthralgia.
Infants in the first 2 wk of life (1) whose mothers have traveled to or resided in an affected area within 2 wk of delivery and (2) have ≥2 of the following manifestations: fever, rash, conjunctivitis, or arthralgia.
§ More information on laboratory testing for Zika virus infection is available at http://www.cdc.gov/zika/state-labs/index.html.
Adapted from Staples JE et al: Interim guidelines for the evaluation and testing of infants with possible congenital Zika virus infection United States, *MMWR Morb Mortal Wkly Rep* 65(3):63-67, 2016.

BOX 2 Recommended Clinical Evaluation and Laboratory Testing for Infants With Possible Congenital Zika Virus Infection

For all infants with possible congenital Zika virus infection, perform the following:
- Comprehensive physical examination, including careful measurement of occipitofrontal circumference, length, weight, and assessment of gestational age.
- Evaluation for neurologic abnormalities, dysmorphic features, splenomegaly, hepatomegaly, and rash or other skin lesions. Full-body photographs and photographic documentation of any rash, skin lesions, or dysmorphic features should be performed. If an abnormality is noted, consultation with an appropriate specialist is recommended.
- Cranial ultrasound, unless prenatal ultrasound results from third trimester demonstrated no abnormalities of the brain.
- Evaluation of hearing by evoked otoacoustic emissions testing or auditory brainstem response testing, either before discharge from the hospital or within 1 mo after birth. Infants with abnormal initial hearing screens should be referred to an audiologist for further evaluation.
- Ophthalmologic evaluation, including examination of the retina, either before discharge from the hospital or within 1 mo after birth. Infants with abnormal initial eye evaluation should be referred to a pediatric ophthalmologist for further evaluation.
- Other evaluations specific to the infant's clinical presentation.

For infants with microcephaly or intracranial calcifications, additional evaluation includes the following:
- Consultation with a clinical geneticist or dysmorphologist.
- Consultation with a pediatric neurologist to determine appropriate brain imaging and additional evaluation (e.g., ultrasound, computerized tomography scan, magnetic resonance imaging, and electroencephalogram).
- Testing for other congenital infections such as syphilis, toxoplasmosis, rubella, cytomegalovirus infection, lymphocytic choriomeningitis virus infection, and herpes simplex virus infections. Consider consulting a pediatric infectious disease specialist.
- Complete blood count with platelet count and liver function and enzyme tests, including alanine aminotransferase, aspartate aminotransferase, and bilirubin.
- Consideration of genetic and other teratogenic causes based on additional congenital anomalies that are identified through clinical examination and imaging studies.

Adapted from Staples, JE et al: Interim guidelines for the evaluation and testing of infants with possible congenital Zika virus infection - United States, *MMWR Morb Mortal Wkly Rep* 65(3):63-67, 2016.

BOX 3 Recommended Long-Term Follow-up for Infants With Possible Congenital Zika Virus Infection

For all infants with possible congenital Zika virus infection, recommended long-term follow-up:
- Report case to state, territorial, or local health department and monitor for additional guidance as it is released.
- Consider conducting additional hearing screen at age 6 mo. Refer any child with developmental delay for an audiologic evaluation. Ensure that appropriate follow-up of abnormal newborn hearing screening has occurred.
- Carefully evaluate occipitofrontal circumference and developmental characteristics and milestones throughout the first year of life, in consultation with appropriate medical specialists (e.g., pediatric neurology, developmental and behavioral pediatrics, physical and speech therapy).

Adapted from Staples, JE et al: Interim guidelines for the evaluation and testing of infants with possible congenital Zika virus infection - United States, *MMWR Morb Mortal Wkly Rep* 65(3):63-67, 2016.

BOX 4 Recommendations for Counseling Persons in Areas of Active Zika Virus Transmission Interested in Attempting Conception

Assess risk of Zika virus exposure
Environment
- Air conditioning, window screens in home
- Work environment
- Residence in area with high mosquito density
- Level of Zika virus transmission in the local area

Personal measures to prevent mosquito bites
- Protective clothing
- Use of EPA-registered insect repellent
- Emptying/removing standing water in containers

Personal measures to prevent sexual transmission
- Willingness to use condoms or abstain from sex throughout pregnancy

Discuss Zika virus infection in pregnancy
- Signs/symptoms of Zika virus disease
- Possible adverse consequences of Zika virus infection during pregnancy
- Unknown duration of epidemic

Explore reproductive life plan
- Fertility
- Age
- Reproductive history
- Medical history
- Personal values, preferences

Discuss risks/benefits of pregnancy at this time with woman and her partner
- If pregnancy not desired now, discuss contraceptive options.

Adapted from Staples JE et al: Interim guidelines for the evaluation and testing of infants with possible congenital Zika virus infection—United States, *MMWR Morb Mortal Wkly Rep* 65(3):63-67, 2016.

BOX 5 Recommendations for Prevention of Sexual Transmission of Zika Virus for Couples in Which a Man Has Traveled to or Resides in an Area with Active Zika Virus Transmission

Couples in which a woman is pregnant
- Couples in which a woman is pregnant should use condoms consistently and correctly or abstain from sex for the duration of the pregnany.

Other couples concerned about sexual transmission*
- Couples in which a man had confirmed Zika virus infection or clinical illness consistent with Zika virus disease should consider using condoms or abstaining from sex for at least 6 months after onset of illness.
- Couples in which a man traveled to an area with active Zika virus transmission but did not develop symptoms of Zika virus disease should consider using condoms or abstaining from sex for at least 8 weeks after departure from the area.
- Couples in which a man resides in an area with active Zika virus transmission but has not developed symptoms of Zika virus disease might consider using condoms or abstaining from sex while active transmission persists.

* Couples who do not desire pregnancy should use the most effective contraception methods that can be used correctly and consistently in addition to condoms, which also reduce the risk for sexually transmitted infections. Couples planning conception have a number of factors to consider, which are discussed in more detail in the following: Petersen EE, et al.: Update: interim guidance for health care providers caring for women of reproductive age with possible Zika virus exposure—United States, 2016, *MMWR* 2016.
From Petersen EE, et al.: Update: interim guidance for health care providers caring for women of reproductive age with possible Zika virus exposure—United States, *MMWR* 65(12):324, 2016.

PREVENTION

- Wear long-sleeved shirts, pants, and hat.
- Insect repellents: Apply to exposed skin in daylight hours when *Aedes* mosquitos are most active:
  1. DEET: Diethyltoluamide 20% to 50% concentration
  2. Icaridin in at least 20% concentration
  3. Lemon eucalyptus extract in at least 30% concentration
- Clothing can be treated with permethrin soak or 1% spray.
- Do not use insect repellents on babies younger than 2 mo and avoid lemon eucalyptus on children younger than 3 yr.
- Recommedations for counseling persons in areas of active Zika virus transmission interested in attempting conception are summarized in Box 4.
- Recommendations for prevention of sexual transmission of Zika virus for couples in which a man has traveled to or resides in an area with active Zika virus transmission are summarized in Box 5.

PATIENT/FAMILY EDUCATION

- Both *Aedes aegypti* and *Aedes albopictus* are daytime biters, so protection is essential during those hours.
- Men who have traveled to areas where Zika virus is present and have developed symptomatic disease should abstain from sexual contact or use a condom for up to 6 mo afterwards.
- Recommendations for counseling persons who live in areas of active Zika virus transmission and are interested in attempting conception.

SUGGESTED READINGS
Available at www.expertconsult.com

RELATED CONTENT
Dengue Fever (Related Key Topic)
Yellow Fever (Related Key Topic)

AUTHOR: **GLENN G. FORT, M.D., M.P.H.**

Differential Diagnosis

SECTION II

Differential Diagnosis

ABDOMINAL DISTENTION

ICD-10CM #	R14.0	Abdominal Distension (Gaseous)

NONMECHANICAL OBSTRUCTION

Excessive intraluminal gas.
Intraabdominal infection.
Trauma.
Retroperitoneal irritation (renal colic, neoplasms, infections, hemorrhage).
Vascular insufficiency (thrombosis, embolism).
Mechanical ventilation.
Extraabdominal infection (sepsis, pneumonia, empyema, osteomyelitis of spine).
Metabolic/toxic abnormalities (hypokalemia, uremia, lead poisoning).
Chemical irritation (perforated ulcer, bile, pancreatitis).
Peritoneal inflammation.
Severe pain, pain medications.

MECHANICAL OBSTRUCTION

Neoplasm (intraluminal, extraluminal).
Adhesions, endometriosis.
Infection (intraabdominal abscess, diverticulitis).
Gallstones.
Foreign body, bezoars.
Pregnancy.
Hernias.
Volvulus.
Stenosis at surgical anastomosis, radiation stenosis.
Fecaliths.
Inflammatory bowel disease.
Gastric outlet obstruction.
Hematoma.
Other: parasites, superior mesenteric artery (SMA) syndrome, pneumatosis intestinalis, annular pancreas, Hirschsprung's disease, intussusception, meconium.

ABDOMINAL PAIN, ADOLESCENCE[50]

ICD-10CM #	R10.817	Generalized Abdominal Tenderness
	R10.827	Generalized Rebound Abdominal Tenderness

Acute gastroenteritis.
Irritable bowel syndrome (IBS).
Anxiety.
Mittelschmerz.
Appendicitis.
Inflammatory bowel disease.
Peptic ulcer disease (PUD).
Cholecystitis.
Neoplasm.
Diabetic ketoacidosis.
Functional abdominal pain.
Pelvic inflammatory disease (PID).
Pregnancy.
Pyelonephritis.
Renal stone.
Trauma.

ABDOMINAL PAIN, CHILDHOOD[50]

ICD-10CM #	R10.817	Generalized Abdominal Tenderness
	R10.827	Generalized Rebound Abdominal Tenderness

Acute gastroenteritis.
Appendicitis.
Constipation.
Cholecystitis, acute.
Intestinal obstruction.
Pancreatitis.
Neoplasm.
Inflammatory bowel disease.
Other:
    Functional abdominal pain.
    Pyelonephritis.
    Pneumonia.
    Diabetic ketoacidosis.
    Heavy metal poisoning.
    Sickle cell crisis.
    Trauma.
    Anxiety.
    Sexual abuse.

ABDOMINAL PAIN, CHRONIC LOWER[72]

ICD-10CM #	R10.814	Left Lower Quadrant Abdominal Tenderness
	R10.824	Left Lower Quadrant Rebound Abdominal Tenderness
	R10.813	Right Lower Quadrant Abdominal Tenderness
	R10.823	Right Lower Quadrant Rebound Abdominal Tenderness
	R10.30	Lower Abdominal Pain, Unspecified

ORGANIC DISORDERS

Common
Gynecologic disease.
Lactase deficiency.
Diverticulitis/diverticulosis.
Crohn's disease.
Intestinal obstruction.
Uncommon
Chronic intestinal pseudoobstruction.
Mesenteric ischemia.
Malignancy (e.g., ovarian carcinoma).
Abdominal wall pain.
Spinal disease.
Testicular disease.
Metabolic diseases (e.g., diabetes mellitus, familial Mediterranean fever, C1 esterase deficiency [angioneurotic edema], porphyria, lead poisoning, tabes dorsalis, renal failure).

FUNCTIONAL DISORDERS

Common
Irritable bowel syndrome.
Functional abdominal bloating.
Uncommon
Functional abdominal pain.

ABDOMINAL PAIN, DIFFUSE

ICD-10CM #	R10.817	Generalized Abdominal Tenderness
	R10.827	Generalized Rebound Abdominal Tenderness

Early appendicitis.
Aortic aneurysm.
Gastroenteritis.
Intestinal obstruction.
Diverticulitis.
Peritonitis.
Mesenteric insufficiency or infarction.
Pancreatitis.
Inflammatory bowel disease.
Irritable bowel.
Mesenteric adenitis.
Metabolic: toxins, lead poisoning, uremia, drug overdose, diabetic ketoacidosis (DKA), heavy metal poisoning.
Sickle cell crisis.
Pneumonia (rare).
Trauma.
Urinary tract infection, PID.
Other: anxiety, acute intermittent porphyria, tabes dorsalis, periarteritis nodosa, Henoch-Schönlein purpura, adrenal insufficiency.

ABDOMINAL PAIN, EPIGASTRIC

ICD-10CM #	R10.816	Epigastric Abdominal Tenderness
	R10.826	Epigastric Rebound Abdominal Tenderness

Gastric: PUD, gastric outlet obstruction, gastric ulcer.
Duodenal: PUD, duodenitis.
Biliary: cholecystitis, cholangitis, biliary dyskinesia.
Hepatic: hepatitis.
Pancreatic: pancreatitis.
Intestinal: high small bowel obstruction, early appendicitis.
Cardiac: angina, MI, pericarditis.
Pulmonary: pneumonia, pleurisy, pneumothorax.
Subphrenic abscess.
Vascular: dissecting aneurysm, mesenteric ischemia.
Psychiatric: anxiety.

ABDOMINAL PAIN, EXTRAABDOMINAL AND SYSTEMIC CAUSES[23]

ICD-10CM #	R10.817	Generalized Abdominal Tenderness

Differential Diagnosis

II

EXTRAABDOMINAL AND SYSTEMIC CAUSES OF ACUTE ABDOMINAL PAIN

Cardiac
Endocarditis
Heart failure
Myocardial ischemia and infarction
Myocarditis

Thoracic
Empyema
Esophageal rupture (Boerhaave's syndrome)
Esophageal spasm
Esophagitis
Pleurodynia (Bornholm's disease)
Pneumonitis
Pneumothorax
Pulmonary embolism and infarction

Hemotologic
Acute leukemia
Hemolytic anemia
Henoch-Schönlein purpura
Sickle cell disease

Metabolic
Acute adrenal insufficiency (Addison's disease)
Diabetes mellitus (especially with ketoacidosis)
Hyperlipidemia
Hyperparathyroidism
Hypersensitivity reactions (e.g., to insect bites, reptile venoms)
Lead poisoning
Porphyria
Toxins
Uremia

Infections
Herpes zoster
Osteomyelitis
Typhoid fever

Neurologic
Abdominal epilepsy
Radiculopathy, spinal cord or peripheral nerve tumors, degenerative arthritis of spine, herniated vertebral disk
Tabes dorsalis

Miscellaneous
Angioedema
Familial Mediterranean fever
Heat stroke
Muscle contusion, hematoma, tumor
Narcotic withdrawal
Psychiatric disorders

ABDOMINAL PAIN, INFANCY[50]

| ICD-10CM # | R10.817 | Generalized Abdominal Tenderness |
| | R10.827 | Generalized Rebound Abdominal Tenderness |

Acute gastroenteritis.
Appendicitis.
Intussusception.
Volvulus.
Meckel diverticulum.
Other: colic, trauma.

ABDOMINAL PAIN, LEFT LOWER QUADRANT

| ICD-10CM # | R10.814 | Left Lower Quadrant Abdominal Tenderness |
| | R10.824 | Left Lower Quadrant Rebound Abdominal Tenderness |

Intestinal: diverticulitis, diverticulosis, intestinal obstruction, perforated ulcer, inflammatory bowel disease, perforated descending colon, inguinal hernia, neoplasm, appendicitis.
Reproductive: ectopic pregnancy, ovarian cyst, torsion of ovarian cyst, tuboovarian abscess, mittelschmerz, endometriosis, seminal vesiculitis.
Renal: renal or ureteral calculi, pyelonephritis, neoplasm.
Vascular: leaking aortic aneurysm.
Psoas abscess.
Trauma.

ABDOMINAL PAIN, LEFT UPPER QUADRANT

| ICD-10CM # | R19.02 | Left Upper Quadrant Abdominal Swelling, Mass, and Lump |

Gastric: PUD, gastritis, pyloric stenosis, hiatal hernia.
Pancreatic: pancreatitis, neoplasm, stone in pancreatic duct or ampulla.
Cardiac: MI, angina pectoris.
Splenic: splenomegaly, ruptured spleen, splenic abscess, splenic infarction.
Renal: calculi, pyelonephritis, neoplasm.
Pulmonary: pneumonia, empyema, pulmonary infarction.
Vascular: ruptured aortic aneurysm.
Cutaneous: herpes zoster.
Trauma.
Intestinal: high fecal impaction, perforated colon, diverticulitis.

ABDOMINAL PAIN, NONSURGICAL CAUSES

| ICD-10CM # | R19.8 | Other Specified Symptoms and Signs Involving the Digestive System and Abdomen |
| | R10.817 | Generalized abdominal tenderness |

Irritable bowel syndrome.
Urinary tract infection, pyelonephritis, salpingitis, PID.
Gastroenteritis, gastritis, peptic ulcer.
Diverticular spasm.
Hepatitis, mononucleosis.
Pancreatitis.
Inferior wall myocardial infarction.
Basilar pneumonia, pulmonary embolism.
Diabetic ketoacidosis.
Strain or hematoma of rectus muscle.
Ruptured Graafian follicle.
Herpes zoster.

Nerve root compression.
Sickle cell crisis.
Acute adrenal insufficiency.
Other: acute porphyria, familial Mediterranean fever, tabes dorsalis, anxiety, sexual abuse.

ABDOMINAL PAIN, PERIUMBILICAL

| ICD-10CM # | R10.815 | Periumbilic Abdominal Tenderness |
| | R10.825 | Periumbilic Rebound Abdominal Tenderness |

Intestinal: small bowel obstruction or gangrene, early appendicitis.
Vascular: mesenteric thrombosis, dissecting aortic aneurysm.
Pancreatic: pancreatitis.
Metabolic: uremia, DKA.
Trauma.

ABDOMINAL PAIN, POORLY LOCALIZED[50]

| ICD-10CM # | R10.819 | Abdominal Tenderness, Unspecified Site |

EXTRAABDOMINAL

Metabolic
DKA, acute intermittent porphyria, hyperthyroidism, hypothyroidism, hypercalcemia, hypokalemia, uremia, hyperlipidemia, hyperparathyroidism.

Hematologic
Sickle cell crisis, leukemia or lymphoma, Henoch-Schönlein purpura.

Infectious
Infectious mononucleosis, Rocky Mountain spotted fever, acquired immunodeficiency syndrome (AIDS), streptococcal pharyngitis (in children), herpes zoster.

Drugs and Toxins
Heavy metal poisoning, black widow spider bites, withdrawal syndromes, mushroom ingestion.

Referred Pain
Pulmonary: pneumonia, pulmonary embolism, pneumothorax.
Cardiac: angina, MI, pericarditis, myocarditis.
Genitourinary: prostatitis, epididymitis, orchitis, testicular torsion.
Musculoskeletal: rectus sheath hematoma.

Functional
Somatization disorder, malingering, hypochondriasis, Münchausen syndrome.

INTRAABDOMINAL

Early appendicitis, gastroenteritis, peritonitis, pancreatitis, abdominal aortic aneurysm, mesenteric insufficiency or infarction, intestinal obstruction, volvulus, ulcerative colitis.

ABDOMINAL PAIN, POST-CHOLECYSTECTOMY[23]

ICD-10CM #	R10.817	Generalized Abdominal Tenderness

CAUSES OF ABDOMINAL PAIN AFTER CHOLECYSTECTOMY

Biliary Causes
Biliary stricture
Biliary tract malignancy
Choledocholithiasis
Choledochocele
Cystic duct remnant
SOD

Pancreatic Causes
Pancreatitis
Pseudocyst
Malignancy

Other GI Disorders
Esophageal motor disorders
GERD
Intestinal malignancy
Intraabdominal adhesions
IBS
Mesenteric ischemia
PUD

Extraintestinal Disorders
Coronary artery disease
Intercostal neuritis
Neurologic disorders
Psychiatric disorders
Wound neuroma

ABDOMINAL PAIN, PREGNANCY

ICD-10CM #	R10.817	Generalized Abdominal Tenderness
	R10.827	Generalized Rebound Abdominal Tenderness

GYNECOLOGIC (GESTATIONAL AGE IN PARENTHESES)

Miscarriage	(<20 wk; 80% <12 wk)
Septic abortion	(<20 wk)
Ectopic pregnancy	(<14 wk)
Corpus luteum cyst rupture	(<12 wk)
Ovarian torsion	(especially <24 wk)
Pelvic inflammatory disease	(<12 wk)
Chorioamnionitis	(>16 wk)
Abruptio placentae	(>16 wk)

NONGYNECOLOGIC

Appendicitis	(Throughout)
Cholecystitis	(Throughout)
Hepatitis	(Throughout)
Pyelonephritis	(Throughout)
Preeclampsia	(>20 wk)

ABDOMINAL PAIN, RIGHT LOWER QUADRANT

ICD-10CM #	R10.813	Right Lower Quadrant Abdominal Tenderness
	R10.823	Right Lower Quadrant Rebound Abdominal Tenderness

Intestinal: acute appendicitis, regional enteritis, incarcerated hernia, cecal diverticulitis, intestinal obstruction, perforated ulcer, perforated cecum, Meckel diverticulitis.
Reproductive: ectopic pregnancy, ovarian cyst, torsion of ovarian cyst, salpingitis, tuboovarian abscess, mittelschmerz, endometriosis, seminal vesiculitis.
Renal: renal and ureteral calculi, neoplasms, pyelonephritis.
Vascular: leaking aortic aneurysm.
Cutaneous: herpes zoster.
Psoas abscess.
Trauma.
Cholecystitis.

ABDOMINAL PAIN, RIGHT UPPER QUADRANT

ICD-10CM #	R10.811	Right Upper Quadrant Abdominal Tenderness
	R10.821	Right Upper Quadrant Rebound Abdominal Tenderness

Biliary: calculi, infection, inflammation, neoplasm.
Hepatic: hepatitis, abscess, hepatic congestion, neoplasm, trauma.
Gastric: PUD, pyloric stenosis, neoplasm, alcoholic gastritis, hiatal hernia.
Pancreatic: pancreatitis, neoplasm, stone in pancreatic duct or ampulla.
Renal: calculi, infection, inflammation, neoplasm, rupture of kidney.
Pulmonary: pneumonia, pulmonary infarction, right-sided pleurisy.
Intestinal: retrocecal appendicitis, intestinal obstruction, high fecal impaction, diverticulitis.
Cardiac: myocardial ischemia (particularly involving the inferior wall), pericarditis.
Cutaneous: herpes zoster.
Trauma.
Fitz-Hugh-Curtis syndrome (perihepatitis).

ABDOMINAL PAIN, RIGHT UPPER QUADRANT, DIFFERENTIAL DIAGNOSIS IN PREGNANCY[27]

ICD-10CM #	R10.811	Right Upper Quadrant Abdominal Tenderness
	R10.821	Right Upper Quadrant Rebound Abdominal Tenderness

DIFFERENTIAL DIAGNOSIS OF RIGHT UPPER QUADRANT ABDOMINAL PAIN DURING PREGNANCY

Hepatic Disorders:
Hepatitis.
Hepatic vascular engorgement.
Hepatic hematoma.
Hepatic malignancy.
Biliary Tract Disease:
Biliary colic.
Choledocholithiasis.
Cholangitis.
Cholecystitis.
Diseases Related to Pregnancy:
Preeclampsia or eclampsia.
Hemolysis, elevated liver enzymes, and low platelet count (HELLP) syndrome.
Acute fatty liver of pregnancy.
Hepatic hemorrhage or rupture.
Renal Disorders:
Pyelonephritis.
Nephrolithiasis.
Gastrointestinal Disorders:
Peptic ulcer disease.
Perforated duodenal ulcer.
Other Conditions in RUQ:
Rib fracture.
Shingles.
Referred Pain from Other Organ Disease:
Pneumonia.
Pulmonary embolus or infarct.
Pleural effusion.
Radiculopathy.
Inferior wall myocardial infarction.
Colon cancer.

ABDOMINAL PAIN, SUPRAPUBIC

ICD-10CM #	R10.30	Lower Abdominal Pain, Unspecified

Intestinal: colon obstruction or gangrene, diverticulitis, appendicitis.
Reproductive system: ectopic pregnancy, mittelschmerz, torsion of ovarian cyst, PID, salpingitis, endometriosis, rupture of endometrioma.
Cystitis, rupture of urinary bladder.

ABDOMINAL WALL MASSES[72]

ICD-10CM #	R19.00	Intraabdominal and Pelvic Swelling, Mass and Lump, Unspecified Site

LUMPS ARISING IN THE SKIN AND SUBCUTANEOUS FAT (THAT COULD OCCUR ANYWHERE ON THE BODY)

Lipoma.
Sebaceous cyst.

Differential Diagnosis

II

LUMPS ARISING IN THE SKIN AND SUBCUTANEOUS FAT (SPECIFIC TO THE ANTERIOR ABDOMINAL WALL)

Tumor nodule of the umbilicus (secondary to the intraperitoneal malignancy, also called *Sister Mary Joseph nodule*).

LUMPS ARISING IN THE FASCIA AND MUSCLE

Rectus sheath hematoma (usually painful).
Desmoid tumor (associated with Gardner's syndrome).

HERNIA

Incisional: It has an overlying scar. The sac may be very much larger than the neck of the hernia.

Umbilical: The hernia is through the umbilical scar. Those presenting at birth commonly resolve in the first years of life.

Paraumbilical: The neck is just lateral to the umbilical scar. Patients usually present later in life.

Epigastric: It occurs in the midline between the xiphoid process and the umbilicus. They are usually small (<2 cm). They result when a knuckle of extraperitoneal fat extrudes through a small defect in the linea alba. Commonly irreducible and without an expansile cough impulse.

Spigelian: A rare hernia found along the linea semilunaris at the lateral edge of the rectus sheath, most commonly a third of the way between the umbilicus and the pubis.

DIVARICATION OF THE RECTI

Supraumbilical elliptical swelling of the attenuated linea alba (no cough impulse).

ABORTION, RECURRENT

ICD-10CM # P01.8   Newborn (Suspected to Be) Affected by Other Maternal Complications of Pregnancy

Congenital anatomic abnormalities.
Adhesions (uterine synechiae).
Uterine fibroids.
Endometriosis.
Endocrine abnormalities (luteal phase insufficiency, hypothyroidism, uncontrolled diabetes mellitus [DM]).
Parenteral chromosome abnormalities.
Maternal infections (cervical mycoplasma, ureaplasma, chlamydia).
DES exposure, heavy metal exposure.
Thrombocytosis.
Allogenic immunity, autoimmunity, lupus anticoagulant.

ACHES AND PAINS, DIFFUSE[44]

ICD-10CM # M25.50   Pain in Unspecified Joint

Postviral arthralgias/myalgias.
Bilateral soft tissue rheumatism.
Overuse syndromes.
Fibrositis.
Hypothyroidism.
Metabolic bone disease.
Paraneoplastic syndrome.
Myopathy (polymyositis, dermatomyositis).
Rheumatoid arthritis (RA).
Sjögren's syndrome.
Polymyalgia rheumatica.
Hypermobility.
Benign arthralgias/myalgias.
Chronic fatigue syndrome.
Hypophosphatemia.

ACIDOSIS, HYPERCHLORIC METABOLIC[74]

ICD-10CM # E87.2   Acidosis

GASTROINTESTINAL BICARBONATE LOSS

Diarrhea.
External pancreatic or small bowel drainage.
Ureterosigmoidostomy, jejunal loop.
Drugs:
  Calcium chloride (acidifying agent).
  Magnesium sulfate (diarrhea).
  Cholestyramine (bile acid diarrhea).

RENAL ACIDOSIS

Hypokalemic:
  Proximal RTA (type 2).
  Distal (classic) RTA (type 1).
  Drug-induced hypokalemia:
  - Acetazolamide (proximal RTA).
  - Amphotericin B (distal RTA).

Hyperkalemic:
  Generalized distal nephron dysfunction (type 4 RTA).
  Mineralocorticoid deficiency or resistance (pseudohypoaldosteronism type 1) PHA-I, PHA-II.
  ↓ Na$^+$ delivery to distal nephron.
  Tubulointerstitial disease.
  Ammonium excretion defect.
  Drug-induced hyperkalemia:
  - Potassium-sparing diuretics (amiloride, triamterene, spironolactone).
  - Trimethoprim.
  - Pentamidine.
  - Angiotensin-converting enzyme inhibitors and angiotensin II receptor blockers.
  - Nonsteroidal anti-inflammatory drugs.
  - Cyclosporine, tacrolimus.

Normokalemic:
  Early renal insufficiency.

OTHER

Acid loads (ammonium chloride, hyperalimentation).

Loss of potential bicarbonate: ketosis with ketone excretion.
Dilution acidosis (rapid saline administration).
Hippurate.
Cation-exchange resins.

ACIDOSIS, LACTIC[74]

ICD-10CM # E87.2   Acidosis

CAUSES OF LACTIC ACIDOSIS

L-Lactic Acidosis
Conditions associated with type A lactic acidosis:
  Poor tissue perfusion.
  Shock:
  ○ Cardiogenic.
  ○ Hemorrhagic.
  ○ Septic.
  Profound hypoxemia:
  ○ Severe asthma.
  ○ Carbon monoxide poisoning.
Conditions associated with type B lactic acidosis:
  Liver disease.
Metformin.
Inborn errors of metabolism.
Pyroglutamic acidosis.
Kombucha tea.
d-Lactic Acidosis
Short bowel syndrome.
Ischemic bowel.
Small bowel obstruction.

ACIDOSIS, METABOLIC

ICD-10CM # E87.2   Acidosis

METABOLIC ACIDOSIS WITH INCREASED ANION GAP (AG ACIDOSIS)

Lactic acidosis.
Ketoacidosis (DM, alcoholic ketoacidosis).
Uremia (chronic renal failure).
Ingestion of toxins (paraldehyde, methanol, salicylate, ethylene glycol).
High-fat diet (mild acidosis).

METABOLIC ACIDOSIS WITH NORMAL AG (HYPERCHLOREMIC ACIDOSIS)

Renal tubular acidosis (including acidosis of aldosterone deficiency).
Intestinal loss of HCO_3^- (diarrhea, pancreatic fistula).
Carbonic anhydrase inhibitors (e.g., acetazolamide).
Dilutional acidosis (as a result of rapid infusion of bicarbonate-free isotonic saline).
Ingestion of exogenous acids (ammonium chloride, methionine, cystine, calcium chloride).
Ileostomy.
Ureterosigmoidostomy.
Drugs: amiloride, triamterene, spironolactone, β-blockers.

ACIDOSIS, RESPIRATORY

ICD-10CM # E87.2   Acidosis

Pulmonary disease (COPD, severe pneumonia, pulmonary edema, interstitial fibrosis).

Airway obstruction (foreign body, severe bronchospasm, laryngospasm).

Thoracic cage disorders (pneumothorax, flail chest, kyphoscoliosis).

Defects in muscles of respiration (myasthenia gravis, hypokalemia, muscular dystrophy).

Defects in peripheral nervous system (amyotrophic lateral sclerosis, poliomyelitis, Guillain-Barré syndrome, botulism, tetanus, organophosphate poisoning, spinal cord injury).

Depression of respiratory center (anesthesia, narcotics, sedatives, vertebral artery embolism or thrombosis, increased intracranial pressure).

Failure of mechanical ventilator.

ACUTE KIDNEY INJURY AND LIVER DISEASE, CAUSES[24,25]

| ICD-10CM # | S37.009A | Unspecified Injury of Unspecified Kidney, Initial Encounter |
| | K76.89 | Other Specified Diseases of Liver |

Prerenal uremia:	Diuretic use, gastrointestinal loss, peritoneal aspiration, hypoalbuminemia
Hepatorenal syndrome	
Acute tubular necrosis:	Hyperbilirubinemia, sepsis, toxic shock syndrome
Drugs:	Acetaminophen (paracetamol), NSAIDs, tetracycline, rifampicin, isoniazid, anesthetic agents, sulfonamides, allopurinol, methotrexate
Infections:	Hepatitis C and cryoglobulinemia, hepatitis B and polyarteritis nodosa, leptospirosis, hantavirus, Epstein-Barr virus, gram-negative sepsis, spontaneous bacterial peritonitis
Other:	Papillary necrosis and obstruction, inhalation of chlorinated hydrocarbons, mushroom poisoning (*Amanita phalloides*)

ACUTE KIDNEY INJURY DUE TO INTRINSIC RENAL DISEASES[51]

| ICD-10CM # | varies with specific diagnosis |

INTRINSIC RENAL DISEASES THAT CAUSE ACUTE KIDNEY INJURY

Vascular Diseases
Large-Vessel Diseases
Renal artery thrombosis or stenosis.
Renal vein thrombosis.
Atheroembolic disease.
Small- and Medium-Vessel Diseases
Scleroderma.

Malignant hypertension.
Hemolytic uremic syndrome.
Thrombotic thrombocytopenic purpura.
HIV-associated microangiopathy.
Glomerular Diseases
Systemic Diseases
Systemic lupus erythematosus.
Infective endocarditis.
Systemic vasculitis (e.g., periarteritis nodosa, Wegener's granulomatosis).
Henoch-Schönlein purpura.
HIV-associated nephropathy.
Essential mixed cryoglobulinemia.
Goodpasture's syndrome.
Primary Renal Diseases
Poststreptococcal glomerulonephritis.
Other postinfectious glomerulonephritis.
Rapidly progressive glomerulonephritis.
Tubulointerstitial Diseases and Conditions
Drugs (many).
Toxins (e.g., heavy metals, ethylene glycol).
Infections.
Multiple myeloma.
Acute Tubular Necrosis
Ischemia
Shock.
Sepsis.
Severe prerenal azotemia.
Nephrotoxins
Antibiotics.
Radiographic contrast agents.
Myoglobinuria.
Hemoglobinuria.
Other Diseases and Conditions
Severe liver disease.
Allergic reactions.
NSAIDs.

ACUTE KIDNEY INJURY, HIV PATIENT, CAUSES[24,25]

| ICD-10CM # | S37.009A | Unspecified Injury of Unspecified Kidney, Initial Encounter with B20 Human Immunodeficiency Virus (HIV) Disease |

Prerenal:	Diarrhea, nausea and vomiting, cirrhosis and hepatorenal syndrome, sepsis
Vascular:	Thrombotic microangiopathy
Glomerular:	Immune complex glomerulonephritis (MPGN secondary to hepatitis C virus, postinfectious glomerulonephritis), HIVAN
Acute tubular necrosis:	Sepsis, hypotension, nephrotoxins (aminoglycosides, amphotericin, acyclovir, cidofovir, tenofovir, pentamidine)
Acute interstitial nephritis:	Drug-induced (co-trimoxazole), rifampicin, foscarnet, nevirapine), CMV infection, DILS
Drug-induced intratubular obstruction:	Sulfadiazine, indinavir, foscarnet, acyclovir

Postrenal obstruction:	Stones, tuberculosis, fungal ball, tumor
Associated with IV drug use:	Sepsis, endocarditis, heroin-associated nephropathy (FSGS), rhabdomyolysis

CMV, Cytomegalovirus; *DILS,* diffusive infiltrative lymphocytosis syndrome; *FSGS,* focal segmental glomerulosclerosis; *HIVAN,* HIV-associated nephropathy; *MPGN,* membranoproliferative glomerulonephritis.

ACUTE KIDNEY INJURY IN SPECIFIC CLINICAL SETTINGS[67]

| ICD-10CM # | N17.9 | Acute Kidney Failure, Unspecified |

MAJOR CAUSES OF ACUTE KIDNEY INJURY IN SPECIFIC CLINICAL SETTINGS

AKI in the Cancer Patient
Prerenal azotemia
　Hypovolemia (e.g., poor intake, vomiting, diarrhea)
Intrinsic AKI
　Exogenous nephrotoxins: chemotherapy, antibiotics, contrast media
　Endogenous toxins: hyperuricemia, hypercalcemia, tumor lysis, paraproteins
　Other: radiation, HUS/TTP, glomerulonephritis, amyloid, malignant infiltration
Postrenal AKI
　Ureteric or bladder neck obstruction
AKI after Cardiac Surgery
Prerenal azotemia
　Hypovolemia (surgical losses, diuretics), cardiac failure, vasodilators
Intrinsic AKI
　Ischemic ATN (even in absence of hypotension)
　Atheroembolic disease after aortic manipulation/intraaortic balloon pump
　Preoperative or perioperative administration of contrast medium
　Allergic interstitial nephritis induced by perioperative antibiotics
Postrenal AKI
　Obstructed urinary catheter, exacerbation of voiding dysfunction
AKI in Pregnancy
Prerenal azotemia
　Acute fatty liver of pregnancy with fulminant hepatic failure
Intrinsic AKI
　Preeclampsia or eclampsia
　Postpartum HUS/TTP
　HELLP syndrome
　Ischemia: postpartum hemorrhage, abruptio placentae, amniotic fluid embolus
　Direct toxicity of illegal abortifacients
Postrenal AKI
　Obstruction with pyelonephritis
AKI after Solid Organ or Bone Marrow Transplantation
Prerenal azotemia
　Intravascular volume depletion (e.g., diuretic therapy)
　Vasoactive drugs (e.g., calcineurin inhibitors, amphotericin B)

Differential Diagnosis

II

Hepatorenal syndrome, venoocclusive disease of liver (BMT)
Intrinsic AKI
Postoperative ischemic ATN (even in absence of hypotension)
Sepsis
Exogenous nephrotoxins: aminoglycosides, amphotericin B, radiocontrast media
HUS/TTP (e.g., cyclosporine or myeloablative radiotherapy related)
Allergic tubulointerstitial nephritis
Postrenal AKI
Obstructed urinary catheter

AKI and Pulmonary Disease (Pulmonary Renal Syndrome)
Prerenal azotemia
Diminished cardiac output complicating pulmonary embolism, severe pulmonary hypertension, or positive-pressure mechanical ventilation
Intrinsic AKI
Vasculitis
Goodpasture's syndrome, ANCA-associated vasculitis, SLE, eosinophilic granulomatosis with polyangiitis, polyarteritis nodosa, cryoglobulinemia, right-sided endocarditis, lymphomatoid granulomatosis, sarcoidosis, scleroderma
Toxins
Ingestion of paraquat or diquat
Infections
Legionnaires' disease, *Mycoplasma* infection, tuberculosis, disseminated viral or fungal infection
AKI from any cause with hypervolemia and pulmonary edema
Lung cancer with hypercalcemia, tumor lysis, or glomerulonephritis

AKI and Liver Disease
Prerenal azotemia
Reduced true (GI hemorrhage, GI losses from lactulose, diuretics, large-volume paracentesis) circulatory volume or effective (hypoalbuminemia, splanchnic vasodilation)
Hepatorenal syndrome type 1 or 2
Tense ascites with abdominal compartment syndrome
Intrinsic AKI
Ischemic (severe hypoperfusion—see earlier) or direct nephrotoxicity and hepatotoxicity of drugs or toxins (e.g., carbon tetrachloride, acetaminophen, tetracyclines, methoxyflurane)
Tubulointerstitial nephritis plus hepatitis caused by drugs (e.g., sulfonamides, rifampin, phenytoin, allopurinol, phenindione), infections (leptospirosis, brucellosis, Epstein-Barr virus infection, cytomegalovirus infection), malignant infiltration (leukemia, lymphoma), or sarcoidosis
Glomerulonephritis or vasculitis (e.g., polyarteritis nodosa, ANCA-associated glomerulonephritis, cryoglobulinemia, SLE, postinfectious hepatitis or liver abscess

AKI and Nephrotic Syndrome
Prerenal azotemia
Intravascular volume depletion (diuretic therapy, hypoalbuminemia)

Intrinsic AKI
Manifestation of primary glomerular disease
Collapsing glomerulopathy (e.g., HIV, pamidronate)
Associated ATN (older hypertensive males)
Associated interstitial nephritis (NSAIDs, rifampin, interferon alfa)
Other—amyloid or light-chain deposition disease, renal vein thrombosis, severe interstitial edema

AKI, Acute kidney injury; ANCA, antineutrophil cytoplasmic antibody; ATN, acute tubular necrosis; BMT, bone marrow transplantation; GI, gastrointestinal; HELLP, hemolysis, elevated liver enzymes, low platelets; HIV, human immunodeficiency virus; HUS, hemolytic uremic syndrome; NSAID, nonsteroidal antiinflammatory drug; SLE, systemic lupus erythematosus; TTP, thrombotic thrombocytopenic purpura.

ACUTE KIDNEY INJURY, PIGMENT INDUCED[51]

ICD-10CM # varies with specific diagnosis

CAUSES OF PIGMENT-INDUCED ACUTE KIDNEY INJURY
Rhabdomyolysis and myoglobinuria.
Vigorous exercise.
Arterial embolization.
Status epilepticus.
Status asthmaticus.
Coma-induced and pressure-induced myonecrosis.
Heat stress.
Diabetic ketoacidosis.
Myopathy.
Alcoholism.
Hypokalemia.
Hypophosphatemia.
Hemoglobinuria.
Transfusion reactions.
Snake envenomation.
Malaria.
Mechanical destruction of RBCs by prosthetic valves.
G6PD deficiency.

G6PD, glucose-6-phosphate dehydrogenase.

ACUTE LUNG INJURY, DISEASE AND DISORDERS ASSOCIATIONS[52]

ICD-10CM # S27.3 Injury, lung

CLINICAL DISORDERS ASSOCIATED WITH ACUTE LUNG INJURY
Infectious Causes
Gram-negative or gram-positive sepsis.
Bacterial pneumonia.
Viral pneumonia.
Fungal pneumonia
Parasitic infections.
Mycobacterial disease.
Aspiration
Gastric acid.
Food and other particulate matter.
Fresh or sea water (near drowning).
Hydrocarbon fluids.

Trauma
Lung contusion.
Fat emboli.
Nonthoracic trauma.
Thermal injury (burns).
Blast injury (explosion, lightning).
Overdistention (mechanical ventilation).
Inhaled gases (phosgene, ammonia).
Hemodynamic Disturbances
Shock of any etiology.
Anaphylaxis.
High-altitude pulmonary edema.
Reperfusion.
Air embolism.
Amniotic fluid embolism.
Drugs
Heroin.
Methadone.
Propoxyphene.
Naloxone.
Cocaine.
Barbiturates.
Colchicine.
Salicylates.
Ethchlorvynol.
Interleukin-2.
Protamine.
Hydrochlorothiazide.
Hematologic Disorders
Disseminated intravascular coagulation.
Incompatible blood transfusion.
Rh incompatibility.
Antileukocyte antibodies.
Leukoagglutinin reactions.
Post–cardiopulmonary bypass, pump oxygenator.
Metabolic Disorders
Pancreatitis.
Diabetic ketoacidosis.
Neurologic Disorders
Head trauma.
Grand mal seizures.
Increased intracranial pressure (any cause).
Subarachnoid or intracerebral hemorrhage.
Miscellaneous Disorders
Lung reexpansion.
Upper airway obstruction.

ACUTE SCROTUM

ICD-10CM # R10.2 Pelvic and Perineal Pain

Testicular torsion.
Epididymitis.
Testicular neoplasm.
Orchitis.
Trauma.

ADNEXAL MASS[50]

ICD-10CM # R19.00 Intraabdominal and Pelvic Swelling, Mass and Lump, Unspecified Site

Ovary (neoplasm, endometriosis, functional cyst).
Fallopian tube (ectopic pregnancy, neoplasm, tuboovarian abscess, hydrosalpinx, paratubal cyst).
Uterus (fibroid, neoplasm).

Retroperitoneum (neoplasm, abdominal wall hematoma or abscess).
Urinary tract (pelvic kidney, distended bladder, urachal cyst).
Inflammatory bowel disease.
GI tract neoplasm.
Diverticular disease.
Appendicitis.
Bowel loop with feces.

ADRENAL CALCIFICATIONS[62]

ICD-10CM #	E27.8	Other Specified Disorder of Adrenal Gland

CAUSES OF ADRENAL CALCIFICATION

Infection
   Tuberculosis
   Histoplasmosis
   Echinococcus
Prior hemorrhage
Neoplasm
   Adrenocortical carcinoma
   Myelolipoma
   Pheochromocytoma
Hemangioma (rare)

ADRENAL CYSTIC LESIONS[62]

ICD-10CM #	E27.8	Other Specified Disorder of Adrenal Gland

CYSTIC ADRENAL LESIONS

Pseudocyst
Endothelial cyst
Epithelial cyst
Infection (*Echinococcus*, abscess)
Necrotic neoplasm
Cystic pheochromocytoma
Lymphangioma

ADRENAL MASSES[70]

ICD-10CM #	C74.90	Malignant Neoplasm of Unspecified Part of Unspecified Adrenal Gland
	E27.8	Other Specified Disorders of Adrenal Gland

UNILATERAL ADRENAL MASSES

Functional Lesions
Adrenal adenoma.
Adrenal carcinoma.
Pheochromocytoma.
Primary aldosteronism, adenomatous type.
Nonfunctional Lesions
Incidentaloma of adrenal.
Ganglioneuroma.
Myelolipoma.
Hematoma.
Adenolipoma.
Metastasis.

BILATERAL ADRENAL MASSES

Functional Lesions
ACTH-dependent Cushing's syndrome.
Congenital adrenal hyperplasia.
Pheochromocytoma.
Conn's syndrome, hyperplastic variety.
Micronodular adrenal disease.
Idiopathic bilateral adrenal hypertrophy.
Nonfunctional Lesions
Infection (tuberculosis, fungi).
Infiltration (leukemia, lymphoma).
Replacement (amyloidosis).
Hemorrhage.
Bilateral metastases.

ADRENAL PSEUDOMASSES[62]

ICD-10CM #	E27.8	Other Specified Disorder of Adrenal Gland

Thickened diaphragmatic crus
Accessory spleen
Gastric fundus
Gastric diverticulum
Renal vein
Retrocrural and retroperitoneal adenopathy
Upper-pole renal cysts and tumors
Pancreatic tumors
Hypertrophied caudate lobe of liver
Fluid-filled colon interposed between stomach and kidney

ADRENOCORTICAL HYPERFUNCTION[3]

ICD-10CM #	E26.9	Hyperaldosteronism, Unspecified

SYNDROMES OF ADRENOCORTICAL HYPERFUNCTION

States of Glucocorticoid Excess
Physiologic states
Stress.
Strenuous exercise.
Last trimester of pregnancy.
Pathologic States
Psychiatric conditions (pseudo-Cushing's disorders):
   Depression.
   Alcoholism.
   Anorexia nervosa.
   Panic disorders.
   Alcohol and drug withdrawal.
ACTH-dependent states:
   Pituitary adenoma (Cushing's disease).
   Ectopic ACTH syndrome.
   Bronchial carcinoid.
   Thymic carcinoid.
   Islet cell tumor.
   Small cell lung carcinoma.
   Ectopic CRH secretion.
ACTH-independent states:
   Adrenal adenoma.
   Adrenal carcinoma.
   Micronodular adrenal disease.

Exogenous Sources
Glucocorticoid intake.
ACTH intake.
States of Mineralocorticoid Excess
Primary Aldosteronism
Aldosterone-secreting adenoma.
Bilateral adrenal hyperplasia.
Aldosterone-secreting carcinoma.
Glucocorticoid-suppressible hyperaldosteronism.
Adrenal Enzyme Deficiencies
11b-Hydroxylase deficiency.
17a-Hydroxylase deficiency.
11b-Hydroxysteroid dehydrogenase, type II.
Exogenous Mineralocorticoids
Licorice.
Carbenoxolone.
Fludrocortisone.
Secondary Hyperaldosteronism
Associated with hypertension:
   Accelerated hypertension.
   Renovascular hypertension.
   Estrogen administration.
   Renin-secreting tumors.
Without hypertension:
   Bartter syndrome.
   Sodium-wasting nephropathy.
   Renal tubular acidosis.
   Diuretic and laxative abuse.
   Edematous states (cirrhosis, nephrosis, congestive heart failure).

ACTH, Adrenocorticotropin hormone; *CRH*, corticotropin-releasing hormone.

ADRENOCORTICAL HYPOFUNCTION

ICD-10CM #	E27.49	Other Adrenocortical Insufficiency

SYNDROMES OF ADRENOCORTICAL HYPOFUNCTION

Primary Adrenal Disorders
Combined Glucocorticoid and Mineralocorticoid Deficiency
Autoimmune:
   Isolated autoimmune disease (Addison disease).
   Polyglandular autoimmune syndrome, type I.
   Polyglandular autoimmune syndrome, type II.
Infectious:
   Tuberculosis.
   Fungal.
   Cytomegalovirus.
   Human immunodeficiency virus.
Vascular:
   Bilateral adrenal hemorrhage.
   Sepsis.
   Coagulopathy.
   Thrombosis; embolism.
   Adrenal infarction.
Infiltration:
   Metastatic carcinoma and lymphoma.
   Sarcoidosis.
   Amyloidosis.
   Hemochromatosis.
Congenital:
   Congenital adrenal hyperplasia.

Differential Diagnosis

II

- 21-Hydroxylase deficiency.
- 3b-ol Dehydrogenase deficiency.
- 20,22-Desmolase deficiency.

Adrenal unresponsiveness to ACTH.
Congenital adrenal hypoplasia.
Adrenoleukodystrophy.
Adrenomyeloneuropathy.

Iatrogenic
Bilateral adrenalectomy.
Drugs:
 Metyrapone, aminoglutethimide, trilostane, ketoconazole, o,p¢-DDD, mifepristone.

Mineralocorticoid deficiency without glucocorticoid deficiency
Cortiscosterone methyl oxidase deficiency.
Isolated zona glomerulosa defect.
Heparin therapy.
Critical illness.
Converting-enzyme inhibitors.

Secondary Adrenal Disorders
Secondary Adrenal Insufficiency
Hypothalamic-pituitary dysfunction.
Exogenous glucocorticoids.
After removal of an ACTH-secreting tumor.
Hyporeninemic Hypoaldosteronism
Diabetic nephropathy.
Tubulointerstitial diseases.
Obstructive uropathy.
Autonomic neuropathy.
Nonsteroidal antiinflammatory drugs.
β-Adrenergic drugs.

ACTH, Adrenocorticotropic hormone.

ADVERSE FOOD REACTIONS, DIFFERENTIAL DIAGNOSIS[46]

ICD-10CM #	T78.1XXA	Other Adverse Food Reactions, Not Elsewhere Classified, Initial Encounter

GASTROINTESTINAL DISORDERS (WITH VOMITING AND/OR DIARRHEA)
Structural abnormalities (pyloric stenosis, Hirschsprung's disease).
Enzyme deficiencies (primary or secondary):
 Disaccharidase deficiency—lactase, fructase, sucrase-isomaltase.
 Galactosemia.
Other: pancreatic insufficiency (cystic fibrosis), peptic disease.

CONTAMINANTS AND ADDITIVES
Flavorings and preservatives—rarely cause symptoms: Sodium metabisulfite, monosodium glutamate, nitrites.
Dyes and colorings—very rarely cause symptoms (urticaria, eczema): Tartrazine.
Toxins: Bacterial, fungal (aflatoxin), fish-related (scombroid, ciguatera).
Infectious organisms:
 Bacteria (*Salmonella, Escherichia coli, Shigella*).
 Virus (rotavirus, enterovirus).
 Parasites (*Giardia, Akis simplex* [in fish]).
Accidental contaminants: Heavy metals, pesticides.

Pharmacologic agents: Caffeine, glycosidal alkaloid solanine (potato spuds), histamine (fish), serotonin (banana, tomato), tryptamine (tomato), tyramine (cheese).

PSYCHOLOGIC REACTIONS
Food phobias.

ADYNAMIC ILEUS[50]

ICD-10CM #	K56.0	Paralytic Ileus
	K56.7	Ileus, Unspecified

Abdominal trauma.
Infection (retroperitoneal, pelvic, intrathoracic).
Laparotomy.
Metabolic disease (hypokalemia).
Renal colic.
Skeletal injury (rib fracture, vertebral fracture).
Medications (e.g., narcotics).

AEROPHAGIA (BELCHING, ERUCTATION)

ICD-10CM #	R14.0	Abdominal Distention (Gaseous)
	R14.1	Gas Pain
	R14.2	Eructation
	R14.3	Flatulence

Anxiety disorders.
Rapid food ingestion.
Carbonated beverages.
Nursing infants (especially when nursing in horizontal position).
Eating or drinking in supine position.
Gum chewing.
Poorly fitting dentures, orthodontic appliances.
Hiatal hernia, gastritis, nonulcer dyspepsia.
Cholelithiasis, cholecystitis.
Ingestion of legumes, onions, peppers.

AIR-SPACE OPACIFICATION ON X-RAY[33]

ICD-10CM #	R91.8	Other nonspecific abnormal finding of lung field

CAUSES OF AIR-SPACE OPACIFICATION
Edema
Cardiogenic.
Non-cardiogenic.
Inflammation/Infection
Wegener's granulomatosis.
Cryptogenic organizing pneumonia.
Blood
Idiopathic pulmonary hemosiderosis.
Antibasement membrane antibody disease.
Systemic lupus erythematosus.
Miscellaneous Causes
Eosinophilic pneumonia.
Alveolar proteinosis.
Alveolar cell carcinoma.
Alveolar microlithiasis.
Lymphoma (MALToma).
Sarcoidosis.

AIRWAY OBSTRUCTION, PEDIATRIC AGE[38]

ICD-10CM #	J44.9	Chronic Obstructive Pulmonary Disease, Unspecified
	T17.900A	Unspecified Foreign Body in Respiratory Tract, Part Unspecified Causing Asphyxiation, Initial Encounter
	T17.908A	Unspecified Foreign Body in Respiratory Tract, Part Unspecified Causing Other Injury, Initial Encounter
	T17.910A	Gastric Contents in Respiratory Tract, Part Unspecified Causing Asphyxiation, Initial Encounter
	T17.918A	Gastric Contents in Respiratory Tract, Part Unspecified Causing Other Injury, Initial Encounter
	T17.920A	Food in Respiratory Tract, Part Unspecified Causing Asphyxiation, Initial Encounter
	T17.928A	Food in Respiratory Tract, Part Unspecified Causing Other Injury, Initial Encounter
	T17.990A	Other Foreign Object in Respiratory Tract, Part Unspecified in Causing Asphyxiation, Initial Encounter
	T17.998A	Other Foreign Object in Respiratory Tract, Part Unspecified Causing Other Injury, Initial Encounter
	J38.5	Laryngeal Spasm
	J68.9	Unspecified Respiratory Condition Due To Chemicals, Gases, Fumes, and Vapors

CONGENITAL CAUSES

Craniofacial dysmorphism.
Hemangioma.
Laryngeal cleft/web.
Laryngoceles, cysts.
Laryngomalacia.
Macroglossia.
Tracheal stenosis.
Vascular ring.
Vocal cord paralysis.

ACQUIRED INFECTIOUS CAUSES

Acute laryngotracheobronchitis.
Epiglottitis.
Laryngeal papillomatosis.
Membranous croup (bacterial tracheitis).
Mononucleosis.
Retropharyngeal abscess.
Spasmodic croup.
Diphtheria.

ACQUIRED NONINFECTIOUS CAUSES

Anaphylaxis.
Foreign body aspiration.
Supraglottic hypotonia.
Thermal/chemical burn.
Trauma.
Vocal cord paralysis.
Angioneurotic edema.

AKINETIC/RIGID SYNDROME[3]

| ICD-10CM # | | R29.8 Akinesis |

Parkinsonism (idiopathic, drug-induced).
Catatonia (psychosis).
Progressive supranuclear palsy.
Multisystem atrophy (Shy-Drager syndrome, olivopontocerebellar atrophy).
Diffuse Lewy-body disease.
Toxins (MPTP, manganese, carbon monoxide).
Huntington's disease and other hereditary neurodegenerative disorders.

ALCOHOL-RELATED SEIZURES[51]

| ICD-10CM # | | F10.232 |

DIFFERENTIAL DIAGNOSIS OF ALCOHOL-RELATED SEIZURES

Withdrawal (alcohol or drugs).
Exacerbation of idiopathic or posttraumatic seizures.
Acute intoxication (amphetamines, anticholinergics, cocaine, isoniazid, organophosphates, phenothiazines, tricyclic antidepressants, salicylates, lithium).
Metabolic (hypoglycemia, hyponatremia, hypernatremia, hypocalcemia, hepatic failure).
Infectious (meningitis, encephalitis, brain abscess).
Trauma (intracranial hemorrhage).
Cerebrovascular accident.
Sleep deprivation.
Noncompliance with anticonvulsants.

ALKALOSIS, METABOLIC

| ICD-10CM # | E87.3 | Alkalosis |

CAUSES OF METABOLIC ALKALOSIS

Exogenous HCO_3- Loads
Acute alkali administration.
Milk-alkali syndrome.
Effective Extracellular Volume Contraction, Normotension, Hypokalemia, and Secondary Hyperreninemic Hyperaldosteronism
Gastrointestinal origin:
  Vomiting.
  Gastric aspiration.
  Congenital chloridorrhea.
  Villous adenoma.
  Combined administration of sodium polystyrene sulfonate (Kayexalate and aluminum hydroxide).
Renal origin:
  Diuretics (especially thiazides and loop diuretics).
  Acute.
  Chronic.
  Edematous states.
  Posthypercapnic state.
  Hypercalcemia-hypoparathyroidism.
  Recovery from lactic acidosis or ketoacidosis.
  Nonreabsorbable anions such as penicillin, carbenicillin.
  Mg^{++} deficiency.
  K^+ depletion.
  Bartter syndrome (loss-of-function mutation of $Cl-$ transport in thick ascending limb of Henle loop).
  Gitelman syndrome (loss-of-function mutation in $Na^+/Cl-$ cotransporter).
  Carbohydrate refeeding after starvation.
Extracellular Volume Expansion, Hypertension, K^+ Deficiency, and Hypermineralocorticoidism
Associated with high renin:
  Renal artery stenosis.
  Accelerated hypertension.
  Renin-secreting tumor.
  Estrogen therapy.
Associated with low renin:
  Primary aldosteronism.
  Adenoma.
  Hyperplasia.
  Carcinoma.
  Glucocorticoid suppressible.
Adrenal enzymatic defects:
  11β-Hydroxylase deficiency.
  17α-Hydroxylase deficiency.
Cushing syndrome or disease:
  Ectopic corticotropin.
  Adrenal carcinoma.
  Adrenal adenoma.
  Primary pituitary.
Other:
  Licorice.
  Carbenoxolone.
  Chewer's tobacco.
  Lydia Pinkham tablets.

Gain-of-Function Mutation of ENaC with Extracellular Fluid Volume Expansion, Hypertension, K^+ Deficiency, and Hyporeninemic Hypoaldosteronism
Liddle syndrome.

ALKALOSIS, RESPIRATORY

| ICD-10CM # | E87.3 | Alkalosis |

Hypoxemia (pneumonia, pulmonary embolism, atelectasis, high-altitude living).
Drugs (salicylates, xanthenes, progesterone, epinephrine, thyroxine, nicotine).
Central nervous system (CNS) disorders (tumor, cerebrovascular accident [CVA], trauma, infections).
Psychogenic hyperventilation (anxiety, hysteria).
Hepatic encephalopathy.
Gram-negative sepsis.
Hyponatremia.
Sudden recovery from metabolic acidosis.
Assisted ventilation.

ALOPECIA[29,55]

ICD-10CM #	L65.9	Nonscarring Hair Loss, Unspecified
	L63.2	Ophiasis
	L63.8	Other Alopecia Areata
	Q84.0	Congenital Alopecia
	Q84.1	Congenital Morphological Disturbances of Hair, Not Elsewhere Classified
	Q84.2	Other Congenital Malformations of Hair
	F54	Psychological and Behavioral Factors Associated with Disorders or Diseases Classified Elsewhere

SCARRING ALOPECIA

Congenital (aplasia cutis).
Tinea capitis with inflammation (kerion).
Bacterial folliculitis.
Discoid lupus erythematosus.
Lichen planopilaris.
Folliculitis decalvans.
Neoplasm.
Trauma.

NONSCARRING ALOPECIA

Cosmetic treatment.
Tinea capitis.
Structural hair shaft disease.
Trichotillomania (hair pulling).
Anagen arrest.
Telogen arrest.
Alopecia areata.
Androgenetic alopecia.

Differential Diagnosis

II

ALOPECIA AND HYPOTRICHOSIS, IN CHILDREN AND ADOLESCENTS

ICD-10CM #	L65.9	Nonscarring Hair Loss, Unspecified
	L63.2	Ophiasis
	L63.8	Other Alopecia Areata
	Q84.0	Congenital Alopecia
	Q84.1	Congenital Morphological Disturbances Of Hair, Not Elsewhere Classified
	Q84.2	Other Congenital Malformations Of Hair

Congenital total alopecia: atrichia with papules, Moynahan alopecia syndrome.

Congenital localized alopecia: aplasia cutis, triangular alopecia, sebaceous nevus.

Hereditary hypotrichosis: Marie-Unna syndrome, hypotrichosis with juvenile macular dystrophy, hypotrichosis–Mari type, ichthyosis with hypotrichosis, cartilage-hair hypoplasia, Hallermann-Streiff syndrome, trichorhinophalangeal syndrome, ectodermal dysplasia ("pure" hair and nail and other ectodermal dysplasias).

Diffuse alopecia of endocrine origin: hypopituitarism, hypothyroidism, hypoparathyroidism, hyperthyroidism.

Alopecia of nutritional origin: marasmus, kwashiorkor, iron deficiency, zinc deficiency (acrodermatitis enteropathica), gluten-sensitive enteropathy, essential fatty acid deficiency, biotinidase deficiency.

Disturbances of the hair cycle: telogen effluvium.

Toxic alopecia: anagen effluvium.

Autoimmune alopecia: alopecia areata.

Traumatic alopecia: traction alopecia, trichotillomania.

Cicatricial alopecia: lupus erythematosus, lichen planopilaris, pseudopelade, morphea (en coup de saber), dermatomyositis, infection (kerion, favus, tuberculosis, syphilis, folliculitis, leishmaniasis, herpes zoster, varicella), acne keloidalis, follicular mucinosis, sarcoidosis.

Hair shaft abnormalities: monilethrix, pili annulati, pili torti, trichorrhexis invaginata, trichorrhexis nodosa, woolly hair syndrome, Menkes disease, trichothiodystrophy, trichodento-osseous syndrome, uncombable hair syndrome (spun-glass hair, pili trianguli et canaliculi).

ALOPECIA, DRUG-INDUCED

ICD-10CM #	L65.9	Nonscarring hair loss, unspecified
	L63.8	Alopecia areata

DRUGS REPORTED TO INDUCE HAIR LOSS

ACE inhibitors (captopril, enalapril, moexipril, ramipril).

Allopurinol.

Amiodarone.

Amphetamines.[1,2]

Analgesics, antiinflammatories (ibuprofen, indomethacin, naproxen).

Androgens.[3]

Anticoagulants (coumarin, dextran, heparin/heparinoids).

Antiepileptics (carbamazepine, hydantoins, lamotrigine, troxidone, valproic acid, vigabatrin).

Antipsychotics (flupenthixol decanoate, fluphenazine decanoate).

Antithyroid drugs (carbimazole, iodine, thiouracil).

Appetite suppressants.

Aromatase inhibitors (fadrozole, 4-OHA, vorozole).

Benzimidazoles (albendazole, mebendazole)

β-Blockers (levobunolol, metoprolol, nadolol, propranolol, timolol).

Bromocriptine.

Buspirone.

Butyrophenones.

Cantharidin.

Chloramphenicol.

Cholestyramine.

Cidofovir.

Cimetidine.

Clonazepam.

Clotrimezole.

Colchicine.

Contraceptives (oral).[4]

Danazol.

Diazoxide.

Diclofenac.

Dixyrazine.

Ethambutol.

Ethionamide.

Fibrates (clofibrate, fenofibrate).

G-CSF (granulocyte-colony stimulating factor)

Gefitinib.[5]

Gentamicin.

Glatiramer acetate.

Glibenclamide.

Gold salts.

Haloperidol.

Immunoglobulins.

Indanediones.

Indinavir.

Interferons.

Isonicotinic acid hydrazide.[6]

Leflunomide.

Levodopa.

Lithium.

Maprotiline.

Mesalazine.

Methyldopa.

Methysergide.

[1]Established by multiple reports or proved by rechallenge.

[†]Hair loss usually severe.

[2]Involvement principally of cancellous bone.

[3]May produce androgenetic alopecia.

[4]May produce telogen effluvium 3 months after discontinuation.

[5]Involvement of cancellous and cortical bone.

[6]May produce anagen effluvium.

Metyrapone.

Minoxidil.

Nicotinic acid.

Nitrofurantoin.

Octreotide.

Olanzapine.

Pentosan polysulfate.

Phenindione.

Potassium thiocyanate.

Pyridostigmine.

Radiation (<700 Gy).

Retinoids (acitretin, etretinate, isotretinoin).

Retinol (vitamin A).

Risperidone.

Salicylates.

Serotonin reuptake inhibitors (fluoxetine, fluvoxamine, paroxetine, sertraline).

Sorafenib.

Spironolactone.

Strontium ranelate.

Sulfasalazine.

Tamoxifen.

Terbinafine.

Terfenadine.

Thiamphenicol.

Thyroxine.

Tocopherol (vitamin E).

Trazodone.

Triazoles (fluconazole, itraconazole).

Tricyclic antidepressants (amitriptyline, desipramine, doxepin, imipramine, maprotiline).

Trimethadione.

Triparanol.

Vasopressin.

ALVEOLAR CONSOLIDATION

ICD-10CM #	J18.2	Hypostatic Pneumonia, Unspecified Organism
	J81.1	Hypostatic Pneumonia, Unspecified Organism

Infection.

Neoplasm (bronchoalveolar carcinoma, lymphoma).

Aspiration.

Trauma.

Hemorrhage (Wegener's, Goodpasture's, bleeding diathesis).

ARDS.

CHF.

Renal failure.

Eosinophilic pneumonia.

Bronchiolitis obliterans.

Pulmonary alveolar proteinosis.

ALVEOLAR HEMORRHAGE[55]

ICD-10CM #	P26.1	Massive Pulmonary Hemorrhage Originating in the Perinatal Period
	K08.8	Alveolar hemorrhage
	P26.8	Other Pulmonary Hemorrhages Originating in the Perinatal Period

Hematologic disorders (coagulopathies, thrombocytopenia).
Goodpasture's syndrome (anti-basement membrane antibody disease).
Granulomatosis with polyangiitis (Wegener's vasculitis).
Immune complex-mediated vasculitis.
Idiopathic pulmonary hemosiderosis.
Drugs (penicillamine).
Lymphangiogram contrast.
Mitral stenosis.

AMENORRHEA

ICD-10CM #	N91.2	Amenorrhea, Unspecified

PREGNANCY

Early Menopause
Hypothalamic Dysfunction
defective synthesis or release of LHRH, anorexia nervosa, stress, exercise.
Pituitary Dysfunction
neoplasm, postpartum hemorrhage, surgery, radiotherapy.
Ovarian Dysfunction
gonadal dysgenesis, 17a-hydroxylase deficiency, premature ovarian failure, polycystic ovarian disease, gonadal stromal tumors.

UTEROVAGINAL ABNORMALITIES

Congenital: imperforate hymen, imperforate cervix, imperforate or absent vagina, Müllerian agenesis.
Acquired: destruction of endometrium with curettage (Asherman's syndrome), closure of cervix or vagina caused by traumatic injury, hysterectomy.

OTHER

Metabolic diseases (liver, kidney), malnutrition, rapid weight loss, exogenous obesity, endocrine abnormalities (Cushing's syndrome, Graves' disease, hypothyroidism).

AMNESIA

ICD-10CM #	F19.96	Other Psychoactive Substance Use, Unspecified With Psychoactive Substance-Induced Persisting Amnestic Disorder
	F44.0	Dissociative Amnesia
	R41.2	Retrograde Amnesia
	G45.4	Transient Global Amnesia

Degenerative diseases (e.g., Alzheimer's, Huntington's disease).
CVA (especially when involving thalamus, basal forebrain, and hippocampus).
Head trauma.
Postsurgical (e.g., mammillary body surgery, bilateral temporal lobectomy).
Infections (herpes simplex encephalitis, meningitis).
Wernicke-Korsakoff syndrome.
Cerebral hypoxia.

Hypoglycemia.
CNS neoplasms.
Creutzfeldt-Jakob disease.
Medications (e.g., midazolam and other benzodiazepines).
Psychosis.
Malingering.

AMNIOTIC FLUID α-FETOPROTEIN ELEVATION[33]

ICD-10CM #	Z36	Encounter for Antenatal Screening of Mother

CAUSES OF ELEVATED AMNIOTIC FLUID α-FETOPROTEIN

Craniospinal defect (open neural tube defect).
Omphalocele.
Gastroschisis.
Duodenal atresia.
Congenital nephrosis.
Cystic hygroma.
Unbalanced D/G dislocation.
Down, Tay-Sachs, Klinefelter's, Turner's syndromes.
Fetal tumors.
Epidermolysis bullosa.
Pilonidal sinus.
Rhesus disease.
Fetal demise.
Incorrect dates.
Multiple pregnancy.

ANAL ABSCESS AND FISTULA[72]

ICD-10CM #	K61.0	Anal Abscess
	K61.1	Rectal Abscess
	K61.3	Ischiorectal Abscess
	K60.3	Anal fistula

Primary anal gland infection.
Secondary abscess:
 Inflammatory bowel disease:
  ■ Crohn's disease.
  ■ Ulcerative colitis.
 Infection:
  ■ Tuberculosis.
  ■ Actinomycosis.
  ■ Threadworm.
 Trauma.
 Leukopenia.
 Immunosuppression:
  ■ HIV.
  ■ Drugs.
 Rectal cancer.
 Diabetes mellitus.

ANAL INCONTINENCE[50]

ICD-10CM #	R15.9	Full Incontinence of Feces

TRAUMATIC

Nerve injured in surgery.
Spinal cord injury.
Obstetric trauma.
Sphincter injury.

NEUROLOGIC

Spinal cord lesions.
Dementia.
Autonomic neuropathy (e.g., DM).
Obstetrics: pudendal nerve stretched during surgery.
Hirschsprung's disease.

MASS EFFECT

Carcinoma of anal canal.
Carcinoma of rectum.
Foreign body.
Fecal impaction.
Hemorrhoids.

MEDICAL

Procidentia.
Inflammatory disease.
Diarrhea.
Laxative abuse.

PEDIATRIC

Congenital.
Meningocele.
Myelomeningocele.
Spina bifida.
After corrective surgery for imperforate anus.
Sexual abuse.
Encopresis.

ANAPHYLAXIS[43]

ICD-10CM #	T78.2	Anaphylactic Shock, Unspecified, Initial Encounter

PULMONARY

Laryngeal edema.
Epiglottitis.
Foreign body aspiration.
Pulmonary embolus.
Asphyxiation.
Hyperventilation.

CARDIOVASCULAR

Myocardial infarction.
Arrhythmia.
Hypovolemic shock.
Cardiac arrest.

CNS

Vasovagal reaction.
CVA.
Seizure disorder.
Drug overdose.

ENDOCRINE

Hypoglycemia.
Pheochromocytoma.
Carcinoid syndrome.
Catamenial (progesterone-induced anaphylaxis).

PSYCHIATRIC

Vocal cord dysfunction syndrome.
Münchausen syndrome.
Panic attack/globus hystericus.

Differential Diagnosis

II

OTHER

Hereditary angioedema.
Cord urticaria.
Idiopathic urticaria.
Mastocytosis.
Serum sickness.
Idiopathic capillary leak syndrome.
Sulfite exposure.
Scombroid poisoning (tuna, blue fish, mackerel).

ANAPHYLAXIS MIMICS[59]

ICD-10CM #	Varies with Specific Diagnosis

CONDITIONS THAT MIMIC ANAPHYLAXIS

Vasovagal episodes
Acute pulmonary events
  Acute asthmatic attacks
  Acute pulmonary edema
  Pulmonary embolus
  Spontaneous pneumothorax
  Foreign body aspiration
Acute cardiac events
  Supraventricular tachycardias
  Acute myocardial infarction/ischemia
Drug overdoses
Insulin shock
Carcinoid attacks

ANAPHYLAXIS, PATHOPHYSIOLOGIC CLASSIFICATION[2]

ICD-10CM #	T78.2	Anaphylactic shock, unspecified, initial encounter

PATHOPHYSIOLOGIC CLASSIFICATION OF ANAPHYLAXIS

IgE Dependent, Immunologic
Foods.
Drugs.
Insect stings and bites.
Exercise (food dependent).
Other causes.
IgE Independent, Immunologic
Immune aggregates.
IgG anti-IgA.
Cytotoxic.
Disturbance of arachidonic acid metabolism:
- Aspirin.
- Other nonsteroidal antiinflammatory drugs.
Activation of kallikrein-kinin contact system:
- Dialysis membranes.
- Radiocontrast media.
Multimediator recruitment:
- Complement.
- Clotting.
- Clot lysis.
- Kallikrein-kinin contact system.
Other causes
Nonimmunologic
Direct mediator release from mast cells and basophils:

- Drugs, e.g., opiates.
- Physical factors, e.g., cold and sunlight.
Exercise
c-kit Mutation (D816V)
Other causes
Idiopathic

ANAPHYLACTOID SYNDROME OF PREGNANCY[1]

ICD-10CM #	088.113

CARDIOVASCULAR COLLAPSE, HYPOTENSION

Acute coronary syndromes, myocardial infarction.
Cardiomyopathy.
Pulmonary embolism.
Anesthesia complications, transfusion reaction.
Sepsis, systemic inflammatory response syndrome.

RESPIRATORY ARREST

Pulmonary embolism, air embolism.
Anesthesia complications, transfusion reaction.
Aspiration.

ALTERED MENTAL STATUS, SEIZURE

Eclampsia.
Cerebrovascular accident.
Hypoglycemia.

COAGULOPATHY

Disseminated intravascular coagulation.
Consumptive coagulopathy from hemorrhage.

ANDROGEN EXCESS, REPRODUCTIVE-AGE WOMAN

ICD-10CM #	E28.1	Androgen Excess

Polycystic ovary syndrome.
Idiopathic.
Medications (e.g., anabolizing agents, testosterone, danazol).
Pregnancy (luteoma, hyperreaction luteinalis).
Sertoli-Leydig ovarian neoplasm.
Adrenal adenoma or hyperplasia.
Cushing's syndrome.
Glucocorticoid resistance.
Hypothyroidism.
Hyperprolactinemia.

ANDROGEN RESISTANCE[53]

ICD-10CM #	E34.5	Androgen resistance syndrome

CONGENITAL OR DEVELOPMENTAL DISORDERS

Uncommon causes:
  Kennedy disease (spinal and bulbar muscular atrophy).
  Partial androgen insensitivity syndrome (AR mutations).
  5α-reductase type 2 deficiency.
  Complete androgen insensitivity syndrome (female phenotype).

ACQUIRED DISORDERS

Common causes:
  AR antagonists (bicalutamide, nilutamide).
  Drugs (spironolactone, cyproterone acetate, marijuana, histamine 2 receptor antagonists).
Uncommon causes:
  Celiac disease.

ANEMIA, APLASTIC[40]

ICD-10CM #	D61.09	Other Constitutional Aplastic Anemia

ACQUIRED APLASTIC ANEMIA

Secondary aplastic anemia.
Irradiation.
Drugs and chemicals.
Regular effects.
Cytotoxic agents.
Benzene.
Idiosyncratic reactions.
Chloramphenicol.
Nonsteroidal antiinflammatory drugs.
Antiepileptics.
Gold.
Other drugs and chemicals.
Viruses.
Epstein-Barr virus (infectious mononucleosis).
Hepatitis virus (non-A, non-B, non-C, non-G hepatitis).
Parvovirus (transient aplastic crisis, some pure red cell aplasia).
Human immunodeficiency virus (acquired immunodeficiency syndrome).
Immune diseases.
Eosinophilic fasciitis.
Hyperimmunoglobulinemia.
Thymoma and thymic carcinoma.
Graft-versus-host disease in immunodeficiency.
Paroxysmal nocturnal hemoglobinuria.
Pregnancy.
Idiopathic aplastic anemia.

INHERITED APLASTIC ANEMIA

Fanconi anemia.
Dyskeratosis congenita.
Shwachman-Diamond syndrome.
Reticular dysgenesis.
Amegakaryocytic thrombocytopenia.
Familial aplastic anemias.
Preleukemia (e.g., monosomy 7).
Nonhematologic syndromes (e.g., Down, Dubowitz, Seckel).

ANEMIA, APLASTIC, DUE TO DRUGS AND CHEMICALS[1]

ICD-10CM #	D61.1	Drug-Induced Aplastic Anemia
	D61.2	Aplastic Anemia Due to Other External Agents
	D61.89	Other Specified Aplastic Anemias and Other Bone Marrow Failure Syndromes

Agents that regularly produce marrow depression as a major toxic effect when used in commonly employed doses or normal exposures:

Cytotoxic drugs used in cancer chemotherapy.

Alkylating agents (busulfan, melphalan, cyclophosphamide).

Antimetabolites (antifolic compounds, nucleotide analogs), antimitotics (vincristine, vinblastine, colchicine).

Some antibiotics (daunorubicin, doxorubicin [Adriamycin]).

Benzene (and less often benzene-containing chemicals); kerosene, carbon tetrachloride, Stoddard's solvent, chlorophenols).

Agents probably associated with aplastic anemia but with a relatively low probability relative to their use:

Chloramphenicol.

Insecticides.

Antiprotozoals (quinacrine and chloroquine).

Nonsteroidal antiinflammatory drugs (including phenylbutazone, indomethacin, ibuprofen, sulindac, diclofenac, naproxen, piroxicam, fenoprofen, fenbufen, aspirin).

Anticonvulsants (hydantoins, carbamazepine, phenacemide, ethosuximide).

Gold, arsenic, and other heavy metals such as bismuth and mercury.

Sulfonamides as a class.

Antithyroid medications (methimazole, methylthiouracil, propylthiouracil).

Antidiabetes drugs (tolbutamide, carbutamide, chlorpropamide).

Carbonic anhydrase inhibitors (acetazolamide, methazolamide, mesalazine).

D-Penicillamine.

2-Chlorodeoxyadenosine.

Agents more rarely associated with aplastic anemia:

Antibiotics (streptomycin, tetracycline, methicillin, ampicillin, mebendazole and albendazole, sulfonamides, flucytosine, mefloquine, dapsone).

Antihistamines (cimetidine, ranitidine, chlorpheniramine).

Sedatives and tranquilizers (chlorpromazine, prochlorperazine, piperacetazine, chlordiazepoxide, meprobamate, methyprylon, remoxipride).

Antiarrhythmics (tocainide, amiodarone).

Allopurinol (can potentiate marrow suppression by cytotoxic drugs).

Ticlopidine.

Methyldopa.

Quinidine.

Lithium.

Guanidine.

Canthaxanthin.

Thiocyanate.

Carbimazole.

Cyanamide.

Deferoxamine.

Amphetamines.

ANEMIA, CAUSES IN PREGNANCY[27]

ICD-10CM #		
	D50.8	Other Iron Deficiency Anemias
	D50.9	Iron Deficiency Anemia, Unspecified
	D51.0	Vitamin B_{12} Deficiency Anemia Due to Intrinsic Factor Deficiency
	D51.1	Vitamin B_{12} Deficiency Anemia Due to Selective Vitamin B_{12} Malabsorption with Proteinuria
	D51.3	Other Dietary Vitamin B_{12} Deficiency Anemia
	D51.8	Other Vitamin B_{12} Deficiency Anemias
	D52.0	Dietary Folate Deficiency Anemia
	D52.1	Drug-Induced Folate Deficiency Anemia
	D52.8	Other Folate Deficiency Anemias
	D52.9	Folate Deficiency Anemia, Unspecified
	D53.1	Other Megaloblastic Anemias, Not Elsewhere Classified
	D53.0	Protein Deficiency Anemia
	D53.2	Scorbutic Anemia
	D53.8	Other Specified Nutritional Anemias
	D53.9	Nutritional Anemia, Unspecified
	D64.0	Hereditary Sideroblastic Anemia
	D64.1	Secondary Sideroblastic Anemia Due to Disease
	D64.2	Secondary Sideroblastic Anemia Due to Drugs and Toxins
	D64.3	Other Sideroblastic Anemias

CAUSES OF ANEMIA DURING PREGNANCY

Common Causes—85% of Anemia:

Physiologic anemia.

Iron deficiency.

Uncommon Causes:

Folic acid deficiency.

Vitamin B_{12} deficiency (due to the rapid increase in bariatric surgery).

Hemoglobinopathies:

- Sickle cell disease.
- Hemoglobin SC.
- β-Thalassemia minor.

Bariatric surgery.

Gastrointestinal bleeding.

Rare Causes:

Hemoglobinopathies:

- β-Thalassemia major.
- α-Thalassemia.

Syndromes of chronic hemolysis:

- Hereditary spherocytosis.
- Paroxysmal nocturnal hemoglobinuria.

Hematologic malignancy.

ANEMIA, DRUG-INDUCED[35]

ICD-10CM #	D61.1	Drug-Induced Aplastic Anemia

DRUGS THAT MAY INTERFERE WITH RED CELL PRODUCTION BY INDUCING MARROW SUPPRESSION OR APLASIA

Alcohol.

Antineoplastic drugs.

Antithyroid drugs.

Antibiotics.

Oral hypoglycemic agents.

Phenylbutazone.

Azidothymidine (AZT).

DRUGS THAT INTERFERE WITH VITAMIN B_{12}, FOLATE, OR IRON ABSORPTION OR UTILIZATION

Nitrous oxide.

Anticonvulsant drugs.

Antineoplastic drugs.

Isoniazid

Cycloserine A.

DRUGS CAPABLE OF PROMOTING HEMOLYSIS

Immune Mediated

Penicillins.

Quinine.

α-methyldopa.

Procainamide.

Mitomycin C.

Oxidative Stress

Antimalarials.

Sulfonamide drugs.

Nalidixic acid.

DRUGS THAT MAY PRODUCE OR PROMOTE BLOOD LOSS

Aspirin.

Alcohol.

Nonsteroidal antiinflammatory agents.

Corticosteroids.

Anticoagulants.

ANEMIA, HYPOCHROMIC[40]

ICD-10CM #		
	D50.8	Other Iron Deficiency Anemias
	D50.9	Iron Deficiency Anemia, Unspecified
	D64.0	Hereditary Sideroblastic Anemia
	D64.1	Secondary Sideroblastic Anemia Due to Disease
	D64.2	Secondary Sideroblastic Anemia Due to Drugs and Toxins
	D64.3	Other Sideroblastic Anemias

Differential Diagnosis

II

DECREASED BODY IRON STORES

Iron-deficiency anemia.

NORMAL OR INCREASED BODY IRON STORES

Impaired iron metabolism.
Anemia of chronic disease.
Defective absorption, transport, or use of iron.
Disorders of globin synthesis:
○ Thalassemia.
○ Other microcytic hemoglobinopathies.
Disorders of heme synthesis: sideroblastic anemias:
○ Hereditary.
○ Acquired.

ANEMIA, LOW RETICULOCYTE COUNT[3]

ICD-10CM # D64.9   Anemia, Unspecified

MICROCYTIC ANEMIA (MCV <80)

Iron deficiency.
Thalassemia minor.
Sideroblastic anemia.
Lead poisoning.

MACROCYTIC ANEMIA (MCV >100)

Megaloblastic anemias.
Folate deficiency.
Vitamin B_{12} deficiency.
Drug-induced megaloblastic anemia.
Nonmegaloblastic macrocytosis.
Liver disease.
Hypothyroidism.

NORMOCYTIC ANEMIA (MCV 80-100)

Early iron deficiency.
Aplastic anemia.
Myelophthisic disorders.
Endocrinopathies.
Anemia of chronic disease.
Uremia.
Mixed nutritional deficiency.

ANEMIA, MEGALOBLASTIC[70]

ICD-10CM #		
D51.0	Vitamin B12 Deficiency Anemia Due to Intrinsic Factor Deficiency
D51.1	Vitamin B12 Deficiency Anemia Due to Selective Vitamin B12 Malabsorption with Proteinuria
D51.3	Other Dietary Vitamin B12 Deficiency Anemia
D51.8	Other Vitamin B12 Deficiency Anemias
D52.0	Dietary Folate Deficiency Anemia
D52.1	Drug-Induced Folate Deficiency Anemia
D52.8	Other Folate Deficiency Anemias
D52.9	Folate Deficiency Anemia, Unspecified
D53.1	Other Megaloblastic Anemias, Not Elsewhere Classified
D53.0	Protein Deficiency Anemia
D53.2	Scorbutic Anemia
D53.8	Other Specified Nutritional Anemias
D53.9	Nutritional Anemia, Unspecified

COBALAMIN (CBL) DEFICIENCY

Nutritional CBL Deficiency (Insufficient CBL Intake)

Vegetarians, vegans, breastfed infants of mothers with pernicious anemia.

Abnormal Intragastric Events (Inadequate Proteolysis of Food CBL)

Atrophic gastritis, partial gastrectomy with hypochlorhydria.

Loss/Atrophy of Gastric Oxyntic Mucosa (Deficient Intrinsic Factor [If] Molecules)

Total or partial gastrectomy, pernicious anemia (PA), caustic destruction (lye).

Abnormal Events in Small Bowel Lumen

Inadequate pancreatic protease (R-CBL not degraded, CBL not transferred to IF).
○ Insufficiency of pancreatic protease—pancreatic insufficiency.
○ Inactivation of pancreatic protease—Zollinger-Ellison syndrome.
Usurping of luminal CBL (inadequate CBL binding to IF).
○ By bacteria—stasis syndromes (blind loops, pouches of diverticulosis, strictures, fistulas, anastomoses); impaired bowel motility (scleroderma, pseudoobstruction), hypogammaglobulinemia.
○ By *Diphyllobothrium latum.*

Disorders of Ileal Mucosa/IF Receptors (IF-CBL not Bound to IF Receptors)

Diminished or absent IF receptors—ileal bypass/resection/fistula.
Abnormal mucosal architecture/function—tropical/nontropical sprue, Crohn's disease, TB ileitis, infiltration by lymphomas, amyloidosis.
IF-/post IF-receptor defects—Imerslund-Graesbeck syndrome, TC II deficiency.
Drug-induced effects (slow K, biguanides, cholestyramine, colchicine, neomycin, PAS).

DISORDERS OF PLASMA CBL TRANSPORT (TC II-CBL NOT DELIVERED TO TC II RECEPTORS)

Congenital TC II deficiency, defective binding of TC II-CBL to TC II receptors (rare).

METABOLIC DISORDERS (CBL NOT UTILIZED BY CELL)

Inborn enzyme errors (rare).
Acquired disorders: (CBL oxidized to cob[III] alamin)—N_2O inhalation.

FOLATE DEFICIENCY

Nutritional Causes

Decreased dietary intake—poverty and famine (associated with kwashiorkor, marasmus), institutionalized individuals (psychiatric/nursing homes), chronic debilitating disease/goats' milk (low in folate), special diets (slimming), cultural/ethnic cooking techniques (food folate destroyed) or habits (folate-rich foods not consumed).
Decreased diet and increased requirements:
○ Physiologic: pregnancy and lactation, prematurity, infancy.
○ Pathologic: intrinsic hematologic disease (autoimmune hemolytic disease), drugs, malaria; hemoglobinopathies (SS, thalassemia), RBC membrane defects (hereditary spherocytosis, paroxysmal nocturnal hemoglobinopathy); abnormal hematopoiesis (leukemia/lymphoma, myelodysplastic syndrome, agnogenic myeloid metaplasia with myelofibrosis); infiltration with malignant disease; dermatologic (psoriasis).

Folate Malabsorption

With normal intestinal mucosa:
○ Some drugs (controversial).
○ Congenital folate malabsorption (rare).
With mucosal abnormalities—tropical and nontropical sprue, regional enteritis.

Defective Cellular Folate Uptake—Familial Aplastic Anemia (Rare), Inadequate Cellular Utilization

Folate antagonists (methotrexate).
Hereditary enzyme deficiencies involving folate.

Drugs (Multiple Effects on Folate Metabolism)

Alcohol, sulfasalazine, triamterene, pyrimethamine, trimethoprim-sulfamethoxazole, diphenylhydantoin, barbiturates.

MISCELLANEOUS MEGALOBLASTIC ANEMIAS (NOT CAUSED BY CBL OR FOLATE DEFICIENCY)

Congenital Disorders of DNA Synthesis (Rare)

Orotic aciduria, Lesch-Nyhan syndrome, congenital dyserythropoietic anemia.

Acquired Disorders of DNA Synthesis

Thiamine-responsive megaloblastosis (rare).
Malignancy—erythroleukemia—refractory sideroblastic anemias—all antineoplastic drugs that inhibit DNA synthesis.
Toxins—alcohol.

ANEMIA, MICROCYTIC, HYPOCHROMIC, DIFFERENTIAL DIAGNOSIS[39]

ICD-10CM #	D50.8	Other Iron Deficiency Anemias
	D50.9	Iron Deficiency Anemia, Unspecified
	D64.0	Hereditary Sideroblastic Anemia
	D64.1	Secondary Sideroblastic Anemia Due to Disease
	D64.2	Secondary Sideroblastic Anemia Due to Drugs and Toxins
	D64.3	Other Sideroblastic Anemias

DIFFERENTIAL DIAGNOSIS OF MICROCYTIC HYPOCHROMIC ANEMIA

Decreased Body Iron Stores
Iron-deficiency anemia.
Normal or Increased Body Iron Stores
Anemia of chronic disease.
Defective absorption, transport, or use of iron.
Iron-refractory, iron-deficiency anemia after parenteral iron.
Atransferrinemia.
Aceruloplasminemia.
Divalent metal transporter 1 (DMT1 or SLC11A2) deficiency.
Ferroportin-associated hemochromatosis with impaired iron export (type 4A).
Heme oxygenase 1 deficiency.
Disorders of globin synthesis.
Decreased Body Iron Stores
Thalassemia.
　○ Other microcytic hemoglobinopathies.
　○ Disorders of heme synthesis:
Sideroblastic anemias.
　○ Hereditary.
　○ Acquired.

ANERGY, CUTANEOUS[70]

| ICD-10CM # | D89.9 | Disorder Involving the Immune Mechanism, Unspecified |

IMMUNOLOGIC

Acquired (AIDS, acute leukemia, carcinoma, CLL, Hodgkin's lymphoma, NHL).
Congenital (ataxia-telangiectasia, Di George's syndrome, severe combined immunodeficiency, Wiskott-Aldrich syndrome).

INFECTIONS

Bacterial (bacterial pneumonia, brucellosis).
Disseminated mycotic infections.
Mycobacterial (lepromatous leprosy, TB).
Viral (varicella, hepatitis, influenza, mononucleosis, measles, mumps).

IMMUNOSUPPRESSIVE MEDICATIONS

Systemic corticosteroids.
Methotrexate, cyclophosphamide.
Rifampin.

OTHER

Alcoholic cirrhosis, biliary cirrhosis, sarcoidosis, rheumatic disease.
Diabetes, Crohn's disease, uremia.
Anemia, pyridoxine deficiency, sickle cell anemia.
Burns, malnutrition, pregnancy, old age, surgery.

ANEURYSMS, THORACIC AORTA

| ICD-10CM # | I71.2 | Thoracic Aortic Aneurysm, Without Rupture |

Trauma.
Infection.
Inflammatory (syphilis, Takayasu's disease).
Collagen vascular disease (RA, ankylosing spondylitis).
Annuloaortic ectasia (Marfan's syndrome, Ehlers-Danlos syndrome).
Congenital.
Coarctation.
Cystic medial necrosis.

ANHIDROSIS

ICD-10CM #	L74.0	Miliaria Rubra
	L74.1	Miliaria Crystallina
	L74.2	Miliaria Profunda

Drugs (anticholinergics).
Dehydration.
Hysteria.
Obstruction of sweat ducts (e.g., inflammation, miliaria).
Local radiant heat or pressure.
CNS lesions (medulla, hypothalamus, pons).
Spinal cord lesions.
Lesions of sympathetic nerves.
Congenital sweat gland disturbances.

ANION GAP ACIDOSIS[74]

| ICD-10CM # | E87.2 | Acidosis |

CLINICAL CAUSES OF HIGH ANION GAP AND NORMAL ANION GAP ACIDOSIS

High Anion Gap
Ketoacidosis:
　Diabetic ketoacidosis (acetoacetate).
　Alcoholic (β-hydroxybutyrate).
　Starvation.
Lactic acid acidosis:
　L-Lactic acid acidosis (types A and B).
　D-Lactic acid acidosis.
　Renal failure: sulfate, phosphate, urate, hippurate.
Ingestions (toxins and their metabolites):

Ethylene glycol → glycolate, oxalate.
Methyl alcohol → formate.
Salicylate → ketones, lactate, salicylate.
Paraldehyde → organic anions.
Toluene → hippurate (commonly presents with normal anion gap).
Propylene glycol → lactate.
Pyroglutamic acidosis (acetaminophen use) → 5-oxoproline.
Normal Anion Gap
Gastrointestinal loss of HCO_3^- (negative urine anion gap):
　Diarrhea.
　Fistula, external.
Renal loss of HCO_3^- or failure to excrete NH_4^+ (positive urine anion gap):
　Proximal renal tubular acidosis (RTA type 2).
　Acetazolamide.
　Classic distal renal tubular acidosis (low serum K^+) RTA type 1.
　Generalized distal renal tubular defect (high serum K^+) RTA type 4.
Miscellaneous:
　NH_4Cl ingestion.
　Sulfur ingestion.
　Dilutional acidosis.
　Late stages in treatment of diabetic ketoacidosis.

ANION GAP INCREASE

| ICD-10CM # | E87.8 | Other Disorders of Electrolyte and Fluid Balance, Not Elsewhere Classified |

Uremia.
Ketoacidosis (diabetic, starvation, alcoholic).
Lactic acidosis.
Ethylene glycol poisoning.
Salicylate overdose.
Methanol poisoning.

ANISOCORIA

| ICD-10CM # | H57.02 | Anisocoria |

Mydriatic or miotic drugs.
Prosthetic eye.
Inflammation (keratitis, iridocyclitis).
Infections (herpes zoster, syphilis, meningitis, encephalitis, TB, diphtheria, botulism).
Subdural hemorrhage.
Cavernous sinus thrombosis.
Intracranial neoplasm.
Cerebral aneurysm.
Glaucoma.
CNS degenerative diseases.
Internal carotid ischemia.
Toxic polyneuritis (alcohol, lead).
Adie's syndrome.
Horner's syndrome.
DM.
Trauma.
Congenital.

Differential Diagnosis

II

ANORECTAL DISEASE, AIDS PATIENT[23]

ICD-10CM #   Varies with Specific Diagnosis

DIFFERENTIAL DIAGNOSIS OF ANORECTAL DISEASE IN PATIENTS WITH AIDS

INFECTIONS
Bacteria
*Chlamydia trachomatis**
Lymphogranuloma venereum
*Neisseria gonorrhoeae**
Shigella flexneri
Mycobacterium tuberculosis
Protozoa
Entamoeba histolytica
Leishmania donovani
Viruses
HSV*
Cytomegalovirus*
Fungi
Candida albicans
Histoplasma capsulatum
NEOPLASMS
Lymphoma*
Kaposi's sarcoma
Squamous cell carcinoma
Cloacogenic carcinoma
Condyloma acuminatum
OTHER
Idiopathic ulcers*
Perirectal abscess, fistula*

*More frequent diagnosis.

ANOREXIA[72]

ICD-10CM #   R63.0   Anorexia

SELECTED CAUSES OF ANOREXIA

Gastrointestinal Tract/Liver
Gastric outlet obstruction or small bowel obstruction.
Gastric cancer.
Hepatic metastases.
Acute viral hepatitis.
Metabolic
Addison's disease.
Hypopituitarism.
Hyperparathyroidism.
Functional
Extremely unpleasant sight/smell.
Systemic
Chronic pain.
Renal failure.
Severe congestive heart failure.
Respiratory failure.
Psychiatric
Depression.
Anorexia nervosa.
Medications
Digoxin.
Narcotic analgesics.
Diuretics.
Antihypertensives.
Chemotherapeutic agents.
Amphetamines.
Miscellaneous
Excessive smoking.
Excessive alcohol intake.
Oral cavity disease.
Thiamine deficiency.
Early pregnancy.
Hypogeusia or dysgeusia.

ANOVULATION

ICD-10CM #   N97.0   Female Infertility Associated with Anovulation

Anorexia and bulimia.
Strenuous exercise.
Weight loss/malnutrition.
Empty sella syndrome.
Pituitary disorders (infarction, infection, trauma, irradiation, surgery, microadenomas, macroadenomas).
Idiopathic hypopituitarism.
Drug induced.
Thyroid dysfunction (hypothyroidism, hyperthyroidism).
Systemic diseases (e.g., liver disease).
Adrenal hyperfunction (Cushing's syndrome, congenital adrenal hyperplasia).
Polycystic ovarian syndrome.
Isolated gonadotropin deficiency.

APPENDICITIS, DIFFERENTIAL DIAGNOSIS IN PREGNANCY[27]

ICD-10CM #   codes vary with specific

DIFFERENTIAL DIAGNOSIS OF APPENDICITIS DURING PREGNANCY

Gynecologic Conditions
Ruptured ovarian cyst.
Adnexal torsion.
Pelvic inflammatory disease or salpingitis.
Endometriosis.
Ovarian cancer.
Obstetrical Causes
Abruptio placentae.
Chorioamnionitis.
Endometritis.
Uterine fibroid degeneration.
Labor (preterm or term).
Viscus perforation after abortion.
Ruptured ectopic pregnancy.
Gastrointestinal Causes
Crohn's disease.
Colonic diverticulitis (right side).
Cholecystitis.
Pancreatitis.
Mesenteric lymphadenitis.
Gastroenteritis.
Colon cancer.
Intestinal obstruction.
Hernia (incarcerated inguinal or internal).
Colonic intussusception.
Ruptured Meckel's diverticulum.
Colonic perforation.
Acute mesenteric ischemia.
Other Causes
Pyelonephritis.
Urolithiasis.

APPETITE LOSS IN INFANTS AND CHILDREN[38]

ICD-10CM #   R63.0   Anorexia
F50.8   Other Eating Disorders
F98.29   Other Feeding Disorders of Infancy and Early Childhood

ORGANIC DISEASE

Infection (Acute or Chronic) Neurologic
Congenital degenerative disease.
Hypothalamic lesion.
Increased intracranial pressure (including a brain tumor).
Swallowing disorders (neuromuscular).
Gastrointestinal
Oral lesions (e.g., thrush or herpes simplex).
Gastroesophageal reflux.
Obstruction (especially with gastric or intestinal distention).
Inflammatory bowel disease.
Celiac disease.
Constipation.
Cardiac
Congestive heart failure (especially associated with cyanotic lesions).
Metabolic
Renal failure and/or renal tubule acidosis.
Liver failure.
Congenital metabolic disease.
Lead poisoning.
Nutritional
Marasmus.
Iron deficiency.
Zinc deficiency.
Fever
RA.
Rheumatic fever.
Drugs
Morphine.
Digitalis.
Antimetabolites.
Methylphenidate.
Amphetamines.
Miscellaneous
Prolonged restriction of oral feedings, beginning in the neonatal period.
Systemic lupus erythematosus (SLE).
Tumor.

PSYCHOLOGIC FACTORS

Anxiety, fear, depression, mania (limbic influence on the hypothalamus).
Avoidance of symptoms associated with meals (abdominal pain, diarrhea, bloating, urgency, dumping syndrome).
Anorexia nervosa.
Excessive weight loss and food aversion in athletes, simulating anorexia nervosa.

ARTERIAL OCCLUSION[30]

| ICD-10CM # | I74.3 | Embolism and Thrombosis of Arteries of the Lower Extremities |
| | I74.2 | Embolism and Thrombosis of Arteries of the Upper Extremities |

Thromboembolism (post-MI, mitral stenosis, rheumatic valve disease, atrial fibrillation, atrial myxoma, marantic endocarditis, bacterial endocarditis, Libman-Sacks endocarditis).
Atheroembolism (microemboli composed of cholesterol, calcium, and platelets from proximal atherosclerotic plaques).
Arterial thrombosis (endothelial injury, altered arterial blood flow, trauma, severe atherosclerosis, acute vasculitis).
Vasospasm.
Trauma.
Hypercoagulable states.
Miscellaneous (irradiation, drugs, infections, necrotizing).

ARTHRITIS AND ABDOMINAL PAIN

ICD-10CM #	M00.9	Pyogenic Arthritis, Unspecified
	R10.817	Generalized Abdominal Tenderness
	M02.9	Reactive arthropathy

Viral syndrome.
Inflammatory bowel disease.
Celiac disease.
Vasculitis.
SLE.
RA.
Scleroderma.
Amyloidosis.
Chronic hepatitis C.
Whipple's disease.
Polyarteritis nodosa.
Behçet's disease.
Familial Mediterranean fever.
Blind loop syndrome.
Babesiosis.
Lyme disease.
Ehrlichiosis.

ARTHRITIS AND DIARRHEA

| ICD-10CM # | M00.9 | Pyogenic Arthritis, Unspecified |
| | R19.7 | Diarrhea, Unspecified |

Viral syndrome.
Inflammatory bowel disease.
Celiac disease.
Whipple's disease.
Enterogenic (bacterial) reactive arthritis.
Collagenous colitis.
Behçet's disease.
Hyperthyroidism.

Spondyloarthropathy.
Blind loop syndrome.

ARTHRITIS AND EYE LESIONS[15]

ICD-10CM #	M00.9	Pyogenic Arthritis, Unspecified
	M02.3	Reiter disease
	M02.9	Reactive arthropathy

SLE.
Sjögren's syndrome.
Behçet's syndrome.
Sarcoidosis.
Subacute bacterial endocarditis (SBE).
Lyme disease.
Granulomatosis with polyangiitis (Wegener's granulomatosis).
Giant cell arteritis.
Takayasu's arteritis.
RA, JRA.
Scleroderma.
Inflammatory bowel disease.
Whipple's disease.
Ankylosing spondylitis.
Reactive arthritis.
Psoriatic arthritis.

ARTHRITIS AND HEART MURMUR[15]

ICD-10CM #	M00.9	Pyogenic Arthritis, Unspecified
	I01.8	Other Acute Rheumatic Heart Disease
	M02.9	Reactive arthropathy

SBE.
Cardiac myxoma.
Ankylosing spondylitis.
Reactive arthritis.
Acute rheumatic fever.
RA.
SLE with Libman-Sacks endocarditis.
Relapsing polychondritis.

ARTHRITIS AND MUSCLE WEAKNESS[17]

ICD-10CM #	M00.9	Pyogenic Arthritis, Unspecified
	M62.9	Disorder of Muscle, Unspecified
	M02.9	Reactive arthropathy

RA.
Ankylosing spondylitis.
Polymyositis.
Dermatomyositis.
SLE, scleroderma, mixed connective tissue disease.
Sarcoidosis.
HIV-associated arthritis.
Whipple's disease.

ARTHRITIS AND RASH[15]

| ICD-10CM # | M00.9 | Pyogenic Arthritis, Unspecified |

| | R21 | Rash and Other Nonspecific Skin Eruption |
| | M02.9 | Reactive arthropathy |

Chronic urticaria.
Vasculitic urticaria.
SLE.
Dermatomyositis.
Polymyositis.
Psoriatic arthritis.
Reactive arthritis.
Chronic sarcoidosis.
Serum sickness.
Sweet's syndrome.
Leprosy.

ARTHRITIS AND SUBCUTANEOUS NODULES[15]

ICD-10CM #	M00.9	Pyogenic Arthritis, Unspecified
	A18.4	Tuberculosis of Skin and Subcutaneous Tissue
	M02.9	Reactive arthropathy

RA.
Gout.
Pseudogout (rare).
Sarcoidosis.
Light chain (LA) amyloidosis (primary, multiple myeloma).
Acute rheumatic fever (ARF).
Hemochromatosis.
Whipple's disease.
Multicentric reticulohistiocytosis.

ARTHRITIS AND WEIGHT LOSS[15]

ICD-10CM #	M00.9	Pyogenic Arthritis, Unspecified
	R63.4	Abnormal Weight Loss
	M02.9	Reactive arthropathy

Severe RA.
RA with vasculitis.
Reactive arthritis.
RA or psoriatic arthritis or ankylosing spondylitis with amyloidosis.
Cancer.
Enteropathic arthritis (Crohn's, ulcerative colitis).
HIV infection.
Whipple's disease.
Blind loop syndrome.
Scleroderma with intestinal bacterial overgrowth.

ARTHRITIS OR EXTREMITY PAIN, IN CHILDREN AND ADOLESCENTS[46]

| ICD-10CM # | M02.9 Reactive arthropathy |

CAUSES OF ARTHRITIS OR EXTREMITY PAIN IN CHILDREN AND ADOLESCENTS

Rheumatic and Inflammatory Diseases
Juvenile idiopathic arthritis.
Systemic lupus erythematosus.
Juvenile dermatomyositis.
Polyarteritis.
Vasculitis.
Scleroderma.
Sjögren syndrome.
Behçet disease.
Overlap syndromes.
Granulomatosis with polyangiitis (Wegener granulomatosis).
Sarcoidosis.
Kawasaki syndrome.
Henoch-Schönlein purpura.
Chronic recurrent multifocal osteomyelitis.

Seronegative Spondyloarthropathies
Juvenile ankylosing spondylitis.
Inflammatory bowel disease.
Psoriatic arthritis.
Reactive arthritis associated with urethritis, iridocyclitis, and mucocutaneous lesions.

Infectious Illnesses
Bacterial arthritis (septic arthritis, Staphylococcus aureus, pneumococcus, gonococcus, Haemophilus influenzae).
Lyme disease.
Viral illness (parvovirus, rubella, mumps, Epstein-Barr virus, hepatitis B).
Fungal arthritis.
Mycobacterial infection.
Spirochetal infection.
Endocarditis.

Reactive Arthritis
Acute rheumatic fever.
Reactive arthritis (postinfectious due to Shigella, Salmonella, Yersinia, Chlamydia, or meningococcus).
Serum sickness.
Toxic synovitis of the hip.
Postimmunization.

Immunodeficiencies
Hypogammaglobulinemia.
Immunoglobulin A deficiency.
Human immunodeficiency virus.

Congenital and Metabolic Disorders
Gout.
Pseudogout.
Mucopolysaccharidoses.
Thyroid disease (hypothyroidism, hyperthyroidism).
Hyperparathyroidism.
Vitamin C deficiency (scurvy).
Hereditary connective tissue disease (Marfan syndrome, Ehlers-Danlos syndrome).
Fabry disease.
Farber disease.
Amyloidosis (familial Mediterranean fever).

Bone and Cartilage Disorders
Trauma.
Patellofemoral syndrome.
Hypermobility syndrome.
Osteochondritis dissecans.
Avascular necrosis (including Legg-Calvé-Perthes disease).
Hypertrophic osteoarthropathy.

Slipped capital femoral epiphysis.
Osteolysis.
Benign bone tumors (including osteoid osteoma).
Histiocytosis.
Rickets.

Neuropathic Disorders
Peripheral neuropathies.
Carpal tunnel syndrome.
Charcot joints.

Neoplastic Disorders
Leukemia.
Neuroblastoma.
Lymphoma.
Bone tumors (osteosarcoma, Ewing sarcoma).
Histiocytic syndromes.
Synovial tumors.

Hematologic Disorders
Hemophilia.
Hemoglobinopathies (including sickle cell disease).

Miscellaneous Disorders
Pigmented villonodular synovitis.
Plant-thorn synovitis (foreign body arthritis).
Myositis ossificans.
Eosinophilic fasciitis.
Tendinitis (overuse injury).
Raynaud phenomenon.

Pain Syndromes
Fibromyalgia.
Growing pains.
Depression (with somatization).
Reflex sympathetic dystrophy.
Regional myofascial pain syndromes.

ARTHRITIS, AXIAL SKELETON

ICD-10CM #		
	M45.9	Ankylosing Spondylitis of Unspecified Sites in Spine
	L40.54	Psoriatic Juvenile Arthropathy
	L40.59	Other Psoriatic Arthropathy
	M15.9	Polyosteoarthritis, Unspecified
	M45.9	Ankylosing Spondylitis of Unspecified Sites in Spine

RA.
Psoriatic arthritis.
Reiter's syndrome (reactive arthritis).
Ankylosing spondylitis.
Juvenile RA.
Degenerative disease of the nucleus pulposus.
Spondylosis deformans.
Diffuse idiopathic skeletal hyperostosis (DISH).
Alkaptonuria.
Infection.

ARTHRITIS, CHRONIC, MONOARTICULAR OR OLIGOARTICULAR, INFECTIOUS CAUSES[9]

ICD-10CM #	varies with specific diagnosis

INFECTIOUS CAUSES OF CHRONIC MONARTICULAR OR OLIGOARTICULAR ARTHRITIS

Bacterial
Borrelia burgdorferi.
Tropheryma whipplei.
Treponema pallidum.
Nocardia spp.

Fungi
Candida spp.
Cryptococcus neoformans.
Blastomyces dermatitidis.
Coccidioides spp.
Paracoccidioides brasiliensis.
Sporothrix schenckii.
Aspergillus spp. and other molds, including Rhizopus, Scedosporium, and Fusarium.

Mycobacteria
Mycobacterium tuberculosis.
M. kansasii.
M. marinum.
M. avium-intracellulare complex.
M. terrae.
M. fortuitum, M. chelonae, M. abscessus.
M. haemophilum.
M. leprae.

Parasites
Helminths.
Filariae.

ARTHRITIS, FEVER, AND RASH[15]

ICD-10CM #	M00.9	Pyogenic Arthritis, Unspecified
	M02.9	Reactive arthropathy
	R21	Rash and Other Nonspecific Skin Eruption
	R50.9	Fever, Unspecified

Rubella, parvovirus B19.
Gonococcemia, meningococcemia.
Secondary syphilis, Lyme borreliosis.
Adult acute rheumatic fever, adult Still's disease, adult Kawasaki disease.
Vasculitic urticaria.
Acute sarcoidosis.
Familial Mediterranean fever.
Hyperimmunoglobulinemia D and periodic fever syndrome.

ARTHRITIS, MONOARTICULAR AND OLIGOARTICULAR[6]

ICD-10CM #	M19.90	Unspecified Osteoarthritis, Unspecified Site
	M01.X0	Direct Infection of Unspecified Joint in Infectious and Parasitic Diseases Classified Elsewhere
	M13.10	Monoarthritis, Not Elsewhere Classified, Unspecified Site

Septic arthritis (*S. aureus, Neisseria gonorrhoeae,* meningococci, streptococci, *Streptococcus pneumoniae,* enteric gram-negative bacilli).

Crystalline-induced arthritis (gout, pseudogout, calcium oxalate, hydroxyapatite and other basic calcium/phosphate crystals).

Traumatic joint injury.

Hemarthrosis.

Monoarticular or oligoarticular flare of an inflammatory polyarticular rheumatic disease (RA, psoriatic arthritis, Reiter's syndrome [reactive arthritis], SLE).

ARTHRITIS, PEDIATRIC AGE[38]

ICD-10CM #		
	M01.X0	Direct Infection of Unspecified Joint in Infectious and Parasitic Diseases Classified Elsewhere
	M08.00	Unspecified Juvenile Rheumatoid Arthritis of Unspecified Site
	M08.3	Juvenile Rheumatoid Polyarthritis (Seronegative)
	M08.40	Pauciarticular Juvenile Rheumatoid Arthritis, Unspecified Site

RHEUMATIC DISEASES OF CHILDHOOD

Acute rheumatic fever.

SLE.

Juvenile ankylosing spondylitis.

Polymyositis and dermatomyositis.

Vasculitis.

Scleroderma.

Psoriatic arthritis.

Mixed connective tissue disease and overlap syndromes.

Kawasaki disease.

Behçet's syndrome.

Familial Mediterranean fever.

Reiter's syndrome (reactive arthritis).

Reflex sympathetic dystrophy.

Fibromyalgia (fibrositis).

INFECTIOUS DISEASES

Bacterial arthritis.

Viral or postviral arthritis.

Fungal arthritis.

Osteomyelitis.

Reactive arthritis.

NEOPLASTIC DISEASES

Leukemia.

Lymphoma.

Neuroblastoma.

Primary bone tumors.

NONINFLAMMATORY DISORDERS

Trauma.

Avascular necrosis syndromes.

Osteochondroses.

Slipped capital femoral epiphysis.

Diskitis.

Patellofemoral dysfunction (chondromalacia patellae).

Toxic synovitis of the hip.

Overuse syndromes.

GENETIC OR CONGENITAL SYNDROMES

Hematologic Disorders

Sickle cell disease.

Hemophilia.

INFLAMMATORY BOWEL DISEASE

Miscellaneous

Growing pains.

Psychogenic arthralgias (conversion reactions).

Hypermobility syndrome.

Villonodular synovitis.

Foreign body arthritis.

ARTHRITIS, POLYARTICULAR

ICD-10CM #		
	M15.0	Primary Generalized (Osteo)Arthritis
	M12.89	Other Specific Arthropathies, Not Elsewhere Classified, Multiple Sites
	M08.3	Juvenile Rheumatoid Polyarthritis (Seronegative)

RA, juvenile (rheumatoid) polyarthritis.

SLE, other connective tissue diseases, erythema nodosum, palindromic rheumatism, relapsing polychondritis.

Psoriatic arthritis, ankylosing spondylitis.

Sarcoidosis.

Lyme arthritis, bacterial endocarditis, *Neisseria gonorrhoeae* infection, rheumatic fever, Reiter's disease (reactive arthritis).

Crystal deposition disease.

Hypersensitivity to serum or drugs.

Hepatitis B, HIV, rubella, mumps.

Other: serum sickness, leukemias, lymphomas, enteropathic arthropathy, Whipple's disease, Behçet's syndrome, Henoch-Schönlein purpura, familial Mediterranean fever, hypertrophic pulmonary osteoarthropathy.

ASCITES

ICD-10CM #		
	R18.0	Malignant Ascites
	C78.6	Secondary Malignant Neoplasm of Retroperitoneum and Peritoneum
	I89.8	Other Specified Noninfective Disorders of Lymphatic Vessels and Lymph Nodes

Hypoalbuminemia: nephrotic syndrome, protein-losing gastroenteropathy, starvation.

Cirrhosis.

Hepatic congestion: CHF, constrictive pericarditis, tricuspid insufficiency, hepatic vein obstruction (Budd-Chiari syndrome), inferior vena cava or portal vein obstruction.

Peritoneal infections: TB and other bacterial infections, fungal diseases, parasites.

Neoplasms: primary hepatic neoplasms, metastases to liver or peritoneum, lymphomas, leukemias, myeloid metaplasia.

Lymphatic obstruction: mediastinal tumors, trauma to the thoracic duct, filariasis.

Ovarian disease: Meigs' syndrome, struma ovarii.

Chronic pancreatitis or pseudocyst: pancreatic ascites.

Leakage of bile: bile ascites.

Urinary obstruction or trauma: urine ascites.

Myxedema.

Chylous ascites.

ASPIRATION LUNG INJURY, CHILDREN[46]

ICD-10CM #		
	P24.8	Neonatal aspiration syndromes

CONDITIONS PREDISPOSING TO ASPIRATION LUNG INJURY IN CHILDREN

Anatomic and Mechanical

Tracheoesophageal fistula.

Laryngeal cleft.

Vascular ring.

Cleft palate.

Micrognathia.

Macroglossia.

Achalasia.

Esophageal foreign body.

Tracheostomy.

Endotracheal tube.

Nasoenteric tube.

Collagen vascular disease (scleroderma, dermatomyositises).

Gastroesophageal reflux disease.

Obesity.

Neuromuscular

Altered consciousness.

Immaturity of swallowing/prematurity.

Dysautonomia.

Increased intracranial pressure.

Hydrocephalus.

Vocal cord paralysis.

Cerebral palsy.

Muscular dystrophy.

Myasthenia gravis.

Guillain-Barré syndrome.

Werdnig-Hoffmann disease.

Ataxia-telangiectasia.

Cerebral vascular accident.

Miscellaneous

Poor oral hygiene.

Gingivitis.

Prolonged hospitalization.

Gastric outlet or intestinal obstruction.

Poor feeding techniques (bottle propping, overfeeding, inappropriate foods for toddlers).

Bronchopulmonary dysplasia.

Viral infection.

Differential Diagnosis

II

ASTHENIA

ICD-10CM #	G93.3	Postviral Fatigue Syndrome
	R53.1	Weakness
	R53.81	Other Malaise
	R53.83	Other Fatigue

Depression.
Chronic fatigue syndrome.
Sleep disorders.
Anemia.
Hypothyroidism.
Sedentary lifestyle.
Medications (e.g., narcotics, sedatives).
Infections.
Dehydration/electrolyte disorders.
COPD and other pulmonary disorders.
Renal failure.
CHF.
Diabetes.
Addison's disease.
Paraneoplastic syndrome.

ASTHMA, CHILDHOOD[8]

ICD-10CM #	J45.20	Mild Intermittent Asthma, Uncomplicated
	J45.22	Mild Intermittent Asthma with Status Asthmaticus

INFECTIONS

Bronchiolitis (RSV).
Pneumonia.
Croup.
Tuberculosis, histoplasmosis.
Bronchiectasis.
Bronchiolitis obliterans.
Bronchitis.
Sinusitis.

ANATOMIC, CONGENITAL

Cystic fibrosis.
Vascular rings.
Ciliary dyskinesia.
B-lymphocyte immune defect.
Congestive heart failure.
Laryngotracheomalacia.
Tumor, lymphoma.
H-type tracheoesophageal fistula.
Repaired tracheoesophageal fistula.
Gastroesophageal reflux.

VASCULITIS, HYPERSENSITIVITY

Allergic bronchopulmonary aspergillosis.
Allergic alveolitis, hypersensitivity pneumonitis.
Churg-Strauss syndrome.
Periarteritis nodosa.

OTHER

Foreign body aspiration.
Pulmonary thromboembolism.
Psychogenic cough.
Sarcoidosis.
Bronchopulmonary dysplasia.
Vocal cord dysfunction.

ATAXIA

ICD-10CM #	R27.0	Ataxia, Unspecified
	R27.8	Other Lack of Coordination
	R27.9	Unspecified Lack of Coordination
	F10.229	Alcohol Dependence with Intoxication, Unspecified
	F10.20	Alcohol Dependence, Uncomplicated
	G11.1	Early-Onset Cerebellar Ataxia
	G31.89	Other Specified Degenerative Diseases of Nervous System
	F44.4	Conversion Disorder with Motor Symptom or Deficit
	F44.6	Conversion Disorder with Sensory Symptom or Deficit

Vertebral-basilar artery ischemia.
Diabetic neuropathy.
Tabes dorsalis.
Vitamin B_{12} deficiency.
Multiple sclerosis and other demyelinating diseases.
Meningomyelopathy.
Cerebellar neoplasms, hemorrhage, abscess, infarct.
Nutritional (Wernicke's encephalopathy).
Paraneoplastic syndromes.
Parainfectious: Guillain-Barré syndrome, acute ataxia of childhood and young adults.
Toxins: phenytoin, alcohol, sedatives, organophosphates.
Wilson's disease (hepatolenticular degeneration).
Hypothyroidism.
Myopathy.
Cerebellar and spinocerebellar degeneration: ataxia/telangiectasia, Friedreich's ataxia.
Frontal lobe lesions: tumors, thrombosis of anterior cerebral artery, hydrocephalus.
Labyrinthine destruction: neoplasm, injury, inflammation, compression.
Hysteria.
AIDS.

ATAXIA, ACUTE OR RECURRENT[20]

ICD-10CM #	R27.0	Ataxia, Unspecified
	R27.8	Other Lack of Coordination
	R27.9	Unspecified Lack of Coordination
	F10.229	Alcohol Dependence with Intoxication, Unspecified
	F10.20	Alcohol Dependence, Uncomplicated
	G11.1	Early-Onset Cerebellar Ataxia

	G31.89	Other Specified Degenerative Diseases of Nervous System
	F44.4	Conversion Disorder with Motor Symptom or Deficit
	F44.6	Conversion Disorder with Sensory Symptom or Deficit

Drug ingestion (e.g., phenytoin, carbamazepine, sedatives, hypnotics, and phencyclidine) or intoxication (e.g., alcohol, ethylene glycol, hydrocarbon fumes, lead, mercury, or thallium).
Postinfectious (cerebellitis [e.g., varicella], acute disseminated encephalomyelitis).
Head trauma.
Basilar migraine.
Benign paroxysmal vertigo (migraine equivalent).
Brain tumor or neuroblastoma (if accompanied by opsoclonus or myoclonus [i.e., "dancing eyes, dancing feet"]).
Hydrocephalus.
Infection (e.g., labyrinthitis, abscess).
Seizure (ictal or postictal).
Vascular events (e.g., cerebellar hemorrhage or stroke).
Miller-Fisher variant of Guillain-Barré syndrome (ataxia, ophthalmoplegia, and areflexia). Warning: If bulbar signs present, disease is likely progressive; patient may lose ability to protect airway and/or ability to breathe.
Inherited ataxias.
Inborn errors of metabolism (e.g., mitochondrial disorders, amino-acidopathies, urea cycle defects).
Conversion reaction.
Multiple sclerosis.

ATAXIA, CEREBELLAR, ADULT ONSET[68]

ICD-10CM #	G11.0	Congenital Nonprogressive Ataxia
	G11.2	Late-Onset Cerebellar Ataxia

CAUSES OF ADULT ONSET CEREBELLAR ATAXIA

Inherited
Later onset SCA syndromes.
Rarely Friedreich's ataxia.
Congenital
Arnold–Chiari malformation (cerebellar ectopia).
Inflammatory
Multiple sclerosis.
Sarcoidosis.
Infections (TB, viral).
Neoplastic
Often metastatic in adults.
Meningioma, neurofibroma.
Hemangioblastoma.
Paraneoplastic
Usually with small cell bronchial carcinoma.
Vascular
Infarction, hemorrhage.

Arteriovenous malformations.
Trauma
Head injury.
Postsurgical.
Toxic
Alcohol, phenytoin, solvent abuse.
Endocrine
Hypothyroidism (very rare).
Degenerative
Multiple system atrophy (MSA).

ATAXIA, CEREBELLAR, CHILDREN[68]

ICD-10CM #	G11.0	Congenital Nonprogressive Ataxia
	G11.2	Late-Onset Cerebellar Ataxia

CAUSES OF CEREBELLAR ATAXIA IN CHILDREN

Congenital Malformations
Cerebellar agenesis/hypoplasia.
Dandy–Walker syndrome.
Arnold–Chiari malformation.
Hereditary Ataxias
Friedreich's ataxia.
Trauma
Birth trauma.
Head injury in childhood.
Infectious
Secondary to bacterial meningitis.
Secondary to encephalitis.
Hydrocephalus
Tumors
Medulloblastoma.
Astrocytoma.
Hemangioblastoma.

ATAXIA, CHRONIC OR PROGRESSIVE[20]

ICD-10CM #	R27.0	Ataxia, Unspecified
	R27.8	Other Lack of Coordination
	R27.9	Unspecified Lack of Coordination
	G11.1	Early-Onset Cerebellar Ataxia
	G11.0	Congenital Nonprogressive Ataxia
	G11.2	Late-Onset Cerebellar Ataxia
	G11.3	Cerebellar Ataxia with Defective DNA Repair
	G11.8	Other Hereditary Ataxia

Hydrocephalus.
Hypothyroidism.
Tumor or paraneoplastic syndrome.
Low vitamin E levels (e.g., cystic fibrosis).
Wilson disease.
Inborn errors of metabolism.
Inherited ataxias (e.g., ataxia-telangiectasia, Friedreich's ataxia).

ATELECTASIS

ICD-10CM #	J98.11	Atelectasis

Lung neoplasm (primary or metastatic).
Infection (pneumonia, TB, fungal, histoplasmosis).
Postoperative (lower lobes).
Sarcoidosis.
Mucoid impaction.
Foreign body.
Postinflammatory (middle lobe syndrome).
Pneumothorax.
Pleural effusion.
Pneumoconiosis.
Interstitial fibrosis.
Bulla.
Mediastinal or adjacent mass.

ATRIAL ENLARGEMENT, LEFT ATRIUM[33]

ICD-10CM #	I51.7	Cardiomegaly

CAUSES OF LARGE LEFT ATRIUM

Causes Due to Volume Overload
Mitral regurgitation (often with left ventricular failure).
Ventricular septal defect.
Patent ductus arteriosus.
Atrial septal defect with shunt reversal (i.e., pulmonary hypertension).
ASD with tricuspid atresia (obligatory shunt reversal).
Aortopulmonary window.
Causes Due to Pressure Overload
Mitral stenosis.
Noncompliant left ventricle: hypertension, hypertrophic cardiomyopathy, aortic stenosis.
Left ventricular failure (often with secondary mitral regurgitation).
Left atrial myxoma.
Other Causes (Both Rare)
Atrial fibrillation.
Isolated/idiopathic.

ATRIAL ENLARGEMENT, RIGHT ATRIUM

ICD-10CM #	I51.7	Cardiomegaly

Right ventricular failure.
Atrial septal defect.
Tricuspid regurgitation.
Tricuspid stenosis.
Pulmonary hypertension.
Restrictive cardiomyopathy.
Right atrial myxoma.
Ebstein's anomaly.
Anomalous pulmonary venous drainage to the right atrium.
Endomyocardial fibrosis.
Sinus of Valsalva fistula.
Arrhythmogenic right ventricular dysplasia.

ATYPICAL LYMPHOCYTOSIS, HETEROPHIL NEGATIVE, INFECTIOUS CAUSES[3]

ICD-10CM #	D72.820	Lymphocytosis (Symptomatic)

MOST COMMON INFECTIOUS CAUSES OF HETEROPHIL-NEGATIVE ATYPICAL LYMPHOCYTOSIS

Babesiosis.
Cytomegalovirus.
Epstein-Barr virus (particularly in children).
Human herpesvirus 6.
Human immunodeficiency virus (especially during acute seroconversion).
Infectious mononucleosis.
Malaria.
Measles.
Toxoplasmosis.
Varicella.
Infectious hepatitis.

AV NODAL BLOCK[30]

ICD-10CM #	I44.30	Unspecified Atrioventricular Block
	I44.2	Atrioventricular Block, Complete

Idiopathic fibrosis (Lenègre's disease).
Sclerodegenerative processes (e.g., Lev's disease with calcification of the mitral and aortic annuli).
AV node radiofrequency ablation procedure.
Medications (e.g., digoxin, beta-blockers, calcium channel blockers, class III antiarrhythmics).
Acute inferior wall MI.
Myocarditis.
Infections (endocarditis, Lyme disease).
Infiltrative diseases (e.g., hemochromatosis, sarcoidosis, amyloidosis).
Trauma (including cardiac surgical procedures).
Collagen vascular diseases.
Aortic root diseases (e.g., spondylitis).
Electrolyte abnormalities (e.g., hyperkalemia).

BACK PAIN

ICD-10CM #	M54.89	Other Dorsalgia
	M54.9	Dorsalgia, Unspecified
	M54.5	Low Back Pain
	F45.42	Pain Disorder with Related Psychological Factors
	M54.08	Panniculitis Affecting Regions of Neck and Back, Sacral and Sacrococcygeal Region
	S23.9XXA	Sprain of Unspecified Parts of Thorax, Initial Encounter
	M43.27	Fusion of Spine, Lumbosacral Region
	M43.28	Fusion of Spine, Sacral and Sacrococcygeal Region

Differential Diagnosis

II

| | M53.2X7 | Spinal Instabilities, Lumbosacral Region |
| | M53.3 | Sacrococcygeal Disorders, Not Elsewhere Classified |

Trauma: injury to bone, joint, or ligament.
Mechanical: pregnancy, obesity, fatigue, scoliosis.
Degenerative: osteoarthritis.
Infections: osteomyelitis, subarachnoid or spinal abscess, TB, meningitis, basilar pneumonia.
Metabolic: osteoporosis, osteomalacia.
Vascular: leaking aortic aneurysm, subarachnoid or spinal hemorrhage/infarction.
Neoplastic: myeloma, Hodgkin's disease, carcinoma of pancreas, metastatic neoplasm from breast, prostate, lung.
GI: penetrating ulcer, pancreatitis, cholelithiasis, inflammatory bowel disease.
Renal: hydronephrosis, calculus, neoplasm, renal infarction, pyelonephritis.
Hematologic: sickle cell crisis, acute hemolysis.
Gynecologic: neoplasm of uterus or ovary, dysmenorrhea, salpingitis, uterine prolapse.
Inflammatory: ankylosing spondylitis, psoriatic arthritis, Reiter's syndrome (reactive arthritis).
Lumbosacral strain.
Psychogenic: malingering, hysteria, anxiety.
Endocrine: adrenal hemorrhage or infarction.

BACK PAIN, CHILDREN AND ADOLESCENTS[46]

| ICD-10CM # | M54.5 | Low Back Pain |
| | M54.9 | Dorsalgia |

INFLAMMATORY OR INFECTIOUS
Diskitis.
Vertebral osteomyelitis (pyogenic, tuberculous).
Spinal epidural abscess.
Pyelonephritis.
Pancreatitis.

RHEUMATOLOGIC
Pauciarticular juvenile rheumatoid arthritis.
Reiter syndrome (reactive arthritis).
Ankylosing spondylitis.
Psoriatic arthritis.

DEVELOPMENTAL
Spondylolysis.
Spondylolisthesis.
Scheuermann disease.
Scoliosis.

TRAUMATIC (ACUTE VERSUS REPETITIVE)
Hip-pelvis anomalies.
Herniated disk.
Overuse syndromes.
Vertebral stress fractures.
Upper cervical spine instability.

NEOPLASTIC
Vertebral Tumors
Benign
Eosinophilic granuloma.
Aneurysmal bone cyst.
Osteoid osteoma.
Osteoblastoma.
Malignant
Osteogenic sarcoma.
Leukemia.
Lymphoma.
Metastatic tumors.
Spinal Cord, Ganglia, and Nerve Roots
Intramedullary spinal cord tumor.
Sympathetic chain.
Ganglioneuroma.
Ganglioneuroblastoma.
Neuroblastoma.

OTHER
Intraabdominal or pelvic pathology.
Following lumbar puncture.
Conversion reaction.
Juvenile osteoporosis.

BACK PAIN, LOW, ACUTE[6]

| ICD-10CM # | M54.5 | Low Back Pain |

DIFFERENTIAL CONSIDERATIONS IN ACUTE LOW BACK PAIN
Emergent
Aortic dissection.
Cauda equina syndrome.
Epidural abscess or hematoma.
Meningitis.
Ruptured/expanding aortic aneurysm.
Spinal fracture or subluxation with cord or root impingement.
Urgent
Back pain with neurologic deficits.
Disk herniation causing neurologic compromise.
Malignancy.
Sciatica with motor nerve root compression.
Spinal fractures without cord impingement.
Spinal stenosis.
Transverse myelitis.
Vertebral osteomyelitis.
Common or Stable
Acute ligamentous injury.
Acute muscle strain.
Ankylosing spondylitis.
Degenerative joint disease.
Intervertebral disk disease without impingement.
Pathologic fracture without impingement.
Seropositive arthritis.
Spondylolisthesis.
Referred or Visceral
Cholecystitis.
Esophageal disease.
Nephrolithiasis.
Ovarian torsion, mass, or tumor.
Pancreatitis.
Peptic ulcer disease.
Pleural effusion.
Pneumonia.
Pulmonary embolism.

Pyelonephritis.
Retroperitoneal hemorrhage or mass.

BACK PAIN, VISCEROGENIC ORIGIN

ICD-10CM #	F45.41	Pain Disorder Exclusively Related to Psychological Factors
	M54	Dorsalgia
	M54.5	Low back pain

Urolithiasis.
Aortic aneurysm.
Colorectal carcinoma.
Endometriosis.
Tubal pregnancy.
Prostatitis.
Peptic ulcer.
Pancreatitis.
Diverticular spasm.
Metastatic neoplasm (e.g., bladder, uterus, ovary, kidney).

BACTERIAL OVERGROWTH, SMALL INTESTINE[72]

| ICD-10CM # | A04.9 | Bacterial intestinal infection, unspecified |

Gastric surgery—Billroth II.
Small bowel diverticula.
Small bowel stricture:
  Crohn's disease.
  Radiation enteritis.
Impaired small intestinal motility:
  Scleroderma.
  Diabetes mellitus.
  Chronic intestinal pseudoobstruction.
Miscellaneous/multifactorial
  Elderly.
  Immune deficiency syndromes.
  Chronic pancreatitis.
  Cirrhosis.

BALLISM[7]

| ICD-10CM # | G25.4 | Drug-Induced Chorea |
| | G25.5 | Other Chorea |

Cerebral infarction or hemorrhage.
Medications (e.g., dopamine agonists, phenytoin).
CNS neoplasm (primary or metastatic).
Nonketotic hyperosmolar state.

---

[7]Violent, flinging, nonpatterned rapid movements

BILE DUCT, DILATED[72]

| ICD-10CM # | K83.1 | Obstruction of bile duct |

Normal variant.
Post-cholecystectomy.
Unsuspected bile duct stone.
Sphincter of Oddi stenosis.
Occult bile duct stricture.
Previous bile duct injury.
Early carcinoma of the pancreas, carcinoma of the bile duct, or carcinoma of the ampulla.

Extrinsic compression of the bile duct by a primary or secondary neoplasm.

BILIARY OBSTRUCTION[62]

ICD-10CM #   varies with specific diagnosis

CAUSES OF BILIARY OBSTRUCTION

Benign Miscellaneous
Choledocholithiasis*
Hemobilia*
Congenital biliary diseases
   Caroli's disease*
   Choledochal cysts
Cholangitis
   Infectious
Acute pyogenic cholangitis*
Biliary parasites*
Recurrent pyogenic cholangitis*
HIV cholangiopathy
   Sclerosing cholangitis
Neoplasms
Cholangiocarcinoma
Gallbladder carcinoma
Locally invasive tumors (esp. pancreatic adeno-carcinoma)
Ampullary tumors
Metastases
Extrinsic compression
Mirizzi syndrome*
Pancreatitis
Adenopathy

---

*Denotes causes of painful jaundice.

BILIARY TREE, REFLUX OF GAS OR BOWEL[75]

ICD-10CM #   varies with specific diagnosis

CAUSES OF REFLUX OF GAS OR BOWEL CONTRAST INTO THE BILIARY TREE

Iatrogenic.
Sphincterotomy.
Choledochojejunostomy.
Gallstone fistula.
Cholecystoduodenal fistula.
Perforated ulcer.
Choledochoduodenal fistula.
Carcinoma.
Choledochoenteric fistula.

BLADDER (URINARY) WALL THICKENING[62]

ICD-10CM #   Varies with Specific Diagnosis

CAUSES OF BLADDER WALL THICKENING

Focal
Neoplasm
Transitional cell carcinoma
Squamous cell carcinoma
Adenocarcinoma

Lymphoma
Metastases
Infectious/Inflammatory
Tuberculosis (acute)
Schistosomiasis (acute)
Cystitis
Malakoplakia
Cystitis cystica
Cystitis glandularis
Fistula
Medical Diseases
Endometriosis
Amyloidosis
Trauma
Hematoma
Diffuse
Neoplasm
Transitional cell carcinoma
Squamous cell carcinoma
Adenocarcinoma
Infectious/Inflammatory
Cystitis
Tuberculosis (chronic)
Schistosomiasis (chronic)
Medical Diseases
Interstitial cystitis
Amyloidosis
Neurogenic Bladder
Detrusor hyperreflexia
Bladder Outlet Obstruction
With muscular hypertrophy

BLEEDING, LOWER GI

ICD-10CM #   K92.2   Gastrointestinal Hemorrhage, Unspecified

(ORIGINATING BELOW THE LIGAMENT OF TREITZ)

Small Intestine
Ischemic bowel disease (mesenteric thrombosis, embolism, vasculitis, trauma).
Small bowel neoplasm: leiomyomas, carcinoids.
Hereditary hemorrhagic telangiectasia (Rendu-Osler-Weber syndrome).
Meckel diverticulum and other small intestine diverticula.
Aortoenteric fistula.
Intestinal hemangiomas: blue rubber-bleb nevi, intestinal hemangiomas, cutaneous vascular nevi.
Hamartomatous polyps: Peutz-Jeghers syndrome (intestinal polyps, mucocutaneous pigmentation).
Infections of small bowel: tuberculous enteritis, enteritis necroticans.
Volvulus.
Intussusception.
Lymphoma of small bowel, sarcoma, Kaposi's sarcoma.
Irradiation ileitis.
AV malformation of small intestine.
Inflammatory bowel disease.
Polyarteritis nodosa.
Other: pancreatoenteric fistulas, Henoch-Schönlein purpura, Ehlers-Danlos syndrome, SLE, amyloidosis, metastatic melanoma.

Colon
Carcinoma (particularly left colon).
Diverticular disease.
Inflammatory bowel disease.
Ischemic colitis.
Colonic polyps.
Vascular abnormalities: angiodysplasia, vascular ectasia.
Radiation colitis.
Infectious colitis.
Uremic colitis.
Aortoenteric fistula.
Lymphoma of large bowel.
Hemorrhoids.
Anal fissure.
Trauma, foreign body.
Solitary rectal/cecal ulcers.
Long-distance running.

BLEEDING, LOWER GI, PEDIATRIC[6]

ICD-10CM #   K92.2   Gastrointestinal Hemorrhage, Unspecified

<3 MO

Swallowed maternal blood.
Infectious colitis.
Milk allergy.
Bleeding diathesis.
Intussusception.
Midgut volvulus.
Meckel diverticulum.
Necrotizing enterocolitis.

<2 YR

Anal fissure.
Infectious colitis.
Milk allergy.
Colitis.
Intussusception.
Meckel diverticulum.
Polyp.
Duplication.
Hemolytic-uremic syndrome.
Inflammatory bowel disease.
Pseudomembranous enterocolitis.

<5 YR

Infectious colitis.
Anal fissure.
Polyp.
Intussusception.
Meckel diverticulum.
Henoch-Schönlein purpura.
Hemolytic-uremic syndrome.
Inflammatory bowel disease.
Pseudomembranous enterocolitis.

5 TO 18 YR

Infectious colitis.
Inflammatory bowel disease.
Pseudomembranous enterocolitis.
Polyp.
Hemolytic-uremic syndrome.
Hemorrhoids.

BLEEDING, RECTAL[72]

ICD-10CM #	K92.2	Gastrointestinal Hemorrhage, Unspecified

IN PATIENTS <40 YR

Very Common
Hemorrhoids.
Anal fissure.
Inflammatory bowel disease (mainly proctitis).
Less Common
Polyps (hamartomatous or adenomatous).
Infective colitis.
Meckel's diverticulum.
Intussusception.
Rare
Colorectal cancer.

IN PATIENTS >40 YR

Hemorrhoids.
Anal fissure.
Colorectal cancer.
Colorectal polyps (mostly adenomas).
Angiodysplasia.
Diverticular disease.
Inflammatory bowel disease.
Ischemic colitis.
Infective colitis.

BLEEDING, THIRD TRIMESTER[1]

ICD-10CM #	N93.9	Abnormal uterine and vaginal bleeding, unspecified

Placental abruption.
Placenta previa.
Bloody show (extrusion of cervical mucus).
Vasa previa.
Disseminated intravascular coagulopathy.
Uterine rupture.
Cervicitis, cervical cancer, or other cervical abnormality.
Vaginal laceration.

BLEEDING, UPPER GI

ICD-10CM #	K92.2	Gastrointestinal Hemorrhage, Unspecified

(ORIGINATING ABOVE THE LIGAMENT OF TREITZ)

Swallowed Hemoptysis
Oral or pharyngeal lesions: swallowed blood from nose or oropharynx.
Esophageal: varices, ulceration, esophagitis, Mallory-Weiss tear, carcinoma, trauma.
Gastric: peptic ulcer (including Cushing and Curling's ulcers), gastritis, angiodysplasia, gastric neoplasms, hiatal hernia, gastric diverticulum, pseudoxanthoma elasticum, Rendu-Osler-Weber syndrome.
Duodenal: peptic ulcer, duodenitis, angiodysplasia, aortoduodenal fistula, duodenal diverticulum, duodenal tumors, carcinoma of

ampulla of Vater, parasites (e.g., hookworm), Crohn's disease.
Biliary: hematobilia (e.g., penetrating injury to liver, hepatobiliary malignancy, endoscopic papillotomy).

BLEEDING, UPPER GI, PEDIATRIC[6]

ICD-10CM #	K92.2	Gastrointestinal Hemorrhage, Unspecified

<3 MO

Swallowed maternal blood.
Gastritis.
Ulcer, stress.
Bleeding diathesis.
Foreign body (NG tube).
Vascular malformation.
Duplication.

<2 YR

Esophagitis.
Gastritis.
Ulcer.
Pyloric stenosis.
Mallory-Weiss syndrome.
Vascular malformation.
Duplication.

<5 YR

Esophagitis.
Gastritis.
Ulcer.
Esophageal varices.
Foreign body.
Mallory-Weiss syndrome.
Hemophilia.
Vascular malformations.

5 TO 18 YR

Esophagitis.
Gastritis.
Ulcer.
Esophageal varices.
Mallory-Weiss syndrome.
Inflammatory bowel disease.
Hemophilia.
Vascular malformation.

BLEEDING, VAGINAL, NON-PREGNANT FEMALE[1]

ICD-10CM #	N93.9	Abnormal uterine and vaginal bleeding, unspecified

TRAUMA

Blunt force.
Penetrating force.
Foreign bodies.

INFECTIOUS

Vaginitis.
Cervicitis.
Endometritis.

DYSFUNCTIONAL UTERINE BLEEDING

Ovulatory.
Anovulatory.
Adenomyosis.

BENIGN GROWTHS

Uterine leiomyomas.
Cervical polyps.

MALIGNANCY

Vulvar.
Cervical.
Uterine.
Ovarian.

SYSTEMIC DISEASE

Medications
Anticoagulation (warfarin [Coumadin], low-molecular-weight heparin, clopidogrel [Plavix]).
Antipsychotics.
Corticosteroids.
Tamoxifen.
Selective serotonin reuptake inhibitors.
Contraceptives (oral, intrauterine devices, intramuscular).

BLINDNESS, GERIATRIC AGE

ICD-10CM #	H54.8	Legal Blindness, as Defined in USA

Cataracts.
Glaucoma.
Diabetic retinopathy.
Macular degeneration.
Trauma.
CVA.
Corneal scarring.
Giant cell arteritis.
Ocular herpes zoster.

BLINDNESS, MONOCULAR, TRANSIENT

ICD-10CM #	H54.41	Blindness, Right Eye, Normal Vision Left Eye
	H54.42	Blindness, Left Eye, Normal Vision Right Eye

Migraine (vasospasm).
Embolic cerebrovascular disease.
Intermittent angle-closure glaucoma.
Partial retinal vein occlusion.
Hyphema.
Optic disc edema.
Giant cell arteritis.
Psychogenic.
Hypotension.
Hypercoagulopathy disorders.
Multiple sclerosis.

BLINDNESS, PEDIATRIC AGE[47]

ICD-10CM #	H54.41	Blindness, Right Eye, Normal Vision Left Eye

| H54.42 | Blindness, Left Eye, Normal Vision Right Eye |

CONGENITAL

Optic nerve hypoplasia or aplasia.
Optic coloboma.
Congenital hydrocephalus.
Hydranencephaly.
Porencephaly.
Microencephaly.
Encephalocele, particularly occipital type.
Morning glory disc.
Aniridia.
Anterior microphthalmia.
Peter's anomaly.
Persistent pupillary membrane.
Glaucoma.
Cataracts.
Persistent hyperplastic primary vitreous.

PHAKOMATOSES

- Tuberous sclerosis.
- Neurofibromatosis (special association with optic glioma).
- Sturge-Weber syndrome.
- von Hippel–Lindau disease.

TUMORS

Retinoblastoma.
Optic glioma.
Perioptic meningioma.
Craniopharyngioma.
Cerebral glioma.
Posterior and intraventricular tumors when complicated by hydrocephalus.
Pseudotumor cerebri.

NEURODEGENERATIVE DISEASES

- Cerebral storage disease.
- Gangliosidoses, particularly Tay-Sachs disease (infantile amaurotic familial idiocy), Sandhoff's variant, generalized gangliosidosis.
- Other lipidoses and ceroid lipofuscinoses, particularly the late-onset amaurotic familial idiocies such as those of Jansky-Bielschowsky and of Batten-Mayou-Spielmeyer-Vogt.
- Mucopolysaccharidoses, particularly Hurler's syndrome and Hunter's syndrome.
- Leukodystrophies (dysmyelination disorders), particularly metachromatic leukodystrophy and Canavan's disease.
- Demyelinating sclerosis (myelinoclastic diseases), especially Schilder's disease and Devic's neuromyelitis optica.
- Special types: Dawson's disease, Leigh's disease, Bassen-Kornzweig syndrome, Refsum's disease.
- Retinal degenerations: retinitis pigmentosa and its variants, Leber's congenital type.
- Optic atrophies: congenital autosomal recessive type, infantile and congenital autosomal dominant types, Leber's disease, and atrophies associated with hereditary ataxias—the types of Behr, of Marie, and of Sanger-Brown.

INFECTIOUS PROCESSES

Encephalitis, especially in the prenatal infection syndromes caused by *Toxoplasma gondii*, cytomegalovirus, rubella virus, *Treponema pallidum*, herpes simplex.
Meningitis, arachnoiditis.
Chorioretinitis.
Endophthalmitis.
Keratitis.

HEMATOLOGIC DISORDERS

Leukemia with central nervous system involvement.

VASCULAR AND CIRCULATORY DISORDERS

Collagen vascular diseases.
Arteriovenous malformations—intracerebral hemorrhage, subarachnoid hemorrhage.
Central retinal occlusion.

TRAUMA

- Contusion or avulsion of optic nerves, chiasm, globe, cornea.
- Cerebral contusion or laceration.
- Intracerebral, subarachnoid, or subdural hemorrhage.

DRUGS AND TOXINS OTHER

- Retinopathy of prematurity.
- Sclerocornea.
- Conversion reaction.
- Optic neuritis.
- Osteopetrosis.

BLISTERS, SUBEPIDERMAL

| ICD-10CM # | T07 | Unspecified Multiple Injuries |

Burns.
Porphyria cutanea tarda.
Bullous pemphigoid.
Bullous drug reaction.
Arthropod bite reaction.
Toxic epidermal necrosis.
Dermatitis herpetiformis.
Polymorphous light eruption.
Variegate porphyria.
SLE.
Epidermolysis bullosa.
Pseudoporphyria.
Acute graft-versus-host reaction.
Linear IgA disease.
Leukocytoclastic vasculitis.
Pressure necrosis.
Urticaria pigmentosa.
Amyloidosis.

BONE AND/OR SOFT TISSUE HYPERTROPHY[60]

| ICD-10CM # | M85.80 | Other specified disorders of bone density and structure, unspecified site |

DISORDERS ASSOCIATED WITH BONE AND/OR SOFT TISSUE HYPERTROPHY

Conditions Associated with Generalized Overgrowth

Pituitary gigantism and acromegaly.
Other endocrine disorders.
Cerebral gigantism (Sotos).

Conditions Associated with Limb Hemihypertrophy

Lipomatosis.
Idiopathic congenital hemihypertrophy (associated with tumors, e.g., Wilms tumor, adrenocortical tumors, hepatoblastoma).
Proteus syndrome (capillary port-wine hemangiomas, lymphangiomas, lipomas, epidermal nevi, hypertrophy hands and feet, macrocephaly).
Maffucci syndrome (enchondromas, exostosis, lymphangiomas, venous angiomas).
Klippel-Trenaunay syndrome (capillary port-wine hemangiomas, varicosities, lymphangiomas).
Parkes Weber syndrome (capillary port-wine hemangiomas, varicosities, arteriovenous fistula).
Blue rubber bleb nevus syndrome (cavernous hemangiomas of skin, gastrointestinal tract).
Other angiodysplasias (e.g., Servelle-Martorell syndrome; venous arterial malformations with limb hypertrophy and bony hypoplasia).
Beckwith-Wiedemann syndrome (macroglossia, visceromegaly, omphaloceles, hemihypertrophy, etc.).

Conditions Associated with Macrodactyly

Neurofibromatosis.
Macrodystrophia lipomatosa.
Proteus syndrome.
Bannayan-Zonana syndrome (lipomatosis, angiomatosis, macrocephaly).
Hemangiomatosis and other vascular malformations (Klippel-Trenaunay and Parkes Weber).
Lymphangiomatosis.
Arteriovenous malformation.
Maffucci syndrome, Ollier disease.
Epidermal nevus syndrome.

BONE DENSITY, DECREASED, GENERALIZED[33]

| ICD-10CM # | M85.80 | Other Specified Disorders of Bone Density and Structure, Unspecified Site |

DISORDERS ASSOCIATED WITH GENERALIZED LOSS OF BONE DENSITY

Disorders of Multiple or Uncertain Cause

Senile osteoporosis.[8]
Juvenile osteoporosis.
Osteogenesis imperfecta.[9]

Secondary Bone Disorders

Endocrine
Adrenal cortex.
  Cushing's disease.
  Addison's disease.
Gonadal disorders.
  Postmenopausal osteoporosis.
  Hypogonadism.
Pituitary.

---

[8]Patients who cannot synthesize Lewis blood group antigens (~5% of the population) do not produce CA-19-9 antigen.
*Common cause of decrease in bone density in adults.
[9]Common cause of decrease in bone density in children.

Acromegaly.
Hypopituitarism.
Pancreas.
Diabetes mellitus.
Thyroid.
Hyperthyroidism.
Hypothyroidism.
Parathyroid.
Hyperparathyroidism.

Marrow Replacement and Expansion
Myeloma.
Leukemia.
Lymphoma.
Metastatic disease.
Gaucher's disease.
Anemias (sickle cell, thalassaemia, hemophilia).

Drugs And Other Substances
Steroids.
Heparin (osteoporosis).
Anticonvulsants (osteomalacia).
Immunosuppressants.
Alcohol.

Chronic Disease
Chronic renal disease.
Hepatic insufficiency.
GI malabsorption syndromes.
Chronic inflammatory polyarthropathies.
Chronic debility or immobilization.

BONE DENSITY, DECREASED, LOCALIZED[33]

ICD-10CM #	Z82.62	Family History of Osteoporosis
	M85.80	Other specified disorders of bone density and structure, unspecified site

DISORDERS ASSOCIATED WITH LOCALIZED LOSS OF BONE DENSITY

Disuse osteoporosis.[10]
Reflex sympathetic dystrophy (Sudeck's).
Osteolytic syndromes.
Acro-osteolysis, primary and secondary.
Massive osteolysis of Gorham.
Carpotarsal osteolysis.
Transient regional osteoporosis.
Neuromuscular disorders.
Infection.
Arthropathies.
Tumors, primary and secondary, myelomatosis.

[10]Common causes.

BONE LESIONS, PREFERENTIAL SITE OF ORIGIN[69]

ICD-10CM #	C41.0	Malignant Neoplasm of Bones of Skull and Face
	C41.1	Malignant Neoplasm of Mandible
	C41.2	Malignant Neoplasm of Vertebral Column
	C41.3	Malignant Neoplasm of Ribs, Sternum and Clavicle
	C40.00	Malignant Neoplasm of Scapula and Long Bones of Unspecified Upper Limb
	C40.10	Malignant neoplasm of Short Bones of Unspecified Upper Limb
	C41.4	Malignant Neoplasm of Pelvic Bones, Sacrum and Coccyx
	C40.20	Malignant Neoplasm of Long Bones of Unspecified Lower Limb
	C40.30	Malignant Neoplasm of Short Bones of Unspecified Lower Limb
	C41.9	Malignant Neoplasm of Bone and Articular Cartilage, Unspecified
	C79.51	Secondary Malignant Neoplasm of Bone
	C79.52	Secondary Malignant Neoplasm of Bone Marrow

EPIPHYSIS

Chondroblastoma.
Giant cell tumor—after fusion of growth plate.
Langerhans' cell histiocytosis.
Clear cell chondrosarcoma.
Osteosarcoma.

METAPHYSIS

Parosteal sarcoma.
Chondrosarcoma.
Fibrosarcoma.
Nonossifying fibroma.
Giant cell tumor—before fusion of growth plate.
Unicameral bone cyst.
Aneurysmal bone cyst.

DIAPHYSIS

Myeloma.
Ewing's tumor.
Reticulum cell sarcoma.

METADIAPHYSEAL

Fibrosarcoma.
Fibrous dysplasia.
Enchondroma.
Osteoid osteoma.
Chondromyofibroma.

BONE MARROW FAILURE SYNDROMES, INHERITED[40]

ICD-10CM #	D61.89	Other Specified Aplastic Anemias and Other Bone Marrow Failure Syndromes

BI-LINEAGE AND TRI-LINEAGE CYTOPENIAS

Fanconi anemia.
Shwachman-Diamond syndrome.
Dyskeratosis congenita.
Amegakaryocytic thrombocytopenia:
Other inherited thrombocytopenia disorders.
Other genetic syndromes:
Down syndrome.
Dubowitz syndrome.
Seckel syndrome.
Reticular dysgenesis.
Schimke immunoosseous dysplasia.
Noonan syndrome.
Cartilage-hair hypoplasia.
Familial marrow failure (non-Fanconi).

UNI-LINEAGE CYTOPENIA

Diamond-Blackfan anemia.
Kostmann syndrome/Congenital neutropenia:
ELA2 mutations.
HAX1 mutations.
GFI1 mutations.
WASP mutations.
Constitutive cell surface G-CSF-R mutations.
Other inherited neutropenia syndromes:
Barth syndrome.
Glycogen storage disease 1b.
Miscellaneous.
Thrombocytopenia with absent radii.
Congenital dyserythropoietic anemias (CDAs):
Types I, II, III, IV.
Variants.
Nonclassifiable CDAs.
Groups IV, V, VI, VII.

BONE MARROW FIBROSIS[29]

ICD-10CM #	D75.9	Disease of Blood and Blood-Forming Organs, Unspecified

MYELOID DISORDERS

Myelofibrosis with myeloid metaplasia.
Metastatic cancer.
Chronic myeloid leukemia.
Myelodysplastic syndrome.
Atypical myeloid disorder.
Acute megakaryocytic leukemia.
Other acute myeloid leukemias.
Gray platelet syndrome.

LYMPHOID DISORDERS

Hairy cell leukemia.
Multiple myeloma.
Lymphoma.

NONHEMATOLOGIC DISORDERS

Connective tissue disorder.
Infections (tuberculosis, kala-azar).
Vitamin D deficiency (rickets).
Renal osteodystrophy.

BONE MASS, LOW[3]

ICD-10CM #	M85.80	Other specified disorders of bone density and structure, unspecified site

SECONDARY CAUSES OF LOW BONE MASS

Endocrine Diseases
Female hypogonadism.
Hyperprolactinemia.
Hypothalamic amenorrhea.
Anorexia nervosa.
Premature and primary ovarian failure.
Female athlete triad.
Male hypogonadism.
Primary gonadal failure (e.g., Klinefelter's syndrome).
Secondary gonadal failure (e.g., idiopathic hypogonadotropic hypogonadism, androgen deprivation therapy for prostate cancer).
Hyperthyroidism.
Hyperparathyroidism.
Hypercortisolism.
Vitamin D insufficiency or deficiency.

Gastrointestinal Diseases
- Subtotal gastrectomy.
- Gastric bypass surgery.
- Malabsorption syndromes.
- Chronic obstructive jaundice.
- Primary biliary cirrhosis and other cirrhoses.

Bone Marrow Disorders
Multiple myeloma.
Monoclonal gammopathy of unknown significance (MGUS).
Lymphoma.
Leukemia.
Hemolytic anemias.
Systemic mastocytosis.
Disseminated carcinoma.

Connective Tissue Diseases
Osteogenesis imperfecta.
Ehlers-Danlos syndrome.
Marfan's syndrome.
Homocystinuria.

Drugs
Alcohol.
Antiseizure medications.
Aromatase inhibitors.
Chemotherapy.
Cyclosporine.
Depo-medroxyprogesterone.
Excess thyroid hormone.
Glucocorticoids.
Gonadotropin-releasing hormone agonists.
Heparin.

Miscellaneous Causes
Immobilization.
Rheumatoid arthritis.
Chronic obstructive pulmonary disease.
Weight loss.

BONE MINERAL DENSITY, INCREASED

ICD-10CM #	M89.30	Hypertrophy of Bone, Unspecified Site

	M89.8X9	Other Specified Disorders of Bone, Unspecified Site
	M94.8X9	Other Specified Disorders of Cartilage, Unspecified Sites

Paget's disease of bone.
Skeletal metastases.
DISH.
Osteonecrosis.
Sarcoidosis.
Hypoparathyroidism, pseudohypoparathyroidism.
Milk-alkali syndrome.
Osteopetrosis.
Hypervitaminosis A or D.
Dysplasias (craniodiaphyseal, craniometaphyseal, frontometaphyseal).
Endosteal hyperostosis.
Fluorosis.
Heavy metal poisoning.
Ionizing radiation.
Other: lymphoma, leukemia, mastocytosis, multiple myeloma, polycythemia vera.

BONE PAIN

ICD-10CM #	M89.8	Pain, bone

Trauma.
Neoplasm (primary or metastatic).
Osteoporosis with compression fracture.
Paget's disease of bone.
Infection (osteomyelitis, septic arthritis).
Osteomalacia.
Viral syndrome.
Sickle cell disease.
Anxiety.

BONE RESORPTION[69]

ICD-10CM #	M89.9	Disorder of Bone, Unspecified
	M94.9	Disorder of Cartilage, Unspecified

DISTAL CLAVICLE

Hyperparathyroidism.
RA.
Scleroderma.
Posttraumatic osteolysis.
Progeria.
Pycnodysostosis.
Cleidocranial dysplasia.

INFERIOR ASPECT OF RIBS

Vascular impression, associated with but not limited to coarctation of the aorta.
Hyperparathyroidism.
Neurofibromatosis.

TERMINAL PHALANGEAL TUFTS

Scleroderma.
Raynaud's phenomenon.
Vascular disease.
Frostbite, electrical burns.
Psoriasis.

Tabes dorsalis.
Hyperparathyroidism.

GENERALIZED RESORPTION

Paraplegia.
Myositis ossificans.
Osteoporosis.

BOWEL WALL THICKENING[75]

ICD-10CM #		varies with specific diagnosis

BENIGN VERSUS MALIGNANT BOWEL WALL THICKENING

Benign
Homogeneous attenuation.
Symmetrical.
Circumferential.
Thickening <1 cm.
Segmental or diffuse involvement.
Double halo sign.
Dark inner ring.
Bright outer ring.
Target sign.
Bright inner ring.
Dark middle ring.
Bright outer ring.

Malignant
Heterogeneous attenuation.
Asymmetrical.
Eccentric.
Thickening >1 to 2 cm.
Focal mass.
Abrupt transition.
Lobulated contour.
Spiculated contour.
Narrowed bowel lumen.
Enlarged lymph nodes.
Liver metastases.

BOW LEGS (GENU VARUM), CLASSIFICATION[46]

ICD-10CM #	E64.3	Genu varum, acquired
	Q74.1	Congenital malformation of knee

PHYSIOLOGIC

Asymmetric Growth
Tibia vara (Blount disease).
  Infantile.
  Juvenile.
  Adolescent.
Focal fibrocartilaginous dysplasia.
Physeal injury.
Trauma.
Infection.
Tumor.

METABOLIC DISORDERS

Vitamin D deficiency (nutritional rickets).
Vitamin D–resistant rickets.
Hypophosphatasia.

SKELETAL DYSPLASIA

Metaphyseal dysplasia.
Achondroplasia.
Enchondromatosis.

Differential Diagnosis

II

BRADYCARDIA, SINUS[30]

| ICD-10CM # | I49.8 | Other Specified Cardiac Arrhythmias |
| | R00.1 | Bradycardia, Unspecified |

Idiopathic.
Degenerative processes (e.g., Lev's disease, Lenègre's disease).

Medications
β-Blockers.
Some calcium channel blockers (diltiazem, verapamil).
Digoxin (when vagal tone is high).
Class I antiarrhythmic agents (e.g., procainamide).
Class III antiarrhythmic agents (amiodarone, sotalol).
Clonidine.
Lithium carbonate.

ACUTE MYOCARDIAL ISCHEMIA AND INFARCTION
Right or left circumflex coronary artery occlusion or spasm.
High vagal tone (e.g., athletes).

BRAIN MASS[1]

ICD-10CM #	C71	Malignant neoplasm of brain
	D33	Benign neoplasm of brain
	I61.9	Intracranial hemorrhage, unspecified

METASTATIC BRAIN TUMOR
Primary brain tumor
Meningioma.
Glioma.
Pituitary adenoma.
Vestibular schwannoma.
Primary or secondary central nervous system lymphoma.
Infections
Abscess.
Toxoplasmosis.
Neurocysticercosis.
Tuberculoma.
Progressive multifocal leukoencephalopathy.

VASCULAR DISEASE
Hemorrhage
Anomalies (arteriovenous malformation).
Intratumoral.
Hypertensive.
Infarct
Embolism.
Thrombosis (sinus venous).
Inflammatory
Multiple sclerosis.
Encephalomyelitis.

BREAST INFLAMMATORY LESION[21]

ICD-10CM #	N61	Inflammatory Disorders of Breast
	N60.19	Diffuse Cystic Mastopathy of Unspecified Breast
	P39.0	Neonatal Infective Mastitis
	P83.4	Breast Engorgement of Newborn

Mastitis (*S. aureus*, β-hemolytic *Streptococcus*).
Trauma.
Foreign body (sutures, breast implants).
Granuloma (TB, fungal).
Fat necrosis post biopsy.
Necrosis or infarction (anticoagulant therapy, pregnancy).
Breast malignancy.

BREAST MASS

| ICD-10CM # | N63 | Unspecified Lump in Breast |

Fibrocystic breasts.
Benign tumors (fibroadenoma, papilloma).
Mastitis (acute bacterial mastitis, chronic mastitis).
Malignant neoplasm.
Fat necrosis.
Hematoma.
Duct ectasia.
Mammary adenosis.

BREATH ODOR[66]

| ICD-10CM # | R19.6 | Halitosis |

Sweet, fruity: DKA, starvation ketosis.
Fishy, stale: uremia (trimethylamines).
Ammonia-like: uremia (ammonia).
Musty fish, clover: fetor hepaticus (hepatic failure).
Foul, feculent: intestinal obstruction/diverticulum.
Foul, putrid: nasal/sinus pathology (infection, foreign body, cancer), respiratory infections (empyema, lung abscess, bronchiectasis).
Halitosis: tonsillitis, gingivitis, respiratory infections, Vincent's angina, gastroesophageal reflux, achalasia, certain foods (garlic, onions, protein drinks, etc.)
Cinnamon: pulmonary TB.

BREATHING, NOISY[66]

ICD-10CM #	R06.00	Dyspnea, Unspecified
	R06.09	Other Forms of Dyspnea
	R06.3	Periodic Breathing
	R06.83	Snoring
	R06.89	Other Abnormalities of Breathing
	R06.1	Stridor

Infection: upper respiratory infection, peritonsillar abscess, retropharyngeal abscess, epiglottitis, laryngitis, tracheitis, bronchitis, bronchiolitis.
Irritants and allergens: hyperactive airway, asthma (reactive airway disease), rhinitis, angioneurotic edema.
Compression from outside of the airway: esophageal cysts or foreign body, neoplasms, lymphadenopathy.
Congenital malformation and abnormality: vascular rings, laryngeal webs, laryngomalacia, tracheomalacia, hemangiomas within the upper airway, stenoses within the upper airway, cystic fibrosis.
Acquired abnormality (at every level of the airway): nasal polyps, hypertrophied adenoids and/or tonsils, foreign body, intraluminal tumors, bronchiectasis.
Neurogenic disorder: vocal cord paralysis.

BRONCHIAL OBSTRUCTION[33]

| ICD-10CM # | J98.0 | Tracheobronchial collapse |

CAUSES OF BRONCHIAL OBSTRUCTION
Outside the Bronchus
Lymph nodes and other masses.
In the Wall of the Bronchus
Tumors
Lung carcinoma (commonly squamous cell).
Bronchial carcinoid.
Metastasis.
Hamartoma.
Inflammation
Tuberculosis.
Sarcoidosis.
Granulomatosis with polyangiitis (Wegener's granulomatosis).
Inflammatory bowel disease.
Bronchomalacia
Broncholith.
Inside the Bronchus
Mucus plug.
Inhaled foreign body.

BRONCHOPLEURAL FISTULA[33]

| ICD-10CM # | J86.0 | Bronchopleural fistula |

CAUSES OF BRONCHOPLEURAL FISTULA
Trauma
Penetrating.
Iatrogenic (especially post-pneumonectomy, post-lobectomy, post-biopsy).
Infection
Necrotizing pneumonia.
Empyema.
Tuberculosis.
Septic embolus.
Infected pulmonary infarct.

BROWN URINE

| ICD-10CM # | R82 | Other abnormal findings in urine |

Bile pigments.
Myoglobin.
Concentrated urine.
Use of multivitamin supplements.

Medications (antimalarials, metronidazole, nitrofurantoin, levodopa, methyldopa, phenazopyridine).
Diet rich in fava beans.
Urinary tract infection.

BRUISING

ICD-10CM #	I99.8	Other Disorder of Circulatory System

Medication-induced (warfarin, aspirin, NSAIDs, prednisone).
Alcohol abuse.
Senile purpura.
Purpura simplex.
Physical abuse.
Vasculitis.
Platelet disorders.
Coagulation factor deficiencies.
Cushing's disease.
Vitamin C deficiency.
Marfan's syndrome.
Ehlers-Danlos syndrome.
Disseminated intravascular coagulation.
Leukemia.
Hereditary hemorrhagic telangiectasia.

BULLOUS DISEASES

ICD-10CM #	L13.9	Bullous Disorder, Unspecified
	L12.0	Bullous Pemphigoid
	L12.8	Other Pemphigoid
	L10.0	Pemphigus Vulgaris
	L10.1	Pemphigus Vegetans
	L10.2	Pemphigus Foliaceous
	L10.4	Pemphigus Erythematosus
	L10.9	Pemphigus, Unspecified
	L10.0	Pemphigus Vulgaris
	L10.1	Pemphigus Vegetans
	L10.2	Pemphigus Foliaceous
	L10.4	Pemphigus Erythematosus
	L10.9	Pemphigus, Unspecified

Bullous pemphigoid.
Pemphigus vulgaris.
Pemphigus foliaceus.
Paraneoplastic pemphigus.
Cicatricial pemphigoid.
Erythema multiforme.
Dermatitis herpetiformis.
Herpes gestationis.
Impetigo.
Erosive lichen planus.
Linear IgA bullous dermatosis.
Epidermolysis bullosa acquisita.

CAFÉ-AU-LAIT SPOTS[46]

ICD-10CM #	L81.3	Cafe au lait spots

Neurofibromatosis types 1 and 2.
McCune-Albright syndrome.
Russell-Silver syndrome.
Ataxia-telangiectasia.

Fanconi anemia.
Tuberous sclerosis.
Bloom syndrome.
Basal cell nevus syndrome.
Gaucher disease.
Chédiak-Higashi syndrome.
Hunter syndrome.
Maffucci syndrome.
Multiple mucosal neuroma syndrome.
Watson syndrome.
Proteus syndrome.
Turner syndrome.
Ring chromosome syndrome.
Jaffe-Campanacci syndrome.

CALCIFICATION ON CHEST X-RAY

ICD-10CM #	J98.4	Calcification of lung
	M51.84	Other Intervertebral Disc Disorders, Thoracic Region
	M51.85	Other Intervertebral Disc Disorders, Thoracolumbar Region

Lung neoplasm (primary or metastatic).
Silicosis.
Idiopathic pulmonary fibrosis.
Tuberculosis.
Histoplasmosis.
Disseminated varicella infection.
Mitral stenosis (end-stage).
Secondary hyperparathyroidism.

CALCIFICATIONS, ABDOMINAL, NONVISCERAL ON X-RAY[33]

ICD-10CM #	M61.9	Calcification and Ossification of Muscle, Unspecified

NONVISCERAL ABDOMINAL CALCIFICATION

Common
Atherosclerosis.
Mesenteric lymph nodes.
Phleboliths.
Aneurysm.
Dermoid cyst.
Differentiate
Rib cartilage.
Injections in the buttocks.
Uncommon
Infestations.
  Armillifer armillatus.
  Cysticercosis.
  Guinea worm.
  Hydatid.
Tumors.
  Lipoma.
  Hemangioma.
  Neuroblastoma.
  Osteo/chondrosarcoma of soft tissues.
  Retroperitoneal sarcoma of soft tissues.
  Peritoneal metastases.
  Pheochromocytoma.

Tuberculosis.
  Peritonitis.
  Psoas abscess.
Meconium peritonitis.
Pseudomyxoma Peritonei
Mesenteric cyst.
Pancreatitis with saponification.
Lithopedion.
Appendices Epiploicae
Ligaments.
Foreign bodies.
Posttraumatic buttock cysts.

CALCIFICATIONS, ADRENAL GLAND ON X-RAY[33]

ICD-10CM #	E27.4	Calcification, adrenal gland

ADRENAL GLAND CALCIFICATION

Common
Idiopathic.
Hemorrhage.
Tuberculosis.
Neuroblastoma/ganglioneuroma.
Pheochromocytoma.
Uncommon
Other tumors:
  Adenoma.
  Carcinoma.
  Dermoid.
Addison's disease.
Cyst.
Histoplasmosis.

CALCIFICATIONS, CARDIAC ON X-RAY[33]

ICD-10CM #	I51.5	Calcification, myocardium
	I25.1	Calcification, arteriosclerotic

CAUSES OF VISIBLE CALCIFICATION WITHIN THE HEART

Coronary Artery
Atherosclerosis.
Aortic Root
Atherosclerotic aorta.
Thrombus.
Syphilis.
Ankylosing spondylitis.
Homograft calcification.
Pericardium
Chronic pericarditis, tuberculosis, hemopericardium, pyogenic or viral pericarditis.
Posttraumatic.
Postoperative.
Uremic pericarditis.
Asbestosis (may be pleural calcification applied to pericardium).
Myocardium
Ventricular aneurysm (may mimic pericardial calcification).
Calcified myocardial infarction.

Postmyocarditis.
Endocardium
Endomyocardial fibrosis.
Thrombus.
Valve Cusps
Calcified valves (particularly mitral and aortic valves).
Mitral annulus calcification.
Homograft calcification.
Old vegetation.
Valve Annulus
Submitral.
Mitral.
Aortic.
Left Atrium
Wall.
Thrombus.
Atrial myxoma.
Pulmonary Artery
Pulmonary hypertension.
Postoperative.
Postoperative Serumoma Calcified Hydatid Cyst

CALCIFICATIONS, CUTANEOUS

| ICD-10CM # | L94.2 | Calcinosis Cutis |
| | L98.8 | Other Specified Disorders of the Skin and Subcutaneous Tissue |

Calcification, Raynaud's phenomenon, esophageal dysmotility, sclerodactyly, and telangiectasia (CREST) syndrome.
Trauma.
Pancreatitis or pancreatic cancer.
Chronic renal failure.
Sarcoidosis.
Hyperparathyroidism.
Milk-alkali syndrome.
Hypervitaminosis D.
Panniculitis.
Idiopathic.
Iatrogenic (e.g., application of calcium alginate dressing to skin).
Multiple myeloma.
Dermatomyositis.
Parasitic infections.
Leukemia.
Lymphoma.

CALCIFICATIONS, GENITAL TRACT, FEMALE ON X-RAY[33]

| ICD-10CM # | E83.59 | Other Disorders of Calcium Metabolism |

FEMALE GENITAL TRACT CALCIFICATION
Uterus
Leiomyomas.
Squamous cell carcinoma.
Adenocarcinoma of endometrium.
Leiomyosarcoma.
Lithopedion.
Fallopian Tubes
Ovary.
Dermoid cyst.

Serous cystadenoma/carcinoma.
Tuberculosis.
Cysts.
Autoamputation.

CALCIFICATIONS, LIVER ON X-RAY[33]

ICD-10CM #	K76.89	Other Specified Diseases of Liver
	NEC	Granuloma, hepatic
	K75.3	

LIVER CALCIFICATION
Common
Granuloma (tuberculosis, histoplasmosis, brucellosis).
  Multiple scattered round densities.
Hydatid cyst.
  Fine curvilinear in wall, or dense and irregular if contracted.
Primary liver tumor (hemangioma, hepatoblastoma, hepatoma, cholangiocarcinoma).
  Irregular patterns or multiple nodules.
Metastases (mucinous primary of colon or breast, cystadenocarcinoma of ovary).
  Finely stippled, may be extensive.
Uncommon
Hepatic artery aneurysm.
Armillifer armillatus infestation.
Chronic granulomatous disease of childhood.
Cyst (congenital or acquired).
Hematoma.
Intrahepatic gallstones.
Old liver abscess.
Portal vein thrombosis.
Differentiate
Hemochromatosis.
Thorotrast, thallium, iron.

CALCIFICATIONS, PANCREAS ON X-RAY[33]

| ICD-10CM # | K86.8 | Calcification, pancreas |

PANCREATIC CALCIFICATION
Common
Chronic pancreatitis.
Uncommon
Acute pancreatitis (saponification).
Tumors.
  Cystadenoma.
  Cystadenocarcinoma.
  Islet cell tumor.
  Metastases.
Hereditary pancreatitis (large clumps).
Hemorrhage.
Hyperparathyroidism.
Pseudocyst.
Cavernous lymphangioma.
Mucoviscidosis.
Kwashiorkor.

CALCIFICATIONS, SPLEEN ON X-RAY[33]

| ICD-10CM # | D73.8 | Calcification, spleen |

SPLENIC CALCIFICATION
Larger than 10 mm
Splenic artery aneurysm.
Splenic artery atheroma.
Cyst.
  Posttraumatic.
  Dermoid.
  Epidermoid.
  Hydatid.
Hematoma.
Infarct.
Abscess.
Tuberculosis.
Smaller than 10 mm
Histoplasmosis.
Tuberculosis.
Phleboliths.
Armillifer armillatus infestation.
Brucellosis.
Infarcts.

CALCIFICATIONS, VALVULAR ON X-RAY[33]

| ICD-10CM # | | I51.5 Calcification, heart |

CAUSES OF RADIOGRAPHICALLY VISIBLE VALVE CALCIFICATION
Aortic Valve
Rheumatic aortic valve disease.
Bicuspid aortic valve.
Age/degenerate aortic valve.
Syphilis.
Ankylosing spondylitis.
Homograft calcification.
Mitral Valve
Rheumatic mitral valve disease.
Mitral annulus calcification.
Old vegetation (may only be visible on CT).
Homograft calcification.
Pulmonary Valve
Congenital pulmonary valve stenosis.
Rheumatic pulmonary valve disease (rare).
Fallot's tetralogy (usually after repair).
Pulmonary hypertension.
Homograft calcification.
Tricuspid Valve
Rheumatic tricuspid valve disease.
Old vegetation (may only be visible on ultrafast CT).

CALCIUM STONES

| ICD-10CM # | N20.9 | Urinary Calculus, Unspecified |

Medications (e.g., antacids, loop diuretics, vitamin D, acetazolamide, glucocorticoids).
Primary hyperparathyroidism.
Hypercalcemia from malignancy.
Sarcoidosis.
Prolonged immobilization.
Hyperoxaluria (e.g., Crohn's disease, celiac disease, chronic pancreatitis).
Hyperuricosuria (e.g., hyperuricemia, excessive dietary purine, allopurinol, probenecid).
Renal tubular acidosis.
Milk-alkali syndrome.

Thyrotoxicosis.
Hypocitraturia (e.g., metabolic acidosis, hypo-magnesemia, hypokalemia).

CARDIAC ARREST, NONTRAUMATIC[50]

ICD-10CM #	I46.9	Cardiac Arrest, Cause Unspecified

Cardiac (coronary artery disease, cardiomyopathies, structural abnormalities, valve dysfunction, arrhythmias).
Respiratory (upper airway obstruction, hypoventilation, pulmonary embolism, asthma, COPD exacerbation, pulmonary edema).
Circulatory (tension pneumothorax, pericardial tamponade, PE, hemorrhage, sepsis).
Electrolyte abnormalities (hypokalemia or hyperkalemia, hypomagnesemia or hypermagnesemia, hypocalcemia).
Medications (tricyclic antidepressants, digoxin, theophylline, calcium channel blockers).
Drug abuse (cocaine, heroin, amphetamines).
Toxins (carbon monoxide, cyanide).
Environmental (drowning/near-drowning, electrocution, lightning, hypothermia or hyperthermia, venomous snakes).

CARDIAC DEATH, SUDDEN[3]

ICD-10CM #	Z86.74	Personal History of Sudden Cardiac Arrest

Ventricular tachycardia.
Bradyarrhythmia, sick sinus syndrome.
Aortic stenosis.
Tetralogy of Fallot.
Pericardial tamponade.
Cardiac tumors.
Complications of infective endocarditis.
Hypertrophic cardiomyopathy (arrhythmia or obstruction).
Myocardial ischemia.
Atherosclerosis.
Prinzmetal's angina.
Kawasaki's arteritis.

CARDIAC ENLARGEMENT[30]

ICD-10CM #	I51.7	Cardiomegaly
	Q23.8	Other Congenital Malformations of Aortic and Mitral Valves
	Q24.8	Other Specified Congenital Malformations of Heart
	I11.9	Hypertensive Heart Disease Without Heart Failure

CHAMBER ENLARGEMENT

Chronic Volume Overload
• Mitral or aortic regurgitation.
• Left-to-right shunt (PDA, VSD, AV fistula).

Cardiomyopathy
Ischemic.
Nonischemic.

Decompensated Pressure Overload
• Aortic stenosis.
• Hypertension.

High-Output States
Severe anemia.
Thyrotoxicosis.

Bradycardia
Severe sinus bradycardia.
Complete heart block.

LEFT ATRIUM

LV failure of any cause.
Mitral valve disease.
Myxoma.

RIGHT VENTRICLE

• Chronic volume overload.
• Tricuspid or pulmonic regurgitation.
• Left-to-right shunt (ASD).
• Decompensated pressure overload:
  ○ Pulmonic stenosis.
  ○ Pulmonary artery hypertension:
    ○ Primary.
    ○ Secondary (PE, COPD).
    ○ Pulmonary venoocclusive disease.

RIGHT ATRIUM

RV failure of any cause.
Tricuspid valve disease.
Myxoma.
Ebstein's anomaly.

MULTICHAMBER ENLARGEMENT

Hypertrophic cardiomyopathy.
Acromegaly.
Severe obesity.

PERICARDIAL DISEASE

Pericardial effusion with or without tamponade.
Effusive constrictive disease.
Pericardial cyst, loculated effusion.

PSEUDOCARDIOMEGALY

Epicardial fat.
Chest wall deformity (pectus excavatum, straight back syndrome).
Low lung volumes.
AP chest x-ray.
Mediastinal tumor, cyst.

CARDIAC MURMURS

ICD-10CM #	R01.0	Benign and Innocent Cardiac Murmurs
	R01.1	Cardiac murmur, unspecified

SYSTOLIC

Mitral regurgitation (MR).
Tricuspid regurgitation (TR).
Ventricular septal defect (VSD).

Aortic stenosis (AS).
Idiopathic hypertrophic subaortic stenosis (IHSS).
Pulmonic stenosis (PS).
Innocent murmur of childhood.
Coarctation of aorta.
Mitral valve prolapse (MVP).

DIASTOLIC

Aortic regurgitation (AR).
Atrial myxoma.
Mitral stenosis (MS).
Pulmonary artery branch stenosis.
Tricuspid stenosis (TS).
Graham Steell murmur (diastolic decrescendo murmur heard in severe pulmonary hypertension).
Pulmonic regurgitation (PR).
Severe mitral regurgitation (MR).
Austin Flint murmur (diastolic rumble heard in severe AR).
Severe VSD and patent ductus arteriosus.

CONTINUOUS

Patent ductus arteriosus.
Pulmonary AV fistula.

CARDIAC TUMORS[31]

ICD-10CM #	C38.0	Malignant Neoplasm of Heart
	D15.1	Benign neoplasm of heart

PRIMARY

Benign.
  Myxoma.
  Lipoma.
  Fibroma.
  Rhabdomyoma.
  Fibroelastoma.
Malignant.
  Sarcoma.
  Mesothelioma.
  Lymphoma.

SECONDARY

Direct Extension
Lung cancer.
Breast cancer.
Mediastinal tumors.

Metastatic Tumors
Malignant melanoma.
Leukemia.
Lymphoma.

Venous Extension
Renal cell cancer.
Adrenal cancer.
Liver cancer.

CARDIOEMBOLISM

ICD-10CM #	I21.3 ST	Elevation (STEMI) Myocardial Infarction of Unspecified Site
	I21.9	Acute myocardial infarction, unspecified

Differential Diagnosis

II

Acute MI.
Atrial fibrillation.
Left ventricular aneurysm.
Valvular heart disease (e.g., rheumatic mitral valve disease, mitral valve prolapse).
Dilated cardiomyopathy.
Atrial septal defect.
Patent foramen ovale.
Cardioversion for atrial fibrillation.
Infective endocarditis.
Atrial septal aneurysm.
Sick sinus syndrome and cardiac arrhythmias.
Nonbacterial thrombotic endocarditis.
Prosthetic heart valves.
Atrial myxoma and other intracardiac tumors.
Cyanotic heart disease.
Balloon angioplasty.
Coronary artery bypass grafting.
Aneurysms of sinus of Valsalva.
Other: VVI pacing, ventricular support devices, heart transplantation, intracardiac defects with paradoxical embolism.

CARDIOGENIC SHOCK

ICD-10CM #	R57.0	Cardiogenic Shock

Myocardial infarction.
Arrhythmias.
Pericardial effusion/tamponade.
Chest trauma.
Valvular heart disease.
Myocarditis.
Cardiomyopathy.
CHF, end-stage.

CATARACTS, PEDIATRIC AGE

ICD-10CM #	H26.0	Infantile, juvenile and presenile cataracts

DEVELOPMENTAL VARIANTS

Prematurity (Y-suture vacuoles) with or without retinopathy of prematurity.

GENETIC DISORDERS

Simple Mendelian Inheritance
Autosomal dominant (most common).
Autosomal recessive.
X-linked.
Major Chromosomal Defects
Trisomy disorders (13, 18, 21).
Turner syndrome (45X).
Deletion syndromes (11p13, 18p, 18q).
Duplication syndromes (3q, 20p, 10q).
Multisystem Genetic Disorders
Alport syndrome (hearing loss, renal disease).
Alström syndrome (nerve deafness, diabetes mellitus).
Apert disease (craniosynostosis, syndactyly).
Cockayne syndrome (premature senility, skin photosensitivity).
Conradi disease (chondrodysplasia punctata).
Crouzon disease (dysostosis craniofacialis).
Hallermann-Streiff syndrome (microphthalmia, small pinched nose, skin atrophy, hypotrichosis).
Hypohidrotic ectodermal dysplasia (anomalous dentition, hypohidrosis, hypotrichosis).

Ichthyosis (keratinizing disorder with thick, scaly skin).
Incontinentia pigmenti (dental anomalies, mental retardation, cutaneous lesions).
Lowe syndrome (oculocerebrorenal syndrome: hypotonia, renal disease).
Marfan syndrome.
Marinesco-Sjögren syndrome (cerebellar ataxia, hypotonia).
Meckel-Gruber syndrome (renal dysplasia, encephalocele).
Myotonic dystrophy.
Nail-patella syndrome (renal dysfunction, dysplastic nails, hypoplastic patella).
Nevoid basal cell carcinoma syndrome (autosomal dominant, basal cell carcinoma erupts in childhood).
Peters anomaly (corneal opacifications with iris-corneal dysgenesis).
Reiger syndrome (iris dysplasia, myotonic dystrophy).
Rothmund-Thomson syndrome (poikiloderma: skin atrophy).
Rubinstein-Taybi syndrome (broad great toe, mental retardation).
Smith-Lemli-Opitz syndrome (toe syndactyly, hypospadias, mental retardation).
Sotos syndrome (cerebral gigantism).
Spondyloepiphyseal dysplasia (dwarfism, short trunk).
Werner syndrome (premature aging in 2nd decade of life).
Inborn Errors of Metabolism
Abetalipoproteinemia (absent chylomicrons, retinal degeneration).
Fabry disease (α-galactosidase A deficiency).
Galactokinase deficiency.
Galactosemia (galactose-1-phosphate uridyl transferase deficiency).
Homocystinemia (subluxation of lens, mental retardation).
Mannosidosis (acid α-mannosidase deficiency).
Niemann-Pick disease (sphingomyelinase deficiency).
Refsum disease (phytanic acid α-hydrolase deficiency).
Wilson disease (accumulation of copper leads to cirrhosis and neurologic symptoms).

ENDOCRINOPATHIES

Hypocalcemia (hypoparathyroidism).
Hypoglycemia.
Diabetes mellitus.

CONGENITAL INFECTIONS

Toxoplasmosis.
Cytomegalovirus infection.
Syphilis.
Rubella.
Perinatal herpes simplex infection.
Measles (rubeola).
Poliomyelitis.
Influenza.
Varicella-zoster.

OCULAR ANOMALIES

Microphthalmia.
Coloboma.
Aniridia.

Mesodermal dysgenesis.
Persistent papillary membrane.
Posterior lenticonus.
Persistent hyperplastic primary vitreous.
Primitive hyaloid vascular system.

MISCELLANEOUS DISORDERS

Atopic dermatitis.
Drugs (corticosteroids).
Radiation.
Trauma.
IDIOPATHIC

CAVITARY LESION ON CHEST X-RAY[32]

ICD-10CM #	R91.8	Other Nonspecific Abnormal Finding of Lung Field

NECROTIZING INFECTIONS

Bacteria: anaerobes, *Staphylococcus aureus*, enteric gram-negative bacteria, *Pseudomonas aeruginosa*, Legionella species, *Haemophilus influenzae*, *Streptococcus pyogenes*, *Streptococcus pneumoniae*, *Rhodococcus*, *Actinomyces*.
Mycobacteria: *Mycobacterium tuberculosis*, *Mycobacterium kansasii*, MAI.
Bacteria-like: *Nocardia* species.
Fungi: *Coccidioides immitis*, *Histoplasma capsulatum*, *Blastomyces hominis*, *Aspergillus* species, *Mucor* species.
Parasitic: *Entamoeba histolytica*, *Echinococcus*, *Paragonimus westermani*.

CAVITARY INFARCTION

Bland infarction (with or without superimposed infection).
Lung contusion.

SEPTIC EMBOLISM

S. aureus, anaerobes, others.

VASCULITIS

Wegener's granulomatosis, periarteritis.

NEOPLASMS

Bronchogenic carcinoma, metastatic carcinoma, lymphoma.

MISCELLANEOUS LESIONS

- Cysts, blebs, bullae, or pneumatocele with or without fluid collections.
- Sequestration.
- Empyema with air-fluid level.
- Bronchiectasis.

CEREBRAL INFARCTION SECONDARY TO INHERITED DISORDERS

ICD-10CM #	I63.50	Cerebral Infarction Due to Unspecified Occlusion or Stenosis of Unspecified Cerebral Artery

Homocystinuria.
Marfan's syndrome.
Ehlers-Danlos syndrome.
Rendu-Osler-Weber syndrome.
Pseudoxanthoma elasticum.
Fabry's disease.

CEREBRAL VASCULITIS, CAUSES[26]

ICD-10CM #	varies with specific diagnosis

PRIMARY CEREBRAL VASCULITIDES

Takayasu arteritis.
Primary cerebral vasculitis.
Polyarteritis nodosa.

SECONDARY VASCULITIDES

Immune Disorders
Systemic lupus erythematosus.
Wegner granulomatosis.
Kawasaki syndrome.
Sarcoidosis.
Henoch-Schönlein purpura.
Primary Intracranial Infections
Bacterial meningitis (especially *Diplococcus pneumoniae*).
Tuberculous meningitis.
Mycotic infections.
Cat-scratch disease.
Human immunodeficiency virus/acquired immunodeficiency syndrome.
Malaria.
Lyme disease.
Rickettsial infections.
Brucellosis.

CEREBROVASCULAR DISEASE, ISCHEMIC[78]

ICD-10CM #	I67.9	Cerebrovascular Disease, Unspecified

VASCULAR DISORDERS

Large-vessel atherothrombotic disease.
Lacunar disease.
Arterial-to-arterial embolization.
Carotid or vertebral artery dissection.
Fibromuscular dysplasia.
Migraine.
Venous thrombosis.
Radiation.
Complications of arteriography.
Multiple, progressive intracranial arterial occlusions.

INFLAMMATORY DISORDERS

Giant cell arteritis.
Polyarteritis nodosa.
SLE.
Granulomatous angiitis.
Takayasu's disease.
Arteritis associated with amphetamine, cocaine, or phenylpropanolamine.
Syphilis, mucormycosis.
Sjögren's syndrome.
Behçet's syndrome.

CARDIAC DISORDERS

Rheumatic heart disease.
Mural thrombus.
Arrhythmias.
Mitral valve prolapse.
Prosthetic heart valve.
Endocarditis.
Myxoma.
Paradoxical embolus.

HEMATOLOGIC DISORDERS

Thrombotic thrombocytopenic purpura.
Sickle cell disease.
Hypercoagulable states.
Polycythemia.
Thrombocytosis.
Leukocytosis.
Lupus anticoagulant.

CERVICAL INSTABILITY, PEDIATRIC

ICD-10CM #	M50	Cervical disc disorders

CONGENITAL

Vertebral (Bony Anomalies)
Craniooccipital defects (occipital vertebrae, basilar impression, occipital dysplasias, condylar hypoplasia, occipitalized atlas).
Atlantoaxial defects (aplasia of atlas arch, aplasia of odontoid process).
Subaxial anomalies (failure of segmentation and/or fusion, spina bifida, spondylolisthesis).
Ligamentous or Combined Anomalies
Found at birth as an element of somatogenic aberration.
Syndromic Disorders
Down syndrome.
Klippel-Feil syndrome.
22q11.2 deletion syndrome.
Larsen syndrome.
Marfan syndrome.
Ehlers-Danlos syndrome.

ACQUIRED

Trauma.
Infection (pyogenic, granulomatous).
Tumor (including neurofibromatosis).
Inflammatory conditions (e.g., juvenile rheumatoid arthritis).
Osteochondrodysplasias (e.g., achondroplasia, diastrophic dysplasia, metatropic dysplasia, spondyloepiphyseal dysplasia).
Storage disorders (e.g., mucopolysaccharidoses).
Metabolic disorders (rickets).
Miscellaneous (including osteogenesis imperfecta, sequela of surgery).

CHEST PAIN, CHILDREN[8]

ICD-10CM #	R07.9	Chest Pain, Unspecified
	R07.82	Intercostal Pain
	R07.89	Other Chest Pain
	R07.1	Chest Pain on Breathing
	R07.81	Pleurodynia

MUSCULOSKELETAL (COMMON)

Trauma (accidental, abuse).
Exercise, overuse injury (strain, bursitis).
Costochondritis (Tietze's syndrome).
Herpes zoster (cutaneous).
Pleurodynia.
Fibrositis.
Slipping rib.
Sickle cell anemia vasoocclusive crisis.
Osteomyelitis (rare).
Primary or metastatic tumor (rare).

PULMONARY (COMMON)

Pneumonia.
Pleurisy.
Asthma.
Chronic cough.
Pneumothorax.
Infarction (sickle cell anemia).
Foreign body.
Embolism (rare).
Pulmonary hypertension (rare).
Tumor (rare).

GASTROINTESTINAL (LESS COMMON)

Esophagitis (gastroesophageal reflux).
Esophageal foreign body.
Esophageal spasm.
Cholecystitis.
Subdiaphragmatic abscess.
Perihepatitis (Fitz-Hugh-Curtis syndrome).
Peptic ulcer disease.

CARDIAC (LESS COMMON)

Pericarditis.
Postpericardiotomy syndrome.
Endocarditis.
Mitral valve prolapse.
Aortic or subaortic stenosis.
Arrhythmias.
Marfan's syndrome (dissecting aortic aneurysm).
Anomalous coronary artery.
Kawasaki disease.
Cocaine, sympathomimetic ingestion.
Angina (familial hypercholesterolemia).

IDIOPATHIC (COMMON)

Anxiety, hyperventilation.
Panic disorder.

OTHER (LESS COMMON)

Spinal cord or nerve root compression.
Breast-related pathologic condition.
Castleman's disease (lymph node neoplasm).

CHEST PAIN, NONPLEURITIC[18]

ICD-10CM #	R07.9	Chest Pain, Unspecified
	R07.82	Intercostal Pain
	R07.89	Other Chest Pain

Cardiac: myocardial ischemia/infarction, myocarditis.
Esophageal: spasm, esophagitis, ulceration, neoplasm, achalasia, diverticula, foreign body.

Referred pain from subdiaphragmatic GI structures.

Gastric and duodenal: hiatal hernia, neoplasm, PUD.

Gallbladder and biliary: cholecystitis, cholelithiasis, impacted stone, neoplasm.

Pancreatic: pancreatitis, neoplasm.

Dissecting aortic aneurysm.

Pain originating from skin, breasts, and musculoskeletal structures: herpes zoster, mastitis, cervical spondylosis.

Mediastinal tumors: lymphoma, thymoma.

Pulmonary: neoplasm, pneumonia, pulmonary embolism/infarction.

Psychoneurosis.

Chest pain associated with mitral valve prolapse.

CHEST PAIN, PLEURITIC

| ICD-10CM # | R07.1 | Chest Pain on Breathing |
| | R07.81 | Pleurodynia |

Cardiac: pericarditis, postpericardiotomy/Dressler's syndrome.

Pulmonary: pneumothorax, hemothorax, embolism/infarction, pneumonia, empyema, neoplasm, bronchiectasis, pneumomediastinum, TB, carcinomatous effusion.

GI: liver abscess, pancreatitis, esophageal rupture, Whipple's disease with associated pericarditis or pleuritis.

Subdiaphragmatic abscess.

Pain originating from skin and musculoskeletal tissues: costochondritis, chest wall trauma, fractured rib, interstitial fibrositis, myositis, strain of pectoralis muscle, herpes zoster, soft tissue and bone tumors.

Collagen vascular diseases with pleuritis.

Psychoneurosis.

Familial Mediterranean fever.

CHEST WALL TUMORS, PRIMARY[14]

| ICD-10CM # | varies with specific diagnosis |

SOFT TISSUE
Benign
Lipoma.
Hemangioma.
Lymphangioma.
Fibroma.
Rhabdomyoma.
Neurofibroma.
Desmoid tumor.
Malignant
Malignant fibrous histiocytoma.
Rhabdosarcoma.
Liposarcoma.
Neurofibrosarcoma.
Leiomyosarcoma.

BONY AND CARTILAGINOUS
Benign
Fibrous dysplasia.
Osteochondroma.

Chondroma.
Askin tumor.
Plasmacytoma.
Malignant
Chondrosarcoma.
Osteogenic sarcoma.
Ewing sarcoma.

CHIASMAL DISEASE[11]

| ICD-10CM # | varies with specific diagnosis |

CAUSES OF CHIASMAL DISEASE
Tumors
Pituitary adenomas.
Craniopharyngioma.
Meningioma.
Glioma.
Chordoma.
Dysgerminoma.
Nasopharyngeal tumors.
Metastases.
Non-neoplastic masses
Aneurysm.
Rathke pouch cysts.
Fibrous dysplasia.
Sphenoidal sinus mucocele.
Arachnoid cysts.
Miscellaneous
Demyelination.
Inflammation (e.g., sarcoidosis).
Trauma.
Radiation-induced necrosis.
Toxicity (e.g., ethambutol).
Vasculitis.

CHILDHOOD EOSINOPHILIA

| ICD-10CM # | D72.1 | Eosinophilia |

PHYSIOLOGIC
Prematurity.
Infants receiving hyperalimentation.
Familial.

INFECTIOUS
Parasitic (with tissue-invasive helminths, e.g., trichinosis, strongyloidiasis, pneumocystosis, filariasis, cysticercosis, cutaneous and visceral larva migrans, echinococcosis).
Bacterial (brucellosis, tularemia, cat-scratch disease, *Chlamydia*).
Fungal (histoplasmosis, blastomycosis, coccidioidomycosis, allergic bronchopulmonary aspergillosis).
Mycobacterial (tuberculosis, leprosy).
Viral (hepatitis A, hepatitis B, hepatitis C, Epstein-Barr virus).

PULMONARY
Allergic (rhinitis, asthma).
Loeffler syndrome.
Hypersensitivity pneumonitis.
Eosinophilic pneumonia.
Pulmonary interstitial eosinophilia.

DERMATOLOGIC
Atopic dermatitis.
Pemphigus.
Dermatitis herpetiformis.
Infantile eosinophilic pustular folliculitis.
Episodic angioedema and urticaria.
Eosinophilic fasciitis (Schulman syndrome).
Eosinophilic cellulitis (Wells syndrome).
Kimura disease.

ONCOLOGIC
Neoplasm (lung, gastrointestinal, uterine).
Hodgkin disease.
Leukemia.
Myelofibrosis.

IMMUNOLOGIC
T-cell immunodeficiencies.
Hyperimmunoglobulin E (Job) syndrome.
Wiskott-Aldrich syndrome.
Graft-versus-host disease.
Drug hypersensitivity.
Post-irradiation.
Post-splenectomy.

ENDOCRINE
Post-adrenalectomy.
Addison disease.
Panhypopituitarism.

CARDIOVASCULAR
Loeffler disease (fibroplastic endocarditis).
Congenital heart disease.
Hypersensitivity vasculitis.

GASTROINTESTINAL
Milk protein allergy.
Inflammatory bowel disease.
Eosinophilic esophagitis.
Eosinophilic gastroenteritis.

CHOLANGITIS, ACUTE[14]

| ICD-10CM # | K83.0 | Cholangitis |

NONIATROGENIC
Benign Conditions
Choledocholithiasis.
 Primary.
 Secondary.
Pancreatitis (chronic/acute), including pancreatic pseudocyst.
Papillary stenosis.
Mirizzi syndrome.
Choledochal cysts (type V, Caroli disease).
Primary sclerosing cholangitis.
Malignancies
Pancreatic cancer.
Cholangiocarcinoma.
Porta hepatis tumor/metastasis.

IATROGENIC
Obstructed biliary endoprosthesis.
Iatrogenic biliary stricture.
Direct surgical trauma.
Ischemia-induced stricture.
Anastomotic stricture (biliobiliary/bilioenteric anastomosis).

CHOLESTASIS[29]

ICD-10CM #	K80.65	Calculus of Gallbladder and Bile Duct with Chronic Cholecystitis with Obstruction

EXTRAHEPATIC

- Choledocholithiasis.
- Bile duct stricture.
- Cholangiocarcinoma.
- Pancreatic carcinoma.
- Chronic pancreatitis.
- Papillary stenosis.
- Ampullary cancer.
- Primary sclerosing cholangitis.
- Choledochal cysts.
- Parasites (e.g., ascaris, clonorchis).
- AIDS.
- Cholangiography.
- Biliary atresia.
- Portal lymphadenopathy.
- Mirizzi's syndrome.

INTRAHEPATIC

- Viral hepatitis.
- Alcoholic hepatitis.
- Drug induced.
- Ductopenia syndromes.
- Primary biliary cirrhosis.
- Benign recurrent intrahepatic cholestasis.
- Byler's disease.
- Primary sclerosing cholangitis.
- Alagille's syndrome.
- Sarcoid.
- Lymphoma.
- Postoperative.
- Total parenteral nutrition.
- α-1-antitrypsin deficiency.

CHOLESTASIS, NEONATAL AND INFANTILE, DIFFERENTIAL DIAGNOSIS[46]

ICD-10CM #	O26.6	Liver disorders in pregnancy, childbirth and the puerperium

INFECTIOUS

- Generalized bacterial sepsis.
- Viral hepatitis.
  Hepatitis A, B, C, D.
  Cytomegalovirus.
  Rubella virus.
  Herpesvirus: herpes simplex, human herpesvirus 6 and 7.
  Varicella virus.
  Coxsackievirus.
  Echovirus.
  Reovirus type 3.
  Parvovirus B19.
  HIV.
  Adenovirus.
- Others.
  Toxoplasmosis.
  Syphilis.

Tuberculosis.
Listeriosis.
Urinary tract infection.

TOXIC

Sepsis.
Parenteral nutrition related.
Drug related.

METABOLIC

Disorders of amino acid metabolism.
  Tyrosinemia.
Disorders of lipid metabolism.
  Wolman disease.
  Niemann-Pick disease (type C).
  Gaucher disease.
Cholesterol ester storage disease.
Disorders of carbohydrate metabolism.
  Galactosemia.
  Fructosemia.
  Glycogenosis IV.
Disorders of bile acid biosynthesis.
Other metabolic defects.
  α1-Antitrypsin deficiency.
  Cystic fibrosis.
  Hypopituitarism.
  Hypothyroidism.
  Zellweger (cerebrohepatorenal) syndrome.
  Neonatal iron storage disease.
  Indian childhood cirrhosis/infantile copper overload.
  Congenital disorders of glycosylation.
  Mitochondrial hepatopathies.
  Citrin deficiency.

GENETIC OR CHROMOSOMAL

Trisomy 17, 18, 21.
Donahue syndrome.

INTRAHEPATIC CHOLESTASIS SYNDROMES

"Idiopathic" neonatal hepatitis.
Alagille syndrome (arteriohepatic dysplasia).
Nonsyndromic bile duct paucity syndrome.
Intrahepatic cholestasis (PFIC):
  FIC-1 deficiency.
  BSEP deficiency.
  MDR3 deficiency.
Familial benign recurrent cholestasis associated with lymphedema (Aagenaes).
Congenital hepatic fibrosis.
Caroli disease (cystic dilatation of intrahepatic ducts).

EXTRAHEPATIC DISEASES

Biliary atresia.
Sclerosing cholangitis.
Bile duct stricture/stenosis.
Choledochal-pancreaticoductal junction anomaly.
Spontaneous perforation of the bile duct.
Choledochal cyst.
Mass (neoplasia, stone).
Bile/mucous plug ("inspissated bile").

MISCELLANEOUS

Shock and hypoperfusion.
Associated with enteritis.
Associated with intestinal obstruction.

Neonatal lupus erythematosus.
Myeloproliferative disease (trisomy 21).
Hemophagocytic lymphohistiocytosis.
Arthrogryposis cholestatic pigmentary syndrome.

CHOLESTATIC LIVER ENZYME ELEVATION, EXTRAHEPATIC CAUSES[23]

ICD-10CM #	Varies with Specific Diagnosis

EXTRAHEPATIC CAUSES OF CHOLESTATIC LIVER ENZYMES IN ADULTS

Intrinsic
Choledocholithiasis
Immune-Mediated Duct Injury
  Autoimmune pancreatitis
  PSC
Malignancy
  Ampullary cancer
  Cholangiocarcinoma
Infections
  AIDS cholangiopathy
    Cytomegalovirus
    Cryptosporidiosis
    Microsporidiosis
  Parasitic infections
    Ascariasis
Extrinsic
Malignancy
  Gallbladder cancer
  Metastases, including portal adenopathy from metastases
  Pancreatic cancer
Mirizzi's Syndrome
Pancreatitis
Pancreatic Pseudocyst

CHOLESTATIC LIVER ENZYME ELEVATION, INTRAHEPATIC CAUSES[23]

ICD-10CM #	Varies with Specific Causes

INTRAHEPATIC CAUSES OF CHOLESTATIC LIVER ENZYME ELEVATIONS IN ADULTS

Drugs[11]
Bland cholestasis
  Anabolic steroids
  Estrogens
Cholestatic hepatitis
  Angiotensin-converting enzyme inhibitors: captopril, enalapril
  Antimicrobials: amoxicillin-clavulanic acid, ketoconazole
  Azathioprine
  Chlorpromazine
  NSAIDs: sulindac, piroxicam
Granulomatous hepatitis
  Allopurinol

---

[11]Categorized by histologic pattern. Drug lists are not meant to be comprehensive.

Antibiotics: sulfonamides
Antiepileptics: carbamazepine, phenytoin
Cardiovascular agents: hydralazine, procainamide, quinidine
Phenylbutazone
Vanishing bile duct syndrome
Amoxicillin-clavulanic acid
Chlorpromazine
Dicloxacillin
Flucloxacillin
Macrolides
PBC
PSC
Granulomatous Liver Disease.
Infections
Brucellosis
Fungal: histoplasmosis, coccidioidomycosis
Leprosy
Q fever
Schistosomiasis
TB, *Mycobacterium avium* complex, bacillus Calmette-Guérin
Sarcoidosis
Idiopathic granulomatous hepatitis
Other
Crohn's disease
Heavy metal exposure: beryllium, copper
Hodgkin's disease
Viral Hepatitis
HAV and HEV
HBV and HCV, including fibrosing cholestatic hepatitis
EBV
Cytomegalovirus
Idiopathic Adulthood Ductopenia
Genetic Conditions
Progressive familial intrahepatic cholestasis
Type 1 (formerly Byler's disease)
Type 2
Type 3
Benign recurrent intrahepatic cholestasis
Type 1
Type 2
CF
Malignancy
Hepatocellular carcinoma
Metastatic disease
Paraneoplastic syndrome
Non-Hodgkin's lymphoma
Prostate cancer
Renal cell cancer
Infiltrative Liver Disease
Amyloidosis
Lymphoma
Intrahepatic Cholestasis of Pregnancy
TPN
Graft-versus-Host Disease
Sepsis

CHOREA

ICD-10CM #   G25.4   Drug-Induced Chorea
              G25.5   Other Chorea

Medications (e.g., neuroleptics, tricyclics, antiparkinsonian drugs).
Cerebral palsy.
Huntington's disease.
Benign hereditary chorea.

Thyroid disorder (hyperthyroidism, hypothyroidism).
Friedreich's ataxia.
Ataxia-telangiectasia.
Hypoglycemia, hyperglycemia.
Electrolyte abnormalities (hyponatremia, hypocalcemia, hypomagnesemia, hypernatremia).
Vitamin B_{12} deficiency.
SLE.
Wilson's disease.
Alcohol.
Cocaine.
Carbon monoxide poisoning.
Mercury poisoning.

CHOREOATHETOSIS[55]

ICD-10CM #   G25.5   Choreoathetosis

SYSTEMIC DISEASES

SLE.
Polycythemia.
Thyrotoxicosis.
Rheumatic fever.
Cirrhosis of the liver (acquired hepatocerebral degeneration).
DM.
Wilson's disease.

PRIMARY DEGENERATIVE BRAIN DISEASES

Huntington's chorea.
Olivopontocerebellar atrophies.
Neuroacanthocytosis.

FOCAL BRAIN DISEASES

Hemichorea.
Stroke.
Tumor.
Arteriovenous malformation.

DRUG-INDUCED CHOREOATHETOSIS

Parkinson's Disease Drugs
Levodopa.

EPILEPSY DRUGS

Phenytoin.
Carbamazepine.
Phenobarbital.
Gabapentin.
Valproate.
Psychostimulant Drugs
Cocaine.
Amphetamine.
Methamphetamine.
Dextroamphetamine.
Methylphenidate.
Pemoline.
Psychotropic Drugs
Lithium.
Tricyclic antidepressant drugs.
Oral Contraceptive Drugs
Cimetidine

CHYLOTHORAX

ICD-10CM #   I89.8   Other Specified Noninfective Disorders of Lymphatic Vessels and Lymph Nodes

Post-lymph node dissection of neck or chest.
Subclavian venous catheterization.
Thoracic aneurysm repair.
Trauma to chest and neck.
Mediastinal tumor resection.
Esophagectomy, pneumonectomy.
Lymphangitis, mediastinitis.
Neoplasms (lymphoma, carcinoma of esophagus, lung, mediastinal malignancies).
Sympathectomy.
Venous thrombosis.
Congenital.

CLOUDY URINE

ICD-10CM #   R82   Other abnormal findings in urine

Concentrated urine.
Use of multivitamin supplements.
Diet high in purine-rich foods.
Pyuria.
Phosphaturia.
Urinary tract infection.
Lipiduria.
Chyluria.
Hyperoxaluria.

CLUBBING

ICD-10CM #   R68.3   Clubbing of Fingers

Pulmonary neoplasm (lung, pleura).
Other neoplasm (GI, liver, Hodgkin's, thymus, osteogenic sarcoma).
Pulmonary infectious process (empyema, abscess, bronchiectasis, TB, chronic pneumonitis).
Extrapulmonary infectious process (subacute bacterial endocarditis, intestinal TB, bacterial or amebic dysentery, arterial graft sepsis).
Pneumoconiosis.
Cystic fibrosis.
Sarcoidosis.
Cyanotic congenital heart disease.
Endocrine (Graves' disease, hyperparathyroidism).
Inflammatory bowel disease.
Celiac disease.
Chronic liver disease, cirrhosis (particularly biliary and juvenile).
Pulmonary AV malformations.
Idiopathic.
Thyroid acropachy.
Hereditary (pachydermoperiostosis).
Chronic trauma (jackhammer operators, machine workers).

COBALAMIN DEFICIENCY[40]

ICD-10CM #   E53.8   Deficiency of Other Specified B Group Vitamins

ETIOPATHOPHYSIOLOGIC CLASSIFICATION OF COBALAMIN DEFICIENCY

Nutritional cobalamin deficiency (i.e., insufficient cobalamin intake):

Vegetarians, poverty-imposed near-vegetarians, breastfed infants of mothers with pernicious anemia.

Abnormal intragastric events (i.e., inadequate proteolysis of food cobalamin):

Atrophic gastritis, partial gastritis with hypochlorhydria, proton-pump inhibitors, H_2 blockers.

Loss or atrophy of gastric oxyntic mucosa (i.e., deficient intrinsic factor [IF] molecules):

Total or partial gastrectomy, pernicious anemia, caustic destruction (lye).

Abnormal events in small bowel lumen:

Inadequate pancreatic protease (e.g., R-cobalamin not degraded, cobalamin not transferred to IF):

- Insufficient pancreatic protease (i.e., pancreatic insufficiency).
- Inactivation of pancreatic protease (i.e., Zollinger–Ellison syndrome).

Usurping of luminal cobalamin (i.e., inadequate cobalamin binding to IF):

By bacteria, during stasis syndromes (e.g., blind loops, pouches of diverticulosis, strictures, fistulas, anastomosis), impaired bowel motility (e.g., scleroderma), hypogammaglobulinemia.

By *Diphyllobothrium latum* (fish tapeworm).

Disorders of ileal mucosa/IF–cobalamin receptors (i.e., IF–cobalamin not bound to IF–cobalamin receptors):

- ○ Diminished or absent IF–cobalamin receptors (e.g., ileal bypass, resection, fistula).
- ○ Abnormal mucosal architecture/function (e.g., tropical or nontropical sprue, Crohn's disease, tuberculosis ileitis, infiltration by lymphomas, amyloidosis).
- ○ IF-/post-IF–cobalamin receptor defects (e.g., Imerslund–Gräsbeck syndrome, transcobalamin II [TC II] deficiency).
- ○ Drug effects (e.g., slow K, metformin, cholestyramine, colchicine, neomycin).
- Disorders of plasma cobalamin transport (i.e., TC II–cobalamin not delivered to TC II receptors):
  - ○ Congenital TC II deficiency, defective binding of TC II–cobalamin to TC II receptors (rare).
- Metabolic disorders (i.e., cobalamin not used by cells):

Inborn enzyme errors (rare).

Acquired disorders (e.g., cobalamin functionally inactivated by irreversible oxidation, N_2O inhalation).

COLIC, ACUTE ABDOMINAL[72]

ICD-10CM # R10.0 Acute Abdomen

Acute gastroenteritis.
Food poisoning.
Nonspecific causes.
Constipation.
Gastric outlet obstruction:
Chronic peptic ulceration.
Gastric cancer.

Small bowel obstruction:
Adhesions:
Postsurgical.
Inflammatory (e.g., diverticular).
Radiation.
Meckel's diverticulum.
Metastatic.
Stricture:
Ischemic.
Radiation.
Inflammatory (e.g., Crohn's disease).
Volvulus intussusception:
Tumor (e.g., Peutz-Jeghers syndrome).
Superior mesenteric artery syndrome.
Intraluminal bolus:
Gallstone.
Bezoar.
Hernia:
Abdominal wall.
Internal.
Neoplasm:
Benign (e.g., leiomyoma).
Malignant (e.g., carcinoid tumor, adenocarcinoma).
Large bowel obstruction:
Colon cancer.
Diverticular disease.
Volvulus.
Uterine:
Missed abortion.
Parturition.
Period pain.

COLON ISCHEMIA[23]

ICD-10CM # Varies with Specific Diagnosis

CAUSES OF COLON ISCHEMIA

Acute pancreatitis
Allergy
Amyloidosis
Heart failure or cardiac arrhythmias
Hematologic disorders and coagulopathies:
Activated protein C resistance
Antithrombin deficiency
Factor V Leiden mutation
Paroxysmal nocturnal hemoglobinuria
Polycythemia vera
Protein C and S deficiencies
Prothrombin G20210A mutation
Sickle cell disease
Infection:
Bacteria (*Escherichia coli* O157:H7)
Parasites (*Angiostrongylus costaricensis*)
Viruses (HBV, HCV, cytomegalovirus)
Inferior mesenteric artery thrombosis
Long-distance running
Medications and toxins:
Alosetron
Cocaine
Danazol
Digitalis compounds
Ergots
Estrogens
Flutamide
Glycerin enema
Gold salts
Immunosuppressive agents

Interferon-α
Methamphetamine
NSAIDs
Penicillin
Phenylephrine
Polyethylene glycol 3350 colon lavage solutions
Pit viper toxin
Progestins
Pseudoephedrine
Psychotropic drugs
Saline laxatives
Sumatriptan
Tegaserod
Vasopressin
Pheochromocytoma
Ruptured ectopic pregnancy
Shock
Strangulated hernia
Surgery/procedures:
Aortic aneurysmectomy
Aortoiliac reconstruction
Barium enema
Colectomy with inferior mesenteric artery ligation
Colon bypass
Colonoscopy
Exchange transfusions
Gynecologic operations
Lumbar aortography
Thromboembolism:
Cholesterol (atheroembolism)
Myxoma (left atrial)
Trauma (blunt or penetrating)
Vasculitis and vasculopathy:
Buerger's disease
Eosinophilic granulomatosis with angiitis
Fibromuscular dysplasia
Kawasaki's disease
Polyarteritis nodosa
Rheumatoid vasculitis
SLE
Takayasu's arteritis
Volvulus

COLOR CHANGES, CUTANEOUS[66]

ICD-10CM # L81.9 Disorder of Pigmentation, Unspecified

BROWN

Generalized: pituitary, adrenal, liver disease, ACTH-producing tumor (e.g., oat cell lung carcinoma).
Localized: nevi, neurofibromatosis.

WHITE

Generalized: albinism.
Localized: vitiligo, Raynaud's syndrome.

RED (ERYTHEMA)

- Generalized: fever, polycythemia, urticaria, viral exanthems.
- Localized: inflammation, infection, Raynaud's syndrome.

YELLOW

- Generalized: liver disease, chronic renal disease, anemia.
- Generalized (except sclera): hypothyroidism, increased intake of vegetables containing carotene.
- Localized: resolving hematoma, infection, peripheral vascular insufficiency.

BLUE

Lips, mouth, nail beds: cardiovascular and pulmonary diseases, Raynaud's.

COMA

ICD-10CM # R40.20 Unspecified Coma

Vascular: hemorrhage, thrombosis, embolism.
CNS infections: meningitis, encephalitis, cerebral abscess.
Cerebral neoplasms with herniation.
Head injury: subdural hematoma, cerebral concussion, cerebral contusion.
Drugs: narcotics, sedatives, hypnotics.
Ingestion or inhalation of toxins: CO, alcohol, lead.
Metabolic disturbances.
Hypoxia.
Acid-base disorders.
Hypoglycemia, hyperglycemia.
Hepatic failure.
Electrolyte disorders.
Uremia.
Hypothyroidism.
Hypothermia, hyperthermia.
Hypotension, malignant hypertension.
Postictal.

COMA, NORMAL COMPUTED TOMOGRAPHY[3]

ICD-10CM # R40.20 Unspecified coma

MENINGEAL DISORDERS

Subarachnoid hemorrhage (uncommon).
Bacterial meningitis.
Encephalitis.
Subdural empyema.

EXOGENOUS TOXINS

Sedative drugs and barbiturates.
Anesthetics and γ-hydroxybutyrate.[12]
Alcohols.
Stimulants:
  ○ Phencyclidines.[13]
  ○ Cocaine and amphetamines.[14]
- Psychotropic drugs:
  ○ Cyclic antidepressants.
  ○ Phenothiazines.
  ○ Lithium.

---

[12]General anesthetic, similar to g-aminobutyric acid; recreational drug and body building aid. Rapid onset, rapid recovery often with myoclonic jerking and confusion. Deep coma (2-3 hr; Glasgow Coma Scale = 3) with maintenance of vital signs.

[13]Coma associated with cholinergic signs: lacrimation, salivation, bronchorrhea, and hyperthermia.

[14]Coma after seizures or status (i.e., a prolonged postictal state).

- Anticonvulsants.
- Opioids.
- Clonidine.[15]
- Penicillins.
- Salicylates.
- Anticholinergics.
- Carbon monoxide, cyanide, and methemoglobinemia.

---

[15]An antihypertensive agent active through the opiate receptor system; frequent overdose when used to treat narcotic withdrawal.

ENDOGENOUS TOXINS/ DEFICIENCIES/DERANGEMENTS

Hypoxia and ischemia.
Hypoglycemia.
Hypercalcemia.
Osmolar:
  Hyperglycemia.
  Hyponatremia.
  Hypernatremia.
Organ system failure:
  Hepatic encephalopathy.
  Uremic encephalopathy.
  Pulmonary insufficiency (carbon dioxide narcosis).

SEIZURES

Prolonged postictal state.
Spike-wave stupor.

HYPOTHERMIA OR HYPERTHERMIA

- Brain stem ischemia.
- Basilar artery stroke.
- Brain stem or cerebellar hemorrhage.
- Conversion or malingering.

COMA, PEDIATRIC POPULATION[61]

ICD-10CM # R40.20 Unspecified coma

ANOXIA

Birth asphyxia.
Carbon monoxide poisoning.
Croup/epiglottitis.
Meconium aspiration.

INFECTION

- Hemolysis.
- Blood loss.
- Hydrops fetalis.
- Infection.
- Meningoencephalitis.
- Sepsis.
- Postimmunization encephalitis.

INCREASED INTRACRANIAL PRESSURE

Anoxia.
Inborn metabolic errors.
Toxic encephalopathy.
Reye's syndrome.
Head trauma/intracranial bleed.
Hydrocephalus.
Posterior fossa tumors.

HYPERTENSIVE ENCEPHALOPATHY

Coarctation of aorta.
Nephritis.
Vasculitis.
Pheochromocytoma.

ISCHEMIA

Hypoplastic left heart.
Shunting lesions.
Aortic stenosis.
Cardiovascular collapse (any cause).

PURPURIC CAUSES

Disseminated intravascular coagulation.
Hemolytic-uremic syndrome.
Leukemia.
Thrombotic purpura.

HYPERCAPNIA

Cystic fibrosis.
Bronchopulmonary dysplasia.
Congenital lung anomalies.

NEOPLASM

Medulloblastoma.
Glioma of brain stem.
Posterior fossa tumors.

DRUGS/TOXINS

Maternal sedation.
Alcohol.
Any drug.
Lead.
Salicylism.
Arsenic.
Pesticides.

ELECTROLYTE ABNORMALITIES

Hypernatremia (diarrhea, dehydration, salt poisoning).
Hyponatremia (SIADH, androgenital syndrome, gastroenteritis).
Hyperkalemia (renal failure, salicylism, androgenitalism).
Hypokalemia (diarrhea, hyperaldosteronism, salicylism, DKA).
Hypocalcemia (vitamin D deficiency, hyperparathyroidism).
Severe acidosis (sepsis, cold injury, salicylism, DKA).

HYPOGLYCEMIA

Birth injury or stress.
Diabetes.
Alcohol.
Salicylism.
Hyperinsulinemia.
Iatrogenic.

POSTSEIZURE

Renal Causes
Nephritis.
Hypoplastic kidneys.
Hepatic Causes
Acute hepatitis.
Fulminant hepatic failure.
Inborn metabolic errors.
Bile duct atresia.

CONGESTIVE HEART FAILURE AND CARDIOMYOPATHY[3]

ICD-10CM #	I50.9	Heart failure, unspecified
	I42.7	Cardiomyopathy due to drug and external agent

CAUSES OF CONGESTIVE HEART FAILURE AND CARDIOMYOPATHY

Coronary Artery Disease
Acute ischemia.
Myocardial infarction.
Ischemic cardiomyopathy with hibernating myocardium.
Idiopathic
Idiopathic dilated cardiomyopathy.
Idiopathic restrictive cardiomyopathy.
Peripartum.
Pressure Overload
Hypertension.
Aortic stenosis.
Volume Overload
Mitral regurgitation.
Aortic insufficiency.
Anemia.
Atrioventricular fistula.
Toxins
Ethanol.
Cocaine.
Doxorubicin (Adriamycin).
Methamphetamine.
Metabolic-Endocrine
Thiamine deficiency.
Diabetes.
Hemochromatosis.
Thyrotoxicosis.
Obesity.
Infiltrative
Amyloidosis.
Inflammatory
Viral myocarditis.
Hereditary
Hypertrophic.
Dilated.

*Genetic bases for these cardiomyopathies have been identified in a large number of individual patients and families. Most of the mutations have been found in cardiac contractile or structural proteins.

CONGESTIVE HEART FAILURE, INFANT[1]

ICD-10CM #	I05.9	Heart failure, unspecified

Critical coarctation of the aorta.
Interrupted aortic arch.
Congenital aortic stenosis.
Hypoplastic left heart syndrome.
Large ventricular septal defect.
Truncus arteriosus.
Unrecognized supraventricular tachycardia.
Cardiac tamponade.
Myocarditis.

CONJUNCTIVAL NEOPLASM

ICD-10CM #	varies with specific diagnosis

MALIGNANT
Squamous cell carcinoma.
Melanoma.
Sebaceous carcinoma.
Kaposi's sarcoma.
Metastatic neoplasms.

BENIGN
Melanocytic nevus.
Squamous papilloma.
Hemangioma.
Lymphangioma.
Myxoma.

CONSCIOUSNESS IMPAIRMENT, ACUTE, IN CRITICALLY ILL PATIENT

ICD-10CM #	F05.9	Delirium, unspecified

GENERAL CAUSES OF ACUTELY IMPAIRED CONSCIOUSNESS IN THE CRITICALLY ILL

Infection
Sepsis encephalopathy.
Central nervous system infection.
Drugs
Narcotics.
Benzodiazepines.
Anticholinergics.
Anticonvulsants.
Tricyclic antidepressants.
Selective serotonin uptake inhibitors.
Phenothiazines.
Steroids.
Immunosuppressants (cyclosporine, FK-506, OKT3).
Anesthetics.
Electrolyte and Acid-Base Disturbances
Hyponatremia.
Hypernatremia.
Hypercalcemia.
Hypermagnesemia.
Severe acidemia and alkalemia.
Organ System Failure
Shock.
Renal failure.
Hepatic failure.
Pancreatitis.
Respiratory failure (hypoxia, hypercapnia).
Endocrine Disorders
Hypoglycemia.
Hyperglycemia.
Hypothyroidism.
Hyperthyroidism.
Pituitary apoplexy.
Drug Withdrawal
Alcohol.
Opiates.
Barbiturates.
Benzodiazepines.
Vascular Causes
Shock.
Hypotension.
Hypertensive encephalopathy.
Central nervous system vasculitis.
Cerebral venous sinus thrombosis.
Central Nervous System Disorders
Hemorrhage.

Stroke.
Brain edema.
Hydrocephalus.
Increased intracranial pressure.
Meningitis.
Ventriculitis.
Brain abscess.
Subdural empyema.
Seizures.
Vasculitis.
Seizures
Convulsive and nonconvulsive status epilepticus.
Miscellaneous
Fat embolism syndrome.
Neuroleptic malignant syndrome.
Thiamine deficiency (Wernicke encephalopathy).
Psychogenic unresponsiveness.

CONSTIPATION

ICD-10CM #	K59.00	Constipation, unspecified

Intestinal obstruction.
Fecal impaction.
Diverticular disease.
GI neoplasm.
Strangulated femoral hernia.
Gallstone ileus.
Tuberculous stricture.
Adhesions.
Ameboma.
Volvulus.
Intussusception.
Inflammatory bowel disease.
Hematoma of bowel wall, secondary to trauma or anticoagulants.
Poor dietary habits: insufficient bulk in diet, inadequate fluid intake.
Change from daily routine: travel, hospital admission, physical inactivity.
Acute abdominal conditions: renal colic, salpingitis, biliary colic, appendicitis, ischemia.
Hypercalcemia or hypokalemia, uremia.
Irritable bowel syndrome, pregnancy, anorexia nervosa, depression.
Painful anal conditions: hemorrhoids, fissure, stricture.
Decreased intestinal peristalsis: old age, spinal cord injuries, myxedema, diabetes, multiple sclerosis, Parkinsonism and other neurologic diseases.
Drugs: codeine, morphine, antacids with aluminum, verapamil, anticonvulsants, anticholinergics, disopyramide, cholestyramine, alosetron, iron supplements.
Hirschsprung's disease, meconium ileus, congenital atresia in infants.

CONSTIPATION, ADULT PATIENT[72]

ICD-10CM #	K59.00	Constipation, unspecified

NO GROSS STRUCTURAL ABNORMALITY
Inadequate fiber intake.
Irritable bowel syndrome (associated with abdominal pain) or functional constipation.

Idiopathic slow-transit constipation.
"Obstructed defecation" pelvic floor dysfunction (or dyssynergia).

STRUCTURAL DISORDERS

Anal fissure, infection, or stenosis.
Colon cancer or stricture.
Aganglionosis and/or abnormal myenteric plexus:
Hirschsprung's disease.
Chagas' disease.
Neuropathic pseudoobstruction.
Abnormal colonic muscle:
Myopathy.
Dystrophia myotonica.
Systemic sclerosis.
Idiopathic megarectum and/or megacolon.
Proximal megacolon.

NEUROLOGIC CAUSES

Diabetic autonomic neuropathy.
Damage to the sacral parasympathetic outflow.
Spinal cord damage or disease (e.g., multiple sclerosis).
Parkinson's disease.
Blunting of consciousness, mental retardation, psychosis.
Pain induced by straining (e.g., sciatic nerve compression).

ENDOCRINE OR METABOLIC CAUSES

Hypothyroidism.
Hypercalcemia.
Porphyria.
Pregnancy.

PSYCHOLOGIC DISORDERS

Depression.
Anorexia nervosa.
Denied bowel habit.

DRUG SIDE EFFECTS

COPD DECOMPENSATION[51]

ICD-10CM # J44.1s

CAUSES OF ACUTE DECOMPENSATION IN THE PATIENT WITH CHRONIC OBSTRUCTIVE PULMONARY DISEASE

Acute Exacerbations
Infectious
Viral.
Rhinovirus, respiratory syncytial virus, coronavirus, influenza virus.
Bacterial.
Haemophilus influenzae, Streptococcus pneumoniae, Moraxella (Branhamella) catarrhalis, Pseudomonas aeruginosa.
Atypical bacteria.
Chlamydia pneumoniae, Legionella.
Air Pollution
Nitrogen dioxide.
Ozone.
Particulates, dust.

Other Critical Events
Pneumothorax.
Pulmonary embolism.
Lobar atelectasis.
Congestive heart failure.
Pneumonia.
Pulmonary compression (e.g., obesity, ascites, gastric distention, pleural effusion).
Trauma (e.g., rib fractures, pulmonary contusion).
Neuromuscular and metabolic disorders.
Unrelated treatable chronic pulmonary disease (bronchiectasis, tuberculosis, sarcoidosis).
Noncompliance with prescribed treatment regimens.
Iatrogenic.
Inadequate therapy.
Inappropriate therapy (e.g., deleterious drugs).

CORNEAL SENSATION, DECREASED

ICD-10CM # H18.899 Other specified disorders of cornea, unspecified eye

Herpes (simplex, zoster).
Contact lens wear.
Topical agents (NSAIDs, anesthetics, beta-blockers).
Diabetes.
Eye trauma.
Postsurgery.

COUGH

ICD-10CM # R05 Cough

Infectious process (viral, bacterial).
Postinfectious.
"Smoker's cough."
Rhinitis (allergic, vasomotor, postinfectious).
Asthma.
Exposure to irritants (noxious fumes, smoke, cold air).
Drug-induced (especially ACE inhibitors, beta-blockers).
GERD.
Interstitial lung disease.
Lung neoplasms.
Lymphomas, mediastinal neoplasms.
Bronchiectasis.
Cardiac (CHF, pulmonary edema, mitral stenosis, pericardial inflammation).
Recurrent aspiration.
Inflammation of larynx, pleura, diaphragm, mediastinum.
Cystic fibrosis.
Anxiety.
Other: pulmonary embolism, foreign body inhalation, aortic aneurysm, Zenker's diverticulum, osteophytes, substernal thyroid, thyroiditis, PMR.

COUGH, CHRONIC, ADULT PATIENT[2]

ICD-10CM #   R05

CAUSES OF CHRONIC COUGH IN ADULTS

Intrathoracic Causes
Lungs and Airways
Asthma.
Nonasthmatic eosinophilic bronchitis.
Chronic bronchitis.
Bronchiectasis.
ACEIs.
Inhaled medications.
Chronic exposure to environmental and occupational irritants.
Bronchogenic and metastatic carcinoma.
Bronchial carcinoid.
Foreign body or endobronchial suture.
Broncholith.
Infectious and noninfectious bronchiolitis.
Chronic infectious pneumonias (e.g., bacterial, tuberculous, fungal, parasitic).
Chronic infectious tracheobronchitis (as in tuberculosis or aspergillosis).
Chronic interstitial lung disease (e.g., sarcoidosis, HSP, IPF, asbestosis).
Pulmonary vasculitis (as in granulomatosis with polyangiitis).
Sjögren syndrome with xerotrachea.
Relapsing polychondritis.
Pleura
Chronic effusion.
Diaphragm
Transvenous pacemaker stimulation.
Mediastinum
Neural tumors.
Thymoma.
Teratoma.
Lymphoma.
Metastatic lymphadenopathy.
Intrathoracic goiter.
Bronchogenic cyst.
Cardiovascular
Mitral stenosis.
Left ventricular failure.
Pulmonary thromboembolism.
Enlarged left atrium.
Vascular ring.
Aberrant innominate artery.
Aortic aneurysm.
Pericardial stimulation by transvenous pacemaker.
Extrathoracic Causes
Head and Neck
Rhinitis and sinusitis.
Nasal polyps.
Rhinolith.
Oropharyngeal dysphagia.
Laryngeal disorders (e.g., vocal fold dysfunction, laryngomalacia).
Postviral vagal neuropathy.
Recurrent aspiration.
Elongated uvula.
Chronically infected tonsils.
Neurilemmoma of vagus nerve.
Neuroma of internal laryngeal nerve.
Ascending palatine artery aneurysm.
Osteophytes of cervical spine.
Mammomonogamus (Syngamus) laryngeus infection.
Thyroiditis.

Upper Gastrointestinal
Gastroesophageal reflux disease.
Esophageal cyst or diverticulum.
Tracheoesophageal fistula.
Central Nervous System
Psychogenic or habit cough.
Tic disorders.
Gilles de la Tourette syndrome.

ACEI, Angiotensin-converting enzyme inhibitor; *HSP*, hypersensitivity pneumonitis; *IPF*, idiopathic pulmonary fibrosis.

CUTANEOUS INFECTIONS, ATHLETES

ICD-10CM #   L08.9   Local infection of the skin and subcutaneous tissue, unspecified

Tinea pedis.
Tinea cruris.
Molluscum contagiosum.
Herpes simplex.
Verruca vulgaris.
Folliculitis.
Impetigo.
Furuncles.
Otitis externa.
Erythrasma.

CYANOSIS[6]

ICD-10CM #   R23.0   Cyanosis

DIFFERENTIAL DIAGNOSIS OF CYANOSIS

Peripheral Cyanosis
Low cardiac output states
Shock.
Left ventricular failure.
Hypovolemia.
Environmental exposure (cold)
Air or water.
Arterial occlusion
Thrombosis.
Embolism.
Vasospasm (Raynaud's phenomenon).
Peripheral vascular disease.
Venous obstruction
Redistribution of blood flow from extremities
Central Cyanosis
Decreased arterial oxygen saturation
High altitude (>8000 ft).
Impaired pulmonary function.
  Hypoventilation.
  Impaired oxygen diffusion.
  Ventilation-perfusion mismatching.
    Pulmonary embolism.
    Acute respiratory distress syndrome.
    Pulmonary hypertension.
  Respiratory compromise.
    Upper airway obstruction.
    Pneumonia.
    Diaphragmatic hernia.
    Tension pneumothorax.
    Polycythemia.

Anatomic Shunts
Pulmonary arteriovenous fistulae and intrapulmonary shunts.
Cerebral, hepatic, peripheral arteriovenous fistulae.
Cyanotic congenital heart disease.
  Endocardial cushion defects.
  Ventricular septal defects.
  Coarctation of aorta.
  Tetralogy of Fallot.
  Total anomalous pulmonary venous drainage.
  Hypoplastic left ventricle.
  Pulmonary vein stenosis.
  Tricuspid atresia and anomalies.
  Premature closure of foramen ovale.
  Dextrocardia.
  Pulmonary stenosis of atrial septal defect.
  Patent ductus arteriosus with reversed shunt.
Abnormal Hemoglobin
Methemoglobinemia.
  Hereditary.
  Acquired.
Sulfhemoglobinemia.
Mutant hemoglobin with low oxygen affinity (e.g., hemoglobin Kansas).

CYANOSIS, NEONATAL[1]

ICD-10CM #   R23.0   Cyanosis

RESPIRATORY

Upper Airway
Choanal atresia.
Macroglossia.
Glossoptosis (secondary to micrognathia).
Laryngomalacia.
Laryngeal web or cyst.
Vascular anomalies (e.g., cystic hygromas, rings).
Subglottic stenosis (commonly secondary to intubation).
Foreign body.
Lower Airway
Pneumonia.
Bronchiolitis.
Pulmonary edema.
Atelectasis.
Bronchopulmonary dysplasia.

SYSTEMIC

Sepsis.
Trauma.
Poisons.

CARDIAC

Cyanotic congenital heart diseases.
Transposition of the great vessels (most common neonatal).
Tetralogy of Fallot.
Truncus arteriosus.
Tricuspid atresia.
Total anomalous pulmonary venous return.
Ebstein anomaly.
Gastrointestinal.
Gastroesophageal reflux.

NEUROLOGIC

Seizures.
Central hypoventilation syndrome (Ondine curse).
Spinal muscular atrophy type I (Werdnig-Hoffmann).
Botulism.
Congenital myopathies.

HEMATOLOGIC

Methemoglobinemia.

DAYTIME SLEEPINESS

ICD-10CM #   R53.82   Chronic fatigue, unspecified

Sleep deprivation.
Medication induced (e.g., benzodiazepines, beta-blockers, narcotics, sedative antidepressants, gabapentin).
Depression.
Obstructive sleep apnea.
Medical illness (e.g., severe anemia, hypothyroidism, COPD, hepatic failure, renal insufficiency, CHF, electrolyte disturbances).
Circadian rhythm abnormalities (e.g., jet lag, shift work sleep disorder).
Restless legs syndrome.
Posttrauma.
Narcolepsy.
Neurologic disorders (e.g., neurodegenerative disorders; parkinsonism; multiple sclerosis; lesions affecting thalamus, hypothalamus, or brain stem).

DELAYED PASSAGE OF MECONIUM[33]

ICD-10CM #   P76.0   Meconium plug syndrome

Ileal atresia.
Meconium ileus.
Functional immaturity of the colon.
Colon atresia.
Anorectal malformations.
Hirschsprung's disease.
Megacystis-microcolon-intestinal hypoperistalsis syndrome.
Extrinsic compression of the distal bowel by a mass lesion.
  Mesenteric cyst.
  Enteric duplication cyst.
Paralytic ileus, sepsis, drugs, and metabolic upset.

DELIRIUM[50]

ICD-10CM #   R40.0   Somnolence
               R40.1   Stupor
               F05   Delirium due to known physiological condition

PHARMACOLOGIC AGENTS

Anxiolytics (benzodiazepines).
Antidepressants (e.g., amitriptyline, doxepin, imipramine).
Cardiovascular agents (e.g., methyldopa, digitalis, reserpine, propranolol, procainamide, captopril, disopyramide).
Antihistamine.
Cimetidine.
Corticosteroids.
Antineoplastics.
Drugs of abuse (alcohol, cannabis, amphetamines, cocaine, hallucinogens, opioids, sedative-hypnotics, phencyclidine).

METABOLIC DISORDERS

Hypercalcemia.
Hypercarbia.
Hypoglycemia.
Hyponatremia.
Hypoxia.

INFLAMMATORY DISORDERS

Sarcoidosis.
SLE.
Giant cell arteritis.

ORGAN FAILURE

Hepatic encephalopathy.
Uremia.

NEUROLOGIC DISORDERS

Alzheimer's disease.
CVA.
Encephalitis (including HIV).
Encephalopathies.
Epilepsy.
Huntington's disease.
Multiple sclerosis.
Neoplasms.
Normal-pressure hydrocephalus.
Parkinson's disease.
Pick's disease.
Wilson's disease.

ENDOCRINE DISORDERS

Addison's disease.
Cushing's disease.
Panhypopituitarism.
Parathyroid disease.
Postpartum psychosis.
Recurrent menstrual psychosis.
Sydenham's chorea.
Thyroid disease.

DEFICIENCY STATES

Niacin.
Thiamine, vitamin B_{12}, and folate.

DELIRIUM AND AGITATION, DRUG-INDUCED

ICD-10CM # F05.9 Delirium, unspecified

COMMONLY USED DRUGS ASSOCIATED WITH DELIRIUM AND AGITATION

Benzodiazepines.
Opiates (especially meperidine).
Anticholinergics.
Antihistamines.
H_2 blockers.
Antibiotics.
Corticosteroids.
Metoclopramide.

DELIRIUM, AGITATED[6]

ICD-10CM # F05 Delirium due to known physiological condition

Metabolic causes:
　Electrolyte abnormalities.
　Hypoglycemia.

Hypoxia.
Uremia/hyperammonemia.
Structural lesions of the CNS:
　Trauma.
　Stroke.
　Hemorrhage.
　Mass.
Endocrine disease:
　Thyrotoxicosis.
Infections:
　Bacterial/viral meningitis/encephalitis.
Toxicologic causes:
　Sympathomimetic/stimulants.
　Cocaine.
　Amphetamines and derivatives.
　Caffeine.
　Phencyclidine/ketamine.
　Anticholinergics.
　Serotonin syndrome.
　Sedative-hypnotic withdrawal.
Heatstroke.
Postictal state.

CNS, Central nervous system.

DELIRIUM, DIALYSIS PATIENT[50]

| **ICD-10CM #** | F05 | Delirium due to known physiological condition |
| | F06.8 | Other specified mental disorders due to known physiological condition |

STRUCTURAL

Cerebrovascular accident (particularly hemorrhage).
Subdural hematoma.
Intracerebral abscess.
Brain tumor.

METABOLIC

Disequilibrium syndrome.
Uremia.
Drug effects.
Meningitis.
Hypertensive encephalopathy.
Hypotension.
Postictal state.
Hypernatremia or hyponatremia.
Hypercalcemia.
Hypermagnesemia.
Hypoglycemia.
Severe hyperglycemia.
Hypoxemia.
Dialysis dementia.

DEMYELINATING DISEASES[78]

ICD-10CM # G37.9 Demyelinating disease of central nervous system, unspecified

MULTIPLE SCLEROSIS

Relapsing and chronic progressive forms.
Acute multiple sclerosis.
Neuromyelitis optica (Devic's disease).

DIFFUSE CEREBRAL SCLEROSIS

Schilder's encephalitis periaxialis diffusa.
Baló's concentric sclerosis.

ACUTE DISSEMINATED ENCEPHALOMYELITIS

After measles, chickenpox, rubella, influenza, mumps.
After rabies or smallpox vaccination.

NECROTIZING HEMORRHAGIC ENCEPHALITIS

Hemorrhagic leukoencephalitis.

LEUKODYSTROPHIES

Krabbe's globoid leukodystrophy.
Metachromatic leukodystrophy.
Adrenoleukodystrophy.
Adrenomyeloneuropathy.
Pelizaeus-Merzbacher leukodystrophy.
Canavan's disease.
Alexander's disease.

DIAPHRAGM ELEVATION, BILATERAL, SYMMETRICAL[33]

ICD-10CM # J98.6 Disorders of diaphragm

CAUSES OF BILATERAL SYMMETRICAL ELEVATION OF THE DIAPHRAGM

Supine position.
Poor inspiration.
Obesity.
Pregnancy.
Abdominal distention (ascites, intestinal obstruction, abdominal mass).
Diffuse pulmonary fibrosis.
Lymphangitis carcinomatosa.
Disseminated lupus erythematosus.
Bilateral basal pulmonary emboli.
Painful conditions (after abdominal surgery).
Bilateral diaphragmatic paralysis.

DIAPHRAGM ELEVATION, UNILATERAL[33]

ICD-10CM # J98.6 Disorders of diaphragm

CAUSES OF UNILATERAL ELEVATION OF THE DIAPHRAGM

Posture—lateral decubitus position (dependent side).
Gaseous distention of stomach or colon.
Dorsal scoliosis.
Pulmonary hypoplasia.
Pulmonary collapse.
Phrenic nerve palsy.
Eventration.
Pneumonia or pleurisy.
Pulmonary thromboembolism.
Rib fracture and other painful conditions.
Subphrenic infection.
Subphrenic mass.

DIARRHEA, ACUTE WATERY AND BLOODY[72]

ICD-10CM #	K52.2	Allergic and dietetic gastroenteritis and colitis
	K52.89	Other specified noninfective gastroenteritis and colitis
	R19.7	Diarrhea, unspecified

ACUTE WATERY DIARRHEA

Gastrointestinal infections:
Protozoal (e.g., *Giardia*).
Bacterial (e.g., enterotoxigenic *Escherichia coli*, cholera).
Viral (e.g., rotavirus, Norwalk virus).
Drugs.
Toxins.
Dietary constituents (e.g., lactose intolerance).
Onset of chronic diarrheal illness.

ACUTE BLOODY DIARRHEA

Infectious colitis:
Confluent proctocolitis (e.g., *Shigella, Campylobacter, Salmonella, Entamoeba histolytica*).
Segmental colitis (e.g., *Campylobacter, Salmonella,* enteroinvasive *E. coli, Aeromonas, E. histolytica*).
Drug-induced colitis (e.g., nonsteroidal anti-inflammatory drugs [NSAIDs]).
Inflammatory bowel disease.
Ischemic colitis (usually elderly patient with underlying heart disease or arrhythmias).
Antibiotic-associated colitis.

DIARRHEA, INFECTIOUS[6]

| ICD-10CM # | A09 | Infectious gastroenteritis and colitis, unspecified |

ETIOLOGIC AGENTS OF INFECTIOUS DIARRHEA

Viral (60% of Cases)
Astrovirus.
Calicivirus.
Coronavirus.
Cytomegalovirus.[16]
Enteric adenovirus.
Hepatitis A through G.
Herpes simplex virus.
HIV enteropathy.
Norwalk-like agents.
Pararotavirus.
Norwalk virus.
Picornavirus.
Rotavirus.
Small round viruses.
Bacterial (20% of Cases)

Invasive
Aeromonas spp.

Campylobacter spp.
Clostridium difficile.
Enteroinvasive *E. coli.*
Mycobacterium spp.
Plesiomonas shigelloides.
Salmonella spp.
Shigella spp.
Vibrio fluvialis.
Vibrio parahaemolyticus.
Vibrio vulnificus.
Yersinia enterocolitica.
Yersinia pseudotuberculosis.

Toxigenic
Food poisoning with preformed toxins.
Bacillus cereus.
Clostridium botulinum.
Staphylococcus aureus.
Toxin formation after colonization.
Aeromonas hydrophila.
Clostridium perfringens.
Enterohemorrhagic *E. coli* O157:H7.
Enterotoxigenic *E. coli.*
Klebsiella pneumoniae.
Shigella spp.
Vibrio cholerae.
Other bacteria
Parasitic (5% of Cases)
Protozoa
Balantidium coli.
Blastocystis hominis.
Cryptosporidium.
Cyclospora.
Dientamoeba fragilis.
Entamoeba histolytica.
Entamoeba polecki.
Enteromonas hominis.
Giardia lamblia.
Isospora belli.
Microsporidia.
Sarcocystis hominis.
Helminths
Angiostrongylus costaricense.
Anisakiasis.
Ascaris lumbricoides.
Diphyllobothrium latum.
Enterobius vermicularis.
Hookworms.
Schistosoma spp.
Strongyloides stercoralis.
Taenia spp.
Trichinella spiralis.
Trichuris trichiura.

DIARRHEA, NONINFECTIOUS[6]

| ICD-10CM # | K59.1 | Functional diarrhea |

CAUSES OF NONINFECTIOUS DIARRHEA

Toxins
Drugs
ACE inhibitors.
Alprazolam.
Antacids (Mg).
Antibiotics.
Antidepressants.
Antiepileptic drugs.
Antihypertensives.

Antiparkinson drugs.
Beta-blockers.
Caffeine.
Cardiac antiarrhythmics.
Chemotherapy agents.
Cholesterol-lowering drugs.
Cholinergic agents.
Cholinesterase inhibitors.
Colchicine.
Digitalis.
Diuretics.
Flurouracil.
Fluoxetine.
Histamine H_2-receptor antagonists.
Hydralazine.
Lactulose.
Laxatives/cathartics.
Levodopa.
Lithium.
NSAIDs.
Neomycin.
Podophyllin.
Procainamide.
Prostaglandins.
Quinidine.
Ricinoleic acid.
Theophylline.
Thyroid hormone.
Valproic acid.
Dietetic foods
Mannitol.
Sorbitol.
Xylitol.
Fish-associated toxins
Amnestic shellfish poisoning.
Ciguatera.
Echinoderms.
Neurotoxic shellfish poisoning.
Paralytic shellfish poisoning.
Scombroid.
Tetroton.
Plant-associated toxins
Herbal preparations.
Horse chestnut.
Mushrooms—*Amanita* spp.
Nicotine.
Other plant toxins:
Pesticides—organophosphates.
Pokeweed.
Rhubarb.
Miscellaneous:
Allergic reactions.
Carbon monoxide poisoning.
Ethanol.
Heavy metals.
Monosodium glutamate (MSG).
Opiate withdrawal.
Gastrointestinal Pathology
Appendicitis.
Autonomic dysfunction.
Bile acid malabsorption.
Blind loop.
Bowel obstruction.
Celiac disease.
Cirrhosis.
Defects in amino acid transport.
Diverticular disease.
Familial dysautonomia.
Fecal impaction.

[16]Associated with fever, abdominal pain, and fecal red blood cells or white blood cells. % indicates the estimated contribution to total cases.

Fecal incontinence.
GI bleed.
GI cancer.
Hirschsprung's disease.
Inflammatory bowel disease (ulcerative colitis, Crohn's disease).
Intussusception.
Irritable bowel syndrome.
Ischemic bowel.
Lactose/fructose intolerance.
Malabsorption syndromes.
Malrotation.
Postsurgical.
Postvagotomy.
Radiation therapy.
Short gut syndrome.
Small bowel resection.
Strictures.
Toxic megacolon.
Tropical sprue.
Volvulus.
Whipple's disease.
Endocrine Related
Carcinoid syndrome (serotonin).
Hormonal hypersecretion.
Hyperthyroidism (thyroid hormone).
Medullary carcinoma of the thyroid (calcitonin).
Pancreatic cholera (VIP).
Somatostatinoma (somatostatin).
Systemic mastocytosis (histamine).
Zollinger-Ellison syndrome (gastrin).
Endocrine pathology
Adrenal insufficiency.
Diabetes enteropathy.
Hypoparathyroidism.
Pancreatic insufficiency.
Systemic Illness/Other
Alcoholism.
Amyloidosis.
Connective tissue disease.
Cystic fibrosis.
Ectopic pregnancy.
Hemolytic-uremic syndrome.
Henoch-Schönlein purpura.
Lymphoma.
Otitis media—infants.
Pelvic inflammatory disease.
Pneumonia/sepsis.
Pyelonephritis.
Scleroderma/SLE.
Severe malnutrition.
Stevens-Johnson syndrome.
Toxic shock syndrome.
Wilson's disease.
Miscellaneous:
○ Factitious diarrhea.
○ Runner's diarrhea.

ACE, Angiotensin-converting enzyme; *GI,* gastrointestinal; *NSAIDs,* nonsteroidal antiinflammatory drugs; *SLE,* systemic lupus erythematosus; *VIP,* vasoactive intestinal polypeptide.

DIARRHEA, TUBE-FED PATIENT[29]

| ICD-10CM # | K91.89 | Other postprocedural complications and disorders of digestive system |

COMMON CAUSES UNRELATED TO TUBE FEEDING
Elixir medications containing sorbitol.
Magnesium-containing antacids.
Antibiotic-induced sterile gut.
Pseudomembranous colitis.

POSSIBLE CAUSES RELATED TO TUBE FEEDING
- Inadequate fiber to form stool bulk.
- High fat content of formula (in the presence of fat malabsorption syndrome).
- Bacterial contamination of enteral products and delivery systems (causal association with diarrhea not documented).
- Rapid advancement in rate (after the GI tract is unused for prolonged periods).

UNLIKELY CAUSES RELATED TO TUBE FEEDING
Formula hyperosmolality (proven not to be the cause of diarrhea).
Lactose (absent from nearly all enteral feeding formulas).

DIPLOPIA, BINOCULAR

| ICD-10CM # | H53.2 | Diplopia |

Cranial nerve palsy (3rd, 4th, 6th).
Thyroid eye disease.
Myasthenia gravis.
Decompensated strabismus.
Orbital trauma with blowout fracture.
Orbital pseudotumor.
Cavernous sinus thrombosis.

DIPLOPIA, MONOCULAR

| ICD-10CM # | H53.2 | Diplopia |

Postoperative corrected longstanding tropia.
Defective contact lenses.
Poorly fitting bifocals.
Trauma to iris.
Corneal disorder (e.g., dry eye, astigmatism).
Cataracts.
Lens subluxation.
Nystagmus.
Eyelid twitching.
Foreign body in aqueous or vitreous media.
Migraine.
Lesions of occipital cortex.
Psychogenic.

DIPLOPIA, VERTICAL

| ICD-10CM # | H53.2 | Diplopia |

- Myasthenia.
- Superior oblique palsy.
- Myositis or pseudotumor with orbital involvement.
- Lymphoma or metastases affecting the orbits.
- Brain stem or cerebellar lesions.
- Hydrocephalus.
- Third nerve palsy.
- Botulism.
- Wernicke's encephalopathy.
- Dysthyroid orbitopathy (muscle infiltration).

DYSENTERY AND INFLAMMATORY ENTEROCOLITIS[9]

| ICD-10CM # | varies with specific diagnosis |

DIFFERENTIAL DIAGNOSIS OF ACUTE BACTERIAL DYSENTERY AND INFLAMMATORY ENTEROCOLITIS
Specific Infectious Processes
Bacillary dysentery (*Shigella dysenteriae, Shigella flexneri, Shigella sonnei, Shigella boydii;* invasive *Escherichia coli*).
Campylobacteriosis (*Campylobacter jejuni*).
Amebic dysentery (*Entamoeba histolytica*).
Ciliary dysentery (*Balantidium coli*).
Vibriosis (*Vibrio parahaemolyticus*).
Salmonellosis (*Salmonella typhimurium*).
Typhoid fever (*Salmonella typhi*).
Enteric fever (*Salmonella choleraesuis, Salmonella paratyphi*).
Yersiniosis (*Yersinia enterocolitica*).
Proctitis
Gonococcal (*Neisseria gonorrhoeae*).
Herpetic (*herpes simplex virus*).
Chlamydial (*Chlamydia trachomatis*).
Syphilitic (*Treponema pallidum*).
Other Syndromes
Necrotizing enterocolitis of the newborn.
Enteritis necroticans.
Pseudomembranous enterocolitis or *Clostridium difficile* colitis without overt pseudomembranes (*C. difficile*).
Diverticulitis.
Typhlitis.
Chronic Inflammatory Processes
Enteropathogenic and enteroaggregative *E. coli.*
Syphilis.
Gastrointestinal tuberculosis.
Gastrointestinal mycosis (including *Basidiobolus ranarum*).
Parasitic enteritis.
Syndromes without Known Infectious Cause
Idiopathic ulcerative colitis.
Crohn's disease.
Radiation enteritis.
Ischemic colitis.
Allergic enteritis.
Brainerd diarrhea.

DIZZINESS

| ICD-10CM # | R42 | Dizziness and giddiness |

- Viral syndrome.
- Anxiety, hyperventilation.
- Benign positional paroxysmal vertigo.
- Medications (e.g., sedatives, antihypertensives, analgesics).
- Withdrawal from medications (e.g., benzodiazepines, SSRIs).
- Alcohol or drug abuse.
- Postural hypotension.
- Hypoglycemia, hyperglycemia.
- Hematologic disorders (e.g., anemia, polycythemia, leukemia).
- Head trauma.
- Menière's disease.

- Vertebrobasilar ischemia.
- Cervical osteoarthritis.
- Cardiac abnormalities (arrhythmias, cardiomyopathy, CHF, pericarditis).
- Multiple sclerosis.
- Peripheral vestibulopathy.
- Air or sea travel.
- Electrolyte abnormalities.
- Eye problems (cornea, lens, retina).
- Migraine.
- Brain stem infarct.
- Autonomic neuropathy.
- Chronic otomastoiditis.
- Complex partial seizures.
- Ramsey Hunt syndrome.
- Arteritis.
- Syncope and presyncope.
- Perilymph fistula.
- Cerebellopontine tumor.
- Hepatic or renal disease.

DRY EYE

ICD-10CM #	H04.129 Dry eye syndrome of unspecified lacrimal gland

Contacts.
Medications (antihistamines, clonidine, beta-blockers, ibuprofen, scopolamine).
Keratoconjunctivitis sicca.
Trauma.
Environmental causes (air conditioning in patient with contacts).

DYSLIPOPROTEINEMIAS, SECONDARY CAUSES[10]

ICD-10CM #	E78.4 Other hyperlipidemia

Cause	Disorder
Metabolic	Diabetes
	Lipodystrophy
	Glycogen storage disorders
Renal	Chronic renal failure
	Glomerulonephritis with nephritic syndrome
Hepatic	Cirrhosis
	Biliary obstruction
	Porphyria
Hormonal	Estrogens
	Progesterones
	Growth hormone
	Thyroid disorders (hypothyroidism) Corticosteroids
Lifestyle	Physical inactivity
	Obesity
	Diet rich in fats, saturated fats
	Alcohol intake
	Smoking

Cause	Disorder
Medications	Retinoic acid derivatives
	Glucocorticoids
	Exogenous estrogens
	Thiazide diuretics
	Beta-adrenergic blockers (non-selective)
	Testosterone and other anabolic steroids
	Immunosuppressive medications (cyclosporine)
	Antiviral medications (human immunodeficiency virus protease inhibitors)
	Antischizophrenic agents

DYSPAREUNIA[21]

ICD-10CM #	N94.1	Dyspareunia
	N44.8	Other noninflammatory disorders of the testis
	N50.8	Other specified disorders of male genital organs
	N53.12	Painful ejaculation
	F52.6	Dyspareunia not due to a substance or known physiological condition

INTROITAL

Vaginismus.
Intact or rigid hymen.
Clitoral problems.
Vulvovaginitis.
Vaginal atrophy: hypoestrogen.
Vulvar dystrophy.
Bartholin or Skene gland infection.
Inadequate lubrication.
Operative scarring.

MIDVAGINAL

Urethritis.
Trigonitis.
Cystitis.
Short vagina.
Operative scarring.
Inadequate lubrication.

DEEP

Endometriosis.
Pelvic infection.
Uterine retroversion.
Ovarian pathology.
GI.
Orthopedic.
Abnormal penile size or shape.

DYSPEPSIA AND PYROSIS, DIFFERENTIAL DIAGNOSIS DURING PREGNANCY[27]

ICD-10CM #	K30	Dyspepsia, atonic
	F45.3	Dyspepsia, psychogenic

DIFFERENTIAL DIAGNOSIS OF DYSPEPSIA OR PYROSIS DURING PREGNANCY

Gastroesophageal reflux disease.
Peptic ulcer disease.
Nausea and vomiting of pregnancy.
Hyperemesis gravidarum.
Pancreatitis.
Biliary colic.
Acute cholecystitis.
Viral hepatitis.
Appendicitis.
Acute fatty liver of pregnancy (in late pregnancy).
Irritable bowel syndrome/nonulcer dyspepsia.

DYSPHAGIA

ICD-10CM #	R13.10 Dysphagia, unspecified

Esophageal obstruction: neoplasm, foreign body, achalasia, stricture, spasm, esophageal web, diverticulum, Schatzki's ring.
Peptic esophagitis with stricture, Barrett's stricture.
External esophageal compression: neoplasms (thyroid neoplasm, lymphoma, mediastinal tumors), thyroid enlargement, aortic aneurysm, vertebral spurs, aberrant right subclavian artery (dysphagia lusoria).
Hiatal hernia, GERD.
Oropharyngeal lesions: pharyngitis, glossitis, stomatitis, neoplasms.
Hysteria: globus hystericus.
Neurologic and/or neuromuscular disturbances: bulbar paralysis, myasthenia gravis, ALS, multiple sclerosis, Parkinsonism, CVA, diabetic neuropathy.
Toxins: poisoning, botulism, tetanus, postdiphtheritic dysphagia.
Systemic diseases: scleroderma, amyloidosis, dermatomyositis.
Candida and herpes esophagitis.
Presbyesophagus.

DYSPHAGIA, ESOPHAGEAL[23]

ICD-10CM #	R13-14 Dysphagia, Pharyngoesophageal phase

COMMON CAUSES OF ESOPHAGEAL DYSPHAGIA

Motility (Neuromuscular) Disorders
Primary
Achalasia
Distal esophageal spasm
Hypercontractile (jackhammer) esophagus
Hypertensive LES
Nutcracker (high-pressure) esophagus
Other peristaltic abnormalities[17]
Secondary
Chagas' disease
Reflux-related dysmotility
Scleroderma and other rheumatologic disorders

---

[17]Peristaltic abnormalities include absent peristalsis and weak peristalsis, as well as hypertensive peristalsis (nutcracker esophagus).

Differential Diagnosis

II

Structural (Mechanical) Disorders
Intrinsic
Carcinoma and benign tumors
Diverticula
Eosinophilic esophagitis
Esophageal rings and webs (other than Schatzki ring)
Foreign body
Lower esophageal (Schatzki) ring
Medication-induced stricture
Peptic stricture
Extrinsic
Mediastinal mass
Spinal osteophytes
Vascular compression

LES, lower esophageal sphincter.

DYSPHAGIA, OROPHARYNGEAL[72]

ICD-10CM #   R13.12   Dysphagia, oropharyngeal phase

FUNCTIONAL DISORDERS

Central Nervous System
Stroke.
Head injury.
Parkinson's disease.
Motor neuron disease.
Multiple sclerosis.
Tumor.
Drugs (e.g., phenothiazines).
Malformations (e.g., syrinx, Arnold–Chiari).
Neural
Motor neuron disease.
Myasthenia gravis.
Radiotherapy.
Poliomyelitis.
Familial dysautonomia.
Muscle
Autoimmune myopathy (polymyositis, dermatomyositis, systemic lupus erythematosus).
Thyrotoxic myopathy.
Guillain-Barré motor neuropathy.
Muscular dystrophies.

STRUCTURAL DISORDERS

Head/neck surgery.
Stricture.
Radiotherapy.
Tumor.
Pharyngeal pouch.
Web.
Extrinsic (e.g., osteophytes).

MISCELLANEOUS

Xerostomia.

DYSPNEA

ICD-10CM #   R06.9   Unspecified abnormalities of breathing

Upper airway obstruction: trauma, neoplasm, epiglottitis, laryngeal edema, tongue retraction, laryngospasm, abductor paralysis of vocal cords, aspiration of foreign body.
Lower airway obstruction: neoplasm, COPD, asthma, aspiration of foreign body.

Pulmonary infection: pneumonia, abscess, empyema, TB, bronchiectasis.
Pulmonary hypertension.
Pulmonary embolism/infarction.
Parenchymal lung disease.
Pulmonary vascular congestion.
Cardiac disease: ASHD, valvular lesions, cardiac dysrhythmias, cardiomyopathy, pericardial effusion, cardiac shunts.
Space-occupying lesions: neoplasm, large hiatal hernia, pleural effusions.
Disease of chest wall: severe kyphoscoliosis, fractured ribs, sternal compression, morbid obesity.
Neurologic dysfunction: Guillain-Barré syndrome, botulism, polio, spinal cord injury.
Interstitial pulmonary disease: sarcoidosis, collagen vascular diseases, DIP, Hamman-Rich pneumonitis, etc.
Pneumoconioses: silicosis, berylliosis, etc.
Mesothelioma.
Pneumothorax, hemothorax, pleural effusion.
Inhalation of toxins.
Cholinergic drug intoxication.
Carcinoid syndrome.
Hematologic: anemia, polycythemia, hemoglobinopathies.
Thyrotoxicosis, myxedema.
Diaphragmatic compression caused by abdominal distention, subphrenic abscess, ascites.
Lung resection.
Metabolic abnormalities: uremia, hepatic coma, DKA.
Sepsis.
Atelectasis.
Psychoneurosis.
Diaphragmatic paralysis.
Pregnancy.

DYSURIA

ICD-10CM #   R30.0   Dysuria
               R30.9   Painful micturition, unspecified

Urinary tract infection.
Estrogen deficiency (in postmenopausal female).
Vaginitis.
Genital infection (e.g., herpes, condyloma).
Interstitial cystitis.
Chemical irritation (e.g., deodorant aerosols, douches).
Meatal stenosis or stricture.
Reiter's syndrome.
Bladder neoplasm.
GI etiology (diverticulitis, Crohn's disease).
Impaired bladder or sphincter action.
Urethral carbuncle.
Chronic fibrosis posttrauma.
Radiation therapy.
Prostatitis.
Urethritis (gonococcal, *Chlamydia*).
Behçet's syndrome.
Stevens-Johnson syndrome.

EARACHE[64]

ICD-10CM #   H92.09   Otalgia, unspecified ear

Otitis media.
Serous otitis media.

Eustachitis.
Otitis externa.
Otitic barotrauma.
Mastoiditis.
Foreign body.
Impacted cerumen.
Referred otalgia, as with TMJ dysfunction, dental problems, and tumors.

ECTOPIC ACTH SECRETION[29]

ICD-10CM #   E34.2   Ectopic hormone secretion, not elsewhere classified

Small cell carcinoma of lung.
Endocrine tumors of foregut origin.
    Thymic carcinoid.
    Islet cell tumor.
    Medullary carcinoid, thyroid.
    Bronchial carcinoid.
Pheochromocytoma.
Ovarian tumors.

EDEMA, CHILDREN[38]

ICD-10CM #   R60.0   Localized edema
               R60.1   Generalized edema
               R60.9   Edema, unspecified

CARDIOVASCULAR

Congestive heart failure.
Acute thrombi or emboli.
Vasculitis of many types.

RENAL

Nephrotic syndrome.
Glomerulonephritis of many types.
End-stage renal failure.

ENDOCRINE OR METABOLIC

Thyroid disease.
Starvation.
Hereditary angioedema.

IATROGENIC

Drugs (diuretics and steroids).
Water or salt overload.

HEMATOLOGIC

Hemolytic disease of the newborn.

GASTROINTESTINAL

Hepatic cirrhosis.
Protein-losing enteritis.
Lymphangiectasis.
Cystic fibrosis.
Celiac disease.
Enteritis of many types.

LYMPHATIC ABNORMALITIES

Congenital (gonadal dysgenesis).
Acquired.

EDEMA, GENERALIZED

ICD-10CM #   R60.0   Localized edema
               R60.1   Generalized edema
               R60.9   Edema, unspecified

Congestive heart failure (CHF).
Cirrhosis.
Nephrotic syndrome.
Pregnancy.
Idiopathic.
Acute nephritic syndrome.
Myxedema.
Medications (NSAIDs, estrogens, vasodilators).

EDEMA, LEG, UNILATERAL[50]

| ICD-10CM # | R60.0 | Localized edema |
| | R60.9 | Edema, unspecified |

WITH PAIN

DVT.
Postphlebitic syndrome.
Popliteal cyst rupture.
Gastrocnemius rupture.
Cellulitis.
Psoas or other abscess.

WITHOUT PAIN

DVT.
Postphlebitic syndrome.
Other venous insufficiency (after saphenous vein harvest, varicosities).
Lymphatic obstruction/lymphedema (carcinoma, lymphoma, sarcoidosis, filariasis, retroperitoneal fibrosis).

EDEMA OF LOWER EXTREMITIES

| ICD-10CM # | R60.0 | Localized edema |
| | R60.9 | Edema, unspecified |

CHF (right-sided).
Hepatic cirrhosis.
Nephrosis.
Myxedema.
Lymphedema.
Pregnancy.
Abdominal mass: neoplasm, cyst.
Venous compression from abdominal aneurysm.
Varicose veins.
Bilateral cellulitis.
Bilateral thrombophlebitis.
Vena cava thrombosis, venous thrombosis.
Retroperitoneal fibrosis.

EJECTION SOUND OR CLICK

| ICD-10CM # | R01.2 | Other cardiac sounds |

Aortic regurgitation.
Aortic root dilatation.
Systemic hypertension.
Chronic pulmonary hypertension.
Tetralogy of Fallot.
Atrial septal defect.
Pulmonary valve stenosis.
Aortic aneurysm.

ELBOW PAIN

| ICD-10CM # | M25.529 | Pain in unspecified elbow |

Trauma.
Infection.

Inflammatory arthritis.
Lateral or medial epicondylitis.
Entrapment neuropathy.
Olecranon bursitis.
Osteoarthritis.
Gout.
Cervical disease (referred pain).
Shoulder disease (referred pain).
Partial subluxation.
Synovial osteochondromatosis.
Loose body.

ELEVATED HEMIDIAPHRAGM

ICD-10CM #	J98.6	Disorders of diaphragm
	Q79.0	Congenital diaphragmatic hernia
	Q79.1	Other congenital malformations of diaphragm

Neoplasm (bronchogenic carcinoma, mediastinal neoplasm, intrahepatic lesion).
Substernal thyroid.
Infectious process (pneumonia, empyema, TB, subphrenic abscess, hepatic abscess).
Atelectasis.
Idiopathic.
Eventration.
Phrenic nerve dysfunction (myelitis, myotonia, herpes zoster).
Trauma to phrenic nerve or diaphragm (e.g., surgery).
Aortic aneurysm.
Intraabdominal mass.
Pulmonary infarction.
Pleurisy.
Radiation therapy.
Rib fracture.

EMBOLI, ARTERIAL[50]

| ICD-10CM # | I74.3 | Embolism and thrombosis of arteries of the lower extremities |
| | I74.2 | Embolism and thrombosis of arteries of the upper extremities |

Myocardial infarction with mural thrombi.
Atrial fibrillation.
Cardiomyopathies.
Prosthetic heart valves.
CHF.
Endocarditis.
Left ventricular aneurysm.
Left atrial myxoma.
Sick sinus syndrome.
Paradoxical embolus from venous thrombosis.
Aneurysms of large blood vessels.
Atheromatous ulcers of large blood vessels.

EMESIS, PEDIATRIC AGE[38]

ICD-10CM #	R11.10	Vomiting, unspecified
	R11.11	Vomiting without nausea
	R11.12	Projectile vomiting

INFANCY

Gastrointestinal Tract

Congenital:

Regurgitation—chalasia, gastroesophageal reflux.
Atresia—stenosis (tracheoesophageal fistula, prepyloric diaphragm, intestinal atresia).
Duplication.
Volvulus (errors in rotation and fixation, Meckel diverticulum).
Congenital bands.
Hirschsprung's disease.
Meconium ileus (cystic fibrosis), meconium plug.

Acquired:

Acute infectious gastroenteritis, food poisoning (staphylococcal, clostridial).
Pyloric stenosis.
Gastritis, duodenitis.
Intussusception.
Incarcerated hernia—inguinal, internal secondary to old adhesions.
Cow's milk protein intolerance, food allergy, eosinophilic gastroenteritis.
Disaccharidase deficiency.
Celiac disease—presents after introduction of gluten in diet; inherited risk.
Adynamic ileus—the mediator for many nongastrointestinal causes.
Neonatal necrotizing enterocolitis.
Chronic granulomatous disease with gastric outlet obstruction.

Nongastrointestinal Tract

Infectious—otitis, urinary tract infection, pneumonia, upper respiratory tract infection, sepsis, meningitis.
Metabolic—aminoaciduria and organic aciduria, galactosemia, fructosemia, adrenogenital syndrome, renal tubular acidosis, diabetic ketoacidosis, Reye's syndrome.
Central nervous system—trauma, tumor, infection, diencephalic syndrome, rumination, autonomic responses (pain, shock).
Medications—anticholinergics, aspirin, alcohol, idiosyncratic reaction (e.g., codeine).

CHILDHOOD

Gastrointestinal Tract

Peptic ulcer—vomiting is a common presentation in children younger than 6 yr old.
Trauma—duodenal hematoma, traumatic pancreatitis, perforated bowel.
Pancreatitis—mumps, trauma, cystic fibrosis, hyperparathyroidism, hyperlipidemia, organic acidemias.
Crohn's disease.
Idiopathic intestinal pseudoobstruction.
Superior mesenteric artery syndrome.

Nongastrointestinal Tract

Central nervous system—cyclic vomiting, migraine, anorexia nervosa, bulimia.

ENCEPHALOMYELITIS, NONVIRAL CAUSES[50]

| ICD-10CM # | G04.81 | Other encephalitis and encephalomyelitis |

Subacute bacterial endocarditis.
Rocky Mountain spotted fever.
Typhus.
Ehrlichia.
Q fever.
Chlamydia.
Mycoplasma.
Legionella.
Brucellosis.
Listeria.
Whipple's disease.
Cat-scratch disease.
Syphilis (meningovascular).
Relapsing fever.
Lyme disease.
Leptospirosis.
Nocardia.
Actinomycosis.
Tuberculosis.
Cryptococcus.
Histoplasma.
Toxoplasma.
Plasmodium falciparum.
Trypanosomiasis.
Behçet's disease.
Vasculitis.
Carcinoma.
Drug reactions.

ENCEPHALOPATHY, HYPERTENSIVE[74]

ICD-10CM #		varies with specific diagnosis

Cerebral infarction.
Subarachnoid hemorrhage.
Intracerebral hemorrhage.
Subdural or epidural hematoma.
Brain tumor or other mass lesion.
Seizure disorder.
Central nervous system vasculitis.
Encephalitis/meningitis.
Drug ingestion.
Drug withdrawal.

ENCEPHALOPATHY, METABOLIC[70]

ICD-10CM #	F10.27	Alcohol dependence with alcohol-induced persisting dementia
	K72.90	Hepatic failure, unspecified without coma
	K72.91	Hepatic failure, unspecified with coma
	G92	Toxic encephalopathy
	T56.0X1A	Toxic effect of lead and its compounds, accidental (unintentional), initial encounter
	T56.0X2A	Toxic effect of lead and its compounds, intentional self-harm, initial encounter

Substrate deficiency: hypoxia/ischemia, carbon monoxide poisoning, hypoglycemia.
Cofactor deficiency: thiamine, vitamin B_{12}, pyridoxine (INH administration).
Electrolyte disorders: hyponatremia, hypercalcemia, carbon dioxide narcosis, dialysis, hypermagnesemia, disequilibrium syndrome.
Endocrinopathies: DKA, hyperosmolar coma, hypothyroidism, hyperadrenocorticism, hyperparathyroidism.
Endogenous toxins: liver disease, uremia, porphyria.
Exogenous toxins: drug overdose (sedative/hypnotics, ethanol, narcotics, salicylates, tricyclic antidepressants), drug withdrawal, toxicity of therapeutic medications, industrial toxins (e.g., organophosphates, heavy metals), sepsis.
Heat stroke.
Epilepsy (postictal).

ENDOMETRIAL THICKENING[62]

ICD-10CM #		Varies with Specific Diagnosis

CAUSES OF ENDOMETRIAL THICKENING

Early intrauterine pregnancy
Incomplete abortion
Ectopic pregnancy
Retained products of conception
Trophoblastic disease
Endometritis
Adhesions
Hyperplasia
Polyps
Carcinoma

ENTHESOPATHY

ICD-10CM #	M46.00	Spinal enthesopathy, site unspecified

Viremia or bacteremia.
Ankylosing spondylitis.
Psoriatic arthritis.
Drug-induced (quinolones, etretinate).
Reactive arthritis.
DISH.
Reiter's syndrome.

EOSINOPHILIA, DISEASE ASSOCIATIONS[49]

ICD-10CM #	D72.1	Eosinophilia NEC
	J82	Eosinophilia, pulmonary

DISEASES, SYNDROMES, AND CONDITIONS COMMONLY ASSOCIATED WITH PERIPHERAL BLOOD EOSINOPHILIA AND/OR TISSUE EOSINOPHILIA

Infectious Agents
Parasitic Infections
Tropical eosinophilia.
Visceral larval migrans (VLM, toxocariasis).
Helminth infections.
Filariasis (*Wuchereria bancrofti, Brugia malay*).
Onchocerciasis.
Schistosomiasis.
Fascioliasis.
Paragonimiasis.
Strongyloidiasis.
Trichinosis.
Hookworm.
Ascariasis.
Echinococcosis/hydatid disease.
Fungal Infections
Coccidioidomycosis.
Cryptococcosis (CSF eosinophilia) in HIV.
Allergic Diseases
Asthma (atopic and intrinsic, nasal polyps, aspirin intolerance syndromes).
Bronchopulmonary aspergillosis.
Allergic rhinitis.
Urticarias (acute allergic and chronic idiopathic).
Atopic dermatitis.
Acute drug (hypersensitivity) reactions (interstitial nephritis, cholestatic hepatitis, exfoliative dermatitis).
Respiratory Tract Disorders
Hypersensitivity pneumonitis (rare).
Allergic bronchopulmonary aspergillosis.
Eosinophilic pneumonia.
Transient pulmonary infiltrates (Löeffler syndrome).
Prolonged pulmonary infiltrates with eosinophilia (PIE syndrome).
Tropical pulmonary eosinophilia (TPE).
Bronchiectasis.
Cystic fibrosis.
Endocrinologic Disorders
Addison disease.
Gastrointestinal Diseases
Inflammatory bowel disease (IBD).
Eosinophilic gastroenteritis, eosinophilic esophagitis (EE).
Allergic gastroenteritis (young children).
Celiac disease (when associated with EE).
Toxic Reactions to Ingested Agents
Eosinophil myalgia syndrome (L-tryptophan).
Toxic oil syndrome.
Reactions to Cytokine Therapies
IL-2 and IL-2 plus lymphokine activated killer (LAK) cells.
GM-CSF therapy.
Cutaneous Disorders
Atopic dermatitis.
Immunologic skin diseases.
Scabies.
Myiasis.
Chlamydial pneumonia of infancy.
Scarlet fever and pneumococcal pneumonia (convalescent phase).

Cat scratch disease.
Eosinophilic cellulitis (Wells syndrome).
Episodic angioedema with eosinophilia.
Chronic idiopathic urticaria.
Bullous pemphigoid.
Herpes gestationis.
Angioblastic lymphoid hyperplasia (Kimura disease).

Immunodeficiency Syndromes
Wiskott-Aldrich syndrome.
Selective IgA deficiency with atopy.
Hyper-IgE recurrent infection syndrome (Job syndrome).
Swiss-type and sex-linked combined immuno-deficiency.
Nezelof syndrome.
Graft-versus-host-disease (GVHD).

Connective Tissue Diseases
- **Vasculitis/Collagen Vascular Disorders**
  Hypersensitivity vasculitis.
  Allergic granulomatosis with angiitis (Churg-Strauss syndrome).
  Serum sickness.
  Eosinophilic fasciitis.
  Sjögren syndrome.
  Rheumatoid arthritis (severe).

Neoplastic, Myeloproliferative, and Ly Neoplasms and Syndromes
- *Neoplastic*
  Ovarian carcinoma.
  Solid tumors (mucin-secreting, epithelial cell origin).
Chronic eosinophil leukemia.
Idiopathic hypereosinophilic syndromes (HES).
Systemic mastocytosis.
Myeloproliferative
  Chronic myelogenous leukemia (CML) acute myelogenous leukemia (AML) and myelo-dysplastic syndrome (MDS).
  Myelomonocytic leukemia with bone marrow eosinophilia (M4Eo, inversion 16).
Lymphoproliferative
  T-cell lymphocytic leukemia.
  Lymphomas (T cell, Hodgkin disease).
  Angioimmunoblastic lymphadenopathy.

Rare Causes
- Chronic active hepatitis.
- Chronic dialysis.
- Acute pancreatitis.
- Postirradiation.
- Hypopituitarism.

EOSINOPHILIA, GI[23]

ICD-10CM # D72.1 Eosinophilia

CAUSES OF GI EOSINOPHILIA

GERD
Eosinophilic GI disorders
  Eosinophilic esophagitis
    Connective tissue disease-associated eosinophilic esophagitis
    Familial eosinophilic esophagitis
  Eosinophilic gastritis
  Eosinophilic enteritis
  Eosinophilic gastroenteritis
Infections
  Schistosomiasis

Anisakiasis
GI basidiobolomycosis
Toxocariasis
Celiac disease
Hypereosinophilic syndrome
Drug hypersensitivity response
IBD
Transplant-associated eosinophilic enteritis
Eosinophilic granulomatosis with polyangiitis
Toxic injury
Graft-versus-host disease

EOSINOPHILIC LUNG DISEASE[33]

ICD-10CM # NEC J82 Eosinophilia, pulmonary

IDIOPATHIC

Simple pulmonary eosinophilia (Löffler's syndrome).
Acute eosinophilic pneumonia.
Chronic eosinophilic pneumonia.
Hypereosinophilic syndrome.

DRUG-INDUCED

Aminosalicylic acid.
Para-aminosalicylic acid.
NSAIDs.
Captopril.
Cocaine.
Minocycline.
Nitrofurantoin.
Phenytoin.

INFECTION

Parasitic (ascariasis, paragonimiasis. tropical eosinophilia).
Fungal (aspergillus).
Bacterial (TB, atypical mycobacterial infection, brucella).
Viral (respiratory syncytial virus).

IMMUNOLOGIC DISEASES

Wegener's granulomatosis.
Churg–Strauss syndrome.
Rheumatoid disease.
Sarcoidosis.

NEOPLASMS

Bronchogenic carcinoma.
Bronchial carcinoid.
Lymphoma (Hodgkin's, non-Hodgkin's).

EOSINOPHILIA, PARASITIC CAUSES[9]

ICD-10CM # varies with specific diagnosis

PARASITIC CAUSES OF EOSINOPHILIA

Widespread Geographic Distribution
Ascariasis (migratory phase).
Hookworm.[†]
Strongyloidiasis.[*‡]

[†]Moderate to marked during larval migration in early infection; most often absent or very mild during chronic infection.

Tropical pulmonary eosinophilia.
Lymphatic filariasis.
Schistosomiasis.
Toxocariasis.
Cysticercosis (*Taenia solium*).
Echinococcosis (cyst rupture).
Trichinosis.
Trichuriasis.
Aberrant helminthiasis from animals.

Limited Geographic Distribution
Clonorchiasis.
Paragonimiasis.
Fascioliasis.
Angiostrongyliasis.
Opisthorchiasis.
Onchocerciasis, loiasis, and other nonlymphatic filariases.
Gnathostomiasis.
Capillariasis.
Trichostrongyliasis.

---

[*]Most frequent parasitic causes of massive eosino-philia (>5000/mm³).
[‡]Absent in disseminated infection in compromised hosts.

EPIGASTRIC PAIN[72]

ICD-10CM #		
	R10.816	Epigastric abdominal tenderness
	R10.826	Epigastric rebound abdominal tenderness

Peptic ulceration (uncomplicated).[18]
Peptic ulceration (perforated).
Biliary colic.
Acute pancreatitis.
Abdominal aortic aneurysm.
Anxiety.
Inferior wall MI.

---

[18]Conditions that also cause right upper quadrant pain

EPILEPSY

ICD-10CM # G40.909 Epilepsy, unspecified, not intractable, without status epilepticus

Psychogenic spells.
Transient ischemic attack.
Hypoglycemia.
Syncope.
Narcolepsy.
Migraine.
Paroxysmal vertigo.
Arrhythmias.
Drug reaction.

EPISTAXIS

ICD-10CM # R04.0 Epistaxis

Trauma.
Medications (nasal sprays, NSAIDs, anticoagulants, antiplatelets).
Nasal polyps.
Cocaine use.

Coagulopathy (hemophilia, liver disease, DIC, thrombocytopenia).
Systemic disorders (hypertension, uremia).
Infections.
Anatomic malformations.
Rhinitis.
Nasal polyps.
Local neoplasms (benign and malignant).
Desiccation.
Foreign body.

ERECTILE DYSFUNCTION, ORGANIC[61]

ICD-10CM #	N52.9	Male erectile dysfunction, unspecified

Neurogenic abnormalities: Somatic nerve neuropathy, central nervous system abnormalities.
Psychogenic causes: Depression, performance anxiety, marital conflict.
Endocrine causes: Hyperprolactinemia, hypogonadotropic hypogonadism, testicular failure, estrogen excess.
Trauma: Pelvic fracture, prostate surgery, penile fracture.
Systemic disease: DM, renal failure, hepatic cirrhosis.
Medications: Diuretics, antidepressants, H_2 blockers, exogenous hormones, alcohol, antihypertensives, nicotine abuse, finasteride, etc.
Structural abnormalities: Peyronie's disease.

EROSIONS, GENITALIA

ICD-10CM #	N36.8	Other specified disorders of urethra

Candidiasis.
Intraepithelial neoplasia.
Squamous cell carcinoma.
Lichen planus.
Pemphigus vulgaris.
Erythema multiforme.
Lichen sclerosus.
Bullous pemphigoid.
Extramammary Paget's disease.
Impetigo.

ERYTHEMATOUS ANNULAR SKIN LESIONS

ICD-10CM #	L53.8	Other specified erythematous conditions

Tinea corporis.
Warfarin plaques.
Erythema multiforme.
Erythema annulare.
Cutaneous lupus.
Cutaneous sarcoidosis.
Trauma.
Acute febrile neutrophilic dermatosis (Sweet's syndrome).

ERYTHROCYTOSIS[40]

ICD-10CM #	D75.0	Familial erythrocytosis

CAUSES OF ERYTHROCYTOSIS

Relative or Spurious Erythrocytosis (Normal Red Cell Mass)
Hemoconcentration secondary to dehydration (diarrhea, diaphoresis, diuretics, water deprivation, emesis, ethanol, hypertension, preeclampsia, pheochromocytoma, carbon monoxide intoxication).
True or Absolute Erythrocytosis
Polycythemia vera.
Primary congenital polycythemia.
Secondary erythrocytosis caused by:
Congenital causes (e.g., activating mutation of erythropoietin receptor).
Hypoxia caused by carbon monoxide poisoning, high oxygen affinity hemoglobin, high-altitude residence, chronic pulmonary disease, hypoventilation syndromes such as sleep apnea, right to left cardiac shunt, neurologic defects involving the respiratory center.
Nonhypoxic causes with pathologic erythropoietin production.
Renal disease (cysts, hydronephrosis, renal artery stenosis, focal glomerulonephritis, renal transplantation).
Tumors (renal cell cancer, hepatocellular carcinoma, cerebellar hemangioblastoma, uterine fibromyoma, adrenal tumors, meningioma, pheochromocytoma).
Drug-associated causes:
Androgen therapy.
Exogenous erythropoietin growth factor therapy.

ERYTHRODERMA

ICD-10CM #	L53.9	Erythematous condition, unspecified

Drug reaction (e.g., allopurinol, ampicillin, phenytoin, vancomycin, dapsone, omeprazole, carbamazepine).
Atopic dermatitis.
Psoriasis.
Contact dermatitis.
Idiopathic.
Pityriasis rubra.
Chronic actinic dermatitis.
Bullous pemphigoid.
Paraneoplastic.
Cutaneous T-cell lymphoma.
Connective tissue disease.
Hypereosinophilia syndrome.

ESOPHAGEAL PERFORATION[50]

ICD-10CM #	K22.3	Perforation of esophagus
	S27.819A	Unspecified injury of esophagus (thoracic part), initial encounter

Trauma.
Caustic burns.
Iatrogenic.
Foreign bodies.
Spontaneous rupture (Boerhaave's syndrome).
Postoperative breakdown of anastomosis.

ESOPHAGEAL STRICTURES[65]

ICD-10CM #		Varies with Specific Diagnosis

BENIGN

Congenital
Esophageal atresia
Tracheoesophageal fistula
Web

ACQUIRED

Peptic
Gastroesophageal reflux
Scleroderma
Schatzki ring
Caustic ingestion
Drug induced
Anticholinergic medications
Aspirin
Ferrous sulfate
Fosamax
Nonsteroidal antiinflammatory
Quinidine
Potassium supplements
Tetracycline
Vitamin C
Eosinophilic esophagitis
Iatrogenic
Variceal ligation/injection
Endoscopic mucosal resection
Ablation therapy (cryotherapy/radiofrequency)
Postoperative (anastomotic)
Radiation
Instrumentation
Nasogastric tube
Infections
Fungal: moniliasis
Bacterial: syphilis
Mycobacterial: tuberculosis
Granulomatous
Crohn disease
Dermatosis
Epidermolysis bullosa dystrophica
Pemphigoid
Behçet disease

MALIGNANT

Primary
Secondary

ESOPHAGEAL TUMORS, BENIGN[65]

ICD-10CM #		Varies with Specific Diagnosis

CLASSIFICATION OF BENIGN ESOPHAGEAL TUMORS

Mucosa (First and Second Esophageal Ultrasound [EUS] Layers)
Squamous papilloma
Fibrovascular polyp
Retention cyst
Submucosa (Third EUS Layer)
Lipoma
Fibroma
Neurofibroma
Granular cell tumor
Hemangiomas
Salivary gland–type tumor
Muscularis Propria (Fourth EUS Layer)
Leiomyoma
Duplication cyst
Periesophageal Tissue (Fifth EUS Layer)
Foregut cyst

ESOPHAGITIS[50]

ICD-10CM #	K20.9	Esophagitis, unspecified

INFECTIOUS

Candidiasis.
Cytomegalovirus.
Herpes simplex virus.
HIV infection, acute.

NONINFECTIOUS

Gastroesophageal reflux.
Mucositis from cancer chemotherapy.
Mucositis from radiation therapy.
Aphthous ulcers.

ESOPHAGUS, SYSTEMIC DISEASES[65]

ICD-10CM #		Varies with Specific Diagnosis

SYSTEMIC DISEASES OF THE ESOPHAGUS

Connective Tissue Disorders
Scleroderma
Systemic lupus erythematosus
Polymyositis
Dermatomyositis
Mixed connective tissue disorder
Raynaud disease
Allergic Disease
Eosinophilic esophagitis
Metabolic Diseases
Amyloidosis
Diabetes mellitus
Hypothyroidism
Hyperthyroidism
Dermatologic Diseases
Epidermolysis bullosa
Pemphigus vulgaris
Pemphigoid
Erythema multiforme
Lichen planus
Behçet disease
Infectious Diseases
Histoplasmosis

Tuberculosis
Actinomycosis
Immunocompromised host
   Fungal: *Candida* species
   Viral: herpes simplex, cytomegalovirus
   Mycobacterial
   Bacterial: *Streptococcus viridans, Staphylococcus,* bacilli, *Treponema pallidum*
   Protozoal
Miscellaneous Disorders
Sarcoidosis
Crohn disease

ESOTROPIA

ICD-10CM #	H50.00	Unspecified esotropia
	H50.43	Accommodative component in esotropia
	H50.05	Alternating esotropia

Congenital.
Accommodative esotropia.
Myasthenia gravis.
Abducens palsy.
Pseudo-sixth nerve palsy.
Medial rectus entrapment (e.g., blowout fracture).
Posterior internuclear ophthalmoplegia.
Wernicke's encephalopathy.
Thyroid myopathy.
Chiari malformation.

EXANTHEMS[55]

ICD-10CM #	R21	Rash and other nonspecific skin eruption

Measles.
Rubella.
Erythema infectiosum (fifth disease).
Roseola exanthema.
Varicella.
Enterovirus.
Adenovirus.
Epstein-Barr virus.
Kawasaki disease.
Staphylococcal scalded skin.
Scarlet fever.
Meningococcemia.
Rocky Mountain spotted fever.

EYELID NEOPLASM

ICD-10CM #	C44.101	Unspecified malignant neoplasm of skin of unspecified eyelid, including canthus

MALIGNANT

Melanoma.
Basal cell carcinoma.
Squamous cell carcinoma.
Bowen's disease.
Sebaceous cell carcinoma.
Metastatic lymphoma/leukemia.

BENIGN

Melanocytic nevus.
Pilar, eccrine, or apocrine tumor.
Neurofibroma.
Keratosis.
Squamous papilloma.
Keratoacanthoma.

EYELID RETRACTION

ICD-10CM #	H02.89	Other specified disorders of eyelid

Congenital.
Graves' ophthalmopathy.
Myasthenia gravis.
Postsurgical.
Guillain-Barré syndrome.
Cerebellar disease.
Horizontal gaze palsy.
Partial palsy of superior rectus muscle.
Encephalitis.
Closed head injury.
Disseminated sclerosis.
Eye trauma.
Contact lens wear.
Proptosis.
Eyelid neoplasm.
Atopic dermatitis.
Herpes zoster ophthalmicus.
Botulinum toxin injection.
Cyclic oculomotor paralysis.
Spheroid wing meningioma.
Hepatic cirrhosis.
Down syndrome.
Essential hypertension.
Meningitis.
Paget's disease of bone.

EYE PAIN

ICD-10CM #	H57.13	Ocular pain, bilateral

Foreign body.
Herpes zoster.
Trauma.
Conjunctivitis.
Iritis.
Iridocyclitis.
Uveitis.
Blepharitis.
Ingrown lashes.
Orbital or periorbital cellulitis/abscess.
Sinusitis.
Headache.
Glaucoma.
Inflammation of lacrimal gland.
Tic douloureux.
Cerebral aneurysm.
Cerebral neoplasm.
Entropion.
Retrobulbar neuritis.
UV light.
Dry eyes.
Irritation or inflammation from eye drops, dust, cosmetics, etc.

FACIAL PAIN

ICD-10CM #	G50.1	Atypical facial pain

Differential Diagnosis

II

Infection, abscess.
Postherpetic neuralgia.
Trauma, posttraumatic neuralgia.
Tic douloureux.
Cluster headache, "lower-half headache."
Geniculate neuralgia.
Anxiety, somatization syndrome.
Glossopharyngeal neuralgia.
Carotidynia.

FACIAL PARALYSIS[55]

ICD-10CM #	G51.0	Bell's palsy

INFECTION

Bacterial: otitis media, mastoiditis, meningitis, Lyme disease.
Viral: herpes zoster, mononucleosis, varicella, rubella, mumps, Bell's palsy.
Mycobacterial: TB, meningitis, leprosy.
Miscellaneous: syphilis, malaria.

TRAUMA

Temporal bone fracture, facial laceration.
Surgery.

NEOPLASM

Malignant: squamous cell carcinoma, basal cell and adenocystic tumors, leukemia, parotid neoplasms, metastatic tumors.
Benign: facial nerve neuroma, vestibular schwannoma, congenital cholesteatoma.

IMMUNOLOGIC

Guillain-Barré syndrome, periarteritis nodosa.
Reaction to tetanus antiserum.

METABOLIC

Pregnancy.
Hypothyroidism.
DM.

FAILURE TO THRIVE

ICD-10CM #	R62.50	Unspecified lack of expected normal physiological development in childhood

PSYCHOSOCIAL/BEHAVIORAL

Inadequate diet because of poverty/food insufficiency, errors in food preparation.
Poor parenting skills (lack of knowledge of sufficient diet).
Child/parent interaction problems (autonomy struggles, coercive feeding, maternal depression).
Food refusal.
Rumination.
Parental cognitive or mental health problems.
Child abuse or neglect; emotional deprivation.

NEUROLOGIC

Cerebral palsy.
Hypothalamic and other CNS tumors (diencephalic syndrome).
Neuromuscular disorders.
Neurodegenerative disorders.

RENAL

Recurrent urinary tract infection.
Renal tubular acidosis.
Renal failure.

ENDOCRINE

Diabetes mellitus.
Diabetes insipidus.
Hypothyroidism/hyperthyroidism.
Growth hormone deficiency.
Adrenal insufficiency.

GENETIC/METABOLIC/CONGENITAL

Sickle cell disease.
Inborn errors of metabolism (organic acidosis, hyperammonemia, storage disease).
Fetal alcohol syndrome.
Skeletal dysplasias.
Chromosomal disorders.
Multiple congenital anomaly syndromes (VATER [vertebral defects, imperforate anus, tracheo-esophageal fistula, radial and renal dysplasia], CHARGE [coloboma, heart disease, atresia choanae, retarded growth and retarded development and/or central nervous system anomalies, genital hypoplasia, ear anomalies and/or deafness]).

GASTROINTESTINAL

Pyloric stenosis.
Gastroesophageal reflux.
Repair of tracheoesophageal fistula.
Malrotation.
Malabsorption syndromes.
Celiac disease.
Milk intolerance: lactose, protein.
Pancreatic insufficiency syndromes (cystic fibrosis).
Chronic cholestasis.
Inflammatory bowel disease.
Chronic congenital diarrhea states.
Short bowel syndrome.
Pseudoobstruction.
Hirschsprung disease.
Food allergy.

CARDIAC

Cyanotic heart lesions.
Congestive heart failure.
Vascular rings.

PULMONARY/RESPIRATORY

Severe asthma.
Cystic fibrosis; bronchiectasis.
Chronic respiratory failure.
Bronchopulmonary dysplasia.
Adenoid/tonsillar hypertrophy.
Obstructive sleep apnea.

MISCELLANEOUS

Collagen vascular disease.
Malignancy.
Primary immunodeficiency.
Transplantation.

INFECTIONS

Perinatal infection (TORCHES [toxoplasma, other, rubella, cytomegalovirus, herpes simplex]).
Occult/chronic infections.

Parasitic infestation.
Tuberculosis.
HIV.

FATIGUE

ICD-10CM #	R53.83	Other fatigue
	F48.0	Neurasthenia

Depression.
Anxiety, emotional stress.
Inadequate sleep.
Chronic fatigue syndrome.
Prolonged physical activity.
Pregnancy and postpartum period.
Anemia.
Hypothyroidism.
Medications (β-blockers, anxiolytics, antidepressants, sedating antihistamines, clonidine, methyldopa).
Viral or bacterial infections.
Sleep apnea syndrome.
Dieting.
Renal failure, CHF, COPD, liver disease.

FATIGUE, CHRONIC

ICD-10CM #	R53.83	Other fatigue
	F48.0	Neurasthenia

CHRONIC INFECTIONS

Hepatitis C.
Lyme disease.
Parasitic and fungal infections.
Tuberculosis.
Human immunodeficiency virus.
Xenotropic murine leukemia retrovirus.

SLEEP DISORDERS

Obstructive sleep apnea.
Restless leg syndrome.
Circadian rhythm disorder.
Upper airway resistance syndrome.
Narcolepsy/parasomnias.
Alpha-delta sleep disorder.

ENDOCRINE/METABOLIC DISORDERS

Addison's disease.
Cushing's syndrome.
Poorly controlled diabetes.
Thyroid disorders.
Hemochromatosis.
Hypopituitarism.
Diabetes insipidus.

GENERAL MEDICAL DISORDERS

Anemia (any cause).
Chronic renal/hepatic failure.
Malnutrition.
Medication side effects.
Chronic pain disorders.

PSYCHOLOGICAL

Mood disorders (depression, anxiety, bipolar).
Schizophrenia.
Posttraumatic stress disorder.
Anorexia nervosa/bulimia.
Childhood abuse and/or neglect.

CHRONIC INFLAMMATION

Rheumatoid arthritis.
Systemic lupus erythematosus.
Sjögren's syndrome.
Polymyositis/dermatomyositis.
Vasculitis.
Sarcoidosis.

CARDIOPULMONARY

Congestive heart failure.
Neurally mediated hypotension.
Postural orthostatic tachycardia syndrome.
Pulmonary hypertension.
Chronic obstructive pulmonary disease.
Mitral valve prolapse.

GASTROINTESTINAL

Celiac disease.
Inflammatory bowel disease.
Autoimmune hepatitis.
Hepatic cirrhosis.

MALIGNANCY

Lymphoma and occult malignancies.
Postchemotherapy syndrome.

NEUROLOGIC DISORDERS

Multiple sclerosis.
Myasthenia gravis.
Muscular dystrophies.
Parkinson's disease.
Early dementia.

LIFESTYLE FACTORS

Chronic overwork.
Persistent unresolved stress.
Inadequate exercise.
Morbid obesity (body mass index >40).
Alcoholism/drug abuse.

FATTY LIVER

| ICD-10CM # | K76.0 | Fatty (change of) liver, not elsewhere classified |
| | K76.89 | Other specified diseases of liver |

Obesity.
Alcohol abuse.
DM.
Acute fatty liver of pregnancy.
Medications (tetracycline, valproic acid, glucocorticoids, amiodarone, estrogen, methotrexate).
Reye's syndrome.
Wilson's disease.
Nonalcoholic steatosis.

FEVER AND CARDIOPULMONARY FAILURE[22]

| ICD-10CM # | R50.9 | Fever, unspecified |

DIFFERENTIAL DIAGNOSIS OF FEVER AND RAPIDLY PROGRESSIVE CARDIOPULMONARY FAILURE

Bacterial Infection

Severe community-acquired pneumonia.
Meningitis, endocarditis.
Rickettsial disease (babesiois, ehrlichiosis, Rocky Mountain spotted fever, scrub typhus, Mediterranean spotted fever).
Q-Fever (*Coxiella burnetii*).
Brucellosis.
Plague (*Yersinia pestis*).
Tularemia (*Francisella tularensis*).
Typhoid fever/salmonellosis.
Leptospirosis (*Leptospira interrogans*).
Anthrax.
Mycobacterial infections.

Viral Infections

Viral pneumonia (influenza, CMV, EBV, VZV, SARS).
Hantavirus.
Dengue fever and yellow fever.
Hemorrhagic fever (Lassa, Marburg, or Ebola viruses).

Fungal infections

Coccidiomycosis.
Cryptococcus.
Histoplasmosis.
Blastomycosis.

Parasitic infections

Malaria.
Leishmaniasis.
Schistosomiasis.
Strongyloides.

Noninfectious causes

Inflammatory:
- Rapid-onset interstitial pneumonia (acute interstitial pneumonia, acute hypersensitivity pneumonitis).
- Acute eosinophilic pneumonia.
- ARDS due to other causes (inhalation injury, drug overdose, trauma).

Rheumatologic disorders:
- Wegener granulomatosis, Churg-Strauss disease, Goodpasture's syndrome.
- Systemic lupus erythematosus, antiphospholipid syndrome.

Other:
- Malignancy, lymphoma, lymphoproliferative disease, leukemia.
- Pulmonary embolism, aortic dissection, acute myocardial infarction.
- Adrenal insufficiency, thyroid storm.

ARDS, acute respiratory distress syndrome; *CMV*, Cytomegalovirus; *EBV*, Epstein-Barr virus; *SARS*, severe acute respiratory syndrome; *VZV*, varicella zoster virus.

FEVER AND JAUNDICE

| ICD-10CM # | R50.9 | Fever, unspecified |
| | R17 | Unspecified jaundice |

Bacterial sepsis.
Cholangitis.
Hepatic abscess.
Leptospirosis.
Malaria.
Viral hepatitis.
Yellow fever.

FEVER AND LYMPHADENOPATHY

| ICD-10CM # | R59.9 | Enlarged lymph nodes, unspecified |
| | R50.9 | Fever, unspecified |

REGIONAL

Cervical
Streptococci.
Tuberculosis.
Viral upper respiratory infection.

Peripheral
Bartonella henselae.
Herpesviruses.
Lymphoma.
Metastatic cancer.
Sporotrichosis.
Streptococci.

Inguinal
Chancroid.
Herpes.
Lymphogranuloma venereum.
Syphilis (primary).

GENERALIZED

Cytomegalovirus.
Epstein-Barr virus.
HIV.
Lymphoma.
Sarcoidosis.
Syphilis (secondary).
Toxoplasmosis.
Viral hepatitis.

FEVER AND RASH

ICD-10CM #	R21	Rash and other nonspecific skin eruption
	R21	Rash and other nonspecific skin eruption
	R50.9	Fever, unspecified

Drug hypersensitivity: penicillin, sulfonamides, thiazides, anticonvulsants, allopurinol.
Viral infection: measles, rubella, varicella, erythema infectiosum, roseola, enterovirus infection, viral hepatitis, infectious mononucleosis, acute HIV.
Other infections: meningococcemia, staphylococcemia, scarlet fever, typhoid fever, *Pseudomonas* bacteremia, Rocky Mountain spotted fever, Lyme disease, secondary syphilis, bacterial endocarditis, babesiosis, brucellosis, listeriosis.
Serum sickness.
Erythema multiforme.
Erythema marginatum.
Erythema nodosum.
SLE.
Dermatomyositis.
Allergic vasculitis.
Pityriasis rosea.
Herpes zoster.

FEVER AND RASH IN ICU[72]

| ICD-10CM # | R21 | Rash and other nonspecific skin eruption |
| | R50.9 | Fever, unspecified |

Differential Diagnosis

DIFFERENTIAL DIAGNOSTIC CLINICAL FEATURES OF FEVER AND RASH IN THE ICU

Rash with Shock

Infectious causes: toxic shock syndrome, meningococcemia, postsplenectomy sepsis, overwhelming *Staphylococcus aureus* bacteremia/acute bacterial endocarditis, arboviral hemorrhagic fevers, hemorrhagic smallpox, *Vibrio vulnificus*, gas gangrene, dengue fever.
Noninfectious cause: systemic lupus erythematosus (on steroids).

RASH WITH MENTAL CHANGES

Infectious causes: Rocky Mountain spotted fever, meningococcemia (with meningitis), *S. aureus* acute bacterial endocarditis, Chikungunya fever, typhus.
Noninfectious cause: systemic lupus erythematosus.

RASH WITH CONJUNCTIVAL SUFFUSION

Infectious causes: Rocky Mountain spotted fever, dengue fever, arboviral hemorrhagic fevers, toxic shock syndrome.
Noninfectious cause: adult Kawasaki's disease.

RASH WITH RELATIVE BRADYCARDIA

Infectious causes: Rocky Mountain spotted fever, typhus, dengue fever, typhoid, arboviral hemorrhagic fevers.
Noninfectious cause: drug rash.

RASH WITH ABDOMINAL PAIN

Infectious causes: *V. vulnificus*, gas gangrene, *Clostridium sordelli*, scarlet fever.
Noninfectious causes: cholesterol emboli syndrome, systemic lupus erythematosus.

RASH ON PALMS AND SOLES

Infectious causes: Rocky Mountain spotted fever, toxic shock syndrome, chickenpox, smallpox, monkeypox, scarlet fever.
Noninfectious cause: drug rash.

RASH WITH DIARRHEA

Infectious causes: *V. vulnificus*, gas gangrene, toxic shock syndrome, dengue fever, arboviral hemorrhagic fevers.
Noninfectious cause: none.

RASH WITH EDEMA OF DORSUM OF HANDS/FEET

Infectious causes: Rocky Mountain spotted fever, toxic shock syndrome.
Noninfectious cause: adult Kawasaki's disease.

RASH WITH BULLAE

Infectious causes: *V. vulnificus*, *S. aureus* complicated skin/skin structure infection, gas gangrene.
Noninfectious cause: none.

RASH WITH HEART MURMUR

Infectious cause: acute bacterial endocarditis.
Noninfectious cause: systemic lupus erythematosus.
Rash with gangrene of nose tip
Infectious cause: *S. aureus* acute bacterial endocarditis.
Noninfectious causes: systemic lupus erythematosus, vasculitis.

RASH WITH CEREBROVASCULAR ACCIDENT

- Infectious causes: cholesterol emboli syndrome, *S. aureus* acute bacterial endocarditis.
- Noninfectious cause: none.

RASH WITH SPLENOMEGALY

Infectious causes: Rocky Mountain spotted fever, typhus.
Noninfectious causes: systemic lupus erythematosus, adult Kawasaki's disease.

RASH WITH DEAFNESS

- Infectious causes: Rocky Mountain spotted fever, typhus, meningococcal meningitis.
- Noninfectious cause: none.

RASH WITH HEPATOSPLENOMEGALY

Infectious causes: Rocky Mountain spotted fever, typhus.
Noninfectious cause: atypical measles.

RASH WITH HEPATOMEGALY

Infectious cause: typhus.
Noninfectious cause: none.

FEVER, AFTER TRAVEL TO THE TROPICS[3]

ICD-10CM # R50.81   Fever presenting with conditions classified elsewhere

CAUSES OF FEVER AFTER TRAVEL TO THE TROPICS

80% of Specific Infections Causing Fever (Includes Respiratory and Urinary Tract Infection)
Malaria.
Viral hepatitis.
Febrile illness unrelated to foreign travel.
Dengue fever.
Enteric fever (typhoid and paratyphoid fevers).
Other Causes
- Gastroenteritis.
- Rickettsia.
- Leptospirosis.
- Schistosomiasis.
- Amebic liver abscess.
- Tuberculosis.
- Acute HIV infection.
- Others.

FEVER, DRUG-INDUCED[31]

ICD-10CM # R50.2   Drug induced fever

SELECTED AGENTS ASSOCIATED WITH DRUG-INDUCED FEVER

Common
- Antimicrobial:
  - Amphotericin B.
  - β-Lactams.
  - Sulfonamides.
- Cardiovascular:
  - Procainamide.
  - Quinidine.
- Central nervous system:
  - Carbamazepine.
  - Phenytoin.
- Miscellaneous:
  - Bleomycin.
  - Interferon-α.
  - Interleukin-2.

Less Common
Antimicrobial:
  Clindamycin.
  Fluoroquinolones.
  Rifampin.
Cardiovascular:
  Diltiazem.
  Hydralazine.
Central nervous system:
  Haloperidol.
  Serotonin reuptake inhibitors.
Miscellaneous:
  Allopurinol.
  Cimetidine.
  Tacrolimus.

FEVER, HOSPITAL ASSOCIATED[31]

ICD-10CM #   R50.2   Drug induced fever
            R50.9   Fever, unspecified

SELECTED CAUSES OF HOSPITAL-ASSOCIATED FEVER

Common
Infectious:
  Clostridium difficile enterocolitis.
  Pneumonia.
  Surgical wound.
  Urinary tract.
  Vascular catheter.
Noninfectious:
  Drug-induced fever.
  Hematoma.
  Immediate postoperative state.
  Transfusion reaction.
  Venous thromboembolism.
Less Common
Infectious:
  Biliary tract disease.
  Endometritis.
  Intraabdominal abscess.
  Mediastinitis.
  Sinusitis.
Noninfectious:
  Adrenal insufficiency.
  Gout.
  Myocardial infarction.
  Organ infarction.
  Pancreatitis.

FEVER IN RETURNING TRAVELERS AND IMMIGRANTS[55]

ICD-10CM # R50.81 Fever presenting with conditions classified elsewhere

COMMON*

Acute respiratory tract infection (worldwide).
Gastroenteritis (worldwide) [foodborne, waterborne, fecal-oral].
Enteric fever, including typhoid (worldwide) [food, water].
Urinary tract infection (worldwide) [sexual contact].
Drug reactions [antibiotics, prophylactic agents, other] {rash frequent}.
Malaria (tropics, limited areas of temperate zones) [mosquitoes].
Arboviruses (Africa; tropics) [mosquitoes, ticks, mites].
Dengue (Asia, Caribbean, Africa) [mosquitoes].
Viral hepatitis (worldwide).
Hepatitis A (worldwide) [food, fecal-oral].
Hepatitis B (worldwide, especially Asia, sub-Saharan Africa) [sexual contact] {long incubation period}.
Hepatitis C (worldwide) [blood or sexual contact].
Hepatitis E (Asia, North Africa, Mexico, others) [food, water].
Tuberculosis (worldwide) [airborne, milk] {long period to symptomatic infection}.
Sexually transmitted diseases (worldwide) [sexual contact].

LESS COMMON*

Filariasis (Asia, Africa, South America) [biting insects] {long incubation period, eosinophilia}.
Measles (developing world) [airborne] {in susceptible individual}.
Amebic abscess (worldwide) [food].
Brucellosis (worldwide) [milk, cheese, food, animal contact].
Listeriosis (worldwide) [foodborne] {meningitis}.
Leptospirosis (worldwide) [animal contact, open fresh water] {jaundice, meningitis}.
Strongyloidiasis (warm and tropical areas) [soil contact] {eosinophilia}.
Toxoplasmosis (worldwide) [undercooked meat].

RARE

Relapsing fever (western Americas, Asia, northern Africa) [ticks, lice].
Hemorrhagic fevers (worldwide) [arthropod and nonarthropod transmitted].

---

*Diagnoses for which particular symptoms are indicative are in *italics*. Exposure to regions of the world that are most likely to be significant to the diagnosis are presented in (parentheses). Vectors, risk behaviors, and sources associated with acquisition are presented in [brackets]. Special clinical characteristics are listed within {braces}.

Yellow fever (tropics) [mosquitoes] {hepatitis}.
Hemorrhagic fever with renal syndrome (Europe, Asia, North America) [rodent urine] {renal impairment}.
Hantavirus pulmonary syndrome (western North America, other) [rodent urine] {respiratory distress syndrome}.
Lassa fever (Africa) [rodent excreta, person to person] {high mortality rate}
Other—chikungunya, Rift Valley, Ebola-Marburg, etc. (various) [insect bites, rodent excreta, aerosols, person to person] {often severe}.
Rickettsial infections {rashes and eschars}.
Leishmaniasis, visceral (Middle East, Mediterranean, Africa, Asia, South America) [biting flies] {long incubation period}.
Acute schistosomiasis (Africa, Asia, South America, Caribbean) [fresh water].
Chagas' disease (South and Central America) [reduviid bug bites] {often asymptomatic}.
African trypanosomiasis (Africa) [tsetse fly bite] {neurologic syndromes, sleeping sickness}.
Bartonellosis (South America) [sandfly bite] {skin nodules}.
HIV infection/AIDS (worldwide) [sexual and blood contact].
Trichinosis (worldwide) [undercooked meat] {eosinophilia}.
Plague (temperate and tropical plains) [animal exposures and fleas].
Tularemia (worldwide) [animal contact, fleas, aerosols] {ulcers, lymph nodes}.
Anthrax (worldwide) [animal, animal product contact] {ulcers}.
Lyme disease (North America, Europe) [tick bites] {arthritis, meningitis, cardiac abnormalities}.

FEVER, NONINFECTIOUS CAUSES[6]

ICD-10CM # R50.9 Fever, unspecified

DIFFERENTIAL DIAGNOSIS—NONINFECTIOUS CAUSES OF FEVER

Critical Diagnoses

Acute myocardial infarction.
Pulmonary embolism/infarction.
Intracranial hemorrhage.
Cerebrovascular accident.
Neuroleptic-malignant syndrome.
Thyroid storm.
Acute adrenal insufficiency.
Transfusion reaction.
Pulmonary edema.

Emergent Diagnoses

Congestive heart failure.
Dehydration.
Recent seizure.
Sickle cell disease.
Transplant rejection.
Pancreatitis.
Deep vein thrombosis.

Nonemergent Diagnoses

Drug fever.
Malignancy.
Gout.
Sarcoidosis.

Crohn's disease.
Postmyocardiotomy syndrome.

FEVER, POSTPARTUM[1]

ICD-10CM # R50.9 Fever, unspecified

MOST COMMON

Metritis.
Urinary tract infection.
Pneumonia.
Wound infection.
Mastitis.
Superficial or deep vein thrombosis.

MOST THREATENING

Toxic shock syndrome.
Necrotizing fasciitis.
Pelvic phlegmon.
Pelvic abscess.
Peritonitis.
Septic pelvic thrombosis.
Breast abscess.

FEVER, PERIODIC[26]

ICD-10CM # R50.9 Fever, unspecified

HEREDITARY

Nonhereditary
Infectious
Hidden infectious focus (e.g., aortoenteric fistula, Caroli's disease).
Recurrent reinfection (e.g., chronic meningococcemia, host defense defect).
Specific infection (e.g., Whipple's disease, malaria).
Noninfectious inflammatory disorder, e.g.:
 Adult-onset Still's disease.
 Juvenile chronic rheumatoid arthritis.
 Periodic fever, aphthous stomatitis, pharyngitis, and adenitis.
 Schnitzler syndrome.
 Behçet's syndrome.
 Crohn's disease.
 Sarcoidosis.
 Extrinsic alveolitis.
 Humidifier lung, polymer fume fever.
 Neoplastic.
Lymphoma (e.g., Hodgkin's disease, angioimmunoblastic lymphoma).
Solid tumor (e.g., pheochromocytoma, myxoma, colon carcinoma).
Vascular (e.g., recurrent pulmonary embolism)
Hypothalamic.
Psychogenic periodic fever.
Factitious or fraudulent.

FEVER, PEDIATRIC, ACUTE[1]

ICD-10CM # R50.9 Fever, unspecified

COMMON VIRAL INFECTIONS

Central Nervous System
Meningitis.
Encephalitis.
Tumor.

Brain abscess.

Head, Ears, Eyes, Nose, and Throat
Otitis media.
Pharyngitis.
Retropharyngeal abscess.
Peritonsillar abscess.
Lateral pharyngeal wall abscess.
Stomatitis.
Influenza.
Sinusitis.
Parotitis.
Cervical adenitis.
Periorbital cellulitis.
Orbital cellulitis or abscess.

Respiratory System
Bronchiolitis.
Croup.
Epiglottitis.
Pneumonia.
Upper respiratory infection.

Cardiovascular System
Myocarditis.
Pericarditis.
Endocarditis.

Genitourinary System
Urinary tract infection.
Tuboovarian abscess.

Gastrointestinal Tract
Acute viral gastroenteritis.
Bacterial enteritis.
Appendicitis.

Focal Soft Tissue Infections
Cellulitis.

Musculoskeletal System
Osteomyelitis.
Septic arthritis.

Rheumatologic Disorders
Acute rheumatic fever.
Juvenile rheumatoid arthritis.
Henoch-Schönlein purpura.

Vasculitis
Behçet syndrome.

Malignancy
Leukemia.
Lymphoma.
Sarcoma.

Systemic Illness
Bacteremia.
Viremia.
Sepsis.
Kawasaki disease.
Toxic shock syndrome.
Rocky Mountain spotted fever.
Meningococcemia.

MISCELLANEOUS DISORDERS

Toxicologic
Anticholinergic toxidromes.
Salicylate overdose.
Amphetamine.
Cocaine.

Endocrine
Thyrotoxicosis.

FEVER, RECURRENT OR PERIODIC, IN CHILDREN[46]

ICD-10CM #	R50.2	Drug induced fever
	R50.9	Fever, unspecified

INFECTIOUS DISEASES

Brucellosis.
Rat-bite fever.
Relapsing fever.

RHEUMATIC DISEASES

Juvenile idiopathic arthritis (systemic onset).
Behçet disease.
Systemic lupus erythematosus.
Relapsing polychondritis.
Crohn's disease.

HEREDITARY AUTOINFLAMMATORY SYNDROMES

Familial Mediterranean fever (FMF).
Cryopyrinopathies:
    Familial cold autoinflammatory syndrome (FCAS).
    Muckle-Wells syndrome (MWS).
    Chronic infantile neurologic cutaneous and articular (CINCA) syndrome, also called neonatal-onset multisystem inflammatory disease (NOMID).
Tumor necrosis factor receptor–associated periodic syndrome (TRAPS).
Hyperimmunoglobulinemia D with periodic fever syndrome (HIDS).

CYCLIC HEMATOPOIESIS

Hereditary form.
Acquired form.

IDIOPATHIC CONDITIONS

Periodic fever with aphthous stomatitis, pharyngitis, and adenitis (PFAPA).

FEVER WITH MACULOPAPULAR OR PETECHIAL RASH[59]

ICD-10CM #	R21	Rash and Nonspecific Skin Eruption
ICD-10CM #	R50.9	Fever, Unspecified

DIFFERENTIAL DIAGNOSIS OF FEVER WITH MACULOPAPULAR OR PETECHIAL RASH

Rocky Mountain spotted fever
Meningococcal disease
Enteroviral infection (echovirus and coxsackievirus)
Human herpesvirus 6 infection (roseola)
Human parvovirus B19 infection (fifth disease)
Epstein-Barr virus infection
Disseminated gonococcal infection
Murine typhus
Ehrlichiosis
Group A streptococcal pharyngitis
Mycoplasma pneumoniae Infection
Leptospirosis
Secondary syphilis
Kawasaki disease
Thrombotic thrombocytopenic purpura (TTP)
Drug reactions
Immune complex–mediated illness
Toxic shock syndrome
Erythema multiforme

Stevens-Johnson syndrome

FINGER LESIONS, INFLAMMATORY

ICD-10CM #	B08.8	Other specified viral infections characterized by skin and mucous membrane lesions
	L03.0	Cellulitis of finger and toe

Paronychia.
Herpes simplex type 1 (herpetic whitlow).
Dyshidrotic eczema (pompholyx).
Herpes zoster.
Bacterial endocarditis (Osler's nodes).
Psoriatic arthritis.

FLACCID PARALYSIS, ACUTE, DIFFERENTIAL DIAGNOSIS[46]

ICD-10CM #	G83.9	Paralytic syndrome, unspecified

Brain stem stroke.
Brain stem encephalitis.
Acute anterior poliomyelitis.
    Caused by poliovirus.
    Caused by other neurotropic viruses.
Acute myelopathy.
    Space-occupying lesions.
    Acute transverse myelitis.
Peripheral neuropathy.
    Guillain-Barré syndrome.
    Post-rabies vaccine neuropathy.
    Diphtheritic neuropathy.
    Heavy metals, biologic toxins, or drug intoxication.
    Acute intermittent porphyria.
    Vasculitic neuropathy.
    Critical illness neuropathy.
    Lymphomatous neuropathy.
Disorders of neuromuscular transmission.
    Myasthenia gravis.
    Biologic or industrial toxins.
    Tic paralysis.
Disorders of muscle.
    Hypokalemia.
    Hypophosphatemia.
    Inflammatory myopathy.
    Acute rhabdomyolysis.
    Trichinosis.
    Periodic paralyses.

FLATULENCE AND BLOATING[64]

ICD-10CM #	R14.0	Abdominal distension (gaseous)
	R14.1	Gas pain
	R14.2	Eructation
	R14.3	Flatulence

Ingestion of nonabsorbable carbohydrates.
Ingestion of carbonated beverages.
Malabsorption: pancreatic insufficiency, biliary disease, celiac disease, bacterial overgrowth in small intestine.
Lactase deficiency.

Irritable bowel syndrome.
Anxiety disorders.
Food poisoning, giardiasis.

FLUSHING[54]

ICD-10CM #	R23.2	Flushing

Physiologic flushing: menopause, ingestion of monosodium glutamate (Chinese restaurant syndrome), ingestion of hot drinks.
Drugs: alcohol (with or without disulfiram, metronidazole, or chlorpropamide), nicotinic acid, diltiazem, nifedipine, levodopa, bromocriptine, vancomycin, amyl nitrate.
Neoplastic disorders: carcinoid syndrome, VIPoma syndrome, medullary carcinoma of thyroid, systemic mastocytosis, basophilic chronic myelocytic leukemia, renal cell carcinoma.
Anxiety.
Agnogenic flushing.

FOLATE DEFICIENCY[40]

ICD-10CM #	D52.0	Dietary folate deficiency anemia
	D52.1	Drug-induced folate deficiency anemia
	D52.8	Other folate deficiency anemias
	D52.9	Folate deficiency anemia, unspecified

ETIOPATHOPHYSIOLOGIC CLASSIFICATION OF FOLATE DEFICIENCY

Nutritional causes:
  Decreased dietary intake:
    Poverty and famine.
    Institutionalized individuals (e.g., psychiatric, nursing homes), chronic debilitating disease.
    Prolonged feeding of infants with goat's milk, special slimming diets or food fads (i.e., folate-rich foods not consumed), cultural or ethnic cooking techniques (i.e., food folate destroyed).
  Decreased diet and increased requirements:
    Physiologic (e.g., pregnancy and lactation, prematurity, hyperemesis gravidarum, infancy).
    Pathologic (e.g., intrinsic hematologic diseases involving hemolysis with compensatory erythropoiesis, abnormal hematopoiesis, or bone marrow infiltration with malignant disease and dermatologic disease such as psoriasis).
Folate malabsorption:
  With normal intestinal mucosa:
    Some drugs (controversial).
    Congenital folate malabsorption (rare).
    With mucosal abnormalities (e.g., tropical and nontropical sprue, regional enteritis).
Defective cellular folate uptake:
  Familial aplastic anemia (rare).
  Acute cerebral folate deficiency.
Inadequate cellular use:
  Folate antagonists (e.g., methotrexate).

Hereditary enzyme deficiencies involving folate.
Drugs:
  Multiple effects on folate metabolism (e.g., alcohol, sulfasalazine, triamterene, pyrimethamine, trimethoprim-sulfamethoxazole, diphenylhydantoin, barbiturates).
Acute folate deficiency:
  Intensive care unit setting.
  Uncertain origin.

FOOT AND ANKLE PAIN[24]

ICD-10CM #	M25.5	Pain in joint
	M25.9	Joint disorder, unspecified

TENDON, LIGAMENT, AND MUSCLE

Gastrocnemius-soleus strain.
Plantaris rupture.
Anterior talofibular ligament tear.
Calcaneofibular ligament tear.
Deltoid ligament tear.
Anterolateral impingement due to complete tear of anterior talofibular ligament and anterior inferior tibiofibular ligament.
Syndesmotic impingement due to tear of syndesmosis.
Sinus tarsi syndrome (lateral hindfoot pain and instability due to injury of contents of the sinus and tarsal tunnel).
Achilles tendinitis.
Achilles rupture.
Plantar fasciitis.
Posterior tibial tendon dysfunction.
Flexor hallucis longus dysfunction.
Tibialis anterior tendon tear.
Peroneus brevis tendon tear.

BONE

Fracture of talus.
Calcaneal fracture.
Navicular fractures.
Lisfranc fracture-dislocation (fracture of the first metatarsal base with dislocation of medial cuneiform).
Metatarsal stress fracture.
Freiberg's infraction (sclerosis and flattening of the second metatarsal head due to trauma or microtrauma).
Avascular necrosis of the talus.
Fracture of the phalanges.
Fracture of the sesamoids.
Sesamoiditis.
Metatarsalgia.

JOINT

Osteoarthritis.
Gout.
Rheumatoid arthritis.
Other inflammatory arthritides.
Charcot's joint.
Osteochondral lesion of the talus.

PERIARTICULAR STRUCTURES

Shin splint (periosteal avulsion and periostitis at the insertion of the medial soleus due to repetitive overuse, such as in running and hiking).
Hallux rigidus.
Hallux valgus.
Ingrown toenail.
Toe deformities.
Turf toe (sprain of the first metatarsophalangeal joint due to hyperextension forces).
Plantar fasciitis.
Plantar fibromatosis.

NERVES

Anterior tarsal tunnel syndrome (involvement of deep peroneal nerve under the superficial fascia of the ankle).
Morton's neuroma.

VESSELS

Atherosclerosis.
Compartment syndrome.

REFERRED PAIN

Complex regional pain syndrome.

FOOT AND ANKLE PAIN, IN DIFFERENT AGE GROUPS[17]

ICD-10CM #	M25.579	Pain in unspecified ankle and joints of unspecified foot

COMMON CAUSES OF FOOT AND ANKLE PAIN IN DIFFERENT AGE GROUPS

Childhood (2-10 yr)
Intraarticular
Club foot.
Congenital midfoot and forefoot deformities.
Septic arthritis.
Periarticular
Osteomyelitis.
Adolescence (10-18 yr)
Intraarticular
Arch disorders (pes cavus, pes planus).
Periarticular
Osteomyelitis.
Tumors.
Early Adulthood (18-30 yr)
Intraarticular
Metatarsalgia.
Hallux valgus.
Hallux rigidus.
Osteochondritis.
Accessory ossicles.
Periarticular
Achilles tendonitis.
Achilles tendon rupture.
Fasciitis.
Referred
Lumbar spine.
Knee.
Adulthood (30-50 yr)
Intraarticular
Osteoarthritis.
Inflammatory arthritis.
Gout.
Metatarsalgia.
Hallux valgus.

Hallux rigidus.
Osteochondritis.
Accessory ossicles.
Periarticular
Ischemic foot pain.
Diabetes.
Bursitis.
Tendonitis.
Plantar fasciitis.
Corns.
Referred
Lumbar spine.
Knee.
Old Age (>50 yr)
Intraarticular
Osteoarthritis.
Inflammatory arthritis.
Gout.
Metatarsalgia.
Hallux valgus.
Hallux rigidus.
Periarticular
Ischemic foot pain.
Diabetes.
Bursitis.
Tendonitis.
Plantar fasciitis.
Corns.
Referred
Lumbar spine.
Knee.

FOOT DERMATITIS

| ICD-10CM # | B35.3 | Tinea pedis |
| | K25 | Unspecified contact dermatitis |

Tinea pedis.
Dyshidrotic eczema.
Tylosis (mechanically induced hyperkeratosis, fissuring, and dryness).
Allergic contact dermatitis.
Psoriasis.
Peripheral vascular insufficiency.
Neuropathic foot ulcers (DM, poorly fitting shoes).
Acquired plantar keratoderma.
Sézary's syndrome.

FOOTDROP

| ICD-10CM # | M21.379 | Foot drop, unspecified foot |

Peripheral neuropathy.
L5 radiculopathy.
Peroneal nerve compression.
Sciatic nerve palsy.
Scapuloperoneal syndromes.
Spasticity.
Peroneal nerve compression.
Myopathy.
Dystonia.

FOOT LESION, ULCERATING

| ICD-10CM # | S90.929A | Unspecified superficial injury of unspecified foot, initial encounter |

	S90.933A	Unspecified superficial injury of unspecified great toe, initial encounter
	S90.936A	Unspecified superficial injury of unspecified lesser toe(s), initial encounter
	L08.89	Other specified local infections of the skin and subcutaneous tissue

Cellulitis.
Plantar wart.
Squamous cell carcinoma.
Actinomycosis (Madura foot).
Plantar fibromatosis.
Pseudoepitheliomatous hyperplasia.

FOOT PAIN

| ICD-10CM # | M25.579 | Pain in unspecified ankle and joints of unspecified foot |

Trauma (fractures, musculoskeletal and ligamentous strain).
Inflammation (plantar fasciitis, Achilles tendonitis or bursitis, calcaneal apophysitis).
Arterial insufficiency, Raynaud's phenomenon, thromboangiitis obliterans.
Gout, pseudogout.
Calcaneal spur.
Infection (cellulitis, abscess, lymphangitis, gangrene).
Decubitus ulcer.
Paronychia, ingrown toenail.
Thrombophlebitis, postphlebitic syndrome.

FOOT PAIN BY AGE[46]

| ICD-10CM # | M25.579 | Pain in unspecified ankle and joints of unspecified foot |

0-6 YEARS
Poorly fitting shoes.
Foreign body.
Fracture.
Osteomyelitis.
Leukemia.
Puncture wound.
Drawing of blood.
Dactylitis.
Juvenile rheumatoid arthritis (JRA).

6-12 YEARS
Poorly fitting shoes.
Sever disease.
Enthesopathy (JRA).
Foreign body.
Accessory navicular.
Tarsal coalition.
Ewing sarcoma.
Hypermobile flatfoot.

Trauma (sprains, fractures).
Puncture wound.

12-20 YEARS
Poorly fitting shoes.
Stress fracture.
Foreign body.
Ingrown toenail.
Metatarsalgia.
Plantar fasciitis.
Osteochondroses (avascular necrosis).
Freiberg infarction.
Köhler disease.
Achilles tendinitis.
Trauma (sprains).
Plantar warts.
Tarsal coalition.

FOREARM AND HAND PAIN

ICD-10CM #	S59.809A	Other specified injuries of unspecified elbow, initial encounter
	S59.919A	Unspecified injury of unspecified forearm, initial encounter
	S69.80XA	Other specified injuries of unspecified wrist, hand and finger(s), initial encounter
	S69.90XA	Unspecified injury of unspecified wrist, hand and finger(s), initial encounter

Epicondylitis.
Tenosynovitis.
Osteoarthritis.
Cubital tunnel syndrome.
Carpal tunnel syndrome.
Trauma.
Herpes zoster.
Peripheral vascular insufficiency.
Infection (cellulitis, abscess).

FOREARM FRACTURES[3A]

| ICD-10CM # | S52 | Fracture of forearm |

TRAUMATIC
Wrist sprain, elbow sprain.
Ligamentous injuries, forearm contusions, hematomas.
Dislocations of the elbow or wrist (including nursemaid's elbow).

INFECTIOUS
Cellulitis of the forearm, abscesses.
Necrotizing fasciitis.

VASCULAR
Acute arterial occlusion.
Venous thrombosis.

NEUROLOGIC

Neurapraxias, carpal tunnel syndrome.
Systemic neurologic syndromes involving the nerves of the upper extremities.

ARTHRITIS

Septic joint, gonococcal arthritis, rheumatoid arthritis, osteoarthritis.
Pseudogout, gout.
Systemic lupus erythematosus, rheumatic fever, viral syndrome.
Reiter syndrome, Lyme disease, serum sickness.

OTHER

Olecranon bursitis, soft tissue masses.
Normal growth plates, nutrient vessels.

GAIT ABNORMALITY

ICD-10CM #	R26.0	Ataxic gait
	R26.1	Paralytic gait
	R26.89	Other abnormalities of gait and mobility
	R26.9	Unspecified abnormalities of gait and mobility

Parkinsonism.
Degenerative joint disease (hips, back, knees).
Multiple sclerosis.
Trauma, foot pain.
CVA.
Cerebellar lesions.
Infections (tabes, encephalitis, meningitis).
Sensory ataxia.
Dystonia, cerebral palsy, neuromuscular disorders.
Metabolic abnormalities.

GALACTORRHEA[55]

ICD-10CM #	N64.3	Galactorrhea not associated with childbirth

Prolonged suckling.
Drugs (INH, phenothiazines, reserpine derivatives, amphetamines, spironolactone and tricyclic antidepressants).
Major stressors (surgery, trauma).
Hypothyroidism.
Pituitary tumors.

GALLBLADDER SONOGRAPHIC NON-VISUALIZATION[62]

ICD-10CM #	Varies with Specific Diagnosis

CAUSES OF SONOGRAPHIC NONVISUALIZATION OF GALLBLADDER

Previous cholecystectomy
Physiologic contraction
Fibrosed gallbladder duct—chronic cholecystitis
Air-filled gallbladder or emphysematous cholecystitis
Tumefactive sludge
Agenesis of gallbladder
Ectopic location

GALLBLADDER WALL THICKENING[62]

ICD-10CM #	Varies with Specific Diagnosis

CAUSES OF GALLBLADDER WALL THICKENING

Generalized Edematous States
Congestive heart failure
Renal failure
End-stage cirrhosis
Hypoalbuminemia
Inflammatory Conditions
Primary
 Acute cholecystitis
 Cholangitis
 Chronic cholecystitis
Secondary
 Acute hepatitis
 Perforated duodenal ulcer
 Pancreatitis
 Diverticulitis/colitis
Neoplastic Conditions
Gallbladder adenocarcinoma
Metastases
Miscellaneous
Adenomyomatosis
Mural varicosities

GASTRIC DILATATION[33]

ICD-10CM #	K31.0	Acute dilatation of stomach

CAUSES OF A MASSIVELY DILATED STOMACH

Mechanical Gastric Outlet Obstruction
Duodenal or pyloric canal ulceration.
Carcinoma of pyloric antrum.
Extrinsic compression.
Paralytic Ileus
Surgery.
Trauma.
Peritonitis.
Pancreatitis.
Cholecystitis.
Diabetes mellitus.
Hepatic coma.
Drugs.
Gastric Volvulus
Intubation.
Air swallowing.

GASTRIC EMPTYING, DELAYED[3]

ICD-10CM #	K30	Functional dyspepsia

CAUSES OF DELAYED GASTRIC EMPTYING

Mechanical Causes
Peptic ulcer disease, scarred pylorus.
Malignancy: gastric cancer, gastric lymphoma, pancreatic cancer.

Gastric surgery: vagotomy, gastric resection, Roux-en-Y anastomosis.
Crohn's disease.
Endocrine and Metabolic Causes
Diabetes mellitus.
Hypothyroidism.
Hypoadrenal states.
Electrolyte abnormalities.
Chronic renal failure.
Medications.
Anticholinergics.
Opiates.
Dopamine agonists.
Tricyclic antidepressants.
Abnormalities of Gastric Smooth Muscle
Scleroderma.
Polymyositis, dermatomyositis.
Amyloidosis.
Pseudoobstruction.
Myotonic dystrophy.
Neuropathy.
Scleroderma.
Amyloidosis.
Autonomic neuropathy.
Central Nervous System or Psychiatric Disorders
Brain stem tumors.
Spinal cord injury.
Anorexia nervosa.
Stress.
Miscellaneous
Idiopathic gastroparesis.
Gastroesophageal reflux disease.
Nonulcer (functional) dyspepsia.
Cancer cachexia or anorexia.

GASTRIC EMPTYING, RAPID

ICD-10CM #	K30	Functional dyspepsia

Pancreatic insufficiency.
Dumping syndrome.
Peptic ulcer.
Celiac disease.
Promotility agents.
Zollinger-Ellison disease.

GENITAL DISCHARGE, FEMALE[21]

ICD-10CM #	N94.9	Unspecified condition associated with female genital organs and menstrual cycle

Physiologic discharge: cervical mucus, vaginal transudation, bacteria, squamous epithelial cells.
Individual variation.
Pregnancy.
Sexual response.
Menstrual cycle variation.
Infection.
Foreign body: tampon, cervical cap, other.
Neoplasm.
Fistula.
IUD.
Cervical ectropion.
Spermicide.

Differential Diagnosis

II

Nongenital causes: urinary incontinence, urinary tract fistula, Crohn's disease, rectovaginal fistula.

GENITAL LESIONS, INFECTIOUS CAUSES[9]

ICD-10CM # varies with specific diagnosis

INFECTIOUS CAUSES OF GENITAL LESIONS

Sexually Transmitted Infections
Syphilis:
- Primary (chancre).
- Secondary (condyloma latum).

Herpes simplex virus types 1 and 2.
Chancroid *(Haemophilus ducreyi)*.
Lymphogranuloma venereum.
Granuloma inguinale (donovanosis).
Human papillomavirus.
Sarcoptes scabiei.
Molluscum contagiosum.

Nonsexually Transmitted Infections
Folliculitis.
Tuberculosis.
Tularemia.
Histoplasmosis.
Candida (balanitis or vaginitis).
Amebiasis.

GENITAL LESIONS, NONINFECTIOUS CAUSES[9]

ICD-10CM # varies with specific diagnosis

NONVENEREAL CAUSES OF GENITAL LESIONS

Trauma.
Malignancies (e.g., squamous cell carcinoma).
Behçet's syndrome.
Lipschütz's vulvar ulcers.
Peyronie's disease.
Fixed-drug eruption.
Eczema.
Psoriasis.
Inflammatory bowel disease.
Contact dermatitis.
Lichen planus.
Hidradenitis suppurativa.
Postinflammatory hypopigmentation.
Aphthous ulcers (associated with human immunodeficiency virus).

GENITAL SORES[3]

ICD-10CM #	A60.9	Anogenital herpesviral infection, unspecified
	A51.0	Primary genital syphilis
	A63.0	Anogenital (venereal) warts
	A57	Chancroid
	A58	Granuloma inguinale
	A55	Chlamydial lymphogranuloma (venereum)

	N94.89	Other specified conditions associated with female genital organs and menstrual cycle
	N50.8	Other specified disorders of male genital organs

Herpes genitalis.
Syphilis.
Chancroid.
Lymphogranuloma venereum.
Granuloma inguinale.
Condyloma acuminatum.
Neoplastic lesion.
Trauma.

GLOMERULONEPHRITIS ASSOCIATED WITH MALIGNANCY[67]

ICD-10CM #	N00.9	Acute Nephritic Syndrome with Unspecified Morphologic Changes

Membranous glomerulonephritis:
Breast cancer
Lung cancer
Colon cancer
Prostate cancer
Graft-versus-host disease
Minimal change disease:
Hodgkin's lymphoma
Non-Hodgkin's lymphoma
Graft-versus-host disease
Case reports
Immunoglobulin A nephritis
Antineutrophil cytoplasmic antibody vasculitis
Focal segmental glomerulosclerosis

GLOMERULONEPHRITIS, RAPIDLY PROGRESSIVE[3]

ICD-10CM #	N05.9	Unspecified nephritic syndrome with unspecified morphologic changes

DIFFERENTIAL DIAGNOSIS OF RAPIDLY PROGRESSIVE GLOMERULONEPHRITIS

Linear Immune Staining
Anti-GBM disease.
Goodpasture's syndrome.
Rarely membranous glomerulonephritis.
Granular Immune Staining
Subacute bacterial endocarditis (past infectious).
Lupus nephritis.
Cryoglobulinemia.
Membranoproliferative glomerulonephritis (type II more than type I).
Immunoglobulin A nephropathy, Henoch-Schönlein purpura.
Idiopathic.

No Immune Staining (Pauci-immune)
Antineutrophil cytoplasmic antibody-associated vasculitis (Wegener granulomatosis, microscopic polyangiitis, Churg-Strauss syndrome).
Idiopathic.

GLOMERULOPATHIES, THROMBOTIC, MICROANGIOPATHIC[3]

ICD-10CM #	M31.1	Thrombotic microangiopathy

THROMBOTIC MICROANGIOPATHIC GLOMERULOPATHIES

Thrombotic thrombocytopenic purpura.
Hemolytic-uremic syndrome.
Malignant hypertension.
Scleroderma renal crisis.
Preeclampsia, eclampsia.
HELLP syndrome (hemolysis, elevated liver enzymes, low platelets).
Antiphospholipid antibody syndrome.
Drugs: oral contraceptives, quinine, cyclosporine, tacrolimus, ticlopidine, clopidogrel.

GLOMERULOSCLEROSIS, FOCAL SEGMENTAL[3]

ICD-10CM #	N03.3	Chronic nephritic syndrome with diffuse mesangial proliferative glomerulonephritis

ETIOLOGY OF FOCAL SEGMENTAL GLOMERULOSCLEROSIS (FSGS)

Primary idiopathic FSGS.
Secondary FSGS.
HIV (usually collapsing variant).
Reflux nephropathy.
Heroin abuse.
Sickle cell disease.
Oligomeganephronia.
Renal dysgenesis or agenesis (low nephron mass).
Radiation nephritis.
Familial podocytopathies.
NPHS1 (nephrin) mutation.
NPHS2 (podocin) mutation.
TRPC6 (cation channel) mutation.
ACTN4 (a-actinin 4 mutation).

GLOSSODYNIA[72]

ICD-10CM #	K14.6	Glossodynia

DENTURE-RELATED

Dentures (ill-fitting, monomer from denture base).
Dental plaque.
Oral parafunction.

INFECTIVE/DERMATOLOGIC

Candidiasis.
Lichen planus.

DEFICIENCY STATES

Iron, B12, folate, B2 (riboflavin), B6 (pyridoxine), zinc.

ENDOCRINE

Diabetes.
Myxedema.
Hormonal changes occurring during menopause.

NEUROLOGICALLY MEDIATED

Referred from tonsils, teeth.
Lingual nerve neuropathy.
Glossopharyngeal neuralgia.
Esophageal reflux.

IATROGENIC

Mouthwash.

XEROSTOMIA

PSYCHOGENIC

IDIOPATHIC

GLUCOCORTICOID DEFICIENCY[29]

ICD-10CM #	E27.1	Primary adrenocortical insufficiency
	E27.3	Drug-induced adrenocortical insufficiency

ACTH-independent causes.
TB.
Autoimmune (idiopathic).
Other rare causes:
    Fungal infection.
    Adrenal hemorrhage.
    Metastases.
    Sarcoidosis.
    Amyloidosis.
    Adrenoleukodystrophy.
    Adrenomyeloneuropathy.
    HIV infection.
    Congenital adrenal hyperplasia.
    Medications (e.g., ketoconazole).
ACTH-dependent causes:
    Hypothalamic-pituitary-adrenal suppression.
    Exogenous.
    Glucocorticoid.
    ACTH.
    Endogenous—cure of Cushing's syndrome.
Hypothalamic-pituitary lesions.
    Neoplasm:
        Primary pituitary tumor.
        Metastatic tumor.
        Craniopharyngioma.
    Infection:
        Tuberculosis.
        Actinomycosis.
        Nocardiosis.
Sarcoid.
Head trauma.
Isolated ACTH deficiency.

GOITER

ICD-10CM #	E01.2	Iodine-deficiency related (endemic) goiter, unspecified
	E04.9	Nontoxic goiter, unspecified
	E04.9	Nontoxic goiter, unspecified
	E07.1	Dyshormogenetic goiter
	E01.2	Iodine-deficiency related (endemic) goiter, unspecified
	E04.9	Nontoxic goiter, unspecified
	E04.2	Nontoxic multinodular goiter
	E04.0	Nontoxic diffuse goiter
	E05.10	Thyrotoxicosis with toxic single thyroid nodule without thyrotoxic crisis or storm

Thyroiditis.
Toxic multinodular goiter.
Graves' disease.
Medications (PTU, methimazole, sulfonamides, sulfonylureas, ethionamide, amiodarone, lithium, etc.).
Iodine deficiency.
Sarcoidosis, amyloidosis.
Defective thyroid hormone synthesis.
Resistance to thyroid hormone.

GRANULOMATOUS DERMATITIDES

ICD-10CM #	L92.9	Granulomatous disorder of the skin and subcutaneous tissue, unspecified

Granuloma annulare.
Sarcoidosis.
Necrobiosis lipoidica diabeticorum.
Cutaneous Crohn's disease.
Rheumatoid nodules.
Annular elastolytic giant cell granuloma (actinic granuloma).
Foreign body granuloma.

GRANULOMATOUS DISORDERS[63]

ICD-10CM #	M31.30	Wegener's granulomatosis without renal involvement
	K75.3	Granulomatous hepatitis
	L92.9	Granulomatous disorder of skin and subcutaneous tissue, unspecified

INFECTIONS

Fungi
Histoplasma.
Coccidioides.
Blastomyces.
Sporothrix.
Aspergillus.
Cryptococcus.
Protozoa
Toxoplasma.
Leishmania.
Metazoa
Toxocara.
Schistosoma.
Spirochetes
Treponema pallidum.
T. pertenue.
T. carateum.
Mycobacteria
M. tuberculosis.
M. leprae.
M. kansasii.
M. marinum.
M. avian.
Bacille Calmette-Guérin (BCG) vaccine.
Bacteria
Brucella.
Yersinia.
Other Infections
Cat-scratch disease.
Lymphogranuloma.

NEOPLASIA

Carcinoma.
Reticulosis.
Pinealoma.
Dysgerminoma.
Seminoma.
Reticulum cell sarcoma.
Malignant nasal granuloma.

CHEMICALS

Beryllium.
Zirconium.
Silica.
Starch.

IMMUNOLOGIC ABERRATIONS

Sarcoidosis.
Crohn's disease.
Primary biliary cirrhosis.
Wegener's granulomatosis.
Giant cell arteritis.
Peyronie's disease.
Hypogammaglobulinemia.
SLE.
Lymphomatoid granulomatosis.
Histiocytosis X.
Hepatic granulomatous disease.
Immune complex disease.
Rosenthal-Melkersson syndrome.
Churg-Strauss allergic granulomatosis.

LEUKOCYTE OXIDASE DEFECT

Chronic granulomatous disease of childhood.

Differential Diagnosis

II

EXTRINSIC ALLERGIC ALVEOLITIS

Farmer's lung.
Bird fancier's.
Mushroom worker's.
Suberosis (cork dust).
Bagassosis.
Maple bark stripper's.
Paprika splitter's.
Coffee bean.
Spatlese lung.

OTHER DISORDERS

Whipple's disease.
Pyrexia of unknown origin.
Radiotherapy.
Cancer chemotherapy.
Panniculitis.
Chalazion.
Sebaceous cyst.
Dermoid.
Sea urchin spine injury.

GRANULOMATOUS LIVER DISEASE

ICD-10CM #	K75.3	Granulomatous hepatitis

Sarcoidosis.
Wegener's granulomatosis.
Vasculitis.
Inflammatory bowel disease.
Allergic granulomatosis.
Erythema nodosum.
Infections (fungal, viral, parasitic).
Primary biliary cirrhosis.
Lymphoma.
Hodgkin's disease.
Drugs (e.g., allopurinol, hydralazine, sulfonamides, penicillins).
Toxins (copper sulfate, beryllium).

GREEN OR BLUE URINE

ICD-10CM #	R82	Other abnormal findings in urine

Pseudomonal urinary tract infection
Medications: triamterene, amitriptyline, IV cimetidine, IV promethazine.
Biliverdin.
Dyes (methylene blue, indigo carmine).

GROIN LUMP[72]

ICD-10CM #	R19.09	Other intraabdominal and pelvic swelling, mass and lump
	R22.9	Localized swelling, mass and lump, unspecified

COMMON CAUSES

Inguinal hernia.
Femoral hernia.
Lymph node.

OTHER CAUSES

Saphena varix.

Femoral artery aneurysm/pseudoaneurysm.
Psoas abscess.
Lipoma of the cord.
Encysted hydrocele of the cord (male).
Testicular maldescent (male).
Hydrocele of canal of Nuck (female).

GROIN MASSES

ICD-10CM #	R22.9	Localized swelling, mass and lump, unspecified
	S39.848A	Other specified injuries of external genitals, initial encounter

Hernia (inguinal, femoral).
Hydrocele.
Varicocele.
Sebaceous cyst.
Hidradenitis of inguinal apocrine glands.
Neoplasm: lymphoma, metastases.
Lipoma.
Hematoma.
Reactive inguinal adenopathy, femoral adenitis.
Folliculitis, psoas abscess.
Epididymitis, testicular torsion, ectopic testes.
Aneurysm or pseudoaneurysm of femoral artery.

GROIN PAIN[14]

ICD-10CM #	R52	Pain, unspecified

DIFFERENTIAL DIAGNOSIS OF GROIN PAIN

Surgery
Workers' Compensation.
Hernia.
Recurrent hernia.
Posthernia.
Orthopedic
Hip disorders.
    Acetabular labral tears.
    Avascular necrosis.
    Chondritis dissecans.
    Legg-Calvé-Perthes disease.
    Osteoarthritis.
    Pelvic stress fractures.
    Slipped femoral capital epiphysis.
    Synovitis.
Urology
Cystitis.
Epididymitis.
Nephrolithiasis.
Prostate cancer.
Prostatitis.
Torsion of testes.
Urethral extravasation.
Urinary tract infection.
Vas granuloma/fibrosis.
Dermatology
Lymphadenitis.
Psoriasis/burn.
Sebaceous cyst/hidradenitis.
Thrombophlebitis/cellulitis.

Neurosurgery
Disk disease.
Spinal injuries, inflammation, tumors.
Spondylolisthesis.
Spondylolysis.
Rheumatology
Connective tissue disorders.
Iliopsoas bursitis.
Osteitis pubis.
Systemic lupus erythematosus.
Neurology
Lumbosacral disorders.
Neurofibromatosis.
Infectious Disease
Herpes zoster.
HIV/tuberculosis.
Lyme disease.
Psoas abscess.
Sports Medicine
"Sports hernia" (adductor strains).
Gilmore's groin.
Vascular
Abscess hematoma.
Post-vein stripping.
Pseudoaneurysm.
Vascular graft.
Gastroenterology
Appendicitis/adhesions.
Diverticulitis.
Inflammatory retroperitoneal phlegmon (pancreatitis).
Meckel diverticulum.
Granulomatous colitis.
Gynecology
Cesarean section.
Cervical cancer.
Endometriosis.
Tubal/ovarian disorders.

GROIN PAIN, ACTIVE PATIENT[71]

ICD-10CM #	S39.848A	Other specified injuries of external genitals, initial encounter
	R52	Pain, unspecified

MUSCULOSKELETAL

Avascular necrosis of the femoral head.
Avulsion fracture (lesser trochanter, anterior superior iliac spine, anterior inferior iliac spine).
Bursitis (iliopectineal, trochanteric).
Entrapment of the ilioinguinal or iliofemoral nerve.
Gracilis syndrome.
Muscle tear (adductors, iliopsoas, rectus abdominis, gracilis, sartorius, rectus femoris).
Myositis ossificans of the hip muscles.
Osteitis pubis.
Osteoarthritis of the femoral head.
Slipped capital femoral epiphysis.
Stress fracture of the femoral head or neck and pubis.
Synovitis.

HERNIA-RELATED

Avulsion of the internal oblique muscle in the conjoined tendon.
Defect at the insertion of the rectus abdominis muscle.
Direct inguinal hernia.
Femoral ring hernia.
Indirect inguinal hernia.
Inguinal canal weakness.

UROLOGIC

Epididymitis.
Fracture of the testis.
Hydrocele.
Kidney stone.
Posterior urethritis.
Prostatitis.
Testicular cancer.
Torsion of the testis.
Urinary tract infection.
Varicocele.

GYNECOLOGIC

Ectopic pregnancy.
Ovarian cyst.
Pelvic inflammatory disease.
Torsion of the ovary.
Vaginitis.

LYMPHATIC ENLARGEMENT IN GROIN

GYNECOMASTIA

ICD-10CM #	N62	Hypertrophy of breast

Physiologic (puberty, newborns, aging).
Drugs (estrogen and estrogen precursors, 5-a reductase inhibitors, digitalis, testosterone and exogenous androgens, clomiphene, cimetidine, spironolactone, ketoconazole, amiodarone, ACE inhibitors, isoniazid, phenytoin, methyldopa, metoclopramide, phenothiazine).
Increased prolactin level (prolactinoma).
Liver disease.
Adrenal disease.
Thyrotoxicosis.
Increased estrogen production (hCG-producing tumor, testicular tumor, bronchogenic carcinoma).
Secondary hypogonadism.
Primary gonadal failure (trauma, castration, viral orchitis, granulomatous disease).
Defects in androgen synthesis.
Testosterone deficiency.
Klinefelter's syndrome.

HAIR LOSS[34]

ICD-10CM #	L63.8	Other alopecia areata
	L63.9	Alopecia areata, unspecified
	L64.0	Drug-induced androgenic alopecia
	L64.8	Other androgenic alopecia

GENERALIZED

Acute blood loss.*
Childbirth.
Crash diets (inadequate protein).
Drugs:
- Coumarin.
- Heparin.
- Propranolol.
- Vitamin A.
- High fever.
Hypothyroidism and hyperthyroidisms.
Physical stress (e.g., surgery).
Physiologic stress (e.g., neonate).
Psychologic stress.
Severe illness (e.g., systemic lupus erythematosis).
Cancer chemotherapeutic agents.
Poisoning:
- Thallium (rat poison).
- Arsenic.
Radiation therapy.
Secondary syphilis: "moth eaten" alopecia.

LOCALIZED

Androgenetic alopecia:†
- Male pattern.
- Female pattern.
Hirsutism.
Alopecia areata.
Trichotillomania.
Traction alopecia.
Scarring alopecia:
- Developmental defects: aplasia cutis.
Physical injury: burns, pressure.
Infection:
- Fungal: kerion.
- Bacterial: folliculitis, furuncle.
- Viral: herpes zoster.
Neoplasms:
- Metastatic carcinoma.
- Sclerosing basal cell carcinoma.
Lupus erythematosus.
Lichen planus.
Cicatricial pemphigoid.
Scleroderma.

*Diffuse, uniform loss, but many hairs left randomly distributed in area of loss.
†Most or all hair missing from involved area.

HALITOSIS

ICD-10CM #	R19.6	Halitosis

Tobacco use.
Alcohol use.
Dry mouth (mouth breathing, inadequate fluid intake).
Foods (onion, garlic, meats, nuts, protein drinks).
Disease of mouth or nose (infections, cancer, inflammation).
Medications (antihistamines, antidepressants).
Systemic disorders (diabetes, uremia).
GI disorders (esophageal diverticula, hiatal hernia, GERD, achalasia).
Sinusitis.
Pulmonary disorders (bronchiectasis, pneumonia, neoplasms, TB).

HAND PAIN AND SWELLING[15]

ICD-10CM #	729.5	Pain in limb

Trauma.
Gout.
Pseudogout.
Cellulitis.
Lymphangitis.
DVT of upper extremity.
Thrombophlebitis.
RA.
Remitting seronegative symmetrical synovitis with pitting edema (RS3PE).
Polymyalgia rheumatica.
Mixed connective tissue disease.
Scleroderma.
Rupture of the olecranon bursa.
Metzger's syndrome (neoplasia).
The puffy hand of drug addiction.
Reflex sympathetic dystrophy.
Eosinophilic fasciitis.
Sickle cell (hand-foot syndrome).
Leprosy.
Factitial (the rubber band syndrome).

HEADACHE[28]

ICD-10CM #	G44.1	Vascular headache, not elsewhere classified
	R51	Headache
	G44.209	Tension-type headache, unspecified, not intractable
	G44.009	Cluster headache syndrome, unspecified, not intractable
	G43.909	Migraine, unspecified, not intractable, without status migrainosus
	G44.1	Vascular headache, not elsewhere classified

Vascular: migraine, cluster headaches, temporal arteritis, hypertension, cavernous sinus thrombosis.
Musculoskeletal: neck and shoulder muscle contraction, strain of extraocular and/or intraocular muscles, cervical spondylosis, temporomandibular arthritis.
Infections: meningitis, encephalitis, brain abscess, sepsis, sinusitis, osteomyelitis, parotitis, mastoiditis.
Cerebral neoplasm.
Subdural hematoma.
Cerebral hemorrhage/infarct.
Pseudotumor cerebri.
Normal-pressure hydrocephalus (NPH).
Postlumbar puncture.
Cerebral aneurysm, arteriovenous malformations.
Posttrauma.
Dental problems: abscess, periodontitis, poorly fitting dentures.

Differential Diagnosis

II

Trigeminal neuralgia, glossopharyngeal neuralgia.

Otitis and other ear diseases.

Glaucoma and other eye diseases.

Metabolic: uremia, carbon monoxide inhalation, hypoxia.

Pheochromocytoma, hypoglycemia, hypothyroidism.

Effort induced: benign exertional headache, cough, headache, coital cephalalgia.

Drugs: alcohol, nitrates, histamine antagonists.

Paget's disease of the skull.

Emotional, psychiatric.

HEADACHE, ACUTE[20]

ICD-10CM # R51 Headache

DIFFERENTIAL DIAGNOSIS OF ACUTE HEADACHE

Evaluation of the first acute headache should exclude pathologic causes listed here before consideration of more common etiologies.

Increased intracranial pressure (ICP): Trauma, hemorrhage, tumor, hydrocephalus, pseudotumor cerebri, abscess, arachnoid cyst, cerebral edema.

Decreased ICP: After ventriculoperitoneal shunt, lumbar puncture, cerebrospinal fluid leak from basilar skull fracture.

Meningeal inflammation: Meningitis, leukemia, subarachnoid or subdural hemorrhage.

Vascular: Vasculitis, arteriovenous malformation, hypertension, cerebrovascular accident.

Bone, soft tissue: Referred pain from scalp, eyes, ears, sinuses, nose, teeth, pharynx, cervical spine, temporomandibular joint.

Infection: Systemic infection, encephalitis, sinusitis, etc.

First migraine.

HEADACHE AND FACIAL PAIN[70]

ICD-10CM # R51 Headache
G44.1 Vascular headache, not elsewhere classified

VASCULAR HEADACHES

Migraine

Migraine with headaches and inconspicuous neurologic features:

Migraine without aura ("common migraine").

Migraine with headaches and conspicuous neurologic features:

With transient neurologic symptoms:

Migraine with typical aura ("classic migraine").

Sensory, basilar, and hemiplegic migraine.

With prolonged or permanent neurologic features ("complicated migraine"):

Ophthalmoplegic migraine.

Migrainous infarction.

Migraine without headaches but with conspicuous neurologic features ("migraine equivalents"):

Abdominal migraine.

Benign paroxysmal vertigo of childhood.

Migraine aura without headache ("isolated auras," transient migrainous accompaniments).

Cluster Headaches

Episodic cluster headache ("cyclic cluster headaches").

Chronic cluster headaches.

Chronic paroxysmal hemicrania.

Other Vascular Headaches

Headaches of reactive vasodilation (fever, drug-induced, postictal, hypoglycemia, hypoxia, hypercarbia, hyperthyroidism).

Headaches associated with arterial hypertension:

Chronic severe hypertension (diastolic 120 mm Hg).

Paroxysmal severe hypertension (pheochromocytoma, some coital headaches).

Headaches caused by cranial arteritis:

Giant cell arteritis ("temporal arteritis").

Other vasculitides.

HEADACHES ASSOCIATED WITH DEMONSTRABLE MUSCLE SPASM

Headache caused by posturally induced or perilesional muscle spasm:

Headaches of sustained or impaired posture (e.g., prolonged close work, driving).

Headaches associated with cervical spondylosis and other diseases of cervical spine.

Myofascial pain dysfunction syndrome (headache or facial pain associated with disorders of teeth, jaws, and related structures, or "TMJ syndrome").

Headaches caused by psychophysiologic muscular contraction ("muscle contraction headaches," or tension-type headache associated with disorder of pericranial muscles).

HEADACHES AND FACIAL PAIN WITHOUT DEMONSTRABLE PHYSICAL SUBSTRATE

Headaches of uncertain etiology:

"Tension headaches" (tension-type headache unassociated with disorder of pericranial muscles).

Some forms of posttraumatic headache.

Psychogenic headaches (e.g., hypochondriacal, conversional, delusional, malingered).

Facial pain of uncertain etiology ("atypical facial pain").

COMBINED TENSION-MIGRAINE HEADACHES

Episodic migraine superimposed on chronic tension headaches.

Chronic daily headaches:

Associated with analgesic and/or ergotamine overuse ("rebound headaches").

Not associated with drug overuse.

HEADACHES AND HEAD PAINS CAUSED BY DISEASES OF EYES, EARS, NOSE, SINUSES, TEETH, OR SKULL

HEADACHES CAUSED BY MENINGEAL INFLAMMATION

Subarachnoid hemorrhage.

Meningitis and meningoencephalitis.

Others (e.g., meningeal carcinomatosis).

HEADACHES ASSOCIATED WITH ALTERED INTRACRANIAL PRESSURE ("TRACTION HEADACHES")

Increased Intracranial Pressure

Intracranial mass lesions (neoplasm, hematoma, abscess, etc.).

Hydrocephalus.

Benign intracranial hypertension.

Venous sinus thrombosis.

Decreased Intracranial Pressure

Post–lumbar puncture headaches.

Spontaneous hypoliquorrheic headaches.

HEADACHES AND HEAD PAINS CAUSED BY CRANIAL NEURALGIAS

Presumed Irritation of Superficial Nerves

Occipital neuralgia.

Supraorbital neuralgia.

Presumed Irritation of Intracranial Nerves

Trigeminal neuralgia ("tic douloureux").

Glossopharyngeal neuralgia.

HEADACHE, CHRONIC[20]

ICD-10CM # R51 Headache

DIFFERENTIAL DIAGNOSIS OF RECURRENT OR CHRONIC HEADACHES

Migraine (with or without aura).

Tension.

Analgesic rebound.

Caffeine withdrawal.

Sleep deprivation (e.g., in children with sleep apnea) or chronic hypoxia.

Tumor.

Psychogenic: Conversion disorder, malingering.

Cluster headache.

HEAD AND NECK, SOFT TISSUE MASSES

ICD-10CM # R22.0 Localized swelling, mass and lump, head
R22.1 Localized swelling, mass and lump, neck

Lipoma.

Pilar cyst.

Epidermal inclusion cyst.

Dermoid cyst.

Bone cyst.

Hemangioma.

Eosinophilic granuloma.

Other: facial nerve neuroma, teratoma, rhabdomyoma, rhabdomyosarcoma, branchial cleft cyst.

HEARING LOSS, ACUTE[50]

ICD-10CM # H91.23 Sudden idiopathic hearing loss, bilateral

Infectious: mumps, measles, influenza, herpes simplex, herpes zoster, CMV, mononucleosis, syphilis.

Vascular: macroglobulinemia, sickle cell disease, Berger's disease, leukemia, polycythemia, fat emboli, hypercoagulable states.

Metabolic: diabetes, pregnancy, hyperlipoproteinemia.

Conductive: cerumen impaction, foreign bodies, otitis media, otitis externa, barotrauma, trauma.

Medications: aminoglycosides, loop diuretics, antineoplastics, salicylates, vancomycin.

Neoplasm: acoustic neuroma, metastatic neoplasm.

HEARTBURN AND INDIGESTION[64]

ICD-10CM #	R12	Heartburn
	K30	Functional dyspepsia

Reflux esophagitis.

Gastritis.

Nonulcer dyspepsia.

Functional GI disorder (anxiety disorder, social/environmental stresses).

Excessive intestinal gas (ingestion of flatulogenic foods, GI stasis, constipation).

Gas entrapment (hepatitis or splenic flexure syndrome).

Neoplasm (adenocarcinoma of stomach or esophagus, lymphoma).

Gallbladder disease.

HEART FAILURE WITH PRESERVED LEFT VENTRICULAR EJECTION FRACTION[31]

ICD-10CM #	I50.9	Heart failure, unspecified

CAUSES OF (AND ALTERNATIVE EXPLANATIONS FOR) HEART FAILURE WITH PRESERVED LEFT VENTRICULAR EJECTION FRACTION (>45%-50%)

Inaccurate diagnosis of heart failure (e.g., pulmonary disease, obesity).

Inaccurate measurements of ejection fraction.

Systolic function overestimated by ejection fraction (e.g., mitral regurgitation).

Episodic, unrecognized systolic dysfunction.

Intermittent ischemia.

Arrhythmia.

Severe hypertension.

Alcohol abuse.

Diastolic dysfunction.

Abnormalities of myocardial relaxation:
Ischemia.
Hypertrophy.

Abnormalities of myocardial compliance:
Hypertrophy.
Aging.
Fibrosis.
Diabetes mellitus.
Infiltrative disease (amyloidosis, sarcoidosis).
Storage disease (hemochromatosis).
Endomyocardial disease (endomyocardial fibrosis, radiation, anthracyclines).

Pericardial disease (constriction, tamponade).

HEART FAILURE, ACUTE[6]

ICD-10CM #	I50.9	Heart failure, unspecified

COMMON PRECIPITATING CAUSES OF ACUTE HF

Systemic hypertension.

Myocardial infarction or ischemia.

Dysrhythmia.

Systemic infection.

Anemia.

Dietary, physical, environmental, and emotional excesses.

Pregnancy.

Thyrotoxicosis or hypothyroidism.

Acute myocarditis.

Acute valvular dysfunction.

Pulmonary embolus.

Pharmacologic complications.

HEART FAILURE, CHRONIC[10]

ICD-10CM #	I50.9	Heart failure, unspecified

Myocardial disease.

Coronary artery disease.
Myocardial infarction.[19]
Myocardial ischemia.

Chronic pressure overload.
Hypertension.
Obstructive valvular disease.

Chronic volume overload.
Regurgitant valvular disease.
Intracardiac (left-to-right) shunting.
Extracardiac shunting.

Nonischemic dilated cardiomyopathy.
Familial or genetic disorders.
Infiltrative disorders.
Toxic or drug-induced damage.
Metabolic disorder.
Viral or other infectious agents.

Disorders of rate and rhythm.
Chronic bradyarrhythmias.
Chronic tachyarrhythmias.

Pulmonary heart disease
Cor pulmonale.
Pulmonary vascular disorders.

High-output states.

Metabolic disorders.
Thyrotoxicosis.
Nutritional disorders (beriberi).

Excessive blood flow requirements.
Systemic arteriovenous shunting.
Chronic anemia.

[19]Indicates conditions that can also lead to HF with a preserved EF.

HEART FAILURE, CONGENITAL HEART DISEASE CAUSES[58]

ICD-10CM #	I50.9	Heart failure, unspecified

CAUSES OF CONGESTIVE HEART FAILURE RESULTING FROM CONGENITAL HEART DISEASE

Age of Onset	Cause
At birth:	HLHS.
	Volume overload lesions:
	• Severe tricuspid or pulmonary insufficiency.
	• Large systemic arteriovenous fistula.
First week	TGA.
	PDA in small premature infants.
	HLHS (with more favorable anatomy).
	TAPVR, particularly those with pulmonary venous obstruction.
	Others.
	Systemic arteriovenous fistula.
	Critical AS or PS.
1-4 wk	COA with associated anomalies.
	Critical AS.
	Large left-to-right shunt lesions (VSD, PDA) in premature infants.
	All other lesions previously listed.
4-6 wk	Some left-to-right shunt lesions such as ECD.
6 wk-4 mo	Large VSD.
	Large PDA.
	Others, such as anomalous left coronary artery from the PA.

AS, Aortic stenosis; *COA*, coarctation of the aorta; *ECD*, endocardial cushion defect; *HLHS*, hypoplastic left heart syndrome; *PA*, pulmonary artery; *PDA*, patent ductus arteriosus; *PS*, pulmonary stenosis; *TAPVR*, total anomalous pulmonary venous return; *TGA*, transposition of the great arteries; *VSD*, ventricular septal defect.

HEART FAILURE, PATHOGENIC CAUSES[31]

ICD-10CM #	I50.9	Heart failure, unspecified

IMPAIRED SYSTOLIC (CONTRACTILE) FUNCTION

Ischemic damage or dysfunction:
Myocardial infarction.
Persistent or intermittent myocardial ischemia.
Hypoperfusion (shock).

Chronic pressure overloading:
Hypertension.
Obstructive valvular disease.

Chronic volume overload:
    Regurgitant valvular disease.
    Intracardiac left-to-right shunting.
    Extracardiac shunting.
Nonischemic dilated cardiomyopathy:
    Familial/genetic disorders.
    Toxic/drug-induced damage
    Immunologically mediated necrosis.
    Infectious agents.
    Metabolic disorders.
    Infiltrative processes.
    Idiopathic conditions.

IMPAIRED DIASTOLIC FUNCTION (RESTRICTED FILLING, INCREASED STIFFNESS)

- Pathologic myocardial hypertrophy:
  Primary (hypertrophic cardiomyopathies).
  Secondary (hypertension).
Aging.
Ischemic fibrosis.
Restrictive cardiomyopathy:
  ○ Infiltrative disorders (amyloidosis, sarcoidosis).
  ○ Storage diseases (hemochromatosis, genetic abnormalities).
- Endomyocardial disorders.

MECHANICAL ABNORMALITIES

Intracardiac:
    Obstructive valvular disease.
    Regurgitant valvular disease.
    Intracardiac shunts.
    Other congenital abnormalities.
Extracardiac:
    Obstructive (coarctation, supravalvular aortic stenosis).
    Left-to-right shunting (patent ductus arteriosus).

DISORDERS OF RATE AND RHYTHM

- Bradyarrhythmias (sinus node dysfunction, conduction abnormalities).
- Tachyarrhythmias (ineffective rhythms, chronic tachycardia).

PULMONARY HEART DISEASE

- Cor pulmonale.
- Pulmonary vascular disorders.

HIGH-OUTPUT STATES

Metabolic disorders:
    Thyrotoxicosis.
    Nutritional disorders (beriberi).
    Excessive blood flow requirements:
        Chronic anemia.
        Systemic arteriovenous shunting.

HEART FAILURE, PREGNANCY

ICD-10CM # I50.9   Heart failure, unspecified

Congenital valvular heart disease exacerbated by pregnancy.
Peripartum cardiomyopathy.
Untreated thyrotoxicosis.

Hypothyroidism.
Pulmonary hypertension.
Myocardial infarction.

HEAT STROKE[1]

ICD-10CM # T67.0   Heatstroke and sunstroke

Sepsis.
Encephalitis.
Meningitis.
Brain abscess.
Malaria (cerebral falciparum).
Typhoid fever.
Tetanus.
Alcohol withdrawal syndrome.
Neuroleptic malignant syndrome (see Tips and Tricks box).
Anticholinergic toxicity.
Salicylate toxicity.
Phencyclidine hydrochloride (PCP), cocaine, or amphetamine toxicity.
Status epilepticus.
Cerebral hemorrhage.
Diabetic ketoacidosis.
Thyroid storm.

HEEL PAIN

ICD-10CM # M25.50   Pain in unspecified joint

Achilles tendonitis/tendinopathy (insertional, noninsertional).
Retrocalcaneal bursitis (superficial, deep).
Plantar fasciopathy.
Neuropathy (tarsal tunnel, posterior tibial nerve [medial calcaneal branch], abductor digiti quinti).
Calcaneal stress fracture.
Puncture wound, foreign body.
Cellulitis.
Spondyloarthropathy.
Fat pad atrophy.
Soft tissue tumor.
S1 radiculopathy.
Paget's disease of bone.
Haglund deformity.
Primary or metastatic bone tumor.

HEEL PAIN, PLANTAR[44]

ICD-10CM # M79.609   Pain in unspecified limb

SKIN

Keratoses.
Verruca.
Ulcer.
Fissure.

CONNECTIVE TISSUE

Fat
Atrophy.
Panniculitis.
Dense Connective Tissue
Inflammatory fasciitis.
Fibromatosis.
Enthesopathy.

Bursitis.
Bone (Calcaneus)
Stress fracture.
Paget's disease.
Benign bone cyst/tumor.
Malignant bone tumor.
Metabolic bone disease (osteopenia).
Nerve
Tarsal tunnel.
Plantar nerve entrapment.
S1 nerve root radiculopathy.
Painful peripheral neuropathy.

INFECTION

Dermatomycoses.
Acute osteomyelitis.
Plantar abscess.

MISCELLANEOUS

Foreign body.
Nonunion calcaneus fracture.
Psychogenic.
Idiopathic.

HEMARTHROSIS

ICD-10CM # T14.90   Injury, unspecified

Trauma.
Anticoagulant therapy.
Thrombocytopenia, thrombocytosis.
Bleeding disorders (e.g., von Willebrand's disease).
Charcot's joint.
Idiopathic.
Other: pigmented villonodular synovitis, hemangioma, synovioma, AV fistula, ruptured aneurysm.

HEMATEMESIS[72]

ICD-10CM # K92.0   Hematemesis

CAUSES OF HEMATEMESIS

Very Common
Gastric or duodenal ulcer or erosions.
Common
Mallory-Weiss tear (a laceration at the gastroesophageal junction).
Ulcerative esophagitis.
Esophageal varices.
Uncommon
Vascular malformations.
Ulcerated gastrointestinal stromal tumor.
Carcinoma of esophagus or stomach.
Aortoenteric fistula.

HEMATURIA

ICD-10CM # R31.9   Hematuria, unspecified

Use the mnemonic TICS:
  T (trauma): blow to kidney, insertion of Foley catheter or foreign body in urethra, prolonged and severe exercise, very rapid emptying of overdistended bladder.
  (tumor): hypernephroma, Wilms' tumor, papillary carcinoma of the bladder, prostatic and urethral neoplasms.

(toxins): turpentine, phenols, sulfonamides and other antibiotics, cyclophosphamide, NSAIDs.

I (infections): glomerulonephritis, TB, cystitis, prostatitis, urethritis, *Schistosoma haematobium,* yellow fever, blackwater fever.

(inflammatory processes): Goodpasture's syndrome, periarteritis, postirradiation.

C (calculi): renal, ureteral, bladder, urethra.

(cysts): simple cysts, polycystic disease.

(congenital anomalies): hemangiomas, aneurysms, AVM.

S (surgery): invasive procedures, prostatic resection, cystoscopy.

(sickle cell disease and other hematologic disturbances): hemophilia, thrombocytopenia, anticoagulants.

(somewhere else): bleeding genitals, factitious (drug addicts).

HEMATURIA, DIFFERENTIAL BASED ON AGE AND SEX

ICD-10CM # R31.9   Hematuria, unspecified

0 TO 20 YR

Acute urinary tract infections.
Acute glomerulonephritis.
Congenital urinary tract anomalies with obstruction.
Trauma to genitals.

20 TO 40 YR

Acute urinary tract infection.
Trauma to genitals.
Urolithiasis.
Bladder cancer.

40 TO 60 YR (WOMEN)

Acute urinary tract infection.
Bladder cancer.
Urolithiasis.

40 TO 60 YR (MEN)

Acute urinary tract infection.
Bladder cancer.
Urolithiasis.

60 YR AND OLDER (WOMEN)

Acute urinary tract infection.
Bladder cancer.
Vaginal trauma or irritation.
Urolithiasis.

60 YR AND OLDER (MEN)

Acute urinary tract infection.
Benign prostatic hyperplasia.
Bladder cancer.
Urolithiasis.
Trauma.

HEMATURIA, IN CHILDREN[6]

ICD-10CM # R31.9   Hematuria, unspecified

EXTRARENAL

Trauma.
Meatal stenosis or posterior urethral valves.

Exercise.
Menstruation or rectal bleeding.
Foreign bodies.
Cystitis, urethritis, or epididymitis.

INTRARENAL

Pyelonephritis.
Renal or bladder stones or tumors.
Poststreptococcal or idiopathic glomerulonephritis.
Acute interstitial nephritis.
Acute tubular necrosis.
Basement membrane glomerular disease.
Renal vein or arterial thrombosis.
Recurrent familial hematuria.
Polycystic kidney disease.

SYSTEMIC

Henoch-Schönlein purpura.
Systemic lupus erythematosus.
Hemolytic-uremic syndrome.
Infectious mononucleosis.
Sickle cell disease or other hemoglobinopathies.
Bacterial endocarditis or artificial cardiac valves.
Bleeding disorders, warfarin, or aspirin.
Medications such as amitriptyline or chlorpromazine, radiocontrast dyes.
Munchausen syndrome or factitious.

HEMIPARESIS/HEMIPLEGIA

| **ICD-10CM #** | G81.00 | Flaccid hemiplegia affecting unspecified side |
| | G81.10 | Spastic hemiplegia affecting unspecified side |

CVA.
Transient ischemic attack.
Cerebral neoplasm.
Multiple sclerosis or other demyelinating disorder.
CNS infection.
Migraine.
Hypoglycemia.
Subdural hematoma.
Vasculitis.
Todd's paralysis.
Epidural hematoma.
Metabolic (hyperosmolar state, electrolyte imbalance).
Psychiatric disorders.
Congenital disorders.
Leukodystrophies.

HEMOLYSIS AND HEMOGLOBINURIA

ICD-10CM #	P55.8	Other hemolytic diseases of newborn
	P55.9	Hemolytic disease of newborn, unspecified
	R82.3	Hemoglobinuria

Erythrocyte trauma (prosthetic cardiac valves, marching and severe trauma, extensive burns).
Infections (malaria, *Bartonella, Clostridium welchii*).

Brown recluse spider bite.
Incompatible blood transfusions.
Hemolytic-uremic syndrome.
Thrombotic thrombocytopenic purpura (TTP).
Paroxysmal nocturnal hemoglobinuria (PNH).
Drugs (penicillins, quinidine, methyldopa, sulfonamides, nitrofurantoin).
Erythrocyte enzyme deficiencies (e.g., exposure to fava beans in patients with glucose-6-phosphate dehydrogenase deficiency).

HEMOLYSIS, INTRAVASCULAR

| **ICD-10CM #** | D59.6 | Hemoglobinuria due to hemolysis from other external causes |
| | D59.8 | Other acquired hemolytic anemias |

- Infections.
- Exertional hemolysis (e.g., prolonged march).
- Valve hemolysis.
- Microangiopathic hemolytic anemia.
- Osmotic and chemical agents.
- Thermal injury.
- Cold agglutinins.
- Venoms (snakes, spiders).
- Paroxysmal nocturnal hemoglobinuria (PNH).

HEMOLYSIS, MECHANICAL

| **ICD-10CM #** | D59.4 | Other nonautoimmune hemolytic anemias |

Prosthetic heart valves.
Aortic stenosis.
Malignant hypertension.
Metastatic adenocarcinoma.
Traumatic exercise.
Renal transplants.
Renal cortical necrosis.
Glomerulonephritis.
Thrombotic thrombocytopenic purpura (TTP), hemolytic-uremic syndrome (HUS).
Renal vasculitis.
Scleroderma.
Diabetes mellitus.

HEMOPERITONEUM

| **ICD-10CM #** | K66.1 | Hemoperitoneum |

Ruptured Graafian follicle.
Ruptured spleen.
Ectopic pregnancy.
Traumatic laceration of liver.
Ruptured aneurysm.
Ruptured bladder.
Traumatic laceration of bowel, pancreas, uterus.

HEMOPTYSIS

| **ICD-10CM #** | R04.2 | Hemoptysis |

CARDIOVASCULAR

Pulmonary embolism/infarction.
Left ventricular failure.
Mitral stenosis.
AV fistula.

Differential Diagnosis

II

Severe hypertension.
Erosion of aortic aneurysm.

PULMONARY

Neoplasm (primary or metastatic).
Infection.
Pneumonia: *Streptococcus pneumoniae, Klebsiella pneumoniae, Staphylococcus aureus, Legionella pneumophila.*
Bronchiectasis.
Abscess.
TB.
Bronchitis.
Fungal infections (aspergillosis, coccidioidomycosis).
Parasitic infections (amebiasis, ascariasis, paragonimiasis).
Vasculitis: Wegener's granulomatosis, Churg-Strauss syndrome, Henoch-Schönlein purpura.
Goodpasture's syndrome.
Trauma (needle biopsy, foreign body, right-sided heart catheterization, prolonged and severe cough).
Cystic fibrosis, bullous emphysema.
Pulmonary sequestration.
Pulmonary AV fistula.
SLE.
Idiopathic pulmonary hemosiderosis.
Drugs: aspirin, anticoagulants, penicillamine.
Pulmonary hypertension.
Mediastinal fibrosis.

OTHER

Epistaxis, trauma.
Laryngeal bleeding (laryngitis, laryngeal neoplasm).
Hematologic disorders (clotting abnormalities, DIC, thrombocytopenia).

HEMORRHAGIC CYSTITIS[76]

ICD-10CM #	N39.0	Urinary Tract Infection

DIFFERENTIAL DIAGNOSIS FOR HEMORRHAGIC CYSTITIS[20]

Infectious
  Bacterial
  Viral (especially BK virus, adenovirus)
  Fungal
  Parasitic
Trauma
  External
  Postsurgical (e.g., transurethral resection of the bladder)
Malignancy
  Bladder primary
  Bladder invasion from local/distant primary
Vascular malformation
Chemical exposure
  Cyclophosphamide
  Ifosfamide
  Busulfan

Thiotepa
Temozolomide
Aniline dye
Ether
Nonoxynol-9 (accidental urethral insertion of vaginal contraceptive)
Radiation therapy history (e.g., prostate cancer, cervical cancer)
Medication induced
  Penicillin and derivatives (via immune reaction)
  Bleomycin
  Danazol
  Tiaprofenic
  Allopurinol
  Phensuximide
  Methenamine mandelate
  Acetic acid
Manifestation of systemic disease
  Amyloidosis
  Rheumatoid arthritis
  Crohn disease

HEPATIC CYSTS[70]

ICD-10CM #	Q44.6	Cystic disease of liver
	B67.8	Echinococcosis, unspecified, of liver

CONGENITAL HEPATIC CYSTS

Parenchymal: solitary cyst, polycystic disease.
Ductal: localized dilatation, multiple cystic dilatations of intrahepatic ducts (Caroli's disease).

ACQUIRED HEPATIC CYSTS

Inflammatory cysts: retention cysts, echinococcal cyst, amebic cyst.
Neoplastic cyst.
Peliosis hepatis.

HEPATIC GRANULOMAS[3]

ICD-10CM #	K75.3	Granulomatous hepatitis

INFECTIONS

Bacterial, spirochetal: TB and atypical mycobacterial infections, tularemia, brucellosis, leprosy, syphilis, Whipple's disease, listeriosis.
Viral: mononucleosis, CMV.
Rickettsial: Q fever.
Fungal: coccidioidomycosis, histoplasmosis, cryptococcal infections, actinomycosis, aspergillosis, nocardiosis.
Parasitic: schistosomiasis, clonorchiasis, toxocariasis, ascariasis, toxoplasmosis, amebiasis.

HEPATOBILIARY DISORDERS

Primary biliary cirrhosis, granulomatous hepatitis, jejunoileal bypass.

SYSTEMIC DISORDERS

Sarcoidosis, Wegener's granulomatosis, inflammatory bowel disease, Hodgkin's disease, lymphoma.

DRUGS/TOXINS

Beryllium, parenteral foreign material (starch, talc, silicone, etc.), phenylbutazone, α-methyldopa, procainamide, allopurinol, phenytoin, nitrofurantoin, hydralazine.

HEPATITIS, ACUTE[50]

ICD-10CM #	B17.8	Acute viral hepatitis, unspecified
	B15	Acute hepatitis A
	B16	Acute hepatitis B
	B17.1	Acute hepatitis C
	B17.2	Acute hepatitis E

Infectious:
  Hepatitis A, B, C, D, E.
  Epstein-Barr virus.
  Cytomegalovirus.
  Herpes simplex virus.
  Yellow fever.
  Leptospirosis.
  Q fever.
  HIV.
  Brucellosis.
  Lyme disease.
  Syphilis.
Noninfectious:
  Drug induced.
  Autoimmune.
  Ischemic.
  Acute fatty liver of pregnancy.
  Acute Budd-Chiari syndrome.
  Wilson's disease.

HEPATITIS, CHRONIC[50]

ICD-10CM #	K73.9	Chronic hepatitis, unspecified
	B18.0	Chronic viral hepatitis B with δ-agent
	B18.2	Chronic viral hepatitis C

Chronic viral hepatitis:
  Hepatitis B.
  Hepatitis C.
  Hepatitis D.
Autoimmune hepatitis and variant syndromes.
Hereditary hemochromatosis.
Wilson's disease.
α_1-Antitrypsin deficiency.
Fatty liver and nonalcoholic steatohepatitis.
Alcoholic liver disease.
Drug-induced liver disease.
Hepatic granulomas:
  Infectious.
  Drug induced.
  Neoplastic.
  Idiopathic.

HEPATITIS, IN CHILDREN[46]

ICD-10CM #	B17.9	Acute viral hepatitis, unspecified
	K73.9	Chronic hepatitis, unspecified

---

[20]Bleeding localized to bladder after diagnostic workup for gross hematuria with cystoscopy, urine cytology, and upper tract imaging is without clear cause of alternative bleeding source

CAUSES AND DIFFERENTIAL DIAGNOSIS OF HEPATITIS IN CHILDREN

Infectious
Hepatotropic viruses:
  HAV.
  HBV.
  HCV.
  HDV.
  HEV.
  Hepatitis non–A-E viruses.
Systemic infection that can include hepatitis:
  Adenovirus.
  Arbovirus.
  Coxsackievirus.
  Cytomegalovirus.
  Enterovirus.
  Epstein-Barr virus.
  "Exotic" viruses (e.g., yellow fever).
  Herpes simplex virus.
  Human immunodeficiency virus.
  Paramyxovirus.
  Rubella.
  Varicella zoster.
Other.

Nonviral liver infections
Abscess.
Amebiasis.
Bacterial sepsis.
Brucellosis.
Fitz-Hugh-Curtis syndrome.
Histoplasmosis.
Leptospirosis.
Tuberculosis.
Other.

Autoimmune
Autoimmune hepatitis.
Sclerosing cholangitis.
Other (e.g., systemic lupus erythematosus, juvenile rheumatoid arthritis).

Metabolic
α1-Antitrypsin deficiency.
Tyrosinemia.
Wilson disease.
Other.

Toxic
Iatrogenic or drug induced (e.g., acetaminophen).
Environmental (e.g., pesticides).

Anatomic
Choledochal cyst.
Biliary atresia.
Other.

Hemodynamic
Shock.
Congestive heart failure.
Budd-Chiari syndrome.
Other.

Nonalcoholic Fatty Liver Disease
Idiopathic.
Reye syndrome.
Other.

HEPATOMEGALY

ICD-10CM # R16.0 Hepatomegaly, not elsewhere classified

FREQUENT JAUNDICE
Infectious hepatitis.
Toxic hepatitis.
Carcinoma: liver, pancreas, bile ducts, metastatic neoplasm to liver.
Cirrhosis.
Obstruction of common bile duct.
Alcoholic hepatitis.
Biliary cirrhosis.
Cholangitis.
Hemochromatosis with cirrhosis.

INFREQUENT JAUNDICE
CHF.
Amyloidosis.
Liver abscess.
Sarcoidosis.
Infectious mononucleosis.
Alcoholic fatty infiltration.
Nonalcoholic steatohepatitis.
Lymphoma.
Leukemia.
Budd-Chiari syndrome.
Myelofibrosis with myeloid metaplasia.
Familial hyperlipoproteinemia type 1.
Other: amebiasis, hydatid disease of liver, schistosomiasis, kala-azar (Leishmania donovani), Hurler's syndrome, Gaucher's disease, kwashiorkor.

HEPATOMEGALY, BY SHAPE OF LIVER[72]

ICD-10CM # R16.0 Hepatomegaly, not elsewhere classified

DIFFUSELY ENLARGED AND SMOOTH

Massive
Metastatic disease.
Alcoholic liver disease with fatty infiltration.
Myeloproliferative diseases (e.g., polycythemia rubra vera, myelofibrosis).

Moderate
The above causes.
Hemochromatosis.
Hematologic disease (e.g., chronic myeloid leukemia, lymphoma).
Fatty liver (e.g., diabetes mellitus, obesity).
Infiltrative disorders (e.g., amyloid).

Mild
The above causes.
Hepatitis (viral, drugs).
Cirrhosis.
Biliary obstruction.
Granulomatous disorders (e.g., sarcoid).
HIV infection.

DIFFUSELY ENLARGED AND IRREGULAR
Metastatic disease.
Cirrhosis.
Hydatid disease.
Polycystic liver disease.

LOCALIZED SWELLINGS
Riedel's lobe (a normal variant—the lobe may be palpable in the right lumbar region).
Metastasis.

Large simple hepatic cyst.
Hydatid cyst.
Hepatoma.
Liver abscess (e.g., amebic abscess).

HERMAPHRODITISM[8]

ICD-10CM # Q56.3 Pseudohermaphroditism, unspecified
Q56.4 Indeterminate sex, unspecified

Female Pseudohermaphroditism
  Androgen exposure:
    Fetal source:
      21-Hydroxylase (P450 c21) deficiency.
      11β-Hydroxylase (P450 c11) deficiency.
      3β-Hydroxysteroid dehydrogenase II (3β-HSD II) deficiency.
      Aromatase (P450arom) deficiency.
      Maternal source.
      Virilizing ovarian tumor.
      Virilizing adrenal tumor.
      Androgenic drugs.
Undetermined origin:
    Associated with genitourinary and GI tract defects.

MALE PSEUDOHERMAPHRODITISM

- Defects in testicular differentiation:
  o Denys-Drash syndrome (mutation in WT1 gene).
  o WAGR syndrome (Wilms tumor, aniridia, genitourinary malformation, retardation).
  o Deletion of 11p13.
  o Camptomelic syndrome (autosomal gene at 17q24.3-q25.1) and SOX 9 mutation.
  o XY pure gonadal dysgenesis (Swyer syndrome).
  o Mutation in SRY gene.
  o Unknown cause.
  o XY gonadal agenesis.
- Deficiency of testicular hormones:
  o Leydig cell aplasia.
  o Mutation in LH receptor.
  o Lipoid adrenal hyperplasia (P450 scc) deficiency; mutation in StAR (steroidogenic acute regulatory protein).
  o 3α-HSD II deficiency.
  o 17-Hydroxylase/17, 20-lyase (P450 c17) deficiency.
  o Persistent Müllerian duct syndrome.
  o Gene mutations, Müllerian-inhibiting substance (MIS).
  o Receptor defects for MIS.
Defect in androgen action:
    5α-Reductase II mutations.
  Androgen receptor defects:
    Complete androgen insensitivity syndrome.
    Partial androgen insensitivity syndrome.
    Reifenstein and other syndromes.
    Smith-Lemli-Opitz syndrome.
Defect in conversion of 7-dehydrocholesterol to cholesterol.

TRUE HERMAPHRODITISM
XX.
XY.
XX/XY chimeras.

HICCUPS[43]

ICD-10CM #	R06.6	Hiccough

TRANSIENT HICCUPS

Sudden excitement, emotion.
Gastric distention.
Esophageal obstruction.
Alcohol ingestion.
Sudden change in temperature.

PERSISTENT OR CHRONIC HICCUPS

Toxic/metabolic: uremia, DM, hyperventilation, hypocalcemia, hypokalemia, hyponatremia, gout, fever.
Drugs: benzodiazepines, steroids, α-methyldopa, barbiturates.
Surgery/general anesthesia.
Thoracic/diaphragmatic disorders: pneumonia, lung cancer, asthma, pleuritis, pericarditis, myocardial infarction, aortic aneurysm, esophagitis, esophageal obstruction, diaphragmatic hernia or irritation.
Abdominal disorders: gastric ulcer or cancer, hepatobiliary or pancreatic disease, IBD, bowel obstruction, intraabdominal or subphrenic abscess, prostatic infection or cancer.
Central nervous system disorders: traumatic, infectious, vascular, structural.
Ear, nose, and throat disorders: pharyngitis, laryngitis, tumor, irritation of auditory canal.
Psychogenic disorders.
Idiopathic disorders.

HILAR AND MEDIASTINAL LYMPH NODE ENLARGEMENT[31]

ICD-10CM #	R59.0	Mediastinal adenopathy

DISORDERS ASSOCIATED WITH HILAR AND MEDIASTINAL LYMPH NODE ENLARGEMENT

Sarcoidosis.
Lymphoma.
Fungal disease.
Tuberculosis.
Metastatic cancer.
Silicosis, coal worker's pneumoconiosis, beryllium lung.

HIP PAIN, CHILDREN[50]

ICD-10CM #	S79.819A	Other specified injuries of unspecified hip, initial encounter
	S79.829A	Other specified injuries of unspecified thigh, initial encounter
	S79.919A	Unspecified injury of unspecified hip, initial encounter

TRAUMA

Hip or pelvis fractures.
Overuse injuries.

INFECTION

Septic arthritis.
Osteomyelitis.

INFLAMMATION

Transient synovitis.
Juvenile RA.
Rheumatic fever.

NEOPLASM

Leukemia.
Osteogenic or Ewing's sarcoma.
Metastatic disease.

HEMATOLOGIC DISORDERS

Hemophilia.
Sickle cell anemia.

MISCELLANEOUS

Legg-Calvé-Perthes disease.
Slipped capital femoral epiphysis.

HIP PAIN, DIFFERENTIAL DIAGNOSIS[37]

ICD-10CM #	M25.559	Pain in unspecified hip

ARTICULAR

Inflammatory joint disease
Rheumatoid arthritis.
Spondyloarthropathies.
Polymyalgia rheumatica.
Degenerative joint disease
Primary osteoarthritis.
Secondary osteoarthritis.
Metabolic joint diseases
Gout.
Pseudogout.
Ochronosis.
Hemochromatosis.
Wilson's disease.
Acromegaly.
Femoroacetabular impingement
Acetabular labral tear
Infections
Tumors
Benign.
Pigmented villonodular sclerosis.
Osteochondromatosis.
Malignant.
Synovial sarcoma.
Synovial metastasis.
Hemarthrosis.
In children:
Toxic synovitis.
Juvenile chronic arthritis.

REFERRED PAIN

Thoracolumbar spine.
Intraabdominal structures.
Retroperitoneal structures.

PERIARTICULAR

Bursitis.
Trochanteric.
Iliopsoas.
Ischiogluteal.
Tendinitis.
Trochanteric.
Adductor.
Acute calcific periarthritis.
Heterotropic ossification.

OSSEOUS

Bone lesions.
Fractures.
Neoplasms.
Infection.
Osteonecrosis of the femoral head.
Paget's disease.
Metabolic bone disease.
Stress fracture.
Transient osteoporosis.
In children:
Congenital dislocation of the hip.
Acetabular dysplasia.
Coxa vara.
Slipped capital femoral epiphysis.
Legg-Calvé-Perthes disease.
Rickets.

NEUROLOGIC

Entrapment neuropathies.
Lateral femoral cutaneous nerve (meralgia paresthetica).
Lumbar nerve root compression.
L2, L3, and L4.

VASCULAR

Atherosclerosis of aorta, iliac vessels.

HIP PAIN, IN DIFFERENT AGE GROUPS[17]

ICD-10CM #	M25.559	Pain in unspecified hip

COMMON CAUSES OF HIP PAIN IN DIFFERENT AGE GROUPS

Childhood (2-10 yr)
Intraarticular
Developmental dislocation of the hip.
Perthes' disease.
Irritable hip.
Rickets.
Periarticular
Osteomyelitis.
Referred
Abdominal.
Adolescence (10-18 yr)
Intraarticular
Slipped upper femoral epiphysis.
Torn labrum.
Periarticular
• Trochanteric bursitis.
• Snapping hip.
• Osteomyelitis.
• Tumors.

Referred

Abdominal.
Lumbar spine.

Early Adulthood (18-30 yr)

Intraarticular

- Inflammatory arthritis.
- Torn labrum.

Periarticular

- Bursitis.

Referred

Abdominal.
Lumbar spine.

Adulthood (30-50 yr)

Intraarticular

Osteoarthritis.
Inflammatory arthritis.
Osteonecrosis.
Transient osteoporosis.

Periarticular

Bursitis.

Referred

Abdominal.
Lumbar spine.

Old Age (>50 yr)

Intraarticular

Osteoarthritis.
Inflammatory arthritis.

Referred

Abdominal.
Lumbar spine.

HIP PAIN WITHOUT OBVIOUS FRACTURE[6]

| ICD-10CM # | R52 | Pain, unspecified |
| | M25.559 | Pain in unspecified hip |

DIFFERENTIAL DIAGNOSIS OF A PAINFUL HIP WITHOUT OBVIOUS FRACTURE

Referred pain (lumbar spine, hip, or knee).
Avascular necrosis of the femoral head.
Degenerative joint disease or osteoarthritis.
Herniation of a lumbar disk.
Diskitis.
Toxic synovitis of the hip.
Septic arthritis.
Bursitis.
Tendonitis.
Ligamentous injuries of the knee or hip.
Occult fracture.
Slipped capital femoral epiphysis.
Perthes' disease.
Tumor (lymphoma).
Deep venous thrombosis.
Arterial insufficiency.
Osteomyelitis.
Iliopsoas abscess.
Retroperitoneal hematoma.
Inguinal hernia.
Inguinal lymphadenopathy.
Genitourinary complaints.
Sports-related hernia.

HIRSUTISM

| ICD-10CM # | L68.0 | Hirsutism |

- Idiopathic: familial, possibly increased sensitivity to androgens.
- Menopause.
- Polycystic ovarian syndrome.
- Drugs: androgens, anabolic steroids, methyl-testosterone, minoxidil, diazoxide, phenytoin, glucocorticoids, cyclosporine.
- Congenital adrenal hyperplasia.
- Adrenal virilizing tumor.
- Ovarian virilizing tumor: arrhenoblastoma, hilus cell tumor.
- Pituitary adenoma.
- Cushing's syndrome.
- Hypothyroidism (congenital and juvenile).
- Acromegaly.
- Testicular feminization.

HIV INFECTION, ANORECTAL LESIONS[50]

| ICD-10CM # | B20 | Human immunodeficiency virus [HIV] disease |
| | Z21 | Asymptomatic human immunodeficiency virus [HIV] infection status |

COMMON CONDITIONS

- Anal fissure.
- Abscess and fistula.
- Hemorrhoids.
- Pruritus ani.
- Pilonidal disease.

COMMON STDs

Gonorrhea.
Chlamydia.
Herpes.
Chancroid.
Syphilis.
Condylomata acuminata.

ATYPICAL CONDITIONS

Infectious: TB, CMV, actinomycosis, cryptococcus.
Neoplastic: lymphoma, Kaposi's sarcoma, squamous cell carcinoma.
Other: idiopathic and ulcer.

HIV INFECTION, CHEST RADIOGRAPHIC ABNORMALITIES[50]

| ICD-10CM # | B20 | Human immunodeficiency virus [HIV] disease |
| | Z21 | Asymptomatic human immunodeficiency virus [HIV] infection status |

DIFFUSE INTERSTITIAL INFILTRATION

Pneumocystis jiroveci.

Cytomegalovirus.
Mycobacterium tuberculosis.
Mycobacterium avium complex.
Histoplasmosis.
Coccidioidomycosis.
Lymphoid interstitial pneumonitis.

FOCAL CONSOLIDATION

Bacterial pneumonia.
Mycoplasma pneumoniae.
Pneumocystis jiroveci.
Mycobacterium tuberculosis.
Mycobacterium avium complex.

NODULAR LESIONS

- Kaposi's sarcoma.
- Mycobacterium tuberculosis.
- Mycobacterium avium complex.
- Fungal lesions.
- Toxoplasmosis.

CAVITARY LESIONS

- Pneumocystis jiroveci.
- Mycobacterium tuberculosis.
- Bacterial infection.

PLEURAL EFFUSION

Kaposi's sarcoma.
(Small effusion may be associated with any infection).

ADENOPATHY

Kaposi's sarcoma.
Lymphoma.
Mycobacterium tuberculosis.
Cryptococcus.

PNEUMOTHORAX

Kaposi's sarcoma.

HIV INFECTION, COGNITIVE IMPAIRMENT[50]

| ICD-10CM # | B20 | Human immunodeficiency virus [HIV] disease |

EARLY TO MID-STAGE HIV DISEASE

Depression.
Alcohol and substance abuse.
Medication-induced cognitive impairment.
Metabolic encephalopathies.
HIV-related cognitive impairment.

ADVANCED HIV DISEASE (CD4+ <100/MM[3])

- Opportunistic infection of CNS.
- Neurosyphilis.
- CNS lymphoma.
- Progressive multifocal leukoencephalopathy.
- Depression.
- Metabolic encephalopathies.
- Medication-induced cognitive impairment.
- Stroke.
- HIV dementia.

HIV INFECTION, CUTANEOUS MANIFESTATIONS[43]

ICD-10CM #	B20	Human immunodeficiency virus [HIV] disease
	Z21	Asymptomatic human immunodeficiency virus [HIV] infection status

BACTERIAL INFECTION

Bacillary angiomatosis: Numerous angiomatous nodules associated with fever, chills, weight loss.

Staphylococcus aureus: Folliculitis, ecthyma, impetigo, bullous impetigo, furuncles, carbuncles.

Syphilis: May occur in different forms (primary, secondary, tertiary); chancre may become painful because of secondary infection.

FUNGAL INFECTION

- Candidiasis: Mucous membranes (oral, vulvovaginal), less commonly candida intertrigo or paronychia.
- Cryptococcoses: Papules or nodules that strongly resemble molluscum contagiosum; other forms include pustules, purpuric papules, and vegetating plaques.
- Seborrheic dermatitis: Scaling and erythema in the hair-bearing areas (eyebrows, scalp, chest, and pubic area).

ARTHROPOD INFESTATIONS

Scabies: Pruritus with or without rash, usually generalized but can be limited to a single digit.

VIRAL INFECTION

Herpes simplex: Vesicular lesion in clusters; perianal, genital, orofacial, or digital; can be disseminated.

Herpes zoster: Painful dermatomal vesicles that may ulcerate or disseminate.

HIV: Discrete erythematous macules and papules on the upper trunk, palms, and soles are the most characteristic cutaneous finding of acute HIV infection.

Human papillomavirus: Genital warts (may become unusually extensive).

Kaposi's sarcoma (herpesvirus): Erythematous macules or papules; enlarge at varying rates; violaceous nodules or plaques; occasionally painful.

Molluscum contagiosum: Discrete umbilicated papules commonly on the face, neck, and intertriginous sites (axilla, groin, or buttocks).

NONINFECTIOUS

Drug reactions: More frequent and severe in HIV patients.

Nutritional deficiencies: Mainly seen in children and patients with chronic diarrhea; diffuse skin manifestations, depending upon the deficiency.

Psoriasis: Scaly lesions; diffuse or localized; can be associated with arthritis.

Vasculitis: Palpable purpuric eruption (can resemble septic emboli).

HIV INFECTION, ESOPHAGEAL DISEASE

ICD-10CM #	B20	Human immunodeficiency virus [HIV] disease
	K21.9	Gastro-esophageal reflux disease without esophagitis

Candida infection.
Cytomegalovirus infection.
Aphthous ulcer.
Herpes simplex.

HIV INFECTION, HEPATIC DISEASE[50]

ICD-10CM #	B20	Human immunodeficiency virus [HIV] disease

VIRUSES

Hepatitis A.
Hepatitis B.
Hepatitis C.
Hepatitis D (with HBV).
Epstein-Barr virus.
Cytomegalovirus.
Herpes simplex virus.
Adenovirus.
Varicella-zoster virus.

MYCOBACTERIA

Mycobacterium avium complex.
Mycobacterium tuberculosis.

FUNGI

Histoplasma capsulatum.
Cryptococcus neoformans.
Coccidioides immitis.
Candida albicans.
Pneumocystis jiroveci.
Penicillium marneffei.

PROTOZOA

Toxoplasma gondii.
Cryptosporidium parvum.
Microsporida.
Schistosoma.

BACTERIA

Bartonella henselae (peliosis hepatis).

MALIGNANCY

Kaposi's sarcoma (HHV-8).
Non-Hodgkin's lymphoma.
Hepatocellular carcinoma.

MEDICATIONS

Zidovudine.
Didanosine.
Ritonavir.
Other HIV-1 protease inhibitors.
Fluconazole.
Macrolide antibiotics.
Isoniazid.
Rifampin.
Trimethoprim-sulfamethoxazole.

HIV INFECTION, LOWER GI TRACT DISEASE[50]

ICD-10CM #	B20	Human immunodeficiency virus [HIV] disease

CAUSES OF ENTEROCOLITIS

Bacteria
Campylobacter jejuni and other spp.
Salmonella spp.
Shigella flexneri.
Aeromonas hydrophila.
Plesiomonas shigelloides.
Yersinia enterocolitica.
Vibrio spp.
Mycobacterium avium complex.
Mycobacterium tuberculosis.
Escherichia coli (enterotoxigenic, enteroadherent).
Bacterial overgrowth.
Clostridium difficile (toxin).

Parasites
Cryptosporidium parvum.
Microsporida (*Enterocytozoon bieneusi, Septata intestinalis*).
Isospora belli.
Entamoeba histolytica.
Giardia lamblia.
Cyclospora cayetanensis.

Viruses
Cytomegalovirus.
Adenovirus.
Calicivirus.
Astrovirus.
Picobirnavirus.
Human immunodeficiency virus.

Fungi
Histoplasma capsulatum.

CAUSES OF PROCTITIS

Bacteria
Chlamydia trachomatis.
Neisseria gonorrhoeae.
Treponema pallidum.

Viruses
Herpes simplex.
Cytomegalovirus.

HIV INFECTION, MUSCULOSKELETAL DISORDERS[60]

ICD-10CM #	B20	Human immunodeficiency virus [HIV] disease

MUSCULOSKELETAL DISORDERS ASSOCIATED WITH HIV INFECTION

Joints, Ligaments, and Soft Tissues
Painful articular syndrome.
HIV-associated arthritis.

Reactive arthritis.
Septic arthritis.
Psoriatic arthritis.
Diffuse infiltrative lymphocytosis syndrome.
Systemic lupus erythematosus.
Rheumatoid arthritis.
Vasculitis (polyarteritis nodosa, drug induced).
Immune reconstitution inflammatory syndrome.
Cellulitis and soft tissue abscesses.
Fasciitis (including necrotizing fasciitis).
Bursitis and tenosynovitis.
Muscles
HIV myopathy.
Nucleoside reverse transcriptase inhibitor (NRTI) myopathy.
Muscle infections (pyomyositis, toxoplasmosis).
Other (rhabdomyolysis, non-Hodgkin's lymphoma, myasthenia gravis, nemaline [rod] myopathy, and inclusion body myositis).
Bones
Osteomyelitis.
Osteopenia and osteoporosis.
Osteonecrosis.
Hypertrophic osteoarthropathy.
Opportunistic Infections, HIV/AIDS-Defining Neoplastic Disorders, and Other Disorders Affecting Any Part of the Musculoskeletal System in HIV Infection
Neoplasia:
- Kaposi sarcoma.
- Non-Hodgkin's lymphoma.
- Hodgkin's lymphoma.
- Leiomyosarcoma.
- Ewing sarcoma.

Infection:
- Tuberculosis.
- Disseminated *Mycobacterium avium* complex infection.
- Coccidioidomycosis.
- Toxoplasmosis.
- Bacillary angiomatosis.

Other:
HIV-related lipodystrophy.
- HIV wasting syndrome.

HIV INFECTION, OCULAR MANIFESTATIONS[70]

| ICD-10CM # | B20 | Human immunodeficiency virus [HIV] disease |
| | Z21 | Asymptomatic human immunodeficiency virus [HIV] infection status |

EYELIDS
Molluscum contagiosum.
Kaposi's sarcoma.

CORNEA/CONJUNCTIVA
Keratoconjunctivitis sicca.
Bacterial/fungal ulcerative keratitis.
Herpes simplex.
Herpes zoster ophthalmicus.

Conjunctival microvasculopathy.
Kaposi's sarcoma.

RETINA, CHOROID, AND VITREOUS
Microvasculopathy.
Endophthalmitis.
Cytomegalovirus retinitis.
Acute retinal necrosis.
Syphilis.
Toxoplasmosis.
Pneumocystis choroidopathy.
Cryptococcosis.
Mycobacterial infection.
Intraocular lymphoma.
Candidiasis.
Histoplasmosis.

DRUGS ASSOCIATED WITH OCULAR TOXICITY
Rifabutin.
Didanosine.

NEUROOPHTHALMIC
Disc edema.
Primary or secondary optic neuropathy.
Cranial nerve palsies.

ORBITAL
Lymphoma.
Infection.
Pseudotumor.

HIV INFECTION, PULMONARY DISEASE[9,50]

| ICD-10CM # | B20 | Human immunodeficiency virus [HIV] disease |
| | I28.8 | Other diseases of pulmonary vessels |

RADIOGRAPHIC APPEARANCE
Diffuse Interstitial Infiltrates
Pneumocystis jiroveci.
Mycobacterium tuberculosis, especially with advanced human immunodeficiency virus disease.
Histoplasma capsulatum.
Coccidioides spp.
Cryptococcus neoformans.
Toxoplasma gondii.
Cytomegalovirus.
Influenza.
Lymphocytic interstitial pneumonitis.
Abacavir hypersensitivity.
Focal Consolidation
Pyogenic bacterial pneumonia from *Streptococcus pneumoniae, Haemophilus influenzae.*
M. tuberculosis.
Legionella spp.
Rhodococcus equi.
Hilar Adenopathy
M. tuberculosis.
H. capsulatum.
Coccidioides spp.
Non-Hodgkin's or Hodgkin's lymphoma.
Mycobacterium avium complex.

Cavitary Disease
Pyogenic bacterial pneumonia from *Pseudomonas aeruginosa, Staphylococcus aureus,* Enterobacteriaceae.
M. tuberculosis.
C. neoformans.
R. equi.
Aspergillus spp.
Nocardia spp.
Mycobacterium avium complex.
P. jiroveci.
Nodules or Masses
M. tuberculosis.
C. neoformans.
Aspergillus spp.
H. capsulatum.
Nocardia spp.
Non-Hodgkin's lymphoma.
Kaposi sarcoma.
Lung cancer.
Normal Radiograph
P. jiroveci.
M. tuberculosis.

CAUSES
Mycobacterial
M. tuberculosis.
M. kansasii.
M. avium complex.
Other nontuberculous mycobacteria.
Other Bacterial
Streptococcus pneumoniae.
Staphylococcus aureus.
Haemophilus influenzae.
Enterobacteriaceae.
Pseudomonas aeruginosa.
Moraxella catarrhalis.
Group A *Streptococcus.*
Nocardia spp.
Rhodococcus equi.
Chlamydia pneumoniae.
Fungal
Pneumocystis carinii.
Cryptococcus neoformans.
Histoplasma capsulatum.
Coccidioides immitis.
Aspergillus spp.
Blastomyces dermatitidis.
Penicillium marneffei.
Viral
Cytomegalovirus.
Herpes simplex virus.
Adenovirus.
Respiratory syncytial virus.
Influenza viruses.
Parainfluenza virus.
Other
Toxoplasma gondii.
Strongyloides stercoralis.
Kaposi's sarcoma.
Lymphoma.
Lung cancer.
Lymphocytic interstitial pneumonitis.
Nonspecific interstitial pneumonitis.
Bronchiolitis obliterans with organizing pneumonia.
Pulmonary hypertension.
Emphysema-like or bullous disease.
Pneumothorax.

Differential Diagnosis

II

Congestive heart failure.
Diffuse alveolar damage.
Pulmonary embolus.

HOARSENESS

ICD-10CM #	R49.8	Other voice and resonance disorders

Allergic rhinitis.
Infections (laryngitis, epiglottitis, tracheitis, croup).
Vocal cord polyps.
Voice strain.
Irritants (tobacco smoke).
Vocal cord trauma (intubation, surgery).
Neoplastic involvement of vocal cord (primary or metastatic).
Neurologic abnormalities (multiple sclerosis, ALS, parkinsonism).
Endocrine abnormalities (puberty, menopause, hypothyroidism).
Other (laryngeal webs or cysts, psychogenic, muscle tension abnormalities).

HYDROCEPHALUS

ICD-10CM #	G91.1	Obstructive hydrocephalus

Head trauma.
Brain neoplasm (primary or metastatic).
Spinal cord tumor.
Cerebellar infarction.
Exudative or granulomatous meningitis.
Cerebellar hemorrhage.
Subarachnoid hemorrhage.
Aqueductal stenosis.
Third ventricle colloid cyst.
Hindbrain malformation.
Viral encephalitis.
Metastases to leptomeninges.

HYPERCALCEMIA

ICD-10CM #	E83.52	Hypercalcemia

Malignancy: increased bone resorption via osteoclast-activating factors, secretion of PTH-like substances, prostaglandin E_2, direct erosion by tumor cells, transforming growth factors, colony-stimulating activity. Hypercalcemia is common in the following neoplasms:
  Solid tumors: breast, lung, pancreas, kidneys, ovary.
  Hematologic cancers: myeloma, lymphosarcoma, adult T-cell lymphoma, Burkitt's lymphoma.
Hyperparathyroidism: increased bone resorption, GI absorption, and renal absorption; etiology:
  Parathyroid hyperplasia, adenoma.
  Hyperparathyroidism or renal failure with secondary hyperparathyroidism.
Granulomatous disorders: increased GI absorption (e.g., sarcoidosis).
Paget's disease: increased bone resorption, seen only during periods of immobilization.
Vitamin D intoxication, milk-alkali syndrome; increased GI absorption.
Thiazides: increased renal absorption.

Other causes: familial hypocalciuric hypercalcemia, thyrotoxicosis, adrenal insufficiency, prolonged immobilization, vitamin A intoxication, recovery from acute renal failure, lithium administration, pheochromocytoma, disseminated SLE.

HYPERCALCEMIA, MALIGNANCY-INDUCED

ICD-10CM #	E83.52	Hypercalcemia

Lung carcinoma	(6% frequency, 35% of hypercalcemic cases)
Breast carcinoma	(10% frequency, 25% of hypercalcemic cases)
Multiple myeloma	(33% frequency, 10% of hypercalcemic cases)
Lymphoma	(4% of hypercalcemic cases)
Genitourinary cancer	(6% of hypercalcemic cases)

HYPERCAPNIA, PERSISTENT[70]

ICD-10CM #	R06.00	Dyspnea, unspecified
	R06.09	Other forms of dyspnea
	R06.89	Other abnormalities of breathing

Hypercapnia with normal lungs: CNS disturbances (CVA, parkinsonism, encephalitis), metabolic alkalosis, myxedema, primary alveolar hypoventilation, spinal cord lesions.
Diseases of the chest wall (e.g., kyphoscoliosis, ankylosing spondylitis).
Neuromuscular disorders (e.g., myasthenia gravis, Guillain-Barré syndrome, amyotrophic lateral sclerosis, muscular dystrophy, poliomyelitis).
COPD.

HYPERCOAGULABLE STATE, ASSOCIATED DISORDERS[40]

ICD-10CM #	D68.69	Other thrombophilia

Systemic lupus erythematosus in association with the presence of a lupus anticoagulant or antiphospholipid antibodies.

MALIGNANCY

Disease-related: includes migratory superficial thrombophlebitis (Trousseau syndrome), nonbacterial thrombotic endocarditis, thrombosis associated with chronic DIC, thrombotic microangiopathy.
Treatment-related: associated with the administration of various chemotherapeutic agents (L-asparaginase, mitomycin, some adjuvant chemotherapeutic agents for treatment of breast cancer, thalidomide or lenalidomide in conjunction with high doses of dexamethasone).
Infusion of prothrombin complex concentrates.

Nephrotic syndrome.
Heparin-induced thrombocytopenia.
Myeloproliferative disorders.
Paroxysmal nocturnal hemoglobinuria.
DIC, Disseminated intravascular coagulopathy.

HYPERGASTRINEMIA

ICD-10CM #	E16.4	Abnormal secretion of gastrin

Decreased gastrin release inhibition from medications (proton pump inhibitors [PPIs], H_2 receptor antagonists), vagotomy.
Chronic renal failure.
Hypochlorhydria due to atrophic gastritis, gastric carcinoma, pernicious anemia.
Gastrinoma (Zollinger-Ellison syndrome).
Pyloric obstruction.
Hyperplasia of antral G cells.
RA.

HYPERHIDROSIS[8]

ICD-10CM #	R61	Generalized hyperhidrosis

CORTICAL

Emotional.
Familial dysautonomia.
Congenital ichthyosiform erythroderma.
Epidermolysis bullosa.
Nail-patella syndrome.
Jadassohn-Lewandowsky syndrome.
Pachyonychia congenita.
Palmoplantar keratoderma.

HYPOTHALAMIC

Drugs
Antipyretics.
Emetics.
Insulin.
Meperidine.
Exercise Infection
Defervescence.
Chronic illness.
Metabolic
Debility.
DM.
Hyperpituitarism.
Hyperthyroidism.
Hypoglycemia.
Obesity.
Porphyria.
Pregnancy.
Rickets.
Infantile scurvy.
Cardiovascular
Heart failure.
Shock.
Vasomotor
Cold injury.
Raynaud phenomenon.
RA.
Neurologic
Abscess.
Familial dysautonomia.
Postencephalitic.
Tumor.

Miscellaneous
Chédiak-Higashi syndrome.
Compensatory.
Phenylketonuria.
Pheochromocytoma.
Vitiligo.
Medullary
Physiologic gustatory sweating.
Encephalitis.
Granulosis rubra nasi.
Syringomyelia.
Thoracic sympathetic trunk injury.
Spinal
Cord transection.
Syringomyelia.
Changes in Blood Flow
Mallucci syndrome.
Arteriovenous fistula.
Klippel-Trenaunay syndrome.
Glomus tumor.
Blue rubber bleb nevus syndrome.

HYPERKALEMIA

ICD-10CM # E87.5 Hyperkalemia

Pseudohyperkalemia.
Hemolyzed specimen.
Severe thrombocytosis (platelet count 0.106 ml).
Severe leukocytosis (white blood cell count 0.105 ml).
Fist clenching during phlebotomy.
Excessive potassium intake (often in setting of impaired excretion).
Potassium replacement therapy.
High potassium diet.
Salt substitutes with potassium.
Potassium salts of antibiotics.
Decreased renal excretion.
Potassium-sparing diuretics (e.g., spironolactone, triamterene, amiloride).
Renal insufficiency.
Mineralocorticoid deficiency.
Hyporeninemic hypoaldosteronism.
Tubular unresponsiveness to aldosterone (e.g., SLE, multiple myeloma, sickle cell disease).
Type 4 RTA.
ACE inhibitors.
Heparin administration.
NSAIDs.
Trimethoprim-sulfamethoxazole.
Beta-blockers.
Pentamidine.
Redistribution (excessive cellular release).
Acidemia (each 0.1 decrease in pH increases the serum potassium by 0.4 to 0.6 mEq/L). Lactic acidosis and ketoacidosis cause minimal redistribution.
Insulin deficiency.
Drugs (e.g., succinylcholine, markedly increased digitalis level, arginine, beta-adrenergic blockers).
Hypertonicity.
Hemolysis.
Tissue necrosis, rhabdomyolysis, burns.
Hyperkalemic periodic paralysis.

HYPERKALEMIA, DRUG-INDUCED[74]

ICD-10CM # E87.5 Hyperkalemia

IMPAIRED RENIN-ALDOSTERONE ELABORATION/FUNCTION

Cyclooxygenase inhibitors (NSAIDs).
β-Adrenergic antagonists.
Spironolactone.
Angiotensin-converting enzyme inhibitors and angiotensin II receptor blockers.
Heparin.

INHIBITORS OF RENAL POTASSIUM SECRETION

Potassium-sparing diuretics (amiloride, triamterene).
Trimethoprim.
Pentamidine.
Cyclosporine.
Digitalis overdose.
Lithium.

ALTERED POTASSIUM DISTRIBUTION

Insulin antagonists (somatostatin, diazoxide).
β-Adrenergic antagonists.
α-Adrenergic agonists.
Hypertonic solutions.
Digitalis.
Succinylcholine.
Arginine hydrochloride, lysine hydrochloride.

HYPERKALEMIA IN CHILDREN[67]

ICD-10CM # E87.5 Hyperkalemia

MOST RELEVANT CAUSES OF HYPERKALEMIA IN PEDIATRIC PATIENTS

Pseudohyperkalemia
Improper collection of blood
Hematologic disorders: leukocytosis, thrombocytosis, spherocytosis
Transcellular Shift of Potassium
Acidosis
Insulin deficiency
Hyperosmolality
Exercise with nonselective β-blockers
Familial hyperkalemic periodic paralysis
Increased Potassium Load
From exogenous origin: pharmacologic supplements
From endogenous origin (cellular lysis): burns, trauma, intravascular hemolysis, rhabdomyolysis, tumor mass destruction
Decreased Urinary Excretion
Renal failure
Mineralocorticoid deficiency
Addison's disease
Hypoaldosteronism
Mineralocorticoid resistance
Type 1 and type 2 pseudohypoaldosteronism
Renal tubular acidosis: type 4 and hyperkalemic form of type 1

"Hyperkalemic" drugs: potassium-sparing diuretics, trimethoprim, calcineurin inhibitors, blockers of the renin angiotensin aldosterone system

HYPERKINETIC MOVEMENT DISORDERS[57]

ICD-10CM #	F90.8	Attention-deficit hyperactivity disorder, other type
	E83.00	Disorder of copper metabolism, unspecified
	E83.01	Wilson's disease
	E83.09	Other disorders of copper metabolism
	G24.02	Drug induced acute dystonia
	G24.1	Genetic torsion dystonia

Chorea, choreoathetosis: drug-induced, Huntington's chorea, Sydenham's chorea.
Tardive dyskinesia (e.g., phenothiazines).
Hemiballismus (lacunar CVA near subthalamic nuclei in basal ganglia, metastatic lesions, toxoplasmosis [in AIDS]).
Dystonia (idiopathic, familial, drug-induced [prochlorperazine, metoclopramide]), Wilson's disease.
Liver failure.
Thyrotoxicosis.
SLE, polycythemia.

HYPERMAGNESEMIA

| ICD-10CM # | E83.40 | Disorders of magnesium metabolism, unspecified |
| | E83.41 | Hypermagnesemia |

Renal failure (decreased GFR).
Decreased renal excretion secondary to salt depletion.
Abuse of antacids and laxatives containing magnesium in patients with renal insufficiency.
Endocrinopathies (deficiency of mineralocorticoid or thyroid hormone).
Increased tissue breakdown (rhabdomyolysis).
Redistribution: acute DKA, pheochromocytoma.
Other: lithium, volume depletion, familial hypocalciuric hypercalcemia.

HYPEROSTOSIS, CORTICAL BONE[33]

| ICD-10CM # | M48.19 | Ankylosing hyperostosis [Forestier], multiple sites in spine |

DISORDERS ASSOCIATED WITH HYPEROSTOSIS OF CORTICAL BONE

Progressive diaphyseal dysplasia.
Endosteal hyperostosis.
Pachydermoperiostosis.
Hypertrophic oseoarthropathy.

Thyroid acropachy.
Hypervitaminosis A.
Paget's disease.
Infantile cortical hyperostosis.

HYPERPHOSPHATEMIA

ICD-10CM # E83.30 Disorder of phosphorus metabolism, unspecified

Excessive phosphate administration.
Excessive oral intake or IV administration.
Laxatives containing phosphate (phosphate tablets, phosphate enemas).
Decreased renal phosphate excretion.
Acute or chronic renal failure.
Hypoparathyroidism or pseudohypoparathyroidism.
Acromegaly, thyrotoxicosis.
Bisphosphonate therapy.
Tumor calcinosis.
Sickle cell anemia.
Transcellular shift out of cells.
Chemotherapy of lymphoma or leukemia, tumor lysis syndrome, hemolysis.
Acidosis.
Rhabdomyolysis, malignant hyperthermia.
Artifact: in vitro hemolysis.
Pseudohyperphosphatemia: hyperlipidemia, paraproteinemia, hyperbilirubinemia.

HYPERPHOSPHATEMIA IN CHILDREN[67]

ICD-10CM # E83.30 Disorder of phosphorus metabolism, unspecified

CAUSES OF HYPERPHOSPHATEMIA

Impaired Renal Excretion of Phosphate
Renal insufficiency
Hypoparathyroidism, pseudohypoparathyroidism
Transient parathyroid resistance of infancy
Acromegaly
Tumoral calcinosis
Hyperthyroidism
Juvenile hypogonadism
High ambient temperature
Heparin
Bisphosphonate etidronate
Increased Phosphate Intake
Exogenous Loads
Phosphate salts: laxatives and enemas
Vitamin D intoxication
Blood transfusion
White phosphorus burns
Liposomal amphotericin B
Fosphenytoin
Parenteral phosphate
Endogenous Loads
Crush injury
Rhabdomyolysis
Cytotoxic therapy of neoplasms: tumor lysis
Hemolysis
Malignant hyperthermia

Catabolic states
Lactic acidosis
Fulminant hepatitis
Transcellular Shift of Phosphate
Cellular shift in diabetes ketoacidosis
Metabolic acidosis
Respiratory acidosis
Miscellaneous
Hyperostosis

HYPERPIGMENTATION[13]

ICD-10CM # L81.4 Other melanin hyperpigmentation

Addison's disease.[21]
Arsenic ingestion.
ACTH- or MSH-producing tumors (e.g., oat cell carcinoma of the lung).
Drug induced (e.g., antimalarials, some cytotoxic agents).
Hemochromatosis ("bronze" diabetes).
Malabsorption syndrome (Whipple's disease and celiac sprue).
Melanoma.
Melanotropic hormone injection.
Pheochromocytoma.
Porphyrias (porphyria cutanea tarda and variegate porphyria).
Pregnancy.
Progressive systemic sclerosis and related conditions.
PUVA therapy (psoralen administration) for psoriasis and vitiligo.

ACTH, Adrenocorticotropic hormone; *MSH,* melanocyte-stimulating hormone; *PUVA,* psoralen plus ultraviolet A.
[21]Accentuation on sun-exposed surfaces.

HYPERPROLACTINEMIA[53]

ICD-10CM # E22.1 Hyperprolactinemia

PHYSIOLOGIC

Pregnancy.
Lactation.
Stress.
Sleep.
Coitus.
Exercise.

PATHOLOGIC

Hypothalamic-Pituitary Stalk Damage
Tumors: craniopharyngioma, suprasellar pituitary mass extension, meningioma, dysgerminoma, hypothalamic metastases.
Granulomas.
Infiltrations.
Rathke's cyst.
Irradiation.
Trauma: pituitary stalk section, sellar surgery, head trauma.
Pituitary
1. Prolactinoma.
2. Acromegaly.
3. Macroadenoma (compressive).
4. Idiopathic.
5. Plurihormonal adenoma.

6. Lymphocytic hypophysitis or parasellar mass.
7. Macroprolactinemia.
Systemic Disorders
Chronic renal failure.
Polycystic ovary syndrome.
Cirrhosis.
Pseudocyesis.
Epileptic seizures.
Cranial irradiation.
Chest: neurogenic chest wall trauma, surgery, herpes zoster.

PHARMACOLOGIC

Neuropeptide
Thyrotropin-releasing hormone.
Drug-Induced Hypersecretion
Dopamine receptor blockers:
  Phenothiazines: chlorpromazine, perphenazine.
  Butyrophenones: haloperidol.
  Thioxanthenes.
  Metoclopramide.
Dopamine synthesis inhibitors:
  α-Methyldopa.
Catecholamine depleters:
  Reserpine.
Cholinergic Agonist
Physostigmine.
Antihypertensives
Labetalol.
Reserpine.
Verapamil.
H_2 Antihistamines
Cimetidine.
Ranitidine.
Estrogens
Oral contraceptives.
Oral contraceptive withdrawal.
Anticonvulsant
Phenytoin.
Anesthetics
Neuroleptics.
Chlorpromazine.
Risperidone.
Promazine.
Promethazine.
Trifluoperazine.
Fluphenazine.
Butaperazine.
Perphenazine.
Thiethylperazine.
Thioridazine.
Haloperidol.
Pimozide.
Thiothixene.
Molindone.
Opiates and Opiate Antagonists
Heroin.
Methadone.
Apomorphine.
Morphine.
Antidepressants
Tricyclic antidepressants: chlorimipramine, amitriptyline.
Selective serotonin reuptake inhibitors: fluoxetine.

HYPERSPLENISM, ASSOCIATED CONDITIONS

ICD-10CM # D73.1   Hypersplenism

Cirrhosis.
Portal vein thrombosis.
Myeloproliferative diseases.
Lymphomas.
Leukemias.
Splenic vein thrombosis.
Autoimmune disease.
Sickle cell disease.
Thalassemias.
Gaucher's disease.
Niemann-Pick disease.

HYPERTENSION, ADRENOCORTICAL CAUSES[53]

ICD-10CM # I15.8   Other secondary hypertension

LOW RENIN AND HIGH ALDOSTERONE

Primary Aldosteronism

Aldosterone-producing adenoma (APA)	35% of cases
Bilateral idiopathic hyperplasia (IHA)	60% of cases
Primary (unilateral) adrenal hyperplasia	2% of cases
Aldosterone-producing adrenocortical carcinoma	<1% of cases
Familial hyperaldosteronism (FH)	
Glucocorticoid-remediable aldosteronism (FH type I)	<1% of cases
FH type II (APA or IHA)—<2% of cases	
Ectopic aldosterone-producing adenoma or carcinoma	<0.1% of cases

LOW RENIN AND LOW ALDOSTERONE

Hyperdeoxycorticosteronism

Congenital adrenal hyperplasia.
 11β-Hydroxylase deficiency.
 17α-Hydroxylase deficiency.
Deoxycorticosterone-producing tumor.
Primary cortisol resistance.
Apparent mineralocorticoid excess (AME)/11β-HSD[22] deficiency.
 Genetic: Type 1 AME.
Acquired: Licorice or carbenoxolone ingestion (type 1 AME), Cushing's syndrome (type 2 AME).

[22]HSD, hydroxysteroid dehydrogenase

Cushing's Syndrome

Exogenous glucocorticoid administration—most common cause.
Endogenous.
 ACTH[23]-dependent—85% of cases: Pituitary, ectopic.
 ACTH-independent—15% of cases: Unilateral adrenal disease (adenoma or carcinoma), bilateral adrenal disease (massive macronodular hyperplasia [rare], primary pigmented nodular adrenal disease [rare]).

[23]ACTH, corticotropin

HYPERTENSION, ENDOCRINE CAUSES[53]

ICD-10CM # I15.8   Other secondary hypertension

ADRENAL-DEPENDENT CAUSES

Pheochromocytoma.
Primary aldosteronism.
Hyperdeoxycorticosteronism.
 Congenital adrenal hyperplasia: 11β-Hydroxylase deficiency, 17α-hydroxylase deficiency.
 Deoxycorticosterone-producing tumor.
 Primary cortisol resistance.
Cushing's syndrome.

AME/11β-HSD (HYDROXYSTEROID DEHYDROGENASE) DEFICIENCY

Genetic.
 Type 1 apparent mineralocorticoid excess (AME).
Acquired.
 Licorice or carbenoxolone ingestion (type 1 AME).
 Cushing's syndrome (type 2 AME).

THYROID-DEPENDENT CAUSES

Hypothyroidism.
Hyperthyroidism.

PARATHYROID-DEPENDENT CAUSES

Hyperparathyroidism.

PITUITARY-DEPENDENT CAUSES

Acromegaly.
Cushing's syndrome.

HYPERTENSION, IN CHILDREN[6]

ICD-10CM # I10   Essential (primary) hypertension

PRIMARY

Essential hypertension.

SECONDARY

Renal

Glomerulonephritis.
Henoch-Schönlein purpura.
Pyelonephritis.
Obstruction of reflux.
Polycystic kidney disease.
Diabetic nephropathy.
Trauma.
Renal transplant or hemodialysis.
Tuberous sclerosis.
Systemic lupus nephritis.

Endocrine

Pheochromocytoma.
Cushing's syndrome.
Congenital adrenal hyperplasia.
Corticosteroid treatment.
Hyperthyroidism.
Neuroblastoma.
Ovarian tumor.

Cardiac

Congestive heart failure.
Coarctation of the aorta.

Vascular

Hemolytic-uremic syndrome.
Kawasaki syndrome.
Renal artery thrombosis or stenosis.

Neurologic

Central nervous system tumor or infection.
Central nervous system trauma or abuse.
Increased intracranial pressure.
Guillain-Barré syndrome.

Neoplastic

Neuroblastoma.
Wilms' tumor.
Pheochromocytoma.
Adrenal carcinoma.

Drugs

Corticosteroids.
Cocaine.
Sympathomimetics.
Oral contraceptives.
Phencyclidine.
Beta-blocker or clonidine withdrawal.
Lead, mercury.

Others

Iatrogenic fluid overload.
Volume overload from end-stage renal disease.

HYPERTENSION, RESISTANT[67]

ICD-10CM # I10   Essential (primary) hypertension
ICD-10CM # I15   Secondary Hypertension

CAUSES OF RESISTANT HYPERTENSION

Pseudoresistance
 White coat hypertension or office elevations
 Pseudohypertension in older patients
 Use of small cuff on very obese arm
Nonadherence to therapeutic regimen
Volume overload
Drug-related causes
 Antihypertensive drug dosage too low
 Wrong type of diuretic
 Inappropriate combinations of antihypertensive drugs
Drug actions and interactions
 Sympathomimetics
 Nasal decongestants
 Appetite suppressants

Cocaine
Caffeine
Oral contraceptives
Adrenal steroids
Licorice (may be found in chewing tobacco)
Cyclosporine, tacrolimus
Erythropoiesis-stimulating agents (ESAs) and
　Erythropoietin
Antidepressants
Nonsteroidal antiinflammatory drugs
Concomitant conditions
　Obesity
　Sleep apnea
　Ethanol intake >1 oz (30 mL)/day
　Anxiety, hyperventilation
Secondary causes of hypertension
　Renovascular hypertension
　Primary aldosteronism
　Pheochromocytoma
　Hypothyroidism
　Hyperthyroidism
　Hyperparathyroidism
　Aortic coarctation
　Renal disease

HYPERTENSIVE CRISIS SYNDROMES[74]

| ICD-10CM # | I13 | Hypertensive heart and renal disease |
| | I15 | Secondary hypertension |

Malignant hypertension.
Nonmalignant hypertension with target organ
　disorders:
　Patient requiring emergency surgery with
　　poorly controlled hypertension.
　Hyperviscosity syndrome.
　Postoperative patient.
　Renal transplant patient: acute rejection,
　　transplant renal artery stenosis.
　Quadriplegic patient with autonomic hyper-
　　reflexia.
　Severe burns.
　Acute aortic dissection.
　Intracranial hemorrhage, ischemic stroke, or
　　subarachnoid hemorrhage.
　Hypertensive encephalopathy.
　Myocardial ischemia/acute left ventricular
　　failure.
　Preeclampsia/eclampsia.
　Antiphospholipid antibody syndrome.
　Acute renal failure:
　　Scleroderma renal crisis.
　　Chronic glomerulonephritis.
　　Reflux nephropathy.
　　Analgesic nephropathy.
　　Acute glomerulonephritis.
　　Radiation nephritis.
　　Ask-Upmark kidney.
　　Chronic lead intoxication.
　Renovascular hypertension:
　　Fibromuscular dysplasia.
　　Atherosclerosis.
　Endocrine hypertension:
　　Congenital adrenal hyperplasia.
　　Pheochromocytoma.
　　Oral contraceptives.
　　Aldosteronism.

Cushing disease.
Systemic vasculitis.
Atheroembolic renal crisis.
Drugs:
　Oral contraceptives.
　Nonsteroidal antiinflammatory agents.
　Atropine.
　Corticosteroids.
　Sympathomimetics.
　Cyclosporine.
　Erythropoietin.
Lead intoxication.
Catecholamine excess states:
　Pheochromocytoma.
　MAO/tyramine interaction.
　Antihypertensive withdrawal.
　Cocaine intoxication, sympathomimetic
　　overdose.

HYPERTRICHOSIS[16]

ICD-10CM #	L68.0	Hirsutism
	L68.1	Acquired hypertrichosis lanuginosa
	L68.3	Polytrichia
	L68.9	Hypertrichosis, unspecified
	Q84.1	Congenital morphological disturbances of hair, not elsewhere classified

DRUGS

Dilantin.
Streptomycin.
Hexachlorobenzene.
Penicillamine.
Diazoxide.
Minoxidil.
Cyclosporine.

SYSTEMIC ILLNESS

Hypothyroidism.
Anorexia nervosa.
Malnutrition.
Porphyria.
Dermatomyositis.

IDIOPATHIC

HYPERTROPHIC OSTEOARTHROPATHY

| ICD-10CM # | M89.40 | Other hypertrophic osteoarthropathy, unspecified site |

Idiopathic.
Pulmonary disease (e.g., pulmonary fibrosis,
　cystic fibrosis, sarcoidosis).
Bronchogenic carcinoma.
AIDS.
GI neoplasm (e.g., esophagus, colon).
Hepatic neoplasm, cirrhosis.
Cardiovascular diseases, aortic aneurysm, aor-
　tic prosthesis.
Congenital cyanotic heart disease, patent duc-
　tus arteriosus.

Pulmonary infections, bacterial endocarditis,
　amebic dysentery.
Inflammatory bowel disease.
Connective tissue diseases.
Lymphomas.
Thyroid acropachy.

HYPERVENTILATION, PERSISTENT[70]

| ICD-10CM # | R06.4 | Hyperventilation |

Fibrotic lung disease.
Metabolic acidosis (e.g., diabetes, uremia).
CNS disorders (midbrain and pontine lesions).
Hepatic coma.
Salicylate intoxication.
Fever.
Sepsis.
Psychogenic (e.g., anxiety).

HYPOCALCEMIA

| ICD-10CM # | E83.51 | Hypocalcemia |

Renal insufficiency: hypocalcemia caused by:
　Increased calcium deposits in bone and
　　soft tissue secondary to increased serum
　　phosphate level.
　Decreased production of 1,25-dihydroxyvi-
　　tamin D.
　Excessive loss of 25-OHD (nephrotic syn-
　　drome).
Hypoalbuminemia: each decrease in serum
　albumin (g/L) will decrease serum calcium
　by 0.8 mg/dl but will not change free (ion-
　ized) calcium.
Vitamin D deficiency:
　Malabsorption (most common cause).
　Inadequate intake.
　Decreased production of 1,25-dihydroxyvi-
　　tamin D (vitamin D–dependent rickets,
　　renal failure).
　Decreased production of 25-OHD (parenchy-
　　mal liver disease).
　Accelerated 25-OHD catabolism (phenytoin,
　　phenobarbital).
　End-organ resistance to 1,25-dihydroxyvi-
　　tamin D.
Hypomagnesemia: hypocalcemia caused by:
　Decreased PTH secretion.
　Inhibition of PTH effect on bone.
Pancreatitis, hyperphosphatemia, osteoblastic
　metastases: hypocalcemia is secondary to
　increased calcium deposits (bone, abdomen).
Pseudohypoparathyroidism (PHP): autosomal
　recessive disorder characterized by short
　stature, shortening of metacarpal bones,
　obesity, and mental retardation; the hypocal-
　cemia is secondary to congenital end-organ
　resistance to PTH.
Idiopathic hypoparathyroidism, surgical removal
　of parathyroids (e.g., neck surgery).
"Hungry bones syndrome": rapid transfer of cal-
　cium from plasma into bones after removal of
　a parathyroid tumor.
Sepsis.
Massive blood transfusion (as a result of EDTA
　in blood).

HYPOCALCEMIA IN PEDIATRIC PATIENTS[67]

ICD-10CM #   E83.51   Hypocalcemia

CAUSES OF HYPOCALCEMIA

Neonatal Hypocalcemia

Early neonatal hypocalcemia (first few days of life)

Maternal hyperparathyroidism
Maternal diabetes mellitus
Toxemia of pregnancy
Sepsis
SGA, IUGR, prematurity
Asphyxia
Transfusion (citrated blood products)
Congenital rubella
Hypomagnesemia
Respiratory or metabolic alkalosis

Late neonatal hypocalcemia (fourth to tenth day of life)

Vitamin D deficiency: nutritional deficiency; VDR loss-of-function mutation; deficient 1α-hydroxylase activity
Phosphate overload: excessive intake of evaporated/whole milk
Nutritional calcium deficiency
Hypomagnesemia
Hypoalbuminemia (nephrotic syndrome)
Transfusion (citrated blood products)
Acute/chronic kidney insufficiency
Diuretics (furosemide)
Organic acidemia
Primary hypoparathyroidism: DiGeorge's syndrome; familial hypoparathyroidism; pseudohypoparathyroidism; Kenny-Caffey syndrome; partial deletion of GCMB; retardation dysmorphism syndrome; Pearson's mitochondriopathy; Kerns-Sayre mitochondriopathy; PTH gene defects; CaSR-activating gene mutation

Hypocalcemia in Childhood

Parathyroid-related hypocalcemia

Primary hypoparathyroidism: DiGeorge's syndrome; familial hypoparathyroidism; pseudohypoparathyroidism; Kenny-Caffey syndrome; Sanjad-Sakati syndrome; partial deletion of GCMB; retardation dysmorphism syndrome; Pearson's mitochondropathy; Kerns-Sayre mitochondropathy; PTH gene defects; CaSR-activating gene mutation; Bartter's syndrome type 5
Secondary hypoparathyroidism: radiation; surgery; infiltration (hemochromatosis, thalassemia, Wilson's disease)
Autoimmune polyglandular syndrome type 1

Vitamin D–related hypocalcemia

Nutritional vitamin D deficiency
Defective 1α-hydroxylase activity
VDR loss-of-function mutation
Nutritional calcium deficiency
Hypomagnesemia
Hyperphosphatemia: kidney failure; rhabdomyolysis; tumor lysis
Hypoalbuminemia (nephrotic syndrome)
Medications: diuretics; chemotherapy; transfusion (citrated blood)
Organic acidemia (IVA, MMA, PPA)

CaSR, Calcium-sensing receptor; GCMB, glial cell missing homolog B (a parathyroid-specific transcription factor); IUGR, intrauterine growth retardation; IVA, isovaleric acidemia; MMA, methylmalonic acidemia; PPA, propionic acidemia; PTH, parathyroid hormone; SGA, small for gestational age; VDR, vitamin D receptor.

HYPOCAPNIA

ICD-10CM #   R06.8   Hypoventilation

Hyperventilation.
Pneumonia, pneumonitis.
Fever, sepsis.
Medications (salicylates, beta-adrenergic agonists, progesterone, methylxanthines).
Pulmonary disease (asthma, interstitial fibrosis).
Pulmonary embolism.
Hepatic failure.
Metabolic acidosis.
High altitude.
CHF.
Pregnancy.
Pain.
CNS lesions.

HYPOGLYCEMIA

ICD-10CM #		
	E16.2	Hypoglycemia, unspecified
	E10.65	Type 1 diabetes mellitus with hyperglycemia
	E15	Nondiabetic hypoglycemic coma
	K91.2	Postsurgical malabsorption, not elsewhere classified
	E16.2	Hypoglycemia, unspecified

Oral hypoglycemics (therapeutic, factitious).
Exogenous insulin (therapeutic, factitious).
Postoperative gastric emptying (alimentary hyperinsulinism).
Severe malnutrition.
Liver disease.
Hypermetabolic state (sepsis).
Ketotic hypoglycemia.
Insulinoma.
Antibodies to endogenous insulin.
Hormone deficiencies (glucagon, growth hormone, hypoadrenalism).
Enzyme disorders in metabolism of glycogen, hexose, glycolysis, and Krebs cycle.
Idiopathic.

HYPOGLYCEMIA, IN INFANTS AND CHILDREN[46]

ICD-10CM #   E16.2   Hypoglycemia, unspecified

CLASSIFICATION OF HYPOGLYCEMIA IN INFANTS AND CHILDREN

Neonatal Transient Hypoglycemia

Associated with Inadequate Substrate or Immature Enzyme Function in Otherwise Normal Neonates

Prematurity.
Small for gestational age.
Normal newborn.

Transient Neonatal Hyperinsulinism Also Present in

Infant of diabetic mother.
Discordant twin.
Birth asphyxia.
Infant of toxemic mother.

NEONATAL, INFANTILE, OR CHILDHOOD PERSISTENT HYPOGLYCEMIAS

Hormonal Disorders

Hyperinsulinism.
Recessive K_{ATP} channel HI.
Recessive HADH (hydroxyl acyl CoA dehydrogenase) mutation HI.
Recessive UCP2 (mitochondrial uncoupling protein 2) mutation HI.
Focal K_{ATP} channel HI.
Dominant K_{ATP} channel HI.
Dominant glucokinase HI.
Dominant glutamate dehydrogenase HI (hyperinsulinism/hyperammonemia syndrome).
Dominant mutation in HNF4A (hepatic nuclear factor 4 alpha) HI with MODY later in life.
Dominant mutation in SLC16A1 (the pyruvate transporter)-exercise-induced hypoglycemia.
Acquired islet adenoma.
Beckwith-Wiedemann syndrome.
Insulin administration (Munchausen syndrome by proxy).
Oral sulfonylurea drugs.
Congenital disorders of glycosylation.

Counter-Regulatory Hormone Deficiency

Panhypopituitarism.
Isolated growth hormone deficiency.
Addison disease.
Epinephrine deficiency.

Glycogenolysis and Gluconeogenesis Disorders

Glucose-6-phosphatase deficiency (GSD 1a).
Glucose-6-phosphate translocase deficiency (GSD 1b).
Amylo-1,6-glucosidase (debranching enzyme) deficiency (GSD 3).
Liver phosphorylase deficiency (GSD 6).
Phosphorylase kinase deficiency (GSD 9).
Glycogen synthetase deficiency (GSD 0).
Fructose-1,6-diphosphatase deficiency.
Pyruvate carboxylase deficiency.
Galactosemia.
Hereditary fructose intolerance.

Lipolysis Disorders

Fatty Acid Oxidation Disorders

Carnitine transporter deficiency (primary carnitine deficiency).
Carnitine palmitoyltransferase-1 deficiency.
Carnitine translocase deficiency.
Carnitine palmitoyltransferase-2 deficiency.
Secondary carnitine deficiencies.
Very long, long-, medium-, short-chain acyl-CoA dehydrogenase deficiency.

OTHER ETIOLOGIES

Substrate-Limited

Ketotic hypoglycemia.
Poisoning—drugs.
Salicylates.
Alcohol.

Differential Diagnosis

II

Oral hypoglycemic agents.
Insulin.
Propranolol.
Pentamidine.
Quinine.
Disopyramide.
Ackee fruit (unripe)—hypoglycin.
Vacor (rat poison).
Trimethoprim-sulfamethoxazole (with renal failure).

Liver Disease
Reye syndrome.
Hepatitis.
Cirrhosis.
Hepatoma.

Amino Acid and Organic Acid Disorders
Maple syrup urine disease.
Propionic acidemia.
Methylmalonic acidemia.
Tyrosinosis.
Glutaric aciduria.
3-Hydroxy-3-methylglutaric aciduria.

Systemic Disorders
Sepsis.
Carcinoma/sarcoma (secreting—insulin-like growth factor II).
Heart failure.
Malnutrition.
Malabsorption.
Anti-insulin receptor antibodies.
Anti-insulin antibodies.
Neonatal hyperviscosity.
Renal failure.
Diarrhea.
Burns.
Shock.
Postsurgical.
Pseudohypoglycemia (leukocytosis, polycythemia).
Excessive insulin therapy of insulin-dependent diabetes mellitus.
Factitious.
Nissen fundoplication (dumping syndrome).
Falciparum malaria.

GSD, Glycogen storage disease; *HI*, hyperinsulinemia; K_{ATP} regulated potassium channel.

HYPOGONADISM

ICD-10CM #	E28.310	Symptomatic premature menopause
	E29.1	Testicular hypofunction
	E28.39	Other primary ovarian failure
	E23.6	Other disorders of pituitary gland

HYPERGONADOTROPIC HYPOGONADISM

Hormone resistance (androgen, LH insensitivity).
Gonadal defects (e.g., Klinefelter's syndrome, myotonic dystrophy).
Drug-induced (e.g., spironolactone, cytotoxins).
Alcoholism, radiation-induced.
Mumps orchitis.
Anatomic defects, castration.

HYPOGONADOTROPIC HYPOGONADISM

Pituitary lesions (neoplasms, granulomas, infarction, hemochromatosis, vasculitis).
Drug-induced (e.g., glucocorticoids).
Hyperprolactinemia.
Genetic disorders (Laurence-Moon-Biedl syndrome, Prader-Willi).
Delayed puberty.
Other: chronic disease, nutritional deficiency, Kallmann's syndrome, idiopathic isolated LH or FSH deficiency.

HYPOKALEMIA

ICD-10CM #	E87.6	Hypokalemia

Cellular shift (redistribution) and undetermined mechanisms.
Alkalosis (each 0.1 increase in pH decreases serum potassium by 0.4 to 0.6 mEq/L).
Insulin administration.
Vitamin B_{12} therapy for megaloblastic anemias, acute leukemias.
Hypokalemic periodic paralysis: rare familial disorder manifested by recurrent attacks of flaccid paralysis and hypokalemia.
Beta-adrenergic agonists (e.g., terbutaline), decongestants, bronchodilators, theophylline, caffeine.
Barium poisoning, toluene intoxication, verapamil intoxication, chloroquine intoxication.
Correction of digoxin intoxication with digoxin antibody fragments (Digibind).
Increased renal excretion.
Drugs:
  Diuretics, including carbonic anhydrase inhibitors (e.g., acetazolamide).
  Amphotericin B.
  High-dose sodium penicillin, nafcillin, ampicillin, or carbenicillin.
  Cisplatin.
  Aminoglycosides.
  Corticosteroids, mineralocorticoids.
  Foscarnet sodium.
RTA: distal (type 1) or proximal (type 2).
Diabetic ketoacidosis (DKA), ureteroenterostomy.
Magnesium deficiency.
Postobstruction diuresis, diuretic phase of ATN.
Osmotic diuresis (e.g., mannitol).
Bartter's syndrome: hyperplasia of juxtaglomerular cells leading to increased renin and aldosterone, metabolic alkalosis, hypokalemia, muscle weakness, and tetany (seen in young adults).
Increased mineralocorticoid activity (primary or secondary aldosteronism), Cushing's syndrome.
Chronic metabolic alkalosis from loss of gastric fluid (increased renal potassium secretion).
GI loss:
  Vomiting, nasogastric suction.
  Diarrhea.
  Laxative abuse.
  Villous adenoma.
  Fistulas.
  Inadequate dietary intake (e.g., anorexia nervosa).

Cutaneous loss (excessive sweating).
High dietary sodium intake, excessive use of licorice.

HYPOKALEMIA IN PEDIATRIC PATIENTS[67]

ICD-10CM #	E87.6	Hypokalemia

MOST RELEVANT CAUSES OF HYPOKALEMIA IN PEDIATRIC PATIENTS

Acute Redistribution of Potassium to the Intracellular Compartment
Metabolic alkalosis
Insulin administration
Hypokalemic periodic paralysis
Prolonged Lack of Intake
Increased Renal Loss
Drugs: diuretics, antibiotics, aminoglycosides, penicillin, amphotericin B, capreomycin
Metabolic acidosis and diabetic ketoacidosis
Increased mineralocorticoid activity
Cushing's syndrome
Congenital adrenal hyperplasia
Primary or secondary hyperaldosteronism
Primary tubulopathies
Bartter's syndrome
Gitelman's syndrome
Liddle's syndrome
Types 1 and 2 renal tubular acidosis
Epilepsy, ataxia, sensorineural deafness, and tubulopathy (EAST) syndrome
Fanconi's syndrome
Increased Gastrointestinal Loss
Vomiting (hypertrophic pyloric stenosis)
Diarrhea

HYPOMAGNESEMIA

ICD-10CM #	E83.40	Disorders of magnesium metabolism, unspecified
	E83.42	Hypomagnesemia

GASTROINTESTINAL AND NUTRITIONAL

Defective GI absorption (malabsorption).
Inadequate dietary intake (e.g., alcoholics).
Parenteral therapy without magnesium.
Chronic diarrhea, villous adenoma, prolonged nasogastric suction, fistulas (small bowel, biliary).

EXCESSIVE RENAL LOSSES

Diuretics.
RTA.
Diuretic phase of ATN.
Endocrine disturbances (DKA, hyperaldosteronism, hyperthyroidism, hyperparathyroidism), SIADH, Bartter's syndrome, hypercalciuria, hypokalemia.
Cisplatin, alcohol, cyclosporine, digoxin, pentamidine, mannitol, amphotericin B, foscarnet, methotrexate.
Antibiotics (gentamicin, ticarcillin, carbenicillin).

Redistribution: hypoalbuminemia, cirrhosis, administration of insulin and glucose, theophylline, epinephrine, acute pancreatitis, cardiopulmonary bypass.

Miscellaneous: sweating, burns, prolonged exercise, lactation, "hungry-bones" syndrome.

HYPOMAGNESEMIA IN PEDIATRIC PATIENTS[67]

ICD-10CM # E83.42 Hypomagnesemia

MAIN CAUSES OF HYPOMAGNESEMIA IN CHILDREN

Primary Inherited Disorders

Familial hypomagnesemia with hypercalciuria and nephrocalcinosis

Hypomagnesemia with secondary hypocalcemia

Autosomal dominant hypomagnesemia

Isolated autosomal recessive hypomagnesemia with normocalciuria

Activating mutations of calcium-sensing receptor

Gitelman's syndrome

Bartter's syndrome

Secondary Disorders

Decreased gastrointestinal absorption
  Malabsorptive syndromes
  Vomiting and diarrhea
Increased urinary excretion
  Extracellular volume expansion
  Polyuric states: obstructive uropathy, kidney transplant
Drugs
  Diuretics
  Calcineurin antagonists
  Others: cisplatinum, aminoglycosides, amphotericin B
  Metabolic acidosis
Miscellaneous: "hungry bone," low-birth-weight newborn, infant of diabetic mother

HYPONATREMIA

ICD-10CM # E87.1 Hypo-osmolality and hyponatremia

Renal loss from renal disease, diuretics.

GI loss (diarrhea, vomiting, suction).

Hypertonic hyponatremia (e.g., increased serum osmolality from hyperglycemia).

Transcutaneous loss (extensive burns, excessive sweating).

Fluid sequestration (e.g., ascites).

Osmotic diuresis (e.g., mannitol, glucose).

Dilutional (psychogenic polydipsia, iatrogenic).

Syndrome of inappropriate antidiuretic hormone secretion.

Edema with water and sodium retention.

Artifact (e.g., severe hyperlipidemia).

Laboratory error.

Adrenal insufficiency.

HYPOPHOSPHATEMIA

ICD-10CM #	E83.30	Disorder of phosphorus metabolism, unspecified
	E83.31	Familial hypophosphatemia

Decreased intake (prolonged starvation [alcoholics], hyperalimentation, or IV infusion without phosphate).

Malabsorption.

Phosphate-binding antacids.

Renal loss:
  RTA.
  Fanconi syndrome, vitamin D–resistant rickets.
  ATN (diuretic phase).
  Hyperparathyroidism (primary or secondary).
  Familial hypophosphatemia.
  Hypokalemia, hypomagnesemia.
  Acute volume expansion.
  Glycosuria, idiopathic hypercalciuria.
  Acetazolamide.
Transcellular shift into cells:
  Alcohol withdrawal.
  DKA (recovery phase).
  Glucose-insulin or catecholamine infusion.
  Anabolic steroids.
  Total parenteral nutrition.
  Theophylline overdose.
  Severe hyperthermia; recovery from hypothermia.
  "Hungry bones" syndrome.

HYPOPHOSPHATEMIA IN PEDIATRIC PATIENTS[67]

ICD-10CM #	E83.30	Disorder of phosphorus metabolism, unspecified

CAUSES OF HYPOPHOSPHATEMIA

Decreased Phosphate Intake

Starvation, inadequate phosphate intake, chronic diarrhea, chronic alcoholism

Total parenteral nutrition with insufficient phosphate content

Increased Loss of Phosphate

Increased renal phosphate excretion
  Primary hyperparathyroidism
  Secondary hyperparathyroidism: vitamin D deficiency or resistance (including 1α-hydroxylase deficiency, VDR mutations, VDDR); imatinib
  Excess FGF-23 or phosphatonins: X-linked hypophosphatemia, AD hypophosphatemic rickets, tumor-induced osteomalacia, epidermal nevus, McCune-Albright syndrome
  Fanconi's syndrome, cystinosis, Wilson's disease, Dent's disease, Lowe's syndrome, multiple myeloma, amyloidosis, heavy-metal toxicity, rewarming of hyperthermia, Na/Pi-IIa and Na/Pi-IIc mutation (HHRH)
  PTHrP-dependent hypercalcemia of malignancy
  Hypomagnesemia
Decreased intestinal absorption
  Vitamin D deficiency or resistance (VDDR I and II)
  Malabsorption
Increased intestinal loss
  Phosphate binding antacids used in treating peptic ulcers
Increased loss from other routes
  Skin: severe burns
  Vomiting

Phosphate Shifting from Extracellular Compartment to Cells and Bones

Diabetic ketoacidosis

Alcohol intoxication

Acute respiratory alkalosis, salicylate intoxication, gram-negative sepsis, toxic shock syndrome, acute gout

Refeeding syndromes from starvation, anorexia nervosa, hepatic failure: acute intravenous glucose, fructose, glycerol

Rapid cellular proliferation: intensive erythropoietin therapy, GM-CSF therapy, leukemic blast crisis

Recovery from hypothermia

Heat stroke

Post parathyroidectomy; "hungry bone" disease: osteoblastic metastases, antiresorptive treatment of severe Paget's disease

Catecholamine (albuterol, dopamine, terbutaline, epinephrine)

Thyrotoxic periodic paralysis

Hypocalcemic periodic paralysis

Miscellaneous

Hyperaldosteronism

Oncogenic hypophosphatemia

Post kidney transplantation

Post partial hepatectomy

High-dose corticosteroids, estrogens

Medications: ifosfamide; toluene; calcitonin; bisphosphonate; tenofovir; paraquat, cisplatin; acetazolamide and other diuretics

Post obstructive diuresis

AD, Autosomal dominant; FGF-23, fibroblast growth factor 23; GM-CSF, granulocyte-macrophage colony-stimulating factor; HHRH, hereditary hypophosphatemic rickets with hypercalciuria; Na/Pi-II, type II sodium-dependent phosphate cotransporter; PTHrP, parathyroid hormone–related peptide; VDR, vitamin D receptor; VDDR, vitamin D–dependent rickets.

HYPOPIGMENTATION

ICD-10CM #	L81.9	Disorder of pigmentation, unspecified

Vitiligo.

Tinea versicolor.

Atopic dermatitis.

Chemical leukoderma.

Idiopathic hypomelanosis.

Sarcoidosis.

SLE.

Scleroderma.

Oculocutaneous albinism.

Phenylketonuria.

Nevoid hypopigmentation.

HYPOTENSION, POSTURAL

ICD-10CM # I95.89 Other hypotension

Antihypertensive medications (especially a-blockers, diuretics, ACE inhibitors).

Volume depletion (hemorrhage, dehydration).

Impaired cardiac output (constrictive pericarditis, aortic stenosis).

Peripheral autonomic dysfunction (DM, Guillain-Barré).

Idiopathic orthostatic hypotension.

Central autonomic dysfunction (Shy-Drager syndrome).

Peripheral venous disease.
Adrenal insufficiency.

HYPOTHYROIDISM, CONGENITAL[46]

ICD-10CM #	E03.0	Congenital hypothyroidism with diffuse goiter
	E03.1	Congenital hypothyroidism without goiter

ETIOLOGIC CLASSIFICATION OF CONGENITAL HYPOTHYROIDISM

Primary Hypothyroidism

Defect of fetal thyroid development (dysgenesis):
Aplasia.
Hypoplasia.
Ectopia.
Defect in thyroid hormone synthesis (dyshormonogenesis):
Iodide transport defect: mutation in thyroglobulin gene.
Thyroid organification, or coupling defect: mutation in thyroid peroxidase gene.
Defects in H_2O_2 generation: mutations in DUOXA2 maturation factor or *DUOX2* gene.
Thyroglobulin synthesis defect: mutation in thyroglobulin gene.
Deiodination defect: mutation in *DEHAL1* gene.
TSH unresponsiveness:
$G_s\alpha$ mutation (e.g., type 1A pseudohypothyroidism).
Mutation in TSH receptor.
Defect in thyroid hormone transport: mutation in monocarboxylate transporter 8 *(MCT8)* gene.
Iodine deficiency (endemic goiter).
Maternal antibodies: thyrotropin receptor–blocking antibody (TRBAb, also termed *thyrotropin-binding inhibitor immunoglobulin*).
Maternal medications:
Iodides, amiodarone.
Propylthiouracil, methimazole.
Radioiodine.

CENTRAL (HYPOPITUITARY) HYPOTHYROIDISM

PIT-1 mutations:
Deficiency of thyroid-stimulating hormone (TSH).
Deficiency of growth hormone.
Deficiency of prolactin.
PROP-1 mutations:
Deficiency of TSH.
Deficiency of growth hormone.
Deficiency of prolactin.
Deficiency of luteinizing hormone.
Deficiency of follicle-stimulating hormone.
±Deficiency of adrenocorticotropic hormone.
TSH deficiency: mutation in TSH β subunit gene (manifests as primary hypothyroidism with elevated TSH level).
Multiple pituitary deficiencies (e.g., craniopharyngioma).

Thyroid-releasing hormone (TRH) deficiency:
Isolated.
Multiple hypothalamic deficiencies (e.g., septooptic dysplasia).
TRH unresponsiveness.
Mutations in TRH receptor.

HYPOTONIA, INFANTILE, DIFFERENTIAL DIAGNOSIS[46]

ICD-10CM #	H44.40	Unspecified hypotony of eye

Cerebral hypotonia.
Benign congenital hypotonia.
Chromosome disorders.
Prader-Willi syndrome.
Trisomy.
Chronic nonprogressive encephalopathy.
Cerebral malformation.
Perinatal distress.
Postnatal disorders.
Peroxisomal disorders.
Cerebrohepatorenal syndrome (Zellweger syndrome).
Neonatal adrenoleukodystrophy.
Other genetic defects.
Familial dysautonomia.
Oculocerebrorenal syndrome (Lowe syndrome).
Other metabolic defects.
Acid maltase deficiency (see "Metabolic Myopathies").
Infantile G_{M_1} gangliosidosis.
Spinal cord disorders.
Spinal muscular atrophies.
Acute infantile.
Autosomal dominant.
Autosomal recessive.
Cytochrome-*c* oxidase deficiency.
X-linked.
Chronic infantile.
• Autosomal dominant.
• Autosomal recessive.
• Congenital cervical spinal muscular atrophy.
• Infantile neuronal degeneration.
• Neurogenic arthrogryposis.
Polyneuropathies.
Congenital hypomyelinating neuropathy.
Giant axonal neuropathy.
Hereditary motor-sensory neuropathies.
Disorders of neuromuscular transmission.
Familial infantile myasthenia.
Infantile botulism.
Transitory myasthenia gravis.
Fiber-type disproportion myopathies.
Central core disease.
Congenital fiber-type disproportion myopathy.
Myotubular (centronuclear) myopathy.
Acute.
Chronic.
Nemaline (rod) myopathy.
Autosomal dominant.
Autosomal recessive.
Metabolic myopathies.
Acid maltase deficiency.

Cytochrome-*c* oxidase deficiency.
Muscular dystrophies.
• Bethlem myopathy.
• Congenital dystrophinopathy.
• Congenital muscular dystrophy.
• Merosin deficiency, primary.
• Merosin deficiency, secondary.
• Merosin positive.
• Congenital myotonic dystrophy.

HYPOTONIC POLYURIA[67]

ICD-10CM #		Varies with Specific Diagnosis

CAUSES OF HYPOTONIC POLYURIA

Central (Neurogenic) Diabetes Insipidus

Congenital (congenital malformations, autosomal dominant, arginine vasopressin [AVP] neurophysin gene mutations)
Drug- or toxin-induced (ethanol, diphenylhydantoin, snake venom)
Granulomatous (histiocytosis, sarcoidosis)
Neoplastic (craniopharyngioma, germinoma, lymphoma, leukemia, meningioma, pituitary tumor; metastases)
Infectious (meningitis, tuberculosis, encephalitis)
Inflammatory, autoimmune (lymphocytic infundibuloneurohypophysitis)
Trauma (neurosurgery, deceleration injury)
Vascular (cerebral hemorrhage or infarction, brain death)
Idiopathic

Osmoreceptor Dysfunction

Granulomatous (histiocytosis, sarcoidosis)
Neoplastic (craniopharyngioma, pinealoma, meningioma, metastases)
Vascular (anterior communicating artery aneurysm or ligation, intrahypothalamic hemorrhage)
Other (hydrocephalus, ventricular or suprasellar cyst, trauma, degenerative diseases)
Idiopathic

Increased AVP Metabolism

Pregnancy

Nephrogenic Diabetes Insipidus.
Congenital (X-linked recessive, AVP V2 receptor gene mutations, autosomal recessive or dominant, aquaporin-2 water channel gene mutations)
Drug-induced (demeclocycline, lithium, cisplatin, methoxyflurane)
Hypercalcemia
Hypokalemia
Infiltrating lesions (sarcoidosis, amyloidosis)
Vascular (sickle cell anemia)
Mechanical (polycystic kidney disease, bilateral ureteral obstruction)
Solute diuresis (glucose, mannitol, sodium, radiocontrast dyes)
Idiopathic

Primary Polydipsia

Psychogenic (schizophrenia, obsessive-compulsive behaviors)
Dipsogenic (downward resetting of thirst threshold, idiopathic or similar lesions, as with central DI)

HYPOVOLEMIA[67]

ICD-10CM #	Varies with Specific Diagnosis

CAUSES OF ABSOLUTE AND RELATIVE HYPOVOLEMIA

Absolute
Extrarenal
Gastrointestinal fluid loss
Bleeding
Skin fluid loss
Respiratory fluid loss
Extracorporeal ultrafiltration
Renal
Diuretics
Obstructive uropathy/postobstructive diuresis
Hormone deficiency
Hypoaldosteronism
Adrenal insufficiency
Na+ wasting tubulopathies
Genetic
Acquired tubulointerstitial disease
Relative
Extrarenal
Edematous states
Heart failure
Cirrhosis
Generalized vasodilation
Sepsis
Drugs
Pregnancy
Third-space loss
Renal
Severe nephrotic syndrome

HYPOVOLEMIC SHOCK, PEDIATRIC POPULATION[26]

ICD-10CM #	R57.1	Hypovolemic shock
	R57.8	Other shock

ETIOLOGIES OF HYPOVOLEMIC SHOCK

Whole blood loss.
Absolute loss: hemorrhage.
External bleeding.
Internal bleeding.
- ○ Gastrointestinal.
- ○ Intraabdominal (spleen, liver).
- ○ Major vessel injury.
- ○ Intracranial (in infants).
- ○ Fractures.
Relative loss.
  Pharmacologic (barbiturates, vasodilators).
  Positive pressure ventilation.
  Spinal cord injury.
  Sepsis.
  Anaphylaxis.
Plasma loss.
Burns.
Capillary leak syndromes.
  Inflammation, sepsis.
  Anaphylaxis.
Protein-losing syndromes.
Fluid and electrolyte loss.
Vomiting and diarrhea.

Excessive diuretic use.
Endocrine:
  Adrenal insufficiency.
  Diabetes insipidus.
  Diabetes mellitus.

HYPOXEMIA AND HYPERCAPNIC RESPIRATORY FAILURE[59]

ICD-10CM #	Varies with Specific Diagnosis

COMMON CAUSES OF HYPOXEMIC AND HYPERCAPNIC RESPIRATORY FAILURE

Brain
Bulbar poliomyelitis
Central alveolar hypoventilation
Cerebrovascular accident
Cerebral malignancy
Drug overdose (e.g., narcotic, sedative/hypnotic)
Elevated intracranial pressure
Encephalitis and meningitis
Pontine herniation
Postoperative anesthetic depression
Spinal Cord
Amyotrophic lateral sclerosis
Cervical cordotomy
Guillain-Barré syndrome
Poliomyelitis
Spinal cord trauma
Neuromuscular System
Acute intermittent porphyria
Botulism
Cholinergic crisis
Curariform drugs
Electrolyte disorders (e.g., hypophosphatemia, hypomagnesemia)
Hypokalemic periodic paralysis
Multiple sclerosis
Myasthenia gravis
Myxedema
Neuromuscular blocking antibiotics (e.g., polymyxin, streptomycin)
Organophosphate insecticides
Peripheral neuritis
Polymyositis
Respiratory muscle fatigue—critical illness polyneuropathy/polymyopathy
Tetanus
Upper Airway
Epiglottitis and laryngotracheitis
Large tonsils and adenoids
Obstructive sleep apnea
Postintubation laryngeal edema
Tracheal obstruction
Vocal cord paralysis
Thorax and Pleura
Chest wall burn with eschar formation
Chest wall trauma—flail chest
Kyphoscoliosis
Massive abdominal distention
Massive obesity
Muscular dystrophy
Large pleural effusion/pleural fibrosis
Pneumothorax

Rheumatoid spondylitis
Thoracoplasty
Cardiovascular System
Cardiogenic pulmonary edema
Left ventricular failure
Mitral stenosis
Biventricular failure
Fat embolism
Snake bite
Uremia
Volume overload
Pulmonary veno-occlusive disease
Lower Airway and Alveoli
Acute respiratory distress syndrome (ARDS)
Aspiration
Asthma
Atelectasis
Bronchiectasis
Bronchiolitis
Chronic obstructive pulmonary disease
Cystic fibrosis
Interstitial lung disease
Massive bilateral pneumonia
Near-drowning
Pancreatitis
Pulmonary contusion
Radiation lung injury
Sepsis
Smoke inhalation
Surgical resection of lung parenchyma

ILIAC FOSSA PAIN, LEFT SIDED[72]

ICD-10CM #	M25.5	Pain in joint

GASTROINTESTINAL CAUSES OF ACUTE LEFT ILIAC FOSSA PAIN

Nonspecific left iliac fossa pain including constipation.
Acute gastroenteritis.
Acute diverticulitis.
Colonic carcinoma.
Colonic ischemia.
Localized small bowel perforation.

ILIAC FOSSA PAIN, RIGHT SIDED[72]

ICD-10CM #	M25.5	Pain in joint

DIFFERENTIAL DIAGNOSIS OF RIGHT ILIAC FOSSA PAIN

Gastrointestinal Causes
Nonspecific right iliac fossa pain.
Acute appendicitis.
Mesenteric adenitis.
Terminal ileitis.
Acute inflammation of Meckel's diverticulum.
Crohn's disease of the terminal ileum.
Cecal carcinoma.
Inflammatory cecal lesion (e.g., diverticulitis in a solitary cecal diverticulum).
Inflammatory lesion of the terminal ileum (e.g., foreign body perforation).
Non-Gastrointestinal Causes
Ruptured ovarian follicle (mittelschmerz).

Acute salpingitis (pelvic inflammatory disease).
Rupture/torsion or hemorrhage of an ovarian cyst.
Endometriosis.
Ectopic pregnancy.
Urinary tract infection.

IMMUNODEFICIENCY, CONGENITAL (PRIMARY)

ICD-10CM #	D80.0	Hereditary hyopgammaglobulinemia
	D80.1	Nonfamilial hypogammaglobulinemia
	D80.2	Selective deficiency of IgA
	D80.3	Selective deficiency of IgG
	D80.4	Selective deficiency of IgM

CONGENITAL (PRIMARY) CAUSES OF IMMUNODEFICIENCY

T-lymphocyte Deficiencies
DiGeorge syndrome (thymic aplasia with reduced CD4 and CD3 cells).
Purine nucleoside phosphorylase deficiency (marked T-cell depletion).

B-lymphocyte Deficiencies
Bruton X-linked agammaglobulinemia (absence of B cells, plasma cells, and antibody).
Selective immunoglobulin G (IgG) subclass deficiencies.
Selective IgA deficiency.
Hyper-IgM immunodeficiency (elevated IgM but reduced IgG and IgA).

Mixed T- and B-lymphocyte Deficiencies
Common variable immunodeficiency (leads to various B-cell activation or differentiation defects and gradual deterioration of T-cell number and function).
Severe combined immunodeficiency (severe reduction in IgG and absence of T cells).
Wiskott-Aldrich syndrome (decreased T-cell number and function, low IgM, occasionally low IgG).
Ataxia-telangiectasia (decreased T-cell number and function; IgA, IgE, IgG_2, and IgG_4 deficiency).

Disorders of Complement
C3 deficiency (congenital absence of C3 or consumption of C3 due to deficiency of C3b inactivator).

Phagocyte Defects
Chronic granulomatous disease (defect in nicotinamide adenine dinucleotide phosphate oxidase in phagocytic cells).
Chédiak-Higashi syndrome (impaired microbicidal activity of phagocytes).
Kostmann syndrome, Shwachman-Diamond syndrome, cyclic neutropenia (low neutrophil count).

IMPOTENCE[54]

| ICD-10CM # | F52.21 | Male erectile disorder |

| | F52.8 | Other sexual dysfunction not due to a substance or known physiological condition |
| | N52.9 | Male erectile dysfunction, unspecified |

Psychogenic.
Endocrine: hyperprolactinemia, DM, Cushing's syndrome, hypothyroidism or hyperthyroidism, abnormality of hypothalamic-pituitary-testicular axis.
Vascular: arterial insufficiency, venous leakage, AV malformation, local trauma.
Medications.
Neurogenic: autonomic or sensory neuropathy, spinal cord trauma or tumor, CVA, multiple sclerosis, temporal lobe epilepsy.
Systemic illness: renal failure, COPD, cirrhosis of liver, myotonic dystrophy.
Peyronie's disease.
Prostatectomy.

INCONTINENCE, FECAL[72]

| ICD-10CM # | R15.9 | Full incontinence of feces |

NORMAL SPHINCTER

Diarrhea.
Anorectal conditions:
  Rectal carcinoma.
  Inflammatory bowel disease.
  Hemorrhoids.
  Mucosal prolapse.
  Fissure-in-ano.
  Abnormal rectal sensation.

ABNORMAL SPHINCTER

Congenital abnormalities.
Anal sepsis.
Neurologic conditions.
Rectal prolapse.
Sphincter trauma.
Neurogenic (idiopathic) incontinence.

INFECTIOUS DIARRHEA IN TROPICS[23]

| ICD-10CM # | R19.7 | Diarrhea, Unspecified |

CAUSES OF INFECTIOUS DIARRHEA IN THE TROPICS

Bacteria
  Aeromonas hydrophila
  Arcobacter butzleri
  Bacteroides fragilis, enterotoxigenic
  Campylobacter jejuni
  Escherichia coli: enterotoxigenic, enteroaggregative, enteroinvasive, enterohemorrhagic
  Laribacter hongkongensis
  Plesiomonas shigelloides
  Salmonella, non-typhoidal
  Shigella species: S. dysenteriae, S. flexneri, S. sonnei, S. boydii
  Vibrio cholerae 01, 0139, non-01 non-0139

  Vibrio parahaemolyticus
  Yersinia enterocolitica
Helminths
  Paracapillaria philippinensis
  Fasciolopsis buski
  Heterophyiasis (Metagonimus yokogawai, Haplorchis taichui)
  Schistosoma mansoni
  Strongyloides stercoralis
Protozoa
  Blastocystis hominis
  Cryptosporidium parvum
  Cyclospora cayetanensis
  Encephalitozoon intestinalis
  Enterocytozoon bieneusi
  Giardia lamblia
  Isospora belli
  Leishmania donovani
Viruses
  Astroviruses
  Caliciviruses: Norovirus and Sapovirus
  Enteric adenoviruses
  HIV
  Picornaviruses
  Rotavirus

INFERTILITY, FEMALE[29]

| ICD-10CM # | N97.9 | Female infertility, unspecified |

FALLOPIAN TUBE PATHOLOGY

PID or puerperal infection.
Congenital anomalies.
Endometriosis.
Secondary to past peritonitis of nongenital origin.
Amenorrhea and anovulation.
Minor anovulatory disturbances.

CERVICAL AND UTERINE FACTORS

Leiomyomas and polyps.
Uterine anomalies.
Intrauterine synechiae (Asherman's syndrome).
Destroyed endocervical glands (postsurgery or postinfection).

VAGINAL FACTORS

Congenital absence of vagina.
Imperforate hymen.
Vaginismus.
Vaginitis.

IMMUNOLOGIC FACTORS

Sperm-immobilizing antibodies.
Sperm-agglutinating antibodies.

NUTRITIONAL AND METABOLIC FACTORS

Thyroid disorders.
DM.
Severe nutritional disturbances.

INFERTILITY, MALE[29]

| ICD-10CM # | N46.9 | Male infertility, unspecified |

DECREASED PRODUCTION OF SPERMATOZOA

Varicocele.
Testicular failure.
Endocrine disorders.
Cryptorchidism.
Stress, smoking, caffeine, nicotine, recreational drugs.

DUCTAL OBSTRUCTION

Epididymal (postinfection).
Congenital absence of vas deferens.
Ejaculatory duct (postinfection).
Postvasectomy.

INABILITY TO DELIVER SPERM INTO VAGINA

Ejaculatory disturbances.
Hypospadias.
Sexual problems (i.e., impotence), medical or psychological.

ABNORMAL SEMEN

Infection.
Abnormal volume.
Abnormal viscosity.
Abnormal sperm motion.

IMMUNOLOGIC FACTORS

Sperm-immobilizing antibodies.
Sperm-agglutinating antibodies.

INSOMNIA[64]

ICD-10CM #		
	780.51	Insomnia with Sleep Apnea
	G47.00	Insomnia, unspecified
	F51.01	Primary insomnia
	F51.03	Paradoxical insomnia
	F51.09	Other insomnia not due to a substance or known physiological condition

Anxiety disorder, psychophysiologic insomnia.
Depression.
Drugs (e.g., caffeine, amphetamines, cocaine), hypnotic-dependent sleep disorder.
Pain, fibromyalgia.
Inadequate sleep hygiene.
Restless leg syndrome.
Obstructive sleep apnea.
Sleep bruxism.
Medical illness (e.g., GERD, sleep-related asthma, parkinsonism and movement disorders).
Narcolepsy.
Other: periodic leg movement of sleep, central sleep apnea, REM behavioral disorder.

INTESTINAL PSEUDOOBSTRUCTION[70]

ICD-10CM #	K56.0	Paralytic ileus
	K56.7	Ileus, unspecified
	K59.9	Functional intestinal disorder, unspecified

"PRIMARY" (IDIOPATHIC INTESTINAL PSEUDOOBSTRUCTION)

Hollow visceral myopathy:
  Familial.
  Sporadic.
Neuropathic:
  Abnormal myenteric plexus.
  Normal myenteric plexus.

SECONDARY

Scleroderma.
Myxedema.
Amyloidosis.
Muscular dystrophy.
Hypokalemia.
Chronic renal failure.
DM.
Drug toxicity caused by:
  Anticholinergics.
  Opiate narcotics.
Ogilvie's syndrome.

INTRAABDOMINAL MASS LESION, NEONATAL[33]

ICD-10CM #	R19.00	Intraabdominal and pelvic swelling, mass and lump, unspecified site

CAUSES OF A NEONATAL INTRA-ABDOMINAL MASS LESION

Complicated meconium ileus.
Dilated bowel proximal to an obstruction.
Mesenteric or duplication cyst.
Abscess.
GU causes:
  Hydronephrosis.
  Renal cystic disease.
  Mesoblastic nephroma.
  Wilms' tumor.
  Adrenal hemorrhage.
  Neuroblastoma.
  Retroperitoneal teratoma.
  Ovarian cyst.
  Hydrometrocolpos.
Hemangioendothelioma.
Hepatoblastoma.
Choledochal, hepatic, or splenic cysts.

INTRACEREBRAL HEMORRHAGE, NONHYPERTENSIVE CAUSES

ICD-10CM #	I61.9	Nontraumatic intracerebral hemorrhage, unspecified

Trauma.
Anticoagulation.
Intracranial tumors.
Vascular malformations.
Bleeding disorders.
Vasculitides (e.g., polyarteritis nodosa, granulomatous angiitis).

Cocaine and other sympathomimetic agents.
Cerebral amyloid angiopathy.

INTRACRANIAL LESION

ICD-10CM #	G93.89	Other specified disorders of brain

Tumor (primary or metastatic).
Abscess.
Stroke.
Intracranial hemorrhage.
Angioma.
Multiple sclerosis (initial single lesion).
Granuloma.
Herpes encephalitis.
Artifact.

INTRAOCULAR NEOPLASM

ICD-10CM #	C69.9	Malignant disorder of eye, unspecified

MALIGNANT

Retinoblastoma.
Melanoma.
Reticulum cell sarcoma.
Metastatic tumor.

BENIGN

Melanocytic nevus.
Hemangioma.
Reactive lymphoid hyperplasia.

IRON OVERLOAD[40]

ICD-10CM #	E83.10	Disorder of iron metabolism, unspecified

HEREDITARY IRON OVERLOAD

Hereditary hemochromatosis:
  HFE-associated (type 1).
  Non–HFE-associated:
    Transferrin receptor 2–associated (type 3).
Juvenile hemochromatosis (type 2):
  Hemojuvelin-associated (type 2A).
  Hepcidin-associated (type 2B).
Autosomal dominant hemochromatosis:
  Ferroportin-associated (type 4).
DMT1-associated hemochromatosis.
Atransferrinemia.
Aceruloplasminemia.

ACQUIRED IRON OVERLOAD

Iron-loading anemias (refractory anemias with hypercellular erythroid marrow).
Chronic liver disease.
Porphyria cutanea tarda.
Insulin resistance–associated hepatic iron overload.
African dietary iron overload.[24]
Medical iron ingestion.
Parenteral iron overload:
  Transfusional iron overload.
  Inadvertent iron overload from therapeutic injections.

---

[24]May have a genetic component.

PERINATAL IRON OVERLOAD

Neonatal hemochromatosis.
Trichohepatoenteric syndrome.
Cerebrohepatorenal syndrome.
GRACILE[25] (Fellman) syndrome.

FOCAL SEQUESTRATION OF IRON

Idiopathic pulmonary hemosiderosis.
Renal hemosiderosis.
Associated with neurologic abnormalities:
    Pantothenate kinase–associated neurode-
        generation (formerly called Hallervorden-
        Spatz syndrome).
    Neuroferritinopathy.
    Friedreich's ataxia.

---

[25]*GRACILE*, Growth retardation, aminoaciduria, cholestasis, iron overload, lactic acidosis, and early
death.

ISCHEMIA, UPPER EXTREMITY, CAUSES[14]

ICD-10CM #	S45.809A	Unspecified injury of other specified blood vessels at shoulder and upper arm level, unspecified arm, initial encounter

VASOSPASM

Raynaud disease.
Medication induced: vasopressors, b-blockers.
Ergot poisoning.

INTRINSIC ARTERIAL DISEASE

- Atherosclerosis.
- Radiation arteritis.
- Azotemic arteriopathy.
- Spontaneous dissection.
- Fibromuscular dysplasia.

INFLAMMATORY DISEASES

Connective tissue disorders.
Buerger disease.
Takayasu arteritis.
Temporal (giant cell) arteritis.
Hypersensitivity angiitis.

NONINFLAMMATORY MEDICAL DISEASE

- Thrombophilic states.
- Myeloproliferative disorders.
- Cold injury.
- Hepatitis-associated vasculitis.
- Cryoglobulinemia.
- Vinyl chloride exposure.

EMBOLISM

Cardiac (most common).
Proximal aneurysm.
Arterial thoracic outlet syndrome.
Atheroembolism.
Paradoxic embolus (with accompanying septal
    defect).

TRAUMA

Iatrogenic.
Blunt arterial injury.
Penetrating arterial injury.
Hypothenar hammer syndrome.
Vibration.

ISCHEMIC BOWEL DISEASE[1]

ICD-10CM #	K55.1	Vascular disorder of intestine
	I99	Other and unspecified disorders of circulatory system

Abdominal aortic aneurysm: rupture or expan-
    sion.
Perforated ulcer or viscus.
Ruptured ectopic pregnancy (woman of child-
    bearing age).
Incarcerated or strangulated hernia.
Septic shock.
Intussusception.
Volvulus.
Salpingitis or tuboovarian abscess.
Torsion of the ovary or testicle.
Appendicitis.
Pelvic mass or torsion.
Pancreatitis.
Diverticulitis.
Ruptured ovarian cyst.
Renal colic.
Biliary colic.
Also consider atypical manifestations of:
    ○ Inferior wall myocardial infarction.
    ○ Pulmonary embolism.
    ○ Pneumonia.
    ○ Diabetic ketoacidosis.
    ○ Acute glaucoma.
Differential diagnoses are listed in order of
    urgency.

ISCHEMIC COLITIS, NONOCCLUSIVE[43]

ICD-10CM #	K55.1	Chronic vascular disorders of intestine

ACUTE DIMINUTION OF COLONIC INTRAMURAL BLOOD FLOW

Small Vessel Obstruction

Collagen-vascular disease.
Vasculitis, diabetes.
Oral contraceptives.

Nonocclusive Hypoperfusion

Hemorrhage.
CHF, MI, arrhythmias.
Sepsis.
Vasoconstricting agents: vasopressin, ergot.
Increased viscosity: polycythemia, sickle cell
    disease, thrombocytosis.

INCREASED DEMAND ON MARGINAL BLOOD FLOW

Increased Motility

Mass lesion, stricture.
Constipation.

Increased Intraluminal Pressure

Bowel obstruction.
Colonoscopy.
Barium enema.

ISCHEMIC NECROSIS OF CARTILAGE AND BONE[29]

ICD-10CM #	M89.9	Disorder of bone, unspecified
	M94.9	Disorder of cartilage, unspecified

ENDOCRINE/METABOLIC

Ethanol abuse.
Glucocorticoid therapy.
Cushing's disease.
DM.
Hyperuricemia.
Osteomalacia.
Hyperlipidemia.

STORAGE DISEASES (E.G., GAUCHER'S DISEASE)

Hemoglobinopathies (e.g., sickle cell disease).
Trauma (e.g., dislocation, fracture).
HIV infection.
Dysbaric conditions (e.g., caisson disease).
Collagen-vascular disorders.
Irradiation.
Pancreatitis.
Organ transplantation.
Hemodialysis.
Burns.
Intravascular coagulation.
Idiopathic, familial.

JAUNDICE

ICD-10CM #	R17	Unspecified jaundice
	K83.8	Other specified diseases of biliary tract
	E80.7	Disorder of bilirubin metabolism, unspecified

PREDOMINANCE OF DIRECT (CONJUGATED) BILIRUBIN

Extrahepatic obstruction.
Common duct abnormalities: calculi, neoplasm,
    stricture, cyst, sclerosing cholangitis.
Metastatic carcinoma.
Pancreatic carcinoma, pseudocyst.
Ampullary carcinoma.
Hepatocellular disease: hepatitis, cirrhosis.
Drugs: estrogens, phenothiazines, captopril,
    methyltestosterone, labetalol.
Cholestatic jaundice of pregnancy.
Hereditary disorders: Dubin-Johnson syndrome,
    Rotor's syndrome.
Recurrent benign intrahepatic cholestasis.

PREDOMINANCE OF INDIRECT (UNCONJUGATED) BILIRUBIN

Hemolysis: hereditary and acquired hemolytic
    anemias.

Inefficient marrow production.

Impaired hepatic conjugation: chloramphenicol.

Neonatal jaundice.

Hereditary disorders: Gilbert's syndrome, Crigler-Najjar syndrome.

JAUNDICE, CLASSIFICATION[3]

ICD-10CM #	R17	Unspecified jaundice

PREHEPATIC (PREDOMINANTLY UNCONJUGATED HYPERBILIRUBINEMIA)

Overproduction

Hemolysis (e.g., spherocytosis, sickle cell disease, hemolysis of the newborn, autoimmune disorders).

Ineffective erythropoiesis (e.g., megaloblastic anemias).

Hematomas.

Pulmonary emboli.

HEPATIC (UNCONJUGATED HYPERBILIRUBINEMIA)

Decreased Hepatic Uptake

Gilbert syndrome.

Drugs (e.g., rifampin, radiographic contrast agents).

Neonatal jaundice.

Posthepatitis.

Decreased cystolic binding proteins (e.g., newborn or premature infants).

Portacaval shunt.

Prolonged fasting.

Decreased Conjugation Due to Limited Glucuronyl Transferase Activity

Gilbert's disease.

Crigler-Najjar syndrome, types I and II.

Neonatal jaundice.

Breast-milk jaundice.

Chronic persistent hepatitis.

Wilson's disease.

Noncirrhotic portal fibrosis.

Drug inhibition (e.g., chloramphenicol).

PREDOMINANTLY CONJUGATED HYPERBILIRUBINEMIA

Impaired Hepatic Excretion

Familial disorders (Dubin-Johnson syndrome, Rotor syndrome, benign recurrent cholestasis, cholestasis of pregnancy).

Hepatocellular infiltrative disorders.

Liver metastasis.

Liver cirrhosis.

Hepatitis (viral, bacterial, parasitic, autoimmune, ethanol, and drug-induced).

Drug-induced cholestasis (especially chlorpromazine, erythromycin estolate, isoniazid, halothane).

Primary biliary cirrhosis.

Primary sclerosing cholangitis.

Pericholangitis.

Congestive heart failure.

Shock.

Toxemia of pregnancy.

Sarcoidosis.

Hepatic trauma.

Amyloidosis.

Autoimmune cholangiopathy.

Vanishing bile duct syndrome.

Sepsis.

Postoperative complications.

EXTRAHEPATIC

Extrahepatic Biliary Obstruction

Gallstones, choledocholithiasis.

Cholecystitis.

Tumors of the head of the pancreas (adenocarcinoma, mucinous duct ectasia, neuroendocrine tumors, metastasis).

Tumors of bile ducts (cholangiocarcinoma, Klatskin tumor: cholangiocarcinoma at the bifurcation).

Gallbladder cancer.

Tumors of the ampulla of Vater (adenoma, adenocarcinoma).

Tumors of the duodenum (adenocarcinoma, lymphoma).

Hemobilia (blood in the biliary tree).

Biliary strictures (postcholecystectomy, post-liver transplantation, primary sclerosing cholangitis).

Congential disorders (biliary atresia, idiopathic dilation of common bile duct, cystic fibrosis).

Metastasis to the hepatic hilum.

Primary bile duct lymphoma.

Cholangiopathy of acquired immunodeficiency syndrome.

Choledochal cysts.

Infectious cholangiopathy (Clonorchis sinensis, Ascaris lumbricoides, Fasciola hepatica).

Chronic pancreatitis (fibrosis of the head of the pancreas).

JAUNDICE, NEONATAL[3]

ICD-10CM #	P59.9	Neonatal jaundice, unspecified

PREHEPATIC

Hereditary spherocytosis.

Nonspherocytic hemolytic anemia (glucose-6-phosphate dehydrogenase deficiency, α-thalassemia, vitamin K_3–induced hemolysis, pyruvate kinase deficiency).

HEPATIC

Crigler-Najjar syndrome, types I and II.

α_1-Antitrypsin deficiency.

Sepsis.

Drug-induced.

Hypothyroidism.

Breast-milk jaundice.

Fetomaternal blood group incompatibility (Rhesus, Landsteiner groups ABO).

POSTHEPATIC

Extrahepatic biliary obstruction.

Biliary atresia.

Bile duct paucity.

Alagille syndrome.

JOINT AND PERIARTICULAR PAIN, ACUTE[24]

ICD-10CM #	M25.50	Joint pain

COMMON ACUTE MONOARTHRITIS

Septic arthritis (nongonococcal, gonococcal).

Crystal arthritis (gout, pseudogout).

Reactive arthritides.

Lyme disease.

Plant thorn synovitis.

Other infections (mycobacterial, viral, soft tissue).

TRAUMA OR INTERNAL DERANGEMENT

Loose bodies.

Stress fractures.

Ischemic necrosis.

Hemarthrosis.

ACUTE MONOARTHRITIS OR POLYARTHRITIS

Psoriatic arthritis.

Enteropathic arthritis.

Rheumatoid arthritis/palindromic rheumatism.

Juvenile inflammatory arthritides.

MONOARTHROPATHIES FROM NONINFLAMMATORY DISEASE

Osteoarthritis.

Charcot's joints.

Storage diseases (hemochromatosis, ochronosis).

SYNOVIAL DISEASES

Pigmented villonodular synovitis.

Lipoma arborescens.

Synovial osteochondromatosis.

Reflex sympathetic dystrophy.

Sarcoidosis.

Amyloid.

ACUTE MONOARTHRITIS OF SYSTEMIC DISEASE

Systemic lupus erythematosus.

Vasculitides (antineutrophil cytoplasmic antibody positive and negative).

Henoch-Schönlein purpura.

Behçet's disease.

Bacterial endocarditis.

Familial Mediterranean fever.

Relapsing polychondritis.

SOFT TISSUE LESIONS

Bone Diseases

Paget's disease.

Osteomyelitis (Brodie's abscess).

Osteogenic/osteoid tumors.

Metastatic disease.

Pulmonary hypertrophic osteoarthropathy.

This table shows the causes of inflammation in any one joint (monoarthritis) and pain around the joint that presents without inflammation (monoarthropathy).

JOINT PAIN, ANTERIOR HIP, MEDIAL THIGH, KNEE[55]

ICD-10CM #	M25.50	Pain in unspecified joint
	M25.559	Pain in unspecified hip
	M25.569	Pain in unspecified knee

ACUTE

Acute rheumatic fever.
Adductor muscle strain.
Avascular necrosis.
Crystal arthritis.
Femoral artery (pseudo) aneurysm.
Fracture (femoral neck or intertrochanteric).
Hemarthrosis.
Hernia.
Herpes zoster.
Iliopectineal bursitis.
Iliopsoas tendinitis.
Inguinal lymphadenitis.
Osteomalacia.
Painful transient osteoporosis of hip.
Septic arthritis.

SUBACUTE AND CHRONIC

Adductory muscle strain.
Amyloidosis.
Acute rheumatic fever.
Femoral artery aneurysm.
Hernia (inguinal or femoral).
Iliopectineal bursitis.
Iliopsoas tendinitis.
Inguinal lymphadenopathy.
Osteochondromatosis.
Osteomyelitis.
Osteitis deformans (Paget's disease).
Osteomalacia (pseudofracture).
Postherpetic neuralgia.
Sterile synovitis (e.g., RA, psoriatic, SLE).

JOINT PAIN, HIP, LATERAL THIGH[55]

ICD-10CM #	S79.919A	Unspecified injury of unspecified hip, initial encounter
	S79.929A	Unspecified injury of unspecified thigh, initial encounter
	M25.9	Joint disorder, unspecified

ACUTE

Herpes zoster.
Iliotibial tendinitis.
Impacted fracture of femoral neck.
Lateral femoral cutaneous neuropathy (meralgia paresthetica).
Radiculopathy: L4-5.
Trochanteric avulsion fracture (greater trochanter).
Trochanteric bursitis.
Trochanteric fracture.

SUBACUTE AND CHRONIC

Lateral femoral cutaneous neuropathy (meralgia paresthetica).
Osteomyelitis.
Postherpetic neuralgia.
Radiculopathy: L4-5.
Tumors.

JOINT PAIN, POLYARTICULAR

ICD-10CM #	M25.50	Pain in unspecified joint

Osteoarthritis.
RA.
Fibromyalgia.
Viral syndrome (e.g., human parvovirus B19 infection).
SLE.
Psoriatic arthritis.
Ankylosing spondylitis.

JOINT PAIN, POSTERIOR HIPS, THIGH, BUTTOCKS[55]

ICD-10CM #	M25.50	Pain in unspecified joint
	M25.559	Pain in unspecified hip
	M25.569	Pain in unspecified knee

ACUTE

Gluteal muscle strain.
Herpes zoster.
Ischial bursitis.
Ischial or sacral fracture.
Osteomalacia (pseudofracture).
Sciatic neuropathy.
Radiculopathy: L5-S1.

SUBACUTE AND CHRONIC

Gluteal muscle strain.
Ischial bursitis.
Lumbar spinal stenosis.
Osteoarthritis of hip.
Osteitis deformans (Paget's disease).
Osteomyelitis.
Osteochondromatosis.
Osteomalacia (pseudofracture).
Postherpetic neuralgia.
Radiculopathy: L5-S1.
Tumors.

JOINT SWELLING

ICD-10CM #	M25.40	Effusion, unspecified joint

Trauma.
Osteoarthritis.
Gout.
Pyogenic arthritis.
Pseudogout.
RA.
Viral syndrome.

JUGULAR VENOUS DISTENTION

ICD-10CM #	I99.8	Other disorder of circulatory system

Right-sided heart failure.
Cardiac tamponade.
Constrictive pericarditis.
Goiter.
Tension pneumothorax.

Pulmonary hypertension.
Cardiomyopathy (restrictive).
Superior vena cava syndrome.
Valsalva maneuver.
Right atrial myxoma.
COPD.

KERATITIS, NONINFECTIOUS

ICD-10CM #	H16.9	Unspecified keratitis

Collagen vascular disease.
Atopic keratoconjunctivitis.
Chemical injury.
Thermal injury.
Ectropion/entropion.
Lid defects.
Exophthalmos.
Keratoconjunctivitis sicca.
Erythema multiforme.
Mucous membrane pemphigoid.
DM (delayed epithelial healing).
Neuroparalytic (cranial nerve VII).
Neurotrophic (diabetes, cranial nerve V).

KIDNEY CYSTIC DISEASE[76]

ICD-10CM #	Varies with Specific Diagnosis

CYSTIC DISEASES OF THE KIDNEY

Inheritable

Autosomal recessive (infantile) polycystic kidney disease
Autosomal dominant (adult) polycystic kidney disease
  Juvenile nephronophthisis and medullary cystic disease complex
  Juvenile nephronophthisis (autosomal recessive)
Medullary cystic disease (autosomal dominant)
Congenital nephrosis (familial nephrotic syndrome) (autosomal recessive)
Familial hypoplastic glomerulocystic disease (autosomal dominant)
Multiple malformation syndromes with renal cysts (e.g., tuberous sclerosis, von Hippel-Lindau disease)

Nonheritable

Multicystic kidney (multicystic dysplastic kidney)
Benign multilocular cyst (cystic nephroma)
Simple cysts
Medullary sponge kidney
Sporadic glomerulocystic kidney disease
Acquired renal cystic disease
Calyceal diverticulum (pyelogenic cyst)

KIDNEY ENLARGEMENT, UNILATERAL[72]

ICD-10CM #	N13.30	Unspecified hydronephrosis

Hydronephrosis (may be bilateral).
Polycystic kidney (may be bilateral).
Simple cyst of kidney.
Renal cell carcinoma.
Pyonephrosis (may be bilateral).
Acute renal vein thrombosis.

KIDNEY INJURY, CANCER PATIENTS[67]

ICD-10CM # Varies with Specific Diagnosis

CAUSES OF ACUTE KIDNEY INJURY IN CANCER PATIENTS

Prerenal
Sepsis
Volume depletion (vomiting, diarrhea, mucositis)
Hepatorenal syndrome (venoocclusive disease of the liver)
Capillary leak syndrome (interleukin-2 administration)
Hypercalcemia
Intrinsic
Acute tubular necrosis
Ischemia (sepsis/shock)
Nephrotoxic (aminoglycosides, amphotericin B, chemotherapy)
Tubulointerstitial nephritis
Tumor lysis syndrome (urate and phosphate nephropathy)
Allergic reaction
Pyelonephritis
Opportunistic infections
Infiltration (lymphoma/leukemia)
Vascular
Thrombotic microangiopathy
Cancer treated
Drug induced
Bone marrow transplantation
Radiation injury
Amyloidosis
Light-chain deposition disease
Paraneoplastic syndromes (membranous, antineutrophil cytoplasmic antibody associated, focal segmental glomerulosclerosis)
Postrenal
Intrarenal (urate, acyclovir, methotrexate)
Extrarenal (retroperitoneal fibrosis, lymphadenopathy, direct invasion)

KNEE PAIN[55]

ICD-10CM #		
	S83.419A	Sprain of medial collateral ligament of unspecified knee, initial encounter
	S83.509A	Sprain of unspecified cruciate ligament of unspecified knee, initial encounter
	M23.50	Chronic instability of knee, unspecified knee
	M23.8X9	Other internal derangements of unspecified knee
	S83.289A	Other tear of lateral meniscus, current injury, unspecified knee, initial encounter
	S83.249A	Other tear of medial meniscus, current injury, unspecified knee, initial encounter
	M25.669	Stiffness of unspecified knee, not elsewhere classified

DIFFUSE
Articular.
Anterior.
Prepatellar bursitis.
Patellar tendon enthesopathy.
Chondromalacia patellae.
Patellofemoral osteoarthritis.
Cruciate ligament injury.
Medial plica syndrome.

MEDIAL
Anserine bursitis.
Spontaneous osteonecrosis.
Osteoarthritis.
Medial meniscal tear.
Medial collateral ligament bursitis.
Referred pain from hip and L3.
Fibromyalgia.

LATERAL
Iliotibial band syndrome.
Meniscal cyst.
Lateral meniscal tear.
Collateral ligament.
Peroneal tenosynovitis.

POSTERIOR
Popliteal cyst (Baker's cyst).
Tendinitis.
Aneurysms, ganglions, sarcoma.

KNEE PAIN, IN DIFFERENT AGE GROUPS[17]

ICD-10CM #	M25.569	Pain in unspecified knee

COMMON CAUSES OF KNEE PAIN IN DIFFERENT AGE GROUPS

Childhood (2-10 yr)
Intraarticular
Juvenile arthritis.
Osteochondritis dissecans.
Infection.
Torn discoid meniscus.
Periarticular
Osteomyelitis.
Referred
Perthes' disease.
Irritable hip.
Adolescence (10-18 yr)
Intraarticular
Osteochondritis dissecans.
Torn meniscus.
Anterior knee pain syndrome.
Patellar instability.

Periarticular
Osgood–Schlatter disease.
Sinding–Larsen–Johansson syndrome.
Osteomyelitis.
Bone tumors.
Referred
Slipped upper femoral epiphysis.
Early Adulthood (18-30 yr)
Intraarticular
Torn meniscus.
Patellar instability.
Anterior knee pain syndrome.
Inflammatory arthritis.
Periarticular
Ligament injuries.
Bursitis.
Adulthood (30-50 yr)
Intraarticular
Degenerate meniscal tears.
Osteoarthritis.
Inflammatory arthritis.
Periarticular
Bursitis.
Referred
Osteoarthritis of hip.
Spinal disorders.
Old Age (>50 yr)
Intraarticular
Osteoarthritis.
Inflammatory arthritis.
Periarticular
Bursitis.
Referred
Osteoarthritis of hip.
Spinal disorders.

LARGE BOWEL STRICTURE[33]

ICD-10CM # S36.5 Injury of colon

CAUSES OF LARGE BOWEL STRICTURES

Physiologic:
  Spasm.
  Distended bladder.
Maligant:
  Annular carcinoma.
  Scirrhous carcinoma.
  Lymphoma.
Diverticular disease:
  Muscle thickening.
  Pericolic abscess.
  Superimposed malignancy.
Ischemia.
Radiation colitis.
Inflammatory bowel disease:
  Ulcerative colitis.
  Crohn's disease.
  Tuberculosis.
  Lymphogranuloma venereum.
  Amebiasis.
Extrinsic disease:
  Intraabdominal masses.
  Metastatic carcinoma.
  Endometriosis.
  Pelvic lipomatosis.
  Cholecystitis.
  Pancreatitis.

Miscellaneous:
  Postoperative anastomosis.
  Trauma.
  Hirschsprung's disease.

LEFT AXIS DEVIATION[45]

ICD-10CM #	I44.7	Left bundle-branch block, unspecified
	I44.4	Left anterior fascicular block
	I44.5	Left posterior fascicular block
	I44.60	Unspecified fascicular block
	I44.69	Other fascicular block

Normal variation.
Left anterior fascicular block (hemiblock).
Left bundle branch block.
Left ventricular hypertrophy.
Mechanical shifts causing a horizontal heart, high diaphragm, pregnancy, ascites.
Some forms of ventricular tachycardia.
Endocardial cushion defects and other congenital heart disease.

LEFT BUNDLE BRANCH BLOCK

ICD-10CM #	I44.7	Left bundle-branch block, unspecified

Ischemic heart disease.
Electrolyte abnormalities (e.g., hyperkalemia).
Cardiomyopathy.
Idiopathic.
LVH.
Pulmonary embolism.
Cardiac trauma.
Bacterial endocarditis.

LEG CRAMPS, NOCTURNAL

ICD-10CM #	R25.2	Cramp and spasm

Diabetic neuropathy.
Medications.
Electrolyte abnormalities (hypokalemia, hyponatremia, hypocalcemia, hyperkalemia, hypophosphatemia).
Respiratory alkalosis.
Uremia.
Hemodialysis.
Peripheral nerve injury.
ALS.
Alcohol use.
Heat cramps.
Vitamin B_{12} deficiency.
Hyperthyroidism.
Contractures.
DVT.
Hypoglycemia.
Peripheral vascular insufficiency.
Baker's cyst.

LEG LENGTH DISCREPANCIES[47]

ICD-10CM #	M21.759	Unequal limb length (acquired), unspecified femur

	M21.769	Unequal limb length (acquired), unspecified tibia and fibula
	Q72.899	Other reduction defects of unspecified lower limb

CONGENITAL
Proximal femoral local deficiency.
Coxa vara.
Hemiatrophy-hemihypertrophy (anisomelia).
Developmental dysplasia of the hip.

DEVELOPMENTAL
Legg-Calvé-Perthes disease.

NEUROMUSCULAR
Polio.
Cerebral palsy (hemiplegia).

INFECTIOUS
Pyogenic osteomyelitis with physeal damage.

TRAUMA
Physeal injury with premature closure.
Overgrowth.
Malunion (shortening).

TUMOR
Physeal destruction.
Radiation-induced physeal injury.
Overgrowth.

LEG MOVEMENT WHEN STANDING, INVOLUNTARY

ICD-10CM #	R25.8	Other abnormal involuntary movements

Benign essential tremor.
Orthostatic tremor.
Spastic ataxia.
Cerebellar truncal tremor.
Postanoxic myoclonus.

LEG PAIN WITH EXERCISE

ICD-10CM #	R25.2	Cramp and spasm

Shin splints.
Arteriosclerosis obliterans.
Neurogenic (spinal cord compression or ischemia).
Venous claudication.
Popliteal cyst.
DVT.
Thromboangiitis obliterans.
Adventitial cysts.
Popliteal artery entrapment syndrome.
McArdle syndrome.

LEG SWELLING[1]

ICD-10CM #	R60.0

Deep vein thrombosis.
Cellulitis.
Baker cyst rupture or inflammation.

Congestive heart failure.
Renal failure.
Liver failure.
Inferior vena cava compression.
Musculoskeletal trauma.
Polyarteritis nodosa.
Erythema nodosum.
Myositis.
Tendinitis.
Lymphedema.
Superficial thrombophlebitis.
Compartment syndrome.

LEG ULCERS[55]

ICD-10CM #	I70.25	Atherosclerosis of native arteries of other extremities with ulceration
	L97.909	Non-pressure chronic ulcer of unspecified part of unspecified lower leg with unspecified severity

VASCULAR
Arterial: arteriosclerosis, thromboangiitis obliterans, AV malformation, cholesterol emboli.
Venous: superficial varicosities, incompetent perforators, DVT, lymphatic abnormalities.

VASCULITIS HEMATOLOGIC
Sickle cell anemia, thalassemia, polycythemia vera, leukemia, cold agglutinin disease.
Macroglobulinemia, protein C and protein S deficiency, cryoglobulinemia, lupus anticoagulant, antiphospholipid syndrome.

INFECTIOUS
Fungal: Blastomycosis, coccidioidomycosis, histoplasmosis, sporotrichosis.
Bacterial: Furuncle, ecthyma, septic emboli.
Protozoal: leishmaniasis.

METABOLIC
Necrobiosis lipoidica diabeticorum.
Localized bullous pemphigoid.
Gout, calcinosis cutis, Gaucher's disease.

TUMORS
Basal cell carcinoma, squamous cell carcinoma, melanoma.
Mycosis fungoides, Kaposi's sarcoma, metastatic neoplasms.

TRAUMA
Burns, cold injury, radiation dermatitis.
Insect bites.
Factitial, excessive pressure.

NEUROPATHIC
Diabetic trophic ulcers.
Tabes dorsalis, syringomyelia.

DRUGS
Warfarin, IV colchicine extravasation, methotrexate, halogens, ergotism, hydroxyurea.

PANNICULITIS

Weber-Christian disease.
Pancreatic fat necrosis, alpha-antitrypsinase deficiency.

LEPTOMENINGEAL LESIONS

ICD-10CM # G03.9 Leptomeningitis

Metastases.
Multiple sclerosis.
Bacterial or viral meningitis.
Vasculitis.
Lyme disease.
Tuberculosis.
Fungal infections (e.g., *Cryptococcus*).
Sarcoidosis.
Wegener's granulomatosis.
Neurocysticercosis.
Rheumatoid nodules.
Histiocytosis.

LEUKOCORIA

ICD-10CM # H57.9 Unspecified disorder of eye and adnexa

Cataract.
Retinal detachment.
Retinoblastoma.
Retinal telangiectasia.
Retrolenticular vascularized membrane.
Familial exudative vitreoretinopathy.

LID RETRACTION, CAUSES[42]

ICD-10CM # H02.539 Eyelid retraction unspecified eye, unspecified lid

Thyroid eye disease.
Neurogenic:
  Contralateral unilateral ptosis.
  Unopposed levator action due to facial palsy.
  3rd nerve misdirection.
  Marcus Gunn jaw-winking syndrome.
  Collier sign of the dorsal midbrain (Parinaud syndrome).
  Infantile hydrocephalus (setting sun sign).
  Parkinsonism.
  Sympathomimetic drops.
Mechanical:
  Surgical over-correction of ptosis.
  Scarring of upper lid skin.
Congenital:
  Isolated.
  Duane retraction syndrome.
  Down syndrome.
  Transient "eye popping" reflex in normal infants.
Miscellaneous:
  Prominent globe (pseudo-lid retraction).
  Uremia (Summerskill sign).
  Idiopathic.

LIGHT-NEAR DISSOCIATION[11]

ICD-10CM # varies with specific diagnosis

CAUSES OF LIGHT-NEAR DISSOCIATION

Unilateral
Afferent conduction defect.
Adie pupil.
Herpes zoster ophthalmicus.
Aberrant regeneration of the third cranial nerve.

Bilateral
Neurosyphilis.
Type 1 diabetes mellitus.
Myotonic dystrophy.
Parinaud (dorsal midbrain) syndrome.
Familial amyloidosis.
Encephalitis.
Chronic alcoholism.

LIMB ISCHEMIA, ACUTE, NONTRAUMATIC[14]

ICD-10CM # Atherosclerosis of arteries of extremities

CAUSES OF NONTRAUMATIC ACUTE LIMB ISCHEMIA

Atherosclerotic
In situ thrombosis.
Atheroembolism from thoracic aortic aneurysm/abdominal aortic aneurysm.
Femoral/popliteal aneurysm with or without compression.
Dissection.

Nonatherosclerotic
Embolism from cardiac thrombosis (atrial fibrillation, post–myocardial infarction akinesis).
Graft thrombosis, graft aneurysm.
Mycotic emboli.
Raynaud syndrome.
Arteritis with thrombosis.
Inherited and acquired hypercoagulable states.
Drug-induced vasospasm.
External compression (Baker cyst, popliteal entrapment).

Mimics
Phlegmasia cerulea dolens.
Acute neuropathy.
Hypovolemia.
Systemic shock.

LIMP

ICD-10CM #		
	R26.0	Ataxic gait
	R26.1	Paralytic gait
	R26.89	Other abnormalities of gait and mobility
	R26.9	Unspecified abnormalities of gait and mobility
	M25.80	Other specified joint disorders, unspecified joint
	F44.4	Conversion disorder with motor symptom or deficit
	F44.6	Conversion disorder with sensory symptom or deficit

Degenerative joint disease, osteochondritis dissecans, chondromalacia patellae.

Trauma to extremities, vertebral disk, hips.
Poorly fitting shoes, foreign body in shoe, unequal leg length.
Splinter in foot.
Joint infection (septic arthritis, osteomyelitis), viral arthritis.
Abdominal pain (e.g., appendicitis, incarcerated hernia), testicular torsion.
Polio, neuromuscular disorders, Guillain-Barré syndrome, multiple sclerosis.
Osgood-Schlatter disease.
Legg-Calvé-Perthes disease.
Factitious, somatization syndrome.
Neoplasm (local or metastatic).
Other: diskitis, periostitis, sickle cell disease, hemophilia.

LIMPING, PEDIATRIC AGE[47]

ICD-10CM #		
	R26.0	Ataxic gait
	R26.1	Paralytic gait
	R26.89	Other abnormalities of gait and mobility
	R26.9	Unspecified abnormalities of gait and mobility

TODDLER (1-3 YR)
Infection:
  Septic arthritis:
    Hip.
    Knee.
  Osteomyelitis.
  Diskitis.
Occult trauma:
  Toddler's fracture.
Neoplasia.

CHILDHOOD (4-10 YR)
Infection:
  Septic arthritis:
    ■ Hip.
    ■ Knee.
  Osteomyelitis.
  Diskitis.
  Transient synovitis, hip.
LCPD.
Tarsal coalition.
Rheumatologic disorder:
  JRA.
Trauma.
Neoplasia.

ADOLESCENCE (11+ YR)
● SCFE.
● Rheumatologic disorder:
  JRA.
Trauma.
Tarsal coalition.
Hip dislocation (DDH).
Neoplasia.

DDH, Developmental dysplasia of the hip; *JRA,* juvenile RA; *LCPD,* Legg-Calvé-Perthes disease; *SCFE,* slipped capital femoral epiphysis.

LIVEDO RETICULARIS

ICD-10CM # L95.0 Livedoid vasculitis

Emboli (SBE, left atrial myxoma, cholesterol emboli).
Thrombocythemia or polycythemia.
Antiphospholipid antibody syndrome.
Cryoglobulinemia, cryofibrinogenemia.
Leukocytoclastic vasculitis.
SLE, RA, dermatomyositis.
Pancreatitis.
Drugs (quinine, quinidine, amantadine, catecholamines).
Physiologic (cutis marmorata).
Congenital.

LIVER DISEASE, PREGNANCY[72]

ICD-10CM #	K75.89	Other specified inflammatory liver diseases

INCIDENTAL TO PREGNANCY

Viral hepatitis.
Alcohol related.
Autoimmune chronic active hepatitis.

RELATED TO PREGNANCY (POSSIBLY INFLUENCED BY HORMONES PRESENT IN PREGNANCY)

- Complicated gallstone disease.
- Hepatic adenoma.
- Focal nodular hyperplasia.
- Budd-Chiari syndrome.

SPECIFIC TO PREGNANCY

- Severe hyperemesis gravidarum.
- Benign intrahepatic cholestasis.
- Acute fatty liver of pregnancy.
- Preeclampsia (HELLP).

LIVER LESIONS, BENIGN, OFTEN CONFUSED WITH MALIGNANCY

ICD-10CM #	K76.1	Chronic passive congestion of liver
	K76.89	Other specified diseases of liver

Fatty infiltration.
Adenoma.
Hemangioma.
Cysts.
Flow artifacts.
Focal nodular hyperplasia.
Nonenhanced vessels.

LOW-VOLTAGE ECG

ICD-10CM #	R94.31	Abnormal electrocardiogram [ECG] [EKG]

Hypothyroidism.
Obesity.
Pericardial effusion.
Anasarca.
Pleural effusion.
Pneumothorax.

Amyloidosis.
Aortic stenosis.

LUNG CANCER, OCCUPATIONAL CAUSES[33]

ICD-10CM #	C34.90	Malignant neoplasm of unspecified part of unspecified bronchus or lung

CAUSES OF OCCUPATIONAL LUNG CANCER

Asbestos	Lagging, insulation
Arsenic	Metal smelting, pesticide manufacture
Beryllium	Electronics, dental prosthetic manufacture
Chromium	Coloring pigment production, electroplating
Nickel	Electroplating
Silica	Grinding, quarrying, sandblasting
Radon	Mining
Uranium	Mining

LUNG DISEASE AND GASTROINTESTINAL AND LIVER INVOLVEMENT[52]

ICD-10CM #	codes vary with specific diagnosis

ESOPHAGEAL REFLUX

Aspiration pneumonia.
Asthma.
Scleroderma.
Bronchitis.
Bronchiectasis.
Cough.
Pulmonary fibrosis.
Mycobacterial disease.

INFLAMMATORY BOWEL DISEASE

Bronchitis.
Bronchiectasis.
Bronchiolitis.
Colobronchial fistula.
Desquamative interstitial lung disease.
Drug reactions for agents that treat inflammatory bowel disease.
Eosinophilic lung disease.
Interstitial lung disease.
Necrobiotic nodules.
Obstructive lung disease.
Organizing pneumonia.
Reduced diffusing capacity.
Sarcoidosis.
Serositis affecting pleura or pericarditis.
Tracheal stenosis.

LIVER

Alpha1-antitrypsin deficiency.
Chronic active hepatitis.
Hepatopulmonary syndrome.
Portapulmonary hypertension.

Primary biliary cirrhosis.
Hepatosplenomegaly.
  Amyloidosis.
  Collagen vascular disease.
  Eosinophilic granulomatosis.
  Lymphatic interstitial pneumonia.
  Sarcoidosis.

LUNG DISEASE AND RENAL INVOLVEMENT[52]

ICD-10CM #	codes vary with specific diagnosis

LUNG DISEASE WITH RENAL INVOLVEMENT

Glomerulonephritis
Systemic vasculitis.
Collagen vascular disease.
Antibasement membrane.
Sarcoidosis.
Nephrotic Syndrome
Amyloidosis.
Disseminated Langerhans cell histiocytosis.
Drug-induced lung disease.
Paraneoplastic syndrome.
Post transplantation.
Pulmonary hydatid disease.
Systemic lupus erythematosus.
Vasculitis.
Venous thrombosis.
Renal Mass
Lymphangioleiomyomatosis.
Metastasis neoplasm.
Renal carcinoid.
Tuberous sclerosis.
Wegener's granulomatosis.
Nephrolithiasis
Alveolar proteinosis.
Cystic fibrosis.
Hypercalcemic syndromes.
Osteolysis from mycobacteria or fungi.
Sarcoidosis.
Systemic Hypertension
Collagen vascular disease.
Diffuse alveolar hemorrhage.
Pulmonary renal syndromes.
Neurofibromatosis.
Sleep apnea.

LUNG DISEASE AND SKIN AND SUBCUTANEOUS LESIONS[52]

ICD-10CM #	codes vary with specific diagnosis

SKIN AND SUBCUTANEOUS LESIONS ASSOCIATED WITH LUNG DISEASE

Skin Lesions
Diffuse pigment change.
  Acanthosis nigricans—lung neoplasm.
  Albinism—Hermansky-Pudlak syndrome.
  Bronze pigmentation—hemosiderosis.
  Gray-brown—Whipple's disease.
Cutaneous draining sinus.

Fungal infections (especially histoplasmosis).
Mycobacterial infections (especially tuberculosis).
Neoplasms (especially mesothelial tumors).
Necrotizing vasculitis.
Other bacterial infections (especially actinomycosis).
Cutaneous ulcers.
Beryllium disease.
Chronic venous insufficiency.
Fungal infections (especially histoplasmosis).
Mycobacterial disease.
Necrotizing vasculitis.
Parasitic disease.
Polycythemia.
Sickle cell disease.
Tularemia.
Cutaneous vasculitis.
Behçet's syndrome.
Churg-Strauss syndrome.
Collagen vascular disease.
Sarcoidosis.
Wegener's granulomatosis.
Erythema multiforme.
Drug reactions.
Fungi (especially coccidiomycosis).
Mycoplasma and other infectious agents.
Neoplasms.
Exfoliative dermatitis.
Adverse drug reactions.
Chemotherapy.
Disseminated malignancy.
Graft-versus-host disease.
Radiation therapy.
Flushing.
Bronchial carcinoid, pheochromocytoma, other neoplasms.
Carbon dioxide, cyanide, and other toxins.
Drugs.
Foods and vasodilatory substances.
Hormones.
Mastocytosis.
Metabolic states (e.g., hyperthyroidism, fever).
Macular rash.
Anti-basement membrane disease.
Café-au-lait spots (neurofibromatosis).
Coal miner's scars.
Collagen vascular disease.
Idiopathic pulmonary fibrosis.
Rose spots (psittacosis).
Sarcoidosis.
Syphilis.
Viral pneumonia.
Maculopapular rash.
Amyloidosis.
Drug-induced lung disease.
Collagen vascular disease.
Gaucher's disease.
Kaposi's sarcoma.
Lung neoplasm.
Lymphomatoid granulomatosis.
Lymphoma.
Parasites.
Sarcoidosis.
Syphilis.
Vasculitis.
Viral pneumonia
Telangiectasia

Arteriovenous malformation.
Ataxia-telangiectasia.
Carcinoid syndrome.
Cushing's disease.
Hepatopulmonary syndrome and other chronic liver diseases.
Hereditary hemorrhagic telangiectasia (Osler-Weber-Rendu).
Mastocytosis.
Systemic sclerosis and other collagen vascular diseases.
Urticaria
Asthma.
Drug reactions.
Cystic fibrosis.
Exercise-induced urticaria.
Food allergy.
Hereditary angioneurotic edema.
Inhaled antigens.
Insect bites and stings.
Infectious agents, such as mycoplasma and helicobacter.
Mastocytosis.
Occupational sensitization.
Parasites.
Vasculitis.

Nail Changes with Lung Disease
Color changes:
Cigarette smoking discoloration.
Splinter hemorrhages.
Yellow nail syndrome.
Beau's lines (any severe illness):
Dermatomyositis.
Sarcoidosis.
Seronegative arthropathies.
Systemic sclerosis.

Lung Disease with Subcutaneous Involvement
Adenopathy:
Environmental mycobacteria.
Fungal infections.
Human immunodeficiency visurs infections.
Metastatic neoplasm.
Leukemia.
Lymphoma.
Sarcoidosis.
Tuberculosis.
Calcinosis:
- Dermatomyositis.
- Metastatic osteosarcoma.
- Mixed connective tissue disease.
- Scleroderma.
- Tuberculosis.
- Uremic metastatic calcification.
Erythema induratum (Bazin's disease):
Aortic stenosis.
Cryoglobulinemia.
Nodular vasculitis.
Panniculitis.
Peripheral neuropathy.
Takayasu's disease.
Streptococcus infection.
Tuberculosis and other mycobacterial disease.
Weber-Christian disease.
Erythema nodosa:
Neoplasm.
Other infectious and inflammatory diseases.
Primary coccidiomycosis, histoplasmosis.

Primary tuberculosis.
Psittacosis.
Sarcoidosis.
Subcutaneous nodules:
Amyloidosis.
Neoplasm.
Neurofibromatosis.
Rheumatoid arthritis.
Tuberous sclerosis (angiofibromas).
von Recklinghausen.
Weber-Christian disease.

Lung Disease with Salivary Gland Enlargement
Bulimia and aspiration.
Gaucher's disease.
Lymphoid interstitial pneumonitis.
Lymphatic carcinoma.
Lymphoma.
Other causes of lymphadenopathy.
Sarcoidosis.
Sjögren disease.

LUNG DISEASE WITH BONE, JOINT, NERVE, AND MUSCLE INVOLVEMENT[52]

ICD-10CM #   codes vary with specific diagnosis

ARTHRITIS
Ankylosing spondylitis.
Collagen vascular diseases.
Reactive arthritis.
Sarcoidosis.
Systemic vasculitis.
Tuberculosis.

BONE LESIONS
Ankylosing spondylitis.
Blastomycosis and other fungal disease.
Collagen vascular diseases.
Eosinophilic granulomatosis.
Fibrous histiocytoma.
Gaucher's disease.
Neoplasm.
Sarcoidosis.
Tuberculosis.

MUSCLE DISEASE
Collagen vascular disease.
L-Tryptophan.
Diabetes insipidus.
Eosinophilic granulomatosis.
Polymyositis.
Sarcoidosis.

NEUROLOGIC DISEASE
Acute inflammatory polyneuropathy.
Amyotrophic lateral sclerosis.
Aspiration.
Botulism.
Lambert-Eaton syndrome.
Myasthenia gravis.
Organophosphate poisoning.
Polio and postpolio syndrome.
Sarcoidosis.
Churg-Strauss syndrome.
Wegener's granulomatosis.

LUNG TUMORS, BENIGN[65]

ICD-10CM # varies with specific disorder

COMMON BENIGN TUMORS OF THE LUNG BASED ON CELLS OF ORIGIN

Tumors of Epithelial Origin
Mucous gland adenoma
Clara cell adenoma
Mucous cystadenoma
Pleomorphic adenoma
Tumors of Mesenchymal Origin
Hamartoma
Inflammatory pseudotumor
Chondroma
Fibroma
Benign endobronchial fibrous histiocytoma
Leiomyoma
Lipoma
Lymphatic lesions
Tumors of Miscellaneous Origin
Nodular pulmonary amyloidosis
Clear cell tumor (sugar tumor)
Thymoma
Granular cell tumor
Teratoma
Pulmonary paraganglioma

LUNG VOLUMES IN DIFFUSE LUNG DISEASE[31]

ICD-10CM # varies with specific disorder

LARGE LUNG VOLUMES

Emphysema.
Chonic asthma.
Diffuse bronchiolitis obliterans.
Highly trained athletes.
Lymphangioleiomyomatosis.

SMALL LUNG VOLUMES

End-stage lung fibrosis.
Bilateral diaphragmatic paralysis.
Massive ascites.

NORMAL LUNG VOLUMES

Sarcoidosis.
Langerhans cell histiocytosis.
Neurofibromatosis.
Emphysema with pulmonary fibrosis.

LYMPHADENOPATHY[29]

ICD-10CM # R59.9 Enlarged lymph nodes, unspecified

GENERALIZED

AIDS.
Lymphoma: Hodgkin's disease, non-Hodgkin's lymphoma.
Leukemias, reticuloendotheliosis.
Infectious mononucleosis, CMV, and other viral infections.
Diffuse skin infection: generalized furunculosis, multiple tick bites.
Parasitic infections: toxoplasmosis, filariasis, leishmaniasis, Chagas' disease.

Serum sickness.
Collagen vascular diseases (RA, SLE).
Dengue (arbovirus infection).
Sarcoidosis and other granulomatous diseases.
Drugs: INH, hydantoin derivatives, antithyroid and antileprosy drugs.
Secondary syphilis.
Hyperthyroidism, lipid-storage diseases.

LOCALIZED

Cervical Nodes
Infections of the head, neck, ears, sinuses, scalp, pharynx.
Mononucleosis.
Lymphoma.
TB.
Malignancy of head and neck.
Rubella.
Scalene/Supraclavicular Nodes
Lymphoma.
Lung neoplasm.
Bacterial or fungal infection of thorax or retroperitoneum.
GI malignancy.
Axillary Nodes
Infections of hands and arms.
Cat-scratch disease.
Neoplasm (lymphoma, melanoma, breast carcinoma).
Brucellosis.
Epitrochlear Nodes
Infections of the hand.
Lymphoma.
Tularemia.
Sarcoidosis, secondary syphilis (usually bilateral).
Inguinal Nodes
Infections of leg or foot, folliculitis (pubic hair).
LGV, syphilis.
Lymphoma.
Pelvic malignancy.
Pasteurella pestis.
Hilar Nodes
Sarcoidosis.
TB.
Lung carcinoma.
Fungal infections, systemic.
Mediastinal Nodes
Sarcoidosis.
Lymphoma.
Lung neoplasm.
TB.
Mononucleosis.
Histoplasmosis.
Abdominal/Retroperitoneal Nodes
Lymphoma.
TB.
Neoplasm (ovary, testes, prostate, and other malignancies).

LYMPHANGITIS[50]

ICD-10CM # I89.1 Lymphangitis

Acute:
  Group A streptococci.
  Staphylococcus aureus.
  Pasteurella multocida.
Chronic:
  Sporothrix schenckii (sporotrichosis).

Mycobacterium marinum (swimming pool granuloma).
Mycobacterium kansasii.
Nocardia brasiliensis.
W. bancrofti.

LYMPHEDEMA[41]

ICD-10CM #	I89.0	Lymphedema, not elsewhere classified
	I97.2	Postmastectomy lymphedema syndrome
	Q82.0	Hereditary lymphedema

CLASSIFICATION OF LYMPHEDEMA

Primary lymphedema
Congenital lymphedema (Milroy's disease).
Lymphedema praecox.
Lymphedema tarda.
Syndromes associated with primary lymphedema
Yellow nail syndrome.
Turner syndrome.
Noonan syndrome.
Pes cavus.
Phakomatosis pigmentovascularis.
Distichiasis-lymphedema.
Emberger syndrome.
WILD syndrome.
Hypotrichosis-telangiectasia-lymphedema syndrome.
Cutaneous disorders sometimes associated with primary lymphedema
Yellow nails.
Hemangiomas.
Xanthomatosis and chylous lymphedema.
Congenital absence of nails.
Secondary lymphedema
Postmastectomy lymphedema.
Melphalan isolated limb perfusion.
Malignant occlusion with obstruction.
Extrinsic pressure.
Factitial lymphedema.
Postradiation therapy.
Following recurrent lymphangitis/cellulitis.
Lymphedema of upper limb in recurrent eczema.
Granulomatous disease.
Rosaceous lymphedema.
Primary amyloidosis.
Complications of lymphedema
Cellulitis of lymphedema.
Elephantiasis nostra verrucosa.
Ulceration.
Lymphangiosarcoma.

LYMPHOCYTOSIS, ATYPICAL[50]

| ICD-10CM # | D72.89 | Other specified disorders of white blood cells |

Epstein-Barr virus primary infection (infectious mononucleosis).
Cytomegalovirus primary infection (heterophile-negative mono).

Human herpesvirus 6 primary infection (roseola).
Primary HIV infection.
Toxoplasmosis.
Acute viral hepatitis.
Rubella, mumps.
Drug reactions (e.g., phenytoin, sulfa).

MACROTHROMBOCYTOPENIA, INHERITED[40]

ICD-10CM #   varies with specific disorder

Bernard-Soulier syndrome.
MHY9-related disorders:
   May-Hegglin anomaly.
   Sebastian syndrome.
   Fechtner syndrome.
   Epstein syndrome.
Gray platelet syndrome.
Montreal platelet syndrome.
Mediterranean macrothrombocytopenia.
Mediterranean stomatocytosis/macrothrombocytemia.
GATA1 mutations.
Sialyl-Lewis-S antigen deficiency.
Paris-Trousseau syndrome.
Platelet-type von Willebrand's disease.

MACULAR CRYSTALS[11]

ICD-10CM #   varies with specific diagnosis

OTHER CAUSES OF MACULAR CRYSTALS

Primary hyperoxaluria.
Bietti corneoretinal crystalline dystrophy.
Cystinosis.
Sjögren–Larsson syndrome.
Gyrate atrophy.
Acquired parafoveal telangiectasis.
Talc-corn starch emboli.
West African crystalline maculopathy.

MADAROSIS[11]

ICD-10CM #   H02.729   Madarosis of unspecified eye, unspecified eyelid and periocular area

CAUSES OF MADAROSIS
Local
Chronic anterior lid margin disease.
Infiltrating lid tumors.
Burns.
Radiotherapy or cryotherapy of lid tumors.
Skin disorders
Generalized alopecia.
Psoriasis.
Systemic diseases.
Myxoedema.
Systemic lupus erythematosus.
Acquired syphilis.
Lepromatous leprosy.
Following removal
Procedures for trichiasis.
Trichotillomania (psychiatric disorder of hair removal).

MALABSORPTION[72]

ICD-10CM #   K90.89   Other intestinal malabsorption

CAUSES OF MALABSORPTION
More Common
Celiac disease.
Chronic pancreatitis.
Post gastrectomy.
Crohn's disease.
Small bowel resection.
Small intestinal bacterial overgrowth.
Lactase deficiency.
Less Common
AIDS (*Myobacterium avium* intracellulare, AIDS enteropathy).
Whipple's disease.
Intestinal lymphoma.
Immunoproliferative small intestinal disease (alpha heavy chain disease).
Radiation enteritis.
Collagenous sprue.
Tropical sprue.
Non-granulomatous ulcerative jejunoileitis.
Eosinophilic gastroenteritis.
Amyloidosis.
Zollinger-Ellison syndrome.
Intestinal lymphangiectasia.
Systemic mastocytosis.
Chronic mesenteric ischemia.
Abetalipoproteinemia (autosomal recessive).

MALABSORPTION SYNDROME IN TROPICS[23]

ICD-10CM #   K90.89   Other intestinal malabsorption

CAUSES OF MALABSORPTION SYNDROME IN THE TROPICS
SIBO
Following ulcer surgery
Secondary to intestinal TB and Crohn's disease
Infections
Bacteria
   Mycobacterium avium intracellulare complex
   Mycobacterium tuberculosis
Helminths
   Paracapillaria philippinensis
   Strongyloides stercoralis
Protozoa
   Cryptosporidium parvum
   Cyclospora cayetanensis
   Encephalitozoon intestinalis
   Enterocytozoon bieneusi
   Giardia lamblia
   Isospora belli
   Leishmania donovani
Lymphatic Obstruction
   Intestinal lymphangiectasia
Mucosal Diseases
   Autoimmune enteropathy
   Celiac disease
   Eosinophilic gastroenteritis
   HIV enteropathy

Immunoproliferative small intestinal disease
Intestinal lymphoma
Primary immunodeficiencies
Tropical sprue
Neonatal Diseases
   Microvillus inclusion disease
   Tufting enteropathy
Pancreatic Insufficiency
   Alcoholic pancreatitis
   CF
   Tropical pancreatitis
Specific Transport Disorders
   Abetalipoproteinemia
   Fructose malabsorption
   Glucose-galactose malabsorption
   Hypolactasia
   Sucrose intolerance

MALNUTRITION, CAUSES IN EARLY LIFE[46]

ICD-10CM #   E46   Unspecified protein-energy malnutrition

0-6 MO
Breastfeeding difficulties.
Improper formula preparation.
Impaired parent/child interaction.
Congenital syndromes.
Prenatal infections or teratogenic exposures.
Poor feeding (sucking, swallowing) or feeding refusal (aversion).
Maternal psychological disorder (depression or attachment disorder).
Congenital heart disease.
Cystic fibrosis.
Neurologic abnormalities.
Child neglect.
Recurrent infections.

6-12 MO
Celiac disease.
Food intolerance.
Child neglect.
Delayed introduction of age-appropriate foods or poor transition to food.
Recurrent infections.
Food allergy.

AFTER INFANCY
Acquired chronic diseases.
Highly distractible child.
Inappropriate mealtime environment.
Inappropriate diet (e.g., excessive juice consumption, avoidance of high-calorie foods).
Recurrent infections.

MEDIASTINAL COMPARTMENTS, ANATOMY AND PATHOLOGY[77]

ICD-10CM #   varies with specific disorder

ANTERIOR
Normal Structures
Lymph nodes.
Connective tissue.
Thymus (remnant in adults).

Differential Diagnosis

II

Masses
Thymoma.
Germ cell neoplasm.
Lymphoma.
Thyroid enlargement (intrathoracic goiter).
Other tumors.

MIDDLE
Normal Structures
Pericardium.
Heart.
Vessels: Ascending aorta, venae cavae, main pulmonary arteries.
Trachea.
Lymph nodes.
Nerves: Phrenic, upper vagus.
Masses
Carcinoma.
Lymphoma.
Pericardial cyst.
Bronchogenic cyst.
Benign lymph node enlargement (granulomatous disease).

POSTERIOR
Normal Structures
Vessels: Descending aorta.
Esophagus.
Vertebral column.
Nerves: Sympathetic chain, lower vagus.
Lymph nodes.
Connective tissue.
Masses
Neurogenic tumor.
Diaphragmatic hernia.

MEDIASTINAL MASSES OR WIDENING ON CHEST X-RAY

| ICD-10CM # | R59.9 | Enlarged lymph nodes, unspecified |
| | J98.5 | Diseases of mediastinum, not elsewhere classified |

Lymphoma: Hodgkin's disease and non-Hodgkin's lymphoma.
Sarcoidosis.
Vascular: aortic aneurysm, ectasia, or tortuosity of aorta or bronchocephalic vessels.
Carcinoma: lungs, esophagus.
Esophageal diverticula.
Hiatal hernia.
Achalasia.
Prominent pulmonary outflow tract: pulmonary hypertension, pulmonary embolism, right-to-left shunts.
Trauma: mediastinal hemorrhage.
Pneumomediastinum.
Lymphadenopathy caused by silicosis and other pneumoconioses.
Leukemias.
Infections: TB, viral (rare), *Mycoplasma* (rare), fungal, tularemia.
Substernal thyroid.
Thymoma.
Teratoma.
Bronchogenic cyst.

Pericardial cyst.
Neurofibroma, neurosarcoma, ganglioneuroma.

MEDIASTINAL MASSES, SITES OF ORIGIN[75]

| ICD-10CM # | varies with specific diagnosis |

DIFFERENTIAL DIAGNOSIS OF MEDIASTINAL MASSES BASED ON COMMON SITES OF ORIGIN
Prevascular space (anterior mediastinum)
Thymic masses.
Thymoma.
Thymic carcinoma.
Thymic neuroendocrine tumor.
Thymolipoma.
Thymic cyst.
Thymic hyperplasia.
Thymic lymphoma.
Germ cell tumors.
Teratoma and dermoid cyst.
Seminoma.
Nonseminomatous germ cell tumors.
Thyroid abnormalities (goiter and neoplasm).
Parathyroid tumor or hyperplasia.
Lymph node masses (particularly Hodgkin's lymphoma).
Vascular abnormalities (aorta and great vessels).
Mesenchymal abnormalities (e.g., lipomatosis, lipoma).
Foregut cyst.
Lymphangioma.
Hemangioma.
Retrosternal space (anterior mediastinum)
Lymph node masses.
Pretracheal space (middle mediastinum)
Lymph node masses.
Lung carcinoma.
Sarcoidosis.
Lymphoma (particularly Hodgkin's disease).
Metastases.
Infections (e.g., tuberculosis).
Foregut cyst.
Tracheal tumor.
Mesenchymal masses (e.g., lipomatosis, lipoma).
Thyroid abnormalities.
Vascular abnormalities (aorta and great vessels).
Lymphangioma and hemangioma.
Aortopulmonary window (middle mediastinum)
Lymph node masses.
Lung carcinoma.
Sarcoidosis.
Lymphoma.
Metastases.
Infections (e.g., tuberculosis).
Mesenchymal masses (e.g., lipomatosis, lipoma).
Vascular abnormalities (aorta or pulmonary artery).
Chemodectoma.
Foregut cyst.
Subcarinal space and azygoesophageal recess (middle mediastinum)
Lymph node masses.
Lung carcinoma.
Sarcoidosis.

Lymphoma.
Metastases.
Infections (e.g., tuberculosis).
Foregut cyst.
Dilated azygos vein.
Esophageal masses.
Varices.
Hernia.
Paravertebral masses (posterior mediastinum)
Neurogenic tumor.
Nerve sheath tumors.
Sympathetic ganglia tumors.
Paraganglioma.
Meningocele.
Foregut cyst.
Neurenteric cyst.
Thoracic spine abnormalities.
Extramedullary hematopoiesis.
Fluid collections and pseudocyst.
Vascular abnormalities.
Hernias.
Esophageal masses.
Varices.
Mesenchymal masses (e.g., lipomatosis, lipoma).
Lymph node masses.
Lymphoma (particularly non-Hodgkin's).
Metastases.
Dilated azygos or hemiazygos vein.
Hernia.
Lymphangioma and hemangioma.
Thymic mass or germ cell tumor.
Anterior cardiophrenic angle masses.
Lymph node masses (particularly lymphoma and metastases).
Pericardial cyst.
Fat pad.
Morgagni hernia.
Thymic masses.
Germ cell tumors.

MEDIASTINITIS, ACUTE[50]

| ICD-10CM # | J98.5 | Diseases of mediastinum, not elsewhere classified |

Esophageal perforation.
Iatrogenic.
EGD, esophageal dilation, esophageal variceal sclerotherapy, nasogastric tube, Sengstaken-Blackmore tube, endotracheal intubation, esophageal surgery, paraesophageal surgery, transesophageal echocardiography, anterior stabilization of cervical vertebral bodies.
Swallowed foreign bodies.
Trauma.
Spontaneous perforation (e.g., emesis, carcinoma).
Head and neck infections (e.g., tonsillitis, pharyngitis, parotitis, epiglottitis, odontogenic).
Infections originating at another site (e.g., TB, pneumonia, pancreatitis, osteomyelitis of sternum, clavicle, ribs).
Cardiothoracic surgery (median sternotomy) (e.g., CABG, valve replacement, other types of cardiothoracic surgery).

MELANONYCHIA

ICD-10CM # NEC   Melanin
             L81.4   hyperpigmentation

Pregnancy.
Trauma.
Medications (e.g., AZT, 5-fluorouracil, doxorubicin, psoralens).
Nail matrix nevus.
HIV infection.
Onychomycosis.
Melanocyte hyperplasia.
Verrucae.
Pustular psoriasis.
Lichen planus.
Basal cell carcinoma.
Nail matrix melanoma.
Subungual keratosis.
Addison's disease.
Bowen's disease.

MEMORY LOSS SYMPTOMS, ELDERLY PATIENTS

ICD-10CM # R41.2   Retrograde amnesia

Age-related mild cognitive impairment.
Depression (pseudodementia).
Medications (e.g., anticholinergics, sedatives).
Hypothyroidism.
Chronic hypoxia.
Cerebrovascular infarcts.
Alzheimer's disease.
Hepatic disease.
Chronic renal failure.
Hyperthyroidism.
Frontotemporal dementia.
Lewy body dementia.

MENINGITIS, CHRONIC[50]

ICD-10CM # G03.1   Chronic meningitis

TB.
Fungal CNS infection.
Tertiary syphilis.
CNS neoplasm.
Metabolic encephalopathies.
Multiple sclerosis.
Chronic subdural hematoma.
SLE cerebritis.
Encephalitides.
Sarcoidosis.
NSAIDs.
Behçet's syndrome.
Anatomic defects (traumatic, congenital, postoperative).
Granulomatous angiitis.

MENINGITIS, RECURRENT[50]

ICD-10CM # G03.2   Benign recurrent
             meningitis [Mollaret]

Drug induced (with rechallenge).
Parameningeal focus.
  Infection (sinusitis, mastoiditis, osteomyelitis, brain abscess).
  Tumor (epidermoid cyst, craniopharyngioma).
Posttraumatic (bacterial).

Mollaret's meningitis.
SLE.
Herpes simplex virus.

MENTAL STATUS CHANGES AND COMA[6]

ICD-10CM # R41.82   Altered mental
              status, unspecified

METABOLIC/SYSTEMIC ETIOLOGY OF ALTERED MENTAL STATUS AND COMA

Hypoxia
Severe pulmonary disease (hypoventilation).
Severe anemia.
Environmental/toxin:
Methemoglobinemia.
  Cyanide.
  Carbon monoxide.
  Decreased atmospheric oxygen (high altitude).
  Near-drowning.

Disorders of Glucose
Hypoglycemia:
  Chronic alcohol abuse and liver disease.
  Excessive use of insulin or other hypoglycemic agents.
  Insulinoma.
Hyperglycemia:
  Diabetic ketoacidosis.
  Nonketotic hyperosmolar coma.

Decreased Cerebral Blood Flow
Hypovolemic shock.
Cardiac:
  Vasovagal syncope.
  Arrhythmias.
  Myocardial infarction.
  Valvular disorders.
  Congestive heart failure.
  Pericardial effusion/tamponade.
  Myocarditis.
Infectious:
  Septic shock.
  Bacterial meningitis.
Vascular/hematologic:
  Hypertensive encephalopathy.
  Pseudotumor cerebri.
  Hyperviscosity (sickle cell, polycythemia).
  Hyperventilation.
  Cerebral lupus vasculitis.
  Thrombotic thrombocytopenic purpura.
  Disseminated intravascular coagulation.

Metabolic Cofactor Deficiency
Thiamine (Wernicke-Korsakoff syndrome).
Pyridoxine (isoniazid overdose).
Folic acid (chronic alcohol abuse).
Cyanocobalamin.
Niacin.

Electrolye/pH Disturbances
Acidosis/alkalosis.
Hypernatremia/hyponatremia.[26]
Hypercalcemia/hypocalcemia.
Hypophosphatemia.
Hypermagnesemia/hypomagnesemia.

---

[26]Can be associated with dilution of formula in infant feeding.

Endocrine Disorders
Myxedema coma, thyrotoxicosis.
Hypopituitarism.
Addison's disease (primary or secondary).
Cushing's disease.
Pheochromocytoma.
Hyperparathyroidism/hypoparathyroidism.
Endogenous Toxins
Hyperammonemia (liver failure).
Uremia (renal disease).
Carbon dioxide narcosis (pulmonary disease).
Porphyria.
Exogenous Toxins
Alcohols:
  Ethanol, isopropyl alcohol, methanol, ethylene glycol.
Acid poisons:
  Salicylates.
  Paraldehyde.
  Ammonium chloride.
Antidepressant medications:
  Lithium.
  Tricyclic antidepressants (TCAs).
  Selective serotonin reuptake inhibitors (SSRIs).
  Monamine oxidase inhibitors (MAOIs).
Stimulants:
  Amphetamines/methamphetamines.
  Cocaine.
  Over-the-counter sympathomimetics.
Narcotics/opiates:
  Morphine.
  Heroin.
  Codeine, oxycodone, meperidine, hydrocodone.
  Methadone.
  Fentanyl.
  Propoxyphene.
Sedative-hypnotics:
  Benzodiazepines.
  Barbiturates.
  Rohypnol.
  Bromide.
Hallucinogens:
  Lysergic acid diethylamide (LSD).
  Marijuana.
  Mescaline, peyote.
  Mushrooms.
  Phencyclidine (PCP).
Herbs/plants:
  Aconite.
  Jimson weed.
  Morning glory.
Volatile substances:
  Hydrocarbons (gasoline, butane, toluene, benzene, chloroform).
  Nitrites.
  Anesthetic agents (nitrous oxide, ether).
Other:
  γ-Hydroxybutyrate (GHB).
  Ketamine.
  Penicillin.
  Cardiac glycosides.
  Anticonvulsants.
  Steroids.
  Heavy metals.
  Cimetidine.
  Organophosphates.

Disorders of Temperature Regulation/ Environmental
- Hypothermia.
- Heat stroke.
- Malignant hyperthermia.
- Neuroleptic malignant syndrome.
- High-altitude cerebral edema (HACE).
- Dysbarism.

Primary Glial or Neuronal Disorders
Adrenoleukodystrophy.
Creutzfeldt-Jakob disease.
Progressive multifocal leukoencephalopathy.
Marchiafava-Bignami disease.
Gliomatosis cerebri.
Central pontine myelinolysis.

Other Disorders of Unknown Etiology
- Seizures.
- Postictal states.
- Reye's syndrome.[27]
- Intussuception.

---

[27]Prominent in the pediatric population.

MENTAL STATUS CHANGES AND COMA, STRUCTURAL CAUSES[1]

ICD-10CM #   R40.1

COMMON AGE-RELATED CAUSES OF ALTERED MENTAL STATUS AND COMA

Infant
Infection.
Trauma, abuse.
Metabolic.

Child
Toxic ingestion.

Adolescent, Young Adult
Toxic ingestion.
Recreational drug use.
Trauma.

Elderly
- Medication changes.
- Over-the-counter medications.
- Infection.
- Alterations in living environment.
- Stroke.
- Trauma.

MENTAL STATUS CHANGES AND COMA, METABOLIC AND SYSTEMIC CAUSES[1]

ICD-10CM #   CM40.1

METABOLIC AND SYSTEMIC CAUSES OF ALTERED MENTAL STATUS AND COMA

Hypoxia, Hypercapnia
- Severe pulmonary disease (hypoventilation).
- Severe anemia.
- Environmental, toxic.
- Methemoglobinemia.
- Cyanide.
- Carbon monoxide.
- Decreased atmospheric oxygen (high altitude).

- Near-drowning.

Glucose Disorders
Hypoglycemia:
  Chronic alcohol abuse and liver disease.
  Excessive dosage of insulin or other hypoglycemic agents.
  Insulinoma.
Hyperglycemia:
  Diabetic ketoacidosis.
  Nonketotic hyperosmolar coma.

Decreased Cerebral Blood Flow
Hypovolemic shock.
Cardiac:
  Vasovagal syncope.
  Arrhythmias.
  Myocardial infarction.
  Valvular disorders.
  Congestive heart failure.
  Pericardial effusion, tamponade.
  Myocarditis.
Infectious
  Septic shock.
  Bacterial meningitis.
Vascular, hematologic
  Hypertensive encephalopathy.
  Pseudotumor cerebri.
  Hyperviscosity (sickle cell, polycythemia).
  Hyperventilation.
  Cerebral vasculitis as a manifestation of systemic lupus erythematosus.
  Thrombotic thrombocytopenic purpura.
  Disseminated intravascular coagulation.

Metabolic Cofactor Deficiency
Thiamine (Wernicke-Korsakoff syndrome).
Pyridoxine (isoniazid overdose).
Folic acid (chronic alcohol abuse).
Cyanocobalamin.
Niacin.

Electrolyte, pH Disturbances
Acidosis, alkalosis.
Hypernatremia, hyponatremia.[28]
Hypercalcemia, hypocalcemia.
Hypophosphatemia.
Hypermagnesemia, hypomagnesemia.

Endocrine Disorders
Myxedema coma, thyrotoxicosis.
Hypopituitarism.
Addison disease (primary or secondary).
Cushing disease.
Pheochromocytoma.
Hyperparathyroidism, hypoparathyroidism.

Endogenous Toxins
Hyperammonemia (liver failure).
Uremia (renal disease).
Carbon dioxide narcosis (pulmonary disease).
Porphyria.

Exogenous Toxins
Alcohols:
  Ethanol, isopropyl alcohol, methanol, ethylene glycol.
Acid poisons:
  Salicylates.
  Paraldehyde.
  Ammonium chloride.
Antidepressant medications:
  Lithium.

---

[28]Can be associated with dilution of formula in infant feeding.

Tricyclic antidepressants.
Selective serotonin reuptake inhibitors.
Monoamine oxidase inhibitors.
Stimulants:
  Amphetamines, methamphetamines.
  Cocaine.
  Over-the-counter sympathomimetics.
Narcotics, opiates:
  Morphine.
  Heroin.
  Codeine, oxycodone, meperidine, hydrocodone.
  Methadone.
  Fentanyl.
  Propoxyphene.
Sedative-hypnotics:
  Benzodiazepines.
  Barbiturates.
  Rohypnol.
  Bromide.
Hallucinogens:
  Lysergic acid diethylamide.
  Marijuana.
  Mescaline, peyote.
  Mushrooms.
  Phencyclidine.
Herbs, plants:
  Aconite.
  Jimsonweed.
  Morning glory.
Volatile substances:
  Hydrocarbons (gasoline, butane, toluene, benzene, chloroform).
  Nitrites.
  Anesthetic agents (nitrous oxide, ether).
Other:
  γ-Hydroxybutyrate.
  Ketamine.
  Penicillin.
  Cardiac glycosides.
  Anticonvulsants.
  Steroids.
  Heavy metals.
  Cimetidine.
  Organophosphates.

Disorders of Temperature Regulation, Environmental
Hypothermia.
Heat stroke.
Malignant hyperthermia.
Neuroleptic malignant syndrome.
High-altitude cerebral edema.
Dysbarism.

Primary Glial or Neuronal Disorders
Adrenoleukodystrophy.
Creutzfeldt-Jakob disease.
Progressive multifocal leukoencephalopathy.
Marchiafava-Bignami disease.
Gliomatosis cerebri.
Central pontine myelinolysis.

Other Disorders with Unknown Etiology
Seizures.
Postictal states.
Reye syndrome.
Intussusception.

MESENTERIC ARTERIAL EMBOLISM, ASSOCIATED FACTORS[6]

ICD-10CM #   I74.09   Other arterial embolism and thrombosis of abdominal aorta

FACTORS ASSOCIATED WITH MESENTERIC ARTERIAL EMBOLISM

Coronary artery disease.
    Post-myocardial infarction mural thrombi.
    Congestive heart failure.
Valvular heart disease.
    Rheumatic mitral valve disease.
    Nonbacterial endocarditis.
Arrhythmias.
    Chronic atrial fibrillation.
Aortic aneurysms or dissections.
Coronary angiography.

MESENTERIC ISCHEMIA, NONOCCLUSIVE[50]

ICD-10CM #	K55.0	Acute vascular disorders of intestine
	K55.1	Chronic vascular disorders of intestine
	S35.8X9A	Unspecified injury of other blood vessels at abdomen, lower back and pelvis level, initial encounter

- Cardiovascular disease resulting in low-flow states (CHF, cardiogenic shock, post cardiopulmonary bypass, dysrhythmias).
- Septic shock.
- Drug induced (cocaine, vasopressors, ergot alkaloid poisoning).

MESENTERIC VENOUS THROMBOSIS[50]

ICD-10CM #   I82.91   Chronic embolism and thrombosis of unspecified vein

Hypercoagulable states (protein C or S deficiency, antithrombin III deficiency, Factor V Leyden, malignancy, polycythemia vera, sickle cell disease, homocystinemia, lupus anticoagulant, cardiolipin antibody).
Trauma (operative venous injury, abdominal trauma, postsplenectomy).
Inflammatory conditions (pancreatitis, diverticulitis, appendicitis, cholangitis).
Other: CHF, renal failure, portal hypertension, decompression sickness.

METASTATIC NEOPLASMS

ICD-10CM #	C79.51	Secondary malignant neoplasm of bone
	C79.52	Secondary malignant neoplasm of bone marrow
	C79.31	Secondary malignant neoplasm of brain
	C78.7	Secondary malignant neoplasm of liver and intrahepatic bile duct
	C78.00	Secondary malignant neoplasm of unspecified lung

To: Bone	To: Brain
Breast	Lung
Lung	Breast
Prostate	Melanoma
Thyroid	GU tract
Kidney	Colon
Bladder	Sinuses
Endometrium	Sarcoma
Cervix	Skin
Melanoma	Thyroid

To: Liver	To: Lung
Colon	Breast
Stomach	Colon
Pancreas	Kidney
Breast	Testis
Lymphomas	Stomach
Bronchus	Thyroid
Lung	Melanoma
Sarcoma	
Choriocarcinoma	
Kidney	

METHAEMOGLOBINAEMIA, DRUG INDUCED[39]

ICD-10CM #   D74   Methaemoglobinaemia

SUBSTANCES ASSOCIATED WITH METHAEMOGLOBINAEMIA

Acetaminophen (nitrobenzene derivative).
Acetanilide.
Local anesthetics.
    Benzocaine.
    Lidocaine.
    Prilocaine.
Aniline dyes.
Celecoxib.
Dapsone.
Flutamide.
Ifosfamide.
Metoclopramide.
Nitric oxide.
Nitrites.
    Amyl nitrite.
    Isobutyl nitrite.
    Sodium nitrite.
    Nitrates (bacterial conversion to nitrites).
Nitrobenzenes/nitrobenzoates.
Nitroethane (nail polish remover).
Nitrofurans.
Nitroglycerin.
Paraquat/monolinuron.
Phenacetin.
Phenazopyridine (pyridium).
Primaquine.
Rasuricase.
Sulfamethoxazole.

MICROCEPHALY[8]

ICD-10CM #   Q02   Microcephaly

PRIMARY (GENETIC)

Familial (autosomal recessive).
Autosomal dominant.
Syndromes:
    Down (21-trisomy).
    Edward (18-trisomy).
    Cri-du-chat (5 p-).
    Cornelia de Lange.
    Rubinstein-Taybi.
    Smith-Lemli-Opitz.

SECONDARY (NONGENETIC)

Radiation.
Congenital infections:
    Cytomegalovirus.
    Rubella.
    Toxoplasmosis.
Drugs:
    Fetal alcohol.
    Fetal hydantoin.
Meningitis/encephalitis.
Malnutrition.
Metabolic.
Hyperthermia.
Hypoxic-ischemic encephalopathy.

MICROPENIS[54]

| ICD-10CM # | N48.89 | Other specified disorders of penis |
| | Q55.62 | Hypoplasia of penis |

HYPOGONADOTROPIC HYPOGONADISM (HYPOTHALAMIC OR PITUITARY DEFICIENCIES)

Kallmann's syndrome: autosomal dominant; associated with hyposmia.
Prader-Willi syndrome: hypotonia, mental retardation, obesity, small hands and feet.
Rud syndrome: hyposomia, ichthyosis, mental retardation.
De Morsier's syndrome (septooptic dysplasia): hypopituitarism, hypoplastic optic discs, absent septum pellucidum.

HYPERGONADOTROPIC HYPOGONADISM

Primary testicular defect: disorders of testicular differentiation or inborn errors of testosterone synthesis.
Klinefelter's syndrome.
Other X polysomies (i.e., XXXXY, XXXY).
Robinow's syndrome: brachymesomelic dwarfism, dysmorphic facies.

PARTIAL ANDROGEN INSENSITIVITY

IDIOPATHIC

Defective morphogenesis of the penis.

MIOSIS

ICD-10CM #   H57.03   Miosis

Medications (e.g., morphine, pilocarpine).
Neurosyphilis.
Congenital.

Iritis.
CNS pontine lesion.
CNS infections.
Cavernous sinus thrombosis.
Inflammation/irritation of cornea or conjunctiva.

MONOARTHRITIS, ACUTE

ICD-10CM #	M13.10	Monoarthritis, not elsewhere classified, unspecified site

Overuse.
Trauma.
Gout.
Pseudogout.
Osteoarthritis.
Infectious arthritis (e.g., gonococcal, Lyme disease, viral, mycobacteria, fungi).
Osteomyelitis.
Avascular necrosis of bone.
Hemarthrosis.
Bowel disease–associated arthritis.
Bone malignancy.
Psoriatic arthritis.
Juvenile RA.
Sarcoidosis.
Hemoglobinopathies.
Vasculitic syndromes.
Behçet's syndrome.
Foreign body synovitis.
Hypertrophic pulmonary osteoarthropathy.
Amyloidosis, familial Mediterranean fever.

MONOCYTOSIS[40]

ICD-10CM #	D72.821	Monocytosis (symptomatic)

Inflammatory diseases:
    Autoimmune/granulomatous.
    Systemic lupus erythematosus.
    Rheumatoid arthritis.
    Giant cell arteritis.
    Myositis.
    Polyarteritis.
    Ulcerative colitis.
    Regional enteritis.
    Sarcoidosis.
Infectious diseases:
    Tuberculosis.
    Syphilis.
    Subacute bacterial endocarditis.
Malignant disorders:
    Preleukemia.
    Nonlymphocytic leukemia.
    Histiocytoses.
    Hodgkin's disease.
    Non-Hodgkin's lymphoma.
    Carcinomas.
Miscellaneous:
    Chronic neutropenia.
    Post splenectomy.

MONONEUROPATHY

ICD-10CM #	G58.9	Mononeuropathy, unspecified

Herpes zoster.
Herpes simplex.

Vasculitis.
Trauma, compression.
Diabetes.
Postinfectious or inflammatory.

MONONEUROPATHY, ISOLATED[6]

ICD-10CM #	G56.90	Unspecified mononeuropathy of unspecified upper limb

UPPER EXTREMITY

Radial nerve.
    Axilla.
    Humerus.
    Elbow (posterior interosseous neuropathy).
    Wrist (superficial cutaneous radial neuropathy).
Ulnar nerve.
    Axilla.
    Humerus.
    Elbow.
    Condylar groove.
    Cubital tunnel.
Wrist (Guyon's canal).
Hand.
    Superficial terminal ulnar neuropathy.
    Deep terminal ulnar neuropathy.
        Proximal hypothenar.
        Distal hypothenar.
Median nerve.
Axilla.
Humerus (musculocutaneous mononeuropathy).
Forearm.
    Anterior interosseus.
    Pronator syndrome.
Wrist (carpal tunnel).
Hand (recurrent motor branch).
Suprascapular mononeuropathy.
    Axillary mononeuropathy.

LOWER EXTREMITY

Sciatic nerve.
Femoral nerve.
    Iliacus compartment (proximal).
    Saphenous mononeuropathy (distal).
Lateral femoral cutaneous (meralgia paresthetica).
Peroneal nerve.
    Common peroneal mononeuropathy (fibular head, popliteal fossa).
    Deep peroneal mononeuropathy (anterior compartment).
Tibial nerve.
    Popliteal fossa (proximal).
    Tarsal tunnel (distal).
Sural nerve.
    Popliteal fossa, calf (proximal).
    Fifth metatarsal base (distal).
Plantar nerve.
    Distal to tarsal tunnel.
    Interdigital neuropathies (Morton's neuroma).
Obturator mononeuropathy.

MONONEUROPATHY MULTIPLEX[51]

ICD-10CM #	G58.9	Mononeuropathy, unspecified

MONONEUROPATHY MULTIPLEX

Vasculitis
Systemic vasculitis:
    Polyarteritis nodosa.
    Rheumatoid arthritis.
    Systemic lupus erythematosus.
    Sjögren's syndrome (keratoconjunctivitis sicca).
Nonsystemic vasculitis
Diabetes mellitus
Neoplastic
Paraneoplastic.
Direct infiltration.
Infectious
Lyme disease.
HIV infection.
Sarcoid
Toxic (lead)
Transient (polycythemia vera).
Cryoglobulinemia (hepatitis C)

MONONUCLEOSIS, MONOSPOT NEGATIVE[3]

ICD-10CM #	B27.90	Infectious mononucleosis, unspecified without complication

DIFFERENTIAL DIAGNOSIS OF MONOSPOT-NEGATIVE MONONUCLEOSIS

Acute HIV infection.
EBV mononucleosis (particularly in children).
Cytomegalovirus.
Acute toxoplasmosis.
Streptococcal pharyngitis.
Acute hepatitis B infection.

EBV, Epstein-Barr virus; *HIV*, human immunodeficiency virus.

MUSCLE DISEASE[68]

ICD-10CM #	M60.009	Infective myositis, unspecified site

CLASSIFICATION OF MUSCLE DISEASE

Muscular Dystrophies
Duchenne.
Becker.
Limb girdle.
Childhood.
Facioscapulohumeral.
Myotonic Disorders
Dystrophia myotonica.
Myotonica congenita.
Inflammatory
Infective: bacterial, viral, parasitic.
Unknown cause: polymyositis, dermatomyositis, sarcoidosis.

Endocrine
Thyroid disease—hyper- and hypothyroidism.
Cushing's disease.
Addison's disease.
Hyperparathyroidism.
Metabolic
- Glycogen storage diseases.
- Periodic paralyses.
- Mitochondrial diseases.

Drug-induced
- Corticosteroids.
- Chloroquine.
- Amiodarone.
- Penicillamine.
- Alcohol.
- Zidovudine.
- Clofibrate.

Other
- Inclusion body myositis.

MUSCLE WEAKNESS

ICD-10CM #   M62.9   Disorder of muscle, unspecified

Physical deconditioning.
Impaired cardiac output (e.g., mitral stenosis, mitral regurgitation).
Uremia, liver failure.
Electrolyte abnormalities (hypokalemia, hyperkalemia, hypophosphatemia, hypercalcemia), hypoglycemia.
Drug induced (e.g., statin myopathy).
Muscular dystrophies.
Steroid myopathy.
Alcoholic myopathy.
Myasthenia gravis, Lambert-Eaton syndrome.
Infections (polio, botulism, HIV, hepatitis, diphtheria, tick paralysis, neurosyphilis, brucellosis, TB, trichinosis).
Pernicious anemia, other anemias, beriberi.
Psychiatric illness (depression, somatization syndrome).
Organophosphate or arsenic poisoning.
Inflammatory myopathies (e.g., collagen vascular disease, RA, sarcoidosis).
Endocrinopathies (e.g., adrenal insufficiency, hypothyroidism), diabetic neuropathy.
Other: motor neuron disease, mitochondrial myopathy, l-tryptophan (eosinophilia-myalgia), rhabdomyolysis, glycogen storage disease, lipid storage disease.

MUSCLE WEAKNESS, LOWER MOTOR NEURON VERSUS UPPER MOTOR NEURON[78]

ICD-10CM #   M62.9   Disorder of muscle, unspecified

LOWER MOTOR NEURON

Weakness, usually severe.
Marked muscle atrophy.
Fasciculations.
Decreased muscle stretch reflexes.
Clonus not present.
Flaccidity.
No Babinski sign.

Asymmetric and may involve one limb only in the beginning to become generalized as the disease progresses.

UPPER MOTOR NEURON

Weakness, usually less severe.
Minimal disuse muscle atrophy.
No fasciculations.
Increased muscle stretch reflexes.
Clonus may be present.
Spasticity.
Babinski sign.
Often initial impairment of only skilled movements.
In the limbs the following muscles may be the only ones weak or weaker than the others: triceps; wrist and finger extensors; interossei; iliopsoas; hamstrings; and foot dorsiflexors, inverters, and extroverters.

MUSCULOSKELETAL BENIGN TUMORS AND TUMOR-LIKE LESIONS[60]

ICD-10CM #   varies with specific diagnosis

Fibrous dysplasia.
Enchondromatosis.
Osteochondromatosis.
Synovial cysts.
Brown tumors in hyperparathyroidism.
Langerhans cell histiocytosis (eosinophilic granuloma).
Hemangiomatosis.
Bone islands, osteoma (Gardner syndrome).
Fibrous cortical defect, nonossifying fibroma.
Giant cell tumor.
Neurofibromatosis.
Amyloidosis.
Mastocytosis.
SAPHO, chronic multifocal osteomyelitis.

SAPHO, Synovitis, acne, pustulosis, hyperostosis, osteitis.

MUSCULOSKELETAL MALIGNANT TUMORS AND TUMOR-LIKE LESIONS[60]

ICD-10CM #   varies with specific diagnosis

Metastases.
Myeloma.
Angiosarcoma.
Leukemia.
Neuroblastoma.
Ewing sarcoma.
Osteosarcomatosis.
Lymphoma.

MYDRIASIS

ICD-10CM #   H57.04   Mydriasis

Coma.
Medications (cocaine, atropine, epinephrine, etc.).

Glaucoma.
Cerebral aneurysm.
Ocular trauma.
Head trauma.
Optic atrophy.
Cerebral neoplasm.
Iridocyclitis.

MYELIN DISORDERS

ICD-10CM #   varies with specific diagnosis

Multiple sclerosis.
Vitamin B_{12} deficiency.
Radiation.
Hypoxia.
Toxicity from carbon monoxide, alcohol, mercury.
Progressive multifocal encephalopathy.
Acute disseminated encephalomyelitis.
Acute hemorrhagic leukoencephalopathy.
Phenylketonuria.
Adrenoleukodystrophy.
Krabbe's disease.

MYELOPATHY AND MYELITIS[70]

ICD-10CM #   M51.9   Unspecified thoracic, thoracolumbar and lumbosacral intervertebral disc disorder
G95.9   Disease of spinal cord, unspecified

INFLAMMATORY

Infectious: spirochetal TB, zoster, rabies, HIV, polio, rickettsial, fungal, parasitic.
Noninfectious: idiopathic transverse myelitis, multiple sclerosis.

TOXIC/METABOLIC

DM, pernicious anemia, chronic liver disease, pellagra, arsenic.

TRAUMA COMPRESSION

Spinal neoplasm, cervical spondylosis, epidural abscess, epidural hematoma.

VASCULAR

AV malformation, SLE, periarteritis nodosa, dissecting aortic aneurysm.

PHYSICAL AGENTS

Electrical injury, irradiation.

NEOPLASTIC

Spinal cord tumors, paraneoplastic myelopathy.

MYOCARDIAL ISCHEMIA[70]

ICD-10CM #   I25.5   Ischemic cardiomyopathy
I25.89   Other forms of chronic ischemic heart disease

Differential Diagnosis

II

I25.9	Chronic ischemic heart disease, unspecified	
I24.8	Other forms of acute ischemic heart disease	

Atherosclerotic obstructive coronary artery disease.
Nonatherosclerotic coronary artery disease:
  Coronary artery spasm.
  Congenital coronary artery anomalies:
    Anomalous origin of coronary artery from pulmonary artery.
    Aberrant origin of coronary artery from aorta or another coronary artery.
    Coronary arteriovenous fistula.
    Coronary artery aneurysm.
Acquired disorders of coronary arteries:
  Coronary artery embolism.
  Dissection:
    Surgical.
    During percutaneous coronary angioplasty.
    Aortic dissection.
    Spontaneous (e.g., during pregnancy).
  Extrinsic compression:
    Tumors.
    Granulomas.
    Amyloidosis.
  Collagen-vascular disease:
    Polyarteritis nodosa.
    Temporal arteritis.
    RA.
    SLE.
    Scleroderma.
  Miscellaneous disorders:
    Irradiation.
    Trauma.
    Kawasaki disease.
  Syphilis.
  Hereditary disorders:
    Pseudoxanthoma elasticum.
    Gargoylism.
    Progeria.
    Homocystinuria.
    Primary oxaluria.
"Functional" causes of myocardial ischemia in absence of anatomic coronary artery disease:
  Syndrome X.
  Hypertrophic cardiomyopathy.
  Dilated cardiomyopathy.
  Muscle bridge.
  Hypertensive heart disease.
  Pulmonary hypertension.
  Valvular heart disease; aortic stenosis, aortic regurgitation.

MYOCLONUS

ICD-10CM # G25.3 Myoclonus

Physiologic (e.g., exercise or anxiety induced).
Renal failure.
Hepatic failure.
Hyponatremia.
Hypoglycemia or severe hyperglycemia.
Postdialysis.
Epileptic myoclonus.
Postencephalitis.
CNS lesion (stroke, neoplasm).

CNS trauma.
Parkinson's disease.
Medications (e.g., tricyclics, L-dopa).
Friedreich's ataxia.
Ataxia-telangiectasia.
Wilson's disease.
Huntington's disease.
Progressive supranuclear palsy.
Heavy metal poisoning.
Benign familial.

MYOPATHIC SYNDROMES, DRUG-INDUCED[37]

ICD-10CM # G72.9 Myopathy, unspecified

TYPE OF MYOPATHY

Necrotizing myopathy.
Inflammatory myopathy.
Mitochondrial myopathy.
Hypokalemic myopathy.
Antimicrotubular myopathy.
Lysosomal storage myopathy.
Corticosteroid myopathy.
Others.

DRUGS

HMG-CoA reductase inhibitors (statins), fibrates, alcohol.
Penicillamine, interferon-a, procainamide.
Zidovudine.
Diuretics, laxatives, licorice, amphotericin B, alcohol.
Colchicine, vincristine.
Chloroquine, hydroxychloroquine, quinacrine, amiodarone, perhexiline.
Corticosteroids, especially fluorinated.
Ipecac syrup, emetine.

MYOPATHIES ASSOCIATED WITH REST PAIN[37]

ICD-10CM # G72.9 Myopathy, unspecified

Childhood dermatomyositis.
Hypothyroid myopathy.
Acute alcoholic myopathy.
Drug-induced myopathies.
Infectious myopathies.
Myopathies associated with metabolic bone disease.
Carnitine palmitoyl transferase deficiency.
Rhabdomyolysis from any cause.

MYOPATHIES, HIV ASSOCIATED[24]

ICD-10CM # R25.2

HIV-Associated Myopathies	Myopathies Secondary to Antiretrovirals	Others
HIV polymyositis.	Zidovudine myopathy.	Opportunistic infections involving muscle (toxoplasmosis).
Inclusion body myositis.	Toxic mitochondrial myopathies related to other NRTIs.	Tumor infiltrations of skeletal muscle.
Nemaline myopathy.		

HIV-Associated Myopathies	Myopathies Secondary to Antiretrovirals	Others
Diffuse infiltrative lymphocytosis syndrome.	HIV-associated lipodystrophy syndrome.	Rhabdomyolysis.
HIV wasting syndrome.	Immune reconstitution syndrome related to ART.	
Vasculitic processes.		
Myasthenia gravis and other myasthenic syndromes.		
Chronic fatigue and fibromyalgia.		

NRTIs, nucleoside reverse transcriptase inhibitors; *ART*, antiretroviral therapy.

MYOPATHIES, INFECTIOUS

ICD-10CM # G72.9 Myopathy, unspecified

HIV.
Viral myositis.
Trichinosis.
Toxoplasmosis.
Cysticercosis.

MYOPATHIES, INFLAMMATORY

ICD-10CM # G72.9 Myopathy, unspecified

SLE, RA.
Sarcoidosis.
Paraneoplastic syndrome.
Polymyositis, dermatomyositis.
Polyarteritis nodosa.
Mixed connective tissue disease.
Scleroderma.
Inclusion body myositis.
Sjögren's syndrome.
Cimetidine, D-penicillamine.

MYOPATHIES, METABOLIC[37]

ICD-10CM # G72.9 Myopathy, unspecified

DISORDERED GLYCOGEN METABOLISM

Myophosphorylase deficiency (McArdle disease).
Phosphorylase b kinase deficiency.
Phosphofructokinase deficiency.
Debrancher enzyme deficiency.
Brancher enzyme deficiency.
Phosphoglycerate kinase deficiency.
Phosphoglycerate mutase deficiency.
Lactate dehydrogenase deficiency.
Acid maltase deficiency.

Aldolase deficiency.
b-Enolase deficiency.

DISORDERED LIPID METABOLISM

Carnitine deficiencies.
Carnitine palmitoyltransferase deficiency.
Fatty acid acyl-CoA dehydrogenase deficiencies.

MITOCHONDRIAL MYOPATHIES

Coenzyme Q10 deficiency.
Respiratory chain complex deficiencies.

ENDOCRINE

Acromegaly.
Hypothyroidism.
Hyperthyroidism.
Hyperparathyroidism.
Cushing disease.
Addison disease.
Hyperaldosteronism.

METABOLIC-NUTRITIONAL

Uremia.
Hepatic failure.
Malabsorption.
Periodic paralysis.
Vitamin D deficiency.
Vitamin E deficiency.

ELECTROLYTE DISORDERS

Sodium: hypernatremia and hyponatremia.
Potassium: hyperkalemia and hypokalemia.
Calcium: hypercalcemia and hypocalcemia.
Phosphate: hypophosphatemia.
Magnesium: hypomagnesemia.

MYOPATHIES, TOXIC[3]

ICD-10CM # G72.2 Myopathy due to other toxic agents

- Inflammatory: cimetidine, D-penicillamine.
- Noninflammatory necrotizing or vacuolar: cholesterol-lowering agents, chloroquine, colchicine.
- Acute muscle necrosis and myoglobinuria: cholesterol-lowering drugs, alcohol, cocaine.
- Malignant hyperthermia: halothane, ethylene, others; succinylcholine.
- Mitochondrial: zidovudine.
- Myosin loss: nondepolarizing neuromuscular blocking agents; glucocorticoids.

MYOSITIS, INFECTIOUS CAUSES[37]

ICD-10CM # M60.009 Infective myositis, unspecified site

VIRAL

Influenza A and B viruses.
Enteroviruses (coxsackieviruses, echoviruses).
Human immunodeficiency virus.
Human T-cell lymphotrophic virus type 1.
Hepatitis B and C viruses.
Cytomegalovirus.
Epstein-Barr virus.
Adenovirus.

Varicella-zoster virus.
Parainfluenza.

PARASITIC

Trichinella species.
Echinococcus species.
Schistosoma species.
Toxoplasma gondii.
Trypanosoma cruzi.
Sarcocystis species.

BACTERIAL

Staphylococcus aureus.
Streptococcus, groups A and B.
Aeromonas hydrophila.
Borrelia burgdorferi.
Clostridium perfringens.
Anaerobic streptococci.
Mycobacterium species.
Rickettsia species.

FUNGAL

Candida species.
Cryptococcus neoformans.
Microsporida.

MYOSITIS, INFLAMMATORY[3]

ICD-10CM #	M60.009	Infective myositis, unspecified site
	M60.9	Myositis, unspecified
	M60.10	Interstitial myositis of unspecified site

INFECTIOUS

Viral myositis:
Retroviruses (HIV, HTLV-I).
Enteroviruses (echovirus, Coxsackievirus).
Other viruses (influenza, hepatitis A and B, Epstein-Barr virus).
Bacterial: pyomyositis.
Parasites: trichinosis, cysticercosis.
Fungi: candidiasis.

IDIOPATHIC

Granulomatous myositis (sarcoid, giant cell).
Eosinophilic myositis.
Eosinophilia-myalgia syndrome.

ENDOCRINE/METABOLIC DISORDERS

- Hypothyroidism.
- Hyperthyroidism.
- Hypercortisolism.
- Hyperparathyroidism.
- Hypoparathyroidism.
- Hypocalcemia.
- Hypokalemia.

METABOLIC MYOPATHIES

- Myophosphorylase deficiency (McArdle's disease).
- Phosphofructokinase deficiency.
- Myoadenylate deaminase deficiency.
- Acid maltase deficiency.
- Lipid storage diseases.
- Acute rhabdomyolysis.

DRUG-INDUCED MYOPATHIES

Alcohol.
d-Penicillamine.
Zidovudine.
Colchicine.
Chloroquine, hydroxychloroquine.
Lipid-lowering agents.
Cyclosporine.
Cocaine, heroin, barbiturates.
Corticosteroids.

NEUROLOGIC DISORDERS

Muscular dystrophies.
Congenital myopathies.
Motor neuron disease.
Guillain-Barré syndrome.
Myasthenia gravis.

NAIL CLUBBING

ICD-10CM # R68.3 Clubbing of nails

COPD.
Pulmonary malignancy.
Cirrhosis.
Inflammatory bowel disease.
Chronic bronchitis.
Congenital heart disease.
Endocarditis.
AV malformations.
Asbestosis.
Trauma.
Idiopathic.

NAIL, HORIZONTAL WHITE LINES (BEAU'S LINES)

ICD-10CM # L60.4 Beau's lines

Malnutrition.
Idiopathic.
Trauma.
Prolonged systemic illnesses.
Pemphigus.
Raynaud's disease.

NAIL KOILONYCHIA

ICD-10CM # L60.8 Other nail disorders

Trauma.
Iron deficiency.
SLE.
Hemochromatosis.
Raynaud's disease.
Nail-patella syndrome.
Idiopathic.

NAIL ONYCHOLYSIS

ICD-10CM # L60.1 Onycholysis

Infection.
Trauma.
Psoriasis.
Connective tissue disorders.
Sarcoidosis.
Hyperthyroidism.
Amyloidosis.
Nutritional deficiencies.

NAIL PITTING

ICD-10CM # L60.8 Other nail disorders

Psoriasis.
Alopecia areata.
Reiter's syndrome.
Trauma.
Idiopathic.

NAIL SPLINTER HEMORRHAGE

ICD-10CM # L60.8 Other nail disorders

SBE.
Trauma.
Malignancies.
Oral contraceptives.
Pregnancy.
SLE.
Antiphospholipid syndrome.
Psoriasis.
RA.
Peptic ulcer disease.

NAIL STRIATIONS

ICD-10CM # L60.8 Other nail disorders

Psoriasis.
Alopecia areata.
Trauma.
Atopic dermatitis.
Vitiligo.

NAIL TELANGIECTASIA

ICD-10CM # L60.8 Other nail disorders

RA.
Scleroderma.
Trauma.
SLE.
Dermatomyositis.

NAIL WHITENING (TERRY'S NAILS)

ICD-10CM # L60.8 Other nail disorders

Malnutrition.
Trauma.
Liver disease (cirrhosis, hepatic failure).
DM.
Hyperthyroidism.
Idiopathic.

NAIL YELLOWING

ICD-10CM # L60.8 Other nail disorders

Tobacco abuse.
Nephrotic syndrome.
Chronic infections (TB, sinusitis).
Bronchiectasis.
Lymphedema.
Raynaud's disease.
RA.
Pleural effusions.
Thyroiditis.
Immunodeficiency.

NASAL AND PARANASAL SINUS TUMORS[33]

ICD-10CM # C30.0 Malignant neoplasm of nasal cavity

BENIGN AND MALIGNANT NASAL AND PARANASAL SINUS TUMORS

Epithelial Tumors

BENIGN

Papilloma.
Adenoma.
Inverting papilloma.

MALIGNANT

Squamous carcinoma.
Adenocarcinoma.
Melanoma.
Adenoid cystic carcinoma.
Malignant salivary tumors.

MESENCHYMAL TUMORS

Benign
Osteoma.
Ossifying fibroma complex.
Angiofibroma.
Chondroma.
Malignant
Osteogenic sarcoma.
Fibrosarcoma.
Angiosarcoma.
Chondrosarcoma.
Lymphoma.
Rhabdomyosarcoma.

NASAL MASSES, CONGENITAL[33]

ICD-10CM # J34.1 Cyst and mucocele of nose and nasal sinus
J34.89 Other specified disorders of nose and nasal sinuses

Dermoid.
Nasal cerebral heterotopia (glioma).
Frontal meningoencephalocele.
Nasolacrimal duct mucocele.
Nasal hamartoma.
Nasal hemangioma.

NAUSEA AND VOMITING

ICD-10CM # R11.2 Nausea with vomiting, unspecified

Infections (viral, bacterial).
Intestinal obstruction.
Metabolic (uremia, electrolyte abnormalities, DKA, acidosis, etc.).
Severe pain.
Anxiety, fear.
Psychiatric disorders (bulimia, anorexia nervosa).
Pregnancy.
Medications (NSAIDs, erythromycin, morphine, codeine, aminophylline, chemotherapeutic agents, etc.).
Withdrawal from substance abuse (drugs, alcohol).

Head trauma.
Vestibular or middle ear disease.
Migraine headache.
CNS neoplasms.
Radiation sickness.
PUD.
Carcinoma of GI tract.
Reye's syndrome.
Eye disorders.
Abdominal trauma.

NAUSEA AND VOMITING, CAUSES DURING PREGNANCY[27]

ICD-10CM # R11.2 Nausea with vomiting, unspecified

DIFFERENTIAL DIAGNOSIS OF NAUSEA AND VOMITING DURING PREGNANCY

Nausea and vomiting of pregnancy.
Hyperemesis gravidarum.
Pancreatitis.
Symptomatic cholelithiasis.
Viral hepatitis.
Peptic ulcer disease.
Gastric cancer.
Intestinal obstruction.
Intestinal pseudoobstruction.
Gastroparesis diabeticorum.
Gastritis.
Gastroesophageal reflux disease.
Acute pyelonephritis.
Drug toxicity.
Vagotomy.
Preeclampsia/eclampsia.
Acute fatty liver of pregnancy.
Hemolysis, elevated liver enzymes, and low platelets (HELLP) syndrome.
Anorexia nervosa/bulimia.
Other neuropsychiatric disorders.

NAUSEA AND VOMITING, CHRONIC[23]

ICD-10CM # R11.2 Nausea with vomiting, unspecified

DIFFERENTIAL DIAGNOSIS OF CHRONIC NAUSEA AND VOMITING

Mechanical GI tract obstruction (pylorus, bile duct, small intestine, colon)
Mucosal inflammation
Peritoneal irritation
Carcinomas (e.g., gastric, ovarian, renal, bronchogenic)
Metabolic/endocrine disorders (diabetic mellitus, hypothyroidism, hyperthyroidism, adrenal insufficiency, uremia)
Medications (anticholinergics, narcotics, L-dopa, progesterone, calcium channel blockers, digitalis, NSAIDs, antidysrhythmic agents, lubiprostone, cannabis, metformin, amylin analogs)
Gastroparesis

Gastric dysrhythmias (tachygastria, bradygastria, mixed)

Central nervous system disorders (tumors, migraine, seizures, stroke, orthostatic intolerance)

Psychogenic disorders (anorexia nervosa, bulimia nervosa)

NECK AND ARM PAIN

| ICD-10CM # | M54.2 | Cervicalgia |
| | S46.919A | Strain of unspecified muscle, fascia and tendon at shoulder and upper arm level, unspecified arm, initial encounter |

Cervical disk syndrome.
Trauma, musculoskeletal strain.
Rotator cuff syndrome.
Bicipital tendonitis.
Glenohumeral arthritis.
Acromioclavicular arthritis.
Thoracic outlet syndrome.
Pancoast tumor.
Infection (cellulitis, abscess).
Angina pectoris.

NECK MASS[55]

| ICD-10CM # | R22.1 | Localized swelling, mass and lump, neck |

CONGENITAL ANOMALIES

Thyroglossal duct cyst.
Bronchial apparatus anomalies.
Teratomas.
Ranula.
Dermoid cysts.
Hemangioma.
Laryngoceles.
Cystic hygroma.

NONNEOPLASTIC INFLAMMATORY ETIOLOGIES

Folliculitis.
Adenopathy secondary to peritonsillar abscess.
Retropharyngeal or parapharyngeal abscess.
Salivary gland infections.
Viral infections (mononucleosis, HIV, CMV).
TB.
Cat-scratch disease.
Toxoplasmosis.
Actinomyces.
Atypical mycobacterium.
Jugular vein thrombus.

NEOPLASM (PRIMARY OR METASTATIC)
LIPOMA

NECK PAIN[55]

| ICD-10CM # | M54.2 | Cervicalgia |

INFLAMMATORY DISEASES

RA.
Spondyloarthropathies.
Juvenile RA.

NONINFLAMMATORY DISEASE

Cervical osteoarthritis.
Diskogenic neck pain.
Diffuse idiopathic skeletal hyperostosis.
Fibromyalgia or myofascial pain.

INFECTIOUS CAUSES

Meningitis.
Osteomyelitis.
Infectious diskitis.

NEOPLASMS

Primary.
Metastatic.

REFERRED PAIN

Temporomandibular joint pain.
Cardiac pain.
Diaphragmatic irritation.
GI sources (gastric ulcer, gallbladder, pancreas).

NECK PAIN FROM RHEUMATOLOGIC DISORDERS[24]

| ICD-10CM # | | M54.2 Cervicalgia |

Rheumatoid arthritis
   Without disease of the C1-C2 joint.
   With structural cervical abnormalities: C1-C2 subluxation, C1-C2 facet involvement.
Spondyloarthropathies.
Reactive arthritis.
Psoriatic arthritis.
Enteropathic arthritis.
Polymyalgia rheumatica.
Osteoarthritis.
Fibromyalgia.
Nonspecific musculoskeletal pain.
Miscellaneous spondyloarthropathies.
   Whipple's disease.
   Behçet's disease.
   Paget's disease.
   Acromegaly.
   Ossification of the posterior longitudinal ligament.
   Diffuse idiopathic skeletal hyperostosis.

NECROTIZING PNEUMONIAS[3]

| ICD-10CM # | J15.8 | Pneumonia due to other specified bacteria |

COMMON

Tuberculosis.
Staphylococcus.
Gram-negative bacilli.
Anaerobes.
Fungi.
Pneumocystis jirovecii.

RARE

Streptococcus pneumoniae.
Legionella.
Viruses.
Mycoplasma pneumoniae.

NEPHRITIC SYNDROME, ACUTE[3]

| ICD-10CM # | N00.8 | Acute nephritic syndrome with other morphologic changes |

LOW SERUM COMPLEMENT LEVEL

Acute postinfectious glomerulonephritis.
Membranoproliferative glomerulonephritis.
SLE.
Subacute bacterial endocarditis.
Visceral abscess "shunt" nephritis.
Cryoglobulinemia.

NORMAL SERUM COMPLEMENT LEVEL

IgA nephropathy.
Antiglomerular basement membrane disease.
Polyarteritis nodosa.
Wegener's glomerulonephritis.
Henoch-Schönlein purpura.
Goodpasture's syndrome.

NEPHROCALCINOSIS

| ICD-10CM # | E83.59 | Other disorders of calcium metabolism |

Sarcoidosis.
Hyperparathyroidism.
Chronic glomerulonephritis.
Milk-alkali syndrome.
Distal renal tubular acidosis.
Medullary sponge kidney.
Bartter's syndrome.
Hypervitaminosis D.
Idiopathic hypercalciuria.
Hyperoxaluria.
Cortical necrosis.
Tuberculosis.
Idiopathic hypercalciuria.
Rapidly progressive osteoporosis.

NEPHROPATHY, OBSTRUCTIVE[76]

| ICD-10CM # | | Varies with Specific Diagnosis |

POSSIBLE CAUSES OF OBSTRUCTIVE NEPHROPATHY

RENAL
Congenital
Polycystic kidney
Renal cyst
Peripelvic cyst
Ureteropelvic junction obstruction

Neoplastic
Wilms tumor
Renal cell carcinoma
Transitional cell carcinoma of the collecting system
Multiple myeloma
Inflammatory
Tuberculosis
Echinococcus infection
Metabolic
Calculi
Miscellaneous
Sloughed papillae
Trauma
Renal artery aneurysm
URETER
Congenital
Stricture
Ureterocele
Obstructing megaureter
Retrocaval ureter
Prune belly syndrome
Neoplastic
Primary carcinoma of ureter
Metastatic carcinoma
Inflammatory
Tuberculosis
Amyloidosis
Schistosomiasis
Abscess
Ureteritis cystica
Endometriosis
Miscellaneous
Retroperitoneal fibrosis
Pelvic lipomatosis
Aortic aneurysm
Radiation therapy
Lymphocele
Trauma
Urinoma
Pregnancy
Radiofrequency ablation
BLADDER AND URETHRA
Congenital
Posterior urethral valve
Phimosis
Hydrocolpos
Neoplastic
Bladder carcinoma
Prostate carcinoma
Carcinoma of urethra
Carcinoma of penis
Inflammatory
Prostatitis
Paraurethral abscess
Miscellaneous
Benign prostatic hypertrophy
Neurogenic bladder
Urethral stricture

NEUROGENIC BLADDER[56]

ICD-10CM #	N31.9	Neuromuscular dysfunction of bladder, unspecified

SUPRATENTORIAL
CVA.
Parkinson's disease.

Alzheimer's disease.
Cerebral palsy.

SPINAL CORD
Spinal cord injury.
Spinal stenosis.
Central cord syndrome.
ALS.
Multiple sclerosis.
Myelodysplasia.

PERIPHERAL NEUROPATHY
Diabetes.
Alcohol.
Shingles.
Syphilis.

NEUROLOGIC DEFICIT, FOCAL[50]

ICD-10CM #	G45.9	Transient cerebral ischemic attack, unspecified
	I67.848	Other cerebrovascular vasospasm and vasoconstriction

TRAUMATIC: INTRACRANIAL, INTRASPINAL
Subdural hematoma.
Intraparenchymal hemorrhage.
Epidural hematoma.
Traumatic hemorrhagic necrosis.

INFECTIOUS
Brain abscess.
Epidural and subdural abscesses.
Meningitis.

NEOPLASTIC
Primary central nervous system tumors.
Metastatic tumors.
Syringomyelia.
Vascular.
Thrombosis.
Embolism.
Spontaneous hemorrhage: arteriovenous malformation, aneurysm, hypertensive.

METABOLIC
Hypoglycemia.
B_{12} deficiency.
Postseizure.
Hyperosmolar nonketotic.

OTHER
Migraine.
Bell's palsy.
Psychogenic.

NEUROLOGIC DEFICIT, MULTIFOCAL[50]

ICD-10CM #	I67.89	Other cerebrovascular disease

	G45.9	Transient cerebral ischemic attack, unspecified
	I67.848	Other cerebrovascular vasospasm and vasoconstriction

Acute disseminated encephalomyelitis: postviral or postimmunization.
Infectious encephalomyelitis: poliovirus, enteroviruses, arbovirus, herpes zoster, Epstein-Barr virus.
Granulomatous encephalomyelitis: sarcoid.
Autoimmune: SLE.
Other: familial spinocerebellar degenerations.

NEUROMUSCULAR JUNCTION DYSFUNCTION[3]

ICD-10CM #	N31.9	Neuromuscular dysfunction of bladder, unspecified

DISORDERS OF THE NEUROMUSCULAR JUNCTION
Autoimmune
Myasthenia gravis.
Lambert-Eaton myasthenic syndrome.
Congenital
Presynaptic defects in ACh resynthesis, packaging, or release.
Synaptic defect: congenital end plate AChE deficiency.
Postsynaptic defects: slow-channel syndromes.
Postsynaptic defects: decreased response to ACh.
Fast-channel syndromes.
AChR deficiency without kinetic abnormality.
Familial limb-girdle myasthenia.
Toxic
Botulism.
Drug-induced disorders.
Organophosphate intoxication.

Ach, Acetylcholine; *AChE,* acetylcholinesterase; *AChR,* acetylcholine receptor.

NEURONOPATHIES, SENSORY (GANGLIONOPATHIES)[6]

ICD-10CM #	G60.0	Hereditary motor and sensory neuropathy

Herpes:
Herpes simplex I and II.
Varicella zoster (shingles).
Inflammatory sensory polyganglionopathy (ISP).
Paraneoplastic.
Primary biliary cirrhosis.
Sjögren's syndrome (keratoconjunctivitis sicca).
Toxin-induced:
Pyridoxine (vitamin B_6) overdose.
Metals:
Platinum (cisplatin).
Methyl mercury.
Vitamin E deficiency.

NEUROPATHIC BLADDER

ICD-10CM # N31.9 Neuromuscular dysfunction of bladder, unspecified

- Diabetes.
- Stroke.
- Multiple sclerosis.
- Parkinson's disease.
- Dementia.
- Encephalopathy.
- Brain trauma.
- Spinal cord trauma.
- Pelvic surgery.
- Spina bifida.

NEUROPATHIES WITH FACIAL NERVE INVOLVEMENT

ICD-10CM # G51.8 Other disorders of facial nerve

- Sarcoidosis.
- HIV.
- Lyme disease.
- Guillain-Barré.
- Others: chronic inflammatory polyneuropathy, Tangier disease, amyloidosis.

NEUROPATHIES, AUTONOMIC[46]

ICD-10CM # G63 Polyneuropathy in diseases classified elsewhere

GUILLAIN-BARRÉ SYNDROME
Non–Guillain-Barré syndrome autoimmunity.
Paraneoplastic (type I antineuronal nuclear antibody).
Lambert-Eaton syndrome.
Antibodies to neuronal nicotinc acetylcholine receptors.
Antibodies to P/Q type calcium channels.
Other autoantibodies.
Systemic lupus erythematosus.

HEREDITARY
Type I autosomal dominant.
Type II autosomal recessive (Morvan disease).
Type III autosomal recessive (Riley-Day).
Type IV autosomal recessive (congenital insensitivity to pain with anhidrosis).
Type V absence of pain.

METABOLIC
Fabry disease.
Diabetes mellitus.
Tangier disease.
Porphyria.

INFECTIOUS
HIV.
Chagas' disease.
Botulism.
Leprosy.
Diphtheria.

OTHER
Triple A (Allgrove) syndrome.
Navajo Indian neuropathy.
Multiple endocrine neoplasia type 2b.

TOXINS

NEUROPATHIES, AUTONOMIC, PERIPHERAL, CAUSES[31]

ICD-10CM # G90.09 Other idiopathic peripheral autonomic neuropathy

METABOLIC
Diabetes mellitus.
Alcohol.
Acute intermittent porphyria.
Uremia.

AUTOIMMUNE
Autoimmune autonomic ganglionopathy.
Guillain-Barré syndrome.
Morvan's syndrome.
Lambert-Eaton myasthenic syndrome.
Chronic inflammatory demyelinating polyradiculoneuropathy.
Sjögren syndrome.
Systemic lupus erythematosus.
Mixed connective tissue diseases.

PARAPROTEINEMIC
Amyloidosis.

NUTRITIONAL
Cyanocobalamin deficiency.
Thiamine deficiency.
Gluten-sensitive neuropathy.

TOXIC
Heavy metals.
Organic solvents.
Organophosphates.
Vacor.
Acrylamide.

DRUG INDUCED
Cisplatin.
Vincristine.
Amiodarone.
Metronidazole.
Perhexiline.
Paclitaxel.

INFECTIOUS
Human immunodeficiency virus.
Leprosy.
Chagas' disease.
Botulism.
Diphtheria.
Lyme disease.

GENETIC
Hereditary sensory and autonomic neuropathies.
   Types I and II.
   Type III (familial dysautonomia).
   Type IV (congenital insensitivity to pain).

Type V.
Fabry disease.

IDIOPATHIC
Adie's syndrome.
Ross' syndrome.
Acute cholinergic neuropathy.
Chronic idiopathic anhidrosis.
Amyotrophic lateral sclerosis.

NEUROPATHIES, PAINFUL[78]

ICD-10CM #		
	G58.9	Mononeuropathy, unspecified
	G62.1	Alcoholic polyneuropathy
	G61.89	Other inflammatory polyneuropathies
	G60.0	Hereditary motor and sensory neuropathy
	G60.0	Hereditary motor and sensory neuropathy
	E11.42	Type 2 diabetes mellitus with diabetic polyneuropathy
	E10.42	Type 1 diabetes mellitus with diabetic polyneuropathy

MONONEUROPATHIES
Compressive neuropathy (carpal tunnel, meralgia paresthetica).
Trigeminal neuralgia.
Ischemic neuropathy.
Polyarteritis nodosa.
Diabetic mononeuropathy.
Herpes zoster.
Idiopathic and familial brachial plexopathy.

POLYNEUROPATHIES
DM.
Paraneoplastic sensory neuropathy.
Nutritional neuropathy.
Multiple myeloma.
Amyloid.
Dominantly inherited sensory neuropathy.
Toxic (arsenic, thallium, metronidazole).
AIDS-associated neuropathy.
Tangier disease.
Fabry's disease.

NEUROPATHIES, PERIPHERAL, ASYMMETRICAL PROXIMAL/ DISTAL[6]

ICD-10CM # G99.0 Autonomic neuropathy in diseases classified elsewhere

BRACHIAL PLEXOPATHY
Open
Direct plexus injury (knife or gunshot wound).
Neurovascular (plexus ischemia).
Iatrogenic (central line insertion).

Differential Diagnosis

II

Closed
Traction injuries:
  "Stingers."
  Traction neurapraxia.
  Partial or complete nerve root avulsion.
Radiation.
Neoplastic.
Idiopathic brachial plexitis.
Throracic outlet.

LUMBOSACRAL PLEXOPATHIES

Open
Closed
Traction injuries:
  Pelvic double vertical shearing fracture.
  Posterior hip dislocation.
  Retroperitoneal hemorrhage.
Vasospastic (deep buttock injection).
Neoplastic.
Radiation.
Idiopathic lumbosacral plexitis.
Infectious:
  Herpesvirus (sacrococcygeal).
  Herpes simplex II.
  Herpes zoster.
Cytomegalovirus (CMV) polyradiculopathy (HIV).

NEUROPATHIES, TOXIC AND METABOLIC[46]

ICD-10CM # NEC G62.2 Toxic neuropathy

METALS

Arsenic (insecticide, herbicide).
Lead (paint, batteries, pottery).
Mercury (metallic, vapor).
Thallium (rodenticides).
Gold.

OCCUPATIONAL OR INDUSTRIAL CHEMICALS

Acrylamide (grouting, flocculation).
Carbon disulfide (solvent).
Cyanide.
Dichlorophenoxyacetate.
Dimethylaminopropionitrite.
Ethylene oxide (gas sterilization).
Hexacarbons (glue, solvents).
Organophosphates (insecticides, petroleum additive).
Polychlorinated biphenyls.
Tetrachlorbiphenyl.
Trichloroethylene.

DRUGS

Amiodarone.
Chloramphenicol.
Chloroquine.
Cisplatin.
Colchicine.
Dapsone.
Ethambutol.
Ethanol.
Gold.
Hydralazine.
Isoniazid.
Metronidazole.
Nitrofurantoin.
Nitrous oxide.

Nucleosides (antiretroviral agents ddC, ddl, d4T, others).
Penicillamine.
Pentamidine.
Phenytoin.
Pyridoxine (excessive).
Statins.
Stilbamidine.
Suramin.
Taxanes (paclitaxel, docetaxel).
Thalidomide.
Tryptophan (eosinophilia-myalgia syndrome).
Vincristine.

METABOLIC DISORDER

Fabry disease.
Krabbe disease.
Leukodystrophies.
Porphyria.
Tangier disease.
Tyrosinemia.
Uremia.

NEUTROPENIA, DRUG-INDUCED[39]

ICD-10CM # D70

DRUGS COMMONLY ASSOCIATED WITH NEUTROPENIA

Antibiotics:
  Vancomycin.
  Semisynthetic penicillins.
  Chloramphenicol.
  Sulfa.
  Linezolid.
Antithyroid drugs:
  Methimazole.
  Propylthiouracil.
Cardiovascular:
  Ticlopidine.
  Procainamide.
Antipsychotics:
  Clozapine.
  Olanzapine.
  Chlorpromazine.
Anticonvulsants:
  Phenytoin.
  Carbamazepine
  Valproic acid.
Antiinflammatory agents:
  Indomethacin.
  Sulfasalazine.
  Phenylbutazone.
H2 blockers:
  Cimetidine.
  Ranitidine.
Analgesics:
  Dipyrone.
Antineoplastic:
  Rituximab.
Anthelminthic:
  Levamisole.

NEUTROPENIA WITH DECREASED MARROW RESERVE[40]

ICD-10CM # D70.8   Other neutropenia

PRIMARY

Severe congenital neutropenia.
Shwachman–Diamond syndrome.
Cyclic neutropenia.

SECONDARY

Lymphoproliferative disorder of granular lymphocytes.
Chemotherapy.
Drug induced (nonimmune).
Nutritional.
Viral infection (varicella, EBV, measles, CMV, hepatitis, HIV).

NEUTROPENIA WITH NORMAL MARROW RESERVE[40]

ICD-10CM # D70.9   Neutropenia, unspecified

Chronic benign neutropenia of infancy and childhood.
Ethnic or benign familial neutropenia.
Autoimmune neutropenia.
Alloimmune neutropenia.
Drug-induced neutropenia.
Infection-related neutropenia.
Hypersplenism.

NEUTROPENIA, IN CHILDHOOD[73]

ICD-10CM # D70.8   Other neutropenia
D70.9   Neutropenia unspecified

ACQUIRED

Infection.
Immune mediated.
Hypersplenism.
Vitamin B_{12}, folate, copper deficiency.
Drugs or toxic substances.
Aplastic anemia.
Malignancies or preleukemic disorders.
Ionizing radiation.

CONGENITAL

Cyclic neutropenia.
Severe congenital neutropenia (Kostmann syndrome).
Chronic benign neutropenia of childhood.
Shwachman-Diamond syndrome.
Fanconi anemia.
Metabolic disorders (amino acidopathies, Barth syndrome, glycogen storage disorders).
Osteopetrosis.
Neutropenia with pigmentation abnormalities, e.g., Chédiak-Higashi.

NEUTROPHILIA[40]

ICD-10CM # D72.0   Neutrophilia, hereditary giant
D71   Functional disorders of polymorphonuclear neutrophils

CLASSIFICATION OF NEUTROPHILIA

Primary (No Other Evident Associated Disease)
Hereditary neutrophilia.
Chronic idiopathic neutrophilia.
Chronic myelogenous leukemia (CML) and other myeloproliferative diseases.
Familial myeloproliferative disease.
Congenital anomalies and leukemoid reaction.
Leukocyte adhesion factor deficiency (LAD).
Familial cold urticaria and leukocytosis.

Secondary
Infection.
Stress neutrophilia.
Chronic inflammation.
Drug induced.
Nonhematologic malignancy.
Generalized marrow stimulation as in hemolysis.
Asplenia and hyposplenism.

NIPPLE LESIONS

ICD-10CM # varies with specific diagnosis

Contact dermatitis.
Trauma.
Paget's disease.
Sebaceous hyperplasia.
Neurofibroma.
Accessory nipple.
Papillary adenoma.
Nevoid hyperkeratosis.
Cellulitis.

NODULAR LESIONS, SKIN

ICD-10CM # R22.9 Localized swelling, mass and lump, unspecified

Lipoma.
Cherry angioma.
Angiokeratoma.
Hemangioma.
Classic Kaposi's sarcoma.
Nodular melanoma.
Pyogenic granuloma.
Angiosarcoma.
Eccrine poroma.

NODULES, PAINFUL

ICD-10CM # R22.9 Localized swelling, mass and lump, unspecified

Arthropod bite or sting.
Erythema nodosum.
Glomus tumor.
Neuroma.
Leiomyoma.
Angiolipoma.
Dermatofibroma.
Osler's node.
Blue rubber bleb nevus.
Vasculitis.
Sweet's syndrome.

NYSTAGMUS

ICD-10CM # H55.00 Unspecified nystagmus

H55.89	Other irregular eye movements

Medications (meperidine, barbiturates, phenytoin, phenothiazines, etc.).
Multiple sclerosis.
Congenital.
Neoplasm (cerebellar, brain stem, cerebral).
Labyrinthine or vestibular lesions.
CNS infections.
Optic atrophy.
Other: Arnold–Chiari malformation, syringobulbia, chorioretinitis, meningeal cysts.

NYSTAGMUS, MONOCULAR

ICD-10CM # H55.09 Other forms of nystagmus
H55.00 Unspecified nystagmus

Amblyopia.
Strabismus.
Multiple sclerosis.
Monocular blindness.
Internuclear ophthalmoplegia.
Lid fasciculations.
Brain stem infarct.

ODYNOPHAGIA[72]

ICD-10CM # varies with specific diagnosis

CAUSES OF ODYNOPHAGIA

Infections
Herpes simplex virus.
Cytomegalovirus.
Candidiasis.

Chemical, Inflammatory
Gastroesophageal reflux.
Drug induced (Slow-K, tetracyclines, quinidine).
Radiation.
Graft-versus-host disease.
Crohn's disease.
Dermatologic diseases (pemphigus and pemphigoid).

OPACIFICATION OF HEMIDIAPHRAGM ON X-RAY[33]

ICD-10CM # varies with specific diagnosis

CAUSES OF OPACIFICATION OF A HEMITHORAX
Pleural effusion.
Consolidation.
Collapse.
Massive tumor.
Fibrothorax.
Combination of above lesions.
Pneumonectomy.
Lung agenesis.

OPHTHALMOPLEGIA[3]

ICD-10CM # H51.9 Unspecified disorder of binocular movement

H49.00	Third [oculomotor] nerve palsy, unspecified eye

BILATERAL
Botulism.
Myasthenia gravis.
Wernicke's encephalopathy.
Acute cranial polyneuropathy.
Brain stem stroke.

UNILATERAL
Carotid-posterior (3rd cranial nerve, pupil involved communicating aneurysm).
Diabetic-idiopathic (3rd or 6th cranial nerve, pupil spared).
Myasthenia gravis.
Brain stem stroke.

OPSOCLONUS[29]

ICD-10CM # H55.89 Other irregular eye movements

Multiple sclerosis.
Encephalitis.
CNS lymphoma.
Hydrocephalus.
Pontine hemorrhage.
Thalamic disorder (glioma, hemorrhage).
Hyperosmolar coma.
Carcinoma, paraneoplastic.
Cocaine.
Medications (e.g., phenytoin, haloperidol, amitriptyline, diazepam, vidarabine).

---

[29]Spontaneous, multivector, chaotic eye movement

OPTIC ATROPHY[68]

ICD-10CM # H47.20 Unspecified optic atrophy

CAUSES OF OPTIC ATROPHY

Optic Nerve Compression
Pituitary tumor.
Carotid aneurysm.
Glaucoma.
Optic nerve tumor.
Sphenoid meningioma.
Olfactory groove meningioma.

Optic Neuritis Following Longstanding Papilledema Central Retinal Artery Occlusion Toxic/Metabolic
Diabetes.
Methyl alcohol.
Tobacco.
Quinine.
Ethambutol.
Lead and arsenic.
Anemia.

Secondary to Retinal Disease
Senile macular degeneration.
Retinitis pigmentosa.
Severe chorioretinitis.

Secondary to Trauma
Orbital fracture.

Hereditary
Leber's optic atrophy.

Hereditary ataxias.
Spinocerebellar degeneration.

OPTIC DISC ELEVATION[11]

ICD-10CM # varies with specific diagnosis

CAUSES OF OPTIC DISC ELEVATION

Papilloedema.
Accelerated hypertension.
Anterior optic neuropathy.
Ischemic.
Inflammatory.
Infiltrative.
Compressive, including orbital disease.
Pseudopapilloedema.
Disc drusen.
Tilted optic disc.
Peripapillary myelinated nerve fibers.
Crowded disc in hypermetropia.
Mitochondrial optic neuropathies.
Leber hereditary optic neuropathy.
Methanol poisoning.
Intraocular disease.
Central retinal vein occlusion.
Uveitis.
Posterior scleritis.
Hypotony.

ORAL MUCOSA, ERYTHEMATOUS LESIONS[18]

ICD-10CM #	K12.2	Cellulitis and abscess of mouth
	K13.70	Unspecified lesions of oral mucosa
	K13.79	Other lesions of oral mucosa

Allergy.
Erythroplakia.
Candidiasis.
Geographic tongue.
Stomatitis areata migrans.
Plasma cell gingivitis.
Pemphigus vulgaris.

ORAL MUCOSA, PIGMENTED LESIONS[18]

ICD-10CM #	K12.2	Cellulitis and abscess of mouth
	K13.70	Unspecified lesions of oral mucosa
	K13.79	Other lesions of oral mucosa
	K13.5	Oral submucous fibrosis

Racial pigmentation.
Oral melanotic macule.
Peutz-Jeghers syndrome.
Neurofibromatosis.
Albright's syndrome.
Addison's disease.
Chloasma.
Drug reaction: quinacrine, Minocin, chlorpromazine, Myleran.
Amalgam tattoo.

Lead line.
Smoker's melanosis.
Nevi.
Melanoma.

ORAL MUCOSA, PUNCTATE EROSIVE LESIONS[18]

ICD-10CM #	K12.2	Cellulitis and abscess of mouth
	K13.70	Unspecified lesions of oral mucosa
	K13.79	Other lesions of oral mucosa

Viral lesion: Herpes simplex, coxsackievirus (A, B, A16), herpes zoster.
Aphthous stomatitis.
Sutton's disease (giant aphthae).
Behçet's syndrome.
Reiter's syndrome.
Neutropenia.
Acute necrotizing ulcerative gingivostomatitis (ANUG).
Drug reaction.
Inflammatory bowel disease.
Contact allergy.

ORAL MUCOSA, WHITE LESIONS[18]

ICD-10CM #	K12.2	Cellulitis and abscess of mouth
	K13.70	Unspecified lesions of oral mucosa
	K13.79	Other lesions of oral mucosa
	K13.5	Oral submucous fibrosis

Leukoplakia.
White, hairy leukoplakia.
Squamous cell carcinoma.
Lichen planus.
Stomatitis nicotinica.
Benign intraepithelial dyskeratosis.
White spongy nevus.
Leukoedema.
Darier-White disease.
Pachyonychia congenital.
Candidiasis.
Allergy.
SLE.

ORAL ULCERS, ACUTE

| ICD-10CM # | K13.70 | Unspecified lesions of oral mucosa |
| | K13.79 | Other lesions of oral mucosa |

Trauma (including thermal trauma).
Aphthous stomatitis.
Syphilis.
Herpes simplex infection.
Herpes zoster.

ORAL VESICLES AND ULCERS[3]

| ICD-10CM # | K13.70 | Unspecified lesions of oral mucosa |

| | K13.79 | Other lesions of oral mucosa |

Aphthous stomatitis.
Primary herpes simplex infection.
Vincent's stomatitis.
Syphilis.
Coxsackievirus A (herpangina).
Fungi (histoplasmosis).
Behçet's syndrome.
SLE.
Reiter's syndrome.
Crohn's disease.
Erythema multiforme.
Pemphigus.
Pemphigoid.

ORBITAL INFLAMMATION[11]

ICD-10CM #	H05.019	Cellulitis of unspecified orbit
	C69.10	Malignant neoplasm of unspecified orbit
	D31.60	Benign neoplasm of unspecified orbit
	H05.029	Osteomyelitis of unspecified orbit
	H05.049	Tenonitis of unspecified orbit
	H05.229	Edema of unspecified orbit
	H05.239	Hemorrhage of unspecified orbit

DIFFERENTIAL DIAGNOSIS OF AN ACUTELY INFLAMED ORBIT

Infection
Bacterial orbital cellulitis.
Fungal orbital infection.
Dacryocystitis.
Infective dacryoadenitis.
Vascular lesions
Acute orbital hemorrhage,
Cavernous sinus thrombosis.
Carotid–cavernous fistula.
Neoplasia
Rapidly progressive retinoblastoma.
Lacrimal gland tumor.
Other neoplasms (e.g., metastatic lesion with inflammation, lymphoma, Waldenström macroglobulinemia).
Rhabdomyosarcoma, leukemia, lymphangioma, or neuroblastoma in children
Endocrine
Thyroid eye disease of rapid onset.
Non-neoplastic inflammation
Idiopathic orbital inflammatory disease.
Tolosa–Hunt syndrome.
Orbital myositis.
Acute allergic conjunctivitis with lid swelling.
Herpes zoster ophthalmicus.
Herpes simplex skin rash.
Sarcoidosis.

Vasculitides: Wegener granulomatosis, polyarteritis nodosa.
Scleritis, including posterior scleritis.
Ruptured dermoid cyst.

ORBITAL LESIONS, CALCIFIED

| ICD-10CM # | H05.89 | Other disorders of orbit |

Chronic inflammation.
Phlebolith.
Dermoid cyst.
Mucocele walls.
Tumors (lacrimal gland, fibro-osseous).
Meningioma (optic sheath).
Lymphangioma.
Orbital varix.

ORBITAL LESIONS, CYSTIC

| ICD-10CM # | H05.9 | Unspecified disorder of orbit |

Sweat gland cyst.
Dermoid cyst.
Lacrimal gland cyst.
Abscess.
Conjunctival cyst.
Lymphangioma.
Schwannoma.

ORGASM DYSFUNCTION[21]

| ICD-10CM # | F52.31 | Female orgasmic disorder |
| | F52.32 | Male orgasmic disorder |

Anorgasmia: inadequate stimulation or learning.
Spinal cord lesion or injury.
Multiple sclerosis.
Alcoholic neuropathy.
Amyotrophic lateral sclerosis.
Spinal cord accident.
Spinal cord trauma.
Peripheral nerve damage.
Radical pelvic surgery.
Herniated lumbar disk.
Hypothyroidism.
Addison's disease.
Cushing's disease.
Acromegaly.
Hypopituitarism.
Pharmacologic agents (e.g., SSRIs, beta-blockers).
Psychogenic.

OROFACIAL PAIN

| ICD-10CM # | R51 | Facial pain |

Dental abscess.
Sinusitis.
Otitis media.
Otitis externa.
Wisdom tooth eruption.
Sialoadenitis.
Herpes zoster.
Trigeminal neuralgia.
Parotitis.

Anxiety disorder.
Malingering.

OSTEOLYTIC BENIGN BONE LESIONS, MULTIPLE[60]

| ICD-10CM # | | varies with specific diagnosis |

COMMON MULTIPLE OSTEOLYTIC BENIGN LESIONS

Cystic lesions in joint disease.
Amyloidosis.
Brown tumors in hyperparathyroidism.
Enchondromatosis.
Fibrous dysplasia.
Osteomyelitis (including tuberculosis, hydatid, sarcoid, etc.).
Massive osteolysis (Gorham disease).
Mastocytosis.
Neurofibromatosis.
Langerhans cell histiocytosis (histiocytosis X).

OSTEOPOROSIS IN CHILDREN[60]

| ICD-10CM # | M81.8 | Other osteoporosis without current pathological fracture |

CAUSES OF OSTEOPOROSIS IN CHILDREN

Systemic long-term oral glucocorticoid therapy.
Chronic inflammatory disease (e.g., juvenile inflammatory arthritis).
Hypogonadism—primary or secondary.
Prolonged immobilization.
Osteogenesis imperfecta.
Idiopathic juvenile osteoporosis.

OSTEOPOROSIS, SECONDARY CAUSES

| ICD-10CM # | M81.0 | Age-related osteoporosis without current pathological fracture |

Medication induced (e.g., glucocorticoids, anticonvulsants, heparin, LHRH agonists or antagonists).
Hyperparathyroidism.
Hyperthyroidism.
Prolonged immobilization.
Chronic renal failure.
Sickle cell disease.
Multiple myeloma.
Myeloproliferative diseases.
Leukemias and lymphomas.
Acromegaly.
Prolactinoma.
DM.
Total parenteral nutrition.
Malabsorption.
Chronic hypophosphatemia.
Connective tissue disorders (e.g., osteogenesis imperfecta, Marfan's syndrome, Ehlers-Danlos).
Hepatobiliary disease.
Postgastrectomy.
Aluminum-containing antacids.

Systemic mastocytosis.
Homocystinuria.

OSTEOSCLEROSIS, DIFFUSE[33]

| ICD-10CM # | Q77.4 | Congenital osteosclerosis |

DISORDERS ASSOCIATED WITH DIFFUSE OSTEOSCLEROSIS

Neoplastic Causes[30]
Prostate carcinoma, breast carcinoma, gastrointestinal adenocarcinoma, carcinoid tumors, transitional cell carcinoma of the bladder, myeloma, lymphoma, leukemia.
Hematologic Causes
Sickle cell disorders, mastocytosis, myelofibrosis, polycythemia vera.
Metabolic Causes
Renal osteodystrophy, primary hyperparathyroidism, familial hypophosphatemic osteomalacia, hypervitaminosis D, fluorosis, hypoparathyroidism, pseudohypoparathyroidism.
Primary Osseous Disorders[31]
Osteoporosis.
Pyknodysostosis.
Paget's disease.

[30]Involvement principally of cancellous bone
[31]Involvement of cancellous and cortical bone

OSTEOSCLEROTIC BENIGN BONE LESIONS, MULTIPLE[60]

| # |

COMMON MULTIPLE OSTEOSCLEROTIC BENIGN LESIONS

Bone infarcts.
Bone islands.
Callus.
Osteomyelitis (chronic, multifocal).
Paget disease.
Fibrous dysplasia.
Enchondromatosis.
Mastocytosis.
Matured benign lesions (e.g., nonossifying fibromas).
Osteomas (Gardner syndrome).
Osteopathia striata.
Osteopoikilosis.

OVULATORY DYSFUNCTION[43]

| ICD-10CM # | N97.0 | Female infertility associated with anovulation |
| | N92.3 | Ovulation bleeding |

HYPERANDROGENIC ANOVULATION

Polycystic ovarian syndrome.
Late-onset congenital adrenal hyperplasias.
Ovarian hyperthecosis.
Androgen-producing ovarian tumors.

Differential Diagnosis

Androgen-producing adrenal tumors.
Cushing's syndrome.

HYPOESTROGENIC ANOVULATION (HYPOTHALAMIC OR PITUITARY ETIOLOGY)

Hypogonadotropic Hypoestrogenic States
Reversible:
  Functional hypothalamic amenorrheas:
    Eating disorders (anorexia nervosa, excessive weight loss).
    Excessive athletic training.
Neoplastic:
  Craniopharyngioma.
  Pituitary stalk compression.
Infiltrative diseases:
  Histiocytosis-X.
  Sarcoidosis.
Hypophysitis.
Pituitary adenomas:
  Hyperprolactinemia.
  Euprolactinemic galactorrhea.
Endocrinopathies:
  Hypothyroidism/hyperthyroidism.
  Cushing's disease.
Irreversible:
  Kallmann's syndrome.
  Isolated gonadotropin deficiency (hypothalamic or pituitary origin).
  Panhypopituitarism/pituitary insufficiency:
    Sheehan's syndrome, pituitary apoplexy.
    Pituitary irradiation or ablation.

Hypergonadotropic Hypoestrogenic States
Physiologic states:
  Menopause.
  Perimenopause.
Premature ovarian failure.
Immune-related:
  Radiation/chemotherapy-induced.
Ovarian dysgenesis.
Turner's syndrome.
46XX with mutations of X.
Androgen insensitivity syndrome.

MISCELLANEOUS
Endometriosis.
Luteal phase defect.

PAIN, MIDFOOT

| ICD-10CM # | M25.579 | Pain in unspecified ankle and joints of unspecified foot |

MEDIAL ASPECT
Tendonitis of posterior tibialis.
Tendonitis of flexor digitorum longus.
Tendonitis of flexor hallucis longus.
Infection (osteomyelitis, septic arthritis, cellulitis) of foot.
Peripheral vascular insufficiency.
Fracture.
Osteoarthritis.
Gout, pseudogout.
Neuropathy.
Tumor.

LATERAL ASPECT
Peroneus longus tendonitis.

Peroneus brevis tendonitis.
Infection (osteomyelitis, septic arthritis, cellulitis) of foot.
Peripheral vascular insufficiency.
Fracture.
Osteoarthritis.
Gout, pseudogout.
Neuropathy.
Tumor.

PAIN, PLANTAR ASPECT, HEEL

| ICD-10CM # | M25.579 | Pain in unspecified ankle and joints of unspecified foot |

Plantar fasciitis.
Tarsal tunnel syndrome.
Neuroma.
Infection (osteomyelitis, septic arthritis, cellulitis) of foot.
Peripheral vascular insufficiency.
Fracture.
Bone cyst.
Osteoarthritis.
Gout, pseudogout.
Neuropathy.
Tumor.
Heel pad atrophy.
Plantar fascia rupture.

PAIN, POSTERIOR HEEL

| ICD-10CM # | M79.609 | Pain in unspecified limb |

Achilles tendonitis.
Retrocalcaneal bursitis.
Retroachilles bursitis.
Infection (osteomyelitis, septic arthritis, cellulitis) of foot.
Peripheral vascular insufficiency.
Fracture.
Osteoarthritis.
Gout, pseudogout.
Neuropathy.
Tumor.

PALINDROMIC RHEUMATISM[15]

ICD-10CM #	M12.30	Palindromic rheumatism, unspecified site
	M12.319	Palindromic rheumatism, unspecified shoulder
	M12.329	Palindromic rheumatism, unspecified elbow
	M12.339	Palindromic rheumatism, unspecified wrist
	M12.349	Palindromic rheumatism, unspecified hand
	M12.359	Palindromic rheumatism, unspecified hip
	M12.369	Palindromic rheumatism, unspecified knee
	M12.379	Palindromic rheumatism, unspecified ankle and foot
	M12.38	Palindromic rheumatism, vertebrae
	M12.39	Palindromic rheumatism, multiple sites

Palindromic RA.
Essential palindromic rheumatism.
Crystal synovitis (gout, CPPD, pseudogout, calcific periarthritis).
Lyme borreliosis, stages 2 and 3.
Sarcoidosis.
Whipple's disease.
Acute rheumatic fever.
Reactive arthritis (rare).

PALMOPLANTAR HYPERKERATOSIS

ICD-10CM #	L85.1	Acquired keratosis [keratoderma] palmaris et plantaris
	L85.2	Keratosis punctata (palmaris et plantaris)
	L87.0	Keratosis follicularis et parafollicularis in cutem penetrans

Superficial skin infection.
Chronic eczema.
Repeated trauma.
Psoriasis.
Reiter's syndrome.
Paraneoplastic acrokeratosis.

PALPITATIONS[64]

| ICD-10CM # | R00.2 | Palpitations |

Anxiety.
Electrolyte abnormalities (hypokalemia, hypomagnesemia).
Exercise.
Hyperthyroidism.
Ischemic heart disease.
Ingestion of stimulant drugs (cocaine, amphetamines, caffeine).
Medications (digoxin, beta-blockers, calcium channel antagonists, hydralazines, diuretics, minoxidil).
Hypoglycemia in type 1 DM.
Mitral valve prolapse.
Wolff-Parkinson-White (WPW) syndrome.
Sick sinus syndrome.

PANCREATIC CALCIFICATIONS

| ICD-10CM # | K86.1 | Other chronic pancreatitis |
| | K86.8 | Other specified diseases of pancreas |

Chronic pancreatitis.
Hyperparathyroidism.
Metastatic neoplasm.
Pseudocyst.
Hereditary pancreatitis.
Cystoadenoma.
Cystoadenocarcinoma.
Cavernous lymphangioma.
Hemorrhage.
Acute pancreatitis (saponification).

PANCREATIC CYSTIC LESIONS[75]

ICD-10CM #	K86.2	Cyst of pancreas
	K86.3	Pseudocyst of pancreas

Pseudocyst.
Serous cystadenoma.
Mucinous cystic neoplasm.
Intraductal papillary mucinous neoplasm.
Solid and papillary epithelial neoplasm.
True epithelial cyst.
Duodenal diverticulum.
Cystic neuroendocrine tumors.
Ductal adenocarcinoma with cystic degeneration.
Cystic metastases.
Cystic degeneration in sarcoma, hemangioma, and paraganglioma.

PANCREATIC SOLID LESIONS[75]

ICD-10CM #	C25.9	Malignant neoplasm of pancreas, unspecified
	D13.6	Benign neoplasm of pancreas

Neoplastic solid tumors.
Ductal adenocarcinoma.
Pancreatic neuroendocrine tumor.
Pancreatic lymphoma.
Metastases to the pancreas.
Solid pseudopapillary tumor.
Pancreaticoblastoma.
Acinar cell carcinoma.
Mesenchymal tumors (sarcoma, fibrous histiocytoma, etc.).
Nonneoplastic solid lesions.
Focal chronic pancreatitis.
Autoimmune pancreatitis.
Groove pancreatitis.
Focal sparing of diffuse pancreatic fatty infiltration.
Intrapancreatic accessory spleen.
Developmental pancreas lobulation.
Sarcoidosis of the pancreas.

PANCREATITIS, ACUTE, IN CHILDREN[46]

ICD-10CM #	K85	Acute pancreatitis

CAUSES OF ACUTE PANCREATITIS IN CHILDREN

Drugs and Toxins

Acetaminophen overdose.

Alcohol.
L-Asparaginase.
Azathioprine.
Carbamazepine.
Cimetidine.
Corticosteroids.
Enalapril.
Erythromycin.
Estrogen.
Furosemide.
Isoniazid.
Lisinopril.
6-Mercaptopurine.
Methyldopa.
Metronidazole.
Organophosphate poisoning.
Pentamidine.
Retrovirals: DDC, DDI, tenofovir.
Sulfonamides: mesalamine, 5-aminosalicylates, sulfasalazine, trimethoprim/sulfamethoxazole.
Sulindac.
Tetracycline.
Thiazides.
Valproic acid.
Venom (spider, scorpion, Gila monster lizard).
Vincristine.

Genetic

Cationic trypsinogen gene *(PRSS1)*.
Chymotrypsin C gene *(CTRC)*.
Cystic fibrosis gene *(CFTR)*.
Trypsin inhibitor gene *(SPINK1)*.

Infectious

Ascariasis.
Coxsackie B virus.
Epstein-Barr virus.
Hepatitis A, B.
Influenza A, B.
Leptospirosis.
Malaria.
Measles.
Mumps.
Mycoplasma.
Reye syndrome: varicella, influenza B.
Rubella.
Rubeola.
Septic shock.

Obstructive

Ampullary disease.
Ascariasis.
Biliary tract malformations.
Choledochal cyst.
Choledochocele.
Cholelithiasis, microlithiasis, and choledocholithiasis (stones or sludge).
Duplication cyst.
Endoscopic retrograde cholangiopancreatography (ERCP) complication.
Pancreas divisum.
Pancreatic ductal abnormalities.
Postoperative.
Sphincter of Oddi dysfunction.
Tumor.

Systemic Disease

Autoimmune pancreatitis.
Brain tumor.
Collagen vascular diseases.
Crohn disease.
Diabetes mellitus.
Head trauma.

Hemochromatosis.
Hemolytic-uremic syndrome.
Hyperlipidemia: type I, IV, V.
Hyperparathyroidism/Hypercalcemia.
Kawasaki disease.
Malnutrition.
Organic acidemia.
Peptic ulcer.
Periarteritis nodosa.
Renal failure.
Systemic lupus erythematosus.
Transplantation: bone marrow, heart, liver, kidney, pancreas.
Vasculitis.

Traumatic

Blunt injury.
Burns.
Child abuse.
Hypothermia.
Surgical trauma.
Total body cast.

PANCREATITIS, DRUG-INDUCED[6]

ICD-10CM #	K85.3	Drug induced acute pancreatitis

DEFINITE

Acetaminophen.
Azathioprine.
Cimetidine.
Cisplatin.
Corticosteroids.
Didanosine.
Erythromycin.
Estrogens.
Ethyl alcohol.
Furosemide.
L-Asparaginase.
Mercaptopurine.
Metronidazole.
Methyldopa.
Nitrofurantoin.
Octreotide.
Organophosphates.
Pentamidine.
Ranitidine.
Tetracycline.
Salicylates.
Sulfonamides, trimethoprim-sulfamethoxazole, sulfasalazine.
Sulindac.
Valproic acid.

POSSIBLE

Bumetanide.
Carbamazepine.
Chlorthalidone.
Clonidine.
Colchicine.
Cyclosporine.
Cytarabine.
Diazoxide.
Enalapril.
Ergotamine.
Ethacrynic acid.
Indomethacin.

Isoniazid.
Isotretinoin.
Mefenamic acid.
Opiates.
Phenformin.
Piroxicam.
Procainamide.
Rifampin.
Thiazides.

PANCYTOPENIA[40]

ICD-10CM #　D61.818　Other pancytopenia

PANCYTOPENIA WITH HYPOCELLULAR BONE MARROW

Acquired aplastic anemia.
Inherited aplastic anemia (Fanconi anemia and others).
Some myelodysplasia syndromes.
Rare aleukemic leukemia (acute myelogenous leukemia).
Some acute lymphoblastic leukemias.
Some lymphomas of bone marrow.

PANCYTOPENIA WITH CELLULAR BONE MARROW

Primary bone marrow diseases.
Myelodysplasia syndromes.
Paroxysmal nocturnal hemoglobinuria.
Myelofibrosis.
Some aleukemic leukemias.
Myelophthisis.
Bone marrow lymphoma.
Hairy cell leukemia.
Secondary to systemic diseases.
Systemic lupus erythematosus, Sjögren syndrome.
Hypersplenism.
Vitamin B_{12}, folate deficiency (familial defect).
Overwhelming infection.
Alcohol.
Brucellosis.
Ehrlichiosis.
Sarcoidosis.
Tuberculosis and atypical mycobacteria.

HYPOCELLULAR BONE MARROW ± CYTOPENIA

Q fever.
Legionnaires disease.
Mycobacteria.
Tuberculosis.[32]
Anorexia nervosa, starvation.
Hypothyroidism.

---

[32]Pancytopenia in tuberculosis only rarely is associated with a hypocellular bone marrow at biopsy or autopsy. Marrow failure in the setting of tuberculosis is almost always fatal; exceptional patients probably had underlying myelodysplasia or acute leukemia.

PANCYTOPENIA SYNDROME, INHERITED[46]

ICD-10CM #　D61.818　Other pancytopenia

Fanconi anemia.
Shwachman-Diamond syndrome.

Dyskeratosis congenita.
Congenital amegakaryocytic thrombocytopenia.
Unclassified inherited bone marrow failure syndromes.
Other genetic syndromes:
　Down syndrome.
　Dubowitz syndrome.
　Seckel syndrome.
　Reticular dysgenesis.
　Schimke immunoosseous dysplasia.
　Familial aplastic anemia (non-Fanconi).
　Cartilage-hair hypoplasia.
　Noonan syndrome.

PAPILLEDEMA

ICD-10CM #　H47.10　Unspecified papilledema

CNS infections (viral, bacterial, fungal).
Medications (lithium, cisplatin, corticosteroids, tetracycline, etc.).
Head trauma.
CNS neoplasm (primary or metastatic).
Pseudotumor cerebri.
Cavernous sinus thrombosis.
SLE.
Sarcoidosis.
Subarachnoid hemorrhage.
Carbon dioxide retention.
Arnold–Chiari malformation and other developmental or congenital malformations.
Orbital lesions.
Central retinal vein occlusion.
Hypertensive encephalopathy.
Metabolic abnormalities.

PAPULOSQUAMOUS DISEASES[29]

ICD-10CM #　L98.8　Other specified disorders of the skin and subcutaneous tissue

Psoriasis.
Pityriasis rubra pilaris.
Pityriasis rosea.
Lichen planus.
Lichen nitidus.
Secondary syphilis.
Pityriasis lichenoides.
Parapsoriasis.
Mycosis fungoides.
Dermatophytosis.
Tinea versicolor.

PARANEOPLASTIC NEUROLOGIC SYNDROMES

ICD-10CM #　G13.0　Paraneoplastic neuromyopathy and neuropathy

Lambert-Eaton myasthenic syndrome.
Myasthenia gravis.
Guillain-Barré syndrome.
Amyotrophic lateral sclerosis.
Dermatomyositis.
Carcinoid myopathy.
Cerebellar degeneration.

Encephalomyelitis.
Optic neuritis, uveitis, retinopathy.
Stiff-man syndrome.
Autonomic neuropathy.
Brachial neuritis.
Sensory neuropathy.
Progressive multifocal leukoencephalopathy.

PARANEOPLASTIC SYNDROMES, ENDOCRINE[70]

ICD-10CM #　G13.0　Paraneoplastic neuromyopathy and neuropathy

Hypercalcemia.
Syndrome of inappropriate secretion of antidiuretic hormone.
Hypoglycemia.
Zollinger-Ellison syndrome.
Ectopic secretion of human chorionic gonadotropin.
Cushing's syndrome.

PARANEOPLASTIC SYNDROMES, NONENDOCRINE[70]

ICD-10CM #　G13.0　Paraneoplastic neuromyopathy and neuropathy

CUTANEOUS

Dermatomyositis.
Acanthosis nigricans.
Sweet's syndrome.
Erythema gyratum repens.
Systemic nodular panniculitis (Weber-Christian disease).

RENAL

Nephrotic syndrome.
Nephrogenic diabetes insipidus.

NEUROLOGIC

Subacute cerebellar degeneration.
Progressive multifocal leukoencephalopathy.
Subacute motor neuropathy.
Sensory neuropathy.
Ascending acute polyneuropathy (Guillain-Barré syndrome).
Myasthenic syndrome (Eaton-Lambert syndrome).

HEMATOLOGIC

Microangiopathic hemolytic anemia.
Migratory thrombophlebitis (Trousseau's syndrome).
Anemia of chronic disease.

RHEUMATOLOGIC

Polymyalgia rheumatica.
Hypertrophic pulmonary osteoarthropathy.

PARAPARESIS, ACUTE OR SUBACUTE[68]

ICD-10CM #　G82.2　Paraparesis

CAUSES OF ACUTE OR SUBACUTE PARAPARESIS

Trauma to a Previously Normal Spine

Vertebral Disease

Metastatic carcinoma.
Cervical spondylosis.
Dorsal disk prolapse.
Paget's disease.
Rheumatoid arthritis.
Pott's disease of spine.

Tumors

Extradural or intradural carcinoma, lymphoma, myeloma, leukemia.
Dorsal meningioma.
Neurofibroma.

Hematologic Disease

Any cause of thrombocytopenia.
Other clotting disorders.
Leukemia.
Anticoagulant treatment.
Epidural or intramedullary hemorrhage.

Infection

Epidural abscess.
TB abscess.
Syphilitic myelitis.
HIV infection.
Vascular myelopathy.

Vascular

Anterior spinal artery occlusion.
Infarction secondary to hypotension.
Embolic infarction.
Infarction secondary to aortic dissection.
Arteriovenous malformation: infarction or hemorrhage.
Primary intramedullary hemorrhage.
Vasculitis—polyarteritis nodosa (PAN).

Inflammatory

Myelitis of unknown cause.
Multiple sclerosis.
Systemic lupus erythematosus.
Sarcoidosis.

Metabolic

Subacute degeneration of the cord.

PARAPARESIS, CHRONIC PROGRESSIVE[68]

ICD-10CM #   G82.2   Paraparesis

CAUSES OF CHRONIC PROGRESSIVE PARAPARESIS

Vertebral Disease

Cervical spondylosis.
Dorsal disk prolapse.
Rheumatoid arthritis.
Pott's disease of spine.
Ankylosing spondylitis.

Tumors

Meningioma.
Neurofibroma.
Glioma.
Ependymoma.
Chordoma.
Lipoma.

Syringomyelia

With Arnold–Chiari malformation.
With tumor.
Posttraumatic.

Infection

Tropical spastic paraparesis (HTLV 1 infection).
Syphilitic myelitis.

Vascular

Arteriovenous malformation.

Inflammatory

Multiple sclerosis.
Sarcoidosis.
Radiation myelopathy.
Arachnoiditis.

Metabolic

• Subacute combined degeneration of the cord.
• Paget's disease.

Degenerative

Motor neuron disease.

Hereditary

• Hereditary spastic paraplegia.

PARAPLEGIA

ICD-10CM #	G82.20	Paraplegia, unspecified
	G80.1	Spastic diplegic cerebral palsy
	I69.969	Other paralytic syndrome following unspecified cerebrovascular disease affecting unspecified side

Trauma: penetrating wounds to motor cortex, fracture-dislocation of vertebral column with compression of spinal cord or cauda equina, prolapsed disk, electrical injuries.

Neoplasm: parasagittal region, vertebrae, meninges, spinal cord, cauda equina, Hodgkin's disease, NHL, leukemic deposits, pelvic neoplasms.

Multiple sclerosis and other demyelinating disorders.

Mechanical compression of spinal cord, cauda equina, or lumbosacral plexus: Paget's disease, kyphoscoliosis, herniation of intervertebral disk, spondylosis, ankylosing spondylitis, RA, aortic aneurysm.

Infections: spinal abscess, syphilis, TB, poliomyelitis, leprosy.

Thrombosis of superior sagittal sinus.

Polyneuritis: Guillain-Barré syndrome, diabetes, alcohol, beriberi, heavy metals.

Heredofamilial muscular dystrophies.

ALS.

Congenital and familial conditions: syringomyelia, myelomeningocele, myelodysplasia.

Hysteria.

PARASELLAR MASSES[53]

ICD-10CM #	code varies with specific diagnosis

GENETIC

Transcription factor mutations (e.g., PROP1[33]).

[33]PROP1, prophet of Pit1 (paired-like homeodomain transcription factor).

CYSTS

Rathke's.
Arachnoid.
Epidermoid.
Dermoid.

TUMORS

• Hormone-secreting or nonfunctional pituitary adenoma.
• Granular cell tumor.
• Craniopharyngioma (cystic components).
• Chordoma.
• Meningioma.
• Sarcoma.
• Glioma.
• Schwannoma.
• Germ cell tumor.
• Vascular tumor.
• Solid or hematological metastasis.

MALFORMATION AND HAMARTOMAS

• Ectopic pituitary, neurohypophyseal, or salivary tissue.
• Hypothalamic hamartoma.
• Gangliocytoma.

MISCELLANEOUS LESIONS

Aneurysms.
Hypophysitis.
Infections.
Sarcoidosis.
Giant cell granuloma.
Histiocytosis X.

PARESTHESIAS

ICD-10CM #	R20.2	Paresthesia of skin
	G54.8	Other nerve root and plexus disorders

Multiple sclerosis.
Nutritional deficiencies (thiamin, vitamin B_{12}, folic acid).
Compression of spinal cord or peripheral nerves.
Medications (e.g., INH, lithium, nitrofurantoin, gold, cisplatin, hydralazine, amitriptyline, sulfonamides, amiodarone, metronidazole, dapsone, disulfiram, chloramphenicol).
Toxic chemicals (e.g., lead, arsenic, cyanide, mercury, organophosphates).
DM.
Myxedema.
Alcohol.
Sarcoidosis.
Neoplasms.
Infections (HIV, Lyme disease, herpes zoster, leprosy, diphtheria).
Charcot-Marie-Tooth syndrome and other hereditary neuropathies.
Guillain-Barré neuropathy.

PARKINSONISM-PLUS SYNDROMES

ICD-10CM #	G21.8	Other secondary parkinsonism

Parkinson's disease.
Shy-Drager syndrome.

Corticobasal degeneration.
Olivo-ponto-cerebellar atrophy.
Dementia with Lewy bodies.
Progressive supranuclear palsy.
Striatonigral degeneration.

PAROTID SWELLING[7]

ICD-10CM #	K11.20	Sialoadenitis, unspecified
	B26.9	Mumps without complication
	K11.8	Other diseases of salivary glands
	K11.5	Sialolithiasis
	K11.3	Abscess of salivary gland

INFECTIOUS

Mumps.
Parainfluenza.
Influenza.
Cytomegalovirus infection.
Coxsackievirus infection.
Lymphocytic choriomeningitis.
Echovirus infection.
Suppuration (bacterial).
Actinomyces infection.
Mycobacterial infection.
Cat-scratch disease.

NONINFECTIOUS

Drug hypersensitivity (thiouracil, phenothiazines, thiocyanate, iodides, copper, isoprenaline, lead, mercury, phenylbutazone).
Sarcoidosis.
Tumors, mixed.
Hemangioma, lymphangioma.
Sialectasis.
Sjögren's syndrome.
Mikulicz's syndrome (scleroderma, mixed connective tissue disease, SLE).
Recurrent idiopathic parotitis.
Pneumoparotitis.
Trauma.
Sialolithiasis.
Foreign body.
Cystic fibrosis.
Malnutrition (marasmus, alcohol cirrhosis).
Dehydration.
DM.
Waldenström's macroglobulinemia.
Reiter's syndrome (reactive arthritis).
Amyloidosis.

NONPAROTID SWELLING

Hypertrophy of masseter muscle.
Lymphadenopathy.
Rheumatoid mandibular joint swelling.
Tumors of jaw.
Infantile cortical hyperostosis.

PELVIC AVULSION FRACTURES[60]

ICD-10CM #	M84.350A	Stress fracture pelvis, initial encounter
	M84.454A	Pathological fracture pelvis, initial encounter

ACUTE AVULSION FRACTURE

Nontraumatic avulsion fracture
Soft tissue injury
Aggressive-looking appearance
Incidental normal variant

Bone metastasis, prior graft harvesting.
Tendon tear, muscle strain.
Osteomyelitis, tumor.
Accessory bone.

CHRONIC AVULSION FRACTURE

Apophyseal avulsion injury
Soft tissue injury

Apophysitis, traction periostitis.
Bursitis, degenerative tendinopathy, calcific tendinitis.

PELVIC MASS

ICD-10CM #	R19.09	Other intraabdominal and pelvic swelling, mass and lump

Hemorrhagic ovarian cyst.
Simple ovarian cyst (follicle or corpus luteum).
Ovarian carcinoma, carcinoma of fallopian tube, colorectal carcinoma, metastatic carcinoma, prostate carcinoma, bladder carcinoma, lymphoma, Hodgkin's disease.
Cystadenoma, teratoma, endometrioma.
Leiomyoma.
Leiomyosarcoma.
Diverticulitis, diverticular abscess.
Appendiceal abscess, tuboovarian abscess.
Ectopic pregnancy, intrauterine pregnancy.
Paraovarian cyst.
Hydrosalpinx.

PELVIC PAIN, CAUSES IN WOMEN[6]

ICD-10CM #	N94	Pain and other conditions associated with female genital organs and menstrual cycle
	G10.2	Pelvic and perineal pain
	G89.4	Chronic pain syndrome

POTENTIAL CAUSES OF PELVIC PAIN IN WOMEN

Reproductive Tract
Ovarian torsion.
Ovarian cyst.
Salpingitis/tubo-ovarian abscess.
Septic pelvic thrombophlebitis.
Endometritis.

Endometriosis.
Uterine perforation.
Uterine fibroids.
Dysmenorrhea.
Pregnancy-related
First Trimester
Ectopic pregnancy.
Threatened abortion.
Nonviable pregnancy.
Ovarian hyperstimulation syndrome.
Second and Third Trimesters
Placenta previa.
Placental abruption.
Round ligament pain.
Intestinal Tract
Appendicitis.
Diverticulitis.
Ischemic bowel.
Perforated viscus.
Bowel obstruction.
Incarcerated/strangulated hernia.
Inflammatory bowel disease.
Gastroenteritis.
Urinary Tract
Pyelonephritis.
Cystitis.
Ureteral stone.

PELVIC PAIN, CHRONIC[16]

ICD-10CM #	N94.89	Other specified conditions associated with female genital organs and menstrual cycle
	R10.2	Pelvic and perineal pain
	R10.10	Upper abdominal pain, unspecified
	R10.2	Pelvic and perineal pain
	R10.30	Lower abdominal pain, unspecified

GYNECOLOGIC DISORDERS

Primary dysmenorrhea.
Endometriosis.
Adenomyosis.
Adhesions.
Fibroids.
Retained ovary syndrome after hysterectomy.
Previous tubal ligation.
Chronic pelvic infection.

MUSCULOSKELETAL DISORDERS

Myofascial pain syndrome.

GASTROINTESTINAL DISORDERS

Irritable bowel syndrome.
Inflammatory bowel disease.

URINARY TRACT DISORDERS

Interstitial cystitis.
Nonbacterial urethritis.

PELVIC PAIN, GENITAL ORIGIN[50]

ICD-10CM #	N94.89	Other specified conditions associated with female genital organs and menstrual cycle
	R10.2	Pelvic and perineal pain
	R10.10	Upper abdominal pain, unspecified
	R10.2	Pelvic and perineal pain
	R10.30	Lower abdominal pain, unspecified

PERITONEAL IRRITATION

Ruptured ectopic pregnancy.
Ovarian cyst rupture.
Ruptured tuboovarian abscess.
Uterine perforation.

TORSION

Ovarian cyst or tumor.
Pedunculated fibroid.

INTRATUMOR HEMORRHAGE OR INFARCTION

Ovarian cyst.
Solid ovarian tumor.
Uterine leiomyoma.

INFECTION

Endometritis.
Pelvic inflammatory disease.
Trichomonas cervicitis or vaginitis.
Tuboovarian abscess.

PREGNANCY-RELATED

First Trimester
Ectopic pregnancy.
Abortion.
Corpus luteum hematoma.
Late Pregnancy
Placental problems.
Preeclampsia.
Premature labor.

MISCELLANEOUS

Endometriosis.
Foreign objects.
Pelvic adhesions.
Pelvic neoplasm.
Primary dysmenorrhea.

PELVIC PAIN, NON-PREGNANT FEMALE[1]

ICD-10CM #	N94.89	Other specified conditions associated with female genital organs and menstrual cycle
	R10.2	Pelvic and perineal pain

	R10.10	Upper abdominal pain, unspecified
	R10.30	Lower abdominal pain, unspecified

DIFFERENTIAL DIAGNOSIS OF PELVIC PAIN IN NONPREGNANT FEMALES

Gynecologic Diagnoses
Infectious:
  Vaginitis.
  Cervicitis.
  Endometritis.
  Tuboovarian abscess.
  Pelvic inflammatory disease.
Ovarian:
  Ovarian torsion.
  Ruptured ovarian cyst.
  Ovarian tumor.
  Degenerating ovarian tumor.
  Mittelschmerz.
Cervical:
  Cervical polyps.
  Cervical stenosis.
  Cervical cancer.
Uterine:
  Uterine fibroids.
  Degenerating uterine fibroids.
  Adenomyosis.
  Endometrial carcinoma.
Extrauterine:
  Endometriosis.
  Adhesions.
  Residual accessory ovary.

Nongynecologic Diagnoses
Gastrointestinal:
  Acute appendicitis.
  Mesenteric lymphadenitis.
  Diverticulitis.
  Inflammatory bowel disease.
  Irritable bowel syndrome.
  Bowel obstruction.
  Intraabdominal abscess.
  Colorectal carcinoma.
Urinary:
  Cystitis.
  Renal colic.
  Bladder cancer.
Musculoskeletal:
  Abdominal wall pain.
  Lumbar back pain.
  Fibromyalgia.
  Muscular strain.
  Piriformis syndrome.
Neurologic:
  Lumbar radiculopathy.
  Shingles.
  Spondylosis.
Psychologic:
  Personality disorders.
  Major depressive disorder.

PENILE RASH

ICD-10CM #	R21	Rash and other nonspecific skin eruption

Herpes simplex 2.
Balanitis (Candida).
Condyloma acuminatum.
Molluscum contagiosum.
Scabies.
Pediculosis pubis.
Pearly penile papules.
Lichen nitidus.
Fox-Fordyce disease (follicular papules).
Trauma.

PERIANAL PAIN[72]

ICD-10CM #	K62.89	Other specified diseases of anus and rectum

Fissure-in-ano
Anal sepsis
  Anal abscess
  Anal fistula
Hemorrhoids
  Internal hemorrhoids
  External hemorrhoids
Pruritus ani
Proctalgia fugax
Chronic perianal pain syndromes
  Coccygodynia
  Descending perineum syndrome
  Levator ani syndrome
  Idiopathic perineal pain

PERICARDIAL EFFUSION

ICD-10CM #	I30.9	Acute pericarditis, unspecified
	I31.3	Pericardial effusion

Pericarditis.
Uremia.
Myxedema.
Neoplasm (leukemia, lymphoma, metastatic).
Hemorrhage (trauma, leakage of thoracic aneurysm).
SLE, rheumatoid disease.
Myocardial infarction.

PERIODIC PARALYSIS, HYPERKALEMIC

ICD-10CM #	G83.9	Paralytic syndrome, unspecified

Chronic renal failure.
Renal insufficiency with excessive potassium supplementation.
Potassium-sparing diuretics.
Endocrinopathies (hypoaldosteronism, adrenal insufficiency).

PERIODIC PARALYSIS, HYPOKALEMIC

ICD-10CM #	G83.9	Paralytic syndrome, unspecified

Chronic diarrhea (laxative abuse, sprue, villous adenoma).
Potassium-depleting diuretics.
Medications (amphotericin B, corticosteroids).
Chronic licorice ingestion.

Thyrotoxicosis.
Renal tubular acidosis.
Conn's syndrome.
Barter's syndrome.
Barium intoxication.

PERITONEAL CARCINOMATOSIS[29]

ICD-10CM # C78.6 Secondary malignant neoplasm of retroperitoneum and peritoneum

PRIMARY DISORDERS OF THE PERITONEUM: MESOTHELIOMA

Metastatic spread from:
 Stomach.
 Colon.
 Pancreas.
 Carcinoid.
Other Intraabdominal Organs
Ovary.
Pseudomyxoma peritonei.
Extraabdominal Primary Tumors
Breast.
Lung.
Hematologic Malignancy
Lymphoma.

PERITONEAL EFFUSION[36]

ICD-10CM # R18 Ascites
 R85.9 Unspecified abnormal finding in specimens from digestive organs and abdominal cavity
 R88.8 Abnormal findings in other body fluids and substances

TRANSUDATES

Increased hydrostatic pressure or decreased plasma oncotic pressure.
Congestive heart failure.
Hepatic cirrhosis.
Hypoproteinemia.

EXUDATES

Increased capillary permeability or decreased lymphatic resorption.
Infections (TB, spontaneous bacterial peritonitis, secondary bacterial peritonitis).
Neoplasms (hepatoma, metastatic carcinoma, lymphoma, mesothelioma).
Trauma.
Pancreatitis.
Bile peritonitis (e.g., ruptured gallbladder).

CHYLOUS EFFUSION

Damage or obstruction to thoracic duct.
Trauma.
Lymphoma.
Carcinoma.
Tuberculosis.
Parasitic infection.

PERIUMBILICAL SWELLING

ICD-10CM # R19.00 Intraabdominal and pelvic swelling, mass and lump, unspecified site

Umbilical hernia.
Lipoma.
Epigastric hernia.
Umbilical granuloma.
Omphalocele.
Gastroschisis.
Caput medusae.

PHARYNGEAL OBSTRUCTION, CAUSES[52]

ICD-10CM # varies with specific diagnosis

CAUSES OF PHARYNGEAL OBSTRUCTION

Malignant or benign tumors (e.g., papillomas, polyps).
Infection (e.g., croup, epiglottitis, tonsillar abscess).
Edema or hypertrophy (e.g., angioneurotic edema, anaphylactic reactions, postradiation therapy, obstructive sleep apnea).
Trauma (e.g., cricoid fracture, cervical subluxation, precervical hematoma).
Burn injury.
Extrinsic compression (e.g., goiter or pregnancy-related thyroid enlargement).
Foreign body.
Congenital web (infants).
Sarcoidosis and other granulomatous diseases.
Amyloid.

PHEOCHROMOCYTOMA-TYPE SPELLS[53]

ICD-10CM # I15.2 Hypertension due to pheochromocytoma

DIFFERENTIAL DIAGNOSIS OF PHEOCHROMOCYTOMA-TYPE SPELLS

Endocrine Causes
Carbohydrate intolerance.
Hyperadrenergic spells.
Hypoglycemia.
Pancreatic tumors (e.g., insulinoma).
Pheochromocytoma.
Primary hypogonadism (menopausal syndrome).
Thyrotoxicosis.
Cardiovascular Causes
Angina.
Cardiovascular deconditioning.
Labile essential hypertension.
Orthostatic hypotension.
Paroxysmal cardiac arrhythmia.
Pulmonary edema.
Renovascular disease.
Syncope (e.g., vasovagal reaction).
Psychologic Causes
Factitious (e.g., drugs, Valsalva).
Hyperventilation.

Severe anxiety and panic disorders.
Somatization disorder.
Pharmacologic Causes
Chlorpropamide-alcohol flush.
Combination of a monoamine oxidase inhibitor and a decongestant.
Illegal drug ingestion (cocaine, phencyclidine, lysergic acid diethylamide).
Sympathomimetic drug ingestion.
Vancomycin ("red man syndrome").
Withdrawal of adrenergic-inhibitor.
Neurologic Causes
Autonomic neuropathy.
Cerebrovascular insufficiency.
Diencephalic epilepsy (autonomic seizures).
Migraine headache.
Postural orthostatic tachycardia syndrome.
Stroke.
Other Causes
Carcinoid syndrome.
 Mast cell disease.
 Recurrent idiopathic anaphylaxis.
 Unexplained flushing spells.

PHOTODERMATOSES[29]

ICD-10CM # L56.0 Drug phototoxic response
 L56.1 Drug photoallergic response
 L56.2 Photocontact dermatitis [berloque dermatitis]

Polymorphous light eruption.
Chronic actinic dermatitis.
Solar urticaria.
Phototoxicity and photoallergy.
Porphyrias.

PHOTOSENSITIVITY

ICD-10CM # L56.0 Drug phototoxic response
 L56.1 Drug photoallergic response
 L56.2 Photocontact dermatitis [berloque dermatitis]

Solar urticaria.
Photoallergic reaction.
Phototoxic reaction.
Polymorphous light eruption.
Porphyria cutanea tarda.
SLE.
Drug induced (e.g., tetracyclines).

PIGMENTURIA[6]

ICD-10CM # R82 Other abnormal findings in urine

HEMOGLOBINURIA

Hemolysis.

HEMATURIA

Renal causes.
Trauma.

ACUTE INTERMITTENT PORPHYRIA

Bilirubinuria
Food
Beets.
Drugs
Vitamin B_{12}.
Rifampin.
Phenytoin.
Laxatives.

PITUITARY REGION TUMORS[33]

ICD-10CM # varies with specific diagnosis

PRIMARY TUMORS IN THE SELLAR AND PARASELLAR REGION

Pituitary macroadenoma.
Meningioma.
Schwannoma (e.g., of fifth nerve).
Chordoma.
Chondrosarcoma.
Crangiopharyngioma.
Rathke's cleft cyst.
Dermoid.
Epidermoid.
Tuber cinereum hamartoma.
Optic glioma.
Germ cell tumors.

PLEURAL EFFUSIONS

ICD-10CM #	J91.8	Pleural effusion in other conditions classified elsewhere

EXUDATIVE

Neoplasm: bronchogenic carcinoma, breast carcinoma, mesothelioma, lymphoma, ovarian carcinoma, multiple myeloma, leukemia, Meigs' syndrome.
Infections: viral pneumonia, bacterial pneumonia, *Mycoplasma,* TB, fungal and parasitic diseases, extension from subphrenic abscess.
Trauma.
Collagen vascular diseases: SLE, RA, scleroderma, polyarteritis, granulomatosis with polyangiitis (Wegener's granulomatosis).
Pulmonary infarction.
Pancreatitis.
Postcardiotomy/Dressler's syndrome.
Drug-induced SLE (hydralazine, procainamide).
Postabdominal surgery.
Ruptured esophagus.
Chronic effusion secondary to congestive failure.

TRANSUDATIVE

CHF.
Hepatic cirrhosis.
Nephrotic syndrome.
Hypoproteinemia from any cause.
Meigs' syndrome.

PLEURAL EFFUSIONS, MALIGNANCY-ASSOCIATED

ICD-10CM #	C78.2	Secondary malignant neoplasm of pleura

Lung cancer	(30% to 40%)
Breast cancer	(20% to 25%)
Lymphoma	(10% to 15%)
Leukemia	(5% to 10%)
GI tract	(5%)
GU tract	(5%)
Reproductive	(3%)

PLEURAL HYPERPLASIA[65]

ICD-10CM #	Varies with Specific Diagnosis

BENIGN CAUSES OF PLEURAL HYPERPLASIA

Pleural infections
Radiation
Surgery
Trauma
Intracavitary treatments (chemotherapy or sclerosing agents)
Collagen vascular diseases
Systemic immune diseases (systemic lupus erythematosus, rheumatoid arthritis, Sjögren syndrome, Wegener granulomatosis)
Subpleural pulmonary abnormalities (infarction, infection, neoplasia)
Pneumothorax
Drug reactions (nitrofurantoin, bromocriptine, methysergide, procarbazine)
Pancreatitis, uremia
Pneumoconiosis (asbestosis)

PLEURAL MASSES[65]

ICD-10CM #	Varies with Specific Diagnosis

CAUSES OF PLEURAL MASSES

- Inflammatory pleural reactions
  - Reactive mesothelial hyperplasia or organizing pleuritis versus atypical mesothelial hyperplasia
  - Nodular pleural plaques
- Pulmonary tumors that may resemble pleural tumors
  - Inflammatory pseudotumor of the lung
- Benign pleural tumors
  - Solitary fibrous tumor
  - Lipomas and lipoblastomas
  - Adenomatous tumors
  - Calcifying fibrous tumors
  - Mesothelial cysts
  - Multicystic mesothelioma
  - Schwannoma
- Pleural tumors with low malignant potential
  - Desmoid tumors
  - Well-differentiated papillary mesothelioma
  - Pleural thymoma
- Primary malignant pleural tumors that may look like benign tumors
  - Malignant solitary fibrous tumor
  - Pleuropulmonary blastoma
- Localized malignant mesothelioma
- Vascular sarcoma
- Liposarcoma
- Pleuropulmonary synovial sarcoma
- Askin tumor or primitive neuroectodermal tumor (PNET)
- Desmoplastic small round cell tumor
- Malignant pleural tumors
  - Metastatic malignancies to the pleura
  - Malignant mesothelioma

PNEUMATOSIS INTESTINALIS IN NEONATE AND OLDER CHILD[33]

ICD-10CM # varies with specific diagnosis

CAUSES OF PNEUMATOSIS INTESTINALIS IN THE NEONATE AND THE OLDER CHILD

- Necrotizing enterocolitis.
- Bowel ischemia, inflammation, and obstruction.
- Cyanotic congenital heart disease.
- Hirschsprung's disease.
- Gastroschisis.
- Anorectal atresia.
- Inflammatory bowel disease.
- Lymphoma.
- Leukemia.
- CMV and rotavirus gastroenteritis.
- Colonoscopy.
- Caustic ingestion.
- Short bowel syndrome.
- Congenital immune deficiency states.
- *Clostridium* infection.
- Chronic steroid use.
- Posthepatic, renal, or bone marrow transplant.
- Collagen vascular disease.
- Graft-versus-host disease.
- AIDS.

PNEUMONIA, CHRONIC[9]

ICD-10CM #	J15.9	Unspecified bacterial pneumonia
	J12.9	Viral pneumonia, unspecified
	B25.0	Cytomegaloviral pneumonitis
	J18.0	Bronchopneumonia, unspecified organism

INFECTIOUS AGENTS THAT TYPICALLY CAUSE CHRONIC PNEUMONIA

Bacteria
Mixed aerobic and anaerobic bacteria.
Actinomyces spp.
Nocardia spp.
Rhodococcus equi.
Burkholderia pseudomallei.
Mycobacteria
Mycobacterium tuberculosis.
Mycobacterium kansasii.
Mycobacterium avium complex.
Mycobacterium abscessus.
Mycobacterium terrae.

Fungi
Aspergillus spp.
Blastomyces dermatitidis.
Coccidioides spp.
Cryptococcus neoformans.
Cryptococcus gattii.
Dark-walled molds.
Emmonsia parvum var. crescens.
Histoplasma capsulatum.
Sporothrix schenckii complex.
Paracoccidioides brasiliensis.
Penicillium marneffei.
Scedosporium apiospermum.
Parasites
Dirofilaria.
    Echinococcus granulosus.
    Filaria (tropical pulmonary eosinophilia).
    Paragonimus westermani.

NONINFECTIOUS CAUSES OF CHRONIC PNEUMONIA

Neoplasia
Carcinoma (primary or metastatic).
Hodgkin's disease and non-Hodgkin's lymphoma.
Other lymphoproliferative disorders.
Cystic Fibrosis
Sarcoidosis
Amyloidosis
Vasculitis (Autoimmune Diseases).
Systemic lupus erythematosus.
Polyarteritis nodosa.
Granulomatosis with polyangiitis (Wegener's granulomatosis).
Allergic angiitis and granulomatosis (Churg-Strauss syndrome).
Goodpasture's syndrome.
Microscopic polyangiitis.
Lymphomatoid granulomatosis.
Progressive systemic sclerosis.
Rheumatoid arthritis.
Mixed connective tissue syndrome (overlap syndrome).
Chemicals, Drugs
Radiation
Recurrent Pulmonary Emboli
Bronchial Obstruction with Atelectasis (e.g., Tumor, Foreign Body)
    Pulmonary Sequestration
    Pulmonary Infiltration with Eosinophilia Syndrome
Löffler's syndrome—usually transient.
Pneumonia plus asthma (e.g., allergic bronchopulmonary aspergillosis).
Bronchocentric granulomatosis.
Chronic eosinophilic pneumonia.
Pneumoconiosis
Asbestosis.
Berylliosis.
Silicosis.
Anthracosilicosis.
Chronic Form of Extrinsic Allergic Alveolitis (Hypersensitivity Pneumonitis)

OTHER LUNG DISEASES: CAUSE UNKNOWN

Chronic Organizing Pneumonia
Chronic Interstitial Pneumonia (Fibrosing Alveolitis, Idiopathic Pulmonary Fibrosis)
Usual interstitial pneumonia (UIP).

Desquamative interstitial pneumonia (DIP).
Lymphocytic interstitial pneumonia (LIP).
Giant cell interstitial pneumonia (GIP).
Eosinophilic granuloma (histiocytosis X).
Lymphangioleiomyomatosis.
Pulmonary alveolar proteinosis.
Pulmonary alveolar microlithiasis.
Idiopathic pulmonary hemosiderosis.
Angiocentric immunoproliferative lesions.

PNEUMONIA MIMICS[12]

ICD-10CM # varies with specific diagnosis

NONINFECTIOUS CAUSES THAT MAY PRESENT AS PNEUMONIA

Radiologic Technique
Inadequate inspiration.
Breast shadow.
Thymus.
Uneven grid on film.
Underpenetrated film.
Primary Pulmonary
Asthma.
Bronchiectasis.
Atelectasis.
Bronchopulmonary dysplasia.
Cystic fibrosis.
Pulmonary sequestration.
Congenital cystic adenomatoid malformation.
α_1-Antitrypsin deficiency.
Aspiration
Foreign body.
Chemical.
Recurrent caused by anatomic or physiologic disorders.
Primary Cardiac
Congenital heart disease.
Congestive heart failure.
Pulmonary Infarction
Sickle cell vasoocclusive crisis.
Pulmonary embolism.
Collagen Vascular Disorders
Acute Respiratory Distress Syndrome
Pleural Effusion
Neoplasm.
From Boyer KM: Nonbacterial pneumonia. In Feigin RD, Cherry JD (eds): Textbook of Pediatric Infectious Diseases, 4th ed. Philadelphia, WB Saunders, 1998, pp 260-273.

PNEUMONIA, NONRESPONDING, CAUSES[52]

ICD-10CM #		
	J15.9	Unspecified bacterial pneumonia
	J12.9	Viral pneumonia, unspecified
	B25.0	Cytomegaloviral pneumonitis
	J18.0	Bronchopneumonia, unspecified organism

CAUSES OF NONRESPONDING PNEUMONIA

Infectious Pneumonia
• Resistant microorganisms:

  ○ Community-acquired pneumonia (e.g., *Streptococcus pneumoniae, Staphylococcus aureus*).
  ○ *Nosocomial pneumonia* (e.g., *Acinetobacter*, methicillin-resistant *Staphylococcus aureus* (MRSA), *Pseudomonas aeruginosa*).
• Uncommon microorganisms (e.g., *Mycobacterium tuberculosis, Nocardia* spp., fungi, *Pneumocystis jirovecii*).
• Complications of pneumonia:
  Empyema.
  Abscess or necrotizing pneumonia.
  Metastatic infection.
Noninfectious Pneumonia
Neoplasms.
Pulmonary hemorrhage.
Pulmonary embolism.
Sarcoidosis.
Eosinophilic pneumonia.
Pulmonary edema.
Acute respiratory distress syndrome.
Bronchiolitis obliterans with organizing pneumonia.
Drug-induced pulmonary disease.
Pulmonary vasculitis.

PNEUMONIA, RECURRENT

ICD-10CM #	J15.9	Unspecified bacterial pneumonia
	J12.9	Viral pneumonia, unspecified
	B25.0	Cytomegaloviral pneumonitis
	J18.0	Bronchopneumonia, unspecified organism

Mechanical obstruction from neoplasm.
Chronic aspiration (tube feeding, alcoholism, CVA, neuromuscular disorders, seizure disorder, inability to cough).
Bronchiectasis.
Kyphoscoliosis.
COPD, CHF, asthma, silicosis, pulmonary fibrosis, cystic fibrosis.
Pulmonary TB, chronic sinusitis.
Immunosuppression (HIV, corticosteroids, leukemia, chemotherapy, splenectomy).

PNEUMOPERITONEUM, NEONATAL[33]

ICD-10CM # varies with specific diagnosis

CAUSES OF NEONATAL PNEUMOPERITONEUM

Necrotizing enterocolitis.
Spontaneous perforation of a hollow viscus.
    Stomach.
    Duodenum.
    Ileum.
    Colon.
Malrotation and volvulus.
Distal obstruction.
Perforation of Meckel's diverticulum.
Anterior abdominal wall defects.
    Pentalogy of Cantrell.
    Omphalocele.
    Gastroschisis.
    Cloacal exstrophy.

Stress and peptic ulcers.
Mechanical ventilation (air leak) or resuscitation ("bagging").
Post-laparotomy.
Iatrogenic gastric perforation with an orogastric tube.
Iatrogenic colon perforation.
   Thermometer.
   During an enema.
Indomethacin.
Dexamethasone treatment.

PNEUMOTHORAX, IN CHILDREN[46]

ICD-10CM #	J93.0	Spontaneous tension pneumothorax
	J93	Pneumothorax
	J93.9	Pneumothorax unspecified

SPONTANEOUS

Primary idiopathic—usually resulting from ruptured subpleural blebs.
Secondary blebs.
Congenital lung disease:
   Congenital cystic adenomatoid malformation.
   Bronchogenic cysts.
   Pulmonary hypoplasia.
Conditions associated with increased intrathoracic pressure:
   Asthma.
   Bronchiolitis.
   Air-block syndrome in neonates.
   Cystic fibrosis.
   Airway foreign body.
Infection:
   Pneumatocele.
   Lung abscess.
   Bronchopleural fistula.
Diffuse lung disease:
   Langerhans cell histiocytosis.
   Tuberous sclerosis.
   Marfan syndrome.
   Ehlers-Danlos syndrome.
Metastatic neoplasm—usually osteosarcoma (rare).

TRAUMATIC

Noniatrogenic.
   Penetrating trauma.
   Blunt trauma.
   Loud music (air pressure).
Iatrogenic.
   Thoracotomy.
   Thoracoscopy, thoracentesis.
   Tracheostomy.
   Tube or needle puncture.
Mechanical ventilation.

POLIOSIS[11]

| ICD-10CM # | varies with specific diagnosis |

CAUSES OF POLIOSIS

Ocular
Chronic anterior blepharitis.

Sympathetic ophthalmitis.
Idiopathic uveitis.
Systemic
Vogt–Koyanagi–Harada syndrome.
Waardenburg syndrome.
Vitiligo.
Marfan syndrome.
Tuberous sclerosis.

POLYCYTHEMIA

| ICD-10CM # | D45 | Polycythemia primary |
| | D75.1 | Polycythemia secondary |

Tobacco abuse.
Chronic lung disease.
High altitude.
Sleep apnea.
Right-to-left cardiac shunts.
Erythropoietin administration.
Androgens/anabolic steroids.
Polycystic kidney disease.
Renal cell carcinoma.
Hepatocellular carcinoma.
Polycythemia vera.
Carbon monoxide exposure.
Primary familial and congenital polycythemia.
High-oxygen–affinity hemoglobins.
Uterine leiomyoma, meningioma, pheochromocytoma, parathyroid carcinoma.
Cobalt exposure.

POLYCYTHEMIAS, DIFFERENTIAL DIAGNOSIS[39]

| ICD-10CM # | D45 | Polycythemia primary |
| | D75.1 | Polycythemia secondary |

DIFFERENTIAL DIAGNOSIS OF THE POLYCYTHEMIAS

Relative or Spurious Polycythemia
Decreased plasma volume—reduced fluid intake, marked loss of body fluids (diaphoresis, vomiting, diarrhea, "third spacing").
Gaisböck syndrome.
Overfilling of blood in collection vacuum tubes.
Absolute polycythemia
Secondary polycythemia.
Acquired.
Hypoxia.
   Pulmonary disease.
   Cyanotic congenital heart disease.
   Hypoventilation syndromes:
      Sleep apnea.
      Pickwickian syndrome.
      High altitude.
      Smokers' polycythemia, hookah polycythemia, carbon monoxide intoxication caused by industrial exposure.
Postrenal transplantation erythrocytosis.
Aberrant erythropoietin production.
Tumors:
   Renal cell carcinoma.
   Wilms tumor.
   Hepatic carcinoma.
   Uterine leiomyomata.

Virilizing ovarian tumors.
Vascular cerebellar tumors.
Miscellaneous renal and hepatic disorders:
   Solitary renal cysts.
   Polycystic kidney disease.
   Renal artery stenosis hydronephrosis.
   Viral hepatitis.
Endocrine disorders:
   Cushing syndrome.
   Primary aldosteronism.
   Androgen use.
   Erythropoietin use.
   Congenital Polycythemias:
      Abnormal high-affinity hemoglobin variants.
      Bisphosphoglycerate deficiency.
      Congenital methemoglobinemia.
      Chuvash polycythemia (von Hippel Lindau mutations).
      Prolyl hydroxylase mutations.
      Hypoxia-inducible factor gene mutations.
Primary polycythemias:
   Primary congenital and familial polycythemia.
   Polycythemia vera.

POLYCYTHEMIA, RELATIVE VERSUS ABSOLUTE[40]

| ICD-10CM # | D75.1 | Secondary polycythemia |

RELATIVE OR SPURIOUS POLYCYTHEMIA

Decreased plasma volume—reduced fluid intake, marked loss of body fluids (diaphoresis, vomiting, diarrhea, "third-spacing").
Gaisböck syndrome.
Overfilling of blood in collection vacuum tubes.

ABSOLUTE POLYCYTHEMIA

Primary Congenital and Familial Polycythemia
Secondary Polycythemia Acquired
Hypoxia:
   Pulmonary disease.
   Cyanotic congenital heart disease.
   Hypoventilation syndromes—sleep apnea, Pickwickian syndrome.
High altitude.
Smokers' polycythemia, carbon monoxide intoxication due to industrial exposure.
Postrenal transplantation erythrocytosis.
Aberrant erythropoietin production
Tumors—renal cell carcinoma, Wilms' tumor, hepatic carcinoma, uterine leiomyomata, virilizing ovarian tumors, vascular cerebellar tumors.
Miscellaneous renal and hepatic disorders—solitary renal cysts, polycystic kidney disease, renal artery stenosis, hydronephrosis, viral hepatitis.
Endocrine disorders—Cushing's syndrome, primary aldosteronism.
Androgen use.
Erythropoietin use.

Differential Diagnosis

II

Congenital:
    Abnormal high-affinity hemoglobin variants.
    Bisphosphoglycerate deficiency.
    Congenital methemoglobinemia.
    Chuvash polycythemia (von Hippel–Lindau
      mutations).
    Prolyl hydroxylase mutations.

POLYCYTHEMIA VERA

POLYMYALGIAS[37]

ICD-10CM #	M35.3	Polymyalgia rheumatica

DISEASE ENTITIES WITH POLYMYALGIAS

Rheumatoid arthritis.
Rotator cuff syndrome.
Osteoarthritis of shoulder and hip joints.
Fibromyalgia.
Polymyositis/dermatomyositis.
Spondyloarthritis.
Systemic lupus erythematosus.
Vasculitides.
Paraneoplastic myalgias.
Infection-associated myalgias.
Statin therapy.
RS3PE (remitting seronegative symmetric synovitis and pitting edema).
Parkinson's disease.
Hypothyroidism.

POLYNEUROPATHY[78]

ICD-10CM #	G61.9	Inflammatory polyneuropathy, unspecified

PREDOMINANTLY MOTOR

- Guillain-Barré syndrome.
- Porphyria.
- Diphtheria.
- Lead.
- Hereditary sensorimotor neuropathy, types I and II.
- Paraneoplastic neuropathy.

PREDOMINANTLY SENSORY

Diabetes.
Amyloidosis.
Leprosy.
Lyme disease.
Paraneoplastic neuropathy.
Vitamin B_{12} deficiency.
Hereditary sensory neuropathy, types I-IV.

PREDOMINANTLY AUTONOMIC

- Diabetes.
- Amyloidosis.
- Alcoholic neuropathy.
- Familial dysautonomias.

MIXED SENSORIMOTOR

- Systemic diseases: renal failure, hypothyroidism, acromegaly, RA, periarteritis nodosa, SLE, multiple myeloma, macroglobulinemia, remote effect of malignancy.
- Medications: isoniazid, nitrofurantoin, ethambutol, chloramphenicol, chloroquine,

vincristine, vinblastine, dapsone, disulfiram, diphenylhydantoin, cisplatin, 1-tryptophan.
- Environmental toxins: *N*-hexane, methyl *N*-butyl ketone, acrylamide, carbon disulfide, carbon monoxide, hexachlorophene, organophosphates.
- Deficiency disorders: malabsorption, alcoholism, vitamin B_1 deficiency, Refsum's disease, metachromatic leukodystrophy.

POLYNEUROPATHY, DEMYELINATING[6]

ICD-10CM #	G37.9	Demyelinating disease of central nervous system, unspecified

Guillain-Barré syndrome.
    Acute inflammatory demyelinating polyradiculoneuropathy (AIDP).
    Acute motor axonal neuropathy (AMAN).
    Acute motor and sensory axonal neuropathy (AMSAN).
    Miller Fisher syndrome.
Chronic inflammatory demyelinating polyradiculoplexo-neuropathy.
Malignancy.
HIV.
Hepatitis B.
Buckthorn.
Diphtheria.

POLYNEUROPATHY, DISTAL SENSORIMOTOR[6]

ICD-10CM #	G63	Polyneuropathy in diseases classified elsewhere

Diabetes mellitus.
Alcoholism.
Neoplastic or paraneoplastic.
Hereditary motor and sensory neuropathies (Charcot-Marie-Tooth).
Cryptogenic sensorimotor polyneuropathies (CSPN).
HIV.
Toxins:
    Organic or industrial agents:
      Acrylamide.
      Allyl chloride.
      Carbon disulfide.
      Ethylene oxide.
      Hexacarbons.
      Methyl bromide.
      Organophosphate-induced delayed polyneuropathy (OPIDP).
      Polychlorinated biphenyls (PCBs).
      Trichloroethylene.
      Vacor.
    Metals:
      Arsenic.
      Gold.
      Mercury (inorganic).
      Thallium.
    Therapeutic agents:
      Amiodarone.
      Antiretrovirals.
      Dapsone.
      Disulfiram.

    Isoniazid.
    Metronidazole.
    Nitrofurantoin.
    Paclitaxel (Taxol).
    Phenytoin.
    Statins (HMG-CoA reductase inhibitors).
    Thalidomide.
    Vinca alkaloids (vincristine, vinblastine).
Nutritional:
    Beriberi (thiamine or vitamin B_1).
    Pellagra (niacin, B vitamins).
    Pernicious anemia (vitamin B_{12}).
    Pyridoxine deficiency (vitamin B_6).
End-organ dysfunction
    ○ Acromegaly.
    ○ Chronic pulmonary disease.
    ○ Hypothyroidism.
    ○ Renal failure (uremic neuropathy).
Paraproteinemias:
    ○ Amyloidosis.
    ○ Monoclonal gammopathy of unknown significance (MGUS).
    ○ Multiple myeloma.
    ○ Waldenström's macroglobulinemia.
Porphyria.

HMG-CoA, Hydroxymethylglutaryl coenzyme A.

POLYNEUROPATHY, DRUG-INDUCED[78]

ICD-10CM #	G62.0	Drug-induced polyneuropathy

DRUGS IN ONCOLOGY

Vincristine.
Procarbazine.
Cisplatin.
Misonidazole.
Metronidazole
Taxol.

DRUGS IN INFECTIOUS DISEASES

Isoniazid.
Nitrofurantoin.
Dapsone.
ddC (dideoxycytidine).
ddI (dideoxyinosine).

DRUGS IN CARDIOLOGY

Hydralazine.
Perhexiline maleate.
Procainamide.
Disopyramide.

DRUGS IN RHEUMATOLOGY

Gold salts.
Chloroquine.

DRUGS IN NEUROLOGY AND PSYCHIATRY

- Diphenylhydantoin.
- Glutethimide.
- Methaqualone.

MISCELLANEOUS

- Disulfiram (Antabuse).
- Vitamin: (pyridoxine in megadoses).

POLYNEUROPATHY, SYMMETRIC[78]

ICD-10CM # G61.9 Inflammatory polyneuropathy, unspecified

ACQUIRED NEUROPATHIES

Toxic:
Drugs.
Industrial toxins.
Heavy metals.
Abused substances.
Metabolic/endocrine:
Diabetes.
Chronic renal failure.
Hypothyroidism.
Polyneuropathy of critical illness.
Nutritional deficiency:
Vitamin B_{12} deficiency.
Alcoholism.
Vitamin E deficiency.
Paraneoplastic:
Carcinoma.
Lymphoma.
Plasma cell dyscrasia:
Myeloma, typical, atypical, and solitary forms.
Primary systemic amyloidosis.
Idiopathic chronic inflammatory demyelinating polyneuropathies.
Polyneuropathies associated with peripheral nerve autoantibodies.
Acquired immunodeficiency syndrome.

INHERITED NEUROPATHIES

Neuropathies with Biochemical Markers
- Refsum's disease.
- Bassen-Kornzweig disease.
- Tangier disease.
- Metachromatic leukodystrophy.
- Krabbe's disease.
- Adrenomyeloneuropathy.
- Fabry's disease.

Neuropathies without Biochemical Markers or Systemic Involvement
Hereditary motor neuropathy.
Hereditary sensory neuropathy.
Hereditary sensorimotor neuropathy.

POLYURIA

ICD-10CM # R35.8 Other polyuria

DM.
Diabetes insipidus.
Primary polydipsia (compulsive water drinking).
Hypercalcemia.
Hypokalemia.
Postobstructive uropathy.
Diuretic phase of renal failure.
Drugs: diuretics, caffeine, alcohol, lithium.
Sickle cell trait or disease, chronic pyelonephritis (failure to concentrate urine).
Anxiety, cold weather.

POPLITEAL SWELLING

ICD-10CM# I87.1 Compression of vein

I72.4	Aneurysm of artery of lower extremity
S85.009A	Unspecified injury of popliteal artery, unspecified leg, initial encounter
I77.3	Arterial fibromuscular dysplasia
M71.20	Synovial cyst of popliteal space [Baker], unspecified knee
I80.3	Phlebitis and thrombophlebitis of lower extremities, unspecified
M66.369	Spontaneous rupture of flexor tendons, unspecified lower leg

Phlebitis (superficial).
Lymphadenitis.
Trauma: fractured tibia or fibula, contusion, traumatic neuroma.
DVT.
Ruptured varicose vein.
Baker's cyst.
Popliteal abscess.
Osteomyelitis.
Ruptured tendon.
Aneurysm of popliteal artery.
Neoplasm: lipoma, osteogenic sarcoma, neurofibroma, fibrosarcoma.

PORTAL HYPERTENSION[3]

ICD-10CM # K76.6 Portal hypertension

INCREASED RESISTANCE TO FLOW

Presinusoidal
Portal or splenic vein occlusion (thrombosis, tumor).
Schistosomiasis.
Congenital hepatic fibrosis.
Sarcoidosis.
Sinusoidal
Cirrhosis (all causes).
Alcoholic hepatitis.
Postsinusoidal
Venoocclusive disease.
Budd-Chiari syndrome.
Constrictive pericarditis.

INCREASED PORTAL BLOOD FLOW

Splenomegaly not caused by liver disease.
Arterioportal fistula.

POSTMENOPAUSAL BLEEDING

ICD-10CM # N95.0 Postmenopausal bleeding

Hormone replacement therapy.
Neoplasm (uterine, ovarian, cervical, vaginal, vulvar).
Atrophic vaginitis.
Vaginal infection.
Polyp.
Extragenital (GI, urinary).
Tamoxifen.
Trauma.

POSTURAL HYPOTENSION, NONNEUROLOGIC CAUSES

ICD-10CM # I95.1 Orthostatic hypotension

Diuretics and hypertensive agents.
GI hemorrhage.
Alcohol.
Excessive heat.
Rapid volume loss from diarrhea, vomiting.
Hemodialysis.
Extensive burns.
Pyrexia.
Aortic stenosis (impaired output).
Constrictive pericarditis, atrial myxoma (impaired cardiac filling).
Adrenal insufficiency.
Diabetes insipidus.
Vasodilatory agents (e.g., nitrates).

PREMATURE GRAYING, SCALP HAIR

ICD-10CM # varies with specific diagnosis

Chemical exposure (e.g., phenol/catechol derivatives, sulfhydryls, arsenic).
Physical agents (e.g., ionizing radiation, lasers).
Hyperthyroidism.
Vitamin B_{12} deficiency.
Down syndrome.
Chronic and severe protein deficiency.
Vitiligo.
Idiopathic.
Myotonic dystrophy.
Ataxia-telangiectasia.
Progeria.
Werner's syndrome.

PREMATURE VENTRICULAR CONTRACTIONS AND VENTRICULAR TACHYCARDIA[6]

ICD-10CM #	I49.40	Unspecified premature depolarization
	I47.2	Ventricular tachycardia

CAUSES OF PREMATURE VENTRICULAR CONTRACTIONS AND VENTRICULAR TACHYCARDIA

Acute or previous myocardial infarction/ischemia.
Hypokalemia.
Hypoxemia.
Ischemic heart disease.
Valvular disease.

Catecholamine excess.[34]
Other drug intoxications (especially cyclic anti-depressants).
Idiopathic causes.[35]
Digitalis toxicity.
Hypomagnesemia.
Hypercapnia.
Class I antidysrhythmic agents.
Ethanol.
Myocardial contusion.
Cardiomyopathy.
Acidosis.
Alkalosis.
Methylxanthine toxicity.

---

[34]Relative increase in sympathetic tone from drugs (direct or indirect) or conditions that augment catecholamine release or decrease parasympathetic tone.

[35]Isolated premature ventricular contractions (PVCs) can occur in up to 50% of young subjects without obvious cardiac or noncardiac disease; however, multiform and repetitive PVCs and ventricular tachycardia are rarely seen in this population.

PRESACRAL MASSES IN CHILDREN[62]

ICD-10CM #	Varies with Specific Diagnosis

PRESACRAL MASSES IN CHILDREN

Solid
Sacrococcygeal teratoma
Neuroblastoma
Rhabdomyosarcoma
Fibroma
Lipoma
Leiomyoma
Lymphoma
Hemangioendothelioma
Sacral bone tumors
Cystic
Abscess
Rectal duplication
Hematoma
Lymphocele
Neurenteric cyst
Sacral osteomyelitis
Ulcerative colitis
Anterior meningocele

PROLONGED QT SYNDROMES[51]

ICD-10CM #	I45.81	Long QT syndrome

CLASSIFICATION AND CAUSES OF PROLONGED QT SYNDROMES THAT PRODUCE TORSADES DE POINTES

Pause Dependent (Acquired)
Drug induced: Class IA and IC antidysrhythmics; many phenothiazines and butyrophenones (notably haloperidol and droperidol), cyclic antidepressants, antibiotics (especially macrolides), organophosphates, antihistamines,

antifungals, antiseizure and antiemetic agents.
Electrolyte abnormalities: hypokalemia, hypomagnesemia, hypocalcemia (rarely).
Diet related: starvation, low protein.
Severe bradycardia or atrioventricular block.
Hypothyroidism.
Contrast injection.
Cerebrovascular accident (especially intraparenchymal).
Myocardial ischemia.
Adrenergic Dependent (Tachycardia Prompted)
Congenital:
    Jervell and Lange-Nielsen syndrome (deafness, autosomal recessive).
    Romano-Ward syndrome (normal hearing, autosomal dominant).
    Sporadic (normal hearing, no familial tendency).
    Mitral valve prolapse.
Acquired (Rare):
    Cerebrovascular disease (especially subarachnoid hemorrhage).
    Autonomic surgery: radical neck dissection, carotid endarterectomy, truncal vagotomy.

PROPTOSIS[57]

ICD-10CM #	H05.20	Unspecified exophthalmos
	H05.2	Ocular proptosis

Thyrotoxicosis.
Orbital pseudotumor.
Optic nerve tumor.
Cavernous sinus AV fistula, cavernous sinus thrombosis.
Cellulitis.
Metastatic tumor to orbit.

PROPTOSIS AND PALATAL NECROTIC ULCERS

ICD-10CM #	K13.70	Unspecified lesions of oral mucosa
	K13.79	Other lesions of oral mucosa
	H05.20	Unspecified exophthalmos

Cavernous sinus thrombosis.
Bacterial orbital cellulitis.
Metastatic neoplasm.
Rhinocerebral mucormycosis.
Ecthyma gangrenosum.
CNS aspergillosis.

PROTEIN-LOSING ENTEROPATHY, PEDIATRIC AGE[46]

ICD-10CM #	E44.0	Moderate protein-energy malnutrition

CAUSES OF PROTEIN-LOSING ENTEROPATHY

Mucosal inflammation:
Infection:

Cytomegalovirus.
Bacterial overgrowth.
Invasive bacterial infection.
Gastric inflammation:
    Ménétrier disease.
    Eosinophilic gastroenteropathy.
Intestinal inflammation:
    Celiac disease.
    Crohn disease.
Eosinophilic gastroenteropathy:
    Tropical sprue.
    Radiation enteritis.
Primary intestinal lymphangiectasia.
Secondary intestinal lymphangiectasia:
    Constrictive pericarditis.
    Congestive heart failure.
    Post–Fontan procedure.
    Malrotation.
    Lymphoma.
    Sarcoidosis.
    Radiation therapy.
Colonic inflammation:
    Inflammatory bowel diseases.
    Necrotizing enterocolitis.
Congenital disorders of glycosylation.

PROTEINURIA

ICD-10CM #	R80.9	Proteinuria, unspecified

'Nephrotic syndrome as a result of primary renal diseases.
Malignant hypertension.
Malignancies: multiple myeloma, leukemias, Hodgkin's disease.
CHF.
DM.
SLE, RA.
Sickle cell disease.
Goodpasture's syndrome.
Malaria.
Amyloidosis, sarcoidosis.
Tubular lesions: cystinosis.
Functional (after heavy exercise).
Pyelonephritis.
Pregnancy.
Constrictive pericarditis.
Renal vein thrombosis.
Toxic nephropathies: heavy metals, drugs.
Radiation nephritis.
Orthostatic (postural) proteinuria.
Benign proteinuria: fever, heat, or cold exposure.

PRURITUS

ICD-10CM #	L29.9	Pruritus, unspecified
	L29.3	Anogenital pruritus, unspecified

Dry skin.
Drug-induced eruption, fiberglass exposure.
Scabies.
Skin diseases.
Myeloproliferative disorders: mycosis fungoides, Hodgkin's lymphoma, multiple myeloma, polycythemia vera.
Cholestatic liver disease.
Endocrine disorders: DM, thyroid disease, carcinoid, pregnancy.

Carcinoma: breast, lung, gastric.
Chronic renal failure.
Iron deficiency.
AIDS.
Neurosis.
Sjögren's syndrome.

PRURITUS ANI[51]

ICD-10CM #   L29.0   Pruritus ani

FECAL IRRITATION

Poor hygiene.
Anorectal conditions (fissure, fistula, hemorrhoids, skin tags, perianal clefts).
Spicy foods, citrus foods, caffeine, colchicine, quinidine.

CONTACT DERMATITIS

Anesthetic agents, topical corticosteroids, perfumed soap.

DERMATOLOGIC DISORDERS

Psoriasis, seborrhea, lichen simplex or sclerosus.

SYSTEMIC DISORDERS

Chronic renal failure, myxedema, DM, thyrotoxicosis, polycythemia vera, Hodgkin's disease.

SEXUALLY TRANSMITTED DISEASES

Syphilis, herpes simplex virus, human papillomavirus.

OTHER INFECTIOUS AGENTS

Pinworms.
Scabies.
Bacterial infection, viral infection.

PRURITUS VULVAE[68]

ICD-10CM #   L29.3   Anogenital pruritus, unspecified

CAUSES OF PRURITUS VULVAE

Diseases Special to Vulval Skin
Lichen sclerosus et atrophicus.
Leukoplakia.
Carcinoma.
Skin Disease
Psoriasis.
Atopic dermatitis.
Irritant and allergic contact dermatitis (especially medicaments).
Infection
Candidiasis.
Trichomonas.
Infestation
Pediculosis.
Psychogenic
Anxiety.
Depression.
Unknown

PSEUDOCYANOSIS, ETIOLOGY

ICD-10CM #   varies with etiology

Medications: amiodarone, minocycline, chlorpromazine.
Heavy metals:
  Gold (systemic absorption).
  Silver (systemic absorption).
Local contact with color dyes, gold, silver.

PSEUDOHERMAPHRODITISM, FEMALE

ICD-10CM #		
	E25.0	Congenital adrenogenital disorders associated with enzyme deficiency
	E25.8	Other adrenogenital disorders
	E25.9	Adrenogenital disorder, unspecified
	Q56.3	Pseudohermaphroditism, unspecified
	Q56.4	Indeterminate sex, unspecified

Congenital adrenal hyperplasia.
Maternal use of testosterone or related steroids.
Virilizing ovarian or adrenal tumor.
Virilizing luteoma of pregnancy.
Disturbances in differentiation of urogenital structures, non-androgen related.
Maternal virilizing adrenal hyperplasia.
Fetal P450 aromatase deficiency.

PSEUDOHERMAPHRODITISM, MALE

ICD-10CM#		
	E25.0	Congenital adrenogenital disorders associated with enzyme deficiency
	E25.8	Other adrenogenital disorders
	E25.9	Adrenogenital disorder, unspecified
	Q56.3	Pseudohermaphroditism, unspecified
	Q56.4	Indeterminate sex, unspecified

Maternal ingestion of progestogens.
End-organ resistance to androgenic hormones.
5-α-reductase-2 deficiency.
XY gonadal dysgenesis.
Testicular regression syndrome.
Defects in testosterone metabolism by peripheral tissues.
Testosterone biosynthesis defects.

PSEUDOINFARCTION[45]

ICD-10CM #   varies with specific diagnosis

Cardiac tumors, primary and secondary.
Cardiomyopathy (particularly hypertrophic and dilated).
Chagas' disease.
Chest deformity.
COPD (particularly emphysema).
HIV infection.
Hyperkalemia.
Left anterior fascicular block.
Left bundle branch block.
Left ventricular hypertrophy.

Myocarditis and pericarditis.
Normal variant.
Pneumothorax.
Poor R wave progression, rotational changes, and lead placement.
Pulmonary embolism.
Trauma to chest (nonpenetrating).
Wolff-Parkinson-White syndrome.
Rare causes: pancreatitis, amyloidosis, sarcoidosis, scleroderma.

PSYCHOSIS[55]

ICD-10CM #	# F29	Unspecified psychosis not due to a substance or known physiological condition
	F29	Unspecified psychosis not due to a substance or known physiological condition
	F10.231	Alcohol dependence with withdrawal delirium
	F01.51	Vascular dementia with behavioral disturbance

PRIMARY

Schizophrenia related.[36]
Major depression.
Dementia.
Bipolar disorder.

SECONDARY

Drug use.[37]
Drug withdrawal.[38]
Drug toxicity.[39]
Charles Bonnet syndrome.
Infections (pneumonia).
Electrolyte imbalance.
Syphilis.
Congestive heart failure.
Parkinson's disease.
Trauma to temporal lobe.
Postpartum psychosis.
Hypothyroidism/hyperthyroidism.
Hypomagnesemia.
Epilepsy.
Meningitis.
Encephalitis.
Brain abscess.
Herpes encephalopathy.
Hypoxia.
Hypercarbia.
Hypoglycemia.
Thiamine deficiency.
Postoperative states.

---

[36]Includes schizophrenia, schizophreniform disorder, brief reactive psychosis.
[37]Includes hypnotics, glucocorticoids, marijuana, phencyclidine, atropine, dopaminergic agents (e.g., amantadine, bromocriptine, l-dopa), immunosuppressants.
[38]Includes alcohol, barbiturates, benzodiazepines.
[39]Includes digitalis, theophylline, cimetidine, anticholinergics, glucocorticoids, catecholaminergic agents.

PSYCHOSIS, MEDICAL DISORDERS-INDUCED[51]

| ICD-10CM # | F29 | Unspecified psychosis not due to a substance or known physiological condition |
| | F53 | Puerperal psychosis |

MEDICAL DISORDERS THAT MAY CAUSE ACUTE PSYCHOSIS

Metabolic Disorders
Hypercalcemia.
Hypercarbia.
Hypoglycemia.
Hyponatremia.
Hypoxia.

Inflammatory Disorders
Sarcoidosis.
Systemic lupus erythematosus.
Temporal (giant cell) arteritis.

Organ Failure
Hepatic encephalopathy.
Uremia.

Neurologic Disorders
Alzheimer's disease.
Cerebrovascular disease.
Encephalitis (including HIV infection).
Encephalopathies.
Epilepsy.
Huntington's disease.
Multiple sclerosis.
Neoplasms.
Normal-pressure hydrocephalus.
Parkinson's disease.
Pick's disease.
Wilson's disease.

Endocrine disorders
Addison's disease.
Cushing's disease.
Panhypopituitarism.
Parathyroid disease.
Postpartum psychosis.
Recurrent menstrual psychosis.
Sydenham's chorea.
Thyroid disease.

Deficiency States
Niacin.
Thiamine.
Vitamin B_{12} and folate.

PSYCHOSIS, MEDICATION-INDUCED[51]

| ICD-10CM # | F10.5 | Psychotic disorder due to psychoactive substance use |

PHARMACOLOGIC AGENTS THAT MAY CAUSE ACUTE PSYCHOSIS

Antianxiety Agents
Alprazolam.
Chlordiazepoxide.
Clonazepam.
Clorazepate.
Diazepam.

Ethchlorvynol.

Antibiotics
Isoniazid.
Rifampin.

Anticonvulsants
Ethosuximide.
Phenobarbital.
Phenytoin.
Primidone.

Antidepressants
Amitriptyline.
Doxepin.
Imipramine.
Protriptyline.
Trimipramine.

Cardiovascular Drugs
Captopril.
Digitalis.
Disopyramide.
Methyldopa.
Procainamide.
Propranolol.
Reserpine.

Drugs of Abuse
Alcohol.
Amphetamines.
Cannabis.
Cocaine.
Hallucinogens.
Opioids.
Phencyclidine.
Sedative-hypnotics.

Miscellaneous Drugs
Antihistamines.
Antineoplastics.
Bromides.
Cimetidine.
Corticosteroids.
Disulfiram.
Heavy metals.

PTOSIS

ICD-10CM #	H02.409	Unspecified ptosis of unspecified eyelid
	Q10.0	Congenital ptosis
	H02.419	Mechanical ptosis of unspecified eyelid
	H02.429	Myogenic ptosis of unspecified eyelid
	H02.439	Paralytic ptosis unspecified eyelid

Third nerve palsy.
Myasthenia gravis.
Horner's syndrome.
Senile ptosis.

PUBERTY, DELAYED[54]

| ICD-10CM # | E30.0 | Delayed puberty |

NORMAL OR LOW SERUM GONADOTROPIN LEVELS

Constitutional delay in growth and development.
Hypothalamic and/or pituitary disorders:
  Isolated deficiency of growth hormone.
  Isolated deficiency of Gn-RH.

Isolated deficiency of LH and/or FSH.
Multiple anterior pituitary hormone deficiencies.
Associated with congenital anomalies: Kallmann's syndrome; Prader-Willi syndrome; Laurence-Moon-Biedl syndrome; Friedreich's ataxia.
Trauma.
Postinfection.
Hyperprolactinemia.
Postirradiation.
Infiltrative disease (histiocytosis).
Tumor.
Autoimmune hypophysitis.
Idiopathic.
Functional:
  Chronic endocrinologic or systemic disorders.
  Emotional disorders.
  Drugs: cannabis.

INCREASED SERUM GONADOTROPIN LEVELS

Gonadal abnormalities:
  Congenital:
    Gonadal dysgenesis.
    Klinefelter's syndrome.
    Bilateral anorchism.
    Resistant ovary syndrome.
    Myotonic dystrophy in males.
    17-Hydroxylase deficiency in females.
    Galactosemia.
  Acquired:
    Bilateral gonadal failure resulting from trauma or infection or after surgery, irradiation, or chemotherapy.
    Oophoritis: isolated or with other autoimmune disorders.
Uterine or vaginal disorders:
  Absence of uterus and/or vagina.
  Testicular feminization: complete or incomplete androgen insensitivity.

PUBERTY, PRECOCIOUS

ICD-10CM #	E25.0	Congenital adrenogenital disorders associated with enzyme deficiency
	E25.8	Other adrenogenital disorders
	E25.9	Adrenogenital disorder, unspecified

Idiopathic.
Congenital virilizing adrenal hyperplasia.
Hypothalamic tumors.
Head trauma.
Hydrocephalus.
Degenerative CNS disease.
Arachnoid cyst.
Sex chromosome abnormalities (e.g., 47, XXY, 48, XXXY).
Perinatal asphyxia.
CNS infection (e.g., meningitis, encephalitis).

PULMONARY CRACKLES

| ICD-10CM # | R09.8 | Friction sounds, chest |

Pneumonia.
Left ventricular failure.
Asbestosis, silicosis, interstitial lung disease.
Chronic bronchitis.
Alveolitis (allergic, fibrosing).
Neoplasm.

PULMONARY CYSTS ON X-RAY[33]

| ICD-10CM # | Q33.0 | Polycystic lungs, congenital |
| | J98.4 | Pulmonary manifestations |

CAUSES OF CYSTS IN THE LUNG ON CHEST RADIOGRAPH

Cystic fibrosis.
Cystic bronchiectasis.
Bronchopulmonary dysplasia (neonate and older).
Tuberculosis (apical thick walled).
Pulmonary abscess (thick wall, fluid level).
Empyema.
Streptococcal pneumatocele (thin wall, postinfective).
Cavitating pneumonia.
Mycetoma (apical cyst with contents).
Cystic congenital adenomatoid malformation (basal cysts of varying size).
Diaphragmatic hernia (cysts of similar size).
Hiatal hernia (posterior).
Morgagni hernia (midline anterior).
Bronchopulmonary sequestration (basal).
Congenital lobar emphysema.
Hydatid disease (in endemic areas).
Kerosene inhalation (pneumatocele).
Histiocytosis and other causes of interstitial disease.

PULMONARY EDEMA, NONCARDIOGENIC[33]

| ICD-10CM # | J81.0 | Acute pulmonary edema |

CAUSES OF NONCARDIOGENIC PULMONARY EDEMA

Adult respiratory distress syndrome.
Drowning.
Asphyxia.
Upper airway obstruction (usually with cardiomegaly).
High altitude.
Increased intracranial pressure.
Postictal.
Noxious gases:
  Smoke.
  Nitrous dioxide (silo filler's disease).
  Sulfur dioxide.
  Nitrogen mustard.
Drugs:
  Aspirin.
  Diazepam, chlordiazepoxide, barbiturates.
  Narcotics (heroin, methadone, morphine).
  β-adrenergic drugs (terbutaline).
  Contrast media.
  Colchicine.

Fluorescein.
Hydrochlorothiazide.
Nitrofurantoin.
Propoxyphene.
Poisons:
  Parathion.
Transfusion reactions.
Renal failure: transplantation.
Bone marrow transplantation.
Fat embolism.
Pancreatitis.

PULMONARY EOSINOPHILIA[2]

| ICD-10CM # | NEC J82 | Eosinophilia, pulmonary |

TYPES AND CAUSES OF PULMONARY EOSINOPHILIA

Drug- and toxin-induced eosinophilic lung diseases.
Helminth and fungal infection-related eosinophilic lung diseases:
  Transpulmonary passage of larvae (i.e., Löffler syndrome): *Ascaris*, hookworm, *Strongyloides.*
  Pulmonary parenchymal invasion: mostly helminths, paragonimiasis.
  Heavy hematogenous seeding with helminths: trichinellosis, disseminated strongyloidiasis, cutaneous and visceral larva migrans, schistosomiasis.
  Tropical pulmonary eosinophilia: filaria.
  Allergic bronchopulmonary aspergillosis.
Chronic eosinophilic pneumonia.
Acute eosinophilic pneumonia.
Churg-Strauss syndrome (vasculitis).
Other: neoplasia, idiopathic hypereosinophilic syndrome, bronchocentric granulomatosis.

PULMONARY HEMORRHAGE, FOCAL[59]

| ICD-10CM # | R04.8 | Pulmonary hemorrhage |

CAUSES OF FOCAL PULMONARY HEMORRHAGE

Iatrogenic Disorders
Bronchoscopy
Lung biopsy
Pulmonary artery catheterization
Transtracheal aspiration
Radiofrequency ablation
Brachytherapy
Infectious Disorders
Lung abscess
Mycetoma
Necrotizing pneumonia (*Staphylococcus aureus*, gram-negative aerobes, *Legionella*, Actinomyces species, *Stenotrophomonas, Kytococcus sedentarius,* Leptospira species, Yersinia pestis, Francisella tularensis)
Parasitic infection (paragonimiasis, amebiasis, ascariasis, clonorchiasis, echinococcosis, hookworm infestation, strongyloidiasis, trichinosis, schistosomiasis)

Parenchymal fungal infection (aspergillosis, mucormycosis, coccidioidomycosis, histoplasmosis, maduromycosis, botryomycosis)
Tuberculosis (active or inactive)
Viral tracheitis
Herpetic tracheobronchitis
Interstitial Lung Diseases
Lymphangioleiomyomatosis
Sarcoidosis
Tuberous sclerosis
Pneumoconiosis
Langerhans cell granulomatosis
Miscellaneous Disorders
Amyloidosis
Bronchogenic cyst
Broncholithiasis
Bronchopleural fistula
Thoracic endometriosis
Foreign body
Tracheopathia osteoplastica
Lipoid pneumonia
Organophosphate aspiration
Chronic pancreatitis
Neoplastic Disorders
Bronchial adenoma
Lung cancer
Tracheal tumors (mucoepidermoid, squamous cell, adenoid cystic, glomus)
Pulmonary blastoma
Pleuropulmonary angiosarcoma
Sarcoma (synovial, myofibroblastic)
Clear cell tumor
Metastatic disease (prostate, renal, breast, ovarian)
Tracheobronchial schwannoma
Pulmonary Airway Diseases
Bronchiectasis
Bronchitis
Granulomatous tracheobronchitis (ulcerative colitis, Crohn's disease, Wegener's granulomatosis)
Cystic fibrosis
Bullous emphysema
Traumatic Injury
Blunt chest trauma
Penetrating injury
Ruptured bronchus
Lightning injury
Thoracic splenosis
Vascular Disorders
Pulmonary embolism, infarction
Systemic cholesterol emboli
Intralobar sequestration
Pulmonary artery aneurysms
Behçet's disease, Hughes-Stovin syndrome, traumatic pseudoaneurysms
Acquired arteriovenous malformations
Osler-Weber-Rendu syndrome (hereditary hemorrhagic telangiectasia)
Takayasu's arteritis
Aortic aneurysms
Trachea–innominate artery fistulas
Scimitar syndrome
Vena cava-bronchial
Dieulafoy's disease of bronchus
Ventriculopulmonary fistulas
Hemangioma (sclerosing, cavernous, tracheal)

Differential Diagnosis

II

PULMONARY HEMORRHAGE, PEDIATRIC AGE

ICD-10CM # P26.9 Pulmonary hemorrhage newborn

CAUSES OF PULMONARY HEMORRHAGE (HEMOPTYSIS)

Focal Hemorrhage

Bronchitis and bronchiectasis (especially cystic fibrosis related).

Infection (acute or chronic), pneumonia, abscess.

Tuberculosis.

Trauma.

Pulmonary arteriovenous malformation.

Foreign body (chronic).

Neoplasm including hemangioma.

Pulmonary embolus with or without infarction.

Bronchogenic cysts.

Diffuse hemorrhage

Idiopathic of infancy.

Congenital heart disease (including pulmonary hypertension, venoocclusive disease, congestive heart failure).

Prematurity.

Cow's milk hyperreactivity (Heiner syndrome).

Goodpasture syndrome.

Collagen vascular diseases (systemic lupus erythematosus, rheumatoid arthritis).

Henoch-Schönlein purpura and vasculitic disorders.

Granulomatous disease (Wegener granulomatosis).

Celiac disease.

Coagulopathy (congenital or acquired).

Malignancy.

Immunodeficiency.

Exogenous toxins.

Hyperammonemia.

Pulmonary hypertension.

Pulmonary alveolar hemosiderosis.

Tuberous sclerosis.

Lymphangiomyomatosis or lymphangioleiomyomatosis.

Physical injury or abuse.

PULMONARY HEMORRHAGIC SYNDROMES, DIFFUSE[33]

ICD-10CM # P26.1 Massive pulmonary hemorrhage originating in the perinatal period
R04.8 Pulmonary hemorrhage

CLASSIFICATION OF DIFFUSE PULMONARY HEMORRHAGE SYNDROMES

Non-immunocompromised patients

Antibasement membrane antibody disease/Goodpasture's syndrome.

Diseases of presumed immune etiology, with or without nephropathy:

Systemic lupus erythematosus.

Rheumatoid arthritis.

Systemic sclerosis.

Systemic necrotizing vasculitis.

Granulomatosis with polyangiitis (Wegener's granulomatosis).

Microscopic polyarteritis.

Diseases with no known immune etiology:

Idiopathic pulmonary hemosiderosis.

Rapidly progressive glomerulonephritis without immune complexes.

Fibrillary glomerulonephritis.

Drug-induced (anticoagulants, trimellitic anhydride, cocaine, lymphangiography).

Valvular heart disease.

Disseminated intravascular coagulation.

Acute lung injury.

Tumors.

Immunocompromised Patients

Blood dyscrasias.

Infection.

Tumors.

PULMONARY INFILTRATES, IMMUNOCOMPROMISED HOST[77]

ICD-10CM # J82 Pulmonary eosinophilia, not elsewhere classified
J98.4 Other disorders of lung

CAUSES OF PULMONARY INFILTRATES IN THE IMMUNOCOMPROMISED HOST

Infections:

Bacteria:

Gram-positive cocci, especially *Staphylococcus.*

Gram-negative bacilli.

Mycobacterium tuberculosis.

Nontuberculous mycobacteria.

Nocardia.

Viruses:

Cytomegalovirus.

Herpesvirus.

Fungi:

Aspergillus.

Cryptococcus.

Candida.

Mucor.

Pneumocystis jiroveci.

Protozoa:

Toxoplasmagondii (rare).

Pulmonary effects of therapy:

1. Chemotherapeutic agents.
2. Radiation therapy.
3. Pulmonary hemorrhage.
4. Congestive heart failure.
5. Disseminated malignancy.
6. Nonspecified interstitial pneumonitis (no defined etiology).

PULMONARY LESIONS

ICD-10CM# J98.4 Other disorders of lung
J70.9 Respiratory conditions due to unspecified external agent

S27.309A Unspecified injury of lung, unspecified, initial encounter

TB.

Legionella pneumonia.

Mycoplasma pneumonia.

Viral pneumonia.

Pneumocystis carinii.

Hypersensitivity pneumonitis.

Aspiration pneumonia.

Fungal disease (aspergillosis, histoplasmosis).

ARDS associated with pneumonia.

Psittacosis.

Sarcoidosis.

Septic emboli.

Metastatic cancer.

Multiple pulmonary emboli.

Rheumatoid nodules.

PULMONARY MASS, SOLITARY, CAUSES[33]

ICD-10CM # R91.1 Solitary pulmonary nodule

CAUSES OF A SOLITARY PULMONARY MASS

Bronchial carcinoma.

Bronchial carcinoid.

Granuloma.

Hamartoma.

Metastasis.

Chronic pneumonia or abscess.

Hydatid cyst.

Pulmonary hematoma.

Bronchocele.

Fungus ball.

Massive fibrosis in coal workers.

Bronchogenic cyst.

Sequestration.

Arteriovenous malformation.

Pulmonary infarct.

Round atelectasis.

PULMONARY MASS, SOLITARY, MIMICS[33]

ICD-10CM # varies with specific diagnosis

SIMULANTS OF A SOLITARY PULMONARY MASS

Extrathoracic artifacts.

Cutaneous masses.

Bony lesions.

Pleural tumors or plaques.

Encysted pleural fluid.

Pulmonary vessels.

PULMONARY NODULE, SOLITARY

ICD-10CM # J98.4 Other disorders of lung

Bronchogenic carcinoma.
Granuloma from histoplasmosis.
TB granuloma.
Granuloma from coccidioidomycosis.
Metastatic carcinoma.
Bronchial adenoma.
Bronchogenic cyst.
Hamartoma.
AV malformation.
Other: fibroma, intrapulmonary lymph node, sclerosing hemangioma, bronchopulmonary sequestration.

PULMONARY–RENAL SYNDROMES, CAUSES[25]

ICD-10CM # varies with specific diagnosis

Systemic vasculitis	Anti-GBM disease (Goodpasture's). ANCA associated: Granulomatosis with polyangiitis (Wegener's granulomatosis). Microscopic polyarteritis. Churg-Strauss syndrome. Drugs (penicillamine, hydralazine, propylthiouracil). Immune complex disease. Lupus erythematosus. Henoch-Schönlein purpura. Mixed cryoglobulinemia. Rheumatoid vasculitis.
Infection	Severe bacterial pneumonia; postinfectious glomerulonephritis; *Legionella;* hantavirus; opportunistic infection in immunocompromised patients; infective endocarditis.
Pulmonary edema and AKI	Volume overload; severe left ventricular failure.
Multiorgan failure	Acute respiratory distress syndrome and AKI.
Other	Paraquat poisoning; renal vein or IVC thrombosis with pulmonary emboli.

AKI, Acute kidney injury; *ANCA,* anti-neutrophil cytoplasmic antibody; *GBM,* glomerular basement membrane; *IVC,* inferior vena cava.

PULSELESS ELECTRICAL ACTIVITY

ICD-10CM # I46.9 Cardiac arrest, cause unspecified

Hypovolemia.
Hypoxia.
Hyperkalemia.
Acidosis.
Cardiac tamponade.
Tension pneumothorax.
Pulmonary embolus.
Drug overdose.
Hypothermia.

PUPILLARY DILATATION, POOR RESPONSE TO DARKNESS

ICD-10CM # H21.569 Pupillary abnormality, unspecified eye

Drugs (narcotics, general anesthetics, cholinergics).
Acute trauma (spasm from prostaglandin release).
Inflammation, infection (interruption of inhibitory fibers to the Edinger-Westphal nucleus).
Old age (loss of inhibition at midbrain from reticular activating formation).
Horner's syndrome (sympathetic neuron interruption).
Adie's syndrome tonic pupil.
Lymphoma.
Congenital miosis.

PURPURA

ICD-10CM #	D69.2	Other nonthrombocytopenic purpura
	D69.0	Allergic purpura
	D69.49	Other primary thrombocytopenia
	M31.1	Thrombotic microangiopathy

THROMBOTIC

Trauma.
Septic emboli, atheromatous emboli.
DIC.
Thrombocytopenia.
Meningococcemia.
Rocky Mountain spotted fever.
Hemolytic-uremic syndrome.
Viral infection: echo, coxsackie.
Scurvy.
Other: left atrial myxoma, cryoglobulinemia, vasculitis, hyperglobulinemic purpura.

PURPURA, NONPALPABLE[40]

ICD-10CM # D69.2 Other nonthrombocytopenic purpura

INCREASED TRANSMURAL PRESSURE GRADIENT

Acute (Valsalva, coughing, vomiting, high altitude, weight lifting).
Chronic—Venous stasis.

DECREASED MECHANICAL INTEGRITY OF MICROCIRCULATION AND SUPPORTING TISSUES

Age related (infancy and actinic purpura).
Glucocorticoid excess—Cushing syndrome and glucocorticoid therapy.
Vitamin C deficiency (scurvy).
Abnormal connective tissue—Ehlers-Danlos syndrome.
Amyloid infiltration of blood vessels.

Colloid milium.
Hormonal—Female easy bruising syndrome (purpura simplex).
Lorenzo's oil.
MELAS syndrome.

TRAUMA TO BLOOD VESSELS

Physical:
  Injuries.
  Child abuse.
  Factitial purpura.
Ultraviolet purpura:
  Purpuric sunburn.
  Solar purpura.
Infectious:
  Bacterial.
  Rickettsial.
  Fungal.
  Viral.
  Parasitic.
Embolic:
  Infectious organisms.
  Atheroemboli (cholesterol crystal emboli).
  Fat emboli.
Allergic and/or inflammatory:
  Serum sickness.
  Pigmented purpuric eruptions.
  Pyoderma gangrenosum.
  Contact dermatitis.
  Familial Mediterranean fever.
Neoplastic.
Metabolic:
  Erythropoietic porphyria.
  Calciphylaxis.
Immunoglobulin related (hyperglobulinemic purpura of Waldenström and light-chain vasculitis).
Drug related.
Thrombotic:
  Disseminated intravascular coagulation.
  Warfarin (Coumadin)-induced skin necrosis.
  Protein C or protein S deficiency, factor V Leiden, prothrombin G20201A.
  Purpura fulminans.
  Paroxysmal nocturnal hemoglobinuria.
  Antiphospholipid antibody syndrome.
  Hemangioma with thrombocytopenia and consumptive coagulopathy (Kasabach-Merritt syndrome).

UNKNOWN CAUSE— PSYCHOGENIC PURPURA

PURPURA, NONPURPURIC DISORDERS SIMULATING PURPURA[3]

ICD-10CM # varies with specific diagnosis

Disorders with telangiectasias:
  Cherry angiomas.
  Hereditary hemorrhagic telangiectasia.
  Chronic actinic telangiectasia.
  Scleroderma.
  CREST syndrome.
  Ataxia-telangiectasia.
  Chronic liver disease.
  Pregnancy-related telangiectasia.
Kaposi sarcoma and other vascular sarcomas.

Fabry disease.
Neonatal extramedullary hematopoiesis.
Angioma serpiginosum.

PURPURA, PALPABLE[40]

ICD-10CM #   D69.2   Other nonthrombocytopenic purpura

Cutaneous vasculitis:
    Systemic vasculitides.
    Paraneoplastic vasculitis.
    Henoch-Schönlein purpura.
    Acute hemorrhagic edema of infancy.
    Livedoid vasculitis.
    Idiopathic.
    Urticarial.
Cryoglobulinemia.
Cryofibrinogenemia.
Primary cutaneous diseases.

QT INTERVAL PROLONGATION[45]

ICD-10CM #   R94.31   Abnormal electrocardiogram [ECG] [EKG]
               I45.81   Long QT syndrome

Drugs:
    Class I antiarrhythmics (e.g., disopyramide, procainamide, quinidine).
    Class III antiarrhythmics.
    Tricyclic antidepressants.
    Phenothiazines.
    Astemizole.
    Terfenadine.
    Adenosine.
    Antibiotics (e.g., erythromycin and other macrolides).
    Antifungal agents.
    Pentamidine, chloroquine.
Ischemic heart disease.
Cerebrovascular disease.
Rheumatic fever.
Myocarditis.
Mitral valve prolapse.
Electrolyte abnormalities.
Hypocalcemia.
Hypothyroidism.
Liquid protein diets.
Organophosphate insecticides.
Congenital prolonged QT syndrome.

RADIATION-INDUCED NEOPLASMS[60]

ICD-10CM #   varies with specific diagnosis

RADIATION-INDUCED NEOPLASMS

Osteochondroma
Benign.
Exclusively with childhood irradiation.
Histologically identical to spontaneous osteochondroma.
Sarcoma
Malignant.
Latent period of 4 years or more.

Histologically identical to spontaneous sarcoma.
Commonly malignant fibrous histiocytoma or osteosarcoma.
Occurs in either bone or soft tissue.
Tumors in Other Organ Systems
Squamous cell cancer of the skin.
Breast cancer.
Leukemia, with shorter latent period than sarcoma.

RECTAL MASS, PALPABLE[72]

ICD-10CM #   R22.9   Localized swelling, mass and lump, unspecified

Rectal carcinoma.
Rectal polyp.
Hypertrophied anal papilla.
Diverticular phlegmon (prolapsing into the pouch of Douglas).
Sigmoid colon carcinoma (prolapsing into the pouch of Douglas).
Metastatic deposits at the pelvic reflection (Blumer's shelf).
Primary pelvic malignancy (uterine, ovarian, prostatic, or cervical).
Mesorectal lymph nodes.
Endometriosis.
Solitary rectal ulcer syndrome.
Foreign body.
Feces.
Presacral cyst.
Amebic granuloma.
Vaginal tampon and even the pubic bone may be mistaken for a rectal mass.

RECTAL PAIN

ICD-10CM #   K62.89   Other specified diseases of anus and rectum

Anal fissure.
Thrombosed hemorrhoid.
Anorectal abscess.
Foreign bodies.
Fecal impaction.
Endometriosis.
Neoplasms (primary or metastatic).
Pelvic inflammatory disease.
Inflammation of sacral nerves.
Compression of sacral nerves.
Prostatitis.
Other: proctalgia fugax, uterine abnormalities, myopathies, coccygodynia.

RED BLOOD CELL APLASIA, ACQUIRED, ETIOLOGY

ICD-10CM #   D61.01   Constitutional (pure) red blood cell aplasia

Idiopathic (>50% of cases).
Medications (most frequent with phenytoin).
Non-Hodgkin's lymphoma.
Viral infections (parvovirus B19, EB virus, mumps, hepatitis).
Myelodysplastic syndromes.
Thymoma.
Autoimmune diseases.

Allogenic bone marrow transplant from ABO incompatible donor.
Pregnancy.

RED BLOOD CELL FRAGMENTATION HEMOLYSIS, CAUSES[39]

ICD-10CM #   varies with specific disorder

CAUSES OF RED BLOOD CELL FRAGMENTATION HEMOLYSIS

Damaged microvasculature.
Thrombotic thrombocytopenic purpura–hemolytic uremic syndrome (TTP–HUS).
Associated with pregnancy: preeclampsia or eclampsia; hemolysis plus elevated liver enzymes plus low platelets (HELLP syndrome).
Associated with malignancy, with or without mitomycin C treatment.
Vasculitis: polyarteritis, Wegener granulomatosis, acute glomerulonephritis, or *Rickettsia*-like infections.
Systemic lupus erythematosus.
Abnormalities of renal vasculature: malignant hypertension, acute glomerulonephritis, scleroderma, or allograft rejection with or without cyclosporine treatment.
Disseminated intravascular coagulation.
Malignant hypertension.
Catastrophic antiphospholipid antibody syndrome.
Atrioventricular malformations.
Kasabach-Merritt syndrome.
Hemangioendotheliomas.
Atrioventricular shunts for congenital and acquired conditions (e.g., stents, coils, transjugular intrahepatic portosystemic shunt, Levine shunts).
Cardiac abnormalities:
    Replaced valve, prosthesis, graft, or patch.
    Aortic stenosis or regurgitant jets (e.g., in ruptured sinus of Valsalva).
Drugs:
    Cyclosporine.
    Mitomycin.
    Ticlopidine.
    Clopidogrel.
    Tacrolimus.
    Cocaine.
Systemic infection:
    Bacterial endocarditis.
    Brucellosis.
    Cytomegalovirus.
    Human immunodeficiency virus.
    Ehrlichiosis.
    Rocky Mountain spotted fever

RED EYE

ICD-10CM #   H57.8   Other specified disorders of eye and adnexa

Infectious conjunctivitis (bacterial, viral).
Allergic conjunctivitis.
Acute glaucoma.
Keratitis (bacterial, viral).

Iritis.
Trauma.

RED EYE, ACUTE[4]

ICD-10CM #   H57.8

Obvious open globe.
Corneal abrasion.
Corneal ulcer.
Subconjunctival hemorrhage.
Hyphema.
Occult open globe.
Herpes simplex virus glaucoma.
Iritis, traumatic iritis.
Scleritis.
Conjunctivitis.
Blepharitis.
Ultraviolet keratitis.
Episcleritis.
Conjunctival foreign body.
Dry eye.
Contact lens overwear syndrome.

RED HOT JOINT

ICD-10CM #   varies with specific diagnosis

Trauma.
Gout.
Infection (septic joint).
Pseudogout (calcium pyrophosphate dehydrate crystal deposition).
Psoriatic arthropathy.
Reactive arthritis.
Palindromic rheumatism.

RED URINE

ICD-10CM #   R39.19   Other difficulties with micturition

Hematuria.
Porphyrins.
Hemoglobinuria.
Myoglobinuria.
Medications (phenazopyridine, aminosalicylic acid, deferoxamine, phenazopyridine, phenolphthalein, NSAIDs, rifampin, phenytoin, methyldopa, doxorubicin, phenacetin).
Foods (beets, berries, maize).
Urate crystalluria.

RENAL ALLOGRAFT DYSFUNCTION[31]

ICD-10CM #   T86.1   Complications of renal allograft

IMMEDIATE/DELAYED GRAFT FUNCTION (1-3 DAYS)

Acute tubular necrosis.
Hyperacute humoral rejection.
Urinary leak or obstruction.
Renal artery or vein thrombosis.
Recurrence of disease (e.g., focal segmental glomerulosclerosis).

EARLY POSTTRANSPLANTATION PERIOD (FIRST MONTH)

Acute cellular rejection.

Acute humoral rejection.
Calcineurin inhibitor toxicity.
Urinary tract obstruction.
Volume depletion.
Recurrence of disease.

Late Acute Dysfunction

Acute rejection.
Cyclosporine or tacrolimus toxicity.
Recurrence of primary disease.
Tubulointerstitial nephritis, drug-induced.
Renal artery stenosis.
Infection (bacterial urinary tract infection [UTI], cytomegalovirus, BK virus).
Hemodynamic (volume; use of angiotensin-converting enzyme inhibitor, angiotensin II receptor blocker).

Chronic Dysfunction

Chronic rejection.
Cyclosporine or tacrolimus toxicity.
Recurrent renal disease.
De novo renal disease.
Urinary tract obstruction.
Bacterial UTI.
Hypertensive nephrosclerosis.

RENAL ARTERY OCCLUSION, CAUSES

ICD-10CM #   N28.0   Ischemia and infarction of kidney

Atrial fibrillation.
Angiography or stent placement.
Abdominal aortic surgery.
Trauma.
Renal artery aneurysm/dissection.
Vasculitis.
Thrombosis in patient with fibromuscular dysplasia.
Atherosclerosis.
Septic embolism.
Mural thrombus thromboembolism.
Atrial myxoma thromboembolism.
Mitral stenosis thromboembolism.
Prosthetic valve thromboembolism.
Renal cell carcinoma.

RENAL COLIC[4]

ICD-10CM #   N23

Vascular:
  Abdominal aortic aneurysm.
  Aortic dissection.
  Renal artery dissection.
  Renal artery stenosis.
  Renal vein thrombosis.
  Renal infarct.
  Mesenteric ischemia.
  Retroperitoneal hemorrhage.
Gastrointestinal:
  Incarcerated hernia.
  Appendicitis.
  Cholecystitis.
  Biliary colic.
  Pancreatitis.
  Bowel obstruction.
  Diverticulitis.
Gynecologic:
  Ectopic pregnancy.

Ovarian torsion.
  Tuboovarian abscess.
  Pelvic inflammatory disease.
  Endometriosis.
Genitourinary:
  Testicular torsion.
  Pyelonephritis.
  Perinephric abscess.
  Urinary tract tumor.
  Renal papillary necrosis.
  Upper urinary tract hemorrhage.
Musculoskeletal:
  Lumbar strain.
  Radiculopathy.
  Disk herniation.
  Vertebral compression fracture.
Dermatologic:
  Herpes zoster.
Miscellaneous:
  Factitious.

RENAL CYSTIC DISORDERS

ICD-10CM #   Q61.01   Congenital single renal cyst

Simple cysts.
Acquired cystic kidney disease.
Autosomal dominant polycystic kidney disease.
Autosomal recessive polycystic kidney disease.
Medullary cystic disease.
Medullary sponge kidney.

RENAL DISEASE, SKIN MANIFESTATIONS[67]

ICD-10CM #   Varies with Specific Diagnosis

SKIN MANIFESTATIONS SECONDARY TO RENAL DISEASE

Nonspecific

Pruritus
Xerosis
Acquired ichthyosis
Pigmentary alteration
  Pallor (secondary to anemia)
  Hyperpigmentation
  Dyspigmentation (yellow tint)
Infections (fungal, bacterial, viral)
Purpura

Somewhat Specific

Acquired perforating dermatosis
Calciphylaxis
Metastatic calcification
Blistering disorders
  Porphyria cutanea tarda
  Pseudoporphyria
Eruptive xanthomas
Pseudo–Kaposi's sarcoma

Specific

Nephrogenic systemic fibrosis
Dialysis-associated steal syndrome
Metastatic renal cell carcinoma
Dialysis-related amyloidosis
Arteriovenous shunt dermatitis
Uremic frost

RENAL FAILURE, ACUTE, PIGMENT-INDUCED[6]

ICD-10CM #   N19   Unspecified kidney failure

CAUSES OF PIGMENT-INDUCED ACUTE RENAL FAILURE

Rhabdomyolysis and myoglobinuria.
Vigorous exercise.
Arterial embolization.
Status epilepticus.
Status asthmaticus.
Coma-induced and pressure-induced myonecrosis.
Heat stress.
Diabetic ketoacidosis.
Myopathy.
Alcoholism.
Hypokalemia.
Hypophosphatemia.
Hemoglobinuria.
Transfusion reactions.
Snake envenomation.
Malaria.
Mechanical destruction of RBCs by prosthetic valves.
G6PD deficiency.

G6PD, Glucose-6-phosphate dehydrogenase; *RBCs,* red blood cells.

RENAL FAILURE, CHRONIC[31]

ICD-10CM #   N18.9   Chronic kidney disease, unspecified

CAUSES OF CHRONIC RENAL FAILURE

Diabetic glomerulosclerosis (systemic disease involving the kidney).
Hypertensive nephrosclerosis.
Glomerular disease:
  Glomerulonephritis.
  Amyloidosis, light chain disease (systemic disease involving the kidney).
  Systemic lupus erythematosus, Wegener granulomatosis (systemic disease involving the kidney).
Tubulointerstitial disease:
  Reflux nephropathy (chronic pyelonephritis).
  Analgesic nephropathy.
  Obstructive nephropathy (stones, benign prostatic hypertrophy).
  Myeloma kidney (systemic disease involving the kidney).
Vascular disease:
  Scleroderma (systemic disease involving the kidney).
  Vasculitis (systemic disease involving the kidney).
  Renovascular renal failure (ischemic nephropathy).
  Atheroembolic renal disease (systemic disease involving the kidney).
Cystic disease:
  Autosomal dominant polycystic kidney disease.
  Medullary cystic kidney disease.

RENAL FAILURE, INTRINSIC OR PARENCHYMAL CAUSES[70]

ICD-10CM #   N17.0   Acute kidney failure with tubular necrosis
        N17.1   Acute kidney failure with acute cortical necrosis
        N17.2   Acute kidney failure with medullary necrosis
        N17.8   Other acute kidney failure
        N17.9   Acute kidney failure, unspecified
        N18.9   Chronic kidney disease, unspecified

ABNORMALITIES OF THE VASCULATURE

Renal arteries: atherosclerosis, thromboembolism, arteritis.
Renal veins: thrombosis.
Microvasculature: vasculitis, thrombotic microangiopathy.

ABNORMALITIES OF GLOMERULI (ACUTE GLOMERULONEPHRITIS)

Antiglomerular membrane disease (Goodpasture's syndrome).
Immune complex glomerulonephritis: SLE, postinfectious, idiopathic, membranoproliferative.

ABNORMALITIES OF INTERSTITIUM (ACUTE INTERSTITIAL NEPHRITIS)

Drugs (e.g., antibiotics, NSAIDs, diuretics, anticonvulsants, allopurinol).
Infectious pyelonephritis.
Infiltrative: lymphoma, leukemia, sarcoidosis.

ABNORMALITIES OF TUBULES

Physical obstruction (uric acid, oxalate, light chains).
Acute tubular necrosis:
  Ischemic.
  Toxic (antibiotics, chemotherapy, immunosuppressives, radiocontrast dyes, heavy metals, myoglobin, hemolyzed RBCs).

RENAL FAILURE, POSTRENAL CAUSES[70]

ICD-10CM #   N17.0   Acute kidney failure with tubular necrosis
        N17.1   Acute kidney failure with acute cortical necrosis
        N17.2   Acute kidney failure with medullary necrosis
        N17.8   Other acute kidney failure
        N17.9   Acute kidney failure, unspecified
        N18.9   Chronic kidney disease, unspecified

URETER AND RENAL PELVIS

Intrinsic obstruction:
  Blood clots.
  Stones.
  Sloughed papillae: diabetes, sickle cell disease, analgesic nephropathy.
  Inflammatory: fungus ball.
Extrinsic obstruction:
  Malignancy.
  Retroperitoneal fibrosis.
  Iatrogenic: inadvertent ligation of ureters.

BLADDER

Prostatic hypertrophy or malignancy.
Neuropathic bladder.
Blood clots.
Bladder cancer.
Stones.

URETHRAL

Strictures.
Congenital valves.

RENAL FAILURE, PRERENAL CAUSES[70]

ICD-10CM #   N17.0   Acute kidney failure with tubular necrosis
        N17.1   Acute kidney failure with acute cortical necrosis
        N17.2   Acute kidney failure with medullary necrosis
        N17.8   Other acute kidney failure
        N17.9   Acute kidney failure, unspecified
        N18.9   Chronic kidney disease, unspecified

DECREASED CARDIAC OUTPUT

CHF.
Arrhythmias.
Pericardial constriction or tamponade.
Pulmonary embolism.

HYPOVOLEMIA

GI tract loss (vomiting, diarrhea, nasogastric suction).
Blood losses (trauma, GI tract surgery).
Renal losses (diuretics, mineralocorticoid deficiency, postobstructive diuresis).
Skin losses (burns).

VOLUME REDISTRIBUTION (DECREASE IN EFFECTIVE BLOOD VOLUME)

Hypoalbuminemic states (cirrhosis, nephrosis).
Sequestration of fluid in "third" space (ischemic bowel, peritonitis, pancreatitis).
Peripheral vasodilation (sepsis, vasodilators, anaphylaxis).

ALTERED RENAL VASCULAR RESISTANCE

Increase in afferent vascular resistance (NSAIDs, liver disease, sepsis, hypercalcemia, cyclosporine).
Decrease in efferent arteriolar tone (ACE inhibitors).

RENAL INFARCTION[25]

ICD-10CM # N28.0   Ischemia and infarction of kidney

CAUSES OF RENAL INFARCTION

Thrombosis: Spontaneous
Atherosclerotic disease of aorta and renal artery.
Fibromuscular dysplasia of renal artery.
Aneurysms of aorta or renal artery.
Dissection of aorta or renal artery.
  Marfan's syndrome.
  Ehlers-Danlos syndrome.
Vasculitis involving renal artery.
  o Polyarteritis nodosa.
  o Takayasu's arteritis.
  o Kawasaki disease.
  o Thromboangiitis obliterans.
  o Other necrotizing vasculitides.
- Inflammatory disease of the aorta or renal artery.
  Syphilis.
  Tuberculosis.
  Mycoses.
Hypercoagulable states.
  o Nephrotic syndrome.
  o Antiphospholipid syndrome.
  o Antithrombin III deficiency.
  o Homocystinuria.
- Thrombotic microangiopathies.
  Hemolytic-uremic syndrome.
  Thrombotic thrombocytopenic purpura.
  Antiphospholipid syndrome.
  Malignant hypertension.
  Scleroderma.
  Sickle cell nephropathy.
  Polycythemia vera.
  Postpartum hemolytic-uremic syndrome.
  Hyperacute vascular allograft rejection.
Thrombosis: Induced
Traumatic.
Following endovascular intervention.
Post renal transplantation.
Embolism
Cardiac source.
  o Atrial fibrillation or other arrhythmias.
  o Native and prosthetic valvular heart disease.
  o Infective endocarditis.
  o Marantic endocarditis.
- Myocardial infarction with mural thrombi.
  o Left atrial myxoma or other tumor.
- Noncardiac sources.
  Atheromatous embolic disease.
  Paradoxical emboli.
  Fat emboli.
  Tumor emboli.
Therapeutic renal embolization.
Segmental renal infarction of childhood.
Cisplatinum and gemcitabine.
Sickle cell disease or sickle cell trait.

RENAL PARENCHYMAL DISEASE, CHRONIC[33]

ICD-10CM # N28.9   Disorder of kidney and ureter, unspecified

DIFFERENTIAL DIAGNOSIS OF CHRONIC RENAL PARENCHYMAL DISEASE

No Papillary/Caliceal Abnormality
Diffuse Parenchymal Loss
Bilateral:
  Chronic glomerulonephritis.
  Diffuse small-vessel disease.
  Hereditary nephropathies.
Unilateral:
  Renal artery stenosis.
  Postirradiation.
  Rare:
    Hypoplastic kidney.
    Postobstructive atrophy.

FOCAL PARENCHYMAL LOSS

Infarct.
Previous trauma.
Papillary/Caliceal Abnormality
Diffuse Parenchymal Loss
Obstructive nephropathy.
Generalized reflux nephropathy.
No Parenchymal Loss
Papillary necrosis.
TB.
Medullary sponge kidney.
Megacalices.
Pelvicaliceal cyst.
Focal Parenchymal Loss
Focal reflux nephropathy (chronic atrophic pyelonephritis).
TB.
Calculus disease.

RENAL VEIN THROMBOSIS, CAUSES

ICD-10CM # I82.3   Embolism and thrombosis of renal vein

Nephrotic syndrome.
Renal cell carcinoma.
Aortic aneurysm causing compression.
Lymphadenopathy.
Retroperitoneal fibrosis.
Estrogen therapy.
Pregnancy.
Renal cell carcinoma with vein invasion.
Severe dehydration.

RESPIRATORY DISTRESS IN THE NEWBORN, CAUSES[27]

ICD-10CM # J96.00   Acute respiratory failure

Respiratory Distress in the Newborn
Noncardiopulmonary
Hypothermia or hyperthermia.
Hypoglycemia.
Metabolic acidosis.
Drug intoxications; withdrawal.
Polycythemia.
Central nervous system insult.
Asphyxia.
Hemorrhage.
Neuromuscular disease.
Werdnig-Hoffman disease.
Myopathies.

Phrenic nerve injury.
Skeletal abnormalities.
Asphyxiating thoracic dystrophy.
Cardiovascular
Left-sided outflow obstruction.
Hypoplastic left heart.
Aortic stenosis.
Coarctation of the aorta.
Cyanotic lesions.
Transposition of the great vessels.
Total anomalous pulmonary venous return
Tricuspid atresia.
Right-sided outflow obstruction.
Pulmonary
Upper airway obstruction.
Choanal atresia.
Vocal cord paralysis.
Meconium aspiration.
Clear fluid aspiration.
Transient tachypnea.
Pneumonia.
Pulmonary hypoplasia.
Primary.
Secondary.
Hyaline membrane disease.
Pneumothorax.
Pleural effusions.
Mass lesions.
Lobar emphysema.
Cystic adenomatoid malformation.

RESPIRATORY FAILURE, HYPOVENTILATORY[55]

ICD-10CM # J96.00   Acute respiratory failure, unspecified whether with hypoxia or hypercapnia
J96.90   Respiratory failure, unspecified, unspecified whether with hypoxia or hypercapnia

ABNORMAL RESPIRATORY CAPACITY (NORMAL RESPIRATORY WORKLOADS)

Acute depression of central nervous system:
  Various causes.
Chronic central hypoventilation syndromes:
  Obesity-hypoventilation syndrome.
  Sleep apnea syndrome.
  Hypothyroidism.
  Shy-Drager syndrome (multisystem atrophy syndrome).
Acute toxic paralysis syndromes:
  Botulism.
  Tetanus.
  Toxic ingestion or bites.
  Organophosphate poisoning.
Neuromuscular disorders (acute and chronic):
  Myasthenia gravis.
  Guillain-Barré syndrome.
  Drugs.
  Amyotrophic lateral sclerosis.
  Muscular dystrophies.
  Polymyositis.
  Spinal cord injury.
  Traumatic phrenic nerve paralysis.

ABNORMAL PULMONARY WORKLOADS

Chronic obstructive pulmonary disease:
  Chronic bronchitis.
  Asthmatic bronchitis.
  Emphysema.
Asthma and acute bronchial hyperreactivity syndromes.
Upper airway obstruction.
Interstitial lung diseases.

ABNORMAL EXTRAPULMONARY WORKLOADS

Chronic thoracic cage disorders:
  Severe kyphoscoliosis.
  After thoracoplasty.
  After thoracic cage injury.
Acute thoracic cage trauma and burns.
Pneumothorax.
Pleural fibrosis and effusions.
Abdominal processes.

RESPIRATORY MUSCLE WEAKNESS[59]

ICD-10CM #	Varies with Specific Diagnosis

CAUSES OF DECREASED RESPIRATORY MUSCLE STRENGTH OR ENDURANCE

Disorders of the phrenic nerve
  Guillain-Barré syndrome
  Poliomyelitis
Respiratory muscle atrophy
Disorders of neuromuscular transmission
  Myasthenia gravis
  Ventilator dependence
  Malnutrition
  Myopathy
  Critical illness polyneuropathy/myopathy
Altered diaphragmatic force-length relationship
  Dynamic hyperinflation and diaphragmatic flattening

RETINOPATHY, HYPERTENSIVE

ICD-10CM #	H35.039	Hypertensive retinopathy, unspecified eye

Retinal venous obstruction.
Diabetic retinopathy.
Ocular ischemic syndrome.
Hyperviscosity.
Tortuosity of retinal artery.

RHINITIS

ICD-10CM #	J31.0	Chronic rhinitis
	J30.0	Vasomotor rhinitis
	J30.1	Allergic rhinitis due to pollen
	J30.2	Other seasonal allergic rhinitis
	J30.5	Allergic rhinitis due to food
	J30.89	Other allergic rhinitis

	J30.9	Allergic rhinitis, unspecified

Allergic rhinitis.
Infectious rhinitis.
Vasomotor rhinitis.
Exercise-induced rhinitis.
Emotional rhinitis.
Rhinitis medicamentosa.
Hormone-mediated rhinitis (menses, pregnancy, oral contraceptives, hypothyroidism).
GERD.
Chemical- or irritant-induced rhinitis.
Rhinitis mimics:
  Deviated septum.
  Enlarged adenoids.
  Nasal polyps/tumors.
  Foreign bodies.
  CSF rhinorrhea.
  Sarcoidosis.
  Midline granuloma.
  Granulomatosis with polyangiitis (Wegener's granulomatosis).
  SLE.
  Sjögren's syndrome.

RHINITIS, CHRONIC[2]

ICD-10CM #	J31.0	Chronic rhinitis

CLASSIFICATION OF CHRONIC RHINITIS

Allergic
Systemic.
Local (entopy).
Work-Related
Irritant.
Corrosive.
Immunologic.
Infectious (Rhinosinusitis)
Allergic.
Nonallergic.
Nonallergic
Idiopathic.
Nonallergic with eosinophilia.
Atrophic.
Primary.
Secondary.
Medication-related.
Topical vasoconstrictors (rhinitis medicamentosa).
Oral medications.
Exercise-induced.
Cold air–induced.
Gustatory.
Hormonal.
Aging.
Systemic diseases.

RHINOSINUSITIS, DIFFERENTIAL DIAGNOSIS[52]

ICD-10CM #	varies with specific diagnosis

DIFFERENTIAL DIAGNOSIS OF RHINOSINUSITIS

Allergic Rhinitis
Seasonal.

Perennial.
Combined seasonal and perennial.
Allergic fungal rhinosinusitis.
Nonallergic Rhinitis
Nonallergic, noninflammatory idiopathic rhinopathy (vasomotor rhinitis).
Nonallergic rhinitis with eosinophilia syndrome (NARES).
Cold dry air–induced rhinitis.
Gustatory rhinitis.
Infectious Rhinosinusitis
Bacterial.
Viral.
Fungal.
Granulomatous.
Drug-Induced Rhinitis
Oral contraceptives.
Various antihypertensives and ocular β-blockers.
Topical decongestants (rhinitis medicamentosa).
Phosphodiesterase-5 antagonists.
Mechanical Causes of Rhinosinusitis
• Septal deviation.
• Nasal foreign body.
• Choanal atresia or stenosis.
• Adenoid hypertrophy.
• Encephalocele.
• Glioma.
• Dermoid.
Innate and Acquired Immunity Disorders
Congenital or acquired immunodeficiencies.
Cystic fibrosis.
Immotile cilia syndrome.
Systemic Inflammatory Disorders
Sarcoidosis.
Wegener's granulomatosis.
Vasculitis.
Neoplastic Causes
Benign:
  Polyps.
  Nasopharyngeal angiofibroma.
  Inverting papilloma.
Malignant:
  Adenocarcinoma.
  Squamous cell carcinoma.
  Aesthesioneuroblastoma.
  Lymphoma.
  Rhabdomyosarcoma.

RIB DEFECTS ON X-RAY[33]

ICD-10CM #	varies with specific diagnosis

CAUSES OF SUPERIOR MARGINAL RIB DEFECTS

Normal
Isolated defects.
Projectional artifacts (due to lordosis).
Neurologic
Paralytic poliomyelitis.
Quadriparesis.
Collagen Vascular Disease
Rheumatoid arthritis.
SLE.
Systemic sclerosis.
Local Pressure
Chest drainage tube.
Osteochondroma.

Neural tumor.
Coarctation of aorta.
Hyperparathyroidism Miscellaneous
Osteogenesis imperfecta.
Marfan's syndrome.

RIB NOTCHING ON X-RAY[33]

ICD-10CM # varies with specific diagnosis

CAUSES OF INFERIOR RIB NOTCHING
ARTERIAL

AORTIC OBSTRUCTION

Aortic coarctation.
Aortic thrombosis.
Aortitis.

SUBCLAVIAN ARTERY OBSTRUCTION

Blalock-Taussig operation.
Arteritis.
Atherosclerotic occlusion.

PULMONARY OLIGEMIA

Pulmonary atresia.
Tetralogy of Fallot.
Multiple pulmonary arterial stenoses.
Venous

CHRONIC SUPERIOR VENA CAVAL OBSTRUCTION

Arteriovenous
Arteriovenous Malformation
Pulmonary.
Chest wall.
Neural
Neurofibromas

RIGHT AXIS DEVIATION[45]

ICD-10CM # varies with specific diagnosis

Normal variation.
Right ventricular hypertrophy.
Left posterior fascicular block.
Lateral myocardial infarction.
Pulmonary embolism.
Dextrocardia.
Mechanical shifts or emphysema causing a vertical heart.

SALIVARY GLAND ENLARGEMENT

ICD-10CM #	K11.1	Hypertrophy of salivary gland

Neoplasm.
Sialolithiasis.
Infection (mumps, bacterial infection, HIV, TB).
Sarcoidosis.
Idiopathic.
Acromegaly.
Anorexia/bulimia.
Chronic pancreatitis.
Medications (e.g., phenylbutazone).
Cirrhosis.
DM.

SALIVARY GLAND SECRETION, DECREASED

ICD-10CM #	K11.7	Disturbances of salivary secretion
	R68.2	Dry mouth, unspecified

Medications (antihistamines, antidepressants, neuroleptics, antihypertensives).
Dehydration.
Anxiety.
Sjögren's syndrome.
Sarcoidosis.
Mumps.
Amyloidosis.
CNS disorders.
Head and neck radiation.

SCLERODERMA-LIKE SYNDROMES[3]

ICD-10CM # varies with specific diagnosis

OTHER DISEASES

Morphea.
Eosinophilic fasciitis.
Scleredema (of Buschke).
Scleromyxedema.
Graft-versus-host disease.
Nephrogenic-fibrosing dermopathy.

ENVIRONMENTAL AGENTS AND DRUGS

Bleomycin.
l-Tryptophan.
Organic solvents.
Pentazocine.
Toxic oil syndrome.
Vinyl chloride disease.
Gadolinium.

SCROTAL CALCIFICATIONS[62]

ICD-10CM #	Varies with Specific Diagnosis

SCROTAL CALCIFICATIONS

Testicular
Solitary, postinflammatory granulomatous, vascular
Microlithiasis
"Burned-out" germ cell tumor
Large-cell calcifying Sertoli cell tumor
Teratoma
Mixed germ cell tumor
Sarcoid
Tuberculosis
Chronic infarct
Extratesticular
Tunica vaginalis "scrotal pearls"
Chronic epididymitis
Schistosomiasis

SCROTAL MASSES, BOYS AND ADOLESCENTS[46]

ICD-10CM #	R22.9	Localized swelling, mass and lump, unspecified

PAINFUL

Testicular torsion.
Torsion of appendix testis.
Epididymitis.
Trauma: ruptured testis, hematocele.
Inguinal hernia (incarcerated).
Mumps orchitis.

PAINLESS

Hydrocele.
Inguinal hernia.[40]
Varicocele.
Spermatocele.
Testicular tumor.
Henoch-Schönlein purpura.
Idiopathic scrotal edema.

---

[40]May be associated with discomfort.

SCROTAL PAIN[55]

ICD-10CM#	S31.30XA	Unspecified open wound of scrotum and testes, initial encounter
	N50.9	Disorder of male genital organs, unspecified
	R10.2	Pelvic and perineal pain
	N49.9	Inflammatory disorder of unspecified male genital organ
	N50.1	Vascular disorders of male genital organs
	N49.9	Inflammatory disorder of unspecified male genital organ

Torsion:
 Appendages.
 Spermatic cord.
Infection:
 Orchitis.
 Abscess.
 Epididymitis.
Neoplasia:
 Benign.
 Malignant.
Incarcerated hernia.
Trauma.
Hydrocele.
Spermatocele.
Varicocele.

SCROTAL PAIN, ADOLESCENT OR PEDIATRIC PATIENT[76]

ICD-10CM #	Varies with Specific Diagnosis

DIFFERENTIAL DIAGNOSIS OF PEDIATRIC ADOLESCENT ACUTE SCROTAL PAIN

Appendage torsion
 Appendix testis
 Other appendage (epididymis, paradidymis, vas aberrans)

Spermatic cord torsion
  Intravaginal, acute or intermittent
  Extravaginal
Epididymitis
  Infectious
    Urinary tract infection
    Sexually transmitted disease
    ?Viral
  Sterile or traumatic
Scrotal edema or erythema
  Diaper dermatitis, insect bite, or other skin lesions
  Idiopathic scrotal edema
Orchitis
  Associated with epididymitis with or without abscess
  Vasculitis (e.g., Henoch-Schönlein purpura)
  Viral illness (mumps)
Trauma
  Hematocele or scrotal contusion or testis rupture
Hernia or hydrocele
  Inguinal hernia with or without incarceration
  Communicating hydrocele
  Encysted hydrocele with or without torsion
  Associated with acute abdominal pathology (e.g., appendicitis, peritonitis)
Varicocele
Intrascrotal mass
  Cystic dysplasia or tumor of testis
  Epididymal cyst, spermatocele or tumor
  Other paratesticular tumors
Musculoskeletal pain from inguinal tendonitis or muscle strain
Referred pain (e.g., ureteral calculus or anomaly)

SCROTAL SWELLING

ICD-10CM #	N50.8	Other specified disorders of male genital organs

Hydrocele.
Varicocele.
Neoplasm.
Acute epididymitis.
Orchitis.
Trauma.
Hernia.
Torsion of spermatic cord.
Torsion of epididymis.
Torsion of testis.
Insect bite.
Folliculitis.
Sebaceous cyst.
Thrombosis of spermatic vein.
Other: lymphedema, dermatitis, fat necrosis, Henoch-Schönlein purpura, idiopathic scrotal edema.

SEIZURE

ICD-10CM #	R56.9	Unspecified convulsions

Syncope.
Alcohol abuse/withdrawal.
TIA.
Hemiparetic migraine.
Psychiatric disorders.
Carotid sinus hypersensitivity.
Hyperventilation, prolonged breath holding.

Hypoglycemia.
Narcolepsy.
Movement disorders (tics, hemiballismus).
Hyponatremia.
Brain tumor (primary or metastatic).
Tetanus.
Strychnine, phencyclidine poisoning.

SEIZURE, PEDIATRIC[6]

ICD-10CM #	R56.9	Unspecified convulsions
	P90	Convulsions of newborn

First Month of Life
First Day
Hypoxia.
Drugs.
Trauma.
Infection.
Hyperglycemia.
Hypoglycemia.
Pyridoxine deficiency.
Day 2-3
Infection.
Drug withdrawal.
Hypoglycemia.
Hypocalcemia.
Developmental malformation.
Intracranial hemorrhage.
Inborn error of metabolism.
Hyponatremia or hypernatremia.
Day >4
Infection.
Hypocalcemia.
Hyperphosphatemia.
Hyponatremia.
Developmental malformation.
Drug withdrawal.
Inborn error of metabolism.

1 TO 6 MO
As above.

6 MO TO 3 YR
Febrile seizures.
Birth injury.
Infection.
Toxin.
Trauma.
Metabolic disorder.
Cerebral degenerative disease.

>3 YR
Idiopathic.
Infection.
Trauma.
Cerebral degenerative disease.

SEIZURE MIMICS[3]

ICD-10CM #	varies with specific diagnosis

NON-EPILEPTIC EPISODIC DISORDERS THAT MAY RESEMBLE SEIZURES

Movement disorders: myoclonus, paroxysmal choreoathetosis, episodic ataxias, hyperexplexia (startle disease).

Migraine: confusional, vertebrobasilar, visual auras.
Syncope.
Behavioral and psychiatric: psychogenic non-epileptic attacks (pseudoseizures), hyperventilation syndrome, panic or anxiety disorder, dissociative states.
Cataplexy (usually associated with narcolepsy).
Transient ischemic attack.
Alcoholic blackouts.
Hypoglycemia.

SEXUAL DIFFERENTIATION ABNORMALITIES[76]

ICD-10CM #	Varies with Specific Diagnosis

ABNORMAL SEXUAL DIFFERENTIATION

1. Disorders of gonadal differentiation
   Seminiferous tubule dysgenesis
   Klinefelter syndrome
   46,XX male
   Syndromes of gonadal dysgenesis
     Turner syndrome
     Pure gonadal dysgenesis
     Mixed gonadal dysgenesis
     Partial gonadal dysgenesis (dysgenetic male pseudohermaphroditism)
     Bilateral vanishing testis, testicular regression syndromes
2. Ovotesticular DSD (true hermaphroditism)
3. 46,XX DSD (masculinized female)
   Congenital adrenal hyperplasia (21-hydroxylase, 11β-hydroxylase, 3β-hydroxysteroid dehydrogenase deficiencies)
   Maternal androgens
4. 46,XY DSD (undermasculinized male)
   Leydig cell agenesis, unresponsiveness
   Disorders of testosterone biosynthesis
   Variants of congenital adrenal hyperplasia affecting corticosteroid and testosterone synthesis
     StAR deficiency (congenital lipoid adrenal hyperplasia)
     Cytochrome P450 oxidoreductase (POR) deficiency
     3β-Hydroxysteroid dehydrogenase deficiency
     17β-Hydroxylase deficiency
   Disorders of testosterone biosynthesis
     17,20-Lyase deficiency
     17β-Hydroxysteroid oxidoreductase deficiency
   Disorders of androgen-dependent target tissue
     Androgen receptor and postreceptor defects
     Syndrome of complete (severe) androgen insensitivity
     Syndrome of partial androgen insensitivity
     Mild androgen insensitivity syndrome (MAIS)
   Disorders of testosterone metabolism by peripheral tissues
     5α-Reductase deficiency
     Disorders of synthesis, secretion, or response to müllerian-inhibiting substance
   Persistent müllerian duct syndrome
5. Unclassified forms
   In females: Mayer-Rokitansky-Küster-Hauser syndrome
   DSD, disorder of sex development.

SEXUAL DYSFUNCTION, FEMALE[3]

ICD-10CM #	R37	Sexual dysfunction, unspecified

FACTORS THAT MAY INFLUENCE SEXUAL FUNCTIONING IN WOMEN

Biological
Medications (e.g., antidepressants, antihypertensives).
Vaginal atrophy, pain with intercourse.
Low testosterone levels (e.g., bilateral oophorectomy).
Illness (e.g., diabetes, hypothyroidism, cerebrovascular accident).
Sleep disturbances, fatigue.
Disability or pain from illness (e.g., arthritis).
Incontinence.
Psychological
Depression.
Body image.
Interpersonal
Marital issues.
Poor communication.
Partner's sexual problems (e.g., erectile dysfunction).
Partner's health problems (e.g., myocardial infarction).
Sociocultural
Ageism ("too old" to want sex).
Multiple other obligations and commitments.
Lack of partner.

SEXUALLY TRANSMITTED DISEASES, ANORECTAL REGION[51]

ICD-10CM #	K62.89	Other specified diseases of anus and rectum

ULCERATIVE

Lymphogranuloma venereum.
Herpes simplex virus.
Early (primary) syphilis.
Chancroid (*Haemophilus ducreyi*).
Cytomegalovirus.
Idiopathic (usually HIV positive).

NONULCERATIVE

Condyloma acuminatum.
Gonorrhea.
Chlamydia (*Chlamydia trachomatis*).
Syphilis.

SEXUAL PRECOCITY[79]

ICD-10CM #	E30.1	Precocious puberty
	E30.8	Other disorders of puberty

TRUE PRECOCIOUS PUBERTY

Premature reactivation of LHRH pulse generator.

INCOMPLETE SEXUAL PRECOCITY

(Pituitary gonadotropin independent).
Males
Chorionic gonadotropin-secreting tumor.
Leydig cell tumor.
Familial testotoxicosis.
Virilizing congenital adrenal hyperplasia.
Virilizing adrenal tumor.
Premature adrenarche.
Females
Granulosa cell tumor (follicular cysts may be manifested similarly).
Follicular cyst.
Feminizing adrenal tumor.
Premature thelarche.
Premature adrenarche.
Late-onset virilizing congenital adrenal hyperplasia.
In Both Sexes
McCune-Albright syndrome.
Primary hypothyroidism.

SHOULDER PAIN

ICD-10CM #	M24.819	Other specific joint derangements of unspecified shoulder, not elsewhere classified
	M75.80	Other shoulder lesions, unspecified shoulder
	S43.409A	Unspecified sprain of unspecified shoulder joint, initial encounter
	S46.919A	Strain of unspecified muscle, fascia and tendon at shoulder and upper arm level, unspecified arm, initial encounter

WITH LOCAL FINDINGS IN SHOULDER

Trauma: contusion, fracture, muscle strain, trauma to spinal cord.
Arthrosis, arthritis, RA, ankylosing spondylitis.
Bursitis, synovitis, tendinitis, tenosynovitis.
Aseptic (avascular) necrosis.
Local infection: septic arthritis, osteomyelitis, abscess, herpes zoster, TB.

WITHOUT LOCAL FINDINGS IN SHOULDER

Cardiovascular disorders: ischemic heart disease, pericarditis, aortic aneurysm.
Subdiaphragmatic abscess, liver abscess.
Cholelithiasis, cholecystitis.
Pulmonary lesions: apical bronchial carcinoma, pleurisy, pneumothorax, pneumonia.
GI lesions: PUD, gastric neoplasm, peptic esophagitis.
Pancreatic lesions: carcinoma, calculi, pancreatitis.
CNS abnormalities: neoplasm, vascular abnormalities.
Multiple sclerosis.
Syringomyelia.
Polymyositis/dermatomyositis.
Psychogenic.
Polymyalgia rheumatica.
Ectopic pregnancy.

SHOULDER PAIN BY LOCATION

ICD-10CM #	M75.80	Other shoulder lesions, unspecified shoulder
	S43.499A	Other sprain of unspecified shoulder joint, initial encounter
	S46.019A	Strain of muscle(s) and tendon(s) of the rotator cuff of unspecified shoulder, initial encounter
	S46.819A	Strain of other muscles, fascia and tendons at shoulder and upper arm level, unspecified arm, initial encounter

TOP OF SHOULDER (C4)

Cervical source.
Acromioclavicular.
Sternoclavicular.
Diaphragmatic.

SUPEROLATERAL (C5)

Rotator cuff tendinitis.
Impingement.
Adhesive capsulitis.
Glenohumeral arthritis.

ANTERIOR

Bicipital tendinitis and rupture.
Glenoid labral tear.
Adhesive capsulitis.
Glenohumeral arthritis.
Osteonecrosis.

AXILLARY

Neoplasm (Pancoast's, mediastinal).
Herpes zoster.

SHOULDER PAIN, IN DIFFERENT AGE GROUPS[17]

ICD-10CM #	M25.519	Pain in unspecified shoulder

Differential Diagnosis

II

COMMON CAUSES OF SHOULDER PAIN IN DIFFERENT AGE GROUPS

Childhood (2-10 yr)
Intraarticular
Instability.
Periarticular
Osteochondromas.
Adolescence (10-18 yr)
Intraarticular
Instability.
Early Adulthood (18-30 yr)
Intraarticular
Instability.
Acromioclavicular joint sprain.
Periarticular
Calcific tendonitis.
Impingement.
Referred
Cervical.
Adulthood (30-60 yr)
Intraarticular
Osteochondritis.
Osteoarthritis.
Frozen shoulder.
Inflammatory arthritis.
Periarticular
Calcific tendonitis.
Impingement.
Rotator cuff tear.
Bicipital tendonitis.
Referred
Cervical.
Old Age (>60 yr)
Intraarticular
Osteochondritis.
Osteoarthritis.
Frozen shoulder.
Inflammatory arthritis.
Periarticular
Impingement.
Rotator cuff tear.
Referred
Cervical.

SINUS NODE DYSFUNCTION[31]

ICD-10CM # varies with specific diagnosis

CAUSES OF SINUS NODE DYSFUNCTION

Intrinsic
- Hypothyroidism.
- Fibrocalcific degeneration.
- Increased vagal tone, especially in sleep apnea.
- Congenital mutations.
- Scleroderma.
- Amyloidosis.
- Chagas disease.

Extrinsic
Trauma, including cardiac surgery.
Drugs:
    Calcium-channel blockers.
    β-Blockers.
    Digoxin.
    Antiarrhythmic medications (amiodarone, dronedarone, sotalol, flecainide, propafenone).
    Lithium.

SINUS OSTIAL OBSTRUCTION[9]

ICD-10CM # Codes vary with specific diagnosis

FACTORS THAT PREDISPOSE TO SINUS OSTIAL OBSTRUCTION

Mucosal Swelling
Systemic factors:
    Viral upper respiratory infection.
    Allergic inflammation.
    Cystic fibrosis.
    Immune disorders.
    Ciliary dyskinesia.
    Tobacco smoke.
Local insult:
    Facial trauma.
    Swimming, diving.
    Rhinitis medicamentosa.
    Nasal intubation.
Mechanical Obstruction
Choanal atresia.
Deviated septum.
Nasal polyps.
Foreign body.
Tumor.
Ethmoid bullae.

SINUS TACHYCARDIA[59]

ICD-10CM # R00.0 Tachycardia, Unspecified

DIFFERENTIAL DIAGNOSIS OF SINUS TACHYCARDIA

Etiologic Category
Specific Disorders
Hemodynamic
    Heart failure—systolic and diastolic heart failure caused by ischemic, valvular, or nonischemic myopathy
    Loss of circulating blood volume—gastrointestinal bleeding, anemia, shifts of intravascular fluid due to changes in colloidal osmotic pressure or inflammation
    Septic shock—dehydration
    Vascular shunts—intracardiac as well as aortovenous malformations, fistulas
    Pulmonary embolism
Metabolic and neurohumoral
    Sepsis—infections and inflammatory conditions
    Hyperthyroidism
    Paget's disease of the bone
    Pheochromocytoma
    Carcinoid syndrome
    Beriberi heart disease
    Carcinoma
    Hyperpyrexia
    Acidosis
    Exercise
Pharmacologic
    Sympathomimetic agents—isoproterenol, epinephrine, or dopamine
    Vagolytic agents, atropine, acopolamine
    Vasodilators—nitrates, angiotensin-converting enzyme inhibitors, angiotensin receptor blockers, hydrazine, as well as centrally acting vasodilators
    Thyroid preparations, caffeine and nicotine
    Bronchodilators, including theophylline and terbutaline
    Anesthetic agents, including spinal anesthetics, causing peripheral vasodilation
    Drugs of abuse—amphetamines, cocaine, "ecstasy," cannabis
Neurologic/psychological
    Pain
    Fear, anxiety, and hysteria
    Hyper-beta adrenergic phase of neurocardiogenic syncope
    Autonomic dysfunction such as with diabetes

SKIN AND RENAL[67]

ICD-10CM # varies with specific diagnosis

SELECTED CONDITIONS WITH CONCURRENT SKIN AND RENAL INVOLVEMENT

More Common
Lupus erythematosus
Leukocytoclastic vasculitis
Henoch-Schönlein purpura
Mixed cryoglobulinemia
Diabetes mellitus
Systemic vasculitis
Less Common
Nail-patella syndrome
Hemolytic-uremic syndrome
Toxic shock syndrome
Mixed connective tissue disease
Dermatomyositis
Rheumatoid arthritis
Sjögren's syndrome
Dermatitis herpetiformis
Sarcoidosis
Systemic sclerosis
Ulcerative colitis
Amyloidosis
Toxic epidermolysis
Hypothyroidism
Graves' disease
Fabry's disease
Neurofibromatosis
Hurler's syndrome
Castleman's disease
Infectious endocarditis
Staphylococcal scalded skin syndrome (in adults)

SKIN INDURATION, CHRONIC[37]

ICD-10CM # varies with specific diagnosis

CONDITIONS ASSOCIATED WITH CHRONIC SKIN INDURATION

Systemic sclerosis.
Localized scleroderma.
Scleroderma variants.
Scleredema.
    ○ Scleredema adultorum of Buschke.
    ○ Scleredema diabeticorum.
    ○ Scleredema neonatorum.
- Scleromyxedema.

- Nephrogenic fibrosing dermopathy.
- Eosinophilic syndromes.
  - Eosinophilic fasciitis (diffuse fasciitis with eosinophilia, Schulman disease).
  - Eosinophilia-myalgia syndrome.
  - Toxic oil syndrome.
- Chronic graft-versus-host disease.
- Pseudoscleroderma (local injection of vitamin K, bleomycin, pentazocine).
- Metabolic diseases.
  Porphyria cutanea tarda.
  Phenylketonuria.
  Werner syndrome.
  Acromegaly.
Pachydermoperiostitis.
Polyneuropathy, organomegaly, endocrinopathy, monoclonal gammopathy (POEMS).
Stiff skin syndrome.
Reflex sympathetic dystrophy.
Hemiplegia.

SMALL BOWEL MASSES[72]

ICD-10CM #   varies with specific diagnosis

Cyst:
  Mesenteric cyst.
Tumor:
  Benign.
  Malignant.
Intussusception.
Inflammation:
  Crohn's disease.

SMALL BOWEL OBSTRUCTION[51]

ICD-10CM # K56.5 Intestinal adhesions [bands] with obstruction (postprocedural) (postinfection)
          Q41.9 Congenital absence, atresia and stenosis of small intestine, part unspecified

INTRINSIC

Congenital (atresia, stenosis).
Inflammatory (Crohn's, radiation enteritis).
Neoplasms (metastatic or primary).
Intussusception.
Traumatic (hematoma).

EXTRINSIC

Hernias (internal and external).
Adhesions.
Volvulus.
Compressing masses (tumors, abscesses, hematomas).

INTRALUMINAL

Foreign body.
Gallstones.
Bezoars.
Barium.
Ascaris infestation.

SMALL INTESTINE ULCERATION

ICD-10CM # K63.3   Ulcer of intestine

Inflammatory bowel disease.
Celiac disease.
Vasculitis, SLE, Behçet's syndrome.
Uremia.
Infections *(Campylobacter,* TB, *Yersinia,* parasites, typhoid, cytomegalovirus [CMV], *Clostridium).*
Mesenteric insufficiency.
Neoplasms.
Radiation.
Drugs (salicylates, potassium, indomethacin, antimetabolites).
Meckel diverticulum.
Zollinger-Ellison syndrome.
Lymphocytic enterocolitis.
Stomal ulceration.

SMELL DISTURBANCE

ICD-10CM # R43.8   Other disturbances of smell and taste

Upper respiratory tract infection.
Nasal or paranasal sinus disease.
Exposure to noxious vapors.
Head trauma.
Idiopathic.
Dental caries, periodontal disease.
Medications.

SODIUM RETENTION, RENAL CAUSES[67]

ICD-10CM #   varies with specific diagnosis

CAUSES OF RENAL SODIUM RETENTION

Primary
Oliguric acute kidney injury
Chronic kidney disease
Glomerular disease
Severe bilateral renal artery stenosis
Na^+-retaining tubulopathies (genetic)
Mineralocorticoid excess
Secondary
Heart failure
Cirrhosis
Idiopathic edema

SOFT TISSUE MASS MIMICKING MALIGNANCY[60]

ICD-10CM #   varies with specific diagnosis

OVERVIEW OF DISEASES THAT CAN PRESENT AS A SOFT TISSUE MASS MIMICKING MALIGNANCY

Etiology	Disease Entity
Trauma:	Muscle contusion.
	Hematoma.
	Muscle herniation.
	Calcific myonecrosis.
	Hypothenar hammer syndrome.
	Myositis ossificans.
Metabolic:	Diabetic myopathy.
	Gout.
	Pseudogout.
	Calcific tendinosis.
Congenital:	Accessory muscle.
Infectious:	Necrotizing fasciitis.
	Abscess.
	Pyomyositis.
	Hydatid cystic disease.
	Cat-scratch disease.
	Actinomycosis.
Inflammation:	Bursitis.
	Sarcoidosis.
	Foreign body reaction.
	Injection granuloma.
	Granuloma annulare.
	Epidermal inclusion cyst.
Vascular:	Adventitial cystic disease.
	Pseudoaneurysm.
	Thrombosed vein.
	Arteriovenous vascular malformation.
Miscellaneous:	Focal myositis.
	Amyloid tumor of soft tissue.

SOFT TISSUE TUMORS, PEDIATRIC PATIENTS[60]

ICD-10CM #   varies with specific diagnosis

PEDIATRIC SOFT TISSUE TUMORS

Vascular lesions:
  Hemangioma of infancy.*
  Congenital hemangioma.
  Hemangioendothelioma (Kasabach-Merritt syndrome).
  Arteriovenous malformation.
  Venous malformations.
  Lymphatic malformation (lymphangioma, cystic hygroma).
  Capillary malformation.
Adipocytic tumors:
  Lipoma.
  Lipoblastoma.
  Liposarcoma.
Fibrohistiocytic tumors:
  Pigmented villonodular synovitis.
  Giant cell tumor of tendon sheath.
Fibroblastic and myofibroblastic tumors:
  Nodular fasciitis.
  Fibrous hamartoma of infancy.
  Myofibroma, myofibromatosis.
  Infantile fibrosarcoma.
  Fibromatosis colli.
Neurogenic tumors:
  Schwannoma.

*Lesions with MR-specific features.

Differential Diagnosis

II

Neurofibroma.
Malignant nerve sheath tumor.
Leiomyoma
Rhabdomyosarcoma
Tumors of uncertain differentiation
Synovial cell sarcoma.
Primitive neuroectodermal tumor (Ewing sarcoma).
Pilomatricoma

SORE THROAT[6]

ICD-10CM #   J02   Acute pharyngitis

DIFFERENTIAL DIAGNOSIS FOR SORE THROAT

Infectious Causes
Aerobes
Common:
Streptococcus pyogenes (GABHS).
GABHS.
Peptostreptococcus spp.
Non–group A streptococcus.
Neisseria gonorrhoeae.
Neisseria meningitides.
Mycoplasma pneumoniae.
Arcanobacterium hemolyticum.
Chlamydia trachomatis.
Staphylococcus aureus.
Uncommon:
Haemophilus influenzae.
Haemophilus parainfluenzae.
Coccidioides spp.
Corynebacterium diphtheriae.
Streptococcus pneumoniae.
Yersinia enterocolitica.
Treponema pallidum.
Francisella tularensis.
Legionella pneumophila.
Mycobacterium spp.

ANAEROBES

Bacteroides spp.
Peptococcus spp.
Clostridium spp.
Fusobacterium spp.
Prevotella spp.

OTHER

Candida spp.

VIRAL

Rhinovirus.
Adenovirus.
Coronavirus.
Herpes simplex 1, 2.
Influenza A, B.
Parainfluenza.
Cytomegalovirus.
Epstein-Barr.
Varicella-zoster.
Hepatitis virus.
Noninfectious Causes

SYSTEMIC

Kawasaki disease.
Stevens-Johnson syndrome.
Cyclic neutropenia.
Thyroiditis.
Connective tissue disease.

TRAUMA, MISCELLANEOUS

Penetrating injury.
Angioneurotic edema.
Retained foreign body.
Anomalous aortic arch.
Laryngeal fracture.
Calcific retropharyngeal tendinitis.
Retropharyngeal hematoma.
Caustic exposure.

TUMOR

Tongue.
Larynx.
Thyroid.
Leukemia.

SPASTIC PARAPLEGIAS

ICD-10CM #   G82.20   Paraplegia, unspecified

Cervical spondylosis.
Friedreich's ataxia.
Multiple sclerosis.
Spinal cord tumor.
HIV.
Tertiary syphilis.
Vitamin B_{12} deficiency.
Spinocerebellar ataxias.
Syringomyelia.
Spinal cord AV malformations.
Adrenoleukodystrophy.

SPINAL CORD COMPRESSION, EPIDURAL

ICD-10CM #   varies with specific diagnosis

Osteoarthritis.
Meningioma.
Spinal epidural abscess.
Spinal epidural hematoma.
Spinal epidural vascular malformations.
RA.
Metastatic cancer (vertebral, intramedullary, leptomeninges).
Radiation myelopathy.
Neurofibroma.
Sarcoidosis.
Paraneoplastic myelopathy.
Histiocytosis.

SPINAL CORD DYSFUNCTION

ICD-10CM #		
	G95.9	Disease of spinal cord, unspecified
	Q07.9	Congenital malformation of nervous system, unspecified
	D51.1	Vitamin B_{12} deficiency anemia due to selective vitamin B_{12} malabsorption with proteinuria
	D51.3	Other dietary vitamin B_{12} deficiency anemia
	D51.8	Other vitamin B_{12} deficiency anemias

	G95.89	Other specified diseases of spinal cord
	G95.19	Other vascular myelopathies

Trauma.
Multiple sclerosis.
Transverse myelitis.
Neoplasm (primary, metastatic).
Syringomyelia.
Spinal epidural abscess.
HIV myelopathy.
Diskitis.
Spinal epidural hematoma.
Spinal cord infarction.
Spinal AV malformation.
Subarachnoid hemorrhage.

SPINAL CORD DYSFUNCTION, NONTRAUMATIC[6]

ICD-10CM #   Q07.9   Congenital malformation of nervous system, unspecified

NONTRAUMATIC ETIOLOGIES OF SPINAL CORD DYSFUNCTION

Processes Affecting the Spinal Cord or Blood Supply Directly
Multiple sclerosis.
Transverse myelitis.
Spinal arteriovenous malformation/subarachnoid hemorrhage.
Syringomyelia.
HIV myelopathy.
Other myelopathies.
Spinal cord infarction.
Compressive Lesions Affecting the Spinal Cord
Spinal epidural abscess.
Spinal epidural hematoma.
Diskitis.
Neoplasm.
Metastatic.
Primary CNS.

HIV, Human immunodeficiency virus; *CNS*, central nervous system.

SPINAL CORD ISCHEMIC SYNDROMES

ICD-10CM #   varies with specific diagnosis

Systemic hypotension.
Venous or arterial occlusion.
Arterial dissection.
Thromboembolism.
Endovascular procedures.
Vasculitis.
Fibrocartilaginous embolism.
Regional hemodynamic compromise.

SPINAL TUMORS[29]

ICD-10CM #   varies with specific diagnosis

EXTRADURAL

Metastases.
Primary bone tumors arising in spine.

INTRADURAL EXTRAMEDULLARY

Meningiomas.
Neurofibromas.
Schwannomas.
Lipomas.
Arachnoid cysts.
Epidermoid cysts.
Metastasis.

INTRAMEDULLARY

Ependymoma.
Glioma.
Hemangioblastoma.
Lipoma.
Metastases.

SPLENIC CYSTS, CLASSIFICATION[14]

ICD-10CM #   D73.4   Cyst of spleen

- Primary (true).
- Parasitic.
- Nonparasitic.
- Congenital.
- Epidermoid.
- Dermoid.
- Mesothelial (serous).
- Transitional.
- Neoplastic.
- Secondary (false): pseudocysts.
- Traumatic.
- Degenerative.
- Inflammatory.
- Hemorrhagic.

SPLENIC MASSES, FOCAL SOLID[62]

ICD-10CM #   Varies with Specific Diagnosis

FOCAL SOLID SPLENIC MASSES

Benign
Hemangioma
Hamartoma
Littoral cell angioma
Lymphangioma
Sclerosing angiomatoid nodular transformation (SANT)
Inflammatory pseudotumor

Malignant
Lymphoma
Metastases
Angiosarcoma
Hemangiopericytoma

Other
Infarct

SPLENIC NODULES[62]

ICD-10CM #   Varies with Specific Diagnosis

CAUSES OF SPLENIC NODULES

Infectious
Tuberculosis/Mycobacterium avium-intracellulare complex
Pyogenic abscesses
Histoplasmosis
Candida abscesses
Cat-scratch disease
Pneumocystis jiroveci (formerly P. carinii pneumonia)

Inflammatory
Sarcoidosis

Malignant
Lymphoma
Metastases

Other
Gamna-Gandy bodies
Gaucher's disease

SPLENIC TUMORS, CLASSIFICATION[14]

ICD-10CM #   C26.1   Malignant neoplasm of spleen

- Malignant.
- Lymphoproliferative disease.
- Non-Hodgkin lymphoma.
- Hodgkin disease.
- Hairy cell leukemia.
- Chronic lymphocytic leukemia.
- Myeloproliferative disease.
- Chronic myelogenous leukemia.
- Myelofibrosis.
- Primary tumors.
- Angiosarcoma.
- Metastatic tumors.
- Benign.
- Hemangiomas.
- Hamartomas.
- Lymphangiomas.
- Sclerosing angiomatoid nodular transformation (SANT).

SPLENOMEGALY

ICD-10CM #   R16.1   Splenomegaly, not elsewhere classified
      D73.2   Chronic congestive splenomegaly
      R16.1   Splenomegaly, not elsewhere classified

Hepatic cirrhosis.
Neoplastic involvement: CML, CLL, lymphoma, multiple myeloma.
Bacterial infections: TB, infectious endocarditis, typhoid fever, splenic abscess.
Viral infections: infectious mononucleosis, viral hepatitis, HIV.
Gaucher's disease and other lipid storage diseases.
Sarcoidosis.
Parasitic infections (malaria, kala-azar, histoplasmosis).
Hereditary and acquired hemolytic anemias.
Idiopathic thrombocytopenic purpura (ITP).
Collagen vascular disorders: SLE, RA (Felty's syndrome), polyarteritis nodosa.
Serum sickness, drug hypersensitivity reaction.

Splenic cysts and benign tumors: hemangioma, lymphangioma.
Thrombosis of splenic or portal vein.
Polycythemia vera, myeloid metaplasia.

SPLENOMEGALY AND HEPATOMEGALY[72]

ICD-10CM #   R16.1   Splenomegaly, not elsewhere classified
      R16.0   Hepatomegaly, not elsewhere classified

CAUSES OF SPLENOMEGALY AND HEPATOSPLENOMEGALY

Massive Splenomegaly
Hematologic disease (e.g., chronic myeloid leukemia, myelofibrosis).

Moderate Splenomegaly
The above causes.
Portal hypertension.
Hematologic disease (e.g., lymphoma, leukemia, thalassemia).
Storage disease (e.g., Gaucher's disease).

Small Splenomegaly
The above causes.
Infective (hepatitis, leptospirosis, malaria, bacterial endocarditis).
Hematologic disease (e.g., hemolytic anemias, essential thrombocythemia, polycythemia rubra vera).
Connective tissue diseases or vasculitis (e.g., rheumatoid arthritis, systemic lupus erythematosus, polyarteritis nodosa).
Solitary cyst, polycystic syndrome, hydatid cyst.
Infiltration (amyloid, sarcoid).

Hepatosplenomegaly
Chronic liver disease with portal hypertension.
Hematologic disease (e.g., myeloproliferative disease, lymphoma).
Infection (e.g., amyloid, sarcoid).
Connective tissue disease (e.g., systemic lupus erythematosus).

SPLENOMEGALY, CHILDREN[40]

ICD-10CM #   R16.1   Splenomegaly, not elsewhere classified

DISORDERS OF THE BLOOD

Hemolytic anemia: congenital/acquired.
Thalassemia.
Sickle cell disease.
Leukemia.
Osteopetrosis.
Myelofibrosis/myeloid metaplasia/thrombocythemia.

INFECTIONS: ACUTE AND CHRONIC

Viral:
     Congenital (e.g., TORCH association).
     Mononucleosis (e.g., EBV, CMV infection).
     Virus-associated hemophagocytic syndrome.
     Human immunodeficiency virus.
Bacterial:
     Sepsis/abscess.
     Brucellosis.

Salmonellosis.
Tularemia.
Tuberculosis.
Subacute bacterial endocarditis.
Syphilis.
Lyme disease.
Fungal:
Histoplasmosis (disseminated).
Rickettsial:
Rocky Mountain spotted fever.
Cat scratch disease.
Parasitic:
Toxoplasmosis.
Malaria.
Leishmaniasis (kala-azar).
Schistosomiasis.
Echinococcosis.

HEPATIC/PORTAL SYSTEM DISORDERS

Acute/chronic active hepatitis.
Cirrhosis/hepatic fibrosis/biliary atresia.
Portal or splenic venous obstruction (Banti syndrome).

AUTOIMMUNE DISEASE

Juvenile rheumatoid arthritis.
Systemic lupus erythematosus.
Autoimmune lymphoproliferative syndrome (Canale–Smith syndrome).

NEOPLASMS/CYSTS

Lymphomas (Hodgkin and non-Hodgkin).
Hemangiomas/lymphangiomas.
Hamartomas.
Congenital or acquired (posttraumatic) cysts.

STORAGE DISEASES/INBORN ERRORS OF METABOLISM

Lipidoses: Gaucher disease, Niemann–Pick disease, others.
Mucopolysaccharidoses.
Defects in carbohydrate metabolism: galactosemia, fructose intolerance.
Sea-blue histiocyte syndrome.

MISCELLANEOUS DISORDERS

Histiocytoses:
Reactive.
Langerhans cell.
Malignant.
Sarcoidosis.
Congestive heart failure.
Familial Mediterranean fever.

CMV, Cytomegalovirus; *EBV*, Epstein-Barr virus; *TORCH*, toxoplasmosis, other infections, rubella, cytomegalovirus infection, herpes simplex.

SPONTANEOUS PNEUMOTHORAX[51]

ICD-10CM #	J93.0	Spontaneous tension pneumothorax
	J93.11	Primary spontaneous pneumothorax
	J93.12	Secondary spontaneous pneumothorax

CAUSES OF SECONDARY SPONTANEOUS PNEUMOTHORAX

Airway Disease
Chronic obstructive pulmonary disease.
Asthma.
Cystic fibrosis.
Infections
Necrotizing bacterial pneumonia, lung abscess.
Pneumocystis jiroveci pneumonia.
Tuberculosis.
Interstitial Lung Disease
Sarcoidosis.
Idiopathic pulmonary fibrosis.
Lymphangiomyomatosis.
Tuberous sclerosis.
Pneumoconioses.
Neoplasms
Primary lung cancers.
Pulmonary or pleural metastases.
Miscellaneous
Connective tissue diseases.
Pulmonary infarction.
Endometriosis, catamenial pneumothorax.

STATURAL OVERGROWTH[53]

| ICD-10CM # | E34.4 |

FETAL OVERGROWTH

Maternal diabetes mellitus.
Cerebral gigantism (Sotos syndrome).
Weaver's syndrome.
Beckwith-Wiedemann syndrome.
Other insulin-like growth factor 2 (IGF2) excess syndromes.

POSTNATAL OVERGROWTH LEADING TO CHILDHOOD TALL STATURE

Familial (constitutional) tall stature.
Cerebral gigantism.
Beckwith-Wiedemann syndrome.
Exogenous obesity.
Excess growth hormone (GH) secretion (pituitary gigantism).
McCune-Albright syndrome or multiple endocrine neoplasia (MEN) associated with excess GH secretion.
Precocious puberty.
Marfan's syndrome.
Klinefelter's syndrome (XXY).
Weaver's syndrome.
Fragile X syndrome.
Homocystinuria.
XYY.
Hyperthyroidism.

POSTNATAL OVERGROWTH LEADING TO ADULT TALL STATURE

Familial (constitutional) tall stature.
Androgen or estrogen deficiency/estrogen resistance (in males).
Testicular feminization.
Excess GH secretion.
Marfan's syndrome.
Klinefelter's syndrome (XXY).
XYY.

STEATOHEPATITIS

| ICD-10CM # | K76.0 | Fatty (change of) liver, not elsewhere classified |
| | K76.89 | Other specified diseases of liver |

Alcohol abuse.
Obesity.
DM.
Parenteral nutrition.
Medications (high-dose estrogen, amiodarone, corticosteroids, methotrexate, nifedipine).
Jejunoileal bypass.
Abetalipoproteinemia.
Wilson's disease, Weber-Christian disease.

STOMATITIS, BULLOUS

| ICD-10CM # | K12.30 | Oral mucositis (ulcerative), unspecified |

Erythema multiforme.
Erosive lichen planus.
Bullous pemphigoid.
SLE.
Pemphigus vulgaris.
Mucous membrane pemphigoid.

STRIDOR IN NEONATES[1]

| ICD-10CM # | R06.1 | Stridor |

INTRINSIC LESIONS

Larynx
Laryngomalacia.
Infection (laryngitis).
Vocal cord paralysis.
Laryngeal web.
Laryngocele or laryngeal cyst.
Laryngotracheal esophageal cleft.
Foreign body.
Trachea
Tracheomalacia.
Tracheal stenosis.
Tracheoesophageal fistula.
Subglottic hemangioma.
Tracheal web.
Extrinsic Compression
Vascular ring.
Anomalous innominate artery.
Mediastinal mass.
Esophageal foreign body.
Other
Macroglossia.
Gastroesophageal reflux.

STRIDOR, PEDIATRIC AGE[8]

| ICD-10CM # | R06.1 | Stridor |

RECURRENT

Allergic (spasmodic) croup.
Respiratory infections in a child with otherwise asymptomatic anatomic narrowing of the large airways.
Laryngomalacia.

PERSISTENT

Laryngeal obstruction:
  Laryngomalacia.
  Papillomas, other tumors.
  Cysts and laryngoceles.
  Laryngeal webs.
  Bilateral abductor paralysis of the cords.
  Foreign body.
Tracheobronchial disease:
  Tracheomalacia.
  Subglottic tracheal webs.
Endotracheal, endobronchial tumors.
Subglottic tracheal stenosis.
Congenital.
Acquired.
Extrinsic masses.
Mediastinal masses.
Vascular ring.
Lobar emphysema.
Bronchogenic cysts.
Thyroid enlargement.
Esophageal foreign body.
Tracheoesophageal fistulas.
Other.
Gastroesophageal reflux.
Macroglossia, Pierre Robin syndrome.
Cri-du-chat syndrome.
Hysterical stridor.
Hypocalcemia.

STROKE[70]

ICD-10CM #	Varies with Specific Diagnosis

STROKE "MIMICS"

Hypoglycemia.
Drug overdose or intoxication.
Hysterical conversion reaction.
Hyperventilation.
Metabolic encephalopathy.
Migraine.
Syncope.
Transient global amnesia.
Seizures.
Vestibular vertigo.

STROKE, PEDIATRIC AGE[47]

ICD-10CM #	I67.89	Other cerebrovascular disease

CARDIAC DISEASE

Congenital:
  Aortic stenosis.
  Mitral stenosis; mitral prolapse.
  Ventricular septal defects.
  Patent ductus arteriosus.
  Cyanotic congenital heart disease involving right-to-left shunt.
Acquired:
  Endocarditis (bacterial, SLE).
  Kawasaki disease.
  Cardiomyopathy.
  Atrial myxoma.
  Arrhythmia.
  Paradoxical emboli through patent foramen ovale.
  Rheumatic fever.
Prosthetic heart valve.

HEMATOLOGIC ABNORMALITIES

Hemoglobinopathies:
  Sickle cell (SS) disease.
  Sickle (SC) disease.
Polycythemia.
Leukemia/lymphoma.
Thrombocytopenia.
Thrombocytosis.
Disorders of coagulation:
  Protein C deficiency.
  Protein S deficiency.
  Factor V Leiden.
  Antithrombin III deficiency.
  Lupus anticoagulant.
Oral contraceptive pill use.
Pregnancy and the postpartum state.
Disseminated intravascular coagulation.
Paroxysmal nocturnal hemoglobinuria.
Inflammatory bowel disease (thrombosis).

INFLAMMATORY DISORDERS

- Meningitis:
  ○ Viral.
  ○ Bacterial.
  ○ Tuberculosis.
- Systemic infection:
  ○ Viremia.
  ○ Bacteremia.
  ○ Local head and neck infections.
- Drug-induced inflammation:
  ○ Amphetamine.
  ○ Cocaine.
- Autoimmune disease:
  ○ SLE.
  ○ Juvenile RA.
  ○ Takayasu's arteritis.
  ○ Mixed connective tissue disease.
  ○ Polyarteritis nodosum.
  ○ Primary CNS vasculitis.
  ○ Sarcoidosis.
  ○ Behçet's syndrome.
  ○ Granulomatosis with polyangiitis (Wegener's granulomatosis).

METABOLIC DISEASE ASSOCIATED WITH STROKE

Homocystinuria.
Pseudoxanthoma elasticum.
Fabry's disease.
Sulfite oxidase deficiency.
Mitochondrial disorders:
  MELAS.
  Leigh syndrome.
Ornithine transcarbamylase deficiency.

INTRACEREBRAL VASCULAR PROCESSES

Ruptured aneurysm.
Arteriovenous malformation.
Fibromuscular dysplasia.
Moyamoya disease.
Migraine headache.
Postsubarachnoid hemorrhage vasospasm.
Hereditary hemorrhagic telangiectasia.
Sturge-Weber syndrome.
Carotid artery dissection.
Postvaricella.

TRAUMA AND OTHER EXTERNAL CAUSES

Child abuse.
Head trauma/neck trauma.
Oral trauma.
Placental embolism.
ECMO therapy.

CNS, Central nervous system; *ECMO,* extracorporeal membrane oxygenation; *MELAS,* mitochondrial encephalomyopathy, lactic acidosis, and stroke.

STROKE, YOUNG ADULT, CAUSES[3]

ICD-10CM #	I64	Stroke
	I67.89	Other cerebrovascular disease

Cardiac factors (ASD, MVP, patent foramen ovale).
Inflammatory factors (SLE, polyarteritis nodosa).
Infections (endocarditis, neurosyphilis).
Drugs (cocaine, heroin, oral contraceptives, decongestants).
Arterial dissection.
Hematolic factors (DIC, TTP, deficiency of protein S, protein C, antithrombin III).
Migraine.
Postpartum angiopathy.
Other: premature atherosclerosis, fibromuscular dysplasia.

ST-SEGMENT DEPRESSION, NONCORONARY CAUSES[10]

ICD-10CM #	R94.31

NONCORONARY CAUSES OF ST-SEGMENT DEPRESSION

Anemia.
Cardiomyopathy.
Digitalis use.
Glucose load.
Hyperventilation.
Hypokalemia.
Intraventricular conduction disturbance.
Left ventricular hypertrophy.
Mitral valve prolapse.
Preexcitation syndrome.
Severe aortic stenosis.
Severe hypertension.
Severe hypoxia.
Severe volume overload (aortic, mitral regurgitation).
Sudden excessive exercise.
Supraventricular tachyarrhythmias.

ST-SEGMENT ELEVATION[1]

ICD-10CM #	R94.31	Abnormal ECG

DIFFERENTIAL DIAGNOSIS OF ST-SEGMENT ELEVATION ON ELECTROCARDIOGRAPHY

ST-segment elevation myocardial infarction.
Pericarditis.
Benign early repolarization.
Left bundle branch block.

Differential
Diagnosis

II

Left ventricular hypertrophy.
Left ventricular aneurysm.
Paced ventricular rhythms.
Prinzmetal angina.
Hyperkalemia.
Hypothermia with Osborne waves.
Intracranial hemorrhage.
Brugada syndrome.
Normal variant.

ST SEGMENT ELEVATIONS, NONISCHEMIC

ICD-10CM # R94.31 Abnormal electrocardiogram [ECG] [EKG]

Early repolarization.
Acute pericarditis.
LVH.
Normal pattern variant.
LBBB.
Pulmonary embolism.
Hyperkalemia.
Postcardioversion.

SUDDEN DEATH, PEDIATRIC AGE[8]

ICD-10CM # R99 Ill-defined and unknown cause of mortality

SIDS AND SIDS "MIMICS"

SIDS.
Long QT syndromes.
Inborn errors of metabolism.
Child abuse.
Myocarditis.
Duct-dependent congenital heart disease.

CORRECTED OR UNOPERATED CONGENITAL HEART DISEASE

Aortic stenosis.
Tetralogy of Fallot.
Transposition of great vessels (postoperative atrial switch).
Mitral valve prolapse.
Hematologic left heart syndrome.
Eisenmenger's syndrome.

CORONARY ARTERIAL DISEASE

Anomalous origin.
Anomalous tract.
Kawasaki disease.
Periarteritis.
Arterial dissection.
Marfan's syndrome.
Myocardial infarction.

MYOCARDIAL DISEASE

Myocarditis.
Hypertrophic cardiomyopathy.
Dilated cardiomyopathy.
Arrhythmogenic right ventricular dysplasia.

CONDUCTION SYSTEM ABNORMALITY/ARRHYTHMIA

Long Q-T syndromes.
Proarrhythmic drugs.

Preexcitation syndromes.
Heart block.
Commotio cordis.
Idiopathic ventricular fibrillation.
Heart tumor.

MISCELLANEOUS

Pulmonary hypertension.
Pulmonary embolism.
Heat stroke.
Cocaine.
Anorexia nervosa.
Electrolyte disturbances.

SIDS, Sudden infant death syndrome.

SUDDEN DEATH, YOUNG ATHLETE

ICD-10CM # R99 Ill-defined and unknown cause of mortality

Hypertrophic cardiomyopathy.
Coronary artery anomalies.
Myocarditis.
Ruptured aortic aneurysm (Marfan's syndrome).
Arrhythmias.
Aortic valve stenosis.
Asthma.
Trauma (cerebral, cardiac).
Drug and alcohol abuse.
Heat stroke.
Cardiac sarcoidosis.
Atherosclerotic coronary artery disease.
Dilated cardiomyopathy.

SWOLLEN LIMB

ICD-10CM # M79.89 Other specified soft tissue disorders

Trauma.
Insect bite.
Abscess.
Lymphedema.
Thrombophlebitis.
Lipoma.
Neurofibroma.
Postphlebitic syndrome.
Myositis ossificans.
Nephrosis, cirrhosis, CHF.
Hypoalbuminemia.
Varicose veins.

TALL STATURE[54]

ICD-10CM # E22.0 Acromegaly and pituitary gigantism

CONSTITUTIONAL (FAMILIAL OR GENETIC)—MOST COMMON CAUSE

ENDOCRINE CAUSES

Growth hormone excess—gigantism.
Sexual precocity (tall as children, short as adults):
  True sexual precocity.
  Pseudosexual precocity.
Androgen deficiency:
  Klinefelter's syndrome.
  Bilateral anorchism.

GENETIC CAUSES

Klinefelter's syndrome.
Syndromes of XYY, XXYY.

MISCELLANEOUS SYNDROMES AND DISORDERS

Cerebral gigantism or Sotos' syndrome: prominent forehead, hypertelorism, high arched palate, dolichocephaly, mental retardation, large hands and feet, and premature eruption of teeth. Large at birth, with most rapid growth in first 4 yr of life.
Marfan's syndrome: disorder of mesodermal tissues, subluxation of the lenses, arachnodactyly, and aortic aneurysm.
Homocystinuria: same phenotype as Marfan's syndrome.
Obesity: tall as infants, children, and adolescents.
Total lipodystrophy: large hands and feet, generalized loss of subcutaneous fat, insulin-resistant DM, and hepatomegaly.
Beckwith-Wiedemann syndrome: neonatal tallness, omphalocele, macroglossia, and neonatal hypoglycemia.
Weaver-Smith syndrome: excessive intrauterine growth, mental retardation, megalocephaly, widened bifrontal diameter, hypertelorism, large ears, micrognathia, camptodactyly, broad thumbs, and limited extension of elbows and knees.
Marshall-Smith syndrome: excessive intrauterine growth, mental retardation, blue sclerae, failure to thrive, and early death.

TARDIVE DYSKINESIA[28]

ICD-10CM # R27.9 Unspecified lack of coordination
F44.4 Conversion disorder with motor symptom or deficit
F44.6 Conversion disorder with sensory symptom or deficit
G24.4 Idiopathic orofacial dystonia

DIFFERENTIAL DIAGNOSIS

Medications (antidepressants, anticholinergics, amphetamines, lithium, l-dopa, phenytoin).
Brain neoplasms.
Ill-fitting dentures.
Huntington's disease.
Idiopathic dystonias (tics, blepharospasm, aging).
Wilson's disease.
Extrapyramidal syndrome (postanoxic or postencephalitic).
Torsion dystonia.

TASTE AND SMELL LOSS[3]

ICD-10CM # R43.0 Anosmia
R43.1 Parosmia
R43.2 Parageusia

TASTE

Local: radiation therapy.

Systemic: cancer, renal failure, hepatic failure, nutritional deficiency (vitamin B_{12}, zinc), Cushing's syndrome, hypothyroidism, DM, infection (influenza), drugs (antirheumatic and antiproliferative).

Neurologic: Bell's palsy, familial dysautonomia, multiple sclerosis.

SMELL

Local: allergic rhinitis, sinusitis, nasal polyposis, bronchial asthma.

Systemic: renal failure, hepatic failure, nutritional deficiency (vitamin B_{12}), Cushing's syndrome, hypothyroidism, DM, infection (viral hepatitis, influenza), drugs (nasal sprays, antibiotics).

Neurologic: head trauma, multiple sclerosis, Parkinson's disease, frontal brain tumor.

TELANGIECTASIA

| ICD-10CM # | I78.8 | Other diseases of capillaries |
| | I78.9 | Disease of capillaries, unspecified |

Oral contraceptive agents.
Pregnancy.
Rosacea.
Varicose veins.
Trauma.
Drug induced (corticosteroids, systemic or topical).
Spider telangiectases.
Hepatic cirrhosis.
Mastocytosis.
SLE, dermatomyositis, systemic sclerosis.

TENDINOPATHY[51]

| ICD-10CM # | M67.90 | Unspecified disorder of synovium and tendon, unspecified site |
| | M71.9 | Bursopathy, unspecified |

INTRINSIC FACTORS

Anatomic Factors
Malalignment.
Muscle weakness or imbalance.
Muscle inflexibility.
Decreased vascularity.

Systemic Factors
Inflammatory conditions (e.g., SLE).
Pregnancy.
Quinolone-induced tendinopathy.

Age-Related Factors
Tendon degeneration.
Increased tendon stiffness.
Tendon calcification.
Decreased vascularity.

EXTRINSIC FACTORS

Repetitive Mechanical Load
Excessive duration.
Excessive frequency.
Excessive intensity.
Poor technique.

Workplace factors.
Equipment Problems
Footwear.
Athletic field surface.
Equipment factors (e.g., racquet size).
Protective gear.

TESTICULAR CYSTIC LESIONS[62]

| ICD-10CM # | | Varies with Specific Diagnosis |

Benign
Tunica albuginea cysts
Tunica vaginalis cysts
Intratesticular cysts
Tubular ectasia of rete testis
Cystic dysplasia
Epidermoid cysts
Abscess
Malignant
Nonseminomatous germ cell tumor
Necrosis or hemorrhage in tumor
Tubular obstruction by tumor
Lymphoma

TESTICULAR FAILURE[19]

| ICD-10CM # | E29 | Testicular dysfunction |

PRIMARY

Klinefelter's syndrome (XXY).
XYY.
Vanishing testes syndrome (in utero or early postnatal torsion).
Noonan's syndrome.
Varicocele.
Myotonic dystrophy.
Orchitis (mumps, gonorrhea).
Cryptorchidism.
Chemical exposure.
Irradiation to testes.
Spinal cord injury.
Polyglandular failure.
Idiopathic oligospermia or azoospermia.
Germinal cell aplasia (Sertoli cell–only syndrome).
Idiopathic testicular failure.
Testicular torsion.
Testicular trauma.
Diethylstilbestrol (maternal use during pregnancy leading to in utero estrogen exposure).
Testicular tumor with subsequent irradiation therapy, chemotherapy, or surgery (retroperitoneal lymph node dissection or orchiectomy).

SECONDARY

Delayed puberty.
Kallmann's syndrome.
Isolated gonadotropin deficiency.
Prader-Labhart-Willi syndrome.
Lawrence-Moon-Biedl syndrome.
Central nervous system irradiation.
Prepubertal panhypopituitarism.
Postpubertal panhypopituitarism.

Hypogonadism secondary to hyperprolactinemia.
Adrenogenital syndrome.
Chronic liver disease.
Chronic renal failure/uremia.
Hemochromatosis.
Cushing's syndrome.
Malnutrition.
Massive obesity.
Sickle cell anemia.
Hyper/hypothyroidism.
Anabolic steroid use.

TESTICULAR PAIN

| ICD-10CM # | N50.9 | Disorder of male genital organs, unspecified |
| | R10.2 | Pelvic and perineal pain |

Testicular torsion.
Trauma.
Epididymitis.
Orchitis.
Neoplasm.
Urolithiasis.
Inguinal hernia.
Infection (cellulitis, abscess, folliculitis).
Anxiety.

TESTICULAR SIZE VARIATIONS[19]

ICD-10CM #	N50.0	Atrophy of testis
	N44.2	Benign cyst of testis
	N44.8	Other noninflammatory disorders of the testis
	N50.3	Cyst of epididymis
	N50.8	Other specified disorders of male genital organs
	N53.12	Painful ejaculation
	E29.1	Testicular hypofunction

SMALL TESTES

Hypothalamic-pituitary dysfunction.
Gonadotropin deficiency.
Growth hormone deficiency.
Normal variant.
Primary hypogonadism.
Autoimmune destruction.
Chemotherapy.
Cryptorchidism.
Irradiation.
Klinefelter's syndrome.
Orchiditis.
Testicular regression syndrome.
Torsion.
Trauma.

LARGE TESTES

Adrenal rest tissue.
Compensatory.
Fragile X syndrome.
Idiopathic.
Tumor.

TETANUS[51]

ICD-10CM #   A35   Other tetanus

TETANUS "MIMICS"

Acute abdomen.
Black widow spider bite.
Dental abscess.
Dislocated mandible.
Dystonic reaction.
Encephalitis.
Head trauma.
Hyperventilation syndrome.
Hypocalcemia.
Meningitis.
Peritonsillar abscess.
Progressive fluctuating muscular rigidity (stiff-man syndrome).
Psychogenic.
Rabies.
Sepsis.
Subarachnoid hemorrhage.
Status epilepticus.
Strychnine poisoning.
Temporomandibular joint syndrome.

THROMBOCYTOPENIA

ICD-10CM #   D47.3   Essential (hemorrhagic) thrombocythemia
D69.59   Other secondary thrombocytopenia
D69.6   Thrombocytopenia, unspecified

INCREASED DESTRUCTION
Immunologic
Drugs: quinine, quinidine, digitalis, procainamide, thiazide diuretics, sulfonamides, phenytoin, aspirin, penicillin, heparin, gold, meprobamate, sulfa drugs, phenylbutazone, nonsteroidal anti-inflammatory drugs (NSAIDs), methyldopa, cimetidine, furosemide, INH, cephalosporins, chlorpropamide, organic arsenicals, chloroquine, platelet glycoprotein IIb/IIIa receptor inhibitors, ranitidine, indomethacin, carboplatin, ticlopidine, clopidogrel.
Idiopathic thrombocytopenic purpura (ITP).
Transfusion reaction: transfusion of platelets with plasminogen activator (PLA) in recipients without PLA-1.
Fetal/maternal incompatibility.
Collagen vascular diseases (e.g., SLE).
Autoimmune hemolytic anemia.
Lymphoreticular disorders (e.g., CLL).
Nonimmunologic
Prosthetic heart valves.
Thrombotic thrombocytopenic purpura (TTP).
Sepsis.
DIC.
Hemolytic-uremic syndrome (HUS).
Giant cavernous hemangioma.

DECREASED PRODUCTION
Abnormal marrow.
Marrow infiltration (e.g., leukemia, lymphoma, fibrosis).
Marrow suppression (e.g., chemotherapy, alcohol, radiation).

Hereditary disorders.
Wiskott-Aldrich syndrome: X-linked disorder characterized by thrombocytopenia, eczema, and repeated infections.
May-Hegglin anomaly: increased megakaryocytes but ineffective thrombopoiesis.
Vitamin deficiencies (e.g., vitamin B_{12}, folic acid).

SPLENIC SEQUESTRATION, HYPERSPLENISM

DILUTIONAL, AS A RESULT OF MASSIVE TRANSFUSION

THROMBOCYTOPENIA, IN PREGNANCY[40]

ICD-10CM #   D69.59   Other secondary thrombocytopenia

Incidental thrombocytopenia of pregnancy (gestational thrombocytopenia).
Preeclampsia/eclampsia.[41]
   Peripartum/postpartum thrombotic microangiopathy.
Disseminated intravascular coagulation (DIC) secondary to:
   Abruptio placentae.
   Endometritis.
   Amniotic fluid embolism.
   Retained fetus.
Thrombotic thrombocytopenic purpura.
Hemolytic-uremic syndrome.

---

[41]Preeclampsia/eclampsia usually is not associated with overt DIC.

THROMBOCYTOPENIA, INHERITED DISORDERS[3]

ICD-10CM #   D47.3   Essential (hemorrhagic) thrombocythemia

Amegakaryocytic thrombocytopenia.
Thrombocytopenia–absent radii.
MYH9-related thrombocytopenia:
May-Hegglin anomaly.
Fechtner syndrome.
Epstein syndrome.
Sebastian syndrome.
X-linked macrothrombocytopenia.
Wiskott-Aldrich syndrome.
X-linked thrombocytopenia.
Thrombocytopenia and radioulnar synostosis.
Familial platelet disorder—AML.
Familial dominant thrombocytopenia.
Paris-Trousseau thrombocytopenia.
Bernard-Soulier syndrome.
Bernard-Soulier carrier/Mediterranean macro-thrombocytopenia.

THROMBOCYTOPENIA IN NEWBORNS, DIFFERENTIAL DIAGNOSIS[39]

ICD-10CM #   D47.3   Essential (hemorrhagic) thrombocythemia

D69.59   Other secondary thrombocytopenia
D69.6   Thrombocytopenia, unspecified

DIFFERENTIAL DIAGNOSIS OF THROMBOCYTOPENIA IN NEWBORNS

Perinatal hypoxemia
Placental insufficiency
Congenital infection
   Sepsis.
   Toxoplasmosis.
   Rubella.
   Cytomegalovirus.
Autoimmune:
   Maternal immune thrombocytopenia.
   Maternal systemic lupus erythematosus.
Disseminated intravascular coagulation
Maternal drug exposure
Congenital heart disease
Hereditary thrombocytopenia
   MYH9 macrothrombocytopenia (including May-Hegglin anomaly).
   Thrombocytopenia absent radii syndrome.
   Amegakaryocytic thrombocytopenia.
   Wiskott-Aldrich syndrome.
   Fanconi anemia.
Hemangioma with thrombocytopenia
   Kasabach-Merritt syndrome.
Bone marrow infiltration
   Congenital leukemia.

THROMBOCYTOSIS

ICD-10CM #   D75.9   Disease of blood and blood-forming organs, unspecified

Iron deficiency.
Posthemorrhage.
Neoplasms (GI tract).
CML.
Polycythemia vera.
Myelofibrosis with myeloid metaplasia.
Infections.
After splenectomy.
Postpartum.
Hemophilia.
Pancreatitis.
Cirrhosis.
Idiopathic.

THROMBOSIS OR THROMBOTIC DIATHESIS[3]

ICD-10CM #   I74.09   Other arterial embolism and thrombosis of abdominal aorta

DIFFERENTIAL DIAGNOSIS OF THE PATIENT PRESENTING WITH THROMBOSIS OR THROMBOTIC DIATHESIS

Inherited (Primary) Hypercoagulable States
Activated protein C resistance caused by factor V Leiden mutation.

Prothrombin gene mutation (G to A transition at position 20210 in the 3-untranslated region).
Antithrombin III deficiency.
Protein C deficiency.
Protein S deficiency.
Dysfibrinogenemias (rare).

Acquired (Secondary) Hypercoagulable States
In association with physiologic or thrombogenic stimuli:
Pregnancy (especially the postpartum period).
Estrogen use (oral contraceptives, hormone replacement therapy).
Immobilization.
Trauma.
Postoperative state.
Advancing age.
Obesity.
Prolonged air travel.
Lupus anticoagulant or antiphospholipid antibody syndrome.
In association with other clinical disorders.

Mixed/Unknown
Activated protein C resistance in the absence of factor V Leiden.
Elevated factor VIII level.
Elevated factor XI level.
Elevated factor IX level.
Elevated thrombin activatable fibrinolysis inhibitor (TAFI) level.
Decreased free tissue factor pathway inhibitor (TFPI) level.
Decreased plasma fibrinolytic activity.

THYMIC MASSES[65]

ICD-10CM # varies with specific diagnosis

THYMIC MASSES
Thymic hyperplasia
Thymoma
Thymic carcinoma
Thymic neuroendocrine tumors
   Carcinoid
   Small-cell carcinoma
Thymic cysts (not rhizomatous)
Thymolipoma
Metastases to the thymus

THYMOMA, DISEASES ASSOCIATIONS[65]

ICD-10CM # varies with specific diagnosis

SYSTEMIC DISEASES MOST COMMONLY ASSOCIATED WITH THYMOMA
Myasthenia gravis
Cytopenias (most commonly red cell hypoplasia)
Nonthymic malignancies
Hypogammaglobulinemia
Systemic lupus erythematosus
Polymyositis
Rheumatoid arthritis
Thyroiditis
Sjögren syndrome
Ulcerative colitis

THYROMEGALY

ICD-10CM # varies with specific diagnosis

Goiter.
Graves' disease.
Thyroiditis (lymphocytic, granulomatous, suppurative).
Toxic adenoma.
Neoplasm (primary, metastatic).

THYROTOXICOSIS[53]

ICD-10CM # E05.80

CAUSES OF THYROTOXICOSIS

Sustained Hormone Overproduction (Hyperthyroidism)
Low TSH, High RAIU:
Graves' disease (von Basedow's disease).
Toxic multinodular goiter.
Toxic adenoma.
Chorionic gonadotropin-induced.
   Gestational hyperthyroidism: physiologic hyperthyroidism of pregnancy, familial gestational hyperthyroidism due to TSH receptor mutations.
   Trophoblastic tumors
Inherited nonimmune hyperthyroidism associated with TSH receptor or G protein mutations.
Low TSH, Low RAIU:
   Iodide-induced hyperthyroidism (Jod-Basedow effect).
   Amiodarone-associated hyperthyroidism due to iodide release.
Struma Ovarii:
   Metastatic functioning thyroid carcinoma.
Normal or Elevated TSH:
   TSH-secreting pituitary tumors.
   Thyroid hormone resistance with pituitary predominance.

Transient Hormone Excess (Thyrotoxicosis)
Low TSH, Low RAIU:
- Thyroiditis.
   Autoimmune: lymphocytic thyroiditis (silent thyroiditis, painless thyroiditis, postpartum thyroiditis), acute exacerbation of Hashimoto's disease.
Viral or postviral.
   ■ Subacute (granulomatous, painful, postviral) thyroiditis.
   ○ Drug-induced or associated thyroiditis.
     Amiodarone.
     Lithium, interferon-α, interleukin-2, GM-CSF.
Infectious thyroiditis.
Exogenous Thyroid Hormone.
   Iatrogenic overreplacement.
   Thyrotoxicosis factitia.
   Ingestion of natural products containing thyroid hormone.
     "Hamburger" thyrotoxicosis.
     Natural foodstuffs.
     Thyromimetic compounds (e.g., tiratricol PLB).
     Occupational exposure to thyroid hormone (e.g., pill manufacturing, veterinary occupations).

GM-CSF, granulocyte-macrophage colony-stimulating factor; *RAIU*, radioactive iodine uptake; *TSH*, thyroid-stimulating hormone.

TICK-RELATED INFECTIONS

ICD-10CM #	A77.0	Spotted fever due to Rickettsia rickettsii
	A93.2	Colorado tick fever
	B60.0	Babesiosis
	A77.8	Other spotted fevers
	A69.20	Lyme disease, unspecified

- Lyme disease.
- Rocky Mountain spotted fever.
- Babesiosis.
- Tularemia.
- Q fever.
- Colorado tick fever.
- Ehrlichiosis.
- Relapsing fever.

TICS

ICD-10CM # F95.9 Tic disorder, unspecified

- Tourette's syndrome.
- Physiologic tic.
- Anxiety disorder.
- Huntington's disease.
- Medications (e.g., antipsychotics, carbamazepine, phenytoin, phenobarbital).
- Encephalitis.
- Head trauma.
- Schizophrenia.
- Carbon monoxide poisoning.
- Stroke.
- Sydenham's chorea.
- Creutzfeldt-Jakob disease.

TORSADES DE POINTES[45]

ICD-10CM # I47.2 Ventricular tachycardia

Antiarrhythmics known to increase the QT interval (e.g., quinidine, procainamide, amiodarone, disopyramide, sotalol).
Tricyclic antidepressants and phenothiazines.
Histamine (H₁) antagonists (e.g., astemizole, terfenadine).
Antiviral and antifungal agents and antibiotics.
Hypokinemia.
Hypomagnesemia.
Insecticide poisoning.
Bradyarrhythmias.
Congenital long QT syndrome.
Subarachnoid hemorrhage.
Chloroquinine, pentamidine.
Cocaine abuse.

TOXIC MEGACOLON, CAUSES[14]

ICD-10CM # K59.3 Megacolon, not elsewhere classified

INFLAMMATORY
Ulcerative colitis.
Crohn's disease.

INFECTIOUS
Bacterial.
Clostridium difficile pseudomembranous colitis.

Salmonella (typhoid and nontyphoid).
Shigella.
Campylobacter.
Yersinia.
Parasitic.
   Entamoeba histolytica.
   Cryptosporidium.
Viral.
   Cytomegalovirus colitis.

OTHER

Ischemia.
Kaposi sarcoma.

TRACHEOBRONCHIAL NARROWING ON X-RAY[33]

ICD-10CM #   varies with specific diagnosis

CAUSES OF TRACHEOBRONCHIAL NARROWING

Long-segment/Diffuse Narrowing
Sarcoidosis.
Amyloidosis.
Granulomatosis with polyangiitis (Wegener's granulomatosis).
Relapsing polychondritis.
Tracheobronchopathia osteochondroplastica.
Pemphigoid.
Short-segment Narrowing
Previous intubation or tracheostomy.
Congenital stenosis or web.
Extrinsic compression (from thyroid).
Adenoid cystic carcinoma.
Squamous carcinoma.

TREMOR

ICD-10CM #	R25.0	Abnormal head movements
	R25.1	Tremor, unspecified
	R25.2	Cramp and spasm
	R25.3	Fasciculation
	R25.9	Unspecified abnormal involuntary movements
	G25.0	Essential tremor
	G25.1	Drug-induced tremor
	G25.2	Other specified forms of tremor

REST TREMORS

Parkinson's disease.
Other parkinsonian syndromes (less commonly).
Midbrain (rubral) tremor: rest <postural <kinetic.
Wilson's disease (also acquired hepatocerebral degeneration).
Essential tremor—only if severe: rest <postural and action.

POSTURAL AND ACTION (TERMINAL) TREMORS

Physiologic tremor.
Exaggerated physiologic tremor (these factors can also aggravate other forms of tremor).

Stress, fatigue, anxiety, emotion.
Endocrine: hypoglycemia, thyrotoxicosis, pheochromocytoma, adrenocorticosteroids.
Drugs and toxins: b-agonists, dopamine agonists, amphetamines, lithium, tricyclic antidepressants, neuroleptics, theophylline, caffeine, valproic acid, alcohol withdrawal, mercury (Hatter's shakes), lead, arsenic, others.
Essential tremor (familial or sporadic)
Primary writing tremor.
With other CNS disorders.
   Parkinson's disease.
   Other akinetic-rigid syndromes.
   Idiopathic dystonia, including focal dystonias.
With peripheral neuropathy.
   Charcot-Marie-Tooth syndrome (controversial whether to call this the Roussy-Levy syndrome).
   Variety of other peripheral neuropathies (especially dysgammaglobulinemia).
Cerebellar tremor.

KINETIC (INTENTION) TREMOR

Disease of cerebellar outflow (dentate nucleus and superior cerebellar peduncle): multiple sclerosis, trauma, tumor, vascular disease, Wilson's acquired hepatocerebral degeneration, drugs, toxins (e.g., mercury), others.

MISCELLANEOUS RHYTHMICAL MOVEMENT DISORDERS

Psychogenic tremor.
Orthostatic tremor.
Rhythmical movements in dystonia (dystonic tremor).
Rhythmical myoclonus (segmental myoclonus—e.g., palatal or branchial myoclonus, spinal myoclonus, limb myorhythmia).
Oscillatory myoclonus.
Asterixis.
Clonus.
Epilepsia partialis continua.
Hereditary chin quivering.
Spasmus nutans.
Head bobbing with third ventricular cysts.
Nystagmus.

TREMOR, IN CHILDREN, CAUSES[46]

ICD-10CM #	R25.0	Abnormal head movements
	R25.1	Tremor, unspecified
	R25.2	Cramp and spasm
	R25.3	Fasciculation
	R25.9	Unspecified abnormal involuntary movements

BENIGN

Enhanced physiologic tremor.
Shuddering attacks.
Jitteriness.
Spasmus nutans.

STATIC INJURY/STRUCTURAL

Cerebellar malformation.
Stroke (particularly in the midbrain or cerebellum).

Multiple sclerosis.

HEREDITARY/DEGENERATIVE

Familial essential tremor.
Fragile X premutation.
Wilson disease.
Huntington disease.
Juvenile parkinsonism (tremor is rare).
Pallidonigral degeneration.

METABOLIC

Hyperthyroidism.
Hyperadrenergic state (including pheochromocytoma and neuroblastoma).
Hypomagnesemia.
Hypocalcemia.
Hypoglycemia.
Hepatic encephalopathy.
Vitamin B_{12} deficiency.
Inborn errors of metabolism.
Mitochondrial disorders.

DRUGS/TOXINS

Valproate, phenytoin, carbamazepine, lamotrigine, gabapentin, lithium, tricyclic antidepressants, stimulants (cocaine, amphetamine, caffeine, thyroxine, bronchodilators), neuroleptics, cyclosporin, toluene, mercury, thallium, amiodarone, nicotine, lead, manganese, arsenic, cyanide, naphthalene, ethanol, lindane, serotonin reuptake inhibitors.

PERIPHERAL NEUROPATHIES
PSYCHOGENIC

TRICHOMEGALY[11]

ICD-10CM #   Not available

CAUSES OF TRICHOMEGALY

Drug-induced: topical prostaglandin analogues, phenytoin and cyclosporine.
Malnutrition.
AIDS.
Porphyria.
Hypothyroidism.
Familial.
Congenital: Oliver–McFarlane, Cornelia de Lange, Goldstein–Hutt, Hermansky–Pudlak syndromes.

TUBULOINTERSTITIAL DISEASE, ACUTE[29]

ICD-10CM #	N17.0	Acute kidney failure with tubular necrosis

DRUGS

Antibiotics, penicillins, cephalosporins, rifampin.
Sulfonamides: cotrimoxazole, sulfamethoxazole.
NSAIDs: propionic acid derivatives.
Miscellaneous: phenytoin, thiazides, allopurinol, cimetidine, ifosfamide.

INFECTIONS

Invasion of renal parenchyma.
Reaction to systemic infections: streptococcal, diphtheria, hantavirus.

SYSTEMIC DISEASES

Immune mediated: SLE, transplanted kidney, cryoglobulinemias.
Metabolic: Urate, oxalate.
Neoplastic: Lymphoproliferative diseases.

IDIOPATHIC

TUBULOINTERSTITIAL KIDNEY DISEASE[29]

ICD-10CM #	N17.0	Acute kidney failure with tubular necrosis

Ischemic and toxic acute tubular necrosis.
Allergic interstitial nephritis.
Interstitial nephritis secondary to immune complex-related collagen vascular disease (e.g., SLE, Sjögren's).
Granulomatous diseases (sarcoidosis, uveitis).
Pigment-related tubular injury (myoglobinuria, hemoglobinuria).
Hypercalcemia with nephrocalcinosis.
Tubular obstruction (drugs such as indinavir, uric acid in tumor lysis syndrome).
Myeloma kidney or cast nephropathy.
Infection-related interstitial nephritis: *Legionella, Leptospira.*
Infiltrative diseases (e.g., lymphoma).

TUMOR MARKERS ELEVATION[72]

ICD-10CM #	R97.8	Other abnormal tumor markers

CAUSES OF ELEVATED LEVELS OF TUMOR MARKERS

Carcinoembryonic Antigen (CEA)
Colonic cancer (higher levels if the tumor is more differentiated or is extensive or has spread to the liver).
Lung or breast cancer; seminoma.
Cigarette smokers.
Cirrhosis, inflammatory bowel disease, rectal polyps, pancreatitis.
Advanced age.

Alpha-Fetoprotein
Hepatocellular cancer: very high titers or a rising titer is strongly suggestive, but >10% of patients do not have an elevated level.
Hepatic regeneration (e.g., cirrhosis, alcoholic or viral hepatitis).
Cancer of the stomach, colon, pancreas, or lung.
Teratocarcinoma or embryonal cell carcinoma (testis, ovary, extragonadal).
Pregnancy.
Ataxia-telangiectasia.
Normal variant.

Prostate-Specific Antigen
Prostate carcinoma (localized disease).
Prostatic hyperplasia.
Prostatitis.
Prostatic infarction.

Cancer-Associated Antigen (CA-19-9)[42]
Pancreatic carcinoma (80% with advanced, well-differentiated cancer have an elevated level).

Other gastrointestinal cancers: colon, stomach, bile duct.
Acute or chronic pancreatitis.
Chronic liver disease.
Biliary tract disease.

UREMIC ENCEPHALOPATHY, DIFFERENTIAL DIAGNOSIS[25]

ICD-10CM #	G93.40	Encephalopathy, unspecified

Differential Diagnosis	Comment
Hypertensive encephalopathy	
Systemic inflammatory response syndrome (SIRS):	Observed in septic patients
Systemic vasculitis:	Vasculitis or lupus with cerebral involvement
Drug-induced neurotoxicity	
Analgesics:	Meperidine, codeine, morphine, gabapentin
Antibiotics:	High-dose penicillins (may cause seizures), acyclovir, ethambutol (optic nerve damage), erythromycin and aminoglycosides (may cause ototoxicity), nitrofurantoin and isoniazid (peripheral neuropathy)
Psychotropics:	Lithium, haloperidol, clonazepam, diazepam, chlorpromazine
Immunosuppressants:	Cyclosporine, tacrolimus
Chemotherapeutics:	Cisplatinum, ifosfamide
Others:	High doses of loop diuretics (ototoxic), ephedrine, methyldopa, aluminum
Cerebral atheroembolic disease:	Follows recent aortic or cardiac angiography; associated with peripheral manifestations, including lower extremity cyanosis, livedo reticularis, and eosinophilia
Subdural hematoma	

Differential Diagnosis	Comment
Posterior leukoencephalopathy:	Observed particularly following renal transplantation due to reversible, abnormal permeability of the blood-brain barrier Often manifests as headache followed by mental depression, visual loss, and seizures in the context of volume expansion, acute hypertension, and often treatment with corticosteroids or calcineurin inhibitors Lesions in the parietal, temporal, and occipital lobes may be seen on imaging studies

URETERAL COLIC[48]

ICD-10CM #	R33.8	Other retention of urine
	N13.8	Other obstructive and reflux uropathy

DIAGNOSTIC DIFFERENTIALS OF RENAL OR URETERAL COLIC

Acute cholecystitis, acute cholelithiasis.
Acute appendicitis.
Pelvic inflammatory disease.
Diverticulosis and/or diverticulitis.
Intestinal obstruction.
Leaking abdominal aortic aneurysm.
Musculoskeletal sprains.
Herniated disk.
Hepes zoster (shingles).
Gastrointestinal dysfunction with ileus and/or toxic colonic dilatation.

URETERAL STRICTURE[76]

ICD-10CM #		Varies with Specific Diagnosis

ETIOLOGY OF URETERAL STRICTURE

Malignancy (e.g., transitional cell carcinoma, cervical cancer)
Ureteral calculus
Radiation
Ischemia or trauma caused by surgical dissection
Periureteral fibrosis caused by abdominal aortic aneurysm or endometriosis
Endoscopic instrumentation

---

[42]Patients who cannot synthesize Lewis blood group antigens (~5% of the population) do not produce CA-19–9 antigen.

Renal ablation injury
Infection (tuberculosis)
Idiopathic condition

URETERIC OBSTRUCTION, CONGENITAL[33]

| ICD-10CM # | N13.8 | Other obstructive and reflux uropathy |
| | N20.9 | Urolithiasis |

CONGENITAL CAUSES OF URETERIC OBSTRUCTION

Primary megaureter.
Ureterocele (ectopic and orthotopic).
Ureteric valve.
Distal ureteric stenosis.
Ureteric atresia.
Circumcaval ureter and variants.
Bladder diverticulum.

URETHRAL BLEEDING[76]

| ICD-10CM # | Varies with Specific Diagnosis |

DIFFERENTIAL DIAGNOSIS FOR URETHRAL BLEEDING

Male
Trauma
　Blunt (straddle injury, kick to perineum)
　Penetrating (foreign body insertion, failed urethral catheterization)
　Intercourse related (penile fracture, masturbation)
Urethritis
　Bacterial (gonococcal, nongonococcal)
　Viral
　Chemical
　Autoimmune (Reiter syndrome)
Malignancy
　Urothelial carcinoma
　Squamous cell carcinoma (meatus/glans)
Condyloma
Calculus disease
Female
Trauma
　Blunt (pelvic fracture)
　Penetrating (foreign body)
Urethral diverticulum
Urethral caruncle
Urethritis
Malignancy
Calculus disease

URETHRAL DISCHARGE AND DYSURIA

ICD-10CM #	R36.0	Urethral discharge without blood
	R36.9	Urethral discharge, unspecified
	N36.9	Urethral disorder, unspecified
	N39.9	Disorder of urinary system, unspecified
	R30.0	Dysuria
	R30.9	Painful micturition, unspecified

Urethritis (gonococcal, chlamydial, trichomonal).
Cystitis.
Prostatitis.
Vaginitis (candidiasis, chemical).
Meatal stenosis.
Interstitial cystitis.
Trauma (foreign body, masturbation, horseback or bike riding).

URETHRAL OBSTRUCTION, CHILDREN[33]

| ICD-10CM # | N13.8 | Other obstructive and reflux uropathy |

CAUSES OF URETHRAL OBSTRUCTION IN CHILDREN

Intrinsic Lesions
Valve (posterior, anterior, saccular diverticulum).
Stenosis, atresia.
Inflammatory stricture.
Traumatic stricture:
　External trauma (saddle injury, and so on).
　Iatrogenic trauma (catheter, cystoscopy, surgery).
Urethral "tumors":
　Girls: leiomyoma.
　Boys: polyp, rhabdomyosarcoma.
Miscellaneous (epidermolysis bullosa).
Extrinsic Lesions
Presacral mass dissecting inferiorly (tumor, cyst).
Fecal impaction (Hirschsprung's, postrepair anal atresia, habitual constipation, neuropathy).
Mass originating in genital organs:
　Boys: utricle cyst, prostate rhabdomyosarcoma, seminal vesicle cyst, Cowper's duct cyst.
　Girls: hydrometrocolpos, hydrocolpos, fused labia.

URIC ACID STONES

| ICD-10CM # | N20.9 | Urolithiasis |

Hyperuricemia.
Excessive dietary purine.
Medications (salicylates, allopurinol, probenecid).
Urine pH <5.5 (e.g., diarrhea, high animal protein diet).
Decreased urine output (dehydration, malabsorption, diarrhea, inadequate fluid intake).
Tumor lysis.
Hemolytic anemia.
Myeloproliferative disorders.

URINARY INCONTINENCE, CHILDREN[46]

| ICD-10CM # | R32 | Unspecified urinary incontinence |

CAUSES OF URINARY INCONTINENCE IN CHILDHOOD

Overactive bladder.
Infrequent voiding.
Detrusor-sphincter dyssynergia.
Non-neurogenic neurogenic bladder (Hinman syndrome).

Vaginal voiding.
Giggle incontinence.
Cystitis.
Bladder outlet obstruction (posterior urethral valves).
Ectopic ureter and fistula.
Sphincter abnormality (epispadias, exstrophy; urogenital sinus abnormality).
Neuropathic.
Overflow incontinence.
Traumatic.
Iatrogenic.
Behavioral.
Combination.

URINARY RETENTION[48]

| ICD-10CM # | R33.9 | Retention of urine, unspecified |

COMMON CAUSES OF URINARY RETENTION

Obstructive Cause
Urethral stricture.
Enlarged prostate.
Lower genitourinary tract malignancy.
Pelvic malignancy.
Bladder stones.
Foreign body.
Blood clot.
Posterior urethral valves.
Ureterocele.
Primary Detrusor Insufficiency
Detrusor areflexia.
Multiple sclerosis.
Iatrogenic injury during abdominal or back surgery.
Spinal cord injury.
Myelomeningocele.

URINARY RETENTION, ACUTE

| ICD-10CM # | R33.9 | Retention of urine, unspecified |

Mechanical obstruction: urethral stone, foreign body, urethral stricture, BPH, prostate carcinoma, prostatitis, trauma with hematoma formation.
Neurogenic bladder.
Neurologic disease (MS, parkinsonism, tabes dorsalis, CVA).
Spinal cord injury.
CNS neoplasm (primary or metastatic).
Spinal anesthesia.
Lower urinary tract instrumentation.
Medications (antihistamines, antidepressants, narcotics, anticholinergics).
Abdominal or pelvic surgery.
Alcohol toxicity.
Pregnancy.
Anxiety.
Encephalitis.
Postoperative pain.
Spina bifida occulta.

URINARY TRACT BLEEDING, UPPER[76]

| ICD-10CM # | Varies with Specific Diagnosis |

DIFFERENTIAL DIAGNOSIS FOR UPPER URINARY TRACT BLEEDING

Renal glomerular diseases
  IgA nephropathy (Berger disease)
  Thin basement membrane disease
  Acute glomerulonephritis (e.g., poststrepto-coccal)
  Lupus nephritis
  Hereditary nephritis (e.g., Alport syndrome)
Renal tubulointerstitial diseases
  Papillary necrosis
  Sickle cell nephropathy
  Analgesic nephropathy
  Polycystic kidney disease
  Medullary sponge kidney
Vasculitis
  Henoch-Schönlein purpura
  Wegener granulomatosis
Infection
  Pyelonephritis
  Xanthogranulomatous pyelonephritis
  Renal tuberculosis
  Fungal infection
Obstruction
  Ureteropelvic junction obstruction
  Ureteral stricture
Nephrolithiasis
Malignancy
  Renal cortical tumors (renal cell carcinoma, benign tumors)
  Upper tract urothelial carcinoma
Fibroepithelial polyp
Vascular diseases
  Renal arteriovenous malformations (congenital, acquired)
  Iliac arterio-ureteral fistula
  Renal artery aneurysm (especially ruptured)
  Renal artery pseudoaneurysm
  Renal artery and/or vein thrombosis
  Hemangioma
  Atheroembolic disease
  Nutcracker syndrome
  Loin-pain hematuria syndrome
Trauma
  Blunt
  Penetrating
Lateralizing essential hematuria

URINARY TRACT OBSTRUCTION[31]

| ICD-10CM # | N21.8 | Other lower urinary tract calculus |
| | N20.9 | Urolithiasis |

INTRARENAL

Uric acid nephropathy.
Sulfonamide precipitates.
Acyclovir, indinavir precipitates.
Multiple myeloma.

URETERAL

Intrinsic
Intraluminal.
  Nephrolithiasis.
  Papillary necrosis.
  Blood clots.

  Fungus balls.
Intramural.
  Ureteropelvic junction dysfunction.
  Ureterovesical junction dysfunction.
  Ureteral valve, polyp, or tumor.
  Ureteral stricture.
    Schistosomiasis.
    Tuberculosis.
    Scarring from instrumentation.
    Drugs (e.g., nonsteroidal anti-inflammatory agents [NSAIDs]).

Extrinsic
Vascular system.
  Aneurysm: abdominal aorta or iliac vessels.
  Aberrant vessels: ureteropelvic junction.
  Venous: retrocaval ureter.
Gastrointestinal tract.
  Crohn's disease.
  Diverticulitis.
  Appendiceal abscess.
  Colon cancer.
  Pancreatic tumor, abscess, or cyst.
Reproductive system.
  Uterus: pregnancy, prolapse, tumor, endometriosis.
  Ovary: abscess, tumor, ovarian remnants.
  Gartner's duct cyst, tuboovarian abscess.
Retroperitoneal disease.
  Retroperitoneal fibrosis: radiation, drugs, idiopathic.
  Inflammatory: tuberculosis, sarcoidosis.
  Hematoma.
  Primary tumor (e.g., lymphoma, sarcoma).
  Metastatic tumor (e.g., cervix, ovarian, bladder, colon).
  Lymphocele.
  Pelvic lipomatosis.

BLADDER

Neurogenic bladder.
  Diabetes mellitus.
  Spinal cord defect.
  Trauma.
  Multiple sclerosis.
  Stroke.
  Parkinson's disease.
  Spinal anesthesia.
  Anticholinergics.
Bladder neck dysfunction.
Bladder calculus.
Bladder cancer.

URETHRA

Urethral stricture.
Prostate hypertrophy or cancer.
Obstruction from instrumentation.

URINARY TRACT OBSTRUCTION, CONGENITAL CAUSES[67]

| ICD-10CM # | | Varies with Specific Diagnosis |

CONGENITAL CAUSES OF URINARY TRACT OBSTRUCTION

Ureteropelvic Junction
Ureteropelvic junction obstruction

Proximal and Middle Ureter
Ureteral folds
Ureteral valves
Strictures
Benign fibroepithelial polyps
Retrocaval ureter
Distal Ureter
Ureterovesical junction obstruction
Vesicoureteral reflux
Prune-belly syndrome
Ureteroceles
Bladder
Bladder diverticula
Neurologic conditions (e.g., spina bifida)
Urethra
Posterior urethral valves
Urethral diverticula
Anterior urethral valves
Urethral atresia
Labial fusion

URINE CASTS

| ICD-10CM # | R82.99 | Other abnormal findings in urine |

Normal finding.
Pyelonephritis.
Chronic renal disease.
Nephrotic syndrome.
Acute tubular necrosis.
Interstitial nephritis.
Nephritic syndrome.
Glomerulonephritis.
Eclampsia.
Heavy metal ingestion.
Allograft rejection.
Hypothyroidism.

URINE COLOR ABNORMALITIES[48]

| ICD-10CM # | R82.5 | Elevated urine levels of drugs, medicaments and biological substances |
| | R82.99 | Other abnormal findings in urine |

COMMON CAUSES OF ABNORMAL URINE COLOR

Colorless

DISEASE

Diabetes mellitus.
Diabetes insipidus.

DRUG

Ethyl alcohol.
Diuretics.

MISCELLANEOUS

Overhydration.
Yellow-orange

DRUG

Tetracycline.
Flutamide.
Pyridium.

Azo Gantrisin (Roche Labs, Nutley, NJ).
Sulfasalazine.
Vitamin B.

MISCELLANEOUS
Dehydration.
Milky White

DISEASE
Urinary tract infection/pyuria.
Blue-green

DISEASE
Pseudomonas urinary tract infection.

DRUG
Methylene blue.
Urised (Polymedica Pharmaceuticals, Woburn, MA).
Indigo carmine.
Doan's pills (Novartis Consumer Health, Parsippany, NJ).
Clorets (Cadbury Adams, Parsippany, NJ).
Amitriptyline.
Red-brown

DISEASE
Hematuria.
Hemolytic anemia.
Hemoglobinuria.
Lead poisoning.
Mercury poisoning.
Porphyria.

DRUG
Rifampin.
Ex-Lax (Novartis Consumer Health, Parsippany, NJ).
Phenolphthalein.
Phenothiazines.
Nitrofurantoin.
Doxorubicin.

MISCELLANEOUS
Beets.
Blackberries.
Rhubarb.
Brown-black

DISEASE
Fecaluria.
Methemoglobinuria.
Melaninuria.

DRUG
Metronidazole.
Methyldopa.
Methocarbamol.

MISCELLANEOUS
Fava beans.
Aloe.

URINE, RED[56]
ICD-10CM #   varies with specific diagnosis

WITH A POSITIVE DIPSTICK
Hematuria.
Hemoglobinuria: negative urinalysis.

Myoglobinuria: negative urinalysis.

WITH A NEGATIVE DIPSTICK
Drugs
Aminosalicylic acid.
Deferoxamine mesylate.
Ibuprofen.
Phenacetin.
Phenolphthalein.
Phensuximide.
Rifampin.
Anthraquinone laxatives.
Doxorubicin.
Methyldopa.
Phenazopyridine.
Phenothiazine.
Phenytoin.
Dyes
Azo dyes.
Eosin.
Foods
Beets, berries, maize.
Rhodamine B.
Metabolic
- Porphyrins.
- *Serratia marcescens* (red diaper syndrome).
- Urate crystalluria.

UROLITHIASIS-LIKE PAIN[67]
ICD-10CM #   Varies with Specific Diagnosis

DIFFERENTIAL DIAGNOSIS OF UROLITHIASIS-LIKE PAIN
Category
Disorders
Renal
  Pyelonephritis
  Blood clot
  Renal infarction
  Tumor (kidney or pelvis)
  Papillary necrosis
Ureteral
  Tumor
  Blood clot
  Stricture
Bladder
  Tumor
  Blood clot
  Urinary retention
Intraabdominal
  Peritonitis
  Appendicitis
  Biliary disease
  Bowel obstruction
  Vascular disorder
  Aortic aneurysm
  Mesenteric insufficiency
Retroperitoneal
  Lymphadenopathy
  Fibrosis
  Tumor
Gynecologic
  Ectopic or tubal pregnancy
  Ovarian torsion, cyst rupture
  Pelvic inflammatory disease
  Cervical cancer
  Endometriosis
  Ovarian vein syndrome

Neuromuscular
  Muscle pain
  Rib fracture
  Radiculitis
Infectious
  Herpes zoster
  Pleuritis, pneumonia
  Fungal bezoar

UROPATHY, OBSTRUCTIVE[70]

| **ICD-10CM #** | N13.9 | Obstructive and reflux uropathy, unspecified |
| | N20.9 | Urolithiasis |

INTRINSIC CAUSES
Intraluminal
Intratubular deposition of crystals (uric acid, sulfas).
Stones.
Papillary tissue.
Blood clots.
Intramural
- Functional.
- Ureter (ureteropelvic or ureterovesical dysfunction).
- Bladder (neurogenic): spinal cord defect or trauma, diabetes, multiple sclerosis, Parkinson's disease, cerebrovascular accidents.
- Bladder neck dysfunction.
Anatomic
Tumors.
Infection, granuloma.
Strictures.

EXTRINSIC CAUSES
Originating in the Reproductive System
Prostate: benign hypertrophy or cancer.
Uterus: pregnancy, tumors, prolapse, endometriosis.
Ovary: abscess, tumor, cysts.
Originating in the Vascular System
Aneurysms (aorta, iliac vessels).
Aberrant arteries (ureteropelvic junction).
Venous (ovarian veins, retrocaval ureter).
Originating in the Gastrointestinal Tract
- Crohn's disease.
- Pancreatitis.
- Appendicitis.
- Tumors.
Originating in the Retroperitoneal Space
- Inflammations.
- Fibrosis.
- Tumor, hematomas.

UROSEPSIS[48]

| **ICD-10CM #** | A41.9 | Sepsis, unspecified organism |

COMMON CAUSES OF UROSEPSIS
Obstructing ureteral stone with pyonephrosis.
Staghorn calculus with urinary tract infection.
Ureteral obstruction with proximal urinary tract infection.
Urinary retention with urinary tract infection.

Acute prostatitis with prostatic abscess.
Perinephric abscess or renal carbuncle.
Urethral stricture with periurethral abscess.
Fournier gangrene.
Foreign body within urinary tract (e.g., Foley catheter).

UTERINE BLEEDING, ABNORMAL[21]

ICD-10CM #	N92.6	Irregular menstruation, unspecified
	N93.9	Abnormal uterine and vaginal bleeding, unspecified

PREGNANCY

Threatened abortion.
Incomplete abortion.
Complete abortion.
Molar pregnancy.
Ectopic pregnancy.
Retained products of conception.

OVULATORY

Vulva: infection, laceration, tumor.
Vagina: infection, laceration, tumor, foreign body.
Cervix: polyps, cervical erosion, cervicitis, carcinoma.
Uterus: fibroids (submucous fibroids most likely to cause abnormal bleeding), polyps, adenomyosis, endometritis, intrauterine device, atrophic endometrium.
Pregnancy complications: ectopic pregnancy; threatened, incomplete, complete abortion; retained products of conception.
Abnormality of clotting system.
Midcycle bleeding.
Halban's disease (persistent corpus luteum).
Menorrhagia.
Pelvic inflammatory disease.

ANOVULATORY

Physiologic causes:
Puberty.
Perimenopausal.
Pathologic causes:
Ovarian failure (FSH over 40 IU/ml).
Hyperandrogenism.
Hyperprolactinemia.
Obesity.
Hypothalamic dysfunction (polycystic ovaries); LH/FSH ratio greater than 2:1.
Hyperplasia.
Endometrial carcinoma.
Estrogen-producing tumors.
Hypothyroidism.

UVEITIS, PEDIATRIC AGE

ICD-10CM #	H20.9	Anterior uveitis

ANTERIOR UVEITIS

Juvenile rheumatoid arthritis (pauciarticular).
Sarcoidosis.
Trauma.

Tuberculosis.
Kawasaki disease.
Ulcerative colitis.
Postinfectious (enteric or genital) with arthritis and rash.
Spirochetal (syphilis, leptospiral).
Heterochromic iridocyclitis (Fuchs).
Viral (herpes simplex, herpes zoster).
Ankylosing spondylitis.
Stevens-Johnson syndrome.
Idiopathic.
Drugs.

POSTERIOR UVEITIS (CHOROIDITIS—MAY INVOLVE RETINA)

Toxoplasmosis.
Parasites (toxocariasis).
Sarcoidosis.
Tuberculosis.
Viral (rubella, herpes simplex, HIV, cytomegalovirus).
Subacute sclerosing panencephalitis.
Idiopathic.

ANTERIOR AND/OR POSTERIOR UVEITIS

Sympathetic ophthalmia (trauma to other eye).
Vogt-Koyanagi-Harada syndrome (uveo-otocutaneous syndrome: poliosis, vitiligo, deafness, tinnitus, uveitis, aseptic meningitis, retinitis).
Behçet syndrome.
Lyme disease.

VAGINAL BLEEDING, PREGNANCY[16]

ICD-10CM #	N93.9	Abnormal uterine and vaginal bleeding, unspecified

FIRST TRIMESTER

Implantation bleeding.
Abortion.
Threatened.
Complete.
Incomplete.
Missed.
Ectopic pregnancy.
Neoplasia.
Hydatidiform mole.
Cervix.

THIRD TRIMESTER

Placenta previa.
Placental abruption.
Premature labor.
Choriocarcinoma.

VAGINAL DISCHARGE, PREPUBERTAL GIRLS[38]

ICD-10CM #	N89.8	Other specified noninflammatory disorders of vagina

Irritative (bubble baths, sand).
Poor perineal hygiene.
Foreign body.

Associated systemic illness (group A streptococci, chickenpox).
Infections.
Escherichia coli with foreign body.
Shigella organisms.
Yersinia organisms.
Infections (consider sexual abuse).
Chlamydia trachomatis.
Neisseria gonorrhoeae.
Trichomonas vaginalis.
Tumor (rare).

VALVULAR HEART DISEASE[3]

ICD-10CM #	varies with specific diagnosis

MAJOR CAUSES OF VALVULAR HEART DISEASE IN ADULTS

Aortic Stenosis
Bicuspid aortic valve.
Rheumatic fever.
Degenerative stenosis.
Aortic Regurgitation
Bicuspid aortic valve.
Aortic dissection.
Endocarditis.
Rheumatic fever.
Aortic root dilation.
Mitral Stenosis
Rheumatic fever.
Mitral Regurgitation

CHRONIC

Mitral valve prolapse.
Left ventricular dilation.
Posterior wall myocardial infarction.
Rheumatic fever.
Endocarditis.

ACUTE

Posterior wall or papillary muscle ischemia.
Papillary muscle or chordal rupture.
Endocarditis.
Prosthetic valve dysfunction.
Systolic anterior motion of mitral valve.

TRICUSPID REGURGITATION

Functional (annular) dilation.
Tricuspid valve prolapse.
Endocarditis.
Carcinoid heart disease.

VASCULAR LESIONS OF GI TRACT[23]

ICD-10CM #	Varies with Specific Diagnosis

Primary Vascular Lesions
Aneurysms of the aorta and its branches
Angioectasia (angiodysplasia, vascular ectasia)
Arteriovenous malformation
Blue rubber bleb nevus
Capillary phlebectasia
Dieulafoy's lesion
Glomus tumor

Hemangioma
Hemangiomatosis
Hemangioendothelioma
Hemangiopericytoma
Hemangiosarcoma
Hemorrhoids
Kaposi's sarcoma
Diseases and Syndromes with Vascular Lesions
Blue rubber bleb nevus syndrome
Ehlers-Danlos syndrome
Hereditary hemorrhagic telangiectasia (Osler-Weber-Rendu disease)
Klippel-Trenaunay or Parkes Weber syndrome
Kohlmeier-Degos syndrome
Marfan's syndrome
Pseudoxanthoma elasticum
PSS (scleroderma, CREST)
Scurvy
Turner's syndrome
von Willebrand's disease
Systemic Disorders Associated with Vascular Lesions
Portal hypertension
    Congestive gastropathy and colopathy
    GAVE (watermelon stomach)
    Spider telangiectasias
    Varices
Renal failure
    GI telangiectasias
    GAVE (watermelon stomach)
Vasculitis (e.g., polyarteritis nodosa)
Iatrogenic lesions
    Radiation telangiectasia

CREST, Calcinosis, Raynaud's phenomenon, esophageal dysmotility, sclerodactyly, telangiectasia; GAVE, gastric antral vascular ectasia

VASCULITIS, CLASSIFICATION[51]

ICD-10CM #   I77.6   Arteritis, unspecified

LARGE VESSEL DISEASE

Arteritis
Giant cell arteritis.
Takayasu's arteritis.
Arteritis associated with Reiter's syndrome (reactive arthritis), ankylosing spondylitis.

MEDIUM AND SMALL VESSEL DISEASE

Polyarteritis Nodosa
Primary (idiopathic).
Associated with viruses (hepatitis B or C, CMV, HIV, herpes zoster).
Associated with malignancy (hairy cell leukemia).
Familial Mediterranean fever.
Granulomatous Vasculitis
Granulomatosis with polyangiitis (Wegener's granulomatosis).
Lymphomatoid granulomatosis.

Behçet's Disease
Kawasaki Disease (Mucocutaneous Lymph Node Syndrome)

PREDOMINANTLY SMALL VESSEL DISEASE

Hypersensitivity Vasculitis (Leukocytoclastic Vasculitis)
Henoch-Schönlein purpura.
Mixed cryoglobulinemia.
Serum sickness.
Vasculitis associated with connective tissue diseases (SLE, Sjögren's syndrome).
Vasculitis associated with specific syndromes:
    Primary biliary cirrhosis.
    Lyme disease.
    Chronic active hepatitis.
    Drug-induced vasculitis.
Churg-Strauss Syndrome
Goodpasture's Syndrome
Erythema Nodosum
Panniculitis. Buerger's Disease (Thrombophlebitis Obliterans)

VASCULITIS (DISEASES THAT MIMIC VASCULITIS)[55]

ICD-10CM #   varies with specific diagnosis

EMBOLIC DISEASE

Infectious or marantic endocarditis.
Cardiac mural thrombus.
Atrial myxoma.
Cholesterol embolization syndrome.

NONINFLAMMATORY VESSEL WALL DISRUPTION

Atherosclerosis.
Arterial fibromuscular dysplasia.
Drug effects (vasoconstrictors, anticoagulants).
Radiation.
Genetic disease (neurofibromatosis, Ehlers-Danlos syndrome).
Amyloidosis.
Intravascular malignant lymphoma.

DIFFUSE COAGULATION

Disseminated intravascular coagulation.
Thrombotic thrombocytopenic purpura.
Hemolytic-uremic syndrome.
Protein C and S deficiencies, factor V/Leiden mutation.
Antiphospholipid syndrome.

VEGETATIVE STATE, PERSISTENT[3]

ICD-10CM #   R40.3   Persistent vegetative state

PERSISTENT VEGETATIVE STATE: COMMON CAUSES[43]

Trauma (diffuse axonal injury).

---

[43]A vegetative state may not necessarily begin with coma but can also develop as the end stage of neurodegenerative diseases (e.g., Alzheimer's disease) of adults or children and can accompany severe congenital developmental abnormalities of the brain such as anencephaly.

Cardiac arrest and hypoperfusion (laminar necrosis of cortical mantle and/or thalamic necrosis).
Bihemispheric infarctions.
Purulent meningitis or encephalitis (cortical injury).
Carbon monoxide.
Prolonged hypoglycemic coma.

VENTILATION–PERFUSION MISMATCH ON LUNG SCAN

ICD-10CM #   varies with specific diagnosis

Pulmonary embolism.
Emphysema.
Irradiation.
Pulmonary hypertension.
AV malformations.
Pulmonary thrombosis.
External compression of pulmonary artery (neoplasm, cysts, fibrosing mediastinitis).
Vasculitis.
Tuberculosis.
Pulmonary thrombosis.
Congenital (pulmonary artery hypoplasia, congenital heart disease with upper lobe diversion).
Sequestered segment.
Parasitic lung disease.
Intraluminal obstruction from catheter fragments.

VENTRICULAR FAILURE

ICD-10CM #   I51.9   Heart disease, unspecified

LEFT VENTRICULAR FAILURE

Systemic hypertension.
Valvular heart disease (AS, AR, MR).
Cardiomyopathy, myocarditis.
Bacterial endocarditis.
Myocardial infarction.
Idiopathic hypertrophic subaortic stenosis.

RIGHT VENTRICULAR FAILURE

Valvular heart disease (mitral stenosis).
Pulmonary hypertension.
Bacterial endocarditis (right-sided).
Right ventricular infarction.

BIVENTRICULAR FAILURE

Left ventricular failure.
Cardiomyopathy.
Myocarditis
Arrhythmias.
Anemia.
Thyrotoxicosis.
Arteriovenous fistula.
Paget's disease.
Beriberi.

VERRUCOUS LESIONS

ICD-10CM #   varies with specific diagnosis

Warts.
Seborrheic keratosis.
Lichen simplex.
Acanthosis nigricans.
Scabies (Norwegian, crusted).

Verrucous carcinoma.
Nevus sebaceous.
Deep fungal infection.

VERTIGO

ICD-10CM #	R42	Dizziness and giddiness
	H81.13	Benign paroxysmal vertigo, bilateral
	H81.49	Vertigo of central origin, unspecified ear
	H81.399	Other peripheral vertigo, unspecified ear
	H81.23	Vestibular neuronitis, bilateral

PERIPHERAL

Otitis media.
Acute labyrinthitis.
Vestibular neuronitis.
Benign positional vertigo.
Meniere's disease.
Ototoxic drugs: streptomycin, gentamicin.
Lesions of the eighth nerve: acoustic neuroma, meningioma, mononeuropathy, metastatic carcinoma.
Mastoiditis.

CNS OR SYSTEMIC

Vertebrobasilar artery insufficiency.
Posterior fossa tumor or other brain tumors.
Infarction/hemorrhage of cerebral cortex, cerebellum, or brain stem.
Basilar migraine.
Metabolic: drugs, hypoxia, anemia, fever.
Hypotension/severe hypertension.
Multiple sclerosis.
CNS infections: viral, bacterial.
Temporal lobe epilepsy.
Arnold–Chiari malformation, syringobulbia.
Psychogenic: ventilation, hysteria.

VERTIGO, CENTRAL[1]

ICD-10CM #	R42

MAJOR CAUSES OF CENTRAL VERTIGO

Demyelination.
  Acquired.
  Leukodystrophies.
  Multiple sclerosis.
Familial disorders.
  Friedreich ataxia.
  Spinocerebellar ataxia.
  Familial episodic ataxia (type 1 and type 2).
  Olivopontocerebellar atrophy.
Central nervous system infections.
  Lyme neuroborreliosis.
  Meningitis.
  Tuberculosis.
Intrinsic brainstem lesion.
  Tumor.
  Arteriovenous malformation.
  Trauma.

Migraine.
  Basilar.
  Benign paroxysmal positional vertigo of childhood.
Toxins.
  Drugs, alcohol.
  Analgesics.
  Anticonvulsants.
  Antihypertensives.
  Hypnotics.
  Tranquilizers.
Metabolic and endocrine disorders.
  Hyperinsulinism.
  Impaired glucose tolerance.
  Diabetes mellitus.
  Hypertriglyceridemia.
  Hypothyroidism.
Systemic conditions.
  Paget disease.
Stroke/ischemia.
  Vertebrobasilar.
  Cerebellar.
  Posterior inferior cerebellar artery syndrome.
  Lateral medullary syndrome.
  Medial medullary infarct.
  Basilar artery syndrome.
  Anterior inferior cerebellar artery.
Other causes of posterior ischemia.
  Subclavian steal syndrome.
  Rotational vertebral artery occlusion syndrome.
  Vertebral artery dissection.
  Vertebral or basilar artery dolichoectasia.
  Neoplasm of the fourth ventricle.
  Chiari malformation.
  Superficial siderosis of the central nervous system.
  Vestibular epilepsy.

VESICULOBULLOUS DISEASES[29]

ICD-10CM #	L94.2	Calcinosis cutis
	L98.8	Other specified disorders of the skin and subcutaneous tissue

IMMUNOLOGICALLY MEDIATED DISEASES

Bullous pemphigoid.
Herpes gestationis.
Mucous membrane pemphigoid.
Epidermolysis bullosa acquisita.
Dermatitis herpetiformis.
Pemphigus (vulgaris, foliaceus, paraneoplastic).

HYPERSENSITIVITY DISEASES

Erythema multiforme minor.
Erythema multiforme major (Stevens-Johnson syndrome).
Toxic epidermal necrolysis.

METABOLIC DISEASES

Porphyria cutanea tarda.
Pseudoporphyria.
Diabetic blisters.

INHERITED GENETIC DISORDERS

Epidermolysis bullosa.
  Simplex.
  Junctional.
  Dystrophic.

INFECTIOUS DISEASES

Impetigo.
Staphylococcal scalded skin syndrome.
Herpes simplex.
Varicella.
Herpes zoster.

VISION LOSS, ACUTE, PAINFUL

ICD-10CM #	H53.139	Sudden visual loss, unspecified eye

Acute angle-closure glaucoma.
Corneal ulcer.
Uveitis.
Endophthalmitis.
Factitious.
Somatization syndrome.
Trauma.

VISION LOSS, ACUTE, PAINLESS

ICD-10CM #	H53.139	Sudden visual loss, unspecified eye

Retinal artery occlusion.
Optic neuritis.
Retinal vein occlusion.
Vitreous hemorrhage.
Retinal detachment.
Exudative macular degeneration.
CVA.
Ischemic optic neuropathy.
Factitious.
Somatization syndrome, anxiety reaction.

VISION LOSS AFTER DIVING[4]

ICD-10CM #	H53.139

DIFFERENTIAL DIAGNOSIS OF DECREASED VISION AFTER DIVING

- Decompression sickness.
- Arterial gas embolism.
- Bubbles under contact lenses.
- Displaced contact lens.
- Antifog agent keratopathy.
- Contact lens adherence syndrome.
- Transdermal scopolamine
- Hyperoxic myopia.
- Oxymetazoline optic neuropathy.
- Diving-induced migraine phenomena.
- Eye disorders not related to diving.

VISION LOSS, CHILDREN

ICD-10CM #	H53.9	Unspecified visual disturbance

Craniopharyngioma.
Hereditary optic atrophy.

Optic nerve glioma.
Glioma of chiasm.
Albinism.
Optic nerve hypoplasia.

VISION LOSS, CHRONIC, PROGRESSIVE

ICD-10CM # H54.7 Unspecified visual loss

- Cataract.
- Macular degeneration.
- Cerebral neoplasm.
- Refractive error.
- Open-angle glaucoma.

VISION LOSS, MONOCULAR, TRANSIENT

ICD-10CM # H54.7 Unspecified visual loss

Thromboembolism.
Vasculitis.
Migraine (vasospasm).
Anxiety reaction.
CNS tumor.
Temporal arteritis.
Multiple sclerosis.

VITREOUS HEMORRHAGE[42]

ICD-10CM # H43.13 Vitreous hemorrhage, bilateral

CAUSES OF VITREOUS HEMORRHAGE

Acute posterior vitreous detachment associated either with a retinal tear or avulsion of a peripheral vessel.
Proliferative retinopathies.
   Diabetic.
   Following retinal vein occlusion.
   Sickle cell disease.
   Eales disease.
   Vasculitis.
Miscellaneous retinal disorders.
   ○ Macroaneurysm.
   ○ Telangiectasis.
   ○ Capillary hemangioma.
Trauma.
   ○ Blunt.
   ○ Penetrating.
   ○ Iatrogenic.
Systemic.
   Bleeding disorders.
   Terson syndrome.

VOCAL CORD PARALYSIS

ICD-10CM #	J38.00	Paralysis of vocal cords and larynx, unspecified
	J38.01	Paralysis of vocal cords and larynx, unilateral
	J38.02	Paralysis of vocal cords and larynx, bilateral

Neoplasm: primary or metastatic (e.g., lung, thyroid, parathyroid, mediastinum).
Neck surgery (parathyroid, thyroid, carotid endarterectomy, cervical spine).
Idiopathic.
Viral, bacterial, or fungal infection.
Trauma (intubation, penetrating neck injury).
Cardiac surgery.
RA.
Multiple sclerosis.
Parkinsonism.
Toxic neuropathy.
CVA.
CNS abnormalities: hydrocephalus, Arnold–Chiari malformation, meningomyelocele.

VOLUME DEPLETION[3]

ICD-10CM # E86.9 Volume depletion, unspecified

GI losses:
   Upper: bleeding, nasogastric suction, vomiting.
   Lower: bleeding, diarrhea, enteric or pancreatic fistula, tube drainage.
Renal losses:
   Salt and water: diuretics, osmotic diuresis, postobstructive diuresis, acute tubular necrosis (recovery phase), salt-losing nephropathy, adrenal insufficiency, renal tubular acidosis.
Water loss: diabetes insipidus.
Skin and respiratory losses:
   Sweat, burns, insensible losses.
Sequestration without external fluid loss:
   Intestinal obstruction, peritonitis, pancreatitis, rhabdomyolysis, internal bleeding.

VOLUME EXCESS[3]

ICD-10CM # varies with specific diagnosis

Primary Renal Sodium Retention (Increased Effective Circulating Volume)
Renal failure, nephritic syndrome, acute glomerulonephritis.
Primary hyperaldosteronism.
Cushing's syndrome.
Liver disease.
Secondary Renal Sodium Retention (Decreased Effective Circulating Volume)
Heart failure.
Liver disease.
Nephrotic syndrome (minimal change disease).
Pregnancy.

VOMITING

ICD-10CM #	R11.10	Vomiting, unspecified
	R11.11	Vomiting without nausea
	R11.12	Projectile vomiting

GI disturbances:
   Obstruction: esophageal, pyloric, intestinal.
   Infections: viral or bacterial enteritis, viral hepatitis, food poisoning, gastroenteritis.
   Pancreatitis.
   Appendicitis.
   Biliary colic.
   Peritonitis.
   Perforated bowel.
   Diabetic gastroparesis.
Other: gastritis, PUD, IBD, GI tract neoplasms.
Drugs: morphine, digitalis, cytotoxic agents, bromocriptine.
Severe pain: MI, renal colic.
Metabolic disorders: uremia, acidosis/alkalosis, hyperglycemia, DKA, thyrotoxicosis.
Trauma: blows to the testicles, epigastrium.
Vertigo.
Reye's syndrome.
Increased intracranial pressure.
CNS disturbances: trauma, hemorrhage, infarction, neoplasm, infection, hypertensive encephalopathy, migraine.
Radiation sickness.
Nausea and vomiting of pregnancy, hyperemesis gravidarum.
Motion sickness.
Bulimia, anorexia nervosa.
Psychogenic: emotional disturbances, offensive sights or smells.
Severe coughing.
Pyelonephritis.
Boerhaave's syndrome.
Carbon monoxide poisoning.

VOMITING, NEONATAL[1]

ICD-10CM # R11.10

CAUSES OF NEONATAL VOMITING

Anatomic Causes
Esophagus, trachea, great vessels:
   Stricture.
   Web.
   Tracheoesophageal fistula.
   Laryngeal cleft.
   Double aortic arch.
Stomach and duodenum:
   Pyloric stenosis.
   Duodenal atresia (usually noted on the first day of life)
Small and large intestine:
   Volvulus secondary to malrotation.
   Incarcerated hernia.
   Hirschsprung disease (secondary to obstipation).
   Necrotizing enterocolitis.
Genitourinary:
   Testicular torsion.
Nonanatomic Causes
Infection:
   Septicemia.
   Meningitis.
   Urinary tract infection.
   Gastroenteritis.
   Otitis media
Increased intracranial pressure:
   Cerebral edema.
   Subdural hematoma.

Hydrocephalus.
Brain tumor.
Congenital adrenal hyperplasia (salt-losing variety).
Inborn errors of metabolism.
Renal disease.

VULVAR LESIONS[21]

ICD-10CM #		
	N77.0	Ulceration of vulva in diseases classified elsewhere
	N90.7	Vulvar cyst
	N90.89	Other specified noninflammatory disorders of vulva and perineum
	D07.1	Carcinoma in situ of vulva
	N90.89	Other specified noninflammatory disorders of vulva and perineum
	N90.5	Atrophy of vulva

RED LESION

Infection/Infestation
Fungal infection:
  Candida.
  Tinea cruris.
  Intertrigo.
  Pityriasis versicolor.
Sarcoptes scabiei.
Erythrasma: Corynebacterium minutissimum.
Granuloma inguinale: Calymmatobacterium granulomatis.
Folliculitis: Staphylococcus aureus.
Hidradenitis suppurativa.
Behçet's syndrome.

Inflammation
Reactive vulvitis.
Chemical irritation:
  Detergent.
  Dyes.
  Perfume.
  Spermicide.
  Lubricants.
  Hygiene sprays.
  Podophyllum.
  Topical 5-FU.
  Saliva.
  Gentian violet.
  Semen.
Mechanical trauma: scratching.
Vestibular adenitis.
Essential vulvodynia.
Psoriasis.
Seborrheic dermatitis.

Neoplasm
Vulvar intraepithelial neoplasia (VIN):
  Mild dysplasia.
  Moderate dysplasia.
  Severe dysplasia.
  Carcinoma-in-situ.
Vulvar dystrophy.
Bowen's disease.
Invasive cancer:
  Squamous cell carcinoma.

Malignant melanoma.
Sarcoma.
Basal cell carcinoma.
Adenocarcinoma.
Paget's disease.
Undifferentiated.

WHITE LESION
Vulvar dystrophy:
  Lichen sclerosus.
  Vulvar dystrophy.
  Vulvar hyperplasia.
  Mixed dystrophy.
VIN.
Vitiligo.
Partial albinism.
Intertrigo.
Radiation treatment.

DARK LESION
Lentigo.
Nevi (mole).
Neoplasm (see "Neoplasm, Vulvar," below).
Reactive hyperpigmentation.
Seborrheic keratosis.
Pubic lice.

ULCERATIVE LESION

Infection
Herpes simplex.
Vaccinia.
Treponema pallidum.
Granuloma inguinale.
Pyoderma.
Tuberculosis.

Noninfectious
Behçet's disease.
Crohn's disease.
Pemphigus.
Pemphigoid.
Hidradenitis suppurativa (see "Neoplasm, Vulvar," below).

Neoplasm
Basal cell carcinoma.
Squamous cell carcinoma.
Vulvar tumor <1 cm:
  Condyloma acuminatum.
  Molluscum contagiosum.
  Epidermal inclusion.
  Vestibular cyst.
  Mesonephric duct.
  VIN.
  Hemangioma.
  Hidradenoma.
  Neurofibroma.
  Syringoma.
  Accessory breast tissue.
  Acrochordon.
  Endometriosis.
  Fox-Fordyce disease.
  Pilonidal sinus.
Vulvar tumor >1 cm:
  Bartholin cyst or abscess.
  Lymphogranuloma venereum.
  Fibroma.
  Lipoma.
  Verrucous carcinoma.
  Squamous cell carcinoma.

Hernia.
Edema.
Hematoma.
Acrochordon.
Epidermal cysts.
Neurofibromatosis.
Accessory breast tissue.

WEAKNESS, ACUTE, EMERGENT[51]

ICD-10CM #	M62.81	Muscle weakness (generalized)

Demyelinating disorders (Guillain-Barré, chronic inflammatory demyelinating polyneuropathy [CIDP]).
Myasthenia gravis.
Infectious (poliomyelitis, diphtheria).
Toxic (botulism, tick paralysis, paralytic shellfish toxin, puffer fish, newts).
Metabolic (acquired or familial hypokalemia, hypophosphatemia, hypermagnesemia).
Metal poisoning (arsenic, thallium).
Porphyria.

WEAKNESS, GRADUAL ONSET

ICD-10CM #	M62.81	Muscle weakness (generalized)

Depression.
Malingering.
Anemia.
Hypothyroidism.
Medications (e.g., sedatives, antidepressants, narcotics).
CHF.
Renal failure.
Liver failure.
Respiratory insufficiency.
Alcoholism.
Nutritional deficiencies.
Disorders of motor unit.
Basal ganglia disorders.
Upper motor neuron lesions.

WEAKNESS, NONNEUROMUSCULAR CAUSES

ICD-10CM #	G93.3	Postviral fatigue syndrome
	R53.1	Weakness
	R53.81	Other malaise
	R53.83	Other fatigue

Anxiety disorder.
Infectious process.
Anemia.
Renal insufficiency.
Hyperventilation.
Malignancy.
Hypothyroidism.
Hypotension.
Hypercapnia.
Hypoglycemia.
Cardiac arrhythmias.
Hepatic insufficiency.

Electrolyte imbalance.
Malnutrition.
Cerebrovascular insufficiency.

WEIGHT GAIN

| ICD-10CM # | R63.5 | Abnormal weight gain |
| | E66.9 | Obesity, unspecified |

Sedentary lifestyle.
Fluid overload.
Discontinuation of tobacco abuse.
Endocrine disorders (hypothyroidism, hyperinsulinism associated with maturity-onset DM, Cushing's syndrome, hypogonadism, insulinoma, hyperprolactinemia, acromegaly).
Medications (nutritional supplements, oral contraceptives, glucocorticoids, etc.).
Anxiety disorders with compulsive eating.
Laurence-Moon-Biedl syndrome, Prader-Willi syndrome, other congenital diseases.
Hypothalamic injury (rare; <100 cases reported in medical literature).

WEIGHT LOSS

| ICD-10CM # | R63.4 | Abnormal weight loss |

Malignancy.
Psychiatric disorders (depression, anorexia nervosa).
New-onset DM.
Malabsorption.
COPD.
AIDS.
Uremia, liver disease.
Thyrotoxicosis, pheochromocytoma, carcinoid syndrome.
Addison's disease.
Intestinal parasites.
Peptic ulcer disease.
Inflammatory bowel disease.
Food faddism.
Postgastrectomy syndrome.

WHEEZING

| ICD-10CM # | R06.2 | Wheezing |

Asthma.
COPD.
Interstitial lung disease.
Infections (pneumonia, bronchitis, bronchiolitis, epiglottitis).
Cardiac asthma.
GERD with aspiration.
Foreign body aspiration.
Pulmonary embolism.
Anaphylaxis.
Obstruction of airway (neoplasm, goiter, edema or hemorrhage from trauma, aneurysm, congenital abnormalities, strictures, spasm).
Carcinoid syndrome.

WHEEZING, PEDIATRIC AGE[8]

| ICD-10CM # | R06.2 | Wheezing |

Reactive airways disease.
Atopic asthma.
Infection-associated airway reactivity.
Exercise-induced asthma.

Salicylate-induced asthma and nasal polyposis.
Asthmatic bronchitis.
Other hypersensitivity reactions:
    Hypersensitivity pneumonitis.
    Tropical eosinophilia.
    Visceral larva migrans.
    Allergic bronchopulmonary aspergillosis.
Aspiration:
    Foreign body.
    Food, saliva, gastric contents.
    Laryngotracheoesophageal cleft.
    Tracheoesophageal fistula, H-type.
    Pharyngeal incoordination or neuromuscular weakness.
Cystic fibrosis.
Primary ciliary dyskinesia.
Cardiac failure.
Bronchiolitis obliterans.
Extrinsic compression of airways:
    Vascular ring.
    Enlarged lymph node.
    Mediastinal tumor.
    Lung cysts.
Tracheobronchomalacia.
Endobronchial masses.
Gastroesophageal reflux.
Pulmonary hemosiderosis.
Sequelae of bronchopulmonary dysplasia.
"Hysterical" glottic closure.
Cigarette smoke, other environmental insults.

WRIST AND HAND PAIN, IN DIFFERENT AGE GROUPS[17]

| ICD-10CM # | S69.80XA | Other specified injuries of unspecified wrist, hand and finger(s), initial encounter |
| | S69.90XA | Unspecified injury of unspecified wrist, hand and finger(s), initial encounter |

COMMON CAUSES OF WRIST AND HAND PAIN IN DIFFERENT AGE GROUPS

Childhood (2-10 yr)
Intraarticular
Infection.
Periarticular.
Fracture.
Osteomyelitis.
Adolescence (10-18 yr)
Intraarticular
Infection.
Periarticular
Trauma.
Osteomyelitis.
Tumors.
Ganglion.
Idiopathic wrist pain.
Early Adulthood (18-30 yr)
Intraarticular
Inflammatory arthritis.
Infection.
Osteoarthritis.

Periarticular
Peripheral nerve entrapment.
Tendonitis.
Referred
Cervical.
Adulthood (30-50 yr)
Intraarticular
Inflammatory arthritis.
Infection.
Osteoarthritis.
Periarticular
Peripheral nerve entrapment.
Tendonitis.
Referred
Cervical.
Chest.
Cardiac.
Old age (>50 yr)
Intraarticular
Inflammatory arthritis.
Osteoarthritis.
Periarticular
Peripheral nerve entrapment.
Tendonitis.
Referred
Cervical.
Chest.
Cardiac.

WRIST PAIN

| ICD-10CM # | S69.80XA | Other specified injuries of unspecified wrist, hand and finger(s), initial encounter |
| | S69.90XA | Unspecified injury of unspecified wrist, hand and finger(s), initial encounter |

MECHANICAL
Osteoarthritis.
Ligament tear.
Fracture.
Ganglion.
De Quervain's tenosynovitis.
Avascular necrosis (scaphoid, lunate).
Nonunion of scaphoid or lunate.
Neoplasm.

METABOLIC
Pregnancy.
Diabetes.
Gout.
Pseudogout.
Paget's disease.
Acromegaly.
Hypothyroidism.
Hyperparathyroidism.

INFECTIOUS
Osteomyelitis.
Septic arthritis.
Cat-scratch disease.
Tick bite (Lyme disease, babesiosis).
Tuberculosis.

NEUROLOGIC

Peripheral neuropathy.
Nerve injury (median, ulnar, radial nerve).
Thoracic outlet compression syndrome.
Distal posterior interosseous nerve syndrome.

RHEUMATOLOGIC

Psoriasis.
RA.
SLE, mixed connective tissue disorder (MCTD).
Scleroderma.

MISCELLANEOUS

Granulomatous (sarcoidosis).
Amyloidosis.
Multiple myeloma.
Leukemia.

XEROPHTHALMIA[55]

ICD-10CM #	H11.149	Conjunctival xerosis, unspecified, unspecified eye

MEDICATIONS

Tricyclic antidepressants: amitriptyline, doxepin.
Antihistamines: diphenhydramine, chlorpheniramine, promethazine, and many cold and decongestant preparations.
Anticholinergic agents: antiemetics such as scopolamine, antispasmodic agents such as oxybutynin chloride.

ABNORMALITIES OF EYELID FUNCTION

Neuromuscular disorders.
Aging.
Thyrotoxicosis.

ABNORMALITIES OF TEAR PRODUCTION

Hypovitaminosis A.
Stevens-Johnson syndrome.
Familial diseases affecting sebaceous secretions.

ABNORMALITIES OF CORNEAL SURFACES

Scarring from past injuries and herpes simplex infection.

XEROSTOMIA[55]

ICD-10CM #	K11.7	Disturbances of salivary secretion
	R68.2	Dry mouth, unspecified

MEDICATIONS

Tricyclic antidepressants: amitriptyline, doxepin.
Antihistamines: diphenhydramine, chlorpheniramine, promethazine, and many cold and decongestant preparations.
Anticholinergic agents: antiemetics such as scopolamine, antispasmodic agents such as oxybutynin chloride.

DEHYDRATION

Debility.
Fever.

POLYURIA

Alcohol intake.
Arrhythmia.
Diabetes.

PREVIOUS HEAD AND NECK IRRADIATION SYSTEMIC DISEASES

Sjögren's syndrome.
Sarcoidosis.
Amyloidosis.
Human immunodeficiency virus (HIV) infection.
Graft-versus-host disease.

YELLOW URINE

ICD-10CM #	R82	Other abnormal findings in urine

Normal coloration.
Concentrated urine.
Use of multivitamin supplements.
Diet rich in carrots.
Use of Cascara.
Urinary tract infection

REFERENCES

1. Adams JG, et al.: *Emergency medicine, clinical essentials*, ed 2, Philadelphia, Elsevier.
2. Adkinson NF, et al.: *Middleton's allergy principles and practice*, ed 8, Philadelphia, 2014, Saunders.
3. Andreoli TE: *Cecil essentials of medicine*, ed 5, Philadelphia, Saunders.
4. Auerbach P: *Wilderness medicine*, Philadelphia, Saunders.
5. Ballinger A: *Kumar & Clark's essentials of clinical medicine*, ed 6, Edinburgh, Saunders.
6. Barkin RM, Rosen P: *Emergency pediatrics: a guide to ambulatory care*, ed 5, St Louis, Mosby.
7. Baude AI: *Infectious diseases and medical microbiology*, ed 2, Philadelphia, Saunders.
8. Behrman RE: *Nelson textbook of pediatrics*, ed 16, Philadelphia, Saunders.
9. Bennett JE, Dolin R, Blaser MJ: *Mandell, Douglas, and Bennett's principles and practice of infectious diseases*, ed 8, Philadelphia, 2015, Saunders.
10. Bonow RO, et al.: *Braunwauld's heart disease*, ed 9, Philadelphia, Elsevier.
11. Bowling B: *Kanski's clinical ophthalmology*, ed 8, Philadelphia, 2016, Elsevier.
12. Boyer KM: Nonbacterial pneumonia. In Feigin RD, Cherry JD, editors: *Textbook of pediatric infectious diseases*, ed 4, Philadelphia, 1998, WB Saunders, pp 260–273.
13. Callen JP: *Color atlas of dermatology*, ed 2, Philadelphia, WB Saunders.
14. Cameron JL, Cameron AM: *Current surgical therapy*, ed 10, Philadelphia, Saunders.
15. Canoso J: *Rheumatology in primary care*, Philadelphia, Saunders.
16. Carlson KJ: *Primary care of women*, ed 2, St Louis, Mosby.
17. Carr A, Hamilton W: *Orthopedics in primary care*, ed 2, Philadelphia, Saunders.
18. Conn R: *Current diagnosis*, ed 9, Philadelphia, Saunders.
19. Copeland LJ: *Textbook of gynecology*, ed 2, Philadelphia, Saunders.
20. Custer JW, Rau RE: *The Harriet Lane handbook*, ed 18, St Louis, Mosby.
21. Danakas G: *Practical guide to the care of the gynecologic/obstetric patient*. St Louis, Mosby.
22. Eberlein M, et al.: A fall in Ghana, *Am J Med* 122:1091, 2009.
23. Feldman M, Friedman LS, Brandt LJ: *Sleisenger and Fordtran's gastrointestinal and liver disease*, ed 10, Philadelphia, 2016, Elsevier.
24. Firestein GS, Budd RC, Gabriel SE, et al.: *Kelly's textbook of rheumatology*, ed 9, Philadelphia, Saunders.
25. Floege J, et al.: *Comprehensive clinical nephrology*, ed 4, Philadelphia, Saunders.
26. Fuhrman BP, et al.: *Pediatric critical care*, ed 4, Philadelphia, Saunders.
27. Gabbe SG: *Obstetrics*, ed 6, Philadelphia, Saunders.
28. Goldberg RJ: *The care of the psychiatric patient*, ed 3, St Louis, Mosby.
29. Goldman L, Ausiello D: *Cecil textbook of medicine*, ed 21, Philadelphia, Saunders.
30. Goldman L, Braunwald E: *Braunwauld Primary cardiology*, Philadelphia, Saunders.
31. Goldman L, Schafer AI: *Goldman's Cecil medicine*, ed 24, Philadelphia, Saunders.
32. Gorbach SL: *Infectious diseases*, ed 2, Philadelphia, Saunders.
33. Grainger RG, Allison D: *Grainger & Allison's diagnostic radiology, a textbook of medical imaging*, ed 4, London, Churchill Livingstone.
34. Habif TP: *Clinical dermatology*, ed 6, Philadelphia, 2016, Elsevier.
35. Harrington J: *Consultation in internal medicine*, ed 2, St Louis, Mosby.
36. Henry JB: *Clinical diagnosis and management by laboratory methods*, ed 20, Philadelphia, Saunders.
37. Hochberg MC, et al.: *Rheumatology*, ed 5, Mosby: St. Louis.
38. Hoekelman R: *Primary pediatric care*, ed 3, St Louis, Mosby.
39. Hoffman R: *Hematology, basic principles and practice*, ed 6, Philadelphia, Saunders.
40. Hoffmann R, et al.: *Hematology: basic principles and practice*, ed 5, Philadelphia, Churchill Livingstone.
41. James WD, et al.: *Andrews' diseases of the skin*, ed 12, Philadelphia, 2016, Saunders.
42. Kanski JJ, Bowling B: *Clinical ophthalmology, a systematic approach*, ed 7, Philadelphia, Saunders.
43. Kassirer J: *Current therapy in adult medicine*, ed 4, St Louis, Mosby.
44. Kassirer J: *Practical rheumatology*, London, Mosby.
45. Khan MG: *Rapid ECG interpretation*, Philadelphia, Saunders.
46. Kliegman RM, et al.: *Nelson textbook of pediatrics*, ed 19, Philadelphia, Saunders.
47. Kliegman R: *Practical strategies in pediatric diagnosis and therapy*, Philadelphia, Saunders.
48. Lipshultz LI, Khera M, Atwal DT: *Urology and the primary care practitioner*, ed 3, Philadelphia, Elsevier.

Differential Diagnosis

II

49. Mahanty S, Nutman TB: Eosinophilia and eosinophil-related disorders. In Middleton EJ, Reed CE, Ellis EF, et al. editors: *Allergy: Principles and practice*, ed 4, Mosby-Year Book: St Louis, p. 1077.

50. Mandell GL: *Mandell, Douglas, and Bennett's principles and practice of infectious diseases*, ed 6, New York, Churchill Livingstone.

51. Marx JA, et al.: *Rosen's emergency medicine*, ed 8, Philadelphia, 2014, Saunders.

52. Mason RJ: *Murray & Nadel's textbook of respiratory medicine*, ed 5, Philadelphia, Saunders.

53. Melmed S, Polonsky KS, Larsen PR, Kronenberg HM: *Williams textbook of endocrinology*, ed 12, Philadelphia, Saunders.

54. Moore WT, Eastman RC: *Diagnostic endocrinology*, ed 2, St Louis, Mosby.

55. Noble J: *Primary care medicine*, ed 3, St Louis, Mosby.

56. Nseyo UO: *Urology for primary care physicians*, Philadelphia, Saunders.

57. Palay D: *Ophthalmology for the primary care physician*, St Louis, Mosby.

58. Park MK: *Park's Pediatric cardiology for practitioners*, ed 6, Philadelphia, 2014, Saunders.

59. Parrillo JE, Dellinger RP: *Critical care medicine, principles of diagnosis and management in the adult*, ed 4, Philadelphia, 2014, Elsevier.

60. Pope TL, Bloem HL, Beltran J, Morrison WB, Wilson DJ: *Musculoskeletal imaging*, ed 2, Philadelphia, 2014, Saunders.

61. Rakel RE: *Principles of family practice*, ed 6, Philadelphia, Saunders.

62. Rumack CM, et al.: *Diagnostic ultrasound*, ed 4, Philadelphia, 2011, Elsevier.

63. Schwarz MI: *Interstitial lung disease*, ed 2, St Louis, Mosby.

64. Seller RH: *Differential diagnosis of common complaints*, ed 4, Philadelphia, Saunders.

65. Sellke FW, del Nido PJ, Swanson SJ: *Sabiston & Spencer surgery of the chest*, ed 9, Philadelphia, 2016, Elsevier.

66. Siedel HM: *Mosby's guide to physical examination*, ed 4, St Louis, Mosby.

67. Skorecki K, et al.: *Brenner & Rector's the kidney*, ed 10, Philadelphia, 2016, Elsevier.

68. Souhami RL, Moxham J: *Textbook of medicine*, ed 4, London, Churchill Livingstone.

69. Specht N: *Practical guide to diagnostic imaging*, St Louis, Mosby.

70. Stein JH: *Internal medicine*, ed 5, St Louis, Mosby.

71. Swain R, Snodgrass JG: Managing groin pain, *Phys Sportmed* 23(56), 1995.

72. Talley NJ, Martin CJ: *Clinical gastroenterology*, ed 2, Sydney, Churchill Livingstone.

73. Tschudy MM, Arcara KM: *The Harriet Lane handbook*, ed 19, Philadelphia, Mosby.

74. Vincent JL, et al.: *Textbook of critical care*, ed 6, Philadelphia, Saunders.

75. Webb WR, Brant WE, Major NM: *Fundamentals of body CT*, ed 4, Philadelphia, 2015, Saunders.

76. Wein AJ, et al.: *Campbell-Walsh urology*, ed 11, Philadelphia, 2016, Elsevier.

77. Weinberg SE, et al.: *Principles of pulmonary medicine*, ed 5, Philadelphia, Saunders.

78. Wiederholt WC: *Neurology for non-neurologists*, ed 4, Philadelphia, Saunders.

79. Wilson JD: *Williams textbook of endocrinology*, ed 9, Philadelphia, Saunders.

Clinical Algorithms

Clinical Algorithms

PLEASE NOTE: These algorithms are designed to assist clinicians in the evaluation and treatment of patients. They may not apply to all patients with a particular disorder and are not intended to replace the clinician's individual judgment.

Additional algorithms available at www.expertconsult.com

Adrenal Incidentaloma (Fig. E11)
Anemia in Newborn (Fig. E25)
Anemia with Reticulocytosis (Fig. E28)
Aspiration, Gastric Contents (Fig. E36)
Aspiration, Oral Contents (Fig. E37)
Bleeding and Bruising Problems (Fig. E42)
Bleeding Disorder, Congenital (Fig. E43)
Bleeding, Early Pregnancy (Fig. E45)
Bleeding, Neonate (Fig. E47)
Bleeding, Variceal (Fig. E50)
Bradycardia, Pediatric Patient (Fig. E52)
Breast, Radiologic Evaluation (Fig. E54)
Breastfeeding Difficulties (Fig. E57)
Bullae on Lower Extremities (Fig. E58)
Cardiomyopathy, Ischemic (Fig. E64)
Convulsive Disorder, Suspected, Pediatric Patient (Fig. E70)
Corneal Disorders (Fig. E71)
Cutaneous Microvascular Occlusion Syndromes (Fig. E73, Tables E8 and E9)
Cystitis, Acute (Fig. E76)
Dehydration Correction, Pediatric Patient (Fig. E79, Tables E10 to E13)
Dementia, Management (Fig. E80, Table E14)
Developmental Delay (Fig. E81)
Diarrhea, Chronic, in Patients with HIV Infection (Fig. E84, Table E15)
Diarrhea, Watery (Fig. E85)
Dilated Pupil (Fig. E86)
Dyspepsia (Fig. E90)
Ear Pain (Fig. E95)
Eosinophilic Dermatoses (Fig. E99)
Erythroderma (Fig. E101, Table E20)
Fever and Infection in High-Risk Hematology Patient without Obvious Source (Fig. E106)
Fever and Neutropenia, Pediatric Patient (Fig. E108)
Flushing (Fig. E110)
Foreign Body, in Wound (Fig. E112)
Fracture, Bone (Fig. E113)
Genitalia, Ambiguous (Fig. E115)
GI Bleeding, Pediatric Patient (Fig. E116)
Goiter Evaluation and Management (Fig. E119)
Hematochezia, Management (Fig. E122)
Hematuria, Pediatric Patient (Fig. E124)
HIV Detection, Patients at Risk (Fig. E130)

Intubation, Pediatric Patient (Fig. E159, Table E31)
Ischemia, Colon Management (Fig. E160)
Knee Dislocation Treatment (Fig. E165)
Liver Mass, Solid (Fig. E169)
Lymphadenopathy, Axillary (Fig. E171)
Lymphadenopathy, Cervical (Fig. E172)
Lymphadenopathy, Epitrochlear (Fig. E173)
Lymphadenopathy, Inguinal (Fig. E175)
Myocardial Ischemia, Suspected (Fig. E186)
Myositis (Fig. E187)
Nail Dystrophy (Fig. E188)
Nutrition Assessment and Intervention in Cancer Patients (Fig. E193)
Nutritional Support (Fig. E194, Box E9)
Onycholysis (Fig. E203)
Pancreatic Islet Cell Tumors (Fig. E205)
Papulosquamous Disorders, Pediatric Patient (Fig. E207)
Pericardial Effusion, Malignant (Fig. E214)
Photosensitivity (Fig. E216)
Pleural Effusion, Malignant (Fig. E220)
Polycythemia (Fig. E224)
Pruritus, Pregnant Patient (Fig. E227)
Pseudohermaphroditism (Fig. E228)
Reactive Erythema, Pediatric Patient (Fig. E232)
Renal Disease, Ischemic, Management (Fig. E234)
Respiratory Distress (Fig. E239)
Rhinorrhea (Fig. E240)
Sexual Dysfunction Evaluation (Fig. E242)
Sexual Precocity, Female Breast Development (Fig. E243)
Sexual Precocity, Female Pubic Hair Development (Fig. E244, Table E54)
Sexual Precocity, Male (Fig. E245, Table E55)
Shin Splints (Fig. E246)
Short Stature (Fig. E248)
Skin Blisters (Fig. E252, Table E57)
Spine Tumor (Fig. E258)
Spondylosis, Cervical (Fig. E262)
Stroke (Fig. E263)
Subcutaneous Ossification, Evaluation (Fig. E264)
Tachycardia, Pediatric Patient (Fig. E268)
Thrombotic Microangiopathies, Differential Diagnosis (Fig. E272)
Unconscious Patient (Fig. E277)
Vaginal Prolapse/Pelvic Organ Prolapse (Fig. E281)

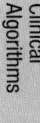

Clinical Algorithms

III

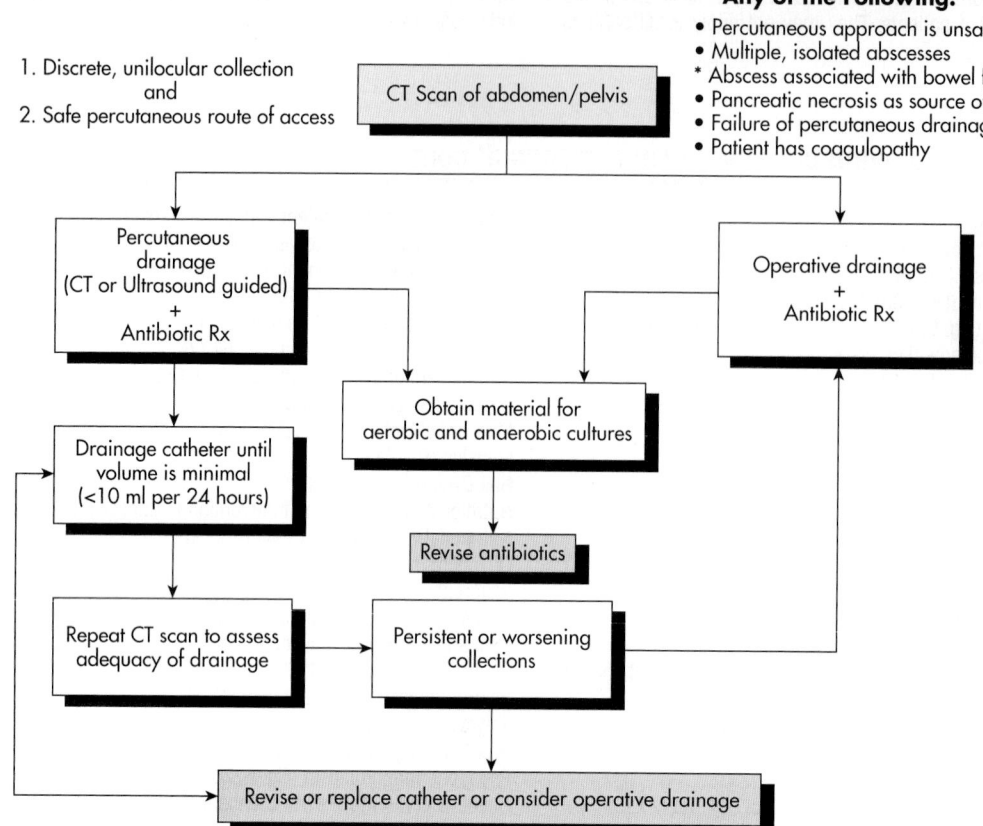

1. Discrete, unilocular collection
  and
2. Safe percutaneous route of access

CT Scan of abdomen/pelvis

Any of the Following:
• Percutaneous approach is unsafe
• Multiple, isolated abscesses
* Abscess associated with bowel fistula
• Pancreatic necrosis as source of abscess
• Failure of percutaneous drainage
• Patient has coagulopathy

Percutaneous drainage (CT or Ultrasound guided) + Antibiotic Rx

Operative drainage + Antibiotic Rx

Obtain material for aerobic and anaerobic cultures

Revise antibiotics

Drainage catheter until volume is minimal (<10 ml per 24 hours)

Repeat CT scan to assess adequacy of drainage

Persistent or worsening collections

Revise or replace catheter or consider operative drainage

FIG. 1 Approach to management of intraabdominal abscesses including indications for consideration of percutaneous versus operative drainage. (Parrillo JE, Dellinger RP: Critical Care Medicine, Principles of Diagnosis and Management in the Adult, 4th ed, ISBN # 978-0-323-08929-6, 2014, Elsevier.)

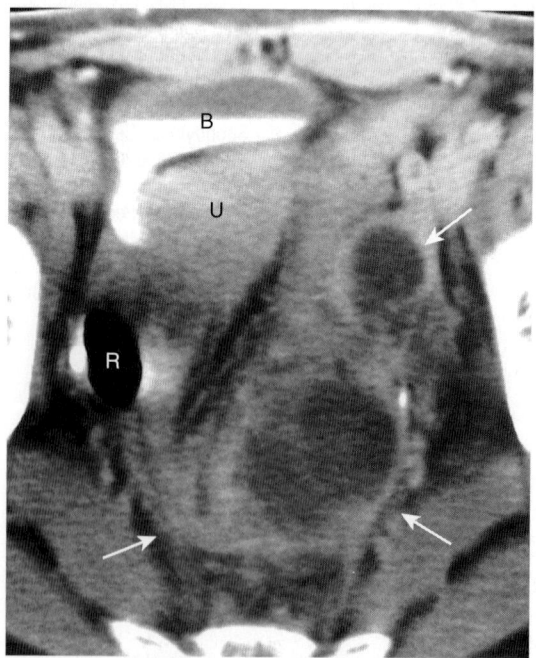

FIG. 2 Tuboovarian abscess. A poorly marginated cystic and solid inflammatory mass (between *arrows*) displaces the rectum (R), uterus (U), and bladder (B) anteriorly and rightward. The left ovary and dilated left fallopian tube are incorporated within the mass but are not definitively identified. The patient was suffering from sepsis and had acute pelvic pain. (Webb WR, Brandt WE, Major NM: Fundamentals of body CT, 4th ed, Philadelphia, Elsevier, 2015, ISBN# 978-0-323-22146-7.)

TABLE 1   Comparison of Common Causes of Acute Abdominal Pain

Cause	Onset	Location	Character	Descriptor	Radiation	Intensity
Appendicitis	Gradual	Periumbilical area early; RLQ late	Diffuse early; localized later	Aching	None	++
Cholecystitis	Acute	RUQ	Localized	Constricting	Scapula	++
Pancreatitis	Acute	Epigastrium, back	Localized	Boring	Midback	++ to +++
Diverticulitis	Gradual	LLQ	Localized	Aching	None	++ to +++
Perforated peptic ulcer	Sudden	Epigastrium	Localized early, diffuse later	Burning	None	+++
Small bowel obstruction	Gradual	Periumbilical area	Diffuse	Cramping	None	++
Mesenteric ischemia, infarction	Sudden	Periumbilical area	Diffuse	Agonizing	None	+++
Ruptured abdominal aortic aneurysm	Sudden	Abdomen, back, flank	Diffuse	Tearing	None	+++
Gastroenteritis	Gradual	Periumbilical area	Diffuse	Spasmodic	None	+ to ++
Pelvic inflammatory disease	Gradual	Either LQ, pelvis	Localized	Aching	Upper thigh	++
Ruptured ectopic pregnancy	Sudden	Either LQ, pelvis	Localized	Sharp	None	++

+, mild; ++, moderate; +++, severe; LLQ, left lower quadrant; LQ, lower quadrant; RLQ, right lower quadrant; RUQ, right upper quadrant.
Feldman M, Friedman LS, Brandt LJ: Sleisenger and Fortran's Gastrointestinal and Liver Disease, 10th ed, ISBN# 978-1-4557-4692-7, 2016, Elsevier.

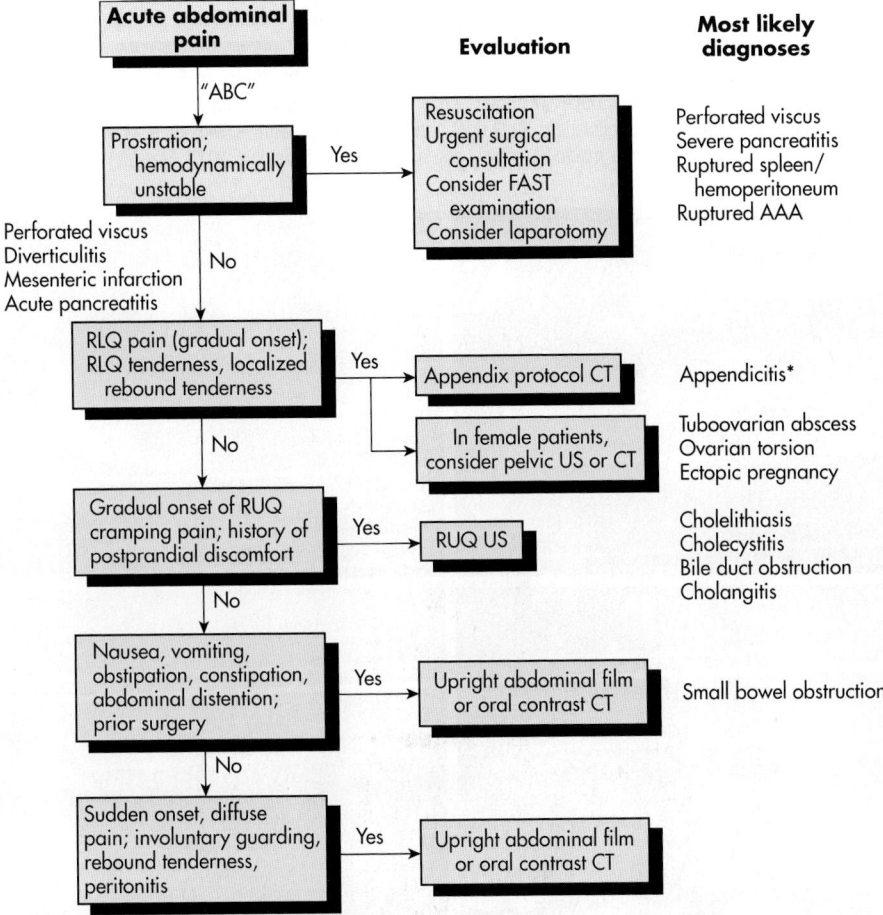

FIG. 3 An approach to the urgent evaluation of abdominal pain. Specific complaints and physical examination findings are coupled with appropriate radiologic imaging. *For left lower quadrant pain, the most likely diagnosis is diverticulitis. *AAA*, abdominal aortic aneurysm; *ABC*, airway, breathing, circulation; *FAST*, focused abdominal sonogram for trauma; *RLQ*, right lower quadrant; *RUQ*, right upper quadrant. (Feldman M, Friedman LS, Brandt LJ: Sleisenger and Fortran's Gastrointestinal and Liver Disease, 10th ed, ISBN# 978-1-4557-4692-7, 2016, Elsevier.)

Clinical Algorithms

III

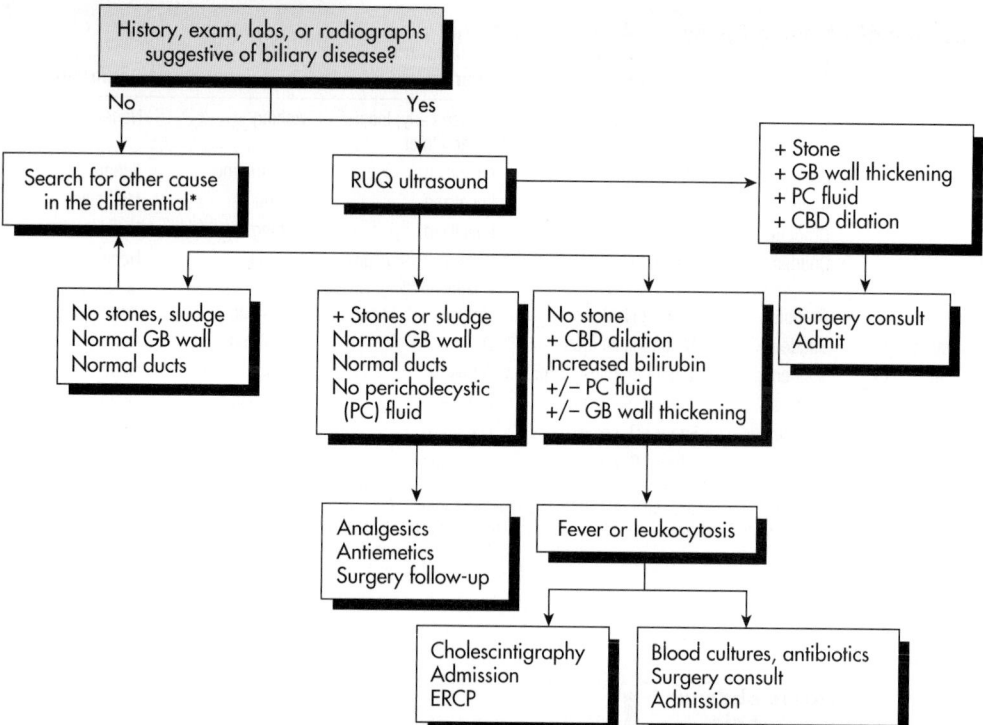

FIG. 4 Treatment algorithm for right upper quadrant (RUQ) pain. *Refer to Section II, Differential Diagnosis, Abdominal Pain Right Upper Quadrant. *CBD*, Common bile duct; *ERCP*, endoscopic retrograde cholangiopancreatography; *GB*, gallbladder; *RUQ*, right upper quadrant; +, with; −, without; ±, with or without. (From Adams JG et al: *Emergency medicine, clinical essentials,* ed 2, Philadelphia, 2013, Elsevier.)

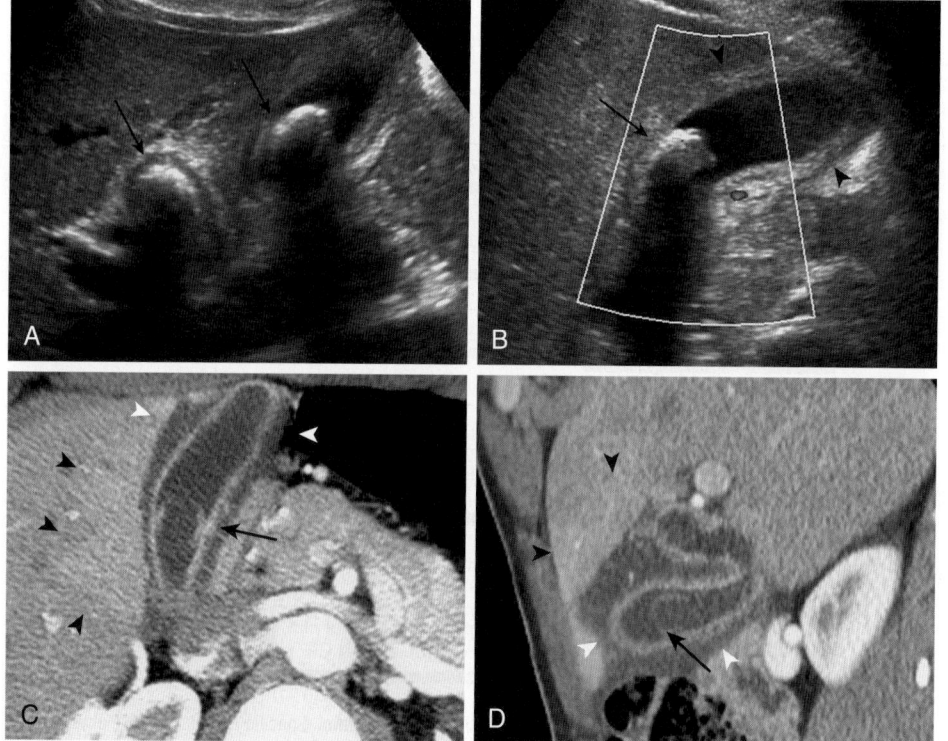

FIG. 5 A 43-year-old man with acute cholecystitis. Ultrasound images **(A** and **B)** demonstrate echogenic, shadowing gallstones *(arrows)* with gallbladder wall thickening *(arrowheads)* in a patient in whom a sonographic Murphy's sign was elicited. Axial **(C)** and sagittal **(D)** portal venous phase computed tomography images reveal a gallstone *(arrows),* as well as a thickened gallbladder wall *(white arrowheads).* Although not acquired in the arterial phase of contrast, hepatic hyperenhancement consistent with secondary inflammation is nevertheless seen *(black arrowheads).*These findings are specific for this life-threatening complication and should be recognized and treated urgently. (Soto JA, Lucey BC: Emergency Radiology, the requisites, 2nd ed, ISBN# 978-0-323-37640-2, 2017, Elsevier.)

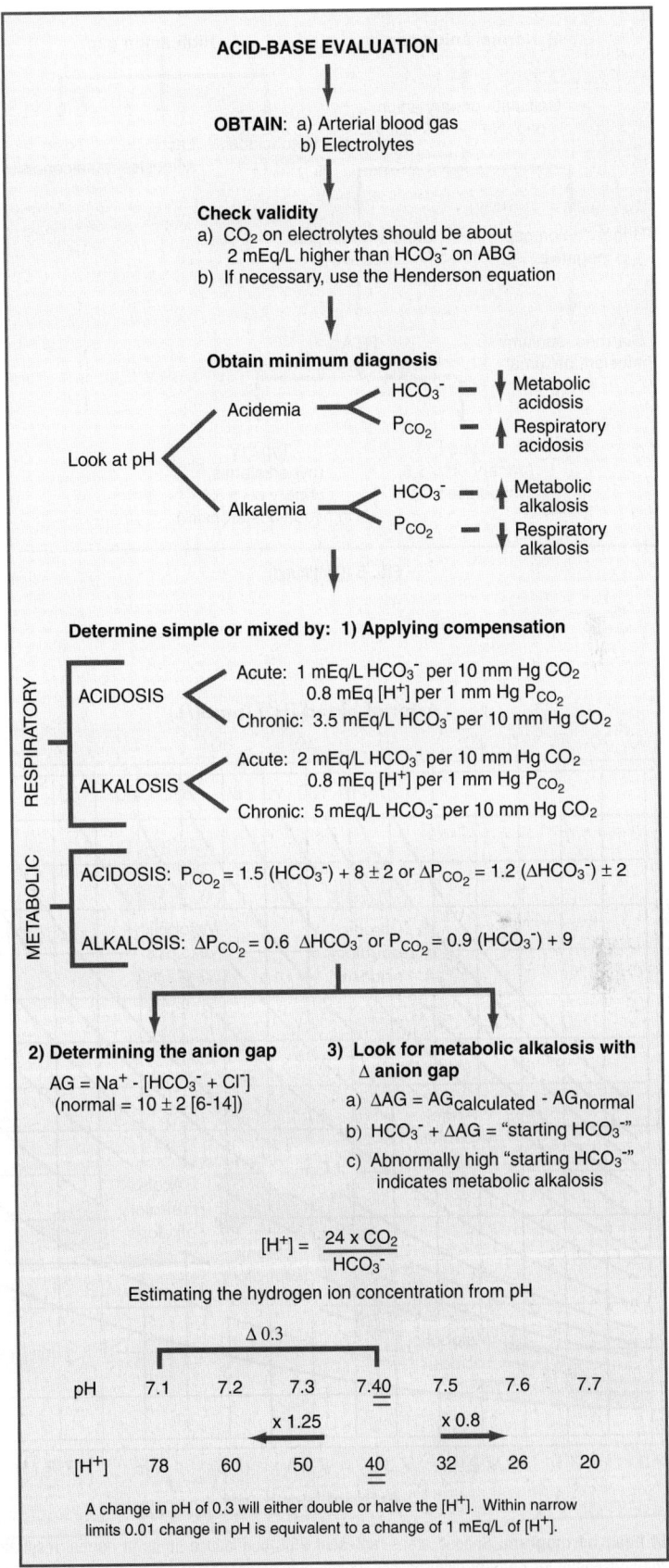

FIG. 6 Scheme for assessing acid-base homeostasis. (Modified from Andreoli TE [ed]: *Cecil essentials of medicine,* ed 7, Philadelphia, 2008, Saunders.)

Continued on next page

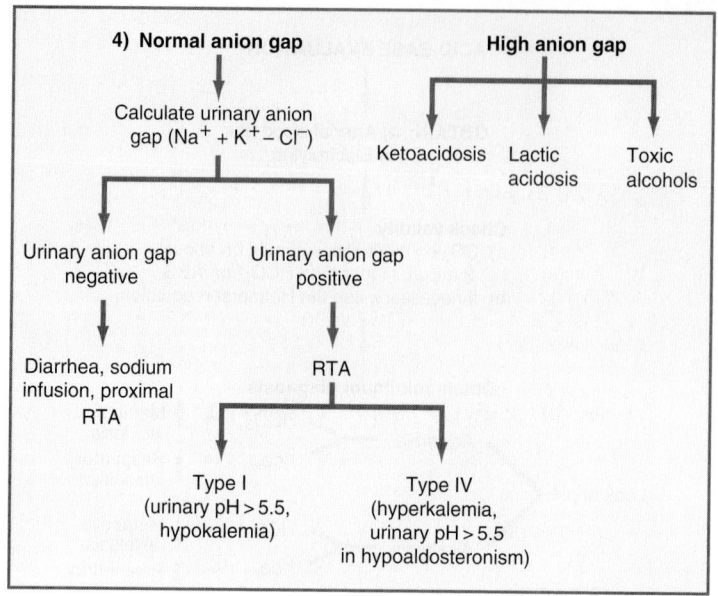

FIG. 6 (Continued)

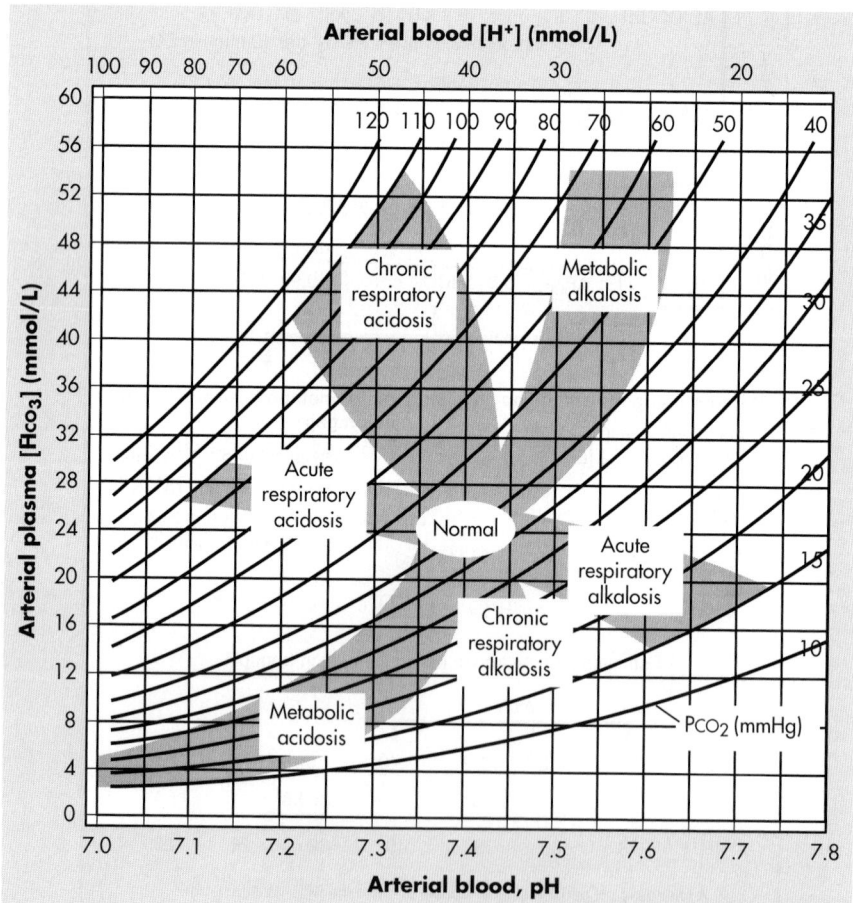

FIG. 7 Acid base normogram. Shaded areas represent 95% confidence limits of normal respiratory and metabolic compensations for primary disturbances. Points outside shaded areas represent a mixed disorder, assuming absence of laboratory error. (From Vincent JL, et al: *Textbook of critical care*, ed 6, Philadelphia, 2011, Saunders.)

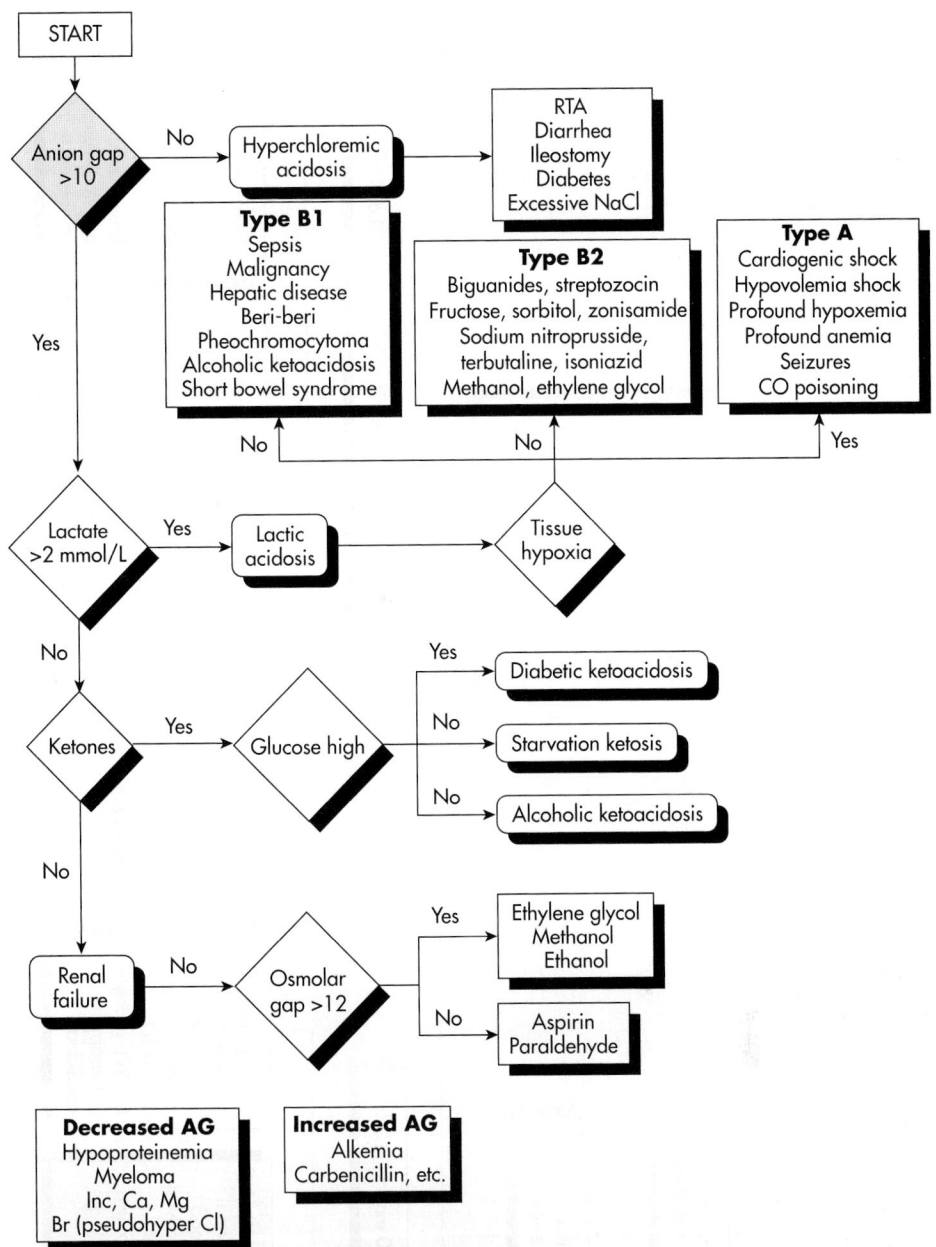

FIG. 8 Diagnostic approach to metabolic acidosis. (Modified from Vincent JL, Ahraham E, Moore FA, et al: *Textbook of critical care*, ed 6, Philadelphia, 2011, Saunders.)

Clinical
Algorithms

III

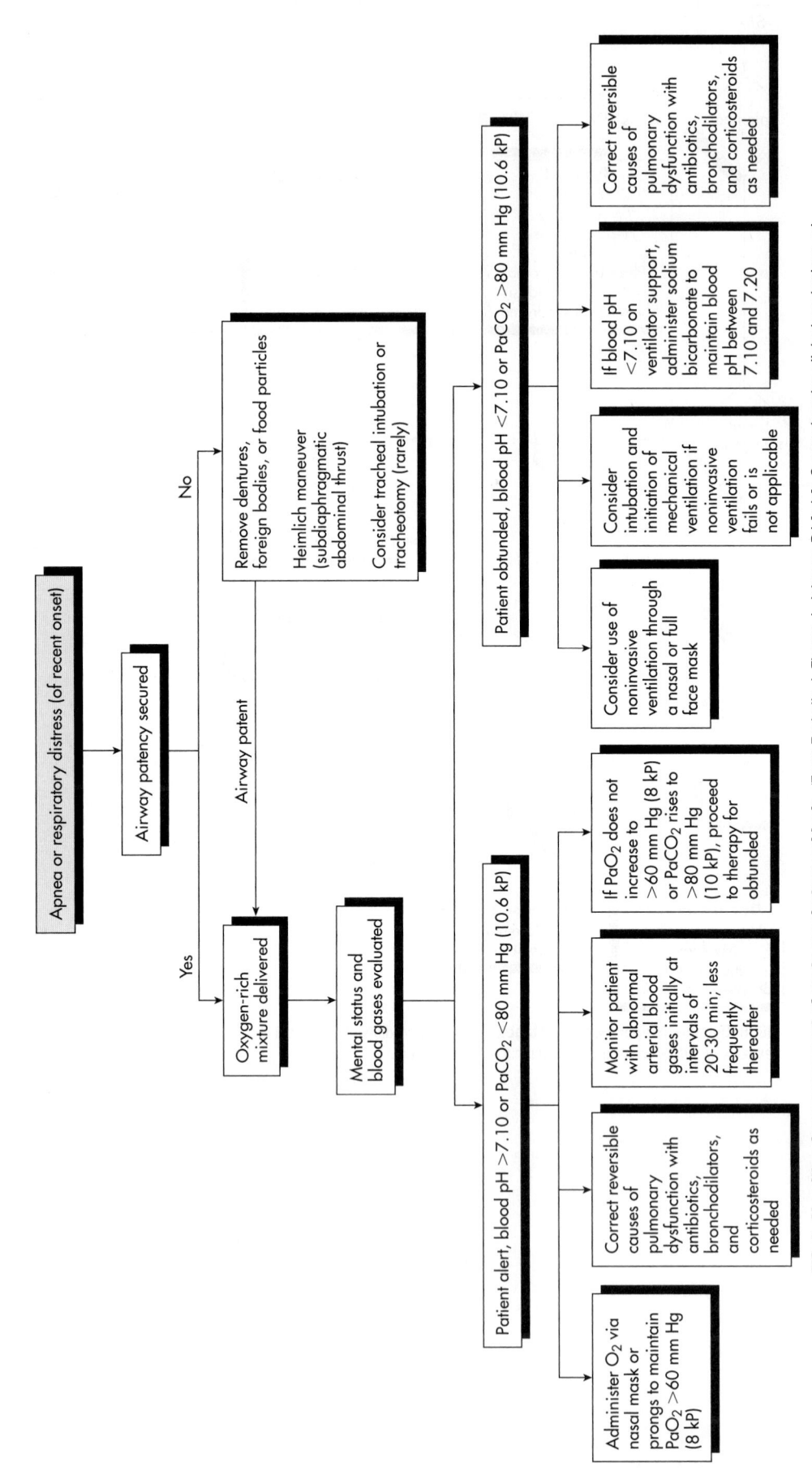

FIG. 9 Algorithm for management of acute respiratory acidosis. (From Feehally J, Floege J, Johnson RJ [eds]: *Comprehensive clinical nephrology*, ed 3, St Louis, 2007, Mosby.)

Apnea or respiratory distress (of recent onset)

Airway patency secured

No → Remove dentures, foreign bodies, or food particles

Heimlich maneuver (subdiaphragmatic abdominal thrust)

Consider tracheal intubation or tracheotomy (rarely)

Yes → Oxygen-rich mixture delivered

Airway patent

Mental status and blood gases evaluated

Patient alert, blood pH >7.10 or PaCO₂ <80 mm Hg (10.6 kP)

Administer O₂ via nasal mask or prongs to maintain PaO₂ >60 mm Hg (8 kP)

Correct reversible causes of pulmonary dysfunction with antibiotics, bronchodilators, and corticosteroids as needed

Monitor patient with abnormal arterial blood gases initially at intervals of 20-30 min; less frequently thereafter

If PaO₂ does not increase to >60 mm Hg (8 kP) or PaCO₂ rises to >80 mm Hg (10 kP), proceed to therapy for obtunded

Patient obtunded, blood pH <7.10 or PaCO₂ >80 mm Hg (10.6 kP)

Consider use of noninvasive ventilation through a nasal or full face mask

Consider intubation and initiation of mechanical ventilation if noninvasive ventilation fails or is not applicable

If blood pH <7.10 on ventilator support, administer sodium bicarbonate to maintain blood pH between 7.10 and 7.20

Correct reversible causes of pulmonary dysfunction with antibiotics, bronchodilators, and corticosteroids as needed

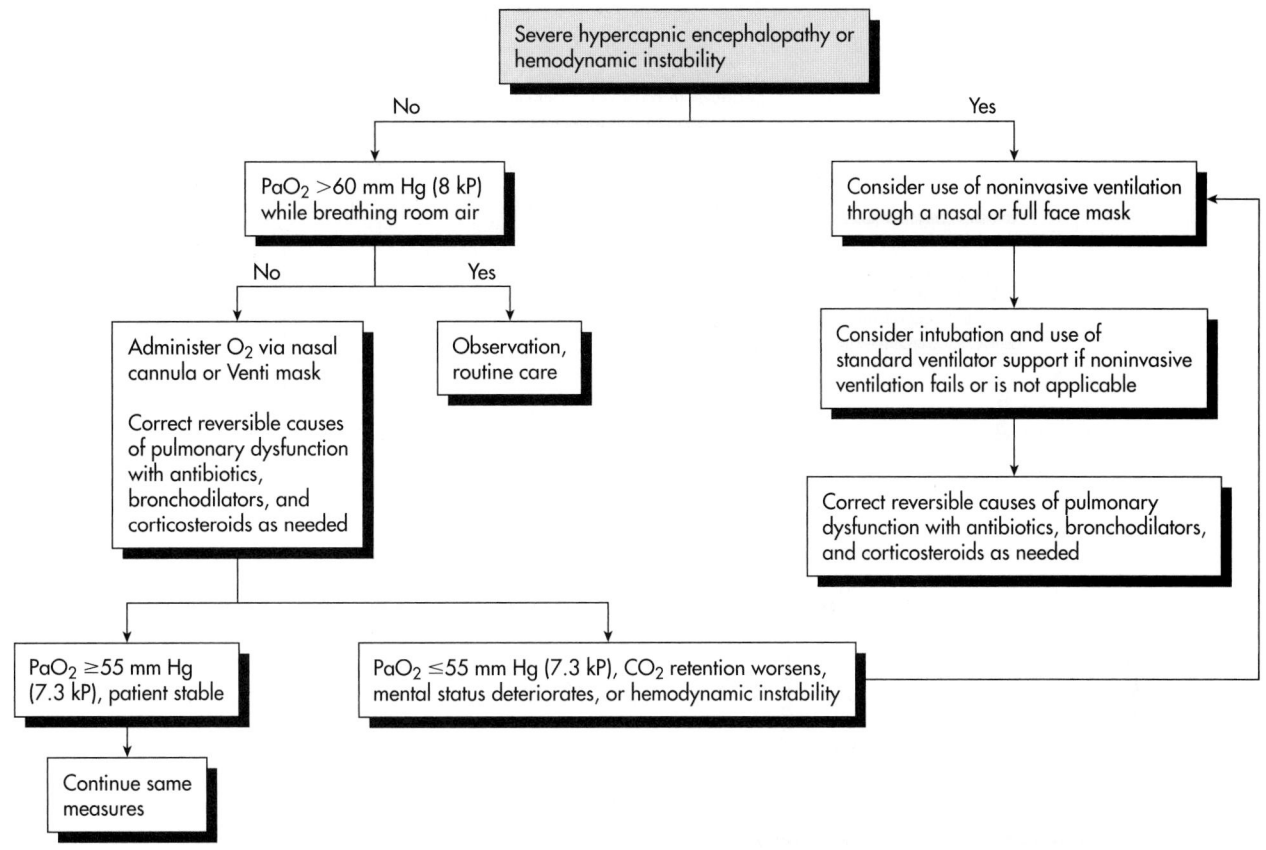

FIG. 10 Algorithm for management of chronic respiratory acidosis. (From Feehally J, Floege J, Johnson RJ [eds]: *Comprehensive clinical nephrology,* ed 3, St Louis, 2007, Mosby.)

ICD-10CM # C74.90 Malignant neoplasm of unspecified part of
unspecified adrenal gland
E27.8 Other specified disorders of adrenal gland

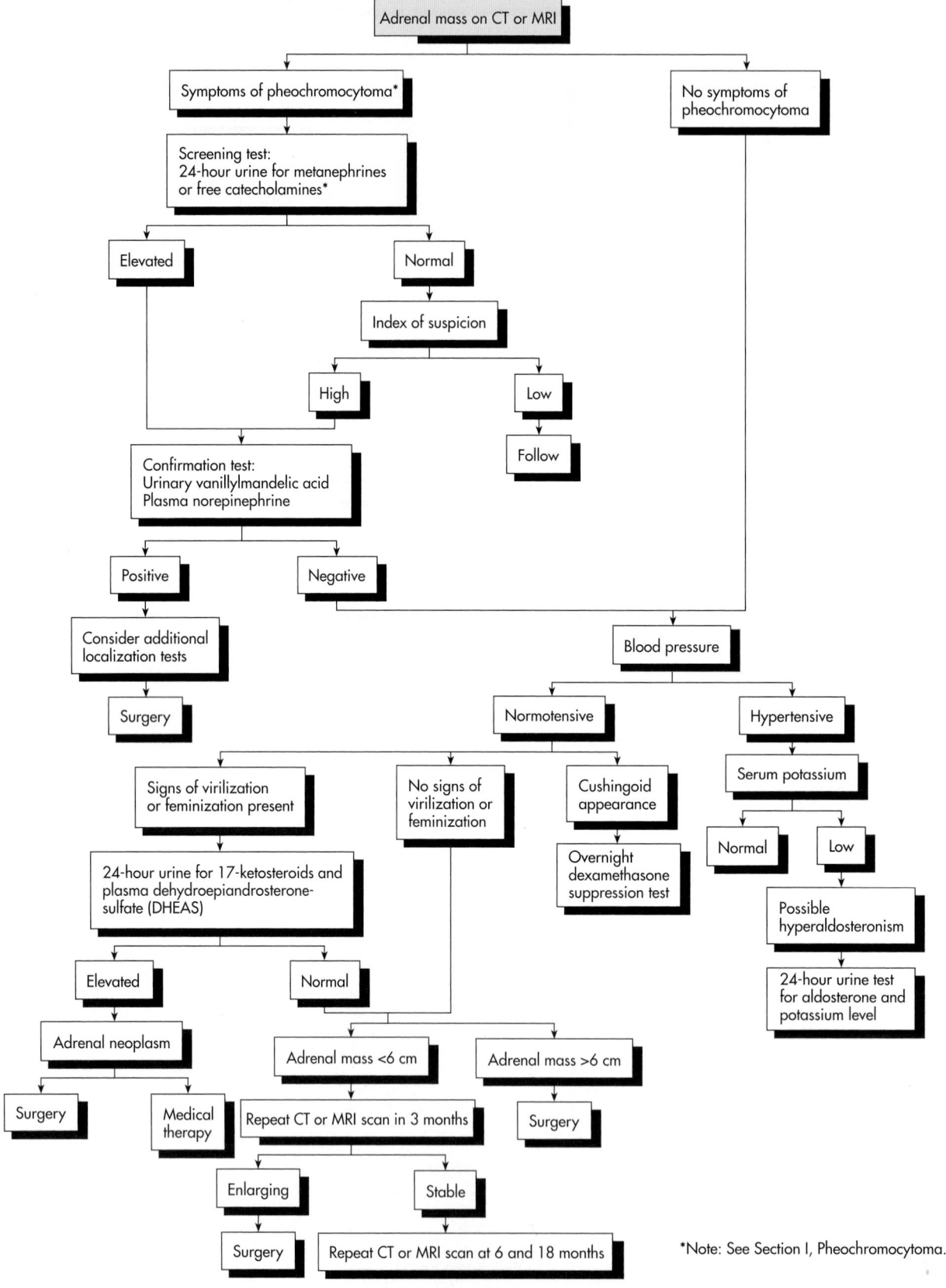

FIG. 12 Evaluation of adrenal mass. *CT,* Computed tomography; *MRI,* magnetic resonance imaging.
(Modified from Greene HL, Johnson WP, Lemcke D [eds]: *Decision making in medicine,* ed 2, St Louis, 1998, Mosby.)

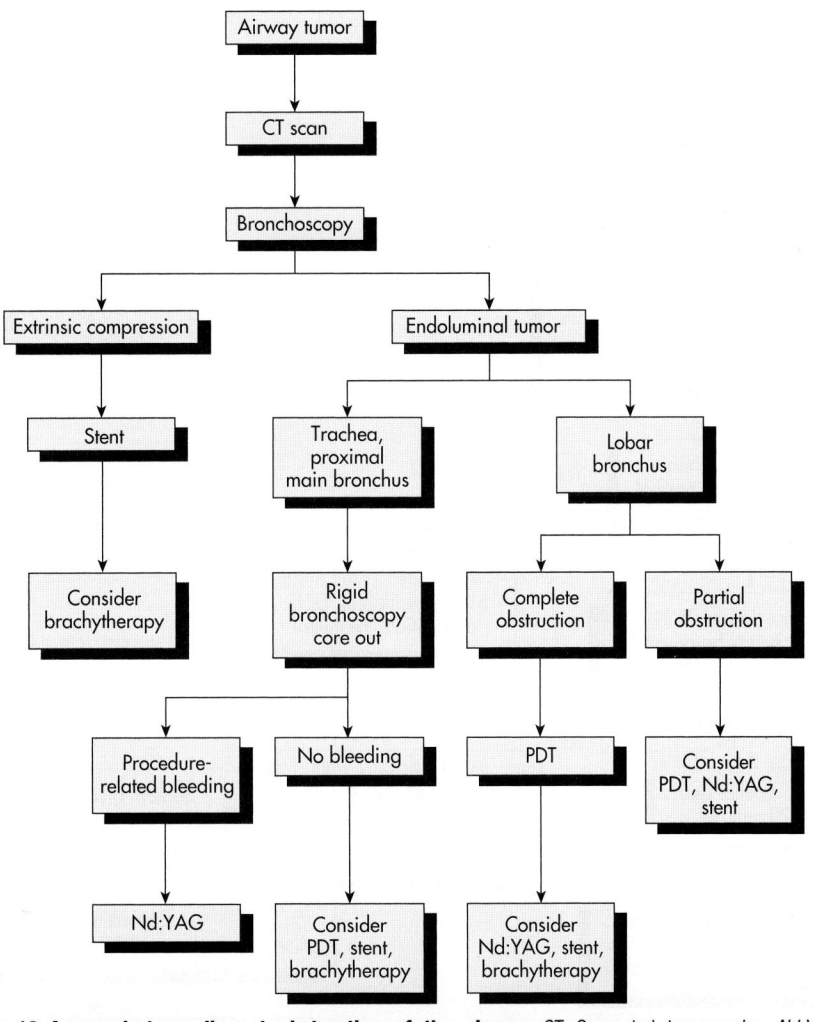

FIG. 13 Approach to malignant obstruction of the airway. *CT,* Computed tomography; *Nd:YAG,* neodymium:yttrium-aluminum-garnet; *PDT,* photodynamic therapy. (Sellke FW, del Nido PJ, Swanson SJ: Sabiston & Spencer Surgery of the Chest, 9th ed. ISBN # 978-0-323-24126-7, 2016, Elsevier.)

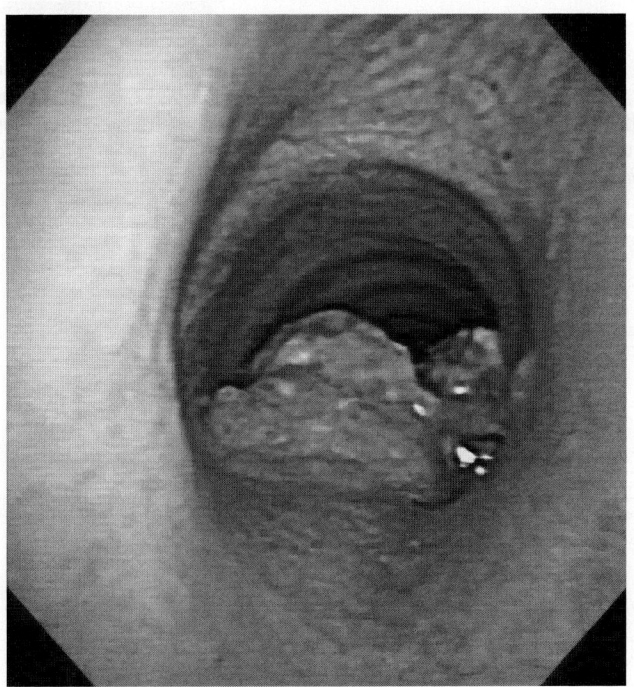

FIG. 14 An exophytic squamous cell carcinoma of the trachea. (Sellke FW, del Nido PJ, Swanson SJ: Sabiston & Spencer Surgery of the Chest, 9th ed. ISBN # 978-0-323-24126-7, 2016, Elsevier.)

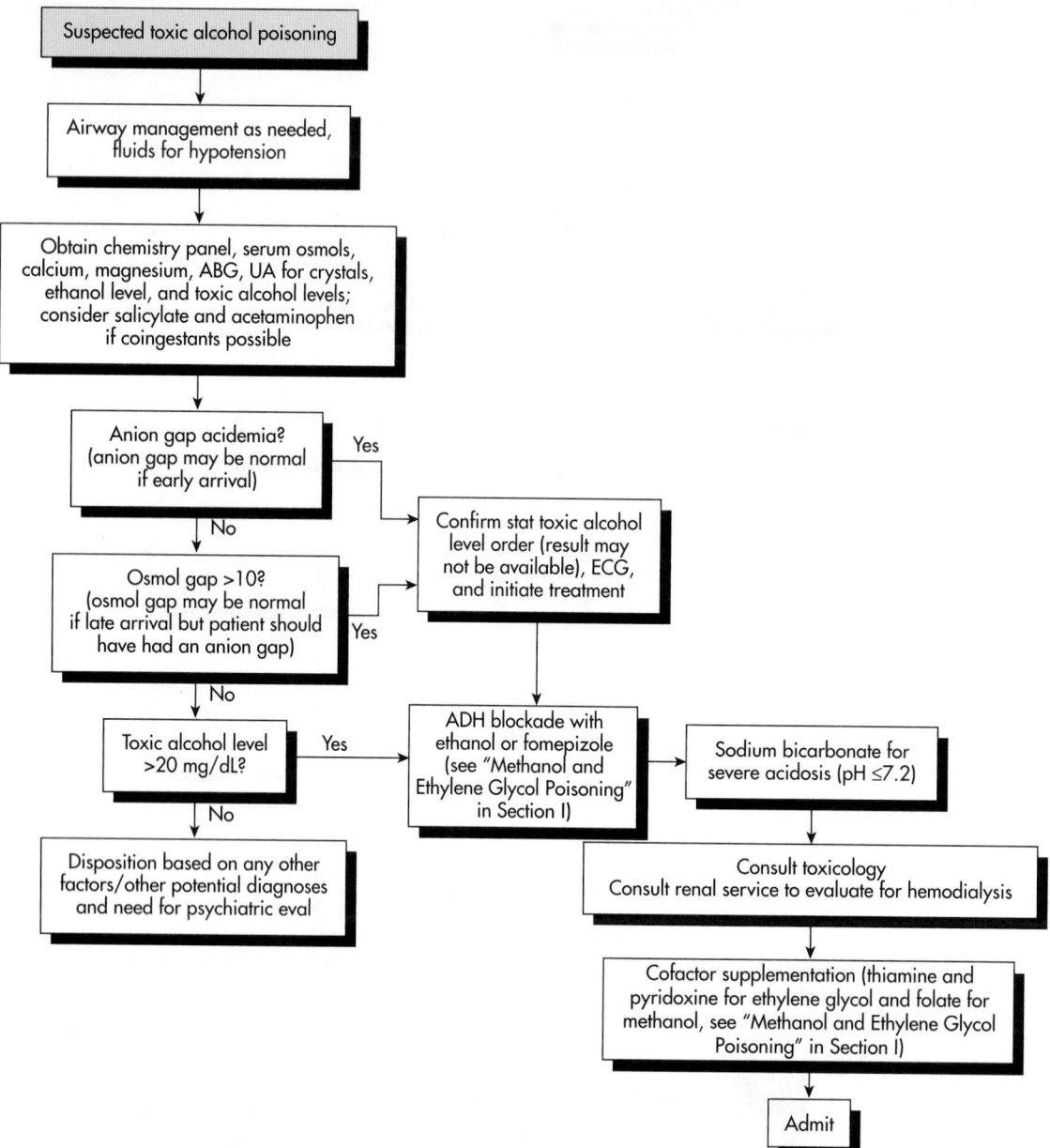

FIG. 15 Treatment algorithm for toxic alcohol poisoning. *ABG*, arterial blood gas measurements; *ADH*, alcohol dehydrogenase; *ECG*, electrocardiography; *UA*, urinalysis. (From Adams JG et al: *Emergency medicine, clinical essentials*, ed 2, Philadelphia, 2013, Elsevier.)

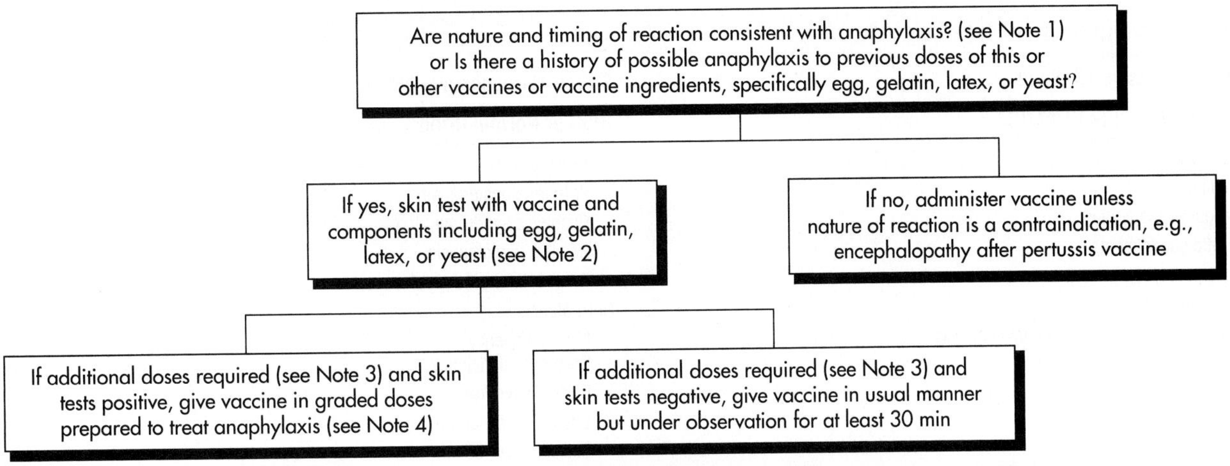

Are nature and timing of reaction consistent with anaphylaxis? (see Note 1) or Is there a history of possible anaphylaxis to previous doses of this or other vaccines or vaccine ingredients, specifically egg, gelatin, latex, or yeast?

If yes, skin test with vaccine and components including egg, gelatin, latex, or yeast (see Note 2)

If no, administer vaccine unless nature of reaction is a contraindication, e.g., encephalopathy after pertussis vaccine

If additional doses required (see Note 3) and skin tests positive, give vaccine in graded doses prepared to treat anaphylaxis (see Note 4)

If additional doses required (see Note 3) and skin tests negative, give vaccine in usual manner but under observation for at least 30 min

FIG. 16 Suggested approach to suspected immediate-type allergic reactions to vaccines.
Note 1. Are nature and timing of reaction consistent with a systemic IgE-mediated reaction? *Probable systemic IgE-mediated reaction:* reaction occurring within 4 hours of vaccine administration to include signs and/or symptoms from more than one of the following systems: *Possible systemic IgE-mediated reaction:*

- Dermatologic: urticaria, flushing, angioedema, pruritus.
- Respiratory: rhinoconjunctivitis (red, watery, itchy eyes, stuffy, runny, itchy nose, sneezing), upper airway edema (change in voice, difficulty swallowing, difficulty breathing, stridor), bronchospasm/asthma (cough, wheeze, shortness of breath, chest tightness).
- Cardiovascular: hypotension, tachycardia, palpitations, light-headedness, loss of consciousness (note: hypotension or loss of consciousness with pallor and bradycardia is much more likely to be due to a vasovagal reaction).
- Gastrointestinal: cramping, nausea, vomiting, diarrhea.

Possible systemic IgE-mediated reaction:
- Signs and/or symptoms from only one system (as previously)
- Signs and/or symptoms from more than one system (as previously) but occurring more than 4 hours after vaccination

Note 2. Skin tests with vaccine and components including egg, gelatin, latex, or yeast. *Vaccine skin tests:*
Vaccine component skin tests:
- Prick test with full-strength vaccine; consider 1 : 10 dilution if patient has a history of life-threatening reaction.
- If results of prick test with full-strength vaccine are negative, perform intradermal testing with 0.02 mL of vaccine at a 1 : 100 dilution.
- Vaccine skin tests may cause false (or clinically irrelevant) positive reactions. Thus, if skin testing gives a positive reaction, also perform on normal control subjects.

Vaccine component skin tests:
- Prick tests with commercial extracts of egg (influenza and yellow fever vaccines) or Saccharomyces cerevisiae yeast (hepatitis B and quadrivalent human papillomavirus vaccines).
- Prick test with sugared gelatin (e.g., Jell-O): dissolve 1 teaspoon of gelatin powder in 5 mL of normal saline.
- Vaccines that contain gelatin: influenza (some brands), measles, mumps, rabies (some brands), rubella, typhoid (capsule), varicella, yellow fever, zoster.
- Prick test with latex: soak 2 fingers of latex glove or a toy balloon in 5 ml of normal saline. Vaccines that contain latex in packaging: available at http://www.cdc.gov/vaccines/pubs/pinkbook/downloads/appendices/B/latex-table.pdf.
- In vitro assays for specific IgE antibody to egg, gelatin, latex, and yeast also are commercially available as an alternative or complement to skin testing.

Note 3. If fewer than the recommended number of doses are received, consider measuring level of IgG antibodies to immunizing agent. If the measured level is associated with protection from disease, consider withholding additional doses, although magnitude and duration of immunity may be less than if all doses received.

Note 4. Vaccine administration in graded doses:
- With a vaccine for which the usual dose is 0.5 mL, administer graded doses of vaccine at 15-minute intervals: 0.05 mL of 1 : 10 dilution, 0.05 mL of full strength, 0.10 mL of full strength, 0.15 mL of full strength, 0.20 Ml of full strength (From Adkinson NF, et al: *Middleton's allergy principles and practice*, ed 8, Philadelphia, 2014, Saunders.)

Clinical Algorithms

Table 2 Diagnosis of Metabolic Alkalosis

Saline-Responsive Alkalosis	Saline-Unresponsive Alkalosis
Low Urinary [Cl⁻] (<10 mEq/L)	**High or Normal Urinary [Cl⁻] (>15-20 mEq/L)**
Normotensive	Hypertensive
Vomiting	Primary aldosteronism
Nasogastric aspiration	Cushing's syndrome
Diuretic use (distant)	Renal artery stenosis
Posthypercapnia	Renal failure plus alkali therapy
Villous adenoma	Normotensive
Bicarbonate treatment of organic acidosis	Mg^{2+} deficiency
	Severe K^+ deficiency
K^+ deficiency	Bartter's syndrome
Hypertensive	Gitelman's syndrome
Liddle's syndrome	Diuretic use (recent)

Skorecki K, Chertow GM, Marsden PA, Taal MW, Yu ASL, Wasser WG: Brenner & Rector's the kidney, ed 10, Elsevier, ISBN # 978-1-4557-4836-5, Philadelphia, 2016.

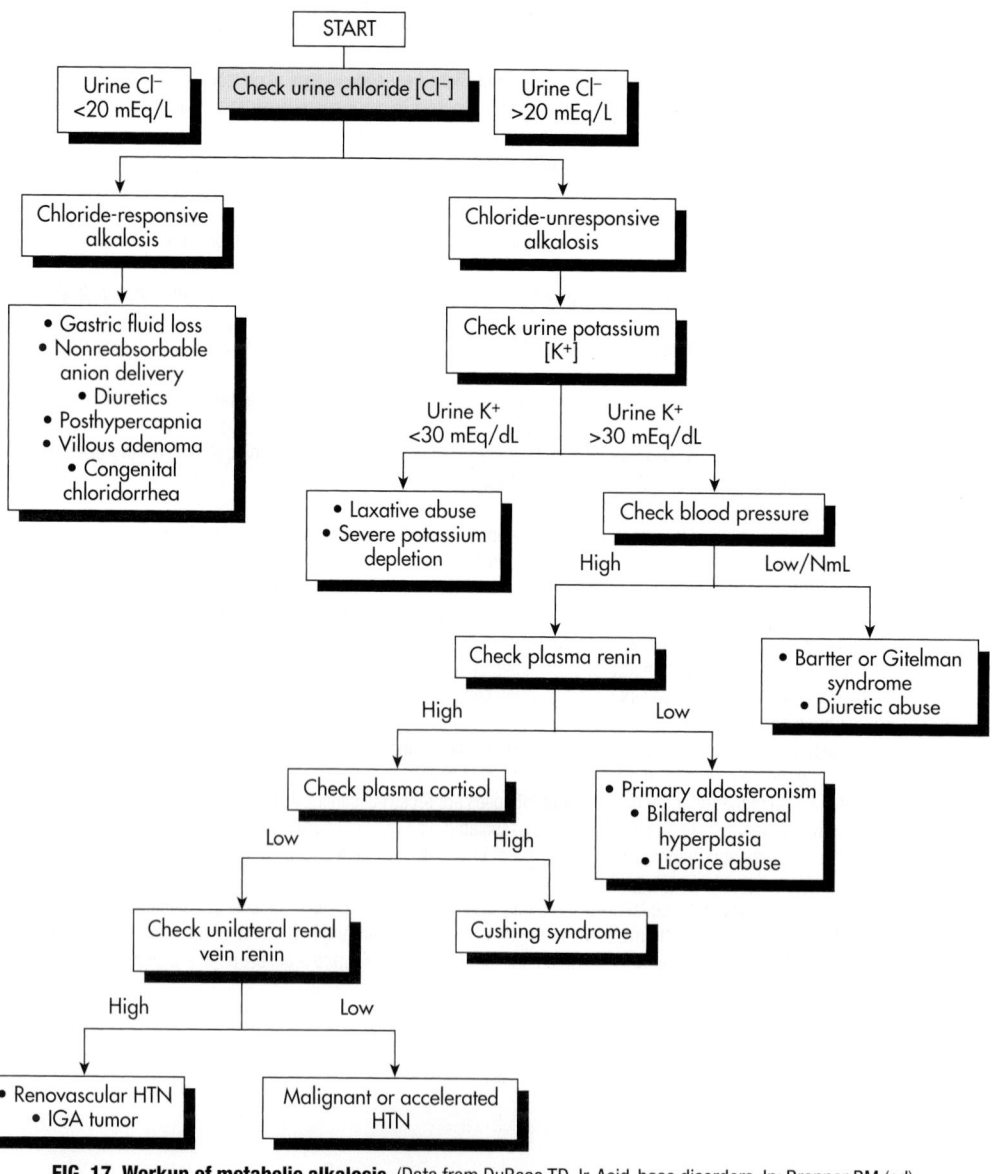

FIG. 17 Workup of metabolic alkalosis. (Data from DuBose TD Jr. Acid-base disorders. In: Brenner BM (ed). *Brenner and Rector's the kidney*, ed 8, Philadelphia, 2008, Saunders, p. 513.)

ALKALOSIS, RESPIRATORY TREATMENT

Respiratory alkalosis

→ Implement cause-specific measures

Hypoxemia
→ Yes → **Oxygen therapy**

Mechanical hyperventilation
→ Yes → Addition of dead space or change mode of ventilation (e.g., assist-control to mandatory ventilation) → If persistent, sedation with or without skeletal muscle paralysis

Salicylate intoxication
→ Yes → Consider: Induced emesis/gastric lavage, activated charcoal with sorbitol, forced diuresis, urinary alkalinization, hemodialysis (severe poisoning)

Psychogenic hyperventilation
→ Yes → Consider having patient rebreathe into a closed system

Acute mountain sickness (preventive treatment)
→ Yes → Slower ascent, acetazolamide, oxygen therapy

Sepsis, circulatory failure, hepatic failure, other causes
→ Yes → Specific measures tailored to the underlying cause

Blood pH ≥7.55
→ Yes → Hemodynamic instability, altered mental status, or cardiac arrhythmias → Yes → Consider measures to correct blood pH ≤7.50 by:

1. Reducing HCO_3^-: acetazolamide; ultrafiltration and isotonic saline replacement; hemodialysis using a low HCO_3^- bath

2. Increasing $PaCO_2$: rebreathing into a closed system; control hypoventilation by ventilator with or without skeletal muscle paralysis

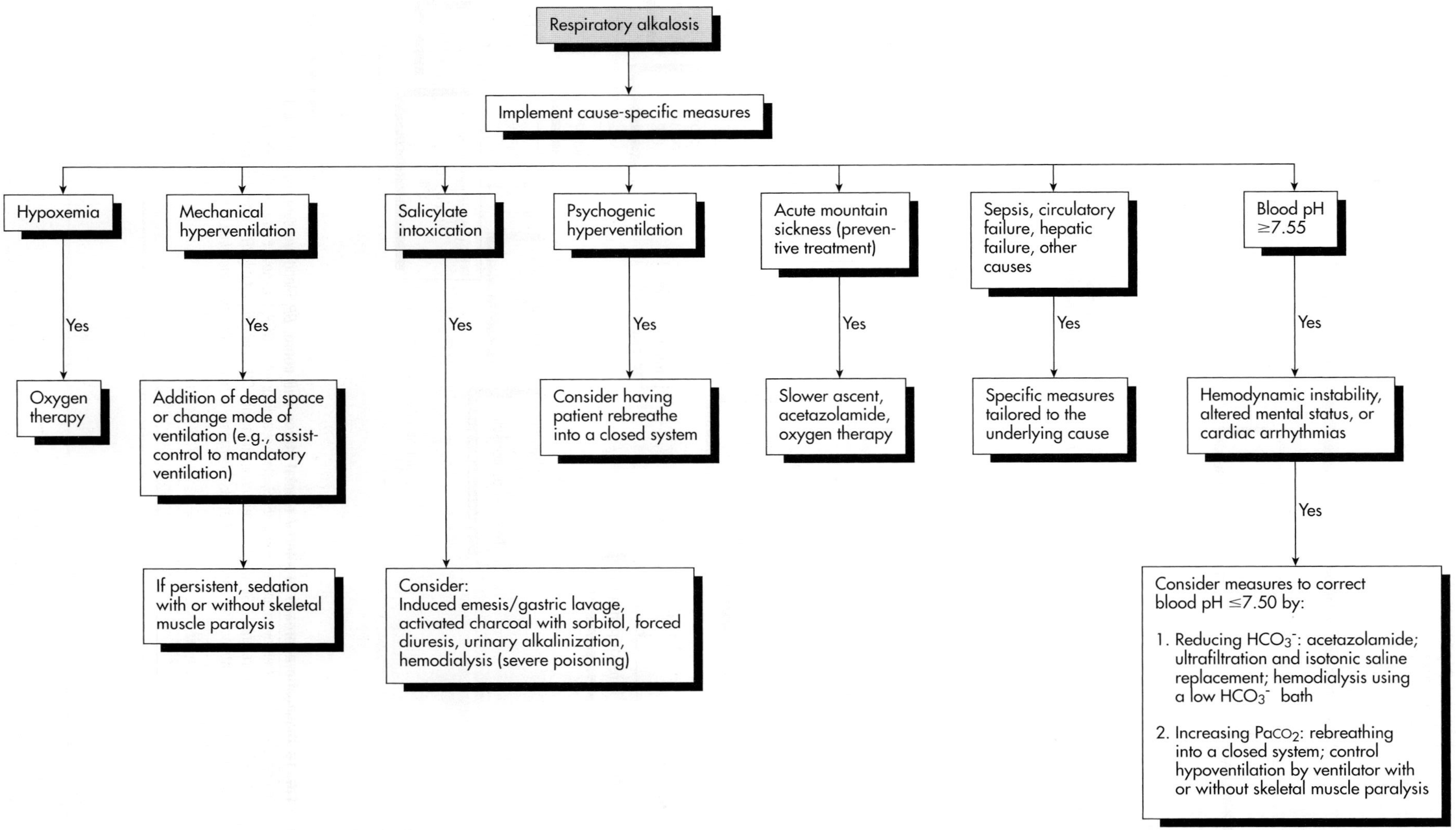

FIG. 18 Recommended treatment of respiratory alkalosis. (From Feehally J, Floege J, Johnson RJ [eds]: *Comprehensive clinical nephrology*, ed 3, St Louis, 2007, Mosby.)

Clinical Algorithms

III

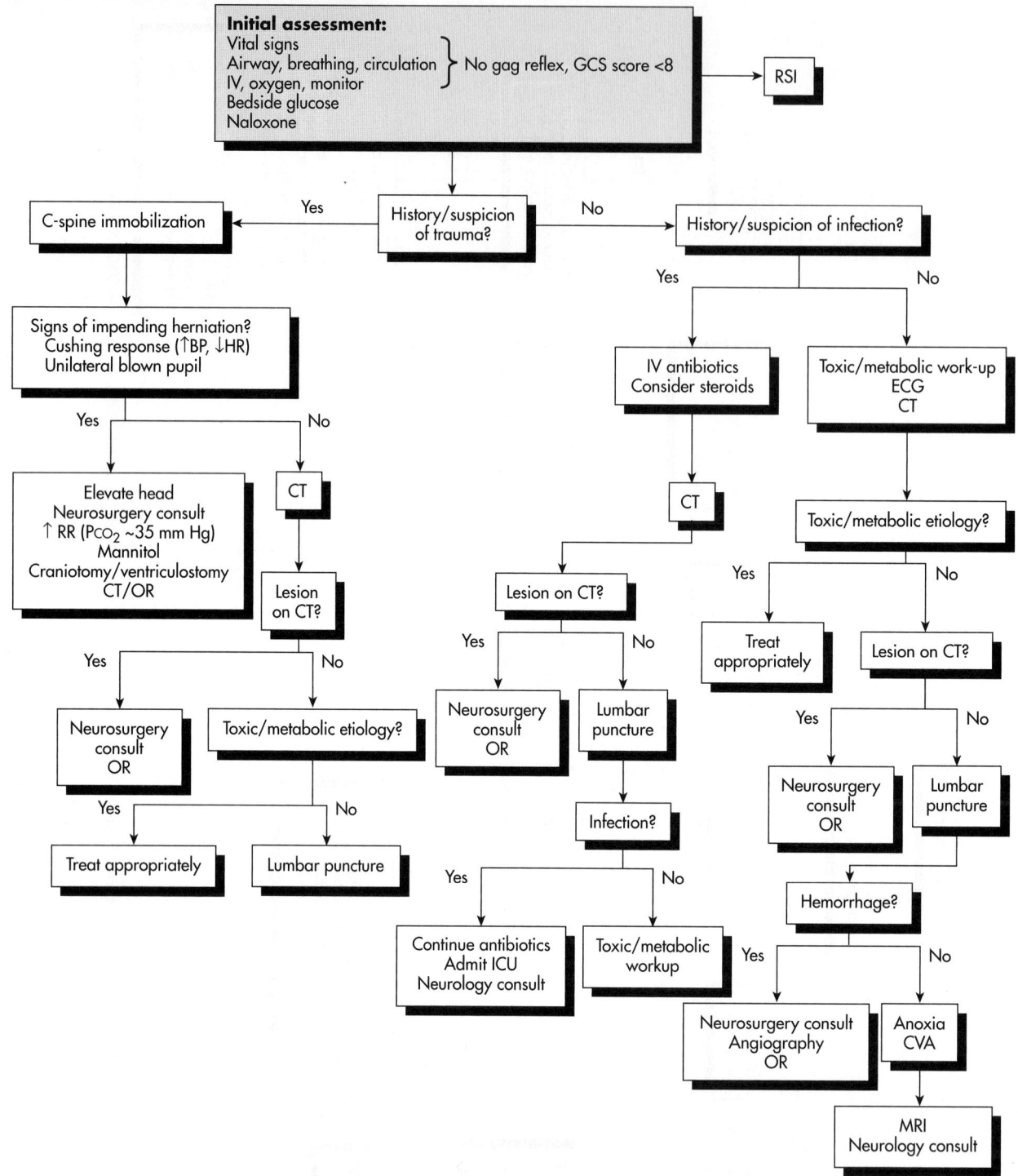

FIG. 19 Diagnostic approach to altered mental status and coma. *BP,* Blood pressure; *CT,* computed tomography; *CVA,* cerebrovascular accident; *ECG,* electrocardiography; *GCS,* Glasgow Coma Scale; *HR,* heart rate; *ICU,* intensive care unit; *MRI,* magnetic resonance imaging; *OR,* operating room; *RR,* respiratory rate; *RSI,* rapid-sequence intubation. (From Adams JG et al: *Emergency medicine, clinical essentials,* ed 2, Philadelphia, 2013, Elsevier.)

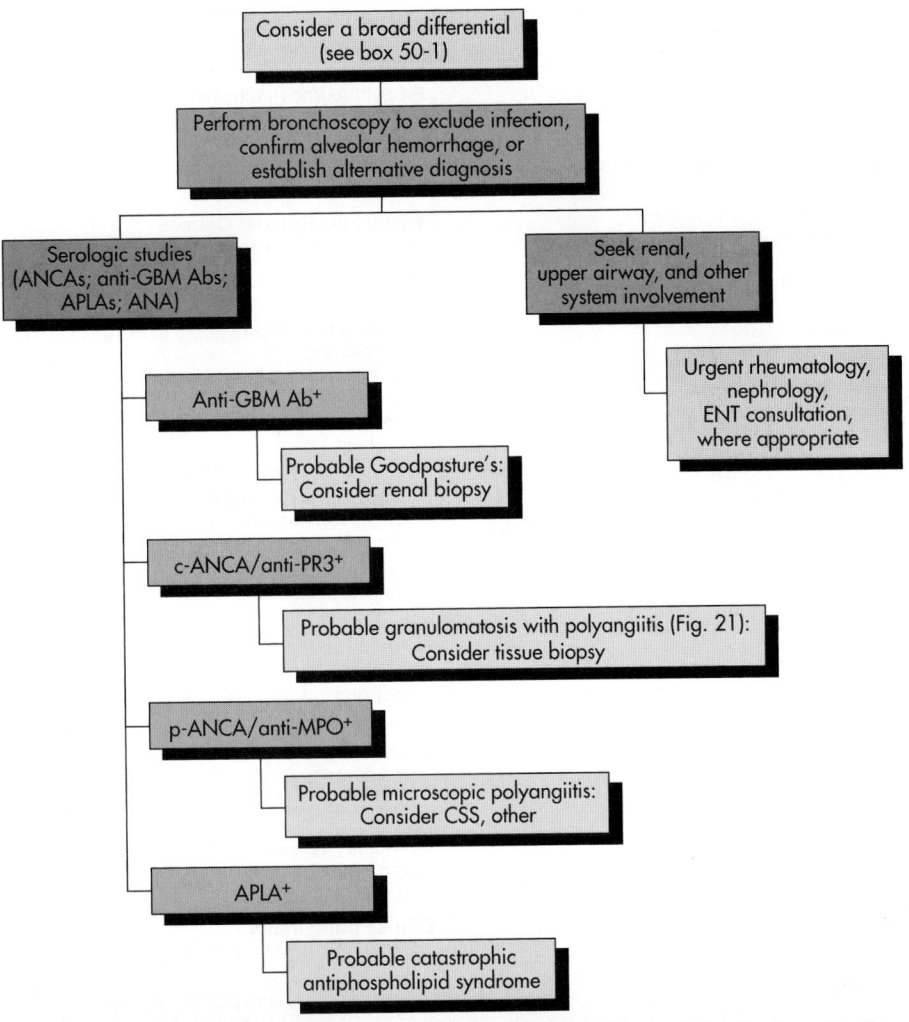

FIG. 20 Diagnosis and management of alveolar hemorrhage syndromes. *ANA*, antinuclear antibodies; *ANCA*, antineutrophil cytoplasmic antibody; *anti-GBM Abs*, anti–glomerular basement membrane antibodies; *anti-MPO*, antimyeloperoxidase antibodies; *anti-PR3*, antiproteinase antibodies; *APLAs*, antiphospholipid antibodies; *CSS*, Churg-Strauss syndrome; *ENT*, ear, nose, and throat. (Parrillo JE, Dellinger RP: Critical Care Medicine, Principles of Diagnosis and Management in the Adult, 4th ed, ISBN # 978-0-323-08929-6, 2014, Elsevier.)

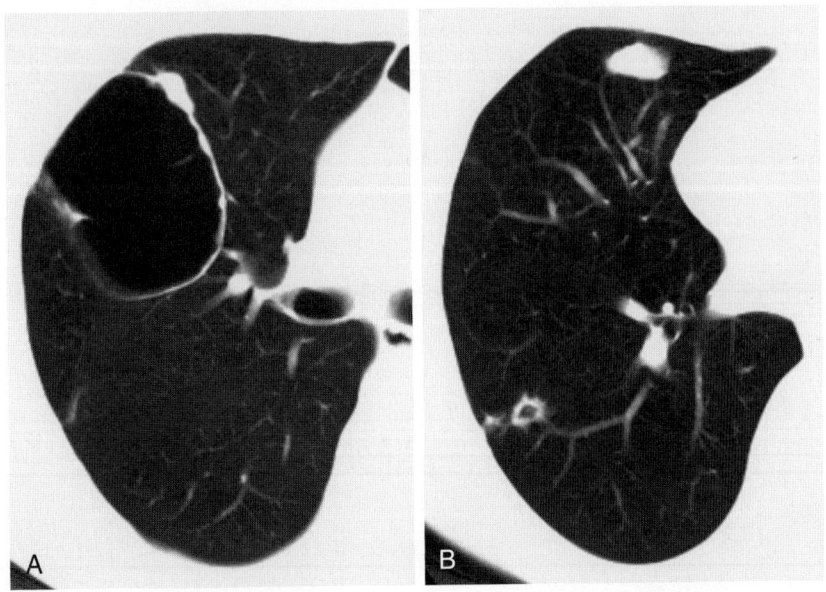

FIG. 21 Granulomatosis with polyangiitis (Wegener's granulomatosis). A and **B**, Thin-walled cavities and nodules are present. (Webb WR, Brandt WE, Major NM: Fundamentals of body CT, 4th ed, Philadelphia, Elsevier, 2015, ISBN# 978-0-323-22146-7.)

BOX 1 Causes of Diffuse Alveolar Hemorrhage

Immunologic Diseases
Anti–glomerular basement membrane antibody disease (Goodpasture's syndrome)
Vasculitides associated with circulating or in situ immune complexes
    Systemic lupus erythematosus
    Mixed connective tissue disease
    Schönlein-Henoch purpura
    Essential mixed cryoglobulinemia
    Tumor-related vasculitis
    Endocarditis-related vasculitis
    Polyarteritis nodosa
    Systemic necrotizing vasculitis
Vasculitides associated with antineutrophil cytoplasmic antibodies
    Granulomatosis with polyangiitis
    Microscopic polyangiitis
    Idiopathic necrotizing crescentic glomerulonephritis
Rapidly progressive glomerulonephritis
Associated with other connective tissue diseases, pathophysiology unknown
    Rheumatoid arthritis
    Progressive systemic sclerosis
    Behçet's disease
Associated with other renal diseases
IgA nephropathy
Diabetic nephropathy
Associated with precipitating antibodies to milk (Heiner's syndrome)
Idiopathic pulmonary hemosiderosis
Primary antiphospholipid antibody syndrome

Chemical or Drug-Related Causes
Amiodarone
D-Penicillamine
Isocyanates
Nitrofurantoin
Retinoic acid
Trimellitic anhydride
"Crack" cocaine
Sirolimus
Everolimus
Propylthiouracil-induced vasculitis
Erlotinib
Bevacizumab
Gemcitabine
Infliximab

Transplant-Related Causes
Bone marrow transplant
Renal transplant
Lung transplant

Bleeding Diathesis
Thrombocytopenia
Leukemia with diffuse alveolar damage
Viral pneumonia
Bacterial or fungal sepsis
Radiation
Chemotherapy toxic to lung
Blast counts >80,000/μL
Extrinsic anticoagulants/thrombolytics
Warfarin overdose
Tissue plasminogen activator
Platelet glycoprotein IIb/IIIa inhibitors
Coagulopathies
Cirrhosis
DIC

Infections
Legionnaires' disease

Pulmonary Venous Hypertension
Mitral stenosis
Mitral regurgitation
Pulmonary capillary hemangiomatosis
Pulmonary venoocclusive disease
Fibrosing mediastinitis
Congenital heart disease

Diffuse Lung Injury
Negative-pressure pulmonary hemorrhage
Breath-hold diving
Postictal neurogenic pulmonary edema

DIC, disseminated intravascular coagulation; *IgA*, immunoglobulin A.
Parrillo JE, Dellinger RP: Critical Care Medicine, Principles of Diagnosis and Management in the Adult, 4th ed, ISBN # 978-0-323-08929-6, 2014, Elsevier.

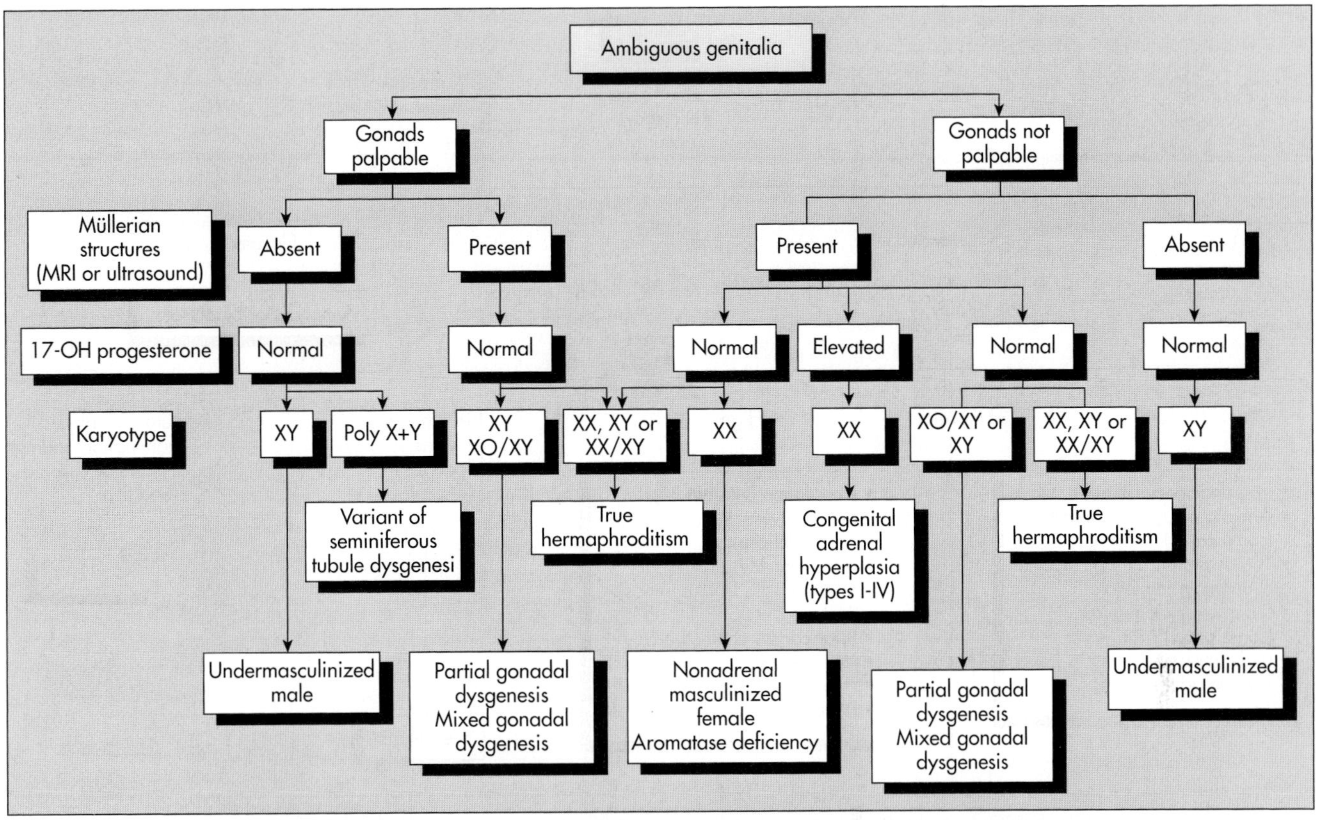

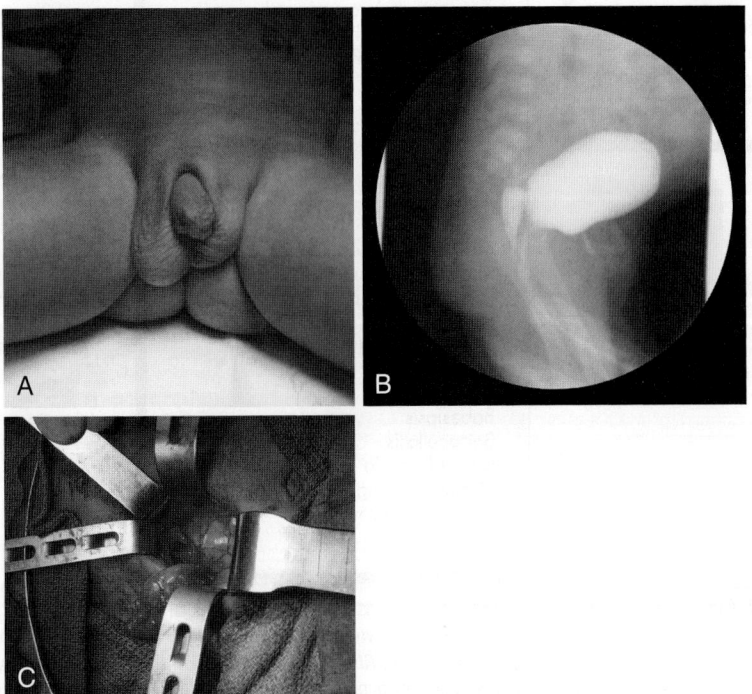

FIG. 22 Diagnostic algorithm for a newborn with ambiguous genitalia based on gonadal palpability, presence or absence of müllerian structures, 17-hydroxyprogesterone concentration, and karyotype. *MRI,* magnetic resonance imaging (Modified from Grumbach MM, Conte FH. Disorders of sex differentiation. In: Wilson JD, Foster DW, editors. Williams textbook of endocrinology. Philadelphia: Saunders; 1998. p. 1401.) (Wein AJ, Kavoussi LR, Partin AW, Peters CA: Campbell-Walsh Urology, 11th ed, ISBN# 978-1-4557-7567-5, 2016, Elsevier.)

FIG. 23 **A,** Patient with mixed gonadal dysgenesis showing asymmetrical anatomy. **B,** Hemiuterus and opacified fallopian tube in left inguinal hernia. **C,** Structures noted in **B** shown at surgical exploration. (Wein AJ, Kavoussi LR, Partin AW, Peters CA: Campbell-Walsh Urology, 11th ed, ISBN# 978-1-4557-7567-5, 2016, Elsevier.)

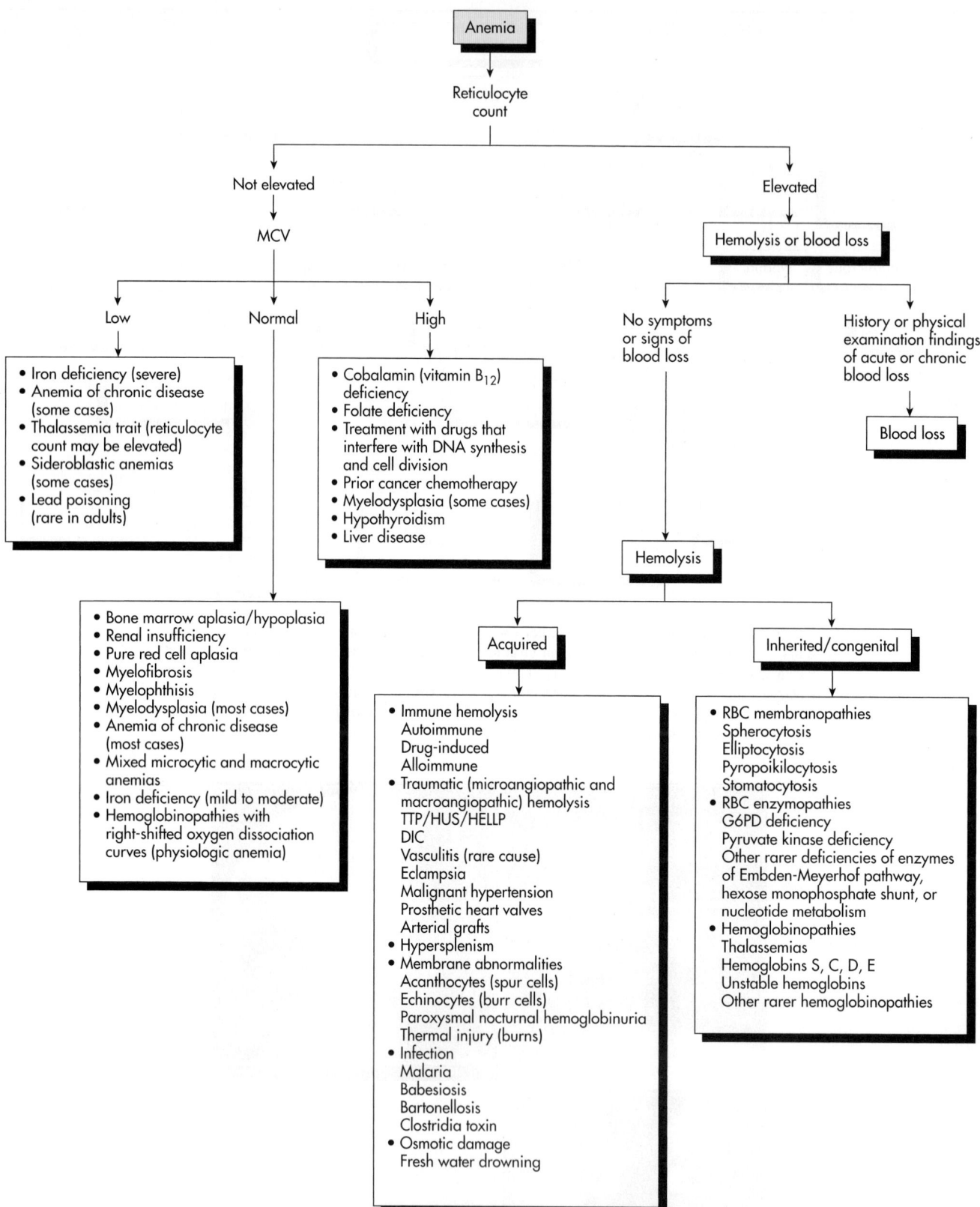

FIG. 24 Algorithm for diagnosis of anemias. *DIC,* Disseminated intravascular coagulation; *G6PD,* glucose-6-phosphate-dehydrogenase; *HELLP,* hepatomegaly-elevated liver (function tests)-low platelets; *HUS,* hemolytic-uremic syndrome; *MCV,* mean corpuscular volume; *RBC,* red blood cell; *TTP,* thrombotic thrombocytopenic purpura. (From Goldman L, Ausiello D [eds]: *Cecil textbook of medicine,* ed 23, Philadelphia, 2008, Saunders.)

Macrocytic anemia

Reticulocyte count, serum B₁₂ level, RBC folate, TSH, ALT, AST

Reticulocyte count elevated

Diagnosis: spurious elevation of MCV

Examine peripheral smear for indices of nonreticulocyte red cells

R/O acute blood loss

Reticulocyte count not elevated

No megaloblastic changes on peripheral blood smear

Abnormal liver function tests → Evaluate for causes of liver disease

Abnormal thyroid function tests → Correct hypothyroidism

Down syndrome → No treatment needed

Megaloblastic changes on peripheral blood smear (hypersegmented neutrophils)

Serum B₁₂ decreased → Diagnosis: B₁₂ deficiency → Evaluate for etiology (see Section I, "Anemia, Pernicious") → Initiate B₁₂ replacement

Serum B₁₂ normal, folate decreased* → Diagnosis: folic acid deficiency → Evaluate for dietary causes

Serum B₁₂ normal or increased, folate normal*

No possible offending medication → Consider serum methylmalonic acid if cobalamin deficiency is suspected and B₁₂ level is normal

Possible medication effect

Improvement with discontinuing medication → Change medication

No improvement with discontinuing medication → Bone marrow aspiration and biopsy to evaluate for myelodysplasia

Normal

Elevated → B₁₂ deficiency → Initiate replacement

*Measure both serum and RBC folate levels.

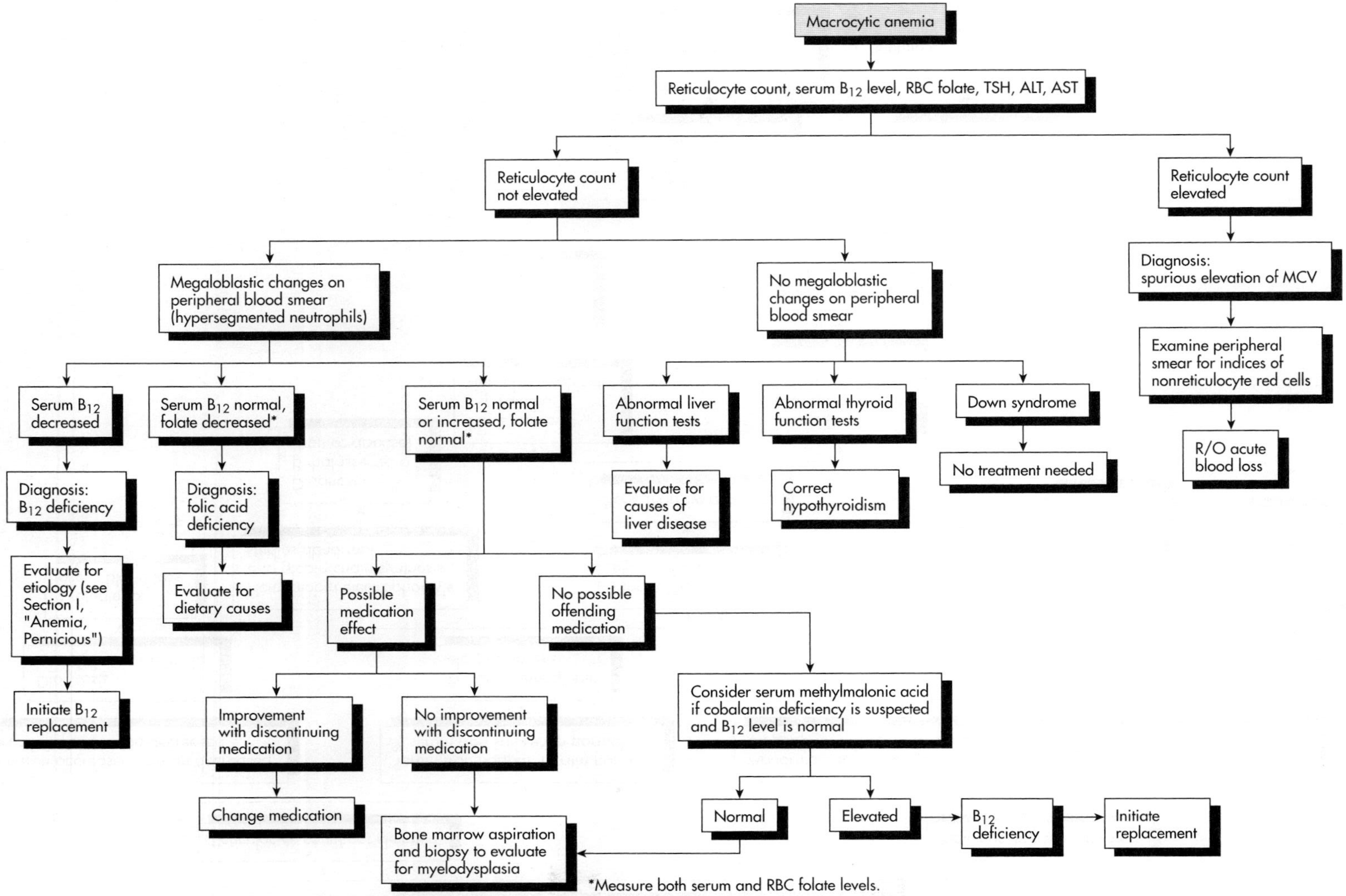

FIG. 26 Differential diagnosis of macrocytic anemia. *MCV,* Mean corpuscular volume. (Modified from Rakel RE [ed]: *Principles of family practice,* ed 7, Philadelphia, 2007, Saunders.)

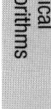

Clinical Algorithms

III

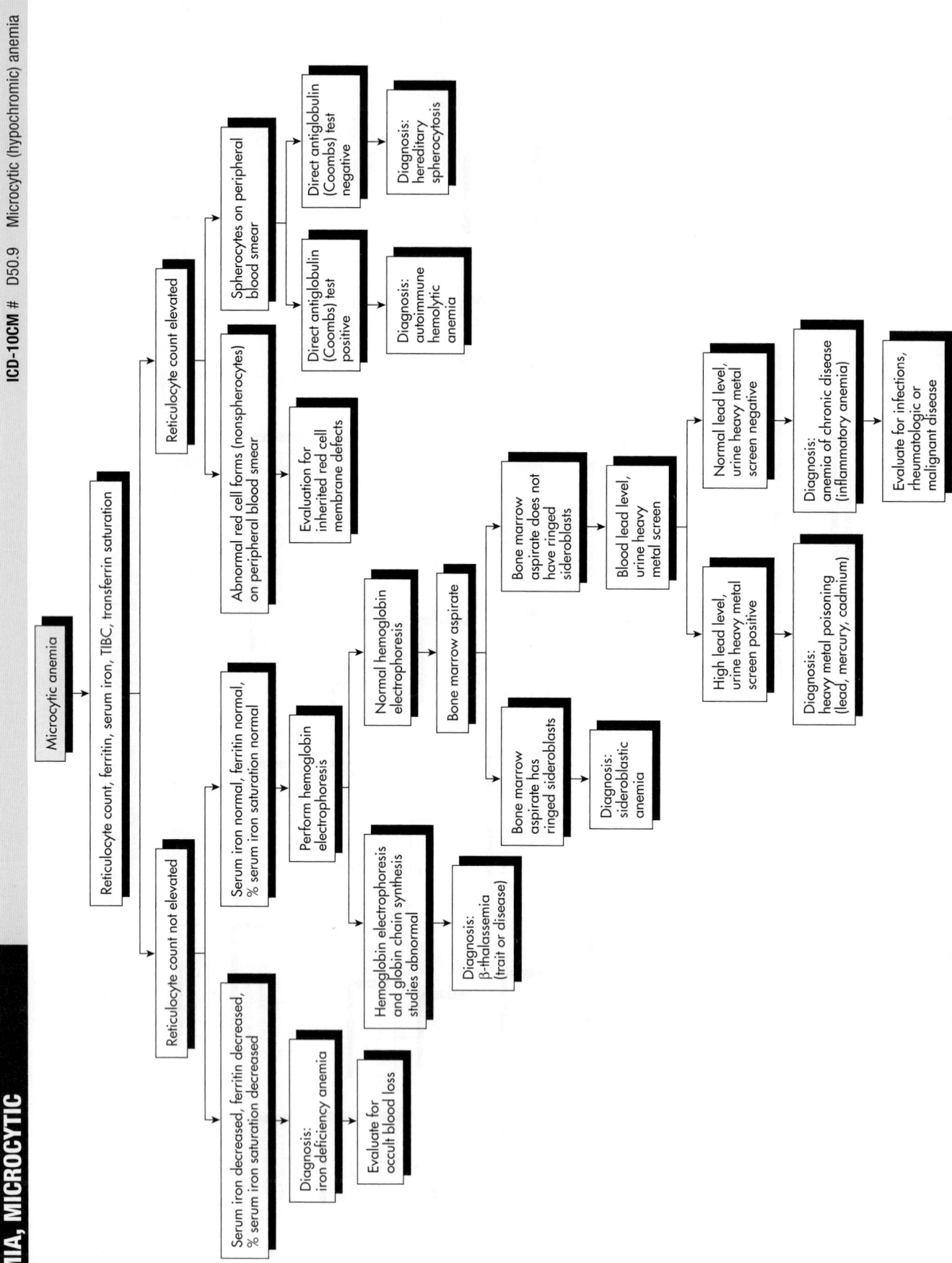

FIG. 27 Differential diagnosis of microcytic anemia. *TIBC,* Total iron binding capacity. (Modified from Rakel RE [ed]: *Principles of family practice,* ed 7, Philadelphia, 2007, Saunders.)

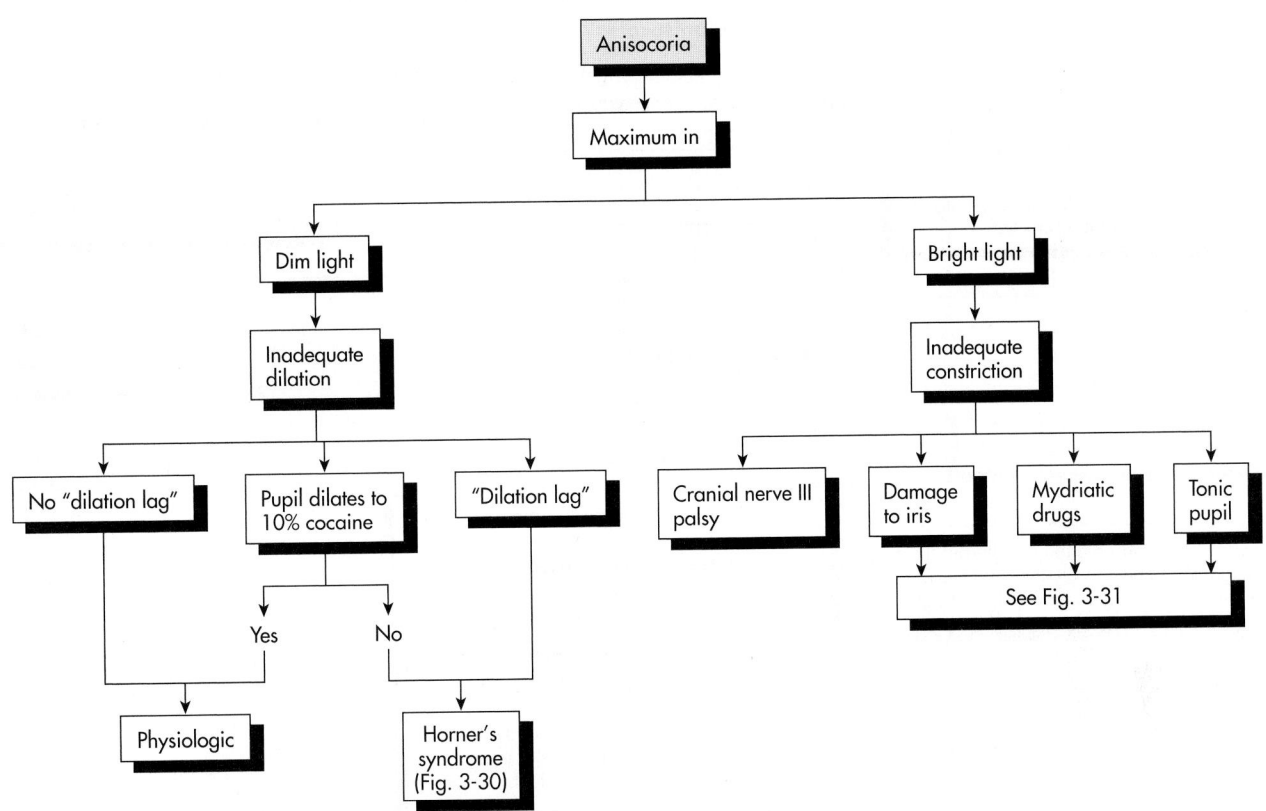

FIG. 29 Algorithm for the approach to unequal pupils (anisocoria). (From Andreoli TE [ed]: *Cecil essentials of medicine,* ed 7, Philadelphia, 2008, Saunders.)

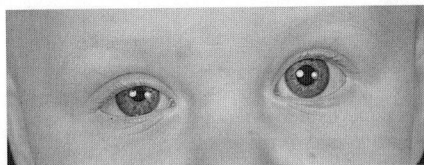

FIG. 30 Horner's syndrome clearly acquired in infancy must be evaluated for neuroblastoma, a treatable tumor. This baby, with a right ptosis and miosis, developed a flush during cycloplegia that made the vasomotor abnormality very clear—the Horner's side remained pale. The baby had no sign of Horner's syndrome during her first 8 months, but at 16 months Horner's syndrome is obvious (ptosis, miosis, and upside-down ptosis). Because the syndrome was acquired, a chest radiograph was ordered; it showed a mass in the pulmonary apex. Magnetic resonance imaging confirmed the lesion. Surgery showed it to be a neuroblastoma. (From Yanoff M, Duker JS: *Ophthalmology,* ed 2, St Louis, 2004, Mosby.)

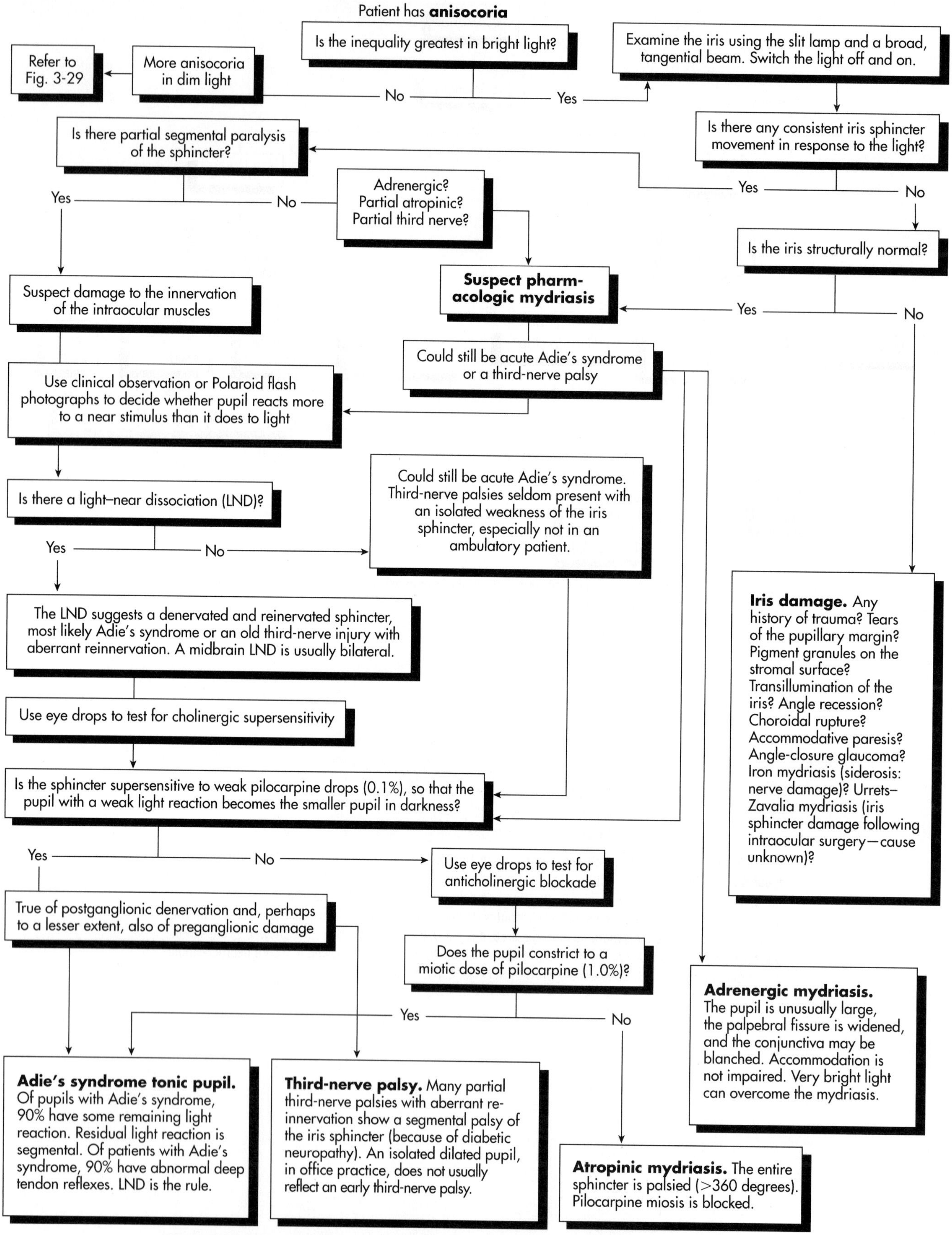

Patient has **anisocoria**

Is the inequality greatest in bright light?

Examine the iris using the slit lamp and a broad, tangential beam. Switch the light off and on.

Refer to Fig. 3-29

More anisocoria in dim light

— No —

— Yes —

Is there partial segmental paralysis of the sphincter?

Is there any consistent iris sphincter movement in response to the light?

— Yes — — No —

Adrenergic? Partial atropinic? Partial third nerve?

— Yes — — No —

Is the iris structurally normal?

Suspect damage to the innervation of the intraocular muscles

Suspect pharmacologic mydriasis

— Yes — — No —

Could still be acute Adie's syndrome or a third-nerve palsy

Use clinical observation or Polaroid flash photographs to decide whether pupil reacts more to a near stimulus than it does to light

Could still be acute Adie's syndrome. Third-nerve palsies seldom present with an isolated weakness of the iris sphincter, especially not in an ambulatory patient.

Is there a light–near dissociation (LND)?

— Yes — — No —

The LND suggests a denervated and reinnervated sphincter, most likely Adie's syndrome or an old third-nerve injury with aberrant reinnervation. A midbrain LND is usually bilateral.

Iris damage. Any history of trauma? Tears of the pupillary margin? Pigment granules on the stromal surface? Transillumination of the iris? Angle recession? Choroidal rupture? Accommodative paresis? Angle-closure glaucoma? Iron mydriasis (siderosis: nerve damage)? Urrets–Zavalia mydriasis (iris sphincter damage following intraocular surgery—cause unknown)?

Use eye drops to test for cholinergic supersensitivity

Is the sphincter supersensitive to weak pilocarpine drops (0.1%), so that the pupil with a weak light reaction becomes the smaller pupil in darkness?

— Yes — — No —

Use eye drops to test for anticholinergic blockade

True of postganglionic denervation and, perhaps to a lesser extent, also of preganglionic damage

Does the pupil constrict to a miotic dose of pilocarpine (1.0%)?

— Yes — — No —

Adrenergic mydriasis. The pupil is unusually large, the palpebral fissure is widened, and the conjunctiva may be blanched. Accommodation is not impaired. Very bright light can overcome the mydriasis.

Adie's syndrome tonic pupil. Of pupils with Adie's syndrome, 90% have some remaining light reaction. Residual light reaction is segmental. Of patients with Adie's syndrome, 90% have abnormal deep tendon reflexes. LND is the rule.

Third-nerve palsy. Many partial third-nerve palsies with aberrant re-innervation show a segmental palsy of the iris sphincter (because of diabetic neuropathy). An isolated dilated pupil, in office practice, does not usually reflect an early third-nerve palsy.

Atropinic mydriasis. The entire sphincter is palsied (>360 degrees). Pilocarpine miosis is blocked.

FIG. 31 Diagnosis of pupillary abnormalities in which anisocoria increases in bright light. Initial pupillary inequality is greater in bright light than in darkness, which indicates that the sphincter of the large pupil is weak or that a parasympathetic lesion is present on that side. (From Yanoff M, Duker JS: *Ophthalmology*, ed 2, St Louis, 2004, Mosby.)

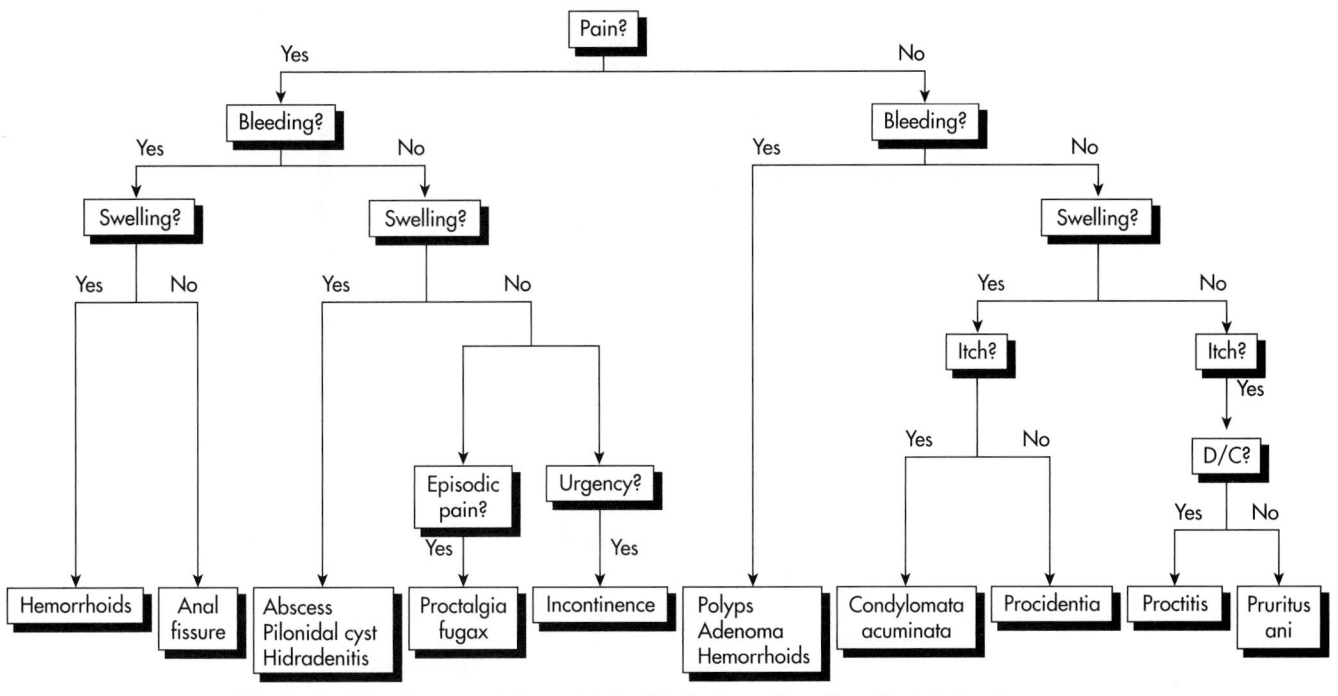

FIG. 32 Algorithm for anorectal complaints. *D/C,* discharge. (From Marx JA, et al: *Rosen's emergency medicine*, ed 8, Philadelphia, 2014, Saunders.)

BOX 2, A The WASH Regimen for Management of Hemorrhoids

- *W*arm water
- *A*nalgesic agents
- *S*tool softeners
- *H*igh-fiber diet

From Marx JA, et al: *Rosen's emergency medicine*, ed 8, Philadelphia, 2014, Saunders.

BOX 2, B Medical History in Diagnosis of Anorectal Disorders

Anorectal History
Pain
Bleeding
Swelling
Itching
Discharge
Urgency

Gastrointestinal History
Change in bowel habits (straining, flatus, color, consistency, frequency)
Nausea or vomiting
Incontinence of stool
Underlying GI disease (Crohn's disease, cancer, polyps)

Systemic Disease History
Diabetes mellitus
Coagulopathy
Cancer
HIV infection

Sexual History of the Anus
Penetration
Known STDs
Assault

GI, Gastrointestinal; *HIV,* human immunodeficiency virus; *STD,* sexually transmitted disease.
From Marx JA, et al: *Rosen's emergency medicine*, ed 8, Philadelphia, 2014, Saunders.

Clinical Algorithms

III

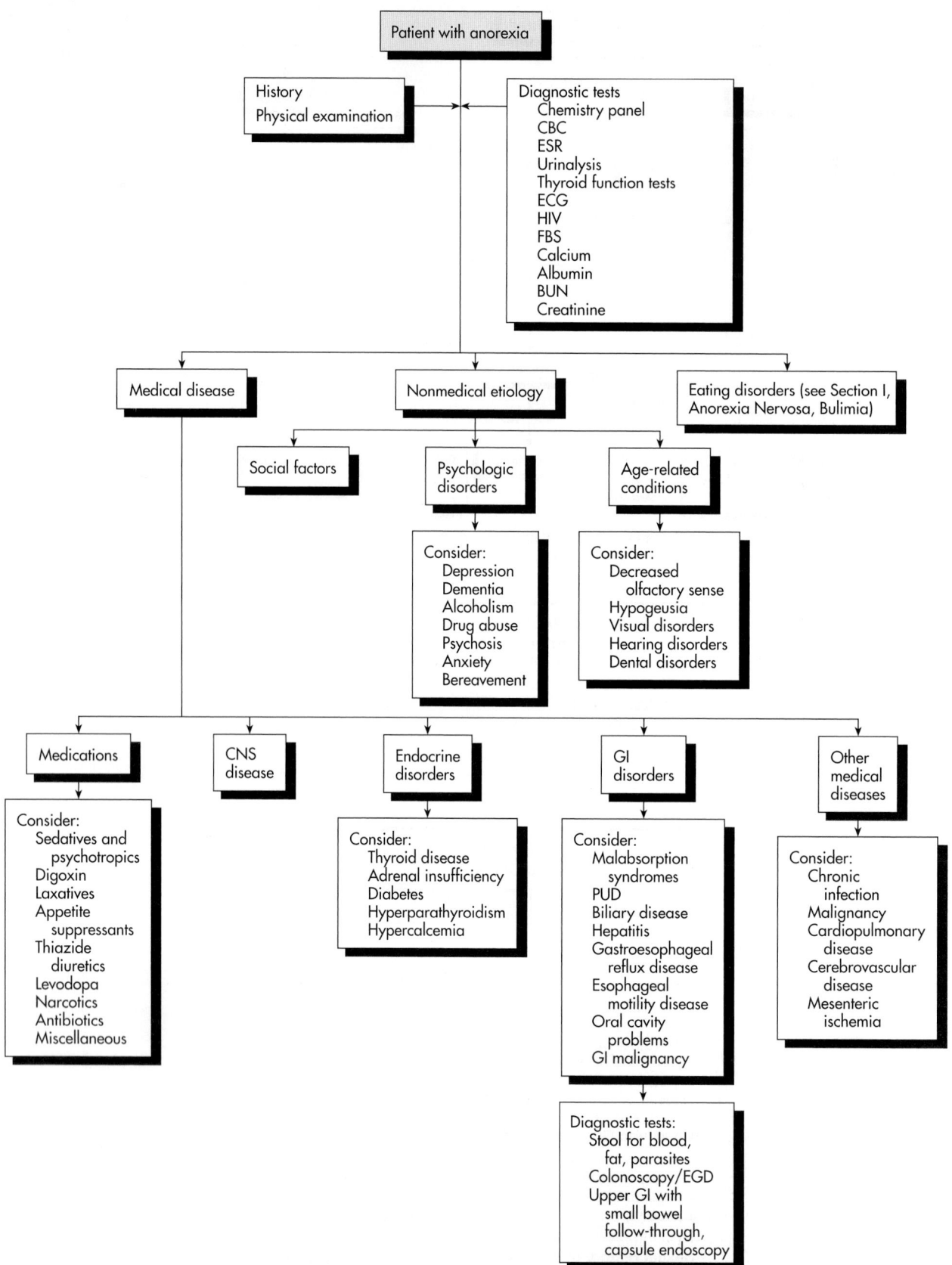

FIG. 33 Evaluation of anorexia. *BUN,* Blood urea nitrogen; *CBC,* complete blood count; *CNS,* central nervous system; *ECG,* electrocardiogram; *ESR,* erythrocyte sedimentation rate; *FBS,* fasting blood sugar; *GI,* gastrointestinal; *PUD,* peptic ulcer disease. (Modified from Greene HL, Johnson WP, Lemcke D [eds]: *Decision making in medicine,* ed 2, St Louis, 1998, Mosby.)

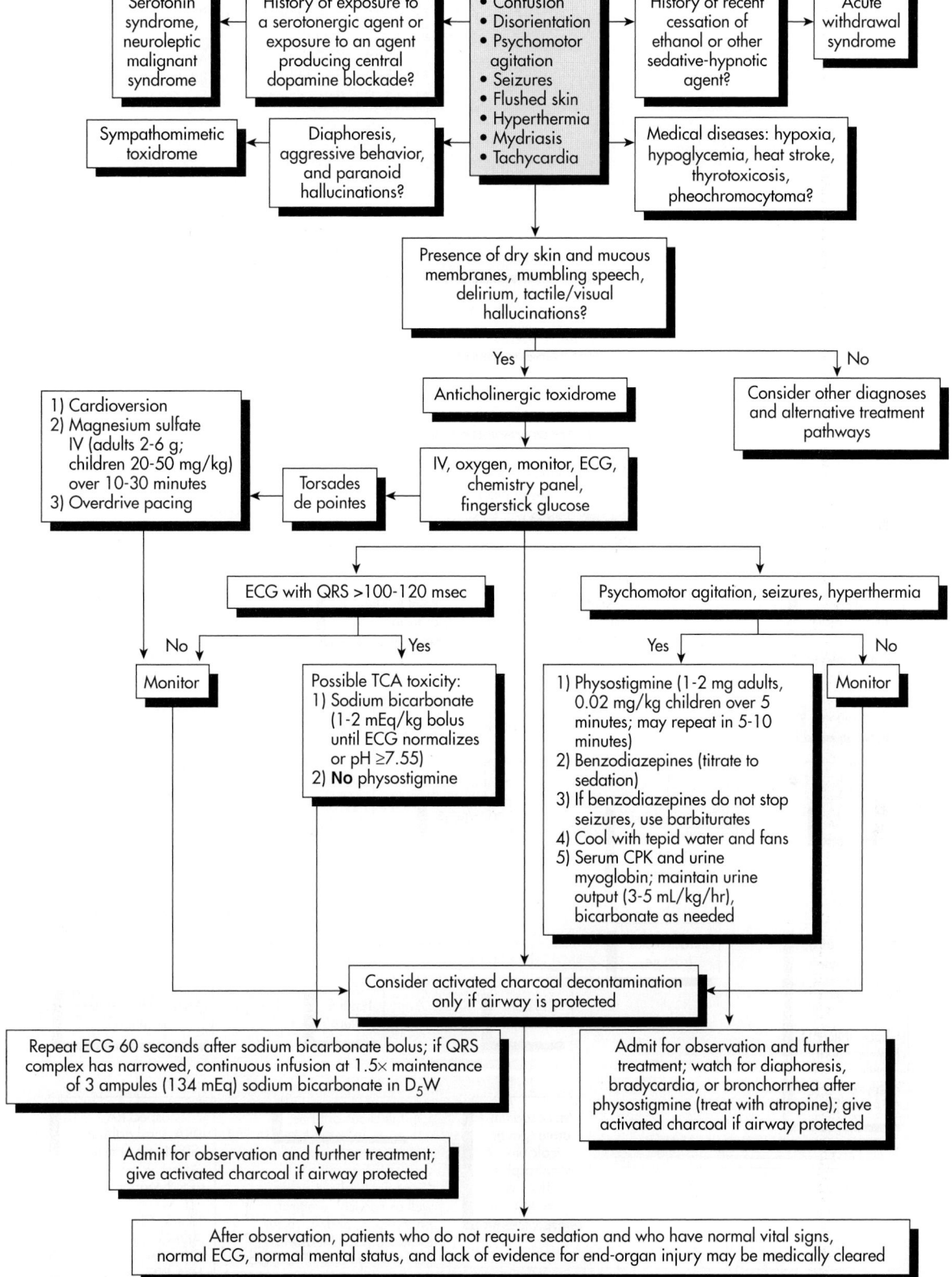

FIG. 34 Algorithm for the recognition and treatment of anticholinergic toxicity. *CPK,* Creatine phosphokinase; *D₅W,* 5% dextrose in water; *ECG,* electrocardiogram; *IV,* intravenous line; *TCA,* tricyclic antidepressant. (From Adams JG et al: *Emergency medicine, clinical essentials,* ed 2, Philadelphia, 2013, Elsevier.)

ICD-10CM #	M25.50	Pain in unspecified joint
	M25.519	Pain in unspecified shoulder
	M25.529	Pain in unspecified elbow
	M25.539	Pain in unspecified wrist
	M79.643	Pain in unspecified hand
	M25.559	Pain in unspecified hip
	M25.569	Pain in unspecified knee
	M25.579	Pain in unspecified ankle and joints of unspecified foot
	M79.646	Pain in unspecified finger(s)

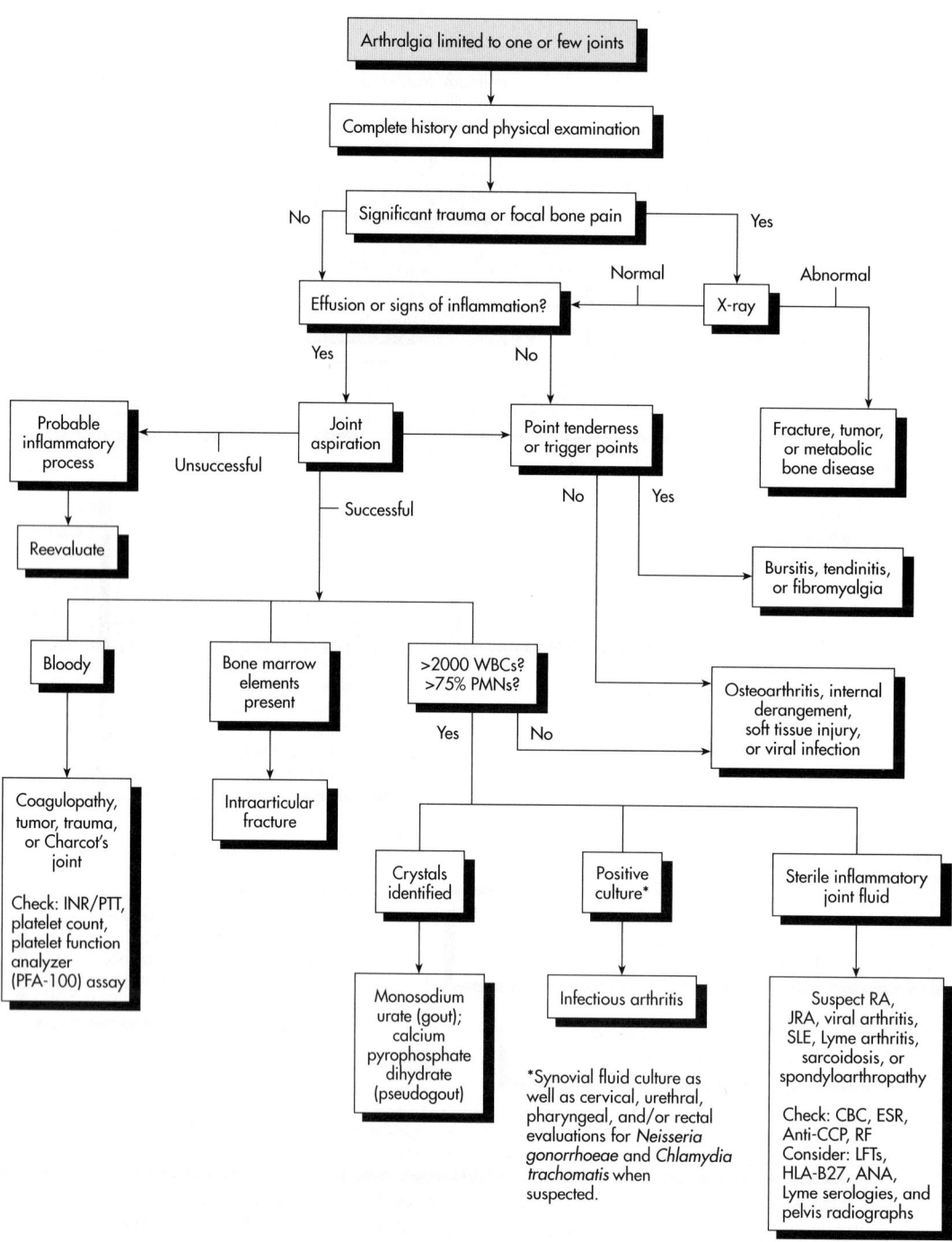

FIG. 35 A diagnostic approach to arthralgia in a few joints. *ANA,* Antinuclear antibodies; *Anti-CCP,* anti-cyclic citrullinated peptide; *CBC,* complete blood count; *ESR,* erythrocyte sedimentation rate; *JRA,* juvenile rheumatoid arthritis; *LFTs,* liver function tests; *PMNs,* polymorphonuclear neutrophils; *PT,* prothrombin time; *PTT,* partial thromboplastin time; *RA,* rheumatoid arthritis; *RF,* rheumatoid factor; *SLE,* systemic lupus erythematosus; *WBCs,* white blood cells. (Modified from American College of Rheumatology Ad Hoc Committee on Clinical Guidelines: *Arthritis Rheum* 39:1, 1996.)

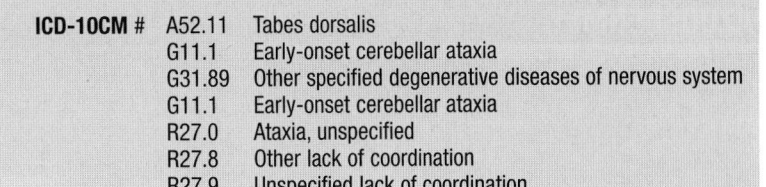

ICD-10CM #

A52.11	Tabes dorsalis
G11.1	Early-onset cerebellar ataxia
G31.89	Other specified degenerative diseases of nervous system
G11.1	Early-onset cerebellar ataxia
R27.0	Ataxia, unspecified
R27.8	Other lack of coordination
R27.9	Unspecified lack of coordination

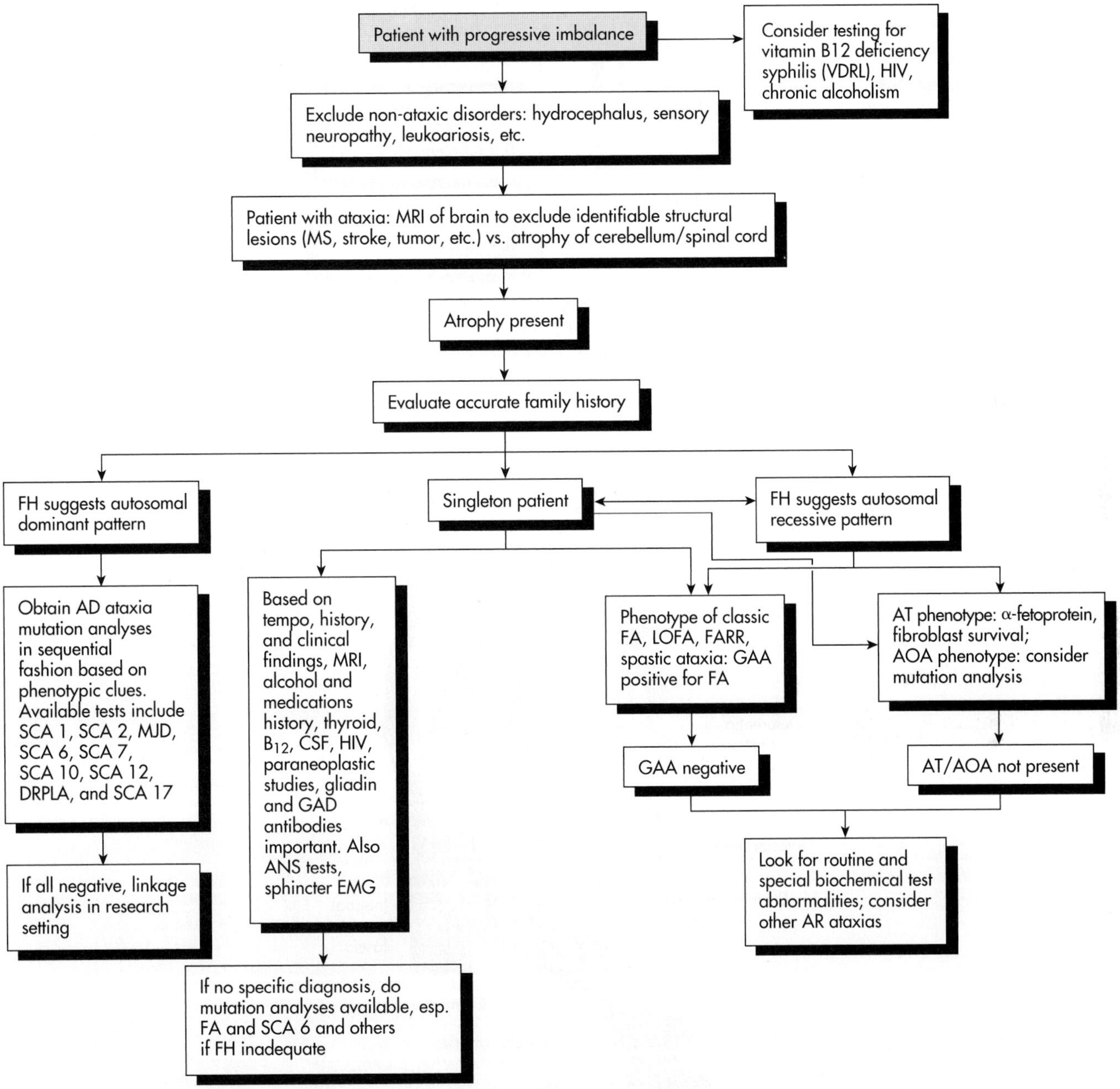

Patient with progressive imbalance → Consider testing for vitamin B12 deficiency syphilis (VDRL), HIV, chronic alcoholism

Exclude non-ataxic disorders: hydrocephalus, sensory neuropathy, leukoariosis, etc.

Patient with ataxia: MRI of brain to exclude identifiable structural lesions (MS, stroke, tumor, etc.) vs. atrophy of cerebellum/spinal cord

Atrophy present

Evaluate accurate family history

FH suggests autosomal dominant pattern

Singleton patient ↔ FH suggests autosomal recessive pattern

Obtain AD ataxia mutation analyses in sequential fashion based on phenotypic clues. Available tests include SCA 1, SCA 2, MJD, SCA 6, SCA 7, SCA 10, SCA 12, DRPLA, and SCA 17

If all negative, linkage analysis in research setting

Based on tempo, history, and clinical findings, MRI, alcohol and medications history, thyroid, B$_{12}$, CSF, HIV, paraneoplastic studies, gliadin and GAD antibodies important. Also ANS tests, sphincter EMG

Phenotype of classic FA, LOFA, FARR, spastic ataxia: GAA positive for FA

AT phenotype: α-fetoprotein, fibroblast survival; AOA phenotype: consider mutation analysis

GAA negative

AT/AOA not present

Look for routine and special biochemical test abnormalities; consider other AR ataxias

If no specific diagnosis, do mutation analyses available, esp. FA and SCA 6 and others if FH inadequate

Clinical Algorithms

III

FIG. 38 An algorithm for a diagnostic approach to patients with progressive ataxia. *AD*, Autosomal dominant; *AOA*, ataxia with oculomotor apraxia; *AR*, autosomal recessive; *AT*, ataxia-telangiectasia; *CSF*, cerebrospinal fluid; *DRPLA*, dentatorubral-pallidoluysian atrophy; *EMG*, electromyelography; *FA*, Friedreich's ataxia; *FH*, family history; *GAD*, glutamate decarboxylase; *HIV*, human immunodeficiency virus; *MRI*, magnetic resonance imaging; *MS*, multiple sclerosis; *SCA*, spinocerebellar ataxia. (Modified from Bradley WG et al [eds]: *Neurology in clinical practice*, ed 4, Philadelphia, 2004, Butterworth Heinemann.)

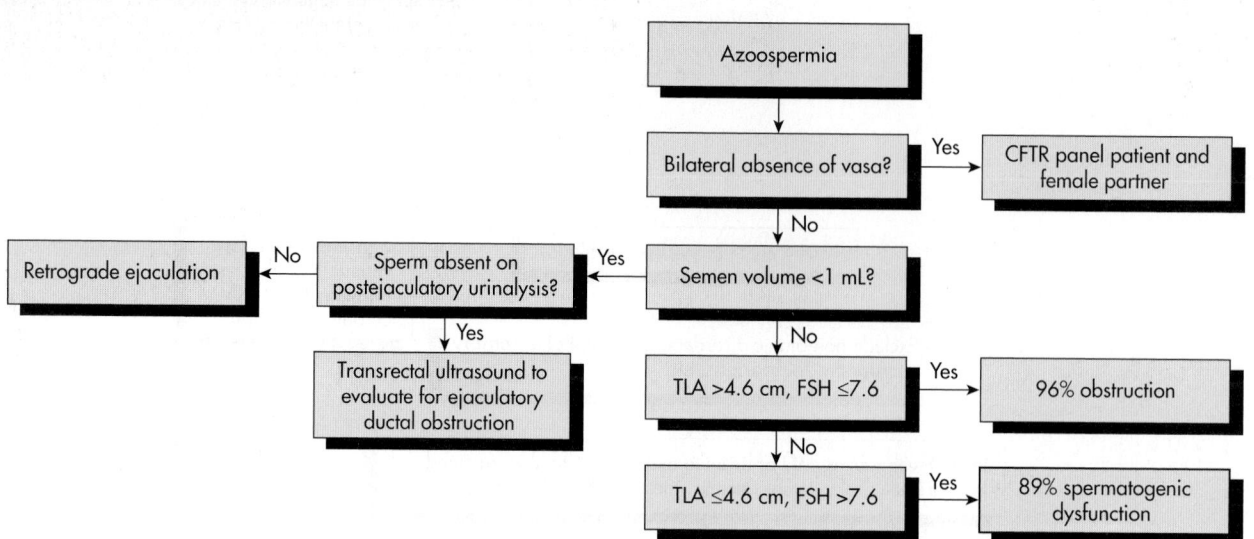

FIG. 39 **Algorithm for evaluation of azoospermia.** *CFTR,* cystic fibrosis transmembrane conductance regulator; *FSH,* follicle-stimulating hormone; *TLA,* testis longitudinal axis measured by caliper orchidometer. (Wein AJ, Kavoussi LR, Partin AW, Peters CA: Campbell-Walsh Urology, 11th ed, ISBN# 978-1-4557-7567-5, 2016, Elsevier.)

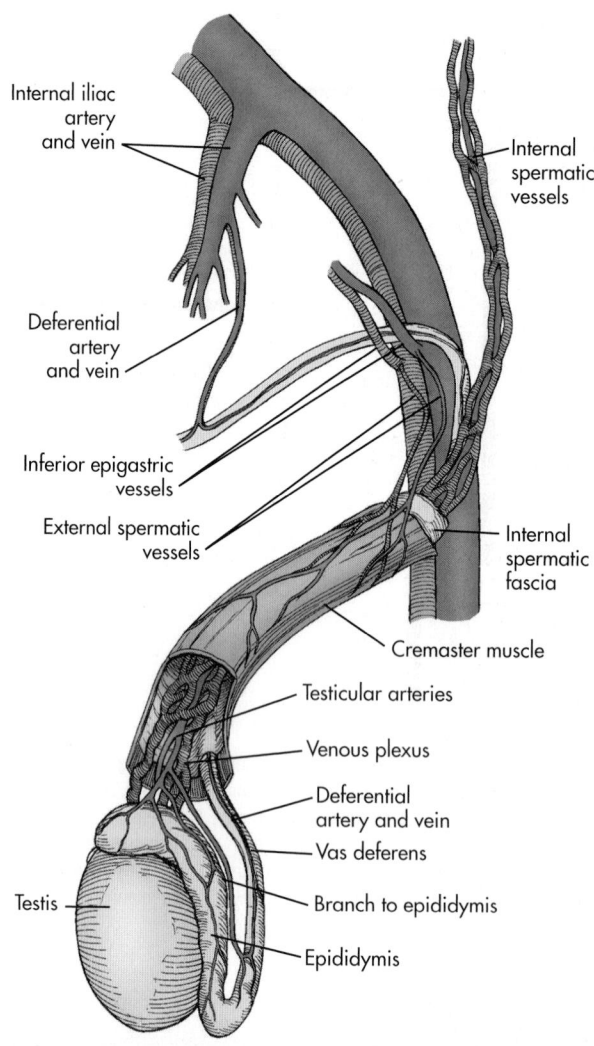

FIG. 40 Schematic illustration of interconnections between internal spermatic, external spermatic (cremasteric), and deferential vessels in the peritesticular region and spermatic cord. (Wein AJ, Kavoussi LR, Partin AW, Peters CA: Campbell-Walsh Urology, 11th ed, ISBN# 978-1-4557-7567-5, 2016, Elsevier.)

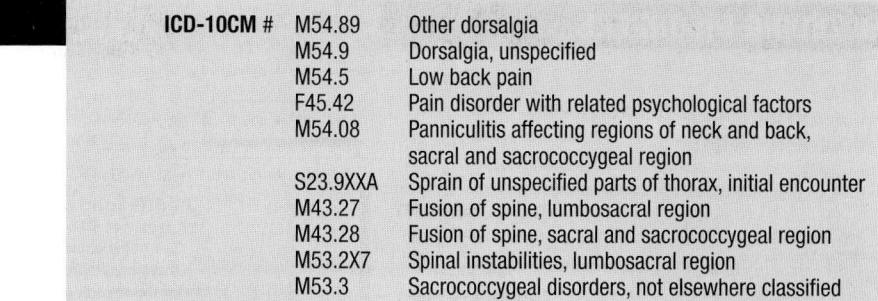

ICD-10CM #		
	M54.89	Other dorsalgia
	M54.9	Dorsalgia, unspecified
	M54.5	Low back pain
	F45.42	Pain disorder with related psychological factors
	M54.08	Panniculitis affecting regions of neck and back, sacral and sacrococcygeal region
	S23.9XXA	Sprain of unspecified parts of thorax, initial encounter
	M43.27	Fusion of spine, lumbosacral region
	M43.28	Fusion of spine, sacral and sacrococcygeal region
	M53.2X7	Spinal instabilities, lumbosacral region
	M53.3	Sacrococcygeal disorders, not elsewhere classified

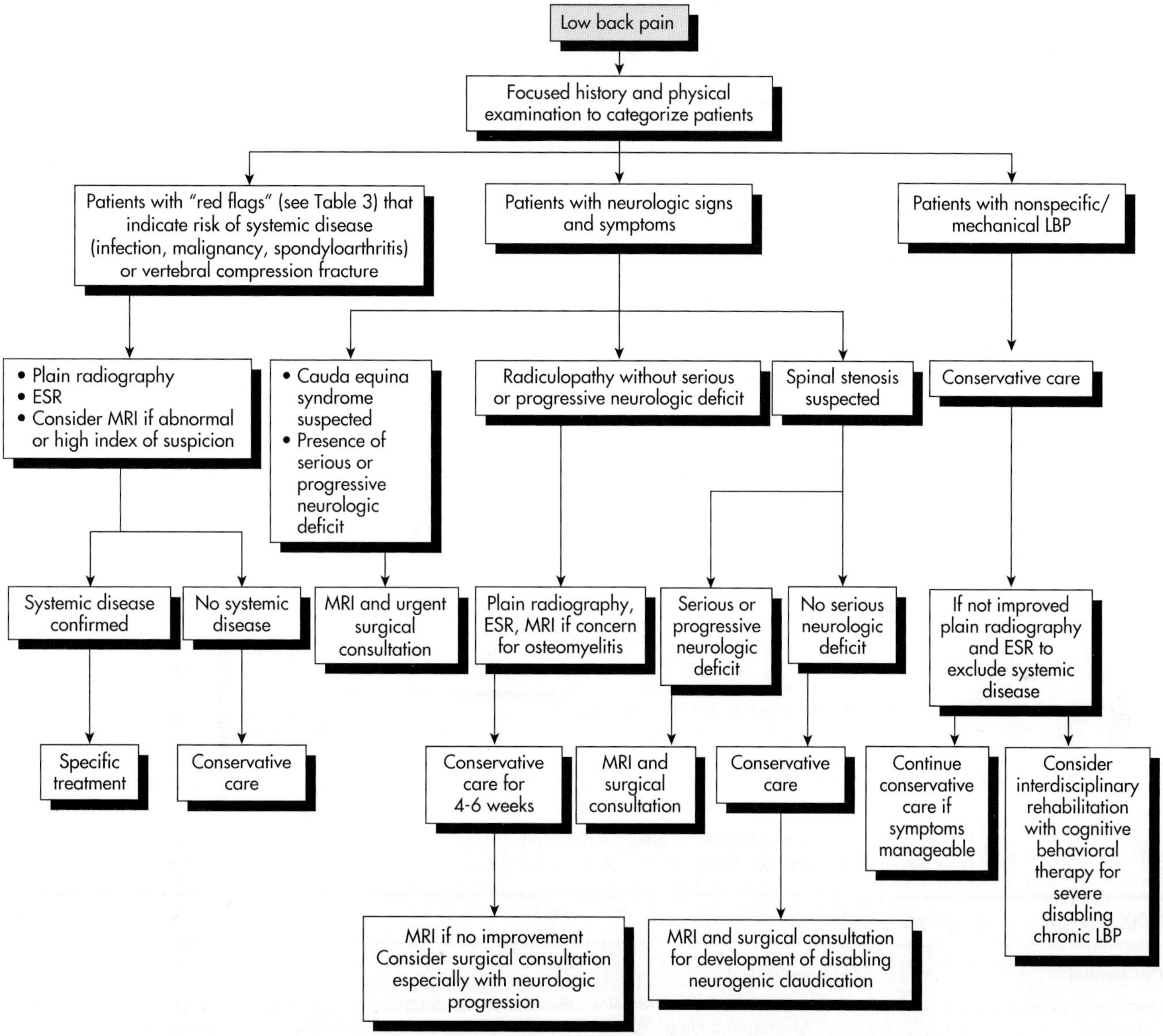

FIG. 41 Algorithm for the differential diagnosis and treatment of low back pain. *ESR*, erythrocyte sedimentation rate; *LBP*, low back pain; *MRI*, magnetic resonance imaging. (From Firestein GS, Budd RC, Gabriel SE, et al: *Kelley's textbook of rheumatology*, ed 9, Philadelphia, 2013, Saunders.)

Clinical Algorithms

TABLE 3 Red Flags for Potentially Serious Conditions

Possible Fracture	Possible Tumor or Infection	Possible Cauda Equina Syndrome
From Medical History		
Major trauma, such as vehicle accident or fall from height	Age over 50 or under 20 yr	Saddle anesthesia
Minor trauma or even strenuous lifting (in older or potentially osteoporotic patient)	History of cancer	Recent onset of bladder dysfunction, such as urinary retention, increased frequency, or overflow incontinence
	Constitutional symptoms, such as recent fever or chills or unexplained weight loss Risk factors for spinal infection: recent bacterial infection (e.g., urinary tract infection), intravenous drug abuse, or immune suppression (from steroids, transplant, or human immunodeficiency virus)	Severe or progressive neurologic deficit in the lower extremity
	Pain that worsens when supine; severe nighttime pain	

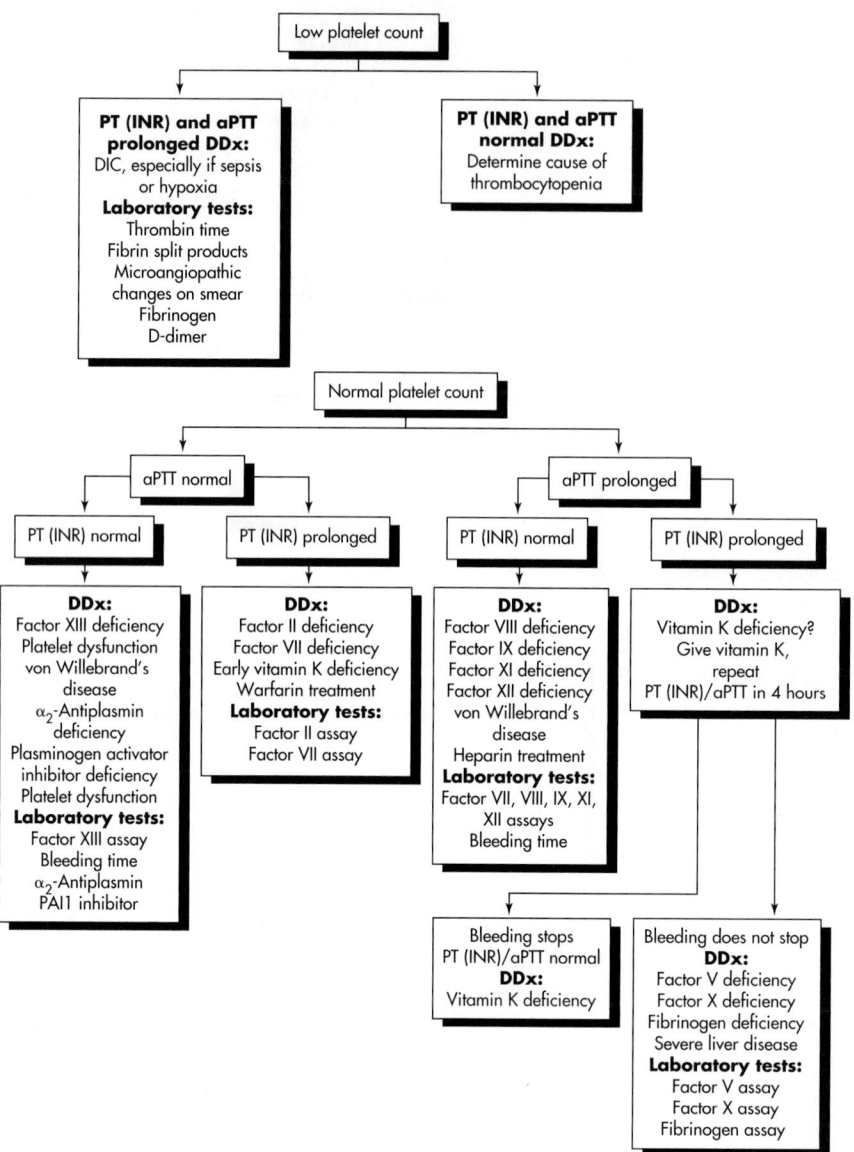

FIG. 44 Differential diagnosis (DDx) of bleeding disorders. (From Cluster JW, Rau RE: *The Harriet Lane handbook,* ed 18, St Louis, 2009, Mosby.)

BOX 3 Bleeding Disorders

Congenital

Disorder of platelet number or function

Thrombocytopenia: Secondary to bone marrow disease or defective megakaryocyte maturation

Disorders of platelet function: Bernard-Soulier syndrome, Glanzmann thrombasthenia, storage pool diseases

Factor VIII deficiency: See text (Section I)

Factor IX deficiency: See text (Section I)

von Willebrand's disease: See text (Section I)

Acquired

Disseminated intravascular coagulation: Characterized by prolonged PT and aPTT, decreased fibrinogen and platelets, increased fibrin degradation products, and elevated D-dimers. Treatment includes identifying and treating underlying disorder. Replacement of depleted coagulation factors with FFP may be necessary in severe cases, especially when bleeding is present; 10-15 ml/kg will raise clotting factors 20%. Fibrinogen, if depleted, can be given as cryoprecipitate. Platelet transfusions may also be necessary.

Liver disease: The liver is the major site of synthesis of factors V, VII, IX, X, XI, XII, XIII, prothrombin, plasminogen, fibrinogen, protein C and S, and ATIII. Treatment with FFP and platelets may be needed, but this will increase hepatic protein load. Vitamin K should be given to patients with liver disease and clotting abnormalities.

Vitamin K deficiency: Factors II, VII, IX, X, protein C, and protein S are vitamin K dependent. Early vitamin K deficiency may present with isolated prolonged PT because factor VII has the shortest half-life. Fibrinogen should be normal.

Hemolytic-uremic syndrome/thrombotic thrombocytopenic purpura (HUS/TTP): Characterized by the triad of microangiopathic hemolytic anemia, uremia, and thrombocytopenia. HUS/TTP is often triggered by bacterial enteritis, especially caused by *Escherichia coli* O157:H7, although there are a variety of causes. HUS does not typically include coagulation abnormalities, such as those seen in DIC. Avoid blood products in patients with HUS thought to be secondary to pneumococcal infection. TTP includes the triad of HUS in addition to fever and CNS changes and is more common in older adolescents and adults.

From Custer JW, Rau RE: *The Harriet Lane handbook,* ed 18, St Louis, 2009, Mosby.

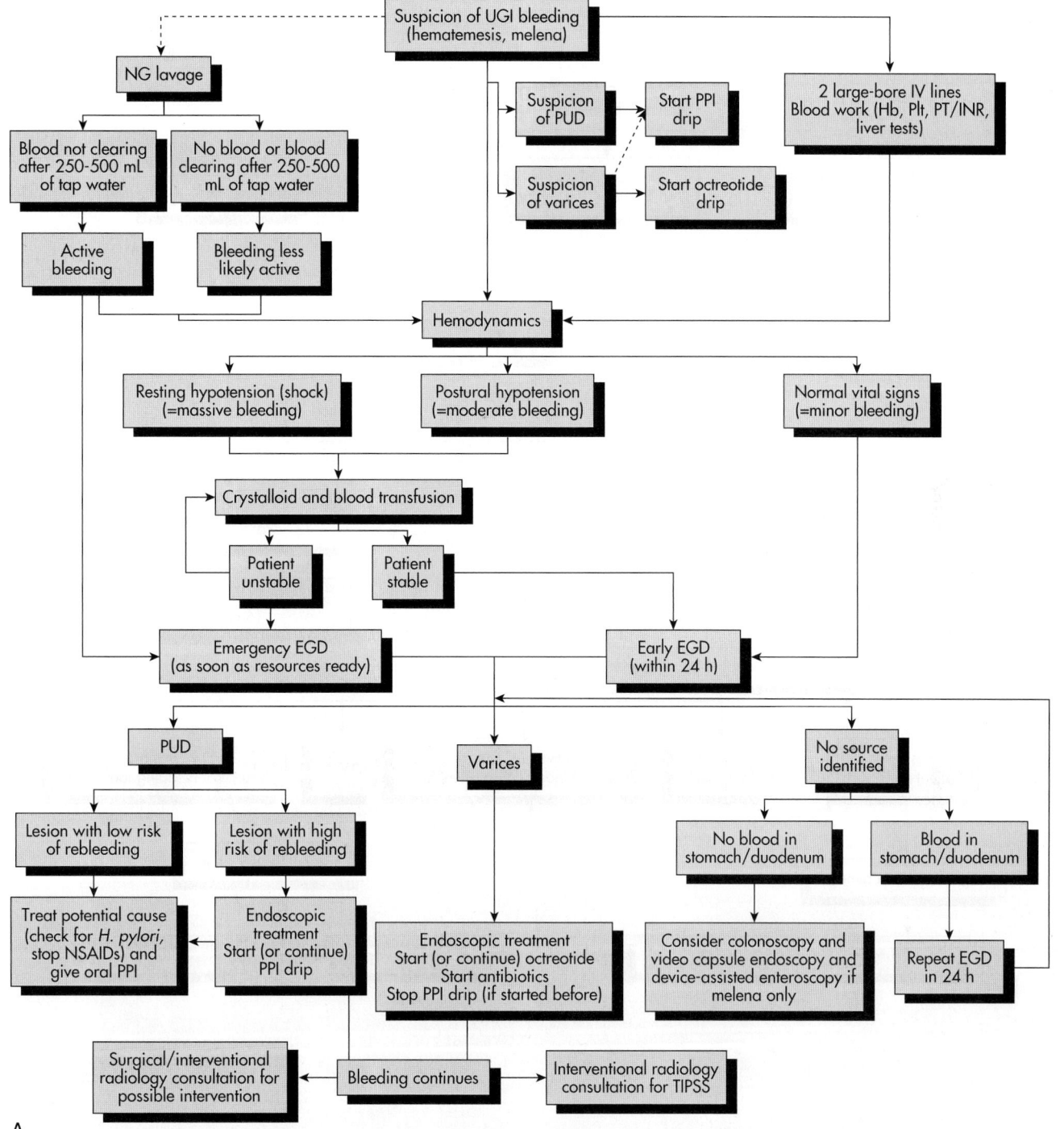

A

FIG. 46　A, Approach to managing upper gastrointestinal bleeding in critical care patients. **B,** Approach to managing lower gastrointestinal bleeding in critical care patients. *AVM,* arteriovenous malformation; *EGD,* esophagogastroduodenoscopy; *Hb,* hemoglobin; *INR,* international normalized ratio; *LGI,* lower gastrointestinal; *NG,* nasogastric; *NSAIDs,* nonsteroidal antiinflammatory drugs; *Plt,* platelets; *PPI,* proton pump inhibitor; *PT,* prothrombin time; *PUD,* peptic ulcer disease; *RBC,* red blood cell; *TIPSS,* transjugular intrahepatic portosystemic stent shunt; *UGI,* upper gastrointestinal. (Parrillo JE, Dellinger RP: Critical Care Medicine, Principles of Diagnosis and Management in the Adult, 4th ed, ISBN # 978-0-323-08929-6, 2014, Elsevier.)

Continued on next page

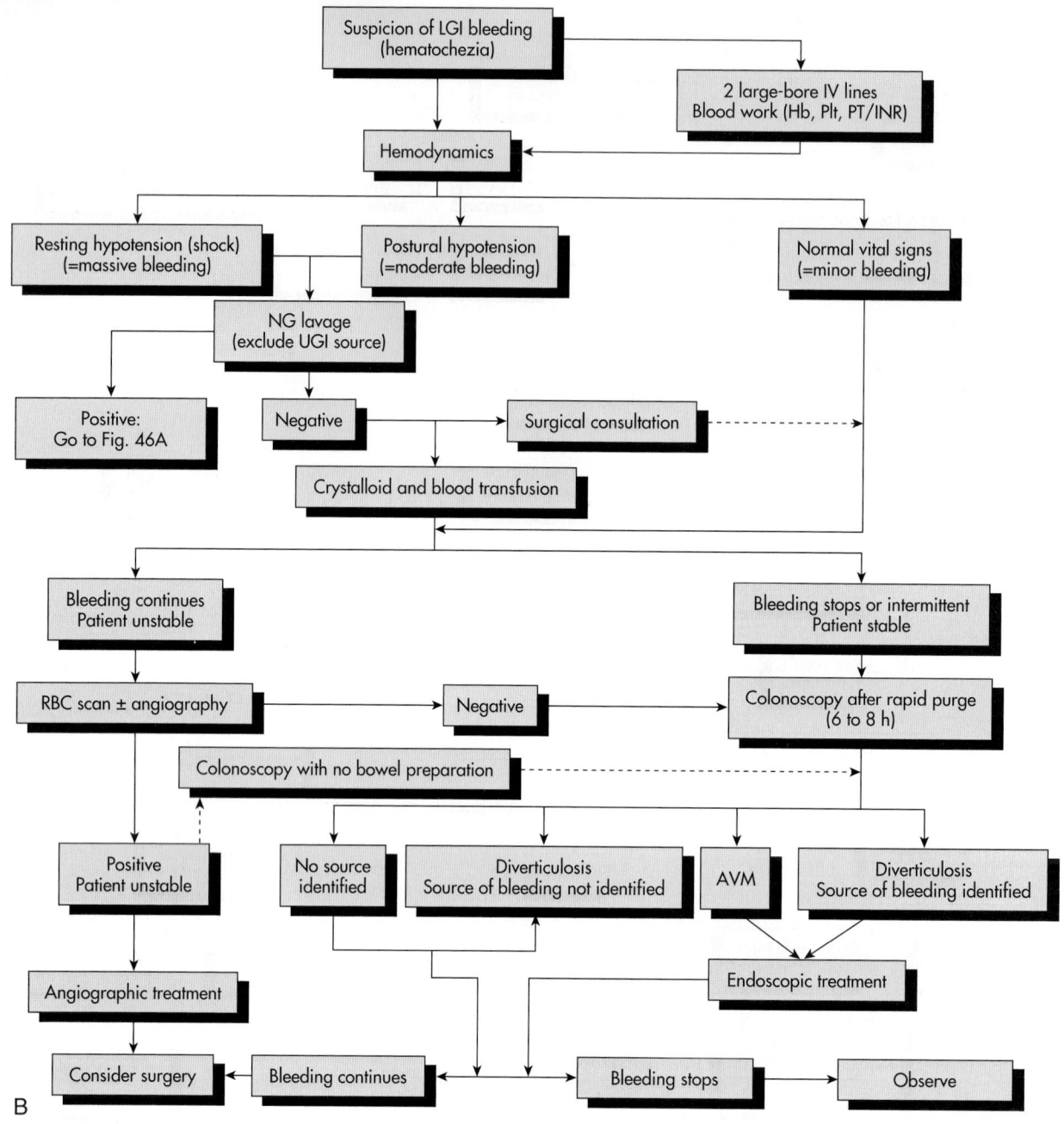

FIG. 46 (Continued)

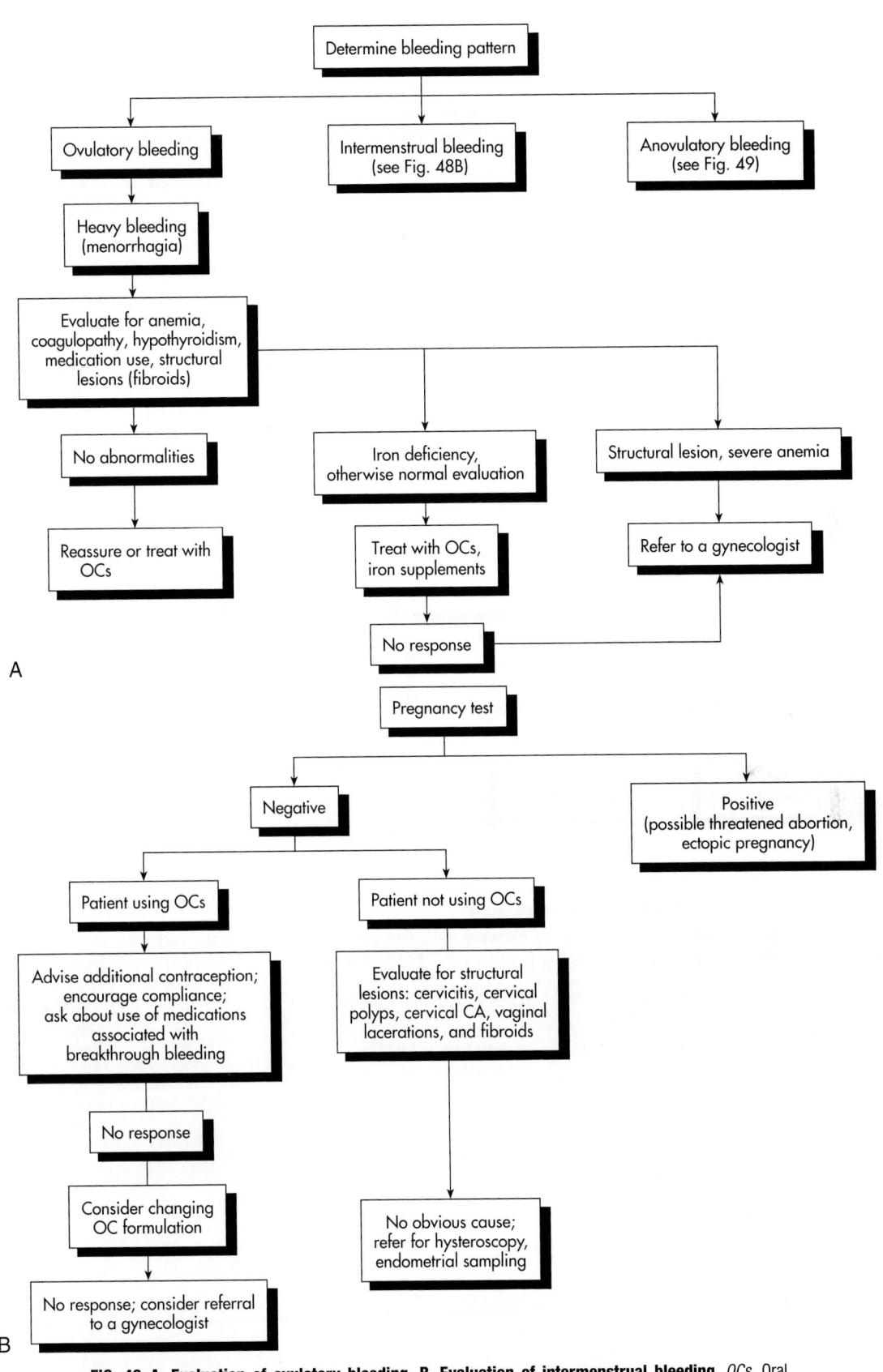

FIG. 48 A, Evaluation of ovulatory bleeding. B, Evaluation of intermenstrual bleeding. *OCs*, Oral contraceptives. (Modified from Appleby J, Henderson M, Wathen PI: *Intern Med* Sept:17, 1996.)

Clinical
Algorithms

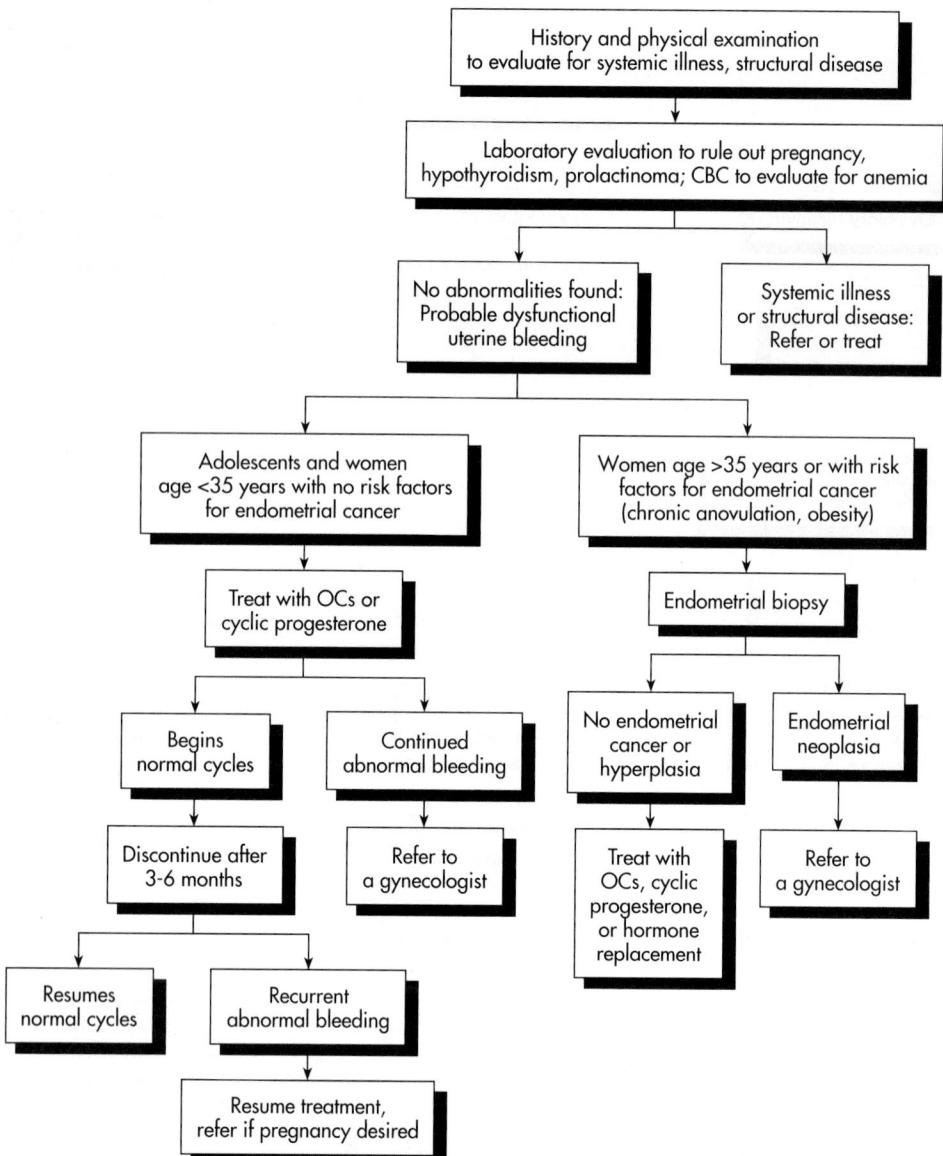

FIG. 49 Evaluation of anovulatory bleeding. *CBC*, Complete blood count; *OCs*, oral contraceptives.
(From Appleby J, Henderson M, Wathen PI: *Intern Med*, Sept:17, 1996.)

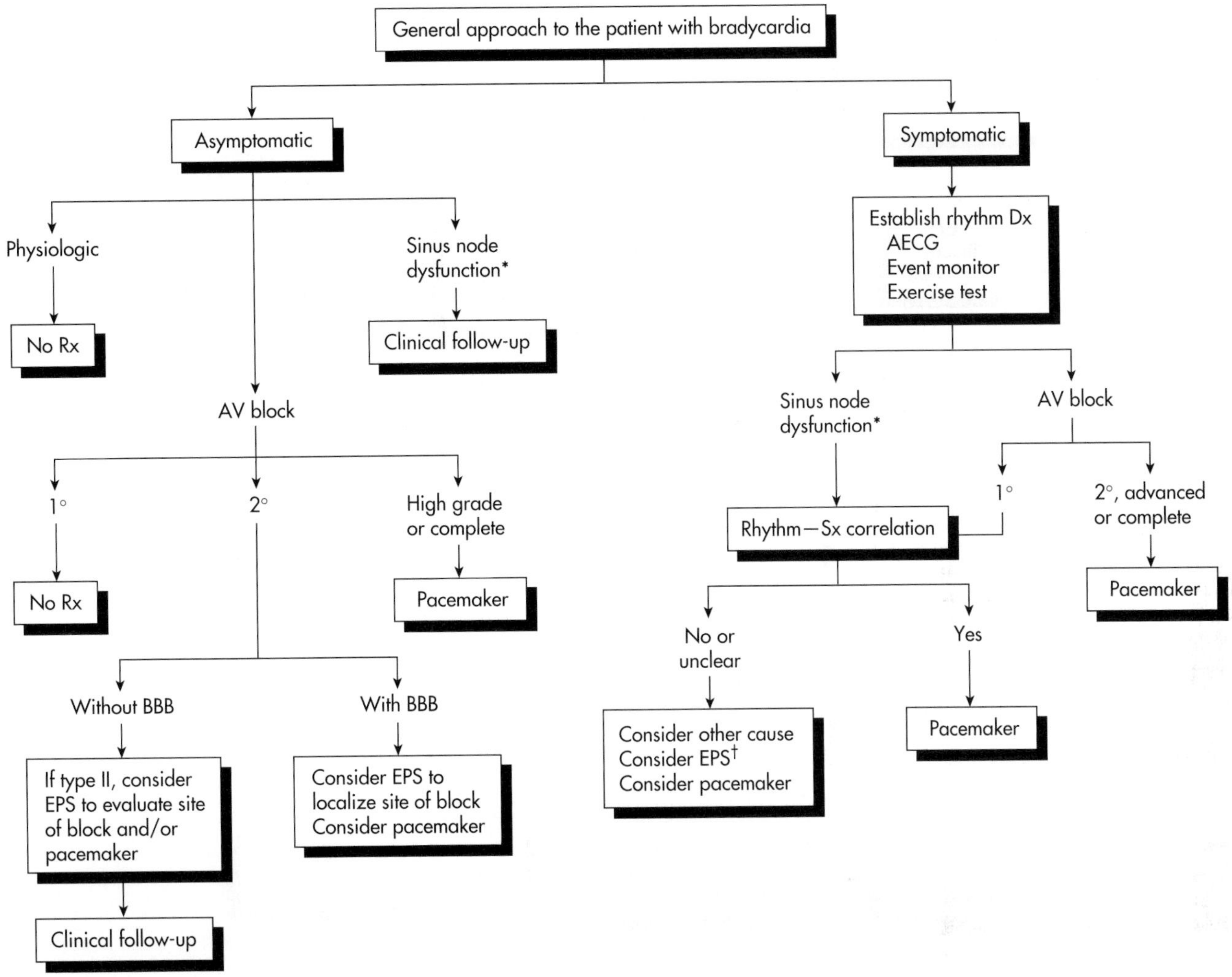

ICD-10CM #	R00.1	Bradycardia	**1585**
	I49.8	Other specified cardiac arrhythmias	
	I49.5	Sick sinus syndrome	

General approach to the patient with bradycardia

Asymptomatic

Physiologic

Sinus node dysfunction*

No Rx

Clinical follow-up

AV block

1°

2°

High grade or complete

No Rx

Pacemaker

Without BBB

With BBB

If type II, consider EPS to evaluate site of block and/or pacemaker

Consider EPS to localize site of block
Consider pacemaker

Clinical follow-up

Symptomatic

Establish rhythm Dx
AECG
Event monitor
Exercise test

Sinus node dysfunction*

AV block

Rhythm—Sx correlation

1°

2°, advanced or complete

No or unclear

Yes

Pacemaker

Consider other cause
Consider EPS†
Consider pacemaker

Pacemaker

*Includes bradycardia-tachycardia syndrome.
†EPS includes sinus node function and ventricular arrhythmia induction studies.

FIG. 51 General approach to the patient with bradycardia. *AECG,* Ambulatory electrocardiography; *AV,* atrioventricular; *BBB,* bundle branch block; *Dx,* diagnostic; *EPS,* electrophysiologic study; *Rx,* treatment; *Sx,* symptoms; *1°,* first-degree; *2°,* second-degree. (From Goldman L, Braunwald E [eds]: *Primary cardiology,* ed 2, Philadelphia, 2003, Saunders.)

Clinical Algorithms

ICD-10CM # N64.52 Nipple discharge
N64.51 Induration of breast
N64.53 Retraction of nipple
N64.59 Other signs and symptoms in breast

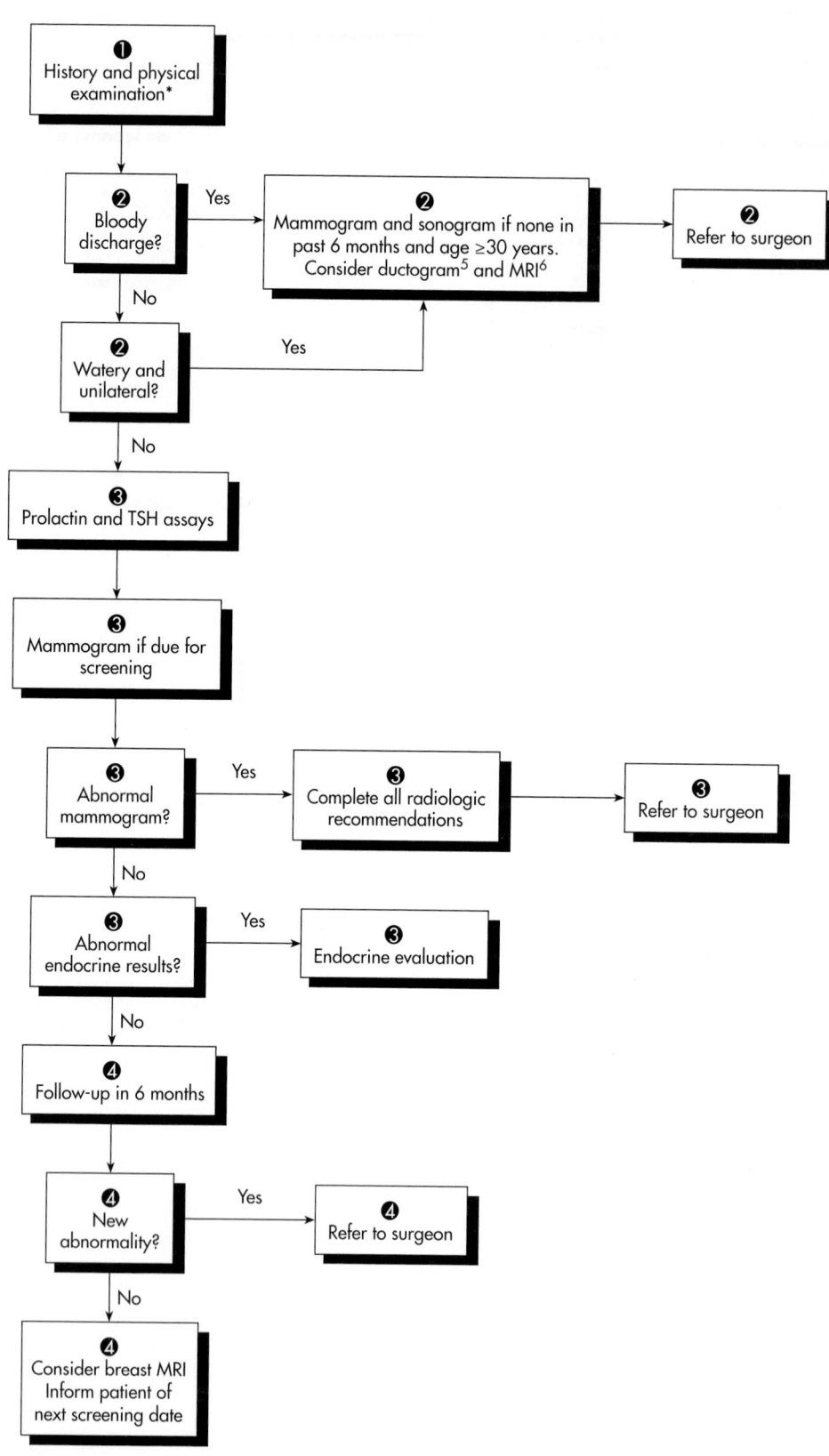

*Without palpable mass.

FIG. 53 Breast cancer screening and evaluation. The primary goal of evaluation and management of nipple discharge is separation of patients with pathological causes of discharge from those with benign

BREAST, NIPPLE DISCHARGE
EVALUATION—cont'd

ICD-10CM #	N64.52	Nipple discharge
	N64.51	Induration of breast
	N64.53	Retraction of nipple
	N64.59	Other signs and symptoms in breast

1587

FIG. 53 (Continued)

physiologic findings. Physiologic discharge is usually bilateral, involves multiple ducts, tests negative for blood regardless of color, and can be associated with nipple stimulation or breast compression. Approximately 50%-80% of women in their reproductive years can express some type of fluid from the breast. During the normal hormonal stimulation caused by pregnancy and breast feeding, the mammary glands often produce physiologic discharge of milk and colostrum. This discharge can be seen for up to 1 year postpartum after the cessation of breastfeeding. Nipple discharge is classified as pathologic if it is spontaneous, unilateral, bloody, serous, clear, or associated with a mass. Common causes of pathologic discharge are intraductal papilloma, duct ectasia, carcinoma, and infection. Of these, the most commonly seen is a benign papilloma, identified in up to 57% of cases of pathologic nipple discharge. A papilloma is a benign epithelial neoplasm that can be a cause of clear or bloody discharge. Papilloma can be classified as a spectrum of lesions that may be associated with atypical cells and low-grade carcinomas. The management of benign papilloma remains controversial. Duct ectasia is another common cause of pathologic discharge, seen in approximately 33% of cases. Malignancy is found in only 5%-15% of cases of pathologic nipple discharge, and is most commonly ductal carcinoma in situ. (Modified from Institute for Clinical Systems Integration, Minneapolis: *Postgrad Med* 100:182, 1996.)

1. **History and physical examination**[1]. Patients who present with a complaint of nipple discharge should be evaluated with breast-related history taking and a physical examination. History taking is aimed at uncovering and characterizing any other breast-related symptom. A risk assessment should also be undertaken for identified risk factors, including patient age over 50 years, any past personal history of breast cancer, history of hyperplasia on previous breast biopsies, and family history of breast cancer in first-degree relatives (mother, sister, daughter). Physical examination should include inspection of the breast for any evidence of ulceration or contour changes and inspection of the nipple for Paget's disease. Palpation should be performed with the patient in both the upright and the supine positions to determine the presence of any palpable mass.

2. **Bloody discharge?** If the discharge appears frankly bloody, the patient should be referred to a surgeon for evaluation. At the time of referral, a mammogram of the involved breast should be obtained if the patient is over 40 years of age and has not had a mammogram within the preceding 6 months. Similarly, patients with a watery, unilateral discharge should be referred to a surgeon for evaluation and possible biopsy.

3. **Endocrine tests. Mammogram**. If the discharge appears frankly milky or is bilateral, serum prolactin and serum thyroid-stimulating hormone (TSH) assays should be performed to rule out the presence of an endocrinologic basis for the symptoms. At the time of that visit, a mammogram should also be performed if the patient is due for routine mammographic screening according to the recommended intervals. Mammography has a low positive predictive value of only 16.7%, and low sensitivity of 59% in the diagnosis of malignant duct pathology associated with nipple discharge.[2] A patient with an abnormal mammogram should be further evaluated radiologically to better characterize the lesion and then be referred to a surgeon if appropriate. Make certain that all recommended additional views, ultrasound examinations, and follow-up studies have been obtained before referral to a surgeon. Should the mammogram appear normal, results of the assays for TSH and prolactin should be reviewed. If the results are abnormal, the patient should undergo appropriate evaluation for etiology, either by a primary care physician or by an endocrinologist.

4. **Six-month follow-up results**. If results of the mammogram and the endocrinologic screening studies are normal, the patient should return for a follow-up visit in 6 months to ensure that there has been no specific change in the character of the discharge, such as development of frank bleeding or Paget's disease, that would warrant surgical evaluation. If the evaluation at that follow-up visit fails to reveal any palpable or visible abnormalities, the patient should be returned to the routine screening process with studies performed at the recommended intervals.

5. **Ultrasound**. Breast ultrasound is complementary to mammography and is noninvasive, free of ionizing radiation, and is extremely useful in the evaluation of patients with nipple discharge. Ultrasound is used primarily to detect masses and determine whether a palpable or mammographically identified mass is cystic, solid, or within a duct. It can also be used to delineate the relationship of the mass within the involved ductal system and the number of ducts involved. It has been reported that a benign physical examination and a negative subareolar ultrasound virtually exclude the possibility of malignancy in patients with pathologic nipple discharge. In patients with pathologic discharge, ultrasound has a reported sensitivity of 97%, specificity of 60%, and positive predictive values of 95%.[2]

6. **Contrast-enhanced MRI**. The role of MRI in the evaluation of nipple discharge is emerging as a preferred, less invasive alternative to ductography. MRI has a high sensitivity (94%-100%) for the detection of breast cancer. MRI requires the intravenous injection of a gadolinium-based contrast agent. As opposed to ductography, MRI is able to characterize lesions and provide a means for histologic diagnosis via percutaneous MRI-guided core biopsy.[2]

---

[1]ICSI health care guidelines are designed to assist clinicians by providing an analytic framework for the evaluation and treatment of patients. They are not intended either to replace a clinician's judgment or to establish a protocol for all patients with a particular condition. A guideline will rarely establish the only approach to a problem. In addition, guidelines are "living documents" that are expected to be imperfect and are subject to annual review and revision.
[2]From Patel BK, Falcon S, Drukteinis J: Management of nipple discharge and the associated imaging findings. *Am J Med* 128(4), 2015.

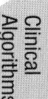

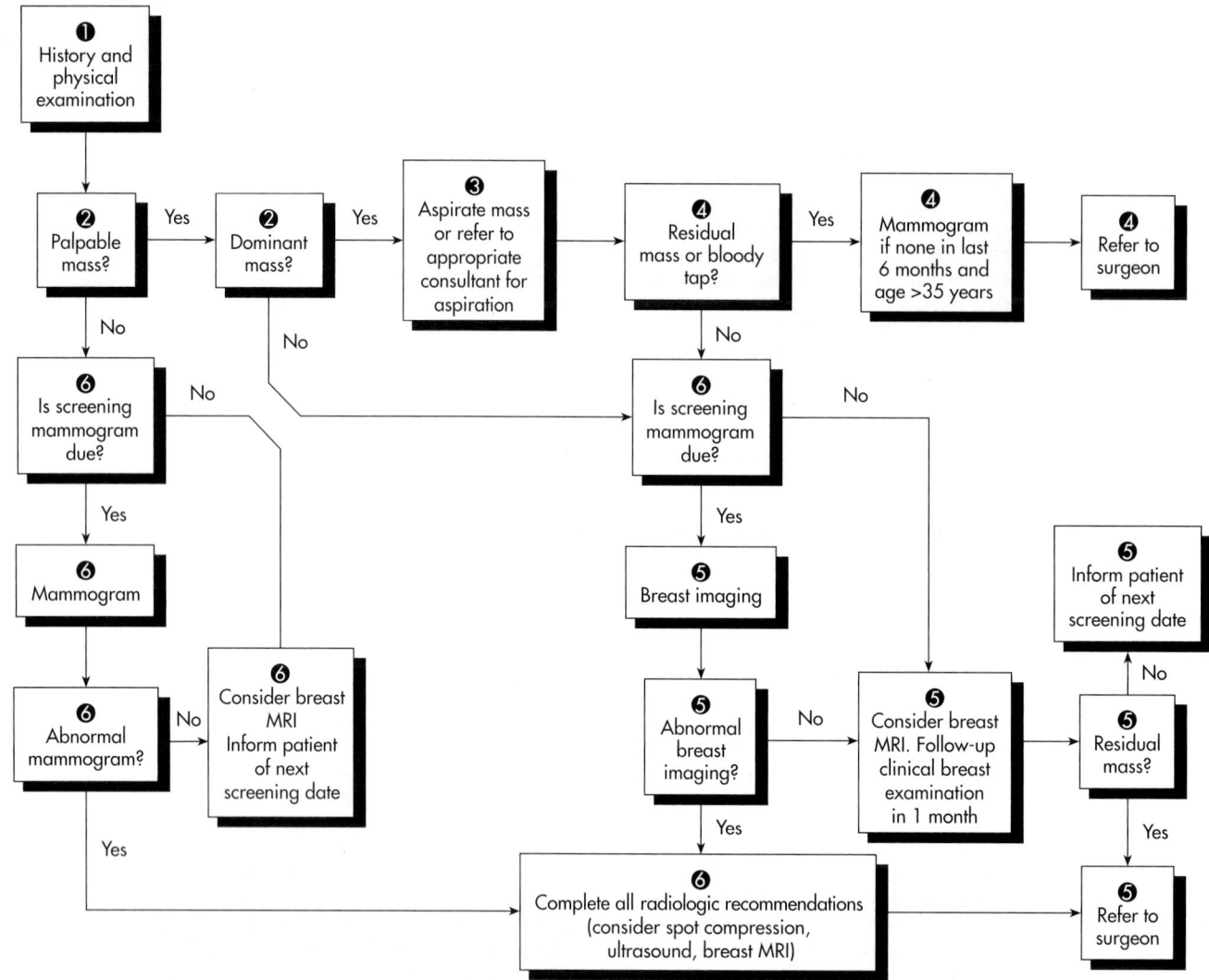

FIG. 55 Breast cancer screening and evaluation. (Modified from Institute for Clinical Systems Integration, Minneapolis: *Postgrad Med* 100:182, 1996.)

1. **History and physical examination.**[3] Primary care evaluation is initiated with history taking aimed at uncovering and characterizing any breast-related symptom. A risk assessment should also be undertaken for identified risk factors, including patient age over 50 years, any past personal history of breast cancer, history of hyperplasia on previous breast biopsies, and family history of breast cancer in first-degree relatives (mother, sister, daughter). Physical examination should include inspection of the breast for any evidence of ulceration or contour changes and inspection of the nipple for Paget's disease. Palpation should be performed with the patient in both the upright and supine positions to determine the presence of any palpable mass.

2. **Palpable mass?** Dominant mass? A dominant mass is a palpable finding that is discrete and clearly different from the surrounding parenchyma. If a palpable mass is identified, it should be determined whether it represents a dominant (i.e., discrete) mass, which requires immediate evaluation. The primary care physician or appropriate consultant should attempt to aspirate any dominant mass because a simple cyst may be uncovered, in which case aspiration completes the evaluation process.

3. **Aspirate mass or refer for aspiration.** Aspiration of a dominant palpable mass should be performed by the primary care physician or by the appropriate consultant. The breast skin is prepped with alcohol. Then, with the lesion immobilized by the nonoperating hand, an 18- to 25-gauge needle mounted on a 10-ml syringe is directed to the central portion of the mass for a single attempt at aspiration. Successful aspiration of a simple cyst would yield a nonbloody fluid with complete resolution of the dominant mass. Typical watery fluid may be discarded. However, cyst fluid that is bloody or unusually tenacious should be examined cytologically.

[3]ICSI health care guidelines are designed to assist clinicians by providing an analytic framework for the evaluation and treatment of patients. They are not intended either to replace a clinician's judgment or to establish a protocol for all patients with a particular condition. A guideline will rarely establish the only approach to a problem. In addition, guidelines are "living documents" that are expected to be imperfect and are subject to annual review and revision.

FIG. 55 (Continued)

4. **Residual mass or bloody tap?** Mammogram if none in past 6 months. Refer to surgeon. Should the mass remain after the attempt at aspiration or should frank blood be aspirated during the process, the presence of a malignant process cannot be ruled out. Patients with a residual mass or bloody tap should be referred to a surgeon for possible biopsy. Before the referral, a mammogram should be obtained for any patient over age 35 years who has not had a mammogram within the preceding 6 months. In patients 35 years and under, obtaining any other breast-imaging studies should be left to the discretion of the surgeon or radiologist.

5. **Is screening mammogram due?** Breast imaging. Follow-up clinical breast examination. Refer to surgeon. Should physical examination demonstrate a palpable mass that is not clearly a discrete and dominant mass, its size, location, and character should be documented in anticipation of a follow-up examination. A screening mammogram should be obtained if one has not been done within the recommended interval. If no mammogram is required or if a required mammogram demonstrates no abnormality, a follow-up examination in 1 month is indicated. Breast MRI should be considered. Should any residual mass be identified, the patient should be referred to a surgeon for possible biopsy. Patients with a persisting nondominant palpable mass that does not resolve within 1 month and those with any recurring cystic mass should be referred for surgical evaluation. If no mass is apparent at the time of the follow-up examination, the patient should then be informed of the appropriate date for her next screening examination, according to the recommended intervals.

6. **Screening mammogram and results.** After completion of the physical examination, the appropriateness of routine screening mammogram should be determined. If a mammogram is done, the radiologist should provide the results to the primary care physician for reporting to the patient. Should any abnormalities be uncovered, it will be the responsibility of the radiologist to complete any additional imaging studies required for the complete radiographic characterization of the lesion. The radiologist should make certain that all recommended additional views, follow-up studies, and ultrasound examinations have been completed before referral to a surgeon. However, it is important that the primary care physician who ordered the mammogram review the results of these studies to understand fully the opinion of the radiologist and to ensure that all recommendations of the radiologist have been completed. Should the radiologist recommend that surgical consultation is warranted, it will be the responsibility of the primary care physician to establish this referral.

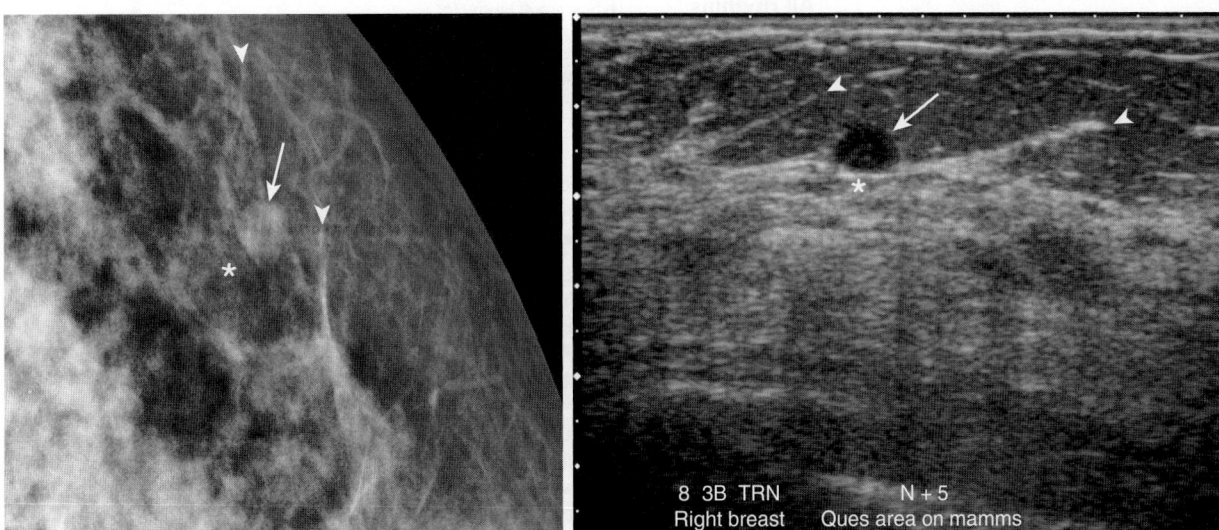

8 3B TRN   N + 5
Right breast   Ques area on mamms

FIG. 56 Mammographic-sonographic correlation of surrounding tissue density. Mammogram shows a nodule projecting between two Cooper's ligaments *(arrowheads)* and bulging anteriorly into the subcutaneous fat *(arrow)* from the mammary zone *(asterisk)* Sonogram shows that the mammographic nodule is a small cyst that protrudes out of fibrous tissue in the mammary zone (asterisk) and into the subcutaneous fat *(arrow)*. It lies between two Cooper's ligaments *(arrowheads)*. (Rumack CM, Wilson SR, Charboneau JW, Levine D: Diagnostic Ultrasound, 4th ed. ISBN# 978-0-323-05397-6, Elsevier, 2011.)

Clinical
Algorithms

III

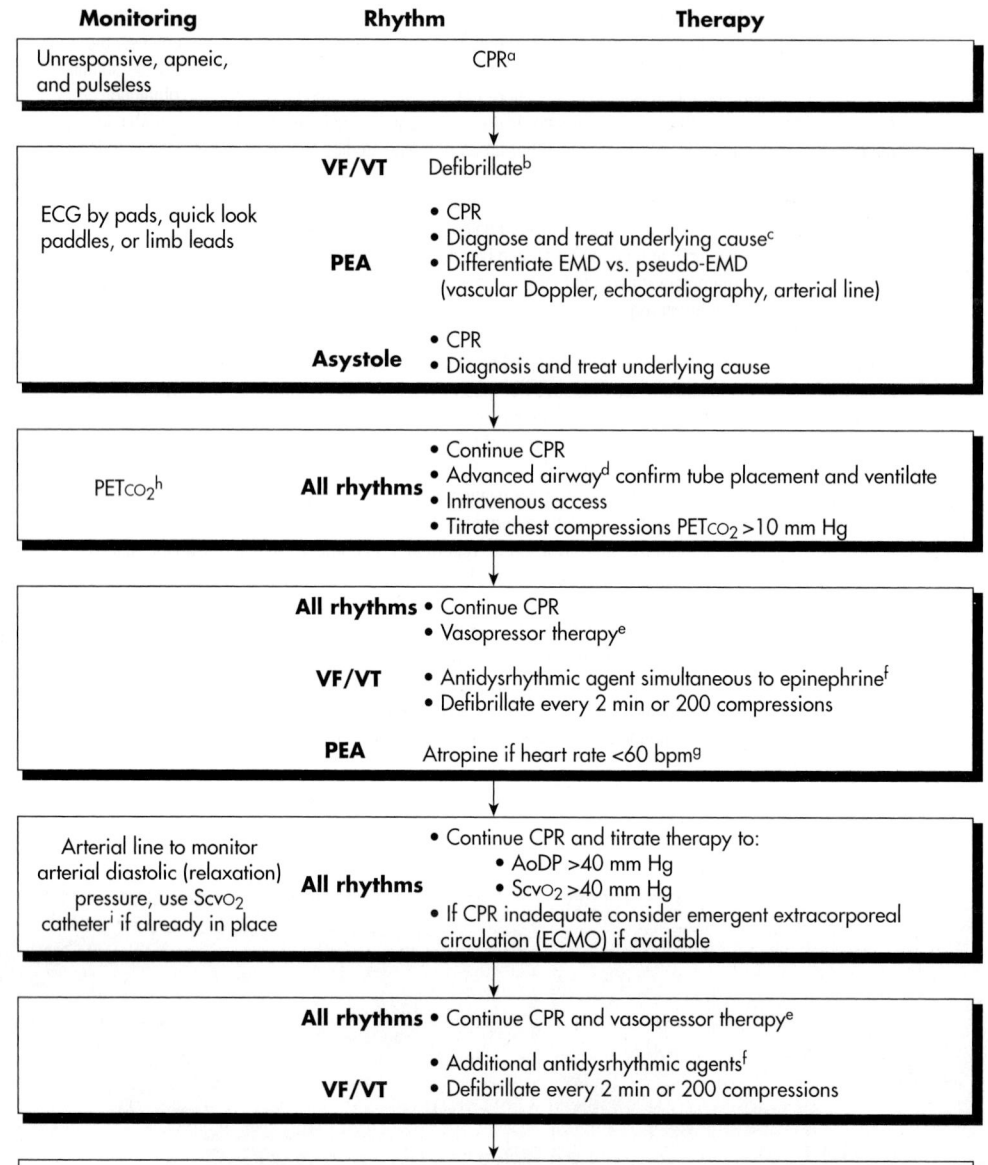

| Monitoring | Rhythm | Therapy |

FIG. 59 Emergency treatment algorithm for treatment of cardiac arrest. [a]If arrest is witnessed and known to be of short duration, immediate rhythm assessment and defibrillation or ventricular fibrillation/ventricular tachycardia (VF/VT) precede cardiopulmonary resuscitation (CPR). In cases of prolonged untreated VF/VT, 1 to 2 minutes of CPR before defibrillation may enhance the ability to achieve return of spontaneous circulation. *EMD,* Electromechanical dissociation; *PEA,* pulseless electrical activity. [b]Biphasic defibrillation should use manufacturer-recommended energy versus monophasic defibrillation (360 J). [c]See Section I, Pulseless Electrical Activity. [d]Endotracheal intubation or supraglottic airway when feasible with minimal interruption in chest compressions. [e]Epinephrine, initial dose of 1 mg intravenously (IV) or intraosseously (IO), or 2.5 mg by endotracheal tube (ETT). Repeat every 3 to 5 minutes. Subsequent doses may be increased up to 0.1 mg/kg. An alternative to epinephrine is vasopressin, 40 U via IV push. Vasopressin is potentially more effective if the presenting rhythm is asystolic. The dose (40 U) can be repeated once in 3 minutes, followed by administration of epinephrine every 3 to 5 minutes. [f]Amiodarone, 300 mg via IV push, followed by 150 mg every 30 minutes. Lidocaine is an alternative antidysrhythmic if amiodarone is not available. Magnesium sulfate, 1 to 2 g via IV push in torsades de pointes or known hypomagnesemia. [g]Atropine, 1 mg via IV push or 2.5 mg by ETT. Repeat dose every 3 to 5 minutes to a total dose of 0.04 mg/kg. *AoDP,* Aortic diastolic pressure; *ECG,* electrocardiogram; *ScvO₂,* central venous oxygen saturation. [h]Changes in the partial pressure of end-tidal carbon dioxide (PETCO₂) may not be predictive of myocardial blood flow in the setting of high-dose vasopressor therapy. [i]Invasive monitoring should be performed only if adequate personnel are available and if it would not delay therapeutic interventions. (From Marx JA, et al: *Rosen's emergency medicine,* ed 8, Philadelphia, 2014, Saunders.)

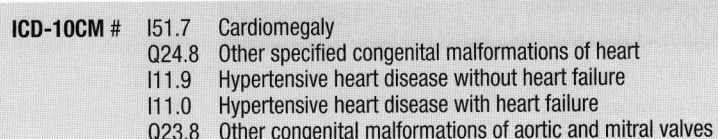

ICD-10CM #	I51.7	Cardiomegaly
	Q24.8	Other specified congenital malformations of heart
	I11.9	Hypertensive heart disease without heart failure
	I11.0	Hypertensive heart disease with heart failure
	Q23.8	Other congenital malformations of aortic and mitral valves

Evaluation of cardiomegaly on chest x-ray

Review history
Examination
ECG

Echocardiogram

Left ventricular dilation

Evaluate for:
  Valvular heart disease
  Coronary artery disease
  Cardiomyopathy

Biventricular dilation

Consider right heart failure secondary to left heart failure from various causes of left ventricular dilation

Right ventricular dilation

Pulmonary hypertension?

Yes

Evaluate for:
  Pulmonary emboli
  Mitral stenosis
  Primary pulmonary hypertension
  Eisenmenger's syndrome

No

Evaluate for:
  Atrial septal defect
  Tricuspid regurgitation

Pericardial effusion/thickening/mass

R/O tamponade

? Pericardiocentesis

? Cause

Consider:
  CT
  MRI
  Surgery/biopsy

No abnormalities

No further workup

FIG. 60 Approach to the patient with cardiomegaly. When cardiomegaly is found on the chest radiograph, the history and physical examination should be reviewed and an electrocardiogram *(ECG)* performed before obtaining a two-dimensional Doppler echocardiographic study. Cardiomegaly may be explained by left ventricular dilation, biventricular dilation, right ventricular dilation, or pericardial abnormalities, or it may be found to be spurious on the echocardiogram. Rarely, isolated abnormalities of the atrium, particularly the left atrium, may cause abnormalities on the chest radiograph but will not cause true cardiomegaly. Depending on the echocardiographic findings, further tests can help elucidate the cause of echocardiographically confirmed cardiomegaly. *CT*, Computed tomography; *MRI*, magnetic resonance imaging; *R/O*, rule out. (From Goldman L, Braunwald E [eds]: *Primary cardiology*, ed 2, Philadelphia, 2003, Saunders.)

Clinical Algorithms

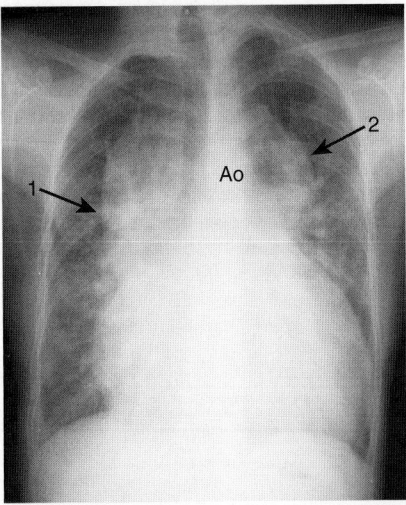

FIG. 61 "Snowman" heart in a 36-year-old man with increasing shortness of breath. Posteroanterior chest film examination shows cardiomegaly and increased pulmonary blood flow. The superior mediastinum is widened, the result of dilatation of the left vertical vein *(arrow 2)* and the right-sided superior vena cava *(arrow 1)*. The trachea is displaced by a normal left-sided aortic arch (Ao). (Boxt LM, Abbara S: The requisites, Cardiac Imaging, 4th ed, ISBN # 978-1-4557-4865-5, Philadelphia, 2016, Elsevier.)

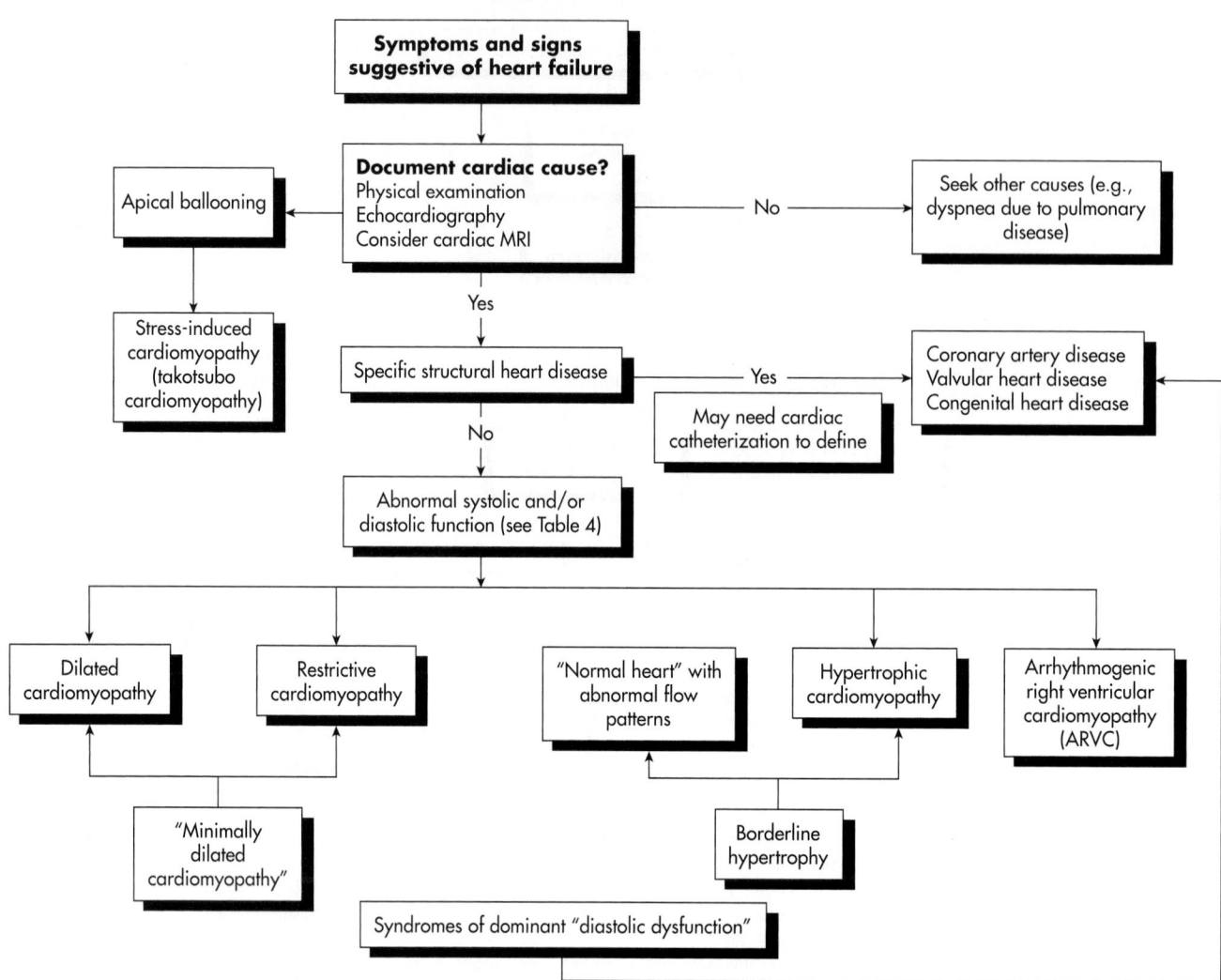

FIG. 62 Initial approach to classification of cardiomyopathy. The evaluation of symptoms or signs consistent with heart failure first includes confirmation that they can be attributed to a cardiac cause. Although this conclusion is often apparent from routine physical examination, echocardiography serves to confirm cardiac disease and provides clues to the presence of other cardiac disease, such as focal abnormalities, suggesting primary valve disease or congenital heart disease. Having excluded these conditions, cardiomyopathy is generally considered to be dilated, restrictive, or hypertrophic. Patients with apparently normal cardiac structure and contraction are occasionally found to demonstrate abnormal intracardiac flow patterns consistent with diastolic dysfunction but should also be evaluated carefully for other causes of their symptoms. Most patients with so-called diastolic dysfunction also demonstrate at least borderline criteria for left ventricular hypertrophy, frequently in the setting of chronic hypertension and diabetes. A moderately decreased ejection fraction without marked dilation or a pattern of restrictive cardiomyopathy is sometimes referred to as "minimally dilated cardiomyopathy," which may represent either a distinct entity or a transition between acute and chronic disease. (From Goldman L, Ausiello D [eds]: *Cecil textbook of medicine,* ed 23, Philadelphia, 2008, Saunders.)

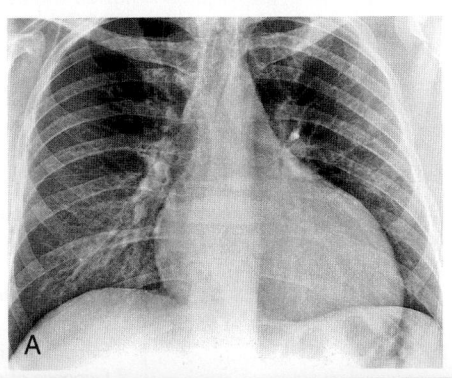

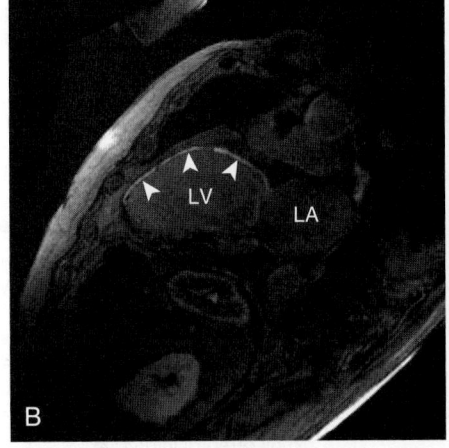
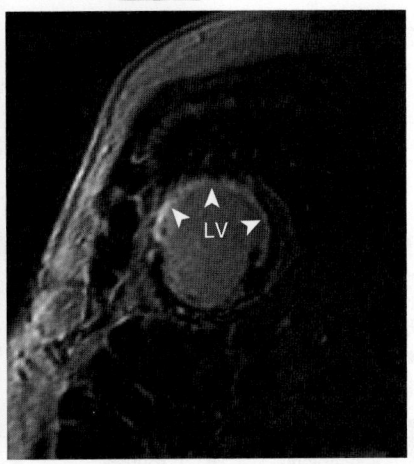

FIG. 63 Dilated cardiomyopathy. A, The heart shows enlargement of all four chambers. The azygos vein and superior vena cava are slightly dilated, reflecting high central venous pressure. **B,** Delayed enhanced magnetic resonance images demonstrate ischemic dilated cardiomyopathy. Extensive subendocardial delayed hyper-enhancement *(arrowheads)* demonstrates features of old myocardial infarction: it follows a vascular territory (the left anterior descending), it is based on the subendocardium, and there is thinning of the affected myo-cardium. *LA,* Left atrium; *LV,* left ventricle. (Boxt LM, Abbara S: The requisites, Cardiac Imaging, 4th ed, ISBN # 978-1-4557-4865-5, Philadelphia, 2016, Elsevier.)

Table 4 Profiles of Myocardial Disease

	Hypertrophic	Dilated	Restrictive	ARVC
Causes	Genetic	Myocarditis Metabolic/endocrine Genetic	Infiltrative or storage diseases Endomyocardial (e.g., Löffler's, carcinoid)	Genetic
Ejection fraction	Increased	Reduced	25%-50%	Normal until end stage 30% regional LV disease
Left ventricular End-diastolic dimension	Usually decreased	Increased	Normal	Normal until end stage Right ventricle dilated
Left ventricular wall thickness	Increased	Normal	Normal or mildly increased	Normal
Atrial size	Increased	Increased	Increased; may be massive	Left atrium normal; right dilated in severe disease
Valvular disease	Mitral regurgitation (SAM)	Mitral (functional); tricuspid regurgitation in late stages	Mitral and tricuspid regurgi-tation, rarely severe	Tricuspid regurgitation in severe disease
Common symptoms	Dyspnea; chest pain, syncope Late: orthopnea, PND	Dyspnea, fatigue Late: orthopnea, PND	Dyspnea Late: orthopnea, PND, right heart failure	Palpitations, syncope Late: right heart failure
Arrhythmia	Atrial fibrillation, ventricular tachycardia; conduction block in PRKAG2, mito-chondrial; Fabry's disease	Ventricular tachyarrhythmias; heart block in Chagas' disease, giant cell myocar-ditis, laminopathies	Atrial fibrillation; conduction block in sarcoid, amyloi-dosis, desminopathy	Ventricular ectopy and tachy-cardia

ARVC, Arrhythmogenic right ventricular cardiomyopathy; *LV,* left ventricular; *SAM,* systolic anterior motion of mitral valve; *PND,* paroxysmal nocturnal dyspnea.
From Goldman L, Schafer AI [eds]: *Goldman's Cecil medicine,* ed 24, Philadelphia, 2012, Saunders.

ICD-10CM # I67.82   Cerebral ischemia
            I67.81   Acute cerebrovascular insufficiency
            I67.89   Other cerebrovascular disease
            I67.848   Other cerebrovascular vasospasm and vasoconstriction
            G45.9   Transient cerebral ischemic attack, unspecified

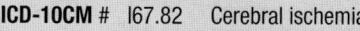

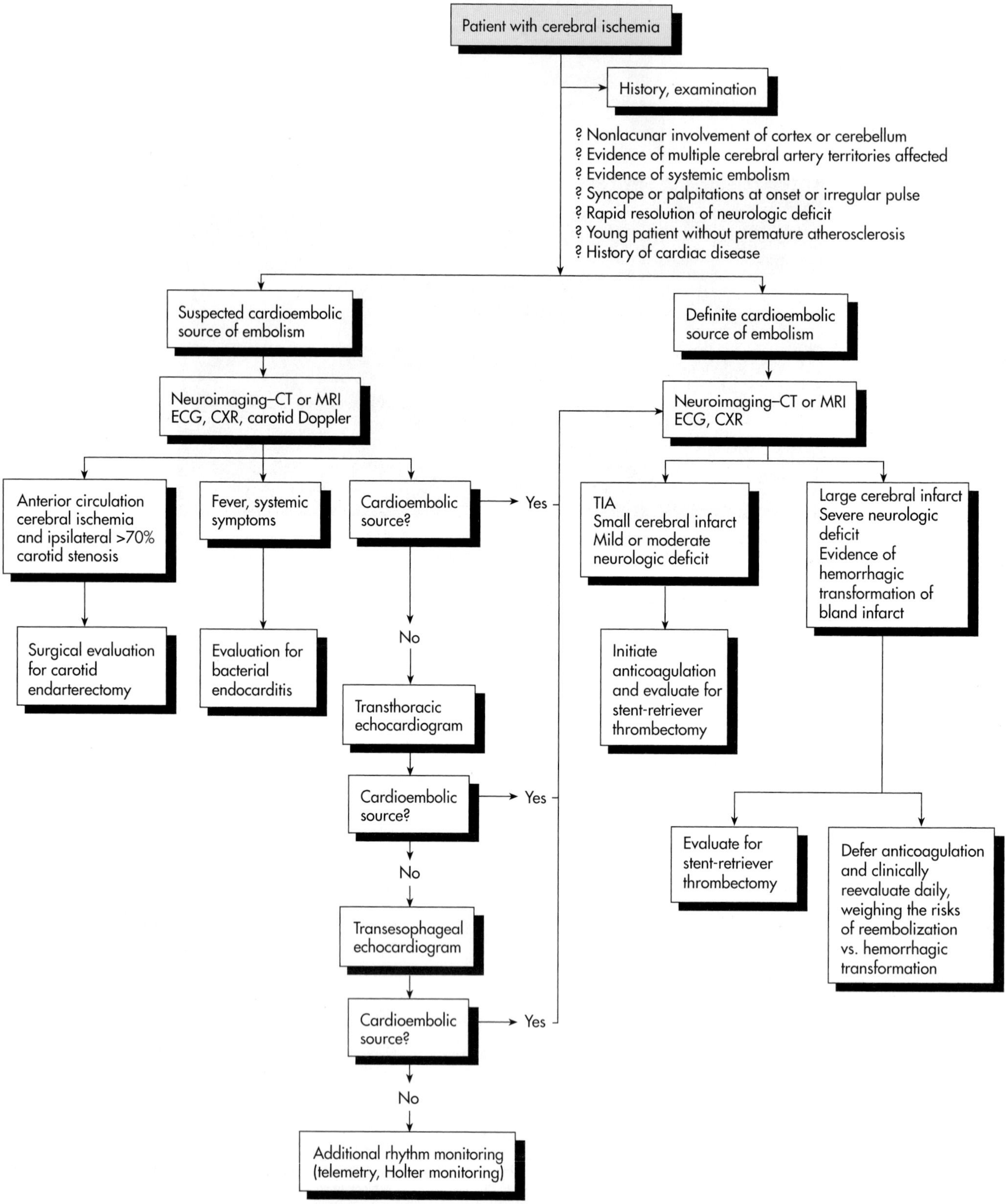

Patient with cerebral ischemia

History, examination

? Nonlacunar involvement of cortex or cerebellum
? Evidence of multiple cerebral artery territories affected
? Evidence of systemic embolism
? Syncope or palpitations at onset or irregular pulse
? Rapid resolution of neurologic deficit
? Young patient without premature atherosclerosis
? History of cardiac disease

Suspected cardioembolic source of embolism

Definite cardioembolic source of embolism

Neuroimaging—CT or MRI ECG, CXR, carotid Doppler

Neuroimaging—CT or MRI ECG, CXR

Anterior circulation cerebral ischemia and ipsilateral >70% carotid stenosis

Fever, systemic symptoms

Cardioembolic source? → Yes

TIA Small cerebral infarct Mild or moderate neurologic deficit

Large cerebral infarct Severe neurologic deficit Evidence of hemorrhagic transformation of bland infarct

Surgical evaluation for carotid endarterectomy

Evaluation for bacterial endocarditis

No

Initiate anticoagulation and evaluate for stent-retriever thrombectomy

Transthoracic echocardiogram

Cardioembolic source? → Yes

No

Transesophageal echocardiogram

Cardioembolic source? → Yes

No

Evaluate for stent-retriever thrombectomy

Defer anticoagulation and clinically reevaluate daily, weighing the risks of reembolization vs. hemorrhagic transformation

Additional rhythm monitoring (telemetry, Holter monitoring)

FIG. 65 Evaluation of patients with cerebral ischemia for a cardioembolic source. *CT,* Computed tomography; *CXR,* chest radiograph; *ECG,* electrocardiogram; *MRI,* magnetic resonance imaging; *TIA,* transient ischemic attack. (Modified from Johnson R [ed]: *Current therapy in neurologic disease,* ed 5, St Louis, 1997, Mosby.)

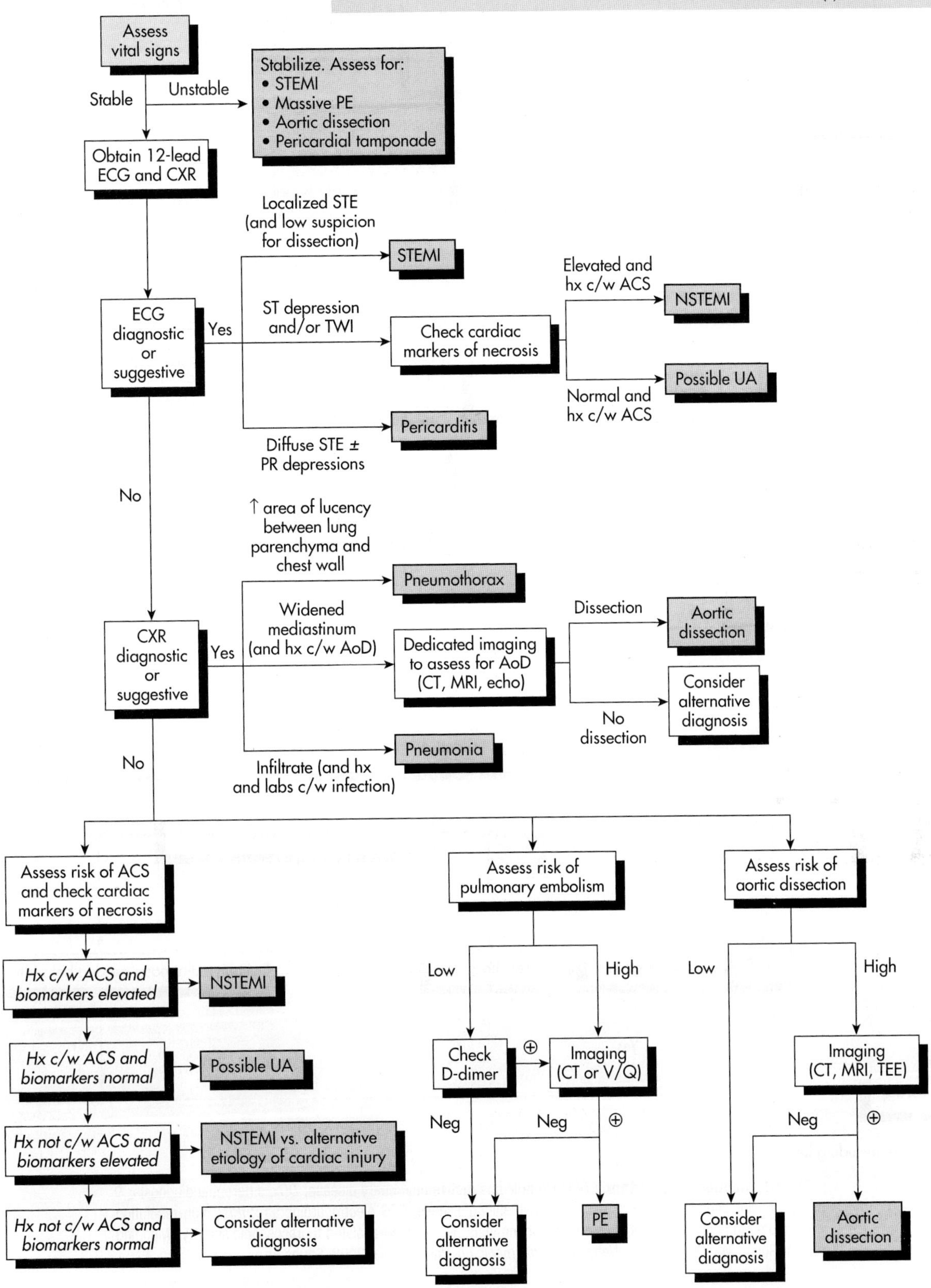

CHEST PAIN

ICD-10CM # R07.2 Pain(s) heart
R07.3 Pain(s) chest anterior wall
R07.4 Pain(s) chest

1595

FIG. 66 **Algorithm for the initial diagnostic approach to a patient with chest pain**. *AoD*, Aortic dissection; *c/w*, consistent with; *CXR*, chest x-ray; *hx*, history; *NSTEMI*, non–ST-segment myocardial infarction; *PE*, pulmonary embolism; *STE*, ST elevation; *STEMI*, ST-segment myocardial infarction; *TEE*, transesophageal echocardiography; *UA*, unstable angina; *V/Q*, ventilation-perfusion scan. (From Bonow RO et al: *Braunwald's heart disease*, ed 9, Philadelphia, 2012, Elsevier.)

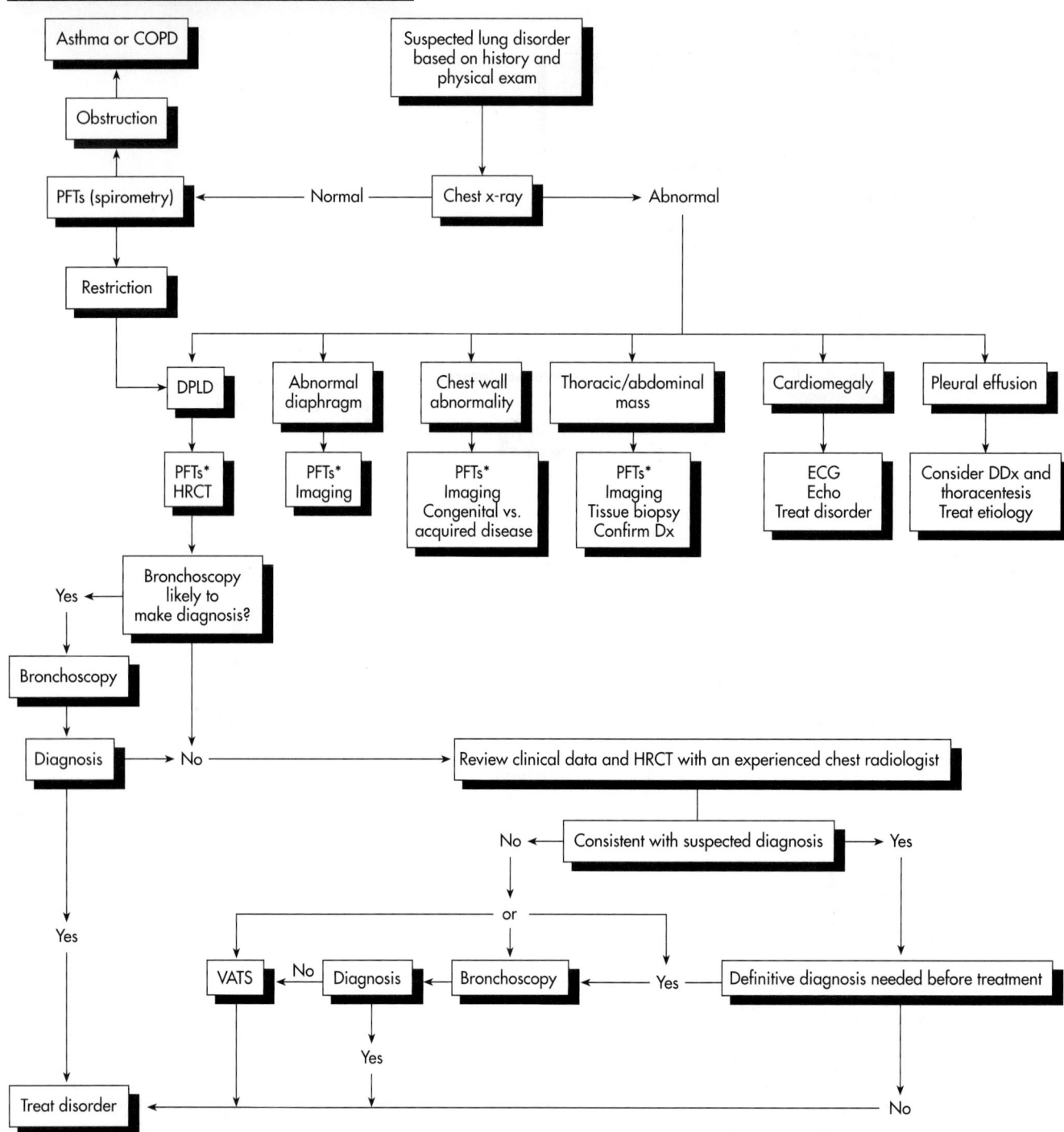

*PFTs = Full set including lung volumes and DLCO

FIG. 67 Diagnostic algorithm. *COPD,* Chronic obstructive pulmonary disease; *DDx,* differential diagnosis; *D*
LCO, diffusion capacity; *DPLD,* diffuse parenchymal lung disease; *ECG,* electrocardiogram; *HRCT,* high-resolution
computed tomography; *PFTs,* pulmonary function tests; *VATS,* video-assisted thoracoscopic surgery. (Modified
from Runge MS, Greganti MA: *Netter's internal medicine,* Philadelphia, 2008, Saunders.)

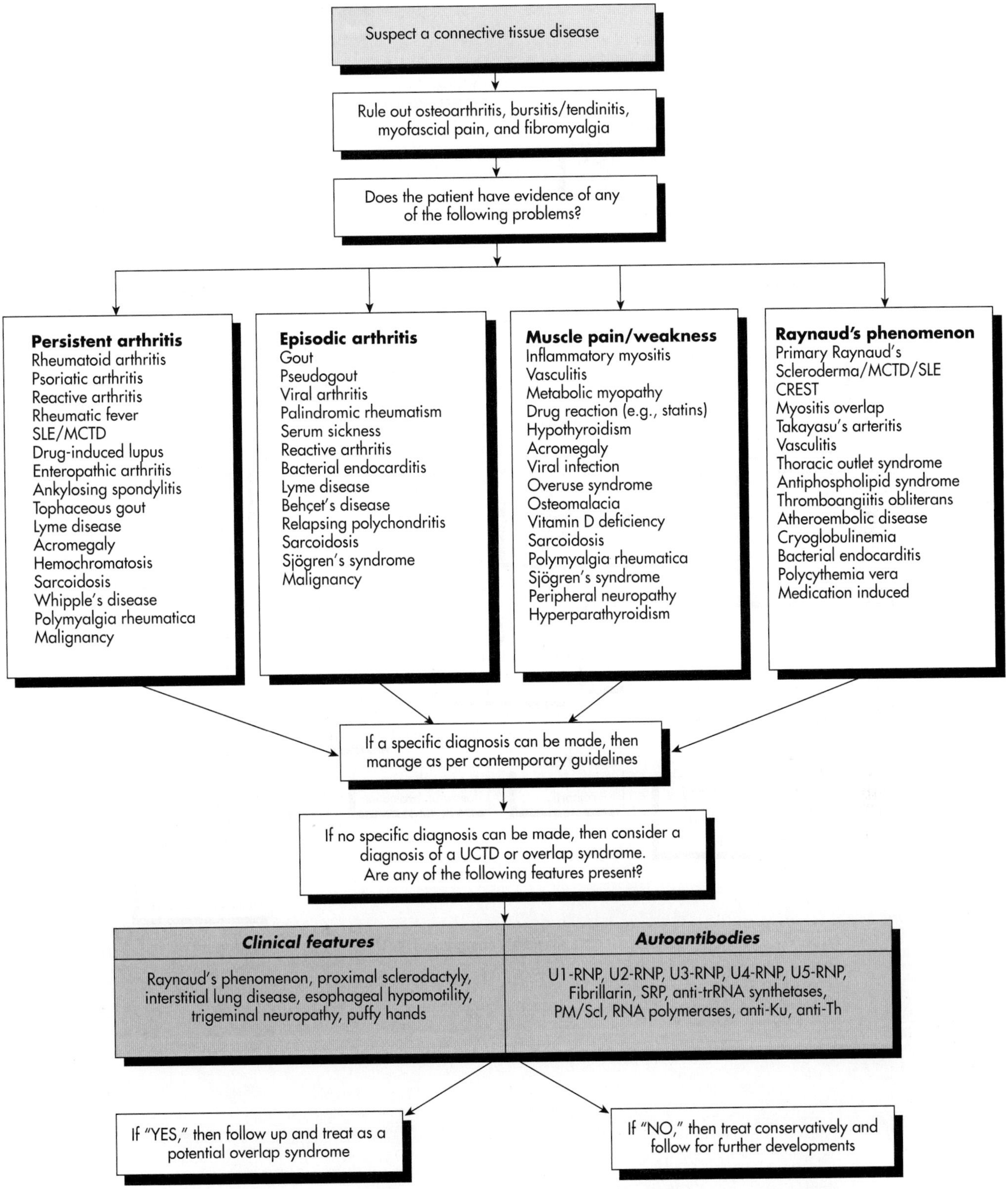

Suspect a connective tissue disease

Rule out osteoarthritis, bursitis/tendinitis, myofascial pain, and fibromyalgia

Does the patient have evidence of any of the following problems?

Persistent arthritis
Rheumatoid arthritis
Psoriatic arthritis
Reactive arthritis
Rheumatic fever
SLE/MCTD
Drug-induced lupus
Enteropathic arthritis
Ankylosing spondylitis
Tophaceous gout
Lyme disease
Acromegaly
Hemochromatosis
Sarcoidosis
Whipple's disease
Polymyalgia rheumatica
Malignancy

Episodic arthritis
Gout
Pseudogout
Viral arthritis
Palindromic rheumatism
Serum sickness
Reactive arthritis
Bacterial endocarditis
Lyme disease
Behçet's disease
Relapsing polychondritis
Sarcoidosis
Sjögren's syndrome
Malignancy

Muscle pain/weakness
Inflammatory myositis
Vasculitis
Metabolic myopathy
Drug reaction (e.g., statins)
Hypothyroidism
Acromegaly
Viral infection
Overuse syndrome
Osteomalacia
Vitamin D deficiency
Sarcoidosis
Polymyalgia rheumatica
Sjögren's syndrome
Peripheral neuropathy
Hyperparathyroidism

Raynaud's phenomenon
Primary Raynaud's
Scleroderma/MCTD/SLE
CREST
Myositis overlap
Takayasu's arteritis
Vasculitis
Thoracic outlet syndrome
Antiphospholipid syndrome
Thromboangiitis obliterans
Atheroembolic disease
Cryoglobulinemia
Bacterial endocarditis
Polycythemia vera
Medication induced

If a specific diagnosis can be made, then manage as per contemporary guidelines

If no specific diagnosis can be made, then consider a diagnosis of a UCTD or overlap syndrome. Are any of the following features present?

Clinical features	*Autoantibodies*
Raynaud's phenomenon, proximal sclerodactyly, interstitial lung disease, esophageal hypomotility, trigeminal neuropathy, puffy hands	U1-RNP, U2-RNP, U3-RNP, U4-RNP, U5-RNP, Fibrillarin, SRP, anti-trRNA synthetases, PM/Scl, RNA polymerases, anti-Ku, anti-Th

If "YES," then follow up and treat as a potential overlap syndrome

If "NO," then treat conservatively and follow for further developments

FIG. 68 Algorithm for evaluating patients with undifferentiated connective tissue disease (UCTD). *CREST,* Calcinosis, Raynaud's phenomenon, esophageal dysmotility, sclerodactyly, and telangiectasia; *MCTD,* mixed connective tissue disease; *SLE,* systemic lupus erythematosus. (From Firestein GS, Budd RC, Gabriel SE, et al: *Kelley's textbook of rheumatology,* ed 9, Philadelphia, 2013, Saunders. [Original credit: Courtesy Dr. George Raj, Non Surgical Spine and Joint Clinic PS, Bellingham, Wash.])

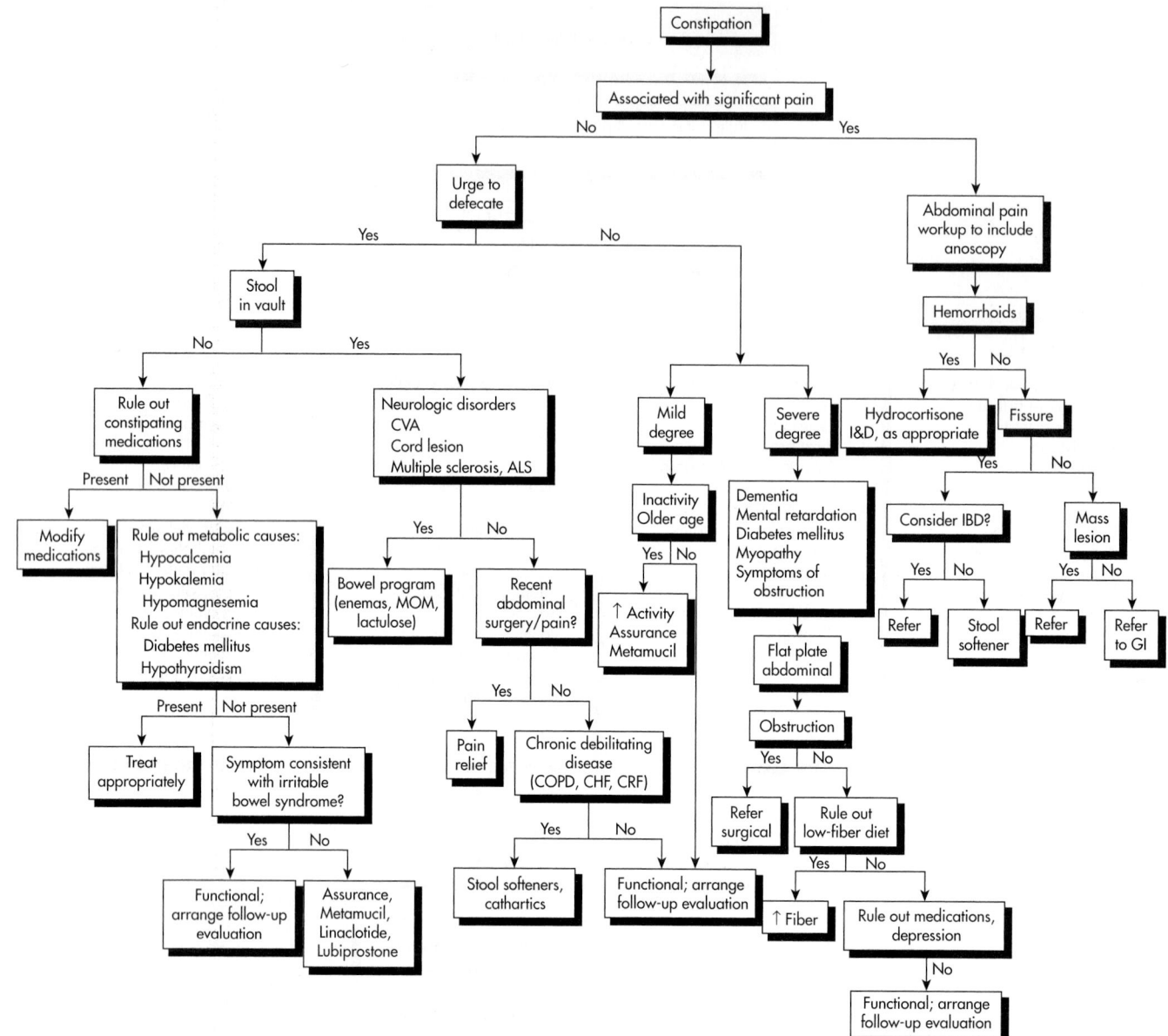

FIG. 69 Algorithmic approach to the diagnosis of constipation. *ALS*, Amyotrophic lateral sclerosis; *CHF*, congestive heart failure; *COPD*, chronic obstructive pulmonary disease; *CRF*, chronic renal failure; *CVA*, cerebrovascular accident; *GI*, gastroenterology; *IBD*, inflammatory bowel disease; *I&D*, incision and drainage; *MOM*, milk of magnesia. (From Marx JA et al: *Rosen's emergency medicine*, ed 8, Philadelphia, 2014, Saunders.)

Table 5 Preparations Used in the Symptomatic Treatment of Constipation

Medication	Maximal Recommended Dose	Onset of Action	Comments
Bulk Laxatives			Indigestible fiber attracts water, which leads to larger, softer fecal mass.
Psyllium (Metamucil)	Titrate up to 20 g	12-72 hr	Natural fiber that undergoes bacterial degradation, which may contribute to bloating and flatus. Should be taken with plenty of water to avoid intestinal obstruction.
Methylcellulose (Citrucel)	Titrate up to 20 g		Semisynthetic cellulose fiber that is relatively resistant to colonic bacterial degradation.
Polycarbophil (Fibercon)	Titrate up to 20 g		Synthetic fiber of polymer of acrylic acid, resistant to bacterial degradation.
Osmotic Laxatives			Draw water into the intestines along osmotic gradient.
Magnesium or Sodium Salts			
Magnesium hydroxide (milk of magnesia)	30-45 ml once daily	1-6 hr	A small percentage of magnesium is absorbed—use caution in patients with renal insufficiency and in children.
Magnesium citrate	150-300 ml as needed	3-6 hr	
Sodium phosphate (Fleet Phospho-soda)	20-45 ml with 12 oz of water as needed		Hyperphosphatemia may result if patient has renal insufficiency. Commonly used before colonoscopy.
Poorly Absorbed Sugars			
Lactulose	15-30 ml once or twice a day	24-48 hr	Synthetic disaccharide not absorbed by the small intestine. Gas and bloating common.
Sorbitol	15-30 ml once or twice a day		Poorly absorbed by small intestine.
Polyethylene glycol and electrolytes (GoLYTELY, MiraLax)	17 g two or three times a day	12-24 hr	Organic polymers that are poorly absorbed and not metabolized by bacteria, thus may cause less bloating and cramping. Can be mixed with noncarbonated beverages.
Stimulant Laxatives			Stimulate intestinal motility or secretion.
Senna (Senokot, Ex-Lax)	8-34 mg daily	6-12 hr	Stimulates secretion and motility of small intestine and colon.
Bisacodyl (Dulcolax, Correctol)	5-10 mg daily		
Stool Softeners			Increase water penetration and soften stool.
Docusate sodium (Colace)	100 mg twice a day; some use higher doses	24-48 hr	In many studies, no better than placebo. Not recommended as first-line or solo therapy.
Mineral oil (Fleet mineral oil)	5-15 ml orally at night		Provides lubrication for the passage of stool. Long-term use is not recommended. Lipid pneumonia can occur in patients predisposed to aspiration.
Newer Agents			
Lubiprostone (Amitiza)	24 µg once or twice per day	1 hr	A chloride channel activator. FDA approved for treatment of chronic idiopathic constipation in adults. Adverse effects: headache, nausea, diarrhea.
Methylnaltrexone (Relistor)	8-12 mg SQ		Used in refractory opioid-induced constipation.
Linaclotide (Linzess)	145 mcg daily 30 min prior to meals	2-6 hr	Peptide agonist of the guanylate cyclase 2C. It increases smooth muscle contractions. Useful in IBS with constipation.

FDA, U.S. Food and Drug Administration; *SQ,* subcutaneously.
From Marx JA et al: *Rosen's emergency medicine*, ed 8, Philadelphia, 2014, Saunders.

BOX 4 General Approach to Treatment of Constipation

For specific agents, dosages, and precautions, see Table 5.

I. Core Program for All Patients
- Adequate intake of fluid and fiber is one key to preventing constipation. Fiber is available primarily from grains and bran cereals. Flatulence, bloating, and cramps are common side effects encountered when bran fiber is introduced.
- Another source of bulk is from synthetic bulk agents (e.g., psyllium). Bulk agents require an adequate amount of fluid intake; otherwise, they may worsen constipation.
- Avoid irritant laxatives as part of a core program because long-term use may decrease bowel motility. Encourage the patient to exercise and respond promptly to the urge to defecate.

II. Individualized Program-Specific Indications and General Comments
- *Stimulant laxatives (e.g., senna, bisacodyl):* Many believe that long-term use of these agents leads to dependency and habituation, but this is not substantiated. When used appropriately, these medications are not harmful and are very effective. Senna is probably the first-line choice among this class of laxatives.

- *Osmotic laxatives (e.g., polyethylene glycol [PEG], lactulose, milk of magnesia, magnesium citrate):* These agents are most commonly used for colonic preparation before bowel procedures. These agents are safe and well tolerated. PEG has been shown to be slightly more effective than lactulose and causes less bloating and flatus.
- *Lubricants and stool softeners:* Oral mineral oil lubricants and stool softeners are particularly helpful in patients who have acute painful perianal lesions. The softening and coating of the stool can make passage much easier and less painful, preventing constipation. Mineral oil is contraindicated in patients with swallowing problems or in those who are particularly debilitated, to prevent aspiration leading to lipid pneumonia.
- *Suppositories and enemas:* These agents may be helpful in patients who tend to have trouble expelling soft stool from the rectum. Glycerin suppositories may have a soothing effect and be helpful in patients with constipation caused by local, painful perianal lesions. Tap-water enemas are helpful when disimpaction is necessary.

From Marx JA et al: *Rosen's emergency medicine*, ed 8, Philadelphia, 2014, Saunders.

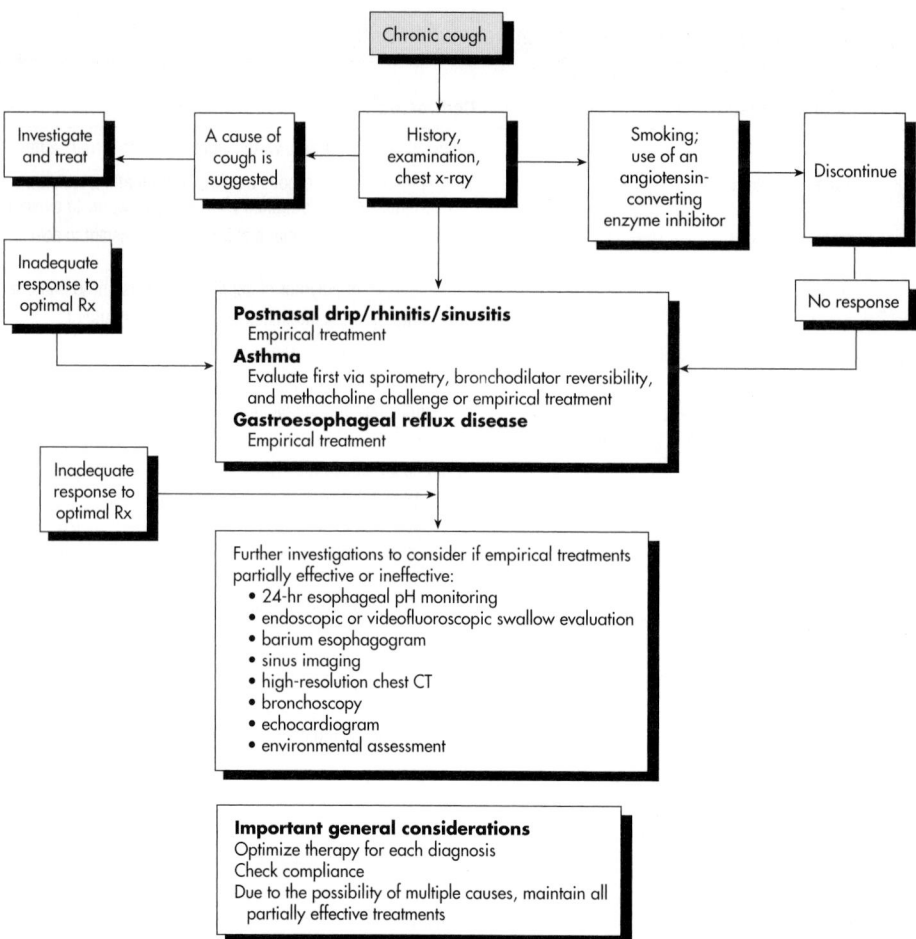

FIG. 72 Algorithm for the management of chronic cough lasting >8 weeks. *CT*, Computed tomography; *Rx*, prescription. (From Goldman L, Schafer AI: *Goldman's Cecil medicine*, ed 24, Philadelphia, 2012, Saunders.)

Table 6 Testing Characteristics of Diagnostic Protocol for Evaluation of Chronic Cough

Tests	Diagnosis	Positive Predictive Value (%)	Negative Predictive Value (%)
Sinus radiograph	Sinusitis	57-81	95-100
Methacholine inhalation challenge	Asthma	60-82	100
Modified barium esophagography	GERD, esophageal stricture	38-63	63-93
Esophageal pH*	GERD	89-100	>100
Bronchoscopy	Endobronchial mass/lesion	50-89	100

*24-Hour esophageal pH monitoring. *GERD*, Gastroesophageal reflux disease.
From Goldman L, Schafer AI [eds]: *Goldman's Cecil medicine*, ed 24, Philadelphia, 2012, Saunders.

Table 7 Definitions and Common Causes of Cough in Adults and Children

Age Group	Type of Cough	Duration	Common Causes
Adults	Acute	<3 weeks	• Common cold • Exacerbation of lung disease (e.g., asthma) • Acute environmental exposure • Acute cardiopulmonary disease
	Subacute	3-8 weeks	• Postinfectious cough • Pertussis infection • Exacerbation of underlying lung disease (e.g., asthma, COPD, bronchiectasis)
	Chronic	>8 weeks	• ACEI therapy • Smoking/chronic bronchitis • Underlying lung disease • UACS • Asthma • NAEB • GERD
Children	Acute	<4 weeks	• Common cold • Exacerbation of underlying lung disease • Acute cardiopulmonary disease
	Chronic	>4 weeks	• Asthma • Protracted bacterial bronchitis • Tracheobronchomalacia • Chronic rhinosinusitis • Recurrent aspiration • GERD • Underlying lung disease (e.g., bronchiectasis) • Pulmonary infections (e.g., pertussis)

ACEI, Angiotensin-converting enzyme inhibitor; *COPD,* chronic obstructive pulmonary disease; *GERD,* gastroesophageal reflux disease; *NAEB,* nonasthmatic eosinophilic bronchitis; *UACS,* upper airway cough syndrome.
From Adkinson NF et al: *Middleton's allergy principles and practice,* ed 8, Philadelphia, 2014, Saunders.

BOX 5 Pitfalls and Errors in the Diagnosis and Management of Chronic Cough in Adults

General Considerations
• Failing to consider that UACS, asthma/NAEB, and/or GERD are likely when the chest radiograph is normal or near-normal in appearance and the patient is a nonsmoker and is not taking an ACEI
• Failing to include UACS, asthma/NAEB, and/or GERD in the differential diagnosis because clinical or radiographic evidence confirms the presence of an "obvious" cause of the patient's cough (e.g., solitary pulmonary nodule, idiopathic pulmonary fibrosis)
• Not recognizing multiple simultaneous causes of cough
• Failing to continue treatment trials long enough to accurately assess their effectiveness
• Prematurely diagnosing "unexplained" cough before a bronchoscopy has been performed to assess for unsuspected airway disease
• Mistakenly diagnosing "unexplained" cough or diagnosing psychogenic cough before a complete evaluation for cough has been performed

Upper Airway Cough Syndrome
• Failing to realize that UACS can manifest as cough productive of phlegm
• Not recognizing that chronic cough can be the sole manifestation of UACS in at least 20% of the cases
• Failing to consider sinusitis as a cause of UACS
• Mistakenly assuming that selective histamine H_1 receptor antagonists are effective in treating nonallergic causes of UACS
• Missing allergic rhinitis because symptoms are perennial
• Missing aspirin-exacerbated disease in a patient with nasal polyps

Asthma/NAEB
• Failing to realize that these conditions can sometimes manifest as cough productive of phlegm

• Not recognizing that chronic cough can sometimes be the sole manifestation of asthma (so-called cough variant asthma)
• Mistakenly assuming that a positive result on bronchial challenge (e.g., methacholine challenge) is diagnostic of asthma when it is merely *consistent* with the diagnosis
• Failing to consider NAEB when the bronchial challenge test yields a negative result
• Not recognizing that inhaled medications can sometimes provoke cough
• Failing to consider occupational and environmental causes of asthma/NAEB

Gastroesophageal Reflux Disease
• Failing to realize that GERD can sometimes manifest as cough productive of phlegm
• Not recognizing that chronic cough can sometimes be the sole manifestation of GERD (so-called silent GERD)
• Mistakenly concluding that cough cannot be due to GERD simply because cough does not resolve with relief of gastrointestinal symptoms
• Not considering nonacid reflux and mistakenly assuming that cough will always respond to acid suppression
• Failing to assess the adequacy of GERD treatment by using 24-hour monitoring of esophageal pH and impedance
• Not recognizing coexisting diseases (e.g., sleep apnea) and medications (e.g., nitrates, progesterone) that may impair the effectiveness of GERD treatment
• Failing to recognize that surgery may help when intensive medical therapy has failed

Angiotensin-Converting Enzyme Inhibitor
• Failing to consider ACEI therapy as a cause of chronic cough simply because the cough predated initiation of the ACEI
• Mistakenly concluding that ACEI therapy is not the cause of chronic cough because the cough did not resolve within 1 to 3 weeks of stopping the ACEI

ACEI, Angiotensin-converting enzyme inhibitor; *GERD,* gastroesophageal reflux disease; *NAEB,* nonasthmatic eosinophilic bronchitis; *UACS,* upper airway cough syndrome.
From Adkinson NF et al: *Middleton's allergy principles and practice,* ed 8, Philadelphia, 2014, Saunders.

Clinical Algorithms

III

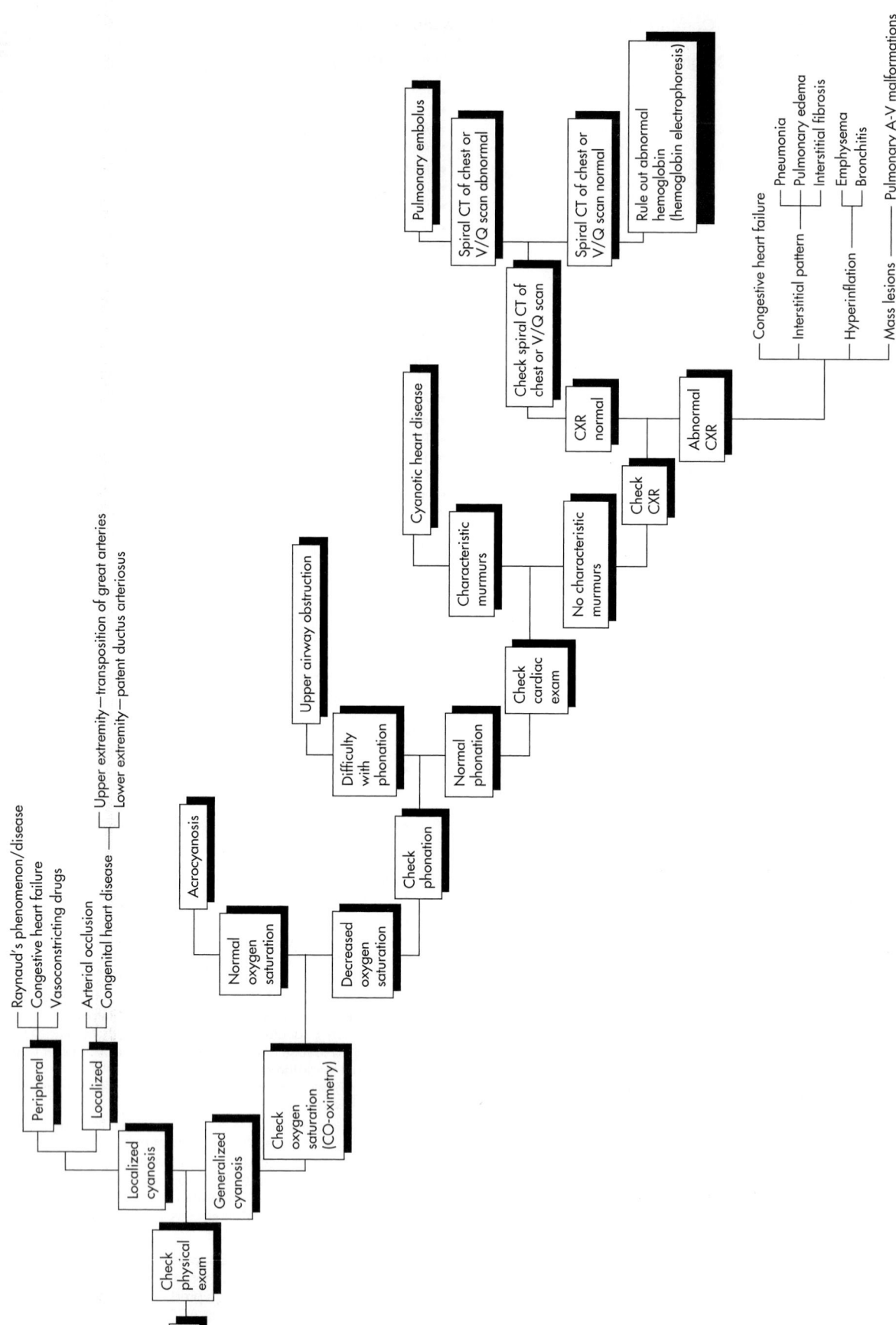

FIG. 74 Cyanosis. *A-V,* Arteriovenous; *CXR,* chest x-ray; *V/Q,* ventilation-perfusion. (From Healey PM: *Common medical diagnosis: an algorithmic approach,* ed 3, Philadelphia, 2000, Saunders.)

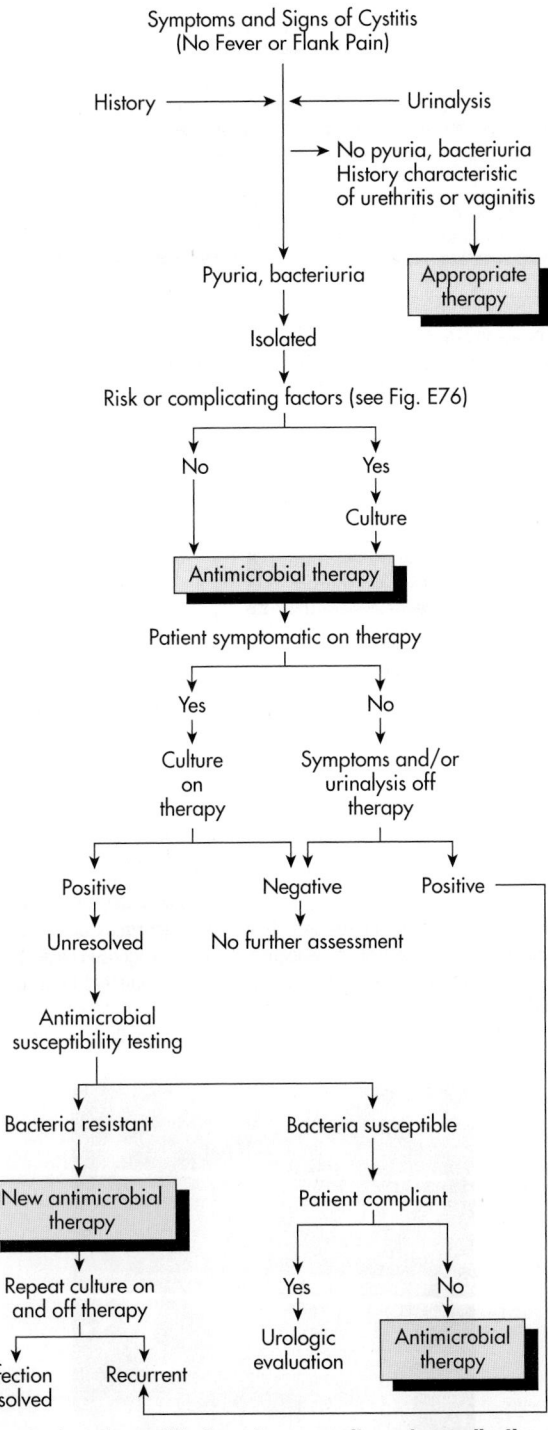

FIG. 75   Management of acute cystitis based on severity and complicating factors. (Wein AJ, Kavoussi LR, Partin AW, Peters CA: Campbell-Walsh Urology, 11th ed, ISBN# 978-1-4557-7567-5, 2016, Elsevier.)

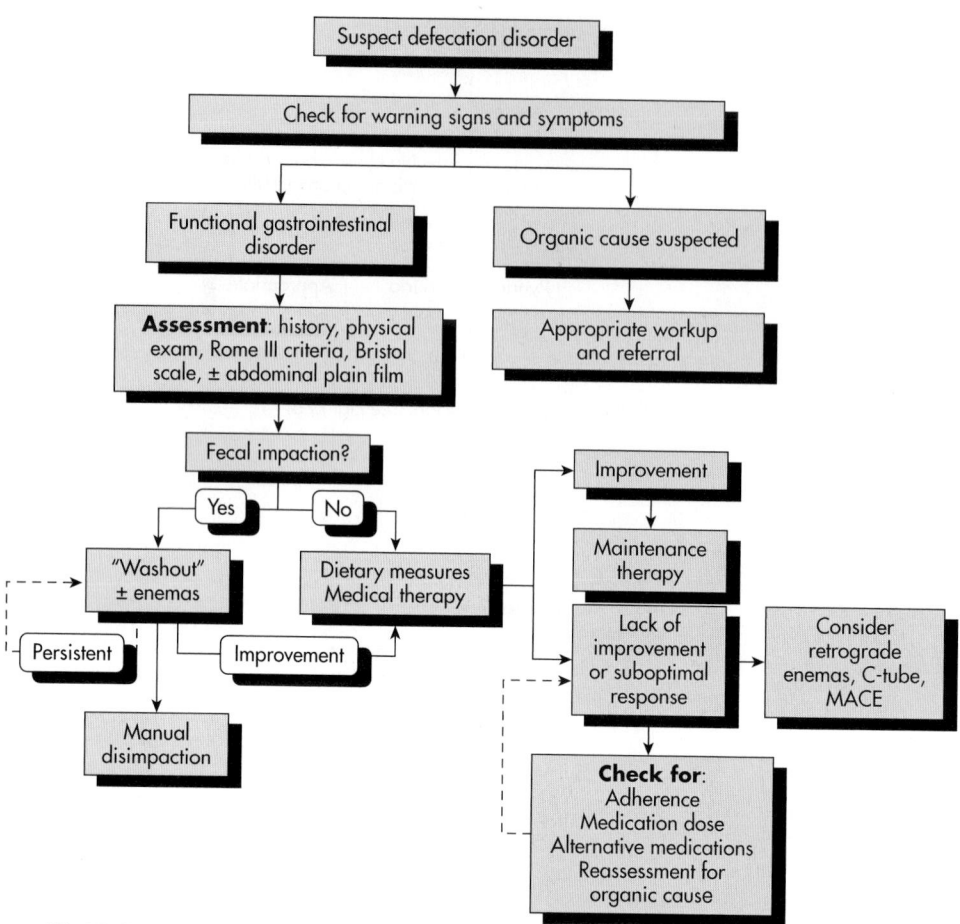

FIG. 77 Management algorithm for childhood defecation disorders seen in a pediatric urology practice. Lack of improvement or intractable constipation should be diagnosed based on worsening response, absence of response, or suboptimal response to adequate medical treatment for at least 3 months. *C-tube,* cecostomy tube; *MACE,* Malone antegrade continence enema procedure. (Wein AJ, Kavoussi LR, Partin AW, Peters CA: Campbell-Walsh Urology, 11th ed, ISBN# 978-1-4557-7567-5, 2016, Elsevier.)

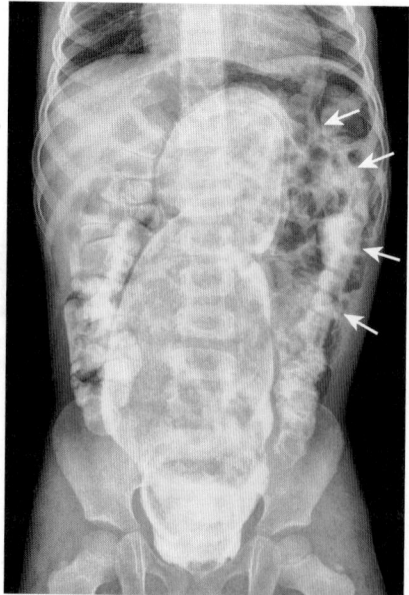

FIG. 78 Soluble contrast enema for evaluation of child with defecation problems since birth. Findings suggestive of Hirschsprung disease, including massively distended colon and rectum that can progress toward more normal-appearing large bowel *(arrows).* This child was subsequently assessed with a rectal biopsy to confirm the diagnosis. (Wein AJ, Kavoussi LR, Partin AW, Peters CA: Campbell-Walsh Urology, 11th ed, ISBN# 978-1-4557-7567-5, 2016, Elsevier.)

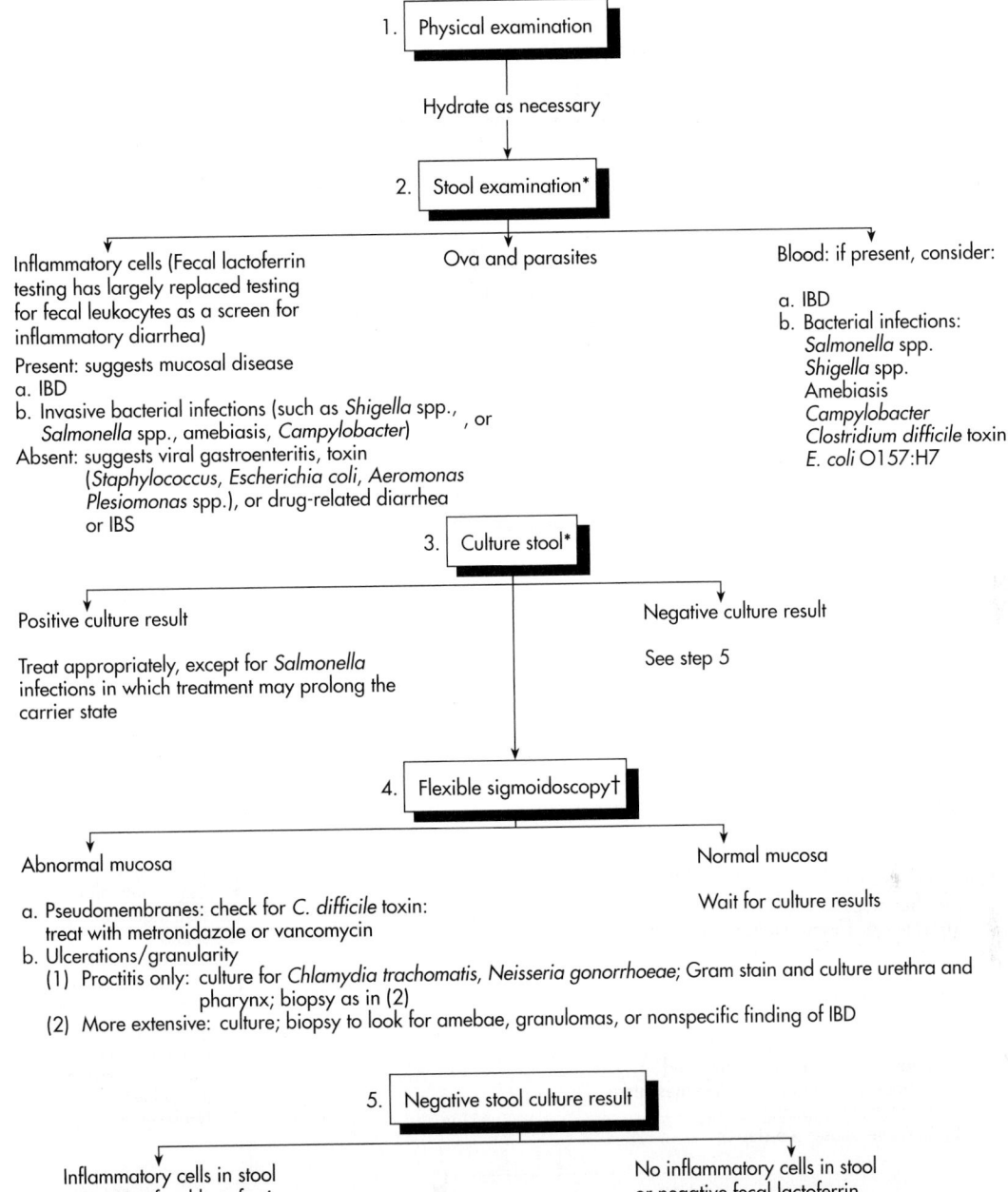

1. Physical examination

Hydrate as necessary

2. Stool examination*

Inflammatory cells (Fecal lactoferrin testing has largely replaced testing for fecal leukocytes as a screen for inflammatory diarrhea)

Present: suggests mucosal disease
a. IBD
b. Invasive bacterial infections (such as *Shigella* spp., *Salmonella* spp., amebiasis, *Campylobacter*) , or
Absent: suggests viral gastroenteritis, toxin (*Staphylococcus, Escherichia coli, Aeromonas Plesiomonas* spp.), or drug-related diarrhea or IBS

Ova and parasites

Blood: if present, consider:

a. IBD
b. Bacterial infections:
Salmonella spp.
Shigella spp.
Amebiasis
Campylobacter
Clostridium difficile toxin
E. coli O157:H7

3. Culture stool*

Positive culture result

Treat appropriately, except for *Salmonella* infections in which treatment may prolong the carrier state

Negative culture result

See step 5

4. Flexible sigmoidoscopy†

Abnormal mucosa

a. Pseudomembranes: check for *C. difficile* toxin: treat with metronidazole or vancomycin
b. Ulcerations/granularity
 (1) Proctitis only: culture for *Chlamydia trachomatis, Neisseria gonorrhoeae*; Gram stain and culture urethra and pharynx; biopsy as in (2)
 (2) More extensive: culture; biopsy to look for amebae, granulomas, or nonspecific finding of IBD

Normal mucosa

Wait for culture results

5. Negative stool culture result

Inflammatory cells in stool or positive fecal lactoferrin

IBD likely

a. Severely ill: rule out toxic megacolon; analyze blood cultures; abdominal x-ray; treat as IBD
b. Not severely ill: colonoscopy after careful and gentle preparation

No inflammatory cells in stool or negative fecal lactoferrin

a. If history is appropriate, with travel to endemic areas, or if patient has hypogammaglobulinemia, evaluate duodenal aspirate for *Giardia*
b. Stop all drugs, stop milk products, rule out malabsorption, observe, and treat symptomatically; if symptoms persist or recur, perform colonoscopy

FIG. 82 Diagnostic steps in the assessment of acute diarrhea. *For most cases of acute diarrhea, testing is not indicated. Stool examination and culture should be reserved for patients with severe illness, bloody stool, severe dehydration, immunosuppression, and for suspected nosocomial infection. †The role of lower endoscopy in acute diarrhea is limited. It should be considered only if the diagnosis is unclear after blood and stool tests in severely symptomatic patients. ‡Acute diarrhea is defined as stool with increased water content, volume, or frequency that lasts less than 14 days. *IBD,* Inflammatory bowel disease; *IBS,* irritable bowel syndrome. (Modified from Stein JH [ed]: *Internal medicine,* ed 5, St Louis, 1998, Mosby.)

Clinical Algorithms

III

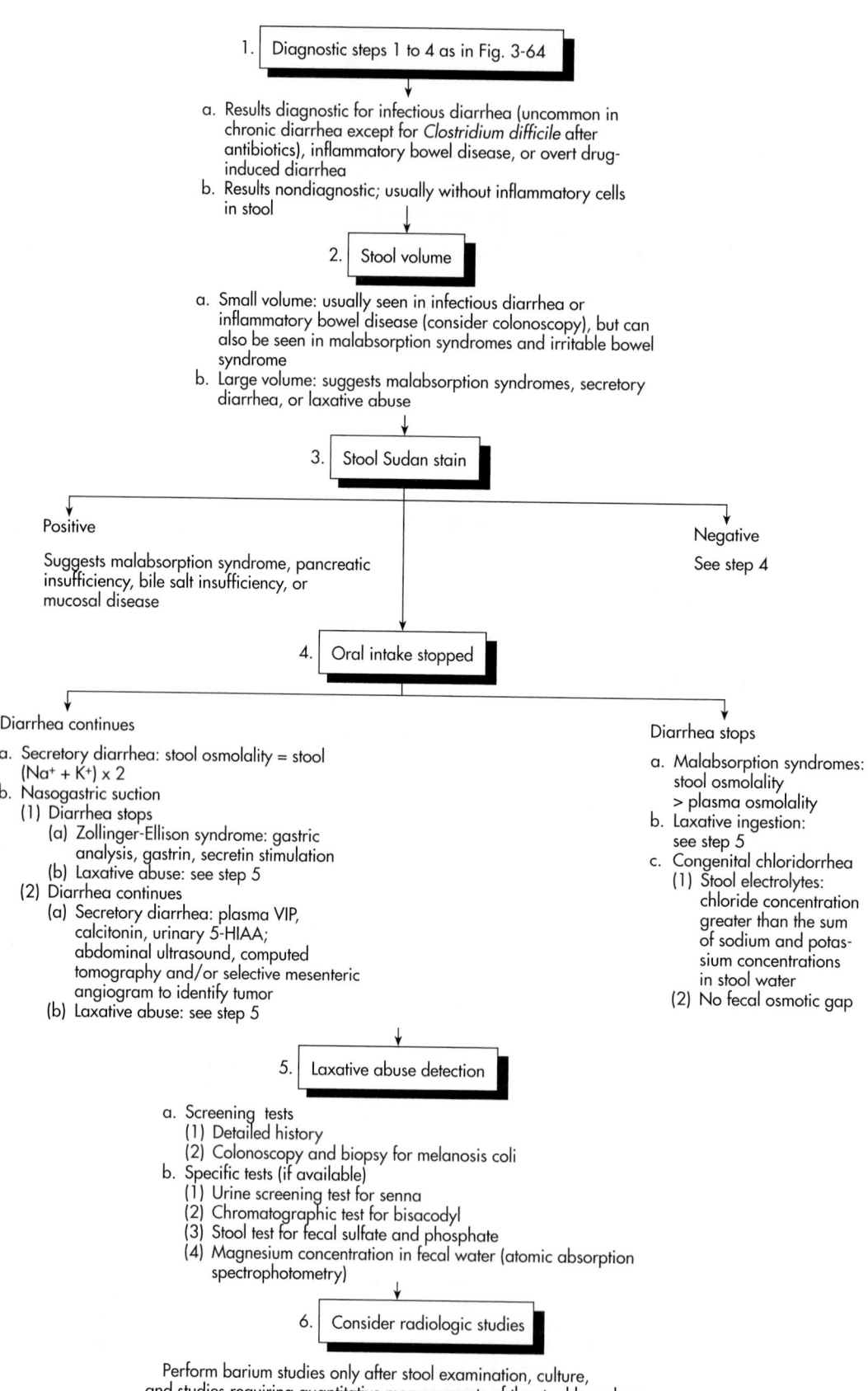

FIG. 83 Diagnostic approach to the patient with chronic diarrhea (patients who are HIV negative).
5-HIAA, 5-Hydroxyindoleacetic acid; *VIP,* vasoactive intestinal polypeptide. (Modified from Stein JH [ed]: *Internal medicine,* ed 5, St Louis, 1998, Mosby.)

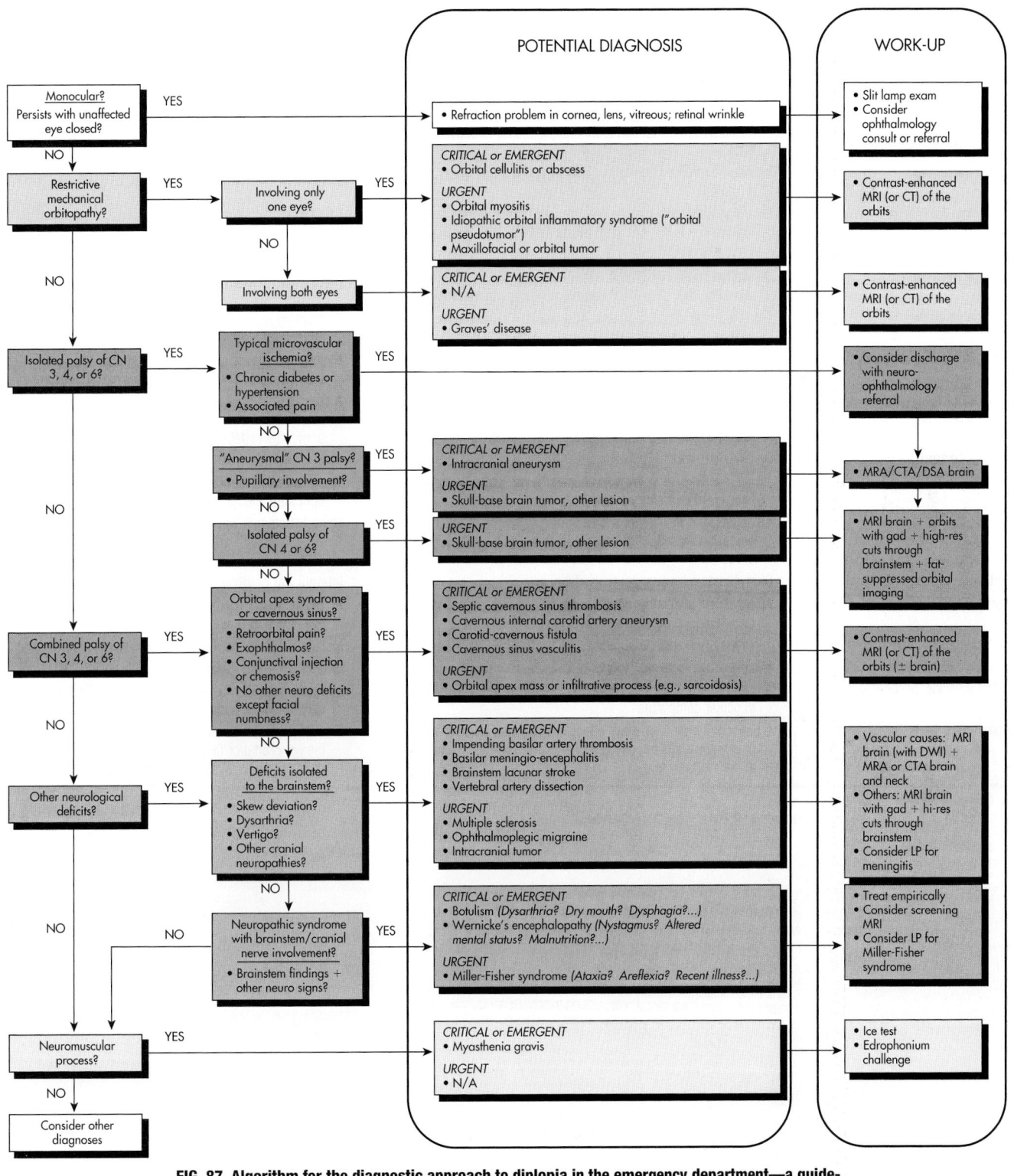

FIG. 87 Algorithm for the diagnostic approach to diplopia in the emergency department—a guide-line. *CN,* Cranial nerve; *CT,* computed tomography; *CTA,* CT angiogram; *DSA,* digital subtraction angiography (conventional angiography); *DWI,* diffusion-weighted imaging; *gad,* gadolinium; *hi-res,* high-resolution; *LP,* lumbar puncture; *MRA,* magnetic resonance angiography; *MRI,* magnetic resonance imaging. (From Marx JA et al: *Rosen's emergency medicine,* ed 8, Philadelphia, 2014, Saunders.)

Clinical
Algorithms

III

TABLE 16   Important Causes of Diplopia

Diplopia-Causing Entity	Mechanism and Mortality	Distinguishing Features
Tier 1—Critical		
Basilar artery thrombosis	Acute thrombosis of the basilar artery with brainstem ischemia; untreated, mortality 70%-90%	Vertigo, dysarthria, other cranial nerve involvement; risk factors for stroke
Botulism	Toxin inhibits of release of acetylcholine (ACh) at cholinergic synapses and presynaptic myoneural junctions; untreated, mortality 60%	Dysarthria, dysphagia, autonomic dysreflexia, pupillary dysfunction
Basilar meningitis	Infection; untreated, mortality close to 100% if bacterial (25%-40% if treated)	Headache, meningismus, fever
Aneurysm	Enlarging aneurysm directly compresses cranial nerve; untreated, rupture risk is 1% per year; mortality 26%-50% per rupture	CN III palsy with pupillary involvement
Tier 2—Emergent		
Vertebral dissection	Dissection causes vertebrobasilar ischemia; acute untreated, mortality 28% (2%-5% if neurologically asymptomatic)	Neck pain, vertigo; risk factors for vertebral dissection
Myasthenia gravis	Autoantibodies develop against ACh nicotinic postsynaptic receptors; untreated, crisis mortality 42% (5% if treated)	Fluctuating muscle weakness, ptosis, and diplopia worsen with activity and improve with rest
Wernicke's encephalopathy	Thiamine-dependent metabolic failure and tissue injury; untreated, mortality 20%	Nystagmus, ataxia, altered mental status, and ophthalmoplegia; risk factors and nutritional deficiency
Orbital apex syndrome, cavernous sinus process	Inflammation or infection in the orbital apex or cavernous sinus directly affects oculomotor cranial nerves; acute mortality low unless infectious and complicated by meningitis	A combination of palsies of CN III, IV, or VI, with retroorbital pain, conjunctival injection, and possible periorbital or facial numbness
Tier 3—Urgent		
Brainstem tumor	Tumor involvement at the supranuclear level; acute mortality low (long-term mortality variable)	Skew deviation vertical diplopia, internuclear ophthalmoplegia
Miller-Fisher syndrome	Autoantibodies develop to a cranial nerve ganglioside, GQ1b; acute mortality low if fully differentiated from GBS; mortality 2%-12% if GBS	Ophthalmoplegia, ataxia, areflexia
Multiple sclerosis	Demyelinating lesions; acute mortality low	Internuclear ophthalmoplegia
Thyroid myopathy (Graves' disease)	Autoimmune myopathy; acute mortality low with regard to ocular complaints	Proptosis, restriction of elevation and abduction of the eye, signs of Graves' disease
Ophthalmoplegic migraine	Inflammatory cranial neuropathy; low mortality—self-limited disease	Ipsilateral headache, CN (usually III) palsy
Ischemic neuropathy	Microvascular ischemia; mortality low—self-limited disease	Isolated CN palsy (pupil-sparing if CN III)
Orbital myositis, pseudotumor	Autoimmune or idiopathic myositis; acute mortality low with regard to ocular complaints	Eye pain, restriction of movement, periorbital edema; exophthalmos and chemosis when more severe
Orbital apex mass	A tumor, infiltration, or mass effect in the orbital apex or cavernous sinus directly compresses oculomotor cranial nerves; acute mortality low	A combination of palsies of CN III, IV, or VI, and possible periorbital or facial numbness, with retroorbital pain, proptosis, signs of venous congestion

CN, Cranial nerve; *GBS,* Guillain-Barre syndrome.
From Marx JA et al: *Rosen's emergency medicine*, ed 8, Philadelphia, 2014, Saunders.

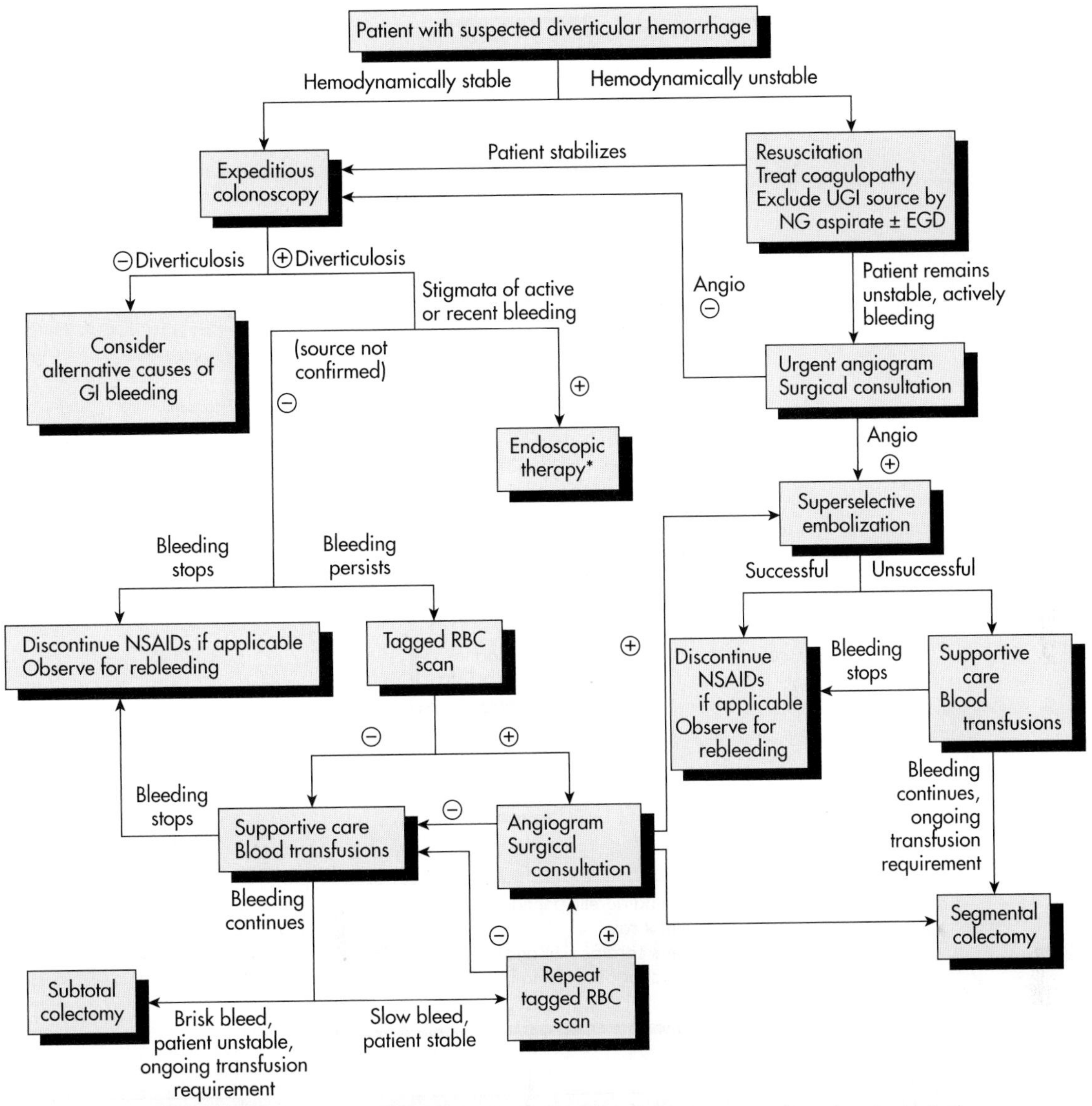

Patient with suspected diverticular hemorrhage

Hemodynamically stable   Hemodynamically unstable

Expeditious colonoscopy   ← Patient stabilizes ←   Resuscitation
                                                      Treat coagulopathy
                                                      Exclude UGI source by
                                                      NG aspirate ± EGD

⊖ Diverticulosis   ⊕ Diverticulosis

                              Stigmata of active   Angio
                              or recent bleeding   ⊖
Consider
alternative causes of   (source not   Patient remains
GI bleeding   confirmed)   unstable, actively
                          ⊖   ⊕   bleeding

                                              Endoscopic   Urgent angiogram
                                              therapy*   Surgical consultation

                                                                         Angio
                                                                          ⊕

                                                                   Superselective
                                                                   embolization

Bleeding   Bleeding   Successful   Unsuccessful
stops   persists

Discontinue NSAIDs if applicable   Tagged RBC   ⊕   Discontinue   Bleeding   Supportive
Observe for rebleeding   scan   NSAIDs   stops   care
                                                             if applicable   Blood
                                                             Observe for   transfusions
                                   ⊖   ⊕   rebleeding

Bleeding   Bleeding
stops   continues,
                                                                                            ongoing
                  Supportive care   ⊖   Angiogram   transfusion
                  Blood transfusions   Surgical   requirement
                                          consultation
                                                                                    Segmental
                  Bleeding   colectomy
                  continues   ⊖   ⊕

Subtotal   Brisk bleed,   Slow bleed,   Repeat
colectomy   patient unstable, patient stable tagged RBC
                  ongoing transfusion   scan
                  requirement

FIG. 88 Algorithm for the management of patients with suspected diverticular hemorrhage. *Angio*, angiogram; *RBC*, red blood cell; *UGI*, upper GI. (Feldman M, Friedman LS, Brandt LJ: Sleisenger and Fortran's Gastrointestinal and Liver Disease, 10th ed, ISBN# 978-1-4557-4692-7, 2016, Elsevier.)
*Endoscopic therapy may consist of epinephrine injection alone or in combination with other therapies such as heater probe coagulation, bipolar coagulation, endoclips (Fig. 84), fibrin sealant, and band lication.

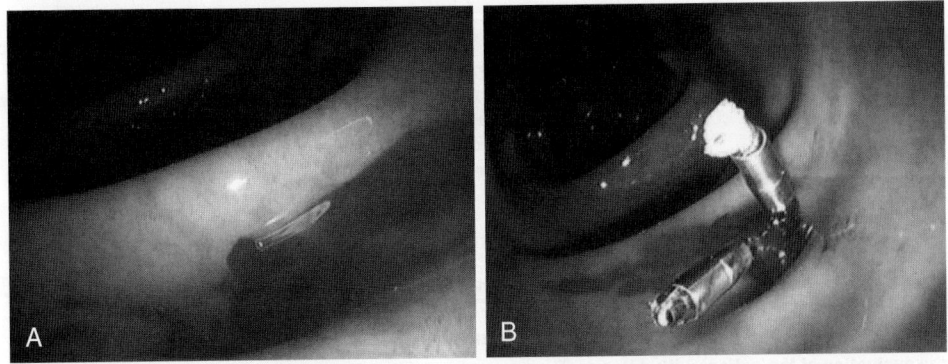

FIG. 89 Colonoscopy in a patient with lower intestinal bleeding from a diverticulum in whom a site of active bleeding was identified *(A)* and treated successfully with placement of 2 endoclips *(B)*. (Courtesy Janak Shah, MD. San Francisco, CA.) (Feldman M, Friedman LS, Brandt LJ: Sleisenger and Fortran's Gastrointestinal and Liver Disease, 10th ed, ISBN# 978-1-4557-4692-7, 2016, Elsevier.)

Clinical Algorithms

III

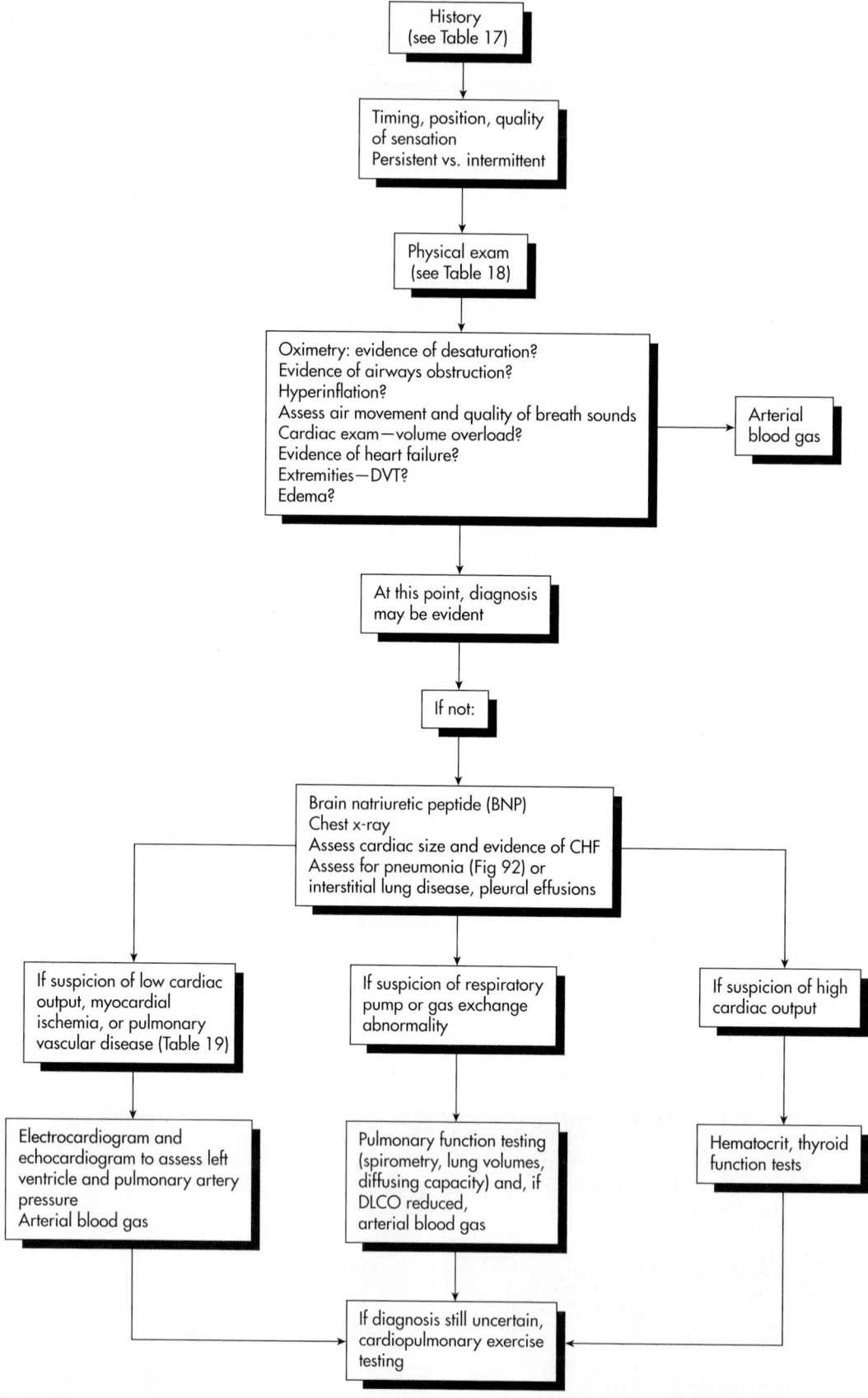

FIG. 91 Algorithm for the evaluation of the patient with dyspnea. The pace and completeness with which one approaches this framework depends on the intensity and acuity of the patient's symptoms. In a patient with severe, acute dyspnea, for example, an arterial blood gas measurement may be one of the first laboratory evaluations, whereas this measurement might not be obtained until much later in the workup in a patient with chronic breathlessness of unclear cause. A therapeutic trial of a medication, for example, a bronchodilator, may be instituted at any point if one is fairly confident of the diagnosis based on the data available at that time. *CHF,* Congestive heart failure; *DLCO,* diffusing capacity of the lung for carbon monoxide; *DVT,* deep venous thrombosis. (Modified from Schwartzstein RM, Feller-Kopman D: Approach to the patient with dyspnea. In Braunwald E, Goldman L [eds]: *Primary cardiology,* ed 2, Philadelphia, 2003, Saunders.)

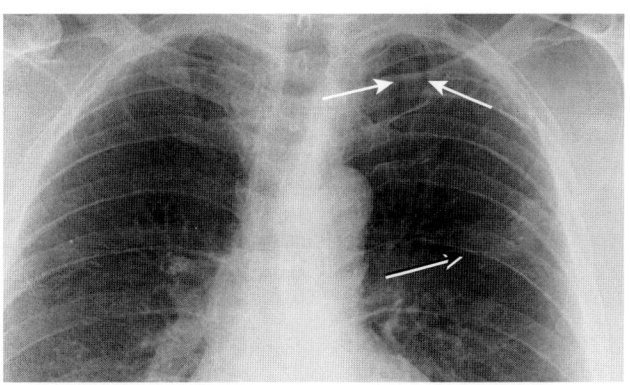

FIG. 92 Chest radiograph of a patient presenting with cough and fever. A faint area of opacification within the left midlung proved to be pneumonia *(black arrow)*. Additionally, a small left apical carcinoma was detected *(white arrows)*. Because of multiple overlying structures, including the first ribs and the clavicles, the pulmonary apices are a "danger" area in terms of risk of missed findings on chest radiographs. Close inspection of the apices is warranted on every chest radiograph. (Soto JA, Lucey BC: Emergency Radiology, the requisites, 2nd ed, ISBN# 978-0-323-37640-2, 2017, Elsevier.)

TABLE 17　Differential Diagnoses for Acute Dyspnea

Organ System	Critical Diagnoses	Emergent Diagnoses	Nonemergent Diagnoses
Pulmonary	Airway obstruction	Spontaneous pneumothorax	Pleural effusion
	Pulmonary embolus	Asthma	Neoplasm
	Noncardiogenic edema	Cor pulmonale	Pneumonia (CAP score ≤ 70)
	Anaphylaxis	Aspiration	COPD
	Ventilatory failure	Pneumonia (CAP score >70)	
Cardiac	Pulmonary edema	Pericarditis	Congenital heart disease
	Myocardial infarction		Valvular heart disease
	Cardiac tamponade		Cardiomyopathy
Primarily Associated with Normal or Increased Respiratory Effort			
Abdominal		Mechanical interference	Pregnancy
		Hypotension, sepsis from ruptured viscus, bowel obstruction, inflammatory or infectious process	Ascites Obesity
Psychogenic			Hyperventilation syndrome
			Somatization disorder
			Panic attack
Metabolic or endocrine	Toxic ingestion	Renal failure	Fever
	DKA	Electrolyte abnormalities	Thyroid disease
		Metabolic acidosis	
Infectious	Epiglottitis	Pneumonia (CAP score >70)	Pneumonia (CAP score ≤70)
Traumatic	Tension pneumothorax	Simple pneumothorax, hemothorax	Rib fractures
	Cardiac tamponade	Diaphragmatic rupture	
	Flail chest		
Hematologic	Carbon monoxide poisoning	Anemia	
	Acute chest syndrome		
Primarily Associated with Decreased Respiratory Effort			
Neuromuscular	CVA, intracranial insult	Multiple sclerosis	ALS
	Organophosphate poisoning	Guillain-Barré syndrome	Polymyositis
		Tick paralysis	Porphyria

ALS, Amyotrophic lateral sclerosis; *CAP,* community-acquired pneumonia; *COPD,* chronic obstructive pulmonary disease; *CVA,* cerebrovascular accident; *DKA,* diabetic ketoacidosis.
From Marx JA et al: *Rosen's Emergency Medicine,* ed 8, Philadelphia, 2014, Saunders.

Clinical Algorithms

III

TABLE 18 Pivotal Findings in Physical Examination

Sign	Physical Finding	Diagnoses to Consider
Vital signs	Tachypnea	Pneumonia, pneumothorax
	Hypopnea	Intracranial insult, drug or toxin ingestion
	Tachycardia	PE, traumatic chest injury
	Hypotension	Tension pneumothorax
	Fever	Pneumonia, PE
General appearance	Cachexia, weight loss	Malignancy, acquired immune disorder, mycobacterial infection
	Obesity	Hypoventilation, sleep apnea, PE
	Pregnancy	PE
	Barrel chest	COPD
	"Sniffing" position	Epiglottitis
	"Tripoding" position	COPD or asthma with severe distress
	Traumatic injury	Pneumothorax (simple, tension), rib fractures, flail chest, hemothorax, pulmonary contusion
Skin and nails	Tobacco stains or odor	COPD, malignancy, infection
	Clubbing	Chronic hypoxia, intracardiac shunts, or pulmonary vascular anomalies
	Pallid skin or conjunctivae	Anemia
	Muscle wasting	Neuromuscular disease
	Bruising	Chest wall: rib fractures, pneumothorax
		Diffuse: thrombocytopenia, chronic steroid use, anticoagulation
	Subcutaneous emphysema	Rib fractures, pneumothorax, tracheobronchial disruption
	Hives, rash	Allergic reaction, infection, tick-borne illness
Neck	Stridor	Upper airway edema or infection, foreign body, traumatic injury, anaphylaxis
	JVD	Tension pneumothorax, COPD or asthma exacerbation, fluid overload or CHF, PE
Lung examination	Wheezes	CHF, anaphylaxis
		Bronchospasm
	Rales	CHF, pneumonia, PE
	Unilateral decrease	Pneumothorax, pleural effusion, consolidation, rib fractures or contusion, pulmonary contusion
	Hemoptysis	Malignancy, infection, bleeding disorder, CHF
	Sputum production	Infection (viral, bacterial)
	Friction rub	Pleurisy
	Abnormal respiratory pattern (e.g., Cheyne-Stokes)	Intracranial insult
Chest examination	Crepitance or pain on palpation	Rib or sternal fractures
	Subcutaneous emphysema	Pneumothorax, tracheobronchial rupture
	Thoracoabdominal desynchrony	Diaphragmatic injury with herniation; cervical spinal cord trauma
	Flail segment	Flail chest, pulmonary contusion
Cardiac examination	Murmur	PE
	S_3 or S_4 gallop	PE
	S_2 accentuation	PE
	Muffled heart sounds	Cardiac tamponade
Extremities	Calf tenderness, Homans' sign	PE
	Edema	CHF
Neurologic examination	Focal deficits (motor, sensory, cognitive)	Stroke, intracranial hemorrhage causing central abnormal respiratory drive; if long-standing, risk of aspiration pneumonia
	Symmetrical deficits	Neuromuscular disease
	Diffuse weakness	Metabolic or electrolyte abnormality (hypocalcemia, hypomagnesemia, hypophosphatemia), anemia
	Hyporeflexia	Hypermagnesemia
	Ascending weakness	Guillain-Barré syndrome

CHF, Congestive heart failure; *COPD,* chronic obstructive pulmonary disease; *JVD,* jugular venous distention; *PE,* pulmonary embolism.
From Marx JA et al: *Rosen's Emergency Medicine*, ed 8, Philadelphia, 2014, Saunders.

TABLE 19 Diagnostic Table: Patterns of Diseases Often Resulting in Dyspnea

Disease	History (Dyspnea)	Associated Symptoms	Signs and Physical Findings	Tests
Pulmonary embolism	• HPI: abrupt onset, pleuritic pain, immobility (travel, recent surgery) • PMH: malignancy, DVT, PE, hypercoagulability, oral contraception, obesity	Diaphoresis, exertional dyspnea	Tachycardia, tachypnea, low-grade fever	• Pulse oximetry, ABG (A-a gradient), D-dimer • ECG (dysrhythmia, right-sided heart strain) • CXR (Westermark sign, Hampton's hump), spiral CT, MRV • Pulmonary angiogram • Ultrasound positive for DVT
Pneumonia	Fever, productive cough, chest pain	Anorexia, chills, nausea, vomiting, exertional dyspnea, cough	Fever, tachycardia, tachypnea, rales or decreased breath sounds	CXR, CBC, sputum and blood cultures
Bacterial	SH: tobacco use			Pulse oximetry Waveform capnography if altered mental status, ABG if capnography unavailable and acid-base derangement or hypercarbia suspected
Viral	Exposure (e.g., influenza, varicella)			
Opportunistic	Immune disorder, chemotherapy			
Fungal or parasitic	Exposure (e.g., birds), indolent onset	Episodic fever, nonproductive cough		
Pneumothorax	Abrupt onset: trauma, chest pain, thin males more likely to have spontaneous pneumothorax	Localized chest pain	Decreased breath sounds, subcutaneous emphysema, chest wall wounds or instability	• CXR: pneumothorax, rib fractures, hemothorax • Ultrasound: pneumothorax, pleural effusion
Simple				Ultrasound positive for pneumothorax
Tension	Decompensation of simple pneumothorax	Diaphoresis	JVD, tracheal deviation, muffled heart sounds, cardiovascular collapse	Clinical diagnosis: requires immediate decompression. May verify via bedside ultrasound
COPD or asthma	Tobacco use, medication noncompliance, URI symptoms, sudden weather change	Air hunger, diaphoresis	• Retractions, accessory muscle use, tripoding, cyanosis • "Shark fin" capnograph	• CXR: rule out infiltrate, pneumothorax, atelectasis (mucus plug) • Ultrasound: distinguish from heart failure
	PMH: environmental allergies FH: asthma			Waveform capnography
Malignancy	Weight loss, tobacco, or other occupational exposure	Dysphagia	Hemoptysis	CXR, chest CT: mass, hilar adenopathy, focal atelectasis
Fluid overload	• Gradual onset, dietary indiscretion or medication noncompliance, chest pain • PMH: recent MI, diabetes, CHF	Worsening orthopnea, PND	JVD, peripheral edema, S_3 or S_4 gallop, new cardiac dysrhythmia, hepatojugular reflux	• CXR and/or ultrasound: pleural effusion, interstitial edema, Kerley B lines, cardiomegaly • ECG: ischemia, dysrhythmia • NT-proBNP
Anaphylaxis	Abrupt onset, exposure to allergen	Dysphagia	Oral swelling, stridor, wheezing, hives	

A-a, Alveolar-arterial; *ABG,* arterial blood gas; *CBC,* complete blood count; *CHF,* congestive heart failure; *CT,* computed tomography; *CXR,* chest x-ray examination; *DVT,* deep vein thrombosis; *ECG,* electrocardiogram; *FH,* family history; *HPI,* history of present illness; *JVD,* jugular venous distention; *MI,* myocardial infarction; *MRV,* magnetic resonance venography; *NT-proBNP,* amino-terminal pro–B–type natriuretic peptide; *PE,* pulmonary embolism; *PMH,* past medical history; *PND,* paroxysmal nocturnal dyspnea; *SH,* social history; *URI,* upper respiratory infection.
From Marx JA et al: Rosen's Emergency Medicine, ed 8, Philadelphia, 2014, Saunders.

Clinical Algorithms

III

DYSURIA AND/OR URETHRAL/ VAGINAL DISCHARGE

ICD-10CM #

R30.0	Dysuria
R30.9	Painful micturition, unspecified
R36.0	Urethral discharge without blood
R36.9	Urethral discharge, unspecified
N89.8	Other specified noninflammatory disorders of vagina

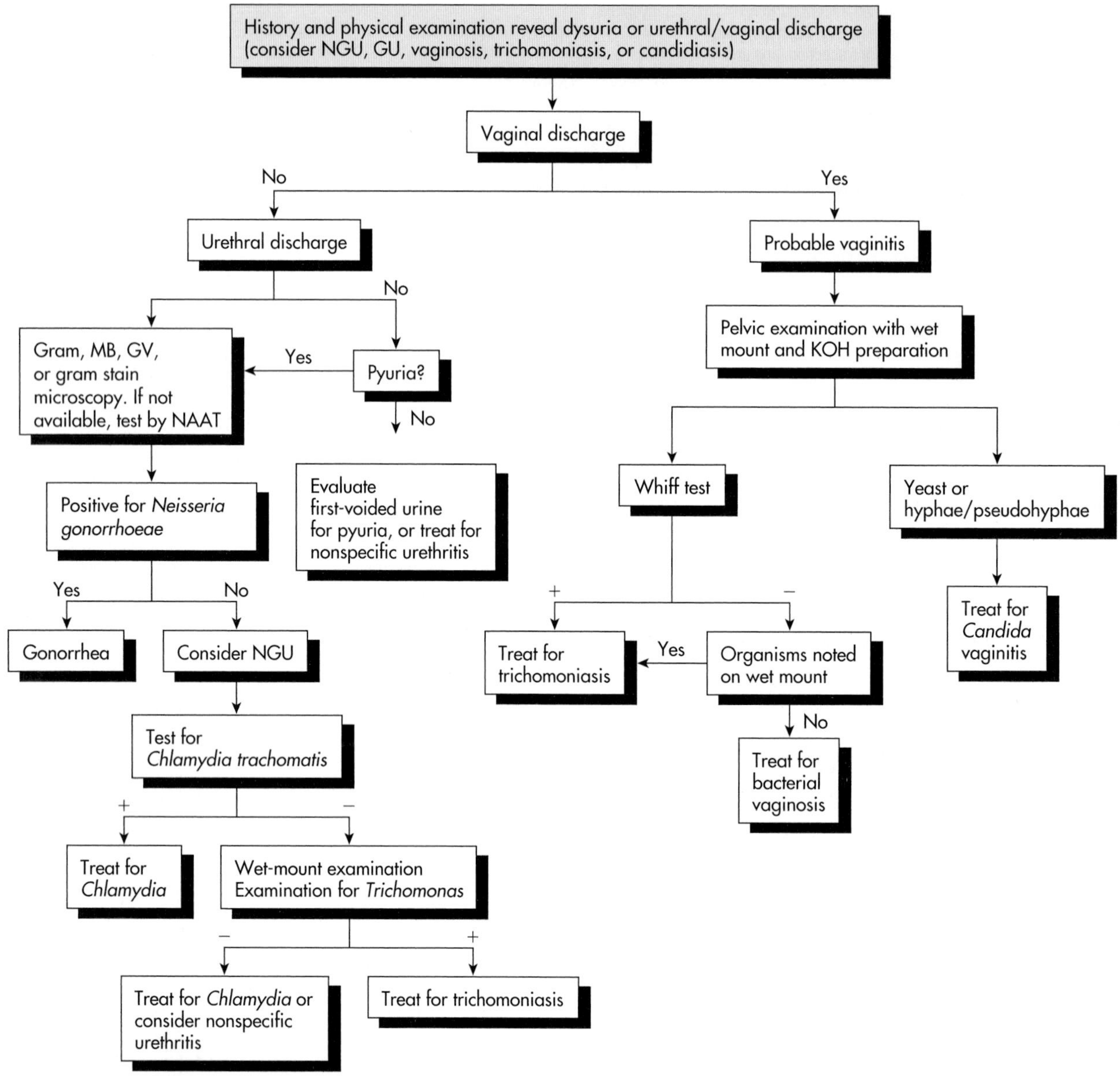

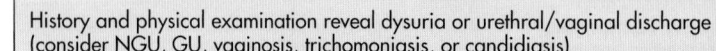

FIG. 93 Evaluation of patients with dysuria and/or urethral/vaginal discharge. *GU,* Gonococcal urethritis; *GV,* gentian violet; *KOH,* potassium hydroxide; *MB,* methylene blue; *NAAT,* nucleic amplification test; *NGU,* nongonococcal urethritis. (Modified from Nseyo UO [ed]: Urology for primary care physicians, Philadelphia, 1999, Saunders.)

Management of Ear Pain

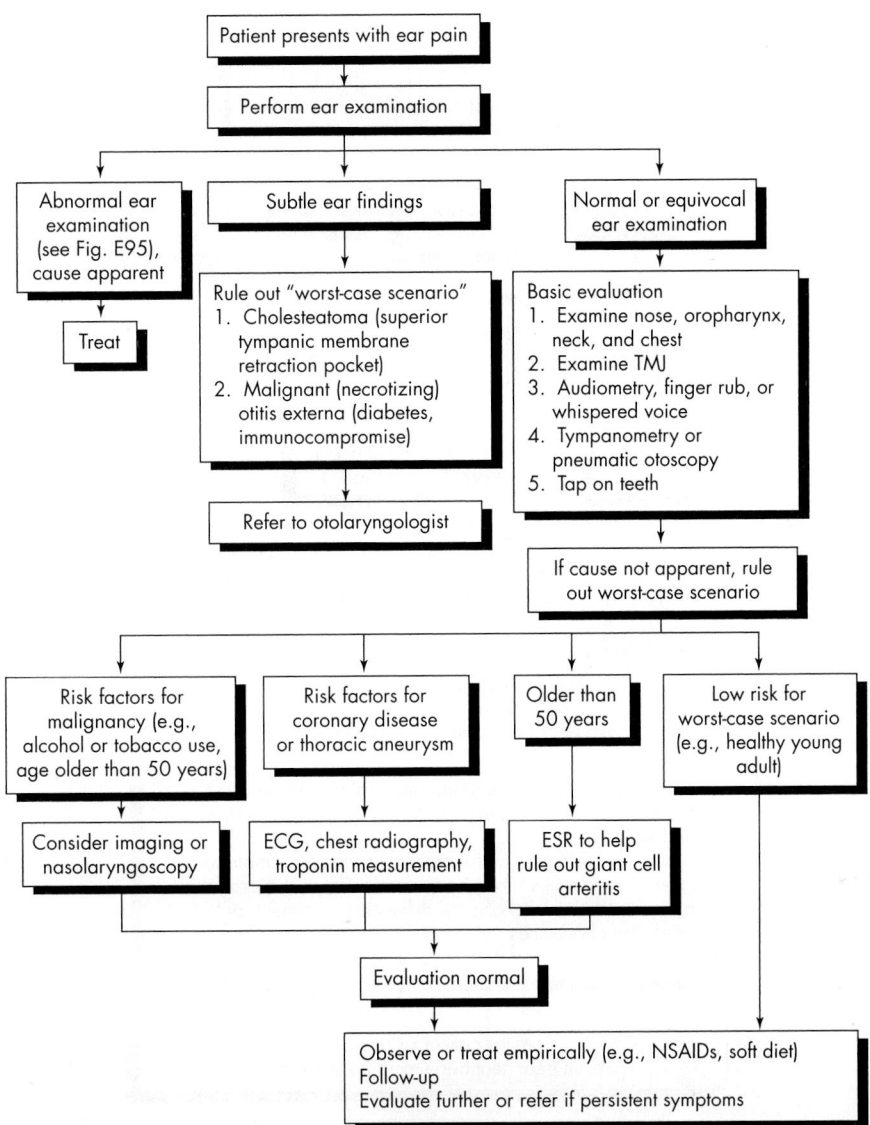

FIG. 94 Management of ear pain. *ECG,* Electrocardiography; *ESR,* erythrocyte sedimentation rate; *NSAIDs,* nonsteroidal antiinflammatory drugs; *TMJ,* temporomandibular joint. (Modified from Ely JW et al: Diagnosis of ear pain, *Am Fam Physician* 77[5]:622, 2008.)

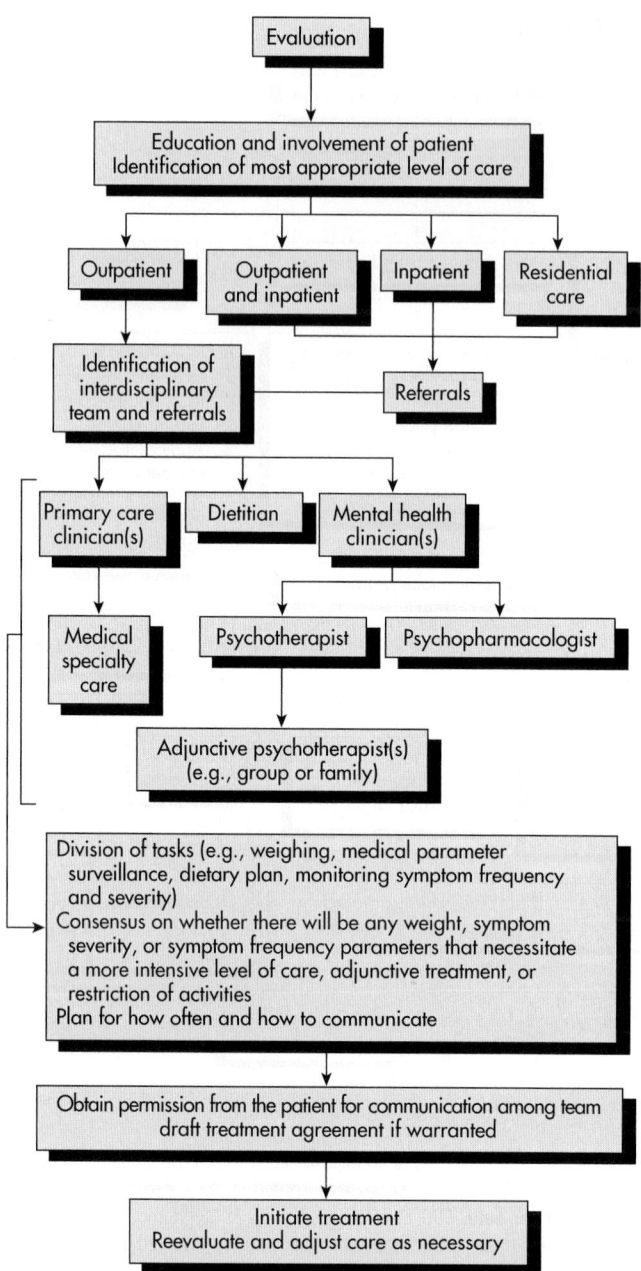

FIG. 96 Algorithm for team management of adult patients with an eating disorder. (Feldman M, Friedman LS, Brandt LJ: Sleisenger and Fortran's Gastrointestinal and Liver Disease, 10th ed, ISBN# 978-1-4557-4692-7, 2016, Elsevier.)

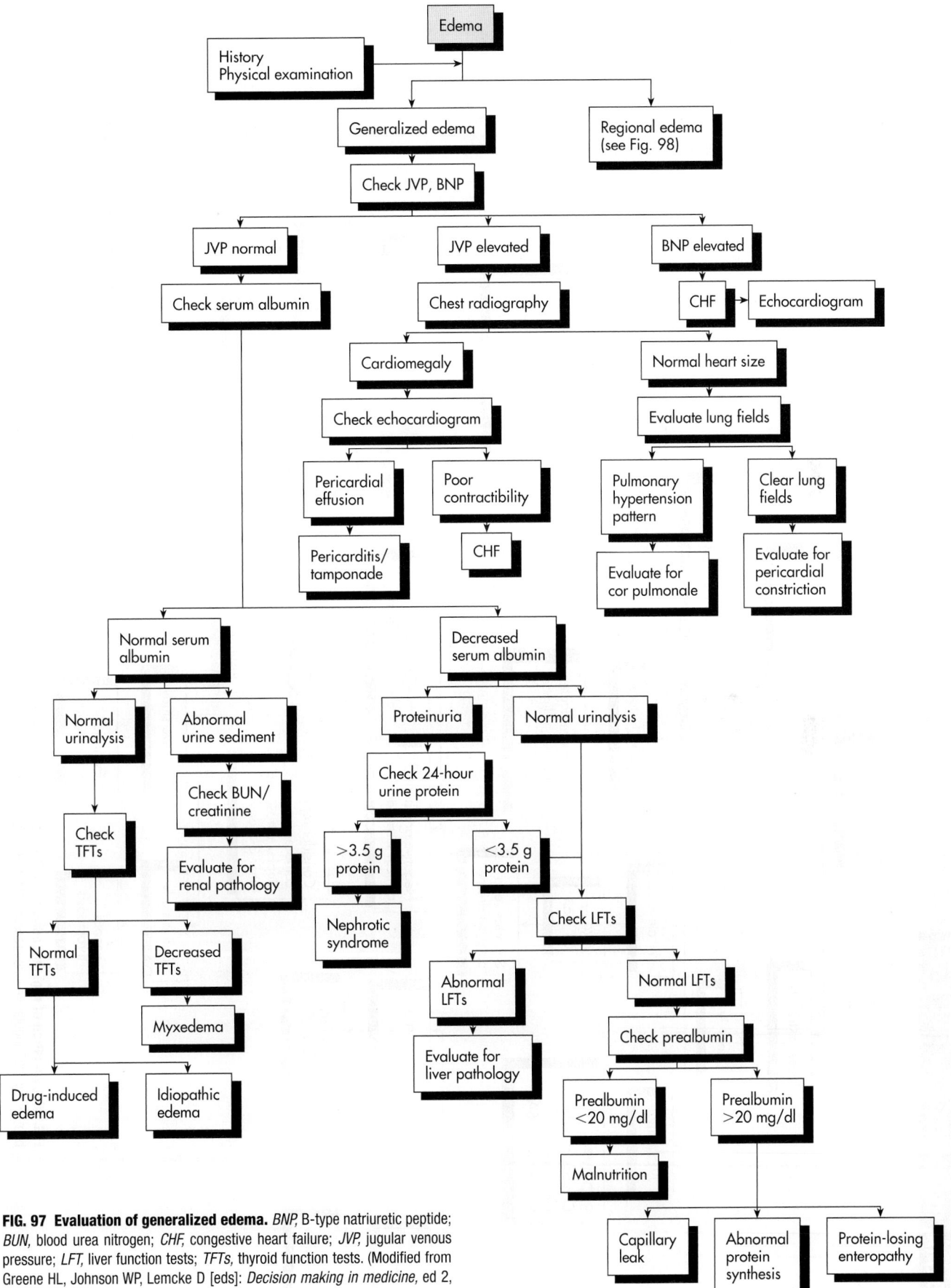

FIG. 97 Evaluation of generalized edema. *BNP,* B-type natriuretic peptide; *BUN,* blood urea nitrogen; *CHF,* congestive heart failure; *JVP,* jugular venous pressure; *LFT,* liver function tests; *TFTs,* thyroid function tests. (Modified from Greene HL, Johnson WP, Lemcke D [eds]: *Decision making in medicine,* ed 2, St Louis, 1998, Mosby.)

Clinical Algorithms

EDEMA, REGIONAL

ICD-10CM # T78.3 Edema, essential, acute

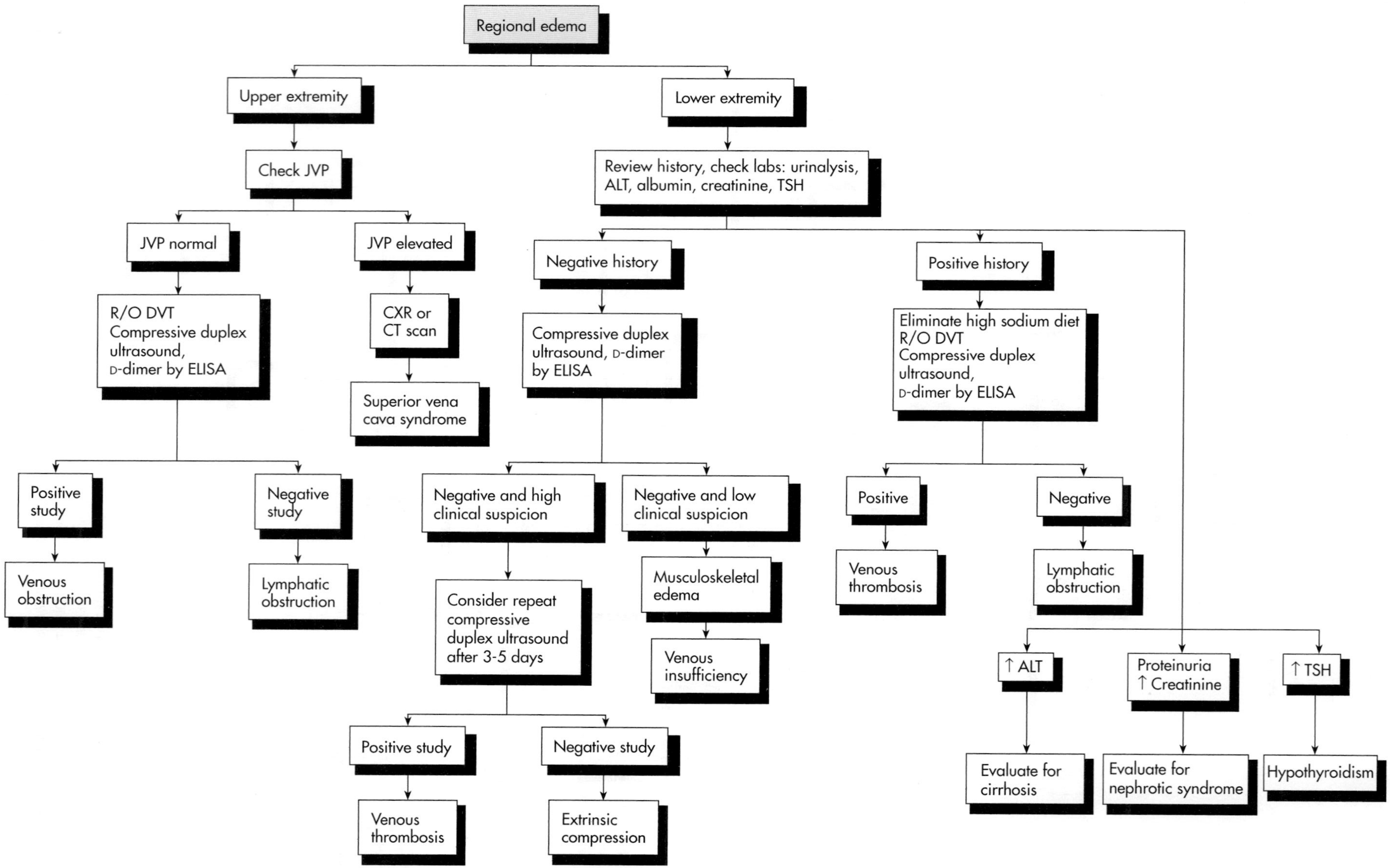

FIG. 98 Evaluation of regional edema. *CT,* Computed tomography; *CXR,* chest x-ray examination; *DVT,* deep venous thrombosis; *ELISA,* enzyme-linked immunosorbent assay; *JVP,* jugular venous pressure. (Modified from Greene HL, Johnson WP, Lemcke D [eds]: *Decision making in medicine,* ed 2, St Louis, 1998, Mosby.)

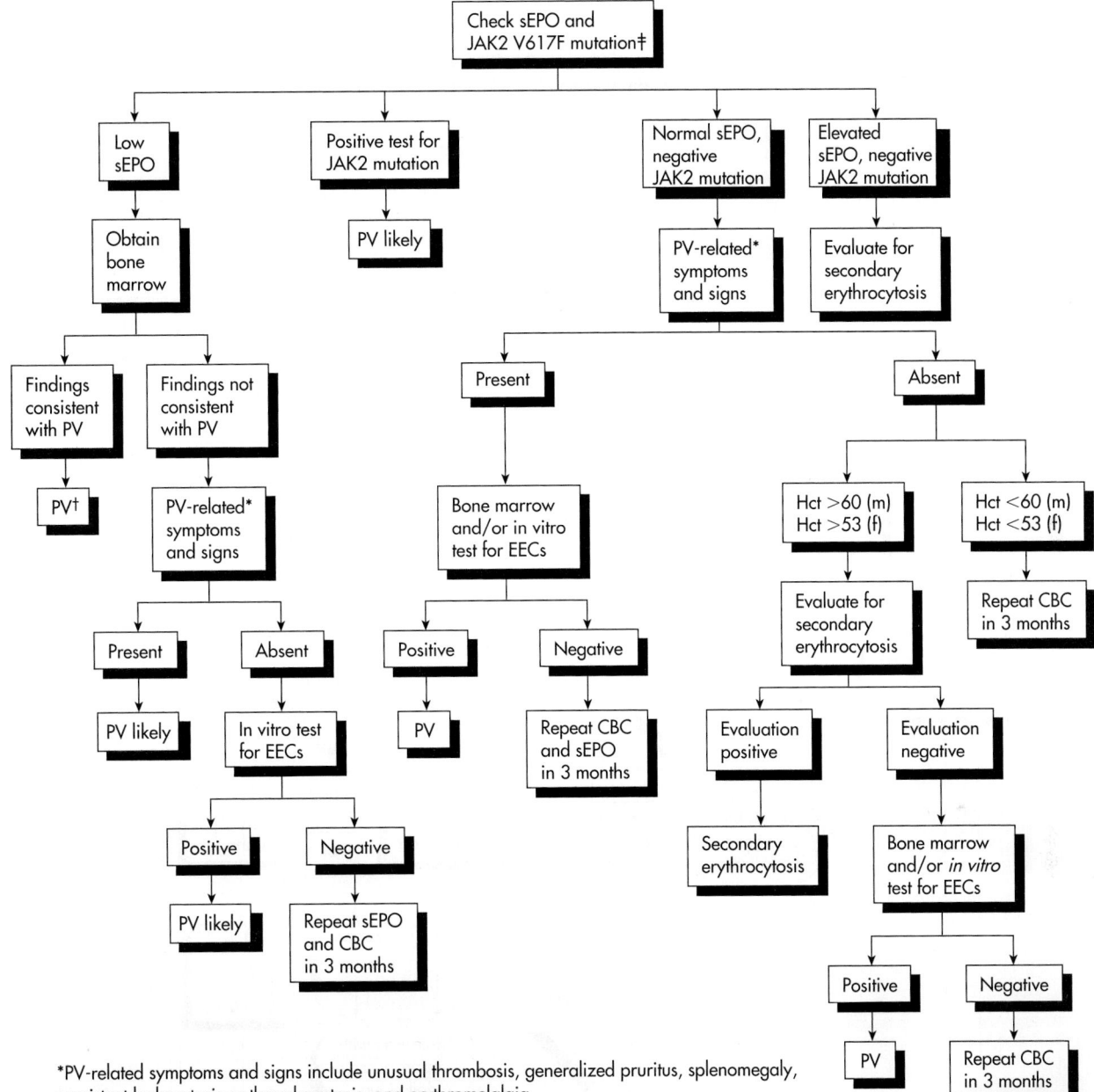

*PV-related symptoms and signs include unusual thrombosis, generalized pruritus, splenomegaly, persistent leukocytosis or thrombocytosis, and erythromelalgia.

†Note: Refer to Section I, Polycythemia Vera, for additional information on this topic.

‡The JAK2 mutation is found in >95% of patients with PV and can be used for diagnostic purposes.

FIG. 100 A diagnostic approach to acquired erythrocytosis. *CBC,* Complete blood cell count; *EEC,* endogenous (spontaneous) erythroid colonies; *f,* female; *Hct,* hematocrit; *m,* male; *PV,* polycythemia vera; *sEPO,* serum erythropoietin level. (Modified from Goldman L, Schafer AL [eds]: *Cecil textbook of medicine,* ed 24, Philadelphia, 2012, Saunders.)

Clinical
Algorithms

III

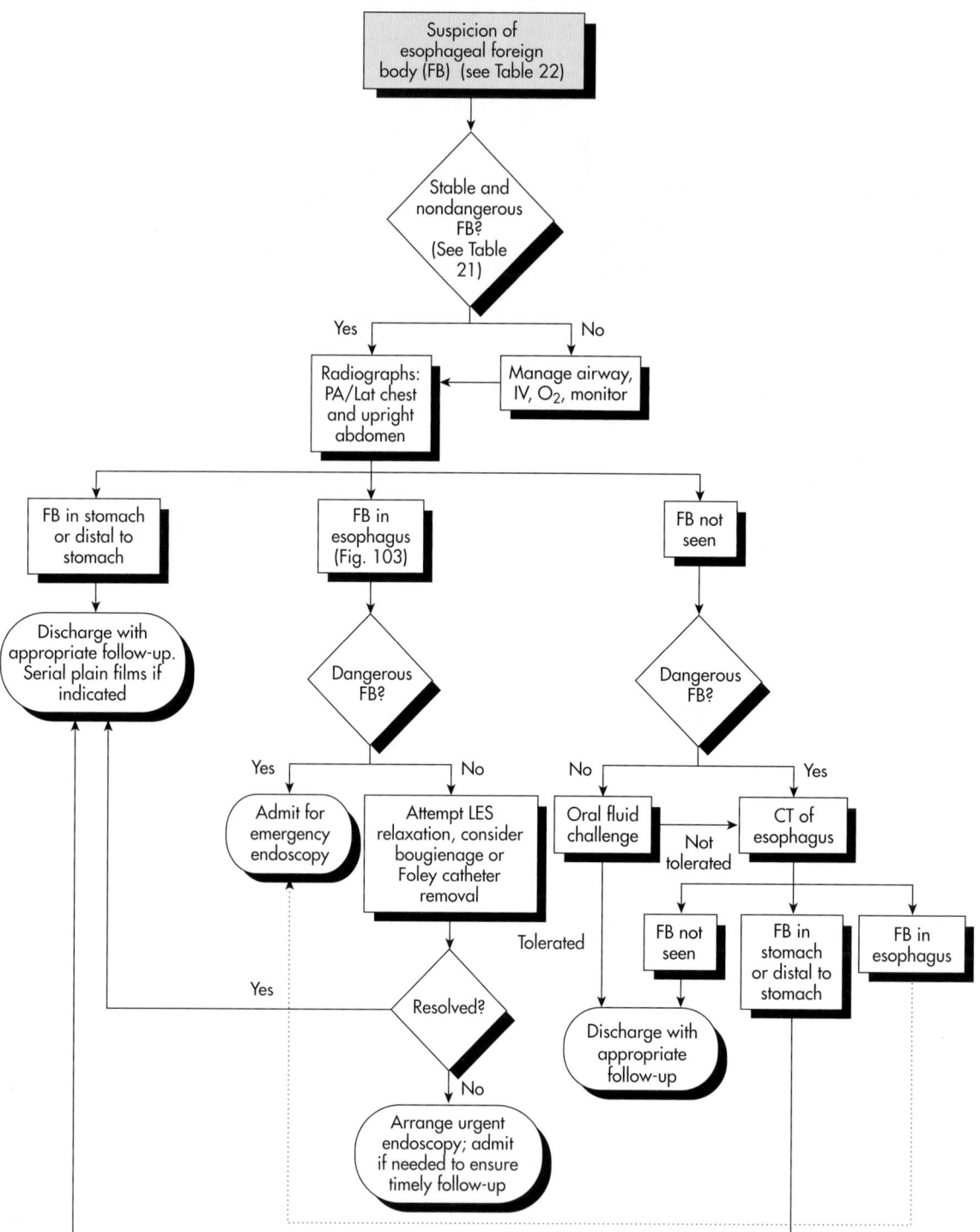

FIG. 102 Diagnostic algorithm for the evaluation of a suspected esophageal foreign body. *CT,* Computed tomography; *IV,* intravenous line; *Lat,* lateral; *LES,* lower esophageal sphincter; *PA,* posteroanterior. (From Adams JG et al: *Emergency medicine, clinical essentials,* ed 2, Philadelphia, 2013, Elsevier.)

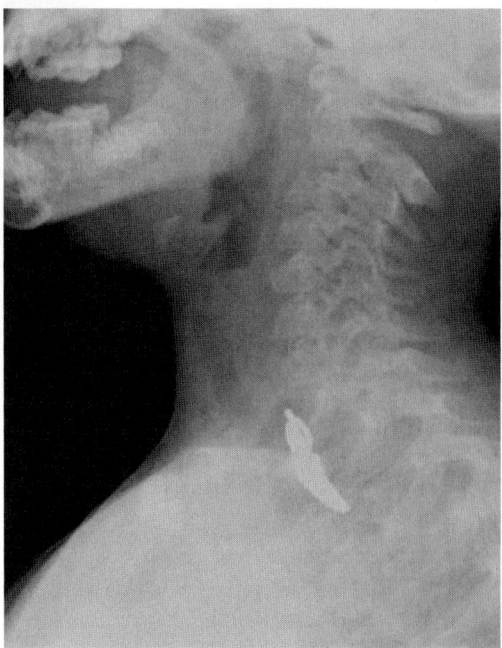

FIG. 103 A lateral radiograph of the neck in a child demonstrates an ingested radio-opaque foreign body lodged within the esophagus posterior to the trachea. (Soto JA, Lucey BC: Emergency Radiology, the requisites, 2nd ed, ISBN# 978-0-323-37640-2, 2017, Elsevier.)

Table 21   Most Threatening and Most Common Esophageal Foreign Bodies

Most Threatening

In Children

Disc batteries
Bones
Needles
Other sharp objects

In Adults

Disc batteries
Bones
Packets of illicit drugs
Toothpicks

Most Common

In Children

Coins
Marbles
Buttons
Toys

In Adults

Food boluses
Bones
Dentures
Oral piercings

From Adams JG, et al: *Emergency medicine, clinical essentials*, ed 2, Philadelphia, 2013, Elsevier.

Table 22   Differential Diagnosis for Esophageal Foreign Bodies

In Children

Perforation
Abrasion or laceration
Airway foreign body
Esophagitis
Epiglottitis
Globus hystericus
Reactive airways disease

In Adults

Perforation
Abrasion or laceration
Spasm
Esophagitis
Diverticulum
Malignancy
Myocardial infarction
Globus hystericus

From Adams JG, et al: *Emergency medicine, clinical essentials*, ed 2, Philadelphia, 2013, Elsevier.

Clinical Algorithms

FATIGUE

ICD-10CM #	R53.83	Other fatigue
	F48.8	Other specified nonpsychotic mental disorders
	R53.83	Other fatigue

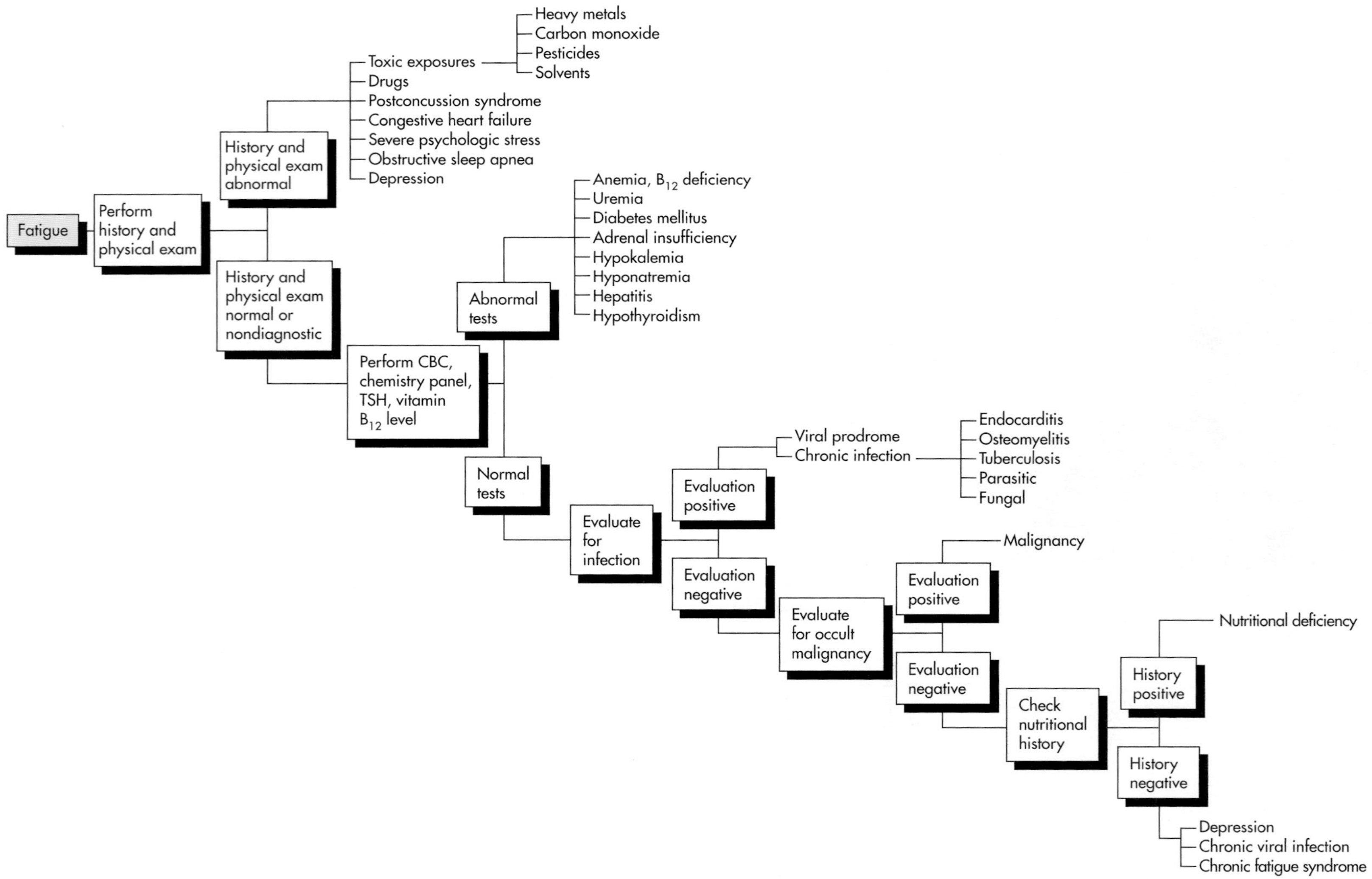

FIG. 104 Evaluation of fatigue. *CBC,* Complete blood count. (Modified from Healey PM: *Common medical diagnosis: an algorithmic approach,* ed 3, Philadelphia, 2000, Saunders.)

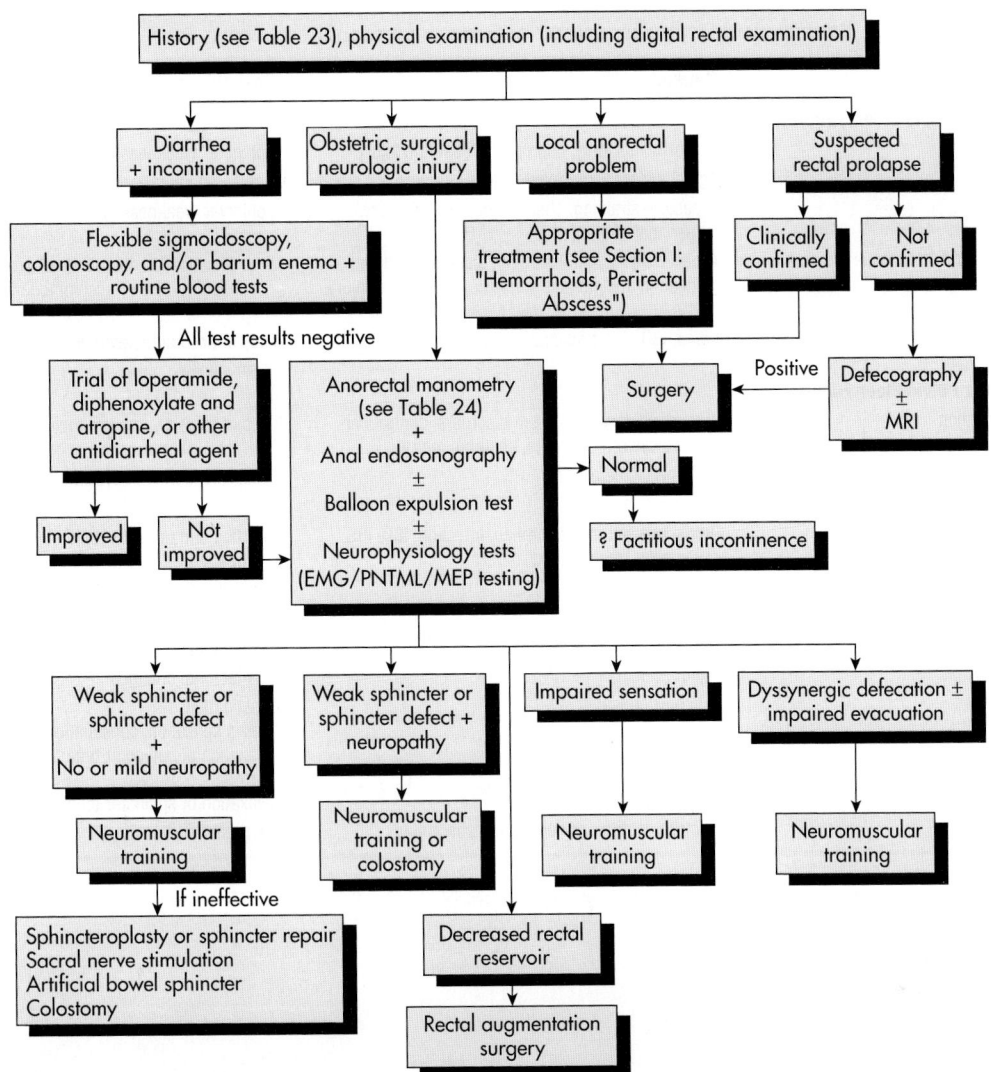

FIG. 105 Algorithm for the evaluation and management of patients with fecal incontinence.
EMG, electromyography; *MEP*, motor evoked potential; *PNTML*, pudendal nerve terminal motor latency.
(Feldman M, Friedman LS, Brandt LJ: Sleisenger and Fortran's Gastrointestinal and Liver Disease, 10th ed,
ISBN# 978-1-4557-4692-7, 2016, Elsevier.)

TABLE 23 Mechanisms, Causes, and Pathophysiology of Fecal Incontinence

Mechanism	Causes	Pathophysiology
Abnormal Anorectal or Pelvic Floor Structures		
Anal sphincter muscles	Hemorrhoidectomy, neuropathy, obstetric injury	Sphincter weakness, loss of sampling reflex
Puborectalis muscle	Aging, excessive perineal descent, trauma	Obtuse anorectal angle, sphincter weakness
Pudendal nerve	Excessive straining, obstetric or surgical injury, perineal descent	Sphincter weakness, sensory loss, impaired reflexes
Nervous system, spinal cord, autonomic nervous system	Avulsion injury, spine surgery, diabetes mellitus, head injury, multiple sclerosis, spinal cord injury, stroke	Loss of sensation, impaired reflexes, secondary myopathy, loss of accommodation
Rectum	Aging, IBD, IBS, prolapse, radiation	Loss of accommodation, loss of sensation, hyper-sensitivity
Abnormal Anorectal or Pelvic Floor Function		
Impaired anorectal sensation	Autonomic nervous system disorders, central nervous system disorders, obstetric injury	Loss of stool awareness, rectoanal agnosia
Fecal impaction	Dyssynergic defecation	Fecal retention with overflow, impaired sensation
Altered Stool Characteristics		
Increased volume and loose consistency	Drugs, bile salt malabsorption, infection, IBD, IBS, laxatives, metabolic disorders	Diarrhea and urgency, rapid stool transport, impaired accommodation
Hard stools, retention	Drugs, dyssynergia	Fecal retention with overflow
Miscellaneous		
Physical mobility, cognitive function	Aging, dementia, disability	Multifactorial changes
Psychosis	Willful soiling	Multifactorial changes
Drugs*	Anticholinergics	Constipation
	Antidepressants	Altered sensation, constipation
	Caffeine	Relaxation of sphincter tone
	Laxatives	Diarrhea
	Muscle relaxants	Relaxation of sphincter tone
Food intolerance	Fructose, lactose, or sorbitol malabsorption	Diarrhea, flatus

*Pathophysiology is noted for each class of drugs.

Feldman M, Friedman LS, Brandt LJ: Sleisenger and Fortran's Gastrointestinal and Liver Disease, 10th ed, ISBN# 978-1-4557-4692-7, 2016, Elsevier.

TABLE 24 Diagnostic Tests for Fecal Incontinence*

| Test | Clinical Use | | Quality of Evidence | Comments |
	Advantages	Disadvantages		
Physiologic				
Anorectal manometry	Quantifies EAS and IAS pressures; identifies rectal hyposensitivity, rectal hypersensitivity, impaired rectal compliance, dyssynergic defecation	Lack of standardization	Good	Useful for detecting anal sphincter weakness, altered rectal sensation and accommodation, and dyssynergia
Needle EMG	Quantifies spike potentials and re-innervation pattern indicating neuropathy or myopathy	Invasive, painful; not widely available	Fair	Useful but used largely in research laboratories
Surface EMG	Displays EMG activity; can provide information on normal or weak muscle tone	Inaccurate, frequent artifacts	Fair	Used largely for neuromuscular training
Pudendal nerve terminal motor latency (PNTML)	Measures latency of the terminal portion of the pudendal nerve, simple to perform	Minimally invasive, low sensitivity, interobserver differences	Fair	Conflicting data; correlation with other tests and surgical outcome unclear
Translumbar and transsacral motor evoked potentials	Quantifies the nerve conduction time of the entire spinoanal and spinorectal pathways; minimally invasive	Lack of standardization, training, controlled studies, and availability	Fair	Promising noninvasive test; more objective and higher yield than PNTML
Colonic transit study with radiopaque markers	Evaluates the presence of fecal retention; inexpensive and widely available	Inconsistent methodology, validity has been questioned	Good	Useful for identifying patients with fecal seepage and older persons with impaction
Balloon expulsion test (BET)	Simple, inexpensive, bedside assessment of ability to expel a simulated stool; identifies dyssynergic defecation	Lack of standardization	Good	Normal BET does not exclude dyssynergia; should be interpreted in the context of other anorectal test results
Imaging				
Anorectal US	Visualizes IAS and EAS defects, thickness, and atrophy and puborectalis muscles	Interobserver bias; scars difficult to identify	Good	Most widely available
Defecography	Detects prolapse, intussusception, obtuse anorectal angle, and pelvic floor weakness, as well as rectoceles and megarectum	Radiation exposure, embarrassment, availability, interobserver bias, inconsistent methodology	Fair	Useful and complementary with other tests
MRI	Simultaneously evaluates global pelvic floor anatomy and dynamic motion; reveals sphincter morphology and pathology outside the anorectum	Expensive, lack of standardization and availability	Fair	Used as an adjunct to other tests
Plain abdominal film	Identifies excessive amount of stool in the colon; simple, inexpensive, widely available	Lack of standardization of interpretation, lack of controlled studies	Poor	Not recommended for routine evaluation but useful in older adults and children with incontinence and fecal impaction
Barium enema	Identifies megacolon, megarectum, stenosis, diverticulosis, extrinsic compression, and intraluminal masses	Lack of standardization, embarrassment, radiation exposure, lack of controlled studies	Poor	Not recommended as part of routine evaluation
Endoscopy				
Flexible sigmoidoscopy and colonoscopy	Directly visualizes the colon to exclude mucosal lesions (e.g., solitary rectal ulcer syndrome, inflammation, malignancy)	Invasive, risks related to procedure (perforation, bleeding) and sedation	Poor	Indicated in patients with unexplained diarrhea and seepage and patients >age 50

EAS, external anal sphincter; *EMG*, electromyography; *IAS*, internal anal sphincter.

*Evidence-based summary.

Feldman M, Friedman LS, Brandt LJ: Sleisenger and Fortran's Gastrointestinal and Liver Disease, 10th ed, ISBN# 978-1-4557-4692-7, 2016, Elsevier.

Clinical Algorithms

III

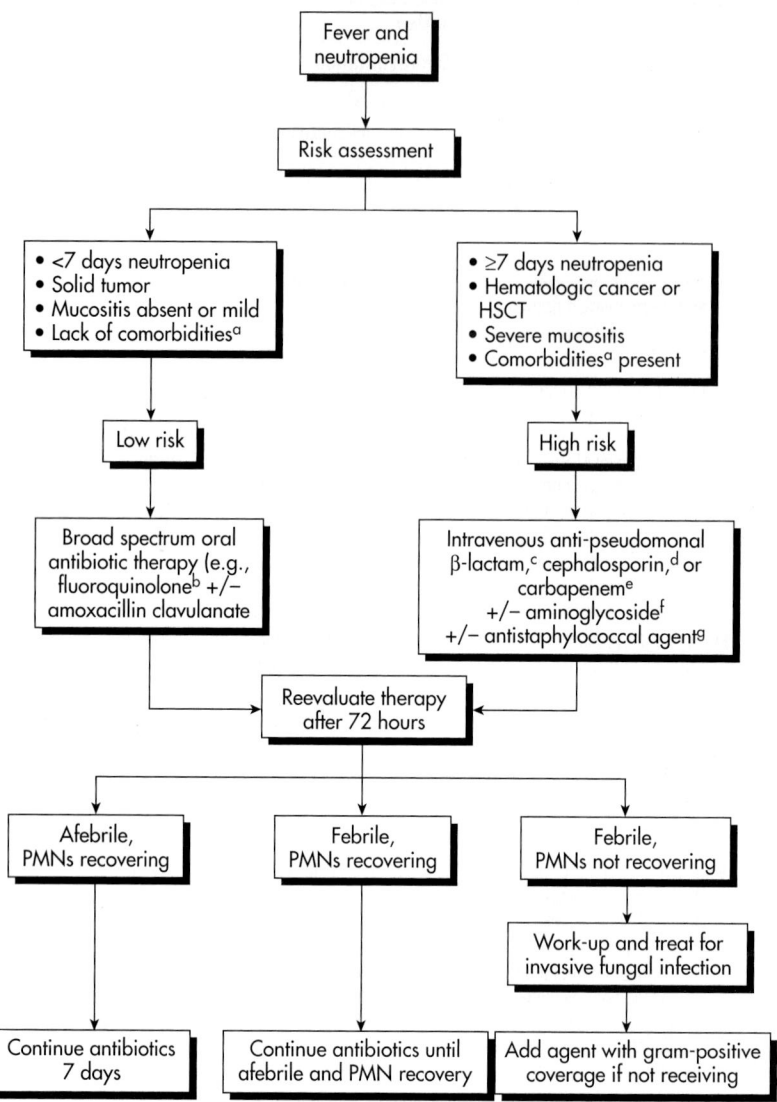

^a Hypotension, altered mental status, neurologic changes, respiratory failure, abdominal pain, hemorrhage, cardiac compromise or new arrythmia, catheter tunnel infection, extensive cellulitis, acute renal or liver failure

^b Institution-sensitivity dependent, ciprofloxacin, levofloxacin, moxifloxacin

^c Drug selection and dosing institution-specific: piperacillin tazobactam, ticarcillin/clavulanate

^d Drug selection and dosing institution-specific: ceftazidime, cefepime, ^eimipenem/cilastatin, meropenem, doripenem

^f Gentamin, tobramycin, or amakacin

^g Drug selection and institution-specific: vancomycin, linezolid, daptomycin, ceftaroline

FIG. 107 Approach to patient with fever and neutropenia. (From Hoffman R: Hematology, basic principles and practice, 6th ed, Philadelphia, Saunders, 2013, Figure 88.3.)

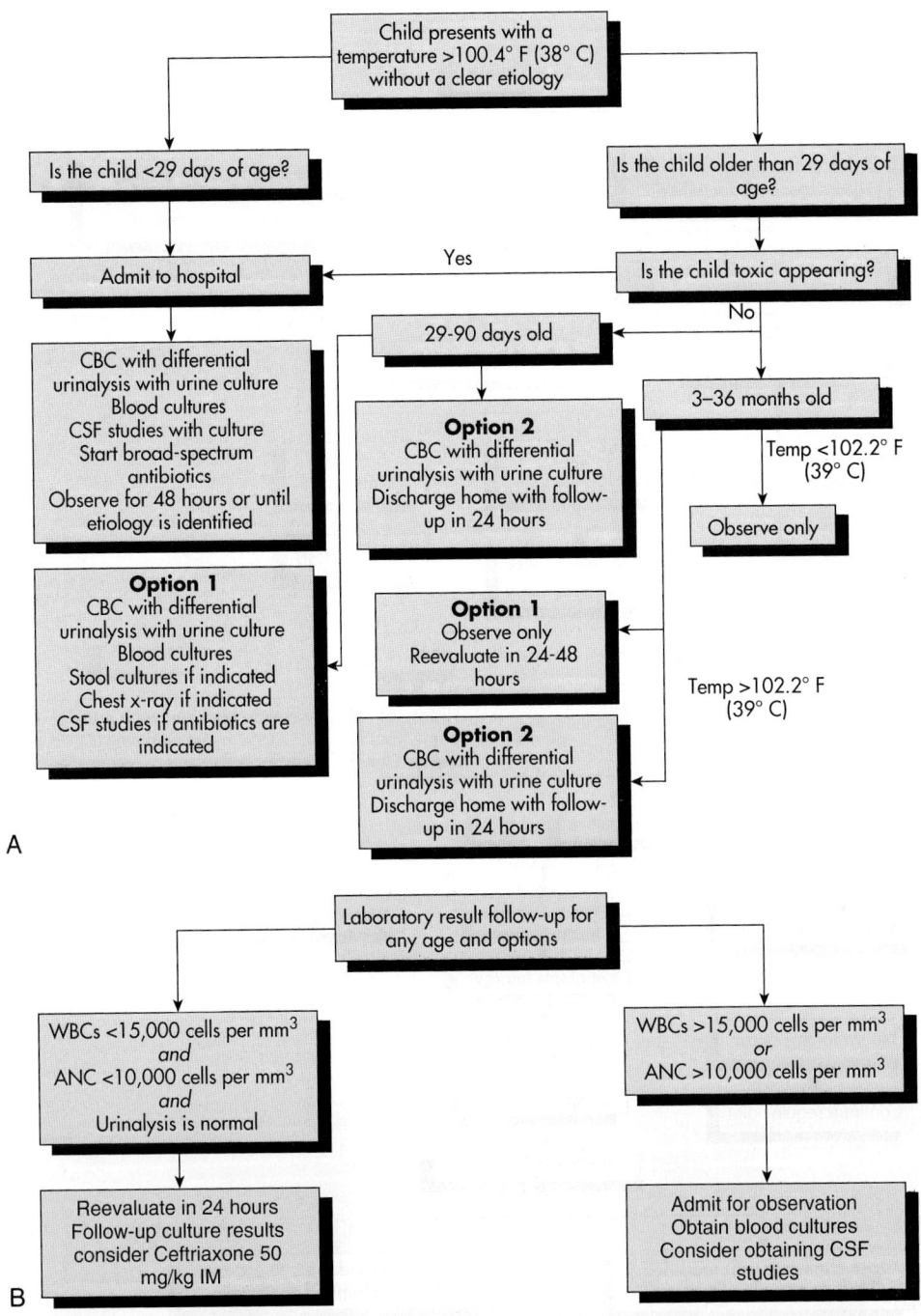

FIG. 109   A, Algorithm for the treatment of a child aged 0 to 36 months with a fever higher than 100.4° F (38° C) with no etiology for the fever. **B,** Continued considerations for the treatment of a child aged 0 to 36 months with a fever higher than 100.4° F (38° C) with no etiology for the fever. *ANC*, absolute neutrophil count; *CBC*, complete blood count; *CSF*, cerebrospinal fluid; *IM*, intramuscular; *WBCs*, white blood cells. (Wein AJ, Kavoussi LR, Partin AW, Peters CA: Campbell-Walsh Urology, 11th ed, ISBN# 978-1-4557-7567-5, 2016, Elsevier.)

Clinical
Algorithms

III

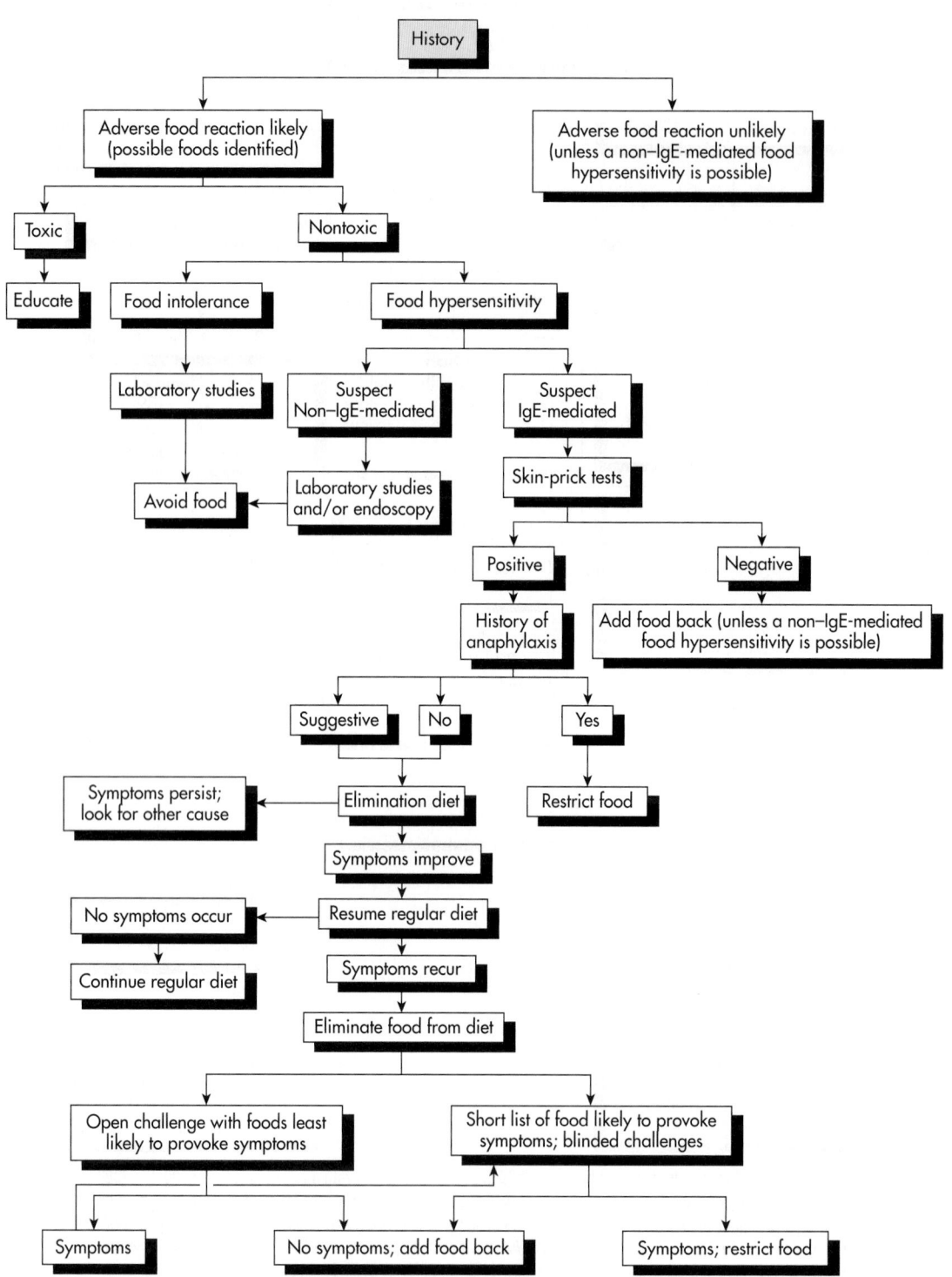

FIG. 111 Algorithm for the evaluation and management of adverse food reactions. (Feldman M, Friedman LS, Brandt LJ: Sleisenger and Fortran's Gastrointestinal and Liver Disease, 10th ed, ISBN# 978-1-4557-4692-7, 2016, Elsevier.)

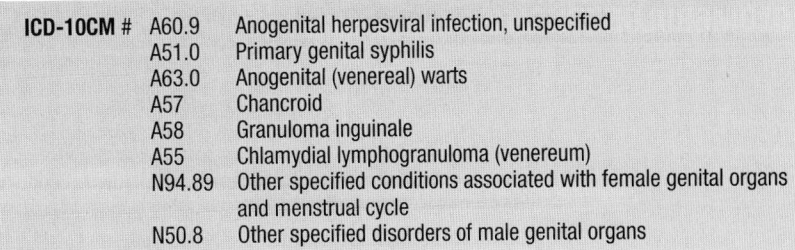

ICD-10CM #	
A60.9	Anogenital herpesviral infection, unspecified
A51.0	Primary genital syphilis
A63.0	Anogenital (venereal) warts
A57	Chancroid
A58	Granuloma inguinale
A55	Chlamydial lymphogranuloma (venereum)
N94.89	Other specified conditions associated with female genital organs and menstrual cycle
N50.8	Other specified disorders of male genital organs

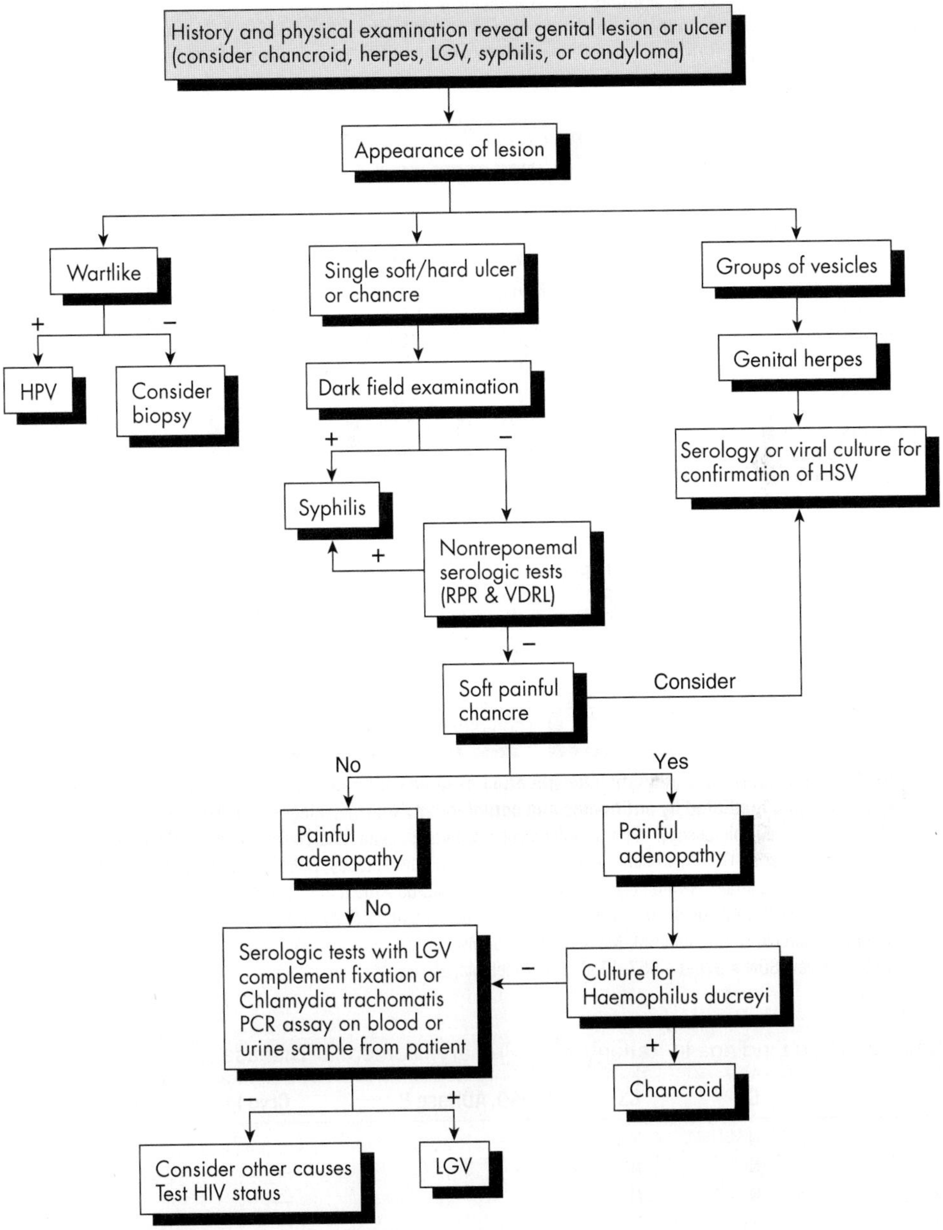

History and physical examination reveal genital lesion or ulcer (consider chancroid, herpes, LGV, syphilis, or condyloma)

Appearance of lesion

Wartlike
+ → HPV
− → Consider biopsy

Single soft/hard ulcer or chancre
Dark field examination
+ → Syphilis
− → Nontreponemal serologic tests (RPR & VDRL)
  + → Syphilis
  − → Soft painful chancre

Groups of vesicles
Genital herpes
Serology or viral culture for confirmation of HSV

Soft painful chancre — Consider → Serology or viral culture for confirmation of HSV

Soft painful chancre
No → Painful adenopathy
  No → Serologic tests with LGV complement fixation or Chlamydia trachomatis PCR assay on blood or urine sample from patient

Yes → Painful adenopathy
  → Culture for Haemophilus ducreyi
    − → Serologic tests with LGV complement fixation or Chlamydia trachomatis PCR assay on blood or urine sample from patient
    + → Chancroid

Serologic tests with LGV...
− → Consider other causes Test HIV status
+ → LGV

FIG. 114 Evaluation of patients with genital lesions or ulcers. *HIV,* Human immunodeficiency virus; *HPV,* human papillomavirus; *HSV,* herpes simplex virus; *LGV,* lymphogranuloma venereum; *RPR,* rapid plasma reagin; *VDRL,* Venereal Disease Research Laboratory. (Modified from Nseyo UO [ed]: *Urology for primary care physicians,* Philadelphia, 1999, Saunders.)

Clinical Algorithms

III

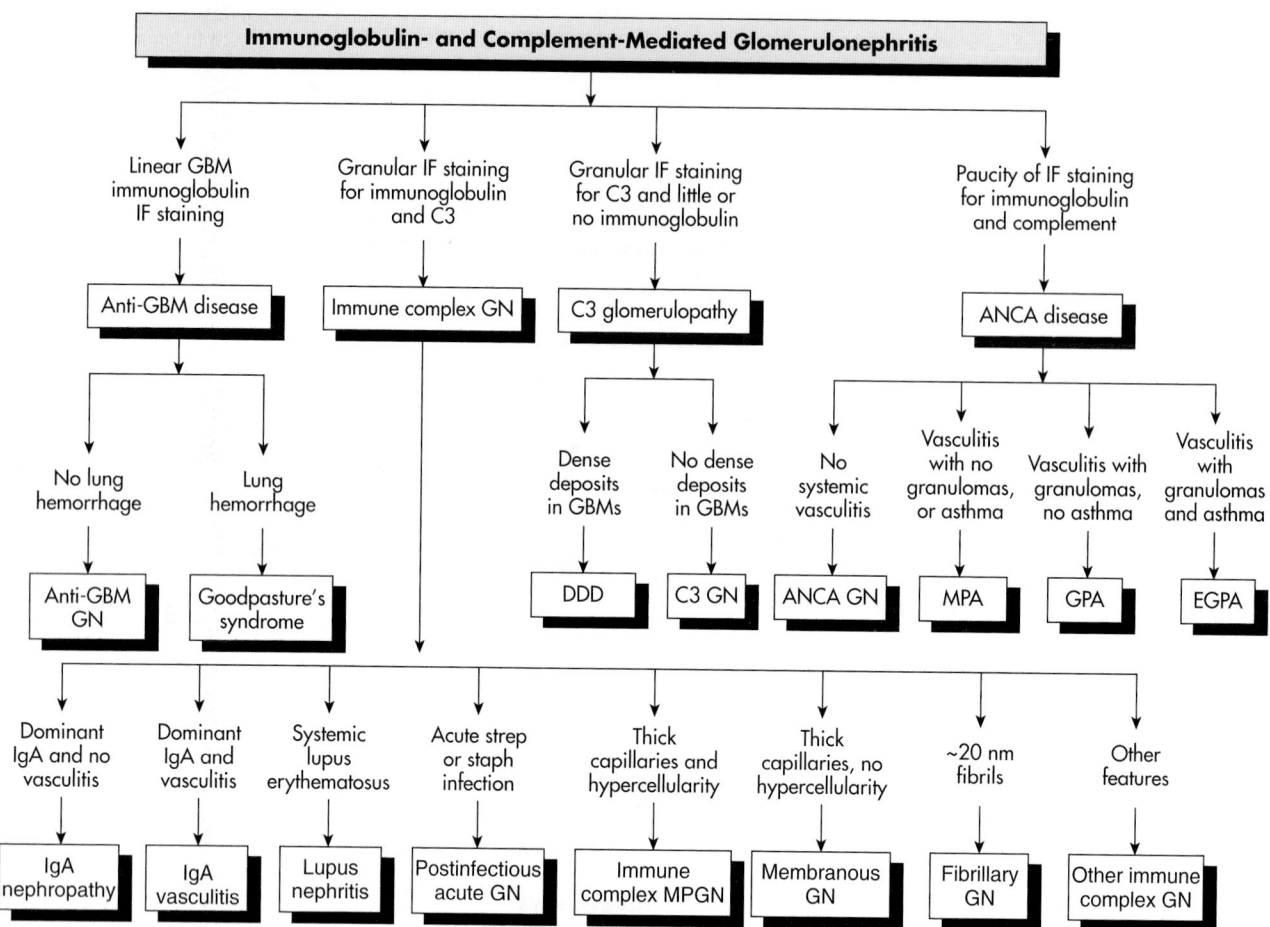

FIG. 117 Algorithm for diagnostic classification of glomerulonephritis (GN) that is known or suspected of being mediated by antibodies and complement. Note that integration of light microcopy, immunofluorescence (IF) microscopy, electron microscopy, laboratory data, and clinical manifestations is required to precisely diagnose GN. *ANCA,* Anti-neutrophil cytoplasmic autoantibody; *DDD,* dense deposit disease; *EGPA,* eosinophilic granulomatosis with polyangiitis; *GBM,* glomerular basement membrane; *GPA,* granulomatosis with polyangiitis; *IgA,* immunoglobulin A; *MPA,* microscopic polyangiitis; *MPGN,* membranoproliferative glomerulonephritis. (Skorecki K, Chertow GM, Marsden PA, Taal MW, Yu ASL, Wasser WG: Brenner & Rector's the Kidney, ed 10, Elsevier, ISBN # 978-1-4557-4836-5, Philadelphia, 2016.)

Table 25 Selected Serologic Findings in Patients with Primary Glomerular Disease

Disease	C4	C3	ASO, ADNase B	Cryo Ig	Anti-GBM	ANCA
Minimal change disease	N	N	—	—	—	—
Focal glomerulosclerosis	N	N	—	—	—	—
Membranous nephropathy	N	N	—	—	—	—
Membranoproliferative GN*						
Type I	N or ↓↓	↓↓	+	++	—	—
Type II	N	↓↓↓	+	—	—	—
Fibrillary GN	N	N	—	—	—	—
IgA nephropathy	N	N	—	—	—	—
Acute poststreptococcal GN	N or ↓	↓↓	+++	++	—	—
Crescentic GN						
Anti-GBM	N	N	—	—	+++	±
Immune complex	N or ↓	N or ↓↓	—	N/++	—	±
ANCA small vessel vasculitis	N	N	—	—	±	+++

ANCA, Antineutrophil cytoplasmic autoantibody; *ADNase B,* anti–deoxyribonuclease B; *ASO,* anti–streptolysin O; *cryo Ig,* cryoglobulins; *GBM,* glomerular basement membrane; *GN,* glomerulonephritis; *N,* normal levels.

*Former membranoproliferative glomerulonephritis classification schema.

Skorecki K, Chertow GM, Marsden PA, Taal MW, Yu ASL, Wasser WG: Brenner & Rector's the Kidney, ed 10, Elsevier, ISBN # 978-1-4557-4836-5, Philadelphia, 2016.

ICD-10CM #   E04.0   Nontoxic diffuse goiter   **1631**
              E04.1   Nontoxic uninodular goiter
              E04.2   Nontoxic multinodular goiter
              E05.0   Toxic goiter

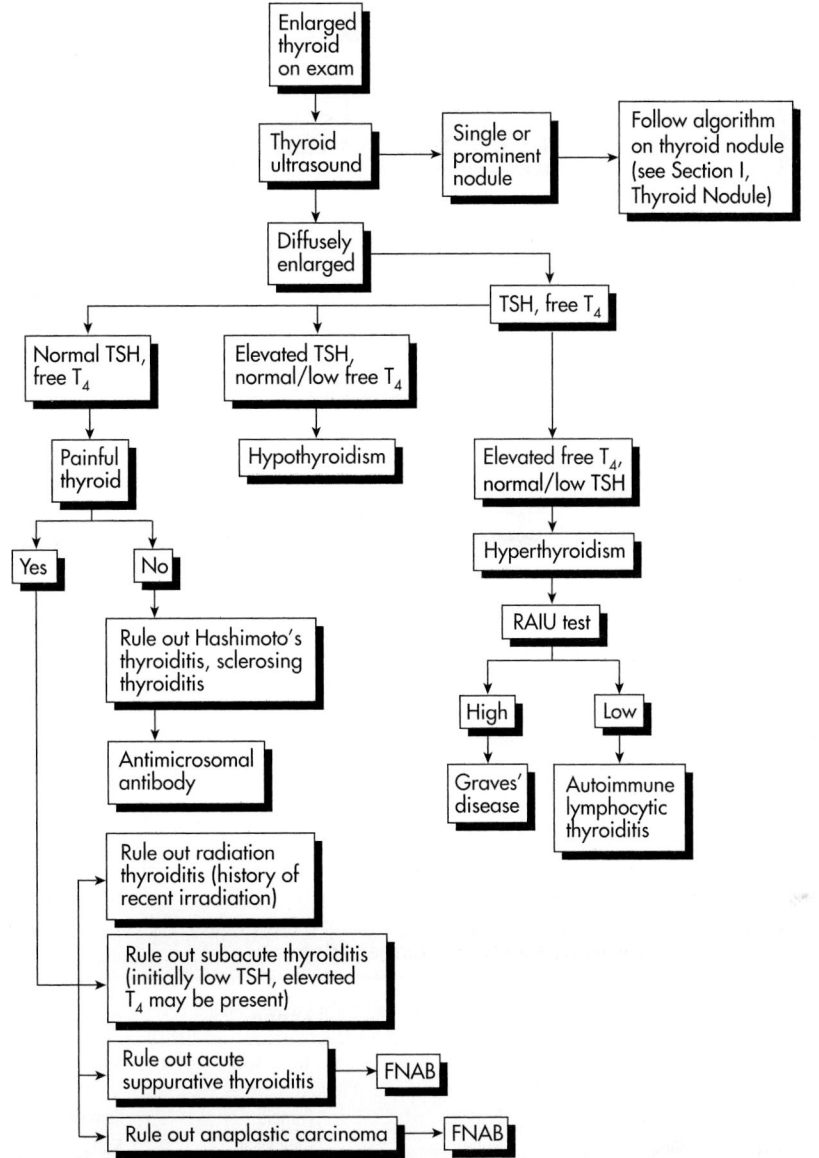

FIG. 118 Diagnostic algorithm. *FNAB,* Fine needle aspiration biopsy. (From Ferri, F: *Ferri's best test: a practical guide to clinical laboratory medicine and diagnostic imaging,* 3rd ed, Philadelphia, Saunders, 2014.)

Diagnostic Imaging	Lab Evaluation
Best Test(s)	***Best Test(s)***
Ultrasound of thyroid	TSH, free T$_4$
Ancillary Tests	***Ancillary Tests***
• RAIU scan of thyroid	CBC with differential
	Antimicrosomal Ab
	Thyroglobulin level

Clinical
Algorithms

III

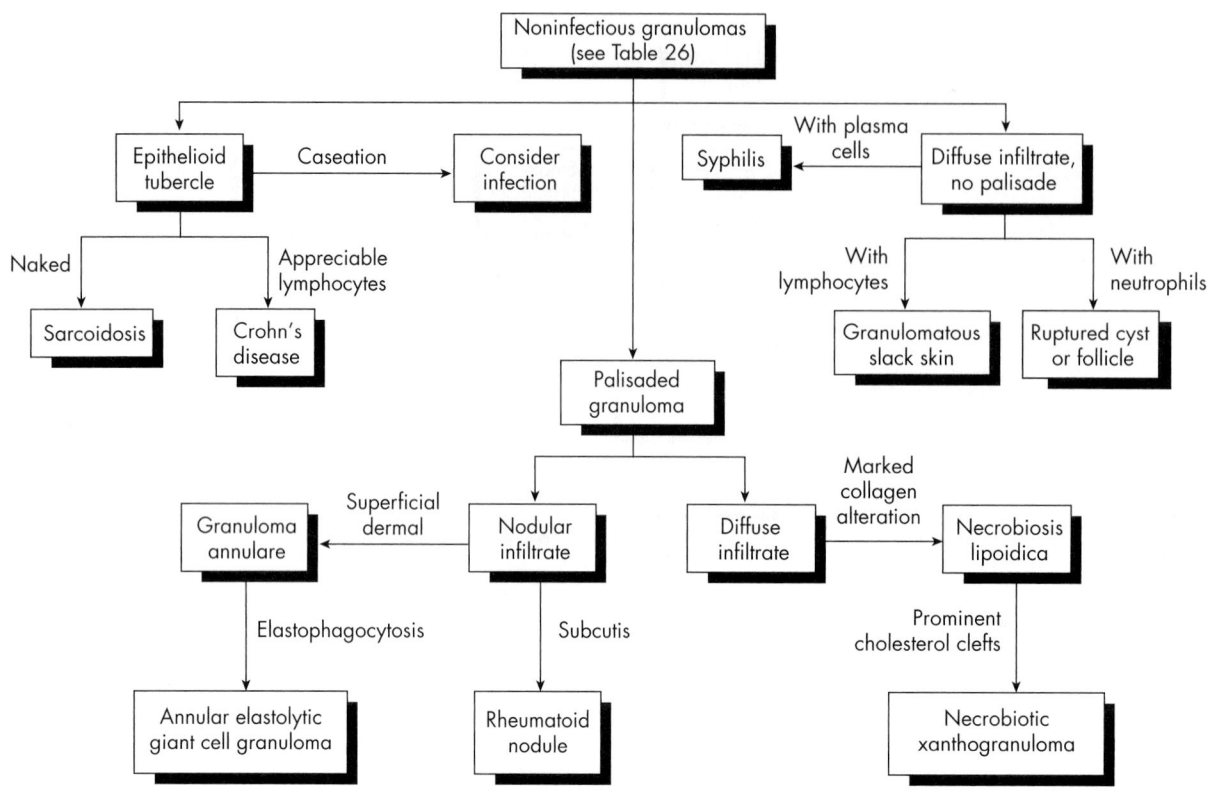

FIG. 120 Noninfectious granulomas. Paradigm for histologic diagnosis.

Table 26 Clinical Features of the Major Granulomatous Dermatitides

	Sarcoidosis	Classic GA*	NLD	AEGCG	Crohn's Disease	Rheumatoid Nodule
Average age (years)	25-35, 45-65	<30		40	35	30-40
Sex	Female	Female	Female	Female	Female	Female
Racial predilection in United States	African American	None	None	Caucasian	None	None
Site	Symmetric on face, neck, upper trunk, extremities	Hands, feet, extremities	Anterior and lateral distal lower extremities	Face, neck, forearms	Genital areas, lower >upper extremities	Juxtaarticular areas, elbows, hands, ankles, feet
Appearance	Red to red-brown papules and plaques	Papules coalescing into annular plaques	Plaques with elevated borders, telangiectasias centrally	Annular plaques	Dusky erythema and swelling, ulceration	Skin-colored, firm, mobile subcutaneous nodules
Size of lesions	1-5 cm	1-2 mm papules, <5 cm annular plaques	>10 cm	1-6 cm	Variable	1-3 cm
Number of lesions	Variable	1-10	1-10	1-10	1-5	1-10
Associations	Systemic manifestations of sarcoidosis	Rare diabetes mellitus, malignancy	Diabetes mellitus	Actinic damage	Intestinal Crohn's disease	Rheumatoid arthritis
Special clinical characteristics	Occasional central atrophy and hypopigmentation	Central hyperpigmentation	Yellow-brown atrophic centers, ulceration	Central atrophy and hypopigmentation	Draining sinuses and fistulae	Occasional ulceration, especially at site of trauma

AEGCG, Annular elastolytic giant cell granuloma; *GA,* granuloma annulare; *NLD,* necrobiosis lipoidica diabeticorum.
*Clinical variants include generalized, micropapular, nodular, perforating, subcutaneous, and patch GA.
From Bolognia JL et al: *Dermatology,* ed 2, St Louis, 2008, Mosby.

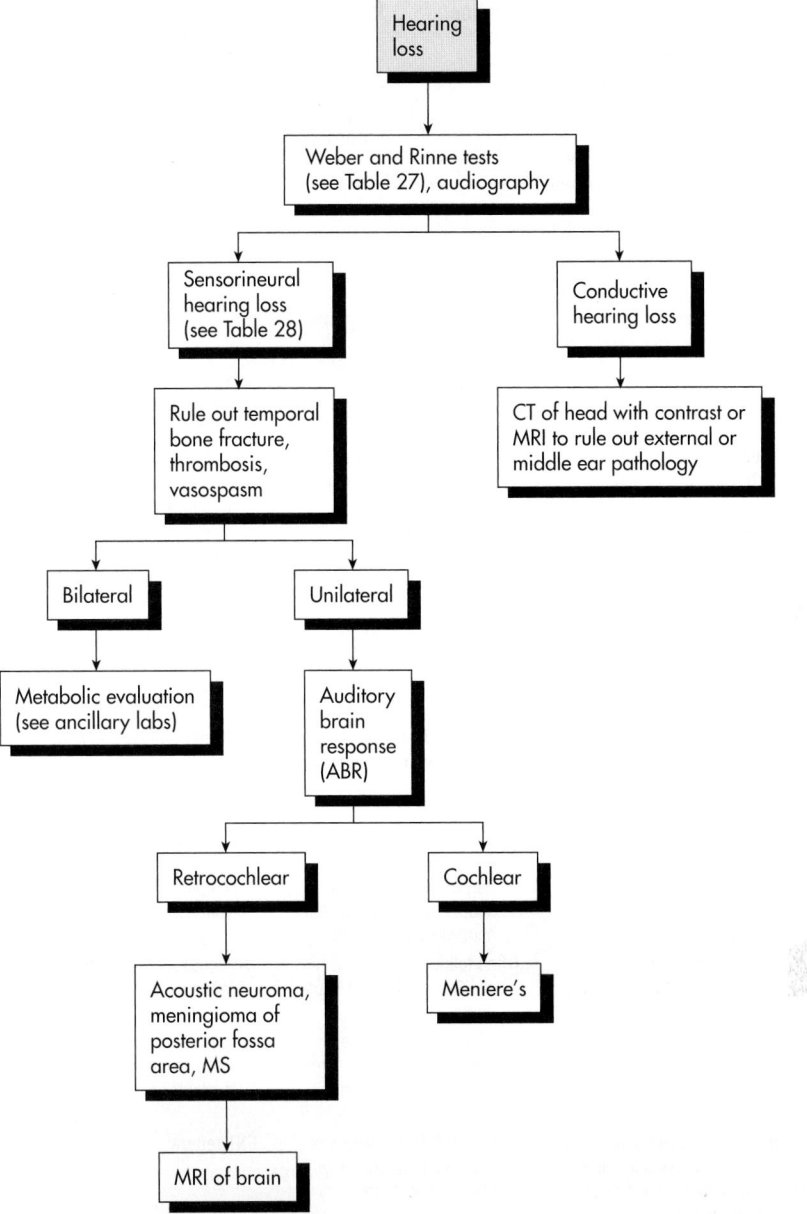

FIG. 121 Evaluation of hearing loss. *CT,* Computed tomography; *MRI,* magnetic resonance imaging; *MS,* multiple sclerosis. (From Ferri FF: *Ferri's best test: a practical guide to clinical laboratory medicine and diagnostic imaging,* ed 3, Philadelphia, 2014, Mosby.)

BOX 6   Hearing Loss

Diagnostic imaging	Lab evaluation
Best test	**Best test**
• None	None
Ancillary tests	**Ancillary tests**
CT of head with contrast or MRI with contrast	CBC
CT of temporal bone without contrast	ALT, AST
	ANA, VDRL
	TSH

ALT, Alanine aminotransferase; *ANA,* antibody to nuclear antigens; *AST,* angiotensin sensitivity test; *CBC,* complete blood count; *CT,* computed tomography; *TSH,* thyroid-stimulating hormone; *VDRL,* Venereal Disease Research Laboratory.
From Ferri FF: *Ferri's best test: a practical guide to clinical laboratory medicine and diagnostic imaging,* ed 3, Philadelphia, 2014, Mosby.

Clinical
Algorithms

Table 27 Interpretation of the Weber and Rinne Tests

	Weber without Lateralization	Weber Lateralizes Right	Weber Lateralizes Left
Rinne both ears: AC >BC	Normal	S/N loss in the left ear	S/N loss in the right ear
Rinne left ear: BC >AC	–	Combined loss: conduction and S/N loss in the left ear	Conduction loss in the left ear
Rinne right ear: BC >AC	–	Conduction loss in the right ear	Combined loss: conduction and S/N loss in the right ear

AC, Air conduction; *BC,* bone conduction; *S/N,* sensorineural.
From Adams JG et al: *Emergency medicine, clinical essentials,* ed 2, Philadelphia, 2013, Elsevier.

Table 28 Lesions That Cause Hearing Loss

	Description of Pathology	Onset/Course	Actions or Treatment	Prognosis
Conductive Lesion				
Foreign body	Mass in external canal blocks sound conduction	Acute onset associated or not with pain, drainage, or odor	Removal. Evaluate for infection. Evaluate for TM perforation	Excellent
Otitis externa	Edema and detritus obstruct external canal	Rapid onset. Pain, edema, swelling. Drainage, odor often present	Aural toilet to remove debris. Topical (± oral) antibiotics. Evaluate for necrotizing otitis	Excellent if treated appropriately
Exostosis	Bony growths obstruct canal. Often seen with prolonged exposure to cold water (divers)	Slow insidious onset. No pain or drainage unless causes complete obstruction	Evaluate for infection. Reassure patient. Refer to ENT	Good
Tympanosclerosis	TM scarring from perforations or infections. Decreased mobility impairs sound conduction	Slow onset following perforations, trauma or infections	ENT referral. Reassurance	Variable
Perforated TM	Disruption of TM integrity results in impaired transmission of sound to ossicle	Acute onset. May follow direct trauma or sudden barotrauma. May have sudden relief from pain if caused by otitis media	Treat infectious causes. Counsel on importance of keeping water out of ear canal. ENT referral	Good
Sterile effusion (barotrauma)	Fluid in middle ear dampens conduction through ossicles	Often following flight, diving, or URI. Bubbles can cause intermittent pain	Decongestants. Evaluate for infection. Follow-up	Excellent
Acute otitis media	Pus (or fluid) in middle ear dampens conduction through ossicles	Acute to subacute onset, often following URI. Often associated with pain ± fever	Antibiotics (unless viral cause suspected), decongestants, pain control	Excellent if treated appropriately
Cholesteatoma	Trapped stratified squamous epithelial mass in middle ear. Interferes with ossicle conduction	Slow onset. Often history of previous perforations or chronic infections	ENT referral	Variable. May destroy ossicles or erode into surrounding structures
Glomus tumor	Vascular tumor occupies middle ear space. Interferes with ossicle conduction	Slow onset. May be associated with rushing pulsatile sensation	ENT referral	Variable
Cancer	Squamous cell most common. Obstructs external canal	Slow onset. Often noticed first by others. Painless unless occlusion causes otitis externa	ENT referral. Evaluate for secondary infection	Variable
Sensorineural Lesion				
Perilymph fistula (inner ear barotrauma)	Disruption of round or oval window allows leakage of perilymph into middle ear	Sudden onset of hearing loss often with tinnitus and vertigo. Frequently follows straining or abrupt change in pressure. Turning in direction of fistula exacerbates symptoms	Complete bed rest. Elevate head of bed and avoid increases in CSF pressure. Severe symptoms or noncompliance may require hospitalization. ENT consultation for possible oval or round window patch	Variable
Viral cochleitis	Cochlear inflammation. Often following URI	Rapid onset. Often following URI	Steroids often used (no good data)	Variable

Table 28   Lesions That Cause Hearing Loss—cont'd

	Description of Pathology	Onset/Course	Actions or Treatment	Prognosis
Presbycusis	Age-related hearing loss. May be related to previous chronic noise exposure	Slow onset. Usually symmetric. High frequencies most affected. Tinnitus may occur	Hearing aid may help with both hearing loss and tinnitus	Variable
Acoustic neuroma	Benign schwannoma of 8th cranial nerve	Slow onset. Usually unilateral. May exhibit tinnitus, vertigo. May exhibit facial hyperesthesias or twitching	May require surgical excision if symptoms debilitating	Variable
Ototoxic agents	Direct toxicity to inner ear structures	Variable onset. High frequency most affected. Exposure to ototoxic drugs. May have associated tinnitus	Stop use of offending agent	Variable. Hearing loss at time of stopping offending agent is usually permanent
Multiple sclerosis	Multiple demyelinating lesions interfere with nerve conduction	Often other associated neurologic findings. May wax and wane	Standard multiple sclerosis treatment (steroids, cytotoxic agents)	Variable
Stroke/CVA	Focal ischemic lesion of auditory nerve or auditory cortex	Sudden onset. Often associated with other neurologic deficits	Treat CVA risk factors (ASA, anticoagulants, glycemic control, BP control)	Variable
Meningitis	Infection enters inner ear through CNS-perilymph connection. Damages organ of Corti	Follows clinical picture of meningitis	Treat infection. Steroids may limit inflammation and damage	Variable
Meniere's disease (endolymphatic hydrops)	Abnormal homeostasis of inner ear fluids (clinical diagnosis; definitive diagnosis made histologically)	Episodic spells of vertigo. Associated sensation of fullness, tinnitus, and SNHL or auditory distortion. Low-frequency ranges most affected	Reduce salt, caffeine, nicotine (vasoconstrictors) intake. Consider diuretics, antihistamines, anticholinergics. ENT referral	Variable
Chronic noise exposure	Direct mechanical damage to cochlear structures and hair cells	Slow onset. Usually high frequency most affected	Prevention measures (earplugs). Stop exposure	Usually permanent
Skull trauma	Interruption of cranial nerve VIII, ossicle disruption, or shearing effects on organ of Corti	Sudden onset after trauma	ENT consultation for possible surgical repair	Variable: ossicle disruption has better prognosis than nerve or organ of Corti damage
Autoimmune causes	Vascular or neuronal inflammatory changes	Bilateral asymmetric SNHL. May be fluctuating or progressive. Often other systemic autoimmune findings	Outpatient autoimmune evaluation. Steroids and cytotoxic agents may slow progression	Variable

ASA, Acetylsalicylic acid; *BP,* blood pressure; *CNS,* central nervous system; *CSF,* cerebrospinal fluid; *CVA,* cerebrovascular accident; *ENT,* ear, nose, and throat; *SNHL,* sensorineural hearing loss; *TM,* tympanic membrane; *URI,* upper respiratory infection.
From Adams JG et al: *Emergency medicine, clinical essentials,* ed 2, Philadelphia, 2013, Elsevier.

Clinical Algorithms

III

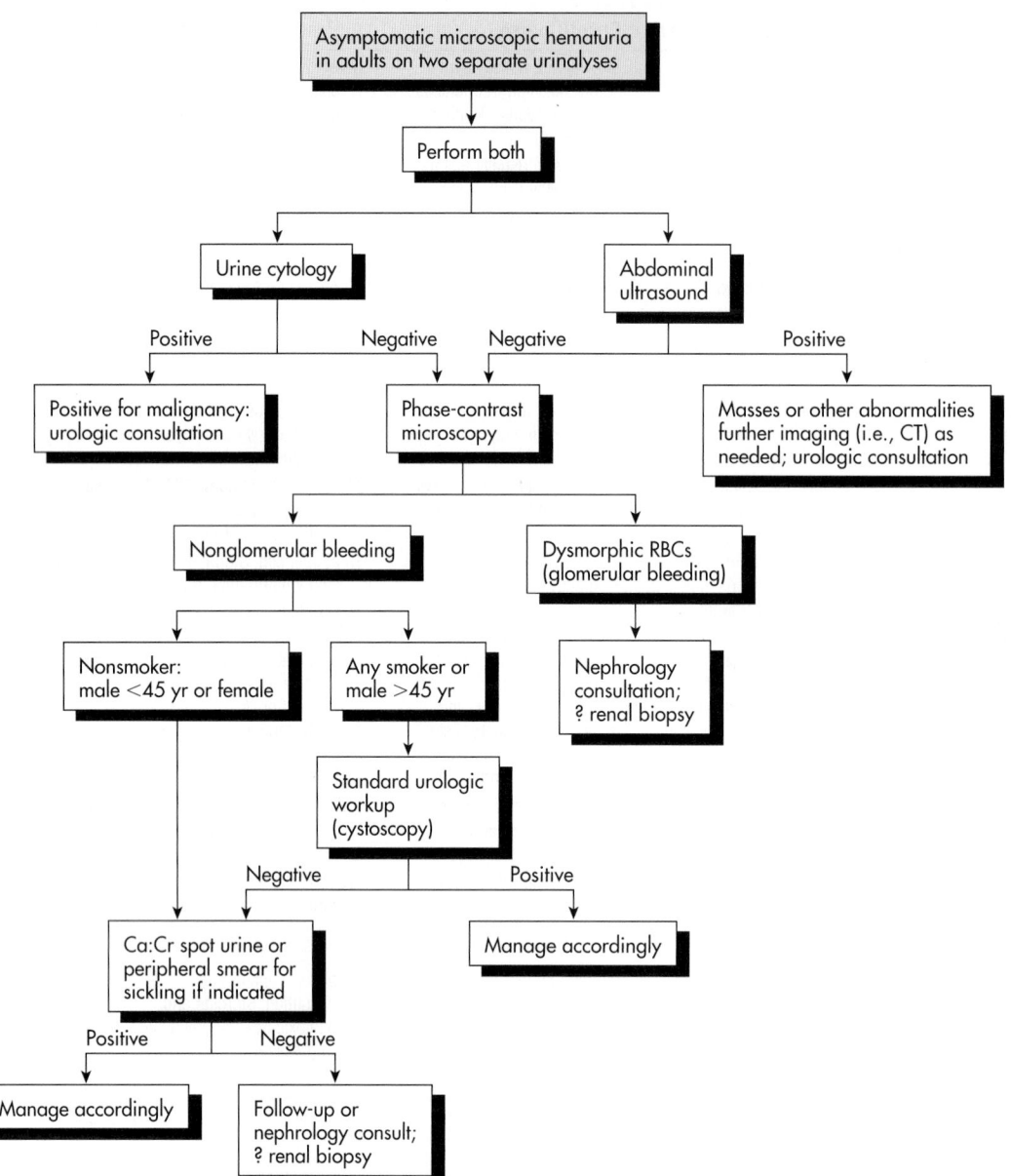

FIG. 123 Suggested algorithm for the evaluation of adult asymptomatic microscopic hematuria.
These patients must have no symptoms referable to the hematuria and a negative urinalysis except for red blood cells *(RBCs)*. Adults with gross hematuria require a full urologic evaluation. *Ca:Cr,* Calcium:creatinine ratio. (Modified from Nseyo UO [ed]: *Urology for primary care physicians,* Philadelphia, 1999, Saunders.)

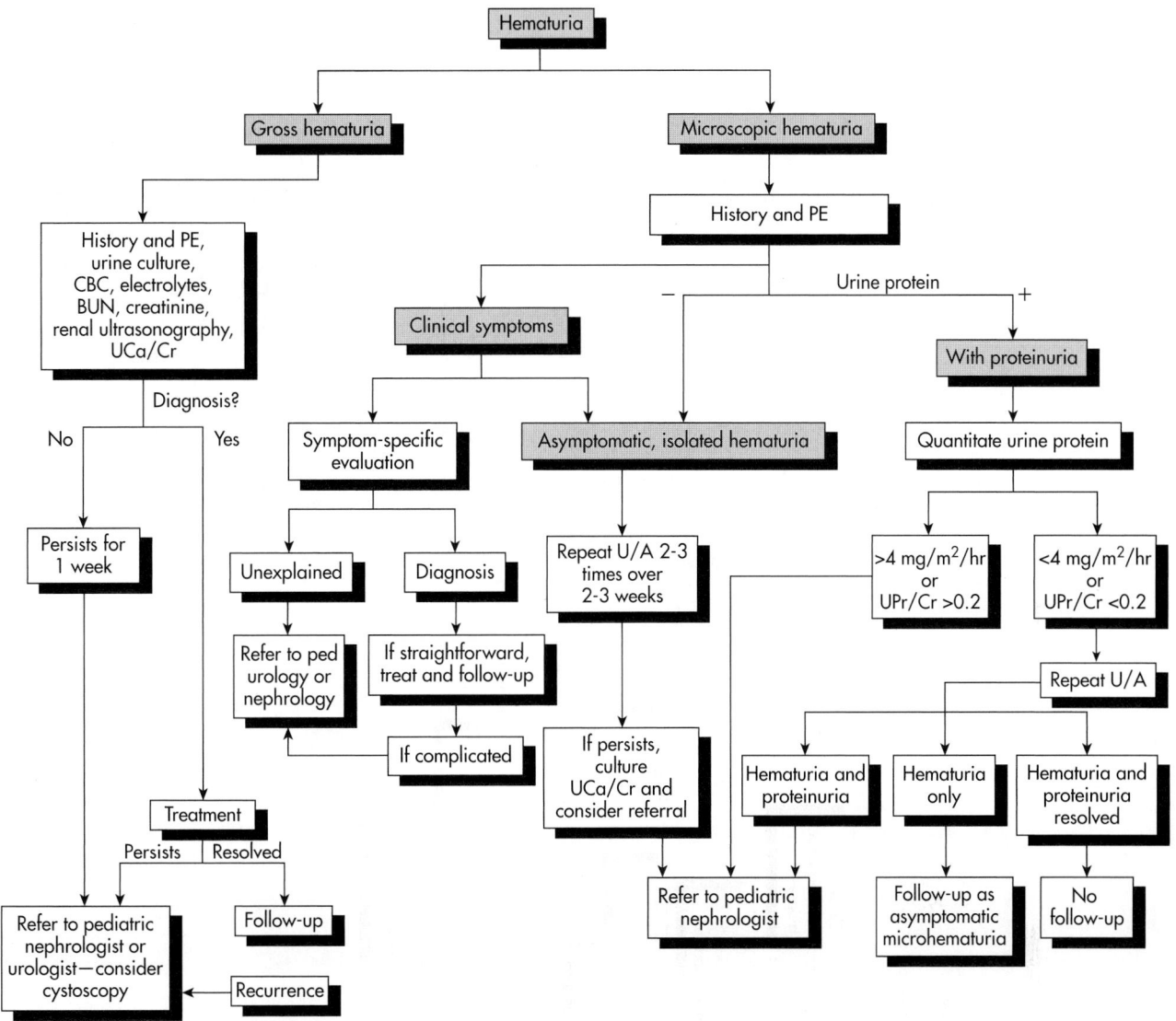

FIG. 125 Algorithm for the treatment of hematuria. *BUN*, blood urea nitrogen; *CBC*, complete blood cell count; *PE*, physical examination; *U/A*, urinalysis; *UCa/Cr*, urinary calcium/creatinine ratio; *UPr/Cr*, urinary protein/creatinine ratio. (Wein AJ, Kavoussi LR, Partin AW, Peters CA: Campbell-Walsh Urology, 11th ed, ISBN# 978-1-4557-7567-5, 2016, Elsevier.)

Clinical
Algorithms

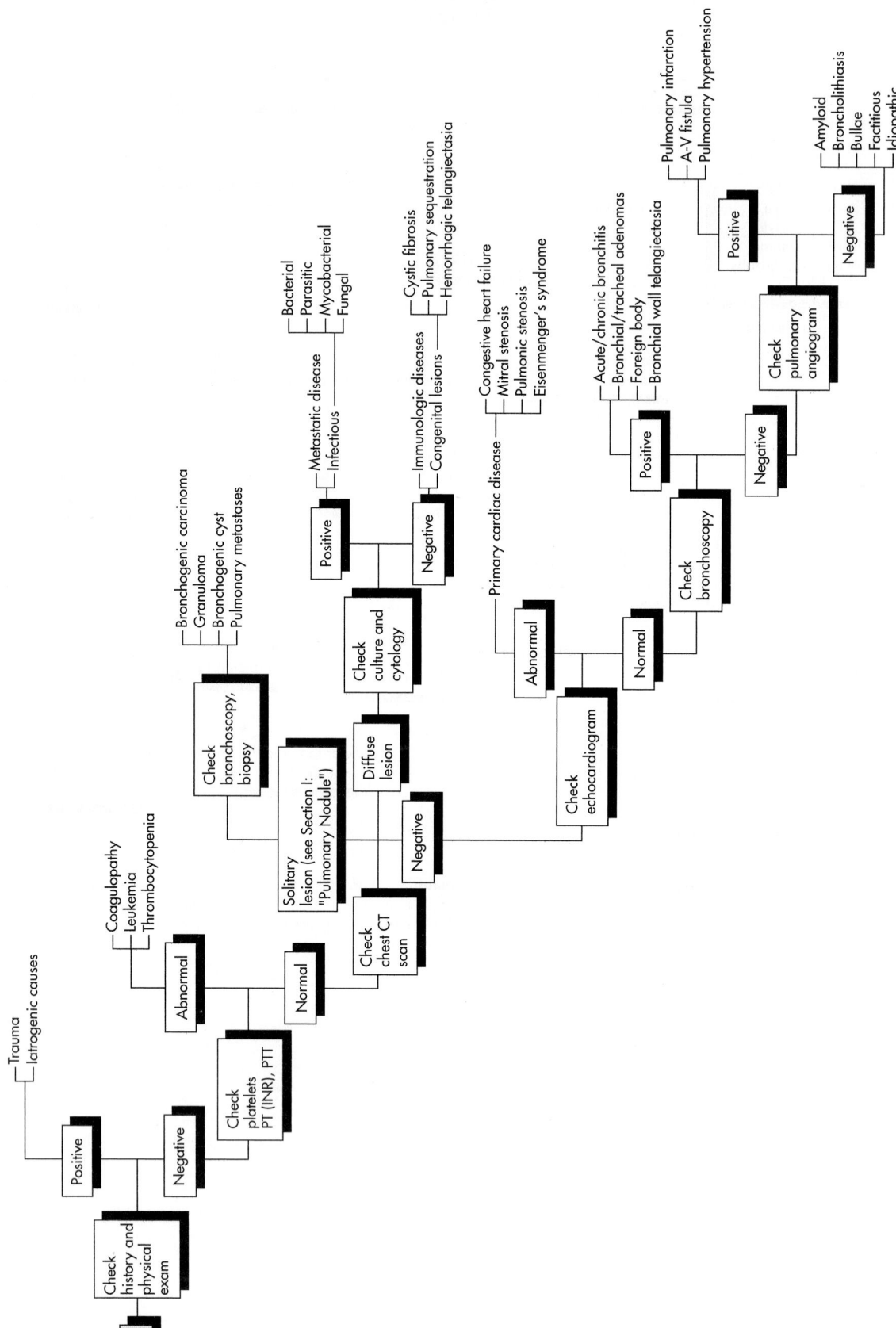

FIG. 126 Evaluation of hemoptysis. *A-V,* Arteriovenous; *CXR,* chest x-ray; *INR,* International Normalized Ratio; *PT,* prothrombin time; *PTT,* partial thromboplastin time. (From Healey PM: *Common medical diagnosis: an algorithmic approach,* ed 3, Philadelphia, 2000, Saunders.)

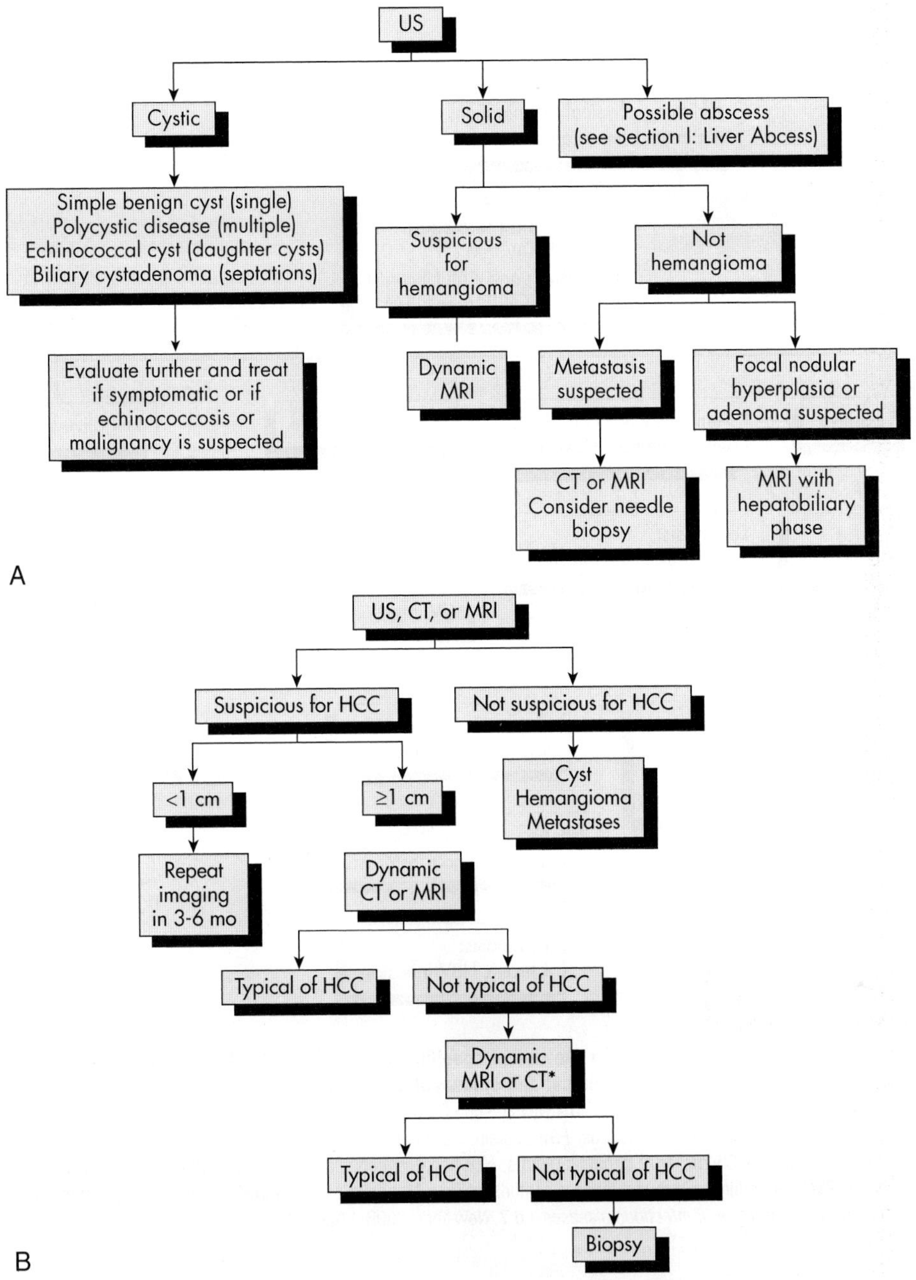

US

Cystic

Solid

Possible abscess
(see Section I: Liver Abcess)

Simple benign cyst (single)
Polycystic disease (multiple)
Echinococcal cyst (daughter cysts)
Biliary cystadenoma (septations)

Suspicious
for
hemangioma

Not
hemangioma

Evaluate further and treat
if symptomatic or if
echinococcosis or
malignancy is suspected

Dynamic
MRI

Metastasis
suspected

Focal nodular
hyperplasia or
adenoma suspected

CT or MRI
Consider needle
biopsy

MRI with
hepatobiliary
phase

A

US, CT, or MRI

Suspicious for HCC

Not suspicious for HCC

<1 cm

≥1 cm

Cyst
Hemangioma
Metastases

Repeat
imaging
in 3-6 mo

Dynamic
CT or MRI

Typical of HCC

Not typical of HCC

Dynamic
MRI or CT*

Typical of HCC

Not typical of HCC

Biopsy

B

FIG. 127 A, Algorithm for the approach to the management of a patient, not known to have cirrhosis, with a hepatic mass (often incidental, possibly symptomatic). **B,** Algorithm for the approach to the management of a patient with known or suspected cirrhosis and a hepatic mass (found on routine surveillance, because of symptoms, or because of an increasing AFP level). *Perform imaging modality not previously performed. HCC, hepatocellular carcinoma. (Feldman M, Friedman LS, Brandt LJ: Sleisenger and Fortran's Gastrointestinal and Liver Disease, 10th ed, ISBN# 978-1-4557-4692-7, 2016, Elsevier.)

Clinical
Algorithms

III

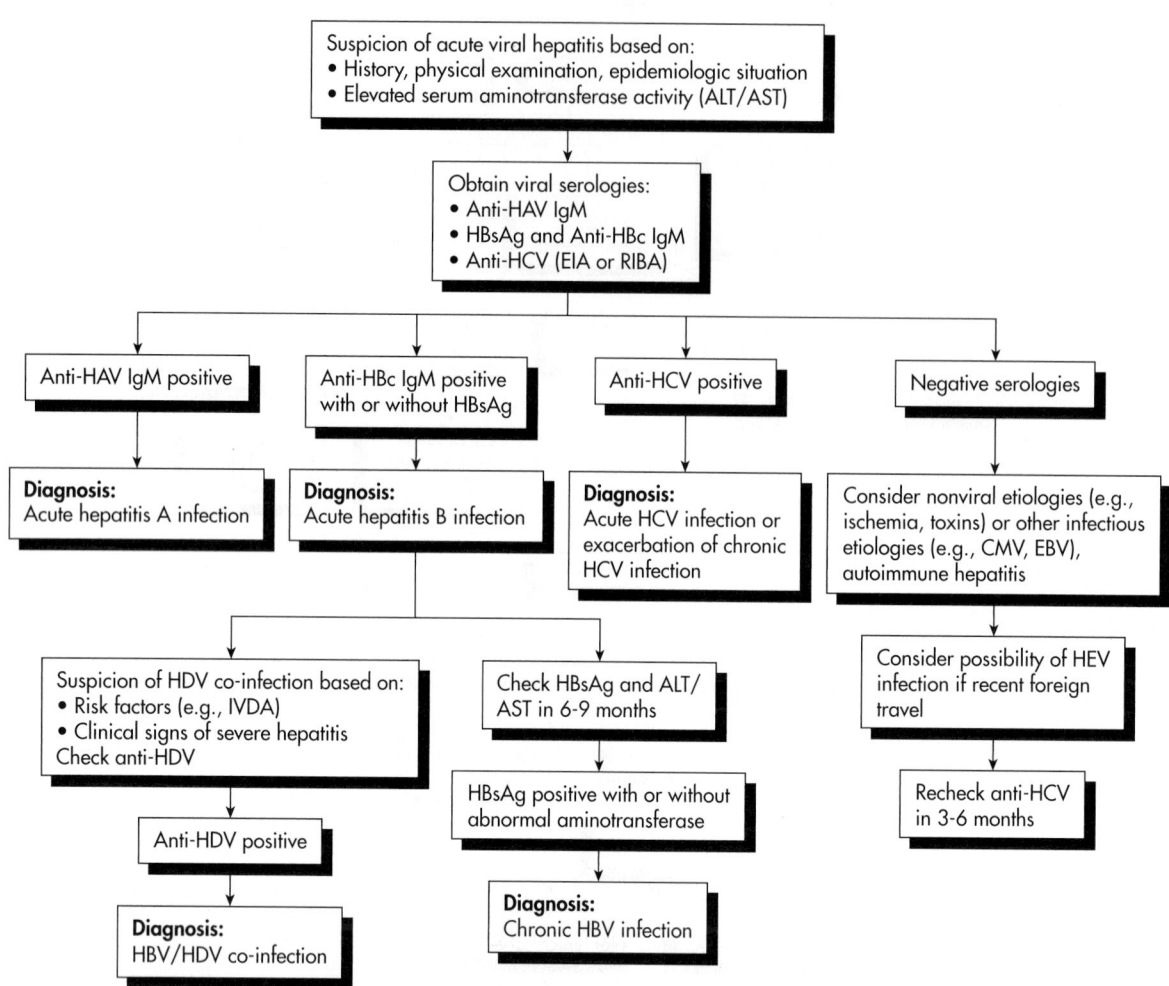

FIG. 128 A flow diagram showing the use of specific serologic tests for the diagnosis of acute viral hepatitis in relation to the clinical and epidemiologic setting. Co-infections and superinfections of chronic hepatitis B or C patients should always be considered in cases that do not fit well with the clinical or serologic picture. *CMV,* Cytomegalovirus; *EBV,* Epstein-Barr virus; *EIA,* enzyme immunoassay; *HBV,* hepatitis B virus; *HCV,* hepatitis C virus; *HDV,* hepatitis D virus; *HEV,* hepatoencephalomyelitis virus; *IVDA,* intravenous drug abuse; *RIBA,* recombinant immunoblot assay. (Modified from Mandell GL et al: *Mandell, Douglas, and Bennett's principles and practice of infectious diseases,* ed 7, New York, 2008, Churchill Livingstone.)

HEPATOMEGALY

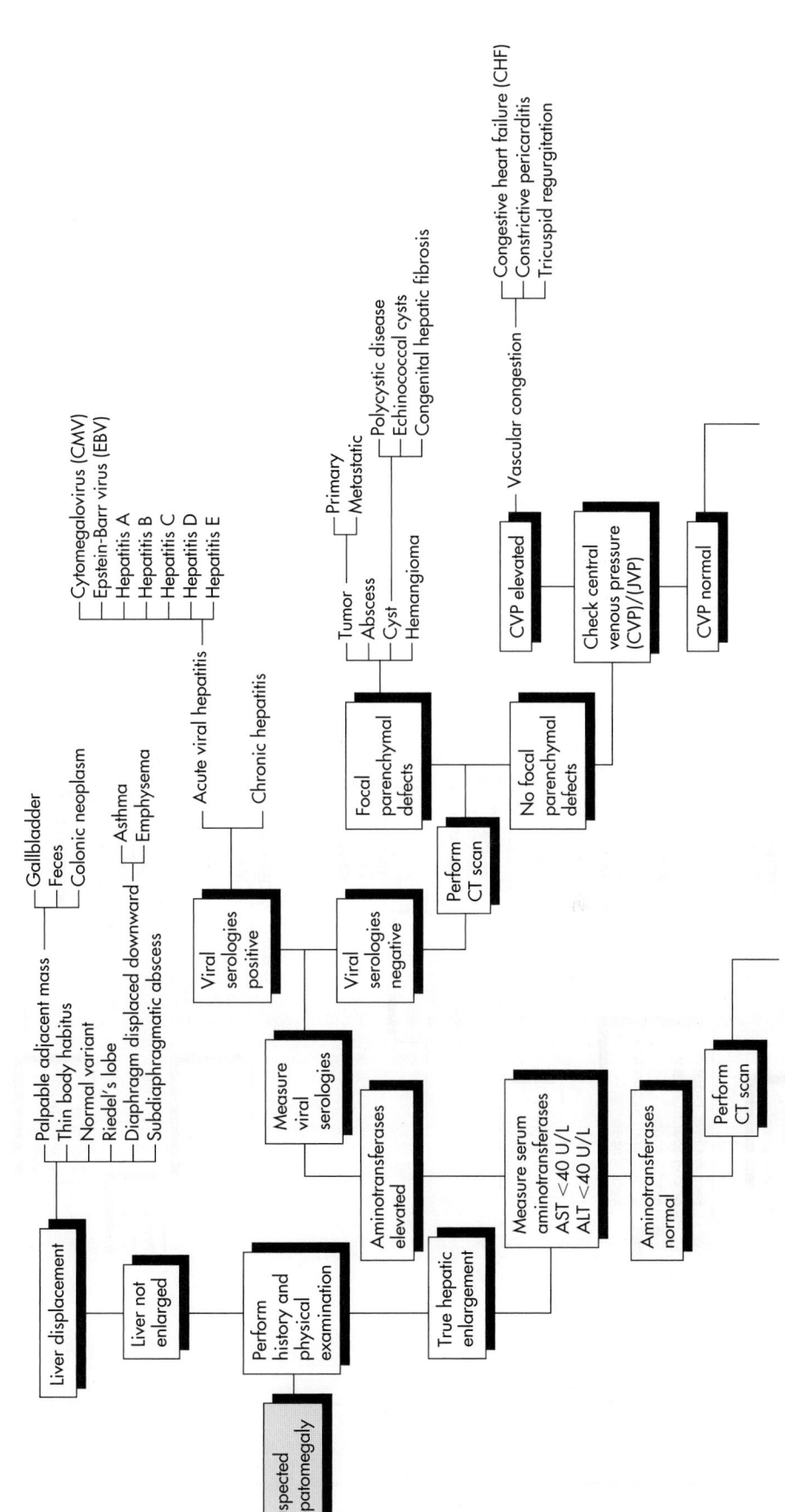

FIG. 129 Hepatomegaly. *ALT,* Alanine aminotransferase; *AST,* aspartate aminotransferase; *CT,* computed tomography; *JVP,* jugular venous pressure. (Modified from Healey PM: *Common medical diagnosis: an algorithmic approach,* ed 3, Philadelphia, 2000, Saunders.)

Continued on next page

Clinical
Algorithms

III

HEPATOMEGALY—cont'd **ICD-10CM #** R16.0 Hepatomegaly, not elsewhere classified

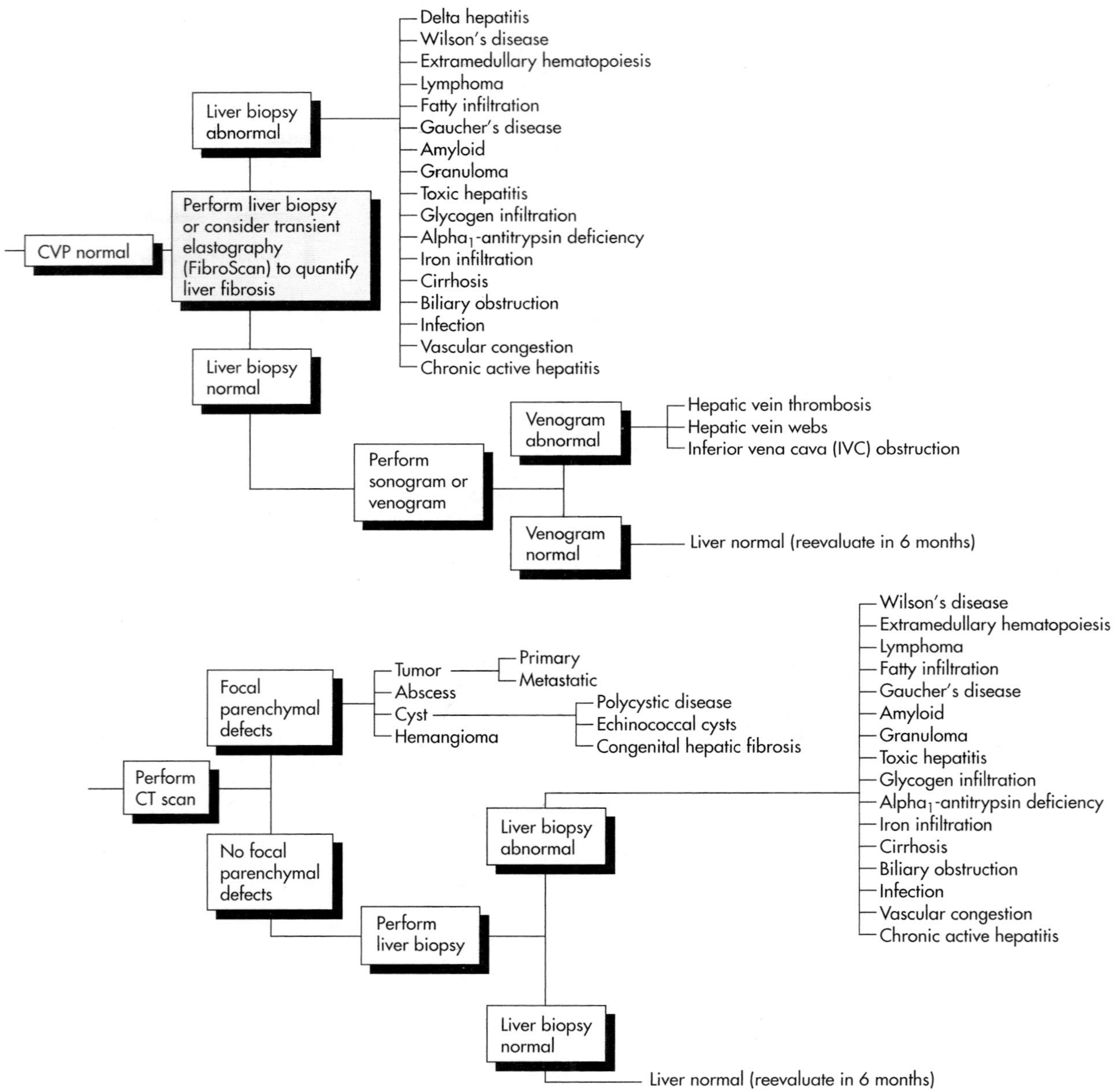
CVP normal
Perform liver biopsy or consider transient elastography (FibroScan) to quantify liver fibrosis
Liver biopsy abnormal
Delta hepatitis
Wilson's disease
Extramedullary hematopoiesis
Lymphoma
Fatty infiltration
Gaucher's disease
Amyloid
Granuloma
Toxic hepatitis
Glycogen infiltration
Alpha$_1$-antitrypsin deficiency
Iron infiltration
Cirrhosis
Biliary obstruction
Infection
Vascular congestion
Chronic active hepatitis
Liver biopsy normal
Perform sonogram or venogram
Venogram abnormal
Hepatic vein thrombosis
Hepatic vein webs
Inferior vena cava (IVC) obstruction
Venogram normal
Liver normal (reevaluate in 6 months)
Perform CT scan
Focal parenchymal defects
Tumor
Primary
Metastatic
Abscess
Cyst
Polycystic disease
Echinococcal cysts
Congenital hepatic fibrosis
Hemangioma
No focal parenchymal defects
Perform liver biopsy
Liver biopsy abnormal
Wilson's disease
Extramedullary hematopoiesis
Lymphoma
Fatty infiltration
Gaucher's disease
Amyloid
Granuloma
Toxic hepatitis
Glycogen infiltration
Alpha$_1$-antitrypsin deficiency
Iron infiltration
Cirrhosis
Biliary obstruction
Infection
Vascular congestion
Chronic active hepatitis
Liver biopsy normal
Liver normal (reevaluate in 6 months)

FIG. 129 (Continued)

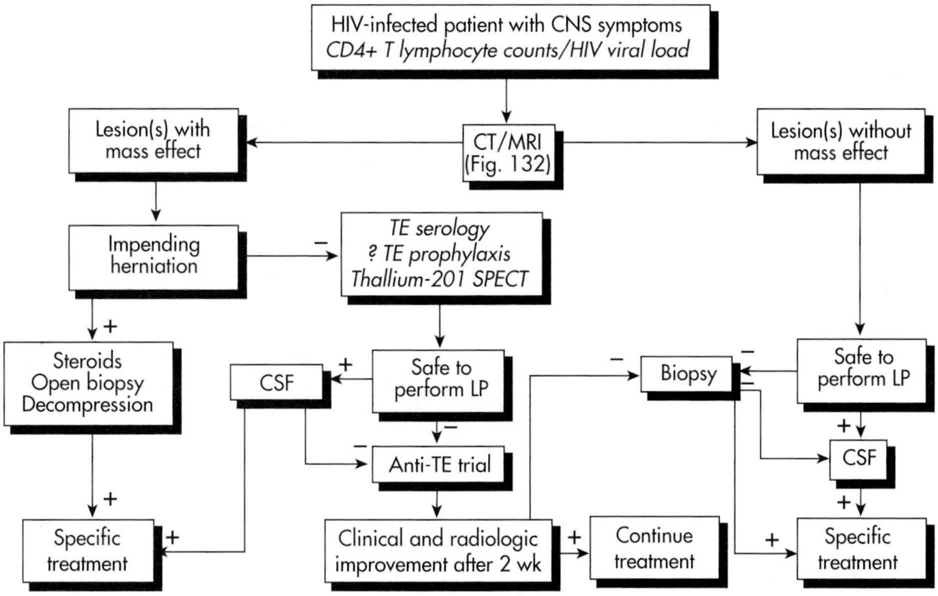

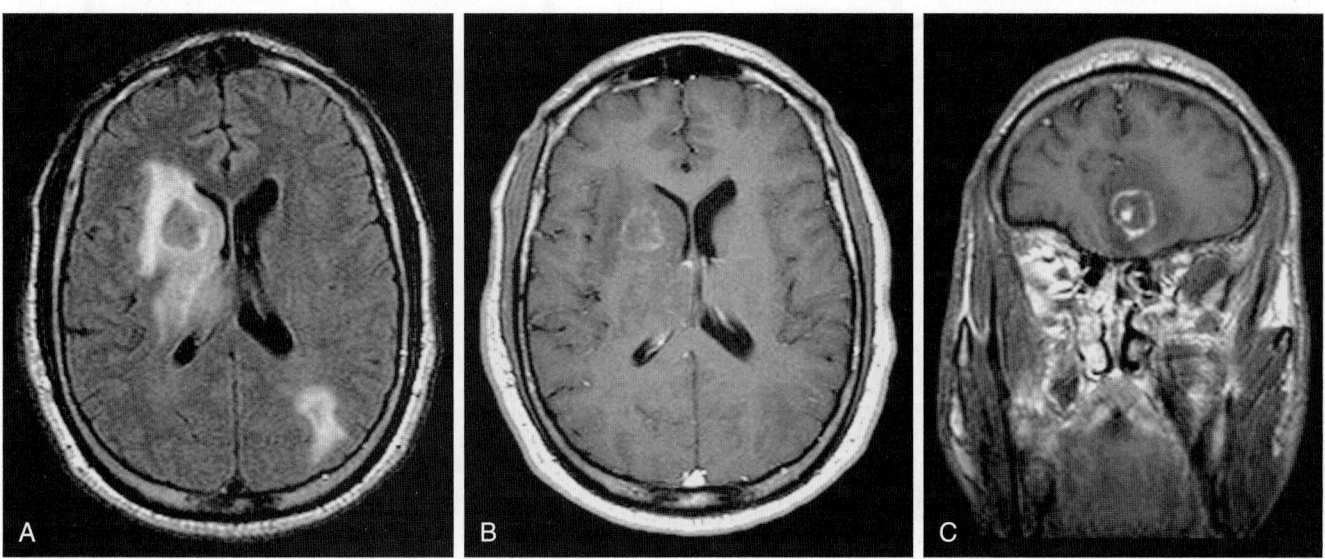

FIG. 131 Management of the human immunodeficiency virus (HIV) type 1–infected patient with central nervous system (CNS) mass lesions. The elements in italics represent data that contribute to the decision-making process (see text for details). *CSF*, Cerebrospinal fluid; *CT*, computed tomography; *LP*, lumbar puncture; *MRI*, magnetic resonance imaging; *SPECT*, single-photon emission computed tomography; *TE*, *Toxoplasma* encephalitis. (From Bennett JE, Dolin R, Blaser MJ: *Mandell, Douglas, and Bennett's principles and practice of infectious diseases*, ed 8, Philadelphia, 2015, Saunders.)

FIG. 132 Toxoplasmosis. A, A fluid-attenuated inversion recovery image shows isointense lesions in the right basal ganglia and left parietal lobe with surrounding edema. **B,** A postgadolinium T1-weighted image shows faint rim enhancement of right basal ganglia lesion. **C,** A postgadolinium T1-weighted image shows a typical "target" sign in a left frontal lobe lesion. (Soto JA, Lucey BC: Emergency Radiology, the requisites, 2nd ed, ISBN# 978-0-323-37640-2, 2017, Elsevier.)

Clinical
Algorithms

III

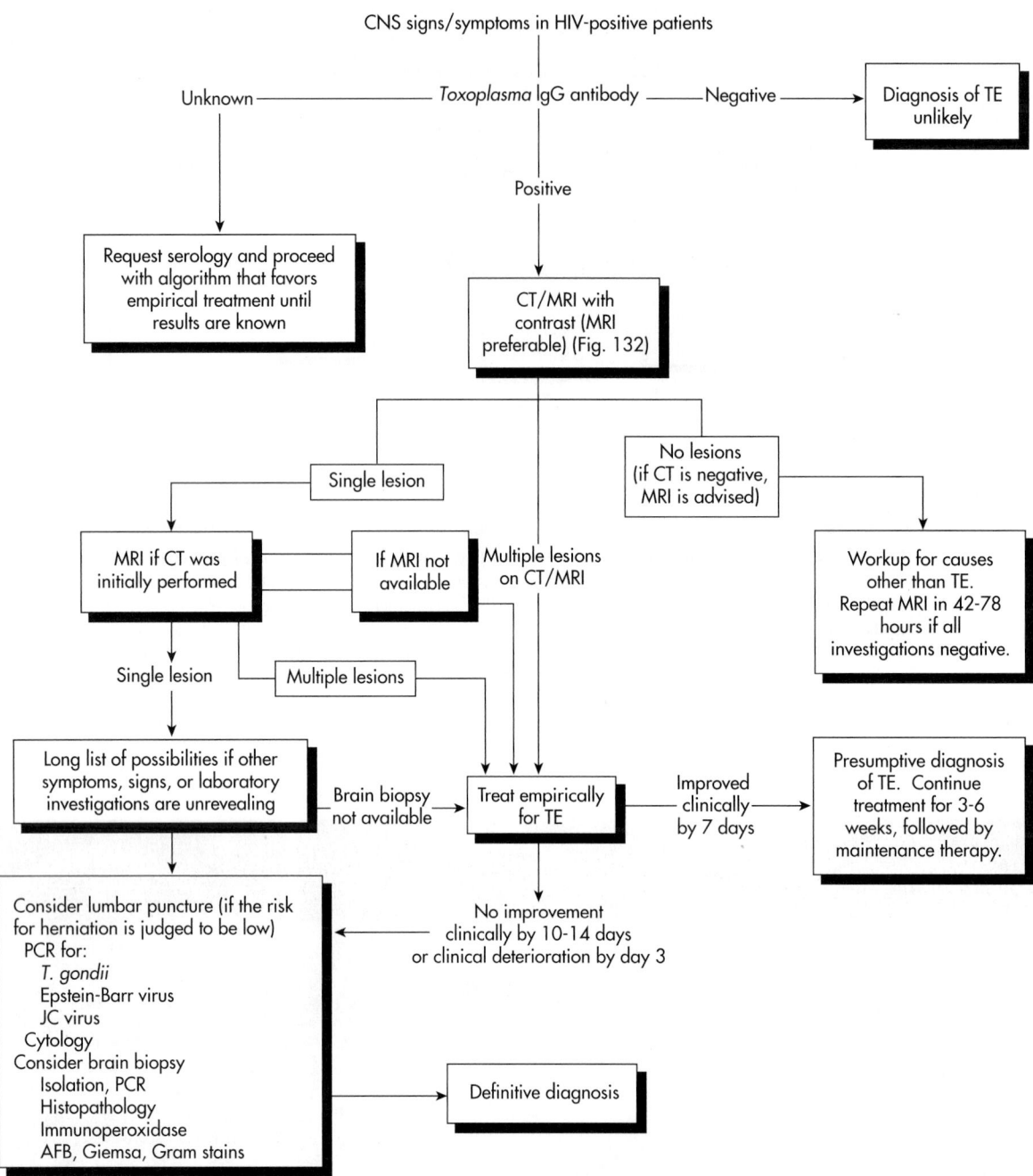

FIG. 133 Diagnostic approach and management algorithm for human immunodeficiency virus (HIV)-infected patients with central nervous system (CNS) symptoms or signs that might potentially be toxoplasmic encephalitis (TE). *AFB,* Acid-fast bacilli; *CT,* computed tomography; *IgG,* immunoglobulin G; *MRI,* magnetic resonance imaging; *PCR,* polymerase chain reaction. (From Bennett JE, Dolin R, Blaser MJ: *Mandell, Douglas, and Bennett's principles and practice of infectious diseases,* ed 8, Philadelphia, 2015, Saunders.)

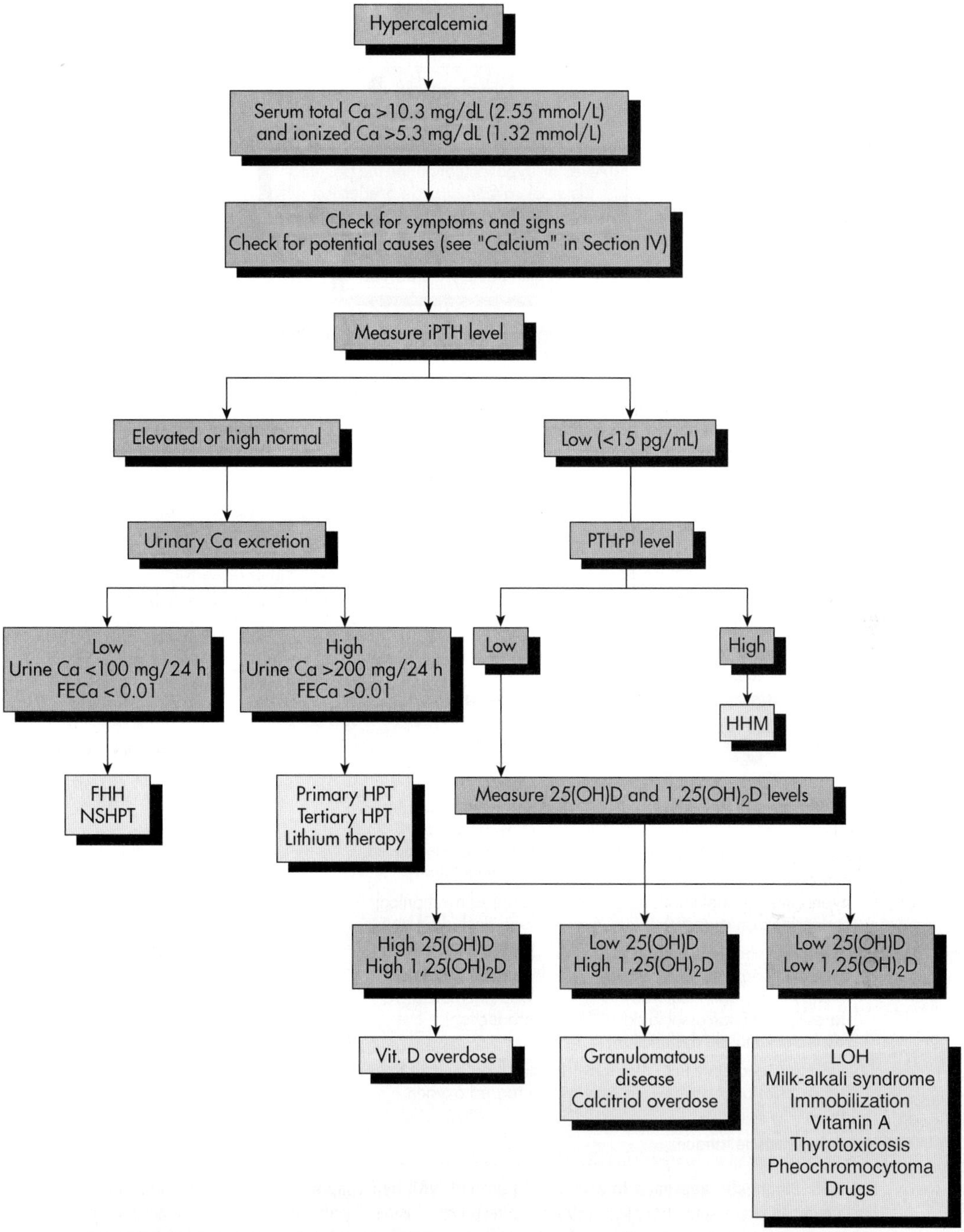

```
                          Hypercalcemia

              Serum total Ca >10.3 mg/dL (2.55 mmol/L)
              and ionized Ca >5.3 mg/dL (1.32 mmol/L)

                    Check for symptoms and signs
              Check for potential causes (see "Calcium" in Section IV)

                        Measure iPTH level

          Elevated or high normal                  Low (<15 pg/mL)

            Urinary Ca excretion                     PTHrP level

       Low                    High              Low            High
  Urine Ca <100 mg/24 h   Urine Ca >200 mg/24 h
  FECa < 0.01             FECa >0.01                            HHM

       FHH                  Primary HPT
       NSHPT                Tertiary HPT   Measure 25(OH)D and 1,25(OH)2D levels
                            Lithium therapy

              High 25(OH)D        Low 25(OH)D        Low 25(OH)D
              High 1,25(OH)2D     High 1,25(OH)2D    Low 1,25(OH)2D

              Vit. D overdose     Granulomatous          LOH
                                  disease           Milk-alkali syndrome
                                  Calcitriol overdose    Immobilization
                                                     Vitamin A
                                                     Thyrotoxicosis
                                                     Pheochromocytoma
                                                     Drugs
```

FIG. 134 Algorithm for evaluation of hypercalcemia. *FECa,* Fractional excretion of calcium; *FHH,* familial hypocalciuric hypercalcemia; *HHM,* humoral hypercalcemia of malignancy; *HPT,* hyperparathyroidism; *iPTH,* intact parathyroid hormone; *LOH,* localized osteolytic hypercalcemia; *NSHPT,* neonatal severe hyperparathyroidism; *PTHrP,* parathyroid hormone–related peptide. (Skorecki K, Chertow GM, Marsden PA, Taal MW, Yu ASL, Wasser WG: Brenner & Rector's the Kidney, ed 10, Elsevier, ISBN # 978-1-4557-4836-5, Philadelphia, 2016.)

Clinical Algorithms

III

Diagnostic Imaging

Best Test(s)
None

Ancillary Tests
Radiograph of painful bones (r/o bone neoplasm, multiple myeloma)
Tc-99m parathyroid scan (r/o parathyroid adenoma)
Ultrasound of parathyroid glands
Ultrasound of kidneys (r/o renal cell carcinoma)

Lab Evaluation

Best Test(s)
Serum calcium level
PTH level

Ancillary Tests
Serum phosphate, magnesium, alkaline phosphatase, albumin
Electrolytes, BUN, creatinine
24-hour urine collection for calcium
Urinary cyclic AMP
PSA (if prostate carcinoma is suspected)
Serum and urine protein immunoelectro-phoresis (if multiple myeloma suspected)

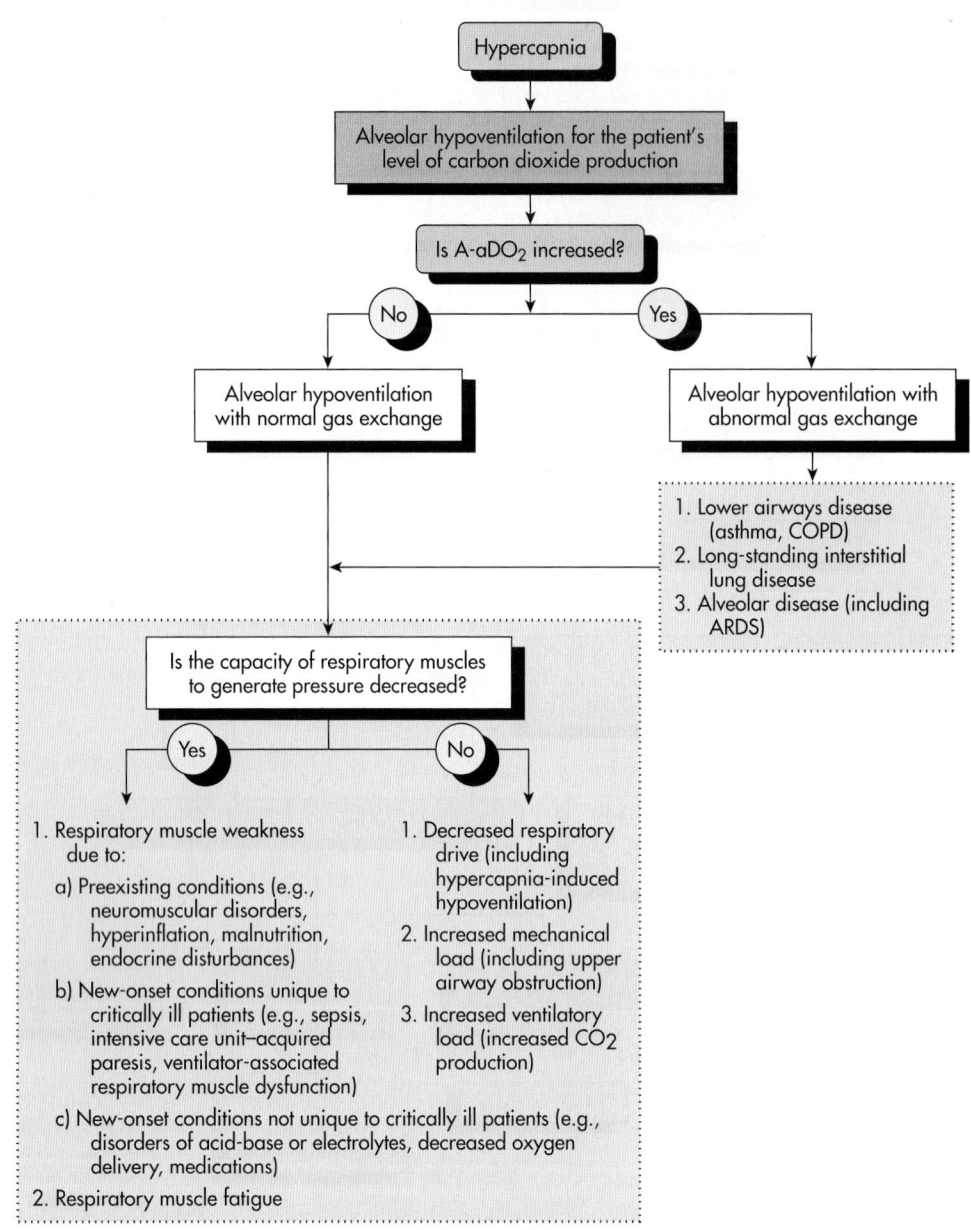

FIG. 135 Diagnostic approach to critically ill patient with hypercapnia. *A-aDo₂*, alveolar-arterial difference in partial pressure of oxygen; *ARDS*, acute respiratory distress syndrome; *COPD*, chronic obstructive pulmonary disease. (Parrillo JE, Dellinger RP: Critical Care Medicine, Principles of Diagnosis and Management in the Adult, 4th ed, ISBN # 978-0-323-08929-6, 2014, Elsevier.)

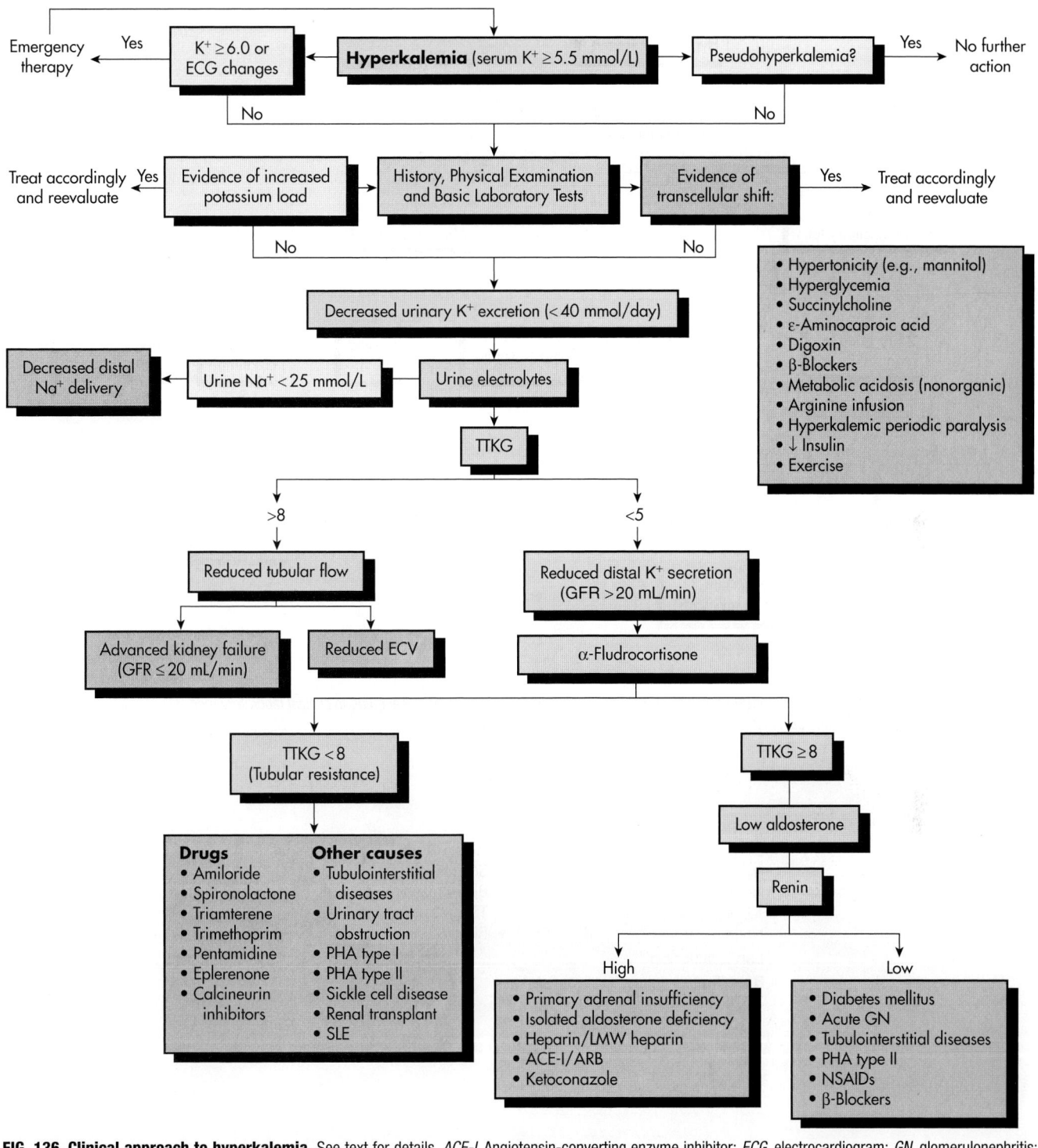

FIG. 136 Clinical approach to hyperkalemia. See text for details. *ACE-I*, Angiotensin-converting enzyme inhibitor; *ECG*, electrocardiogram; *GN*, glomerulonephritis; *ARB*, angiotensin II receptor blocker; *CCD*, cortical collecting duct; *ECV*, effective circulatory volume; *GFR*, glomerular filtration rate; *HIV*, human immunodeficiency virus; *LMW heparin*, low-molecular-weight heparin; *NSAIDs*, nonsteroidal antiinflammatory drugs; *PHA*, pseudohypoaldosteronism; *SLE*, systemic lupus erythematosus; *TTKG*, transtubular potassium gradient. (Skorecki K, Chertow GM, Marsden PA, Taal MW, Yu ASL, Wasser WG: Brenner & Rector's the Kidney, ed 10, Elsevier, ISBN # 978-1-4557-4836-5, Philadelphia, 2016.)

Diagnostic Imaging

Best Test(s)
None

Ancillary Tests
None

Lab Evaluation

Best Test(s)
Heparinized potassium level

Ancillary Tests
- Serum electrolytes, BUN, plasma osmolality, urine osmolality creatinine, urine potassium, calculation of TTKG
- Glucose, CBC
- CPK (when rhabdomyolysis is suspected)

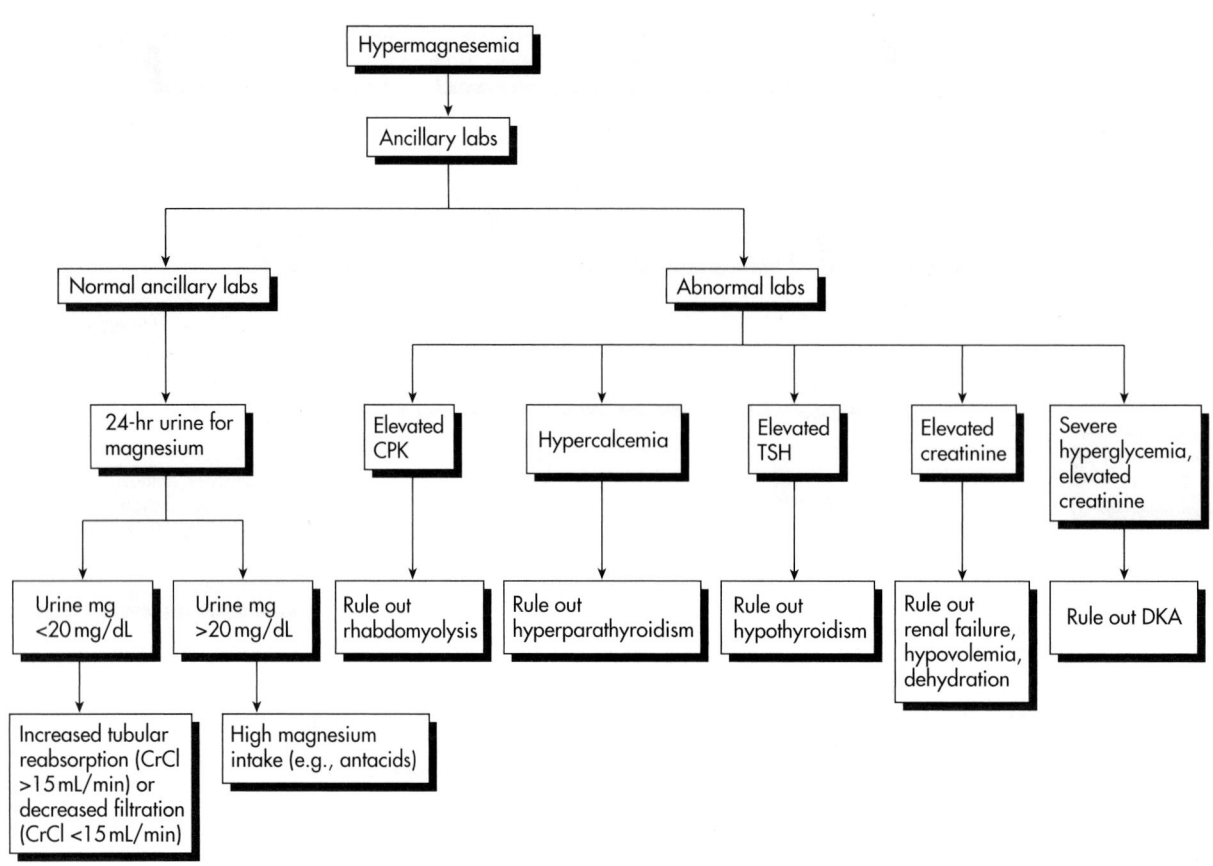

FIG. 137 Diagnostic algorithm. (From Ferri, F: *Ferri's best test: a practical guide to clinical laboratory medicine and diagnostic imaging,* ed 3, Philadelphia, 2014, Saunders.)

Diagnostic Imaging
Best Test(s)
None
Ancillary Tests
None
Lab Evaluation
Best Test(s)
24-hour urine magnesium level

Ancillary Tests
- Serum electrolytes, calcium
- BUN, creatinine, glucose
- TSH
- CPK

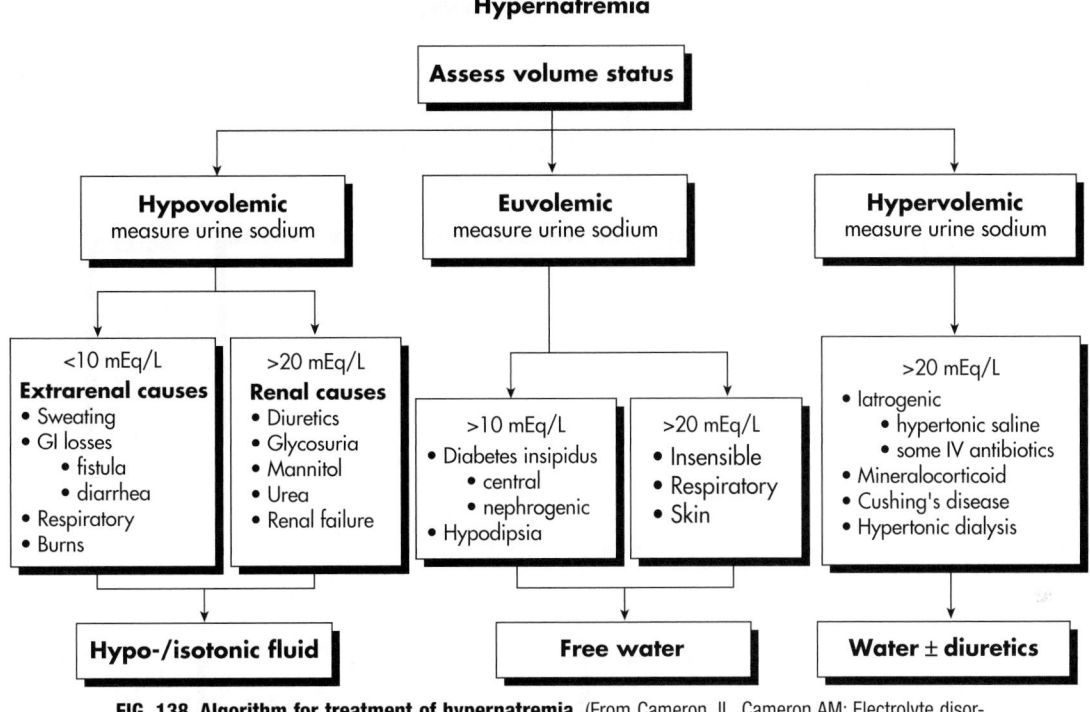

FIG. 138 Algorithm for treatment of hypernatremia. (From Cameron JL, Cameron AM: Electrolyte disorders, Current surgical therapy, ed 10, Philadelphia, 2011, Saunders.)

Diagnostic Imaging	Lab Evaluation
Best Test(s)	***Best Test(s)***
None	Serum electrolytes, urine sodium
Ancillary Tests	***Ancillary Tests***
None	Urine osmolality
	BUN, creatinine

ICD-10CM # L81.4 Other melanin hyperpigmentation

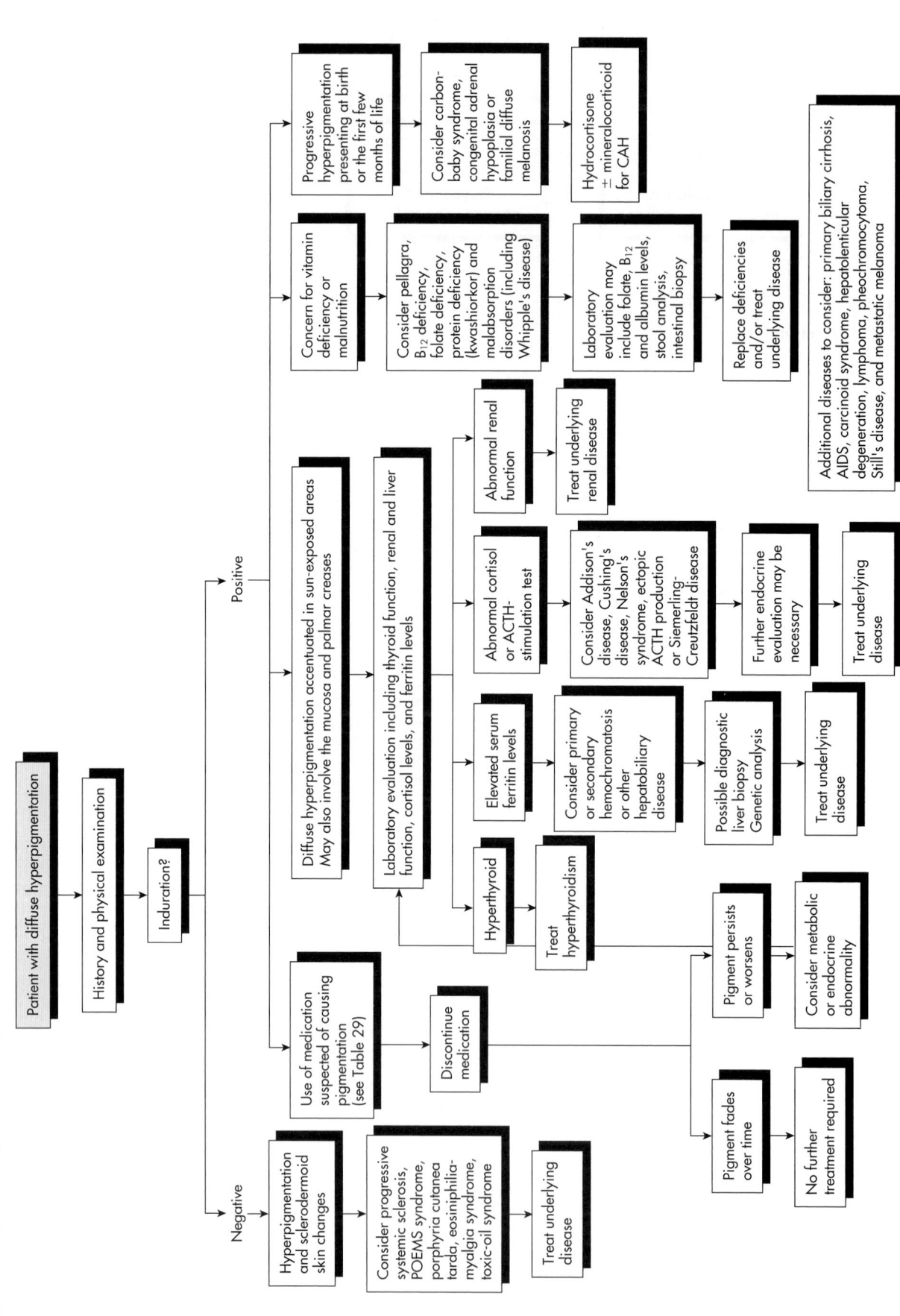

FIG. 139 Approach to the adult patient with diffuse hyperpigmentation. *ACTH,* Adrenocorticotropic hormone; *AIDS,* acquired immunodeficiency syndrome; *CAH,* congenital adrenal hyperplasia; *POEMS,* polyneuropathy, organomegaly, endocrinopathy, monoclonal gammopathy, skin changes. (From Bolognia JL et al [eds]: *Dermatology,* ed 2, St Louis, 2008, Mosby.)

Table 29 Drugs and Chemicals Associated with Hyperpigmentation

Drug or Chemical	Clinical Features	Histopathology/Comment
Cancer Chemotherapeutic Agents		
BCNU (Topical)	• Hyperpigmentation at site of application (no reaction seen with parenteral administration)	• Hyperplasia of basal melanocytes consistent with postinflammatory hyperpigmentation
Bleomycin	• Linear, flagellate bands, associated with minor trauma • Nails may be involved • Hyperpigmentation overlying joints	Increased epidermal melanin Little dermal pigment incontinence No increase in epidermal melanocytes
Busulfan	• Generalized hyperpigmentation resembling Addison's disease; sometimes-seen in association with drug-induced pulmonary fibrosis	• Increased melanin in basal keratinocytes and in dermal macrophages
Cyclophosphamide	• Diffuse hyperpigmentation of the skin and mucous membranes • Localized pigment of the nails (transverse or longitudinal bands), palms and soles, or teeth	• Pigmentation usually regresses within 6 to 12 months after therapy is discontinued
Dactinomycin	• Generalized hyperpigmentation, most prominent on the face	• Pigmentation fades after treatment discontinued
Daunorubicin	• Hyperpigmentation of light-exposed areas • Transverse brown-black nail bands	• Structurally similar to doxorubicin
Doxorubicin	• Pigmentation of the nails; hyperpigmentation of the palmar creases, palms, soles, buccal mucosa, dorsae of the knuckles and tongue	• Increased epidermal melanin • Increased number of melanocytes
5-Fluorouracil	• Hyperpigmentation in sun-exposed areas • Increased pigmentation of skin overlying veins used for infusion, dorsae of the hands and trunk	• Synergistic hyperpigmentation of irradiation portal sites
Hydroxyurea	• Reversible hyperpigmentation over pressure points and the back • Nails may be involved	• Lichenoid eruption with secondary hyperpigmentation
Mechlorethamine (nitrogen mustard)	• Topical use for cutaneous lymphoma may result in generalized hyperpigmentation • More intense in lesional skin	• Disaggregation of melanosomes within keratinocytes • Increased number of melanocytes
Methotrexate	• Uniform hyperpigmentation in sun-exposed areas	• Uncommon • May be postinflammatory hyperpigmentation secondary to photosensitivity reaction
Antimalarials		
Amino quinolones (chloroquine, hydroxychloroquine, amodiaquine)	• Yellow-brown or gray to blue-black pigment, usually in pretibial areas; face, hard palate, and subungual areas may be involved	• Dyspigmentation in up to 25% of patients • Dermal deposition of melanin-drug complexes; hemosiderin around capillaries • May fade, but rarely resolves, upon discontinuation of drug
Heavy Metals		
Arsenic	• Areas of bronze hyperpigmentation ± superimposed raindrops • Keratoses on the palms and soles associated with pigmentation	• May appear 1-20 years after exposure • Dermal and epidermal deposition of arsenic • Increased epidermal melanin synthesis
Bismuth	• Generalized blue-gray discoloration of face, neck, dorsal hands • Oral mucosa and gingivae may be involved	• Bismuth granules in the papillary and reticular dermis
Gold	• Permanent blue-gray discoloration in sun-exposed areas, mostly around the eyes (chrysiasis)	• Gold particles within macrophage lysosomes in the dermis
Iron	• Permanent brown pigment at injection or application sites	• Pigment coats collagen fibers and is deposited in dermal macrophages
Lead	• "Lead line" in gingival margin • Nail pigmentation	• Lead line is due to subepithelial deposition of lead granules
Mercury	• Slate-gray pigmentation, particularly in skin folds	• Brown-black granules free in dermis, in association with elastic fibers, and within macrophages
Silver	• Generalized slate-gray pigmentation, increased in sun-exposed areas • Nails and sclerae may also be involved • Localized at sites of application	• Silver granules in the basement membrane and on the membrana propria of eccrine glands
Hormones		
Oral contraceptives	• Melasma; increased pigment of nipples and nevi	• Increased melanocytes and increased melanin synthesis
ACTH/MSH	• Diffuse brown or bronze pigmentation; seen in Addison's disease and Cushing's syndrome	• Increased melanin synthesis
Miscellaneous Compounds		
Amiodarone	• Slate-gray to violaceous discoloration of sun-exposed skin	• Yellow-brown granules in dermis, mostly perivascular • Lysosomal inclusions with a lipid-like substance
Azidothymidine (zidovudine, AZT)	• Nail and mucocutaneous hyperpigmentation	• Skin biopsy shows increased epidermal and dermal melanin
Clofazimine	• Diffuse red to red-brown discoloration of skin • Violet-brown to bluish discoloration, especially lesional skin	• Redness secondary to drug in fat • Phagolysosomes with lipofuscin material

Continued on next page

Clinical Algorithms

Table 29 Drugs and Chemicals Associated with Hyperpigmentation—cont'd

Drug or Chemical	Clinical Features	Histopathology/Comment
Dioxins	• Chloracne most common skin finding • Hyperpigmentation may occur in sun-exposed areas	• Rare, except in accidental exposure
Hydroquinone	• Hyperpigmentation in areas of application due to exogenous ochronosis	• Yellow-brown banana-shaped fibers in papillary dermis
Minocycline	• Blue-black discoloration in old acne scars or sites of inflammation as well as lower extremities • May also involve nails, sclerae, oral mucosa, bones, and teeth • Generalized "muddy brown" pigmentation pattern in some patients	• Iron-containing granules and/or increased melanin, depending on clinical type
Psoralens	• Increased pigmentation after exposure to UVA light (PUVA)	• Proliferation of follicular melanocytes • Increased synthesis and transfer of melanin
Psychotropic drugs (phenothiazine, chlorpromazine, imipramine, desipramine)	• Slate-gray discoloration in sun-exposed areas	• Golden-brown granules in the upper dermis • Electron-dense inclusion bodies

From Bolognia JL et al [eds]: *Dermatology,* ed 2, St Louis, 2008, Mosby.

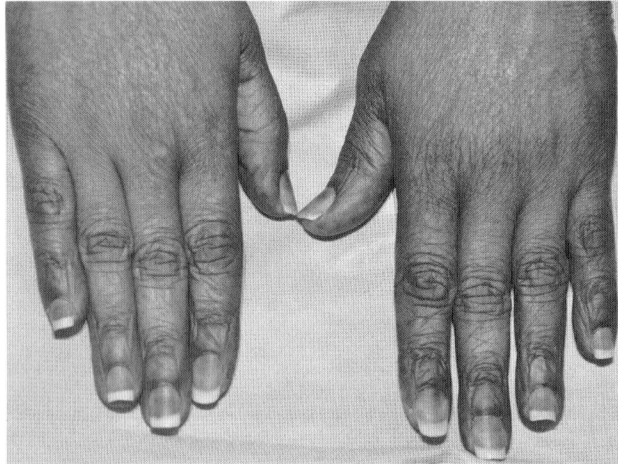

FIG. 140 Hyperpigmentation of the nails in a 61-year-old woman receiving paclitaxel for breast cancer (Callen JP, Jorizzo JL et al: Dermatologic Signs of Systemic Disease, 5th ed, ISBN # 978-0-323-35829-3, 2017, Elsevier.)

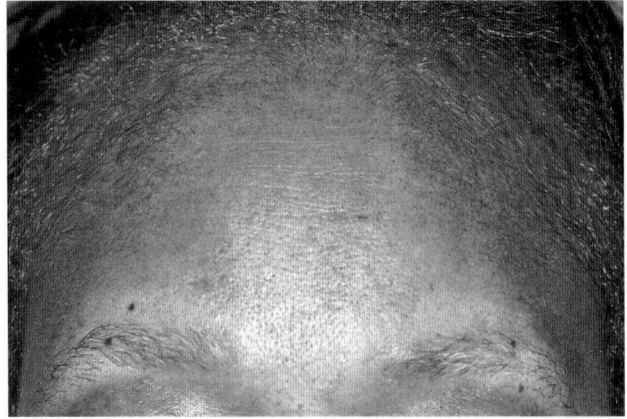

FIG. 141 Grade 1 skin (facial) hyperpigmentation in a 62-year-old woman, during treatment with imatinib for a gastrointestinal stromal tumor. (Callen JP, Jorizzo JL et al: Dermatologic Signs of Systemic Disease, 5th ed, ISBN # 978-0-323-35829-3, 2017, Elsevier.)

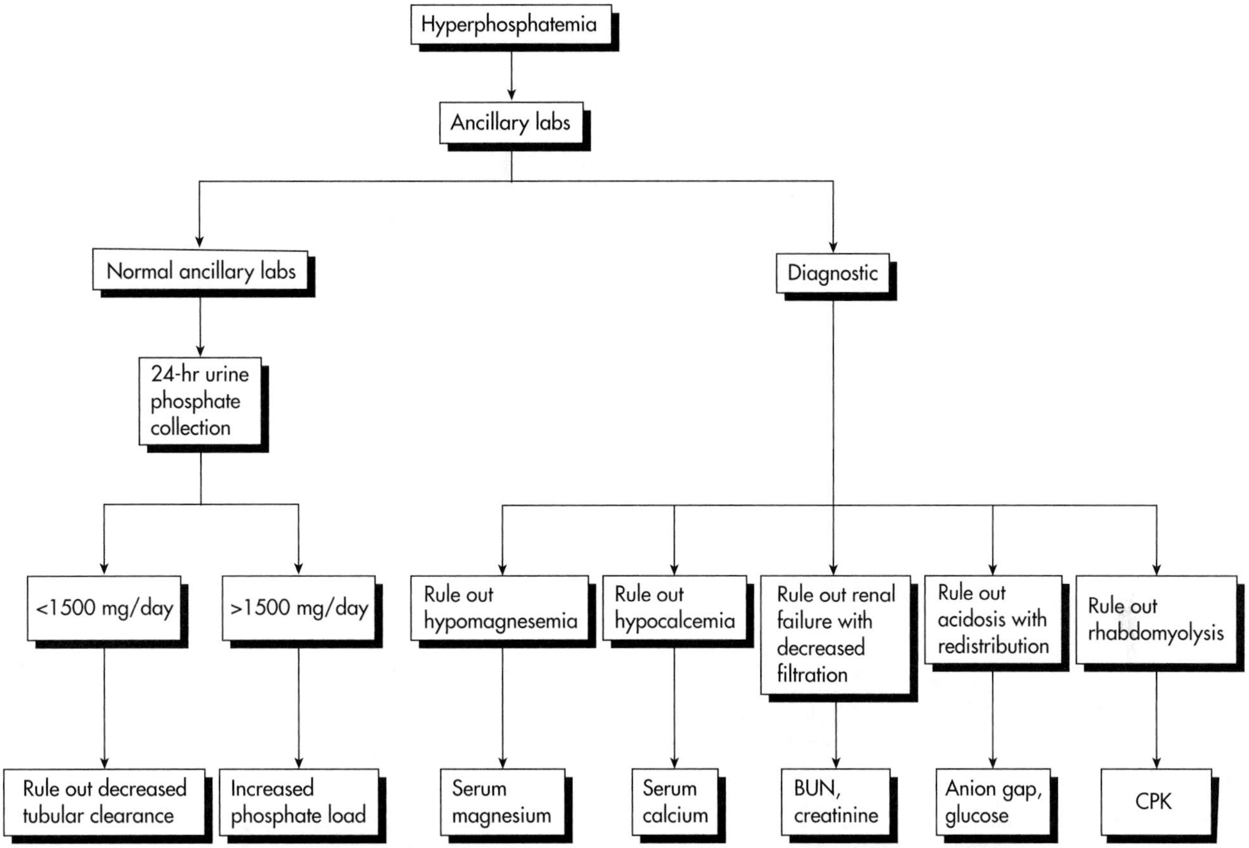

```
                          ┌──────────────────────┐
                          │  Hyperphosphatemia   │
                          └──────────┬───────────┘
                                     │
                          ┌──────────┴───────────┐
                          │    Ancillary labs    │
                          └──────────┬───────────┘
                 ┌───────────────────┴───────────────────┐
        ┌────────┴─────────┐                      ┌───────┴────────┐
        │ Normal ancillary │                      │   Diagnostic   │
        │      labs        │                      └───────┬────────┘
        └────────┬─────────┘
        ┌────────┴─────────┐
        │    24-hr urine   │
        │    phosphate     │
        │    collection    │
        └────────┬─────────┘
```

<1500 mg/day	>1500 mg/day	Rule out hypomagnesemia	Rule out hypocalcemia	Rule out renal failure with decreased filtration	Rule out acidosis with redistribution	Rule out rhabdomyolysis
Rule out decreased tubular clearance	Increased phosphate load	Serum magnesium	Serum calcium	BUN, creatinine	Anion gap, glucose	CPK

FIG. 142 Diagnostic algorithm. (From Ferri, F: *Ferri's best test: a practical guide to clinical laboratory medicine and diagnostic imaging,* ed 3, Philadelphia, 2014, Saunders.)

Diagnostic Imaging
Best Test(s)
- None
Ancillary Tests
- None
Lab Evaluation
Best Test(s)
- 24-hour urine phosphate collection

Ancillary Tests
- Serum electrolytes, BUN, creatinine, magnesium, calcium, glucose
- Urinalysis, CPK

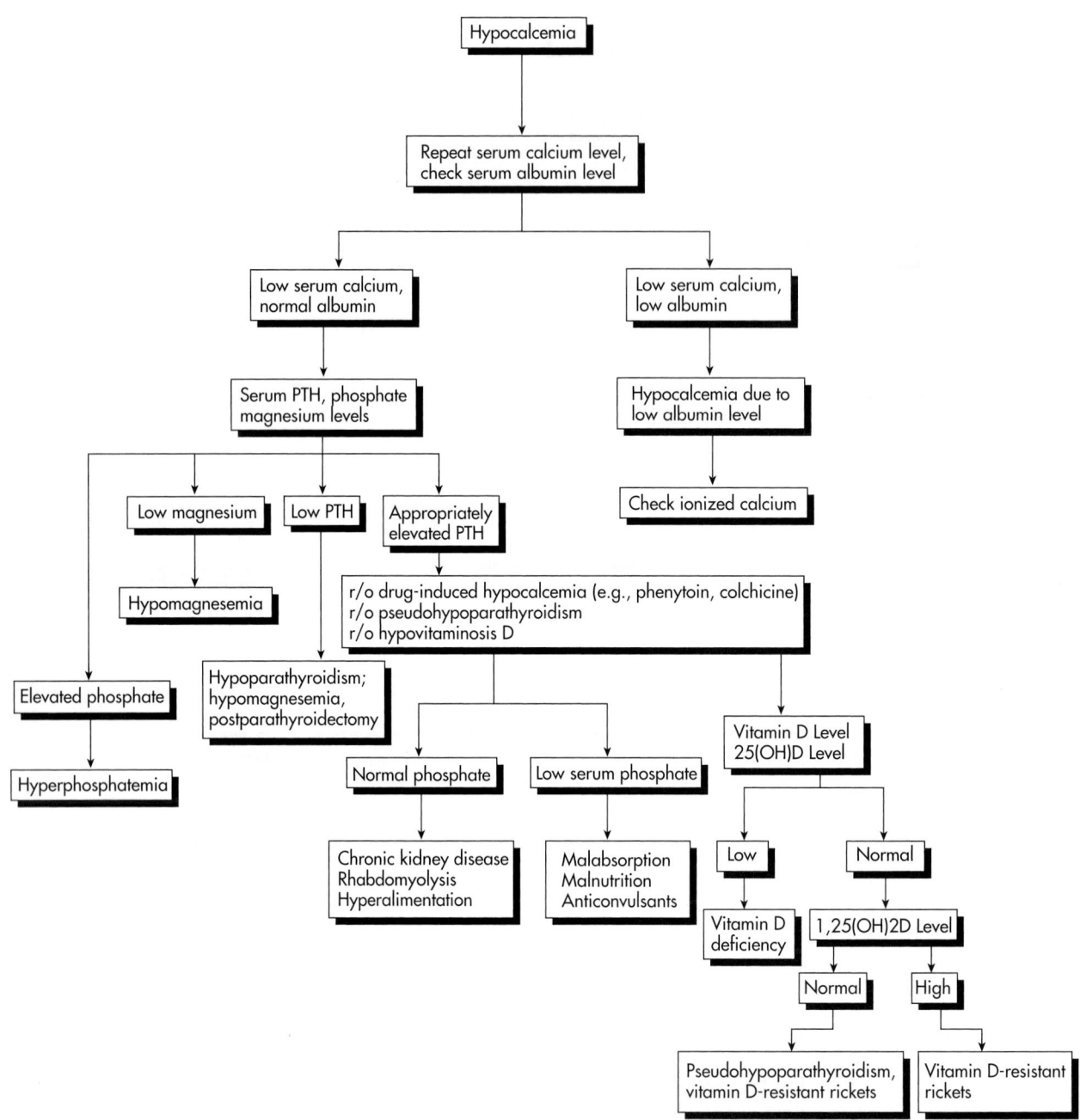

FIG. 143 Diagnostic algorithm. (From Ferri, F: *Ferri's best test: a practical guide to clinical laboratory medicine and diagnostic imaging,* ed 3, Philadelphia, 2014, Saunders.)

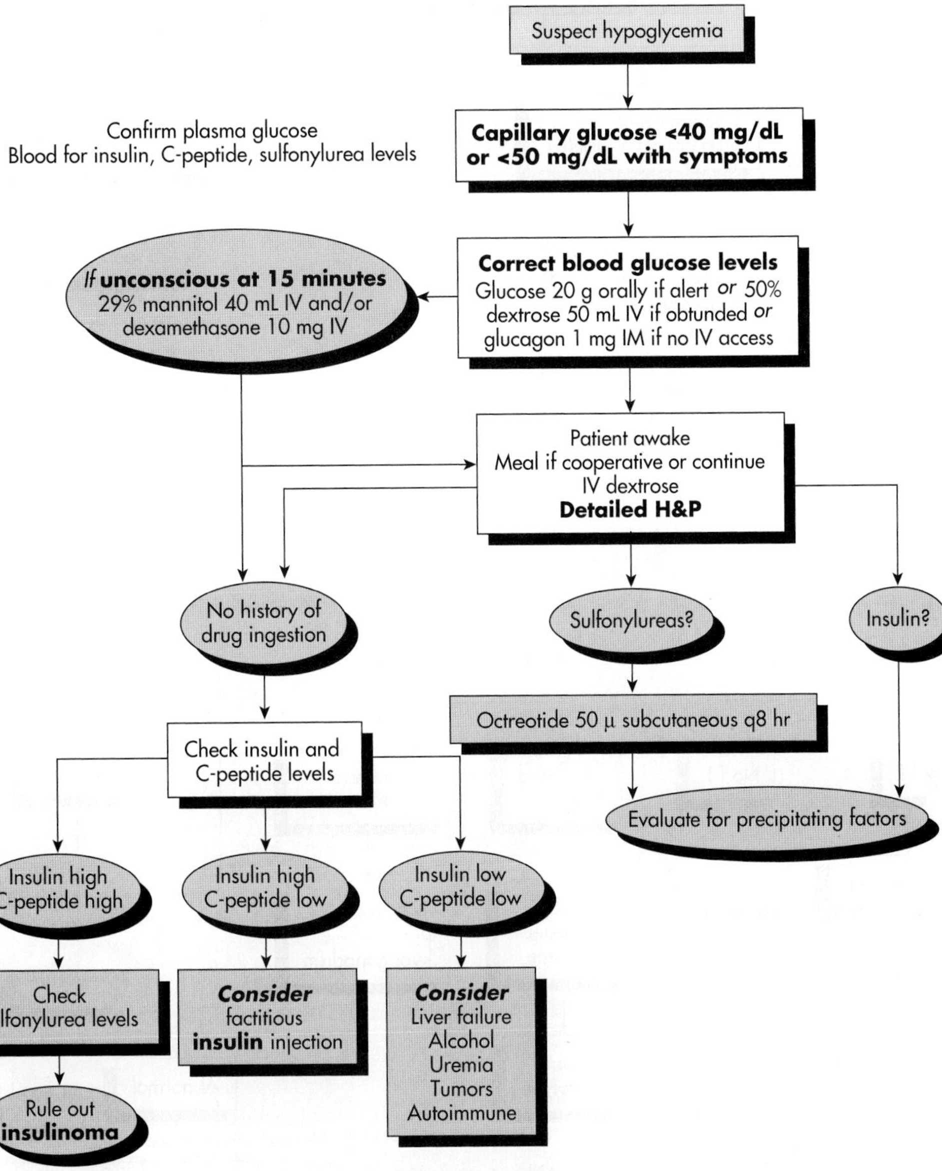

HYPOGLYCEMIA

ICD-10CM # E16.2 Hypoglycemia, spontaneous
E16.0 Hypoglycemia, drug-induced
E16.1 Hypoglycemia, reactive
E16.3 Hypersecretion, glucagon

1655

Suspect hypoglycemia

**Capillary glucose <40 mg/dL
or <50 mg/dL with symptoms**

Confirm plasma glucose
Blood for insulin, C-peptide, sulfonylurea levels

Correct blood glucose levels
Glucose 20 g orally if alert *or* 50%
dextrose 50 mL IV if obtunded *or*
glucagon 1 mg IM if no IV access

If **unconscious at 15 minutes**
29% mannitol 40 mL IV and/or
dexamethasone 10 mg IV

Patient awake
Meal if cooperative or continue
IV dextrose
Detailed H&P

No history of
drug ingestion

Sulfonylureas?

Insulin?

Check insulin and
C-peptide levels

Octreotide 50 µ subcutaneous q8 hr

Evaluate for precipitating factors

Insulin high
C-peptide high

Insulin high
C-peptide low

Insulin low
C-peptide low

Check
sulfonylurea levels

Consider
factitious
insulin injection

Consider
Liver failure
Alcohol
Uremia
Tumors
Autoimmune

Rule out
insulinoma

FIG. 144 Decision tree for suspected hypoglycemia in adults. (From Vincent JL, Abraham E, Moore FA, et al: *Textbook of critical care*, ed 6, Philadelphia, 2011, Saunders.)

Clinical
Algorithms

III

ICD-10CM # E28.310 Symptomatic premature menopause
E29.1 Testicular hypofunction
E28.39 Other primary ovarian failure
E23.6 Other disorders of pituitary gland

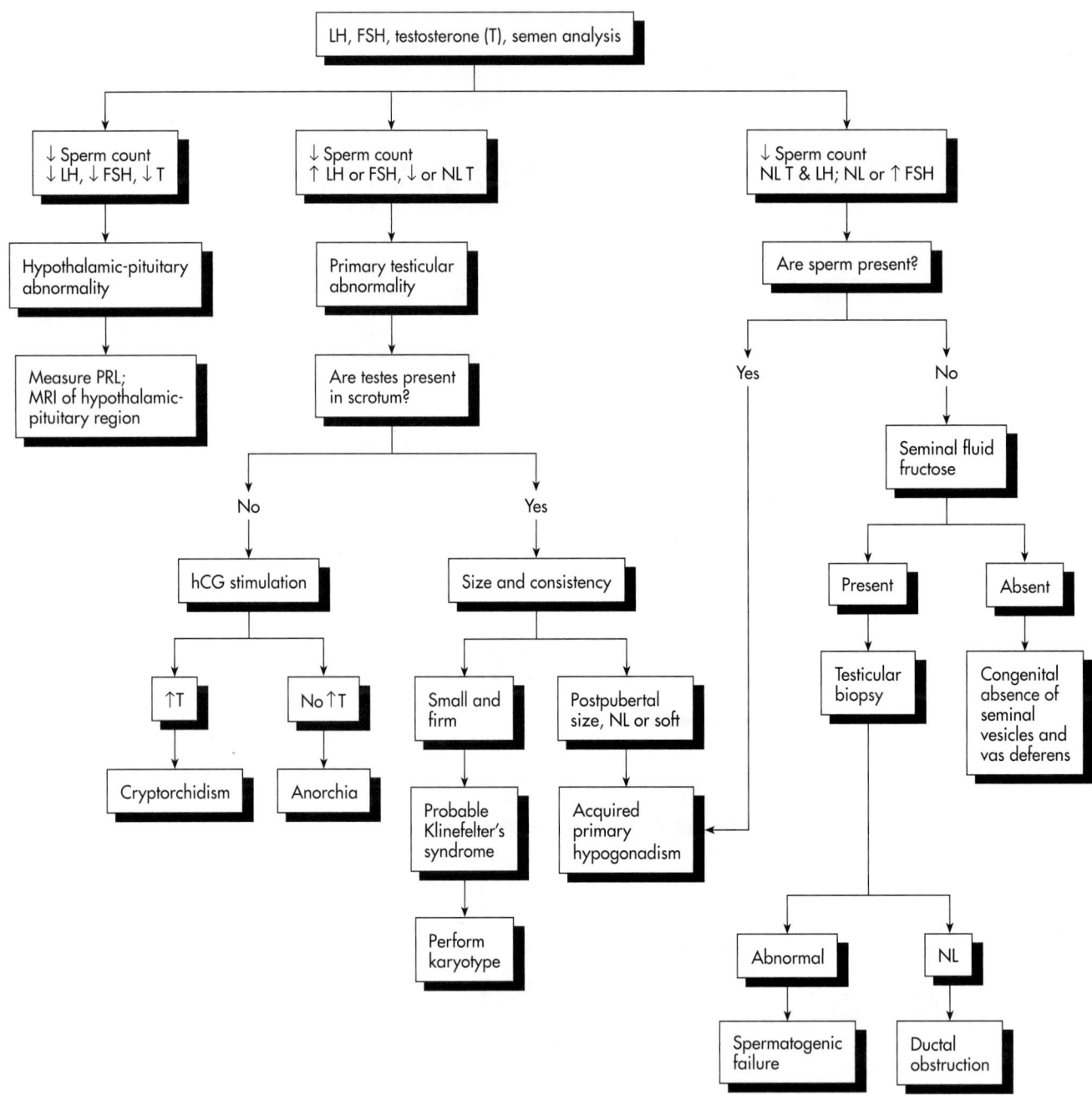

FIG. 145 Laboratory evaluation of hypogonadism in men. *FSH,* Follicle-stimulating hormone; *hCG,* human chorionic gonadotropin; *LH,* luteinizing hormone; *MRI,* magnetic resonance imaging; *NL,* normal; *PRL,* prolactin; ↑, elevated; ↓, decreased or low. (From Andreoli TE [ed]: *Cecil essentials of medicine,* ed 7, Philadelphia, 2008, Saunders.)

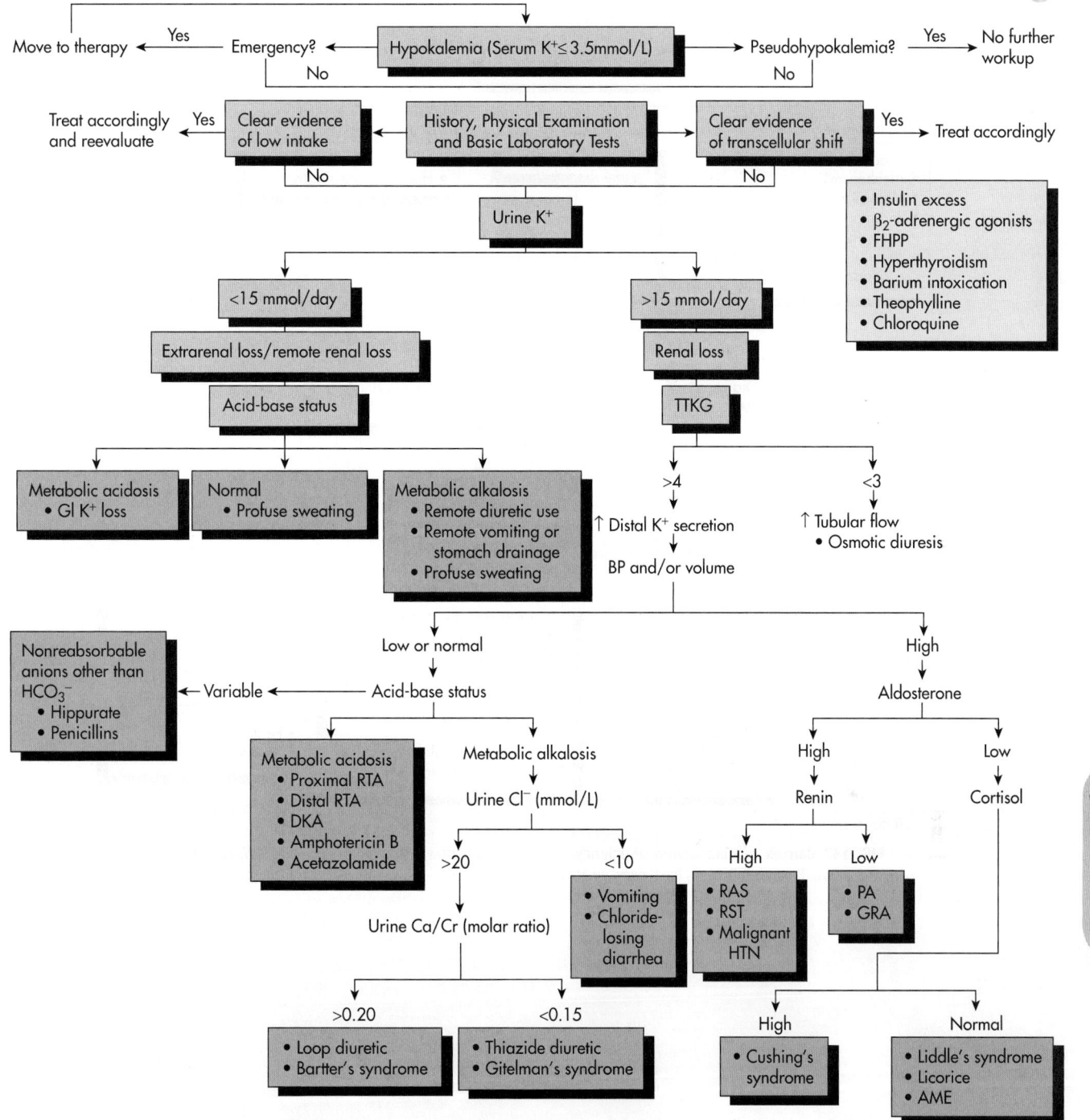

FIG. 146 The clinical approach to hypokalemia. See text for details. *AME*, Apparent mineralocorticoid excess; *BP*, blood pressure; *CCD*, cortical collecting duct; *DKA*, diabetic ketoacidosis; *FHPP*, familial hypokalemic periodic paralysis; *GI*, gastrointestinal; *GRA*, glucocorticoid-remediable aldosteronism; *HTN*, hypertension; *PA*, primary aldosteronism; *RAS*, renal artery stenosis; *RST*, renin-secreting tumor; *RTA*, renal tubular acidosis; *TTKG*, transtubular potassium gradient. (Skorecki K, Chertow GM, Marsden PA, Taal MW, Yu ASL, Wasser WG: Brenner & Rector's the Kidney, ed 10, Elsevier, ISBN # 978-1-4557-4836-5, Philadelphia, 2016.)

Clinical Algorithms

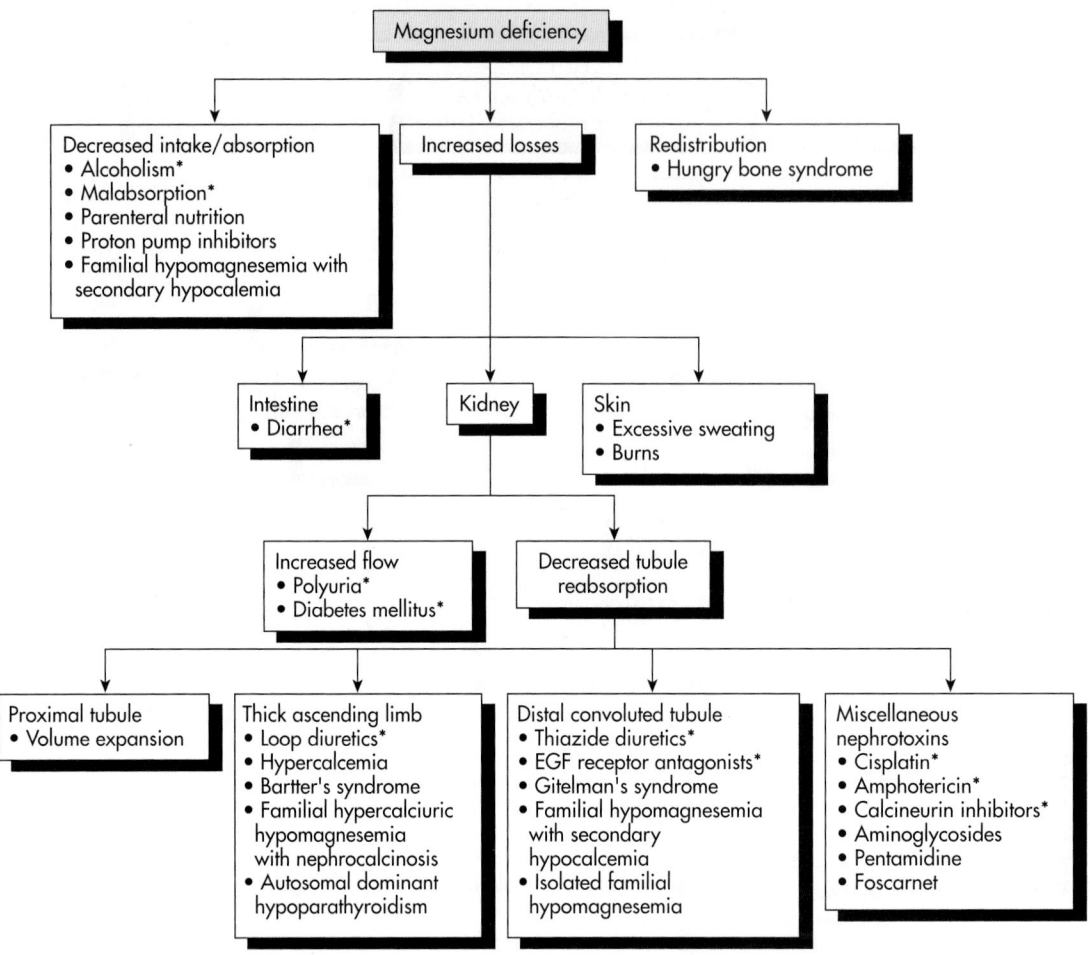

FIG. 147 Causes of magnesium deficiency. (Skorecki K, Chertow GM, Marsden PA, Taal MW, Yu ASL, Wasser WG: Brenner & Rector's the Kidney, ed 10, Elsevier, ISBN # 978-1-4557-4836-5, Philadelphia, 2016.)

Hyponatremia

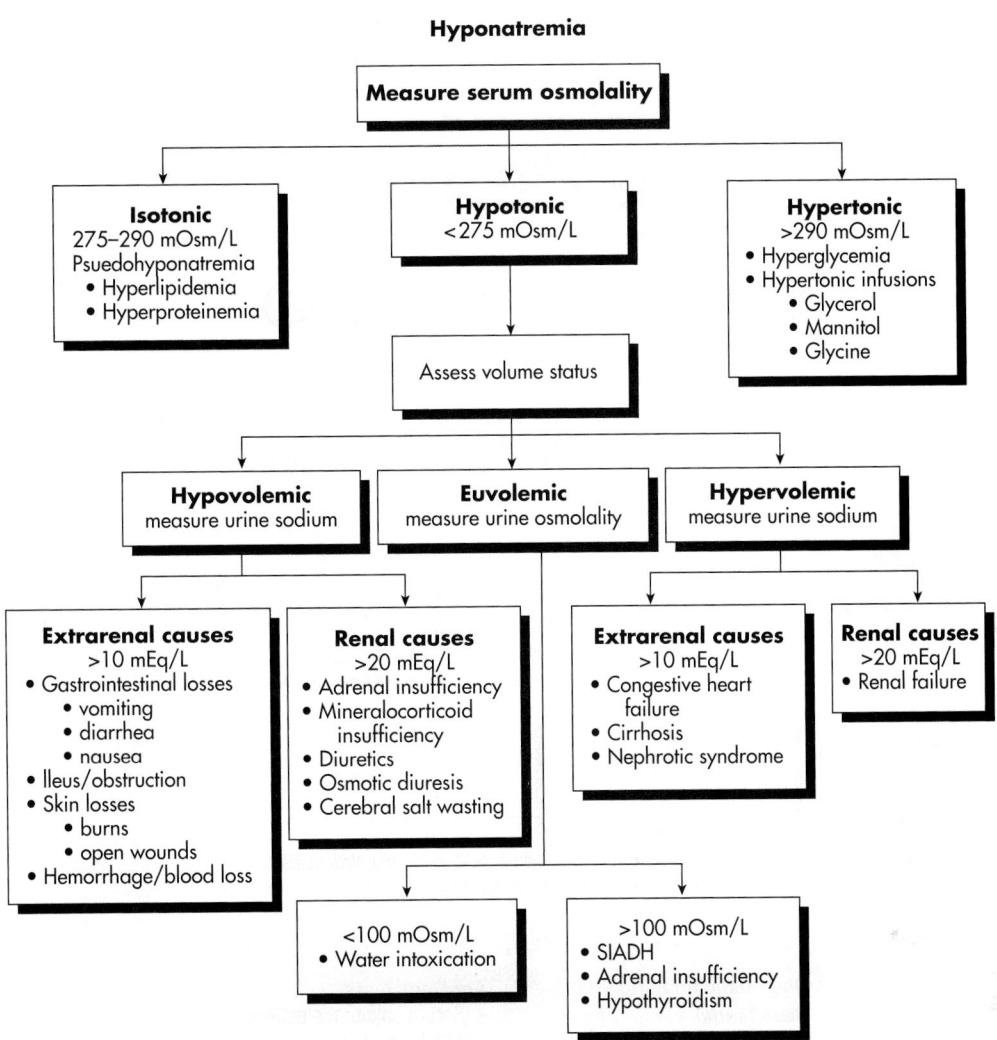

FIG. 148 **Algorithm for treatment of hyponatremia.** *SIADH*, Syndrome of inappropriate antidiuretic hormone. (From Cameron JL, Cameron AM: Electrolyte disorders. Current surgical therapy, ed 10, Philadelphia, Saunders, 2011.)

ICD-9CM #   Hypophosphatemia
ICD-10CM #   E83.30   Disorder of phosphorus metabolism, unspecified
            E83.31   Familial hypophosphatemia

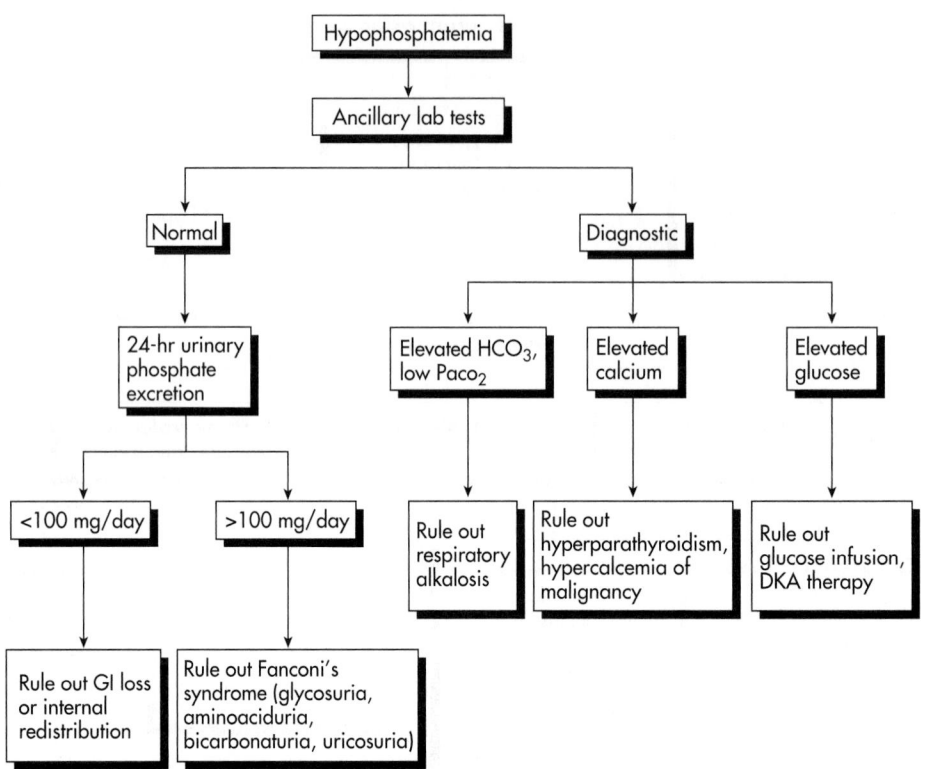

FIG. 149 **Diagnostic algorithm.** (From Ferri, F: *Ferri's best test: a practical guide to clinical laboratory medicine and diagnostic imaging,* ed 3, Philadelphia, 2014, Saunders.)

Diagnostic Imaging
Best Test(s)
- None

Ancillary Tests
- None

Lab Evaluation
Best Test(s)
- 24-hour urine phosphate excretion

Ancillary Tests
- Serum calcium, electrolytes, creatinine, glucose
- ABGs
- PTH, vitamin D level

HYPOTENSION

ICD-10CM #	
I95.9	Hypotension, unspecified
I95.89	Other hypotension
I95.3	Hypotension of hemodialysis
I95.1	Orthostatic hypotension

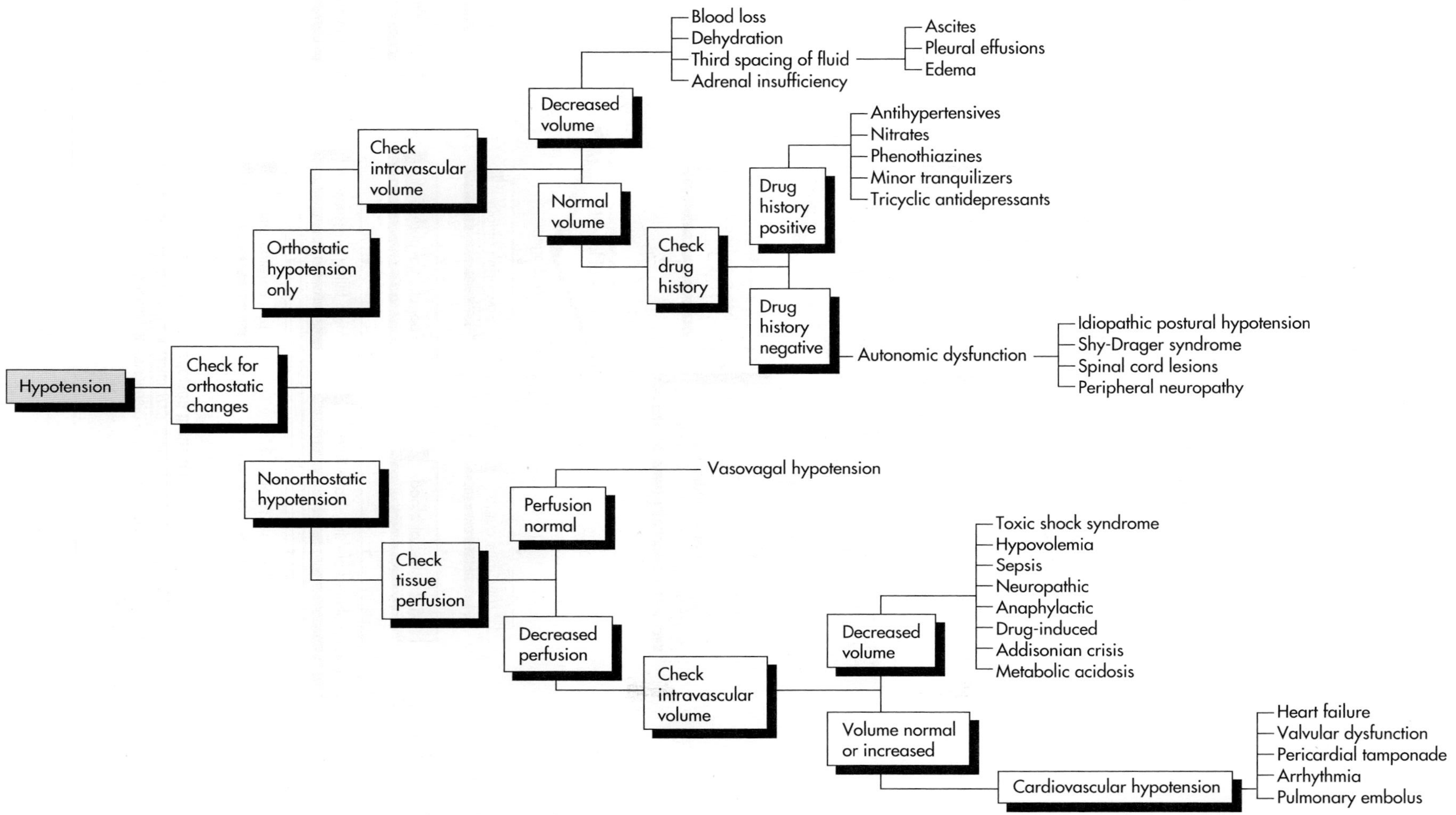

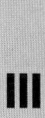

FIG. 150 Hypotension. (From Healey PM: *Common medical diagnosis: an algorithmic approach*, ed 3, Philadelphia, 2000, Saunders.)

Clinical Algorithms

III

Hypotension

Check for orthostatic changes

Orthostatic hypotension only

Nonorthostatic hypotension

Check intravascular volume

Check tissue perfusion

Decreased volume
- Blood loss
- Dehydration
- Third spacing of fluid — Ascites, Pleural effusions, Edema
- Adrenal insufficiency

Normal volume

Check drug history

Drug history positive
- Antihypertensives
- Nitrates
- Phenothiazines
- Minor tranquilizers
- Tricyclic antidepressants

Drug history negative

Autonomic dysfunction
- Idiopathic postural hypotension
- Shy-Drager syndrome
- Spinal cord lesions
- Peripheral neuropathy

Perfusion normal

Vasovagal hypotension

Decreased perfusion

Check intravascular volume

Decreased volume
- Toxic shock syndrome
- Hypovolemia
- Sepsis
- Neuropathic
- Anaphylactic
- Drug-induced
- Addisonian crisis
- Metabolic acidosis

Volume normal or increased

Cardiovascular hypotension
- Heart failure
- Valvular dysfunction
- Pericardial tamponade
- Arrhythmia
- Pulmonary embolus

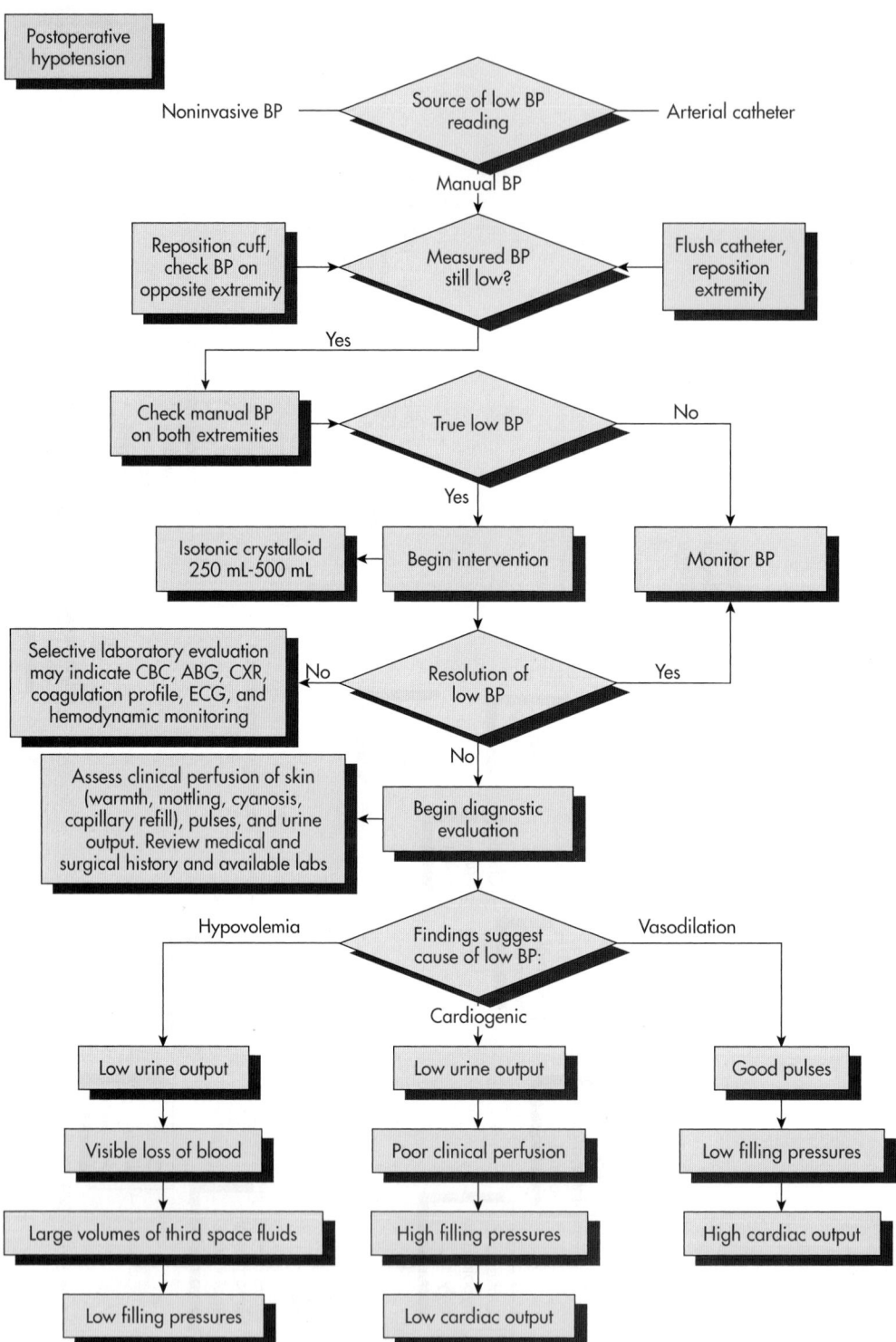

FIG. 151 Approach to managing postoperative hypotension. *ABG*, arterial blood gases; *BP*, blood pressure; *CBC*, complete blood count; *CXR*, chest x-ray study; *ECG*, electrocardiogram. (Parrillo JE, Dellinger RP: Critical Care Medicine, Principles of Diagnosis and Management in the Adult, 4th ed, ISBN # 978-0-323-08929-6, 2014, Elsevier.)

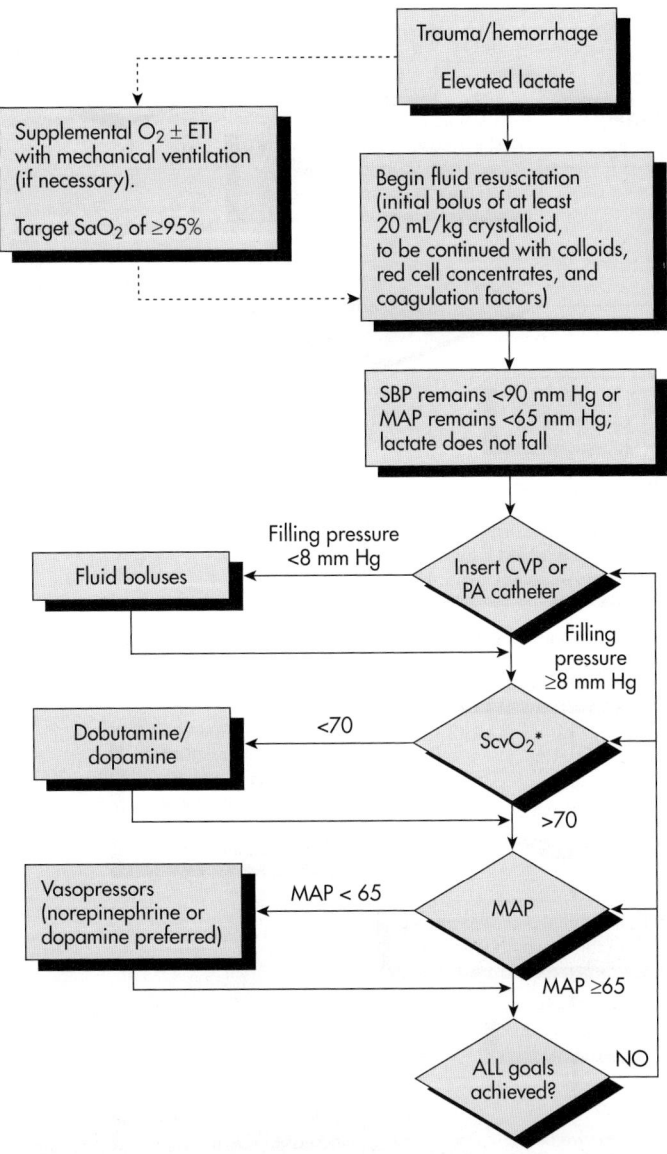

*If pulmonary artery catheter is used a mixed venous O₂ saturation is an acceptable surrogate, and 65% would be the target.

FIG. 152 Hypovolemic shock management protocol. *CVP*, central venous pressure; *ETI*, endotracheal intubation; *MAP*, mean arterial pressure; *PA*, pulmonary artery; *Sao₂*, oxygen saturation; *SBP*, systolic blood pressure; *Scvo₂*, central venous oxygen saturation. (Parrillo JE, Dellinger RP: Critical Care Medicine, Principles of Diagnosis and Management in the Adult, 4th ed, ISBN # 978-0-323-08929-6, 2014, Elsevier.)

Table 30 Clinical Classification of Severity of Posthemorrhagic Hypovolemic Shock

Feature	Class I	Class II	Class III	Class IV
Blood loss				
mL	<750	750-1500	>1500-2000	>2000
%	<15	15-30	>30-40	>40
Heart rate (beats/min)	<100	>100	>120	>140
Blood pressure	Normal	Normal	Decreased	Decreased
Pulse pressure	Normal	Decreased	Decreased	Decreased
Respiratory rate	14-20	20-30	30-40	>40
Urinary output (mL/h)	>30	20-30	5-15	Negligible
Mental status	Slightly anxious	Mildly anxious	Anxious, confused	Confused, lethargic
Fluid replacement (mL/h)	Crystalloid	Crystalloid/colloid	Crystalloid and blood	Crystalloid and blood

Parrillo JE, Dellinger RP: Critical Care Medicine, Principles of Diagnosis and Management in the Adult, 4th ed, ISBN # 978-0-323-08929-6, 2014, Elsevier.

Clinical
Algorithms

III

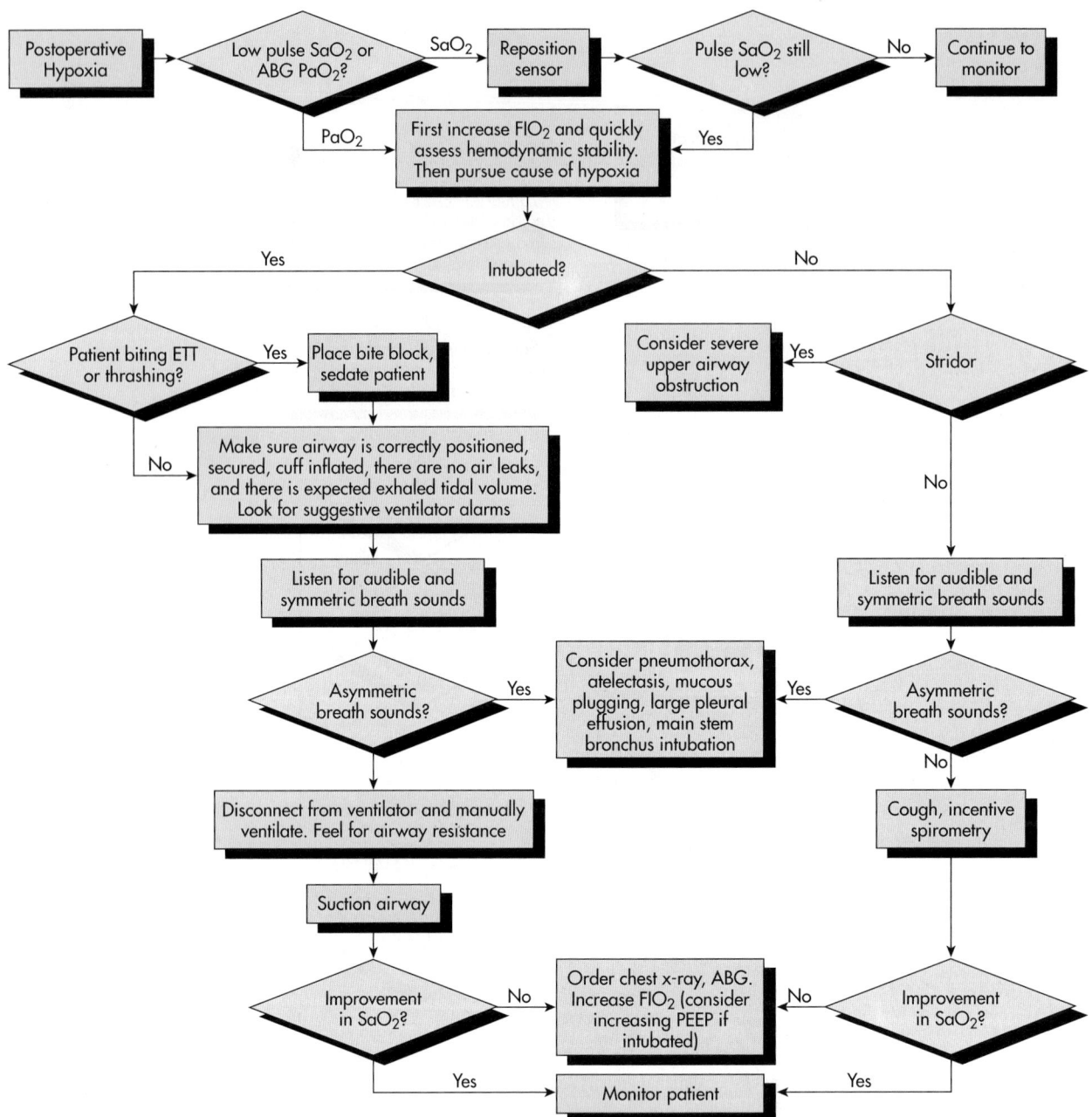

FIG. 153 Approach to managing postoperative hypoxemia. *ABG*, arterial blood gas; *ETT*, endotracheal tube; *FIO₂*, fraction of inspired oxygen; *PaO₂*, arterial oxygen tension; *PEEP*, positive end-expiratory pressure; *SaO₂*, arterial oxygen saturation. (Parrillo JE, Dellinger RP: Critical Care Medicine, Principles of Diagnosis and Management in the Adult, 4th ed, ISBN # 978-0-323-08929-6, 2014, Elsevier.)

INFECTIONS OF SOFT TISSUE, JOINTS, AND BONE

ICD-10CM #	M00.9	Pyogenic arthritis, unspecified	**1665**
	M86.9	Osteomyelitis unspecified	
	T84.3	Infection and inflammatory reaction	
	M79.9	Soft tissue disorder, unspecified	

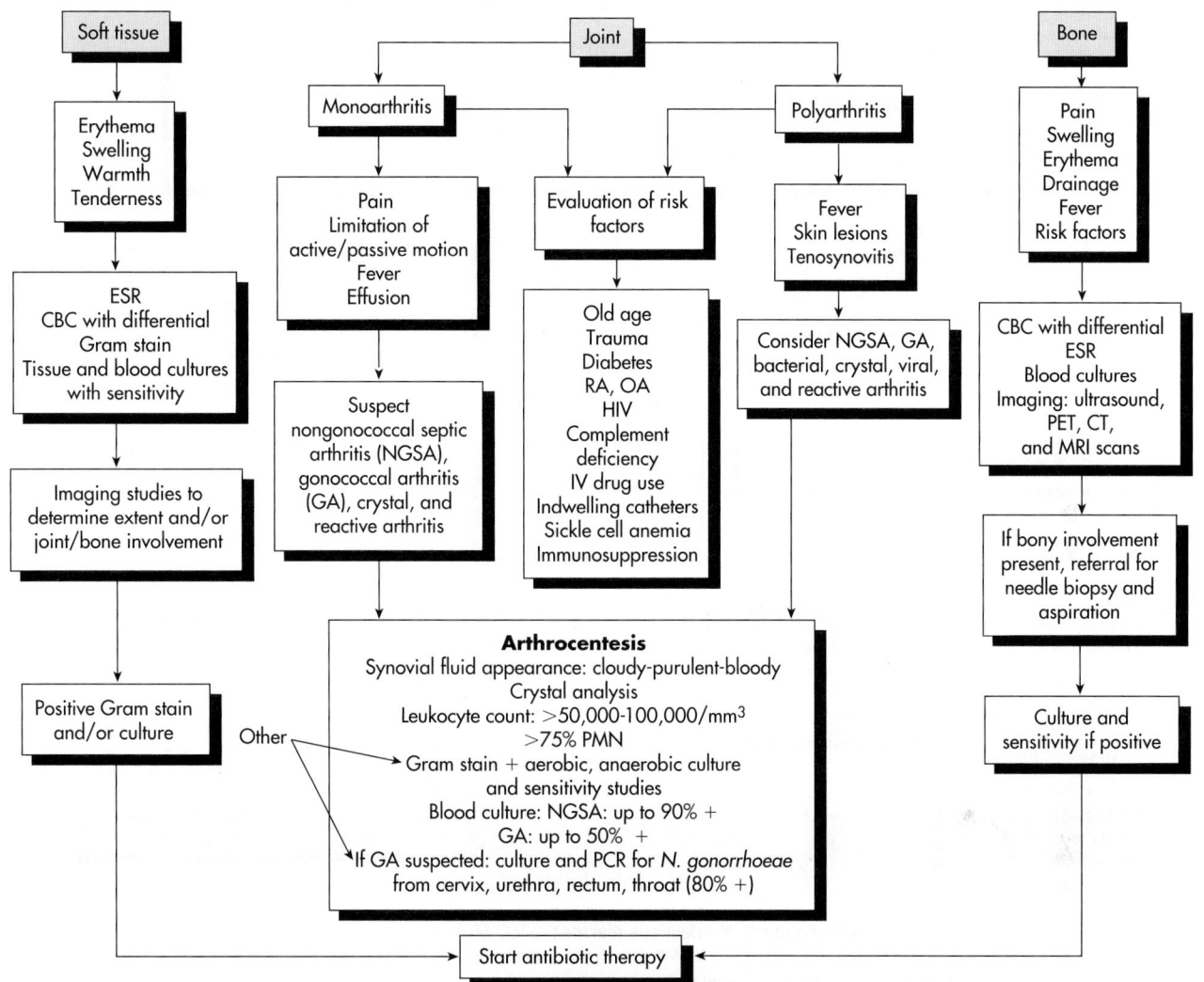

FIG. 154 Clinical evaluation of infections of soft tissues, joints, and bone. *CBC,* Complete blood count; *CT,* computed tomography; *ESR,* erythrocyte sedimentation rate; *GA,* gonococcal arthritis; *HIV,* human immunodeficiency virus; *IV,* intravenous; *MRI,* magnetic resonance imaging; *NGSA,* nongonococcal septic arthritis; *OA,* osteoarthritis; *PCR,* polymerase chain reaction; *PET,* positron emission tomography; *PMN,* polymorphonuclear leukocyte; *RA,* rheumatoid arthritis. (From Goldman L, Schafer AI: *Goldman's Cecil medicine,* ed 24, Philadelphia, 2012, Saunders.)

Clinical Algorithms

IIII

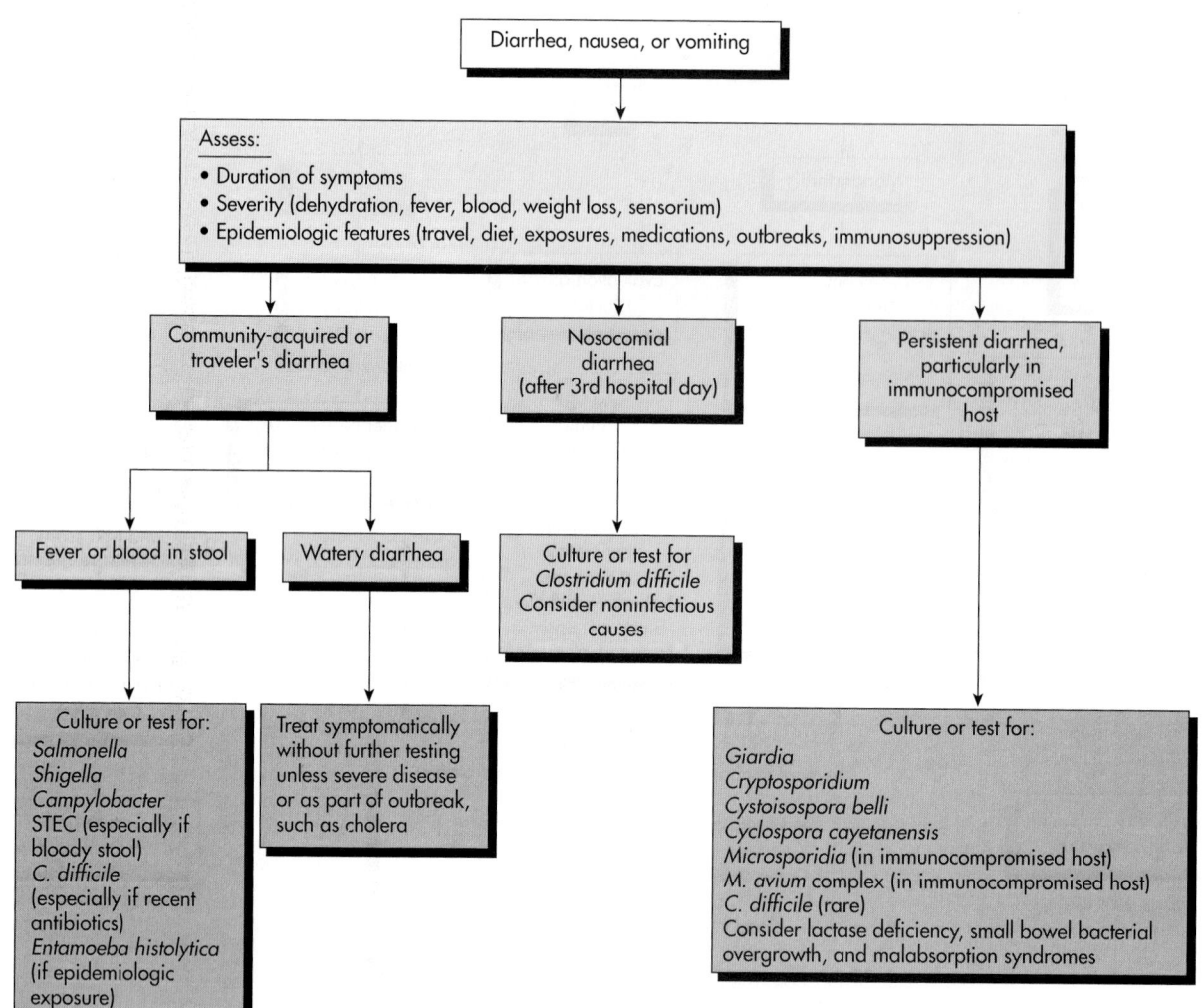

FIG. 155 Approach to diagnosis of infectious diarrhea. *STEC*, Shiga toxin–producing *Escherichia coli*. (From Bennett JE, Dolin R, Blaser MJ: *Mandell, Douglas, and Bennett's principles and practice of infectious diseases*, ed 8, Philadelphia, 2015, Saunders.)

ICD-10CM #
M00.9 Pyogenic arthritis, unspecified
M01.1 Tuberculous arthritis
M01.2 Arthritis in Lyme disease
M01.5 Arthritis in viral disease
M02.9 Reactive arthropathy, unspecified
M08.9 Juvenile arthritis, unspecified
M10.9 Gout, unspecified

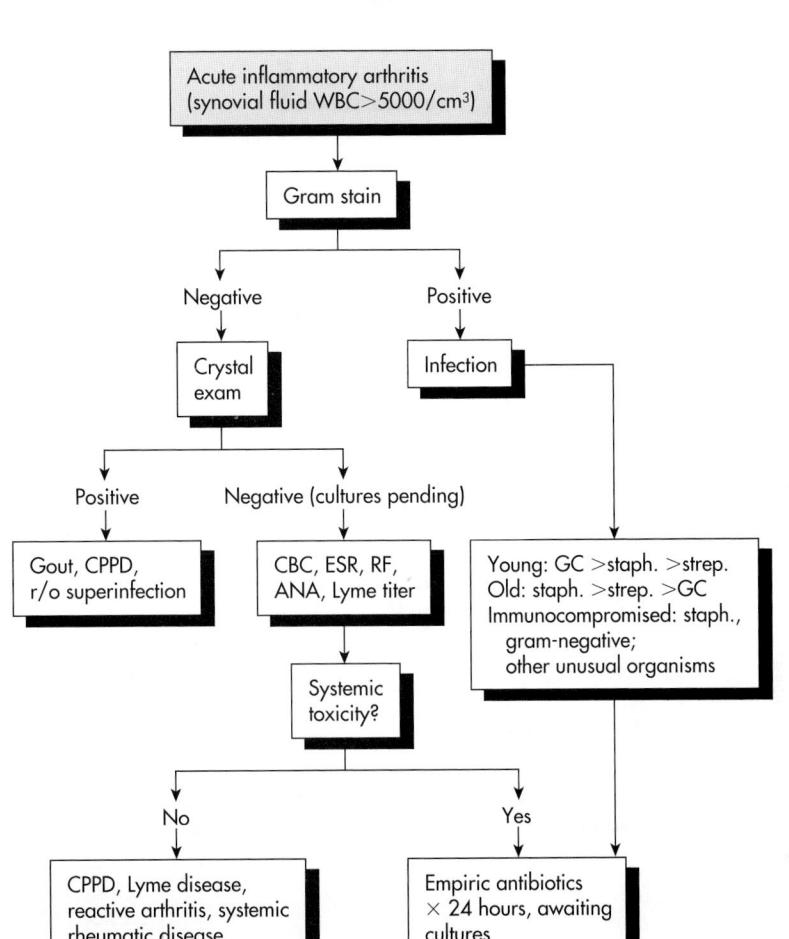

FIG. 156 Approach to acute inflammatory arthritis. *ANA,* Antinuclear antibody test; *CBC,* complete blood count; *CPPD;* calcium pyrophosphate deposition disease; *ESR,* erythrocyte sedimentation rate; *F/U,* follow-up; *GC,* gonococcal infection; *RF,* rheumatoid factor; *r/o,* rule out; *staph.,* staphylococcal infection; *strep.,* streptococcal infection; *WBC,* white blood cell count. (From Harris ED et al [eds]: *Kelley's textbook of rheumatology,* ed 7, Philadelphia, 2005, Saunders.)

Clinical
Algorithms

III

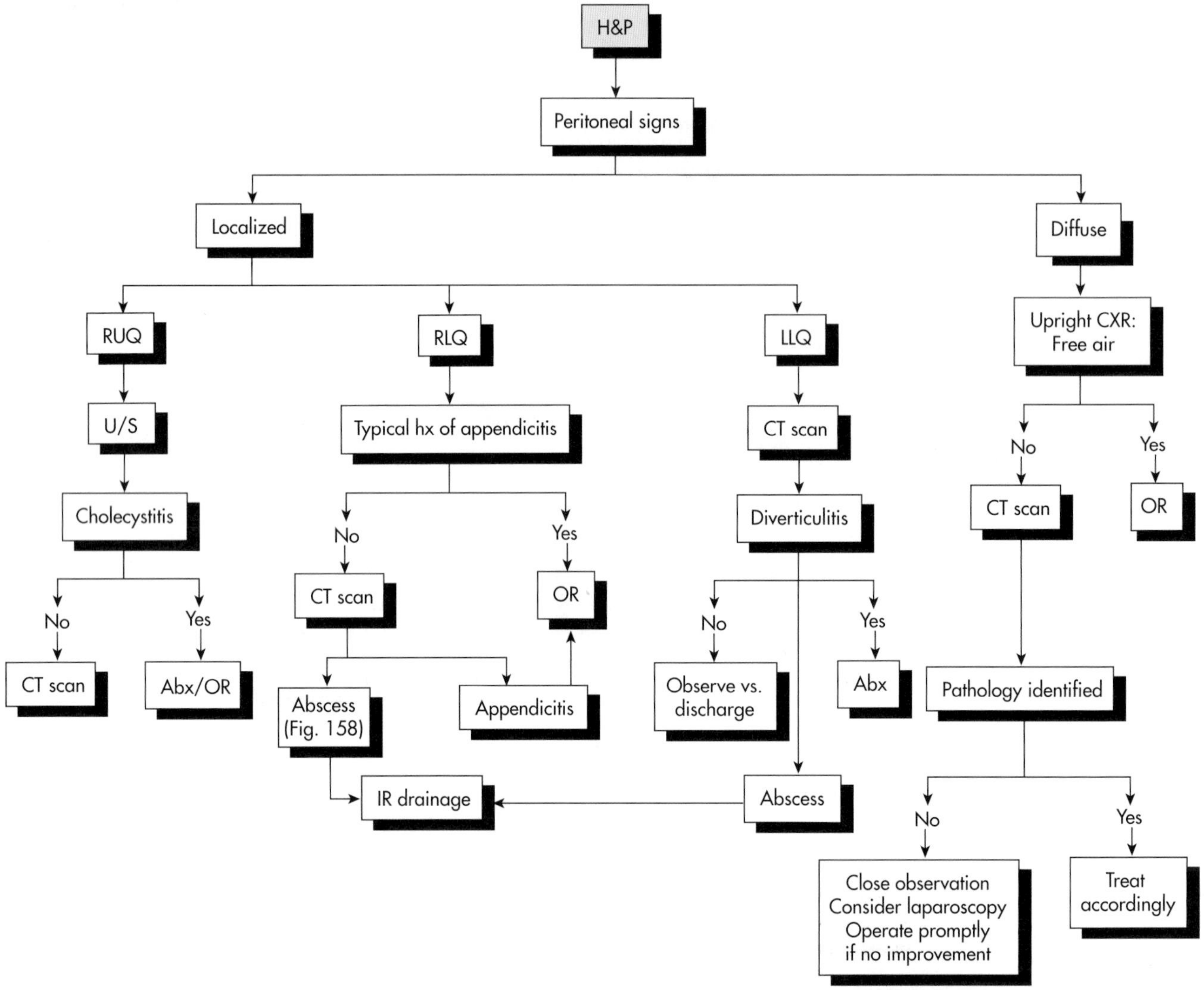

H&P

↓

Peritoneal signs

Localized   Diffuse

Localized:

RUQ   RLQ   LLQ

RUQ → U/S → Cholecystitis
- No → CT scan
- Yes → Abx/OR

RLQ → Typical hx of appendicitis
- No → CT scan → Abscess (Fig. 158) → IR drainage
- No → CT scan → Appendicitis
- Yes → OR → Appendicitis

LLQ → CT scan → Diverticulitis
- No → Observe vs. discharge
- Yes → Abx
- → Abscess → IR drainage

Diffuse:

Upright CXR: Free air
- No → CT scan → Pathology identified
  - No → Close observation, Consider laparoscopy, Operate promptly if no improvement
  - Yes → Treat accordingly
- Yes → OR

FIG. 157 Algorithm for the diagnosis and management of patients with suspected intraabdominal infection. *H&P,* History and physical exam; *Abx,* antibiotics; *CXR,* chest radiograph; *hx,* history; *IR,* interventional radiology; *LLQ,* left lower quadrant; *RLQ,* right lower quadrant; *RUQ,* right upper quadrant; *U/S,* ultrasound. (From Cameron JL, Cameron AM: *Current surgical therapy,* ed 10, Philadelphia, 2011, Saunders.)

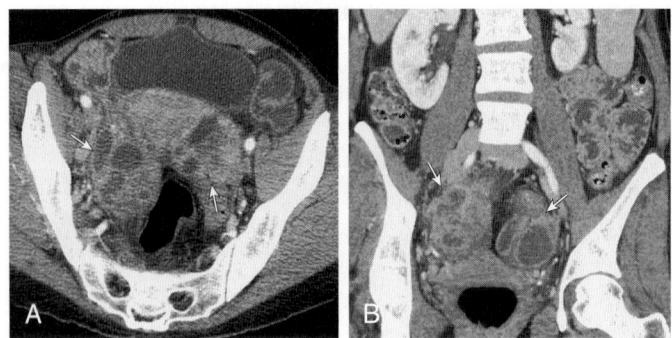

FIG. 158 Axial (A) and coronal (B) postcontrast computed tomographic images showing bilateral tuboovarian abcesses *(arrow).* (Fielding JR et al: *Gynecologic Imaging,* Philadelphia, 2011, Saunders ISBN #978-1-4377-1575-0.)

ICD-10CM# R17   Unspecified jaundice
           K83.2 Other specified diseases of biliary tract
           E80.7 Disorder of bilirubin metabolism, unspecified

1669

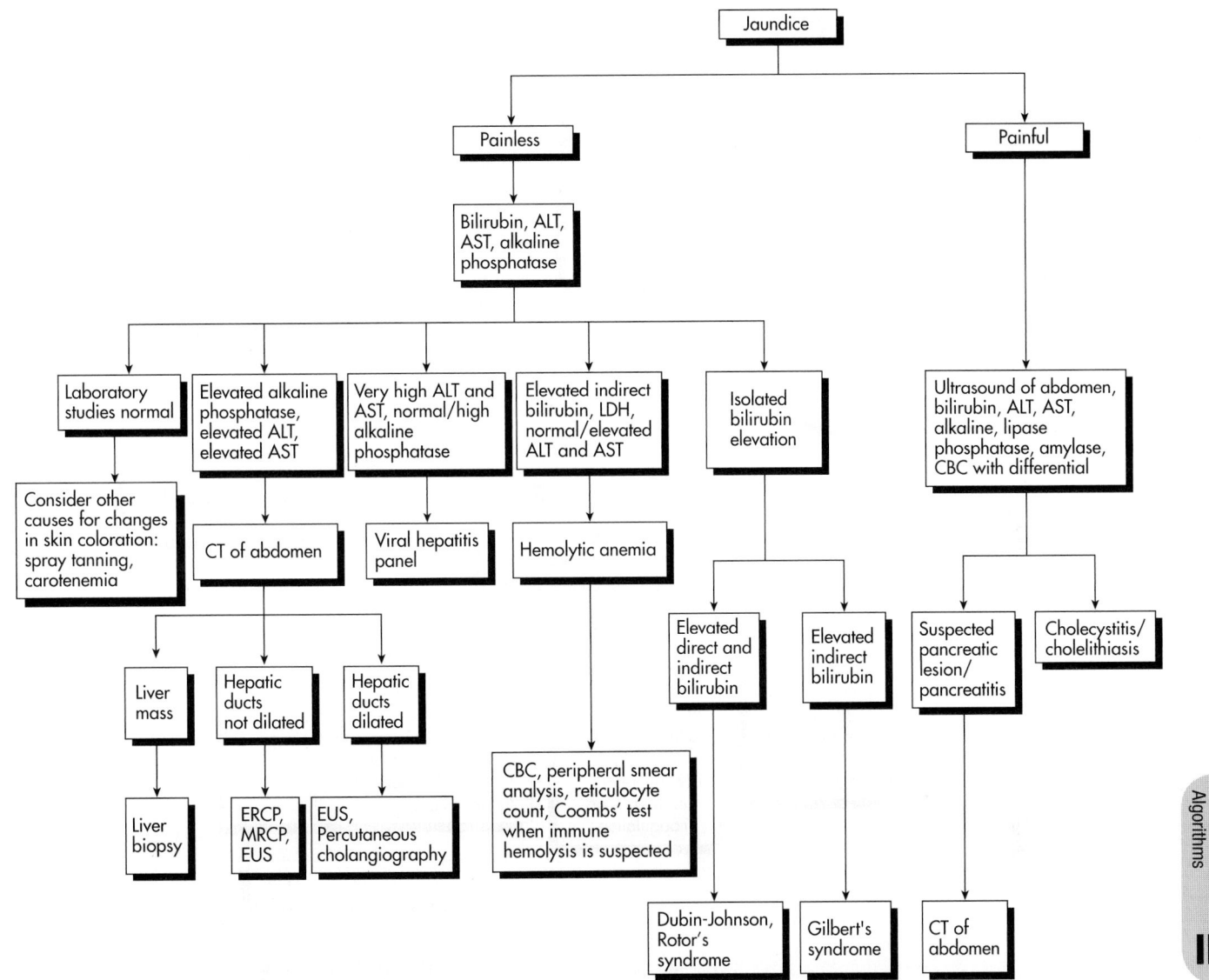

FIG. 161 Diagnostic algorithm. (From Ferri, F: *Ferri's best test: a practical guide to clinical laboratory medicine and diagnostic imaging,* ed 3, Philadelphia, 2014, Saunders.)

Diagnostic Imaging	Lab Evaluation
Best Test(s) • CT of abdomen with contrast if painless jaundice • Ultrasound of abdomen if painful jaundice	**Best Test(s)** • Bilirubin with fractionation • Alkaline phosphatase, ALT, AST • Viral hepatitis panel
Ancillary Tests • MRCP • ERCP • EUS	**Ancillary Tests** • Serum amylase, lipase, LDH • CBC, reticulocyte count, Coombs' test • BUN, creatinine, electrolytes • Liver biopsy

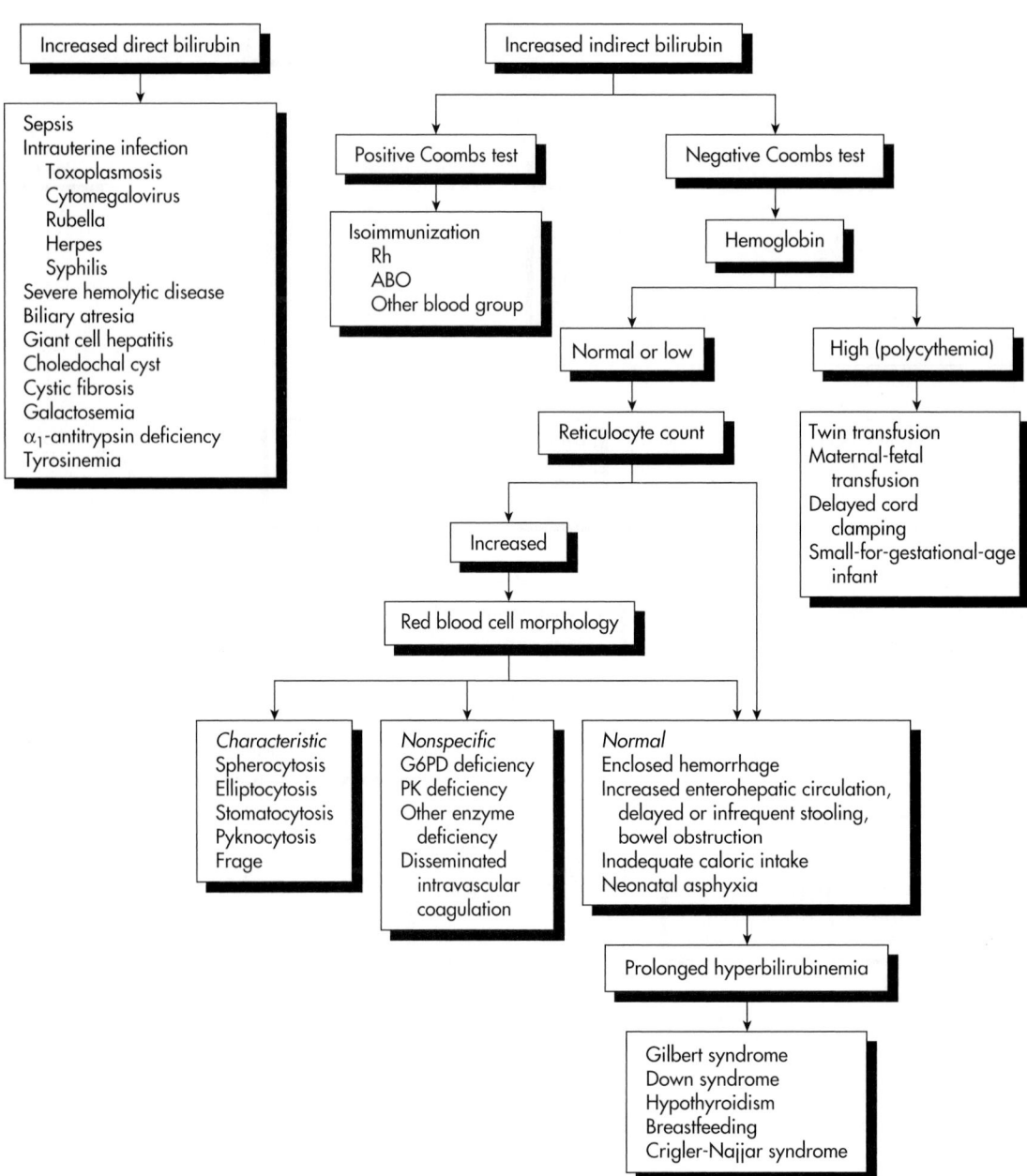

FIG. 162 Schematic approach to the diagnosis of neonatal jaundice. *G6PD,* Glucose-6-phosphate dehydrogenase; *PK,* pyruvate kinase. (From Oski FA: Differential diagnosis of jaundice. In Taeusch HW, Ballard RA, Avery MA [eds]: *Schaffer and Avery's diseases of the newborn,* ed 6, Philadelphia, 1991, Saunders.)

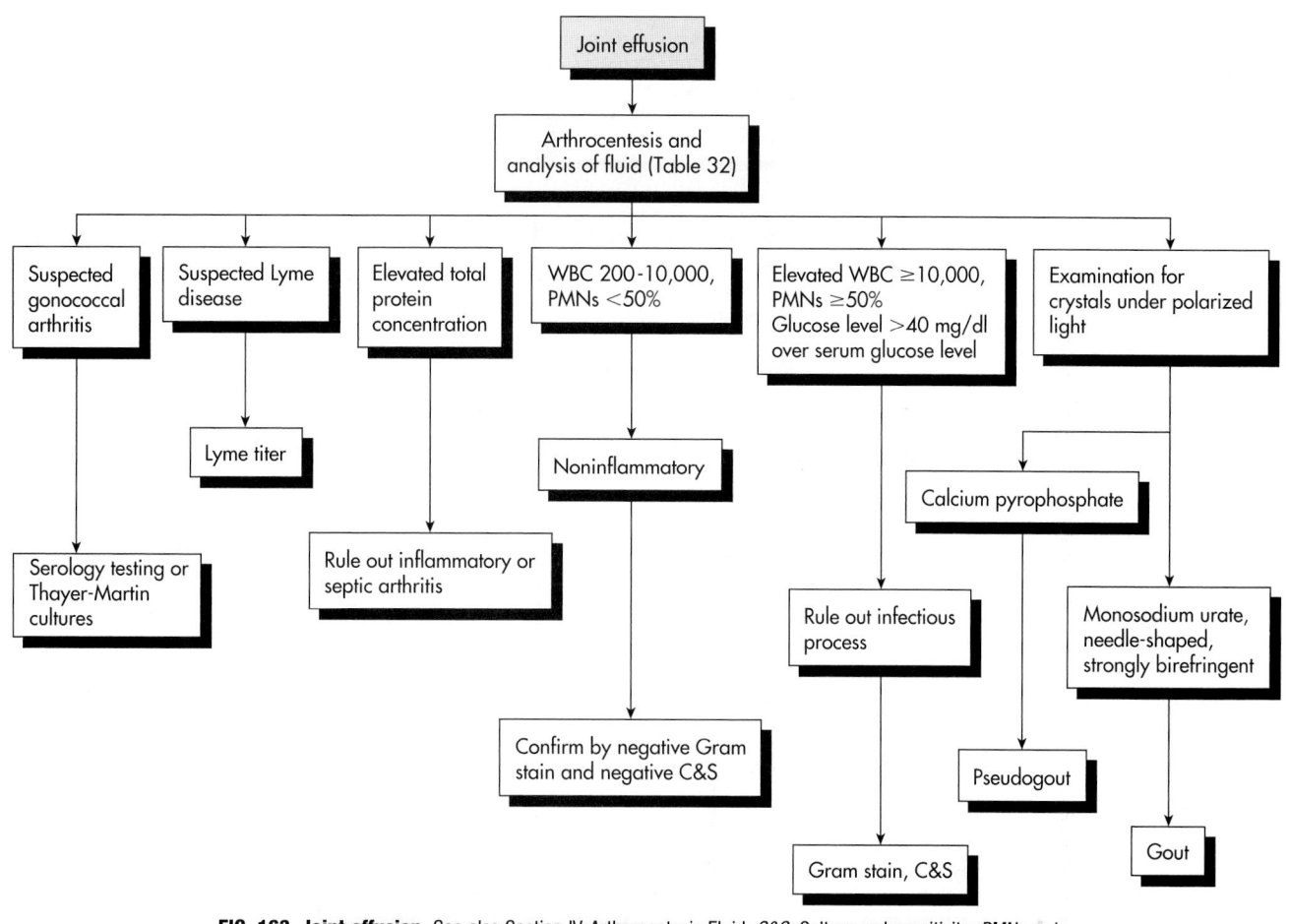

FIG. 163 Joint effusion. See also Section IV, Arthrocentesis Fluid. *C&S,* Culture and sensitivity; *PMNs,* polymorphonuclear leukocytes; *WBC,* white blood cell count.

Table 32   Indications for Arthrocentesis

Undiagnosed Arthritis with Effusion

Characterize type of arthritis
    Noninflammatory (WBC <2000/mm³)
    Inflammatory (WBC >2000/mm³)
    Septic (WBC >50,000/mm³)
Definitive diagnosis
    Gout (urate crystals)
    Pseudogout (calcium pyrophosphate dihydrate crystals)
    Septic arthritis (Gram stain [rare] or culture)

Undiagnosed Arthritis without Effusion

May be definitive in gout (knee, first metatarsophalangeal joint)

Patient with Known Diagnosis

Septic arthritis (repeated taps for adequate drainage)
Other types of arthritis for symptomatic relief (with or without injection)*

WBC, white blood cells.
*Most studies show improved effect if fluid aspirated before injection.
Firestein: Kelley's textbook of rheumatology / Gary S. Firestein ... [et al.].—9th ed. ISBN
    978-1-4377-1738-9 , 2013, Saunders.

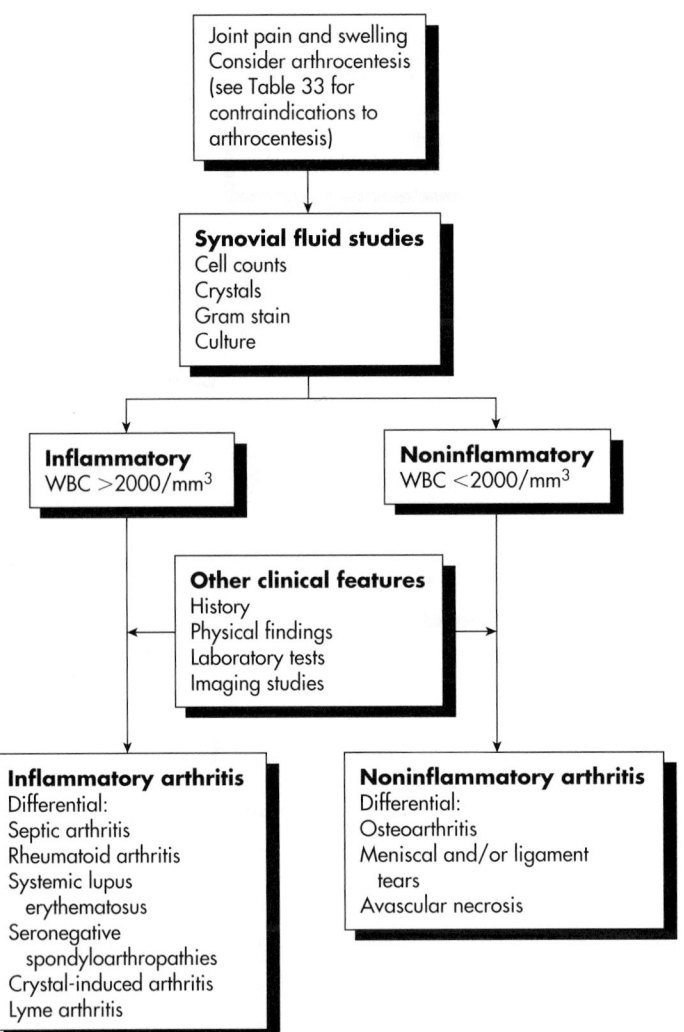

FIG. 164 Diagnostic approach for swollen joints. *WBC,* White blood cell count. (From Goldman L, Schafer AL [eds]: *Cecil textbook of medicine,* ed 24, Philadelphia, 2012, Saunders.)

Table 33   Contraindications to Arthrocentesis and Joint Injection

Contraindication	Comment
Established infection in nearby structures (e.g., cellulitis, septic bursitis)	Sometimes gout mimics cellulitis, creating a confusing picture
Septicemia (theoretic risk of introducing organism into joint)	Need to tap suspected septic joints in septic patients
Disrupted skin barrier (e.g., psoriasis)	Do not tap through lesions
Bleeding disorder (not absolute, but use more care)	Risk of bleeding very low, even in patients taking warfarin
Septic joint	Steroid injection contraindicated
Prior lack of response	Relative contraindication
Difficult-to-access joint	Relative contraindication without imaging aid

Firestein: Kelley's textbook of rheumatology / Gary S. Firestein … [et al.].—9th ed. ISBN 978-1-4377-1738-9 , 2013, Saunders.

ICD-10CM #   M12.9   Arthropathy, unspecified
S99.919A   Unspecified injury of unspecified ankle, initial encounter
M25.669   Stiffness of unspecified knee, not elsewhere classified
M25.469   Effusion, unspecified

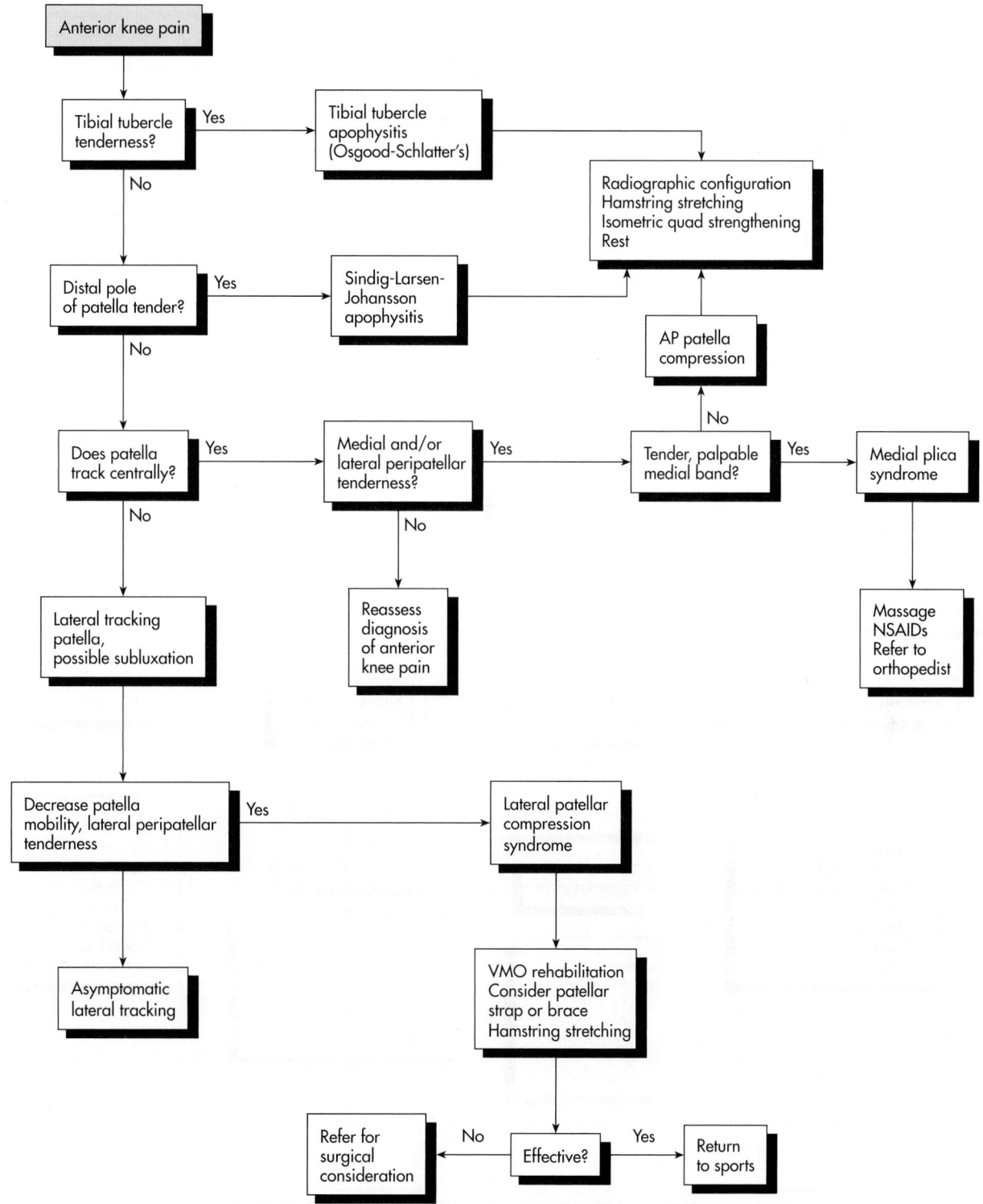

FIG. 166 **Evaluation and management of knee extensor mechanism pain. Focused treatment based on specific etiology will prevent recurrence.** *AP,* Anteroposterior; *NSAIDs,* nonsteroidal antiinflammatory drugs; *VMO,* vastus medialis obliquus muscle. (From Scudieri G [ed]: *Sports medicine, principles of primary care,* St Louis, 1997, Mosby.)

Clinical
Algorithms

ICD-10CM #   I70.25   Atherosclerosis of native arteries of other extremities
                          with ulceration
             L97.909   Non-pressure chronic ulcer of unspecified part of
                          unspecified lower leg with unspecified severity
             L98.499   Non-pressure chronic ulcer of skin of other sites with
                          unspecified severity
             L89.90   Pressure ulcer of unspecified site, unspecified stage

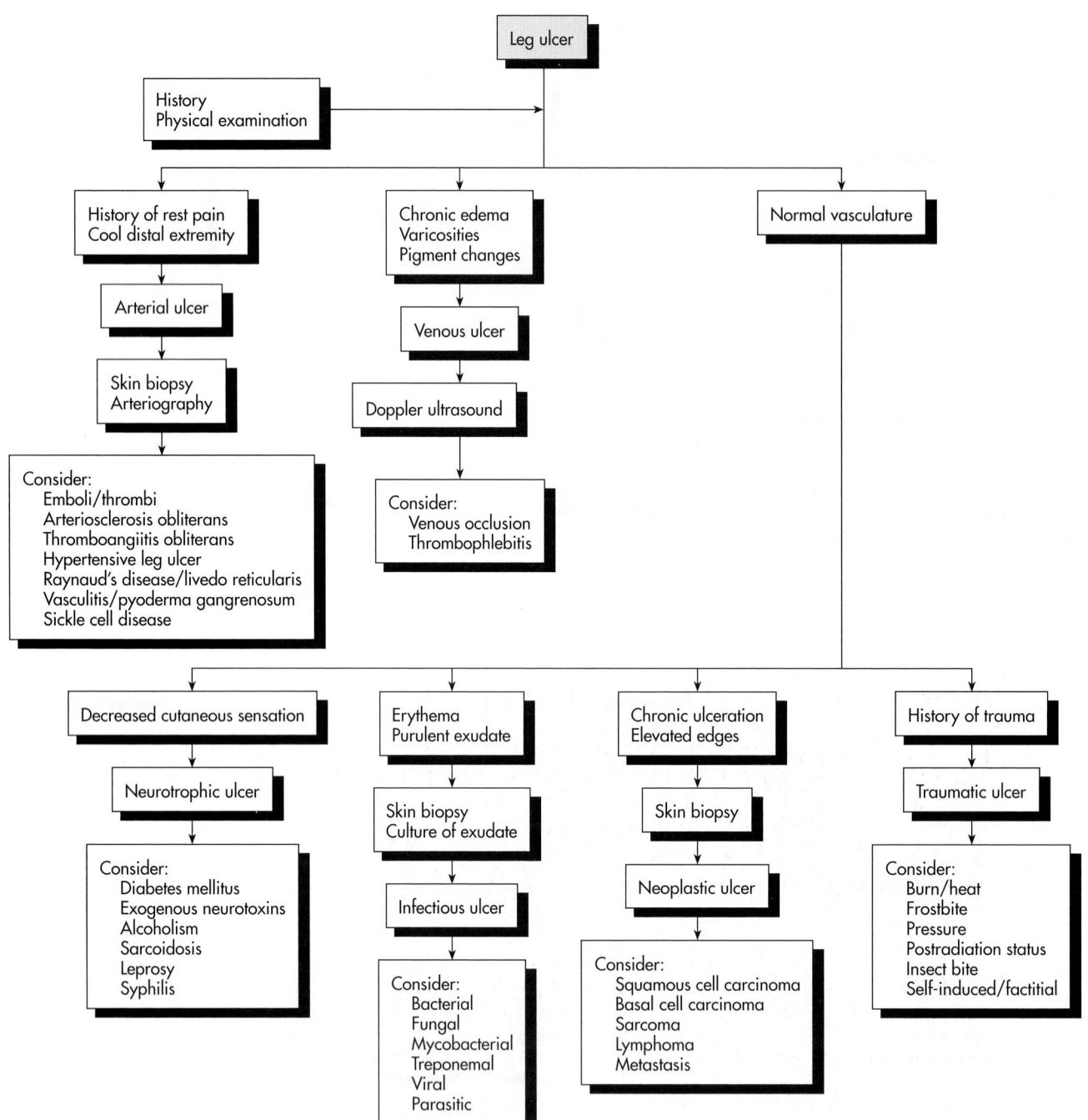

FIG. 167 Leg ulcer. (From Greene HL, Johnson WP, Lemcke D [eds]: *Decision making in medicine,* ed 2, St Louis, 1998, Mosby.)

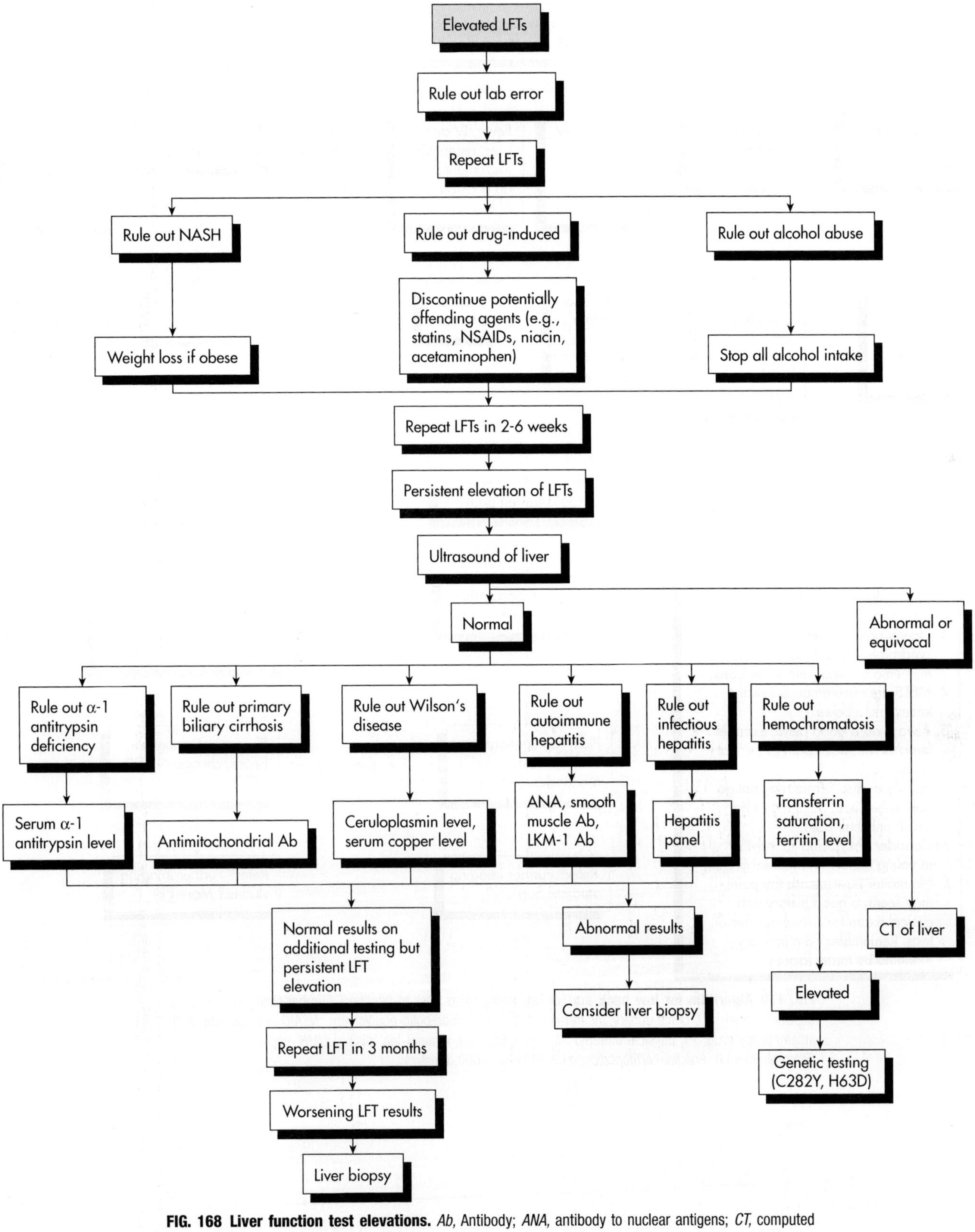

Elevated LFTs

↓

Rule out lab error

↓

Repeat LFTs

```
Rule out NASH          Rule out drug-induced          Rule out alcohol abuse
      ↓                          ↓                              ↓
Weight loss if obese   Discontinue potentially        Stop all alcohol intake
                       offending agents (e.g.,
                       statins, NSAIDs, niacin,
                       acetaminophen)
```

↓

Repeat LFTs in 2-6 weeks

↓

Persistent elevation of LFTs

↓

Ultrasound of liver

```
                Normal                              Abnormal or
                                                    equivocal
```

```
Rule out α-1    Rule out primary   Rule out Wilson's   Rule out        Rule out       Rule out
antitrypsin     biliary cirrhosis  disease             autoimmune      infectious     hemochromatosis
deficiency                                             hepatitis       hepatitis
    ↓                ↓                  ↓                  ↓               ↓              ↓
Serum α-1       Antimitochondrial  Ceruloplasmin      ANA, smooth     Hepatitis      Transferrin
antitrypsin     Ab                 level,             muscle Ab,      panel          saturation,
level                              serum copper       LKM-1 Ab                       ferritin level
                                   level
```

Normal results on additional testing but persistent LFT elevation

↓

Repeat LFT in 3 months

↓

Worsening LFT results

↓

Liver biopsy

Abnormal results

↓

Consider liver biopsy

CT of liver

Elevated

↓

Genetic testing (C282Y, H63D)

FIG. 168 Liver function test elevations. *Ab,* Antibody; *ANA,* antibody to nuclear antigens; *CT,* computed tomography; *IEP,* immunoelectrophoresis; *LFTs,* liver function tests; *LKM,* liver-kidney microsome; *NASH,* non-alcoholic steatohepatitis; *NSAIDs,* nonsteroidal antiinflammatory drugs.

Clinical Algorithms

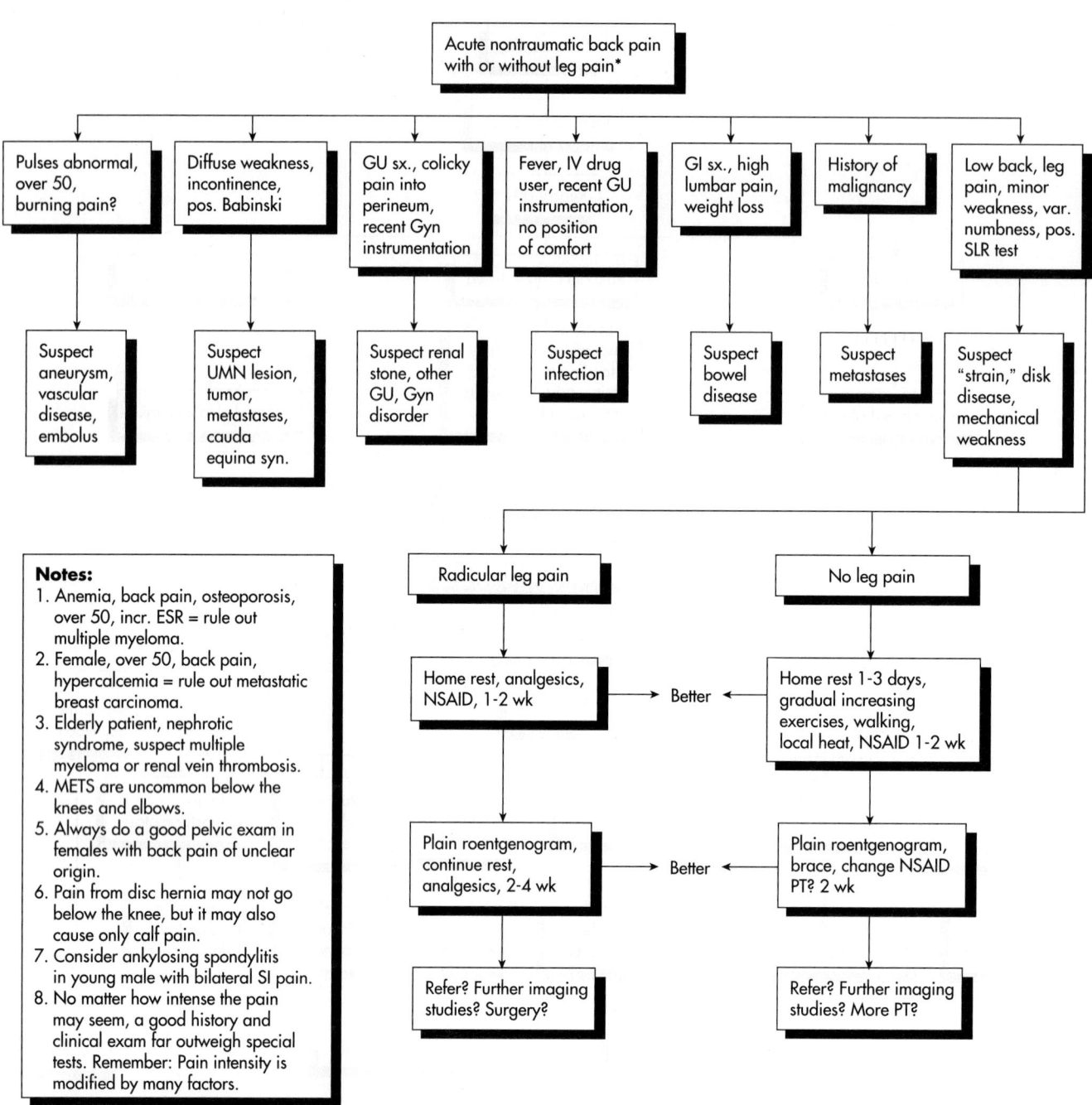

Notes:
1. Anemia, back pain, osteoporosis, over 50, incr. ESR = rule out multiple myeloma.
2. Female, over 50, back pain, hypercalcemia = rule out metastatic breast carcinoma.
3. Elderly patient, nephrotic syndrome, suspect multiple myeloma or renal vein thrombosis.
4. METS are uncommon below the knees and elbows.
5. Always do a good pelvic exam in females with back pain of unclear origin.
6. Pain from disc hernia may not go below the knee, but it may also cause only calf pain.
7. Consider ankylosing spondylitis in young male with bilateral SI pain.
8. No matter how intense the pain may seem, a good history and clinical exam far outweigh special tests. Remember: Pain intensity is modified by many factors.

FIG. 170 Algorithm for low back and/or leg pain. *Also refer to Section I, Lumbar Disk Syndrome. GI, Gastrointestinal; GU, genitourinary; IV, intravenous; METS, metabolic equivalents; NSAID, nonsteroidal anti-inflammatory drug; PT, physical therapy; SI, sacroiliac; SLR, straight-leg raising; UMN, upper motor neuron. (From Mercier LR: Practical orthopedics, ed 2, St Louis, 2000, Mosby.)

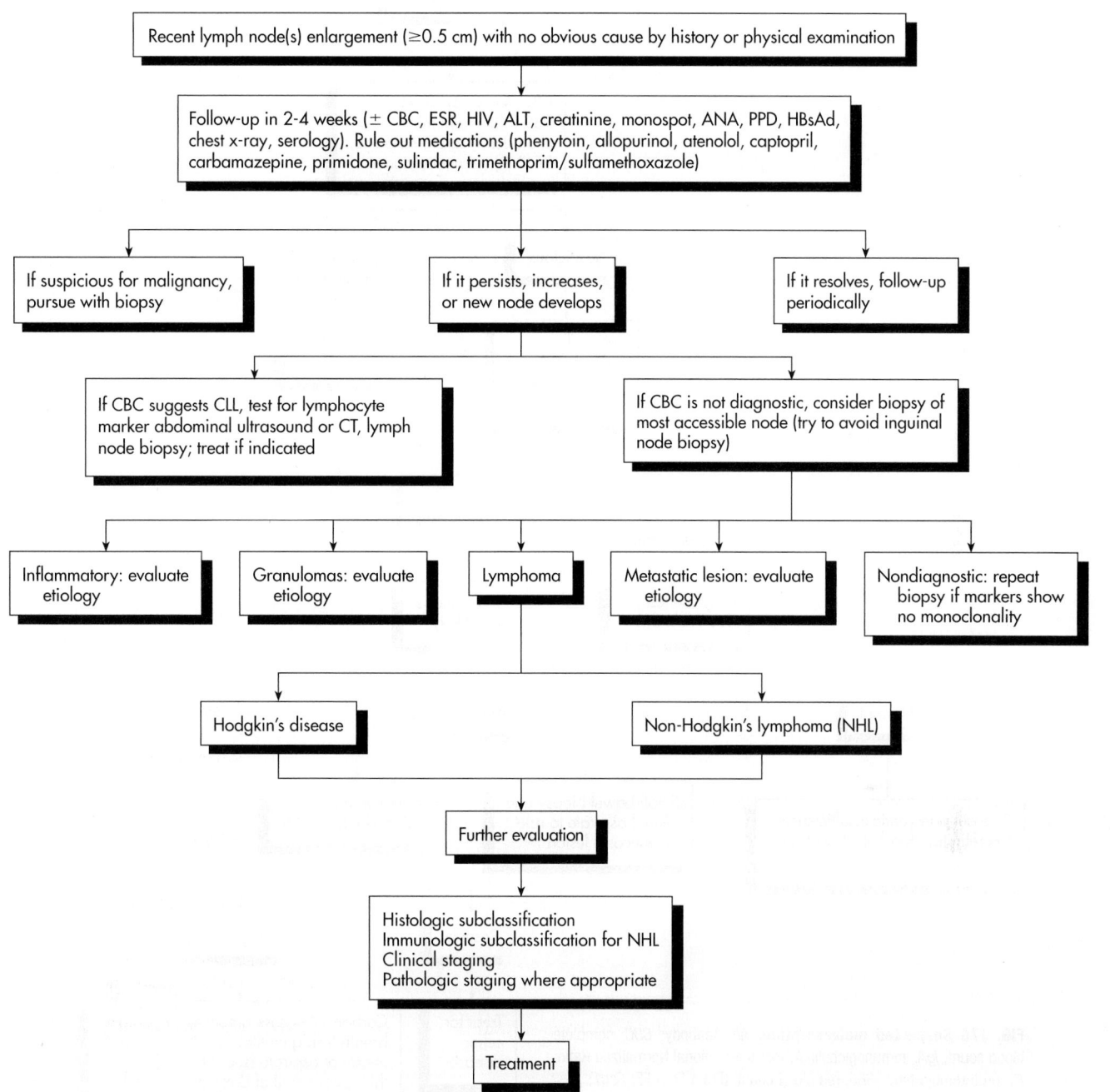

FIG. 174 Workup of lymphadenopathy. *ALT,* Alanine aminotransferase; *CBC,* complete blood count; *CLL,* chronic lymphocytic leukemia; *CT,* computed tomography; *ESR,* erythrocyte sedimentation rate. (Modified from Noble J [ed]: *Primary care medicine,* ed 3, St Louis, 2001, Mosby.)

Clinical
Algorithms

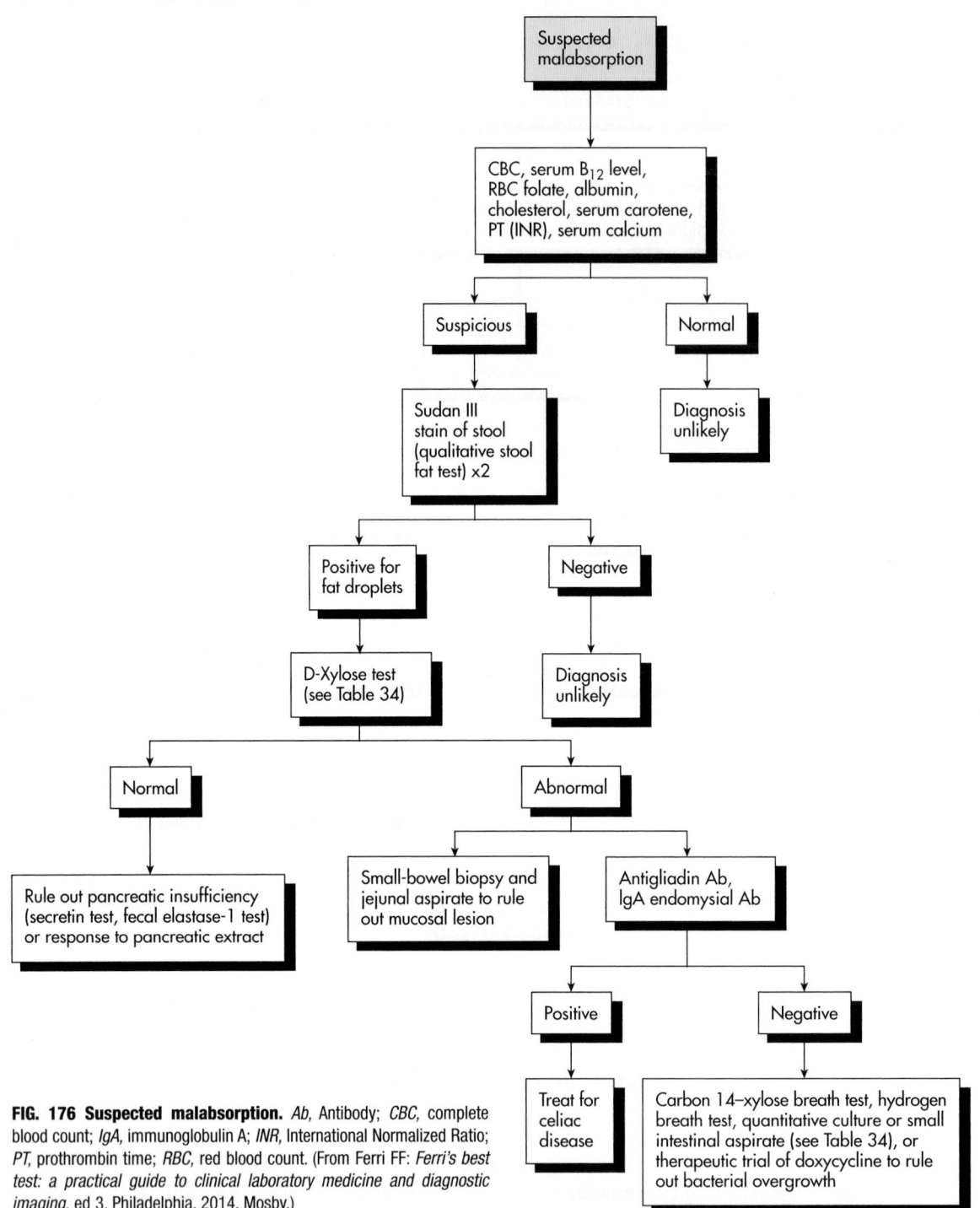

FIG. 176 Suspected malabsorption. *Ab*, Antibody; *CBC*, complete blood count; *IgA*, immunoglobulin A; *INR*, International Normalized Ratio; *PT*, prothrombin time; *RBC*, red blood count. (From Ferri FF: *Ferri's best test: a practical guide to clinical laboratory medicine and diagnostic imaging*, ed 3, Philadelphia, 2014, Mosby.)

BOX 7   Malabsorption, Suspected

Diagnostic Imaging
Best Test
Small-bowel series
Ancillary Test
CT of pancreas with IV contrast

Lab Evaluation
Best Test
Biopsy of small bowel

Ancillary Tests
Albumin, total protein
ALT, AST, PT
Serum lytes, BUN, creatinine
Sudan III stain of stool for fecal leukocytes
CBC, RBC folate, serum iron, serum carotene, cholesterol, serum calcium
Hydrogen 14-C xylose breath test
D-Xylose test, secretin test
Quantitative fecal test
Antigliadin antibody, IgA endomysial antibody

ALT, Alanine aminotransferase; *AST*, aspartate aminotransferase; *BUN*, blood urea nitrogen; *CBC*, complete blood count; *CT*, computed tomography; *IgA*, immunoglobulin A; *IV*, intravenous; *PT*, prothrombin time; *RBC*, red blood count.
From Ferri FF: *Ferri's best test: a practical guide to clinical laboratory medicine and diagnostic imaging*, ed 3, Philadelphia, 2014, Elsevier Mosby.

Table 34   Tests for the Evaluation of Malabsorption*

Test	Comments
General Tests of Absorption	
Quantitative stool fat test	Gold standard test of fat malabsorption, with which all other tests are compared. Requires ingestion of a high-fat diet (100 g) for 2 days before and during the collection. Stool is collected for 3 days. Normally, <7 g/24 hr is excreted on a high-fat diet. Borderline abnormalities of 8-14 g/24 hr may be seen in secretory or osmotic diarrheas that are not caused by malabsorption. There are false-negative findings if fat intake is inadequate. False-positive results can occur if mineral oil laxatives or rectal suppositories (e.g., cocoa butter) are given to the patient before stool collection.
Qualitative stool fat test	Sudan stain of a stool sample for fat. Many fat droplets per medium-power field (×40) constitute a positive test result. The nuclear magnetic resonance method determines the percentage of fat in the stool (normal, <20%). The test depends on an adequate fat intake (100 g/day). There is high sensitivity (90%) and specificity (90%) with fat malabsorption of >10 g/24 hr. Sensitivity drops with stool fat in the range of 6-10 g/24 hr.
D-Xylose test	A test of small intestinal mucosal absorption, used to distinguish mucosal malabsorption from malabsorption due to pancreatic insufficiency. An oral dose of D-xylose (24 g/500 ml water) is administered, and D-xylose excretion is measured in a 5-hr urine collection. Normally, >4 g of D-xylose is excreted in the urine over 5 hr. The test also may be positive in bacterial overgrowth owing to metabolism of D-xylose by bacteria in the intestinal lumen. False-positive test results occur with renal failure, ascites, and an incomplete urine collection. Blood levels at 1 and 3 hr improve sensitivity. May be normal with mild or limited mucosal disease.
Hydrogen breath test	Most useful in the diagnosis of lactase deficiency. An oral dose of lactose (1 g/kg body weight) is administered after measurement of basal breath H_2 levels. The sole source of H_2 in the mammal is bacterial fermentation; unabsorbed lactose makes its way to colonic bacteria, resulting in excess breath H_2. A *late peak* (within 3-6 hr) of >20 ppm of exhaled H_2 after lactose ingestion suggests lactose malabsorption. Absorption of other carbohydrates (e.g., sucrose, glucose, fructose) also can be tested.
Specific Tests for Malabsorption	
Tests for Pancreatic Function	
Secretin stimulation test	The gold standard test of pancreatic function. Requires duodenal test intubation with a double-lumen tube and collection of pancreatic juice in response to IV secretin. Allows measurement of bicarbonate (HCO_3-) and pancreatic enzymes. A sensitive test of pancreatic function, but labor intensive and invasive.
Fecal elastase-1 test	Stool test for pancreatic function. Equal sensitivity to the secretin stimulation test for the diagnosis of moderate-to-severe pancreatic insufficiency. More specific than the fecal chymotrypsin test. Unreliable with mild insufficiency. False-positive results occur with increased stool volume and intestinal mucosal diseases.
Tests for Bacterial Overgrowth	
Quantitative culture of small intestinal aspirate	Gold standard test for bacterial overgrowth. Greater than 10^5 colony-forming units (CFU)/ml in the jejunum suggests bacterial overgrowth. Requires special anaerobic sample collection, rapid anaerobic and aerobic plating, and care to avoid oropharyngeal contamination. False-negative results occur with focal jejunal diverticula and when overgrowth is distal to the site aspirated.
Hydrogen breath test	The 50-g glucose breath test has a sensitivity of 90% for growth of 10^5 colonic-type bacteria in the small intestine. If bacterial overgrowth is present, increased H_2 is excreted in the breath. A hydrogen level (within 2 hr) of >20 ppm suggests bacterial overgrowth. False-negative results occur with non-hydrogen-producing organisms.
^{14}C-D-xylose breath test	This test uses 1 g of carbon 14–labeled D-xylose. It has a sensitivity and specificity >90% for growth of 10^5 test colonic-type bacteria in the small intestine. Bacteria metabolize D-xylose with release of $^{14}CO_2$, which is absorbed and exhaled. Non-degraded D-xylose is absorbed in the small bowel and does not reach the colon, yielding a greater specificity than the lactulose H_2 breath test. A nonradioactive ^{13}C-D-xylose breath test is suitable for children and pregnant women.
Tests for Mucosal Disease	
Small bowel biopsy	Obtained for a specific diagnosis when there is a high index of suspicion for small intestinal disease. Several biopsy specimens (4-5) must be obtained to maximize the diagnostic yield. Distal duodenal biopsy specimens are usually adequate for diagnosis, but occasionally enteroscopy with jejunal biopsy specimens is necessary. Small intestinal biopsy provides a specific diagnosis in some diseases (e.g., intestinal infection, Whipple's disease, abetalipoproteinemia, agammaglobulinemia, lymphangiectasia, lymphoma, amyloidosis). In other conditions, such as celiac disease and tropical sprue, the biopsy specimens show characteristic findings, but the diagnosis is made on improvement after treatment.
Tests of Ileal Function	
Schilling test	A test of vitamin B_{12} absorption
^{75}SeHCAT test	This is a test of bile acid absorption. Seven days after ingestion of radiolabeled synthetic selenium-homocholic acid conjugated with taurine (^{75}SeHCAT), whole body retention is measured by a gamma-counting device. The result is expressed as a fraction of baseline ingestion. Retention values of less than 10% are abnormal and indicate bile acid malabsorption with a sensitivity of 80%-90% and specificity of 70%-100%. The radiation dose is equivalent to a plain chest x-ray. Liver disease and bacterial overgrowth may give false results. Not approved for use in the United States.

*Not all these tests are readily available. A strong suspicion for any disease may warrant forgoing an extensive work-up and obtaining the test with highest diagnostic yield. In some cases, empirical treatment, such as removing lactose from the diet of an otherwise healthy individual with lactose intolerance, is warranted without any testing.

From Goldman L, Schafer AI: *Goldman's Cecil Medicine,* ed 24, Philadelphia, 2012, Saunders.

Clinical Algorithms

III

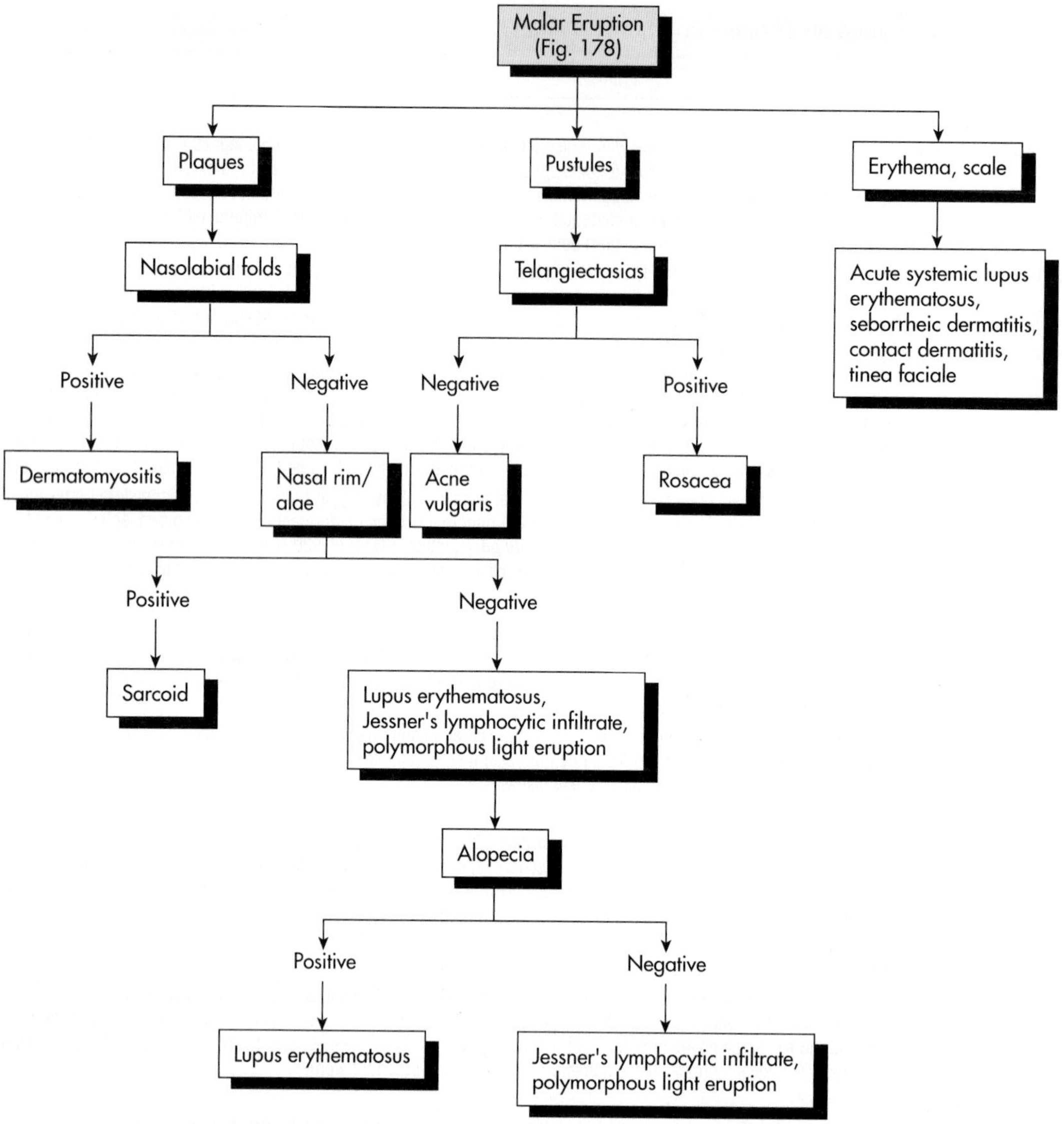

```
                        ┌──────────────────┐
                        │  Malar Eruption  │
                        │    (Fig. 178)    │
                        └──────────────────┘
```

Malar Eruption (Fig. 178)

— Plaques
— Pustules
— Erythema, scale

Plaques → Nasolabial folds
- Positive → Dermatomyositis
- Negative → Nasal rim/alae
  - Positive → Sarcoid
  - Negative → Lupus erythematosus, Jessner's lymphocytic infiltrate, polymorphous light eruption
    → Alopecia
    - Positive → Lupus erythematosus
    - Negative → Jessner's lymphocytic infiltrate, polymorphous light eruption

Pustules → Telangiectasias
- Negative → Acne vulgaris
- Positive → Rosacea

Erythema, scale → Acute systemic lupus erythematosus, seborrheic dermatitis, contact dermatitis, tinea faciale

FIG. 177 Clinical algorithm for diagnosis of a malar eruption, which must be confirmed by appropriate cultures, serology, and biopsy. (From Harris ED et al [eds]: *Kelley's textbook of rheumatology,* ed 7, Philadelphia, 2005, Saunders.)

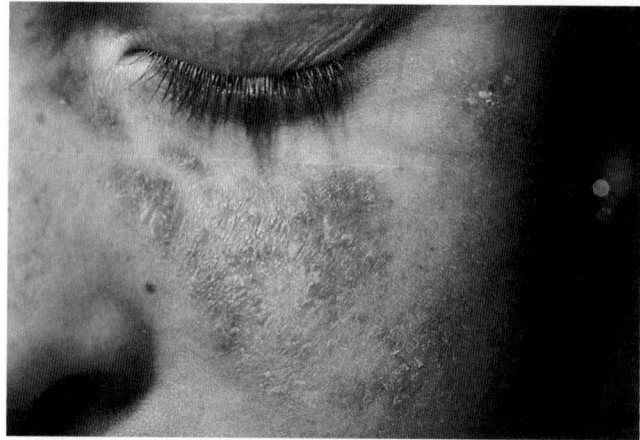

FIG. 178 Systemic lupus erythematosus. Mild scaling and erythema of the malar rash. (Paller AS, Mancini AJ: Hurwitz Clinical pediatric Dermatology, 5th ed, Elsevier, Philadelphia, 2016, ISBN# 978-0-323-24475-6.)

EVALUATION OF THE DISTRESSED PATIENT ON MECHANICAL VENTILATION

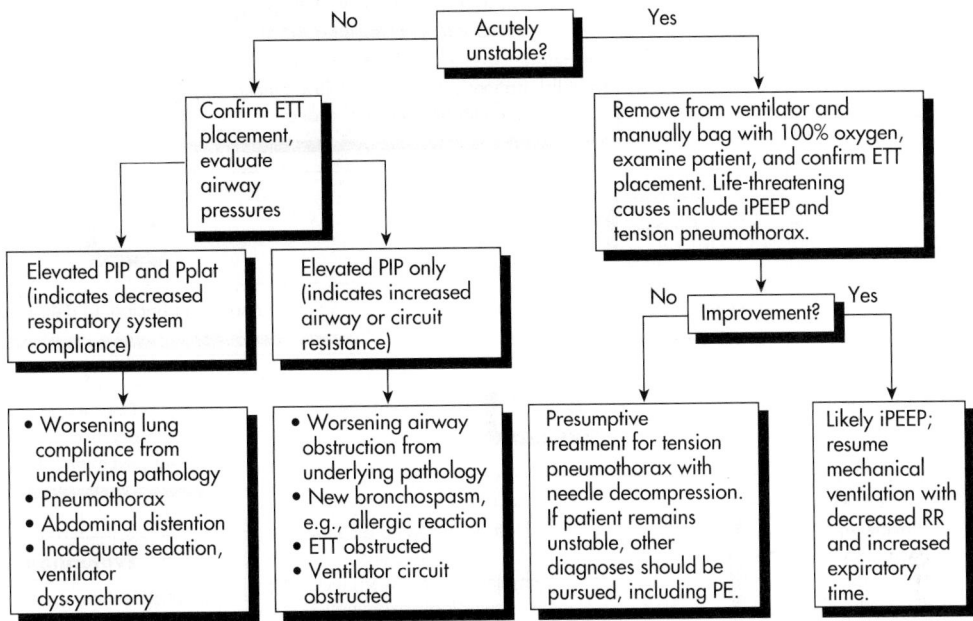

FIG. 179 Algorithm for evaluation of the distressed patient on mechanical ventilation. (From Marx JA et al: *Rosen's emergency medicine*, ed 8, Philadelphia, 2014, Saunders.)

Table 35 Troubleshooting the Ventilator: Potential Causes of Acute Respiratory Distress

With Hemodynamic Compromise: Immediately Discontinue Mechanical Ventilation

Increased intrinsic positive end-expiratory pressure (iPEEP)

Tension pneumothorax

Massive pulmonary embolus

Without Hemodynamic Compromise: Search for Underlying Cause

Mechanical	Physiologic
Endotracheal tube migration into bronchus	Worsening lung compliance
Endotracheal tube obstruction	Worsening airway obstruction
Endotracheal tube cuff leak	Abdominal distention
Inadvertent extubation	Pulmonary embolus
Discontinuity in ventilator circuit	Pain or inadequate sedation

From Marx JA et al: *Rosen's emergency medicine*, ed 8, Philadelphia, 2014, Saunders.

Clinical Algorithms

III

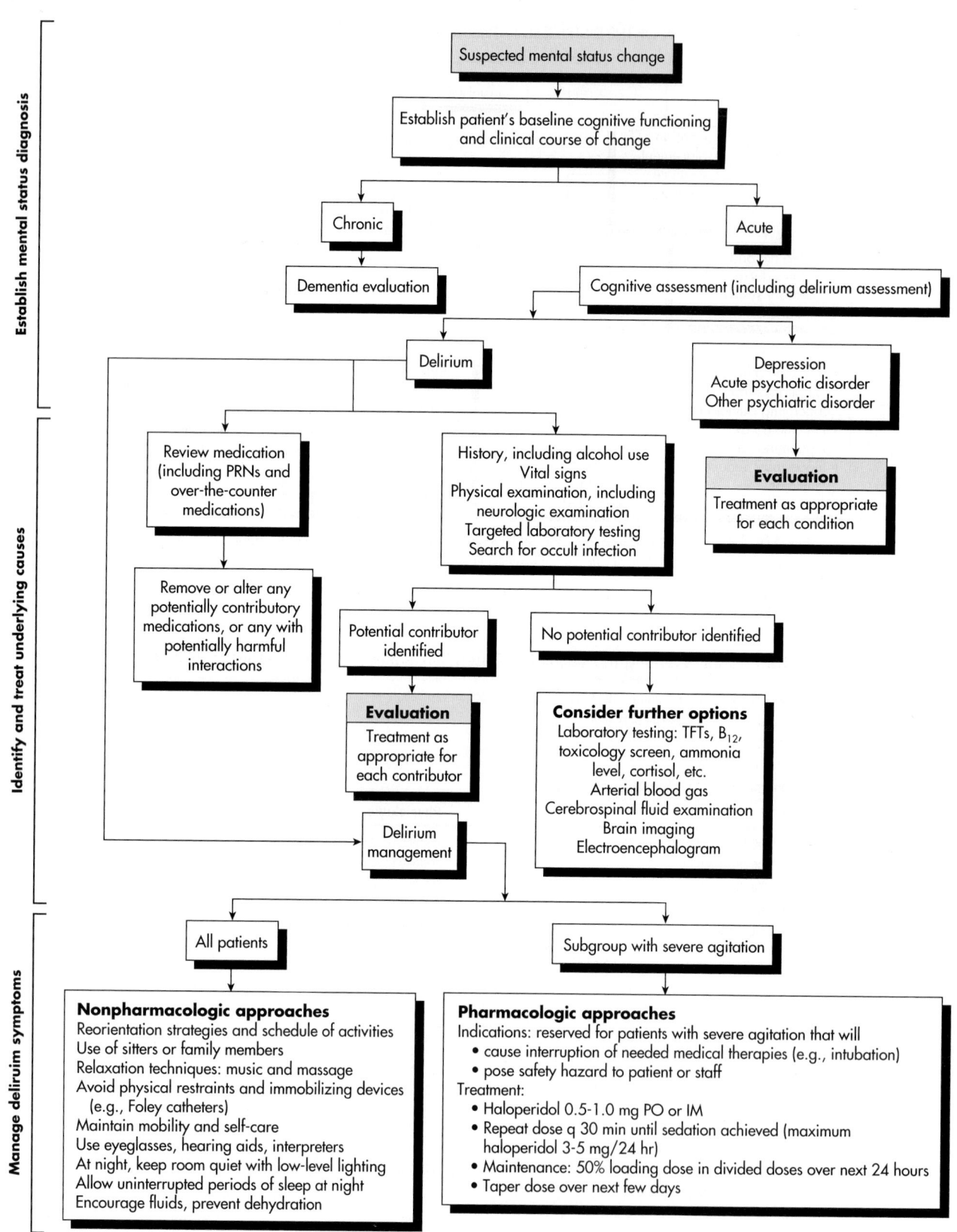

FIG. 180 Algorithm for the evaluation of suspected mental status change in older patients. *PRN,*
As needed; *TFTs,* thyroid function tests. (From Goldman L, Schafer AI: *Goldman's Cecil medicine,* ed 24,
Philadelphia, 2012, Saunders.)

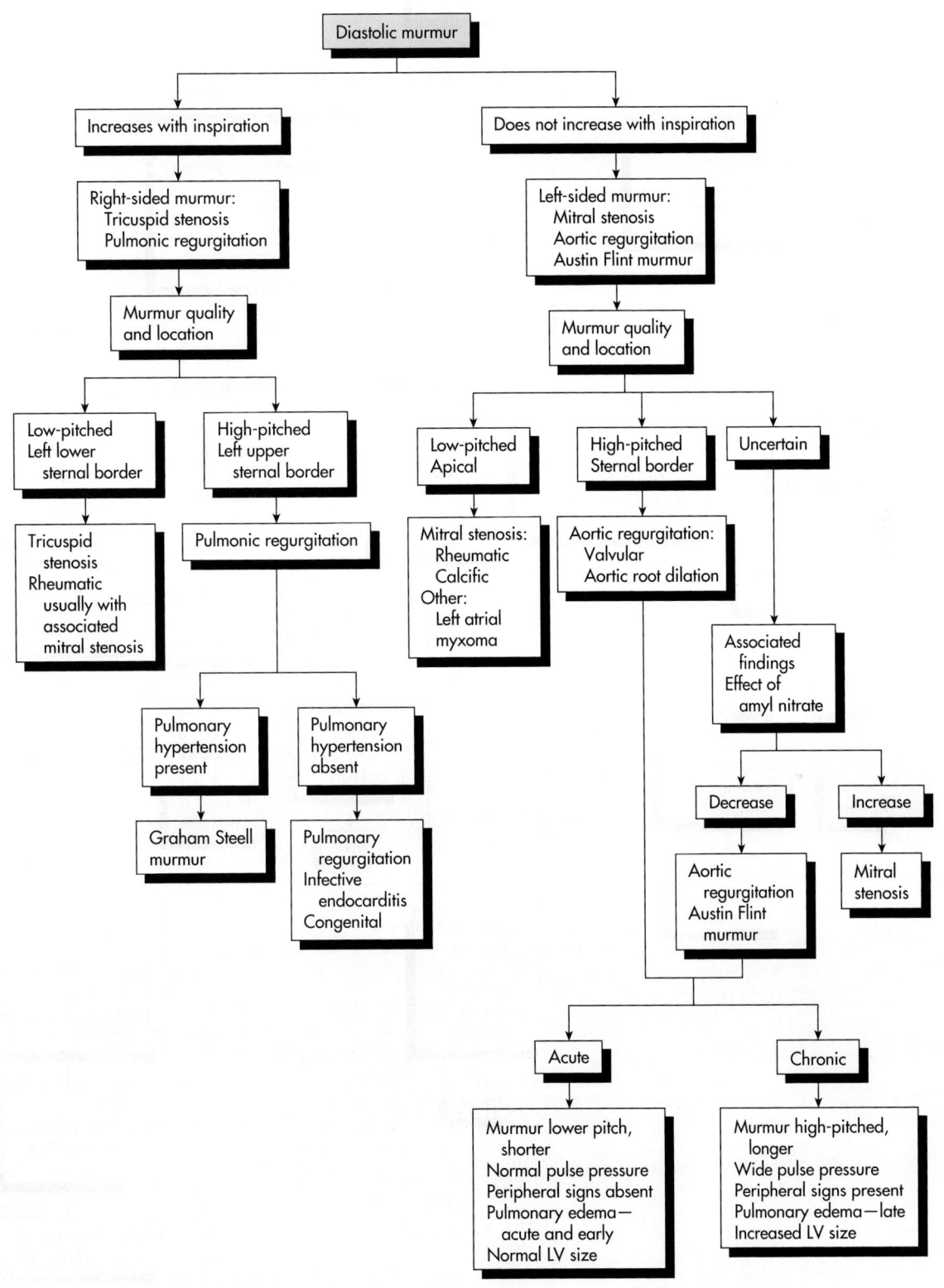

FIG. 181 Diastolic murmur. *LV,* Left ventricle. (From Greene HL, Johnson WP, Lemcke DL [eds]: *Decision making in medicine,* ed 2, St Louis, 1998, Mosby.)

Clinical Algorithms

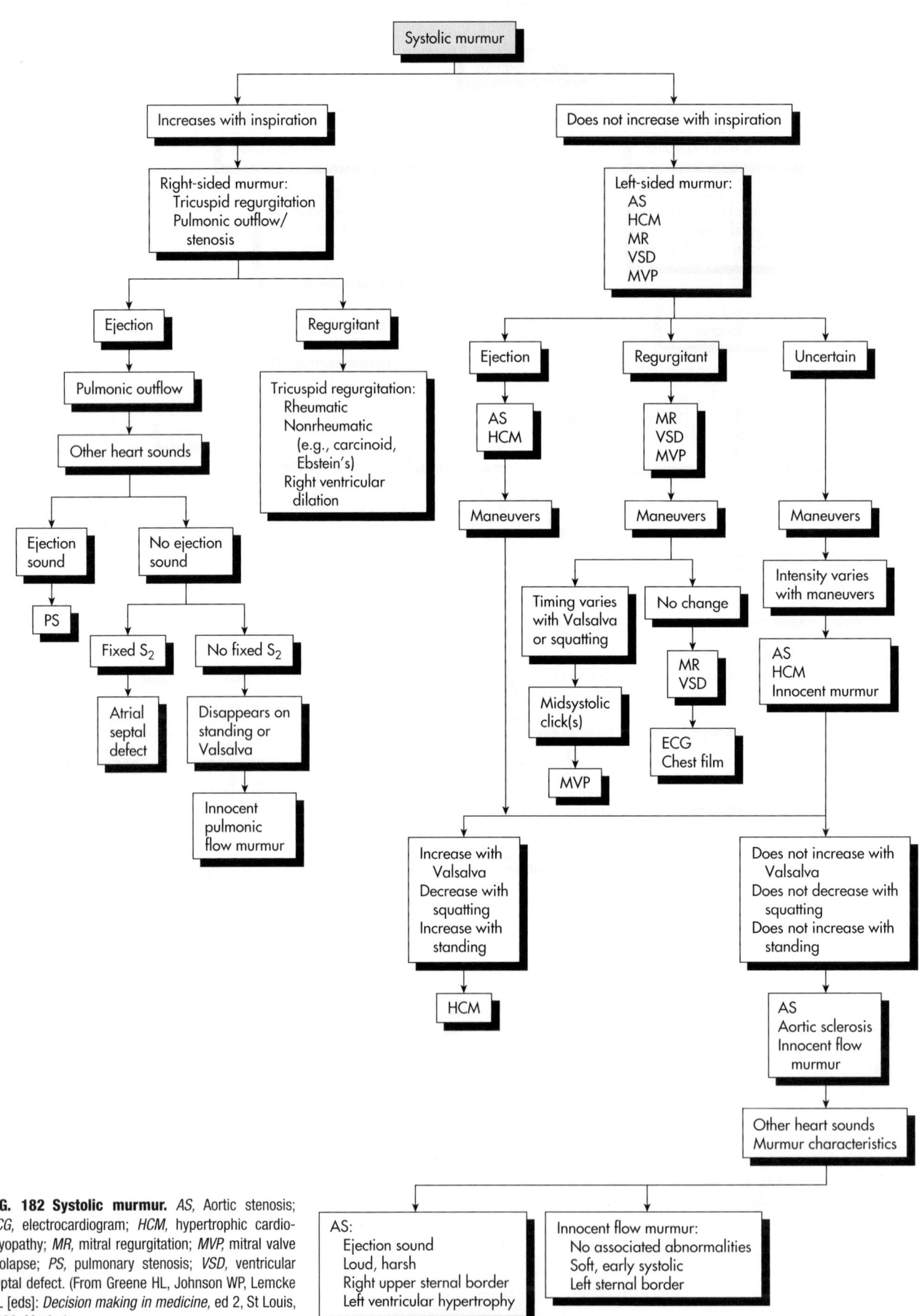

FIG. 182 Systolic murmur. *AS,* Aortic stenosis; *ECG,* electrocardiogram; *HCM,* hypertrophic cardiomyopathy; *MR,* mitral regurgitation; *MVP,* mitral valve prolapse; *PS,* pulmonary stenosis; *VSD,* ventricular septal defect. (From Greene HL, Johnson WP, Lemcke DL [eds]: *Decision making in medicine,* ed 2, St Louis, 1998, Mosby.)

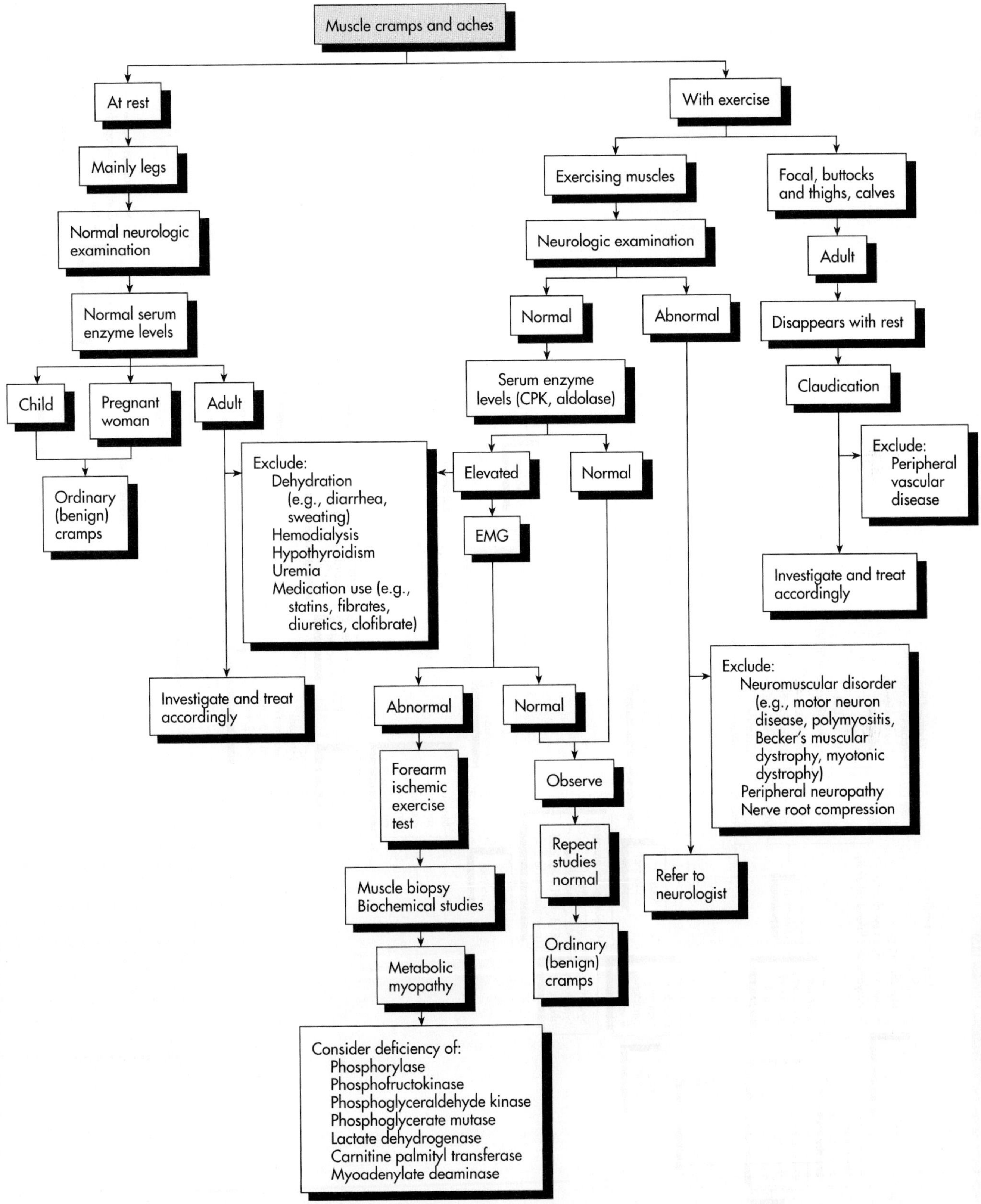

Muscle cramps and aches

At rest

Mainly legs

Normal neurologic examination

Normal serum enzyme levels

Child | Pregnant woman | Adult

Ordinary (benign) cramps

Exclude:
  Dehydration (e.g., diarrhea, sweating)
  Hemodialysis
  Hypothyroidism
  Uremia
  Medication use (e.g., statins, fibrates, diuretics, clofibrate)

Investigate and treat accordingly

With exercise

Exercising muscles

Neurologic examination

Normal | Abnormal

Serum enzyme levels (CPK, aldolase)

Elevated | Normal

EMG

Abnormal | Normal

Forearm ischemic exercise test

Muscle biopsy Biochemical studies

Metabolic myopathy

Consider deficiency of:
  Phosphorylase
  Phosphofructokinase
  Phosphoglyceraldehyde kinase
  Phosphoglycerate mutase
  Lactate dehydrogenase
  Carnitine palmityl transferase
  Myoadenylate deaminase

Observe

Repeat studies normal

Ordinary (benign) cramps

Exclude:
  Neuromuscular disorder (e.g., motor neuron disease, polymyositis, Becker's muscular dystrophy, myotonic dystrophy)
  Peripheral neuropathy
  Nerve root compression

Refer to neurologist

Focal, buttocks and thighs, calves

Adult

Disappears with rest

Claudication

Exclude:
  Peripheral vascular disease

Investigate and treat accordingly

FIG. 183 Evaluation of muscle cramps and aches. *CPK,* Creatine phosphokinase; *EMG,* electromyography. (From Greene HL, Johnson WP, Lemcke D [eds]: *Decision making in medicine,* ed 2, St Louis, 1998, Mosby.)

Clinical Algorithms

MUSCLE WEAKNESS

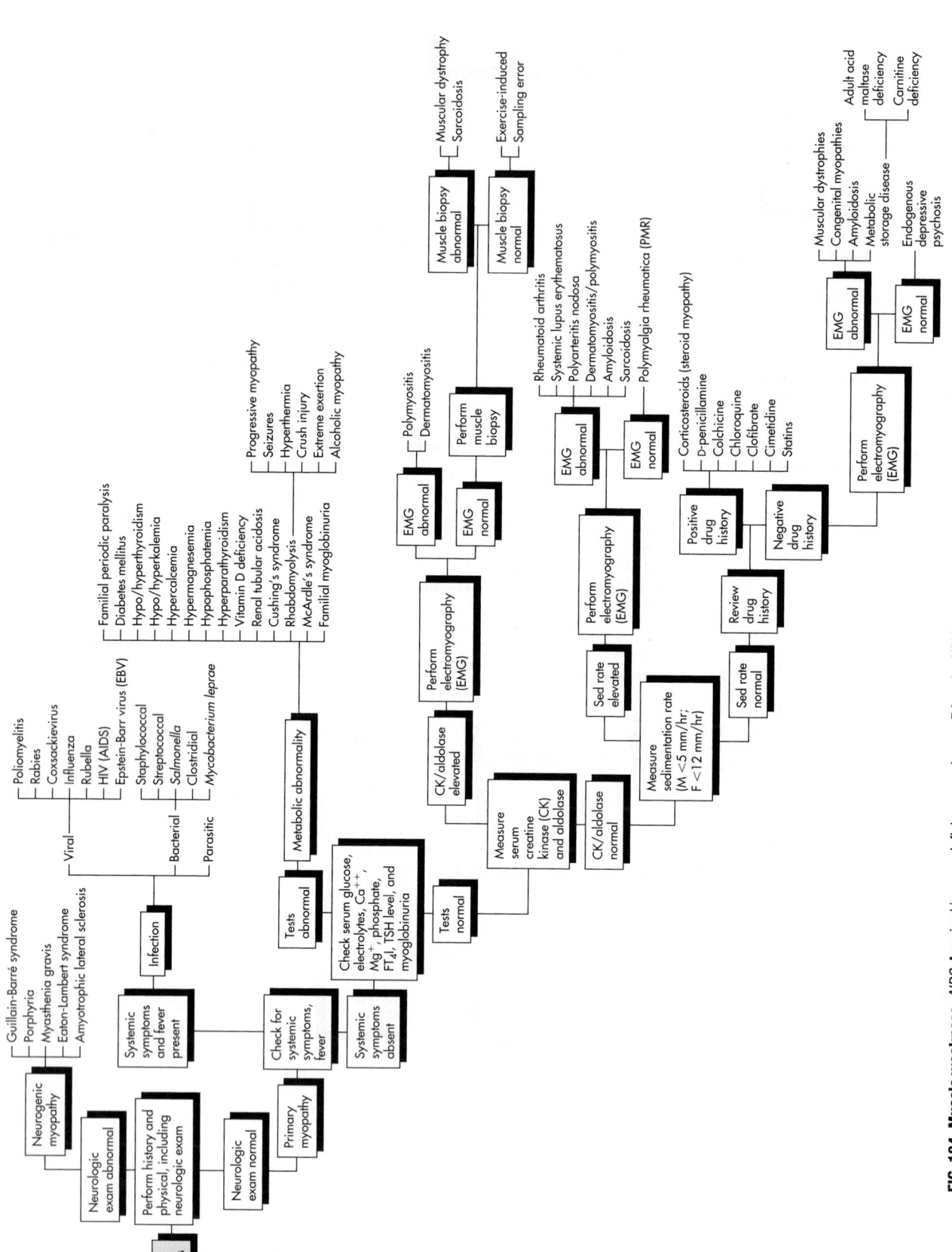

FIG. 184 Muscle weakness. *AIDS,* Acquired immunodeficiency syndrome; *F,* female; *HIV,* human immunodeficiency virus; *M,* male. (From Healey PM: *Common medical diagnosis: an algorithmic approach,* ed 3, Philadelphia, 2000, Saunders.)

MUSCULOSKELETAL COMPLAINTS

ICD-10CM # M25.50 -Pain(s) joint
-Arthralgia (allergic)
-Arthrodynia
-Polyarthralgia

1687

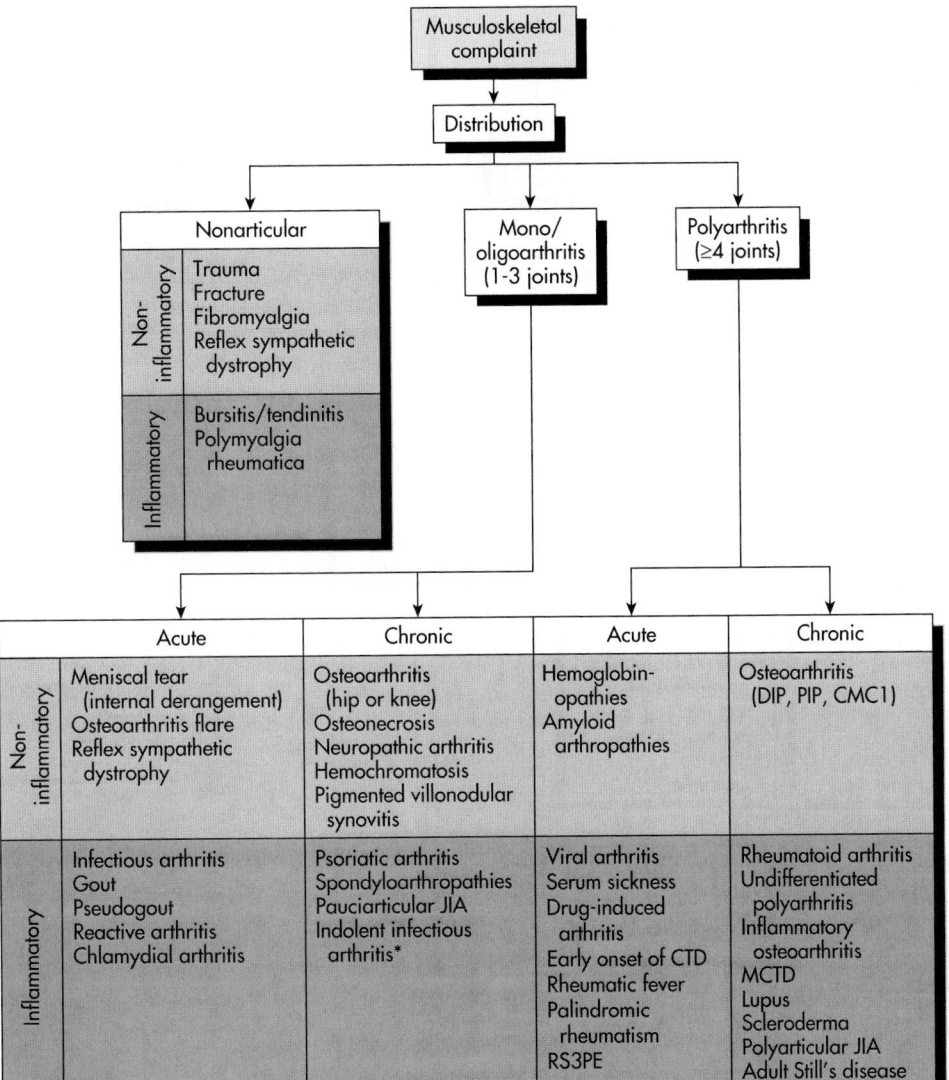

FIG. 185 Algorithm for assessing initial history and examination. *CMC*, Carpometacarpal; *CTD*, connective tissue disease; *DIP*, distal interphalangeal; *JIA*, juvenile idiopathic arthritis; *MCTD*, mixed connective tissue disease; *PIP*, proximal interphalangeal. (Firestein GS, Budd RC, Gabriel SE, et al: *Kelley's textbook of rheumatology*, ed 9, Philadelphia, 2013, Saunders.)

Clinical Algorithms

III

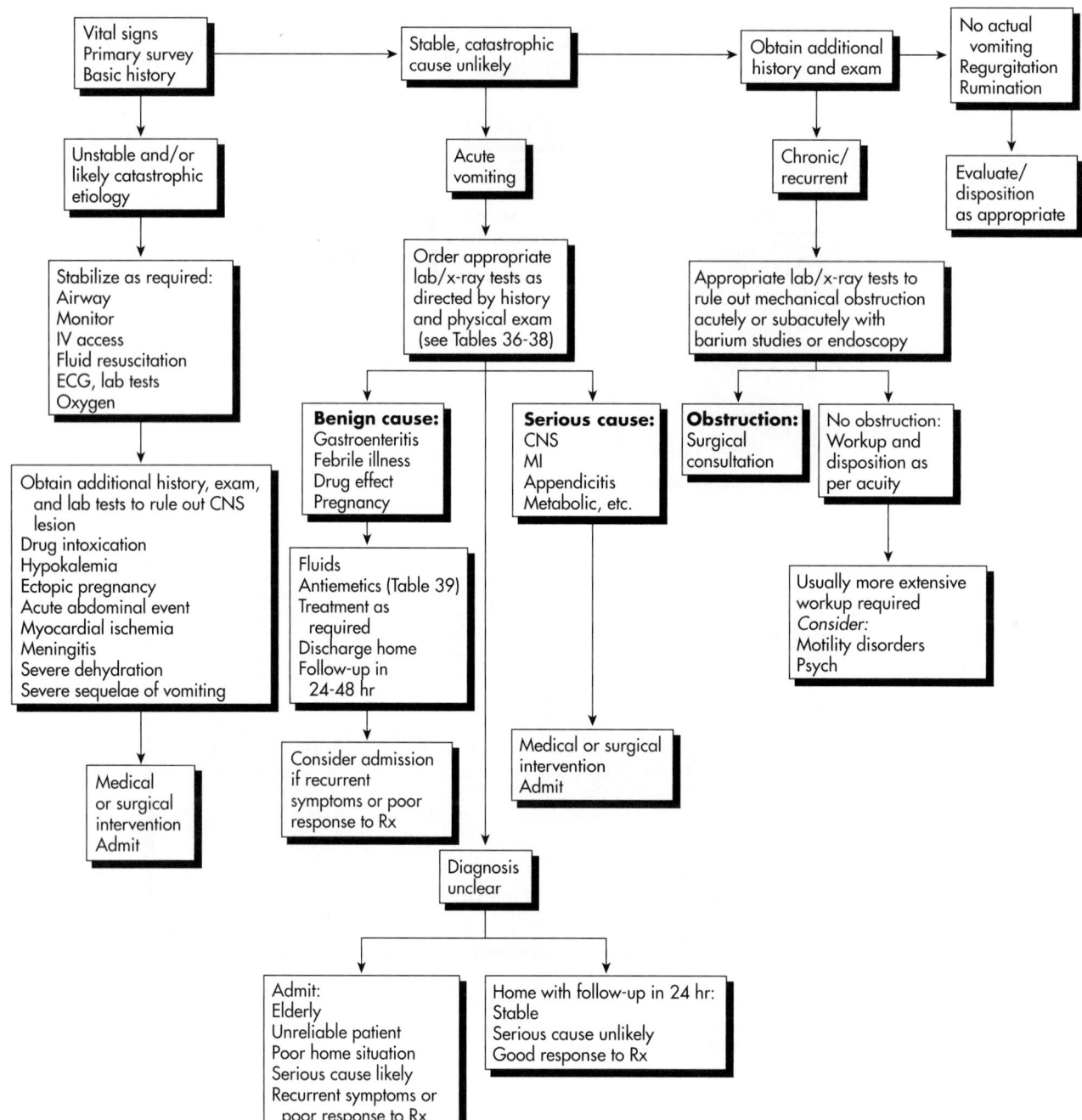

FIG. 189 Approach to the patient with nausea and vomiting. *CNS,* Central nervous system; *ECG,* electrocardiogram; *IV,* intravenous; *MI,* myocardial infarction; *Psych,* psychogenic; *Rx,* treatment. (From Marx JA et al: *Rosen's emergency medicine,* ed 8, Philadelphia, 2014, Saunders.)

Table 36   Differential Diagnosis of Nausea and Vomiting

Etiologic Category	Critical Diagnoses	Emergent Diagnoses	Nonemergent Diagnoses
Gastrointestinal (GI)	• Boerhaave's syndrome • Ischemic bowel • GI bleeding	• Gastric outlet obstruction • Pancreatitis • Cholecystitis or cholangitis • Bowel obstruction or ileus • Ruptured viscus • Appendicitis • Peritonitis • Spontaneous bacterial peritonitis	• Gastritis • Gastroparesis • Peptic ulcer disease • Inflammatory bowel disease • Biliary colic • Hepatitis • Gastroenteritis
Neurologic	• Intracerebral bleed • Meningitis	• Migraine • CNS tumor • Raised ICP	
Endocrine	• DKA	• Adrenal insufficiency • Uremia	• Thyroid
Pregnancy		Hyperemesis gravidarum	• Nausea and vomiting of pregnancy
Drug toxicity		• Acetaminophen • Digoxin • Aspirin • Theophylline	
Therapeutic drug use			• Aspirin • Antibiotics • Erythromycin • Ibuprofen • Chemotherapy
Drugs of abuse			Narcotics Narcotic withdrawal Alcohol
Genitourinary		Gonadal torsion	Urinary tract infection Poisoning Nephrolithiasis
Miscellaneous	Myocardial infarction Sepsis	• Carbon monoxide • Electrolyte disorders • Organophosphate poisoning	• Motion sickness • Labyrinthitis

CNS, Central nervous system; *DKA,* diabetic ketoacidosis; *ICP,* intracranial pressure.
From Marx JA et al: *Rosen's emergency medicine,* ed 8, Philadelphia, 2014, Saunders.

Clinical
Algorithms

III

Table 37   Disorders Commonly Associated with Vomiting

Disorder	History	Prevalence	Physical Examination	Useful Tests	Comments
Nausea and vomiting of pregnancy (NVP)	Vomiting occurs predominantly in the morning. Associated breast tenderness. NVP typically starts in weeks 4-7, peaks in weeks 10-16, and disappears by week 20. Vomiting that begins after week 12 or continues past week 20 should prompt a search for another cause.	Very common Affects 75% of all pregnancies	Benign abdomen	Urine pregnancy test Serum electrolytes, urine ketones to exclude hyperemesis gravidarum	Consider NVP in all females of childbearing age. Prognosis for mother and infant is excellent. NVP is associated with a decreased risk of miscarriage, fetal growth retardation, and fetal mortality.
Hyperemesis gravidarum	Severe, protracted form of NVP. No universally accepted definition of the disease. Generally accepted hallmarks include 5% weight loss, ketonuria, and electrolyte disturbance. Hyperemesis is associated with multiple gestation, molar pregnancy, and nulliparity.	Uncommon Affects <1% of pregnancies	Signs of dehydration Benign abdomen	β-hCG Urinalysis for ketones Serum electrolytes Ultrasound examination to exclude molar pregnancy or multiple gestation	Most studies have found no adverse outcomes for the fetus. A few studies, however, have shown a correlation with fetal growth retardation.

Continued on next page

Table 37   Disorders Commonly Associated with Vomiting—cont'd

Disorder	History	Prevalence	Physical Examination	Useful Tests	Comments
Gastroenteritis	Fever, diarrhea, and crampy abdominal pain. Vomiting and pain occur early, usually followed by diarrhea within 24 hr.	Very common	Benign abdomen	Usually not necessary	Early gastroenteritis, when only vomiting and periumbilical pain are present, may be confused with early appendicitis. Diarrhea is usually in the diagnosis of gastroenteritis.
Gastritis	Epigastric pain, belching, bloating, fullness, heartburn, and food intolerance. Use of NSAIDs or ETOH common.	Very common	Mild epigastric tenderness may be present.	Lipase and pregnancy test may be necessary to exclude other diagnoses.	Removal of inciting agent along with antacid therapy will resolve symptoms in most patients.
Peptic ulcer disease (PUD)	Epigastric pain present in 90% of cases. Classically, duodenal ulcer pain is relieved by food whereas gastric ulcer pain is made worse. Presence of severe pain should raise suspicion of perforation.	Very common	Mild epigastric tenderness	Hemoglobin if bleeding is suspected Heme-positive stool Upright abdominal film if perforation is suspected	Three major causes of PUD are NSAIDs, *Helicobacter pylori* infection, and hypersecretory states.
Biliary disease	Abdominal pain may be midepigastric or right upper quadrant (RUQ). Onset frequently after a fatty meal. May have history of similar episodes in the past.	Very common	RUQ tenderness present in most cases. If instructed to breathe deeply during palpation in the RUQ, the patient experiences heightened tenderness and inspiratory arrest (Murphy's sign).	WBCs Lipase Serum bilirubin Alkaline phosphatase RUQ ultrasound examination ERCP	Normal temperature, WBCs, and spontaneous resolution of symptoms suggest biliary colic. Fever, Murphy's sign, elevated WBCs, and suggestive ultrasound indicate cholecystitis.
Myocardial infarction (MI)	Patients typically have substernal chest pain that may radiate to left arm or jaw. Often associated with dyspnea, diaphoresis, or dizziness.	Common	Patients often are anxious and in distress from pain. No diagnostic examination findings.	ECG (new Q waves, ST segment changes, or T wave inversions) troponin	Not all patients have chest pain. A subset of patients, particularly diabetics and elders, may have only nausea, vomiting, and epigastric discomfort.
Diabetic ketoacidosis (DKA)	Polydipsia and polyuria occur early. Without treatment, altered mental status and coma may develop. In patients with long-standing diabetes, DKA may be triggered by infection, trauma, MI, or surgery.	Common	"Fruity" breath odor results from serum acetone. Tachypnea occurs with attempts to "blow off" carbon dioxide to compensate for metabolic acidosis. Signs of dehydration may be present. Severe cases often manifest with altered mental status or coma.	Serum glucose, urine ketones, ABGs	DKA may be the first manifestation of diabetes in some patients. These patients often do not recognize the importance of polydipsia and polyuria. They often report only nausea, vomiting, and epigastric pain.

Table 37   Disorders Commonly Associated with Vomiting—cont'd

Disorder	History	Prevalence	Physical Examination	Useful Tests	Comments
Pancreatitis	Presenting symptom is epigastric pain, which often radiates to the back. Most cases are caused by gallstones or alcoholism. Other causes include hypercalcemia, hyperlipidemia, drugs (sulfas and thiazides), ERCP.	Common	Epigastric tenderness is present. Associated paralytic ileus may cause abdominal distention and decreased bowel sounds. Frank shock may be present in severe cases.	Lipase WBCs, serum glucose, LDH, AST Hematocrit, BUN, calcium, ABGs	Criteria correlating with higher mortality: *At admission*—age >55 yr, WBCs >16,000/mm^3, glucose >200 dL, base deficit >4, LDH >350 IU/L, AST >250 U/L *Within 48 hours*—Hct drop of 10%, BUN >2 mg/dL, Po$_2$ <60 mm Hg, calcium <8 mg, fluid sequestration >4 L
Appendicitis	Abdominal pain classically begins in periumbilical region and later moves to right lower quadrant. Anorexia is common.	Common	Localized tenderness over right lower quadrant. Low-grade fever may be present.	WBCs Ultrasound Abdominal CT	Early appendicitis can be a difficult diagnosis to make. It is still frequently missed on the first physician encounter.
Bowel obstruction	Classically, abdominal pain consists of intermittent cramps occurring at regular intervals. The frequency of the cramps varies with the level of the obstruction; the higher the level, the more frequent the cramps. The location of the pain also varies with the level of the obstruction; high obstruction causes epigastric pain, midlevel obstruction causes periumbilical pain, colonic obstruction causes hypogastric pain.	Common	Abdominal distention, mild diffuse tenderness, and high-pitched "tinkling" bowel sounds may be present. Thorough search for hernias should be performed.	Supine and upright plain abdominal films Abdominal CT	Adhesions, hernias, and tumors account for 90% of bowel obstructions. Other causes include intussusception, volvulus, foreign bodies, gallstone ileus, inflammatory bowel disease, stricture, cystic fibrosis, and hematoma.
Carbon monoxide (CO) poisoning	Headache is usually present. CO poisoning often occurs during winter months when furnaces are turned on. Family members may have similar symptoms if they also have been exposed.	Uncommon	No reliable signs of early CO poisoning	CO level	Because CO is a tasteless, odorless gas, patients may not realize they have been exposed. It is important to keep a high index of suspicion during the cold months.
Boerhaave's syndrome	Patients may have neck, chest, or epigastric pain. Forceful, protracted vomiting usually causes the tear. Most cases follow a bout of heavy eating and drinking. Other reported causes include childbirth, defecation, seizures, and heavy lifting.	Uncommon	Tachypnea, tachycardia, and hypotension may be present. Escaped air from the esophagus may produce subcutaneous emphysema. Air in the mediastinum produces a "crunching" sound as the heart beats (Hamman's sign).	CXR may show pleural effusion, widened mediastinum, pneumothorax, or pneumomediastinum. Esophagogram with water-soluble contrast is definitive.	The classic presentation includes forceful vomiting, severe chest pain, subcutaneous emphysema, and multiple CXR findings. There is a growing body of evidence that most cases do not have this "classic" picture. In more subtle presentations, the diagnosis can be difficult to make.

ABGs, arterial blood gases; *AST*, aspartate aminotransferase; β-*hCG*, β-human chorionic gonadotropin; *BUN*, blood urea nitrogen; *CT*, computed tomography; *CXR*, chest radiography; *ECG*, electrocardiogram; *ERCP*, endoscopic retrograde cholangiopancreatography; *ETOH*, ethyl alcohol; *Hct*, hematocrit; *LDH*, lactate dehydrogenase; *NSAID*, nonsteroidal anti-inflammatory drug; *Po$_2$*, partial pressure of oxygen; *WBC*, white blood cell.

Marx JA et al: *Rosen's Emergency Medicine*, ed 8, Philadelphia, 2014, Saunders. ISBN:978-1-4557-0605-1.

Clinical Algorithms

III

Table 38 Etiology of Nausea and Vomiting in Pediatric Age Groups

Etiologic Category	Newborn	Infant	Child	Adolescent
Infectious	Sepsis, meningitis, UTI, thrush	Pneumonia, otitis media, thrush	Gastroenteritis	Gastroenteritis, URI
Anatomic	Atresia and webs, malrotation, stenosis, meconium ileus, Hirschsprung's disease	Pyloric stenosis, intussusception, Hirschsprung's disease	Bezoars, chronic granulomatous disease	PUD, superior mesenteric syndrome
Gastrointestinal	Reflux, overfeeding, gastric outlet obstruction, volvulus	Reflux, gastritis, milk intolerance	Appendicitis, pancreatic, hepatitis, other food intolerance	Achalasia, hepatitis
Neurologic	Subdural hematoma, hydrocephalus	Subdural hematoma	Neoplasia, migraine, Reye's syndrome, motion sickness, hypertension	Neoplasia, migraine, motion sickness, hypertension
Metabolic	Organic or amino acidemias, urea cycle defects, galactosemia, hypercalcemia, phenylketonuria, kernicterus	Hereditary fructose intolerance, disorders of fatty acid metabolism, uremia, adrenal hyperplasia, kernicterus	Diabetes, vitamin A excess	Diabetes, pregnancy, acute intermittent porphyria
Other	Idiopathic, cardiac failure	Rumination, cardiac failure	Cyclic vomiting syndrome, toxins, food poisoning, Munchausen syndrome by proxy	Psychogenic, anorexia

PUD, peptic ulcer disease; *URI,* upper respiratory infection; *UTI,* urinary tract infection.
Adapted from Li HK, Sunku BK: Vomiting and nausea. In Wyllie R, Hyams JS, eds: Pediatric Gastrointestinal and Liver Disease: Pathophysiology, Diagnosis, Management. Philadelphia: WB Saunders; 2005:127-149.
Marx JA et al: *Rosen's Emergency Medicine*, ed 8, Philadelphia, 2014, Saunders. ISBN:978-1-4557-0605-1.

Table 39 Commonly Used Medications for the Treatment of Nausea and Vomiting

Medication	Dose	Comments
Promethazine (Phenergan)	*Adult:* 12.5-25 mg IV, IM, PO, or by rectum *Pediatric:* 0.25-1 mg/kg/dose q4-6h prn IV, IM, PO, or by rectum; max 25 mg/dose	May be repeated every 4-6 hr until cessation of vomiting. May cause dry mouth, dizziness, blurred vision. Boxed warning for use under 2 yr old.
Prochlorperazine (Compazine)	*Adult:* 5-10 mg IM or PO; 2.5-10 mg IV; 25 mg by rectum *Pediatric:* 0.4 mg/kg/24 hr tid-qid PO or by rectum; 0.1-0.15 mg/kg/dose tid-qid IM; max 40 mg/24 hr	May be repeated every 4 hr IV or IM or every 12 hr by rectum until cessation of vomiting. May cause lethargy, hypotension, extrapyramidal effects.
Metoclopramide (Reglan)	*Adult:* 10 mg IM or IV, may repeat q6h *Pediatric:* 1-2 mg/kg/dose q2-6h IV q2-3h	May cause dystonic reactions, tardive dyskinesia, neuroleptic malignant syndrome.
Ondansetron (Zofran)	*Adult:* 4 mg IV single dose *Pediatric:* up to 40 kg: 0.1 mg/kg; >40 kg: 4 mg/dose IV single dose	May cause headache, dizziness, and musculoskeletal pain.

IM, intramuscularly; *IV,* intravenously; *PO,* orally; *prn,* as needed.
Marx JA et al: *Rosen's Emergency Medicine*, ed 8, Philadelphia, 2014, Saunders. ISBN:978-1-4557-0605-1.

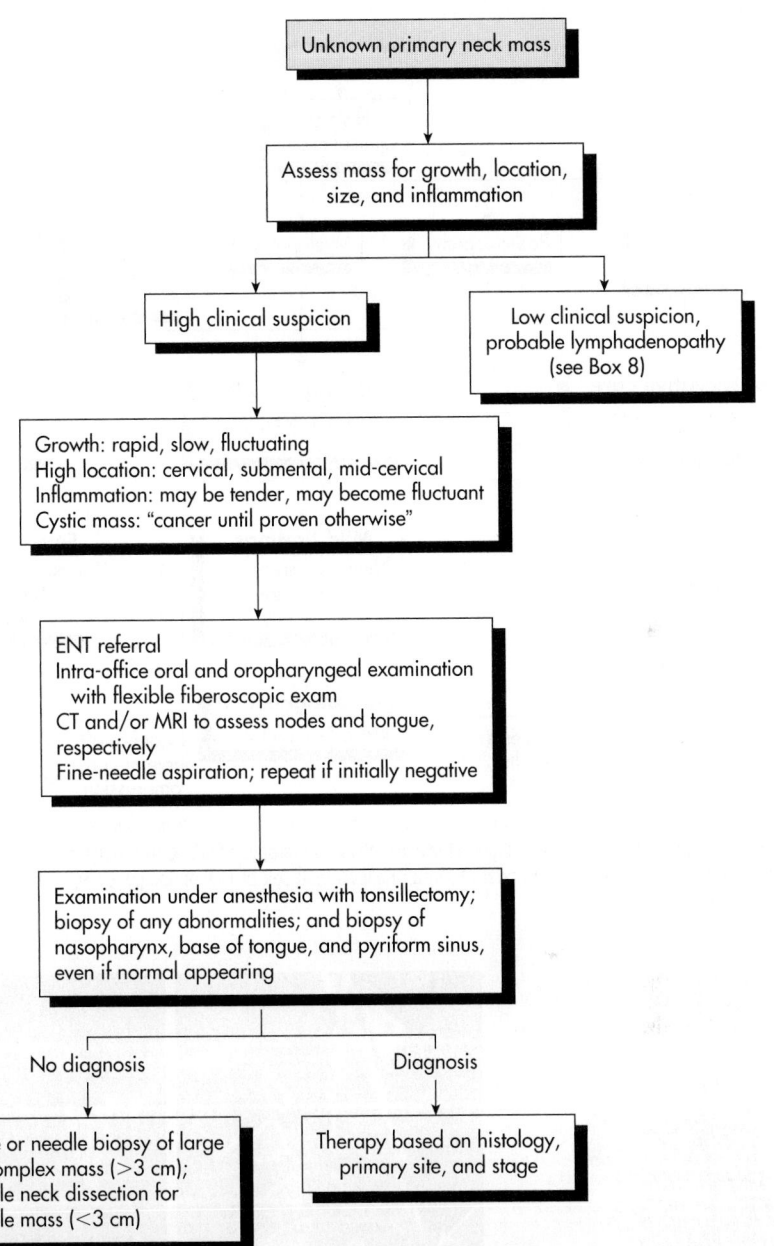

FIG. 190 Evaluation of an unknown primary neck mass. *CT,* Computed tomography; *ENT,* ear, nose, and throat; *MRI,* magnetic resonance imaging. (From Goldman L, Schafer AL [eds]: *Cecil textbook of medicine,* ed 24, Philadelphia, 2012, Saunders.)

Clinical
Algorithms

BOX 8   An Approach to the Patient with Lymphadenopathy

- Does the patient have a known illness that causes lymphadenopathy? Treat and monitor for resolution.
- Is there an obvious infection to explain the lymphadenopathy (e.g., infectious mononucleosis)? Treat and monitor for resolution.
- Are the nodes very large and/or very firm and thus suggestive of malignancy? Perform a biopsy.
- Is the patient very concerned about malignancy and unable to be reassured that malignancy is unlikely? Perform a biopsy.
- If none of the preceding are true, perform a complete blood cell count and if it is unrevealing, monitor for a predetermined period (usually 2 to 6 weeks). If the nodes do not regress or if they increase in size, perform a biopsy.

From Goldman L, Ausiello D (eds): *Cecil textbook of medicine,* ed 23, Philadelphia, 2008, Saunders.

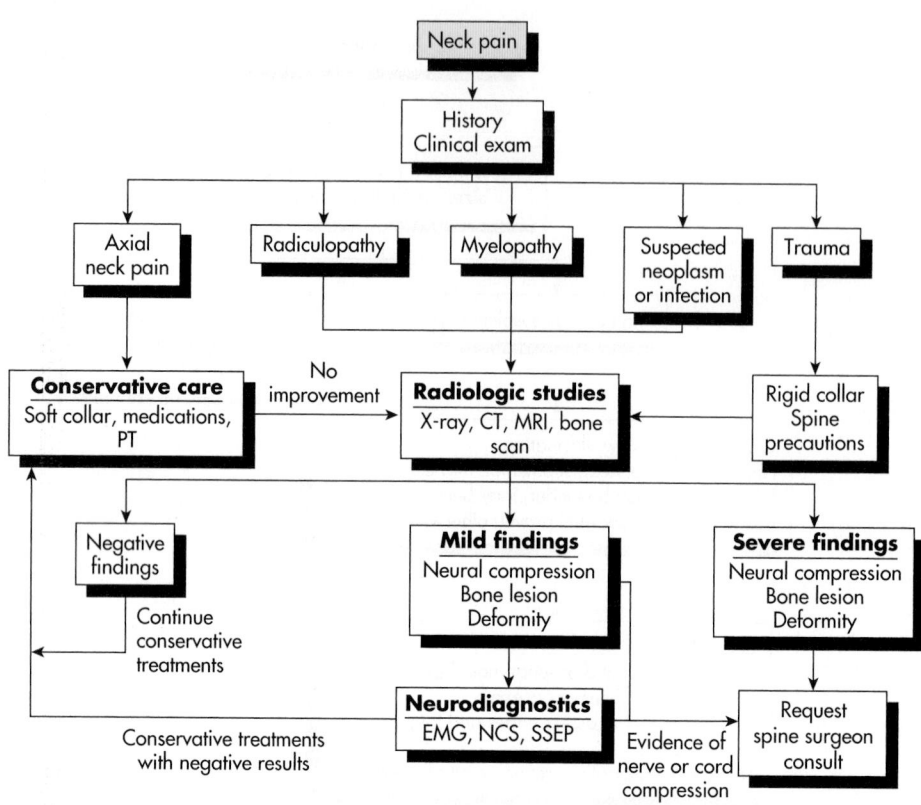

FIG. 191 Algorithm of neck pain. *CT,* Computed tomography; *EMG,* electromyogram; *MRI,* magnetic resonance imaging; *NCS,* nerve conduction study; *PT,* physical therapy; *SSEP,* somatosensory evoked potentials. (From Firestein GS, Budd RC, Gabriel SE, et al: Kelley's textbook of rheumatology, ed 9, Philadelphia, 2013, Saunders.)

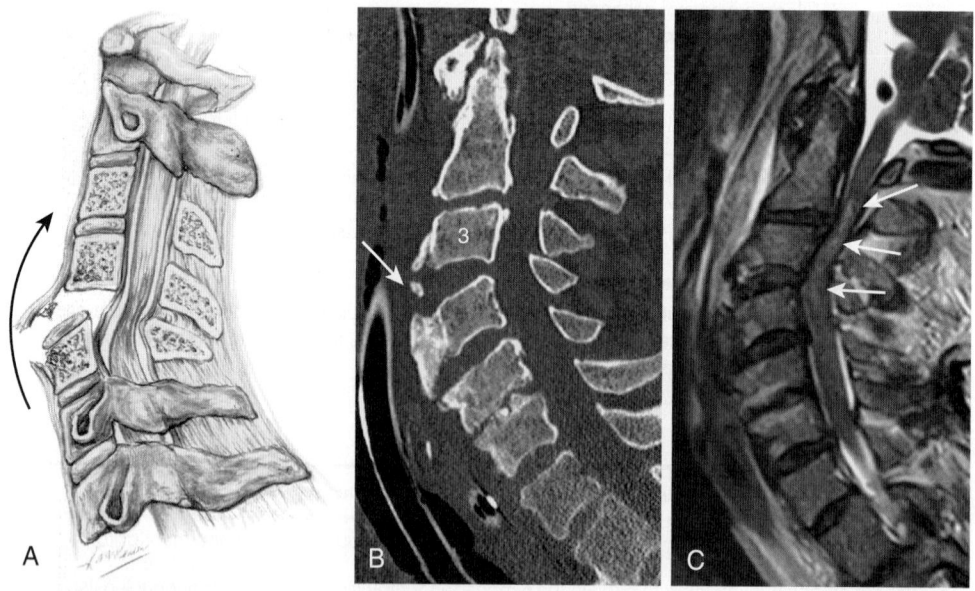

FIG. 192 Extension injury. A, Drawing shows mechanism and injury. There is a small avulsion from the anterosuperior margin of the vertebra immediately below the affected level. Note the wide disk space and retrolisthesis, hallmarks of this injury. The spinal cord is frequently injured in this setting. **B,** Sagittal reconstructed CT image shows widening of the C3 disk space with an avulsed fragment of bone *(arrow)* and retrolisthesis. **C,** T2-weighted MR image shows cord hemorrhage *(arrows).* The patient is quadriplegic. (Pope TL, Bloem HL et al: *Musculoskeletal imaging,* ed 2, Elsevier 2015, ISBN :978-1-4557-0813-0.)

ICD-10CM #	H55.00	Unspecified nystagmus
	H81.13	Benign paroxysmal vertigo, bilateral
	H81.49	Vertigo of central origin, unspecified ear
	H55.89	Other irregular eye movements

Identification of Types of Nystagmus (Fig. 200)

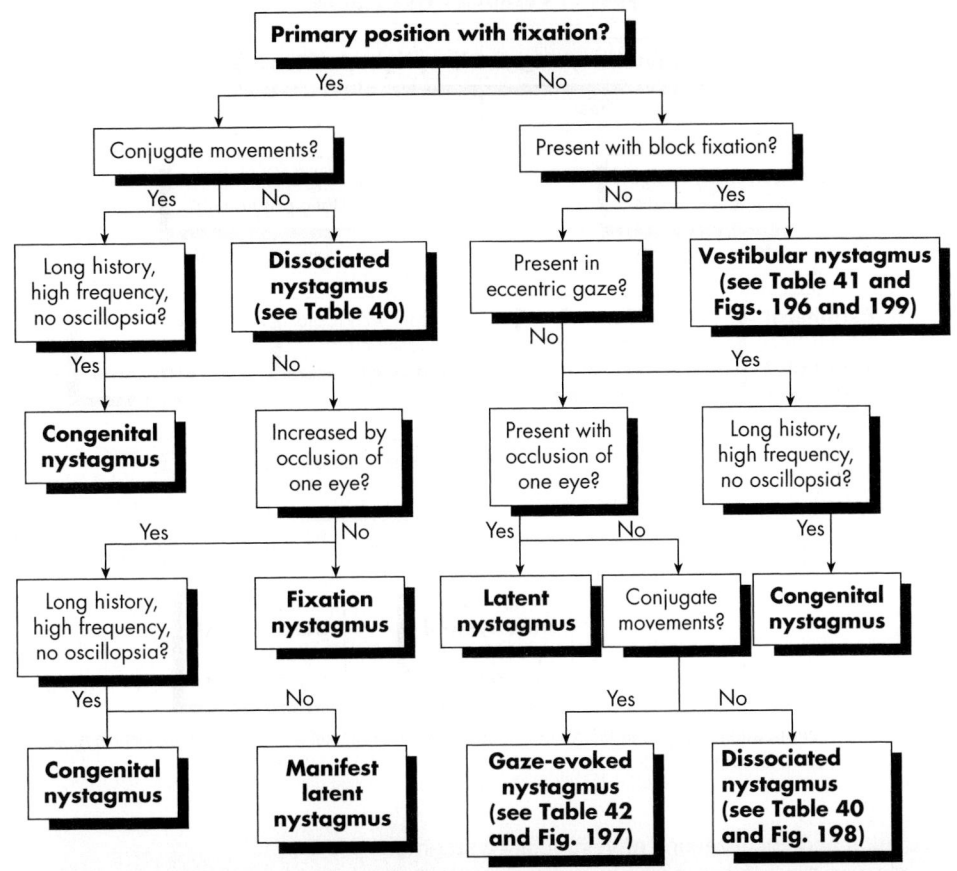

FIG. 195 Identification of types of nystagmus. (From Yanoff M, Duker JS: *Ophthalmology,* ed 2, St Louis, 2004, Mosby.)

Table 40 Characteristics and Localizations of Dissociated Nystagmus

Nystagmus	Characteristics	Localization
Acquired pendular in adults	Pendular, horizontal, vertical, torsional, disconjugate (coexisting palatal myoclonus)	Brain stem, cerebellum
Superior oblique myokymia	Pendular, jerk, torsional, vertical, high frequency, small amplitude, monocular	Trochlear nucleus
See-saw	Pendular, vertical, torsional, rising eye intorts, falling eye extorts; rarely jerk	Midbrain (interstitial nucleus of Cajal)
Abducting "nystagmus" of internuclear ophthalmoplegia	Jerk, horizontal, decreasing velocity slow components, larger in abducting eye	Medial longitudinal fasciculus in pons, midbrain horizontal gaze
Abducting nystagmus of myasthenia gravis	Gaze-paretic nystagmus in horizontal gaze, greater paresis of medial rectus muscle	Myoneural junction—myasthenia gravis

From Yanoff M, Duker JS: *Ophthalmology,* ed 2, St Louis, 2004, Mosby.

Clinical Algorithms

III

ICD-10CM #
H55.00	Unspecified nystagmus
H81.13	Benign paroxysmal vertigo, bilateral
H81.49	Vertigo of central origin, unspecified ear
H55.89	Other irregular eye movements

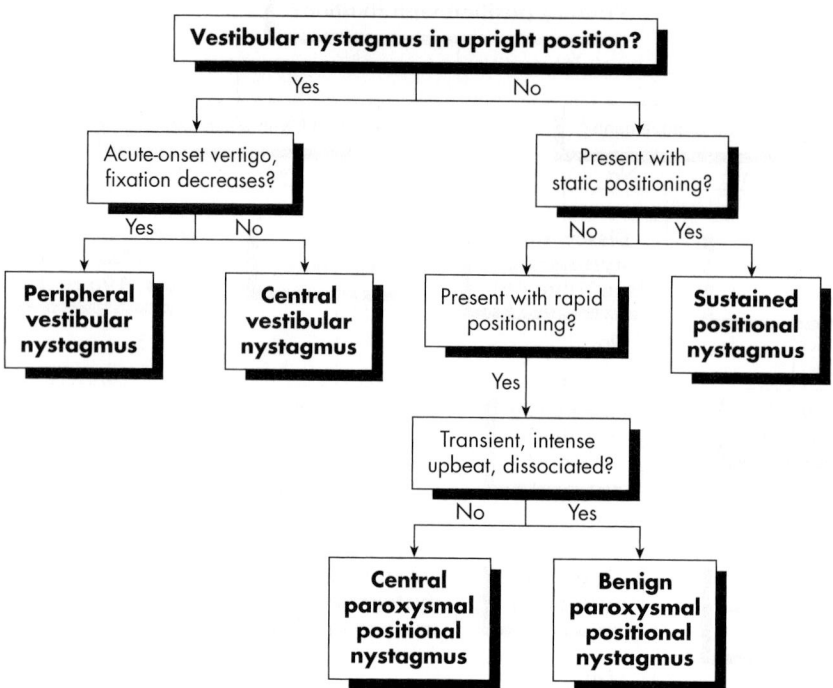

FIG. 196 Identification of types of vestibular nystagmus. (From Yanoff M, Duker JS: *Ophthalmology*, ed 2, St Louis, 2004, Mosby.)

Table 41   Characteristics and Localizations of Vestibular Nystagmus

Nystagmus	Characteristics	Localization
Spontaneous peripheral vestibular	Jerk, horizontal, small torsional, inhibited by fixation	Labyrinth, eighth nerve (acute)
Central vestibular (fixation) nystagmus	Jerk, pendular, horizontal, vertical, torsional, not inhibited by fixation	Brain stem, cerebellum
Sustained positional vestibular	Jerk, horizontal, small torsional, direction fixed, direction changing (static positioning)	Labyrinth, eighth nerve or brain stem, cerebellum
Benign paroxysmal positional	Jerk, dissociated upbeat, latency, not inhibited by fixation, fatigue (Nylen–Barany maneuver)	Posterior vertical canal
Central paroxysmal positional	Jerk, symmetric, upbeat, downbeat	Brain stem, cerebellum

From Yanoff M, Duker JS: *Ophthalmology*, ed 2, St Louis, 2004, Mosby.

Table 42   Characteristics and Localizations of Gaze-Evoked Nystagmus

Nystagmus	Characteristics	Localization
Physiologic, endpoint	Jerk, small amplitude, intermittent, extremes of horizontal and up gaze	Physiologic
Gaze-paretic (symmetric)	Jerk (decreasing velocity slow components) at 30° eccentric gaze	Nonlocalizing (drugs, mental fatigue)
Gaze-paretic (asymmetric)	Jerk (decreasing velocity slow components), horizontal, at 30° eccentric gaze, larger amplitude toward side of lesion	Lesions of brain stem, cerebellum, cerebral hemisphere
Rebound	Jerk, horizontal, decreases and direction can reverse in eccentric gaze, transient jerk nystagmus on return to primary gaze, fast components beating toward eccentric gaze	Cerebellum
Myasthenia gravis	Jerk, horizontal or vertical, gradual onset in prolonged eccentric gaze	Myoneural junction (fatigue—increasing transmission block)

From Yanoff M, Duker JS: *Ophthalmology*, ed 2, St Louis, 2004, Mosby.

NYSTAGMUS—cont'd

ICD-10CM #   H55.00   Unspecified nystagmus
             H81.13   Benign paroxysmal vertigo, bilateral
             H81.49   Vertigo of central origin, unspecified ear
             H55.89   Other irregular eye movements

1697

**Identification
of Types of Gaze-Evoked Nystagmus**

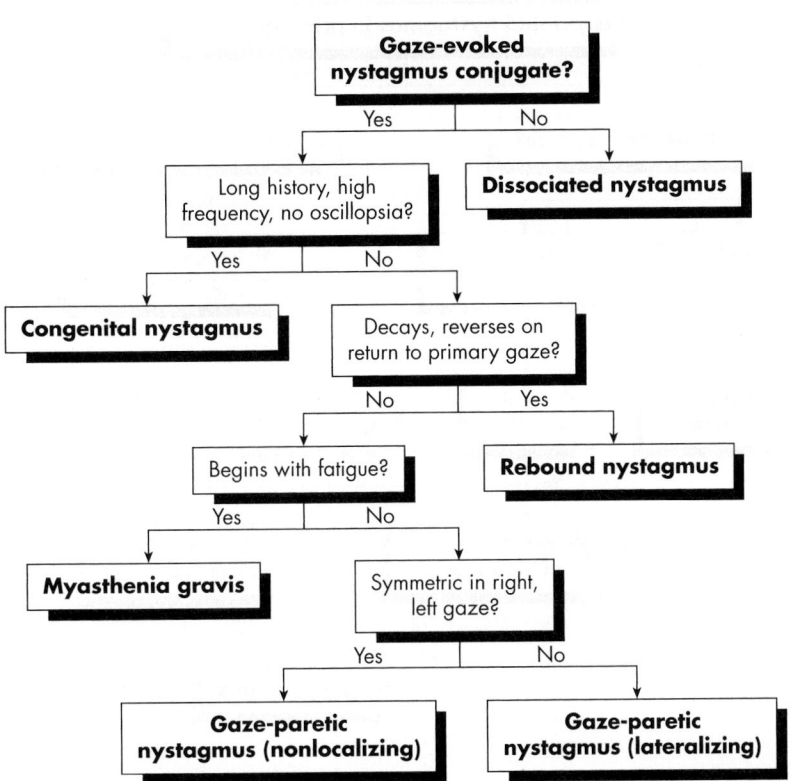

FIG. 197 **Identification of types of gaze-evoked nystagmus.** (From Yanoff M, Duker JS: *Ophthalmology,* ed 2, St Louis, 2004, Mosby.)

Clinical
Algorithms

III

ICD-10CM # H55.00 Unspecified nystagmus
H81.13 Benign paroxysmal vertigo, bilateral
H81.49 Vertigo of central origin, unspecified ear
H55.89 Other irregular eye movements

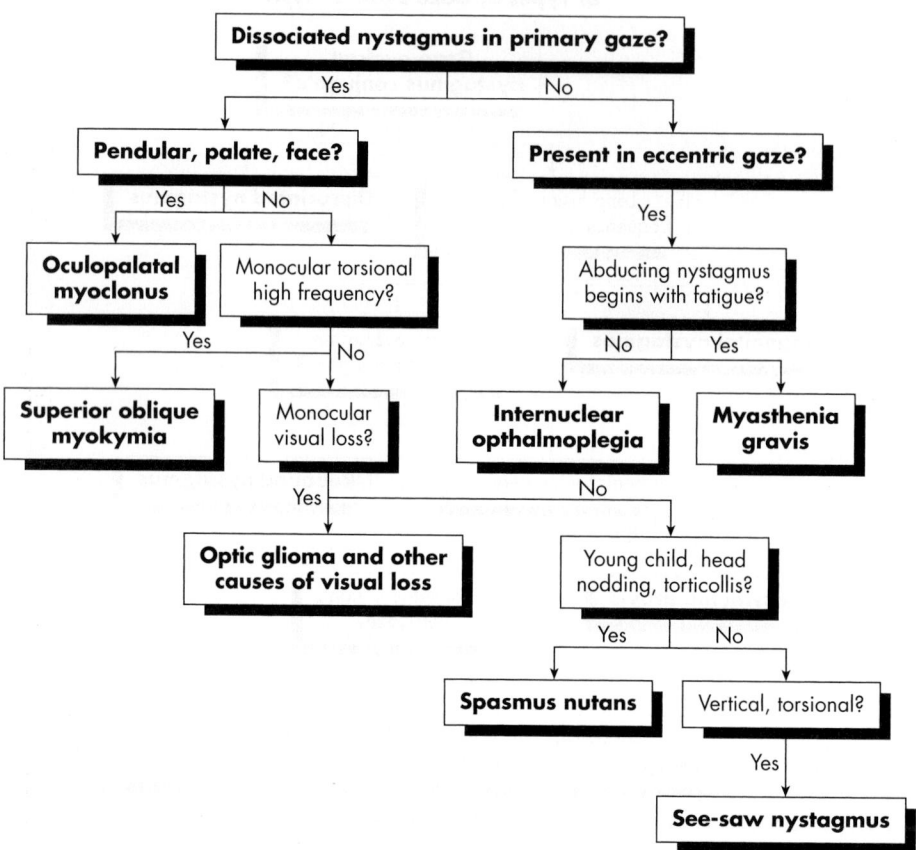

FIG. 198 Identification of types of dissociated nystagmus. (From Yanoff M, Duker JS: *Ophthalmology,* ed 2, St Louis, 2004, Mosby.)

ICD-10CM # H55.00 Unspecified nystagmus
H81.13 Benign paroxysmal vertigo, bilateral
H81.49 Vertigo of central origin, unspecified ear
H55.89 Other irregular eye movements

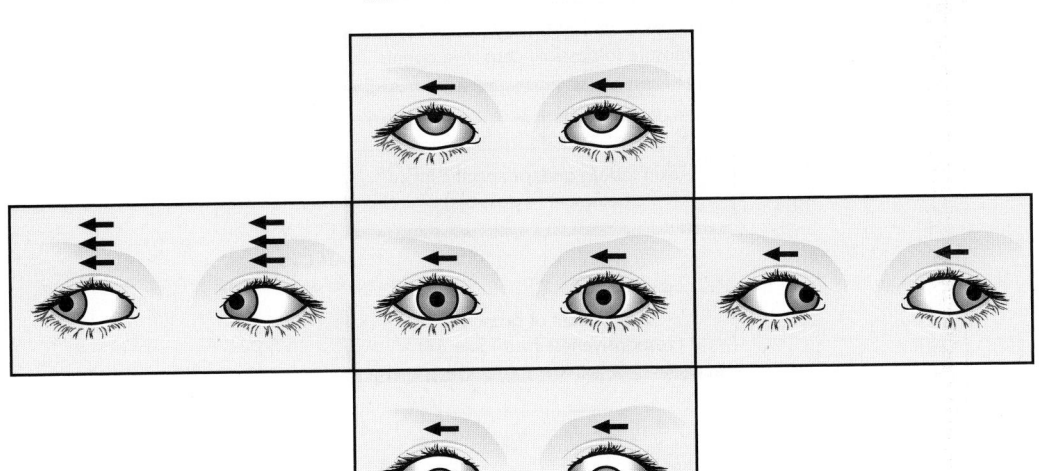

FIG. 199 Peripheral vestibular nystagmus (Courtesy of JJ Kanski, *Signs in Ophthalmology: Causes and Differential Diagnosis*, Mosby 2010) (Bowling B: *Kanski's Clinical ophthalmology, a systemic approach*, 8th ed, Elsevier, 2016, ISBN # 978-0-7020-5572-0.)

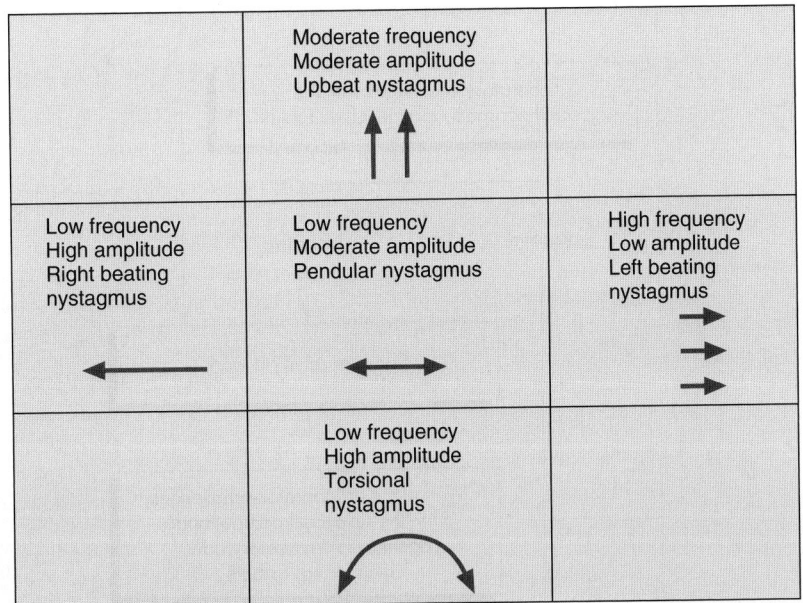

FIG. 200 Schematic for documenting nystagmus (Courtesy of JJ Kanski, *Signs in Ophthalmology: Causes and Differential Diagnosis*, Mosby 2010) (Bowling B: *Kanski's Clinical ophthalmology, a systemic approach*, 8th ed, Elsevier, 2016, ISBN # 978-0-7020-5572-0.)

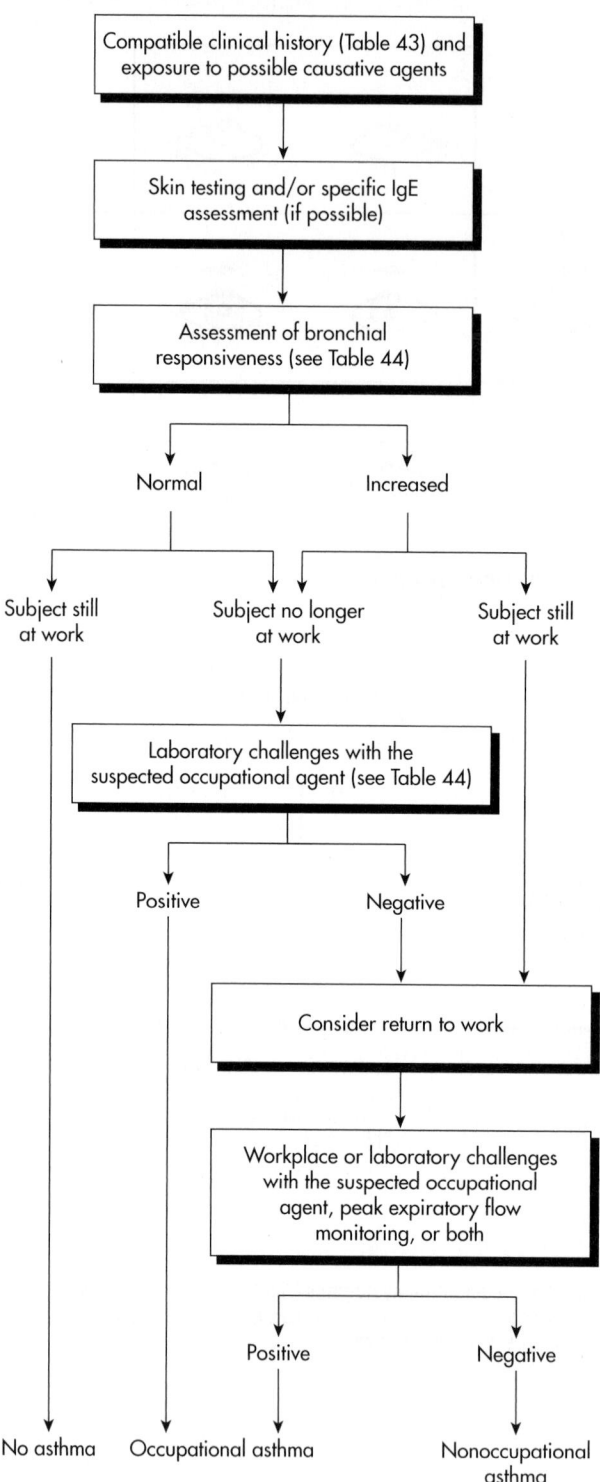

FIG. 201 Algorithm for the investigation of occupational asthma. *IgE,* Immunoglobulin E. (From Adkinson NF et al: *Middleton's allergy principles and practice*, ed 8, Philadelphia, 2014, Saunders.)

TABLE 43 Differences between Occupational Asthma with a Latency Period and Irritant-Induced Asthma

	OA with a Latency period	IrIA
Latency period	Variable but at least a matter of weeks	Onset of symptoms within minutes or hours
Mechanisms	Immunologic sensitization	?
Physiopathology	Like common asthma	Massive epithelial desquamation with early deposition of collagen. No role of eosinophils. Oxidative process.
Frequency	85%–90% of all cases of OA	10%–15% of all cases of OA
Symptoms	Wheeze predominant	Cough predominant
Function	The degree of airway hyperresponsiveness to methacholine reflects severity.	Severity not reflected by the degree of responsiveness to methacholine.
Response to bronchodilator	+++	++
Response to inhaled steroids	+++	++
Improvement with time	Good in general	Moderate, little or absent

IrIA, irritant-induced asthma; *OA*, occupational asthma.
Mason RJ, Broaddus CV et al: Murray & Nadel's Textbook of Respiratory Medicine, 5th ed, ISBN: 978-1-4160-4710-0, Philadelphia, Saunders 2010.

Table 44 Advantages and Limitations of Diagnostic Tests Used in the Investigation of Occupational Asthma (OA)

Diagnostic Test(s)	Advantages/Limitations
Assessment of bronchial responsiveness	• Simple, low cost • Allow to confirm the diagnosis of asthma • Low specificity for diagnosis of OA. The lack of NSBHR does not allow discarding the diagnosis of OA in subjects who have been removed from the workplace.
Immunologic tests	• Easy to perform, low cost • Commercial extracts are available (skin-prick tests or specific IgE for HMW agents). • Lack of standardization for a majority of occupational allergens except latex • Measure of specific IgE available for some LMW agents (anhydrides, acids, isocyanates, aldehydes), but low sensitivity • Identify the sensitization but not the disease itself
PEF monitoring	• Low cost • Requires the worker's collaboration • Low adherence (<60%) • Possible falsification of the results • Requires 2 weeks at and away from work, which are not always possible for the workers • Impossible to perform when the worker has already been removed from exposure • No standardized method for interpreting the results • Interpretation of the results requires experience
Specific inhalation challenges in the laboratory	• Confirmation of the diagnosis of OA when the test is positive • False-negative tests are possible. • Costly • Available in a small number of centers worldwide
Specific inhalation challenges at the workplace	• Exclude diagnosis if response is negative when performed in the usual work conditions • Requires usual work condition • Costly
Noninvasive measures of airway inflammation	Sputum cell counts • Impossible to falsify • Bring additional evidence to the diagnosis of OA • Costly • Not widely available • Does not allow to confirm or discard the diagnosis of OA by itself Exhaled NO measurement • Easy to perform • Inconsistent results • Difficult to interpret • Affected by many different factors

HMW, High-molecular-weight; *IgE*, immunoglobulin E; *LMW*, low-molecular-weight; *NO*, nitric oxide; *NSBHR*, nonspecific bronchial hyperresponsiveness; *PEF*, peak expiratory flow.
From Adkinson NF et al: *Middleton's allergy principles and practice*, ed 8, Philadelphia, 2014, Saunders.

Clinical Algorithms

III

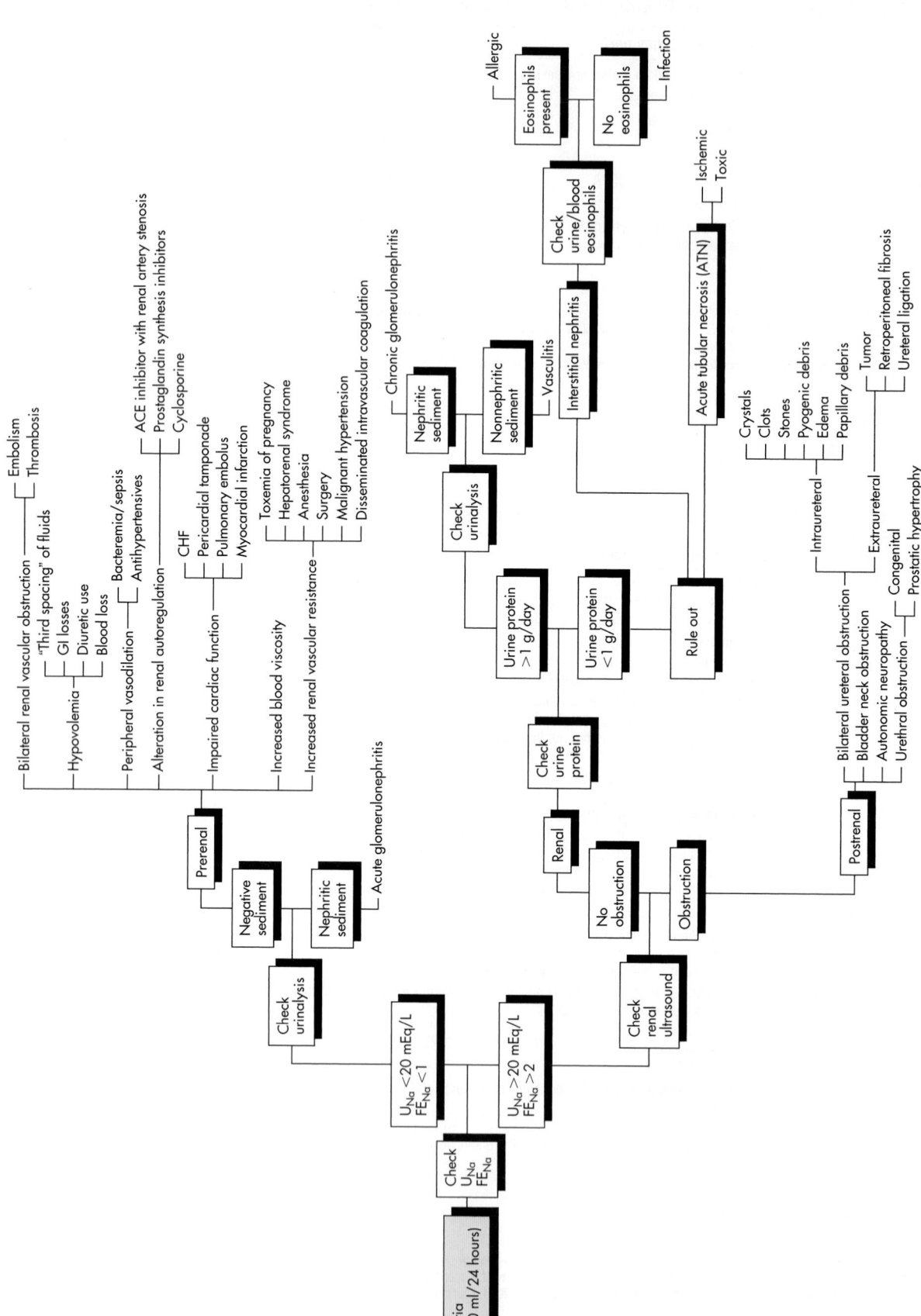

FIG. 202 Evaluation of oliguria. *ACE,* Angiotensin-converting enzyme; *CHF,* congestive heart failure; *GI,* gastrointestinal. (Modified from Healey PM: *Common medical diagnosis: an algorithmic approach,* ed 3, Philadelphia, 2000, Saunders.)

Evaluation of Patients with Palpitations, Dizziness, and/or Syncope

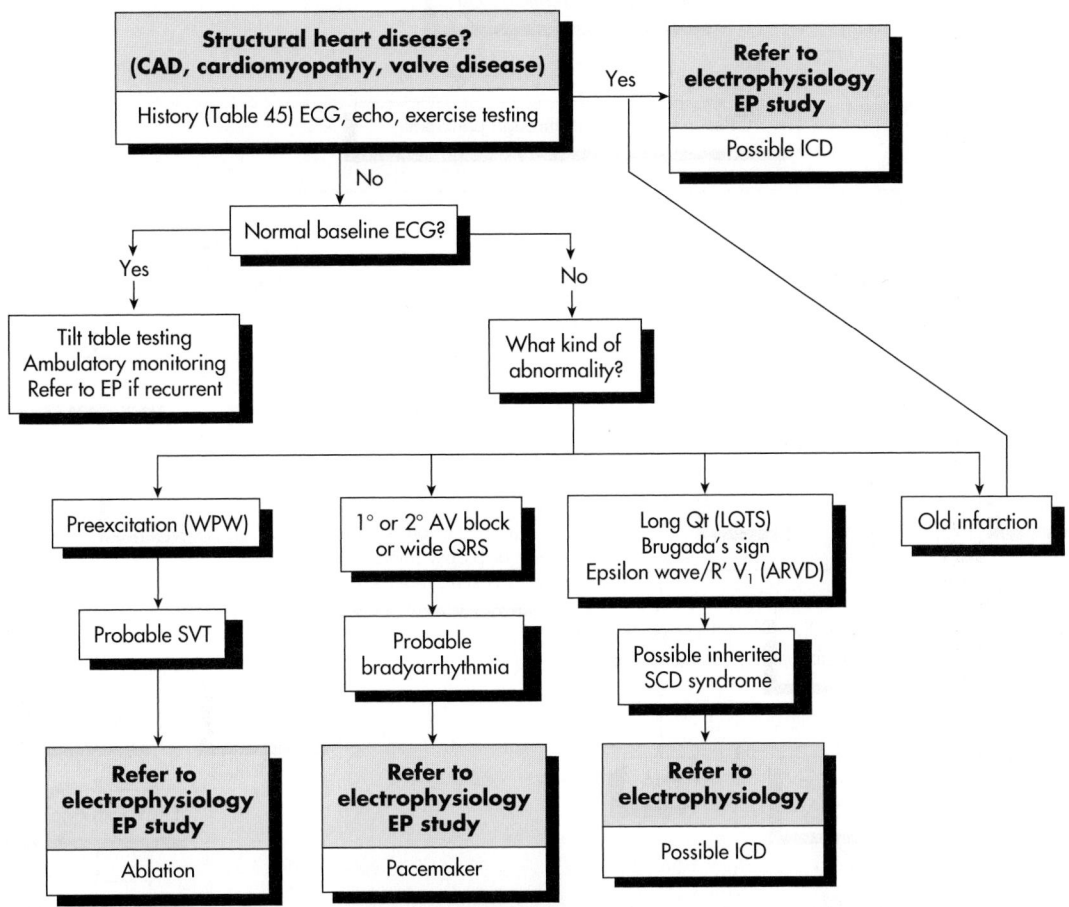

FIG. 204 Algorithm for evaluating patients with symptoms of palpitation, dizziness, or syncope. *ARVD,* Arrhythmogenic right ventricular dysplasia; *AV,* atrioventricular; *CAD,* coronary artery disease; *ECG,* electrocardiogram; *echo,* echocardiogram; *EP,* electrophysiology; *ICD,* implantable cardioverter-defibrillator; *LQTS,* long QT syndrome; *SCD,* sudden cardiac death; *SVT,* supraventricular tachycardia; *WPW,* Wolff-Parkinson-White syndrome. (From Goldman L, Schafer AI: *Goldman's Cecil medicine,* ed 24, Philadelphia, 2012, Saunders.)

Table 45 Items to Be Covered in History of Patient with Palpitation

Does the Palpitation Occur:	If So, Suspect:
As isolated "jumps" or "skips"?	Extrasystoles
In attacks known to be of abrupt beginning, with a heart rate of 120 beats/min or over, with regular or irregular rhythm?	Paroxysmal rapid heart action
Independent of exercise or excitement adequate to account for the symptom?	Atrial fibrillation, atrial flutter, thyrotoxicosis, anemia, febrile states, hypoglycemia, anxiety state
In attacks developing rapidly though not absolutely abruptly, unrelated to exertion or excitement?	Hemorrhage, hypoglycemia, tumor of the adrenal medulla
In conjunction with the taking of drugs?	Tobacco, coffee, tea, alcohol, epinephrine, ephedrine, aminophylline, atropine, thyroid extract, monoamine oxidase inhibitors
On standing?	Postural hypotension
In middle-aged women, in conjunction with flushes and sweats?	Menopausal syndrome
When the rate is known to be normal and the rhythm regular?	Anxiety state

From Goldman L, Braunwald E: Chest discomfort and palpitation. In Isselbacher KJ, Braunwald E et al [eds]: *Harrison's principles of internal medicine,* ed 13, New York, 1994, McGraw-Hill.

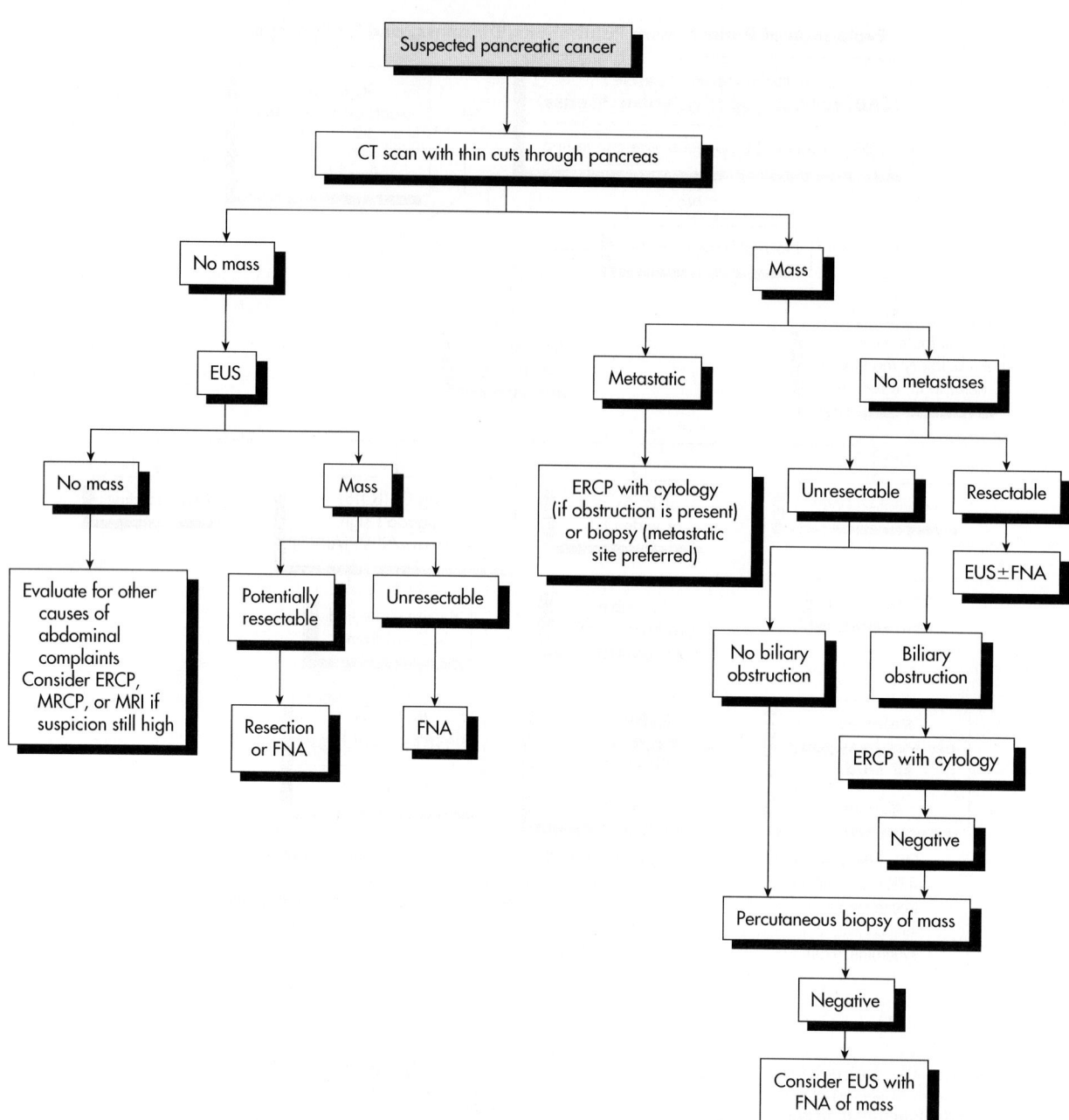

FIG. 206 Diagnostic algorithm for pancreatic cancer. Intraoperative fine-needle aspiration (FNA) if found inoperable during surgery. *CT,* Computed tomography; *ERCP,* endoscopic retrograde cholangiopancreatography; *EUS,* endoscopic ultrasonography; *MRI,* magnetic resonance imaging. (From Goldman L, Schafer AL [eds]: *Cecil textbook of medicine,* ed 24, Philadelphia, 2012, Saunders.)

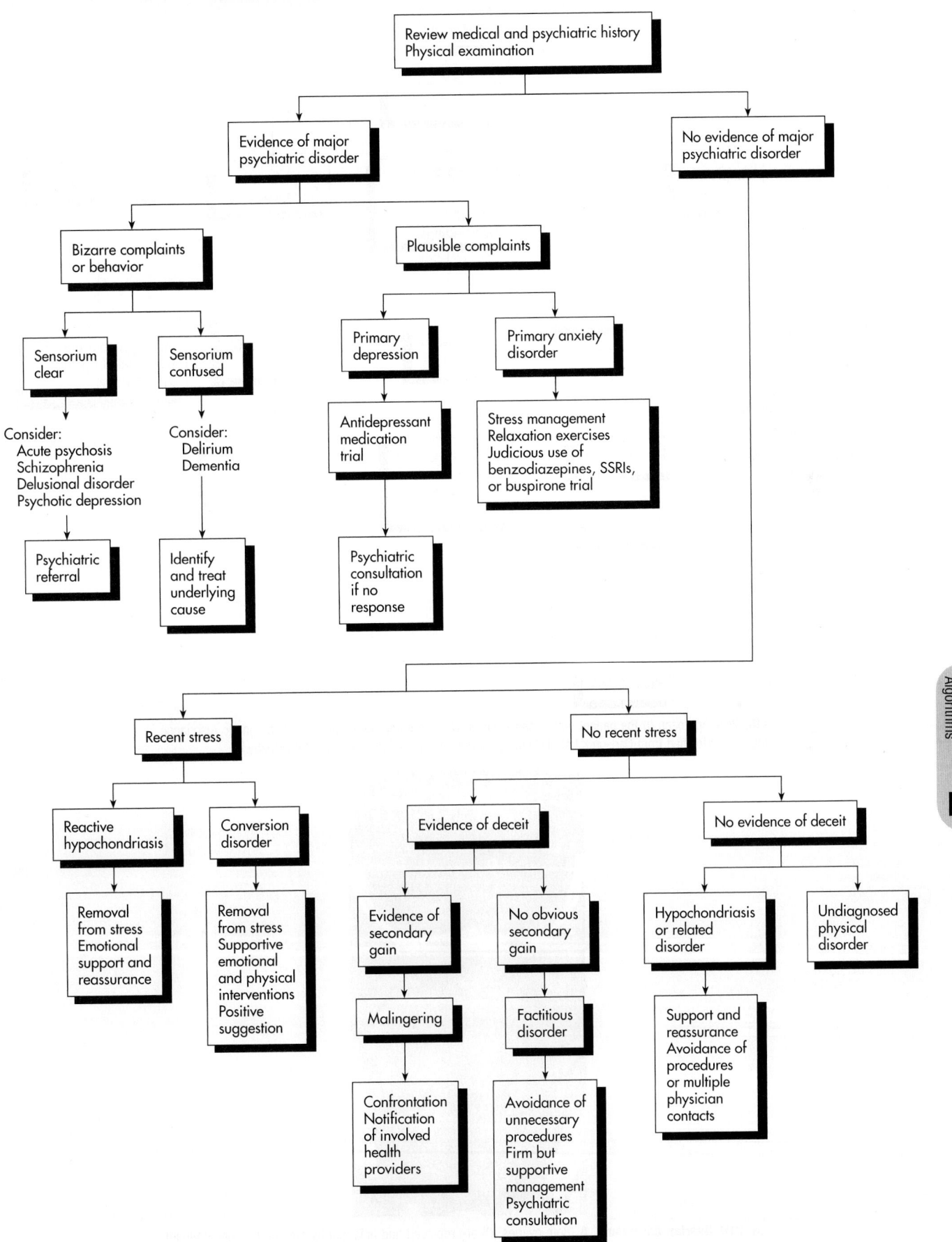

FIG. 208 Patient with ill-defined physical complaints. Previous or recent evaluations are noncontributory. *SSRIs,* Selective serotonin reuptake inhibitors. (From Greene H, Johnson WP, Lemcke D [eds]: *Decision making in medicine,* ed 2, St Louis, 1998, Mosby.)

Clinical Algorithms

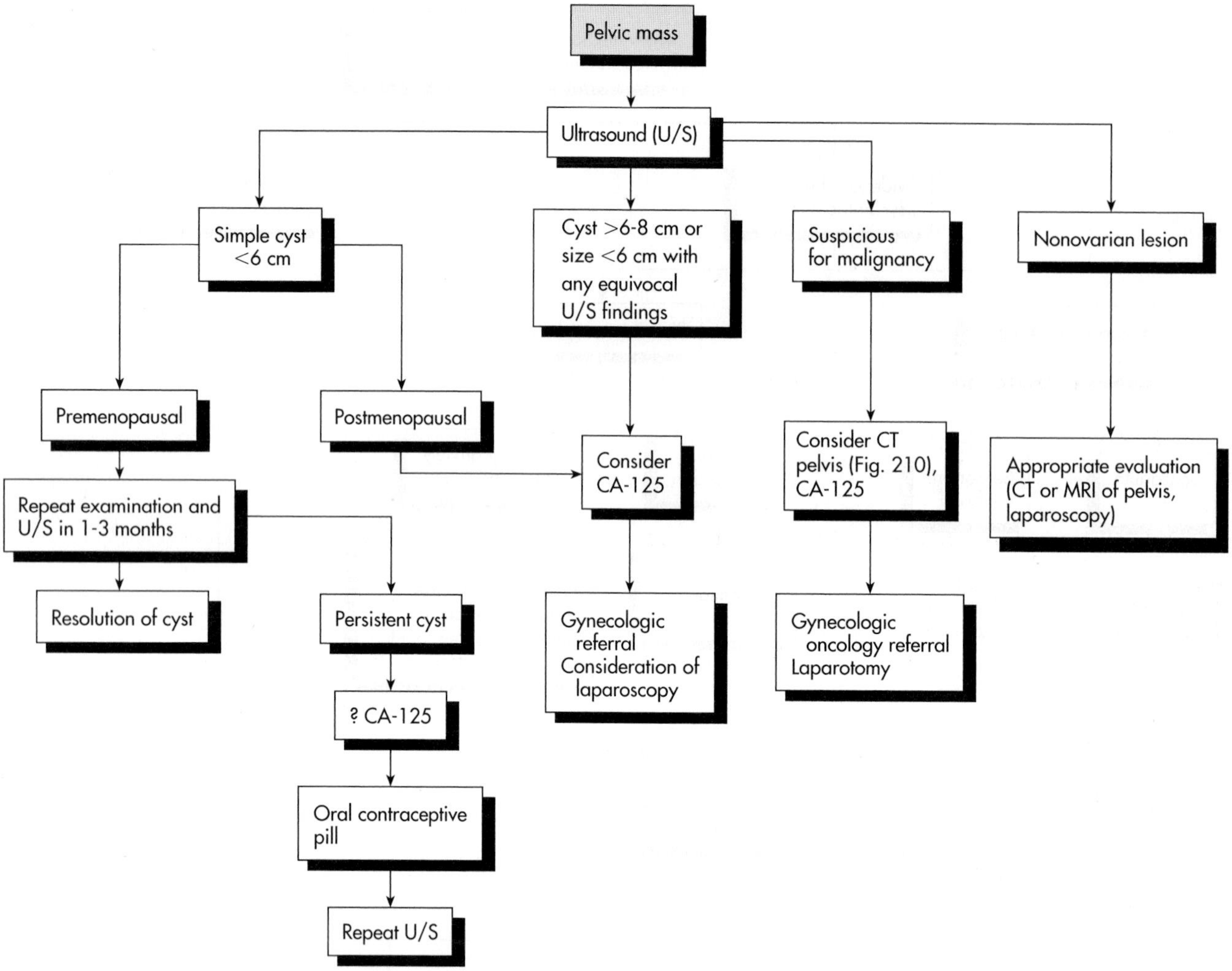

```
                              ┌─────────────┐
                              │ Pelvic mass │
                              └──────┬──────┘
                              ┌──────┴──────┐
                              │ Ultrasound  │
                              │    (U/S)    │
                              └─────────────┘
```

Pelvic mass → Ultrasound (U/S)

Ultrasound (U/S) branches to:

Simple cyst <6 cm →
- Premenopausal → Repeat examination and U/S in 1-3 months → Resolution of cyst
- Postmenopausal → Consider CA-125

Repeat examination and U/S in 1-3 months → Persistent cyst → ? CA-125 → Oral contraceptive pill → Repeat U/S

Cyst >6-8 cm or size <6 cm with any equivocal U/S findings → Consider CA-125 → Gynecologic referral Consideration of laparoscopy

Suspicious for malignancy → Consider CT pelvis (Fig. 210), CA-125 → Gynecologic oncology referral Laparotomy

Nonovarian lesion → Appropriate evaluation (CT or MRI of pelvis, laparoscopy)

FIG. 209 Approach to the patient with a pelvic mass. *CT,* Computed tomography; *MRI,* magnetic resonance imaging. (Modified from Carlson KJ et al: *Primary care of women,* ed 2, St Louis, 2002, Mosby.)

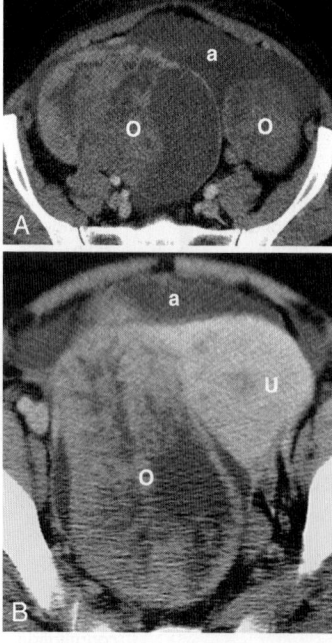

FIG. 210 Ovarian carcinoma. A, Both ovaries (O) are replaced and enlarged by tumors with predominant solid components. Ascites (a) is present providing strong evidence of tumor spread to the peritoneal cavity. **B,** A large mass (O) with predominant solid components arises from the right ovary and displaces the uterus (U) anteriorly and leftward. Ascites (a) is present. (From Webb WR, Brant WE, Major NM: *Fundamentals of body CT,* ed 4, Philadelphia, 2015, Saunders.)

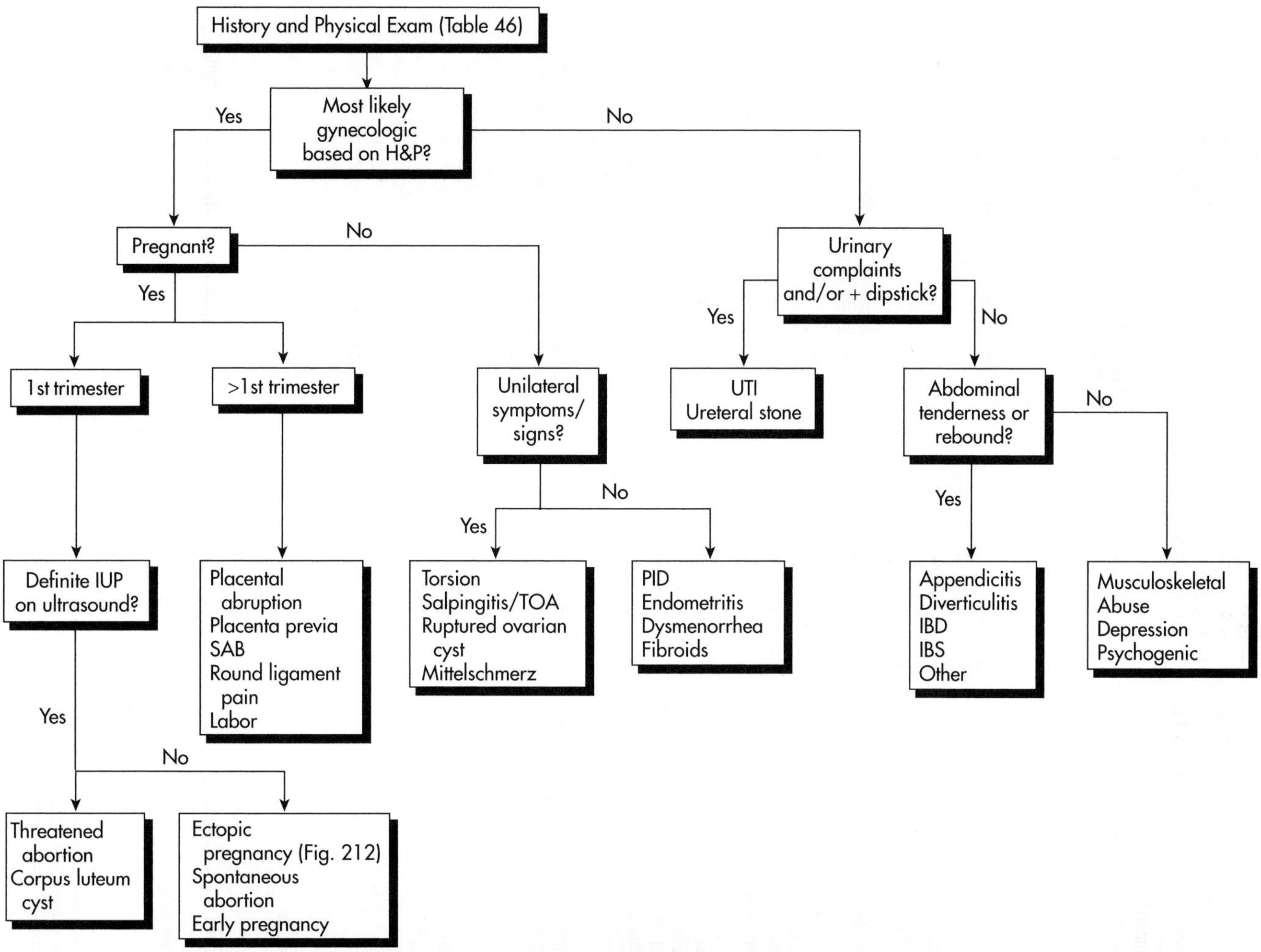

History and Physical Exam (Table 46)

Most likely gynecologic based on H&P?

— Yes → Pregnant?

— No → Urinary complaints and/or + dipstick?

Pregnant?
- Yes
- No

Urinary complaints and/or + dipstick?
- Yes → UTI / Ureteral stone
- No → Abdominal tenderness or rebound?

1st trimester

>1st trimester

Unilateral symptoms/signs?

Abdominal tenderness or rebound?
- Yes → Appendicitis / Diverticulitis / IBD / IBS / Other
- No → Musculoskeletal / Abuse / Depression / Psychogenic

1st trimester
→ Definite IUP on ultrasound?
- Yes → Threatened abortion / Corpus luteum cyst
- No → Ectopic pregnancy (Fig. 212) / Spontaneous abortion / Early pregnancy

>1st trimester
→ Placental abruption / Placenta previa / SAB / Round ligament pain / Labor

Unilateral symptoms/signs?
- Yes → Torsion / Salpingitis/TOA / Ruptured ovarian cyst / Mittelschmerz
- No → PID / Endometritis / Dysmenorrhea / Fibroids

FIG. 211 Diagnostic algorithm for acute pelvic pain. *H&P,* History and physical; *IBD,* inflammatory bowel disease; *IBS,* irritable bowel syndrome; *IUP,* intrauterine pregnancy; *PID,* pelvic inflammatory disease; *SAB,* spontaneous abortion; *TOA,* tubo-ovarian abscess; *UTI,* urinary tract infection. (From Marx JA et al: *Rosen's emergency medicine,* ed 8, Philadelphia, 2014, Saunders.)

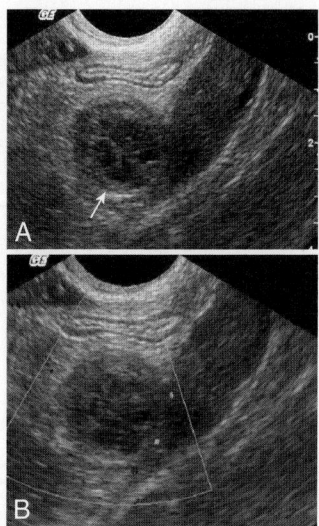

FIG. 212 Ectopic pregnancy seen as mixed-echogenicity mass. A 30-year-old woman presented with left lower quadrant pain at 7 weeks' gestation and β-hCG of 500 mIU/mL and falling over a 3-day period. **A,** In the left adnexa, medial to the left ovary, there was a 2-cm mass *(arrow)* with mixed echogenicity, and **B,** only minimal peripheral vascularity. A left ectopic pregnancy was confirmed and based on a falling β-hCG was treated expectantly and resolved without complication. (Rumack CM, Wilson SR, Charboneau JW, Levine D: Diagnostic Ultrasound, 4th ed . ISBN# 978-0-323-05397-6, Elsevier 2011.)

Table 46 Differentiation of Common or Potentially Catastrophic Causes of Pelvic Pain

Causative Disorder or Condition	Pain History	Associated Symptoms	Supporting History	Prevalence in ED	Physical Examination	Useful Tests	Atypical or Additional Aspects
Ectopic pregnancy (critical if ruptured)	Classically severe, sharp, lateral pelvic pain, but severity, location, and quality highly variable.	Vaginal bleeding (often mild, can be absent).	Missed period; history of previous ectopic pregnancy, infertility, pelvic surgery, PID, or IUD use.	Common	Classically unilateral adnexal tenderness, adnexal mass, and CMT.	Pelvic US, quantitative β-hCG, T&C, laparoscopy.	Cannot reliably exclude diagnosis based on history and physical examination. Severe pain, hypotension, or peritonitis suggests rupture.
Ruptured ovarian cyst (emergent—critical with significant hemorrhage; otherwise, urgent)	Abrupt moderate to severe lateral pain.	Light-headedness if bleeding is severe; rectal pain arises from fluid in cul-de-sac.		Uncommon	Hypotension and tachycardia if blood loss is significant; possible peritonitis.	Pelvic US, CBC, T&C.	Physical examination findings often do not correlate with volume of blood in pelvis at US.
Ovarian torsion (emergent)	Acute onset of moderate to severe lateral pain.	Nausea and vomiting.	History of ovarian mass or cyst.	Uncommon	Adnexal mass and tenderness, possible peritonitis.	US with Doppler flow studies, laparoscopy.	Torsion can be intermittent.
Appendicitis (emergent)	Duration often <48 hr, generalized followed by localized RLQ pain.	Low-grade fever, nausea, anorexia.	Migration of pain to RLQ from center, abdominal pain before vomiting.	Common	RLQ tenderness, possible peritonitis.	US or CT in unclear cases.	Early in course, tenderness may be minimal or poorly localized.
PID, TOA (TOA: emergent; PID: urgent-emergent)	Without TOA, pain usually bilateral. May manifest acutely within 48 hr or subacutely with up to 3 wk of pain.	Fever, vaginal discharge.	Vaginal discharge, history of PID, history of unprotected intercourse or multiple partners.	PID: common TOA: uncommon	Pus from cervical os, CMT, adnexal tenderness. Peritonitis suggests severe PID or TOA.	CBC, ESR, CRP, pelvic US, laparoscopy, cervical cultures, cervical smear for WBCs.	History and physical examination may be inaccurate for diagnosis, particularly in patients with subacute presentation.
UTI (urgent)	Pain with urination. Patient may have flank pain from associated pyelonephritis.	Urinary urgency and frequency; fever and vomiting if patient has associated pyelonephritis.	Recent urologic procedure, prior history of UTI.	Common	Suprapubic tenderness, flank tenderness and fever with pyelonephritis.	Urinalysis, urine culture (if recurrent or complicated).	WBCs can be present in urine with PID and appendicitis. RBCs present in urine with hemorrhagic cystitis.
Ureteral colic (urgent)	Acute onset, manifests within hours. Pain is lateral, usually moderate to severe. Often radiates into the groin or costovertebral angle or flank.	Nausea and vomiting.	Prior history of stones.	Common	Patient often appears uncomfortable, but physical examination can be otherwise unremarkable.	Urinalysis: hematuria present in approximately 80% of cases. Renal ultrasound for hydronephrosis. Abdominal CT.	If stone is at ureterovesicular junction, patient can have localized pain that can mimic appendicitis or other acute pelvic pathology.
Unruptured ovarian cyst or tumor	Lateral ache, gradual onset.	Often minimal.	Prior history of similar pain.	Common	Lateral pelvic tenderness, with or without a mass.	Pelvic US.	
Endometriosis	Unilateral or bilateral pelvic pain, often recurrent.	Dysmenorrhea, dyspareunia.	Prior history of same type of pain in association with menstrual cycle.	Common	Unilateral or bilateral adnexal tenderness, occasionally pelvic mass present, peritoneal findings uncommon.	Pelvic US, laparoscopy.	Symptoms can mimic other types of pelvic pathology; laparoscopy often is needed for confirmation.

β-hCG, β-Human chorionic gonadotropin; CBC, complete blood count; CMT, cervical motion tenderness; CRP, C-reactive protein; CT, computed tomography; ED, emergency department; ESR, erythrocyte sedimentation rate; IUD, intrauterine device; PID, pelvic inflammatory disease; RBC, red blood cell; RLQ, right lower quadrant; T&C, type and crossmatch; TOA, tubo-ovarian abscess; US, ultrasonography; UTI, urinary tract infection; WBC, white blood cell.
From Marx JA et al: *Rosen's emergency medicine*, ed 8, Philadelphia, 2014, Saunders.

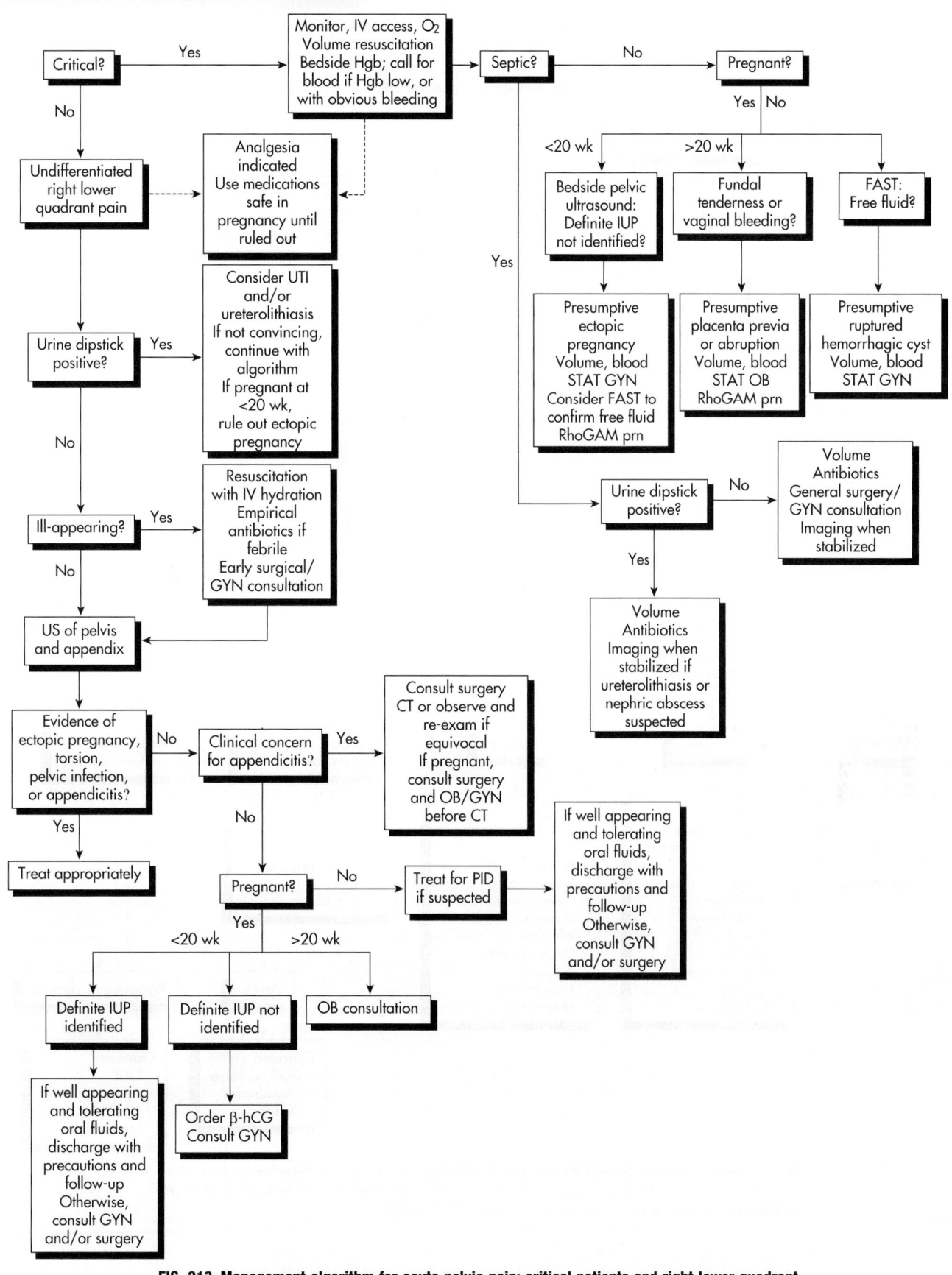

FIG. 213 Management algorithm for acute pelvic pain: critical patients and right lower quadrant pain presentations. β-hCG, β-Human chorionic gonadotropin; CT, computed tomography; FAST, focused assessment with sonography for trauma; GYN, gynecology; Hgb, hemoglobin; IUP, intrauterine pregnancy; IV, intravenous; OB, obstetrics; PID, pelvic inflammatory disease; STAT, immediately; US, ultrasound; UTI, urinary tract infection. (From Marx JA et al: *Rosen's emergency medicine*, ed 8, Philadelphia, 2014, Saunders.)

Clinical Algorithms

ICD-10CM # G60.9   Hereditary and idiopathic neuropathy, unspecified
G57.10 Meralgia paresthetica, unspecified lower limb
G90.09 Other idiopathic peripheral autonomic neuropathy

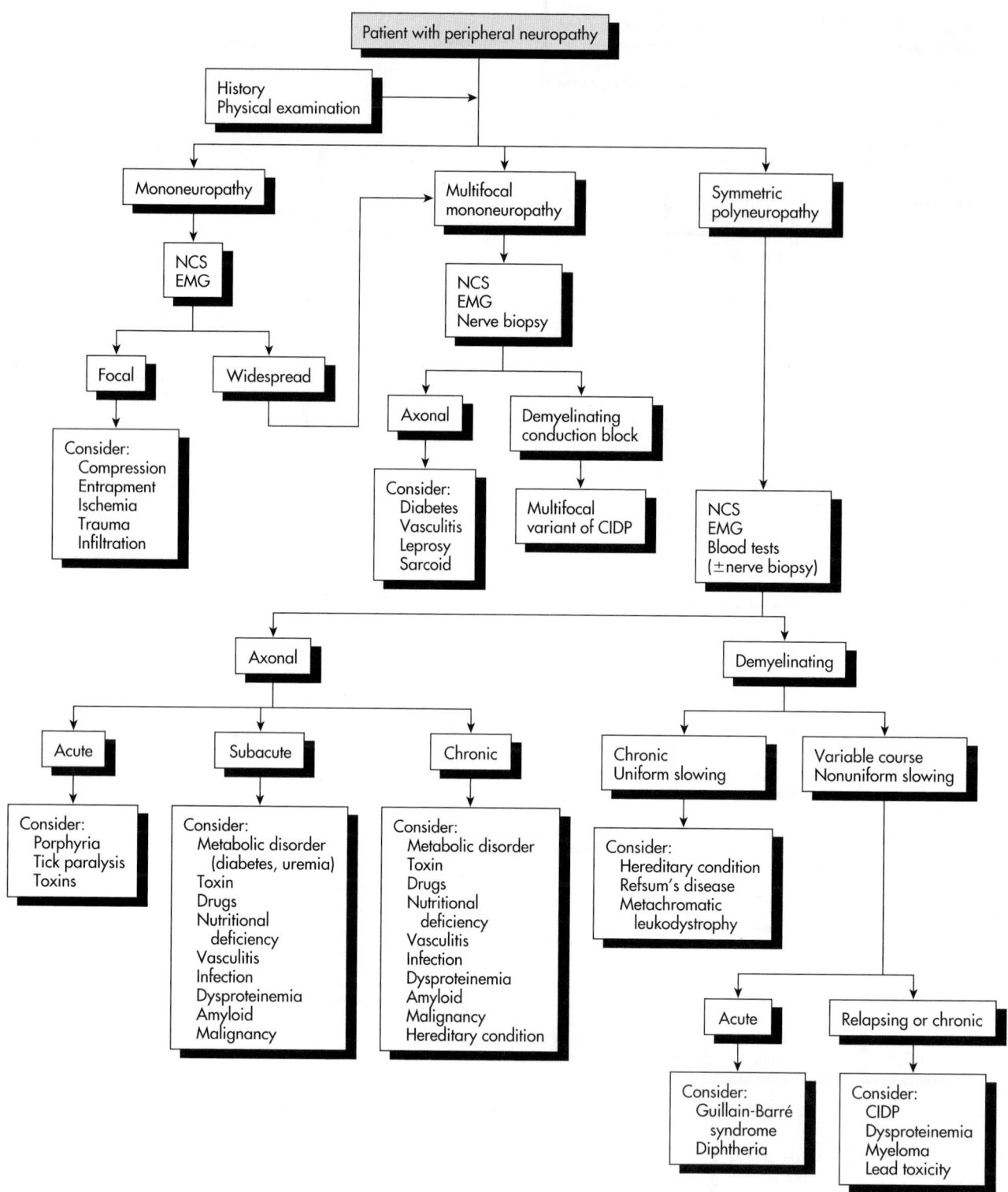

FIG. 215 Approach to the patient with peripheral neuropathy. *CIDP*, Chronic inflammatory demyelinating polyradiculopathy; *EMG*, electromyogram; *NCS*, nerve conduction studies. (From Greene HL, Johnson WP, Lemcke DL: *Decision making in medicine*, ed 2, St Louis, 1988, Mosby.)

PITUITARY TUMOR

ICD-10CM # D44.3 Neoplasm of uncertain behavior of pituitary gland
E22.8 Other hyperfunction of pituitary gland
E22.0 Acromegaly and pituitary gigantism

1711

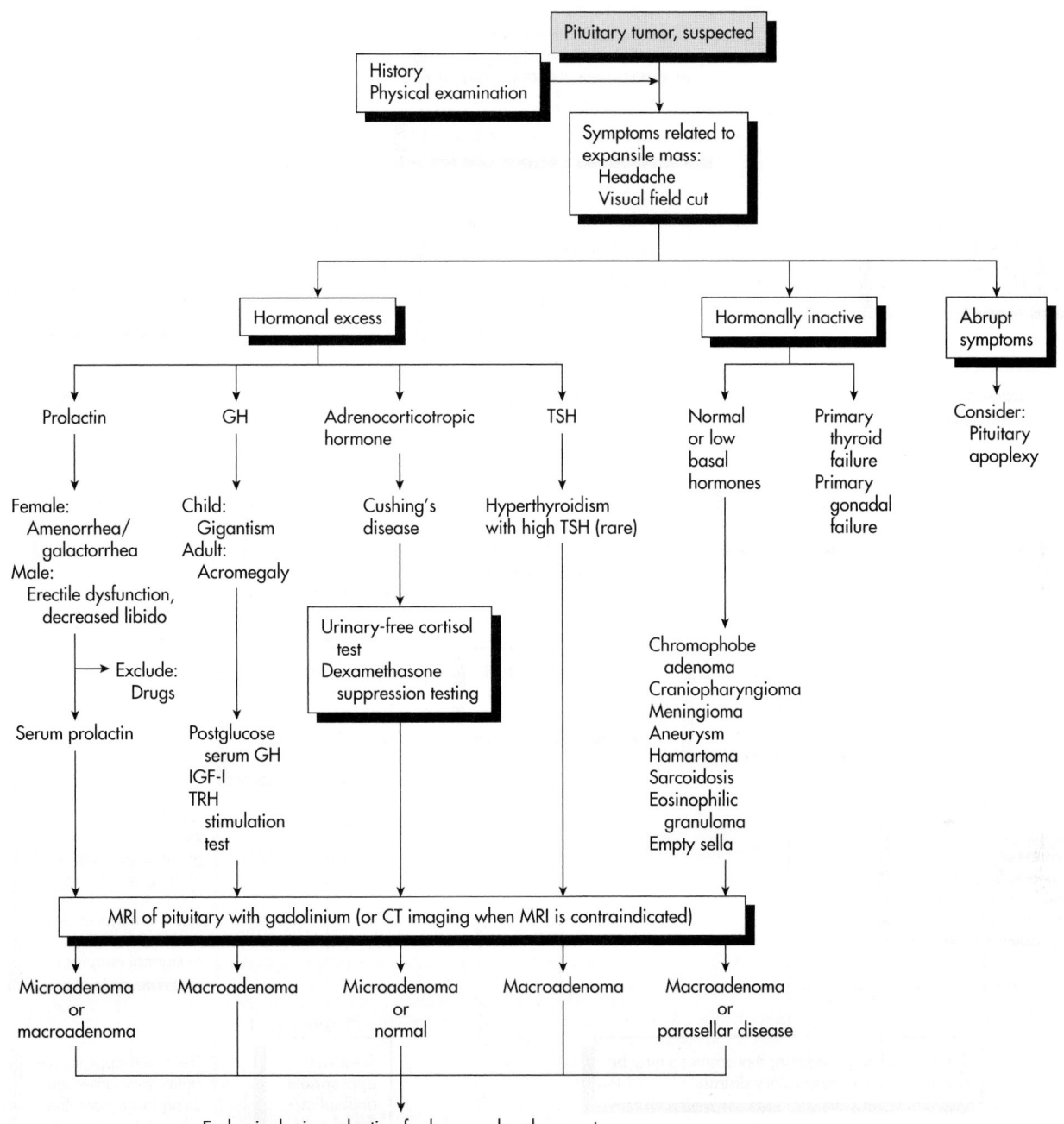

FIG. 217 Evaluation of suspected pituitary tumor. *CT,* Computed tomography; *GH,* growth hormone; *IGF-I,* one of the insulin-like growth factors; *MRI,* magnetic resonance imaging; *TRH,* thyrotropin-releasing hormone; *TSH,* thyroid-stimulating hormone. (Modified from Greene HL, Johnson WP, Lemcke DL: *Decision making in medicine,* ed 2, St Louis, 1998, Mosby.)

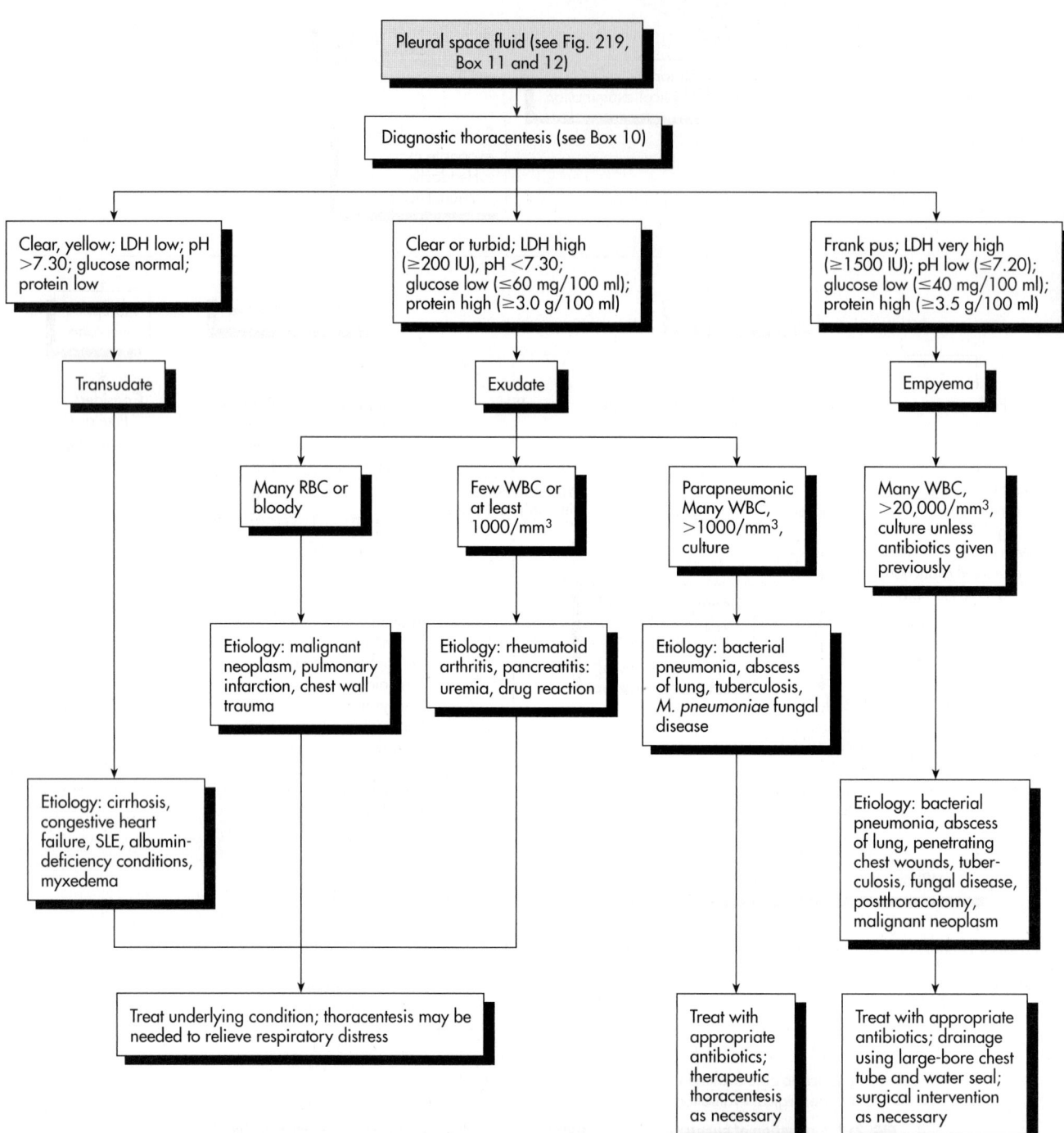

FIG. 218 Evaluation, common etiologies, and management of pleural effusion and empyema.
Additional information on empyema is available in Section I, Empyema. *LDH,* Lactate dehydrogenase; *RBC,* red
blood cells; *SLE,* systemic lupus erythematosus; *WBC,* white blood cells. (From Kassirer J [ed]: *Current therapy
in adult medicine,* ed 4, St Louis, 1998, Mosby.)

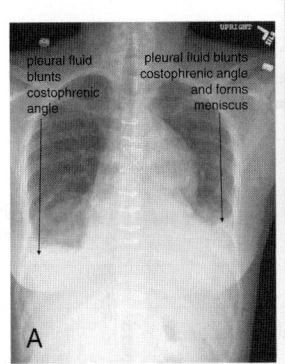

FIG. 219 Pleural effusions: Posterior-anterior (PA) and lateral upright views. A, A PA upright view, where a pleural effusion is most evident on this patient's left side. Both costophrenic angles are blunted. The pleural effusion forms a meniscus against the left lateral chest wall. **B,** The lateral upright view shows two meniscus densities, suggesting bilateral pleural effusions. The posterior diaphragmatic recess is filled with pleural fluid, which forms a meniscus with the posterior chest wall. (From Broder JS: *Diagnostic imaging for the emergency physician*, Philadelphia, 2011, Saunders.)

BOX 10   Light Criteria for Classification of Pleural Effusions

In 1972, Light et al. developed the currently accepted benchmark for classifying pleural fluid, as follows:
Pleural fluid protein-to-serum protein ratio >0.5:1
Pleural fluid lactate dehydrogenase (LDH)-to-serum LDH ratio >0.6:1
Pleural fluid LDH greater than two thirds the upper limit of normal for serum LDH (a cutoff value of 200 IU/L was used previously)
Pleural fluid is classified as an exudate if it meets any of the aforementioned criteria. Conversely, if all three characteristics are absent, the fluid is classified as a transudate. These researchers achieved a diagnostic sensitivity of 99% and a specificity of 98% for classification of an exudate.

From Adams JG, et al: *Emergency medicine, clinical essentials*, ed 2, Philadelphia, 2013, Elsevier.

BOX 11   Signs and Symptoms of Effusion[5]

Dyspnea
Cough (dry, nonproductive)
Chest pain (pleuritic or nonpleuritic)
Chest wall discomfort
Decreased breath sounds
Dullness to percussion
Egophony, tactile fremitus
Pleural friction rub
   Disease-specific signs and symptoms may include:
Orthopnea
Paroxysmal nocturnal dyspnea
Fever
Night sweats

[5]A detailed past medical history may uncover the cause of the effusion.
From Adams JG, et al: *Emergency medicine, clinical essentials*, ed 2, Philadelphia, 2013, Elsevier.

BOX 12   Causes of Pleural Effusions

Transudates
Atelectasis (early)
Congestive heart failure
Cirrhosis
Glomerulonephritis
Hypoalbuminemia
Myxedema
Nephrotic syndrome
Peritoneal dialysis
Pulmonary embolism
Superior vena cava syndrome

Exudates
Infectious
Bacterial infection
Bronchiectasis
Fungal infection
Lung abscess
Parasitic infection
Traumatic hemothorax
Tuberculosis
Viral illness

Malignancies
Lymphoma
Mesothelioma
Primary lung cancer
Pulmonary metastasis

Connective Tissue Disease
Rheumatoid arthritis
Systemic lupus erythematosus

Abdominal/Gastrointestinal
Esophageal rupture
Pancreatic disorders
Subphrenic abscess

Other
Atelectasis (chronic)
Chylothorax
Drug reactions (amiodarone)
Postpartum state
Pulmonary infarction or embolism
Uremia

From Adams JG, et al: *Emergency medicine, clinical essentials*, ed 2, Philadelphia, 2013, Elsevier.

Clinical
Algorithms

III

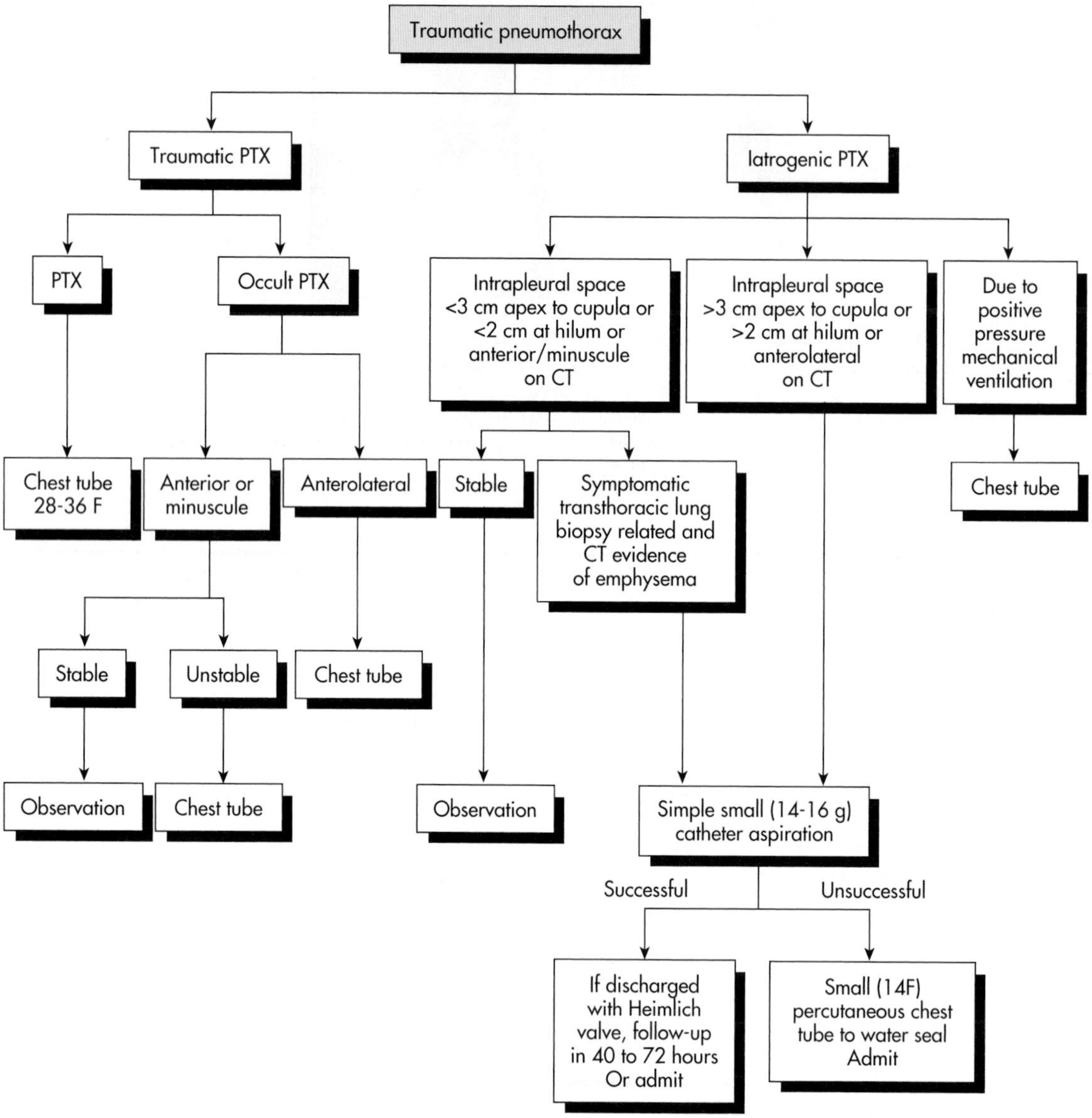

Traumatic pneumothorax

Traumatic PTX | Iatrogenic PTX

PTX | Occult PTX

Intrapleural space <3 cm apex to cupula or <2 cm at hilum or anterior/minuscule on CT | Intrapleural space >3 cm apex to cupula or >2 cm at hilum or anterolateral on CT | Due to positive pressure mechanical ventilation

Chest tube 28-36 F | Anterior or minuscule | Anterolateral | Stable | Symptomatic transthoracic lung biopsy related and CT evidence of emphysema | Chest tube

Stable | Unstable | Chest tube

Observation | Chest tube | Observation | Simple small (14-16 g) catheter aspiration

Successful　　　Unsuccessful

If discharged with Heimlich valve, follow-up in 40 to 72 hours Or admit | Small (14F) percutaneous chest tube to water seal Admit

FIG. 221 Algorithmic approach to the treatment of traumatic pneumothorax. *CT*, Computed tomography; *PTX*, pneumothorax. (From Adams JG, et al: *Emergency medicine, clinical essentials*, ed 2, Philadelphia, 2013, Elsevier.)

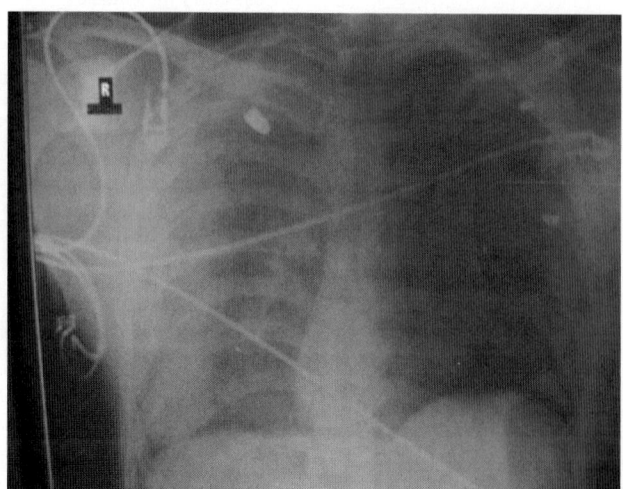

FIG. 222 Hemothorax secondary to gunshot wound. Note haziness over right hemithorax with bullet seen in right upper lobe. (Marx JA et al: *Rosen's Emergency Medicine*, ed 8, Philadelphia, 2014, Saunders.)

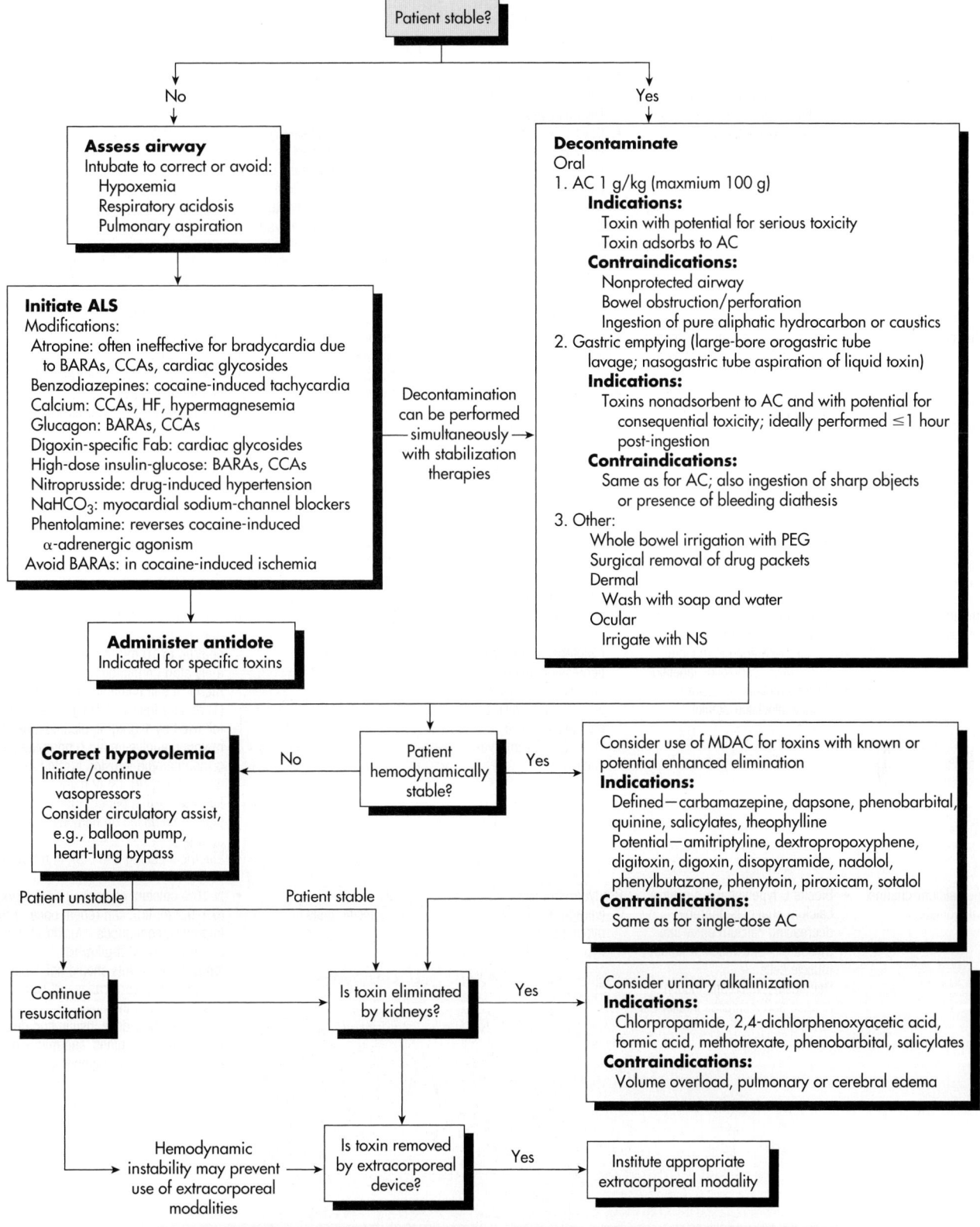

FIG. 223 Algorithm for the management of acute poisoning. See also Table 47. *AC,* Activated charcoal; *ALS,* advanced life support; *BARAs,* β-adrenergic receptor antagonists; *CCAs,* L-type calcium-channel antagonists; *HF,* hydrofluoric acid; *MDAC,* multidose activated charcoal; *NS,* 0.9% saline solution; *PEG,* nonabsorbable polyethylene glycol solution. (From Goldman L, Schafer AI: *Goldman's Cecil medicine,* ed 24, Philadelphia, 2012, Saunders.)

Clinical
Algorithms

Table 47 Pathophysiology, Clinical Effects, and Management of Specific Drugs and Toxicants

Drug or Toxicant	Pathophysiology	Clinical Effects	Laboratory	Specific Therapy
Acetaminophen	NAPQI (toxic metabolite) binds hepatic and renal tubular cells; acetaminophen itself induces transient decrease in functional factor VII	• Initial: nausea, vomiting, coma, lactic acidosis in severe cases • Days 1-3: elevated INR, aminotransferase, and bilirubin levels; RUQ tenderness; increased creatinine level in severe cases • Days 4-14: gradual recovery or continued increase in INR and creatinine, lactic acidosis, coma, cerebral edema, death	• Potentially toxic level ≥150 μg/ml 4 hr after ingestion* • INR may be transiently elevated in first 24 hr because of decrease in functional factor VII; further increases indicate hepatic necrosis; elevated aminotransferase and bilirubin levels not predictive of hepatic failure • Creatinine elevated in severe cases	NAC can increase INR but not aPTT†
Amphetamines	• Increased release of presynaptic norepinephrine and dopamine • Increased serotonin release (especially MDMA, PMA, DOB, other synthetic amphetamines)	• Mild: euphoria, decreased appetite, repetitive behavior • Moderate: vomiting, agitation, hypertension, tachycardia, mydriasis, bruxism, diaphoresis • Severe: hypertension or hypotension, arrhythmias, hyperthermia, seizures, coma, hepatotoxicity, rhabdomyolysis, DIC, hyponatremia (SIADH), renal failure, cerebral infarction or hemorrhage	Not helpful; many false-positives and false-negatives on screening tests	IV crystalloids External cooling Benzodiazepines or barbiturates to control agitation or seizures Benzodiazepines or nitroprusside for hypertension See SSRIs/SRIs for features and treatment of serotonin syndrome
β-Adrenergic receptor antagonists	Blocks catecholamines from β-adrenergic receptors • α- and β-adrenergic receptor antagonism: carvedilol, labetalol • Delayed rectifier potassium-channel blockade: sotalol	Bradyarrhythmias, decreased myocardial contractility, hypotension, respiratory depression, decreased consciousness with seizures or coma (lipophilic agents, e.g., propranolol), prolonged QT interval (sotalol)	• ECG • No specific tests	• IV glucagon, 3.5-5 mg over 2-min period; if no increase in BP or HR, can repeat up to 10 mg; if effective, immediately start continuous infusion at 2-10 mg/hr; if still unstable, options include (1) regular insulin, 1 U/kg by IV bolus, followed by 1 U/kg/hr, plus dextrose to maintain euglycemia; (2) norepinephrine or dobutamine infusion titrated to desirable BP and HR; (3) IV milrinone, 50 μg/kg over 10-min period, then 0.375-0.75 μg/kg/min based on hemodynamic status‡ • Electrical pacing and IABP in refractory cases
L-type calcium-channel antagonists	• Blocks L-type voltage-sensitive calcium channels, thereby decreasing calcium entry into myocardial and vascular smooth muscle cells • Decreases pancreatic insulin release and increases insulin resistance	Bradyarrhythmias (verapamil, diltiazem), hypotension, hyperglycemia	• ECG • No specific tests	• IV 10% calcium chloride, 10-20 mg/kg (0.1-0.2 ml/kg); can repeat once; if BP improves, continuous infusion at 0.2-0.5 ml/kg/hr (20-50 mg/kg/hr) • Ionized Ca^{2+} levels should not exceed 2× normal (severe cases will be refractory to calcium therapy) • Glucagon, high-dose insulin and dextrose, catecholamines, and milrinone (as for β-adrenergic antagonists)

Table 47 Pathophysiology, Clinical Effects, and Management of Specific Drugs and Toxicants—cont'd

Drug or Toxicant	Pathophysiology	Clinical Effects	Laboratory	Specific Therapy
Cardiac glycosides, including digoxin, bufadienolides (toxic toad venom), or cardenolides (e.g., oleander, lily of the valley, dogbane)	• Inhibits Na^+, K^+-ATPase • Decreased CNS sympathetic output • Decreased baroreceptor sensitivity • Increased vagal acetylcholine discharge	Bradyarrhythmias, including second- and third-degree AV block and asystole Ventricular ectopy, tachycardia, fibrillation Junctional tachycardia, paroxysmal atrial tachycardia with block Weakness, visual disturbances, nausea, vomiting	• Serum digoxin level • Serum potassium (hyperkalemia occurs in acute poisoning; hypokalemia may be present in chronic poisoning), magnesium, and creatinine levels	• Correct hypokalemia and hypomagnesemia; do not give calcium • Digoxin-specific antibody fragments (Fab) indicated if patient has hemodynamically significant arrhythmias, serum potassium ≥5 mg/L, Mobitz II or third-degree AV block, ingestion of bufadienolide- or cardenolide-containing agents, or renal insufficiency • Empirical dose • Chronic: 2-5 vials • Acute: 10-20 vials • Calculated dose • Chronic: number of vials = 2 × serum digoxin level (ng/ml) × 5.6 × weight (kg)/1000 • Acute: number of vials = 2 × oral digoxin dose (mg) × 0.8
Cyclic antidepressants	Myocardial sodium- and potassium-channel blockade Blockade of α-adrenergic and cholinergic muscarinic receptors Inhibition of norepinephrine reuptake	• Decreased level of consciousness (can develop rapidly), myoclonus, seizures, coma • Anticholinergic toxidrome • Sinus tachycardia, ventricular conduction delays, ventricular arrhythmias, asystole • Hypotension	Serum levels not helpful in management	• Intermittent IV boluses of $NaHCO_3$ (1 mEq/kg) to maintain arterial pH at 7.5 because acidemia can worsen cardiovascular complications • Intubation and neuroparalytic drugs may be useful to ameliorate acidemia from muscular hyperactivity while seizures are being treated • Contraindicated drugs: types IA and IC antiarrhythmic agents; physostigmine, flumazenil
Ethylene glycol, methanol (e.g., antifreeze, window cleaners, camping stove fuels)	• Ethylene glycol: toxic metabolites produce cytotoxicity in CNS, kidneys, lungs, heart, liver, muscles; metabolic acidosis is due to glycolate accumulation; oxalate complexes with calcium, so hypocalcemia can develop • Methanol: metabolized to formic acid, which is responsible for metabolic acidosis and inhibition of cytochrome aa_3; target organs include retina, optic nerve, CNS	• Ethylene glycol: CNS depression, cerebral edema, seizures, anion gap metabolic acidosis, renal failure with acute tubular necrosis, pulmonary edema, myositis • Methanol: nausea, vomiting; cerebral edema, hemorrhage, infarcts; necrosis of thalamus and putamen; anion gap metabolic acidosis; visual disturbances, papilledema, hyperemic optic disc, nonreactive pupils	• Serum ethylene glycol and methanol levels; levels may be low or undetectable if significant metabolism has occurred • Ethylene glycol: serum calcium, creatinine, BUN levels; examine urine for calcium oxalate crystals; false hyperlactatemia occurs with certain analyzers using L-lactate oxidase, which cross-reacts with glycolic and glyoxylic acids	• For both: fomepizole (which inhibits alcohol dehydrogenase and blocks formation of toxic metabolites), 15 mg/kg IV loading dose, then 10 mg/kg IV for 4 doses during the next 48 hr, then 15 mg/kg for subsequent doses; interval dosing is q12h (q4h during hemodialysis, with dosing interval adjustments at start and finish); continue until ethylene glycol or methanol is no longer detectable • Use of ethanol is no longer recommended • Hemodialysis: initiate if level is ≥50 mg/dl or metabolic acidosis with end-organ toxicity; continue until acidosis resolves and serum level of ethylene glycol or methanol is undetectable • Monitor for cerebral edema with possible herniation • Ethylene glycol: IV calcium for symptomatic hypocalcemia • Methanol: folinic acid, 50 mg IV q4h until methanol not detectable and acidosis cleared
γ-Hydroxybutyrate (GHB) and its precursors (γ-butyrolactone and 1,4-butanediol [1,4-BD])	Agonist effect on CNS GHB receptors; indirect action with opioid receptors (may increase proenkephalins); metabolized to GABA, interacts with $GABA_B$ receptors; decreases dopamine release	• CNS: rapid loss of consciousness, with recovery typical within 2-4 hr; myoclonus (possible seizures) • Respiratory depression; bradycardia; nausea, vomiting	No specific tests	• Supportive care, including respiratory support as needed • Withdrawal resembles sedative-hypnotic withdrawal and can be treated with benzodiazepines or pentobarbital

Clinical Algorithms

III

Continued on next page

Table 47   Pathophysiology, Clinical Effects, and Management of Specific Drugs and Toxicants—cont'd

Drug or Toxicant	Pathophysiology	Clinical Effects	Laboratory	Specific Therapy
Lithium	Decreases brain inositol; alters CNS serotonin, dopamine, and norepinephrine; inhibits adenylate cyclases, including those that mediate vasopressin-induced renal concentration and thyroid function	• Chronic toxicity usually more severe than acute toxicity: tremor, hyperreflexia, drowsiness, incoordination, clonus, confusion, ataxia; in severe cases, seizures, coma, death; recovery may take weeks, and CNS deficits may persist • Sinus node dysfunction, QT prolongation, T wave abnormalities, U waves • Nephrogenic diabetes insipidus, hypothyroidism, hyperthyroidism, hypercalcemia, pseudotumor cerebri • Acute toxicity: nausea, vomiting, diarrhea, and milder neurologic findings	• Peak serum levels: • Normal dose 2-3 hr; up to 5 hr for sustained-release lithium • Acute overdose: peak may be delayed ≥4-12 hr	• Replenish intravascular volume, maintain urinary output at 1-2 ml/kg/hr • Consider GI decontamination with oral polyethylene glycol electrolyte solution within 1-2 hr after acute overdose of sustained-release drug • Hemodialysis§ in patients with altered mental status, ataxia, seizures, or coma or in patients with mild symptoms in the setting of acute overdose or renal insufficiency • Ineffective or contraindicated therapies include oral activated charcoal, diuretics, and aminophylline
Opioids (e.g., heroin, morphine, oxycodone, fentanyl)	Agonist effect at CNS μ, κ, and δ opioid receptors; result is cell hyperpolarization and decreased neurotransmitter release	• CNS depression, respiratory depression, miosis • Dextromethorphan increases CNS serotonin and inhibits NMDA receptors, which causes hallucinations • Propoxyphene and its metabolite norpropoxyphene block sodium channels and can cause seizures and wide-complex arrhythmias similar to cyclic antidepressants; NaHCO₃ treats arrhythmias • Seizure risk with tramadol, meperidine, propoxyphene • Rapid, powerful heroin-like effect when sustained-release oxycodone is crushed before ingestion, snorting, or smoking • QTc prolongation and torsades de pointes with methadone	Rapid urine drug screens detect morphine and codeine but may not detect semisynthetic and synthetic opioids; some interferents/irrelevants	• IV naloxone, 0.4-2 mg; can repeat up to 10 mg if no response • Continuous infusion for recurrent symptoms or sustained-release opioid ingestion; give 50% of dose that produces desired effect 15 min after initial effect is obtained, then infuse two thirds of this dose every hr; infusion rate can be increased or decreased to maintain normal respiration and avoid withdrawal symptoms • Contraindicated therapies: nalmefene and naltrexone should not be used for acute opioid reversal
Organophosphorus compounds and carbamates (e.g., diazinon, mevinphos, fenthion, aldicarb)	Inhibits acetylcholinesterase, resulting in excessive acetylcholine stimulation of nicotinic and muscarinic receptors in autonomic and somatic motor nervous systems and CNS	• Nicotinic-mediated effects: tachycardia, mydriasis, hypertension, delirium, coma, seizures, muscle weakness, fasciculations • Muscarinic-mediated effects: salivation, lacrimation, urination, vomiting, defecation, miosis, bronchorrhea, bronchospasm, bradycardia	• Serum (butyrylcholinesterase) or RBC (acetylcholinesterase) activity <50% of normal • Clinical recovery occurs before serum cholinesterase levels normalize	• Atropine, 1-2 mg by initial IV bolus; double the dose every 5 min (2 mg, 4 mg, 8 mg, 16 mg, etc.) until drying of bronchial secretions, adequate oxygenation, pulse >80 bpm, systolic blood pressure >80 mm Hg achieved; continuous infusion at 10%-20% of total stabilizing dose per hr; stop infusion if patient develops any signs or symptoms of anticholinergic toxidrome; restart infusion at lower rate when signs or symptoms abate • Pralidoxime‖ chloride 30 mg/kg (maximum 2 g) IV bolus over 30 min, then 8-10 mg/kg/hr (maximum 650 mg/hr) continuous infusion; administer as soon as possible after poisoning; continue 12-24 hr after atropine no longer required and symptoms resolve

POISONING, ACUTE—cont'd

ICD-10CM #   Z13.88   Encounter for screening for disorder due to exposure
to contaminants
E865.8   Accidental poisoning from other specified foods

1719

Table 47   Pathophysiology, Clinical Effects, and Management of Specific Drugs and Toxicants—cont'd

Drug or Toxicant	Pathophysiology	Clinical Effects	Laboratory	Specific Therapy
Salicylates	Inhibits cyclooxygenase; decreases formation of prostaglandins and thromboxane A_2; stimulates CNS medullary respiratory receptor and chemoreceptor trigger zone; impairs platelet function; disrupts carbohydrate metabolism; uncouples oxidative phosphorylation; increases vascular permeability	• Acute toxicity • Mild: nausea, vomiting, diaphoresis, tinnitus, decreased hearing, hyperpnea, tachypnea • Moderate–severe: confusion, delirium, coma, seizures, hyperthermia, ALI; death can occur within hours of overdose • Chronic toxicity: same as acute, but may not have diaphoresis or vomiting • Consider diagnosis in patients with new-onset confusion, anion gap metabolic acidosis, or ALI	• Serum salicylate level: toxic ≥30 mg/dl; level ≥100 mg/dL indicates life-threatening toxicity with possible sudden, rapid clinical deterioration; in chronic toxicity, levels may be minimally elevated (>30 mg/dl), and clinical evaluation is more reliable for gauging degree of toxicity • Arterial blood gases: respiratory alkalosis with metabolic acidosis • Anion gap metabolic acidosis • Prolonged PT and PTT, ketonuria, ketonemia	Multidose activated charcoal q2-3h in acute overdose with progressive symptoms or rising salicylate level
SSRIs/SRIs	• Inhibits re-uptake of serotonin • SRIs have additional effects (e.g., duloxetine inhibits norepinephrine re-uptake, nefazodone inhibits serotonergic 5-HT2 receptors, trazodone inhibits peripheral α-adrenergic receptors, venlafaxine inhibits norepinephrine and dopamine re-uptake)	• Vomiting, blurred vision, CNS depression, tachycardia • Seizures and coma rare • Torsades de pointes reported with citalopram • Serotonin syndrome: clonus, agitation, tremor, diaphoresis, hyperreflexia; hyperthermia and hypertonicity in severe cases	• No specific tests • If serotonin syndrome suspected: electrolytes, BUN, glucose, liver enzymes, coagulation panel, blood gases, chest radiograph	• Respiratory support as needed • Benzodiazepines for agitation or seizures • Serotonin syndrome: consider cyproheptadine, 12 mg PO initial dose then 2 mg PO q2h (to a maximum of 32 mg/day) until symptoms resolve • Critical care therapies for hyperthermia, rhabdomyolysis, DIC, ARDS, renal and hepatic dysfunction, torsades de pointes

ALI, Acute lung injury; *aPTT,* activated partial thromboplastin time; *ARDS,* acute respiratory distress syndrome; *AV,* atrioventricular; *BP,* blood pressure; *bpm,* beats per minute; *BUN,* blood urea nitrogen; *CNS,* central nervous system; *DIC,* disseminated intravascular coagulation; *DOB,* 4-bromo-2,5-dimethoxyamphetamine; *ECG,* electrocardiogram; *GABA,* α-aminobutyric acid; *GI,* gastrointestinal; *HR,* heart rate; *IABP,* intra-aortic balloon counterpulsation; *INR,* international normalized ratio; *IV,* intravenous; *MDMA,* 3,4-methylenedioxymethamphetamine; *Na¹,K¹-ATPase,* sodium, potassium adenosine triphosphatase; *NAC,* N-acetylcysteine; *NAPQI,* N-acetyl-p-benzoquinone imine; *NMDA,* N-methyl-ᴅ-aspartate; *PMA,* paramethoxyamphetamine; *PT,* prothrombin time; *PTT,* partial thromboplastin time; *RBC,* red blood cell; *RUQ,* upper right quadrant (abdomen); *SIADH,* syndrome of inappropriate antidiuretic secretion; *SRI,* serotonin re-uptake inhibitor; *SSRI,* selective serotonin re-uptake inhibitor.

*A nomogram to evaluate the potential toxicity of levels drawn more than 4 hours after ingestion is provided in Fig. 7, from Rumack BH, Matthew H: Acetaminophen poisoning and toxicity, *Pediatrics* 1975;55):871-876. The nomogram is valid only for levels drawn after a single acute ingestion.

†NAC can be discontinued in patients with uncomplicated disease after a loading dose plus six maintenance doses if hepatic aminotransferase levels are normal and acetaminophen is not detected; otherwise, the full regimen should be administered.

‡Adjust infusion for reduced renal function.

§Continue hemodialysis until the serum lithium level is less than 1 mEq/L. Recheck the level 8 hr after dialysis, and restart hemodialysis if the level is higher than 1 mEq/L. Repeat this cycle until the serum lithium level remains lower than 1 mEq/L.

ˡA double-blind, randomized, placebo-controlled trial of pralidoxime in acute organophosphorus poisoning found no significant difference in mortality rates or need for intubation.

Clinical Algorithms

III

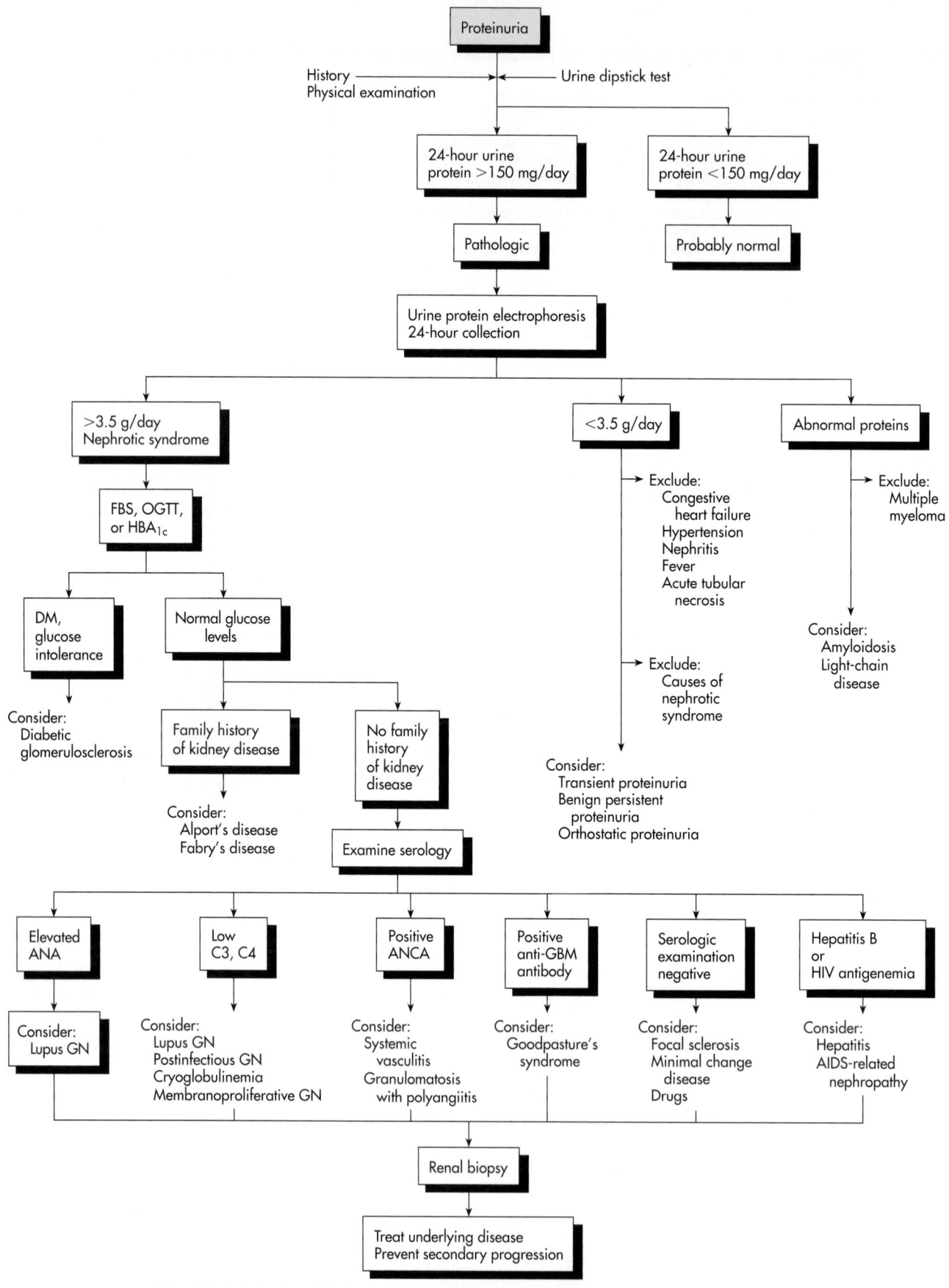

FIG. 225 Proteinuria. *AIDS,* Acquired immunodeficiency syndrome; *ANA,* antinuclear antibody; *ANCA,* antineutrophil cytoplasmic autoantibody; *anti-GBM,* anti-glomerular basement membrane; *FBS,* fasting blood sugar; *GN,* glomerulonephritis; *OGTT,* oral glucose tolerance test. (Modified from Greene HL, Johnson WP, Lemcke DL [eds]: *Decision making in medicine,* ed 2, St Louis, 1998, Mosby.)

ICD-10CM # L29.9　Pruritus, unspecified

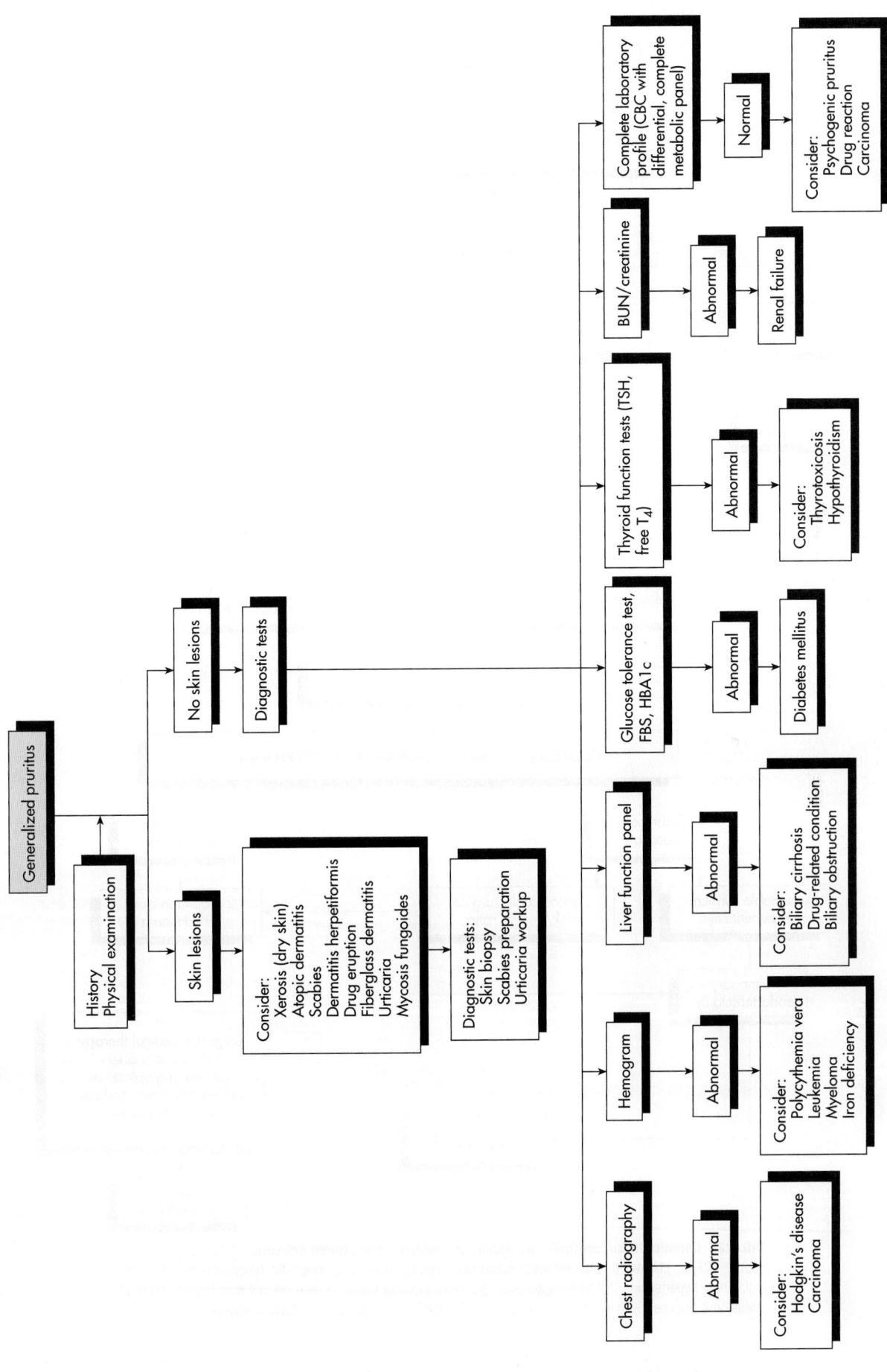

FIG. 226　Evaluation of generalized pruritus. *BUN,* Blood urea nitrogen; *CBC,* complete blood count; *FBS,* fasting blood sugar; *HBA1c,* hemoglobin A1c; *T₄,* thyroxine; *TSH,* thyroid-stimulating hormone. (From Greene HL, Johnson WP, Lemcke DL [eds]: *Decision making in medicine,* ed 2, St Louis, 1998, Mosby.)

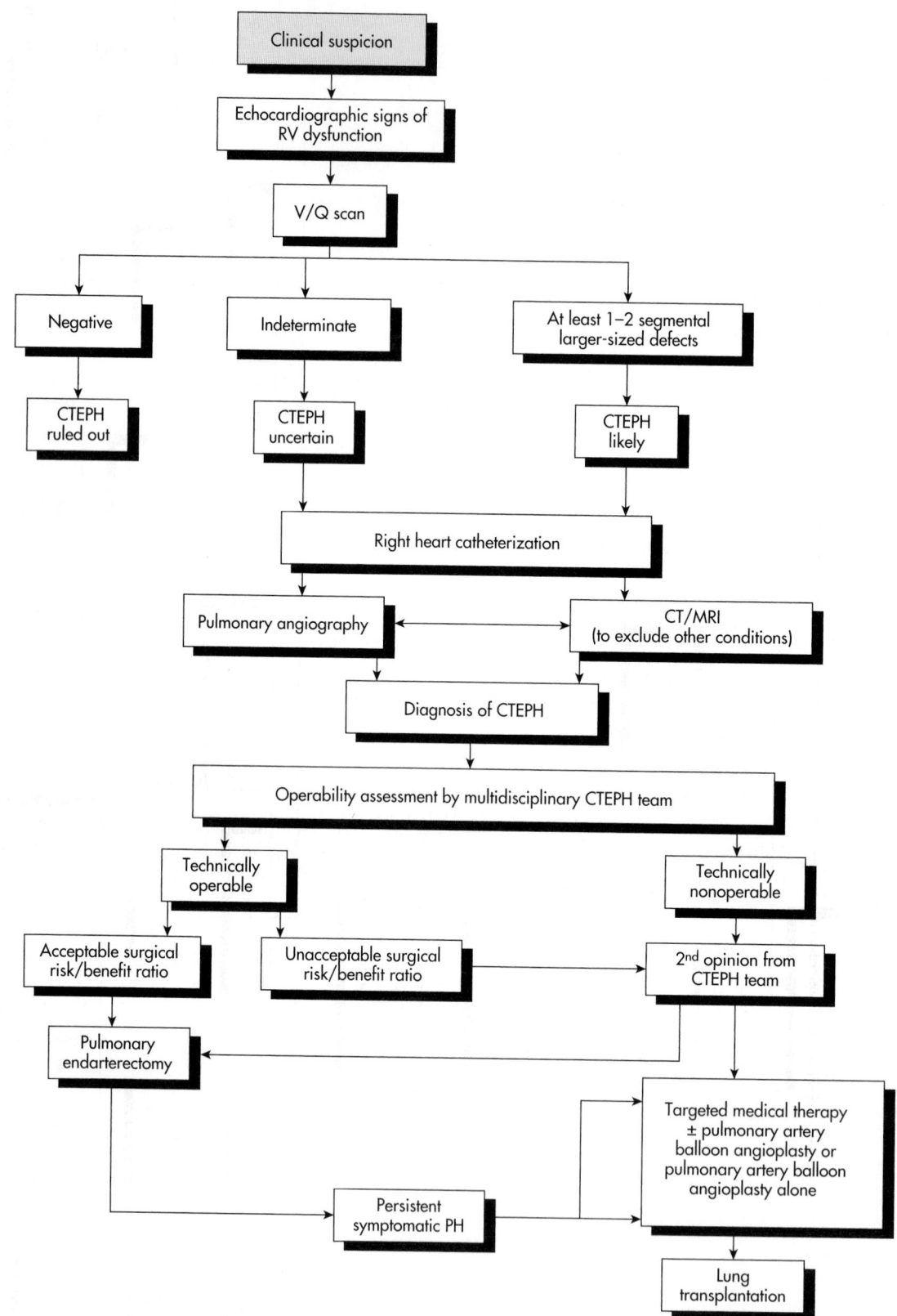

FIG. 229 Chronic thromboembolic pulmonary hypertension treatment scheme. *CT,* Computed tomography; *CTEPH,* chronic thromboembolic pulmonary hypertension; *MRI,* magnetic resonance imaging; *PH,* pulmonary hypertension; *RV,* right ventricular; *V/Q,* ventilation-perfusion. (Sellke FW, del Nido PJ, Swanson SJ: Sabiston & Spencer Surgery of the Chest, 9th ed. ISBN # 978-0-323-24126-7, 2016, Elsevier.)

SOLID & PART-SOLID NODULES

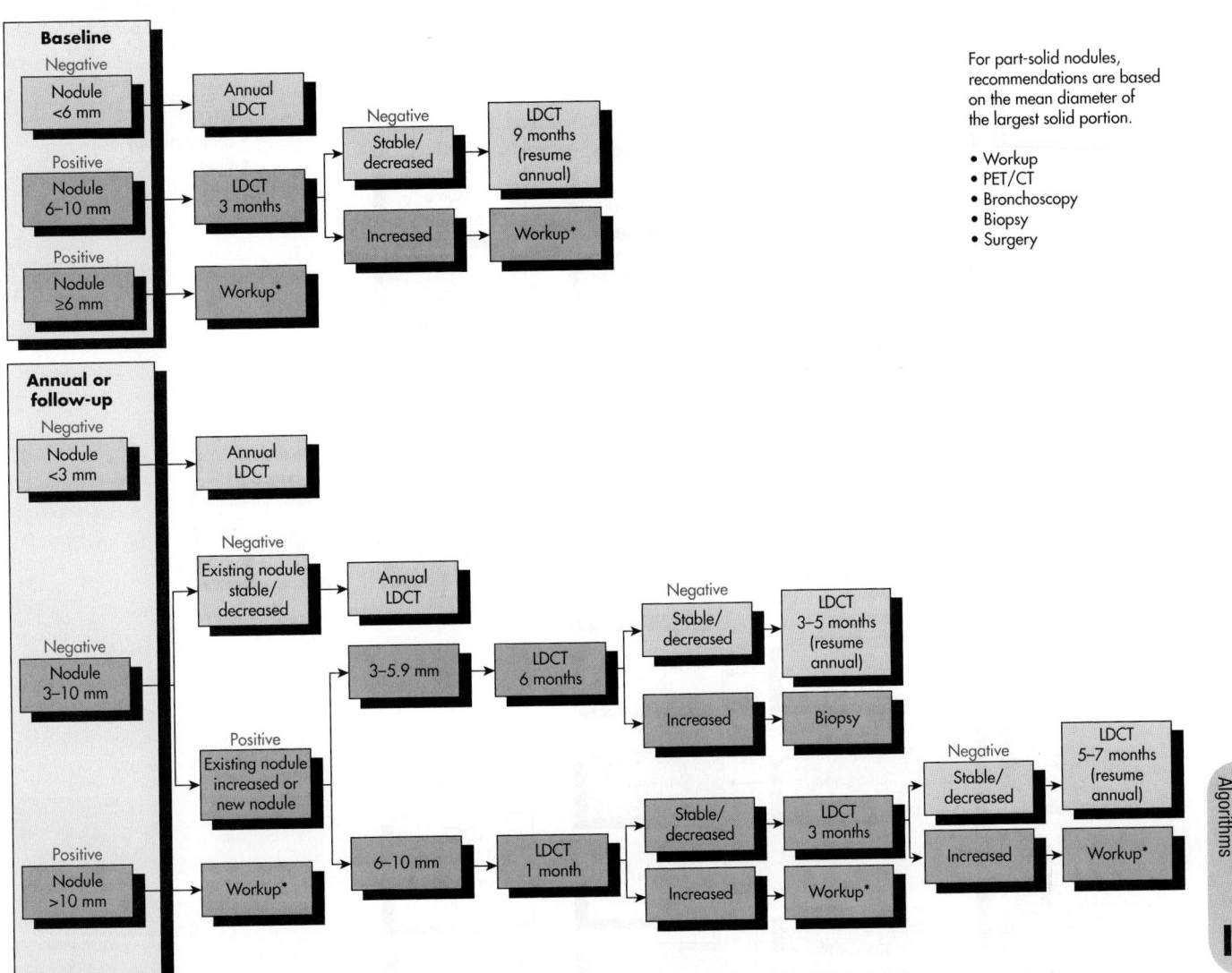

For part-solid nodules, recommendations are based on the mean diameter of the largest solid portion.

- Workup
- PET/CT
- Bronchoscopy
- Biopsy
- Surgery

A

FIG. 230 The diagnostic algorithm for (A) solid or part-solid nodules and (B) nonsolid nodules. This algorithm was created through discussion by a multidisciplinary group composed of thoracic surgeons, radiologists, pulmonologists, oncologists, and pathologists. *Workup is at the discretion of the treating physicians but typically consists of a PET/CT and tissue diagnosis, either by bronchoscopy, CT-guided biopsy, or for highly suspicious nodules, minimally invasive surgery. *CT,* Computed tomography; *LDCT,* low-dose computed tomography; *PET,* positron emission tomography. (Sellke FW, del Nido PJ, Swanson SJ: Sabiston & Spencer Surgery of the Chest, 9th ed. ISBN # 978-0-323-24126-7, 2016, Elsevier.) The Fleishner Society recommendations for computed tomography follow-up of pulmonary nodules are summarized in Tables 48-50.

Continued on next page

NONSOLID NODULES

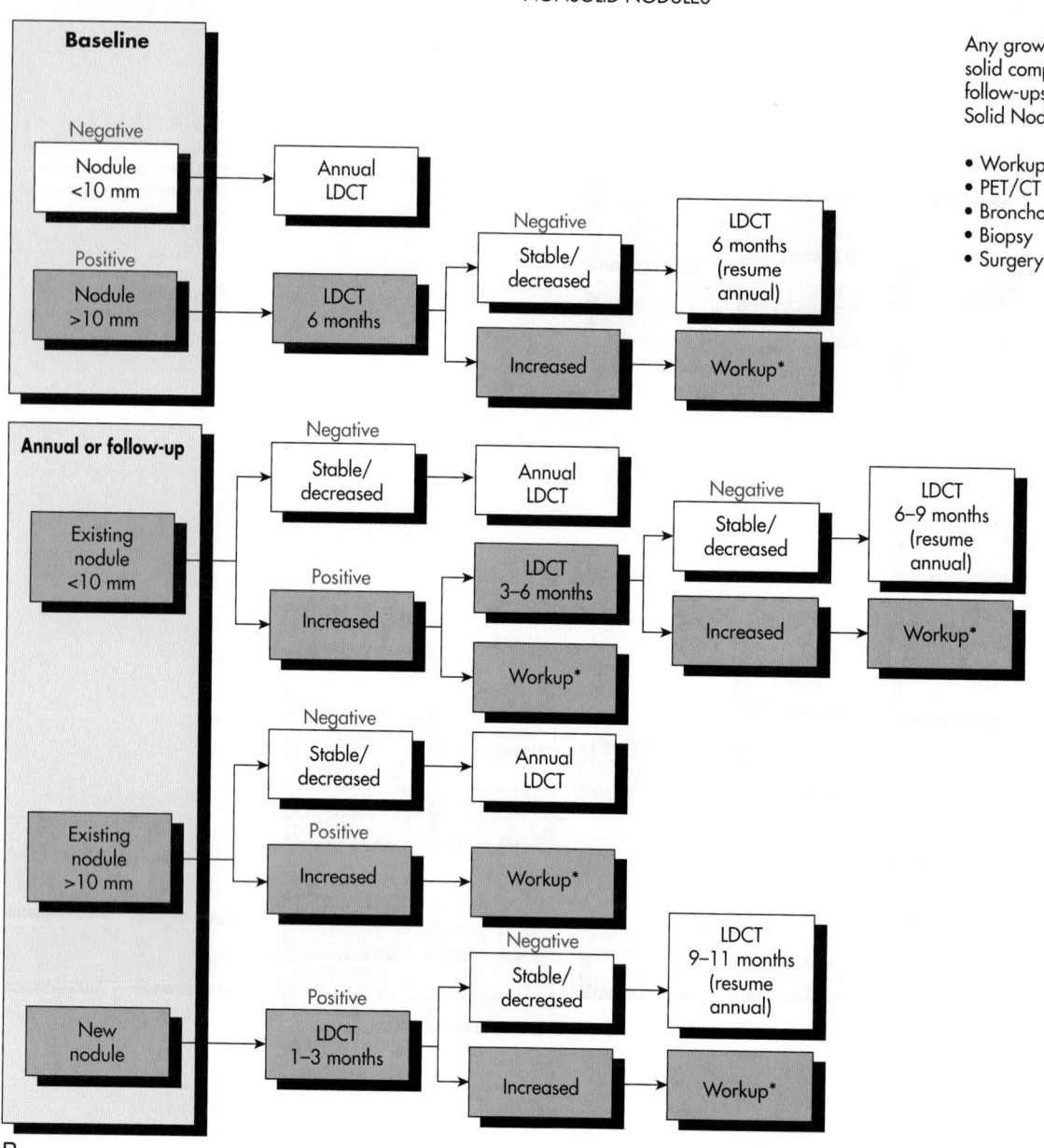

Any growth or development of solid components prompts follow-ups as per Solid & Part-Solid Nodule algorithm.

- Workup
- PET/CT
- Bronchoscopy
- Biopsy
- Surgery

B

FIG. 230 (Continued)

Table 48 Fleischner Society Recommendations for Computed Tomography (CT) Follow-up (FU) of Solid Nodules*

Nodule Size	Low-Risk Patient	High-Risk patient
≤ 4 mm	No FU CT needed (FU is optional)	FU CT at 12 months; if unchanged, no further FU
> 4–6 mm	FU CT at 12 months; if unchanged, no further FU	FU CT at 6–12 months, then at 18–24 months if no change
> 6–8 mm	FU CT at 6–12 months, then at 18–24 months if no change	FU CT at 3–6 months, then at 9–12 and 24 months if no change
> 8 mm	Options: FU CT at 3, 9, and 24 months; positron emission tomography; biopsy; video-assisted thoracic surgery	

*Nodule size is average of length and width. Low-risk patient, minimal or absent history of smoking or other known risk factors; high-risk patient, history of smoking or other known risk factors.
From Webb WR, Brant WE, Major NM: *Fundamentals of body CT*, ed 4, Philadelphia, 2015, Saunders.

Table 49 Fleischner Society Recommendations for Computed Tomography (CT) Follow-up (FU) of Solitary Ground-Glass Opacity (GGO) or Part-GGO Nodules

Nodule Type	Recommendation	Additional Remarks
Solitary pure GGO ≤ 5 mm	No FU CT required	Use 1-mm slices to confirm nodule is pure GGO
Solitary pure GGO > 5 mm	FU CT at 3 months; if persistent, yearly FU for at least 3 years	Positron emission tomography of limited value and not recommended
Solitary part-solid nodules	FU CT at 3 months; if persistent and solid component < 5 mm, yearly FU for at least 3 years; if persistent and solid component ≥ 5 mm, then biopsy or resection	Consider positron emission tomography if nodule >1 cm

From Webb WR, Brant WE, Major NM: *Fundamentals of body CT*, ed 4, Philadelphia, 2015, Saunders.

Table 50 Fleischner Society Recommendations for Computed Tomography (CT) Follow-up (FU) of Multiple Ground-Glass Opacity (GGO) or Part-GGO Nodules

Nodule Type	Recommendation	Additional Remarks
Multiple pure GGO ≤ 5 mm	FU CT at 2 and 4 years	Consider alternate cause for GGO nodules
Multiple pure GGO > 5 mm; no dominant lesion	FU CT at 3 months; if persistent, yearly FU for at least 3 years	Positron emission tomography of limited value and not recommended
Dominant part-solid nodule(s)	FU CT at 3 months; if persistent, then biopsy or resection, particularly if solid component ≥ 5 mm	Consider lung-sparing surgery in patients with a dominant lesion suspicious for lung cancer

From Webb WR, Brant WE, Major NM: *Fundamentals of body CT*, ed 4, Philadelphia, 2015, Saunders.

Clinical
Algorithms

III

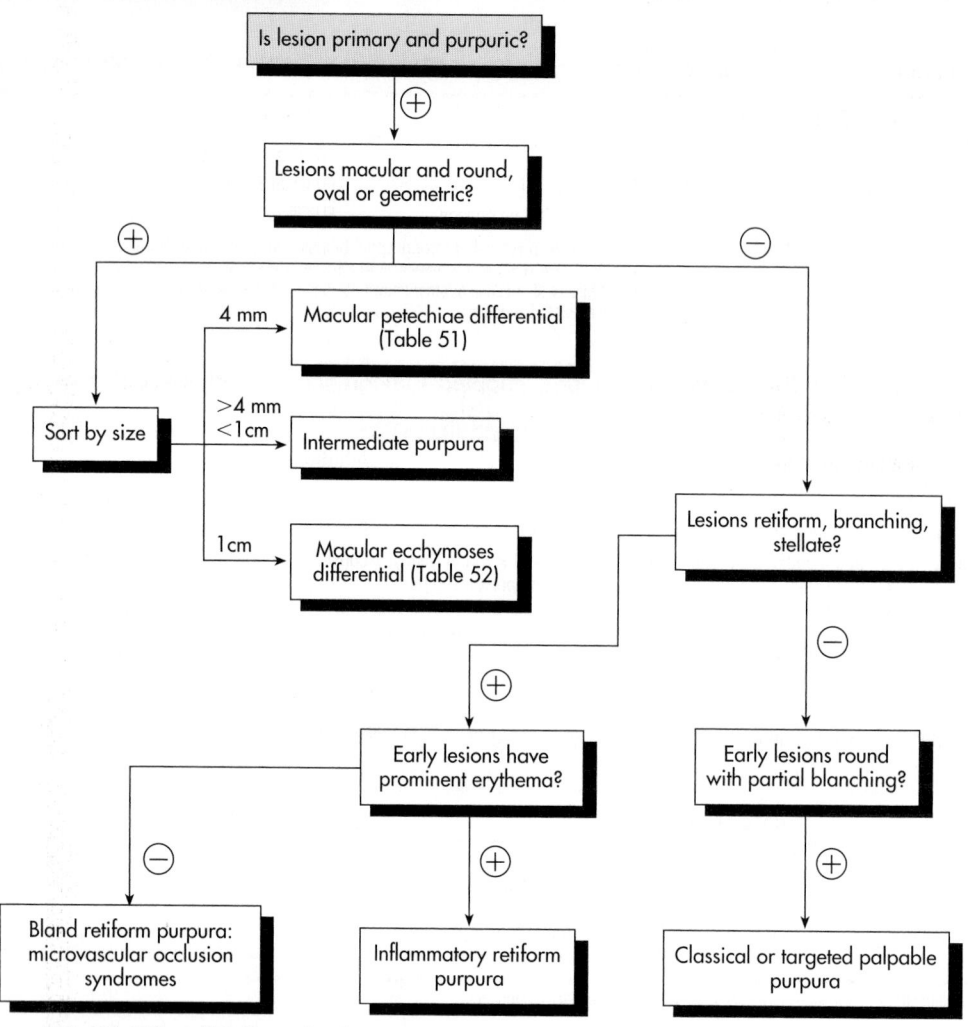

FIG. 231 Differential diagnosis of purpura. (From Bolognia JL, Jorizzo JL, Rapini RP: *Dermatology,* St Louis, 2003, Mosby.)

Table 51 Differential Diagnosis of Petechial Hemorrhage—Non-Palpable, Non-Retiform and ≤4 mm in Diameter

Pathophysiology: Hemostatically Relevant Thrombocytopenia (<550,000/mm³) **

Major etiologies*
Idiopathic thrombocytopenic purpura
Thrombotic thrombocytopenic purpura
Disseminated intravascular coagulation
Other acquired thrombocytopenias, including drug-related
    Peripheral destruction (e.g., quinine, quinidine)
    Decreased production, idiosyncratic or dose-related (e.g., chemotherapy)
    Bone marrow infiltration, fibrosis or failure

Pathophysiology: Abnormal Platelet Function

Major etiologies*
Congenital or hereditary platelet function defects
Acquired platelet function defects
    Aspirin, nonsteroidal antiinflammatory drugs
    Renal insufficiency
    Monoclonal gammopathy
Thrombocytosis in myeloproliferative disease (often >1,000,000/mm³)

Pathophysiology: Non-Platelet Etiologies

- Major etiologies*
- Spiking elevations of intravascular venous pressure (Valsalva maneuver-like, e.g., repetitive vomiting, childbirth, paroxysmal coughing, seizure)
- Fixed increased pressure (e.g., stasis, ligatures)
- Trauma (often linear)
- Perifollicular (vitamin C deficiency)
- Mildly inflammatory conditions
    ○ Chronic pigmented purpura
    ○ Hypergammaglobulinemic purpura of Waldenström

Table 52 Differential Diagnosis for Macular Purpura and Ecchymoses—Non-Palpable and Non-Retiform

Intermediate Macular Purpura (>4 mm, <1 cm in diameter)
- Major etiologies*
- Hypergammaglobulinemic purpura of Waldenström
- Infection/inflammation in patients with thrombocytopenia
- Rarely, minimally inflamed immune complex vasculitis (usually dependent distribution)

Ecchymoses (≥1 cm in diameter)
Pathophysiology: procoagulant defect plus minor trauma*
    ○ Anticoagulant use
    ○ Hepatic insufficiency with poor procoagulant synthesis
    ○ Vitamin K deficiency
    ○ Disseminated intravascular coagulation (some)

Pathophysiology: poor dermal support of vessels plus minor trauma*
    ○ Actinic (solar, senile) purpura
    ○ Corticosteroid therapy, topical or systemic
    ○ Vitamin C deficiency (scurvy)
    ○ Systemic amyloidosis (light chain-related, some familial types)
    ○ Ehlers-Danlos syndrome (primarily type IV)

Pathophysiology: other causes plus minor trauma*
    ○ Hypergammaglobulinemic purpura of Waldenström
    ○ Platelet function defects, including von Willebrand disease, medications, metabolic diseases
    ○ Acquired or congenital thrombocytopenia

*Partial list.
**Most patients do not have petechiae until platelets ≤20,000/mm³.

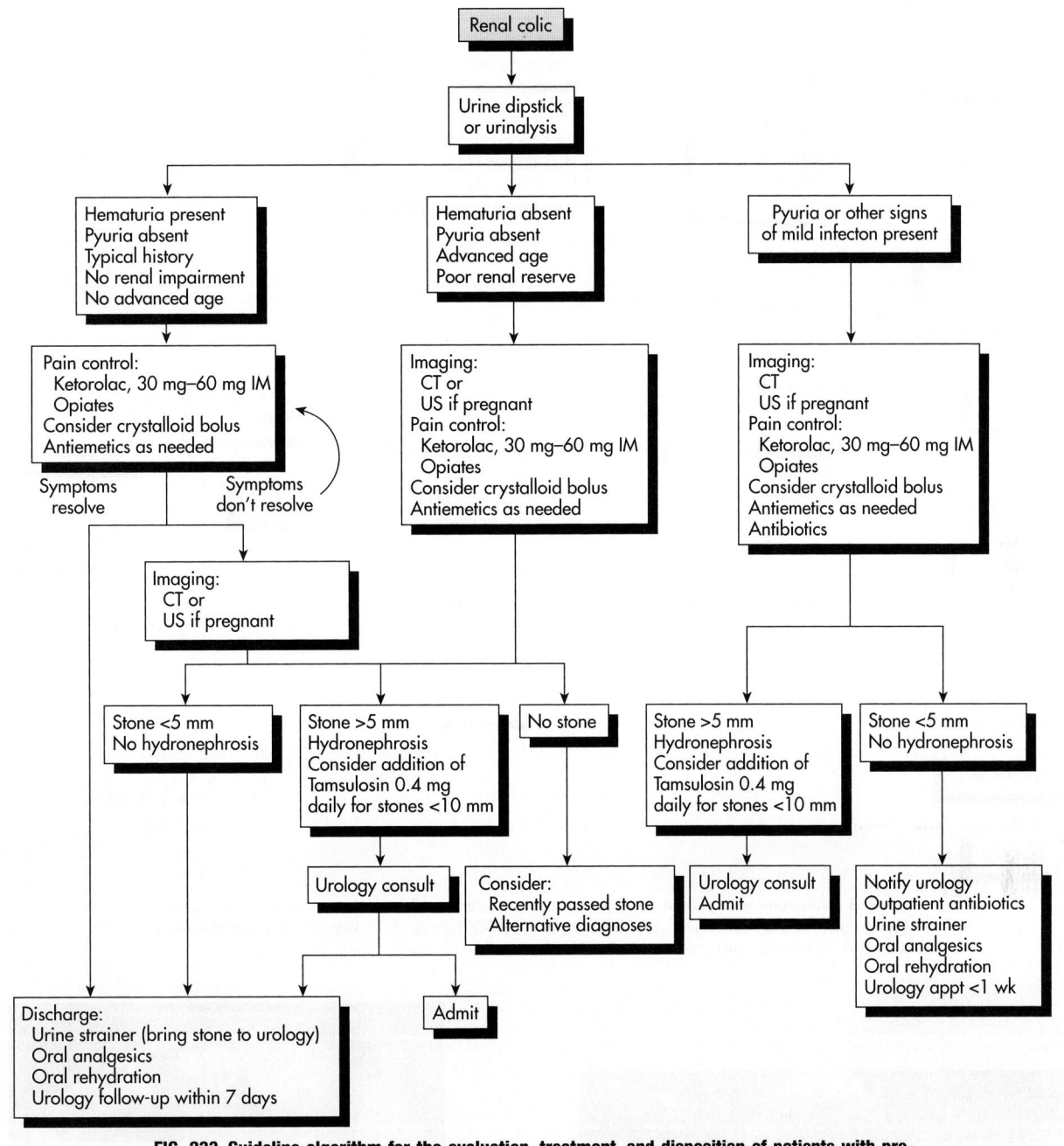

FIG. 233 Guideline algorithm for the evaluation, treatment, and disposition of patients with presumed renal colic. *CT*, Computed tomography; *IV*, intravenously; *US*, ultrasonography. (Modified from Adams JG, et al: *Emergency medicine, clinical essentials*, ed 2, Philadelphia, 2013, Elsevier.)

```
┌─────────────────┐        ┌──────────────────┐        ┌────────────────────────┐
│ Cystic          │◄───────│ Renal ultrasound │───────►│ Mass not identified    │
│ Smooth wall     │        └──────────────────┘        │ (confirmed with CT scan)│
│ No internal echoes│              │                    └────────────────────────┘
└─────────────────┘              │                              │
        │                        ▼                              ▼
        ▼                 ┌──────────────┐           ┌────────────────────────┐
  ┌─────────┐            │ Solid/complex│           │ Hypoechoic mass suspicious│
  │ Observe │            │ Internal echoes│          │ for abscess (Fig. 236) │
  └─────────┘            │ Irregular wall│           └────────────────────────┘
                         └──────────────┘
```

Flowchart (FIG. 235):

- Renal ultrasound → Cystic / Smooth wall / No internal echoes → Observe
- Renal ultrasound → Solid/complex / Internal echoes / Irregular wall → CT scan
- Renal ultrasound → Mass not identified (confirmed with CT scan) → Hypoechoic mass suspicious for abscess (Fig. 236) → CT scan
- CT scan → Negative CT number / Fat density / Angiomyolipoma → Observe
- CT scan → Complex mass / No contrast enhancement / Indeterminate → Renal arteriogram
  - Renal arteriogram → Avascular Inconclusive → Needle aspiration → Malignant cells → Surgery
  - Renal arteriogram → Neovascularity → Surgery
- CT scan → Solid / Contrast enhancement / Vascular tumor → Surgery; → Suspected caval thrombus → MRI → Surgery
- CT scan → Decreased attenuation suspicious for abscess (Fig. 237) → IV antibiotic

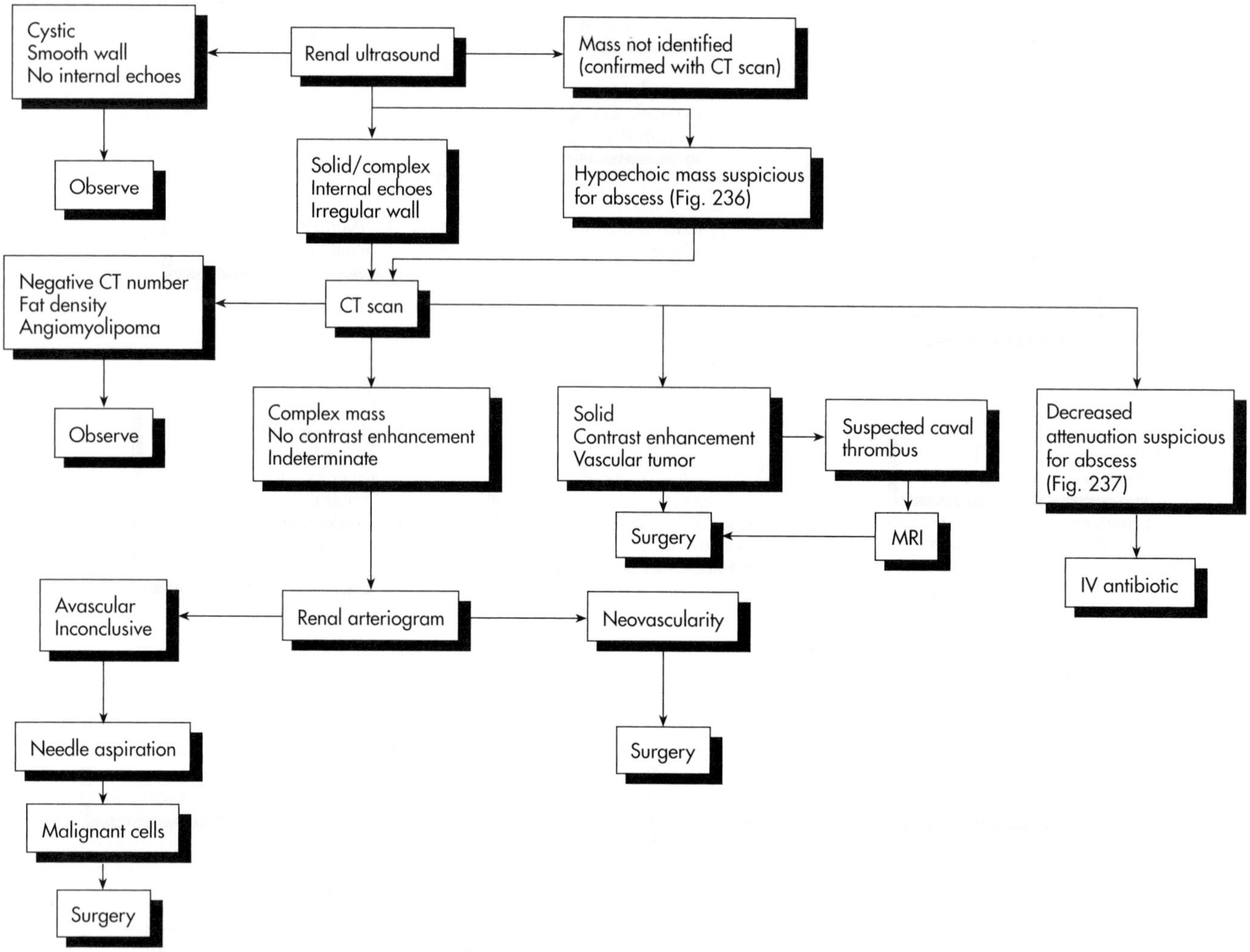

FIG. 235 Evaluation of a patient with a renal mass on renal ultrasound. *CT,* Computed tomography; *MRI,* magnetic resonance imaging. (Modified from Williams RD: Tumors of the kidney, ureter, and bladder. In Goldman L, Schafer AL [eds]: *Cecil textbook of medicine,* ed 23, Philadelphia, 2008, Saunders.)

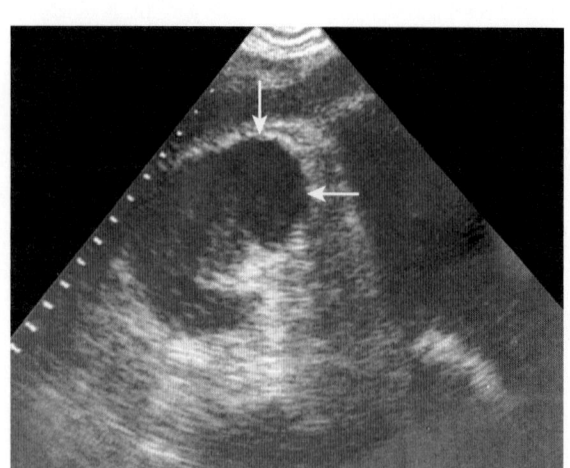

FIG. 236 Acute renal abscess. Transverse ultrasound image of the right kidney demonstrates a poorly marginated rounded focal hypoechoic mass *(arrows)* in the anterior portion of the kidney. (Wein AJ, Kavoussi LR, Partin AW, Peters CA: Campbell-Walsh Urology, 11th ed, ISBN# 978-1-4557-7567-5, 2016, Elsevier.)

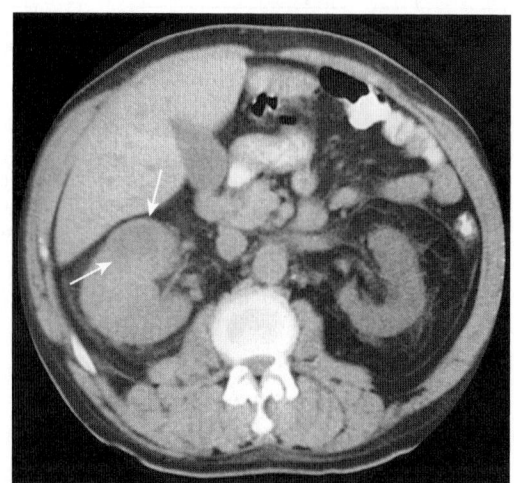

FIG. 237 Acute renal abscess. Nonenhanced computed tomography scan through the mid pole of the right kidney demonstrates right renal enlargement and an area of decreased attenuation *(arrows).* After antimicrobial therapy, a follow-up scan showed complete regression of these findings. (Wein AJ, Kavoussi LR, Partin AW, Peters CA: Campbell-Walsh Urology, 11th ed, ISBN# 978-1-4557-7567-5, 2016, Elsevier.)

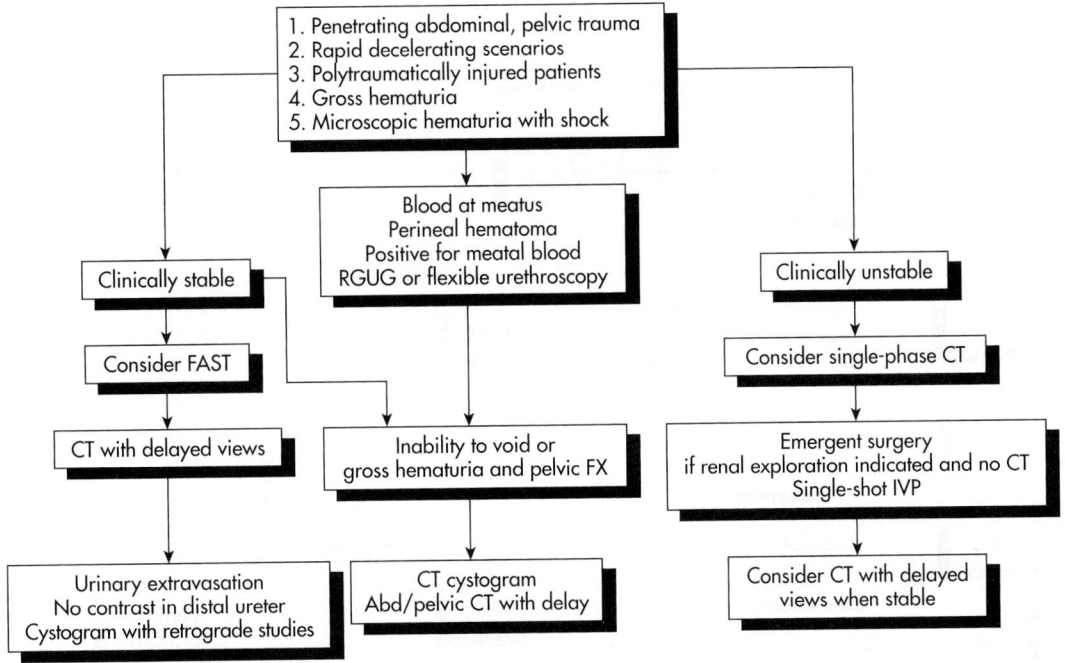

FIG. 238 Recommended evaluation protocol for patients with a medical history or physical findings consistent with possible genitourinary injury. *Abd*, abdominal; *CT*, computed tomography; *FAST*, focused assessment with sonography for trauma; *FX*, fracture; *IVP*, intravenous pyelography; *RGUG*, retrograde urethrogram. (Wein AJ, Kavoussi LR, Partin AW, Peters CA: Campbell-Walsh Urology, 11th ed, ISBN# 978-1-4557-7567-5, 2016, Elsevier.)

TABLE 53 Consensus Recommendations for Management of Renal Trauma

Clinical Findings and/or Grade of Renal Injury	Recommended Treatment
Grade 1 or 2 renal injury irrespective of traumatic etiology*	Nonoperative
Isolated grade 3, grade 4, and hemodynamically stable grade 5 renal injuries	Nonoperative
Uncontrollable renal hemorrhage/vascular instability; occasionally grade 4 "shattered" kidneys and a high percentage of grade 5 injuries	Absolute requirement for surgical intervention
Persistent or delayed hemorrhage not responding to angiographic embolization	Absolute requirement for surgical intervention
Expanding pulsatile retroperitoneal mass found on surgical exploration for coexisting intraabdominal injuries	Absolute requirement for surgical intervention (verify contralateral renal function prior to exploration)
Penetrating trauma, inadequate preoperative radiographic staging because of vascular instability of patient, retroperitoneal hemorrhage found on exploration	Retroperitoneal (renal) exploration recommended (verify contralateral renal function prior to exploration)
Blunt trauma; inadequate preoperative radiographic staging because of vascular instability of patient; no duodenal, pancreatic, or colonic injuries with retroperitoneal hemorrhage found on exploration	Observation—if FAST with bilateral blood flow. If no FAST obtained, consider intraoperative single-shot IVP/US with renal blood flow assessment or CT immediately following stabilization of patient
Blunt trauma; inadequate preoperative radiographic staging because of vascular instability of patient; duodenal, pancreatic, or colonic injuries with retroperitoneal hemorrhage found on exploration	Surgical interventions with renorrhaphy an option (verify contralateral renal function prior to exploration) *or* Drain intra-abdominal injuries. Observation—if FAST with bilateral blood flow. If no FAST obtained, consider intraoperative single-shot IVP/US with renal blood flow assessment or CT immediately following stabilization of patient
Blunt/penetrating trauma; radiographic screening studies reveal grade 3 renal injury with devitalized renal fragments, grade 4 or 5 renal injury, coexisting intraabdominal injuries—especially duodenum, pancreas, and colon	Retroperitoneal (renal) exploration with renorrhaphy and repair recommended

CT, computed tomography; *FAST*, focused assessment with sonography for trauma; *IVP*, intravenous pyelography; *US*, ultrasound.
*Blunt or penetrating trauma.
Wein AJ, Kavoussi LR, Partin AW, Peters CA: Campbell-Walsh Urology, 11th ed, ISBN# 978-1-4557-7567-5, 2016, Elsevier.

Clinical Algorithms

III

ICD-10CM # N44.2 Benign cyst of testis
N44.8 Other noninflammatory disorders of the testis
N50.3 Cyst of epididymis
N50.8 Other specified disorders of male genital organs

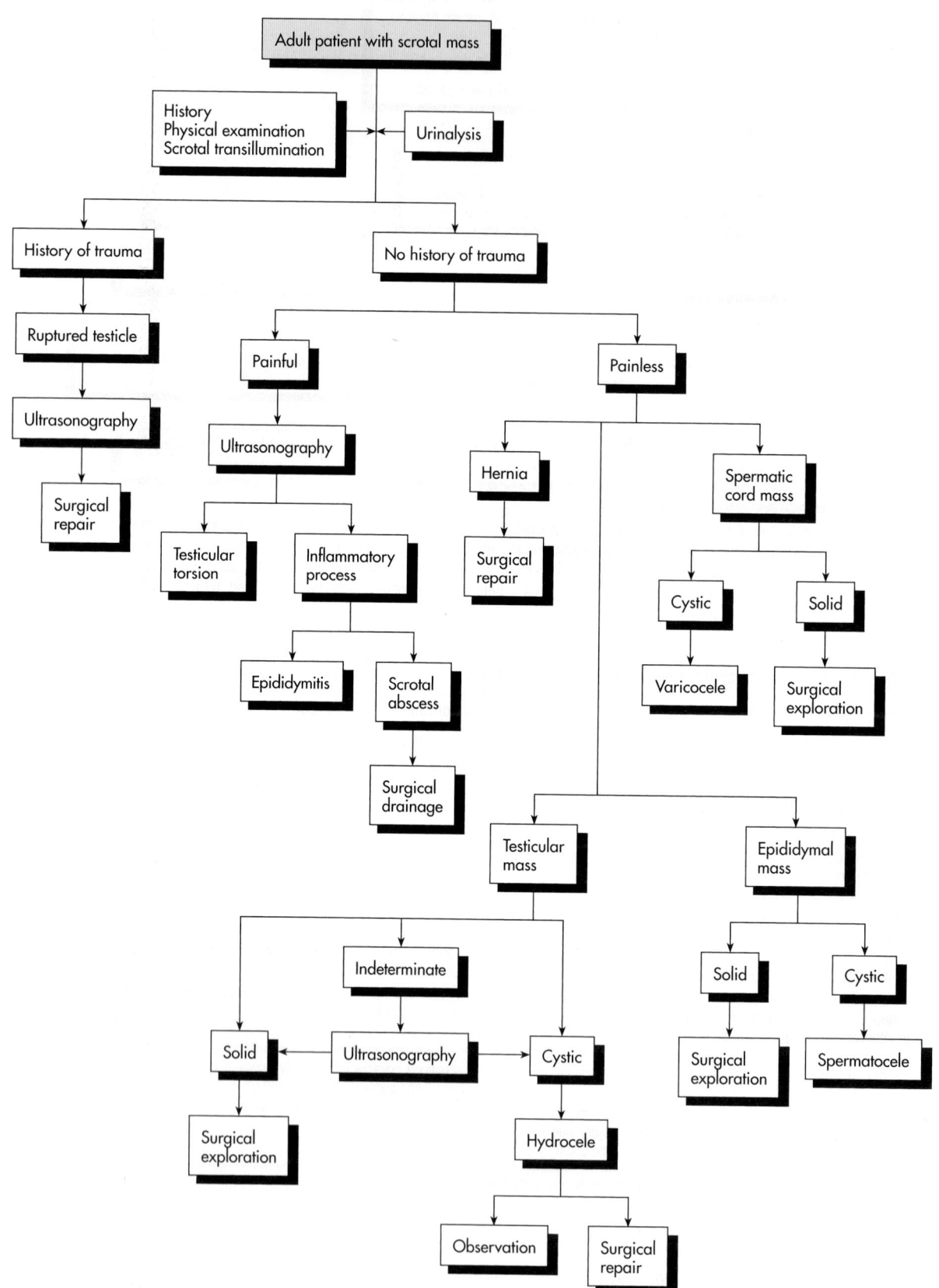

FIG. 241 Evaluation of scrotal mass. (From Greene HL, Johnson WP, Lemcke DL [eds]: *Decision making in medicine*, ed 2, St Louis, 1998, Mosby.)

SHOCK

ICD-10CM #	R57.9	Shock, unspecified	1731
	R57.0	Cardiogenic shock	
	R57.1	Hypovolemic shock	
	R57.8	Other shock	

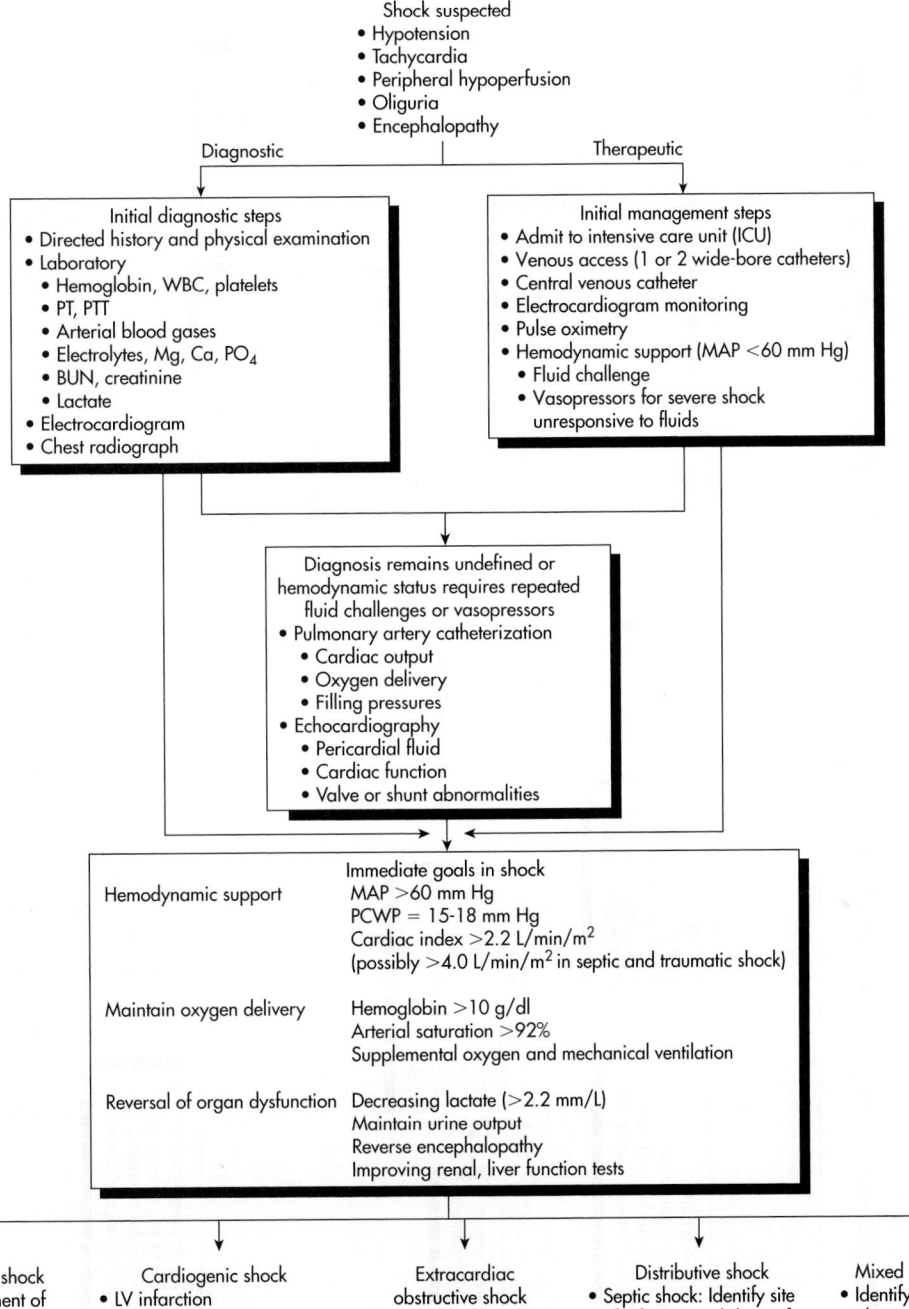

FIG. 247 An approach to the diagnosis and treatment of shock. *BUN,* Blood urea nitrogen; *CT,* computed tomography; *LV,* left ventricular; *MAP,* mean arterial pressure; *MRI,* magnetic resonance imaging; *PA,* pulmonary arterial; *PCWP,* pulmonary capillary wedge pressure; *PT,* prothrombin time; *PTT,* partial thromboplastin time; *RV,* right ventricular; *WBC,* white blood cell count. (From Goldman L, Ausiello D [eds]: *Cecil textbook of medicine,* ed 24, Philadelphia, 2012, Saunders.)

Clinical Algorithms

III

SHOULDER PAIN

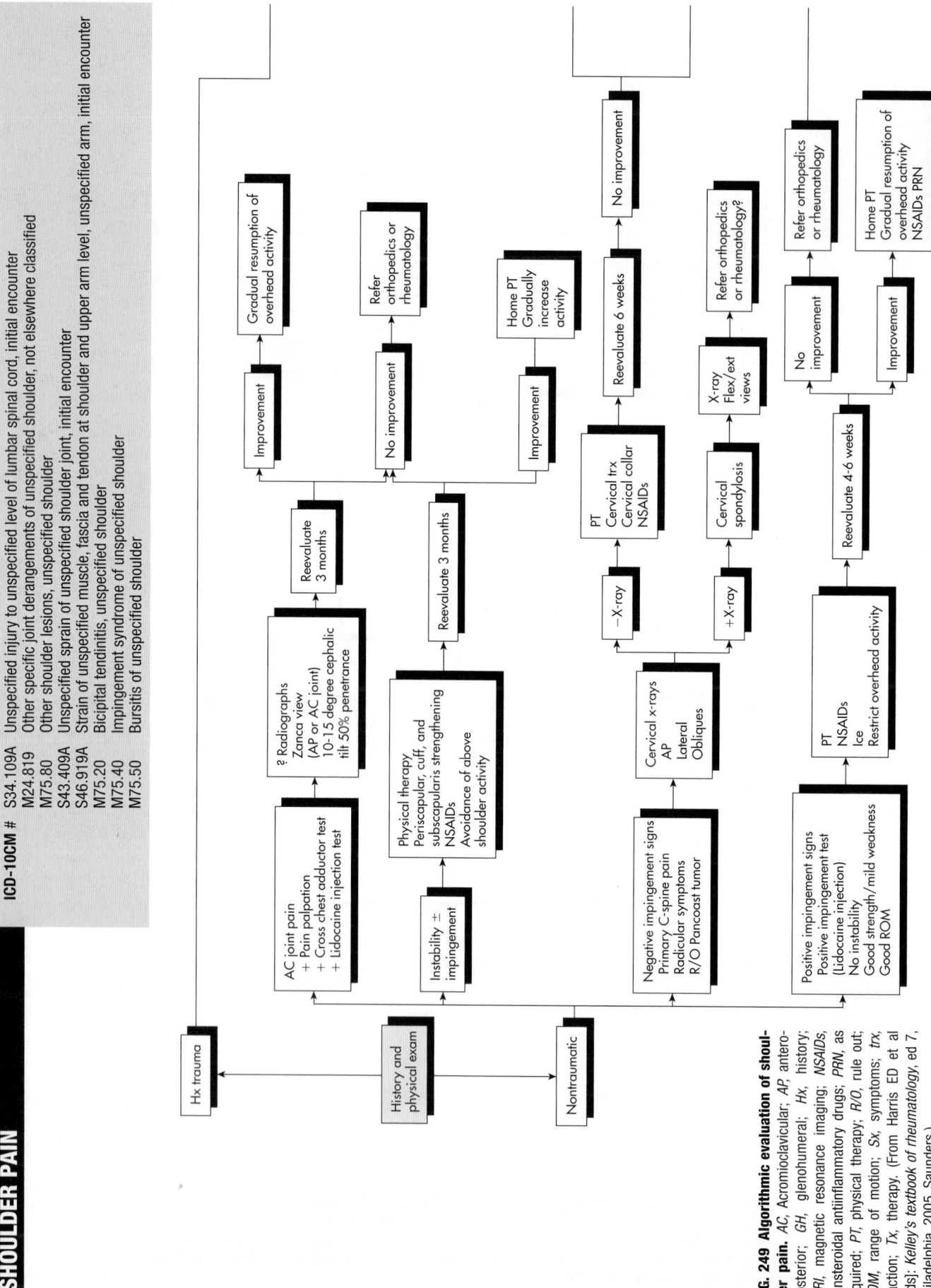

ICD-10CM #	
S34.109A	Unspecified injury to unspecified level of lumbar spinal cord, initial encounter
M24.819	Other specific joint derangements of unspecified shoulder, not elsewhere classified
M75.80	Other shoulder lesions, unspecified shoulder
S43.409A	Unspecified sprain of unspecified shoulder joint, initial encounter
S46.919A	Strain of unspecified muscle, fascia and tendon at shoulder and upper arm level, unspecified arm, initial encounter
M75.20	Bicipital tendinitis, unspecified shoulder
M75.40	Impingement syndrome of unspecified shoulder
M75.50	Bursitis of unspecified shoulder

FIG. 249 Algorithmic evaluation of shoulder pain. *AC,* Acromioclavicular; *AP,* anteroposterior; *GH,* glenohumeral; *Hx,* history; *MRI,* magnetic resonance imaging; *NSAIDs,* nonsteroidal antiinflammatory drugs; *PRN,* as required; *PT,* physical therapy; *R/O,* rule out; *ROM,* range of motion; *Sx,* symptoms; *trx,* traction; *Tx,* therapy. (From Harris ED et al [eds]: *Kelley's textbook of rheumatology,* ed 7, Philadelphia, 2005, Saunders.)

SHOULDER PAIN—cont'd

ICD-10CM #	
S34.109A	Unspecified injury to unspecified level of lumbar spinal cord, initial encounter
M24.819	Other specific joint derangements of unspecified shoulder, not elsewhere classified
M75.80	Other shoulder lesions, unspecified shoulder
S43.409A	Unspecified sprain of unspecified shoulder joint, initial encounter
S46.919A	Strain of unspecified muscle, fascia and tendon at shoulder and upper arm level, unspecified arm, initial encounter
M75.20	Bicipital tendinitis, unspecified shoulder
M75.40	Impingement syndrome of unspecified shoulder
M75.50	Bursitis of unspecified shoulder

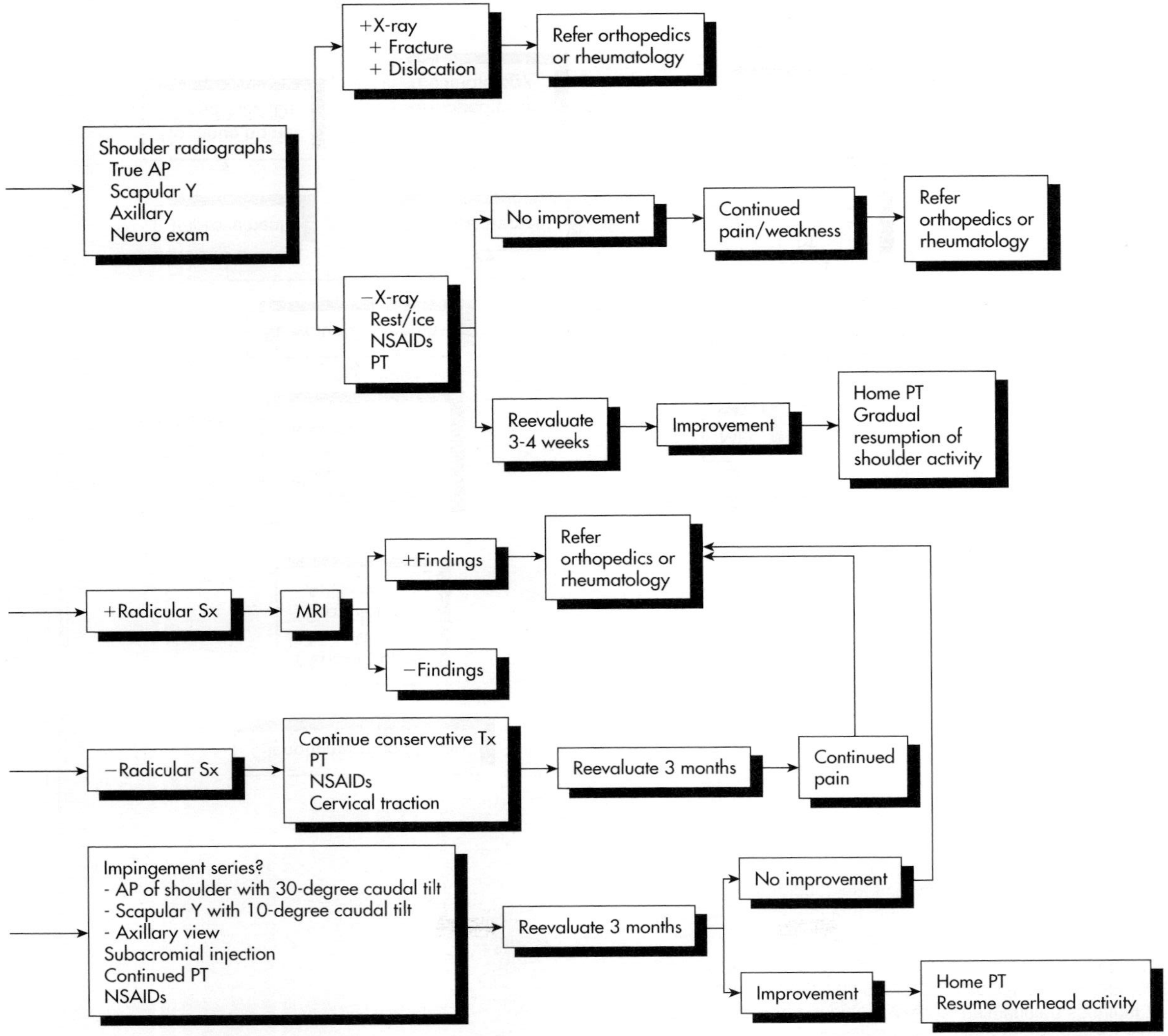

Shoulder radiographs
True AP
Scapular Y
Axillary
Neuro exam

+X-ray
+ Fracture
+ Dislocation
→ Refer orthopedics or rheumatology

−X-ray
Rest/ice
NSAIDs
PT

No improvement → Continued pain/weakness → Refer orthopedics or rheumatology

Reevaluate 3-4 weeks → Improvement → Home PT
Gradual resumption of shoulder activity

+Radicular Sx → MRI

+Findings → Refer orthopedics or rheumatology

−Findings

−Radicular Sx → Continue conservative Tx
PT
NSAIDs
Cervical traction

Reevaluate 3 months → Continued pain → Refer orthopedics or rheumatology

Impingement series?
- AP of shoulder with 30-degree caudal tilt
- Scapular Y with 10-degree caudal tilt
- Axillary view
Subacromial injection
Continued PT
NSAIDs

Reevaluate 3 months → No improvement

→ Improvement → Home PT
Resume overhead activity

FIG. 249 (Continued)

Clinical
Algorithms

III

Continued on next page

SHOULDER PAIN—cont'd

ICD-10CM #	
S34.109A	Unspecified injury to unspecified level of lumbar spinal cord, initial encounter
M24.819	Other specific joint derangements of unspecified shoulder, not elsewhere classified
M75.80	Other shoulder lesions, unspecified shoulder
S43.409A	Unspecified sprain of unspecified shoulder joint, initial encounter
S46.919A	Strain of unspecified muscle, fascia and tendon at shoulder and upper arm level, unspecified arm, initial encounter
M75.20	Bicipital tendinitis, unspecified shoulder
M75.40	Impingement syndrome of unspecified shoulder
M75.50	Bursitis of unspecified shoulder

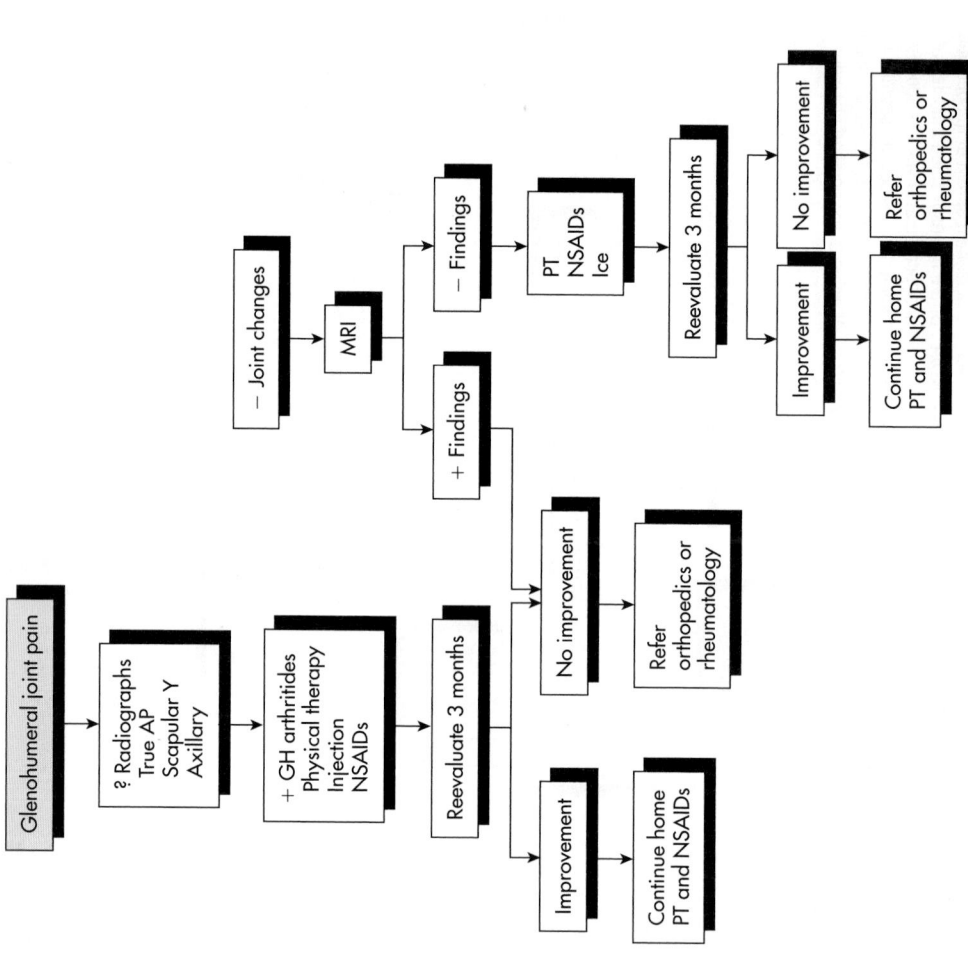

FIG. 249 (Continued)

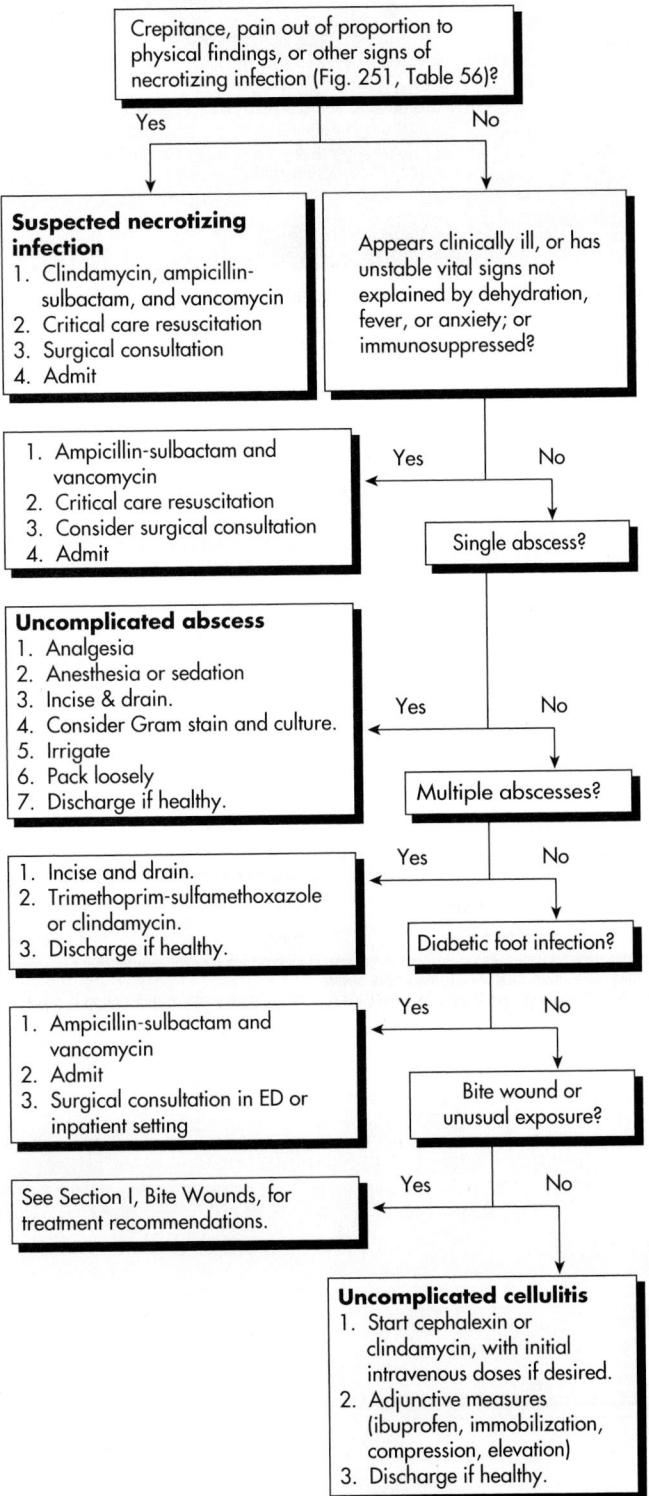

FIG. 250 Universal algorithm for skin and soft tissue infections (assuming no prior treatment).
(From Marx JA et al: *Rosen's emergency medicine*, ed 8, Philadelphia, 2014, Saunders.)

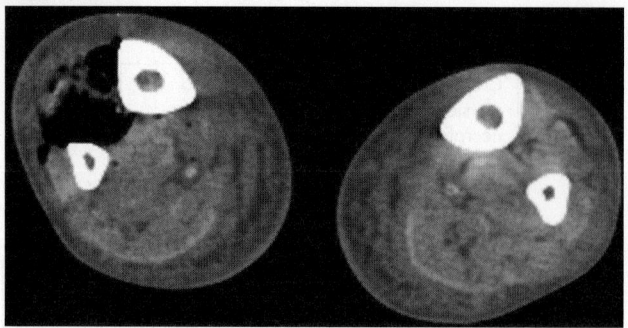

FIG. 251 Necrotizing fasciitis. Axial computed tomography through the lower extremities demonstrates gas in the anterior soft tissues. Necrotizing fasciitis is a clinical diagnosis. Imaging may lead to a delay in treatment. (Webb WR, Brandt WE, Major NM: Fundamentals of body CT, 4th ed, Philadelphia, Elsevier, 2015, ISBN# 978-0-323-22146-7)

Table 56 Differentiating Features of Necrotizing Skin and Soft Tissue Infections

Feature	Progressive Bacterial Synergistic Gangrene	Nonclostridial Anaerobic Cellulitis	Clostridial Myonecrosis (Gas Gangrene)	Necrotizing Fasciitis Type 1	Necrotizing Fasciitis Type 2
Risk factors	Surgery, ileostomy, colostomy, chronic ulceration	Diabetes mellitus	Trauma, surgery	Diabetes mellitus, surgery, perineal infection	Trauma, surgery, none
Microbiology	Microaerophilic streptococci plus *Staphylococcus aureus*	Non–spore-forming anaerobes ± coliforms, streptococci, *S. aureus*	*Clostridium* spp.	Polymicrobial (Enterobacteriaceae plus anaerobes)	Group A streptococci
Course	Slow	Slow or rapid	Very rapid	Rapid	Very rapid
Pain	++++	++/+++	++++	+++/++++	++++
Gas formation	−	++++	++	++	−
Appearance	Central necrotic ulcer, erythematous periphery	Erythematous skin necrosis	Bullae, necrosis	Bullae, skin	Bullae, necrotic skin and tissue
Drainage	Purulent if present	Purulent	Serosanguineous	"Dishwater," seropurulent	Serous if present
Depth of involvement	Skin, soft tissue	Skin, soft tissue	Muscle	Fascia	Fascia
Systemic toxicity	±	+++/++++	++++	+++/++++	++++

−, absent; ±, occasionally present; +, minimal; ++, mild; +++, moderate; ++++, marked or severe.
Parrillo JE, Dellinger RP: Critical Care Medicine, Principles of Diagnosis and Management in the Adult, 4th ed, ISBN # 978-0-323-08929-6, 2014, Elsevier.

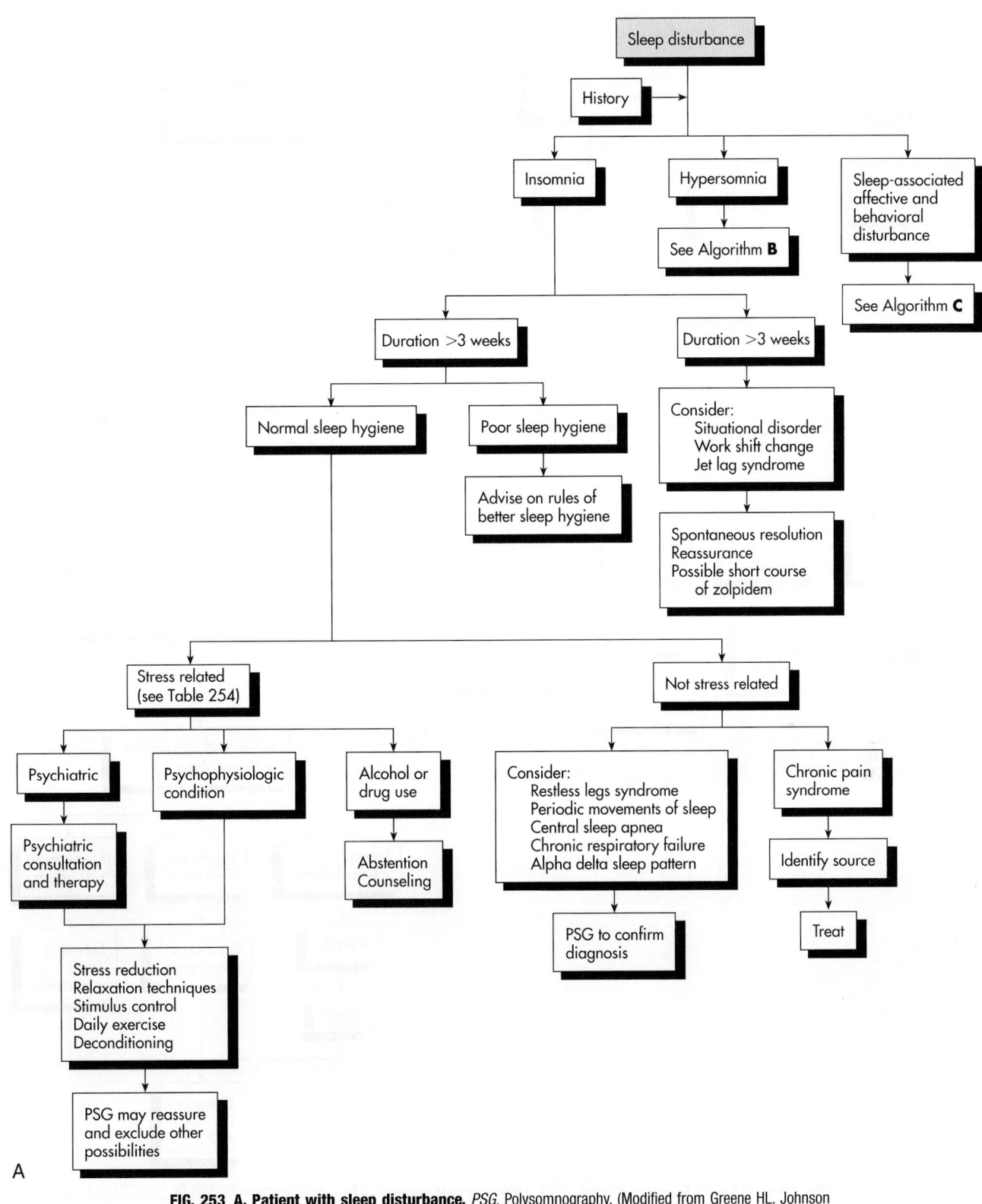

FIG. 253 A, Patient with sleep disturbance. *PSG,* Polysomnography. (Modified from Greene HL, Johnson WP, Lemcke DL [eds]: *Decision making in medicine,* ed 2, St Louis, 1998, Mosby.)

Continued on next page

Clinical Algorithms

III

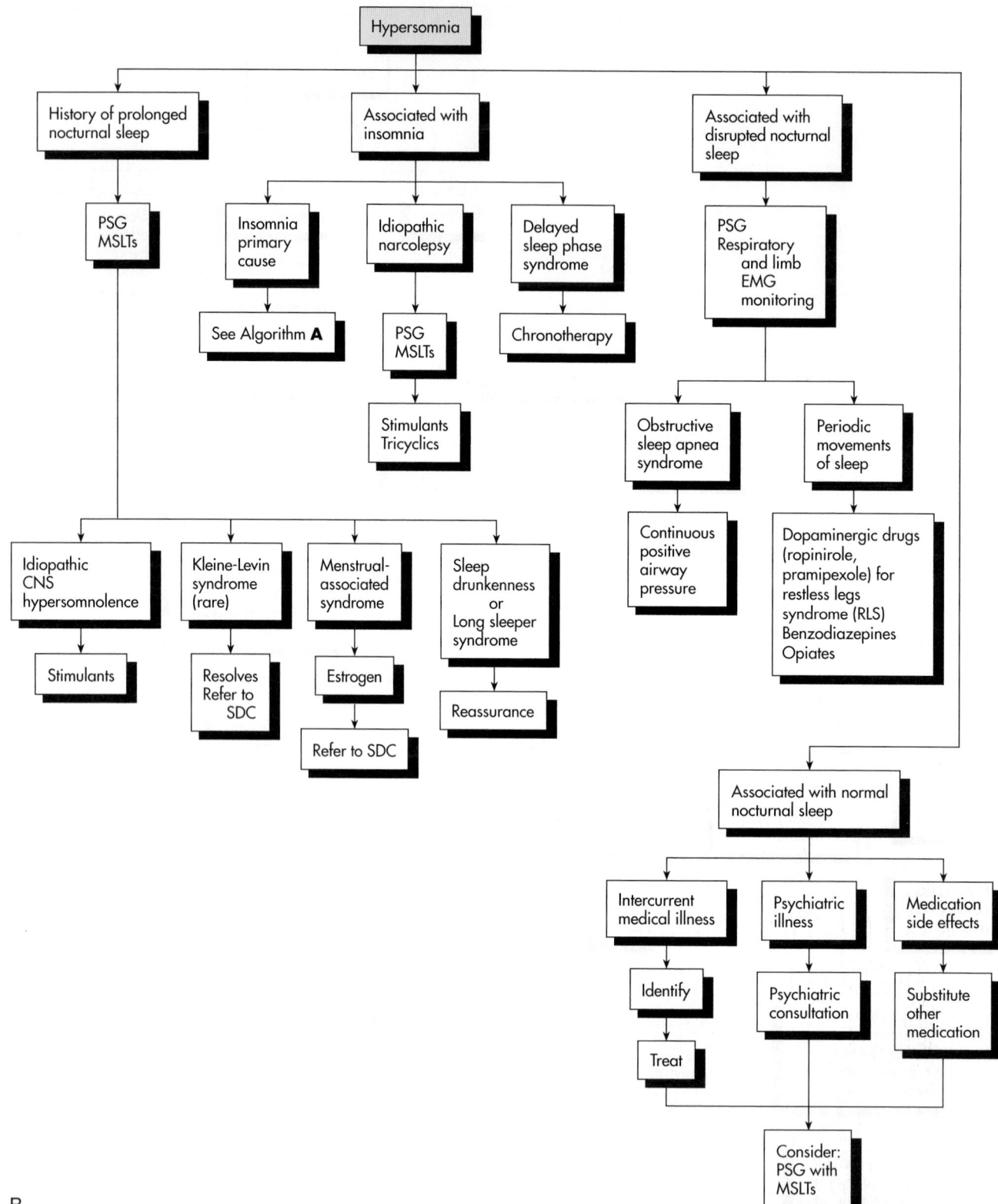

FIG. 253 (Continued) **B, Hypersomnia.** *CNS,* Central nervous system; *EMG,* electromyogram; *MSLTs,* multiple sleep latency tests; *PSG,* polysomnography; *SDC,* sleep disorders clinic. (Modified from Greene HL, Johnson WP, Lemcke DL [eds]: *Decision making in medicine,* ed 2, St Louis, 1998, Mosby.)

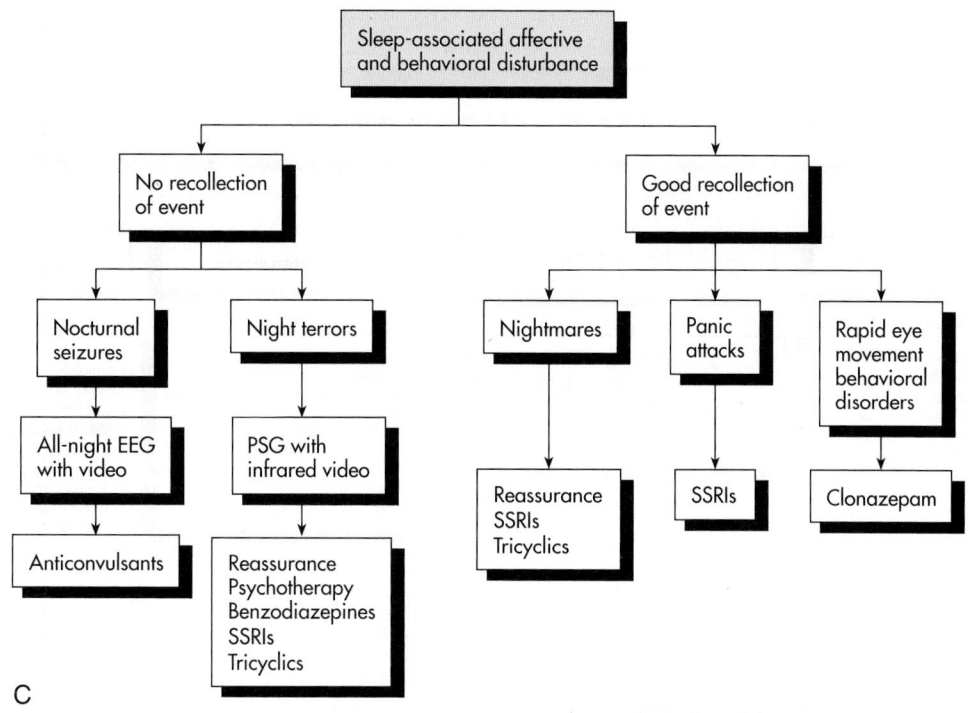

FIG. 253 (Continued) **C, Sleep-associated affective and behavioral disturbance.** *EEG,* Electroencephalogram; *PSG,* polysomnography; *SSRIs,* selective serotonin reuptake inhibitors. (Modified from Greene HL, Johnson WP, Lemcke DL [eds]: *Decision making in medicine,* ed 2, St Louis, 1998, Mosby.)

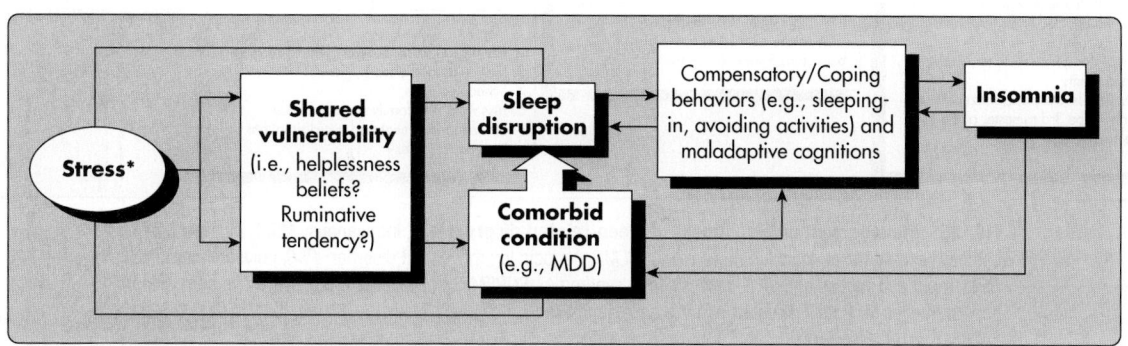

FIG. 254 Possible etiologic pathways for comorbid insomnia. *Stress may be in the form of an internal (e.g., hormonal change) or external (e.g., interpersonal conflict) event that can directly cause either sleep disruption or a comorbid condition. Compensatory behaviors or arousing cognitions are thought to play a role in causing or maintaining the insomnia. The stressor may also operate through a moderator variable (i.e., a shared vulnerability trait) of insomnia and the comorbid illness. *MDD,* Major depressive disorder. (Kryger M, Roth T, Dement WC: Principles and Practice of Sleep Medicine, 6th ed, ISBN # 978-0-323-24288-2, 2017, Elsevier.)

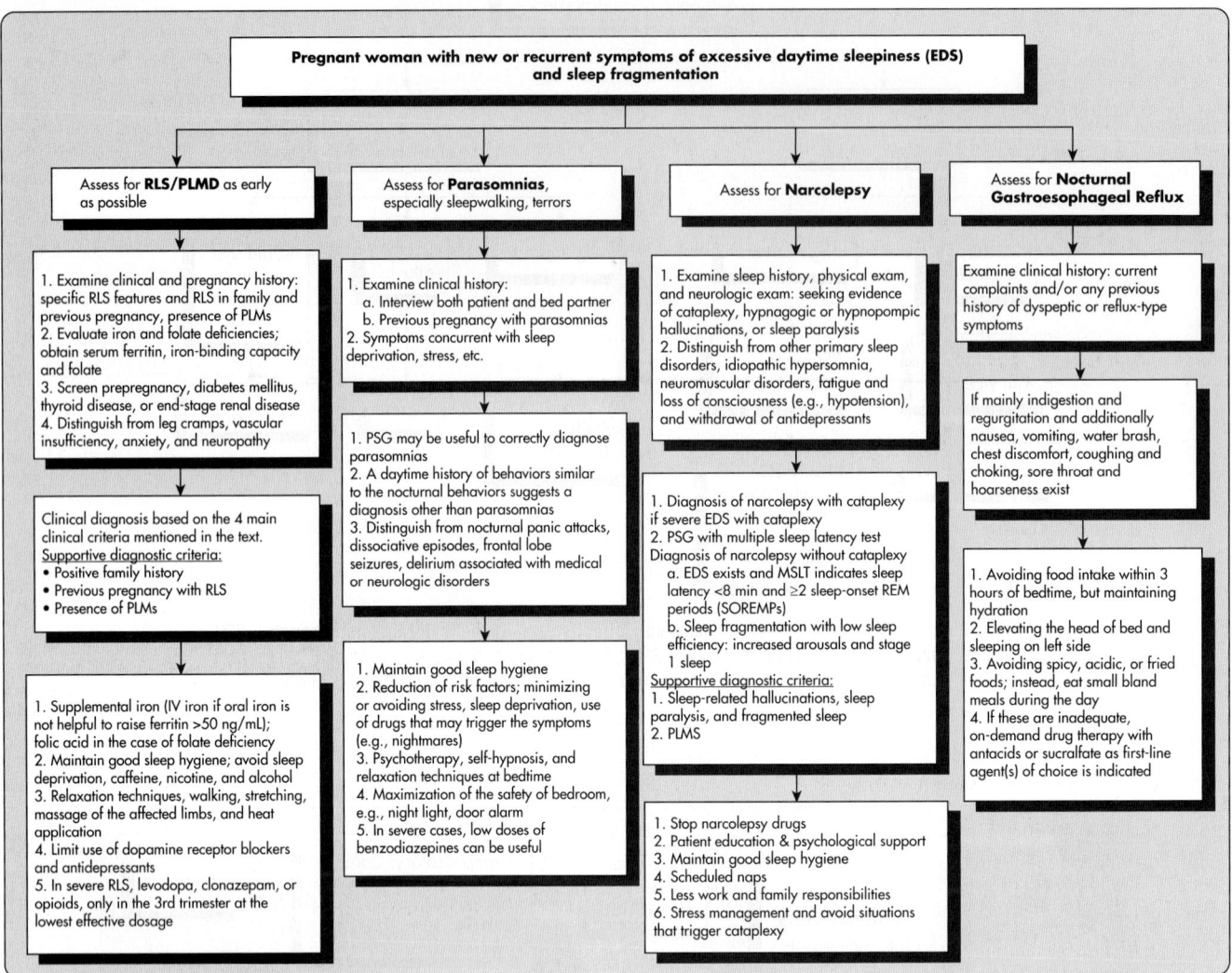

FIG. 255 Management and treatment of sleep-related disorders. *IV*, Intravenous; *MSLT*, Multiple Sleep Latency Test; *PLMs*, periodic leg movements; *PLMD*, periodic leg movement disorder; *PSG*, polysomnography; *REM*, rapid eye movement; *RLS*, restless legs syndrome; *SOREMP*, sleep-onset rapid eye movement sleep period. (Kryger M, Roth T, Dement WC: Principles and Practice of Sleep Medicine, 6th ed, ISBN # 978-0-323-24288-2, 2017, Elsevier.)

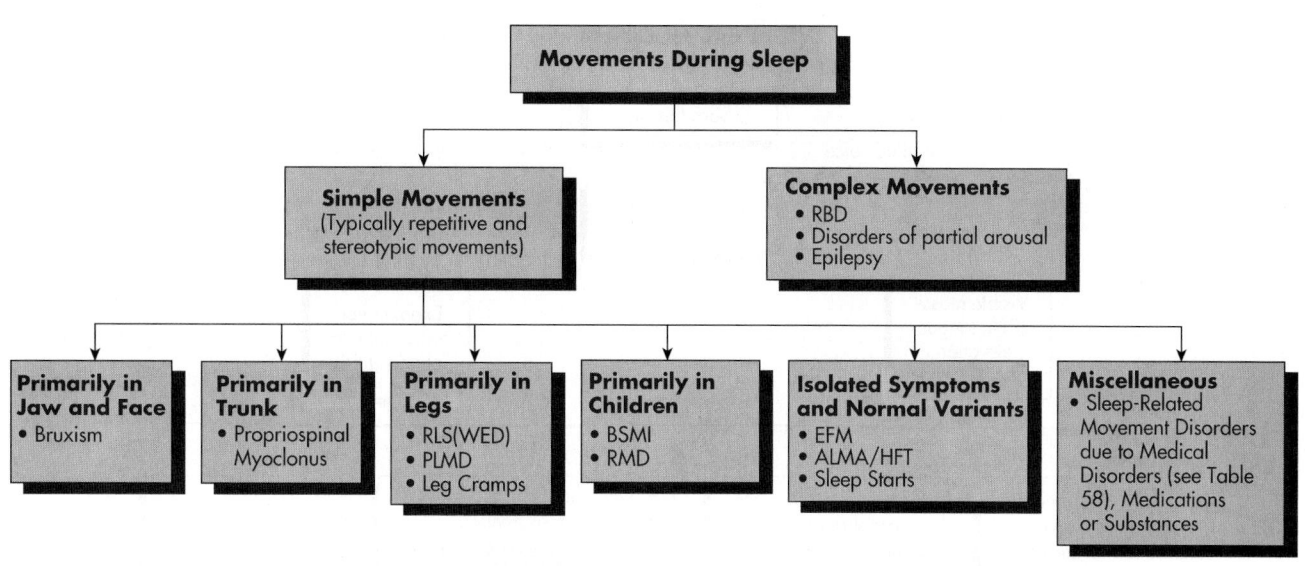

FIG. 256 Flow chart for the approach to the differential diagnosis of sleep-related movement disorders. *ALMA,* Alternating leg muscle activation; *BSMI,* benign sleep myoclonus of infancy; *EFM,* excessive fragmentary myoclonus; *HFT,* hypnagogic foot tremor; *PLMD,* periodic limb movement disorder; *RBD,* rapid eye movement (REM) sleep behavior disorder; *RLS (WED),* restless legs syndrome (Willis-Ekbom disease); *RMD,* rhythmic movement disorder. (Kryger M, Roth T, Dement WC: Principles and Practice of Sleep Medicine, 6th ed, ISBN # 978-0-323-24288-2, 2017, Elsevier.)

Table 58 Distinguishing Features of Nocturnal Events

Feature	Disorders of Arousal	Sleep-Related Eating Disorder	REM Behavior Disorder	Recurrent Isolated Sleep Paralysis	Exploding Head Syndrome	Psychogenic Events	Nocturnal Seizures
Behavior	Confused; semipurposeful movement with eyes open	Eating typically high-calorie foods; eyes open	Sometimes combative with eyes closed	Episodes of inability to move	Painless sensation of explosion inside the head	Variable	Dependent on the portion of brain involved
Age of onset	Childhood and adolescence	Variable	Older adult	Variable	Adult	Adolescence to adulthood	Variable
Time of occurrence	First third of night	First half of night	During REM	Typically on awakening	Usually near sleep onset but can be variable	Anytime	Anytime
Frequency of events	Less than one per night	Variable	Multiple per night	Variable less than weekly	Rare	Variable	Frontal seizures—multiple per night
Duration	Minutes	Minutes	Seconds to minute	Seconds to minutes	Seconds	Variable minutes or longer	Usually under 3 minutes
Memory of event	Usually none	Usually none or limited	Dream recall	Yes	Yes	None	Usually none
Stereotypical movements	No	No	No	No	Similar sensation	No	Yes
Polysomnogram findings	Arousals from slow wave sleep	Arousal from NREM sleep	Excessive electromyogram tone during REM sleep	Arousal from REM sleep	Usually occurs in light sleep	Occur from awake state	Potentially epileptiform activity

Kryger M, Roth T, Dement WC: Principles and Practice of Sleep Medicine, 6th ed, ISBN # 978-0-323-24288-2, 2017, Elsevier.

Clinical Algorithms

III

DIAGNOSTIC ALGORITHM

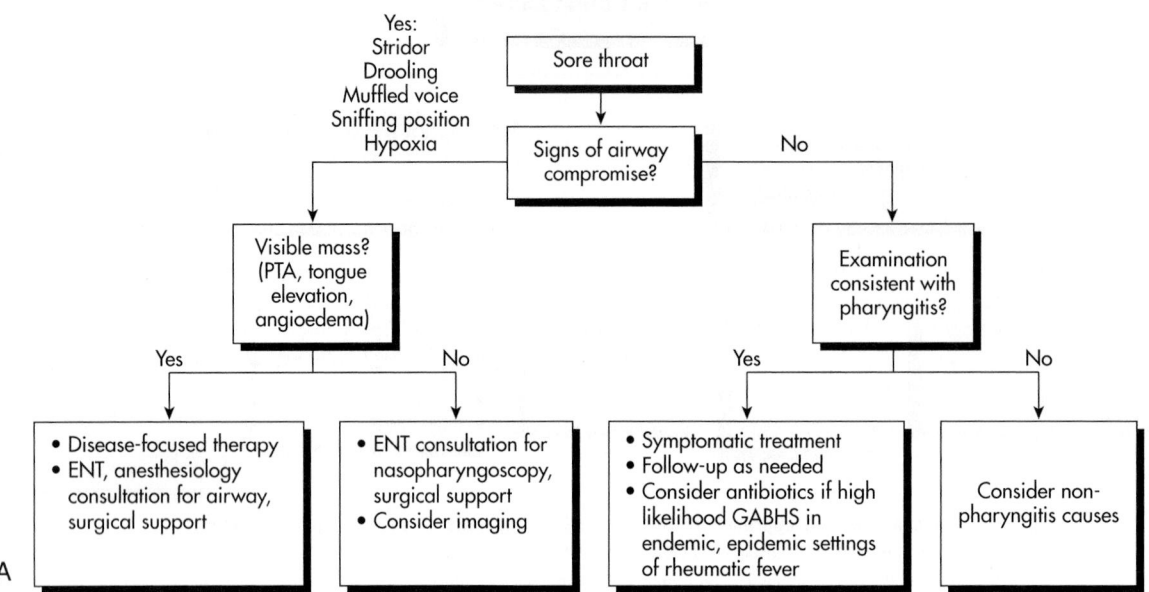

MANAGEMENT ALGORITHM

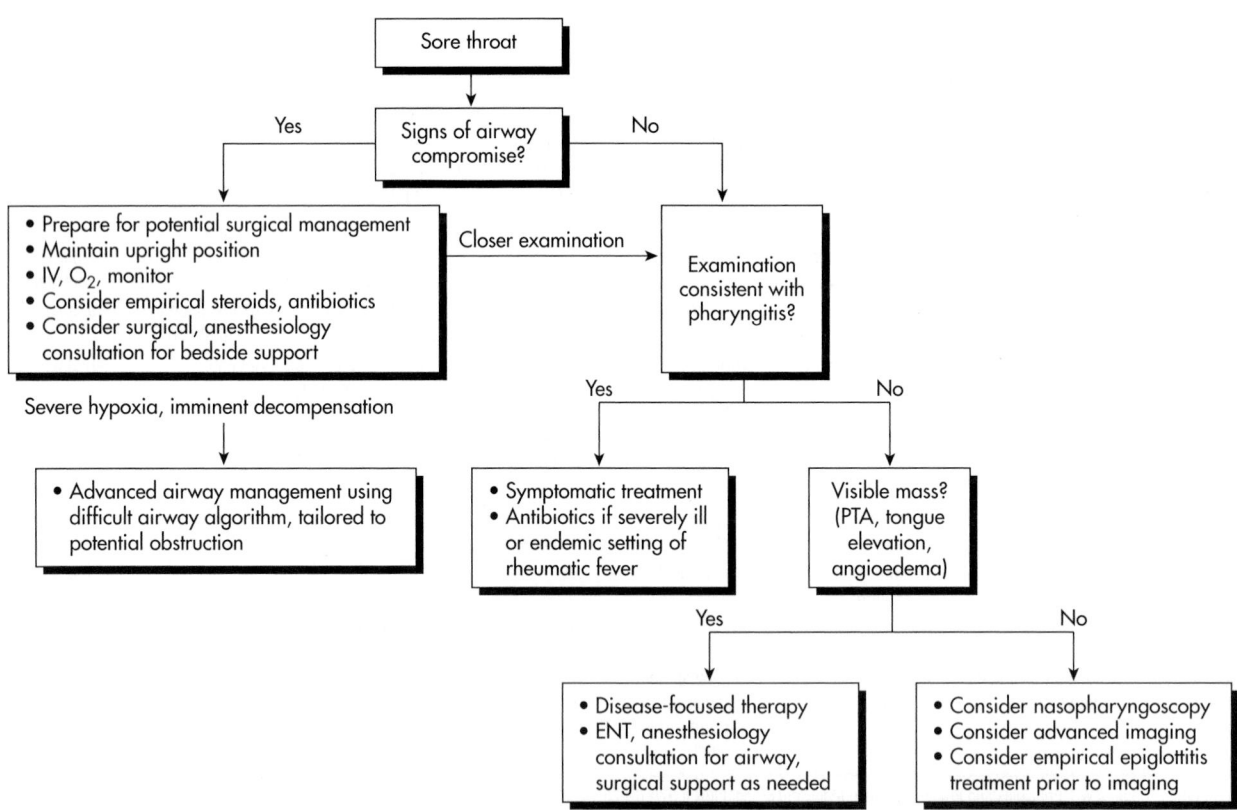

FIG. 257 Clinical approach to the patient with sore throat—diagnosis and management. Refer to Section I, Pharyngitis/Tonsillitis and Epiglottitis, for additional information on this matter. *ENT,* Ear-nose-throat; *GABHS,* group A beta-hemolytic streptococcus; *IV,* intravenous; *PTA,* peritonsillar abscess. (From Marx JA et al: *Rosen's emergency medicine,* ed 8, Philadelphia, 2014, Saunders.)

SPLENOMEGALY

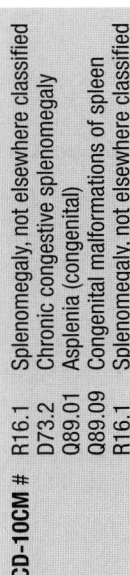

ICD-10CM #
R16.1   Splenomegaly, not elsewhere classified
D73.2   Chronic congestive splenomegaly
Q89.01   Asplenia (congenital)
Q89.09   Congenital malformations of spleen
R16.1   Splenomegaly, not elsewhere classified

Splenomegaly

With lymphadenopathy
See Section III algorithm,
Lymphadenopathy,
Generalized

Without lymphadenopathy

Confirm
Spleen ultrasound or CT

Exclude
Portal hypertension
Congestive heart failure
Subacute bacterial endocarditis

Splenic cyst or
displacement of normal-
sized spleen excluded

Evaluate for immunologic disorders
Systemic lupus erythematosus
Rheumatoid arthritis
Felty's syndrome

Immunologic causes
excluded

Examine peripheral blood smear
Hematologic malignancies
Nonmalignant hematologic disease
Parasitemia

Results negative
or equivocal

Bone marrow aspiration, biopsy, and cultures
Hematologic conditions
Chronic fungal and mycobacterial infections
Gaucher's disease
Amyloidosis

Bone marrow nondiagnostic,
cultures negative

Asymptomatic:
Follow

Symptomatic:
Consider splenectomy for diagnosis

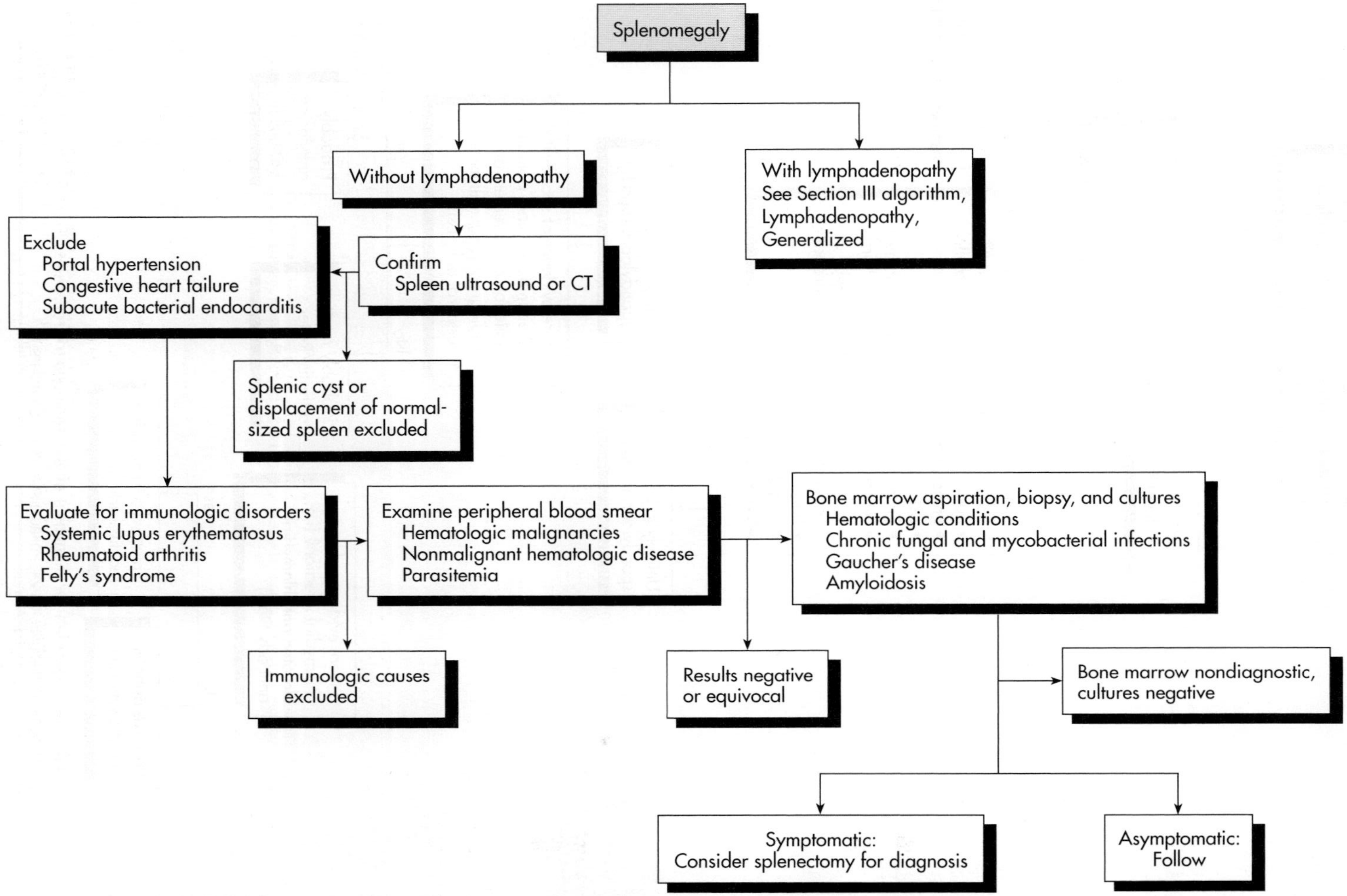

FIG. 259 Clinical approach to patient with splenomegaly. *CT,* Computed tomography. (Modified from Stein JH [ed]: *Internal medicine,* ed 5, St Louis, 1998, Mosby.)

Clinical
Algorithms

III

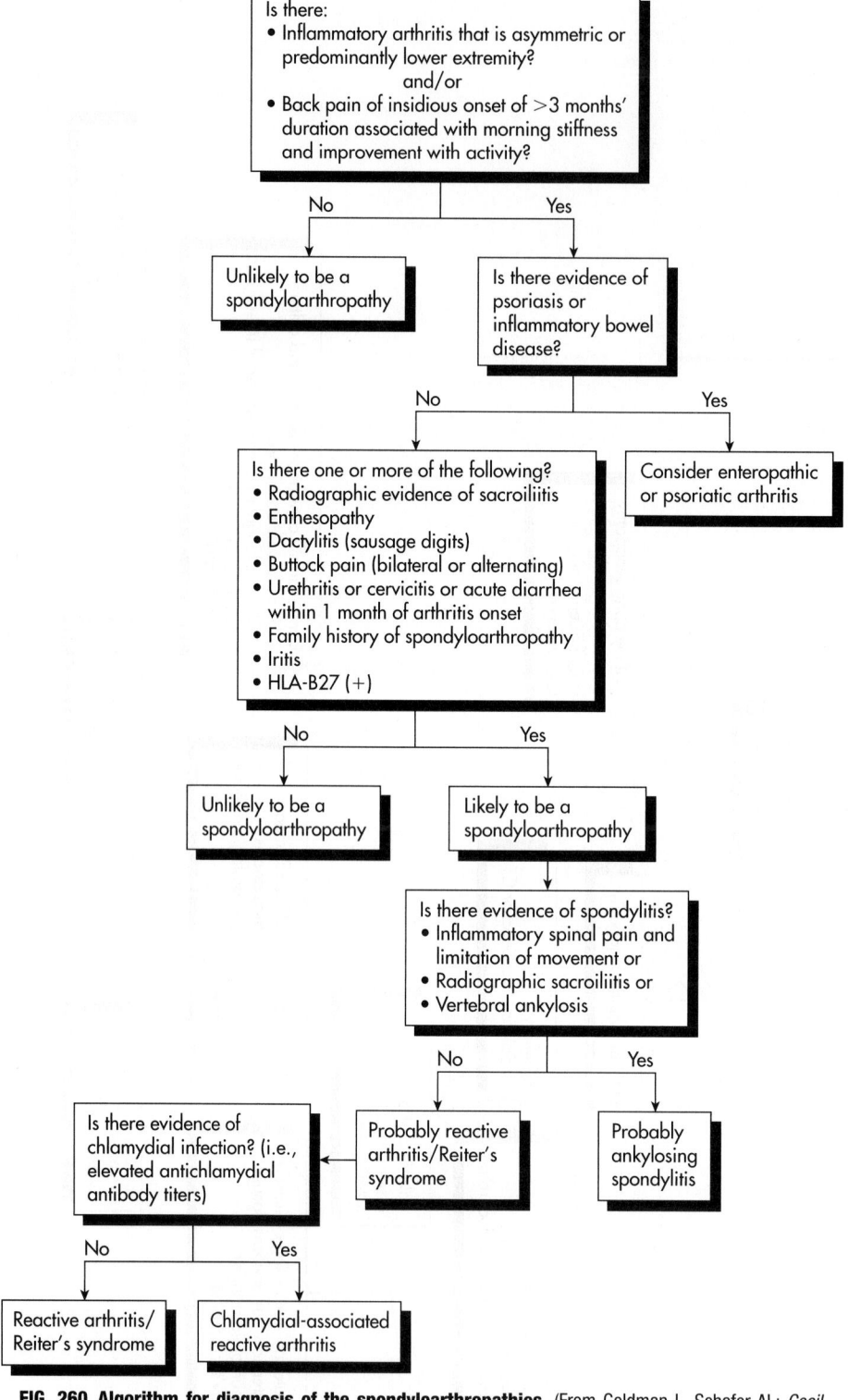

FIG. 260 Algorithm for diagnosis of the spondyloarthropathies. (From Goldman L, Schafer AL: *Cecil textbook of medicine,* ed 24, Philadelphia, 2012, Saunders.)

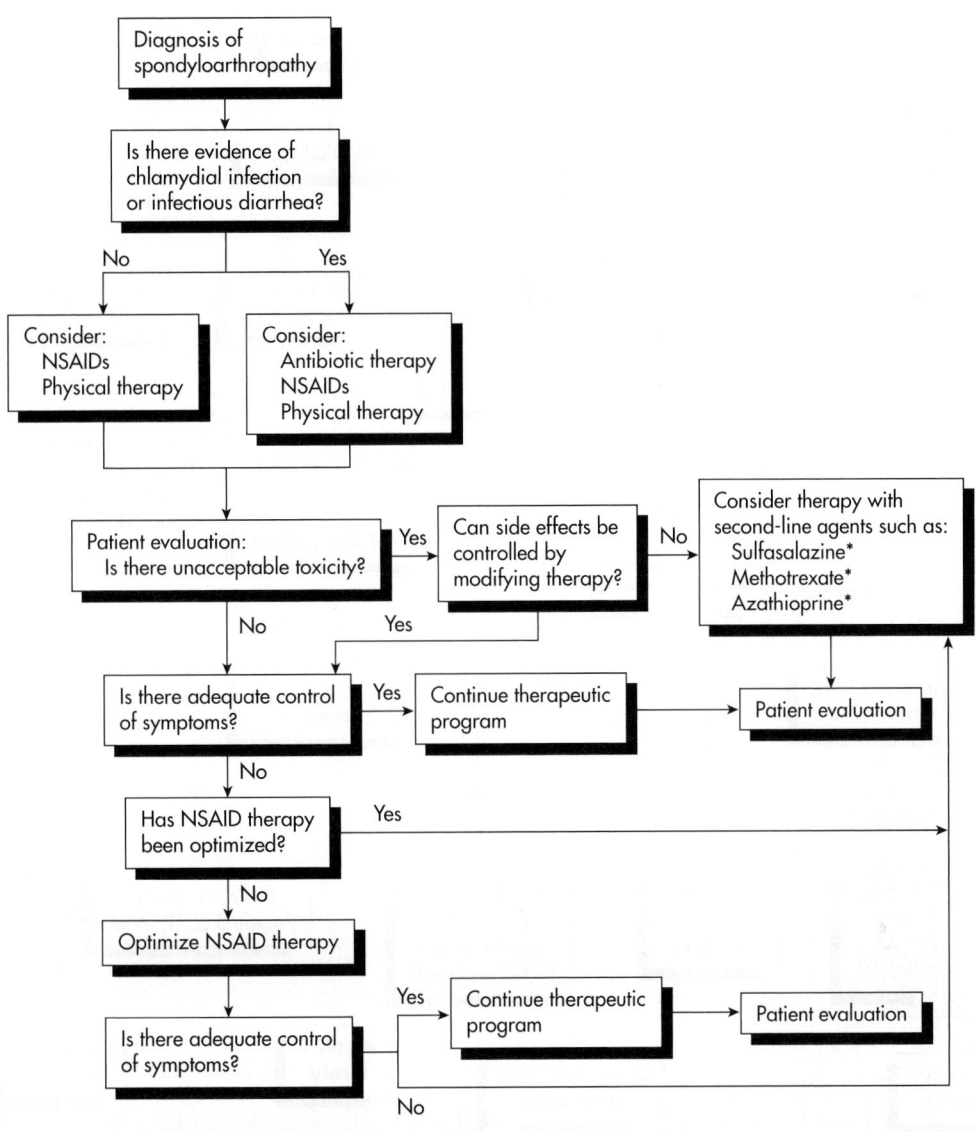

*Not approved by the FDA for treatment of spondyloarthropathies.

FIG. 261 Treatment algorithm for patients with a spondyloarthropathy. *FDA,* Food and Drug Administration; *NSAID,* nonsteroidal antiinflammatory drug. (From Goldman L, Schafer AL: *Cecil textbook of medicine,* ed 24, Philadelphia, 2012, Saunders.)

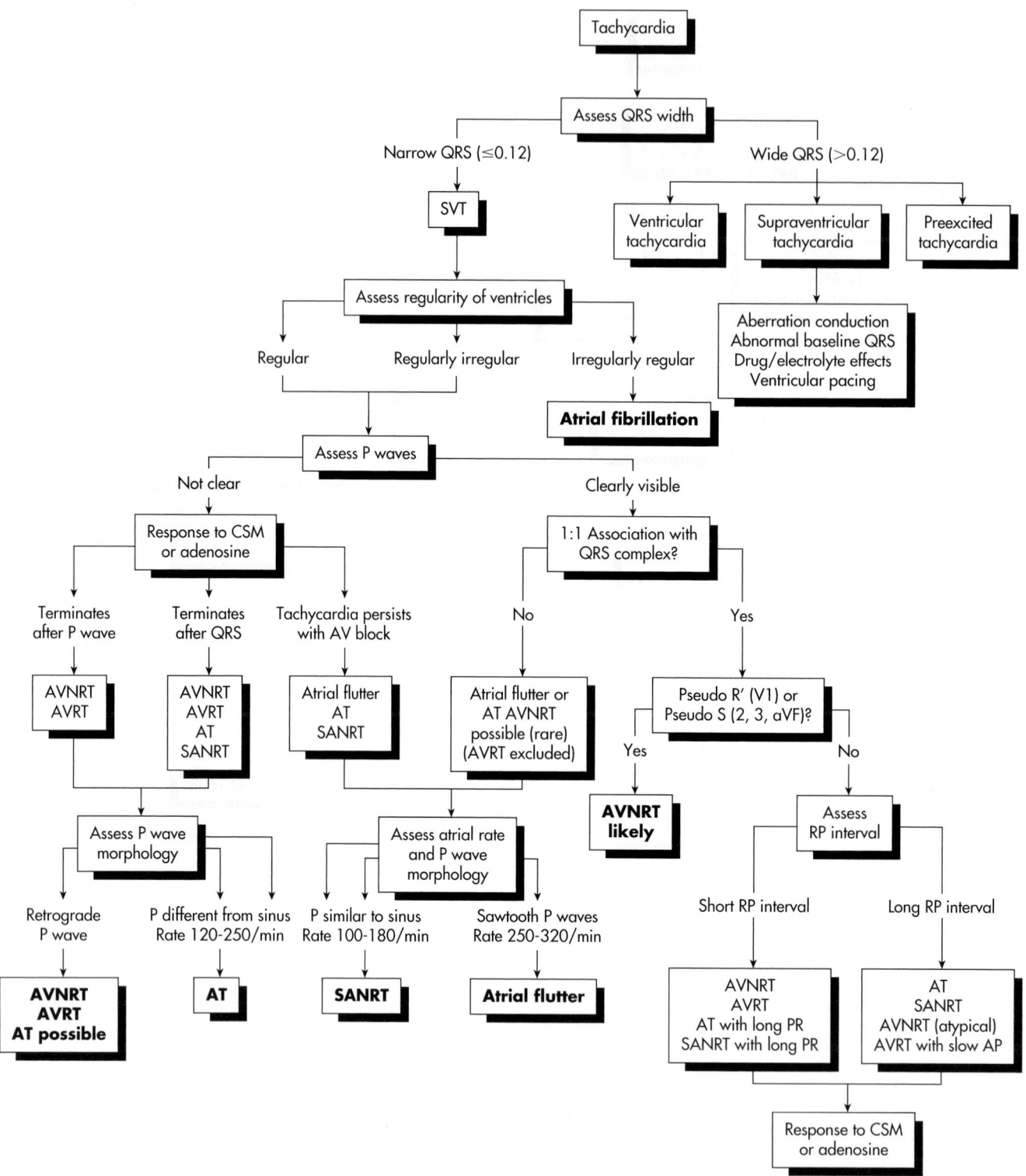

FIG. 265 Stepwise approach to the diagnosis of type of tachycardia based on 12-lead electrocardiogram during the episode. The initial step is to determine whether the tachycardia has a wide or narrow QRS complex (see Fig.266). For wide complex tachycardia, see Fig. 269; the remainder of the algorithm is helpful in diagnosing the type of narrow-complex tachycardia. *AP,* Accessory pathway; *AT,* atrial tachycardia; *AV,* atrioventricular; *AVNRT,* AV nodal reentrant tachycardia; *AVRT,* AV reciprocating tachycardia; *CSM,* carotid sinus massage; *SANRT,* sinoatrial nodal reentry tachycardia; *SVT,* supraventricular tachycardia. (From Zipes DP, Libby P, Bonow RO, Braunwald E [eds]: *Braunwald's heart disease,* ed 7, Philadelphia, 2005, Saunders.)

TACHYCARDIA, NARROW COMPLEX

ICD-10CM #	I49.02	Ventricular flutter
	I49.8	Other specified cardiac arrhythmias
	R00.1	Bradycardia, unspecified

1747

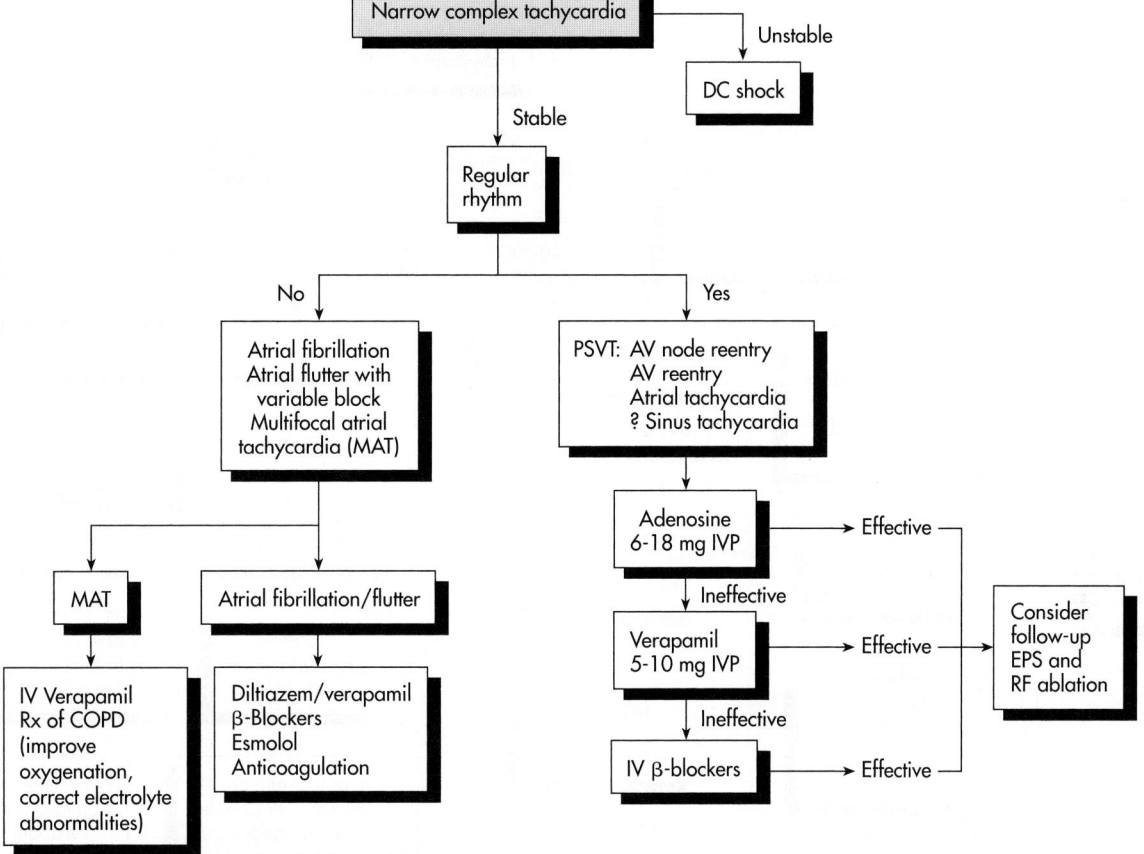

FIG. 266 Evaluation and management of narrow complex tachycardia. *AV,* Atrioventricular; *COPD,* chronic obstructive pulmonary disease; *EPS,* electrophysiologic studies; *IV,* intravenous; *IVP,* intravenous push; *PSVT,* paroxysmal supraventricular tachycardia; *RF,* radiofrequency.

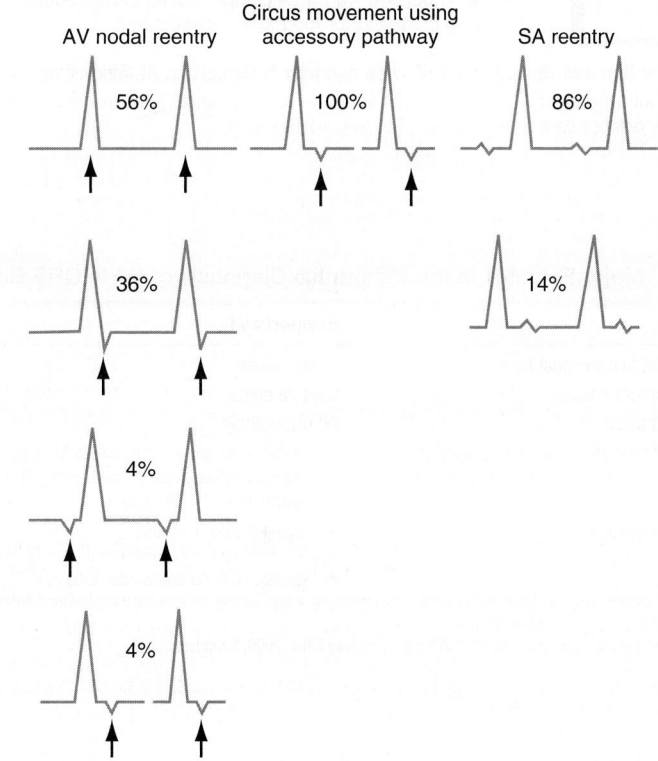

FIG. 267 Location of P waves in common causes of regular narrow-complex tachycardia. *AV,* atrioventricular; *SA,* sinoatrial. (From Marriott HJL, Conover MB: Advanced Concepts in Dysrhythmias, 2nd ed. St Louis, Mosby, 1989.) (Marx JA et al: *Rosen's Emergency Medicine,* ed 8, Philadelphia, 2014, Saunders.)

ICD-10CM # I49.02 Ventricular flutter
I49.8 Other specified cardiac arrhythmias
R00.1 Bradycardia, unspecified

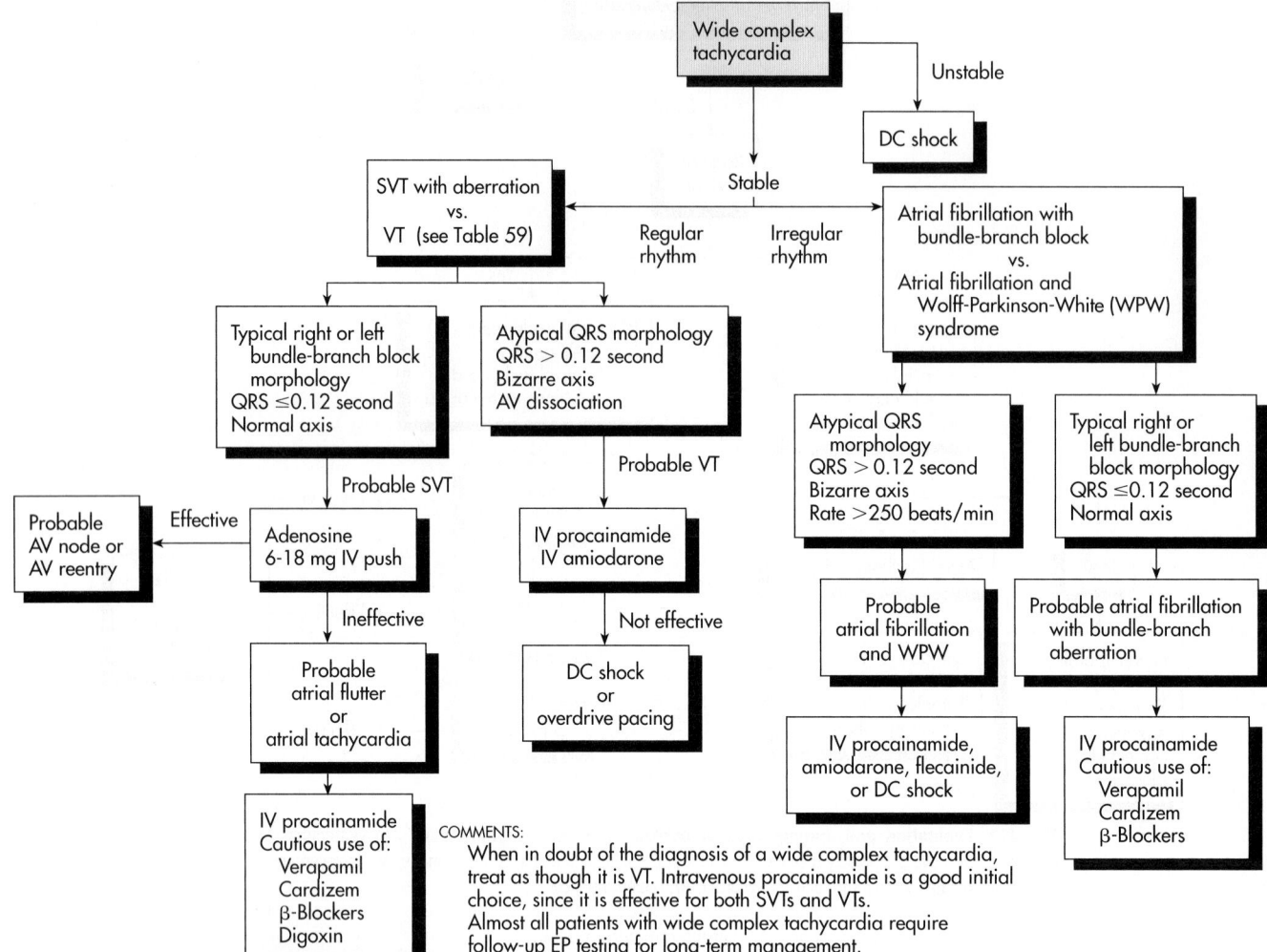

FIG. 269 Evaluation and management of wide complex tachycardia. *AV,* Atrioventricular; *EP,* electrophysiologic; *IV,* intravenous; *SVT,* supraventricular tachycardia; *VT,* ventricular tachycardia. (From Driscoll CE et al: *The family practice desk reference,* ed 3, St Louis, 1996, Mosby.)

Table 59 Major Features in the Differential Diagnosis of Wide QRS Beats	
Supports SVT	**Supports VT**
Slowing or termination by vagal tone	Fusion beats
Onset with premature P wave	Capture beats
RP interval <100 msec	AV dissociation
P and QRS rate and rhythm linked to suggest that ventricular activation depends on atrial discharge, e.g., 2:1 AV block rSR′ V1	P and QRS rate and rhythm linked to suggest that atrial activation depends on ventricular discharge, e.g., 2:1 VA block
Long-short cycle sequence	• "Compensatory" pause
	• Left axis deviation; QRS duration >140 msec
	• Specific QRS contours (see text)

SVT, Supraventricular tachycardia; *VT,* ventricular tachycardia.
From Zipes DP et al [eds]: *Braunwauld's heart disease,* ed 7, Philadelphia, 2005, Saunders.

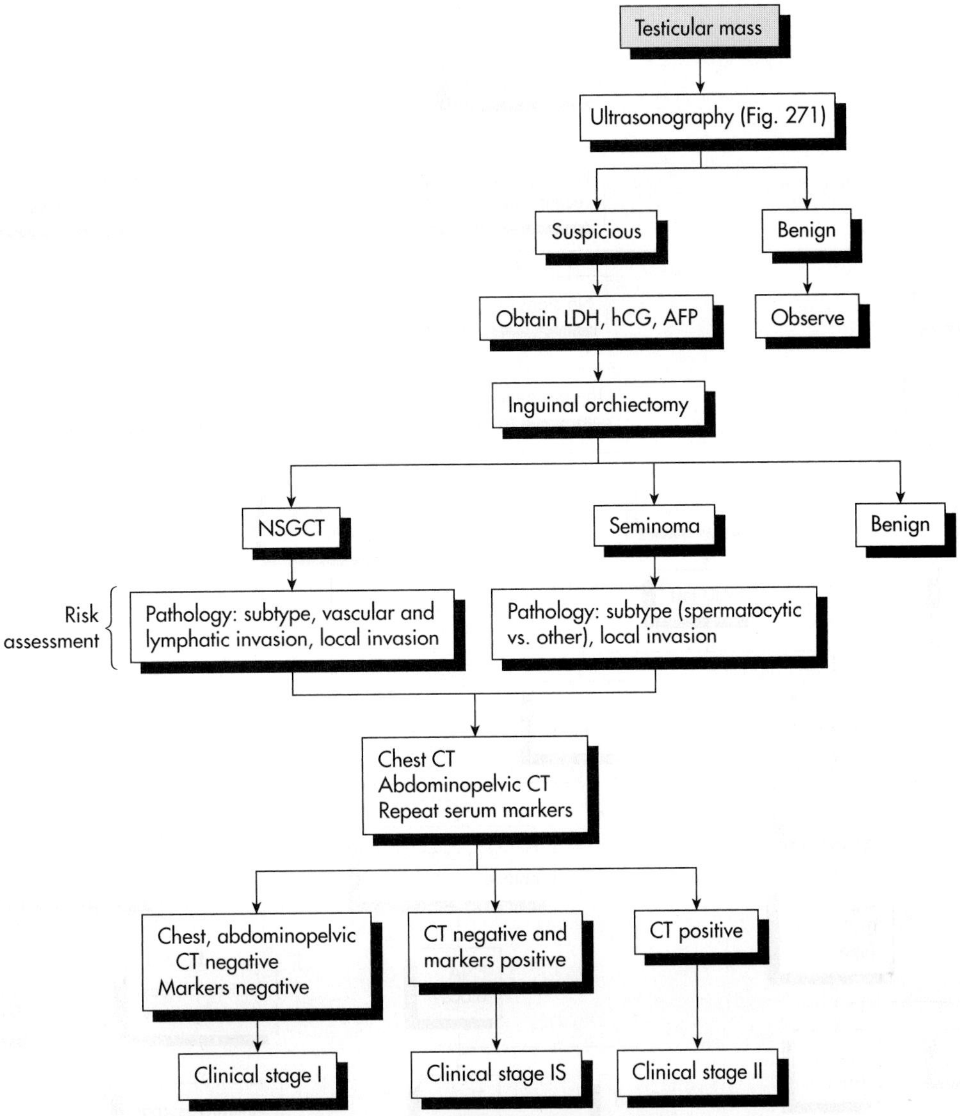

```
                        ┌─────────────────┐
                        │ Testicular mass │
                        └─────────────────┘
                                 │
                        ┌──────────────────────┐
                        │ Ultrasonography (Fig. 271) │
                        └──────────────────────┘
                           │                │
                   ┌────────────┐      ┌─────────┐
                   │ Suspicious │      │ Benign  │
                   └────────────┘      └─────────┘
                         │                  │
                ┌──────────────────┐   ┌─────────┐
                │ Obtain LDH, hCG, AFP │ │ Observe │
                └──────────────────┘   └─────────┘
                         │
                ┌──────────────────┐
                │ Inguinal orchiectomy │
                └──────────────────┘
              │               │              │
         ┌────────┐      ┌──────────┐    ┌────────┐
         │ NSGCT  │      │ Seminoma │    │ Benign │
         └────────┘      └──────────┘    └────────┘
```

Risk assessment

| Pathology: subtype, vascular and lymphatic invasion, local invasion | Pathology: subtype (spermatocytic vs. other), local invasion |

```
                ┌──────────────────────┐
                │ Chest CT             │
                │ Abdominopelvic CT    │
                │ Repeat serum markers │
                └──────────────────────┘
          │                 │              │
┌──────────────────┐ ┌────────────────┐ ┌───────────┐
│ Chest, abdominopelvic │ CT negative and │ │ CT positive │
│ CT negative      │ │ markers positive │ └───────────┘
│ Markers negative │ └────────────────┘
└──────────────────┘
        │                   │               │
┌──────────────┐    ┌──────────────┐  ┌──────────────┐
│ Clinical stage I │  │ Clinical stage IS │ │ Clinical stage II │
└──────────────┘    └──────────────┘  └──────────────┘
```

FIG. 270 Diagnosis, staging, and risk assessment of patients with testicular germ cell tumor. See Section I, Testicular Cancer, for additional information. *AFP,* α-Fetoprotein; *CT,* computed tomography; *hCG,* human chorionic gonadotropin; *LDH,* lactic dehydrogenase; *NSGCT,* nonseminoma germ cell tumor. (From Abeloff MD: *Clinical oncology,* ed 4, New York, 2007, Churchill Livingstone.)

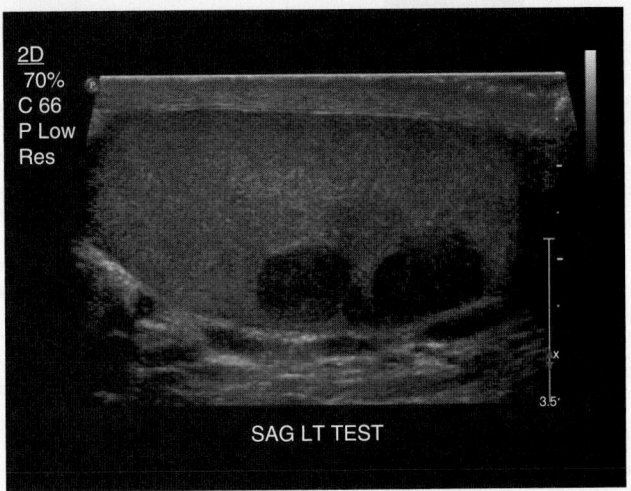

FIG. 271 Sagittal view of ultrasound of left testis showing multinodular hypoechoic intratesticular lesion confirmed to be pure seminoma at orchiectomy. (Wein AJ, Kavoussi LR, Partin AW, Peters CA: Campbell-Walsh Urology, 11th ed, ISBN# 978-1-4557-7567-5, 2016, Elsevier.)

Clinical
Algorithms

III

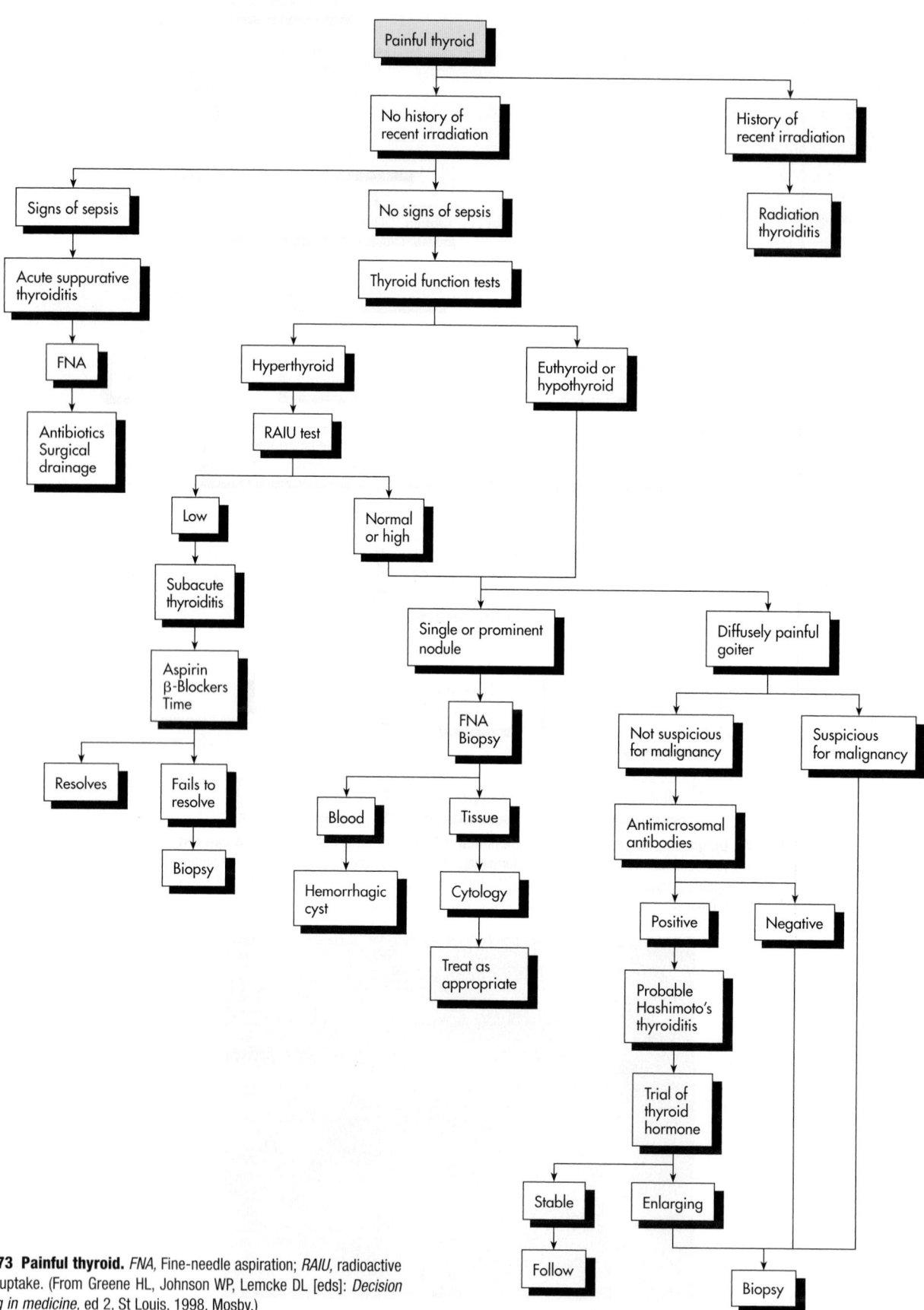

FIG. 273 Painful thyroid. *FNA,* Fine-needle aspiration; *RAIU,* radioactive iodine uptake. (From Greene HL, Johnson WP, Lemcke DL [eds]: *Decision making in medicine,* ed 2, St Louis, 1998, Mosby.)

Patient with symptoms and signs suggesting thyrotoxicosis, no amiodarone; serum TSH <0.2 mU/L, free T₄ or T₃ elevated

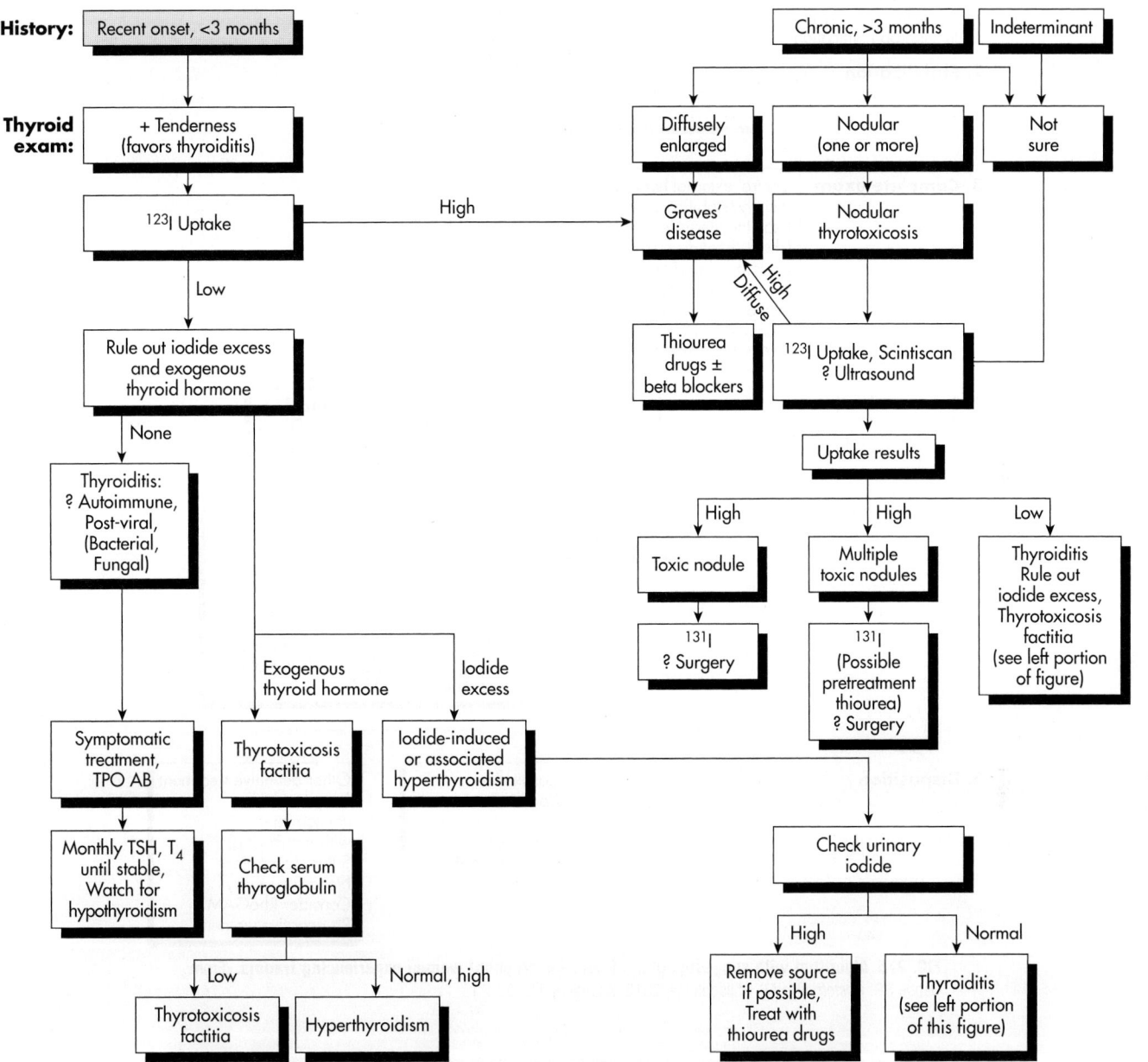

FIG. 274 Algorithm for determining the cause of thyrotropin-independent thyrotoxicosis. Additional information on thyrotoxicosis is available in Section I, topics Hyperthyroidism, Thyroid Nodule, Thyroiditis, Thyroid Storm, and Graves Disease. *T₃*, Triiodothyronine; *T₄*, thyroxine; *TPO AB*, thyroid peroxidase antibody; *TSH*, thyroid-stimulating hormone (thyrotropin). (From Melmed S, Polonsky KS, Larsen PR, Kronenberg HM, *Williams textbook of endocrinology*, ed 12, Philadelphia, 2011, Saunders.)

Clinical
Algorithms

III

EMERGENCY DEPARTMENT MANAGEMENT: TRAUMA IN PREGNANCY

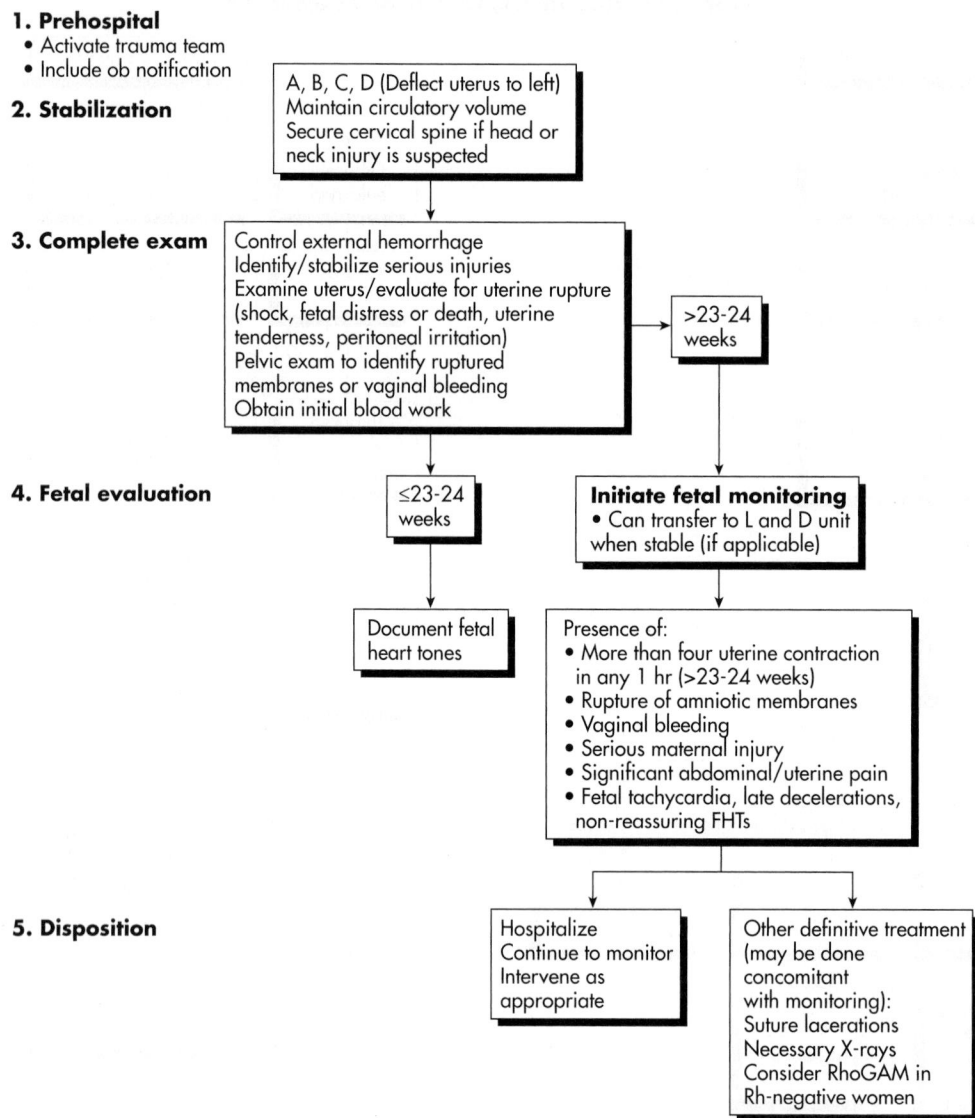

1. Prehospital
- Activate trauma team
- Include ob notification

2. Stabilization

A, B, C, D (Deflect uterus to left)
Maintain circulatory volume
Secure cervical spine if head or
neck injury is suspected

3. Complete exam

Control external hemorrhage
Identify/stabilize serious injuries
Examine uterus/evaluate for uterine rupture
(shock, fetal distress or death, uterine
tenderness, peritoneal irritation)
Pelvic exam to identify ruptured
membranes or vaginal bleeding
Obtain initial blood work

>23-24
weeks

4. Fetal evaluation

≤23-24
weeks

Initiate fetal monitoring
- Can transfer to L and D unit
when stable (if applicable)

Document fetal
heart tones

Presence of:
- More than four uterine contraction
in any 1 hr (>23-24 weeks)
- Rupture of amniotic membranes
- Vaginal bleeding
- Serious maternal injury
- Significant abdominal/uterine pain
- Fetal tachycardia, late decelerations,
non-reassuring FHTs

5. Disposition

Hospitalize
Continue to monitor
Intervene as
appropriate

Other definitive treatment
(may be done
concomitant
with monitoring):
Suture lacerations
Necessary X-rays
Consider RhoGAM in
Rh-negative women

FIG. 275 Algorithm with suggested plan of care for pregnant women experiencing trauma. (From Gabbe SG: *Obstetrics,* ed 6, Philadelphia, 2012, Saunders, Fig. 25-2.)

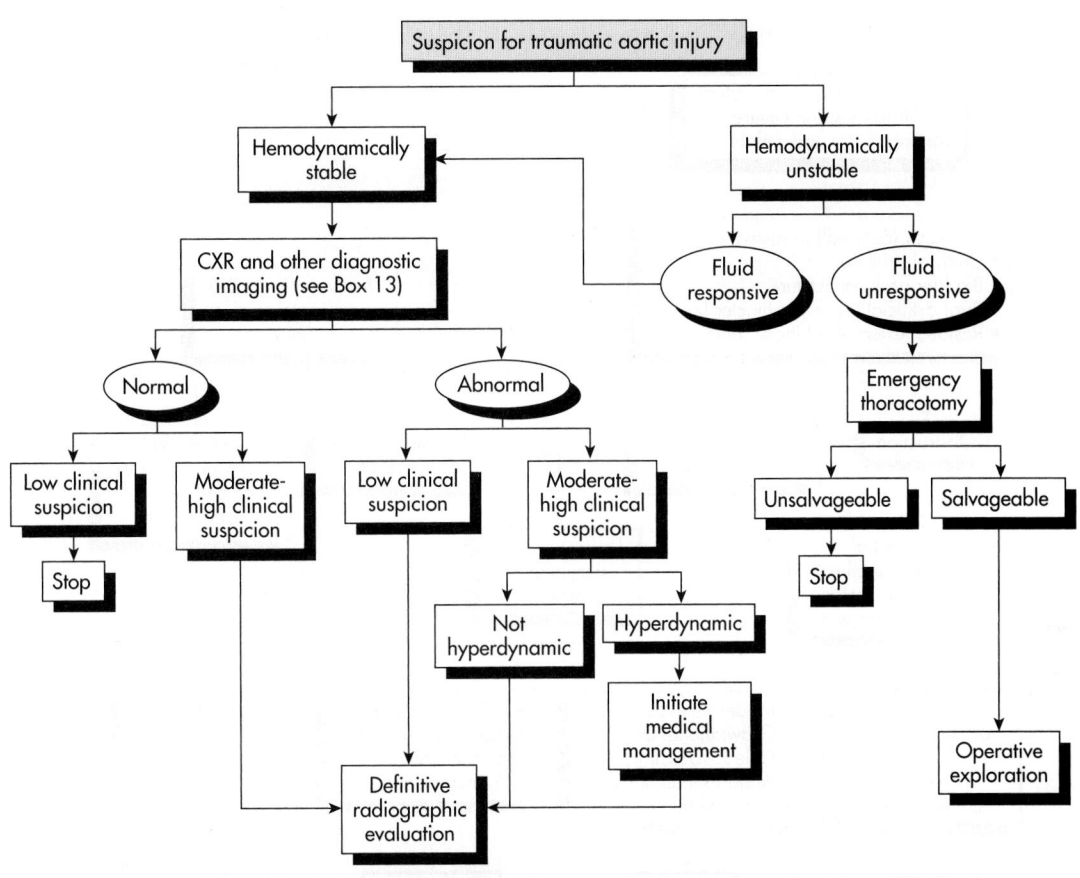

FIG. 276 Diagnostic management algorithm for suspected traumatic aortic injury. *CXR,* Chest radiograph. (Modified from Adams JG, et al: *Emergency medicine, clinical essentials,* ed 2, Philadelphia, 2013, Elsevier.)

BOX 13   Pros and Cons of Imaging Modalities for Great Vessel Injury

Chest Radiography
Pros
Inexpensive
Performed at the bedside
Easy to interpret
Cons
Nonspecific
False-negative rate of 7% to 10% for traumatic aortic injury

Computed Tomographic Angiography
Pros
Identifies mediastinal hematoma and differentiates its causes
Identifies aortic injury, including intimal tears
Sensitivity and specificity approaching 100% for traumatic aortic injury
Cons
Poor delineation of nonaortic vascular injuries
Requires relative hemodynamic stability to obtain

Aortography
Pros
Traditional "gold standard"
Beneficial in the diagnosis of branch vessel injuries
Delineates equivocal computed tomographic angiographic findings
Cons
Difficult to obtain on an emergency basis
Requires relative hemodynamic stability

Transesophageal Echocardiography
Pros
May be performed at the bedside
Not limited by body habitus
Cons
Poor availability on an emergency basis
Contraindicated in patients with an unstable cervical spine or suspected esophageal trauma

MALE SPHINCTERIC URINARY INCONTINENCE (UI)

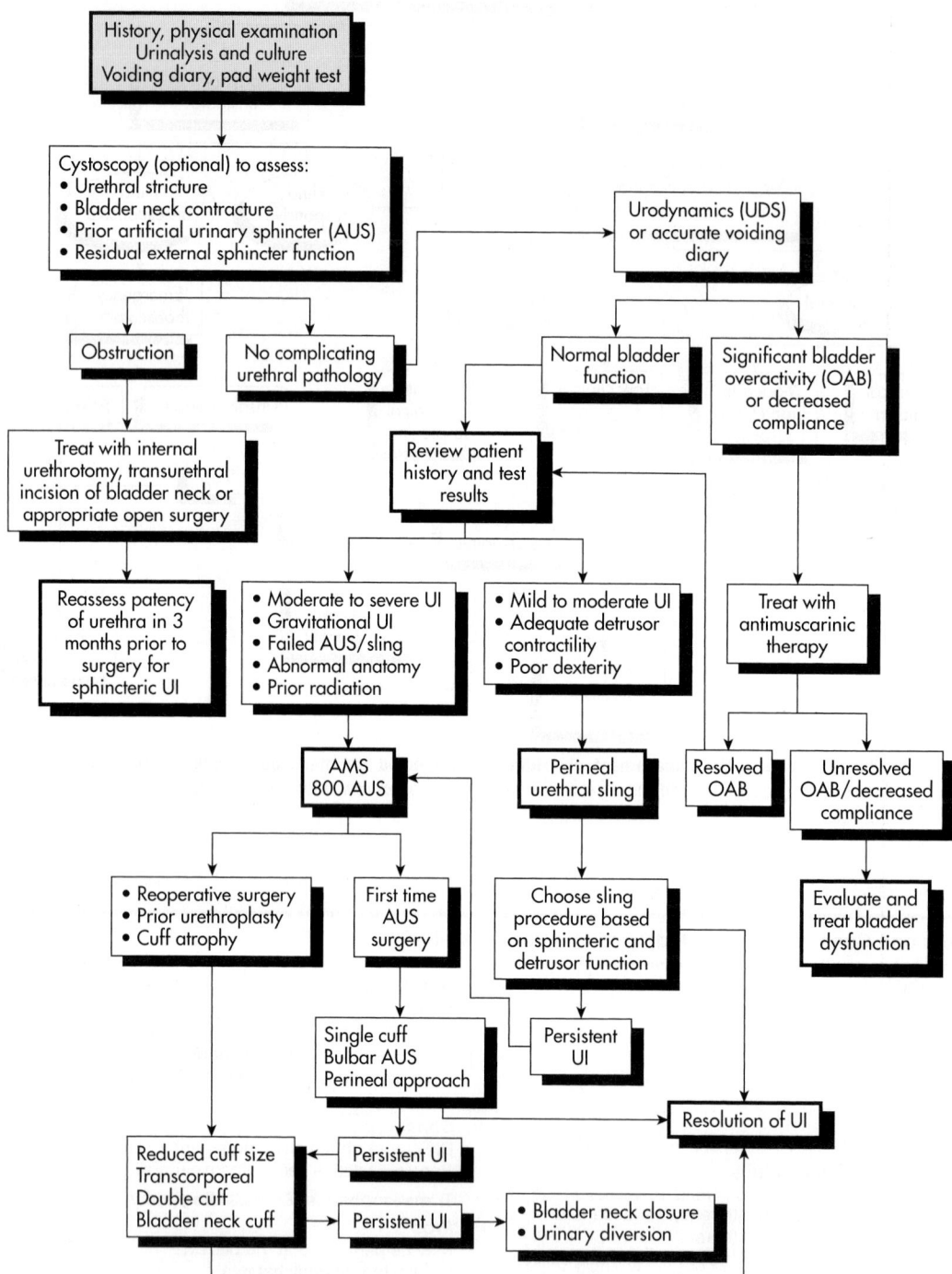

FIG. 278 Algorithm for the evaluation and management of sphincteric urinary incontinence. OAB, overactive bladder; UI, urinary incontinence. (Wein AJ, Kavoussi LR, Partin AW, Peters CA: Campbell-Walsh Urology, 11th ed, ISBN# 978-1-4557-7567-5, 2016, Elsevier.)

Investigation and Management of Suspected Urinary Tract Obstruction

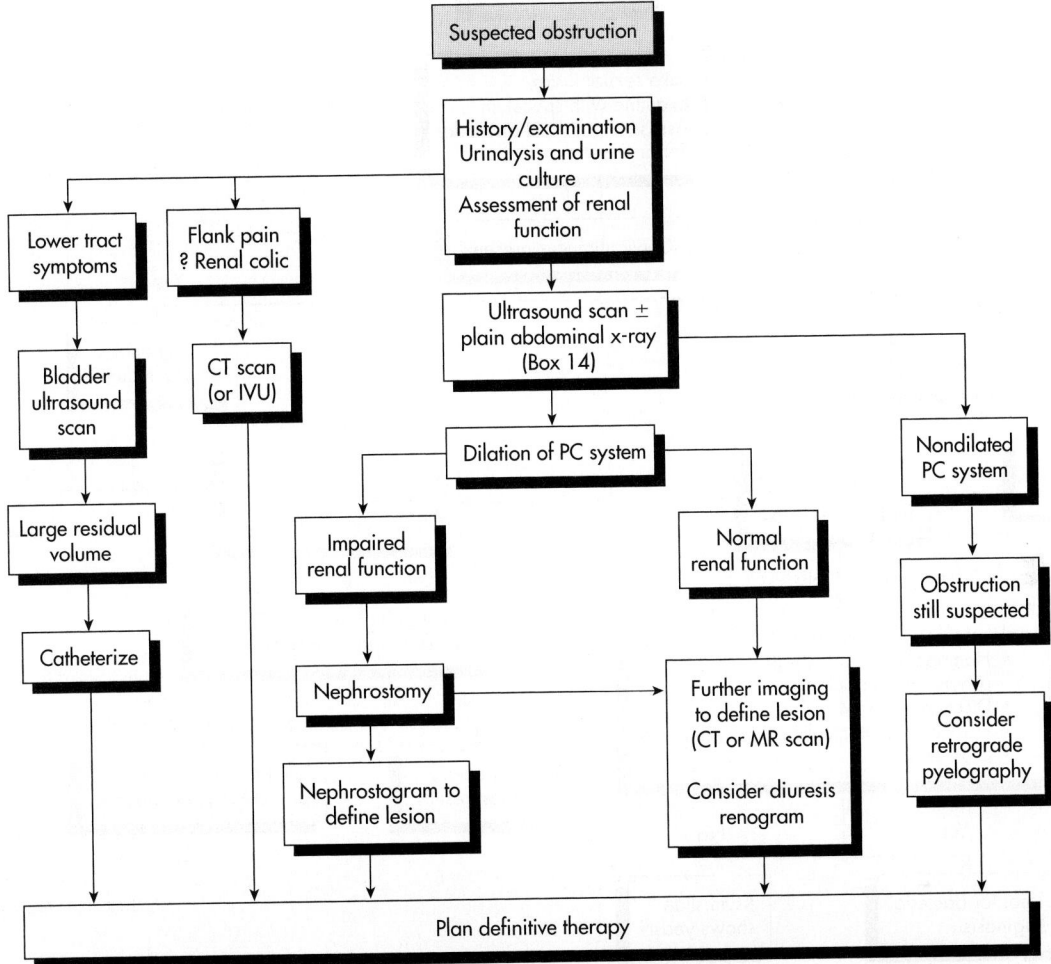

FIG. 279 Investigation and management of suspected urinary tract obstruction. A full history and examination should be performed together with urinalysis, urine microscopy and culture, and measurement of renal function and serum electrolytes. Ultrasound is a useful first-line investigation for any patient with suspected urinary tract obstruction. Helical (spiral) computed tomography (CT) is now the preferred imaging technique when renal calculi are suspected. Either CT or magnetic resonance (MRI) urography can accurately diagnose both the site and the cause of obstruction in most cases. If there is renal impairment, insertion of a nephrostomy allows the effective relief of the obstruction and time for renal function to recover while definitive therapy is planned. *IVU,* Intravenous urography; *PC,* pelvicalyceal. (From Floege J et al: *Comprehensive clinical nephrology,* ed 4, Philadelphia, 2010, Saunders.)

BOX 14   Diagnostic Tests Used in Obstructive Uropathy

Upper Urinary Tract Obstruction
Sonography (ultrasound)
Plain films of the abdomen (KUB)
Excretory or intravenous pyelography
  (very rarely needed)
Retrograde pyelography
Isotopic renography
Computed tomography (helical CT)
Magnetic resonance imaging
Pressure flow studies (the Whitaker test)

Lower Urinary Tract Obstruction
- Some of the tests listed at left
- Cystoscopy
- Voiding cystourethrogram
- Retrograde urethrography
- Urodynamic tests
- Debimetry
- Cystometrography
- Electromyography
- Urethral pressure profile

KUB, Kidneys, ureter, bladder.

Clinical Algorithms

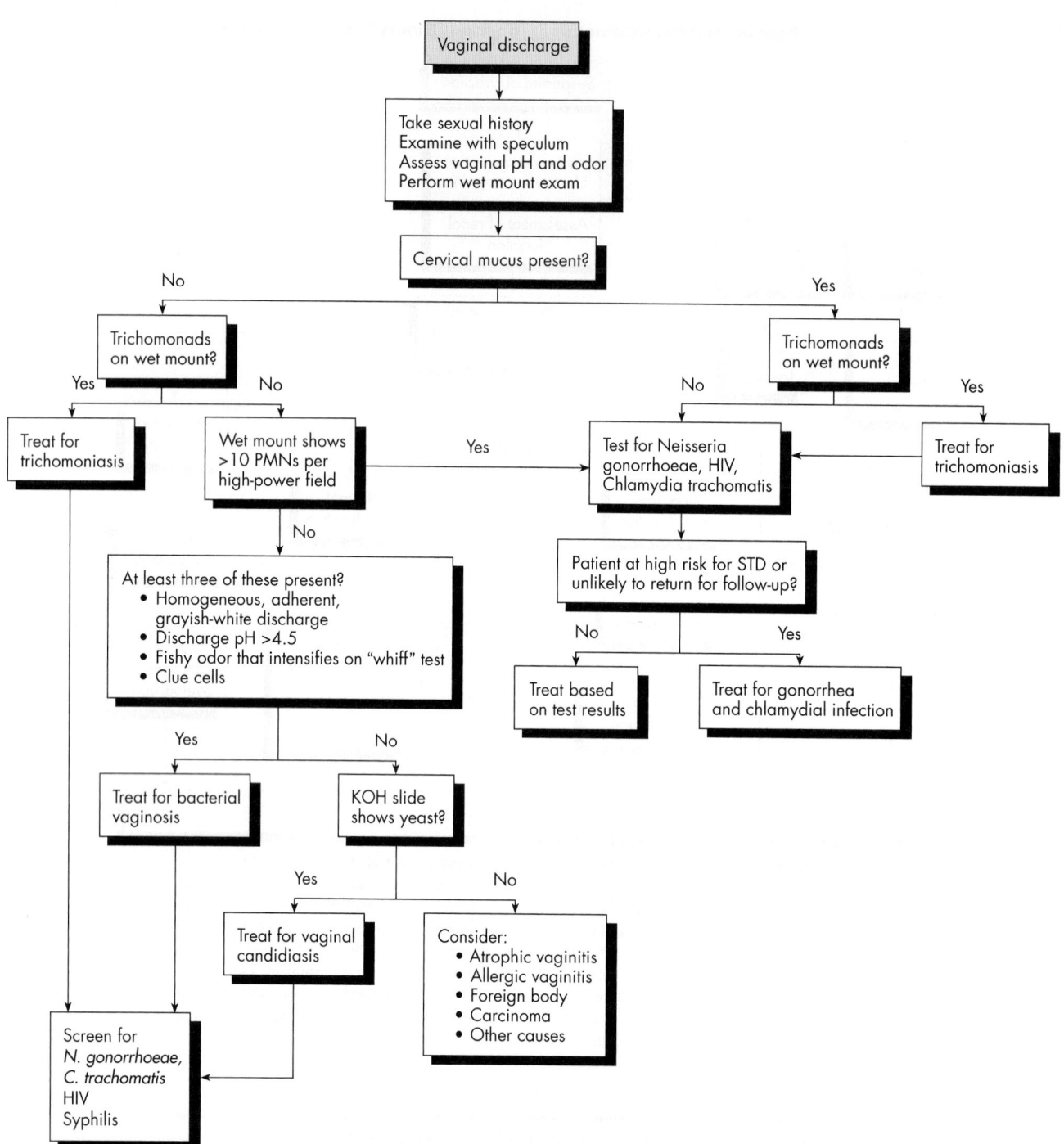

FIG. 280 Evaluation of vaginal discharge. See Section I, Vaginitis, Fungal, and Vaginitis Trichomonas for additional information on vaginal discharge evaluation. *HIV,* Human immunodeficiency virus; *KOH,* potassium hydroxide; *PMN,* polymorphonuclear leukocyte; *STD,* sexually transmitted disease.

Critical questions and priority actions for pediatric vaginitis

Any concerns of possible sexual abuse require further evaluation

Prominent discharge?

Prepuberty: Consider physiologic leukorrhea

Newborn? Consider maternal estrogen effect

Foul smelling? Look for foreign body; consider saline irrigation of vagina if suspected (toilet paper)

Genital warts present? If age < 18 months, possible vertical transmission; inquire about maternal HPV. Age > 18 months, consider sexual abuse

Vaginal or abdominal mass? Refer for evaluation by surgery or gynecology

Bleeding?

Hypopigmented labia and perianal area? Refer to dermatology for possible lichen sclerosus

Doughnut-shaped dark red mucosa at urethral meatus? Consider urethral prolapse; treatment is sitz baths, estrogen cream, and referral

Physical exam reveals precocious puberty? Palpate abdomen for masses; refer for pediatric endocrine evaluation

Trauma? Tense hematoma may be drained or large lacerations may need closure in OR. Ensure that the patient can urinate

Can you see the source of bleeding? Consider exam under anesthesia

Irritation or itching?

Itching? Nighttime symptoms? Look for pinworms; do tape test for ova

Fever or dark erythema? Swab for group A streptococcus infection

May be caused by poor hygiene, tight clothing, perfumes and bubble baths, or overzealous wiping

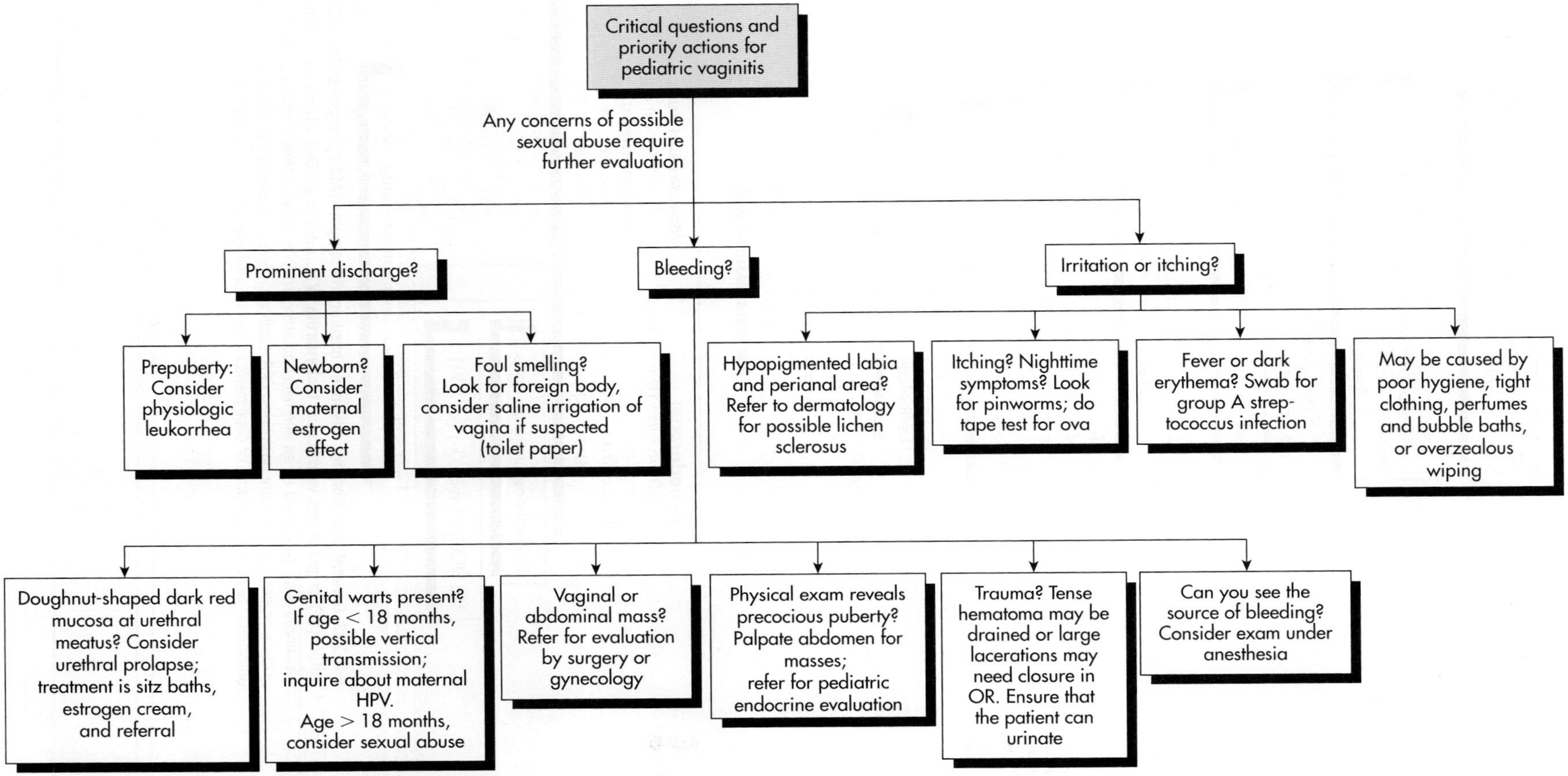

FIG. 282 Algorithm showing critical questions and priority actions for pediatric vaginitis. Additional information on pediatric vaginitis is available in Section I, Vaginitis, Prepubescent. *HPV,* Human papillomavirus; *OR,* operating room. (From Adams JG, et al: *Emergency medicine, clinical essentials,* ed 2, Philadelphia, 2013, Elsevier.)

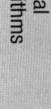

Clinical Algorithms

III

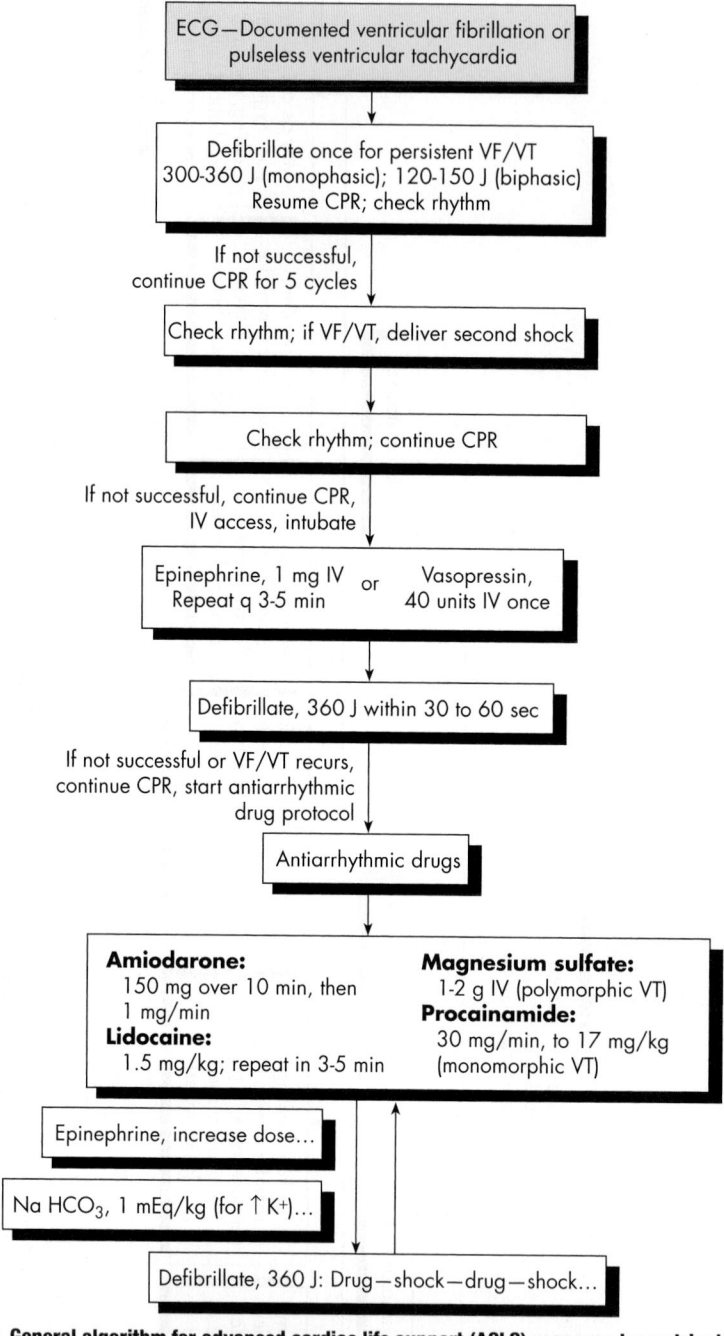

FIG. 283 General algorithm for advanced cardiac life support (ACLS) response to ventricular fibrillation (VF) or pulseless ventricular tachycardia (VT). *Note:* In a 2008 advisory, 200 compression-only sequences were suggested as an alternative to standard CPR cycles between shocks, and this approach is under consideration for future guidelines. *CPR,* Cardiopulmonary resuscitation; *ECG,* electrocardiogram. (From Goldman L, Schafer AI: *Goldman's Cecil medicine,* ed 24, Philadelphia, 2012, Saunders.)

ICD-10CM #	R42	Dizziness and giddiness	**1759**
	H81.13	Benign paroxysmal vertigo, bilateral	
	H81.49	Vertigo of central origin, unspecified ear	
	H81.399	Other peripheral vertigo, unspecified ear	
	H81.23	Vestibular neuronitis, bilateral	

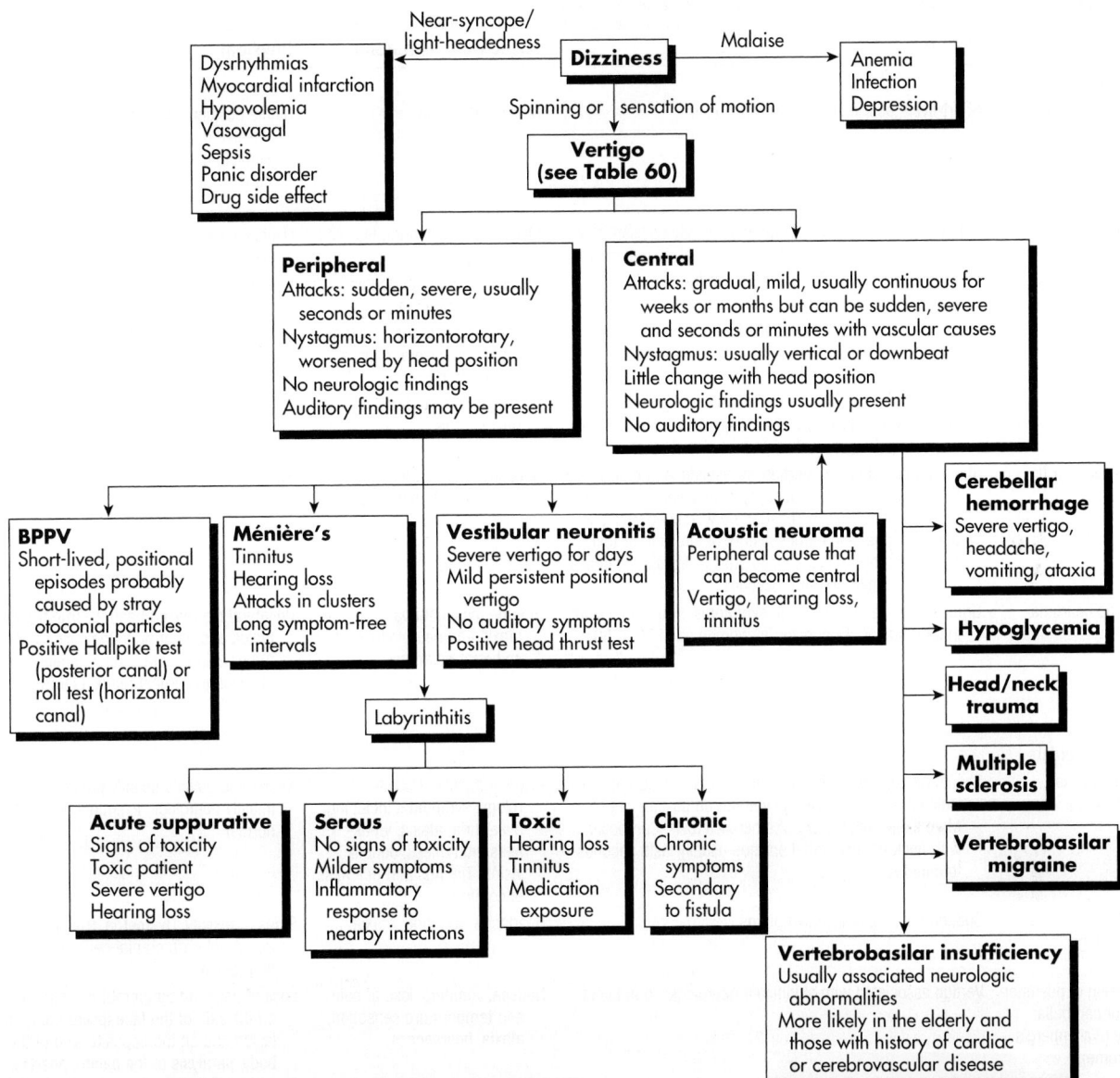

FIG. 284 Diagnostic algorithm for dizziness and vertigo. Additional topics Vestibular Neuronitis, Acoustic Neuroma, Labyrinthitis, Meniere's Disease, and Benign Paroxysmal Positional Vertigo are available in Section I. *BPPV*, Benign paroxysmal positional vertigo. (From Marx JA et al: *Rosen's emergency medicine*, ed 8, Philadelphia, 2014, Saunders.)

Clinical
Algorithms

III

ICD-10CM #	R42	Dizziness and giddiness
	H81.13	Benign paroxysmal vertigo, bilateral
	H81.49	Vertigo of central origin, unspecified ear
	H81.399	Other peripheral vertigo, unspecified ear
	H81.23	Vestibular neuronitis, bilateral

Table 60 Differential Diagnosis of Patients with True Vertigo

Cause	History	Associated Symptoms	Physical
Peripheral			
1. Benign paroxysmal positional vertigo	Short-lived, positional, fatigable episodes	Nausea, vomiting	Single position can precipitate vertigo. Positive result on Hallpike test (posterior semicircular canal) or Roll test (horizontal canal).
2. Labyrinthitis			
A. Serous	Mild to severe positional symptoms. Usually coexisting or antecedent infection of ear, nose, throat, or meninges.	Mild to severe hearing loss can occur	Usually nontoxic patient with minimal fever elevation
B. Acute suppurative	Coexisting acute exudative infection of the inner ear. Severe symptoms.	Usually severe hearing loss, nausea, vomiting	Febrile patient showing signs of toxicity. Acute otitis media.
C. Toxic	Gradually progressive symptoms: Patients on medication causing toxicity.	Hearing loss that may become rapid and severe, nausea and vomiting	Hearing loss. Ataxia common feature in chronic phase.
3. Ménière's disease	Recurrent episodes of severe rotational vertigo usually lasting hours. Onset usually abrupt. Attacks may occur in clusters. Long symptom-free remissions.	Nausea, vomiting, tinnitus, hearing loss	Positional nystagmus not present
4. Vestibular neuritis	Sudden onset of severe vertigo, increasing in intensity for hours, then gradually subsiding over several days but can last weeks to months. Can be worsened with positional change. Sometimes history of infection or toxic exposure that precedes initial attack. Highest incidence is found in third and fifth decades.	Nausea, vomiting. Auditory symptoms do not occur.	Spontaneous nystagmus toward the involved ear may be present.
5. Acoustic neuroma	Gradual onset and increase in symptoms. Neurologic signs in later stages. Most occur in women aged 30 to 60.	Hearing loss, tinnitus. True ataxia and neurologic signs as tumor enlarges.	Unilateral decreased hearing. True truncal ataxia and other neurologic signs when tumor enlarges. May have diminution or absence of corneal reflex. Eighth cranial nerve deficit may be present.
Central			
1. Vascular disorders			
A. Vertebrobasilar insufficiency	Should be considered in any patient of advanced age with isolated new-onset vertigo without an obvious cause. More likely with history of atherosclerosis. Can occur with neck trauma. Initial episode usually lasts seconds to minutes.	Often headache. Usually neurologic symptoms including dysarthria, ataxia, weakness, numbness, double vision. Tinnitus and deafness uncommon.	Neurologic deficits usually present, but initially neurologic examination can be normal
B. Cerebellar hemorrhage	Sudden onset of severe symptoms	Headache, vomiting, ataxia	Signs of toxicity. Dysmetria, true ataxia. Ipsilateral sixth cranial nerve palsy may be present.
C. Occlusion of posterior inferior cerebellar artery (Wallenberg's syndrome)	Vertigo associated with significant neurologic complaints	Nausea, vomiting, loss of pain and temperature sensation, ataxia, hoarseness	Loss of pain and temperature sensation on the side of the face ipsilateral to the lesion and on the opposite side of the body, paralysis of the palate, pharynx, and larynx. Horner's syndrome (ipsilateral ptosis, miosis, and decreased facial sweating).
2. Head trauma	Symptoms begin with or shortly after head trauma. Positional symptoms most common type after trauma. Self-limited symptoms that can persist weeks to months.	Usually mild nausea	Occasionally, basilar skull fracture
3. Vertebrobasilar migraine	Vertigo almost always followed by headache. Patient has usually had similar episodes in past. Most patients have a family history of migraine. Syndrome usually begins in adolescence.	Dysarthria, ataxia, visual disturbances, or paresthesias usually precede headache	No residual neurologic or otologic signs are present after attack
4. Multiple sclerosis	Vertigo presenting symptom in 7%-10% and appears in the course of the disease in a third. Onset may be severe and suggest labyrinth disease. Disease onset usually between ages 20 and 40. Often history of other attacks with varying neurologic signs or symptoms.	Nausea and vomiting, which may be severe	May have horizontal, rotary, or vertical nystagmus. Nystagmus may persist after the vertiginous symptoms have subsided. Bilateral internuclear ophthalmoplegia and ataxic eye movements suggest multiple sclerosis.
5. Temporal lobe epilepsy	Can be initial or prominent symptom in some patients with the disorder	Memory impairment, hallucinations, trancelike states, seizures	May have aphasia or convulsions
6. Hypoglycemia	Should be considered in diabetics and any other patient with unexplained symptoms	Sweating, anxiety	Tachycardia, mental status change may be present

From Marx JA et al: *Rosen's emergency medicine*, ed 8, Philadelphia, 2014, Saunders.

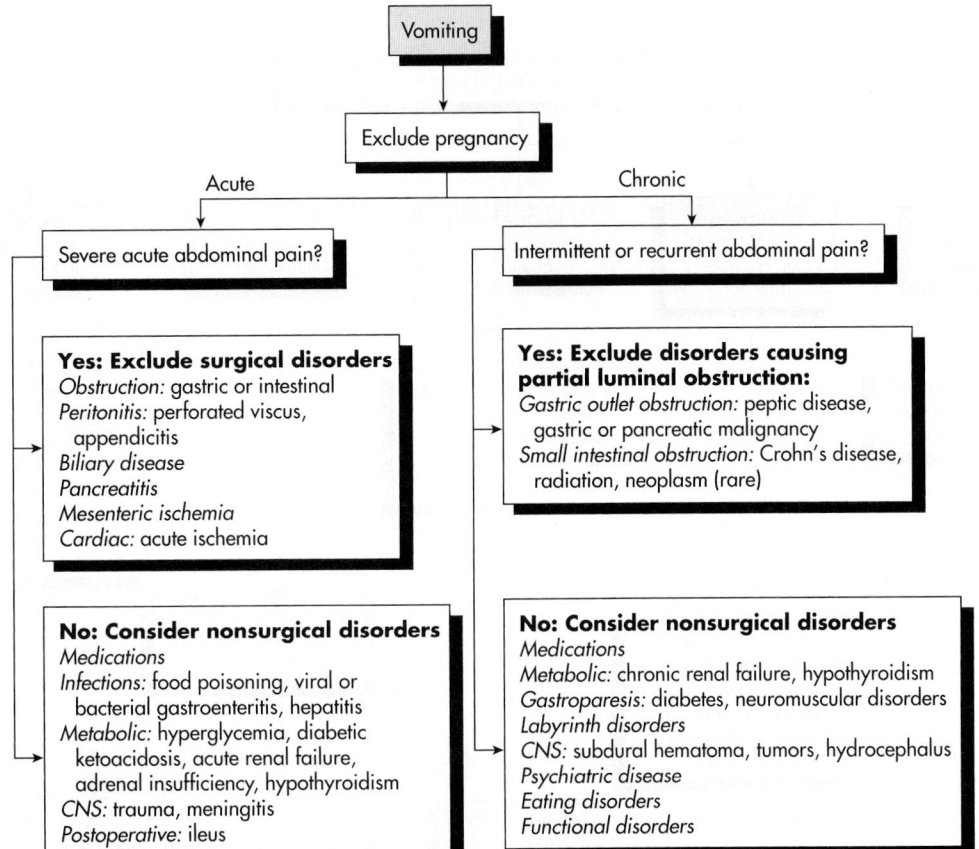

FIG. 285 Approach to the patient with vomiting. *CNS,* Central nervous system. (From Goldman L, Schafer AI: *Goldman's Cecil medicine,* ed 24, Philadelphia, 2012, Saunders.)

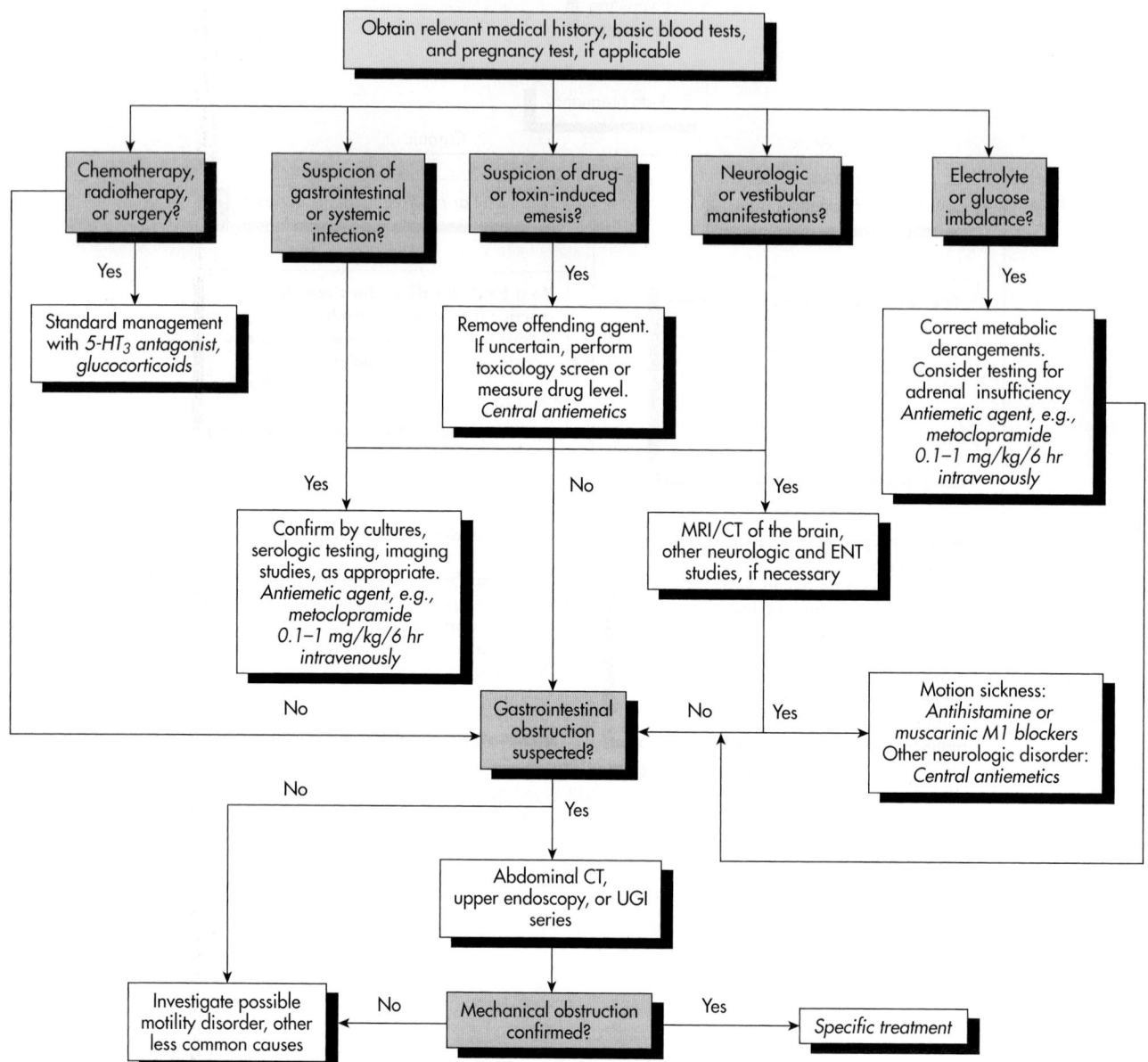

FIG. 286 Algorithm for management of a patient with acute vomiting. Possible treatments are italicized. *ENT*, ear, nose, and throat; *5-HT*, 5-hydroxytryptamine; *UGI*, upper GI. Potential treatments are shown in italics. (Feldman M, Friedman LS, Brandt LJ: Sleisenger and Fortran's Gastrointestinal and Liver Disease, 10th ed, ISBN# 978-1-4557-4692-7, 2016, Elsevier.)

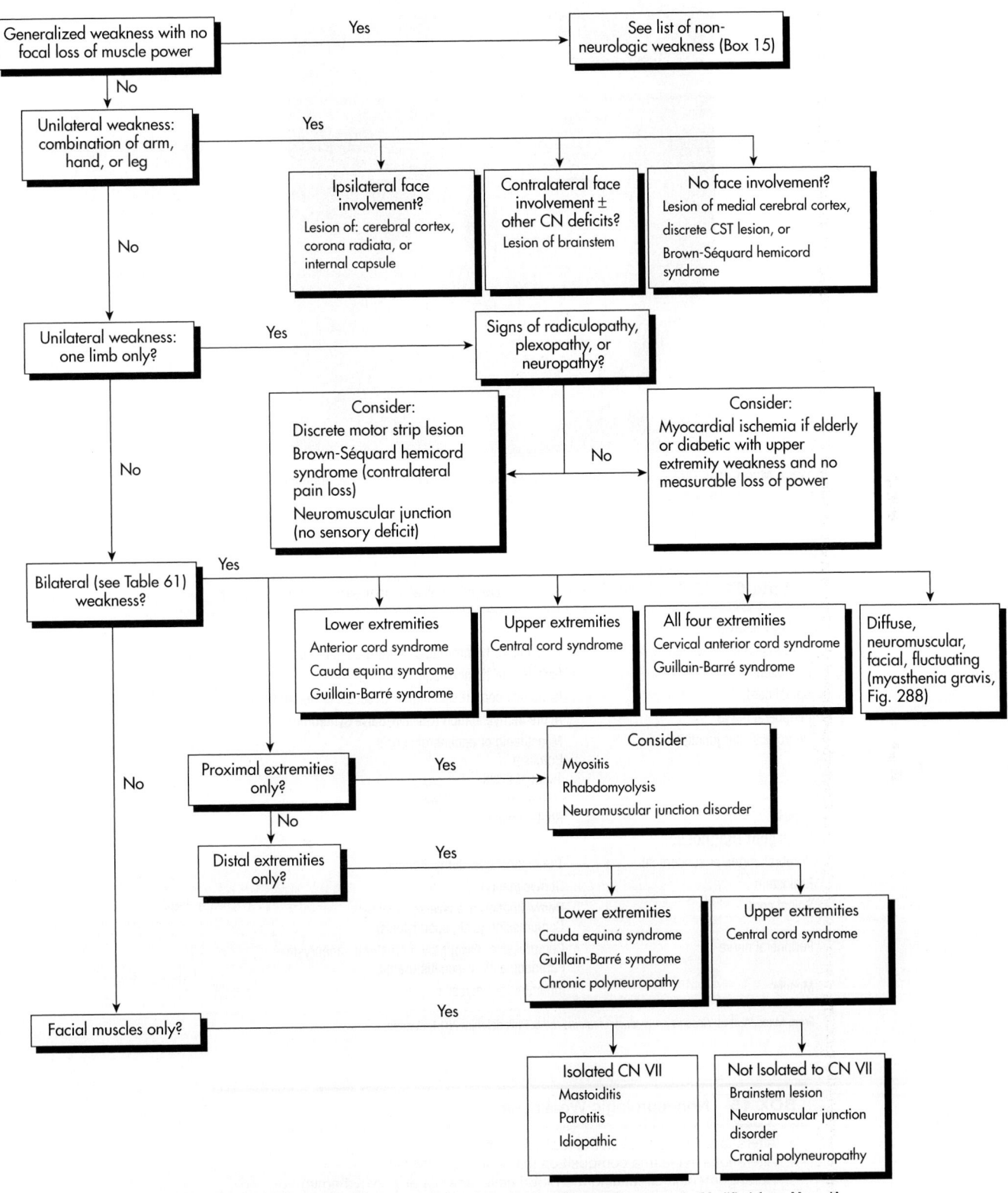

FIG. 287 Common clinical patterns of weakness, classified and assessed. (Modified from Marx JA et al: *Rosen's emergency medicine*, ed 8, Philadelphia, 2014, Saunders.)

Clinical Algorithms

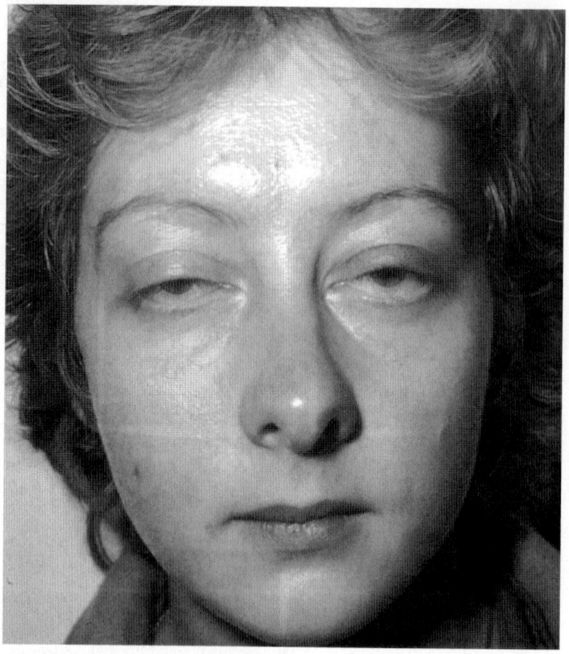

FIG. 288 Myopathic facies in myasthenia gravis (Bowling B: Kanski's Clinical ophthalmology, a systemic approach, 8th ed, Elsevier, 2016, ISBN # 978-0-7020-5572-0.)

Table 61 Critical and Emergent Causes of Neuromuscular Weakness

Critical Diagnoses

Cerebral cortex or subcortical	Ischemic or hemorrhagic cerebrovascular accident (CVA)
Brainstem	Ischemic or hemorrhagic CVA
Spinal cord	Ischemia, compression (disk, abscess, or hematoma)
Peripheral nerve	Acute demyelination (Guillain-Barré syndrome)
Neuromuscular junction	Myasthenic or cholinergic crisis
	Botulism
	Tick paralysis
	Organophosphate poisoning
Muscle	Rhabdomyolysis

Emergent Diagnoses

Cerebral cortex or subcortical	Tumor, abscess, demyelination
Brainstem	Demyelination
Spinal cord	Demyelination (transverse myelitis)
	Compression (disk, spondylosis)
Peripheral nerve	Compressive plexopathy (hematoma, aneurysm)
	Paraneoplastic vasculitis uremia
Muscle	Inflammatory myositis

From Marx JA et al: *Rosen's emergency medicine*, ed 8, Philadelphia, 2014, Saunders.

BOX 15 Nonneurologic Weakness

- Alterations in plasma volume (dehydration)
- Alterations in plasma composition (glucose, electrolytes).
- Derangement in circulating red blood cells (anemia or polycythemia)
- Decrement in cardiac pump function (myocardial ischemia)
- Drop in systemic vascular resistance (vasodilatory shock from any cause)
- Increased metabolic demand (local or systemic infection, endocrinopathy, toxin)
- Mitochondrial dysfunction (severe sepsis or toxin-mediated)
- Global depression of the central nervous system (sedatives, stimulant withdrawal)

From Marx JA et al: *Rosen's emergency medicine*, ed 8, Philadelphia, 2014, Saunders.

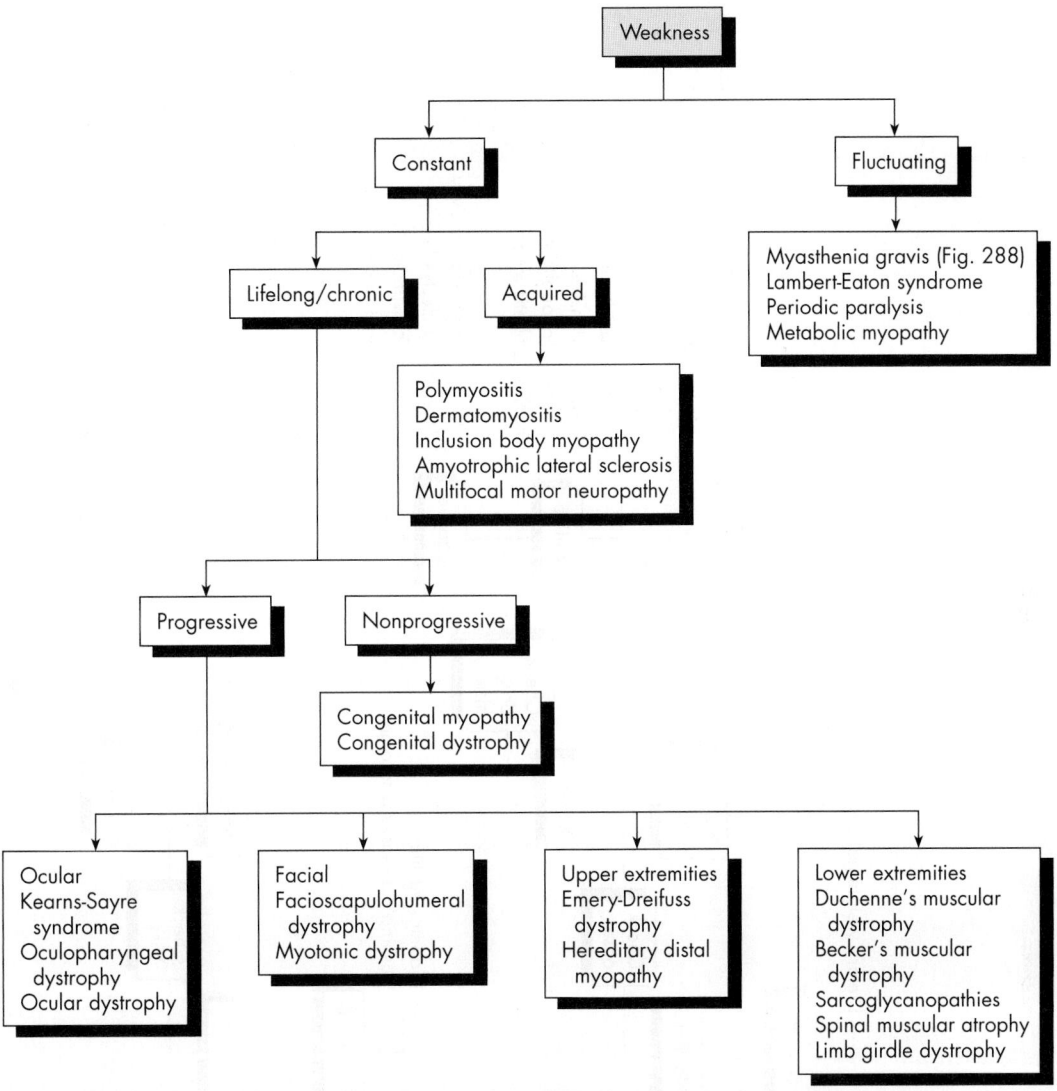

FIG. 289 An algorithm for the approach to the patient with weakness. (From Bradley WG, Daroff RB, Fenichel GM, Jankovic J [eds]: *Neurology in clinical practice,* ed 4, Philadelphia, 2004, Butterworth Heinemann.)

Clinical Algorithms

III

ICD-10CM #
R63.5 Abnormal weight gain
E66.9 Obesity, unspecified

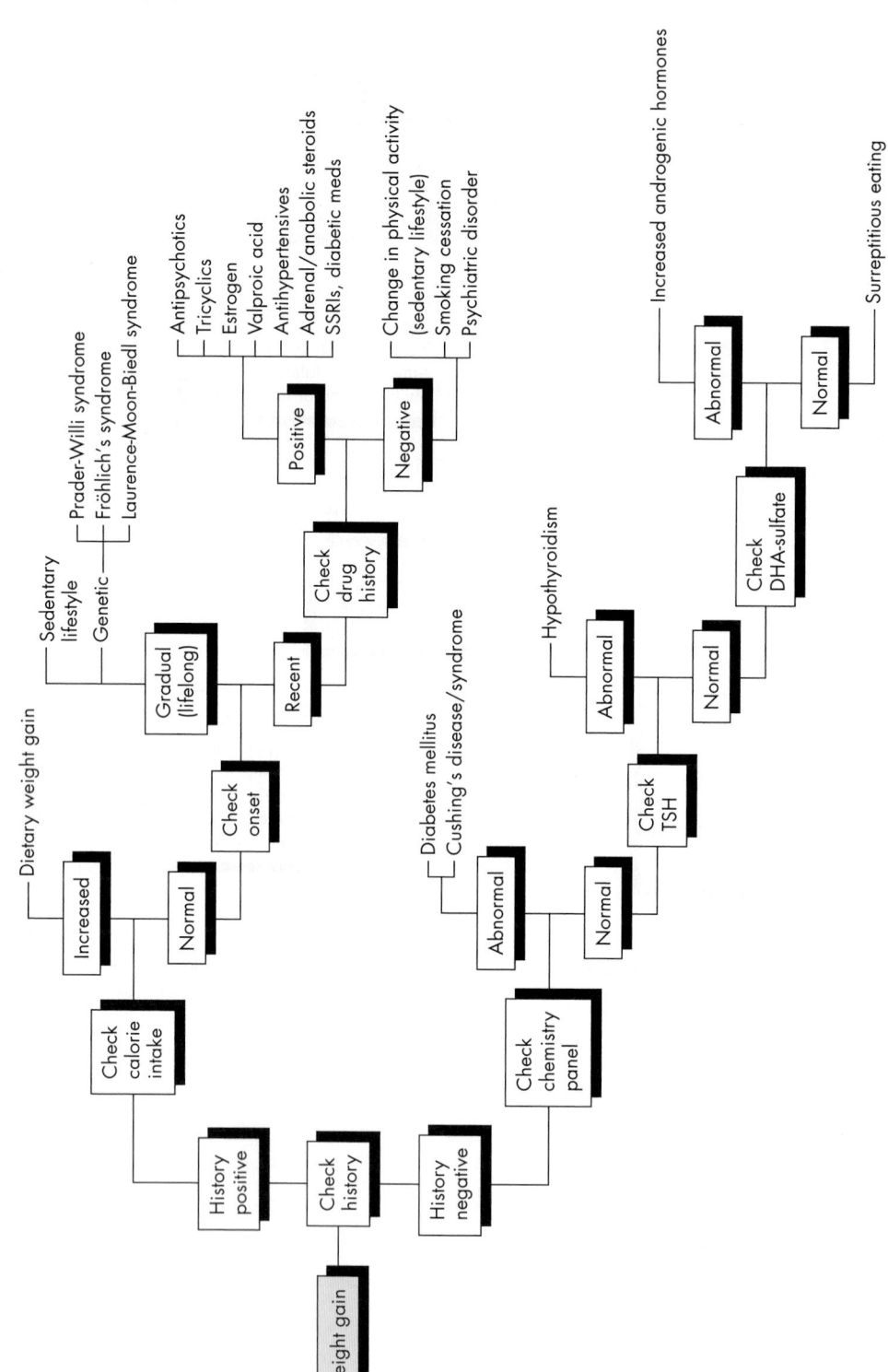

FIG. 290 Weight gain. *DHA,* Dehydroepiandrosterone; *SSRIs,* serotonin reuptake inhibitors; *TSH,* thyroid-stimulating hormone. (Modified from Healey PM: *Common medical diagnosis: an algorithmic approach,* ed 3, Philadelphia, 2000, Saunders.)

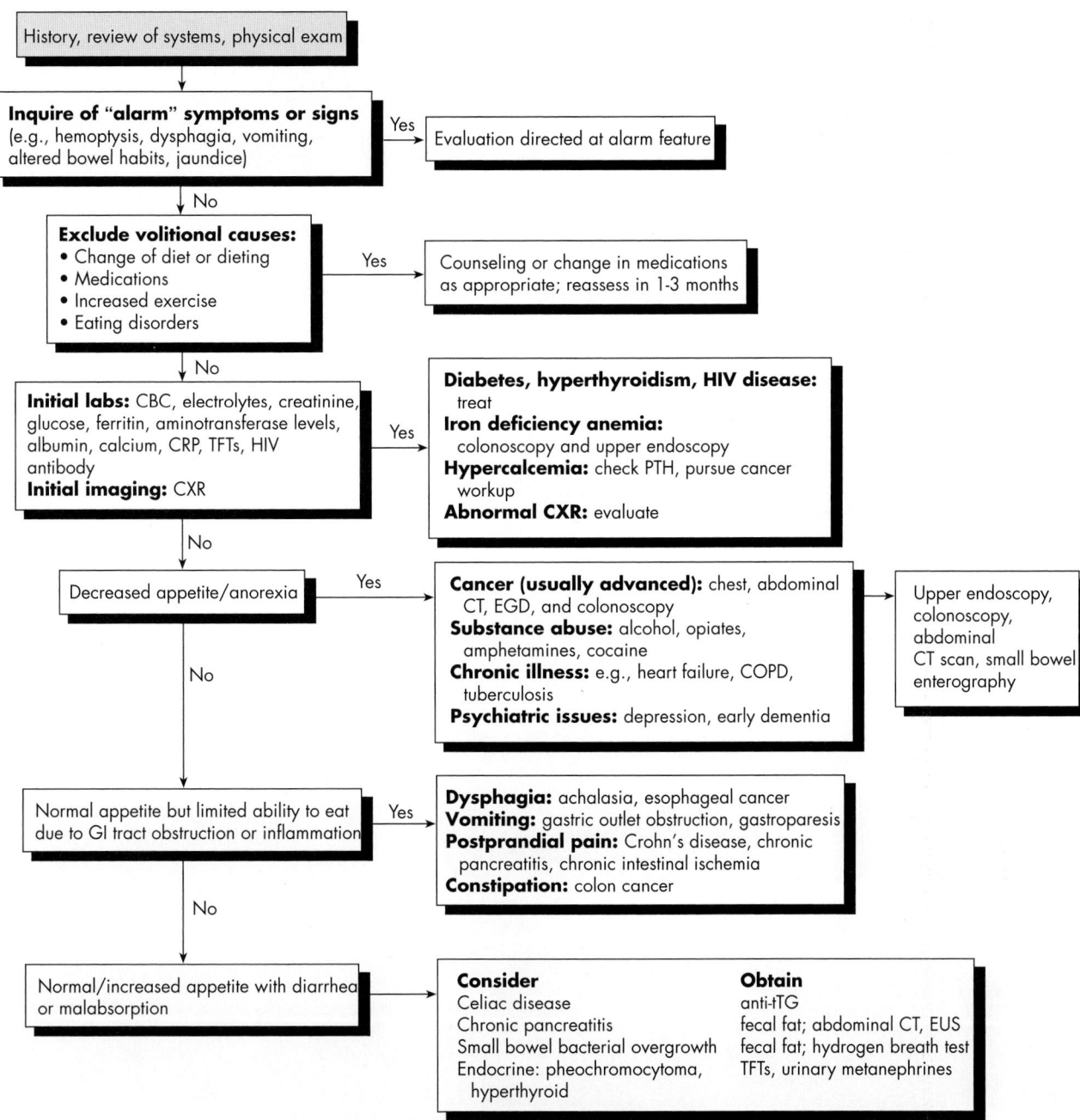

FIG. 291 Approach to the patient with unintentional weight loss greater than 5%. *CBC*, Complete blood count; *COPD*, chronic obstructive pulmonary disease; *CRP*, C-reactive protein; *CT*, computed tomography; *CXR*, chest radiograph; *EGD*, esophagogastroduodenoscopy; *EUS*, endoscopic ultrasound; *GI*, gastrointestinal; *HIV*, human immunodeficiency virus; *PTH*, parathyroid hormone; *TFTs*, thyroid function tests; *tTG*, tissue transglutaminase; *U/A*, urinalysis. (From Goldman L, Schafer AI: *Goldman's Cecil medicine*, ed 24, Philadelphia, 2012, Saunders.)

Clinical Algorithms

Laboratory Tests and Interpretation of Results

INTRODUCTION

This section contains more than 300 commonly performed laboratory tests. In general, the tests are discussed in the following format:

1. Laboratory test.
2. Normal range in adult patients. Normal values are given using the present (traditional) reference interval, followed by the Système Internationale (SI) reference interval, the conversion factor (CF), and the suggested minimum increment (SMI).
3. Common abnormalities, such as positive test, increased, or decreased value.
4. Causes of abnormal result.

The normal ranges may differ slightly, depending on the laboratory. The reader should be aware of the "normal range" of the particular laboratory performing the test. Every attempt has been made to present current laboratory test data, with emphasis on practical considerations.

ACE LEVEL
See ANGIOTENSIN-CONVERTING ENZYME

ACETONE (serum or plasma)
Normal: Negative
Elevated in: DKA, starvation, isopropanol ingestion

ACETYLCHOLINE RECEPTOR (AChR) ANTIBODY
Normal: <0.03 nmol/L
Elevated in: Myasthenia gravis. Changes in AChR concentration correlate with the clinical severity of myasthenia gravis following therapy and during therapy with prednisone and immunosuppressants. False-positive AChR antibody results may be found in patients with Eaton-Lambert syndrome.

ACID-BASE REFERENCE VALUES
See Tables 1 and 2.

ACID PHOSPHATASE (serum)
Normal range: 0-5.5 U/L (0-90 nkat/L [CF: 16.67; SMI:2 nkat/L])
Elevated in: Carcinoma of prostate, other neoplasms (breast, bone), Paget's disease, osteogenesis imperfecta, malignant invasion of bone, Gaucher's disease, multiple myeloma, myeloproliferative disorders, benign prostatic hypertrophy, prostatic palpation or surgery, hyperparathyroidism, liver disease, chronic renal failure, idiopathic thrombocytopenic purpura, bronchitis

ACID SERUM TEST
See HAM TEST

ACTIVATED CLOTTING TIME (ACT)
Normal: This test is used to determine the dose of protamine sulfate to reverse the effect of heparin as an anticoagulant during angioplasty, cardiac surgery, and hemodialysis. The accepted goal during cardiopulmonary bypass surgery is usually 400-500 sec.

ACTIVATED PARTIAL THROMBOPLASTIN TIME (APTT, aPTT)
See PARTIAL THROMBOPLASTIN TIME

ADRENOCORTICOTROPIC HORMONE
Normal: 9-52 pg/ml. Table 3 describes patterns of serum levels of ACTH and cortisol in different adrenal gland disorders.
Elevated in: Addison's disease, ectopic ACTH-producing tumors, congenital adrenal hyperplasia, Nelson's syndrome, pituitary-dependent Cushing's disease
Decreased in: Secondary adrenocortical insufficiency, hypopituitarism, adrenal adenoma or adrenal carcinoma

ALANINE AMINOPEPTIDASE
Normal
Male: 1.11-1.71 mcg/ml
Female: 0.96-1.52 mcg/ml
Elevated in: Liver or pancreatic disease, ethanol use, oral contraceptives use, malignancy, tobacco use, pregnancy
Decreased in: Abortion

ALANINE AMINOTRANSFERASE (ALT, SGPT)
See Fig. 1, an algorithm for evaluation of elevated ALT. Table 4 describes patterns of liver function tests in liver disorders.
Normal range: 0-35 U/L (0.058 µkat/L [CF: 0.02 µkat/L])
Elevated in: Liver disease (hepatitis, cirrhosis, Reye's syndrome), hepatic congestion, infectious mononucleosis, myocardial infarction, myocarditis, severe muscle trauma, dermatomyositis/polymyositis, muscular dystrophy, drugs (antibiotics, narcotics, antihypertensive agents, heparin, labetalol, statins, NSAIDs, amiodarone, chlorpromazine, phenytoin), malignancy, renal and pulmonary infarction, seizures, eclampsia, shock liver

TABLE 1 Commonly Used Acid-Base Reference Values for Arterial and Venous Plasma or Serum (Averaged from Various Sources)

	ARTERIAL		VENOUS	
	Conventional Units	SI Units*	Conventional Units	SI Units*
pH	7.40 (7.35-7.45)	7.40 (7.35-7.45)	7.37 (7.32-7.42)	7.37 (7.32-7.42)
Pco_2	40 mm Hg (35-45)	5.33 kPa (4.67-6.10)	45 mm Hg (45-50)	6.10 kPa (5.33-6.67)
Po_2	80-100 mm Hg	10.66-13.33 kPa	40 mm Hg (37-43)	5.33 kPa (4.93-5.73)
HCO_3 (CO_2 combining power)	24 mEq/L (20-28)	24 mmol/L (20-28)	26 mEq/L (22-30)	26 mmol/L (22-30)
CO_2 content	25 mEq/L (22-28)	25 mmol/L (22-28)	27 mEq/L (24-30)	27 mmol/L(24-30)

From Ravel R: *Clinical laboratory medicine,* ed 6, St Louis, 1995, Mosby.
*International system.

TABLE 2 Summary of Laboratory Findings in Primary Uncomplicated Respiratory and Metabolic Acid-Base Disorders*

Disorder	Pco_2	pH	Base Excess
Acute primary respiratory hypoactivity (respiratory acidosis)	Increase	Decrease	Normal/positive
Acute primary respiratory hyperactivity (respiratory alkalosis)	Decrease	Increase	Normal/negative
Uncompensated metabolic acidosis	Normal	Decrease	Negative
Uncompensated metabolic alkalosis	Normal	Increase	Positive
Partially compensated metabolic acidosis	Decrease	Decrease	Negative
Partially compensated metabolic alkalosis	Increase	Increase	Positive
Chronic primary respiratory hypoactivity (compensated respiratory acidosis)	Increase	Normal	Positive
Fully compensated metabolic alkalosis	Increase	Normal	Positive
Chronic primary respiratory hyperactivity (compensated respiratory alkalosis)	Decrease	Normal	Negative
Fully compensated metabolic acidosis	Decrease	Normal	Negative

From Ravel R: *Clinical laboratory medicine,* ed 6, St Louis, 1995, Mosby.
*Base excess results refer to negative (–) values more than 22 and positive (+) values more than 12.

Laboratory Tests

IV

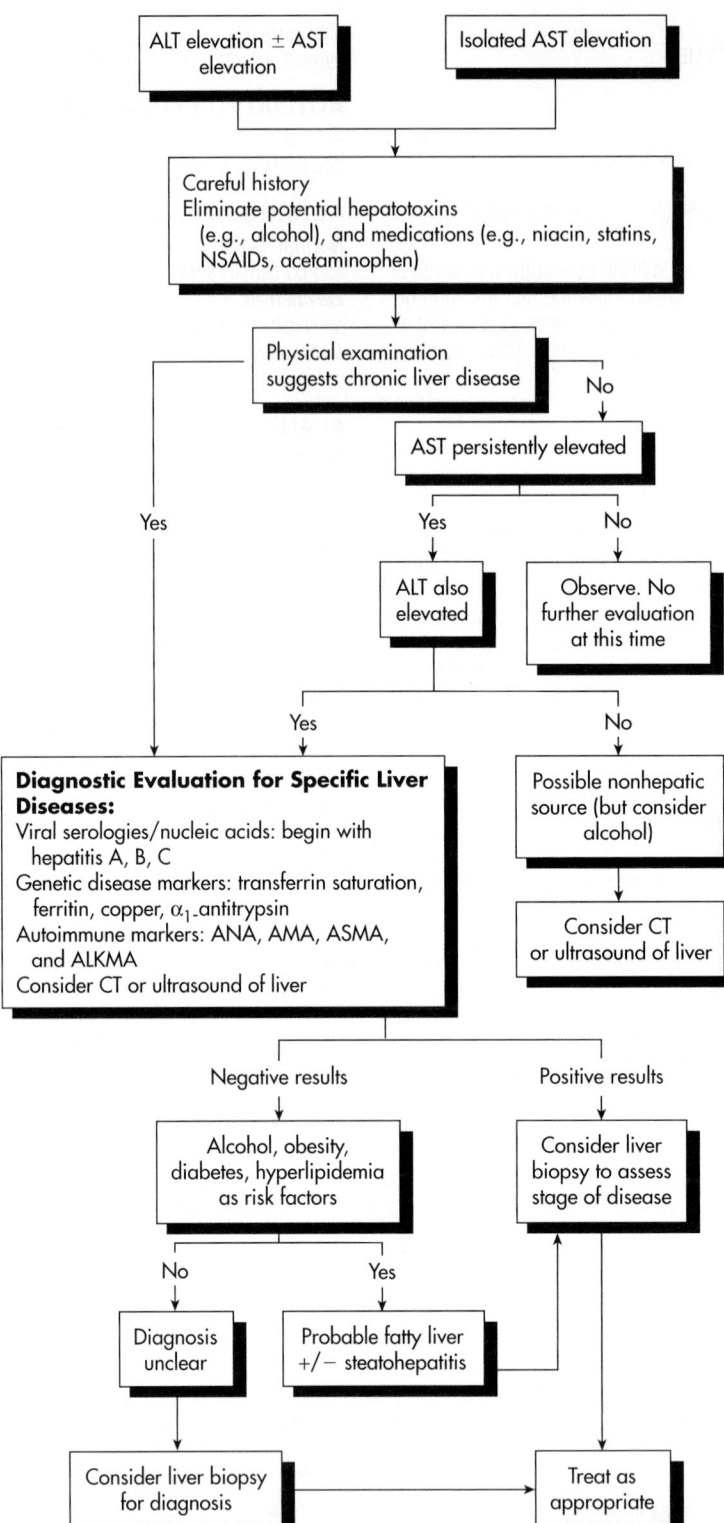

FIG. 1 Approach to the evaluation of isolated elevated levels of serum alanine aminotransferase *(ALT)* and/or aspartate aminotransferase *(AST)* in the asymptomatic patient. *ALKMA,* Anti–liver/kidney microsomal antibody; *AMA,* antimitochondrial antibody; *ANA,* antinuclear antibody; *ASMA,* anti–smooth muscle antibody; *NSAIDs,* nonsteroidal anti-inflammatory drugs. (Modified from Goldman L, Ausiello D [eds]: *Cecil textbook of medicine,* ed 24, Philadelphia, 2012, Saunders.)

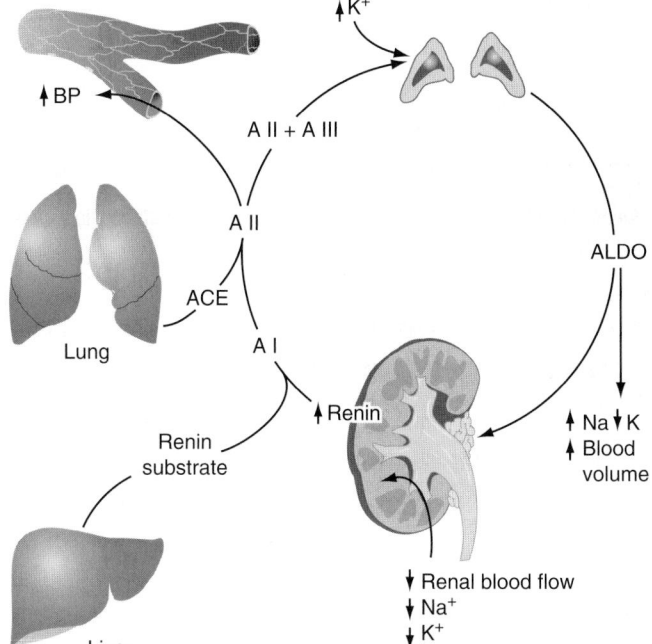

FIG. 2 The normal renin-angiotensin-aldosterone axis. Renin, secreted by the kidney, cleaves angiotensin I from renin substrate (angiotensinogen) produced by the liver. Angiotensin I is converted to angiotensin II by angiotensin-converting enzyme (ACE), mainly in the lung. Angiotensin II increases peripheral vascular resistance and, together with angiotensin III, stimulates aldosterone (ALDO) secretion, which results in sodium retention and increased plasma volume. (Adapted from Stewart PM: The adrenal cortex. In Larsen PR, Kronenberg HM, Melmed S, et al, editors: *Williams textbook of endocrinology,* ed 10, Philadelphia, 2003, Saunders, p 499.)

(McPherson RA, Pincus MR: Henry's Clinical Diagnosis and Management by Laboratory Methods, 23rd ed, ISBN # 978-0323-29568-0, 2017, Elsevier)

ALBUMIN (serum)
Normal range: 4-6 g/dl (40-60 g/L [CF:10; SMI: 1 g/L])
Elevated in: Dehydration (relative increase)
Decreased in: Liver disease, nephrotic syndrome, poor nutritional status, rapid IV hydration, protein-losing enteropathies (e.g., inflammatory bowel disease), severe burns, neoplasia, chronic inflammatory diseases, pregnancy, oral contraceptives, prolonged immobilization, lymphomas, hypervitaminosis A, chronic glomerulonephritis

ALCOHOL DEHYDROGENASE
Normal: 0-7 U/L
Elevated in: Drug-induced hepatocellular damage, obstructive jaundice, malignancy, inflammation, infection

ALDOLASE (serum)
Normal range: 0-6 U/L (0-100 nkat/L [CF: 16.67; SMI: 20 nkat/L])
Elevated in: Muscular dystrophy, rhabdomyolysis, dermatomyositis/polymyositis, trichinosis, acute hepatitis and other liver diseases, myocardial infarction, prostatic carcinoma, hemorrhagic pancreatitis, gangrene, delirium tremens, burns
Decreased in: Loss of muscle mass, late stages of muscular dystrophy

ALDOSTERONE
Normal range
Recumbent: 50-150 ng/L
Upright: 150-300 ng/L
(Highest levels in neonates, decreasing over time to adult levels). The normal renin-angiotensin-aldosterone axis is illustraded in Fig. 2.
Elevated in: Primary aldosteronism, secondary aldosteronism, pseudoprimary aldosteronism. Table 5 differentiates the various causes of hyperaldosteronism.
Decreased in
Patient with hypertension: diabetes mellitus, Turner's syndrome, acute alcohol intoxication, excess secretion of deoxycorticosterone, corticosterone, and 18-hydroxycorticosterone
Patient without hypertension: Addison's disease, hypoaldosteronism resulting from renin deficiency, isolated aldosterone deficiency. Table 6 differentiates the various causes of hypoaldosteronism.

TABLE 3 Patterns of Serum Levels of ACTH and Cortisol in Different Adrenal Gland Conditions

Condition	Cortisol	ACTH	Dexamethasone Suppression, Low Dose	Dexamethasone Suppression, High Dose	Site of Disease
Normal adrenal	Normal	Normal	N/A	N/A	None
Primary hypoadrenalism	Low	High	N/A	N/A	Adrenal gland
Secondary hypoadrenalism	Low	Low	N/A	N/A	Pituitary
Primary hyperadrenalism—high cortisol, low ACTH	High	Low	N/A	N/A	Adrenal
Primary hyperadrenalism—high cortisol, borderline low ACTH	High	Borderline low	Positive	N/A	Adrenal
Primary hyperadrenalism due to adrenal hyperplasia—high cortisol, borderline low ACTH	High	Borderline low	Negative	Positive	Adrenal
Primary hyperadrenalism due to adrenal adenoma/carcinoma—high cortisol, borderline low ACTH	High	Borderline low	Negative	Negative	Adrenal
Secondary hyperadrenalism	High	High	N/A	N/A	Pituitary

(McPherson RA, Pincus MR: Henry's Clinical Diagnosis and Management by Laboratory Methods, 23rd ed, ISBN # 978-0323-29568-0, 2017, Elsevier)

TABLE 4 Six Fundamental Patterns of Liver Function Tests

Condition	AST	ALT	LD	AP	TP	Albumin	Bilirubin	Ammonia
1. Hepatitis	H	H	H	H	N	N	H	N
2. Cirrhosis	N	N	N	N–sl H	L	L	H	H
3. Biliary obstruction	N	N	N	H	N	N	H	N
4. Space-occupying lesion	N or H	N or H	H	H	N	N	N–H	N
5. Passive congestion	Sl H	sl H	sl H	N–sl H	N	N	N–sl H	N
6. Fulminant failure	Very H	H	H	H	L	L	H	H

H, High; *N,* normal; *L,* low; *sl,* slightly; *AST,* aspartate aminotransferase; *ALT,* alanine aminotransferase; *LD,* lactate dehydrogenase; *AP,* alkaline phosphatase; *TP,* total protein.
(McPherson RA, Pincus MR: Henry's Clinical Diagnosis and Management by Laboratory Methods, 23rd ed, ISBN # 978-0323-29568-0, 2017, Elsevier)

Laboratory Tests

IV

TABLE 5 Differentiating the Various Causes of Hyperaldosteronism

Disorder	Aldosterone	Renin	Serum K+
Primary hyperaldosteronism	↑	↓	↓
Renin-secreting tumor	↑	↑	↓—N
Dexamethasone-suppressible hyperaldosteronism	↑	↓	↓
Renovascular hypertension	N—↑	N—↑	↓—N
Bartter's syndrome	↑	↑	↓
Diuretics, congestive heart failure, cirrhosis, nephrotic syndrome	↑	↑	N—↓

N, Normal.
(McPherson RA, Pincus MR: Henry's Clinical Diagnosis and Management by Laboratory Methods, 23rd ed, ISBN # 978-0323-29568-0, 2017, Elsevier)

TABLE 6 Differentiating the Various Causes of Hypoaldosteronism

Disorder	Aldosterone	Renin	Serum K+
Addison's disease	↓	↑	↑
Cushing's syndrome	↓	↓	N or ↓
Liddle's syndrome	↓	↓	↓
Hyporeninemic hypoaldosteronism	↓	↓	↑
Apparent mineralocorticoid excess	↓	↓	↓
Isolated hypoaldosteronism	↓	↑	↑

N, Normal.
(McPherson RA, Pincus MR: Henry's Clinical Diagnosis and Management by Laboratory Methods, 23rd ed, ISBN # 978-0323-29568-0, 2017, Elsevier)

ALKALINE PHOSPHATASE (ALP) (serum)

See Fig. E3 for approach to elevated ALP.
Normal range: 30-120 U/L (0.5-2 μkat/L [CF:0.01667; SMI: 0.1 μkat/L])
Elevated in
LIVER AND BILIARY TRACT ORIGIN
Extrahepatic bile duct obstruction
Intrahepatic biliary obstruction
Liver cell acute injury
Liver passive congestion
Drug-induced liver cell dysfunction
Space-occupying lesions
Primary biliary cirrhosis
Sepsis
BONE ORIGIN (OSTEOBLAST HYPERACTIVITY)
Physiologic (rapid) bone growth (childhood and adolescence)
Metastatic tumor with osteoblastic reaction
Fracture healing
Paget's disease of bone
CAPILLARY ENDOTHELIAL ORIGIN
Granulation tissue formation (active)
PLACENTAL ORIGIN.
Pregnancy
Some parenteral albumin preparations
OTHER
Thyrotoxicosis
Benign transient hyperphosphatasemia
Primary hyperparathyroidism
Decreased in: Hypothyroidism, pernicious anemia, hypophosphatemia, hypervitaminosis D, malnutrition

ALPHA-1-ANTITRYPSIN (serum)

Normal range: 110-140 mg/dl
Decreased in: Homozygous or heterozygous deficiency

ALPHA-1-FETOPROTEIN (serum)

See α-1 FETOPROTEIN

ALT

See ALANINE AMINOTRANSFERASE

ALUMINUM (serum)

Normal range: 0-6 ng/ml
Elevated in: Chronic renal failure on dialysis, parenteral nutrition, industrial exposure

AMA

See ANTIMITOCHONDRIAL ANTIBODY

AMEBIASIS SEROLOGIC TEST

Test description: Test is used to support diagnosis of amebiasis caused by *Entamoeba histolytica*. Serum acute and convalescent titers are drawn 1-3 weeks apart. A fourfold increase in titer is the most indicative result.

AMINOLEVULINIC ACID (δ-ALA) (24-HR URINE COLLECTION)

Normal: 1.5-7.5 mg/day
Elevated in: Acute porphyrias, lead poisoning, DKA, pregnancy, anticonvulsant drugs, hereditary tyrosinemia
Decreased in: Alcoholic liver disease

AMMONIA (serum)

See Fig. E4 for approach to hyperammonemia in pediatric patients.
Normal range: 10-80 μg/dl (5-50 μmol/L [CF: 0.5872; SMI:5 μmol/L])
Elevated in: Hepatic failure, hepatic encephalopathy, Reye's syndrome, portacaval shunt, drugs (diuretics, polymyxin B, methicillin)
Decreased in: Drugs (neomycin, lactulose, tetracycline), renal failure

AMYLASE (serum)

Normal range: 0-130 U/L (0-2.17 μkat/L [CF: 0.01667; SMI: 0.01 μkat/L])
Elevated in: Acute pancreatitis, pancreatic neoplasm, abscess, pseudocyst, ascites, macroamylasemia, perforated peptic ulcer, intestinal obstruction, intestinal infarction, acute cholecystitis, appendicitis, ruptured ectopic pregnancy, salivary gland inflammation, peritonitis, burns, diabetic ketoacidosis, renal insufficiency, drugs (morphine), carcinomatosis (of lung, esophagus, ovary), acute ethanol ingestion, mumps, prostate tumors, post-endoscopic retrograde cholangiopancreatography, bulimia, anorexia nervosa
Decreased in: Advanced chronic pancreatitis, hepatic necrosis, cystic fibrosis

AMYLASE, URINE

See URINE AMYLASE

AMYLOID A PROTEIN (serum)

Normal: <10 mcg/ml
Elevated in: Inflammatory disorders (acute phase–reacting protein), infections, acute coronary syndrome, malignancies

ANA

See ANTINUCLEAR ANTIBODY

ANCA

See ANTINEUTROPHIL CYTOPLASMIC ANTIBODY

ANDROSTENEDIONE (serum)

Normal
Male: 75-205 ng/dl
Female: 85-275 ng/dl
Elevated in: Congenital adrenal hyperplasia, polycystic ovary syndrome, ectopic ACTH-producing tumor, Cushing's syndrome, hirsutism, hyperplasia of ovarian stroma, ovarian neoplasm
Decreased in: Ovarian failure, adrenal failure, sickle cell anemia

ANGIOTENSIN II

Normal: 10-60 pg/ml
Elevated in: Hypertension, CHF, cirrhosis, renin-secreting renal tumor, volume depletion
Decreased in: ACE inhibitor drugs, ARB drugs, primary aldosteronism, Cushing's syndrome

ANGIOTENSIN-CONVERTING ENZYME (ACE level)

Normal range: <40 nmol/ml/min (<670 nkat/L [CF: 16.67; SMI: 10 nkat/L])
Elevated in: Sarcoidosis, primary biliary cirrhosis, alcoholic liver disease, hyperthyroidism, hyperparathyroidism, diabetes mellitus, amyloidosis, multiple myeloma, lung disease (asbestosis, silicosis, berylliosis, allergic alveolitis, coccidioidomycosis), Gaucher's disease, leprosy

ANH

See ATRIAL NATRIURETIC HORMONE

ANION GAP

Normal range: 9-14 mEq/L
Elevated in: Lactic acidosis, ketoacidosis (diabetes, alcoholic starvation), uremia (chronic renal failure), ingestion of toxins (paraldehyde, methanol, salicylates, ethylene glycol), hyperosmolar nonketotic coma, antibiotics (carbenicillin)
Decreased in: Hypoalbuminemia, severe hypermagnesemia, IgG myeloma, lithium toxicity, laboratory error (falsely decreased sodium or overestimation of bicarbonate or chloride), hypercalcemia of parathyroid origin, antibiotics (e.g., polymyxin)

ANTICARDIOLIPIN ANTIBODY (ACA)

Normal range: Negative. Test includes detection of IgG, IgM, and IgA antibodies to phospholipid, cardiolipin
Present in: Antiphospholipid antibody syndrome, chronic hepatitis C

ANTICOAGULANT

See CIRCULATING ANTICOAGULANT

ANTIDIURETIC HORMONE

Normal range: mOsm/kg 295-300 (4-12 pg/ml)
Elevated in: SIADH, antipsychotic medications, ectopic ADH from systemic neoplasm, Guillain-Barré syndrome, CNS infections, brain tumors, nephrogenic diabetes insipidus
Decreased in: Central diabetes insipidus, nephritic syndrome, psychogenic polydipsias, demeclocycline, lithium, phenytoin, alcohol. Table 7 describes

---

TABLE 7 Water Deprivation Test for Diagnosing and Classifying Diabetes Insipidus

Patients with mild polyuria may be instructed to withhold all fluid intake from 10 PM onward. For those with more severe polyuria (8 to 10 L/day), water deprivation should be started early in the morning under close observation.

1. During testing, the patient is forbidden to take in anything by mouth.
2. Obtain the following baseline parameters: urine volume (Uvol) and urinary osmolality (Uosm), plasma osmolality (Posm), and plasma sodium (PNa). Also record the weight and blood pressure (BP)/pulse (P) seated and standing.
3. Urine and plasma are collected hourly for Uvol, Uosm, and Posm. Weight, BP, and P are also recorded. Record requests for fluid.
4. When the Uosm has plateaued (e.g., hourly increase <30 mOsm/kg for 3 consecutive hours), or when body weight has decreased by 3% to 5%, or the patient develops a >20–mm Hg drop in systolic BP, obtain samples for Uvol, Uosm, Posm, PNa, and AVP (plasma).
5. Administer 1 mcg of desmopressin IV or IM, or 5 mcg of AVP SC Uosm; urine output and Posm are recorded at 30, 60, and 120 minutes after the injection. The highest Uosm value is used to evaluate the patient's response to AVP.

Precautions

When possible, discontinue any medications that can influence ADH secretion. Observe for hypotension and nausea, which may stimulate ADH secretion. The patient should not be permitted to smoke during the test.

Interpretation

Normal	Final Uosm before AVP challenge is higher than Posm. Following AVP challenge, the Uosm is less than 10% higher than the maximal Uosm achieved with water restriction alone.
Neurogenic DI	Final Uosm before AVP challenge is less than Posm. Following AVP administration, there is a greater than 50% increase in Uosm.
Nephrogenic DI	Final Uosm before AVP challenge is less than Posm. Following AVP administration, there is a less than 10% increase in Uosm.
Partial central DI	Uosm may be higher than Posm following dehydration; however, there is only a 10% to 50% increase in Uosm following administration of AVP.
Partial nephrogenic DI	Uosm may be higher than Posm following dehydration; however, there is a greater than 10% increase in Uosm following administration of AVP.

Plotting basal and postdehydration Uosm and plasma ADH on the nomograms from Zerbe and Robertson will permit further distinction between partial nephrogenic DI, partial central DI, and primary polydipsia

ADH, Antidiuretic hormone; *AVP*, arginine vasopressin; *DI*, diabetes insipidus; *IM*, intramuscular; *IV*, intravenous; *SC*, subcutaneous.
(McPherson RA, Pincus MR: Henry's Clinical Diagnosis and Management by Laboratory Methods, 23rd ed, ISBN # 978-0323-29568-0, 2017, Elsevier)

TABLE 8 Tests in the Differential Diagnosis of Disorders of Water Homeostasis

Disorder	BASELINE			AFTER 12-HOUR FLUID RESTRICTION			Urine Osmolality Post-AVP Challenge
	Serum Na+ and Osmolality	Urine Na+ and Osmolality	Serum ADH	Serum Na+ and Osmolality	Urine Na+ and Osmolality	Serum ADH	
Normal control	N	N	N	N	High	High	Same
SIADH	Low	N-High	High	Low-N	High	High	—
Neurogenic DI	N-High	Low	Low	High	Low-N	Low	Increased
Nephrogenic DI	N-High	Low	N-High	High	Low-N	High	Same
Psychogenic polydipsia	Low–N	Low	Low	N	N-High	N-High	Same

ADH, Antidiuretic hormone; *AVP*, arginine vasopressin; *DI*, diabetes insipidus; *N*, normal; *SIADH*, syndrome of inappropriate secretion of ADH.
(McPherson RA, Pincus MR: Henry's Clinical Diagnosis and Management by Laboratory Methods, 23rd ed, ISBN # 978-0323-29568-0, 2017, Elsevier)

BOX 1   Causes of Polyuria Due to Water Diuresis

Lack of ADH
Central diabetes insipidus (DI): congenital or acquired (idiopathic cell degeneration, tumors and granulomas, surgery, trauma, infarction, and infection of the pituitary gland or hypothalamus)
Dipsogenic: psychogenic, organic brain disease, iatrogenic
Gestational DI: Excess vasopressinase

Failure of the Kidney to Respond to ADH (Nephrogenic DI)
Congenital nephrogenic DI: a defect in ADH receptor, a defect in aquaporin expression.
Chronic renal failure.
Acquired nephrogenic DI: lithium toxicity, demeclocycline toxicity, methoxyflurane toxicity, amyloidosis, light chain nephropathy, hypercalcemia, hypokalemia, obstructive uropathy

(McPherson RA, Pincus MR: Henry's Clinical Diagnosis and Management by Laboratory Methods, 23rd ed, ISBN # 978-0323-29568-0, 2017, Elsevier)

the water deprivation test used for diagnosing and classifying diabetes insipidus. Table 8 summarizes tests in the differential diagnosis of water homeostasis. Causes of polyuria due to water diuresis are described in Box 1.

ANTI-DNA

Normal range: Absent
Present in: Systemic lupus erythematosus, chronic active hepatitis, infectious mononucleosis, biliary cirrhosis

ANTI-DS DNA

Normal: <25 U
Elevated in: Systemic lupus erythematosus

ANTIGLOBULIN TEST

See COOMBS TEST

ANTIGLOMERULAR BASEMENT ANTIBODY

See GLOMERULAR BASEMENT MEMBRANE ANTIBODY

ANTIHISTONE

Normal: <1 U
Elevated in: Drug-induced lupus erythematosus

ANTIMITOCHONDRIAL ANTIBODY (AMA, Mitochondrial antibody)

Normal range: <1:20 titer
Elevated in: Primary biliary cirrhosis (85%-95%), chronic active hepatitis (25%-30%), cryptogenic cirrhosis (25%-30%)

ANTINEUTROPHIL CYTOPLASMIC ANTIBODY (ANCA)

Positive test: Cytoplasmic pattern (cANCA): positive in Wegener's granulomatosis (see Fig. E5 and Table E9 for approach to patient with positive c-ANCA)

    Perinuclear pattern (pANCA): positive in inflammatory bowel disease, primary biliary cirrhosis, primary sclerosing cholangitis, autoimmune chronic active hepatitis, crescentic glomerulonephritis (see Table E9 for approach to patient with positive P-ANCA)

ANTINUCLEAR ANTIBODY (ANA)

Fig. E6 describes an algorithm for the use of antinuclear antibodies in the diagnosis of connective tissue disorders. See Fig. E7 for approach to positive ANA pattern

Normal range: <1:20 titer

    Positive test: Systemic lupus erythematosus (more significant if titer >1:160), drugs (phenytoin, ethosuximide, primidone, methyldopa, hydralazine, carbamazepine, penicillin, procainamide, chlorpromazine, griseofulvin, thiazides), chronic active hepatitis, autoimmune thyroid disease (positive ANA is found in up to 45% of patients), idiopathic thrombocytopenic purpura, multiple sclerosis, rheumatoid arthritis, scleroderma, mixed connective tissue disease, necrotizing vasculitis, Sjögren's syndrome,

---

TABLE 10   Disease-Associated ANA Subtypes

Nuclear Location	Disease(s)
"Native" DNA (dsDNA, or dsDNA/ssDNA complex)	SLE (60%-70%; range, 35%-75%) Also PSS (5%-55%), MCTD (11%-25%), RA (5%-40%), DM (5%-25%), SS (5%)
sNP	SLE (50%) Also other collagen diseases
DNP (DNA-histone complex)	SLE (52%) Also MCTD (8%), RA (3%)
Histones	Drug-induced SLE (95%) Also SLE (30%), RA (15%-24%)
ENA Sm	SLE (30%-40%; range, 28%-40%) Also MCTD (0%-8%); RNP (U1-RNP) MCTD (in high titer without any other ANA subtype present: 95%-100%) Also SLE (26%-50%), PSS (11%-22%), RA (10%), SS (3%)
SS-A (Ro)*	SS without RA (60%-70%) Also SLE (26%-50%), neonatal SLE (over 95%), PSS (30%), MCTD (50%), SS with RA (9%), PBC (15%-19%)
SS-B (La)	SS without RA (40%-60%) Also SLE (5%-15%), SS with RA (5%)
Scl-70*	PSS (15%-43%)
Centromere*	CREST syndrome (70%-90%; range, 57%-96%) Also PSS (4%-20%), PBC (12%)
Nucleolar	PSS (scleroderma) (54%-90%) Also SLE (25%-26%), RA (9%)
RAP (RANA)	SS with RA (60%-76%) Also SS without RA (5%)
Jo-1	Polymyositis (30%)
PM-1	Polymyositis or PMS/PSS overlap syndrome (60%-90%) Also DM (17%)
ssDNA	SLE (60%-70%) Also CAH, infectious mononucleosis, RA, chronic GN, chronic infections, PBC

Cytoplasmic Location	Disease(s)
Mitochondrial	PBC (90%-100%) Also CAH (7%-30%), cryptogenic cirrhosis (30%), acute hepatitis, viral hepatitis (3%), other liver diseases (0%-20%), SLE (5%), SS and PSS (8%)
Microsomal†	Chronic active hepatitis (60%-80%), Hashimoto's thyroiditis (97%)
Ribosomal	SLE (5%-12%)
Smooth muscle‡	Chronic active hepatitis (60%-91%)

CAH, Chronic active hepatitis; *DM,* dermatomyositis; *GN,* glomerulonephritis; *MS,* multiple sclerosis; *PBC,* primary biliary cirrhosis; *SS,* Sjögren's syndrome.
*Not detected using rat or mouse liver or kidney tissue method.
†Not detected by cultured cell method.
‡Detected by cultured cells but better with rat or mouse tissue.
From Ravel R: *Clinical laboratory medicine,* ed 6, St Louis, 1995, Mosby.

TABLE 11   Assay Measurements in Heterozygous Antithrombin (ATIII) Deficiency for Diagnosis

	ACTIVITY		
Type	Antigen	Heparin Cofactor	Progressive ATIII
I	Low	Low	Low
II			
Active site defect	Normal	Low	Low
Heparin-binding site defect	Normal	Low	Normal

From Hoffman R et al: *Hematology: basic principles and practice,* ed 5, Philadelphia, 2009, Churchill Livingstone.

tuberculosis, pulmonary interstitial fibrosis. Positive ANA results are nonspecific and can be found in healthy individuals (13.8% of the adult general population). Table 10 describes diseases associated with ANA subtypes. Fig. 8 illustrates various fluorescent ANA test patterns.

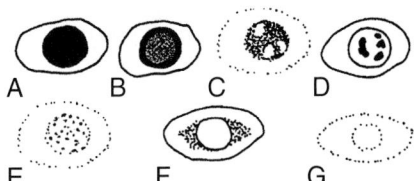

FIG. 8 Fluorescent antinuclear antibody test patterns (HEP-2 cells). **A,** Solid (homogeneous). **B,** Peripheral (rim). **C,** Speckled. **D,** Nucleolar. **E,** Anticentromere. **F,** Antimitochondrial. **G,** Normal (nonreactive). (From Ravel R [ed]: *Clinical laboratory medicine,* ed 6, St Louis, 1995, Mosby.)

ANTI-RNP ANTIBODY

See EXTRACTABLE NUCLEAR ANTIGEN

ANTI-SCL-70

Normal: Absent
Elevated in: Scleroderma

ANTI-SM (anti-Smith) ANTIBODY

See EXTRACTABLE NUCLEAR ANTIGEN

ANTI-SMOOTH MUSCLE ANTIBODY

See SMOOTH MUSCLE ANTIBODY

ANTISTREPTOLYSIN O TITER (Streptozyme, ASLO titer)

Normal range for adults: <160 Todd units
Elevated in: Streptococcal upper airway infection, acute rheumatic fever, acute glomerulonephritis, increased levels of β-lipoprotein

NOTE: A fourfold increase in titer between acute and convalescent specimens is diagnostic of streptococcal upper airway infection regardless of the initial titer.

ANTITHROMBIN III

See Table 11.
Normal range: 81%-120% of normal activity; 17-30 mg/dl
Decreased in: Hereditary deficiency of antithrombin III, disseminated intravascular coagulation, pulmonary embolism, cirrhosis, thrombolytic therapy, chronic liver failure, postsurgery, third trimester of pregnancy, oral contraceptives, nephrotic syndrome, IV heparin >3 days, sepsis, acute leukemia, carcinoma, thrombophlebitis
Elevated in: Warfarin drugs, post-myocardial infarction

APOLIPOPROTEIN A-1 (Apo A-1)

Normal: Desirable >120 mg/dl
Elevated in: Familial hyperalphalipoproteinemia, statins, niacin, estrogens, weight loss, familial cholesteryl ester transfer protein (CETP) deficiency
Decreased in: Familial hypoalphalipoproteinemia, Tangier disease, diuretics, androgens, cigarette smoking, hepatocellular disorders, chronic renal failure, nephritic syndrome, coronary heart disease, cholestasis

APOLIPOPROTEIN B (Apo B)

Normal: Desirable <100 mg/dl; high risk >120 mg/dl
Elevated in: High saturated fat diet, high-cholesterol diet, hyperapobetalipoproteinemia, familial combined hyperlipidemia, anabolic steroids, diuretics, beta-blockers, corticosteroids, progestins, diabetes, hypothyroidism, chronic renal failure, liver disease, Cushing's syndrome, coronary heart disease
Decreased in: Statins, niacin, low-cholesterol diet, malnutrition, abetalipoproteinemia, hypobetalipoproteinemia, hyperthyroidism

ARTERIAL BLOOD GASES

Normal range:
Po$_2$: 75-100 mm Hg
Pco$_2$: 35-45 mm Hg
HCO$_3$: 24-28 mEq/L
pH: 7.35-7.45
Abnormal values: Acid-base disturbances (see the following)

BOX 2 Causes of Metabolic Acidosis by Net Acid Excretion

Renal Acidosis: Absolute or Relative Reduction in Net Acid Excretion
Uremic acidosis
Renal tubular acidosis
- Distal renal tubular acidosis (type I)
- Proximal renal tubular acidosis (type II)
- Aldosterone deficiency or unresponsiveness (type IV)

Extrarenal Acidosis: Increase in Net Acid Excretion
Gastrointestinal loss of bicarbonate
Ingestion of acids or acid precursors: ammonium chloride, sulfur-containing compounds
Acid precursors or toxins: salicylate, ethylene glycol, methanol, toluene, acetaminophen, paraldehyde
Organic acidosis
- L-lactic acidosis
- D-lactic acidosis
- Ketoacidosis
- Pyroglutamic acidosis

(McPherson RA, Pincus MR: Henry's Clinical Diagnosis and Management by Laboratory Methods, 23rd ed, ISBN # 978-0323-29568-0, 2017, Elsevier)

BOX 3 Causes of L-Lactic Acidosis

Type A Lactic Acidosis Due to Tissue Hypoxia
Circulatory shock
Severe hypoxemia
Heart failure
Severe anemia
Grand mal seizure

Type B Lactic Acidosis, No Tissue Hypoxia
Acute alcoholism
Drugs and toxins (e.g., metformin, antiretroviral drugs, salicylate intoxication)
Diabetes mellitus
Leukemia
Deficiency of thiamin or riboflavin
Idiopathic

(McPherson RA, Pincus MR: Henry's Clinical Diagnosis and Management by Laboratory Methods, 23rd ed, ISBN # 978-0323-29568-0, 2017, Elsevier)

METABOLIC ACIDOSIS
Causes of metabolic acidosis by net acid excretion are summarized in Box 2.
Metabolic acidosis with increased AG (AG acidosis)
Lactic acidosis (see Box 3)
Ketoacidosis (diabetes mellitus, alcoholic ketoacidosis)
Uremia (chronic renal failure)
Ingestion of toxins (paraldehyde, methanol, salicylate, ethylene glycol)
High-fat diet (mild acidosis)
Metabolic acidosis with normal AG (hyperchloremic acidosis)
Renal tubular acidosis (including acidosis of aldosterone deficiency)
Intestinal loss of HCO$_3^-$ (diarrhea, pancreatic fistula)
Carbonic anhydrase inhibitors (e.g., acetazolamide)
Dilutional acidosis (as a result of rapid infusion of bicarbonate-free isotonic saline)
Ingestion of exogenous acids (ammonium chloride, methionine, cystine, calcium chloride)
Ileostomy
Ureterosigmoidostomy
Drugs: amiloride, triamterene, spironolactone, β-blockers
RESPIRATORY ACIDOSIS
Pulmonary disease (COPD, severe pneumonia, pulmonary edema, interstitial fibrosis)
Airway obstruction (foreign body, severe bronchospasm, laryngospasm)
Thoracic cage disorders (pneumothorax, flail chest, kyphoscoliosis)
Defects in muscles of respiration (myasthenia gravis, hypokalemia, muscular dystrophy)

TABLE 12   Reference Intervals for Synovial Fluid Constituents

Constituent	Synovial Fluid	Plasma
Total protein	1-3 g/dL	6-8 g/dL
Albumin	55%-70%	50%-65%
α_1-Globulin	6%-8%	3%-5%
α_2-Globulin	5%-7%	7%-13%
β-Globulin	8%-10%	8%-14%
γ-Globulin	10%-14%	12%-22%
Hyaluronic acid	0.3-0.4 g/dL	
Glucose	70-110 mg/dL	70-110 mg/dL
Uric acid	2-8 mg/dL	2-8 mg/dL
Lactate	9-29 mg/dL	9-29 mg/dL

Modified from Kjeldsberg CR, Knight JA: *Body fluids: laboratory examination of amniotic, cerebrospinal, seminal, serous and synovial fluids*, ed 3, Chicago, 1993, © American Society for Clinical Pathology, with permission.

(McPherson RA, Pincus MR: Henry's Clinical Diagnosis and Management by Laboratory Methods, 23rd ed, ISBN # 978-0323-29568-0, 2017, Elsevier)

Defects in peripheral nervous system (amyotrophic lateral sclerosis, polio-myelitis, Guillain-Barré syndrome, botulism, tetanus, organophosphate poisoning, spinal cord injury)

Depression of respiratory center (anesthesia, narcotics, sedatives, vertebral artery embolism or thrombosis, increased intracranial pressure)

Failure of mechanical ventilator

METABOLIC ALKALOSIS. Divided into chloride-responsive (urinary chloride <15 mEq/L) and chloride-resistant forms (urinary chloride level >15 mEq/L)

Chloride-responsive

Vomiting

Nasogastric (NG) suction

Diuretics

Posthypercapnic alkalosis

Stool losses (laxative abuse, cystic fibrosis, villous adenoma)

Massive blood transfusion

Exogenous alkali administration

Chloride-resistant

Hyperadrenocorticoid states (Cushing's syndrome, primary hyperaldosteronism, secondary mineralocorticoidism [licorice, chewing tobacco])

Hypomagnesemia

Hypokalemia

Bartter's syndrome

RESPIRATORY ALKALOSIS

Hypoxemia (pneumonia, pulmonary embolism, atelectasis, high-altitude living)

Drugs (salicylates, xanthines, progesterone, epinephrine, thyroxine, nicotine)

Central nervous system (CNS) disorders (tumor, cerebrovascular accident [CVA], trauma, infections)

Psychogenic hyperventilation (anxiety, hysteria)

Hepatic encephalopathy

Gram-negative sepsis

Hyponatremia

Sudden recovery from metabolic acidosis

Assisted ventilation

ARTHROCENTESIS FLUID

Reference intervals for synovial fluid constituents are described in Table 12.

Interpretation of results:

1. **Color:** Normally it is clear or pale yellow; cloudiness indicates inflammatory process or presence of crystals, cell debris, fibrin, or triglycerides.

2. **Viscosity:** Normally it has a high viscosity because of hyaluronate; when fluid is placed on a slide, it can be stretched to a string >2 cm in length before separating (low viscosity indicates breakdown of hyaluronate [lysosomal enzymes from leukocytes] or the presence of edema fluid).

3. **Mucin clot:** Add 1 ml of fluid to 5 ml of a 5% acetic acid solution and allow 1 minute for the clot to form; a firm clot (does not fragment on shaking) is normal and indicates the presence of large molecules of hyaluronic acid (this test is nonspecific and infrequently done).

4. **Glucose:** Normally it approximately equals serum glucose level; a difference of more than 40 mg/dl is suggestive of infection.

5. **Protein:** Total protein concentration is <2.5 g/dl in the normal synovial fluid; it is elevated in inflammatory and septic arthritis.

6. Microscopic examination for crystals
   a. **Gout:** Monosodium urate crystals
   b. **Pseudogout:** Calcium pyrophosphate dihydrate crystals

ASLO TITER

See ANTISTREPTOLYSIN O TITER

ASPARTATE AMINOTRANSFERASE (AST, SGOT)

Normal range: 0-35 U/L (0-0.58 μkat/L [CF: 0.01667, SMI: 0.01μkat/L])

Elevated in

HEART.

Acute myocardial infarction

Pericarditis (active: some cases)

LIVER.

Hepatitis virus, Epstein-Barr, or cytomegalovirus infection

Active cirrhosis

Liver passive congestion or hypoxia

Alcohol- or drug-induced liver dysfunction

Space-occupying lesions (active)

Fatty liver (severe)

Extrahepatic biliary obstruction (early)

Drug-induced

SKELETAL MUSCLE.

Acute skeletal muscle injury

Muscle inflammation (infectious or noninfectious)

Muscular dystrophy (active)

Recent surgery

Delirium tremens

KIDNEY.

Acute injury or damage

Renal infarct

OTHER.

Intestinal infarction

Shock

Cholecystitis

Acute pancreatitis

Hypothyroidism

Heparin therapy (60%-80% of cases)

Fig. 1 describes an approach to the evaluation of AST elevation.

ATRIAL NATRIURETIC HORMONE (ANH)

Normal: 20-77 pg/ml

Elevated in: CHF, volume overload, cardiovascular disease with high filling pressure

Decreased with: Prazosin and other alpha blockers

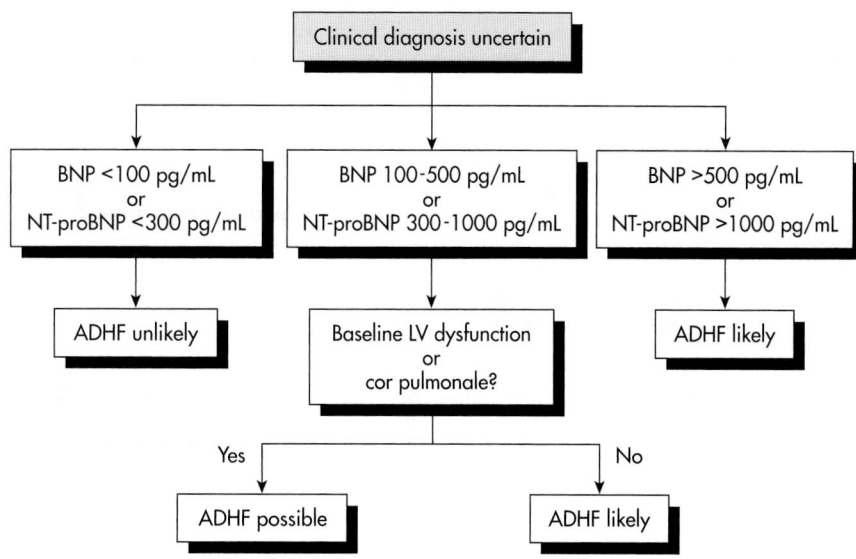

FIG. 9 Interpretation of natriuretic peptide levels. *ADHF*, Acute decompensated heart failure; *BNP*, B-type natriuretic peptide; *NT-proBNP*, inactive N-terminal fragment of BNP. (From Adams JG, et al: *Emergency medicine, clinical essentials*, ed 2, Philadelphia, 2013, Elsevier.)

B-TYPE NATRIURETIC PEPTIDE (BNP)

Normal range: up to 100 mcg/L. Natriuretic peptides are secreted to regulate fluid volume, blood pressure, and electrolyte balance. They have activity in both the central and peripheral nervous systems. In humans the main source of circulatory BNP is the heart ventricles.

Elevated in: Heart failure. This test is useful to differentiate heart failure patients from those with chronic obstructive pulmonary disease presenting with dyspnea. Levels are also increased in asymptomatic left ventricular dysfunction, arterial and pulmonary hypertension, cardiac hypertrophy, valvular heart disease, arrhythmia, and acute coronary syndrome. See Fig. 9.

BASOPHIL COUNT

Normal range:

a. 0.4%-1% of total WBC; 40-100/mm^3

Elevated in: Leukemia, inflammatory processes, polycythemia vera, Hodgkin's lymphoma, hemolytic anemia, after splenectomy, myeloid metaplasia, myxedema

Decreased in: Stress, hypersensitivity reaction, steroids, pregnancy, hyperthyroidism, postirradiation

BICARBONATE

Normal:

Arterial: 21-28 mEq/L

Venous: 22-29 mEq/L

Elevated in: Metabolic alkalosis, compensated respiratory acidosis, diuretics, corticosteroids, laxative abuse

Decreased in: Metabolic acidosis, compensated respiratory alkalosis, acetazolamide, cyclosporine, cholestyramine, methanol or ethylene glycol poisoning

BILE, URINE

See URINE BILE

BILIRUBIN, DIRECT (conjugated bilirubin)

Normal range:

0-0.2 mg/dl (0-4 μmol/L [CF: 17.10; SMI: 2 μmol/L])

Elevated in: Hepatocellular disease, biliary obstruction, drug-induced cholestasis, hereditary disorders (Dubin-Johnson syndrome, Rotor's syndrome)

BILIRUBIN, INDIRECT (unconjugated bilirubin)

Normal range:

0-1.0 mg/dl (2-18 μmol/L [CF: 17.10; SMI: 2 μmol/L])

Elevated in:

Increased bilirubin production (if normal liver, serum unconjugated bilirubin is usually less than 4 mg/100 ml)

Hemolytic anemia
  Acquired
  Congenital
Resorption from extravascular sources
  Hematomas
  Pulmonary infarcts
Excessive ineffective erythropoiesis
  Congenital (congenital dyserythropoietic anemias)
  Acquired (pernicious anemia, severe lead poisoning; if present, bilirubinemia is usually mild)
Defective hepatic unconjugated bilirubin clearance (defective uptake or conjugation)
Severe liver disease
Gilbert's syndrome
Crigler-Najjar type I or II
Drug-induced inhibition
Portacaval shunt
Congestive heart failure
Hyperthyroidism (uncommon)

BILIRUBIN, TOTAL

See Fig. 10 and Table 13, for evaluation of hyperbilirubinemia and liver disease.

Normal range:

0-1.0 mg/dl (2-18 μmol/L [CF: 17.10, SMI: 2 μmol/L])

Elevated in: Liver disease (hepatitis, cirrhosis, cholangitis, neoplasm, biliary obstruction, infectious mononucleosis), hereditary disorders (Gilbert's disease, Dubin-Johnson syndrome), drugs (steroids, statins, niacin, acetaminophen, diphenylhydantoin, phenothiazines, penicillin, erythromycin, clindamycin, captopril, amphotericin B, sulfonamides, azathioprine, isoniazid, 5-aminosalicylic acid, allopurinol, methyldopa, indomethacin, halothane, oral contraceptives, procainamide, tolbutamide, labetalol), hemolysis, pulmonary embolism or infarct, hepatic congestion secondary to congestive heart failure

BILIRUBIN, URINE

See URINE BILE

BLADDER TUMOR ASSOCIATED ANTIGEN

Normal:

≤14 U/ml. Test is used to detect bladder cancer recurrence. Sensitivity 57%-83% and specificity 68%-72%.

Elevated in: Bladder cancer, renal stones, nephritis, UTI, hematuria, renal cancer, cystitis, recent bladder or urinary tract trauma

BLEEDING TIME (modified Ivy method)

See Fig. E11 for evaluation of patients with prolonged bleeding time.

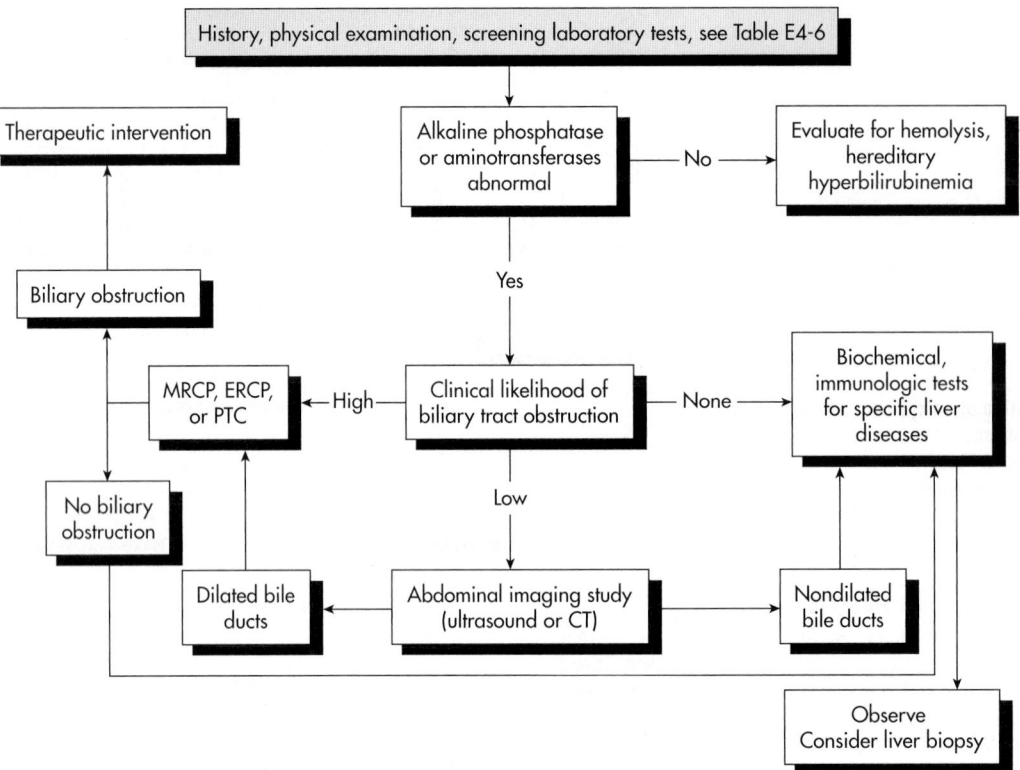

FIG. 10 Diagnosis algorithm for the evaluation of hyperbilirubinemia and other liver test abnormalities and/or signs and symptoms suggestive of liver disease. CT, Computed tomography; ERCP, endoscopic retrograde cholangiopancreatography; MRCP, magnetic resonance cholangiopancreatography; PTC, percutaneous cholangiogram. (From Goldman L, Ausiello D [eds]: *Cecil textbook of medicine,* ed 24, Philadelphia, 2012, Saunders. Modified from Lidofsky SD, Scharschmidt BF: Jaundice. In Feldman M, Scharschmidt BF, Sleisenger MH [eds]: *Gastrointestinal and liver disease,* ed 6, Philadelphia, 1998, Saunders.)

TABLE 13   Obstructive Jaundice versus Cholestatic Liver Disease

Feature	Suggests Obstructive Jaundice	Suggests Parenchymal Liver Disease
History	Abdominal pain Fever, rigors Prior biliary surgery Older age Acholic stools	Anorexia, malaise, myalgias, suggestive of viral prodrome Known infectious exposure Receipt of blood products, use of intravenous drugs Exposure to known hepatotoxin Family history of jaundice
Physical examination	High fever Abdominal tenderness Palpable abdominal mass Abdominal scar	Ascites Other stigmata of liver disease (e.g., prominent abdominal veins, gynecomastia, spider angiomata, asterixis, encephalopathy, Kayser-Fleischer rings)
Laboratory studies	Predominant elevation of serum bilirubin and alkaline phosphatase Prothrombin time that is normal or normalizes with vitamin K administration Elevated serum amylase	Predominant elevation of serum aminotransferases Prolonged prothrombin time that does not correct with vitamin K administration Blood tests indicative of specific liver disease

From Goldman L, Ausiello D (eds): *Cecil textbook of medicine,* ed 24, Philadelphia, 2012, Saunders.

Normal range: 2 to 9.5 min

Elevated in: Thrombocytopenia, capillary wall abnormalities, platelet abnormalities (Bernard-Soulier disease, Glanzmann's disease), drugs (aspirin, warfarin, antiinflammatory medications, streptokinase, urokinase, dextran, β-lactam antibiotics, moxalactam), disseminated intravascular coagulation, cirrhosis, uremia, myeloproliferative disorders, von Willebrand's disease.

Bleeding time tests are no longer performed at many hospitals and have been replaced by the platelet function analyzer (PFA-100) assay.

BLOOD VOLUME, TOTAL

Normal: 60-80 ml/kg

Elevated in: Polycythemia vera, pulmonary disease, CHF, renal insufficiency, pregnancy, acidosis, thyrotoxicosis

Decreased in: Anemia, hemorrhage, vomiting, diarrhea, dehydration, burns, starvation

BNP

See B-TYPE NATRIURETIC PEPTIDE

BORDETELLA PERTUSSIS SEROLOGY

Test description: PCR of nasopharyngeal aspirates or secretions is used to identify *Bordetella pertussis,* the organism responsible for whooping cough.

BRCA ANALYSIS
DESCRIPTION OF ANALYSIS
Comprehensive BRCA analysis

BRCA1: Full sequence determination in both forward and reverse directions of approximately 5500 base pairs comprising 22 coding exons and one noncoding exon (exon 4) and approximately 800 adjacent base pairs in the noncoding intervening sequence (intron). Exon 1, which is noncoding, is not analyzed. The wild-type *BRCA1* gene encodes a protein comprising 1863 amino acids.

BRCA2: Full sequence determination in both forward and reverse directions of approximately 10,200 base pairs comprising 26 coding exons and approximately 900 adjacent base pairs in the noncoding intervening sequence (intron). Exon 1, which is noncoding, is not analyzed. The wild-type *BRCA2* gene encodes a protein comprising 3418 amino acids.

The noncoding intronic regions of *BRCA1* and *BRCA2* that are analyzed do not extend more than 20 base pairs proximal to the 5' end and 10 base pairs distal to the 3' end of each exon.

Single-site BRCA analysis: DNA sequence analysis for a specified mutation in *BRCA1* and/or *BRCA2.*

Multisite 3 BRCA analysis: DNA sequence analysis of specific portions of *BRCA1* exon 2, *BRCA1* exon 20, and *BRCA2* exon 11 designed to detect only mutations 187delAG and 5385insC in *BRCA1* and 6174delT in *BRCA2.*

Interpretive Criteria

"Positive for a deleterious mutation": Includes all mutations (nonsense, insertions, deletions) that prematurely terminate ("truncate") the protein product of *BRCA1* at least 10 amino acids from the C-terminus, or the protein product of *BRCA2* at least 110 amino acids from the C-terminus (based on documentation of deleterious mutations in *BRCA1* and *BRCA2).*

In addition, specific missense mutations and noncoding intervening sequence (IVS) mutations are recognized as deleterious on the basis of data derived from linkage analysis of high-risk families, functional assays, biochemical evidence, and/or demonstration of abnormal mRNA transcript processing.

"Genetic variant, suspected deleterious": Includes genetic variants for which the available evidence indicates a likelihood, but not proof, that the mutation is deleterious. The specific evidence supporting such an interpretation will be summarized for individual variants on each such report.

"Genetic variant, favor polymorphism": Includes genetic variants for which available evidence indicates that the variant is highly unlikely to contribute substantially to cancer risk. The specific evidence supporting such an interpretation will be summarized for individual variants on each such report.

"Genetic variant of uncertain significance": Includes missense mutations and mutations that occur in analyzed intronic regions whose clinical significance has not yet been determined, as well as chain-terminating mutations that truncate *BRCA1* and *BRCA2* distal to amino acid positions 1853 and 3308, respectively.

"No deleterious mutation detected": Includes nontruncating genetic variants observed at an allele frequency of approximately 1% of a suitable control population (providing that no data suggest clinical significance), as well as all genetic variants for which published data demonstrate absence of substantial clinical significance. Also includes mutations in the protein-coding region that neither alter the amino acid sequence nor are predicted to significantly affect exon splicing, and base pair alterations in noncoding portions of the gene that have been demonstrated to have no deleterious effect on the length or stability of the mRNA transcript.

There may be uncommon genetic abnormalities in *BRCA1* and *BRCA2* that will not be detected by *BRCA* analysis. This analysis, however, is believed to rule out the majority of abnormalities in these genes, which are believed responsible for most hereditary susceptibility to breast and ovarian cancer.

"Specific variant/mutation not identified": Specific and designated deleterious mutations or variants of uncertain clinical significance are not present in the individual being tested. If one (or rarely two) specific deleterious mutations have been identified in a family member, a negative analysis for the specific mutation(s) indicates that the tested individual is at the general population risk of developing breast or ovarian cancer.

BREATH HYDROGEN TEST (hydrogen breath test)

Normal: This test is for bacterial overgrowth. H_2 excretion fasting: 4.6 ± 5.1, after lactulose, early increase <12. Lactulose usually results in a colonic response >30 min after ingestion.

Elevated in: A high fasting breath H_2 level and an increase of at least 12 ppm within 30 min after lactulose challenge indicate presence of bacterial overgrowth in the small intestine. The increase must precede the colonic response.

False positives in: Accelerated gastric emptying, laxative use

False negatives in: Use of antibiotics and patients who are nonhydrogen producers

BUN

See UREA NITROGEN, BLOOD

C282Y AND H63D MUTATION ANALYSIS

Procedure: Detection of the C282Y and H63D mutations is accomplished by amplification of exons 2 and 4 of the *HFE* gene on chromosome 6 by polymerase chain reaction (PCR) followed by allele-specific hybridization and chemiluminescent detection of hybridized probes. H63D is viewed by some as a polymorphism rather than a mutation because of its prevalence in the population, because 15% of the individuals affected with hereditary hemochromatosis (HH) are compound heterozygotes for C282Y and H63D and about 1% of patients are H63D homozygotes, which suggests that H63D may be causative in the development of the disorder at reduced penetrance.

Interpretation: Homozygosity for the C282Y mutation has been associated with an increased risk of being affected with HH compared with the general population. The genotype is observed in 60%-90% of individuals affected with HH and occurs in less than 1% of the general population. However, approximately 25% of asymptomatic individuals with this genotype do not develop the disorder.

C3

See COMPLEMENT

C4

See COMPLEMENT

CALCITONIN (serum)

Normal range: <100 pg/ml (<100 ng/L [CF: 1; SMI: 10 ng/L])

Elevated in: Medullary carcinoma of the thyroid (particularly if level >1500 pg/ml), carcinoma of the breast, apudomas, carcinoids, renal failure, thyroiditis

CALCIUM (serum)

Normal range: 8.8-10.3 mg/dl (2.2-2.58 μmol/L [CF: 0.2495; SMI: 0.02 μmol/L])

ELEVATED

Relatively common:

Neoplasia
Bone primary
Myeloma
Acute leukemia
Nonbone solid tumors
Breast
Lung
Squamous nonpulmonary
Kidney
Neoplasm secretion of parathyroid hormone-related protein (PTHrP, "ectopic PTH")
Primary hyperparathyroidism
Thiazide diuretics
Tertiary (renal) hyperparathyroidism
Idiopathic
Spurious (artifactual) hypercalcemia
Dehydration
Serum protein elevation
Laboratory technical problem (lab error)

Relatively uncommon:

Sarcoidosis
Hyperthyroidism
Immobilization (mostly seen in children and adolescents)
Diuretic phase of acute renal tubular necrosis
Vitamin D intoxication
Milk-alkali syndrome
Addison's disease
Lithium therapy
Idiopathic hypercalcemia of infancy
Acromegaly
Theophylline toxicity

Table 14 describes the laboratory differential diagnosis of hypercalcemia.

DECREASED

Artifactual
Hypoalbuminemia
Hemodilution
Primary hypoparathyroidism
Pseudohypoparathyroidism
Vitamin D related
Vitamin D deficiency
Malabsorption
Renal failure
Magnesium deficiency
Sepsis
Chronic alcoholism
Tumor lysis syndrome
Rhabdomyolysis
Alkalosis (respiratory or metabolic)
Acute pancreatitis
Drug-induced hypocalcemia
Large doses of magnesium sulfate
Anticonvulsants
Mithramycin
Gentamicin
Cimetidine

Table 15 describes the laboratory differential diagnosis of hypocalcemia.

CALCIUM, URINE

See URINE CALCIUM

CANCER ANTIGEN 15-3 (CA 15-3)

Normal: <30 U/ml

Elevated in: Approximately 80% of women with metastatic breast cancer. Clinical sensitivity is 0.60, specificity 0.87, positive predictive value 0.91. This test is generally used to predict recurrence of breast cancer and evaluate response to therapy. May also be elevated in liver cancer, pancreatic cancer, ovarian cancer, colorectal cancer. Elevations can also occur with benign breast and liver disease.

TABLE 14   Laboratory Differential Diagnosis of Hypercalcemia

Diagnosis	PLASMA TESTS					URINE TESTS			Comments
	Ca	PO₄	PTH	25(OH)D	1,25(OH)₂D	cAMP	TmP/GFR	Ca	
Primary hyperparathy-roidism	↑	N/↓	↑	N	N/↑	↑	↓	↑	Parathyroid adenoma most common
MEN I									Parathyroid hyperplasia; also includes pituitary and pancreatic neoplasms
MEN IIa									Parathyroid hyperplasia; also includes medullary thyroid carcinoma and pheochromocytoma
MEN IIb									Parathyroid disease uncommon, primarily medullary thyroid carcinoma and pheochromocytoma
FHH	↑	N	N/↑	N	N	N/↑	N/↓	↓↓	Autosomal dominant inheritance; hypercalcemia present within first decade; benign
Malignancy									
Solid tumor, humoral	↑	N/↓	↓	N	N	↑	↓	↑↑	Primarily epidermoid tumors; PTH-related protein(s) is mediator
Solid tumor, osteolytic	↑	N/↑	↓	N	N	↓	↑	↑↑	
Lymphoma	↑	N/↑	↓	N/↓	↑	↓	↑	↑↑	
Granulomatous disease	↑	N/↑	↓	N/↓	↑↑	↓	↑	↑↑	Sarcoid most common etiology
Vitamin D intoxication	↑	N/↑	↓	↑↑	N	↓	↑	↑↑	
Hyperthyroidism	↑	N	↓	N	N	N	N	↑↑	Plasma concentrations of T₄ and/or T₃ are elevated

From Moore WT, Eastman RC: *Diagnostic endocrinology,* ed 2, St Louis, 1996, Mosby.

Ca, Calcium; *cAMP,* cyclic adenosine monophosphate; *FHH,* familial hypocalciuric hypercalcemia; *GFR,* glomerular filtration rate; *MEN,* multiple endocrine neoplasia; *25(OH)D,* 25 hydroxyvitamin D; *PO₄,* phosphate; *PTH,* parathyroid hormone; *T₃,* triiodothyronine; *T₄,* thyroxine; *TmP,* renal threshold for phosphorus.

TABLE 15 Laboratory Differential Diagnosis of Hypocalcemia

Diagnosis	PLASMA TESTS					URINE TESTS					Comments
	Ca	PO$_4$	PTH	25(OH)D	1,25(OH)$_2$D	cAMP	cAMP after PTH	TmP/GFR	TmP/GFR after PTH	Ca	
Hypoparathyroidism	↓	↑	N/↓	N	↓	↓	↑↑	↑	↓↓	N/↓	Deficiency of PTH
Pseudohypoparathyroidism											
Type I	↓	↑	↑↑	N	↓	↓	NC	↑	↑	N/↓	Resistance to PTH; patients may have Albright's hereditary osteodystrophy and resistance to multiple hormones
Type II	↓	N	↑↑	N	↓	↓	↑	↑	↑	N/↓	Renal resistance to cAMP
Vitamin D deficiency	↓	N/↓	↑↑	↓↓	N/↓	↑	↑	↓	↓	↓↓	Deficient supply (e.g., nutrition) or absorption (e.g., pancreatic insufficiency) of vitamin D
Vitamin D–dependent Rickets											
Type I	↓	N/↓	↑↑	N	↓	↑↑		↓		↓↓	Deficient activity of renal 25(OH) D-1α-hydroxylase
Type II	↓	N/↓	↑↑	N	↑↑	↑		↓		↓↓	Resistance to 1,25(OH)$_2$D

From Moore WT, Eastman RC: *Diagnostic endocrinology,* ed 2, St Louis, 1996, Mosby.

Ca, Calcium; *cAMP,* cyclic adenosine monophosphate; *FHH,* familial hypocalciuric hypercalcemia; *GFR,* glomerular filtration rate; *MEN,* multiple endocrine neoplasia; *NC,* no change or small increase; *(OH)D,* hydroxycalciferol D; *PO$_4$,* phosphate; *PTH,* parathyroid hormone; *T$_3$,* triiodothyronine; *T$_4$,* thyroxine; *TmP,* renal threshold for phosphorus.

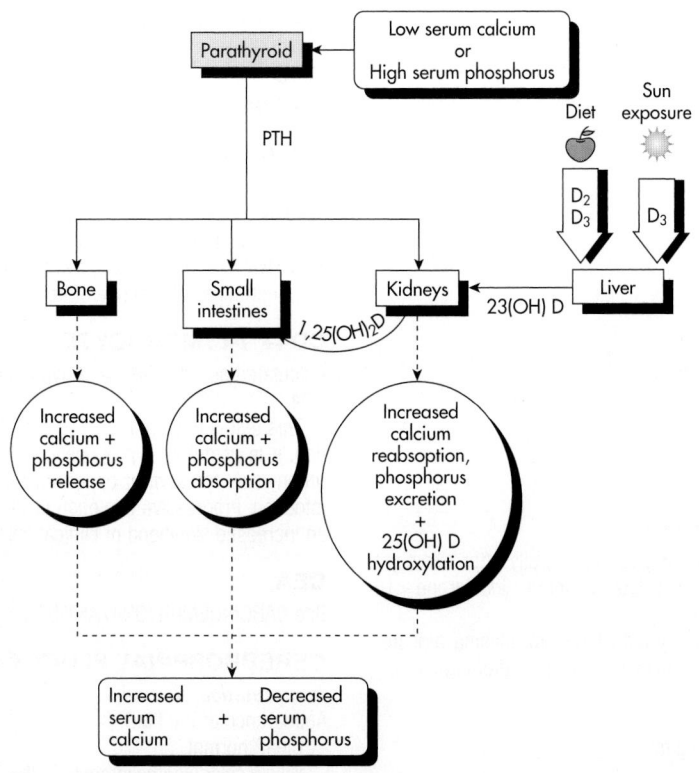

FIG. 12 Calcium homeostasis. Parathyroid hormone (PTH) is released from the parathyroid glands in response to hypocalcemia and hyperphosphatemia. PTH acts on bone, the small intestines, and the kidneys to effect a rise in serum calcium and a net decrease in serum phosphorus. Hydroxylation of inactive forms of vitamin D occurs in the liver and kidneys. 1,25(OH)2D facilitates intestinal absorption of calcium and phosphorus. *1,25(OH)2D,* 1,25-Dihydroxyvitamin D; *25(OH) D,* 25-hydroxyvitamin D; *D2,* vitamin D2; *D3,* vitamin D3. (From Adams JG, et al: *Emergency medicine, clinical essentials,* ed 2, Philadelphia, 2013, Elsevier.)

CANCER ANTIGEN 27-29 (CA 27-29)

Normal: <38 U/ml
Elevated in: Approximately 75% of women with metastatic breast cancer. Clinical sensitivity is 0.57, specificity 0.97, positive predictive value 0.83, negative predictive value 0.92. This test is generally used to predict recurrence of breast cancer and evaluate response to therapy. May also be elevated in liver cancer, pancreatic cancer, ovarian cancer, colorectal cancer. Elevations can also occur with benign breast and liver disease.

CANCER ANTIGEN 72-4 (CA 72-4)

Normal: <4.0 ng/ml
Elevated in: Gastric cancer (elevated in >50% of patients). Often used in combination with CA 72-4, CA 19-9, and CEA to monitor gastric cancer after treatment.

CANCER ANTIGEN 125 (CA 125)

Normal range: <1.4%

This test uses an antibody against antigen from tissue culture of an ovarian tumor cell line. Various published evaluations report sensitivity of about 75%-80% in patients with ovarian carcinoma. There is also an appreciable incidence of elevated values in nonovarian malignancies and in certain benign conditions (see below). Test values may transiently increase during chemotherapy.

MALIGNANT
Epithelial ovarian carcinoma, 75%-80% (range, 25%-92%; better in serous than mucinous cystadenocarcinoma)
Endometrial carcinoma, 25%-48% (2%-90%)
Pancreatic carcinoma, 59%
Colorectal carcinoma, 20% (15%-56%)
Endocervical adenocarcinoma, 83%
Squamous cervical or vaginal carcinoma, 7%-14%
Lung carcinoma, 32%
Breast carcinoma, 12%-40%
Lymphoma, 35%

BENIGN
Cirrhosis, 40%-80%
Acute pancreatitis, 38%
Acute peritonitis, 75%
Endometriosis, 88%
Acute pelvic inflammatory disease, 33%
Pregnancy first trimester, 2%-24%
During menstruation (occasionally)
Renal failure (?frequency)
Normal persons, 0.6%-1.4%

CAPTOPRIL STIMULATION TEST

Normal: Test performed by giving 25 mg captopril orally after overnight fast. Patient should be seated during test. After captopril, aldosterone <15 ng/dl, renin >2 ng angiotensin L/ml/hr.
Interpretation: In patients with primary aldosteronism, plasma aldosterone remains high and plasma renin activity remains low after captopril.

CARBAMAZEPINE (Tegretol)

Normal therapeutic range: 4-12 mcg/ml

CARBOHYDRATE ANTIGEN 19-9

Normal: <37.0 U/ml
Elevated in: GI cancer, most frequently pancreatic cancer. Amount of elevation has no relation to tumor mass. Elevations can also occur with cirrhosis, cholangitis, and chronic or acute pancreatitis.

CARBON DIOXIDE, PARTIAL PRESSURE

Normal
Male: 35-48 mm Hg
Female: 32-45 mm Hg
Elevated in: Respiratory acidosis
Decreased in: Respiratory alkalosis

CARBON MONOXIDE

See CARBOXYHEMOGLOBIN

CARBOXYHEMOGLOBIN

Normal range: Saturation of hemoglobin <2%; smokers <9%
Elevated in: Smoking, exposure to smoking, exposure to automobile exhaust fumes, malfunctioning gas-burning appliances

CARCINOEMBRYONIC ANTIGEN (CEA)

Normal range
Nonsmokers: 0-2.5 ng/ml (0-2.5 μg/L [CF: 1; SMI: 0.1 μg/L])
Smokers: 0-5 ng/ml (0-5 μg/L [CF: 1; SMI: 0.1 μg/L])
Elevated in
Colorectal carcinomas, pancreatic carcinomas, and metastatic disease (usually produce higher elevations: >20 ng/ml)
Carcinomas of the esophagus, stomach, small intestine, liver, breast, ovary, lung, and thyroid (usually produce lesser elevations)
Benign conditions (smoking, inflammatory bowel disease, hypothyroidism, cirrhosis, pancreatitis, infections) (usually produce levels <10 ng/ml)

CAROTENE (serum)

Normal range: 50-250 μg/dl (0.9-4.6 μmol/L [CF: 0.01863; SMI: 0.1 μmol/L])
Elevated in: Carotenemia, chronic nephritis, diabetes mellitus, hypothyroidism, nephrotic syndrome, hyperlipidemia
Decreased in: Fat malabsorption, steatorrhea, pancreatic insufficiency, lack of carotenoids in diet, high fever, liver disease

CATECHOLAMINES, URINE

See URINE CATECHOLAMINES

CBC

See COMPLETE BLOOD COUNT

CD40 LIGAND

Normal: <5 mcg/L. CD40 ligand is a soluble protein that is shed from activated leukocytes and platelets and used in risk stratification for acute coronary syndrome.
Elevated in: Acute coronary syndrome. Increased CD40 ligand is associated with higher incidence of death or nonfatal MI.

CD4+ T-LYMPHOCYTE COUNT (CD4+ T-cells)

Calculated as total WBC × % lymphocytes × % lymphocytes stained with CD4.

This test is used primarily to evaluate immune dysfunction in HIV infection. It is useful as a prognostic indicator and as a criterion for initiating prophylaxis for several opportunistic infections that are sequelae of HIV infection. Progressive depletion of CD4+ T-lymphocytes is associated with an increased likelihood of clinical complications (Table 16).

CEA

See CARCINOEMBRYONIC ANTIGEN

CEREBROSPINAL FLUID (CSF)

Interpretation of results
Appearance of the fluid
Clear: normal.
Yellow color (xanthochromia) in the supernatant of centrifuged CSF within 1 hour or less after collection is usually the result of previous bleeding (subarachnoid hemorrhage); it may also be caused by increased CSF protein, melanin from meningeal melanosarcomas, or carotenoids.
Pinkish color is usually the result of a bloody tap; the color generally clears progressively from tubes 1 to 4 (the supernatant is usually crystal clear in traumatic taps).
Turbidity usually indicates the presence of leukocytes (bleeding introduces approximately 1 WBC/500 RBCs into the CSF).
CSF pressure: elevated pressure can be seen with meningitis, meningoencephalitis, pseudotumor cerebri, mass lesions, and intracerebral bleeding.
Cell count: in the adult the CSF is normally free of cells (although up to 5 mononuclear cells/mm^3 is considered normal); the presence of granulocytes is never normal.

TABLE 16 Relation of CD4 Lymphocyte Counts to the Onset of Certain HIV-Associated Infections and Neoplasms in North America

CD4 Count (Cells/mm³)*	Opportunistic Infection or Neoplasm	Frequency (%)†
>500	Herpes zoster, polydermatomal	5-10
200-500	*Mycobacterium tuberculosis* infection, pulmonary and extrapulmonary	2-20
	Oral hairy leukoplakia	40-70
	Candida pharyngitis (thrush)	40-70
	Recurrent *Candida* vaginitis	15-30 (F)
	Kaposi's sarcoma, mucocutaneous	15-30 (M)
	Bacterial pneumonia, recurrent	15-20
	Cervical neoplasia	1-2 (F)
100-200	*Pneumocystis carinii* pneumonia	15-60
	Herpes simplex, chronic, ulcerative	5-10
	Histoplasma capsulatum infection, disseminated	0-20
	Kaposi's sarcoma, visceral	3-8 (M)
	Progressive multifocal leukoencephalopathy	2-3
	Lymphoma, non-Hodgkin's	2-5
<100	*Candida* esophagitis	15-20
	Mycobacterium avium-intracellulare, disseminated	25-40
	Toxoplasma gondii encephalitis	5-25
	Cryptosporidium enteritis	2-10
	CMV retinitis	20-35
	Cryptococcus neoformans encephalitis	2-5
	CMV esophagitis or colitis	6-12
	Lymphoma, central nervous system	4-8

From Andreoli TE (ed): *Cecil essentials of medicine*, ed 5, Philadelphia, 2000, Saunders.
CMV, Cytomegalovirus; *F*, exclusively in women; *HIV*, human immunodeficiency virus; *M*, almost exclusively in men.
*Table indicates CD4 count at which specific infections or neoplasms generally begin to appear. Each infection may recur or progress during the subsequent course of HIV disease.
†Even within the United States, great regional differences in the incidence of specific opportunistic infections are apparent. For example, disseminated histoplasmosis is common in the Mississippi River drainage area but very rare in individuals who have lived exclusively on the East or West Coast.

Neutrophils: seen in bacterial meningitis, early viral meningoencephalitis, and early tuberculosis (TB) meningitis. Box 4 summarizes causes of increased CSF neutrophils.

Increased lymphocytes: TB meningitis, viral meningoencephalitis, syphilitic meningoencephalitis, fungal meningitis. Causes of CSF lymphocytosis are summarized in Box 5.

CSF plasmacytosis: Box 6 describes inflammatory and infectious causes of CSF plasmacytosis.

CSF eosinophilia: Causes of CSF eosinophilic pleocytosis are summarized in Box 7.

Protein: serum proteins are generally too large to cross the normal blood–CSF barrier; however, increased CSF protein is seen with meningeal inflammation, traumatic tap, increased CNS synthesis, tissue degeneration, obstruction to CSF circulation, and Guillain-Barré syndrome. Mean concentrations of plasma and CSF proteins are summarized in Table 18. Conditions associated with increased CSF total protein are summarized in Box 8.

Glucose
Decreased glucose is seen with bacterial meningitis, TB meningitis, fungal meningitis, subarachnoid hemorrhage, and some cases of viral meningitis.
A mild increase in CSF glucose can be seen in patients with very elevated serum glucose levels.

Table 17 describes CSF findings in central nervous system disorders. Causes of xanthochromia are summarized in Table 19.

CERULOPLASMIN (serum)

Normal range: 20-35 mg/dl (200-350 mg/L [CF: 10; SMI: 10 mg/L])

Elevated in: Pregnancy, estrogens, oral contraceptives, neoplastic diseases (leukemias, Hodgkin's lymphoma, carcinomas), inflammatory states, systemic lupus erythematosus, primary biliary cirrhosis, rheumatoid arthritis

Decreased in: Wilson's disease (values often <10 mg/dl), nephrotic syndrome, advanced liver disease, malabsorption, total parenteral nutrition, Menkes' syndrome

CHLAMYDIA GROUP ANTIBODY SEROLOGIC TEST

Test description: Acute and convalescent sera is drawn 2-4 weeks apart. A fourfold increase in titer between acute and convalescent sera is necessary for confirmation. A single titer ≥1:64 is considered indicative of psittacosis or LGV.

CHLAMYDIA TRACHOMATIS PCR

Test description: Test is performed on endocervical swab, urine, and intraurethral swab (see Table 20)
Normal: Negative

CHLORIDE (serum)

Normal range: 95-105 mEq/L (95-105 mmol/L [CF: 1; SMI: 1 mmol/L])
Elevated in: Dehydration, excessive infusion of normal saline solution, cystic fibrosis (sweat test), hyperparathyroidism, renal tubular disease, metabolic acidosis, prolonged diarrhea, drugs (ammonium chloride administration, acetazolamide, boric acid, triamterene)
Decreased in: Congestive heart failure, syndrome of inappropriate antidiuretic hormone secretion, Addison's disease, vomiting, gastric suction, salt-losing nephritis, continuous infusion of D_5W, thiazide diuretic administration, diaphoresis, diarrhea, burns, diabetic ketoacidosis

CHLORIDE (sweat)

Normal: 0-40 mmol/L
Borderline/indeterminate: 41-60 mmol/L
Consistent with cystic fibrosis: >60 mmol/L
False low results can occur with edema, excessive sweating, and hypoproteinemia.

CHLORIDE, URINE

See URINE CHLORIDE

CHOLECYSTOKININ-PANCREOZYMIN (CCK, CCK-PZ)

Normal: <80 pg/ml
Elevated in: Pancreatic disease, celiac disease, gastric ulcer, postgastrectomy, IBS, fatty food intolerance

CHOLESTEROL, HIGH-DENSITY LIPOPROTEIN

See HIGH-DENSITY LIPOPROTEIN CHOLESTEROL

CHOLESTEROL, LOW-DENSITY LIPOPROTEIN

See LOW-DENSITY LIPOPROTEIN CHOLESTEROL

CHOLESTEROL, TOTAL

Normal range: Varies with age
Generally <200 mg/dl (<5.20 mmol/L [CF: 0.02586; SMI: 0.05 mmol/L])
Elevated in: Primary hypercholesterolemia, biliary obstruction, diabetes mellitus, nephrotic syndrome, hypothyroidism, primary biliary cirrhosis, high-cholesterol diet, pregnancy third trimester, myocardial infarction, drugs (steroids, phenothiazines, oral contraceptives). Classic hyperlipidemia phenotypes are summarized in Table 21.
Decreased in: Medications (statins, niacin), starvation, malabsorption, sideroblastic anemia, thalassemia, abetalipoproteinemia, hyperthyroidism, Cushing's syndrome, hepatic failure, multiple myeloma, polycythemia vera, chronic myelocytic leukemia, myeloid metaplasia, Waldenström's macroglobulinemia, myelofibrosis

CHORIONIC GONADOTROPINS, HUMAN (serum) (HCG)

Normal range, serum:
Female, premenopausal: <0.8 IU/L; postmenopausal <3.3 IU/L
Male: <0.7 IU/L

TABLE 17   Cerebrospinal Fluid Findings in Central Nervous System Disorders

Condition	Pressure (mm H$_2$O)	Leukocytes (mm^3)	Protein (mg/dl)	Glucose (mg/dl)	Comments
Normal	50-80	<5, ≥75% lymphocytes	20-45	>50 (or 75% serum glucose)	
Common Forms of Meningitis					
Acute bacterial meningitis	Usually elevated (100-300)	100-10,000 or more; usually 300-2000; PMNs predominate	Usually 100-500	Decreased, usually <40 (or <66% serum glucose)	Organisms usually seen on Gram stain and recovered by culture; latex agglutination of CSF usually positive
Partially treated bacterial meningitis	Normal or elevated	5-10,000; PMNs usual but mononuclear cells may predominate if pretreated for extended period	Usually 100-500	Normal or decreased	Organisms may be seen on Gram stain; latex agglutination CSF may be positive; pretreatment may render CSF sterile
Viral meningitis or meningoencephalitis	Normal or slightly elevated (80-150)	Rarely >1000 cells; eastern equine encephalitis and lymphocytic choriomeningitis may have cell counts of several thousand; PMNs early but mononuclear cells predominate through most of the course	Usually 50-200	Generally normal; may be decreased to <40 in some viral diseases, particularly mumps (15%-20% of cases)	HSV encephalitis is suggested by focal seizures or by focal findings on CT or MRI scans or EEG. Enteroviruses and HSV infrequently recovered from CSF. HSV and enteroviruses may be detected by PCR of CSF.
Uncommon Forms of Meningitis					
Tuberculous meningitis	Usually elevated	10-500; PMNs early but lymphocytes predominate through most of the course	100-3000; may be higher in presence of block	<50 in most cases; decreases with time if treatment is not provided	Acid-fast organisms almost never seen on smear; organisms may be recovered in culture of large volumes of CSF; *Mycobacterium tuberculosis* may be detected by PCR of CSF
Fungal meningitis	Usually elevated	5-500; PMNs early but mononuclear cells predominate through most of the course; cryptococcal meningitis may have no cellular inflammatory response	25-500	<50; decreases with time if treatment is not provided	Budding yeast may be seen; organisms may be recovered in culture; cryptococcal antigen (CSF and serum) may be positive in cryptococcal infection
Syphilis (acute) and leptospirosis	Usually elevated	50-500; lymphocytes predominate	50-200	Usually normal	Positive CSF serology; spirochetes not demonstrable by usual techniques of smear or culture; darkfield examination may be positive
Amebic (*Naegleria*) meningoencephalitis	Elevated	1000-10,000 or more; PMNs predominate	50-500	Normal or slightly decreased	Mobile amebae may be seen by hanging-drop examination of CSF at room temperature
Brain and Parameningeal Abscesses					
Brain abscess	Usually elevated (100-300)	5-200; CSF rarely acellular; lymphocytes predominate; if abscess ruptures into ventricle, PMNs predominate and cell count may reach >100,000	75-500	Normal unless abscess ruptures into ventricular system	No organisms on smear or culture unless abscess ruptures into ventricular system
Subdural empyema	Usually elevated (100-300)	100-5000; PMNs predominate	100-500	Normal	No organisms on smear or culture of CSF unless meningitis also present; organisms found on tap of subdural fluid
Cerebral epidural abscess	Normal to slightly elevated	10-500; lymphocytes predominate	50-200	Normal	No organisms on smear or culture of CSF
Spinal epidural abscess	Usually low, with spinal block	10-100; lymphocytes predominate	50-400	Normal	No organisms on smear or culture of CSF
Chemical (drugs, dermoid cysts, myelography dye)	Usually elevated	100-1000 or more; PMNs predominate	50-100	Normal or slightly decreased	Epithelial cells may be seen within CSF by use of polarized light in some children with dermoids
Noninfectious Causes					
Sarcoidosis	Normal or elevated slightly	0-100; mononuclear	40-100	Normal	No specific findings
Systemic lupus erythematosus with CNS involvement	Slightly elevated	0-500; PMNs usually predominate; lymphocytes may be present	100	Normal or slightly decreased	No organisms on smear or culture; LE preparation may be positive; positive neuronal and ribosomal P protein antibodies in CSF
Tumor, leukemia	Slightly elevated to very high	0-100 or more; mononuclear or blast cells	50-1000	Normal to decreased (20-40)	Cytology may be positive

From Behrman RE: *Nelson textbook of pediatrics*, ed 17, Philadelphia, 2004, Saunders.
CNS, Central nervous system; *CSF*, cerebrospinal fluid; *CT*, computed tomography; *EEG*, electroencephalogram; *HSV*, herpes simplex virus; *MRI*, magnetic resonance imaging; *PCR*, polymerase chain reaction; *PMN*, polymorphonuclear neutrophils.

BOX 4   Causes of Increased CSF Neutrophils

Meningitis
    Bacterial meningitis
    Early viral meningoencephalitis
    Early tuberculous meningitis
    Early mycotic meningitis
    Amebic encephalomyelitis
Other infections
    Cerebral abscess
    Subdural empyema
    AIDS-related CMV radiculopathy
Following seizures
Following CNS hemorrhage
    Subarachnoid
    Intracerebral
Following CNS infarct
Reaction to repeated lumbar punctures
Injection of foreign material in subarachnoid space (e.g., metho-
    trexate, contrast media)
Metastatic tumor in contact with CSF

AIDS, Acquired immunodeficiency syndrome; *CMV,* cytomegalovirus; *CNS,* central nervous system; *CSF,* cerebrospinal fluid.
(McPherson RA, Pincus MR: Henry's Clinical Diagnosis and Management by Laboratory Methods, 23rd ed, ISBN # 978-0323-29568-0, 2017, Elsevier)

BOX 5   Causes of CSF Lymphocytosis

Meningitis
Viral meningitis
Tuberculous meningitis
Fungal meningitis
Syphilitic meningoencephalitis
Leptospiral meningitis
Bacterial due to uncommon organisms
Early bacterial meningitis where leukocyte counts are relatively low
Parasitic infestations (e.g., cysticercosis, trichinosis, toxoplasmosis)
Aseptic meningitis due to septic focus adjacent to meninges

Degenerative Disorders
Subacute sclerosing panencephalitis
Multiple sclerosis
Drug abuse encephalopathy
Guillain-Barré syndrome
Acute disseminated encephalomyelitis

Other Inflammatory Disorders
Handl syndrome (headache with neurologic deficits and CSF
    lymphocytosis)
Sarcoidosis
Polyneuritis
CNS periarteritis

CNS, Central nervous system; *CSF,* cerebrospinal fluid.
(McPherson RA, Pincus MR: Henry's Clinical Diagnosis and Management by Laboratory Methods, 23rd ed, ISBN # 978-0323-29568-0, 2017, Elsevier)

BOX 6   Inflammatory and Infectious Causes of CSF Plasmacytosis

Acute viral infections
Guillain-Barré syndrome
Multiple sclerosis
Parasitic CNS infestations
Sarcoidosis
Subacute sclerosing panencephalitis
Syphilitic meningoencephalitis
Tuberculous meningitis

CNS, Central nervous system; *CSF,* cerebrospinal fluid.
(McPherson RA, Pincus MR: Henry's Clinical Diagnosis and Management by Laboratory Methods, 23rd ed, ISBN # 978-0323-29568-0, 2017, Elsevier)

BOX 7   Causes of CSF Eosinophilic Pleocytosis

Commonly associated with:	**Infrequently associated with:**
Acute polyneuritis	
CNS reaction to foreign material (drugs, shunts)	Bacterial meningitis
Fungal infections	Leukemia/lymphoma
Idiopathic eosinophilic meningitis	Myeloproliferative disorders
Idiopathic hypereosinophilic syndrome	Neurosarcoidosis
Parasitic infections	Primary brain tumors
	Tuberculous meningoencephalitis
	Viral meningitis

CNS, Central nervous system; *CSF,* cerebrospinal fluid.
Modified from Kjeldsberg CR, Knight JA: *Body fluids: laboratory examination of amniotic, cerebrospinal, seminal, serous and synovial fluids,* ed 3, Chicago, 1993, © American Society for Clinical Pathology, with permission.
(McPherson RA, Pincus MR: Henry's Clinical Diagnosis and Management by Laboratory Methods, 23rd ed, ISBN # 978-0323-29568-0, 2017, Elsevier)

BOX 8   Conditions Associated with Increased CSF Total Protein

Traumatic Spinal Puncture
Increased Blood-CSF Permeability
Arachnoiditis (e.g., following methotrexate therapy)
Meningitis (bacterial, viral, fungal, tuberculous)
Hemorrhage (subarachnoid, intracerebral)
Endocrine/metabolic disorders
    Milk-alkali syndrome with hypercalcemia
    Diabetic neuropathy
    Hereditary neuropathies and myelopathies
    Decreased endocrine function (thyroid, parathyroid)
    Other disorders (uremia, dehydration)

Drug Toxicity
Ethanol, phenothiazines, phenytoin

CSF Circulation Defects
Mechanical obstruction (tumor, abscess, herniated disk)
Loculated CSF effusion

Increased Immunoglobulin (Ig)G Synthesis
Multiple sclerosis

Neurosyphilis
Subacute sclerosing panencephalitis

Increased IgG Synthesis and Blood-CSF Permeability
Guillain-Barré syndrome
Collagen vascular diseases (e.g., lupus, periarteritis)
Chronic inflammatory demyelinating polyradiculopathy

CSF, Cerebrospinal fluid.
(McPherson RA, Pincus MR: Henry's Clinical Diagnosis and Management by Laboratory Methods, 23rd ed, ISBN # 978-0323-29568-0, 2017, Elsevier)

TABLE 18   Mean Concentrations of Plasma and CSF Proteins

Protein	CSF, mg/L	Plasma/CSF Ratio
Prealbumin	17.3	14
Albumin	155.0	236
Transferrin	14.4	142
Ceruloplasmin	1.0	366
Immunoglobulin (Ig)G	12.3	802
IgA	1.3	1346
α_2-Microglobulin	2.0	1111
Fibrinogen	0.6	4940
IgM	0.6	1167
β-Lipoprotein	0.6	6213

Adapted from Felgenhauer K: Protein size and cerebrospinal fluid composition, *Klin Wochenschr* 52:1158, 1974, with permission.
CSF, Cerebrospinal fluid.
(McPherson RA, Pincus MR: Henry's Clinical Diagnosis and Management by Laboratory Methods, 23rd ed, ISBN # 978-0323-29568-0, 2017, Elsevier)

TABLE 19 Xanthochromia and Associated Diseases/Disorders

CSF Supernatant Color	Associated Diseases/Disorders
Pink	RBC lysis/hemoglobin breakdown products
Yellow	RBC lysis/hemoglobin breakdown products Hyperbilirubinemia CSF protein >150 mg/dL (1.5 g/L)
Orange	RBC lysis/hemoglobin breakdown products Hypervitaminosis A (carotenoids)
Yellow-green	Hyperbilirubinemia (biliverdin)
Brown	Meningeal metastatic melanoma

CSF, Cerebrospinal fluid; *RBC,* red blood cell.
(McPherson RA, Pincus MR: Henry's Clinical Diagnosis and Management by Laboratory Methods, 23rd ed, ISBN # 978-0323-29568-0, 2017, Elsevier)

TABLE 20 Specimens for Detection of *Chlamydia trachomatis**

Disease	Specimen
Mucopurulent cervicitis	Endocervical swab, urine
Acute urethral syndrome (women)	Urethral swab, urine
Acute endometritis	Endometrial aspirate
Acute salpingitis	Fallopian tube biopsy
Nongonococcal urethritis (men)	Urethral swab, urine
Inclusion conjunctivitis	Conjunctival scrapings/swab
Trachoma	Conjunctival scrapings/swab
Lymphogranuloma venereum	Lymph node aspirate, biopsy of ulcerated lesion, serum
Pneumonitis (infants)	Serum, tracheobronchial aspirate, nasopharyngeal swab

*Urine is acceptable for some enzyme-linked immunoassays and for the commercial nucleic acid amplification tests.
(McPherson RA, Pincus MR: Henry's Clinical Diagnosis and Management by Laboratory Methods, 23rd ed, ISBN # 978-0323-29568-0, 2017, Elsevier)

TABLE 21 Classic Hyperlipidemia Phenotypes

WHO ICD and OMIM Numbers	Type	Particle	Triglycerides	Cholesterol	Comments
E78.3 238600	1 (familial chylomicronemia or LPL deficiency)	CM	High	Normal	Low cardiac risk; hereditary, found mostly in pediatric patients and young adults; autosomal recessive mutation in *LPL* or *APOC2; APOA5, LMF-1,* and *GPIHBP1* mutations are linked to this phenotype.
E78.0 143890	2A (heterozygous and homozygous familial hypercholesterolemia)	LDL	Normal	High	High cardiac risk; mostly polygenic disease; about 10% are monogenic; heterozygous form is due to mutations in *LDLR, APOB,* or *PCSK9;* homozygous form is due to mutations in *LDLR* or *LDLRAP1* (ARH).
E78.4 144250	2B (combined hyperlipoproteinemia)	VLDL, LDL	High	High	High cardiac risk; polygenic disease; links to mutations in *USF1, APOB,* and *LPL*
E78.2 107741	3 (dysbetalipoproteinemia)	IDL	High	High	High cardiac risk; mutations in *APOE* gene or homozygous for E2 allele of *APOE*
E78.1 144600, 145750	4 (primary hypertriglyceridemia)	VLDL	High	Normal	Lower cardiac risk than type 2 or 3; polygenic disease
E78.3 144650	5 (mixed hyperlipidemia)	VLDL, CM	High	High	Low cardiac risk; polygenic disease; 10% of patients have mutations in *LPL, APOC2,* and *APOA5;* mutations in *APOE, TRIB1, CHREBP, GALNT2, GCKR,* and *ANGPTL3* are thought to contribute to this disease.

ANGPTL3, Angiopoietin-like 3; *APOA5,* apolipoprotein A-V; *APOB,* apolipoprotein B; *APOC2,* apolipoprotein C-II; *APOE,* apolipoprotein E; *CHREBP,* carbohydrate response element binding protein (or *MLXIPL*); *CM,* chylomicron; *GALNT2,* UDP-N'-acetyl-alpha-ᴅ-galactosamine-polypeptide *N*-acetylgalactosaminyltransferase 2; *GCKR,* glucokinase regulator; *ICD,* International Classification of Diseases; *IDL,* intermediate-density lipoprotein; *LDL,* low-density lipoprotein; *LDLRAP1,* LDLR adaptor protein 1 (also known as ARH); *OMIM,* Online Mendelian Inheritance in Man; *TRIB1,* tribbles homologue 1; *USF1,* upstream transcription factor 1; *VLDL,* very-low-density lipoprotein; *WHO,* World Health Organization.
(McPherson RA, Pincus MR: Henry's Clinical Diagnosis and Management by Laboratory Methods, 23rd ed, ISBN # 978-0323-29568-0, 2017, Elsevier)

Elevated in
Pregnancy, choriocarcinoma, gestational trophoblastic neoplasia (including molar gestations), placental site trophoblastic tumors; human antimouse antibodies (HAMA) can produce false serum assay for hCG.

The principal use of this test is to diagnose pregnancy. The concentration of hCG increases significantly during the initial 6 weeks of pregnancy.

Normal range: Varies with gestational stage:
1 wk: 5-50 mU/ml 1-2 wk: 50-550 mU/ml
2-3 wk: up to 5000 mU/ml
3-4 wk: up to 10,000 mU/ml
4-5 wk: up to 50,000 mU/ml
2-3 mo: 10,000-100,000 mU/ml

Peak values approaching 100,000 IU/L occur 60-70 days following implantation.

hCG levels generally double every 1-3 days. In patients with concentration <2000 IU/L, an increase of serum hCG <66% after 2 days is suggestive of spontaneous abortion or ruptured ectopic gestation.

CHYMOTRYPSIN

Normal: <10 mcg/L
Elevated in: Acute pancreatitis, chronic renal failure, oral enzyme preparations, gastric cancer, pancreatic cancer
Decreased in: Chronic pancreatitis, late cystic fibrosis

CIRCULATING ANTICOAGULANT (lupus anticoagulant)

Normal: Negative
Detected in: Systemic lupus erythematosus, drug-induced lupus, long-term phenothiazine therapy, multiple myeloma, ulcerative colitis, rheumatoid arthritis, postpartum, hemophilia, neoplasms, chronic inflammatory states, AIDS, nephrotic syndrome

NOTE: The name is a misnomer because these patients are prone to hypercoagulability and thrombosis.

CK
See CREATINE KINASE

CLONIDINE SUPPRESSION TEST

Interpretation: Clonidine inhibits neurogenic catecholamine release and will cause a decrease in plasma norepinephrine into the reference interval in hypertensive subjects without pheochromocytoma. Test is performed by giving 4.3 mcg clonidine/kg orally after overnight fast. Norepinephrine is measured at 3 hr. Result should be within established reference range and decrease to <50% of baseline concentration. Lack of decrease in norepinephrine is suggestive of pheochromocytoma.

CLOSTRIDIUM DIFFICILE TOXIN ASSAY (stool)

Normal: Negative
Detected in: Antibiotic-associated diarrhea and pseudomembranous colitis

CO
See CARBOXYHEMOGLOBIN

COAGULATION FACTORS

See Table 22 for characteristics of coagulation factors.
See Table 23 for differential diagnosis of low factor VIII.

Factor reference ranges

a. V: >10%
b. VII: >10%
c. VIII: 50%-170%
d. IX: 60%-136%
e. X: >10%
f. XI: 50%-150%
g. XII: >30%

Table 24 describes screening laboratory results in coagulation factor deficiencies. Characterization of coagulation factors and their deficiencies is summarized in Table 25.

COBALAMIN, SERUM

See VITAMIN B$_{12}$

COLD AGGLUTININS TITER

Normal range: <1:32

TABLE 22 Characteristics of Coagulation Factors

Factor	Descriptive Name	Source	Approximate Half-Life (hr)	Function
I	Fibrinogen	Liver	120	Substrate for fibrin clot (CP)
II	Prothrombin	Liver (VKD)	60	Serine protease (CP)
V	Proaccelerin, labile factor	Liver	12-36	Cofactor (CP)
VII	Serum prothrombin conversion accelerator, pro-convertin	Liver (VKD)	6	(?) Serine protease (EP)
VIII	Antihemophilic factor or globulin	Endothelial cells and (?) elsewhere	12	Cofactor (IP)
IX	Plasma thromboplastin component, Christmas factor	Liver (VKD)	24	Serine protease (IP)
X	Stuart-Prower factor	Liver (VKD)	36	Serine protease (CP)
XI	Plasma thromboplastin antecedent	(?) Liver	40-84	Serine protease (IP)
XII	Hageman factor	(?) Liver	50	Serine protease contact activation (IP)
XIII	Fibrin-stabilizing factor	(?) Liver	96-180	Transglutaminase (CP)
Prekallikrein	Fletcher factor	(?) Liver	?	Serine protease contact activation (IP)
High-molecular-weight kininogen	Fitzgerald factor, Flaujeac or Williams factor	(?) Liver	?	Cofactor, contact activation (IP)

From Noble J (ed): *Primary care medicine,* ed 3, St Louis, 2001, Mosby.
CP, Common pathway; *EP,* extrinsic pathway; *IP,* intrinsic pathway; *VKD,* vitamin K dependent.

TABLE 23 Differential Diagnosis of a Low Factor VIII Level

1. FVIII <10%
   1. Severe or moderately severe hemophilia A
   2. Severe type 1 vWD
   3. Type 3 vWD
   4. Type 2N vWD
   5. Acquired hemophilia A
   6. Acquired vWD
2. FVIII: 10% to 50%
   1. Mild hemophilia A
   2. Type 1 vWD
   3. Type 2N vWD
   4. Combined FVIII and FV deficiency

From Hoffman R: *Hematology: basic principles and practice,* ed 6, Philadelphia, Saunders, 2013.
FV, Factor V; *FVIII,* factor VIII; *VWD,* von Willebrand disease.

TABLE 24 Screening Laboratory Results in Coagulation Factor Deficiencies

Deficient Factor	Frequency	PT	PTT	TT
I (fibrinogen)	Rare	↑	↑	↑
II (prothrombin)	Very rare	↑	↑	↑
V 1:1,000,000	↑		↑	NL
VII	1:500,000	↑	NL	NL
VIII	1:5000 (male)	NL	↑	NL
IX	1:30,000 (male)	NL	↑	NL
X 1:500,000	↑		↑	NL
XI	Rare*	NL	↑	NL
XII or HMWK or PK†	Rare	NL	↑	NL
XIII	Rare	NL	NL	↑

From Andreoli TE (ed): *Cecil essentials of medicine,* ed 5, Philadelphia, 2001, Saunders.
↑Increased over normal range; *HMWK,* high-molecular-weight kininogen; *NL,* normal; *PK,* prekallikrein; *PT,* prothrombin time; *PTT,* partial thromboplastin time; *TT,* thrombin time.
*Except in those of Ashkenazi Jewish descent (approximately 4% are heterozygous for factor XI deficiency).
†Not associated with clinical bleeding.

Laboratory Tests

IV

Elevated in:

Primary atypical pneumonia (*Mycoplasma* pneumonia), infectious mononucleosis, CMV infection

Others: hepatic cirrhosis, acquired hemolytic anemia, frostbite, multiple myeloma, lymphoma, malaria

COMPLEMENT

Normal range:

C3: 70-160 mg/dl (0.7-1.6 g/L [CF: 0.01; SMI: 0.1 g/L])

C4: 20-40 mg/dl (0.2-0.4 g/L [CF: 0.01; SMI: 0.1 g/L])

Abnormal values:

Decreased C3: Active SLE, immune complex disease, acute glomerulonephritis, inborn C3 deficiency, membranoproliferative glomerulonephritis, infective endocarditis, serum sickness, autoimmune/chronic active hepatitis

Decreased C4: Immune complex disease, active SLE, infective endocarditis, inborn C4 deficiency, hereditary angioedema, hypergammaglobulinemic states, cryoglobulinemic vasculitis Note: The complement system has daunting nomenclature; accordingly, some basic definitions are given in Box 9.

COMPLEMENT DEFICIENCY

Table 26 describes complement deficiency states.

COMPLETE BLOOD COUNT (CBC)

See Fig. 13, which describes an algorithm for the evaluation of patients with neutropenia.

White blood cells 3200-9800/mm^3 (3.2-9.8 × 10^9/L [CF: 0.001; SMI: 0.1 × 10^9/L])

Red blood cells

　Male: 4.3-5.9 × 10^6/mm^3 (4.3-5.9 × 10^{12}/L [CF: 0.001; SMI: 0.1 × 10^{12}/L])

　Female: 3.5-5 × 10^6/mm^3 (3.5-5 × 10^{12}/L [CF: 0.001; SMI: 0.1 × 10^{12}/L])

Hemoglobin

Male: 13.6-17.7 g/dl (136-172 g/L [CF: 10; SMI: 1 g/L])

Female: 12-15 g/dl (120-150 g/L [CF: 10; SMI: 1 g/L])

Hematocrit

　Male: 39%-49% (0.39-0.49 [CF: 0.01; SMI: 0.01])

　Female: 33%-43% (0.33-0.43 [CF: 0.01; SMI: 0.01])

Mean corpuscular volume (MCV): 76-100 μm^3 (76-100 fL [CF: 1; SMI: 1 fL])

Mean corpuscular hemoglobin (MCH): 27-33 pg (27-33 pg [CF: 1; SMI: 1 pg])

BOX 9   Definitions

Classical pathway: C1, C4, C2, C3, and the terminal components.

Alternative pathway: Factor B, factor D, properdin, and the terminal components.

Lectin activation pathway: MBL, MASP1, MASP2, C3, and the terminal components.

Anaphylatoxins: C3a, C4a, C5a. These are mediators of smooth muscle contraction, degranulation of mast cells, enhanced neutrophil aggregation, increased vascular permeability.

Opsonization: Renders a particle more easily phagocytosed.

C3 tickover: This term occasionally is used to describe spontaneous C3 hydrolysis.

Membrane attack complex (terminal components): C5, C6, C7, C8, C9.

CH50: Used to define the dilution of serum capable of lysing 50% of sensitized sheep red cells. This assay measures the intactness of the classical pathway through the terminal components.

AH50: Used to define the dilution of serum capable of lysing 50% of nonsensitized rabbit red cells. This assay measures the intactness of the alternative pathway through the terminal components.

From Adkinson NF et al: *Middleton's allergy principles and practice*, ed 8, Philadelphia, 2014, Saunders.

BOX 10   Factors That May Alter Serum Creatinine (Cr) Level

Endogenous

Reduced muscle mass: ↓

Hyperbilirubinemia: ↓

Exogenous

Medications inhibiting tubular secretion (trimethoprim, cimetidine): ↑

Medications Interfering with Laboratory Assays*

Flucytosine and cefoxitin: ↑

Catecholamines: ↓

(Parrillo JE, Dellinger RP: Critical Care Medicine, Principles of Diagnosis and Management in the Adult, 4th ed, ISBN # 978-0-323-08929-6, 2014, Elsevier)

*Varies by assay type used.

TABLE 25   Characterization of Coagulation Factors and Their Deficiencies

Factor	Molecular Weight, kDa	Gene Location	Normal Circulating Half-Life	Incidence	Inheritance	Bleeding Severity
Fibrinogen	330	4q31.3-q32.1	2-4 days	1:1 million	Recessive	Mild–severe*
II	72	11p11.2	3-4 days	Very rare	Recessive	Mild–moderate
V	330	1q24.2	36 hours	1:1 million	Recessive	Moderate
V and VIII combined	—	LMAN1:18q21.32 MCFD2:2p21	36 hours for FV; 10-14 hours for FVIII	1:2 million	Recessive	Mild–moderate
VII	50	13q34	3-6 hours	1:500,000	Recessive	Mild–severe
VIII	330	Xq28	10-14 hours	1:10,000	Sex-linked	Mild–severe
IX	56	Xq27	18-24 hours	1:30,000	Sex-linked	Mild–severe
X	58	13q34	40-60 hours	1:500,000	Recessive	Mild–severe
XI	160	4q35.2	40-70 hours	Rare†	Recessive	Mild–moderate
XII	80	5q33-qter	50-70 days	Rare	Recessive	No bleeding
PK	88	4q33-q35	Not known	Very rare	Recessive	No bleeding
HK	120	3q27	9-10 hours	Extremely rare	Recessive	No bleeding
XIII	320	A:6p25.1 B:1q31.3	11-14 days	<1:1 million	Recessive	Moderate–severe

HK, High molecular weight kininogen; *PK,* prekallikrein.

*May be associated with thrombosis.

†Rare except in those of Ashkenazi Jewish descent.

(McPherson RA, Pincus MR: Henry's Clinical Diagnosis and Management by Laboratory Methods, 23rd ed, ISBN # 978-0323-29568-0, 2017, Elsevier)

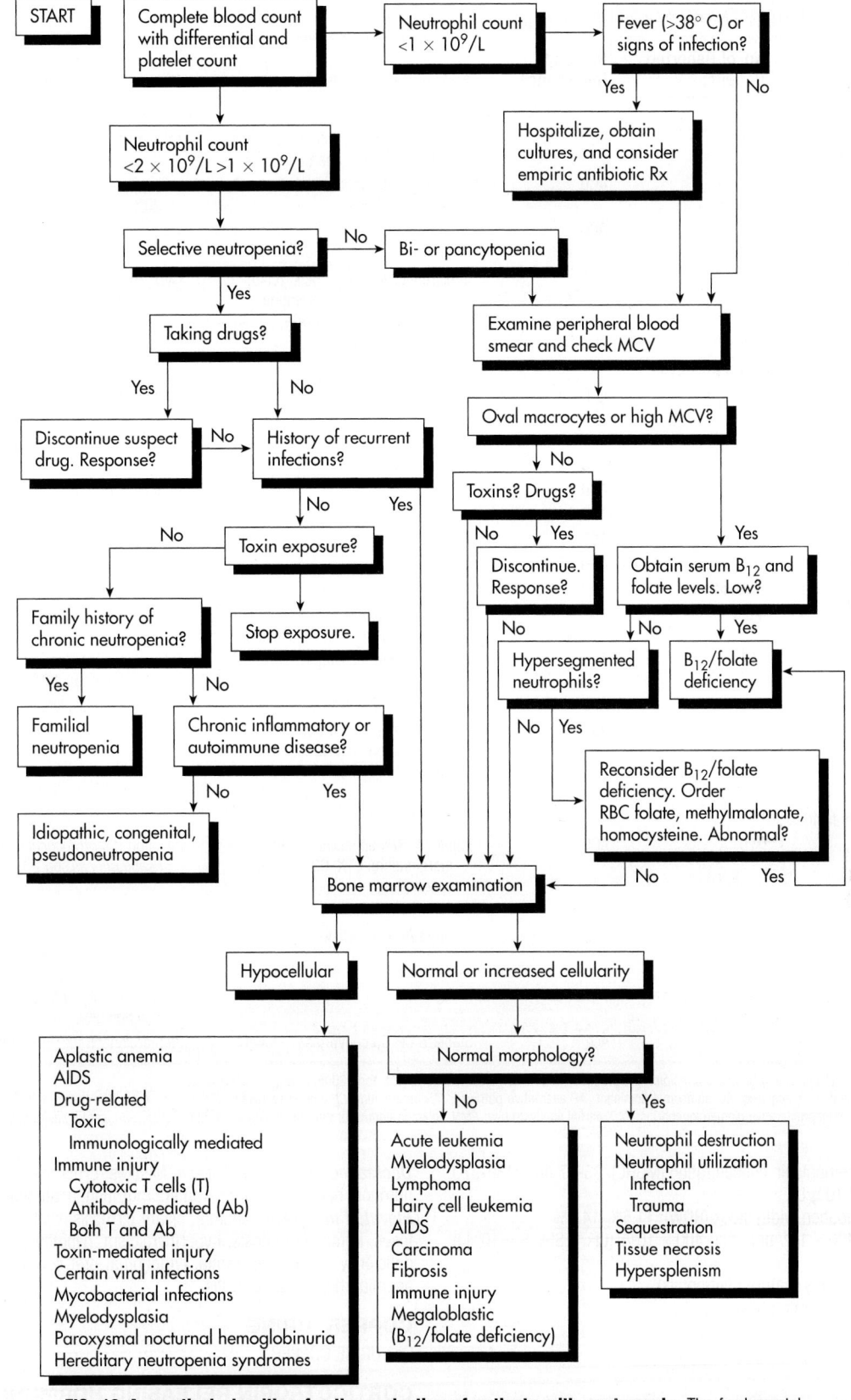

FIG. 13 A practical algorithm for the evaluation of patients with neutropenia. The fundamental diagnostic principle is that for patients with severe neutropenia or for those with bicytopenia or pancytopenia, bone marrow examination will likely be necessary unless the following diagnoses are made: (1) a nutritional (folate or vitamin B_{12}) deficiency or (2) drug- or toxin-induced neutropenia in a patient whose neutropenia resolves after discontinuation of the offending agent. *AIDS,* Acquired immunodeficiency syndrome; *MCV,* mean corpuscular volume; *RBC,* red blood cell. (From Goldman L, Ausiello D [eds]: *Cecil textbook of medicine,* ed 24, Philadelphia, 2012, Saunders.)

TABLE 26   Complement Deficiency States

Component	No. of Reported Patients	Mode of Inheritance	Functional Defects	Disease Associations
Classic Pathway				
C1qrs	31	ACD	Impaired IC handling, delayed C' activation, impaired immune response	CVD, 48%; infection (encapsulated bacteria), 22%; both, 18%; healthy, 12%
C4	21	ACD	Impaired C' activation in absence of specific antibody	Infection (meningococcal), 74%; healthy, 26%
C2	109	ACD		
Alternative Pathway				
D	3	ACD	Impaired IC handling, opson/phag; granulocytosis, CTX, immune response and absent SBA	CVD, 79%; recurrent infection (encapsulated bacteria), 71%
P	70	XL		
Junction of Classic and Alternative Pathways				
C3	19	ACD	Impaired CTX; absent SBA	Infection (*Neisseria*, primarily meningococcal), 58%; CVD, 4%
Terminal Components				
C5	27	ACD	Absent SBA	Both, 1%
C6	77	ACD		Healthy, 25%
C7	73	ACD		
C8	73	ACD		
C9	165	ACD	Impaired SBA	Healthy, 91%; infection, 9%
Plasma Proteins Regulating C' Activation				
C1-INH	Many	AD	Uncontrolled generation of an inflammatory mediator on C' activation	Hereditary angioedema
H	13	Acq	Uncontrolled AP activation → low C3	CVD, 40%; CVD plus infection (encapsulated bacteria), 40%; healthy, 20%
I	14	ACD	Uncontrolled AP activation → low C3	Infection (encapsulated bacteria), 100%
Membrane proteins regulating C' activation	Many	Acq	Impaired regulation of C3b and C8 deposited on host RBCs; PMN, platelets → cell lysis	Paroxysmal nocturnal hemoglobinuria
Decay-accelerating factor				
Homologous restriction factor				
CD59	>20	ACD	Impaired PMN adhesive functions (i.e., margination), CTX, C3bi-mediated opson/phag	Infection (*Staphylococcus aureus, Pseudomonas* spp.), 100%
CR3 autoantibodies				
C3 nephritic factors	>59	Acq	Stabilize AP, convertase → low C3	MPGN, 41%; PLD, 25%; infection (encapsulated bacteria), 16%; MPGN plus PLD, 10%; PLD plus infection, 5%; MPGN plus PLD plus infection, 3%; MPGN plus infection, 2%
C4 nephritic factor		Acq	Stabilize CP, C3 convertase → low C3	Glomerulonephritis, 50%; CVD, 50%

From Mandell GL: *Mandell, Douglas, and Bennett's principles and practice of infectious diseases*, ed 6, New York, 2005, Churchill Livingstone.
ACD, Autosomal codominant; *Acq,* acquired; *AD,* autosomal dominant; *AP,* alternative pathway; *C,* complement; *CP,* classic pathway; *CTX,* chemotaxis; *CVD,* collagen-vascular disease; *IC,* immune complex, *MPGN,* membranoproliferative glomerulonephritis; *PLD,* partial lipodystrophy; *PMN,* polymorphonuclear neutrophil; *RBCs,* red blood cells; *SBA,* serum bactericidal activity; *XL,* X-linked.

Mean corpuscular hemoglobin concentration (MCHC): 33-37 g/dl (330-370 g/L [CF: 10; SMI: 10 g/L])
Red blood cell distribution width index (RDW): 11.5%-14.5%
Platelet count: 130-400 × 10^3/mm^3 (130-400 × 10^9/L [CF: 1; SMI: 5 × 10^9/L])
Differential:
    2-6 stabs (bands, early mature neutrophils)
    60-70 segs (mature neutrophils)
    1-4 eosinophils
    0-1 basophils
    2-8 monocytes
    25-40 lymphocytes

CONJUGATED BILIRUBIN
See BILIRUBIN, DIRECT

COPPER (serum)
Normal range: 70-140 µg/dl (11-22 µmol/L [CF: 0.1574, SMI: 0.2 µmol/L])

Decreased in: Wilson's disease, Menkes' syndrome, malabsorption, malnutrition, nephrosis, total parenteral nutrition, acute leukemia in remission
Elevated in: Aplastic anemia, biliary cirrhosis, systemic lupus erythematosus, hemochromatosis, hyperthyroidism, hypothyroidism, infection, iron deficiency anemia, leukemia, lymphoma, oral contraceptives, pernicious anemia, rheumatoid arthritis

COPPER, URINE
See URINE COPPER

CORTICOTROPIN RELEASING HORMONE (CRH) STIMULATION TEST
Normal: A dose of 0.5 mg of dexamethasone is given every 6 hours for 2 days; 2 hours after last dose 1 mcg/kg CRH is given IV. Samples are drawn after 15 min. Normally there is a twofold to fourfold increase in mean baseline concentration of ACTH or cortisol. Cortisol >1.4 mcg/L is virtually 100% specific and 100% diagnostic.

Interpretation

Normal or exaggerated response: Pituitary Cushing's disease

No response: Ectopic ACTH-secreting tumor

A positive response to CRH or a suppressed response to high-dose dexamethasone has a 97% positive predictive value for Cushing's disease. However, a lack of response to either test excludes Cushing's disease in only 64%-78% of patients. When the tests are considered together, negative responses from both have a 100% predictive value for ectopic ACTH secretion.

CORTISOL, PLASMA

Normal range

Varies with time of collection (circadian variation):

8 AM: 4-19 µg/dl (110-520 nmol/L [CF: 27.59; SMI: 10 nmol/L])

4 PM: 2-15 µg/dl (50-410 nmol/L [CF: 27.59; SMI: 10 nmol/L])

Elevated in: Ectopic adrenocorticotropic hormone production (i.e., oat cell carcinoma of lung), loss of normal diurnal variation, pregnancy, chronic renal failure, iatrogenic, stress, adrenal or pituitary hyperplasia, or adenomas

Decreased in: Primary adrenocortical insufficiency, anterior pituitary hypofunction, secondary adrenocortical insufficiency, adrenogenital syndromes

C-PEPTIDE

Elevated in: Insulinoma, sulfonylurea administration

Decreased in: Insulin-dependent diabetes mellitus, factitious insulin administration

COOMBS DIRECT

See DIRECT ANTIGLOBULIN

COOMBS INDIRECT

See INDIRECT ANTIGLOBULIN

CPK

See CREATINE KINASE

C-REACTIVE PROTEIN

Normal range: 6.8-820 µg/dl (68-8200 µg/L [CF: 10; SMI: 10 µg/L])

Elevated in: Rheumatoid arthritis, rheumatic fever, inflammatory bowel disease, bacterial infections, myocardial infarction, oral contraceptives, third trimester of pregnancy (acute phase reactant), inflammatory and neoplastic diseases. Table 27 shows a comparison of erythrocyte sedimentation rate and C-reactive protein, and Table 28 shows conditions associated with elevated C-reactive protein levels.

C-REACTIVE PROTEIN, HIGH SENSITIVITY (hs-CRP, cardio-CRP)

This is a cardiac risk marker. It is increased in patients with silent atherosclerosis years before a cardiovascular event and is independent of cholesterol level and other lipoproteins. It can be used to help stratify cardiac risk.

INTERPRETATION OF RESULTS

Cardio-CRP result (mg/L)	Risk
0.6	Lowest risk
0.7-1.1	Low risk
1.2-1.9	Moderate risk
2.0-3.8	High risk
3.9-4.9	Highest risk
≥5.0	Results may be confounded by acute inflammatory disease. If clinically indicated, a repeat test should be performed in 2 or more weeks.

CREATINE KINASE (CK, CPK)

Fig. E14 describes a diagnostic approach to creatine kinase elevation.

Normal range: 0-130 U/L (0-2.16 µkat/L [CF: 0.01667; SMI: 0.01 µkat/L])

Elevated in: Myocardial infarction, myocarditis, rhabdomyolysis, myositis, crush injury/trauma, polymyositis, dermatomyositis, vigorous exercise, muscular dystrophy, myxedema, seizures, malignant hyperthermia

TABLE 27 Comparison of Erythrocyte Sedimentation Rate and C-Reactive Protein

	Erythrocyte Sedimentation Rate	C-Reactive Protein
Advantages	• Much clinical information in the literature • May reflect overall health status	• Rapid response to inflammatory stimuli • Wide range of clinically relevant values are detectable • Unaffected by age and gender • Reflects value of a single acute phase protein • Can be measured on stored sera • Quantitation is precise and reproducible
Disadvantages	• Affected by age and gender • Affected by red blood cell morphology • Affected by anemia and polycythemia • Reflects levels of many plasma proteins, not all of which are acute phase proteins • Responds slowly to inflammatory stimuli • Requires fresh sample • May be affected by drugs	• None

From Firestein GS, Budd RC, Gabriel SE, et al: *Kelley's textbook of rheumatology*, ed 9, Philadelphia, 2013, Saunders.

TABLE 28 Conditions Associated with Elevated C-Reactive Protein Levels

Normal or Minor Elevation (<1 mg/dL)	Moderate Elevation (1-10 mg/dL)	Marked Elevation (>10 mg/dL)
• Vigorous exercise • Common cold • Pregnancy • Gingivitis • Seizures • Depression • Insulin resistance and diabetes • Several genetic polymorphisms • Obesity	• Myocardial infarction • Malignancies • Pancreatitis • Mucosal infection (bronchitis, cystitis) • Most connective tissue diseases • Rheumatoid arthritis	• Acute bacterial infection (80%-85%) • Major trauma • Systemic vasculitis

From Firestein GS, Budd RC, Gabriel SE, et al: *Kelley's textbook of rheumatology*, ed 9, Philadelphia, 2013, Saunders.

Laboratory Tests

IV

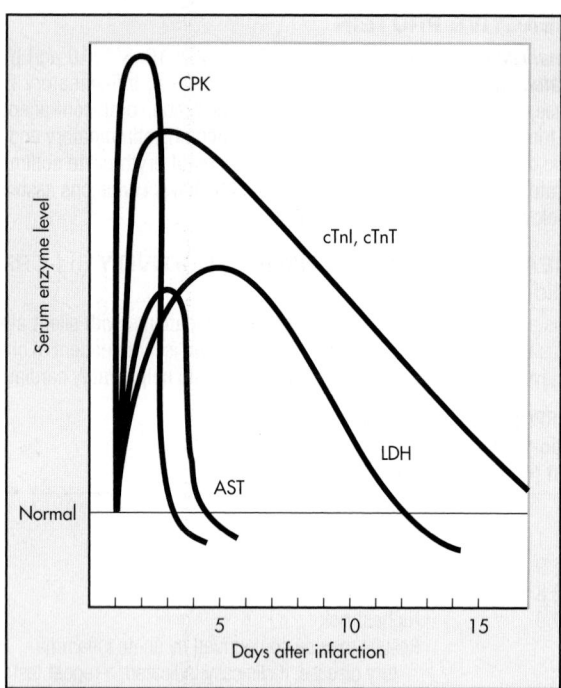

FIG. 15 Evaluation of creatine kinase elevation. *AST,* Aspartate aminotransferase; *CPK,* creatine kinase; *cTnI,* cardiac troponin I; *cTnT,* cardiac troponin T; *LDH,* lactate dehydrogenase. (From Greene HL, Johnson WP, Lemcke D [eds]: *Decision making in medicine,* ed 2, St Louis, 1998, Mosby.)

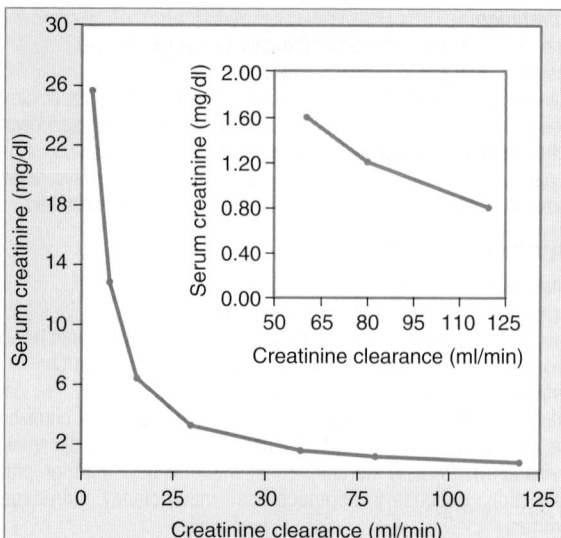

FIG. 16 Relationship between creatinine clearance and serum creatinine. In steady state, serum creatinine should increase twofold for each 50% reduction in creatinine clearance. *Inset* represents enlarged view of changes in serum creatinine as creatinine clearance decreases from 120 to 60 ml/min. If serum creatinine is 0.8 mg/dl when creatinine clearance is 120 ml/min, creatinine clearance can decrease by 33% such that increased serum creatinine is still within normal range. (From Vincent JL et al: *Textbook of critical care,* ed 6, Philadelphia, 2011, Saunders.)

syndrome, IM injections, cerebrovascular accident, pulmonary embolism and infarction, acute dissection of aorta

Decreased in: Corticosteroid use, decreased muscle mass, connective tissue disorders, alcoholic liver disease, metastatic neoplasms

CREATINE KINASE ISOENZYMES

CK-BB
Elevated In: Cerebrovascular accident, subarachnoid hemorrhage, neoplasms (prostate, gastrointestinal tract, brain, ovary, breast, lung), severe shock, bowel infarction, hypothermia, meningitis

CK-MB
Elevated In: Myocardial infarction (MI), myocarditis, pericarditis, muscular dystrophy, cardiac defibrillation, cardiac surgery, extensive rhabdomyolysis, strenuous exercise (marathon runners), mixed connective tissue disease, cardiomyopathy, hypothermia

NOTE: CK-MB exists in the blood in two subforms. MB_2 is released from cardiac cells and converted in the blood to MB_1. Rapid assay of CK-MB subforms can detect MI (CK-MB_2 ≥1.0 U/L, with a ratio of CK-MB_2/CK-MB_1 ≥1.5) within 6 hours of onset of symptoms.

Fig. 15 illustrates the time course of CK, AST, troponins, and LDH activity after acute MI.

CK-MM
Elevated In: Crush injury, seizures, malignant hyperthermia syndrome, rhabdomyolysis, myositis, polymyositis, dermatomyositis, vigorous exercise, muscular dystrophy, IM injections, acute dissection of aorta

CREATININE (serum)

Normal range: 0.6-1.2 mg/dl (50-110 µmol/L [CF: 88.4; SMI: 10 µmol/L]). Fig. 16 illustrates the relationship between creatinine clearance and serum creatinine. Factors that may alter serum creatinine level are described in Box 10.

Elevated in: Renal insufficiency (acute and chronic), decreased renal perfusion (hypotension, dehydration, congestive heart failure), urinary tract infection, rhabdomyolysis, ketonemia

Drugs (antibiotics [aminoglycosides, cephalosporins], hydantoin, diuretics, methyldopa)

The RIFLE criteria for acute kidney injury is summarized in Table 29. A classification of acute kidney injury (AKI) is described in Table 30.

Falsely elevated in: Diabetic ketoacidosis, administration of some cephalosporins (e.g., cefoxitin, cephalothin)

TABLE 29 RIFLE Criteria for Acute Kidney Injury

	GFR and Serum Creatinine Changes	Urine Volume Changes
R (Risk)	Increase in SCreat >1.5×	Urine volume <0.5 mL/kg/hr >6 hr
	Decrease in GFR >25%	
I (Injury)	Increase in SCreat >2×	Urine volume <0.5 mL/kg/hr >12 hr
	Decrease in GFR >50%	
F (Failure)	Increase in SCreat >3×	Urine volume <0.3 mL/kg/hr >24 hr
	Decrease in GFR >75%	Anuria >12 hr
	SCreat >4 mg/dL	
L (Loss)	Complete loss of kidney function >4 weeks	
E (ESRD)	End-stage kidney disease >3 months	

SCreat, Serum creatinine.
(McPherson RA, Pincus MR: Henry's Clinical Diagnosis and Management by Laboratory Methods, 23rd ed, ISBN # 978-0323-29568-0, 2017, Elsevier)

TABLE 30 New Classification for Acute Kidney Injury (AKI) Criteria

Stage	Serum Creatinine Criteria	Urine Output Criteria
1	>0.3 mg/dL (26.4 µmol/L) or >150% to 200%	<0.5 mL/kg for >6 hr
2	>200% to 300%	<0.5 mL/kg for >12 hr
3	>300%, 4 mg/dL (354 µmol/L) or acute increase of >0.5 mg/dL	<0.3 mL/kg for >24 hr or anuria >12 hr

(McPherson RA, Pincus MR: Henry's Clinical Diagnosis and Management by Laboratory Methods, 23rd ed, ISBN # 978-0323-29568-0, 2017, Elsevier)

BOX 11   Calculation of Creatinine Clearance

$C_{cr} = U_{cr} \times V/P_{cr}$
where C_{cr}= clearance of creatinine (ml/min)
U_{cr} = urine creatinine (mg/dl)
V= volume of urine (ml/min) (for 24-hr volume: divide by 1440)
P_{cr} = plasma creatinine (mg/dl)
    Normal range: 95 to 105 ml/min/1.75m²

BOX 12   Cockcroft-Gault Formula to Calculate Creatinine Clearance (C_{cr})

$$C_{cr} = \frac{(140 - \text{age in year}) \times (\text{lean body weight in kg})}{S_{cr} \text{inmg/dl} - 72}$$

Decreased in: Decreased muscle mass (including amputees and older persons), pregnancy, prolonged debilitation

CREATININE CLEARANCE

Normal range: 75-124 ml/min (1.24-2.08 ml/sec [CF: 0.01667; SMI: 0.02 ml/sec])
   Box 11 describes a formula for calculation of creatinine clearance.
   The Cockcroft-Gault formula to calculate creatinine clearance is described in Box 12
Elevated in: Pregnancy, exercise
Decreased in: Renal insufficiency, drugs (cimetidine, procainamide, antibiotics, quinidine)

CREATININE, URINE

See URINE CREATININE

CRYOGLOBULINS (serum)

Normal range: Not detectable
Present in: Collagen vascular diseases, chronic lymphocytic leukemia, hemolytic anemias, multiple myeloma, Waldenström's macroglobulinemia, chronic active hepatitis, Hodgkin's disease

CRYPTOSPORIDIUM ANTIGEN BY EIA (stool)

Normal range: Not detected
Present in: Cryptosporidiosis

CSF

See CEREBROSPINAL FLUID

CYSTATIN C

Normal: Cystatin C is a cysteine protease inhibitor that is produced at a constant rate by all nucleated cells. It is freely filtered by the glomerulus and reabsorbed (but not secreted) by the renal tubules with no extrarenal excretion. Its concentration is not affected by diet, muscle mass, or acute inflammation. Normal range when measured by particle-enhanced nephelometric immunoassay (PENIA) is <0.28 mg/L.
Elevated in: Renal disorders. Good predictor of the severity of acute tubular necrosis. Cystatin C increases more rapidly than creatinine in the early stages of GFR impairment. The cystatin C concentration is an independent risk factor for heart failure in older adults and appears to provide a better measure of risk assessment than the serum creatinine concentration.

CYSTIC FIBROSIS PCR

Test description: Test can be performed on whole blood or tissue. Common mutations in the cystic fibrosis transmembrane regulator (CFTR) gene can be used to detect 75%-80% of mutant alleles.

CYTOMEGALOVIRUS BY PCR

Test description: Test can be performed on whole blood, plasma, or tissue. Qualitative PCR is highly sensitive but may not be able to differentiate between latent and active infection.

D-DIMER

Normal range
<0.5 mcg/ml
Elevated in
DVT, pulmonary embolism, high levels of rheumatoid factor, activation of coagulation and fibrolytic system from any cause
D-dimer assay by ELISA assists in the diagnosis of DVT and pulmonary embolism. This test has significant limitations because it can be elevated whenever the coagulation and fibrinolytic systems are activated and can also be falsely elevated with high rheumatoid factor levels.
A positive d-dimer is not diagnostic for PE. Patients with positive d-dimer and clinical suspicion for PE need additional tests such as chest CT to confirm diagnosis.
PE might be ruled out in patients with negative d-dimer and low pretest probability for PE.

DEHYDROEPIANDROSTERONE SULFATE

Normal
Males:

Ages 19-30:	125-619 mcg/dl
31-50:	59-452 mcg/dl
51-60:	20-413 mcg/dl
61-83:	10-285 mcg/dl

Females:

Ages 19-30:	29-781 mcg/dl
31-50:	12-379 mcg/dl
Postmenopausal:	30-260 mcg/dl

Elevated in: Hirsutism, congenital adrenal hyperplasia, adrenal carcinomas, adrenal adenomas, polycystic ovary syndrome, ectopic ACTH-producing tumors, Cushing's disease, spironolactone

DEHYDROTESTOSTERONE (serum, urine)

Normal
Serum: Males: 30-85 ng/dl; females: 4-22 ng/dl
Urine, 24 h: Males: 20-50 mcg/day; females: <8 mcg/day
Elevated in
Hirsutism
Decreased in
5-α-reductase deficiency, hypogonadism

DEOXYCORTICOSTERONE (11-DEOXYCORTICOSTERONE, DOC) (serum)

Normal: 2-19 ng/dl. Normal secretion depends on ACTH and is suppressible by dexamethasone.
Elevated in
Adrenogenital syndromes due to 17- and 11-hydroxylase deficiencies, pregnancy
Decreased in
Preeclampsia

DEXAMETHASONE SUPPRESSION TEST, OVERNIGHT

Normal: Test is performed by giving 1 mg dexamethasone orally at 11 PM and measuring serum cortisol at 8 AM the following morning. Normal response is cortisol suppression to <3 mcg/dl; If dose of 4 mg dexamethasone is given, cortisol suppression will be to <50% of baseline.
Interpretation: Cushing's syndrome (<10 mcg/dl), endogenous depression (half of patients suppress test values <5 mcg/dl). Most patients with pituitary Cushing's disease demonstrate suppression, whereas patients with adrenal adenoma, carcinoma, and ectopic ACTH-producing tumors do not.

DIGOXIN

Normal therapeutic range
0.5-2 ng/ml
Elevated in: Impaired renal function, excessive dosing, concomitant use of quinidine, amiodarone, verapamil, fluoxetine, nifedipine. Toxicity may occur at a lower blood concentration in the presence of hypokalemia, hypomagnesemia, and hypercalcemia.

Laboratory Tests

IV

TABLE 31   Applications for Direct and Indirect Antiglobulin Techniques

	Applications	Purpose	What Is Detected
Direct antiglobulin test (DAT)	Investigation of HTR	To detect circulating donor red cells that are sensitized with recipient antibody. A positive DAT is the first immunohematologic evidence of a hemolytic reaction after transfusion	DAT positive owing to IgG and/or C3d depending on the antibodies responsible
	Diagnosis of HDFN	To detect maternal antibodies that have crossed the placenta to sensitize fetal red cells	DAT almost always positive as a result of IgG; occasionally C3d if ABO antibodies involved
	Diagnosis of AIHA	To detect autoantibody sensitizing a patient's own red cells	Warm autoantibodies: DAT almost always positive owing to IgG Cold autoantibodies: DAT may be due to C3d only
	Investigation of drug-induced hemolysis	To detect antidrug/red cell antibodies and/or subsequent activation of the complement system	DAT may be positive owing to IgG, C3d, or both, depending on the mechanism involved (see under Investigation of Autoimmune Hemolytic Anemia section) Indirect antiglobulin test
	Antibody detection (or antibody screen)	To detect clinically significant IgG alloantibodies in the recipient	Recipient IgG antibodies bound to reagent screening cells*
	Antibody identification	To specifically identify those antibodies detected by reagent screening cells or by donor red cells	Recipient IgG antibodies bound to reagent cells from a panel of 10-12 donors*
	Crossmatching	To detect antibodies that may have been missed by the antibody screen because of absence of the corresponding antigen or presence of a dosing antibody	Recipient IgG antibodies bound to donor red cells*
	Red cell antigen typing	To type patient or donor red cells for antigens that can be detected by IgG antisera reactive only by the AGT. A common example of this would be the weak D test	Specific binding of reagent IgG antibodies to red cells positive for the corresponding antigen

AGT, Antihuman globulin test; *AIHA,* autoimmune hemolytic anemia; *HDFN,* hemolytic disease of the fetus and newborn; *HTR,* hemolytic transfusion reaction; *Ig,* immunoglobulin.
*If complement is fixed in vitro, it may be detected if polyspecific antiglobulin is used.
(McPherson RA, Pincus MR: Henry's Clinical Diagnosis and Management by Laboratory Methods, 23rd ed, ISBN # 978-0323-29568-0, 2017, Elsevier)

DILANTIN
See PHENYTOIN

DIRECT ANTIGLOBULIN (Coombs Direct)

Normal: Negative
Positive: Autoimmune hemolytic anemia, erythroblastosis fetalis, transfusion reactions, drugs (α-methyldopa, penicillins, tetracycline, sulfonamides, levodopa, cephalosporins, quinidine, insulin)
False-positive: May be seen with cold agglutinins

DISACCHARIDE ABSORPTION TESTS

Normal: Test is used to diagnose malabsorption due to disaccharide deficiency. It is performed by giving disaccharide orally 1 g/kg body weight to a total of 25 g. Blood is drawn at 0, 30, 60, 90, and 120 min. Normal response is a change in glucose from fasting value >30 mg/dl, inconclusive when increase is 20-30 mg/dl, abnormal when increase is >20 mg/dl. Test can also be performed by measuring air at 0, 30, 60, 90, and 120 min. Normal is H_2 >20 ppm above baseline level before a colonic response.
Decreased in: Disaccharide deficiency (lactose, fructose, sorbitol), celiac disease, sprue, acute gastroenteritis

DOC
See DEOXYCORTICOSTERONE

DONATH-LANDSTEINER (D-L) TEST FOR PAROXYSMAL COLD HEMOGLOBINURIA

Normal: No hemolysis
Interpretation: Hemolysis indicates presence of bithermic cold hemolysins or Donath-Landsteiner antibodies (D-L Ab)

DOPAMINE

Normal range
175 pg/ml
Elevated in: Pheochromocytomas, neuroblastomas, stress, vigorous exercise, certain foods (bananas, chocolate, coffee, tea, vanilla)

D-XYLOSE ABSORPTION

Normal range
21%-31% excreted in 5 hours
Decreased in
Malabsorption syndrome

D-XYLOSE ABSORPTION TEST

Normal range
URINE: ≥4 g/5 hours (5-hour urine collection in adults >12 years [25-g dose])
SERUM: ≥25 mg/dl (adult, 1 hour, 25-g dose, normal renal function)
Normal results: In patients with malabsorption, normal results suggest pancreatic disease as an etiology of the malabsorption.
Abnormal results: Celiac disease, Crohn's disease, tropical sprue, surgical bowel resection, AIDS. False-positives can occur with decreased renal function, dehydration/hypovolemia, surgical blind loops, decreased gastric emptying, vomiting.

ELECTROPHORESIS, HEMOGLOBIN
See HEMOGLOBIN ELECTROPHORESIS

ELECTROPHORESIS, PROTEIN
See PROTEIN ELECTROPHORESIS

ENA COMPLEX
See EXTRACTABLE NUCLEAR ANTIGEN

ENDOMYSIAL ANTIBODIES

Normal: Not detected
Present in
Celiac disease, dermatitis herpetiformis

EOSINOPHIL COUNT

Normal range
1%-4% eosinophils (0-440/mm^3)

TABLE 32 Eosinophilia Investigation in Returning Travelers

History	Allergies
	Drugs and vitamins (L-tryptophan)
	Regions, localities, and duration of exposure
Physical examination	Skin, subcutaneous tissues
	Liver/spleen
	Signs of other systemic disease
Initial investigations	Full blood count and differential white blood cell count
	Stool examination for ova and parasites (×3) Urine analysis
	Examination of midday urine for ova and parasites (×3) (in those who have traveled to Africa or the Middle East)
Further investigations as suggested by travel and exposure from history	*Strongyloides* culture and serologic testing Duodenal aspirate (strongyloidiasis, hookworm)
	Serologic testing (schistosomiasis, filariasis) Day/night blood films (filariasis)
Further studies if suggested by history and physical examination	Skin snips (onchocerciasis)
	Chest x-ray examination (hydatid cyst, tropical pulmonary eosinophilia, paragonimiasis)
	Soft tissue x-ray examination (cysticercosis) Sputum examination for ova and parasites (paragonimiasis)
	Abdominal ultrasound examination (hydatid cyst)
	Cystoscopy with or without biopsy (schistosomiasis)
	Rectal snips (schistosomiasis)

From Hoffman R: *Hematology: basic principles and practice*, ed 6, Philadelphia, Saunders, 2013.

Elevated in
HELMINTHIC PARASITES
Ascaris lumbricoides (invasive larval stage)
Hookworms (invasive larval stage)
Strongyloides stercoralis (initial infection and autoinfection)
Trichinosis
Filariasis
Echinococcus granulosus and *E. multilocularis*
Toxocara species
Animal hookworms
Angiostrongylus cantonensis and *A. costaricensis*
Schistosomiasis
Liver flukes
Fasciolopsis buski
Anisakiasis
Capillaria philippinensis
Paragonimus westermani
"Tropical eosinophilia" (unidentified microfilariae)
Note: Table 32 describes an approach to investigation of eosinophilia in returning travelers
OTHER INFECTIONS/INFESTATIONS
Pulmonary aspergillosis
Severe scabies
ALLERGIES
Asthma
Hay fever
Drug reactions
Atopic dermatitis
AUTOIMMUNE AND RELATED DISORDERS
Polyarteritis nodosa
Necrotizing vasculitis
Eosinophilic fasciitis
Pemphigus
NEOPLASTIC DISEASES
Hodgkin's disease
Mycosis fungoides
Chronic myelocytic leukemia

Eosinophilic leukemia
Polycythemia vera
Mucin-secreting adenocarcinomas
IMMUNODEFICIENCY STATES
Hyperimmunoglobulin E with recurrent infection
Wiskott-Aldrich syndrome
OTHER
Addison's disease
Inflammatory bowel disease
Dermatitis herpetiformis
Toxic/chemical syndrome
Eosinophilic myalgia syndrome, tryptophan, toxic oil syndrome
Hypereosinophilic syndrome (unknown etiology)

EPINEPHRINE, PLASMA
Normal range
0-90 pg/ml
Elevated in: Pheochromocytomas, neuroblastomas, stress, vigorous exercise, certain foods (bananas, chocolate, coffee, tea, vanilla), hypoglycemia

EPSTEIN-BARR VIRUS SEROLOGY (Box 13)
Normal range: IgG anti-VCA <1:10 or negative>
Abnormal
IgG anti-VCA >1:10 or positive indicates either current or previous infection
IgM anti-VCA >1:10 or positive indicates current or recent infection
Anti-EBNA ≥1.5 or positive indicates previous infection
Table 33 and Fig. 17 describe test interpretation.

BOX 13 Epstein-Barr Virus–Associated Malignancies

Malignancy	Epstein-Barr Virus Frequency
Hodgkin disease	≈40%
Non-Hodgkin lymphomas	
Burkitt lymphoma	20%-95%
Diffuse large B-cell lymphoma and CD30⁺ Ki-1⁺ anaplastic large cell lymphoma	10%-35%
Lymphomatoid granulomatosis	80%-95%
T cell–rich B-cell lymphoma	20%
Angioimmunoblastic lymphoma	>80%
T-cell, NK cell, and T/NK-cell lymphomas	30%-90%
Nasopharyngeal carcinoma	>95%
Gastric adenocarcinoma	5%-10%
Pyothorax-associated lymphoma	>95%
Leiomyosarcoma in immunocompromised patients	>95%

From Hoffman R: *Hematology: basic principles and practice,* ed 6, Philadelphia, Saunders, 2013.

ERYTHROCYTE SEDIMENTATION RATE (ESR, sed rate, sedimentation rate)
Normal range
Male: 0-15 mm/hr
Female: 0-20 mm/hr
Elevated in: Collagen vascular diseases, infections, myocardial infarction, neoplasms, inflammatory states (acute phase reactant), hyperthyroidism, hypothyroidism, rouleaux formation
Decreased in: Sickle cell disease, polycythemia, corticosteroids, spherocytosis, anisocytosis, hypofibrinogenemia, increased serum viscosity

ERYTHROPOIETIN (EP)
Normal: 3.7-16.0 IU/L by radioimmunoassay
Erythropoietin is a glycoprotein secreted by the kidneys that stimulates RBC production by acting on erythroid-committed stem cells.
Increased in
Extremely high: Generally seen in patients with severe anemia (Hct, <25; Hb<7) such as in cases of aplastic anemia, severe hemolytic anemia, hematologic cancers
Very high: Patients with mild to moderate anemia (Hct, 25-35; Hb, 7-10)

Laboratory Tests

IV

TABLE 33 Antibody Tests in Epstein-Barr Viral Infection

	Appearance	Peak	Disappears
Heterophil Ab	3-5 days after onset of Sx (range, 0-21 days)	During second wk after onset of Sx (1-4 wk)	2-3 mo after onset of Sx (still found at 1 yr in 20% of cases)
VCA-IgM	Beginning of Sx (1 wk before to 1 wk after Sx begin)	During first wk after onset of Sx (0-21 days)	2-3 mo after onset of Sx (1-6 mo)
VCA-IgG	3 days after onset of Sx (0-2 wk)	During second wk after onset of Sx (1-3 wk)	Decline to lower level, then persists for life
EBNA-IgG	3 wk after onset of Sx (1-4 wk)	8 mo after appearance (3-12 mo)	Lifelong
EA-D	5 days after onset of Sx (during first 1-2 wk after onset of Sx)	14-21 days after onset of Sx (1-4 wk)	9 wk after appearance (2-6 mo)
EBNA-IgM	Same as VCA-IgM	Same as VCA-IgM	Same as VCA-IgM

From Ravel R: *Clinical laboratory medicine*, ed 6, St Louis, 1995, Mosby.
Ab, Antibody; *EA*, early antigen; *EBNA*, Epstein-Barr virus nuclear antigen; *Sx*, symptoms; *VCA*, viral capsid antigen.

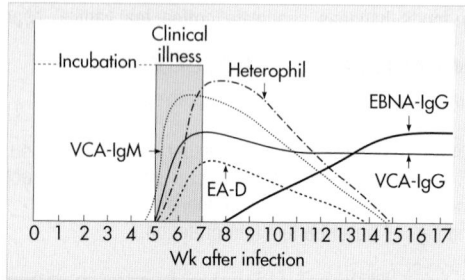

FIG. 17 Tests in Epstein-Barr viral infection. See Table 33 for abbreviations. (From Ravel R [ed]: *Clinical laboratory medicine*, ed 6, St Louis, 1995, Mosby.)

High: Patients with mild anemia (e.g., AIDS, myelodysplasia)

Erythropoietin can be inappropriately elevated in patients with malignant neoplasms, renal cysts, postrenal transplant, meningioma, hemangioblastoma, and leiomyoma.

Decreased in: Renal failure, polycythemia vera, autonomic neuropathy

ESTRADIOL (serum)

Normal range

Female, premenopausal: 30-400 pg/ml, depending on phase of menstrual cycle

Female, postmenopausal: 0-30 pg/ml

Male, adult: 10-50 pg/ml

Decreased in: Ovarian failure

Elevated in: Tumors of ovary, testis, adrenal, or nonendocrine sites (rare)

ESTROGEN

Normal range (serum)

Males:	20-80 pg/ml
Females:	
Follicular:	60-200 pg/ml
Luteal:	160-400 pg/ml
Postmenopausal:	<130 pg/ml

Normal Range (urine)

Males:	4-23 μg/g creatinine
Females:	
Follicular:	7-65 μg/g creatinine
Midcycle:	32-104 μg/g creatinine
Luteal:	8-135 μg/g creatinine

Elevated in: Hyperplasia of adrenal cortex, ovarian tumors producing estrogen, granulosa and thecal cell tumors, testicular tumors

Decreased in: Menopause, hypopituitarism, primary ovarian malfunction, anorexia nervosa, hypofunction of adrenal cortex, ovarian agenesis, psychogenic stress, gonadotropin-releasing hormone deficiency

ETHANOL (blood)

Normal range:

Negative (values <10 mg/dl are considered negative)

Ethanol is metabolized at 10-25 mg/dl/hr. Levels ≥80 mg/dl are considered evidence of impairment for driving. Fatal blood concentration is considered to be >400 mg/dl. Table 34 summarizes the influence of acute ethanol ingestion on ethanol levels and behavior.

TABLE 34 Influence of Acute Ethanol Ingestion on Ethanol Levels and Behavior

Ounces	Blood Concentration	Influence
1-2	10-50 mg/dL (2.2-10.9 mmol/L)	None to mild euphoria
3-4	50-100 mg/dL (10.9-21.7 mmol/L or greater)	Mild influence on stereoscopic vision and dark adaptation
	100 mg/dL (21.7 mmol/L)	Legally intoxicated
4-6	100-150 mg/dL (21.7-32.6 mmol/L)	Euphoria; disappearance of inhibition; prolonged reaction time
6-7	150-200 mg/dL (32.6-43.4 mmol/L)	Moderately severe poisoning; reaction time greatly prolonged; loss of inhibition and slight disturbances in equilibrium and coordination
8-9	200-250 mg/dL (43.4-54.3 mmol/L)	Severe degree of poisoning; disturbances of equilibrium and coordination; retardation of the thought processes and clouding of consciousness
10-15	250-400 mg/dL (54.3-86.8 mmol/L)	Deep, possibly fatal, coma

(McPherson RA, Pincus MR: Henry's Clinical Diagnosis and Management by Laboratory Methods, 23rd ed, ISBN # 978-0323-29568-0, 2017, Elsevier)

EXTRACTABLE NUCLEAR ANTIGEN (ENA COMPLEX, ANTI-RNP ANTIBODY, ANTI-SM, ANTI-SMITH)

Normal: Negative

Present in

Systemic lupus erythematosus, rheumatoid arthritis, Sjögren's syndrome, mixed connective tissue disease

FACTOR V LEIDEN
Test description: PCR test performed on whole blood or tissue. This single mutation, found in 2%-8% of the general Caucasian population, is the single most common cause of hereditary thrombophilia.

FASTING BLOOD SUGAR
See GLUCOSE, FASTING

FBS
See GLUCOSE, FASTING

FDP
See FIBRIN DEGRADATION PRODUCT

FECAL FAT, QUANTITATIVE (72-hr collection)
Normal range
2-6 g/24 hr (7-21 mmol/dl [CF: 3.515; SMI: 1 mmol/dl])
Elevated in
Malabsorption syndrome

FECAL GLOBIN IMMUNOCHEMICAL TEST
Normal: Negative. This test is performed by immunochromatography on a cellulose strip that has been impregnated with various antibodies. The test uses a small amount of toilet water as the specimen and is placed onto absorbent pads of card similar to traditional OB card. There is no direct handling of stool. This test is specific for the globin portion of the hemoglobin molecule, which confers lower GI bleeding specificity. It specifically detects blood from the lower GI tract; guaic tests are not lower GI specific. It is more sensitive than typical Hemoccult test (detection limit 50 mcg Hb/g feces versus >500 mcg Hb/g feces for Hemoccult). It has no dietary restrictions and gives no false-positives due to plant peroxidases and red meats. It has no medication restrictions. Iron supplements and NSAIDs do not cause false-positives. Vitamin C does not cause false-negatives.
Positive in
Lower GI bleeding

FERRITIN (serum)
Normal range
18-300 ng/ml (18-300 µg/L [CF: 1; SMI: 10 µg/L])
Elevated in: Hyperthyroidism, inflammatory states, liver disease (ferritin elevated from necrotic hepatocytes), neoplasms (neuroblastomas, lymphomas, leukemia, breast carcinoma), iron replacement therapy, hemochromatosis, hemosiderosis. Table 35 summarizes hereditary iron overload disorders.
Decreased in: Iron deficiency anemia

α-1 FETOPROTEIN
Normal range
0-20 ng/ml (0-20 µg/L [CF: 1; SMI: 1 µg/L])

Table 35 Hereditary Iron Overload Disorders

Disorder	Gene, Chromosome Location	Inheritance	Plasma Transferrin Saturation	Plasma Ferritin	Iron Deposition Sites	Clinical Manifestations
Hereditary hemochromatosis, *HFE*-associated (type 1; OMIM 235200)	HFE, 6p21	Autosomal recessive	Early increase; >45%	Later increase after third decade	Parenchymal iron overload affecting hepatocytes, heart, pancreas, other organs	Liver and heart disease, diabetes, gonadal failure, arthritis, skin pigmentation
Hereditary hemochromatosis, TfR2-associated (type 3; OMIM 604250)	TFR2, 7q22	Autosomal recessive	Early increase; >45%	Later increase after third decade	Parenchymal iron overload affecting hepatocytes, heart, pancreas, other organs	Liver and heart disease, diabetes, gonadal failure, arthritis, skin pigmentation
Juvenile hemochromatosis, hemojuvelin-associated (type 2A; OMIM 602390)	HJV, 1q21	Autosomal recessive	Early increase; >45%	Increased by second decade	Parenchymal iron overload affecting hepatocytes, heart, pancreas, other organs	As for hereditary hemochromatosis, but liver involvement less prominent
Juvenile hemochromatosis, hepcidin-associated (type 2B; OMIM 613313)	HAMP, 19q13	Autosomal recessive	Early increase; >45%	Increased by second decade	Parenchymal iron overload affecting hepatocytes, heart, pancreas, other organs	As for hereditary hemochromatosis, but liver involvement less prominent
Hemochromatosis, DMT1-associated (OMIM 206100)	SCL11A2, 12q13	Autosomal recessive	Early increase; >45%	Normal to moderately elevated	Hepatic iron overload, predominantly in hepatocytes	Severe microcytic anemia, liver dysfunction
Atransferrinemia (OMIM 209300)	TF, 3q22	Autosomal recessive	No plasma transferrin	Increased	Parenchymal iron overload affecting hepatocytes, heart, pancreas; no iron in bone marrow or spleen	Transfusion-dependent iron deficiency anemia, growth retardation, poor survival
Aceruloplasminemia (OMIM 604290)	CP, 3q24-q25	Autosomal recessive	Decreased	Increased	Marked iron accumulation in basal ganglia, liver, pancreas	Diabetes, progressive neurologic disease, retinal degeneration
Hemochromatosis, ferroportin-associated, with impaired iron export (type 4A; OMIM 606069)	SLC40A1, 2q32	Autosomal dominant	Remains normal or low	Early increase	Predominantly macrophage iron deposition	None
Hemochromatosis, ferroportin-associated, with hepcidin resistance (type 4B; OMIM 606069)	SLC40A1, 2q32	Autosomal dominant	Early increase; >45%	Early increase	Parenchymal iron overload affecting hepatocytes, heart, pancreas, other organs	Similar to HFE-associated hemochromatosis

From Hoffman R, et al: *Hematology, basic principles and practice*, ed 6, Philadelphia, 2013, Saunders.

Laboratory Tests

IV

Elevated in: Hepatocellular carcinoma (usually values >1000 ng/ml), germinal neoplasms (testis, ovary, mediastinum, retroperitoneum), liver disease (alcoholic cirrhosis, acute hepatitis, chronic active hepatitis), fetal anencephaly, spina bifida, basal cell carcinoma, breast carcinoma, pancreatic carcinoma, gastric carcinoma, retinoblastoma, esophageal atresia

FIBRIN DEGRADATION PRODUCT (FDP)

Normal range:

<10 µg/ml

Elevated in: Disseminated intravascular coagulation, primary fibrinolysis, pulmonary embolism, severe liver disease

NOTE: The presence of rheumatoid factor may cause falsely elevated FDP.

FIBRINOGEN

Normal range

200-400 mg/dl (2-4 g/L [CF: 0.01; SMI: 0.1 g/L])

Elevated in: Tissue inflammation or damage (acute phase protein reactant), oral contraceptives, pregnancy, acute infection, myocardial infarction

Decreased in: Disseminated intravascular coagulation, hereditary afibrinogenemia, liver disease, primary or secondary fibrinolysis, cachexia

FOLATE (folic acid)

Normal range

Plasma: 2-10 ng/ml (4-22 nmol/L [CF: 2.266; SMI: 2 nmol/L])

Red blood cells: 140-960 ng/ml (550-2200 nmol/L [CF: 2.266; SMI: 10 nmol/L])

Decreased in: Folic acid deficiency (inadequate intake, malabsorption), alcoholism, drugs (methotrexate, trimethoprim, phenytoin, oral contraceptives, Azulfidine), vitamin B_{12} deficiency (defective red cell folate absorption), hemolytic anemia. Box 14 summarizes an etiophysiologic classification of folate deficiency.

Elevated in: Folic acid therapy

BOX 14 **Etiopathophysiologic Classification of Folate Deficiency**

Nutritional causes
  Decreased dietary intake—poverty and famine, institutionalized individuals (psychiatric/nursing homes)/chronic debilitating disease, prolonged feeding of infants with goat's milk, special slimming diets or food fads (folate-rich foods not consumed), cultural/ethnic cooking techniques (food folate destroyed)
  Decreased diet and increased requirements
    Physiologic—pregnancy and lactation, prematurity, hyperemesis gravidarum, infancy
    Pathologic
    Intrinsic hematologic diseases involving hemolysis with compensatory erythropoiesis, abnormal hematopoiesis, or bone marrow infiltration with malignant disease
    Dermatologic disease—psoriasis
Folate malabsorption
With normal intestinal mucosa
Drugs—sulfasalazine, pyrimethamine, proton pump inhibitors (via inhibition of proton-coupled folate transporter [PCFT])
  Hereditary folate malabsorption (mutations in PCFTs) (rare)
  With mucosal abnormalities—tropical and nontropical sprue, regional enteritis
Defective cerebral spinal fluid folate transport—cerebral folate deficiency (mutation or autoantibodies to folate receptors) (rare)
Inadequate cellular utilization
  Folate antagonists (methotrexate)
  Hereditary enzyme deficiencies involving folate
Drugs (multiple effects on folate metabolism)—alcohol, sulfasalazine, triamterene, pyrimethamine, trimethoprim-sulfamethoxazole, diphenylhydantoin, barbiturates

FOLLICLE-STIMULATING HORMONE (FSH)

Normal range

5-20 mIU/ml

Elevated in: Menopause, primary gonadal failure, alcoholism, castration, Klinefelter's syndrome, gonadotropin-secreting pituitary hormones

Decreased in: Pregnancy, polycystic ovary disease, anorexia nervosa, anterior pituitary hypofunction

FREE T4

See T_4, FREE

FREE THYROXINE INDEX

Normal range

1.1-4.3

INCREASED THYROXINE OR FREE THYROXINE VALUES

Laboratory error

Primary hyperthyroidism (T4/T3 type)

Severe thyroxine-binding globulin elevation

Excess therapy of hypothyroidism

Excessive dose of levothyroxine

Active thyroiditis (subacute, painless, early active Hashimoto's disease)

Familial dysalbuminemic hyperthyroxinemia (some FT4 kits, especially analog types)

Peripheral resistance to T4 syndrome

Amiodarone or propranolol

Postpartum transient toxicosis

Factitious hyperthyroidism

Jod-Basedow (iodine-induced) hyperthyroidism

Severe nonthyroid illness

Acute psychosis (especially paranoid schizophrenia)

T4 sample drawn 2-4 hr after levothyroxine dose

Struma ovarii

Pituitary thyroid-stimulating hormone–secreting tumor

Certain x-ray contrast media (Telepaque and Oragrafin)

Acute porphyria

Heparin effect (some T4 and FT4 kits)

Amphetamine, heroin, methadone, and phencyclidine abuse

Perphenazine or 5-fluorouracil

Antithyroid or anti-IgG heterophil (HAMA) autoantibodies

"T4" hyperthyroidism

Hyperemesis gravidarum; about 50% of patients

High altitudes

DECREASED THYROXINE OR FREE THYROXINE VALUES

Laboratory error

Primary hypothyroidism

Severe nonthyroid illness

Lithium therapy

Severe thyroxine-binding globulin decrease (congenital, disease, or drug-induced) or severe albumin decrease

Dilantin, Depakene, or high-dose salicylate drugs

Pituitary insufficiency

Large doses of inorganic iodide (e.g., saturated solution of potassium iodide)

Moderate or severe iodine deficiency

Cushing's syndrome

High-dose glucocorticoid drugs

Pregnancy, third trimester (low normal or small decrease)

Addison's disease; some patients (30%)

Heparin effect (a few FT4 kits)

Desipramine or amiodarone drugs

Acute psychiatric illness

FTA-ABS (serum)

Normal

Nonreactive

Reactive in

Syphilis, other treponemal diseases (yaws, pinta, bejel), SLE, pregnancy

FUROSEMIDE STIMULATION TEST

Normal: Test is performed by giving 60 mg furosemide orally after overnight fast. Patient should be on a normal diet without medications the week before the test. Normal results: renin 1-6 ng angiotensin L/ml/hr.

Elevated in: Renovascular hypertension, Barrter's syndrome, high-renin essential hypertension, pheochromocytoma

No response in: Primary aldosteronism, low-renin essential hypertension, hyporeninemic hypoaldosteronism

GAMMA-GLUTAMYL TRANSFERASE (GGT)

See γ-GLUTAMYL TRANSFERASE

GASTRIN (serum)

Normal range: 0-180 pg/ml (0-180 ng/L [CF: 1; SMI: 10 ng/L])

Elevated in: Zollinger-Ellison syndrome (gastrinoma), pernicious anemia, hyperparathyroidism, retained gastric antrum, chronic renal failure, gastric ulcer, chronic atrophic gastritis, pyloric obstruction, malignant neoplasms of the stomach, H_2-blockers, omeprazole, calcium therapy, ulcerative colitis, rheumatoid arthritis

GASTRIN STIMULATION TEST

Normal: Gastrin stimulation test after calcium infusion is performed by giving a calcium infusion (15 mg/kg in 500 ml normal saline over 4 hours). Serum is drawn in fasting state before infusion and at 1, 2, 3, and 4 hr. Normal response is little or no increase over baseline gastrin level.

Elevated in: Gastrinoma (gastrin >400 pg/ml), duodenal ulcer (gastrin level increase <400 ng/L)

Decreased in: Pernicious anemia, atrophic gastritis

GLIADIN ANTIBODIES, IGA AND IGG

Normal: <25 U, equivocal 20-25 U, positive >25 U. Test is useful to monitor compliance with gluten-free diet in patients with celiac disease.

Elevated in: Celiac disease with dietary noncompliance

GLOMERULAR BASEMENT MEMBRANE (GBM) ANTIBODY

Normal: Negative

Present in: Goodpasture's syndrome

GLOMERULAR FILTRATION RATE

See Box 15 for a summary of common equations for calculating GFR or creatinine clearance. Chronic kidney disease stages based on GFR are summarized in Table 36.

Normal

Ages 20-29	116 ml/min/1.73 m²
Ages 30-39	107 ml/min/1.73 m²
Ages 40-49	99 ml/min/1.73 m²
Ages 50-59	93 ml/min/1.73 m²
Ages 60-69	85 ml/min/1.73 m²
Ages >75	75 ml/min/1.73 m²

Decreased in: Renal insufficiency, decreased renal blood flow

GLUCAGON

Normal: 20-100 pg/ml

Elevated in: Glucagonoma (900-7800 pg/ml), chronic renal failure, diabetes mellitus, glucocorticoids, insulin, nifedipine, danazol, sympathomimetic amines

Decreased in: Hyperlipoproteinemia (types III, IV), beta-blockers, secretin

GLUCOSE, FASTING (FBS, fasting blood sugar)

Fig. E18 describes the approach to hypoglycemia. An algorithm for evaluation of hypoglycemia in children is described in Fig. E19.

Normal range: 60-99 mg/dl (3.8-6.0 mmol/L [CF: 0.05551; SMI: 0.1 mmol/L])

Elevated in: Diabetes mellitus, stress, infections, myocardial infarction, cerebrovascular accident, Cushing's syndrome, acromegaly, acute pancreatitis, glucagonoma, hemochromatosis, drugs (glucocorticoids, diuretics [thiazides, loop diuretics]), glucose intolerance, impaired fasting glucose

---

BOX 15   Common Equations for Estimating Glomerular Filtration Rate or Creatinine Clearance

Cockcoft-Gault ($C_{Cr} \cdot BSA/1.73$ m²)
For men: $C_{Cr} = [(140 - age) \cdot weight\ (kg)]/S_{Cr} \cdot 72$
For women: $C_{Cr} = ([(140 - age) \cdot weight\ (kg)]/S_{Cr} \cdot 72) \cdot 0.85$

MDRD (1)
$GFR = 170 \cdot [S_{Cr}]^{-0.999} \cdot [age]^{-0.176} \cdot [0.762$ if patient is female$] \cdot [1.18$ if patient is black$] \cdot [BUN]^{-0170} \cdot [Alb]^{0.318}$

MDRD (2)
$GFR = 186 \cdot [S_{Cr}]^{-1.154} \cdot [age]^{-0.203} \cdot [0.742$ if patient is female$] \cdot [1.212$ if patient is black$]$

Jellife (1) ($C_{Cr} \cdot BSA/1.73$ m²)
For men: $(98 - [0.8 \cdot (age - 20)])/S_{Cr}$
For women: $(98 - [0.8 \cdot (age - 20)])S_{Cr} \cdot 0.90$

Jellife (2)
For men: $(100/S_{Cr}) - {}^{12}$
For women: $(80/S_{Cr}) - {}^{7}$

Mawer
For men: $weight \cdot [29.3 - (0.203 \cdot age)] \cdot [1 - (0.03 \cdot S_{Cr})]$
For women: $weight \cdot [25.3 - (0.175 \cdot age)] \cdot [1 - (0.03 \cdot S_{Cr})]$

Bjornsson
For men: $[27 - (0.173 \cdot age)] \cdot weight \cdot 0/S_{Cr}$
For women: $[25 - (0.175 \cdot age)] \cdot weight \cdot 0.07/S_{Cr}$

Gates
For men: $(89.4 \cdot S_{Cr}^{-1.2}) + (55 - age) \cdot (0.447 \cdot S_{Cr}^{-1.1})$
For women: $(89.4 \cdot S_{Cr}^{-1.2}) + (55 - age) \cdot (0.447 \cdot S_{Cr}^{-1.1})$

Salazar-Corcoran
For men: $[137 - age] \cdot [(0.285 \cdot weight) + (12.1 \cdot height^2)]/(51 \cdot S_{Cr})$
For women: $[146 - age] \cdot [(0.287 \cdot weight) + (9.74 \cdot height^2)]/(60 \cdot S_{Cr})$

From Vincent JL et al: *Textbook of critical care,* ed 6, Philadelphia, 2011, Saunders.

Table 36   Chronic Kidney Disease Stages

Stage	eGFR (mL/min/1.73 m²)	Urinalysis Findings
1	≥90	Hematuria, proteinuria, or imaging abnormalities at >3 months
2	60-89	Hematuria, proteinuria, or imaging abnormalities at >3 months
3	30-59	↑ or normal
4	15-29	↑ or normal
5	0-14	↑ or normal

eGFR, estimated glomerular filtration rate.
(Parrillo JE, Dellinger RP: Critical Care Medicine, Principles of Diagnosis and Management in the Adult, 4th ed, ISBN # 978-0-323-08929-6, 2014, Elsevier)

Decreased in: Sulfonylurea therapy, insulin therapy, reactive hypoglycemia (e.g., subtotal gastrectomy), starvation, insulinoma, glycogen storage disorders, severe liver disease or renal disease, ethanol-induced hypoglycemia, mesenchymal tumors that secrete insulin-like hormones

GLUCOSE, POSTPRANDIAL

Normal range: <140 mg/dl (<7.8 mmol/L [CF: 0.05551; SMI: 0.1 mmol/L])

Elevated in: Diabetes mellitus, glucose intolerance

Decreased in: Post-gastrointestinal resection, reactive hypoglycemia, hereditary fructose intolerance, galactosemia, leucine sensitivity

GLUCOSE TOLERANCE TEST

Normal values above fasting

30 min: 30-60 mg/dl (1.65-3.3 mmol/L [CF: 0.05551; SMI: 0.1 mmol/L])
60 min: 20-50 mg/dl (1.1-2.75 mmol/L [CF: 0.05551; SMI: 0.1 mmol/L])

TABLE 37   Glycemic Goals in Adults*

	Hemoglobin A$_{1c}$ (%)	PREPRANDIAL GLUCOSE		POSTPRANDIAL GLUCOSE**	
		mg/dL	mmol/L	mg/dL	mmol/L
ADA[†]: Adults	<7.0[‡]	80-130	4.4-7.2	<180	<10.0
Pregnant adults	<6.0	60-99	3.3-5.5	100-129	5.6-7.2
Older adults:					
Healthy	<7.5	90-130	5.0-7.2	90-150	5.0-8.3
Intermediate	<8.0	90-150	5.0-8.3	100-180	5.6-10.0
Poor health	<8.5	100-180	5.6-10.0	110-200	6.1-11.1
AACE[§,¶]	≤6.5	≤110	≤6.1	≤140	<7.8

*Youth <18 years of age: goal hemoglobin A$_{1c}$ <7.5%.
**1 to 2 hours after beginning a meal for adults, except bedtime for older adults.
[†]American Diabetes Association (2015); Chiang et al (2014).
[‡]Lower goals may be appropriate for selected individuals if this can be accomplished safely (without significant hypoglycemia). Higher goals may be appropriate in some individuals (e.g., with a history of severe hypoglycemia, limited life expectancy, advanced complications, extensive comorbid conditions, or long-standing diabetes in whom the goal is difficult to achieve with appropriate education, monitoring, and therapies, including insulin).
[§]AACE, American Association of Clinical Endocrinologists, 2015.
[¶]For patients without concurrent serious illness and at low hypoglycemia risk.
(McPherson RA, Pincus MR: Henry's Clinical Diagnosis and Management by Laboratory Methods, 23rd ed, ISBN # 978-0323-29568-0, 2017, Elsevier)

120 min: 5-15 mg/dl (0.28-0.83 mmol/L [CF: 0.05551; SMI: 0.1 mmol/L])
180 min: fasting level or below
Abnormal in: Glucose intolerance, diabetes mellitus, Cushing's syndrome, acromegaly, pheochromocytoma, gestational diabetes

GLUCOSE-6-PHOSPHATE DEHYDROGENASE (G6PD) SCREEN (blood)

Normal: G6PD enzyme activity detected
Abnormal: If a deficiency is detected, quantitation of G6PD is necessary; a G6PD screen may be falsely interpreted as "normal" after an episode of hemolysis because most G6PD-deficient cells have been destroyed.

γ-GLUTAMYL TRANSFERASE (GGT)

Normal range: 0-30 U/L (0.050 μkat/L [CF: 0.01667; SMI: 0.01 μkat/L])
Elevated in: Chronic alcoholic liver disease, neoplasms (hepatoma, metastatic disease to the liver, carcinoma of the pancreas), systemic lupus erythematosus, congestive heart failure, trauma, nephrotic syndrome, sepsis, cholestasis, drugs (phenytoin, barbiturates)

GLYCOHEMOGLOBIN (glycated glycosylated] hemoglobin), (HbA1c)

Normal range: 4.0%-5.9%. Glycemic goals in adults are summarized in Table 37.
Elevated in: Uncontrolled diabetes mellitus (glycated hemoglobin levels reflect the level of glucose control over the preceding 120 days), lead toxicity, alcoholism, iron deficiency anemia, hypertriglyceridemia
Decreased in: Hemolytic anemias, decreased red blood cell survival, pregnancy, acute or chronic blood loss, chronic renal failure, insulinoma, congenital spherocytosis, hemoglobin S, C, and D diseases

GROWTH HORMONE

Normal: Male: 1-9 ng/ml; female: 1-16 ng/ml
Elevated in: Pituitary gigantism, acromegaly, ectopic GH secretion, cirrhosis, renal failure, anorexia nervosa, stress, exercise, prolonged fasting, amphetamines, beta-blockers, insulin, levodopa, metoclopramide, clonidine, vasopressin, human growth hormone (HGH) supplementation
Decreased in: Hypopituitarism, pituitary dwarfism, adrenocortical hyperfunction, bromocriptine, corticosteroids, glucose

GROWTH HORMONE RELEASING HORMONE (GHRH)

Normal: <50 pg/ml
Elevated in: Acromegaly caused by GHRH secretion by neoplasms

GROWTH HORMONE SUPPRESSION TEST (after glucose)

Normal: Test is done by giving 1.75 g glucose/kg orally after overnight fast. Blood is drawn at baseline, after 60 min, and after 120 min of glucose load. Normal response is growth hormone suppression to <2 ng/ml or undetectable levels.
Abnormal: There is no or incomplete suppression from the high basal level in gigantism or acromegaly.

HAM TEST (acid serum test)

Normal: Negative
Positive in: Paroxysmal nocturnal hemoglobinuria
False-positive in: Hereditary or acquired spherocytosis, recent transfusion with aged red blood cells, aplastic anemia, myeloproliferative syndromes, leukemia, hereditary dyserythropoietic anemia type II

HAPTOGLOBIN (serum)

Normal range: 50-220 mg/dl (0.50-2.2 g/L [CF: 0.01; SMI: 0.01 g/L])
Elevated in: Inflammation (acute phase reactant), collagen vascular diseases, infections (acute phase reactant), drugs (androgens), obstructive liver disease
Decreased in: Hemolysis (intravascular more than extravascular), megaloblastic anemia, severe liver disease, large tissue hematomas, infectious mononucleosis, drugs (oral contraceptives)

HBA$_{1C}$

See GLYCOHEMOGLOBIN

HDL

See HIGH-DENSITY LIPOPROTEIN CHOLESTEROL

HELICOBACTER PYLORI (serology, stool antigen)

Normal range: Not detected
Detected in: H. pylori infection. Positive serology can indicate current or past infection. Positive stool antigen test indicates acute infection (sensitivity and specificity >90%). Stool testing should be delayed at least 4 weeks after eradication therapy.

HEMATOCRIT

Normal range
Male: 39%-49% (0.39-0.49 [CF: 0.01; SMI: 0.01])
Female: 33%-43% (0.33-0.43 [CF: 0.01; SMI: 0.01])
Elevated in: Polycythemia vera, smoking, chronic obstructive pulmonary disease, high altitudes, dehydration, hypovolemia
Decreased in: Blood loss (gastrointestinal, genitourinary) anemia

TABLE 38 Neonatal Hemoglobin (Hb) Electrophoresis Patterns*

FA	Fetal Hb and adult normal Hb; the normal newborn pattern.
FAV	Indicates the presence of both HbF and HbA. However, an anomalous band (V) is present, which does not appear to be any of the common Hb variants.
FAS	Indicates fetal Hb, adult normal HbA, and HbS, consistent with benign sickle cell trait.
FS	Fetal and sickle HbS without detectable adult normal HbA. Consistent with clinically significant homozygous sickle Hb genotype (S/S) or sickle β-thalassemia, with manifestations of sickle cell anemia during childhood.
FC†	Designates the presence of HbC without adult normal HbA. Consistent with clinically significant homozygous HbC genotype (C/C), resulting in a mild hematologic disorder presenting during childhood.
FSC	HbS and HbC present. This heterozygous condition could lead to the manifestations of sickle cell disease during childhood.
FAC	HbC and adult normal HbA present, consistent with benign HbC trait.
FSA	Heterozygous HbS/β-thalassemia, a clinically significant sickling disorder.
F†	Fetal HbF is present without adult normal HbA. Although this may indicate a delayed appearance of HbA, it is also consistent with homozygous β-thalassemia major, or homozygous hereditary persistence of fetal HbF.
FV†	Fetal HbF and an anomalous Hb variant (V) are present.
AF	May indicate prior blood transfusion. Submit another filter paper blood specimen when the infant is 4 mo of age, at which time the transfused blood cells should have been cleared.

From Tschudy MM, Arcara KM: *The Harriet Lane handbook,* ed 19, Philadelphia, 2012, Mosby.
NOTE: HbA: α2β2; HbF: α2γ2; HbA2: α2δ2.
*Hemoglobin variants are reported in order of decreasing abundance; for example, FA indicates more fetal than adult hemoglobin.
†Repeat blood specimen should be submitted to confirm the original interpretation.

HEMOGLOBIN

Normal range
Male: 13.6-17.7 g/dl (136-172 g/L [CF: 10; SMI: 1 g/L])
Female: 12.0-15.0 g/dl (120-150 g/L [CF: 10; SMI: 1 g/L])
Elevated in: Hemoconcentration, dehydration, polycythemia vera, chronic obstructive pulmonary disease, high altitudes, false elevations (hyperlipemic plasma, white blood cells >50,000/mm^3), stress
Decreased in: Hemorrhagic (gastrointestinal, genitourinary) anemia

HEMOGLOBIN A$_{1C}$

See GLYCOHEMOGLOBIN

HEMOGLOBIN ELECTROPHORESIS

Table 38 describes neonatal hemoglobin electrophoresis patterns, Table 39 summarizes types of hemoglobin, and Table 40 describes classifications of hemoglobinopathies.
Normal range
HbA$_1$: 95%-98%
HbA$_2$: 1.5%-3.5%
HbF: <2%
HbC: absent
HbS: absent

HEMOGLOBIN, GLYCATED

See GLYCOHEMOGLOBIN

HEMOGLOBIN, GLYCOSYLATED

See GLYCOHEMOGLOBIN

HEMOGLOBIN H

See Table 39.
Normal: Negative

TABLE 39 Types of Hemoglobin

	Hemoglobin	Structure	Comment
Normal	A	$\alpha_2\beta_2$	97% of adult hemoglobin
	A$_2$	$\alpha_2\delta_2$	2% of adult Hb; elevated in β-thalassemia
	F	$\alpha_2\gamma_2$	Normal Hb in fetus from 3rd to 9th month; increased in β-thalassemia
Abnormal chain production	H	β_4	Found in α-thalassemia, biologically useless
	Barts	γ_4	Found in α-thalassemia, biologically useless
Abnormal chain structure	S	$\alpha_2\beta_2$	Substitution of valine for glutamic acid in position 6 of β chain
	C	$\alpha_2\beta_2$	Substitution of lysine for glutamic acid in position 6 of β chain

From Ballinger A: *Kumar & Clark's essentials of clinical medicine,* ed 6, Edinburgh, 2012, Saunders.

TABLE 40 Classification of Hemoglobinopathies

Structural hemoglobinopathies—hemoglobins with altered amino acid sequences that result in deranged function or altered physical or chemical properties
Abnormal Hemoglobin Polymerization—HBS
Altered Oxygen Affinity
High affinity—polycythemia
Low affinity—cyanosis, pseudoanemia
Hemoglobins That Oxidize Readily
Unstable hemoglobins, hemolytic anemia, jaundice
M hemoglobins—methemoglobinemia, cyanosis
Thalassemias—Defective Production of Globin Chains
α-Thalassemias
β-Thalassemias
δβ-, γδβ-, αβ-Thalassemias
Structural hemoglobinopathies—structurally abnormal Hb associated with coinherited thalassemia phenotype
HbE
Hb Constant Spring
Hb Lepore
Hereditary Persistence of Fetal Hemoglobin—Persistence of High Levels of Hbf Into Adult Life
Pancellular—all red blood cells contain elevated HbF levels
Nondeletion forms
Deletion forms
Hb Kenya
Heterocellular—only specific subpopulation of red blood cells contain elevated levels of HbF
Acquired Hemoglobinopathies
Methemoglobin due to toxic exposures
Sulfhemoglobin due to toxic exposures
Carboxyhemoglobin
HbH in erythroleukemia
Elevated HbF in states of erythroid stress and bone marrow dysplasia, usually heterocellular

From Hoffman R: *Hematology: basic principles and practice,* ed 6, Philadelphia, 2013, Saunders.
Hb, Hemoglobin.

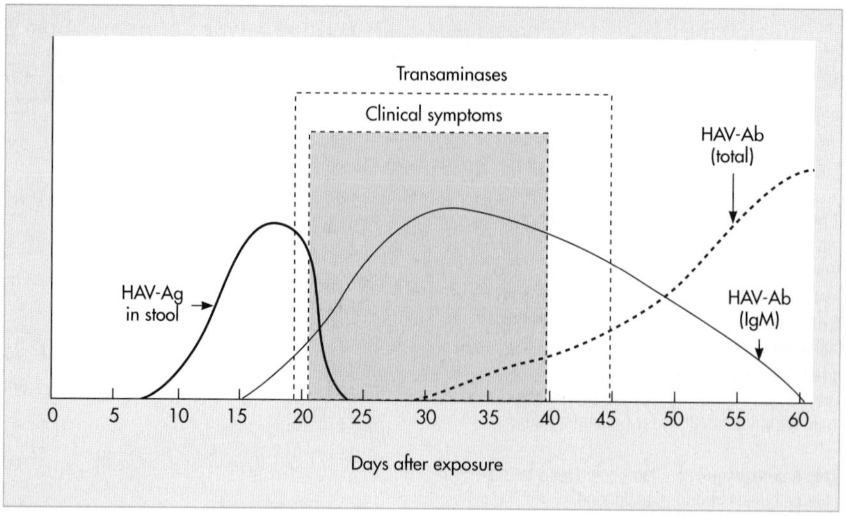

FIG. 20 Serologic tests in HAV infection. (From Ravel R [ed]: *Clinical laboratory medicine,* ed 6, St Louis, 1995, Mosby.)

Present in

Hemoglobin H disease, alpha-thalassemia trait, unstable hemoglobin disorders

HEMOGLOBIN, URINE

See URINE HEMOGLOBIN, FREE

HEMOSIDERIN, URINE

See URINE HEMOGLOBIN, FREE

HEPARIN-INDUCED THROMBOCYTOPENIA ANTIBODIES

Normal: Antigen assay: Negative, <0.45; weak, 0.45-1.0; strong, >1.0
Elevated in: Heparin-induced thrombocytopenia

HEPATITIS A ANTIBODY

Normal: Negative
Present in: Viral hepatitis A; can be IgM or IgG (if IgM, acute hepatitis A; if IgG, previous infection with hepatitis A)
   See Fig. 20 for serologic tests in HAV infection.

HAV-IgM ANTIBODY

Appearance: About the same time as clinical symptoms (3-4 weeks after exposure; range, 14-60 days), or just before beginning of AST/ALT elevation (range, 10 days before to 7 days after)
Peak: About 3-4 weeks after onset of symptoms (1-6 weeks)
Becomes nondetectable: 3-4 months after onset of symptoms (1-6 months). In a few cases HAV-IgM antibody can persist as long as 12-14 months.

HAV TOTAL ANTIBODY

Appearance: About 3 weeks after IgM becomes detectable (therefore about the middle of clinical symptom period to early convalescence)
Peak: About 1-2 months after onset
Becomes nondetectable: Remains elevated for life but can somewhat slowly fall

HEPATITIS A VIRAL INFECTION

Best all-purpose test(s) to diagnose acute HAV infection = HAV-Ab (IgM)
Best all-purpose test(s) to demonstrate past HAV infection/immunity = HAV-Ab (total)

HEPATITIS B SURFACE ANTIGEN (HBsAg)

Normal: Not detected
Detected in: Acute viral hepatitis type B, chronic hepatitis B
Appearance: 2-6 weeks after exposure (range, 6 days to 6 months); 5%-15% of patients are negative at onset of jaundice

TABLE 41   Serologic Markers of Hepatitis B Infection

	HBsAg	anti-HBc	anti-HBs	IgM anti-HBc
Susceptible to infection	Negative	Negative	Negative	Negative
Immune due to natural infection	Negative	Positive	Positive	Negative
Immune due to hepatitis B vaccination	Negative	Negative	Positive	Negative
Acutely infected	Positive	Positive	Negative	Positive
Chronically infected	Positive	Positive	Negative	Negative

From Ballinger A: *Kumar & Clark's essentials of clinical medicine,* ed 6, Edinburgh, 2012, Saunders.

Peak: 1-2 weeks before to 1-2 weeks after onset of symptoms
Becomes nondetectable: 1-3 months after peak (range, 1 week to 5 months)

HEPATITIS B VIRAL INFECTION

See Table 41
   Figs. 21, 22, and 23 illustrate antigens and antibodies in hepatitis B infection.
HB$_s$
-Ag
HB$_S$Ag: shows current active HBV infection.
Persistence over 6 months indicates carrier/chronic HBV infection.
HBV nucleic acid probe: present before and longer than HB$_S$Ag.
More reliable marker for increased infectivity than HB$_S$Ag and/or HB$_e$Ag.
-Ab
HB$_S$Ab-total: shows previous healed HBV infection and evidence of immunity.
HB$_c$
-Ab
HB$_C$Ab-IgM: shows either acute or very recent infection by HBV.
In convalescent phase of acute HBV, may be elevated when HB$_S$Ag has disappeared (core window).
Negative HB$_C$Ab-IgM with positive HB$_S$Ag suggests either very early acute HBV or carrier/chronic HBV.
HB$_C$Ab-total: only useful to show past HBV infection if HB$_S$Ag and HB$_C$Ab-IgM are both negative.
HB$_e$
-Ag
HB$_e$-AbAg: when present, especially without HB$_e$Ab, suggests increased patient infectivity.
HB$_e$Ab-total: when present, suggests less patient infectivity.
   HB$_S$Ag positive, HB$_C$Ab negative

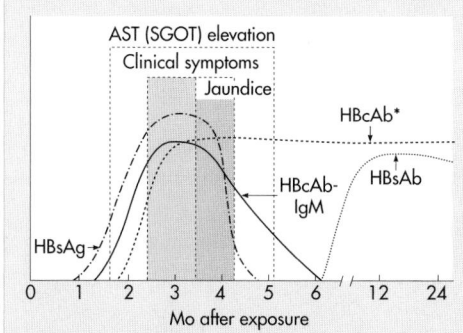

FIG. 21 HBV surface antigen-antibody and core antibodies. Note "core window." *HB$_C$Ab = HB$_C$Ab-IgM + HBCAb-IgG (combined). (From Ravel R [ed]: *Clinical laboratory medicine,* ed 6, St Louis, 1995, Mosby.)

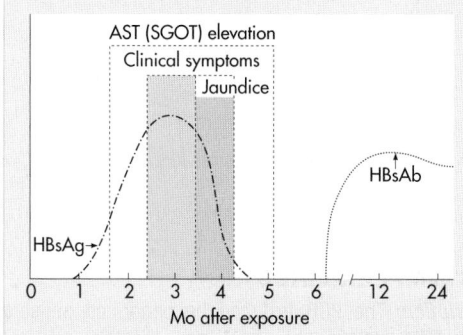

FIG. 22 HBV surface antigen and antibody (HB$_S$Ag and HB$_S$Ab-total). (From Ravel R [ed]: *Clinical laboratory medicine,* ed 6, St Louis, 1995, Mosby.)

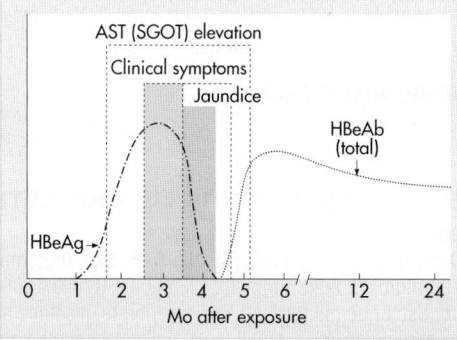

FIG. 23 HBVe antigen and antibody. (From Ravel R [ed]: *Clinical laboratory medicine,* ed 6, St Louis, 1995, Mosby.)

About 5% (range, 0%-17%) of patients with early-stage HBV acute infection (HB$_C$Ab rises later)

HB$_S$Ag positive, HB$_C$Ab positive, HB$_S$Ab negative
  Most of the clinical symptom stage
  Chronic HBV carriers without evidence of liver disease ("asymptomatic carriers")
  Chronic HBV hepatitis (chronic persistent type or chronic active type)

HB$_S$Ag negative, HB$_C$Ab positive,* HB$_S$Ab negative
  Late clinical symptom stage or early convalescence stage (core window)
  Chronic HBV infection with HB$_S$Ag below detection levels with current tests
  Old previous HBV infection

HB$_S$Ag negative, HB$_C$Ab positive, HB$_S$Ab positive
  Late convalescence to complete recovery
  Old infection

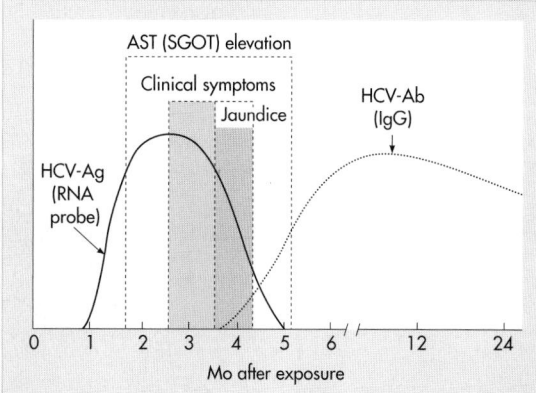

FIG. 24 HCV antigen and antibody. (From Ravel R [ed]: *Clinical laboratory medicine,* ed 6, St Louis, 1995, Mosby.)

TABLE 42	Interpretation of Patterns of HCV Markers		
Interpretation	**Anti-HCV**	**RIBA**	**HCV RNA**
Acute HCV infection	−	−	+
Active HCV infection	+	+	+
Possible HCV clearance	+	+	−
False-positive HCV test	+	−	−
Requires further study	+	Indeterminate*	−

HCV, Hepatitis C; *RIBA,* recombinant immunoassay.
*Indeterminate result: only one band positive, or more than one band and nonspecific reactivity.
(McPherson RA, Pincus MR: Henry's Clinical Diagnosis and Management by Laboratory Methods, 23rd ed, ISBN # 978-0323-29568-0, 2017, Elsevier.)

HEPATITIS C VIRAL INFECTION

Fig. 24 illustrates antigens and antibodies in hepatitis C infection. Table 42 summarizes interpretation of patterns of HCV markers.

HEPATITIS C RNA

Normal: Negative

Elevated in: Hepatitis C. Detection of hepatitis C-RNA is used to confirm current infection and to monitor treatment. Quantitative assays (viral load) are needed before treatment to assess response (<2 log decrease after 12-week treatment indicates lack of response).

HCV
-Ag
HCV nucleic acid probe: shows current infection by HCV (especially with PCR amplification).
-Ab
HCV-Ab (IgG): current, convalescent, or old HCV infection.

HAV
-Ag
HAV-Ag by EM: shows presence of virus in stool early in infection.
-Ab
HAV-Ab (IgM): current or recent HAV infection.
HAV-Ab (total): convalescent or old HAV infection.

HEPATITIS D VIRAL INFECTION

Fig. 25 illustrates antigens and antibodies in hepatitis D infection.
Best current all-purpose screening test = HDV-Ab (total)
Best test to differentiate acute from chronic infection = HDV-Ab (IgM)

DELTA HEPATITIS COINFECTION (ACUTE HDV1 ACUTE HBV) OR SUPERINFECTION (ACUTE HDV1 CHRONIC HBV)

HDV
-Ag
HDV-Ag: shows current infection (acute or chronic) by HDV.
HDV nucleic acid probe: detects antigen before and longer than HDV-Ag by EIA.

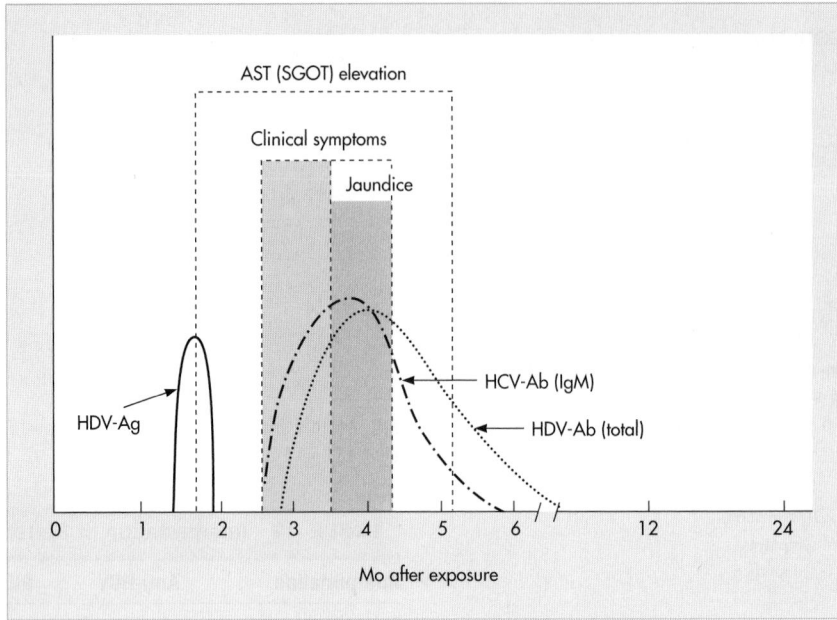

FIG. 25 HDV antigen and antibodies. (From Ravel R [ed]: *Clinical laboratory medicine,* ed 6, St Louis, 1995, Mosby.)

-Ab

HDV-Ab (IgM): high elevation in acute HDV; does not persist.

Low or moderate elevation in convalescent HDV; does not persist.

Low to high persistent elevation in chronic HDV (depends on degree of cell injury and sensitivity of the assay).

HDV-Ab (total): high elevation in acute HDV; does not persist.

High persistent elevation in chronic HDV.

HDV-Ag

Detected by DNA probe, less often by immunoassay

Appearance: Prodromal stage (before symptoms); just at or after initial rise in ALT (about a week after appearance of HB_SAg and about the time HB_CAb-IgM level begins to rise)

Peak: 2-3 days after onset

Becomes nondetectable: 1-4 days (may persist until shortly after symptoms appear)

HDV-Ab (IgM)

Appearance: About 10 days after symptoms begin (range, 1-28 days)

Peak: About 2 weeks after first detection

Becomes nondetectable: About 35 days (range, 10-80 days) after first detection (most other IgM antibodies take 3-6 months to become nondetectable)

HDV-Ab (total)

Appearance: About 50 days after symptoms begin (range, 14-80 days); about 5 weeks after HDV-Ag (range, 3-11 weeks)

Peak: About 2 weeks after first detection

Becomes nondetectable: About 7 months after first detection (range, 4-14 months)

HER-2/*NEU*

Normal: Negative

Present in: 25%-30% of primary breast cancers. It can also be found in other epithelial tumors, including lung, hepatocellular, pancreatic, colon, stomach, ovarian, cervical, and bladder cancer. Trastuzumab (Herceptin) is a humanized monoclonal antibody against Her-2/*neu*. This test is useful to identify patients with metastatic; recurrent; and/or treatment-refractory, unresectable, locally advanced breast cancer for trastuzumab treatment.

HERPES SIMPLEX VIRUS (HSV)

Test description: The PCR test can be performed on serum biopsy samples, CSF, vitreous humor.

HFE SCREEN FOR HEREDITARY HEMOCHROMATOSIS

Test description: PCR test can be performed on whole blood or tissue. One mutation (C282Y) and two polymorphisms (H63D, S65C) account for the majority of alleles associated with this disease.

HETEROPHIL ANTIBODY

Normal: Negative

Positive in: Infectious mononucleosis

HIGH-DENSITY LIPOPROTEIN (HDL) **CHOLESTEROL**

Normal range

Male: 40-70 mg/dl (0.8-1.8 mmol/L [CF: 0.02586; SMI: 0.05 mmol/L])

Female: 50-90 mg/dl (1.1-2.35 mmol/L [CF: 0.02586; SMI: 0.05 mmol/L])

Increased in: Use of gemfibrozil, statins, fenofibrate, nicotinic acid, estrogens, regular aerobic exercise, small (1 oz) daily alcohol intake

Decreased in: Deficiency of apoproteins, liver disease, probucol ingestion, Tangier disease

NOTE: A cholesterol/HDL ratio >4.0 is associated with increased risk of coronary artery disease. Table 43 summarizes significant human apolipoproteins.

HLA ANTIGENS

Associated disorders: see Table 44

HOMOCYSTEINE (plasma)

Normal range

0-30 years: 4.6-8.1 mcmol/L

30-59 years: 6.3-11.2 mcmol/L (males), 4.5-7.9 mcmol/L (females)

>59 years: 5.8-11.9 mcmol/L

Increased: Thrombophilic states, B_6, B_{12}, folic acid, riboflavin deficiency, pregnancy, homocystinuria

NOTE: An increased homocysteine level is an independent risk factor for atherosclerosis.

TABLE 43   Significant Human Apolipoproteins

Apolipoprotein	Major Lipoproteins	Mr* (kDa)	Amino Acids	Chromosome	PLASMA CONCENTRATION mmol/L	mg/dL
A-I	HDL	29	243-245	11	32-46	90-130
A-II	HDL	17.4	154	1	18-29	30-50
A-IV	HDL, LDL	44.5	396	11		
(a)	Lp(a)	350-700	Variable	6		
B-100	VLDL, IDL, LDL	512.7	4536	2	1.5-1.8	80-100
B-48	CM	240.8	2152	2	<0.2	<5
C-I	CM, LDL	6.6	57	19	6.1-10.8	4-7
C-II	CM, LDL	8.9	78 or 79	19	3.4-9.1	3-8
C-III	CM	8.8	79	11	9.1-17.1	8-15
D	HDL	19	169	3		
E	CM, LDL, IDL	34.1	299	19	0.8-1.6	3-6
F	HDL, LDL, VLDL	29	162	12		8.35
H	VLDL	50	326	17		20
J	HDL	80	449	8		
L	HDL	39-42	383	22	Not present in plasma	
M	HDL, LDL, VLDL, CM	26	188	6		2-15
0	HDL, LDL, VLDL	22.3	198	X		

CM, Chylomicron; *HDL*, high-density lipoprotein; *IDL*, intermediate-density lipoprotein; *LDL*, low-density lipoprotein; *Lp(a)*, lipoprotein A; *VLDL*, very-low-density lipoprotein.
*Relative molecular mass.
(McPherson RA, Pincus MR: Henry's Clinical Diagnosis and Management by Laboratory Methods, 23rd ed, ISBN # 978-0323-29568-0, 2017, Elsevier)

TABLE 44   HLA Antigens Associated with Specific Diseases

Antigen	Condition	Antigen	Condition
HLA-B27	Ankylosing spondylitis	HLA-B8, Dw3	Celiac disease
	Reiter's syndrome	HLA-B8, Dw3	Dermatitis herpetiformis
	Psoriatic arthritis	HLA-B8	Myasthenia gravis
HLA-A10, B18, Dw2	C2 deficiency	HLA-B8	Chronic active hepatitis in children
HLA-A2, B40, Cw3	C4 deficiency	HLA-Drw4	Active chronic hepatitis in adults
HLA-B7, Dw2	Multiple sclerosis	HLA-B13, Bw17	Psoriasis
HLA-A3	Hemochromatosis		

From Cerra FB: *Manual of critical care*, St Louis, 1987, Mosby.
HLA, Human leukocyte antigen.

HUMAN CHORIONIC GONADOTROPIN (hCG)

Normal range: Varies with gestational stage:

1 wk:	5-50 mU/ml
1-2 wk:	50-550 mU/ml
2-3 wk:	up to 5000 mU/ml
3-4 wk:	up to 10,000 mU/ml
4-5 wk:	up to 50,000 mU/ml
2-3 mo:	10,000-100,000 mU/ml

Elevated in: Normal pregnancy, hydatidiform mole, choriocarcinoma, germ cell tumors of testicle, some nontrophoblastic neoplasms (e.g., neoplasms of cervix, gastrointestinal tract, ovary, lung, breast)

HUMAN HERPES VIRUS 8 (HHV8)

Test description: PCR test can be performed on whole blood, tissue, bone marrow, and urine. HHV8 is found in all forms of Kaposi's sarcoma.

HUMAN IMMUNODEFICIENCY VIRUS ANTIBODY, TYPE 1 (HIV-1)

Normal range: Not detected

Abnormal result: HIV antibodies usually appear in the blood 1-4 months after infection.

Testing sequence

ELISA is the recommended initial screening test. Sensitivity and specificity are >99%. False-positive ELISA may occur with autoimmune disorders, administration of immune globulin manufactured before 1985, within 6 weeks of testing, in the presence of rheumatoid factor, in the presence of DLA-DR antibodies in multigravida female, with administration of influenza vaccine within 3 months of testing, with hemodialysis, with positive plasma reagin test, and with certain medical disorders (hemophilia, hypergammaglobulinemia, alcoholic hepatitis).

A positive ELISA is confirmed with Western blot (Fig. 26). False-positive Western blot may result from connective tissue disorders, human leukocyte antigen antibodies, polyclonal gammopathies, hyperbilirubinemia, presence of antibody to another human retrovirus, or cross-reaction with other non-virus-derived proteins in healthy persons. Undetermined Western blot may occur in AIDS patients with advanced immunodeficiency (caused by loss of antibodies) and in recent HIV infections.

PCR is used to confirm indeterminate Western blot results or negative results in persons with suspected HIV infection.

Fig. 27 describes tests in HIV infection; indications for plasma HIV RNA testing are described in Table 45.

HUMAN IMMUNODEFICIENCY VIRUS TYPE 1 (HIV-1) ANTIGEN (P24), QUALITATIVE (P24 ANTIGEN)

Normal range: Negative. This test detects uncomplexed HIV-1 p24 antigen. The core protein p24 is the first detectable protein encoded by the group-specific antigen *(gag)* gene. This protein is a marker for viremia. This test should not be used in place of HIV-1 antibody testing as a screen for HIV-1 infection. HIV-1 p24 may be detectable in the first month of acute HIV-1 infection and generally falls to undetectable levels during the asymptomatic stage of HIV-1 infection. A negative result does not exclude the possibility of infection or exposure to HIV-1. It is recommended that a negative result be followed with repeat testing at least 8 weeks after the

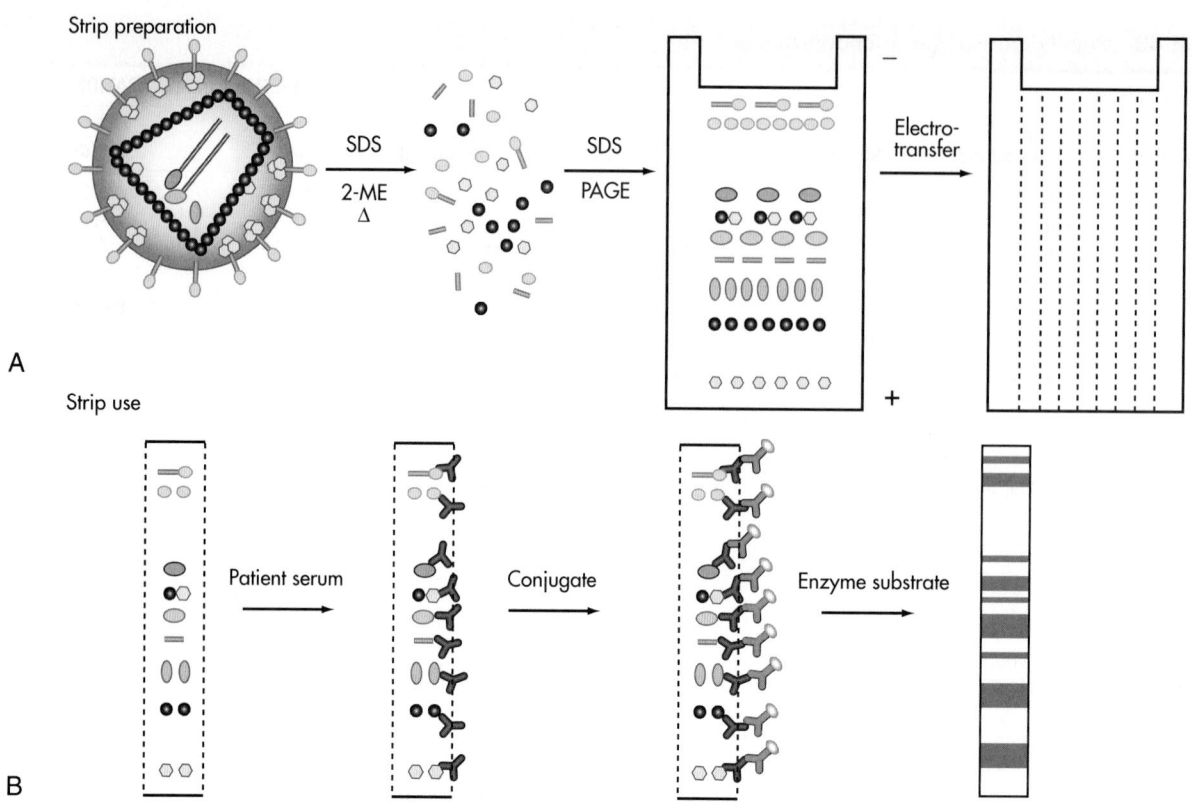

FIG. 26 Human immunodeficiency virus (HIV) Western blot. A, Western blot strips are prepared with purified HIV virions that are disrupted with ionic detergent and reducing agent, subjected to sodium dodecyl sulfate–polyacrylamide gel electrophoresis (SDS-PAGE), and electrotransferred to solid strips, typically of nitrocellulose. **B,** Strips are sequentially incubated with patient sample (serum, plasma, saliva, or urine); enzyme-conjugated antihuman IgG; and enzyme substrate. The positions of enzymes bound identify the presence of antibody to individual HIV proteins. (From Bennett JE , Dolin R, Blaser MJ: *Mandell, Douglas, and Bennett's principles and practice of infectious diseases,* ed 8, Philadelphia, 2015, Saunders.)

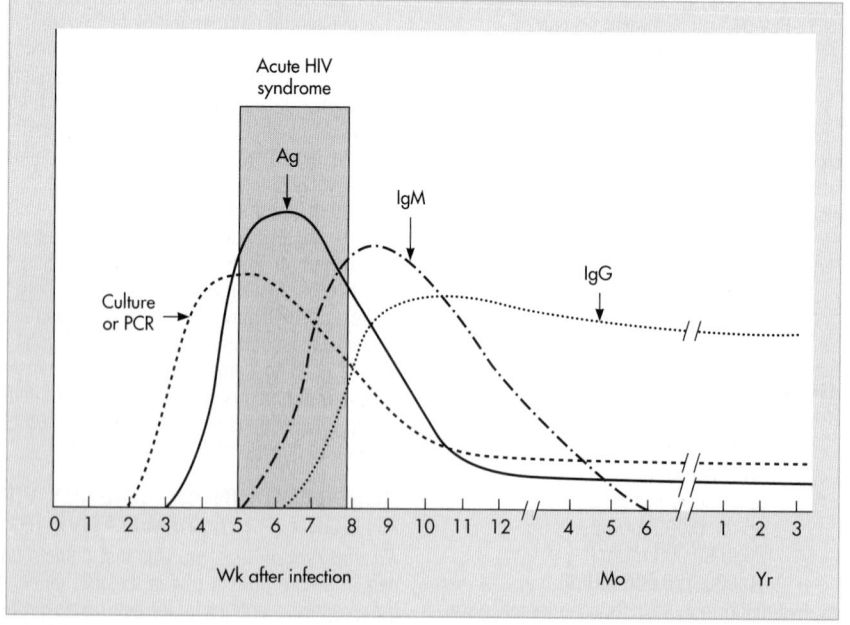

FIG. 27 Tests in HIV-1 infection. (From Ravel R [ed]: *Clinical laboratory medicine,* ed 6, St Louis, 1995, Mosby.)

TABLE 45 Indications for Plasma HIV RNA Testing*

Clinical Indication	Information	Use
Syndrome consistent with acute HIV infection	Establishes diagnosis when HIV antibody test is negative or indeterminate	Diagnosis[†]
Initial evaluation of newly diagnosed HIV infection	Baseline viral load set point	Decision to start or defer therapy
Every 3-4 mo in patients not on therapy	Changes in viral load	Decision to start therapy
4-8 wk after initiation of antiretroviral therapy	Initial assessment of drug efficacy	Decision to continue or change therapy
3-4 mo after start of therapy	Maximal effect of therapy	Decision to continue or change therapy
Every 3-4 mo in patients on therapy	Durability of antiretroviral effect	Decision to continue or change therapy
Clinical event or significant decline in CD4+ T cells	Association with changing or stable	Decision to continue, initiate, or change

From Report of the NIH Panel to Define Principles of Therapy of HIV Infection, *MMWR Recomm Rep* 47(RR-5):1-41, 1998.
*Acute illness (e.g., bacterial pneumonia, tuberculosis, HSV, PCP) and immunizations can cause increase in plasma HIV RNA for 2-4 wk; viral load testing should not be performed during this time. Plasma HIV RNA results should usually be verified with a repeat determination before starting or making changes in therapy. HIV RNA should be measured using the same laboratory and the same assay.
[†]Diagnosis of HIV infection determined by HIV RNA testing should be confirmed by standard methods (e.g., Western blot serology) performed 2-4 mo after the initial indeterminate or negative test.

original test. This test is used primarily for screening of donated blood and plasma and as an aid for the prognosis of HIV-1 infection.

HUMAN IMMUNODEFICIENCY VIRUS TYPE 1 (HIV-1) VIRAL LOAD

Normal range: HIV-1 RNA, quant. bDNA 3: less than 50 copies/ml or less than 1.7 log copies/ml

This test should be used only in individuals with documented HIV-1 infection for monitoring the progression of infection, response to antiretroviral therapy, and disease prognosis. It is not indicated for diagnosis of HIV infection.

HUMAN PAPILLOMA VIRUS (HPV)

Test description: PCR test can be performed on cervical smears, biopsies, scrapings, liquid cytology specimen, and anogenital tissues.

HUNTINGTON'S DISEASE PCR

Test description: PCR can be performed on whole blood. Huntington's disease is caused by the expansion of the trinucleotide repeat CAG within IT 15 (huntingtin). Pre- and post-test counseling should be performed when ordering this test.

HYDROGEN BREATH TEST

See BREATH HYDROGEN TEST

5-HYDROXYINDOLE-ACETIC ACID, URINE

See URINE 5-HYDROXYINDOLE-ACETIC ACID

IMMUNE COMPLEX ASSAY

Normal: Negative
Detected in: Collagen vascular disorders, glomerulonephritis, neoplastic diseases, malaria, primary biliary cirrhosis, chronic acute hepatitis, bacterial endocarditis, vasculitis

IMMUNOGLOBULINS

Normal range

IgA:	50-350 mg/dl (0.5-3.5 g/L [CF: 0.01; SMI: 0.01 g/L])
IgD:	<6 mg/dl (<60 mg/L [CF: 0.01; SMI: 0.01 g/L])
IgE:	<25 μg/dl (<0.00025 g/L [CF: 0.01; SMI: 0.01 g/L])
IgG:	800-1500 mg/dl (8-15 g/L [CF: 0.01; SMI: 0.01 g/L])
IgM:	45-150 mg/dl (0.45-1.5 g/L [CF: 0.01; SMI: 0.01 g/L])

Table 46 summarizes biologic properties of human immunoglobulin isotopes. Box 18 summarizes selected conditions associated with monoclonal immunoglobulins. Disease states associated with polyclonal hyperimmunoglobulinemia are described in Table 47.
Elevated in
IgA: Lymphoproliferative disorders, Berger's nephropathy, chronic infections, autoimmune disorders, liver disease

IgE: Allergic disorders, parasitic infections, immunologic disorders, IgE myeloma (see Box 16 for summary of nonallergic diseases associated with high levels of IgE. Box 17 summarizes conditions with very high IgE levels)
IgG: Chronic granulomatous infections, infectious diseases, inflammation, myeloma, liver disease
IgM: Primary biliary cirrhosis, infectious diseases (brucellosis, malaria), Waldenström's macroglobulinemia, liver disease
Decreased in:
IgA: Nephrotic syndrome, protein-losing enteropathy, congenital deficiency, lymphocytic leukemia, ataxia-telangiectasia, chronic sinopulmonary disease
IgE: Hypogammaglobulinemia, neoplasms (breast, bronchial, cervical), ataxia-telangiectasia, primary biliary cirrhosis (see Box 16)
IgG: Congenital or acquired deficiency, lymphocytic leukemia, phenytoin, methylprednisolone, nephrotic syndrome, protein-losing enteropathy
IgM: Congenital deficiency, lymphocytic leukemia, nephrotic syndrome

INDIRECT ANTIGLOBULIN (Coombs Indirect)

Normal: Negative
Positive: Acquired hemolytic anemia, incompatible cross-matched blood, anti-Rh antibodies, drugs (methyldopa, mefenamic acid, levodopa)
Fig. 28 illustrates the mechanism of Coombs test.

INFLUENZA A AND B TESTS

Test description: PCR can be performed on nasopharyngeal swab, wash, or aspirate
Normal: Negative

INSULIN AUTOANTIBODIES

Normal: Negative
Present in: Exogenous insulin from insulin therapy. The presence of islet cell antibodies indicates ongoing beta cell destruction. This test is useful in the early diagnosis of type 1a diabetes mellitus and in the identification of patients at high risk for type 1a diabetes.

INSULIN, FREE

Normal: <17 mcU/ml
Elevated in: Insulin overdose, insulin resistance syndromes, endogenous hyperinsulinemia
Decreased in: Inadequately treated type 1 diabetes mellitus

INSULIN-LIKE GROWTH FACTOR-1 (IGF-1) (Serum)

Normal range

Ages 16-24:	182-780 ng/ml
Ages 25-39:	114-492 ng/ml
Ages 40-54:	90-360 ng/ml
Ages >55:	71-290 ng/ml

Elevated in: Adolescence, acromegaly, pregnancy, precocious puberty, obesity
Decreased in: Malnutrition, delayed puberty, diabetes mellitus, hypopituitarism, cirrhosis, old age

TABLE 46 Selected Biologic Properties of Human Immunoglobulin Isotypes

Characteristics	IgG1	IgG2	IgG3	IgG4	IgM	IgA1	IgA2	IgD	IgE
Physical Properties									
Molecular weight (kD)	146	146	165	146	970*	160	160	170	190
Serum half-life (days)	29	27	7	16	5	6	6	–	2
Anatomic Distribution									
Mean serum level (mg/mL)	5-12	2-6	0.5-1.0	0.2-1.0	0.5-1.5	0.5-2.0	0-0.2	0-0.4	0-0.002
Transport across placenta	+++	+	++	±	–	–	–	–	–
Transport across epithelium	–	–	–	–	+	+++†	+++†	–	–
Extravascular diffusion	+++	+++	+++	+++	±	++‡	++‡	+	+
Functional Activity									
Antigen neutralization	++	++	++	++	++	++	++	–	–
Complement fixation	++	+	++	–	+++	+	+	–	–
ADCC	+	+	+	±	–	–	–	–	+
Immediate hypersensitivity	–	–	–	–	–	–	–	–	+++

From Adkinson NF et al: *Middleton's allergy principles and practice*, ed 8, Philadelphia, 2014, Saunders.
ADCC, Antibody-dependent cellular cytotoxicity; –, no effect; ±, no effect or negligible degree; +, small degree; ++, moderate degree; +++, large degree.
*Pentameric IgM plus J chain.
†Dimer.
‡Monomer.

BOX 16 Nonallergic Diseases Associated with Altered Total Serum Immunoglobulin E Levels

Increased Levels (≥500 IU/ml)

Parasitic Diseases
Ascariasis
Visceral larva migrans
Capillariasis
Paragonimiasis
Fascioliasis
Schistosomiasis
Hookworm
Trichinosis
Filariasis
Strongyloidiasis
Echinococcosis
Onchocerciasis
Malaria

Infections
Allergic bronchopulmonary mycosis
Systemic candidiasis
Coccidioidomycosis
Leprosy
Epstein-Barr virus mononucleosis
Cytomegalovirus mononucleosis
Viral respiratory infections
Human immunodeficiency virus (HIV) type 1 infections
Pertussis

Cutaneous Diseases
Alopecia areata
Bullous pemphigoid
Chronic acral dermatitis
Streptococcal erythema nodosum

Other Diseases and Disorders
Nephrotic syndrome
Drug-induced interstitial nephritis

Liver disease
Cystic fibrosis
Kawasaki disease
Infantile polyarteritis nodosa
Primary pulmonary hemosiderosis
Guillain-Barré syndrome
Burns
Rheumatoid arthritis
Bone marrow transplantation
Cigarette smoking
Alcoholism

Neoplastic Diseases
Hodgkin disease
Immunoglobulin E (IgE) myeloma
Bronchial carcinoma

Immunodeficiency Diseases
Wiskott-Aldrich syndrome
Hyper-IgE syndrome
Thymic hypoplasia (DiGeorge syndrome)
Cellular immunodeficiency with immunoglobulins (Nezelof syndrome)
Selective IgA deficiency

Medications
Enfuvirtide
Pholcodine

Decreased Levels (<5 IU/ml)
Familial IgE deficiency and recurrent sinopulmonary infections
Human T cell lymphotropic virus type 1 infections
Primary biliary cirrhosis

From Adkinson NF et al: *Middleton's allergy principles and practice*, ed 8, Philadelphia, 2014, Saunders.

INSULIN-LIKE GROWTH FACTOR-II

Normal range: 288-736 ng/ml
Elevated in: Hypoglycemia associated with non–islet cell tumors, hepatoma, and Wilms' tumor
Decreased in: Growth hormone deficiency

INTERNATIONAL NORMALIZED RATIO (INR)

The INR is a comparative rating of prothrombin time (PT) ratios. The INR represents the observed PT ratio adjusted by the International Reference Thromboplastin. It provides a universal result indicative of what the patient's PT result would have been if measured using the primary World

---

BOX 17 Conditions Associated with Unusually High Serum Immunoglobulin E Concentrations (≥500 IU/ml)

Allergic bronchopulmonary mycosis
Allergic fungal sinusitis
Atopic dermatitis
Human immunodeficiency virus (HIV) infection
Hyperimmunoglobulin E (hyper-IgE) syndrome
Immunoglobulin E myeloma
Kimura disease
Lymphoma
Netherton syndrome
Systemic helminthic parasitosis
Tuberculosis

From Adkinson NF et al: *Middleton's allergy principles and practice*, ed 8, Philadelphia, 2014, Saunders.

BOX 18 Selected Conditions Associated with Monoclonal Immunoglobulins

- Multiple myeloma
- Macroglobulinemia of Waldenström
- Chronic lymphocytic leukemia
- Other leukemias
- Lymphomas
- "Benign" monoclonal gammopathy
- Systemic capillary leak syndrome
- Amyloidosis
- Chronic liver disease such as chronic active hepatitis, primary biliary cirrhosis
- Autoimmune disorders, including rheumatoid arthritis, systemic lupus erythematosus, thyroiditis, pernicious anemia, polyarteritis nodosa, Sjögren's syndrome
- Gaucher's disease
- Malignancies of various types
- Hereditary spherocytosis
- HIV infection, including AIDS

AIDS, Acquired immune deficiency syndrome; *HIV,* human immunodeficiency virus. (McPherson RA, Pincus MR: Henry's Clinical Diagnosis and Management by Laboratory Methods, 23rd ed, ISBN # 978-0323-29568-0, 2017, Elsevier)

Health Organization International Reference reagent. For proper interpretation of INR values, the patient should be on stable anticoagulant therapy.
RECOMMENDED INR RANGES:

Proximal deep vein thrombosis:	2-3
Pulmonary embolism:	2-3
Transient ischemic attacks:	2-3
Atrial fibrillation:	2-3
Mechanical prosthetic valves:	2.5-3.5
Recurrent venous thromboembolic disease:	2.5-3.5

INTRINSIC FACTOR ANTIBODIES

Normal: Negative
Present in: Pernicious anemia (>50% of patients). Cyanocobalamin may give false-positive results.

IRON (Serum)

Normal: Male: 65-175 mcg/dl; female: 50-1170 mcg/dl
Elevated in: Hemochromatosis, excessive iron therapy, repeated transfusions, lead poisoning, hemolytic anemia, aplastic anemia, pernicious anemia
Decreased in: Iron deficiency anemia, hypothyroidism, chronic infection

IRON-BINDING CAPACITY, TOTAL (TIBC)

Normal range: 250-460 µg/dl (45-82 µmol/L [CF: 0.1791; SMI: 1 µmol/L])

TABLE 47 Polyclonal Hyperimmunoglobulinemias: Some Associated Disease States

Condition	Immunoglobulin (Ig) Classes
Immunodeficiency Diseases	
Hyperimmunoglobulin E and recurrent infections	IgE
Wiskott-Aldrich syndrome	IgA, IgE
"Dysgammaglobulinemia type I"	IgM
Hyperimmunoglobulin A and recurrent infections	IgA
Acquired immune deficiency syndrome (AIDS)	All classes
Infections	
Congenital infections (syphilis, toxoplasmosis, rubella, cytomegalovirus)	IgM
Infectious mononucleosis	IgM or all
Trypanosomiasis	IgM or all
Intestinal parasitism	All classes
Several helminthic infections	IgE
Visceral larva migrans	All classes
Chronic granulomatous disease of childhood	All classes
Leprosy	All classes
Chronic infection in general	All classes, with a preference for IgG
Liver Diseases	
Chronic active hepatitis	IgG predominates
Acute hepatitis	IgG predominates
Biliary cirrhosis	IgM predominates
Lupoid hepatitis	All classes
Pulmonary Disorders	
Pulmonary hypersensitivity syndrome	All classes
Sarcoidosis	All classes
Berylliosis	All classes
"Autoimmune" Disorders	
Systemic lupus erythematosus	All classes
Rheumatoid arthritis	IgA or all
Many "autoimmune" states such as thyroiditis	All classes
Scleroderma	All classes
Cold agglutinin disease	IgM
Anaphylactoid purpura	IgA
Miscellaneous	
Down syndrome	All classes
Amyloidosis	All classes
Narcotic addiction	IgM
Renal tubular disease	All classes

(McPherson RA, Pincus MR: Henry's Clinical Diagnosis and Management by Laboratory Methods, 23rd ed, ISBN # 978-0323-29568-0, 2017, Elsevier)

Elevated in: Iron deficiency anemia, pregnancy, polycythemia, hepatitis, weight loss
Decreased in: Anemia of chronic disease, hemochromatosis, chronic liver disease, hemolytic anemias, malnutrition (protein depletion)
Table 48 describes TIBC and serum iron abnormalities.

IRON SATURATION (% Transferrin Saturation)

Normal:
Male: 20%-50%
Female: 15%-50%
Elevated in: Hemochromatosis, excessive iron intake, aplastic anemia, thalassemia, vitamin B_6 deficiency
Decreased in: hypochromic anemias, GI malignancy

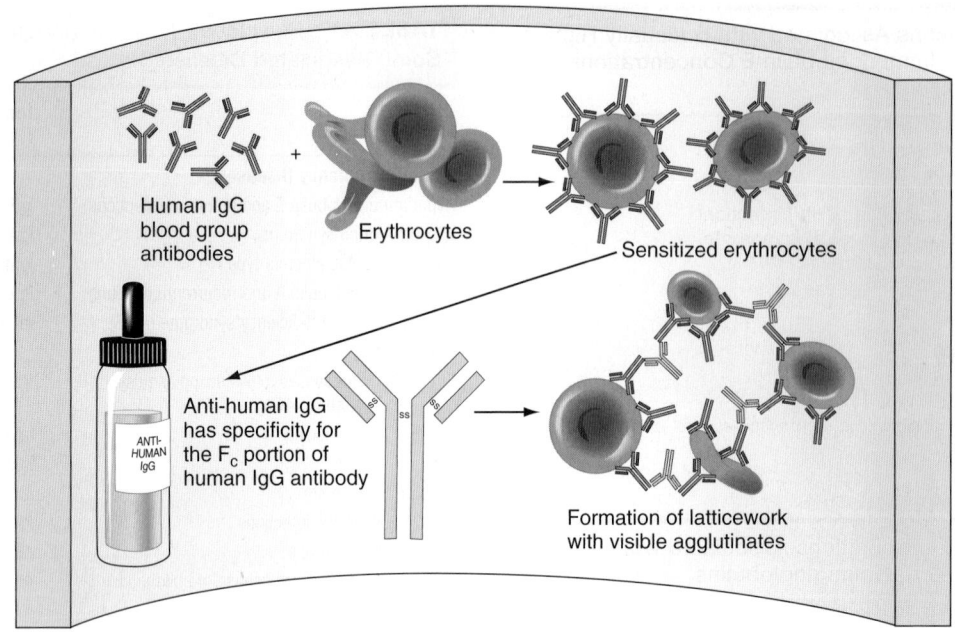

FIG. 28 Antihuman globulin antibodies form a bridge between adjacent erythrocytes sensitized with human immunoglobulin (Ig)G or complement components (McPherson RA, Pincus MR: Henry's Clinical Diagnosis and Management by Laboratory Methods, 23rd ed, ISBN # 978-0323-29568-0, 2017, Elsevier)

TABLE 48   Serum Iron and Total Iron-Binding Capacity Patterns

SI↓	TIBC↓	Chronic diseases Uremia
SI↓	TIBC↑	Chronic iron deficiency anemia Pregnancy in third trimester
SI↑	TIBC↓	Hemachromatosis iron therapy overload (TIBC may be normal) Hemolytic anemia; thalassemia; lead poisoning; megaloblastic anemia; aplastic, pyridoxine deficiency, or other sideroblastic anemias
SI↑	TIBC↑	Oral contraceptives Acute hepatitis (some report TIBC is low normal) Chronic hepatitis (some patients)
SI↑	TIBCNL	B$_{12}$ or folate deficiency
SI↓	TIBCNL	Chronic iron deficiency (some patients) Acute infection, surgery, tissue damage
SI NL	TIBC↑	B$_{12}$/folate deficiency plus iron deficiency

From Ravel R: *Clinical laboratory medicine*, ed 6, St Louis, 1995, Mosby.
NL, Normal; *SI*, serum iron; *TIBC*, total iron-binding capacity.

LACTATE (blood)

Normal range: 0.5-2.0 mEq/L
Elevated in: Tissue hypoxia (shock, respiratory failure, severe CHF, severe anemia, carbon monoxide or cyanide poisoning), systemic disorders (liver or renal failure, seizures), abnormal intestinal flora (d-lactic acidosis), drugs or toxins (salicylates, ethanol, methanol, ethylene glycol), G6PD deficiency

LACTATE DEHYDROGENASE (LDH)

Normal range: 50-150 U/L (0.82-2.66 μkat/L [CF: 0.01667; SMI: 0.02 μkat/L])
Elevated in:
Infarction of myocardium, lung, kidney
Diseases of cardiopulmonary system, liver, collagen, central nervous system
Hemolytic anemias, megaloblastic anemias, transfusions, seizures, muscle trauma, muscular dystrophy, acute pancreatitis, hypotension, shock, infectious mononucleosis, inflammation, neoplasia, intestinal obstruction, hypothyroidism

LACTATE DEHYDROGENASE ISOENZYMES

Normal range

LDH$_1$:   22%-36% (cardiac, red blood cell) (0.22-0.36 [CF: 0.01, SMI: 0.01])
LDH$_2$:   35%-46% (cardiac, red blood cell) (0.35-0.46)
LDH$_3$:   13%-26% (pulmonary) (0.15-0.26)
LDH$_4$:   3%-10% (striated muscle, liver) (0.03-0.1)
LDH$_5$:   2%-9% (striated muscle, liver) (0.02-0.09)
Normal ratios
LDH$_1$ <LDH$_2$
LDH$_5$ <LDH$_4$
Abnormal values
LDH$_1$ >LDH$_2$: Myocardial infarction (can also be seen with hemolytic anemias, pernicious anemia, folate deficiency, renal infarct)
LDH$_5$ >LDH$_4$: Liver disease (cirrhosis, hepatitis, hepatic congestion)

LACTOSE TOLERANCE TEST (serum)

Normal: Test is performed by giving 2 g/kg body weight lactose orally and drawing glucose level at 0, 30, 45, 60, and 90 min. Normal response is change in glucose from fasting value to >30 mg/dl. Inconclusive response is increase of 20-30 mg/dl, abnormal response is increase <20 mg/dl. Table 49 summarizes laboratory tests in the differential diagnosis of diarrhea.
Abnormal in: Lactase deficiency

LAP SCORE

See LEUKOCYTE ALKALINE PHOSPHATASE

LEAD

Normal: Child, <10 mcg/dl; adult, <25 mcg/dl; acceptable for industrial exposure, <50 mcg/dl
Elevated in: Lead exposure, lead poisoning

LDH

See LACTATE DEHYDROGENASE

LDL

See LOW-DENSITY LIPOPROTEIN CHOLESTEROL

TABLE 49 Laboratory Tests in the Differential Diagnosis of Diarrhea

Test	Method	Use
Initial Screening Tests		
Fecal leukocytes	Wright's stain or methylene blue	Identify inflammatory diarrhea
Fecal occult blood test	Immunochemical	Detect blood
Fecal osmotic gap	$290 - 2 \times$ (fecal $Na^+ + K^+$)	Distinguish secretory vs. osmotic diarrhea
Stool alkalinization	Color change after adding NaOH to stool/urine	Phenolphthalein laxative ingestion
Infectious Causes		
Stool bacterial culture	Routine culture and sensitivity	Identify *Shigella, Salmonella*
Stool special culture	Specialized culture and serotyping	Identify *E. coli* 0157:H7, *Yersinia, Campylobacter*
Stool *C. difficile* toxin assay	EIA for toxins A and B	Pseudomembranous colitis
HIV serology	EIA, Western blot	HIV enteritis
Stool rotavirus screen	EIA for antigen	Rotavirus enteritis
Stool ova and parasites	Concentration and stains	Enteric parasitic infection
Stool mycobacteria	Acid-fast stain, culture and sensitivity, PCR	*Mycobacterium*, antibiotic selection
Stool *E. histolytica* Ag	EIA for antigen	*Entameoba histolytica*
Stool *Giardia* Ag	EIA for antigen	*Giardia lamblia*
Stool *Cryptosporidium* Ag	EIA for antigen	*Cryptosporidium parvum*
Endocrine Causes		
Urine 5-HIAA or blood serotonin	HPLC	Carcinoid syndrome
Serum VIP	RIA	VIPoma
Serum TSH, free T4	Immunoassay	Hyperthyroidism
Serum gastrin	RIA	Zollinger-Ellison syndrome
Serum calcitonin	RIA	Hypocalcemia-related diarrhea
Serum somatostatin	RIA	Somatostatinoma
Malabsorption		
Lactose tolerance test	See text	Lactase deficiency
Stool reducing sugars	Clinitest tablets	Carbohydrate intolerance
Sweat chloride	See text	Cystic fibrosis
D-Xylose absorption test	See text	Evaluate pancreatic and jejunal function
Fecal fat stain	Fat stain	Lipid malabsorption
Serum carotene	Spectrophotometry	Lipid malabsorption
^{14}C-glyceryl trioleate test malabsorption	See text	Lipid malabsorption
Serum IgA	Nephelometry	Rule out IgA deficiency
Antitissue transglutaminase antibody	EIA	Celiac disease
Hydrogen breath test	Electrochemical hydrogen monitorinomatography g	Carbohydrate malabsorption
Bacterial colony count	Small bowel aspirate and quantitative culture	Bacterial overgrowth
Other		
Serum ionized calcium	Ion-specific electrode	Hypocalcemia-related diarrhea
Serum protein and albumin	Nephelometry, photometry	IBD, protein-losing enteropathy
Stool alpha-1-antitrypsin	Nephelometry	Protein-losing enteropathy
Quantitative immunoglobulins	Nephelometry	Agammaglobulinemia
7α-Hydroxy-4-cholestin-3-one	HPLC	Bile salt malabsorption
Fecal elastase or pancreolauryl test	EIA	Pancreatic insufficiency
Intestinal biopsy	Endoscopic or open biopsy	Whipple's disease, MAI, abetalipoproteinemia, neoplasia, lymphoma, amyloidosis, eosinophilic gastroenteritis, agammaglobulinemia, intestinal lymphangiectasia, Crohn's disease, tuberculosis, graft-versus-host disease, *Giardia*, other parasitic infections, collagenous colitis, microscopic colitis
Extraintestinal causes	See text	Hyperthyroidism, diabetes, hypoparathyroidism, adrenal cortical insufficiency, hormone-secreting tumors

5-HIAA, 5-Hydroxyindoleacetic acid; *Ab*, antibody; *Ag*, amtigen; *EIA*, enzyme immunoassay; *HIV*, human immunodeficiency virus; *HPLC*, high-performance liquid chromatography; *IBD*, inflammatory bowel disease; *MAI*, *Mycobacterium avium-intracellulare*; *PCR*, polymerase chain reaction; *RIA*, radioimmunoassay; *TSH*, thyroid-stimulating hormone; *VIP*, vasoactive intestinal peptide.
(McPherson RA, Pincus MR: Henry's Clinical Diagnosis and Management by Laboratory Methods, 23rd ed, ISBN # 978-0323-29568-0, 2017, Elsevier)

Laboratory Tests

IV

LEGIONELLA PNEUMOPHILA PCR

Test description: PCR can be performed on lung tissue, water sputum, bronchoalveolar lavage, and other respiratory fluids.

LEGIONELLA TITER

Normal: Negative
Positive in: Legionnaire's disease (presumptive: ≥1:256 titer; definitive: fourfold titer increase to ≥1:128)

LEUKOCYTE ALKALINE PHOSPHATASE (LAP)

Normal range: 13-100 (33-188 U)
Elevated in: Leukemoid reactions, neutrophilia secondary to infections (except in sickle cell crisis—no significant increase in LAP score), Hodgkin's disease, polycythemia vera, hairy cell leukemia, aplastic anemia, Down syndrome, myelofibrosis
Decreased in: Acute and chronic granulocytic leukemia, thrombocytopenic purpura, paroxysmal nocturnal hemoglobinuria, hypophosphatemia, collagen disorders

LEUKOCYTE COUNT

See COMPLETE BLOOD COUNT

LIPASE

Normal range: 0-160 U/L (0-2.66 μkat/L [CF: 0.01667; SMI: 0.02 μkat/L])
Elevated in: Acute pancreatitis, perforated peptic ulcer, carcinoma of pancreas (early stage), pancreatic duct obstruction, bowel infarction, intestinal obstruction

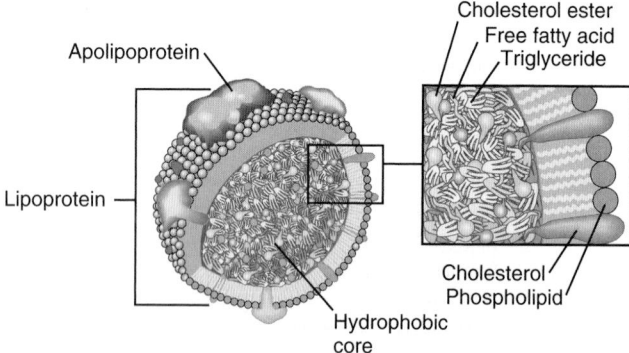

FIG. 29 Lipoprotein structure. Lipoproteins are spherical particles with a hydrophobic core and an amphiphilic surface. The surface consists of a single layer of phospholipids. This surface layer also contains proteins and free cholesterol. The hydrophobic core mainly contains triglycerides and cholesterol esters (McPherson RA, Pincus MR: Henry's Clinical Diagnosis and Management by Laboratory Methods, 23rd ed, ISBN # 978-0323-29568-0, 2017, Elsevier)

LIPOPROTEIN(a)

Normal: Male: 1.35-19.6 mg/dl; female: 1.24-20.1 mg/dl. Fig. 29 illustrates lipoprotein structure. Table 50 summarizes the major classes of human plasma lipoproteins. The chemical composition of major classes of plasma lipoproteins is described in Table 51.
Elevated in: Coronary artery disease, uncontrolled diabetes, hypothyroidism, chronic renal failure, pregnancy, tobacco use, infections, nephritic syndrome
Decreased in: Niacin, omega-3 fatty acids, estrogens, tamoxifen, statins

LIPOPROTEIN CHOLESTEROL, HIGH-DENSITY

See HIGH-DENSITY LIPOPROTEIN CHOLESTEROL

LIPOPROTEIN CHOLESTEROL, LOW-DENSITY

See LOW-DENSITY LIPOPROTEIN CHOLESTEROL

LIVER KIDNEY MICROSOME TYPE 1 ANTIBODIES (LKM1)

Normal: <20 U
Elevated in: Autoimmune hepatitis type 2

LKM1

See LIVER KIDNEY MICROSOME TYPE 1 ANTIBODIES

LOW-DENSITY LIPOPROTEIN (LDL) CHOLESTEROL

Normal range: 50-130 mg/dl (1.30-1.68 mmol/L [CF: 0.02586; SMI: 0.05 mmol/L]). Fig. 30 illustrates the LDL receptor pathway and regulation of cholesterol metabolism.

<70	Optimal in diabetics, prior MI, and patients with cardiac risk factors
100-129	Near or above optimal
130-159	Borderline high
160-189	High
≥190	Very high

LUPUS ANTICOAGULANT

See CIRCULATING ANTICOAGULANT

LUTEINIZING HORMONE

Normal range: 5-25 mIU/ml
Elevated in: Postmenopause, pituitary adenoma, primary gonadal dysfunction, polycystic ovary syndrome
Decreased in: Severe illness, anorexia nervosa, malnutrition, pituitary or hypothalamic impairment, severe stress

LYME DISEASE ANTIBODY TITER

Normal range: Negative

TABLE 50 Major Classes of Human Plasma Lipoproteins: Physicochemical Characteristics

Particle	Electrophoretic Mobility*	Major Apolipoproteins	Diameter (Å)	Density (kg/L)	Sf†
Chylomicrons	Origin	ApoA-I, A-IV, B-48, C-I, C-II, C-III, E	750-12,000	<0.95	>400
VLDL	Pre-β	ApoB-100, C-I, C-II, C-III, E	300-700	0.95-1.006	20-400
IDL	β or pre-β	ApoB-100, E1.006–1.019	12-20		
LDL	B	ApoB-100	180-300	1.019-1.063	0-12
HDL₂	A	ApoA-I, A-II, E	50-120	1.063-1.125	
HDL₃	A	ApoA-II, A-I, E	50-120	1.125-1.210	
Lp(a)	Pre-β	ApoB-100, Apo(a)		1.045-1.080	

HDL₂, Ultracentrifugation subclass of high-density lipoprotein; *HDL₃*, ultracentrifugation subclass of high-density lipoprotein; *IDL,* intermediate-density lipoprotein; *LDL,* low-density lipoprotein; *Lp(a),* lipoprotein A; *VLDL,* very-low-density lipoprotein.
*Agarose gel electrophoresis.
†Svedberg flotation rate.
(McPherson RA, Pincus MR: Henry's Clinical Diagnosis and Management by Laboratory Methods, 23rd ed, ISBN # 978-0323-29568-0, 2017, Elsevier)

Positive result: FIG. 31 illustrates the usual serologic response in Lyme disease.

A serologic test is not necessary or helpful for several days after a tick bite because it is only 40%-50% sensitive in this stage, and a negative test does not rule out the diagnosis.

LYMPHOCYTES

Normal range
15%-40%
Total lymphocyte count = 800-2600/mm^3
Total T lymphocyte = 800-2200/mm^3
CD4 lymphocytes = ≥ 400/mm^3
CD8 lymphocytes = 200-800/mm^3

Normal CD4/CD8 ratio is 2.0.

Elevated in: Chronic infections, infectious mononucleosis and other viral infections, chronic lymphocytic leukemia, Hodgkin's disease, ulcerative colitis, hypoadrenalism, idiopathic thrombocytopenia

Decreased in
AIDS, bone marrow suppression from chemotherapeutic agents or chemotherapy, aplastic anemia, neoplasms, steroids, adrenocortical hyperfunction, neurologic disorders (multiple sclerosis, myasthenia gravis, Guillain-Barré syndrome)

CD4 lymphocytes are calculated as total white blood cells × % lymphocytes × % lymphocytes stained with CD4. They are decreased in AIDS and other immune dysfunction.

Table 52 describes various lymphocyte abnormalities in peripheral blood. Box 19 summarizes key causes of lymphocytopenia.

TABLE 51 Chemical Composition of Major Classes of Plasma Lipoproteins

	Protein (%)*	Free Cholesterol (%)	Cholesterol Esters (%)	Triglyceride (%)	Phospholipid (%)
Chylomicrons	1-2	1-3	2-4	80-95	3-6
VLDL	6-10	4-8	16-22	45-65	15-20
IDL	Intermediate between VLDL and LDL				
LDL	18-22	6-8	45-50	4-8	18-24
HDL	45-55	3-5	15-20	2-7	26-32

Data from Albers (1974), Gaubatz et al (1983), Fless et al (1984), Gotto et al (1986), Gries et al (1988), and Hegele (2009).
HDL, High-density lipoprotein; *IDL,* intermediate-density lipoprotein; *LDL,* low-density lipoprotein; *VLDL,* very-low-density lipoprotein.
*Percentage of dry weight.
(McPherson RA, Pincus MR: Henry's Clinical Diagnosis and Management by Laboratory Methods, 23rd ed, ISBN # 978-0323-29568-0, 2017, Elsevier)

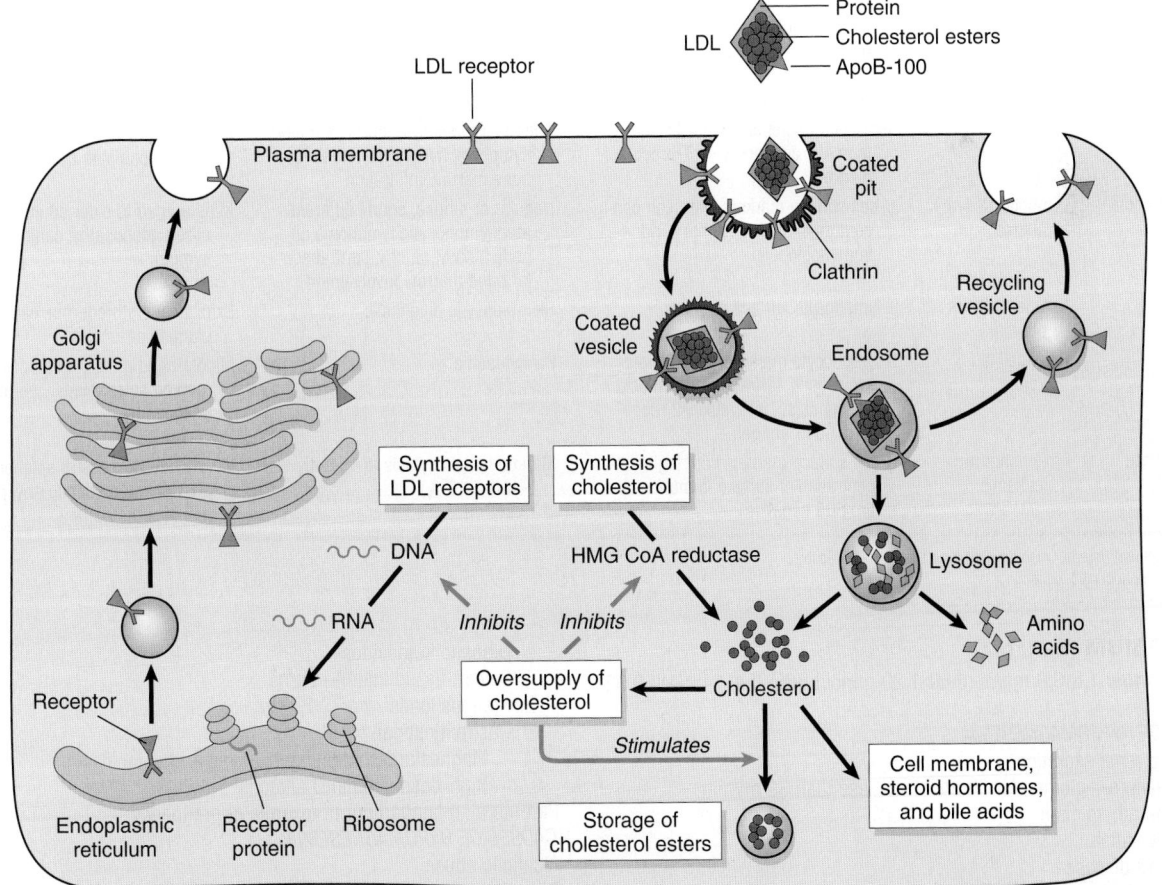

FIG. 30 The low-density lipoprotein (LDL) receptor pathway and regulation of cholesterol metabolism. (McPherson RA, Pincus MR: Henry's Clinical Diagnosis and Management by Laboratory Methods, 23rd ed, ISBN # 978-0323-29568-0, 2017, Elsevier)

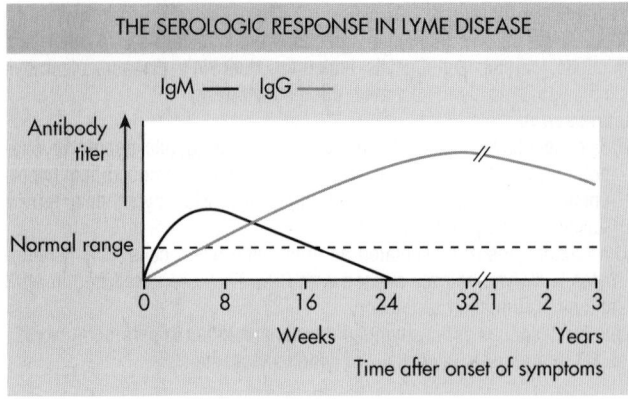

THE SEROLOGIC RESPONSE IN LYME DISEASE

IgM —— IgG ——

Antibody titer

Normal range

0   8   16   24   32   1   2   3

Weeks   Years

Time after onset of symptoms

FIG. 31 IgM and IgG responses in Lyme disease.

BOX 19 Key Causes of Lymphocytopenia

- Destructive—radiation, chemotherapy, corticosteroids
- Debilitative—starvation, aplastic anemia, terminal cancer, collagen vascular disease, renal failure
- Infectious—viral hepatitis, influenza, typhoid fever, TB
- AIDS-associated—HIV cytopathic effect, nutritional imbalance, drug effect
- Congenital immunodeficiency—Wiskott-Aldrich syndrome
- Abnormal lymphatic circulation—intestinal lymphangiectasia, obstruction, thoracic duct drainage/rupture, CHF

AIDS, Acquired immunodeficiency syndrome; *CHF,* congestive heart failure; *HIV,* human immunodeficiency virus; *TB,* tuberculosis.
(McPherson RA, Pincus MR: Henry's Clinical Diagnosis and Management by Laboratory Methods, 23rd ed, ISBN # 978-0323-29568-0, 2017, Elsevier)

TABLE 52 Differential Diagnosis of Abnormal Lymphocytes in Peripheral Blood

Lymphocyte Type	Usual Disease Association	Cytologic Features	Laboratory Features	Clinical Features
Small lymphocyte	Chronic lymphocytic leukemia	B-cell surface markers with low concentration of surface immunoglobulin, CD5 antigen	Hypogammaglobulinemia in 50%; positive direct Coombs test in 15%; on node biopsy, diffuse, well-differentiated lymphocytic infiltrate	Elderly adults; presentation runs gamut from asymptomatic with lymphocytosis only to bulky disease with adenopathy, splenomegaly, and "packed" bone marrow
Atypical lymphocyte	Infectious mononucleosis, other viral illnesses	Suppressor T-cell markers	Heterophil agglutinin; positive serology for Epstein-Barr virus, cytomegalovirus, toxoplasma, HBsAg	Pharyngitis, fever, adenopathy, rash, splenomegaly, palatal petechiae, jaundice
Plasmacytoid lymphocyte	Waldenström's macroglobulin anemia	Cytoplasmic IgM, periodic acid-Schiff positivity	IgM paraprotein, rouleaux, cryoglobulins	Adenopathy, splenomegaly, absence of bone lesions, hyperviscosity syndrome, cryopathic phenomena
Lymphoblast	ALL	Terminal transferase positivity, common ALL antigen, B- or T-precursor markers	Anemia, granulocytopenia, thrombocytopenia, hyperuricemia, diffuse bone marrow infiltration	Peak incidence in childhood, acute onset, bone pain frequent
Lymphosarcoma cell	Lymphocytic lymphoma	B-cell surface markers with high concentration of monoclonal surface immunoglobulin	Nodular or diffuse, poorly differentiated lymphocytic lymphoma on node biopsy, patchy, peritrabecular bone marrow involvement	Middle-aged to older adults, generalized adenopathy, constitutional symptoms
Sézary cell	Cutaneous lymphomas	T-lymphocyte surface markers	Skin biopsy is diagnostic	Exfoliative erythroderma, cutaneous plaques or tumors
Hairy cell	Hairy cell leukemia	B-lymphocyte markers, cytoplasmic projections, tartrate-resistant acid phosphatase, interleukin-2 receptors, CD11 antigen	Pancytopenia	Middle-aged males, moderate to marked splenomegaly without adenopathy
Prolymphocyte	Prolymphocytic leukemia	B-cell surface markers with high concentration of surface immunoglobulin, CD5 negative	Marked lymphocytosis (frequently >100 × 10^9/L)	Elderly adults, massive splenomegaly, minimum adenopathy, poor response to therapy

From Stein JH (ed): *Internal medicine,* ed 5, St Louis, 1998, Mosby.
ALL, Acute lymphoblastic leukemia.

MAGNESIUM (Serum)

Normal range: 1.8-3.0 mg/dl (0.80-1.20 mmol/L [CF: 0.4114; SMI: 0.02 mmol/L])

CAUSES OF HYPERMAGNESEMIA

Decreased renal excretion
  Renal failure—glomerular filtration rate less than 30 ml/min
  Hyperparathyroidism
  Hypothyroidism
  Addison's disease
  Lithium intoxication
  Familial hypocalciuric hypercalcemia
Other causes: usually in association with decrease in glomerular filtration rate
  Endogenous loads

    Diabetic ketoacidosis
    Severe tissue injury—burns
  Exogenous loads
    Gastrointestinal
      Magnesium-containing laxatives and antacids
      High-dose vitamin D analogs
Parenteral: management of toxemia of pregnancy

CAUSES OF HYPOMAGNESEMIA

Alcoholic abuse
Diuretic use
Renal losses
Acute and chronic renal failure
Postobstructive diuresis

TABLE 53 Clinical Conditions Not to Be Confused With Megaloblastosis

Macrocytosis* Without Megaloblastosis†

Reticulocytosis
Liver disease
Aplastic anemia
Myelodysplastic syndromes (especially 5q-)
Multiple myeloma
Hypoxemia
Smokers

Spurious Increases In MCV Without Macro-Ovalocytosis‡

Cold agglutinin disease
Marked hyperglycemia
Leukocytosis
Older individuals

From Hoffman R: *Hematology: basic principles and practice*, ed 6, Philadelphia, 2013, Saunders. *MCV,* Mean corpuscular volume.

*The central pallor that normally occupies about one-third of the normal red blood cell is decreased in macro-ovalocytes. This contrasts with the finding of thin macrocytes, in which the central pallor is increased.

†Although megaloblastosis implies that a bone marrow test has been performed, with the addition of highly sensitive tests for the specific diagnosis of cobalamin and folate deficiency, the need for a bone marrow test is often dictated by the urgency to make the diagnosis.

‡When the Coulter counter readings of a high MCV are not confirmed by looking at the peripheral smear.

Acute tubular necrosis
Chronic glomerulonephritis
Chronic pyelonephritis
Interstitial nephropathy
Renal transplantation
Gastrointestinal losses
Chronic diarrhea
Nasogastric suctioning
Short bowel syndrome
Protein-calorie malnutrition
Bowel fistula
Total parenteral nutrition
Acute pancreatitis
Endocrine
Diabetes mellitus
Hyperaldosteronism
Hyperthyroidism
Hyperparathyroidism
Acute intermittent porphyria
Pregnancy
Drugs
Aminoglycosides
Amphotericin
β-agonists
Cisplatin
Cyclosporine
Diuretics
Foscarnet
Pentamidine
Theophylline
Congenital disorders
Familial hypomagnesemia
Maternal diabetes
Maternal hypothyroidism
Maternal hyperparathyroidism

MEAN CORPUSCULAR VOLUME (MCV)

Normal range: 76-100 μm³ (76-100 fL) (76-100 fL [CF: 1; SMI: 1 fL])

Table 53 summarizes clinical conditions not to be confused with megaloblastosis. See Tables 54, 55, and 56 for descriptions of MCV abnormalities.

METANEPHRINES, URINE

See URINE METANEPHRINES

TABLE 54 Some Causes of Increased Mean Corpuscular Volume (Macrocytosis)

Causes	% of all Macrocytosis Patients*	% of Macrocytosis in Each Disease†
Common		
Folate or B₁₂ deficiency	20-30 (5-50)‡	80-90 (4-100)
Chronic liver disease	15-20 (6-28)	25-30 (8-65)
Chronic alcoholism	10-12 (3-15)	60 (26-90)
Cytotoxic chemotherapy	10-15 (2-20)	30-40 (13-82)
Cardiorespiratory abnormality	8 (7-9.5)	?
Reticulocytosis	6-7 (0-15)	Depends on severity
Myelodysplastic syndromes	Frequent over age 40 yr	>60 in RAEB and RARS
Unexplained	25 (22.5-27)	—
Normal newborn		
Less Common	<4%	
Noncytotoxic drugs		
> Zidovudine		
Phenytoin		30 (14-50)
Azathioprine		
Hypothyroidism		20-30 (8-55)
Chronic leukemia/myelo-fibrosis		
Radiotherapy for malignancy		
Chronic renal disease (occasional patients)		
Distance-runner macrocytosis (some persons)		
Down syndrome		
Artifactual (e.g., cold agglutinins)		

From Ravel R: *Clinical laboratory medicine*, ed 6, St Louis, 1995, Mosby.

RAEB, Refractory anemia with excessive blasts; *RARS,* refractory anemia with ring sideroblasts (formerly called "IASA," or idiopathic acquired sideroblastic anemia).

*Percentage of all patients with macrocytosis.
†Percentage of patients with each condition listed who have macrocytosis.
‡Numbers in parentheses are literature range.

TABLE 55 Some Causes of Decreased Mean Corpuscular Volume (Microcytosis)

Common	Less Common
Chronic iron deficiency	Some cases of polycythemia
α- or β-thalassemia (minor)	Some cases of lead poisoning
Anemia of chronic disease	Some cases of congenital spherocytosis Some cases of sideroblastic anemia Certain abnormal hemoglobins (HbE, Hb Lepore)

From Ravel R: *Clinical laboratory medicine*, ed 6, St Louis, 1995, Mosby.

METHYLMALONIC ACID (Serum)

Normal: <0.2 mcmol/L
Elevated in: Vitamin B₁₂ deficiency, pregnancy, methylmalonic acidemia

MITOCHONDRIAL ANTIBODY (AMA)

Normal: Negative
Present in: Primary biliary cirrhosis (>90% of patients)

MONOCYTE COUNT

Normal range: 2%-8%
Elevated in: Viral diseases, parasites, infections, neoplasms, inflammatory bowel disease, monocytic leukemia, lymphomas, myeloma, sarcoidosis
Decreased in: Aplastic anemia, lymphocytic leukemia, glucocorticoid administration
See Table 57 for changes in monocyte number.

MYCOPLASMA PNEUMONIAE PCR

Test description: PCR can be performed on sputum, bronchoalveolar lavage, nasopharyngeal and throat swabs, other respiratory fluids, and lung tissue

MYELIN BASIC PROTEIN, CEREBROSPINAL FLUID

Normal: <2.5 ng/ml
Elevated in: Multiple sclerosis, CNS trauma, stroke, encephalitis

MYOGLOBIN, URINE

See URINE MYOGLOBIN

TABLE 56 Differential Diagnosis of Microcytic Hypochromic Anemia

Decreased Body Iron Stores

Iron-deficiency anemia

Normal or Increased Body Iron Stores

Anemia of chronic disease

Defective absorption, transport, or use of iron

Iron-refractory, iron-deficiency anemia after parenteral iron

Atransferrinemia

Aceruloplasminemia

Divalent metal transporter 1 (DMT1 or SLC11A2) deficiency

Ferroportin-associated hemochromatosis with impaired iron export (type 4A)

Heme oxygenase 1 deficiency

Disorders of globin synthesis
   Thalassemia
   Other microcytic hemoglobinopathies

Disorders of heme synthesis: sideroblastic anemias
   Hereditary
   Acquired

From Hoffman R, et al: *Hematology, basic principles and practice*, ed 6, Philadelphia, 2013, Saunders.

TABLE 57 Changes in Monocyte Number

Monocytosis

Infections: tuberculosis, granulomatous infection, brucellosis, subacute bacterial endocarditis

Connective tissue disorder

Recovery from myelosuppression

Hematologic malignancies
   MDS, MPD, MDS–MPD overlap, CMML
   Acute and chronic monocytic leukemia, myelomonocytic leukemia
   Hodgkin and non-Hodgkin lymphomas

Monocytopenia

Hairy cell leukemia

MonoMAC syndrome

Aplastic anemia

Drugs: chemotherapy, IFN-α, glucocorticoids (transient)

Radiation therapy

From Hoffman R: Hematology, basic principles and practice, ed 6, Philadelphia, 2013, Saunders. *CMML*, Chronic myelomonocytic leukemia; *IFN*, interferon; *MDS*, myelodysplastic syndrome; *monoMAC*, monocytopenia and mycobacterium avium complex syndrome; *MPD*, myeloproliferative disorder.

NEISSERIA GONORRHOEAE PCR

Test description: Test can be performed on endocervical swab, urine, and intraurethral swab
Normal: Negative

NEUTROPHIL COUNT

Normal range: 50%-70%
Subsets:
   l.   Stabs (bands, early mature neutrophils): 2%-6%
   m. Segs (mature neutrophils): 60%-70%
Elevated in: Acute bacterial infections, acute myocardial infarction, stress, neoplasms, myelocytic leukemia
Decreased in: Viral infections, aplastic anemias, immunosuppressive drugs, radiation therapy to bone marrow, agranulocytosis, drugs (antibiotics, antithyroidals, clopidogrel), lymphocytic and monocytic leukemias
Box 20 describes various drugs that can cause neutropenia. Table 58 describes miscellaneous inherited neutropenia disorders.

NOREPINEPHRINE

Normal range: 0-600 pg/ml
Elevated in: Pheochromocytomas, neuroblastomas, stress, vigorous exercise, certain foods (bananas, chocolate, coffee, tea, vanilla)

BOX 20 Drugs That Cause Neutropenia

Antiarrhythmics: tocainide, procainamide, propranolol, quinidine
Antibiotics: chloramphenicol, penicillins, sulfonamides, p-aminosalicylic acid (PAS), rifampin, vancomycin, isoniazid, nitrofurantoin
Antimalarials: dapsone, quinine, pyrimethamine
Anticonvulsants: phenytoin, mephenytoin, trimethadione, ethosuximide, carbamazepine
Hypoglycemic agents: tolbutamide, chlorpropamide
Antihistamines: cimetidine, brompheniramine, tripelennamine
Antihypertensives: methyldopa, captopril
Antiinflammatory agents: aminopyrine, phenylbutazone, gold salts, ibuprofen, indomethacin
Antithyroid agents: propylthiouracil, methimazole, thiouracil
Diuretics: acetazolamide, hydrochlorothiazide, chlorthalidone
Phenothiazines: chlorpromazine, promazine, prochlorperazine
Immunosuppressive agents: antimetabolites
Cytotoxic agents: alkylating agents, antimetabolites, anthracyclines, *Vinca* alkaloids, cisplatin, hydroxyurea, dactinomycin
Other agents: recombinant interferons, allopurinol, ethanol, levamisole, penicillamine, zidovudine, streptokinase, carbamazepine, clopidogrel, ticlopidine

Modified from Goldman L, Ausiello D (eds): *Cecil textbook of medicine*, ed 22, Philadelphia, 2004, Saunders.

5′-NUCLEOTIDASE

Normal range: 2-16 IU/L (3-27 × 10^8 kat/L [CF: 1.67 × 10^8; SMI: 1 × 10^8 kat/L])
Elevated in: Biliary obstruction, metastatic neoplasms to liver, primary biliary cirrhosis, renal failure, pancreatic carcinoma, chronic active hepatitis

OSMOLALITY (serum)

Normal range: 280-300 mOsm/kg (280-300 mmol/kg [CF: 1; SMI: 1 mmol/kg])
It can also be estimated by the following formula:

$$2\,([Na] + [K] + glucose/18 + BUN/2.8)$$

The relationship between plasma osmolality and plasma arginine vasopressin is illustrated in Fig. 32.
Elevated in: Dehydration, hypernatremia, diabetes insipidus, uremia, hyperglycemia, mannitol therapy, ingestion of toxins (ethylene glycol, methanol, ethanol), hypercalcemia, diuretics
Decreased in: Syndrome of inappropriate diuretic hormone secretion, hyponatremia, overhydration, Addison's disease, hypothyroidism

TABLE 58 Miscellaneous Inherited Neutropenia Disorders

Diagnosis	Genetics	Mapping	Mutant Gene	Additional Features
Hyper IgM syndrome, type 1	X-L	Xq26	CD40L	↓IgG, IgA, IgE, autoimmune cytopenias
Hermansky-Pudlak syndrome, type 2	AR	5q14.1	AP3B1	↓IgG, partial albinism, platelet dysfunction
Griscelli syndrome, type 1	AR	15q21	MYO5A	Neurologic dysfunction, partial albinism
Griscelli syndrome, type 2	AR	15q21	RAB27A	Same as type 1 plus hemophagocytosis
Chediak-Higashi syndrome	AR	1q42.1-q42.2	LYST (CHSI)	Immunodeficiency, partial albinism
Poikiloderma with neutropenia	AR	16q13	C16ORF57	Rash, short stature, dystrophic nails
P14 deficiency	AR	1q22	MAPBPIP	Immunodeficiency, hypopigmentation
Cohen syndrome	AR	8q22-q23	VPS13B/COH1	Retinopathy, retardation, skeletal anomalies
Charcot-Marie-Tooth syndrome, type 2	AD	19p13.2	DMN2	Axonal demyelinating neuropathy

AD, Autosomal dominant; *AR*, autosomal recessive; *Ig*, immunoglobulin; *X-L*, X-linked recessive.
Data compiled from Online Mendelian Inheritance in Man (http://ncbi.nlm.nih.gov/omim); From Hoffman R: *Hematology: basic principles and practice*, ed 6, Philadelphia, 2013, Saunders.

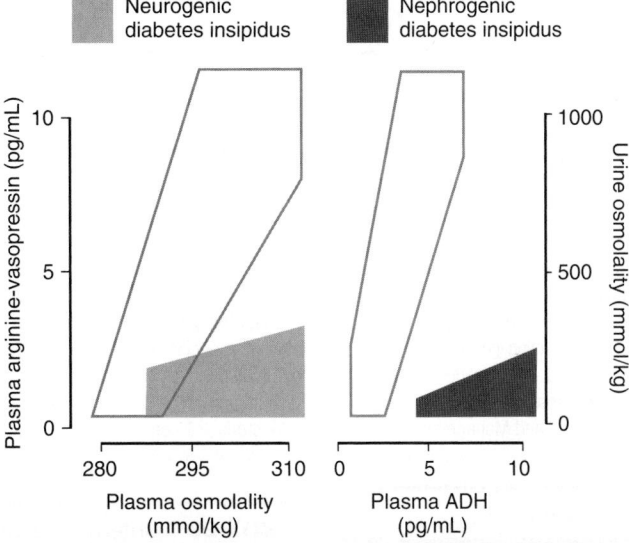

FIG. 32 *Left,* Relationship between plasma arginine vasopressin (AVP/ADH) and plasma osmolality during the infusion of hypertonic saline. Patients with primary polydipsia and nephrogenic diabetes insipidus (DI) have values within the normal range *(open area),* in contrast to patients with neurogenic DI, who show a subnormal plasma ADH response to a rise in osmolality *(pink).* *Right,* Relationship between urine osmolality and plasma ADH during dehydration and water loading. Patients with primary polydipsia and neurogenic DI have values within the normal range *(open area),* in contrast to patients with nephrogenic DI, who have hypotonic urine despite high plasma ADH *(green).* (Redrawn from Bichet DG: Diabetes insipidus and vasopressin. In Moore TW, Eastman RC, editors: *Diagnostic endocrinology,* ed 2, St Louis, 1996, Mosby, p 168, with permission.) (McPherson RA, Pincus MR: Henry's Clinical Diagnosis and Management by Laboratory Methods, 23rd ed, ISBN # 978-0-323-29568-0, 2017, Elsevier)

OSMOLALITY, URINE

Normal range: 50-1200 mOsm/kg (50-1200 mmol/kg [CF: 1; SMI: 1 mmol/kg])

Elevated in: Syndrome of inappropriate antidiuretic hormone secretion, dehydration, glycosuria, adrenal insufficiency, high-protein diet

Decreased in: Diabetes insipidus, excessive water intake, IV hydration with D₅W, acute renal insufficiency, glomerulonephritis

The relationship between plasma urine osmolality and plasma arginine vasopressin in patients with polyuria is illustrated in Fig. 32.

OSMOTIC FRAGILITY TEST

Normal: Hemolysis begins at 0.50, w/v [5.0 g/L] and is complete at 0.30, w/v [3.0 g/L] NaCl.

Elevated in: Hereditary spherocytosis, hereditary stomatocytosis, spherocytosis associated with acquired immune hemolytic anemia

Decreased in: Iron deficiency anemia, thalassemias, liver disease, leptocytosis associated with asplenia

PARACENTESIS FLUID

Testing and evaluation of results
Process the fluid as follows:
Tube 1: LDH, glucose, albumin
Tube 2: protein, specific gravity
Tube 3: cell count and differential
Tube 4: save until further notice
Draw serum LDH, protein, albumin.
Gram stain, AFB stain, bacterial and fungal cultures, amylase, and triglycerides should be ordered only when clearly indicated; bedside inoculation of blood-culture bottles with ascitic fluid improves sensitivity in detecting bacterial growth.
If malignant ascites is suspected, consider a carcinoembryonic antigen level on the paracentesis fluid and cytologic evaluation.
In suspected spontaneous bacterial peritonitis (SBP) the incidence of positive cultures can be increased by injecting 10 to 20 ml of ascitic fluid into blood culture bottles.
Peritoneal effusion can be subdivided as exudative or transudative based on its characteristics (see Section II).
The serum-ascites albumin gradient (serum albumin level–ascitic fluid albumin level [SAAG]) correlates directly with portal pressure and can also be used to classify ascites. Patients with gradients ≥1.1 g/dl have portal hypertension, and those with gradients ≤1.1 g/dl do not; the accuracy of this method is >95%.
For the differential diagnosis of ascites, refer to Section II.
An ascitic fluid polymorphonuclear leukocyte count >500/μl is suggestive of SBP.

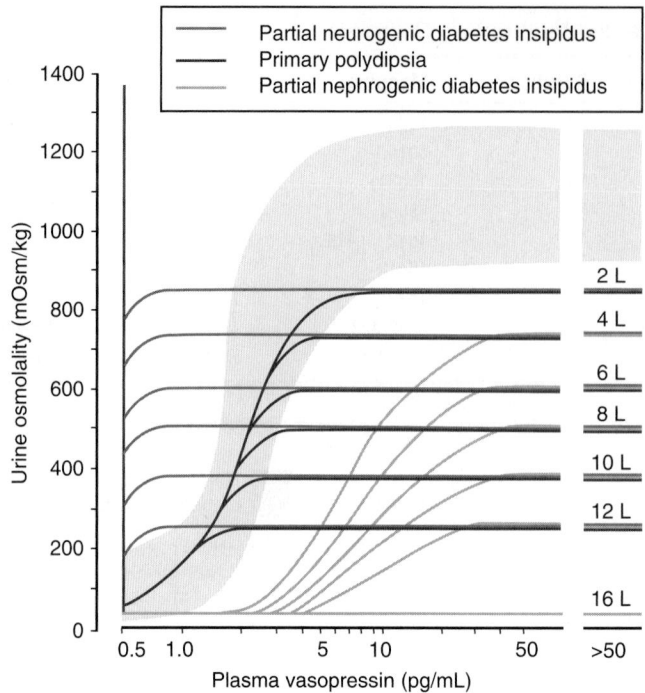

FIG. 33 The relationship between urine osmolality (Uosm) and plasma arginine vasopressin (AVP/ADH) in patients with polyuria of diverse causes and severity. Each of the three categories of polyuria is described by its own family of sigmoid curves of differing heights. Differences in height within a family reflect differences in maximum concentrating capacity caused by "washout" of the medullary concentration gradient. They are proportional to the severity of the polyuria (indicated in liters per day at the right end of each plateau). The normal response is depicted in yellow. The three categories of polyuria differ principally in the ascending portion of the dose-response curve. In patients with partial neurogenic diabetes insipidus (DI), the curve lies to the left of normal, reflecting increased sensitivity to the antidiuretic effects of very low concentrations of plasma ADH. In contrast, in patients with partial nephrogenic DI, the curve lies to the right of normal, reflecting decreased sensitivity to ADH. In primary polydipsia, the relationship of Uosm to ADH remains relatively normal. (Redrawn from Bichet DG: Diabetes insipidus and vasopressin. In Moore WT, Eastman RC, editors: *Diagnostic endocrinology,* ed 2, St Louis, 1996, Mosby, p 158, with permission.) (McPherson RA, Pincus MR: Henry's Clinical Diagnosis and Management by Laboratory Methods, 23rd ed, ISBN # 978-0323-29568-0, 2017, Elsevier)

BOX 21   Causes of Peritoneal Effusions

Transudates: Increased Hydrostatic Pressure or Decreased Plasma Oncotic Pressure
Congestive heart failure
Hepatic cirrhosis
Hypoproteinemia (e.g., nephrotic syndrome)

Exudates: Increased Capillary Permeability or Decreased Lymphatic Resorption
Infections
　　Primary bacterial peritonitis
　　Secondary bacterial peritonitis (e.g., appendicitis, bowel rupture)
　　Tuberculosis
Neoplasms
　　Hepatoma
　　Lymphoma
　　Mesothelioma
　　Metastatic carcinoma
　　Ovarian carcinoma
　　Prostate cancer
Trauma
Pancreatitis
Bile peritonitis (e.g., ruptured gallbladder)

Chylous Effusion
Damage to or obstruction of thoracic duct (e.g., trauma, lymphoma, carcinoma, tuberculosis and other granulomas [e.g., sarcoidosis, histoplasmosis], parasitic infestation)

(McPherson RA, Pincus MR: Henry's Clinical Diagnosis and Management by Laboratory Methods, 23rd ed, ISBN # 978-0323-29568-0, 2017, Elsevier)

A blood-ascitic fluid albumin gradient. Box 21 summarizes causes of peritoneal effusions. Useful criteria for evaluation of peritoneal lavage is summarized in Box 22. Recommended tests in peritoneal effusions are summarized in Box 23.

BOX 22   Criteria for Evaluation of Peritoneal Lavage

Positive Result
Aspiration of >15 mL gross blood on catheter placement
Grossly bloody lavage fluid
RBC >100,000/μL after blunt trauma
RBC >50,000/μL after penetrating trauma
WBC >500/μL
Amylase >110 U/dL

Indeterminate Result
Small amount of gross blood on catheter placement
RBC 50,000-100,000/μL after blunt trauma
RBC 1000-50,000/μL after penetrating trauma
WBC 100-500/μL

Negative Result
RBC <50,000/μL after blunt trauma
RBC <1000/μL after penetrating trauma
WBC <100/μL

Modified from Feied CF: Diagnostic peritoneal lavage, *Postgrad Med* 85:40, 1989, with permission.
RBC, Red blood cells; *WBC,* white blood cells.
(McPherson RA, Pincus MR: Henry's Clinical Diagnosis and Management by Laboratory Methods, 23rd ed, ISBN # 978-0323-29568-0, 2017, Elsevier)

PARATHYROID HORMONE (PTH)
Normal
Serum, intact molecule 10-65 pg/ml
Plasma 1.0-5.0 pmol/L
Elevated in: Hyperparathyroidism (primary or secondary), pseudohypoparathyroidism, anticonvulsants, corticosteroids, lithium, INH,

BOX 23 Recommended Tests in Peritoneal Effusions

Useful in Most Patients
Gross examination
Cytology
Stains and culture for microorganisms
Serum-ascites albumin concentration gradient

Useful in Selected Disorders
Total leukocyte and differential cell counts
RBC count (lavage)
Bilirubin
Creatinine/urea nitrogen
Enzymes (ADA, ALP, amylase, LD, telomerase)
Lactate
Cholesterol (malignant ascites)
Fibronectin
Tumor markers (CEA, PSA, CA 19-9, CA 15-3, CA-125)
Immunocytology/flow cytometry
Tuberculostearic acid

ADA, Adenosine deaminase; *ALP,* alkaline phosphatase; *CEA,* carcinoembryonic antigen; *LD,* lactate dehydrogenase; *PSA,* prostate-specific antigen; *RBC,* red blood cell.
Modified from Kjeldsberg CR, Knight JA: *Body fluids: Laboratory examination of amniotic, cerebrospinal, seminal, serous and synovial fluids,* ed 3, Chicago, 1993, © American Society for Clinical Pathology, with permission.
(McPherson RA, Pincus MR: Henry's Clinical Diagnosis and Management by Laboratory Methods, 23rd ed, ISBN # 978-0323-29568-0, 2017, Elsevier)

TABLE 59 Clinical Peculiarities of Coagulation Protein Screening Tests

Long aPTT, normal or long PT, no bleeding	Normal aPTT, PT, *with bleeding*
Long aPTT Only	
Factor XII deficiency	Factor XIII deficiency or inhibitor
Prekallikrein deficiency	α_2-Antiplasmin deficiency or defect
High-molecular-weight kininogen	Plasminogen activator inhibitor deficiency or defect
Lupus anticoagulant	α_1-Antitrypsin Pittsburgh defect
Long aPTT and PT	
Dysfibrinogenemia with fibrinopeptide B release	
Lupus anticoagulant	

From Hoffman R et al: *Hematology: basic principles and practice,* ed 5, Philadelphia, 2009, Churchill Livingstone.

rifampin, phosphates, Zollinger-Ellison syndrome, hereditary vitamin D deficiency
Decreased in: Hypoparathyroidism, sarcoidosis, cimetidine, beta-blockers, hyperthyroidism, hypomagnesemia

PARIETAL CELL ANTIBODIES

Normal: Negative
Present in: Pernicious anemia (>90%), atrophic gastritis (up to 50%), thyroiditis (30%), Addison's disease, myasthenia gravis, Sjögren's syndrome, type 1 DM

PARTIAL THROMBOPLASTIN TIME (PTT), ACTIVATED PARTIAL THROMBOPLASTIN TIME (APTT)

See Table 59 for interpretation of coagulation protein screening tests.
Normal range: 25-41 sec
Elevated in: Heparin therapy, coagulation factor deficiency (I, II, V, VIII, IX, X, XI, XII), liver disease, vitamin K deficiency, disseminated intravascular coagulation, circulating anticoagulant, warfarin therapy, specific factor inhibition (PCN reaction, rheumatoid arthritis), thrombolytic therapy, nephrotic syndrome
NOTE: Useful to evaluate the intrinsic coagulation system.

PEPSINOGEN I

Normal: 124-142 ng/ml
Elevated in: ZE syndrome, duodenal ulcer, acute gastritis
Decreased in: Atrophic gastritis, gastric carcinoma, myxedema, pernicious anemia, Addison's disease

PH, BLOOD

Normal values
Arterial: 7.35-7.45
Venous: 7.32-7.42
For abnormal values, refer to ARTERIAL BLOOD GASES.

PH, URINE

See URINE pH

PHENOBARBITAL

Normal therapeutic range: 15-30 mcg/ml for epilepsy control

PHENYTOIN (Dilantin)

Normal therapeutic range: 10-20 mcg/ml

PHOSPHATASE, ACID

See ACID PHOSPHATASE

PHOSPHATASE, ALKALINE

See ALKALINE PHOSPHATASE

PHOSPHATE (serum)

Normal range: 2.5-5 mg/dl (0.8-1.6 mmol/L [CF: 0.3229; SMI: 0.05 mmol/L])
DECREASED
Parenteral hyperalimentation
Diabetic acidosis
Alcohol withdrawal
Severe metabolic or respiratory alkalosis
Antacids that bind phosphorus
Malnutrition with refeeding using low-phosphorus nutrients
Renal tubule failure to reabsorb phosphate (Fanconi's syndrome; congenital disorder; vitamin D deficiency)
Glucose administration
Nasogastric suction
Malabsorption
Gram-negative sepsis
Primary hyperthyroidism
Chlorothiazide diuretics
Therapy of acute severe asthma
Acute respiratory failure with mechanical ventilation
INCREASED
Renal failure
Severe muscle injury
Phosphate-containing antacids
Hypoparathyroidism
Tumor lysis syndrome

PLASMINOGEN

Normal: Immunoassay (antigen): <20 mg/dl
Elevated in: Infection, trauma, neoplasm, myocardial infarction (acute phase reactant), pregnancy, bilirubinemia
Decreased in: DIC, severe liver disease, thrombolytic therapy with streptokinase or urokinase, alteplase

PLATELET AGGREGATION

Normal: Full aggregation (generally >60%) in response to epinephrine, thrombin, ristocetin, ADP, collagen
Elevated in: Heparin, hemolysis, lipemia, nicotine, hereditary and acquired disorders of platelet adhesion, activation, and aggregation
Decreased in: Aspirin, some penicillins, chloroquine, chlorpromazine, clofibrate, captopril, Glanzmann's thrombasthenia, Bernard-Soulier syndrome,

Wiskott-Aldrich syndrome, cyclooxygenase deficiency. In von Willebrand's disease there is normal aggregation with ADP, collagen, and epinephrine but abnormal agglutination with ristocetin.

PLATELET ANTIBODIES

Normal: Absent

Present in: ITP (>90% of patients with chronic ITP). Patients with nonimmune thrombocytopenias may have false-positive results.

PLATELET COUNT

See Fig. E34 for evaluation of thrombocytosis. Box E24 describes testing for thrombocytopenia. See Table 60 for differential diagnosis.

Normal range: 130-400 × 103/mm3 (130-400 × 109/L [CF: 1; SMI: 5 × 109/L])

Elevated in

REACTIVE THROMBOCYTOSIS

Infections or inflammatory states: vasculitis, allergic reactions, etc.

Surgery and tissue damage: myocardial infarction, pancreatitis, etc.

Postsplenectomy state

Malignancy: solid tumors, lymphoma

Iron deficiency anemia, hemolytic anemia, acute blood loss

Uncertain etiology

Rebound effect after chemotherapy or immune thrombocytopenia

Renal disorders: renal failure, nephrotic syndrome

MYELOPROLIFERATIVE DISORDERS

Chronic myeloid leukemia

Primary thrombocythemia

Polycythemia vera

Idiopathic myelofibrosis

Decreased

Increased destruction (see Table 61)

Immunologic

Drugs: quinine, quinidine, digitalis, procainamide, thiazide diuretics, sulfonamides, phenytoin, aspirin, penicillin, heparin, gold, meprobamate, cimetidine, furosemide, INH, cephalosporins, chlorpropamide, organic arsenicals, chloroquine

Idiopathic thrombocytopenic purpura

Transfusion reaction: transfusion of platelets with platelet antigen HPA-1a (PL^{A1}) in recipients without PL^{A1}

Fetal/maternal incompatibility

Vasculitis (e.g., systemic lupus erythematosus)

Autoimmune hemolytic anemia

Lymphoreticular disorders (e.g., chronic lymphocytic leukemia)

Nonimmunologic

Prosthetic heart valves

Thrombotic thrombocytopenic purpura

Sepsis

Disseminated intravascular coagulation

Hemolytic-uremic syndrome

Giant cavernous hemangioma

Decreased production

Abnormal marrow

Marrow infiltration (e.g., leukemia, lymphoma, fibrosis)

Marrow suppression (e.g., chemotherapy, alcohol, radiation)

Hereditary disorders (see Table 62)

Wiskott-Aldrich syndrome: X-linked disorder characterized by thrombocytopenia, eczema, and repeated infections

May-Hegglin anomaly: increased megakaryocytes but ineffective thrombopoiesis

Vitamin deficiencies (e.g., vitamin B$_{12}$, folic acid)

Splenic sequestration, hypersplenism

Dilutional, secondary to massive transfusion

PLATELET FUNCTION ANALYSIS 100 ASSAY (PFA)

Normal: This test is a two-component assay where blood is aspirated through two capillary tubes, one of which is coated with collagen and ADP (COL/ADP) and the other with collagen and epinephrine (COL/EPI). The test measures the ability of platelets to occlude an aperture in a biologically active membrane treated with COL/ADP and COL/EPI. During the test, the platelets

TABLE 60 Differential Diagnosis of Thrombocytopenia in Suspected Disseminated Intravascular Coagulation

Differential Diagnosis	Additional Diagnostic Clues
DIC	Prolonged aPTT and PT, increased FDP, low levels of AT or protein C
Sepsis without DIC	Positive (blood) cultures, positive sepsis criteria, hematophagocytosis in BM aspirate
Massive blood loss	Major bleeding, low hemoglobin, prolonged aPTT and PT
Thrombotic microangiopathy	Schistocytes in blood smear, Coombs-negative hemolysis, fever, neurologic symptoms, renal insufficiency, coagulation test results usually normal, ADAMTS13 levels decreased
Heparin-induced thrombocytopenia	Use of heparin, venous or arterial thrombosis, positive HIT test (usually immunoassay for heparin-platelet factor 4 antibodies), increase in platelet count after cessation of heparin; coagulation tests usually normal
Immune thrombocytopenia	Antiplatelet antibodies, normal or increased number of megakaryocytes in BM aspirate, TPO decreased; coagulation tests usually normal
Drug-induced thrombocytopenia	Decreased number of megakaryocytes in BM aspirate or detection of drug-induced antiplatelet antibodies, increase in platelet count after cessation of drug; coagulation test results usually normal

From Hoffman R: *Hematology, basic principles and practice,* ed 6, Philadelphia, Saunders, 2013. *ADAMTS13,* A disintegrin and metalloproteinase with a thrombospondin type 1 motif, member 13; *aPTT,* activated partial thromboplastin time; *AT,* antithrombin; *BM,* bone marrow; *DIC,* disseminated intravascular coagulation; *FDP,* fibrin degradation product; *HIT,* heparin-induced thrombocytopenia; *PT,* prothrombin time; *TPO,* thrombopoietin.

adhere to the surface of the tube and cause blood flow to cease. The closing time refers to the cessation of blood flow and is reported in conjunction with the hematocrit and platelet count. Hematocrit count must be >25% and platelet count >50 K/microliter for the test to be performed.

COL/ADP: 70-120 sec

COL/EPI: 75-120 sec

Elevated in: Acquired platelet dysfunction, von Willebrand's disease, anemia, thrombocytopenia, use of aspirin and NSAIDs

PLEURAL FLUID

Testing and evaluation of results

Pleural effusion fluid should be differentiated in exudate or transudate. The initial laboratory studies should be aimed only at distinguishing an exudate from a transudate.

Tube 1: protein, LDH, albumin.

Tubes 2, 3, 4: save the fluid until further notice. In selected patients with suspected empyema, a pH level may be useful (generally ≤7.0). See following for proper procedure to obtain a pH level from pleural fluid.

A serum/effusion albumin gradient of ≤1.2 g/dl is indicative of exudative effusions, especially in patients with congestive heart failure (CHF) treated with diuretics.

Note the appearance of the fluid:

A grossly hemorrhagic effusion can be a result of a traumatic tap, neoplasm, or an embolus with infarction.

A milky appearance indicates either of the following:

Chylous effusion: caused by trauma or tumor invasion of the thoracic duct; lipoprotein electrophoresis of the effusion reveals chylomicrons and triglyceride levels >115 mg/dl.

Pseudochylous effusion: often seen with chronic inflammation of the pleural space (e.g., TB, connective tissue diseases).

If transudate, consider CHF, cirrhosis, chronic renal failure, and other hypoproteinemic states and perform subsequent workup accordingly.

TABLE 61 Mechanisms of Platelet Destruction

Type of Thrombocytopenia	Specific Example(s)
Immune Mediated	
Autoantibody-mediated platelet destruction by reticuloendothelial system (RES)	Primary immune thrombocytopenic purpura; secondary immune thrombocytopenia associated with lymphoproliferative disease; collagen vascular disease; infections such as infectious mononucleosis; human immunodeficiency virus syndrome
Alloantibody-mediated platelet destruction by RES	Neonatal alloimmune thrombocytopenia; posttransfusion purpura; passive alloimmune thrombocytopenia; alloimmune platelet transfusion refractoriness
Drug-dependent, antibody-mediated platelet destruction by RES	Drug-induced immune thrombocytopenic purpura (e.g., quinine)
Platelet activation by binding of immunoglobulin G (IgG) Fc of drug-dependent IgG to platelet FcγIIa receptors	Heparin-induced thrombocytopenia
Non–Immune Mediated	
Platelet activation by thrombin or proinflammatory cytokines	Disseminated intravascular coagulation; septicemia/systemic inflammatory response syndromes
Platelet destruction via ingestion by macrophages (hemophagocytosis)	Infections; certain malignant lymphoproliferative disorders
Platelet destruction through platelet interactions with altered von Willebrand factor	Thrombotic thrombocytopenic purpura; hemolytic-uremic syndrome; aortic stenosis
Platelet losses on artificial surfaces	Cardiopulmonary bypass surgery; use of intravascular catheters
Decreased platelet survival associated with cardiovascular disease	Congenital and acquired heart disease; cardiomyopathy; pulmonary embolism

Modified with permission from Warkentin TE, Kelton JG: Thrombocytopenia due to platelet destruction and hypersplenism. In Hoffman R, Benz EJ Jr, Shattil SJ, et al, editors: *Hematology: basic principles and practice.* Philadelphia, 2005, Elsevier Churchill Livingstone, pp 2305–2325.
(McPherson RA, Pincus MR: Henry's Clinical Diagnosis and Management by Laboratory Methods, 23rd ed, ISBN # 978-0-323-29568-0, 2017, Elsevier)

If exudate, consider ordering these tests on the pleural fluid:
Cytologic examination for malignant cells (for suspected neoplasm).
Gram stain, cultures (aerobic and anaerobic), and sensitivities (for suspected infectious process).
AFB stain and cultures (for suspected TB).
pH: a value <7.0 suggests parapneumonic effusion or empyema; a pleural fluid pH must be drawn anaerobically and iced immediately; the syringe should be prerinsed with 0.2 ml of 1:1000 heparin.
Glucose: a low glucose level suggests parapneumonic effusions and rheumatoid arthritis.
Amylase: a high amylase level suggests pancreatitis or ruptured esophagus.
Perplexing pleural effusions are often a result of malignancy (e.g., lymphoma, malignant mesothelioma, ovarian carcinoma), TB, subdiaphragmatic processes, prior asbestos exposure, and postcardiac injury syndrome.
Box 25 Describes a cellular differential of pleural effusions. Features differentiating exudative from transudative pleural effusion are summarized in Table 63.

POTASSIUM (serum)

Normal range: 3.5-5 mEq/L (3.5-5 mmol/L [CF: 1; SMI: 0.1 mmol/L])
CAUSES OF HYPERKALEMIA
See Fig. E35 for evaluation and treatment of hyperkalemia, and Fig. E36 for electrocardiographic changes in hyperkalemia.)

TABLE 62 Classification of Inherited Thrombocytopenias by Platelet Size

SMALL PLATELETS (MPV <7 FL)	Normal-Sized Platelets (MPV 7-11 fL)	Large Platelets (MPV >11 fL)
Wiskott-Aldrich syndrome	Congenital amegakaryocytic thrombocytopenia	*MYH9*-related disorders
X-linked thrombocytopenia	Thrombocytopenia absent radius syndrome	Bernard-Soulier syndrome
	Radioulnar synostosis with amegakaryocytic thrombocytopenia	Gray platelet syndrome
	RUNX1 mutations (FPD/AML)	Velocardiofacial syndrome
	ANKRD26-related thrombocytopenia	*GATA*-1 mutations
	CYCS-related thrombocytopenia	Type 2B von Willebrand disease
		Platelet-type von Willebrand disease
		Paris-Trousseau (Jacobsen) syndrome
		TUBB1-related macrothrombocytopenia Thrombocytopenia associated with sitosterolemia

Modified with permission from Kumar R, Kahr WHA: Congenital thrombocytopenia: Clinical manifestations, laboratory abnormalities, and molecular defects of a heterogeneous group of conditions. In Rao AK, editor: *Hematology/oncology Clinics of North America: disorders of the platelets* (vol 27), Philadelphia, 2013, Elsevier, pp 465–494.
(McPherson RA, Pincus MR: Henry's Clinical Diagnosis and Management by Laboratory Methods, 23rd ed, ISBN # 978-0323-29568-0, 2017, Elsevier)

BOX 25 Cellular Differential of Pleural Effusions

Neutrophilia (>50%)
Bacterial pneumonia (parapneumonic effusion)
Pulmonary infarction
Pancreatitis
Subphrenic abscess
Early tuberculosis
Transudates (>10%)

Lymphocytosis (>50%)
Tuberculosis
Viral infection
Malignancy (lymphoma, other neoplasms)
True chylothorax
Rheumatoid pleuritis
Systemic lupus erythematosus
Uremic effusions
Transudates (≈30%)

Eosinophilia (>10%)
Pneumothorax (air in pleural space)
Trauma
Pulmonary infarction
Congestive heart failure
Infection (especially parasitic, fungal)
Hypersensitivity syndromes
Drug reaction
Rheumatologic diseases
Hodgkin's disease
Idiopathic

(McPherson RA, Pincus MR: Henry's Clinical Diagnosis and Management by Laboratory Methods, 23rd ed, ISBN # 978-0-323-29568-0, 2017, Elsevier)

Laboratory Tests

IV

TABLE 63 Features Differentiating Exudative from Transudative Pleural Effusion

Feature	Transudate	Exudate
Appearance	Serous	Cloudy
Leukocyte count	<10,000/mm^3	>50,000/mm^3
pH	>7.2	<7.2
Protein	<3.0 g/dL	>3.0 g/dL
Ratio of pleural fluid protein to serum	<0.5	>0.5
Lactate dehydrogenase (LDH)	<200 IU/L	>200 IU/L
Ratio of pleural fluid LDH to serum	<0.6	>0.6
Glucose	≥60 mg/dL	<60 mg/dL

From Bennett JE, Dolin R, Blaser MJ: *Mandell, Douglas, and Bennett's principles and practice of infectious diseases*, ed 8, Philadelphia, 2015, Saunders.

Pseudohyperkalemia
 Hemolysis of sample
 Thrombocytosis
 Leukocytosis
 Laboratory error
Increased potassium intake and absorption
 Potassium supplements (oral and parenteral)
 Dietary: salt substitutes
 Stored blood
 Potassium-containing medications
Impaired renal excretion
 Acute renal failure
 Chronic renal failure
 Tubular defect in potassium secretion
  1 Renal allograft
  2 Analgesic nephropathy
  3 Sickle cell disease
  4 Obstructive uropathy
 Hypoaldosteronism
  ▪ Primary (Addison's disease)
  ▪ Secondary
  • Hyporeninemic hypoaldosteronism (type IV RTA)
  • Congenital adrenal hyperplasia
  • Drug-induced
   ○ NSAIDs
   ○ ACE inhibitors
   ○ Heparin
   ○ Cyclosporine
Transcellular shifts
 ○ Acidosis
 ○ Hypertonicity
 ○ Insulin deficiency
 ○ Drugs
  ▪ β-blockers
  ▪ Digitalis toxicity
  ▪ Succinylcholine
 ○ Exercise
 ○ Hyperkalemic periodic paralysis
Cellular injury
 ○ Rhabdomyolysis
 ○ Severe intravascular hemolysis
 ○ Acute tumor lysis syndrome
 ○ Burns and crush injuries

CAUSES OF HYPOKALEMIA
• Decreased intake
 ○ Decreased dietary potassium
 ○ Impaired absorption of potassium
 ○ Clay ingestion
 ○ Kayexalate
• Increased loss
 ○ Renal
  Hyperaldosteronism
   Primary
    (1) Conn's syndrome
    (2) Adrenal hyperplasia
   Secondary
    (1) Congestive heart failure
    (2) Cirrhosis
    (3) Nephrotic syndrome
    (4) Dehydration
  Bartter's syndrome
  Glycyrrhizic acid (licorice, chewing tobacco)
  Excessive adrenal corticosteroids
   a. Cushing's syndrome
   b. Steroid therapy
   c. Adrenogenital syndrome
  Renal tubular defects
   a. Renal tubular acidosis
   b. Obstructive uropathy
   c. Salt-wasting nephropathy
  Drugs
   a. Diuretics
   b. Aminoglycosides
   c. Mannitol
   d. Amphotericin
   e. Cisplatin
   f. Carbenicillin
 ○ Gastrointestinal
  1. Vomiting
  2. Nasogastric suction
  3. Diarrhea
  4. Malabsorption
  5. Ileostomy
  6. Villous adenoma
  7. Laxative abuse
 ○ Increased losses from the skin
  1. Excessive sweating
  2. Burns
• Transcellular shifts
 A. Alkalosis
  1. Vomiting
  2. Diuretics
  3. Hyperventilation
  4. Bicarbonate therapy
 B. Insulin
  1. Exogenous
  2. Endogenous response to glucose
 C. β$_2$-Agonists (albuterol, terbutaline, epinephrine)
 D. Hypokalemia periodic paralysis
  1. Familial
  2. Thyrotoxic
• Miscellaneous
 A. Anabolic state
 B. Intravenous hyperalimentation
 C. Treatment of megaloblastic anemia
 D. Acute mountain sickness

POTASSIUM, URINE
See URINE POTASSIUM

PROCAINAMIDE
Normal therapeutic range: 4-10 mcg/ml

PROGESTERONE (serum)
Normal
Female: Follicular phase: 15-70 ng/dl
Luteal phase: 200-2500 ng/dl

Male: 15-70 ng/dl

Elevated in: Congenital adrenal hyperplasia, clomiphene, corticosterone, 11-deoxycortisol, dihydroprogesterone, molar pregnancy, lipoid ovarian tumor

Decreased in: Primary or secondary hypogonadism, oral contraceptives, ampicillin, threatened abortion

PROLACTIN

See Fig. E37 for the evaluation of hyperprolactinemia.

Normal range: <20 ng/ml (<20 μg/L [CF: 1; SMI: 1 μg/L])

Elevated in: Prolactinomas (level >200 micrograms/L highly suggestive), drugs (phenothiazines, cimetidine, tricyclic antidepressants, metoclopramide, estrogens, antihypertensives [methyldopa], verapamil, haloperidol), postpartum, stress, hypoglycemia, hypothyroidism, chronic liver disease, end-stage renal disease, brain radiation therapy, polycystic ovary syndrome, seizures, exercise, coitus, lactation. Mild hyperprolactinemia (<100 micrograms/L) can also be caused by large sellar masses, including nonfunctioning pituitary adenoma.

PROSTATE-SPECIFIC ANTIGEN (PSA)

Normal range: 0-4 ng/ml

Table 64 describes age-specific reference ranges for PSA.

Elevated in: Benign prostatic hypertrophy, carcinoma of prostate, prostatitis, postrectal examination, prostate trauma.

Factors affecting serum PSA are described in Table 65.

NOTE: Measurement of free PSA is useful to assess the probability of prostate cancer in patients with normal digital rectal examination and total PSA between 4 and 10 ng/ml. In these patients, the global risk of prostate cancer is 25%; however, if the free PSA is >25%, the risk of prostate cancer decreases to 8%, whereas if the free PSA is <10%, the risk of cancer increases to 56%. Free PSA is also useful to evaluate the aggressiveness

of prostate cancer. A low free PSA percentage generally indicates a high-grade cancer, whereas a high free PSA percentage is generally associated with a slower-growing tumor.

Decreased in: 5-α reductase inhibitors (finasteride, dutasteride), saw palmetto use, antiandrogens

PROSTATIC ACID PHOSPHATASE

Normal: 0-0.8 U/L

Elevated in: Prostate cancer (especially in metastatic prostate cancer), BPH, prostatitis, post-prostate surgery or manipulation, hemolysis, androgens, clofibrate

Decreased in: Ketoconazole

PROTEIN (serum)

Normal range: 6-8 g/dl (60-80 g/L [CF: 10; SMI: 1 g/L])

Elevated in: Dehydration, multiple myeloma, Waldenström's macroglobulinemia, sarcoidosis, collagen vascular diseases

Decreased in: Malnutrition, low-protein diet, overhydration, malabsorption, pregnancy, severe burns, neoplasms, chronic diseases, cirrhosis, nephrosis

PROTEIN C ASSAY

See Table 66.

Normal: 70%-140%

Elevated in: Oral contraceptives, stanozol

Decreased in: Congenital protein C deficiency, warfarin therapy, Vitamin K deficiency, renal insufficiency, consumptive coagulopathies

PROTEIN ELECTROPHORESIS (serum)

Normal range

Albumin: 60%-75% (0.6-0.75 [CF: 0.01; SMI: 0.01])

α-1: 1.7%-5% (0.02-0.05)
α-2: 6.7%-12.5% (0.07-0.13)
β: 8.3%-16.3% (0.08-0.16)
γ: 10.7%-20% (0.11-0.2)

Albumin: 3.6-5.2 g/dl (36-52 g/L [CF: 0.01; SMI: 1 g/L])

α-1: 0.1-0.4 g/dl (1-4 g/L)
α-2: 0.4-1 g/dl (4-10 g/L)
β: 0.5-1.2 g/dl (5-12 g/L)
γ: 0.6-1.6 g/dl (6-16 g/L)

Elevated in

Albumin: dehydration

α-1: neoplastic diseases, inflammation

α-2: neoplasms, inflammation, infection, nephrotic syndrome

β: hypothyroidism, biliary cirrhosis, diabetes mellitus

γ: See IMMUNOGLOBULINS

Decreased in

Albumin: malnutrition, chronic liver disease, malabsorption, nephrotic syndrome, burns, systemic lupus erythematosus

α-1: emphysema (α-1 antitrypsin deficiency), nephrosis

α-2: hemolytic anemias (decreased haptoglobin), severe hepatocellular damage

β: hypocholesterolemia, nephrosis

γ: See IMMUNOGLOBULINS

Fig. 38 describes serum protein electrophoretic patterns.

TABLE 64 Age-Specific Reference Ranges for PSA

	SERUM PSA (NG/ML)		
Age (yr)	Whites	Japanese	African Americans
40-49	0-2.5	0-2.0	0-2.0
50-59	0-3.5	0-3.0	0-4.0
60-69	0-4.5	0-4.0	0-4.5
70-79	0-6.5	0-5.0	0-5.5

From Nseyo UO (ed): *Urology for primary care physicians,* Philadelphia, 1999, Saunders. *PSA,* Prostate-specific antigen.

TABLE 65 Factors Affecting Serum PSA

Factors Affecting Serum PSA	Duration of Effect
Prostate cell number	NA
Prostate size	NA
Recent ejaculation	6-48 hours
Prostate manipulation	
Vigorous massage	1 week
Cystoscopy	1 week
Prostate biopsy	4-6 weeks
Prostatitis	
Acute	3-6 months
Chronic	Unknown
Prostate cancer	NA
Drugs: finasteride*	3-6 months

NA, Not applicable; *PSA,* prostate-specific antigen.
*Lowers PSA for as long as patient is on the medication.
From Nseyo UO (ed): *Urology for primary care physicians,* Philadelphia, 1999, Saunders.

TABLE 66 Assay Measurement in Heterozygote Protein C Deficiency

	ACTIVITY		
Type	Antigen	Amidolytic	Coagulant
I	Low	Low	Low
II	Normal	Low	Low
	Normal	Normal	Low

From Hoffman R et al: *Hematology: basic principles and practice,* ed 5, Philadelphia, 2009, Churchill Livingstone.

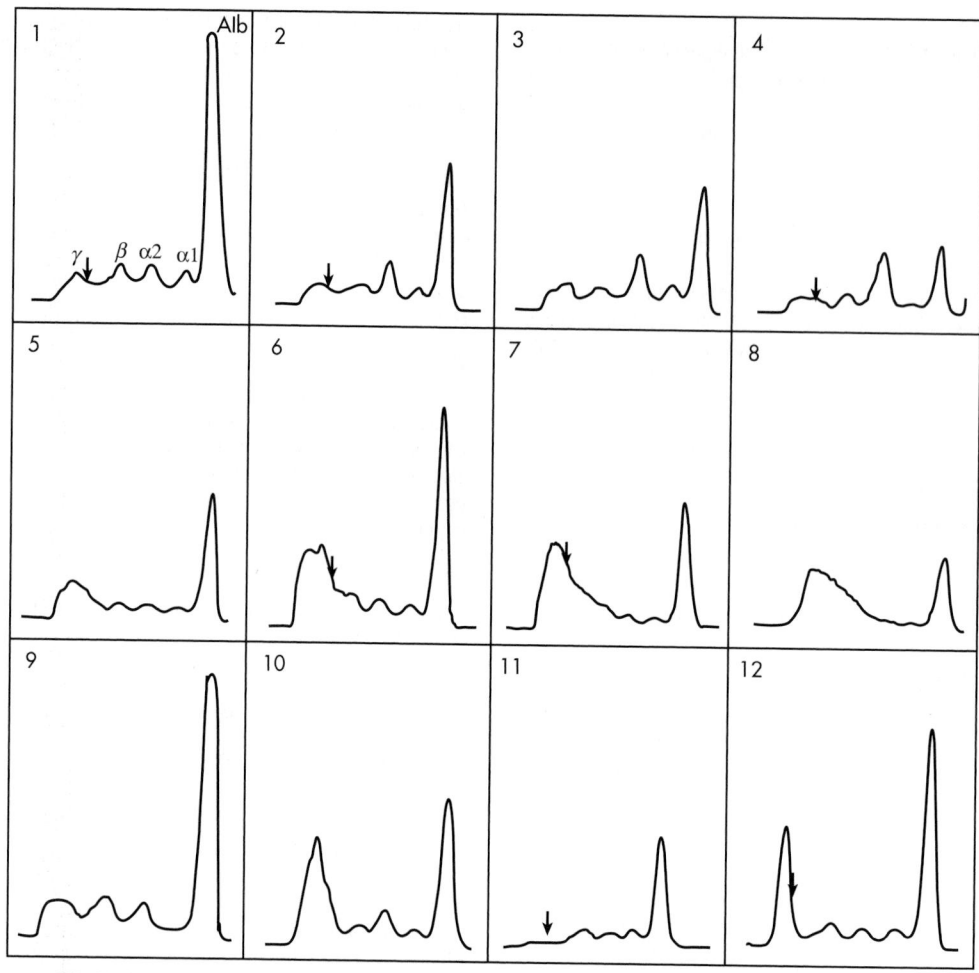

FIG. 38 Typical serum protein electrophoretic patterns. 1, Normal (*arrow* near γ region indicates serum application point). **2,** Acute reaction pattern. **3,** Acute reaction or nephrotic syndrome. **4,** Nephrotic syndrome. **5,** Chronic inflammation, cirrhosis, granulomatous diseases, rheumatoid-collagen group. **6,** Same as 5, but γ elevation is more pronounced. There is also partial (but not complete) β-γ fusion. **7,** Suggestive of cirrhosis but could be found in the granulomatous diseases or the rheumatoid-collagen group. **8,** Characteristic pattern of cirrhosis. **9,** α-1 Antitrypsin deficiency with mild γ elevation suggesting concurrent chronic disease. **10,** Same as 5, but the γ elevation is marked. The configuration of the γ peak superficially mimics that of myeloma, but is more broad-based. There are superimposed acute reaction changes. **11,** Hypogammaglobulinemia or light-chain myeloma. **12,** Myeloma, Waldenström's macroglobulinemia, idiopathic or secondary monoclonal gammopathy. (From Ravel R [ed]: *Clinical laboratory medicine,* ed 6, St Louis, 1995, Mosby.)

PROTEIN S ASSAY

See Table 67.

Normal: 65%-140%

Elevated in: Presence of lupus anticoagulant

Decreased in: Hereditary deficiency, acute thrombotic events, DIC, surgery, oral contraceptives, pregnancy, hormone replacement therapy, l-asparaginase treatment

PROTHROMBIN TIME (PT)

Normal range: 10-12 sec

Elevated in: Liver disease, oral anticoagulants (warfarin), heparin, factor deficiency (I, II, V, VII, X), disseminated intravascular coagulation, vitamin K deficiency, afibrinogenemia, dysfibrinogenemia, drugs (salicylate, chloral hydrate, diphenylhydantoin, estrogens, antacids, phenylbutazone, quinidine, antibiotics, allopurinol, anabolic steroids). Table 68 describes a differential diagnosis of abnormal coagulation screening tests.

Decreased in: Vitamin K supplementation, thrombophlebitis, drugs (glutethimide, estrogens, griseofulvin, diphenhydramine)

PROTOPORPHYRIN (Free erythrocyte)

Normal range: 16-36 μg/dl of red blood cells (0.28-0.64 μmol/L [CF: 0.0177; SMI: 0.02 μmol/L])

Elevated in: Iron deficiency, lead poisoning, sideroblastic anemias, anemia of chronic disease, hemolytic anemias, erythropoietic protoporphyria

PSA

See PROSTATE-SPECIFIC ANTIGEN

PT

See PROTHROMBIN TIME

PTH

See PARATHYROID HORMONE

PTT

See PARTIAL THROMBOPLASTIN TIME

TABLE 67 Assay Measurements in Heterozygote Protein S Deficiency

Type	ACTIVITY		
	Protein S Total Antigen	Protein S Free Antigen	Protein S Activity
I (classic)	Low	Low	Low
II	Normal	Normal	Low
III	Normal	Low	Low

From Hoffman R et al: *Hematology: basic principles and practice,* ed 5, Philadelphia, 2009, Churchill Livingstone.

TABLE 68 Differential Diagnosis of Abnormal Coagulation Screening Tests

Abnormal Activated Partial Thromboplastin Time (APTT) Alone

Associated with bleeding: VIII, IX, and XI defects

Not associated with bleeding: XII, prekallikrein (PK), high molecular weight kininogen, lupus anticoagulants

Abnormal Prothrombin Time (PT) Alone

Factor VII defects

Combined Abnormal APTT and PT

Medical conditions: Anticoagulants, disseminated intravascular coagulation (DIC), liver disease, vitamin K deficiency, massive transfusion

Rarely dysfibrinogenemia; factor X, V, and II defects

(McPherson RA, Pincus MR: Henry's Clinical Diagnosis and Management by Laboratory Methods, 23rd ed, ISBN # 978-0323-29568-0, 2017, Elsevier)

RAPID PLASMA REAGIN (RPR)

Description: Non-treponemal test traditionally used as a screening test for syphilis. It is a quantitative test and antibody titers can be monitored to assess treatment response.

Normal: Negative

Positive: Syphilis. False-positive results may occur with pregnancy, autoimmune diseases, tuberculosis, and other inflammatory conditions. Positive results should be confirmed with treponemal serologic tests (e.g., T-pallidum enzyme immunoassay [TP-EIA])

RDW

See RED BLOOD CELL DISTRIBUTION WIDTH

RED BLOOD CELL (RBC) COUNT

Normal range

Male: $4.3\text{-}5.9 \times 10^6/mm^3$ ($4.3\text{-}5.9 \times 10^{12}/L$ [CF: 1; SMI: $0.1 \times 10^{12}/L$])
Female: $3.5\text{-}5 \times 10^6/mm^3$ ($3.5\text{-}5 \times 10^{12}/L$ [CF: 1; SMI: $0.1 \times 10^{12}/L$])

Elevated in: Polycythemia vera, smokers, high altitude, cardiovascular disease, renal cell carcinoma and other erythropoietin-producing neoplasms, stress, hemoconcentration/dehydration

Decreased in: Anemias, hemolysis, chronic renal failure, hemorrhage, failure of marrow production

RED BLOOD CELL DISTRIBUTION WIDTH (RDW)

Measures variability of red cell size (anisocytosis)

Normal range: 11.5-14.5

Normal RDW and elevated mean corpuscular volume (MCV): Aplastic anemia, preleukemia

Normal MCV: Normal, anemia of chronic disease, acute blood loss or hemolysis, chronic lymphocytic leukemia (CLL), chronic myelocytic leukemia, nonanemic enzymopathy or hemoglobinopathy

Decreased MCV: Anemia of chronic disease, heterozygous thalassemia

Elevated RDW and elevated MCV: Vitamin B_{12} deficiency, folate deficiency, immune hemolytic anemia, cold agglutinins, CLL with high count, liver disease

Normal MCV: Early iron deficiency, early vitamin B_{12} deficiency, early folate deficiency, anemic globinopathy

Decreased MCV: Iron deficiency, red blood cell fragmentation, HbH disease, thalassemia intermedia

RED BLOOD CELL FOLATE

See FOLATE

RED BLOOD CELL MASS (volume)

Normal range:

Male: 20-36 ml/kg body weight ($1.15\text{-}1.21$ L/m^2 body surface area)
Female: 19-31 ml/kg body weight ($0.95\text{-}1.00$ L/m^2 body surface area)

Elevated in: Polycythemia vera, hypoxia (smokers, high altitude, cardiovascular disease), hemoglobinopathies with high oxygen affinity, erythropoietin-producing tumors (renal cell carcinoma)

Decreased in: Hemorrhage, chronic disease, failure of marrow production, anemias, hemolysis

RED BLOOD CELL MORPHOLOGY

See Figs. 39 and 40. Table 69 summarizes peripheral blood film evaluation in a patient with red cell membrane disorder.

RENIN (serum)

Elevated in: Drugs (thiazides, estrogen, minoxidil), chronic renal failure, Bartter's syndrome, pregnancy (normal), pheochromocytoma, renal hypertension, reduced plasma volume, secondary aldosteronism

Decreased in: Adrenocortical hypertension, increased plasma volume, primary aldosteronism, drugs (propranolol, reserpine, clonidine)

Table 70 describes typical renin-aldosterone patterns in various conditions.

RESPIRATORY SYNCYTIAL VIRUS (RSV) SCREEN

Test description: PCR test can be performed on nasopharyngeal swab, wash, or aspirate

RETICULOCYTE COUNT

See Fig. E41 and Table 71.

Normal range: 0.5%-1.5%

Elevated in: Hemolytic anemia (sickle cell crisis, thalassemia major, autoimmune hemolysis), hemorrhage, postanemia therapy (folic acid, ferrous sulfate, vitamin B_{12}), chronic renal failure

Decreased in: Aplastic anemia, marrow suppression (sepsis, chemotherapeutic agents, radiation), hepatic cirrhosis, blood transfusion, anemias of disordered maturation (iron deficiency anemia, megaloblastic anemia, sideroblastic anemia, anemia of chronic disease)

RHEUMATOID FACTOR

Normal: Negative. Present in titer >1:20

RHEUMATIC DISEASES

Rheumatoid arthritis

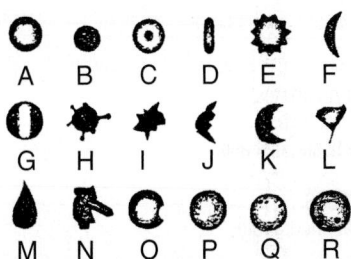

FIG. 39 Abnormal red blood cells (RBCs). **A,** Normal RBC. **B,** Spherocyte. **C,** Target cell. **D,** Elliptocyte. **E,** Echinocyte. **F,** Sickle cell. **G,** Stomatocyte. **H,** Acanthocyte. **I** to **L,** Schistocytes. **M,** Teardrop RBC. **N,** Distorted RBC with Hb C crystal protruding. **O,** Degmacyte. **P,** Basophilic stippling. **Q,** Pappenheimer bodies. **R,** Howell-Jolly body. (From Ravel R [ed]: *Clinical laboratory medicine,* ed 6, St Louis, 1995, Mosby.)

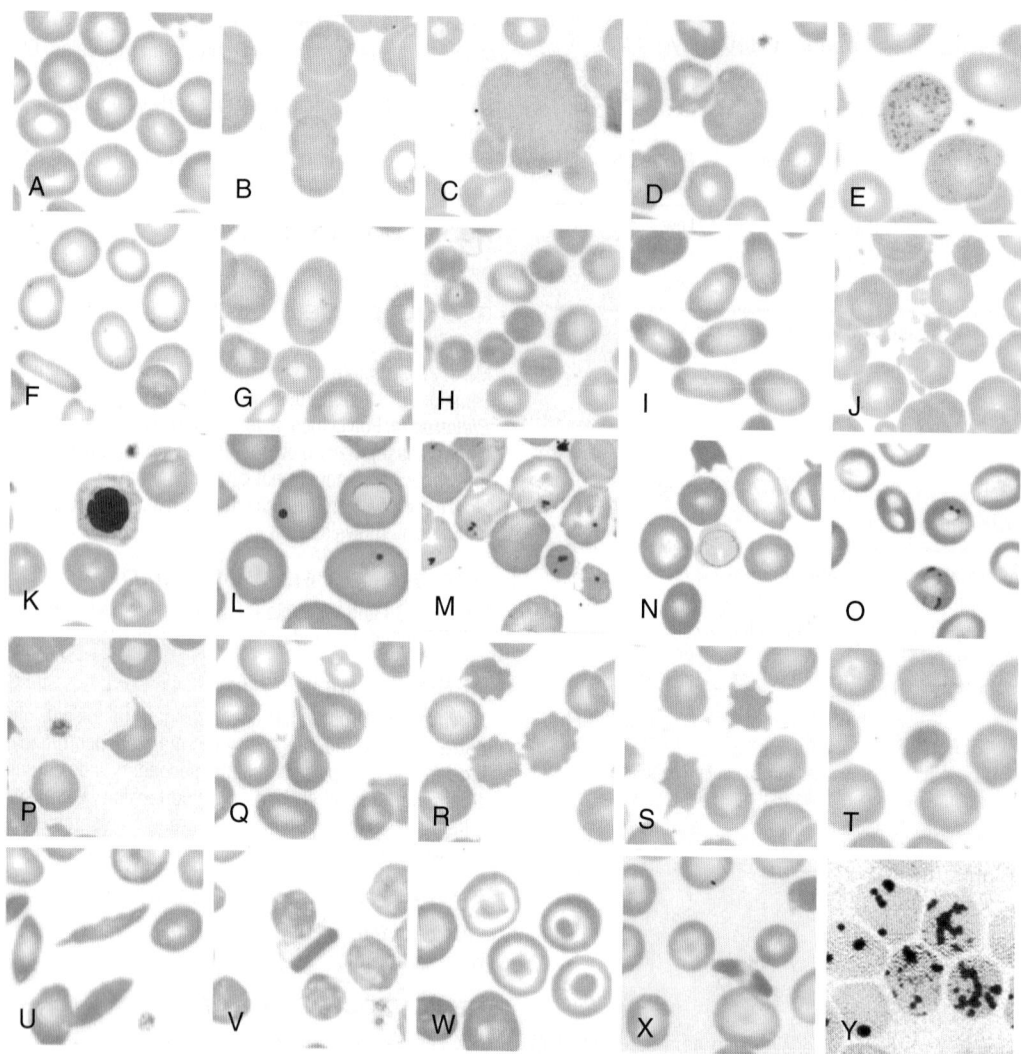

FIG. 40 Useful peripheral blood and red blood cell features in the evaluation of anemia. **A,** Normal red blood cells (RBCs). Note the central pallor is one-third the diameter of the entire cell. **B,** Rouleaux formation is indicative of increased plasma protein. **C,** Agglutination indicates an antibody-mediated process such as cold agglutinin disease. **D,** Polychromatophilic cell. The gray-blue color is attributable to RNA and the cell is equivalent to a reticulocyte, which must be identified with a reticulocyte stain. **E,** Basophilic stippling. This also is attributable to increased RNA caused either by a left shift in erythroid cells or lead toxicity. **F,** Hypochromic microcytic cells typical of iron-deficiency anemia. Note the widened central pallor and the "pencil" cell in the lower left. **G,** Macroovalocyte as can be seen in either megaloblastic anemia or myelodysplastic syndrome. **H,** Microspherocytes typical of hereditary spherocytosis. **I,** Elliptocytes (ovalocytes) from a patient with hereditary elliptocytosis. **J,** RBC fragments from thermal injury (burn patient). **K,** Nucleated RBC. **L,** Howell-Jolly bodies indicative of splenic dysfunction or absence. **M,** Pappenheimer bodies from a patient with sideroblastic anemia. **N,** Cabot ring, as can be seen in megaloblastic anemia or myelodysplastic syndromes. **O,** Malarial parasites *(Plasmodium falciparum).* **P,** Schistocyte typical of a microangiopathic hemolytic anemia. **Q,** Tear-drop form indicates marrow fibrosis and extramedullary hematopoiesis. **R,** Echinocyte (Burr cell) with rounded edges. **S,** Acanthocyte (spur cell) with more irregular pointed ends. This was from a patient with neuroacanthocytosis. They can also be seen in patients with liver disease and lipid abnormalities. **T,** "Bite" cell from a patient with glucose-6-phosphate dehydrogenase (G6PD) deficiency. **U,** Sickle cell, from a patient with homozygous sickle cell disease. **V,** Hemoglobin C crystal. **W,** Target cells. **X,** Hemoglobin C disease. Note that the RBC in center has condensed hemoglobin at each pole. **Y,** Heinz body preparation (supravital stain) from a patient with G6PD deficiency. Note that the cells to the right have increased precipitated hemoglobin. From Hoffman R, et al: *Hematology, basic principles and practice,* ed 6, Philadelphia, 2013, Saunders.

Sjögren's syndrome
Systemic lupus erythematosus
Polymyositis/dermatomyositis
Mixed connective tissue disease
Scleroderma
INFECTIOUS DISEASES
Subacute bacterial endocarditis
Tuberculosis
Infectious mononucleosis
Hepatitis
Syphilis
Leprosy
Influenza
MALIGNANCIES

Lymphoma
Multiple myeloma
Waldenström's macroglobulinemia
Postradiation or postchemotherapy
MISCELLANEOUS
Normal adults, especially the elderly
Sarcoidosis
Chronic pulmonary disease (interstitial fibrosis)
Chronic liver disease (chronic active hepatitis, cirrhosis)
Mixed essential cryoglobulinemia
Hypergammaglobulinemic purpura

RNP

See EXTRACTABLE NUCLEAR ANTIGEN

TABLE 69 Peripheral Blood Film Evaluation in a Patient with Red Cell Membrane Disorder

Shape	Pathobiology	Diagnosis
Microspherocytes	Loss of membrane lipids leading to a reduction of surface area resulting from deficiencies of spectrin, ankyrin, or band 3 and protein 4.2 Removal of membrane material from antibody-coated red cells by macrophages Removal of membrane-associated Heinz bodies, with the adjacent membrane lipids, by the spleen	HS Immunohemolytic anemias Heinz body hemolytic anemias
Elliptocytes	Permanent red cell deformation resulting from a weakening of skeletal protein interactions (such as the spectrin dimer-dimer contact). This facilitates disruption of existing protein contacts during shear stress–induced elliptical deformation. Subsequently, new protein contacts are formed that stabilize elliptical shape Unknown	Mild common HE Iron deficiency, megaloblastic anemias, myelofibrosis, myelophthisic anemias, myelodysplastic syndrome, thalassemias
Poikilocytes/Fragments	Weakening of skeletal protein contacts resulting from skeletal protein mutations Unknown	Hemolytic HE/HPP Iron deficiency, megaloblastic anemias, myelofibrosis, myelophthisic anemias, myelodysplastic syndrome, thalassemias
Schistocytes, fragmented red cells	Red cells "torn" by mechanical trauma (fibrin strands, turbulent flow)	"Microangiopathic" hemolytic anemia associated with disseminated intravascular coagulation, thrombotic thrombocytopenic purpura, vasculitis, heart valve prostheses
Acanthocytes	Uptake of cholesterol and its preferential accumulation in the outer leaflet of the lipid bilayer Selective accumulation of sphingomyelin in the outer lipid leaflet Unknown	Spur cell hemolytic anemia in severe liver disease Abetalipoproteinemia, Chorea-acanthocytosis syndrome, malnutrition, hypothyroidism McLeod phenotype
Echinocytes	Expansion of the surface area of the outer hemileaflet of lipid bilayer relative to the inner hemileaflet Unknown	Hemolytic anemia associated with hypomagnesemia and hypophosphatemia in malnourished patients, pyruvate kinase deficiency; in vitro artifact of low blood storage (ATP depletion), contact with glass or elevated pH Hemolysis in long-distance runners, renal failure
Stomatocytes	Expansion of the surface area of the inner hemileaflet of the bilayer relative to the outer leaflet Unknown	Exposure of red cells to cationic anesthetics in vitro; in vivo the drug concentrations may not be sufficient to produce similar effect Alcoholism, inherited disorders of membrane permeability (hereditary stomatocytosis)
Target cells	Absolute excess of membrane lipids (both cholesterol and phospholipids: "symmetric" lipid gain), followed by an increase of cell surface area Relative excess of surface area because of a decrease in cell volume	Obstructive jaundice, liver disease with intrahepatic cholestasis Thalassemias and some hemoglobinopathies (C, D, E)

From Hoffman R, et al: *Hematology, basic principles and practice*, ed 6, Philadelphia, 2013, Saunders.
ATP, Adenosine triphosphate; *HE,* hereditary elliptocytosis; *HPP,* hereditary pyropoikilocytosis; *HS,* hereditary spherocytosis.

TABLE 70 Typical Renin-Aldosterone Patterns in Various Conditions

	Plasma Renin	Aldosterone
Primary aldosteronism	Low	High
"Low-renin" essential hypertension	Low	Normal
Cushing's syndrome	Low	Low-normal
Licorice ingestion syndrome	Low	Low
High-salt diet	Low	Low
Oral contraceptives	High	Normal
Cirrhosis	High	High
Malignant hypertension	High	High
Unilateral renal disease	High	High
"High-renin" essential hypertension	High	High
Pregnancy	High	High
Diuretic overuse	High	High
Juxtaglomerular tumor (Bartter's syndrome)	High	High
Low-salt diet	High	High
Addison's disease	High	Low
Hypokalemia	High	Low

From Ravel R: *Clinical laboratory medicine*, ed 6, St Louis, 1995, Mosby.

TABLE 71 Combining the Reticulocyte Count and Red Blood Cell Parameters for Diagnosis

MCV, RDW	Reticulocyte Count <75,000/µL	Reticulocyte Count >100,000/µL
Low, Normal	Anemia of chronic disease	
Normal, Normal	Anemia of chronic disease	
High, Normal	Chemotherapy/antivirals/alcohol Aplastic anemia	Chronic liver disease
Low, High	Iron deficiency anemia	Sickle cell-β-thalassemia
Normal, High	Early iron, folate, vitamin B_{12} deficiency Myelodysplasia	Sickle cell anemia, sickle cell disease
High, High	Folate or vitamin B_{12} deficiency Myelodysplasia	Immune hemolytic anemia Chronic liver disease

From Hoffman R et al: *Hematology: basic principles and practice*, ed 5, Philadelphia, 2009, Churchill Livingstone.
MCV, Mean corpuscular volume; *RDW,* red blood cell distribution width.

Laboratory Tests

IV

RPR

See RAPID PLASMA REAGIN

ROTAVIRUS SEROLOGY

Test description: PCR test is performed on stool specimen
Normal: Negative

SED RATE

See ERYTHROCYTE SEDIMENTATION RATE

SEDIMENTATION RATE

See ERYTHROCYTE SEDIMENTATION RATE

TABLE 72 Semen Analysis Reference Ranges

Color	Grayish white
pH	7.3-7.8 (literature range, 7.0-7.8)
Volume	2.0-5.0 ml (literature range, 1.5-6.0 ml)
Sperm count	20-250 million/ml (literature range for upper limit varies from 100-250 million/ml)
Motility	>60% motile <3 hours after specimen is obtained (literature range, >40% to >70%)
% Normal sperm	>60% (literature range, >60% to >70%)
Viscosity	Can be poured from a pipet in droplets rather than a thick strand

From Ravel R (ed): *Clinical laboratory medicine,* ed 6, St Louis, 1995, Mosby.

SEMEN ANALYSIS

Table 72 describes semen analysis reference ranges.

SGOT

See ASPARTATE AMINOTRANSFERASE

SGPT

See ALANINE AMINOTRANSFERASE

SICKLE CELL TEST

Normal: Negative
Positive in: Sickle cell anemia, sickle cell trait, combination of *Hb S* gene with other disorders such as alpha-thalassemia, beta-thalassemia.

SMOOTH MUSCLE ANTIBODY

Normal: Negative
Present in: Chronic acute hepatitis, primary sclerosing cholangitis, primary biliary cirrhosis, autoimmune hepatitis, infectious mononucleosis

SODIUM (serum)

Normal range: 135-147 mEq/L (135-147 mmol/L [CF: 1; SMI: 1 mmol/L]). Electrolyte concentrations in extracellular and intracellular fluid are summarized in Table 73.
HYPONATREMIA
Common causes of hyponatremia and electrolyte patterns in serum and urine with normal renal function are described in Table 74. Table E75 describes drugs associated with hyponatremia.

TABLE 73 Electrolyte Concentrations in Extracellular and Intracellular Fluids

	PLASMA		INTERSTITIAL FLUID		PLASMA WATER		CELL WATER (MUSCLE)	
	(mmol/L)	(mmol/L)	(mmol/L)	(mmol/L)	(mmol/L)	(mmol/L)	(mmol/L)	(mmol/L)
Na^+	140	140	145.3	145.3	149.8	149.8	13	13
K^+	4.5	4.5	4.7	4.7	4.8	4.8	140	140
Ca^{++}	5.0	2.5	2.8	1.4	5.3	5.3	10^{-7}	0.5×10^{-7}
Mg^{++}	1.7	0.85	1.0	0.5	1.8	0.9	7.0	3.5
Cl^-	104	104	114.7	114.7	111.4	111.4	3	3
$HCO3^-$	24	24	26.5	26.5	25.7	25.7	10	10
$SO42^-$	1.0	0.5	1.2	0.6	1.1	0.55	–	–
P	2.1	1.2+	2.1++	1.2+	2.2	1.25+	107	57+++
Protein	15	1	8	0.5	16	1	40	2.5*
Organic anion	5	5	5.6	5.6	5.3	5.3	–	–

+The calculation is based on the assumption that the pH of the extracellular fluid is 7.4 and the pK of inorganic $H2PO4^-$ is 6.8.
++The concentration of P in the interstitial fluid would be increased by the Donnan effect, but reduced by the lower protein-bound phosphate, and these two opposing effects keep interstitial phosphate concentration about equal to that of plasma.
+++The intracellular molal concentration of phosphate is calculated with the assumption that the pK of organic phosphates in the cell is 6.1 and the intracellular pH 7.0.
*The calculation is based on the assumption that each mmol of intracellular protein has an average of 15 mEq.
(McPherson RA, Pincus MR: Henry's Clinical Diagnosis and Management by Laboratory Methods, 23rd ed, ISBN # 978-0323-29568-0, 2017, Elsevier)

TABLE 74 Common Causes of Hyponatremia and Electrolyte Patterns in Serum and Urine with Normal Renal Function*

Cause	Serum Na	Urine Na (UNa)	Urine Osmolality	Serum K	24-Hour UNa
1. Overhydration	Low	Low	Low	Normal or low	Low
2. Diuretics	Low	Low	Low	Low	High
3. SIADH†	Low	High	High	Normal or low	High
4. Adrenal failure	Low	Mildly elevated	Normal	High	High
5. Bartter's syndrome	Low	Low	Low	Low	High
6. Diabetic hyperosmolarity‡	Low	Normal	Normal	High	Normal

*All Na and K values are concentrations, except for 24-hour UNa, which is the total number of milliequivalents of Na excreted in 24 hours in the urine.
†Secretion of inappropriate levels of antidiuretic hormone.
‡In this condition, serum glucose is markedly elevated.
(McPherson RA, Pincus MR: Henry's Clinical Diagnosis and Management by Laboratory Methods, 23rd ed, ISBN # 978-0323-29568-0, 2017, Elsevier)

Sodium and water depletion (deficit hyponatremia)
  Loss of gastrointestinal secretions with replacement of fluid but not electrolytes
    Vomiting
    Diarrhea
    Tube drainage
  Loss from skin with replacement of fluids but not electrolytes
    Excessive sweating
    Extensive burns
  Loss from kidney
    Diuretics
    Chronic renal insufficiency (uremia) with acidosis
  Metabolic loss
    Starvation with acidosis
    Diabetic acidosis
  Endocrine loss
    Addison's disease
    Sudden withdrawal of long-term steroid therapy
  Iatrogenic loss from serous cavities
    Paracentesis or thoracentesis
  Excessive water (dilution hyponatremia)
    Excessive water administration
    Congestive heart failure
    Cirrhosis
    Nephrotic syndrome
    Hypoalbuminemia (severe)
    Acute renal failure with oliguria
Inappropriate antidiuretic hormone (IADH) syndrome
Intracellular loss (reset osmostat syndrome)
False hyponatremia (actually a dilutional effect)
    Marked hypertriglyceridemia
    Marked hyperproteinemia
    Severe hyperglycemia

HYPERNATREMIA

Common causes of hypernatremia and electrolyte patterns in serum and urine with normal renal function are summarized in Table 76.

Dehydration is the most frequent overall clinical finding in hypernatremia.

Deficient water intake (either orally or intravenously)

Excess kidney water output (diabetes insipidus, osmotic diuresis)

Excess skin water output (excess sweating, loss from burns)

Excess gastrointestinal tract output (severe protracted vomiting or diarrhea without fluid therapy)

Accidental sodium overdose

High-protein tube feedings

STREPTOZYME

See ANTISTREPTOLYSIN O TITER

SUCROSE HEMOLYSIS TEST (sugar water test)

Normal: Absence of hemolysis
Positive in: Paroxysmal nocturnal hemoglobinuria
False-positive: autoimmune hemolytic anemia, megaloblastic anemias
False-negative: may occur with use of heparin or EDTA

SUDAN III STAIN (qualitative screening for fecal fat)

Normal: Negative. Test should be preceded by diet containing 100-150 g of dietary fat/day for 1 week, avoidance of high-fiber diet, and avoidance of suppositories or oily material before specimen collection.
Positive in: Steatorrhea, use of castor oil or mineral oil droplets

SYNOVIAL FLUID ANALYSIS

Table 77 describes the classification and interpretation of synovial fluid analysis. An algorithm for analysis of joint fluid is illustrated in Fig. 42.

TABLE 76 Common Causes of Hypernatremia and Electrolyte Patterns in Serum and Urine with Normal Renal Function*

Cause	Serum Na	Urine Na (UNa)	Urine Osmolality	Serum K	24-Hour UNa
1. Dehydration	High	High	High	Normal	Varies
2. Diabetes insipidus	High	Low	Low	Normal	Low
3. Cushing's disease or syndrome	High	Low	Normal	Low	Low

*All Na and K values are concentrations, except for 24-hour UNa, which is the total number of milliequivalents of Na excreted in 24 hours in the urine.
(McPherson RA, Pincus MR: Henry's Clinical Diagnosis and Management by Laboratory Methods, 23rd ed, ISBN # 978-0323-29568-0, 2017, Elsevier)

TABLE 77 Classification and Interpretation of Synovial Fluid Analysis

Group	Diseases	Appearance	Viscosity	Mucin Clot	WBC/mm³	% PMN	Glucose (mg/dl) (Blood-Synovial Fluid)	Protein (g/dl)
Normal	—	Clear	↑	Firm	<200	<25	<10	<2.5
I (noninflammatory)	Osteoarthritis, aseptic necrosis, traumatic arthritis, erythema nodosum, osteochondritis dissecans	Clear, yellow (may be xanthochromic if traumatic arthritis)	↑	Firm	↑ Up to 10,000	<25	<10	<2.5
II (inflammatory)	Crystal-induced arthritis, rheumatoid arthritis, Reiter's syndrome, collagen vascular disease, psoriatic arthritis, serum sickness, rheumatic fever	Clear, yellow, turbid	↓	Friable	↑↑ Up to 100,000	40-90	<40	<2.5
III (septic)	Bacterial (staphylococcal, gonococcal, tuberculosis)	Turbid	↓/↑	Friable	↑↑↑ Up to 5 million	40-100	20-100	>2.5

↑, Elevated; ↑↑ >markedly high; ↓, decreased; *PMN*, polymorphonuclear leukocytes. Note that there is considerable overlap in the numbers listed above.

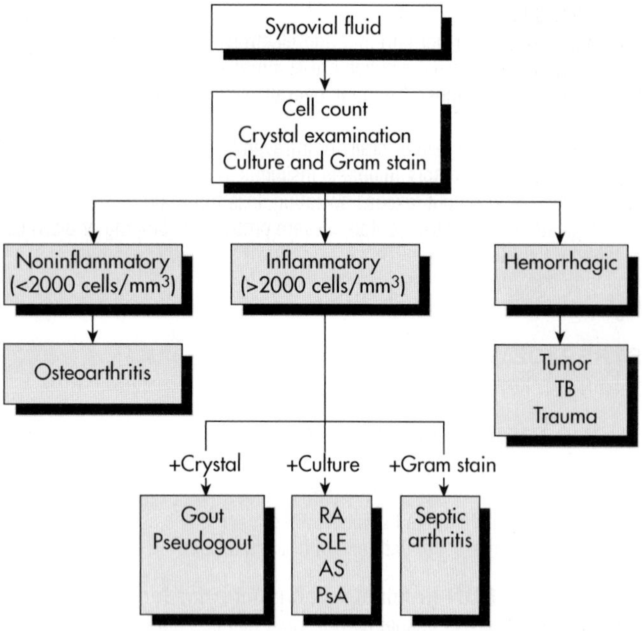

FIG. 42 Algorithm for analysis of joint fluid. Examples of inflammatory arthritis are indicated, although many conditions can produce these findings. *AS,* ankylosing spondylitis; *PsA,* psoriatic arthritis; *RA,* rheumatoid arthritis; *SLE,* systemic lupus erythematosus; *TB,* tuberculosis. (From Goldman L, Schafer AI: *Goldman's Cecil medicine,* ed 24, Philadelphia, 2012, Saunders.)

T₃ (triiodothyronine)

See Table 78 for T₃ abnormalities.

Normal range: 75-220 ng/dl (1.2-3.4 nmol/L [CF: 0.01536; SMI: 0.1 nmol/L])

Abnormal values:

Elevated in hyperthyroidism (usually earlier and to a greater extent than serum T₄).

Useful in diagnosing:

T₃ hyperthyroidism (thyrotoxicosis): increased T₃, normal FTI.

Toxic nodular goiter: increased T₃, normal or increased T₄.

Iodine deficiency: normal T₃, possibly decreased T₄.

Thyroid replacement therapy with liothyronine (Cytomel): normal T₄, increased T₃ if patient is symptomatically hyperthyroid.

Not ordered routinely but indicated when hyperthyroidism is suspected and serum-free T₄ or FTI inconclusive.

T₃ RESIN UPTAKE (T₃RU)

Normal range: 25%-35%

Abnormal values: Increased in hyperthyroidism. T₃ resin uptake (T₃RU or RT₃U) measures the percentage of free T₄ (not bound to protein); it does not measure serum T₃ concentration; T₃RU and other tests that reflect thyroid hormone binding to plasma protein are also known as *thyroid hormone-binding ratios* (THBR).

T₄, FREE (Free thyroxine)

Normal range: 0.8-2.8 ng/dl

Elevated in

Graves' disease, toxic multinodular goiter, toxic adenoma, iatrogenic and factitious causes, transient hyperthyroidism

Serum-free T₄ directly measures unbound thyroxine. Free T₄ can be measured by equilibrium dialysis (gold standard of free T₄ assays) or by immunometric techniques (influenced by serum levels of lipids, proteins, and certain drugs). The free thyroxine index (FTI) can also be easily calculated by multiplying T₄ times T₃RU and dividing the result by 100; the FTI corrects for any abnormal T₄ values secondary to protein binding: $FTI = T_4 \times T_3RU/100$.

Normal values equal 1.1 to 4.3.

T₄, SERUM T₄

Normal range: 0.8-2.8 ng/dl (10-36 pmol/L [CF: 12.87; SMI: 1 pmol/L])

Abnormal values: Serum thyroxine (T₄)

Elevated in:

Graves' disease

Toxic multinodular goiter

Toxic adenoma

Iatrogenic and factitious

Transient hyperthyroidism

Subacute thyroiditis

Hashimoto's thyroiditis

Silent thyroiditis

Rare causes: hypersecretion of TSH (e.g., pituitary neoplasms), struma ovarii, ingestion of large amounts of iodine in a patient with preexisting thyroid hyperplasia or adenoma (Jod-Basedow phenomenon), hydatidiform mole, carcinoma of thyroid, amiodarone therapy of arrhythmias.

Serum thyroxine test measures both circulating thyroxine bound to protein (represents >99% of circulating T₄) and unbound (free) thyroxine. Values vary with protein binding; changes in the concentration of T₄ secondary

Condition	T₄	FT₄I	T₃	FT₃I	TSH	TSI	TRH Stimulation
Hyperthyroidism							
Graves' disease	↑	↑	↑	↑	↓	+	↓
Toxic nodular goiter	↑	↑	↑	↑	↓	−	↓
Pituitary TSH-secreting tumors	↑	↑	↑	↑	↑	−	↓
T₃ thyrotoxicosis	N	N	↑	↑	↓	+, −	↓
T₄ thyrotoxicosis	↑	↑	N	N	↓	+, −	↓
Hypothyroidism							
Primary	↓	↓	↓	↓	↑	+, −	↑
Secondary	↓	↓	↓	↓	↓ N	−	↓
Tertiary	↓	↓	↓	↓	↓, N	−	N
Peripheral unresponsiveness	↑, N	↑, N	↑, N	↑	↑, N	−	N, ↑

TABLE 78   Findings in Thyroid Function Tests in Various Clinical Conditions

From Tilton RC, Barrows A: *Clinical laboratory medicine,* St Louis, 1992, Mosby.
↑, Increased; ↓, decreased; +, − variable; *N,* normal.

to changes in thyroxine-binding globulin (TBG) can be caused by the following:

Increased TBG (↑T4)	Decreased TBG (↓T4)
Pregnancy	Androgens, glucocorticoids
Estrogens	Nephrotic syndrome, cirrhosis
Acute infectious hepatitis	Acromegaly
Oral contraceptives	Hypoproteinemia
Familial	Familial
Fluorouracil, clofibrate	Phenytoin, ASA and other NSAIDs, heroin, methadone, high-dose penicillin, asparaginase, chronic debilitating illness

To eliminate the suspected influence of protein binding on thyroxine values, two additional tests are available: T_3 resin uptake and serum free thyroxine. Table 79 summarizes the effects of pregnancy on thyroid physiology, and Table 80 describes changes in thyroid hormone levels during illness.

TEGRETOL

See CARBAMAZEPINE.

TESTOSTERONE (total testosterone)

Normal range: Variable with age and sex. Testosterone circulates in plasma mostly bound to plasma proteins and sex hormone-binding globulin (SHBG). Approximately 2% of testosterone circulates in free form (biologically active form). Low testosterone levels in obese patients may be due to reduced levels of SHBG; therefore, it is essential to measure free testosterone when evaluating androgen deficiency in obese patients.

Serum/plasma
Males: 280-1100 ng/dl   Females: 15-70 ng/dl
Urine
Males: 50-135 μg/day   Females: 2-12 μg/day
Elevated in: Testicular tumors, ovarian masculinizing tumors, testosterone replacement therapy
Decreased in: Hypogonadism, obesity, insulin resistance, sleep apnea. Fig. 43 illustrates testosterone level changes with age. The diagnosis of androgen deficiency should be based on at least 2 morning testosterone measurements (collected on separate days) in a symptomatic patient.

THEOPHYLLINE

Normal therapeutic range: 10-20 mcg/ml

THORACENTESIS FLUID

See PLEURAL FLUID

THROMBIN TIME (TT)

Normal range: 11.3-18.5 sec
Elevated in: Thrombolytic and heparin therapy, disseminated intravascular coagulation, hypofibrinogenemia, dysfibrinogenemia

THYROGLOBULIN

Normal: 3-40 ng/ml. Thyroglobulin is a tumor marker for monitoring the status of patients with papillary or follicular thyroid cancer following resection.
Elevated in: Papillary or follicular thyroid cancer, Hashimoto's thyroiditis, Graves' disease, subacute thyroiditis

THYROID MICROSOMAL ANTIBODIES

Normal: Undetectable. Low titers may be present in 5%-10% of normal individuals
Elevated in: Hashimoto's disease, thyroid carcinoma, early hypothyroidism, pernicious anemia

THYROID-STIMULATING HORMONE (TSH)

See Fig. 44 for an algorithmic approach to thyroid testing.

TABLE 79 Effects of Pregnancy on Thyroid Physiology

Physiologic Change	Thyroid-Related Consequences
↑ Serum thyroxine-binding globulin	↑ Total T_4 and T_3; ↑ T_4 production
↑ Plasma volume	↑ T_4 and T_3 pool size; ↑ T_4 production; ↑ cardiac output
D3 expression in placenta and (?) uterus	↑ T_4 production
First-trimester ↑ in hCG	↑ Free T_4; ↓ basal thyrotropin; ↑ T_4 production
↑ Renal I− clearance	↑ Iodine requirements
↑ T_4 production; fetal T_4 synthesis during second and third trimesters	
↑ Oxygen consumption by fetoplacental unit, gravid uterus, and mother	↑ Basal metabolic rate; ↑ cardiac output

From Melmed S, Polonsky KS, Larsen PR, Kronenberg HM: *Williams textbook of endocrinology,* ed 12, Philadelphia, 2011, Saunders.
D3, type 3 iodothyronine deiodinase; *I−,* plasma iodide; *hCG,* human chorionic gonadotropin; T_3, triiodothyronine; T_4, thyroxine.

TABLE 80 Changes in Thyroid Hormone Levels during Illness

Severity of Illness	Free T_3	Free T_4	Reverse T_3	TSH	Probable Cause
Mild	↓	N	↑	N	↓ D2, D1
Moderate	↓↓	N, ↑↓	↑↑	N, ↓	↓↓ D2, D1,?↑ D3
Severe	↓↓↓	↓	↑	↓↓	↓↓ D2, D1, ↑D3
Recovery	↓	↓	↑	↑	?

From Melmed S, Polonsky KS, Larsen PR, Kronenberg HM: *Williams textbook of endocrinology,* ed 12, Philadelphia, 2011, Saunders.
D1 through *D3,* iodothyronine deiodinases; *N,* no change; T_3, triiodothyronine; T_4, thyroxine; *TSH,* thyroid-stimulating hormone.

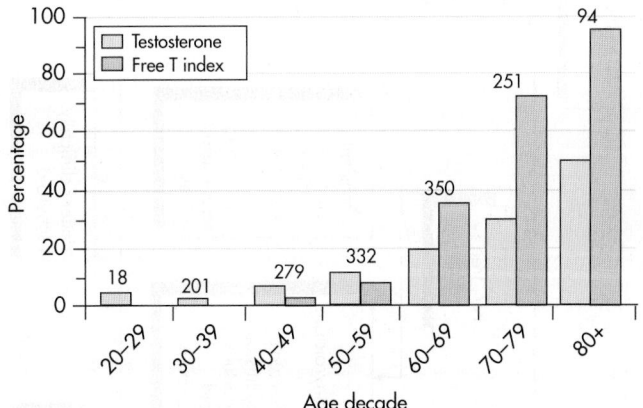

FIG. 43 Hypogonadism in aging men. Bar height indicates the percentage of men in each 10-year interval, from the third to the ninth decades, with at least one testosterone value in the hypogonadal range. The criteria used for these determinations are total testosterone less than 11.3 nmol/L (325 ng/dL) and testosterone and sex hormone–binding globulin (free T index) less than 0.153 nmol/nmol. The numbers above each pair of bars indicate the number of men studied in the corresponding decade. The fraction of men who are hypogonadal increases progressively after age 50 years by either criterion. More men are hypogonadal by free T index than by total testosterone after 50 years, and there seems to be a progressively greater difference with increasing age between the two criteria. (From Goldman L, Schafer AI: *Goldman's Cecil medicine,* ed 24, Philadelphia, 2012, Saunders.)

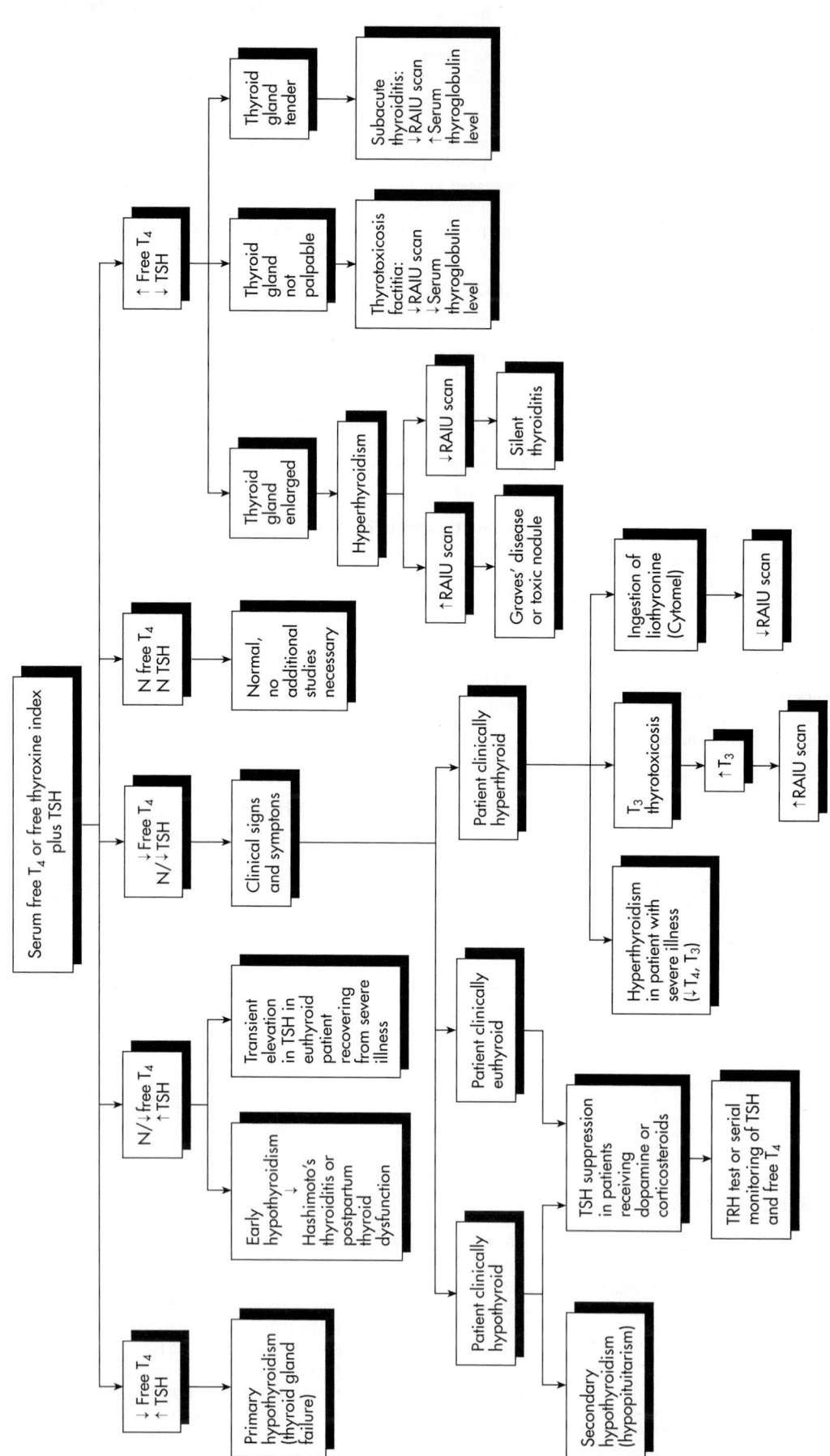

FIG. 44 Diagnostic approach to thyroid testing. *N*, Normal; *RAIU*, radioactive iodine uptake; *TRH*, thyrotropin–releasing hormone; *TSH*, thyroid-stimulating hormone. (From Ferri FF: *Practical guide to the care of the medical patient*, ed 8, St Louis, 2011, Mosby.)

Normal range: 2-11 µU/ml (2-11 mU/L [CF: 1; SMI: 1 mU/L])
CONDITIONS THAT INCREASE SERUM THYROID-STIMULATING HORMONE VALUES
Laboratory error
Primary hypothyroidism
Synthroid therapy with insufficient dose
Lithium or amiodarone; some patients
Hashimoto's thyroiditis in later stage
Large doses of inorganic iodide (e.g., SSKI)
Severe nonthyroid illness in recovery phase
Iodine deficiency (moderate or severe)
Addison's disease
TSH specimen drawn in evening (peak of diurnal variation)
Pituitary TSH-secreting tumor
Therapy of hypothyroidism (3-6 wk after beginning therapy [range, 1-8 wk]; sometimes longer when pretherapy TSH is over 100 µU/ml)
Acute psychiatric illness
Peripheral resistance to T_4 syndrome
Antibodies (e.g., HAMA) interfering with monoclonal sandwich method of TSH assay
Telepaque (iopanoic acid) and Oragrafin (ipodate) x-ray contrast media
Amphetamines
High altitudes
CONDITIONS THAT DECREASE SERUM THYROID-STIMULATING HORMONE VALUES
Laboratory error
T_4/T_3 toxicosis (diffuse or nodular etiology)
Excessive therapy for hypothyroidism
Active thyroiditis (subacute, painless, or early active Hashimoto's disease)
Multinodular goiter containing areas of autonomy
Severe nonthyroid illness (especially acute trauma, dopamine, or glucocorticoid)
T_3 toxicosis
Pituitary insufficiency
Cushing's syndrome (and some patients on high-dose glucocorticoid)
Jod-Basedow (iodine-induced) hyperthyroidism
Thyroid-stimulating hormone drawn 2-4 hr after levothyroxine dose
Postpartum transient toxicosis
Factitious hyperthyroidism
Struma ovarii
Radioimmunoassay, surgery, or antithyroid drug therapy for hyperthyroidism 4-6 weeks (range, 2 wk to 2 yr) after the treatment
Interleukin-2 drugs (3%-6% of cases) or α-interferon therapy (1% of cases)
Hyperemesis gravidarum
Amiodarone therapy.
See Table 80 for changes in thyroid hormone levels during illness.

THYROTROPIN (TSH) RECEPTOR ANTIBODIES

Normal: <130% of basal activity
Elevated in: Values between 1.3 and 2.0 are found in 10% of patients with thyroid disease other than Graves' disease. Values >2.8 have been found only in patients with Graves' disease.

THYROTROPIN-RELEASING HORMONE (TRH) STIMULATION TEST

Normal: Baseline TSH <11 microU/ml; Stimulated TSH: more than double the baseline.

In primary hypothyroidism the TSH increase is 2× to 3× the normal result. In secondary hypothyroidism no TSH response occurs. In tertiary hypothyroidism (hypothalamic failure) there is a delayed rise in the TSH level.

THYROXINE (T_4)

Normal range: 4-11 µg/dl (51-142 nmol/L [CF: 12.87; SMI: 1 nmol/L])
Elevated: Hyperthyroidism (see Fig. 44)

TIBC

See IRON-BINDING CAPACITY, TOTAL

TISSUE TRANSGLUTAMINASE ANTIBODY

Normal: Negative
Present in: Celiac disease (specificity; 94%-97%, sensitivity, 90%-98%), dermatitis herpetiformis

TRANSFERRIN

Normal range: 170-370 mg/dl (1.7-3.7 g/L [CF: 0.01; SMI: 0.01 g/L])
Elevated in: Iron deficiency anemia, oral contraceptive administration, viral hepatitis, late pregnancy
Decreased in: Nephrotic syndrome, liver disease, hereditary deficiency, protein malnutrition, neoplasms, chronic inflammatory states, chronic illness, thalassemia, hemochromatosis, hemolytic anemia

TRIGLYCERIDES

Normal range: <150 mg/dl (<1.80 mmol/L [CF: 0.01129; SMI: 0.02 mmol/L])
Elevated in: Hyperlipoproteinemias (types I, IIb, III, IV, V), hypothyroidism, pregnancy, estrogens, acute myocardial infarction, pancreatitis, alcohol intake, nephrotic syndrome, diabetes mellitus, glycogen storage disease
Decreased in: Malnutrition, congenital abetalipoproteinemias, drugs (e.g., gemfibrozil, fenofibrate, nicotinic acid, clofibrate)

TRIIODOTHYRONINE

See T_3

TROPONINS (serum)

See Box 26 for causes of troponin elevations.
Normal range: 0-0.4 ng/ml (negative). If there is clinical suspicion of evolving acute MI or ischemic episode, repeat testing in 5-6 hours is recommended.
Indeterminate: 0.05-0.49 ng/ml. Suggest further tests. In a patient with unstable angina and this troponin I level, there is an increased risk of a cardiac event in the near future.
Strong probability of acute MI: ≥0.05 ng/ml
Cardiac troponin T (cTnT) is a highly sensitive marker for myocardial injury for the first 48 hours after MI and for up to 5-7 days (see Fig. 16, under "Creatine Kinase Isoenzymes"). It may also be elevated in renal failure, chronic muscle disease, and trauma.

BOX 26	Causes of Serum Troponin T and I Elevations, Including Both Acute Coronary Syndromes, Noncoronary Cardiac Events, and Noncardiac Ailments

Acute coronary syndrome/acute myocardial infarction
Shock of any form (cardiogenic, obstructive, distributive)
Myocarditis and myopericarditis
Cardiomyopathies
Acute congestive heart failure (pulmonary edema)
Sepsis
Pulmonary embolism
Renal failure
Sympathomimetic ingestions
Polytrauma
Burns
Acute CNS event
Rhabdomyolysis
Cardiac neoplasm, inflammatory syndromes, and infiltrative diseases
Congenital coronary anomalies
Extreme physical exertion

From Vincent JL et al: *Textbook of critical care,* ed 6, Philadelphia, 2011, Saunders.

Laboratory Tests

IV

Cardiac troponin I (cTnI) is highly sensitive and specific for myocardial injury (≥CK-MB) in the initial 8 hours, peaks within 24 hours and lasts up to 7 days. With progressively higher levels of cTnI, the risk of mortality increases because the amount of necrosis increases.

TSH
See THYROID-STIMULATING HORMONE

TT
See THROMBIN TIME

TUBERCULIN TEST (PPD)
Abnormal results: see Box 27. Box 28 describes factors associated with false-negative tuberculin tests.

UNCONJUGATED BILIRUBIN
See BILIRUBIN, DIRECT

UREA NITROGEN, BLOOD (BUN)
Normal range: 8-18 mg/dl (3-6.5 mmol/L [CF: 0.357; SMI: 0.5 mmol/L])

Box 29 describes factors affecting BUN level independent of renal function.

Elevated in: Dehydration, drugs (aminoglycosides and other antibiotics, diuretics, lithium, corticosteroids), gastrointestinal bleeding, decreased renal blood flow (shock, congestive heart failure, myocardial infarction), renal disease (glomerulonephritis, pyelonephritis, diabetic nephropathy), urinary tract obstruction (prostatic hypertrophy)

Decreased in: Liver disease, malnutrition, third trimester of pregnancy, overhydration, acromegaly, celiac disease

URIC ACID (serum)
Normal range: 2-7 mg/dl

Elevated in: Renal failure, gout, excessive cell lysis (chemotherapeutic agents, radiation therapy, leukemia, lymphoma, hemolytic anemia), hereditary enzyme deficiency (hypoxanthine-guanine-phosphoribosyl transferase), acidosis, myeloproliferative disorders, diet high in purines or protein, drugs (diuretics, low doses of ASA, ethambutol, nicotinic acid), lead poisoning, hypothyroidism, Addison's disease, nephrogenic diabetes insipidus, active psoriasis, polycystic kidneys

Decreased in: Drugs (allopurinol, febuxostat, high doses of ASA, probenecid, warfarin, corticosteroid), deficiency of xanthine oxidase, syndrome of inappropriate antidiuretic hormone secretion, renal tubular deficits (Fanconi's syndrome), alcoholism, liver disease, diet deficient in protein or purines, Wilson's disease, hemochromatosis

URINALYSIS
Normal range
Color: light straw
Appearance: clear
Ketones: absent
pH: 4.5-8 (average, 6)
Protein: absent
Glucose: absent
Specific gravity: 1.005-1.030
Occult blood absent
Microscopic examination:
    Red blood cells: 0-5 (high-power field)
    White blood cells: 0-5 (high-power field)
    Bacteria (spun specimen): absent
    Casts: 0-4 hyaline (low-power field)

Abnormalities in the microscopic examination of urine are described in Table 81. Causes of abnormal appearance and color of urine are described in Table 82. Urine color changes with commonly used drugs are summarized in Table 83.

BOX 27   PPD Reaction Size Considered "Positive" (Intracutaneous 5 TU Mantoux Test at 48 hr)

5 mm or More
HIV infection or risk factors for HIV
Close recent contact with active TB case
Persons with chest x-ray consistent with healed TB

10 mm or More
Foreign-born persons from countries with high TB prevalence in Asia, Africa, and Latin America
IV drug users
Medically underserved low-income population groups (including Native Americans, Hispanics, and blacks)
Residents of long-term care facilities (nursing homes, mental institutions)
Medical conditions that increase risk for TB (silicosis, gastrectomy, undernourishment, diabetes mellitus, high-dose corticosteroids or immunosuppression Rx, leukemia or lymphoma, other malignancies)
Employees of long-term care facilities, schools, child care facilities, health care facilities

15 mm or More
All others not already listed

TB, Tuberculosis; *TU,* tuberculin units.

BOX 28   Factors Associated with False-Negative Tuberculin Tests

Technical Errors
Improper administration
Inaccurate reading
Loss of potency of antigen
Patient-Related Factors (Anergy)
Age (elderly)
Nutritional status
Medications: corticosteroids, immunosuppressive agents
Severe tuberculosis
Coexisting diseases
    HIV infection
    Viral illness or vaccination
    Lymphoreticular malignances
    Sarcoidosis
    Solid tumors
    Lepromatous leprosy
    Sjögren's syndrome
    Ataxia telangiectasia
    Uremia
    Primary biliary cirrhosis
    Systemic lupus erythematosus
Severe systemic disease of any etiology

From Stein JH (ed): *Internal medicine,* ed 4, St Louis, 1994, Mosby.

BOX 29   Factors Affecting Blood Urea Nitrogen Level Independent of Renal Function

Disproportionate Increase in Blood Urea Nitrogen
Volume depletion ("prerenal azotemia")
Gastrointestinal hemorrhage
Corticosteroid or cytotoxic agents
High-protein diet
Obstructive uropathy
Sepsis
Catabolic states, tissue breakdown

Disproportionate Decrease in Blood Urea Nitrogen
Low-protein diet
Liver disease

From Andreoli TE (ed): *Cecil essentials of medicine,* ed 5, Philadelphia, 2001, Saunders.

TABLE 81	Microscopic Examination of the Urine
Finding	**Associations**
Casts	
Red blood cell	Glomerulonephritis, vasculitis
White blood cell	Interstitial nephritis, pyelonephritis
Epithelial cell	Acute tubular necrosis, interstitial nephritis, glomerulonephritis
Granular	Renal parenchymal disease (nonspecific)
Waxy, broad	Advanced renal failure
Hyaline	Normal finding in concentrated urine
Fatty	Heavy proteinuria
Cells	
Red blood cell	Urinary tract infection, urinary tract inflammation
White blood cell	Urinary tract infection, urinary tract inflammation
Eosinophil	Acute interstitial nephritis
(Squamous) epithelial cell	Contaminants
Crystals	
Uric acid	Acid urine, acute uric acid nephropathy, hyperuricosuria
Calcium phosphate	Alkaline urine
Calcium oxalate	Acid urine, hyperoxaluria, ethylene glycol poisoning
Cystine	Cystinuria
Sulfur	Sulfa-containing antibiotics

From Andreoli TE (ed): *Cecil essentials of medicine*, ed 5, Philadelphia, 2001, Saunders.

URINE AMYLASE

Normal range: 35-260 U Somogyi/hr (6.5-48.1 U/hr [CF: 0.185; SMI: 1 U/hr])
Elevated in: Pancreatitis, carcinoma of the pancreas

URINE BILE

Normal: Absent
Abnormal
Urine bilirubin: hepatitis (viral, toxic, drug-induced), biliary obstruction
Urine urobilinogen: hepatitis (viral, toxic, drug-induced), hemolytic jaundice, liver cell dysfunction (cirrhosis, infection, metastases)

URINE CALCIUM

Normal range: <250 mg/24 hr (<6.2 mmol/dl [CF: 0.02495; SMI: 0.1 mmol/dl])
Elevated in: Primary hyperparathyroidism, hypervitaminosis D, bone metastases, multiple myeloma, increased calcium intake, steroids, prolonged immobilization, sarcoidosis, Paget's disease, idiopathic hypercalciuria, renal tubular acidosis
Decreased in: Hypoparathyroidism, pseudohypoparathyroidism, vitamin D deficiency, vitamin D–resistant rickets, diet low in calcium, drugs (thiazide diuretics, oral contraceptives), familial hypocalciuric hypercalcemia, renal osteodystrophy, potassium citrate therapy

URINE CAMP

Elevated in: Hypercalciuria, familial hypocalciuric hypercalcemia, primary hyperparathyroidism, pseudohypoparathyroidism, rickets
Decreased in: Vitamin D intoxication, sarcoidosis

URINE CATECHOLAMINES

Normal range
Norepinephrine: <100 µg/24 hr (<590 nmol/day [CF: 5.911; SMI: 10 nmol/day])
Epinephrine: <10 µg/24 hr (55 nmol/day [CF: 5.458; SMI: 5 nmol/day])
Elevated in: Pheochromocytoma, neuroblastoma, severe stress

TABLE 82	Appearance and Color of Urine	
Appearance	**Cause**	**Remarks**
Colorless Cloudy	Very dilute urine	Polyuria, diabetes insipidus
	Phosphates, carbonates	Soluble in dilute acetic acid
	Urates, uric acid	Dissolve at 60° C and in alkali
	Leukocytes	Insoluble in dilute acetic acid
	Red blood cells ("smoky")	Lyse in dilute acetic acid
	Bacteria, yeasts	Insoluble in dilute acetic acid
	Spermatozoa	Insoluble in dilute acetic acid
	Prostatic fluid	
	Mucin, mucous threads	May be flocculent
	Calculi, "gravel"	Phosphates, oxalates
	Clumps, pus, tissue	
	Fecal contamination	Rectovesical fistula
	Radiographic dye	In acid urine
Milky	Many neutrophils (pyuria)	Insoluble in dilute acetic acid
	Fat	Nephrosis, crush injury – soluble in ether
	Lipiduria, opalescent	Lymphatic obstruction- soluble in ether
	Chyluria, milky	Vaginal creams
	Emulsified paraffin	
Yellow	Acriflavine	Green fluorescence
Yellow-orange	Concentrated urine	Dehydration, fever
	Urobilin in excess	No yellow foam
	Bilirubin	Yellow foam if sufficient bilirubin
Yellow-green	Bilirubin-biliverdin	Yellow foam
Yellow-brown	Bilirubin-biliverdin	"Beer" brown, yellow foam
Red	Hemoglobin	Positive
	Erythrocytes	Positive } Reagent strip for blood
	Myoglobin	Positive
	Porphyrin	May be colorless
	Fuscin, aniline dye	Foods, candy
	Beets	Yellow alkaline, genetic
	Menstrual contamination	Clots, mucus
Red-purple	Porphyrins	May be colorless
Red-brown	Erythrocytes	
	Hemoglobin on standing	
	Methemoglobin	Acid pH
	Myoglobin	Muscle injury
	Bilifuscin (dipyrrole)	Result of unstable hemoglobin
Brown-black	Methemoglobin	Blood, acid pH
	Homogentisic acid	On standing, alkaline; alkaptonuria
	Melanin	On standing, rare
Blue-green	Indicans	Small intestine infections
	Pseudomonas infections	
	Chlorophyll	Mouth deodorants

(McPherson RA, Pincus MR: Henry's Clinical Diagnosis and Management by Laboratory Methods, 23rd ed, ISBN # 978-0323-29568-0, 2017, Elsevier).

URINE CHLORIDE

Normal range: 110-250 mEq/day (110-250 mmol/day [CF: 1; SMI: 1 mmol/day])
Elevated in: Corticosteroids, Bartter's syndrome, diuretics, metabolic acidosis, severe hypokalemia
Decreased in: Chloride depletion (vomiting), colonic villous adenoma, chronic renal failure, renal tubular acidosis

URINE COPPER

Normal range: <40 µg/24 hr (<0.6 µmol/day [CF: 0.01574; SMI: 0.2 µmol/day])

URINE CORTISOL, FREE

Normal range: 10-110 µg/24 hr (30-300 nmol/day [CF: 2.759; SMI: 10 nmol/day])
Elevated: See CORTISOL, PLASMA

TABLE 83   Urine Color Changes with Commonly Used Drugs*

Drug	Color
Alcohol, ethyl	Pale, diuresis
Anthraquinone laxatives (senna, cascara)	Reddish, alkaline; yellow-brown, acid
Chlorzoxazone (Paraflex) (muscle relaxant)	Red
Deferoxamine mesylate (Desferal) (chelates iron)	Red
Ethoxazene (Serenium) (urinary analgesic)	Orange, red
Fluorescein sodium (given IV)	Yellow
Furazolidone (Furoxone) (Tricofuron) (an antibacterial, antiprotozoal nitrofuran)	Brown
Indigo carmine dye (renal function, cytoscopy)	Blue
Iron sorbitol (Jectofer) (possibly other iron compounds forming iron sulfide in urine)	Brown on standing
Levodopa (L-dopa) (for parkinsonism)	Red then brown, alkaline
Mepacrine (Atabrine) (antimalarial) (intestinal worms, *Giardia*)	Yellow
Methocarbamol (Robaxin) (muscle relaxant)	Green-brown
Methyldopa (Aldomet) (antihypertensive)	Darkens; if oxidizing agents present, red to brown
Methylene blue (used to delineate fistulas)	Blue, blue-green
Metronidazole (Flagyl) (for *Trichomonas* infection, amebiasis, *Giardia*)	Darkening, reddish brown
Nitrofurantoin (Furadantin) (antibacterial)	Brown-yellow
Phenazopyridine (Pyridium) (urinary analgesic), also compounded with sulfonamides (e.g., Azo Gantrisin)	Orange-red, acid pH
Phenindione (Hedulin) (anticoagulant) (important to distinguish from hematuria)	Orange, alkaline; color disappears on acidifying
Phenol poisoning	Brown; oxidized to quinones (green)
Phenolphthalein (purgative)	Red-purple, alkaline pH
Phenolsulfonphthalein (also sulfobromophthalein)	Pink-red, alkaline pH
Rifampin (Rifadin, Rimactane) (tuberculosis therapy)	Bright orange-red
Riboflavin (multivitamins)	Bright yellow
Sulfasalazine (Azulfidine) (for ulcerative colitis)	Orange-yellow, alkaline pH

*Other commonly used drugs have been noted to produce color change once or occasionally: amitriptyline (Elavil)—blue-green; phenothiazines—red; triamterene (Dyrenium)—pale blue (blue fluorescence in acid urine).
(McPherson RA, Pincus MR: Henry's Clinical Diagnosis and Management by Laboratory Methods, 23rd ed, ISBN # 978-0323-29568-0, 2017, Elsevier).

URINE CREATININE (24 hr)

Normal range
Male: 0.8-1.8 g/day (7-16 mmol/day [CF: 8.840; SMI: 0.1 mmol/day])
Female: 0.6-1.6 g/day (5.3-14 mmol/day)
NOTE: Useful test as an indicator of completeness of 24-hr urine collection.

URINE CRYSTALS

Uric acid: acid urine, hyperuricosuria, uric acid nephropathy
Sulfur: antibiotics containing sulfa
Calcium oxalate: ethylene glycol poisoning, acid urine, hyperoxaluria
Calcium phosphate: alkaline urine
Cystine: cystinuria

URINE EOSINOPHILS

Normal: Absent
Present in: Interstitial nephritis, acute tubular necrosis, urinary tract infection, kidney transplant rejection, hepatorenal syndrome

URINE GLUCOSE (qualitative)

Normal: Absent
Present in: Diabetes mellitus, renal glycosuria (decreased renal threshold for glucose), glucose intolerance

URINE HEMOGLOBIN, FREE

Normal: Absent
Present in: Hemolysis (with saturation of serum haptoglobin binding capacity and renal threshold for tubular absorption of hemoglobin)

URINE HEMOSIDERIN

Normal: Absent
Present in: Paroxysmal nocturnal hemoglobinuria, chronic hemolytic anemia, hemochromatosis, blood transfusion, thalassemias

URINE 5-HYDROXYINDOLE-ACETIC ACID (urine 5-HIAA)

Normal range: 2-8 mg/24 hr (10-40 μmol/day [CF: 5.23; SMI: 5 μmol/day])
Elevated in: Carcinoid tumors, after ingestion of certain foods (bananas, plums, tomatoes, avocados, pineapples, eggplant, walnuts), drugs (monoamine oxidase inhibitors, phenacetin, methyldopa, glycerol guaiacolate, acetaminophen, salicylates, phenothiazines, imipramine, methocarbamol, reserpine, methamphetamine). See Table 84.

URINE INDICAN

Normal: Absent
Present in: Malabsorption secondary to intestinal bacterial overgrowth

URINE KETONES (semiquantitative)

Normal: Absent
Present in: Diabetic ketoacidosis, alcoholic ketoacidosis, starvation, isopropanol ingestion

URINE METANEPHRINES

Normal range: 0-2.0 mg/24 hr (0-11.0 μmol/day [CF: 5.458; SMI: 0.5 μmol/day])
Elevated in: Pheochromocytoma, neuroblastoma, drugs (caffeine, phenothiazines, monoamine oxidase inhibitors), stress. Table 85 summarizes medications that may increase metanephrine levels.

URINE MYOGLOBIN

Normal: Absent
Present in: Severe trauma, hyperthermia, polymyositis/dermatomyositis, carbon monoxide poisoning, drugs (narcotic and amphetamine toxicity), hypothyroidism, muscle ischemia
Table 86 differentiates hematuria and hemoglobinuria from myoglobinuria.

URINE NITRITE

Normal: Absent
Present in: Urinary tract infections

URINE OCCULT BLOOD

Normal: Negative
Positive in: Trauma to urinary tract, renal disease (glomerulonephritis, pyelonephritis), renal or ureteral calculi, bladder lesions (carcinoma, cystitis), prostatitis, prostatic carcinoma, menstrual contamination, hematopoietic disorders (hemophilia, thrombocytopenia), anticoagulants, ASA

URINE OSMOLALITY

See OSMOLALITY, URINE

URINE pH

Normal range: 4.6-8 (average, 6)
Elevated in: Bacteriuria, vegetarian diet, renal failure with inability to form ammonia, drugs (antibiotics, sodium bicarbonate, acetazolamide)

TABLE 84 Factors That Interfere with Determination of Urinary 5-HIAA

Foods	Drugs
Factors That Produce False-Positive Results	
Avocado	Acetaminophen
Banana	Acetanilid
Chocolate	Caffeine
Coffee	Fluorouracil
Eggplant	Guaifenesin
Pecan	l-Dopa
Pineapple	Melphalan
Plum	Mephenesin
Tea	Methamphetamine
Walnuts	Methocarbamol
	Methysergide maleate
	Phenmetrazine
	Reserpine
	Salicylates
Factors That Cause False-Negative Results	
None	Corticotropin
	p-Chlorophenylalanine
	Chlorpromazine
	Heparin
	Imipramine
	Isoniazid
	Methenamine mandelate
	Methyldopa
	Monoamine oxidase inhibitors
	Phenothiazine
	Promethazine

From Melmed S, Polonsky KS, Larsen PR, Kronenberg HM: *Williams textbook of endocrinology*, ed 12, Philadelphia, 2011, Saunders.
5-HIAA, 5-hydroxyindoleacetic acid.

TABLE 85 Medications That May Increase Measured Levels of Fractionated Catecholamines and Metanephrines

Tricyclic antidepressants (including cyclobenzaprine)
Levodopa
Drugs containing adrenergic receptor agonists (e.g., decongestants)
Amphetamines
Buspirone and antipsychotic agents
Prochlorperazine
Reserpine
Withdrawal from clonidine and other drugs (e.g., illicit drugs)
Illicit drugs (e.g., cocaine, heroin)
Ethanol

From Melmed S, Polonsky KS, Larsen PR, Kronenberg HM: *Williams textbook of endocrinology*, ed 12, Philadelphia, 2011, Saunders.

Decreased in: Acidosis (metabolic, respiratory), drugs (ammonium chloride, methenamine mandelate), diabetes mellitus, starvation, diarrhea

URINE PHOSPHATE

Normal range: 0.8-2.0 g/24 hr
Elevated in: Acute tubular necrosis (diuretic phase), chronic renal disease, uncontrolled diabetes mellitus, hyperparathyroidism, hypomagnesemia, metabolic acidosis, metabolic alkalosis, neurofibromatosis, adult-onset vitamin D–resistant hypophosphatemic osteomalacia
Decreased in: Acromegaly, acute renal failure, decreased dietary intake, hypoparathyroidism, respiratory acidosis

TABLE 86 Differentiation of Hematuria, Hemoglobinuria, and Myoglobinuria

Condition	Plasma Findings	Urine Findings
Hematuria	Color—normal	Color—normal, smoky, pink, red, brown
		Erythrocytes—many
		Renal—red blood cell casts
		Protein—marked increase
		Lower urinary tract—no casts
		Protein—present or absent
Hemoglobinuria	Color—pink (early)	Color—pink, red, brown
	Haptoglobin—low	Erythrocytes—occasional
		Pigment casts—occasional
		Protein—present or absent
		Hemosiderin—late
Myoglobinuria	Color—normal	Color—red, brown
	Haptoglobin—normal	Erythrocytes—occasional
	Creatine kinase—marked increase	Dense brown casts—occasional
	Aldolase—increased	Protein—present or absent

(McPherson RA, Pincus MR: *Henry's Clinical Diagnosis and Management by Laboratory Methods*, 23rd ed, ISBN # 978-0323-29568-0, 2017, Elsevier).

URINE POTASSIUM

Normal range: 25-100 mEq/24 hr (25-100 mmol/day [CF: 1; SMI: 1 mmol/day])
Elevated in: Aldosteronism (primary, secondary), glucocorticoids, alkalosis, renal tubular acidosis, excessive dietary potassium intake
Decreased in: Acute renal failure, potassium-sparing diuretics, diarrhea, hypokalemia

URINE PROTEIN (quantitative)

Normal range: <150 mg/24 hr (<0.15 g/day [CF: 0.001; SMI: 0.01 g/day])
Elevated in
Nephrotic syndrome as a result of primary renal diseases
Malignant hypertension
Malignancies: multiple myeloma, leukemias, Hodgkin's disease
Congestive heart failure
Diabetes mellitus
Systemic lupus erythematosus, rheumatoid arthritis
Sickle cell disease
Goodpasture's syndrome
Malaria
Amyloidosis, sarcoidosis
Tubular lesions: cystinosis
Functional (after heavy exercise)
Pyelonephritis
Pregnancy
Constrictive pericarditis
Renal vein thrombosis
Toxic nephropathies: heavy metals, drugs
Radiation nephritis
Orthostatic (postural) proteinuria
Benign proteinuria: fever, heat or cold exposure

URINE SEDIMENT

See Fig. 45 for visual evaluation of common abnormalities. Table 87 summarizes characteristics of amorphous and crystalline urinary sediments.

URINE SODIUM (quantitative)

See Table 88 for use of urine electrolytes in the differential diagnosis of hypokalemia. Table 89 describes urine sodium findings in acute kidney injury (AKI).

TABLE 87 Characteristics of Amorphous and Crystalline Urinary Sediments

Substance	Description	Acid	Neutral	Alkaline	Solubility Characteristics and Comments
		URINE pH WHERE FOUND			
Ampicillin	Uncommon—from high dose; colorless; long prisms that form clusters, sheaves	+	−	−	
Bilirubin	Reddish brown; amorphous needles, rhombic plates, or cubes; may color uric acid crystals	+	−	−	Soluble in alkali, acid, acetone, and chloroform
Cholesterol	Rare; colorless; flat plate with corner notch; accompanies fatty casts and oval fat bodies	+	+	−	Very soluble in chloroform, ether, and hot alcohol
Calcium carbonate	Colorless; small granules in pairs, fours; spheres; rarely needles	−	+	+	Soluble in acetic acid with effervescence
Calcium oxalate	Dihydrate—common; colorless; small refractile octahedron Monohydrate—uncommon; dumbbell and ovoid rectangle	+	+	−	Soluble in dilute HCl
Cystine	Colorless; hexagonal plates, often laminated; rapidly destroyed by bacteria; may be confused with uric acid, but cystine is soluble in dilute hydrochloric acid	+	−	−	Soluble in alkali (especially ammonia) and dilute HCl; insoluble in boiling water, acetic acid, alcohol, ether; apply cyanide-nitroprusside reaction
Hematin	Small, biconvex "whetstone" seen with hemoglobinuria	+	−	−	
Hemosiderin	Golden brown; granules in clumps, in cells, casts	+	+	−	Blue with Prussian blue
Hippuric acid	Rare; colorless, needles, rhombic plates and four-sided prisms; distinguish from phosphates	+	+	+	Soluble with hot water and alkali; insoluble in acetic acid
Indigotin	Rare; blue; amorphous or small crystals; colors other crystals	+	+	+	Very soluble in chloroform; soluble in ether; insoluble in acetone
Phosphates					
Amorphous phosphate (magnesium, calcium)	Colorless; fine, granular precipitate	−	+	+	Insoluble with heat; soluble with acetic acid, dilute HCl
Calcium hydrogen phosphate	Less common; colorless, star-shaped or long, thin prisms or needles; form rosettes	sl	+	sl	Slightly soluble in dilute acetic acid, soluble in dilute HCl
Triple phosphate (ammonium, magnesium)	Common form: colorless; three- to six-sided prisms, "coffin lids" Less often: Flat, fern leaf form, sheets, flakes	−	+	+	Soluble in dilute acetic acid
Radiographic media (meglumine diatrizoate)	Intravenous: Colorless; thin, rhombic plates, some with notch, resemble cholesterol plates; elongated crystals Retrograde: Colorless; long, pointed crystals	+	−	−	Soluble in 10% NaOH: Insoluble in ether and chloroform; high specific gravity in urine: polarizes with interference colors
Sulfonamides					
Acetylsulfadiazine	Wheat sheaves with eccentric binding	+	−	−	
Acetylsulfamethoxazole	Brown; dense spheres or irregular divided spheres	+	−	−	
Sulfadiazine	Brown; dense globules	+	−	−	Soluble in acetone
Tyrosine	Rare; colorless or yellow, appears black with focusing; fine silky needles in sheaves or rosettes	+	−	−	Soluble in alkali, dilute mineral acid, relatively heat soluble; insoluble in alcohol, ether
Urates					
Amorphous (calcium, magnesium, sodium, potassium)	Common; colorless to yellow-brown; amorphous, granular precipitate	+	+	−	Soluble in dilute alkali; soluble at 60° C or lower; change to uric acid crystal with concentrated HCl or acetic acid
Monosodium urate	Colorless; needles or amorphous precipitate	+	−	−	
Urates (sodium, potassium, ammonium)	Brown; small, spherical; clusters resemble biurates	sl	+	−	Soluble at 60° C; change to uric acid with glacial acetic acid
Ammonium biurate	Common in "old" urine; dark yellow or brown; spheres or "thorn apples" (spheres with horns)	−	+	+	Soluble at 60° C with acetic acid; soluble strong alkali; change to uric acid with concentrated hydrochloric or acetic acid
Uric acid	Common; yellow, red-brown, brown; large variety of shapes—rhombic, four-sided plates, rosettes, "whetstones" lemon shapes; rarely, colorless hexagonals	+	−	−	Soluble in alkali: Insoluble in alcohol and acids; polarizes with interference colors
Xanthine	Rare; colorless; small, rhombic plates	+	+	−	Soluble in alkali; soluble with heat; insoluble in acetic acid

sl, Slight.

(McPherson RA, Pincus MR: Henry's Clinical Diagnosis and Management by Laboratory Methods, 23rd ed, ISBN # 978-0323-29568-0, 2017, Elsevier).

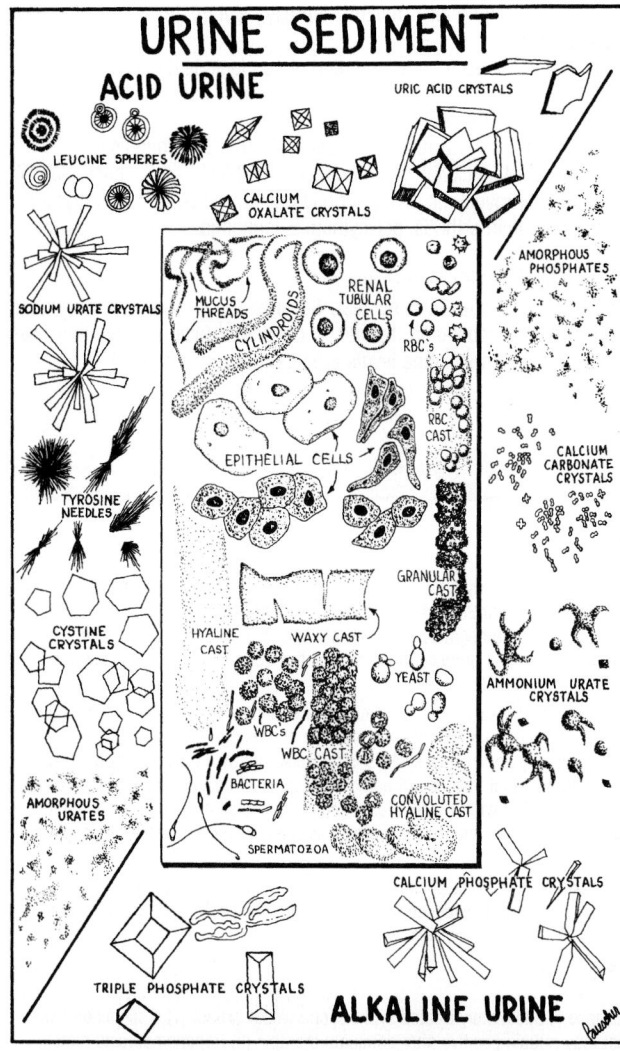

URINE SEDIMENT

ACID URINE

URIC ACID CRYSTALS

LEUCINE SPHERES

CALCIUM OXALATE CRYSTALS

AMORPHOUS PHOSPHATES

SODIUM URATE CRYSTALS

MUCUS THREADS

RENAL TUBULAR CELLS

CYLINDROIDS

RBC's

EPITHELIAL CELLS

RBC CAST

CALCIUM CARBONATE CRYSTALS

TYROSINE NEEDLES

GRANULAR CAST

CYSTINE CRYSTALS

HYALINE CAST

WAXY CAST

YEAST

AMMONIUM URATE CRYSTALS

WBCs

WBC CAST

BACTERIA

AMORPHOUS URATES

CONVOLUTED HYALINE CAST

SPERMATOZOA

CALCIUM PHOSPHATE CRYSTALS

TRIPLE PHOSPHATE CRYSTALS

ALKALINE URINE

FIG. 45 Microscopic examination of urinary sediment. (From Grigorian Greene M: *The Harriet Lane handbook: a manual for pediatric house officers*, ed 17, St Louis, 2007, Mosby.)

Normal range: 40-220 mEq/day (40-220 mmol/day [CF: 1; SMI: 1 mmol/day])
Elevated in: Diuretic administration, high sodium intake, salt-losing nephritis, acute tubular necrosis, vomiting, Addison's disease, syndrome of inappropriate antidiuretic hormone secretion, hypothyroidism, congestive heart failure, hepatic failure, chronic renal failure, Bartter's syndrome, glucocorticoid deficiency, interstitial nephritis caused by analgesic abuse, mannitol, dextran, or glycerol therapy, milk-alkali syndrome, decreased renin secretion, postobstructive diuresis
Decreased In: Increased aldosterone, glucocorticoid excess, hyponatremia, prerenal azotemia, decreased salt intake

URINE SPECIFIC GRAVITY
Normal range: 1.005-1.030
Elevated in: Dehydration, excessive fluid losses (vomiting, diarrhea, fever), x-ray contrast media, diabetes mellitus, congestive heart failure, syndrome of inappropriate antidiuretic hormone secretion, adrenal insufficiency, decreased fluid intake
Decreased in: Diabetes insipidus, renal disease (glomerulonephritis, pyelonephritis), excessive fluid intake or IV hydration

URINE VANILLYLMANDELIC ACID (VMA)
Normal range: <6.8 mg/24 hr (<35 μmol/day [CF: 5.046; SMI: 1 μmol/day])

TABLE 88 Urine Electrolytes* in the Differential Diagnosis of Hypokalemia

Condition	URINE ELECTROLYTE	
	Na+	Cl-
Vomiting		
Recent	High†	Low‡
Remote	Low	Low
Diuretics		
Recent	High	High
Remote	Low	Low
Diarrhea or Laxative Abuse	Low	High
Bartter's or Gitelman's Syndrome	High	High

From Vincent JL et al: *Textbook of critical care*, ed 6, Philadelphia, 2011, Saunders.
*Do not use the urine electrolytes in this fashion during polyuric states.
†High = urine concentration >15 mmol/L.
‡Low = urine concentration <15 mmol/L.

TABLE 89 Urinalysis Findings in Acute Kidney Injury (AKI)

Etiologic Disorder	Urine Chemistry	Urine Sediment
Prerenal	U_{Na} <20 mmol/L FE_{Na} <1% FE_{urea} <35%	Normal or nearly normal (hyaline casts and rare granular casts)
Acute tubular necrosis	U_{Na} >40 mmol/L FE_{Na} >2% FE_{urea} >60%	Renal tubular epithelial cells, epithelial cell casts, coarse pigmented (muddy brown) casts
Acute interstitial nephritis	Variable; U_{Na} may be >40 mmol/L, FE_{Na} may be >2%	Red blood cells, white blood cells, white blood cell casts, eosinophils
Acute glomerulonephritis	Variable; U_{Na} may be <20 mmol/L, FE_{Na} may be <1%	Red blood cells (dysmorphic), red blood cell casts
Acute vascular disease	Variable; U_{Na} may be <20 mmol/L, FE_{Na} may be <1%	Red blood cells, red blood cell casts in HUS/TTP, eosinophils in atheroembolic disease
Crystal-associated AKI	Variable	Crystalluria Uric acid crystals in tumor lysis syndrome Calcium oxalate crystals in ethylene glycol ingestion Drug crystals (acyclovir, methotrexate, indinavir, triamterene, sulfadiazine)
Obstructive	Variable; early U_{Na} may be <20 mmol/L, FE_{Na} may be <1%; late U_{Na} may be >40 mmol/L, FE_{Na} may be >2%	Normal or red blood cells, white blood cells and crystals

FE_{Na}, fractional excretion of sodium; FE_{urea}, fractional excretion of urea; HUS, hemolytic-uremic syndrome; TTP, thrombotic thrombocytopenic purpura; U_{Na}, urine sodium concentration.
(Parrillo JE, Dellinger RP: Critical Care Medicine, Principles of Diagnosis and Management in the Adult, 4th ed, ISBN # 978-0-323-08929-6, 2014, Elsevier)

Elevated in: Pheochromocytoma, neuroblastoma, ganglioblastoma, drugs (isoproterenol, methocarbamol, levodopa, sulfonamides, chlorpromazine), severe stress, after ingestion of bananas, chocolate, vanilla, tea, coffee
Decreased in: Drugs (monoamine oxidase inhibitors, reserpine, guanethidine, methyldopa)

Laboratory Tests

IV

VARICELLA-ZOSTER VIRUS (VZV) SEROLOGY

Test description: Test can be performed on whole blood, tissue, skin lesions, and CSF

VASOACTIVE INTESTINAL PEPTIDE (VIP)

Normal: <50 pg/ml
Elevated in: Pancreatic VIP-omas, neuroblastoma, pancreatic islet cell hyperplasia, liver disease, MEN I, ganglioneuroma, ganglioneuroblastoma

VDRL

Normal range: Negative
Positive test: Syphilis, other treponemal diseases (yaws, pinta, bejel)
   NOTE: A false-positive test may be seen in patients with systemic lupus erythematosus and other autoimmune diseases, infectious mononucleosis, HIV, atypical pneumonia, malaria, leprosy, typhus fever, rat-bite fever, relapsing fever.
   NOTE: See Table 90 for interpretation of serologic tests for syphilis.

VISCOSITY (serum)

Normal range: 1.4-1.8 relative to water (1.10-1.22 centipoise)
Elevated in: Monoclonal gammopathies (Waldenström's macroglobulinemia, multiple myeloma), hyperfibrinogenemia, systemic lupus erythematosus, rheumatoid arthritis, polycythemia, leukemia

VITAMIN B$_{12}$ (cobalamin)

See Fig. E46 for the Schilling test. See Box 30 for etiopathophysiologic classification of cobalamin deficiency. Causes of false-positive and false-negative serum cobalamine levels are summarized in Table 91.

TABLE 90 Interpretation of Serologic Tests for Syphilis*

Nontreponemal Tests	Treponemal Tests	Interpretation of Finding: Is Syphilis Present?*
Nonreactive	Nonreactive	Early primary syphilis is not ruled out by negative serologic tests. Early syphilis is present in 13%-30% of patients who have a negative microhemagglutination *Treponema pallidum* test; in about 30% of patients who present with chancre but have a nonreactive reagin test; and in about 10% of patients who have a negative FTA-ABS test. Late syphilis is present in a very small fraction of patients. Adequately treated syphilis in remote past may produce these results, but treponemal tests usually remain reactive.
	Reactive	Observed in about 10% of patients with chancre. The treponemal tests may turn positive shortly before the reagin tests. Reagin tests repeated after several days are generally positive. In adequately treated early syphilis, the reagin test may return to nonreactive within 1-2 yr, whereas the treponemal tests generally do not. Late syphilis is not ruled out by a negative reagin test. The sensitivity of the reagin tests is lower than that of treponemal tests in untreated late syphilis. In secondary syphilis, rarely, a highly reactive serum appears negative when tested undiluted with a reagin test because flocculation is inhibited by relative antibody excess. Not reported to occur with treponemal tests. Quantitative reagin tests are positive. False-positive treponemal tests occur in 40% of patients with Lyme disease.
Reactive	Nonreactive borderline (FTA-ABS)	Finding is not diagnostic of syphilis but constitutes a classic biologic false-positive reaction. Not diagnostic of syphilis; most patients (90%) with this pattern do not develop clinical or serologic evidence of syphilis. Repeat test is indicated. Chronic borderline results are associated with a variety of conditions other than syphilis.
	Beaded (FTA-ABS)	Not diagnostic of syphilis. Seen with collagen vascular disease.
	Reactive	Findings diagnostic of syphilis or other treponemal disease. In adequately treated syphilis, one would expect (1) a sustained four-fold drop in titer of reagin test, although reagin test may remain positive after adequate therapy; (2) treponemal tests remain positive after adequate therapy. Concurrent false-positive results on both nontreponemal and treponemal tests could occur in rare instances. It may be impossible to rule out syphilis in an individual with this test profile.

From Stein JH (ed): *Internal medicine*, ed 4, St Louis, 1994, Mosby.
FTA-ABS, Fluorescent treponemal antibody, absorbed.
*Serologic data must always be interpreted in the light of a total clinical evaluation. Diagnosis based on serologic criteria alone is fraught with error. Serologic tests apparently in conflict with clinical diagnosis should be confirmed by repetition or possibly referral to a reference laboratory.

BOX 30 Etiopathophysiologic Classification of Cobalamin Deficiency

Nutritional cobalamin deficiency (insufficient cobalamin intake)—vegetarians, poverty-imposed near-vegetarians, breastfed infants of mothers with pernicious anemia
Abnormal intragastric events (inadequate proteolysis of food cobalamin)—atrophic gastritis, hypochlorhydria, proton pump inhibitors, H$_2$ blockers
Loss/atrophy of gastric oxyntic mucosa (deficient intrinsic factor [IF] molecules)—total or partial gastrectomy, adult and juvenile pernicious anemia, caustic destruction (lye)
Abnormal events in the small bowel lumen
   Inadequate pancreatic protease (R factor–cobalamin not degraded, cobalamin not transferred to IF)
   Insufficient pancreatic protease—pancreatic insufficiency
   Inactivation of pancreatic protease—Zollinger-Ellison syndrome
   Usurping of luminal cobalamin (inadequate binding of cobalamin to IF)
   By bacteria-stasis syndromes (blind loops, pouches of diverticulosis, strictures, fistulas, anastomosis), impaired bowel motility (scleroderma), hypogammaglobulinemia

   By *Diphyllobothrium latum* (fish tapeworm)
Disorders of ileal mucosa/IF-cobalamin receptors (IF-cobalamin not bound to IF-cobalamin receptors [cubam receptors])
   Diminished or absent cubam receptors—ileal bypass/resection/fistula
   Abnormal mucosal architecture/function—tropical/nontropical sprue, Crohn disease, tuberculous ileitis, amyloidosis
   Cubam receptor defects—Imerslund-Gräsbeck syndrome
   Drug-effects—metformin, cholestyramine, colchicine, neomycin
Disorders of plasma cobalamin transport (transcobalamin [TCII]-cobalamin not delivered to TCII receptors)—congenital TCII deficiency, defective binding of TCII-cobalamin to TCII receptors (rare)
Metabolic disorders (cobalamin not used by cell)
Inborn enzyme errors—cblA to cblG disorders
Acquired disorders (cobalamin inactivated by irreversible oxidation)—nitrous oxide

From Hoffman R: *Hematology: basic principles and practice*, ed 6, Philadelphia, Saunders, 2013.

Normal
190-900 ng/ml
Causes of vitamin B$_{12}$ deficiency:

   a. Pernicious anemia (antibodies against intrinsic factor and gastric parietal cells)

   b. Dietary (strict lacto-ovovegetarians, food faddists)

   c. Malabsorption (achlorhydria, gastrectomy, ileal resection, pancreatic insufficiency, drugs [omeprazole, cholestyramine])

Falsely low levels occur in patients with severe folate deficiency, in patients using high doses of ascorbic acid, and when cobalamin levels are measured after nuclear medicine studies (radioactivity interferes with cobalamin radioimmunoassay).

Falsely high or normal levels in patients with cobalamin deficiency can occur in severe liver disease and chronic granulocytic leukemia.

The absence of anemia or macrocytosis does not exclude the diagnosis of cobalamin deficiency.

VITAMIN D, 1,25 DIHYDROXY CALCIFEROL

Normal: 16-65 pg/ml
Elevated in: Tumor calcinosis, primary hyperparathyroidism, sarcoidosis, tuberculosis, idiopathic hypercalciuria
Decreased in: Nutritional deficiency, postmenopausal osteoporosis, chronic renal failure, hypoparathyroidism, tumor-induced osteomalacia, rickets, elevated blood lead levels. Table 92 compares vitamin D levels in various disorders.

VITAMIN K

Normal: 0.10-2.20 ng/ml
Decreased in: Primary biliary cirrhosis, anticoagulants, antibiotics, cholestyramine, GI disease, pancreatic disease, cystic fibrosis, obstructive jaundice, hypoprothrombinemia, hemorrhagic disease of the newborn

---

TABLE 91   Serum Cobalamin: False-Positive and False-Negative Test Results

Falsely Low Serum Cobalamin in the Absence of True Cobalamin Deficiency

Folate deficiency (one-third of patients)
Multiple myeloma
TCI deficiency
Megadose vitamin C therapy

Falsely Raised Cobalamin Levels in the Presence of True Deficiency*

Cobalamin binders (TCI and II) increased (e.g., myeloproliferative states, hepatomas, and fibrolamellar hepatic tumors)
TCII-producing macrophages are activated (e.g., autoimmune diseases, monoblastic leukemias and lymphomas)
Release of cobalamin from hepatocytes (e.g., active liver disease)
High serum anti-IF antibody titer

From Hoffman R, et al: *Hematology, basic principles and practice*, ed 6, Philadelphia, 2013, Saunders.
IF, Intrinsic factor; *TC,* transcobalamin.
*Although a low serum cobalamin level is not synonymous with cobalamin deficiency, 5% of patients with true cobalamin deficiency have low-normal cobalamin levels, a potentially serious problem because the patient's underlying cobalamin deficiency will progress if uncorrected.

VON WILLEBRAND FACTOR

Normal: Levels vary according to blood type; blood type O: 50-150 U/dl; blood type non-O: 90-200 U/dl
Decreased in: von Willebrand's disease (however, in type II von Willebrand's disease the antigen may be normal but the function is impaired)

TABLE 92   Serum Calcium, Phosphate, and Vitamin D Levels in Various Disorders

Disorder	Calcium	25(OH)D	1,25(OH)D	Phosphate
25(OH)D intoxication	High	High	Low, normal	Normal, high
Primary hyperparathyroidism	High	Normal	Normal, high	Low
Secondary hyperparathyroidism	Low	Low, normal, high	Low, normal, high	Low, normal, high
Tertiary hyperparathyroidism	Normal, high*	Low, normal, high	Low, normal, high	Low, normal, high
Malignancy	High	Normal	Low, normal	Low
Vitamin D deficiency	Low	Low	Low, normal, high	Low
Renal failure	Low	Normal	Low	High
Hyperphosphatemia	Low	Normal	Low	High
Vitamin D rickets type I, II	Low	Normal, high	Low, normal, high	Low
Granulomatous diseases (sarcoid/TB)	High	Low, normal, high	High	Normal, high
Postmenopausal osteoporosis	Normal	Normal	Normal	Normal
Senile osteoporosis	Normal	Normal	Normal	Normal
Osteomalacia	Low, normal	Low, normal	Low	Low, normal, high

*Calcium may be normal in the setting of concurrent 1,25(OH)$_2$D$_3$ deficiency.
(McPherson RA, Pincus MR: Henry's Clinical Diagnosis and Management by Laboratory Methods, 23rd ed, ISBN # 978-0323-29568-0, 2017, Elsevier)

Laboratory Tests

IV

Clinical Practice Guidelines

PART A

THE PERIODIC HEALTH EXAMINATION

*Age-Specific Charts, 1849

TABLE 1   Birth to 10 years, 1849
TABLE 2   Ages 11 to 24 years, 1851
TABLE 3   Ages 25 to 64 years, 1853
TABLE 4   Ages 65 and older, 1855
TABLE 5   Pregnant women, 1857
TABLE 6   Cervical cancer screening guidelines, 1858

PART B

IMMUNIZATIONS AND CHEMOPROPHYLAXIS

Childhood and Adolescent Immunizations, 1859

TABLE 7 Recommended immunization schedule for children and adolescents aged 18 years or younger—United States, 1859
TABLE 8 Catch-up immunization schedule for persons aged 4 months through 18 years who start late or who are more than 1 month behind—United States, 1860

General Recommendations on Immunization, 1865

TABLE 9 Recommended and minimum ages and intervals between vaccine doses, 1865
TABLE 10 Guidelines for spacing of live and inactivated antigens, 1866
TABLE 11 Guidelines for administering antibody-containing products and vaccines, 1866

TABLE 12 Recommended intervals between administration of antibody-containing products and measles- or varicella-containing vaccine, by product and indication for vaccination, 1867
TABLE 13 Contraindications and precautions to commonly used vaccines, 1868
TABLE 14 Conditions commonly misperceived as contraindications to vaccination, 1870
Vaccine administration (includes Figs. E1 through E5), 1872
TABLE 15 Treatment of anaphylaxis in children and adults with drugs administered intramuscularly or orally, 1872
TABLE 16 Vaccination of persons with primary and secondary immunodeficiencies, 1873
TABLE 17 Immunizations for pediatric oncology patients, 1874
TABLE 18 Approaches to the evaluation and vaccination of persons vaccinated outside the United States who have no (or questionable) vaccination records, 1875

Immunizations for Adults, 1876

TABLE 19 Recommended immunization schedule for adults aged 19 years or older by age group, United States, 1877
TABLE 20A Recommended immunization schedule for adults aged 19 years or older by medical condition and other indications, United States, 1878
TABLE 20B Contraindications and precautions for vaccines recommended for adults aged 19 years or older, 1882
TABLE 21 Immunization and pregnancy, 1883
TABLE 22 Immunizing agents and immunization schedules for health care workers (HCWs), 1884
TABLE 23 Recommendations for persons with medical conditions requiring special vaccination considerations, 1887
TABLE 24 Vaccinations for international travel, 1888

---

*Data modified from U.S. Preventive Services Task Force: *Guide to clinical preventive services: report of the U.S. Preventive Services Task Force*, ed 2, Washington, DC, 1996 (revised 2001), U.S. Department of Health and Human Services. Text downloaded from http://text.nlm.nih.gov

Recommendations and Implementation Strategies for Hepatitis B Vaccination of Adults, 1889

BOX 1 Adults recommended to receive hepatitis B vaccination, 1889
BOX 2 Hepatitis B vaccine schedules for adults (aged ≥20 yr), 1889
TABLE 25 Recommended doses of currently licensed formulations of adult hepatitis B vaccine by group and vaccine type, 1890
TABLE 26 Recommended HIV/AIDS, sexually transmitted disease (STD), and viral hepatitis prevention services by risk population, 1890
TABLE 27 Guidelines for postexposure prophylaxis of persons with non-occupational exposures to blood or body fluids that contain blood by exposure type and vaccination status, 1891
TABLE 28 Typical interpretation of serologic test results for hepatitis B virus infection, 1891

Hepatitis A Prophylaxis, 1892

TABLE 29 Recommended dosages of hepatitis A immune globulin, 1892
TABLE 30 Licensed dosages of hepatitis A vaccines, 1892

Influenza Treatment and Prophylaxis, 1893

BOX 3 Summary of seasonal influenza vaccination recommendations, 1893
TABLE 31 Live, attenuated influenza vaccine (LAIV) compared with inactivated influenza vaccine (TIV) for seasonal influenza, United States formulations, 1894
Indications for use of antivirals, 1895
FIGURE 6 Algorithm for determining recommended influenza immunization actions for children, 1896

HIV Testing and Postexposure Prophylaxis, 1897

Recommendations for HIV testing of adults, adolescents, and pregnant women, 1897
FIGURE 7 Algorithm for evaluation and treatment of possible nonoccupational HIV exposure, 1899
TABLE 32 HIV exposure, estimated per-act risk, 1899

TABLE 33 Regimens for 28-day postexposure prophylaxis for HIV infection, 1900
TABLE 34 Antiretroviral therapy medications, adult dosage, and side effects, 1901
TABLE 35 Laboratory tests generally recommended for persons after exposure to HIV, 1902
BOX 4 Situations for which expert consultation for HIV postexposure prophylaxis is advised, 1902
BOX 5 Occupational exposure management resources, 1903
BOX 6 Management of occupational blood exposures, 1904

Endocarditis Prophylaxis, 1905

TABLE 36 Cardiac conditions associated with the highest risk of adverse outcome from endocarditis for which prophylaxis with dental procedures is recommended, 1905
TABLE 37 Dental procedures for which endocarditis prophylaxis is recommended for patients in Table 36, 1905
TABLE 38 Regimens for a dental procedure, 1905
TABLE 39 Summary of major changes in updated recommendations, 1906

Hepatitis C Testing, 1907

BOX 7 Recommendations for prevention and control of hepatitis C virus (HCV) infection and HCV-related chronic diseases, 1907
FIGURE 8 Analytic framework for guiding HCV testing among persons born during 1945-1965, 1908

Hepatitis B Virus Postexposure Protection for Health Care Personnel, 1909

TABLE 40 Postexposure management of health care personnel after occupational percutaneous and mucosal exposure to blood and body fluids, by health care personnel HepB vaccination and response status, 1909

PART A • THE PERIODIC HEALTH EXAMINATION

Age-Specific Charts

TABLE 1 Birth to 10 Years

Interventions considered and recommended for the Periodic Health Examination

Leading causes of death
Conditions originating in perinatal period
Congenital anomalies
Sudden infant death syndrome
Unintentional injuries (non–motor vehicle)
Motor vehicle injuries

INTERVENTIONS FOR THE GENERAL POPULATION

Screening
Height and weight
Blood pressure
Vision screen (ages 3-4 yr)
Hemoglobinopathy screen (birth)[1]
Phenylalanine level (birth)[2]
Thyroxine and/or thyroid-stimulating hormone (birth)[3]
Lead level

Counseling
Injury prevention
Child safety car seats (age <5 yr)
Lap/shoulder belts (age ≥5 yr)
Bicycle helmet; avoid bicycling near traffic
Smoke detector, flame-retardant sleepwear
Hot water heater temperature <120°-130° F
Window/stair guards, pool fence
Safe storage of drugs, toxic substances, firearms, and matches
Syrup of ipecac, poison control phone number
CPR training for parents/caretakers

Diet and exercise
Breastfeeding, iron-enriched formula and foods (infants and toddlers)
Limit fat and cholesterol; maintain caloric balance; emphasize grains, fruits, vegetables (age ≥2 yr)
Regular physical activity*

Substance use
Effects of passive smoking*
Antitobacco message*

Dental health
Regular visits to dental care provider*
Floss, brush with fluoride toothpaste daily*
Advice about baby bottle tooth decay*

Immunizations
Diphtheria-tetanus-pertussis (DTaP)[4]
Inactivated poliovirus vaccine (IPV)[5]
Measles-mumps-rubella (MMR)[6]
Haemophilus influenzae type b (Hib) conjugate[7]
Hepatitis A vaccine (HR4)
Hepatitis B[8]
Varicella[9]
Pneumococcal vaccine[10]
Influenza[11]
Meningococcal conjugate vaccine (MCV)[12]
Rotavirus (RV)[13]
Human papillomavirus vaccine (HPV)[14]

Chemoprophylaxis
Ocular prophylaxis (birth)

INTERVENTIONS FOR HIGH-RISK POPULATIONS

Population	Potential Interventions (see detailed high-risk definitions)
Preterm or low birth weight	Hemoglobin/hematocrit (HR1)
Infants of mothers at risk for HIV	HIV testing (HR2)
Low income; immigrants	Hemoglobin/hematocrit (HR1); PPD (HR3)
TB contacts	PPD (HR3)
Native American/Alaska Native	Hemoglobin/hematocrit (HR1); PPD (HR3); pneumococcal vaccine (HR5)
Residents of long-term care facilities	PPD (HR3); hepatitis A vaccine (HR4); influenza vaccine (HR6)
Certain chronic medical conditions	PPD (HR3); pneumococcal vaccine (HR5); influenza vaccine (HR6)
Increased individual or community lead exposure	Blood lead level (HR7)
Inadequate water fluoridation	Daily fluoride supplement (HR8)
Family history of skin cancer; nevi; fair skin, eyes, hair	Avoid excess/midday sun, use protective clothing* (HR9)

CPR, Cardiopulmonary resuscitation; *HR,* high risk; *PPD,* purified protein derivative; *STDs,* sexually transmitted diseases; *TB,* tuberculosis.
[1]Whether screening should be universal or targeted to high-risk groups depends on the proportion of high-risk individuals in the screening area and other considerations. [2]If done during first 24 hr of life, repeat by age 2 wk. [3]Optimally between day 2 and 6, but in all cases before newborn nursery discharge. [4]2, 4, 6, and 12-18 mo; once between age 4-6 yr. [5]2, 4, 6-18 mo; once between age 4-6 yr. [6]12-15 mo and 4-6 yr. [7]2, 4, 6 and 12-15 mo; no dose needed at 6 mo if PRP-OMP vaccine is used for first 2 doses. [8]Birth, 1 mo, 6 mo; or, 0-2 mo, 1-2 mo later, and 6-18 mo. If not done in infancy: current visit, and 1 and 6 mo later. [9]12-18 mo; or any child without history of chickenpox or previous immunization. Include information on risk in adulthood, duration of immunity, and potential need for booster doses. Administer a second dose of varicella vaccine at age 4-6 yr. [10]Pneumococcal polysaccharide vaccine (PPSV) can be administered at the same time as the other childhood vaccines at a separate site. [11]Influenza vaccine is recommended in children 6 mo-18 yr of age. [12]Administer meningococcal conjugate vaccine (MCV) to children aged 2 through 10 yr with terminal complement component deficiency, anatomic or functional asplenia, and certain other high-risk groups (see *MMWR* 54[RR-7], 2005). Persons who received MPSV 3 or more years previously and who remain at increased risk for meningococcal disease should be revaccinated with MCV. [13]Administer first dose at 2 mo. If Rotarix® is administered at ages 2 and 4 mo, a dose at 6 mo is not indicated. [14]HPV4 may be administered in a 3-dose series to males aged 9 through 26 yr and females aged 11 to 26 yr to reduce the likelihood of acquiring genital warts.
*The ability of clinician counseling to influence this behavior is unproven.

HR1: Infants aged 6-12 mo who are living in poverty, black, Native American or Alaska Native, immigrants from developing countries, preterm and low-birth-weight infants, infants whose principal dietary intake is unfortified cow's milk.

HR2: Infants born to high-risk mothers whose HIV status is unknown. Women at high risk include past or present injection drug users; persons who exchange sex for money or drugs and their sex partners; injection drug–using, bisexual, or HIV-positive sex partners currently or in past; persons seeking treatment for STDs; persons who received a blood transfusion between 1978 and 1985.

HR3: Persons infected with HIV, close contacts of persons with known or suspected TB, persons with medical risk factors associated with TB, immigrants from countries with high TB prevalence, medically underserved low-income populations (including homeless), residents of long-term care facilities.

HR4: Hepatitis A vaccine (Hep A) is recommended for all children at 1 yr of age (i.e., 12-23 mo). The two doses in the series should be administered at least 6 mo apart. Children who are not vaccinated by 2 yr of age can be vaccinated at subsequent visits.

HR5: Immunocompetent persons ≥2 yr with certain medical conditions, including chronic cardiac or pulmonary disease, diabetes mellitus, and anatomic asplenia, as well as cochlear implant candidates and recipients. Immunocompetent persons ≥2 yr living in high-risk environments or social settings (e.g., certain Native American and Alaska Native populations).

HR6: Annual vaccinations of children ≥6 mo who are residents of chronic care facilities or who have chronic cardiopulmonary disorders, metabolic diseases (including diabetes mellitus), hemoglobinopathies, immunosuppression, or renal dysfunction.

HR7: Children approximately age 12 mo who (1) live in communities in which the prevalence of lead levels requiring individual intervention, including residential lead hazard control or chelation, is high or undefined; (2) live in or frequently visit a home built before 1950 with dilapidated paint or with recent or ongoing renovation or remodeling; (3) have close contact with a person who has an elevated lead level; (4) live near lead industry or heavy traffic; (5) live with someone whose job or hobby involves lead exposure; (6) use lead-based pottery; or (7) take traditional ethnic remedies that contain lead.

HR8: Children living in areas with inadequate water fluoridation (<0.6 ppm).

HR9: Persons with a family history of skin cancer; a large number of moles; atypical moles; poor tanning ability; or light skin, hair, and eye color.

TABLE 2 Ages 11 to 24 Years

Interventions considered and recommended for the Periodic Health Examination	Leading causes of death
	Motor vehicle accidents/other unintentional injuries
	Homicide
	Suicide
	Malignant neoplasms
	Heart diseases

INTERVENTIONS FOR THE GENERAL POPULATION

Screening
Height and weight
Blood pressure[1]
Papanicolaou (Pap) test[2] (females)
Chlamydia and *Gonorrhea* screen[3]
HIV screening
Lipid panel (in high-risk young adults only)
Rubella serology or vaccination history[4] (females >12 yr)
Assess for problem drinking
Lead level

Counseling

Injury prevention
Lap/shoulder belts
Bicycle/motorcycle/ATV helmets*
Smoke detector*
Safe storage/removal of firearms*

Substance use
Avoid tobacco use
Avoid underage drinking and illicit drug use*
Avoid alcohol/drug use while driving, swimming, boating, etc.*

Sexual behavior
STD prevention: abstinence*; avoid high-risk behavior*;
    condoms/female barrier with spermicide*
Unintended pregnancy: contraception

Diet and exercise
Limit fat and cholesterol; maintain caloric balance; emphasize grains, fruits,
    vegetables
Folic acid daily supplements 0.4 to 0.8 mg/day for all women planning or capable
    of pregnancy
Adequate calcium intake (females)
Regular physical activity*

Dental health
Regular visits to dental care provider*
Floss, brush with fluoride toothpaste daily

Immunizations
Tetanus, diphtheria, pertussis†
Hepatitis B[5]
Measles-mumps-rubella (MMR) (11-12 yr)[6]
Varicella (11-12 yr)[7]
Rubella (females >12 yr)[4]
Meningococcal[8]
Human papilloma virus (females 11-26 yr, males 9-26 yr)[9]
Influenza[10]
Pneumococcal polysaccharide vaccine (PPSV)[11]

Chemoprophylaxis
Multivitamin with folic acid (females)

INTERVENTIONS FOR HIGH-RISK POPULATIONS

Population	*Potential Interventions (see detailed high-risk definitions)*
High-risk sexual behavior	RPR/VDRL (HR1); screen for gonorrhea (female) (HR2), HIV (HR3), chlamydia (female) (HR4); hepatitis A vaccine (HR5)
Injection or street drug use	RPR/VDRL (HR1); HIV screen (HR3); hepatitis A vaccine (HR5); PPD (HR6); advice to reduce infection risk (HR7)
TB contacts; immigrants; low income	PPD (HR6)
Native Americans/Alaska Natives	Hepatitis A vaccine (HR5); PPD (HR6); pneumococcal vaccine (HR8)
Travelers to developing countries	Hepatitis A vaccine (HR5)
Certain chronic medical conditions	PPD (HR6); pneumococcal vaccine (HR8); influenza vaccine (HR9)
Settings where adolescents and young adults congregate	Second MMR (HR10)
Susceptible to varicella, measles, mumps	Varicella vaccine (HR11); MMR (HR12)
Institutionalized persons; health care/lab workers	Hepatitis A vaccine (HR5); PPD (HR6); influenza vaccine (HR9)
Family history of skin cancer; nevi; fair skin, eyes, hair	Avoid excess/midday sun, use protective clothing* (HR13)
Prior pregnancy with neural tube defect	Folic acid 0.4-0.8 mg/day (HR14)
Inadequate water fluoridation	Daily fluoride supplement (HR15)
Pregnancy	HIV screen, Tdap vaccine (given in second or early third trimester of pregnancy)
Infants 6-11 mo of age travelling internationally	MMR

ATV, All-terrain vehicle; *HR*, high risk; *PPD*, purified protein derivative; *RPR*, rapid plasmin reagin; *STD*, sexually transmitted disease; *TB*, tuberculosis; *VDRL*, Venereal Disease Research Laboratory.
[1]Periodic blood pressure for persons aged ≥21 yr. [2]Screening for cervical cancer should begin at 21 years of age, regardless of sexual behaviors and risk factors. Cytology without HPV testing should be performed every 3 years. [3]If sexually active, Table 6 summarizes cervical cancer screening guidelines. [4]Serologic testing, documented vaccination history, and routine vaccination against rubella (preferably with MMR) are equally acceptable alternatives. [5]If not previously immunized: current visit and 1 and 6 mo later. [6]If no previous second dose of MMR. [7]If susceptible to chickenpox. [8]Meningococcal conjugate vaccine (MCV) can be administered at 11-12 yr visit, at high school entry, or at beginning of college (especially indicated in students living in college dormitories). Meningococcal group B vaccine (Trumenba) is approved for use in individuals 10 through 25 years of age for active immunization to prevent invasive disease caused by *Neisseria meningitidis* serogroup B. [9]Quadrivalent human papillomavirus (types 6, 11, 16, 18) recombinant vaccine (Gardasil) should be given to all females aged 11-26 yr who have not been previously vaccinated. The vaccine is indicated for the prevention of cervical cancer and genital warts caused by the human papilloma virus (HPV) 6, 11, 16, or 18. Gardasil is an intramuscular injection for administration to the thigh or upper arm. The schedule consists of two doses if first dose is given at 11-12 years of age and second dose given 6-12 months later. If second dose is given less than 5 months apart, will need third dose. In patients with weakened immune system or if vaccination started between ages 15 to 26 three 0.5-ml doses are recommended, with the second dose given 2 mo after the first, and the final dose administered 6 mo after the initial dose. HPV4 may also be administered in a 3-dose series to males aged 9 through 26 years to reduce their likelihood of acquiring genital warts. A bivalent HPV vaccine is available for prevention of cervical dysplasia in females. [10]Influenza vaccine is recommended for children 6 mo to 18 yr of age and all adults. [11]Administer to children with certain underlying medical conditions (see *MMWR* 46[RR-8], 1997), including a cochlear implant. A single revaccination should be administered to children with functional or anatomic asplenia or other immunocompromising condition after 5 yr.
*The ability of clinician counseling to influence this behavior is unproven.
†Tdap vaccine is recommended for adolescents aged 11-12 yr who have completed the recommended childhood DTP/DTaP vaccination series and have not received a Td booster dose. Adolescents aged 13-18 yr who missed the 11-12-yr Td/Tdap booster dose should also receive a single dose of Tdap if they have completed the recommended childhood DTP/DTaP vaccination series. A 5-yr interval from the last Td dose is encouraged when Tdap is used as a booster drug; however, a shorter interval may be used if pertussis immunity is needed. For pregnant patients, the Tdap vaccine is recommended with each pregnancy between 27 and 36 weeks of gestation.

HR1: Persons who exchange sex for money or drugs and their sex partners, persons with other STDs (including HIV), and sexual contacts of persons with active syphilis. Clinicians should also consider local epidemiology.

HR2: Females who have had two or more sex partners in the last year or a sex partner with multiple sexual contacts; exchanged sex for money or drugs; or have a history of repeated episodes of gonorrhea. Clinicians should also consider local epidemiology.

HR3: Males who had sex with males; past or present injection drug users; persons who exchange sex for money or drugs and their sex partners; injection drug–using, bisexual, or HIV-positive sex partner currently or in the past; recipients of a blood transfusion between 1978 and 1985; persons seeking treatment for STDs. Clinicians should also consider screening for HIV in general population.

HR4: Sexually active females with multiple risk factors, including history of prior STD, new or multiple sex partners, age <25 yr, nonuse or inconsistent use of barrier contraceptives, or cervical ectopy. Clinicians should consider local epidemiology of the disease in identifying other high-risk groups.

HR5: Persons living in, traveling to, or working in areas where the disease is endemic and where periodic outbreaks occur (e.g., countries with high or intermediate endemicity; certain Alaska Native, Pacific Island, Native American, and religious communities); men who have sex with men; injection or street drug users; persons with clotting factor disorders or chronic liver disease, diabetics. Vaccine may be considered for institutionalized persons and workers in these institutions; military personnel; and daycare, hospital, and laboratory workers. Clinicians should also consider local epidemiology.

HR6: HIV-positive, close contacts of persons with known or suspected TB, health care workers, persons with medical risk factors associated with TB, immigrants from countries with high TB prevalence, medically underserved low-income populations (including homeless), alcoholics, injection drug users, and residents of long-term care facilities.

HR7: Persons who continue to inject drugs.

HR8: Immunocompetent persons with certain medical conditions, including chronic cardiac, renal, or pulmonary disease; diabetes mellitus; cochlear implant candidates and recipients; and anatomic asplenia. Immunocompetent persons who live in high-risk environments or social settings (e.g., certain Native American and Alaska Native populations). Adults who smoke cigarettes, persons with asymptomatic or symptomatic HIV infection.

HR9: Annual vaccination of residents of chronic care facilities; persons with chronic cardiopulmonary disorders, metabolic diseases (including diabetes mellitus), hemoglobinopathies, immunosuppression, or renal dysfunction; and health care providers for high-risk patients.

HR10: Adolescents and young adults in settings where such individuals congregate (e.g., high schools and colleges) if they have not previously received a second dose.

HR11: Healthy persons aged ≥13 yr without a history of chickenpox or previous immunization. Consider serologic testing for presumed susceptible persons aged ≥13 yr.

HR12: Persons born after 1956 who lack evidence of immunity to measles or mumps (e.g., documented receipt of live vaccine on or after the first birthday, laboratory evidence of immunity, or a history of physician-diagnosed measles or mumps).

HR13: Persons with a family or personal history of skin cancer; a large number of moles; atypical moles; poor tanning ability; or light skin, hair, and eye color.

HR14: Women with prior pregnancy affected by neural tube defect who are planning pregnancy and any woman planning or capable of pregnancy.

HR15: Persons aged <17 yr living in areas with inadequate water fluoridation (<0.6 ppm).

TABLE 3 Ages 25 to 64 Years

Interventions considered and recommended for the Periodic Health Examination	Leading causes of death
	Malignant neoplasms
	Heart diseases
	Motor vehicle and other unintentional injuries
	HIV infection
	Suicide and homicide

INTERVENTIONS FOR THE GENERAL POPULATION

Screening

Blood pressure

Height and weight

Lipid panel (men aged 35-64 yr, women aged 45-64 yr)

HIV screening

Papanicolaou (Pap) test (women)[1]

Cytology without HPV testing starting at age 21

Cytology with HPV testing starting at 30 years of age

Fecal occult blood test[2] and/or colonoscopy (≥50 yr)

Mammogram ± clinical breast examination[3] (women 40-69 yr)[8]

Bone density scan in postmenopausal women

Assess for problem drinking

Rubella serology or vaccination history[4] (women of childbearing age)

Counseling

Substance use

Tobacco cessation

Avoid alcohol/drug use while driving, swimming, boating, etc.*

Diet and exercise

Limit fat and cholesterol; maintain caloric balance; emphasize grains, fruits, vegetables

Adequate calcium intake (women)

Regular physical activity*

Injury prevention

Lap/shoulder belts

Motorcycle/bicycle/ATV helmets*

Smoke detector*

Safe storage/removal of firearms*

Sexual behavior

STD prevention: avoid high-risk behavior*; condoms/female barrier with spermicide*

Unintended pregnancy: contraception

Dental health

Regular visits to dental care provider*

Floss, brush with fluoride toothpaste daily*

Immunizations

Tetanus-diphtheria-pertussis (Tdap) booster[7]

Rubella[4] (women of childbearing age)

Influenza vaccine†

Human papillomavirus[5]

Herpes zoster (≥60 yr)[6]

Chemoprophylaxis

Multivitamin with folic acid 0.4-0.8 mg/day (women planning or capable of pregnancy)

INTERVENTIONS FOR HIGH-RISK POPULATIONS

Population	Potential Interventions (see detailed high-risk definitions)
High-risk sexual behavior	RPR/VDRL (HR1); screen for gonorrhea (female) (HR2), HIV (HR3), chlamydia (female) (HR4); hepatitis B vaccine (HR5); hepatitis A vaccine (HR6)
Injection or street drug use	RPR/VDRL (HR1); HIV screen (HR3); hepatitis B vaccine (HR5); hepatitis A vaccine (HR6); PPD (HR7); advice to reduce infection risk (HR8)
Low income; TB contacts; immigrants; alcoholics	PPD (HR7)
Native Americans/Alaska Natives	Hepatitis A vaccine (HR6); PPD (HR7); pneumococcal vaccine (HR9)
Travelers to developing countries	Hepatitis B vaccine (HR5); hepatitis A vaccine (HR6)
Certain chronic medical conditions	PPD (HR7); pneumococcal vaccine (HR9); influenza vaccine (HR10)
Blood product recipients	HIV screen (HR3); hepatitis B vaccine (HR5); hepatitis C screen
Susceptible to measles, mumps, or varicella	MMR (HR11); varicella vaccine (HR12)
Institutionalized persons	Hepatitis A vaccine (HR6); PPD (HR7); pneumococcal vaccine (HR9); influenza vaccine (HR10)
Health care/lab workers	Hepatitis B vaccine (HR5); hepatitis A vaccine (HR6); PPD (HR7); influenza vaccine (HR10)
Family history of skin cancer; fair skin, eyes, hair	Avoid excess/midday sun, use protective clothing* (HR13)
Previous pregnancy with neural tube defect	Folic acid 0.4-0.8 mg/day (HR14)
Cardiovascular risk factors	Lipid panel (HR 15)
Pregnancy	HIV screen, Tdap vaccine (in second or early third trimester of pregnancy)
Diabetes mellitus	Hepatitis B vaccine (HR5)

ATV, All-terrain vehicle; *HPV,* human papillomavirus; *HR,* high risk; *MMR,* measles-mumps-rubella; *PPD,* purified protein derivative; *RPR,* rapid plasma reagin; *STD,* sexually transmitted disease; *TB,* tuberculosis; *Tdap,* tetanus and diphtheria toxoids and acellular pertussis; *VDRL,* Venereal Disease Research Laboratory.

[1]Women who are or have been sexually active and who have a cervix: q ≤3 yr. Routine Pap smear screening is unnecessary for women who have undergone a complete hysterectomy for benign disease. The American College of Obstetricians and Gynecologists (ACOG) recommends that routine Pap smears should start at age 21. Women 30 and older should wait 3 yrs between paps once they have had three consecutive clear tests. For women 21-29 years old, cervical cytology alone should be performed every 3 years. For women 30-65 years old, co-testing with cervical cytology and human papilloma virus (HPV) testing should be performed every 5 years. Screening should occur more frequently in women who have established risk factors for cervical cancer (including immunocompromised status, HIV infection, history of cervical intraepithelial neoplasia, exposure to diethylstilbestrol in utero). [2]Annually. [3]Mammogram q1-2 yr, or mammogram q1-2 yr with annual clinical breast examination. [4]Serologic testing, documented vaccination history, and routine vaccination (preferably with MMR) are equally acceptable. [5]Quadrivalent human papillomavirus (types 6, 11, 16, 18) recombinant vaccine (Gardasil) should be given to all females aged 9-26 yr who have not been previously vaccinated. The vaccine is indicated for the prevention of cervical cancer and genital warts caused by the human papillomavirus (HPV) 6, 11, 16, or 18. Gardasil is an intramuscular injection for administration to the thigh or upper arm. The schedule consists of three 0.5-ml doses, with the second dose given 2 mo after the first, and the final dose administered 6 mo after the initial dose. Gardasil is also indicated in males aged 9 to 26 yr for prevention of genital warts. A bivalent HPV vaccine is available for prevention of cervical dysplasia in females. [6]Herpes zoster vaccine (Zostavax) is indicated for prevention of herpes zoster (shingles) in individuals 60 yr or older. Zostavax is administered as a single dose subcutaneously. It is a lyophilic preparation of the Oka/Merck strain of live, attenuated varicella-zoster virus (VZV). It should not be administered to individuals with a history of primary or acquired immunodeficiency states, persons on immunosuppressive therapy (including high-dose corticosteroids), those with active untreated tuberculosis, and those who may be pregnant. [7]For pregnant patients, the Tdap is recommended with each pregnancy between 27 and 36 weeks of gestation. [8]American Cancer Society guidelines for average risk women recommend optional annual screening mammography at age 40-44, screening (strong recommendation) beginning at age 45, annual screening 45-54, biannual screening with option to continue annual screening, continue screening as long as overall health is good and life expectancy is ≥10 years. Clinical breast examination for screening is not recommended.

*The ability of clinician counseling to influence this behavior is unproven.

†A live attenuated influenza vaccine (LAIV, FluMist) administered intranasally is available for healthy persons aged 2 to 49 yr.

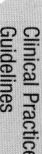

Clinical Practice Guidelines

V

HR1: Persons who exchange sex for money or drugs and their sex partners, persons with other STDs (including HIV), and sexual contacts of persons with active syphilis. Clinicians should also consider local epidemiology.

HR2: Women who exchange sex for money or drugs or who have had repeated episodes of gonorrhea. Clinicians should also consider local epidemiology.

HR3: Men who had sex with men after 1975; past or present injection drug users; persons who exchange sex for money or drugs and their sex partners; persons with current or past injection drug–using, bisexual, or HIV-positive sex partners; recipients of a blood transfusion between 1978 and 1985; persons seeking treatment for STDs. Clinicians should also consider local epidemiology and HIV screening in the general population.

HR4: Sexually active women with multiple risk factors, including history of STD, new or multiple sex partners, nonuse or inconsistent use of barrier contraceptives, or cervical ectopy. Clinicians should also consider local epidemiology.

HR5: Blood product recipients (including hemodialysis patients), persons with frequent occupational exposure to blood or blood products, men who have sex with men, injection drug users and their sex partners, persons with multiple recent sex partners, persons with other STDs (including HIV), travelers to countries with endemic hepatitis B, all diabetics age 19 to 59. In 2017 hepatitis B vaccination was expanded to all adults with chronic liver disease, including, but not limited to, hepatitis C virus infection, cirrhosis, fatty liver disease, alcoholic liver disease, autoimmune hepatitis, and an alanine aminotransferase (ALT) or aspartate aminotransferase (AST) level greater than twice the upper limit of normal.

HR6: Persons living in, traveling to, or working in areas where the disease is endemic and where periodic outbreaks occur (e.g., countries with high or intermediate endemicity; certain Alaska Native, Pacific Island, Native American, and religious communities); men who have sex with men; injection or street drug users; patients with clotting factor disorders or chronic liver disease. Consider for institutionalized persons and workers in these institutions; military personnel; and day-care, hospital, and laboratory workers. Clinicians should also consider local epidemiology.

HR7: HIV-positive, close contacts of persons with known or suspected TB, health care workers, persons with medical risk factors associated with TB, immigrants from countries with high TB prevalence, medically underserved low-income populations (including homeless), alcoholics, injection drug users, and residents of long-term care facilities.

HR8: Persons who continue to inject drugs.

HR9: Immunocompetent institutionalized persons and immunocompetent persons with certain medical conditions, including chronic cardiac, renal, or pulmonary disease; anatomic asplenia; diabetes mellitus; or cochlear implant candidates and recipients. Immunocompetent persons who live in high-risk environments or social settings (e.g., certain Native American and Alaska Native populations), adults who smoke cigarettes, persons with asymptomatic or symptomatic HIV infection.

HR10: Annual vaccination of residents of long-term care facilities; persons with chronic cardiopulmonary disorders, metabolic diseases (including diabetes mellitus), hemoglobinopathies, immunosuppression, or renal dysfunction; and health care providers of high-risk patients.

HR11: Persons born after 1956 who lack evidence of immunity to measles or mumps (e.g., documented receipt of live vaccine on or after the first birthday, laboratory evidence of immunity, or a history of physician-diagnosed measles or mumps).

HR12: Healthy adults without a history of chickenpox or previous immunization. Consider serologic testing for presumed susceptible adults.

HR13: Persons with a family or personal history of skin cancer; a large number of moles; atypical moles; poor tanning ability; or light skin, hair, and eye color.

HR14: Women with previous pregnancy affected by neural tube disorder who are planning pregnancy.

HR15: Clinicians should consider a fasting serum lipid panel on a case-by-case basis.

TABLE 4   Ages 65 and Older

Interventions considered and recommended for the Periodic Health Examination	Leading causes of death
	Heart diseases
	Malignant neoplasms (lung, colorectal, breast)
	Cerebrovascular disease
	Chronic obstructive pulmonary disease
	Pneumonia and influenza

INTERVENTIONS FOR THE GENERAL POPULATION

Screening

Blood pressure

Height and weight

Fecal occult blood test[1] and/or colonoscopy

Mammogram ± clinical breast examination[2] (women ≤69 yr)

Papanicolaou (Pap) test (women)[3]

Bone density scan in postmenopausal patients

Vision screening

Assess for hearing impairment

Assess for problem drinking

Offer HIV screen

Counseling

Substance use

Tobacco cessation

Avoid alcohol/drug use while driving, swimming, boating, etc.*

Diet and exercise

Limit fat and cholesterol; maintain caloric balance; emphasize grains, fruits, vegetables

Adequate calcium intake (women)

Regular physical activity*

Injury prevention

Lap/shoulder belts

Motorcycle and bicycle helmets*

Fall prevention*

Safe storage/removal of firearms*

Smoke detector*

Set hot water heater to <120°-130° F

CPR training for household members

Dental health

Regular visits to dental care provider*

Floss, brush with fluoride toothpaste daily*

Sexual behavior

STD prevention: avoid high-risk sexual behavior*; use condoms

Immunizations

Pneumococcal vaccine[5]

Influenza[1]

Tetanus-diphtheria (Td) boosters every 10 years, with 1 substitute Tdap dose

Herpes zoster[4]

INTERVENTIONS FOR HIGH-RISK POPULATIONS

Population	Potential Interventions (see detailed high-risk definitions)
Institutionalized persons	PPD (HR1); hepatitis A vaccine (HR2); amantadine/rimantadine (HR4)
Chronic medical conditions; TB contacts; low income; immigrants; alcoholics	PPD (HR1)
Persons ≥75 yr or ≥70 yr with risk factors for falls	Fall prevention intervention (HR5)
Cardiovascular disease risk factors	Consider lipid screening (HR6)
Family history of skin cancer; nevi; fair skin, eyes, hair	Avoid excess/midday sun, use protective clothing* (HR7)
Native Americans/Alaska Natives	PPD (HR1); hepatitis A vaccine (HR2)
Travelers to developing countries	Hepatitis A vaccine (HR2); hepatitis B vaccine (HR8)
Blood product recipients	HIV screen (HR3); hepatitis B vaccine (HR8)
High-risk sexual behavior	Hepatitis A vaccine (HR2); HIV screen (HR3); hepatitis B vaccine (HR8); RPR/VDRL (HR9)
Injection or street drug use	PPD (HR1); hepatitis A vaccine (HR2); HIV screen (HR3); hepatitis B vaccine (HR8); RPR/VDRL (HR9); advice to reduce infection risk (HR10)
Health care/lab workers	PPD (HR1); hepatitis A vaccine (HR2); amantadine/rimantadine (HR4); hepatitis B vaccine (HR8)
Persons susceptible to varicella	Varicella vaccine (HR11)
Men aged 65 to 75 who have ever smoked	Ultrasound of abdominal aorta (HR12)

HR, High risk; *PPD*, purified protein derivative; *RPR*, rapid plasma reagin; *STD*, sexually transmitted disease; *TB*, tuberculosis; *VDRL*, Venereal Disease Research Laboratory.

[1]Annually. [2]Mammogram q1-2 yr, or mammogram q1-2 yr with annual clinical breast exam. [3]The American Cancer Society (ACS) recommends that Pap testing can be discontinued at age 65 after three negative Pap tests or two negative HPV tests in past three years. ACOG (American College of Obstetricians and Gynecologists) recommends discontinuing Pap testing at age 65 to 70 after three negative tests in preceding 10 years. [4]Herpes zoster vaccine (Zostavax) is indicated for prevention of herpes zoster (shingles) in individuals age ≥60 yr. Zostavax is administered as a single dose subcutaneously. It is a lyophilic preparation of the Oka/Merck strain of live, attenuated varicella zoster virus (VZV). It should not be administered to individuals with a history of primary or acquired immunodeficiency states, persons on immunosuppressive therapy (including high-dose corticosteroids), those with active untreated tuberculosis, and those who may be pregnant. [5]Healthy adults 65 years and older receiving a pneumococcal vaccine for the first time should receive PCV13 and then PPSV23 6 to 12 months later. If a patient has already received the PPSV23 vaccine after 65 years of age, the PCV13 dose should be administered at least one year after the PPSV23 dose.
*The ability of clinician counseling to influence this behavior is unproven.

HR1: HIV-positive persons, close contacts of persons with known or suspected TB, health care workers, persons with medical risk factors associated with TB, immigrants from countries with high TB prevalence, medically underserved low-income populations (including homeless), alcoholics, injection drug users, and residents of long-term care facilities.

HR2: Persons living in, traveling to, or working in areas where the disease is endemic and where periodic outbreaks occur (e.g., countries with high or intermediate endemicity; certain Alaska Native, Pacific Island, Native American, and religious communities); men who have sex with men; injection or street drug users; persons with clotting factor disorders or chronic liver disease. Consider for institutionalized persons and workers in these institutions and day care, hospital, and laboratory workers. Clinicians should also consider local epidemiology and HIV screening in the general population.

HR3: Men who had sex with men after 1975; past or present injection drug users; persons who exchange sex for money or drugs and their sex partners; persons with current or past injection drug–using, bisexual, or HIV-positive sex partners; recipients of a blood transfusion between 1978 and 1985; persons seeking treatment for STDs. Clinicians should also consider local epidemiology.

HR4: Consider for persons who have not received influenza vaccine or are vaccinated late, when the vaccine may be ineffective because of major antigenic changes in the virus; for unvaccinated persons who provide home care for high-risk persons; as supplemental protection in persons who are expected to have a poor antibody response; and for high-risk persons in whom the vaccine is contraindicated.

HR5: Persons aged ≥75 yr or 70-74 yr with one or more additional risk factors, including use of certain psychoactive and cardiac medications (e.g., benzodiazepines, antihypertensives); use of four or more prescription medications; impaired cognition, strength, balance, or gait. Intensive individualized, home-based multifactorial fall prevention intervention is recommended in settings where adequate resources are available to deliver such services.

HR6: Clinicians should consider fasting lipid panel screening on a case-by-case basis for persons aged 65 to 75 yr, especially in those with additional risk factors (e.g., smoking, diabetes, or hypertension).

HR7: Persons with a family or personal history of skin cancer; a large number of moles; atypical moles; poor tanning ability; or light skin, hair, and eye color.

HR8: Blood product recipients (including hemodialysis patients), persons with frequent occupational exposure to blood or blood products, men who have sex with men, injection drug users and their sex partners, persons with multiple recent sex partners, persons with other STDs (including HIV), travelers to countries with endemic hepatitis B. In 2017 hepatitis B vaccination was expanded to all adults with chronic liver disease, including, but not limited to, hepatitis C virus infection, cirrhosis, fatty liver disease, alcoholic liver disease, autoimmune hepatitis, and an alanine aminotransferase (ALT) or aspartate aminotransferase (AST) level greater than twice the upper limit of normal.

HR9: Persons who exchange sex for money or drugs and their sex partners, persons with other STDs (including HIV), and sexual contacts of persons with active syphilis. Clinicians should also consider local epidemiology.

HR10: Persons who continue to inject drugs.

HR11: Healthy adults without a history of chickenpox or previous immunization. Consider serologic testing for presumed susceptible adults.

HR12: Consider ultrasound of abdominal aorta to screen for abdominal aortic aneurysm in all men aged 65 to 75 yr who have ever smoked.

TABLE 5 Pregnant Women*

Interventions considered and recommended for the Periodic Health Examination

INTERVENTIONS FOR THE GENERAL POPULATION

Screening

First visit

Blood pressure

Hemoglobin/hematocrit

Hepatitis B surface antigen (HBsAg)

RPR/VDRL

Chlamydia screen (<25 yr)

Rubella serology or vaccination history

D(Rh) typing, antibody screen

Offer CVS (<13 wk)[1] or amniocentesis (15-18 wk)[1] (age ≥35 yr)

Offer hemoglobinopathy screening

Assess for problem or risk drinking

Offer HIV screening[2]

Follow-up visits

Blood pressure

Urine culture (12-16 wk)

Offer amniocentesis (15-18 wk)[1] (age ≥35 yr)

Offer multiple marker testing[1] (15-18 wk)

Offer serum α-fetoprotein[1] (16-18 wk)

Counseling

Tobacco cessation; effects of passive smoking

Alcohol/other drug use

Nutrition, including adequate calcium intake

Encourage breastfeeding

Lap/shoulder belts

Infant safety car seats

STD prevention: avoid high-risk sexual behavior†; use condoms†

Chemoprophylaxis

Multivitamin with folic acid[3]

Immunizations

Influenza

Tdap[4]

INTERVENTIONS FOR HIGH-RISK POPULATIONS

Population	*Potential Interventions (see detailed high-risk definitions)*
High-risk sexual behavior	Screen for chlamydia (first visit) (HR1), gonorrhea (first visit) (HR2), HIV (first visit) (HR3); HBsAg (third trimester) (HR4); RPR/VDRL (third trimester) (HR5)
Blood transfusion between 1978 and 1985	HIV screen (first visit) (HR3)
Injection drug use	HIV screen (HR3); HBsAg (third trimester) (HR4); advice to reduce infection risk (HR6)
Unsensitized D-negative women	D(Rh) antibody testing (24-28 wk) (HR7)
Risk factors for Down syndrome	Offer CVS (first trimester), amniocentesis (15-18 wk)1 (HR8)
Prior pregnancy with neural tube defect	Offer amniocentesis (15-18 wk),1 folic acid 4.0 mg3 (HR9)

CVS, Chorionic villus sampling; *HR,* high risk; *RPR,* rapid plasma reagin; *VDRL,* Venereal Disease Research Laboratory.

[1]Women with access to counseling and follow-up services, reliable standardized laboratories, skilled high-resolution ultrasound and, for those receiving serum marker testing, amniocentesis capabilities. [2]Universal screening is recommended. [3]Beginning at least 1 mo before conception and continuing through the first trimester. [4]For pregnant patients, the Tdap vaccine is recommended with each pregnancy between 27 and 36 weeks of gestation.

*See Tables 2 and 3 for other preventive services recommended for women of this age group.

†The ability of clinician counseling to influence this behavior is unproven.

HR1: Women with history of STD or new or multiple sex partners. Clinicians should also consider local epidemiology. Chlamydia screen should be repeated in third trimester if at continued risk.

HR2: Women younger than 25 yr with two or more sex partners in the last year or whose sex partner has multiple sexual contacts, women who exchange sex for money or drugs, and women with a history of repeated episodes of gonorrhea. Clinicians should also consider local epidemiology. Gonorrhea screen should be repeated in the third trimester if at continued risk.

HR3: Universal screening for HIV infection is recommended for all pregnant women. It is especially important in women with the following individual risk factors: past or present injection drug use; history of exchanging sex for money or drugs; injection drug–using, bisexual, or HIV-positive sex partner currently or in the past; recipients of a blood transfusion between 1978 and 1985; persons seeking treatment for STDs.

HR4: Women who are initially HBsAg negative who are at high risk because of injection drug use, who have suspected exposure to hepatitis B during pregnancy, and who have had multiple sex partners.

HR5: Women who exchange sex for money or drugs, women with other STDs (including HIV), and sexual contacts of persons with active syphilis. Clinicians should also consider local epidemiology.

HR6: Women who continue to inject drugs.

HR7: Unsensitized D-negative women.

HR8: Prior pregnancy affected by Down syndrome, advanced maternal age (≥35 yr), known carriage of chromosome rearrangement.

HR9: Women with previous pregnancy affected by neural tube defect.

TABLE 6 Cervical Cancer Screening Guidelines*			
Group	**ACOG 2009**	**USPSTF 2012**	**ACS 2012**
Women age <21	No screening	No screening	No screening
Women age 21-29	Cytology every 2 years; HPV testing not recommended	Cytology every 3 years; HPV testing not recommended	Cytology every 3 years; HPV testing not recommended
Women age 30-65	Cytology every 3 years if three consecutive normal results; addition of HPV testing also appropriate	Cytology every 3 years or cytology plus HPV testing every 5 years	Cytology plus HPV every 5 years (preferred) or cytology alone every 3 years; both are regardless of screening history
Women age <65	Following three normal screening results and no abnormal results in the last 10 years, screening may be discontinued	If adequately screened in the past, screening should be discontinued	If adequately screened in the past, screening should be discontinued
Women with total hysterectomy and no prior history of high-grade CIN	No need to continue screening if hysterectomy was for benign indication	Screening should be discontinued	Screening should be discontinued

ACOG, American College of Obstetricians and Gynecologists; *ACS,* American Cancer Society; *CIN,* Cervical intraepithelial neoplasia; *HPV,* human papillomavirus; *USPSTF,* U.S. Preventive Services Task Force.

*The American College of Physicians (ACP) recommends the following: (1) Cytology without HPV testing every three years starting at age 21; (2) cytology with HPV testing may be performed starting at 30 years of age once every 5 years in average-risk women 30 years or older who prefer longer screening intervals; and (3) screening should stop after 65 years of age in the setting of three consecutive negative cytology results or two consecutive negative cytology plus HPV cotesting results, with the most recent test performed within the previous five years.

PART B • IMMUNIZATIONS AND CHEMOPROPHYLAXIS

Childhood and Adolescent Immunizations

TABLE 7 Recommended Immunization Schedule for Children and Adolescents Aged 18 Years or Younger—United States, 2017. (For those who fall behind or start late, see that catch-up schedule [Table 8])

These recommendations must be read with the footnotes that follow. For those who fall behind or start late, provide catch-up vaccination at the earliest opportunity as indicated by the divided bars. To determine minimum intervals between doses, see the catch-up schedule (Table 8). School entry and adolescent vaccine age groups are shaded in gray.

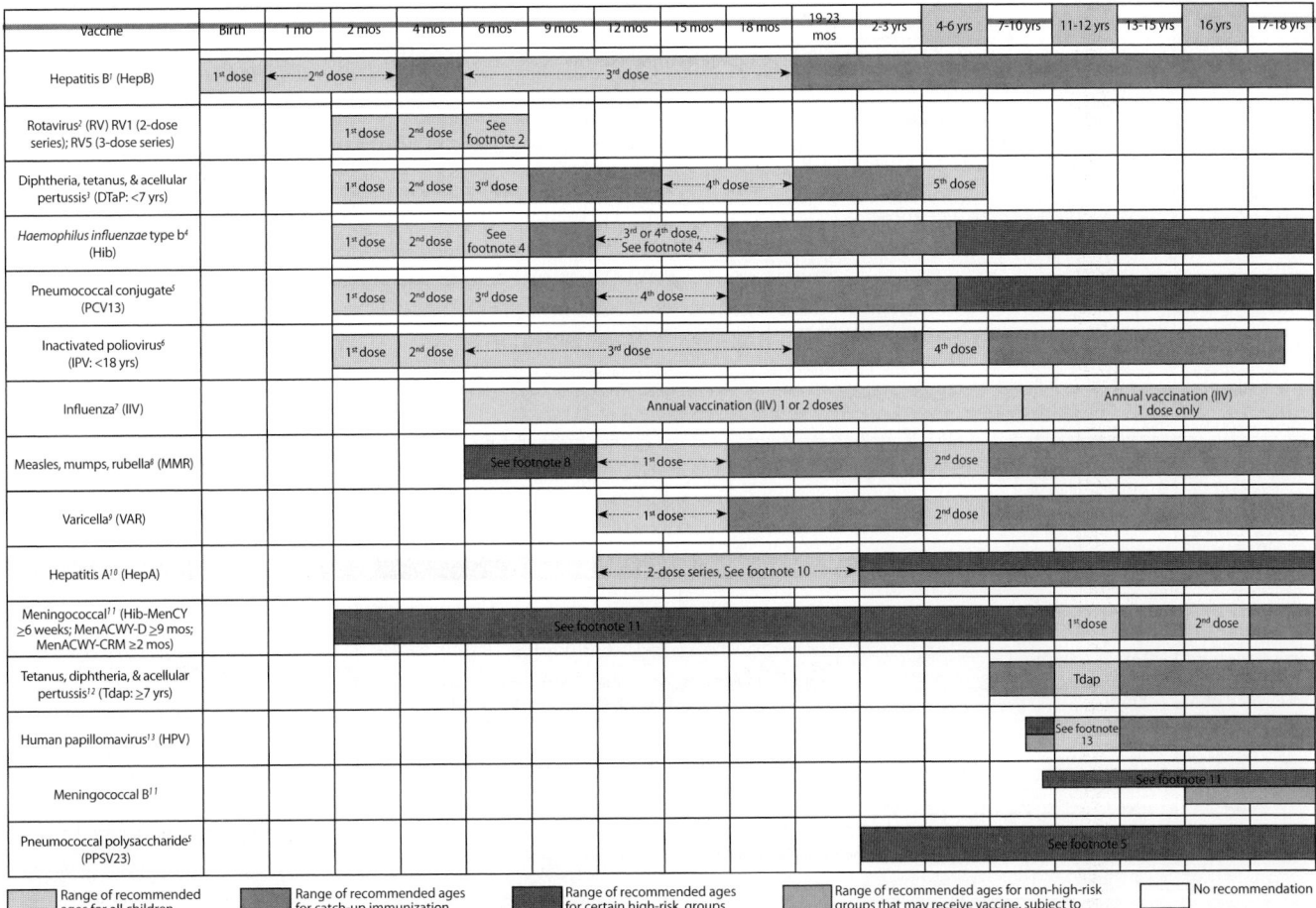

Vaccine	Birth	1 mo	2 mos	4 mos	6 mos	9 mos	12 mos	15 mos	18 mos	19-23 mos	2-3 yrs	4-6 yrs	7-10 yrs	11-12 yrs	13-15 yrs	16 yrs	17-18 yrs
Hepatitis B[1] (HepB)	1st dose	◄───2nd dose───►			◄────────────────3rd dose────────────────►												
Rotavirus[2] (RV) RV1 (2-dose series); RV5 (3-dose series)			1st dose	2nd dose	See footnote 2												
Diphtheria, tetanus, & acellular pertussis[3] (DTaP: <7 yrs)			1st dose	2nd dose	3rd dose		◄──────4th dose──────►					5th dose					
Haemophilus influenzae type b[4] (Hib)			1st dose	2nd dose	See footnote 4		3rd or 4th dose, See footnote 4										
Pneumococcal conjugate[5] (PCV13)			1st dose	2nd dose	3rd dose		◄──────4th dose──────►										
Inactivated poliovirus[6] (IPV: <18 yrs)			1st dose	2nd dose	◄────────────3rd dose────────────►							4th dose					
Influenza[7] (IIV)					Annual vaccination (IIV) 1 or 2 doses									Annual vaccination (IIV) 1 dose only			
Measles, mumps, rubella[8] (MMR)					See footnote 8		◄──────1st dose──────►					2nd dose					
Varicella[9] (VAR)							◄──────1st dose──────►					2nd dose					
Hepatitis A[10] (HepA)							◄──────2-dose series, See footnote 10──────►										
Meningococcal[11] (Hib-MenCY ≥6 weeks; MenACWY-D ≥9 mos; MenACWY-CRM ≥2 mos)				See footnote 11										1st dose		2nd dose	
Tetanus, diphtheria, & acellular pertussis[12] (Tdap: ≥7 yrs)														Tdap			
Human papillomavirus[13] (HPV)														See footnote 13			
Meningococcal B[11]														See footnote 11			
Pneumococcal polysaccharide[5] (PPSV23)												See footnote 5					

▢ Range of recommended ages for all children	▢ Range of recommended ages for catch-up immunization	▢ Range of recommended ages for certain high-risk groups	▢ Range of recommended ages for non-high-risk groups that may receive vaccine, subject to individual clinical decision making	▢ No recommendation

This schedule includes recommendations in effect as of January 1, 2017. Any dose not administered at the recommended age should be administered at a subsequent visit, when indicated and feasible. The use of a combination vaccine generally is preferred over separate injections of its equivalent component vaccines. Vaccination providers should consult the relevant Advisory Committee on Immunization Practices (ACIP) statement for detailed recommendations, available online at http://www.cdc.gov/vaccines/hcp/acip-recs/index.html. Clinically significant adverse events that follow vaccination should be reported to the Vaccine Adverse Event Reporting System (VAERS) online (http://www.vaers.hhs.gov) or by telephone (800-822-7967). Suspected cases of vaccine-preventable diseases should be reported to the state or local health department. Additional information, including precautions and contraindications for vaccination, is available from CDC online (http://www.cdc.gov/vaccines/hcp/admin/contraindications.html) or by telephone (800-CDC-INFO [800-232-4636]).

This schedule is approved by the Advisory Committee on Immunization Practices (http://www.cdc.gov/vaccines/acip), the American Academy of Pediatrics (http://www.aap.org), the American Academy of Family Physicians (http://www.aafp.org), and the American College of Obstetricians and Gynecologists (http://www.acog.org).

NOTE: The above recommendations must be read along with the footnotes of this schedule.

TABLE 8 Catch-up Immunization Schedule for Persons Aged 4 Months Through 18 Years Who Start Late or Who Are More Than 1 Month Behind—United States, 2017

The table below provides catch-up schedules and minimum intervals between doses for children whose vaccinations have been delayed. A vaccine series does not need to be restarted, regardless of the time that has elapsed between doses. Use the section appropriate for the child's age. Always use this table in conjunction with Table 7 and the footnotes that follow.

Vaccine	Minimum Age for Dose 1	Minimum Interval Between Doses			
		Dose 1 to Dose 2	Dose 2 to Dose 3	Dose 3 to Dose 4	Dose 4 to Dose 5
		Children age 4 months through 6 years			
Hepatitis B[1]	Birth	4 weeks	8 weeks *and* at least 16 weeks after first dose. Minimum age for the final dose is 24 weeks.		
Rotavirus[2]	6 weeks	4 weeks	4 weeks[2]		
Diphtheria, tetanus, and acellular pertussis[3]	6 weeks	4 weeks	4 weeks	6 months	6 months[3]
Haemophilus influenzae type b[4]	6 weeks	4 weeks if first dose was administered before the 1st birthday. 8 weeks (as final dose) if first dose was administered at age 12 through 14 months. No further doses needed if first dose was administered at age 15 months or older.	4 weeks[4] if current age is younger than 12 months **and** first dose was administered at younger than age 7 months, **and** at least 1 previous dose was PRP-T (ActHib, Pentacel, Hiberix) or unknown. 8 weeks *and* age 12 through 59 months (as final dose)[4] • if current age is younger than 12 months **and** first dose was administered at age 7 through 11 months; OR • if current age is 12 through 59 months **and** first dose was administered before the 1st birthday, **and** second dose administered at younger than age 15 months; OR • if both doses were PRP-OMP (PedvaxHIB; Comvax) **and** were administered before the 1st birthday. No further doses needed if previous dose was administered at age 15 months or older.	8 weeks (as final dose) This dose only necessary for children age 12 through 59 months who received 3 doses before the 1st birthday.	
Pneumococcal[5]	6 weeks	4 weeks if first dose administered before the 1st birthday. 8 weeks (as final dose for healthy children) if first dose was administered at the 1st birthday or after. No further doses needed for healthy children if first dose was administered at age 24 months or older.	4 weeks if current age is younger than 12 months and previous dose given at <7 months old. 8 weeks (as final dose for healthy children) if previous dose given between 7-11 months (wait until at least 12 months old); OR if current age is 12 months or older and at least 1 dose was given before age 12 months. No further doses needed for healthy children if previous dose administered at age 24 months or older.	8 weeks (as final dose) This dose only necessary for children aged 12 through 59 months who received 3 doses before age 12 months or for children at high risk who received 3 doses at any age.	
Inactivated poliovirus[6]	6 weeks	4 weeks[6]	4 weeks[6]	6 months[6] (minimum age 4 years for final dose).	
Measles, mumps, rubella[8]	12 months	4 weeks			
Varicella[9]	12 months	3 months			
Hepatitis A[10]	12 months	6 months			
Meningococcal[11] (Hib-MenCY ≥6 weeks; MenACWY-D ≥9 mos; MenACWY-CRM ≥2 mos)	6 weeks	8 weeks[11]	See footnote 11	See footnote 11	
		Children and adolescents age 7 through 18 years			
Meningococcal[11] (MenACWY-D ≥9 mos; MenACWY-CRM ≥2 mos)	Not Applicable (N/A)	8 weeks[11]			
Tetanus, diphtheria; tetanus, diphtheria, and acellular pertussis[12]	7 years[12]	4 weeks	4 weeks if first dose of DTaP/DT was administered before the 1st birthday. 6 months (as final dose) if first dose of DTaP/DT or Tdap/Td was administered at or after the 1st birthday.	6 months if first dose of DTaP/DT was administered before the 1st birthday.	
Human papillomavirus[13]	9 years	Routine dosing intervals are recommended.[13]			
Hepatitis A[10]	N/A	6 months			
Hepatitis B[1]	N/A	4 weeks	8 weeks **and** at least 16 weeks after first dose.		
Inactivated poliovirus[6]	N/A	4 weeks	4 weeks[6]	6 months[6]	
Measles, mumps, rubella[8]	N/A	4 weeks			
Varicella[9]	N/A	3 months if younger than age 13 years. 4 weeks if age 13 years or older.			

NOTE: The above recommendations must be read along with the footnotes of this schedule.

Footnotes — Recommended immunization schedule for persons aged 0 through 18 years—United States, 2016

For further guidance on the use of the vaccines mentioned below, see: http://www.cdc.gov/vaccines/hcp/acip-recs/index.html.
For vaccine recommendations for persons 19 years of age and older, see the adult immunization schedule.

Additional information

- For information on contraindications and precautions for the use of a vaccine and for additional information regarding that vaccine, vaccination providers should consult the ACIP General Recommendations on Immunization and the relevant ACIP statement, available online at http://www.cdc.gov/vaccines/hcp/acip-recs/index.html.
- For purposes of calculating intervals between doses, 4 weeks = 28 days. Intervals of 4 months or greater are determined by calendar months.
- Vaccine doses administered ≤4 days before the minimum interval are considered valid. Doses of any vaccine administered ≥5 days earlier than the minimum interval or minimum age should not be counted as valid doses and should be repeated as age-appropriate. The repeat dose should be spaced after the invalid dose by the recommended minimum interval. For further details, Table 1, *Recommended and minimum ages and intervals between vaccine doses, in MMWR, General Recommendations on Immunization and Reports/Vol. 60/No. 2*, available online at http://www.cdc.gov/mmwr/pdf/rr/rr6002.pdf.
- Information on travel vaccine requirements and recommendations is available at http://wwwnc.cdc.gov/travel/.
- For vaccination of persons with primary and secondary immunodeficiencies, see Table 13, *Vaccination of persons with primary and secondary immunodeficiences, in General Recommendations on Immunization* (ACIP), available at http://www.cdc.gov/mmwr/pdf/rr/rr6002.pdf.; and Immunization in Special Clinical Circumstances, (American Academy of Pediatrics). In: Kimberlin DW, Brady MT, Jackson MA, Long SS, eds. *Red Book: 2015 report of the Committee on Infectious Diseases. 30th ed.* Elk Grove Village, IL: American Academy of Pediatrics, 2015:68-107.
- The National Vaccine Injury Compensation Program (VICP) is a no-fault alternative to the traditional legal system for resolving vaccine injury petitions. Created by the National Childhood Vaccine Injury Act of 1986, it provides compensation to people found to be injured by certain vaccines. All vaccines within the recommended childhood immunization schedule are covered by VICP except for pneumococcal polysaccharide vaccine (PPSV23). For more information; see http://www.hrsa.gov/vaccinecompensation/index.html.

1. **Hepatitis B (HepB) vaccine. (Minimum age: birth)**
   Routine vaccination:
   At birth:
   - Administer monovalent HepB vaccine to all newborns within 24 hours of birth.
   - For infants born to hepatitis B surface antigen (HBsAg)-positive mothers, administer HepB vaccine and 0.5 mL of hepatitis B immune globulin (HBIG) within 12 hours of birth. These infants should be tested for HBsAg and antibody to HBsAg (anti-HBs) at age 9 through 12 months (preferably at the next well-child visit) or 1 to 2 months after completion of the HepB series if the series was delayed.
   - If mother's HBsAg status is unknown, within 12 hours of birth administer HepB vaccine regardless of birth weight. For infants weighing less than 2,000 grams, administer HBIG in addition to HepB vaccine within 12 hours of birth. Determine mother's HBsAg status as soon as possible and, if mother is HBsAg-positive, also administer HBIG to infants weighing 2,000 grams or more as soon as possible, but no later than age 7 days.
   Doses following the birth dose:
   - The second dose should be administered at age 1 or 2 months. Monovalent HepB vaccine should be used for doses administered before age 6 weeks.
   - Infants who did not receive a birth dose should receive 3 doses of a HepB-containing vaccine on a schedule of 0, 1 to 2 months, and 6 months, starting as soon as feasible. See Table 8.
   - Administer the second dose 1 to 2 months after the first dose (minimum interval of 4 weeks), administer the third dose at least 8 weeks after the second dose AND at least 16 weeks after the **first** dose. The final (third or fourth) dose in the HepB vaccine series should be administered **no earlier than age 24 weeks.**
   - Administration of a total of 4 doses of HepB vaccine is permitted when a combination vaccine containing HepB is administered after the birth dose.
   Catch-up vaccination:
   - Unvaccinated persons should complete a 3-dose series.
   - A 2-dose series (doses separated by at least 4 months) of adult formulation Recombivax HB is licensed for use in children aged 11 through 15 years.
   - For other catch-up guidance, see Table 8.

2. **Rotavirus (RV) vaccines. (Minimum age: 6 weeks for both RV1 [Rotarix] and RV5 [RotaTeq])**
   Routine vaccination:
   Administer a series of RV vaccine to all infants as follows:
   - If Rotarix is used, administer a 2-dose series at ages 2 and 4 months.
   - If RotaTeq is used, administer a 3-dose series at ages 2, 4, and 6 months.
   - If any dose in the series was RotaTeq or vaccine product is unknown for any dose in the series, a total of 3 doses of RV vaccine should be administered.

   Catch-up vaccination:
   - The maximum age for the first dose in the series is 14 weeks, 6 days; vaccination should not be initiated for infants aged 15 weeks, 0 days or older.
   - The maximum age for the final dose in the series is 8 months, 0 days.
   - For other catch-up guidance, see Table 8.

3. **Diphtheria and tetanus toxoids and acellular pertussis (DTaP) vaccine. (Minimum age: 6 weeks. Exception: DTaP-IPV [Kinrix, Quadracel]: 4 years)**
   Routine vaccination:
   - Administer a 5-dose series of DTaP vaccine at ages 2, 4, 6, 15 through 18 months, and 4 through 6 years. The fourth dose may be administered as early as age 12 months, provided at least 6 months have elapsed since the third dose.
   - Inadvertent administration of fourth DTaP dose early: If the fourth dose of DTaP was administered at least 4 months after the third dose of DTaP and the child was 12 months of age or older, it does not need to be repeated.
   Catch-up vaccination:
   - The fifth dose of DTaP vaccine is not necessary if the fourth dose was administered at age 4 years or older.
   - For other catch-up guidance, see Table 8.

4. ***Haemophilus influenzae* type b (Hib) conjugate vaccine. (Minimum age: 6 weeks for PRP-T [ActHIB, DTaP-IPV/Hib (Pentacel), Hiberix, and Hib-MenCY (MenHibrix)], PRP-OMP [PedvaxHIB])**
   Routine vaccination:
   - Administer a 2- or 3-dose Hib vaccine primary series and a booster dose (dose 3 or 4 depending on vaccine used in primary series) at age 12 through 15 months to complete a full Hib vaccine series.
   - The primary series with ActHIB, MenHibrix, Hiberix, or Pentacel consists of 3 doses and should be administered at ages 2, 4, and 6 months. The primary series with PedvaxHib consists of 2 doses and should be administered at ages 2 and 4 months; a dose at age 6 months is not indicated.
   - One booster dose (dose 3 or 4 depending on vaccine used in primary series) of any Hib vaccine should be administered at age 12 through 15 months.
   - For recommendations on the use of MenHibrix in patients at increased risk for meningococcal disease, refer to the meningococcal vaccine footnotes and also to *MMWR* February 28, 2014 / 63(RR01);1-13, available at http://www.cdc.gov/mmwr/PDF/rr/rr6301.pdf.

   Catch-up vaccination:
   - If dose 1 was administered at ages 12 through 14 months, administer a second (final) dose at least 8 weeks after dose 1, regardless of Hib vaccine used in the primary series.

- If both doses were PRP-OMP (PedvaxHIB or COMVAX), and were administered before the first birthday, the third (and final) dose should be administered at age 12 through 59 months and at least 8 weeks after the second dose.
- If the first dose was administered at age 7 through 11 months, administer the second dose at least 4 weeks later and a third (and final) dose at age 12 through 15 months or 8 weeks after second dose, whichever is later.
- If first dose is administered before the first birthday and second dose administered at younger than 15 months, a third (and final) dose should be administered 8 weeks later.
- For unvaccinated children aged 15–59 months, administer only 1 dose.
- For other catch-up guidance, see Table 8. For catch-up guidance related to MenHibrix, please see the meningococcal vaccine footnotes and also *MMWR* February 28, 2014 / 63(RR01);1-13, available at http://www.cdc.gov/mmwr/PDF/rr/rr6301.pdf.

Vaccination of persons with high-risk conditions:

Children aged 12 through 59 months who are at increased risk for Hib disease, including chemotherapy recipients and those with anatomic or functional asplenia (including sickle cell disease), human immunodeficiency virus (HIV) infection, immunoglobulin deficiency, or early component complement deficiency, who have received either no doses or only 1 dose of Hib vaccine before age 12 months, should receive 2 additional doses of Hib vaccine 8 weeks apart; children who received 2 or more doses of Hib vaccine before age 12 months should receive 1 additional dose.

- For patients younger than age 5 years undergoing chemotherapy or radiation treatment who received a Hib vaccine dose(s) within 14 days of starting therapy or during therapy, repeat the dose(s) at least 3 months following therapy completion.
- Recipients of hematopoietic stem cell transplant (HSCT) should be revaccinated with a 3-dose regimen of Hib vaccine starting 6 to 12 months after successful transplant, regardless of vaccination history; doses should be administered at least 4 weeks apart.
- A single dose of any Hib-containing vaccine should be administered to unimmunized* children and adolescents 15 months of age and older undergoing an elective splenectomy; if possible, vaccine should be administered at least 14 days before procedure.
- Hib vaccine is not routinely recommended for patients 5 years or older. However, 1 dose of Hib vaccine should be administered to unimmunized* persons aged 5 years or older who have anatomic or functional asplenia (including sickle cell disease) and unimmunized* persons 5 through 18 years of age with HIV infection.
  Patients who have not received a primary series and booster dose or at least 1 dose of Hib vaccine after 14 months of age are considered unimmunized.

5. **Pneumococcal vaccines. (Minimum age: 6 weeks for PCV13, 2 years for PPSV23)**

Routine vaccination with PCV13:

- Administer a 4-dose series of PCV13 vaccine at ages 2, 4, and 6 months and at age 12 through 15 months.

Catch-up vaccination with PCV13:

- Administer 1 dose of PCV13 to all healthy children aged 24 through 59 months who are not completely vaccinated for their age.
- For other catch-up guidance, see Table 8.

Vaccination of persons with high-risk conditions with PCV13 and PPSV23:

- All recommended PCV13 doses should be administered prior to PPSV23 vaccination if possible.
- For children aged 2 through 5 years with any of the following conditions: chronic heart disease (particularly cyanotic congenital heart disease and cardiac failure); chronic lung disease (including asthma if treated with high-dose oral corticosteroid therapy); diabetes mellitus; cerebrospinal fluid leak; cochlear implant; sickle cell disease and other

hemoglobinopathies; anatomic or functional asplenia; HIV infection; chronic renal failure; nephrotic syndrome; diseases associated with treatment with immunosuppressive drugs or radiation therapy, including malignant neoplasms, leukemias, lymphomas, and Hodgkin disease; solid organ transplantation; or congenital immunodeficiency:
1. Administer 1 dose of PCV13 if any incomplete schedule of 3 doses of PCV13 was received previously.
2. Administer 2 doses of PCV13 at least 8 weeks apart if unvaccinated or any incomplete schedule of fewer than 3 doses of PCV13 was received previously.
3. The minimum interval between doses of PCV13 is 8 weeks.
4. For children with no history of PPSV23 vaccination, administer PPSV23 at least 8 weeks after the most recent dose of PCV13.

- For children aged 6 through 18 years who have cerebrospinal fluid leak; cochlear implant; sickle cell disease and other hemoglobinopathies; anatomic or functional asplenia; congenital or acquired immunodeficiencies; HIV infection; chronic renal failure; nephrotic syndrome; diseases associated with treatment with immunosuppressive drugs or radiation therapy, including malignant neoplasms, leukemias, lymphomas, and Hodgkin disease; generalized malignancy; solid organ transplantation; or multiple myeloma:
1. If neither PCV13 nor PPSV23 has been received previously, administer 1 dose of PCV13 now and 1 dose of PPSV23 at least 8 weeks later.
2. If PCV13 has been received previously but PPSV23 has not, administer 1 dose of PPSV23 at least 8 weeks after the most recent dose of PCV13.
3. If PPSV23 has been received but PCV13 has not, administer 1 dose of PCV13 at least 8 weeks after the most recent dose of PPSV23.

- For children aged 6 through 18 years with chronic heart disease (particularly cyanotic congenital heart disease and cardiac failure), chronic lung disease (including asthma if treated with high-dose oral corticosteroid therapy), diabetes mellitus, alcoholism, or chronic liver disease, who have not received PPSV23, administer 1 dose of PPSV23. If PCV13 has been received previously, then PPSV23 should be administered at least 8 weeks after any prior PCV13 dose.
- A single revaccination with PPSV23 should be administered 5 years after the first dose to children with sickle cell disease or other hemoglobinopathies; anatomic or functional asplenia; congenital or acquired immunodeficiencies; HIV infection; chronic renal failure; nephrotic syndrome; diseases associated with treatment with immunosuppressive drugs or radiation therapy, including malignant neoplasms, leukemias, lymphomas, and Hodgkin disease; generalized malignancy; solid organ transplantation; or multiple myeloma.

6. **Inactivated poliovirus vaccine (IPV). (Minimum age: 6 weeks)**

Routine vaccination:

- Administer a 4-dose series of IPV at ages 2, 4, 6 through 18 months, and 4 through 6 years. The final dose in the series should be administered on or after the fourth birthday and at least 6 months after the previous dose.

Catch-up vaccination:

- In the first 6 months of life, minimum age and minimum intervals are only recommended if the person is at risk of imminent exposure to circulating poliovirus (i.e., travel to a polio-endemic region or during an outbreak).
- If 4 or more doses are administered before age 4 years, an additional dose should be administered at age 4 through 6 years and at least 6 months after the previous dose.
- A fourth dose is not necessary if the third dose was administered at age 4 years or older and at least 6 months after the previous dose.
- If both oral polio vaccine (OPV) and IPV were administered as part of a series, a total of 4 doses should be administered, regardless of the child's current age. If only OPV were administered, and all doses were given prior to 4 years of age, 1 dose of IPV should be given at 4 years or older, at least 4 weeks after the last OPV dose.
- IPV is not routinely recommended for U.S. residents aged 18 years or older.
- For other catch-up guidance, see Table 8.

7. **Influenza vaccines. (Minimum age: 6 months for inactivated influenza vaccine [IIV], 18 years for recombinant influenza vaccine [RIV])**

Routine vaccination:
- Administer influenza vaccine annually to all children beginning at age 6 months. For the 2016–17 season, use of live attenuated influenza vaccine (LAIV) is not recommended.

For children aged 6 months through 8 years:
- For the 2016–17 season, administer 2 doses (separated by at least 4 weeks) to children who are receiving influenza vaccine for the first time or who have not previously received ≥2 doses of trivalent or quadrivalent influenza vaccine before July 1, 2016. For additional guidance, follow dosing guidelines in the 2016–17 ACIP influenza vaccine recommendations (see *MMWR* August 26, 2016;65(5):1-54, available at http://www.cdc.gov/mmwr/volumes/65/rr/pdfs/rr6505.pdf).
- For the 2017–18 season, follow dosing guidelines in the 2017–18 ACIP influenza vaccine recommendations.

For persons aged 9 years and older:
- Administer 1 dose.

8. **Measles, mumps, and rubella (MMR) vaccine. (Minimum age: 12 months for routine vaccination)**

Routine vaccination:
- Administer a 2-dose series of MMR vaccine at ages 12 through 15 months and 4 through 6 years. The second dose may be administered before age 4 years, provided at least 4 weeks have elapsed since the first dose.
- Administer 1 dose of MMR vaccine to infants aged 6 through 11 months before departure from the United States for international travel. These children should be revaccinated with 2 doses of MMR vaccine, the first at age 12 through 15 months (12 months if the child remains in an area where disease risk is high), and the second dose at least 4 weeks later.
- Administer 2 doses of MMR vaccine to children aged 12 months and older before departure from the United States for international travel. The first dose should be administered on or after age 12 months and the second dose at least 4 weeks later.

Catch-up vaccination:
- Ensure that all school-aged children and adolescents have had 2 doses of MMR vaccine; the minimum interval between the 2 doses is 4 weeks.

9. **Varicella (VAR) vaccine. (Minimum age: 12 months)**

Routine vaccination:
- Administer a 2-dose series of VAR vaccine at ages 12 through 15 months and 4 through 6 years. The second dose may be administered before age 4 years, provided at least 3 months have elapsed since the first dose. If the second dose was administered at least 4 weeks after the first dose, it can be accepted as valid.

Catch-up vaccination:
- Ensure that all persons aged 7 through 18 years without evidence of immunity (see *MMWR* 2007;56 [No. RR-4], available at http://www.cdc.gov/mmwr/pdf/rr/rr5604.pdf) have 2 doses of varicella vaccine. For children aged 7 through 12 years, the recommended minimum interval between doses is 3 months (if the second dose was administered at least 4 weeks after the first dose, it can be accepted as valid); for persons aged 13 years and older, the minimum interval between doses is 4 weeks.

10. **Hepatitis A (HepA) vaccine. (Minimum age: 12 months)**

Routine vaccination:
- Initiate the 2-dose HepA vaccine series at ages 12 through 23 months; separate the 2 doses by 6 to 18 months.
- Children who have received 1 dose of HepA vaccine before age 24 months should receive a second dose 6 to 18 months after the first dose.
- For any person aged 2 years and older who has not already received the HepA vaccine series, 2 doses of HepA vaccine separated by 6 to 18 months may be administered if immunity against hepatitis A virus infection is desired.

Catch-up vaccination:
- The minimum interval between the 2 doses is 6 months.

Special populations:
- Administer 2 doses of HepA vaccine at least 6 months apart to previously unvaccinated persons who live in areas where vaccination programs target older children, or who are at increased risk for infection. This includes persons traveling to or working in countries that have high or intermediate endemicity of infection; men having sex with men; users of injection and non-injection illicit drugs; persons who work with HAV-infected primates or with HAV in a research laboratory; persons with clotting-factor disorders; persons with chronic liver disease; and persons who anticipate close personal contact (e.g., household or regular babysitting) with an international adoptee during the first 60 days after arrival in the United States from a country with high or intermediate endemicity. The first dose should be administered as soon as the adoption is planned, ideally 2 or more weeks before the arrival of the adoptee.

11. **Meningococcal vaccines. (Minimum age: 6 weeks for Hib-MenCY [MenHibrix], 2 months for MenACWY-CRM [Menveo], 9 months for MenACWY-D [Menactra], 10 years for serogroup B meningococcal [MenB] vaccines: MenB-4C [Bexsero] and MenB-FHbp [Trumenba])**

Routine vaccination:
- Administer a single dose of Menactra or Menveo vaccine at age 11 through 12 years, with a booster dose at age 16 years.
- For children aged 2 months through 18 years with high-risk conditions, see "Meningococcal conjugate ACWY vaccination of persons with high-risk conditions and other persons at increased risk" and "Meningococcal B vaccination of persons with high-risk conditions and other persons at increased risk of disease" below.

Catch-up vaccination:
- Administer Menactra or Menveo vaccine at age 13 through 18 years if not previously vaccinated.
- If the first dose is administered at age 13 through 15 years, a booster dose should be administered at age 16 through 18 years with a minimum interval of at least 8 weeks between doses.
- If the first dose is administered at age 16 years or older, a booster dose is not needed.
- For other catch-up guidance, see Table 8.

Clinical discretion:
- Young adults aged 16 through 23 years (preferred age range is 16 through 18 years) who are not at increased risk for meningococcal disease may be vaccinated with a 2-dose series of either Bexsero (0, ≥1 month) or Trumenba (0, 6 months) vaccine to provide short-term protection against most strains of serogroup B meningococcal disease. The two MenB vaccines are not interchangeable; the same vaccine product must be used for all doses.
- If the second dose of Trumenba is given at an interval of <6 months, a third dose should be given at least 6 months after the first dose; the minimum interval between the second and third doses is 4 weeks.

Meningococcal conjugate ACWY vaccination of persons with high-risk conditions and other persons at increased risk of disease: Children with anatomic or functional asplenia (including sickle cell disease), children with HIV infection, or children with persistent complement component deficiency (includes persons with inherited or chronic deficiencies in C3, C5-9, properdin, factor D, factor H, or taking eculizumab [Soliris]):

- **Menveo**
  - *Children who initiate vaccination at 8 weeks.* Administer doses at ages 2, 4, 6, and 12 months.
  - *Unvaccinated children who initiate vaccination at 7 through 23 months.* Administer 2 primary doses, with the second dose at least 12 weeks after the first dose AND after the first birthday.
  - *Children 24 months and older who have not received a complete series.* Administer 2 primary doses at least 8 weeks apart.

- **MenHibrix**
  - *Children who initiate vaccination at 6 weeks:* Administer doses at ages 2, 4, 6, and 12 through 15 months.

o If the first dose of MenHibrix is given at or after age 12 months, a total of 2 doses should be given at least 8 weeks apart to ensure protection against serogroups C and Y meningococcal disease.

- **Menactra**

   o **Children with anatomic or functional asplenia or HIV infection**

   – *Children 24 months and older who have not received a complete series.* Administer 2 primary doses at least 8 weeks apart. If Menactra is administered to a child with asplenia (including sickle cell disease) or HIV infection, do not administer Menactra until age 2 years and at least 4 weeks after the completion of all PCV13 doses.

   o **Children with persistent complement component deficiency**

   – *Children 9 through 23 months.* Administer 2 primary doses at least 12 weeks apart.

   – *Children 24 months and older who have not received a complete series.* Administer 2 primary doses at least 8 weeks apart.

   o **All high-risk children**

   – If Menactra is to be administered to a child at high risk for meningococcal disease, it is recommended that Menactra be given either before or at the same time as DTaP.

Meningococcal B vaccination of persons with high-risk conditions and other persons at increased risk of disease:
Children with anatomic or functional asplenia (including sickle cell disease) or children with persistent complement component deficiency (includes persons with inherited or chronic deficiencies in C3, C5-C9, properdin, factor D, factor H, or taking eculizumab [Soliris]):

- **Bexsero or Trumenba**

   o *Persons 10 years or older who have not received a complete series.* Administer a 2-dose series of Bexsero, with doses at least 1 month apart, or a 3-dose series of Trumenba, with the second dose at least 1-2 months after the first and the third dose at least 6 months after the first. The two MenB vaccines are not interchangeable; the same vaccine product must be used for all doses.

For children who travel to or reside in countries in which meningococcal disease is hyperendemic or epidemic, including countries in the African meningitis belt or the Hajj:

- Administer an age-appropriate formulation and series of Menactra or Menveo for protection against serogroups A and W meningococcal disease. Prior receipt of MenHibrix is not sufficient for children traveling to the meningitis belt or the Hajj because it does not contain serogroups A or W.

For children at risk during an outbreak attributable to a vaccine serogroup:

- For serogroup A, C, W, or Y: Administer or complete an age- and formulation-appropriate series of MenHibrix, Menactra, or Menveo.
- For serogroup B: Administer a 2-dose series of Bexsero, with doses at least 1 month apart, or a 3-dose series of Trumenba, with the second dose at least 1-2 months after the first and the third dose at least 6 months after the first. The two MenB vaccines are not interchangeable; the same vaccine product must be used for all doses.

For MenACWY booster doses among persons with high-risk conditions, refer to *MMWR* 2013;62(RR02);1-22, available at http://www.cdc.gov/mmwr/preview/mmwrhtml/rr6202a1.htm, *MMWR* June 20, 2014/63(24):527-530, at http://www.cdc.gov/mmwr/pdf/wk/mm6324.pdf, and *MMWR* November 4, 2016;65(43):1189-1194, at http://www.cdc.gov/mmwr/volumes/65/wr/pdfs/mm6543a3.pdf.

For other catch-up recommendations for these persons, and complete information on use of meningococcal vaccines, including guidance related to vaccination of persons at increased risk of infection, see meningococcal *MMWR* publications, available at: http://www.cdc.gov/vaccines/hcp/acip-recs/vacc-specific/mening.html.

12. **Tetanus and diphtheria toxoids and acellular pertussis (Tdap) vaccine. (Minimum age: 10 years for both Boostrix and Adacel)**
   Routine vaccination:
   - Administer 1 dose of Tdap vaccine to all adolescents aged 11 through 12 years.
   - Tdap may be administered regardless of the interval since the last tetanus and diphtheria toxoid-containing vaccine.
   - Administer 1 dose of Tdap vaccine to pregnant adolescents during each pregnancy (preferably during the early part of gestational weeks 27 through 36), regardless of time since prior Td or Tdap vaccination.

   Catch-up vaccination:
   - Persons aged 7 years and older who are not fully immunized with DTaP vaccine should receive Tdap vaccine as 1 dose (preferably the first) in the catch-up series; if additional doses are needed, use Td vaccine. For children 7 through 10 years who receive a dose of Tdap as part of the catch-up series, an adolescent Tdap vaccine dose at age 11 through 12 years may be administered.
   - Persons aged 11 through 18 years who have not received Tdap vaccine should receive a dose followed by tetanus and diphtheria toxoids (Td) booster doses every 10 years thereafter.
   - Inadvertent doses of DTaP vaccine:
     - If administered inadvertently to a child aged 7 through 10 years, the dose may count as part of the catch-up series. This dose may count as the adolescent Tdap dose, or the child may receive a Tdap booster dose at age 11 through 12 years.
     - If administered inadvertently to an adolescent aged 11 through 18 years, the dose should be counted as the adolescent Tdap booster.
   - For other catch-up guidance, see Table 8.

13. **Human papillomavirus (HPV) vaccines. (Minimum age: 9 years for 4vHPV [Gardasil] and 9vHPV [Gardasil 9])**
   Routine and catch-up vaccination:
   - Administer a 2-dose series of HPV vaccine on a schedule of 0, 6-12 months to all adolescents aged 11 or 12 years. The vaccination series can start at age 9 years.
   - Administer HPV vaccine to all adolescents through age 18 years who were not previously adequately vaccinated. The number of recommended doses is based on age at administration of the first dose.
   - For persons initiating vaccination before age 15, the recommended immunization schedule is 2 doses of HPV vaccine at 0, 6-12 months.
   - For persons initiating vaccination at age 15 years or older, the recommended immunization schedule is 3 doses of HPV vaccine at 0, 1-2, 6 months.
   - A vaccine dose administered at a shorter interval should be readministered at the recommended interval.
     - In a 2-dose schedule of HPV vaccine, the minimum interval is 5 months between the first and second dose. If the second dose is administered at a shorter interval, a third dose should be administered a minimum of 12 weeks after the second dose and a minimum of 5 months after the first dose.
     - In a 3-dose schedule of HPV vaccine, the minimum intervals are 4 weeks between the first and second dose, 12 weeks between the second and third dose, and 5 months between the first and third dose. If a vaccine dose is administered at a shorter interval, it should be readministered after another minimum interval has been met since the most recent dose.

   Special populations:
   - For children with history of sexual abuse or assault, administer HPV vaccine beginning at age 9 years.
   - Immunocompromised persons*, including those with human immunodeficiency virus (HIV) infection, should receive a 3-dose series at 0, 1-2, and 6 months, regardless of age at vaccine initiation.
   - Note: HPV vaccination is not recommended during pregnancy, although there is no evidence that the vaccine poses harm. If a woman is found to be pregnant after initiating the vaccination series, no intervention is needed; the remaining vaccine doses should be delayed until after the pregnancy. Pregnancy testing is not needed before HPV vaccination.

*See *MMWR* December 16, 2016;65(49):1405-1408, available at http://www.cdc.gov/mmwr/volumes/65/wr/pdfs/mm6549a5.pdf.

General Recommendations on Immunization

TABLE 9 Recommended and Minimum Ages and Intervals between Vaccine Doses*†

Vaccine and Dose Number	Recommended Age for this Dose	Minimum Age for this Dose	Recommended Interval to Next Dose	Minimum Interval to Next Dose
HepB-1§	Birth	Birth	1-4 months	4 weeks
HepB-2	1-2 months	4 weeks	2-17 months	8 weeks
HepB-3¶	6-18 months	24 weeks	—	—
DTaP-1§	2 months	6 weeks	2 months	4 weeks
DTaP-2	4 months	10 weeks***	2 months	4 weeks
DTaP-3	6 months	14 weeks	6-12 months	6 months**††
DTaP-4	15-18 months	12 months	3 years	6 months**
DTaP-5	4-6 years	4 years	—	—
Hib-1§§§	2 months	6 weeks	2 months	4 weeks
Hib-2	4 months	10 weeks	2 months	4 weeks
Hib-3¶¶	6 months	14 weeks	6-9 months	8 weeks
Hib-4	12-15 months	12 months	—	—
IPV-1§	2 months	6 weeks	2 months	4 weeks
IPV-2	4 months	10 weeks	2-14 months	4 weeks
IPV-3	6-18 months	14 weeks	3-5 years	6 months
IPV-4***	4-6 years	4 years	—	—
PCV-1§§	2 months	6 weeks	8 weeks	4 weeks
PCV-2	4 months	10 weeks	8 weeks	4 weeks
PCV-3	6 months	14 weeks	6 months	8 weeks
PCV-4	12-15 months	12 months	—	—
MMR-1†††	12-15 months	12 months	3-5 years	4 weeks
MMR-2†††	4-6 years	13 months	—	—
Varicella-1†††	12-15 months	12 months	3-5 years	12 weeks§§§
Varicella-2†††	4-6 years	15 months	—	—
HepA-1	12-23 months	12 months	6-18 months**	6 months**
HepA-2	≥18 months	18 months	—	—
Influenza inactivated¶¶¶	≥6 months	6 months****	1 month	4 weeks
LAIV (intranasal)¶¶¶	2-49 years	2 years	1 month	4 weeks
MCV4-1††††	11-12 years	2 years	5 years	8 weeks
MCV4-2	16 years	11 years (+8 weeks)	—	—
MPSV4-1††††	—	2 years	5 years	5 years
MPSV4-2	—	7 years	—	—
Td	11-12 years	7 years	10 years	5 years
Tdap§§§§	≥11 years	7 years	—	—
PPSV-1	—	2 years	5 years	5 years
PPSV-2¶¶¶¶	—	7 years	—	—
HPV-1*****	11-12 years	9 years	2 months	4 weeks
HPV-2	11-12 years (+2 months)	9 years (+4 weeks)	4 months	12 weeks†††††
HPV-3†††††	11-12 years (+6 months)	9 years (+24 weeks)	—	—
Rotavirus-1§§§§§	2 months	6 weeks	2 months	4 weeks
Rotavirus-2	4 months	10 weeks	2 months	4 weeks
Rotavirus-3¶¶¶¶¶	6 months	14 weeks	—	—
Herpes zoster******	≥60 years	60 years	—	—
Pneumococcal vaccine††††††	—	—	—	—

DTaP, Diphtheria and tetanus toxoids and acellular pertussis; *HepA*, hepatitis A; *HepB*, hepatitis B; *Hib*, Haemophilus influenzae type b; *HPV*, human papillomavirus; *IPV*, inactivated poliovirus; *LAIV*, live, attenuated influenza vaccine; *MCV4*, quadrivalent meningococcal conjugate vaccine; *MMR*, measles, mumps, and rubella; *MMRV*, measles, mumps, rubella, and varicella; *MPSV4*, quadrivalent meningococcal polysaccharide vaccine; *PCV*, pneumococcal conjugate vaccine; *PPSV*, pneumococcal polysaccharide vaccine; *PRP-OMB*, polyribosylribitol phosphate-meningococcal outer membrane protein conjugate; *Td*, tetanus and diphtheria toxoids; *Tdap*, tetanus toxoid, reduced diphtheria toxoid, and acellular pertussis.

*Combination vaccines are available. Use of licensed combination vaccines is generally preferred to separate injections of their equivalent component vaccines. When administering combination vaccines, the minimum age for administration is the oldest age for any of the individual components; the minimum interval between doses is equal to the greatest interval of any of the individual components.

†Information on travel vaccines, including typhoid, Japanese encephalitis, and yellow fever, is available at http://www.cdc.gov/travel. Information on other vaccines that are licensed in the United States but not distributed, including anthrax and smallpox, is available at http://www.bt.cdc.gov.

§Combination vaccines containing the hepatitis B component are available. These vaccines should not be administered to infants aged <6 weeks because of the other components (i.e., Hib, DTaP, HepA, and IPV).

¶HepB-3 should be administered at least 8 weeks after HepB-2 and at least 16 weeks after HepB-1 and should not be administered before age 24 weeks.

**Calendar months.

††The minimum recommended interval between DTaP-3 and DTaP-4 is 6 months. However, DTaP-4 need not be repeated if administered at least 4 months after DTaP-3.

§§For Hib and PCV, children receiving the first dose of vaccine at age ≥7 months require fewer doses to complete the series.

TABLE 9 Recommended and Minimum Ages and Intervals between Vaccine Doses*†—cont'd

¶¶If PRP-QMP (Pedvax-Hib, Merck Vaccine Division) was administered at ages 2 and 4 months, a dose at age 6 months is not necessary.
***A fourth dose is not needed if the third dose was administered at ≥4 years and at least 6 months after the previous dose.
†††Combination MMRV vaccine can be used for children aged 12 months to 12 years.
§§§The minimum interval from Varicella-1 to Varicella-2 for persons beginning the series at age ≥13 years is 4 weeks.
¶¶¶One dose of influenza vaccine per season is recommended for most persons. Children aged <9 years who are receiving influenza vaccine for the first time or who received only 1 dose the previous season (if it was their first vaccination season) should receive 2 doses this season.
****The minimum age for inactivated influenza vaccine varies by vaccine manufacturer. See package insert for vaccine-specific minimum ages.
††††Revaccination with meningococcal vaccine is recommended for previously vaccinated persons who remain at high risk for meningococcal disease. (Source: CDC. Updated recommendations from the Advisory Committee on Immunization Practices (ACIP) for revaccination of persons at prolonged increased risk for meningococcal disease. *MMWR* 2009;58:[1042-3]).
§§§§Only 1 dose of Tdap is recommended. Subsequent doses should be given as Td. For one brand of Tdap, the minimum age is 11 years. For management of a tetanus-prone wound in persons who have received a primary series of tetanus-toxoid–containing vaccine, the minimum interval after a previous dose of any tetanus-containing vaccine is 5 years.
¶¶¶¶A second dose of PPSV 5 years after the first dose is recommended for persons aged ≤65 years at highest risk for serious pneumococcal infection and those who are likely to have a rapid decline in pneumococcal antibody concentration. (Source: CDC. Prevention of pneumococcal disease: recommendations of the Advisory Committee on Immunization Practices [ACIP]. *MMWR* 1997;46[No. RR-8]).
*****Bivalent HPV vaccine is approved for females aged 10-25 years. Quadrivalent HPV vaccine is approved for males and females aged 9-26 years.
††††††The minimum age for HPV-3 is based on the baseline minimum age for the first dose (i.e., 108 months) and the minimum interval of 24 weeks between the first and third dose. Dose 3 need not be repeated if it is administered at least 16 weeks after the first dose.
§§§§§The first dose of rotavirus must be administered at age 6 weeks through 14 weeks and 6 days. The vaccine series should not be started for infants aged ≥15 weeks, 0 days. Rotavirus should not be administered to children older than 8 months, 0 days of age regardless of the number of doses received between 6 weeks and 8 months, 0 days of age.
¶¶¶¶¶If 2 doses of Rotarix (GlaxoSmithKline) are administered as age appropriate, a third dose is not necessary.
******Herpes zoster vaccine is recommended as a single dose for persons aged ≥60 years.

TABLE 10 Guidelines for Spacing of Live and Inactivated Antigens

Antigen Combination	Recommended Minimum Interval between Doses
Two or more inactivated*	May be administered simultaneously or at any interval between doses
Inactivated and live	May be administered simultaneously or at any interval between doses
Two or more live intranasal or injectable†	28 days minimum interval, if not administered simultaneously

From Centers for Disease Control and Prevention: General recommendations on immunization: recommendations of the Advisory Committee on Immunization Practices (ACIP), *MMWR* 60(2):38, 2011.
*Certain experts suggest a 28-day interval between tetanus toxoid, reduced diphtheria toxoid, and acellular pertussis (Tdap) vaccine and tetravalent meningococcal conjugate vaccine if they are not administered simultaneously.
†Live oral vaccines (e.g., Ty21a typhoid vaccine and rotavirus vaccine) may be administered simultaneously or at any interval before or after inactivated or live injectable vaccines.

TABLE 11 Guidelines for Administering Antibody-Containing Products* and Vaccines

Type of Administration	PRODUCTS ADMINISTERED		Recommended Minimum Interval Between Doses
Simultaneous (during the same office visit)	Antibody-containing products and inactivated antigen		Can be administered simultaneously at different anatomic sites or at any time interval between doses
	Antibody-containing products and live antigen		Should not be administered simultaneously.† If simultaneous administration of measles-containing vaccine or varicella vaccine is unavoidable, administer at different sites and revaccinate or test for seroconversion after the recommended interval
Nonsimultaneous	**Administered First**	**Administered Second**	
	Antibody-containing products	Inactivated antigen	No interval necessary
	Inactivated antigen	Antibody-containing products	No interval necessary
	Antibody-containing products	Live antigen	Dose related†‡
	Live antigen	Antibody-containing products	2 weeks†

From Centers for Disease Control and Prevention: General recommendations on immunization: recommendations of the Advisory Committee on Immunization Practices (ACIP), *MMWR* 60: (RR-2), 2011.
*Blood products containing substantial amounts of immune globulin include intramuscular and intravenous immune globulin, specific hyperimmune globulin (e.g., hepatitis B immune globulin, tetanus immune globulin, varicella zoster immune globulin, and rabies immune globulin), whole blood, packed red blood cells, plasma, and platelet products.
†Yellow fever vaccine; rotavirus vaccine; oral Ty21a typhoid vaccine; live, attenuated influenza vaccine; and zoster vaccine are exceptions to these recommendations. These live, attenuated vaccines can be administered at any time before or after or simultaneously with an antibody-containing product.
‡The duration of interference of antibody-containing products with the immune response to the measles component of measles-containing vaccine, and possibly varicella vaccine, is dose related.

TABLE 12 Recommended Intervals between Administration of Antibody-Containing Products and Measles- or Varicella-Containing Vaccine, by Product and Indication for Vaccination

Product/Indication	Dose (mg IgG/kg) and Route*	Recommended Interval before Measles- or Varicella-Containing Vaccine[†] Administration (months)
Tetanus IG	250 units (10 mg IgG/kg) IM	3
Hepatitis A IG		
Contact prophylaxis	0.02 ml/kg (33 mg IgG/kg) IM	3
International travel	0.06 ml/kg (10 mg IgG/kg) IM	3
Hepatitis B IG	0.06 ml/kg (10 mg IgG/kg) IM	3
Rabies IG	20 IU/kg (22 mg IgG/kg) IM	4
Varicella IG	125 units/10 kg (60–200 mg IgG/kg) IM, maximum 625 units	5
Measles prophylaxis IG		
Standard (i.e., nonimmunocompromised) contact	0.25 ml/kg (40 mg IgG/kg) IM	5
Immunocompromised contact	0.50 ml/kg (80 mg IgG/kg) IM	6
Blood transfusion		
RBCs, washed	10 ml/kg negligible IgG/kg IV	None
RBCs, adenine-saline added	10 ml/kg (10 mg IgG/kg) IV	3
Packed RBCs (hematocrit 65%)[§]	10 ml/kg (60 mg IgG/kg) IV	6
Whole blood (hematocrit 35%-50%)[§]	10 ml/kg (80-100 mg IgG/kg) IV	6
Plasma/platelet products	10 ml/kg (160 mg IgG/kg) IV	7
Cytomegalovirus IGIV	150 mg/kg maximum	6
IGIV		
Replacement therapy for immune deficiencies[¶]	300-400 mg/kg IV[¶]	8
Immune thrombocytopenic purpura treatment	400 mg/kg IV	8
Postexposure varicella prophylaxis**	400 mg/kg IV	8
Immune thrombocytopenic purpura treatment	1000 mg/kg IV	10
Kawasaki disease	2 g/kg IV	11
Monoclonal antibody to respiratory syncytial virus	15 mg/kg IM	None
F protein (Synagis [MedImmune])[††]		

HIV, human immunodeficiency virus; *IG*, immune globulin; *IgG*, immune globulin G; *IGIV*, intravenous immune globulin; *mg IgG/kg*, milligrams of immune globulin G per kilogram of body weight; *IM*, intramuscular; *IV*, intravenous; *RBCs*, red blood cells.

*This table is not intended for determining the correct indications and dosages for using antibody-containing products. Unvaccinated persons might not be protected fully against measles during the entire recommended interval, and additional doses of IG or measles vaccine might be indicated after measles exposure. Concentrations of measles antibody in an IG preparation can vary by manufacturer's lot. Rates of antibody clearance after receipt of an IG preparation also might vary. Recommended intervals are extrapolated from an estimated half-life of 30 days for passively acquired antibody and an observed interference with the immune response to measles vaccine for 5 months after a dose of 80 mg IgG/kg.

[†]Does not include zoster vaccine. Zoster vaccine may be given with antibody-containing blood products.

[§]Assumes a serum IgG concentration of 16 mg/ml

[¶]Measles and varicella vaccinations are recommended for children with asymptomatic or mildly symptomatic HIV infection but are contraindicated for persons with severe immunosuppression from HIV or any other immunosuppressive disorder.

**The investigational VariZIG, similar to licensed varicella-zoster IG (VZIG), is a purified human IG preparation made from plasma containing high levels of antivaricella antibodies (IgG). The interval between VariZIG and varicella vaccine (Var or MMRV) is 5 months.

[††]Contains antibody only to respiratory syncytial virus.

From Centers for Disease Control and Prevention: General recommendations on immunization: recommendations of the Advisory Committee on Immunization Practices (ACIP), *MMWR* 60: (RR-2), 2011.

TABLE 13 Contraindications and Precautions* to Commonly Used Vaccines

Vaccine	Contraindications	Precautions
DTaP	Severe allergic reaction (e.g., anaphylaxis) after a previous dose or to a vaccine component Encephalopathy (e.g., coma, decreased level of consciousness, or prolonged seizures), not attributable to another identifiable cause, within 7 days of administration of previous dose of DTP or DTaP	Progressive neurologic disorder, including infantile spasms, uncontrolled epilepsy, progressive encephalopathy; defer DTaP until neurologic status clarified and stabilized Temperature of ≥105° F (≥40° C) within 48 hours after vaccination with a previous dose of DTP or DTaP Collapse or shock-like state (i.e., hypotonic hyporesponsive episode) within 48 hours after receiving a previous dose of DTP/DTaP Seizure ≤3 days after receiving a previous dose of DTP/DTaP Persistent, inconsolable crying lasting ≥3 hours within 48 hours after receiving a previous dose of DTP/DTaP GBS <6 weeks after previous dose of tetanus toxoid-containing vaccine History of Arthus-type hypersensitivity reactions after a previous dose of tetanus toxoid-containing vaccine; defer vaccination until at least 10 years have elapsed since the last tetanus-toxoid–containing vaccine Moderate or severe acute illness with or without fever
DT, Td	Severe allergic reaction (e.g., anaphylaxis) after a previous dose or to a vaccine component	GBS <6 weeks after previous dose of tetanus toxoid-containing vaccine History of Arthus-type hypersensitivity reactions after a previous dose of tetanus toxoid-containing vaccine; defer vaccination until at least 10 years have elapsed since the last tetanus-toxoid–containing vaccine Moderate or severe acute illness with or without fever
Tdap	Severe allergic reaction (e.g., anaphylaxis) after a previous dose or to a vaccine component Encephalopathy (e.g., coma, decreased level of consciousness, or prolonged seizures), not attributable to another identifiable cause, within 7 days of administration of previous dose of DTP, DTaP, or Tdap	GBS <6 weeks after a previous dose of tetanus toxoid-containing vaccine Progressive or unstable neurologic disorder, uncontrolled seizures, or progressive encephalopathy until a treatment regimen has been established and the condition has stabilized History of Arthus-type hypersensitivity reactions after a previous dose of tetanus toxoid-containing vaccine; defer vaccination until at least 10 years have elapsed since the last tetanus toxoid-containing vaccine Moderate or severe acute illness with or without fever
IPV	Severe allergic reaction (e.g., anaphylaxis) after a previous dose or to a vaccine component	Pregnancy Moderate or severe acute illness with or without fever
MMR†§	Severe allergic reaction (e.g., anaphylaxis) after a previous dose or to a vaccine component Pregnancy: Known severe immunodeficiency (e.g., from hematologic and solid tumors, receipt of chemotherapy, congenital immunodeficiency, or long-term immunosuppressive therapy¶ or patients with HIV infection who are severely immunocompromised)§	Recent (≤11 months) receipt of antibody-containing blood product (specific interval depends on product) History of thrombocytopenia or thrombocytopenic purpura Need for tuberculin skin testing†† Moderate or severe acute illness with or without fever
Hib	Severe allergic reaction (e.g., anaphylaxis) after a previous dose or to a vaccine component Age <6 weeks	Moderate or severe acute illness with or without fever
Hepatitis B	Severe allergic reaction (e.g., anaphylaxis) after a previous dose or to a vaccine component	Infant weight <2000 g§§ Moderate or severe acute illness with or without fever
Hepatitis A	Severe allergic reaction (e.g., anaphylaxis) after a previous dose or to a vaccine component	Pregnancy: Moderate or severe acute illness with or without fever
Varicella	Severe allergic reaction (e.g., anaphylaxis) after a previous dose or to a vaccine component Known severe immunodeficiency (e.g., from hematologic and solid tumors, receipt of chemotherapy, congenital immunodeficiency, or long-term immunosuppressive therapy¶ or patients with HIV infection who are severely immunocompromised)§ Pregnancy	Recent (≤11 months) receipt of antibody-containing blood product (specific interval depends on product)¶¶ Moderate or severe acute illness with or without fever
PCV	Severe allergic reaction (e.g., anaphylaxis) after a previous dose (of PCV7, PCV13, or any diphtheria toxoid-containing vaccine) or to a component of a vaccine (PCV7, PCV13, or any diphtheria toxoid-containing vaccine)	Moderate or severe acute illness with or without fever
TIV	Severe allergic reaction (e.g., anaphylaxis) after a previous dose or to vaccine component, including egg protein	GBS <6 weeks after a previous dose of influenza vaccine Moderate or severe acute illness with or without fever
LAIV	Severe allergic reaction (e.g., anaphylaxis) after a previous dose or to vaccine component, including egg protein Pregnancy Immunosuppression Certain chronic medical conditions***	GBS <6 weeks after a previous dose of influenza vaccine Moderate or severe acute illness with or without fever

TABLE 13 Contraindications and Precautions* to Commonly Used Vaccines—cont'd

Vaccine	Contraindications	Precautions
PPSV	Severe allergic reaction (e.g., anaphylaxis) after a previous dose or to a vaccine component	Moderate or severe acute illness with or without fever
MCV4	Severe allergic reaction (e.g., anaphylaxis) after a previous dose or to a vaccine component	Moderate or severe acute illness with or without fever
MPSV4	Severe allergic reaction (e.g., anaphylaxis) after a previous dose or to a vaccine component	Moderate or severe acute illness with or without fever
HPV	Severe allergic reaction (e.g., anaphylaxis) after a previous dose or to a vaccine component	Pregnancy: Moderate or severe acute illness with or without fever
Rotavirus	Severe allergic reaction (e.g., anaphylaxis) after a previous dose or to a vaccine component SCID	Altered immunocompetence other than SCID: History of intussusception Chronic gastrointestinal disease[†††] Spina bifida or bladder exstrophy[†††] Moderate or severe acute illness with or without fever
Zoster	Severe allergic reaction (e.g., anaphylaxis) after a previous dose or to a vaccine component Substantial suppression of cellular immunity Pregnancy	Moderate or severe acute illness with or without fever

DT, diphtheria and tetanus toxoids; *DTaP*, diphtheria and tetanus toxoids and acellular pertussis; *GBS*, Guillain-Barré syndrome; *HBsAg*, hepatitis B surface antigen; *Hib*, *Haemophilus influenzae* type b; *HIV*, human immunodeficiency virus; *HPV*, human papillomavirus; *IPV*, inactivated poliovirus; *LAIV*, live, attenuated influenza vaccine; *MCV4*, quadrivalent meningococcal conjugate vaccine; *MMRV* measles, mumps, rubella; *MPSV4*, quadrivalent meningococcal polysaccharide vaccine; *PCV*, pneumococcal conjugate vaccine; *PPSV*, pneumococcal polysaccharide vaccine; *SCID*, severe combined immunodeficiency; *Td*, tetanus and diphtheria toxoids; *Tdap*, tetanus toxoid, reduced diphtheria toxoid, and acellular pertussis; *TIV*, trivalent inactivated influenza vaccine.

*Events or conditions listed as precautions should be reviewed carefully. Benefits of and risks for administering a specific vaccine to a person under these circumstances should be considered. If the risk from the vaccine is believed to outweigh the benefit, the vaccine should not be administered. If the benefit of vaccination is believed to outweigh the risk, the vaccine should be administered. Whether and when to administer DTaP to children with proven or suspected underlying neurologic disorders should be decided on a case-by-case basis.

[†]HIV-infected children may receive varicella and measles vaccine if CD4+ T-lymphocyte count is <15%. (Source: Adapted from American Academy of Pediatrics. Passive immunization. In: Pickering LK, ed. *Red book: 2009 report of the committee on infectious diseases*. 28th ed. Elk Grove Village. IL: American Academy of Pediatrics: 2009.)

[§]MMR and varicella vaccines can be administered on the same day. If not administered on the same day, these vaccines should be separated by at least 28 days.

[¶]Substantially immunosuppressive steroid dose is considered to be ≥2 weeks of daily receipt of 20 mg or 2 mg/kg body weight of prednisone or equivalent.

[††]Measles vaccination might suppress tuberculin reactivity temporarily. Measles-containing vaccine can be administered on the same day as tuberculin skin testing. If testing cannot be performed until after the day of MMR vaccination, the test should be postponed for ≥4 weeks after the vaccination. If an urgent need exists to skin test, do so with the understanding that reactivity might be reduced by the vaccine.

[§§]Hepatitis B vaccination should be deferred for infants weighing <2000 g if the mother is documented to be HBsAg-negative at the time of the infant's birth. Vaccination can commence at chronological age 1 month or at hospital discharge. For infants born to HBsAg-positive women, hepatitis B immune globulin and hepatitis B vaccine should be administered within 12 hours after birth, regardless of weight.

[¶¶]Vaccine should be deferred for the appropriate interval if replacement immune globulin products are being administered.

[***]Source: CDC. Prevention and control of seasonal influenza with vaccines: recommendations of the Advisory Committee on Immunization Practices (ACIP), 2010. *MMWR* 2010;59(No. RR-8).

[†††]For details see CDC. Prevention of rotavirus gastroenteritis among infants and children: recommendations of the Advisory Committee on Immunization Practices. *MMWR* 2009;58(No. RR-2).

From Centers for Disease Control and Prevention: General recommendations on immunization: recommendations of the Advisory Committee on Immunization Practices (ACIP), *MMWR* 60: (RR-2), 2011.

TABLE 14 Conditions Commonly Misperceived as Contraindications to Vaccination

Vaccine	Conditions Commonly Misperceived as Contraindications (i.e., Vaccination May be Administered under These Conditions)
General for all vaccines, including DTaP, pediatric DT, adult Td, adolescent-adult Tdap, IPV, MMR, Hib, hepatitis A, hepatitis B, varicella, rotavirus, PCV, TIV, LAIV, PPSV, MCV4, MPSV4, HPV, and herpes zoster	Mild acute illness with or without fever
	Mild-to-moderate local reaction (i.e., swelling, redness, soreness); low-grade or moderate fever after previous dose
	Lack of previous physical examination in well-appearing person
	Current antimicrobial therapy*
	Convalescent phase of illness
	Preterm birth (hepatitis B vaccine is an exception in certain circumstances)†
	Recent exposure to an infectious disease
	History of penicillin allergy, other nonvaccine allergies, relatives with allergies, or receiving allergen extract immunotherapy
DTaP	Fever of <105° F (<40° C), fussiness or mild drowsiness after a previous dose of DTP/DTaP
	Family history of seizures
	Family history of sudden infant death syndrome
	Family history of an adverse event after DTP or DTaP administration
	Stable neurologic conditions (e.g., cerebral palsy, well-controlled seizures, or developmental delay)
Tdap	Fever of ≥105° F (≥40° C) for <48 hours after vaccination with a previous dose of DTP or DTaP
	Collapse or shock-like state (i.e., hypotonic hyporesponsive episode) within 48 hours after receiving a previous dose of DTaP
	Seizure <3 days after receiving a previous dose of DTP/DTaP
	Persistent, inconsolable crying lasting <3 hours within 48 hours after receiving a previous dose of DTP/DTaP
	History of extensive limb swelling after DTP/DTaP/Td that is not an Arthus-type reaction
	Stable neurologic disorder
	History of brachial neuritis
	Latex allergy that is not anaphylactic
	Breastfeeding
	Immunosuppression
IPV	Previous receipt of ≥1 dose of oral polio vaccine
MMR§,¶	Positive tuberculin skin test
	Simultaneous tuberculin skin testing**
	Breastfeeding
	Pregnancy of recipient's mother or other close or household contact
	Recipient is female of childbearing age
	Immunodeficient family member or household contact
	Asymptomatic or mildly symptomatic HIV infection
	Allergy to eggs
Hepatitis B	Pregnancy
	Autoimmune disease (e.g., systemic lupus erythematosus or rheumatoid arthritis)
Varicella	Pregnancy of recipient's mother or other close or household contact
	Immunodeficient family member or household contact††
	Asymptomatic or mildly symptomatic HIV infection
	Humoral immunodeficiency (e.g., agammaglobulinemia)
TIV	Nonsevere (e.g., contact) allergy to latex, thimerosal, or egg
	Concurrent administration of Coumadin or aminophylline
LAIV	Health care providers that see patients with chronic diseases or altered immunocompetence (an exception is providers for severely immunocompromised patients requiring care in a protected environment)
	Breastfeeding
	Contacts of persons with chronic disease or altered immunocompetence (an exception is contacts of severely immunocompromised patients requiring care in a protected environment)
PPSV	History of invasive pneumococcal disease or pneumonia
HPV	Immunosuppression
	Previous equivocal or abnormal Papanicolaou test
	Known HPV infection
	Breastfeeding
	History of genital warts
Rotavirus	Prematurity
	Immunosuppressed household contacts
	Pregnant household contacts

TABLE 14 Conditions Commonly Misperceived as Contraindications to Vaccination—cont'd

Vaccine	Conditions Commonly Misperceived as Contraindications (i.e., Vaccination May be Administered under These Conditions)
Zoster	Therapy with low-dose methotrexate (≤0.4 mg/kg/week), azathioprine (≤3.0 mg/kg/day), or 6-mercaptopurine (≤1.5 mg/kg/day) for treatment of rheumatoid arthritis, psoriasis, polymyositis, sarcoidosis, inflammatory bowel disease, or other conditions
	Health care providers of patients with chronic diseases or altered immunocompetence
	Contacts of patients with chronic diseases or altered immunocompetence
	Unknown or uncertain history of varicella in a U.S.-born person

DT, Diphtheria and tetanus toxoids; *DTP*, diphtheria toxoid, tetanus toxoid, and pertussis; *DTaP*, diphtheria and tetanus toxoids and acellular pertussis; *HBsAg*, hepatitis B surface antigen; *Hib, Haemophilus influenzae* type b; *HPV*, human papillomavirus; *IPV*, inactivated poliovirus; *LAIV*, live, attenuated influenza vaccine; *MCV4*, quadrivalent meningococcal conjugate vaccine; *MMR*, measles, mumps, and rubella; *MPSV4*, quadrivalent meningococcal polysaccharide vaccine; *PCV*, pneumococcal conjugate vaccine; *PPSV*, pneumococcal polysaccharide vaccine; *Td*, tetanus and diphtheria toxoids; *Tdap*, tetanus toxoid, reduced diphtheria toxoid, and acellular pertussis; *TIV*, trivalent inactivated influenza vaccine.

*Antibacterial drugs might interfere with Ty21a oral typhoid vaccine, and certain antiviral drugs might interfere with varicella-containing vaccines and LAIV.

†Hepatitis B vaccination should be deferred for infants weighing <2000 g if the mother is documented to be HBsAg-negative at the time of the infant's birth. Vaccination can commence at chronologic age 1 month or at hospital discharge. For infants born to HBsAg-positive women, hepatitis B immune globulin and hepatitis B vaccine should be administered within 12 hours after birth, regardless of weight.

§MMR and varicella vaccines can be administered on the same day. If not administered on the same day, these vaccines should be separated by at least 28 days.

¶HIV-infected children should receive immune globulin after exposure to measles. HIV-infected children can receive varicella and measles vaccine if CD4+ T-lymphocyte count is >15%. (Source: Adapted from American Academy of Pediatrics. Passive immunization. In: Pickering LK, ed. *Red book: 2009 report of the Committee on Infectious Diseases*, 28th ed. Elk Grove Village, IL: American Academy of Pediatrics; 2009.)

**Measles vaccination might suppress tuberculin reactivity temporarily. Measles-containing vaccine can be administered on the same day as tuberculin skin testing. If testing cannot be performed until after the day of MMR vaccination, the test should be postponed for at least 4 weeks after the vaccination. If an urgent need exists to skin test, do so with the understanding that reactivity might be reduced by the vaccine.

††If a vaccinee experiences a presumed vaccine-related rash 7-25 days after vaccination, the person should avoid direct contact with immunocompromised persons for the duration of the rash.

From Centers for Disease Control and Prevention: General recommendations on immunization: recommendations of the Advisory Committee on Immunization Practices (ACIP), *MMWR* 60: (RR-2), 2011.

VACCINE ADMINISTRATION*

INFECTION CONTROL AND STERILE TECHNIQUE

Persons administering vaccines should follow appropriate precautions to minimize risk for spread of disease. Hands should be cleansed with an alcohol-based, waterless antiseptic hand rub or washed with soap and water between each patient contact. Occupational Safety and Health Administration (OSHA) regulations do not require that gloves be worn when administering vaccinations unless persons administering vaccinations are likely to come into contact with potentially infectious body fluids or have open lesions on their hands. Needles used for injections must be sterile and disposable to minimize the risk for contamination. A separate needle and syringe should be used for each injection. Changing needles between drawing vaccine from a vial and injecting it into a recipient is not necessary. Different vaccines should never be mixed in the same syringe unless specifically licensed for such use, and no attempt should be made to transfer between syringes.

For all intramuscular injections, the needle should be long enough to reach the muscle mass and prevent vaccine from seeping into subcutaneous tissue, but not so long as to involve underlying nerves, blood vessels, or bone. Vaccinators should be familiar with the anatomy of the area where they are injecting vaccine. Intramuscular injections are administered at a 90-degree angle to the skin, preferably into the anterolateral aspect of the thigh or the deltoid muscle of the upper arm depending on the age of the patient.

Decision on needle size and site of injection must be made for each person on the basis of the size of the muscle, the thickness of adipose tissue at the injection site, the volume of the material to be administered, injection technique, and the depth below the muscle surface into which the material is to be injected (Fig. E1). Aspiration before injection of vaccines or toxoids (i.e., pulling back on the syringe plunger after needle insertion before injection) is not required because no large blood vessel exists at the recommended injection sites.

INFANTS (AGED <12 MONTHS)

For the majority of infants, the anterolateral aspect of the thigh is the recommended site for injection because it provides a large muscle mass (Fig. E2). The muscles of the buttock have not been used for administration of vaccines in infants and children because of concern about potential injury to the sciatic nerve, which is well documented after injection of antimicrobial agents into the buttock. If the gluteal muscle must be used, care should be taken to define the anatomic landmarks.† Injection technique is the most important parameter to ensure efficient intramuscular vaccine delivery. If the subcutaneous and muscle tissue are bunched to minimize the chance of striking bone, a 1-inch needle is required to ensure intramuscular administration in infants. For the majority of infants, a 1-inch, 22- to 25-gauge needle is sufficient to penetrate muscle in an infant's thigh. For newborn (first 28 days of life) and premature infants, a 5/8-inch-long needle usually is adequate if the skin is stretched flat between thumb and forefinger and the needle inserted at a 90-degree angle to the skin.

TODDLERS AND OLDER CHILDREN (AGED 12 MONTHS TO 10 YEARS)

The deltoid muscle should be used if the muscle mass is adequate. The needle size for deltoid site injections can range from 22 to 25 gauge and from 5/8 to 1 inch on the basis of the size of the muscle and the thickness of adipose tissue at the injection site (Fig. E3). A 5/8-inch needle is adequate only for the deltoid muscle and only if the skin is stretched flat between the thumb and forefinger and the needle inserted at a 90-degree angle to the skin. For toddlers, the anterolateral thigh can be used, but the needle should be at least 1 inch in length.

ADOLESCENTS AND ADULTS (AGED >11 YEARS)

For adults and adolescents, the deltoid muscle is recommended for routine intramuscular vaccinations. The anterolateral thigh also can be used. For men and women weighing <130 lb (<60 kg) a 5/8- to 1-inch needle is sufficient to ensure intramuscular injection. For women weighing 130 to 200 lb (60 to 90 kg) and men 130 to 260 lb (60 to 118 kg), a 1- to 1½-inch needle is needed. For women weighing >200 lb (>90 kg) or men weighing >260 lb (>118 kg), a 1½-inch needle is required.

SUBCUTANEOUS INJECTIONS

Subcutaneous injections are administered at a 45-degree angle, usually into the thigh for infants younger than 12 months and in the upper-outer triceps area of persons aged 12 months and older. Subcutaneous injections can be administered into the upper-outer triceps area of an infant if necessary. A 5/8-inch, 23- to 25-gauge needle should be inserted into the subcutaneous tissue (Figs. E4 and E5).

TABLE 15 Treatment of Anaphylaxis in Children and Adults with Drugs Administered Intramuscularly or Orally

Drug	Dosage
Children	
Primary Regimen	
Epinephrine 1:1000 (aqueous) (1 mg/ml)*	0.01 mg/kg up to 0.5 mg (administer 0.01 ml/kg/dose up to 0.5 mL) IM repeated every 10-20 minutes up to 3 doses
Secondary Regimen	
Diphenhydramine	1-2 mg/kg oral, IM, or IV, every 4-6 hours (100 mg, maximum single dose)
Hydroxyzine	0.5-1 mg/kg oral, IM, every 4-6 hours (100 mg, maximum single dose)
Prednisone	1.5-2 mg/kg oral (60 mg, maximum single dose); use corticosteroids as long as needed
Adults	
Primary Regimen	
Epinephrine 1:1000 (aqueous)*	0.01 mg/kg up to 0.5 mg (administer 0.01 ml/kg/dose up to 0.5 ml) IM repeated every 10-20 minutes up to 3 doses
Secondary Regimen	
Diphenhydramine	1-2 mg/kg up to l00 mg IM or oral, every 4-6 hours

IM, Intramuscular; *IV,* intravenous.
*If the agent causing the anaphylactic reaction was administered by injection, epinephrine may be injected into the same site to slow absorption.
From Centers for Disease Control and Prevention: General recommendations on immunization: recommendations of the Advisory Committee on Immunization Practices (ACIP), *MMWR* 60:(RR-2), 2011. Adapted from American Academy of Pediatrics. Passive immunization. In: Pickering LK, Baker CJ, Kimberlin DW, Long SS, eds: *Red book: 2009 report of the Committee on Infectious Diseases,* 28th ed. Elk Grove Village, IL: American Academy of Pediatrics, 2009:66-7; Immunization Action Coalition. Medical management of vaccine reactions in adult patients (available at www.immunize.org/catg.d/p3082.pdf); and *Mosby's drug consult,* St Louis, 2005, Mosby.

TABLE 16 Vaccination of Persons with Primary and Secondary Immunodeficiencies

Primary	Specific Immunodeficiency	Contraindicated Vaccines*	Risk-Specific Recommended Vaccines*	Effectiveness and Comments
B-lymphocyte (humoral)	Severe antibody deficiencies (e.g., X-linked agammaglobulinemia and common variable immunodeficiency)	OPV[†] Smallpox LAIV BCG Ty21a (live typhoid) Yellow fever	Pneumococcal Consider measles and varicella vaccination	The effectiveness of any vaccine is uncertain if it depends only on the humoral response (e.g., PPSV or MPSV4). IVIG interferes with the immune response to measles vaccine and possibly varicella vaccine.
	Less severe antibody deficiencies (e.g., selective IgA deficiency and IgG subclass deficiency)	OPV[†] BCG Yellow fever Other live vaccines appear to be safe.	Pneumococcal	All vaccines likely effective; immune response might be attenuated.
T-lymphocyte (cell-mediated and humoral)	Complete deficits (e.g., severe combined immunodeficiency [SCID] disease, complete DiGeorge syndrome)	All live vaccines[§,¶,**]	Pneumococcal	Vaccines might be ineffective.
	Partial defects (e.g., most patients with DiGeorge syndrome, Wiskott-Aldrich syndrome, ataxia-telangiectasia)	All live vaccines[§,¶,**]	Pneumococcal Meningococcal Hib (if not administered in infancy)	Effectiveness of any vaccine depends on degree of immune suppression.
Complement	Persistent complement, properdin, or factor B deficiency	None	Pneumococcal Meningococcal	All routine vaccines likely effective.
Phagocytic function	Chronic granulomatous disease, leukocyte adhesion defect, and myeloperoxidase deficiency	Live bacterial vaccines[§]	Pneumococcal[††]	All inactivated vaccines safe and likely effective. Live viral vaccines likely safe and effective.
Secondary	HIV/AIDS	OPV[†] Smallpox BCG LAIV Withhold MMR and varicella in severely immunocompromised persons. Yellow fever vaccine might have a contraindication or a precaution depending on clinical parameters of immune function***	Pneumococcal Consider Hib (if not administered in infancy) and meningococcal vaccination.	MMR, varicella, rotavirus, and all inactivated vaccines, including inactivated influenza, might be effective.[§§]
	Malignant neoplasm, transplantation, immunosuppressive or radiation therapy	Live viral and bacterial, depending on immune status[§,¶]	Pneumococcal	Effectiveness of any vaccine depends on degree of immune suppression.
	Asplenia	None	Pneumococcal Meningococcal Hib (if not administered in infancy)	All routine vaccines likely effective.
	Chronic renal disease	LAIV	Pneumococcal Hepatitis B[¶¶]	All routine vaccines likely effective.

AIDS, acquired immunodeficiency syndrome; *BCG*, bacille Calmette-Guérin; *Hib*, *Haemophilus influenzae* type b; *HIV*, human immunodeficiency virus; *Ig*, immunoglobulin; *IGIV*, immune globulin intravenous; *LAIV*, live, attenuated influenza vaccine; *MMR*, measles, mumps, and rubella; *MPSV4*, quadrivalent meningococcal polysaccharide vaccine; *OPV*, oral poliovirus polysaccharide vaccine; *PPSV*, pneumococcal polysaccharide vaccine.

*Other vaccines that are universally or routinely recommended should be given if not contraindicated.

[†]OPV is no longer available in the United States.

[§]Live bacterial vaccines: BCG and oral Ty21a *Salmonella typhi* vaccine.

[¶]Live viral vaccines: MMR, MMRV, OPV, LAIV, yellow fever, zoster, rotavirus, varicella, and vaccinia (smallpox). Smallpox vaccine is not recommended for children or the general public.

[**]Regarding T-lymphocyte immunodeficiency as a contraindication for rotavirus vaccine, data exist only for severe combined immunodeficiency.

[††]Pneumococcal vaccine is not indicated for children with chronic granulomatous disease beyond age-based universal recommendations for PCV. Children with chronic granulomatous disease are not at increased risk for pneumococcal disease.

[§§]HIV-infected children should receive IG after exposure to measles and may receive varicella and measles vaccine if CD4+ T-lymphocyte count is ≥15%.

[¶¶]Indicated based on the risk from dialysis-based bloodborne transmission.

[***]Symptomatic HIV infection or CD4+ T-lymphocyte count of <200/mm[3] or <15% of total lymphocytes for children aged <6 years is a contraindication to yellow fever vaccine administration. Asymptomatic HIV infection with CD4+ T-lymphocyte count of 200–499/mm[3] for persons aged ≥6 years or 15%–24% of total lymphocytes for children aged <6 years is a precaution for yellow fever vaccine administration. Details of yellow fever vaccine recommendations are available from CDC. (CDC. Yellow fever vaccine recommendations of the Advisory Committee on Immunization Practices [ACIP]. *MMWR* 2010;59[No. RR-7].)

From Centers for Disease Control and Prevention: General recommendations on immunization: recommendations of the Advisory Committee on Immunization Practices (ACIP), *MMWR* 60:(RR-2), 2011. Adapted from American Academy of Pediatrics. Passive immunization. In: Pickering LK, Baker CJ, Kimberlin DW, Long SS, eds: *Red book: 2009 report of the Committee on Infectious Diseases*, 28th ed. Elk Grove Village, IL: American Academy of Pediatrics; 2009:74–5.

TABLE 17 Immunizations for Pediatric Oncology Patients

Vaccine	Indications and Comments
DTaP	Indicated for incompletely immunized children <7 yr, even during active chemotherapy
Td	Indicated 1 yr after completion of therapy in children 7 yr
Hib	Indicated for incompletely immunized children if <7 yr
HBV	Indicated for incompletely immunized children
23PS	Indicated for asplenic patients
PCV13	Indicated for incompletely immunized children <5 yr
Meningococcus	Consider in asplenic patients
IPV	Indicated for incompletely immunized children; also recommended for all household contacts requiring immunization to reduce the risk of vaccine-associated polio
MMR	Contraindicated until child is in remission and finished with all chemotherapy for 3-6 mo; may need to reimmunize after chemotherapy if titers have fallen below protective levels
Influenza	Defer in active chemotherapy; may give as early as 3-4 wk after remission and off chemotherapy if during influenza season; peripheral granulocyte and lymphocyte counts should be >1000/µL; should also be given to household contact of children with cancer
Varicella	Consider immunizing children who have remained in remission and have finished chemotherapy for >1 yr; with absolute lymphocyte count of >700/µl and platelet count of >100,000/µL within 24 hr of immunization; check titers of previously immunized children to verify protective levels of antibodies

DTaP, Diphtheria, tetanus, and pertussis; *HBV,* hepatitis B virus; *Hib, Haemophilus influenzae* type b; *IPV,* inactivated polio vaccine; *MMR,* measles, mumps, rubella; *PCV13,* pneumococcal conjugate vaccine; *Td,* tetanus, diphtheria; *23PS,* 23-valent pneumococcal polysaccharide vaccine.
From *MMWR* 49(RR-10):1-147, 2000.

TABLE 18 Approaches to the Evaluation and Vaccination of Persons Vaccinated Outside the United States Who Have No (or Questionable) Vaccination Records

Vaccine	Recommended Approach	Alternative Approach*
MMR	Revaccination with MMR	Serologic testing for IgG antibodies to measles, mumps, and rubella
Hib	Age-appropriate revaccination	—
Hepatitis A	Age-appropriate revaccination	Serologic testing for IgG antibodies to hepatitis A
Hepatitis B	Age-appropriate revaccination and serologic testing for HBsAg[†]	—
Poliovirus	Revaccinate with inactivated poliovirus vaccine	Serologic testing for neutralizing antibody to poliovirus types 1, 2, and 3 (limited availability)
DTaP	Revaccination with DTaP, with serologic testing for specific IgG antibody to tetanus and diphtheria toxins in the event of a severe local reaction	Persons whose records indicate receipt of ≥3 doses: serologic testing for specific IgG antibody to diphtheria and tetanus toxins before administering additional doses, or administer a single booster dose of DTaP, followed by serologic testing after 1 month for specific IgG antibody to diphtheria and tetanus toxins with revaccination as appropriate
Tdap	Age-appropriate vaccination of persons who are candidates for Tdap vaccine on the basis of time since last diphtheria and tetanus-toxoid–containing vaccines.	—
Varicella	Age-appropriate vaccination of persons who lack evidence of varicella immunity	—
Pneumococcal conjugate	Age-appropriate vaccination	—
Rotavirus	Age-appropriate vaccination	—
HPV	Age-appropriate vaccination	—
Zoster	Age-appropriate vaccination	—

DTaP, Diphtheria and tetanus toxoids and acellular pertussis; *HBsAg,* hepatitis B surface antigen; *Hib, Haemophilus influenzae* type b; *HPV,* human papillomavirus; *IgG,* immune globulin G; *MMR,* measles, mumps, and rubella; *Tdap,* tetanus toxoid, reduced diphtheria toxoid, and acellular pertussis.

*There is a recommended approach for all vaccines and an alternative approach for some vaccines.

[†]In rare instances, hepatitis B vaccine can give a false-positive HBsAg result up to 18 days after vaccination; therefore, blood should be drawn to test for HBsAg before vaccinating. (Source: CDC. A comprehensive immunization strategy to eliminate transmission of hepatitis B virus infection in the United States: recommendations of the Advisory Committee on Immunization Practices [ACIP]; Part I: Immunization in infants, children, and adolescents, *MMWR* 2005;54(No. RR-16.])

From Centers for Disease Control and Prevention: General recommendations on immunization: recommendations of the Advisory Committee on Immunization Practices (ACIP), *MMWR* 60:(RR-2), 2011.

Immunizations for Adults

RECOMMENDED IMMUNIZATION SCHEDULE FOR ADULTS AGED 19 YEARS OR OLDER, UNITED STATES, 2017

In February 2017, the *Recommended Immunization Schedule for Adults Aged 19 Years or Older, United States, 2017* became effective, as recommended by the Advisory Committee on Immunization Practices (ACIP) and approved by the Centers for Disease Control and Prevention (CDC). The 2017 adult immunization schedule was also reviewed and approved by the following professional medical organizations:

- American College of Physicians (www.acponline.org)
- American Academy of Family Physicians (www.aafp.org)
- American College of Obstetricians and Gynecologists (www.acog.org)
- American College of Nurse-Midwives (www.midwife.org)

CDC announced the availability of the 2017 adult immunization schedule at www.cdc.gov/vaccines/schedules/hcp/index.html in the *Morbidity and Mortality Weekly Report (MMWR)*.[1] The schedule is published in its entirety in the *Annals of Internal Medicine*.[2]

The adult immunization schedule describes the age groups and medical conditions and other indications for which licensed vaccines are recommended. The 2017 adult immunization schedule consists of:

- Table 19. Recommended immunization schedule for adults by age group
- Table 20A. Recommended immunization schedule for adults by medical condition and other indications
- Footnotes that accompany each vaccine containing important general information and considerations for special populations
- Table 20B. Contraindications and precautions for vaccines routinely recommended for adults

Consider the following information when reviewing the adult immunization schedule:

- The tables in the adult immunization schedule should be read with the footnotes that contain important general information and information about vaccination of special populations.
- When indicated, administer recommended vaccines to adults whose vaccination history is incomplete or unknown.
- Increased interval between doses of a multi-dose vaccine does not diminish vaccine effectiveness; therefore, it is not necessary to restart the vaccine series or add doses to the series because of an extended interval between doses.
- Adults with immunocompromising conditions should generally avoid live vaccines, e.g., measles, mumps, and rubella vaccine. Inactivated vaccines, e.g., pneumococcal or inactivated influenza vaccines, are generally acceptable.
- Combination vaccines may be used when any component of the combination is indicated and when the other components of the combination vaccine are not contraindicated.
- The use of trade names in the adult immunization schedule is for identification purposes only and does not imply endorsement by the ACIP or CDC.

Details on vaccines recommended for adults and complete ACIP statements are available at www.cdc.gov/vaccines/hcp/acip-recs/index.html. Additional CDC resources include:

- A summary of information on vaccination recommendations, vaccination of persons with immunodeficiencies, preventing and managing adverse reactions, vaccination contraindications and precautions, and other information can be found in *General Recommendations on Immunization* at www.cdc.gov/mmwr/preview/mmwrhtml/rr6002a1.htm.
- Vaccine Information Statements that explain benefits and risks of vaccines are available at www.cdc.gov/vaccines/hcp/vis/index.html.
- Information and resources regarding vaccination of pregnant women are available at www.cdc.gov/vaccines/adults/rec-vac/pregnant.html.
- Information on travel vaccine requirements and recommendations is available at wwnc.cdc.gov/travel/destinations/list.
- *CDC Vaccine Schedules App* for clinicians and other immunization service providers to download is available at www.cdc.gov/vaccines/schedules/hcp/schedule-app.html.
- *Recommended Immunization Schedule for Children and Adolescents Aged 18 Years or Younger* is available at www.cdc.gov/vaccines/schedules/hcp/index.html.

Report suspected cases of reportable vaccine-preventable diseases to the local or state health department.

Report all clinically significant post-vaccination reactions to the Vaccine Adverse Event Reporting System at www.vaers.hhs.gov or by telephone, 800-822-7967. All vaccines included in the 2017 adult immunization schedule except herpes zoster and 23-valent pneumococcal polysaccharide vaccines are covered by the Vaccine Injury Compensation Program. Information on how to file a vaccine injury claim is available at www.hrsa.gov/vaccinecompensation or by telephone, 800-338-2382.

Submit questions and comments regarding the 2017 adult immunization schedule to CDC through www.cdc.gov/cdc-info or by telephone, 800-CDC-INFO (800-232-4636), in English and Spanish, 8:00am–8:00pm ET, Monday–Friday, excluding holidays.

The following acronyms are used for vaccines recommended for adults:

HepA	hepatitis A vaccine
HepA-HepB	hepatitis A and hepatitis B vaccines
HepB	hepatitis B vaccine
Hib	*Haemophilus influenzae* type b conjugate vaccine
HPV vaccine	human papillomavirus vaccine
HZV	herpes zoster vaccine
IIV	inactivated influenza vaccine
LAIV	live attenuated influenza vaccine
MenACWY	serogroups A, C, W, and Y meningococcal conjugate vaccine
MenB	serogroup B meningococcal vaccine
MMR	measles, mumps, and rubella vaccine
MPSV4	serogroups A, C, W, and Y meningococcal polysaccharide vaccine
PCV13	13-valent pneumococcal conjugate vaccine
PPSV23	23-valent pneumococcal polysaccharide vaccine
RIV	recombinant influenza vaccine
Td	tetanus and diphtheria toxoids
Tdap	tetanus toxoid, reduced diphtheria toxoid, and acellular pertussis vaccine
VAR	varicella vaccine

[1] MMWR Morb Mortal Wkly Rep. 2017;66(5). Available at www.cdc.gov/mmwr/volumes/66/wr/mm6605e2.htm?s_cid=mm6605e2_w.

[2] Ann Intern Med. 2017;166:209-218. Available at annals.org/aim/article/doi/10.7326/M16-2936.

TABLE 19 Recommended Immunization Schedule for Adults Aged 19 Years or Older by Age Group, United States, 2017

These recommendations must be read with the footnotes that follow.

Vaccine	19–21 years	22–26 years	27–59 years	60–64 years	≥ 65 years
Influenza[1]	1 dose annually				
Td/Tdap[2]	Substitute Tdap for Td once, then Td booster every 10 yrs				
MMR[3]	1 or 2 doses depending on indication				
VAR[4]	2 doses				
HZV[5]				1 dose	
HPV–Female[6]	3 doses				
HPV–Male[6]	3 doses				
PCV13[7]					1 dose
PPSV23[7]	1 or 2 doses depending on indication				1 dose
HepA[8]	2 or 3 doses depending on vaccine				
HepB[9]	3 doses				
MenACWY or MPSV4[10]	1 or more doses depending on indication				
MenB[10]	2 or 3 doses depending on vaccine				
Hib[11]	1 or 3 doses depending on indication				

Recommended for adults who meet the age requirement, lack documentation of vaccination, or lack evidence of past infection

Recommended for adults with additional medical conditions or other indications

No recommendation

TABLE 20A Recommended Immunization Schedule for Adults Aged 19 Years or Older by Medical Condition and Other Indications, United States, 2017

These recommendations must be read with the footnotes that follow.

Vaccine	Pregnancy[1-6,9]	Immuno-compromised (excluding HIV infection)[3-7,11]	HIV infection CD4+ count (cells/µL)[3-7,9-11] < 200	≥ 200	Asplenia, persistent complement deficiencies[7,10,11]	Kidney failure, end-stage renal disease, on hemodialysis[7,9]	Heart or lung disease, chronic alcoholism[7]	Chronic liver disease[7,9]	Diabetes[7,9]	Healthcare personnel[3,4,9]	Men who have sex with men[6,8,9]
Influenza[1]	1 dose annually										
Td/Tdap[2]	1 dose Tdap each pregnancy	Substitute Tdap for Td once, then Td booster every 10 yrs									
MMR[3]	contraindicated			1 or 2 doses depending on indication							
VAR[4]	contraindicated			2 doses							
HZV[5]	contraindicated			1 dose							
HPV–Female[6]				3 doses through age 26 yrs							
HPV–Male[6]		3 doses through age 26 yrs		3 doses through age 21 yrs							3 doses through age 26 yrs
PCV13[7]				1 dose							
PPSV23[7]						1, 2, or 3 doses depending on indication					
HepA[8]						2 or 3 doses depending on vaccine					
HepB[9]						3 doses					
MenACWY or MPSV4[10]	1 or more doses depending on indication										
MenB[10]	2 or 3 doses depending on vaccine										
Hib[11]		3 doses post-HSCT recipients only		1 dose							

Legend:
- Recommended for adults who meet the age requirement, lack documentation of vaccination, or lack evidence of past infection
- Recommended for adults with additional medical conditions or other indications
- Contraindicated
- No recommendation

Footnotes. Recommended immunization schedule for adults aged 19 years or older, United States, 2017

1. **Influenza vaccination**
   General information
   - All persons aged 6 months or older who do not have a contraindication should receive annual influenza vaccination with an age-appropriate formulation of inactivated influenza vaccine (IIV) or recombinant influenza vaccine (RIV).
   - In addition to standard-dose IIV, available options for adults in specific age groups include: high-dose or adjuvanted IIV for adults aged 65 years or older, intradermal IIV for adults aged 18 through 64 years, and RIV for adults aged 18 years or older.
   - Notes: Live attenuated influenza vaccine (LAIV) should not be used during the 2016–2017 influenza season. A list of currently available influenza vaccines is available at www.cdc.gov/flu/protect/vaccine/ vaccines.htm.

   Special populations
   - Adults with a history of egg allergy who have only hives after exposure to egg should receive age-appropriate IIV or RIV.
   - Adults with a history of egg allergy other than hives, e.g., angioedema, respiratory distress, lightheadedness, or recurrent emesis, or who required epinephrine or another emergency medical intervention, may receive age-appropriate IIV or RIV. The selected vaccine should be administered in an inpatient or outpatient medical setting and under the supervision of a healthcare provider who is able to recognize and manage severe allergic conditions.
   - Pregnant women and women who might become pregnant in the upcoming influenza season should receive IIV.

2. **Tetanus, diphtheria, and acellular pertussis vaccination**
   General information
   - Adults who have not received tetanus and diphtheria toxoids and acellular pertussis vaccine (Tdap) or for whom pertussis vaccination status is unknown should receive 1 dose of Tdap followed by a tetanus and diphtheria toxoids (Td) booster every 10 years. Tdap should be administered regardless of when a tetanus or diphtheria toxoid-containing vaccine was last received.
   - Adults with an unknown or incomplete history of a 3-dose primary series with tetanus and diphtheria toxoid-containing vaccines should complete the primary series that includes 1 dose of Tdap. Unvaccinated adults should receive the first 2 doses at least 4 weeks apart and the third dose 6–12 months after the second dose.
   - Notes: Information on the use of Td or Tdap as tetanus prophylaxis in wound management is available at www.cdc.gov/mmwr/preview/mmwrhtml/rr5517a1.htm.

   Special populations
   - Pregnant women should receive 1 dose of Tdap during each pregnancy, preferably during the early part of gestational weeks 27–36, regardless of prior history of receiving Tdap.

3. **Measles, mumps, and rubella vaccination**
   General information
   - Adults born in 1957 or later without acceptable evidence of immunity to measles, mumps, or rubella (defined below) should receive 1 dose of measles, mumps, and rubella vaccine (MMR) unless they have a medical contraindication to the vaccine, e.g., pregnancy or severe immunodeficiency.
   - Notes: Acceptable evidence of immunity to measles, mumps, or rubella in adults is: born before 1957, documentation of receipt of MMR, or laboratory evidence of immunity or disease. Documentation of healthcare provider-diagnosed disease without laboratory confirmation is not acceptable evidence of immunity.

Special populations

- Pregnant women who do not have evidence of immunity to rubella should receive 1 dose of MMR upon completion or termination of pregnancy and before discharge from the healthcare facility; nonpregnant women of childbearing age without evidence of rubella immunity should receive 1 dose of MMR.
- Adults with primary or acquired immunodeficiency including malignant conditions affecting the bone marrow or lymphatic system, systemic immunosuppressive therapy, or cellular immunodeficiency should not receive MMR.
- Adults with human immunodeficiency virus (HIV) infection and CD4+ T-lymphocyte count ≥200 cells/µl for at least 6 months who do not have evidence of measles, mumps, or rubella immunity should receive 2 doses of MMR at least 28 days apart. Adults with HIV infection and CD4+ T-lymphocyte count <200 cells/µl should not receive MMR.
- Adults who work in healthcare facilities should receive 2 doses of MMR at least 28 days apart; healthcare personnel born before 1957 who are unvaccinated or lack laboratory evidence of measles, mumps, or rubella immunity, or laboratory confirmation of disease should be considered for vaccination with 2 doses of MMR at least 28 days apart for measles or mumps, or 1 dose of MMR for rubella.
- Adults who are students in postsecondary educational institutions or plan to travel internationally should receive 2 doses of MMR at least 28 days apart.
- Adults who received inactivated (killed) measles vaccine or measles vaccine of unknown type during years 1963–1967 should be revaccinated with 1 or 2 doses of MMR.
- Adults who were vaccinated before 1979 with either inactivated mumps vaccine or mumps vaccine of unknown type who are at high risk for mumps infection, e.g., work in a healthcare facility, should be considered for revaccination with 2 doses of MMR at least 28 days apart.

4. Varicella vaccination
General information

- Adults without evidence of immunity to varicella (defined below) should receive 2 doses of single-antigen varicella vaccine (VAR) 4–8 weeks apart, or a second dose if they have received only 1 dose.
- Persons without evidence of immunity for whom VAR should be emphasized are: adults who have close contact with persons at high risk for serious complications, e.g., healthcare personnel and household contacts of immunocompromised persons; adults who live or work in an environment in which transmission of varicella zoster virus is likely, e.g., teachers, childcare workers, and residents and staff in institutional settings; adults who live or work in environments in which varicella transmission has been reported, e.g., college students, residents and staff members of correctional institutions, and military personnel; nonpregnant women of childbearing age; adolescents and adults living in households with children; and international travelers.
- Notes: Evidence of immunity to varicella in adults is: U.S.-born before 1980 (for pregnant women and healthcare personnel, U.S.-born before 1980 is not considered evidence of immunity); documentation of 2 doses of VAR at least 4 weeks apart; history of varicella or herpes zoster diagnosis or verification of varicella or herpes zoster disease by a healthcare provider; or laboratory evidence of immunity or disease.

Special populations

- Pregnant women should be assessed for evidence of varicella immunity. Pregnant women who do not have evidence of immunity should receive the first dose of VAR upon completion or termination of pregnancy and before discharge from the healthcare facility, and the second dose 4–8 weeks after the first dose.
- Healthcare institutions should assess and ensure that all healthcare personnel have evidence of immunity to varicella.
- Adults with malignant conditions, including those that affect the bone marrow or lymphatic system or who receive systemic immunosuppressive therapy, should not receive VAR.
- Adults with human immunodeficiency virus (HIV) infection and CD4+ T-lymphocyte count ≥200 cells/µl may receive 2 doses of VAR 3 months apart. Adults with HIV infection and CD4+ T-lymphocyte count <200 cells/µl should not receive VAR.

5. Herpes zoster vaccination
General information

- Adults aged 60 years or older should receive 1 dose of herpes zoster vaccine (HZV), regardless of whether they had a prior episode of herpes zoster.

Special populations

- Adults aged 60 years or older with chronic medical conditions may receive HZV unless they have a medical contraindication, e.g., pregnancy or severe immunodeficiency.
- Adults with malignant conditions, including those that affect the bone marrow or lymphatic system or who receive systemic immunosuppressive therapy, should not receive HZV.
- Adults with human immunodeficiency virus (HIV) infection and CD4+ T-lymphocyte count <200 cells/µl should not receive HZV.

6. Human papillomavirus vaccination
General information

- Adult females through age 26 years and adult males through age 21 years who have not received any human papillomavirus (HPV) vaccine should receive a 3-dose series of HPV vaccine at 0, 1-2, and 6 months. Males aged 22 through 26 years may be vaccinated with a 3-dose series of HPV vaccine at 0, 1–2, and 6 months.
- Adult females through age 26 years and adult males through age 21 years (and males aged 22 through 26 years who may receive HPV vaccination) who initiated the HPV vaccination series before age 15 years and received 2 doses at least 5 months apart are considered adequately vaccinated and do not need an additional dose of HPV vaccine.
- Adult females through age 26 years and adult males through age 21 years (and males aged 22 through 26 years who may receive HPV vaccination) who initiated the HPV vaccination series before age 15 years and received only 1 dose, or 2 doses less than 5 months apart, are not considered adequately vaccinated and should receive 1 additional dose of HPV vaccine.
- Notes: HPV vaccination is routinely recommended for children at age 11 or 12 years. For adults who had initiated but did not complete the HPV vaccination series, consider their age at first HPV vaccination (described above) and other factors (described below) to determine if they have been adequately vaccinated.

Special populations

- Men who have sex with men through age 26 years who have not received any HPV vaccine should receive a 3-dose series of HPV vaccine at 0, 1-2, and 6 months.
- Adult females and males through age 26 years with immunocompromising conditions (described below), including those with human immunodeficiency virus (HIV) infection, should receive a 3-dose series of HPV vaccine at 0, 1–2, and 6 months.
- Pregnant women are not recommended to receive HPV vaccine, although there is no evidence that the vaccine poses harm. If a woman is found to be pregnant after initiating the HPV vaccination series, delay the remaining doses until after the pregnancy. No other intervention is needed. Pregnancy testing is not needed before administering HPV vaccine.
- Notes: Immunocompromising conditions for which a 3-dose series of HPV vaccine is indicated are primary or secondary immunocompromising conditions that might reduce cell-mediated or humoral immunity, e.g., B-lymphocyte antibody deficiencies, complete or partial T-lymphocyte defects, HIV infection, malignant neoplasm, transplantation, autoimmune disease, and immunosuppressive therapy.

7. Pneumococcal vaccination
General information

- Adults who are immunocompetent and aged 65 years or older should receive 13-valent pneumococcal conjugate vaccine (PCV13) followed by 23-valent pneumococcal polysaccharide vaccine (PPSV23) at least 1 year after PCV13.
- Notes: Adults are recommended to receive 1 dose of PCV13 and 1, 2, or 3 doses of PPSV23 depending on indication. When both PCV13 and PPSV23 are indicated, PCV13 should be administered first; PCV13 and PPSV23 should not be administered during the same visit. If PPSV23 has previously been administered, PCV13 should be administered at least 1

year after PPSV23. When two or more doses of PPSV23 are indicated, the interval between PPSV23 doses should be at least 5 years. Supplemental information on pneumococcal vaccine timing for adults aged 65 years or older and adults aged 19 years or older at high risk for pneumococcal disease (described below) is available at www.cdc.gov/vaccines/vpd-vac/pneumo/downloads/adult-vax-clinician-aid.pdf. No additional doses of PPSV23 are indicated for adults who received PPSV23 at age 65 years or older. When indicated, PCV13 and PPSV23 should be administered to adults whose pneumococcal vaccination history is incomplete or unknown

Special populations

- Adults aged 19 through 64 years with chronic heart disease including congestive heart failure and cardiomyopathies (excluding hypertension); chronic lung disease including chronic obstructive lung disease, emphysema, and asthma; chronic liver disease including cirrhosis; alcoholism; or diabetes mellitus; or who smoke cigarettes should receive PPSV23. At age 65 years or older, they should receive PCV13 and another dose of PPSV23 at least 1 year after PCV13 and at least 5 years after the most recent dose of PPSV23.
- Adults aged 19 years or older with immunocompromising conditions or anatomical or functional asplenia (described below) should receive PCV13 and a dose of PPSV23 at least 8 weeks after PCV13, followed by a second dose of PPSV23 at least 5 years after the first dose of PPSV23. If the most recent dose of PPSV23 was administered before age 65 years, at age 65 years or older, administer another dose of PPSV23 at least 8 weeks after PCV13 and at least 5 years after the most recent dose of PPSV23.
- Adults aged 19 years or older with cerebrospinal fluid leak or cochlear implant should receive PCV13 followed by PPSV23 at least 8 weeks after PCV13. If the most recent dose of PPSV23 was administered before age 65 years, at age 65 years or older, administer another dose of PPSV23 at least 8 weeks after PCV13 and at least 5 years after the most recent dose of PPSV23.
- Notes: Immunocompromising conditions that are indications for pneumococcal vaccination are congenital or acquired immunodeficiency including B- or T-lymphocyte deficiency, complement deficiencies, and phagocytic disorders excluding chronic granulomatous disease; human immunodeficiency virus (HIV) infection; chronic renal failure and nephrotic syndrome; leukemia, lymphoma, Hodgkin disease, generalized malignancy, and multiple myeloma; solid organ transplant; and iatrogenic immunosuppression including long-term systemic corticosteroid and radiation therapy. Anatomical or functional asplenia that are indications for pneumococcal vaccination are sickle cell disease and other hemoglobinopathies, congenital or acquired asplenia, splenic dysfunction, and splenectomy. Pneumococcal vaccines should be given at least 2 weeks before immunosuppressive therapy or an elective splenectomy, and as soon as possible to adults who are diagnosed with HIV infection.

8. Hepatitis A vaccination
General information

- Adults who seek protection from hepatitis A virus infection may receive a 2-dose series of single antigen hepatitis A vaccine (HepA) at either 0 and 6–12 months (Havrix) or 0 and 6–18 months (Vaqta). Adults may also receive a combined hepatitis A and hepatitis B vaccine (HepA-HepB) (Twinrix) as a 3-dose series at 0, 1, and 6 months. Acknowledgment of a specific risk factor by those who seek protection is not needed.

Special populations

- Adults with any of the following indications should receive a HepA series: have chronic liver disease, receive clotting factor concentrates, men who have sex with men, use injection or non-injection drugs, or work with hepatitis A virus-infected primates or in a hepatitis A research laboratory setting.
- Adults who travel in countries with high or intermediate levels of endemic hepatitis A infection or anticipate close personal contact with an international adoptee, e.g., reside in the same household or regularly babysit, from a country with high or intermediate level of endemic hepatitis A infection within the first 60 days of arrival in the United States should receive a HepA series.

9. Hepatitis B vaccination
General information

- Adults who seek protection from hepatitis B virus infection may receive a 3-dose series of single-antigen hepatitis B vaccine (HepB) (Engerix-B, Recombivax HB) at 0, 1, and 6 months. Adults may also receive a combined hepatitis A and hepatitis B vaccine (HepA-HepB) (Twinrix) at 0, 1, and 6 months. Acknowledgment of a specific risk factor by those who seek protection is not needed.

Special populations

- Adults at risk for hepatitis B virus infection by sexual exposure should receive a HepB series, including sex partners of hepatitis B surface antigen (HBsAg)-positive persons, sexually active persons who are not in a mutually monogamous relationship, persons seeking evaluation or treatment for a sexually transmitted infection, and men who have sex with men (MSM).
- Adults at risk for hepatitis B virus infection by percutaneous or mucosal exposure to blood should receive a HepB series, including adults who are recent or current users of injection drugs, household contacts of HBsAg-positive persons, residents and staff of facilities for developmentally disabled persons, incarcerated, healthcare and public safety workers at risk for exposure to blood or blood-contaminated body fluids, younger than age 60 years with diabetes mellitus, and age 60 years or older with diabetes mellitus at the discretion of the treating clinician.
- Adults with chronic liver disease including, but not limited to, hepatitis C virus infection, cirrhosis, fatty liver disease, alcoholic liver disease, autoimmune hepatitis, and an alanine aminotransferase (ALT) or aspartate aminotransferase (AST) level greater than twice the upper limit of normal should receive a HepB series.
- Adults with end-stage renal disease including those on pre-dialysis care, hemodialysis, peritoneal dialysis, and home dialysis should receive a HepB series. Adults on hemodialysis should receive a 3-dose series of 40 μg Recombivax HB at 0, 1, and 6 months or a 4-dose series of 40 μg Engerix-B at 0, 1, 2, and 6 months.
- Adults with human immunodeficiency virus (HIV) infection should receive a HepB series.
- Pregnant women who are at risk for hepatitis B virus infection during pregnancy, e.g., having more than one sex partner during the previous six months, been evaluated or treated for a sexually transmitted infection, recent or current injection drug use, or had an HBsAg-positive sex partner, should receive a HepB series.
- International travelers to regions with high or intermediate levels of endemic hepatitis B virus infection should receive a HepB series.
- Adults in the following settings are assumed to be at risk for hepatitis B virus infection and should receive a HepB series: sexually transmitted disease treatment facilities, HIV testing and treatment facilities, facilities providing drug-abuse treatment and prevention services, healthcare settings targeting services to persons who inject drugs, correctional facilities, healthcare settings targeting services to MSM, hemodialysis facilities and end-stage renal disease programs, and institutions and nonresidential day care facilities for developmentally disabled persons.

10. Meningococcal vaccination
Special populations

- Adults with anatomical or functional asplenia or persistent complement component deficiencies should receive a 2-dose primary series of serogroups A, C, W, and Y meningococcal conjugate vaccine (MenACWY) at least 2 months apart and revaccinate every 5 years. They should also receive a series of serogroup B meningococcal vaccine (MenB) with either a 2-dose series of MenB-4C (Bexsero) at least 1 month apart or a 3-dose series of MenB-FHbp (Trumenba) at 0, 1–2, and 6 months.
- Adults with human immunodeficiency virus (HIV) infection who have not been previously vaccinated should receive a 2-dose primary series of MenACWY at least 2 months apart and revaccinate every 5 years. Those who previously received 1 dose of MenACWY should receive a second dose at least 2 months after the first dose. Adults with HIV infection are not routinely recommended to receive MenB because meningococcal disease in this population is caused primarily by serogroups C, W, and Y.

- Microbiologists who are routinely exposed to isolates of *Neisseria meningitidis* should receive 1 dose of MenACWY and revaccinate every 5 years if the risk for infection remains, and either a 2-dose series of MenB-4C at least 1 month apart or a 3-dose series of MenB-FHbp at 0, 1–2, and 6 months.
- Adults at risk because of a meningococcal disease outbreak should receive 1 dose of MenACWY if the outbreak is attributable to serogroup A, C, W, or Y, or either a 2-dose series of MenB-4C at least 1 month apart or a 3-dose series of MenB-FHbp at 0, 1–2, and 6 months if the outbreak is attributable to serogroup B.
- Adults who travel to or live in countries with hyperendemic or epidemic meningococcal disease should receive 1 dose of MenACWY and revaccinate every 5 years if the risk for infection remains. MenB is not routinely indicated because meningococcal disease in these countries is generally not caused by serogroup B.
- Military recruits should receive 1 dose of MenACWY and revaccinate every 5 years if the increased risk for infection remains.
- First-year college students aged 21 years or younger who live in residence halls should receive 1 dose of MenACWY if they have not received MenACWY at age 16 years or older.
- Young adults aged 16 through 23 years (preferred age range is 16 through 18 years) who are healthy and not at increased risk for serogroup B meningococcal disease (described above) may receive either a 2-dose series of MenB-4C at least 1 month apart or a 2-dose series of MenB-FHbp at 0 and 6 months for short-term protection against most strains of serogroup B meningococcal disease.

- For adults aged 56 years or older who have not previously received serogroups A, C, W, and Y meningococcal vaccine and need only 1 dose, meningococcal polysaccharide serogroups A, C, W, and Y vaccine (MPSV4) is preferred. For adults who previously received MenACWY or anticipate receiving multiple doses of serogroups A, C, W, and Y meningococcal vaccine, MenACWY is preferred.
- Notes: MenB-4C and MenB-FHbp are not interchangeable, i.e., the same vaccine should be used for all doses to complete the series. There is no recommendation for MenB revaccination at this time. MenB may be administered at the same time as MenACWY but at a different anatomic site, if feasible.

11. *Haemophilus influenzae* type b vaccination
Special populations

- Adults who have anatomical or functional asplenia or sickle cell disease, or are undergoing elective splenectomy should receive 1 dose of *Haemophilus influenzae* type b conjugate vaccine (Hib) if they have not previously received Hib. Hib should be administered at least 14 days before splenectomy.
- Adults with a hematopoietic stem cell transplant (HSCT) should receive 3 doses of Hib in at least 4 week intervals 6–12 months after transplant regardless of their Hib history.
- Notes: Hib is not routinely recommended for adults with human immunodeficiency virus infection because their risk for *Haemophilus influenzae* type b infection is low.

The Advisory Committee on Immunization Practices (ACIP) recommendations and package inserts for vaccines provide information on contraindications and precautions related to vaccines. Contraindications are conditions that increase chances of a serious adverse reaction in vaccine recipients and the vaccine should not be administered when a contraindication is present. Precautions should be reviewed for potential risks and benefits for vaccine recipient. For a person with a severe allergy to latex, e.g., anaphylaxis, vaccines supplied in vials or syringes that contain natural rubber latex should not be be administered unless the benefit of vaccination clearly outweighs the risk for a potential allergic reaction. For latex allergies other than anaphylaxis, vaccines supplied in vials or syringes that contain dry, natural rubber or natural rubber latex may be administered.

TABLE 20B Contraindications and Precautions for Vaccines Recommended for Adults Aged 19 Years or Older*

Contraindications and precautions for vaccines routinely recommended for adults

Vaccine	Contraindications	Precautions
All vaccines routinely recommended for adults	• Severe reaction, e.g., anaphylaxis, after a previous dose or to a vaccine component	• Moderate or severe acute illness with or without fever

Additional contraindications and precautions for vaccines routinely recommended for adults

Vaccine	Additional Contraindications	Additional Precautions
IIV[1]		• History of Guillain-Barré Syndrome within 6 weeks after previous influenza vaccination • Egg allergy other than hives, e.g., angioedema, respiratory distress, lightheadedness, or recurrent emesis; or required epinephrine or another emergency medical intervention (IIV may be administered in an inpatient or outpatient medical setting and under the supervision of a healthcare provider who is able to recognize and manage severe allergic conditions)
RIV[1]		• History of Guillain-Barré Syndrome within 6 weeks after previous influenza vaccination
LAIV[1]	• LAIV should not be used during 2016–2017 influenza season	• LAIV should not be used during 2016–2017 influenza season
Tdap/Td	• For pertussis-containing vaccines: encephalopathy, e.g., coma, decreased level of consciousness, or prolonged seizures, not attributable to another identifiable cause within 7 days of administration of a previous dose of a vaccine containing tetanus or diphtheria toxoid or acellular pertussis	• Guillain-Barré Syndrome within 6 weeks after a previous dose of tetanus toxoid-containing vaccine • History of Arthus-type hypersensitivity reactions after a previous dose of tetanus or diphtheria toxoid-containing vaccine. Defer vaccination until at least 10 years have elapsed since the last tetanus toxoid-containing vaccine • For pertussis-containing vaccine, progressive or unstable neurologic disorder, uncontrolled seizures, or progressive encephalopathy (until a treatment regimen has been established and the condition has stabilized)
MMR[2]	• Severe immunodeficiency, e.g., hematologic and solid tumors, chemotherapy, congenital immunodeficiency or long-term immunosuppressive therapy[3], human immunodeficiency virus (HIV) infection with severe immunocompromise • Pregnancy	• Recent (within 11 months) receipt of antibody-containing blood product (specific interval depends on product)[4] • History of thrombocytopenia or thrombocytopenic purpura • Need for tuberculin skin testing[5]
VAR[2]	• Severe immunodeficiency, e.g., hematologic and solid tumors, chemotherapy, congenital immunodeficiency or long-term immunosuppressive therapy[3], HIV infection with severe immunocompromise • Pregnancy	• Recent (within 11 months) receipt of antibody-containing blood product (specific interval depends on product)[4] • Receipt of specific antiviral drugs (acyclovir, famciclovir, or valacyclovir) 24 hours before vaccination (avoid use of these antiviral drugs for 14 days after vaccination)
HZV[2]	• Severe immunodeficiency, e.g., hematologic and solid tumors, chemotherapy, congenital immunodeficiency or long-term immunosuppressive therapy[3], HIV infection with severe immunocompromise • Pregnancy	• Receipt of specific antiviral drugs (acyclovir, famciclovir, or valacyclovir) 24 hours before vaccination (avoid use of these antiviral drugs for 14 days after vaccination)
HPV vaccine		• Pregnancy
PCV13	• Severe allergic reaction to any vaccine containing diphtheria toxoid	

1. For additional information on use of influenza vaccines among persons with egg allergy, see: CDC. Prevention and control of seasonal influenza with vaccines: recommendations of the Advisory Committee on Immunization Practices—United States, 2016–17 influenza season. MMWR 2016;65(RR-5):1–54. Available at www.cdc.gov/mmwr/volumes/65/rr/rr6505a1.htm.
2. MMR may be administered together with VAR or HZV on the same day. If not administered on the same day, separate live vaccines by at least 28 days.
3. Immunosuppressive steroid dose is considered to be daily receipt of 20 mg or more prednisone or equivalent for two or more weeks. Vaccination should be deferred for at least 1 month after discontinuation of immunosuppressive steroid therapy. Providers should consult ACIP recommendations for complete information on the use of specific live vaccines among persons on immune-suppressing medications or with immune suppression because of other reasons.
4. Vaccine should be deferred for the appropriate interval if replacement immune globulin products are being administered. See: CDC. General recommendations on immunization: recommendations of the Advisory Committee on Immunization Practices (ACIP). MMWR 2011;60(No. RR-2). Available at www.cdc.gov/mmwr/preview/mmwrhtml/rr6002a1.htm.
5. Measles vaccination may temporarily suppress tuberculin reactivity. Measles-containing vaccine may be administered on the same day as tuberculin skin testing, or should be postponed for at least 4 weeks after vaccination.

* Adapted from: CDC. Table 6. Contraindications and precautions to commonly used vaccines. General recommendations on immunization: recommendations of the Advisory Committee on Immunization Practices. MMWR 2011;60(No. RR-2):40–41 and from: Hamborsky J, Kroger A, Wolfe S, eds. Appendix A. Epidemiology and prevention of vaccine preventable diseases. 13th ed. Washington, DC: Public Health Foundation, 2015. Available at www.cdc.gov/vaccines/pubs/pinkbook/index.html.

Acronyms of vaccines recommended for adults

HepA	hepatitis A vaccine	LAIV	live attenuated influenza vaccine	PCV13	13-valent pneumococcal conjugate vaccine
HepA-HepB	hepatitis A and hepatitis B vaccines	MenACWY	serogroups A, C, W, and Y meningococcal conjugate vaccine	PPSV23	23-valent pneumococcal polysaccharide vaccine
HepB	hepatitis B vaccine			RIV	recombinant influenza vaccine
Hib	*Haemophilus influenzae* type b conjugate vaccine	MenB	serogroup B meningococcal vaccine	Td	tetanus and diphtheria toxoids
HPV vaccine	human papillomavirus vaccine	MMR	measles, mumps, and rubella vaccine	Tdap	tetanus toxoid, reduced diphtheria toxoid, and acellular pertussis vaccine
HZV	herpes zoster vaccine	MPSV4	serogroups A, C, W, and Y meningococcal polysaccharide vaccine		
IIV	inactivated influenza vaccine			VAR	varicella vaccine

TABLE 21 Immunization and Pregnancy

Vaccine	Before Pregnancy	During Pregnancy	After Pregnancy	Type of Vaccine	Route
Hepatitis A	If at high risk for disease	If at high risk for disease	If at high risk for disease	Inactivated	IM
Hepatitis B	Yes, if at risk	Yes, if at risk	Yes, if at risk	Inactivated	IM
Human papillomavirus (HPV)	Yes, if 9 to 26 years of age	No, under study	Yes, if 9 to 26 years of age	Inactivated	IM
Influenza TIV	Yes	Yes	Yes	Inactivated	IM
Influenza LAIV	Yes, if <50 years and healthy; avoid conception for 4 weeks	No	Yes, if <50 years and healthy; avoid conception for 4 weeks	Live	Nasal spray
MMR	Yes, avoid conception for 4 weeks	No	Yes, give immediately postpartum if susceptible to rubella	Live	SC
Meningococcal:	If indicated	If indicated	If indicated		
Polysaccharide				Inactivated	SC
Conjugate				Inactivated	IM
Pneumococcal polysaccharide	If indicated	If indicated	If indicated	Inactivated	IM or SC
Tetanus/diphtheria Td	Yes, Tdap preferred	If indicated	Yes, Tdap preferred	Toxoid	IM
Tdap, one dose only	Yes, preferred	If high risk of pertussis; otherwise, Td preferred	Yes, preferred	Toxoid/inactivated	IM
Varicella	Yes, avoid conception for 4 weeks	No	Yes, give immediately postpartum if susceptible	Live	SC

IM, Intramuscular; *LAIV,* live, attenuated influenza vaccine; *SC,* subcutaneous; *Tdap,* tetanus and diphtheria toxoids and acellular pertussis; *TIV,* trivalent inactivated influenza vaccine.

TABLE 22   Immunizing Agents and Immunization Schedules for Health Care Workers (HCWs)*

Generic Name	Primary Schedule and Booster(s)	Indications	Major Precautions and Contraindications	Special Considerations
Immunizing Agents Strongly Recommended for Health Care Workers				
Hepatitis B (HB) recombinant vaccine	Two doses IM 4 wk apart; third dose 5 mo after second; booster doses not necessary	**Preexposure:** HCWs at risk for exposure to blood or body fluids	Based on limited data no risk of adverse effects to developing fetuses is apparent. Pregnancy should *not* be considered a contraindication to vaccination of women. Previous anaphylactic reaction to common baker's yeast is a contraindication to vaccination.	The vaccine produces neither therapeutic nor adverse effects on HB-infected persons. Prevaccination serologic screening is not indicated for persons being vaccinated because of occupational risk. HCWs who have contact with patients or blood should be tested 1-2 mo after vaccination to determine serologic response.
Hepatitis B immune globulin (HBIG)	0.06 ml/kg IM as soon as possible after exposure. A second dose of HBIG should be administered 1 mo later if the HB vaccine series has not been started.	**Postexposure prophylaxis:** For persons exposed to blood or body fluids containing HBsAg and who are not immune to HBV infection—0.06 ml/kg IM as soon as possible (but no later than 7 days after exposure)		
Influenza vaccine (inactivated whole-virus and split-virus vaccines)	Annual vaccination with current vaccine Administered IM	HCWs who have contact with patients at high risk for influenza or its complications; HCWs who work in long-term care facilities; HCWs with high-risk medical conditions or who are aged ≥65 yr	History of anaphylactic hypersensitivity to egg ingestion	No evidence exists of risk to mother or fetus when the vaccine is administered to a pregnant woman with an underlying high-risk condition. Influenza vaccination is recommended during second and third trimesters of pregnancy because of increased risk for hospitalization.
Measles live-virus vaccine	One dose SC; second dose at least 1 mo later	HCWs† born during or after 1957 who do not have documentation of having received two doses of live vaccine on or after the first birthday **or** a history of physician-diagnosed measles or serologic evidence of immunity. Vaccination should be considered for all HCWs who lack proof of immunity, including those born before 1957.	Pregnancy; immunocompromised persons,‡ including HIV-infected persons who have evidence of severe immunosuppression; anaphylaxis after gelatin ingestion or administration of neomycin; recent administration of immune globulin	MMR is the vaccine of choice if recipients are likely to be susceptible to rubella and/or mumps as well as measles. Persons vaccinated between 1963 and 1967 with a killed measles vaccine alone, killed vaccine followed by live vaccine, or with a vaccine of unknown type should be revaccinated with two doses of live measles virus vaccine.
Mumps live-virus vaccine	One dose SC; second dose at least 1 mo later	HCWs† believed to be susceptible can be vaccinated. Adults born before 1957 can be considered immune.	Pregnancy; immunocompromised persons,‡ history of anaphylactic reaction after gelatin ingestion or administration of neomycin	MMR is the vaccine of choice if recipients are likely to be susceptible to measles and rubella, as well as mumps.
Hepatitis A virus (HAV) vaccine	Two doses of vaccine either 6-12 mo apart (HAVRIX), or 6 mo apart (VAQTA)	Not routinely indicated for HCWs in the United States. Persons who work with HAV-infected primates or with HAV in a research laboratory setting should be vaccinated.	History of anaphylactic hypersensitivity to alum or, for HAVRIX, the preservative 2-phenoxyethanol. The safety of the vaccine in pregnant women has not been determined; the risk associated with vaccination should be weighed against the risk for hepatitis A in women who may be at high risk for exposure to HAV.	

TABLE 22 Immunizing Agents and Immunization Schedules for Health Care Workers (HCWs)*—cont'd

Generic Name	Primary Schedule and Booster(s)	Indications	Major Precautions and Contraindications	Special Considerations
Meningococcal vaccine	One dose in volume and by route specified by manufacturer; single booster for adults 19 to 21 years of age if the first dose was given before age 16	Laboratory personnel and others with exposure risk.	The safety of the vaccine in pregnant women has not been evaluated; it should not be administered during pregnancy unless the risk for infection is high.	
Typhoid vaccine, IM, SC, and oral	IM vaccine: One 0.5-ml/dose, booster 0.5 ml every 2 yr SC vaccine: Two 0.5-ml doses, ≥4 wk apart, booster 0.5 ml SC or 0.1 ID every 3 yr if exposure continues Oral vaccine: Four doses on alternate days. The manufacturer recommends revaccination with the entire 4-dose series every 5 yr	Workers in microbiology laboratories who frequently work with *Salmonella typhi*	Severe local or systemic reaction to a previous dose. Ty21a (oral) vaccine should not be administered to immunocompromised persons[†] or to persons receiving antimicrobial agents.	Vaccination should not be considered an alternative to the use of proper procedures when handling specimens and cultures in the laboratory.
Vaccinia vaccine (smallpox)	One dose administered with a bifurcated needle; boosters administered every 10 yr	Laboratory workers who directly handle cultures with vaccinia, recombinant vaccinia viruses, or orthopox viruses that infect human beings	The vaccine is contraindicated in pregnancy, in persons with eczema or a history of eczema, and in immunocompromised persons[†] and their household contacts.	Vaccination may be considered for HCWs who have direct contact with contaminated dressings or other infectious material from volunteers in clinical studies involving recombinant vaccinia virus.
Other Vaccine-Preventable Diseases				
Tetanus and diphtheria and pertussis (Tdap)	Two IM doses 4 wk apart or tetanus and diphtheria toxoid for adults with uncertain or incomplete primary vaccination; third dose 6-12 mo after second dose; booster every 10 yr. Substitute a one-time dose of Tdap for one of the doses of Td, either in the primary series or for the routine booster, whichever comes first.	All adults	Except in the first trimester, pregnancy is not a precaution. History of a neurologic reaction or immediate hypersensitivity reaction after a previous dose. History of severe local (Arthus-type) reaction after a previous dose. Such persons should not receive further routine or emergency doses of Td for 10 yr.	Tetanus prophylaxis in wound management[‡]
Pneumococcal polysaccharide vaccine (23 valent)	One dose, 0.5 ml, IM or SC; revaccination recommended for those at highest risk ≥5 yr after the first dose	Adults who are at increased risk of pneumococcal disease and its complications because of underlying health conditions; older adults, especially those age ≥65 who are healthy	The safety of vaccine in pregnant women has not been evaluated; it should not be administered during pregnancy unless the risk for infection is high. Previous recipients of any type of pneumococcal polysaccharide vaccine who are at highest risk for fatal infection or antibody loss may be revaccinated ≥5 yr after the first dose.	

Continued

TABLE 22 Immunizing Agents and Immunization Schedules for Health Care Workers (HCWs)*—cont'd

Generic Name	Primary Schedule and Booster(s)	Indications	Major Precautions and Contraindications	Special Considerations
Rubella live-virus vaccine	One dose SC; second dose at least 1 mo later	Indicated for HCWs,[†] both men and women, who do not have documentation of having received live vaccine on or after their first birthday **or** laboratory evidence of immunity. Adults born before 1957, **except women who can become pregnant,** can be considered immune.	Pregnancy; immunocompromised persons[†]; history of anaphylactic reaction after administration of neomycin	The risk for rubella vaccine–associated malformations in the offspring of women pregnant when vaccinated or who become pregnant within 3 mo after vaccination is negligible. Such women should be counseled regarding the theoretic basis of concern for the fetus. MMR is the vaccine of choice if recipients are likely to be susceptible to measles or mumps as well as rubella.
Varicella-zoster live-virus vaccine	Two 0.5-ml doses SC 4-8 wk apart if ≥13 yr	Indicated for HCWs[†] who do not have either a reliable history of varicella or serologic evidence of immunity	Pregnancy, immunocompromised persons,[‡] history of anaphylactic reaction after receipt of neomycin or gelatin. Avoid salicylate use for 6 wk after vaccination.	Vaccine is available from the manufacturer for certain patients with acute lymphocytic leukemia in remission. Because 71%-93% of persons without a history of varicella are immune, serologic testing before vaccination is likely to be cost effective.
Varicella-zoster immune globulin (VZIG)	Persons <50 kg: 125 μg/10 kg IM; persons ≥50 kg: 625 μg[§]	Persons known or likely to be susceptible (particularly those at high risk for complications, e.g., pregnant women) who have close and prolonged exposure to a contact case or to an infectious hospital staff worker or patient		Serologic testing may help in assessing whether to administer VZIG. If use of VZIG prevents varicella disease, patient should be vaccinated subsequently.

BCG Vaccination

Generic Name	Primary Schedule and Booster(s)	Indications	Major Precautions and Contraindications	Special Considerations
Bacille Calmette-Guérin (BCG) vaccine (TB)	One percutaneous dose of 0.3 ml; no booster dose recommended	Should be considered only for HCWs in areas where multidrug TB is prevalent, a strong likelihood of infection exists, and where comprehensive infection control precautions have failed to prevent TB transmission to HCWs	Should not be administered to immunocompromised persons,[‡] pregnant women	In the United States TB-control efforts are directed toward early identification, treatment of cases, and preventive therapy with isoniazid.

Other Immunobiologics That Are or May Be Indicated for HCWs

Generic Name	Primary Schedule and Booster(s)	Indications	Major Precautions and Contraindications	Special Considerations
Immune globulin (hepatitis A)	**Postexposure**—One IM dose of 0.02 ml/kg administered ≤2 wk after exposure	Indicated for HCWs exposed to feces of infectious patients	Contraindicated in persons with IgA deficiency; do not administer within 2 wk after MMR vaccine or 3 wk after varicella vaccine. Delay administration of MMR vaccine for ≥3 mo and varicella vaccine ≥5 mo after administration of immune globulin	Administer in large muscle mass (deltoid, gluteal).

HBsAg, Hepatitis B surface antigen; *HBV,* hepatitis B virus; *HIV,* human immunodeficiency virus; *IM,* intramuscular; *MMR,* measles, mumps, rubella vaccine; *SC,* subcutaneous; *TB,* tuberculosis.
*Persons who provide health care to patients or work in institutions that provide patient care (e.g., physicians, nurses, emergency medical personnel, dental professionals and students, medical and nursing students, laboratory technicians, hospital volunteers, and administrative and support staff in health care institutions).
[†]All HCWs (i.e., medical or nonmedical, paid or volunteer, full time or part time, student or nonstudent, with or without patient-care responsibilities) who work in health care institutions (e.g., inpatient and outpatient, public and private) should be immune to measles, rubella, and varicella.
[‡]Persons immunocompromised because of immune deficiency diseases, HIV infection, leukemia, lymphoma or generalized malignancy, or immunosuppressed as a result of therapy with corticosteroids, alkylating drugs, antimetabolites, or radiation.
[§]Some experts recommend 125 μg/10 kg regardless of total body weight.
Modified from *MMWR* 46(RR-18), 1998.

TABLE 23 Recommendations for Persons with Medical Conditions Requiring Special Vaccination Considerations

Condition	Tdap	MMR	Varicella	HBV	HAV	Pneumovax[a]	Influenza[b]	HbCV	Meningococcal	IPV	Other Live Vaccines[c]	Other Killed Vaccines[d]
HIV infection	Rou	Rou/Contr[e]	Contr[f]	Rou[g]	Rou	Rec	Rec	Cons	Rou	Rou	Contr	Rou
Severe immunocompromise[h]	Rou	Contr	Contr[f]	Rou[g]	Rou	Rec	Rec	Rou[i]	Rou	Rou	Contr	Rou
Renal failure	Rou	Rou	Rou	Rec[g]	Rou	Rec	Rec	Rou	Rou	Rou	Rou	Rou
Diabetes	Rou	Rou	Rou	Rou	Rou	Rec	Rec	Rou	Rou	Rou	Rou	Rou
Chronic liver disease	Rou	Rou	Rou	Rou	Rec	Rec	Rec	Rou	Rou	Rou	Rou	Rou
Cardiac disease	Rou	Rou	Rou	Rou	Rou	Rec	Rec	Rou	Rou	Rou	Rou	Rou
Pulmonary disease	Rou	Rou	Rou	Rou	Rou	Rec	Rec	Rou	Rou	Rou	Rou	Rou
Alcoholism	Rou	Rou	Rou	Rou	Rou	Rec	Rec	Rou	Rou	Rou	Rou	Rou
Functional/anatomic asplenia	Rou	Rou	Rou	Rou	Rou	Rec[j]	Rec	Rec[j]	Rec[j]	Rou	Rou	Rou
Terminal complement deficiency	Rou	Rou	Rou	Rou	Rou	Rou	Rou	Rou	Rec	Rou	Rou	Rou
Clotting factor disorders	Rou	Rou	Rou	Rec	Rec	Rou	Rou	Rou	Rou	Rou	Rou	Rou

Cons, Consider vaccination; *Contr*, contraindicated; *HAV*, hepatitis A virus; *HbCV*, *Haemophilus influenzae* conjugate vaccine; *HBV*, hepatitis B virus; *IPV*, inactivated poliomyelitis vaccine; *MMR*, measles-mumps-rubella; *Rec*, recommended; *Rou*, routine as outlined for all adults; *Tdap*, tetanus and diphtheria toxoids and acellular pertussis.

aPneumovax should be repeated in 5 yr for patients in whom vaccine is recommended. Asthma without chronic obstructive pulmonary disease is not an indication for the vaccine.
bInfluenza vaccine should also be given to caregivers and household members.
cIncludes bacille Calmette-Guérin, vaccinia, oral typhoid, yellow fever (if exposure cannot be avoided, persons with HIV can be given yellow fever vaccine; see text).
dIncludes rabies (check postvaccination titers in HIV or severely immunocompromised persons), Lyme disease, inactivated typhoid, cholera, plague, and anthrax.
eFor asymptomatic, nonseverely immunocompromised persons with HIV, MMR can be used; it is contraindicated in severely immunocompromised persons. MMR can be considered in symptomatic HIV patients without severe immunocompromise.
fVaricella can be given to household members and caregivers, but if varicella-like rash develops after vaccination, contact should be avoided.
gRecommended for persons with severe chronic renal failure approaching or already receiving dialysis, and higher doses should be given. Antibody titers should be measured after vaccination in these patients and in those with HIV or severe immunocompromise (who may require higher doses) to ensure adequate response. Yearly titers should be measured in dialysis patients.
hSevere immunocompromise can result from congenital immunodeficiency, leukemia, lymphoma, malignancy, organ transplant, chemotherapy, radiation therapy, or high-dose corticosteroids.
iOnly for persons with Hodgkin's disease.
jGive at least 2 wk in advance of elective splenectomy.
Modified and updated from *MMWR* 42(RR-4):16, 1993.

TABLE 24 Vaccinations for International Travel

Disease*	Areas Affected†	Prophylaxis Recommended	Ideal Time between Last Vaccine Dose and Travel
Tetanus	All	All travelers; vaccine series/booster	Probably 30 days for series; anamnestic response to booster
Measles	All	If born after 1956; ensure immunity by antibody titer, diagnosed measles, or two doses of vaccine	As MMR, 7-14 days
Rubella	All	If born after 1956 and any female of childbearing age; rubella titer or one dose of vaccine	As MMR, 7-14 days
Mumps	All	If born after 1956; ensure immunity by antibody titer, diagnosed mumps, or one dose of vaccine	As MMR, 7-14 days
Varicella	All	All travelers; antibody titer, reported illness, or vaccine series	7-14 days
Hepatitis B	5%-20% of population are carriers in Africa, Middle East except Israel, all Southeast Asia, Amazon basin, Haiti, and Dominican Republic; 1%-5% of population are carriers in south-central and southwest Asia, Israel, Japan, Americas, Russia, and eastern and southern Europe	Travelers for more than 6 mo in close contact with population or for less time but with high-risk activities (close household contact, seeking dental or medical care, sex); vaccine series	Probably 30 days
Hepatitis A	Developing countries	Travelers to rural areas; eating and drinking in settings of poor sanitation; vaccine or pooled immune globulin	Vaccine, 30 days Pooled IG, 2 days
Influenza	Tropics throughout the year; southern hemisphere from April to September	Travelers for whom vaccine is otherwise indicated; give current vaccine and revaccinate in fall as usual	7-14 days
Meningococcus*	Sub-Saharan Africa "belt" (Senegal to Ethiopia) from December to June; required for pilgrims to Saudi Arabia during Hajj; epidemics reported in other African nations, India, Nepal, and Mongolia	All travelers; vaccine	7-10 days
Rabies	Endemic dog rabies exists in Mexico, El Salvador, Guatemala, Peru, Colombia, Ecuador, India, Nepal, Philippines, Sri Lanka, Thailand, and Vietnam	Travelers staying for more than 30 days or at high risk of exposure to domestic or wild animals; vaccine series/booster	7-14 days
Poliomyelitis	Developing countries not in western hemisphere; at risk all year in tropics; in temperate zones, incidence increases in summer and fall	All travelers; vaccine series/booster	Parenteral vaccine series, 28 day
Typhoid fever	Many countries in Asia, Africa, Central America, and South America	Travelers with prolonged stay in rural areas with poor sanitation; vaccine series/booster	Oral vaccine, 7 days Parenteral vaccine, probably 14 days
Yellow fever*	North and central South America, forest-savannah zones of Africa; some countries in Africa, Asia, and Middle East require travelers from endemic areas to be vaccinated	All travelers; vaccine/booster at approved yellow fever vaccination center.	10 days
Japanese encephalitis	Seasonally in most areas of Asia, Indian subcontinent, and western Pacific islands; in temperate zones, incidence increases in summer and early fall; in tropics, year-round incidence	Travelers staying for more than 30 days in high-risk rural areas; staying outdoors during transmission season; vaccine series	10 days
Cholera*	Certain undeveloped countries	If required by local authorities, one dose usually suffices; primary series only for those living in high-risk areas under poor sanitary conditions or those with compromised gastric defense mechanisms (achlorhydria, antacid therapy, previous ulcer surgery); booster every 6 mo	Probably 30 days
Plague	Africa, Asia, and Americas in rural mountainous or upland areas	Travelers whose research or field activities bring them in contact with rodents; vaccine series/booster; consider taking tetracycline (500 mg four times a day) for chemoprophylaxis (inferred from clinical experience in treating plague)	Probably 30 days

IG, Immune globulin; *MMR,* measles-mumps-rubella.

*Only yellow fever vaccine is required for entry by any country; cholera vaccine may be required by some local authorities. Meningococcus vaccine is required for pilgrims to Mecca, in Saudi Arabia, during Hajj. However, it is important to follow Centers for Disease Control and Prevention (CDC) recommendations for all vaccines to prevent disease. If a required vaccine is contraindicated or withheld for any reason, attempts should be made to obtain a waiver from the country's consulate or embassy.

†Because areas affected can change, and for more specific details, consult the CDC's traveler's hotline.

From Noble J: *Primary care medicine,* ed 3, St Louis, 2001, Mosby.

Recommendations and Implementation Strategies for Hepatitis B Vaccination of Adults

BOX 1 Adults Recommended to Receive Hepatitis B Vaccination

Persons at Risk for Infection by Sexual Exposure
Sex partners of persons who are HBsAg positive
Sexually active persons who are not in a long-term, mutually monogamous relationship (e.g., persons who have had more than one sex partner during the previous 6 months)
Persons seeking evaluation or treatment for a sexually transmitted disease
Men who have sex with men

Persons at Risk for Infection by Percutaneous or Mucosal Exposure to Blood
Current or recent users of injection drugs
Household contacts of persons who are HBsAg positive
Residents and staff of facilities for developmentally disabled persons

Health care and public safety workers with reasonably anticipated risk for exposure to blood or blood-contaminated body fluids
Persons with end-stage renal disease, including predialysis, hemodialysis, peritoneal dialysis, and home dialysis patients

Others
International travelers to regions with high or intermediate levels (HBsAg prevalence of ≥2%) of endemic HBV infection
Persons with chronic liver disease including, but not limited to, hepatitis C virus infection, cirrhosis, fatty liver disease, alcoholic liver disease, autoimmune hepatitis, and an alanine aminotransferase (ALT) or aspartate aminotransferase (AST) level greater than twice the upper limit of normal.
Persons with HIV infection
All other persons seeking protection from HBV infection

From CDC: A comprehensive immunization strategy to eliminate transmission of hepatitis B virus infection in the United States: recommendations of the Advisory Committee on Immunization Practices (ACIP), *MMWR* 55(RR-16):15, 2006.
HBsAg, Hepatitis B surface antigen; *HBV,* hepatitis B virus.

BOX 2 Hepatitis B Vaccine Schedules for Adults (Aged ≥20 yr)[1]

0, 1, and 6 months
0, 1, and 4 months
0, 2, and 4 months
0, 1, 2, and 12 months[2]

From CDC: A comprehensive immunization strategy to eliminate transmission of hepatitis B virus infection in the United States: recommendations of the Advisory Committee on Immunization Practices (ACIP), *MMWR* 55(RR-16):15, 2006.
[1]All schedules are applicable to single-antigen hepatitis B vaccines; Twinrix (combined hepatitis A and hepatitis B vaccine) may be administered at 0, 1, and 6 months.
[2]A 4-dose schedule of Engerix-B is licensed for all age groups.

TABLE 25 Recommended Doses of Currently Licensed Formulations of Adult Hepatitis B Vaccine by Group and Vaccine Type

| | SINGLE-ANTIGEN VACCINE | | | | COMBINATION VACCINE | |
| | RECOMBIVAX HB[a] | | ENGERIX-B[b] | | TWINRIX[b,c] | |
Group	Dose (μg)[d]	Vol. (ml)	Dose (μg)[d]	Vol. (ml)	Dose (μg)[d]	Vol. (ml)
Adults (aged ≥20 yr)	10	1.0	20	1.0	20	1.0
Hemodialysis patients and other immunocompromised persons aged ≥20 yr	40[e]	1.0	40[f]	2.0	—[g]	—

HB, Hepatitis B.
[a]Merck & Co., Inc., Whitehouse Station, New Jersey.
[b]GlaxoSmithKline Biologicals, Rixensart, Belgium.
[c]Combined hepatitis A and hepatitis B vaccine, recommended for persons aged >18 yr who are at increased risk for both hepatitis B virus and hepatitis A virus infections.
[d]Recombinant hepatitis B surface antigen protein dose.
[e]Dialysis formulation administered on a 3-dose schedule at 0, 1, and 6 mo.
[f]Two 1.0-ml doses administered in 1 or 2 injections on a 4-dose schedule at 0, 1, 2, and 6 mo.
[g]Not applicable.
From Centers for Disease Control and Prevention: A comprehensive immunization strategy to eliminate transmission of hepatitis B virus infection in the United States: recommendations of the Advisory Committee on Immunization Practices (ACIP), *MMWR* 55(RR-16):10, 2006.

TABLE 26 Recommended HIV/AIDS, Sexually Transmitted Disease (STD), and Viral Hepatitis Prevention Services by Risk Population

Risk Population[a]	Recommended Services
High-Risk Heterosexuals	
Persons seeking sexually transmitted disease evaluation or treatment	Hepatitis B vaccination
	Testing for HIV infection[b]
	Testing for syphilis, gonorrhea, and chlamydia, as clinically indicated[c]
Sexually active men not in a long-term, mutually monogamous relationship	Hepatitis B vaccination
	Annual testing for HIV infection[b,d]
Sexually active women not in a long-term, mutually monogamous relationship	Hepatitis B vaccination[e]
	Annual testing for HIV infection[b,d]
	Annual testing for chlamydia (NOTE: Also recommended for all sexually active females aged <25 yr)[c]
Men Who Have Sex with Men (MSM)	
All MSM	Hepatitis A vaccination
	Hepatitis B vaccination[e]
Sexually active MSM not in a long-term, mutually monogamous relationship	Hepatitis A vaccination
	Hepatitis B vaccination[e]
	Annual testing for HIV infection[b]
	Annual testing for syphilis, gonorrhea, and chlamydia[c]
Injection-Drug Users	
	Hepatitis A vaccination[f]
	Hepatitis B vaccination
	Testing for hepatitis C virus infection[g]
	Annual testing for HIV infection[b]
	Substance-abuse treatment[h]

[a]Testing for HIV infection, chlamydia, gonorrhea, syphilis, and hepatitis B surface antigen also is recommended for pregnant women. (CDC: Revised recommendations for HIV testing of adults, adolescents, and pregnant women in health care settings, *MMWR* 55(RR-14], 2006; CDC: Sexually transmitted diseases treatment guidelines, *MMWR* 55(RR-11], 2006; CDC: A comprehensive immunization strategy to eliminate transmission of hepatitis B virus infection in the United States: recommendations of the Advisory Committee on Immunization Practices [ACIP]. Part 1: immunization of infants, children, and adolescents, *MMWR* 54[RR-16], 2005.)
[b]CDC: Revised recommendations for HIV testing of adults, adolescents, and pregnant women in health care settings, *MMWR* 55(RR-14), 2006.
[c]CDC: Sexually transmitted diseases treatment guidelines 2006, *MMWR* 55(RR-11), 2006.
[d]HIV screening is recommended for all persons aged 13-64 yr. Repeat screening is recommended at least annually for persons likely to be at high risk for HIV infection, including MSM or heterosexuals who themselves or whose sex partners have had more than one partner since their most recent HIV test.
[e]Hepatitis B vaccination is recommended for persons who have had more than one sex partner during the previous 6 mo.
[f]CDC: Prevention of hepatitis A through active or passive immunization: recommendations of the Advisory Committee on Immunization Practices (ACIP), *MMWR* 55(RR-7), 2006.
[g]CDC: Recommendations for prevention and control of hepatitis C virus (HCV) infection and HCV-related chronic disease, *MMWR* 47(RR-19), 1998. Recommended frequency of testing for hepatitis C virus infection has not been determined.
[h]CDC: *Substance abuse treatment for injection drug users: a strategy with many benefits*, Atlanta, 2002, U.S. Department of Health and Human Services, CDC. Available at http://www.cdc.gov/idu/facts/treatment.htm.
From Centers for Disease Control and Prevention (CDC): A comprehensive immunization strategy to eliminate transmission of hepatitis B virus infection in the United States: recommendations of the Advisory Committee on Immunization Practices (ACIP), *MMWR* 55(RR-16):17, 2006.

TABLE 27 Guidelines for Postexposure Prophylaxis* of Persons with Nonoccupational Exposures† to Blood or Body Fluids That Contain Blood by Exposure Type and Vaccination Status

	TREATMENT	
Exposure	**Unvaccinated Person‡**	**Previously Vaccinated Person§**
HBsAg-Positive Source		
Percutaneous (e.g., bite or needlestick) or mucosal exposure to HBsAg-positive blood or body fluids	Administer hepatitis B vaccine series and hepatitis B immune globulin (HBIG)	Administer hepatitis B vaccine booster dose
Sex or needle-sharing contact with a person who is HBsAg positive	Administer hepatitis B vaccine series and HBIG	Administer hepatitis B vaccine booster dose
Victim of sexual assault/abuse by a perpetrator who is HBsAg positive	Administer hepatitis B vaccine series and HBIG	Administer hepatitis B vaccine booster dose
Source with Unknown HBsAg Status		
Victim of sexual assault/abuse by a perpetrator with unknown HBsAg status	Administer hepatitis B vaccine series	No treatment
Percutaneous (e.g., bite or needlestick) or mucosal exposure to potentially infectious blood or body fluids from a source with unknown HBsAg status	Administer hepatitis B vaccine series	No treatment
Sexual or needle-sharing contact with person with unknown HBsAg status	Administer hepatitis B vaccine series	No treatment

HBsAg, Hepatitis B surface antigen.
*When indicated, immunoprophylaxis should be initiated as soon as possible, preferably within 24 hours. Studies are limited on the maximum interval after exposure during which postexposure prophylaxis is effective, but the interval is unlikely to exceed 7 days for percutaneous exposures or 14 days for sexual exposures. The hepatitis B vaccine series should be completed.
†These guidelines apply to nonoccupational exposures. Guidelines for management of occupational exposures have been published separately and also can be used for management of nonoccupational exposures if feasible.
‡A person who is in the process of being vaccinated but has not completed the vaccine series should complete the series and receive treatment as indicated.
§A person who has written documentation of a complete hepatitis B vaccine series and did not receive postvaccination testing.
From Centers for Disease Control and Prevention: A comprehensive immunization strategy to eliminate transmission of hepatitis B virus infection in the United States: recommendations of the Advisory Committee on Immunization Practices (ACIP), *MMWR* 55(RR-16):30, 2006.

TABLE 28 Typical Interpretation of Serologic Test Results for Hepatitis B Virus Infection

SEROLOGIC MARKER				
HBsAg	**Total Anti-HBc**	**IgM Anti-HBc**	**Anti-HBs**	**Interpretation**
−*	−	−	−	Never infected
+†‡	−	−	−	Early acute infection; transient (up to 18 days) after vaccination
+	+	+	−	Acute infection
−	+	+	+ or −	Acute resolving infection
−	+	−	+	Recovered from past infection and immune
+	+	−	−	Chronic infection
−	+	−	−	False-positive (i.e., susceptible), past infection, "low-level" chronic infection,§ or passive transfer of anti-HBc to infant born to mother who is HBsAg positive
−	−	−	+	Immune if concentration is >10 mIU/ml after vaccine series completion‖; passive transfer after hepatitis B immune globulin administration

HBc, Antibody to hepatitis B core antigen; *HBs,* antibody to HBsAg; *HBsAg,* hepatitis B surface antigen; *Ig,* immunoglobulin.
*Negative test result.
†Positive test result.
‡To ensure that an HBsAg-positive test result is not a false-positive, samples with reactive HBsAg results should be tested with a licensed neutralizing confirmatory test if recommended in the manufacturer's package insert.
§Persons positive only for anti-HBc are unlikely to be infectious except under unusual circumstances in which they are the source for direct percutaneous exposure of susceptible recipients to large quantities of virus (e.g., blood transfusion or organ transplant).
‖Milli-international units per milliliter.
From Centers for Disease Control and Prevention: A comprehensive immunization strategy to eliminate transmission of hepatitis B virus infection in the United States: recommendations of the Advisory Committee on Immunization Practices (ACIP), *MMWR* 55(RR-16):4, 2006.

Hepatitis A Prophylaxis

TABLE 29   Recommended Dosages of Hepatitis A Immune Globulin

Setting	Duration of Coverage	Dose
Preexposure prophylaxis	Short term (<3 mo)	0.02 ml/kg
	Long term (3-5 mo)*	0.06 ml/kg
Postexposure prophylaxis	—	0.02 ml/kg

NOTE: Immune globulin should be administered intramuscularly into the deltoid or gluteal muscle in children younger than 24 mo; it may be administered in the anterolateral thigh muscle.
*Repeat every 5 mo if continued exposure to hepatitis A virus occurs.
Modified from Centers for Disease Control and Prevention: Prevention of hepatitis A through active or passive immunization: recommendations of the Advisory Committee on Immunization Practices (ACIP), *MMWR* 55(RR-07):9, 2006.

TABLE 30   Licensed Dosages of Hepatitis A Vaccines

Vaccine	Patient's Age	Dose	Volume (ml)	Number of Doses	Schedule (mo)*
Hepatitis A vaccine, inactivated (Havrix)	12 mo to 18 yr	720 EL.U.	0.5	2	0, 6-12
	≥19 yr	1440 EL.U.	1.0	2	0, 6-12
Hepatitis A vaccine, inactivated (Vaqta)	12 mo to 18 yr	25 U	0.5	2	0, 6-18
	≥19 yr	50 U	1.0	2	0, 6-18
Combined hepatitis A and hepatitis B vaccine (Twinrix)	≥18 yr	720 EL.U. of hepatitis A antigen and 20 mcg of hepatitis B surface antigen protein	1.0	3	0, 1, and 6

*Zero represents the timing of the initial dose; subsequent numbers represent months after the initial dose.
Modified from Centers for Disease Control and Prevention: Prevention of hepatitis A through active or passive immunization: recommendations of the Advisory Committee on Immunization Practices (ACIP), *MMWR* 55(RR-07):10, 2006.

Influenza Treatment and Prophylaxis

BOX 3 Summary of Seasonal Influenza Vaccination Recommendations

Children	Adults
All children aged 6 months to 18 years should be vaccinated annually. Children and adolescents at higher risk for influenza complications should continue to be a focus for vaccination efforts as providers and programs transition to routinely vaccinating all children and adolescents, including those who: 　are aged 6 months to 4 years (59 months) 　have chronic pulmonary (including asthma), cardiovascular (except hypertension), renal, hepatic, cognitive, neurologic/neuromuscular, hematologic, or metabolic disorders (including diabetes mellitus) 　are immunosuppressed (including immunosuppression caused by medications or by human immunodeficiency virus) 　are receiving long-term aspirin therapy and therefore might be at risk for experiencing Reye's syndrome after influenza virus infection 　are residents of long-term care facilities 　will be pregnant during the influenza season **Note:** Children aged <6 months cannot receive influenza vaccination. Household and other close contacts (e.g., day-care providers) of children aged <6 months, including older children and adolescents, should be vaccinated.	Annual vaccination against influenza is recommended for any adult who wants to reduce the risk of becoming ill with influenza or of transmitting it to others. Vaccination is recommended for all adults without contraindications in the following groups, because these persons either are at higher risk for influenza complications, or are close contacts of the persons at higher risk: 　persons aged ≥50 years 　women who will be pregnant during the influenza season 　persons who have chronic pulmonary (including asthma), cardiovascular (except hypertension), renal, hepatic, cognitive, neurologic/neuromuscular, hematologic, or metabolic disorders (including diabetes mellitus) 　persons who have immunosuppression (including immunosuppression caused by medications or by human immunodeficiency virus) 　residents of nursing homes and other long-term care facilities 　health care personnel 　household contacts and caregivers of children aged <5 years and adults aged ≥50 years, with particular emphasis on vaccinating contacts of children aged <6 months 　household contacts and caregivers of persons with medical conditions that put them at higher risk for severe complications from influenza

Modified from *MMWR* 58:(RR-8), 2009.

TABLE 31 Live, Attenuated Influenza Vaccine (LAIV) Compared with Inactivated Influenza Vaccine (TIV) for Seasonal Influenza, United States Formulations

Factor	LAIV	TIV
Route of administration	Intranasal spray	Intramuscular injection
Type of vaccine	Live virus	Noninfectious virus (i.e., inactivated)
Number of included virus strains	3 (2 influenza A, 1 influenza B)	3 (2 influenza A, 1 influenza B)
Vaccine virus strains updated	Annually	Annually
Frequency of administration	Annually*	Annually*
Approved age	Persons aged 2-49 yr	Persons aged ≥6 mo
Interval between 2 doses recommended for children aged ≥6 mo to 8 yr who are receiving influenza vaccine for the first time	4 wk	4 wk
Can be administered to persons with medical risk factors for influenza-related complications[†]	No	Yes
Can be administered to children with asthma or children aged 2-4 yr with wheezing during the preceding year[§]	No	Yes
Can be administered to family members or close contacts of immunosuppressed persons not requiring a protected environment	Yes	Yes
Can be administered to family members or close contacts of immunosuppressed persons requiring a protected environment (e.g., hematopoietic stem cell transplant recipient)	No	Yes
Can be administered to family members or close contacts of persons at high risk but not severely immunosuppressed	Yes	Yes
Can be simultaneously administered with other vaccines	Yes[¶]	Yes**
If not simultaneously administered, can be administered within 4 wk of another live vaccine	Prudent to space 4 wk apart	Yes
If not simultaneously administered, can be administered within 4 wk of an inactivated vaccine	Yes	Yes

*Children aged 6 months to 8 years who have never received influenza vaccine before should receive 2 doses. Those who only receive 1 dose in their first year of vaccination should receive 2 doses in the following year, spaced 4 weeks apart.

[†]Persons at higher risk for complications of influenza infection because of underlying medical conditions should not receive LAIV. Persons at higher risk for complications of influenza infection because of underlying medical conditions include adults and children with chronic disorders of the pulmonary or cardiovascular systems; adults and children with chronic metabolic diseases (including diabetes mellitus), renal dysfunction, hemoglobinopathies, or immunosuppression; children and adolescents receiving long-term aspirin therapy (at risk for developing Reye's syndrome after wild-type influenza infection); persons who have any condition (e.g., cognitive dysfunction, spinal cord injuries, seizure disorders, or other neuromuscular disorders) that can compromise respiratory function or the handling of respiratory secretions or that can increase the risk for aspiration; pregnant women; and residents of nursing homes and other chronic-care facilities that house persons with chronic medical conditions.

[§]Clinicians and immunization programs should screen for possible reactive airways diseases when considering use of LAIV for children aged 2-4 years and should avoid use of this vaccine in children with asthma or a recent wheezing episode. Health care providers should consult the medical record, when available, to identify children aged 2-4 years with asthma or recurrent wheezing that might indicate asthma. In addition, to identify children who might be at greater risk for asthma and possibly at increased risk for wheezing after receiving LAIV, parents or caregivers of children aged 2-4 years should be asked: "In the past 12 months, has a health care provider ever told you that your child had wheezing or asthma?" Children whose parents or caregivers answer "yes" to this question and children who have asthma or who had a wheezing episode noted in the medical record during the preceding 12 months should not receive LAIV.

[¶]LAIV coadministration has been evaluated systematically only among children aged 12-15 months who received measles, mumps, and rubella vaccine or varicella vaccine.

**TIV coadministration has been evaluated systematically only among adults who received pneumococcal polysaccharide or zoster vaccine.

Modified from *MMWR* 56(RR-6), 2007.

INDICATIONS FOR USE OF ANTIVIRALS

PERSONS FOR WHOM ANTIVIRAL TREATMENT SHOULD BE CONSIDERED

If possible, antiviral treatment should be started within 48 hours of influenza illness onset. The effectiveness of initiating antiviral treatment more than 48 hours after illness onset has not been established. Persons for whom antiviral treatment should be considered include:

- Persons hospitalized with laboratory-confirmed influenza (limited data suggest benefit even for persons whose antiviral treatment is initiated more than 48 hours after illness onset)
- Persons with laboratory-confirmed influenza pneumonia
- Persons with laboratory-confirmed influenza and bacterial coinfection
- Persons with laboratory-confirmed influenza infection who are at higher risk for influenza complications
- Persons presenting to medical care with laboratory-confirmed influenza within 48 hours of influenza illness onset who want to decrease the duration or severity of their symptoms and transmission of influenza to others at higher risk for complications

PERSONS FOR WHOM ANTIVIRAL CHEMOPROPHYLAXIS SHOULD BE CONSIDERED DURING PERIODS OF INCREASED INFLUENZA ACTIVITY IN THE COMMUNITY

Persons at high risk during the 2 weeks after influenza vaccination (after the second dose for children younger than 9 years who have not previously been vaccinated) if influenza viruses are circulating in the community

Persons at high risk for whom influenza vaccine is contraindicated

Family members or health care providers who are unvaccinated and are likely to have ongoing, close exposure to persons at high risk or unvaccinated persons or infants younger than 6 months

Persons and their family members and close contacts and health care workers when circulating strains of influenza virus in the community are not matched with vaccine strains

Persons with immune deficiencies or those who might not respond to vaccination (e.g., persons infected with HIV or other immunosuppressed conditions or who are receiving immunosuppressive medications)

Unvaccinated staff and persons during response to an outbreak in a closed institutional setting with residents at high risk (e.g., extended-care facilities)

Modified from *MMWR* 57(RR-7), 2008.

NOTE: Recommended antiviral medications (neuraminidase inhibitors) are not licensed for chemoprophylaxis of children younger than 1 year (oseltamivir) or younger than 5 years (zanamivir). Updates or supplements to these recommendations (e.g., expanded age or risk group indications for licensed vaccines) might be required. Health care providers should be alert to announcements of recommendation updates and should check the CDC influenza website periodically for additional information (http://www.cdc.gov/flu).

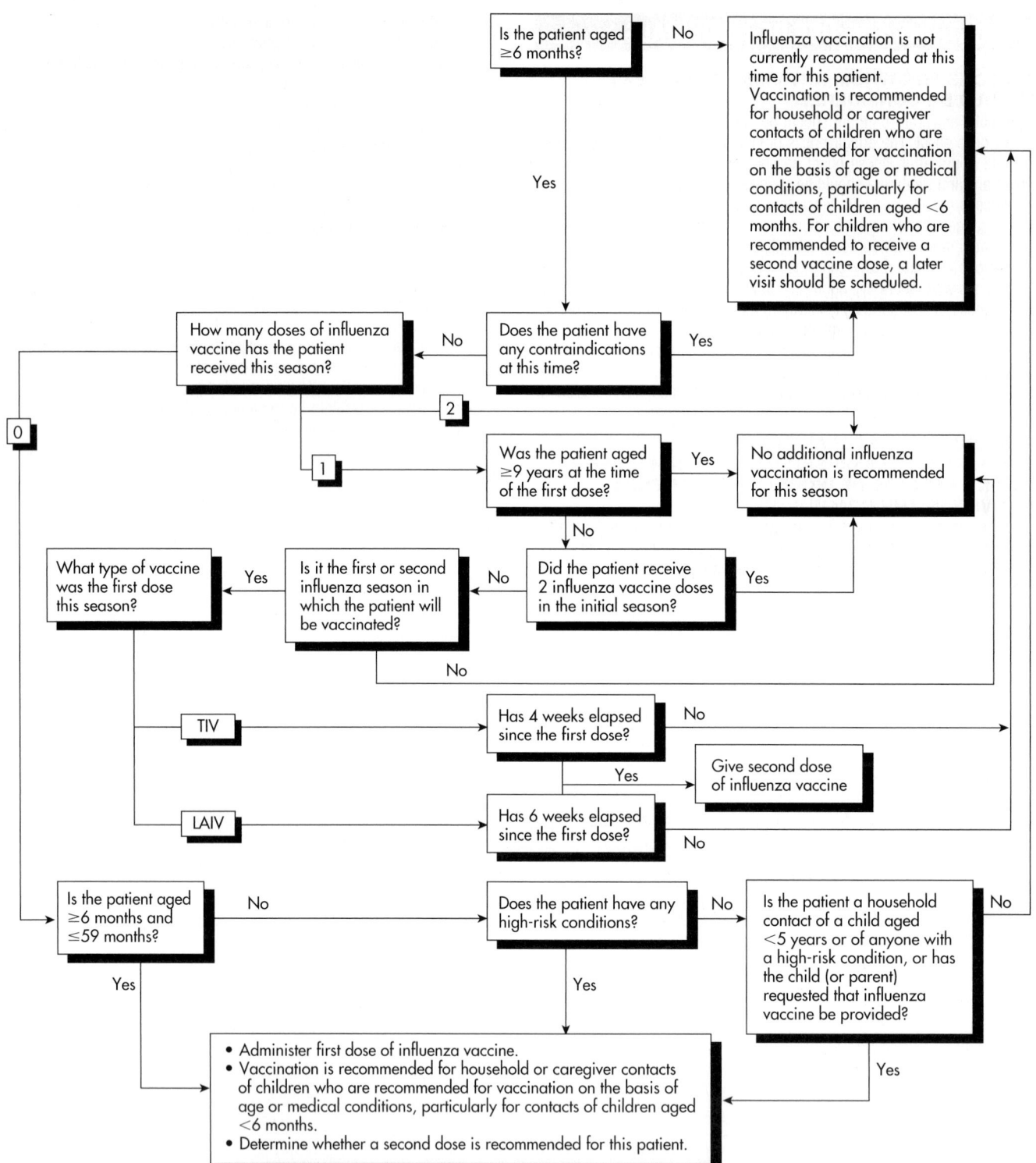

FIG. 6 Algorithm for determining recommended influenza immunization actions for children. *TIV,* Trivalent inactivated influenza vaccine; *LAIV,* Live attenuated influenza vaccine. (Modified with permission from the American Academy of Pediatrics' Committee on Infectious Diseases: Prevention of influenza: recommendations for influenza immunization of children, 2006-2007, *Pediatrics* 119:846-51, 2007.)

HIV Testing and Postexposure Prophylaxis

RECOMMENDATIONS FOR HIV TESTING OF ADULTS, ADOLESCENTS, AND PREGNANT WOMEN

RECOMMENDATIONS FOR ADULTS AND ADOLESCENTS

The CDC recommends that diagnostic human immunodeficiency virus (HIV) testing and opt-out HIV screening be a part of routine clinical care in all health care settings while also preserving the patient's option to decline HIV testing and ensuring a provider-patient relationship conducive to optimal clinical and preventive care. The recommendations are intended for providers in all health care settings, including hospital emergency departments, urgent-care clinics, inpatient services, sexually transmitted disease (STD) clinics or other venues offering clinical STD services, tuberculosis (TB) clinics, substance abuse treatment clinics, other public health clinics, community clinics, correctional health care facilities, and primary care settings. The guidelines address HIV testing in health care settings only; they do not modify existing guidelines concerning HIV counseling, testing, and referral for persons at high risk for HIV who seek or receive HIV testing in nonclinical settings (e.g., community-based organizations, outreach settings, or mobile vans).[4]

SCREENING FOR HIV INFECTION

- In all health care settings, screening for HIV infection should be performed routinely for all patients aged 13 to 64 years. Health care providers should initiate screening unless prevalence of undiagnosed HIV infection in their patients has been documented to be less than 0.1%. In the absence of existing data for HIV prevalence, health care providers should initiate voluntary HIV screening until they establish that the diagnostic yield is less than 1 per 1000 patients screened, at which point such screening is no longer warranted.
- All patients initiating treatment for TB should be screened routinely for HIV infection.
- All patients seeking treatment for STDs, including all patients visiting STD clinics, should be screened routinely for HIV during each visit for a new complaint, regardless of whether the patient is known or suspected to have specific behavior risks for HIV infection.

REPEAT SCREENING

- Health care providers should subsequently test all persons likely to be at high risk for HIV at least annually. Persons likely to be at high risk include users of injection drugs and their sex partners, persons who exchange sex for money or drugs, sex partners of persons who are HIV infected, and men who have sex with men (MSM) or heterosexual persons who themselves or whose sex partners have had more than one sex partner since their most recent HIV test.
- Health care providers should encourage patients and their prospective sex partners to be tested before initiating a new sexual relationship.
- Repeat screening of persons not likely to be at high risk for HIV should be performed on the basis of clinical judgment.
- Unless recent HIV test results are immediately available, any person whose blood or body fluid is the source of an occupational exposure for a health care provider should be informed of the incident and tested for HIV infection at the time the exposure occurs.

CONSENT AND PRETEST INFORMATION

- Screening should be voluntary and undertaken only with the patient's knowledge and understanding that HIV testing is planned.
- Patients should be informed orally or in writing that HIV testing will be performed unless they decline (opt-out screening). Oral or written information should include an explanation of HIV infection and the meanings of positive and negative test results, and the patient should be offered an opportunity to ask questions and decline testing. With such notification, consent for HIV screening should be incorporated into the patient's general informed consent for medical care on the same basis as are other

[4]Data from *MMWR* 57(RR-10), 2008.

screening or diagnostic tests; a separate consent form for HIV testing is not recommended.
- Easily understood informational materials should be made available in the languages of the commonly encountered populations within the service area. The competence of interpreters and bilingual staff to provide language assistance to patients with limited English proficiency must be ensured.
- If a patient declines an HIV test, this decision should be documented in the medical record.

DIAGNOSTIC TESTING FOR HIV INFECTION

- All patients with signs or symptoms consistent with HIV infection or an opportunistic illness characteristic of acquired immunodeficiency syndrome (AIDS) should be tested for HIV.
- Clinicians should maintain a high level of suspicion for acute HIV infection in all patients who have a compatible clinical syndrome and who report recent high-risk behavior. When acute retroviral syndrome is a possibility, a plasma RNA test should be used in conjunction with an HIV antibody test to diagnose acute HIV infection.
- Patients or persons responsible for the patient's care should be notified orally that testing is planned, advised of the indication for testing and the implications of positive and negative test results, and offered an opportunity to ask questions and decline testing. With such notification, the patient's general consent for medical care is considered sufficient for diagnostic HIV testing.

HIV SCREENING FOR PREGNANT WOMEN AND THEIR INFANTS*
Universal Opt-Out Screening

- All pregnant women in the United States should be screened for HIV infection.
- Screening should occur after a woman is notified that HIV screening is recommended for all pregnant patients and that she will receive an HIV test as part of the routine panel of prenatal tests unless she declines (opt-out screening).
- HIV testing must be voluntary and free from coercion. No woman should be tested without her knowledge.
- Pregnant women should receive oral or written information that includes an explanation of HIV infection, a description of interventions that can reduce HIV transmission from mother to infant, and the meanings of positive and negative test results. They should be offered an opportunity to ask questions and decline testing.
- No additional process or written documentation of informed consent beyond what is required for other routine prenatal tests should be required for HIV testing.
- If a patient declines an HIV test, this decision should be documented in the medical record.

ADDRESSING REASONS FOR DECLINING TESTING

- Providers should discuss and address reasons for declining an HIV test (e.g., lack of perceived risk, fear of the disease, and concerns regarding partner violence or potential stigma or discrimination).
- Women who decline an HIV test because they have had a previous negative test result should be informed of the importance of retesting during each pregnancy.
- Logistical reasons for not testing (e.g., scheduling) should be resolved.
- Certain women who initially decline an HIV test might accept at a later date, especially if their concerns are discussed. Certain women will continue to decline testing, and their decisions should be respected and documented in the medical record.

Timing of HIV Testing

- To promote informed and timely therapeutic decisions, health care providers should test women for HIV as early as possible during each pregnancy. Women who decline the test early in prenatal care should be encouraged to be tested at a subsequent visit.
- A second HIV test during the third trimester, preferably less than 36 weeks of gestation, is cost effective even in areas of low HIV prevalence and may be considered for all pregnant women. A second HIV test during

the third trimester is recommended for women who meet one or more of the following criteria:

1. Women who receive health care in jurisdictions with elevated incidence of HIV or AIDS among women aged 15 to 45 years. In 2004, these jurisdictions included Alabama, Connecticut, Delaware, the District of Columbia, Florida, Georgia, Illinois, Louisiana, Maryland, Massachusetts, Mississippi, Nevada, New Jersey, New York, North Carolina, Pennsylvania, Puerto Rico, Rhode Island, South Carolina, Tennessee, Texas, and Virginia.[5]
2. Women who receive health care in facilities in which prenatal screening identifies at least one pregnant woman who is infected with HIV per 1000 women screened.
3. Women who are known to be at high risk for acquiring HIV (e.g., users of injection drugs and their sex partners, women who exchange sex for money or drugs, women who are sex partners of persons who are infected with HIV, and women who have had a new or more than one sex partner during this pregnancy).
4. Women who have signs or symptoms consistent with acute HIV infection. When acute retroviral syndrome is a possibility, a plasma RNA test should be used in conjunction with an HIV antibody test to diagnose acute HIV infection.

Rapid Testing During Labor

- Any woman with undocumented HIV status at the time of labor should be screened with a rapid HIV test unless she declines (opt-out screening).

---

[5]A second HIV test in the third trimester is as cost effective as other common health interventions when HIV incidence among women of childbearing age is =17 HIV cases per 100,000 person-years. In 2004, in jurisdictions with available data on HIV case rates, a rate of 17 new HIV diagnoses per year per 100,000 women aged 15 to 45 years was associated with an AIDS case rate of at least nine AIDS diagnoses per year per 100,000 women aged 15 to 45 years (CDC, unpublished data, 2005). As of 2004, the jurisdictions listed above exceeded these thresholds. The list of specific jurisdictions where a second test in the third trimester is recommended will be updated periodically based on surveillance data.

- Reasons for declining a rapid test should be explored (see "Addressing Reasons for Declining Testing").
- Immediate initiation of appropriate antiretroviral prophylaxis should be recommended to women on the basis of a reactive rapid test result without waiting for the result of a confirmatory test.

Postpartum/Newborn Testing

- When a woman's HIV status is still unknown at the time of delivery, she should be screened immediately postpartum with a rapid HIV test unless she declines (opt-out screening).
- When the mother's HIV status is unknown postpartum, rapid testing of the newborn as soon as possible after birth is recommended so that antiretroviral prophylaxis can be offered to infants exposed to HIV. Women should be informed that identifying HIV antibodies in the newborn indicates that the mother is infected.
- For infants whose HIV exposure status is unknown and who are in foster care, the person legally authorized to provide consent should be informed that rapid HIV testing is recommended for infants whose biologic mothers have not been tested.
- The benefits of neonatal antiretroviral prophylaxis are best realized when it is initiated within 12 hours after birth.

Confirmatory Testing

- Whenever possible, uncertainties regarding laboratory test results indicating HIV infection status should be resolved before final decisions are made regarding reproductive options, antiretroviral therapy, cesarean delivery, or other interventions.
- If the confirmatory test result is not available before delivery, immediate initiation of appropriate antiretroviral prophylaxis should be recommended to any pregnant patient whose HIV screening test result is reactive to reduce the risk for perinatal transmission.

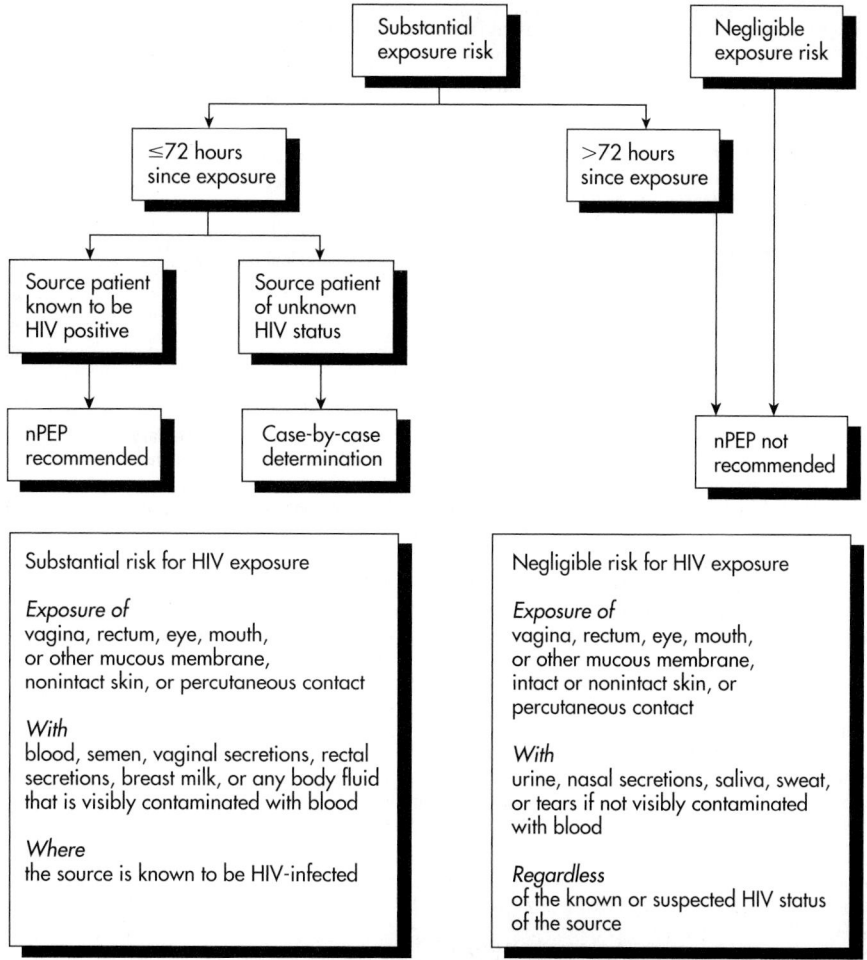

FIG. 7 Algorithm for evaluation and treatment of possible nonoccupational HIV exposure. *nPEP,* Nonoccupational postexposure prophylaxis. (Modified from *MMWR* 54[RR-2], 2005.)

TABLE 32   HIV Exposure, Estimated Per-Act Risk

Exposure Route	Risk per 10,000 Exposures to an Infected Source
Blood transfusion	9000
Needle-sharing injection drug use	67
Receptive anal intercourse	50
Percutaneous needle stick	30
Receptive penile-vaginal intercourse	10
Insertive anal intercourse	6.5
Insertive penile-vaginal intercourse	5
Receptive oral intercourse	1
Insertive oral intercourse	0.5

NOTE: Estimates of risk for transmission from sexual exposures assume no condom use. Source refers to oral intercourse performed on a man.
Modified from *MMWR* 54(RR-2), 2005.

TABLE 33 Regimens for 28-Day Postexposure Prophylaxis for HIV Infection*

Regimen	Dose	Daily Pill Burden[†]no.	Advantages	Disadvantages
Two-Drug Regimens				
Tenofovir–emtricitabine (Truvada)[‡]	One tablet (300 mg of tenofovir with 200 mg of emtricitabine) once daily	1	Well-tolerated; once-daily dosing	Potential nephrotoxicity
Zidovudine–lamivudine (Combivir)[§]	One tablet (300 mg of zidovudine with 150 mg of lamivudine) twice daily	2	Preferred in pregnancy	Twice-daily dosing; less well-tolerated than tenofovir–emtricitabine (nausea, asthenia, neutropenia, anemia, abnormal liver-enzyme levels)
Three-Drug Regimens[‖]				
Ritonavir–lopinavir (Kaletra) (plus either tenofovir–emtricitabine or zidovudine–lamivudine)	Two tablets (50 mg of ritonavir with 200 mg of lopinavir per tablet) twice daily, or four tablets once daily	5 or 6	Either once-daily or twice-daily dosing; one copayment; no refrigeration required; most experience in pregnancy; high genetic barrier to resistance	Gastrointestinal side effects such as diarrhea; may cause elevated liver-enzyme levels or hepatitis
Ritonavir plus atazanavir (plus either tenofovir–emtricitabine or zidovudine–lamivudine)	100 mg of ritonavir plus 300 mg of atazanavir once daily	3 or 4	Once-daily dosing; well tolerated	Ritonavir must be refrigerated; potential for asymptomatic jaundice, renal stones; may cause elevated liver-enzyme levels or hepatitis
Ritonavir plus darunavir (plus either tenofovir–emtricitabine or zidovudine–lamivudine)	100 mg of ritonavir plus two tablets, each containing 400 mg of darunavir, once daily	4 or 5	Once-daily dosing; high genetic barrier to resistance	Ritonavir must be refrigerated; gastrointestinal side effects; may cause elevated liver-enzyme levels or hepatitis

*Tenofovir, emtricitabine, and lamivudine all have activity against hepatitis B. Patients with chronic active hepatitis B (i.e., patients who are positive for hepatitis B surface antigen) may have flares of hepatitis on withdrawal of these agents at the completion of postexposure prophylaxis treatment. Referral to a hepatitis specialist or serial monthly monitoring of liver-enzyme levels for up to 6 months after treatment should be considered.

[†]The daily pill burden in the three-drug regimens depends on which two-drug regimen is chosen.

[‡]The dose of tenofovir–emtricitabine should be reduced to one tablet every 48 hours in patients with a creatinine clearance of 30 to 49 ml per minute. Tenofovir–emtricitabine is not recommended in patients with a creatinine clearance of less than 30 ml per minute or in patients who are undergoing hemodialysis; see the guidelines from the Department of Health and Human Services for considerations regarding doses of individual agents in patients with advanced renal dysfunction.

[§]Zidovudine–lamivudine is not recommended in patients with a creatinine clearance of less than 50 ml per minute; see the guidelines from the Department of Health and Human Services for considerations regarding doses of individual agents in patients with renal dysfunction.

[‖]The boosting agent ritonavir is not considered to be an active drug in tabulating the number of agents in the three-drug regimen.

From Landovitz RJ, Currier JS: Postexposure prophylaxis for HIV infection, *N Engl J Med* 361:1768-75, 2009.

TABLE 34 Antiretroviral Therapy Medications, Adult Dosage, and Side Effects

Medication	Adult Dosage*	Side Effects and Toxicities
Combination Tablets		
Lopinavir/ritonavir (Kaletra)‡	3 tablets twice daily 400 mg lopinavir/100 mg ritonavir	Diarrhea, nausea, vomiting; asthenia; elevated transaminases; hyperglycemia; fat redistribution; lipid abnormalities; possible increased bleeding in persons with hemophilia; pancreatitis
Zidovudine/lamivudine (Combivir)	1 tablet twice daily 300 mg zidovudine/150 mg lamivudine	See following individual medications
Zidovudine/lamivudine/abacavir (Trizivir)	1 tablet twice daily 300 mg zidovudine/150 mg lamivudine/300 mg abacavir	See following individual medications
Lamivudine/abacavir (Epzicom)	1 tablet once daily 300 mg lamivudine/600 mg abacavir	See following individual medications
Emtricitabine/tenofovir (Truvada)	1 tablet once daily 200 mg emtricitabine/300 mg tenofovir	See following individual medications
Single Agents		
Nucleoside and nucleotide reverse transcriptase inhibitors (side effects as a class: lactic acidosis, severe hepatomegaly with steatosis, including some fatal cases)		
Abacavir (Ziagen, ABC)‡	300 mg twice daily or 600 mg once daily	Severe hypersensitivity reaction (can be fatal); nausea; vomiting
Didanosine (Videx, ddl)‡	>60 kg (132 lb) body weight: 200 mg twice daily or 400 mg daily; if with tenofovir, 250 mg/daily	Pancreatitis; nausea, diarrhea; peripheral neuropathy
	<60 kg (132 lb): 125 mg twice daily or 250 mg daily; if with tenofovir, dose not established	
	Do not use with stavudine (d4T, Zerit) during pregnancy; avoid ddl/d4T combination in general because of increased risk for adverse events (e.g., neuropathy, pancreatitis, and hyperlactatemia)	
Emtricitabine (Emtriva, FTC)	200 mg once daily	Minimal toxicity; lactic acidosis and hepatic steatosis a rare but possibly life-threatening event
Lamivudine (Epivir, 3TC)‡	150 mg twice daily or 300 mg once daily	Minimal toxicity; lactic acidosis and hepatic steatosis a rare but possibly life-threatening event
Stavudine (Zerit, d4T)‡	>60 kg (132 lb) body weight: 40 mg twice daily	Pancreatitis; peripheral neuropathy; rapidly progressive ascending neuromuscular weakness (rare)
	<60 kg (132 lb) body weight: 30 mg twice daily	
	Do not use with didanosine (ddl, Videx) during pregnancy; avoid ddl/d4T combination in general because of increased risk of adverse events (e.g., neuropathy, pancreatitis, and hyperlactatemia)	
Tenofovir (Viread)	300 mg daily	Nausea, vomiting, diarrhea; headache; asthenia; flatulence; renal impairment
Zidovudine (Retrovir, AZT)‡	200 mg three times daily or 300 mg twice daily	Bone marrow suppression (anemia, neutropenia); gastrointestinal intolerance; headache; insomnia; asthenia; and myopathy
Nonnucleoside reverse transcriptase inhibitors (side effects as a class: Stevens-Johnson syndrome)		
Efavirenz (Sustiva)	600 mg daily at bedtime	Rash; central nervous system symptoms (e.g., dizziness, impaired concentration, insomnia, and abnormal dreams); transaminase elevation; false-positive cannabinoid test
Protease inhibitors (side effects as a class: gastrointestinal intolerance, hyperlipidemia, hyperglycemia, diabetes, fat redistribution, and possible increased bleeding in hemophiliacs; do not use during known or possible pregnancy)		
Atazanavir (Reyataz)	400 mg once daily; if administered with tenofovir plus ritonavir, 300 mg once daily	Indirect hyperbilirubinemia; prolonged PR interval (use caution in patients with underlying cardiac conduction defects or on concomitant medications that can cause PR prolongation)
Fosamprenavir (Lexiva)‡	1400 mg twice daily	Gastrointestinal intolerance, nausea, vomiting, diarrhea; rash; elevated transaminases; headache
Indinavir (Crixivan)	800 mg q8h	Gastrointestinal intolerance, nausea; nephrolithiasis; headache; asthenia; blurred vision; metallic taste; thrombocytopenia; hemolytic anemia; indirect hyperbilirubinemia (inconsequential)
	With ritonavir (might increase risk for renal adverse events): 800 mg indinavir and 100 mg ritonavir q12h or 800 mg indinavir and 200 mg ritonavir every q12h	
Nelfinavir (Viracept)‡	750 mg three times daily or one 250 mg twice daily	Diarrhea; elevated transaminases
Ritonavir (Norvir)‡	See doses used in combination with other specific protease inhibitors	Gastrointestinal intolerance; nausea, vomiting, diarrhea; paresthesias; hepatitis; pancreatitis; asthenia; taste perversion; many drug interactions
Saquinavir (hard-gel capsule) (Invirase)	With ritonavir: 400 mg saquinavir and 400 mg ritonavir twice daily or 1000 mg saquinavir and 100 mg ritonavir twice daily	Gastrointestinal intolerance; nausea, diarrhea; headache; elevated transaminases
Saquinavir (soft-gel capsule) (Fortovase)	With ritonavir: 400 mg saquinavir and 400 mg ritonavir twice daily or 1000 mg saquinavir and 100 mg ritonavir twice daily	Gastrointestinal intolerance; nausea, diarrhea; abdominal pain; dyspepsia; headache; elevated transaminases

Sources: Modified from U.S. Department of Health and Human Services and the Henry J. Kaiser Family Foundation: *Guidelines for the use of antiretroviral agents in HIV-infected adults and adolescents.* Available at http://www.aidsinfo.nih.gov/guidelines/default_db2.asp?id=50 (refer to website for updated versions); Bartlett JG, Finkbeiner AK: HIV drugs: the guide to living with HIV infection, 2001. Available at http://www.thebody.com/jh/bartlett/drugs.html.

*For pediatric dosing information, see *Guidelines for use of antiretroviral agents in pediatric HIV infection.* Available at http://www.aidsinfo.nih.gov/guidelines/default_db2.asp?id=51.

‡Pediatric formulation available.

TABLE 35 Laboratory Tests Generally Recommended for Persons after Exposure to HIV*

Test	RECOMMENDED DURING TREATMENT		RECOMMENDED AT FOLLOW-UP		
	Baseline	Symptom-Directed†	4-6 wk	12 wk	24 wk
ELISA for HIV antibodies	Yes	Yes	Yes	Yes	Yes
Creatinine, liver function, and complete blood count with differential count	Yes	Yes	No	No	No
HIV viral load	No	Yes	No	No	No
Anti-HBs antibodies	Yes‡	No	No	No	No
HBsAg	Yes‡§	No	No	No	No
HCV antibodies	Yes	No	Yes	Yes	Yes
HCV RNA‖	No	Yes	Yes	Yes	Yes
Screening, including rapid plasma reagin test, for other sexually transmitted infections¶	Yes	Yes	No	Yes	No

Anti-HBs antibodies, Hepatitis B virus surface antibodies; *ELISA,* enzyme-linked immunosorbent assay; *HBsAg,* hepatitis B surface antigen; *HCV,* hepatitis C virus.

*Patients who receive zidovudine plus lamivudine–based regimens should have a complete blood count and measurement of liver-enzyme levels at 2 weeks of treatment, irrespective of the presence or absence of clinical symptoms. Tenofovir plus emtricitabine–based regimens generally involve few side effects, and symptom-directed assessment of serum creatinine or liver-enzyme levels should be considered. The addition of a ritonavir-boosted protease inhibitor should be followed by symptom-directed assessment of liver-enzyme levels, serum glucose levels, or both.

†Symptom-directed tests are for signs or symptoms of toxic effects (rash, nausea, vomiting, or abdominal pain) or HIV seroconversion (fever, fatigue, lymphadenopathy, rash, or oral or genital ulcers).

‡If tests for anti-HBs antibodies and HBsAg are both negative, a vaccination series against HBV infection should be initiated and completed.

§If the patient is HBsAg-positive, he or she should have monthly follow-up of liver function tests after discontinuation of postexposure prophylactic regimens containing tenofovir, lamivudine, or emtricitabine; referral to a specialist in viral hepatitis should be considered.

‖HCV RNA testing may identify early HCV seroconversion; early detection and treatment during acute HCV infection may avert or ameliorate chronic disease. Data are from Dienstag and McHutchison.

¶Rapid plasma reagin testing and testing of urethral-swab and rectal-swab specimens for gonorrhea and chlamydia and of pharyngeal-swab specimens for gonorrhea should be performed as appropriate, according to the patient's sexual risk-taking behaviors and the type of exposure to HIV.

From Landovitz RJ, Currier JS: Postexposure prophylaxis for HIV infection, *N Engl J Med* 361:1768-1775, 2009.

BOX 4 Situations for Which Expert Consultation for HIV Postexposure Prophylaxis Is Advised[6]

- Delayed (i.e., later than 24-36 hours) exposure report
  1. The interval after which there is no benefit from postexposure prophylaxis (PEP) is undefined
- Unknown source (e.g., needle in sharps disposal container or laundry)
  1. Decide use of PEP on a case-by-case basis
  2. Consider the severity of the exposure and the epidemiologic likelihood of HIV exposure
  3. Do not test needles or other sharp instruments for HIV
- Known or suspected pregnancy in the exposed person
  1. Does not preclude the use of optimal PEP regimens
  2. Do not deny PEP solely on the basis of pregnancy
- Resistance of the source virus to antiretroviral agents
  1. Influence of drug resistance on transmission risk is unknown
  2. Selection of drugs to which the source person's virus is unlikely to be resistant is recommended if the source person's virus is known or suspected to be resistant to one or more of the drugs considered for the PEP regimen
  3. Resistance testing of the source person's virus at the time of the exposure is not recommended
- Toxicity of the initial PEP regimen
  1. Adverse symptoms such as nausea and diarrhea are common with PEP
  2. Symptoms often can be managed without changing the PEP regimen by prescribing antimotility and/or antiemetic agents
  3. Modification of dose intervals (i.e., administering a lower dose of drug more frequently throughout the day, as recommended by the manufacturer) in other situations might help alleviate symptoms

[6]Local experts and/or the National Clinicians' Postexposure Prophylaxis Hotline (PEPline [888-448-4911]).

BOX 5 Occupational Exposure Management Resources

National Clinicians' Postexposure Prophylaxis Hotline (PEPline)
Run by University of California–San Francisco/San Francisco General Hospital staff; supported by the Health Resources and Services Administration, Ryan White CARE Act, HIV/AIDS Bureau, AIDS Education and Training Centers, and CDC

Phone: 888-448-4911
Internet: http://www.ucsf.edu/hivcntr

Needlestick!
A website to help clinicians manage and document occupational blood and body fluid exposures. Developed and maintained by the University of California, Los Angeles (UCLA), Emergency Medicine Center, UCLA School of Medicine, and funded in part by CDC and the Agency for Healthcare Research and Quality

Internet: http://www.needlestick.mednet.ucla.edu

Hepatitis Hotline

Phone: 888-443-7232
Internet: http://www.cdc.gov/ncidod/diseases/hepatitis/index.htm

Reporting to CDC: Occupationally acquired HIV infections and failures of PEP

Phone: 800-893-0485

HIV Antiretroviral Pregnancy Registry

Phone: 800-258-4263
Fax: 800-800-1052
Address: 1410 Commonwealth Dr., Suite 215, Wilmington, NC 28405
Internet: http://www.glaxowellcome.com/preg_reg/antiretroviral

Food and Drug Administration Report unusual or severe toxicity to antiretroviral agents

Phone: 800-332-1088
Address: MedWatch, HF-2, FDA, 5600 Fishers Lane, Rockville, MD 20857
Internet: http://www.fda.gov/medwatch

HIV/AIDS Treatment Information Service

Internet: http://www.hivatis.org

BOX 6   Management of Occupational Blood Exposures

Provide Immediate Care to the Exposure Site
- Wash wounds and skin with soap and water
- Flush mucous membranes with water

Determine Risk Associated with Exposure
- Type of fluid (e.g., blood, visibly bloody fluid, other potentially infectious fluid or tissue, and concentrated virus)
- Type of exposure (e.g., percutaneous injury, mucous membrane or nonintact skin exposure, and bites resulting in blood exposure)

Evaluate Exposure Source
- Assess the risk of infection using available information
- Test known sources for HBsAg, anti-HCV, and HIV antibodies (consider using rapid testing)
- For unknown sources, assess risk of exposure to HBV, HCV, or HIV infection
- Do not test discarded needles or syringes for virus contamination

Evaluate the Exposed Person
- Assess immune status for HBV infection (i.e., by history of hepatitis B vaccination and vaccine response)

Give PEP for Exposures Posing Risk of Infection Transmission
- HBV: See Table 27
- HCV: PEP not recommended
- HIV: See Tables 33, 34, and 35 and Fig. 7
  1. Initiate PEP as soon as possible, preferably within hours of exposure
  2. Offer pregnancy testing to all women of childbearing age not known to be pregnant
  3. Seek expert consultation if viral resistance is suspected
  4. Administer PEP for 4 weeks if tolerated

Perform Follow-up Testing and Provide Counseling
- Advise exposed persons to seek medical evaluation for any acute illness occurring during follow-up

HBV Exposures
- Perform follow-up anti-HBs testing in persons who receive hepatitis B vaccine
  1. Test for anti-HBs 1 to 2 months after last dose of vaccine
  2. Anti-HBs response to vaccine cannot be ascertained if HBIG was received in the previous 3 to 4 months

HCV Exposures
- Perform baseline and follow-up testing for anti-HCV and alanine aminotransferase 4 to 6 months after exposure
- Perform HCV RNA at 4 to 6 weeks if earlier diagnosis of HCV infection desired
- Confirm repeatedly reactive anti-HCV enzyme immunoassays with supplemental tests

HIV Exposures
- Perform HIV-antibody testing for at least 6 months after exposure (e.g., at baseline, 6 weeks, 3 months, and 6 months)
- Perform HIV-antibody testing if illness compatible with an acute retroviral syndrome occurs
- Advise exposed persons to use precautions to prevent secondary transmission during the follow-up period
- Evaluate exposed persons taking PEP within 72 hr after exposure and monitor for drug toxicity for at least 2 weeks

HBIG, Hepatitis B immune globulin; *HBsAg,* hepatitis B surface antigen; *HBV,* hepatitis B virus; *HCV,* hepatitis C virus; *HIV,* human immunodeficiency virus; *PEP,* postexposure prophylaxis; *RNA,* ribonucleic acid.

Endocarditis Prophylaxis[7]

TABLE 36 Cardiac Conditions Associated with the Highest Risk of Adverse Outcome from Endocarditis for Which Prophylaxis with Dental Procedures Is Recommended

Prosthetic cardiac valve

Previous infective endocarditis

CHD*

Unrepaired cyanotic CHD, including palliative shunts and conduits

Completely repaired congenital heart defect with prosthetic material or device, whether placed by surgery or by catheter intervention, during the first 6 mo after the procedure[†]

Repaired CHD with residual defects at the site or adjacent to the site of a prosthetic patch or prosthetic device (that inhibit endothelialization)

Cardiac transplant recipients who develop cardiac valvulopathy

CHD, Congenital heart disease.
*Except for the conditions listed above, antibiotic prophylaxis is no longer recommended for any other form of CHD.
[†]Prophylaxis is recommended because endothelialization of prosthetic material occurs within 6 mo after the procedure.

TABLE 37 Dental Procedures for Which Endocarditis Prophylaxis Is Recommended for Patients in Table 36

All dental procedures that involve manipulation of gingival tissue or the periapical region of teeth or perforation of the oral mucosa*

*The following procedures and events do not need prophylaxis: routine anesthetic injections through noninfected tissue, taking dental radiographs, placement of removable prosthodontic or orthodontic appliances, adjustment of orthodontic appliances, placement of orthodontic brackets, shedding of deciduous teeth, and bleeding from trauma to the lips or oral mucosa.

TABLE 38 Regimens for a Dental Procedure

| Situation | Agent | REGIMEN: SINGLE DOSE 30-60 MIN BEFORE PROCEDURE | |
		Adults	Children
Oral	Amoxicillin	2 g	50 mg/kg
Unable to take oral medication	Ampicillin	2 g IM or IV	50 mg/kg IM or IV
	OR		
	Cefazolin or ceftriaxone*	1 g IM or IV	50 mg/kg IM or IV
Allergic to penicillins or ampicillin, oral	Cephalexin*[†]	2 g	50 mg/kg
	OR		
	Clindamycin	600 mg	20 mg/kg
	OR		
	Azithromycin or clarithromycin	500 mg	15 mg/kg
Allergic to penicillins or ampicillin and unable to take oral medicine	Cefazolin or ceftriaxone[†]	1 g IM or IV	50 mg/kg IM or IV
	OR		
	Clindamycin	600 mg IM or IV	20 mg/kg IM or IV

IM, Intramuscular; *IV,* intravenous.
*Or other first-generation or second-generation oral cephalosporin in equivalent adult or pediatric dosage.
[†]Cephalosporins should not be used in an individual with a history of anaphylaxis, angioedema, or urticaria with penicillins or ampicillin.

[7]From Prevention of infective endocarditis. A guideline from the American Heart Association Rheumatic Fever, Endocarditis, and Kawasaki Disease Committee, Council on Cardiovascular Disease in the Young, and the Council on Clinical Cardiology, Council on Cardiovascular Surgery and Anesthesia, and the Quality of Care and Outcomes Research Interdisciplinary Working Group. Circulation published online Apr 19, 2007, DOI: 10.1161/CIRCULATIONAHA.106.183095. Copyright © 2007 American Heart Association. All rights reserved. Print ISSN: 0009-7322. Online ISSN: 1524-4539.

Clinical Practice Guidelines

V

TABLE 39 Summary of Major Changes in Updated Recommendations

We concluded that bacteremia resulting from daily activities is much more likely to cause IE than bacteremia associated with a dental procedure.

We concluded that only an extremely small number of cases of IE might be prevented by antibiotic prophylaxis even if prophylaxis is 100% effective.

Antibiotic prophylaxis is not recommended based solely on an increased lifetime risk of acquisition of IE.

Limit recommendations for IE prophylaxis only to those conditions listed in Table 36.

Antibiotic prophylaxis is no longer recommended for any other form of CHD, except for the conditions listed in Table 36.

Antibiotic prophylaxis is recommended for all dental procedures that involve manipulation of gingival tissues or periapical region of teeth or perforation of oral mucosa only for patients with underlying cardiac conditions associated with the highest risk of adverse outcome from IE (see Table 36).

Antibiotic prophylaxis is recommended for procedures on respiratory tract or infected skin, skin structures, or musculoskeletal tissue only for patients with underlying cardiac conditions associated with the highest risk of adverse outcome from IE (see Table 36).

Antibiotic prophylaxis solely to prevent IE is not recommended for GU or GI tract procedures.

The writing group reaffirms the procedures noted in the 1997 prophylaxis guidelines for which endocarditis prophylaxis is not recommended and extends this to other common procedures, including ear and body piercing, tattooing, and vaginal delivery and hysterectomy.

NOTE: A guide to the clinical preventive services described is available online at http://www.ahrq.gov/clinic/pocketgd07/. *CHD*, Congenital heart disease; *GI*, gastrointestinal; *GU*, genitourinary; *IE*, infective endocarditis.

Hepatitis C Testing

BOX 7 Recommendations for Prevention and Control of Hepatitis C Virus (HCV) Infection and HCV-Related Chronic Diseases

Recommendations for the Identification of Chronic Hepatitis C Virus Infection Among Persons Born During 1945–1965[8]
- Adults born during 1945-1965 should receive one-time testing for HCV without prior ascertainment of HCV risk.
- All persons with identified HCV infection should receive a brief alcohol screening and intervention as clinically indicated, followed by referral to appropriate care and treatment services for HCV infection and related conditions.[9,10]

Guidelines for Prevention and Treatment of Opportunistic Infections in HIV-Infected Adults and Adolescents[9,10]
- HIV-infected patients should be tested routinely for evidence of chronic HCV infection. Initial testing for HCV should be performed using the most sensitive immunoassays licensed for detection of antibody to HCV (anti-HCV) in blood.

Recommendations for Prevention and Control of Hepatitis C Virus (HCV) Infection and HCV-Related Chronic Disease
Routine HCV testing is recommended for
- Persons who ever injected illegal drugs, including those who injected once or a few times many years ago and do not consider themselves drug users.
- Persons with selected medical conditions, including:
  1. persons who received clotting factor concentrates produced before 1987;
  2. persons who were ever on chronic (long-term) hemodialysis;
  3. persons with persistently abnormal alanine aminotransferase levels.
- Prior recipients of transfusions or organ transplants, including:
  1. persons who were notified that they received blood from a donor who later tested positive for HCV infection;
  2. persons who received a transfusion of blood or blood components before July 1992; and
  3. persons who received an organ transplant before July 1992.

Routine HCV testing is recommended for persons with recognized exposures, including
- Health care, emergency medical, and public safety workers after needle sticks, sharps, or mucosal exposures to HCV-positive blood.
- Children born to HCV-positive women.

From Centers for Disease Control and Prevention: Recommendations for the identification of chronic hepatitis C virus infection among persons born during 1945-1965. *MMWR* 2012:61(4).
[8]Source: Centers for Disease Control and Prevention: Recommendations for the identification of chronic hepatitis C virus infection among persons born during 1945–1965. *MMWR* 2012;61(No. RR–4).
[9]Source: Centers for Disease Control and Prevention: Recommendations for prevention and control of hepatitis C virus (HCV) infection and HCV-related chronic disease. *MMWR* 1998;47(No. RR–19).
[10]Source: Centers for Disease Control and Prevention: Guidelines for prevention and treatment of opportunistic infections in HIV-infected adults and adolescents: Recommendations from CDC, the National Institutes of Health, and the HIV Medicine Association of the Infectious Diseases Society of America. *MMWR* 2009;58(No. RR–4).

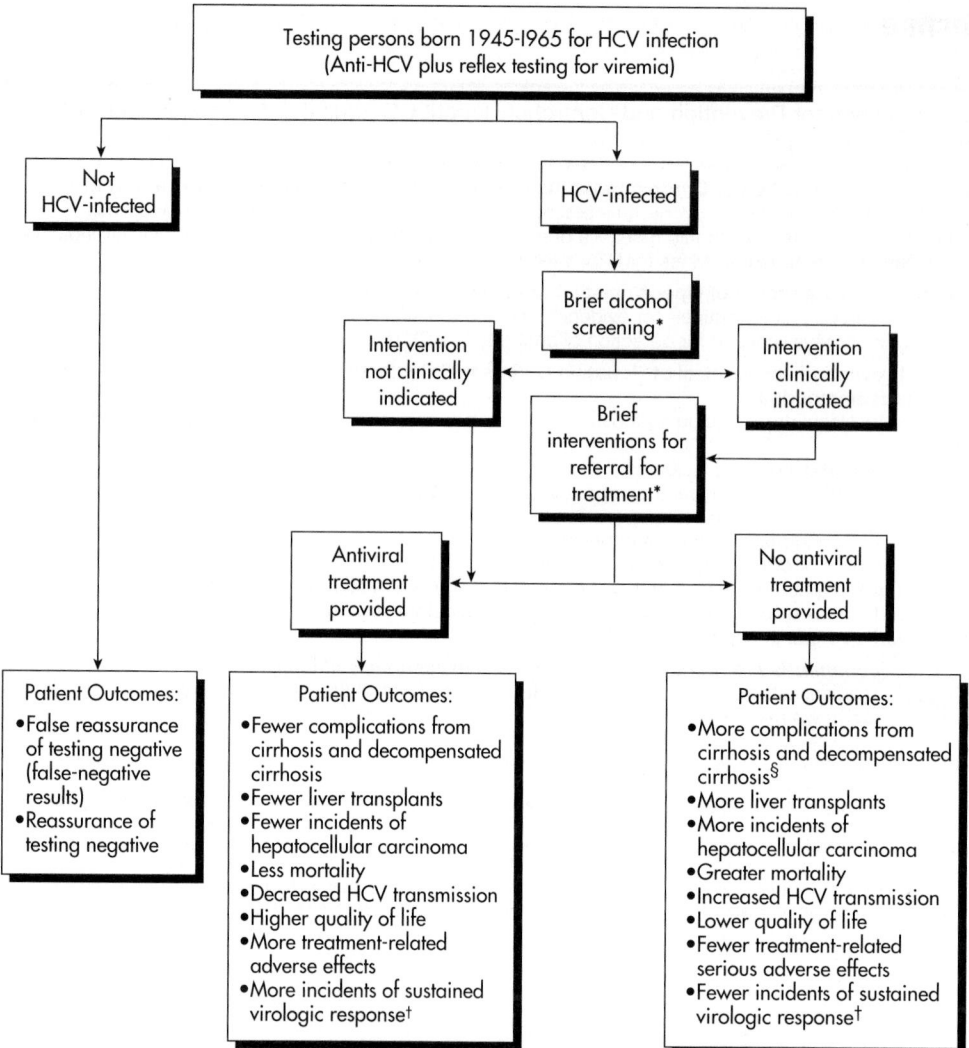

FIG. 8 Analytic Framework for Guiding HCV Testing Among Persons Born During 1945-1965
*Together, these interventions are known as alcohol screening and brief interventions (SBI) For referral for treatment. †Viral eradication after treatment completion. §Cirrhosis with the diagnosis of at least one of the following: ascites, variceal bleeding, encephalopathy, or impaired hepatitis synthetic function.

From Centers for Disease Control and Prevention: Recommendations for the identification of chronic hepatitis C virus infection among persons born during 1945-1965. *MMWR* 2012:61(4).

Hepatitis B Virus Postexposure Protection for Health Care Personnel

TABLE 40 Postexposure Management of Health Care Personnel After Occupational Percutaneous and Mucosal Exposure to Blood and Body Fluids, by Health Care Personnel HepB Vaccination and Response Status

| Health Care Personnel Status | POSTEXPOSURE TESTING | | POSTEXPOSURE PROPHYLAXIS | | Postvaccination Serologic Testing[†] |
	Source Patient (HBsAg)	HCP Testing (anti-HBs)	HBIG*	Vaccination	
Documented responder[‡] after complete series (≥3 doses)	No action needed				
Documented nonresponder[§] after 6 doses	Positive/unknown	—‖	HBIG ×2 separated by 1 mo	—	No
	Negative	No action needed			
Response unknown after 3 doses	Positive/unknown	<10 mIU/mL‖	HBIG ×1	Initiate revaccination	Yes
	Negative	<10 mIU/mL	None		
	Any result	≥10 mIU/mL	No action needed		
Unvaccinated/incompletely vaccinated or vaccine refusers	Positive/unknown	—‖	HBIG ×1	Complete vaccination	Yes
	Negative	—	None	Complete vaccination	Yes

anti-HBs, Antibody to hepatitis B surface antigen; *HBIG*, hepatitis B immune globulin; *HBsAg*, hepatitis B surface antigen; *HCP*, health care personnel.

*HBIG should be administered transmuscularly as soon as possible after exposure when indicated. The effectiveness of HBIG when administered >7 d after percutaneous, mucosal, or nonintact skin exposures is unknown. HBIG dosage is 0.06 mL/kg.

[†]Should be performed 1-2 mo after the last dose of the HepB vaccine series (and 4-6 mo after administration of HBIG to avoid detection of passively administered anti-HBs) using a quantitative method that allows detection of the protective concentration of anti-HBs (≥10 mIU/mL).

[‡]A responder is defined as a person with anti-HBs ≥10 mIU/mL after ≥3 doses of HepB vaccine.

[§]A nonresponder is defined as a person with anti-HBs <10 mIU/mL after ≥6 doses of HepB vaccine.

[‖]HCP who have anti-HBs <10 mIU/mL, or who are unvaccinated or incompletely vaccinated, and sustain an exposure to a source patient who is HBsAg-positive or has unknown HBsAg status, should undergo baseline testing for HBV infection as soon as possible after exposure, and follow-up testing approximately 6 mo later. Initial baseline tests consist of total anti-HBc; testing at approximately 6 months consists of HBsAg and total anti-HBc.

From Centers for Disease Control and Prevention: CDC guidance for evaluating health-care personnel for hepatitis B virus protection and for administering post-exposure management. *MMWR* 2013;62(10).

I. Complementary and Alternative Medicine

II. Nutrition

III. Acute Poisoning

IV. Impairment and Disability Issues

V. Primary Care Procedures (available online)

VI. Patient Teaching Guides (available online)

Definitions of Complementary and Alternative Medicine Terms

Acupuncture   Thin needles are inserted superficially on the skin at locations throughout the body. These points are located along "channels" of energy. Heat can be applied by burning (moxibustion), electric current (electroacupuncture), or pressure (acupressure). Healing is proposed by the restoration of a balance of energy flow called *Qi.* Another explanation suggests that, possibly, the stimulation activates endorphin receptors.

Alexander Technique   A bodywork technique in which rebalancing of "postural sets" (i.e., physical alignment) is taught by mentally focusing on the way correct alignments should look and feel and through verbal and tactile guidance by the practitioner.

Applied Kinesiology   A form of treatment that uses nutrition, physical manipulation, vitamins, diets, and exercise to restore and energize the body. Weak muscles are proposed as a source of dysfunctional health.

Aromatherapy   A form of herbal medicine that uses various oils from plants. Route of administration can be through absorption in the skin or inhalation. The aromatic biochemical structures of certain herbs are thought to act in areas of the brain related to past experiences and emotions (e.g., limbic system).

Ayurveda   A major health system that originated in India and incorporates the body, mind, and spirit to prevent and treat disease. Includes special types of diets, herbs, and minerals.

Biofeedback   A mind-body therapy procedure in which sensors are placed on the body to measure muscle tension, heart rate, and sweat responses or neural activity. Information is provided by visual, auditory, or body-muscle cell activation so as to teach either to increase or decrease physiologic activity, which, when reconstituted, is proposed to improve health problems (e.g., pain, anxiety, or high blood pressure). In some cases, relaxation exercises complement this procedure.

Chelation Therapy   Involves the removal—through intravenous infusion of a chelating agent (synthetic amino acid ethylenediamine tetraacetic acid [EDTA])—of heavy metals, including lead, nickel, and cadmium, as a way to treat certain diseases. Ancillary treatments include the use of vitamins, changes in diet, and exercise.

Cognitive Therapy   Psychological therapy in which the major focus is altering and changing irrational beliefs through a type of Socratic dialogue and self-evaluation of certain illogical thoughts. Conditioning and learning are important components of this therapy.

Craniosacral Therapy   A form of gentle manual manipulation used for diagnosis and for making corrections in a system made up of cerebrospinal fluid, cranial and dural membranes, cranial bones, and sacrum. This system is proposed to be dynamic, with its own physiologic frequency. Through touch and pressure, tension is proposed to be reduced and cranial rhythms normalized, leading to improvement in health and disease.

Diathermy   The use of high-frequency electrical currents as a form of physical therapy and in surgical procedures. The term *diathermy,* derived from the Greek words *dia* and *therma,* literally means "heating through." The three forms of diathermy used by physical therapists are short wave, ultrasound, and microwave.

Eye Movement Desensitization and Reprocessing (EMDR)   A technique that proposes to remove painful memories by behavioral techniques. Rhythmic, multisaccadic eye movements are produced by allowing the patient to track and follow a moving object while imagining a stressful memory or event. By using deconditioning, including verbal interaction with the therapist, the painful memory is extinguished and health improved.

Feldenkrais Method   A bodywork technique that integrates physics, judo, and yoga. The practitioner directs sequences of movement using verbal or hands-on techniques or teaches a system of self-directed exercise to treat physical impairments through the learning of new movement patterns.

Hatha Yoga   The branch of yoga practice that involves physical exercise, breathing practices, and movement. These exercises are designed to have a salutary effect on posture, flexibility, and strength and are intended ultimately to prepare the body to remain still for long periods of meditation.

Hellerwork   A bodywork technique that treats and improves proper body alignment through the development of a more complete awareness of the physical body. The goal is to realign fascia for improvement of standing, sitting, and breathing using "body energy," verbal feedback, and changing emotions and attitudes.

Homeopathy   A form of treatment in which substances (minerals, plant extracts, chemicals, or disease-producing germs), which in sufficient doses would produce a set of illness symptoms in healthy individuals, are given in microdoses to produce a "cure" of those same symptoms. The *symptom* is not thought to be part of the illness but part of a curative process.

Hyperbaric Oxygen   A therapy in which 100% oxygen is given at or above atmospheric pressure. An increase in oxygen in the tissue is proposed to increase blood circulation and improve healing and health and influence the course of disease.

Jin Shin Jyutsu   An ancient bodywork technique to harmonize body, mind, and spirit by gentle touch that uses specific "healing points" at the body surface. The points are proposed to overlie flowing energy (Qi). The therapist's fingers are used to "redirect, balance, and provide a more efficient energy flow" to and throughout the body.

Light Therapy   Natural light or light of specified wavelengths is used to treat disease. This may include ultraviolet light, colored light, or low-intensity laser light. Generally, the eye is the initial entry point for the light because of its direct connection to the brain.

Magnetic Therapy   Magnets are placed directly on the skin, theoretically stimulating living cells and increasing blood flow by ionic currents that are created from polarities on the magnets.

Modified from Spencer JW: *Complementary/alternative medicine: an evidence-based approach,* St Louis, 1999, Mosby.

Mediterranean Diet   A diet that is thought to provide optimal distribution of daily caloric intake of different nutrients and includes 50% to 60% carbohydrates, 30% fats, and 10% proteins. The diet is derived from the eating habits of people in the Mediterranean area, who were shown to have reduced rates of cardiovascular disease.

Mind-Body Therapies   A group of therapies that emphasize using the mind or brain in conjunction with the body to assist healing. Mind-body therapies can involve varying degrees of levels of consciousness, including *hypnosis,* in which selective attention is used to induce a specific altered state (trance) for memory retrieval, relaxation, or suggestion; *visual imagery,* in which the focus is on a target visual stimulus; *yoga,* which involves integration of posture and controlled breathing, relaxation, and/or meditation; *relaxation,* which includes lighter levels of altered states of consciousness through indirect or direct focus; and *meditation,* in which there is an intentional use of posture, concentration, contemplation, and visualization.

Muscle Energy Technique   A manual therapy in osteopathic medicine that includes both passive mobilization and muscle reeducation. Diagnosis of somatic dysfunction is performed by the practitioner, after which the patient is guided to provide corrective muscle contraction.

Music Therapy   The use of music in an either active or passive mode. Used mainly to reduce stress, anxiety, and pain.

Naturopathy   A major health system that includes practices that emphasize diet, nutrition, homeopathy, acupuncture, herbal medicine, manipulation, and various mind-body therapies. Focal points include self-healing and treatment through changes in lifestyle and emphasis on health prevention.

Ornish Diet   A life-choice program based on eating a vegetarian diet containing less than 10% fat. The diet is high in complex carbohydrates and fiber. Meat and fish are generally avoided.

Oslo Diet   An eating plan that emphasizes increased intake of fish and reduced total fat intake. Diet is combined with regular endurance exercise.

Pilates   An educational and exercise approach using the proper body mechanics, movements, truncal and pelvic stabilization, coordinated breathing, and muscle contractions to promote strengthening. Attention is paid to the entire musculoskeletal system.

Prayer   The use of prayer(s) that are offered to "some higher being" or authority to heal and/or arrest disease. May be practiced by the individual patient, by groups, or by other(s) with or without the patient's knowledge (e.g., intercessory).

Pritikin Diet   A weight management plan that is based on a vegetarian framework. Meals are low in fat, high in fiber, and high in complex carbohydrates.

Qi Gong   A form of Chinese exercise-stimulation therapy that proposes to improve health by redirecting mental focus, breathing, coordination, and relaxation. The goal is to "rebalance" the body's own healing capacities by activating proposed electrical or energetic currents that flow along meridians located throughout the body. These meridians, however, do not follow conventional nerve or muscle pathways. In Chinese medical training and practice this therapy includes "external Qi," which is energy transmitted from one person to another so as to heal.

Raja Yoga   Yoga practice that includes all of the other forms of yoga. The practitioner is instructed to follow moral directives, physical exercises, breathing exercises, meditation, devotion, and service to others to facilitate religious awakening.

Reflexology   A bodywork technique that uses reflex points on the hands and feet. Pressure is applied at points that correspond to various body parts, to eliminate blockages thought to produce pain or disease.

Reiki   Comes from the Japanese word meaning "universal life force energy." The practitioner serves as a conduit for healing energy directed into the body or energy field of the recipient without physical contact with the body.

Rolfing   A bodywork technique that involves the myofascia. The body is realigned by using the hands to apply deep pressure and friction that allow more sufficient posture, movement, and the "release" of emotions from the body.

Shiatsu   A Japanese bodywork technique involving finger pressure at specific points on the body mainly to balance "energy" in the body. The major focus is on prevention by keeping the body healthy. The therapy uses more than 600 points on the skin that are proposed to be connected to pathways through which energy flows.

T'ai Chi   A technique that uses slow, purposeful motor-physical movements of the body to control and achieve a more balanced physiologic and psychological state.

Therapeutic Touch   A body energy field technique in which hands are passed over the body without actually touching to recreate and change proposed "energy imbalances" for restoring innate healing forces. Verbal interaction between patient and therapist helps maximize effects.

Traditional Chinese Medicine   An ancient form of medicine that focuses on prevention and secondarily treats disease with an emphasis on maintaining balance through the body by stimulating a constant, smooth-flowing Qi energy. Herbs, acupuncture, massage, diet, and exercise are also used.

Trager Psychophysical Integration   A bodywork technique in which the practitioner enters a meditative state and guides the client through gentle, light, rhythmic, nonintrusive movements. "Mentastics" exercises using self-healing movements are taught to the clients.

AUTHOR: **ANNE L. HUME, PHARM.D.**

Relaxation Techniques

Relaxation Techniques

Relaxation Technique	Summary	Further Resources
Breathing exercise	This is the foundation of most relaxation techniques. Have patients place one hand on the chest and the other on the abdomen. Instruct them to take a slow, deep breath, as if they were sucking in all the air in the room. While doing this, the hand on the abdomen should rise higher than the hand on the chest. This promotes diaphragmatic breathing that increases alveolar expansion in the bases of the lungs. Have them hold the breath for a count of 7 and then exhale. Exhalation should take twice as long as inhalation. Repeat this for a total of five breaths, and encourage patients to do this three times a day.	*Conscious Breathing* by Gay Hendricks is one of many good resources on using breathing for relaxation and health.
Meditation		
Transcendental/The relaxation response	To prevent distracting thoughts, the subject repeats a mantra (a word or sound) over and over again while sitting in a comfortable position. If a distracting thought comes to mind, it is accepted and let go, with the mind focusing again on the mantra.	www.mindbody.harvard.edu or *The Relaxation Response* by Herbert Benson; www.tm.org for information on transcendental meditation.
Mindful meditation	This represents the philosophy of living in the present or in the moment. The *body scan* is one technique where the subject uses breathing to obtain a relaxed state while lying or sitting. The mind progressively focuses on different parts of the body, where it feels any and all sensations intentionally but nonjudgmentally before moving on to another part of the body. A patient with back pain may focus on the quality and characteristics of the pain as if to better understand it and bring it under control.	*Full Catastrophe Living* by Jon Kabat-Zinn describes this technique in full and the program for stress reduction at the University of Massachusetts Medical Center.
Centering prayer	This is a form similar to transcendental meditation that has a more religious foundation. The subject repeats a "sacred word" similar to a mantra. As thoughts come to mind, they are accepted and let go, clearing the mind to become more centered on the spirit within, as if the mind's preoccupied thoughts are the layers of an onion that are peeled away, allowing better understanding of the spirit at the core.	www.centeringprayer.com; look under "method of centering prayer" for a nondenominational discussion.
Progressive muscle relaxation (PMR)	A form of relaxation in which the subject is attuned to the difference in feeling when the muscles are tensed and then relaxed. In a comfortable position, start by tensing the whole body from head to toe. While doing this, notice the feelings of tightness. Take a deep breath in and as you let it out, let the tension release and the muscles relax. This is then followed by progressive tension and relaxation throughout the body. One may start by clenching the fists and then tensing the arms, shoulders, chest, abdomen, hips, legs, and so on, with each step followed by relaxation.	www.uaex.edu/publications/pub/fshei28.htm is a good review of PMR as well as other relaxation exercises. It is sponsored by the University of Arkansas. *You Must Relax* is a book by the founder of this technique, Edmund Jacobson.
Visualization/Self-hypnosis	The subject uses visualization to recruit images that create a relaxed state. For example, if a person is anxious, visualizing images of a place and a time that were peaceful and comforting would help induce relaxation. This is best used in conjunction with a breathing exercise.	There are many CDs, MP3s, and DVDs that can guide people through a visualization "script" that can result in relaxation. Emmett Miller is one well-known author.
Autogenic training	This induces a physiologic response by using simple phrases. For example, "My legs are heavy and warm" is meant to increase the blood flow to this area, resulting in relaxation. This is done progressively from head to toe with the use of deep breathing and repetition of the phrase. After completing this, focus attention on any body part that may still be tense, and then focus the breath and phrase to that area until the whole body is relaxed.	The British Autogenic Society at www.autogenictherapy.org.uk is a good resource for more information.

Continued on following page

Relaxation Techniques—cont'd

Relaxation Technique	Summary	Further Resources
Exercise/Movement		
Aerobic	While performing an aerobic exercise, focus attention on a phrase, sound, word, or prayer and passively disregard other thoughts that may enter the mind. Some may focus on their breathing, saying to themselves, "In" with inhalation and "Out" with exhalation, or repeating "one-two, one-two" with each step they take with jogging. Doing this will help the mind focus, preventing other thoughts that may cause tension.	*Beyond the Relaxation Response* by Herbert Benson includes discussion of his research on inducing the relaxation response while exercising.
Yoga	This has been practiced for thousands of years in India. In America, it has been divided into three aspects: breathing (pranayama yoga), bodily postures or asanas (hatha yoga), and meditation to maintain balance and health. Regular practice induces relaxation.	For Yoga, t'ai chi, and qi gong therapies, it is best to encourage patients to take a class at a local community center or gym and to pick up an introductory book at a library or bookstore.
T'ai chi	An ancient Chinese martial art that uses slow, graceful movements combined with inner mindfulness and breathing techniques to help bring balance between the mind and body.	See above.
Qi gong	A traditional Chinese practice that uses movement, meditation, and controlled breathing to balance the body's vital energy force, Qi.	See above.

From Rakel RE (ed): *Principles of family practice*, ed 6, Philadelphia, 2002, Saunders.

Overview of Selected Natural Products

This table includes a few of the common uses and side effects of selected natural products. The evidence supporting the uses and side effects of these products varies considerably and may be based on anecdotal information or theoretical concerns with the natural products.

Natural Products	Common Use(s)	Adverse Effects/Potential Concerns
African plum (Pygeum)	Benign prostatic hyperplasia	Nausea and abdominal pain have been reported, but pygeum is generally well tolerated. Pygeum does not decrease prostate size or influence PSA concentrations.
Black cohosh	Management of hot flashes in peri- and postmenopausal women	Dyspepsia, rash, weight gain, headache, and cramping have been reported. Concern exists that black cohosh causes liver toxicity, although the botanical was part of a multiingredient blend. The potential development of mild estrogen-like adverse effects, especially endometrial hyperplasia, is of concern.
Butterbur	Prevention of migraine headaches and supported by 2012 American Academy of Neurology; allergic rhinitis	Diarrhea, stomach upset, fatigue, belching, headache, and drowsiness may occur. Due to concern about hepatotoxicity, butterbur products should be free of pyrrolizidine alkaloids. Products should be standardized to 15% petasin and isopetasin.
Chamomile (German)	Motion sickness, anxiety, insomnia; gastrointestinal spasms; mucositis	Allergic reactions occur on rare occasion. Patients with a ragweed allergy should use chamomile with caution.
Chasteberry	Premenstrual dysphoric disorder, premenstrual syndrome, menopausal symptoms, female infertility, mastalgia	Gastrointestinal upset, headache, rash, acne, weight gain, and menstrual bleeding have been reported.
Chitosan	Weight loss, Crohn's disease, hypercholesterolemia, anemia	Gastrointestinal upset, nausea, flatulence, and constipation have been reported. Patients with a shellfish allergy should avoid the use of chitosan.
Chondroitin sulfate	Osteoarthritis, osteoporosis, hyperlipidemia	Gastrointestinal upset, nausea, diarrhea, constipation, and alopecia. Concern exists that chondroitin may have anticoagulant activity due to its structural similarity to part of heparin.
Cinnamon	Type 2 diabetes mellitus, flatulence, gastrointestinal spasms, anorexia, menopausal symptoms, impotence	Cassia cinnamon is one of three types of cinnamon in commercial food products; this is the only type that may have minor effects to improve blood glucose concentrations.
Coenzyme Q10	Chronic heart failure, angina, dilated cardiomyopathy, statin-induced myopathy, Parkinson's disease	Nausea, vomiting, diarrhea, anorexia, heartburn, and rash have been reported. Coenzyme Q10 is structurally similar to vitamin K; concern exists about potential interaction with warfarin.
Cranberry	Prevention and treatment of urinary tract infections; type 2 diabetes mellitus; chronic fatigue syndrome; pleurisy	Gastrointestinal upset and diarrhea have been reported with large doses of cranberry. Uric acid kidney stone formation is also possible with large doses of cranberry over prolonged periods of time.
Dehydroepiandrosterone (DHEA)	Slow or reverse aging, weight loss, metabolic syndrome, erectile dysfunction, immune stimulant, osteoporosis, systemic lupus erythematosus, multiple sclerosis, depression, schizophrenia	Acne and other androgenic effects commonly occur in women. Alopecia, insulin resistance, hepatic dysfunction, and hypertension have been reported. Ingested wild yam and soy cannot be converted into DHEA by humans.
Devil's claw	Osteoarthritis, atherosclerosis, gout, myalgias, fever, migraines	Diarrhea, nausea, and vomiting, as well as allergic reactions, have been reported.
Echinacea	Prevention and treatment of viral respiratory infections; urinary tract infections; chronic fatigue syndrome; attention deficit hyperactivity disorder	Nausea, vomiting, diarrhea, heartburn, headaches, dizziness, arthralgias, and allergic reactions have been reported with echinacea. Patients with a ragweed allergy should avoid use of Echinacea.
Eleuthero (Siberian ginseng)	Maintenance of a normal blood pressure; atherosclerosis; Alzheimer's disease; chronic fatigue syndrome; diabetes; herpes simplex infections	Drowsiness, anxiety, and irritability have been reported.

Continued on following page

Natural Products	Common Use(s)	Adverse Effects/Potential Concerns
Evening primrose oil (EPO)	Premenstrual syndrome, mastalgia, osteoporosis, asthma, menopausal symptoms, eczema, chronic fatigue syndrome	EPO is well tolerated.
Fenugreek	Type 2 diabetes mellitus, anorexia, atherosclerosis; also used as galactogogue	Gastrointestinal upset, flatulence, and hypoglycemia are possible side effects. Patients with a peanut allergy (and an allergy to related plants) should use fenugreek with caution. Nursing mothers who use fenugreek may notice a "maple syrup" smell in their sweat and in the urine of their infants. This may be mistaken to be maple syrup urine disease in the infant.
Feverfew	Prevention of migraines; fever; menstrual-related problems; arthritis; infertility; asthma	Gastrointestinal side effects are the most common with feverfew. A "post-feverfew syndrome" has been reported in individuals who have taken feverfew for prolonged periods of time and then have abruptly stopped the herbal.
Fish oil	Hypertriglyceridemia, coronary heart disease, hypertension, asthma, depression, rheumatoid arthritis, osteoporosis, psoriasis	Heartburn, nausea, rash, and a "fishy" aftertaste can occur. Contamination with pesticides (as well as with mercury and other heavy metals) is a potential concern, although this is unlikely.
Garlic	Hyperlipidemia, hypertension, peripheral arterial disease, type 2 diabetes mellitus	Nausea, vomiting, heartburn, and body odor are most common. "Deodorized" garlic products may lack the active ingredient, allicin.
Ginger	Nausea and vomiting secondary to pregnancy, chemotherapy, motion sickness, surgery	Heartburn, belching, and dermatitis have been reported. In overdoses, ginger has been associated with central nervous system depression and arrhythmias. Efficacy for hyperemesis gravidarum is unknown, and use is not recommended.
Ginkgo	Alzheimer's disease, vascular dementias, tinnitus, acute mountain sickness, intermittent claudication	Gastrointestinal side effects, headaches, dizziness, and allergic skin reactions. Seizures have been reported in several case reports. Products should contain 24% ginkgo flavone glycosides and 6% terpenoids.
Ginseng (Panax)	Increased resistance to stress and improved well-being; increased physical stamina; depression; diabetes; erectile dysfunction	Insomnia has been reported with ginseng. Vaginal bleeding, mastalgia, and amenorrhea have also been reported.
Glucosamine sulfate	Osteoarthritis	Nausea, heartburn, skin reactions, and headache have been reported. Increased glucose concentrations have been a concern but have not been documented. Patients with a shellfish allergy should use glucosamine with caution.
Green tea	Improve cognitive performance; prevention of breast, prostate, and colon cancer; hyperlipidemia; Parkinson's disease; obesity; diabetes; cardiovascular disease	Nausea, vomiting, dyspepsia, dizziness, insomnia, and nervousness have been reported. Side effects may be a result of the large amount of caffeine in green tea products. Hepatotoxicity has been a potential concern with green tea.
Hawthorn	Mild heart failure, angina, arrhythmias, hypertension	Mild gastrointestinal effects, dizziness, rash, palpitations, and nervousness have been reported.
Hoodia	Obesity	Side effects have not been reported. Many products have been adulterated and lack the actual ingredient.
Horse chestnut	Chronic venous insufficiency, including varicose veins; benign prostate hyperplasia; diarrhea	Mild nausea, vomiting, dizziness, headache, and itching. Products are standardized to 16%-20% aescin.
Huperzine	Alzheimer's disease, increased alertness and energy, myasthenia gravis, memory enhancement	Nausea, vomiting, diarrhea, sweating, and blurred vision as a result of the cholinergic effects of huperzine have been reported.
Kava	Anxiety, insomnia, restlessness, seizure disorders, depression, chronic fatigue syndrome	Gastrointestinal upset, headache, dizziness, "kava" dermopathy, and allergic skin reactions. Hepatotoxicity is the primary concern with kava; some countries have banned the use of kava.
Melatonin	Jet lag, insomnia, migraine, chronic fatigue syndrome, breast cancer, gastritis/PUD, osteoporosis; also used for insomnia in children with ADHD	Daytime drowsiness, headache, and dizziness have been reported. Vaginal bleeding has occurred in perimenopausal women. Melatonin from animal sources should be avoided.
Melissa	Cold sores (topically), anxiety, insomnia, Alzheimer's disease, hypertension, dyspepsia	Nausea, vomiting, dizziness, and wheezing have occurred with oral melissa.
Methylsulfonylmethane (MSM)	Chronic pain, arthritis, diabetes, osteoporosis, allergies, obesity, premenstrual syndrome	Nausea, bloating, diarrhea, fatigue, and insomnia have been associated with MSM. This substance is used frequently in combination with glucosamine and chondroitin.
Milk thistle	Protective agent against liver damage due to alcohol, acetaminophen, and carbon tetrachloride; hepatitis C	Nausea, abdominal fullness, diarrhea, and allergic reactions. Patients with a ragweed allergy should use milk thistle with caution.
Peppermint	Irritable bowel syndrome, sinusitis, morning sickness, dysmenorrhea	Heartburn has been reported, as well as laryngeal and bronchial spasm in infants and children.
Policosanol	Hyperlipidemia, intermittent claudication, atherosclerosis	Migraines, insomnia, dizziness, skin rash, and bleeding have been reported with policosanol. The product has antiplatelet effects.
Probiotics	Treatment and prevention of diarrhea including antibiotic-associated diarrhea; irritable bowel syndrome; atopic dermatitis; Crohn's disease	Theoretically, probiotic products may increase risk of infections in immunocompromised individuals.
Red clover phytoestrogens	Menopausal symptoms, premenstrual syndrome, asthma	Rash, myalgias, headaches, and vaginal bleeding have been reported. Theoretically, endometrial hyperplasia is an adverse effect from the use of these compounds.
Red yeast rice	Hyperlipidemia, indigestion, diarrhea, circulatory conditions	Gastrointestinal upset and dizziness may occur. Red yeast rice may contain lovastatin-like compounds and potentially cause rhabdomyolysis.
S-adenosylmethionine (SAM-e)	Depression, anxiety, dementia, osteoarthritis, heart disease	Nausea, vomiting, diarrhea, headache, and nervousness have been reported. Concern exists that SAM-e raises homocysteine levels.

Natural Products	Common Use(s)	Adverse Effects/Potential Concerns
St. John's wort	Depression, anxiety, chronic fatigue syndrome, HIV/AIDS	Anxiety, gastrointestinal upset, vaginal bleeding, neuropathy, and rash can occur. Hypomania has been induced by St. John's wort.
Tea tree oil	Topical use for acne, fungal infections, lice, scabies	Local inflammation and contact dermatitis may occur.
Valerian	Insomnia, depression, chronic fatigue syndrome, menstrual cramps	Headaches, gastrointestinal upset, and drowsiness can occur. Hepatotoxicity is a potential concern with valerian.

AIDS, Acquired immune deficiency syndrome; *HIV*, human immunodeficiency virus.

AUTHOR: **ANNE L. HUME, PHARM.D.**

Natural Products and Drug Interactions

This table lists interactions between selected natural products and prescription and nonprescription drugs. Many of the listed interactions are theoretical in nature and have not been documented to occur in humans. However, interactions with St. John's wort are potentially life threatening in nature. Other interactions are based on small studies of healthy volunteers and use pharmaceutical-quality natural products that may or may not be commercially available.

Natural Products	Drugs	Interactions
Black cohosh	Hepatotoxic drugs	Concern exists that the risk of hepatotoxicity with black cohosh is increased in the presence of hepatotoxic drugs.
	Cisplatin	Animal studies suggest that the efficacy of cisplatin against breast cancer cells may be decreased by black cohosh.
	CYP2D6 substrates	Black cohosh may modestly inhibit CYP2D6 enzyme activity to result in higher drug concentrations.
Butterbur	CYP3A4 inducers (rifampin, carbamazepine, etc.)	Drugs that induce the activity of CYP3A4 increase the risk of the formation of hepatotoxic metabolites from pyrrolizidine alkaloids from some butterbur products.
Chamomile	CNS depressants	Chamomile may have additive CNS depressant effects.
	CYP1A2 substrates	Chamomile may inhibit CYP1A2 enzyme activity to result in higher drug concentrations.
	CYP3A4 substrates	Chamomile may inhibit CYP3A4 enzyme activity to result in higher drug concentrations.
	Estrogens	Chamomile may compete for estrogen receptors.
	Tamoxifen	Chamomile may interfere with the effects of tamoxifen because of its estrogenic effects.
Chaste tree berry	Antipsychotic agents	Chaste tree berry may antagonize the effects of antipsychotic agents through its dopaminergic activity.
	Metoclopramide	Chaste tree berry may antagonize the effects of metoclopramide through its dopaminergic activity.
	Dopamine agonists	Chaste tree berry may possess additive effects to drugs such as levodopa through its dopaminergic activity.
	Oral contraceptives/estrogens	Chaste tree berry may possess additive hormonal effects.
Chondroitin	Warfarin	High-dose chondroitin has structural similarity to a heparinoid and may possess weak anticoagulant effects.
Cinnamon	Hypoglycemic agents	Cinnamon may possess additive effects on blood glucose to those of hypoglycemic agents.
Coenzyme Q10	Antihypertensive agents	Coenzyme Q10 may possess additive effects on blood pressure to those of antihypertensive agents.
	Warfarin	Coenzyme Q10 may lessen the anticoagulant effects of warfarin because of its structural similarity to vitamin K.
	Chemotherapy	The antioxidant effects of coenzyme Q10 may blunt the efficacy of chemotherapeutic agents that depend on the formation of free radicals.
Cranberry	CYP2C9 substrates (warfarin)	Cranberry may inhibit CYP2C9 enzyme activity to result in higher drug concentrations although evidence with warfarin is contradictory.
Dehydroepiandrosterone (DHEA)	Tamoxifen and aromatase inhibitors such as anastrozole.	DHEA may interfere with the antiestrogenic effects of these drugs.
	CYP3A4 substrates	DHEA may slightly inhibit CYP3A4 enzyme activity to result in higher drug concentrations.

Natural Products	Drugs	Interactions
Devil's claw	Antihypertensive agents	Devil's claw may possess additive effects on blood pressure to those of antihypertensive agents.
	Hypoglycemic agents	Devil's claw may possess additive effects on blood glucose to those of hypoglycemic agents.
	H_2 antagonists and PPIs	Devil's claw may raise gastric pH and blunt the efficacy of H_2 antagonists and PPIs.
	CYP3A4 substrates	Devil's claw may inhibit CYP3A4 enzyme activity to result in higher drug concentrations.
	CYP2C9 substrates	Devil's claw may inhibit CYP2C9 enzyme activity to result in higher drug concentrations.
	CYP2C19 substrates	Devil's claw may inhibit CYP2C19 enzyme activity to result in higher drug concentrations.
	Warfarin	Devil's claw may inhibit CYP2C9 enzyme activity to result in higher concentrations of warfarin; purpura has been reported.
Echinacea	Immune suppressants	Echinacea may stimulate immune function, potentially decreasing the effectiveness of drugs such as cyclosporine and prednisone.
	CYP3A4 substrates	Echinacea may modestly induce hepatic CYP3A4 enzyme activity to result in lower drug concentrations.
	CYP1A2 substrates	Echinacea may inhibit CYP1A2 enzyme activity to result in higher drug concentrations.
Eleuthero (Siberian ginseng)	CNS depressants	Eleuthero may have additive CNS depressant effects.
	Antiplatelet and anticoagulant agents	Eleuthero may have antiplatelet activity, potentially increasing the risk of bleeding.
	CYP3A4 substrates	Eleuthero may inhibit CYP3A4 enzyme activity to result in higher drug concentrations.
	CYP1A2 substrates	Eleuthero may modestly inhibit CYP1A2 enzyme activity to result in higher drug concentrations.
	CYP2C9 substrates	Eleuthero may modestly inhibit CYP2C9 enzyme activity to result in higher drug concentrations.
	CYP2D6 substrates	Eleuthero may inhibit CYP2D6 enzyme activity to result in higher drug concentrations.
	Digoxin	Concentration of digoxin has been reported to increase but without evidence of toxicity.
Evening primrose oil (EPO)	Antiplatelet and anticoagulant agents	EPO may have anticoagulant activity, potentially increasing the risk of bleeding.
Fenugreek	Antiplatelet and anticoagulant agents	Fenugreek may have antiplatelet activity, potentially increasing the risk of bleeding.
	Hypoglycemic agents	Fenugreek may potentially lower blood glucose concentrations and have additive effects with hypoglycemic agents.
Feverfew	Antiplatelet and anticoagulant agents	Feverfew may have antiplatelet activity, potentially increasing the risk of bleeding.
	CYP3A4 substrates	Feverfew may inhibit CYP3A4 enzyme activity to result in higher drug concentrations.
	CYP1A2 substrates	Feverfew may inhibit CYP1A2 enzyme activity to result in higher drug concentrations.
	CYP2C9 substrates	Feverfew may inhibit CYP2C9 enzyme activity to result in higher drug concentrations.
	CYP2C19 substrates	Feverfew may inhibit CYP2C19 enzyme activity to result in higher drug concentrations.
Fish oils (omega-3 fatty acids)	Antiplatelet and anticoagulant agents	Fish oils may have antiplatelet activity, potentially increasing the risk of bleeding, although this has not been documented in humans.
	Antihypertensive agents	Fish oils may possess additive effects on blood pressure to those of antihypertensive agents.
	Oral contraceptives	Oral contraceptives may potentially interfere with the triglyceride-lowering effects of fish oil.
Garlic	Antiplatelet and anticoagulant agents	Garlic may have antiplatelet activity, potentially increasing the risk of bleeding.
	CYP3A4 substrates	Garlic may potentially induce CYP3A4 enzyme activity to result in lower drug concentrations; evidence is contradictory.
	CYP2E1 substrates	Garlic may modestly inhibit CYP2E1 enzyme activity to result in higher drug concentrations.
Ginger	Antiplatelet and anticoagulant agents	Ginger may have antiplatelet activity, potentially increasing the risk of bleeding.
	Hypoglycemic agents	Ginger may potentially lower blood glucose concentrations and have additive effects with hypoglycemic agents.
Ginkgo	Antiplatelet and anticoagulant agents	Ginkgo may have antiplatelet activity, potentially increasing the risk of bleeding.
	CYP2C19 substrates	Ginkgo may induce CYP2C19 enzyme activity to result in lower drug concentrations.
	CYP1A2 substrates	Ginkgo may modestly inhibit CYP1A2 enzyme activity to result in higher drug levels.
	CYP2C9 substrates	Ginkgo may modestly inhibit CYP2C9 enzyme activity to result in higher drug concentrations.
	CYP2D6 substrates	Ginkgo may inhibit CYP2D6 enzyme activity to result in higher drug concentrations.
Ginseng (Panax)	Antiplatelet and anticoagulant agents	Panax ginseng may have antiplatelet properties; American ginseng may decrease the effectiveness (international normalized ratio [INR]) of warfarin.
	CYP2D6 substrates	Panax ginseng may modestly inhibit CYP2D6 enzyme activity to result in higher drug concentrations.
	Immune suppressants	Panax ginseng may stimulate immune function, potentially decreasing the effectiveness of drugs such as cyclosporine and prednisone.
	Hypoglycemic agents	Panax ginseng may potentially lower blood glucose levels and have additive effects with hypoglycemic agents.
Glucosamine	Warfarin	High-dose glucosamine (along with high-dose chondroitin) may have additive effects to those of warfarin because of structural similarity to heparin. Evidence is lacking.

Continued on following page

Natural Products	Drugs	Interactions
Green tea extract	Antiplatelet agents	Green tea possesses compounds that may have antiplatelet activity, potentially increasing the risk of bleeding.
	Amphetamines	Caffeine in green tea may increase the risk of CNS toxicity.
	Cocaine	Caffeine in green tea may increase the risk of CNS toxicity.
	Oral contraceptives	Oral contraceptives may decrease the clearance of caffeine in green tea.
	Warfarin	Small amounts of vitamin K have been reported to be present in green tea, potentially decreasing the effectiveness of warfarin.
	Theophylline	Caffeine potentially decreases theophylline clearance.
	Verapamil	Verapamil decreases caffeine clearance, resulting in increased concentrations.
	Quinolone antibiotics	Some quinolone antibiotics decrease the clearance of caffeine.
	Hepatotoxic drugs	Concern exists that the risk of hepatotoxicity with green tea is increased in the presence of hepatotoxic drugs.
Hawthorn	β-Blockers	Hawthorn and β-blockers may have additive effects on blood pressure and heart rate.
	CCBs, nitrates	Hawthorn and CCBs (or nitrates) may have additive effects due to coronary vasodilation.
	Digoxin	Hawthorn may have additive effects to those of digoxin.
	Phosphodiesterase inhibitors	Hawthorn may have additive vasodilatory and hypotensive effects with these drugs.
Horse chestnut seed extract (HCSE)	Antiplatelet and anticoagulant agents	HCSE may have antiplatelet activity, potentially increasing the risk of bleeding.
	Hypoglycemic agents	HCSE may potentially lower blood glucose concentrations and have additive effects with hypoglycemic agents.
Huperzine	AChE inhibitors (donepezil, etc.)	Huperzine may have additive effects when combined with AChE inhibitors.
	Anticholinergic drugs	The effectiveness of huperzine and/or the anticholinergic drug may be decreased by their concomitant administration.
	Cholinergic drugs (bethanechol, etc.)	Huperzine may have additive effects when combined with cholinergic drugs.
Kava	CYP3A4 substrates	Kava may inhibit CYP3A4 enzyme activity to result in higher drug concentrations.
	CYP1A2 substrates	Kava may inhibit CYP1A2 enzyme activity to result in higher drug concentrations.
	CYP2C9 substrates, CYP2C19 substrates	Kava may inhibit CYP2C9 and CYP2C19 enzyme activity to result in higher drug concentrations.
	CYP2D6 substrates	Kava may inhibit CYP2D6 enzyme activity to result in higher drug concentrations.
	P-glycoprotein substrates (digoxin; itraconazole; diltiazem, verapamil; and many other drugs)	Kava may inhibit P-glycoprotein transporter systems.
	Hepatotoxic drugs	Concern exists that the risk of hepatotoxicity from kava is increased in the presence of hepatotoxic drugs.
Melatonin	Antiplatelet and anticoagulant agents	Melatonin may potentiate the effects of antiplatelets and anticoagulants, although the mechanism is unknown.
	CNS depressants	Melatonin may have additive CNS depressant effects.
	Fluvoxamine	Fluvoxamine may increase levels of melatonin.
	Immune suppressants	Melatonin may stimulate immune function, potentially decreasing the effectiveness of drugs such as cyclosporine and prednisone.
	Hypoglycemic agents	Melatonin may impair glucose utilization and may decrease the efficacy of hypoglycemic agents.
Milk thistle	Estrogens (and other drugs that undergo glucuronidation)	Silymarin may increase the clearance of estrogens.
	CYP2C9 substrates	Milk thistle may modestly inhibit CYP2C9 enzyme activity to result in higher drug concentrations.
Peppermint oil	H₂ antagonists and proton pump inhibitors	Peppermint oil may raise gastric pH and blunt efficacy of H₂ antagonists and PPIs.
	CYP3A4 substrates	Peppermint oil may modestly inhibit CYP3A4 enzyme activity to result in higher drug concentrations.
	CYP1A2 substrates	Peppermint oil may modestly inhibit CYP1A2 enzyme activity to result in higher drug concentrations.
	CYP2C9 substrates, CYP2C19 substrates	Peppermint oil may modestly inhibit CYP2C9 and CYP2C19 enzyme activity to result in higher drug concentrations.
Policosanol	Antiplatelet and anticoagulant agents	Policosanol may have antiplatelet activity, potentially increasing the risk of bleeding.
Probiotics	Antibiotics	Antibiotics may kill the live organisms in different probiotic preparations.
	Immune suppressants	Theoretically, probiotics may cause bacterial or fungal infections in patients who are taking immune suppressants chronically.
Red clover phytoestrogens	Antiplatelet and anticoagulant agents	Theoretically, red clover may possess coumarins, which increase the risk of bleeding with antiplatelet and anticoagulants. Evidence is lacking.
	CYP3A4 substrates	Red clover may inhibit CYP3A4 enzyme activity to result in higher drug concentrations.
	CYP2C9 substrates, CYP2C19 substrates	Red clover may inhibit CYP2C9 and CYP2C19 enzyme activity to result in higher drug concentrations.
	CYP1A2 substrates	Red clover may inhibit CYP1A2 enzyme activity to result in higher drug concentrations.

Natural Products	Drugs	Interactions
Red yeast rice	CYP3A4 inhibitors	Drugs that inhibit CYP3A4 may decrease the metabolism of lovastatin in red yeast rice.
	Statins	Red yeast rice contains lovastatin and increases the risk of myopathy.
	Fibrates and niacin	Fibrates and niacin may increase concentrations of lovastatin in red yeast rice.
S-adenosylmethionine (SAM-e)	Antidepressants (including MAOIs)	Additive effects are possible, and there is potential for toxicity.
	Serotonergic drugs (triptans, SSRIs, tramadol, dextromethorphan, etc.)	SAM-e may increase the risk of development of serotonin syndrome when used concomitantly.
Soy phytoestrogens	Estrogens	Soy potentially may inhibit the effects of estrogen.
	Tamoxifen/aromatase inhibitors	Soy's estrogenic effects may antagonize the antitumor effects of tamoxifen/aromatase inhibitors.
	MAOIs	Fermented soy products may contain tyramine.
St. John's wort	CYP3A4 substrates	St. John's wort strongly induces CYP3A4 enzyme activity to result in lower drug concentrations.
	CYP1A2 substrates	St. John's wort modestly induces CYP1A2 enzyme activity to result in lower drug levels.
	CYP2C9 substrates	St. John's wort induces CYP2C9 enzyme activity to result in lower drug concentrations.
	P-glycoprotein substrates (digoxin; itraconazole; diltiazem, verapamil; and many other drugs)	St. John's wort induces P-glycoprotein transporter systems.
	Serotonergic drugs (triptans, SSRIs, tramadol, dextromethorphan, etc.)	St. John's wort may increase the risk of development of serotonin syndrome when used concomitantly.
Valerian	CNS depressants	Valerian may increase the sedative effects of CNS depressants.
	CYP3A4 substrates	Valerian may modestly inhibit the CYP3A4 enzyme activity.

AChE, Acetylcholinesterase; *CCBs,* calcium channel blockers; *CNS,* central nervous system; *MAOIs,* monoamine oxidase inhibitor; *PPIs,* proton pump inhibitors; *SSRIs,* selective serotonin reuptake inhibitors.

EXAMPLES OF DRUGS METABOLIZED BY CYP ENZYMES

The following are examples of drugs that are metabolized through the different cytochrome P450 isoenzymes:

CYP1A2 substrates: theophylline, imipramine, clozapine, naproxen
CYP2C9 substrates: warfarin, tamoxifen, irbesartan, ibuprofen, glipizide
CYP2C19 substrates: omeprazole and other proton pump inhibitors, phenytoin, phenobarbital, cyclophosphamide
CYP2D6 substrates: S-metoprolol, propafenone, paroxetine, risperidone, tramadol
CYP2E1 substrates: acetaminophen, alcohol
CYP3A4 substrates: most statins, indinavir, amlodipine, verapamil, alprazolam, buspirone

AUTHOR: **ANNE L. HUME, PHARM.D.**

Commonly Ingested Plants with Significant Toxic Potential

Plant	Symptoms	Management
Autumn crocus (*Colchicum autumnale*)	Vomiting Diarrhea Initial leukocytosis followed by bone marrow failure Multisystem organ failure	Activated charcoal decontamination Aggressive fluid resuscitation and supportive care
Belladonna alkaloids: jimson weed (*Datura stramonium*) Belladonna ("deadly nightshade"; *Atropa belladonna*)	Anticholinergic toxidrome Seizures	Supportive care, benzodiazepines Consider physostigmine if patient is a threat to self or others; only use if no conduction delays on ECG
Cardiac glycoside–containing plants (foxglove, lily of the valley, oleander, yellow oleander, etc.)	Nausea Vomiting Bradycardia Dysrhythmias (AV block, ventricular ectopy) Hyperkalemia	Digoxin-specific Fab fragments
Jequirity bean and other abrin-containing species (e.g., rosary pea, precatory bean)	Oral pain Vomiting Diarrhea Shock Hemolysis Renal failure	Supportive care, including aggressive volume resuscitation and correction of electrolyte abnormalities
Monkshood (*Aconitum* species)	Numbness and tingling of lips/tongue Vomiting Bradycardia	Atropine for bradycardia Supportive care
Oxalate-containing plants: *Philodendron, Diffenbachia, Colocasia* ("elephant ear")	Local tissue injury Oral pain Vomiting	Supportive care, pain control
Poison hemlock (*Conium maculatum*)	Vomiting Agitation followed by CNS depression Paralysis Respiratory failure	Supportive care
Pokeweed	Hemorrhagic gastroenteritis Burning of mouth and throat	Supportive care
Rhododendron	Vomiting Diarrhea Bradycardia	Atropine for symptomatic bradycardia Supportive care
Tobacco	Vomiting Agitation Diaphoresis Fasciculations Seizures	Supportive care
Water hemlock (*Cicuta* species)	Abdominal pain Vomiting Delirium Seizures	Supportive care, including benzodiazepines for seizures
Yew (*Taxus* species)	GI symptoms QRS widening Hypotension CV collapse	Supportive care Atropine for bradycardia Sodium bicarbonate does not appear to be effective

AV, Atrioventricular; *CNS,* central nervous system; *CV,* cardiovascular; *ECG,* electrocardiogram; *Fab,* fragment, antigen binding; *GI,* gastrointestinal.
From Kliegman RM et al: *Nelson textbook of pediatrics,* ed 19, Philadelphia, 2011, Saunders.

Herbs Associated with Toxicity

Herbal Product	Toxic Chemicals	Toxic Effects
Aconite (*Aconitum* spp.)	Aconitine alkaloids	Nausea, vomiting, paresthesias, weakness, hypotension, asystole, arrhythmias, bradycardia
Chamomile (*Matricaria chamomilla, Anthemis nobilis*)	Allergens	Anaphylaxis, contact dermatitis
Chapparal (*Larrea divaricate, Larrea tridentate*)	Nordihydroguaiaretic acid	Nausea, vomiting, lethargy, hepatitis
Cinnamon oil (*Cinnamomum* spp.)	Cinnamaldehyde	Dermatitis, abuse syndrome
Coltsfoot (*Tussilago farfara*)	Pyrrolizidines	HVOD
Comfrey (*Symphytum officinale*)	Pyrrolizidines	HVOD
Crotalaria spp.	Pyrrolizidines	HVOD
Echinacea (*Echinacea angustifolia*, Compositae spp.)	Polysaccharides	Asthma, atopy, angioedema, anaphylaxis, urticaria
Eucalyptus (*Eucalyptus globulus*)	1,8-cineole	Drowsiness, ataxia, nausea, vomiting, seizures, coma, respiratory failure
Garlic (*Allium sativum*)	Allicin	Dermatitis, chemical burns, oxidizing agent
Germander (*Teucrium chamaedrys*)		Hepatotoxicity
Ginseng (*Panax ginseng*)	Ginsenoside	Ginseng abuse, diarrhea, anxiety, insomnia, hypertension
Glycerated asafetida	Oxidants	Methemoglobinemia
Groundsel (*Senecio longilobus*)	Pyrrolizidines	HVOD
Heliotrope, turnsole (*Crotalaria fulva, Heliotropium, Cynoglossum officinale*)	Pyrrolizidines	HVOD
Jin bu huan (*Stephania* spp., *Corydalis* spp.)	L-Tetrahydropalmitine	Hepatitis, lethargy, coma
Kava-kava (*Piper methysticum*)	Kawain, methysticin	Hepatic failure, "kavaism," neurotoxicity
Kelp	Iodine	Thyroid dysfunction
Laetrile	Cyanide	Coma, seizures, death
Licorice (*Glycyrrhiza glabra*)	Glycyrrhetic acid	Hypertension, cardiac arrhythmias, hypokalemia
Ma huang (*Ephedra sinica*)	Ephedrine	Cardiac arrhythmias, seizures, stroke, hypertension
Monkshood (*Aconitum napellus, A. columbianum*)	Aconite	Cardiac arrhythmias, weakness, coma, shock, paresthesias, vomiting, seizures
Nutmeg (*Myristica fragrans*)	Myristicin, eugenol	Hallucinations, emesis, headache
Nux vomica	Strychnine	Seizures, abdominal pain, respiratory arrest
Pennyroyal (*Mentha pulegium* or *Hedeoma* spp.)	Pulegone	Centrilobular liver necrosis, fetotoxicity, seizures, shock
Ragwort (golden) (*Senecio aureus, Echium*)	Pyrrolizidines	HVOD
Wormwood (*Artemisia* spp.)	Thujone	Seizures, dementia, tremors, headache

HVOD, Hepatic venoocclusive disease.
From Fuhrman BP et al: *Pediatric critical care,* ed 4, Philadelphia, 2011, Saunders.

Websites Providing Data on Herbal Therapy Hazards

Web Address	Website
http://www.fda.gov or http://www.vmcfsan.fda.gov/-dms/aems/html	On the U.S. Food and Drug Administration website under the title "Medwatch," some herb warnings can be found ("special adverse event monitoring system" link)
http://www.faseb.org/aspet/H&MIG3.htm#top	ASPET Herbal and Medicinal Plant Interest Group: a site for an herb discussion group with pharmacologists
http://www.nnlm.nlm.nih.gov/pnr/uwmhg/	University of Washington Medicinal Herb Garden
http://www.nim.nih.gov/medlineplus/herbalmedicine.html	Provides an update on ongoing clinical studies involving herbal products, news, and many links
http://www.update-software.com/abstracts/mainindex.html	The Cochrane Collaboration maintains an updated international database of clinical trials involving complementary and alternative medicine
http://www.amfoundation.org/	Providing consumers and professionals with responsible evidence-based information on the integration of alternative and conventional medicine
http://www.herbmed.org/	An interactive electronic herbal database provides hyperlinked access to scientific data underlying the use of herbs for health; an evidence-based information resource for professionals, researchers, and the general public
http://nccam.nih.gov/	The National Center for Complementary and Alternative Medicine is 1 of 27 institutes and centers that make up the U.S. National Institutes of Health; their mission is to support rigorous research on complementary and alternative medicine, train researchers, and disseminate information to the general public and professionals
http://toxnet.nlm.nih.gov/	A cluster of databases on toxicology, hazardous chemicals, and related areas

From Floege J et al: *Comprehensive clinical nephrology,* ed 4, Philadelphia, 2010, Saunders.

Dietary Supplements: What Every Primary Care Provider Should Know

Primary care providers must be knowledgeable regarding the safety, efficacy, and drug interactions associated with common dietary supplements because of the following:

- An estimated 38% of adults ages 18 years and older reported the use of at least one form of complementary and alternative medicine (CAM) according to the National Health Interview Survey in 2007.
- Almost 17.8% of adults specifically reported the use of dietary supplements, with fish oil, glucosamine, echinacea, flaxseed, and ginseng most frequently used.
- Although the use of dietary supplements has plateaued as a result of consumer concerns about effectiveness and potential adverse effects, usage remains common and potentially dangerous.

COMMON TERMINOLOGY

- A *dietary supplement* is defined as an oral product containing vitamins, minerals, herbs, or other botanicals; amino acids; dietary substances used to supplement the diet by increasing the total dietary intake; or a concentrate, metabolite, constituent, extract, or combination.
- *CAM* refers to the broad domain of healing practices that include diverse health systems, modalities, and practices and their accompanying theories and beliefs (see glossary of terms in Appendix Ia).
- *Complementary therapies* are those that are used *in addition to* conventional therapies, whereas *alternative therapies* are those that are used *instead of* conventional therapies. Most consumers in the United States use dietary supplements as a complementary therapy.
- *Standardization* refers to the practice of producing dietary supplements with a specific amount of a given compound that may or may not include the actual active ingredient. For example, feverfew has been standardized to its parthenolide content.

LEGISLATION

The U.S. Food and Drug Administration (FDA) is frequently criticized for not closely regulating dietary supplements and monitoring their safety. However, although the agency regulates prescription drugs and over-the-counter (OTC) products, the FDA has limited regulatory authority over dietary supplements. This is because the Dietary Supplement and Health Education Act (DSHEA) of 1994 and its resulting regulations limit the FDA's authority. As a result of DSHEA, the FDA is able to act only when a dietary supplement has been documented to contain a prescription drug, as was the case with glyburide in a natural treatment for diabetes and diazepam in an osteoarthritis preparation. In addition, the FDA can act when safety issues related to a product have been clearly documented, although these cases are frequently challenged in the courts.

HEALTH CLAIMS

Dietary supplements generally are marketed under three types of health claims. The first category is the "nutrient content" claim, in which the product is identified as an excellent source of, typically, a mineral such as calcium, based on recommended daily values. The second type is the "significant scientific agreement" claim; these claims are used when some evidence of the product's efficacy exists (e.g., fish oil supplements). The third and most common type of health claim is called a "structure/function" claim; these claims state that the product has some effect on health—for example, "helps to maintain a healthy heart." However, dietary supplements are not permitted to carry claims stating that they are effective in preventing, treating, or curing diseases.

INFORMATION RESOURCES

Appendix Ic provides a brief overview of common dietary supplements. Until recently, few evidence-based resources on dietary supplements were available. Clinical studies and systematic reviews on dietary supplements are now widely available through PubMed, EMBASE, and the Cochrane Database of Systematic Reviews. Although more information is available, references on specific products vary in their interpretation of the available evidence and may exhibit an unintentional bias, either pro or con, regarding the safety and efficacy of dietary supplements.

"Gold standard" evidence-based databases on dietary supplements (subscription required) include the following:

- Natural Medicines Comprehensive Database (http://www.naturaldatabase.com): This database includes listings for many dietary supplements and is organized in a clinician-friendly manner. Monographs include the different common and scientific names; uses and likely effectiveness for different uses; chemical constituents; interactions with drugs, diseases, foods, and laboratory tests; adverse effects; and cautions. The information is extensively referenced and is updated on a daily basis. The primary limitation is that the evaluation of data on clinical effectiveness could be more rigorous.
- Natural Standard (http://www.naturalstandard.com): This database includes listings for dietary supplements and other forms of complementary and alternative medicine. The evidence supporting the assessments in this database is critically evaluated and rigorous in nature. The primary limitation is that many fewer dietary supplements are included in this database.

Evidence-based free websites on dietary supplements include the following:

- National Center for Complementary and Alternative Medicine (NCCAM) (http://nccam.nih.gov)
- Office of Dietary Supplements International Bibliographic Information on Dietary Supplements (http://dietary-supplements.info.nih.gov/Health_Information/IBIDS.aspx)
- Memorial Sloan-Kettering Cancer Center (http://www.mskcc.org/mskcc/html/11570.cfm)

DRUG INTERACTIONS

Clinically significant interactions have been documented between dietary supplements and prescription or OTC drugs. The challenge for primary care providers is to identify real, clinically relevant interactions versus potential or theoretical interactions. Data on interactions with dietary supplements are usually based on isolated case reports or on studies enrolling healthy volunteers. As with drug-drug interactions, the likelihood of an interaction and its severity are influenced especially by concomitant medical conditions, such as heart failure and presence or absence of impaired kidney and liver function.

Appendix Id lists interactions between selected natural products and prescription and nonprescription drugs. The following two broad interactions are particularly important in primary care practice:

- St. John's wort, commonly used for depression, is a potent inducer of cytochrome P450 3A4 isoenzymes and has been documented to increase the clearance of many drugs that are metabolized through this (and other) pathways. (For a list of common drugs cleared in this manner, readers should consult http://medicine.iupui.edu/flockhart/clinlist.htm.) In addition, St. John's wort may induce P-glycoprotein transporter systems that are important for digoxin and some chemotherapeutic agents. St. John's wort has also been associated with the development of serotonin syndrome when used with drugs that have significant serotonergic activity.
- Dietary supplements such as garlic, ginkgo, and feverfew, as well as many others, have been purported to either have antiplatelet activity or have effects on the clotting cascade. This may be important for adults also taking aspirin (and other platelet-active agents) or warfarin.

COUNSELING POINTS

The single most important counseling point related to dietary supplements is always to ask patients about their use of these products and to do so in an open, nonjudgmental manner. The approach should emphasize that many consumers have been interested in vitamins, minerals, herbs, teas, and so on, to maintain their health or to treat illness. If the clinician is unaware of the safety, efficacy, and interactions of a specific product, several websites are available to quickly scan for information. Also, access to drug information centers at colleges of pharmacy is almost always available, and some hospitals now offer programs in integrative medicine.

Patients should be asked about their goals in using the product, as well as how long they have taken it and in what dosage. Allergies to plants should be documented because cross-allergies are common. Clinicians should appreciate that individuals who use dietary supplements may be interested in making lifestyle changes and potentially decreasing their use of prescription drugs. In addition, if an individual is also consulting an alternative medicine practitioner, clinicians should recognize that some alternative health systems discourage the use of established therapies such as vaccines.

Although problems with safety and efficacy have been identified, many dietary supplements are benign except for their cost. Some patients are at higher risk for adverse outcomes from the use of dietary supplements (e.g., those with chronic kidney and liver disease). Patients should be counseled specifically to avoid purchasing dietary supplements over the Internet.

RESEARCH ISSUES

Many clinical and observational studies of dietary supplements have been published. In the past, clinicians frequently stated either that published studies of dietary supplements did not exist or that only a few were available. The reason for this finding was that until recently the National Library of Medicine did not abstract from the peer-reviewed alternative medicine literature. Fortunately, much more research is now readily available. As with all research, the more rigorous the study methodology, the less likely the dietary supplement is to demonstrate clinical benefit.

In evaluating published studies of dietary supplements, the following should be considered:

- Has the correct plant and part of the plant (root, stem, leaf) been used? This critical information may not be known to many clinicians. Consulting a resource such as the National Medicines Comprehensive Database can usually provide the needed information to judge this component of the study.
- Has the content of active ingredients been verified throughout the study? In a recent review of 81 major randomized controlled trials of herbal products, only 12 (15%) reported performing tests to quantify actual contents, and 3 (4%) provided adequate data to compare actual with expected content values of at least one chemical constituent.
- Is the severity of the disease appropriate for study? Negative studies with dietary supplements sometimes inappropriately enroll participants who have moderate-to-severe disease (e.g., those with depression or benign prostatic hyperplasia) when only mild disease would be appropriate.
- Is the duration of the study appropriate? Early studies comparing glucosamine and nonsteroidal antiinflammatory agents (NSAIAs) demonstrated greater efficacy with the NSAIAs because of an inadequate study duration for glucosamine to show any benefit.
- Is a placebo group included? Recent studies with dietary supplements for menopausal symptoms and osteoarthritis have demonstrated placebo responses over 40% to 50%.
- Was the blinding maintained throughout the study? Some dietary supplements, such as saw palmetto, have distinctive odors and tastes that are not easily masked.
- Is the preparation commercially available? Most important, when a study with dietary supplements does show benefit, it frequently is difficult to use the product in practice because the specific formulation studied is not commercially available.

AUTHOR: **ANNE L. HUME, PHARM.D.**

Vitamins and Their Functions

	Biochemistry and Physiology	Deficiency [RDA*]	Toxicity [TUL†]	Assessment of Status
Fat-Soluble Vitamins				
Vitamin A	A family of the retinoid compounds, each member having biologic activity qualitatively similar to retinol. Carotenoids are structurally related to retinoids. Some carotenoids, most notably β-carotene, are metabolized into compounds with vitamin A activity and are therefore considered to be provitamin A compounds. Vitamin A is an integral component of rhodopsin and iodopsins, light-sensitive proteins in rod and cone cells in the retina. *Additional functions:* induction and maintenance of cellular differentiation in certain tissues; signal for appropriate morphogenesis in the developing embryo; maintenance of cell-mediated immunity. One microgram of retinol = 3.33 IU of vitamin A.	Follicular hyperkeratosis and night blindness are early indicators. Conjunctival xerosis, degeneration of the cornea (keratomalacia), and de-differentiation of rapidly proliferating epithelia are later indications of deficiency. *Bitot spots* (focal areas of the conjunctiva or cornea with foamy appearance) are an indication of xerosis. Blindness, due to corneal destruction and retinal dysfunction, ensues if left uncorrected. Increased susceptibility to infection is also a consequence. [F: 700 μg; M: 900 μg]	In adults, >150,000 μg may cause acute toxicity: fatal intracranial hypertension, skin exfoliation, and hepatocellular necrosis. *Chronic* toxicity may occur with habitual daily intake of >10,000 μg: alopecia, ataxia, bone and muscle pain, dermatitis, cheilitis, conjunctivitis, pseudotumor cerebri, hepatocellular necrosis, hyperlipidemia, and hyperostosis are common. Single, large doses of vitamin A (30,000 μg), or habitual intake of >4500 μg/day in early pregnancy can be teratogenic. Excessive intake of carotenoids causes a benign condition characterized by yellowish discoloration of the skin. Habitually large doses of canthaxanthin, a carotenoid, have the additional capability of inducing a retinopathy. [3000 μg]	Retinol concentration in the plasma and vitamin A concentrations in the milk and tears are reasonably accurate measures of adequate status. Toxicity is best assessed by elevated levels of retinyl esters in plasma. A quantitative measure of dark adaptation for night vision or an electroretinogram are useful functional tests.
Vitamin D	A group of sterol compounds whose parent structure is cholecalciferol (vitamin D_3). Cholecalciferol is formed in the skin from 7-dehydrocholesterol (provitamin D_3) by exposure to UVB radiation. A plant sterol, ergocalciferol (provitamin D_2) can be similarly converted into vitamin D_2 and has similar vitamin D activity. The vitamin undergoes sequential hydroxylations in the liver and kidney at the 25 and 1 positions, respectively, producing the most bioactive form of the vitamin, 1,25-dihydroxy vitamin D. Maintains intracellular and extracellular concentrations of calcium and phosphate by enhancing intestinal absorption of the two ions and, in conjunction with PTH, promoting their mobilization from bone mineral. Retards proliferation and promotes differentiation in certain epithelia. One microgram = 40 IU.	Deficiency results in disordered bone modeling called *rickets* in childhood and *osteomalacia* in adults. Expansion of the epiphyseal growth plates and replacement of normal bone with unmineralized bone matrix are the cardinal features of rickets; the latter feature also characterizes osteomalacia. Deformity of bone and pathologic fractures occur. Decreased serum concentrations of calcium and phosphate may occur. [15 μg, ages 19-70 yr; 20 μg, age >70 yr]	Excess amounts result in abnormally high concentrations of calcium and phosphate in the serum: metastatic calcifications, renal damage, and altered mentation may occur. [50 μg]	The serum concentration of the major circulating metabolite, 25-hydroxyvitamin D, is an excellent indicator of systemic status except in chronic renal failure, in which the impairment of renal L-hydroxylation results in disassociation of the mono- and dihydroxyvitamin concentrations. Measuring the serum concentration of 1,25-dihydroxyvitamin D is then necessary.

Continued on following page

	Biochemistry and Physiology	Deficiency [RDA*]	Toxicity [TUL†]	Assessment of Status
Vitamin E	A group of at least 8 naturally occurring compounds, some of which are tocopherols and some of which are tocotrienols. At present, the only dietary form that is thought to be biologically active in humans is α-tocopherol. Acts as an antioxidant and free radical scavenger in lipophilic environments, most notably in cell membranes. Acts in conjunction with other antioxidants such as selenium.	Deficiency due to dietary inadequacy rare. Usually seen in (1) premature infants, (2) individuals with fat malabsorption, and (3) individuals with abetalipoproteinemia. Red blood cell fragility occurs and can produce a hemolytic anemia. Neuronal degeneration produces peripheral neuropathies, ophthalmoplegia, and destruction of posterior columns of spinal cord. Neurologic disease is frequently irreversible if deficiency is not corrected early enough. May contribute to the hemolytic anemia and retrolental fibroplasia seen in premature infants. Reported to suppress cell-mediated immunity. [15 mg]	Depressed levels of vitamin K-dependent procoagulants and potentiation of oral anticoagulants have been reported, as has impaired WBC function. Doses of 800 mg/day have been reported to increase slightly the incidence of hemorrhagic stroke. [1000 mg]	Plasma or serum concentration of α-tocopherol is most commonly used. Additional accuracy is obtained by expressing this value per mg of total plasma lipid. RBC peroxide hemolysis test is not entirely specific but is a useful functional measure of the antioxidant potential of cell membranes.
Vitamin K	A family of naphthoquinone compounds with similar biologic activity. Phylloquinone (vitamin K_1) is derived from plants; a variety of menaquinones (vitamin K_2) is derived from bacterial sources. Serves as an essential cofactor in the post-translational γ-carboxylation of glutamic acid residues in many proteins. These proteins include several circulating procoagulants and anticoagulants as well as proteins in a variety of tissues.	Deficiency syndrome, uncommon except in (1) breast-fed newborns, in whom it may cause "hemorrhagic disease of the newborn," (2) adults with fat malabsorption or who are taking drugs that interfere with vitamin K metabolism (e.g., coumarin, phenytoin, broad-spectrum antibiotics), and (3) individuals taking large doses of vitamin E and anticoagulant drugs. Excessive hemorrhage is the usual manifestation. [F: 90 μg; M: 120 μg]	Rapid intravenous infusion of K_1 has been associated with dyspnea, flushing, and cardiovascular collapse; this is likely related to the dispersing agents in the solution. Supplementation may interfere with coumarin-based anticoagulation. Pregnant women taking large amounts of the provitamin menadione may deliver infants with hemolytic anemia, hyperbilirubinemia, and kernicterus. [no TUL established]	Prothrombin time is typically used as a measure of functional K status; it is neither sensitive nor specific for vitamin K deficiency. Determination of undercarboxylated prothrombin in the plasma is more accurate but less widely available.

Water-Soluble Vitamins

	Biochemistry and Physiology	Deficiency [RDA*]	Toxicity [TUL†]	Assessment of Status
Thiamine (vitamin B_1)	A water-soluble compound containing substituted pyrimidine and thiazole rings and a hydroxyethyl side chain. The coenzyme form is thiamine pyrophosphate (TPP). Serves as a coenzyme in many α-ketoacid decarboxylation and transketolation reactions. Inadequate thiamine availability leads to impairments of above reactions, resulting in inadequate adenosine triphosphate synthesis and abnormal carbohydrate metabolism, respectively. May have an additional role in neuronal conduction independent of aforementioned actions.	Classic deficiency syndrome ("beriberi") described in Asian populations consuming polished rice diet. Alcoholism and chronic renal dialysis are also common precipitants. High carbohydrate intake increases need for B_1. *Mild deficiency:* irritability, fatigue, and headaches. *More severe deficiency:* combinations of peripheral neuropathy, cardiovascular dysfunction, and cerebral dysfunction. Cardiovascular involvement ("wet beriberi"): congestive heart failure and low peripheral vascular resistance. Cerebral disease: nystagmus, ophthalmoplegia, and ataxia (Wernicke's encephalopathy); hallucinations, impaired short-term memory, and confabulation ("Korsakoff's psychosis"). Deficiency syndrome responds within 24 hr to parenteral thiamine but is partially or wholly irreversible after a certain stage. [F: 1.1 mg; M: 1.2 mg]	Excess intake is largely excreted in the urine, although parenteral doses of > 400 mg/day are reported to cause lethargy, ataxia, and reduced tone of the gastrointestinal tract. [TUL not established]	The most effective measure of B_1 status is the erythrocyte transketolase activity coefficient, which measures enzyme activity before and after addition of exogenous TPP: RBCs from a deficient individual express a substantial increase in enzyme activity with addition of TPP. Thiamine concentrations in blood or urine are also used.
Riboflavin (vitamin B_2)	Consists of a substituted isoalloxazine ring with a ribitol side chain. Serves as a coenzyme for a diverse array of biochemical reactions. The primary coenzymatic forms are flavin mononucleotide (FMN) and flavin adenine dinucleotide (FAD). Riboflavin holoenzymes participate in oxidation-reduction reactions in a myriad of metabolic pathways.	Deficiency is usually seen in conjunction with deficiencies of other B vitamins. Isolated deficiency of riboflavin produces hyperemia and edema of nasopharyngeal mucosa, cheilosis, angular stomatitis, glossitis, seborrheic dermatitis, and a normochromic, normocytic anemia. [F: 1.1; M: 1.3]	Toxicity not reported in humans. [TUL not established]	The most common method of assessment is determining the activity coefficient of glutathione reductase in RBCs (the test is invalid for individuals with glucose-6-phosphate dehydrogenase [G6PD] deficiency). Measurements of blood and urine concentrations are less desirable methods.

	Biochemistry and Physiology	Deficiency [RDA*]	Toxicity [TUL†]	Assessment of Status
Niacin (vitamin B₃)	Refers to nicotinic acid and the corresponding amide, nicotinamide. The active coenzymatic forms are composed of nicotinamide affixed to adenine dinucleotide, forming NAD or NADP. More than 200 apoenzymes use these compounds as electron acceptors or hydrogen donors, either as a coenzyme or as a co-substrate. The essential amino acid tryptophan is a precursor of niacin; 60 mg of dietary tryptophan yields approximately 1 mg of niacin. Dietary requirements thus depend partly on tryptophan intake. Requirement is often determined on basis of caloric intake (i.e., niacin equivalents/1000 kcal). Large doses of nicotinic acid (1.5-3 g/day) effectively lower low-density lipoprotein cholesterol and elevate high-density lipoprotein cholesterol.	Pellagra is the classic deficiency syndrome and is often seen in populations in which corn is the major source of energy. Still endemic in parts of China, Africa, and India. Diarrhea, dementia (or associated symptoms of anxiety or insomnia), and a pigmented dermatitis that develops in sun-exposed areas are typical features. Glossitis, stomatitis, vaginitis, vertigo, and burning dysesthesias are early signs. Reported to occasionally occur in carcinoid syndrome because tryptophan is diverted to other synthetic pathways. [F: 14 mg; M: 16 mg]	Human toxicity known largely through studies examining hypolipidemic effects. Includes vasomotor phenomenon (flushing), hyperglycemia, parenchymal liver damage, and hyperuricemia. [35 mg]	Assessment of status is problematic: blood levels of vitamin not reliable. Measurement of urinary excretion of the niacin metabolites, N-methylnicotinamide and 2-pyridone, is thought to be the most effective means of assessment at present.
Vitamin B₆	Refers to several derivatives of pyridine, including pyridoxine (PN), pyridoxal (PL), and pyridoxamine (PM), which are interconvertible in the body. The coenzymatic forms are pyridoxal-5-phosphate (PLP) and pyridoxamine-5-phosphate (PMP). As a coenzyme, B₆ is involved in many transamination reactions (and thereby in gluconeogenesis), in the synthesis of niacin from tryptophan, in the synthesis of several neurotransmitters, and in the synthesis of δ-aminolevulinic acid (and therefore in heme synthesis). It also has functions unrelated to coenzymatic activity: PL and PLP bind to hemoglobin and alter O_2 affinity; PLP also binds to steroid receptors, inhibiting receptor affinity to DNA and thereby modulating steroid activity.	Deficiency usually seen in conjunction with other water-soluble vitamin deficiencies. Stomatitis, angular cheilosis, glossitis, irritability, depression, and confusion occur in moderate to severe depletion; normochromic, normocytic anemia has been reported in severe deficiency. Abnormal electroencephalograms and, in infants, convulsions have also been observed. Some sideroblastic anemias respond to B₆ administration. Isoniazid, cycloserine, penicillamine, ethanol, and theophylline can inhibit B₆ metabolism. [Ages 19-50 yr: 1.3 mg; >50 yr: 1.5 mg for women, 1.7 mg for men]	Long-term use with doses exceeding 200 mg/day (in adults) may cause peripheral neuropathies and photosensitivity. [100 mg]	Many useful laboratory methods of assessment exist. The plasma or erythrocyte PLP levels are most common. Urinary excretion of xanthurenic acid after an oral tryptophan load or activity indices of RBC alanine or aspartic acid transaminases (ALT and AST, respectively) are all functional measures of B₆-dependent enzyme activity.
Folate	A group of related pterin compounds. More than 35 forms of the vitamin are found naturally. The fully oxidized form, folic acid, is not found in nature but is the pharmacologic form of the vitamin. All folate functions relate to its ability to transfer one-carbon groups. It is essential in the *de novo* synthesis of nucleotides and in the metabolism of several amino acids, and is an integral component for the regeneration of the "universal" methyl donor, S-adenosylmethionine. Inhibition of bacterial and cancer cell folate metabolism is the basis for the sulfonamide antibiotics and chemotherapeutic agents such as methotrexate and 5-fluorouracil, respectively.	Women of childbearing age are most likely to be deficient. *Classic deficiency syndrome:* megaloblastic anemia, diarrhea. The hematopoietic cells in bone marrow become enlarged and have immature nuclei, reflecting ineffective DNA synthesis. The peripheral blood smear demonstrates macro-ovalocytes and polymorphonuclear leukocytes with an average of more than 3.5 nuclear lobes. Megaloblastic changes also occur in other epithelia that proliferate rapidly (e.g., oral mucosa, gastrointestinal tract), producing glossitis and diarrhea, respectively. Sulfasalazine and diphenytoin inhibit absorption and predispose to deficiency. [400 µg of dietary folate equivalents (DFE); 1 DFE = 1 µg food folate = 0.6 µg folic acid]	Doses >1000 µg/day may partially correct the anemia of B₁₂ deficiency and may therefore mask (and perhaps exacerbate) the associated neuropathy. Large doses also reported to lower seizure threshold in individuals prone to seizures. Parenteral administration is rarely reported to cause allergic phenomena, which is probably due to dispersion agents. [1000 µg]	Serum folate measures short-term folate balance, whereas RBC folate is a better reflection of tissue status. Serum homocysteine rises early in deficiency but is nonspecific because B₁₂ or B₆ deficiency, renal insufficiency, and older age may also cause elevations.

Continued on following page

	Biochemistry and Physiology	Deficiency [RDA*]	Toxicity [TUL†]	Assessment of Status
Vitamin C (ascorbic and dehydroascorbic acid)	Ascorbic acid readily oxidizes to dehydroascorbic acid in aqueous solution. The latter can be reduced in vivo, so it possesses vitamin C activity. Total vitamin C is therefore the sum of ascorbic and dehydroascorbic acid content. It serves primarily as a biologic antioxidant in aqueous environments. Biosyntheses of collagen, carnitine, bile acids, and norepinephrine, as well as proper functioning of the hepatic mixed-function oxygenase system, depend on this property. Vitamin C in foodstuffs increases the intestinal absorption of nonheme iron.	Overt deficiency is uncommon in developed countries. The classic deficiency syndrome is scurvy: fatigue, depression, and widespread abnormalities in connective tissues, such as inflamed gingivae, petechiae, perifollicular hemorrhages, impaired wound healing, coiled hairs, hyperkeratosis, bleeding into body cavities. In infants, defects in ossification and bone growth may occur. Tobacco smoking lowers plasma and leukocyte vitamin C levels. [F: 75 mg; M: 90 mg; increase requirement for cigarette smokers by 35 mg/day]	≥500 mg/day (in adults) may cause nausea and diarrhea. >1 g/day modestly increases risk for oxalate kidney stones. Supplementation may interfere with laboratory tests based on redox potential (e.g., fecal occult blood testing, serum cholesterol, and glucose). Withdrawal from chronic ingestion of high doses of vitamin C supplements should be done gradually because accommodation appears to occur, raising a concern of "rebound scurvy." [2 g]	Plasma ascorbic acid concentration reflects recent dietary intake, whereas WBC levels more closely reflect tissue stores. Women's plasma levels are approximately 20% higher than men's for any given dietary intake.
Vitamin B_{12}	A group of closely related cobalamin compounds composed of a corrin ring (with a cobalt atom in its center) connected to a ribonucleotide through an aminopropanol bridge. Microorganisms are the ultimate source of all naturally occurring B_{12}. The two active coenzyme forms are deoxyadenosylcobalamin and methylcobalamin. These coenzymes are needed for the synthesis of succinyl coenzyme A (CoA), which is essential in lipid and carbohydrate metabolism, and for the synthesis of methionine. The latter reaction is essential for amino acid metabolism, for purine and pyrimidine synthesis, for many methylation reactions, and for the intracellular retention of folates.	Dietary inadequacy is a rare cause of deficiency except in strict vegetarians. Most deficiencies arise from loss of intestinal absorption, which may occur with pernicious anemia, pancreatic insufficiency, atrophic gastritis, small bowel bacterial overgrowth, or ileal disease. Megaloblastic anemia and megaloblastic changes in other epithelia (see "Folate") are the result of sustained depletion. Demyelination of peripheral nerves, posterior and lateral columns of spinal cord, and nerves within the brain may occur. Altered mentation, depression, and psychoses occur. Hematologic and neurologic complications may occur independently. Folate supplementation, in doses of 1000 μg/day, may partly correct the anemia, thereby masking (or perhaps exacerbating) the neuropathic complication. [2.4 μg]	A few allergic reactions have been reported to crystalline B_{12} preparations and are probably due to impurities, not the vitamin. [TUL not established]	Serum, or plasma, concentrations are generally accurate. Subtle deficiency with neurologic complications, as described in the "Deficiency" column, can best be established by concurrently measuring the concentration of plasma B_{12} and serum methylmalonic acid because the latter is a sensitive indicator of cellular deficiency.
Biotin	A bi-cyclic compound consisting of a ureido ring fused to a substituted tetrahydrothiophene ring. Endogenous synthesis by intestinal flora may contribute significantly to biotin nutriture. Most dietary biotin is linked to lysine, a compound called biotinyl lysine, or biocytin. The lysine must be hydrolyzed by an intestinal enzyme called biotinidase before intestinal absorption occurs. Acts primarily as a coenzyme for several carboxylases; each holoenzyme catalyzes an ATP-dependent CO_2 transfer. The carboxylases are critical enzymes in carbohydrate and lipid metabolism.	Isolated deficiency is rare. Deficiency in humans has been produced by prolonged total parenteral nutrition lacking the vitamin and by ingestion of large quantities of raw egg white, which contains avidin, a protein that binds biotin with such high affinity that it renders it bio-unavailable. Alterations in mental status, myalgias, hyperesthesias, and anorexia occur. Later, a seborrheic dermatitis and alopecia develop. Deficiency is usually accompanied by lactic acidosis and organic aciduria. [30 μg]	Toxicity has not been reported in humans with doses as high as 60 mg/day in children. [TUL not established]	Plasma and urine concentrations of biotin are diminished in the deficient state. Elevated urine concentrations of methyl citrate, 3-methylcrotonylglycine, and 3-hydroxyisovalerate are also observed in deficiency.

	Biochemistry and Physiology	Deficiency [RDA*]	Toxicity [TUL†]	Assessment of Status
Pantothenic acid	Consists of pantoic acid linked to β-alanine through an amide bond. An essential component of CoA and phosphopantetheine, which are essential for synthesis and β-oxidation of fatty acids, as well as synthesis of cholesterol, steroid hormones, vitamins A and D, and other isoprenoid derivatives. CoA is also involved in the synthesis of several amino acids and δ-aminolevulinic acid, a precursor for the corrin ring of vitamin B_{12}, the porphyrin ring of heme, and of cytochromes. CoA is also necessary for the acetylation and fatty acid acylation of a variety of proteins.	Deficiency rare: only reported as a result of feeding semisynthetic diets or an antagonist to the vitamin. Experimental, isolated deficiency in humans produces fatigue, abdominal pain, vomiting, insomnia, and paresthesias of the extremities. [5 mg]	In doses of 10 g/day, diarrhea is reported to occur. [TUL not established]	Whole blood and urine concentrations of pantothenate are indicators of status; serum levels are not thought to be accurate.

PTH, Parathyroid hormone; *UVB*, ultraviolet B.

*Recommended daily allowance (RDA) established for female (F) and male (M) adults by the U.S. Food and Nutrition Board, 1999-2001. In some instances, insufficient data exist to establish an RDA, in which case the adequate intake (AI) established by the board is listed.

†Tolerated upper intake (TUL) established for adults by the U.S. Food and Nutrition Board, 1999-2001.

From Goldman L, Schafer AI: *Goldman's Cecil medicine,* ed 24, Philadelphia, 2012, Saunders.

Nutritional Trace Elements and Their Clinical Implications

	Biochemistry and Physiology	Deficiency [RDA*]	Toxicity [TUL†]	Assessment of Status
Chromium	Dietary chromium consists of both inorganic and organic forms. Its primary function in humans is to potentiate insulin action. It accomplishes this function as a circulating complex called *glucose tolerance factor,* thereby affecting carbohydrate, fat, and protein metabolism.	Deficiency in humans only described in long-term total parenteral nutrition (TPN) patients receiving insufficient chromium. Hyperglycemia or impaired glucose tolerance occurs. Elevated plasma-free fatty acid concentrations, neuropathy, encephalopathy, and abnormalities in nitrogen metabolism are also reported. Whether supplemental chromium may improve glucose tolerance in glucose-intolerant individuals remains controversial. [F: 25 µg; M: 35 µg]	Toxicity after oral ingestion is uncommon and seems confined to gastric irritation. Airborne exposure may cause contact dermatitis, eczema, skin ulcers, and bronchogenic carcinoma. [no TUL established]	Plasma or serum concentration of chromium is a crude indicator of chromium status; it appears to be meaningful when the value is markedly above or below the normal range.
Copper	Copper is absorbed by a specific intestinal transport mechanism. It is carried to the liver where it is bound to ceruloplasmin, which circulates systemically and delivers copper to target tissues in the body. Excretion of copper is largely through bile, and then into the feces. Absorptive and excretory processes vary with the levels of dietary copper, providing a means of copper homeostasis. Copper serves as a component of many enzymes, including amine oxidases, ferroxidases, cytochrome c oxidase, dopamine β-hydroxylase, superoxide dismutase, and tyrosinase.	Dietary deficiency is rare; it has been observed in premature and low-birthweight infants fed exclusively a cow's milk diet and in individuals on long-term TPN without copper. Clinical manifestations include depigmentation of skin and hair, neurologic disturbances, leukopenia, hypochromic microcytic anemia, and skeletal abnormalities. Anemia arises from impaired utilization of iron and is therefore a conditioned form of iron deficiency anemia. The deficiency syndrome, except the anemia and leukopenia, is also observed in Menkes' disease, a rare inherited condition associated with impaired copper utilization. [900 µg]	Acute copper toxicity has been described after excessive oral intake and with absorption of copper salts applied to burned skin. Milder manifestations include nausea, vomiting, epigastric pain, and diarrhea; coma and hepatic necrosis may ensue in severe cases. Toxicity may be seen with doses as low as 70 µg/kg/day. Chronic toxicity is also described. Wilson's disease is a rare, inherited disease associated with abnormally low ceruloplasmin levels and accumulation of copper in the liver and brain, eventually leading to damage to these two organs. [10 mg]	Practical methods for detecting marginal deficiency are not available. Marked deficiency is reliably detected by diminished serum copper and ceruloplasmin concentrations as well as low red blood cell (RBC) superoxide dismutase activity.
Fluorine	Known more commonly by its ionic form, fluoride. It is incorporated into the crystalline structure of bone, thereby altering its physical characteristics.	Intake of <0.1 mg/day in infants and <0.5 mg/day in children is associated with an increased incidence of dental caries. Optimal intake in adults is between 1.5 and 4 mg/day. [F: 3 mg; M: 4 mg]	Acute ingestion of >30 mg/kg body weight is likely to cause death. Excessive chronic intake (0.1 mg/kg/day) leads to mottling of teeth (dental fluorosis), calcification of tendons and ligaments, and exostoses and may increase the brittleness of bones. [10 mg]	Estimates of intake or clinical assessment are used because no good laboratory test exists.

	Biochemistry and Physiology	Deficiency [RDA*]	Toxicity [TUL†]	Assessment of Status
Iodine	Readily absorbed from the diet, concentrated in the thyroid, and integrated into the thyroid hormones, thyroxine (T_4) and triiodothyronine (T_3). These hormones circulate largely bound to thyroxine-binding globulin. They modulate resting energy expenditure and, in the developing human, growth and development.	In the absence of supplementation, populations relying primarily on food from soils with low iodine content have endemic iodine deficiency. Maternal iodine deficiency leads to fetal deficiency, which produces spontaneous abortions, stillbirths, hypothyroidism, cretinism, and dwarfism. Permanent cognitive deficits may result from iodine deficiency during first 2 years of life. In the adult, compensatory hypertrophy of the thyroid goiter occurs along with varying degrees of hypothyroidism. [150 µg]	Large doses (>2 mg/day in adults) may induce hypothyroidism by blocking thyroid hormone synthesis. Supplementation with >100 mg/day to an individual who was formerly deficient occasionally induces hyperthyroidism. [1.1 mg]	Iodine status of a population can be estimated by the prevalence of goiter. Urinary excretion of iodine is an effective laboratory means of assessment. Thyroid-stimulating hormone (TSH) blood level is an indirect, and therefore not entirely specific, means of assessment.
Iron	Conveys the capacity to participate in redox reactions to a number of metalloproteins such as hemoglobin, myoglobin, cytochrome enzymes, and many oxidases and oxygenases. Primary storage form is ferritin and, to a lesser degree, hemosiderin. Intestinal absorption is 15%-20% for "heme" iron and 1%-8% for iron contained in vegetables. Absorption of the latter form is enhanced by the ascorbic acid in foodstuffs; by poultry, fish, or beef; and by an iron-deficient state. It is decreased by phytate and tannins.	The most common micronutrient deficiency in the world. Women of childbearing age are the highest-risk group because of menstrual blood losses, pregnancy, and lactation. The classic deficiency syndrome is hypochromic, microcytic anemia. Glossitis and koilonychia ("spoon" nails) are also observed. Easy fatigability often is an early symptom, before anemia appears. In children, mild deficiency of insufficient severity to cause anemia is associated with behavioral disturbances and poor school performance. [postmenopausal F and M: 8 mg; premenopausal F: 18 mg]	Iron overload typically occurs when habitual dietary intake is extremely high, intestinal absorption is excessive, repeated parenteral administration occurs, or a combination of these factors exists. Excessive iron stores usually accumulate in the reticuloendothelial tissues and cause little damage ("hemosiderosis"). If overload continues, iron eventually begins to accumulate in tissues such as the hepatic parenchyma, pancreas, heart, and synovium, causing hemochromatosis. Hereditary hemochromatosis results from homozygosity of a common recessive trait. Excessive intestinal absorption of iron is seen in homozygotes. [45 mg]	Negative iron balance initially leads to depletion of iron stores in the bone marrow: a bone marrow biopsy and the concentration of serum ferritin are accurate indicators of early depletion. As the severity of deficiency proceeds, serum iron (SI) decreases and total iron-binding capacity (TIBC) increases: an iron saturation (SI/TIBC) of <16% suggests iron deficiency. Microcytosis, hypochromia, and anemia ensue. Elevated levels of serum ferritin or an iron saturation of >60% suggest iron overload, although systemic inflammation elevates serum ferritin regardless of iron status.
Manganese	A component of several metalloenzymes. Most manganese is in mitochondria, where it is a component of manganese superoxide dismutase.	Manganese deficiency in the human has not been conclusively demonstrated. It is said to cause hypocholesterolemia, weight loss, hair and nail changes, dermatitis, and impaired synthesis of vitamin K–dependent proteins. [F: 1.8 mg; M: 2.3 mg]	Toxicity by oral ingestion is unknown in humans. Toxic inhalation causes hallucinations, other alterations in mentation, and extrapyramidal movement disorders. [11 mg]	Until the deficiency syndrome is better defined, an appropriate measure of status will be difficult to develop.
Molybdenum	A cofactor in several enzymes, most prominently xanthine oxidase and sulfite oxidase.	A probable case of human deficiency is described as being secondary to parenteral administration of sulfite and resulted in hyperoxypurinemia, hypouricemia, and low sulfate excretion. [45 µg]	Toxicity not well described in humans, although it may interfere with copper metabolism at high doses. [2 mg]	Laboratory means of assessment not meaningful until deficiency syndrome is better described.
Selenium	Most dietary selenium is in the form of an amino acid complex. Nearly complete absorption of such forms occurs. Homeostasis is largely performed by the kidney, which regulates urinary excretion as a function of selenium status. Selenium is a component of several enzymes, most notably glutathione peroxidase and superoxide dismutase. These enzymes protect against oxidative and free radical damage of various cell structures. The antioxidant protection conveyed by selenium apparently operates in conjunction with vitamin E because deficiency of one seems to potentiate damage induced by a deficiency of the other. Selenium also participates in the enzymatic conversion of thyroxine to its more active metabolite, triiodothyronine.	Deficiency is rare in North America but has been observed in individuals on long-term TPN lacking selenium. Such individuals have myalgias and/or cardiomyopathies. Populations in some regions of the world, most notably some parts of China, have marginal intake of selenium. In these regions Keshan's disease, a condition characterized by cardiomyopathy, is endemic; it can be prevented (but not treated) by selenium supplementation. [55 µg]	Toxicity is associated with nausea, diarrhea, alterations in mental status, peripheral neuropathy, loss of hair and nails: such symptoms were observed in adults who inadvertently consumed 27-2400 mg. [400 µg]	Erythrocyte glutathione peroxidase activity and plasma, or whole blood, selenium concentrations are the most commonly used methods of assessment. They are moderately accurate indicators of status.

Continued on following page

	Biochemistry and Physiology	Deficiency [RDA*]	Toxicity [TUL†]	Assessment of Status
Zinc	Intestinal absorption occurs by a specific process that is enhanced by pregnancy and corticosteroids and diminished by coingestion of phytates, phosphates, iron, copper, lead, or calcium. Diminished intake of zinc leads to an increased efficiency of absorption and decreased fecal excretion, providing a means of zinc homeostasis. Zinc is a component of more than 100 enzymes, among which are DNA polymerase, RNA polymerase, and transfer RNA synthetase.	Zinc deficiency has its most profound effect on rapidly proliferating tissues. *Mild deficiency:* growth retardation in children. *More severe deficiency:* growth arrest, teratogenicity, hypogonadism and infertility, dysgeusia, poor wound healing, diarrhea, dermatitis on the extremities and around orifices, glossitis, alopecia, corneal clouding, loss of dark adaptation, and behavioral changes. Impaired cellular immunity is observed. Excessive loss of gastrointestinal secretions through chronic diarrhea and fistulas may precipitate deficiency. Acrodermatitis enteropathica is a rare, recessively inherited disease in which intestinal absorption of zinc is impaired. [F: 8 mg; M: 11 mg]	Acute zinc toxicity can usually be induced by ingestion of >200 mg of zinc in a single day (in adults). It is manifested as epigastric pain, nausea, vomiting, and diarrhea. Hyperpnea, diaphoresis, and weakness may follow inhalation of zinc fumes. Copper and zinc compete for intestinal absorption: long-term ingestion of >25 mg/day of zinc may lead to copper deficiency. Long-term ingestion of >150 mg/day has been reported to cause gastric erosions, low high-density lipoprotein cholesterol levels, and impaired cellular immunity. [40 mg]	No accurate indicators of zinc status exist for routine clinical use. Plasma, RBC, and hair zinc concentrations are often misleading. Acute illness, in particular, is known to diminish plasma zinc levels, in part by inducing a shift of zinc out of the plasma compartment and into the liver. Functional tests that determine dark adaptation, taste acuity, and rate of wound healing lack specificity.

*Recommended daily allowance (RDA) established for female (F) and male (M) adults by the U.S. Food and Nutrition Board, 1999-2001. In some instances, insufficient data exist to establish an RDA, in which case the adequate intake (AI) established by the board is listed.

†Tolerated upper limit (TUL) established for adults by the U.S. Food and Nutrition Board, 1999-2001.

From Goldman L, Schafer AI: *Goldman's Cecil medicine,* ed 24, Philadelphia, 2012, Saunders.

Summary of Vitamin and Mineral Deficiencies

Vitamin and Mineral Deficiencies	Neurologic Syndrome or Syndromes	Supporting Tests	Treatment	Causes (Other Than Malnutrition)
A (retinol)	Blindness from retinal or corneal damage	Visual fields, visual acuity Serum level <30-65 µg/dl	30,000 IU vitamin A daily × 1 wk	Hypothyroidism, diabetes, renal or liver failure
B_1 (thiamine)	Wernicke's encephalopathy: ataxia, nystagmus, ophthalmoparesis, confusion, delirium Korsakoff's syndrome: amnesia, confabulation Beriberi: axonal neuropathy	MRI: symmetric lesions of midbrain (periaqueductal area), pons, hypothalamus, thalamus, cerebellum MRI: necrosis of mammillary bodies, dorsomedial and anterior thalamus Nerve conduction tests: decreased amplitude Serum thiamine level <20 ng/dl Erythrocyte transketolase	Prevent by 100 mg PO daily before and 1 year after bariatric surgery, 100 mg IV before glucose administration or refeeding Treat Wernicke's encephalopathy with 5 days of thiamine, 100-500 mg IV or IM daily, then PO 100 mg daily Antioxidants (N-acetylcysteine)	Alcoholism, bariatric or other major GI surgery, prolonged vomiting, hemodialysis, diuretic treatment of heart failure, cachexia, 5-fluorouracil, other blockers of thiamine phosphate production
B_3 (niacin)	Pellagra: confusion, dementia, weakness, ataxia, spasticity, myoclonus, glossitis, dermatitis, photosensitivity	Erythrocyte NAD, plasma niacin, urinary N_1-methylnicotinamide	Nicotinic acid, 50 mg PO tid or 25 mg IV tid; nicotinamide, 50-100 mg IM or PO tid	Alcoholism, corn- or cereal-based diet, Hartnup's syndrome, carcinoid syndrome
B_5 (pantothenic acid)	Dysesthesias, foot paresthesias	Deficient coenzyme A	5 mg PO daily	Severe malnutrition
B_6 (pyridoxine)	Neuropathy, sensory ataxia, depression Infantile pyridoxine-deficient epilepsy	Plasma PLP <27 nmol/L; urinary 4-pyridoxic acid, <3 nmol ↑ Homocysteine after methionine loading challenge ↑ α-AASA in urine, plasma, CSF	50-100 mg PO daily for neuropathy (preventive use if taking B_6 antagonist) 100-200 mg daily for adult epilepsy	Diverticulosis, isoniazid, cycloserine, other antagonists Genetic defects in antiquitin (aldehyde dehydrogenase), pyridoxal synthesis
B_{12} (cobalamin)	Myelopathy with spastic paraparesis and sensory ataxia, peripheral neuropathy, optic neuropathy, memory loss, dementia; indirect contributor to stroke	Blood level <200 pg/ml ↑ Methylmalonic acid >145 nmol/L Intrinsic factor antibodies Schilling test, megaloblastic anemia Delayed somatosensory evoked potentials ↑ Homocysteine, total >12.5 µmol/L	IM B_{12}, 1000 µg daily for 1 week, then weekly for 1 month, then monthly or oral B_{12}, 1000 µg daily, or nasal B_{12}, 500 µg weekly for lifetime if abnormal absorption, 50-100 µg daily if normal absorption	Achlorhydria, gastric or ileal resection, blind loop syndrome, sprue, HIV infection, nitrous oxide anesthesia (especially abuse), fish tapeworm, vegan diet
D (calciferol)	Proximal myopathy, often painful; cognitive impairment Secondary compression of spinal cord, plexus, or peripheral nerves from rickets or osteomalacia	25-(OH) vitamin D_3 level <10 ng/ml in urine Serum calcium ↑ PTH >54 pg/ml Osteopenia/porosis on bone densitometry	Daily supplementation with 400 IU, >50,000 IU 3 times per wk if malabsorption; use blood level or urine calcium excretion to guide (should be >100 mg/day)	Lack of exposure to sunlight, including sunblock protection; chronic antiepileptic drug use
E (tocopherol)	Spinal and cerebellar ataxia, Babinski's sign, ophthalmoplegia, peripheral neuropathy, retinitis pigmentosa	Vitamin E level <2.5 mg/L (normal, 6-15 with normal lipid level) ↑ A-β-lipoprotein levels, antigliadin antibodies Genetic analysis to rule out other spinocerebellar ataxias such as Friedreich's ataxia	Supplement with 6-800 IU, 5-10 mg/kg twice daily, for ataxia of genetic causes, water-soluble 200 mg/kg/day or IM α-tocopherol for malabsorption	Biliary atresia, celiac sprue, Genetic: ↓ α-tocopherol transport protein (8q13), microsomal triglyceride transfer protein

Continued on following page

Summary of Vitamin and Mineral Deficiencies

Vitamin and Mineral Deficiencies	Neurologic Syndrome or Syndromes	Supporting Tests	Treatment	Causes (Other Than Malnutrition)
Folate	Dementia, B$_{12}$ deficiency, stroke	↑ Homocysteine, plasma level <2.5 µg/L	1 mg 3 times per day until normal level, then maintenance of 1 mg/day Pregnancy: additional 0.4 mg/day if taking a folate antagonist	Malabsorption or use of antagonist (methotrexate) or antiepileptic medication
K (phytonadione)	Intracranial hemorrhage	INR or PT elevation	IM phytonadione at birth, maternal vitamin K for last month of pregnancy	Medication use that increases metabolism, such as phenytoin
Copper	Myelopathy, neuropathy	Serum Cu <75 µg/dl, ↓ urinary Cu, ceruloplasmin <23 mg/dl MRI: ↑ T$_2$ signal in cervical cord, dorsal column Mutation in ATP7A gene (Menkes' disease)	Elemental Cu, 8 mg/day PO week 1, 6 mg/day week 2, 4 mg/day week 3, 2 mg/day ongoing malabsorption Menkes' disease: 250 mg SC bid	Wilson's disease, Menkes' disease, alcoholism, malabsorption, gastric bypass, zinc toxicity
Magnesium	Seizures, encephalopathy	Serum magnesium <1.5 mg/dl, correct for low albumin	Magnesium sulfate IV or PO Avoid magnesium-wasting drugs	Alcoholism, especially beer
Potassium	Muscle weakness, chronic, acute	Serum potassium <3.5 mEq/L, ECG	IV or PO KCl until normalized	Diuretic use, bulimia

AASA, Aminoadipic semialdehyde; *CSF,* cerebrospinal fluid; *ECG,* electrocardiography; *GI,* gastrointestinal; *HIV,* human immunodeficiency virus; *IM,* intramuscularly; *INR,* international normalized ratio; *IU,* international units; *IV,* intravenously; *MRI,* magnetic resonance imaging; *NAD,* nicotinamide adenine dinucleotide; *PLP,* pyridoxal-5-phosphate (active coenzyme of pyridoxine); *PO,* by mouth; *PT,* prothrombin time; *PTH,* parathyroid hormone; *tid,* three times a day.

From Goldman L, Schafer AI: *Goldman's Cecil medicine,* ed 24, Philadelphia, 2012, Saunders.

Historical and Physical Findings in Poisoning

Sign	Toxin
Odor	
Bitter almonds	Cyanide
Acetone	Isopropyl alcohol, methanol, paraldehyde, salicylates
Alcohol	Ethanol
Wintergreen	Methyl salicylate
Garlic	Arsenic, thallium, organophosphates, selenium
Ocular Signs	
Miosis	Opioids (except propoxyphene, meperidine, and pentazocine), organophosphates and other cholinergics, clonidine, phenothiazines, sedative-hypnotics, olanzapine
Mydriasis	Atropine, cocaine, amphetamines, antihistamines, TCAs, carbamazepine, serotonin syndrome, PCP, LSD, postanoxic encephalopathy
Nystagmus	Phenytoin, barbiturates, sedative-hypnotics, alcohols, carbamazepine, PCP, ketamine, dextromethorphan
Lacrimation	Organophosphates, irritant gas or vapors
Retinal hyperemia	Methanol
Cutaneous Signs	
Diaphoresis	Organophosphates, salicylates, cocaine and other sympathomimetics, serotonin syndrome, withdrawal syndromes
Alopecia	Thallium, arsenic
Erythema	Boric acid, elemental mercury, cyanide, carbon monoxide, disulfiram, scombroid, anticholinergics
Cyanosis (unresponsive to oxygen)	Methemoglobinemia (e.g., benzocaine, dapsone, nitrites, phenazopyridine), amiodarone, silver
Oral Signs	
Salivation	Organophosphates, salicylates, corrosives, ketamine, PCP, strychnine
Oral burns	Corrosives, oxalate-containing plants
Gum lines	Lead, mercury, arsenic, bismuth
Gastrointestinal Signs	
Diarrhea	Antimicrobials, arsenic, iron, boric acid, cholinergics, colchicine, withdrawal
Hematemesis	Arsenic, iron, caustics, NSAIDs, salicylates
Cardiac Signs	
Tachycardia	Sympathomimetics (e.g., amphetamines, cocaine), anticholinergics, antidepressants, theophylline, caffeine, antipsychotics, atropine, salicylates, cellular asphyxiants (cyanide, carbon monoxide, hydrogen sulfide), withdrawal
Bradycardia	β-Blockers, calcium channel blockers, digoxin, clonidine and other central α_2 agonists, organophosphates, opioids, sedative-hypnotics
Hypertension	Sympathomimetics (amphetamines, cocaine, LSD), anticholinergics, clonidine (early), monoamine oxidase inhibitors
Hypotension	β-Blockers, calcium channel blockers, cyclic antidepressants, iron, phenothiazines, barbiturates, clonidine, theophylline, opioids, arsenic, amatoxin mushrooms, cellular asphyxiants (cyanide, carbon monoxide, hydrogen sulfide), snake envenomation
Respiratory Signs	
Depressed respirations	Opioids, sedative-hypnotics, alcohol, clonidine, barbiturates
Tachypnea	Salicylates, amphetamines, caffeine, metabolic acidosis (ethylene glycol, methanol, cyanide), carbon monoxide, hydrocarbons

1939

Continued on following page

Sign	Toxin
Central Nervous System Signs	
Ataxia	Alcohol, anticonvulsants, benzodiazepines, barbiturates, lithium, dextromethorphan, carbon monoxide, inhalants
Coma	Opioids, sedative-hypnotics, anticonvulsants, cyclic antidepressants, antipsychotics, ethanol, anticholinergics, clonidine, GHB, alcohols, salicylates, barbiturates
Seizures	Sympathomimetics, anticholinergics, antidepressants (especially TCAs, bupropion, venlafaxine), isoniazid, camphor, lindane, salicylates, lead, organophosphates, carbamazepine, tramadol, lithium, ginkgo seeds, water hemlock, withdrawal
Delirium/psychosis	Sympathomimetics, anticholinergics, LSD, PCP, hallucinogens, lithium, dextromethorphan, steroids, withdrawal
Peripheral neuropathy	Lead, arsenic, mercury, organophosphates

GHB, Gamma hydroxybutyrate; *LSD,* lysergic acid diethylamide; *NSAID,* nonsteroidal anti-inflammatory drug; *PCP,* phencyclidine; *TCA,* tricylic antidepressant.
From Goldman L, Schafer AI: *Goldman's Cecil medicine,* ed 24, Philadelphia, 2012, Saunders.

Recognizable Poison Syndromes

Poison Syndrome	SIGNS						Possible Toxins
	Vital	Mental Status	Pupils	Skin	Bowel Sounds	Other	
Sympathomimetic	Hypertension, tachycardia, hyperthermia	Agitated, psychosis, delirium	Dilated	Diaphoretic	Normal to increased		Amphetamines, cocaine, Ecstasy, pseudoephedrine, caffeine, theophylline
Anticholinergic	Hypertension, tachycardia, hyperthermia	Agitation, delirium, mumbling speech	Dilated	Dry	Decreased		Antihistamines, tricyclic antidepressants, atropine, jimson weed, phenothiazines
Cholinergic	Bradycardia (although may show tachycardia), BP and temp typically normal	Confusion, coma, fasciculations	Small	Diaphoretic	Hyperactive	Diarrhea, urination, bronchorrhea, bronchospasm, emesis, lacrimation, salivation	Organophosphates, nerve gases, Alzheimer medications
Opioids	Respiratory depression (hallmark of toxicity), bradycardia, hypotension, hypothermia	Depression, coma	Pinpoint	Normal	Normal to decreased		Methadone, suboxone, morphine, oxycodone, heroin, etc.
Sedative-hypnotics	Respiratory depression, HR normal to decreased, BP normal to decreased, temp normal to decreased	Somnolence, coma	Small	Normal	Normal		Barbiturates, benzodiazepines, ethanol
Serotonin syndrome	Hyperthermia, tachycardia, hypertension or hypotension (autonomic instability)	Agitation, confusion, coma	Dilated	Diaphoretic	Increased	Neuromuscular hyperexcitability: clonus, hyperreflexia (lower extremities > upper extremities)	SSRIs, lithium, MAOIs, linezolid, tramadol, meperidine, dextromethorphan
Salicylates	Tachypnea, hyperpnea, tachycardia, hyperthermia	Agitation, confusion, coma	Normal	Diaphoretic	Normal	Nausea, vomiting, tinnitus, ABG with primary respiratory alkalosis and primary metabolic acidosis	Aspirin, bismuth subsalicylate (Pepto-Bismol), methylsalicylates
Withdrawal	Tachycardia, tachypnea, hyperthermia	Lethargy, confusion, delirium	Dilated	Diaphoretic	Increased		Withdrawal from opioids, sedative-hypnotics, ethanol

ABG, Arterial blood gas; *BP,* blood pressure; *HR,* heart rate; *MAOI,* monoamine oxidase inhibitor; *SSRI,* selective serotonin reuptake inhibitor; *temp,* temperature.
From Kliegman RM et al: *Nelson textbook of pediatrics,* ed 19, Philadelphia, 2011, Saunders.

Antidotes and Indications for Use

Antidote	Indication for Use	Dose*	Treatment End Point	Comments
Antivenom (Fab)[†]	Crotalines	4-6 vials; repeat for persistent or worsening clinical condition; repeat doses of 2 vials at 6, 12, and 18 hr after initial antivenom dose(s) are recommended	Halt in progression of circumferential and proximal swelling Resolving systemic effects	Better safety profile than equine-derived antivenom Repetitive dosing indicated for recurrent soft tissue swelling
Antivenom, *Latrodectus* (equine)[†]	Black widow spider (*Latrodectus* sp.)	1 vial diluted in 100 ml NS, infused over 1 hr; can repeat	Resolution of symptoms, vital signs normal	Dilution and slow infusion rate are critical to avoid anaphylactoid reaction Indications include severe pain unresponsive to opioids and severe hypertension Serum sickness can occur IV calcium is ineffective
Atropine	Carbamates Nerve agents Organophosphorus compounds	2 mg IV; double the dose every 5 min to achieve atropinization and hemodynamic stability; then start continuous infusion of 10%-20% of total stabilizing dose per hr	Cessation of excessive oral and pulmonary secretions, >80 bpm, systolic blood pressure >80 mm Hg	Doubling of the dose every 5 min (e.g., 2 mg, 4 mg, 8 mg, 16 mg) estimated to achieve atropinization within 30 min Stop infusion if patient develops any signs or symptoms of anticholinergic toxidrome; restart infusion at lower rate when signs or symptoms abate
Calcium[‡]	Calcium-channel antagonists	Calcium chloride 10%, 20-50 mg (0.2-0.5 ml)/kg/hr	Reversal of hypotension; may not reverse bradycardia	All indications: Monitor ionized calcium levels IV extravasation causes tissue necrosis, especially with calcium chloride Can administer at faster than stated rates for immediate, life-threatening conditions Taper infusions and monitor for relapse of toxicity when discontinuing therapy Calcium chloride contains three times more elemental calcium than calcium gluconate does Calcium-channel antagonists may be ineffective in severe toxicity
	Hydrofluoric acid	Systemic toxicity: calcium gluconate 10%, 1-3 g (10-30 ml) per dose IV over 10-min period; repeat as needed every 5-10 min	Reversal of life-threatening manifestations of hypocalcemia and hyperkalemia	Can dilute and give intraarterially or IV with a Bier block for extremity exposures and burns
	Hyperkalemia (except cardiac glycosides)	Calcium gluconate 10%, 1 g (10 ml) per dose IV over 10-min period; repeat as needed every 5-10 min	Reversal of myocardial depression and conduction delays	May precipitate ventricular arrhythmias
	Hypermagnesemia	Calcium gluconate 10%, 1-2 g (10-20 ml) per dose IV over 10-min period; repeat as needed every 5-10 min	Reversal of respiratory depression, hypotension, and cardiac conduction blocks	Simultaneous therapies to increase magnesium elimination should be instituted
	Hypocalcemia (e.g., ethylene glycol)	Calcium gluconate 10%, 0.5-1.0 g (5-10 ml) per dose over 10-min period; repeat as needed every 10 min	Reversal of tetany	Correct symptomatic hypocalcemia; avoid excessive administration that may increase production of calcium oxalate crystals in ethylene glycol poisoning

Antidote	Indication for Use	Dose*	Treatment End Point	Comments
L-Carnitine	Valproate-induced hyperammonemia or hepatotoxicity	100 mg/kg (maximum 6 g) IV over 30 min, then 15 mg/kg IV over 30-min period q4h (max 6 g/day)	Treat until clinical improvement occurs	Levocarnitine is active form Adjust dose for end-stage renal disease
Cyanide antidote kit	Cyanide		Resolution of lactic acidosis and moderate to severe clinical signs and symptoms: seizures, coma, dyspnea, apnea, hypotension, bradycardia	
Amyl nitrate		Amyl nitrite: 0.3-ml pearls, crush and inhale over 30-sec period		Coordinate amyl nitrite with continued oxygenation and give only until sodium nitrite infusion is begun; nitrites may produce hypotension and excess methemoglobinemia
Sodium nitrite		Sodium nitrite 3%: 10 ml IV over 10-min period		Sodium nitrite dose must be adjusted if patient has hemoglobin <12 g/dl
Sodium thiosulfate		Sodium thiosulfate 25%: 50 ml (12.5 g) IV over 10-min period		Sodium thiosulfate dosing can be repeated
Deferoxamine	Iron	15 ml/kg/hr IV (max 8 g/day) Mild to moderate: administer for 6-12 hr Severe toxicity: administer 24 hr	Resolution of clinical signs and symptoms Do not use urine color, which is an unreliable marker for iron clearance	Indications: symptomatic patients with lethargy, severe abdominal pain, hypovolemia, acidosis, shock; any symptomatic patient with peak serum iron level >350 g/dl Prolonged therapy can cause pulmonary toxicity
Digoxin-specific antibody fragments (Fab)	Digoxin Digitalis Other cardiac glycosides (e.g., bufodienalides [*Bufo toads*], oleander)	Unknown digoxin dose or serum level or for plant or toad source: acute toxicity—10-20 vials; chronic toxicity—3-6 vials Digoxin dose known: number of vials = (mg ingested × 0.8) ÷ 0.5 Digoxin serum level known: number of vials = [serum level (ng/ml) × weight (kg)] ÷ 100	Resolution of hyperkalemia, symptomatic bradydysrhythmias, ventricular arrhythmias, Mobitz II or third-degree heart block	Each vial binds 0.5 mg of digoxin or digitoxin Monitor ECG and potassium levels Digoxin serum levels unreliable after antidote administered unless test is specific for free serum digoxin
Dimercaprol (BAL)	Arsenic Lead Mercury, elemental and inorganic salts	Arsenic: 3-5 mg/kg IM q4h Lead: 75 mg/m² (4 mg/kg) IM q4h for 5 days Inorganic mercury: 5 mg/kg IM, then 2.5 mg/kg IM q12h for 10 days or until patient clinically improved	Arsenic: 24-hr urinary arsenic <50 μg/L Lead: encephalopathy resolved, blood lead level <100 μg/dl, and succimer therapy can be started Mercury, elemental and inorganic: 24-hr urinary mercury <20 μg/L	Maximum adult dose is 3 g/day BAL started 4 hr before initiation of concomitant CaNa₂EDTA for lead encephalopathy Dosing not well established for arsenic and elemental or inorganic mercury toxicity; not used for organic mercury poisoning Adverse effects: painful injections, fever, diaphoresis, agitation, headache, salivation, nausea and vomiting, hemolysis in G6PD-deficient patients, chelation of essential metals Check essential metal levels if chelation is prolonged Succimer is replacing BAL for many indications except lead encephalopathy Treatment end points for arsenic and mercury include improving clinical condition
Edetate calcium disodium (CaNa₂EDTA)	Lead	1500 mg/m²/24 hr (max 3 g) by continuous infusion	Treat for 5 days, followed by 2-day hiatus; repeat until encephalopathy resolved, lead level <100 μg/dl, and succimer therapy can be started	Use in patients with lead encephalopathy or lead level >100 g/dl Administer BAL 4 hr before initiating CaNa₂EDTA Hydrate patient and establish good urinary output before starting therapy Avoid thrombophlebitis by diluting in NS or D₅W to a concentration ≤0.5% Substitution of Na₂EDTA can cause fatal hypocalcemia
Flumazenil	Benzodiazepines Venlafaxine	0.1 mg/min IV to a total dose of 1 mg	Reversal of respiratory depression	Limit use to reversal of inadequate respiration in benzodiazepine-toxic patients Increases intracranial pressure and risk for seizures in presence of underlying seizure disorder or ingestion of seizure-producing toxicants Monitor for resedation up to 2 hr after last dose

Continued on following page

Antidote	Indication for Use	Dose*	Treatment End Point	Comments
Folinate (tetrahydrofolic acid [leuco-vorin])	Methanol Methotrexate	Methanol: 50 mg IV q4h Methotrexate: 100 mg/m² IV q3-6h	Methanol: methanol undetectable, metabolic acidosis cleared Methotrexate: serum level <1 × 10⁻⁸ mol/L	Essential therapy for both toxicants Methotrexate: large ingestions may require increased dose Glucarpidase administered 2-4 hr before or after folinate
Fomepizole	Ethylene glycol Methanol	Dose 1: 15 mg/kg IV Doses over next 48 hr: 10 mg/kg IV All subsequent doses: 15 mg/kg IV Administer q12h, except when HD performed: HD initiation: ½ next dose if >6 hr since last dose HD ongoing: q4h End of HD (based on time of last dose): <1 hr, no dose; 1-3 hr, ½ next dose; >3 hr, next dose	For both: serum level <20 mg/dl and metabolic acidosis resolved	Start immediately if toxic alcohol suspected, without waiting for confirmatory levels Dose amount is not affected by interval timing of doses
Glucagon	β-Adrenergic receptor antagonists Calcium-channel antagonists	Bolus of 3.5-5 mg IV; can repeat to achieve clinical effect, then infusion of 2-10 mg/hr	Reversal of hypotension and bradycardia; taper infusion	Can precipitate vomiting; be prepared to protect airway Mild hyperglycemia occurs Maximum dosing amounts unknown; bolus doses up to 30 mg reported Duration of effect is 15 min; thus infusion must be started immediately
Hydroxocobalamin	Cyanide	Initial: 5 g IV over 15-min period Second dose: 5 g IV over 15 min–2 hr; maximum total dose is 10 g Follow each hydroxocobalamin dose with sodium thiosulfate 25%: 50 ml (12.5 g) IV over 10-min period	Resolution of lactic acidosis and moderate to severe clinical signs and symptoms: seizures, coma, dyspnea, apnea, hypotension, bradycardia	Can be administered IV push if patient is in cardiac arrest Do not give hydroxocobalamin and sodium thiosulfate through the same IV line Adverse effects: red discoloration of plasma, urine, mucous membranes, skin; transient hypertension Interference with laboratory colorometric assays: Levels increased: bilirubin; creatinine; glucose; hemoglobin; magnesium; co-oximetry total Hb, COHb%, MetHb% Levels decreased: AST, ALT, creatinine, co-oximetry O₂Hb%
Hyperbaric oxygen (HBO)	Carbon monoxide Experimental: carbon tetrachloride, cyanide, hydrogen sulfide	3.0 atm pressure for 60 min (25 min O₂, 5 min air, 25 min O₂, 5 min air), then 2.0 atm for 65 min (30 min O₂, 5 min air, 30 min O₂), then "surface" to 1.0 atm	One treatment Second treatment rarely administered (controversial)	Carbon monoxide: treatment protocols may vary HBO indicated for loss of consciousness; seizures; cerebellar dysfunction; impaired cognition; headache, nausea/vomiting persisting after 4 hr O₂ therapy regardless of carboxyhemoglobin level Experimental indications: treatment protocols not established
Insulin-glucose	Calcium-channel antagonists β-Adrenergic receptor antagonists	Regular insulin, 1 U/kg bolus, followed by 0.5-1 U/kg/hr Titrate 50% dextrose IV to avoid hypoglycemia	Reversal of myocardial depression	Beneficial in case series and reports Initiate if glucagon and vasopressor or inotropic drugs fail to reverse myocardial depression; more effective if used before onset of cardiogenic shock Monitor glucose and potassium; hypoglycemia can occur during and after therapy Hyperglycemia results from toxicant-induced insulin resistance, and initial dextrose requirements may be less than anticipated Recovery may be heralded by normalization of glucose levels, with increased dextrose required to avoid hypoglycemia
Intralipid	Cardiac toxicity from local anesthetics (e.g., bupivacaine, ropivacaine) Experimental: verapamil, diltiazem, tricyclic antidepressants, bupropion, propranolol	Use 20% formulation Initial bolus: 1.5 ml/kg IV over 1 min, followed immediately by infusion of 0.25 ml/kg/min for 30-60 min Can repeat bolus for asystole	Return of hemodynamic stability	Use based on animal experiments and human case reports; numerous dosing regimens have been used Use if advanced life support measures fail; continue CPR as needed during drug administration

Antidote	Indication for Use	Dose*	Treatment End Point	Comments
Methylene blue	Methemoglobin-producing agents	1-2 mg/kg body weight (0.1-0.2 ml/kg) of 1% methylene blue is administered over 5-min period; repeat dose for persistent or recurrent symptoms or signs	Resolution of dyspnea and altered mental status	Use if patient is symptomatic (i.e., dyspneic, altered mental status) Maximum dose should not exceed 7 mg/kg (0.7 ml/kg) Contraindicated in G6PD-deficient patients; may cause hemolysis Some toxicants (e.g., dapsone) may require prolonged therapy
N-Acetylcysteine (NAC)	Acetaminophen Experimental: carbon tetrachloride, chloroform, pennyroyal oil	Oral: Load—140 mg/kg Maintenance (starting 4 hr after load)—70 mg/kg q4h IV: Load—150 mg/kg over 1-hr period Maintenance infusion—12.5 mg/kg over 4-hr period, then 6.25 mg/kg per hour as continuous infusion	Administer 24 hr of NAC and repeat AST and APAP levels: if AST normal and APAP not detected, stop NAC; if AST normal and APAP detected, continue NAC for 12 hr, then reassess AST and APAP levels; if AST elevated, continue NAC for total of 72 hr of therapy After 72 hr of therapy, if INR <2.0, stop NAC After patient has received 72 hr of therapy, if INR ≥2.0 or severe hepatotoxicity present, continue NAC until INR <2.0	Most effective if initiated within 8 hr after ingestion; may be started any time after ingestion and is beneficial in severe hepatotoxic states Use IV in patients unable to tolerate PO or with severe hepatotoxicity; the dose and timing differ from the oral regimen Dosage and administration of FDA-approved IV formulation assume early treatment of acute overdose without hepatotoxicity; longer duration of treatment required in patients with hepatotoxicity Treatment end points simplified for ease of use INR result not valid indicator if FFP recently administered
Naloxone	Opioids	Bolus: 0.4-2 mg via IV, sublingual injection, or endotracheal instillation; 0.4-0.8 mg SC Continuous infusion: establish bolus dose required to reverse respiratory depression Begin infusing two thirds of reversal dose every hour, and titrate to maintain adequate respirations Rebolus with half of reversal dose 15 min after reversing respiratory depression	Initial: reversal of respiratory depression with resolution of hypoxia and hypercapnia Final: resolution of CNS and respiratory depression	Preventilate patients with respiratory depression by bag-valve mask or intubation before administration Use smaller doses in opioid-dependent patients; some opioids (e.g., propoxyphene, pentazocine, fentanyls) may require larger doses of naloxone; use continuous infusion for recurrent symptoms and prolonged action of some formulations (e.g., sustained-release morphine, methadone) Resedation can occur Do not use nalmefene or naltrexone to reverse acute toxicity
Octreotide	Sulfonylureas	50 mg SC q6h	Resolution of hypoglycemia and dextrose not required	Maintain dextrose infusion as needed
Physostigmine	Anticholinergic agents (e.g., diphenhydramine, jimsonweed [Datura sp.], scopolamine)	1-2 mg IV over 5-min period; can repeat once after 10-15 min if no effect	Reversal of anticholinergic effects	Duration of effect is 60-90 min Benzodiazepine used for subsequent treatment of agitation and seizures; additional physostigmine used rarely (e.g., refractory seizures or agitation) Adverse effects include seizures, excessive oral secretions, bradyarrhythmias; contraindicated in cyclic antidepressant toxicity
Pralidoxime chloride	Organophosphorus compounds Nerve agents—sarin, VX	30 mg/kg IV bolus (max 2 g) over 30 min, followed by continuous infusion of 8-10 mg/kg/hr (max 650 mg/hr)	Resolution of signs and symptoms, atropine no longer required	Can give initial dose over 2-min period for life-threatening clinical effects Administer early when diagnosis known or strongly suspected Efficacy variable, depending on the organophosphate Fat-soluble organophosphates may require prolonged treatment
Pyridoxine	Ethylene glycol (theoretical efficacy) Isoniazid Monomethylhydrazine mushrooms	100 mg IV 5 g IV, repeat for refractory seizures	One dose Resolution of seizures	Efficacy theoretical Pyridoxine may stop seizures, but patient can remain comatose (isoniazid, mushrooms); use benzodiazepines and phenobarbital concomitantly to manage seizures Excessive dosing can cause neuropathy

Continued on following page

Antidote	Indication for Use	Dose*	Treatment End Point	Comments
Sodium bicarbonate (NaHCO₃)	Reversal of myocardial sodium-channel blockers (e.g., cyclic antidepressants, cocaine, propoxyphene, sodium-channel-blocking antiarrhythmics with $\tau_{recovery}$ >1 sec, piperidine phenothiazines (thioridazine, mesoridazine)	1-2 mEq NaHCO₃/kg via intermittent bolus; repeat as needed	Narrowing of prolonged QRS, resolution of ventricular arrhythmias, reversal of hypotension	Monitor blood pH (optimal pH approximately 7.50); avoid pH >7.55
	Altered tissue distribution or enhanced elimination of salicylates; may be used in chlorophenoxy herbicides, chlorpropamide, formic acid, methotrexate, phenobarbital	1-2 mEq NaHCO₃/kg, followed by 3 ampules (150 ml) NaHCO₃ (44 mEq per 50 ml) in 850 ml of D₅W, infused at 2-3 times normal maintenance fluid rate	Serum salicylate <30 mg/dl and patient clinically stable	Monitor urinary pH hourly; adjust infusion to maintain urine pH of 7.5-8.0 (avoid blood pH >7.55) Monitor ABGs Maintain normokalemia
Succimer (DMSA)	All forms: Arsenic Lead Mercury	10 mg/kg/dose q8h for 5 days, followed by q12h for 14 days Drug holiday for 2 wk; repeat if treatment end point not reached	Arsenic: 24-hr urinary arsenic <50 μg/L Lead: resolution of encephalopathy, gastrointestinal symptoms, neuropathy, nephropathy, arthralgias, myalgias, and blood lead level <70 μg/dl Mercury, elemental and inorganic: 24-hr urinary mercury <20 μg/L Mercury, organic: end point not well established	Oral chelator; adverse effects include rash, transient AST and alkaline phosphatase elevations, and gastrointestinal distress; minimal chelation of essential metals occurs Dosing for arsenic and mercury not well established Therapeutic end point for organic mercury not established; neurotoxicity not responsive to chelation therapy; suggest chelation until blood mercury level within normal value range for reference laboratory
Vitamin K	Anticoagulants (e.g., warfarin, long-acting anticoagulant rodenticides [LAARs])	Subcutaneous: AquaMEPHYTON (K₁), 10-25 mg, repeat every 6-12 hr until oral vitamin K₁ started Oral: 25-50 mg q6h; larger doses may be required	INR is normal 48-72 hr after stopping vitamin K₁ therapy Can also monitor factor VII activity	Anaphylactoid reaction can occur with IV administration Severe bleeding may also require FFP or factor concentrates Base decision to treat on finding of elevated INR; do not administer prophylactic vitamin K₁ Oral therapy has been required for months with LAAR poisoning because of lipophilicity of toxicant, with slow body clearance

ABG, Arterial blood gas; *ALT,* alanine aminotransferase; *APAP,* acetyl-para-aminophenol (acetaminophen); *AST,* aspartate aminotransferase; *BAL,* British antilewisite; *bpm,* beats per minute; *CNS,* central nervous system; *COHb%,* percent carboxyhemoglobin; *CPR,* cardiopulmonary resuscitation; *D₅W,* 5% dextrose in water; *DMSA,* 2,3-dimercaptosuccinic acid; *ECG,* electrocardiogram; *FDA,* Food and Drug Administration; *FFP,* fresh-frozen plasma; *G6PD,* glucose-6-phosphate dehydrogenase; *Hb,* hemoglobin; *HD,* hemodialysis; *IM,* intramuscular; *INR,* international normalized ratio; *IV,* intravenous; *MetHb%,* percent methemoglobinemia; *NS,* normal saline; *O₂Hb%,* percent oxyhemoglobin; *PO,* per os (by mouth); *SC,* subcutaneous; $\tau_{recovery}$, drug blockade recovery rate.

*Dose concentrations and infusion times are not given. Drug dosages may require adjustment in patients with renal or hepatic failure.

†Administer antivenom in a monitored setting; antivenom must be reconstituted and then diluted; initially infuse at a rate of 2 to 5 ml/hr, and double the infusion rate every 5 minutes as tolerated to administer antivenom over a 1-hour period.

‡Ten percent calcium chloride solution = 100 mg/ml (27.2 mg/ml elemental calcium); 10% calcium gluconate solution = 100 mg/ml (9 mg/ml elemental calcium).

From Goldman L, Schafer AI: *Goldman's Cecil medicine,* ed 24, Philadelphia, 2012, Saunders.

Impairment and Disability Issues

Impairment describes harm to anatomy and physiology, whereas *disability* denotes the difficulty a person has performing a function. Reporting disability for different sectors of society has its own nuances. Proper evaluation of impairment/disability starts with knowing who is asking for what. It is an area of practice in which an understanding of some basic concepts can make it rewarding rather than distressing.

- Ultimately, disability is a measure of function. Functional outcomes are becoming increasingly important in medicine, mirroring the shift towards patient-centeredness. All practitioners should have some facility with documenting the effects of an intervention on a patient's physical, psychological, and social functioning. For example, the continuation of an opioid analgesic should be predicated on meeting functional goals negotiated between the patient and physician before initiation of treatment. Even a brief comment on walking distance or work tolerance is better than nothing.
- Some concepts apply to all venues of disability. Primary care providers should rarely be in the position to determine whether a patient can be on or off a specific job. Rather, their task is to give general parameters about which physical exertions are medically dangerous. Try to be specific and use objective criteria where appropriate, but don't be intimidated by a form. Ballpark estimates can often suffice. For example, many chronic low back pain patients may conservatively and safely be described as able to lift/carry up 10 lbs, push/pull 25 lbs, and change positions as needed to keep comfortable. Have thorough medical records and be consistent; lawyers may focus on contradictions in your documentation to help their clients.
- Rehabilitation centers across the country are required to monitor function using a standardized set of criteria called the "Functional Independence Measure (FIM)," which categorizes activities of daily living into divisions such as mobility, transfers, feeding, grooming/hygiene, dressing, bathing, and toileting. In therapy notes, you may come across scores in these categories rating patients on a seven-point scale from totally dependent to moderate-assistance (mod A; patient can perform 50% of task) to modified-independent (patient requires an assistive device) to independent.
- Psychosocial contributing factors such as medicolegal issues can profoundly influence patients' presentations through somatization from secondary gain. However, it is important to differentiate this from malingering, Munchausen's syndrome, or "gaming the system," which are remarkably less prevalent.
- The number of stakeholders expands in the disability system to include the employer, the government, the legal system, and the payer. Each sector has its own regulations. You may be required to fill out disability questionnaires as a condition of accepting payment for clinical services from a payer, such as in the workers' compensation system. Much more commonly, you will be seeing patients for clinical services paid for by an evaluation and management code. In these cases, you are not obligated to provide free medicolegal assessments. Settling payment issues in advance can avoid misunderstanding. Again, before assessing disability, understand who is asking and why.

GOVERNMENT-ADMINISTERED DISABILITY

State Temporary Disability Insurance (TDI) programs, the Family Medical Leave Act of 1993 (FMLA), the Social Security Administration (SSA), and the Department of Veterans Affairs offer disability benefits through the state and federal government.

- State TDI forms must be filled out for the patient to receive any income. They are generally very basic and just engage the social support network for a patient. This may not be the best venue to stipulate partial disability.
- The FMLA provides unpaid leave for qualified medical and family reasons. Because it is a federal program, the forms involved are standard across states and employers. They can be intimidating at first, but are reasonably easy to complete once the basic definitions used are understood. It is recommended that you familiarize yourself with this paperwork the first few times it is encountered. Completing the form for subsequent patients should not be overly burdensome.
- The SSA and the Department of Veterans Affairs have their own internal mechanisms for quantifying disability, but they may subpoena your records or request a summary narrative as part of their processes. If you've kept good clinical notes, your existing documentation should satisfy their requirements. Many patients choose to apply for Social Security Disability Insurance (SSDI) and/or Supplemental Security Income (SSI) through a legal representative. These lawyers may send you a lengthy questionnaire to prepare their case. There are physicians whose practices perform these services and who can be hired by attorneys to facilitate patients' applications. If this nonclinical work appeals to you, consider affiliating with the SSA or contracting your time to lawyers under separate indenture. If not, you may want to recommend the law office contact a suitable practice.

WORKERS' COMPENSATION

In workers' compensation, the payer and employer join the provider in trying to rehabilitate the injured worker. Confidentiality issues are handled differently because these stakeholders may have a right to protected health information.

- Each state has their own laws regarding reporting requirements, and the U.S. Department of Labor governs injured federal employees. If you plan on accepting workers' compensation patients, you must familiarize yourself with the necessary paperwork. Typically, this is a standard, short form that includes measures of function. It may make sense to copy your state's parameters and create a "work note" to be used uniformly in your practice for cases both inside and outside of the workers' compensation system. Functional limitations should pertain to any task, not just to the employee's vocation. In general, employees should not be labeled "on" or "off."
- A notification that an employee has reached "maximal medical improvement" should be made once an employee's condition is expected to change over months/years rather than days/weeks. At this juncture they will transition from temporary disability benefits to permanent disability benefits, possibly including vocational rehabilitation. If ongoing sequelae exist, a permanent impairment rating may be needed to resolve an employee's claim and allow them to progress to the next stage of their life. These are more sophisticated determinations, usually directed by the American Medical Association's (AMA) *Guides to the Evaluation of Permanent Impairment*, now in its sixth edition. Analysis of permanent impairment, causation, and apportionment generally fall out-

side of workers' compensation reporting requirements. Someone with appropriate training may be best suited to complete this task. Consider providing these more detailed services under a separate indenture, such as a consultation arrangement with the employee's attorney. Your state workers' compensation board may have specific guidelines governing these reports. In any case, the work should be done under a clear written agreement, not based on a verbal request by the employee. Very complex cases may also require a formal functional capacity evaluation through an appropriate rehabilitation resource.

PERSONAL INJURY

Patients hurt in car accidents or other personal injuries often are involved in legal cases covering medical care, personal damages, and pain and suffering. Most commonly, you will be helping these patients with their clinical issues under their regular medical insurance, although some providers agree to provide services under a legal lien on the claim. Regardless of your role in a personal injury case, it is helpful to document objective details about the injury and functional parameters. If you are asked to keep someone out of work, try to delineate functional limitations as you would in a workers' compensation employee.

- Similar to the workers' compensation system, it is helpful to state when a patient has reached maximal medical improvement. Personal injury claims can take longer to resolve than in the workers' compensation system, as the employer and insurance company are strongly incentivized to reach a resolution in those cases. In general, an ongoing legal case may hinder a patient from achieving a healthful balance of wellness. It is in the patient's best interest to move the claim toward completion.
- Quantifying permanent disability is a key component of resolving these cases. If a clinician is providing services under a legal lien, there may be a conflict of interest in having that provider quantify the permanent impairment. There may be financial implications to the degree of disability awarded, and this may influence whether or not the clinician will receive payment on their lien. These cases are almost always contentious, and may be best handled by providers with special training, such as an independent medical examiner. Again, the determination typically follows the AMA's *Guides to the Evaluation of Permanent Impairment*. A clinician's role is to manage the patient's injuries, not to negotiate medicolegal issues. If you are not appropriately trained, consider deferring questions regarding disability to someone who is.

PRIVATE DISABILITY

Some patients purchase private insurance plans to provide income in addition to that offered through the government in the case of long-term disability. These forms vary by insurance carrier and change over time. They may need to be filled out periodically to maintain benefits. Many providers opt to charge a separate fee for the completion of this type of paperwork.

CONCLUSION

In summary, impairment and disability are measures of function and should be followed by all good doctors as part of patient-centered care. Providers can be most effective interacting with the various disability systems if they know when they are acting as clinicians and when they are acting as legal consultants. Understanding the principles involved with the different sectors will help you avoid confusion between obligations and opportunities when doing this work.

SUGGESTED READINGS

American Academy of Physical Medicine and Rehabilitation: Disability evaluation. Accessed March 7, 2014, at http://now.aapmr.org/rehab-essentials/special-assessment-mgmt-strategy/Pages/Disability-evaluation.aspx.

Holmes EB: Impairment rating and disability determination. Accessed March 7, 2014, at http://emedicine.medscape.com/article/314195-overview#a1.

Rondinelli R.D.. In: *Guides to the evaluation of permanent impairment*. American Medical Association: Arlington, VA.

AUTHOR: **MATTHEW J. SMITH, M.D.**

A

AA. *See* Secondary amyloidosis
AAA. *See* Abdominal aortic aneurysm
AATD. *See* Alpha-1-antitrypsin, deficiency of
Abacavir
  for acquired immunodeficiency syndrome, 18
  dosing of, 1901t
Abatacept
  for juvenile idiopathic arthritis, 733
  for rheumatoid arthritis, 1127
  for systemic lupus erythematosus, 1242
Abdomen, 489t
Abdominal angiostrongyliasis, 350.e5t
Abdominal aortic aneurysm, 3–6.e2, 4f–5f
Abdominal calcifications, nonvisceral, on x-ray, 1415
Abdominal compartment syndrome, 7–8.e1
  causes of, 7t
  classification of, 8t
  postinjury primary and secondary, 8t
Abdominal distention, 1387–1407
Abdominal pain
  in adolescence, 1387
  arthritis and, 1403
  childhood, 121, 1387
  chronic lower, 1387
  diffuse, 1387
  epigastric, 1387
  fever and rash with, 1440
  in infancy, 1388
  in left lower quadrant, 1388
  in left upper quadrant, 1388
  nonsurgical causes of, 1388
  periumbilical, 1388
  poorly localized, 1388
  post-cholecystectomy, 1389
  in pregnancy, 1389
  rash and fever with, 1440
  recurrent, 722
  in right lower quadrant, 1389
  in right upper quadrant, 1389, 1550–1578, 1552f
  suprapubic, 1389
Abdominal pregnancy, 430, 430f, 431.e1f
Abdominal ultrasound. *See also* Ultrasound
  for abdominal aortic aneurysm, 4, 4f
  for acute pancreatitis, 944
  for cholangiocarcinoma, 284, 284f
  for epiploic appendagitis, 463.e3
  for portal vein thrombosis, 1034, 1034f
  for premature rupture of membranes, 1052
Abdominal wall masses, 1389–1390
ABGs. *See* Arterial blood gases
ABI. *See* Ankle-brachial index
Ablation therapy
  for atrial fibrillation, 151
  for atrial flutter, 154
  for hyperparathyroidism, 656
ABLC. *See* Amphotericin B lipid complex
ABMT. *See* Allogeneic bone marrow transplantation
Abnormal uterine bleeding, 817, 1539
Abortion, recurrent, 1390
ABPA. *See* Allergic bronchopulmonary aspergillosis
Abrasion, corneal, 338–338.e1, 338f
Abruptio placentae, 9–10, 9f–10f
Abscess
  amebic liver, 760, 760b, 761f
  anal, 1397
  anorectal, 978, 978f
  Bartholin's gland, 175–176.e1, 176f
  brain, 207–208.e1, 207t, 208f, 848
  breast, 214–214.e1, 214f
  corticomedullary, 1099

Abscess *(Continued)*
  epidural, 460–460.e1
  hepatic, 289f
  liver, 760–761, 760b, 760t, 761f
  lung, 767–768.e1, 767t, 768f
  mastoid, 801
  nail bed, 958
  pancreatic, 946
  parapharyngeal, 982f
  pelvic, 962.e1f, 962–962.e1
  perinephric, 1099, 1106, 1106f
  perirectal, 978–978.e1, 978f
  peritonsillar, 981–982.e1, 981f, 981t
  pilonidal, 995
  renal, 1099, 1106, 1106f
  retropharyngeal, 1117–1118.e1, 1117f–1118f
  spinal epidural, 1200–1201.e1, 1200f–1201f
  tubo-ovarian, 962–963
Absence seizures, 1153–1153.e1
ABSSSIs. *See* Acute bacterial skin and skin structure
  infections
Abuse
  alcohol, 55
  child, 277–279.e2, 278t, 279b, 279.e1f–279.e2f
  drug, 405–407.e1, 405t–406t
  elder, 437–438.e1, 438f
Abusive head trauma, 277, 1171
ABVD, for Hodgkin lymphoma, 624–625
ACA. *See* Anticardiolipin antibody
Acalculous biliary disease, 504
Acalculous cholecystitis, 290.e1t
Acamprosate, for alcohol abuse, 56t, 58, 407
Acanthosis nigricans, 1028.e3f
Acarbose
  for diabetes mellitus, 381
  for dumping syndrome, 412.e3
Acceleration flexion-extension neck injury, 1376.e7
Accident bowel leakage, 699
Accidental hypothermia, 688
Acclimatization, for high-altitude sickness, 612–613
ACD. *See* Anemia, of chronic disease
ACE. *See* Angiotensin-converting enzyme
ACE inhibitors. *See* Angiotensin-converting enzyme
  inhibitors
ACE wrap, 99.e8f
Aceruloplasminemia, 1799t
Acetaminophen
  for Charcot-Marie-Tooth syndrome, 273
  chronic hepatitis caused by, 410.e2t
  for migraine headache, 546t
  pathophysiology, clinical effects, and management of,
    1716t–1719t
  poisoning caused by, 11–11.e2, 11.e1t, 11.e2f
  for roseola, 1133
  for varicella, 1347
  for whiplash injury, 1376.e7
  for yellow fever, 1378.e2
  for Zika virus, 1379–1380
Acetazolamide
  for acute mountain sickness, 612–613
  for high-altitude cerebral edema, 612–613
  for idiopathic intracranial hypertension, 690.e5
Acetone, serum or plasma, 1771
Acetylcholine receptor antibody, 1771
Acetylsalicylic acid, for cocaine overdose, 313
ACG. *See* Angle-closure glaucoma
Achalasia, 12–13.e1, 12t, 13f
Aches and pains. *See also* Pain
  diffuse, 1390
  muscle cramps and aches, 1685, 1685b, 1685f
Achilles tendinitis, 1105
Achilles tendon rupture, 13.e2–13.e4, 13.e2f
Acid phosphatase, serum, 1771
Acid serum test, 1771
Acid-base system. *See also* Acidosis; Alkalosis
  homeostasis of, 1553–1554, 1553f–1554f
  reference values for, 1771t, 1776.e2t

Acidosis
  anion gap, 1401
  differential diagnosis of, 1390
  lactic, 737–737.e1, 1390, 1777b
  metabolic
    arterial blood gases, 1777
    causes of, 1777b
    diagnostic approach to, 1555, 1555f
    differential diagnosis of, 1390
    hyperchloric, 1390
    in hypothermia, 688
    laboratory findings in, 1771t
  renal tubular, 1113–1114.e1, 1113t, 1114f
  respiratory
    acute, 1555, 1556f
    arterial blood gases, 1777–1778
    chronic, 1557, 1557f
    differential diagnosis of, 1390–1391
    in hypothermia, 688
    laboratory findings in, 1771t
Acinetobacter sp., 849–849.e1
Acitretin, 756
Aclidinium, 301
ACM. *See* Alcoholic cardiomyopathy
Acne inversa, 610
Acne rosacea, 1131
Acne vulgaris, 14–15.e1, 14f–15f
Acoustic neuroma, 16–16.e1
  differential diagnosis of, 187t
  magnetic resonance imaging with gadolinium for, 16, 16f
ACPE. *See* Acute cardiogenic pulmonary edema
ACPO. *See* Acute colonic pseudo-obstruction
Acquired amyloid polyneuropathy, 899t
Acquired aplastic anemia, 1398
Acquired clonal sideroblastic anemia, 90.e3
Acquired erythrocytosis, 1619, 1619f
Acquired immunodeficiency syndrome, 17–24.e7,
    24.e1f–24.e7f. *See also* Human immunodeficiency virus
  acutely ill patient with, 24.e2f
  aspergillosis in, 18t–24t
  bacterial respiratory diseases in, 18t–24t
  cardiac dysfunction in, 24.e7f
  CNS infection in, 24.e5f
  CNS lesion in, 24.e6f
  coccidioidomycosis in, 18t–24t
  cryptococcosis in, 18t–24t
  cytomegalovirus disease in, 18t–24t
  definition of, 630
  diarrhea in, 24.e1f
  disseminated MAC disease in, 18t–24t
  herpes simplex virus disease in, 18t–24t
  histoplasmosis in, 18t–24t, 619–620
  Kaposi's sarcoma in, 735–735.e1, 735f, 735.e1f
  mucocutaneous candidiasis in, 18t–24t
  Pneumocystis jiroveci pneumonia in, 17, 18t–24t, 24.e4f
  progressive multifocal leukoencephalopathy in, 18t–24t
  respiratory complaints in, 24.e3f–24.e4f
  salmonellosis in, 18t–24t
  Toxoplasma gondii encephalitis in, 18t–24t
  vaccines/vaccinations in patients with, 17
  varicella-zoster virus disease in, 18t–24t
Acquired iron overload, 1471–1472
Acquired red blood cell aplasia, 1731.e1
Acquired red cell aplasia, 1096.e2
Acquired reversible sideroblastic anemia, 90.e3
ACR. *See* Albumin to creatinine ratio
Acral lentiginous melanoma, 805
Acrodermatitis chronica atrophicans, 774
Acromegaly, 24.e8–24.e9, 24.e8f, 997–999.e1
Acromioclavicular joint pain, 1133.e4t
Acrophobia, 993
ACS. *See* Abdominal compartment syndrome; Acute coronary
  syndromes
Actinic cheilitis, 25, 99–99.e1, 99f
Actinic cheilosis, 99
Actinic keratosis, 25–26.e1, 25f, 26t
Actinomyces infection, 26.e2

Page numbers followed by "b", "f" and "t" indicate boxes, figures and tables respectively.

Actinomycosis, 26.e2–26.e3, 26.e2f
Action tremors, 1534
Activated charcoal, for acetaminophen poisoning, 11
Activated clotting time, 1771
Activated partial thromboplastin time, 1771, 1821
Acupuncture, 1037
Acute abdomen, 979
Acute abdominal colic, 1423
Acute aortic syndromes, 113f
Acute appendicitis, 121–122.e2
Acute bacterial nephritis, 1097
Acute bacterial prostatitis, 1077–1077.e1
Acute bacterial sinusitis, 1184–1185.e1
Acute bacterial skin and skin structure infections, 265
Acute bronchitis, 27–28.e1
Acute cardiogenic pulmonary edema, 1086
Acute chest syndrome, 1182
Acute cholangitis, 290
Acute cholecystitis, 290.e1t
Acute colonic pseudo-obstruction, 29–30.e1, 29b–30b, 29f
Acute confusional state, 364, 364t, 366.e1t
    algorithm for, 365f
    classification, 364
    delirium, 444
    evaluation of, 365f
    risk factors for, 364t
    theories regarding, 364
Acute conjunctivitis, 326
Acute cor pulmonale, 335, 335f–336f, 337t
Acute coronary syndromes, 31–36.e1, 31t, 33f–35f
Acute cystitis, 1603f, 1603–1603.e1
Acute decompensated heart failure, 553–555, 557–560
Acute diarrhea, 1605, 1605f
Acute diastolic heart failure with pulmonary edema, 1086
Acute diffuse otitis externa, 928–929.e1
Acute endocarditis, 446
Acute eosinophilic pneumonia
    description of, 458.e7
    idiopathic, 458.e7
Acute fatty liver of pregnancy, 485–485.e1
Acute flaccid myelitis, 1020.e2
Acute glomerulonephritis, 522–524.e1, 523t–524t
Acute gout, 529, 530.e3f
Acute headache, 1639–1640
Acute hearing loss, 1661–1662
Acute heart failure with pulmonary edema, 1086
Acute hematogenous osteomyelitis, 924
Acute hemolytic transfusion reaction, 1291, 1291t
Acute hepatic necrosis, 42
Acute hepatitis
    differential diagnosis of, 1454
    drug-induced, 410.e3t
Acute hyponatremia, 681–682
Acute inflammatory demyelinating polyradiculoneuropathy, 537
Acute intermittent porphyria, 1505, 1736.e1t
Acute interstitial nephritis
    characteristics of, 718–719.e1, 719f
    renal failure with, 1518
Acute interstitial pneumonia, 692t
Acute ischemic stroke, 1215–1218.e1, 1215b, 1216f, 1216t, 1217b, 1218f
Acute kidney injury
    characteristics of, 37–41.e2, 37t–38t, 39f, 40t
    classification, 1794t
    contrast-induced, 333–334.e1, 333t, 334b
    diagnosis of, 37t, 39f
    in HIV-infected patient, 1391
    intrinsic renal diseases as cause of, 1391
    liver disease and, 1391
    pigment-induced, 1392
    RIFLE criteria for, 1794t
Acute labyrinthitis, 736
Acute laryngitis, 739–739.e1
Acute limb ischemia
    description of, 975
    nontraumatic, 1477, 1477, 1523
Acute liver failure, 42–44.e1, 42b–44b, 42t, 43f, 44t
Acute low back pain, 1408
Acute lung injury, 45t, 1392
Acute lymphangitis, 776
Acute lymphoblastic leukemia, 743–745.e1, 743t–745t, 745.e1f, 1816f
Acute lymphocytic leukemia, 743
Acute lymphonodular pharyngitis, 604.e2
Acute mediastinitis, 802, 1482

Acute megacolon, 29
Acute mesenteric ischemia, 819–820.e1, 819t, 820.e1f
Acute mesenteric lymphadenitis, 818–818.e1
Acute monoarthritis, 1486
Acute mountain sickness, 612–613.e2, 613b, 613.e1t, 613.e2b
Acute myelogenous leukemia, 746–749.e1, 746t–748t
Acute myeloid leukemia, 746, 748t, 749.e1f
Acute myocardial infarction. See also Myocardial infarction
    cocaine overdose and, 312, 312t, 313.e1f
    description of, 31, 867
Acute necrosis of liver, 42
Acute necrotizing encephalitis, 442
Acute necrotizing ulcerative gingivitis, 518.e2
Acute nephritic syndrome, 522, 1491
Acute neuritis, 1365
Acute nonlymphocytic leukemia, 746
Acute oral ulcers, 1496
Acute otitis media, 928–930, 928f
Acute pancreatitis
    in children, 1711–1712
    description of, 943–946.e1, 943t, 944f, 945t–946t
Acute paronychia, 958–958.e1, 958f
Acute polyneuropathy, 537
Acute primary pulmonary histoplasmosis, 619
Acute promyelocytic leukemia, 748–749
Acute pulmonary artery surgical embolectomy, 1091
Acute pulmonary embolism, 1088t
Acute pyelonephritis, 1097–1100.e1
Acute radiation syndrome, 1100.e13–1100.e14
Acute red eye, 1737–1740
Acute renal failure, 37, 1309. See also Acute kidney injury
    pigment-induced, 1518
Acute renal insufficiency syndrome, 37
Acute respiratory distress syndrome, 45–48.e1, 45t, 46f, 47t
Acute rheumatic fever, 1124.e2
Acute scrotum, 459.e1t, 1392
Acute silicosis, 1183
Acute sinusitis, 1184–1185.e1
Acute streptococcal pharyngitis, 1124.e2
Acute stress disorder, 49–50.e1
Acute subclavian vein thrombosis, 1317f
Acute suppurative otitis media, 930
Acute suppurative sialadenitis, 1176
Acute systolic heart failure with pulmonary edema, 1086
Acute tubo-interstitial nephritis, 718
Acute tubular injury, 1309
Acute tubular necrosis, 600, 1309
Acute ulcerative gingivitis, 518.e1–518.e2
Acute urinary retention, 51–51.e1, 1536
Acute uveitis, 1334
Acute vestibular neuronopathy, 736
Acute viral encephalitis, 442–443.e1, 443t
Acute vision loss
    painful, 1541
    painless, 1541
Acute/subacute decompensated heart failure, 253
Acyclovir
    for acute viral encephalitis, 443
    for herpes simplex, 607t
    for herpes zoster, 609
    for oral hairy leukoplakia, 755
    for Ramsay Hunt syndrome, 1101–1101.e1
    for varicella, 1347
AD. See Alzheimer's disease
AD-32, for bladder cancer, 201
Adalimumab
    for Crohn's disease, 345
    for enteropathic arthritis, 456
    for hidradenitis suppurativa, 611
ADAM 33 gene, 132
Adapalene, 15
ADCA. See Autosomal dominant cerebellar ataxia
Addiction
    drug, 405
    opioid, 405t, 911–913.e1, 912t–913t, 913.e1t
Addison disease, 52, 1829t
Addison-Biermer anemia, 89
Addyi. See Flibanserin
Adenocarcinoma, 232t, 472. See also Cancer; Carcinoma; Tumors/neoplasms
    bladder, 200
    gastric, 506
    lung, 769
    vaginal, 1338
    vulvar, 1372.e2

Adenoidectomy, 931
Adenoma
    aldosterone-secreting, 62.e2f
    pituitary, 997–999.e1, 998t, 999f
Adenopathy, 1457. See also Lymphadenopathy
Adenosarcomas, uterine, 1333
Adenosine
    for atrial flutter, 153
    for supraventricular tachycardia, 1231–1232, 1232f
    for Wolff-Parkinson-White syndrome, 1378
Adenosine diphosphate antagonists, 1055.e4
Adenoviruses
    acute bronchitis caused by, 27t
    croup caused by, 345.e3
ADHD. See Attention deficit hyperactivity disorder
Adhesive capsulitis, 503.e2f
Adnexal masses, 934–934.e1, 1392–1393
Adnexitis, 963
Adolescents. See also Children; Pediatric patients
    abdominal pain in, 1387
    alopecia in, 1396
    altered mental status and coma in, 1484
    arthritis in, extremity pain and, 1403–1404
    back pain in, 1408
    drug abuse in, 406, 406t
    foot and ankle pain in, 1443
    gender dysphoria in, 512.e4
    hand pain in, 1771
    hip pain in, 1456–1457
    human immunodeficiency virus in, 633t
    hypotrichosis in, 1396
    immunizations, 1859–1865
    knee pain in, 1475
    limp in, 1477
    Osgood-Schlatter disease in, 920–920.e1, 920f
    periodic health examination, 1872
    scrotal masses in, 1751–1752
    scrotal pain in, 1521–1522
    shoulder pain in, 1524
    vaccination and infection control for, 1872
    wrist pain in, 1771
ADPKD. See Autosomal dominant polycystic kidney disease
Adrenal calcifications, 1393
Adrenal cystic lesions, 1393
Adrenal enzyme deficiencies, 1393
Adrenal gland calcifications, on x-ray, 1585–1586
Adrenal hyperplasia, congenital, 325.e2–325.e4, 325.e2f
    diagnosis and treatment of, 325.e4t
    non-salt-wasting form of, 325.e2
    prevention of, 325.e3
    salt-wasting form of, 325.e2
Adrenal incidentaloma, 1557.e1, 1557.e1f
Adrenal insufficiency, 52–53.e2, 52t, 53f, 53.e1f–53.e2f
Adrenal mass
    differential diagnosis of, 1393
    evaluation of, 1558f
Adrenal neuroblastoma, 891.e2f
Adrenal pseudomasses, 1393
Adrenal virilism, 325.e2, 325.e2f, 325.e4t
Adrenalectomy, 61, 998–999
Adrenocortical hyperfunction, 1393
Adrenocortical hypofunction, 1393–1394
Adrenocorticotropic hormone, 1771
    deficiency of, 687
    ectopic secretion of, 1616–1617
    patterns of, 1773t
Adrenocorticotropin stimulation test, 325.e3
Adrenogenital syndrome, 325.e2, 325.e2f, 325.e4t
Adriamycin. See Doxorubicin
ADT. See Androgen deprivation therapy
Adult(s)
    foot and ankle pain in, 1443
    in gender dysphoria, 512.e4
    hip pain in, 1457
    immunization for, 1872
    influenza vaccines in, 1860t–1864t
    knee pain in, 1475
    periodic health examination, 1872
    ventricular septal defect in, 1359
Adult onset, cerebellar ataxia, 1406–1407
Adult polycystic kidney disease, 1023
Adult respiratory distress syndrome, 45
Adult Still's disease, 54
Adult-onset congenital adrenal hyperplasia, 73
Adult-onset idiopathic gynecomastia, 539.e1t
Adult-onset Still's disease, 54–54.e1

Adverse drug events, 960.e5–960.e6
Adverse food reactions, 1394
Adynamic ileus, 1394
Aedes aegypti, 369.e2, 369.e2f
Aeromonas hydrophila, 265
Aerophagia, 1394
Affective disturbance, sleep-associated, 1737f–1739f
AFLP. *See* Acute fatty liver of pregnancy
African histoplasmosis, 620
Ag acidosis, 1390
Agammaglobulinemia, 1065.e3t
Agenerase, 18
Agenesis, Müllerian, 73, 74t, 76
Age-related cataracts, 259.e7f
Age-related macular degeneration, 783–784.e1
Age-related senile cataracts, 259.e6
Aggressive systemic mastocytosis, 799t
Agitated delirium, 1610–1614
Agitation, 366.e1t, 1609–1610
α2-Agonist, for ascites, 129t
Agoraphobia, 949–950.e1, 993
AH. *See* Alcoholic hepatitis
AHTR. *See* Acute hemolytic transfusion reaction
AI. *See* Aortic insufficiency
Aicardi-Goutieres syndrome, 423t
AIDS. *See* Acquired immunodeficiency syndrome
AIDS dementia complex, 621
AIH. *See* Autoimmune hepatitis
AIHA. *See* Autoimmune hemolytic anemia
AION. *See* Arteritic anterior ischemic optic neuropathy
AIP. *See* Autoimmune pancreatitis
Airflow reversibility, 133
Air-space opacification, on x-ray, 1012f, 1394
AKC. *See* Atopic keratoconjunctivitis
AKI. *See* Acute kidney injury
Akinetic mutism, 445
Akinetic/rigid syndrome, 1395
Alanine aminopeptidase, 1771
Alanine aminotransferase
    for eosinophilic granulomatosis with polyangiitis, 458.e4
    for hepatitis C, 587
    reference values for, 1771, 1773f
ALARA. *See* As low as reasonably achievable
Alarcon-Segovia criteria, for mixed connective tissue disease,
    840.e2t
Albendazole
    for ascariasis, 126
    for cutaneous larva migrans, 350.e6
    for cysticercosis, 354
    for echinococcosis, 428
    for hookworms, 627
    for microsporidiosis, 831
    for tapeworms, 1250
    for trichinosis, 1301.e3
Albiglutide, 379
Albumin
    for ascites, 129t
    in cirrhosis, 304
    for hepatorenal syndrome, 601
    serum, 1773
Albumin to creatinine ratio, 377
Albuterol
    for acute bronchitis, 28
    for anaphylaxis, 79
    for carcinoid syndrome, 239.e3
    for chronic obstructive pulmonary disease, 301
    for status asthmaticus, 139
Alcohol
    seizures caused by, 1395
    stroke risks, 1222
Alcohol abuse, 55–58.e2, 407
Alcohol dehydrogenase, 1773
Alcohol poisoning, 1560, 1560f
Alcohol withdrawal, 56, 57b, 58.e2f
Alcohol withdrawal syndrome, 367
Alcoholic cardiomyopathy, 242
Alcoholic delirium, 367
Alcoholic hepatitis, 59–60.e1, 60f, 1033t
Alcoholic polyneuritic psychosis, 735.e8
Alcohol-induced liver disease, 902
Alcoholism
    characteristics of, 55–58.e2, 56f, 56t, 57b, 58.e2f
    vaccination considerations for, 1887t
Alcohol-like liver disease, 902
Aldolase, 1773

Aldosterone, 674, 1773, 1829t
Aldosterone antagonists
    for cardiorenal syndrome, 254
    for dilated cardiomyopathy, 245
    for myocardial infarction, 874
Aldosterone receptor antagonists, for heart failure, 559
Aldosterone-secreting adenoma, 62.e2f
Aldosteronism, 61f–62f, 62.e2f, 61–62.e2, 1829t
Aldosteronism with normal blood pressure, 176.e2
Alendronate, for osteoporosis, 926
Alginates, for venous ulcers, 1354
ALI. *See* Acute limb ischemia
Aliskiren
    for Bartter syndrome, 176.e2
    for hypertension, 663
Alkali, 230.e1t, 230–230.e1
Alkaline phosphatase
    in cirrhosis, 304
    leukocyte, 1814
    serum, 1774
Alkalosis
    metabolic
        arterial blood gases, 1778
        differential diagnosis of, 1395
        laboratory findings in, 1771t
        workup of, 1562, 1562f
    respiratory
        arterial blood gases, 1778
        differential diagnosis of, 1395
        laboratory findings in, 1771t
        treatment of, 1563, 1563f
ALL. *See* Acute lymphoblastic leukemia
Allergic alveolitis, extrinsic, 1448
Allergic angiitis, 458.e4
Allergic aspergillosis, 130
Allergic asthma, 132
Allergic bronchopulmonary aspergillosis, 130, 458.e7
Allergic conjunctivitis, 326f, 327t
Allergic contact dermatitis, 329, 1020.e1f–1020.e2f
Allergic granulomatosis, 458.e4
Allergic purpura, 573
Allergic rhinitis, 63–63.e1
Allergy, food, 496–499.e1, 497f, 498t–499t
Allevyn. *See* Foam dressings, for venous ulcers
Alloantibodies, for hemophilia A, 569
Allodynia, 897
Allogeneic bone marrow transplantation
    for acute lymphoblastic leukemia, 744
    for chronic lymphocytic leukemia, 752
    for myelodysplastic syndromes, 865
Allogeneic hematopoietic stem cell transplantation
    for pure red cell aplasia, 1096.e3
    for sickle cell disease, 1181
Allograft dysfunction, renal, 1742–1743
Allopurinol
    for angina pectoris, 95
    for gout, 529, 530t
    granulomatous hepatitis caused by, 410.e3t
    for tumor lysis syndrome prevention, 1311
Almotriptan, for migraine headache, 546t
Alogliptin, for diabetes mellitus, 379
Alopecia
    characteristics of, 64–66.e2, 65f, 66.e2f
    in children and adolescents, 1396
    differential diagnosis of, 1395
    drug-induced, 1396
Alopecia areata, 64, 65f, 1270t
Alpha-1-antitrypsin
    deficiency of, 67–67.e1
    serum, 1774
Alpha-/beta-adrenergic receptor blockers, 663
Alpha-blockers
    for acute urinary retention, 51
    for benign prostatic hyperplasia, 1076
    for hypertension, 663
Alpha-fetoprotein, 305, 1397
Alpha-1-fetoprotein, 1774, 1799–1800
Alpha-thalassemia, 87t, 1256–1257.e1, 1256t–1257t
Alprazolam, for panic disorder, 950
ALS. *See* Amyotrophic lateral sclerosis
ALT. *See* Alanine aminotransferase
Alteplase, for myocardial infarction, 872t
Alitretinoin, for lichen simplex chronicus, 758
Aluminum, serum, 1774
Aluminum carbonate, for radiation exposure,
    1100.e14t–1100.e16t

Aluminum hydroxide, for radiation exposure,
    1100.e14t–1100.e16t
Alveolar consolidation, 1396
Alveolar echinococcosis, 427
Alveolar hemorrhage, 1396–1397
Alveolar PaO₂, 613.e2f
Alveolar-arteriolar oxygen gradient, 1088
Alveolitis, extrinsic allergic, 1448
Alzheimer's disease, 68–69.e1, 69t, 832, 892–893.e1. *See
    also* Dementia
Amanita poisoning, 862, 862t
Amantadine
    cocaine overdose and, 313
    for Huntington's disease, 639
    for influenza, 709t
    for neuroleptic malignant syndrome, 896
    for Parkinson's disease, 957
Amaurosis fugax, 70, 70f, 1294, 1295f
Ambiguous genitalia, 1629.e1b, 1815f
Amblyopia, 71–71.e1, 71f
Ambulatory phlebectomy, for varicose veins, 1349
Amebiasis
    characteristics of, 72–72.e1, 72t, 760
    serologic test for, 1774
Amebic dysentery, 72
Amebic hepatic abscess, 760, 760b, 761f
Amebic liver abscess, 760, 760b, 761f
Amenorrhea, 73–76.e2, 74t, 75f, 76.e2b, 76.e2f, 1397
American College of Rheumatology FM Classification Criteria,
    491
American trypanosomiasis, 272.e2
AMI. *See* Acute mesenteric ischemia; Acute myocardial
    infarction
Amiloride, for ascites, 127
Aminocaproic acid, for hemophilia A, 570
Aminoglutethimide, 999
Aminoglycosides, for pyelonephritis, 1099
Aminolevulinic acid, 1774
Aminolevulinic acid dehydratase-deficient porphyria,
    1736.e1t
Aminophylline
    for anaphylaxis, 79.e2t
    for carcinoid syndrome, 239.e3
    for chronic obstructive pulmonary disease, 301
Amiodarone
    for arrhythmogenic right ventricular dysplasia, 123
    for atrial fibrillation, 150, 151f
    for atrial flutter, 154
    hyperpigmentation with, 1651t–1652t
    parenchymal lung disease caused by, 411, 412.e2f
    pneumonitis caused by, 412.e2f
    for ventricular fibrillation, 1356–1357
    for ventricular tachycardia, 1362
    for Wolff-Parkinson-White syndrome, 1378
Amitriptyline
    for burning mouth syndrome, 226.e4
    for postherpetic neuralgia, 1037
AML. *See* Acute myelogenous leukemia
Amlodipine, for coronary artery disease, 342
Ammonia
    in hepatic encephalopathy, 577–578
    serum, 1774
Ammonium tetrathiomolybdate, for Wilson's disease, 1376.e9
Amnesia
    differential diagnosis of, 1397
    transient global, 1293–1293.e1
Amnestic disorders. *See* Neurocognitive disorders
Amniocentesis, for cervical insufficiency, 271.e2
Amniotic fluid alpha-fetoprotein elevation, 1397
Amniotic fluid dye test, 1053
Amoxicillin
    for acute bronchitis, 28
    for Chlamydia genital infections, 282
    for pharyngitis, 989
    for prepubescent vaginitis, 1342
    for tick bite, 194
    for tonsillitis, 989
    for typhoid fever, 1312.e4
Amoxicillin-clavulanate
    for anaerobic infections, 78
    for bite wounds, 192
    for chronic obstructive pulmonary disease, 301
    for diabetic foot, 385
    for impetigo, 697
    for perirectal abscess, 978
    for peritonsillar abscess, 982

Amoxicillin-clavulanate *(Continued)*
  for prepubescent vaginitis, 1342
  for sialadenitis, 1176
  for urinary tract infection, 1320t
Amoxicillin-clavulanic acid, for perirectal abscess, 978
Amphetamines
  for attention deficit hyperactivity disorder, 161
  pathophysiology, clinical effects, and management of,
    1716t–1719t
Amphotericin B
  for blastomycosis, 202.e3
  for coccidioidomycosis, 313.e3
  for cryptococcosis, 347
  for fungal meningitis, 813.e2–813.e3
  for histoplasmosis, 620
  for invasive candidiasis, 237
  for mucormycosis, 848
  for sporotrichosis, 1205.e3
Amphotericin B lipid complex, for aspergillosis, 131
Ampicillin
  for actinomycosis, 26.e3
  for bacterial meningitis, 813
  for listeriosis, 759
  for peritonsillar abscess, 982
  for pyelonephritis, 1099
Ampicillin-sulbactam
  for anaerobic infections, 78
  for appendicitis, 122
  for bite wounds, 192
  for diverticular disease, 403
  for epididymitis, 459
  for lung abscess, 768
  for orchitis, 917
  for pelvic abscess, 962
  for perirectal abscess, 978
  for peritonsillar abscess, 982
  for retropharyngeal abscess, 1118
Amprenavir, 18
Ampulla cardiomyopathy, 1247
AMS. *See* Acute mountain sickness
Amylase, 944
  serum, 1774
  urine, 1774, 1837
Amyloid A protein, serum, 1774
Amyloid polyneuropathy, 899t
Amyloidosis, 845.e1t, 890f
  characteristics of, 76.e3–76.e6, 76.e3f, 76.e5f,
    76.e5t–76.e6t
  classification of, 76.e4t
  in familial Mediterranean fever, 484
Amyotrophic lateral sclerosis, 77.e1t, 77–77.e1
ANA. *See* Antinuclear antibodies
Anabolic steroid-induced cardiomyopathy, 242
Anaerobic infections, 78–78.e1
Anakinra, 1079
  for adult-onset Still's disease, 54
  for pericarditis, 973
Anal abscess, 1397
Anal fissure, 78.e2–78.e3, 78.e3f
Anal fistula, 1397
Anal incontinence, 699, 1397
Anal neurodermatitis, 1077.e2
Anal ulcer, 78.e2
Analgesics, for neuropathic pain, 899
Anankastic personality disorder, 622.e2
Anaphylactic shock, 79.e1t
Anaphylactoid purpura, 573
Anaphylactoid reaction, 79
Anaphylactoid syndrome, of pregnancy, 1398
Anaphylaxis
  characteristics of, 79.e1t, 79–79.e2
  differential diagnosis of, 1397–1398
  mimics of, 1398
  pathophysiologic classification of, 1398
  treatment of, 1872t
Anaplasia, 888.e2
Anaplasma phagocytophilum, 432, 434.e1f
Anaplasmosis, 432–434.e1, 433t
Anaplastic carcinoma, 1264–1265.e2
Anarthritic rheumatoid syndrome, 1031
Anatomic asplenia, 1887t
ANCA. *See* Antineutrophil cytoplasmic antibodies
ANCA-associated vasculitis, 524t
Ancylostoma duodenale, 126.e1t, 627
Andexanet alfa, 1220
AndroGel, for male hypogonadism, 679

Androgen(s)
  for angioedema, 98
  deficiency of, 539.e1t, 678f
  excess of
    hirsutism caused by, 616, 617b
    in reproductive-age woman, 1398
Androgen deprivation therapy, for prostate cancer, 1073
Androgen insensitivity, partial, micropenis with, 1485
Androgen insensitivity syndrome, 73, 74t, 76
Androgen resistance, 539.e1t, 1398
Androgenetic alopecia, 64, 66.e2f
Androstenedione, serum, 1774
Anejaculation, 435
Anemia
  Addison-Biermer, 89
  algorithm for, 1568, 1568f
  aplastic
    acquired, 1398
    characteristics of, 80–81.e1, 80t, 81f, 81.e1f
    differential diagnosis of, 1398
    drugs and chemicals as cause of, 80t, 1398–1399
    inherited, 1398
  autoimmune hemolytic, 82–84.e2, 82t, 83f, 84t,
    84.e1f–84.e2f, 958.e3t
  of chronic disease, 85, 86f
  diagnosis of, 1568, 1568f
  drug-induced, 1399
  in familial adenomatous polyposis, 482
  hypochromic, 1399–1400
  inflammatory, 85–86.e2, 85f, 86t, 86.e1f–86.e2f
  iron deficiency, 86t, 87–88.e1, 87f–88f
  with low reticulocyte count, 1400
  macrocytic, 1400, 1569, 1569f
  megaloblastic, 89
    with cobalamin deficiency, 1400
    differential diagnosis of, 1400
    with folate deficiency, 1400
    miscellaneous, 1400
  microcytic, 88t, 1401, 1570, 1570f
  in newborn, 1568.e1f
  normocytic, 1400
  pernicious, 89–90.e2, 89t–90t, 90.e1f–90.e2f
  with reticulocytosis, 1570.e1, 1570.e1f
  sickle cell, 1180f
  sideroblastic, 90.e3–90.e4, 90.e3f–90.e4f, 90.e3t
  Waldenström's macroglobulin, abnormal lymphocytes
    with, 1816t
Anergy, cutaneous, 1401
Anergy antigen testing, for pulmonary tuberculosis, 1307
Aneurysms
  abdominal aortic, 3–6.e2, 4f–5f
  dissecting aortic, 113
  thoracic aorta, 1401
Angiitis
  central nervous system, 266.e5
  primary angiitis of the central nervous system,
    1061–1062.e1, 1061t–1062t, 1062.e1f
Angina pectoris
  characteristics of, 91–96.e3, 93f–94f, 96.e2f–96.e3f
  unstable, 31, 91
Angioedema, 97–98.e3, 97f–98f, 98.e2f–98.e3f
Angiofibromas, 1308.e3f, 1308.e4t
Angiography. *See also* Cerebral angiography; Computed
    tomography angiography; Magnetic resonance
    angiography
  for abdominal aortic aneurysm, 5f
  for claudication, 308, 309.e1f
  for eosinophilic granulomatosis with polyangiitis, 458.e4
  for primary angiitis of the central nervous system, 1061
  for pulmonary embolism, 1090
  for renal artery stenosis, 1109, 1109f
  for Takayasu's arteritis, 1245, 1246.e2f
  for thromboangiitis obliterans, 1259.e2b, 1259.e2f
Angioneurotic edema, 97
Angioplasty
  balloon
    for aortic coarctation, 112
    for Budd-Chiari syndrome, 224
  coronary, 96.e2f
Angiotensin II, 1775
Angiotensin receptor blockers
  for cardiorenal syndrome, 254
  for chronic kidney disease, 297
  for dilated cardiomyopathy, 245
  for hypertension, 663
  for renal artery stenosis, 1110

Angiotensin receptor blockers, for heart failure, 558–559
Angiotensin receptor-neprilysin inhibitor, for heart failure, 559
Angiotensin-converting enzyme, 1775
Angiotensin-converting enzyme inhibitors
  for aldosteronism, 61
  for angina pectoris, 95
  for Bartter syndrome, 176.e2
  for cardiorenal syndrome, 254
  for chronic kidney disease, 297
  contraindications for, 558–559
  for coronary artery disease, 342
  for dilated cardiomyopathy, 245
  for heart failure, 558–559
  for hypertension, 663
  for myocardial infarction, 35, 873–874
  for renal artery stenosis, 1110
Angle-closure glaucoma, 521
  acute, 521, 521.e1f
Angular blepharitis, 202.e5
Angular stomatitis, 99–99.e1
ANH. *See* Atrial natriuretic hormone
Anhidrosis, 1401
Anicteric leptospirosis, 742.e8–742.e9
Anidulafungin, for invasive candidiasis, 237
Anion gap, 1775
  acidosis, 1401
  increase, 1401
Anisocoria, 628
  algorithm for, 1571f
  diagnosis of, 1572f
  differential diagnosis of, 1401
ANKH gene, 1078
Ankle
  fracture of, 99.e2–99.e5, 99.e2f–99.e3f, 99.e2t, 99.e3b
  neuropathic, 898f
Ankle pain, 1443–1444, 1456–1457
Ankle sprain, 99.e6–99.e9, 99.e6f–99.e7f, 99.e6t–99.e7t
Ankle-brachial index
  claudication and, 308–309
  description of, 976, 976f, 1259.e1
Ankylosing hyperostosis, 394, 394f–395f
Ankylosing spondylitis
  characteristics of, 100–101.e1, 100f–101f, 101t
  HLA antigens associated with, 1807t
Ann Arbor staging system, for lymphomas, 779, 780t
Annuloplasty, for tricuspid regurgitation, 1301.e5
Anogenital warts, 324, 324f
Anorectal abscess, 978, 978f
Anorectal disease, 1402
Anorectal fissure, 78.e2
Anorectal fistula, 102–102.e1
Anorectal lesions, 1457
Anorectal ulcers, sexually transmitted diseases with, 1523
Anorexia
  differential diagnosis of, 1402
  evaluation of, 1574, 1574f
Anorexia nervosa, 103–104.e1, 103t–104t, 226t
Anorgasmia, 435
Anovulation, 703
  differential diagnosis of, 1402
  hyperandrogenic, 1497–1498
  hypoestrogenic, 1498
Anoxia, coma and, 1424
Anoxic brain injury, 105–106.e1, 105f–106f, 106t
Anoxic encephalopathy, 105
Antacids, 511
Antegrade ureterogram, for hydronephrosis, 644
Anterior chest wall syndrome, 343, 343t
Anterior cord syndrome, 1197–1199.e1, 1198t
Anterior drawer test, 99.e6f
Anterior interosseous nerve syndrome, 1070.e2, 1070.e2f
Anterior nasal packing, 463.e8
Anterior necrotizing scleritis, 1146–1146.e1
Anterior nonnecrotizing scleritis, 1146–1146.e1
Anterior scleritis, 1146
Anterior uveitis, 1334
Anthracycline-induced cardiomyopathy, 242
Anthralin, for psoriasis, 1080
Anthrax, 106.e2f–106.e7, 106.e2f–106.e5f, 106.e6b–106.e7b
Antiandrogens, 512.e6
  for hirsutism, 618
  for paraphilic disorders, 955.e5
Antibiotic-induced colitis, 310
Antibiotics
  for acute bronchitis, 28
  for bacterial pneumonia, 1008, 1010b

Antibiotics *(Continued)*
for Bartholin's gland cyst and abscess, 175
for bronchiectasis, 219
for cavernous sinus thrombosis, 261–262
for conjunctivitis, 326
for hidradenitis suppurativa, 611
for impetigo, 697
for interstitial cystitis, 714
for laryngitis, 739
for mediastinitis, 803
for multidrug-resistant gram-negative rods, 849
for necrotizing fasciitis, 887
for orchitis, 917
for otitis externa, 929
for otitis media, 931
for perirectal abscess, 978
for pertussis, 983
for pyelonephritis, 1099
for Q fever, 1100.e7
for rosacea, 1131
for secondary peritonitis, 979
for sepsis, 1159, 1160t
for septic arthritis, 1161–1162.e3
for severe acute respiratory syndrome, 1164.e3
for shigellosis, 1172
for sinusitis, 1185
for small bowel bacterial overgrowth, 1194–1194.e1
for toxic shock syndrome, 1286
Antibody
acetylcholine receptor, 1771
antimitochondrial, 1776
antinuclear. *See* Antinuclear antibodies
Epstein-Barr virus-specific, 465t
hepatitis A, 1804f, 1804
heterophil, 1806
intrinsic factor, 1811
liver kidney microsome type 1, 1814
mitochondrial, 1817
parietal cell, 1821
platelet, 1822
smooth muscle, 1830
thyroid microsomal, 1833
thyrotropin receptor, 1835
tissue transglutaminase, 1835
Antibody-containing products, 1866t
Anticardiolipin antibody, 1775
Anticholinergics
for Parkinson's disease, 957
poisoning caused by, 1575, 1575f
for urge incontinence, 700–701
Anticholinesterase agents, 738.e2
Anticoagulants
for brain metastases, 210
for heparin-induced thrombocytopenia, 576
for myocardial infarction, 873
preoperative use of, 1055.e4
for pulmonary embolism, 1090–1091, 1091.e3t
for Raynaud's phenomenon, 1104
for renal vein thrombosis, 1115
for venous thrombosis, 650
Anticoagulation
for Budd-Chiari syndrome, 224
for deep vein thrombosis, 359–360
Anticonvulsants
for chronic pain, 939t
for diabetic polyneuropathy, 389
for restless legs syndrome, 1116
Antidepressants
for binge eating disorder, 189
for chronic fatigue syndrome, 291
for chronic pain, 939t
cyclic. *See* Tricyclic antidepressants
for diabetic polyneuropathy, 389
for hypochondriasis, 674.e1
for insomnia, 712
for irritable bowel syndrome, 724
for major depression, 372
for neuropathic pain, 898
for obesity, 907–908
for obsessive-compulsive disorder, 910
for postherpetic neuralgia, 1037
SSRIs. *See* Selective serotonin reuptake inhibitors
tricyclic. *See* Tricyclic antidepressants
Antidiuretic hormone, 1775–1776. *See also*
Syndrome of inappropriate antidiuretic hormone
secretion

Anti-DNA, 522, 1776
Anti-ds DNA, 1776
Antiemetics
for hyperemesis gravidarum, 651
for migraine headache, 546t
Antiepileptics
for brain metastases, 210
for generalized tonic clonic seizures, 1156
for neuropathic pain, 898–899
for obesity, 908
for partial seizures, 1157
Antifibrinolytic agents, for angioedema, 98
Antifreeze, 826
Antifungals
for mucormycosis, 848
for seborrheic dermatitis, 1152
for tinea pedis, 1273
Antigens
human leukocyte, 1807t
live and inactivated, guidelines for, 1866t
Antiglomerular basement antibody, 1776
Anti-glomerular basement membrane disease, 528
Antihistamines
for allergic rhinitis, 63
for anaphylaxis, 79.e2t
for angioedema, 98
for atopic dermatitis, 148
for chronic urticaria, 1328
for conjunctivitis, 326
for contact dermatitis, 329
for food allergies, 496
for insect stings, 195
for lichen simplex chronicus, 758
for nonallergic rhinitis, 904–905
for urticaria, 1326
for Zika virus-related rash, 1380
Antihistone, 1776
Antihypertensive therapy, for diabetes mellitus, 381–382
Anti-LKM antibodies, 595
Antimicrobial therapy, for cholera, 290.e2
Antimitochondrial antibody, 1776
Antineutrophil cytoplasmic antibodies
description of, 1773t, 1776
vasculitis associated with, 1351, 532t
Antinuclear antibodies
in autoimmune hepatitis, 595
description of, 1776, 1776t
in primary biliary cirrhosis, 1064
in rheumatoid arthritis, 1126
Antioxidants, for Friedreich's ataxia, 501.e3
Antiphospholipid antibody syndrome, 107–109.e1, 107f,
107t–108t, 648t, 649
Antiplatelet therapy
for acute ischemic stroke, 1217–1218
for carotid stenosis, 257
for transient ischemic attack, 1294
Antipsychotics
for borderline personality disorder, 205.e2
for delusional parasitosis, 367.e2, 367.e2t
for insomnia, 712
for major depression, 372
for posttraumatic stress disorder, 1044
for psychosis, 1084
for schizophrenia, 1144–1145
for serotonin syndrome, 1164
for tardive dyskinesia, 1251–1251.e1
Antirachitic factor, 1366
Antireflux surgery, for gastroesophageal reflux disease, 174
Antiretroviral therapy
for human immunodeficiency virus, 622, 632–635,
635t–636t
for oral hairy leukoplakia, 755
Anti-RNP antibody, 1777
Anti-Scl 70, 1777
Anti-SM, 1777
Anti-SMAs, 595
Anti-Smith, 1777
Anti-smooth muscle antibody, 1777
Antistreptolysin O titer, 1777
Antithrombin deficiency, 648t–649t, 649–650
Antithrombin III, 1776t, 1777
Antithyroid drugs
for Graves' disease, 535
for hyperthyroidism, 666–667
Antitoxin, botulinum, 206
Antivenom, for snake bites, 198–199

Antiviral agents
for herpes zoster, 609
indications for use, 1895–1897
for influenza, 709t
Antiviral chemotherapy, for herpes simplex, 607t
ANUG. *See* Acute necrotizing ulcerative gingivitis
Anxiety, 110–110.e1
Anxiety attacks, 949
Anxiety neurosis, 110
AOM. *See* Acute otitis media
Aortic aneurysm
abdominal, 1–6.e2, 4f–5f
dissecting, 113
Aortic arch arteritis, 1244
Aortic coarctation
anomalies associated with, 112b
characteristics of, 111–112.e3, 112.e1f–112.e3f, 112b
definition of, 111
hypertension caused by, 112, 660t
imaging of, 111, 112.e1f–112.e2f
rib notching in, 111, 112.e1f
treatment of, 111–112
Aortic dissection, 113–115.e1, 113f–115f
Aortic injury, traumatic, 1753f
Aortic insufficiency, 116
Aortic regurgitation, 113, 116–117.e1, 116f–117f, 117.e1f,
1539
Aortic root dilation, in Marfan's syndrome, 795.e3
Aortic stenosis, 118–120.e1, 118f–120f, 1539
Aortic valve calcification, 1416
Aortic valvular stenosis, 118
Aortitis syndrome, 1244
Aortography, of abdominal aortic aneurysm, 4
AOSD. *See* Adult-onset Still's disease
Apathetic hyperthyroidism, 667
Apathy, 369
Apatite-associated destructive arthritis, 179
Aperistalsis of esophagus, 12
Aphasia, 444
Apixaban
for atrial fibrillation, 152
for pulmonary embolism, 1090
for transient ischemic attack, 1294
Aplasia
acquired red blood cell, 1731.e1
drugs that cause, 1399
pure red cell, 1096.e2–1096.e4, 1096.e2t–1096.e4t,
1096.e4f
Aplastic anemia, 1096.e2
acquired, 1398
characteristics of, 80–81.e1, 80t, 81.e1f
differential diagnosis of, 1398
drugs and chemicals that cause, 80t, 1398–1399
inherited, 1398
Apligraf, for venous ulcers, 1354
APML. *See* Acute promyelocytic leukemia
Apnea-hypopnea index, 1189
Apocrinitis, 610
Apolipoprotein A-1 (Apo A-1), 1777
Appendage torsion, 1255t
Appendagitis, 463.e3
Appendicitis, 818, 818f
characteristics of, 121–122.e2, 121f–122f, 122t
in pregnancy, 1402
Appendicitis epiploica, 463.e3
Appendix torsion, 459.e1t
Appetite loss, in infants and children, 1402
Apremilast, 1080, 1083
APS. *See* Antiphospholipid antibody syndrome
Aquaretics, for ascites, 129t
AR. *See* Aortic regurgitation
Arachnid bites and stings, 194–194.e1, 194.e1f
Arachnodactyly, 795.e4f
Arachnophobia, 993
Arboviral encephalitis, 442
Arboviruses, 442
ARDS. *See* Acute respiratory distress syndrome
ARF. *See* Acute rheumatic fever
Argatroban, for heparin-induced thrombocytopenia, 576
Argentaffinoma syndrome, 239.e2
Argus II retinal implant, 1116.e6
Argyll Robertson pupils, 1243.e5
Aripiprazole, for bipolar disorder, 191
Arm pain, 1491
Armodafinil, for narcolepsy, 884
Aromatic amino acid decarboxylase deficiency, 423t

Arrhenoblastoma, 617f
Arrhythmias. *See also* Tachycardia. *specific arrhythmia*
  sudden death with, 1530
  in Wolff-Parkinson-White syndrome, 1377
Arrhythmogenic right ventricular cardiomyopathy, 123
Arrhythmogenic right ventricular dysplasia, 123–124.e1,
  123f, 124t, 124.e1f
ARS. *See* Acute radiation syndrome
Arsenic, hyperpigmentation with, 1651t–1652t
Arsenic poisoning, 899t
Artemether-lumefantrine, for malaria, 790
Arterial blood gases
  for chronic obstructive pulmonary disease, 299
  description of, 1777–1778
Arterial embolism
  differential diagnosis of, 1433
  mesenteric, factors associated with, 1485
Arterial occlusion, 1403
Arteriosclerosis obliterans, 975
Arteriovenous malformations, cerebral, 164–165.e1,
  164f–165f, 165.e1t
Arteritic anterior ischemic optic neuropathy,
  727–728.e1
Arteritis, 1540
  cerebral, 266.e5
  giant cell, 830t, 1031.e1f
  Takayasu's, 830t, 1244–1246.e2, 1244t–1245t, 1245f,
    1246.e2f
Artesunate, for malaria, 790
Arthralgias
  in Henoch-Schönlein purpura, 573
  limited to one or few joints, 1576, 1576f
Arthritis
  abdominal pain and, 1403
  in axial skeleton, 1404
  in children and adolescents, 1403–1404
  chronic, 1404
  diarrhea and, 1403
  enteropathic, 455–456.e1, 455t
  eye lesions and, 1403
  fever and, 1404
  gouty, 670, 671.e1f
  granulomatous, 534.e2
  heart murmur and, 1403
  in Henoch-Schönlein purpura, 573
  inflammatory, 1667b, 1667f, 1818
  juvenile idiopathic, 732–734.e2, 732t,
    733f–734f, 734.e2f
  monoarticular, 1404–1405
  muscle weakness and, 1403
  oligoarticular, 1404–1405
  osteoarthritis, 921–922.e4, 922f, 922.e4f, 1126t
  in pediatric patients, 1405
  polyarticular, 1405
  psoriatic, 101t, 732, 732t, 1082–1083.e1, 1082b, 1082t,
    1083f, 1083.e1f
    HLA antigens associated with, 1807t
  rash and, 1403
  reactive, 101t, 1105–1105.e1, 1105.e1f
  rheumatoid, 922.e4f, 1125–1128.e3, 1125f, 1126t,
    1127f–1128f
  septic, 1161–1162.e3, 1162f, 1162.e1f–1162.e2f,
    1162.e2t
  subcutaneous nodules and, 1403
  systemic, 732t
  in systemic lupus erythematosus, 1243
  weight loss and, 1403
Arthrocentesis
  for osteoarthritis, 921
  for pseudogout, 1078
  for temporomandibular joint syndrome, 1252
Arthrocentesis fluid, 1778
Arthrochalasia Ehlers-Danlos syndrome, 431.e3
Arthropathy, enteropathic, 101t
Arthropod infestations, 1458
Arthrosis, 921
Articular hip pain, 1456
ARVD. *See* Arrhythmogenic right ventricular dysplasia
ARX gene mutation, 423t
AS. *See* Aortic stenosis
As low as reasonably achievable, 1100.e14
Asbestosis, 125.e2f, 125–125.e2
Ascariasis, 126–126.e1, 126.e1f
Ascaris lumbricoides, 126, 126.e1f, 126.e1t
Ascending cholangitis, 286
Ascending paralysis, 537

Ascites
  characteristics of, 127–129.e2, 127f–129f, 128t–129t,
    129.e1f–129.e2f
  differential diagnosis of, 1405
  pancreatic, 946
  portal hypertension as cause of, 1032f
Ascorbic acid deficiency, 1368
ASD. *See* Acute stress disorder; Atrial septal defect; Autism
  spectrum disorder
Aseptic meningitis, 735.e2, 814
Aseptic necrosis, 166, 922.e5
ASH. *See* Asymmetric septal hypertrophy
"Ash leaf" spots, 1308.e3f, 1308.e4t
Asherman's syndrome, 74
Aspartate aminotransferase
  for eosinophilic granulomatosis with polyangiitis, 458.e4
  reference values for, 1778
Asperger's disorder, 162
Aspergillomas, 130
Aspergillosis
  in acquired immunodeficiency syndrome, 18t–24t
  characteristics of, 130–131.e1, 130f–131f
Aspergillus fumigatus, 458.e7f
Asphyxiation, 404
Aspiration
  of gastric contents, 1576.e1, 1576.e1f
  of oral contents, 1576.e2, 1576.e2f
Aspiration lung injury, in children, 1405
Aspiration pneumonia, 767t, 1006–1006.e1
Aspirin
  for acute coronary syndromes, 32, 34
  for amaurosis fugax, 70
  for angina pectoris, 94
  for antiphospholipid antibody syndrome, 109
  for atrial fibrillation, 152
  for atrial flutter, 154
  for Budd-Chiari syndrome, 224
  for carotid stenosis, 258
  for claudication, 308
  for colorectal cancer, 316
  for coronary artery disease, 342
  for diabetes mellitus, 381
  for Kawasaki disease, 735.e4
  for myocardial infarction, 873
  for pericarditis, 972
  for preeclampsia prophylaxis, 1051
  in pregnancy, 934.e2t
  preoperative use of, 1055.e4
  for pulmonary embolism prophylaxis, 1091
  for transient ischemic attack, 1294
Assisted reproductive technologies, 703
Associated pulmonary arterial hypertension, 1092
Asthenia, 1406
Asthma, 132–141.e4
  ADAM 33 gene associated with, 132
  algorithms for, 141.e3f–141.e4f
  allergic, 132
  anti-IL-13 therapy for, 135
  azithromycin for, 137–139
  bronchial thermoplasty for, 137, 139–140
  in children, 132, 135t–139t, 1406
  chronic obstructive pulmonary disease versus, 140
  classification of, 133, 133t, 136t, 138t
  clinical presentation of, 132
  corticosteroids for, 139–140
  definition of, 132
  demographics of, 132
  diagnosis of, 132–134, 141.e3f
  drug-induced, 132
  epidemiology of, 132
  etiology of, 132
  exacerbations of, 141f
  exercise-induced, 132
  home managed with, 141.e4f
  imaging of, 134
  laboratory testing for, 133–134
  leukotriene modifiers for, 140
  long-acting beta-agonists for, 134–135, 140
  mepolizumab for, 135
  National Asthma Education and Prevention Program
    guidelines, 134t–139t
  omalizumab for, 135
  physical findings in, 132
  reslizumab for, 135
  risk factors for, 132t
  severe, 139–140

Asthma *(Continued)*
  severity of, 133, 133t, 136t, 138t
  short-acting beta-selective adrenergic agonists for,
    134–135
  specialist referral for, 137b, 140
  spirometry for, 133
  tiotropium for, 137
  treatment of, 134–135, 137–140, 141.e3f–141.e4f
Asthma-COPD overlap syndrome, 142–143.e1
Asthmatic bronchitis, 132, 142
Astrocytoma, 144–145.e1, 144f–145f, 212.e2f
Astroglial neoplasms, 144
Asymmetric septal hypertrophy, 246
Asymptomatic inflammatory prostatitis, 1077–1077.e1
AT. *See* Ataxia telangiectasia
Ataque de nervios, 949
Ataxia, 145.e2–145.e4, 145.e3f
  acute, 1406
  cerebellar
    adult onset, 1406–1407
    in children, 1407
  chronic, 1407
  classification of, 1203.e3b
  differential diagnosis of, 1406
  episodic, 1203.e2–1203.e3
  Friedreich's, 501.e3f, 1203.e2–1203.e4
  progressive, 1407, 1577, 1577f
  recurrent, 1406
  spastic, 1203.e3
  spinocerebellar, 1203.e2–1203.e3, 1203.e2f, 1203.e3b
Ataxia telangiectasia, 145.e5–145.e6, 145.e5f
Atazanavir, 18, 1901t
Atazanavir and ritonavir, 634
Atelectasis, 146, 146f, 1407
Atenolol
  for alcohol abuse, 56t
  for atrial fibrillation, 150
  for coronary artery disease, 342
Atherosclerosis of the extremities, 975
Atherosclerotic artery disease, 339, 340f, 341b, 342.e4f
Atherosclerotic cardiovascular disease, 645, 647t
Atherosclerotic disease of the carotid artery, 257
Atherosclerotic occlusive disease, 975
Atherosclerotic renal artery stenosis, 1107
Athletes
  cutaneous infections in, 1427
  sudden death in, 1530
Athlete's foot, 1273, 1273f
Atlantoaxial inflammation, 1125
ATN. *See* Acute tubular necrosis
Atomoxetine, 161
Atopic dermatitis, 147–148.e1, 147b, 148f, 148.e1f, 1077.e4
Atopic eczema, 147
Atopic keratoconjunctivitis, 327t
Atopic neurodermatitis, 147
Atopy patch test, for food allergies, 496
Atorvastatin, for hyperlipidemia, 654.e4t
Atovaquone, for babesiosis, 170
Atovaquone-proguanil, for malaria, 790
Atransferrinemia, 1799t
Atrial enlargement
  left, 1407
  right, 1407
Atrial fibrillation
  atrial septal defect and, 158
  characteristics of, 149–152.e2, 150f–151f
  hypertrophic cardiomyopathy and, 248
  in mitral stenosis, 836
  paroxysmal, 149, 151f
  permanent, 149
  persistent, 149, 151f
  restrictive cardiomyopathy and, 251
  in Wolff-Parkinson-White syndrome, 1377
Atrial flutter, 153–154.e1, 154f
Atrial myxoma, 155–155.e1, 155.e1f
Atrial natriuretic hormone, 1778
Atrial septal defect
  characteristics of, 156–158.e1, 156f–157f, 158.e1f
  coronary sinus septal defect, 156
  primum, 156
  secundum, 156
  sinus venosus defect, 156
Atrial septostomy
  for cor pulmonale, 337
  description of, 1094
Atrial tachycardia, 1230–1232.e1

Atrioventricular block. *See also* AV nodal block
  high-grade, 549f
  pacing for, 550t
  second-degree, 551f–552f
  third-degree, 549, 549f
Atrioventricular dissociation, 159–159.e1, 159f
Atrophic rhinitis, 904
Atrophic vaginitis, 1340
Atrophie blanche, 1352, 1352f
Atrophy
  multiple system, 857.e2–857.e4, 857.e2t–857.e3t, 956,
    1068.e4
  optic, 913.e4, 913.e4f, 1495–1496
  vulvovaginal, 1340
Atropine
  for anaphylaxis, 79.e2t
  for carcinoid syndrome, 239.e3
  intubation and, 1668.e2t
  for second-degree heart block, 552
Attention deficit disorder, 160
Attention deficit hyperactivity disorder, 160–161.e1, 160t
Atypical atrial flutter, 153
Atypical glandular cells, 269
Atypical lymphocyte, 1816t
Atypical lymphocytosis, heterophil negative, 1407
Atypical Parkinsonism, 857.e2
Atypical pneumonia, 1015
Atypical sexual behavior, 955.e4
Atypical squamous cell, 269
AUR. *See* Acute urinary retention
Austin-Flint murmur, 116
Autism, 162
Autism spectrum disorder, 162–163.e1, 162t
Autistic disorder, 162
Autoantibodies
  in autoimmune hepatitis, 595
  in systemic lupus erythematosus, 1241t
Autoeczematization, 690.e4
Autoimmune cholangiopathy, 1063
Autoimmune cholangitis, 595–596
Autoimmune chronic active hepatitis, 595
Autoimmune disease, splenomegaly with, 1528
Autoimmune disease theory, 452
Autoimmune hemolytic anemia, 82–84.e2, 82t, 83f, 84t,
    84.e1f–84.e2f, 958.e3t
Autoimmune hepatitis, 595–596.e1, 595t
Autoimmune pancreatitis, 946–947
Autoimmune polyglandular syndrome type 1, 683
Autologous bone marrow transplantation, 891.e3
Autologous stem cell transplantation
  for multiple myeloma, 852, 854
  for scleroderma, 1149
Autonomic neuropathies, 377, 1493
  peripheral, 1493
Autosomal dominant cerebellar ataxia, 1203.e2
Autosomal dominant polycystic kidney disease,
    1023–1024.e1
AV dissociation. *See* Atrioventricular dissociation
AV nodal block, 1407
AV nodal reentrant tachycardia, 1230–1232.e1
AV reentrant tachycardia
  characteristics of, 1230–1232.e1, 1230f
  in Wolff-Parkinson-White syndrome, 1377
Avascular necrosis, 166–168.e1, 166t, 167f–168f, 922.e5
Avastin. *See* Bevacizumab
Avian influenza, 709.e2–709.e3
AVMs. *See* Arteriovenous malformations
AVN. *See* Avascular necrosis
Avoidant personality disorder, 993
Avulsion fractures, pelvic, 1502
Axial skeleton, arthritis in, 1404
Axillary lymphadenopathy, 1676.e1b, 1676.e1f
Ayurvedic herbal medicine, 410.e1t–410.e2t
Azacitidine
  for acute myelogenous leukemia, 748
  for myelodysplastic syndromes, 865
Azathioprine
  for autoimmune hemolytic anemia, 83
  for autoimmune hepatitis, 596
  for Behçet's disease, 182.e3
  for bullous pemphigoid, 226.e2
  for chronic inflammatory demyelinating polyneuropathy,
    293
  for cirrhosis, 306
  for Cogan's syndrome, 313.e5
  for Crohn's disease, 345

Azathioprine *(Continued)*
  for discoid lupus erythematosus, 396
  for enteropathic arthritis, 456
  for eosinophilic granulomatosis with polyangiitis, 458.e5
  for Henoch-Schönlein purpura, 574
  for inflammatory myopathies, 705
  for Lambert-Eaton myasthenic syndrome, 738.e2
  for paroxysmal cold hemoglobinuria, 958.e2
  for pemphigus vulgaris, 969
  for pericarditis, 973
Azelaic acid, for acne vulgaris, 15
Azelastine hydrochloride
  for allergic rhinitis, 63
  for conjunctivitis, 328t
Azidothymidine, 1651t–1652t
Azithromycin
  for asthma, 137–139
  for babesiosis, 170
  for bacterial pneumonia, 1008
  for cat-scratch disease, 260
  for cervicitis, 272
  for chancroid, 272.e5
  for Chlamydia genital infections, 280
  for cholera, 290.e2
  for chronic obstructive pulmonary disease, 301
  for cystic fibrosis, 352
  for erysipelas, 468
  for gonococcal urethritis, 1318
  for gonorrhea, 527
  for granuloma inguinale, 531.e1
  for impetigo, 697
  for laryngitis, 739
  for Lyme disease, 775
  for mycoplasma pneumonia, 1012
  for nongonococcal urethritis, 1319
  for pertussis, 984, 984t
  for prepubescent vaginitis, 1342
  for shigellosis, 1172
  for typhoid fever, 1136
AZT. *See* Azidothymidine
Aztreonam, for diabetic foot, 385

B

B cells
  deficiencies of, 1065.e3t, 1470
  immune function of, 1065.e3b
  immunodeficiency, vaccination for, 1873t
Babesia spp., 170f
  B. divergens, 169t
  B. microti, 169t
Babesiosis, 169–170.e1, 169t, 170f
Bacillary dysentery, 1172
Bacillus anthracis, 106.e2, 106.e3f
Bacillus Calmette-Guérin vaccine
  for bladder cancer, 201, 202b
  for health care workers, 1884t–1886t
Bacillus cereus, 500t
Bacitracin
  for balanitis, 171
  for burns, 228
Back pain
  in adolescents, 1408
  in children, 1408
  differential diagnosis of, 1407–1415
  low, 1676b
    acute, 1408
    algorithm for, 1676f
    differential diagnosis and treatment of,
      1579–1589.e2, 1798f
    red flags for potentially serious conditions, 1797t
    with viscerogenic origin, 1408
Baclofen, 1196.e1t, 1296
Bacterial arthritis, 1161
Bacterial conjunctivitis, 326f, 328
Bacterial endocarditis, 446, 840
Bacterial gastroenteritis, 509
Bacterial infection
  anaerobic, 78–78.e1
  brain abscess, 207
  epidural abscess, 460
  in HIV infection
    cutaneous manifestations of, 1458
    in hepatic disease, 1458
    in lower gastrointestinal tract disease, 1458
    in pulmonary disease, 1459

Bacterial infection *(Continued)*
  lung abscess and, 767
  myositis with, 1489
  pelvic abscess, 962
  perirectal abscess, 978
  peritonsillar abscess, 981
  renal abscess, 1106
  retropharyngeal abscess, 1117
Bacterial keratitis with ulceration, 338.e2, 338.e2f
Bacterial meningitis, 811–813.e1, 811f–812f, 812t–813t
Bacterial overgrowth
  description of, 785
  small bowel, 1194–1194.e1, 1408
Bacterial pneumonia, 1007–1010.e4, 1008b–1010b, 1008t,
    1009f, 1010.e4f
Bacterial tonsillitis, 981t
Bacterial tracheitis, 345.e4t, 463–463.e2
Bacterial tracheobronchitis, 1290.e2
Bacterial vaginosis, 1343t, 1345–1345.e1, 1345f, 1345.
    e1f
Baden Walker Halfway System, 966b
"Bag of worms", 1347.e2–1347.e3, 1347.e2f, 1347.e2t
Baker's cyst, 170.e2–170.e3, 170.e2f, 229.e5
BAL. *See* Bronchoalveolar lavage
Balance, loss of, 145.e2
Balanitis, 171–171.e1, 171f
Balanitis xerotica obliterans, 757
Balding, 64
BALI Score, 943
Ballism, 1408
Balloon angioplasty
  for aortic coarctation, 112
  for Budd-Chiari syndrome, 224
Balloon mitral valvotomy, for mitral stenosis, 838, 838t
Balloon valvuloplasty, for tricuspid stenosis, 1301.e7
Balo's concentric sclerosis, 855
Balsalazide, for ulcerative colitis, 1314
Bamboo spine, 100, 101f
Band keratopathy, 734.e2f
Bang's disease, 220.e2
Bannayan-Ruvalcaba-Riley syndrome, 985
Bannworth's syndrome, 774
BAONJ. *See* Bisphosphonate-associated osteonecrosis of
    the jaw
Barakol, 410.e1t–410.e2t
Bariatric surgery
  in diabetes mellitus patients, 382
  for obesity, 824, 907–908, 909.e7f, 1190
Barium esophagography, for dysphagia, 420
Barium sulfate, for radiation exposure, 1100.e14t–1100.
    e16t
Barium swallow, for dysphagia, 420, 421.e1f
Barlow's syndrome, 839
Barrett esophagus, 172–174.e1, 173f
Bartholin's gland
  carcinoma of, 1372.e2
  cyst and abscess of, 175–176.e1, 176f
Bartonellosis, 636t
Bartter syndrome, 176.e2–176.e3, 176.e3t, 1829t
Basal body temperature contraception method, 330
Basal cell carcinoma
  characteristics of, 177–178.e1, 177f
  vulvar, 1372.e2
Basic calcium phosphate crystal deposition disease,
    179–180.e1, 179f–180f, 180t
Basophil count, 1779
Bat bites, 1100.e10
Battered child syndrome, 277
Battered elder syndrome, 437
BCC. *See* Basal cell carcinoma
BCP crystal-associated destructive arthropathies, 179
BCPCDD, 179
BCR-ABL fusion oncogene, 753
BDD. *See* Body dysmorphic disorder
Beau's lines, 735.e2, 1688
Becker muscular dystrophy, 860–861, 860f
Becker's sign, 116
Beck's triad, 240
Beckwith-Wiedemann syndrome, 888.e2, 888.e2t
Beclomethasone dipropionate, for allergic rhinitis, 63
BED. *See* Binge eating disorder
Bedaquiline, for pulmonary tuberculosis, 1308
Bedbug(s), 181, 181f–182f
Bedbug bite, 181–182.e1, 181f
Bedsores, 1056
Bedwetting, 457

Bee stings, 195
Beers criteria, 1031.e2
Behavioral disturbance, sleep-associated, 1737f
Behavioral weight loss, 188
Behçet's disease, 182.e2–182.e3, 182.e2f
Behçet's syndrome, 182.e2
Belching, 1394
Belimumab, for systemic lupus erythematosus, 1242
Bell's palsy, 183–184.e1, 183f–184f
Benign essential tremor, 476
Benign hereditary chorea, 639
Benign inoculation lymphoreticulosis, 260
Benign intracranial hypertension, 690.e5
Benign ovarian neoplasms, 934–934.e1, 934f
Benign paroxysmal peritonitis, 484
Benign paroxysmal positional vertigo, 185–187.e1, 185b, 186f, 187t
Benign paroxysmal torticollis, 423t
Benign prostatic hyperplasia, 1075–1076.e2, 1075t, 1076.e2f
Benzalcuronium solution, for bite wounds, 192
Benzathine penicillin, for Scarlet fever, 1143
Benznidazole, for Chagas' disease, 272.e3
Benzodiazepines
    for acute respiratory distress syndrome, 46–48
    for acute stress disorder, 49
    for alcohol withdrawal, 56–57, 56t, 367, 407
    for burning mouth syndrome, 226.e4
    for chemical-induced cardiomyopathy, 243
    for chemotherapy-induced nausea and vomiting, 276
    for generalized anxiety disorder, 110
    for insomnia, 712
    for neuroleptic malignant syndrome, 896
    for panic disorder, 950
    for phobias, 993
    for posttraumatic stress disorder, 1044
    for premenstrual dysphoric disorder, 1053.e2
    for serotonin syndrome, 1164
    for social anxiety disorder, 1194.e4
Benzyl alcohol, for pediculosis, 961
Beraprost, for pulmonary hypertension, 1094
Berger's disease, 693
Beriberi, cerebral, 1376.e3
Bernhardt-Roth syndrome, 817.e2
Beta human chorionic growth hormone, 841
Beta hypersensitivity orthostatic tachycardia syndrome, 1044.e2
Beta natriuretic peptide, cardiorenal syndrome and, 253–254
Beta-blockers
    for angina pectoris, 94
    for aortic dissection, 115
    for aortic regurgitation, 117
    for aortic root dilation in Marfan's syndrome, 795.e3
    for chemical-induced cardiomyopathy, 243
    for cirrhosis, 305
    for claudication, 309
    for cocaine dose, 313
    for dilated cardiomyopathy, 245
    for esophageal varices, 475
    for Graves' disease, 535
    for heart failure, 558–559
    for hypertension, 663
    for hypertrophic cardiomyopathy, 247–248
    for long QT syndrome, 766
    for mitral valve prolapse, 839–840
    for myocardial infarction, 35, 873
    for open-angle glaucoma, 519
    pathophysiology, clinical effects, and management of, 1716t–1719t
    for portal hypertension, 1033
    for posttraumatic stress disorder, 1044
    preoperative use of, 1055.e4
    for social anxiety disorder, 1194.e4
    for thyrotoxic storm, 1268.e2
    for torsade de pointes, 1279–1280
    for ventricular fibrillation, 1356–1357
Betamethasone
    for abruptio placentae, 10
    for Behçet's disease, 182.e3
    for vitiligo, 1370
Beta-thalassemia, 87t, 1256–1257.e1, 1256t–1257t
Bethesda 2001 updated classification, for cervical dysplasia, 269–270
Bevacizumab
    for acoustic neuroma, 16
    for astrocytoma, 145

Bevacizumab (Continued)
    for colorectal cancer, 315
    for Osler-Rendu-Weber syndrome, 920.e2
    for ovarian cancer, 933
Bicarbonate, 1779
    for diabetic ketoacidosis, 388
    gastrointestinal loss of, 1390
    for renal tubular acidosis, 1114
Biceps tendinosis, 187.e2
Biceps tendonitis, 187.e2–187.e4, 187.e2f–187.e4f
Bichloracetic acid, for warts, 1376
Bicipital tendinitis, 1133.e4t
Bicipital tendonitis, 187.e2
Bicipital tenosynovitis, 187.e2
Bilateral acoustic neurofibroma, 894
Bilateral hilar lymphadenopathy, 1138.e1f
Bilateral inferior petrosal sinus sampling, 349
Bilateral optic atrophy, 913.e4
Bile, urine, 1779, 1837
Bile acid malabsorption, 785
Bile acid sequestrants
    for hyperlipidemia, 654.e4t
    lipoprotein metabolism affected by, 647.e1t
Bile duct
    carcinoma of, 283
    dilated, 1408–1409
Bile salts, for cholelithiasis, 290
Bilharziasis, 1143.e1
Biliary cirrhosis, 1063
Biliary colic, 290.e1t
Biliary decompression, for cholangitis, 286
Biliary dyskinesia, 504
Biliary obstruction, 1409
Biliary sepsis, 286
Biliary tree, reflux of gas or bowel, 1409
Bilirubin
    in cirrhosis, 304
    direct, 1670–1671, 1779
    indirect, 1671–1672, 1779
    total, 1779
    urine, 1779
Binge eating disorder, 103t, 188–189.e1, 225
Binge-eating/purging anorexia nervosa, 103
Binocular diplopia, 1430
Biological therapy
    for juvenile idiopathic arthritis, 733
    for mycosis fungoides, 863.e4
Biomarkers
    cardiac
        in acute coronary syndrome, 32, 34f
        for dilated cardiomyopathy, 244
    hypertrophic cardiomyopathy, 247
BIONJ. See Bisphosphonate-induced osteonecrosis of the jaw
Biopsy
    bone marrow
        for acute lymphoblastic leukemia, 745.e1f
        for hairy cell leukemia, 754.e4f
        for hypereosinophilic syndrome, 651.e1, 651.e2f
        for myelodysplastic syndrome, 864, 866.e2f
        for non-Hodgkin lymphomas, 779, 781.e1f
        for polycythemia vera, 1030.e1f
    for eosinophilic granulomatosis with polyangiitis, 458.e4
    for hepatocellular carcinoma, 597
    for histoplasmosis, 620.e1f
    for hypereosinophilic syndrome, 651.e1, 651.e2f
    for inclusion body myositis, 698, 698.e1f
    for inflammatory myopathies, 704
    for interstitial nephritis, 719
    for Langerhans cell histiocytosis, 618.e2–618.e3
    liver
        for hemochromatosis, 565, 566f
        for primary sclerosing cholangitis, 1068
    lung, for hypersensitivity pneumonitis, 658
    for melanoma, 805
    for mucormycosis, 848
    muscle, for inclusion body myositis, 698, 698.e1f
    for mycosis fungoides, 863.e2
    for non-Hodgkin lymphomas, 779, 781.e1f
    for primary angiitis of the central nervous system, 1062, 1062.e1f
    for primary biliary cirrhosis, 1064
    for prostate cancer, 1072
    for thyroid nodule, 1266
Bioresorbable stents, for ST-segment elevation myocardial infarction, 869

Bipolar disorder
    borderline personality disorder and, 205.e2
    characteristics of, 190–191.e1
BIPSS. See Bilateral inferior petrosal sinus sampling
Bird fancier's lung, 657
Bird flu, 709.e2
Birth, breech, 218.e8–218.e9
Birth control, 330
Bismuth, hyperpigmentation with, 1651t
Bisoprolol, for dilated cardiomyopathy, 245
Bisphosphonate(s)
    for Charcot's joint, 274
    for hyperparathyroidism, 656
    for hypertrophic osteoarthropathy, 669
    for osteoporosis, 926
    for Paget's disease of bone, 935
Bisphosphonate-associated osteonecrosis of the jaw, 191.e2
Bisphosphonate-induced osteonecrosis of the jaw, 191.e2
Bisphosphonate-related osteonecrosis of the jaw, 191.e2–191.e3, 927
Bite(s)
    animal, 1100.e10–1100.e11
    arachnid, 194–194.e1, 194.e1f
    bat, 1100.e10
    bedbug, 181–182.e1, 181f
    insect, 181, 195–196.e1, 195f–196f, 196.e1f
    snake, 197–199.e1
Bite wounds, 192–193.e1, 193b, 193t
Bivalirudin
    for acute coronary syndromes, 35
    for heparin-induced thrombocytopenia, 576
Biventricular failure, 1540
Black cohosh, 410.e1t–410.e2t
Black widow spider bites, 194, 194.e1f
Bladder
    neurogenic, 1501
    neuropathic, 1502
    normal position of, 701.e3f
    overactive, 700
    renal failure caused by, 1518
    urinary incontinence, 700–701.e3, 701t, 701.e3f
    urinary tract obstruction caused by, 1537
Bladder cancer, 200–202.e1, 202b, 202f
Bladder pain syndrome, 713
Bladder pressure, 7
Bladder tumor associated antigen, 1779
Bladder wall thickening, 1409
Blastomyces dermatitidis, 202.e2
Blastomycosis, 202.e2–202.e4, 202.e2f–202.e3f
Bleeding. See also Hemorrhage
    dysfunctional uterine, 413–414.e1, 413b–414b, 414t
    evaluation of, 1579.e1, 1579.e1f
    gastrointestinal, 1629.e2, 1629.e2b
        approach to patient with, 1581f, 1581–1582
        evaluation of, 1816f
        lower, 1409
        upper, 1410
    neonate, 1582.e1, 1582.e1f
    postmenopausal, 1509
    rectal, 1410
    in third trimester of pregnancy, 1410
    vaginal
        anovulatory, evaluation of, 1584f
        in non-pregnant female, 1410
        ovulatory, evaluation of, 1583-1584
        in pregnancy, 1335–1335.e1, 1539–1543, 1580.e1f
    variceal, 1584.e1, 1584.e1f
    varicose veins and, 1348
    in Von Willebrand's disease, 1371
Bleeding disorder, 1580b
    congenital, 1579.e2, 1579.e2f
    differential diagnosis of, 1580, 1580f
Bleeding time (modified Ivy method), 1779, 1780.e1f
Bleomycin
    for craniopharyngioma, 343.e2
    hyperpigmentation with, 1651t–1652t
    pneumonitis caused by, 412.e1f
    for warts, 1376
Blepharitis, 202.e5, 202.e5f
Blepharospasm, 422
Blindness. See also Vision loss
    in geriatric age, 1410
    monocular, transient, 1410
    in pediatric age, 1410–1411
Blisters, subepidermal, 1411
Bloating, 1442

Blood
  occult, urine, 1838
  pH of, 1821
Blood disorders, splenomegaly with, 1527
Blood flow, cerebral, 1484
Blood gases, arterial, 299, 1777
Blood loss. *See also* Bleeding; Hemorrhage
  in abruptio placentae, 9
  drugs promoting, 1399
Blood pressure
  in chronic kidney disease, 296
  elevated. *See* Hypertension
  normal, 660
Blood products, 1041b
Blood transfusion
  recommended intervals between administration, 1867t
  for sepsis, 1159
  for sickle cell disease, 1180t, 1181
  for yellow fever, 1378.e2
Blood urea nitrogen, 1836
  cardiorenal syndrome and, 253
  factors affecting level, 1836b
Blood vessels, 1350
Blood volume
  renal failure caused by, 1518
  total, 1781
Bloodstream infections, healthcare-associated, 548.e3–548.e4
Bloody diarrhea, 1429
Blue, cutaneous color changes to, 1424
"Blue blebs", 1348
Blue light, for acne vulgaris, 14–15
Blue urine, 1448
BMI. *See* Body mass index
BNP. *See* Beta natriuretic peptide; Brain natriuretic peptide
BODE index, for chronic obstructive pulmonary disease,
  302–303
Body dysmorphic disorder, 203–203.e1
Body fluids, 1604.e3t
Body mass index, 906
Body ringworm, 1271
Body temperature
  measurement of, 688t
  regulation of, mental changes and coma caused by, 1484
Boeck's sarcoid, 1137
Bone
  diffuse idiopathic skeletal hyperostosis effects on
    formation of, 394
  in foot and ankle pain, 1443
  heel pain and, 1452
  ischemic necrosis of, 1472
  Paget's disease of, 935–935.e1, 935.e1f
  resorption of, 1413
Bone density
  generalized loss of, 1411–1412
  increased, 1413
  localized loss of, 1412
Bone fracture, 1628.e2b, 1628.e2f, 1628.e2–1628.e3
Bone infection, 923, 1665, 1665b, 1665f
Bone lesions
  in histiocytosis X, 618.e2
  osteolytic benign, 1497
  osteosclerotic benign, 1497
  preferential site of origin of, 1412
Bone marrow
  biopsy of
    for acute lymphoblastic leukemia, 745.e1f
    for hairy cell leukemia, 754.e4f
    for hypereosinophilic syndrome, 651.e1, 651.e2f
    for myelodysplastic syndrome, 864, 866.e2f
    for non-Hodgkin lymphomas, 779, 781.e1f
    for polycythemia vera, 1030.e1f
  drugs that suppress, 1399
  fibrosis, 1412
  inherited failure syndromes of, 1412
Bone marrow transplantation
  allogeneic
    for acute lymphoblastic leukemia, 744
    for chronic lymphocytic leukemia, 752
    for myelodysplastic syndromes, 865
  autologous, 891.e3
  for thalassemia, 1257
Bone marrow trephine biopsy section, in hairy cell leukemia,
  754.e4f
Bone mass, low, 1413
Bone mineral density, 925t–926t, 926f–927f, 1369.e1f
Bone pain, 1413

Bone sarcomas, 1140, 1140f
Bone scintigraphy
  for complex regional pain syndrome, 320
  for Paget's disease of bone, 935
Bone tumor, primary malignant, 204–205.e1, 205f
Borborygmi, 509
Borderline personality disorder, 205.e2–205.e4, 205.e3f
Bordetella pertussis
  acute bronchitis caused by, 27t
  serology, 1781
Boric acid, for fungal vaginitis, 1341
Borrelia burgdorferi, 774–775.e1
Botulinum immunoglobulin, 206
Botulinum toxin
  for achalasia, 13
  for anal fissure, 78.e2
  for Bell's palsy, 184
  for bruxism, 222.e2
  food poisoning caused by, 206
  for headache, 547
  for migraine headache, 547
  for urinary incontinence, 701
  for vaginismus, 1339
Botulism, 206–206.e1
Bouchard's nodes, 921, 922.e4f
Boutonniere deformity, 1125, 1125f
Bovine spongiform encephalopathy, 343.e3
Bow legs, 1413
Bowel incontinence, 699–699.e1, 699.e1b
Bowel obstruction, 1525
Bowel wall thickening, 1413
Bowenoid papulosis, 324f
BPD. *See* Borderline personality disorder
BPH. *See* Benign prostatic hyperplasia
BPPV. *See* Benign paroxysmal positional vertigo
Brachial plexopathy, 1493
Brachytherapy, for retinoblastoma, 1116.e8
Bradycardia
  fever and rash with, 1440
  general approach to, 1585, 1585f
  in pediatric patient, 1585.e1, 1585.e1f
  sinus, 1414
Bradycardia-tachycardia syndrome, 1178
Brain abscess, 207–208.e1, 207t, 208f, 848
Brain arteriovenous malformation, 164
Brain attack, 1215, 1221
Brain infarct, 1221
Brain injury
  anoxic, 105–106.e1, 105f–106f, 106t
  traumatic, 1297–1299.e1, 1297b, 1298t, 1299f
Brain mass, 1414
Brain metastases, 209–210.e1, 209f, 210.e1f
Brain natriuretic peptide, 250–251
Brain neoplasms
  benign, 211–212.e2, 211t, 212.e2f
  glioblastoma, 213–213.e1
Brain stem encephalitis, 442
BRCA1, 602
BRCA2, 602
BRCA analysis, 1781
Breast
  abscess of, 214–214.e1, 214f
  engorgement of, 796t
  fibrocystic disease, 490
  nipple discharge evaluation of, 1586f, 1586–1587
  radiologic evaluation of, 1587.e1, 1587.e1–1587.e2
Breast cancer
  characteristics of, 215–218.e7, 215t, 218.e4f–218.e7f
  in pregnancy, 217
Breast diseases
  fibrocystic disease, 490
  galactorrhea, 1070.e1f
  gynecomastia, 1070.e1f
  mastitis, 796–797.e1, 796t
  mastodynia, 800
  Paget's disease, 936–936.e1, 936f
Breast lesion, inflammatory, 1414
Breast mass
  differential diagnosis of, 1414
  differentiation of, 490t
  screening and evaluation of, 1588f, 1588–1589
Breast pain, 800
Breastfeeding difficulties, 1589.e1, 1589.e1f
Breath hydrogen test, 1533
Breath odor, 1414

Breathing, noisy, 1414
Breech birth, 218.e8–218.e9, 218.e8f
Broken heart syndrome, 1247
Bromocriptine
  for acromegaly, 24.e8, 999
  for cocaine overdose, 313
  for mastodynia, 800
  for neuroleptic malignant syndrome, 896
  for premenstrual syndrome, 1055
  for prolactinoma, 999, 1069
Bronchial obstruction, 1414
Bronchial thermoplasty, for asthma, 137, 139–140
Bronchiectasis
  characteristics of, 219–220.e1, 220t
  cystic fibrosis and, 352
Bronchitis, acute, 27–28.e1
Bronchoalveolar carcinoma, 769
Bronchoalveolar lavage
  description of, 348.e2
  for hypersensitivity pneumonitis, 657–658
Bronchodilators
  for atelectasis, 146
  for bronchiectasis, 219
  for chronic obstructive pulmonary disease, 301
  for status asthmaticus, 139
Bronchogenic carcinoma, 769t
Bronchopleural fistula, 1414
Bronchoscopic balloon tamponade, for hemoptysis, 571
Bronchoscopic lavage, for hemoptysis, 571
Bronchoscopy
  for bronchiectasis, 219
  for hemoptysis, 571
  for hypersensitivity pneumonitis, 658
  for lung abscess, 768
  for sarcoidosis, 1138
Bronchospasm, 132, 142
BRONJ. *See* Bisphosphonate-related osteonecrosis of the jaw
Bronze diabetes, 565
Bropirimine, for bladder cancer, 201
Brown, cutaneous color changes to, 1507
Brown recluse spider bites, 194, 194.e1f
Brown urine, 1414
Brown-Séquard syndrome, 1197–1199.e1, 1198t
Brucellosis, 220.e2–220.e3, 220.e2f, 220.e3t
Brugada syndrome, 221–222.e1, 221f, 221t–222t, 424–425,
  426f, 1356–1357
Brugia sp., 776, 778
Bruising, 1579.e1, 1579.e1f
Bruxism, 222.e2, 222.e2f
B-type natriuretic peptide, 555, 1086, 1779–1781
Buccal cellulitis, 266t
Budd-Chiari syndrome, 223–224.e1, 224.e1f, 1033t
Budesonide
  for allergic rhinitis, 63
  for autoimmune hepatitis, 596
  for chronic obstructive pulmonary disease, 301
  for Crohn's disease, 345
  for croup, 345.e3, 345.e4t
Buerger's disease, 1259.e1–1259.e3, 1259.e2b, 1259.e2f
Bulimia nervosa, 103t, 225–226.e1, 226t
Bullae
  fever and rash with, 1440
  on lower extremities, 1589.e2, 1589.e2f
Bullous impetigo, 697
Bullous pemphigoid, 226.e2–226.e3, 226.e2f, 969t
Bullous stomatitis, 1528
BUN. *See* Blood urea nitrogen
Bupivacaine, for cluster headaches, 543
Buprenorphine, 407, 912–913
Bupropion
  for attention deficit hyperactivity disorder, 161
  for bipolar disorder, 191
  for hypoactive sexual desire disorder, 673
  for obesity, 908
  for sexual dysfunction in women, 1169
Burkitt lymphoma, 781
Burn(s), 227–229.e4, 228t, 229.e4f
  care phases for, 229.e2t
  categorization of, by depth, 227t
  classification of, 227
  complications in, 229.e3b
  follow-up care for, 229
  Mayes equations for, 229b
  modified Brooke resuscitation formula for, 229b
  resuscitation for, 228
    formula for, 229b

Burn(s) (Continued)
  "rule of nines" for, 227, 229.e4f
  second-degree, 229.e4f
  "6 Cs" of, 228
  third-degree, 229.e4f
  treatment for, 228–229, 229.e4f
  wound care for, 228–229
Burning mouth syndrome, 226.e4–226.e5
Burr hole evacuation, 462
Bursitis, 229.e5–229.e6
"Bush tea", 410.e1t–410.e2t
Buspirone, 110
Busulfan, hyperpigmentation with, 1651t–1652t
Butenafine
  for tinea corporis, 1271
  for tinea cruris, 1272
  for tinea pedis, 1273
Buttocks, joint pain in, 1474
Bypass tract, in Wolff-Parkinson-White syndrome, 1377,
  1377f, 1378b

C

C2 deficiency, 1807t
C4 deficiency, 1807t
CA-1, 169t
CA-2, 169t
CA-125, 932
CA 15-3, 1782
CA 27-29, 1784
CA 72-4, 1784
CA 125, 452, 1784
Cabergoline, 999
  for acromegaly, 24.e8
  for prolactinoma, 1069
Cabozantinib, 1112
CAD. See Coronary artery disease
Café-au-lait macules/spots, 894, 894f, 1415–1427
Cafergot, for cluster headaches, 543
CAGE-AID, 912, 912t
CAH. See Chronic active hepatitis
Calcaneus, heel pain and, 1452
Calcific periarthritis, 179
Calcific tendinitis, 1133.e4t
Calcific tendonitis, 179
Calcifications
  in breast cancer, 218.e4f
  extraskeletal, in chronic kidney disease, 298.e6f
  pancreatic, 1709.e1
  x-rays of
    adrenal gland, 1585–1586
    cardiac, 1588–1589
    chest, 1579.e1–1579.e2
    cutaneous, 1416
    female genital tract, 1416
    liver, 1416
    nonvisceral abdominal, 1579.e2
    pancreatic, 1416
    splenic, 1416
    valvular, 1416
Calcified orbital lesions, 1497
Calcineurin inhibitors
  for seborrheic dermatitis, 1152
  for vitiligo, 1370
Calcipotriene, for psoriasis, 1080
Calcipotriol, for vitiligo, 1370
Calcitonin
  for hyperparathyroidism, 656
  serum, 1781
Calcitriol
  for hypoparathyroidism, 684
  for renal osteodystrophy, 297
Calcium
  for hypoparathyroidism, 684
  for osteoporosis, 926
  serum, 1783f, 1782, 1843t
  testing of, for hyperparathyroidism, 655
  urine, 1782, 1837
Calcium carbonate
  for radiation exposure, 1100.e14t–1100.e16t
  for renal osteodystrophy, 297
Calcium channel blockers
  for angina pectoris, 95
  for aortic dissection, 115
  for chemical-induced cardiomyopathy, 243
  for cor pulmonale, 337

Calcium channel blockers (Continued)
  for coronary artery disease, 342
  for hypertension, 663–664
  for myocardial infarction, 35
  pathophysiology, clinical effects, and management of,
    1716t–1719t
  for pheochromocytoma, 992.e2t
  for preterm labor, 1060t
  for pulmonary arterial hypertension, 1094
  for Raynaud's phenomenon, 1103
  side effects of, 1060t
Calcium disodium EDTA, 741t
Calcium gluconate
  for hypoparathyroidism, 684
  for radiation exposure, 1100.e14t–1100.e16t
Calcium phosphate, for radiation exposure, 1100.e14t–1100.e16t
Calcium pyrophosphate dihydrate crystal deposition disease,
    1079.e1b, 1079.e2f–1079.e3f, 1078, 1078t, 1079f
Calcium stones, 1325, 1416
Calcium-alkali syndrome, 230.e1t, 230–230.e1
Calculi-related infections, 1099
Caliectasis, 643
Calprotectin, in Crohn's disease, 344
Cameron's lesion, 609.e3
cAMP, urine, 1837
Campylobacter jejuni food poisoning, 500
Campylobacter pylori. See Helicobacter pylori
CA-MRSA. See Community-acquired methicillin-resistant
    Staphylococcus aureus
Cancer. See also Adenocarcinoma; Carcinoma; Tumors/
    neoplasms
  bladder, 200–202.e1, 202b, 202f
  brain, 209
  cervical, 267–268.e1, 267f–268f, 268t
    screening guidelines for, 1858t
    staging of, 268t
  colorectal, 314–316.e1, 316f, 985–986, 985t
    classification and staging of, 314, 314t
    screening and surveillance recommendations, 315t
    survival rates for, 316t
    wall thickening associated with, 316f
  endometrial, 450–451.e1, 450t, 451f
  esophageal, 474.e1f
    algorithm for staging, 473f
    classification of, 472t
    TNM staging system for, 473t
  gastric, 506–507.e2, 507t
  hereditary nonpolyposis colon cancer, 314
  nutrition assessment and intervention in, 1694.e1, 1694.e1f
  oral, 915–916.e1, 915f
  ovarian, 932–933.e1, 932t, 933.e1f
  pancreatic, 941–942.e1, 941f, 942t
  prostate. See Prostate cancer
  risk for, celiac disease and, 264
  testicular, 1253–1254.e1, 1253f, 1254t
  uterine, 450, 450t, 451f
  vaginal, 1338–1338.e1, 1338f
  vulvar, 1372.e2–1372.e3, 1372.e2f–1372.e3f, 1372.e2t
Cancer NOS, 231
Cancer of unknown primary, 231–233.e1, 231b, 232t–233t
Cancer unspecified site, 231
Candida albicans, 1214
Candida balanitis, 234
Candida esophagitis, 235
Candida peritonitis, 236
Candidal infections
  central nervous system, 236
  musculoskeletal, 236
Candidemia, 236
Candidiasis, 1343t
  chronic mucocutaneous, 234
  cutaneous, 234–235.e1, 234f–235f
  disseminated, 236
  hepatosplenic, 236
  in human immunodeficiency virus, 636t
  invasive, 236–237.e1, 237f
  mucosal, 636t
  vulvovaginal, 234, 1341
Candidosis, 234, 234f
Candigas. See Caspofungin
Cangrelor, for myocardial infarction, 873
Cannabinoids, for chronic pain, 939t
CAP. See Community-acquired pneumonia
Capecitabine
  for colorectal cancer, 315
  of esophageal tumors, 474

Capillariasis, 350.e5t
Capital femoral osteochondrosis, 742
Capsaicin
  for burning mouth syndrome, 226.e4
  for chronic pain, 939t
  for postherpetic neuralgia, 609, 1037
Capsule endoscopy, for celiac disease, 264
Capsulitis, 1133.e4t
Captopril, for coronary artery disease, 342
Captopril stimulation test, 1784
Carbamates, 1716t–1719t
Carbamazepine, 1784
  for alcohol abuse, 56t
  for bipolar disorder, 191
  for Charcot-Marie-Tooth syndrome, 275
  for chronic pain, 939t
  granulomatous hepatitis caused by, 410.e3t
  for intermittent explosive disorder, 712.e4t
  for neuropathic pain, 899
  for partial seizures, 1157
  for trigeminal neuralgia, 1302
Carbapenem-resistant Enterobacteriaceae, 849–849.e1
Carbapenems, for necrotizing fasciitis, 887
Carbohydrate antigen 19-9, 1784
Carbohydrate malabsorption, 738, 785
Carbon dioxide, partial pressure of, 1781
Carbon monoxide
  description of, 1784
  poisoning caused by, 238–239.e1, 238t, 239f
Carbonic anhydrase inhibitors, for open-angle
    glaucoma, 519
Carboplatin, 1040t
Carboxyhemoglobin, 238, 238t, 1784
Carcinoembryonic antigen
  colorectal cancer and, 314
  description of, 1784
Carcinoid disease, 239.e2f
Carcinoid syndrome, 239.e2–239.e3, 239.e2f–239.e3f
Carcinoma. See also Cancer
  Bartholin gland, 1372.e2
  basal cell
    characteristics of, 177–178.e1, 177f
    vulvar, 1372.e2
  breast, 215, 215t, 218.e4f
  bronchogenic, 769t
  cholangiocarcinoma. See Cholangiocarcinoma
  endometrial, 450
  hepatocellular, 597f–598f, 598.e1f, 597–598.e1, 598t
  laryngeal, 738.e4–738.e5
  renal cell, 1111–1112.e1, 1111f–1112f, 1112t
  squamous cell. See Squamous cell carcinoma
  thyroid, 1264–1265.e2, 1264t–1265t, 1265.e2f
  tongue, 915f
Carcinomatosis, peritoneal, 1504
Cardia, achalasia of, 12
Cardiac arrest, nontraumatic, 1417
Cardiac biomarkers, in acute coronary syndrome,
    32, 34f
Cardiac calcifications, 1588–1589
Cardiac catheterization. See also Catheterization
  for aortic coarctation, 112.e3f, 111
  for aortic stenosis, 118–119
  for atrial septal defect, 157
  for cardiac tamponade, 240–241
  for dilated cardiomyopathy, 244
  for heart failure, 556–557
  for mitral regurgitation, 834
  for mitral stenosis, 837
  for myocarditis, 876
  for patent ductus arteriosus, 959
  for restrictive cardiomyopathy, 251
  for tetralogy of Fallot, 1255.e6
  for ventricular fibrillation, 1356–1357
Cardiac chamber enlargement, 1417
Cardiac computed tomography, for angina pectoris, 94
Cardiac computed tomography angiography, for coronary
    artery disease, 339
Cardiac death, sudden. See Sudden cardiac death
Cardiac disease. See also Heart disease
  stroke with, 1529
  vaccination considerations for, 1887t
Cardiac enlargement, 1417
Cardiac glycosides
  pathophysiology, clinical effects, and management of,
    1716t–1719t
  toxicity caused by, 395.e2, 395.e3f–395.e4f

Cardiac magnetic resonance imaging
  for angina pectoris, 94
  for dilated cardiomyopathy, 245
  for heart failure, 557
  for mitral regurgitation, 834
  for myocarditis, 876, 877.e1f
  for patent ductus arteriosus, 959
  for restrictive hypertrophic cardiomyopathy, 251
  for Takotsubo cardiomyopathy, 1247
  for tetralogy of Fallot, 1255.e6
Cardiac murmurs, 1417
Cardiac myxoma, 155
Cardiac output, 1518
Cardiac pacing, for carotid sinus syndrome, 256
Cardiac resynchronization therapy
  for cardiorenal syndrome, 254
  for heart failure, 559–560
  for intraventricular conduction delay, 720–721
Cardiac tamponade, 973
  characteristics of, 240–241.e1, 240f–241f, 241.e1f
  constrictive pericarditis and, 240t
  echocardiogram findings in, 240
Cardiac transplantation
  for heart failure, 560
  for myocarditis, 877
Cardiac tumors, 155, 1417
Cardioembolic stroke, 1221
Cardioembolism, 1417
Cardiogenic pulmonary edema, 1086
Cardiogenic shock
  in acute decompensated heart failure, 558
  differential diagnosis of, 1418
Cardiomegaly, 1590–1603.e1, 1591f
Cardiomyopathy
  arrhythmogenic right ventricular, 123, 1593t
  causes of, 1459–1460
  chemical-induced, 242–243.e1, 243f
  classification of, 1592f, 1592–1593
  dilated
    characteristics of, 244–245.e1, 245t
    with Duchenne muscular dystrophy, 245.e1f
    idiopathic, 245
    profile of, 1593t
  hypertrophic, 246–249.e1, 247f–248f, 1593t
  ischemic, 1593.e1, 1593.e1f
  restrictive
    characteristics of, 250–252.e1, 250f
    constrictive pericarditis and, 252.e1t, 252f
    profile of, 1593t
Cardiopulmonary failure, fever and, 1439
Cardiorenal syndrome, 253–254.e1, 254.e1f, 254f
Cardiospasm, achalasia and, 12
Cardioversion
  for atrial fibrillation, 152
  for atrial flutter, 153–154
Carnitine, for cyclic vomiting syndrome, 350.e7–350.e8
Carotene, serum, 1784
Carotid angioplasty and stenting, 258
Carotid bruit, 257
Carotid endarterectomy, for carotid stenosis, 258
Carotid sinus hypersensitivity, 255
Carotid sinus massage, 255
Carotid sinus syncope, 255
Carotid sinus syndrome, 255–256.e1, 255f
Carotid stenosis, 257–258.e1, 257t–258t
Carpal tunnel syndrome
  characteristics of, 259–259.e5, 259.e3f–259.e4f
  electrodiagnostic studies, 259
  imaging studies of, 259
  Phalen's sign in, 259, 259f
  Tinel's sign in, 259, 259f
Carvedilol
  for coronary artery disease, 342
  for dilated cardiomyopathy, 245
Cascara, 410.e1t–410.e2t
Caspofungin
  for aspergillosis, 131
  for invasive candidiasis, 237
Cat bites, 192–193.e1, 193b, 193t
Catamenial pneumothorax, 1019
Cataplexy, 883–884
Cataracts, 259.e6–259.e8, 259.e6f–259.e7f
  congenital infections in, 1418
  developmental variants in, 1418
  differential diagnosis of, 1418
  endocrinopathies in, 1418

Cataracts (Continued)
  genetic disorders in, 1418
  ocular anomalies in, 1418
Catastrophic antiphospholipid antibody syndrome, 107,
    108t, 109
Catecholamines
  for complete heart block, 550
  urine, 1837, 1839t
Catheter angiography, for acute ischemic stroke, 1216–1218,
    1216t, 1218f
Catheter-directed thrombolysis, for deep vein thrombosis,
    359
Catheterization. See also Cardiac catheterization
  for aortic stenosis, 118
  for tricuspid stenosis, 1301.e7
  for urinary retention, 51
  for ventricular septal defect, 1359
Cat-scratch disease, 260.e1f, 260–260.e1
Cat-scratch fever, 260
Cauda equina syndrome, 1197–1199.e1, 1198t
Cavernous sinus thrombosis, 261–262.e1, 262f
Cavitary infarction, 1418
Cavitary lesions
  on chest x-ray, 1418
  in human immunodeficiency virus, 1457
Cavotricuspid atrial flutter, 153
CBC. See Complete blood count
CBT. See Cognitive-behavioral therapy
CC. See Chondrocalcinosis
CCA. See Cholangiocarcinoma
CCBs. See Calcium channel blockers
CCK-PZ. See Cholecystokinin-pancreozymin
CCR5 inhibitors, for human immunodeficiency virus, 633
CD4 count, 631
CD40 ligand, 1784
CD4+ T cells, 1784, 1785t
CDT. See Catheter-directed thrombolysis
^{14}C-D-xylose breath test, 1833t
CEA. See Carcinoembryonic antigen
Cefazolin
  for breast abscess, 214
  for cellulitis, 266
  for osteomyelitis, 924t
Cefepime
  for brain abscess, 208
  for diabetic foot, 385
  for septic arthritis, 1161–1162.e3
Cefixime
  for gonococcal urethritis, 1318
  for gonorrhea, 527
  for nongonococcal urethritis, 1319
  for prostatitis, 1077
  for typhoid fever, 1136
Cefotaxime
  for bacterial pneumonia, 1008
  for brain abscess, 208
  for spontaneous bacterial peritonitis, 980
Cefotetan
  for anaerobic infections, 78
  for pelvic abscess, 962
  for perirectal abscess, 978
Cefoxitin
  for anaerobic infections, 78
  for bite wounds, 192
  for pelvic abscess, 962
  for pelvic inflammatory disease, 964
Ceftaroline, 828
Ceftazidime
  for brain abscess, 208
  for epidural abscess, 460
  for pyelonephritis, 1099
Ceftriaxone
  for bite wounds, 192
  for brain abscess, 208
  for cervicitis, 272
  for chancroid, 272.e5
  for diabetic foot, 385
  for epididymitis, 459
  for epidural abscess, 460
  for gonococcal urethritis, 1318
  for gonorrhea, 527
  for leptospirosis, 742.e8
  for lung abscess, 767
  for Lyme disease, 775
  for nongonococcal urethritis, 1319
  for orchitis, 917

Ceftriaxone (Continued)
  for pelvic inflammatory disease, 964
  for prepubescent vaginitis, 1342
  for prostatitis, 1077
  for renal abscess, 1106
  for septic arthritis, 1161–1162.e3
  for shigellosis, 1172
  for spontaneous bacterial peritonitis, 980
  for tracheitis, 1290.e2
  for typhoid fever, 1136, 1312.e4
  for Whipple's disease, 1376.e8
Cefuroxime
  for acute bronchitis, 28
  for bite wounds, 192
  for chronic obstructive pulmonary disease, 301
  for Lyme disease, 775
Celecoxib, for Gardner's syndrome, 483
Celiac disease, 1203.e2
  characteristics of, 263–264.e1, 263f
  clinical spectrum of, 263t
  HLA antigens associated with, 1807t
Celiac sprue, 263
Cellulitis, 265–266.e2, 266.e2f
  anatomic variants of, 266t
  Haemophilus influenzae, 265
  staphylococcal, 265
Central alpha-antagonists, for hypertension, 663
Central cord syndrome, 1197–1199.e1, 1198t
Central nervous system
  angiitis, 266.e5
  bacterial meningitis of, 811–813.e1, 811f–812f,
    812t–813t
  herpes simplex virus infections of, 607t
  histiocytosis X manifestations of, 618.e2
  histoplasmosis of, 620
  infection, in AIDS-infected patients, 24.e5f
  mumps involvement of, 858
  primary angiitis of the, 1061–1062.e1, 1061t–1062t,
    1062.e1f
  tumors, frequency of, 211t
  vasculitis, 1061
Central spinal stenosis, 1202
Cephalexin
  for balanitis, 171
  for breast abscess, 214
  for impetigo, 697
  for urinary tract infection, 1320t
Cephalic tetanus, 1255.e3
Cephalosporins. See also specific drug
  for bacterial meningitis, 813
  for diabetic foot, 385
  for epididymitis, 459
  for liver abscess, 761
  for salmonellosis, 1136t
Cerclage
  abdominal, 271.e3f
  for cervical insufficiency, 271.e2, 271.e2f
  prophylactic, 271.e2
Cerebellar ataxia
  adult onset, 1406–1407
  in children, 1407
Cerebellar hemorrhage, 187t
Cerebellar tremor, 476
Cerebelloretinal hemangioblastomatosis, 1370.e2
Cerebral amyloid angiopathy, 1061
Cerebral angiography
  for cerebral vasculitis, 266.e6
  for primary angiitis of the central nervous system, 1062.e1
Cerebral arteriovenous malformations, 164–165.e1,
    164f–165f, 165.e1t
Cerebral arteritis, 266.e5
Cerebral beriberi, 1376.e3
Cerebral blood flow decrease, mental changes and coma
    with, 1484
Cerebral catheter angiography, for acute ischemic stroke,
    1216–1218, 1216t, 1218f
Cerebral edema
  in diabetic ketoacidosis, 388
  in hepatic encephalopathy, 578
  high-altitude, 613.e1t, 613.e2b, 612–613.e2, 613b
Cerebral hemorrhage, 1221
Cerebral hypoxia, 105
Cerebral infarct/infarction
  secondary to inherited disorders, 1418–1419
  silent, 1181
Cerebral ischemia, 1594f

Cerebral malaria, 789
Cerebral palsy, 266.e3–266.e4, 266.e3f
Cerebral thrombosis, 1221
Cerebral vasculitis, 266.e5–266.e8, 1061t
    causes of, 1419
    classification of, 266.e5, 266.e6f
Cerebritis, 759
Cerebrospinal fluid, 1784, 1786t
    abnormalities of, in normal-pressure hydrocephalus,
        641–642.e1, 641f, 642.e1f
    analysis of, for chronic inflammatory demyelinating
        polyneuropathy, 292
    bacterial meningitis findings, 812, 812f
    lymphocytosis in, 1787b
    myelin basic protein, 1818
    neutrophils in, 1787b
    plasmacytosis, 1787b
    protein concentrations in, 1787t
    shunting of, for idiopathic intracranial hypertension, 690.e5
Cerebrovascular accident, 1215, 1440. See also Stroke
Cerebrovascular disease
    ischemic, 1419
    preoperative considerations for, 1055.e5
Certolizumab, for enteropathic arthritis, 456
Ceruloplasmin, serum, 1785
Cervarix, 325
Cervical cancer
    characteristics of, 267–268.e1, 267f–268f, 268t
    screening guidelines for, 1858t
    staging of, 268t
Cervical disc syndromes, 268.e2–268.e4, 268.e3f
Cervical dysplasia, 269–271.e1
    grading systems for, 269f
    management of, 270
    recommendations for, 269, 271t
    risk factors of, 270
Cervical instability, pediatric
    acquired, 1419
    congenital, 1419
Cervical insufficiency, 271.e2–271.e3, 271.e2f
Cervical intraepithelial neoplasia, 267
Cervical lymphadenopathy
    characteristics of, 1676.e2, 1676.e2b, 1676.e2f
    in Kawasaki disease, 735.e2
Cervical myelopathy, 268.e2
Cervical polyps, 271.e4, 271.e4f
Cervical pregnancy, 430, 430f, 431.e1f
Cervical radiculopathy, 268.e2
Cervical spondylopathy, 268.e2
Cervical spondylosis, 1745.e1f, 1133.e4t
Cervicitis, 272.e1f, 272–272.e1, 281t
Cervix, infertility and, 1470
Cesarean section
    for abruptio placentae, 10
    for breech birth, 218.e8–218.e9
Cestodes, 1249t
Cetirizine
    for mastocytosis, 798
    for urticaria, 1326
Cetuximab, 315
Cevimeline, for Sjögren's syndrome, 1187
CF. See Cystic fibrosis
Chagas' disease, 272.e2–272.e4, 272.e2f–272.e3f
Chancroid, 272.e5–272.e6, 272.e5f
Change of life, 815
Chaparral leaf, 410.e1t–410.e2t
Charcot neuroosteoarthropathy, 273f
Charcot neuropathic osteoarthropathy, 273
Charcot osteoarthropathy, 273, 273f
Charcot-Marie-Tooth disease, 273–274.e1, 275, 275f, 900–901
Charcot's joint
    characteristics of, 273f, 275–275.e1
    inflammatory theory for, 273
    neurotraumatic theory for, 273
    neurovascular theory for, 273
Chaso/onshido, 410.e1t–410.e2t
CHB. See Complete heart block
Cheilitis, actinic, 25, 99–99.e1, 99f
ChEIs. See Cholinesterase inhibitors
Chelation therapy
    for lead poisoning, 740, 741t
    for thalassemia, 1257
    for Wilson's disease, 1376.e9
Chemical injury, 227, 228t, 229.e4f
    care phases for, 229.e2
    categorization of, by depth, 227t

Chemical injury (Continued)
    classification of, 227
    complications in, 229.e3b
    follow-up care for, 229
    Mayes equations for, 229b
    resuscitation for, 228
        formula for, 229b
    "6 Cs" of, 228
    treatment for, 228–229, 229.e4f
    wound care for, 228–229
Chemicals, granulomatous disorders from, 1447
Chemoprophylaxis
    from age 11 to 24 years, 1851t
    from age 25 to 64 years, 1865t
    birth to 10 years, 1849t
    for influenza, 709
    pregnant women, 1857t
Chemotherapy
    for benign brain neoplasms, 212
    for brain metastases, 210
    for cervical cancer, 267
    for chronic lymphocytic leukemia, 752
    for coccidioidomycosis, 313.e3
    for colorectal cancer, 315
    for glioblastoma, 213
    for hairy cell leukemia, 754.e2
    for head and neck squamous cell carcinoma, 542
    for herpes simplex virus, 607t
    for Hodgkin lymphoma, 624–626
    for invasive breast cancer, 216
    for Langerhans cell histiocytosis, 618.e3–618.e4
    for meningioma, 810
    mucositis caused by, 1214.e2f
    for multiple myeloma, 852
    for mycosis fungoides, 863.e4–863.e5
    for myelodysplastic syndromes, 865
    for nephroblastoma, 888.e2
    for neuroblastoma, 891.e3
    for non-Hodgkin lymphomas, 779–781, 781t
    for non-small cell lung cancer, 771–772
    for oral cancer, 916
    for ovarian cancer, 933, 933.e1f
    for pancreatic cancer, 942
    for prostate cancer, 1073
    pulmonary toxicities caused by, 412t
    for renal cell carcinoma, 1112
    for retinoblastoma, 1116.e8
    for sarcoma, 1140
    toxicities caused by, 412t
Chemotherapy-induced emesis, 276
Chemotherapy-induced nausea and vomiting, 276–276.e1
Cherry-red epiglottitis, 463
Chest cold, 27
Chest pain
    in children, 1419
    diagnostic approach to, 1595, 1595f
    musculoskeletal, 343t
    nonpleuritic, 1419–1420
    pleuritic, 1420
Chest wall pain syndrome, 343, 343t
Chest wall tumors, 1420
Chest x-rays
    abnormality on, 1596, 1596f
    for acute primary pulmonary histoplasmosis, 620
    for acute respiratory distress syndrome, 45, 46f
    for aortic coarctation, 111, 112.e1f
    for aortic stenosis, 118
    for asbestosis, 125, 125.e2f
    for bacterial pneumonia, 1007, 1009f
    calcification on, 1579.e1–1579.e2
    for cardiomegaly, 1590–1603.e1, 1591f
    for cavitary lesion, 1418
    for chronic pulmonary histoplasmosis, 620.e1f, 620
    for dilated cardiomyopathy, 244
    for drug-induced parenchymal lung disease, 411, 412.e2f
    for eosinophilic granulomatosis with polyangiitis, 458.
        e4, 458.e5f
    for heart failure, 556, 557f
    for high-altitude pulmonary edema, 613.e1f
    for histoplasmosis, 620.e1f, 620
    for hypersensitivity pneumonitis, 657
    for hypertrophic osteoarthropathy, 669f
    for idiopathic pulmonary fibrosis, 691, 691f
    for interstitial lung disease, 716, 717t
    for interstitial pneumonia, 1016.e1f
    for liver abscess, 760

Chest x-rays (Continued)
    for lung abscess, 768f
    for lung neoplasms, 773.e6f, 770
    for malignant mesothelioma, 822, 823.e1f, 823f
    for mitral regurgitation, 834
    for mitral stenosis, 837
    for mycoplasma pneumonia, 1011, 1012f
    for patent ductus arteriosus, 959
    for pericarditis, 973f
    for Pneumocystis jiroveci pneumonia, 24.e4f, 1013, 1013f
    for primary lung neoplasms, 770, 773.e6f
    for pulmonary arterial hypertension, 1093, 1093f
    for pulmonary edema, 1086, 1087f
    for pulmonary embolism, 1089
    for restrictive cardiomyopathy, 251
    for sarcoidosis, 1137–1138, 1138.e2f
    for spontaneous pneumothorax, 1017, 1018f, 1019.e2f
    for tension pneumothorax, 1018f
    for tetralogy of Fallot, 1255.e6
    for ventricular septal defect, 1359
Cheyne-Stokes respiration, 554
CHF. See Congestive heart failure
Chiasmal disease, 1420
Chickenpox
    description of, 1347, 1347f
    herpes zoster caused by, 608–609.e1, 608f
Child abuse, 277–279.e2, 278t, 279b, 279.e1f,
        1171–1171.e1, 1171.e1f–1171.e2f
Child maltreatment syndrome, 277
Childhood absence epilepsy, 1153
Childhood autism, 162
Childhood-onset fluency disorder, 1222.e4
Childhood-onset schizophrenia, 162
Child-Pugh staging criteria, for cirrhosis, 306t
Children. See also Adolescents; Infant(s); Neonates; Pediatric
        patients
    abdominal pain in, 1387
    absence seizures in, 1153–1153.e1
    acute lymphoblastic leukemia in, 743
    acute pancreatitis in, 1711–1712
    alopecia in, 1396
    altered mental status and coma, 1484
    anaphylaxis in, 1872t
    ankle pain in, 1443
    appetite loss in, 1402
    arthritis in, extremity pain and, 1403–1404
    aspiration lung injury in, 1405
    asthma in, 132, 135t–139t, 1406
    ataxia telangiectasia in, 145.e5
    back pain in, 1408
    cerebellar ataxia in, 1407
    chest pain in, 1419
    convulsive disorder in, 1599.e1, 1599.e1f
    edema in, 1617–1618
    emesis in, 1433
    eosinophilia, 1420
    febrile seizures in, 1154–1155.e1, 1155f
    fever in, 1441–1442
    foot pain in, 1443–1444
    gender dysphoria in, 512.e4
    hand pain in, 1771
    hematuria in, 1453
    hepatitis in, 1449
    hip pain in, 1456
    hydronephrosis in, 643–644
    hyperkalemia in, 1461
    hyperphosphatemia in, 1462
    hypertension in, 1463
    hypocalcemia in, 1465
    hypoglycemia in, 1465–1466
    hypokalemia in, 1466
    hypomagnesemia in, 1467
    hypophosphatemia in, 1467
    hypotrichosis in, 1396
    hypovolemic shock in, 1469
    immunizations in, 1859
        infection control and, 1872, 1872.e1f
        recommended schedule for, 1860t–1864t
    impetigo in, 697–697.e1, 697f
    influenza vaccine in, 1860t–1864t
    juvenile idiopathic arthritis in, 732–734.e2, 732t,
        733f–734f, 734.e2f
    Kawasaki disease in, 735.e2–735.e4, 735.e2f–735.e3f
    knee pain in, 1473
    lead poisoning in, 740–741, 741t
    limp in, 1475

Children *(Continued)*
long QT syndrome in, 764
medication errors in, 960.e5–960.e6
neuroblastoma in, 891.e3
neutropenia in, 1494
Osgood-Schlatter disease in, 920–920.e1, 920f
osteoporosis in, 1497
pneumatosis intestinalis in, 1505
pneumothorax in, 1507
presacral masses in, 1510
pruritus vulvae in, 1077.e4–1077.e6, 1077.e4f
recurrent or periodic fever in, 1441–1442
retinal hemorrhage in, 1116.e4–1116.e5
retinoblastoma in, 1116.e8–1116.e10, 1116.e8f
rheumatic diseases of, 1405
rickets in, 1128.e4–1128.e5, 1128.e4f
shoulder pain in, 1524
slipped capital femoral epiphysis in, 1191.e2–1191.e3
soft tissue tumors in, 1525–1526
splenomegaly in, 1527–1528
tremor in, 1534
urethral obstruction in, 1536
urinary incontinence in, 1536
ventricular septal defect in, 1358–1359
vision loss in, 1541–1542
wrist pain in, 1771
Zika virus in, 1379–1384.e1, 1380f–1382f, 1383b–1384b
Chimeric antigen receptor T-cell therapy, for acute
lymphoblastic leukemia, 745
Chinese herbal medicines, 410.e1t–410.e2t
Chlamydia genital infections, 280–282.e1
Chlamydia group antibody serologic test, 1785
Chlamydia pneumoniae, 27t
Chlamydia trachomatis, 280
cervical cancer and, 267
lymphogranuloma venereum caused by, 778.e2–778.e3
PCR, 1785
pelvic inflammatory disease and, 963–964.e1
specimens for diagnosing, 1788t
Chlamydophila psittaci, 1079.e4–1079.e5
Chlorambucil, for Behçet's disease, 182.e3
Chloramphenicol
for anaerobic infections, 78
for Rocky Mountain spotted fever, 1130
Chlordiazepoxide
for alcohol abuse, 56t, 58
for alcohol withdrawal, 58
Chlorfenapyr, 182
Chlorhexidine
for bisphosphonate-related osteonecrosis of the jaw, 191.e3
for linear gingival erythema, 518.e1
Chloride
serum, 1785
sweat, 1785
urine, 1785, 1837
Chloroquine
for discoid lupus erythematosus, 396
for malaria, 789–790
Chlorpheniramine, for bedbug bite, 182
Chlorpromazine, for migraine headache, 546t
Cholangiocarcinoma, 1068
algorithm for, 284f
clinical presentation of, 283
definition of, 283
diagnosis of, 283–284
endoscopic retrograde cholangiopancreatography for,
284, 285.e2f
epidemiology of, 283
extrahepatic, 285.e2f
imaging of, 284, 285.e1f
intraductal intrahepatic, 283, 285.e1f
laboratory testing for, 284
perihilar, 284f, 285b
physical findings of, 283
referral for, 285
risk factors for, 283
staging of, 285.e3t–285.e4t
TNM staging of, 285.e3t–285.e4t
treatment of, 284–285
unresectable, 285b
Cholangiography, for primary sclerosing cholangitis,
1067–1068, 1067f
Cholangitis, 286–286.e1
acute, 1420
primary sclerosing, 1067–1068.e1, 1067f, 1067t
Cholecalciferol deficiency, 1366

Cholecystectomy
for cholecystitis, 287
for cholelithiasis, 290, 290t
for salmonellosis, 1136
Cholecystitis, 287–287.e1, 287.e1f
Cholecystokinin-pancreozymin, 1785
Cholecystokinin-stimulated cholescintigraphy, for functional
gallbladder disorder, 504
Choledocholithiasis, 288–289.e1, 288f–289f
Cholelithiasis, 290–290.e1, 290.e1f, 290.e1t
Cholera, 290.e2–290.e4, 290.e3f
outbreaks of, 290.e2
stools of, electrolyte concentration of, 290.e4t
vaccine for, 1888
Cholestasis
differential diagnosis of, 1421
neonatal and infantile, 1421
Cholestatic liver disease, 1780t
Cholestatic liver enzymes, 1421
Cholesterol
in gallstones, 290
hypercholesterolemia, 645–647.e3, 645t, 647.e1t, 647b,
647t
total, 1785
Cholestyramine
for hyperlipidemia, 654.e4t
for primary biliary cirrhosis, 1064–1065
Cholinesterase inhibitors, for Alzheimer's disease, 69
Chondrocalcinosis, 1078, 1079.e2f
Chondroitin, for osteoarthritis, 921
Chondrosarcoma, 204
Chordee, 687.e1
Chorea, 290.e5–290.e6
benign hereditary, 639
complementary medicine for, 290.e5
differential diagnosis of, 1422
in Huntington's disease, 639
in rheumatic fever, 1124.e2
Sydenham's, 639
Chorea gravidarum, 639
Choreoathetosis
differential diagnosis of, 1422
drug-induced, 1422
Chorioamnionitis, 1053
Chorionic gonadotropin, human, 1785–1788, 1807
Chorionic villus sampling, for congenital adrenal hyperplasia,
325.e2
Choroid, HIV infection manifestations in, 1459
Choroid plexus papilloma, 212.e2f
Choroiditis, 1334
Christmas disease, 569
Chromosomal disorders
Down syndrome, 403.e2–403.e3, 403.e2f
Klinefelter's syndrome, 735.e7, 735.e7t
Chromosome constitution disorders, 1312.e2
Chronic acalculous, 504
Chronic acalculous cholecystitis, 504
Chronic active hepatitis, 595
Chronic anxiety, 110
Chronic arthropathy, 1079.e1f
Chronic atrial rhythm, 850
Chronic atrial tachycardia, 850
Chronic bacterial prostatitis, 1077–1077.e1
Chronic bronchitis, 299, 299t–300t, 300f, 302t, 303b
Chronic cholecystitis, 290.e1t
Chronic conjunctivitis, 326
Chronic constrictive pericarditis, 973
Chronic cor pulmonale, 335, 335f–336f, 337t
Chronic cough
diagnostic protocol for, 1600
management algorithm for, 1426–1427, 1600–1601,
734.e2f
Chronic critical limb ischemia, 975
Chronic cutaneous lupus erythematosus, 65, 396, 396f
Chronic cystic mastitis, 490
Chronic diarrhea
diagnostic approach to, 1606, 1606f
with HIV infection, 1606.e1, 1606.e1f
Chronic eosinophilic pneumonia, 458.e7
Chronic Epstein-Barr syndrome, 291
Chronic fatigue, 1438–1439
Chronic fatigue syndrome, 291–291.e1
Chronic fibrosing mediastinitis, 803
Chronic granulocytic leukemia, 753
Chronic headache, 1658
Chronic heart failure, 88, 253

Chronic hepatitis
differential diagnosis of, 1454
drug-induced, 410.e2t
Chronic hepatosplenic suppurative brucellosis, 220.e2
Chronic hiccups, 1456
Chronic hives, 1328
Chronic hydrocephalus, 641
Chronic idiopathic urticaria, 1328
Chronic infectious epididymitis, 459
Chronic inflammatory demyelinating polyneuropathy,
292–293.e1, 292t, 293f
Chronic inflammatory demyelinating polyradiculoneuropathy,
1493
Chronic interstitial nephritis, 718–719.e1
Chronic kidney disease, 298.e6f–298.e7f, 294–298.e7
classification of, 295t
continuing assessment in, 298t
criteria for referral in, 297t
definition of, criteria for, 294t
extraskeletal calcification in, 298.e6f
hypertension caused by, 660t
management plans for, 296t
nutritional recommendations in, 296t
pathophysiology of, 294t
stages of, 1801t
Chronic laryngitis, 739–739.e1
Chronic liver disease, 1887t
Chronic low-dose exposure produces stochastic effects,
1100.e12
Chronic lymphocytic leukemia
abnormal lymphocytes with, 1816t
characteristics of, 750–752.e1, 750–751t, 751f
Chronic meningitis, 1417
Chronic mucocutaneous candidiasis, 234
Chronic myelogenous leukemia, 753–754.e1, 753t, 754f
Chronic myeloid leukemia, 753
Chronic myofascial pain, 879
Chronic nonallergic rhinitis, 904
Chronic obliterative cholangitis, 1067
Chronic obstructive pulmonary disease, 299–303.e4,
299t–300t, 300f, 302t, 303.e4f
abdominal aortic aneurysm and, 6
acute exacerbation of, 299
asthma versus, 140
asthma-COPD overlap syndrome, 142–143.e1
blue bloaters, 299
decompensation for, 1461
pink puffers, 299
Chronic open-angle glaucoma, 519, 520.e2f–520.e3f
Chronic osteomyelitis, 923–924.e1
Chronic otitis externa, 928–929.e1
Chronic pain, 937–940.e4, 938f, 939t–940t, 940.e2f,
940.e3b–940.e4b, 940.e3t
Chronic pancreatitis, 947–948.e2, 948.e1f–948.e2f
Chronic paronychia, 958–958.e1
Chronic periaortitis, 1116.e11
Chronic plaque psoriasis, 1081, 1081f
Chronic pneumonia, 1505–1506
Chronic productive nephritis without exudation, 718
Chronic progressive vision loss, 1542
Chronic prostatitis/chronic pelvic pain syndrome,
1077–1077.e1
Chronic pulmonary histoplasmosis, 619, 620.e1f
Chronic renal failure, 294, 1518
Chronic renal insufficiency, 294
Chronic renal parenchymal disease, 1519
Chronic rhinitis, 1520
Chronic rhinosinusitis with nasal polyps, 885
Chronic silicosis, 1183
Chronic sinusitis, 1184–1185.e1
Chronic skin induration, 1524–1525
Chronic stable angina, 339, 340f, 341b, 342.e4f
Chronic stable ischemic heart disease, 91
Chronic subdural hematoma, 1227
Chronic tophaceous gout, 529, 530.e3f
Chronic urticaria, 98.e2f, 1328–1330.e1, 1329f, 1330t
Chronic uveitis, 1334
Chronic venous disorder, 1348, 1348f, 1348t
Chronic venous insufficiency, 1042, 1352–1353.e1,
1352f–1353f
CHRPE. *See* Congenital hypertrophy of the retinal pigment
epithelium
Churg-Strauss syndrome. *See* Eosinophilic granulomatosis
with polyangiitis
Chylothorax, 1422
Chylous effusion, peritoneal, 1504

Chyluria, 494.e2
Chymotrypsin, 1788
CI-AKI. *See* Contrast-induced acute kidney injury
Cicatricial pemphigoid, 518.e1f
Ciclopirox
    for cutaneous candidiasis, 235
    for tinea pedis, 1273
Cidofovir, for cytomegalovirus infection, 355
Cigarette smoking. *See* Smoking
Ciliary neuralgia, 543
Ciliary neurotrophic factor, 1116.e6
Cilostazol, for claudication, 309, 977
Cimetidine
    for alopecia, 65
    for anaphylaxis, 79.e2t
Cimex lectularius, 181, 181f–182f
Cinacalcet, for hyperparathyroidism, 656
CINV. *See* Chemotherapy-induced nausea and vomiting
Ciprofloxacin
    for anthrax, 106.e3
    for bacterial meningitis, 813
    for balanitis, 171
    for blepharitis, 202.e5
    for brucellosis, 220.e3
    for chancroid, 272.e5
    for diverticular disease, 403
    for epididymitis, 459
    for granuloma inguinale, 531.e1
    for perirectal abscess, 978
    for prostatitis, 1077
    for pyelonephritis, 1099
    for shigellosis, 1172
    for spontaneous bacterial peritonitis, 980
    for tularemia, 1309.e2
    for typhoid fever, 1136, 1312.e4
Circadian rhythm disturbances, 711
Circulating anticoagulant (lupus anticoagulant), 1788
Circulatory disorders, blindness caused by, 1411
Circumscribe neurodermatitis, 758
Cirrhosis
    characteristics of, 304–306.e1, 305f, 306t
    in esophageal varices, 475
    hepatitis B as cause of, 597
    hepatitis C as cause of, 586, 586t
    of kidney, 718
    liver transplantation for, 762–763.e1
    portal hypertension caused by, 305f, 1032, 1033t
    primary biliary, 595–596, 1063–1065.e1, 1064f
    renin-aldosterone pattern in, 1829t
Cisatracurium, 46–48
Cisplatin
    for bladder cancer, 201
    for cervical cancer, 267
    for esophageal tumors, 474
Citalopram, for Alzheimer's disease, 69t
CIU. *See* Chronic idiopathic urticaria
Cladribine
    for hairy cell leukemia, 754.e2
    for mastocytosis, 798
Clap. *See* Gonorrhea
Clarithromycin
    for bacterial pneumonia, 1008
    for gastritis, 508
    for laryngitis, 739
    for mycoplasma pneumonia, 1012
    for pertussis, 984, 984t
    for Q fever, 1100.e7
Classic dengue fever
    characteristics of, 369.e2, 369.e2f, 369.e4f
    classification of, 369.e3b
    distribution of, 369.e2f
    skin manifestations of, 369.e4f
Classic hemophilia, 569
Claudication, 307–309.e1, 307t–308t, 309.e1f–309.e2f, 977
Clavicle, bone resorption in, 1413
Clenbuterol, cocaine overdose and, 312–313
CLI. *See* Critical limb ischemia
Click, ejection, 1433
Climacteric ovarian failure, 815
Clindamycin
    for acne vulgaris, 15
    for actinomycosis, 26.e3
    for anaerobic infections, 78
    for aspiration pneumonia, 1006
    for babesiosis, 170
    for bacterial vaginosis, 1345

Clindamycin *(Continued)*
    for bite wounds, 192
    for gingivitis, 518.e1–518.e2
    for hidradenitis suppurativa, 611
    for lung abscess, 767
    for lymphangitis, 776
    for methicillin-resistant *Staphylococcus aureus*, 828
    for necrotizing fasciitis, 887
    for pelvic abscess, 962
    for pelvic inflammatory disease, 964
    for perirectal abscess, 978
    for peritonsillar abscess, 982
    for retropharyngeal abscess, 1118
    for rosacea, 1131
Clindamycin phosphate/tretinoin, for acne vulgaris, 15
Clinical depression, 371, 372t
Clinical Institute Withdrawal Assessment-Alcohol, 367
Clinical tumor lysis syndrome, 1310
Clinically isolated syndrome, in multiple sclerosis, 857
CLL. *See* Chronic lymphocytic leukemia
CLM. *See* Cutaneous larva migrans
Clobetasol propionate
    for contact dermatitis, 329
    for lichen sclerosus, 757
Clofazimine, hyperpigmentation with, 1651t
Clomiphene citrate
    for dysfunctional uterine bleeding, 414
    for infertility, 703
Clomipramine, for cataplexy, 884
Clonal thrombocytosis, 1260
Clonazepam
    for bipolar disorder, 191
    for burning mouth syndrome, 226.e4
    for myoclonus, 878
Clonidine
    for alcohol abuse, 56t
    for alcohol withdrawal, 56t
    for ascites, 129t
    for attention deficit hyperactivity disorder, 161
    for hot flashes, 629
    for hypertension, 663
    for opioid withdrawal, 407
    for Tourette's syndrome, 1282
Clonidine suppression test, 1789
Clopidogrel
    for acute coronary syndrome, 34
    for angina pectoris, 94
    for antiphospholipid antibody syndrome, 109
    for carotid stenosis, 257
    for claudication, 308
    for coronary artery disease, 342
    for peripheral arterial disease, 976
    for transient ischemic attack, 1294
Clostridial cellulitis, 887, 888t
Clostridial myonecrosis, 888t
Clostridium botulinum food poisoning, 206, 500
Clostridium difficile infection, 310–311.e2, 310f–311f, 548.e3
Clostridium difficile toxin
    assay for, 1789
    description of, 310
Clostridium perfringens, 500
Clostridium tetani, 1255.e3–1255.e4, 1255.e3f
Clotrimazole
    for balanitis, 171
    for fungal vaginitis, 1341
Clotting factor disorders, 1502t
Cloudy urine, 1458
Clozapine, for schizophrenia, 1144–1145
Clubbing
    differential diagnosis of, 1422
    nails, 1489–1495
Clue cells, 1345f
Cluster headache, 543–544.e1, 1644–1645
Clutter, 622.e2
CML. *See* Chronic myelogenous leukemia
CMP. *See* Chronic myofascial pain
CMRI. *See* Cardiac magnetic resonance imaging
CMT. *See* Charcot-Marie-Tooth disease
CMV. *See* Cytomegalovirus
CNS vasculitis, 1061
CNTF. *See* Ciliary neurotrophic factor
Coagulation factors, 1789, 1789t, 1790t
Coagulation profile, in abruptio placentae, 9
Coagulopathy, in hemorrhagic stroke, 1220
Coarctation of the aorta. *See* Aortic coarctation

Coat's syndrome, 1116.e4
Cobalamin
    absorption mechanisms for, 90.e1f
    deficiency of
        diagnosis of, 89t
        differential diagnosis of, 1422–1423
        etiopathophysiologic classification of, 1423, 1842b
        laboratory testing for, 89
        megaloblastic anemia with, 1400
        metabolic disorders and, 1400
        plasma transport disorders and, 1400
        treatment of, 90
Cobb angle, 1150, 1151f
Cobicistat, 18
Cocaine overdose, 312–313.e1, 312t, 313.e1f
Cocaine-induced cardiomyopathy, 242
Coccidioides immitis, 813.e2
Coccidioidomycosis, 313.e2–313.e4, 636t–638t
    in acquired immunodeficiency syndrome, 18t–24t
    risk factors for, 313.e4t
Codeine
    for acute bronchitis, 28
    for chronic pain, 940.e3t, 940t
Coelomic metaplasia theory, 452
Coenzyme Q10, for cyclic vomiting syndrome, 350.e7–350.e8
Cogan's syndrome, 313.e5–313.e6, 313.e5t
Cognitive dysfunction, HIV-related, 621–622.e1, 621f, 621t
Cognitive impairment, 1457
Cognitive-behavioral therapy
    for binge eating disorder, 188
    for body dysmorphic disorder, 203
    for chronic fatigue syndrome, 291
    for compulsive hoarding, 622.e2–622.e3
    for conversion disorder, 334.e2
    for hypochondriasis, 674.e1
    for insomnia, 711
    for intermittent explosive disorder, 712.e4
    for irritable bowel syndrome, 724
    for major depression, 371–372
    for narcissistic personality disorder, 882
    for obsessive-compulsive disorder, 910
    for panic disorder, 950
    for paranoid personality disorder, 955.e2
    for seasonal affective disorder, 1151.e2
    for sexual dysfunction in women, 1169
    for social anxiety disorder, 1194.e4
Colchicine
    for Behçet's disease, 182.e3
    for familial Mediterranean fever, 484
    for gout, 529, 530t
    for hypertrophic osteoarthropathy, 669
    for pericarditis, 973
    for pseudogout, 1079
Cold agglutinin disease, 82
Cold agglutinins titer, 1789
Cold-induced tissue injury, 502–503.e1, 502f, 503b
Colectomy, short bowel resection with, 1173
Colesevelam, for hyperlipidemia, 654.e4t
Colestipol, for hyperlipidemia, 654.e4t
Colic
    acute abdominal, 1423
    renal, 1872.e1f
Colitis
    ischemic, 1472
    ulcerative, 1313–1315.e1, 1315f
        Crohn's disease compared with, 344t, 1313t
        enteropathic arthritis associated with, 455–456.e1, 455t
        infectious agents mimicking, 1314t
        toxic megacolon caused by, 1283, 1284f
Collapse, in elderly, 480, 480t, 481.e1f
Collecting, 622.e2
Colloids
    for abdominal compartment syndrome, 8
    for anaphylaxis, 79.e2t
    for ascites, 129t
    for burns, 229b
Colon
    bleeding in, 1409
    ischemia of, 1423, 1668.e1b, 1668.e3f
Colon cancer, hereditary nonpolyposis, 314
Colonic pseudo-obstruction, acute, 29–30.e1, 29b–30b, 29f
Colonoscopic decompression, for acute colonic pseudo-obstruction, 30

Colonoscopy with biopsy, for colorectal cancer, 315
Colony-stimulating factors, for radiation exposure, 1100.e14
Color changes, cutaneous, 1423–1424
Color Doppler, for Budd-Chiari syndrome, 223–224
Colorado tick fever, 313.e7, 313.e7f
  in children, 313.e7
  pathogenesis of, 313.e7
Colorectal cancer, 314–316.e1, 316f, 985–986, 985t
  classification and staging of, 314, 314t
  screening and surveillance recommendations, 315t
  survival rates for, 316t
  wall thickening associated with, 316f
Coma
  altered mental status, 1564, 1564f
  computed tomography scan and, 1424
  differential diagnosis of, 1424
  mental status changes and, 1483
  in pediatric patients, 1424
Combined hyperlipidemia, 654
Combivir, 634
Comfrey, 410.e1t–410.e2t
Commissural cheilitis, 99
Common bile duct stone(s), 288
Common warts, 1376.e1f, 1375
Commotio cordis, 1356
Communicating hydrocele, 640
Community-acquired aspiration pneumonia, 1006–1006.e1
Community-acquired methicillin-resistant *Staphylococcus aureus*, 548.e3, 828
Community-acquired pneumonia, 1008b–1010b, 1008t
Compartment syndrome
  abdominal, 7–8.e1
    causes of, 7t
    classification of, 8t
    postinjury primary and secondary, independent predictors of, 8t
  causes of, 317
  characteristics of, 317–319.e1, 317f–319f
Complement, 1790
Complement deficiencies, 1790, 1792t, 1065.e5t
Complement disorders, 1470
Complementary and alternative medicine
  for chronic fatigue syndrome, 291
  for chronic pain, 938
  hepatotoxic, 410.e1t–410.e2t
  for hot flashes, 629
  for IgA nephropathy, 694
  for infertility, 703
  for insomnia, 712
  for interstitial cystitis, 714
  for mastitis, 797
  for pain, 938
  for postherpetic neuralgia, 1037
  for pressure injury, 1058
  for statin-induced muscle syndromes, 1209
Complete AV block, 159, 549
Complete blood count, 1790
  for chronic obstructive pulmonary disease, 299
  for *Clostridium difficile* infection, 310
  for Colorado tick fever, 313.e7
Complete decongestive therapy, for lymphedema, 777–778
Complete heart block, 550.e1t, 159, 549–550.e1, 549f, 550t
Complete molar pregnancy, 841–842, 842f
Complex regional pain syndrome, 320.e1f–320.e2f, 320–320.e2, 423t
Complicated grief, 536.e2
Comprehensive ultrasonography, for deep vein thrombosis, 357
Compression, spinal cord, 1526
Compression fractures, vertebral, 1363–1364.e1, 1363f, 1364b
Compression stockings
  for chronic venous insufficiency, 1042, 1353
  for deep vein thrombosis, 359
  for postthrombotic syndrome, 1042
Compression ultrasonography
  for deep vein thrombosis, 357–359
  for upper extremity deep vein thrombosis, 1316, 1317f
Compulsive hoarding, 622.e2
Compulsive overeating, 188
Computed tomography
  for abdominal aortic aneurysm, 3, 4, 4f
  for acute ischemic stroke, 1216, 1216f, 1216t
  for acute mesenteric ischemia, 820.e1f, 820
  for acute pancreatitis, 944–945, 944f, 945t
  for adrenal neuroblastoma, 891.e2f

Computed tomography (Continued)
  for bronchiectasis, 219, 219f
  for cavernous sinus thrombosis, 261
  for cholangiocarcinoma, 285.e1f, 284
  for cholangitis, 286
  for choledocholithiasis, 289, 289f
  for cirrhosis, 305
  contrast-enhanced, for Budd-Chiari syndrome, 224
  for cysticercosis, 353
  for diverticular disease, 403
  for drug-induced parenchymal lung disease, 411, 412.e1f–412.e2f
  for endometriosis, 453f
  for epiploic appendagitis, 463.e3, 463.e3f
  for head and neck squamous cell carcinoma, 541, 542.e1f
  for hepatocellular carcinoma, 597, 597f
  for hiatal hernia, 609.e3f
  for Hodgkin lymphoma, 625f
  for hydrocephalus, 641, 642.e1f
  for hydronephrosis, 644, 644.e1f
  for hypersensitivity pneumonitis, 658, 658f
  for hypertrophic cardiomyopathy, 247
  for idiopathic pulmonary fibrosis, 691, 691f
  for interstitial lung disease, 716, 716f
  for invasive candidiasis, 236
  for jaundice, 730
  for labyrinthitis, 736
  for liver abscess, 760, 761f
  for lumbar spinal stenosis, 1202
  for lung abscess, 768f
  for lung cancer, 772
  for lung neoplasms, 770, 770f
  for meningioma, 809f, 810
  for mesenteric adenitis, 818, 818f
  for nasal polyps, 885, 885.e1f
  for otosclerosis, 931.e2, 931.e2f
  for ovarian cancer, 932, 933.e1f
  for pancreatic cancer, 941f
  for parapharyngeal abscess, 981f
  for patent ductus arteriosus, 959
  for pelvic abscess, 962.e1f
  for pericarditis, 972
  for pheochromocytoma, 992, 992.e1f
  for *Pneumocystis jiroveci* pneumonia, 1014.e1f
  for portal hypertension, 1033.e1f
  for pulmonary embolism, 1088, 1090f
  for renal cell carcinoma, 1112f
  for renal vein thrombosis, 1115f
  for retroperitoneal fibrosis, 1116.e12f
  for retropharyngeal abscess, 1118, 1118f
  for sinusitis, 1185
  for small bowel obstruction, 1192–1193, 1193f
  for subarachnoid hemorrhage, 1224, 1225f
  for subdural hematoma, 1227, 1227f
  for superior vena cava syndrome, 1228–1229, 1229f
  for thromboembolic pulmonary hypertension, 1093f
  for toxic megacolon, 1283, 1284f
Computed tomography angiography
  for acute ischemic stroke, 1216t
  for claudication, 308
  for coronary artery calcification, 342.e4f
  for mesenteric venous thrombosis, 821
  for pulmonary embolism, 1089
  for renal artery stenosis, 1109
Computed tomography colonoscopy, with biopsy, and colorectal cancer, 315
Computed tomography enterography, for small bowel obstruction, 1193
Concentration camp syndrome, 1043
Concussion
  characteristics of, 321–322.e1, 321t–322t, 322f, 1297, 1297b, 1298t, 1299f
  postconcussive syndrome, 1035–1036.e1
Condom
  female, 330
  male, 330
Conduct disorder, 323–323.e1
Conduction system abnormality, sudden death with, 1530
Conductive hearing loss, 931.e2–931.e3, 931.e2f, 931.e2t
Condyloma acuminatum, 324–325.e1, 324f, 1375, 1375f
Condylomata lata, 1238f
"Confetti-like" macules, 1308.e4t
Congenital adrenal hyperplasia, 325.e2–325.e4, 325.e2f
  diagnosis and treatment of, 325.e4t
  non-salt-wasting form of, 325.e2

Congenital adrenal hyperplasia (Continued)
  prevention of, 325.e3
  salt-wasting form of, 325.e2
Congenital cataracts, 259.e6
Congenital erythropoietic porphyria, 1736.e1t
Congenital heart disease
  preoperative considerations for, 1055.e5
  sudden death with, 1530
Congenital hypertrophy of the retinal pigment epithelium, 482
Congenital hypoplasia of aortic arch, 111
Congenital hypoplastic anemia, 1096.e2
Congenital immunodeficiency, 1470
Congenital nasal masses, 1490
Congenital rubella syndrome, 1133.e7–1133.e8, 1133.e8t
Congenital sideroblastic anemia, 90.e3
Congenital spastic paralysis, 266.e3
Congenital static encephalopathy, 266.e3
Congenital syphilis, 1239
Congenital toxoplasmosis, 1287, 1289f
Congenital tricuspid atresia, 1301.e7
Congestive cardiomyopathy, 245
Congestive heart failure, 553, 876. *See also* Heart failure
  cardiorenal syndrome with, 253
  causes of, 1425
  with Chagas' disease, 272.e4
Conivaptan, for syndrome of inappropriate antidiuresis, 1237
Conjugated bilirubin, 1670–1671, 1793
Conjugated estrogen vaginal cream, for estrogen-deficient vaginitis, 1340
Conjugated hyperbilirubinemia, 1473
Conjunctiva
  with fever of undetermined origin, 489t
  human immunodeficiency virus infection manifestations in, 1459
Conjunctival neoplasm, 1425
Conjunctival suffusion, fever and rash with, 1440
Conjunctivitis, 326–328
  allergic, 326f, 327t
  bacterial, 326f, 328
  characteristics of, 281t
  definition of, 326
  demographics of, 326
  diagnosis of, 326
  epidemiology of, 326
  etiology of, 326
  laboratory testing for, 327t
  red eye versus, 328
  referral for, 328
  treatment of, 326–328, 328t
  types of, 327t
Connective tissue, heel pain and, 1452
Connective tissue diseases
  algorithm for evaluating, 1597f
  types of, 397t
Conn's syndrome, 61
Consciousness impairment, acute, in critically ill patient, 1425
Consolidation
  alveolar, 1396
  in human immunodeficiency virus, 1457
Constipation
  in adult patient, 1425–1426
  differential diagnosis of, 1425
  with encopresis, 445.e2
  evaluation of, 1598–1599, 1598f
Constrictive pericarditis
  chronic, 973
  illustration of, 974f
  restrictive cardiomyopathy and, 252.e1t, 252f
Consumptive coagulation, 399.e1f, 399f
  differential diagnostic algorithm for, 399f
  scoring system for, 399.e2b
  testing and diagnosis of, 399f
  underlying conditions with, 399.e1b
Consumptive coagulopathy, 398
Contact dermatitis
  characteristics of, 329–329.e2, 329.e2f
  pruritus ani with, 1511
Continuous murmurs, 1417
Continuous positive airway pressure
  for obstructive sleep apnea, 1190–1191
  for pulmonary edema, 1086
Continuous renal replacement therapy, for acute kidney injury, 41
Continuous subcutaneous insulin infusion, for diabetes mellitus, 381

Contraception
  bleeding irregularities during, 332.e7f
  characteristics of, 330–332.e7, 331t,
    332.e2t–332.e5t, 332.e4f–332.e7f
  emergency, 440.e2–440.e3, 440.e2t, 1166
Contraceptive patch, 330, 332
Contracted kidney, 718
Contrast nephropathy, 333
Contrast venography, for deep vein thrombosis, 359
Contrast-induced acute kidney injury, 333–334.e1, 333t,
  334b
Contrast-induced nephropathy, 333
Contrave, for obesity, 908
Conus medullaris syndrome, 1197–1199.e1, 1198t
Conversion disorder, 334.e2–334.e4
Convulsive disorder, 1599.e1, 1599.e1f
Convulsive seizures, 1156
Convulsive status epilepticus, 1210
Cooley's anemia, 1256
Cooling methods
  for heat exhaustion, 561, 562.e1t
  for heat stroke, 561, 562.e1t
Coombs test, 82
  direct, 1796, 1291
  indirect, 1802, 1291
COPD. See Chronic obstructive pulmonary disease
Copper
  IUD, 440.e2
  serum, 1792
  urine, 1792, 1837
Copperhead snake bites, 197–199.e1
Cor pulmonale, 335–337.e1, 335f–336f, 337t
Coral snake bites, 197–199.e1
Cord prolapse, in breech birth, 218.e8
Cornea
  abrasion of, 338f
  contusion of, 338, 338f
  disorders involving, 1599.e2, 1599.e2f
  erosion of, 338, 338f
  human immunodeficiency virus manifestations in, 1459
  ulceration of, 338.e2–338.e3, 338.e2f
Corneal epithelial defect, 338
Corneal sensation, decreased, 1426
Coronary aneurysms, 735.e4
Coronary angiography
  for angina pectoris, 94
  for coronary artery disease, 339
  for myocardial infarction, 872
Coronary angioplasty
  for myocardial infarction, 874.e1f
  procedure for, 96.e2f
Coronary artery bypass grafting
  for angina pectoris, 95–96
  for myocardial infarction, 872
Coronary artery calcification, 342.e4f
Coronary artery calcium score, 94, 339
Coronary artery disease, 339–342.e4, 340f, 341b,
  342.e4f
  in acute coronary syndromes, 31
  in angina pectoris, 91
  sudden death with, 1530
Coronary artery revascularization, 342
Coronary occlusion, 867
Coronary sinus septal defect, 156
Coronary stent, 95–96, 96.e3f
Coronary thrombosis, 867
Coronaviruses
  acute bronchitis caused by, 27t
  severe acute respiratory syndrome-associated,
    1164.e2–1164.e3
Corrigan's pulse, 116
Cortical bone hyperostosis, 1461
Cortical hyperhidrosis, 1460
Cortical Lewy body disease, 368, 368b, 368f–369f
Corticobasal degeneration, 956, 1068.e4
Corticobasal ganglionic degeneration, 857.e2
Corticomedullary abscess, 1099
Corticosteroids
  for acute respiratory distress syndrome, 48
  for acute viral encephalitis, 443
  for allergic rhinitis, 63
  for anaphylaxis, 79.e2t
  for angioedema, 98
  for arteritic anterior ischemic optic neuropathy, 728
  for atopic dermatitis, 148
  for autoimmune hemolytic anemia, 83

Corticosteroids (Continued)
  for bacterial meningitis, 813
  for bacterial pneumonia, 1008
  for Behçet's disease, 182.e3
  for biceps tendonitis, 187.e2
  for brain metastases, 210
  for bullous pemphigoid, 226.e2
  for carpal tunnel syndrome, 259, 259.e5f
  cataracts caused by, 259.e6
  for cerebral vasculitis, 266.e6
  for chronic obstructive pulmonary disease, 301
  for chronic pain, 939t
  for chronic venous insufficiency, 1353
  for Cogan's syndrome, 313.e5
  for contact dermatitis, 329
  for Crohn's disease, 345
  for croup, 345.e3
  for cysticercosis, 354
  for De Quervain's tenosynovitis, 356–356.e1
  for discoid lupus erythematosus, 396
  for Dupuytren's contracture, 412.e5
  for eosinophilic granulomatosis with polyangiitis, 458.e5
  for erythema nodosum, 471
  for Felty's syndrome, 485.e2
  for giant cell arteritis, 516
  for glioblastoma, 213
  for gout, 529
  for granuloma annulare, 531
  for HELLP syndrome, 564.e2
  for Henoch-Schönlein purpura, 574
  for herpes zoster, 609
  for hidradenitis suppurativa, 611
  for hypereosinophilic syndrome, 651.e1
  for inflammatory myopathies, 705
  for insect stings, 195
  for interstitial nephritis, 719
  for ischemic optic neuropathy, 728
  for lichen planus, 756
  for microscopic polyangiitis, 830
  for miliary tuberculosis, 1305
  for mononucleosis, 846
  for Morton neuroma, 846.e3–846.e4, 846.e4f
  for mycosis fungoides, 863.e3–863.e4
  for myocarditis, 877
  for nasal polyps, 885
  for pemphigus vulgaris, 969
  for pericarditis, 973
  for plantar fasciitis, 1003–1004, 1003f
  for preterm labor, 1060
  for primary sclerosing cholangitis, 1068
  for psoriasis, 1080
  for retroperitoneal fibrosis, 1116.e12, 1116.e12f
  for rheumatic fever, 1124.e3
  for rheumatoid arthritis, 1127
  for sarcoidosis, 1138, 1138t
  for scabies, 1142
  for seborrheic dermatitis, 1152
  for sepsis, 1159
  for severe acute respiratory syndrome, 1164.e3
  for spinal cord compression, 1199
  for squamous cell hyperplasia, 1077.e4
  for status asthmaticus, 139
  for superior vena cava syndrome, 1229
  for systemic vasculitis, 1351
  for thrombotic thrombocytopenic purpura, 1263
  for thyrotoxic storm, 1268.e2
  for transverse myelitis, 1296
  for trichinosis, 1301.e3
  for ulcerative colitis, 1315
  for urticaria, 1326
  for uveitis, 1334
  for vestibular neuronitis, 1365
Cortico-striatal-thalamo-cortical pathways, 1281f
Corticotropin deficiency, 685
Corticotropin releasing hormone
  for Cushing's disease and syndrome, 349
  stimulation test, 1792
Cortisol
  plasma, 1793
  urine, free, 1837
Costochondritis, 343–343.e1, 343t
Costosternal syndrome, 343, 343t
Cottonmouth snake bites, 197–199.e1
Cough
  in asbestosis, 125
  chronic

Cough (Continued)
  diagnostic protocol for, 1600t
  management algorithm for, 1600f, 1600–1601
  differential diagnosis of, 1426
Counseling
  for ages 65 and older, 1855t
  for ages 11 to 24 years, 1860t–1864t
  for ages 25 to 64 years, 1853t
  from birth to 10 years, 1849t
  pregnant women, 1857t
Courvoisier's sign, 288
Cowden's disease, 985–986
Coxa plana, 742
Coxiella burnetii, 1100.e6–1100.e7
Cox-Maze III surgical procedure, for atrial fibrillation, 151
Coxsackie virus infection, 540
CP. See Cerebral palsy
CPA. See Cyproterone acetate
CPAP. See Continuous positive airway pressure
CP/CPPS. See Chronic prostatitis/chronic pelvic pain
  syndrome
C-peptide, 1793
CPH. See Chronic pulmonary histoplasmosis
CPP crystal deposition disease, 1078
CPPD. See Calcium pyrophosphate dihydrate crystal
  deposition disease
Crack overdose, 312, 312t, 313.e1f
Crackles, 1512–1513
Cradle cap, 1152, 1152.e1f
CRAFFT, 912, 912t
Cramps and aches
  leg, nocturnal, 1676.e1–1676.e2
  muscle, 1685, 1685b, 1685f
Cranial arteritis, 515, 515f, 515t
Cranial nerve palsies, 261
Cranial neuralgias, 1655–1656
Craniopharyngioma, 343.e2, 343.e2f
CRE. See Carbapenem-resistant Enterobacteriaceae
C-reactive protein, 1793, 1793t
  high sensitivity, 1793
Creatine kinase, 704, 1122, 1793, 1793.e1f, 1794f
  isoenzymes, 1780.e1f, 1794
Creatine kinase-MB, 869
Creatinine
  clearance, 1795, 1795b
  in eosinophilic granulomatosis with polyangiitis, 458.e4
  serum, 1790b, 1794
  urine, 1795, 1838
Creeping eruption, 350.e5, 350.e5f
Creeping verminous dermatitis, 350.e5, 350.e5f
CREST syndrome, 1148
Creutzfeldt-Jakob disease, 343.e3–343.e4
CRH. See Corticotropin releasing hormone
Critical incident stress debriefing, 50
Critical limb ischemia, 975
"Crocodile tongue", 1186f
CroFab, 199
Crohn's disease, 344–345.e2, 345.e1f, 345.e2t, 345f
  endoscopic evaluation of, 345
  enteropathic arthritis associated with, 455–456.e1,
    455t
  fistulas in, 345f
  imaging studies for, 345
  toxic megacolon caused by, 1283
  ulcerative colitis and, 344t, 345, 1313t
Cromolyn sodium
  for allergic rhinitis, 63
  for conjunctivitis, 328t
Cronkhite-Canada syndrome, 985–986
Crossed eyes, 1214.e4
Crotalid bites, 197–199.e1
Crotamiton, for scabies, 1142t
Crotch itch, 1272
Croup, 345.e3–345.e5, 345.e3f–345.e4f, 345.e4t,
  463–463.e2, 463.e1f
Crowned-dens syndrome, 1078
CRPS. See Complex regional pain syndrome
CRT. See Cardiac resynchronization therapy
Crusted scabies, 1141t
Cryoglobulinemia, 346–346.e1, 346f, 346.e1t
Cryoglobulinemic vasculitis, 346, 346f, 346.e1t, 1351.e2t
Cryoglobulins, serum, 1795
Cryoproteinemia, 346
Cryosurgery
  for basal cell carcinoma, 178t
  for genital warts, 1376

Cryotherapy
  for keloids, 735.e5–735.e6
  with liquid nitrogen
    for cutaneous larva migrans, 350.e6
    or cryoprobe, for condyloma acuminatum, 324
  for warts, 1376
Cryptococcal meningitis, 813.e2, 636t
Cryptococcosis
  in acquired immunodeficiency syndrome, 18t–24t
  characteristics of, 347–347.e1, 347f
Cryptococcus albidus infection, 347
Cryptococcus gattii infection, 347
Cryptococcus laurentii infection, 347
Cryptococcus neoformans, 813.e2, 265
Cryptococcus neoformans infection, 347
Cryptogenic fibrosing alveolitis, 691
Cryptogenic organizing pneumonia, 412f, 692t
Cryptorchidism, 347.e2f, 687.e1–687.e4, 1253
Cryptosporidiosis, 348, 348.e1f
Cryptosporidium antigen by EIA, 1795
Cryptosporidium hominis, 348
Cryptosporidium infection, 348–348.e1, 348.e1f
Crystalloids
  for anaphylaxis, 79.e2t
  for burns, 229b
Crystals, urine, 1796
CST. *See* Cavernous sinus thrombosis
CU. *See* Chronic urticaria
Cubital tunnel syndrome, 348.e2–348.e4, 348.e2f
Cullen's sign, 943
CUP. *See* Cancer of unknown primary
Cuprimine. *See* d-Penicillamine
Cushing's disease/syndrome, 73, 349–350.e4, 350.e2t,
    350.e1f, 350f, 350t, 953–955.e1, 953t, 997–999.e1
  hypertension caused by, 660t
  renin-aldosterone pattern in, 1838t
Cutaneous anergy, 1401
Cutaneous anthrax, 106.e2, 106.e2f
Cutaneous B-cell lymphoma, 863.e5t
Cutaneous calcifications, on x-ray, 1416
Cutaneous candidiasis, 234–235.e1, 234f–235f
Cutaneous color changes, 1423–1424
Cutaneous diphtheria, 395.e5
Cutaneous (discoid) lupus erythematosus, 66
Cutaneous infections, in athletes, 1427
Cutaneous larva migrans, 350.e5–350.e6, 350.e5f, 350.e5t
Cutaneous leishmaniasis, 742.e2
Cutaneous leukocytoclastic angitis, 830t, 1245t
Cutaneous lichen planus, 756–756.e1
Cutaneous lymphomas, 1816
Cutaneous mastocytosis, 799t
Cutaneous microvascular occlusion syndromes,
    1601.e1–1601.e2, 1601.e1f, 1601.e2t
Cutaneous mucormycosis, 848
Cutaneous neurofibromatosis, 895f
Cutaneous paraneoplastic syndromes, 1500
Cutaneous scleroderma, 397t
Cutaneous sporotrichosis, 1205.e2–1205.e4
Cutaneous T-cell lymphoma, 863.e2–863.e5, 863.e2f–863.
    e3f, 863.e5t
CVS. *See* Cyclic vomiting syndrome
C282Y and H63D mutation analysis, 1781–1795
Cyanosis, 1427, 1602, 1602f
Cyclic hematopoiesis, recurrent or periodic fever and, 1442
Cyclic vomiting syndrome, 350.e7–350.e8,
    350.e7b–350.e8b
Cycloid psychosis, 190
Cyclooxygenase inhibitors, 1060t
Cyclopentolate, for uveitis, 1334
Cyclophosphamide
  for amyloidosis, 76.e4
  for aplastic anemia, 81
  for autoimmune hemolytic anemia, 83
  for Behçet's disease, 182.e3
  for breast cancer, 216
  for cerebral vasculitis, 266.e6
  for chronic inflammatory demyelinating polyneuropathy,
    293
  for Cogan's syndrome, 313.e5
  for eosinophilic granulomatosis with polyangiitis, 458.e5
  for granulomatosis with polyangiitis, 533
  for hemophilia B, 570
  hyperpigmentation with, 1651t
  for inflammatory myopathies, 705
  for pemphigus vulgaris, 969
  for polyarteritis nodosa, 1022

Cyclophosphamide *(Continued)*
  for primary angiitis of the central nervous system, 1062
  for systemic lupus erythematosus, 1242
  for transverse myelitis, 1296
  for Waldenström's macroglobulinemia, 1374
Cyclosporine
  for chronic urticaria, 1329
  for enteropathic arthritis, 456
  for Sjögren's syndrome, 1187
Cyclosporine A
  for aplastic anemia, 81
  for Behçet's disease, 182.e3
  for inflammatory myopathies, 705
Cyproheptadine, for serotonin syndrome, 1164
Cyproterone acetate
  for hirsutism, 618
  for pedophilic disorder, 961.e2
Cyst(s)
  Baker's, 170.e2–170.e3, 170.e2f, 229.e5
  Bartholin's gland, 175–176.e1, 176f
  hepatic, 1454
  hepatic echinococcal, 428t
  pulmonary, 1513
  splenic, classification of, 1527
Cystatin C, 1795
  cardiorenal syndrome and, 253
  chronic kidney disease and, 295
Cystectomy, for bladder cancer, 201, 202b
Cystic changes, 490
Cystic disorders, renal, 1745.e3
Cystic duct syndrome, 504
Cystic echinococcosis, 427
Cystic fibrosis, 351–352.e2, 351t, 352f
  bronchiectasis and, 219
  PCR, 1795
Cystic fibrosis transmembrane conductance regulator
    protein, 352
Cystic orbital lesions, 1497
Cysticerciasis, 353, 354f
Cysticercosis, 353–354.e1, 354f, 1249–1250
Cystine stones, 1325
Cystitis, 1322.e2f
  acute, 1603–1603.e1, 1603f
  interstitial, 713–714.e1, 713f
Cystoid macular edema, 1116.e6
Cystourethropexy, for stress incontinence, 700
Cytarabine, 748
Cytogenetics, in ataxia telangiectasia, 145.e5
Cytomegalic inclusion disease virus, 355
Cytomegalovirus, 355–355.e1, 1015–1016
  in acquired immunodeficiency syndrome, 18t–24t
  IGIV, 1867t
  in immunocompromised patients, 355
  by PCR, 1795
  ventriculitis, 443t
Cytomegalovirus retinitis, 636t
Cytopenia
  bi-lineage and tri-lineage, 1412
  uni-lineage, 1412
Cytosponge, 172

D

DA. *See* Dissociative amnesia
Dabigatran
  for atrial fibrillation, 152
  for pulmonary embolism, 1090
  for transient ischemic attack, 1294
Daclatasvir, 588
Daclizumab, 1334
Dactinomycin, hyperpigmentation with, 1651t
Dactylitis, 1082, 1182
DAL-1, 809
Dalbavancin, 828
Dalfampridine, 857
Danazol
  for aplastic anemia, 81
  for autoimmune hemolytic anemia, 83
  for dysfunctional uterine bleeding, 414
  for mastodynia, 800
  for premenstrual syndrome, 1054
  for uterine fibroids, 1332
Dandruff, 1152
Dandy criteria, for idiopathic intracranial hypertension,
    690.e5
Danis-Weber classification, of ankle fractures, 99.e2f

Dantrolene
  chronic hepatitis caused by, 410.e2t
  for malignant hyperthermia, 793
  for neuroleptic malignant syndrome, 896
  for spasticity, 1196.e1t
Dapsone
  for Behçet's disease, 182.e3
  for chronic urticaria, 1328–1329
  for dermatitis herpetiformis, 373
  for erythema elevatum diutinum, 469
  for leprosy, 742.e6
Daptomycin
  for cellulitis, 266
  for erysipelas, 468
  for methicillin-resistant *Staphylococcus aureus*, 828
  for vancomycin-resistant *Enterococcus*, 1346
Darbepoetin alfa
  for chronic kidney disease, 297
  for inflammatory anemia, 85
Darier's disease, 1214
Darunavir, 18
Darunavir and ritonavir, 634
DAT. *See* Direct antiglobulin test
Daunorubicin, 1651t
Daytime sleepiness, 1604–1605
DCIS. *See* Ductal carcinoma in situ
DD. *See* Dissociative disorders
DDAVP. *See* Desmopressin acetate
DDI. *See* Didanosine
D-dimer assays
  for deep vein thrombosis, 358–359
  description of, 1089, 1795–1796
de Musset's sign, 116
De Quervain's disease, 356, 356f
De Quervain's stenosing tenosynovitis, 356, 356f
De Quervain's tendonitis, 356, 356f
De Quervain's tenosynovitis, 356–356.e1, 356f
Deafness, fever and rash with, 1440
Death, sudden
  differential diagnosis of, 1417
  heart failure and, 560
  long QT syndrome and, 764
  mitral valve prolapse and, 840
  in pediatric age, 1530
  risk assessment for, in myocardial infarction, 874
  in young athlete, 1530
DEC. *See* Diethylcarbamazine citrate
Decitabine, 748
Decubitus ulcers, 1056
Deep brain stimulation, for Tourette's syndrome, 1282
Deep frostbite, 502, 502f
Deep gluteal syndrome, 996.e1
Deep vein thrombosis, 357–360.e5, 358f, 360.e4f–360.e5f,
    1042
  prophylaxis of, 360
  recurrent, 360
  upper extremity, 360, 1316–1317.e1, 1316f–1317f
Deerfly fever, 1309.e1, 1309.e1f
DEET. *See* Diethyltoluamide
Deferasirox, for hemochromatosis, 566
Deferoxamine
  for hemochromatosis, 566
  for lead poisoning, 741t
  for radiation exposure, 1100.e14t–1100.e16t
Defibrination syndrome, 398, 399.e1f
  differential diagnostic algorithm for, 399f
  scoring system for, 399.e2b
  testing and diagnosis of, 399f
  underlying conditions with, 399.e1b
Degarelix, 1073
Degenerative disorders, paraparesis with, 1501
Degenerative joint disease, 921, 1243.e5
Dehydration
  in pediatric patients
    clinical observations of, 1801t
    correction of, 1604.e1–1604.e3
  xerostomia with, 1779
Dehydroepiandrosterone sulfate, 1795
  for adrenal insufficiency, 53
  in hirsutism, 617
Dehydrotestosterone, 1795
Delavirdine, 18
Delayed gastric emptying, 1445
Delayed hemolytic transfusion reaction, 1291
Delayed puberty, 361–363.e3, 361f–363f,
    363.e1t–363.e3t, 1512

Delirium, 364–366.e1, 364t, 366.e1t
  acute confusional state, 444
  agitated, 1610–1614
  algorithm for, 365f
  classification, 364
  dementia versus, 366t
  in dialysis patient, 1614
  differential diagnosis of, 1604.e4–1604.e5
  drug-induced, 1609–1610
  in elderly patient, 1682f
  evaluation of, 365f
  management of, 1682f
  psychiatric illness versus, 366t
  risk factors for, 366.e1t, 364t
  theories regarding, 364
Delirium tremens, 367–367.e1
"DELIRIUMS" mnemonic, 481
Delta agent, 590
Delta hepatitis coinfection, 1805
Delta virus, 590
Deltamethrin, 182
Delusional parasitosis, 367.e2–367.e3, 367.e2t
Dementia, 68, 444
  delirium versus, 366t
  with Lewy bodies, 368–369.e1, 368b, 368f–369f, 956,
    1068.e4
  management of, 1604.e4, 1604.e4f
  screening tests for, 1604.e4t
Dementia praecox, 1144
Dementia pugilistica, 956
Demodex folliculorum, 1132
Demyelinating diseases, 1428
Demyelinating polyneuropathy, 1508
Dengue, 369.e2
Dengue fever
  characteristics of, 369.e2–369.e4, 369.e2f,
    369.e4f
  classification of, 369.e3b
  distribution of, 369.e2f
  skin manifestations of, 369.e4f
Dengue hemorrhagic fever, 369.e2, 369.e4f
  classification of, 369.e3b
  distribution of, 369.e2f
  skin manifestations of, 369.e4f
Dengue shock syndrome, 369.e2, 369.e4f
  classification of, 369.e3b
  distribution of, 369.e2f
  skin manifestations of, 369.e4f
Denosumab
  osteonecrosis of the jaw caused by, 191.e2
  for osteoporosis, 926–927
Dense connective tissue, heel pain and, 1452
Dental health
  in ages 65 and older, 1855t
  in ages 11 to 24 years, 1850t
  in ages 25 to 64 years, 1853t
  from birth to 10 years, 1849t
Dental procedures
  prophylaxis with, 1905t
  regimens for, 1905t
Dentatorubral-pallidoluysian atrophy, 1203.e2
Denture-related glossodynia, 1446
Denys-Drash syndrome, 888.e2, 888.e2t
Deoxycorticosterone, 1795
Dependence, substance, 405
Dependent personality disorder, 370–370.e1
Depersonalization disorder, 400
Depo Medrol, 543
Depo-Provera, 330, 332
Depot Medroxyprogesterone acetate, 332.e5t
Depression
  major, 371–372.e1, 372t
  manic-depression, 190
  postpartum, 1039–1039.e1
Depressive episode, 371
Deprivation amblyopia, 71, 71
Dermatitis
  atopic, 147–148.e1, 147b, 148.e1f, 148f
  contact
    characteristics of, 329–329.e2, 329.e2f
    pruritus ani with, 1511
  foot, 1444
  granulomatous
    clinical features of, 1632t
    differential diagnosis of, 1447
  poison ivy, 1020–1020.e1, 1020.e1f

Dermatitis *(Continued)*
    pruritus ani with, 1511
    seborrheic, 1152–1152.e1, 1152.e1f, 1152f, 1269
Dermatitis herpetiformis
    characteristics of, 373–374.e1, 373f–374f
    HLA antigens associated with, 1807t
Dermatoblepharitis, 202.e5
Dermatologic disorders, pruritus ani with, 1511
Dermatomes, 1197f
Dermatomyositis, 397t, 698.e1t, 704, 705t, 706f, 706.e1f
    juvenile, 706.e1f
Dermatoses, eosinophilic, 1618.e1, 1618.e1f
Dermatosparaxis Ehlers-Danlos syndrome, 431.e3
Dermoscopy
    for contact dermatitis, 329
    for melanoma, 805
Descovy, 633–634
Desipramine
    for attention deficit hyperactivity disorder, 161
    for cataplexy, 884
    for postherpetic neuralgia, 1037
Desloratadine, 1328
Desmopressin acetate
    for antidiuretic hormone deficiency, 1235
    for diabetes insipidus, 375, 618.e3
    for enuresis, 457, 458t
    for hemophilia A, 570
    for hyponatremia, 682
    for Von Willebrand's disease, 1372
Desonide, 1370
Desquamative interstitial pneumonia, 692t
Developmental delay, 1604.e5f
Developmental dysfluency, 1222.e4
Device-associated infections, 548.e3
Devic's disease, 855
Dexamethasone
    for acute mountain sickness, 612–613
    for amyloidosis, 76.e4
    for anaphylaxis, 79
    for astrocytoma, 144
    for bacterial meningitis, 813
    for Behçet's disease, 182.e3
    for brain abscess, 208
    for chemotherapy-induced nausea and vomiting, 276
    for chronic inflammatory demyelinating polyneuropathy,
      293
    for cluster headaches, 543
    for congenital adrenal hyperplasia, 325.e3
    for corneal abrasion, 338
    for croup, 345.e4t
    for Cushing's syndrome, 954
    for cysticercosis, 354
    for high-altitude cerebral edema, 612–613
    for high-altitude pulmonary edema, 612–613
    for hirsutism, 618
    for migraine headache, 546
    for thyrotoxic storm, 1268.e2
    for typhoid fever, 1312.e4
    for Waldenström's macroglobulinemia, 1374
Dexamethasone suppression test
    for Cushing's disease and syndrome, 349
    overnight, 1795
Dexmedetomidine, 46–48
Dexrazoxane, 243
Dextroamphetamine
    for attention deficit hyperactivity disorder, 161
    for narcolepsy, 884
Dextromethorphan, for acute bronchitis, 28
DF. *See* Dissociative fugue
DHTR. *See* Delayed hemolytic transfusion reaction
Diabetes hepatitis, 902
Diabetes insipidus, 375–375.e3, 375.e1t, 375.e2f, 375.e3t,
    618.e3
Diabetes mellitus, 376–383.e11
    antihyperglycemic therapy for, 380t
    clinical evaluation of, 383.e11f
    comparison of therapies for, 379t
    criteria for diabetes screening, 378t
    diagnostic categories of, 377t
    insulin for, 381, 381t
    necrobiosis lipoidica with, 377, 383.e11f
    neuropathy of the hindfoot and, 383.e11f
    preoperative management of, 1055.e4–1055.e5
    stroke risks, 1222
    types of, 376t
    vaccination considerations for, 1887t

Diabetic foot, 384–385.e1, 384f–385f
Diabetic foot ulcer, 384, 384f–385f
Diabetic gastroparesis, 382
Diabetic hyperosmolar syndrome, 624
Diabetic ketoacidosis, 386–388.e1, 387f
Diabetic macular edema, 392
Diabetic nephropathy, 1115
Diabetic neuropathy, 376–377, 382
Diabetic peripheral neuropathy, 389, 390f–391f, 391t
Diabetic polyneuropathy, 389–391.e1, 390f–391f, 391t, 899t
Diabetic retinopathy, 376, 382, 392–393.e3, 392t,
    393.e1f–393.e3f, 393f
Dialectical behavior therapy, for borderline personality
    disorder, 205.e2
Dialysis
    for chronic kidney disease, 297
      conflict resolution in shared decision about starting,
        298f
      initiation of, 297t
      principles underlying withdrawal of, 298t
    delirium and, 1614
    for Goodpasture syndrome, 528
    for yellow fever, 1378.e2
3,4-Diaminopyridine, 738.e2
Diaphragm and cervical cap, 331
Diaphragm elevation
    bilateral, symmetrical, 1428
    unilateral, 1428–1429
Diaphragmatic hernia, 609.e2
Diaphysis, bone lesions at, 1412
Diarrhea
    in acquired immunodeficiency syndrome, 24.e1f
    acute, 1605, 1605f
    acute bloody, 1429
    acute watery, 1429
    arthritis and, 1403
    in carcinoid syndrome, 239.e2
    chronic, 1606, 1606f
    Clostridium difficile-associated, 310
    fever and rash with, 1440
    gastrointestinal disorders with, as adverse food reaction,
      1394
    infectious, 510, 1300, 1429, 1470
    laboratory testing for, 1813t
    noninfectious, 1429–1430
    traveler's. *See* Traveler's diarrhea
    in tube-fed patient, 1430
    watery, 1606.e2, 1606.e2f
Diastolic heart failure, 553, 554t
Diastolic murmur, 1417, 1683, 1683b, 1683f
Diazepam
    for alcohol abuse, 56t, 57–58
    for alcohol withdrawal, 367
    for cocaine overdose, 313
    for Ménière's disease, 808
    for spasticity, 1196.e1t
Diazoxide, 712.e2
DIC. *See* Disseminated intravascular coagulation
Diclofenac sodium
    for actinic keratosis, 26
    chronic hepatitis caused by, 410.e2t
Dicloxacillin
    for bursitis, 229.e5
    for cellulitis, 265
    for erysipelas, 468
    for impetigo, 697
Dicyclomine, for opioid withdrawal, 407
DID. *See* Dissociative identity disorder
Didanosine
    for acquired immunodeficiency syndrome, 18
    dosing of, 1901t
Diet
    for ages 11 to 24 years, 1851t
    for ages 25 to 64 years, 1853t
    from birth to 10 years, 1849t
    gluten-free, for dermatitis herpetiformis, 373
    low-salt, 1829t
    modification, for dumping syndrome, 412.e3
Diet-controlled gestational diabetes, 513
Diethylcarbamazine citrate, 494.e3
Diethylpropion, for obesity, 907–908
Diethylstilbestrol exposure, 1338
Diethyltoluamide, 182
DIF. *See* Direct immunofluorescence
Differentiation syndrome, 749
Differin. *See* Adapalene

Diffuse aches and pains, 1390
Diffuse cerebral sclerosis, 1428
Diffuse coagulation, vasculitis mimicked by, 1540
Diffuse cystic mastopathy, 490
Diffuse esophageal spasm, 12t
Diffuse fasciitis with eosinophilia, 458.e2
Diffuse goiter, nontoxic, 1631.e1f
Diffuse idiopathic skeletal hyperostosis, 394–395.e1, 394f–395f
Diffuse interstitial infiltration, in human immunodeficiency virus, 1457
Diffuse large B-cell lymphoma, 779
Diffuse Lewy body disease, 368, 368b, 368f–369f
Diffuse nodular, necrotizing scleritis, 1146
Diffuse osteosclerosis, 1497
Diffuse otitis externa, 928
Diffuse parenchymal lung disease, 715
Diffuse pulmonary hemorrhage syndromes, 1514
DigiFab. *See* Digoxin-specific Fab fragments
Digit(s)
    clubbing of, 668–669.e1, 668f–669f
    gangrene of, 1149.e3f
Digital index, 668f
Digital rectal examination, for prostate cancer, 1071
Digital stenosing tenosynovitis, 1302.e2, 1302.e2f–1302.e3f
Digital subtraction angiography, for subarachnoid hemorrhage, 1225
Digitalis overdose, 395.e2–395.e4, 395.e3f–395.e4f
Digoxin, 1795
    for atrial fibrillation, 150
    for cor pulmonale, 337
    for heart failure, 559
    for supraventricular tachycardia, 1232
Digoxin-specific Fab fragments, 395.e3
Dihydroergotamine
    for cluster headaches, 543
    for migraine headache, 546t
Dilantin, 1796
Dilatation
    gastric, 1631
    pupillary, 1515
Dilatation and curettage, for molar pregnancy, 842
Dilated bile duct, 1408–1409
Dilated cardiomyopathy
    characteristics of, 244–245.e1, 245t
    with Duchenne muscular dystrophy, 245.e1f
    idiopathic, 245
Dilated pupil, 1606.e3, 1606.e3f
DILD. *See* Drug-induced parenchymal lung disease
Diloxanide furoate, 72t
Diltiazem
    for anal fissure, 78.e2
    for atrial fibrillation, 150
    for hypertrophic cardiomyopathy, 248
Dimenhydrinate, 546t
Dimercaprol
    for lead poisoning, 741t
    for radiation exposure, 1100.e14t–1100.e16t
Dimethyl fumarate, 857
Dimethyl sulfoxide, 714
Diogenes syndrome, 437
Dioxins, hyperpigmentation with, 1651t
Diphenhydramine
    for anaphylaxis, 79, 79.e2t
    for carcinoid syndrome, 239.e3
Diphtheria, 395.e5–395.e6
Diphtheria and tetanus toxoids and acellular pertussis vaccine
    catch-up schedule, 1859, 1860t–1864t
    conditions misperceived as contraindications to, 1868t–1871t
    contraindications and precautions, 1868t–1869t
    for pediatric oncology patients, 1874t
    recommended immunization schedule, 1860t–1864t
Diphtheria and tetanus toxoids vaccine, 1868t–1869t
Diphtheria antitoxin, for diphtheria, 395.e5
Diphtheria toxoid, vaccination with, 395.e5
Diphtheric cardiomyopathy, 395.e5
Diphtheric polyneuropathy, 395.e5
Diphyllobothrium latum, 1249t
Diplopia
    binocular, 1430
    monocular, 1430
    vertical, 1430
Dipyridamole
    for angina pectoris, 94
    for carotid stenosis, 257

Direct antiglobulin test, 82, 1291
Direct bilirubin, 1779
Direct Coombs test, 1291, 1793, 1796
Direct immunofluorescence, 373
Direct thrombin inhibitors, 576
Directly observed therapy, for leprosy, 742.e6
Discharge, vaginal
    dysuria and, 1614, 1614f
    evaluation of, 1756f
    in prepubertal girls, 1767
Discitis, 923f
Discoid lupus erythematosus, 396–397.e1, 396f, 397.e1f, 397t, 1214, 1240f
Disease-modifying antirheumatic drugs
    for Felty's syndrome, 485.e2
    for juvenile idiopathic arthritis, 733
    for psoriatic arthritis, 1083
    for rheumatoid arthritis, 1126–1127
DISH. *See* Diffuse idiopathic skeletal hyperostosis
Disimpaction, for encopresis, 445.e2
Dislocation, glenohumeral, 521.e2–521.e3, 521.e2f
Disopyramide, 248
Disruptive mood dysregulation disorder, 191
Dissecting aortic aneurysm, 113
Disseminated candidiasis, 236
Disseminated intravascular coagulation, 398–399.e2, 399.e1f, 1040
    differential diagnosis of, 108t, 399f
    scoring system for, 399.e2b
    testing and diagnosis of, 399f
    underlying conditions with, 399.e1b
Disseminated mucormycosis, 848
Disseminated sclerosis, 855
Disseminated TB, 1304
Dissociated nystagmus
    characteristics and localizations of, 1695t
    types of, 1698f
Dissociative amnesia, 400
Dissociative disorders, 400–401.e1
Dissociative fugue, 400, 1293
Dissociative identity disorder, 400
Distal sensorimotor polyneuropathy, 376
Distal symmetric polyneuropathy, 389, 390f–391f, 391t
Disulfiram, 56t, 407
Diuretic renography, for hydronephrosis, 644
Diuretics
    for ascites, 127, 129.e2f, 129t, 1032
    for Bartter syndrome, 176.e2
    for cardiorenal syndrome, 254
    for dilated cardiomyopathy, 245
    loop, for heart failure, 558
    overuse, 1829t
Divarication of recti, 1390
Diverticular disease, 402–403.e1, 402f
Diverticulitis, 402–403.e1, 402f
Diverticulosis, 402–403.e1, 402f
Diverticulum, Zenker's, 1378.e4–1378.e5, 1378.e4f
Dix-Hallpike maneuver, 185
Dizziness
    algorithm for, 186f, 1872.e1f
    differential diagnosis of, 1430
DKA. *See* Diabetic ketoacidosis
DLBCL. *See* Diffuse large B-cell lymphoma
DMARDs. *See* Disease-modifying antirheumatic drugs
DMDD. *See* Disruptive mood dysregulation disorder
DME. *See* Diabetic macular edema
DMPA. *See* Depot Medroxyprogesterone acetate
DMPS, for lead poisoning, 741t
DNA methyltransferase inhibitors, 865
Dobutamine
    for heart failure, 558
    for pulmonary edema, 1087
Docetaxel, 1073
Docosahexaenoic acid, 1116.e6
Dofetilide
    for atrial fibrillation, 151f
    for atrial flutter, 154
Dog bites, 192–193.e1, 193b, 193t
Dolasetron, 276
Dolutegravir
    for acquired immunodeficiency syndrome, 18
    for human immunodeficiency virus, 634
Domestic violence, 437
Donath-Landsteiner antibody, 958.e2

Donath-Landsteiner hemoglobinuria, 958.e2
Donath-Landsteiner test, for paroxysmal cold hemoglobinuria, 1796
Donepezil, for Alzheimer's disease, 69t
Donovanosis, 531.e1
Dopamine, 1796
    for anaphylaxis, 79, 79.e2t
    for pulmonary edema, 1087
Dopamine agonists
    for Parkinson's disease, 957
    for Tourette's syndrome, 1282
Dopa-response dystonia, 423t
Doppler echocardiography
    for aortic stenosis, 118–119
    for sickle cell disease, 1180
Doppler ultrasound
    for renal artery stenosis, 1108–1109
    for thyroid nodule, 1267.e1f
Doripenem, for anaerobic infections, 78
Double-contrast esophagogram, of esophageal tumors, 473, 474.e2f
Double-crush syndrome, 268.e3
Dowager's hump, 925, 1363f
Down syndrome, 403.e2–403.e3, 403.e2f
Doxazosin, 992.e2t
Doxepin
    for atopic dermatitis, 148
    for chronic urticaria, 1328
    for urticaria, 1326
Doxorubicin
    for amyloidosis, 76.e4
    for breast cancer, 216
    cardiomyopathy induced by, 242
    hyperpigmentation with, 1651t
Doxycycline
    for acne vulgaris, 15
    for actinomycosis, 26.e3
    for acute bronchitis, 28
    for anaplasmosis, 432
    for anthrax, 106.e3
    for bite wounds, 192
    for blepharitis, 202.e5
    for brucellosis, 220.e3
    for cellulitis, 266
    for cervicitis, 272
    for Chlamydia genital infections, 280
    for cholera, 290.e2
    for chronic obstructive pulmonary disease, 301
    for ehrlichiosis, 432
    for epididymitis, 459
    for gonococcal urethritis, 1318
    for gonorrhea, 527
    for granuloma inguinale, 531.e1
    for leptospirosis, 742.e8
    for Lyme disease, 775
    for lymphogranuloma venereum, 778.e2
    for malaria, 790
    for methicillin-resistant *Staphylococcus aureus*, 828
    for nongonococcal urethritis, 1319
    for pelvic abscess, 962
    for pelvic inflammatory disease, 964
    for prostatitis, 1077
    for psittacosis, 1079.e4
    for Q fever, 1100.e7
    for Rocky Mountain spotted fever, 1130
    for tick bite, 194
    for tularemia, 1309.e2
    for Whipple's disease, 1376.e8
DPD. *See* Depersonalization disorder
D-Penicillamine
    for lead poisoning, 740, 741t
    for radiation exposure, 1100.e14t–1100.e16t
DPLD. *See* Diffuse parenchymal lung disease
DRD. *See* Dopa-response dystonia
Dronedarone, 151f
Drop arm test, 1133.e2
Drospirenone/ethinyl estradiol, 15
Drowning, 404–404.e1, 404.e1f
Droxidopa, 857.e3, 857.e3t, 919
Drug(s), 539.e1t. *See also* Medication(s). *specific drug*
    acute pancreatitis from, 1713.e1
    agitation induced by, 1609–1610
    alopecia induced by, 1396
    androgen action affected by, 539.e1t
    anemia induced by, 1399
        aplastic, 80, 1398–1399

Drug(s) (Continued)
  cataracts induced by, 259.e6
  chorea induced by, 639
  choreoathetosis induced by, 1422
  coma induced by, 1424
  consciousness impairment from, 1461
  delirium and, 364, 1609–1610
  diarrhea induced by, 1429
  dystonia induced by, 423t
  eosinophilic lung disease induced by, 1435
  eosinophilic pneumonia induced by, 458.e8
  fever induced by, 1440
  hemolytic anemia induced by, 82
  hepatic granulomas caused by, 1454
  hyperkalemia induced by, 1461
  hypertrichosis from, 1464
  immune thrombocytopenia induced by, 576.e1f
  interstitial nephritis caused by, 718
  leg ulcers with, 1476
  lipoprotein metabolism affected by, 647.e1t
  liver injury induced by, 408–410.e4, 408t–409t,
    410.e1t–410.e3t
  lupus erythematosus induced by, 397t
  methemoglobinemia induced by, 1485
  myopathic syndromes induced by, 1488
  nausea and vomiting induced by, 276
  neuropathies caused by, 1494
  neutropenia induced by, 1494
  ocular toxicity from, 1459
  pancreatitis induced by, 1721.e1–1721.e2
  polyneuropathy induced by, 1508
  polypharmacy, 1031.e2–1031.e3
  scleroderma-like syndromes induced by, 1749–1750
  thrombocytopenia induced by, 1532
  toxic epidermal necrolysis caused by, 1213–1213.e1,
    1282.e2–1282.e3, 1282.e2f, 1282.e2t–1282.e3t
  tremor induced by, 476
  urine color abnormalities induced by, 1537–1538
Drug abuse, 405–407.e1, 405t–406t
Drug Abuse Screening Test, 912, 912t
Drug-induced parenchymal lung disease, 411–412.e2,
  412.e1f–412.e2f, 412f, 412t
Dry ejaculate, 435
Dry eye, 1186, 1431
DSPN. See Distal symmetric polyneuropathy
D4T. See Stavudine
DT vaccine. See Diphtheria and tetanus toxoids vaccine
DTaP vaccine. See Diphtheria and tetanus toxoids and
  acellular pertussis vaccine
DTPA, for radiation exposure, 1100.e14t–1100.e16t
DTs. See Delirium tremens
DU. See Duodenal ulcer
Dual-chamber pacing, for hypertrophic cardiomyopathy,
  248
Dual-energy x-ray absorptiometry, for osteoporosis, 925,
  926t, 927.e5f
Duavee, for hot flashes, 629
DUB. See Dysfunctional uterine bleeding
Duchenne muscular dystrophy
  characteristics of, 860–861, 860f–861f, 861t
  with dilated cardiomyopathy, 245.e1f
Duck hunter's itch, 350.e5, 350.e5f
Ductal carcinoma in situ, 216–217, 218t
Ductal obstruction, 1471
Duhring disease, 373, 373f–374f
Dulaglutide, 379
Duloxetine
  for chronic pain, 939t
  for neuropathic pain, 898
Dumping syndrome, 412.e3–412.e4
Duodenal ulcer, 970
Duplex ultrasound, for claudication, 308
Dupuytren's contracture, 412.e5–412.e7, 412.e5f, 412.e6t,
  987–988
Dural sinus thrombosis, 261
Durie-Salmon staging, of multiple myeloma, 852t
Dutasteride, 1076
D-Xylose absorption, 1796
D-Xylose absorption test, 1796, 1833t
Dysautonomia, 857.e2
Dysautonomic postural orthostatic tachycardia syndrome,
  1044.e2
Dysentery
  amebic, 72
  inflammatory enterocolitis and, 1430
Dysfunctional tear syndrome, 1186

Dysfunctional uterine bleeding, 413–414.e1, 413b–414b,
  414t, 817
Dyskinesia
  differential diagnosis of, 1530
  tardive, 1530
Dyslipidemia, 645, 654.e3t, 1028t
Dyslipoproteinemias, 1431
Dysmenorrhea, 415–415.e2
Dysmorphophobia, 203
Dyspareunia, 416–418.e1, 417f
  differential diagnosis of, 1431, 416
  historical factors of, 416
  vaginismus and, 1339f
Dyspepsia
  approach to patient with, 1609.e1, 1609.e1f
  functional, 419
  nonulcerative, 419–419.e1
  during pregnancy, 1431
Dysphagia
  characteristics of, 420–421.e1, 421.e1f, 421f, 1431
  complications of, 421
  differential diagnosis of, 421f
  esophageal, 420, 1431
  oropharyngeal, 420, 1432
  pathogenesis of, 420
Dysplasia
  arrhythmogenic right ventricular, 123–124.e1, 123f,
    124.e1f, 124t
  cervical. See Cervical dysplasia
Dyspnea, 1432
  algorithm for, 1610–1613, 1610f
  in asbestosis, 125
  in heart failure, 554
  in mitral stenosis, 836
Dysraphism, 1196.e2
Dysrhythmias, 1055.e5
Dysthymia, borderline personality disorder and, 205.e2
Dystonia, 422–423.e1, 422f, 423t
Dystonia-deafness optic neuropathy syndrome, 423t
Dystrophinopathies, 860
Dystrophy, nail, 1836b, 1841f
Dysuria, 1432, 1536, 1614, 1614f
DYT1 dystonia, 423t

E

EAA. See Extrinsic allergic alveolitis
Eale's syndrome, 1116.e4
Ear disorders
  otitis externa, 928–929.e1, 928f
  otitis media, 930–931.e1, 930f
  tinnitus, 1277–1277.e2, 1277.e2f
Ear pain, 1615–1615.e1, 1615f
Earache, 1432–1437
Early infantile autism, 162
Early repolarization pattern, 424–426.e1, 424f–426f, 1356
Early repolarization syndrome, 424
Eating disorders
  anorexia nervosa, 103–104.e1, 103t–104t
  binge eating, 103t
  bulimia nervosa, 103t, 225–226.e1, 226t
Eaton-Lambert syndrome, 738.e2
Eaton's pneumonia, 1011
EBV. See Epstein-Barr virus
EC. See Endometrial cancer
Ecallantide, 98.e3t
Ecchymoses, macular purpura and, 1726t
Echinococcosis, 427–428.e1, 427f–428f, 428.e1f, 428t
Echinococcus granulosus, 1249t
Echinococcus multilocularis, 1249t
Echocardiography
  for angina pectoris, 93
  for aortic coarctation, 111
  for aortic stenosis, 118
  for arrhythmogenic right ventricular dysplasia, 123
  for atrial septal defect, 157, 157f
  for carcinoid syndrome, 239.e3
  for chemical-induced cardiomyopathy, 242–243
  for cor pulmonale, 336
  for dilated cardiomyopathy, 244, 245.e1f
  Doppler, of aortic stenosis, 118–119
  for heart failure, 556
  for hypertrophic cardiomyopathy, 247, 247f
  for interstitial lung disease, 716
  for long QT syndrome, 765
  low-voltage, 1478

Echocardiography (Continued)
  for mitral regurgitation, 833, 833f
  for mitral stenosis, 836–837, 837f
  for mitral valve prolapse, 839, 839f
  for myocarditis, 876
  for patent ductus arteriosus, 959
  for pericarditis, 972, 973f
  for pulmonary arterial hypertension, 1093
  for pulmonary edema, 1086
  for pulmonary embolism, 1090
  for restrictive cardiomyopathy, 251, 251f
  for Takotsubo cardiomyopathy, 1247
  for tetralogy of Fallot, 1255.e6
  for tricuspid stenosis, 1301.e7
  for ventricular septal defect, 1359
Eclampsia, 429–429.e1
ECMO. See Extracorporeal membrane oxygenation
Ectocervicitis, 272
Ectopic adrenocorticotropic hormone secretion, 1616–1617
Ectopic adrenocorticotropic hormone syndrome, 350.e2t
Ectopic pregnancy, 430–431.e1, 430f, 431.e1f
Ectopic testis, 347.e2f
Eculizumab
  for hemolytic-uremic syndrome, 567
  for paroxysmal nocturnal hemoglobinuria, 958.e4
Eczema, 147, 496, 1077.e4
  eyelid, 202.e5
  seborrheic, 1152
  varicose, 1352, 1352f
Eczematous otitis externa, 928
ED. See Erectile dysfunction
Edema. See also Angioedema
  angioneurotic, 97
  cerebral
    in hepatic encephalopathy, 578
    high-altitude, 612–613.e2, 613.e1t, 613.e2b, 613b
  in children, 1617–1618
  generalized, 1432–1433, 1617, 1617f
  leg, unilateral, 1433
  lower extremity, 1433
  lymphedema, 776–778, 777f–778f
  noncardiogenic pulmonary, 1513
  pulmonary, 1087.e1f, 1086–1087.e1, 1087f
    in acute decompensated heart failure, 558
    acute noncardiac, 412.e2f
    high-altitude, 612–613.e2, 613.e1f, 613.e1t,
      613.e2b, 613b
    in mitral stenosis, 836
    noncardiogenic, 1513
  regional, 1618, 1618f
EDH. See Epidural hematoma
Edoxaban, 152
Edrophonium test, for myasthenia gravis, 863, 863.e1f
EDS. See Ehlers-Danlos syndrome
EDTA
  for lead poisoning, 740
  for radiation exposure, 1100.e14t–1100.e16t
EED. See Erythema elevatum diutinum
EF. See Eosinophilic fasciitis
Efavirenz, 1901t
  for acquired immunodeficiency syndrome, 18
  for human immunodeficiency virus, 634
Effort syndrome, 1043
Effusions
  joint, 1671, 1671f
  pericardial, 1503
  peritoneal, 1504
  pleural
    differential diagnosis of, 1505
    in human immunodeficiency virus infection, 1457
    infected, 441
    malignancy-associated, 1505
    purulent, 441
Effusive-constrictive pericarditis, 974
Eflornithine, for hirsutism, 617–618
EGD. See Esophagogastroduodenoscopy
Egg allergy, 496–497
EGPA. See Eosinophilic granulomatosis with polyangiitis
EHEC. See Enterohemorrhagic E. coli
Ehlers-Danlos syndrome, 431.e2–431.e4, 431.e2t, 431.e3f
Ehrlichia phagocytophila, 432
Ehrlichiosis, 432–434.e1, 433t, 434.e1t
EIEC. See Enteroinvasive E. coli
Eisenmenger's complex, 1360
EITB assay. See Enzyme-linked immunoelectrotransfer blot
  assay

Ejaculation disorders, 435–436.e1, 436f
Ejaculatory dysfunction, 435
Ejection sound, 1433
Ekbom syndrome, 367.e2, 367.e2t
Elapid bites, 197–199.e1
Elbow pain, 1433
Elbow tendinitis, 458.e10
Elbow tendinopathy, 458.e10
Elbow tendinosis, 458.e10
Eldepryl, 884
Elderly patients
    abuse of, 437–438.e1, 438f
    acute myeloid leukemia in, 748t
    altered mental status and coma in, 1484
    bowel incontinence in, 699–699.e1, 699.e1b
    delirium in, 1682f
    falls by, 480–481.e2, 480t, 481.e1f
    fecal incontinence in, 699–699.e1, 699.e1b
    fragility hip fractures in, 615
    hip pain in, 1457
    memory loss symptoms in, 1483
    mental status change in, 1682, 1682b, 1682f
    mistreatment of, 437
Electrical dissociation, 1096
Electrical injury, 227, 228t, 229.e4f, 439–440.e1, 439f
    care phases for, 229.e2t
    categorization of, by depth, 227t
    classification of, 227
    complications in, 229.e3b
    follow-up care for, 229
    Mayes equations for, 229b
    resuscitation for, 228
        formula for, 229b
    "6 Cs" of, 228
    treatment for, 228–229, 229.e4f
    wound care for, 228–229
Electrocardiography
    for atrioventricular dissociation, 159f
    for Brugada syndrome, 221
    for chemical-induced cardiomyopathy, 242
    for coronary artery disease, 339
    for early repolarization pattern, 424, 424f–426f
    for heart failure, 556
    for hyperkalemia, 1823.e2f
    for hypertrophic cardiomyopathy, 246, 247f
    for infective endocarditis, 447
    for long QT syndrome, 765f, 1280f
    for mitral regurgitation, 834
    for mitral stenosis, 837
    for multifocal atrial tachycardia, 850f
    for myocardial infarction, 868–869, 868f
    for myocarditis, 876
    for pericarditis, 972, 973f
    for pulmonary embolism, 1089
    for pulseless electrical activity, 1096–1096.e1, 1096f
    for restrictive cardiomyopathy, 251
    for short QT syndrome, 1174, 1175f
    for sick sinus syndrome, 1178–1178.e1, 1178f
    for supraventricular tachycardia, 1231
    for tachycardia-bradycardia syndrome, 1178–1178.e1,
        1178f
    for Takotsubo cardiomyopathy, 1247
    for ventricular tachycardia, 1362.e1f, 1361f
Electrocautery
    for condyloma acuminatum, 325
    description of, 463.e8
Electrocochleography, 808
Electroconvulsive therapy
    for major depression, 372
    for neuroleptic malignant syndrome, 896
Electrodissection
    for basal cell carcinoma, 178t
    for squamous cell carcinoma, 1206
Electrolytes
    abnormalities involving
        coma and, 1424
        mental changes and coma with, 1484
        metabolic myopathies and, 1489
    deficits of, in severe dehydration, 1604.e3t
    replacement of, for diabetic ketoacidosis, 388
Electrophoresis, serum protein, 1825, 1826f
Electrophysiology study, for Brugada syndrome, 222
Elephantiasis, 494.e2, 494.e2f, 776–777, 898f
Elephantiasis nervosa, 894f
Eletriptan, for migraine headache, 546t
Elevated hemidiaphragm, 1433

Elevated liver enzymes, 564.e2
Eloxatin. See Oxaliplatin
Eltrombopag, 81
Eluxadoline, 723
Elvitegravir
    for acquired immunodeficiency syndrome, 18
    for human immunodeficiency virus, 634
EM. See Erythema multiforme
Embolectomy, 1091
Embolic disease, vasculitis mimicked by, 1540
Embolism
    arterial, 1433, 1485
    pulmonary, 1088–1091.e3, 1088t, 1089f–1090f,
        1091.e2f, 1091.e3t
    septic, cavitary lesion with, 1418
EMD. See Electrical dissociation
Emedastine difumarate, 328t
Emergency contraception, 440.e2–440.e3, 440.e2t, 1166
Emery-Dreifuss muscular dystrophy, 860, 861t
Emesis. See also Nausea and vomiting
    chemotherapy-induced, 276
    in pediatric age, 1433
Emphysema
    alpha-1-antitrypsin deficiency and, 67
    characteristics of, 299, 299t–300t, 300f, 302t, 303b
Emphysematous cholecystitis, 290.e1t
Emphysematous pyelonephritis, 1106
Empyema, 441–441.e1, 441f, 1009
Emtricitabine
    for acquired immunodeficiency syndrome, 18
    dosing of, 1901t
Emtricitabine/tenofovir, 1901
ENA complex. See Extractable nuclear antigen
Enalapril
    for chemical-induced cardiomyopathy, 243
    for coronary artery disease, 342
Enalaprilat, 664t
Encephalitis
    acute viral, 442–443.e1, 443t
    mumps and, 858
    necrotizing hemorrhagic, 1428
    Toxoplasma gondii, 18t–24t, 636t–638t, 1290f
    West Nile virus, 1376.e5
Encephalitis lethargica, 442
Encephalitozoon sp., 831
Encephalocutaneous angiomatosis, 1222.e2
Encephalomyelitis
    acute disseminated, 1428
    nonviral causes of, 1433–1434
Encephalopathy, 444–445.e1
    grades of, 42t
    hepatic, 577–579.e1, 577t–578t, 579b
    hypertensive, 1434
    metabolic, 1434
    uremic, 1535
    Wernicke, 735.e8, 1376.e3
Encopresis, 445.e2–445.e3
Endocarditis, 237, 620
    bacterial, 446, 840
    cardiac conditions associated with the highest risk of
        adverse outcome from, 1905t
    dental procedures, 1905t
    infective, 446–449.e3
        clinical manifestations of, 447t
        diagnostic algorithm for, 448f
        modified Duke criteria for diagnosis of, 446b
    prophylaxis, 1905
    tricuspid valve, 446f
    ventricular septal defect and, 1360
Endocervical polyps, 271.e4, 271.e4f
Endocervicitis, 272
Endocrine disorders, 539.e1t
    chronic fatigue from, 1428
    mental changes and coma with, 1484
    myopathy and, 1489
Endocrine paraneoplastic, 1500
Endocrine tests, for nipple discharge, 1586f
Endocrine therapy, for invasive breast cancer, 216
Endocrine tumors, 1370.e2t
Endodermal sinus tumor, 1338
Endogenous toxins
    coma and, 1424
    mental changes and coma with, 1484
Endolymphatic hydrops, 808
Endometrial cancer, 450–451.e1, 450t, 451f
Endometrial hyperplasia, 817

Endometrial stromal sarcoma, 1333
Endometrial thickening, 1434
Endometriosis, 452–453.e1, 452f–453f
Endometritis, 454, 454f, 454t
Endomyometritis, 454
Endomysial antibodies, 1796
Endophthalmitis, 236
Endoscopic mucosal resection, for Barrett esophagus, 174
Endoscopic radiofrequency heating, 512
Endoscopic retrograde cholangiopancreatography
    acute pancreatitis and, 945–946
    for cholangiocarcinoma, 284, 285.e2f
    for cholangitis, 286
    for cholecystitis, 287
    for choledocholithiasis, 289
    chronic pancreatitis and, 947
    for cirrhosis, 305
    for jaundice, 730
    for primary biliary cirrhosis, 1064f
Endoscopic submucosal dissection, for Barrett esophagus,
    174
Endoscopic ultrasonography
    for acute pancreatitis, 945
    for chronic pancreatitis, 948.e2f
    for esophageal tumors, 473, 474.e1f
Endoscopy
    for hiatal hernia, 609.e2
    for Mallory-Weiss tear, 795, 795.e1f
    for nonulcerative dyspepsia, 419
    variceal ligation, for esophageal varices, 1.e2f, 475
Endothelin receptor blockers, for cor pulmonale, 337
Endovascular aneurysm repair, 4–6, 6f
Endovenous ablation, for varicose veins, 1349
End-stage renal disease, 294
    in IgA nephropathy, 694
    kidney transplantation for, 694
    in preeclampsia, 1051
    preoperative management of, 1055.e5
Enfuvirtide, 18
Enoxaparin
    for acute coronary syndrome, 34
    for deep vein thrombosis, 359
    for pulmonary embolism, 1091.e3t
Entamoeba histolytica, 72, 760, 1300
Entecavir, for hepatitis B, 584
Enteric fever, 1312.e4, 1135
Enterically transmitted non-A non-B hepatitis. See Hepatitis
    E virus
Enterobiasis, 996
Enterobius vermicularis, 126.e1t, 996, 996f
Enteroclysis, 1192
Enterococcus, vancomycin-resistant, 1346
Enterococcus faecium, vancomycin-resistant, 548.e3
Enterocolitis, 1458
Enterocytozoon bieneusi, 831
Enterohemorrhagic E. coli food poisoning, 500
Enteroinvasive E. coli, 501
Enteropathic arthritis, 455–456.e1, 455t
Enteropathic arthropathy, 101t
Enteropathy
    gluten-sensitive, 263
    protein-losing, 1510
    tropical, 1303.e2
Enterotoxigenic E. coli
    food poisoning caused by, 500
    traveler's diarrhea caused by, 501, 1300
Enterotoxin-poisoning, 500, 500t
Enterovirus, 814
Enterovirus infection, 540
Enthesitis, 1082
Enthesitis-related arthritis, 732, 732t
Enthesopathy, 1434
Enuresis, 457–458.e1, 458f, 458t
Environmental regulation, mental changes and coma caused
    by, 1484
Enzalutamide, for prostate cancer, 1073
Enzyme-linked immunoelectrotransfer blot assay, for
    cysticercosis, 353
Enzyme-linked immunospot assay, for pulmonary
    tuberculosis, 1307
Eosinophil(s), urine, 1838
Eosinophil count, 1796, 1797t
Eosinophilia, 651.e2b
    childhood, 1420
    diffuse fasciitis with, 458.e2
    disease associated with, 1434–1435

Eosinophilia *(Continued)*
   gastrointestinal, 1435
   pulmonary, 1513
Eosinophilic dermatoses, 1618.e1, 1618.e1f
Eosinophilic fasciitis, 458.e2–458.e3, 458.e2f
Eosinophilic gastroenteritis, 350.e5t
Eosinophilic granuloma, 618.e2
Eosinophilic granulomatosis with polyangiitis, 458.e4–458.e6, 458.e4t, 458.e5f, 458.e8, 830t, 1245t, 1351.e2t
Eosinophilic lung disease, 1435
Eosinophilic meningitis, 350.e5t
Eosinophilic pleocytosis, cerebrospinal fluid, 1787b
Eosinophilic pneumonias, 458.e7–458.e9, 692t
Epicondylalgia, 458.e10
Epicondylitis, 458.e10–458.e12, 458.e10f
Epidemic vomiting disease, 500, 500t
Epidermoid carcinoma. *See* Squamous cell carcinoma
Epididymitis, 281t, 459–459.e1, 917t, 1255t
Epididymoorchitis, 858, 917, 1347.e2t
Epidural abscess, 460–460.e1
Epidural hematoma, 461–462.e1, 461f–462f, 462b
Epidural spinal cord compression, 1526
Epigastric abdominal pain, 1387, 1435
Epiglottitis, 345.e4t, 463–463.e2, 463.e1f, 463f, 981t
Epilepsy
   antiepileptics for. *See* Antiepileptics
   childhood absence, 1153
   differential diagnosis of, 1435
   status epilepticus, 1210–1212, 1210b, 1210t, 1211f–1212f
Epileptic myoclonus, 878
Epinastine hydrochloride, 328t
Epinephrine
   for anaphylaxis, 79, 79.e2t
   for croup, 345.e4t
   for insect stings, 195
   plasma, 1797
   for urticaria, 1327.e2f
Epiphysis, bone lesions at, 1412
Epiploic appendagitis, 463.e3–463.e4, 463.e3f
Epiplopericolitis, 463.e3
Episcleritis, 463.e5–463.e6, 463.e5f, 463.e6t
Episodic ataxias, 1203.e2–1203.e3
Epistaxis, 463.e7–463.e8, 463.e7f, 1435–1436
Epithelial cell, 1837t
Epithelial ovarian cancer, 932
Epitrochlear lymphadenopathy, 1676.e3, 1676.e3b, 1676.e3f
Eplerenone, for heart failure, 559
Epley's maneuver, 185–186
Epodyl, for bladder cancer, 201
Epoetin alfa
   for chronic kidney disease, 297
   for inflammatory anemia, 85
Epoprostenol, 1094
Epstein-Barr virus, 846–846.e2, 846.e1f–846.e2f
   antibodies associated with, 465t
   encephalitis, 443t
   infection with, 464–465, 464f
   malignancies associated with, 464t
   serology, 1797, 1797b, 1798f, 1798t
Eptifibatide, 34
Epworth Sleepiness Scale, 883, 884t, 1190f
Epzicom, 634
Equine heptavalent botulinum antitoxin, 206
Erbitux. *See* Cetuximab
ERCP. *See* Endoscopic retrograde cholangiopancreatography
Erdheim Chester disease, 618.e2
Erectile dysfunction, 466–467.e1, 467.e1t, 467f, 1436
Erection, 1060.e2t
Ergonovine, 1040t
Ergotamine
   for cluster headaches, 543
   for migraine headache, 546, 546t
Erosions, genitalia, 1436
Erosive gastritis, 508
ERP. *See* Early repolarization pattern
ERT. *See* Estrogen replacement therapy
Ertapenem
   for anaerobic infections, 78
   for lung abscess, 768
Eructation, 1394
Eruptive hemangioma, 1100.e4
Erysipelas, 265, 266.e2f, 468, 468f, 928
Erysipelothrix rhusiopathiae, 265
Erythema, reactive, 1872.e1f
Erythema elevatum diutinum, 469–469.e1, 469f

Erythema infectiosum, 493, 493f–494f
Erythema marginatum, 1124.e2
Erythema migrans, 774f
Erythema multiforme, 470, 470f
   herpes simplex virus associated with, 607t
   Stevens-Johnson syndrome, 1213–1213.e1, 1213f
Erythema nodosum, 471, 471f, 952f, 1138, 1138.e1f
Erythematotelangiectatic rosacea, 1131
Erythematous annular skin lesions, 1436
Erythematous lesions, oral mucosa, 1496
Erythematous plaque, 468f
Erythrocyte sedimentation rate, 1797
Erythrocytosis
   acquired, 1619, 1619f
   causes of, 1436
Erythroderma
   differential diagnosis of, 1436, 1619.e1–1619.e2
   drugs associated with, 1807t
Erythrodermic psoriasis, 1081f
Erythromelalgia of the head, 543
Erythromycin
   for acne vulgaris, 15
   for actinomycosis, 26.e3
   for chancroid, 272.e5
   for Chlamydia genital infections, 282
   for cholera, 290.e2
   for granuloma inguinale, 531.e1
   for lymphangitis, 776
   for lymphogranuloma venereum, 778.e2
   for pertussis, 984, 984t
   for pharyngitis, 989
   for respiratory diphtheria, 395.e5
   for Scarlet fever, 1143
   for tonsillitis, 989
Erythroplakia, 915
Erythropoiesis-stimulating agents, for inflammatory anemia, 85
Erythropoietic protoporphyria, 1736.e1t
Erythropoietin, 865, 1797–1798
Erythroprosopalgia of Bing, 543
ESA. *See* Erythropoiesis-stimulating agents
ESBL. *See* Extended-spectrum beta-lactamases
Escherichia coli
   0157:H7, hemolytic-uremic syndrome caused by, 567
   traveler's diarrhea caused by, 1300, 1300t, 1301.e1t
   urinary tract infection caused by, 1320–1321
Esmolol
   for atrial fibrillation, 150
   for hypertension, 664t
   for pheochromocytoma, 992.e2t
Esophageal cardiospasm, 12
Esophageal dysphagia, 1431
Esophageal motor disorders, 12t
Esophageal tumors
   barium swallow for, 474.e2f
   benign, 1436–1437
   characteristics of, 472–474.e2, 473f, 474.e1f–474.e2f
Esophageal varices, 475–475.e2, 475.e1f–475.e2f
Esophagitis
   differential diagnosis of, 1437
   treatment of, 237
Esophagogastroduodenoscopy
   of esophageal tumors, 473, 474.e1f
   for esophageal varices, 475
Esophagogastroscopy, 1034
Esophagus
   achalasia of, 12
   anatomy of, 173f
   Barrett, 172–174.e1, 173f
   disease of, in human immunodeficiency virus infection, 1458
   foreign body in, 1620–1621, 1620f, 1621t
   perforation of, 1436
   strictures of, 1436
   systemic diseases of, 1432
Esotropia, 1214.e4, 1419
ESR. *See* Erythrocyte sedimentation rate
ESRD. *See* End-stage renal disease
Essential cryoglobulinemia, 346, 346f
Essential cryoglobulinemic vasculitis, 830t
Essential hypertension, 660
Essential myoclonus, 878
Essential thrombocythemia, 1260–1261.e1, 1260b, 1261f, 1261.e1f
Essential thrombocythemia, 1260
Essential tremor, 476–476.e1, 476t

Estar. *See* Tar products
Estimated glomerular filtration rate, for cardiorenal syndrome, 253
Estraderm patch, 1340
Estradiol
   for gender dysphoria disorder, 512.e6
   serum, 1798
Estradiol vaginal cream, 1340
Estradiol vaginal tablets, 1340
EstroGel, 816
Estrogen
   description of, 1796
   for dysfunctional uterine bleeding, 413–414
Estrogen agonists, 539.e1t
Estrogen receptor agonists, 539.e1t
Estrogen replacement therapy. *See also* Hormone replacement therapy
   for amenorrhea, 76
   for endometriosis, 453
   for hot flashes, 629
   for menopause, 815–816, 816b
   for osteoporosis, 927
   for Turner syndrome, 1312.e2
Estrogen-deficient vaginitis, 1340–1340.e1, 1340f
Estrogen-secreting tumors, 539.e1t
Estropipate, for menopause, 816
ESWT. *See* Extracorporeal shock wave lithotripsy
ET. *See* Essential thrombocythemia
Etanercept
   for enteropathic arthritis, 456
   for psoriasis, 1081
   for Still's disease, 54
Ethambutol
   for granulomatous arthritis, 534.e2
   for pulmonary tuberculosis, 1308
Ethanol, 1798
Ethinyl estradiol, 331–332
Ethosuximide, 1153–1153.e1
Ethylene glycol
   pathophysiology, clinical effects, and management of, 1716t–1719t
   poisoning caused by, 826–827.e2, 826b, 827.e2f
Etomidate, 1668.e2t
Etonogestrel, 330
Etravirine
   for acquired immunodeficiency syndrome, 18
   for human immunodeficiency virus, 634
Etretinate
   chronic hepatitis caused by, 410.e2t
   for lichen planus, 756
Eugonadism, 73
EVAR. *See* Endovascular aneurysm repair
Everolimus, 507.e4
Ewing's sarcoma, 204
Exanthem subitum, 1133
Exanthems, 1419
Excessive daytime somnolence, 884
Exenatide, 379
Exercise
   in ages 11 to 24 years, 1851t
   in ages 25 to 64 years, 1853t
   from birth to 10 years, 1849t
   for chronic fatigue syndrome, 291
   for diabetes mellitus, 378
   for dilated cardiomyopathy, 245
   for glenohumeral dislocation, 521.e2
   for heart failure, 557
   with leg pain, 1476
   walking, for claudication, 308
Exercise testing
   for heart failure, 556
   for hypertrophic cardiomyopathy, 247
   treadmill, for coronary artery disease, 339
Exercise-induced asthma, 132
Exertional heat stroke, 562t
Exocrine pancreatic cancer, 941–942.e1, 941f, 942t
Exogenous toxins
   coma and, 1424
   mental changes and coma with, 1484
Exotropia, 1214.e4
Exposure therapy, for panic disorder, 950
Exserohilum rostratum, 813.e2
Extended-spectrum beta-lactamases, 849–849.e1
Extensively drug-resistant tuberculosis, 1306
External hemorrhoids, 572.e2–572.e4, 572.e2f–572.e3f
Extracapsular fracture, 614

Extracellular fluid
  composition of, 1604.e3t
  volume of, 1235
Extracorporeal membrane oxygenation
  for acute respiratory distress syndrome, 48
  for cor pulmonale, 336
  for hantavirus pulmonary syndrome, 540.e3
  for pulmonary arterial hypertension, 1094
Extracorporeal shock wave lithotripsy
  for cholelithiasis, 290
  for Peyronie's disease, 987
  for plantar fasciitis, 1004
Extracorporeal ultrafiltration, for cardiorenal
  syndrome, 254
Extractable nuclear antigen, 1798
Extradural hematoma/hemorrhage, 461, 462f
Extrahepatic biliary tree, 731.e1f
Extrahepatic jaundice, 1473
Extramedullary plasmacytoma, 851t
Extrasphincteric fistula, 102
Extraurethral incontinence, 701
Extraurethral urinary incontinence, 700
Extraventricular obstructive hydrocephalus, 641
Extremity pain, 1403–1404
Extrinsic allergic alveolitis, 657, 1448
Exudates, peritoneal effusion with, 1504
Exudative pleural effusions, 1505
Exudative retinal detachment, 1116.e2
Eye(s)
  dry, 1431
  foreign body in, 910.e2, 910.e2f
  herpetic infections of, 607t
  hypertensive retinopathy, 1520
  jaundice manifestations in, 731.e1f
  lesions involving, arthritis and, 1403
  multiple sclerosis manifestations of, 855, 855f
  red, 1736.e1
  Sturge-Weber syndrome manifestations of,
    1222.e2
  sympathetic pathways to, 628.e1f, 628
  vitreous hemorrhage, 1542
Eye disorders
  conjunctivitis. See Conjunctivitis
  Horner's syndrome, 628.e1f, 628–628.e1, 628f
  macular degeneration, 783–784.e1
  optic atrophy, 913.e4, 913.e4f
  optic neuritis, 914.e1f, 913.e4, 914–914.e1, 914f
  strabismus, 1214.e4–1214.e6, 1214.e5f–1214.e6f
  stye, 1223–1223.e1, 1223f
Eye pain, 1419
Eyelid
  HIV infection manifestations in, 1424
  infection or inflammation of, 202.e5
  neoplasm, 1419
  retraction, 1437, 1475
Ezetimibe
  for hyperlipidemia, 654.e4t
  lipoprotein metabolism affected by, 647.e1t

F

F protein, 1867t
FAB classification system, 864
Fabry's disease, 899t
Facial angiofibromas, 1308.e3f, 1308.e4t
Facial erysipelas, 468
Facial nerve palsy, 183
Facial pain, 1437–1445
  headache and, 1639–1640
Facial paralysis, 1623–1627
  idiopathic, 183
Facioscapulohumeral muscular dystrophy, 860, 861t
Factitious disorder, 477–477.e1, 899
Factor IX concentrates, 570
Factor IX hemophilia, 569
Factor V Leiden, 1799–1801
Factor V Leiden mutation, 648–649, 648t
Factor VIII concentrates, 569, 570t
Factor VIII deficiency hemophilia, 569
Factor Xa inhibitors, 152
Fadrozole, 1332
Failure of emission, 435
Failure to thrive
  differential diagnosis of, 1628
  pediatric, 478–479.e1, 478f
Fallopian tube, infertility and, 1470

Falls
  in elderly, 480–481.e2, 480t, 481.e1f
  prevention of, 481.e1f
Faltering growth, 478
Famciclovir
  for herpes simplex, 607t
  for herpes zoster, 609
  for Ramsay Hunt syndrome, 1101–1101.e1
Familial adenomatous polyposis, 482–483.e1, 985t, 986f
Familial amyloid polyneuropathy, 899t
Familial apoprotein CII deficiency, 654
Familial dysbetalipoproteinemia, 654.e3t
Familial hypercholesterolemia, 654, 654.e3t
Familial hyperchylomicronemia, 654.e3t
Familial hyperlipemia, 654.e3
Familial hypertriglyceridemia, 654
Familial hypertrophic cardiomyopathy, 246
Familial hypophosphatemic rickets, 1128.e5
Familial lipoprotein lipase deficiency, 654
Familial Mediterranean fever, 484–484.e1, 484.e1f
Familial paroxysmal polyserositis, 484
Familial testotoxicosis, 1046t
Familial tremor, 476
Familial type 3 hyperlipoproteinemia, 654
Family planning, 330
Famotidine, for anaphylaxis, 79
FAP. See Familial adenomatous polyposis
Farmer's lung, 657
Fasciotomy
  for compartment syndrome, 318
  description of, 1123
  for necrotizing fasciitis, 887
FASD. See Fetal alcohol spectrum disorder
Fasting blood sugar, 1799
  for diabetic polyneuropathy, 389
Fasting plasma glucose, 376
Fat
  fecal, qualitative screening for, 1831
  heel pain and, 1452
  malabsorption of, 785
Fatigue, 1622
  chronic, 1438–1439
  differential diagnosis of, 1438
  evaluation of, 1812f
Fatty liver
  differential diagnosis of, 1439
  of pregnancy, acute, 485–485.e1
Fatty liver hepatitis, 902
FBS. See Fasting blood sugar
FCD. See Fibrocystic breast disease
FDA pregnancy risk classification system, 934.e2t
Fear attacks, 949
Febrile convulsions, 1154
Febrile mucocutaneous syndrome, 1213
Febrile seizures, 485.e2–485.e3, 1154–1155.e1, 1155f
Febuxostat, for gout, 530
Fecal DNA testing, for colorectal cancer, 314
Fecal elastase-1 test, 1833t
Fecal fat
  qualitative screening for, 1831
  quantitative, 1799
Fecal globin immunochemical test, 1799
Fecal immunochemical test, for colorectal cancer, 314
Fecal incontinence, 445.e2, 699–699.e1, 699.e1b,
  1470
Fecal irritation, pruritus ani with, 1511
Fecal microbiota transplantation, 310
Fecal occult blood test, for colorectal cancer, 314
Felty's syndrome, 485.e2–485.e3, 1125
Female genital tract calcifications, on x-ray, 1416
Female genitalia, discharge, 1445–1446
Female infertility, 1470
Female pseudohermaphroditism, 1455, 1511
Female sexual dysfunction, 1168–1170.e1, 1168t, 1169f,
  1523
Femoral fractures
  head, 614f
  intertrochanteric, 614f–615f
  neck, 614, 614f–615f, 614t, 615.e3f
Femring vaginal ring, 816
Fenofibrate, 654.e3t
Fenoldopam mesylate, 664, 664t
Fentanyl
  for chronic pain, 940.e3t, 940t
  intubation and, 1668.e2t
Ferriman-Gallwey scale, for hirsutism, 616

Ferritin
  in hemochromatosis, 565–566
  serum, 1799
Ferrous sulfate, 87–88
Fetal alcohol spectrum disorder, 486, 486t–487t
Fetal alcohol syndrome, 486–487, 486t–487t
Fetal heart monitoring, in abruptio placentae, 9
Fetal hydantoin syndrome, 1312.e2
α-Fetoprotein. See Alpha-1-fetoprotein
FEV1. See Forced expiratory volume, for chronic obstructive
  pulmonary disease
Fever, 1626, 1626f
  arthritis and, 1404
  Brugada syndrome and, 222
  cardiopulmonary failure and, 1439
  in children, 1441–1442, 1626.e1b, 1626.e1f, 1627, 1627f
  Colorado tick, 313.e7, 313.e7f
    in children, 313.e7
    pathogenesis of, 313.e7
  deerfly, 1309.e1
  drug-induced, 1440
  enteric, 1312.e4
  in high-risk hematology patient, 1625.e1, 1625.e1b, 1625.e1f
  hospital-associated, 1440
  in immigrants, 1441
  jaundice and, 1439
  lymphadenopathy and, 1439
  maculopapular rash with, 1442
  noninfectious causes of, 1437
  in pediatric patients, 1626.e1b, 1626.e1f, 1627, 1627f
  periodic, 1437
  petechial rash with, 1442
  postpartum, 1437
  rabbit, 1309.e1
  rash and, 1439
  recurrent, 1441–1442
  after travel to tropics, 1440
  typhoid, 1312.e4–1312.e7, 1312.e4f
  West Nile virus, 1376.e5
Fever of undetermined origin, 488–489.e3, 489.e2f–489.
  e3f, 489f
Fever of unknown origin, 488, 488t
Fexofenadine, 1326, 1328
Fiber, 722
Fibric acid derivatives, 654.e4t
Fibric acids, 647.e1t
Fibrillation
  atrial. See Atrial fibrillation
  ventricular. See Ventricular fibrillation
  in Wolff-Parkinson-White syndrome, 1377
Fibrin degradation product, 1800
Fibrinogen, 1800
Fibrinolytic therapy, for myocardial infarction, 869, 871–872,
  872t
Fibrocystic breast disease, 490
Fibrocystic mastopathy, 490
Fibroids, uterine, 1331–1332.e1, 1331f–1332f
Fibroma, in Meigs' syndrome, 804.e1f
Fibromuscular dysplasia, 1107–1110.e1, 1107f
Fibromyalgia, 343t, 491–492.e2, 492.e2f, 491f, 879t
Fibrosarcoma, 204, 1139f
Fibrosing cholangitis, 1067
Fibrosing mediastinitis, 802
Fibrosis
  bone marrow, 1412
  nephrogenic systemic, 888.e3–888.e4, 888.e3f
"Fibrositis", 491
Fibulin-3, 822
Fidaxomicin, 311
Fifth disease, 493–494.e1, 493f–494f
FIGO staging
  for cervical cancer, 268t
  for ovarian cancer, 932t
  for vulvar cancer, 1372.e2t
Filariasis, 494.e2–494.e3, 494.e2f, 778
Filiform warts, 1375
Financial abuse, elder, 437
Finasteride
  for alopecia, 65
  for benign prostatic hyperplasia, 1076
  for hirsutism, 618
Fine needle aspiration biopsy, for thyroid nodule, 1266
Finger lesions, inflammatory, 1442
Fingolimod, 856
Finkelstein's test, 356f
Fire ant stings, 196f

First heart sound, 836
First visit, pregnant women, 1857t
Fisher grade, of subarachnoid hemorrhage, 1224b
Fissure, anal, 78.e2–78.e3, 78.e3f
Fistula
    anal, 1397
    anorectal, 102–102.e1
    bronchopleural, 1414
    in Crohn's disease, 345f
    vaginal, 1336–1337.e1, 1336f–1337f
Fistula-in-ano, 102
Fistulization, for Bartholin's gland cyst and abscess, 175
Fistulotomy and curettage, for pilonidal disease, 995
FIT. *See* Fecal immunochemical test, for colorectal cancer
5-α reductase inhibitors, for acute urinary retention, 51
Flaccid paralysis, acute, 1442
Flat warts, 1375
Flatulence, 1442–1443
Flecainide
    for atrial fibrillation, 151f
    for atrial flutter, 154
    for Wolff-Parkinson-White syndrome, 1378
Flesh-eating bacteria, 887. *See also* Necrotizing fasciitis
Flexible fiberoptic bronchoscopy, for primary lung neoplasms,
    770
Flibanserin, 673, 1170
Floating eye, 1214.e4
Floppy infant, 701.e4
FloSeal hemostatic matrix, 463.e8
Flow cytometry
    for acute myelogenous leukemia, 746, 746t
    for immunodeficiency assessments, 1065.e6t
Flu, 707. *See also* Influenza
Fluconazole
    for balanitis, 171
    for blastomycosis, 202.e3
    for coccidioidomycosis, 313.e3
    for cryptococcosis, 347
    for cutaneous candidiasis, 235
    for fungal vaginitis, 1341
    for glossitis, 525
    for invasive candidiasis, 237
    for tinea capitis, 1270
    for tinea corporis, 1271
    for tinea versicolor, 1276
Flucytosine
    for cryptococcosis, 347
    for invasive candidiasis, 237
Fludrocortisone
    for adrenal insufficiency, 53
    for congenital adrenal hyperplasia, 325.e3
    for hypoaldosteronism, 674
    for orthostatic hypotension, 857.e3t, 919
Fluid, in peritoneal cavity, 127
Fluid contrast ultrasound, for dysfunctional uterine bleeding,
    413
Fluid replacement
    for cholera, 290.e2
    for diabetic ketoacidosis, 386
    for heat exhaustion, 561
    for heat stroke, 561
    for hyperglycemic hyperosmolar syndrome, 652
    for hyperparathyroidism, 656
    for rhabdomyolysis, 1123
Flunisolide, 63
Fluocinonide, 756
Fluoroquinolones
    for brucellosis, 220.e3
    for otitis externa, 929
    for otitis media, 931
    for prostatitis, 1077–1077.e1
    for psittacosis, 1079.e4
    for pyelonephritis, 1099
    for salmonellosis, 1136t
    for urinary tract infection, 1322, 1322.e2f
5-Fluorouracil
    for actinic keratosis, 26, 26t
    for basal cell carcinoma, 178t
    for bladder cancer, 201
    for breast cancer, 216
    for carcinoid syndrome, 239.e3
    for colorectal cancer, 315
    for condyloma acuminatum, 324
    for gastric cancer, 506
    hyperpigmentation with, 1651t
    for invasive candidiasis, 237

5-Fluorouracil *(Continued)*
    for keloids, 735.e6
    for pancreatic cancer, 942
    for warts, 1376
Fluoxetine
    for cataplexy, 884
    for intermittent explosive disorder, 712.e4t
    for obesity, 908
    for premenstrual dysphoric disorder, 1053.e2
    for premenstrual syndrome, 1055
Flurbiprofen, 546t
Flush syndrome, 239.e2
Flushing, 1627.e1
    carcinoid syndrome and, 239.e2, 239.e2f
    differential diagnosis of, 1443
    evaluation of, 1627.e1f
Flutamide
    for alopecia, 65
    for hirsutism, 618
Fluticasone
    for allergic rhinitis, 63
    for chronic obstructive pulmonary disease, 301
Flutter, atrial, 153–154.e1, 154f
Fluvastatin, 654.e4t
FM. *See* Fibromyalgia
FMD. *See* Fibromuscular dysplasia
FMF. *See* Familial Mediterranean fever
Foam dressings, for venous ulcers, 1354
FOBT. *See* Fecal occult blood test, for colorectal cancer
Focal anaplasia, 888.e2
Focal consolidation, in human immunodeficiency virus
    infection, 1457
Focal neurologic deficit, 1492
Focal segmental glomerulonephrosis, 889–891, 890t
Focal segmental glomerulosclerosis, 1446
Focal seizures, 1157
Focal sequestration, of iron, 1472
Fogo selvagem, 968
Folate, 1800, 1801b
    deficiency of
        diagnosis of, 89t
        differential diagnosis of, 1443
        megaloblastic anemia with, 1400
    drugs interfering with, 1399
    intake of, in pregnancy, 814.e2, 1196.e4
Folic acid
    for chemical-induced cardiomyopathy, 243
    deficiency of, 1368, 1369f
    for pernicious anemia, 90
    for tropical sprue, 1303.e2
Follicle-stimulating hormone, 1800
    deficiency of, 685
    in hirsutism, 617
    in hot flashes, 629
Follicular carcinoma, 1264–1265.e2
Follicular conjunctivitis, 326
Follicular cysts, 1028.e4f, 1046t
Folliculitis, 495, 495f
Fomepizole, 827
Fondaparinux
    for acute coronary syndromes, 34
    for deep vein thrombosis, 359
    for heparin-induced thrombocytopenia, 576
    for pulmonary embolism, 1091.e3t
Fontaine classification, of peripheral arterial disease, 975,
    976t
Food allergies, 496–499.e1, 497f, 498t–499t
Food poisoning
    bacterial, 500–501.e2, 500t
    botulism, 206–206.e1
Food reactions, adverse, 1394
Foot
    dermatitis, 1444
    diabetic, 384–385.e1, 384f–385f
    rash with edema of, 1440
Foot lesion, ulcerating, 1444
Foot pain, 1443, 1443–1444, 1444
Foot ulcer, 377
    diabetic, 384, 384f–385f
Footdrop, 1444
Foramen ovale, patent, 960.e2–960.e4, 960.e2f–960.e3f,
    960.e3t, 1221
Forced elbow extension test, for epicondylitis,
    458.e10f
Forced expiratory volume, for chronic obstructive
    pulmonary disease, 299–300

Forearm
    fracture of, 1444–1445
    pain involving, 1444
Forehead fibrous plaque, 1308.e4t
Foreign body
    esophageal, 1620, 1620f, 1621t
    ocular, 910.e2, 910.e2f
    in wound, 1628.e1, 1628.e1b, 1628.e1f
Forestier disease, 394, 394f–395f
Formaldehyde, 826
Formic acid, 826
47,XXY hypogonadism, 735.e7
Fosamprenavir, 1901
Fosamprenavir and ritonavir, 634
Foscarnet, 355
Fosfomycin, 1322.e2f
Four Corners disease, 540.e2
Fournier's gangrene, 887, 888t
Fractures
    ankle, 99.e2–99.e5, 99.e2f–99.e3f, 99.e2t, 99.e3b
    bone, 1627b, 1627f, 1628.e2
    forearm, 1444–1445
    hip, 614–615.e3, 614f–615f, 614t, 615.e3f
    pelvic avulsion, 1502
    vertebral, 1199t
    vertebral compression, 1363–1364.e1, 1363f, 1364b
Fragile X–associated tremor ataxia syndrome, 857.e2,
    1203.e2
Fragility hip fractures, 615
Fragmented QRS complex, 720
Francisella tularensis, 1309.e1, 776
FRAX calculator, 925
Free insulin, 1809
Free thyroxine index, 1800, 1832
Free triiodothyronine, in Graves' disease, 535
Free urine cortisol, 1837
Free urine hemoglobin, 1838
Freebase overdose, 312, 312t
Fresh frozen plasma, for disseminated intravascular
    coagulation, 398
Friedreich's ataxia, 1203.e2–1203.e4, 501.e3f
Froment's sign, 348.e2
Frontotemporal disorder, 892–893.e1
Frostbite, 502–503.e1, 502f, 503b
Frovatriptan, 546t
Frozen shoulder, 503.e2–503.e3, 503.e2f, 1133.e4t
FS. *See* Felty's syndrome
FSH. *See* Follicle-stimulating hormone
FTA-ABS, serum, 1800
FTT. *See* Failure to thrive
Fulminant hepatic failure, 42, 42b–43b, 578t
Fulminant hepatic necrosis, 42
Fulminant hepatitis, 42
Fumagillin, 831
Functional assays, for heparin-induced thrombocytopenia,
    576.e2t, 576
Functional disorders, abdominal pain and, 1387
Functional dyspepsia, 419
Functional gallbladder disorder, 504–504.e1
Functional impairment, 145.e2
Functional incontinence, 700
Functional syndrome, 1195
Functional tricuspid regurgitation, 1301.e4
Fundi, 489t
Fungal infections
    central nervous system, 813.e2
    histoplasmosis, 619–620.e1, 620.e1f
    in HIV-infected patients
        cutaneous manifestations of, 1458
        hepatic disease and, 1422
        lower gastrointestinal tract disease, 1458
        pulmonary disease, 1459
    lung abscess and, 767
    mucormycosis, 848–848.e1
    myositis with, 1489
    nocardiosis, 901.e1–901.e3, 901.e1f–901.e2f
Fungal keratitis with ulceration, 338.e2, 338.e2f
Fungal meningitis, 813.e2–813.e3, 813.e2t
Fungal vaginitis, 1341–1341.e1
"Fungus balls", 130, 131f
FUO. *See* Fever of undetermined origin
Furosemide
    for ascites, 127, 129.e2f, 129t
    for cor pulmonale, 337
    for hypoaldosteronism, 674
    for idiopathic intracranial hypertension, 690.e5

Furosemide *(Continued)*
for pulmonary edema, 1086
for syndrome of inappropriate antidiuresis, 1237
Furosemide stimulation test, 1801
Furunculosis, 928
Fusion inhibitors, for human immunodeficiency virus, 632–633
Fusospirochetal gingivitis, 518.e2

G

GA. *See* Granuloma annulare
Gabapentin
for burning mouth syndrome, 226.e4
for Charcot-Marie-Tooth syndrome, 275
for chronic pain, 939t
for hot flashes, 629
for neuropathic pain, 898
for postherpetic neuralgia, 609
for transverse myelitis, 1296
Gabapentinoids, 1037
GAD. *See* Generalized anxiety disorder
Gadolinium-associated systemic fibrosis, 888.e3
Gait abnormality, 1445–1449
Gait instability, 145.e2
Galactorrhea, 505–505.e1, 505f, 1070.e1f, 1629.e1–1629.e2
Galantamine, 69t
Gallbladder
perforation of, 290.e1t
sonographic nonvisualization of, 1629.e2
Gallbladder aspiration, for cholecystitis, 287
Gallbladder attack, 287, 287.e1f
Gallbladder disorder, functional, 504–504.e1
Gallbladder dyskinesia, 504
Gallbladder spasm, 504
Gallbladder wall thickening, 1631
Gallium-67 scan, for sarcoidosis, 1138
Gallstone pancreatitis, 944f
Gallstones, 288, 290
Gamma-glutamyl transferase, 1801, 1802
Gamma-glutamyl transpeptidase, 304
Ganciclovir, 355
Ganglia, 505.e2, 505.e2f, 1101f
Ganglion, 505.e2, 505.e2f
Ganglionectomy, 505.e2
Ganglionopathies, 1492
Gardasil, 325
Garden's classification, of femoral neck fractures, 614t, 615.e3f
Gardnerella vaginalis vaginitis, 1345
Gardner's syndrome, 482–483.e1
GAS. *See* Group A streptococci
Gastrectomy, gastric cancer, 507
Gastric adenocarcinoma, 506, 507.e2t
Gastric banding, laparoscopic adjustable, 909.e7f
Gastric cancer, 506–507.e2, 506f, 507t
Gastric contents, aspiration of, 1576.e1, 1576.e1f
Gastric dilatation, 1631
Gastric emptying
delayed, 1445
rapid, 1445
Gastric outlet obstruction, 507.e2f
Gastric prolapse, 909.e7f
Gastric ulcer, 970
malignant, 482f
Gastric volvulus, 609.e3, 1445
Gastrin, serum, 1801
Gastrin stimulation test, 1801
Gastrinoma, 507.e3–507.e6, 507.e3t, 507.e5f–507.e6f
Gastritis, 508
Gastrocnemius-semimembranosus bursa, 170.e2, 229.e5
Gastroenteritis, 509–510.e1
management of, 510f
Salmonella, 1136, 1136t
Gastroesophageal reflux disease, 511–512.e3
in Barrett esophagus, 172, 174
complications of, 609.e3
drug therapy for, 512t
heartburn treatment of, 512.e3f
in hiatal hernia, 609.e2
laryngitis associated with, 739
pathogenesis of, 511f
Gastrointestinal anthrax, 106.e2
Gastrointestinal bicarbonate loss, 1390

Gastrointestinal bleeding, 1629.e2, 1629.e2b
evaluation of, 1816f
lower
differential diagnosis of, 1409
pediatric, 1409
upper
differential diagnosis of, 1410
pediatric, 1410
Gastrointestinal disorders
adverse food reactions and, 1394
pelvic pain in, 1502
Gastrointestinal mucormycosis, 848
Gastrointestinal tract
candidiasis of, 234–235
vascular lesions of, 1539–1540
Gayet-Wernicke encephalopathy, 1376.e3
Gaze-evoked nystagmus, 1696t, 1697f
GBS. *See* Guillain-Barré Syndrome
GCA. *See* Giant cell arteritis
GDM. *See* Gestational diabetes mellitus
Gélineau syndrome, 883
Gemfibrozil, for hyperlipidemia, 654.e4t
Gender dysphoria disorder, 512.e4–512.e7
Gender nonconformity, 512.e4–512.e7
Generalized anxiety disorder, 110–110.e1, 993
Generalized edema, 1617, 1617f
Generalized lymphadenopathy, 1677b, 1677f
Generalized tetanus, 1255.e3
Generalized tonic clonic seizures, 1156
Genetic screening, for hypertrophic cardiomyopathy, 249
Genetics, in autism spectrum disorder, 162
Geniculate ganglion, 1101f
Geniculate herpes, 1101
Genital discharge, female, 1445–1446
Genital herpes, 605, 607t
Genital lesions or ulcers, 1446, 1629–1632, 1814f, 1816b
Genital prolapse, 965–967.e1, 965t, 966b, 967f, 967t
Genital psoriasis, 1081f
Genital sores, 1445–1446
Genital tract, female, calcifications of, on x-ray, 1416
Genital ulcers, 1629–1632, 1814f, 1816b
Genital warts, 1376.e2f, 324, 324f, 1375
Genitalia
ambiguous, 1629.e1f, 1815f
erosions of, 1436
with fever of undetermined origin, 489t
pelvic pain in, 1503
Genitourinary tract candidiasis, 234–235
Gentamicin
for bacterial meningitis, 813
for brucellosis, 220.e3
for granuloma inguinale, 531.e1
for listeriosis, 759
for pelvic abscess, 962
for pelvic inflammatory disease, 964
for tularemia, 1309.e2
Genu varum, 1413
GERD. *See* Gastroesophageal reflux disease
Gerhard's sign, 116
Geriatric abuse, 438f
Geriatric age, blindness in, 1410
Germ cell tumor, 932
German measles, 1133.e7
Germander, 410.e1t–410.e2t
Gestational diabetes mellitus, 377, 513–514.e1, 514.e1t
Gestational hypertension, 1049
Gestational trophoblastic neoplasia, 842t
"Get up and go test", 481
GGT. *See* Gamma-glutamyl transferase
GH. *See* Growth hormone
GHRH. *See* Growth hormone releasing hormone
Giant cell arteritis, 515–516.e1, 515f–516f, 515t, 830t, 1031.e1f, 1351
Giant papillary conjunctivitis, 327t
Giardia duodenalis, 517, 517t
Giardia intestinalis, 517, 517t
Giardiasis, 517–517.e1, 517t
Giemsa banded karyotype, for Turner syndrome, 1312.e2
Gilbert's disease, 518
Gilbert's syndrome, 518, 518t
Gilles de la Tourette syndrome, 1281
Gingivitis, 518.e1
definition of, 518.e1
illustration of, 518.e1f
necrotizing ulcerative, 518.e2

Gingivostomatitis, herpetic, 1214.e3f
Ginkgo biloba
for Alzheimer's disease, 69
for claudication, 309
Gitelman syndrome, 176.e2–176.e3, 176.e3t
Glasgow Coma Scale, 59, 1036
Glatiramer acetate, 856
Glaucoma
angle-closure, 521–521.e1, 521.e1f
narrow-angle, 521, 521.e1f
open-angle, 519–520.e3, 520.e2f–520.e3f, 520f
primary angle-closure, 521–521.e1, 521.e1f
secondary angle-closure, 521
in Sturge-Weber syndrome manifestations of, 1222. e2–1222.e3
Glenohumeral dislocation, 521.e2–521.e3, 521.e2f
Glenohumeral joint
instability of, 1133.e4t
osteoarthrosis of, 1133.e4t
Gliadin, 263
Gliadin antibodies, 1801
Glioblastoma, 213–213.e1
Glioneuronal tumor, 211
Global longitudinal strain imaging, for chemical-induced cardiomyopathy, 242–243
Glomerular basement membrane antibody
description of, 1801
in Goodpasture syndrome, 528
Glomerular filtration rate, 1801, 1801b
for chronic kidney disease, 294–295
classification of, 295t
in contrast-induced acute kidney injury, 333
Glomerulonephritis
acute, 522–524.e1, 523t–524t
antigens identified in, 524t
malignancy associated with, 1446
membranoproliferative, 524t
poststreptococcal, 523t–524t
rapidly progressive, 1446, 523t
renal failure with, 1518
Glomerulopathies, thrombotic, microangiopathic, 1446
Glomerulosclerosis, focal segmental, 1446
Glossitis, 525–525.e1, 525.e1f
Glossodynia, 226.e4, 1446-1447
Glossopyrosis, 226.e4
Glucagon, 79.e2t, 1801
Glucagon-like peptide-1 agonists, 379
Glucagonoma, 507.e3t
Glucocorticoid-induced transcript 1 gene, 140
Glucocorticoids
for alcoholic hepatitis, 60
for Bell's palsy, 184
for blepharitis, 202.e5
for cirrhosis, 306
for congenital adrenal hyperplasia, 325.e3
deficiency of, 1393–1394, 1447
for hypersensitivity pneumonitis, 657–658
for hypocomplementemic urticarial vasculitis, 675
for interstitial lung disease, 717
for lumbar spinal stenosis, 1203
for myxedema coma, 881.e1
for polyarteritis nodosa, 1022
for polymyalgia rheumatica, 1031
for primary angiitis of the central nervous system, 1062
for rhabdomyolysis, 1123
for Still's disease, 54
for Takayasu's arteritis, 1246
for vestibular neuronitis, 1365
Glucosamine, for osteoarthritis, 921
Glucose
fasting, 1801, 1801.e1f, 1801.e2f
mental changes and coma with disorders involving, 1483
postprandial, 1801
urine, 1838
Glucose tolerance test
description of, 1801
for gestational diabetes mellitus, 513
Glucose-6-phosphate dehydrogenase screen, 1802
Glucuronyl transferase, jaundice and, 1473
Glutaric aciduria type 1, 423t
Gluten, celiac disease and, 263
Gluten-free diet
for celiac disease, 264
for dermatitis herpetiformis, 373
Gluten-sensitive enteropathy, 263

Glyburide, 514
Glycemic index, 378
Glyceryl trinitrate, 78.e2
Glycoaldehyde, 826
Glycogen metabolism, disordered, metabolic myopathies and, 1488-1489
Glycohemoglobin, 1802
Glycoprotein IIb/IIIa inhibitors, 34, 873
GM1 gangliosidosis, 423t
GnRH. *See* Gonadotropin-releasing hormone agonists
Goeckerman regimen, 1081
Goiter, 1631, 1631f
  differential diagnosis of, 1447
  evaluation and management of, 1631, 1631.e1, 1631.e1f
  nodular
    evaluation and management of, 1631.e1
    thyroid function test findings in, 1832t
  nontoxic diffuse, 1631.e1
  toxic multinodular, 666
Gold, hyperpigmentation with, 1651t
Gold salt, for Felty's syndrome, 485.e2
Golfer's elbow, 458.e10
Golimumab, for enteropathic arthritis, 456
Gonadal dysgenesis, 1066
Gonadotropin
  deficiency of, 685
  delayed puberty and, 1512
Gonadotropin-releasing hormone
  for paraphilic disorders, 955.e4
  for uterine fibroids, 1332
Gonadotropin-releasing hormone agonists
  for endometriosis, 453
  for hirsutism, 618
  for premenstrual dysphoric disorder, 1053.e2
Gonococcal bartholinitis, 526
Gonococcal cervicitis, 526
Gonococcal urethritis, 526, 526f, 1318-1318.e1
Gonococcal vulvovaginitis, 526
Gonorrhea, 526-527.e1, 963-964.e1
  purulent urethral discharge, 526f
  skin lesions, 527f
Goodpasture syndrome, 523t, 528-528.e1, 528f, 528t, 692t
Goodsall's rule, 102
"Gorlin sign", 431.e2, 431.e3f
Gorlin's syndrome, 211
Gottron's papules, 706.e1f
Gout, 529-530.e3
  episcleritis and, 463.e5f
  hyperuricemia and, 529, 670, 671.e1f
  pseudogout, 1078-1079.e3, 1078t, 1079.e1b, 1079.e1f-1079.e3f, 1079b, 1079f
  treatment of, 530t
Gout flares, 529t
Gouty arthritis, 670, 671.e1f
Gouty kidney, 718
Gower's maneuver, 861f
GPC. *See* Giant papillary conjunctivitis
Graham Steell murmur, 836
Grand mal seizures, 1156
Granisetron, 276
Granular kidney, 718
Granulation tissue-type hemangioma, 1100.e4
Granulocyte colony-stimulating factor, 485.e2
Granulocyte-macrophage colony-stimulating factor, 485.e2
Granuloma, 1632
  hepatic, 1454
  noninfectious, 1632f
Granuloma annulare, 531, 531f
Granuloma inguinale, 529-530.e3, 531.e1, 531.e1f
Granuloma pyogenicum, 1100.e4
Granulomatosis, Wegener's, 532-534.e1, 532f-534f, 534.e1f
Granulomatosis infantisepticum, 759
Granulomatosis with polyangiitis, 458.e4-458.e5, 532-534.e1, 532f-534f, 532t, 534.e1f, 1350
Granulomatous arthritis, 534.e2
Granulomatous dermatitides, 1447, 1632t
Granulomatous disorders, 1447
Granulomatous hepatitis, drug-induced, 410.e3t
Granulomatous liver disease, 1448
Granulomatous mastitis, 796
Granulomatous mediastinitis, 802
Granulomatous uveitis, 1334
Granulomatous vasculitis, 1540
Granulosa cell tumor, 1046t
Graves' disease, 535-536.e1, 535f, 1832t
Graves' ophthalmopathy, 535f-536f, 536f

Graves' orbitopathy, 666, 667.e2f
Gray, 1100.e12
Great vessel injury, 1753b
Greater celandine, 410.e1t-410.e2t
Greater occipital nerve block, for migraine headache, 546
Greater trochanter fracture, 614f
Greater trochanteric bursitis, 1303, 1303f
Greater trochanteric pain syndrome, 1303, 1303f
Green tea leaf extract, 410.e1t-410.e2t
Green urine, 1448
Grey Turner's sign, 943
Grief, complicated or prolonged, 536.e2
Griseofulvin, for tinea capitis, 66, 1269
Groin lump, 1448
Groin masses, 1448
Groin pain, 1448, 1448-1449
Groin ringworm, 1272
Ground-glass opacity
  in hypersensitivity pneumonitis, 658, 658f
  in *Pneumocystis jiroveci* pneumonia, 1014.e1f
Group A streptococci, 989
Group I pulmonary arterial hypertension, 1092
Growth failure, 478
Growth hormone, 1802
  in acromegaly, 24.e8
  deficiency of, 685, 687
Growth hormone releasing hormone, 1802
Growth hormone suppression test, 1802
GSLI. *See* Global longitudinal strain imaging, for chemical-induced cardiomyopathy
GTPS. *See* Greater trochanteric pain syndrome
GU. *See* Gastric ulcer
Guaifenesin
  for acute bronchitis, 28
  for chronic obstructive pulmonary disease, 302
  for laryngitis, 739
  in pregnancy, 934.e2t
Guanfacine
  for attention deficit hyperactivity disorder, 161
  for Tourette's syndrome, 1282
Guanidine hydrochloride, 738.e2
Guanylate cyclase stimulators, 1094
Guar, for dumping syndrome, 412.e3
Guillain-Barré syndrome, 501, 537-538.e1, 1493
Gustatory rhinitis, 904
Gut endocrine tumors, 1370.e2t
Guttate psoriasis, 1081f
Gynecologic disorders, 1502
Gynecomastia, 539-539.e2, 539.e1t, 539f, 1070.e1f-1070.e2f, 1449
Gyromitra poisoning, 862, 862.e1t

H

HACE. *See* High-altitude cerebral edema
HAE. *See* Hereditary angioedema
Haemophilus influenzae type B
  conjugate vaccine for
    catch-up schedule, 1860t-1864t
    contraindication and precautions, 1868t-1869t
    indicated for adults based on medical and other indications, 1878t-1881t
    recommended immunization schedule, 1860t-1864t, 1878t-1881t
  description of, 463
Hair
  hirsutism, 616-618.e1, 616f-617f, 617b
  loss of, 64
    drug-induced, 1396
  premature graying of scalp, 1509
Hairy cell, 1816t
Hairy cell leukemia, 754.e2-754.e4, 754.e3f-754.e4f, 754.e4t-754.e4t
  abnormal lymphocytes with, 1816t
  diagnostic features of, 754.e3t
Hairy leukoplakia, 1214
HAIs. *See* Healthcare-associated infections
Halitosis, 1414, 1449-1469, 1636.e1
Haloperidol
  for delirium, 366
  for Tourette's syndrome, 1282
HAM test, 1802-1809
Hamartomatous polyp, 985
Hampton's hump, 1089
HAND. *See* HIV-associated neurocognitive disorder

Hand pain
  causes of, 1771
  swelling and, 1638-1639
Hand-foot-mouth disease, 540-540.e1, 540.e1f
Hands, rash with edema of, 1440
Hand-Schüller-Christian disease, 618.e2
Hansen's disease, 742.e5-742.e7, 742.e5f-742.e6f
Hantavirus cardiopulmonary syndrome, 540.e2, 540.e2b
Hantavirus pulmonary syndrome, 540.e2-540.e3, 540.e2b
HAPE. *See* High-altitude pulmonary edema
Haptoglobin, serum, 1802
Hashimoto's thyroiditis, 690, 1268-1268.e1
HAV. *See* Hepatitis A virus
HAV total antibody, 1804
HAV-IGM antibody, 1804
Hawkins-Kennedy sign, 1133.e2-1133.e3
Hay fever, 63
HBAT. *See* Heptavalent botulinum antitoxin
HBOC. *See* Hereditary breast and ovarian cancer syndrome
HBsAg, 584, 1891t
HBsAg-positive source, postexposure prophylaxis for, 1877t
HBV. *See* Hepatitis B virus
HCC. *See* Hepatocellular carcinoma
hCG. *See* Human chorionic gonadotropin
HCL. *See* Hairy cell leukemia
HCPS. *See* Hantavirus cardiopulmonary syndrome
HCQ. *See* Hydroxychloroquine
HCTZ. *See* Hydrochlorothiazide
HCV. *See* Hepatitis C virus
HDV. *See* Hepatitis D virus
HDV-Ab. *See* Hepatitis D antibody
HDV-Ag. *See* Hepatitis D antigen
Head
  entrapment of, in breech birth, 218.e8
  with fever of undetermined origin, 489t
  trauma to, 187t
Head and neck cancer, 541, 738.e4, 915
Head and neck squamous cell carcinoma, 541-542.e2, 541f-542f, 542.e1f
Head injury, 1297, 1297b, 1298t, 1299b, 1299f
Head masses, soft tissue, 1659
Head roll test, for benign paroxysmal positional vertigo, 185
Headaches
  acute, 1639-1640
  in benign brain neoplasms, 211
  in cavernous sinus thrombosis, 261
  chronic, 1658
  cluster, 543-544.e1, 1644-1645
  combined tension-migraine, 1648
  differential diagnosis of, 1449
  facial pain and, 1641-1643
  high-altitude, 612, 613.e1t
  migraine, 545-547.e1, 1643-1644
    combined tension-migraine, 1648
    therapy for, 546t
  in postconcussive syndrome, 1035
  in subarachnoid hemorrhage, 1225
  tension-type, 548-548.e1
Head-up tilt test, 1044.e3f, 1234, 1234f
Health examination, periodic, 1849-1858
  adolescents, 1872
  adult, 1872
  age-specific charts of, 1849t, 1851t, 1853t, 1855t, 1857t, 1858t
  of pregnant women, 1857t
Healthcare-associated infections, 548.e2-548.e9
Hearing loss, 931.e2-931.e3, 931.e2f, 931.e2t, 1633, 1633b, 1633-1664
  acute, 1661-1662
  evaluation of, 1633f
  lesions causing, 1817t
  vertigo with and without, 185b, 187t
Heart
  calcification of, on x-ray, 1589.e1-1589.e2
  candidal infections of, 236
  dysfunction of, in AIDS-infected patients, 24.e7f
  enlargement of, 1417
  with fever of undetermined origin, 489t
Heart attack, 867
Heart block
  complete, 159, 549-550.e1, 549f, 550.e1t, 550t
  second-degree, 551-552
Heart catheterization
  for cor pulmonale, 336
  for ventricular septal defect, 1359

Heart disease. *See also* Cardiac disease
   risk factors for, 645t
   valvular, 1539
Heart failure, 553–560.e2
   acute, 1451
   acute decompensated, 553–555, 557–560
   algorithm for, 555f
   cardiac transplantation for, 560
   chronic, 1451
   classification of, 553
   clinical presentation of, 554–555
   compensatory mechanisms in, 553t
   congenital causes of, 1451
   congestive, 1425
   definition of, 553
   demographics of, 554
   diagnosis of, 555–557
   diastolic, 553, 554t
   epidemiology of, 554
   etiology of, 555
   evaluation of, 555f
   exercise for, 557
   hospitalization for, 560
   iron deficiency in, 88
   left ventricular assist device for, 560
   left ventricular failure as cause of, 555
   left-sided, 553
   mortality in, 560
   nonpharmacologic treatment of, 557
   pathogenic causes of, 1451-1452
      high-output states as, 1452
      impaired diastolic function as (restricted filling,
         increased stiffness), 1452
      impaired systolic (contractile) function as,
         1451-1452
      mechanical abnormalities as, 1452
      pulmonary heart disease as, 1452
      rate and rhythm disorders as, 1452
   physical findings of, 554–555
   in pregnancy, 1452
   preserved ejection fraction with, 553
   preserved left ventricular ejection fraction with,
      1663–1664
   preserved systolic function with, 560
   reduced ejection fraction with, 553
   right ventricular failure as cause of, 555
   right-sided, 553
   stages of, 556f
   sudden cardiac death in, 560
   systolic, 553, 554t, 560
   treatment of, 557–560
Heart murmur
   arthritis and, 1403
   fever and rash with, 1440
Heart sounds, 836
Heart transplantation
   for dilated cardiomyopathy, 245
   for heart failure, 560
   for myocarditis, 877
Heartburn
   differential diagnosis of, 1662–1663
   treatment of, 512.e3f
Heat exhaustion, 561–562.e1, 561t–562t, 562.e1t, 562b
Heat illness, 561
Heat stroke, 561–562.e1, 561t–562t, 562b, 562.e1f, 562.e1t,
   896.e1t, 1452
Heberden's nodes, 921, 922.e4f
Heel pain, 1452
   plantar, 1452, 1704.e1
   posterior, 1705–1706
Heel spur syndrome, 1003
Heerfordt syndrome, 1137
Helicobacter pylori
   gastritis, 506, 508
   infection caused by, 563–564.e1, 563f
   peptic ulcer disease caused by, 970–971
   proton pump inhibitors for, 564, 971
   screening for, 173
   serology, stool antigen, 1802
   treatment of, 971
HELLP syndrome, 564.e2–564.e3, 564.e2b, 564.e3f, 1049
Helminthic infections
   hookworms, 627–627.e1, 627f
   syndromes associated with, 350.e5t
   tapeworms, 1249–1250.e1, 1249t, 1250f
Hemangiomas, 165.e1t

Hemarthrosis
   differential diagnosis of, 1452
   in hemophilia, 569f, 570t
   knee, 569f, 570t
Hematemesis, 1452
Hematochezia, 1635.e1, 1635.e1f
Hematocrit, 1802
Hematologic disorders
   blindness caused by, 1411
   deep vein thrombosis and, 357
   stroke with, 1529
Hematologic paraneoplastic syndromes, 1500
Hematologic vasculitis, leg ulcers with, 1476
Hematoma
   epidural, 461–462.e1, 462b, 461f–462f
   extradural, 461, 462f
Hematopoietic stem cell transplantation, allogeneic
   for pure red cell aplasia, 1096.e3
   for sickle cell disease, 1181
Hematospermia, 435
Hematuria, 1504, 1839t
   asymptomatic, 1636, 1636f
   based on age and sex, 1453
   in children, 1453
   differential diagnosis of, 1452-1453
   in hemophilia, 570t
   in pediatric patients, 1636.e1, 1636.e1–1637, 1636.e1f
Hemidiaphragm
   elevated, 1433
   opacification on x-ray, 1495
Hemiparesis, 1222.e2, 1453
Hemiplegia
   alternating, of childhood, 423t
   differential diagnosis of, 1453
Hemochromatosis, 565–566.e1, 565f–566f, 566t, 1799t
Hemodialysis, 41, 827
Hemoglobin, 1803
   in abruptio placentae, 9
   carbon monoxide and, 238
   urine, free, 1838
Hemoglobin A$_{1C}$, 1803
Hemoglobin electrophoresis, 1803, 1803t
Hemoglobin H, 1803, 1803t
Hemoglobin S, 1179
Hemoglobin S disease, 1179
Hemoglobinopathies, 1803t
Hemoglobinuria, 1453, 1504, 1839t
Hemolysis, 564.e2
   differential diagnosis of, 1453
   drugs promoting, 1399
   elevated liver function, and low platelet count. *See* HELLP
      syndrome
   intravascular, 1453
   mechanical, 1453
Hemolytic anemia, 1096.e2
   autoimmune, 82–84.e2, 82t, 83f, 84.e1f–84.e2f, 84t,
      958.e3t
Hemolytic streptococcal gangrene, 887
Hemolytic transfusion reaction, 1291–1292, 1291t
Hemolytic-uremic syndrome, 567–568.e1
Hemoperitoneum, 1453
Hemophagocytic lymphohistiocytosis, 618.e2, 618.e3t
Hemophilia, 569–570.e1, 569f, 570t
Hemophilia A, 569–570.e1, 569f, 570t
Hemophilia B, 569–570.e1, 569f, 570t
Hemophilic arthropathy, 569f
Hemoptysis, 571–572.e1, 836, 1453–1454, 1638
   causes of, 1514
   evaluation of, 1638f
Hemorrhage. *See also* Bleeding
   alveolar, 1396–1397
   diffuse pulmonary syndromes, 1514
   diverticular, 403
   in HELLP syndrome, 564.e3
   intracerebral, 1471
   pelvic pain with, 1503
   petechial, 1890t
   postpartum, 1040–1041.e1, 1040t, 1041b, 1041f
   pulmonary, 1514
   retinal, 1116.e4–1116.e5, 1116.e4f, 1171–1171.e1,
      1171.e1f
   subarachnoid, 1219, 1224–1225.e2, 1224b, 1225.e2t,
      1225f
   subdural, 1227
   vaginal, 1335
   variceal, 475

Hemorrhage fevers, 1378.e2t
Hemorrhagic cystitis, 1454
Hemorrhagic epiploitis, 463.e3
Hemorrhagic gastritis, 508
Hemorrhagic stroke, 1219–1220.e1, 1219f, 1220b
Hemorrhoidopexy, stapled, 572.e4
Hemorrhoids, 572.e2–572.e4, 572.e2f–572.e3f, 572.e2t
Hemosiderin, urine, 1838
Henoch-Schönlein purpura, 573–574.e1, 573f, 574t, 830t,
   1245t, 1350, 1351.e2t
Heparin. *See also* Low-molecular-weight heparin;
      Unfractionated heparin
   for acute coronary syndrome, 34
   for antiphospholipid antibody syndrome, 109
   for Behçet's disease, 182.e3
   for Budd-Chiari syndrome, 224
   for disseminated intravascular coagulation, 398
   for pulmonary embolism, 1090, 1091.e3t
   for Raynaud's phenomenon, 1104
   for transient ischemic attack, 1294
Heparin-associated immune thrombocytopenia, 575
Heparin-induced thrombocytopenia
   antibodies for, 1804
   characteristics of, 575–576.e2, 575t, 576.e1f, 576.e2t
Heparin-induced thrombocytopenia and thrombosis, 575
Hepatic abscess, 289f, 760
Hepatic coma, 577
Hepatic cyst disease, 427t
Hepatic cysts, 1454
Hepatic disease and disorders
   in human immunodeficiency virus infection, 1458
   splenomegaly with, 1528
Hepatic echinococcal cysts, 428t
Hepatic encephalopathy, 577–579.e1, 577t–578t, 579b
Hepatic granulomas, 1454
Hepatic jaundice, neonatal, 1473
Hepatic mass, 1639, 1639f
Hepatic necrosis, 726
Hepatic nephropathy, 600
Hepatic vein thrombosis, 223
Hepatitis
   acute, 1454
   alcoholic, 59–60.e1, 60f, 1033t
   autoimmune, 595–596.e1, 595t
   in children, 1454-1455
   chronic
      active, 1807t
      differential diagnosis of, 1449
   ischemic, 726–726.e1, 726.e1f, 726t
   viral, 582f, 1640, 1640b, 1640f
Hepatitis A antibody, 1804, 1804f
Hepatitis A immune globulin, 1892t
Hepatitis A vaccine
   for adults, 1882t
   catch-up schedule, 1859, 1860t–1864t
   contraindications and precautions, 1868t–1869t
   for health care workers, 1884t–1886t
   indications for, 1878t–1881t
   for international travel, 1888t
   licensed dosages of, 1892t
   during pregnancy, 1883t
   recommended intervals between administration, 1867t
   recommended schedule for, 1860t–1864t, 1878t–1881t
Hepatitis A virus, 580–581.e1, 581f, 637t–638t, 1804
Hepatitis B hyperimmune globulin, 584
Hepatitis B surface antigen (HBsAg), 1804, 59
Hepatitis B vaccine
   for adults, 1882t, 1889
   adults recommended to receive, 1877t
   catch-up schedule, 1859, 1860t–1864t
   conditions misperceived as contraindications to,
      1870t–1871t
   contraindication and precautions, 1868t–1869t
   doses of, 1890t
   for health care workers, 1884t–1886t
   indications for, 1878t–1881t
   for international travel, 1888t
   for pediatric oncology patients, 1874T
   during pregnancy, 1883T
   recommendations and implementation strategies for, 1889
   recommended intervals between administration, 1867t
   schedule for, 1860t–1864t, 1877t, 1878t–1881t, 1889b
Hepatitis B virus, 582–585.e1, 582f–583f, 583t, 585f, 585t,
   592f, 637t–638t, 1804, 1804t, 1805t
   post-exposure protection, 1909, 1909t
   serologic test results for, 1891t

Hepatitis C RNA, 1805
Hepatitis C testing, 1907
Hepatitis C virus
    analytic framework for guiding, 1908f
    cirrhosis caused by, 586, 586t
    human immunodeficiency virus and, 630
    infection caused by, 588–589.e1, 587t, 1805, 1805f
    prevention and control of, 1907
Hepatitis D antibody, 1806
    IgM, 1806f
    total, 1806, 1806f
Hepatitis D antigen, 1806, 1806f
Hepatitis D virus, 590–592.e1
    carriers of, 591b
    clinical presentation of, 590
    definition of, 590
    diagnosis of, 590–591, 592t
    epidemiology of, 590, 590f
    etiology of, 590
    genotypes of, 591t
    hepatitis B virus and, 592f
    infection caused by, 1805
    physical findings in, 590
    prevalence of, 590, 592.e1f
    risk factors for, 590
    treatment of, 591
Hepatitis E virus, 590f, 593–594.e1, 593f, 593t–594t, 594b
Hepatobiliary disorders, hepatic granulomas from, 1454
Hepatocellular carcinoma
    characteristics of, 597–598.e1, 597f–598t, 598.e1f, 598t
    liver transplantation for, 589, 762–763.e1
Hepatoerythropoietic porphyria, 1736.e1t
Hepatoma, 597f
Hepatomegaly
    characteristics of, 1641, 1641–1642, 1641f
    differential diagnosis of, 1455
    fever and rash with, 1440
    in hepatitis B, 582
    by shape of liver, 1455
    splenomegaly and, 1527
Hepatopulmonary syndrome, 599–599.e1, 599.e1f
Hepatorenal failure, 600
Hepatorenal syndrome, 600–601.e1, 600f, 600t–601t, 1033
Hepatosplenic candidiasis, 236
Hepatosplenic schistosomiasis, 1143.e1
Hepatosplenomegaly, 1527
    fever and rash with, 1440
Hepatotoxicity, 11
Hepcidin, 85–86
Heptavalent botulinum antitoxin, 206
Herbalife, 410.e1t–410.e2t
Hereditary amyloidosis, 76.e3
Hereditary angioedema, 97
Hereditary autoinflammatory syndromes, recurrent or
    periodic fever and, 1442
Hereditary autonomic neuropathies, 1493
Hereditary breast and ovarian cancer syndrome, 602–604.
    e1, 602f
Hereditary cancer syndrome, 602
Hereditary cataracts, 259.e6
Hereditary coproporphyria, 1736.e1t
Hereditary disorders, paraparesis with, 1501
Hereditary hemochromatosis, 565, 565f, 566t, 1799t
Hereditary hemorrhagic telangiectasia, 920.e2
Hereditary iron overload, 1471
Hereditary motor and sensory neuropathy, 275, 275f,
    900–901
Hereditary neuropathy, 900–901
Hereditary neuropathy with liability to pressure-sensitive
    palsies, 900–901
Hereditary nonpolyposis colorectal cancer, 314, 602, 782,
    985t
Hereditary site-specific colon cancer, 782
Heritable pulmonary arterial hypertension, 1092
Hermaphroditism
    differential diagnosis of, 1455
    female pseudohermaphroditism, 1511, 1455
    male pseudohermaphroditism, 1511, 1455
    true, 1455
Her-2/neu, 1806
Hernia
    in abdominal wall masses, 1390
    hiatal, 609.e2–609.e4, 609.e2f–609.e3f
    inguinal, 687.e1, 1347.e2t
Herpangina, 604.e2, 604.e2f
Herpes digitalis, 605

Herpes encephalitis, 443.e1f
Herpes gladiatorum, 605, 606
Herpes iris, 1213
Herpes labialis, 605
Herpes simplex, 605–607.e1, 605f, 607t, 607.e1f, 814
Herpes simplex encephalitis, 443t
Herpes simplex virus, 18t–24t, 1806
Herpes zoster, 608–609.e1, 608f
    postherpetic neuralgia, 1037–1038.e1, 1038f
    Ramsay Hunt syndrome, 1101–1101.e1, 1101f
Herpes zoster oticus, 1101
Herpetic geniculate ganglionitis, 1101
Herpetic gingivostomatitis, 1214.e3f
Herpetic whitlow, 607t
Herpetiformis, dermatitis, 1807t
Hertoghe sign, 148f
HES. *See* Hypereosinophilic syndrome
Heterophil antibody, 1806
Heterophil negative, atypical lymphocytosis, 1407
Heterophil-negative mononucleosis, 355
Heterosexuals, high-risk, 1890t
Heterotropia, 1214.e4
Heterozygote protein C deficiency, 1825t
Heterozygote protein S deficiency, 1825t
HEV. *See* Hepatitis E virus
HF. *See* Heart failure; Hot flashes
HFE gene testing, 565–566
HFE screen for hereditary hemochromatosis, 1806
HFMD. *See* Hand-foot-mouth disease
HGA. *See* Human granulocytic anaplasmosis
HGE. *See* Human granulocytic ehrlichiosis
HHS. *See* Hyperosmolar hyperglycemic syndrome
HHT. *See* Hereditary hemorrhagic telangiectasia
HHV-6. *See* Human herpesvirus-6
HHV-7. *See* Human herpesvirus-7
HHV-8. *See* Human herpesvirus-8
Hiatal hernia, 609.e2–609.e4, 609.e2f–609.e3f
Hiatus hernia, 609.e2
Hiccups
    persistent or chronic, 1456
    transient, 1456
Hidradenitis suppurativa, 610–611.e1, 610f
High anion gap acidosis, 1401
High blood pressure, 660
High-altitude cerebral edema, 612–613.e2, 613.e1t, 613.
    e2b, 613b
High-altitude pulmonary edema, 612–613.e2, 613.e1f, 613.
    e1t, 613.e2b, 613b
High-altitude sickness, 612–613.e2, 613.e1t, 613.e2b, 613b
High-density lipoprotein, 647b
High-density lipoprotein cholesterol, 1806
High-grade squamous intraepithelial lesion, 269
High-output states, heart failure and, 1452
High-risk conditions
    with PC13 and PPSV23, vaccination of persons with,
        recommended immunization schedule, 1860t–1864t
    vaccination of persons with, recommended immunization
        schedule, 1860t–1864t
High-risk populations, interventions for
    ages 65 and older, 1855t
    ages 11 to 24 years, 1851t
    ages 25 to 64 years, 1853t
    birth to 10 years, 1849t
    pregnant women, 1857t
High-voltage electrical injuries, lightning injury compared
    with, 439t
Hilar lymph node enlargement, 1456
Hill's sign, 116
Hip
    aseptic necrosis of, 167f
    fracture of, 614–615.e3, 614f–615f, 614t, 615.e3f
Hip disease, in juvenile idiopathic arthritis, 733f
Hip pain
    in adolescence, 1456
    in adulthood, 1457
    in childhood, 1456
    in different age groups, 1456-1457
    differential diagnosis of, 1456
    in joint, 1474
    in old age, 1457
    without fracture, 1457
Hippel-Lindau syndrome, 1370.e2
Hirschberg test, 1214.e4, 1214.e6f
Hirsutism, 616–618.e1, 616f–617f, 617b, 1026, 1457
Histiocytosis X, 618.e2–618.e4, 618.e3f, 618.e3t, 692t
Histoplasma capsulatum, 619–620.e1, 636t–638t, 803

Histoplasmoma, 619
Histoplasmosis
    in AIDS-infected patients, 18t–24t
    characteristics of, 619–620.e1, 620.e1f
Histrionic personality disorder, 620.e2–620.e3
HIT. *See* Heparin-induced thrombocytopenia
HITT. *See* Heparin-induced thrombocytopenia and thrombosis
HIV cognitive dysfunction, 621–622.e1, 621f, 621t
HIV dementia, 621
HIV-1 encephalopathy, 621
HIV-associated dementia, 621
HIV-associated neurocognitive disorder, 621
Hives, 1326, 1327.e1f–1327.e2f, 1327f
HLA-DQ2, 264
HLA-DQ8, 264
HME. *See* Human monocytic ehrlichiosis
HMG-CoA reductase inhibitors
    for claudication, 308–309
    for hyperlipidemia, 654.e4t
    lipoprotein metabolism affected by, 647.e1t
HMSN. *See* Hereditary motor and sensory neuropathy
H1N1, 709.e2
H5N1, 709.e2, 707
HNC. *See* Head and neck cancer
HNPCC. *See* Hereditary nonpolyposis colorectal cancer
HNPP. *See* Hereditary neuropathy with liability to pressure-
    sensitive palsies
HNSCC. *See* Head and neck squamous cell carcinoma
HOA. *See* Hypertrophic osteoarthropathy
Hoarding disorder, 622.e2–622.e4
Hoarseness, 1460
HOCM. *See* Hypertrophic obstructive cardiomyopathy
Hodgkin lymphoma, 623–626.e2
    chemotherapy for, 624–626
    clinical presentation of, 623
    complications of, 626t
    Cotswolds staging of, 624t
    definition of, 623
    demographics of, 623
    diagnosis of, 623–624
    epidemiology of, 623
    imaging of, 623–624, 625f
    morphology of, 626.e1f–626.e2f
    neoplasms secondary to, 626t
    nodular sclerosis, 623–624, 626.e1f–626.e2f
    physical findings of, 623
    prognostic factors for, 626t
    staging of, 623, 624b
    treatment of, 624–625, 625t–626t
Hollenhorst plaque, 727f
Holter monitor, for hypertrophic cardiomyopathy, 247
Holt-Oram syndrome, 156
Homatropine
    for corneal abrasion, 338
    for uveitis, 1334
Homocysteine, plasma, 1806
Hookworm, 126.e1t, 627–627.e1, 627f
Hookworm folliculitis, 350.e5
Hookworm-related cutaneous larva migrans, 350.e5, 350.e5f
Hordeolum, 1223–1223.e1, 1223f
Hormonal implants, for contraception, 332
Hormone replacement therapy. *See also* Estrogen
        replacement therapy
    for dyspareunia, 417
    for estrogen-deficient vaginitis, 1340
    for invasive breast cancer, 216
    for menopause, 815–816, 816b
Hormone-induced rhinitis, 905
Horner's syndrome
    characteristics of, 628–628.e1, 628.e1f, 628f, 769
    neuroblastoma with, 1571f
Horse chestnut seed extract, for chronic venous insufficiency,
    1353
Horton's disease, 515, 515f, 515t
Horton's headache, 543
Hospital addiction syndrome, 477
Hospital-acquired aspiration pneumonia, 1006–1006.e1
Hospital-acquired methicillin-resistant *Staphylococcus
    aureus*, 828
Hospital-associated fever, 1440
Hospitalization
    for heart failure, 560
    for hyperparathyroidism, 656
Hot flashes, 629–629.e1
"Hot tub" folliculitis, 495
Hot tub lung, 657

Housemaid's knee, 229.e5
HP. *See* Hypersensitivity pneumonitis
HPNCC. *See* Hereditary nonpolyposis colorectal cancer
HPS. *See* Hepatopulmonary syndrome
HPV. *See* Human papillomavirus
HPV4. *See* Quadrivalent HPV vaccine
HRS. *See* Hepatorenal syndrome
HSDD. *See* Hypoactive sexual desire disorder
HSIL. *See* High-grade squamous intraepithelial lesion
HSP. *See* Henoch-Schönlein purpura
HSV. *See* Herpes simplex virus
HTGP. *See* Hypertriglyceridemic pancreatitis
HTN. *See* Hypertension
Human bites, 192–193.e1, 193b, 193t
Human chorionic gonadotropin, 1807
    for cryptorchidism, 347.e2
    level, for galactorrhea, 505
    tumors secreting, 539.e1t
Human granulocytic anaplasmosis, 432, 433t
Human granulocytic ehrlichiosis, 432, 433t
Human herpesvirus-6, 1133
Human herpesvirus-8, 1807
Human immunodeficiency virus, 630–638.e1. *See also*
    Acquired immunodeficiency syndrome
    acute, 630
    acute kidney injury and, 1391
    acutely ill patient with, 24.e2f
    in adolescents, 633t
    anorectal lesions in, 1457
    antiretroviral therapy for, 622, 632–635, 635t–636t, 1900t
    cardiac dysfunction in, 24.e7f
    CD4 count in, 631
    central nervous system infection in, 24.e5f
    chest radiographic abnormalities in, 1457
    chronic, 630, 632–635
    clinical presentation of, 630
    cognitive dysfunction and impairment caused by, 1457,
        621–622.e1, 621f, 621t
    congenital, 630
    cutaneous manifestations of, 1458
    definition of, 630
    demographics of, 630
    diagnosis of, 631–632
    diarrhea in, 24.e1f
    differential diagnosis of, 631
    enzyme-linked immunosorbent assay for, 631–632
    epidemiology of, 630
    esophageal disease in, 1458
    etiology of, 630
    exposure to
        estimated per-act risk, 1899t
        expert consultation, 1902b
        postexposure prophylaxis for, 637, 1900t, 1902b
        preexposure prophylaxis for, 637
    gastrointestinal pathogens associated with, 1606.e1t
    genetics of, 630
    hepatic disease and, 1458
    hepatitis C and, 630
    Kaposi's sarcoma in, 732–734.e2, 735.e1f
    laboratory tests for, 631–632
    lower gastrointestinal tract disease and, 1458
    musculoskeletal disorders associated with, 1458–1459
    myopathies associated with, 1488
    neonatal, 630
    neurocognitive deficits caused by, 893
    neuromuscular syndromes in, 632t
    ocular manifestations of, 1658
    opportunistic infections associated with, 636t–638t
    physical findings in, 630
    plasma RNA testing, 1809t
    Pneumocystis jiroveci pneumonia in, 17
    postexposure prophylaxis for, 637, 1900t, 1902b
    preexposure prophylaxis for, 637
    in pregnancy, 635
    prevention of, 637
    pulmonary disease in, 1459
    Reiter's syndrome and, 1105
    respiratory complaints in, 24.e3f–24.e4f
    risk factors for, 630, 632t
    screening for, 1897
        pregnant women and infants, 1897
        repeat, 1897
    serologic tests for, 631
    staging of, 630t, 634t
    structure of, 631f
    testing for, 1897

Human immunodeficiency virus *(Continued)*
    consent and pretest information, 1897
    diagnostic, 1897
    treatment of, 632–637, 635t
    type 1 (HIV-1)
        antibody, 1807
        antigen, 1807
        tests in infection, 1808f
        viral load, 1809
        vaccinations, 1887t, 637b
        viral structure of, 631f
        Western blot for, 1808f
        WHO immunologic classification for, 632t
        workup for, 631
Human leukocyte antigen, 471, 1807t
Human metapneumovirus, 27t
Human monocytic ehrlichiosis, 432, 433t, 434.e1f, 434.
    e1t, 434f
Human papillomavirus, 1809
    cervical cancer caused by, 267–268
    condyloma acuminatum and, 324, 324f
    in human immunodeficiency virus, 637t–638t
    vaccine for, 325, 1376
        catch-up schedule, 1859, 1859t
        conditions misperceived as contraindications to,
            1870t–1871t
        contraindications and precautions, 1868t–1869t
        indications for, 1878t–1881t, 1882
        during pregnancy, 1883t
        recommended schedule, 1860t–1864t, 1878t–1881t
    warts, 1375
Human tetanus immunoglobulin, 1255.e4
Humoral hypercalcemia of malignancy, 954
Hunner's ulcers, 714
Hunt and Hess classification, for subarachnoid hemorrhage,
    1224b
Huntington's chorea, 639
Huntington's disease, 423t, 639–639.e1, 639t, 893
    chorea and, 290.e5
    PCR, 1809
HUS. *See* Hemolytic-uremic syndrome
HUV. *See* Hypocomplementemic urticarial vasculitis
Hyaluronan, 921
Hybrid capture 2 DNA test, 271
Hydatid disease, 427, 427f–428f, 428.e1f, 428t
Hydralazine
    granulomatous hepatitis caused by, 410.e3t
    for hypertension, 664t
    isosorbide dinitrate and, 559
    for preeclampsia, 1051
Hydration, for tumor lysis syndrome prevention, 1310
Hydrocele, 640, 640f, 687.e1, 1347.e2t
Hydrocephalus
    differential diagnosis of, 1460
    normal pressure, 641–642.e1, 641f, 642.e1f
Hydrochlorothiazide, 375
Hydrocodone, 940.e3t, 940t
Hydrocolloids, for venous ulcers, 1354
Hydrocortisone
    for adrenal insufficiency, 53
    for anaphylaxis, 79.e2t
    for atopic dermatitis, 148
    for congenital adrenal hyperplasia, 325.e3
    for De Quervain's tenosynovitis, 356
    for thyrotoxic storm, 1268.e2
Hydrogels (DuoDerm hydrogel), for venous ulcers, 1354
Hydrogen breath test, 1833t
Hydromorphone, 940.e3t, 940t
Hydronephrosis, 643–644.e1, 643f, 644.e1f
Hydroperitoneum, 127
Hydroperitonia, 127
Hydrophobia, 1100.e10
Hydropneumothorax, 1018f
Hydrops abdominis, 127
Hydroquinone
    hyperpigmentation with, 1651t–1652t
    for vitiligo, 1370
Hydroxocobalamin, 239
Hydroxyapatite deposition, 179
τ-Hydroxybutyrate, 1716t–1719t
Hydroxychloroquine
    for chronic urticaria, 1329
    for inflammatory myopathies, 705
    for Q fever, 1100.e7
    for sarcoidosis, 1138
    for Sjögren's syndrome, 1187

Hydroxychloroquine sulfate
    for antiphospholipid antibody syndrome, 109
    for discoid lupus erythematosus, 396
    for Whipple's disease, 1376.e8
Hydroxycut, 410.e1t–410.e2t
5-Hydroxyindoleacetic acid, 239.e2
    urine, 1838, 1839t
11ß-Hydroxylase deficiency, 325.e2, 325.e2f, 325.e4t
17-Hydroxylase deficiency, 325.e2, 325.e2f, 325.e4t
21-Hydroxylase deficiency, 325.e2, 325.e2f, 325.e4t
17α-Hydroxyprogesterone
    for cervical insufficiency, 271.e2
    for congenital adrenal hyperplasia, 325.e3
    in hirsutism, 617
3ß-Hydroxysteroid dehydrogenase deficiency, 325.e2, 325.
    e2f, 325.e4t
Hydroxyurea
    for Budd-Chiari syndrome, 224
    hyperpigmentation with, 1651t–1652t
    for polycythemia vera, 1029
    for sickle cell disease, 1180–1181
    for thrombocytosis, 1261
Hydroxyzine
    for contact dermatitis, 329
    for lichen planus, 756
    for lichen sclerosus, 757
    for lichen simplex chronicus, 758
Hymen, imperforate, 73, 74t
Hymenolepis nana, 1249t
Hyperactivity, 160
Hyperadrenergic postural orthostatic tachycardia syndrome,
    1044.e2
Hyperaldosteronism, 61, 1393, 1774t
    with hypokalemic alkalosis, 176.e2
    without hypertension, 176.e2
Hyperalgesia, 897
Hyperammonemia, 1774
Hyperandrogenic anovulation, 1497-1498
Hyperandrogenism, 1027t
Hyperbaric oxygen. *See also* Oxygen therapy
    for carbon monoxide poisoning, 238
    for diabetic foot, 385
    for pressure injury, 1058
Hyperbilirubinemia
    conjugated, 1473
    diagnosis algorithm for, 1780f
    unconjugated, 1473
Hypercalcemia, 1645, 1645f
    in calcium-alkali syndrome, 230–230.e1
    differential diagnosis of, 1460
    laboratory diagnosis of, 1782T
    malignancy-induced, 1460
    in multiple myeloma, 854
Hypercalcemia of malignancy, 953–955.e1, 953t–954t
Hypercalciuria, hypokalemic alkalosis with, 176.e2
Hypercapnia
    coma and, 1424
    permissive, 46
    persistent, 1460
Hypercapnic respiratory failure, 1469
Hyperchloremic acidosis, 1390
Hyperchloric metabolic acidosis, 1390
Hypercholesteremia, 645
Hypercholesterolemia, 645–647.e3, 645t, 646b, 647.e1t,
    647t
Hypercoagulability workup, for cerebral palsy, 266.e3
Hypercoagulable state, 648–650.e1, 648t, 650.e1b, 650.
    e1f, 650.e1t
    associated disorders with, 1460
Hyperemesis gravidarum, 651
Hypereosinophilic syndrome, 651.e1–651.e2, 651.e2b, 458.e8
Hyperesthesia, 897
Hypergastrinemia, 1460
Hyperglycemia
    in acute ischemic stroke, 1217
    for hyperglycemic hyperosmolar syndrome, 652
Hyperglycemic hyperosmolar syndrome, 652–653.e1
Hyperglycemic hyperosmolar nonketotic coma, 652
Hyperglycemic hyperosmolar nonketotic syndrome, 652
Hypergonadotropic hypoestrogenic states, 1498
Hypergonadotropic hypogonadism, 73, 1066, 1466
    micropenis with, 1485
Hyperhidrosis, 1460–1461
Hyper-IgM syndromes, 1065.e3t
Hyperinsulinemia, 1025
Hyperinsulinemic hypoglycemia, 712.e3t

Hyperkalemia, 1566b, 1647, 1647f
  causes of, 1823
  in children, 1461
  diagnostic approach to, 1823.e1f
  differential diagnosis of, 1461
  drug-induced, 1461
  electrocardiographic changes in, 1823.e2f
  evaluation and treatment of, 1823.e1f
  tumor lysis syndrome and, 1310
Hyperkalemic periodic paralysis, 1503
Hyperkeratosis, palmoplantar, 1707–1709
Hyperkinetic disorder, 160
Hyperkinetic movement disorders, 1461
Hyperlactatemia, 737
Hyperleukocytic leukemia, 744
Hyperlipidemia, 654, 654.e3t, 824
  phenotypes of, 1788t
  in primary biliary cirrhosis, 1064–1065
  stroke risks, 1222
Hyperlipoproteinemia, primary, 654–654.e4, 654.e2f, 654.e2t–654.e4t
Hypermagnesemia, 1461, 1568, 1648f, 1816
Hypermobility Ehlers-Danlos syndrome, 431.e2
Hypernatremia, 1648b, 1649, 1649f, 1831, 1831t
Hypernephroma, 1111
Hyperosmolar hyperglycemic state, 652
Hyperostosis, of cortical bone, 1461–1462
Hyperparathyroidism, 656.e1f, 655–656.e1
Hyperphosphatemia, 1653, 1653b, 1653f
  in children, 1462
  differential diagnosis of, 1462
  tumor lysis syndrome and, 1310
Hyperpigmentation, 1352, 1352f, 1650–1652
  approach to, 1650f
  differential diagnosis of, 1462
  drugs and chemicals associated with, 1651t–1652t
Hyperprolactinemia, 74, 685
  causing androgen deficiency, 539.e1t
  differential diagnosis of, 1462
Hyperreactive airways, 142
Hyperreninemic hypoaldosteronism, 674
Hypersensitivity pneumonitis, 657–658.e1, 658.e1f, 658f, 658t, 692t
Hypersensitivity reactions, 199
Hypersensitivity vasculitis, 1540
Hypersensitivity vesiculobullous diseases, 1541
Hyperserotonemia, 1163
Hypersexuality, 955.e4
Hypersomnia, 1737f
Hypersomnia of central origin, 883
Hypersplenism, 659–659.e1, 1463
Hypertension
  acute decompensated heart failure-associated, 557
  in acute ischemic stroke, 1217
  adrenocortical causes of, 1463
  aortic coarctation as cause of, 112, 660t
  characteristics of, 660–665.e5, 660t–662t, 664t, 665.e2f, 665.e4f–665.e5f, 665.e5t, 665f
  in children, 1463
  clinical presentation of, 660
  definition of, 660
  demographics of, 660
  diagnosis of, 661–662
  endocrine, 665.e2f, 665.e3b, 1463
  epidemiology of, 660
  etiology of, 660, 660t
  gestational, 1049
  in hemorrhagic stroke, 1219–1220, 1220b
  idiopathic intracranial, 690.e5–690.e6
  intraabdominal, 7t
  laboratory testing for, 662
  malignant, 664–665, 1829
  physical findings in, 660
  portal, 1032–1033.e1, 1032f–1033f, 1033.e1f, 1033t, 1509
  in pregnancy, 663–664, 664t
  pregnancy-induced, 1049
  pseudohypertension, 665
  pulmonary, 1092–1095.e2, 1092t, 1093f, 1182
  referrals for, 665.e5t, 665
  renin-aldosterone pattern in, 1829
  renovascular, 663, 1107
  resistant, 665, 1463, 665.e4f
  in retroperitoneal fibrosis, 1116.e11
  secondary causes of, 665.e5f

Hypertension *(Continued)*
  stroke and, 1219–1220, 1220b, 1222
  treatment of, 662–665, 664t
  workup for, 661
Hypertensive crisis syndromes, 1464
Hypertensive emergencies, 664–665, 664t
Hypertensive encephalopathy
  coma and, 1424
  differential diagnosis of, 1434
Hypertensive retinopathy, 1520
Hypertensive urgencies, 664–665
Hyperthermia, 561
  coma and, 1424
  malignant, 792–794.e1, 792b–794b
Hyperthyroidism, 666–667.e2, 667.e1f–667.e2f, 1832
Hypertonic hyponatremia, 681
Hypertonicity, 1196
Hypertrichosis, 1464
Hypertriglyceridemia, 654
Hypertriglyceridemic pancreatitis, 946
Hypertrophic actinic keratosis, 25
Hypertrophic cardiomyopathy, 246–249.e1, 247f–248f
Hypertrophic obstructive cardiomyopathy, 246
Hypertrophic osteoarthropathy, 668–669.e1, 668f–669f, 1464
Hypertropia, 1214.e4
Hyperuricemia
  characteristics of, 670–671.e1, 671.e1f, 671f
  gout and, 529
Hyperventilation, persistent, 1464
Hyperviscosity syndrome, 1373f
Hypnagogic hallucinations, 883–884
Hypnopompic hallucinations, 883–884
Hypoactive sexual desire disorder, 672–673.e1, 672f, 1168
Hypoaldosteronism, 674, 1774t
Hypocalcemia, 1654, 1654b, 1654f
  differential diagnosis of, 1464
  laboratory diagnosis of, 1783t
  in pediatric patients, 1465
  tumor lysis syndrome and, 1310–1311
Hypocapnia, 1465
Hypochondriasis, 674.e1–674.e2. *See also* Illness anxiety disorder
Hypochromic anemia, 1399–1400
Hypocomplementemic urticarial vasculitis, 675–676.e1
Hypocomplementemic urticarial vasculitis syndrome, 675
Hypocretin-1, 883
Hypocretin-2, 883
Hypoestrogenic anovulation, 1498
Hypogammaglobulinemia, 752, 1065.e3t
Hypoglycemia, 1655, 1655f
  in acute ischemic stroke, 1217
  coma and, 1424
  differential diagnosis of, 187t, 1465
  in infants and children, 1465
Hypogonadism, 1656
  differential diagnosis of, 1466
  laboratory evaluation of, 1656f
Hypogonadism, male, 677–679.e1, 678f
Hypogonadotropic hypoestrogenic states, 1498
Hypogonadotropic hypogonadism, 73, 677, 1466
  micropenis with, 1485
Hypokalemia, 1657, 1657f
  causes of, 1824
  differential diagnosis of, 1466
  in pediatric patients, 1466
  renin-aldosterone pattern in, 1829t
Hypokalemic alkalosis, with hypercalciuria, 176.e2
Hypokalemic periodic paralysis, 1503-1504
Hypomagnesemia, 1658, 1658f
  differential diagnosis of, 1466-1467
  in pediatric patients, 1467
Hypomelanotic macules, 1308.e3f, 1308.e4t
Hyponatremia, 680–682.e1, 1235–1237, 1659, 1659f, 1830
  acute, 681–682
  chronic, 680, 682
  clinical presentation of, 680
  definition of, 680
  demographics of, 680
  diagnosis of, 680–681
  differential diagnosis of, 1467
  drugs associated with, 1830.e1t
  epidemiology of, 680
  etiology of, 680

Hyponatremia *(Continued)*
  evaluation of, 1832f
  hypertonic, 681
  physical findings of, 680
  prevention of, 682
  recurrence of, 682
  referral for, 682
  treatment of, 681–682
Hypo-osmolality, 680
Hypoparathyroidism, 683–684.e1, 683t
Hypoparathyroidism-deafness-renal dysplasia syndrome, 683
Hypoparathyroidism-retardation-dysmorphism syndrome, 683
Hypophosphatemia, 1467, 1660, 1660f
Hypopigmentation, 1467
Hypopituitarism
  in acromegaly, 24.e8
  characteristics of, 685–687, 686f, 686t–687t
Hypoplastic anemia, 80
Hypopnea, 1191t
Hyporeninemic hypoaldosteronic renal tubular acidosis, 1113
Hyporeninemic hypoaldosteronism, 674, 1394
Hypospadias, 687.e1–687.e2, 687.e2f
Hypotension, 1661, 1661f
  in acute ischemic stroke, 1217
  orthostatic, 660, 918–919.e1, 918t
    in multiple system atrophy, 857.e2, 857.e3t
    in parkinsonism, 857.e3, 857.e3t
    syncope caused by, 1234
  postural, 1467-1468, 1509
Hypothalamic hyperhidrosis, 1460
Hypothermia
  for anoxic brain injury, 105–106
  characteristics of, 688–689.e1, 688b–689b, 688t, 689.e1b, 689f
  coma and, 1424
  in frostbite, 502
Hypothyroidism, 73, 690–690.e3, 690.e2f, 1046f, 1832t
Hypotonia, infantile, 701.e4, 701.e4t, 1468
Hypotonic polyuria, 1468
Hypotrichosis, 1396
Hypotropia, 1214.e4
Hypouricemic agents, for gout, 530t
Hypoventilatory respiratory failure, 1519-1520
Hypovitaminosis, 1368–1369.e1, 1369f
Hypovolemia
  description of, 1469
  renal failure caused by, 1518
Hypovolemic postural orthostatic tachycardia syndrome, 1044.e2
Hypovolemic shock, 1469
Hypoxemia
  in hepatopulmonary syndrome, 599, 599.e1f
  hypercapnic respiratory failure and, 1469
  polycythemia vera and, 1029
Hypoxia
  of brain, 105
  mental changes and coma with, 1484
Hypoxic hepatitis, 726
Hypoxic-ischemic injury, 105
Hy's rule, 410
Hysterical neurosis, 334.e2
Hysterical personality disorder, 620.e2
Hysterosalpingogram, for infertility, 702f, 703
  HZ. *See* Herpes zoster

I

IAI. *See* Intraabdominal infection
Ibandronate, for osteoporosis, 926
IBD. *See* Inflammatory bowel disease
IBD-related spondyloarthropathy, 455
IBM. *See* Inclusion body myositis
Ibrutinib, for Waldenström's macroglobulinemia, 1374
IBS. *See* Irritable bowel syndrome
Ibuprofen
  for dysmenorrhea, 415
  for migraine headache, 546t
  for opioid withdrawal, 407
  in pregnancy, 934.e2t
  for roseola, 1133
  for transverse myelitis, 1296
Ibutilide, for atrial flutter, 154
IC. *See* Interstitial cystitis
Icatibant, 98.e3t
ICD. *See* Implantable cardioverter-defibrillator

Icteric leptospirosis, 742.e8
Icterus, 729
ID reaction, 690.e4, 690.e4f
Idarucizumab, 1220
IDDM. *See* Insulin-dependent diabetes mellitus
Idebenone, 501.e3
Idiopathic anterior knee pain, 958.e6
Idiopathic cardiomyopathy, 244
Idiopathic clubbing, 668
Idiopathic destructive arthritis of the shoulder, 179
Idiopathic dyspepsia, 419
Idiopathic endolymphatic hydrops, 808
Idiopathic facial paralysis, 183
Idiopathic hypereosinophilic syndrome, 651.e1
Idiopathic hypertension, 660. *See also* Hypertension
Idiopathic hypertrophic subaortic stenosis, 246
Idiopathic inflammatory myopathies, 704, 886
Idiopathic intestinal pseudoobstruction, 1471
Idiopathic intracranial hypertension, 690.e5–690.e6
Idiopathic pleuroparenchymal fibroelastosis, 692t
Idiopathic priapism, 1060.e2
Idiopathic proctocolitis, 1313, 1313t–1314t, 1315f
Idiopathic pulmonary arterial hypertension, 1092
Idiopathic pulmonary fibrosis, 691–692.e1, 691f, 692t
Idiopathic rapidly progressive glomerulonephritis, 523t
Idiopathic restrictive cardiomyopathy, 250
Idiopathic retroperitoneal fibrosis, 1116.e11
Idiopathic rhinitis, 904
Idiopathic subarachnoid hemorrhage, 1224
Idiopathic transverse myelitis, 1296
Idiopathic ventricular fibrillation, 1356
IEA. *See* Intracranial epidural abscess
IED. *See* Intermittent explosive disorder
IgA antiendomysial antibodies test, 264
IgA monoclonal gammopathy, 845t
IgA nephropathy, 522b, 523–524t, 693–694.e1
IgAN. *See* IgA nephropathy
IgE-mediated rhinitis, 63
IGF-I. *See* Insulin-like growth factor-I
IgG monoclonal gammopathy, 845t
IgM MGUS, 844
IgM monoclonal gammopathy, 845t
IGRAs. *See* Interferon gamma release assays
IHES. *See* Idiopathic hypereosinophilic syndrome
IHSS. *See* Idiopathic hypertrophic subaortic stenosis
II. *See* Integrase inhibitors
IIH. *See* Idiopathic intracranial hypertension
IIM. *See* Idiopathic inflammatory myopathies
ILD. *See* Interstitial lung disease
Ileus, adynamic, 1394
ILI. *See* Influenza-like illness
Iliac fossa pain
    left sided, 1469–1472
    right sided, 1668
Iliopsoas hemorrhage, 570t
Illness anxiety disorder, 674.e1–674.e2
Iloprost, for pulmonary hypertension, 1094
IM. *See* Infectious mononucleosis
Imipenem
    for actinomycosis, 26.e3
    for anaerobic infections, 78
    for diverticular disease, 403
    for perirectal abscess, 978
    for secondary peritonitis, 979
Imipramine
    for attention deficit hyperactivity disorder, 161
    for cataplexy, 884
    for enuresis, 458t
Imiquimod
    for actinic keratosis, 26
    for basal cell carcinoma, 177–178, 178t
    for condyloma acuminatum, 325
    for vulvar cancer, 1372.e2
    for warts, 1376
Immigrants, fever in, 1441
Immune complex assay, 1809–1812
Immune reconstitution syndrome, 347
Immune thrombocytopenia, drug-induced, 576.e1f
Immune thrombocytopenic purpura, 695–696.e1, 696.e1f, 696f
Immune-mediated necrotizing myopathy, 886
Immunizations, 1860t–1864t
    administration of, 1866t, 1872
        infection control and sterile technique, 1872
    for adults, 1872
    for ages 65 and older, 1855t

Immunizations *(Continued)*
    for ages 11 to 24 years, 1851t
    for ages 25 to 64 years, 1853t
    for birth to 10 years, 1849t
    childhood, 1860t–1864t
        catch-up, 1860t–1864t
    contraindications and precautions, 1868t–1869t
    for health care workers, 1884t–1886t
    for hepatitis A, 581
    infection control and, 1872
        adolescents and adults, 1872
        infants, 1872, 1872.e1f
        subcutaneous injections, 1872, 1872.e1f
        toddlers and older children, 1872.e1f, 1872
    licensed formulations of, for adults, 1890t
    for pediatric oncology patients, 1874t
    in pregnancy, 1883t
    recommendations for, 1872.e1f, 1865
    schedule intervals, 1887t
Immunoassays, for heparin-induced thrombocytopenia, 576, 576.e2t
Immunocompromised patients
    blastomycosis treatment in, 202.e3
    diffuse pulmonary hemorrhage syndromes in, 1514
    pulmonary infiltrates in, 1514
    recommended immunization schedule for, 1878t–1881t
Immunodeficiency. *See also* Acquired immunodeficiency syndrome
    congenital causes of, 1470
    vaccinations with, 1873t
Immunofluorescence, for Goodpasture syndrome, 528
Immunoglobulin, 1809. *See also* Intravenous immunoglobulins
Immunologic disorders
    eosinophilic lung disease with, 1435
    granulomatous disorders from, 1447
Immunologically mediated vesiculobullous diseases, 1541
Immunomodulators
    for chronic urticaria, 1328–1329
    for enteropathic arthritis, 456
    for myelodysplastic syndromes, 865
    for pericarditis, 973
Immunosuppressive therapy
    for chronic urticaria, 1329–1330
    for eosinophilic granulomatosis with polyangiitis, 458.e5
    for Goodpasture syndrome, 528
    for nephrotic syndrome, 890–891
    for renal cell carcinoma, 1112
    for scleritis, 1146–1146.e1
    for systemic lupus erythematosus, 1242, 1242t–1243t
    for Takayasu's arteritis, 1246
Impaired consciousness, in critically ill patient, 1425
Impella, 1087
Imperforate hymen, 73, 74t
Impetigo, 697–697.e1, 697f, 928
Impetigo contagiosa, 697
Impetigo vulgaris, 697
Impila, 410.e1t–410.e2t
Impingement tests, 1133.e3f
Implanon, 330, 332
Implantable cardioverter-defibrillators
    for Brugada syndrome, 222, 222.e1f
    for heart failure, 560
    for hypertrophic cardiomyopathy, 248
    for long QT syndrome, 766
    for myocardial infarction, 874
    for ventricular fibrillation, 1356–1357
    for ventricular tachycardia, 1362
Impotence, 466, 1470
In vitro fertilization, 703
In vitro testing, for food allergies, 496
Inability to urinate AUR, 51
Inactivated influenza vaccine, 1894t
Inactivated poliovirus vaccine
    catch-up schedule, 1859, 1860t–1864t
    conditions misperceived as contraindications to, 1870t–1871t
    contraindications and precautions, 1868t–1869t
    for pediatric oncology patients, 1874t
    recommended schedule for, 1860t–1864t
Inappropriate secretion of antidiuretic hormone, 1235
Inborn errors of metabolism, splenomegaly with, 1528
Incidentaloma, adrenal, 1557.e1, 1557.e1f
Incisional hernia, 1193f
Inclusion body myositis, 698–698.e1, 698.e1f, 698.e1t, 705t
Incompetent cervix, 271.e2

Incontinence
    anal, 1397
    bowel, 699–699.e1, 699.e1b, 1470
    extraurethral, 701
    fecal, 699–699.e1, 699.e1b, 1470
    urinary
        characteristics of, 457, 700–701.e3, 701.e3f, 701.e3t, 701t
        in children, 1536
Indacaterol, for chronic obstructive pulmonary disease, 301
Indican, urine, 1838
Indigestion, 1662–1663
Indinavir, 18, 1901t–1902t
Indirect antiglobulin, 1809
Indirect bilirubin, 1779
Indirect Coombs test, 1291, 1809
Indocyanine green fluorescent lymphography, for lymphedema, 777
Indolent systemic mastocytosis, 799t
Indomethacin
    for cluster headaches, 543
    for pleurisy, 1005
Industrial chemicals, neuropathies caused by, 1494
Infant(s). *See also* Children; Neonates; Pediatric patients
    abdominal pain in, 1388
    altered mental status and coma in, 1484
    appetite loss in, 1402
    cholestasis in, 1421
    congestive heart failure in, 1425
    cradle cap in, 1152.e1f
    emesis in, 1433
    hypoglycemia in, 1465
    hypotonia in, 701.e4, 701.e4t
    infection control and, 1872, 1872.e1f
    roseola in, 1133–1133.e1, 1133.e1f
    scabies in, 1142.e1f
    ventricular septal defect in, 1358
    Zika virus in, 1379–1384.e1, 1380f–1382f, 1383b–1384b
Infantile autism, early, 162
Infantile botulism, 206
Infantile hypotonia, 701.e4, 701.e4t, 1468
Infantile paralysis, 1020.e2
Infantile polyarteritis, 735.e2
Infarction
    cavitary, 1418
    cerebral, 1418–1419
    pelvic pain with, 1503
    renal, 1519
Infected pleural effusion, 441
Infected pleuritis, 441
Infections. *See also specific infection*
    in acquired immunodeficiency syndrome, 17
    acute pancreatitis with, 1715–1716
    anaerobic, 78–78.e1
    autonomic neuropathies with, 1493
    bacterial. *See* Bacterial infection
    blindness caused by, 1411
    bone, 1665, 1665b, 1665f
    cataracts caused by, 1418
    cavitary lesion with, 1418
    childhood eosinophilia caused by, 1420
    cholestasis caused by, 1421
    chronic fatigue from, 1438
    coma and, 1424
    consciousness impairment from, 1425
    control of
        in adolescents and adults, 1872
        in infants, 1872, 1872.e1f
        in toddlers and older children, 1872, 1872.e1f
    cutaneous, in athletes, 1427
    device-associated, 548.e3
    eosinophilic lung disease with, 1435
    with Epstein-Barr virus, 464–465, 464f
    in erythema nodosum, 471
    eyelid, 202.e5
    facial paralysis and, 1625.e1
    failure to thrive and, 1438
    fever with, 488
    focal neurologic deficit with, 1492
    fungal. *See* Fungal infections
    glossodynia from, 1446–1447
    granulomatous disorders from, 1447
    healthcare-associated, 548.e2–548.e9
    heel pain and, 1452
    Helicobacter pylori, 563–564.e1, 563f
    hepatic granulomas and, 1454

Infections (Continued)
  heterophil negative atypical lymphocytosis caused by, 1407
  in high-risk hematology patient, 1625.e1f, 1625.e1
  intraabdominal, 1668, 1668f
  joints, 1665, 1665f, 1665b
  leg length discrepancy with, 1475
  leg ulcers with, 1476
  myositis with, 1489
  oral-labial herpes simplex virus, 607t
  osteomyelitis, 923–924.e1, 923f, 924t
  paraparesis with, 1498
  parasitic. See Parasitic infections
  parotid swelling with, 1502
  parvovirus B19, 493–494.e1, 493f–494f
  pelvic pain with, 1503
  post-splenectomy, 659
  pruritus ani with, 1511
  pulmonary-renal syndromes with, 1515t
  recurrent or periodic fever from, 1437, 1442
  soft tissue, 1665, 1665f
  splenomegaly with, 1527
  tick-related, 1533
  toxic megacolon with, 1533–1534
  urinary tract, 1320–1322.e2, 1320t, 1321f, 1322.e1b, 1322.e2f
  vesiculobullous disease with, 1541
  viral. See Viral infection
Infectious arthritis, 1161
Infectious diarrhea, 1300, 1429, 1470
  in gastroenteritis, 510
Infectious endocarditis, 835
Infectious hepatitis, 580
Infectious keratitis with ulceration, 338.e2, 338.e2f
Infectious mononucleosis, 464, 464f, 846–846.e2, 846.e1f–846.e2f
  abnormal lymphocytes with, 1816t
  vaccine, for health care workers, 1884t–1886t
Infectious myopathies, 1488
Infectious rhinitis, 904
Infectious thyroiditis, 1268
Infective endocarditis, 446–449.e3
  algorithm for, 448f
  clinical manifestations of, 447t
  diagnosis of, 446b, 448f
  modified Duke criteria for, 446b
Inferior vena cava filters, 1091
Infertility, 702–703.e2, 702f, 703.e2b, 703.e2f
  cervicitis and, 272
  endometriosis-associated, 453
  female, 1470
  male, 1470–1471
Infiltrates, pulmonary, in immunocompromised host, 1514
Infiltrative cardiomyopathy, 250
Inflammation
  eyelid, 202.e5
  meningeal, headaches caused by, 1649
  orbital, 1496
  paraparesis with, 1501
  toxic megacolon with, 1533
Inflammatory anemia, 85–86.e2, 85f, 86.e1f–86.e2f, 86t
Inflammatory arthritis, 1667, 1667f, 1818
Inflammatory bowel disease, 344, 344t, 345.e1f, 345.e2t, 345f, 1313, 1313t–1314t, 1315f
Inflammatory breast lesion, 1414
Inflammatory carcinoma, 217
Inflammatory disorders, stroke with, 1529
Inflammatory enterocolitis, 1430
Inflammatory finger lesions, 1442
Inflammatory myopathies, 704–706.e2, 705t, 706.e1f–706.e2f, 706f, 1488
Inflammatory psoriasis, 1081f
Infliximab
  for Behçet's disease, 182.e3
  for Crohn's disease, 345
  for enteropathic arthritis, 456
  for Still's disease, 54
  for ulcerative colitis, 1315
Influenza, 707–709.e1
  acute bronchitis caused by, 27t
  antiviral agents for, 709t, 1895
  avian, 709.e2–709.e3
  chemoprophylaxis for, 1895
  clinical presentation of, 707
  definition of, 707
  diagnosis of, 707

Influenza (Continued)
  epidemiology of, 707
  pandemics, 709.e2
  physical findings of, 707
  pneumonia caused by, 1015–1016.e1
  prevention of, 708–709
  prophylaxis for, 1893
  pulmonary radiographic findings in, 708t
  signs and symptoms of, 707
  treatment of, 707–708, 709t, 1016, 1893
  vaccine
    for adults, 1882t
    antiviral medications with, 1895
    concurrent administration with other vaccines, 1870t–1871t
    description of, 708–709
    for different age groups, 1859
    for health care workers, 1884t–1886t
    indications for, 1878t–1881t
    for international travel, 1888t
    for pediatric oncology patients, 1874t
    recommended schedule for, 1860t–1864t, 1879t
Influenza A and B tests, 1809
Influenza-like illness, 707
Infrapiriform foramen syndrome, 996.e1
Ingenol mebutate, 26
Inguinal hernia, 687.e1, 1347.e2t
Inguinal lymphadenopathy, 1677, 1677.e1, 1677.e1f
Inguinal orchiopexy, 347.e3f
Inhalation anthrax, 106.e2
Inhalational botulism, 206
Inherited aplastic anemia, 1398
Inherited bone marrow failure syndromes, 1412
Inherited macrothrombocytopenia, 1481
Inherited pancytopenia syndrome, 1500
Inherited thrombocytopenia, 1532
Inhibitory learning, for panic disorder, 950
Injectables, for contraception, 332
Injection drug users
  endocarditis in, 446
  prevention services for, 1890t
Injectional anthrax, 106.e2
Injury prevention
  in ages 65 and older, 1855t
  in ages 11 to 24 years, 1851t
  in ages 25 to 64 years, 1853t
  from birth to 10 years, 1849t
Innominate artery stenosis or occlusion, 1226
Inotropes. See also specific types
  for cardiorenal syndrome, 254
  for cor pulmonale, 336
  for heart failure, 558
  for pulmonary edema, 1087
INR. See International normalized ratio
Insect bites and stings, 181, 195–196.e1, 195f–196f, 196.e1f
Insomnia, 710–712.e1, 711b, 1471
Insulin
  autoantibodies, 1809
  for diabetic ketoacidosis, 386
  free, 1809
  for gestational diabetes mellitus, 514
  for hyperglycemic hyperosmolar syndrome, 652–653
Insulin resistance syndrome, 824
Insulin-dependent diabetes mellitus, 376–383.e11
  antihyperglycemic therapy for, 380t
  clinical evaluation of, 383.e11f
  criteria for diabetes screening, 378t
  diagnostic categories of, 377t
  insulin for, 381, 381t
  necrobiosis lipoidica with, 377, 383.e11f
  neuropathy of the hindfoot and, 383.e11f
  therapies for, 379t
  types of, 376t
Insulin-like growth factor-I
  in acromegaly, 24.e8
  serum, 1809
Insulin-like growth factor-II, 1810
Insulinoma, 507.e3t, 712.e2–712.e3, 712.e3f, 712.e3t
Integrase inhibitors, 18, 632
Intensive care unit
  fever and rash in, 1439–1440
  for hantavirus pulmonary syndrome, 540.e3
Intention tremor, 1534
Interatrial septal defect, 156
Interdigital neuroma, 846.e3

Interferon
  for bladder cancer, 201
  for condyloma acuminatum, 325
Interferon alfa, for cryoglobulinemia, 346
Interferon alfa-2a, for Behçet's disease, 182.e3
Interferon alfa-2b
  for Behçet's disease, 182.e3
  for melanoma, 807
  for West Nile virus infection, 1376.e5
Interferon beta-1a, for multiple sclerosis, 856
Interferon gamma release assays, 1307
Interleukin-2, for bladder cancer, 201
Intermittent claudication, 307, 308t
Intermittent explosive disorder, 712.e4, 712.e4t
Intermittent hemodialysis, for acute kidney injury, 41
Internal hemorrhoids, 572.e2–572.e4, 572.e2f–572.e3f, 572.e2t
International normalized ratio, 1810–1811
International Prognostic Score for Essential Thrombocythemia, 1261
International Prostate Symptom Score, 1075t
Intersexuality, 1815f
Intersphincteric fistula, 102
Interstitial cystitis, 713–714.e1, 713f
Interstitial lung disease, 412t, 715–717.e1, 715t–717t, 716f, 1147
Interstitial nephritis, 718–719.e1, 719.e1f, 719f
Interstitial pneumonia, 715, 1016.e1f
Interstitial pregnancy, 430, 430f, 431.e1f
Interstitial pulmonary disease, 715
Intertrochanteric fracture, 614, 614f–615f
Intestinal lipodystrophy, 1376.e8
Intestinal microbiota transplantation, 311
Intestinal pseudoobstruction, 1471
Intraabdominal hypertension, 7t
Intraabdominal infection, 1668, 1668f
Intraabdominal mass lesion, neonatal, 1471
Intraabdominal pressure, 7
Intraaortic balloon pump, for pulmonary edema, 1087
Intraarticular steroids, for gout, 530t
Intracapsular fracture, 614
Intracellular fluid composition, 1604.e3t
Intracerebral hemorrhage, 1219, 1221–1222, 1471
Intracompartmental pressure, 318
Intracranial atherosclerosis, 1221
Intracranial confusion, 1297
Intracranial contusion, 1297, 1297b, 1298t, 1299f
Intracranial epidural abscess, 460
Intracranial hemorrhage, 1219
Intracranial hypertension, idiopathic, 690.e5–690.e6
Intracranial lesion, 1471
Intracranial pressure
  altered, headaches associated with, 1650–1653
  coma and, 1424
  increased, in hemorrhagic stroke, 1220
Intracranial venous sinus thrombosis, 261
Intracytoplasmic sperm injection, 703
Intraductal intrahepatic cholangiocarcinoma, 283, 285.e1f
Intralesional steroids, for keloids, 735.e5
Intramuscular needle insertion, 1872.e1f
  in adolescents and adults, 1872
  in infants, 1872, 1872.e1f
  in toddlers and older children, 1872, 1872.e1f
Intranuclear ophthalmoplegia, 855, 855f
Intraocular neoplasm, 1471
Intraoperative floppy iris syndrome, 259.e7
Intrapartum asphyxia, 105
Intrarenal abscess, 1106
Intraspinal abscess, 460
Intraurethral alprostadil, for erectile dysfunction, 467
Intrauterine device, 330, 332
Intravascular hemolysis, 1453
Intravenous immunoglobulins
  for immune thrombocytopenic purpura, 695
  for inflammatory myopathies, 705
  for Kawasaki disease, 735.e4
  for myasthenia gravis, 863
  for necrotizing fasciitis, 887–888
  for pericarditis, 973
  for respiratory syncytial virus prophylaxis, 1115.e1
  for toxic shock syndrome, 1286
  for West Nile virus infection, 1376.e5
Intraventricular block, 720
Intraventricular conduction defect, 720
Intraventricular conduction delay, 720–721.e1, 720f
Intrinsic factor antibodies, 1811

Intrinsic rhinitis, 904
Intubation, pediatric, 1668.e1–1668.e2
  rapid-sequence medications for, 1668.e2t
  treatment algorithm for, 1668.e1f
Invasive aspergillosis, 130
Invasive candidiasis, 236–237.e1, 237f
Invasive mechanical ventilation, 303b
Involuntary leg movement, when standing, 1476
Iodine, radioactive, 535
Iodine-123–labeled somatostatin, for carcinoid tumor, 239.e3
Iodoquinol, for amebiasis, 72t
Ionizing radiation exposure, 1100.e12–1100.e17, 1100.
  e12t–1100.e16t
IPAH. See Idiopathic pulmonary arterial hypertension
IPF. See Idiopathic pulmonary fibrosis
Ipratropium
  for anaphylaxis, 79.e2t
  for chronic obstructive pulmonary disease, 301
IPV. See Inactivated poliovirus vaccine
Iridocyclitis, 1334
Irinotecan
  for astrocytoma, 145
  for colorectal cancer, 315
Iritis, 1334
Iron
  decreased stores of, 1401
  drugs interfering with absorption of, 1399
  hyperpigmentation with, 1651t–1652t
  iron deficiency anemia treated with, 87–88
  serum, 1811, 1816t
  storage of, 85, 1401
Iron deficiency, 1736.e1t
  anemia caused by, 86t–88t, 87–88.e1, 87f–88f
  dietary, 87
Iron overload, 1471, 1799t
  hemochromatosis, 565–566.e1, 565f–566f, 566t
Iron saturation (% transferrin saturation), 1811–1812
Iron-binding capacity, total, 1811, 1816t
Irreversible transition, 512.e6
Irritable bowel syndrome, 722–725.e3, 723f, 724t, 725f,
  1675f
Irritable colon, 722
Irritant contact dermatitis, 329, 329.e2f
Isavuconazole, for aspergillosis, 131
Ischemia
  in brain injury, 105
  cerebral, 1594f
  colonic, 1668.e3, 1668.e3f
  coma and, 1424
  limb, nontraumatic, 1477, 1477
  myocardial, 1487–1488, 1687.e1, 1687.e1f
  nonocclusive mesenteric, 1485
  renal disease, 1872.e1f
  retinal, 70
  spinal cord, 1526
  upper extremity, 1472
Ischemic acute renal failure, 1308.e3, 1309
Ischemic bowel diseases, 819t, 821t, 1472
Ischemic cardiomyopathy, 1593.e1, 1593.e1f
Ischemic cerebrovascular disease, 1419
Ischemic colitis, 1472
Ischemic heart disease, 1055.e5
Ischemic hepatitis, 726.e1f, 726–726.e1, 726t
Ischemic hepatopathy, 726
Ischemic necrosis
  of cartilage and bone, 1472
  description of, 922.e5
Ischemic nephropathy, 1107
Ischemic optic neuropathy, 727–728.e1, 727f
Ischemic skin ulcer, 975f
Ischemic stroke, acute, 1215–1218.e1, 1215b, 1216f, 1216t,
  1217b, 1218f
Ischial gluteal bursitis, 229.e5
Isometric neck exercises, for cervical disc syndromes, 268.e3f
Isoniazid
  chronic hepatitis caused by, 410.e2t
  for granulomatous arthritis, 534.e2
  for pulmonary tuberculosis, 1308
Isoproterenol
  for Brugada syndrome, 222
  for torsade de pointes, 1279
Isosorbide dinitrate
  for achalasia, 13
  for coronary artery disease, 342
  hydralazine and, 559
Isospora belli, 636t

Isotretinoin
  for acne vulgaris, 14–15
  for hidradenitis suppurativa, 611
  for rosacea, 1131
Isoxsuprine, 1060b
Isthmus-dependent atrial flutter, 153
ITP. See Immune thrombocytopenic purpura
Itraconazole
  for aspergillosis, 131
  for blastomycosis, 202.e3
  for coccidioidomycosis, 313.e3
  for histoplasmosis, 620
  for invasive candidiasis, 237
  for sporotrichosis, 1205.e3
  for tinea capitis, 1270
  for tinea versicolor, 1276
IUD. See Intrauterine device
Ivabradine, 245
Ivacaftor, 352
IVC thrombosis, 223
IVCD. See Intraventricular conduction delay
Ivermectin
  for ascariasis, 126
  for cutaneous larva migrans, 350.e6
  for filariasis, 494.e3
  for pediculosis, 961
  for scabies, 1141, 1142t
IVF. See In vitro fertilization
IVIG. See Intravenous immunoglobulin

J

J point elevation, 424, 425f
J waves, 689f
Jadelle implant, 330
Janeway lesions, 449.e3f
Japanese encephalitis vaccine, 1888t
Jarisch-Herxheimer reaction, 1239
Jaundice, 1669–1672.e1, 1820b, 1826f
  in adults, 729–731.e1, 730f, 731t, 731.e1f
  classification of, 1672
  differential diagnosis of, 1472–1474
  fever and, 1439
  hepatomegaly and, 1455
  neonatal, 1473, 1670, 1670f
Jaw osteonecrosis, 927
  bisphosphonate-related, 191.e2–191.e3
JC virus, 1068.e2–1068.e3
Jeep disease, 995
Jervell and Lange-Nielsen syndrome, 764, 764t. See also
  Long QT syndrome
JIA. See Juvenile idiopathic arthritis
Jin bu huan, 410.e1t–410.e2t
Jock itch, 1272, 1272f
Joint(s)
  in foot and ankle pain, 1443
  infection of, 1665, 1665f
  red hot, 1740–1741
  swelling of, 1474, 1672, 1672f
Joint effusion, 1671, 1671f
Joint pain, 1672
  acute, 1474
  in anterior hip, 1473–1474
  in buttocks, 1474
  diagnostic approach to, 1823.e2f
  in hip, 1474
  in knee, 1474
  in lateral thigh, 1474
  in medial thigh, 1474
  polyarticular, 1474
  in posterior hips, 1474
  in thigh, 1474
Joseph-Blackfan-Diamond syndrome, 1096.e2
JRA. See Juvenile rheumatoid arthritis
Jugular vein suppurative thrombophlebitis, 1117
Jugular venous distention, 1474
Juvenile dermatomyositis, 704, 706.e1f
Juvenile hemochromatosis, 1799t
Juvenile idiopathic arthritis, 732–734.e2, 732t, 734.e2f,
  733f–734f
Juvenile osteochondrosis, 920
Juvenile polyposis, 985–986, 985t
Juvenile polyps, 985
Juvenile rheumatoid arthritis, 732
Juvenile xanthogranuloma, 618.e2
Juxtaglomerular tumor, 1829t

K

Kahn criteria, for mixed connective tissue disease, 840.e2t
Kala azar, 742.e2
Kallmann's syndrome, 74, 361
Kanner's autism, 162
Kaposi's sarcoma, 735–735.e1, 735.e1f, 735f
Katayama fever, 1143.e1
Kava, 410.e1t–410.e2t
Kawasaki disease, 735.e2–735.e4, 735.e2f–735.e3f
Kayser-Fleischer rings, 304, 1063, 1376.e9, 1376.e10f
KD. See Kawasaki disease
Keloids, 735.e5–735.e6, 735.e5f–735.e6f
Keratitis, noninfectious, 1474–1475
Keratoconjunctivitis, in microsporidiosis, 831
Keratoconjunctivitis sicca, 1186
Keratolytics, for seborrheic dermatitis, 1152
Keratosis, actinic, 25–26.21, 25f, 26t
Kerion, 65, 1269f
Kerley's B lines, 717t
Kernicterus, 423t
Ketamine
  intubation and, 1668.e2t
  for major depression, 372
  for posttraumatic stress disorder, 1044
Ketoconazole
  for Cushing's disease and syndrome, 349, 999
  for fungal vaginitis, 1341
  for precocious puberty, 1045
  for tinea versicolor, 1276
Ketones, urine, 1838
Ketorolac, 546
Ketorolac tromethamine, 328t
Ketotifen fumarate, 328t
Keyhole-limpet hemocyanin, 201
Kidney abscess, 1106
Kidney biopsy, for acute glomerulonephritis, 522
Kidney calculi, 1323
Kidney cystic disease, 1673
Kidney enlargement, unilateral, 1474
Kidney injury, acute
  characteristics of, 37–41.e2, 37t–38t, 39f, 40t
  classification for, 1474
  contrast-induced, 333–334.e1, 333t, 334b
  diagnosis of, 37t, 39f
  in HIV-infected patients, 1391
  intrinsic renal diseases as cause of, 1391
  liver disease and, 1391
  pigment-induced, 1392
  RIFLE criteria for, 1794
Kidney stones, 1323
Kidney transplantation, for end-stage renal disease, 694
Kiesselbach's plexus, 463.e8
Kinetic tremor, 1534
Kissing disease, 464
Klinefelter's syndrome, 735.e7, 735.e7t, 997
Klippel-Trenaunay-Weber syndrome, 1222.e3
Knee
  dislocation of, 1826f
  hemarthrosis of, 569f
Knee pain
  anterior, 1672.e1, 1672.e1f, 1673
  in different age groups, 1475
  differential diagnosis of, 1475
  in joint, 1473–1474
Koebner's phenomenon, 756
Koilonychia, nail, 1693–1694
Kombucha, 410.e1t–410.e2t
Koplik spots, 801.e2, 801.e2f
Korsakoff's psychosis, 735.e8
Korsakoff's syndrome, 735.e8
KP. See Korsakoff's psychosis
Kraurosis vulvae, 757
KS. See Kaposi's sarcoma
Kyphoplasty, for vertebral compression fractures, 1364
Kyphoscoliotic Ehlers-Danlos syndrome, 431.e2

L

LA. See Lactic acidosis
LABA. See Long-acting beta-agonist
Labetalol
  for hypertension, 664t
  for pheochromocytoma, 992.e2t
Labor, preterm, 1059–1060.e1, 1059b–1060b
Laboratory tumor lysis syndrome, 1310

Labyrinthitis, 187t, 736
Lacosamide, 1157
Lacrimal gland enlargement, 1138.e1f
Lactase deficiency, 738
Lactate, 737–737.e1, 1812–1816
Lactate dehydrogenase, 1812
  in cirrhosis, 304
  isoenzymes, 1812
Lactated Ringer's solution, for burns, 229b
Lactation, breast cancer during, 217
Lactation amenorrhea method, 330–331
Lactational abscess, 214
Lactic acidosis, 737–737.e1, 1390, 1777b
Lactose breath hydrogen test, 738
Lactose intolerance, 738–738.e1, 785
Lactose malabsorption, 738
Lactose tolerance test, serum, 1812
Lactulose
  for fulminant hepatic failure, 578
  for hepatic encephalopathy, 578
Laënnec's disease, 902
LAF. *See* Lone atrial fibrillation
L-AMB. *See* Liposomal amphotericin B
Lambert-Eaton myasthenic syndrome, 738.e2–738.e3, 769, 953–955.e1, 953t
Lamivudine
  for acquired immunodeficiency syndrome, 18
  dosing of, 1901t–1902t
  for hepatitis B, 584
Lamivudine/abacavir, 1901t–1902t
Lamotrigine
  for absence seizures, 1153–1153.e1
  for bipolar disorder, 191
  for intermittent explosive disorder, 712.e4t
  for partial seizures, 1157
Langerhans cell histiocytosis, 618.e2–618.e4, 618.e3f, 618.e3t
Lanreotide, for carcinoid syndrome, 239.e3
LAP. *See* Leukocyte alkaline phosphatase
Laparoscopy
  adjustable gastric banding, 909.e7f
  adrenalectomy, for pheochromocytoma, 992
  for hepatocellular carcinoma, 598.e1f
  nephrectomy, for renal cell carcinoma, 1111
  for pelvic abscess, 962
Large bowel stricture, 1475–1481
Large cell lung carcinoma, 769
Larsen-Johansson disease, 920
Laryngeal cancer, 738.e4
Laryngeal carcinoma, 738.e4–738.e5
Laryngitis, 739–739.e1
Laryngotracheobronchitis. *See* Croup
Laser therapy
  for benign prostatic hyperplasia, 1076
  for condyloma acuminatum, 324
  for retinal hemorrhage, 1116.e4
  for warts, 1376
Latent syphilis, 1238–1239.e1
Lateral axillary hiatus syndrome, 1100.e8
Lateral epicondylitis, 458.e10, 458.e10f
Lateral facet compression syndrome, 958.e6
Lateral femoral cutaneous nerve
  entrapment of, 817.e2
  illustration of, 817.e3f
Lateral pillar classification, for Legg-Calvé-Perthes disease, 742f
Lateral spinal stenosis, 1202
Lazy eye, 71, 1214.e4
LBP. *See* Low back pain
LCD. *See* Tar products
LCH. *See* Langerhans cell histiocytosis
LCPD. *See* Legg-Calvé-Perthes disease
LcSSc, 1148
LD50. *See* Lethal dose of radiation
LDH. *See* Lactate dehydrogenase
L-Dopa, for dementia with Lewy bodies, 369
LE. *See* Limbic encephalitis
Lead, 1812
  hyperpigmentation with, 1651t–1652t
  poisoning caused by, 740–741, 741t, 1736.e1t
Ledipasvir/sofosbuvir, 588
Left atrial enlargement, 1407, 1417
Left axis deviation, 1675.e1
Left bundle branch block, 720, 720f, 1676–1677
Left iliac fossa pain, 1469–1472
Left ventricular apical ballooning syndrome, 1247

Left ventricular assist device
  for cardiorenal syndrome, 254
  for heart failure, 560
Left ventricular failure, 555, 1540
Leg edema, unilateral, 1433
Leg length discrepancies, 1676.e2–1676.e3
Leg movement, involuntary, when standing, 1476
Leg pain, 1676
  algorithm for, 1676f
  with exercise, 1476
Leg swelling, 1476
Leg ulcer, 1476–1477, 1674–1677.e1, 1674b, 1674f
Legg-Calvé-Perthes disease, 742–742.e1, 742f
Legionella pneumophila
  description of, 1007–1008, 1010.e4f
  PCR, 1814
Legionella titer, 1814
Leigh syndrome, 423t
Leiomyomas, uterine, 1331
Leiomyosarcomas, uterine, 1333
Leishmania spp
  characteristics of, 742.e2–742.e4
  L. brasiliensis, 776
Leishmaniasis, 742.e2–742.e4
Lemierre's syndrome, 1117
LEMS. *See* Lambert-Eaton myasthenic syndrome
Lenalidomide
  for amyloidosis, 76.e4
  for myelodysplastic syndromes, 865
Lenticular opacities, 259.e6
Lentigo maligna melanoma, 805, 806f
Lepromatous leprosy, 742.e5–742.e6, 742.e6f
Leprosy, 742.e5–742.e7, 742.e5f–742.e6f
Leptomeningeal angioma, 1222.e2
Leptomeningeal lesions, 1477
Leptospira interrogans, 742.e8–742.e9
Leptospirosis, 742.e8–742.e9, 742.e8t
Lermoyez's syndrome, 808
LES. *See* Lower esophageal sphincter
Lesch-Nyhan syndrome, 423t
Lesinurad, for gout, 530
Lesions
  anorectal, 1457
  bone, 1412
  breast, inflammatory, 1414
  cavitary
    on chest x-ray, 1418
    in human immunodeficiency virus, 1457
  eye, arthritis and, 1403
  finger, inflammatory, 1442
  foot, ulcerating, 1444
  genital, 1629–1632, 1814f, 1816b
  hepatic, 1639
  intracranial, 1471
  leptomeningeal, 1477
  liver, 1478
  nodular, 1457
  oral mucosa
    erythematous, 1496
    pigmented, 1496
    punctate erosive, 1496
    white, 1496
  orbital
    calcified, 1497
    cystic, 1497
  pulmonary, 1514
  skin, erythematous annular, 1436
  subcutaneous, lung disease and, 1478–1479
  verrucous, 1540–1541
Lesser occipital nerve block, for migraine headache, 546
Lesser trochanter fracture, 614f
Lethal dose of radiation, 1100.e12
Letrozole
  for dysfunctional uterine bleeding, 414
  for infertility, 703
Letterer-Siwe disease, 618.e2
Leucovorin, 1290
Leukemia
  acute lymphoblastic, 743–745.e1, 743t–745t, 745.e1f
  acute myelogenous, 746–749.e1, 746t–748t
  acute myeloid, 748t, 749.e1f
  acute nonlymphocytic, 746
  acute promyelocytic, 748–749
  chronic lymphocytic, 750–752.e1, 750t–751t, 751f, 1816t
  chronic myelogenous, 753–754.e1, 753t, 754f

Leukemia *(Continued)*
  hairy cell, 754.e2–754.e4, 754.e3f–754.e4f, 754.e3t–754.e4t
    abnormal lymphocytes with, 1816t
    diagnostic features of, 754.e3t
  prolymphocytic, 1816t
Leukemic reticuloendotheliosis, 754.e2, 754.e3t
Leukocoria, 1116.e8, 1116.e8f, 1477
Leukocyte alkaline phosphatase, 1814
Leukocyte count. *See* Complete blood count
Leukocyte oxidase defect, 1447
Leukocytoclastic vasculitis, 469, 1350f, 1540
Leukodystrophies, 1428
Leukoedema, 1214
Leukoplakia, oral
  description of, 915, 915f, 1214
  oral hairy, 755, 755f
Leuprolide, 1045
Levamisole
  for ascariasis, 126
  cocaine overdose and, 312–313
  for erythema multiforme, 470
Levetiracetam, 1156
Levitra. *See* Vardenafil
Levocabastine hydrochloride, 328t
Levocetirizine, 1326
Levodopa, 957
Levofloxacin
  for anthrax, 106.e3
  for *Chlamydia* genital infections, 282
  for chronic obstructive pulmonary disease, 301
  for diverticulitis, 403
  for epididymitis, 459
  for gastritis, 508
  for lymphangitis, 776
  for orchitis, 917
  for perirectal abscess, 978
  for prostatitis, 1077
  for pyelonephritis, 1099
  for shigellosis, 1172
  for typhoid fever, 1136
Levonorgestrel, 440.e2–440.e3, 1166
Levonorgestrel intrauterine system, 330, 332, 817.e1b
Levosimendan, 1087
Levothyroxine
  for hypopituitarism, 687
  for hypothyroidism, 690, 690.e3t
  for myxedema coma, 881.e1
Lewy body dementia, 368, 368b, 368f–369f, 956
Lewy body disease, 857.e2, 892–893.e1
Lewy body type senile dementia, 368, 368b, 368f–369f
Leydig cell tumor, 1046f
LGG. *See* Low-grade glioma
LGV. *See* Lymphogranuloma venereum
Lhermitte's sign, 855
Lice infestation, 961–961.e1, 961f
Lichen planus, 64, 756–756.e1, 756.e1f, 1214
Lichen planus vulva, 1077.e4f
Lichen sclerosus, 757–757.e1, 757f, 1077.e5
Lichen sclerosus et atrophicus, 756–757
Lichen simplex, 1270t
Lichen simplex chronicus, 758, 758f, 1077.e4
Lichenoid actinic keratosis, 25
Licorice ingestion syndrome, 1829t
Lidocaine
  for cluster headaches, 543
  for cocaine overdose, 313
  for diabetic polyneuropathy, 389
  intubation and, 1668.e2t
  for pheochromocytoma, 992.e2t
  for postherpetic neuralgia, 609, 1037
Lifestyle modifications
  for alcoholic hepatitis, 59
  for claudication, 308
  for coronary artery disease, 339–342
Li-Fraumeni syndrome, 211
Ligament, in foot and ankle pain, 1443
Light chain MGUS, 844
Light therapy, for seasonal affective disorder, 1151.e2
Light-chain monoclonal gammopathy, 845t
Light-near dissociation, 1477
Lightning injury
  characteristics of, 439–440.e1, 439f, 440.e1b, 440.e1f
  high-voltage electrical injuries versus, 439t
  mechanisms of, 440b

Limb, swollen, 1530
Limb ischemia, nontraumatic, 1477, 1497
Limb-girdle muscular dystrophy, 860, 861t
Limbic encephalitis, 953–955.e1, 953t
Limbrel, 410.e1t–410.e2t
Limp
  differential diagnosis of, 1477
  in pediatric age, 1477
Linaclotide, 723
Linagliptin, 379
Lindane, 1142t
Linear gingival erythema, 518.e1
Linezolid
  for bursitis, 229.e5
  for erysipelas, 468
  for methicillin-resistant *Staphylococcus aureus*, 828
  for vancomycin-resistant *Enterococcus*, 1346
Linitis plastica, 506
Linzess. *See* Linaclotide
Lipase, 1814
Lipase inhibitors, for obesity, 907–908
Lipid metabolism, disordered, 1489
Lipid-lowering drugs, 95
Lipodermatosclerosis, 1352, 1352f
Lipodystrophy, intestinal, 1376.e8
α-Lipoic acid, for ataxia telangiectasia, 145.e6
Lipoid adrenal hyperplasia, 325.e2, 325.e2f, 325.e4t
Lipokinetix, 410.e1t–410.e2t
Lipoprotein
  classification of, 1814t–1815t, 1815t
  composition of, 654.e2t
  drugs that affect metabolism of, 647.e1t
  high-density, 647b
  plasma, 1815t
  structure of, 654.e2
Lipoprotein(a), 1814
Liposarcoma, 204
Liposomal amphotericin B
  for aspergillosis, 131
  for fungal meningitis, 813.e2–813.e3
Liquid nitrogen therapy, for molluscum contagiosum, 843
Liraglutide, 379
Lisdexamfetamine, 161, 189
Listeria monocytogenes, 759–759.e1
Listerial infection, 759
Listeriosis, 759–759.e1
Lisuride maleate, 800
Lithium
  for bipolar disorder, 191
  for cluster headaches, 543
  for intermittent explosive disorder, 712.e4t
  pathophysiology, clinical effects, and management of, 1716t–1719t
Litigation, myths commonly cited as facts in, 440b
Little's disease, 266.e3
Live, attenuated influenza vaccine
  compared with inactivated influenza vaccine, 1894t
  conditions misperceived as contraindications to, 1870t–1871t
  contraindications and precautions, 1868t–1869t
  persons who should not be vaccinated with, 1984t
  during pregnancy, 1883t
Livedo reticularis, 1477–1478
Liver. *See also* Hepatitis
  abscess of, 760–761, 760b, 760t, 761f
  acetaminophen poisoning, 11.e1t, 11.e2f, 11–11.e2
  calcifications of, on x-ray, 1416
  cirrhosis of, 304–306.e1, 305f, 306t
  fulminant failure of, 578t
  hairy cell leukemia in, 754.e3f
  histiocytosis X manifestations of, 618.e2
  lesions of, 1478
  mass, 1675.e1, 1675.e1b, 1675.e1f
  metastases to, from colorectal cancer, 315
Liver abscess, 760–761, 760b, 760t, 761f
Liver biopsy
  for alcoholic hepatitis, 59
  for Budd-Chiari syndrome, 224
  for cirrhosis, 305
  for hemochromatosis, 565, 566f
  for primary sclerosing cholangitis, 1068
Liver diseases and disorders
  acute kidney injury, 1391
  hepatopulmonary syndrome, 599.e1f, 599–599.e1
  hepatorenal syndrome, 600–601.e1, 600f, 600t–601t
  in pregnancy, 1478

Liver enzymes, elevated, 564.e2
Liver failure, acute, 42–44.e1, 42b–44b, 42t, 43f, 44t
Liver function tests
  elevations in, 1675, 1675b, 1675f
  patterns of, 518t, 1773t
Liver injury
  acute postoperative, 410.e1t
  drug-induced, 408–410.e4, 408t–409t, 410.e1t–410.e3t
Liver kidney microsome type 1 antibodies (LKM1), 1814
Liver transplantation
  for alcoholic hepatitis, 60
  for autoimmune hepatitis, 596
  for Budd-Chiari syndrome, 224
  for cirrhosis, 306
  contraindications for, 762b
  deceased donor, 763
  definition of, 762
  differential diagnosis of, 762
  epidemiology of, 762
  etiology of, 762
  for fulminant hepatic failure, 579b
  for hepatitis C, 589
  for hepatocellular carcinoma, 597–598, 598t
  for hepatopulmonary syndrome, 599
  for hepatorenal syndrome, 601
  indications for, 762b
  living donor, 763
  for nonalcoholic fatty liver disease, 903
  pretransplantation treatment, 763
  for primary biliary cirrhosis, 1065
  for primary sclerosing cholangitis, 1068
  risk factors in, 762
LMWH. *See* Low-molecular-weight heparin
Lobar nephronia, 1097
Lobular capillary hemangioma, 1100.e4
Lobular carcinoma in situ, 218t
Localized amyloidosis, 76.e3
Localized scleroderma, 1147t
Localized tetanus, 1255.e3
Locked-in syndrome, 445
Lockjaw, 1255.e3
Lodoxamide tromethamine, 328t
Löffler's syndrome, 458.e7
Lomitapide, 654
Lone atrial fibrillation, 149
Long incubation hepatitis, 582
Long QT syndrome, 764–766.e1, 764t, 765f, 766t, 1278, 1280, 1280f, 1356
Long-acting beta-agonists
  for asthma, 134–135, 140
  for asthma-COPD overlap syndrome, 143
Long-acting muscarinic antagonists, for asthma-COPD overlap syndrome, 143
Loop diuretics, for heart failure, 558
Loperamide
  for gastroenteritis, 510
  for irritable bowel syndrome, 723
Lopinavir/ritonavir
  for acquired immunodeficiency syndrome, 18
  dosing of, 1901t
  for human immunodeficiency virus, 634
Loratadine, 1326, 1328
Lorazepam
  for alcohol abuse, 56t
  for alcohol withdrawal, 56, 56t, 367
  for bipolar disorder, 191
  for cocaine overdose, 313
  for insomnia, 712
  for serotonin syndrome, 1164
Lorcaserin, 907–908
Loss, 1204
Loss of appetite, in infants and children, 1402
Loss of balance, 145.e2
Lou Gehrig's disease, 77
Lovastatin, 654.e4t
Lovenox, 1294
Low back pain, 766.e2, 766.e3t, 1676b
  acute, 1408
  algorithm for, 1676f
  differential diagnosis of, 1408, 1579–1589.e2, 1798f
  mechanical, 766.e3t
  red flags for, 766.e3t
  treatment of, 1579–1589.e2, 1798f
Low platelet syndrome, 564.e2
Low serum sodium concentration, 680
Low-density lipoprotein cholesterol, 1814

Lower esophageal sphincter, 173f, 511
Lower extremities
  edema of, 1433
  with fever of undetermined origin, 489t
  mononeuropathy of, 1486
Lower gastrointestinal bleeding
  differential diagnosis of, 1409
  pediatric, 1409
Lower gastrointestinal tract disease, 1458
Lower motor neuron, muscle weakness and, 1487
Low-grade glioma, 211
Low-grade squamous intraepithelial lesion, 269
Low-molecular-weight heparin. *See also* Heparin
  for acute coronary syndrome, 34
  for antiphospholipid antibody syndrome, 109
  for deep vein thrombosis, 359
  for pulmonary embolism, 1090, 1091.e3t
  for upper extremity deep vein thrombosis, 1316
  for venous thrombosis, 650
Lown-Ganong-Levine syndrome, 1377
Low-voltage ECG, 1478
LQTS. *See* Long QT syndrome
LS. *See* Lichen sclerosus
L5/S1, 766.e2f
LSIL. *See* Low-grade squamous intraepithelial lesion
LSS. *See* Lumbar spinal stenosis
L-thyroxine, for hypothyroidism, 690, 690.e3t
Lubiprostone, for irritable bowel syndrome, 722–723
Lues, 1238
Lumbago, 766.e2
Lumbar disk syndrome, 766.e2–766.e5, 766.e2f–766.e3f, 766.e3t–766.e4t
Lumbar puncture
  for cavernous sinus thrombosis, 261
  for cerebral vasculitis, 266.e6
  for Guillain-Barré syndrome, 537
  for migraine headache, 545
  for multiple sclerosis, 856
  for subarachnoid hemorrhage, 1224
  for syphilis, 1239
  for tabes dorsalis, 1243.e5
Lumbar spinal stenosis, 766.e2, 1202–1203.e1, 1202f–1203f, 1202t
Lumbosacral plexopathies, 1494
Lump, groin, 1448
Lumpy jaw, 26.e2
Lung abscess, 767–768.e1, 767t, 768f
Lung atelectasis, 146, 146f
Lung biopsy, for hypersensitivity pneumonitis, 658
Lung cancer, 769, 770f
  cancer of unknown primary metastasis to, 231b
  occupational causes of, 1478
Lung disease
  with bone, joint, nerve, and muscle involvement, 1479
  diffuse, lung volumes in, 1480
  eosinophilic, 1435
  gastrointestinal and liver involvement and, 1478
  parenchymal, drug-induced, 411–412.e2, 412.e1f–412.e2f, 412f, 412t
  renal involvement and, 1478
  skin and subcutaneous lesions and, 1478–1479
Lung injury
  acute, 45t
  aspiration, in children, 1405
Lung neoplasms, primary, 769–773.e7, 769t, 770f, 773.e6f
Lung parenchyma infection, 441
Lung resection, for bronchiectasis, 220
Lung scan, ventilation-perfusion mismatch on, 1540
Lung transplantation
  for cor pulmonale, 337
  for cystic fibrosis, 352
  for histiocytosis X, 618.e4
  for idiopathic pulmonary fibrosis, 692
  for interstitial lung disease, 717
  for pulmonary arterial hypertension, 1094
Lung tumors, benign, 1480
Lung volume reduction surgery, for chronic obstructive pulmonary disease, 302
Lupoid hepatitis, 595
Lupus, 1240
Lupus erythematosus. *See* Discoid lupus erythematosus; Systemic lupus erythematosus
Lupus nephritis, 1243t
Lupus pernio, 1138.e1f

Luteinizing hormone, 1814
  deficiency of, 685
  for gender dysphoria disorder, 512.e5
  in hirsutism, 617
  in hot flashes, 629
Luteinizing hormone-releasing hormone agonists, for
    pedophilic disorder, 961.e3
Lutembacher syndrome, 836
LVABS. See Left ventricular apical ballooning syndrome
Lyell's syndrome, 1282.e2
Lyme disease, 774–775.e1, 774f, 775t, 1816f
Lyme disease antibody titer, 1814–1815, 1816f
Lymph node dissection, for melanoma, 807
Lymph node enlargement, hilar and mediastinal, 1456
Lymphadenopathy, 717t
  axillary, 1676.e1b, 1676.e2f
  cervical, 1676.e2, 1676.e2b, 1676.e2f
  differential diagnosis of, 1480
  epitrochlear, 1676.e3, 1676.e3b, 1676.e3f
  fever and, 1439
  generalized, 1677f, 1677b
  in histiocytosis X, 618.e2
  in impetigo, 697
  inguinal, 1677, 1677.e1b, 1677.e1f
  in Kaposi's sarcoma, 735
  in Kawasaki disease, 735.e2
  in sarcoidosis, 1138.e1f–1138.e2f
  vaginal cancer with, 1338f
Lymphangiosarcoma, 778
Lymphangitis, 776, 1480
Lymphatic filariasis, 494.e2, 494.e2f
Lymphatoid granulomatosis, 618.e3t
Lymphedema, 776–778, 777f–778f, 1480
Lymphoblast, 1816t
Lymphoblastic lymphoma, 743
Lymphocutaneous sporotrichosis, 1205.e2–1205.e4
Lymphocyte-depleted Hodgkin lymphoma, 623–624, 626.e1f
Lymphocytes, 1815, 1816t
Lymphocytic interstitial pneumonia, 692t
Lymphocytic leukemia, chronic, 1816t
Lymphocytic lymphoma, 1816t
Lymphocytopenia, 1816b
Lymphocytosis, 846
  atypical, 1480
  cerebrospinal fluid, 1787b
  heterophil negative atypical, infectious causes of, 1407
Lymphogranuloma venereum, 281t, 778.e2–778.e3
Lymphoid disorders, bone marrow fibrosis and, 1412
Lymphoma
  Burkitt, 781
  cutaneous, abnormal lymphocytes with, 1816t
  cutaneous B-cell, 863.e5t
  cutaneous T-cell, 863.e2–863.e5, 863.e5t,
      863.e2f–863.e3f
  diffuse large B-cell, 779
  Hodgkin. See Hodgkin lymphoma
  lymphoblastic, 743
  lymphocytic, abnormal lymphocytes with, 1816t
  lymphoplasmacytic, 1373
  non-Hodgkin, 779–781.e1, 780t–781t, 781.e1f,
      781.e1t, 1188
  primary cutaneous, 863.e5t
Lymphoplasmacytic lymphoma, 1373
Lymphosarcoma cell, 1816t
Lynch syndrome, 602–603, 782–782.e1

M
M2 autoantigens, 1063
Ma huang, 410.e1t–410.e2t
Machado-Joseph disease, 1203.e2
Macitentan, 1094
Macroadenomas, 998
Macrocytic anemia, 1400, 1569, 1569f
Macrocytosis, 1817t
Macroglobulinemia, Waldenström's, 1373–1374.e1, 1373f,
    1374t
Macroglossia, in amyloidosis, 76.e3f
Macrolides
  for bacterial pneumonia, 1008
  for psittacosis, 1079.e4
  for salmonellosis, 1136t
Macro-ovalocytes, 90.e2f
Macrothrombocytopenia, inherited, 1481–1489
Macular crystals, 1680–1681
Macular degeneration, 783–784.e1

Macular edema, diabetic, 392
Macular purpura and ecchymoses, 1726t
Maculopapular rash, 464
  with fever, 1442
Mad cow disease, 343.e3
Madarosis, 1682–1683
Maddrey Discriminant Function, 59
Magnesium
  for Bartter syndrome, 176.e2
  for diabetic ketoacidosis, 388
  for dysmenorrhea, 415
  hypermagnesemia, 1816
  for hyperglycemic hyperosmolar syndrome, 653
  hypomagnesemia, 1816–1817
  for hypoparathyroidism, 684
  serum, 1816–1818
Magnesium sulfate
  for abruptio placentae, 10
  for eclampsia, 429
  for preeclampsia, 1051
  for premature rupture of membranes, 1053
  for preterm labor, 1060b
  side effects of, 1060t
  for torsade de pointes, 1279
Magnetic resonance angiography
  for acute ischemic stroke, 1216t, 1218f
  for acute mesenteric ischemia, 820
  for claudication, 308
  for Cogan's syndrome, 313.e5
  for mesenteric venous thrombosis, 821
  for portal hypertension, 1033f
  for pulmonary embolism, 1090
  for renal artery stenosis, 1109
Magnetic resonance cholangiopancreatography, 945
  for cholangiosarcoma, 284
  for choledocholithiasis, 289
  for jaundice, 730
  for primary sclerosing cholangitis, 1068
Magnetic resonance direct thrombus imaging, for deep vein
    thrombosis, 359
Magnetic resonance imaging
  for Achilles tendinopathy, 13.e2, 13.e3f
  for acute ischemic stroke, 1216, 1216t
  for aortic coarctation, 111, 112.e2f
  for appendicitis, 122
  for arrhythmogenic right ventricular dysplasia, 123,
      124.e2f
  for atrial myxoma, 155.e1f
  for basic calcium phosphate crystal deposition disease,
      180f
  for breast cancer screening, 215
  cardiac. See Cardiac magnetic resonance imaging
  for cavernous sinus thrombosis, 261, 262f
  for cerebral vasculitis, 266.e5–266.e6, 266.e7f
  for cervical cancer, 268
  for Charcot's joint, 273
  for chronic inflammatory demyelinating polyneuropathy,
      293f
  for craniopharyngioma, 343.e2, 343.e2f
  for Creutzfeldt-Jakob disease, 343.e3
  for cysticercosis, 353
  for enteropathic arthritis, 456
  gadolinium-enhanced
    for acoustic neuroma, 16, 16f
    for Budd-Chiari syndrome, 224, 224.e1f
    for Cogan's syndrome, 313.e5
  for hydrocephalus, 641, 642.e1f
  for hydronephrosis, 644
  for hypertrophic cardiomyopathy, 247
  for insulinoma, 712.e3f
  for labyrinthitis, 736
  for lumbar spinal stenosis, 1202, 1203f
  for meningioma, 809f, 810
  for Milwaukee shoulder syndrome, 180f
  for Morton neuroma, 846.e3
  for multiple sclerosis, 856, 856f
  for osteochondritis dissecans, 922.e5, 922.e5f
  for osteomyelitis, 923, 923f
  for pericarditis, 972, 974f
  for pheochromocytoma, 992
  for pituitary adenoma, 999.e1f
  for pleomorphic adenoma, 1134f
  for spinal cord compression, 1199.e1f
  for spinal epidural abscess, 1200, 1200f
  for Sturge-Weber syndrome, 1222.e3f
  for syringomyelia, 1239.e2f

Magnetic resonance imaging (Continued)
  for tarsal tunnel syndrome, 1251.e4f
  for tuberculous spinal osteomyelitis, 1305f
Major depression, 371–372.e1, 372t, 536.e2
Malabsorption, 785–786, 786t, 1678–1679
  causes of, 1687
  evaluation tests for, 1833t
  failure to thrive and, 478
  suspected, 1833f
Malabsorption syndrome, 1481
Malakoplakia, 1106
Malar eruption, 1681f, 1836b
Malaria, 787–791.e1, 787t–788t, 788f, 791t
Malassezia furfur, 1276
Malathion
  for pediculosis, 961
  for scabies, 1142t
Maldigestion, 785
Male erectile disorder, 466
Male hypogonadism, 677–679.e1, 678f
Male infertility, 703, 1470–1471
Male pseudohermaphroditism, 1455, 1511
Malignancy
  esophageal, 472, 472t, 473f, 474.e1f
  with fever of undetermined origin, 488
  glomerulonephritis associated with, 1446
  primary bone tumors, 204–205.e1, 205f
  soft tissue mass mimicking, 1525
  uterine, 1333.e1f, 1333–1333.e1, 1333b
  vaginal, 1338–1338.e1, 1338f
Malignancy unspecified site, 231
Malignancy-associated pleural effusions, 1505
Malignancy-induced hypercalcemia, 1460
Malignant bone lesions, 1140f
Malignant hyperpyrexia, 792
Malignant hypertension, 664–665, 1829t
Malignant hyperthermia, 792–794.e1, 792b–794b, 896.e1t
Malignant mesothelioma, 822–823.e1, 823f, 823.e1f
Malignant mixed Müllerian tumors, 1333
Malignant otitis externa, 928–929.e1, 928f
Malingering, 899
Mallory-Weiss syndrome, 795
Mallory-Weiss tear, 795–795.e1, 795f, 795.e1f
Malnutrition, 1481
Malt worker's lung, 657
Malta fever, 220.e2
Mammalian target of rapamycin, 507.e4
Mammary dysplasia, 490
Mammogram
  for breast cancer screening, 1f–2f, 215, 217f,
      1588f–1589f
  for gynecomastia, 539
  for nipple discharge, 1586f–1587f
Mandibular advancement devices, for obstructive sleep
    apnea, 1190–1191
Manic-depression, 190
Manic-depressive illness, depressed type, 371, 372t
Mannitol
  for ascites, 129t
  for brain abscess, 208
  for hemolytic transfusion reaction, 1291
Maple bark stripper's lung, 657
Maraviroc, 18
Marburg variant, of multiple sclerosis, 855
Marcus Gunn pupil, 855, 914
Marfan's syndrome, 795.e2–795.e4, 795.e2t,
    795.e3f–795.e4f
Marie's disease, 24.e8
Marie-Strümpell disease, 100
Marsupialization
  for Bartholin's gland cyst and abscess, 175
  for pilonidal disease, 995
Masses
  abdominal wall, 1389–1390
  adnexal, 1392–1393
  adrenal, 1393, 1558f
  brain, 1414
  breast
    differential diagnosis of, 1414
    screening and evaluation of, 1588f–1589f, 1797
  groin, 1448
  head and neck, soft tissue, 1659
  hepatic, 1639, 1639f
  liver, 1675.e1, 1675.e1b, 1675.e1f
  mediastinal, on x-ray, 1482
  nasal, congenital, 1490

Masses (Continued)
  neck, 1491, 1693, 1693b, 1693f
  parasellar, 1501
  pelvic, 1502, 1896f
  pulmonary, solitary, 1514
  rectal, palpable, 1730.e7
  red blood cell, 1827
  renal, 1872.e1f
  scrotal, 1751–1752, 1730f
  small bowel, 1525
  testicular, 1749f
Masse's sign, 348.e2
Massive hemoptysis, 571–572.e1
Massive pulmonary embolism, 1091, 1091.e2f
Mast cell leukemia, 799t
Mast cell sarcoma, 799t
Mast cell stabilizers, for allergic conjunctivitis, 326
Mastalgia, 800
Mastectomy, for hereditary breast and ovarian cancer
  syndrome, 603
Mastitis, 796–797.e1, 796t, 797f
Mastocytosis, 798–799.e2, 799t, 799.e1f, 799.e2f
"Mastocytosis in the skin", 798
Mastodynia, 800
Mastoid abscess, 801
Mastoidectomy, 801
Mastoiditis, 801–801.e1
MAT. See Multifocal atrial tachycardia
Maternal estrogen exposure, 539.e1t
Matles test, 13.e2
Mauriceau Smellie Veit maneuver, 218.e8
Mayne's sign, 116
MC. See Molluscum contagiosum
McBurney's point, 121
McCune-Albright syndrome, 1046t
McDonald criteria, for multiple sclerosis, 855, 855t
MCI. See Mild cognitive impairment
McKenzie method, 766.e3
MCTD. See Mixed connective tissue disease
MCV. See Mean corpuscular volume
MCV4. See Quadrivalent meningococcal conjugate vaccine
MD. See Meckel diverticulum; Muscular dystrophy
MDR-GNRs. See Multidrug-resistant gram-negative rods
MDRO. See Multidrug-resistant organisms
MDS. See Myelodysplastic syndromes
Mean corpuscular volume, 1817, 1817t
  increased, 1817t
Measles
  acute bronchitis caused by, 27t
  characteristics of, 801.e2–801.e3, 801.e2f, 801.e3t,
    1015–1016
Measles, mumps, and rubella vaccine, 859, 1133.e7–1133.
    e8
  for adults, 1882t
  catch-up schedule, 1859–1865, 1860t–1864t
  conditions misperceived as contraindications to,
    1870t–1871t
  contraindications and precautions, 1868t–1869t
  indications for, 1878t–1881t
  for international travel, 1888t
  for pediatric oncology patients, 1874t
  during pregnancy, 1883t
  recommended intervals between administration,
    1867t
  recommended schedule for, 1860t–1864t,
    1878t–1881t
Measles live-virus vaccine, for health care workers,
    1884t–1886t
Mebendazole
  for ascariasis, 126
  for hookworms, 627
  for pinworms, 996, 1077.e5
  for trichinosis, 1301.e3
Mechanical heart failure, 1452
Mechanical hemolysis, 1453
Mechanical vacuum devices, 466
Mechanical ventilation
  for abdominal compartment syndrome, 8
  for acute respiratory distress syndrome, 46, 47t
  for Guillain-Barré syndrome, 538
  for hantavirus pulmonary syndrome, 540.e3
Mechlorethamine, 1651t–1652t
Meckel diverticulum, 801.e4, 801.e4f
Meclizine
  for labyrinthitis, 736
  for Ménière's disease, 808

Meclofenamate, 546t
Meconium, delayed passage of, 1604.e1–1604.e4
Medial epicondylitis, 458.e10
Mediastinal compartments, 1481
  anterior, 1482
  middle, 1482
  posterior, 1482
Mediastinal fibrosis, 619
Mediastinal lymph node enlargement, 1456
Mediastinal masses
  sites of origin, 1482
  on x-ray, 1482
Mediastinitis, 802–803.e1, 802t–803t, 803f
  acute, 1482
Mediastinoscopy, for sarcoidosis, 1138
Medically unexplained symptoms, 1195
Medication(s). See also Drug(s)
  atrial fibrillation from, 149
  hepatic disease from, in HIV infections, 1458
  xerostomia and, 1779
Medication Appropriateness Index, 1031.e2
Medication errors, pediatric, 960.e5–960.e6
Medication-related osteonecrosis of the jaw (MRONJ), 191.e2
Medications without a prescription, 934.e2
Medication-treated gestational diabetes, 513
Mediplast. See Salicylic acid plaster
Mediterranean anemia, 1256
Medroxyprogesterone acetate
  for dysfunctional uterine bleeding, 413
  for endometriosis, 453
  for pedophilic disorder, 961.e2
Medullary thyroid carcinoma, 1264–1265.e2
Mefenamic acid, 1055
Megaesophagus, 12
Megaloblastic anemia, 89
  with cobalamin deficiency, 1400
  differential diagnosis of, 1400
  with folate deficiency, 1400
  miscellaneous, 1400
Megaloblastosis, 1817t
Megestrol acetate
  for dysfunctional uterine bleeding, 413
  for hot flashes, 629
Meibomianitis, 1223
Meigs' syndrome, 804–804.e1, 804.e1f
Melancholia, 371
Melanoma
  characteristics of, 805–807.e1, 805f–806f
  vaginal, 1338
  vulvar, 1372.e2
Melanonychia, 1483
Melatonin, for insomnia, 712
MELD score. See Model for End-Stage Liver Disease score
Meleney's synergistic gangrene, 888t
Melphalan, 76.e4
Memantine
  for Alzheimer's disease, 69, 69t
  for dementia with Lewy bodies, 369
Membranoproliferative glomerulonephritis, 524t
Membranous laryngotracheobronchitis, 1290.e2
Membranous nephropathy, 524t, 889–891, 1243t
Memory loss, in elderly, 1483
Men who have sex with men, prevention services for,
    1890t
Menactra, for bacterial meningitis, 813
Ménière's disease, 187t, 808–808.e1, 808t, 1277–1277.e2
Meningeal disorders, coma and, 1424
Meningeal inflammation, headaches caused by, 1649
Meningioma, 211, 809–810.e1, 809f, 809t
Meningitis
  bacterial, 811–813.e1, 811f–812f, 812t–813t
  chronic, 1483
  eosinophilic, 350.e5t
  fungal, 813.e2–813.e3, 813.e2t
  mumps and, 858
  recurrent, 1483
  viral, 814, 814t
Meningocele, 1196.e2–1196.e5, 1196.e2f–1196.e3f
Meningococcal conjugate vaccines
  for adults, 1882t
  for health care workers, 1884t–1886t
  indications for, 1878t–1881t
  for international travel, 1888t
  for pediatric oncology patients, 1874t
  during pregnancy, 1883t
  recommended schedule for, 1860t–1864t

Meningococcal disease
  immunization schedule and intervals, 1859
Meningococcal meningitis, 811f
Meningococcal purpura fulminans, 811f
Meningococcal sepsis, 811f
Meningococcal vaccination
  for international travel, 1888t
  recommended schedule for, 1878t–1881t
Meningoencephalitis, 442, 443t, 759
Meningomyelocele, 814.e1–814.e2, 814.e1f–814.e2f,
    1196.e2–1196.e5
Menometrorrhagia, 413, 817
Menopause, 815–816.e1, 816b
  early, 1397
Menorrhagia, 413, 817.e1b, 817–817.e1
Menstrual cramps, 415
Menstruation, absence of, 73
Mental changes, fever and rash with, 1440
Mental status, altered, 1564, 1564f
Mental status changes
  coma and, 1483–1484
    age-related causes of, 1484
    metabolic and systemic causes of, 1484
    structural causes of, 1484
  in elderly patient, 1682, 1682b, 1682f
Mental status testing, for Alzheimer's disease, 68
Mepolizumab, for asthma, 135
Meralgia paresthetica, 817.e2–817.e3,
    817.e2f–817.e3f
6-Mercaptopurine, for enteropathic arthritis, 456
Merci clot retrieval system, 1216–1217
Mercury, hyperpigmentation with, 1651t–1652t
Meropenem
  for anaerobic infections, 78
  for brain abscess, 208
  for diabetic foot, 385
  for diverticular disease, 403
  for lung abscess, 768
  for perirectal abscess, 978
Mesenteric adenitis, 818–818.e1, 818.e1t, 818f
Mesenteric arterial embolism, 819, 1485
Mesenteric arterial thrombosis, 819
Mesenteric ischemia
  acute, 819–820.e1, 819t, 820.e1f
  nonocclusive, 1485
Mesenteric lymphadenitis, 818
Mesenteric venous thrombosis, 819, 819t, 821–821.e1,
    821b, 821t, 1485
Mesothelioma, 1504
Mesothelioma, malignant, 822–823.e1, 823.e1f, 823f
Mestinon, 857.e3t
Metabolic acidosis
  arterial blood gases, 1777
  causes of, 1777b
  diagnostic approach to, 1555, 1555f
  differential diagnosis of, 1390
  hyperchloric, 1390
  in hypothermia, 688
  laboratory findings in, 1771t
Metabolic alkalosis
  arterial blood gases, 1778
  differential diagnosis of, 1395
  laboratory findings in, 1771t
  workup of, 1562, 1562f
Metabolic cataracts, 259.e6
Metabolic cofactor deficiency, mental changes and coma
  with, 1484
Metabolic disorders
  autonomic neuropathies with, 1493
  chronic fatigue from, 1438
  focal neurologic deficit with, 1492
  neuropathies caused by, 1494
  paraparesis with, 1501
  stroke with, 1529
Metabolic encephalopathy, 364, 364t, 366.e1t, 1434. See
    also Delirium
  algorithm for evaluation of, 365f
  classification, 364
  risk factors for, 364t, 366.e1t
  theories regarding, 364
Metabolic myopathies, 1488–1489
Metabolic neuropathies, 1494
Metabolic syndrome, 824–825.e1, 824t, 825f
  in hidradenitis suppurativa, 610
  in hypercholesterolemia, 647
  in polycystic ovary syndrome, 1028t

Metabolic vesiculobullous diseases, 1541
Metadiaphyseal bone lesions, 1412
Metals, neuropathies caused by, 1494
Metanephrines, urine, 1838, 1839t
Metaphysis, bone lesions at, 1412
Metaproterenol, 28
Metastases
    brain, 209–210.e1, 209f, 210.e1f
    breast cancer, 218.e5f
Metastatic castration-resistant prostate cancer,
    1074t
Metastatic neoplasms, 1485
Metatarsal neuralgia, 846.e3
Metatarsalgia, 825.e2–825.e3, 825.e2f
Metformin
    for diabetes mellitus, 379
    for gestational diabetes mellitus, 514
    for hidradenitis suppurativa, 611
    for hirsutism, 618
Methadone, 912–913
    for chronic pain, 940.e3t, 940t
    for opioid withdrawal, 407
Methanol poisoning, 827.e2f, 826–827.e2, 826b
Methemoglobinemia, drug-induced, 1485
Methicillin-resistant Staphylococcus aureus, 548.e3, 796,
    828–828.e1
Methimazole
    for Graves' disease, 535
    for hyperthyroidism, 666
    for thyrotoxic storm, 1268.e2
Methotrexate
    for Behçet's disease, 182.e3
    for bladder cancer, 201
    for breast cancer, 216
    for Cogan's syndrome, 313.e5
    for Crohn's disease, 345
    for enteropathic arthritis, 456
    for eosinophilic granulomatosis with
        polyangiitis, 458.e5
    for Felty's syndrome, 485.e2
    for granulomatosis with polyangiitis, 534
    hyperpigmentation with, 1651t–1652t
    for inflammatory myopathies, 705
    mucositis caused by, 1214.e2f
    for psoriasis, 1080
    for rheumatoid arthritis, 1127
    for sarcoidosis, 1138
    for Still's disease, 54
Methylcellulose eye drops, 535–536
Methyldopa
    chronic hepatitis caused by, 410.e2t
    for hypertension, 664t
Methylergonovine, 1040t
Methylmalonic acid, serum, 89, 1817
Methylnaltrexone, 30
Methylphenidate
    for attention deficit hyperactivity disorder, 161
    for narcolepsy, 884
Methylprednisolone
    for acute respiratory distress syndrome, 48
    for anaphylaxis, 79
    for chemotherapy-induced nausea and vomiting, 276
    for giant cell arteritis, 516
    for granulomatosis with polyangiitis, 533
    for Henoch-Schönlein purpura, 574
    for immune thrombocytopenic purpura, 695
    for labyrinthitis, 736
    for severe acute respiratory syndrome, 1164.e3
    for spinal cord compression, 1199
Methysergide, 543
Metoclopramide
    for gastroesophageal reflux disorder, 511
    for migraine headache, 546t
Metoprolol
    for atrial fibrillation, 150
    for coronary artery disease, 342
    for dilated cardiomyopathy, 245
    for hypertension, 664t
    for supraventricular tachycardia, 1232
Metrifonate, 1143.e2
Metritis, 454
Metronidazole
    for amebiasis, 72t
    for anaerobic infections, 78
    for bacterial vaginosis, 1345
    for balanitis, 171

Metronidazole (Continued)
    for bite wounds, 192
    for botulism, 206
    for brain abscess, 208
    for breast abscess, 214
    for cavernous sinus thrombosis, 262
    for Clostridium difficile infection, 310–311
    for Crohn's disease, 345
    for diverticulitis, 403
    for epidural abscess, 460
    for gastroenteritis, 510
    for giardiasis, 517
    for Helicobacter pylori, 564
    for liver abscess, 761
    for lung abscess, 767–768
    for pelvic abscess, 962
    for pelvic inflammatory disease, 964
    for perirectal abscess, 978
    for peritonsillar abscess, 982
    for prepubescent vaginitis, 1342
    for retropharyngeal abscess, 1118
    for rosacea, 1131
    for Trichomonas vaginalis, 1343
Metrorrhagia, 413, 817
Metyrapone, 999
Mexiletine
    for long QT syndrome, 766
    for ventricular tachycardia, 1362
MG. See Myasthenia gravis
MGUS. See Monoclonal gammopathy of undetermined
        significance
MH. See Malignant hyperthermia
MI. See Myocardial infarction
Micafungin, 237
Miconazole, 1341
Microangiopathies, thrombotic, 1749.e1f
Microcephaly, 1485
Microcytic anemia, 88t, 1400, 1570, 1570f
Microcytosis, 1817t
Micrometastases, 217
Micropenis, 1485
Microscopic polyangiitis, 829–830.e1,
        829t–830t, 830.e1f
Microscopic polyarteritis, 829
Microsporidiosis, 636t, 831–831.e1
Microsporum spp., 1269–1271
Microvascular angina, 91
Microvascular decompression, for trigeminal neuralgia, 1302
Midazolam
    for alcohol withdrawal, 58, 367
    intubation and, 1668.e2t
Middle East respiratory syndrome, 707
Midfoot pain, 1498–1516
Midodrine
    for ascites, 129t
    for hepatorenal syndrome, 601, 601t
    for orthostatic hypotension, 857.e3t, 919
Mifepristone
    for Cushing's disease and syndrome, 349
    for uterine fibroids, 1332
Miglitol, 381
Migraine headache, 545–547.e1, 1643–1644
    combined tension-migraine, 1648
    therapy for, 546t
Mild cognitive impairment, 832–832.e1
Mild male factor infertility, 703
Mild neurocognitive disorder, 621, 832
Mild traumatic brain injury, 1035b
Miliary tuberculosis, 1304–1305.e2, 1305f
Milk allergy, 496
Milk intolerance, 738
Milrinone, 558
Miltefosine, 742.e2
Milwaukee shoulder syndrome, 179
Mineralocorticoids
    deficiency of, 1393–1394
    excess of, 1393
    exogenous, 1393
Mini pill, 330, 332
Minimal change disease, 889–891, 890t
Minimal hepatic encephalopathy, 577
"Mini-stroke", 1294
Minocycline
    for acne vulgaris, 15
    chronic hepatitis caused by, 410.e2t
    hyperpigmentation with, 1651t–1652t

Minor cognitive–motor disorder, 621f
Minoxidil, 65
Miosis
    differential diagnosis of, 1485–1486
    in Horner's syndrome, 628
Mipomersen, 654
MIS. See Mullerian inhibiting substance
Miscarriage, spontaneous, 1204–1205.e1
Misoprostol, 971, 1040t
Mistletoe, 410.e1t–410.e2t
Mitochondrial antibody, 1817
Mitochondrial DNA mutations, in cyclic vomiting syndrome,
        350.e7
Mitochondrial myopathies, 1489
Mitomycin C, 201, 202b
Mitral annular calcification, 836
Mitral click murmur syndrome, 839
Mitral insufficiency, 833
Mitral regurgitation, 833–835.e1, 833f, 834t, 835f, 840,
        1539–1543
Mitral stenosis, 836–838.e1, 837f, 838t, 1539
Mitral valve
    calcification of, 1416
    repair of, for mitral regurgitation, 834–835, 835f
Mitral valve prolapse, 839–840.e1, 839f, 839t–840t
Mixed connective tissue disease, 840.e2–840.e3, 840.e2f,
        840.e2t
Mixed cryoglobulinemia, 346, 346f, 346.e1t
Mixed lobular and septal panniculitis, 952f
Mixed T- and B-lymphocyte deficiencies, 1470
Mixed urinary incontinence, 700
MMR vaccine. See Measles, mumps, and rubella vaccine
MO-1, 169t
Mobitz type I block, 551, 551f
Mobitz type II block, 551, 552f
Modafinil, for narcolepsy, 884
Model for End-Stage Liver Disease score, 59
Modified Ashworth Scale, 1196t
Modified Brooke resuscitation formula, 229b
Modified Medical Research Council dyspnea questionnaire,
        for chronic obstructive pulmonary disease, 302–303
Mohs' surgery
    for basal cell carcinoma, 178t
    description of, 1206
Molar pregnancy, 841–842.e1, 841f–842f, 842.e1f, 842t
Molluscum contagiosum, 843, 843f
Molluscum pendulum, 1308.e4t
Mongolism, 403.e2
Monilial vulvovaginitis, 1341
Moniliasis, 234
Monoamine oxidase inhibitors, 1194.e4
Monoarthritis, acute, 1486
Monoarticular arthritis, 1404–1405
Monoarticular pseudogout, 1079
Monobenzyl ether, for vitiligo, 1370
Monoclonal antibodies
    for chronic lymphocytic leukemia, 752
    Clostridium difficile infection, 311
    for hepatocellular carcinoma, 598
    for neuroblastoma, 891.e3
    to respiratory syncytial virus, 1867t
Monoclonal gammopathy of undetermined significance,
        844–845.e1, 845.e1f, 845.e1t, 845t, 851t
Monoclonal immunoglobulin protein, in Waldenström's
        macroglobulinemia, 1374t
Monoclonal macroglobulinemia, 1373
Monocular blindness, transient, 1410
Monocular diplopia, 1430
Monocular nystagmus, 1495
Monocular vision loss, 1542
Monocyte count, 1818
Monocytosis, 1486
Monomorphic VT, 1361
Mononeuropathy, 1486
    isolated, 1486
    painful, 1493
Mononeuropathy multiplex, 1486
Mononucleosis
    characteristics of, 846–846.e2, 846.e1f–846.e2f
    infectious, abnormal lymphocytes with, 1816t
    monospot negative, 1486
Monosymptomatic nocturnal enuresis, 458t
Montelukast, 63
Moonshine, 826
Morbilliform rash, 464
Morbillivirus, 801.e2

Morgellons disease, 367.e2, 367.e2t
Morning-after pill, 440.e2
Morphea, 1147
Morphine sulfate
  for acute coronary syndrome, 35
  for chronic pain, 940.e3t, 940t
  for heart failure, 558
  milligram equivalent dosing for, 940.e3t
  for myocardial infarction, 872–873
  for neuropathic pain, 899
  for pulmonary edema, 1086
Morton metatarsalgia, 846.e3
Morton neuroma, 846.e3–846.e5, 846.e3f–846.e4f
Mosaic warts, 1375
Mosquirix, 791
Motesanib, 1265
Motion sickness, 847, 847f
Mouth, trench, 518.e2
Movement disorders, hyperkinetic, 1461
Moxifloxacin
  for anaerobic infections, 78
  for bite wounds, 192
MPA. See Microscopic polyangiitis
MPSV4. See Quadrivalent meningococcal polysaccharide
  vaccine
MR. See Mitral regurgitation
MRCP. See Magnetic resonance cholangiopancreatography
MRDTI. See Magnetic resonance direct thrombus imaging,
  for deep vein thrombosis
MRSA. See Methicillin-resistant Staphylococcus aureus
MS. See Mitral stenosis; Multiple sclerosis
MSA. See Multiple system atrophy
mTOR. See Mammalian target of rapamycin
Mucocutaneous candidiasis, 18t–24t
Mucocutaneous lymph node syndrome, 735.e2
Mucolytic agents, for atelectasis, 146
Mucopurulent cervicitis, 272
Mucormycosis, 848–848.e1
Mucosa-associated lymphoid tissue lymphoma,
  563–564
Mucosal leishmaniasis, 742.e2
Mucositis, 1214–1214.e3, 1214.e1f–1214.e3f
Mueller's sign, 116
Müllerian agenesis, 73, 74t, 76
Mullerian inhibiting substance (MIS), 347.e2
Multibacillary leprosy, 742.e5–742.e6
Multichamber enlargement, 1417
Multidetector computed tomography, of appendicitis,
  121–122, 121f
Multidrug-resistant gram-negative rods, 849–849.e1
Multidrug-resistant organisms, 849
Multidrug-resistant Staphylococcus aureus, 828
Multidrug-resistant tuberculosis, 1306
Multifocal atrial tachycardia, 850–850.e1, 850f
Multifocal neurologic deficit, 1492
Multiple endocrine neoplasia type 1, 1370.e2t
Multiple lipoprotein-type hyperlipidemia, 654
Multiple myeloma, 204, 845.e1t, 851–854.e1, 851f–853f,
  851t–852t
Multiple sclerosis
  characteristics of, 855–857.e1, 855f–856f, 855t–856t,
    1428
  differential diagnosis of, 187t
  HLA antigens associated with, 1807t
Multiple sleep latency test, 883
Multiple solitary plasmacytomas, 851t
Multiple system atrophy, 857.e2–857.e4, 857.e2t–857.e3t,
  956, 1068.e4
Multivitamins, for chemical-induced cardiomyopathy, 243
Mumps, 858–859.e1, 858f, 917–917.e1, 1176
Mumps live-virus vaccine
  for health care workers, 1884t–1886t
  for international travel, 1888t
Munchausen by proxy, 477
Munchausen syndrome, 477–477.e1
Mupirocin ointment, for impetigo, 697
Murmur
  diastolic, 1683, 1683b, 1683f
  systolic, 1684, 1684b, 1684f
  tricuspid stenosis and, 1301.e7
Muscle diseases, 1486–1487
Muscle relaxants
  for chronic pain, 939t
  for myofascial pain, 880
  for temporomandibular joint syndrome, 1252
Muscle spasms, 1646–1647

Muscle weakness, 1686, 1686b, 1686f
  arthritis and, 1403
  differential diagnosis of, 1487
  lower motor neuron, 1487
  neuromuscular, 1765f
  upper motor neuron, 1487
Muscular dystrophy, 860–861, 860f–861f, 861t, 1456,
  1486
Musculoskeletal complaints, 1687, 1687b, 1687f
Musculoskeletal disorders, pelvic pain in, 1502
Musculoskeletal tumors
  benign, 1487
  malignant, 1487
Mushroom poisoning, 862–862.e1, 862t, 862.e1t
MUTYH-associated polyposis, 985t
MVP. See Mitral valve prolapse
MVT. See Mesenteric venous thrombosis
MWT. See Mallory-Weiss tear
My Medication Action Plan, 1031.e3
Myasthenia gravis, 863.e1f, 863–863.e1, 953–955.e1, 953t,
  1807
Mycetoma
  Aspergillus as cause of, 131f
  description of, 901.e1
Mycobacterial infection
  in hepatic disease, 1458
  in pulmonary disease, 1459
Mycobacterium avium complex disease, 636t–638t
Mycobacterium leprae, 742.e5–742.e6
Mycobacterium tuberculosis infection
  in human immunodeficiency virus, 636t–638t
  in miliary tuberculosis, 1304
  in pulmonary tuberculosis, 1306
Mycophenolate mofetil
  for chronic inflammatory demyelinating polyneuropathy,
    293
  for chronic urticaria, 1329
  for inflammatory myopathies, 705
  for pemphigus vulgaris, 969
  topical, for bullous pemphigoid, 226.e2
Mycoplasma pneumoniae, 1011–1012.e1, 1011t, 1012f,
  1213f
  acute bronchitis caused by, 27t
  laryngitis caused by, 739
  PCR, 1818
Mycosis fungoides, 863.e2–863.e5, 863.e2f–863.e3f, 863.
  e5t
Mydriasis, 1487
Myelin basic protein, cerebrospinal fluid, 1818
Myelin disorders, 1487
Myelitis
  myelopathy and, 1487
  transverse, 1296–1296.e1, 1296.e1f
Myelodysplastic syndromes, 866.e1t, 866.e1t, 866.e2b, 866.e2f,
  864–866.e2, 864t, 865f–866f, 866t, 1096.e2
Myelofibrosis, primary, 1065.e8–1065.e10, 1065.e8f,
  1065.e9t, 1065.e10b
Myeloid disorders, bone marrow fibrosis and, 1412
Myeloid growth factors, for myelodysplastic syndromes,
  865
Myelomeningocele, 1196.e2–1196.e4, 1196.e3f
Myelopathy
  from cervical spondylosis, 268.e3
  myelitis and, 1487
Myeloproliferative disorders, platelet count in, 1822
Myocardial disease
  profiles of, 1593t
  sudden death with, 1530
Myocardial fibrosis, 249
Myocardial infarction
  acute, 31
  clinical presentation of, 868
  complications of, 874
  coronary angioplasty for, 874.e1f
  definition of, 867
  diagnosis of, 868–869, 868f
  electrocardiography of, 868–869, 868f
  epidemiology of, 867–868
  etiology of, 868
  incidence of, 867–868
  non-ST-segment elevation, 871f, 867–874.e1
  pericarditis after, 874
  physical findings of, 868
  prevalence of, 867–868
  primary coronary angioplasty for, 874.e1f
  prognosis after, 874

Myocardial infarction (Continued)
  risk assessment for, 869
  ST-segment elevation, 867–868, 870f
  sudden cardiac death risks, 874
  treatment of, 869–874, 870f–871f, 872t, 874.e1f
Myocardial ischemia, 1487–1488, 1687.e1, 1687.e1b,
  1687.e1f
Myocarditis, 237, 875–877.e1, 876t, 877.e1f, 877f
Myoclonus, 878–878.e1, 1488
Myoclonus dystonia, 423t, 878
Myofascial pain syndrome, 491, 879–880.e1, 879f–880f,
  879t, 1252
Myoglobin, urine, 1838
Myoglobinuria, 1839t
Myomas, uterine, 1331
Myonecrosis, 888t
Myopathic syndromes, drug-induced, 1488
Myopathies
  with human immunodeficiency virus, 1488
  infectious, 1488
  inflammatory, 1488
  metabolic, 1488–1489
  mitochondrial, 1489
  with rest pain, 1488
  toxic, 1489
  types of, 1488
Myopericarditis, 974
Myositis, 1687.e2, 1687.e2b
  drug management of, 1832f
  infectious causes of, 1489
  inflammatory, 1489
  necrotizing autoimmune, 886–886.e1, 886f
Myositis syndromes, 704
Myotonia, 881, 881f
Myotonic disorders, 1486
Myotonic dystrophy, 860, 861t, 881, 881f
Myringotomy, 801, 931
Myxedema, 690
Myxedema coma, 881.e1, 881.e1f
Myxoma, atrial, 155.e1f, 155–155.e1

N

NAATs. See Nucleic acid amplification tests
N-Acetylcysteine
  for acute liver failure, 43–44
  for APAP poisoning, 11, 410
  for binge eating disorder, 191
  contrast-induced nephropathy and, 41
  for Raynaud's phenomenon, 1104
Nadolol, 1033
Nafcillin
  for brain abscess, 208
  for breast abscess, 214
  for bursitis, 229.e5
  for cystic fibrosis, 352
  for epidural abscess, 460
  for erysipelas, 468
  for osteomyelitis, 924t
  for renal abscess, 1106
NAFLD. See Nonalcoholic fatty liver disease
Naftidrofuryl, 309, 977
Nail(s)
  Beau's lines, 735.e2, 1688
  clubbing, 1489–1495
  dystrophy of, 1836b, 1841f
  with fever of undetermined origin, 489t
  koilonychia, 1693–1694
  onycholysis, 1694–1695
  pitting, 1694.e1–1694.e2
  splinter hemorrhage, 1694.e2
  striations, 1695–1699
  telangiectasia, 1490
  whitening (Terry's), 1490
  yellowing, 1490
Nail bed abscess, 958
Nail bed infection, 958
Nail disorders
  paronychia, 958–958.e1, 958f
  tinea unguium, 1274–1275.e1, 1274f
NAION. See Non-arteritic anterior ischemic optic
  neuropathy
Naltrexone
  for alcohol abuse, 56t, 58, 407
  description of, 912
NAM. See Necrotizing autoimmune myositis

Naphazoline hydrochloride, 328t
Naproxen
  for dysmenorrhea, 415
  for lumbar spinal stenosis, 1203
  for migraine headache, 546t
  in pregnancy, 934.e2t
  for premenstrual syndrome, 1055
  for transverse myelitis, 1296
NAR. *See* Nonallergic rhinitis
Naratriptan, 546t
Narcissistic personality disorder, 882–882.e1
Narcolepsy, 883–884.e1, 884t
Narcolepsy with cataplexy, 883
Narcolepsy with hypocretin deficiency, 883
Narcolepsy-cataplexy syndrome, 883
Narcotic abuse, 911. *See also* Opioids
Narcotic addiction, 911. *See also* Opioids
NARES. *See* Nonallergic rhinitis with eosinophilia
    syndrome
Narrow complex tachycardia, 1747f
Narrow-angle glaucoma, 521, 521.e1f
Nasal masses, congenital, 1490
Nasal packing, 463.e8
Nasal polypectomy, 885
Nasal polyps, 885–885.e1, 885.e1f, 885b
Nasal sinus tumors, 1490
NASH. *See* Nonalcoholic steatohepatitis
Natalizumab
  for Crohn's disease, 345
  for multiple sclerosis, 857
National Asthma Education and Prevention Program, 132,
    134t–139t
Natroba. *See* Spinosad
Nausea and vomiting. *See also* Vomiting
  approach to patient with, 1761f
  causes of, during pregnancy, 1490
  chronic, 1490–1491
  differential diagnosis of, 1490
NDM-1. *See* New Delhi metallo-beta-lactamase-1
Necator americanus, 126.e1t, 627
Neck injury, acceleration flexion-extension, 1376.e7
Neck masses, 1491, 1693, 1693b
  evaluation of, 1693f
  soft tissue, 1659
Neck pain, 1491, 1496–1497, 1694, 1694b
  algorithm for, 1694f
  from rheumatologic disorders, 1491
Neck trauma, 187t
Necrobiosis lipoidica diabeticorum, 383.e11f, 377
Necrosis
  avascular, 166–168.e1, 166t, 167f–168f
  tubular, 1309
Necrotic ulcers, palatal, 1510
Necrotizing arteritis, 1021
Necrotizing autoimmune myositis, 886–886.e1, 886f
Necrotizing fasciitis, 887–888.e1, 887f–888f, 888t
Necrotizing hemorrhagic encephalitis, 1428
Necrotizing infections, cavitary lesion with, 1418
Necrotizing otitis externa, 928–929.e1
Necrotizing pancreatitis, 945
Necrotizing pneumonia, 1491
Necrotizing ulcerative gingivitis, 518.e2
Nedocromil sodium, 328t
Negative pressure devices, for pressure injury, 1058
Negative pressure wound therapy, for diabetic foot, 385
Neglect
  child, 277
  elder, 437
Neisseria gonorrhoeae, 526, 963–964.e1
  PCR, 1818
  urethritis, 1318
Neisseria meningitidis, 811
Nelfinavir, 18, 1901t
Nematodes, 126.e1t
Neomycin
  for fulminant hepatic failure, 578
  for hepatic encephalopathy, 578
Neonatal pneumoperitoneum, 1506–1507
Neonates
  anemia in, 1568.e1f
  bleeding in, 1582.e1, 1582.e1f
  cholestasis in, 1421
  cyanosis in, 1427
  encephalitis in, 443t
  intraabdominal mass lesions in, 1471
  jaundice in, 1473, 1670, 1670f

Neonates *(Continued)*
  lupus erythematosus in, 397t
  pneumatosis intestinalis in, 1505
  tetanus in, 1255.e3, 1255.e3f
Neoplasms. *See* Tumors/neoplasms
Neosporin, 171
Neostigmine, 30
Nephrectomy, for renal cell carcinoma, 1111–1112
Nephritic syndrome
  acute, 1491
  renal vein thrombus in, 1115f
Nephritis
  interstitial, 718–719.e1, 719f, 719.e1f
  renal failure with, 1518
Nephroblastoma, 888.e2, 888.e2t
Nephrocalcinosis, 1491
Nephrogenic diabetes insipidus, 375, 375.e2f
Nephrogenic fibrosing dermopathy, 888.e3
Nephrogenic systemic fibrosis, 888.e3–888.e4, 888.e3f
Nephrolithiasis, 1323–1325.e6, 1323t–1324t, 1324f, 1325.
    e2b, 1325.e3f–1325.e6f, 1325.e5b, 1325.e6t
Nephropathy
  diabetes mellitus and, 382
  IgA, 693–694.e1
  obstructive, 1491–1492
Nephrotic syndrome, 889–891.e1, 890t–891t, 891.e1f
Nephrotoxic acute renal failure, 1308.e3, 1309
Neprilysin inhibition, for dilated cardiomyopathy, 245
Nerve biopsy specimens, for chronic inflammatory
    demyelinating polyneuropathy, 292
Nerve conduction studies
  for chronic inflammatory demyelinating polyneuropathy,
    292, 293f
  for Guillain-Barré syndrome, 537
Nerves
  in foot and ankle pain, 1443
  heel pain and, 1452
Nesiritide, 558, 1087
Neural tube disorders, 1196.e2
Neuralgia
  cranial, headaches from, 1655–1656
  description of, 897
Neuraminidase inhibitors, 707
Neuritis, vestibular, 1365
Neuroacanthocytosis, 423t
Neuroblastoma, 891.e2–891.e3, 891.e2f, 891.e3t
  with Horner's syndrome, 1571f
Neurocognitive disorders, 892–893.e1
Neurocysticercosis, 353, 354f
Neurodegenerative diseases, 1411
Neurodermatitis, 758
Neurofibroma, 894f
Neurofibromatosis, 211, 894–895.e1, 894f–895f, 1370.e2t
Neurogenic bladder, 1492
Neurogenic diabetes insipidus, 375, 375.e2f
Neurogenic quadrilateral space syndrome, 1100.e8
Neurogenic stuttering, 1222.e4
Neuroinvasive West Nile virus infection, 1376.e5
Neurolabyrinthitis, 1365
Neuroleptic malignant syndrome, 794b, 896–896.e1, 896.
    e1t, 1163
Neuroleptics
  for acute stress disorder, 49
  for Huntington's disease, 639
Neurologic deficit
  focal, 1492
  multifocal, 1492
Neurologic hip pain, 1456
Neurologic paraneoplastic syndromes, 1726
Neuroma, acoustic, 16–16.e1, 16f
Neuromuscular junction dysfunction, 1492
Neuromuscular weakness, 1765f
Neuromyelitis optica, 855
Neuronal disorders, mental changes and coma caused by,
    1484
Neuronitis, vestibular, 1365–1365.e1
Neuropathic arthropathy, 273, 273f, 897t
Neuropathic bladder, 1493
Neuropathic pain, 897–899.e1, 897t, 898f, 899t
Neuropathic postural orthostatic tachycardia syndrome,
    1044.e2
Neuropathies
  autonomic, 1493, 1418
    with facial nerve involvement, 1493
    hereditary, 900–901
    painful, 1493

Neuropathies *(Continued)*
  peripheral
    asymmetrical proximal/distal, 1493–1494
    neurogenic bladder and, 1492
    sensory, 1492
    toxic and metabolic, 1494
Neurosyphilis, 1239
Neutropenia, 1626f, 1626.e1
  in childhood, 1494
  with decreased marrow reserve, 1494
  drug-induced, 1494
  drugs that cause, 1818b
  miscellaneous inherited disorders, 1823t
  with normal marrow reserve, 1494
  in pediatric patient, 1626.e1, 1626.e1f, 1626.e1b, 1627f
Neutrophil count, 1818, 1818b
Neutrophilia, 1494–1495
Neutrophils, hypersegmented, 90.e2f
Nevirapine
  for acquired immunodeficiency syndrome, 18
  for human immunodeficiency virus, 634
New Delhi metallo-beta-lactamase-1, 849
New World leishmaniasis, 742.e2
Newborn conjunctivitis, 326
Nexplanon, 330, 332
NF. *See* Necrotizing fasciitis; Neurofibromatosis
NF1, 894, 895f
NF2, 894
NGU. *See* Nongonococcal urethritis
NHL. *See* Non-Hodgkin lymphoma
Niacin
  deficiency of, 1368, 1369f
  for hyperlipidemia, 654.e4
  therapy for carcinoid syndrome, 239.e3
Niaspan, 654.e4t
Nicotinamide, 1065.e2
Nicotine, in pregnancy, 934.e2t
Nicotine stomatitis, 1214
Nicotinic acetylcholine receptor, 863
Nicotinic acid
  for hyperlipidemia, 654.e4t
  lipoprotein metabolism affected by, 647.e1t
NIDDM. *See* Non-insulin-dependent diabetes mellitus
Niemann-Pick type C disorder, 423t
Nifedipine
  for achalasia, 13
  for high-altitude pulmonary edema, 612–613
  for hypertension, 664t
  for Raynaud's phenomenon, 1103
Nikolsky sign, 969
Nintedanib, 692
Nipple
  discharge from, 1586–1587, 1586f–1587f
  lesions of, 1495
  Paget's disease of, 936f, 936–936.e1
NIPPV. *See* Noninvasive positive pressure ventilation, for
    chronic obstructive pulmonary disease
Nitazoxanide
  for ascariasis, 126
  for cryptosporidium infection, 348
  for giardiasis, 517
Nitrates
  for angina pectoris, 94–95
  for chemical-induced cardiomyopathy, 243
  for pulmonary edema, 1086
Nitric oxide donors, 1060t
Nitrite, urine, 1838
Nitrofurantoin
  chronic hepatitis caused by, 410.e2t
  for urinary tract infection, 1320t
Nitroglycerin
  for acute coronary syndrome, 35
  for cocaine overdose, 313
  for heart failure, 558
  for hypertension, 664t
  for myocardial infarction, 872–873
  for pulmonary edema, 1086
Nitroglycerin ointment, for anal fissure, 78.e2
Nitroprusside
  for aortic dissection, 115
  for pheochromocytoma, 992.e2t
  for pulmonary edema, 1086–1087
Nivolumab, 1112
NMS. *See* Neuroleptic malignant syndrome
NNRTI. *See* Nonnucleoside reverse transcriptase inhibitors
Nocardia spp., 901.e1–901.e3, 901.e1f–901.e2f

Nocardiosis, 901.e1–901.e3, 901.e1f–901.e2f
Nocturia, 457
Nocturnal angina, in heart failure, 554
Nocturnal enuresis, 701
Nocturnal polysomnography, 883
Nodular goiter
    illustration of, 1631.e1f
    toxic, 1832t
Nodular lesions
    in human immunodeficiency virus infections, 1457
    skin, 1495
Nodular lymphangitis, 776
Nodular melanoma, 805, 805f
Nodular plexiform neurofibroma, 894f
Nodular scabies, 1141t
Nodular sclerosis Hodgkin lymphoma, 623–624, 626.
    e1f–626.e2f
Nodules
    painful, 1495
    pulmonary, solitary, 1514–1515
    subcutaneous, arthritis and, 1403
Noisy breathing, 1414
Nonaccidental head injury, 1171
Nonalcoholic fatty liver disease, 902–903.e1, 902f, 1028t
Nonalcoholic steatohepatitis, 902
Nonallergic rhinitis, 904–905.e1
Nonallergic rhinitis with eosinophilia syndrome, 904
Nonallergic-noninfectious chronic rhinitis, 904
Non-arteritic anterior ischemic optic neuropathy, 727–728.e1
Nonbacterial pneumonia, 1015
Nonbacterial regional lymphadenitis, 260
Nonbullous impetigo, 697
Noncommunicating hydrocele, 640
Nonconvulsive status epilepticus, 1210
Nonepileptic seizure, 334.e2
Nongonococcal urethritis, 281t, 1318–1319, 1319.e1f
Nongranulomatous uveitis, 1334
Nonhematologic disorders, bone marrow fibrosis and, 1412
Non-Hodgkin lymphoma, 779–781.e1, 780t–781t, 1188,
    781.e1f, 781.e1t
Non-IgM MGUS, 844
Noninfectious granuloma, 1632f
Noninfectious inflammatory disease with fever of
    undetermined origin, 488
Non-insulin-dependent diabetes mellitus, 376–383.e11
    antihyperglycemic therapy for, 380t
    clinical evaluation of, 383.e11f
    comparison of therapies for, 379t
    criteria for diabetes screening, 378t
    diagnostic categories of, 377t
    insulin for, 381, 381t
    necrobiosis lipoidica with, 377, 383.e11f
    neuropathy of the hindfoot and, 383.e11f
    types of, 376t
Noninvasive positive pressure ventilation, for chronic
    obstructive pulmonary disease, 301
Nonketotic hyperosmolar syndrome, 652
Nonmalignant chronic pain, 937
Nonneuroinvasive West Nile virus infection, 1376.e5
Nonnucleoside reverse transcriptase inhibitors
    description of, 18, 1901t
    for human immunodeficiency virus, 632, 634
Nonocclusive mesenteric ischemia, 819, 819t
Nonorganic symptoms, 1195
Nonpleuritic chest pain, 1419–1420
Nonproliferative diabetic retinopathy, 376, 392, 392t,
    393.e1f–393.e3f, 393f
Nonscarring alopecia, 64, 1395
Nonsecretory myeloma, 851t
Nonsecretory pituitary adenoma, 997–999.e1
Nonseminoma, 1254
Non-small cell lung cancer, 769–771
Nonspecific aortoarteritis, 1244
Nonspecific bacterial epididymitis, 459
Nonspecific febrile illness, 434t
Nonspecific interstitial pneumonia, 412f
Nonspecific intraventricular conduction disturbance, 720
Nonspecific vaginitis, 1345
Non-ST-elevation myocardial infarction, 31
Nonsteroidal anti-inflammatory drugs
    for acute coronary syndrome, 35
    for ankylosing spondylitis, 101
    for Bartter syndrome, 176.e2
    for Behçet's disease, 182.e3
    for chronic fatigue syndrome, 291
    for corneal abrasion, 338

Nonsteroidal anti-inflammatory drugs (Continued)
    for De Quervain's tenosynovitis, 356
    for enteropathic arthritis, 456
    for erythema nodosum, 471
    for Gardner's syndrome, 483
    for hidradenitis suppurativa, 611
    for high-altitude sickness prophylaxis, 612–613
    for hypertrophic osteoarthropathy, 669
    for juvenile idiopathic arthritis, 733
    for lumbar spinal stenosis, 1203
    for mastitis, 796
    for mastodynia, 800
    for migraine headache, 546
    for myofascial pain, 880
    for osteoarthritis, 921
    for patellofemoral pain syndrome, 958.e6
    peptic ulcer disease caused by, 970t
    for pleurisy, 1005
    preoperative use of, 1055.e4
    for psoriatic arthritis, 1083
    for Reiter's syndrome, 1105
    for rheumatoid arthritis, 1127
    for temporomandibular joint syndrome, 1252
    for whiplash injury, 1376.e7
Nonsuppurative destructive cholangitis, 1063
Nonsustained paroxysmal ventricular tachycardia, 1361
Nontoxic diffuse goiter, 1631.e1f
Nontropical sprue, 263
Nonulcerative dyspepsia, 419–419.e1
Non–vitamin K oral anticoagulants, 1220
Noonan syndrome, 1301.e7, 1312.e2
Norepinephrine
    for hepatorenal syndrome, 601, 601t
    laboratory testing for, 1818
Norgestimate/ethinyl estradiol, for acne vulgaris, 15
Normal anion gap acidosis, 1401
Normal-pressure hydrocephalus, 642.e1f, 641–642.e1, 641f
Normocytic anemia, 1400
Norovirus, 548.e3
North American histoplasmosis, 619
Nortriptyline
    for attention deficit hyperactivity disorder, 161
    for burning mouth syndrome, 226.e4
Norwegian scabies, 1141t, 1142, 1142.e1f
Nose tip gangrene, 1440
Nosebleed, 463.e7, 463.e7f
Nosocomial bacterial meningitis, 813
Nosocomial endocarditis, 446
Nosocomial infections, 548.e2
Nosocomial sinusitis, 1185
Novacet. See Sulfacetamide-sulfa lotions
NP. See Nasal polyps
NPD. See Narcissistic personality disorder
NPDR. See Nonproliferative diabetic retinopathy
NPH. See Normal-pressure hydrocephalus
nQSS. See Neurogenic quadrilateral space syndrome
NRTIs. See Nucleoside/nucleotide reverse transcriptase
    inhibitors
NSAIDs. See Nonsteroidal antiinflammatory drugs
NSTEMI. See Non-ST-elevation myocardial infarction
NSVT. See Nonsustained paroxysmal ventricular tachycardia
Nuchal arm, breech birth, 218.e8
Nuclear imaging
    for cholecystitis, 287
    for cholelithiasis, 290
Nuclear renography, for renal artery stenosis, 1110
Nucleic acid amplification tests, 526
    for cervicitis, 272
    for chlamydia genital infections, 272
Nucleoside reverse transcriptase inhibitors, 1901t
Nucleoside/nucleotide reverse transcriptase inhibitors, 632
5-Nucleotidase, 1818
NUG. See Necrotizing ulcerative gingivitis
Nutritional deficiency syndromes, 1376.e3t
Nutritional disorders, 539.e1t
Nutritional support
    for alcoholic hepatitis, 59
    description of, 1694.e2, 1694.e2b, 1694.e2f
Nystagmus, 1495, 1695b
    dissociated
        characteristics and localizations of, 1695t
        identification of types of, 1698f
    gaze-evoked
        characteristics and localizations of, 1696t
        identification of types of, 1697f
    identification of types of, 1695f

Nystagmus (Continued)
    monocular, 1495
    vestibular
        characteristics and localizations of, 1696t
        identification of types of, 1696f
Nystatin
    for cutaneous candidiasis, 235
    for invasive candidiasis, 237

O

OA. See Osteoarthritis
OAG. See Open-angle glaucoma
Oasis, for venous ulcers, 1354
Oat cell carcinoma. See Small cell lung cancer
Obesity
    bariatric surgery for, 824, 907–908, 909.e7f
    clinical presentation of, 906
    comorbidities, 906
    definition of, 906
    demographics of, 906
    diagnosis of, 906–907, 909.e8f
    endocrine evaluation of, 909.e8f
    epidemiology of, 906
    etiology of, 906
    exercise for, 907, 909
    laparoscopic adjustable gastric banding for, 909.e7f
    physical findings of, 906
    in polycystic ovary syndrome, 1028t
    prevention of, 909
    prostate cancer and, 1071
    referral for, 908–909
    stroke risks, 1222
    treatment of, 824–825, 907–909
    weight-loss guidelines, 907t
Obesity dyslipidemia syndrome, 824
Obliterative endophlebitis of the hepatic veins, 223
Obliterative hepatocavopathy, 223
Obsession, 203
Obsessive-compulsive disorder, 622.e2, 910–910.e1
Obsessive-compulsive personality disorder, 622.e2,
    910–910.e1
Obstetric hemorrhage, 1040
Obstruction
    acute pancreatitis with, 1719.e1
    airway, 1394–1395
    bronchial, 1414
    ductal, male infertility and, 1471
    extrahepatic biliary, 1473
    of right atrial emptying, 1301.e7
    small bowel, 1525
    ureteric, congenital, 1762
    urinary tract, 1537
Obstructive jaundice, 1780t
Obstructive nephropathy, 1491–1492
Obstructive sleep apnea, 1189–1191.e1
    clinical presentation of, 1189
    definition of, 1189, 1191t
    demographics of, 1189
    diagnosis of, 1189–1190
    epidemiology of, 1189
    etiology of, 1189
    hypertension caused by, 660t
    imaging of, 1190
    in multiple system atrophy, 857.e2
    physical findings of, 1189
    polysomnography for, 1189, 1190f
    surgery for, 1191
    treatment of, 1190–1191
Obstructive sleep apnea syndrome, 1189
Obstructive sleep apnea–hypopnea syndrome,
    1189
Obstructive uropathy, 1538
Obturator sign, 121
Occipital nerve block, for migraine headache, 546
Occlusion, renal artery, 1745.e1–1745.e2
Occlusion amblyopia, 71
Occult blood, urine, 1838
Occult hydrocephalus, 641
Occult lymph-node metastases, breast cancer and, 217
Occupational chemicals, neuropathies caused by, 1494
Occupational exposures, 1903b
    blood, 1903b
Occupational lung cancer, 1478
OCD. See Obsessive-compulsive disorder; Osteochondritis
    dissecans

Octreotide
  for acromegaly, 24.e8
  for ascites, 129t
  for carcinoid syndrome, 239.e3
  for cluster headaches, 543
  for dumping syndrome, 412.e3
  for hypertrophic osteoarthropathy, 669
  for orthostatic hypotension, 857.e3t, 919
Ocular cicatricial pemphigoid, 463.e6t
Ocular foreign body, 910.e2, 910.e2f
Ocular rosacea, 1131
Oculopharyngeal muscular dystrophy, 860, 861t
Oculosympathetic paresis, 628
ODD. *See* Oppositional defiant disorder
Odor, breathing, 1414
Odynophagia, 1495–1498
Offloading, for Charcot's joint, 274
Ofloxacin
  for blepharitis, 202.e5
  for Chlamydia genital infections, 282
  for corneal abrasion, 338
  for epididymitis, 459
  for Q fever, 1100.e7
Ogilvie's syndrome, 29–30.e1, 29f, 29b–30b
OGTT. *See* Oral glucose tolerance test
OH. *See* Orthostatic hypotension
O'Hara's disease, 1309.e1, 1309.e1f
Ohio Valley fever, 619
OHL. *See* Oral hairy leukoplakia
Oidiomycosis, 234
Oil of cloves, 410.e1t–410.e2t
Olanzapine
  for Alzheimer's disease, 69t
  for schizophrenia, 1144–1145
Old age. *See* Elderly patients
Old World leishmaniasis, 742.e2
Olecranon bursitis, 229.e5
Oligoarthritis, 732t
Oligoarticular arthritis, 1404–1405
Oligoarticular juvenile idiopathic arthritis, 732, 733f
Oligomenorrhea, 413, 817
Oligoovulation, 703
Oliguria, 1702f
Oliguric renal failure of cirrhosis, 600
Olivopontocerebellar atrophy, 857.e2
Olopatadine hydrochloride, 328t
Olsalazine, 1314
Omalizumab
  for asthma, 135
  for chronic urticaria, 1329
  for urticaria, 1326
Omega-3 fatty acids
  for bipolar disorder, 191
  for hyperlipidemia, 654.e4t
  lipoprotein metabolism affected by, 647.e1t
Omphalotus poisoning, 862
OMS. *See* Opsoclonus-myoclonus syndrome
Onabotulinum toxin A, for urinary incontinence, 700–701
Ondansetron, for chemotherapy-induced nausea and
  vomiting, 276
Onycholysis
  causes of, 1702.e1f
  nail, 1694–1695
Onychomycosis, 234, 1274, 1274f. *See also* Tinea unguium
Onychomycosis Severity Index, 1274
Oophoritis, 858, 963
Opacification, air-space, on x-ray, 1394
Open-angle glaucoma, 519, 520.e2f–520.e3f, 520f
Ophthalmoplegia, 1495
Opiate abuse, 911
Opiate addiction, 911
Opioids
  addiction/dependence on, 405t, 911–913.e1, 912t–913t,
    913.e1t
  chronic pain managed with, 940.e3b, 940t
  pathophysiology, clinical effects, and management of,
    1716t–1719t
  prescribing guidelines for, 940.e3b
Opportunistic infections. *See also* specific infection
  in acquired immunodeficiency syndrome, 17, 18t–24t
  human immunodeficiency virus-related, 636t–638t
  prophylaxis for, 636t–638t
Oppositional defiant disorder, 913.e2–913.e3
Opsoclonus, 1495
Opsoclonus-myoclonus syndrome, 891.e2
Optic atrophy, 913.e4, 913.e4f, 1495–1496

Optic disc elevation, 1496
Optic nerve fenestration, for idiopathic intracranial
  hypertension, 690.e5
Optic neuritis, 913.e4, 914–914.e1, 914f, 914.e1f
Optic papillitis, 914
Oral cancer, 915–916.e1, 915f
Oral contents, aspiration of, 1576.e2, 1576.e2f
Oral contraceptives, 330
  for acne vulgaris, 15
  combination, 331–332, 332.e4t, 332.e6f
  for dysfunctional uterine bleeding, 413
  for emergency contraception, 440.e2
  formulations of, 332.e3t
  for hidradenitis suppurativa, 611
  for hirsutism, 617–618
  hyperpigmentation with, 1651t–1652t
  renin-aldosterone pattern in, 1829t
Oral dysesthesia, 226.e4
Oral glucose challenge test, for dumping syndrome, 412.e3
Oral glucose tolerance test
  in diabetes mellitus, 376
  for diabetic polyneuropathy, 389
Oral hairy leukoplakia
  characteristics of, 755, 755f
  mucocutaneous, 464
Oral hypoglycemics, 514
Oral malignant neoplasm, 915
Oral mucosa lesions
  erythematous, 1496
  pigmented, 1496
  punctate erosive, 1496
  white, 1496
Oral splints, for bruxism, 222.e2, 222.e2f
Oral ulcers
  acute, 1496
  vesicles and, 1496
Oral vaccine, for health care workers, 1884t–1886t
Oral vesicles, ulcers and, 1496
Oral-labial herpes simplex virus infections, 607t
Orbit
  human immunodeficiency virus manifestations of, 1459
  inflammation of, 1496–1497
Orbital decompression surgery, for Graves' orbitopathy, 667
Orbital lesions
  calcified, 1497
  cystic, 1497
Orbitopathy, Graves', 667.e2f
Orchiopexy
  for cryptorchidism, 347.e2–347.e4
  inguinal, 347.e3f
Orchitis, 917–917.e1, 917t
Orexin receptor antagonists, for insomnia, 712
Organ failure, 539.e1t
Organic disorders, 1387
Organic erectile dysfunction, 1436
Organophosphorus compounds, 1716t–1719t
Orgasm disorders, 435–436.e1, 436f
Orgasm dysfunction, 1497
Orlistat, 907–908
Ormond's disease, 1116.e11
Ornithosis, 1079.e4
Orofacial dyskinesia, 1251
Orofacial pain, 1497
Oromandibular (orofacial) dystonia, 422, 422f, 423t
Oropharyngeal candidiasis, 234
Oropharyngeal dysphagia, 1432
Oropharynx
  with fever of undetermined origin, 489t
  tumor of, 542.e1f
Ortho Tri-Cyclen. *See* Norgestimate/ethinyl estradiol
Orthopnea, in heart failure, 554
Orthopoxvirus, 1194.e2
Orthostatic hypotension, 660, 918–919.e1, 918t
  in multiple system atrophy, 857.e2, 857.e3t
  in parkinsonism, 857.e3, 857.e3t
  syncope caused by, 1234
Orthostatic intolerance, 1044.e2
Orthostatic tachycardia, 1044.e2
Ortner's syndrome, 335
OSA. *See* Obstructive sleep apnea
Osborne waves, 689f
Oseltamivir, for influenza, 707, 709t, 709.e2
Osgood-Schlatter disease, 920–920.e1, 920f
OSI. *See* Onychomycosis Severity Index
Osler nodes, 449.e2f
Osler-Rendu-Weber syndrome, 920.e2–920.e3, 920.e2f

Osler's disease, 920.e2
Osmolality
  serum, 1818
  urine, 1838
Osmotic fragility test, 1819
Ospemifene, 417
Osseous hip pain, 1456
Ossification, 1745.e3f
Osteitis deformans, 935
Osteoarthritis, 921–922.e4, 922.e4f, 922f, 1126t
Osteoarthropathy, hypertrophic, 1464
Osteoarthrosis, 921
Osteochondritis dissecans, 922.e5–922.e6, 922.e5f
Osteochondrosis, 922.e5
Osteolytic benign bone lesions, 1497
Osteomalacia, 1128.e4, 1366
Osteomas, in familial adenomatous polyposis, 482
Osteomyelitis, 384, 923–924.e1, 923f, 924t
  fungal, 237
  paronychia as cause of, 958
  tuberculous spinal, 1305f
  vertebral, 534.e2
Osteonecrosis, 166, 166t, 167f–168f
  of jaw, 191.e2–191.e3, 927
  of proximal femoral epiphysis, 742
Osteoporosis, 925–927.e5, 925t, 927f, 927.e5f, 1068
  causes of, secondary, 1497
  in children, 1497
  fractures caused by, 1363
Osteosarcoma, 204, 205f
Osteosclerosis, diffuse, 1497
Osteosclerotic benign bone lesions, multiple, 1497
Otitis externa, 928–929.e1, 928f
Otitis media, 930–931.e1, 930f
  with effusion, 928–929.e1, 928f
Otomycosis, 928–929.e1
Otosclerosis, 931.e2–931.e3, 931.e3, 931.e2f, 931.e2t
Otospongiosis, 931.e2–931.e3
Ottawa ankle rules, 99.e7, 99.e7t
Ovarian cancer, 933.e1f, 932–933.e1, 932t
Ovarian insufficiency, primary, 1066–1066.e1, 1066t
Ovarian neoplasm, benign, 934–934.e1, 934f
Ovarian pregnancy, 430, 430f, 431.e1f
Ovarian tumor of low malignant potential, 932
Overactive bladder, 700
Overdose
  digoxin, 395.e2–395.e4, 395.e3f–395.e4f
  tricyclic antidepressant, 1301.e9–1301.e11, 1301.e9f,
    1301.e9t–1301.e10t, 1301.e11f
Overdrive pacing, for atrial flutter, 154
Overflow incontinence, 700
Overlap syndrome, 705–706
Over-the-counter medications, in pregnancy, 934.e2–934.
  e3, 934.e2t
Ovulation suppression, 1054
Ovulatory dysfunction, 1497–1498
Oxacillin
  for breast abscess, 214
  for erysipelas, 468
Oxacillin-resistant *Staphylococcus aureus*, 828
Oxaliplatin, 315
Oxamniquine, 1143.e2
Oxandrolone, 362
Oxazepam, 56t
Oxcarbamazepine
  for bipolar disorder, 191
  for neuropathic pain, 899
  for trigeminal neuralgia, 1302
Oxycodone
  for chronic pain, 940t, 940.e3t
  for neuropathic pain, 899
Oxygen saturation, 613.e2f
Oxygen therapy. *See also* Hyperbaric oxygen
  for acute coronary syndrome, 35
  for chronic obstructive pulmonary disorder, 336
  for cor pulmonale, 336
Oxymorphone, 940t, 940.e3t
Oxytocic drugs, 1040t
Oxytocin, 1040t
Oxytocin receptor antagonists, 1060t
Oxyuriasis, 996

P

PA. *See* Pernicious anemia
PAC. *See* Perennial allergic conjunctivitis

Pacemakers. See also Implantable cardioverter-defibrillators
  for complete heart block, 549, 550t, 550.e1t
  preoperative considerations for, 1055.e5
  for sinus node dysfunction, 1178t
PACG. See Primary angle-closure glaucoma
Pachydermoperiostosis, 668
Pachymeningitis, 534.e1f
PACNS. See Primary angiitis of the central nervous system
PAD. See Peripheral arterial disease
Paget's disease
  of bone, 935–935.e1, 935.e1f
  of breast, 936–936.e1, 936f
Paget-Schroetter syndrome, 360
PAH. See Pulmonary arterial hypertension
Pain
  abdominal. See Abdominal pain
  back. See Back pain
  bone, 1413
  breast, 800
  chest. See Chest pain
  chronic, 940.e2f, 940.e3b–940.e4b, 940.e3t, 937–940.e4,
    938f, 939t–940t
  complex regional pain syndrome, 320.e1f–320.e2f,
    320–320.e2
  diffuse, 1390
  edema with, 1433
  elbow, 1433
  epigastric, 1435
  extremity, 1403–1404
  facial, 1437–1445
    headache and, 1641–1643
  foot, 1444, 1444, 1528
    and ankle, 1443
    midfoot, 1498–1516
  forearm, 1444
  hand, 1444
    in different age groups, 1771
    and swelling, 1638–1639
  heel, 1452
    plantar, 1452, 1704.e1
    posterior, 1705–1706
  iliac fossa, 1469–1472
  knee, 1475, 1475, 1500
  leg, 1676b
    algorithm for, 1676f
    with exercise, 1476
  low back, 766.e2, 766.e3t
  management of, 940.e2f, 937–940.e4, 938f, 939t–940t
  midfoot, 1498–1516
  myofascial, 879–880.e1, 879f–880f, 879t, 1252
  neck, 1491, 1694, 1694b
    algorithm for, 1694f
    from rheumatologic disorders, 1491
  neuropathic, 897t, 898f, 899t, 897–899.e1
  orofacial, 1497
  pelvic
    chronic, 1502
    genital origin, 1503
    in non-pregnant female, 1503
    in women, 1502
  perianal, 1503
  pleuritic, 1005
  rectal, 1731–1732
  scrotal, 1521–1522
  shoulder, 1133.e4t
    in different age groups, 1523–1524
    differential diagnosis of, 1523
    evaluation of, 1732f–1734f
    by location, 1524
  testicular, 1531
  thyroid, 1750f
  urolithiasis-like, 1538
  wrist, 1540
    causes of, 1771
    in different age groups, 1771
Pain syndrome, trochanteric, 1303–1303.e1, 1303f
Painful arc sign, 1133.e2
Painful bladder syndrome, 713, 713f
Painful ejaculation, 435
Painful intercourse, 416, 417f
Painful nodules, 1495
Painful periods, 415
Painful subacute thyroiditis, 1268–1268.e1
Painful temporomandibular joint, 1252
Painful tics/spasms, 1302
Painless postpartum thyroiditis, 1268

PAIR. See Percutaneous aspiration-injection-reaspiration
Palatal myoclonus, 878
Palatal necrotic ulcers, proptosis and, 1510
Palindromic rheumatism, 1706–1707
Pallidal deep-brain stimulation, for Parkinson's
  disease, 957
Palmaris longus tendon, 259.e4f
Palmar rash, 1440
Palmoplantar hyperkeratosis, 1707–1709
Palonosetron, 276
Palpitation, 1709–1710
  algorithm for, 1872.e1f
  history of, 1851t
PAN. See Polyarteritis nodosa
Pancoast tumor, 769
Pancolitis, 1313, 1313t–1314t, 1315f
Pancreas
  abscess of, 946
  calcifications of, 948.e1f, 1416, 1709.e1
  endocrine tumors of, 507.e3t
  mumps involvement of, 858
Pancreatic ascites, 946
Pancreatic cancer, 941–942.e1, 941f, 942t
  diagnostic algorithm for, 1872.e1f
  Lynch syndrome and, 782
Pancreatic cystic lesions, 1710–1711
Pancreatic duct, dilated, 948.e2f
Pancreatic endocrine tumors, 1370.e2t
Pancreatic insufficiency, 785
Pancreatic islet cell tumors, 1872.e1f
Pancreatic solid lesions, 1710.e1–1710.e3
Pancreatitis
  acute
    characteristics of, 943–946.e1, 943t, 944f,
      945t–946t
    in children, 1711–1712
  chronic, 948.e1f–948.e2f, 947–948.e2
  drug-induced, 1721.e1–1721.e2
Pancytopenia, 1723–1724
  in aplastic anemia, 81.e1f
  with cellular bone marrow, 1500
  hypocellular bone marrow, 1500
    cytopenia, 1500
  syndrome, inherited, 1500
Pandemic flu, 709.e2
Panhypopituitarism, 685
Panic attack, 949–950.e1, 949t, 993
Panic disorder, 949–950.e1, 949t
Panitumumab, 315
Panniculitis
  alpha-1-antitrypsin deficiency and, 67
  characteristics of, 951–952, 951t, 952f
  leg ulcers with, 1477
Pannus, 1126
Pantothenic acid deficiency, 1368
Pap cytology, for cervical dysplasia, 269
Pap smear, for cervical polyps, 271.e4
Papillary carcinoma, 1264–1265.e2, 1265.e2f
Papillary conjunctivitis, 326
Papilledema, 690.e5, 1500
Papulopustular rosacea, 1131
Papulosquamous diseases, 1500
Papulosquamous disorders, 1872.e1f
Paracentesis, for ascites, 127, 1032
Paracentesis fluid, 1819–1820
Paracetamol poisoning, 11
Parachute valve, 836
Paraesophageal hiatal hernia, 609.e2, 609.e2f
Paraganglioma, 991, 991t
Parainfluenza viruses, 1015–1016
  acute bronchitis caused by, 27t
  croup caused by, 345.e3
Paralysis
  acute flaccid, 1442
  facial, 183
  periodic
    hyperkalemic, 1503
    hypokalemic, 1503–1504
  vocal cord, 1542
Paralysis agitans, 956
Paralytic ileus, 1445
Paramyotonia congenita, 881
Paranasal sinus tumors, 1490
Paraneoplastic cerebellar degeneration, 953–955.e1, 953t
Paraneoplastic erythrocytosis, 953–955.e1, 953t
Paraneoplastic neuropathy, 899t

Paraneoplastic syndromes, 769t, 953–955.e1, 953t–954t,
  954b
  endocrine, 1500
  neurologic, 1726
  nonendocrine, 1500
Paraneoplastic thrombocytosis, 953–955.e1, 953t
Paranoid personality disorder, 955.e2–955.e3
Paraparesis
  acute or subacute, 1500–1501
  chronic progressive, 1501
Parapharyngeal abscess, 982t
Paraphilic disorders, 961.e2–961.e3
Paraplegias, 1501
  spastic, 1526
Parapneumonic effusion, 1009
Parasellar masses, 1501
Parasitemia, 790
Parasitic infections
  hookworm, 627–627.e1, 627f
  in human immunodeficiency virus infection, 1458
  leishmaniasis, 742.e2–742.e4
  in lower gastrointestinal tract disease, 1458
  lung abscess and, 767
  malaria, 787–791.e1, 787t–788t, 788f
  myositis with, 1489
  pediculosis, 961–961.e1, 961f
  pinworms, 996, 996f
  schistosomiasis, 1143.e1–1143.e3, 1143.e1f
Parasternal chondrodynia, 343, 343t
Parathyroid autotransplantation, for hypoparathyroidism, 684
Parathyroid hormone, 1820–1821
  in hyperparathyroidism, 655–656.e1
  in hypoparathyroidism, 683–684.e1, 683t
Parathyroidectomy, for hyperparathyroidism, 656
Paratyphoid fever, 1135, 1135t
Parenchymal lung disease, drug-induced, 412.e1f–412.e2f,
  411–412.e2, 412f, 412t
Paresthesias, 1501
Paricalcitol, 297
Parietal cell antibodies, 1821
Paritaprevir/ritonavir/ombitasvir, 588
Parkinsonian syndrome, 956f
Parkinsonism
  in multiple system atrophy, 857.e2–857.e3
  myoclonus with, 878
  orthostatic hypotension in, 857.e3, 857.e3t
Parkinsonism-plus syndromes, 1501–1502
Parkinson's disease, 476, 857.e2, 957.e2f, 892–893.e1,
  956–957.e2, 956f
Parks classification, of anorectal abscess, 978f
Paromomycin
  for amebiasis, 72t
  for giardiasis, 517
Paronychia, 234, 958–958.e1, 958f
Parotid gland
  in mumps, 858, 858f
  pleomorphic adenoma of, 1134, 1134f
Parotid swelling, 1502
Parotitis, 858
Paroxetine
  for acute stress disorder, 49
  for premenstrual dysphoric disorder, 1053.e2
  for premenstrual syndrome, 1055
Paroxysmal atrial fibrillation, 149, 151f
Paroxysmal atrial tachycardia, 1231
Paroxysmal cold hemoglobinuria, 958.e2–958.e3, 958.e3t
Paroxysmal nocturnal dyspnea
  in heart failure, 554
  in mitral stenosis, 836
Paroxysmal nocturnal hemoglobinuria, 958.e4–958.e5,
  958.e5f
Paroxysmal positional vertigo, benign, 185–187.e1, 185b,
  186f, 187t
Paroxysmal supraventricular tachycardia, 1230
Parrot pneumonia, 1079.e4
Pars planitis, 1334
Partial lung resection, for bronchiectasis, 220
Partial molar pregnancy, 841–842
Partial seizures, 1157
Partial thromboplastin time, 1821, 1821t
  activated, 1821, 1821t
Partially reversible transition, 512.e5–512.e6
Parvovirus B19 infection, 493–494.e1, 493f–494f
Patch testing, for contact dermatitis, 329
Patellofemoral pain syndrome, 958.e6–958.e7
Patent ductus arteriosus, 959–960.e1, 959f–960f

Patent foramen ovale, 960.e2–960.e4, 960.e2f–960.e3f, 960.e3t, 1221
Paucibacillary leprosy, 742.e5–742.e6
Pautrier microabscesses, 863.e2
PBC. *See* Primary biliary cirrhosis
PCD. *See* Paraneoplastic cerebellar degeneration
PCH. *See* Paroxysmal cold hemoglobinuria
PCI. *See* Percutaneous coronary intervention
PCOS. *See* Polycystic ovary syndrome
PCP, 1013
PCR. *See* Polymerase chain reaction
PCS. *See* Postconcussive syndrome
PCSK9 inhibitors, 342
PCV13. *See* Pneumococcal conjugate vaccine
PD. *See* Parkinson's disease
PDA. *See* Patent ductus arteriosus
PDD NOS, 162
PDH. *See* Progressive disseminated histoplasmosis
PDR. *See* Proliferative diabetic retinopathy
PE. *See* Pulmonary embolism
PEA. *See* Pulseless electrical activity
Pectin, for dumping syndrome, 412.e3
Pediatric enuresis, 458f
Pediatric medication errors, 960.e5–960.e6
Pediatric patients. *See also* Adolescents; Children; Infant(s); Toddlers
    airway obstruction in, 1394–1395
    anal incontinence in, 1397
    arthritis in, 1405
    blindness in, 1410–1411
    bradycardia in, 1585.e1, 1585.e1f
    cataracts in
        congenital infections in, 1418
        developmental variants in, 1418
        differential diagnosis of, 1418
        endocrinopathies in, 1418
        genetic disorders in, 1418
        ocular anomalies in, 1418
    cervical instability in
        acquired, 1419
        congenital, 1419
    coma in, 1424
    dehydration in
        clinical observations of, 1801t
        correction of, 1604.e1–1604.e3
    emesis in, 1433
    failure to thrive in, 478–479.e1, 478f
    fever in, 1626.e1b, 1626.e1f, 1627, 1627f
    gastrointestinal bleeding in, 1629.e2, 1629.e2b
        evaluation of, 1816f
        lower, 1409
        upper, 1410
    hematuria in, 1636.e1, 1636.e1b, 1636.e1f
    hypokalemia in, 1466
    hypomagnesemia, 1467
    hypophosphatemia in, 1467
    hypovolemic shock in, 1469
    immunizations, 1860t–1864t
        catch-up schedule, 1859–1865, 1860t–1864t
    intubation in, 1668.e1–1668.e2, 1668.e1b
        rapid-sequence medications for, 1668.e2t
        treatment algorithm for, 1668.e1f
    limp in, 1477
    neutropenia in, 1626.e1, 1626.e1b, 1626.e1f, 1627f
    protein-losing enteropathy in, 1510
    pulmonary hemorrhage in, 1514
    reactive erythema in, 1872.e1f
    respiratory distress in, 1908f
    seizures in, 1522
    soft tissue tumors in, 1525–1526
    stridor in, 1528–1529
    stroke in, 1529
    sudden death in, 1530
    tachycardia in, 1747.e1f
    undernutrition in, 478
    wheezing in, 1771
Pediculosis, 961–961.e1, 961f
Pediculus spp., 961–961.e1, 961f
Pedophilic disorder, 961.e2–961.e3
Pegloticase, 530
Pegvisomant, 24.e8
Pegylated interferon alpha, 584
Pelvic abscess, 962–962.e1, 962.e1f
Pelvic avulsion fractures, 1502
Pelvic floor muscle training, for stress incontinence, 700–701

Pelvic inflammatory disease, 272, 281t, 963–964.e1, 964.e1f
Pelvic mass, 1502, 1896f
Pelvic organ prolapse, 965–967.e1, 965t, 966b, 967f, 967t
Pelvic outlet syndrome, 996.e1
Pelvic pain
    chronic, 1502
    genital origin, 1503
    in non-pregnant female, 1503
    in women, 1502
Pelvic ultrasound
    for molar pregnancy, 842, 842.e1f
    for polycystic ovary syndrome, 1025, 1028.e3f
Pelviectasis, 643
Pelvocaliectasis, 643
Pembrolizumab, 771
Pemirolast potassium, 328t
Pemphigoid, 226.e2
Pemphigus, 968
Pemphigus erythematosus, 968
Pemphigus foliaceus, 968
Pemphigus vulgaris, 968–969, 968f, 969t
Penicillamine
    for urolithiasis, 1325
    for Wilson's disease, 1376.e9
Penicillin
    for actinomycosis, 26.e3
    for aspiration pneumonia, 1006
    for botulism, 206
    for cellulitis, 266
    for gingivitis, 518.e2
    for leptospirosis, 742.e8
    for lung abscess, 767–768
    for lymphangitis, 776
    for osteomyelitis, 924t
    for peritonsillar abscess, 982
    for retropharyngeal abscess, 1118
    in rheumatic fever, 1124.e3
    for Scarlet fever, 1143
    for syphilis, 1239
    for tabes dorsalis, 1243.e5
Penicillin G
    for brain abscess, 208
    for erysipelas, 468
    for peritonsillar abscess, 981
    for Whipple's disease, 1376.e8
Penicillin V
    for erysipelas, 468
    for pharyngitis, 989
    for prepubescent vaginitis, 1342
    for sickle cell disease, 1181
    for tonsillitis, 989
Penicillin VK
    for actinomycosis, 26.e3
    for anaerobic infections, 78
    for gingivitis, 518.e1
    for lung abscess, 767–768
    for peritonsillar abscess, 982
Penile fibromatosis, 987
Penile plethysmography, 961.e2
Penile rash, 1503
Penis
    curvature of, 687.e1
    hypospadias, 687.e1–687.e2, 687.e2f
    lichen planus of, 756.e1f
    lichen sclerosus of, 757
Pennyroyal, 410.e1t–410.e2t
Pentamidine, 1013–1014
Pentavalent antimonials, 742.e2
Pentosan polysulfate sodium, 714
Pentoxifylline, 977
    for Behçet's disease, 182.e3
    for claudication, 309
    for venous ulcers, 1354
Peptic esophagitis, 511
    heartburn treatment, 512.e3f
    pathogenesis of, 511f
    therapy for, 512t
Peptic ulcer disease
    characteristics of, 970–971.e2, 970t, 970b
    Helicobacter pylori as cause of, 563–564, 970
Perampanel, 1156
Percutaneous aortic balloon valvuloplasty, for aortic stenosis, 119
Percutaneous aspiration-injection-reaspiration, for echinococcosis, 428
Percutaneous balloon mitral valvotomy, 838

Percutaneous coronary intervention
    for angina pectoris, 96
    for heart failure, 560
    for myocardial infarction, 869
Percutaneous embolization, for carcinoid syndrome, 239.e3
Percutaneous endoscopic gastrostomy
    for dysphagia, 421
    for failure to thrive, 479
Percutaneous heart valve replacement, 119
Percutaneous nephrostomy tubes, for hydronephrosis, 644
Percutaneous transhepatic cholangiography
    for cirrhosis, 305
    for jaundice, 730
Percutaneous transluminal coronary angioplasty, for cocaine overdose, 313
Percutaneous vertebroplasty, for vertebral compression fractures, 1364
Perennial allergic conjunctivitis, 327t
Perforation, esophageal, 1436
Perfusion scintigraphy, for cor pulmonale, 336
Perianal abscess, 978, 978f
Perianal cellulitis, 266t
Perianal pain, 1503
Periarteritis nodosa, 1021
Periarticular pain
    acute, 1473
    hip, 1456
Periarticular structures, in foot and ankle pain, 1443
Pericardial disease, cardiac enlargement with, 1417
Pericardial effusion
    description of, 240f–241f, 1503
    malignant, treatment approach to, 1709.e1f
Pericardiocentesis
    for cardiac tamponade, 241
        with draining catheter, 241
Pericarditis, 972–974.e1, 973f–974f
    constrictive, and restrictive cardiomyopathy, 252.e1t, 252f
    treatment of, 237
Periductal mastitis, 796
Perinatal asphyxia, 105
Perinatal iron overload, 1472
Perinephric abscess, 1099, 1106
Period of Purple Crying, 1171
Periodic fever, 484, 787, 1441
Periodic health examination, 1849–1858
    adolescents, 1872
    adult, 1872
    age-specific charts of, 1837t, 1849t, 1851t, 1853t, 1855t, 1857t–1858t, 1858t
    summary of major changes in, 1906t
Periodic paralysis
    hyperkalemic, 1503
    hypokalemic, 1503–1504
Periorbital cellulitis, 266t
Peripheral aromatase activity, 539.e1t
Peripheral arterial disease
    characteristics of, 975–977.e2, 975f–976f, 977.e2f
    claudication in, 307, 307t–308t
Peripheral arterial stenosis, 975
Peripheral nerve vasculitis, 899t
Peripheral neuropathies
    approach to, 1710f
    neurogenic bladder and, 1492
Peripheral tibial nerve stimulation, for urinary incontinence, 701
Peripheral ulcerative keratitis, 463.e6t
Peripheral vascular disease, 975, 1202t
Peripubertal youth, 512.e6
Perirectal abscess, 978–978.e1, 978f
Peritoneal carcinomatosis, 1504
Peritoneal effusion, 1504
Peritoneal irritation, pelvic pain with, 1503
Peritonitis
    secondary, 979
    spontaneous bacterial, 980–980.e1
Peritonsillar abscess, 981–982.e1, 981f–982f, 981t
Periumbilical abdominal pain, 1388
Periumbilical swelling, 1504
Periungual fibromas, 1308.e4t
Perleche, 99
Permanent atrial fibrillation, 149
Permanent pacemaker, for second-degree heart block, 552
Permethrin
    for pediculosis, 961
    for scabies, 1141, 1142t
Permethrin spray, for bedbugs, 182

Permissive hypercapnia, for acute respiratory distress syndrome, 46
Pernicious anemia, 89–90.e2, 89t–90t, 90.e1f–90.e2f
Peroneal muscular atrophy, 275, 275f
Persistent atrial fibrillation, 149, 151f
Persistent complex bereavement disorder, 536.e2
Persistent hiccups, 1456
Persistent juvenile pattern, 424
Persistent prepubertal macromastia, 539.e1t
Persistent vegetative state, 1540
Personality disorders, 620.e2. *See also specific disorders*
  borderline, 205.e2–205.e4, 205.e3f
  dependent, 370–370.e1
  histrionic, 620.e2–620.e3
  narcissistic, 882–882.e1
  obsessive-compulsive, 910–910.e1
  paranoid, 955.e2–955.e3
Perthes disease, 742
Pertussis, 983–984.e1, 983b, 984t
Pervasive developmental disorder, 162
Petechial hemorrhage, 1890t
Petechial rash with fever, 1442
Petit mal epilepsy, 1153
Peutz-Jeghers syndrome, 941, 985–986, 985t, 986f
Peyronie's disease, 987–988, 987b, 988f
PF. *See* Pemphigus foliaceus
PFO. *See* Patent foramen ovale
PFPS. *See* Patellofemoral pain syndrome
PG. *See* Pyoderma gangrenosum
PGU. *See* Postgonococcal urethritis
pH
  blood, 1821
  disturbances, mental changes and coma with, 1484
  urine, 1838–1839
Phagocyte defects, 1470
Phagocytic function, immunodeficiency, vaccination for, 1873t
Phakomatoses, 1411
Phalangeal tufts, 1413
Phalen's sign, 259, 259f
Pharyngeal cancer, 916
Pharyngeal diphtheria, 395.e5
Pharyngeal obstruction, 1504
Pharyngitis, 981t, 989–990.e1, 989t, 1124.e2
Pharyngoesophageal diverticulum, 1378.e4–1378.e5, 1378.e4f–1378.e5f
Phenobarbital, 1821
  for cocaine overdose, 313
  for Gilbert's syndrome, 518
Phenoxybenzamine, 992.e2t
Phentolamine
  for cocaine overdose, 313
  for hypertension, 664t
  for pheochromocytoma, 992.e2t
Phenylbutazone, 410.e3t
Phenylephrine, 248
Phenytoin, 1821
  for cocaine overdose, 313
  for intermittent explosive disorder, 712.e4t
Pheochromocytoma, 991t, 991–992.e2, 992f, 992.e1f, 992.e2t
  hypertension caused by, 660t
  -type spells, 1504
Philadelphia chromosome, 753, 754f, 1261
Phlebotomy
  for cor pulmonale, 336
  for hemochromatosis, 565–566
  for polycythemia vera, 1030b
Phlegmon, 946
PHN. *See* Postherpetic neuralgia
Phobias, 993–994.e1, 994f
Phosphatase
  acid, 1771
  alkaline, 1774
  leukocyte alkaline, 1814
Phosphate
  decreased, 1821
  increased, 1821
  serum, 1821, 1843t
  urine, 1839
Phosphate replacement
  for diabetic ketoacidosis, 388
  for hyperglycemic hyperosmolar syndrome, 653
Phosphodiesterase inhibitors
  for pulmonary edema, 1087
  for Raynaud's phenomenon, 1104

Phosphodiesterase-5 inhibitors
  for erectile dysfunction, 467
  for pulmonary arterial hypertension, 1094
Photocoagulation, for diabetic retinopathy, 393
Photodermatoses, 1504
Photodynamic therapy
  for basal cell carcinoma, 178t
  for macular degeneration, 783
Photoepilation, for hirsutism, 617
Photosensitivity, 1504, 1f–3f
Phototherapy
  for chronic urticaria, 1330
  for seasonal affective disorder, 1151.e2
Phthirus pubis, 961–961.e1
Phymatosis, 1131, 1131f
Physical abuse
  child, 277
  elder, 437
Physical complaints, ill-defined, 1872.e1f
Physical therapy
  for cervical disc syndromes, 268.e3
  for myofascial pain, 880
  for piriformis syndrome, 996.e1–996.e2
Physiologic myoclonus, 878
Physiologic vertigo, 847
PI. *See* Protease inhibitors
PID. *See* Pelvic inflammatory disease. *See also* Primary immunodeficiency disease
PIDDs. *See* Primary immunodeficiency diseases
Pigment stones, 290
Pigmentation, hyperpigmentation, 1650f
Pigmented oral mucosa lesions, 1496
Pigment-induced acute kidney injury, 1392
Pigment-induced acute renal failure, 1518
Pigmenturia, 1504–1505
Piles, 572.e2
"Pill-rolling" tremor, 956f
Pills, contraceptive, 440.e2, 440.e2t
Pilocarpine, 1606.e3f
Pilocarpine iontophoresis test, for cystic fibrosis, 351, 351t
Pilonidal abscess, 995
Pilonidal cyst, 995
Pilonidal disease, 995–995.e1, 995.e1b, 995.e1f
Pilonidal sinus, 995, 995.e1b
Pimecrolimus
  for atopic dermatitis, 148
  for vitiligo, 1370
Pimozide, 1282
PIMs. *See* Potentially inappropriate medications
Pink eye, 326
Pinworms, 126.e1t, 996, 996f, 1077.e5
Pioglitazone, 381
Piperacillin/tazobactam
  for actinomycosis, 26.e3
  for anaerobic infections, 78
  for appendicitis, 122
  for aspiration pneumonia, 1006
  for diabetic foot, 385
  for diverticular disease, 403
  for epididymitis, 459
  for lung abscess, 767
  for necrotizing fasciitis, 887
  for perirectal abscess, 978
  for peritonsillar abscess, 982
  for secondary peritonitis, 979
Piperazine citrate, 126
Pirfenidone, 691
Piriformis syndrome, 996.e1–996.e2, 996.e1f–996.e2f
Pit viper bites, 197, 197t, 199.e1f
Pitting, of nails, 1694.e1–1694.e2
Pituitary adenoma, 686f, 997–999.e1, 998t, 999f
Pituitary apoplexy, 685
Pituitary insufficiency, 685
Pituitary irradiation, for Cushing's disease and syndrome, 349
Pituitary tumors, 685, 1069–1070.e1, 1505
  evaluation of, 1711f
  TSH-secreting, 1832t
Pityriasis amiantacea, 1270t
Pityriasis capitis, 1152
Pityriasis rosea, 1000–1000.e1, 1000f
Pityriasis versicolor, 1276
Pityrosporum orbiculare, 1276
PIVSD. *See* Postinfarct ventricular septal defect
PJP. *See* Pneumocystis jiroveci pneumonia
PKD. *See* Polycystic kidney disease
Placenta previa, 1001–1002.e1, 1001f–1002f

Placental separation, premature, 9
Plague vaccine, 1888t
Plantar fascia, 1003, 1003f
Plantar fasciitis, 1003–1004.e1, 1003f, 1105
Plantar heel pain, 1452, 1704.e1
Plantar neuroma, 846.e3
Plantar warts, 1375
Plaque brachytherapy, for retinoblastoma, 1116.e8
Plaque psoriasis, 1081, 1081f
Plasma
  acid-base reference values for, 1771t
  protein concentrations in, 1787t
Plasma cell hepatitis, 595
Plasma cell myeloma, 204
Plasma exchange
  for hemolytic-uremic syndrome, 567
  for Lambert-Eaton myasthenic syndrome, 738.e2
  for transverse myelitis, 1296
Plasmacytoid lymphocyte, 1816t
Plasmacytoma, 204
Plasmacytosis, cerebrospinal fluid, 1787b
Plasma-derived nanofiltered C1/NH, 98.e3t
Plasmapheresis
  for Guillain-Barré syndrome, 538
  for microscopic polyangiitis, 830
  for myasthenia gravis, 863
  for parasitemia, 790
Plasminogen, 1821
Plasmodium falciparum, 787–791.e1, 787t
Plasmodium knowlesi, 787t
Plasmodium malariae, 787t, 789
Plasmodium ovale, 787t, 788
Plasmodium vivax, 787t, 788f
Plastic induration of the penis, 987
Platelet aggregation, 1821–1822
Platelet antibodies, 1822
Platelet count, 1822.e1f, 1822, 1822t
Platelet destruction, 1823t
Platelet function analysis 100 assay, 1822
Pleomorphic adenoma, 1134, 1134f
Pleural disease, 717t
Pleural effusion, 1505
  causes of, 1713b
  cellular differential of, 1823b
  in human immunodeficiency virus infections, 1457
  infected, 441
  light criteria for classification of, 1713b
  malignancy-associated, 1505, 1713.e1f
  purulent, 441
  signs and symptoms of, 1713b
Pleural hyperplasia, 1505
Pleural masses, 1505
Pleurisy, 1005
Pleuritic chest pain, 1005, 1420
Pleuritis, 1005
Plexopathies
  brachial, 1493–1494
  lumbosacral, 1494
Plumber's itch, 350.e5, 350.e5f
Plumbism, 740
PMDD. *See* Premenstrual dysphoric disorder
PMF. *See* Primary myelofibrosis
"P-mitrale", 837
PML. *See* Progressive multifocal leukoencephalopathy
PMR. *See* Polymyalgia rheumatica
PMS. *See* Premenstrual syndrome
Pneumatic dilation, for achalasia, 13
Pneumatosis intestinalis, in neonate and older child, 1505
Pneumococcal conjugate vaccine, 1010
  for adults, 1882t
  catch-up schedule, 1859–1865, 1860t–1864t
  contraindications and precautions, 1868t–1869t
  indications for, 1878t–1881t
  recommended schedule for, 1878t–1881t
Pneumococcal polysaccharide vaccine
  for adults, 1882t
  conditions misperceived as contraindications to, 1870t–1871t
  contraindications and precautions, 1868t–1869t
  for health care workers, 1884t–1886t
  during pregnancy, 1883t
  recommended immunization schedule, 1878t–1881t
Pneumococcal vaccines
  catch-up schedule, 1859–1865, 1860t–1864t
  recommended ages and intervals, 1865t–1866t
  recommended schedule for, 1860t–1864t

Pneumoconiosis, 1183
Pneumocystis jiroveci pneumonia
  in AIDS-infected patients, 17, 24.e4f
  characteristics of, 636t–638t, 830, 854, 1013–1014.e1,
    1013f–1014f, 1014t, 1014.e1f
  treatment of, 18t–24t
Pneumonia
  aspiration, 767t, 1006–1006.e1
  bacterial, 1007–1010.e4, 1008b–1010b, 1008t, 1009f,
    1010.e4f
  chronic, 1505–1506
  community-acquired, 1008t, 1008b–1010b
  eosinophilic, 458.e7–458.e9
  healthcare-associated, 548.e5
  interstitial, 1016.e1f
  mimics of, 1506
  mycoplasma, 1011–1012.e1, 1011t, 1012f
  necrotizing, 1491
  Nocardia, 901.e1f–901.e2f
  nonresponding, 1506
  Pneumocystis jiroveci
    in AIDS-infected patients, 17, 18t–24t, 24.e4f
    characteristics of, 636t–638t, 830, 854, 1013–1014.e1,
      1013f–1014f, 1014t, 1014.e1f
  recurrent, 1506
  usual interstitial, 691f
  viral, 1015–1016.e1, 1016.e1f
Pneumonia Severity Index, 1007
Pneumoperitoneum, neonatal, 1506–1507
Pneumothorax
  in children, 1507
  spontaneous, 1017–1019.e2, 1017f–1019f, 1019.e2f,
    1528
  tension, 1018, 1018f
PNH. *See* Paroxysmal nocturnal hemoglobinuria
POAG. *See* Primary open-angle glaucoma
Pocket sciatica, 996.e1
Podofilox
  for condyloma acuminatum, 324
  for warts, 1376
Podophyllin
  for condyloma acuminatum, 324
  resin, for warts, 1376
Poison ivy dermatitis, 329, 1020–1020.e1, 1020.e1f
Poisoning
  acetaminophen, 11–11.e2, 11.e2f, 11.e1t
  acute, 1715f
  alcohol, 1560, 1560f
  anticholinergic, 1575, 1575f
  arsenic, 899t
  botulism, 206–206.e1
  carbon monoxide, 238–239.e1, 238t, 239f
  ethylene glycol, 826b, 826–827.e2, 827.e2f
  food, bacterial, 500t, 500–501.e2
  lead, 740–741, 741t, 1736.e1t
  methanol, 826b, 826–827.e2, 827.e2f
  mushroom, 862t, 862–862.e1, 862.e1t
Polio, 1020.e2
Poliomyelitis
  description of, 1020.e2–1020.e3, 1041.e2–1041.e3
  vaccine for, 1888t
Poliosis, 1507
Poloxamer, 1182
Poly(adenosine diphosphate) polymerase inhibitor, 1073
Polyangiitis, microscopic, 1351.e2t
Polyarteritis nodosa, 830t, 1021t, 1022f, 1021–1022.e1,
  1245t, 1350, 1540, 1821
Polyarthralgias, in fifth disease, 493
Polyarthritis, 732, 732t
  in fifth disease, 493
  symmetric, 1083f
Polyarticular arthritis, 1405
Polyarticular joint pain, 1474
Polyarticular pseudogout, 1079
Polycystic echinococcosis, 427
Polycystic kidney disease, 1023–1024.e1
Polycystic ovary syndrome
  characteristics of, 1025–1028.e4, 1025t, 1026f,
    1027t–1028t, 1028.e3f–1028.e4f
  hirsutism caused by, 616, 616f
Polycythemia
  absolute, 1507–1508
  diagnostic algorithm for, 1719.e1f
  differential diagnosis of, 1507
  relative or spurious, 1398, 1507, 1507
Polycythemia vera, 1029–1030.e1, 1029f, 1030b, 1030.e1f

Polygenic hyperalphalipoproteinemia, 654
Polygenic hypercholesterolemia, 654
Polymenorrhea, 413
Polymerase chain reaction
  brucellosis, 220.e2
  Chlamydia trachomatis, 1785
  cystic fibrosis, 1795
  cytomegalovirus, 1795
  Huntington's disease, 1809
  Legionella pneumophila, 1814
  Mycoplasma pneumoniae, 1818
  Neisseria gonorrhoeae, 1818
Polymorphic ventricular tachycardia, 1361
Polymorphous exanthem, in Kawasaki disease, 735.e3f
Polymyalgia rheumatica, 1031b, 1031t, 1031–1031.e1,
  1031.e1f
Polymyalgias, 1508
Polymyositis, 397t, 698.e1t, 704, 705t, 706f, 706.e1f
Polyneuropathy
  chronic inflammatory demyelinating, 292–293.e1
  demyelinating, 1508
  distal sensorimotor, 1508
  drug-induced, 1508
  mixed sensorimotor, 1508
  painful, 1493
  predominantly autonomic, 1508
  predominantly motor, 1508
  predominantly sensory, 1508
  symmetric, 1509
Polyp(s)
  cervical, 271.e4, 271.e4f
  endocervical, 271.e4, 271.e4f
  nasal, 885b, 885–885.e1, 885.e1f
Polypharmacy, 1031.e2–1031.e3
Polypoid gastric cancer, 507.e1f
Polyposis syndrome, 985–986
Polysomnography
  for insomnia, 711
  for narcolepsy, 883
  for obstructive sleep apnea, 1189, 1190f
Polyuria, 1509
  hypotonic, 1468
  water diuresis as cause of, 1776b
  xerostomia with, 1779
POP. *See* Pelvic organ prolapse
Popeye deformity, 187.e3, 187.e4f
Popliteal swelling, 1509
Popliteal synovial cyst, 170.e2
Poradenitis inguinalis, 778.e2
Pork tapeworm, 353, 354f
Porphyria
  acute intermittent, 1736.e1t
  aminolevulinic acid dehydratase-deficient, 1736.e1t
  congenital erythropoietic, 1736.e1t
  diagnostic tests for, 1736.e1t
  hepatoerythropoietic, 1736.e1t
  variegate, 1736.e1t
Porphyria cutanea tarda, 1736.e1t
Portal hypertension, 1032–1033.e1, 1033.e1f, 1032f–1033f,
  1033t
  cirrhosis with, 305f
  differential diagnosis of, 1509
Portal system disorders, splenomegaly with, 1528
Portal systemic shunts, for Budd-Chiari syndrome, 224
Portal vein thrombosis, 1034–1034.e1, 1034f
Port-wine stain, 1222.e2–1222.e3, 1222.e2f
Posaconazole
  for aspergillosis, 131
  for blastomycosis, 202.e3
  for Chagas' disease, 272.e4
  for coccidioidomycosis, 313.e3
  for histoplasmosis, 620
  for invasive candidiasis, 237
Positive ice test, for myasthenia gravis, 863, 863.e1f
Positron emission tomography
  for Hodgkin lymphoma, 625f
  for pheochromocytoma, 992
  for primary lung neoplasms, 770
Postcoital contraception, 330, 332, 440.e2
Postconcussion syndrome, 1035
Postconcussive syndrome, 1035–1036.e1, 1035b
Postconfusion syndrome or encephalopathy, 1035
Postductal coarctation of the aorta, 111
Posterior cerebral artery transient ischemic attack, 1293
Posterior fossa meningioma, 809f
Posterior heel pain, 1705–1706

Posterior ischemic optic neuropathy, 727–728.e1
Posterior malleolus, 99.e2
Posterior scleritis, 1146–1146.e1
Posterior spinal sclerosis, 1243.e5
Posterior tibial nerve neuralgia, 1251.e2
Postgastrectomy syndrome, 412.e3
Postgonococcal urethritis, 1318
Posthepatic jaundice, neonatal, 1473
Postherpetic neuralgia, 609, 1037–1038.e1, 1038f
Postinfarct ventricular septal defect, 1358
Postinfectious irritable bowel syndrome, 1300
Postinfectious polyneuritis, 537
Postinfectious tropical malabsorption, 1303.e2
Post–kala azar dermal leishmaniasis, 742.e2
Post-Lyme disease syndrome, 775
Postmenopausal bleeding, 1509
Postpartum blues, 1039–1039.e1
Postpartum depression, 1039–1039.e1
Postpartum fever, 1441
Postpartum hemorrhage, 1040–1041.e1, 1040t, 1041b,
  1041f
Postpartum psychosis, 1039–1039.e1
Post-phlebitic syndrome, 1042
Postpolio syndrome, 1020.e2, 1041.e2
Postpoliomyelitis syndrome, 1041.e2–1041.e3
Poststreptococcal glomerulonephritis, 523t–524t
Postthrombotic syndrome, 360, 1042, 1042f, 1352
Posttraumatic nervous instability or brain injury, 1035
Posttraumatic stress disorder
  borderline personality disorder and, 205.e2
  description of, 536.e2, 993, 1043–1044.e1
Postural drainage, for bronchiectasis, 219
Postural hypotension, 660, 918, 1467–1468, 1509
Postural orthostatic tachycardia syndrome, 1044.e2–1044.
  e3, 1044.e3f
Postural tachycardia syndrome, 1044.e2
Postural tremors, 1534
Postvoid dribble, 701
Potassium. *See also* Hyperkalemia
  for Bartter syndrome, 176.e2
  hyperkalemic periodic paralysis, 1503
  hypokalemic periodic paralysis, 1503–1504
  serum levels, 1823–1824
  urine, 1839
Potassium citrate, for urolithiasis, 1325
Potassium hydroxide (KOH), for contact dermatitis, 329
Potassium iodide, for radiation exposure, 1100.e14t–1100.
  e16t
Potassium phosphate, for radiation exposure, 1100.
  e14t–1100.e16t
Potassium replacement, for hyperglycemic hyperosmolar
  syndrome, 653
Potentially inappropriate medications, 1031.e2
POTS. *See* Postural orthostatic tachycardia syndrome
Pott's disease, 534.e2
PPD. *See* Paranoid personality disorder
PPH. *See* Postpartum hemorrhage
PPI. *See* Proton pump inhibitors
PPM. *See* Permanent pacemaker
PPoma, 507.e3t
PPS. *See* Postpoliomyelitis syndrome
Pramipexole, 957
Pramlintide, 381
Prasugrel
  for acute coronary syndrome, 34
  for coronary artery disease, 342
Pravastatin, 654.e4t
Praziquantel
  for cysticercosis, 354
  for schistosomiasis, 1143.e2
  for tapeworms, 1250
Prazosin
  for acute stress disorder, 49
  for pheochromocytoma, 992.e2t
PRCA. *See* Pure red cell aplasia
Precocious puberty, 1046t, 1047f–1048f, 1045–1048.e1,
  1512
Precocity, sexual, 1523
Prednisolone
  for autoimmune hepatitis, 596
  for Bell's palsy, 184
  for corneal abrasion, 338
Prednisone
  for amaurosis fugax, 70
  for amyloidosis, 76.e4
  for anaphylaxis, 79

Prednisone (Continued)
for angioedema, 98
for aspergillosis, 131
for autoimmune hemolytic anemia, 83
for autoimmune hepatitis, 596
for Behçet's disease, 182.e3
for Bell's palsy, 184f
for bullous pemphigoid, 226.e2
for celiac disease, 264
for cerebral vasculitis, 266.e6
for chronic inflammatory demyelinating polyneuropathy, 293
for chronic obstructive pulmonary disease, 301
for chronic pain, 939t
for cirrhosis, 306
for cluster headaches, 543
for Cogan's syndrome, 313.e5
for contact dermatitis, 329
for Crohn's disease, 345
for cystic fibrosis, 352
for Duchenne muscular dystrophy, 860
for eosinophilic granulomatosis with polyangiitis, 458.e5
for erythema multiforme, 470
for giant cell arteritis, 516
for hemophilia B, 570
for Henoch-Schönlein purpura, 574
for hypereosinophilic syndrome, 651.e1
for hypersensitivity pneumonitis, 657–658
for immune thrombocytopenic purpura, 695
for inflammatory myopathies, 705
for Lambert-Eaton myasthenic syndrome, 738.e2
for lichen planus, 756
for paroxysmal nocturnal hemoglobinuria, 958.e4
for pemphigus vulgaris, 969
for pityriasis rosea, 1000
for *Pneumocystis jiroveci* pneumonia, 1013
for polyarteritis nodosa, 1022
for polymyalgia rheumatica, 1031
for Ramsay Hunt syndrome, 1101–1101.e1
for rheumatic fever, 1124.e3
for sarcoidosis, 1138
for systemic lupus erythematosus, 1243t
for systemic vasculitis, 1351
for thrombotic thrombocytopenic purpura, 1263
for ulcerative colitis, 1315
for uveitis, 1334
Preductal coarctation of the aorta, 111
Preeclampsia, 1049–1051.e1, 1049b, 1049t–1050t, 1050f–1051f
Preexcitation syndrome, 1377
Pregabalin
for chronic pain, 939t
for diabetic polyneuropathy, 389
for neuropathic pain, 899
Pregnancy
abdominal pain in, 1389
acute fatty liver of, 485–485.e1
amenorrhea during, 1397
anaphylactoid syndrome of, 1398
antivenom use during, 199
atrial septal defect and, 158
breast cancer during, 217
causes of nausea and vomiting in, 1490
ectopic, 430–431.e1, 430f, 431.e1f
effects on thyroid physiology, 1833t
epulis in, 1100.e4
fatty liver of, 485–485.e1
folate intake in, 814.e2, 1196.e4
follow-up visits in, 1857t
gingivitis in, 518.e1
heart failure in, 1452
HELLP syndrome in, 564.e2–564.e3, 564.e2b, 564.e3f
HIV screening in, 1897
human immunodeficiency virus in, 635
hyperemesis gravidarum in, 651
hypertension in, 663–664, 664t
immunizations and, 1883t
liver disease in, 1478
molar, 841–842.e1, 841f, 842t, 842.e1f
nongonococcal urethritis in, 1319
over-the-counter medications in, 934.e2–934.e3, 934.e2t
periodic health examination in, 1857t
in polycystic ovary syndrome patients, 1026
pyelonephritis in, 1322
renin-aldosterone pattern in, 1829t
Rh incompatibility, 1120f–1121f, 1119–1121.e1

Pregnancy (Continued)
seizures of, 429
from sexual assault, 1166
spontaneous, 1204–1205.e1
in Takayasu's arteritis patients, 1246
test for, 440.e3
thrombocytopenia in, 1532
toxemia of, 1049
toxoplasmosis in, 1287–1290.e1, 1288f–1289f
trauma in, 1752f
vaginal bleeding during, 1335–1335.e1, 1539–1543
ventricular septal defect and, 1360
Zika virus in, 1379–1384.e1, 1380f–1382f, 1383b–1384b
Pregnancy-induced hypertension, 1049
Prehepatic jaundice, neonatal, 1473
Preleukemia, 864
Premarin, for dysfunctional uterine bleeding, 413
Premature adrenarche, 1046t
Premature ejaculation, 435
Premature graying, of scalp hair, 1509
Premature labor, 1059
Premature menopause, 1066
Premature ovarian failure, 1066
Premature rupture of membranes, 1052–1053.e1, 1052f
Premature separation, of placenta, 9
Premature ventricular contractions, 1509–1510
Premenstrual dysphoric disorder, 1052–1053.e3
Premenstrual syndrome, 1054–1055.e1, 1054t, 1055f
Preoperative clearance, 1055.e2
Preoperative evaluation, 1055.e2–1055.e6, 1055.e2b, 1055.e3f, 1055.e3t
Preoperative evaluation and risk reduction, 1055.e2
Prepatellar bursitis, 229.e5
Prepubertal lichen sclerosus, 757
Prepubescent vaginitis, 1342–1342.e1
Prerenal azotemia, 600
Preretinal hemorrhage, 1116.e4
Presacral masses, in children, 1510
Presenile gangrene, 1259.e1
Pressure dressing, for corneal abrasion, 338
Pressure injury, 1056–1058.e1, 1056f
Pressure Sore Status Tool, 1058
Pressure sores, 1056
Pressure Ulcer Scale for Healing, 1058
Pressure ulcers, 1056
Pre-stroke, 1294, 1295f
Presumed ocular histoplasmosis syndrome, 619
Preterm birth syndrome, 271.e2
Preterm labor, 1059b–1060b, 1059–1060.e1
Preterm premature rupture of membranes, 1052f, 1052–1053.e1
Priapism, 1060.e2–1060.e3, 1060.e2t
Primaquine, 789
Primary adrenal disorders, 1393–1394
Primary adrenocortical insufficiency, 52
Primary aldosteronism, 61, 1393
hypertension caused by, 660t
Primary amenorrhea, 73
Primary amyloidosis, 845.e1t, 76.e3
Primary angiitis of the central nervous system, 266.e5, 266.e5t, 266.e7t, 1061–1062.e1, 1062.e1f, 1061t–1062t
Primary angle-closure glaucoma, 521–521.e1
Primary atypical pneumonia, 1011
Primary biliary cirrhosis, 595–596, 1063–1065.e1, 1064f
Primary brain tumor, 211
Primary central nervous system tumors, 211t
Primary choledocholithiasis, 288
Primary coronary angioplasty, for myocardial infarction, 874.e1f
Primary cutaneous lymphoma, 863.e5t
Primary empty sella syndrome, 685
Primary focal segmental glomerulonephrosis, 890t
Primary glial disorders, mental changes and coma caused by, 1484
Primary hyperlipoproteinemia, 654–654.e4, 654.e2f, 654.e2t–654.e4t
Primary hyperparathyroidism, 656.e1f, 655–656.e1
Primary hypertrophic osteoarthropathy, 668–669.e1
Primary hyperuricemia, 529
Primary hypothyroidism, 690.e2f, 690–690.e3, 1046t
Primary immunodeficiency diseases
characteristics of, 1065.e2–1065.e7, 1065.e2f, 1065.e3b–1065.e4b, 1065.e3t–1065.e6t
vaccination of, 1873t
Primary intestinal pseudoobstruction, 1471
Primary lung abscess, 767

Primary lymphedema, 777
Primary malignant bone tumor, 205f, 204–205.e1
Primary membranous nephropathy, 890t
Primary myelofibrosis, 1065.e8–1065.e10, 1065.e8f, 1065.e9t, 1065.e10b
Primary open-angle glaucoma, 519, 520.e2f–520.e3f
Primary osteoporosis, 925–927.e5, 925t, 927f, 927.e5f
Primary ovarian insufficiency, 73–74, 1066–1066.e1, 1066t
Primary peritonitis, 980
Primary polycythemia, 1029
Primary Raynaud's phenomenon, 1102–1104.e1, 1102f–1103f
Primary sclerosing cholangitis, 595–596, 1067–1068.e1, 1067f, 1067t
Primary Sjögren's syndrome, 1186–1188.e2
Primary spontaneous pneumothorax, 1017
Primary syphilis, 1238–1239.e1, 1238f
Primary tricuspid regurgitation, 1301.e4
Primidone, 476
Prinzmetal's variant, of angina, 91
Prion disease, 343.e3, 893
Prion protein, 343.e3
Probenecid, 964
Probenemid, 530
Probiotics
for *Clostridium difficile* infection, 310
for fulminant hepatic failure, 578
for hepatic encephalopathy, 578
for irritable bowel syndrome, 724
Procainamide, 1824
Procaine hydrochloride, 192
Prochlorperazine
for Ménière's disease, 808
for migraine headache, 546t
Procidentia, 1104.e2
Proctitis
characteristics of, 281t
herpes simplex virus, 607t
in HIV infection, 1458
Proctocolectomy, for ulcerative colitis, 1315
Prodromal symptoms, 470
Progestasert, 330
Progesterone
for amenorrhea, 76
for dysfunctional uterine bleeding, 413
for gender dysphoria disorder, 512.e6
serum, 1824
Progestins
for endometriosis, 453
for menopause, 816
Program death receptor, 807
Progressive disseminated histoplasmosis, 619
Progressive hepatolenticular degeneration, 1376.e9
Progressive multifocal leukoencephalopathy, 18t–24t, 443t, 1068.e2–1068.e3
Progressive postpoliomyelitis muscular atrophy, 1041.e2
Progressive relapsing multiple sclerosis, 855
Progressive supranuclear ophthalmoplegia, 1068.e4
Progressive supranuclear palsy, 956, 857.e2, 1068.e4–1068.e5, 1068.e4f
Prolactin, 1825
in hirsutism, 617
level for galactorrhea, 505
Prolactinoma
characteristics of, 997–999.e1, 1069–1070.e1, 1070f, 1070.e1f
galactorrhea from, 505, 505f
Proliferative actinic keratosis, 25
Proliferative diabetic retinopathy, 393.e1f–393.e3f, 392, 392t, 393f
Proliferative retinopathy, 376
Prolonged grief disorder, 536.e2
Prolonged QT syndromes, 1510
Prolymphocyte, 1816t
Prolymphocytic leukemia, abnormal lymphocytes with, 1816t
PROM. *See* Premature rupture of membranes
Promethazine
for Ménière's disease, 808
for migraine headache, 546t
Pronator syndrome, 1070.e2, 1070.e2f
Propafenone
for atrial fibrillation, 151f
for atrial flutter, 154
for Wolff-Parkinson-White syndrome, 1378

Propranolol
for alcohol abuse, 56t
for aortic dissection, 115
for essential tremor, 476
for hyperthyroidism, 667
for portal hypertension, 1033
Proptosis, 1510
palatal necrotic ulcers and, 1510
Propylthiouracil
for Graves' disease, 535
for hyperthyroidism, 666
for radiation exposure, 1100.e14t–1100.e16t
for thyrotoxic storm, 1268.e2
Prostaglandin analogs, for open-angle glaucoma, 519
Prostaglandin F2α, dysmenorrhea and, 415
Prostanoids
for cor pulmonale, 337
for pulmonary arterial hypertension, 1094
Prostate, 410.e1t–410.e2t
Prostate cancer
classification of, 1071
clinical presentation of, 1071
definition of, 1071
demographics of, 1071
diagnosis of, 1071–1072
epidemiology of, 1071
Gleason classification of, 1071–1072
laboratory tests for, 1071–1072
metastatic castration-resistant, 1074t
pain syndromes in, 1074t
physical findings of, 1071
risk groups for, 1071t
treatment of, 1072–1074, 1072t
Prostate-specific antigen, 1825
for benign prostatic hyperplasia, 1075–1076
for prostate cancer, 1071–1074.e9
serum, factors that affect, 1825t
Prostatic acid phosphatase, 1825
Prostatic hyperplasia, benign, 1075–1076.e2, 1075t,
1076.e2f
Prostatic hypertrophy, 1075
Prostatitis, 1077–1077.e1
Prosthetic valve endocarditis, 446
Protease inhibitors, 18
dosing of, 1901t
for human immunodeficiency virus, 632, 634
Protein
serum, 1825
urine, quantitative, 1839
Protein C
assay, 1825
deficiency of, 648, 648t–649t, 650, 1825t
Protein C anticoagulant pathway, 1292t
Protein electrophoresis, serum, 1825, 1826f
Protein malabsorption, 785
Protein S
assay, 1826, 1827t
deficiency of, 648, 648t–649t, 1827t
Protein-losing enteropathy, in pediatric age, 1510
Proteinuria
algorithm for, 1720f
differential diagnosis of, 1510
nephrotic-range, 890, 891.e1f
Prothrombin concentrate complex, 1220
Prothrombin G20210A mutation, 648, 648t
Prothrombin time, 1826
Prothrombotic states, 648t
Proton pump inhibitors
for gastrinoma, 507.e4
for gastritis, 508
for gastroesophageal reflux disease, 173, 511
for *Helicobacter pylori*, 564, 971
for nonulcerative dyspepsia, 419
Protoporphyrin, free erythrocyte, 1826
Protozoa, 1458
Protriptyline, 884
Proximal femur fracture, 614
Proximal subclavian artery stenosis or occlusion, 1226
PrP. *See* Prion protein
Prurigo nodularis, 298.e6f
Pruritus
differential diagnosis of, 1510–1511
generalized, evaluation of, 1721f
in pregnancy, 1721.e1f
sequential approach to, 298.e7f
Pruritus ani, 1077.e2–1077.e3, 1511

Pruritus vulvae, 1077.e4–1077.e6, 1077.e4f, 1511
Prussian blue, for radiation exposure, 1100.e14t–1100.e16t
PSA. *See* Prostate-specific antigen
PSC. *See* Primary sclerosing cholangitis
Pseudocardiomegaly, 1417
Pseudoclaudication, 307, 307t
Pseudocyanosis, 1511
Pseudocyst, 945
Pseudoepistaxis, 463.e7
Pseudogout, 1079.e1b, 1079.e1f–1079.e3f, 1078–1079.e3,
1078t, 1079b, 1079f
Pseudohemophilia, 1371
Pseudohermaphroditism
differential diagnosis of, 1455, 1721.e2
female, 1511
male, 1511
Pseudohypertension, 665
Pseudohyponatremia, 680–681
Pseudohypoparathyroidism, 683, 683t–684t
Pseudoinfarction, 1511
Pseudomembranous colitis, 310
Pseudomembranous conjunctivitis, 326
Pseudomembranous croup, 1290.e2
Pseudoobstruction, intestinal, 1471
"Pseudo-polymyalgia rheumatica", 1078
Pseudopseudohypoparathyroidism, 683t
Pseudorheumatoid nodule-subcutaneous granuloma
annulare, 531, 531f
Pseudorubella, 1133
Pseudothrombophlebitis syndrome, 170.e2
Pseudotumor cerebri, 690.e5
Psittacosis, 1079.e4–1079.e5
Psoas sign, 121
Psoralens, hyperpigmentation with, 1651t–1652t
Psoriasis, 1080–1081.e1, 1081f, 1807t, 1269
Psoriatic arthritis, 1807t, 1083.e1f, 101t, 732, 732t,
1082–1083.e1, 1082b, 1082t, 1083f
PsoriGel. *See* Tar products
PSP. *See* Progressive supranuclear palsy
PSVT. *See* Paroxysmal supraventricular tachycardia
Psychodynamic psychotherapy, for dependent personality
disorder, 370
Psychoeducation, for delusional parasitosis, 367.e2
Psychogenic impotence, 467
Psychogenic movement disorder, 334.e2
Psychogenic stuttering, 1222.e4
Psycho-infantile personality disorder, 620.e2
Psychological abuse, elder, 437
Psychosexual desire disorder, situational hypoactive, 672
Psychosexual dysfunction associated with inhibited libido,
672
Psychosexual dysfunction with inhibited libido, 672
Psychosexual therapy, 466
Psychosis, 445, 1084–1085.e1, 1085f. *See also* specific
psychosis
cycloid, 190
differential diagnosis of, 1511
Korsakoff's, 735.e8
medical disorders-induced, 1512
medication-induced, 1512
postpartum, 1039–1039.e1
Psychotherapy
for anorexia nervosa, 103
for binge eating disorder, 188
for borderline personality disorder, 205.e2
for bulimia nervosa, 225
for Crohn's disease, 345
for dissociative disorders, 400
for hypochondriasis, 674.e1
for paranoid personality disorder, 955.e2
Psychotropic drugs, hyperpigmentation with,
1651t–1652t
PT. *See* Prothrombin time
PTA. *See* Peritonsillar abscess
PTEN hamartoma tumor syndrome, 986
PTH. *See* Parathyroid hormone
Ptosis
asymmetric, 863.e1f
differential diagnosis of, 1512
in Horner's syndrome, 628
PTS. *See* Postthrombotic syndrome
PTSD. *See* Posttraumatic stress disorder
PTT. *See* Partial thromboplastin time
PTU. *See* Propylthiouracil
Pubertal delay, 361, 361f–363f, 363.e1t–363.e3t
Pubertas praecox, 1045

Puberty
delayed, 361, 361f–363f, 363.e1t–363.e3t, 1512
precocious, 1045–1048.e1, 1046t, 1047f–1048f, 1512
PUD. *See* Peptic ulcer disease
Puerperal abscess, 214
Pulmonary abscess, 767
Pulmonary arterial hypertension, 840.e3, 1092–1095.e2,
1093f
Pulmonary artery enlargement, 303
Pulmonary clearing, for chronic obstructive pulmonary
disease, 300
Pulmonary crackles, 1512–1513
Pulmonary cysts, 1513
Pulmonary disease, in human immunodeficiency virus
infection, 1459–1460
Pulmonary edema, 1086–1087.e1, 1087f, 1087.e1f
in acute decompensated heart failure, 558
acute noncardiac, 412.e2f
high-altitude, 613.e1f, 613.e1t, 613.e2b, 612–613.e2, 613b
in mitral stenosis, 836
noncardiogenic, 1513
Pulmonary embolism, 1091.e2f, 1091.e3t, 1088–1091.e3,
1088t, 1089f–1090f
Pulmonary eosinophilia, 1513
Pulmonary fibrosis, idiopathic, 691–692.e1, 691f, 692t
Pulmonary function tests, for sarcoidosis, 1138
Pulmonary heart disease, heart failure and, 1452
Pulmonary hemorrhage
diffuse syndromes, 1514
focal, 1513
in microscopic polyangiitis, 830.e1f
in pediatric age, 1514
Pulmonary hypertension
characteristics of, 1092t, 1093f, 1092–1095.e2, 1182
in mitral stenosis, 836
Pulmonary infiltrates, in immunocompromised patients,
1514
Pulmonary lesions, 1514
Pulmonary mass, solitary
causes of, 1514
mimics of, 1514
Pulmonary mucormycosis, 848
Pulmonary nodule
diagnostic algorithm for, 1723f–1724f
solitary, 1514–1515
tests for, 1722b
Pulmonary rehabilitation, for chronic obstructive pulmonary
disease, 300
Pulmonary sporotrichosis, 1205.e2
Pulmonary thromboembolism, 1088
Pulmonary thromboendarterectomy, for cor pulmonale, 337
Pulmonary tuberculosis, 1306–1308.e2, 1308.e2f
Pulmonary valve calcification, 1416
Pulmonary vasoconstriction, 335
Pulmonary vein isolation, for atrial fibrillation, 151
Pulmonary-renal syndromes, 1515
Pulsed Solu-Medrol, 293
Pulseless disease, 1244
Pulseless electrical activity, 1096–1096.e1, 1096f, 1515
Pulseless ventricular tachycardia, 1758f
Pulsion diverticulum, 1378.e4
Pulsus paradoxus, 132
Punctate erosive oral mucosa lesions, 1496
Pupillary block glaucoma, 521
Pupillary dilatation, poor response to darkness, 1515
Pure gonadal dysgenesis, 73
Pure red cell aplasia, 1096.e2–1096.e4, 1096.e2t–1096.
e4t, 1096.e4f
Purpura
differential diagnosis of, 1726f
Henoch-Schönlein, 573–574.e1, 573f, 574t, 1245t
hyperglobulinemic, 1373f
immune thrombocytopenic, 696.e1f, 695–696.e1, 696f
nonpalpable, 1515
nonpurpuric disorder simulating, 1515–1516
palpable, 1516
petechial hemorrhage, 1890t
thrombotic, 1515
thrombotic thrombocytopenic, 1263–1263.e1, 1263.e1f
Purulent conjunctivitis, 326
Purulent otitis media, 930
Purulent pleural effusion, 441
Pustular psoriasis, 1081f
PUVA phototherapy
for mycosis fungoides, 863.e4
for psoriasis, 1080

PV. *See* Pemphigus vulgaris; Polycythemia vera
PVD. *See* Peripheral vascular disease
PVT. *See* Portal vein thrombosis
Pyelocaliectasis, 643
Pyelonephritis, 1097–1100.e1, 1322
Pylethrombosis, 1034
Pyoderma, 697
Pyoderma gangrenosum, 1100.e2–1100.e3, 1100.e2f
Pyogenic arthritis, 1161
Pyogenic granuloma, 1100.e4–1100.e5, 1100.e4f
Pyogenic hepatic abscess, 760
Pyogenic liver abscess, 760, 761f
Pyonephrosis, 1097
Pyosalpinx, 963, 964.e1f
Pyrantel pamoate
    for ascariasis, 126
    for hookworms, 627
    for pinworms, 996
Pyrazinamide
    for granulomatous arthritis, 534.e2
    for pulmonary tuberculosis, 1308
Pyridostigmine
    for Lambert-Eaton myasthenic syndrome, 738.e2
    for myasthenia gravis, 863
    for orthostatic hypotension, 919
Pyridoxine, 90.e3
Pyrimethamine, 1290
Pyrophosphate arthropathy, 1078
Pyrosis, during pregnancy, 1431

Q

Q fever, 1100.e6–1100.e7, 1100.e6f, 1100.e6t
QSS. *See* Quadrilateral space syndrome
QT interval prolongation, 1516
Quadrilateral space syndrome, 1100.e8–1100.e9, 1100.e8f
Quadrivalent HPV vaccine, 1376
Quadrivalent meningococcal conjugate vaccine, 1868t–1869t, 1868t–1869t
Quadrivalent meningococcal polysaccharide vaccine, 1868t–1869t
Quantaferon test, for pulmonary tuberculosis, 1307
Quartan malaria, 787
Quetiapine
    for Alzheimer's disease, 69t
    for bipolar disorder, 191
Quick clot hemostatic agent, 463.e8
Quincke's sign, 116
Quinidine
    for Brugada syndrome, 222
    for malaria, 790
Quinine sulfate
    for babesiosis, 170
    granulomatous hepatitis caused by, 410.e3t
    for malaria, 790
Quinsy, 981
Quinupristin-dalfopristin, for vancomycin-resistant *Enterococcus*, 1346

R

RA. *See* Rheumatoid arthritis
Rabbit fever, 1309.e1, 1309.e1f
Rabies
    characteristics of, 1100.e10–1100.e11, 1100.e11f
    vaccinations for, 1888t
Radiation exposure, 1100.e12–1100.e17, 1100.e12t–1100.e16t
Radiation injury, 227, 228t, 229.e4f
    categorization of, by depth, 227t
    classification of, 227
    complications in, 229.e3b
    follow-up care for, 229
    Mayes equations for, 229b
    resuscitation for, 228
        formula for, 229b
    "6 Cs" of, 228
    treatment for, 228–229, 229.e4f
    wound care for, 228–229
Radiation sickness, 1100.e12
Radiation therapy
    for basal cell carcinoma, 178t
    for brain metastases, 210
    for head and neck squamous cell carcinoma, 542
    for meningioma, 810

Radiation therapy *(Continued)*
    mucositis caused by, 1214.e1f
    for neuroblastoma, 891.e3
    for oral cancer, 916
    for pituitary adenoma, 999
    for prostate cancer, 1072–1073
Radiation-induced neoplasms, 1516–1521
Radical prostatectomy, 1072
Radioactive iodine
    for Graves' disease, 535
    for hyperthyroidism, 666–667, 667.e1f
Radiocontrast-induced nephropathy, 333
Radiofrequency ablation
    for Brugada syndrome, 222
    for supraventricular tachycardia, 1232
Radiography. *See* X-rays
Radiolabeled octreotide, for carcinoid tumor, 239.e3, 239.e3f
Radionuclide imaging, for chemical-induced cardiomyopathy, 243, 243f
Raeder's paratrigeminal syndrome, 628
RAI. *See* Radioactive iodine
Raloxifene
    for osteoporosis, 926
    for uterine fibroids, 1332
Raltegravir, 18
Ramelteon, 712
Ramipril
    for chemical-induced cardiomyopathy, 243
    for claudication, 309
Ramsay Hunt syndrome, 1101–1101.e1, 1101f
Ramucirumab, 474
Ranibizumab, 783
Ranitidine, 79.e2t
Ranolazine
    for angina pectoris, 95
    for coronary artery disease, 342
Rapamycin, 1308.e4
Rape, 1165–1166
Rapid gastric emptying, 412.e3, 1445
Rapid onset dystonia parkinsonism, 423t
Rapidly progressive glomerulonephritis, idiopathic, 523t
RARS. *See* Refractory anemia with ring sideroblasts
RAS. *See* Renal artery stenosis
Rasagiline, 957
Rasburicase, 1311
Rash
    arthritis and, 1403
    erythema migrans, 774f
    in familial Mediterranean fever, 484, 484.e1f
    with fever, 1442
    fever and, 1439
    in herpes zoster, 608, 608f
    in ID reaction, 690.e4, 690.e4f
    in juvenile idiopathic arthritis, 734.e2f
    in Lyme disease, 774f
    in measles, 801.e2, 801.e2f
    penile, 1503
    in Rocky Mountain spotted fever, 1129f–1130f
    in rubella, 1133.e8f
    in Scarlet fever, 1143f
    in smallpox, 1194.e3f
    in systemic lupus erythematosus, 1240f
    in urticaria, 1326
Rasmussen encephalitis, 442
Rattlesnake bites, 197–199.e1
Raxibacumab, 106.e3
Raynaud's phenomenon, 1102–1104.e1, 1102f–1103f, 1104b, 1148, 1149t
RB1 gene, 1116.e8
RBCs. *See* Red blood cells
RCC. *See* Renal cell carcinoma
RCMD-RS. *See* Refractory cytopenia with multilineage dysplasia and ring sideroblasts
RCVS. *See* Reversible cerebral vasoconstriction syndrome
RDW. *See* Red blood cell distribution width
Reactiv. *See* Nitroglycerin ointment
Reactive airway disease, 132, 142
Reactive arthritis, 101t, 1105–1105.e1, 1105.e1f
Reactive erythema, in pediatric patient, 1872.e1f
Reactive thrombocytosis, 1260, 1822
Recombinant activated factor VII, for hemophilia A, 570
Recombinant human C1/NH, 98.e3t
Recombinant human deoxyribonuclease, for cystic fibrosis, 146, 352
Rectal abscess, 978
Rectal bleeding, 1410

Rectal intussusception, 1104.e2
Rectal mass, palpable, 1730.e7
Rectal pain, 1731–1732
Rectal prolapse, 1104.e2–1104.e3, 1104.e2f
Recti, divarication of, 1390
Rectovaginal fistulas, 1336
Rectum, 489t
Recurrent abdominal pain, 722
Recurrent fever, 1441–1442
Recurrent meningitis, 1483
Recurrent pneumonia, 1506
Recurrent polyserositis, 484
Red blood cell distribution width, 1827
Red blood cells
    abnormal, 1827f
    count, 1827
    drugs interfering with, 1399
    mass, 1827
    morphology, 1827
    reticulocyte count and, 1829t
    urine, microscopic examination of, 1837t
Red cell fragmentation hemolysis, 1732–1735
Red cell sensitization, 1119–1121.e1, 1120f–1121f
Red eye, 1736.e1, 326, 328
    acute, 1737–1740
Red hot joint, 1740–1741
Red pigmentation anomaly, cutaneous, 1423
Red urine, 694, 1741–1742, 1538
Reed-Sternberg cells, 623, 626.e2f
Reese-Ellsworth classification system, for retinoblastoma, 1116.e8
Referred hip pain, 1456
Reflex sympathetic dystrophy, 320, 320.e1f
Reflux and direct implantation theory, 452
Reflux esophagitis, 511
    heartburn treatment, 512.e3f
    pathogenesis of, 511f
    therapy for, 512t
Refractive amblyopia, 71
Refractory anemia, 80
Refractory anemia with ring sideroblasts, 90.e3t, 90.e4
Refractory angina, 91
Refractory cytopenia with multilineage dysplasia and ring sideroblasts, 90.e3t, 90.e4
Regional edema, 1618f, 1802, 1805f,
Regional enteritis, 344, 344t, 345f, 345.e1f
Regional osteoporosis, 927.e5f
Regurgitation
    aortic, 113, 116f–117f, 116–117.e1, 117.e1f, 1539
    tricuspid, 1301.e4–1301.e6, 1301.e4f, 1539
Rehydration, 510
Reiter's disease, 1105
Reiter's syndrome, 1105–1105.e1
    characteristics of, 1105.e1f
    food poisoning and, 501
    HLA antigens associated with, 1807t
Relapsing meningitis, 443t
Relapsing-remitting multiple sclerosis, 855
Renal abscess, 1099, 1106, 1106f
Renal acidosis, 1390
Renal allograft dysfunction, 1742–1743
Renal arteriograms, 1109f
Renal artery occlusion, 1745.e1–1745.e2
Renal artery stenosis, 1107–1110.e1, 1107f–1109f
Renal biopsy, for acute glomerulonephritis, 522
Renal carbuncle, 1097
Renal cell carcinoma, 1111–1112.e1, 1111f–1112f, 1112t
Renal colic
    algorithm for, 1872.e1f
    differential diagnosis of, 1745.e2–1745.e3
Renal cystic disorders, 1745.e3
Renal diseases and disorders
    hydronephrosis, 644.e1f, 643–644.e1, 643f
    ischemic, 1872.e1f
    skin manifestations of, 1517
    tubulointerstitial, 1535
    unilateral, 1829t
Renal dysfunction, abdominal aortic aneurysm and, 6
Renal failure
    acute, 37, 1309
    chronic, 1518
    intrinsic or parenchymal causes of, 1518
    pigment-induced acute, 1518
    postrenal causes of, 1518
    prerenal causes of, 1518
    vaccination considerations for, 1887t

Renal infarction, 1519
Renal mass, 1872.e1f
Renal papillary necrosis, 1099
Renal paraneoplastic syndromes, 1500
Renal parenchymal disease, chronic, 1519
Renal pelvis, renal failure caused by, 1518
Renal replacement therapy, for heart failure, 558
Renal sclerosis, 718
Renal tubular acidosis, 1113–1114.e1, 1113t, 1114f
Renal vein thrombosis, 1115, 1115f, 1519
Renin, serum, 1827
Renin inhibitors
    for cardiorenal syndrome, 254
    for hypertension, 663
Renin-aldosterone patterns, 1829t
Renovascular disease, 660t, 1107
Renovascular hypertension, 663, 1107
Reperfusion therapy, for myocardial infarction, 869
Repetitive multifocal paroxysmal atrial tachycardia, 850
Resin uptake (T₃), 1832
Resistant hypertension, 1463
Resisted wrist extension test, for epicondylitis, 458.e10f
Reslizumab, 135
Resorption, bone, 1413
Respiratory acidosis
    acute, 1556, 1556f
    arterial blood gases, 1777–1778
    chronic, 1557, 1557f
    differential diagnosis of, 1390–1391
    in hypothermia, 688
    laboratory findings in, 1771t
Respiratory alkalosis
    arterial blood gases, 1778
    differential diagnosis of, 1395
    laboratory findings in, 1771t
    treatment of, 1563, 1563f
Respiratory bronchiolitis-associated interstitial lung disease, 692t
Respiratory diphtheria, 395.e5
Respiratory distress
    acute respiratory distress syndrome, 45–48.e1, 45t, 46f, 47t
    in newborn, 1519
    in pediatric patient, 1908f
Respiratory effort-related arousal, 1191t
Respiratory failure, hypoventilatory, 1519–1520
Respiratory infections, in acquired immunodeficiency syndrome, 17
Respiratory muscle weakness, 1520
Respiratory syncytial virus, 1115.e1–1115.e2, 1015–1016
    acute bronchitis caused by, 27t
    croup caused by, 345.e3
    screen, 1827
Respiratory tract candidiasis, 234
Rest pain, with myopathies, 1488
Rest tremors, 1534
Restless legs syndrome, 1116–1116.e1, 1116t
Restrictive cardiomyopathy, 250–252.e1, 250f
    classification of, 250
    and constrictive pericarditis, 252.e1t, 252f
Restrictive eye movement, 1214.e4
Retapamulin, 697
Retention, urinary, 51–51.e1
Reteplase, 872t
Reticulocyte count, 1827
    anemia with low, 1400
    differential diagnosis of elevated, 1828.e1f
    red blood cell parameters and, 1829t
Reticulocytosis, anemia with, 1570.e1, 1570.e1f
Retina
    human immunodeficiency virus infection manifestations in, 1459
    tears of, 1116.e2f
Retin-A Micro. *See* Tretinoin microsphere
Retinal breaks, 1116.e3f
Retinal detachment, 1116.e2–1116.e3, 1116.e2f–1116.e3f
Retinal hemorrhage, 1171.e1f, 1116.e4–1116.e5, 1116.e4f, 1171–1171.e1
Retinal ischemia, 70
Retinal migraine, amaurosis fugax and, 70
Retinitis pigmentosa, 1116.e6–1116.e7, 1116.e7f
Retinoblastoma, 1116.e8–1116.e10, 1116.e8f, 211
Retinocerebellar angiomatosis, 1370.e2
Retinoids
    for acne vulgaris, 15
    for actinic keratosis, 26
    for psoriasis, 1080

Retinopathy
    diabetic, 392–393.e3, 392t, 393f, 393.e1f–393.e3f
    hypertensive, 1520
Retraction, eyelid, 1477
Retrobulbar neuritis, 914
Retrograde ejaculation, 435
Retrograde ureterogram, for hydronephrosis, 644
Retropatellar pain syndrome, 958.e6
Retroperitoneal fibrosis, 1116.e11–1116.e12, 1116.e12f
Retropharyngeal abscess, 1117–1118.e1, 1117f–1118f
Rett syndrome, 162, 423t
Revascularization
    for claudication, 308–309
    for heart failure, 560
    for peripheral arterial disease, 977
    for renal artery stenosis, 1110
Reversible cerebral vasoconstriction syndrome, 266.e5, 266.e5t, 266.e7t, 1061–1062
Reversible transition, 512.e5–512.e6
Revised Atlanta Criteria, for acute pancreatitis, 943
Rewarming, for hypothermia, 689
Reye's syndrome, 1118.e2, 1118.e2t
Rh incompatibility, 1120f–1121f, 1119–1121.e1
Rhabdomyolysis, 1122–1124.e1, 1122t, 1123b, 1123f–1124f
Rhagades, 99
Rhegmatogenous retinal detachment, 1116.e2
Rheumatic carditis, 1124.e2
Rheumatic diseases
    childhood, 1405
    recurrent or periodic fever from, 1442
Rheumatic fever
    characteristics of, 1124.e2–1124.e3
    mitral stenosis caused by, 836
Rheumatic heart disease, 836, 1301.e7
Rheumatism, palindromic, 1706–1707
Rheumatoid arthritis, 922.e4f, 1125–1128.e3, 1125f, 1126t, 1127f–1128f
    juvenile, 732
Rheumatoid factor, 1827–1828
Rheumatoid nodules, 1125
Rheumatologic paraneoplastic syndromes, 1500
Rhinitis
    allergic, 63–63.e1
    atrophic, 904
    chronic, 1520
    differential diagnosis of, 1520
    gustatory, 904
    hormone-induced, 905
    infectious, 904
    nonallergic, 904–905.e1
    vasomotor, 904
Rhinitis medicamentosa, 904
Rhinocerebral-rhinoorbital-paranasal syndrome, 848
Rhinorrhea, 1729.e2f
Rhinosinusitis, 1520, 1184
Rhinovirus, 27t
Rhombencephalitis, 759
Rhus, 1020–1020.e1, 1020.e1f
Rhus dermatitis, 329, 1020
Rhythm disorder. *See* Arrhythmias
Rhythm method of contraception, 330–331
Rhythmical movement disorders, 1534
Rib(s)
    bone resorption in, 1413
    defects of, on x-ray, 1520–1521
    notching of, on x-ray, 1521
Ribavirin
    for hepatitis E virus, 594
    for measles, 801.e3
    for respiratory syncytial virus, 1115.e1
    for West Nile virus infection, 1376.e5
Riboflavin deficiency, 1368
Rickets, 1367.e2f, 1128.e4–1128.e5, 1128.e4f, 1366
Rickettsia rickettsii, 1129–1130
Riedel's thyroiditis, 1268–1268.e1
Rifampin
    for anaplasmosis, 432
    for bacterial meningitis, 813
    for brucellosis, 220.e3
    for ehrlichiosis, 432
    for granulomatous arthritis, 534.e2
    for miliary tuberculosis, 1305
    for pulmonary tuberculosis, 1308

Rifapentine, 1308
Rifaximin
    for fulminant hepatic failure, 578
    for hepatic encephalopathy, 578
    for spontaneous bacterial peritonitis, 980
Right atrium enlargement, 1407, 1417
Right axis deviation, 1521
Right bundle branch block, 720
Right heart catheterization, for pulmonary edema, 1086
Right heart diastolic dysfunction, 1301.e7
Right iliac fossa pain, 1667–1668
Right ventricle
    enlargement of, 1417
    extrinsic compression of, 1301.e7
Right ventricular failure, 555, 1540
Right ventricular outflow tract obstruction, 1255.e7
Right ventricular systolic pressure, 1095
Rilpivirine
    for acquired immunodeficiency syndrome, 18
    for human immunodeficiency virus, 634
Riluzole (Rilutek), 77
Rimantadine, 709t
Ring sideroblasts, 90.e4f
Ringing in the ears, 1277
Ringworm, 1269, 1271–1272, 1271f, 1274
Rinne test, 1817t
Riociguat, 1094
Risedronate, 926
Risk reduction in patients undergoing invasive procedures, 1055.e2
Risperidone
    for bipolar disorder, 191
    for delirium, 366
Risus sardonicus, 1255.e3, 1255.e3f
Ritodrine, 1060b
Ritonavir, 1901t, 18
Rituximab
    for granulomatosis with polyangiitis, 533–534
    for immune thrombocytopenic purpura, 695
    for microscopic polyangiitis, 830
    for non-Hodgkin lymphomas, 779
    for paroxysmal cold hemoglobinuria, 958.e2
    for pemphigus vulgaris, 969
    for rheumatoid arthritis, 1127
    for Sjögren's syndrome, 1187
    for systemic vasculitis, 1351
    topical, for bullous pemphigoid, 226.e2
    for Waldenström's macroglobulinemia, 1374
Rivaroxaban
    for atrial fibrillation, 152
    for pulmonary embolism, 1090
    for transient ischemic attack, 1294
Rivastigmine
    for Alzheimer's disease, 69t
    for dementia with Lewy bodies, 369
Rizatriptan, for migraine headache, 546t
RLS. *See* Restless legs syndrome
RMSF. *See* Rocky Mountain spotted fever
Rocky Mountain spotted fever, 1129–1130, 1129f–1130f, 1130b
Rocuronium, 1668.e2t
Roentgen, 1100.e12
Roflumilast, 301
Rokitansky's disease, 223
Rolling hiatal hernia, 609.e2
Romaña's sign, 272.e2
Romano-Ward syndrome, 764, 764t. *See also* Long QT syndrome
ROME II diagnostic criteria, for cyclic vomiting syndrome, 350.e8b
Root compression syndromes, 766.e3t
Ropinirole, 957
Rosacea, 1131–1132.e1, 1131f
Rosai Dorfman disease, 618.e2
Rosenbach's sign, 116
Roseola, 1133.e1f, 1133–1133.e1
Roseola infantum, 1133.e1f, 1133
Rosiglitazone, 381
Rosuvastatin, 654.e4t
Rotator cuff disease, 1133.e2–1133.e6, 1133.e2f–1133.e3f, 1133.e4t, 1133.e5f
Rotator cuff syndrome, 1133.e2
Rotator cuff tears, 1133.e2–1133.e6, 1133.e2f, 1133.e4t
Rotator cuff tendinitis, 1133.e4t
Rotavirus serology, 1830

Rotavirus vaccines
  conditions misperceived as contraindications to, 1870t–1871t
  contraindication and precautions, 1868t–1869t
  recommended schedule for, 1860t–1864t
Roth spots, 1116.e4
Rotterdam BCS Index, 224
Rouleaux formation, 851, 851f
Round worms, 126
Rovsing's sign, 121
RP. *See* Raynaud's phenomenon; Retinitis pigmentosa
RPF. *See* Retroperitoneal fibrosis
RRMS. *See* Relapsing-remitting multiple sclerosis
RSV. *See* Respiratory syncytial virus
RTA. *See* Renal tubular acidosis
RT-QuIC, for prion disease, 343.e3
Rubella, 1133.e7–1133.e8, 1133.e7f–1133.e8f, 1133.e8t
Rubella live-virus vaccine
  for health care workers, 1884t–1886t
  for international travel, 1888t
Rubeola, 801.e2. *See also* Measles
"Rule of nines," 227, 229.e4f
Rumack-Matthew nomogram, 11
Runner's knee, 958.e6
Russula poisoning, 862
Rutherford's classification, of peripheral arterial disease, 975–976
Ruxolitinib, 1029

S

SABAs. *See* Short-acting beta-selective adrenergic agonists
SAC. *See* Seasonal allergic conjunctivitis
Sacral neuromodulation, for urinary incontinence, 701
Sacroiliitis, 455t
Sacubitril/valsartan, 559
SAD. *See* Seasonal affective disorder; Social anxiety disorder
Saddle-nose deformity, in granulomatosis with polyangiitis, 532f
SAH. *See* Subarachnoid hemorrhage
Saint Vitus dance, 290.e5
Salicylates
  pathophysiology, clinical effects, and management of, 1716t–1719t
  for trichinosis, 1301.e3
Salicylic acid
  for acne vulgaris, 15
  for warts, 1376
Salicylic acid plaster, for warts, 1376
Saline, hypertonic, 352
Salivary calculus, 1177
Salivary gland stone, 1177
Salivary glands
  decreased secretion by, 1747–1748
  enlargement of, 1521–1530
  neoplasms of, 1134, 1134f
  sialadenitis of, 1176–1176.e1, 1176.e1f
  sialolithiasis of, 1177–1177.e1, 1177.e1f, 1177f
Salmeterol
  for chronic obstructive pulmonary disease, 301
  for high-altitude pulmonary edema, 613
Salmonella spp., 1135–1136.e1, 1135t
  food poisoning caused by, 500
  S. typhi infection, 1312.e4
Salmonellosis
  in acquired immunodeficiency syndrome, 18t–24t
  characteristics of, 1135–1136.e1, 1135t–1136t
  treatment of, 18t–24t
Salpingectomy, for ectopic pregnancy, 431
Salpingitis, 963
Salpingostomy, for ectopic pregnancy, 431
Salt
  high-salt diet, 1829t
  low-salt diet, 1829t
San Joaquin Valley fever, 313.e2, 313.e4t
Sand worm eruption, 350.e5, 350.e5f
Saquinavir, 18, 1901t
Saquinavir and ritonavir, 634
SAR. *See* Allergic rhinitis; Seasonal allergic rhinitis
Sarcoidosis, 692t, 899t, 1137–1138.e2, 1138.e1f–1138.e2f, 1138t
Sarcoma
  characteristics of, 1139–1140.e1, 1139f–1140f
  Kaposi's, 735–735.e1, 735.e1f, 735f
  uterine, 1333.e1f

Sarcoma *(Continued)*
  vaginal, 1338
  vulvar, 1372.e2
Sarcomere protein gene mutation screening, in hypertrophic cardiomyopathy, 247
Sarcoptes scabiei, 1141–1142.e1, 1142.e1f
SARS. *See* Severe acute respiratory syndrome
Sassafras, 410.e1t–410.e2t
SAT. *See* Serum agglutination test
Sauna taker's lung, 657
Saving, 622.e2
Saw palmetto, 1076
Saxagliptin, 379
SBE. *See* Subacute bacterial endocarditis
SBP. *See* Spontaneous bacterial peritonitis
SBS. *See* Short bowel syndrome
SC. *See* Stress cardiomyopathy
SC vaccine, for health care workers, 1884t–1886t
SCA. *See* Sickle cell anemia; Spinocerebellar ataxia
Scabies, 1141–1142.e1, 1141t–1142t, 1142.e1f
Scalp hair, premature graying of, 1509
Scalp scabies, 1141t
Scapulothoracic bursitis, 229.e5
Scarlatina, 1143
Scarlet fever, 1143, 1143f
Scarring alopecia, 64, 1270t, 1395
SCC. *See* Squamous cell carcinoma
SCD. *See* Sickle cell disease
SCFE. *See* Slipped capital femoral epiphysis
Schilder's diffuse sclerosis, 855
Schilling test, 90, 1833t, 1842.e1f
Schirmer's test, 1186, 1187f
Schistocytes, 1263.e1f
Schistosomes, 1143.e1–1143.e3, 1143.e1f
Schistosomiasis, 1032, 1143.e1–1143.e3, 1143.e1f
Schizophrenia, 1144–1145.e1
  borderline personality disorder and, 205.e2
  childhood-onset, autism spectrum disorder and, 162
Schwannoma, vestibular, 16
Schwannomatosis, 894
Sciatic nerve, 996.e1f
Sciatica, 766.e2
Scintigraphy
  bone
    for complex regional pain syndrome, 320
    for Paget's disease of bone, 935
    for pheochromocytoma, 992
Scleral melt syndrome, 1146
Sclerederma, 1147
Scleritis, 463.e5f, 463.e6t, 1146–1146.e1, 1146f
Sclerodactyly, 1149.e1f–1149.e2f
Scleroderma, 12t, 397t, 1147–1149.e3, 1147b, 1147t, 1149.e1f–1149.e3f, 1149f, 1149t
Scleroderma-like syndromes, 1747.e1
Scleromalacia perforans, 1146–1146.e1
Sclerosing mediastinitis, 802–803
Sclerosing pancreatitis, 947
Sclerosis, tuberous, 1308.e3–1308.e5, 1308.e3f, 1308.e3t–1308.e4t
Sclerotherapy
  for varicocele, 1347.e3
  for varicose veins, 1349
Scoliosis, 1150–1151.e1, 1150f–1151f
Scorpion stings, 194
"Scratch collapse" test, for cubital tunnel syndrome, 348.e2
Screenings
  for ages 65 and older, 1855t
  for ages 11 to 24 years, 1851t
  for ages 25 to 64 years, 1853t
  from birth to 10 years, 1849t
  for cervical cancer, 268
  for hepatocellular carcinoma, 597–598
  for hepatopulmonary syndrome, 599
  for hirsutism, 616–617
  for hypercholesterolemia, 645
  for lung cancer, 772
  for ovarian cancer, 933
  for pancreatic cancer, 942
  for pituitary adenoma, 998t
  in pregnant women, 1857t
  for primary immunodeficiency diseases, 1065.e5
  for renal artery stenosis, 1108
  for schistosomiasis, 1143.e2
  for scoliosis, 1150, 1151f
  for thrombosis, 650.e1b
Scrotal calcifications, 1749.e1

Scrotal masses
  in boys and adolescents, 1751–1752
  evaluation of, 1730f
Scrotal pain, 1521–1522
Scrotal swelling, 1521
Scrotum, acute, 459.e1t, 1392
SCT. *See* Stem cell transplantation
SD. *See* Seborrheic dermatitis
SDH. *See* Subdural hematoma
SEA. *See* Spinal epidural abscess
Seasonal affective disorder, 1151.e2–1151.e3
Seasonal allergic conjunctivitis, 327t
Seasonal allergic rhinitis, 63
Seasonal depression, 1151.e2
Sebopsoriasis, 1152
Seborrhea, 1152
Seborrheic dermatitis, 1152–1152.e1, 1152.e1f, 1152f, 1269
Seborrheic eczema, 1152
Seborrheic otitis externa, 928
Secondary adrenal disorders, 1394
Secondary amenorrhea, 73
Secondary amyloidosis, 76.e3
Secondary angle-closure glaucoma, 521
Secondary focal segmental glomerulonephrosis, 890t
Secondary hyperaldosteronism, 1393
Secondary hyperparathyroidism, 655–656.e1
Secondary hypertrophic osteoarthropathy, 668–669.e1
Secondary hyperuricemia, 529
Secondary hypothyroidism, 690–690.e3
Secondary immunodeficiencies, 1873t
Secondary lung abscess, 767
Secondary lymphedema, 777
Secondary membranous nephropathy, 890t
Secondary open-angle glaucoma, 519
Secondary osteoporosis, 925–927.e5, 925t, 927.e5f, 927f
Secondary peritonitis, 979
Secondary prevention of stroke, 1221–1222.e1, 1222f
Secondary priapism, 1060.e2
Secondary progressive multiple sclerosis, 855
Secondary pulmonary hypertension, 1092
Secondary Raynaud's phenomenon, 1102–1104.e1, 1102f–1103f
Secondary spontaneous pneumothorax, 1017
Secondary syphilis, 1238–1239.e1, 1238f
Second-degree burns, 229.e4f
Second-degree heart block, 551–552, 551f
Secretin stimulation test, 1833t
Secukinumab, 1083
Sed rate. *See* Erythrocyte sedimentation rate
Sedative-hypnotics, for insomnia, 712
Sedimentation rate. *See* Erythrocyte sedimentation rate
[75]SeHCAT test, 1833t
Seizures
  absence, 1153–1153.e1
  alcohol-related, 1395
  in benign brain neoplasms, 211
  coma and, 1424
  differential diagnosis of, 1522
  febrile, 485.e2–485.e3, 1154–1155.e1, 1155f
  generalized tonic clonic, 1156
  in hemorrhagic stroke, 1220
  in infants, 1211f–1212f
  mimics of, 1522
  partial, 1157
  pediatric, 1522
  of pregnancy, 429
  in Sturge-Weber syndrome, 1222.e2–1222.e3
  in subarachnoid hemorrhage, 1225
  tonic clonic, 1156
Selective estrogen receptor modulators, for breast cancer, 218
Selective internal radiation therapy, for hepatocellular carcinoma, 598
Selective renal vein venography, 1115
Selective serotonin reuptake inhibitors
  for acute stress disorder, 49
  for bulimia nervosa, 225
  for compulsive hoarding, 622.e2
  for dependent personality disorder, 370
  for enuresis, 457
  for generalized anxiety disorder, 110
  for intermittent explosive disorder, 712.e4
  for irritable bowel syndrome, 724
  for major depression, 372
  for narcissistic personality disorder, 882
  for panic disorder, 950
  for paraphilic disorders, 955.e5

Selective serotonin reuptake inhibitors *(Continued)*
    for pedophilic disorder, 961.e2
    for postpartum depression, 1039
    for posttraumatic stress disorder, 1044
    for premenstrual dysphoric disorder, 1053.e2
    for seasonal affective disorder, 1151.e2
    for serotonin syndrome, 1164
    for social anxiety disorder, 1194.e4
Selegiline, 957
Selenium, 535–536
Selenium sulfide, 1276
Selexipag, 1094
Self-monitoring of blood glucose, for diabetes mellitus, 378
Self-murder, 1227.e1
Semen
    analysis of, 1830, 1830t
        for varicocele, 1347.e3
    infertility and, 1471
Seminoma, 1254
Semont's maneuvers, 185–186
Senear-Usher syndrome, 968
Senile chorea, 639
Senile keratosis, 25
Senna, 410.e1t–410.e2t
Sensipar. *See* Cinacalcet
Sensorineural hearing loss, 931.e2–931.e3, 931.e2f, 931.e2t
Sensory neuropathies, 1492
Sentinel lymph nodes
    in breast cancer, 215
    excision of, for melanoma, 805
Sepsis, 106.e6b, 1158–1160.e1, 1158t, 1160t
Sepsis syndrome, 1158
Septal ablation, for hypertrophic cardiomyopathy, 249, 249f
Septic arthritis, 237, 1161–1162.e3, 1162.e1f–1162.e2f,
    1162.e2t, 1162f
Septic embolism, cavitary lesion with, 1418
Septic shock, 1158, 1160t
Septicemia, 1158
Serelaxin, 1087
SERMs. *See* Selective estrogen receptor modulators
Seronegative spondyloarthropathies, 1082, 1105
    ankylosing spondylitis, 100–101.e1, 100f–101f, 101t, 1807t
    Reiter's syndrome, 1807t
Serotonergic syndrome, 1163
Serotonin syndrome, 896.e1t, 1163–1164.e1, 1163b, 1163t
Serotonin toxicity, 1163
Serotonin-norepinephrine reuptake inhibitors
    for chronic pain, 939t
    for generalized anxiety disorder, 110
SERPINA Z allele, cystic fibrosis and, 352
Serrated polyposis syndrome, 986
Sertraline
    for acute stress disorder, 49
    for Alzheimer's disease, 69t
    for cataplexy, 884
    for premenstrual syndrome, 1055
Serum, acid-base reference values for, 1771t
Serum agglutination test, for brucellosis, 220.e2
Serum creatinine, 1790b
    for acute glomerulonephritis, 522
    for cardiorenal syndrome, 253
    for granulomatosis with polyangiitis, 533
Serum hepatitis, 582
Serum protein electrophoresis
    for monoclonal gammopathy of undetermined significance,
        844, 845.e1f
    for multiple myeloma, 852, 852f
Serum sickness, 199
Serum T4, 1832–1833
Serum troponins, 1835–1836
Serum viscosity, 1842
Sevelamer, 1100.e14t–1100.e16t
Seventh nerve palsy, 1138.e1f
Severe acute respiratory syndrome, 707, 1164.e2–1164.e3
Severe acute respiratory syndrome-associated coronavirus,
    1164.e2–1164.e3
Severe croup, 463.e1f
Severe immunocompromise, vaccination considerations for,
    1887t
Severe sepsis, 106.e6b, 1158–1160.e1, 1160t
Sex cord stromal tumor, 932
Sex hormone binding globulin, 616, 677
Sexual abuse
    child, 277
    elder, 437
Sexual assault, 1165–1167.e1, 1165b–1166b, 1167f

Sexual behavior
    in ages 65 and older, 1855t
    in ages 11 to 24 years, 1851t
    in ages 25 to 64 years, 1853t
Sexual differentiation abnormalities, 1522
Sexual dysfunction, 466
    evaluation of, 1730.e1f
    orgasm dysfunction, 1497
    in women, 1168–1170.e1, 1168t, 1169f, 1523
Sexual impulsivity disorder, 955.e4
Sexual precocity, 1523
    female
        differential diagnosis of, 1730.e4t
        pubic hair development in, 1730.e3f
Sexual response cycle, 1169f
Sexually active men, prevention services for, 1890t
Sexually active women, prevention services for, 1890t
Sexually transmitted diseases, 1165–1166
    in anorectal region, 1523
    lymphogranuloma venereum, 778.e2–778.e3
    prevention services for, 1890t
    pruritus ani with, 1511
    syphilis, 1238–1239.e1, 1238f
Sexually transmitted epididymitis, 459
Sézary cells, 863.e3f, 1816t
Sézary syndrome, 863.e3f–863.e4f
SF. *See* Scarlet fever
Shagreen patches, 1308.e3f, 1308.e4t
Shaken baby syndrome, 277, 1171–1171.e1, 1171.e1f
Shaken impact syndrome, 277
Shaken infant syndrome, 1171
Sheehan's syndrome, 74, 1171.e2–1171.e3
Shell shock, 1043
Shigella spp
    characteristics of, 1172–1172.e1
    food poisoning caused by, 500
Shigellosis, 1172–1172.e1
Shin splints, 1730.e7f
Shingles, 608
Shock
    anaphylactic, 79.e1t
    cardiogenic, 1418
    diagnosis and treatment of, 1731f
    hypovolemic, 1469
    rash with, fever and, 1440
Shock liver, 726
Short bowel, 1173
Short bowel resection with colectomy, 1173
Short bowel syndrome, 1173–1173.e1, 1173t
Short incubation hepatitis, 580
Short QT syndrome, 1174–1175.e1, 1174t, 1175f, 1356
Short stature
    differential diagnosis of, 1731.e1f
    in Turner syndrome, 1312.e2, 1312.e2f
Short-acting beta-selective adrenergic agonists, for asthma,
    134–135
Shortened cervix, 271.e2
Shoulder hand syndrome, 320
Shoulder impingement, 1133.e2–1133.e6, 1133.e5f
Shoulder impingement syndrome, 1133.e2
Shoulder pain, 1133.e4t
    in different age groups, 1523–1524
    differential diagnosis of, 1523
    evaluation of, 1732f–1734f
    by location, 1524
Shou-wu-pian, 410.e1t–410.e2t
Shulman's syndrome, 458.e2
Shy-Drager syndrome, 857.e2
SIAD. *See* Syndrome of inappropriate antidiuresis
SIADH. *See* Syndrome of inappropriate antidiuretic hormone
Sialadenitis, 1176–1176.e1, 1176.e1f
Sialography, 1177
Sialolithiasis, 1177–1177.e1, 1177.e1f, 1177f
SIBO. *See* Small bowel bacterial overgrowth
Sicca complex, 1186
Sicca syndrome, 1065, 1186
Sick sinus syndrome, 1178–1178.e1, 1178f, 1178t
Sickle cell anemia, 1179, 1180f
Sickle cell disease, 1179–1182.e1, 1179t–1181t, 1180f
Sickle cell test, 1830
Sickle cell trait, 1179
Sideroblastic anemia, 90.e3–90.e4, 90.e3f–90.e4f, 90.e3t
SIDS, 1530
Sigmoidoscopy
    for *Clostridium difficile* infection, 310
    description of, 482

Sildenafil, 467
    for achalasia, 13
    for cor pulmonale, 337
    for pulmonary arterial hypertension, 1092
    for sexual dysfunction in women, 1169
Silent cerebral infarcts, 1181
Silicosis, 1183, 1183b, 1183f
Silver, hyperpigmentation with, 1651t–1652t
Silver sulfadiazine, 228
Simeprevir/sofosbuvir, 588
Simple partial seizures, 1157
Simple phobia, 993
Simple pulmonary eosinophilia, 458.e7
SIMS. *See* Statin-induced muscle syndromes
Simvastatin, for hyperlipidemia, 654.e4t
Sin Nombre virus, 540.e2
Sinecatechin
    for condyloma acuminatum, 324
    for warts, 1376
Sinoatrial exit block, 1178
Sinus
    computed tomography scans, 534f
    vaginal, 1336
Sinus arrest, 1178
Sinus bradycardia, 1414
Sinus histiocytosis with massive lymphadenopathy, 618.e3t
Sinus node dysfunction, 1524
Sinus ostial obstruction, 1524
Sinus pause, 1178
Sinus tachycardia, 1524
Sinus tumors, nasal and paranasal, 1490
Sinus venosus defect, 156
Sinusitis, 1184–1185.e1
Sirolimus, 1308.e4
Sitagliptin, 379
Situational hypoactive sexual desire disorder, 672
Sitz baths, for Bartholin's gland cyst and abscess, 175
Sixth disease, 1133
Sjögren's syndrome, 397t, 1125, 1186–1188.e2,
    1186f–1188f
SJS. *See* Stevens-Johnson syndrome
Skin
    blisters of, 1736.e1f
    with fever of undetermined origin, 489t
    heel pain and, 1452
    Henoch-Schönlein purpura manifestations of, 573, 573f
    histiocytosis X manifestations of, 618.e2
    human immunodeficiency virus manifestations of, 1459
    lung disease and, 1478–1479
    mycosis fungoides manifestations of, 863.e2–863.e5,
        863.e2f–863.e3f
    neurofibromatosis manifestations of, 894–895.e1,
        894f–895f
    nodular lesions of, 1495
    Sturge-Weber syndrome manifestations of, 1222.e2,
        1222.e2f
Skin and skin structure infections, 265
Skin biopsy
    for bullous pemphigoid, 226.e2
    for dermatitis herpetiformis, 373
Skin disorders
    hidradenitis suppurativa, 610–611.e1, 610f
    impetigo, 697–697.e1, 697f
    pemphigus vulgaris, 968–969, 968f, 969t
    pityriasis rosea, 1000–1000.e1, 1000f
    psoriasis, 1080–1081.e1, 1081f
    rosacea, 1131–1132.e1, 1131f
Skin induration, chronic, 1524–1525
Skin lesions
    erythematous annular, 1436
    gonorrhea, 527f
Skin testing, 496
Skinny pants syndrome, 817.e2
Skullcap, 410.e1t–410.e2t
SLE. *See* Systemic lupus erythematosus
Sleep apnea, 1189–1191.e1
    clinical presentation of, 1189
    definition of, 1189, 1191t
    demographics of, 1189
    diagnosis of, 1189–1190
    epidemiology of, 1189
    etiology of, 1189
    imaging of, 1190
    in multiple system atrophy, 857.e2
    physical findings of, 1189
    polysomnography for, 1189, 1190f

Sleep apnea *(Continued)*
    surgery for, 1191
    treatment of, 1190–1191
Sleep apnea syndrome, 1189
Sleep disorders
    algorithm for, 1737f–1739f
    chronic fatigue from, 1438
    hypersomnia, 1737f–1739f
Sleep hygiene, 711, 711b
Sleep paralysis, 883
Sleep-associated affective and behavioral disturbance, 1737f–1739f
Sleep-disordered breathing, 1189
Sliding hiatal hernia, 609.e2, 609.e2f–609.e3f
Slipped capital femoral epiphysis, 1191.e2–1191.e3
Slipped upper femoral epiphysis, 1191.e2
Slipping rib syndrome, 343t
Small bowel bacterial overgrowth, 1194–1194.e1, 1408
Small bowel carcinoid, 239.e3f
Small bowel masses, 1525
Small bowel obstruction, 1192–1193, 1192f–1193f, 1525
Small bowel volvulus, 1193f
Small cell lung cancer, 769, 772
Small intestine
    bleeding in, 1409
    ulceration, 1525
Small lymphocyte, 1816t
Smallpox, 1194.e2–1194.e3, 1194.e2b, 1194.e3f
Smell
    disturbance of, 1525
    loss of, 1530–1531
Smoking
    alpha-1-antitrypsin deficiency and, 67
    cessation of, for abdominal aortic aneurysm prevention, 5
    diabetes mellitus and, 383
    stroke and, 1222
    thromboangiitis obliterans and, 1259.e1
Smoldering multiple myeloma, 845.e1t, 851t
Smooth muscle antibody, 1830
Snail fever, 1143.e1
Snake bites, 197–199.e1, 197t–198t, 199.e1f
SNL. *See* Sentinel lymph nodes
Snoring, 1414
SNRIs. *See* Serotonin-norepinephrine reuptake inhibitors
Social anxiety disorder, 993, 1194.e4–1194.e5
Social phobia disorder, 1194.e4
Social (pragmatic) communication disorder, 162
Sodium
    serum, 1830–1831
    urine, quantitative, 1839–1841, 1841t
Sodium alginate, for radiation exposure, 1100.e14t–1100.e16t
Sodium amobarbital, for eclampsia, 429
Sodium bicarbonate
    contrast-induced nephropathy and, 41
    for lactic acidosis, 737
    for radiation exposure, 1100.e14t–1100.e16t
    for renal tubular acidosis, 1114
Sodium glycerophosphate, for radiation exposure, 1100.e14t–1100.e16t
Sodium iodide, for thyrotoxic storm, 1268.e2
Sodium nitroprusside
    for cocaine overdose, 313
    for heart failure, 558
    for hypertension, 664, 664t
Sodium oxybate, for narcolepsy, 884
Sodium phosphate, for radiation exposure, 1100.e14t–1100.e16t
Sodium retention, 1525
Sodium-glucose co-transporter 2
    description of, 381
    inhibitors of, for diabetes mellitus, 381
Soft chancre, 272.e5
Soft tissue gangrene, 887
Soft tissue infections, 1665
    clinical evaluation of, 1820f
    healthcare-associated, 548.e4
    surgical, 548.e4
Soft tissue lesions, in familial adenomatous polyposis, 482
Soft tissue masses, of head and neck, 1659
Soft tissue tumors, in pediatric patients, 1525–1526
Soiling, 445.e2
Solar keratosis, 25
Soldier's heart, 1043
Soles, rash on, fever and, 1440
Solesta, 699

Solitary plasmacytoma of bone, 851t
Solitary pulmonary mass
    causes of, 1514
    mimics of, 1514
Solitary pulmonary nodules, 1514–1515
Soluble fiber, for irritable bowel syndrome, 722
Somatic symptom disorder, 1195–1195.e1
Somatization disorder. *See* Somatic symptom disorder
Somatization syndrome, 1195
Somatostatin receptor scintigraphy, 712.e3f
Somatostatinoma, 507.e3t
Sore throat, 989, 1526. *See also* Pharyngitis
Sores, genital, 1445–1446
Sotalol
    for atrial fibrillation, 151f
    for atrial flutter, 154
    for ventricular tachycardia, 1362
Soy protein, for hot flashes, 629
SP. *See* Spontaneous pneumothorax
Spasmodic (limb or axial) dystonia, 422, 422f, 423t
Spasmodic torticollis, 1280.e1
Spasms, painful, 1302
Spastic ataxias, 1203.e3
Spastic colon, 722
Spastic paraplegias, 1526
Spasticity, 1196–1196.e1, 1196.e1t, 1196t
Speech and Language Therapy, 1222.e4
Speed's test, 187.e2
Spells, pheochromocytoma-type, 1504
Spermatic cord torsion, 1255
Spermatic vein dysfunction, 1347.e2
Spermatozoa, decreased production of, 1471
Spermicide, 330
Sphenoid wing meningioma, 809f
Sphincteroplasty, 699
Spider bites and stings. *See* Arachnid bites and stings
Spider veins, 1348
Spina bifida, 1196.e2–1196.e5, 1196.e2f–1196.e3f
Spina bifida cystica, 814.e1–814.e5, 1196.e2f–1196.e3f
Spina bifida occulta, 1196.e2–1196.e5, 1196.e2f–1196.e3f
Spinal cord
    compression of, 1199.e1f, 1197–1199.e1, 1197f, 1198t–1199t, 1526
    dysfunction of, 1526
    injuries to, 1199t
    ischemic syndromes involving, 1526
    neurogenic bladder and, 1492
Spinal epidural abscess, 460, 1200–1201.e1, 1200f–1201f
Spinal manipulation therapy, for lumbar disk syndrome, 766.e3
Spinal meningitis, 811
Spinal stenosis, lumbar, 766.e4t, 1202–1203.e1, 1202f–1203f, 1202t
Spinal tumors, 1526–1527
Spinocerebellar ataxia, 1203.e2–1203.e3, 1203.e2f, 1203.e3b
Spinocerebellar ataxia 17, 423t
Spinosad, 961
Spirometra mansonoides, 1249t
Spirometry
    for asthma, 133
    for chronic obstructive pulmonary disease, 299–300
Spironolactone
    for aldosteronism, 61
    for alopecia, 65
    for ascites, 127, 129.e2f, 129t
    for heart failure, 559
    for hirsutism, 618
    for premenstrual syndrome, 1055
Splanchnic arterial vasodilation, 1032
Spleen
    calcifications of, on x-ray, 1416
    hairy cell leukemia in, 754.e3f
    histiocytosis X manifestations of, 618.e2
    hypersplenism, 659–659.e1
Splenectomy
    for Felty's syndrome, 485.e2
    for hypersplenism, 659
    for immune thrombocytopenic purpura, 695–696
Splenic cysts, 1527
Splenic masses, 1527
Splenic nodules, 1527
Splenic tumors, 1527
Splenomegaly
    in children, 1527–1528
    clinical approach to, 1743f

Splenomegaly *(Continued)*
    differential diagnosis of, 1527
    fever and rash with, 1440
    in hairy cell leukemia, 754.e2
    hepatomegaly and, 1527
Splinter hemorrhage, 1116.e4, 1694.e2
SPMS. *See* Secondary progressive multiple sclerosis
Spondylitis, 455t
    ankylosing, 100–101.e1, 100f–101f, 101t
Spondyloarthritis, 1082
Spondyloarthropathies
    algorithm for diagnosis of, 1744f
    seronegative, 1082, 1105
        ankylosing spondylitis, 100–101.e1, 100f–101f, 101t, 1807t
        Reiter's syndrome, 1807t
    treatment algorithm for, 1745f
Spondylolisthesis, 766.e4t
Spondylosis
    cervical, 1745.e1f
    description of, 1202
Spontaneous abortion, 1204
Spontaneous bacterial peritonitis, 980–980.e1
Spontaneous miscarriage, 1204–1205.e1
Spontaneous pneumothorax
    characteristics of, 1017–1019.e2, 1017f–1019f, 1019.e2f, 1528
    in children, 1507
Sporothrix schenckii, 776, 1205.e2–1205.e4
Sporotrichoid lymphangitis, 776
Sporotrichosis, 1205.e2–1205.e4, 1205.e2f
Sports-related mild traumatic brain injury, 321
Sprain, ankle, 99.e6–99.e9, 99.e6f–99.e7f, 99.e6t–99.e7t
Spray and stretch technique, for myofascial pain, 880
Spreading pigmented actinic keratosis, 25
Sprue, tropical, 1303.e2
Spurious thrombocytosis, 1260
SQTS. *See* Short QT syndrome
Squamous cell carcinoma
    in actinic keratosis, 25, 26
    bladder, 200
    characteristics of, 232t, 473, 1206–1207.e1, 1206f–1207f, 1207.e1b
    head and neck, 541–542.e2, 541f–542f, 542.e1f
    lip, 1206f
    lung, 769
    oral, 542.e1f, 915–916.e1, 915f
    vaginal, 1338
    vulvar, 1372.e2, 1372.e2f
Squamous cell hyperplasia, 1077.e4
Squint, 1214.e4
SS. *See* Serotonin syndrome; Sjögren's syndrome
SSc. *See* Systemic sclerosis
SSRIs. *See* Selective serotonin reuptake inhibitors
SSS. *See* Sick sinus syndrome
SSSIs. *See* Skin and skin structure infections
St. Anthony's fire, 468, 468f
Stable ischemic heart disease, 339, 340f, 341b
Staging
    of chronic lymphocytic leukemia, 751
    of hepatocellular carcinoma, 597
    of Hodgkin lymphoma, 623, 624b
    of lymphomas, 779, 780t
    of melanoma, 806
    of multiple myeloma, 852t
    of mycosis fungoides, 863.e2, 863.e5
    of neuroblastoma, 891.e2t
    of pancreatic cancer, 941–942, 942t
    of renal cell carcinoma, 1112t
Stapedectomy, 931.e3
Stapedotomy, 931.e3
Staphylococcal toxic shock syndrome, 1285–1286.e1, 1285t
Staphylococcus aureus
    food poisoning, 500
    glomerulonephritis associated with, 524t
    impetigo caused by, 697–697.e1
    methicillin-resistant, 548.e3, 796, 828–828.e1
    toxic shock syndrome caused by, 1285–1286.e1
Stapled hemorrhoidopexy, 572.e4
Stasis dermatitis, 1352
Stasis ulcers, 1354, 1354f–1355f
Statin-associated autoimmune myopathy, 1208
Statin-induced muscle syndromes, 1208–1209.e1, 1209b
Statin-induced myalgias, 1208
Statin-induced myopathies, 1208
Statin-induced myositis, 1208

Statin-induced rhabdomyolysis, 1123, 1208
Statins
    for coronary artery disease, 342
    for hypercholesterolemia, 645–647, 647t
    for hyperlipidemia, 654.e4t
    for IgA nephropathy, 694
    lipoprotein metabolism affected by, 647.e1t
    for myocardial infarction, 874
    preoperative use of, 1055.e4
Statural overgrowth, 1528
Stature
    short, 1731.e1f
    tall, 1530–1535
Status asthmaticus, 132, 139
Status epilepticus, 1210–1212, 1210b, 1210t, 1211f–1212f
Status post commotio cerebri, 1035
Stavudine, 18, 1901t
Staxyn. See Vardenafil
STDs. See Sexually transmitted diseases
Steatohepatitis, 1528
Steatorrhea, 947
Steele-Richardson-Olszewski syndrome, 1068.e4
Steinberg test, 795.e3f
Stein-Leventhal syndrome, 1025
Stem cell transplantation
    for aplastic anemia, 81
    for multiple myeloma, 852, 854
    for scleroderma, 1149
STEMI. See ST-segment elevation myocardial infarction
Stenosing cholangitis, 1067
Stenosing flexor tenosynovitis, 1302.e2
Stenosing tendovaginitis, 1302.e2
Stenosing tenosynovitis, of the radial styloid process, 356,
    356f
Stenosing tenovaginitis, of the first dorsal compartment,
    356, 356f
Stenosis
    aortic, 118–120.e1, 118f–120f, 1539
    carotid, 257–258.e1
Stenotrophomonas maltophilia, 849–849.e1
Stents/stenting
    for abdominal aortic aneurysm, 6, 6f
    for angina pectoris, 95–96, 96.e3f
    for Budd-Chiari syndrome, 224
    for claudication, 309
    for superior vena cava syndrome, 1229
Stereotactic core needle biopsy, for breast cancer, 215
Stereotactic radiosurgery
    for acromegaly, 24.e8
    for hypopituitarism, 687
    for prolactinoma, 1069
Sterility, 702. See also Infertility
Sterilization, for contraception, 331
Stevens-Johnson syndrome, 1213–1213.e1, 1213f
Still's disease
    adult-onset, 54–54.e1
    juvenile, 732
Stimulants, for attention deficit hyperactivity disorder, 161
Stings
    insect, 195–196.e1, 195f–196f, 196.e1f
    scorpion, 194
Stomach cancer, 506, 507t
Stomatitis, 1214–1214.e3, 1214.e1f–1214.e3f
    bullous, 1528
Stomatodynia, 226.e4
Stones, kidney, 1323
Stool antigen test
    description of, 508
    for Helicobacter pylori, 564, 971
Stool fat test, 1833t
Stool incontinence, 445.e2
STOPP, 1031.e2
Storage diseases, 1528
Strabismus, 1214.e4–1214.e6, 1214.e5f–1214.e6f
Strabismus amblyopia, 71
Strattera. See Atomoxetine
Strawberry tongue, 735.e2f, 1143f
Streptococcal myonecrosis, 888t
Streptococcal pharyngitis, 1124.e2, 1143
Streptococcal toxic shock syndrome, 1285–1286.e1, 1285t
Streptococcus spp
    impetigo caused by, 697–697.e1
    S. pneumoniae, 637t–638t, 1009f
Streptokinase
    for deep vein thrombosis, 359
    for myocardial infarction, 872t

Streptomycin, 1309.e2
Streptozocin, 239.e3
Streptozyme. See Antistreptolysin O titer
Stress cardiomyopathy, 1247–1248.e1, 1247f–1248f
Stress disorder, acute, 49–50.e1
Stress incontinence, 700, 701.e3f, 701.e3t, 967f
Stress test algorithm, 93f
Striations, nails, 1695–1699
Striatonigral degeneration, 857.e2
Stridor
    causes of, 1414
    in neonates, 1528
    in pediatric age, 1528–1529
Stroke, 1215, 1221
    acute ischemic, 1215–1218.e1, 1215b, 1216f, 1216t,
        1217b, 1218f
    cardioembolic, 1221
    cigarette smoking and, 1222
    differential diagnosis of, 1529
    emergency evaluation of, 1745.e2f
    hemorrhagic, 1219–1220.e1, 1219f, 1220b
    long-term complications of, 1222
    in pediatric patients, 1529
    risk factors for, 1222
    secondary prevention of, 1221–1222.e1, 1222f
    thromboembolism as cause of, 149
    in young adults, 1529
Strongyloides stercoralis, 126.e1t
Struvite stones, 1325
ST-segment depression, 1529
ST-segment elevation
    differential diagnosis of, 1529–1530
    nonischemic, 1530
ST-segment elevation myocardial infarction, 31, 867–874.
    e1, 870f
Student's elbow, 229.e5
Sturge (-Weber) (-Dimitri) disease or syndrome, 1222.e2
Sturge-Weber syndrome, 1222.e2–1222.e3,
    1222.e2f–1222.e3f
Stuttering, 1222.e4–1222.e5
Stye, 1223–1223.e1, 1223f
Styloid tenovaginitis, 356
Subacute bacterial endocarditis, 446
Subacute conjunctivitis, 326
Subacute cutaneous lupus erythematosus, 397t
Subacute endocarditis, 446
Subacute necrosis of liver, 42
Subarachnoid hemorrhage, 1219, 1224–1225.e2, 1224b,
    1225.e2t, 1225f
Subareolar abscess, 214
Subchorionic abruption, of placenta, 10f
Subclavian steal syndrome, 187t, 1226
Subclavian vein thrombosis, 1317f
Subclinical hyperthyroidism, 667
Subclinical hypothyroidism, 690
Subcortical dementia, 621
Subcutaneous injections, 1872, 1872.e1f
Subcutaneous lesions, 1478–1479
Subcutaneous nodules, 1403
Subcutaneous ossification, 1745.e3f
Subdural hematoma, 1227, 1227f
Subdural hemorrhage, 1227
Subepidermal blisters, 1411
Sublingual gland neoplasms, 1134
Subluxation. See Glenohumeral dislocation
Submandibular gland
    neoplasms of, 1134
    sialolithiasis of, 1177.e1f
Submucosal fistula, 102
Subretinal hemorrhage, 1116.e4
Subset of nonadenomatous pituitary tumors, 343.e2
Substance abuse, 55, 405
    alcohol, 55
    borderline personality disorder and, 205.e2
Substance dependence, 205.e2, 405
Substance use
    in ages 65 and older, 1855t
    in ages 11 to 24 years, 1851t
    in ages 25 to 64 years, 1853t
    from birth to 10 years, 1849t
Substance use disorder, 405
Substance-induced neurocognitive disorder, 893
Subsumed in female sexual interest/arousal disorder, 672
Subtotal thyroidectomy, for hyperthyroidism, 667
Subtrochanteric fractures, 614f
Subungual melanoma, 806f

Succimer, 740, 741t
Succinylcholine, 1668.e2t
Sucrose hemolysis test, 1831
Sudan III stain, 1831
Sudden cardiac death
    differential diagnosis of, 1417
    heart failure and, 560
    long QT syndrome and, 764
    mitral valve prolapse and, 840
    in pediatric age, 1530
    risk assessment for, in myocardial infarction, 874
    in young athlete, 1530
Sudden unexpected nocturnal death syndrome, 221
Suffocation, 404
Sugar water test, 1831
Suicide, 1227.e1–1227.e2, 1227.e1t
    in Huntington's disease patients, 639
    in schizophrenia patients, 1145
Sulfacet. See Sulfacetamide-sulfa lotions
Sulfacetamide, 338
Sulfacetamide-sulfa lotions, for acne vulgaris, 15
Sulfadiazine, 1290
Sulfapyridine, 374
Sulfasalazine
    for ankylosing spondylitis, 101
    for Behçet's disease, 182.e3
    for chronic urticaria, 1329
    for enteropathic arthritis, 456
    for Reiter's syndrome, 1105
    for ulcerative colitis, 1314
Sulfonylureas, 381
"Sulfur granules", 26.e3
Sulindac, for Gardner's syndrome, 483
Sumatriptan
    for cluster headaches, 543
    for migraine headache, 546t
SumLimer, 1100.e14t–1100.e16t
SUNDS. See Sudden unexpected nocturnal death syndrome
Sunitinib, for gastrinoma, 507.e4
Sunshine vitamin, 1366
Superficial episcleral plexus, 463.e5f
Superficial frostbite, 502, 502f
Superficial phlebitis, 1262
Superficial spreading melanoma, 805, 805f
Superficial suppurative thrombophlebitis, 1262–1262.e1
Superficial venous thrombophlebitis, 1262–1262.e1, 1348
Superior mesenteric arteriogram, 1022f
Superior mesenteric artery
    embolism of, 821t
    obstruction of, 820.e1f
Superior sagittal sinus thrombosis, 262f
Superior vena cava syndrome, 769, 1228–1229,
    1228f–1229f, 1229t
Supine head roll test, for benign paroxysmal positional
    vertigo, 185
Supplemental oxygen, for chronic obstructive pulmonary
    disease, 300
Suppurative cholangitis, 286
Suppurative thrombophlebitis, 1262
Suppurative thyroiditis, 1268–1268.e1
Supraglottitis, 463
Suprapubic abdominal pain, 1389
Suprasellar tumors, 685
Suprasphincteric fistula, 102
Supraspinatus syndrome, 1133.e2
Supraventricular tachycardia
    characteristics of, 1230–1232.e1, 1230f, 1231t
    in Wolff-Parkinson-White syndrome, 1377
Surfactant, 48
Surgery
    for abdominal compartment syndrome, 8
    for Achilles tendinopathy, 13.e3
    for aortic coarctation, 111
    for Bartholin's gland cyst and abscess, 175
    for basal cell carcinoma, 178t
    for benign prostatic hyperplasia, 1076
    for bowel incontinence, 699
    for cervical polyps, 271.e4
    for chronic pancreatitis, 947
    for Graves' orbitopathy, 667
    for headache, 547
    for hemorrhoids, 572.e3f
    for hepatocellular carcinoma, 597–598
    for hiatal hernia, 609.e2
    for hydrocele, 640
    for hydronephrosis, 644

Surgery *(Continued)*
  for hyperparathyroidism, 656
  for hyperthyroidism, 667
  for hypospadias, 687.e1
  for idiopathic intracranial hypertension, 690.e5
  for keloids, 735.e5
  for lumbar spinal stenosis, 1202–1203
  for lung abscess, 768
  for lymphedema, 778
  for Meckel diverticulum, 801.e4
  for mediastinitis, 802
  for melanoma, 807
  for meningioma, 810
  for meningomyelocele, 814.e1
  for mitral regurgitation, 834–835, 835f
  for mitral stenosis, 838, 838t
  for nasal polyps, 885
  for nephroblastoma, 888.e2
  for neuroblastoma, 891.e3
  for neuropathic pain, 899
  for non-small cell lung cancer, 771–772
  for obesity, 907–908, 909.e7f
  for oral cancer, 916
  for osteoarthritis, 922
  for osteomyelitis, 924
  for pancreatic cancer, 942
  for Parkinson's disease, 957
  for partial seizures, 1157
  for patent ductus arteriosus, 959–960
  for patent foramen ovale, 960.e2–960.e3, 960.e3f
  for pelvic abscess, 962
  for peptic ulcer disease, 971
  for pilonidal disease, 995
  for priapism, 1060.e2
  for primary hyperparathyroidism, 656
  for Raynaud's phenomenon, 1104
  for renal cell carcinoma, 1111–1112
  for retinal detachment, 1116.e2
  for retropharyngeal abscess, 1118
  for sarcoma, 1140
  for short bowel syndrome, 1173
  for sinusitis, 1185
  for sleep apnea, 1191
  for spinal epidural abscess, 1201
  for stress incontinence, 701.e3t
  for subdural hematoma, 1227
  for tetralogy of Fallot, 1255.e6–1255.e7
  for thromboangiitis obliterans, 1259.e2
Surgical abdomen, 979
Surgical valve replacement, for aortic stenosis, 119
Surreptitious illness, 477
Sustained monomorphic VT, 1361
Suvorexant, 712
SVC syndrome. *See* Superior vena cava syndrome
SVT. *See* Superficial venous thrombophlebitis;
  Supraventricular tachycardia
Swan-neck deformity, 1125, 1125f
Sweat test, for cystic fibrosis, 351, 351t
Swelling
  hand pain and, 1638–1639
  joint, 1474, 1820–1821, 1823.e2f, 1823b
  parotid, 1502
  periumbilical, 1504
  popliteal, 1509
  scrotal, 1521
Swimmer's ear, 928
Swimmer's itch, 350.e5t, 1143.e1
Swollen limb, 1530
SWS. *See* Sturge-Weber syndrome
Sycosis barbae, 495, 495f
Sydenham's chorea, 290.e5, 639, 1124.e2, 1281
Sydney funnel web spider bites, 194
Symmer's pipestem fibrosis, 1143.e2
Symmetric polyarthritis, 1083f
Symmetric polyneuropathy, 1509
Symmetric skin lesions, 470
Symmetrical lymphadenopathy, 464
Sympathectomy, for Raynaud's phenomenon, 1104
Sympathetic blocks, for postherpetic neuralgia, 609
Sympathomimetics, for obesity, 907–908
Syncope, 1233–1234.e2, 1234.e2b, 1234.e2f, 1234f
  algorithm for, 1872.e1f
  in elderly, 480, 480t, 481.e1f
  in long QT syndrome, 766
  mild, 256
  severe, 256

Syndrome of inappropriate antidiuresis, 953–955.e1,
  1235–1237.e1, 1236t
Syndrome of inappropriate antidiuretic hormone, 953t
Syndrome of inappropriate antidiuretic hormone secretion,
  1235
Syndrome X, 824
Synercid. *See* Quinupristin-dalfopristin
Synovial fluid
  analysis of, 1078, 1831, 1833t
  description of, 1778t
Synucleinopathies, 857.e2
Syo-saiko-to, 410.e1t–410.e2t
Syphilis, 1238–1239.e1, 1238f, 1842t
Syphilitic myeloneuropathy, 1243.e5
Syringomyelia
  characteristics of, 1239.e2–1239.e3, 1239.e2f
  paraparesis with, 1501
Syrinx, 1239.e2
Systemic adjuvant therapy, for breast cancer, 217
Systemic candidiasis, 236
Systemic disorders, hepatic granulomas from, 1454
Systemic inflammatory response syndrome, 1158
Systemic lupus erythematosus, 1240–1243.e4
  arthritis in, 1243
  autoantibodies in, 1241t
  characteristics of, 397t
  clinical presentation of, 1240, 1240f
  definition of, 1240
  demographics of, 1240
  diagnosis of, 1241, 1241t
  epidemiology of, 1240
  etiology of, 1240–1241
  immunosuppressive therapy for, 1242, 1242t–1243t
  laboratory tests for, 1241, 1241t
  lupus nephritis, 1243t
  physical findings in, 1240
  treatment of, 1242–1243, 1242t–1243t
Systemic mastocytosis, 798–799.e2
Systemic sclerosis, 1147–1149.e3, 1147t, 1149f,
  1149.e1f–1149.e3f, 1149t
Systemic vasculitis, 1350–1351.e3, 1350f, 1350t, 1351.e2t,
  1351.e3f
Systolic heart failure, 553, 554t
Systolic murmurs, 1417, 1684, 1684b, 1684f
Systolic pressures, segmental, 308

T

T3. *See* Triiodothyronine
T4. *See* Thyroxine
Tabes dorsalis, 1243.e5–1243.e6, 1243.e5f
Tabetic neurosyphilis, 1243.e5
Tabletop test of Hueston, 412.e5, 412.e5f
TACE. *See* Transarterial chemoembolization
T-ACE questions, 487t
Tachycardia
  atrial, 1230–1232.e1
  AV reentrant
    characteristics of, 1230–1232.e1, 1230f
    in Wolff-Parkinson-White syndrome, 1377
  diagnosis of, 1746f
  multifocal atrial, 850–850.e1, 850f
  narrow complex, 1747f
  in pediatric patient, 1747.e1f
  sinus, 1524
  supraventricular
    characteristics of, 1230–1232.e1, 1230f, 1231t
    in Wolff-Parkinson-White syndrome, 1377
  ventricular
    in arrhythmogenic right ventricular dysplasia, 123
    characteristics of, 1361–1362.e1, 1361f, 1361t,
     1362.e1f
    differential diagnosis of, 1509–1510
    pulseless, 1758f
  wide complex, 1748f
  wide QRS beats and, 1748t
Tachycardia-bradycardia syndrome, 1178–1178.e1, 1178f
Tacrolimus
  for atopic dermatitis, 148
  for vitiligo, 1370
Tadalafil, 467
  for benign prostatic hyperplasia, 1076
  for cor pulmonale, 337
  for high-altitude pulmonary edema, 613
Taenia spp., 1249–1250.e1, 1249t, 1250f
Taeniasis, 353, 354f

Takayasu's arteritis, 830t, 1244–1246.e2, 1244t–1245t,
  1245f, 1246.e2f
Takotsubo cardiomyopathy, 1247–1248.e1, 1247f–1248f
Talar tilt test, 99.e7f
Tall stature, 1530–1535
Tamoxifen
  for gynecomastia, 539
  for mastodynia, 800
TAO. *See* Thromboangiitis obliterans
Tapentadol, 940.e3t
Tapeworm infestation, 1249–1250.e1, 1249t, 1250f
Tar products, 1080
Tardive dyskinesia, 1145, 1251–1251.e1, 1530
Tardive syndrome, 1251
Tarsal tunnel syndrome, 1251.e2–1251.e4, 1251.e2f–1251.
  e4f
Taste, loss of, 1530–1531
Tazarotene (Tazorac), 15
TB. *See* Tuberculosis
TBI. *See* Traumatic brain injury
TCAs. *See* Tricyclic antidepressants
TCCa. *See* Transitional cell carcinoma
T-cell immunity, 1065.e4b
TD. *See* Tardive dyskinesia
Td. *See* Tetanus and diphtheria toxoids
Tdap vaccine. *See* Tetanus and diphtheria toxoids and
  acellular pertussis vaccine
TdP. *See* Torsade de pointes
Tear production abnormalities, 1781
Technetium-99m bone scans
  for osteomyelitis, 923, 923f
  for Paget's disease of bone, 935.e1f
Technetium-99m sulfur colloid scanning, for cirrhosis, 305
TEE. *See* Transesophageal echocardiography
Teenagers. *See* Adolescents
Teeth grinding, 222.e2
Telangiectasia
  ataxia, 145.e5–145.e6, 145.e5f
  differential diagnosis of, 1531
  nail, 1490
  in Osler-Rendu-Weber syndrome, 920.e2, 920.e2f
  in scleroderma, 1149.e3f
Telavancin
  for cellulitis, 266
  for methicillin-resistant *Staphylococcus aureus*, 828
Telbivudine, 584
Telmisartan, 243
Telogen effluvium, 64, 66.e2f
Temozolomide
  for astrocytoma, 145
  for glioblastoma, 213
Temporal arteritis, 515, 515f, 515t
Temporal artery, 489t
Temporal lobe epilepsy, 187t
Temporomandibular disorders, 1252
Temporomandibular dysfunction, 1252
Temporomandibular joint syndrome, 1252–1252.e2,
  1252.e1f–1252.e2f
TEN. *See* Toxic epidermal necrolysis
Tender points, 880
Tendinopathy, 1531
Tendinosis, biceps, 187.e2
Tendon
  Achilles, rupture of, 13.e2–13.e4, 13.e2f
  in foot and ankle pain, 1443
Tendonitis, 356, 356f
  biceps, 187.e2–187.e4, 187.e2f–187.e4f
Tenecteplase, 872t
Tennis elbow, 458.e10
Tenofovir
  for acquired immunodeficiency syndrome, 18
  dosing of, 1901t
  for hepatitis B, 584
Tenosynovitis
  biceps, 187.e2
  digital stenosing, 1302.e2, 1302.e2f–1302.e3f
Tensilon test, for myasthenia gravis, 863, 863.e1f
Tension pneumothorax, 1018, 1018f
Tension-migraine headaches, 1648
Tension-type headache, 548–548.e1
Terazosin, 992.e2t
Terbinafine
  for tinea capitis, 1270
  for tinea corporis, 1271
  for tinea cruris, 1272
  for tinea pedis, 1273

Terbutaline, 1060b
Teriflunomide, 857
Teriparatide
  for bisphosphonate-related osteonecrosis of the jaw, 191.e3
  for osteoporosis, 926
Terlipressin, 601, 601t
Terminal complement deficiency, 1887t
Terminal tremors, 1534
Terry's nails, 1490
Tertian malaria, 787
Tertiary syphilis, 1238–1239.e1
Testicular appendix torsion, 1347.e2t
Testicular cancer, 1253–1254.e1, 1253f, 1254t
Testicular cystic lesions, 1531
Testicular disorders
  hydrocele, 640, 640f
  male hypogonadism, 677–679.e1, 678f
  orchitis, 917–917.e1, 917t
Testicular dysfunction, 677
Testicular failure, 1531
Testicular infection, 917
Testicular inflammation, 917
Testicular mass, 1749f
Testicular neoplasms, 1253
Testicular pain, 1531
Testicular size variations, 1531
Testicular torsion, 459.e1t, 1255–1255.e2, 1255.e1f–1255.e2f, 1255t
Testicular tumor, 1253, 1347.e2t
Testis, undescended, 347.e2, 347.e2f
Testosterone
  for gender dysphoria disorder, 512.e6
  for hypoactive sexual desire disorder, 673
  in male hypogonadism, 677–679.e1, 678f
  in men, 467
  replacement therapy, for male hypogonadism, 678–679
  total, 1833
Testosterone 1% gels, for male hypogonadism, 679
Testosterone enanthate
  for hypopituitarism, 687
  for male hypogonadism, 679
"Tet" spells, 1255.e5, 1255.e6f
Tetanus, 503, 1255.e3–1255.e4, 1255.e3f, 1255.e4t, 1532
Tetanus and diphtheria toxoids
  contraindications and precautions, 1868t–1869t
  for international travel, 1888t
  for pediatric oncology patients, 1874t
  during pregnancy, 1883t
Tetanus and diphtheria toxoids and acellular pertussis vaccine
  for adults, 1882t
  catch-up schedule, 1859–1865, 1860t–1864t
  conditions misperceived as contraindications to, 1870t–1871t
  contraindications and precautions, 1868t–1869t
  for health care workers, 1884t–1886t
  indications for, 1878t–1881t
  for international travel, 1888t
  recommended immunization schedule, 1860t–1864t, 1878t–1881t
  recommended intervals between administration, 1867t
Tetrabenazine
  for chorea, 290.e5
  for Huntington's disease, 639
  for Tourette's syndrome, 1282
Tetracycline
  for acne vulgaris, 15
  for actinomycosis, 26.e3
  for Behçet's disease, 182.e3
  for blepharitis, 202.e5
  for cholera, 290.e2
  for psittacosis, 1079.e4
  for tropical sprue, 1303.e2
Tetralogy of Fallot, 1255.e5–1255.e7, 1255.e5f–1255.e6f
TEVAR. See Thoracic endovascular repair
Thalassemias, 87, 1256–1257.e1, 1256t–1257t, 1257.e1f
Thalidomide
  for amyloidosis, 76.e4
  for Behçet's disease, 182.e3
  for discoid lupus erythematosus, 396
Theca lutein cyst, 842.e1f
Theophylline, 1833
Therapeutic hypothermia, for myocardial infarction, 872
Therapeutic plasma exchange, for Guillain-Barré syndrome, 538

Thermal injury, 227, 228t, 229.e4f
  categorization of, by depth, 227t
  classification of, 227
  complications in, 229.e3b
  follow-up care for, 229
  Mayes equations for, 229b
  resuscitation for, 228
    formula for, 229b
  "6 Cs" of, 228
  treatment for, 228–229, 229.e4f
  wound care for, 228–229
Thiabendazole, for cutaneous larva migrans, 350.e6
Thiamine
  for alcohol withdrawal, 57–58, 367
  for chemical-induced cardiomyopathy, 243
  deficiency of, 1368, 1376.e3
  for Korsakoff's psychosis, 735.e8
  for Wernicke syndrome, 1376.e3–1376.e4
Thiazide diuretics
  for hypertension, 663, 664t
  for hypoparathyroidism, 684
Thiazolidinediones
  for diabetes mellitus, 381
  for hirsutism, 618
Thigh, joint pain in, 1474
Thiopental, 1668.e2t
Thiotepa, 201
Third-degree AV block, 159, 549, 549f
Third-degree burns, 229.e4f
Thompson's test, 13.e2, 13.e2f
Thoracic aorta aneurysms, 1401
Thoracic endovascular repair, for aortic dissection, 114
Thoracic outlet syndrome, 1316, 1133.e4t, 1258–1259, 1258f–1259f
Thoracolumbar vertebral compression fractures, 1363
Thoracostomy, for empyema, 441
Thoracotomy, for empyema, 441
Thrive, failure to, 1628
Throat, sore, 1526
Thrombectomy, for cor pulmonale, 336
Thrombin time, 1833
Thromboangiitis obliterans, 1259.e1–1259.e3, 1259.e2b, 1259.e2f
Thrombocytopenia
  differential diagnosis of, 1532, 1822t
  drugs that cause, 1532
  heparin-induced, 575–576.e2, 575t, 576.e1f, 576.e2t
  in hypersplenism, 659
  inherited, 1823t
  inherited disorders, 1532
  in newborns, 1532
  in pregnancy, 1532
Thrombocytosis
  characteristics of, 1260–1261.e1, 1260b, 1261f, 1261.e1f
  diagnosis of, 1822.e1f
  differential diagnosis of, 1532
  reactive, platelet count in, 1822
Thrombocythemia, 1260
Thromboembolism. See Venous thromboembolism
Thrombolysis, for Budd-Chiari syndrome, 224
Thrombolytic therapy
  for acute ischemic stroke, 1216
  contraindications for, 873t
  for frostbite, 503
  for myocardial infarction, 870, 872, 872t–873t
  for pulmonary embolism, 1090–1091
  for renal vein thrombosis, 1115
Thrombophilia, 648, 650
Thrombophlebitis, superficial venous, 1262–1262.e1
Thrombosis, 648. See also Hypercoagulable state
  arterial, 650
  cavernous sinus, 261–262.e1, 262f
  differential diagnosis of, 1532–1533
  mesenteric arterial, 819
  mesenteric venous, 819, 819t, 821–821.e1, 821b, 821t, 1485
  portal vein, 1034–1034.e1, 1034f
  renal infarction with, 1519
  renal vein, 1115, 1115f, 1519
  sites of, 650.e1t
  superior sagittal sinus, 262f
  venous, 650
Thrombotic diathesis, 1532–1533
Thrombotic microangiopathic glomerulopathies, 1446
Thrombotic microangiopathies, 1749.e1f

Thrombotic thrombocytopenic purpura, 108t, 1263–1263.e1, 1263.e1f. See also Hemolytic-uremic syndrome
Thrombus, 650.e1f
Thymic masses, 1533
Thymoma, 1533
Thymomatous myasthenia gravis, 863
Thyroglobulin, 1833
Thyroid carcinoma, 1264–1265.e2, 1264t–1265t, 1265.e2f
Thyroid disorders
  hyperthyroidism, 666–667.e2, 667.e1f–667.e2f
  hypothyroidism, 690–690.e3, 690.e2f
Thyroid function testing, 1832t
Thyroid gland
  fever of undetermined origin and, 489t
  painful, 1750f
Thyroid microsomal antibodies, 1833
Thyroid nodule, 1266–1267.e1, 1267.e1f, 1267f, 1267t
Thyroid storm, 1268.e2
Thyroidectomy, 1265.e2f
Thyroiditis, 1268–1268.e1, 1268.e1t
Thyroid-stimulating hormone, 1833–1835, 1833t
  in hirsutism, 617
  in hypothyroidism, 690
Thyroid-stimulating hormone receptors, in Graves' disease, 535
Thyroid-stimulating hormone-secreting tumors, 1832t
Thyromegaly, 1533
Thyrotoxic periodic paralysis, 667
Thyrotoxic storm, 1268.e2
Thyrotoxicosis, 535, 666. See also Graves' disease; Hyperthyroidism
  causes of, 1533, 1751f
  thyroid function test findings in, 1832t
Thyrotropin deficiency, 685
Thyrotropin receptor antibodies, 1835
Thyrotropin-releasing hormone stimulation test, 1835
Thyrotropin-secreting pituitary adenoma, 997–999.e1
Thyroxine, 1835
  free index, 1832
    in Graves' disease, 535
  serum, 1832–1833
TIA. See Transient ischemic attack
TIBC. See Total iron-binding capacity
Tibia, Paget's disease of, 935.e1f
Tibial nerve entrapment neuropathy, 1251.e2
Tibiotalar dislocation, 99.e7f
Tic douloureux, 713, 1302, 1302b, 1302f
Ticagrelor
  for acute coronary syndrome, 34
  for angina pectoris, 94
  for coronary artery disease, 342
Ticarcillin-clavulanate
  for anaerobic infections, 78
  for bite wounds, 192
  for diverticular disease, 403
  for epididymitis, 459
  for peritonsillar abscess, 982
Tick bites, 194
Tick-related infections, 1533
Tics
  characteristics of, 423t, 1281–1282
  differential diagnosis of, 1533
  painful, 1302
Tietze's syndrome, 343t
Tigecycline
  for Clostridium difficile infection, 311
  for diabetic foot, 385
  for methicillin-resistant Staphylococcus aureus, 828
Tilt-table testing, for syncope, 1234
Tinea, 64
Tinea capitis, 66, 1269–1270.e1, 1269f, 1270t
Tinea circinata, 1271
Tinea corporis, 1271, 1271f
Tinea cruris, 1272, 1272f
Tinea pedis, 1273, 1273f
Tinea unguium, 1274–1275.e1, 1274f
Tinea versicolor, 1276, 1276f
Tinel's sign, 259, 259f
Tinidazole
  for amebiasis, 72t
  for giardiasis, 517
  for Trichomonas vaginalis, 1343
Tinnitus, 1277–1277.e2, 1277.e2f
Tinzaparin, 1091.e3t
Tioconazole, 1341

Tiopronin, 1325
Tiotropium
    for asthma, 137
    for chronic obstructive pulmonary disease, 301
TIPS. See Transjugular intrahepatic portosystemic shunt
Tissue eosinophilia, 651.e2b
Tissue injury, cold-induced, 502–503.e1, 502f, 503b
Tissue plasminogen activator
    for acute ischemic stroke, 1216, 1217b
    for myocardial infarction, 871–872, 872t
Tissue transglutaminase antibody, 1835
TIV. See Trivalent inactivated influenza vaccine
Tizanidine
    for spasticity, 1196.e1t
    for transverse myelitis, 1296
T-lymphocyte (cell-mediated and humoral),
        immunodeficiency, vaccination for, 1873t
T-lymphocyte deficiencies, 1470
TM. See Transverse myelitis
TMD. See Temporomandibular disorders
TMJ, 1252
TMJ syndrome. See Temporomandibular joint syndrome
TMP-SMX. See Trimethoprim-sulfamethoxazole
TNF inhibitors. See Tumor necrosis factor inhibitors
TOA. See Tubo-ovarian abscess
Tocilizumab
    for adult-onset Still's disease, 54
    for rheumatoid arthritis, 1127
Tocolytic agents
    for preterm labor, 1060, 1060b
    side effects of, 1060t
Toddlers. See also Children; Pediatric patients
    limp in, 1477
    vaccinations and infection control for, 1872, 1872.e1f
Toe-brachial index, 976
TOF. See Tetralogy of Fallot
Tofacitinib, 1127
Tofranil. See Imipramine
Tolnaftate, 1273
Tolvaptan, 1024
Tongue
    carcinoma of, 915f
    glossitis of, 525
    mucositis of, 1214.e2f
    oral hairy leukoplakia of, 755, 755f
Tonic clonic seizures, 1156
Tonsillectomy, 982
Tonsillitis, 981t, 989–990.e1, 989t
Tonsillopharyngitis, 989
Tophi, 671.e1f
Topical aloe vera, for frostbite, 503
Topical apraclonidine test, for Horner's syndrome, 628
Topical cocaine test, for Horner's syndrome, 628
Topical hydroxyamphetamine test, for Horner's syndrome,
    628
Topical retinoids, for oral hairy leukoplakia, 755
Topical testosterone, for male hypogonadism, 679
Topiramate
    for alcohol abuse, 407
    for chronic pain, 939t
    for cluster headaches, 543
    for essential tremor, 476
    for idiopathic intracranial hypertension, 690.e5
    for intermittent explosive disorder, 712.e4t
    for obesity, 908
Torsade de pointes, 1278–1280, 1278f, 1279t, 1280f, 1533
Torsades, 1278
Torsion
    pelvic pain with, 1503
    testicular, 459.e1t–459.e2t, 1255–1255.e2, 1255.e1f–
        1255.e2f, 1255t
Torticollis, 422, 423t, 1280.e1, 1280.e1f
TOS. See Thoracic outlet syndrome
Total abdominal hysterectomy, 450
Total abdominal hysterectomy and bilateral salpingo-
    oophorectomy, 933
Total iron-binding capacity, 1811, 1816t
Total testosterone, 1833
Touraine-Solente-Golé syndrome, 668
Tourette's disorder, 1281
Tourette's syndrome, 1281–1282.e1, 1281f
Toxemia, 429
    of pregnancy, 1049
Toxic alcohols, 826
Toxic cataracts, 259.e6
Toxic dilation of the colon, 1283

Toxic encephalopathy, 364, 364t, 366.e1t
    algorithm for evaluation of, 365f
    classification, 364
    risk factors for, 364t, 366.e1
    theories regarding, 364
Toxic epidermal necrolysis, 1213–1213.e1, 1282.e2–1282.e3,
    1282.e2f, 1282.e3t
Toxic megacolon, 1283–1284.e1, 1283b, 1284f, 1533–1534
Toxic multinodular goiter, 666
Toxic myopathies, 1489
Toxic neuropathies, 1494
Toxic nodular goiter, 1832t
Toxic shock syndrome, 1285–1286.e1, 1285t
Toxicodendron, 1020–1020.e1
Toxicodendron dermatitis, 1020
Toxicology screen (urine), cocaine overdose and, 313
Toxin-induced eosinophilic pneumonia, 458.e8
Toxins. See also Poisoning
    acute pancreatitis induced by, 1713.e1
    aplastic anemia from, 80
    atrial fibrillation from, 149
    botulinum, 206
    Clostridium difficile, 310
    diarrhea and, 1429
    hepatic granulomas caused by, 1454
Toxoplasma gondii
    description of, 1287–1290.e1, 1290.e1f
    encephalitis caused by, 636t–638t, 1290f
    in AIDS-infected patients, 18t–24t
Toxoplasmosis
    in AIDS-infected patients, 24.e6f
    characteristics of, 1287–1290.e1, 1288f–1290f, 1290.e1f
TPA. See Tissue plasminogen activator
TPE. See Therapeutic plasma exchange
TPP. See Thyrotoxic periodic paralysis
TR. See Tricuspid regurgitation
Tracheitis, 345.e4t, 463–463.e2, 1290.e2
Tracheobronchial narrowing, 1534
Tracheobronchitis, bacterial, 1290.e2
Tracheostomy, for acute respiratory distress syndrome, 48
Traction headaches, 1650–1653
Tramadol
    for diabetic polyneuropathy, 389
    for neuropathic pain, 899
Tranexamic acid
    for dysfunctional uterine bleeding, 414
    for uterine fibroids, 1332
Transabdominal ultrasound, for placenta previa, 1002f
Transarterial chemoembolization, for hepatocellular
    carcinoma, 598
Transcatheter aortic valve replacement, 119
Transcobalamin I deficiency, 89
Transcranial Doppler ultrasonography, for sickle cell disease,
    1180
Transcranial magnetic stimulation, for conversion disorder,
    334.e2
Transesophageal echocardiography
    for atrial septal defect, 157, 157f
    for infective endocarditis, 447
    for patent ductus arteriosus, 959
    for patent foramen ovale, 960.e2f, 960.e3
Transferrin, 1835
Transfusion reaction, hemolytic, 1291–1292, 1291t
Transfusion therapy, for thalassemia, 1257. See also Blood
    transfusion
Transfusion-related non-A, non-B hepatitis, 586
Transgender, 512.e4
Transient epileptic amnesia, 1293
Transient global amnesia, 1293–1293.e1
Transient hiccups, 1456
Transient insomnia, 712
Transient ischemic attack, 1294–1295.e1, 1295f
    in carotid stenosis, 257
    in mitral valve prolapse, 840
Transient monocular vision loss, 1542
Transitional cell carcinoma, 200
Transjugular intrahepatic portosystemic shunt, 1032
    for Budd-Chiari syndrome, 224
    for cirrhosis, 305, 306f
    for portal hypertension, 1032
Transmissible spongiform encephalopathy, 343.e3
Transrectal ultrasound, for benign prostatic hyperplasia, 1076
Transsexual, 512.e4
Transsphenoidal microadenomectomy, for Cushing's disease
    and syndrome, 349
Transsphenoidal pituitary surgery, 998t

Transsphincteric fistula, 102
Transthoracic echocardiography, for amaurosis fugax, 70
Transudates, peritoneal effusion with, 1504
Transudative pleural effusions, 1505
Transurethral radical prostatectomy, for benign prostatic
    hyperplasia, 1076
Transurethral resection of bladder tumor, 201, 202f
Transvaginal ultrasound
    for placenta previa, 1002f
    for polycystic ovary syndrome, 1028.e3f
Transvaginal ultrasound, for cervical insufficiency, 271.e2,
    271.e2f
Transverse cord syndrome, 1198t
Transverse myelitis, 1296–1296.e1, 1296.e1f
Transverse vaginal septum, 73, 74t
Trastuzumab
    cardiotoxicity from, 242
    for esophageal tumors, 474
Traube's sign, 116
Trauma
    abusive head, 277
    acute pancreatitis with, 1721–1722
    aortic injury caused by, 1753f
    blindness caused by, 1411
    facial paralysis from, 1626
    focal neurologic deficit and, 1492
    leg length discrepancies with, 1476
    leg ulcers with, 1476
    in pregnancy, 1752f
    sore throat with, 1526
    stroke and, 1529
Traumatic alopecia, 64
Traumatic brain injury, 892–893.e1, 1035, 1035b, 1044,
    1297–1299.e1, 1297b, 1298t, 1299b, 1299f
Traumatic cataracts, 259.e6
Traumatic pneumothorax
    algorithm for, 1714f
    in children, 1507
Travel, fever after, 1440
Traveler's diarrhea, 1300–1301.e1
    definition of, 1300
    enterotoxigenic E. coli as cause of, 501, 1300, 1301.e1t
    epidemiology of, 1300, 1300t
    etiology of, 1301.e1t
    in gastroenteritis, 510
    pathogens that cause, 1300t
Tremor
    in children, 1534
    differential diagnosis of, 1534
    essential, 476–476.e1, 476t
    in Parkinson's disease, 956, 956f
Trench mouth, 518.e2. See also Necrotizing ulcerative
    gingivitis
Treponema pallidum, 1842t
Treprostinil, 1094
Tretinoin
    for acne vulgaris, 15
    for warts, 1376
Tretinoin microsphere, for acne vulgaris, 15
TRH. See Thyrotropin-releasing hormone
Triamcinolone
    for acne vulgaris, 15
    for chronic obstructive pulmonary disease, 301
    for cluster headaches, 543
    for contact dermatitis, 329
    for pruritus vulvae, 1077.e5
    for vitiligo, 1370
Triazoles, 272.e4
Trichinella nativa, 1301.e3
Trichinella spiralis, 1301.e3f
Trichinella spiralis muscle infection, 1301.e2
Trichinellosis, 1301.e2, 1301.e2f
Trichinosis, 1301.e2–1301.e3, 1301.e2f–1301.e3f,
    1301.e2t
Trichloroacetic acid
    for condyloma acuminatum, 324
    for molluscum contagiosum, 843
    for warts, 1376
Trichomegaly, 1534
Trichomonas vaginalis, 1343
Trichomoniasis, 1077.e4, 1343
Trichophyton spp., 1269–1271
Trichotillomania, 65f, 1270f
Trichuris trichiura, 126.e1t
Tricuspid incompetence, 1301.e4, 1301.e4f
Tricuspid insufficiency, 1301.e4, 1301.e4f

Tricuspid regurgitation, 1539
  characteristics of, 1301.e4–1301.e6, 1301.e4f
  cor pulmonale and, 335
Tricuspid stenosis, 1301.e7–1301.e8
Tricuspid surgery, 1301.e8
Tricuspid valve
  calcification of, 1416
  endocarditis of, 446f
  replacement, 1301.e4–1301.e5
Tricuspid valve stenosis, 1301.e7
Tricyclic antidepressants
  for burning mouth syndrome, 226.e4
  for Charcot-Marie-Tooth syndrome, 275
  for chronic pain, 939t
  for enuresis, 457
  intoxication or poisoning caused by, 1301.e9
  for neuropathic pain, 898
  overdose, 1301.e9–1301.e11, 1301.e9f, 1301.e9t–1301.
    e10t, 1301.e11f
  pathophysiology, clinical effects, and management of,
    1716t–1719t
  for postherpetic neuralgia, 1037
  for tension-type headaches, 548
Trigeminal neuralgia, 1302–1302.e1, 1302b, 1302f
Trigger finger, 1302.e2–1302.e3, 1302.e2f–1302.e3f
Trigger points, 880, 880f
Triglycerides, 1835
Triiodothyronine
  abnormalities, 1832t
  free, in Graves' disease, 535
Triiodothyronine resin uptake (T₃RU), 1832
Trimethobenzamide, 546t
Trimethoprim-sulfamethoxazole
  for balanitis, 171
  for bite wounds, 192
  for brucellosis, 220.e3
  for cellulitis, 266
  for chronic obstructive pulmonary disease, 301
  for diverticular disease, 403
  for granuloma inguinale, 531.e1
  for granulomatosis with polyangiitis, 534
  for listeriosis, 759
  for methicillin-resistant Staphylococcus aureus, 828
  for nocardiosis, 901.e2
  for otitis media, 931
  for perirectal abscess, 978
  for pertussis, 984t
  for Pneumocystis jiroveci pneumonia, 1013
  for prostatitis, 1077
  for renal abscess, 1106
  for salmonellosis, 1136
  for urinary tract infection, 1322, 1322.e2f
  for Whipple's disease, 1376.e8
Triptans, 546, 546t
Trisomy 21, 403.e2, 403.e2f
Trivalent inactivated influenza vaccine
  conditions misperceived as contraindications to,
    1870t–1871t
  contraindications and precautions, 1868t–1869t
  during pregnancy, 1883t
Trochanteric bursitis, 1303
Trochanteric pain syndrome, 1303–1303.e1, 1303f
Trochanteric tendinitis, 1303
Tropheryma whippelii, 1376.e8
Tropical bubo, 778.e2
"Tropical enteropathy", 1303.e2
Tropical hemorrhagic fever from YFV, 1378.e2
Tropical pulmonary eosinophilia, 458.e7–458.e8, 494.e2
Tropical splenomegaly, 787
Tropical sprue, 1303.e2
Tropics, fever after travel to, 1440
Troponins
  description of, 869, 1089
  I, 1836
  serum, 1835–1836
  T, 869, 1835
True hermaphroditism, 1455
Truvada, for human immunodeficiency virus, 633
Trypanosoma cruzi, 272.e2–272.e3, 272.e3f
  life cycle of, 272.e3
  vertebrate host of, 272.e3
TS. See Tourette's syndrome; Tricuspid stenosis; Tuberous
    sclerosis
TSC. See Tuberous sclerosis complex
TSH. See Thyroid-stimulating hormone

TSS. See Toxic shock syndrome
TT. See Thrombin time
TTH. See Tension-type headache
TTN truncating mutations, dilated cardiomyopathy
    and, 244
TTP. See Thrombotic thrombocytopenic purpura
Tubal factor infertility, 703
Tubal ligation, 330
Tubal pregnancy, 430, 430f, 431.e1f
Tube feeding, diarrhea and, 1430
Tuberculin test
  description of, 1836
  for pulmonary tuberculosis, 1307
Tuberculoid leprosy, 742.e5–742.e6
Tuberculosis, 692t
  in AIDS-infected patients, 17
  miliary, 1304–1305.e2, 1305f
  pulmonary, 1306–1308.e2, 1308.e2f
Tuberculous arthritis, 534.e2
Tuberculous epididymitis, 459
Tuberculous osteomyelitis, 534.e2, 1305f
Tuberous sclerosis, 1370.e2t–1370.e4t, 1308.e3–1308.e5,
    1308.e3f, 211
Tuberous sclerosis complex, 1308.e3, 1308.e3f, 1308.
    e3t–1308.e4t
Tubo-ovarian abscess, 962–963
Tubular necrosis, acute, 1309
Tubulointerstitial disease, acute, 1534–1535
Tubulointerstitial kidney disease, 1535
Tularemia, 1309.e1–1309.e2, 1309.e1f
Tumor lysis syndrome, 744, 745t, 747, 752, 1310–1312.e1,
    1310b
Tumor markers, 1535
Tumor necrosis factor inhibitors
  for ankylosing spondylitis, 101
  for psoriasis, 1081
Tumor of pregnancy, 1100.e4
Tumor-like lesions, 1487, 1527
Tumors/neoplasms. See also Adenocarcinoma; Cancer;
    Carcinoma, specific tumors
  AIDS-related, 17
  astroglial, 144
  blindness caused by, 1411
  bone, primary, 204–205.e1, 205f
  brain
    benign, 211–212.e2, 211t, 212.e2f
    glioblastoma, 213–213.e1
    metastases, 209
  cardiac, 155, 1417
  cavitary lesion with, 1418
  chest wall, 1420
  coma and, 1424
  conjunctival, 1425
  eosinophilic lung disease with, 1435
  esophageal, 472–474.e2, 473f, 474.e1f–474.e2f
  eyelid, 1437
  facial paralysis from, 1626
  granulomatous disorders from, 1447
  intraocular, 1471
  juxtaglomerular, 1829t
  leg length discrepancies with, 1476
  leg ulcers with, 1476
  metastatic, 1485
  ovarian, benign, 934–934.e1, 934f
  paraparesis with, 1501
  pituitary, 1505, 1832t
  primary lung, 769–773.e7, 769t, 770f, 773.e6f–773.e7f
  salivary gland, 1134, 1134f
  sore throat with, 1526
  spinal, 1526–1527
  splenic, 1527
  splenomegaly with, 1528
  in Von Hippel-Lindau disease, 1370.e2–1370.e4, 1370.
    e2t–1370.e3t, 1370.e3f
Turmeric, 504
Turner syndrome, 73, 1312.e2–1312.e3, 1312.e2f
TWEAK questions, 487t
Twisted neck, 1280.e1
Two-question screener, for major depression, 372
Tympanocentesis, for otitis media, 931
Tympanostomy tubes, 931
Type 1 diabetes mellitus, 376. See also Insulin-dependent
    diabetes mellitus
Type 2 diabetes mellitus, 376. See also Non-insulin-
    dependent diabetes mellitus

Type A hepatitis, 580
Type II familial hyperlipoproteinemia, 645
Type II heparin-induced thrombocytopenia, 575
Typhoid, 1312.e4
Typhoid fever, 1135–1136.e1, 1135t–1136t, 1312.e4–1312.
    e7, 1312.e4f, 1888t
Typhoid vaccine, for health care workers, 1884t–1886t
Tyrosine hydroxylase deficiency, 423t
Tyrosine kinase inhibitors
  for hepatocellular carcinoma, 598
  for non-small cell lung cancer, 771
  for renal cell carcinoma, 1112
Tyrosinemia, 1736.e1t

U

UDCA. See Ursodeoxycholic acid
UEDVT. See Upper extremity deep vein thrombosis
UFH. See Unfractionated heparin
Uhl's anomaly, 123
Uhthoff's phenomenon, 855, 914
Ulcer(s)
  anal, 78.e2
  anorectal, sexually transmitted diseases with, 1523
  Barrett's, 172
  in Behçet's disease, 182.e2
  corneal, 338.e2–338.e3, 338.e2f
  genital, 1629–1632, 1814f, 1816b
  leg, 1674–1677.e1, 1674b, 1674f
  oral
    acute, 1496
    vesicles and, 1496
  palatal necrotic, 1510
  small intestine, 1525
  venous, 1354–1355.e1, 1354f–1355f
Ulcerating foot lesion, 1444
Ulcerative colitis, 1313–1315.e1, 1315f
  Crohn's disease compared with, 344t, 1313t
  enteropathic arthritis associated with, 455–456.e1, 455t
  infectious agents mimicking, 1314t
  toxic megacolon caused by, 1283, 1284f
Ulcus molle, 272.e5
Ulipristal
  description of, 332, 440.e2, 440.e2t, 1166
  for uterine fibroids, 1332
Ultrasound. See also Abdominal ultrasound; Compression
    ultrasonography
  for abruptio placentae, 9–10, 9f–10f
  for Achilles tendinopathy, 13.e2
  for appendicitis, 122, 122f
  for benign ovarian neoplasms, 934, 934f
  for breast cancer screening, 217f
  for breech birth, 218.e8
  for Budd-Chiari syndrome, 223–224
  for cholangiocarcinoma, 285.e1f, 284
  for cholangitis, 286
  for choledocholithiasis, 289
  for cirrhosis, 305
  for claudication, 308
  for compartment syndrome, 318
  for cubital tunnel syndrome, 348.e3
  for enteropathic arthritis, 456
  for gallbladder imaging, 287, 290
  for hepatocellular carcinoma, 597
  for hydrocele, 640, 640f
  for hydronephrosis, 643–644, 643f
  for invasive candidiasis, 236
  for jaundice, 729, 731.e1f
  for liver abscess, 760, 761f
  for molar pregnancy, 842, 842.e1f
  for Morton neuroma, 846.e3, 846.e4f
  for osteoarthritis, 973f
  for pericarditis, 973f
  for polycystic ovary syndrome, 1025, 1028.e3f
  for portal vein thrombosis, 1034, 1034f
  for premature rupture of membranes, 1052
  for renal cell carcinoma, 1111f
  for thyroid nodule, 1266, 1267.e1f
  for venous ulcers, 1355
Umbilical flexural psoriasis, 1081f
Unclassified types, EDS, 431.e3
Unconjugated bilirubin, 1671–1672
Unconjugated hyperbilirubinemia, 1473
Undernutrition, pediatric, 478
Undescended testis, 347.e2, 347.e3f

Undulant fever, 220.e2
Unfractionated heparin. *See also* Heparin
  for acute coronary syndrome, 34
  for antiphospholipid antibody syndrome, 109
  for pulmonary embolism, 1090, 1091.e3t
  for Raynaud's phenomenon, 1104
  for upper extremity deep vein thrombosis, 1316
Unilateral optic atrophy, 913.e4
Unintentional weight loss, 1767f
Unipolar affective disorder, 371
Unna gel paste gauze boot, for chronic venous insufficiency,
  1353
Unspecific intraventricular conduction disturbance, 720
Unstable angina, 31
Upper airway obstruction, 463.e1f
Upper esophageal manometry, for dysphagia, 420, 421.e1f
Upper extremity
  ischemia of, 1472
  mononeuropathy of, 1486
Upper extremity deep vein thrombosis, 1316–1317.e1,
  1316f–1317f
Upper gastrointestinal bleeding
  differential diagnosis of, 1410
  pediatric, 1410
Upper gastrointestinal imaging, for hiatal hernia, 609.e2,
  609.e3f
Upper motor neuron, muscle weakness and, 1487
Upper respiratory tract infections, 604.e2, 604.e2f
Urate, 671.e1f
Urea breath test, 508
  for *Helicobacter pylori*, 563–564, 971
Urease, 563
Uremic encephalopathy, 1535–1539
Ureter
  renal failure caused by, 1518
  urinary tract obstruction caused by, 1537
Ureteral calculi, 1323
Ureteral colic, 1756.e1
Ureteral stenting, for hydronephrosis, 644
Ureteral stones, 1323
Ureteral stricture, 1758–1759
Ureteric obstruction, congenital, 1762
Ureterolithiasis, 1323
Urethra
  bleeding, 1536
  obstruction of, in children, 1536
  renal failure caused by, 1518
  urinary tract obstruction caused by, 1537
Urethral cystoscopy, for benign prostatic hyperplasia, 1076
Urethral discharge, 1536
  dysuria and, 1614, 1614f
  purulent, in gonorrhea, 526f
Urethritis, 281t
  gonococcal, 1318–1318.e1
  nongonococcal, 281t, 1318–1319, 1319.e1f
Urge incontinence, 857
Urgency urinary incontinence, 700
Uric acid, 670–671.e1, 671.e1f, 671f
  serum, 1836
    gout and, 529
Uric acid calculi, 1325
Uric acid stones, 1536
Uricosuric agents, for gout, 530t
Urinalysis, 1836, 1837t
  for acute glomerulonephritis, 522
  for enuresis, 457
  for epididymitis, 459
  for galactorrhea, 505
  for Goodpasture syndrome, 528
  for granulomatosis with polyangiitis, 533
Urinary incontinence
  characteristics of, 457, 700–701.e3, 701.e3f, 701.e3t, 701t
  in children, 1536
Urinary retention
  acute, 51–51.e1, 1536
  causes of, 1536
Urinary schistosomiasis, 1143.e1
Urinary tract bleeding, upper, 1536
Urinary tract disorders, pelvic pain in, 1502
Urinary tract infection, 1320–1322.e2, 1320t, 1321f,
  1322.e1b, 1322.e2f
  healthcare-associated, 548.e3
Urinary tract obstruction
  congenital causes of, 1537
  diagnostic tests for, 1755b

Urinary tract obstruction *(Continued)*
  differential diagnosis of, 1537
  investigation and management of, 1755f
Urinate, inability to, 51
Urine
  abnormalities in renal failure, 40t
  blue-green, 1538
  brown, 1414
  brown-black, 1538
  cloudy, 1422
  color abnormalities in, 1537–1538
  colorless, 1537
  green or blue, 1448
  microscopic examination of, 1837t
  milky white, 1538
  red, 694, 1538, 1741–1742
  red-brown, 1538
  specific gravity of, 1841
  yellow-orange, 1537
Urine amylase, 1837
Urine bile, 1837
Urine calcium, 1837
Urine cAMP, 1837
Urine casts, 1537
Urine catecholamines, 1837, 1839t
Urine chloride, 1837
Urine copper, 1837
Urine cortisol, free, 1837
Urine creatinine, 1838
Urine crystals, 1838
Urine culture, for epididymitis, 459
Urine eosinophils, 1838
Urine glucose, qualitative, 1838
Urine hemoglobin, free, 1838
Urine hemosiderin, 1838
Urine 5-hydroxyindole-acetic acid (urine 5-HIAA), 1838,
  1839t
Urine indican, 1838
Urine ketones, semiquantitative, 1838
Urine metanephrines, 1838, 1839t
Urine myoglobin, 1838
Urine nitrite, 1838
Urine occult blood, 1838
Urine osmolality, 1838
Urine pH, 1838–1839
Urine phosphate, 1839
Urine potassium, 1839
Urine protein, quantitative, 1839
Urine sediment, 1839, 1841f
Urine sodium, quantitative, 1839–1841, 1841t
Urodynamic testing, for urinary incontinence, 682
Uroflowmetry, for benign prostatic hyperplasia, 1076
Urolithiasis, 1323–1325.e6, 1323t–1324t, 1324f, 1325.e2b,
  1325.e3f–1325.e6f, 1325.e5b, 1325.e6t
Urolithiasis-like pain, 1538
Uropathy, obstructive, 1538
Urosepsis, 1538
Ursodeoxycholic acid, 1068
Ursodiol
  for cirrhosis, 306
  for primary biliary cirrhosis, 1064–1065
Urticaria
  acute, 1330
  characteristics of, 1326–1327.e2, 1327.e1f–1327.e2f, 1327f
  chronic, 98.e2f, 1328–1330.e1, 1329f, 1330t
Urticaria pigmentosa, 798
Urticarial vasculitis, 675–676.e1
Urushiol, 1020
U.S. Preventive Services Task Force (USPSTF), 217
Ustekinumab, 1083
Usual interstitial pneumonia, 412f, 691, 691f
Uterine bleeding
  abnormal, 817, 1539
  dysfunctional, 413–414.e1, 413b–414b, 414t, 817
Uterine cancer, 450, 450t, 451f
Uterine fibroids, 1331–1332.e1, 1331f–1332f
Uterine leiomyomas, 1331
Uterine malignancy, 1333–1333.e1, 1333.e1f, 1333b. *See
  also* Endometrial cancer
Uterine myomas, 1331
Uterine prolapse, 965–967.e1, 966b, 967f
Uterosacral ligament hysteropexy, 967
Uterus, infertility and, 1470
UTI. *See* Urinary tract infection
Uveitis, 463.e6t, 1334–1334.e2, 1334.e2f, 1334f, 1539

V

Vaccinations. *See also specific vaccine*
  administration of, 1872
    infection control and sterile technique, 1872
  ages between, recommended, 1865t–1866t
  approaches to evaluation and, 1875t
  for cervical cancer, 268
  children, catch-up schedule, 1859–1865
  conditions commonly misperceived as, 1870t–1871t
  contraindications and precautions to, 1868t–1869t
  for health care workers, 1884t–1886t
  for hepatitis A, 581
  for hepatitis B, 598
  for herpes zoster, 609
  H1N1, 709.e2
  in human immunodeficiency virus, 637b
  infection control with, 1872, 1872.e1f
    adolescents and adults, 1872
    infants and, 1872, 1872.e1f
    needle for, 1872.e1f
    subcutaneous injections, 1872, 1872.e1f,
      1580.e1f
    toddlers and older children, 1872, 1872.e1f
  intervals between, recommended, 1867t
  for malaria, 791
  medical conditions and, 1887t
  for mumps, 859
  for persons with high-risk conditions, 1860t–1864t
  for pertussis, 983–984
  for poliomyelitis, 1020.e2–1020.e3
  for Q fever, 1100.e7
  for rabies, 1100.e10–1100.e11
  for rubella, 1133.e7–1133.e8
  for smallpox, 1194.e3
  for tetanus, 1255.e4
  for typhoid fever, 1312.e5
  for varicella-zoster virus, 1037
  YF-Vax, 1378.e2–1378.e3
Vaccinia, 1194.e3
Vaccinia vaccine, 1884t–1886t
Vagifem. *See* Estradiol vaginal tablets
Vagina, infertility and, 1470
Vaginal bleeding
  in non-pregnant female, 1410
  in pregnancy, 1335–1335.e1, 1580.e1f,
    1763–1765
Vaginal creams, 816
Vaginal cuff abscess, 962
Vaginal delivery, for breech birth, 218.e8
Vaginal discharge
  dysuria and, 1614, 1614f
  evaluation of, 1756f
  in prepubertal girls, 1767
Vaginal fistulas, 1336–1337.e1, 1336f–1337f
Vaginal malignancy, 1338–1338.e1, 1338f
Vaginal prolapse, 1756.e1f
Vaginal ring, 330, 332, 332.e6f
Vaginal sinus, 1336
Vaginal ultrasound, of molar pregnancy, 842.e1f
Vaginismus, 1339, 1339f
Vaginitis
  estrogen-deficient, 1340–1340.e1, 1340f
  fungal, 1341–1341.e1
  pediatric, 1757f
  prepubescent, 1342–1342.e1
  Trichomonas, 1343–1344.e1, 1343f, 1343t
Vaginosis, bacterial, 1343t, 1345–1345.e1, 1345.e1f, 1345f
Vagotomy, for hypertrophic osteoarthropathy, 669
Valacyclovir
  for Bell's palsy, 184, 184f
  for herpes simplex, 607t
  for herpes zoster, 609
  for Ramsay Hunt syndrome, 1101–1101.e1
Valerian, 410.e1t–410.e2t
Valproate, 712.e4t
Valproic acid, 1153–1153.e1
Valsartan/sacubitril, 559
Valvotomy
  for mitral stenosis, 838t
  for tricuspid stenosis, 1301.e7
Valvular calcifications, on x-ray, 1416
Valvular heart disease, 1539
Valvular vegetations, 449.e3f
Valvuloplasty, percutaneous aortic balloon, 119

Vancomycin
  for bacterial meningitis, 813
  for blepharitis, 202.e5
  for brain abscess, 208
  for breast abscess, 214
  for bursitis, 229.e5
  for cavernous sinus thrombosis, 261–262
  for *Clostridium difficile* infection, 311
  for diabetic foot, 385
  for epidural abscess, 460
  for erysipelas, 468
  for listeriosis, 759
  for methicillin-resistant *Staphylococcus aureus*, 828
  for osteomyelitis, 924t
  for primary sclerosing cholangitis, 1068
  for pyelonephritis, 1099
  for renal abscess, 1106
  for septic arthritis, 1161–1162.e3
  for tracheitis, 1290.e2
Vancomycin-resistant *Enterococcus*, 1346
Vancomycin-resistant *Enterococcus faecium*, 548.e3
Vanderbilt disease, 619
Vandetanib, 1265
Vanillylmandelic acid, 1841
Vaquez disease, 1029
Vardenafil, 467
Variceal bleeding, 1584.e1, 1584.e1f
Variceal hemorrhage, 475, 1032
Varicella, 1347–1347.e1, 1347f
Varicella (VAR) vaccine, 1347
  for adults, 1882t
  catch-up schedule for, 1859–1865
  conditions misperceived as contraindications to,
    1870t–1871t
  contraindication and precaution, 1868t–1869t
  indications for, 1878t–1881t
  for international travel, 1888t
  for pediatric oncology patients, 1874t
  during pregnancy, 1883t
  recommended intervals between administration, 1867t
  recommended schedule for, 1860t–1864t, 1878t–1881t
Varicella-zoster immune globulin, 1347, 1884t–1886t
Varicella-zoster live-virus vaccine, 1884t–1886t
Varicella-zoster virus, 1015–1016
  in acquired immunodeficiency syndrome, 18t–24t
  in human immunodeficiency virus, 637t–638t
  serology, 1842–1848
  vaccine, 1037
Varicocele, 1347.e2–1347.e3, 1347.e2f, 1347.e2t
Varicocelectomy, 1347.e3
Varicose eczema, 1352, 1352f
Varicose veins, 1348–1349.e1, 1348f, 1348t
Variegate porphyria, 1736.e1t
VariZIG. *See* Varicella-zoster immune globulin
Vascular disorders
  blindness caused by, 1411
  paraparesis with, 1501
Vascular dissemination theory, 452
Vascular EDS, 431.e2
Vascular endothelial growth factor, for macular degeneration,
  783
Vascular headaches, 1642.e1–1642.e2
Vascular hip pain, 1456
Vascular malformations
  hemangiomas and, 165.e1t
  types of, 165.e1t
Vascular processes, intracerebral, 1529
Vascular quadrilateral space syndrome, 1100.e8
Vascular resistance, renal failure caused by, 1518
Vascular rosacea, 1131–1132
Vasculature abnormalities, renal failure with, 1518
Vasculitides
  Henoch-Schönlein purpura, 573–574.e1, 573f, 574t
  microscopic polyangiitis, 829–830.e1, 829t–830t, 830.e1f
Vasculitis. *See also* specific forms
  cavitary lesion with, 1418
  central nervous system, 1061
  cerebral, 266.e5–266.e8, 1419
  classification of, 1540
  cryoglobulinemic, 346, 346f
  hematologic, leg ulcers with, 1476
  hypocomplementemic urticarial, 675–676.e1
  large vessel, 1540
  medium and small vessel, 1540
  mimics of, 1540
  predominantly small vessel disease, 1540

Vasculitis *(Continued)*
  pulmonary-renal syndromes with, 1515t
  systemic, 1350–1351.e3, 1350f, 1350t, 1351.e2t,
    1351.e3f
Vasectomy, 330–331
Vasoactive intestinal peptide, 1842
Vasoconstrictors, for ascites, 129t
Vasodilators
  for aortic regurgitation, 117
  for cardiorenal syndrome, 254
  for frostbite, 503
  for heart failure, 558
  for hypertension, 664t, 835
  for pulmonary edema, 1086
  for Raynaud's phenomenon, 1103–1104
Vasomotor rhinitis, 904
Vasomotor symptoms, 629, 815
Vasoocclusive disease of the legs, 975
Vasopressin
  for cocaine overdose, 313
  for diabetes insipidus, 375
Vasopressin receptor antagonists, for syndrome of
  inappropriate antidiuresis, 1237
Vasopressors, for lactic acidosis, 737
Vasospasm, in subarachnoid hemorrhage, 1225
VATS. *See* Video-assisted thoracoscopic surgery
VCFs. *See* Vertebral compression fractures
VDRL test, 1842, 1842t
VDRR. *See* Vitamin D-resistant rickets
Vectibix. *See* Panitumumab
Vecuronium, intubation and, 1668.e2t
Vegetative state, persistent, 1540
Veins, varicose, 1348–1349.e1, 1348f, 1348t
Veltin gel. *See* Clindamycin phosphate/tretinoin
Vemurafenib, 807
Venereal warts, 324, 324f, 1375
Venlafaxine
  for cataplexy, 884
  for chronic pain, 939t
  for hot flashes, 629
Venography, for Budd-Chiari syndrome, 224
Venom allergy, 195
Veno-occlusive disease, 1033t
Venous insufficiency, chronic, 1352–1353.e1, 1352f–1353f
Venous plasma or serum, 1771t
Venous thromboembolism
  characteristics of, 357, 360.e4f
  preoperative considerations for, 1055.e5
  stroke caused by, 149
Venous thrombosis
  description of, 650
  mesenteric, 1485
Venous ulcers, 1354–1355.e1, 1354f–1355f
"Ventilation" pneumonitis, 657
Ventilation/perfusion lung scan, for pulmonary embolism,
  1088–1090, 1091.e2f
Ventilation-perfusion mismatch, 1540
Ventricular failure, 1540
Ventricular fibrillation, 1356–1357.e1
Ventricular septal defect, 1358–1360.e1, 1358f–1359f
Ventricular tachycardia. *See also* Supraventricular
  tachycardia
  in arrhythmogenic right ventricular dysplasia, 123
  characteristics of, 1361–1362.e1, 1361f, 1361t,
    1362.e1f
  differential diagnosis of, 1509–1510
  pulseless, 1758f
Ventriculomegaly, 641, 641f
Ventriculoperitoneal shunting, for hydrocephalus, 642
Verapamil
  for atrial fibrillation, 150
  for cluster headaches, 543
  for coronary artery disease, 342
  for hypertrophic cardiomyopathy, 248
  for supraventricular tachycardia, 1232
  for tachycardia, 1747f
  for Wolff-Parkinson-White syndrome, 1378
Vernal keratoconjunctivitis, 327t
Verneuil's disease, 610
Verruca plana, 843, 1375
Verruca plantaris, 1375
Verruca vulgaris, 1375
Verrucous carcinoma, vulvar, 1372.e2
Verrucous lesions, 1540–1541
Vertebral compression fractures, 1363–1364.e1, 1363f,
  1364b

Vertebral disease, paraparesis with, 1501
Vertebral fractures, 1199t
Vertebral osteomyelitis, 534.e2
Vertebrobasilar insufficiency, 187t
Vertebrobasilar migraine, 187t
Vertebroplasty, for vertebral compression fractures, 1364
Verteporfin, 783–784.e1
Vertical diplopia, 1430
Vertigo
  benign paroxysmal positional, 185–187.e1, 185b, 186f,
    187t
  central, 1541
  differential diagnosis of, 1541
  evaluation of, 1759f
  physiologic, 847
Vesicles, oral, 1496
Vesicular stomatitis
  description of, 604.e2
  with exanthema, 540
Vesiculobullous diseases, 1541
Vessel wall disruption, vasculitis mimicked by, 1540
Vestibular neuritis, 1365
Vestibular neuronitis, 187t, 736, 1365–1365.e1
Vestibular neuropathy, 1365
Vestibular nystagmus
  characteristics and localizations of, 1696t
  types of, 1696f
Vestibular schwannoma, 16
Vestibular-evoked myogenic potential, 808
VF. *See* Ventricular fibrillation
VHL. *See* Von Hippel-Lindau disease
Vibrio spp
  V. cholerae food poisoning, 500, 500t
  V. parahaemolyticus, 500–501
  V. vulnificus, 265, 501
Video-assisted thoracoscopic surgery, 441, 1018
Videofluoroscopy, for dysphagia, 420
Vigabatrin, 1308.e4
Vildagliptin, 379
Vinblastine, 201
Vincent's stomatitis, 518.e2
"Violin string" adhesions, 964.e1f
VIP. *See* Vasoactive intestinal peptide
VIPoma, 507.e3t
Viral encephalitis, acute, 442–443.e1, 443t
Viral gastroenteritis, 509
Viral hemorrhage fevers, 540.e2t, 1378.e2t
Viral hepatitis, 582f, 1640, 1640b, 1640f
Viral infection
  in human immunodeficiency virus infection
    cutaneous manifestations, 1458
    and lower gastrointestinal tract disease, 1458
    and pulmonary disease, 1461
  myositis with, 1489
Viral keratitis with ulceration, 338.e2, 338.e2f
Viral meningitis, 814, 814t
Viral neurolabyrinthitis, 736
Viral orchitis, 917–917.e1
Viral parotitis, 858
Viral pharyngitis, 981t
Viral pneumonia, 1015–1016.e1, 1016.e1f
Virilizing adrenal hyperplasia, 325.e2, 325.e2f,
  325.e4t
Virilizing congenital adrenal hyperplasia, 1046t
Visceral larva migrans, 350.e5t
Visceral leishmaniasis, 742.e2
Viscerogenic back pain, 1408
Viscerotrophic leishmaniasis, 742.e2
Viscosity, serum, 1842
Vision loss. *See also* Blindness
  acute
    painful, 1541
    painless, 1541
  amblyopia and, 71–71.e1, 71f
  in children, 1541–1542
  chronic progressive, 1542
  after diving, 1541
  transient monocular, 1542
Vismodegib, for basal cell carcinoma, 178, 178t
Visual field defects, 914.e1f
Visual hallucinations, 369
Vitamin A
  deficiency of, 1368, 1369f
  for measles, 801.e3
Vitamin B$_1$ deficiency, 1368, 1369f
Vitamin B$_2$ deficiency, 1368, 1369f

Vitamin B₃ deficiency, 1368
Vitamin B₅ deficiency, 1368
Vitamin B₆ deficiency, 1368, 1369f
Vitamin B₉ deficiency, 1368
Vitamin B₁₂, 1842–1843, 1842.e1f, 1842b
   deficiency, 90, 1368, 1369f
   drugs interfering with, 1399
Vitamin C deficiency, 1368, 1369f
Vitamin D
   1,25 dihydroxy calciferol, 1843
   deficiency of
      characteristics of, 1366–1367.e2, 1366f, 1367.e2f
      rickets caused by, 1128.e4
   in disorders, 1843t
   for hypoparathyroidism, 684
   metabolism of, 1366f
   natural sources of, 1367
   for osteoporosis, 926
   supplementation, 1367
Vitamin deficiency, 785
Vitamin D–resistant rickets, 1128.e4
Vitamin E
   for ataxia telangiectasia, 145.e6
   deficiency, 1368, 1369f
   for Friedreich's ataxia, 501.e3
   for hot flashes, 629
Vitamin K, 1843
   for anticoagulation reversal, 360
   deficiency
      characteristics of, 1368, 1369f
      disseminated intravascular coagulation and, 398
Vitiligo, 1370–1370.e1, 1370f
Vitreous hemorrhage, 1542
Vitreous humor, 1459
VKC. See Vernal keratoconjunctivitis
VMA. See Vanillylmandelic acid
Vocal cord paralysis, 1542
Voiding cystourethrogram, for hydronephrosis, 644
Volume depletion, 1542
Volume excess, 1542
Volume redistribution, renal failure caused by, 1518
Volvulus
   gastric, 1445
   small bowel, 1193f
Vomiting, 1502, 1542. See also Nausea and vomiting
   cyclic vomiting syndrome, 350.e7–350.e8,
      350.e7b–350.e8b
   gastrointestinal disorders with, as adverse food reaction,
      1394
   neonatal, 1542–1543
Von Hippel-Lindau disease, 1370.e2–1370.e4, 1370.
   e2t–1370.e3t, 1370.e3f, 1370.e3f, 211
von Recklinghausen disease, 894–895.e1
von Willebrand factor, 1371, 1843
von Willebrand's disease, 1371–1372.e1, 1371f, 1372f
Voriconazole
   for aspergillosis, 131
   for fungal meningitis, 813.e2–813.e3
   for histoplasmosis, 620
   for invasive candidiasis, 237
vQSS. See Vascular quadrilateral space syndrome
VRE. See Vancomycin-resistant Enterococcus
VREF. See Vancomycin-resistant Enterococcus faecium
VSD. See Ventricular septal defect
VT. See Ventricular tachycardia
VTE. See Venous thromboembolism
Vulva
   cancer of, 1372.e2–1372.e3, 1372.e2f–1372.e3f,
      1372.e2t
   lesions of, 1543
   lichen planus of, 1077.e4f
   lichen sclerosus of, 757
   melanoma of, 806f
   pruritus vulvae, 1077.e4–1077.e6, 1077.e4f
   sarcoma of, 1372.e2
Vulvovaginal atrophy, 1340
Vulvovaginal candidiasis, 234–235, 1341
Vulvovaginitis
   estrogen-deficient, 1340
   fungal, 1341
   prepubescent, 1342
   Trichomonas, 1343
VVC. See Vulvovaginal candidiasis
vWd. See von Willebrand's disease
Vyvanse. See Lisdexamfetamine
VZV. See Varicella-zoster virus

W

WA-1, 169t
WAGR syndrome, 888.e2
Waldenström's macroglobulinemia, 845.e1t, 1373–1374.e1,
   1373f, 1374t
Walker-Murdoch test, 795.e3f
Walking pneumonia, 1011
Wallenberg's syndrome, 187t
Wallet sciatica, 996.e1
Walleye, 1214.e4
Wandering pacemaker, 850
Warfarin
   for antiphospholipid antibody syndrome, 109
   for atrial fibrillation, 152
   for atrial flutter, 154
   for Behçet's disease, 182.e3
   for Budd-Chiari syndrome, 224
   for cor pulmonale, 337
   for deep vein thrombosis, 359
   skin necrosis caused by, 650
   for transient ischemic attack, 1294
   for upper extremity deep vein thrombosis, 1316
Warm autoimmune hemolytic anemia, 82
Wartenberg's sign, 348.e2
Warts
   characteristics of, 1375–1376.e2, 1375f,
      1376.e1f–1376.e2f
   genital, 324, 324f, 1375, 1376.e2f
Water
   deficits of, in severe dehydration, 1604.e3t
   homeostasis of, 1775t
Water deprivation test, for diabetes insipidus, 375, 375.e1t,
   1775t
Water diuresis, 1776b
Watery diarrhea, 1429, 1606.e2, 1606.e2f
WE. See Wernicke encephalopathy
Weakness
   acute emergent, 1543–1545
   gradual onset, 1771
   nonneuromuscular causes of, 1771
Weaver's bottom, 229.e5
Weber test, 1817t
Wegener's granulomatosis, 532–534.e1, 532f–534f, 830t,
   1245t, 1351.e2t
Weight faltering, 478
Weight gain, 1766f, 1771
Weight loss, 1771
   arthritis and, 1403
   for diabetes mellitus, 378–379
   unintentional, 1767f
Weil's disease, 742.e8
Weil's syndrome, 742.e8
Wells prediction rules, 1088
Wenckebach block, 551, 551f
Wernicke encephalopathy, 735.e8, 1376.e3
Wernicke syndrome, 1376.e3–1376.e4, 1376.e3t
Wernicke-Korsakoff syndrome, 735.e8
Wernicke's superior hemorrhagic polioencephalitis, 1376.e3
West Nile virus
   characteristics of, 1376.e5–1376.e6
   encephalitis caused by, 443t, 1376.e5
West Nile virus encephalitis, 443
Wheals, 1326, 1327.e1f–1327.e2f, 1327f
Wheat allergy, 497
Wheezing, 1771
Whiplash, 1376.e7, 1376.e7t
Whipple's disease, 1376.e8
Whipworms, 126.e1t
White blood cells, 1837t
White oral mucosa lesions, 1496
White pigmentation anomaly, cutaneous, 1423
White sponge nevus, 1214
White urine, 1538
Whitening, nails, 1490
WHO. See World Health Organization
Whooping cough, 983
Wide complex tachycardia, 1748f
Wide QRS beats, tachycardia and, 1748t
Wilms' tumor, 888.e2–888.e3, 888.e2t–888.e3t
Wilson's disease, 476, 639, 731, 1203.e2, 1376.e9–1376.e10,
   1376.e10f
Winter depression, 1151.e2
Wintertime blues, 1151.e2
Wissler-Fanconi syndrome, 54
Wissler's syndrome, 54

Withdrawal
   alcohol, 56, 57b, 58.e2f
   for contraception, 330–331
Withdrawal delirium, 367
Wittmaack-Ekbom syndrome, 1116
WM. See Waldenström's macroglobulinemia
Wolff-Parkinson-White syndrome, 1356, 1377–1378.e1,
   1377f, 1378b
Women
   sexual dysfunction in, 1168–1170.e1, 1168t, 1169f
   ventricular septal defect in, 1360
Wood alcohol, 826
World Health Organization
   filariasis, 494.e3
   immunologic classification for human immunodeficiency
      virus, 632t
   polycythemia vera diagnostic criteria, 1029t
Worms, 126
Wound, foreign body in, 1628.e1, 1628.e1f
Wound botulism, 206
Wound diphtheria, 395.e5
WPW. See Wolff-Parkinson-White syndrome
Wrist pain, 1540, 1771
Writer's cramp, 422
"Wry neck", 1280.e1
Wuchereria bancrofti, 778

X

Xanthochromia, 1788t
Xeloda. See Capecitabine
Xenodiagnosis, for Chagas' disease, 272.e3
Xerophthalmia, 1545
Xerostomia, 1186, 1779
Xiaflex, for Dupuytren's contracture, 412.e5
X-linked lymphoproliferative syndrome, 618.e3t
X-rays
   for abdominal aortic aneurysm, 3
   air-space opacification on, 1394
   for basic calcium phosphate crystal deposition disease,
      179f
   calcification on
      adrenal gland, 1415
      cardiac, 1415–1416
      chest, 1415
      cutaneous, 1416
      female genital tract, 1416
      liver, 1416
      nonvisceral abdominal, 1415
      pancreatic, 1416
      splenic, 1416
      valvular, 1416
   chest. See Chest x-rays
   for chest cavitary lesions, 1418
   for croup, 345.e3, 345.e4f
   for gout, 530.e3f
   for hemidiaphragm, 1495
   for Osgood-Schlatter disease, 920, 920f
   for osteoarthritis, 921, 922.e4f
   for psoriatic arthritis, 1082, 1083.e1f
   for pulmonary cysts, 1513
   for pulmonary tuberculosis, 1307–1308
   for retropharyngeal abscess, 1117–1118, 1118f
   rib defects on, 1520–1521
   rib notching on, 1521
   for rickets, 1367.e2f
   for septic arthritis, 1161–1162.e3, 1162.e2f
   for sinusitis, 1185
   for small bowel obstruction, 1192, 1192f
   for toxic megacolon, 1283, 1284f
   tracheobronchial narrowing on, 1534
   for tricuspid stenosis, 1301.e7
   for vitamin D–deficiency rickets, 1367.e2f
47,XXY hypogonadism, 735.e7

Y

Yasmin. See Drospirenone/ethinyl estradiol
Yeast infection, 234, 1077.e4
Yellow fever
   characteristics of, 1378.e2–1378.e3, 1378.e2t
   vaccine for, 1378.e2–1378.e3, 1888t
Yellow pigmentation anomaly, cutaneous, 1424
Yellow urine, 1545
Yellowing, nails, 1490
Yellow-orange urine, 1537

Yergason's test, 187.e2
Yersinia enterocolitica
    description of, 500
    mesenteric adenitis caused by, 818, 818.e1t
Yersinia pseudotuberculosis, 500
Yersiniosis, 818.e1t
Yuppie flu, 291
Yuzpe regimen, 1166

Z

Zanamivir, 707, 709t
ZD. *See* Zenker's diverticulum
ZE syndrome. *See* Zollinger-Ellison syndrome
Zenker's diverticulum, 1378.e4–1378.e5,
    1378.e4f–1378.e5f

ZES. *See* Zollinger-Ellison syndrome
Ziana. *See* Clindamycin phosphate/tretinoin
Zidovudine. *See also* Azidothymidine
    for acquired immunodeficiency syndrome, 18
    dosing of, 1901t
    for human immunodeficiency virus, 635
Zidovudine/lamivudine, 1901t
Zidovudine/lamivudine/abacavir, 1901t
Zika fever, 1379
Zika virus, 1379–1384.e1, 1380f–1382f, 1383b–1384b
Zika virus disease, 1379
Zinc, for Wilson's disease, 1376.e9
Ziprasidone, 191
Zoledronic acid
    for breast cancer, 217
    for osteoporosis, 926

Zollinger-Ellison syndrome, 507.e3, 507.e3t,
    507.e5f, 971
Zolmitriptan
    for cluster headaches, 543
    for migraine headache, 546t
Zonisamide, 907–908
Zoster vaccination
    for adults, 1882t
    conditions misperceived as contraindications to,
        1870t–1871t
    contraindication and precautions, 1868t–1869t
    indicated for adults based on medical and other
        indications, 1878t–1881t
    recommended immunization schedule, 1878t–1881t
Z-thumb deformity, 1125
Zygomycosis, 848

Methanol and ethylene glycol poisoning — I
Opioid dependence — I
Paraneoplastic syndromes — I
Pleurisy — I
Postthrombotic syndrome — I
Sarcoma — I
Sore throat — II
Statin-induced muscle syndromes — I
Tracheobronchial narrowing on x-ray — II
Upper extremity deep vein thrombosis — I
Vitamin D deficiency — I
Vitamin deficiency (hypovitaminosis) — I

NEPHROLOGY
Acid-base homeostasis — III
Acidosis, metabolic, algorithm — III
Acute kidney injury
Acute tubular necrosis — I
Acute urinary retention (AUR) — I
Alkalosis, metabolic, algorithm — III
AV malformations, cerebral
Calcium-alkali syndrome — I
Calcium stones — II
Cardiorenal syndrome — I
Chronic kidney disease — I
Contrast-induced acute kidney injury (CI-AKI) — I
Dehydration correction, pediatric patient — III
Edema, generalized, algorithm — III
Glomerulonephritis, acute — I
Glomerulonephritis, rapidly progressive — II
Glomerulopathies, thrombotic, microangiopathic — II
Glomerulosclerosis, focal segmental — II
Goodpasture's syndrome — I
Hematuria, in children — II
Hemolytic-uremic syndrome — I
Hepatorenal syndrome — I
Hydronephrosis — I
Hypercalcemia, algorithm — IV
Hyperkalemia, differential diagnosis — II
Hyperkalemia, evaluation and treatment, algorithm — IV
Hypermagnesemia, algorithm — IV
Hypernatremia, algorithm — IV
Hyperuricemia — I
Hypocalcemia, laboratory differential diagnosis — II
Hypokalemia, algorithm — IV
Hypokalemia, differential diagnosis — II
Hypomagnesemia, algorithm — IV
Hypomagnesemia, differential diagnosis — II
Hyponatremia — I, II
Hyponatremia, algorithm — IV
Hypoparathyroidism — I
Hypophosphatemia, algorithm — IV
IgA nephropathy — I
Interstitial nephritis — I
Kidney enlargement, unilateral — II
Microscopic polyangiits — I
Nephrocalcinosis — II
Nephrotic syndrome — I
Oliguria, algorithm — III
Pigmenturia — II
Pyelonephritis — I
Renal abscess — I
Renal artery stenosis — I
Renal cell adenocarcinoma — I
Renal cystic disorders — II
Renal disease, ischemic management — III
Renal failure, acute, pigment-induced — II
Renal mass — III
Renal parenchymal disease, chronic — II
Renal tubular acidosis — I
Renal vein thrombosis — I
Rhabdomyolysis — I
Statin-induced muscle syndromes — I
Tension-type headache — I
Tumor lysis syndrome — I
Uric acid stones — II
Urinary retention — II
Urine color abnormalities — II
Urolithiasis — I

NEUROLOGY
Absence seizures — I
Acoustic neuroma — I
Alzheimer's disease — I
Amaurosis fugax — I
Amblyopia — I
Amyotrophic lateral sclerosis — I
Anisocoria — III
Anoxic brain injury — I
Astrocytoma — I
Ataxia, acute or recurrent — II
Ataxia, cerebellar, adult onset — II
Ataxia, cerebellar, children — II
Ataxia, chronic or progressive — II
Ataxia, progressive — III
Autistic spectrum disorders — I
AV malformations, cerebral — II
Ballism — II
Bell's palsy — I

Benign paroxysmal positional vertigo — I
Blindness, monocular, transient — II
Brain neoplasm — I
Brain neoplasm, benign — I
Brain neoplasm, glioblastoma — I
Carotid stenosis — I
Carpal tunnel syndrome — I
Cerebral infarction secondary to inherited disorders — II
Cerebrospinal fluid (CSF) — IV
Charcot-Marie-Tooth disease — I
Chronic inflammatory demyelinating polyneuropathy — I
Complex regional pain syndrome — I
Concussion — I
Convulsive disorder, pediatric age — III
Daytime sleepiness — I
Delirium — I
Delirium, agitated — II
Delirium, dialysis patient — II
Dementia, algorithm — III
Dementia with Lewy bodies — I
Diabetic polyneuropathy — I
Dilated pupil — III
Diplopia, monocular — II
Diplopia, vertical — II
Dissociative disorders — I
Dizziness — II
Dystonia — I
Elbow pain — II
Encephalomyelitis, nonviral causes — II
Encephalopathy — I
Epidural abscess — I
Epidural hematoma — I
Esotropia — II
Essential tremor — I
Febrile seizures — I
Footdrop — II
Generalized tonic-clonic seizures — I
Guillain-Barré syndrome — I
Headache, acute — II
Headache, chronic — II
Hearing loss, algorithm — III
Hereditary neuropathy — I
HIV cognitive dysfunction — I
Horner's syndrome — I
Huntington's chorea — I
Hydrocephalus, normal pressure — I
Inclusion body myositis — I
Inflammatory myopathies
Intracerebral hemorrhage, nonhypertensive causes — II
Labyrinthitis — I
Leg movement when standing, involuntary — II
Leptomeningeal lesions — II
Memory loss symptoms, elderly patients — II
Meniere's disease — I
Meningioma — I
Mental status changes and coma — II
Migraine headache — I
Mild cognitive impairment — I
Mononeuropathies, isolated — II
Motion sickness — I
Multiple sclerosis — I
Muscle disease — II
Muscle weakness, algorithm — III
Muscular dystrophy — I
Myasthenia gravis — I
Myelin disorders — II
Myoclonus — I
Myotonia — I
Narcolepsy — I
Neurocognitive disorders — I
Neuromuscular junction dysfunction — II
Neuronopathies, sensory (ganglionopathies) — II
Neuropathic bladder — II
Neuropathic pain — I
Neuropathies, peripheral, asymmetrical proximal/distal — II
Neuropathies with facial nerve involvement — II
Nystagmus, monocular — II
Opsoclonus — II
Optic atrophy — II
Optic neuritis — II
Osteosclerosis, diffuse — II
Paraneoplastic neurologic syndromes — II
Paraparesis, acute or subacute — II
Paraparesis, chronic progressive — II
Parkinsonism-plus syndromes — II
Parkinson's disease — I
Partial seizures — I
Polyneuropathies, demyelinating — II
Polyneuropathies, distal, sensorimotor — II
Postconcussive syndrome — I
Postherpetic neuralgia — I
Primary angiitis of the central nervous system — I
Ramsay Hunt syndrome — II
Restless legs syndrome — I
Seizures, mimics — II

Shaken baby syndrome — I
Smell disturbance — II
Spasticity — I
Spinal cord compression — I
Spinal cord compression, epidural — II
Spinal cord dysfunction, non-traumatic — II
Spinal cord ischemic syndromes — II
Spinal stenosis — II
Status epilepticus — I
Stroke, acute ischemic — I
Stroke, hemorrhagic — I
Stroke, secondary prevention — I
Subarachnoid hemorrhage — I
Subclavian steal syndrome — I
Subdural hematoma — I
Syncope — I
Tardive dyskinesia — I
Tension-type headache — I
Tics — II
Tinnitus — I
Transient ischemic attack — I
Transverse myelitis — I
Traumatic brain injury (TBI) — I
Tremors — II
Trigeminal neuralgia — I
Unconscious patient — III
Vegetative state, persistent — II
Vertigo, algorithm — III
Vestibular neuronitis — I
Weakness, neuromuscular — III
Whiplash — I

OPHTHALMOLOGY
Amaurosis fugax — I
Amblyopia — I
Anisocoria — III
Blindness, monocular, transient — II
Conjunctival neoplasm — II
Conjunctivitis — I
Corneal abrasion — I
Corneal disorders — III
Corneal sensation, decreased — II
Cytomegalovirus infection — I
Diabetic retinopathy — I
Dilated pupil — III
Diplopia, monocular — II
Diplopia, vertical — II
Esotropia — II
Eyelid neoplasm — II
Eyelid retraction — II
Glaucoma, open-angle — I
Glaucoma, primary angle-closure — I
Horner's syndrome — I
Intraocular neoplasm — II
Ischemic optic neruopathy — II
Keratitis, noninfectious — II
Macular degeneration — I
Nystagmus, diagnosis — III
Nystagmus, monocular — II
Opsoclonus — II
Optic atrophy — I, II
Optic neuritis — II
Orbital lesions, calcified — II
Orbital lesions, cystic — II
Pupillary dilatation, poor response to darkness — I
Ramsay Hunt syndrome — III
Red eye, acute — I
Reiter's syndrome (reactive arthritis) — II
Retinopathy, hypertensive — II
Scleritis — I
Sjögren's syndrome — I
Stye (hordeolum) — I
Uveitis — I

ORTHOPEDICS
Ankylosing spondylitis — I
Arthralgia limited to one or few joints — III
Aseptic necrosis — II
Back pain, algorithm — III
Back pain, low, acute — II
Back pain, viscerogenic origin — II
Bone tumor, primary malignant — I
Carpal tunnel syndrome — I
Charcot's joint — I
Compartment syndrome — I
Complex regional pain syndrome — I
Concussion — I
Costochondritis — I
De Quervain's tenosynovitis — I
Diffuse idiopathic skeletal hyperostosis (DISH) — I
Elbow pain — I
Enteropathic arthritis — I
Fibromyalgia — I
Foot and ankle pain, in different age groups — I
Footdrop — II
Foot lesion, ulcerating — II
Fracture, bone — III
Gout — I
Heel pain — II

Hip fracture — I
Hip pain, in different age groups — II
Hip pain without obvious fracture — II
Hypertrophic osteoarthropathy — I
Inflammatory arthritis — III
Juvenile idiopathic arthritis — I
Knee pain, anterior — III
Knee pain, in different age groups — II
Legg-Calvé-Perthes disease — I
Muscle cramps and aches — III
Muscle weakness, algorithm — III
Myofascial pain syndrome — I
Osgood-Schlatter disease — I
Osteoarthritis — I
Osteomyelitis — I
Osteoporosis — I
Osteoporosis, secondary causes — II
Paget's disease of the bone — I
Plantar fasciitis — I
Psoriatic arthritis — I
Pseudogout — I
Rheumatoid arthritis — I
Rib defects on x-ray — II
Rib notching on x-ray — II
Scoliosis — I
Septic arthritis — I
Shin splints — III
Shoulder pain — III
Shoulder pain, in different age groups — II
Spinal cord compression — I
Spinal cord compression, epidural — II
Spinal stenosis, lumbar — I
Spine tumor — III
Spondyloarthropathy, diagnosis — III
Spondyloarthropathy, treatment — III
Spondylosis, cervical — III
Temporomandibular joint syndrome — I
Thoracic outlet syndrome — I
Trochanteric bursitis — I
Vertebral compression fractures — I
Whiplash — I
Wrist and hand pain, in different age groups — II
Wrist pain — II

OTORHINOLARYNGOLOGY (ENT)
Acoustic neuroma — I
Allergic rhinitis — I
Epiglottitis — I
Glossitis — I
Goiter evaluation and management — III
Head and neck, soft tissue masses — II
Hearing loss — III
Hemoptysis, algorithm — III
Labyrinthitis — I
Laryngitis — I
Mastoiditis — I
Meniere's disease — I
Mononucleosis — I
Motion sickness — I
Mucormycosis — I
Mumps — I
Nasal polyps — I
Nonallergic rhinitis — I
Oral cancer — I
Otitis externa — I
Otitis media — I
Peritonsillar abscess — I
Pharyngitis/tonsillitis — I
Rhinorrhea — III
Salivary gland neoplasms — I
Sialadenitis — I
Sialolithiasis — I
Sinusitis — I
Sleep apnea — I
Smell disturbance — II
Stomatitis — I
Temporomandibular joint syndrome — I
Thyroid carcinoma — I
Thyroid nodule — I
Thyroid, painful — III
Thyroiditis — I
Tinnitus — I
Vertigo, algorithm — III

PEDIATRICS
Absence seizures — I
Anemia in newborn — III
Asthma — I
Ataxia, cerebellar, children — II
Attention deficit hyperactivity disorder — I
Autistic spectrum disorders — I
Bleeding neonate — III
Bone marrow failure syndromes, inherited — II
Breastfeeding difficulties — III
Child abuse — I
Childhood and adolescent immunizations — V
Colic, acute abdominal — II
Convulsive disorder, pediatric age — III
Cystic fibrosis — I

Dehydration correction, pediatric patient — III
Developmental delay — III
Ear pain — III
Enuresis — I
Epiglottitis — I
Failure to thrive — I
Febrile seizures — I
Fetal alcohol syndrome — I
Fever and neutropenia, pediatric patient — III
Fifth disease (parvovirus infection) — I
Food allergies — I
Generalized tonic-clonic seizures — I
Genitalia, ambiguous — III
Glomerulonephritis, acute — I
Hand-foot-mouth disease — I
Hematuria, pediatric patient — II, III
Hemophilia — I
HIV: Recommended immunization schedule for HIV-infected children — V
Hypertension, in children — II
Hypogonadism, algorithm — III
Hypogonadism, differential diagnosis — II
Immunizations, childhood, accelerated schedule — V
Immunizations, childhood and adolescent schedule — V
Immunizations, contraindications and precautions — V
Immunizations, immunocompromised infants and children — V
Impetigo — I
Intubation, pediatric patient — III
Jaundice, neonatal, algorithm — III
Juvenile rheumatoid arthritis — I
Mononucleosis — I
Mumps — I
Murmur, diastolic — III
Murmur, systolic — III
Muscular dystrophy — I
Nephrotic syndrome — I
Osgood-Schlatter disease — I
Otitis media — I
Papulosquamous disorders, pediatric patient — III
Patent ductus arteriosus — I
Partial seizures — I
Pediculosis — I
Pertussis — I
Pharyngitis/tonsillitis — I
Pinworms — I
Precocious puberty — I
Pseudohermaphroditism, female — II
Pseudohermaphroditism, male — II
Puberty, delayed, differential diagnosis — II
Puberty, precocious — II
Reactive erythema, pediatric patient — III
Retropharyngeal abscess — I
Rh incompatibility — I
Roseola — I
Scabies — I
Scarlet fever — I
Sexual precocity, female breast development — III
Sexual precocity, female pubic hair development — III
Sexual precocity, male — III
Shaken baby syndrome — I
Short stature — III
Splenomegaly, children — II
Status epilepticus — I
Stevens-Johnson syndrome — I
Thrombocytopenia, inherited disorders — II
Tourette's syndrome — I
Urethral obstruction, children — II
Vaginitis, prepubescent — I
Varicella — I
Ventricular septal defect — I
Vision loss, children — II

PSYCHIATRY
Abuse, child — I
Acute stress disorder — I
Alcoholism — I
Anorexia nervosa — I
Anxiety (generalized anxiety disorder) — I
Autistic spectrum disorders — I
Binge eating disorder — I
Bipolar disorder — I
Body dysmorphic disorder — I
Bulimia nervosa — I
Conduct disorder — I
Conversion disorder — I
Delirium — I
Delirium tremens — I
Dementia — III
Dependent personality disorder — I
Depression, major — I
Drug abuse — I
Dyspareunia — I
Elder abuse — I
Enuresis — I
Erectile dysfunction — I
Fatigue, algorithm — III

Factitious disorder (including Munchausen's syndrome) — I
Hypoactive sexual desire disorder — I
Insomnia — I
Memory loss symptoms, elderly patients — II
Narcissistic personality disorder — I
Neurocognitive disorders — I
Neuroleptic malignant syndrome — I
Obsessive-compulsive disorder (OCD) — I
Opioid dependence — I
Panic disorder, with or without agoraphobia — I
Patient with ill-defined physical complaints, algorithm — III
Phobias — I
Postpartum depression — I
Posttraumatic stress disorder — I
Premenstrual syndrome — I
Schizophrenia — I
Serotonin syndrome — I
Sexual assault — I
Sexual dysfunction — III
Sexual dysfunction, female — II
Sleep disorders — III
Somatic symptom disorder — I
Tardive dyskinesia — I
Tourette's syndrome — I
Transient global amnesia — I

PULMONARY DISEASE
Acid-base homeostasis — III
Acidosis, respiratory, acute — III
Acidosis, respiratory, chronic — III
Acute bronchitis — I
Acute respiratory distress syndrome — I
Air-space opacification on x-ray — II
Alkalosis, respiratory, treatment — III
Alpha-1-antitrypsin deficiency — I
Asbestosis — I
Aspergillosis — I
Aspiration, gastric contents — III
Aspiration, oral contents — III
Asthma — I
Asthma-COPD overlap syndrome — I
Atelectasis — I
Bronchial obstruction — II
Bronchiectasis — I
Bronchopleural fistula — II
Chronic obstructive pulmonary disease — I
Churg-Strauss syndrome — I
Chylothorax — II
Cor pulmonale — I
Cough, chronic, algorithm — III
Cyanosis — II
Cyanosis, algorithm — III
Cystic fibrosis — I
Deep vein thrombosis — I
Diaphragm elevation, bilateral, symmetrical — II
Diaphragm elevation, unilateral — II
Drug-induced parenchymal lung disease — I
Dyspnea, diagnosis — III
Empyema — I
Eosinophilic lung disease — II
Goodpasture's syndrome — I
Hemoptysis — I
Hemoptysis, algorithm — III
Hepatopulmonary syndrome — I
High-altitude sickness — I
Hypersensitivity pneumonitis — I
Idiopathic pulmonary fibrosis — I
Interstitial lung disease — I
Lung abscess — I
Lung cancer, occupational causes — II
Lung neoplasms, primary — I
Mesothelioma, malignant — I
Necrotizing pneumonias — II
Neurofibromatosis — I
Opacification of hemidiaphragm on x-ray — II
Pertussis — I
Pleural effusion, malignant — III
Pleural effusions, malignancy-associated — II
Pleural space fluid — III
Pleurisy — I
Pneumonia, aspiration — I
Pneumonia, bacterial — I
Pneumonia, *mycoplasma* — I
Pneumonia, *pneumocystis jiroveci* — I
Pneumonia, viral — I
Postthrombotic syndrome — I
Pulmonary cysts on x-ray — II
Pulmonary edema, non-cardiogenic — II
Pulmonary embolism — I
Pulmonary hemorrhagic syndromes, diffuse — II
Pulmonary hypertension — I
Pulmonary mass, solitary, causes — II
Pulmonary mass, solitary, mimics — II
Pulmonary nodule, algorithm — III
Pulmonary nodule, solitary, differential diagnosis — II
Sarcoidosis — I
Silicosis — I